Textbook of Pediatric Infectious Diseases

Textbook of Pediatric Infectious Diseases

Edition

4

Volume 2

Ralph D. Feigin, M.D.
President and Chief Executive Officer, Baylor College of Medicine
J. S. Abercrombie Professor and Chairman
Department of Pediatrics, and
Distinguished Service Professor
Baylor College of Medicine
Physician-in-Chief
Texas Children's Hospital
Pediatrician-in-Chief
Ben Taub General Hospital
Chief, Pediatric Service
The Methodist Hospital
Houston, Texas

James D. Cherry, M.D., M.S.C.
Professor of Pediatrics
University of California at Los Angeles
School of Medicine
Chief, Division of Infectious Diseases
UCLA Children's Hospital
Los Angeles, California

W.B. SAUNDERS COMPANY
A Division of Harcourt Brace & Company
Philadelphia London Toronto Montreal Sydney Tokyo

W.B. SAUNDERS COMPANY
A Division of Harcourt Brace & Company

The Curtis Center
Independence Square West
Philadelphia, Pennsylvania 19106

Library of Congress Cataloging-in-Publication Data

Textbook of pediatric infectious diseases / [edited by] Ralph D. Feigin,
James D. Cherry.—4th ed.

p. cm.

Includes bibliographical references and indexes.

ISBN 0–7216–6448–2

1. Communicable diseases in children. I. Feigin, Ralph D. II. Cherry, James D. (James Donald). [DNLM: 1. Communicable Diseases—in infancy & childhood. WC 100 T355 1998]

RJ401.T49 1998

618.92′9—dc20

DNLM/DLC 96–26904

ISBN 0–7216–7162–4 Volume 1
0–7216–7163–2 Volume 2
0–7216–6448–2 Set

TEXTBOOK OF PEDIATRIC INFECTIOUS DISEASES

Printed in the United States of America.

Last digit is the print number: 9 8 7 6 5 4 3 2 1

To our wives—Judith *and* Jeanne
our children—Susan, Michael, and Debra, *and*
James, Jeffrey, Susan, and Kenneth
and our grandchildren—Rebecca, Matthew, and Sarah, *and* Ferguson

CONTRIBUTORS

❑ ❑ ❑

Richard D. Aach, B.A., M.D.
Professor, Vice Chairman, and Associate Dean, Case Western Reserve University School of Medicine; Director, Department of Medicine, Mt. Sinai Medical Center, Cleveland, Ohio
Viral Hepatitis Due to Hepatitis Viruses A–E and GB Virus; Cholangitis and Cholecystitis

John G. Aaskov, B.Sc., Ph.D., FRCPath
Senior Lecturer—Immunology, School of Life Science, and Director, WHO Collaborating Centre for Arbovirus Reference and Research, Queensland University of Technology, Brisbane, Queensland, Australia
Alphaviruses; Flaviviruses

Walid Abuhammour, M.D.
Assistant Professor of Pediatrics, Wayne State University School of Medicine; Infectious Diseases Physician, Children's Hospital of Michigan, Detroit, Michigan
Antimicrobial Prophylaxis

David W. K. Acheson, M.D.
Assistant Professor of Medicine, Tufts University School of Medicine; Member, Division of Geographic Medicine and Infectious Diseases, Department of Medicine, New England Medical Center, Boston, Massachusetts
Diarrhea- and Dysentery-Causing Escherichia coli

Christoph Aebi, M.D.
Infectious Disease Fellow, Department of Pediatrics, University of Texas Southwestern Medical Center, Dallas, Texas
Flaviviruses

Laura K. Aguilar, M.D., Ph.D.
Pediatric Resident, Baylor College of Medicine, Texas Children's Hospital, Houston, Texas
Diphtheria

Joshua J. Alexander, M.D., FAAP, FAAPMR
Assistant Professor, Department of Physical Medicine and Rehabilitation and Department of Pediatrics, University of North Carolina School of Medicine, Chapel Hill, North Carolina
Otitis Externa

Miriam J. Alter, Ph.D.
Chief, Epidemiology Section, Hepatitis Branch, Centers for Disease Control and Prevention, Atlanta, Georgia
Hepatitis C Virus

Marvin E. Ament, M.D.
Professor of Pediatrics, University of California, Los Angeles, School of Medicine; Chief, Division of Pediatric Gastroenterology and Nutrition, UCLA Medical Center, Los Angeles, California
Esophagitis

Donald C. Anderson, M.D.
Professor of Pediatrics, Baylor College of Medicine, Houston, Texas; Vice President, Discovery Research Council, Pharmacia & Upjohn Inc., Kalamazoo, Michigan
Leptospirosis; Pneumocystis carinii *Pneumonia*

Marsha S. Anderson, M.D.
Fellow, Pediatric Infectious Disease, University of Colorado, The Children's Hospital, Denver, Colorado
Meningococcal Disease

Stephen S. Arnon, M.D.
Senior Investigator and Chief, Infant Botulism Prevention Program, California Department of Health Services, Berkeley, California
Infant Botulism

Antonio C. Arrieta, M.D.
Associate Director, Pediatric Infectious Diseases, Children's Hospital of Orange County, Orange, California
Urinary Tract Infections

Jane T. Atkins, M.D.
Assistant Professor, Pediatrics, University of Texas–Houston Health Science Center, Houston, Texas
Cryptosporidiosis, Cyclospora *Infection, Isosporiasis, and Microsporidiosis*

Robert L. Atmar, M.D.
Assistant Professor, Departments of Medicine and Microbiology & Immunology, Division of Molecular Virology, Baylor College of Medicine; Assistant Attending, Section of Infectious Diseases, Department of Medicine, Ben Taub General Hospital, Houston, Texas
Coronaviruses

Carol J. Baker, M.D.
Professor of Pediatrics and Microbiology & Immunology and Head, Section of Infectious Diseases, Department of Pediatrics, Baylor College of Medicine; Attending Physician, Infectious Diseases Service, Texas Children's Hospital, Houston, Texas
Cervical Lymphadenitis; Group B Streptococcal Infections

Stephen J. Barenkamp, M.D.
Associate Professor of Pediatrics, St. Louis University School of Medicine; Director, Division of Pediatric Infectious Diseases, Cardinal Glennon Children's Hospital, St. Louis, Missouri
Other Haemophilus *Species*

John G. Bartlett, M.D.
Professor of Medicine, Johns Hopkins University School of Medicine; Chief, Division of Infectious Diseases, Johns Hopkins Hospital, Baltimore, Maryland
Mediastinitis

Robert D. Basow, M.D.
General Pediatrics, Southboro, Massachusetts
Streptobacillus moniliformis *(Rat-Bite Fever);* Spirillum minus *(Rat-Bite Fever)*

Craig W. Beachler, M.D.
Retired; former Active Staff, Washington Hospital, Fremont, California
Nonvenereal Treponematoses

William R. Beisel, M.D., F.A.C.P.
Adjunct Professor, Department of Molecular Microbiology and Immunology, The Johns Hopkins School of Hygiene and Public Health, Baltimore, Maryland
Metabolic Response of the Host to Infections

Beth P. Bell, M.D., M.P.H.
Medical Epidemiologist, Hepatitis Branch, National Center for Infectious Diseases, Centers for Disease Control and Prevention, Atlanta, Georgia
Hepatitis A Virus

Michael L. Bennish, M.D.
Associate Professor of Pediatrics, Medicine, and Community Health, Tufts University School of Medicine; Member, Division of Geographic Medicine and Infectious Diseases, Department of Medicine, New England Medical Center, Boston, Massachusetts
Cholera

David I. Bernstein, M.D.
Professor of Pediatrics, University of Cincinnati; Associate Director, Division of Infectious Diseases, Children's Hospital Medical Center, Cincinnati, Ohio
Rotaviruses

Alison A. Bertuch, M.D., Ph.D.
Postdoctoral Fellow, Hematology-Oncology Section, Department of Pediatrics, Baylor College of Medicine; Postdoctoral Fellow, Texas Children's Cancer Center; Texas Children's Hospital, Houston, Texas
Bacterial Skin Infections

Charles D. Bluestone, M.D.
Eberly Professor of Pediatric Otolaryngology, University of Pittsburgh School of Medicine; Director, Department of Pediatric Otolaryngology, Children's Hospital of Pittsburgh, Pittsburgh, Pennsylvania
Otitis Media

Michael D. Blum, M.D.
Director, Vaccine Infectious Diseases Clinical Research, Merck & Company, Inc., West Point, Pennsylvania
Aspergillus *Infections*

Robert Bortolussi, M.D.
Professor of Pediatrics and Associate Professor of Microbiology, Dalhousie University; Chief of Research and Pediatric Infectious Disease Specialist, IWK–Grace Health Centre, Halifax, Nova Scotia, Canada
Listeriosis

John A. Bosso, Pharm.D.
Professor of Pharmacy and Pediatrics, Colleges of Pharmacy and Medicine, Medical University of South Carolina; Clinical Specialist in Pediatrics, Children's Hospital, Charleston, South Carolina
Fundamentals of Pharmacokinetics, Anti-infective Pharmacodynamics, and Therapeutic Drug Monitoring

Kenneth M. Boyer, M.D.
Professor and Associate Chairman, Department of Pediatrics, Rush Medical College; Director, Section of Pediatric Infectious Diseases, Rush-Presbyterian-St. Luke's Medical Center; Director, Pediatric HIV Programs, Cook County Hospital, Chicago, Illinois
Nonbacterial Pneumonia; Bartonella *(Cat-Scratch Disease);* Borrelia *(Relapsing Fever); Toxoplasmosis*

Michael T. Brady, M.D.
Professor of Pediatrics and Preventive Medicine, College of Medicine, The Ohio State University; Physician Director of HIV Program and Physician Director of Department of Epidemiology, Children's Hospital, Columbus, Ohio
Pseudomonas *and Related Species*

William J. Britt, M.D.
Professor of Pediatrics and Microbiology, University of Alabama School of Medicine; Staff Physician, Children's Hospital, Birmingham, Alabama
Slow Viruses

David A. Bruckner, Sc.D.
Professor, Department of Pathology and Laboratory Medicine, University of California, Los Angeles, School of Medicine; Chief, Clinical Microbiology, UCLA Medical Center, Los Angeles, California
Nomenclature of Aerobic and Anaerobic Bacteria

Yvonne J. Bryson, M.D.
Professor of Pediatrics, University of California, Los Angeles, School of Medicine, and Member, Division of Infectious Diseases, UCLA Children's Hospital, Los Angeles, California
Antiviral Agents

Karina M. Butler, M.B., B.Ch., D.C.H.
Consultant in Pediatric Infectious Diseases, Our Lady's Hospital for Sick Children, The Children's Hospital and the Eastern Health Board, Dublin, Ireland
Cervical Lymphadenitis

Carrie L. Byington, M.D.
Assistant Professor, Departments of Pediatrics and Infectious Diseases, University of Utah School of Medicine and Health Sciences Center, Salt Lake City, Utah
Streptobacillus moniliformis *(Rat-Bite Fever);* Spirillum minus *(Rat-Bite Fever)*

Enrique Caceres, M.D.
Fellow, Pediatric Infectious Diseases, University of Texas–Houston Health Science Center, Houston, Texas
Bacillus cereus; Vibrio parahaemolyticus; *Cryptosporidiosis,* Cyclospora *Infection, Isosporiasis, and Microsporidiosis*

Judith R. Campbell, M.D.
Assistant Professor of Pediatrics, Baylor College of Medicine; Attending Physician, Texas Children's Hospital and Ben Taub Hospital, Houston, Texas
Parotitis

Kathleen A. Campbell, M.D.
Houston Pediatric Associates, Houston, Texas
Coagulase-Positive Staphylococcal Infections

K. Lynn Cates, M.D.
Associate Professor of Pediatrics, Division of Infectious Diseases, Case Western Reserve University, Rainbow Babies and Children's Hospital, Cleveland, Ohio
Immunologic and Phagocytic Responses to Infection; Immunomodulating Agents

Mariam R. Chacko, M.D., M.B., B.S.
Associate Professor, Department of Pediatrics, Baylor College of Medicine; Staff, Texas Children's Hospital, Houston, Texas
Gynecologic Infections in Childhood and Adolescence; Calymmatobacterium granulomatis; Trichomonas *Infections*

Louisa E. Chapman, M.D., M.S.P.H.
Clinical Assistant Professor, Emory University School of Medicine; Medical Epidemiologist, Retrovirus Diseases Branch, Division of AIDS, STD, and TB Laboratory Research, National Center for Infectious Diseases, Centers for Disease Control and Prevention, Atlanta, Georgia
Hantaviruses

Ronni M. Chen, M.D.
Pediatric Ophthalmologist, Kantor Eye Institute, Sarasota; Brandon Eye Clinic, Brandon; and Eye Institute of West Florida, Largo, Florida
Ocular Infections

P. Joan Chesney, M.D.
Professor of Pediatrics, University of Tennessee, Memphis; Active Member, Le Bonheur Children's Medical Center, Memphis, Tennessee
Toxic Shock Syndrome

H. Fred Clark, D.V.M., Ph.D.
Research Professor of Pediatrics, Department of Pediatrics, University of Pennsylvania School of Medicine, Philadelphia, Pennsylvania
Rabies Virus

Thomas G. Cleary, M.D.
Professor of Pediatrics and Director, Pediatric Infectious Diseases, University of Texas–Houston Health Science Center, Houston, Texas
Approach to Patients with Gastrointestinal Tract Infections and Food Poisoning; Bacillus cereus; Shigella; Salmonella; Vibrio parahaemolyticus; Campylobacter jejuni; *Cryptosporidiosis,* Cyclospora *Infection, Isosporiasis, and Microsporidiosis*

Armando G. Correa, M.D.
Assistant Professor of Pediatrics, Baylor College of Medicine; Attending Physician, Texas Children's Hospital and Ben Taub General Hospital, Houston, Texas
Acinetobacter

J. Thomas Cross, Jr., M.D., M.P.H.
Assistant Professor, Division of Infectious Diseases, Department of Internal Medicine and Pediatrics, Louisiana State University School of Medicine and Medical Center—Shreveport, Shreveport, Louisiana
Fungal Meningitis; Other Mycobacteria

Adnan S. Dajani, M.D.
Professor of Pediatrics, Wayne State University School of Medicine; Director, Division of Infectious Diseases, Children's Hospital of Michigan, Detroit, Michigan
Antimicrobial Prophylaxis

Toni Darville, M.D.
Assistant Professor of Pediatrics, University of Arkansas for Medical Sciences; Assistant Professor of Pediatrics, Department of Pediatric Infectious Diseases, Arkansas Children's Hospital, Little Rock, Arkansas
Nocardia

Jeffrey P. Davis, M.D.
Chief Medical Officer and State Epidemiologist for Communicable Diseases, Bureau of Public Health, Wisconsin Division of Health; Adjunct Professor, Departments of Pediatrics and Preventive Medicine, University of Wisconsin Medical School, Madison, Wisconsin
Toxic Shock Syndrome

Gail J. Demmler, M.D.
Associate Professor, Departments of Pediatrics and Pathology, Baylor College of Medicine; Director, Diagnostic Virology Laboratory, Texas Children's Hospital; Attending Physician, Texas Children's Hospital and Ben Taub General Hospital, Houston, Texas
Human Papillomaviruses; Cytomegaloviruses

Penelope H. Dennehy, M.D.
Associate Professor of Pediatrics, Brown University School of Medicine; Associate Director, Division of Pediatric Infectious Diseases, Rhode Island Hospital, Providence, Rhode Island
Active Immunizing Agents

Rosamond Dewart, B.A.
Chief, Travelers' Health Section, Program Operations Branch, Division of Quarantine, National Center for Infectious Diseases, Centers for Disease Control and Prevention, Atlanta, Georgia
Health Information for International Travel

Elliot C. Dick, Ph.D.
Professor of Preventive Medicine (Retired), University of Wisconsin Medical School, Madison, Wisconsin
Rhinoviruses; Coronaviruses

Philip R. Dodge, M.D.
Emeritus Professor of Pediatrics and of Neurology, Washington University School of Medicine; Lecturer in Pediatrics, St. Louis Children's Hospital, St. Louis, Missouri
Parameningeal Infections; Transverse Myelitis or Myelopathy

Desmond F. Duff, M.B., FRCPI, FAAP
Consultant Paediatric Cardiologist, Our Lady's Hospital for Sick Children, Dublin, Ireland
Myocarditis

Lisa M. Dunkle, M.D.
Executive Director, HIV Clinical Research, Bristol-Myers Squibb Pharmaceutical Research Institute, Wallingford, Connecticut
Anaerobic Infections

Paul H. Edelstein, M.D.
Professor of Pathology and Laboratory Medicine, University of Pennsylvania School of

Medicine; Director of Clinical Microbiology, University of Pennsylvania Medical Center, Philadelphia, Pennsylvania
Legionnaires' Disease, Pontiac Fever, and Related Illnesses

Jane C. Edmond, M.D.
Assistant Professor, Department of Ophthalmology, Baylor College of Medicine and Texas Children's Hospital, Houston, Texas
Ocular Infections

Morven S. Edwards, M.D.
Professor of Pediatrics, Baylor College of Medicine; Attending Physician, Texas Children's Hospital and Ben Taub General Hospital, Houston, Texas
Anthrax; Rickettsial Diseases; Animal Bites

B. Keith English, M.D.
Associate Professor, Department of Pediatrics, University of Tennessee College of Medicine; Chief, Division of Infectious Diseases, Le Bonheur Children's Medical Center, Memphis, Tennessee
Enterococcal and Viridans Streptococcal Infections

George D. Ferry, M.D.
Professor of Pediatrics, Baylor College of Medicine; Chief, Gastroenterology and Nutrition Clinic, Texas Children's Hospital, Houston, Texas
Antibiotic-Associated Colitis; Viral Hepatitis Due to Viruses Other than Hepatitis Viruses A–E; Cholangitis and Cholecystitis

Randall G. Fisher, M.D.
Fellow, Pediatric Infectious Diseases, Vanderbilt University Medical Center and Pediatric Infectious Disease Clinic, Vanderbilt University Hospital, Nashville, Tennessee
Miscellaneous Gram-Positive Cocci; Citrobacter; Enterobacter; Klebsiella; Morganella morganii; Proteus; Providencia; Serratia; *Miscellaneous Enterobacteria;* Vibrio vulnificus; *Miscellaneous Non-Enterobacteriaceae Fermentative Bacilli;* Alcaligenes; Eikenella corrodens; Flavobacterium; Stenotrophomonas (Xanthomonas) maltophilia; Erysipelothrix rhusiopathiae

Coy D. Fitch, M.D.
Drefs Professor and Chairman, Department of Internal Medicine, St. Louis University School of Medicine, St. Louis, Missouri
Malaria

Patricia M. Flynn, M.D.
Associate Professor, Department of Pediatrics, University of Tennessee—Memphis; Associate Member, Department of Infectious Diseases, St. Jude Children's Research Hospital, Memphis, Tennessee
Candidiasis

Thomas R. Flynn, D.M.D.
Assistant Professor, Department of Dentistry, Albert Einstein College of Medicine, Yeshiva University; Associate Attending Physician, Montefiore Medical Center, New York, New York
Infections of the Oral Cavity

John P. Fox, M.D., Ph.D. (Deceased)
Formerly Professor Emeritus of Epidemiology, School of Public Health and Community Medicine, University of Washington, Seattle, Washington
Epidemiology of Infectious Diseases

David W. Fraser, M.D.
Adjunct Professor of Medicine, University of Pennsylvania School of Medicine, Philadelphia, Pennsylvania
Public Health Considerations

Lisa M. Frenkel, M.D.
Associate Professor, Department of Pediatrics, Division of Infectious Diseases, University of Washington School of Medicine

and Children's Hospital and Medical Center, Seattle, Washington
Dientamoeba fragilis Infection

Richard A. Friedman, M.D.
Associate Professor of Pediatrics, Baylor College of Medicine; Chief, Arrhythmia and Pacing Services, and Chief, Pediatric Cardiology Outpatient Clinic, Texas Children's Hospital, Houston, Texas
Infectious Pericarditis; Myocarditis

David R. Fulton, M.D.
Professor of Pediatrics, Tufts University School of Medicine; Chief, Pediatric Cardiology, Floating Hospital for Children, Boston, Massachusetts
Noninfectious Carditis

Stacey E. Gallas, M.D.
Private Practice, Houston, Texas
Viral and Fungal Skin Infections

Lynne S. Garcia, M.S., M.T., F(AAM)
Manager, Brentwood Facility, UCLA Clinical Laboratories, Department of Pathology and Laboratory Medicine, UCLA Medical Center, Los Angeles, California
Classification/Nomenclature of Human Parasites

W. Lance George, M.D.
University of California, Los Angeles, School of Medicine; Director, Ambulatory Services, West Los Angeles VA Medical Center, Los Angeles, California
Peritonitis and Intra-abdominal Abscess; Retroperitoneal Infection; Clostridial Intoxication and Infection

Michael A. Gerber, M.D.
University of Connecticut School of Medicine, Farmington; Director, Division of Pediatric Infectious Diseases, Connecticut Children's Medical Center, Hartford, Connecticut
Group A, Group C, and Group G Beta-Hemolytic Streptococcal Infections

Anne A. Gershon, M.D.
Professor of Pediatrics, Columbia University College of Physicians and Surgeons; Attending Physician, Babies' and Children's Hospital, New York, New York
Varicella-Zoster Virus

Mark A. Gilger, M.D.
Assistant Professor of Pediatrics, Baylor College of Medicine; Attending Physician in Gastroenterology and Nutrition, Texas Children's Hospital, Houston, Texas
Whipple Disease; Helicobacter pylori

Daniel G. Glaze, M.D.
Associate Professor, Department of Pediatrics, Section of Neurology; Department of Neurology, Section of Neurophysiology, Baylor College of Medicine, Houston, Texas
Guillain-Barré Syndrome

W. Paul Glezen, M.D.
Professor and Head, Preventive Medicine Section, Departments of Microbiology and Immunology and Pediatrics, Baylor College of Medicine; Adjunct Professor of Epidemiology, School of Public Health, University of Texas Health Science Center; Attending Pediatrician, Harris County Hospital District and Ben Taub General Hospital; Courtesy Staff in Infectious Diseases, Texas Children's Hospital, Houston, Texas
Rhinoviruses; Influenza Viruses

Mary P. Glodé, M.D.
Professor of Pediatrics, University of Colorado Health Sciences Center and the Children's Hospital, Denver, Colorado
Meningococcal Disease

Donald A. Goldmann, M.D.
Professor of Pediatrics, Harvard Medical School; Associate in

Infectious Diseases; Hospital Epidemiologist; Chief, Charles Janeway Medical Service; Director, Bacteriology Laboratory, Children's Hospital, Boston, Massachusetts
Nosocomial Infections; Prevention and Control of Nosocomial Infections in Hospitalized Children

Ellie J. C. Goldstein, M.D.
Clinical Professor of Medicine, University of California, Los Angeles, School of Medicine, Los Angeles; Director, R. M. Alden Research Laboratory, Santa Monica–UCLA Medical Center, Santa Monica, California
Human Bites

Maria D. Goldstein, M.D.
Clinical Associate Professor of Pediatrics, University of New Mexico Health Science Center; District Health Officer, New Mexico Department of Health, Public Health Division, Albuquerque, New Mexico
Plague (Yersinia pestis)

Henry F. Gomez, M.D.
Assistant Professor, Pediatrics, University of Texas–Houston Health Science Center, Houston, Texas
Shigella; Salmonella

Edmond T. Gonzales, Jr., M.D.
Professor of Urology, Scott Department of Urology, Baylor College of Medicine; Head, Department of Surgery, and Chief, Urology Service, Texas Children's Hospital, Houston, Texas
Renal Abscess; Prostatitis

Charles Grose, M.D.
Professor of Pediatrics and Professor of Microbiology, University of Iowa College of Medicine; Director of Infectious Diseases, Department of Pediatrics, University of Iowa Hospital, Iowa City, Iowa
Bacterial Myositis and Pyomyositis; Human Herpesviruses 6, 7, and 8

William C. Gruber, M.D.
Associate Professor, Vanderbilt University School of Medicine; Attending Physician, Vanderbilt University Medical Center, Nashville, Tennessee
Miscellaneous Gram-Positive Cocci; Erysipelothrix rhusiopathiae; *Miscellaneous Gram-Positive Bacilli;* Citrobacter; Enterobacter; Klebsiella; Morganella morganii; Proteus; Providencia; Serratia; *Miscellaneous Enterobacteria;* Vibrio vulnificus; *Miscellaneous Non-Enterobacteriaceae Fermentative Bacilli;* Alcaligenes; Eikenella corrodens; Flavobacterium; Stenotrophomonas (Xanthomonas) maltophilia

Duane J. Gubler, Sc.D.
Adjunct Professor, Department of International Health, Johns Hopkins University School of Hygiene and Public Health, Baltimore, Maryland; Department of Microbiology, Colorado State University, Fort Collins, Colorado; Director, Division of Vector-Borne Infectious Diseases, National Center for Infectious Diseases, Centers for Disease Control and Prevention, Fort Collins, Colorado
Flaviviruses

Roberto A. Guerrero, M.D.
Fellow, Pediatric Gastroenterology and Nutrition, Baylor College of Medicine, Houston, Texas
Whipple Disease

Laura T. Gutman, M.D.
Associate Professor of Pediatrics and Director, Duke STD Program, Duke University Medical Center, Durham, North Carolina
Sexually Transmitted Diseases; Gonorrhea; Syphilis

Caroline Breese Hall, M.D.
Professor of Pediatrics and Medicine in Infectious Diseases, University of Rochester Medical School and Strong Memorial Hospital, Rochester, New York
Parainfluenza Viruses; Respiratory Syncytial Virus

Scott B. Halstead, B.A., M.D.
Senior Scientist, Department of Molecular Microbiology and Immunology, School of Hygiene and Public Health, Baltimore; Scientific Director, Infectious Diseases, Naval Medical Research and Development Command, Bethesda, Maryland
Alphaviruses; Flaviviruses

Margaret R. Hammerschlag, M.D.
Professor of Pediatrics and Medicine, State University of New York Health Science Center at Brooklyn; Co-Director, Pediatric Infectious Diseases, University Hospital of Brooklyn and Kings County Hospital Center, Brooklyn, New York
Peritonsillar, Retropharyngeal, and Parapharyngeal Abscesses; Chlamydia *Pneumonia*

Paul E. Hammerschlag, M.D., F.A.C.S.
Clinical Associate Professor of Otolaryngology, Department of Otolaryngology, New York University School of Medicine; Associate Attending, Tisch Hospital, New York University Medical Center, and Bellevue Hospital, New York, New York
Peritonsillar, Retropharyngeal, and Parapharyngeal Abscesses

I. Celine Hanson, M.D.
Associate Professor of Pediatrics, Baylor College of Medicine and Texas Children's Hospital, Allergy/Immunology Section, Houston, Texas
Chronic Bronchitis; AIDS and Other Acquired Immunodeficiency Diseases

Rick E. Harrison, M.D.
Associate Clinical Professor of Pediatrics, University of California at Los Angeles School of Medicine; Co-Director, Pediatric Intensive Care Unit, and Medical Director, Pediatric Transplant Services, UCLA Medical Center, Los Angeles, California
Tetanus

Ulrich Heininger, M.D.
Assistant Professor of Pediatrics, School of Medicine, Friedrich-Alexander University Nürnberg-Erlangen; Attending Physician, Division of Pediatric Infectious Diseases, Universitätsklinik für Kinder und Jugendliche, Erlangen, Germany
Pertussis and Other Bordetella *Infections*

Gloria P. Heresi, M.D.
Assistant Professor, University of Texas–Houston Health Science Center, Houston, Texas
Campylobacter jejuni

Peter W. Hiatt, M.D.
Assistant Professor of Pediatrics and Director, Cystic Fibrosis Center, Baylor College of Medicine; Director, Infant Pulmonary Function Laboratory, Texas Children's Hospital, Houston, Texas
Cystic Fibrosis; Adult Respiratory Distress Syndrome in Children

Sheila M. Hickey, M.D.
Assistant Professor of Pediatrics, Division of Infectious Diseases, University of New Mexico Health Sciences Center; Attending Physician, Children's Hospital of New Mexico, Albuquerque, New Mexico
Antibacterial Therapeutic Agents

Harry R. Hill, M.D.
Professor of Pediatrics and Pathology, Head, Division of Clinical Immunology and Allergy, University of Utah School of Medicine, Salt Lake City, Utah
Immunomodulating Agents

Peter J. Hotez, M.D., Ph.D.
Associate Professor of Pediatrics, Yale University School of Medicine, New Haven, Connecticut
Amebiasis; Blastocystis hominis *Infection;* Entamoeba coli *Infection;* Balantidium coli; *Parasitic Nematode Infections*

Dexter H. Howard, Ph.D.
Professor Emeritus, Microbiology and Immunology, University of California, Los Angeles, School of Medicine, Los Angeles, California
Classification of Fungi

Walter T. Hughes, M.D.
Professor of Pediatrics, University of Tennessee College of Medicine; Arthur Ashe Chair for Pediatric AIDS Research, St. Jude Children's Research Hospital, Memphis, Tennessee
Candidiasis; Cryptococcosis; Pneumocystis carinii *Pneumonia*

W. Charles Huskins, M.D.
Instructor in Pediatrics, Harvard Medical School; Assistant in Infectious Diseases, Children's Hospital, Boston, Massachusetts
Nosocomial Infections; Prevention and Control of Nosocomial Infections in Hospitalized Children

Sandy T. Hwang, M.D.
Fellow, Division of Pediatric Gastroenterology and Nutrition, Baylor College of Medicine, Houston, Texas
Viral Hepatitis Due to Viruses Other than Hepatitis Viruses A–E

Stanley L. Inhorn, M.D.
Professor of Pathology and Laboratory Medicine and Preventive Medicine, University of Wisconsin Medical School; Pathology Staff, University Hospital, and Clinics Medical Director, Wisconsin State Laboratory of Hygiene, Madison, Wisconsin
Rhinoviruses; Coronaviruses

Richard F. Jacobs, M.D.
Professor of Pediatrics, University of Arkansas for Medical Sciences; Chief, Division of Pediatric Infectious Disease, Arkansas Children's Hospital, Little Rock, Arkansas
Lung Abscess; Other Mycobacteria; Nocardia; Actinobacillus actinomycetemcomitans; *Actinomycosis; Fungal Meningitis; Pleural Effusions and Empyema*

Karl M. Johnson, M.D.
Adjunct Professor, Microbiology, Montana State University, Bozeman, Montana
Arenaviral and Filoviral Hemorrhagic Fevers

Erica E. Jost, M.D., M.P.H.
Clinical Assistant Professor of Pediatrics, Brown University School of Medicine; Assistant Physician, Division of Pediatric Infectious Diseases, Rhode Island Hospital, Providence, Rhode Island
Active Immunizing Agents

David P. Jubelirer, M.D.
Associate Clinical Professor of Pediatrics, University of Oklahoma–Tulsa Medical School, Tulsa, Oklahoma
Infectious Pericarditis

Edward L. Kaplan, M.D.
Professor of Pediatrics, University of Minnesota Medical School; Professor, Division of Epidemiology, School of Public Health, University of Minnesota, Minneapolis, Minnesota
Group A, Group C, and Group G Beta-Hemolytic Streptococcal Infections

Sheldon L. Kaplan, M.D.
Professor and Vice-Chairman for Clinical Affairs, Department of Pediatrics, Baylor College of Medicine; Chief, Infectious Diseases Service, Texas Children's Hospital, Houston, Texas
Microbial Virulence Factors; Pyogenic Liver Abscess; Bacteremia and Septic Shock; Arthropods; Use of the Bacteriology, Mycology, and Parasitology Laboratories

Michael Katz, M.D.
Reuben S. Carpentier Professor, Emeritus, of Pediatrics;

Professor, Emeritus, of Public Health, College of Physicians and Surgeons, Columbia University, New York; Vice President for Research, March of Dimes Birth Defects Foundation, White Plains, New York
Parasitic Nematode Infections

James P. Keating, M.D.
Professor of Pediatrics, Washington University School of Medicine, St. Louis, Missouri
Reye Syndrome; Giardiasis

William A. Kennedy, M.D.
Assistant Professor of Pediatrics and Assistant Professor of Microbiology and Immunology, Dalhousie University, Halifax, Nova Scotia, Canada
Listeriosis

Gerald T. Keusch, M.D.
Professor of Medicine, Tufts University School of Medicine; Chief, Division of Geographic Medicine and Infectious Diseases, Department of Medicine, New England Medical Center, Boston, Massachusetts
Diarrhea- and Dysentery-Causing Escherichia coli; *Cholera*

Jerome O. Klein, M.D.
Professor of Pediatrics, Boston University School of Medicine; Director, Division of Pediatric Infectious Diseases, Boston Medical Center, Boston, Massachusetts
Otitis Media; Bacterial Pneumonias

Mark W. Kline, M.D.
Associate Professor of Pediatrics, Baylor College of Medicine; Attending Physician, Texas Children's Hospital, Houston, Texas
Cystic Fibrosis; Congenital Immune Deficiency

Steve Kohl, M.D.
Professor of Pediatrics, University of California, San Francisco; Chief of Pediatric Infectious Diseases, Attending Pediatrician, Moffitt Long Memorial Hospital and San Francisco General Hospital, San Francisco, California
Herpes Simplex Virus

Heidi M. Kokkinos, B.S., M.T.(ASCP)
Clinical Laboratory Scientist, University of California, Los Angeles, Medical Center, Clinical Microbiology, Los Angeles, California
Classification of Fungi

Peter J. Krause, M.D.
Professor of Pediatrics, University of Connecticut School of Medicine, Farmington; Attending Physician, Division of Pediatric Infectious Diseases, Connecticut Children's Medical Center, Hartford, Connecticut
Babesiosis

Paul Krogstad, B.S., M.S., M.D.
Assistant Professor of Pediatrics, University of California, Los Angeles, School of Medicine, and Member, Division of Infectious Diseases, UCLA Children's Hospital, Los Angeles, California
Osteomyelitis and Septic Arthritis

Thomas L. Kuhls, M.D.
Associate Professor, University of Oklahoma College of Medicine; Attending Physician, Children's Hospital of Oklahoma, Oklahoma City, Oklahoma
Appendicitis and Pelvic Abscess; Pancreatitis; Kingella

Timothy R. La Pine, M.D.
Fellow, Division of Neonatology, Department of Pediatrics, University of Utah School of Medicine, Salt Lake City, Utah
Immunomodulating Agents

Ching C. Lau, M.D., Ph.D.
Assistant Professor, Department of Pediatrics, Baylor College of Medicine, Houston, Texas
Tularemia

Robert J. Leggiadro, M.D.
Clinical Professor of Pediatrics, New York University School of Medicine, New York; Chairman, Department of Pediatrics, St. Vincent's Medical Center of Richmond, Staten Island, New York
Other Campylobacter *Species*

Diana Lennon, M.B.Ch.B, FRACP
Professor of Community Paediatrics, University of Auckland School of Medicine, South Auckland Division; Paediatrician in Infectious Diseases, Starship Children's Hospital, Auckland, New Zealand
Acute Rheumatic Fever

Moise L. Levy, M.D.
Associate Professor of Dermatology/Pediatrics, Baylor College of Medicine; Chief, Dermatology Service, Texas Children's Hospital, Houston, Texas
Viral and Fungal Skin Infections

Karen Lewis, M.D.
Pediatric Infectious Disease Consultant, Phoenix Children's Hospital, Phoenix, Arizona
Mastoiditis

Christine A. Lindsay, Pharm.D.
Clinical Assistant Professor, University of Texas School of Pharmacy, Austin; Clinical Coordinator, Children's Medical Center of Dallas, Dallas, Texas
Fundamentals of Pharmacokinetics, Anti-infective Pharmacodynamics, and Therapeutic Drug Monitoring

Martin I. Lorin, M.D.
Professor of Pediatrics, Baylor College of Medicine; Attending Physician, Texas Children's Hospital, Houston, Texas
Fever: Pathogenesis and Treatment; Fever Without Localizing Signs and Fever of Unknown Origin

Harold S. Margolis, M.D.
Chief, Hepatitis Branch, National Center for Infectious Diseases, Centers for Disease Control and Prevention, Atlanta, Georgia
Hepatitis A Virus; Hepatitis C Virus

Melvin I. Marks, M.D.
Professor and Vice Chair, Department of Pediatrics, University of California, Irvine; Executive Director, Memorial Miller Children's Hospital, Long Beach, California
Urinary Tract Infections

Edward O. Mason, Jr., Ph.D.
Professor of Pediatrics, Microbiology, and Immunology, Baylor College of Medicine; Director, Infectious Disease Laboratory, Texas Children's Hospital, Houston, Texas
Use of the Bacteriology, Mycology, and Parasitology Laboratories; Use of the Serology Laboratory

Eric E. Mast, M.D., M.P.H.
Chief, Surveillance Unit, Epidemiology Section, Hepatitis Branch, Centers for Disease Control and Prevention, Atlanta, Georgia
Hepatitis C Virus

David O. Matson, M.D., Ph.D.
Associate Professor of Pediatrics, Eastern Virginia Medical School; Attending Physician, Children's Hospital of The King's Daughters and Sentara Norfolk General Hospital, Norfolk, Virginia
Caliciviruses, Including Hepatitis E Virus

Suzanne Maxson, M.D.
Pediatric Infectious Diseases, Cook Children's Medical Center, Fort Worth, Texas
Actinobacillus actinomycetemcomitans; *Actinomycosis*

George H. McCracken, Jr., M.D.
Professor of Pediatrics, The Sarah M. and Charles E. Seay Chair in Pediatric Infectious Diseases, University of Texas Southwestern Medical Center; Attending Physician, Children's Medical Center, Dallas, Texas
Perinatal Bacterial Diseases; Antibacterial Therapeutic Agents

James E. McJunkin, M.D.
Professor of Pediatrics, Robert C. Byrd Health Sciences Center of West Virginia, Charleston Division; Medical Staff, Pediatrics, Charleston Area Medical Center, Women and Children's Division, Charleston, West Virginia
California/La Crosse Encephalitis

Kelly T. McKee, Jr., M.D., M.P.H.
Chief, Preventive Medicine Service, Womack Army Medical Center, Ft. Bragg, North Carolina
Hantaviruses

Rima L. McLeod, M.D.
Jules and Doris Stein Research to Prevent Blindness Professor, Departments of Visual Sciences, Medicine, and Pathology, University of Chicago Pritzker School of Medicine; Attending Physician, University of Chicago Hospitals and Michael Reese Hospital and Medical Center, Chicago, Illinois
Toxoplasmosis

Marian E. Melish, M.D.
Professor of Pediatrics, Tropical Medicine, and Medical Microbiology, John A. Burns School of Medicine, University of Hawaii; Infectious Diseases Consultant and Attending Pediatrician, Kapiolani Medical Center for Women and Children, Honolulu, Hawaii
Bacterial Skin Infections; Kawasaki Disease; Coagulase-Positive Staphylococcal Infections

Joseph L. Melnick, Ph.D., M.D.(Hon.), D.Sc.
Distinguished Service Professor, Division of Molecular Virology, Baylor College of Medicine, Houston, Texas
Nomenclature and Classification of Viruses

Wayne M. Meyers, M.D., Ph.D., D.Sc.(Hon.)
Research Affiliate, Tulane Regional Primate Research Center, Tulane University, Covington, Louisiana; Chief, Mycobacteriology Branch, and Registrar, Leprosy Registry, American Registry of Pathology, Armed Forces Institute of Pathology, Washington, D.C.
Leprosy

James N. Miller, Ph.D.
Professor of Microbiology and Immunology, University of California, Los Angeles, School of Medicine, Los Angeles, California
Nonveneral Treponematoses

Marjorie J. Miller, Dr.P.H.
Senior Specialist, Clinical Virology, Clinical Laboratories–Microbiology, UCLA Medical Center, Los Angeles, California
Use of the Diagnostic Virology Laboratory

Linda L. Minnich, M.S., S.M.(HAM)
Clinical Virologist, Charleston Area Medical Center, Charleston, West Virginia
California/La Crosse Encephalitis

Sudipta L. Misra, M.B., B.S., M.D., D.M.
Resident, Department of Pediatrics, Maimonides Medical Center, Brooklyn, New York
Esophagitis

Lynne M. Mofenson, M.D.
Associate Branch Chief for Clinical Research, Pediatric, Adolescent, and Maternal AIDS Branch, Center for Research for Mothers and Children, National Institute of Child Health and Human

Development, National Institutes of Health, Rockville, Maryland
Human Retroviruses

David M. Morens, A.B., M.D.
Professor and Head, Epidemiology Program, School of Public Health, University of Hawaii; Professor of Tropical Medicine, School of Medicine, University of Hawaii; Director of Laboratories, Diamond Head Health Center; Staff Physician, Tripler Army Medical Center, Honolulu, Hawaii
Kawasaki Disease

Edward A. Mortimer, Jr., M.D.
Elisabeth Geverance Prentiss Professor Emeritus, Department of Epidemiology and Biostatistics, School of Medicine, Case Western Reserve University; Associate Pediatrician, University Hospitals of Cleveland, Cleveland, Ohio
Epidemiology of Infectious Diseases

Mark S. Munsey, M.S.
Manager, Clinical Operations, Sepracor Pharmaceuticals, Inc., Marlborough, Massachusetts
Other Anaerobic Infections

Anita Newman, M.D., FACS
Attending Staff Surgeon, Children's Hospital of Los Angeles, Los Angeles, California
Sinusitis; Mastoiditis

Karin Nielsen, M.D., M.P.H.
Clinical Instructor, University of California at Los Angeles School of Medicine; Member, Division of Infectious Diseases, UCLA Children's Hospital, Los Angeles, California
Hepatitis B and D Viruses

Michael R. Nihill, M.D., M.B., B.S., M.S., MRCP
Professor, Department of Pediatrics, Baylor College of Medicine; Consultant, Pediatric Cardiology, Texas Children's Hospital, Methodist Hospital, and Harris County Hospital District, Houston, Texas
Infectious Pericarditis

James C. Overall, Jr., M.D.
Professor of Pediatrics and Pathology, University of Utah School of Medicine; Medical Director, Diagnostic Virology Laboratory, Associated Regional and University Pathologists; Consultant in Pediatric Infectious Diseases, Primary Children's and University of Utah Medical Centers, Salt Lake City, Utah
Viral Infections of the Fetus and Neonate

Kelvin S. Panesar, M.D.
Pediatric Pulmonology Fellow, Baylor College of Medicine, Houston, Texas
Interaction of Infection and Nutrition

Christian C. Patrick, M.D., Ph.D.
Associate Professor, Department of Pediatrics, The University of Tennessee, Memphis, College of Medicine; Director of Academic Programs, Director of Clinical Microbiology and Molecular Microbiology, and Associate Member, St. Jude Children's Research Hospital, Memphis, Tennessee
Opportunistic Infections in the Compromised Host; Coagulase-Negative Staphylococcal Infections

Eric M. Pearlman, M.D., Ph.D.
Resident in Pediatric Neurology, Johns Hopkins University School of Medicine, Baltimore, Maryland
Bacterial Meningitis Beyond the Neonatal Period

Georges Peter, M.D.
Professor of Pediatrics, Brown University School of Medicine; Director, Division of Pediatric Infectious Diseases, Rhode

Island Hospital, Providence, Rhode Island
Active Immunizing Agents

C. J. Peters, M.D.
Chief, Special Pathogens Branch, Centers for Disease Control and Prevention, Atlanta, Georgia
Hantaviruses

Larry K. Pickering, M.D.
Professor of Pediatrics, Eastern Virginia Medical School; Director, Center for Pediatric Research, Children's Hospital of The King's Daughters, Norfolk, Virginia
Approach to Patients with Gastrointestinal Tract Infections and Food Poisoning

Joseph F. Piecuch, D.M.D., M.D.
Clinical Professor, Department of Oral and Maxillofacial Surgery, University of Connecticut School of Dental Medicine, Farmington, Connecticut
Infections of the Oral Cavity

Francisco P. Pinheiro, M.D., Ph.D.
Advisor on Viral Diseases, Pan American Health Organization, World Health Organization, Communicable Diseases Program, Division of Disease Prevention and Control, Washington, D.C.
Other Bunyaviruses

William W. Pinsky, M.D.
Associate Dean for Clinical Affairs, Wayne State University School of Medicine; Senior Vice President for Clinical Affairs and Managed Care, Detroit Medical Center, Detroit, Michigan
Infectious Pericarditis

Stanley A. Plotkin, M.D.
Professor Emeritus of Pediatrics, University of Pennsylvania School of Medicine; Professor Emeritus, Wistar Institute, Philadelphia, Pennsylvania; Medical and Scientific Director, Pasteur Mérieux Connaught, Marnes-La-Coquette, France
Rabies Virus

Scott L. Pomeroy, M.D., Ph.D.
Assistant Professor of Neurology, Harvard Medical School; Assistant in Neurology, Boston Children's Hospital, Boston, Massachusetts
Parameningeal Infections; Transverse Myelitis or Myelopathy

Joan S. Purcell, M.D.
Assistant Professor, Department of Obstetrics and Gynecology/Pediatrics, University of Texas Medical Branch, Galveston, Texas
Trichomonas *Infections*

Jack S. Remington, M.D.
Professor of Medicine, Division of Infectious Diseases, Stanford University School of Medicine; Chairman, Department of Immunology and Infectious Diseases, Marcus A. Krupp Research Chair, Research Institute, Palo Alto Medical Foundation, Palo Alto, California
Toxoplasmosis

Angela Restrepo-Moreno, Ph.D.
Head of the Mycology Laboratory, Corporación para Investigaciones Biológica, Medellin, Colombia
Paracoccidioidomycosis

Michael G. Rinaldi, Ph.D.
Professor of Pathology, Medicine, Microbiology, and Clinical Laboratory Sciences, Director, Fungus Testing Laboratory, University of Texas Health Science Center at San Antonio; Chief, Clinical Microbiology Laboratories, Director, Department of Veterans Affairs, Mycology Reference Laboratory, Audie L. Murphy Division,

South Texas Veterans Health Care System, San Antonio, Texas
Antifungal Agents

John W. Rippon, Ph.D.
Retired; formerly Associate Professor Emeritus of Medicine/Dermatology, University of Chicago Pritzker School of Medicine, Chicago, Illinois
Miscellaneous Mycoses

Judith L. Rowen, M.D.
Assistant Professor, Department of Pediatrics, Infectious Diseases Division, University of Texas Medical Branch, Galveston, Texas
Group B Streptococcal Infections

Xavier Sáez-Llorens, M.D.
Professor of Pediatrics and Infectious Diseases, University of Panama School of Medicine, Panama City; Chief, Pediatric Infectious Disease Division, Hospital del Niño, Panama City, Panama
Perinatal Bacterial Diseases

Pablo J. Sánchez, M.D.
Associate Professor of Pediatrics, Divisions of Neonatal-Perinatal Medicine and Pediatric Infectious Diseases, The University of Texas Southwestern Medical Center at Dallas; Attending Physician, Parkland Memorial Hospital, Children's Medical Center, and St. Paul's Medical Center, Dallas, Texas
Miscellaneous Infections of the Newborn

Jane G. Schaller, M.D.
Professor of Pediatrics, Tufts University School of Medicine; Pediatrician-in-Chief, The Floating Hospital, New England Medical Center, Boston, Massachusetts
Noninfectious Carditis

Ann O. Scheimann, B.S., M.D.
Assistant Professor, Pediatric Gastroenterology and Nutrition, Baylor College of Medicine, Houston, Texas
Cholangitis and Cholecystitis

Kenneth O. Schowengerdt, M.D.
Assistant Professor of Pediatrics (Cardiology), Baylor College of Medicine; Associate in Pediatric Cardiology, Texas Children's Hospital, Houston, Texas
Myocarditis

Gordon E. Schutze, M.D.
Associate Professor of Pediatrics and Pathology, University of Arkansas for Medical Sciences and Arkansas Children's Hospital, Little Rock, Arkansas
Blastomycosis

James S. Seidel, M.D., Ph.D.
Professor of Pediatrics, University of California, Los Angeles, School of Medicine, Los Angeles; Chief, Division of General and Emergency Pediatrics, Harbor-UCLA Medical Center, Torrance, California
Naegleria, Acanthamoeba *and Leptomyxid Ameba*

Craig N. Shapiro, M.D.
Deputy Chief, Epidemiology Section, Hepatitis Branch, National Center for Infectious Diseases, Centers for Disease Control and Prevention, Atlanta, Georgia
Hepatitis A Virus

Eugene D. Shapiro, M.D.
Professor of Pediatrics and of Epidemiology, Yale University School of Medicine and Children's Clinical Research Center; Attending Pediatrician, Children's Hospital at Yale–New Haven, New Haven, Connecticut
Epidemiology and Biostatistics

William T. Shearer, M.D., Ph.D.
Professor of Pediatrics and of Microbiology and Immunology,

Baylor College of Medicine; Chief, Allergy and Immunology Service, Texas Children's Hospital, Houston, Texas
Chronic Bronchitis; Congenital Immune Deficiency; AIDS and Other Acquired Immunodeficiency Diseases

Ziad M. Shehab, M.D.
Professor of Clinical Pediatrics and Pathology, The University of Arizona, Tucson, Arizona
Coccidioidomycosis

Jerry L. Shenep, M.D.
Professor, Department of Pediatrics, University of Tennessee, Memphis, College of Medicine; Associate Member, Department of Infectious Diseases, St. Jude Children's Research Hospital, Memphis, Tennessee
Enterococcal and Viridans Streptococcal Infections

W. Donald Shields, M.D.
Professor of Neurology and Pediatrics, University of California, Los Angeles, School of Medicine; Chief, Division of Pediatric Neurology, UCLA Children's Hospital, Los Angeles, California
Encephalitis and Meningoencephalitis

Robert E. Shope, M.D.
Professor of Pathology, Center for Tropical Diseases, University of Texas Medical Branch, Galveston, Texas
Other Bunyaviruses

Raymond G. Slavin, M.D.
Professor of Internal Medicine and Microbiology, St. Louis University School of Medicine; Director, Division of Allergy and Immunology, St. Louis University Health Sciences Center, St. Louis, Missouri
Hypersensitivity Pneumonitis and Chronic Interstitial Pneumonitis

Karen S. Slobod, M.D., C.M.
Assistant Professor, University of Tennessee, Memphis, College of Medicine; Assistant Member, St. Jude Children's Research Hospital, Memphis, Tennessee
Opportunistic Infections in the Compromised Host

Arnold L. Smith, B.S., M.S., M.D.
Professor and Chairman, Department of Molecular Microbiology, University of Missouri School of Medicine, Columbia, Missouri
Indigenous Flora; Osteomyelitis and Septic Arthritis; Meningococcal Disease

Margaret H. D. Smith, M.D.
Faculty, Tulane University Medical School, New Orleans, Louisiana
Tuberculosis

Steven L. Solomon, M.D.
Assistant Clinical Professor, Division of Infectious Disease, Emory University School of Medicine; Chief, Special Studies Activity, Hospital Infections Program, National Center for Infectious Diseases, Centers for Disease Control and Prevention, Atlanta, Georgia
Public Health Considerations

Jeffrey R. Starke, M.D.
Associate Professor of Pediatrics, Baylor College of Medicine; Director, Infection Control, Texas Children's Hospital, Houston, Texas
Infective Endocarditis; Tuberculosis

Barbara W. Stechenberg, M.D.
Associate Professor of Pediatrics, Tufts University School of Medicine, Boston; Vice Chairman and Director of Pediatric Infectious Diseases, Department of Pediatrics, Baystate Medical Center Children's Hospital, Springfield, Massachusetts
Eosinophilic Meningitis; Moraxella catarrhalis; *Diphtheria;* Pasteurella multocida; *Bartonellosis;* Borrelia *(Lyme Disease)*

Paul G. Steinkuller, M.D.
Assistant Professor, Department of Ophthalmology, Baylor College of Medicine; Chief of Ophthalmology, Texas Children's Hospital, Houston, Texas
Ocular Infections

E. Richard Stiehm, M.D.
Professor of Pediatrics and Chief, Division of Immunology, Department of Pediatrics, University of California, Los Angeles, School of Medicine; Attending Pediatrician, UCLA Children's Hospital, UCLA Medical Center, Los Angeles, California
Passive Immunization

Alan D. Strickland, B.S., M.S., M.D., D.Chem.
Staff Researcher, Discovery Group, Freeport, Texas
Amebiasis

Ciro V. Sumaya, M.D., M.P.H.T.M.
Professor of Pediatrics and Pathology, Division of Infectious Diseases, and Associate Medical Dean, University of Texas Health Science Center; Attending Physician, Medical Center Hospital and Santa Rosa Children's Hospital, San Antonio, Texas
Chronic Fatigue Syndrome; Epstein-Barr Virus

Mary E. Sutton, M.D.
Instructor in Neurology, Harvard Medical School and Boston Children's Hospital, Boston, Massachusetts
Parameningeal Infections; Transverse Myelitis or Myelopathy

David W. Teele, B.A., M.D.
Professor of Paediatrics, Christchurch School of Medicine, University of Otago; Clinical Director, Department of Paediatrics, Christchurch Hospital, Christchurch, New Zealand
Pneumococcal Infections

Robert B. Tesh, B.S., M.S., M.D.
Professor of Pathology and Professor of Microbiology and Immunology, Center for Tropical Diseases, University of Texas Medical Branch, Galveston, Texas
Other Bunyaviruses

Margaret A. Tipple, M.D.
Medical Officer, Office of Health and Safety, Centers for Disease Control and Prevention, Atlanta, Georgia
Health Information for International Travel

Richard G. Topazian, D.D.S.
Professor, Department of Oral and Maxillofacial Surgery, University of Connecticut School of Dental Medicine, Farmington, Connecticut
Infections of the Oral Cavity

Michael F. Tosi, M.D.
Associate Professor of Pediatrics, Case Western Reserve University; Rainbow Babies and Childrens Hospital, Cleveland, Ohio
Immunologic and Phagocytic Responses to Infection

Jeffrey A. Towbin, M.D.
Associate Professor of Pediatrics (Cardiology), Molecular and Human Genetics, Baylor College of Medicine; Pediatric Cardiologist and Director, Heart Failure Clinic, Texas Children's Hospital, Houston, Texas
Myocarditis

Amelia P. A. Travassos da Rosa, Pharmacist
Chief, Arbovirus Service, Instituto Evandro Chagas, Fundação Nacional de Saude, Ministry of Health, Belem, Para, Brazil
Other Bunyaviruses

Theodore F. Tsai, M.D., M.P.H.
Medical Officer, Centers for Disease Control and Prevention, Ft. Collins, Colorado
Orbiviruses and Coltiviruses; Alphaviruses; Flaviviruses; California/La Crosse Encephalitis

Jerrold A. Turner, M.D.
Professor of Medicine and Microbiology and Immunology, University of California, Los Angeles, School of Medicine, Los Angeles; Chief, Section of Parasitic Diseases; Associate Medical Director; and Director of Medical Education, Harbor–UCLA Medical Center, Torrance, California
Cestodes; Trematodes

Jesus G. Vallejo, M.D.
Assistant Professor of Pediatrics, Section of Infectious Disease, Baylor College of Medicine, Houston, Texas
Myocarditis

Jorge Vargas, M.D.
Associate Professor of Pediatrics, University of California at Los Angeles School of Medicine and Division of Pediatric Gastroenterology and Nutrition, UCLA Children's Hospital, Los Angeles, California
Hepatitis B and D Viruses

Pedro F. C. Vasconcelos, M.D.
Infectologist, Arbovirus Service, Instituto Evandro Chagas, Fundação Nacional de Saude, Ministry of Health, Belem, Para, Brazil
Other Bunyaviruses

Ellen R. Wald, M.D.
Professor of Pediatrics and Otolaryngology, University of Pittsburgh School of Medicine; Division Chief, Allergy, Immunology, and Infectious Diseases, Children's Hospital of Pittsburgh, Pittsburgh, Pennsylvania
Uvulitis; Infections in Day Care Environments

Joel I. Ward, M.D.
Professor of Pediatrics, University of California at Los Angeles School of Medicine; Chief, Pediatric Infectious Disease; Director, UCLA Center for Vaccine Research; Harbor–UCLA Medical Center, Torrance, California
Haemophilus influenzae

Richard L. Ward, Ph.D.
Professor of Pediatrics, University of Cincinnati School of Medicine and Children's Hospital Medical Center, Cincinnati, Ohio
Rotaviruses

Louis Weinstein, M.D., Ph.D.
Retired; former lecturer in Medicine, Harvard Medical School, Cambridge; Senior Consultant in Medicine, Brigham and Women's Hospital, Boston, Massachusetts
Tetanus

Robert C. Welliver, M.D.
Professor of Pediatrics, Division of Infectious Diseases, and Co-Director, Division of Infectious Diseases, State University of New York and Children's Hospital, Buffalo, New York
Bronchiolitis and Infectious Asthma

J. Gary Wheeler, M.D.
Associate Professor, Department of Pediatrics, Divisions of Allergy, Clinical Immunology, and Infectious Diseases, University of Arkansas for Medical Sciences; Attending Staff, Arkansas Children's Hospital, Little Rock, Arkansas
Pleural Effusions and Empyema; Lung Abscess

Bernhard L. Wiedermann, M.D.
Associate Professor of Pediatrics, The George Washington University School of Medicine and Health Sciences; Attending in Infectious Diseases and Director, Pediatric Residency Training Program, Children's National Medical Center, Washington, DC
Microbial Virulence Factors; Miscellaneous Causes of Myositis; Aspergillus *Infections; Histoplasmosis; Sporotrichosis; Zygomycosis*

Murray Wittner, M.D., Ph.D.
Professor of Pathology and Parasitology, Albert Einstein College of Medicine; Director, Parasitology and Tropical Diseases Clinic and Laboratory, Jacobi Medical Center, Bronx, New York
Leishmaniasis; Trypanosomiasis

Charles R. Woods, Jr., M.D.
Assistant Professor of Pediatrics, Bowman Gray School of Medicine, Wake Forest University, and Brenner Children's Hospital, Winston-Salem, North Carolina
Gynecologic Infections in Childhood and Adolescence; Other Yersinia *Species*

Edward J. Young, M.D.
Professor of Medicine and Professor of Microbiology and Immunology, Baylor College of Medicine; Chief of Staff, Veterans Affairs Medical Center, Houston, Texas
Brucellosis

Kenneth M. Zangwill, M.D.
Assistant Professor of Pediatrics, Harbor–UCLA Medical Center, University of California at Los Angeles School of Medicine; Member, Division of Infectious Diseases and UCLA Center for Vaccine Research, Harbor–UCLA Medical Center, Los Angeles, California
Haemophilus influenzae

PREFACE

❑ ❑ ❑

Despite the dramatic reduction in morbidity and mortality rates related to infectious diseases that followed the introduction of antimicrobial therapy, as well as active and passive immunization efforts, infectious diseases remain the leading cause of morbidity in infants and children. Children experience an average of six respiratory infections per year, requiring visits to a physician that outnumber the visits made for the purpose of well-child care. Infectious diseases also are the most common cause of school absenteeism.

The first edition of our text was written because we and many of our colleagues were concerned that no single reference existed that comprehensively covered infectious diseases in children. With each subsequent edition, including this one, our goal has been to provide comprehensive coverage of all subjects pertinent to the study of infectious diseases in children. Any attempt to summarize our present understanding of infectious diseases for serious students of the subject is a formidable task. In many areas, new information is accruing so rapidly that material becomes dated before it can appear in a text of this magnitude. Nevertheless, we have endeavored with the help of our many colleagues to provide the most comprehensive and up-to-date discussion of this field.

To provide a text as comprehensive and authoritative as possible, we have enlisted contributions from a large number of individuals, whose collective expertise is responsible for whatever success we may have had in meeting our objective. We offer our deepest appreciation to the 224 fellow contributors from universities or institutions in 10 countries for their professional expertise and devoted scholarship. Their cooperation and willingness to work with us leave us deeply in their debt.

Once again, infectious diseases are discussed according to organ systems that may be affected as well as individually by microorganisms. In all sections in which diseases related to specific agents are discussed, emphasis has been placed to the greatest extent possible on the specificity of clinical manifestations that may be related to the organism causing disease. Detailed information regarding the best means to establish a diagnosis and explicit recommendations for therapy are provided.

The entire text has been revised extensively. This edition also presents a new format for the discussion of infections caused by specific microorganisms. In the past, the various organisms causing disease were alphabetized within each section, offering the reader no particular advantage, as reference to the index still was required to locate a subject by specific page number.

In this edition, the infections with specific microorganisms have been reorganized to more appropriately emphasize the common features that may relate specific microorganisms to each other. Thus, all gram-positive coccal organisms are presented sequentially, followed by gram-negative cocci, gram-positive bacilli, enterobacteria, gram-negative coccobacilli, Treponemataceae, anaerobic bacteria, etc.

In addition, special sections of the text have been devoted to discussions of each of the following: microbial virulence factors; immunologic and phagocytic responses to infection; metabolic response of the host to infections; interaction of infection and nutrition; pathogenesis and treatment of fever; indigenous flora in host economy and pathogenesis; epidemiology of infectious diseases; congenital immune deficiency; AIDS and other acquired immunodeficiency diseases; opportunistic infections in the compromised host; Kawasaki disease; chronic fatigue syndrome; health information for the international traveler; nosocomial infections; prevention and control of infections in hospitalized children; pharmacology and pharmacokinetics of infectious agents; antibacterial, antiviral, antifungal, and antiparasitic agents; public health considerations; infections in day care environments; and use of the bacteriology, mycology, parasitology, virology, and serology laboratories.

A new section on immunomodulating agents and their potential use in the treatment of infectious diseases has been included because information on this subject has become most extensive since the publication of the last edition. Specific sections also are devoted to human bites and animal bites. In addition, the subject of biostatistics as applicable to the subspecialty of infectious diseases has been included for the first time. Other sections that make their first appearance as complete chapters include esophagitis; Whipple disease; infectious hepatitis due to viruses other than hepatitis viruses A through E; *Arcanobacterium haemolyticum; Erysipelothrix rhusiopathiae; Vibrio parahaemolyticus; Acinetobacter; Alcaligenes; Eikenella corrodens; Flavobacterium; Stenotrophomonas (Xanthomonas) maltophilia; Calymmatobacterium granulomatis; Kingella*; caliciviruses, including hepatitis E virus; and orbiviruses and coltiviruses. A chapter also has been devoted to the appropriate and inappropriate uses of prophylactic antimicrobial agents.

This book could not have been brought to fruition without the help and assistance of many individuals whose names do not appear in the text. Words are inadequate to convey our gratitude appropriately; we hope that they know they have our heartfelt thanks.

We would like to single out certain individuals for specific mention. We cannot adequately convey our appreciation for the thousands of hours devoted by Pamela Berea, who edited and also proofread every word of the text that was submitted, either in typed format or on computer disk, as well as the galley and page proofs of this manuscript. We are equally indebted to Mary Campbell, who spent an equivalent amount of time and who was specifically responsible for the coordination of the editorial effort, correspondence with our contributors and with the publisher, and coordination of the manuscript preparation process. We also appreciate the assistance provided to Mary Campbell and to the Editors by Carol Collins, Leslie Spring, Ruthi Stevens, and Sue Yancey, as well as the help provided by Carrel Briley and Sheila Walton.

We also appreciate the help and support of Judith Fletcher, Melissa Messersmith, Sandra Won and Michael Carcel (both formerly of W.B. Saunders), and Tom Stringer at W.B. Saunders, as well as the advice and editorial guidance of Lisette Bralow, who has helped us with every edition of this book.

Finally, we would like to thank the Baylor College of Medicine and Texas Children's Hospital in Houston, Texas, and the University of California School of Medicine at Los Angeles and the UCLA Children's Hospital for providing an environment that is supportive of intellectual pursuits.

RALPH D. FEIGIN, M.D.
JAMES D. CHERRY, M.D.

CONTENTS

❑ ❑ ❑

Color plates appear on pp. 724–729 and 2443–2446.

Volume 1

Part 1

HOST-PARASITE RELATIONSHIPS AND THE PATHOGENESIS OF INFECTIOUS DISEASES

Part 2

INFECTIONS OF SPECIFIC ORGAN SYSTEMS

SECTION ONE
UPPER RESPIRATORY TRACT INFECTIONS

SECTION TWO
LOWER RESPIRATORY TRACT INFECTIONS

SECTION THREE
INFECTIONS OF THE HEART

❑ ❑ ❑

SUBSECTION SIX
TREPONEMATACEAE

❑ ❑ ❑

SUBSECTION SEVEN
ANAEROBIC BACTERIA

SECTION SEVENTEEN
VIRAL INFECTIONS

❑ ❑ ❑

DNA VIRUSES

❑ ❑ ❑

SUBSECTION ONE
PARVOVIRIDAE

❑ ❑ ❑

SUBSECTION TWO
PAPILLOVIRIDAE

❑ ❑ ❑

SUBSECTION FOUR
TOGAVIRIDAE

❑ ❑ ❑

SUBSECTION FIVE
FLAVIVIRIDAE

❑ ❑ ❑

SUBSECTION SIX
ORTHOMYXOVIRIDAE

❑ ❑ ❑

SUBSECTION SEVEN
PARAMYXOVIRIDAE

Part 7

GUIDES TO THE DIAGNOSIS OF INFECTION

Part 8

BIOSTATISTICS APPLICABLE TO THE SUBSPECIALITY OF INFECTIOUS DISEASES

❑ ❑ ❑

SUBSECTION FIVE

GRAM-NEGATIVE COCCOBACILLI

131

ACTINOBACILLUS ACTINOMYCETEMCOMITANS

Suzanne Maxson and Richard F. Jacobs

Actinobacillus actinomycetemcomitans is a fastidious, gram-negative rod that frequently complicates actinomycosis caused by *Actinomyces israelii*. In addition to being associated with actinomycosis, it has been implicated as a pathogen in periodontal disease and is part of the oral flora. This organism is characterized by slow growth in culture and the need for incubation in an atmosphere enhanced with carbon dioxide.[1] Other bacterial species isolated concomitantly in human actinomycosis are *Eikenella corrodens, Fusobacterium, Bacteroides, Capnocytophaga, Staphylococcus, Streptococcus*, and Enterobacteriaceae.

A. actinomycetemcomitans is a pathogen in at least 30 per cent of actinomycotic infections (see Chapter 155).[1] Failure to recognize this organism and treat it adequately has resulted in clinical relapse and deterioration in infected patients with actinomycosis.[2, 4] Severe forms of periodontitis, particularly localized juvenile periodontitis, also are associated with this pathogen, and studies have shown that it strongly is related to children in the 10- to 19-year-old age group.[3] Additionally, it is one of the HACEK (HACEK also includes *Haemophilus aphrophilus, Cardiobacterium hominis, E. corrodens*, and *Kingella kingae*) organisms that has a propensity for infecting heart valves. Endocarditis caused by this organism usually is insidious, with fever occurring in less than 50 per cent of cases.[1] This organism also has been reported to cause pericarditis, meningitis, brain abscess, parotitis, synovitis, osteomyelitis, urinary tract infection, pneumonia, and empyema.[1]

A. actinomycetemcomitans can be cultured on blood and chocolate agar but grows poorly on MacConkey agar. The cultures require incubation in an enhanced carbon dioxide atmosphere.

References

1. McGowan, J. E., and Steinberg, J. P.: Other gram-negative bacilli. *In* Mandell, G. L., Bennett, J. E., and Dolin, R. (eds.): Principles and Practices of Infectious Disease. New York, Churchill Livingstone, 1995, pp. 2106–2107.
2. Morris, J. F., and Sewell, D. L.: Necrotizing pneumonia caused by mixed infection with *Actinobacillus actinomycetemcomitans* and *Actinomyces israelii:* Case report and review. Clin. Infect. Dis. *18*:450–452, 1994.
3. Savitt, E. D., and Kent, R. L.: Distribution of *Actinobacillus actinomycetemcomitans* and *Porphyromonas gingivalis*. J. Periodontol. *62*:490–494, 1991.
4. Tyrrell, J., Noone, P., and Prichard, J. S.: Thoracic actinomycosis complicated by *Actinobacillus actinomycetemcomitans:* Case report and review of literature. Respir. Med. *86*:341–343, 1992.

132

BARTONELLOSIS

Barbara W. Stechenberg

Bartonellosis is a disease unusual in its manifestations and rich in its history. The organism, *Bartonella bacilliformis*, causes two illnesses that are distinctive both clinically and temporally. Besides producing subclinical asymptomatic infections, this organism can cause Oroya fever, a disease characterized by a severe febrile hemolytic anemia, or verruga peruana, an eruption of hemangioma-like lesions. The eponym Carrión disease is used to designate the two forms collectively. The disease is restricted in its distribution to an area in South America including parts of Peru, Ecuador, and Colombia.

The origin of this disease in the history of the region probably precedes considerably the first written documentation of the disorder. The first written account of bartonellosis is attributed to Gago de Vadillo, who published a treatise on the subject in 1630, a century after the arrival of the first Spaniards. In 1764, Cosme Bueno first described the vector of this disease and cutaneous leishmaniasis as the uta or sand fly.[8] The era of the mid-1800s was a period of increasing wealth in Peru because of a new industry, the mining of guano, or bird manure. With this came the building of a railroad from Callao to Oroya and nearly 10,000 workers from Chile, Bolivia, and China. None had previous contact or immunity to Carrión disease. An epidemic that took the lives of hundreds of workers ensued. A cavalry unit of black soldiers sent to round up deserters quickly fell ill with the disease. A physician caring for them was so impressed with the rapidity and the profound anemia of the disease that he said, "It turned the blacks to whites," a remark henceforth frequently associated with the disease.[14]

In 1885, a Peruvian medical student (Carrión) was collecting data on the geographic distribution and clinical features of verruga peruana. Because of concern about the difficulty in diagnosing the pre-eruption period of verruga, he inoculated himself with material taken from a patient with verruga. He experienced his first symptoms 21 days after the inoculation, and then went on to exhibit the classic signs and symptoms of Oroya fever. He realized the significance of his experiment 3 days before he died; he had proved the unitary etiology of the two illnesses.

In 1905, Alberto Barton, a Peruvian physician, described

the etiologic agent *(B. bacilliformis)*, but it was several years before this organism was accepted as the cause of Oroya fever and named in his honor.

THE ORGANISM

B. bacilliformis is small, 0.2 to 1.0 μm wide by 0.3 to 2.0 μm long. It stains easily with Giemsa (purple) and is gram-negative and motile, with a brush of 10 or more unipolar flagella. On electron microscopy, the contrast between *B. bacilliformis* organisms and other members of their genus (*Bartonella*) is striking. Cultured *B. bacilliformis* show the retracted cytoplasm and cell walls typical of bacteria.[10] They are rod-shaped in young culture and become mostly coccoid in older culture. They are obligate aerobes that grow best at 28° C in semisolid nutrient agar with 10 per cent rabbit serum and 0.5 per cent rabbit hemoglobin. Growth is subsurface, usually in 7 to 10 days. The organism is pathogenic only for human beings and other primates. There is one antigenic type. The 16S rRNA sequence analyses show that *B. bacilliformis* is in the $alpha_2$ subgroup of proteobacteria and that its closest relatives are *Bartonella quintana* and *Brucella abortus*.[3]

EPIDEMIOLOGY

The distribution of the disease has been restricted to mountain valleys of the Andes mountains in Peru, Ecuador, and Colombia. Within these regions, it usually is seen only between altitudes of 2500 and 8000 feet above sea level and primarily in valleys that are at right angles to the prevailing wind. This interesting geographic distribution reflects the habits of the sand fly vectors that are seen only at these altitudes. One usually acquires the disease at twilight or soon thereafter because of the feeding habits of the insects. Within the region, the disease is endemic, with sporadic epidemic outbreaks that continue to occur.[7] There have been several isolated reports of anemia with *Bartonella*-like organisms—three cases from Thailand in 1966 and one case from the Sudan in 1969.

PATHOPHYSIOLOGY

After inoculation by the sand fly, *Bartonella* organisms enter the endothelial cells of the blood vessels, where they proliferate during the incubation period. Microscopically, masses of organisms may be noted within the cytoplasm of the cells lining the blood vessels and lymph channels, which causes them to bulge into the lumen of the vessel. The organisms may be found within the reticuloendothelial cells, particularly in the lymph nodes, but also in the liver, spleen, bone marrow, kidneys, adrenals, pancreas, and, more rarely, skin, heart, and lungs.

The organisms then re-enter the blood stream and parasitize the erythrocytes. *B. bacilliformis* organisms bind to the erythrocytes and induce indentations and deformation of the membrane, cause membrane fusion, and then enter into intracellular vacuoles, where they replicate.[2] The resulting anemia primarily is the result of destruction of these parasitized cells. Because as many as 90 per cent of the cells may be infected, profound, rapid anemia is common; the life span of the red blood cells is shortened markedly, particularly in the first few days. All parasitized cells are not destroyed. No hemolysins or agglutinins have been recovered.[12] *B. bacilliformis* can be demonstrated easily with Giemsa stain. In earlier studies, there was considerable controversy over whether the parasites were within or on the surface of red blood cells; Cuadra and Takano[5] have shown that they predominantly are within the cells.

In the recovery phase of the anemia, the rod-shaped organisms change to a more coccoid form and rapidly disappear from the blood.

The patient who survives the acute phase of Oroya fever may or may not develop cutaneous manifestations of the disease. These appear as nodular, hemangiomatous lesions ranging in size from a few millimeters to several centimeters. Light microscopy reveals angioblastic and histiocytic hyperplasia of the dermis. There are numerous newly formed small vessels with endothelial cell proliferation. Mast cells, lymphocytes, and macrophages are present.[1] Electron microscopy demonstrates that the bacterial organisms are in the verruga; the organisms are extracellular in the fine fibrous interstitium. Two types of histiocytic cells make up the verruga—a more numerous one, clear and with many lysosomes, ribosomes, mitochondria, and cytoplasm; and a darker one, with numerous lamellar membranous structures in the cytoplasm.[11] Studies have substantiated the presence of an activity in *B. bacilliformis* that stimulates endothelial cells in vitro and is angiogenic in vivo. This may explain the similar pathogenesis of the verruca and bacillary angiomatosis produced by other *Bartonella* species.[6]

CLINICAL MANIFESTATIONS

The incubation period varies from 2 to 14 weeks with a mean of 3 weeks. The difficulty in determining the duration of the incubation period is the result of the variable symptoms of the disease. Some patients totally are asymptomatic, and disease is detected only by blood culture. Other patients are not anemic but develop symptoms, such as headache, malaise, and occasional fever, and *B. bacilliformis* is recovered from blood cultures. Still others have severe anemia (Oroya fever). Patients with hemolytic anemia are febrile, and organisms may parasitize the erythrocytes. The anemia develops rapidly. Patients are deeply apathetic and have a peculiar discoloration to the skin and sclerae secondary to the combination of slight icterus and severe anemia.[13] Tachycardia and soft hemic murmurs are noted; occasionally, there is peripheral vascular collapse. Headache, vertigo, restlessness, tinnitus, and, occasionally, angina pectoris may be present. Clouding of the sensorium and delirium are rather common; usually these are mild but may progress to overt psychosis. The temperature usually fluctuates between 37.5° and 38.5° C (99.5° and 101.3° F); higher elevation may be caused by intercurrent infection. Physical examination discloses generalized lymphadenopathy.

The anemia is macrocytic and usually hypochromic, with anisocytosis and poikilocytosis. The erythrocyte count may drop to as low as $500{,}000/mm^3$ in the first 2 to 4 weeks of illness. Reticulocytes may increase to 50 per cent. The pathognomonic sign of the disease is the presence of the organism, *B. bacilliformis*, within Giemsa-stained erythrocytes as red-violet rods. The leukocyte count may be normal, low, or elevated.

The "critical stage" of the anemia is the period of transition when the organism suddenly disappears from the red blood cells.[13] During this time, the *Bartonella* organisms change from the rod shape to more coccoid forms, there is a decrease in the number of parasitized erythrocytes, and the anemia decreases so that there is an increase in the red cell count and less hyperbilirubinemia. Clinically, the fever decreases and the patient stabilizes.[13] In some cases, illness may become more severe, which suggests the development of intercurrent infection (usually with *Salmonella*). Although this complication may occur at any time, it is most common during the transition period and may be noted in up to 40 per cent of patients.[4]

In the pre-eruptive stage, patients may complain of pain in their joints, bones, and muscles and of cramps and paresthesias. Inflammatory reactions, such as phlebitis, parotitis, pleuritis, erythema nodosum, and encephalitis, may occur. The anemia and lymphadenopathy of the invasive stage disappear.

The appearance of red cutaneous nodules, verruga, is pathognomonic of the disease in the eruptive stage. Usually, these are in the skin but may be found in mesenchymatous tissue. They vary greatly in number and size, from small nodules to disfiguring zonular (hemangioma-like) lesions. They rarely cause symptoms; however, larger ones may require surgical excision. This stage may last from several months to a year.

DIAGNOSIS

The diagnosis is based on the clinical manifestations, in conjunction with a blood smear showing typical organisms, or on blood cultures. In the preanemic stage or in patients without the typical anemia who reside in an endemic area, the diagnosis can be based on blood cultures alone. The presence of typical verruga in patients from the endemic area is pathognomonic for the disease. IgM antibody may be present in both stages of disease as well as in some healthy persons.[9] Persons with typical Oroya fever treated with antibiotics may not show an antibody response.[7, 9]

TREATMENT

The *B. bacilliformis* organism is sensitive to many antibiotics, including penicillin, tetracycline, streptomycin, and chloramphenicol. With treatment, fever usually abates by 24 hours; the rod-shaped organisms change to more coccoid forms and soon disappear from the blood.

The choice of antibiotic may be guided by considerations other than simple eradication of *B. bacilliformis*, including the risk of intercurrent infection. Chloramphenicol is considered to be the drug of choice because it also is useful in the treatment of salmonellosis.[15] Blood transfusions may be helpful during the period of severe anemia, especially if blood is obtained from patients who have recovered recently from the disease.[12]

Treatment for the verruga peruana usually is not necessary unless particularly large zonular lesions interfere with function; in these persons, surgery may be necessary. Oral tetracycline may be used to aid in healing of the cutaneous lesions.

PROGNOSIS

The mortality rate in untreated bartonellosis has been estimated at about 40 per cent. In untreated patients with intercurrent *Salmonella* infection, the mortality rate has been as high as 90 per cent. With the use of chloramphenicol, prognosis is much improved. Most patients develop permanent immunity.

PREVENTION

DDT has been effective in controlling the disease by eliminating the vector *Phlebotomus*. Persons can protect themselves by leaving endemic areas at night and by using insect repellents. There is no vaccine of demonstrated efficacy.

References

1. Arias-Stella, J., Lieberman, P. H., Erlandson, R. A., et al.: Histology, immunohistochemistry and ultrastructure of the verruga in Carrión's disease. Am. J. Surg. Pathol. *10*:595–610, 1986.
2. Benson, N. A., Kar, S., McLaughlin, G., et al.: Entry of *Bartonella* into erythrocytes. Infect. Immun. *54*:347–353, 1986.
3. Brenner, D. J., O'Connor, S. P., Hollis, D. G., et al: Molecular characterization and proposal of a neotype strain for *Bartonella bacilliformis*. J. Clin. Microbiol. *29*:1299–1302, 1991.
4. Cuadra, M.: Salmonellosis complication in human bartonellosis. Texas Rep. Biol. Med. *14*:97–113, 1956.
5. Cuadra, M., and Takano, J.: The relationship of *Bartonella* to the red blood cell as revealed by electron microscopy. Blood *33*:708–716, 1969.
6. Garcia, F. U., Wojta, J., and Hoover, R. L.: Interactions between live *Bartonella bacilliformis* and endothelial cells. J. Infect. Dis. *165*:1138–1141, 1992.
7. Gray, G. C., Johnson, A. A., Thornton, S. A., et al.: An epidemic of Oroya fever in the Peruvian Andes. Am. J. Trop. Hyg. *42*:215–221, 1990.
8. Herrer, A., and Christensen, H.: Implication of *Phlebotomus* sand flies as vectors of bartonellosis and leishmaniasis as early as 1764. Science *190*:154–155, 1975.
9. Knobloch, J., Solano, L., Alvarez, O., et al.: Antibodies to *Bartonella* as determined by fluorescence antibody test, indirect hemagglutination and ELISA. Trop. Med. Parasitol. *36*:183–185, 1985.
10. Peters, D., and Wigand, R.: Bartonellaceae. Bacteriol. Rev. *19*:150–155, 1955.
11. Recavarren, S., and Lumbreras, H.: Pathogenesis of the verruga of Carrión's disease. Am. J. Pathol. *66*:461–464, 1972.
12. Reynafarje, C., and Ramos, J.: The hemolytic anemia of human bartonellosis. Blood *17*:562–578, 1961.
13. Ricketts, W. E.: Clinical manifestations of Carrión's disease. Arch. Intern. Med. *84*:751–781, 1949.
14. Schultz, M. G.: A history of bartonellosis (Carrión's disease). Am. J. Trop. Med. Hyg. *17*:503–515, 1968.
15. Urteaga, O., and Payne, E.: Treatment of the acute febrile phase of Carrión's disease with chloramphenicol. Am. J. Trop. Med. *4*:507–511, 1955.

133

BRUCELLOSIS

Edward J. Young

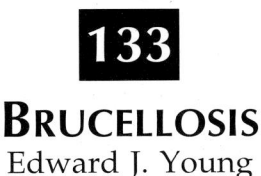

Brucellosis is an infection of domestic and wild animals (zoonosis) that is transmittable to humans. Humans are accidental hosts, playing no role in maintaining the disease in nature. In the United States, a cooperative federal/state program to control bovine brucellosis has reduced dramatically the incidence of human infection. Nevertheless, brucellosis remains enzootic in many parts of the world, notably in the Mediterranean basin, the Arabian peninsula, the Indian subcontinent, and parts of Mexico and Central and South America.[37] The World Health Organization has called for the eradication of brucellosis worldwide; however, a general lack of political conviction makes the achievement of this objective unlikely in the near future.[28]

HISTORY

Brucellosis probably has existed since the time humans first domesticated animals, and Hippocrates mentions a disease compatible with brucellosis (ca. 450 B.C.).[114] The first accurate description of human brucellosis is credited to J. A. Marston, an assistant surgeon in the Royal Army Medical Corps.[127] In 1863, Marston described an illness in troops stationed in Malta during the Crimean War. Marston's report includes a poignant depiction of his own suffering with brucellosis.[82] During the 19th century, brucellosis was known by various names, including Mediterranean fever, Malta fever, gastric remittent fever, and undulant fever.[43] Although the disease caused considerable morbidity and mortality for British military personnel stationed throughout the Mediterranean, the etiology was not apparent immediately. In 1886, David Bruce, another Royal Army Medical Corps surgeon, isolated a microorganism from spleen tissue of victims of Malta fever.[23] He called the bacterium *Micrococcus* (later *Brucella*) *melitensis* and showed that it was present in the blood, urine, and feces of patients. Later, Bruce was appointed head of the Mediterranean Fever Commission (1904 to 1907), which investigated the disease in Malta. Themistocle Zammit, a Maltese physician working with the Commission, identified native goats as the principal source of brucellosis in Malta. The goats were shown to shed the bacteria in their milk, and when fresh goat's milk was replaced with tinned condensed milk in the military mess, the incidence of brucellosis declined dramatically. In 1897, Almroth Wright applied the newly discovered agglutination test to the serologic diagnosis of Malta fever.[129]

Unlike *B. melitensis,* which originally was isolated from human tissues, other *Brucella* species were recognized for the disease they caused in animals (contagious abortion). In 1897, Bernhard Bang, a Danish veterinarian and physician, isolated the "abortion bacillus" (later *Brucella abortus*) from the tissues of diseased cattle.[17] To this day, veterinarians refer to bovine brucellosis as Bang disease. Around 1914, Jacob Traum, a bacteriologist with the Bureau of Animal Industry, isolated an organism from an aborted swine fetus. Initially thought to be the agent of Bang disease, this bacterium later was shown to be a separate species (*Brucella suis*).[59]

The bacteriologist Alice Evans finally recognized the relatedness of these disparate microorganisms in 1918.[46] Evans' work was confirmed by others, and in 1920, K. F. Meyer and E. B. Shaw proposed the name *Brucella* for the genus to honor Bruce.[57, 87]

Additional *Brucella* species were isolated from sheep (*Brucella ovis*) and from desert wood rats (*Brucella neotomae*), but to date they have not been shown to cause human illness. The most recent addition to the genus, *Brucella canis,* was isolated from kennel-bred beagles by Carmichael and Brunner in 1968.[26, 90] Human infection due to *B. canis* was reported first in 1972,[119] but this species is a less common cause of human infection than *B. melitensis, B. abortus,* or *B. suis.*[98] Nevertheless, *B. canis* has been isolated from children and adults,[123] especially among laboratory workers and persons exposed to dogs or other canines.

ETIOLOGY

The organisms of the genus *Brucella* are small, fastidious, nonmotile, non–spore-forming, gram-negative coccobacilli and lack native plasmids. Their metabolism is oxidative, and all strains are aerobic. Many species require carbon dioxide for growth, especially for primary isolation. *Brucella* strains always are catalase-positive, but oxidase activity varies. Although most strains reduce nitrate to nitrite, some do not. The production of hydrogen sulfide also varies, as does urease activity.[39] A variety of media support the growth of *Brucella,* including serum dextrose agar, trypticase soy agar, and chocolate agar. Selective media are not required, except when one is attempting isolation from feces or other contaminated material. Growth of *Brucella* in vitro is fairly slow, and primary isolation may require prolonged incubation. When brucellosis is suspected, cultures should not be discarded before a minimum of 28 days.

There are seven recognized biovars of *B. abortus,* three biovars of *B. melitensis,* and five biovars of *B. suis.* Identification of species and differentiation of biovars are based on the results of oxidative metabolism tests and bacteriophage lysis patterns.[38] Preliminary identification can be made by means of the use of cross-absorbed polyclonal antisera or monoclonal antibodies specific for the A and M epitopes of smooth *Brucella* strains or the R antigen of nonsmooth strains. Caution is advised when using automated bacterial identification schemes because some commercial products lack the profiles for *Brucella* species.[18] Identification tests using polymerase chain reaction are under development.[49, 60] The results of DNA hybridization studies reveal a high degree of genetic relatedness among all *Brucella* species. Nevertheless, it has been recommended that the existing nomenclature be retained for taxonomic purposes and to avoid confusion.[40] Because of the risk of laboratory-acquired brucellosis, special precautions are recommended for the handling of specimens, including the use of biohazard safety cabinets.[88]

EPIDEMIOLOGY

Brucellosis is found worldwide in domestic and wild animals, and nearly all human infections derive directly or indirectly from animal sources.[37] Despite a wide range of susceptible animals, each *Brucella* species has a principal or preferred host: *B. abortus,* cattle; *B. melitensis,* goats; *B. suis,* swine; *B. ovis,* sheep; *B. neotomae,* desert wood rats; *B. canis,* dogs. These associations are not absolute, and secondary hosts are numerous.[100] In the Middle East, for example, camels appear to be an important reservoir of brucellosis[64, 91]; however, the course of infection in camels is understood poorly. Similarly, the role of wildlife in the epidemiology of brucellosis remains unclear.[44, 84]

Historically, brucellosis has been an occupational risk for farmers, ranchers, veterinarians, meat inspectors, abattoir workers, and laboratory personnel. Transmission commonly occurs by direct contact with diseased animals or their carcasses through cuts and abrasions in the unprotected skin.[58] Another route of transmission is aerosols of blood or other secretions through the respiratory tract or the conjunctival sac of the eye. This method of infection especially is common in abattoirs.[63, 124] Veterinarians immunizing cattle with *B. abortus* strain 19 vaccine are at some risk of infection by accidental self-inoculation.[106]

The most common route of transmission of *B. melitensis* is ingestion of unpasteurized goat's milk or cheese.[117, 121, 133] *Brucella* organisms can remain viable in cheese for considerable periods, depending on the time of curing, the salt content, the pH, and the presence of other bacteria.[94] Raw milk products are a particular hazard for travelers to countries in which brucellosis is enzootic, where the disease can be contracted in food without direct animal contact.[16] The meat of infected animals is harmless when cooked adequately[105]; however, the custom of eating raw meat or bone marrow has been linked to outbreaks of human brucellosis.[29]

The epidemiology of human brucellosis has changed in some areas of the country. For example, in Texas between 1977 and 1982, most cases occurred in Caucasian men, with documented exposure to cattle or swine in the course of their occupations. In contrast, between 1982 and 1986, most cases occurred in Hispanics of both sexes, and the principal source of infection was the ingestion of unpasteurized goat's milk cheese.[120] A shift from occupationally acquired brucellosis to food-borne transmission also has been reported in California.[30]

Brucellosis once was believed to be uncommon in children, but it now is recognized that persons of all ages are susceptible.[108] Conditions for transmission of the disease from animals to humans vary from country to country and from culture to culture. Where farm animals traditionally are raised in the home, contact between animals and children is frequent, providing an opportunity for the transmission of zoonoses. Moreover, food-borne brucellosis is not limited to any age or sex and can occur without direct contact with animals.[135] Childhood brucellosis is more common where brucellosis is enzootic and where *B. melitensis* is the prevalent species.[48] The clinical manifestations of brucellosis in children do not differ from those in adults,[55, 118] although unfamiliarity with the disease can delay the diagnosis in children who are not exposed occupationally.[4, 31]

Human-to-human transmission of brucellosis is thought not to occur, although rare cases suggesting venereal transmission have been reported[103, 115] and *Brucella* has been isolated from banked sperm.[126] Brucellosis has been reported in pregnant women and can result in abortion[107]; however, there is little evidence that brucellosis causes abortion more commonly than other bacteremic infections.[99] Pregnant women can be treated successfully for brucellosis without terminating pregnancy or impairing their ability to conceive again. Transplacental transmission of *Brucella* leading to neonatal infection has been suggested but appears to be rare.[75]

PATHOGENESIS

Brucella species are facultative, intracellular pathogens that can survive and replicate within phagocytic cells of the host.[21] Shortly after inoculation into a susceptible host, brucellae are ingested by polymorphonuclear leukocytes. However, neutrophils have a limited ability to destroy phagocytized bacteria, and within this protected environment, the organisms multiply.[134] The mechanisms by which *Brucella* evades intracellular killing are understood only partly but include inhibition of neutrophil granules and inhibition of the peroxidase–hydrogen peroxide–halide bactericidal system.[101, 109] Brucellae also localize within organs of the reticuloendothelial system (liver, spleen, bone marrow), where they multiply in macrophages and monocytes. As the disease progresses, the microbicidal activity of macrophages increases coincidentally with the development of cell-mediated immunity. Macrophage activation involves the action of cytokines (e.g., interferon, tumor necrosis factor), elaborated by specifically committed T lymphocytes.[66] Coincidental to the development of acquired cellular resistance, the host demonstrates dermal sensitivity to a variety of *Brucella* antigens.[62, 80]

The host response to infection with *B. abortus* is characterized by the development of tissue granulomas indistinguishable from sarcoidosis.[22] In contrast, infection with the more virulent species (*B. melitensis* and *B. suis*) more commonly results in visceral microabscesses.[40, 128, 132]

CLINICAL MANIFESTATIONS

The spectrum of human brucellosis ranges from subclinical (diagnosed serologically) to chronic (often manifested by recurrent symptoms over many years).[136] Symptoms are nonspecific, usually occurring within 2 to 3 weeks of inoculation. The onset of disease is insidious in approximately one-half of cases. The disease is characterized by a multitude of somatic complaints, such as fever, sweats, anorexia, fatigue, weight loss, and depression. In contrast with the multiple subjective complaints, there often is a paucity of abnormal physical findings, of which fever and mild lymphadenopathy are the most common. Acute brucellosis is a systemic illness involving multiple organs or organ systems. Occasionally, patients feel well in the morning, with symptoms worsening as the day progresses. Brucellosis can present as fever of undetermined origin,[31] and when untreated, the fever assumes an undulating pattern. Occasionally, symptoms related to a single organ predominate, in which case the disease is called localized.[36] Not unexpectedly, localization often involves organs rich in elements of the reticuloendothelial system.

Arthritis is said to be the most frequent localized complication of brucellosis,[53, 78, 92] and in children, monarticular disease of the hips, knees, and sacroiliac is common.[81] Spondylitis and osteomyelitis also have been reported but are less common in children than adults.[71]

Neurobrucellosis comprises a variety of complications, including meningoencephalitis, myelitis and myelopathies, peripheral and cranial neuropathies, and psychiatric manifestations.[86] Fortunately, direct invasion of the central nervous system is rare, occurring in less than 2 per cent of cases, predominantly caused by *B. melitensis*.[20, 93] Analysis of cerebrospinal fluid in brucella meningitis reveals elevated proteins, normal or reduced glucose, and a lymphocytic pleocytosis. Brucellae rarely are isolated from cerebrospinal fluid, but antibodies to *Brucella* are present in the serum and cerebrospinal fluid in most cases.[9]

Brucellosis, like typhoid fever, can be an enteric infection in which systemic symptoms predominate over gastrointestinal findings. Nevertheless, 30 to 60 per cent of patients with brucellosis complain of anorexia, nausea, vomiting, abdominal discomfort, and weight loss.[48, 55, 61, 89, 108] Rare cases of ileitis[96] and colitis[68, 116] caused by *B. melitensis* have been reported, as have cases of spontaneous peritonitis.[2] Because the liver is the largest organ of the reticuloendothelial system, it probably is involved in most cases of brucellosis. Liver function test values often are normal or elevated only mildly; however, hepatic involvement has been documented by liver biopsy, even when liver function test results were normal.[35] Occasionally, transaminase levels resemble acute viral hepatitis.[74] The histopathology of the liver in *B. abortus* infection is characterized by noncaseating granulomas indistinguishable from sarcoidosis.[112] The spectrum of hepatic lesions caused by *B. melitensis* ranges from small aggregates of mononuclear cells resembling viral hepatitis to collections of cells including histiocytes and epithelioid cells resembling loose granulomas.[132] Infection with *B. suis* can be associated with chronic suppurative liver abscesses.[128] In spite of the extent of liver involvement, the lesions generally resolve with treatment and cirrhosis is extremely rare.[85]

In the genitourinary tract, the testicles are the organs most frequently involved in brucellosis. Acute orchitis or epididymo-orchitis can be the presenting complaint, but more often it occurs in the course of systemic infection.[50, 70]

The respiratory tract is known to be a portal of inoculation in abattoir-associated brucellosis[69]; however, pulmonary complications are relatively uncommon. In a study of 1100 children and 400 adults with brucellosis in Kuwait, Lubani and associates[77] described five adults and four children with pulmonary complications. Hilar and peritracheal lymphadenopathy, pneumonia, lung nodules, pleural effusions, and empyema all have been noted in patients with brucellosis.

Despite the frequency of bacteremia in brucellosis, endocarditis, a potentially lethal complication, fortunately is rare.[7] *Brucella* usually affects previously damaged valves; however, infection with more virulent species (*B. melitensis* and *B. suis*) can involve previously normal valves. Delays in making the diagnosis can lead to complications, such as myocardial abscesses and sinus of Valsalva fistulas. Hence, a combination of antimicrobial drugs and valve replacement surgery often is required to achieve a cure.[65] Other complications include myocarditis, pericarditis, and aneurysms of the aorta and cerebral vessels.

A variety of ocular lesions have been described in patients with brucellosis, of which uveitis is the most common.[110] The pathogenesis of such lesions is a matter of some speculation.[102]

Cutaneous lesions that have been attributed to brucellosis include contact lesions, rashes, abscesses, ulcers, and vasculitis.[19] Subcutaneous papules, from which *Brucella* has been cultured, have been reported in children[52] and adults.[15]

DIAGNOSIS

The symptoms of brucellosis are nonspecific. Therefore, the importance of a detailed history, including occupation, avocations, travel, exposure to animals, and food habits, cannot be overemphasized.[130] Routine laboratory tests generally are not helpful in the diagnosis of brucellosis; however, a variety of hematologic abnormalities have been reported and may suggest the need for more specific tests.[6] For example, unlike most infections, the white blood cell count in brucellosis usually is normal or depressed, rarely exceeding 10,000 cells/mm^3.[27] Anemia is reported in 75 per cent and thrombocytopenia in 40 per cent of cases.[40] Pancytopenia was reported in 6 per cent of children with brucellosis in one series.[5] Examination of the bone marrow may reveal erythrophagocytosis.[83, 125] Microangiopathic hemolytic anemia,[45] thrombocytopenic purpura,[122] and Coombs-positive hemolytic anemia[79] have been associated with brucellosis.

Brucellosis is diagnosed definitively by isolating a *Brucella* species from blood, bone marrow, or other tissues. The rate of isolation from blood varies from 15 to 70 per cent, depending on the methods used and the length of incubation. In some series, the recovery rate from bone marrow exceeded the recovery from blood.[54] Rapid isolation techniques in use in most clinical laboratories, such as Bactec and DuPont Isolator, are adequate when maintained for at least 30 days.[111]

In the absence of bacteriologic confirmation, a presumptive diagnosis can be made by measuring the titer of specific antibodies in the serum.[137] A variety of methods have been applied to the serologic diagnosis of brucellosis. The serum agglutination test (SAT), using antigen from *B. abortus* strain 1119, remains the standard against which others are compared. The SAT detects cross-reacting antibodies against smooth species (*B. abortus*, *B. melitensis*, and *B. suis*) but does not detect antibodies to rough species, such as *B canis*. For the detection of antibodies to *B. canis*, antigen prepared from *B. canis* or *B. ovis* is required.[97]

Human brucellosis is characterized by initial production of IgM antibodies, followed by a switch to IgG antibody synthesis within the second week of infection.[47] After treatment, IgG antibody concentration declines more rapidly than IgM antibody concentration, and, in some patients, low titers of IgM antibodies can persist for many years in the absence of active disease.[24] The prompt decline in IgG antibody concentration is prognostic of a successful outcome of therapy,[51] whereas persistence of a high titer of IgG antibodies presages a clinical relapse.[95]

The SAT measures the total quantity (IgM + IgG) of agglutinins; therefore, a method is needed to differentiate between antibody isotypes. A simple method employs 0.05 M 2-mercaptoethanol treatment of serum, which destroys the agglutinability of IgM without affecting IgG.[25] No single SAT titer *always* is diagnostic, but most patients with active infection have titers greater than or equal to 1:160. False-negative SAT results can occur because of a prozone or the rare presence of so-called "blocking" antibodies. The prozone can be avoided by routinely diluting serum beyond 1:320, and blocking antibodies can be detected by the Coombs test. Among the newer serologic tests, the enzyme-linked immunosorbent assay appears to be the most sensitive.[10] However, more experience is required before it replaces the SAT as the method of choice.

TREATMENT

Antimicrobial chemotherapy lessens morbidity, shortens the course of illness, and reduces the incidence of complications of brucellosis.[56] A variety of drugs are active against *Brucella* species. However, the results of sensitivity tests do not correlate always with clinical effectiveness. For example, β-lactam antibiotics are active in vitro, but treatment with these agents rarely is curative.[73, 131]

Because brucellae are intracellular pathogens, it is believed that penetration into cells is a prerequisite for an effective anti-*Brucella* drug. In addition, the rate of relapse is high unless prolonged treatment is given, usually 4 to 6 weeks.[136]

The tetracyclines are among the most effective antibiotics for treating brucellosis, with a mean minimal inhibitory concentration of less than 1 μg/mL. Traditionally, tetracycline hydrogen chloride (2 g/day orally for 6 weeks) in combination with streptomycin (1 g/day intramuscularly for 2 to 3 weeks) was the recommended treatment for human brucellosis in adults. With good compliance, this combination yielded relapse rates of less than 5 per cent.[56] Because of its longer half-life and fewer side effects, doxycycline (200 mg/day) has replaced tetracycline hydrogen chloride as the preferred analogue. Streptomycin has been shown to enhance in vitro killing of *B. melitensis* by a number of antibiotics,[104] and the effectiveness of doxycycline and streptomycin has been well documented.[33] Gentamicin is as efficacious as streptomycin in vitro and is less toxic; however, clinical trials with gentamicin are limited.

In 1986, the World Health Organization recommended the combination of doxycycline (200 mg/day) plus rifampin (600 to 900 mg/day) as the treatment of choice in adults, with both drugs continued for 6 weeks.[67] Comparative studies of doxycycline-rifampin and doxycycline-streptomycin generally have shown equivalent efficacy when given for 6 weeks, although the latter may be more effective for complications such as spondylitis.[12, 13]

Because tetracyclines are contraindicated for pregnant women and children younger than 9 years of age because of the risk of irreversible staining of deciduous teeth, alternative treatments have been sought. Lubani and associates[76] reported a 6-year multicenter study of childhood brucellosis in Kuwait. They recommended that children younger than 8 years of age receive trimethoprim-sulfamethoxazole (TMP-SMZ) (10/50 mg/kg/day) given twice daily for 3 weeks plus gentamicin (5 mg/kg/day) twice daily for the first 5 days. In a study from Saudi Arabia involving 102 children 45 days to 14 years of age, Al-Eissa and associates[3] reported a high relapse rate (87 per cent) when various combinations of antibiotics were given for only 3 weeks. In contrast, the rate of relapse fell to 8 per cent for patients treated for at least 6 weeks. They reported no relapses among nine patients treated with TMP-SMZ plus rifampin for 8 to 12 weeks.

The fluoroquinolones, especially ofloxacin, are active in vitro against *Brucella* species. However, high relapse rates were reported when quinolones were used alone.[72] A study from Turkey reported that the results of a 6-week course of ofloxacin (400 mg) plus rifampin (600 mg) were comparable with those of doxycycline (200 mg) plus rifampin (600 mg).[1] Although these findings are encouraging, additional experience is needed to determine the role of quinolones in the treatment of brucellosis.

The optimal treatment for complications of brucellosis, such as meningitis and endocarditis, has not been defined with certainty. Doxycycline crosses the blood-brain barrier more effectively than does generic tetracycline, and it has been used in combination with rifampin and TMP-SMZ for neurobrucellosis.[86, 93] Third-generation cephalosporins also achieve high concentrations in cerebrospinal fluid, but the sensitivity of *Brucella* species varies, and in vitro susceptibility should be ensured for the specific isolates before they are used. Although individual cases of brucella endocarditis have been cured using antibiotics alone,[32] most cases have required valve replacement as well.[8]

The vast majority of patients with brucellosis recover completely within a few weeks to months after receiving adequate treatment. Despite appropriate therapy, some patients suffer a relapse characterized by the recurrence of symptoms and the reisolation of brucellae from their blood.[14] Obviously, relapse is more frequent when less than a full 6-week course of antibiotics is given. It is important to recognize that continuing oral antibiotics for 6 weeks taxes the compliance of patients once their symptoms resolve. With few exceptions, relapse is *not* caused by the emergence of antibiotic-resistant strains of *Brucella*.[11]

RELAPSE AND CHRONIC BRUCELLOSIS

In the pre-antibiotic era, the course of brucellosis often was unremitting and chronic infection was common.[114] Since the advent of effective treatment, chronic brucellosis has become rare. Chronic brucellosis usually involves a focus of infection in the bone or other tissues that requires surgical drainage as well as antibiotics for cure. Patients with chronic brucellosis often experience recurrent episodes of fever and other symptoms, and IgG agglutinins remain elevated.[51, 95] Scanning techniques (e.g., technetium-99m bone scan, gallium-67, computed tomography, magnetic resonance imaging) can be useful adjuncts for diagnosing an occult focus of infection.

Even with adequate treatment, convalescence is delayed in some proportion of patients with brucellosis. Such patients continue to complain of ill health, despite the absence of objective evidence of active disease, a decline in the titers of agglutinins, and negative cultures for *Brucella*. It was believed that these patients suffered from psychoneurosis or neurasthenia made worse by the infection.[113] Whether or not this phenomenon is a variant of the chronic fatigue syndrome is not clear.[34] What is clear is that these patients do not benefit from repeated treatment with antibiotics.[137]

References

1. Akova, M., Ozun, O., Akalin, H. E., et al.: Quinolones in treatment of human brucellosis: Comparative trial of ofloxacin-rifampin versus doxycycline-rifampin. Antimicrob. Agents Chemother. *37*:1831–1834, 1993.
2. Al Faraj, S.: Acute abdomen as atypical presentation of brucellosis: Report of two cases and review of literature. J. R. Soc. Med. *88*:91–92, 1995.
3. Al-Eissa, Y. A., Kambal, A. M., Al-Nasser, M. N., et al.: Childhood brucellosis: A study of 102 cases. Pediatr. Infect. Dis. J. *9*:74–79, 1990.
4. Al-Eissa, Y. A.: Unusual suppurative complications of brucellosis in children. Acta Pediatr. *82*:987–992, 1993.
5. Al-Eissa, Y. A., Assuhaimi, S. A., Al-Fawaz, I. M., et al.: Pancytopenia in children with brucellosis: Clinical manifestations and bone marrow findings. Acta Haematol. *89*:132–136, 1993.
6. Al-Eissa, Y., and Al-Nasser, M.: Haematological manifestations of childhood brucellosis. Infection *21*:23–26, 1993.
7. Al-Harthi, S. S.: The morbidity and mortality pattern of *Brucella* endocarditis. Int. J. Cardiol. *25*:321–324, 1989.
8. Al-Kasab, S., Al-Fagih, M. R., Al-Yousef, S., et al.: Brucella infective endocarditis: Successful combined medical and surgical therapy. J. Thorac. Surg. *95*:862–870, 1988.
9. Araj, G. F., Lulu, A. R., Saadah, M. A., et al.: Rapid diagnosis of central nervous system brucellosis by ELISA. J. Neuroimmunol. *12*:173–182, 1986.
10. Araj, G. F., Lulu, A. R., Mustafa, M. Y., et al.: Evaluation of ELISA in the diagnosis of acute and chronic brucellosis. J. Hyg. *97*:457–469, 1986.
11. Ariza, J., Bosch, J., Gudiol, F., et al.: Relevance of in vitro antimicrobial susceptibility of *Brucella melitensis* to relapse rate in human brucellosis. Antimicrob. Agents Chemother. *30*:958–960, 1986.
12. Ariza, J., Gudiol, F., Pallares, R., et al.: Comparative trial of rifampin-doxycycline versus tetracycline-streptomycin in the therapy of human brucellosis. Antimicrob. Agents Chemother. *28*:548–551, 1985.
13. Ariza, J., Gudiol, F., Pallares, R., et al.: Treatment of human brucellosis with doxycycline plus rifampin or doxycycline plus streptomycin: A randomized, double-blind study. Ann. Intern. Med. *117*:25–30, 1992.
14. Ariza, J., Corredoira, J., Pallares, R., et al.: Characteristics of and risk factors for relapse of brucellosis in humans. Clin. Infect. Dis. *20*:1241–1249, 1995.
15. Ariza, J., Servite, O., Pallares, R., et al.: Characteristic cutaneous lesions in patients with brucellosis. Arch. Dermatol. *125*:380–383, 1989.
16. Arnow, P. M., Smaron, M., and Ormiste, V.: Brucellosis in a group of travelers to Spain. J. A. M. A. *251*:505–507, 1984.
17. Bang, B.: The etiology of epizootic abortion. J. Comp. Pathol. Ther. *10*:125, 1897.
18. Barham, W. B., Church, P., Brown, J. E., et al.: Misidentification of *Brucella* species with use of rapid bacterial identification systems. Clin. Infect. Dis. *17*:1068–1069, 1993.
19. Berger, T. G., Guill, M. A., and Gotte, D. K.: Cutaneous lesions in brucellosis. Arch. Dermatol. *117*:40–42, 1981.
20. Bouza, E., Garcia-de-la-Torre, M., Parras, F., et al.: Brucellar meningitis. Rev. Infect. Dis. *9*:810–822, 1987.
21. Braude, A. I.: Studies in the pathology and pathogenesis of experimental brucellosis. I. A comparison of the pathogenicity of *Brucella abortus*, *Brucella melitensis*, and *Brucella suis* for guinea pigs. J. Infect. Dis. *89*:76–82, 1951.
22. Braude, A. I.: Studies in the pathology and pathogenesis of experimental brucellosis. II. Formation of hepatic granuloma and its evolution. J. Infect. Dis. *89*:87–94, 1951.
23. Bruce, D.: Note on the discovery of a micro-organism in Malta fever. Practitioner *39*:161, 1887.
24. Buchanan, T. M., Faber, L. C., and Feldman, R. A.: Brucellosis in the United States, 1960–1972: An abattoir-associated disease. Part I. Clinical features and therapy. Medicine *53*:403–413, 1974.
25. Buchanan, T. M., and Faber, L. C.: 2-mercaptoethanol *Brucella* agglutination test: Usefulness for predicting recovery from brucellosis. J. Clin. Microbiol. *11*:691–693, 1980.
26. Carmichael, L. E., and Brunner, D. W.: Characteristics of a newly recognized species of *Brucella* responsible for infectious canine abortion. Cornell Vet. *58*:579–592, 1968.
27. Castaneda, M. R., and Guerrero, G.: Studies on the leukocyte picture in brucellosis. J. Infect. Dis. *78*:43–48, 1946.
28. Centers for Disease Control: Recommendations of the International Task Force for Disease Eradication. M. M. W. R. *42*:28, 1993.
29. Chan, J., Baxter, C., and Wennman, W. M.: Brucellosis in an Inuit child, probably related to caribou meat consumption. Scand. J. Infect. Dis. *21*:337–338, 1989.
30. Chomel, B. B., De Bess, E. E., Mangiamele, D. M., et al.: Changing trends in the epidemiology of human brucellosis in California from 1973 to 1992: A shift toward foodborne transmission. J. Infect. Dis. *170*:1216–1223, 1994.
31. Chusid, M. J., Perzigian, R. W., Dunne, M., et al.: Brucellosis: An unusual cause of a child's fever of unknown origin. Wisc. Med. J. *88*:11–13, 1989.
32. Cisneros, J. M., Pachon, J., Cuello, J. A., et al.: *Brucella* endocarditis cured by medical treatment. J. Infect. Dis. *160*:907, 1989.
33. Cisneros, J. M., Viciana, P., Colmenero, J., et al.: Multicenter prospective study of treatment of *Brucella melitensis* brucellosis with doxycycline for 6 weeks plus streptomycin for 2 weeks. Antimicrob. Agents Chemother. *34*:881–883, 1990.
34. Cluff, L. E.: Medical aspects of delayed convalescence. Rev. Infect. Dis. *13*(Suppl. 1):S138–S140, 1991.
35. Cohen, F. B., Robins, B., and Lipstein, W.: Isolation of *Brucella abortus* by percutaneous liver biopsy. N. Engl. J. Med. *257*:228–230, 1957.

36. Colmenero, J. D., Regnera, J. M., Martos, F., et al.: Complications associated with *Brucella melitensis* infection: A study of 530 cases. Medicine *75*:195–211, 1996.
37. Corbel, M. J.: Brucellosis: Epidemiology and prevalence worldwide. *In* Young, E. J., and Corbel, M. J. (eds.): Brucellosis: Clinical and Laboratory Aspects. Boca Raton, CRC Press, 1989, pp. 26–40.
38. Corbel, M. J.: Brucella-phages: Advances in the development of a reliable phage typing system for smooth and non-smooth *Brucella* isolates. Ann. Inst. Pasteur Microbiol. *138*:70–75, 1987.
39. Corbel, M. J.: Microbiology of the genus *Brucella. In* Young, E. J., and Corbel, M. J. (eds.): Brucellosis: Clinical and Laboratory Aspects. Boca Raton, CRC Press, 1989, pp. 53–72.
40. Corbel, M. J.: International committee on systematic bacteriology, subcommittee on the taxonomy of *Brucella*. Int. J. Sys. Bacteriol. *38*:450–452, 1988.
41. Crosby, E., Llosa, L., Quesada, M. M., et al.: Hematologic changes in brucellosis. J. Infect. Dis. *150*:419–424, 1984.
42. Crow, J. B., Tormey, D. M., Redner, W. J., et al.: Caseation necrosis in human brucellosis. Am. Rev. Tuberc. *67*:859–868, 1953.
43. Dalrymple-Champneys, W.: Brucella Infection and Undulant Fever in Man. London, Oxford University Press, 1960, pp. 3–9.
44. Davis, D. S., Templeton, J. W., Ficht, T. A., et al.: *Brucella abortus* in captive bison. I. Serology, bacteriology, pathogenesis, and transmission to cattle. J. Wildl. Dis. *26*:360–371, 1990.
45. DiMario, A., Sica, S., Zini, G., et al.: Microangiopathic hemolytic anemia and severe thrombocytopenia in *Brucella* infection. Ann. Haematol. *70*:59–60, 1995.
46. Evans, A. C.: Further studies on *Bacterium abortus* and related bacteria. II. A comparison of *Bacterium abortus* with *Bacterium bronchosepticus* and with the agent which causes Malta fever. J. Infect. Dis. *22*:580–587, 1918.
47. Farrell, J. D., Robertson, L., and Hinchliffe, P. M.: Serum antibody responses in acute brucellosis. J. Hyg. (Lond.) *74*:23–28, 1975.
48. Feiz, J., Sabbaghian, H., and Mirali, M.: Brucellosis due to *B. melitensis* in children. Clin. Pediatr. *12*:904–907, 1978.
49. Fekete, A., Bantle, J. A., Halling, S. M., et al.: Preliminary development of a diagnostic test for *Brucella* using polymerase chain reaction. J. Appl. Bacteriol. *69*:216–227, 1990.
50. Forbes, K. A., Lowry, E. G, Gibson, T. E., et al.: Brucellosis of the genitourinary tract: Review of the literature and report of a case in a child. Urol. Surv. *4*:391–412, 1954.
51. Gazapo, E., Lahoz, J. G., Subiza, J. L., et al.: Changes in IgM and IgG antibody concentrations in brucellosis over time: Importance for diagnosis and follow-up. J. Infect. Dis. *159*:219–225, 1989.
52. Gee-Law, B. M., Nicholas, E. A., Hirose, F. M., et al.: Unusual skin manifestations of brucellosis. Arch. Dermatol. *119*:56–58, 1983.
53. Gotuzzo, E., Alarcon, G. S., and Bocanegra, T. S.: Articular involvement in human brucellosis: A retrospective analysis of 304 cases. Semin. Arthr. Rheum. *12*:245–255, 1982.
54. Gotuzzo, E., Carrillo, C., Guerra, J., et al.: An evaluation of diagnostic methods for brucellosis: The value of bone marrow culture. J. Infect. Dis. *153*:122–125, 1986.
55. Hagenbusch, O. E., and Frei, C. F.: Undulant fever in children. Am. J. Clin. Pathol. *11*:497–515, 1947.
56. Hall, W. H.: Modern chemotherapy for brucellosis in humans. Rev. Infect. Dis. *12*:1060–1099, 1990.
57. Hall, W. H.: History of *Brucella* as a human pathogen. *In* Young, E. J., and Corbel, M. J. (eds.): Brucellosis: Clinical and Laboratory Aspects. Boca Raton, CRC Press, 1989, pp. 1–9.
58. Hardy, A. V., Hudson, M. G., and Jordan, C. F.: The skin as a portal of entry in *B. melitensis* infections. J. Infect. Dis. *45*:271–282, 1929.
59. Hayes, F. M., and Traum, J.: Preliminary report of abortion in swine caused by Br. abortus (Bang). Mod. Vet. Pract. *1*:58–65, 1929.
60. Herman, L., and DeRidder, H.: Identification of *Brucella* spp. by using the polymerase chain reaction. Appl. Environ. Microbiol. *58*:2099–2101, 1992.
61. Ho, H., Zuckerman, M. J., Schaeffer, L., et al.: Brucellosis: Atypical presentation with abdominal pain. Am. J. Gastroenterol. *81*:375–377, 1986.
62. Holland, J. J., and Pickett, M. J.: A cellular basis of immunity in experimental *Brucella* infection. J. Exp. Med. *108*:343–359, 1958.
63. Howe, C., Miller, E. S., Kelly, E. H., et al.: Acute brucellosis among laboratory workers. N. Engl. J. Med. *236*:741–747, 1947.
64. Ismaily, S. I. N., Harby, H. A. M., and Nicoletti, P.: Prevalence of brucella antibodies in four animal species in the Sultanate of Oman. Trop. Anim. Health Prod. 209–270, 1988.
65. Jacobs, F., Abramowicz, D., Vereerstraeten, P., et al.: *Brucella* endocarditis: The role of combined medical and surgical treatment. Rev. Infect. Dis. *12*:740–744, 1990.
66. Jiang, X., and Baldwin, C. L.: Effects of cytokines on intracellular growth of *Brucella abortus*. Infect. Immun. *61*:124–134, 1993.
67. Joint FAO/WHO Expert Committee on Brucellosis, Sixth Report, WHO technical report series. Geneva, World Health Organization, 1986.
68. Jorens, P. G., Michielsen, P. P., Van den Enden, E. J., et al.: A rare cause of colitis: *Brucella melitensis*. Dis. Colon Rectum *34*:194–196, 1991.
69. Kaufmann, A. F., Fox, M. D., Boyce, J. M., et al.: Airborne spread of brucellosis. Ann. N. Y. Acad. Sci. *353*:105–114, 1989.
70. Khan, M. S., Humayoon, M. S., and Al Manee, M. S.: Epididymo-orchitis and brucellosis. Br. J. Urol. *63*:87–89, 1989.
71. Khateeb, M. I., Araj, G. F., Majeed, S. A., et al.: *Brucella* arthritis: A study of 96 cases in Kuwait. Ann. Rheum. Dis. *49*:994–998, 1990.
72. Lang, R., and Rubinstein, E.: Quinolones for the treatment of brucellosis. J. Antimicrob. Agents Chemother. *29*:357–360, 1992.
73. Lang, R., Dagan, R., Potasman, I., et al.: Failure of ceftriaxone in the treatment of acute brucellosis. Clin. Infect. Dis. *14*:506–509, 1992.
74. Losurdo, G., Timitilli, A., Tasso, L., et al.: Acute hepatitis due to *Brucella* in a 2-year-old child. Arch. Dis. Child. *71*:387, 1994.
75. Lubani, M. M., Dudin, K. I., Sharda, D. C., et al.: Neonatal brucellosis. Eur. J. Pediatr. *147*:520–522, 1988.
76. Lubani, M. M., Dudin, K. I., Sharda, D. C., et al.: A multicenter therapeutic study of 1100 children with brucellosis. Pediatr. Infect. Dis. J. *8*:75–78, 1989.
77. Lubani, M. M, Lulu, A. R., Araj, G. F., et al.: Pulmonary brucellosis. Q. J. Med. *71*:319–324, 1989.
78. Lubani, M. M., Sharda, D., and Helin, I.: *Brucella* arthritis in children. Infection *14*:233–236, 1986.
79. Lynch, E. C., McKechnie, J. C., and Alfrey, C. P.: Brucellosis with pancytopenia. Ann. Intern. Med. *69*:319–322, 1968.
80. Mackaness, G. B.: The immunological basis of acquired cellular resistance. J. Exp. Med. *120*:105–120, 1964.
81. Madkour, M. M.: Childhood brucellosis. *In* Madkour, M. M. (ed.): Brucellosis. Boston, Butterworths, 1989, pp. 205–218.
82. Marston, J. A.: Report of fever (Malta). R. Army Med. Dept. Rep. *3*:520–521, 1863.
83. Martin-Moreno, S., Soto-Guzman, O., Bernaldo-de-Quiros, J., et al.: Pancytopenia due to hemophagocytosis in patients with brucellosis: A report of four cases. J. Infect. Dis. *147*:445–449, 1983.
84. McCorquodale, S. M., and DiGiacomo, R. F.: The role of wild North American ungulates in the epidemiology of bovine brucellosis: A review. J. Wildl. Dis. *21*:351–357, 1985.
85. McCullough, N. B., and Eisele, C. W.: *Brucella* hepatitis leading to cirrhosis of the liver. Arch. Intern. Med. *88*:793–802, 1951.
86. McLean, D. R., Russell, N., and Khan, M. Y.: Neurobrucellosis: Clinical and therapeutic features. Clin. Infect. Dis. *15*:582–590, 1992.
87. Meyer, K. F., and Shaw, E. B.: A comparison of the morphological, cultural, and biochemical characteristics of *B. abortus* and *B. melitensis*: Studies of the genus *Brucella* nov. gen. I. J. Infect. Dis. *27*:173–184, 1920.
88. Miller, C. D., Songer, J. R. and Sullivan, J. F.: A twenty-four year review of laboratory-acquired human infections at the National Animal Disease Center. Am. Ind. Hyg. Assoc. J. *48*:271–275, 1987.
89. Mohamed, A. E. S., Ven, D., Madkour, M. M., et al.: Alimentary tract presentations of brucellosis. Ann. Saudi Med. *6*:27–31, 1986.
90. Moore, J. A., and Bennett, M.: A previously undescribed organism associated with canine abortion. Vet. Rec. *80*:604–605, 1967.
91. Mousa, A. R. M., Elhag, K. M., Khogali, M., et al.: The nature of brucellosis in Kuwait: Study of 379 cases. Rev. Infect. Dis. *10*:211–217, 1988.
92. Mousa, A. R. M., Muhtaseb, S. A., Almudallal, D. S., et al.: Osteoarticular complications of brucellosis: A study of 169 cases. Rev. Infect. Dis. *9*:531–543, 1987.
93. Mousa, A. R. M., Koshy, T. S., Araj, G. F., et al.: *Brucella* meningitis: Presentation, diagnosis, and treatment: A prospective study of ten cases. Q. J. Med. *60*:873–885, 1986.
94. Nicoletti, P.: Relationship between animal and human disease. *In* Young, E. J., and Corbel, M. J. (eds.): Brucellosis: Clinical and Laboratory Aspects. Boca Raton, CRC Press, 1989, pp. 41–51.
95. Pellicer, T., Ariza, J., Foz, A., et al.: Specific antibodies detected during relapse of human brucellosis. J. Infect. Dis. *157*:918–924, 1988.
96. Petrella, R., and Young, E. J.: Acute *Brucella* ileitis. Am. J. Gastroenterol. *83*:80–82, 1988.
97. Polt, S. S., and Schaefer, J.: A microagglutination test for human *Brucella canis* antibodies. Am. J. Clin. Pathol. *77*:740–744, 1082.
98. Polt, S. S., Dismukes, W. E., Flint, A., et al.: Human brucellosis caused by *Brucella canis*. Ann. Intern. Med. *97*:717–719, 1982.
99. Porreco, R. P., and Haverkamp, A. D.: Brucellosis in pregnancy. Obstet. Gynecol. *44*:597–602, 1974.
100. Ray, W. C.: Brucellosis (due to *Brucella abortus* and *B. suis*). *In* Steele, J. H. (ed.): Handbook Series in Zoonoses. Vol. I. Boca Raton, CRC Press, 1979, pp. 99–194.
101. Riley, L. D., and Robertson, D. C.: Brucellacidal activity of human and bovine polymorphonuclear leukocyte granule extracts against smooth and rough strains of *Brucella abortus*. Infect. Immun. *46*:231–236, 1984.
102. Rolando, I. M., Carbone, A. O., Gotuzzo, E., et al.: Circulating immune complexes in the pathogenesis of human *Brucella uveitis*. Chibret. Int. J. Ophthalmol. *3*:30–38, 1985.
103. Rubin, B., Band, J. D., Wong, P., et al.: Person-to-person transmission of *Brucella melitensis*. Lancet *337*:14–15, 1991.
104. Rubinstein, E., Lang, R., Shasha, B., et al.: In vitro susceptibility of *Brucella melitensis* to antibiotics. Antimicrob. Agents Chemother. *35*:1925–1927, 1991.
105. Sadler, W. W.: Present evidence on the role of meat in the epidemiology of human brucellosis. Am. J. Public Health *50*:504–514, 1960.
106. Sadusk, J. F., Browne, A. S., and Born, J. L.: Brucellosis in man, resulting from Brucella abortus (strain 19) vaccine. J. A. M. A. 164:1325–1328, 1957.
107. Sarrum, M., Feiz, J., Foruzandeh, M., et al.: Intra uterine fetal infection

with *Brucella melitensis* as a possible cause of second trimester abortion. Am. J. Obstet. Gynecol. *119*:657–660, 1974.
108. Sharda, D. C., and Lubani, M.: A study of brucellosis in childhood. Clin. Pediatr. *25*:492–495, 1986.
109. Smith, L. D., and Ficht, T. A.: Pathogenesis of *Brucella*. Crit. Rev. Microbiol. *17*:209–230, 1990.
110. Solanes, M. P., Heatley, J., Arenas, F., et al.: Ocular complications in brucellosis. Am. J. Ophthalmol. *36*:657–689, 1953.
111. Solomon, H. M., and Jackson, D.: Rapid diagnosis of *Brucella melitensis* in blood: Some operational characteristics of the BACTEC/ALERT. J. Clin. Microbiol. *30*:222–224, 1992.
112. Spink, W. W., Hoffbauer, W., Walker, W. W., et al.: Histopathology of the liver in human brucellosis. J. Lab. Clin. Med. *34*:40–58, 1949.
113. Spink, W. W.: What is chronic brucellosis? Ann. Intern. Med. *35*:358–374, 1951.
114. Spink, W. W.: The Nature of Brucellosis. Minneapolis, University of Minnesota Press, 1956.
115. Stantic-Pavlinic, M., Cec, V., and Mehk, J.: Brucellosis in spouses and the possibility of interhuman infection. Infection *11*:313–314, 1983.
116. Stermer, E., Levy, N., Potasman, I., et al.: Brucellosis as a cause of severe colitis. Am. J. Gastroenterol. *86*:917–919, 1991.
117. Stiles, G. W.: Brucellosis in goats: Recovery of *Brucella melitensis* from cheese manufactured from unpasteurized goat's milk. Rocky Mt. Med. J. *42*:18–25, 1945.
118. Street, L., Grant, W. W., and Alva, J. D.: Brucellosis in childhood. Pediatrics *55*:416–421, 1975.
119. Swenson, R. M., Carmichael, L. E., and Cundy, K. R.: Human infection with *Brucella canis*. Ann. Intern. Med. *76*:435–438, 1972.
120. Taylor, P. M., and Perdue, J. N.: The changing epidemiology of human brucellosis in Texas, 1977–1986. Am. J. Epidemiol. *130*:160–165.
121. Thapar, M. K., and Young, E. J.: Urban outbreak of goat cheese brucellosis. Pediatr. Infect. Dis. J. *5*:640–643, 1986.
122. Todd, K. H., and Lyde, P. D.: Brucellosis and thrombocytopenic purpura: Case report and review. Texas Med. *85*:37–38, 1989.
123. Tosi, M. F., and Nelson, T. J.: *Brucella canis* infection in a 17-month-old child successfully treated with moxalactam. J. Pediatr. *101*:725–727, 1982.
124. Trout, D., Gomez, T. M., Bernard, B. P., et al.: Outbreak of brucellosis at a United States pork packing plant. J. Occup. Environ. Med. *37*:697–703, 1995.
125. Ullrich, C. H., Fader, R., Fahner, J. B., et al.: Brucellosis presenting as prolonged fever and hemophagocytosis. Am. J. Dis. Child. *147*:1037–1038, 1993.
126. Vandercam, B., Zech, F., de Cooman, S., et al.: Isolation of *Brucella melitensis* from banked sperm. Eur. J. Clin. Microbiol. Infect. Dis. *9*:303–304, 1990.
127. Vassallo, D. J.: The Corps disease: Brucellosis and its historical association with the Royal Army Medical Corps. J. R. Army Med. Corps *138*:140–150, 1992.
128. Williams, R. K., and Crossley, K.: Acute and chronic hepatic involvement of brucellosis. Gastroenterology *83*:455–458, 1982.
129. Wright, A. E., and Semple, D.: On the employment of dead bacteria in the serum diagnosis of typhoid and Malta fever. Br. Med. J. *1*:1214–1215, 1897.
130. Young, E. J.: *Brucella* species. *In* Mandell, G. L., Bennett, J. E., and Dolin, R. (eds.): Principles and Practice of Infectious Diseases. New York, Churchill Livingstone, 1995, pp. 2053–2060.
131. Young, E. J.: Brucellosis. *In* Kaplan, S. L. (ed.): Current Therapy in Pediatric Infectious Disease. 3rd ed. St. Louis, B. C. Decker, 1993, pp. 188–189.
132. Young, E. J.: *Brucella melitensis* hepatitis: The absence of granulomas. Ann. Intern. Med. *91*:414–415, 1979.
133. Young, E. J., and Suvannoparrat, U.: Brucellosis outbreak attributed to ingestion of unpasteurized goat cheese. Arch. Intern. Med. *135*:240–243, 1975.
134. Young, E. J., Borchert, M., Kretzer, F. L., et al.: Phagocytosis and killing of *Brucella* by human polymorphonuclear leukocytes. J. Infect. Dis. *151*:682–690, 1985.
135. Young, E. J.: Human brucellosis. Rev. Infect. Dis. *5*:821–842, 1983.
136. Young, E. J.: An overview of human brucellosis. Clin. Infect. Dis. *21*:283–290, 1995.
137. Young, E. J.: Serologic diagnosis of human brucellosis: Analysis of 214 cases by agglutination tests and review of the literature. Clin. Infect. Dis. *13*:359–372, 1991.

134

PERTUSSIS AND OTHER *BORDETELLA* INFECTIONS

James D. Cherry and Ulrich Heininger

Pertussis (whooping cough) is an acute infectious illness of the respiratory tract caused by *Bordetella pertussis* and, less frequently, by *B. parapertussis*.[41, 42, 50] The illness occurs worldwide and affects all age groups, but it is recognized primarily in children; it is most serious in young, unprotected infants.

Effective whole-cell pertussis vaccines became available in the 1940s, and the rate of pertussis was reduced dramatically in countries in which universal immunization of infants and children was implemented. However, even with vaccine use, occasional local epidemics still occur, and there is growing evidence for widespread, frequently atypical, and therefore unrecognized illness in children, adolescents, and adults.[66, 105, 146, 147, 175, 176, 219, 266] *B. pertussis* is one of the major causes of cough illness.

HISTORY

Pertussis was noted as *the kink* (a Scottish term synonymous with fit or paroxysm) and *kindhoest* (a Teutonic word meaning child's cough) in the Middle Ages.[115] The clinical picture of pertussis was presented first in 1640 by Guillaume de Baillou, who described cases in an epidemic in Paris in 1578.[56] The term pertussis was not used until 1670. The isolation of *B. pertussis*, the main causative agent of pertussis, was reported by Bordet and Gengou in 1906,[24] and *B. parapertussis* was recognized 30 years later by Eldering and Kendrick as a different species causing a similar illness in humans.[70, 71]

Vaccines consisting of killed whole *B. pertussis* organisms were developed shortly after the bacterium was isolated, and the first results of protection were reported by Madsen in 1925.[153] The mouse protection test, developed and reported by Kendrick and collaborators in 1947,[127] allowed the standardization of vaccine production. Comprehensive studies conducted by the British Medical Council in the 1940s and 1950s demonstrated a good correlation between the potency of pertussis vaccines as determined in the mouse protection test and their clinical efficacy in children.[163] As a consequence, immunization against pertussis, most commonly in combination with diphtheria and tetanus toxoids (DTP), became part of routine vaccination programs in many countries throughout the world.

Concerns about a relationship between pertussis vaccination and temporally associated serious adverse events (e.g., sudden infant death syndrome) and a variety of neurologic illnesses led to a sharp decline of vaccination rates in Japan and several European countries during the 1970s.[42] These concerns along with well-documented high rates of unpleasant local and systemic reactions led to the development of new acellular vaccines. These vaccines cause less frequent reactions and have been used in Japan since 1981.[131] However, clinical efficacy for acellular vaccines when used in infancy has been demonstrated only recently.

MICROBIOLOGY

The genus *Bordetella* contains six species: *B. pertussis, B. parapertussis, B. bronchiseptica, B. avium, B. hinzii,* and *B. holmesii*.[42, 59, 80, 85, 95, 141, 195, 202, 204, 244, 254, 262] *B. pertussis* exclusively infects humans. *B. parapertussis* also is a human pathogen, but it has been recovered from sheep as well.[202] Both *B. pertussis* and *B. parapertussis* are respiratory pathogens. *B. bronchiseptica* primarily is an animal pathogen that causes atrophic rhinitis and pneumonia in pigs, kennel cough in dogs, pneumonia in cats, and respiratory illnesses in other animals[42, 86, 236]; this organism also is the occasional cause of respiratory illness in humans.[63, 95, 191, 214, 237, 262] *B. avium* is an important cause of respiratory illness in turkeys and other birds.[129]

Two additional species of *Bordetella* have been recognized (*B. holmesii* and *B. hinzii*) that cause human illness; these agents are unique in that they have been isolated from blood cultures and in humans they are not associated with respiratory illnesses.[59, 141, 254]

Bordetella are gram-negative, pleomorphic, aerobic bacilli that are grouped together on the basis of genotypic characteristics and are differentiated as to species by phenotypic characteristics. *B. pertussis* and *B. parapertussis* are closely related organisms with a genetic homology of 98.5 per cent.[7] However, they are listed as distinct species because of important differences. The most important difference is the lack of production of pertussis toxin (PT) by *B. parapertussis*.

Etiology of Pertussis (Whooping Cough)

B. pertussis and *B. parapertussis* are the etiologic agents that cause pertussis; 95 per cent of illnesses are due to *B. pertussis*.[87, 107, 204] In rare instances, *B. bronchiseptica*, which normally is enzootic in pigs, dogs, cats, rodents, and other animals, has been isolated from humans with pertussis-like cough illnesses.[63, 95, 191, 214, 236, 237, 262]

Adenoviruses have been isolated from children with pertussis, and it has been suggested that several adenoviral types on occasion may cause a pertussis-like illness.[8, 55, 57, 188] However, the data of Nelson and associates[188] and Baraff and coworkers[8] as well as our own observations led us to believe that mixed infections are occurring and that classic symptoms are due to *B. pertussis* and not infection with an adenovirus. In young infants, however, co-infection may lead to more severe disease.[13, 140]

It often is suggested that *Chlamydia trachomatis* can cause a pertussis-like illness. However, in our opinion, the repetitive cough of *C. trachomatis* distinctly is different from the paroxysmal cough of *B. pertussis* infection, and so illnesses due to the two agents usually should not be confused clinically.

Antigenic and Biologically Active Components of *Bordetella pertussis*

B. pertussis contains a variety of components that are antigenic or biologically active (Table 134–1).[6, 42, 46, 60, 69, 84, 101, 111, 112, 145, 148, 154, 158, 172, 178, 184, 189, 200, 201, 215, 220, 240, 242, 248, 257, 271] With the exception of tracheal cytotoxin and lipo-oligosaccharide (LOS), all known virulence factors produced by *B. pertussis* are regulated by the single genetic locus *bvgAS*.[252] Under certain conditions, such as environmental temperature of 37° C, *bvgAS* is active, toxins and adhesins are produced, and the organism is virulent in a mouse model (bvg^+ phase). In the bvg^- phase, a different set of genes (*vrg, vir* repressed genes) are expressed. However, *B. pertussis* is avirulent in mice in this phase.[253] The switch from bvg^+ to bvg^- is a phenomenon common to all *Bordetella* species and goes along with a change of phenotype.

Fimbriae (Pili)

Fimbriae are protein projections on the surface of *B. pertussis*.[178, 204, 211] They are highly immunogenic, and antibody to them as well as to other antigens causes agglutination of the

TABLE 134–1. Biologically Active and Antigenic Components of *Bordetella pertussis*

Component	Characteristics
Fimbriae	Two serologic types (types 2 and 3). Antibody to specific types cause agglutination of the organism. Organisms may contain fimbriae 2, fimbriae 3, fimbriae 2 and 3, or neither fimbriae 2 nor fimbriae 3. Fimbriae may play a role as adhesins.
Filamentous hemagglutinin	A cell-surface protein. It functions as an adhesin.
Pertussis toxin (also called lymphocytosis-promoting factor)	A classic bacterial toxin with an enzymatically active A subunit and a B oligomer-binding protein. Effects in animal model systems include histamine sensitization, lymphocytosis promotion, stimulation of insulin secretion, and adjuvant and mitogenic activity. It is an envelope protein that is an important adhesin. It adversely affects host immune cell functions.
Adenylate cyclase toxin	An extracytoplasmic enzyme that impairs host immune cell functions and may contribute to local tissue damage in the respiratory tract. It is a hemolysin.
Heat-labile toxin (also called dermonecrotic toxin)	Cytoplasmic protein that causes skin necrosis in laboratory animals. It may contribute to local tissue damage in the respiratory tract.
Lipo-oligosaccharide	An envelope toxin with activities similar to endotoxins of other gram-negative bacteria. A significant cause of reactions to whole-cell pertussis vaccines. Antibody to lipo-oligosaccharide causes agglutination of the organism.
Tracheal cytotoxin	A disaccharide-tetrapeptide derived from peptidoglycan. Causes local tissue damage in the respiratory tract.
Pertactin	A 69-kDa outer-membrane protein that is an important adhesin. Antibody to pertactin causes agglutination of the organism.

organism. Two fimbrial antigens (fimbriae 2 and 3) are the main agglutinogens; endotoxin and pertactin also are agglutinogens.[173, 211]

In the past, *B. pertussis* strains have been typed based upon the agglutination patterns noted with specific antisera.[42, 72, 211] Six specific agglutinogens were recognized, and organisms specially were typed based upon the presence or absence of agglutination by each specific antiserum. More recently, it has been recognized that two of the agglutinogens (agglutinogens 2 and 3) are fimbrial in location (fimbriae 2 and 3) and that agglutinogens 4, 5, and 6 are minor antigens.[204, 211] All *B. pertussis* strains contain agglutinogen 1, and this agglutinogen may be endotoxin. Another agglutinogen is pertactin, but where this fits in the original typing scheme is unknown.

Fimbriae function as adhesins, but studies suggest that in infection they are not the primary adhesins but serve to sustain attachment established by other attachment factors.[42, 212, 240, 251] In the mouse model system, immunization with purified fimbriae resulted in protection against infection when challenged with *B. pertussis*.[126]

Filamentous Hemagglutinin

Filamentous hemagglutinin (FHA) is a component of the cell wall of *B. pertussis* that in infection acts as an adhesin.[19, 42, 240] Immunization of mice with FHA results in protection against respiratory challenge with *B. pertussis*.[215, 221]

Pertussis Toxin

PT is a classic bacterial adenosine diphosphate–ribosylating toxin with an enzymatically active A subunit (S_1) and a B oligomer (S_{2-5}) binding portion.[42, 81, 121, 184, 200, 201, 241] In animal model systems, the effects of PT include histamine sensitization, lymphocytosis promotion, stimulation of insulin secretion, and adjuvant and mitogenic activity. Pertussis toxin is an envelope protein that is an important adhesin; its enzymatic activity adversely affects host immune cell functions.

In 1979, it was suggested that pertussis was a single PT toxin disease, and this led to the idea that pertussis could be prevented by a PT toxoid vaccine in a manner similar to the success with diphtheria toxoid in diphtheria.[46, 200, 201] Although there are convincing arguments to the contrary, this idea still is prevalent.[209] The most compelling evidence that pertussis due to *B. pertussis* infection is not a PT disease is that identical illness results from *B. parapertussis* infection and this organism does not express PT.[46, 107]

Adenylate Cyclase Toxin

Adenylate cyclase is an extracytoplasmic enzyme that impairs host immune cell functions and may contribute to local tissue damage in the respiratory tract.[42, 112] Mutant *B. pertussis* strains without adenylate cyclase result in avirulence in the murine respiratory infection model.[130]

Heat-Labile Toxin or Dermonecrotic Toxin

This toxin was described by Bordet and Gengou in 1909.[24] It is a cytoplasmic protein that causes skin necrosis in laboratory animals.[186] It may contribute to local tissue damage in the respiratory tract.

Lipo-oligosaccharide

LOS of *B. pertussis* is similar to endotoxins of other gram-negative bacteria.[38, 42] Its function in disease, if any, is unknown. It is a major cause of reactions to whole-cell pertussis vaccines.[10] LOS is a significant agglutinogen. Antibody to LOS has been found to reduce colonization of *B. pertussis* in the lungs and trachea of mice after aerosol challenge.[183]

Tracheal Cytotoxin

Tracheal cytotoxin is a disaccharide-tetra peptide derived from peptidoglycan.[84] It causes local damage to the respiratory epithelium and may affect host neutrophil function adversely.[61, 84]

Pertactin

Pertactin is a 69-kDa outer-membrane protein that is an important adhesin.[19, 138, 195, 196] Antibody to pertactin had a strong protective effect in aerosol challenge studies in mice.[40, 220] Pertactin is an agglutinogen.

Culture, Antigen Detection, and Serology

A laboratory diagnosis of pertussis due to either *B. pertussis* or *B. parapertussis* can be made by culturing the organisms on appropriate media, by identifying their presence using direct fluorescent antibody testing or by polymerase chain reaction (PCR), and by demonstrating the production of specific antibodies. *Bordetella* species can be recovered from nasopharyngeal specimens with the highest rate of isolation within the first 3 weeks of cough.[106, 233] Specimens for culture can be collected by swabbing the nasopharynx, by nasal wash, or by nasal aspiration.[42, 97]

B. pertussis and *B. parapertussis* are recovered most easily by direct plating of the specimen from the patient onto selective media.[42, 116] Specific swabs (calcium alginate) and media (Regan-Lowe or Bordet-Gengou agar and modified Stainer-Scholte broth) are required, and the laboratory should be experienced in isolating the organisms. If cultures cannot be inoculated directly, the use of Regan-Lowe transport medium is recommended. In classic disease, the culture or a direct fluorescent antibody study will be positive in about 80 per cent of cases if the specimen was obtained within 2 weeks of onset of cough and antibiotics had not been administered previously.[106, 198]

PCR has been used to identify *B. pertussis* and *B. parapertussis* from nasopharyngeal specimens.[208, 216, 217, 268] This diagnostic tool has the advantage of a much higher sensitivity compared with conventional culture. In a prospective study, in which swabs for PCR and culture were obtained simultaneously from 555 subjects with cough illnesses, the use of PCR increased the identification of *B. pertussis* infections almost fourfold from 28 to 111.[217] However, because it is more expensive than culture and subject to easy contamination, it has not been used widely as a routine procedure.[161]

Natural infection with *B. pertussis* is followed by a rise in serum concentrations of IgA, IgG, and IgM antibodies to specific antigens of the organism as well as to preparations of the whole organism.[58, 79, 155, 166, 198] In contrast to natural infection, immunization induces mainly IgM and IgG antibodies. A serologic diagnosis of pertussis may be established by demonstration of an agglutinin titer rise or by use of enzyme-linked immunosorbent assay (ELISA) with demonstration of an increase in IgA or IgG antibody to PT, FHA, pertactin, fimbriae, or the sonicated whole organism.[66, 98, 146, 147, 175, 176, 219, 266] In addition, if age-specific control values for a population are determined, the diagnosis of pertussis can be established by high antibody values on single serum samples.[64, 175, 219, 225, 266]

The use of a battery of serologic tests allows the diagnosis of pertussis in many patients with negative cultures for *B. pertussis*.[100, 175] Conversely, some culture-positive patients, particularly children who are younger than 3 months of age, fail to develop measurable antibodies.[246]

An ELISA also has been developed for the detection of IgA antibody to *B. pertussis* in nasopharyngeal secretions as an indicator of recent infections.[85, 89, 267] *B. pertussis* IgA appears in nasopharyngeal secretions during the second or third week of illness and persists for at least 3 months.[85] However, the appearance of secretory IgA may be delayed in children younger than 1 year of age.[185] This antibody is not induced by parenteral *B. pertussis* vaccination. The detection of *B. pertussis* IgA in secretions by use of ELISA may be a diagnostic aid in culture-negative patients whose symptoms have persisted for more than 3 weeks.

EPIDEMIOLOGY

Pertussis is one of the most highly communicable diseases; when it has been introduced into a susceptible population, attack rates of 100 per cent in susceptible individuals have been recorded.[136] The highest risk of disease is among infants and young children.

Incidence

The incidence of pertussis and its mortality are affected markedly by pertussis vaccine use. In the prevaccine era in the United States, the average attack rate of reported pertussis was 157 per 100,000 population compared with 230 per 100,000 population in England and Wales (Fig. 134–1).[41] Previous studies, however, have suggested that reported cases represent only between 15 and 25 per cent of cases that actually occur.[103, 124, 125, 229]

With the introduction and widespread use of pertussis vaccines, the attack rate in the United States fell about 150-fold from 1943 to 1976. A similar but less pronounced decrease of illness was noted in England and Wales. For the 7-year period 1976 to 1982, the attack rate in the United States remained between 0.5 and 1.0 per 100,000 population (Fig. 134–2).[37] From 1982 to 1993, the attack rate curve was modestly upward, reaching a rate of 2.3 per 100,000. The reason for this upward trend is unknown, but it most likely is due to a heightened awareness of the disease and perhaps due to the decreased efficacy of one of the vaccines widely used in the United States.[52, 91, 96]

Pertussis epidemics in the prevaccine era occurred at 2- to 5-year intervals (average, 3.2 years), and these cycles have continued in the vaccine era. As noted by Fine and Clarkson,[75, 76] this continuation of the same cycles today as in the prevaccine era indicates that although immunization has controlled disease, it has not reduced the transmission of the organism in the population.[41]

In the prevaccine era, about 85 per cent of all cases in the United States were noted in children from 1 to 9 years of age.[41] In contrast, today 41 per cent of cases are reported in infants and 28 per cent are in persons 10 years of age or older. Today, pertussis in adults is an important source of *B. pertussis* infection in unimmunized or partially immunized children.[44, 134, 143, 144, 179, 187, 243] Disease in adults usually is not recognized as pertussis, even though the cough frequently is paroxysmal and the illness persists for weeks.[203, 219]

In a study in university students, it was found by members of our group that 26 per cent of students with cough illnesses of 6 days' duration or longer had *B. pertussis* infections and none was clinically diagnosed correctly.[175] The findings in this study led to the suggestion that *B. pertussis* infections are endemic in adults and are responsible for cyclic outbreaks in susceptible children. More recent studies in the United States and Germany support this hypothesis.[61, 66, 176, 219, 266]

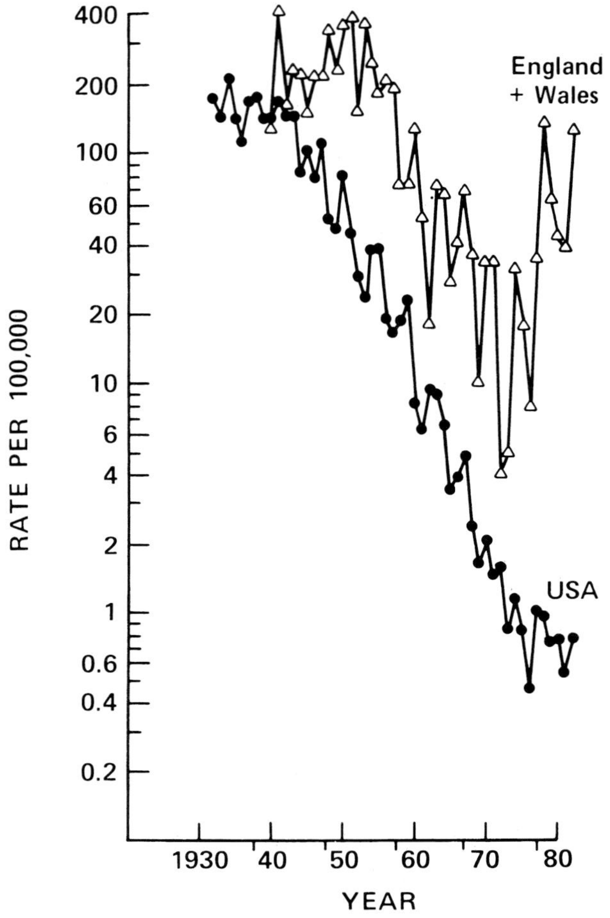

FIGURE 134–1. *Pertussis attack rates by year for the United States and England and Wales. (From Cherry, J. D.: The epidemiology of pertussis and pertussis immunization in the United Kingdom and the United States: A comparative study. Curr. Probl. Pediatr.* 14*:1–78, 1984.)*

Morbidity and Mortality

During the first 30 years of the twentieth century, pertussis was an important cause of death in the United States and Great Britain.[135] There were 36,013 deaths from pertussis in the United States between 1926 and 1930.[87] Most of these deaths occurred in children younger than 1 year of age. The pertussis death rate curve in the United States has declined throughout this century. In infants, the mortality rate declined about fivefold from 1900 to 1944. During the next 35 years, it decreased more than 85-fold.[180, 181] Today, the majority of deaths due to pertussis occur in unimmunized infants younger than 6 months of age.[36] During 1992 and 1993, 23 deaths attributed to pertussis were reported in the United States.[265] Of these 23 patients, 18 were younger than 6 months of age and 11 were younger than 2 months of age. Young maternal age and preterm delivery were risk factors for fatal disease. Presently in the United States, there are about 10 reported deaths per year.[37]

It is important to point out that deaths due to pertussis frequently are misdiagnosed as deaths due to other respira-

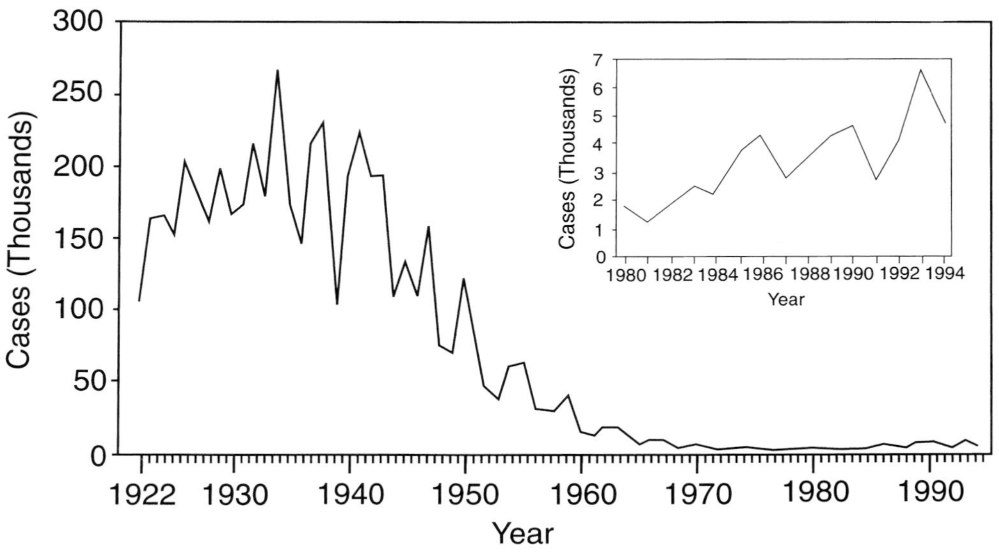

FIGURE 134–2. *Number of reported pertussis cases by year, United States, 1922–1994. (Data for 1994 are provisional.) (From Centers for Disease Control and Prevention: Pertussis: United States, January 1992–June 1995. M. M. W. R. 44:525–529, 1995.)*

tory infectious illnesses.[41, 105, 192] For example, in England and Wales during the epidemic from 1977 to 1979 and at the beginning of the epidemic in 1982, there were 32 reported deaths due to pertussis.[41] However, when excess deaths due to other respiratory infectious illnesses are examined, it appears that there were about 362 additional deaths due to pertussis.

Morbidity due to pertussis in recent years can be gleaned from a number of reports. The number of pertussis-related hospitalizations, complications, and deaths in the United States in 1992 through 1994 is presented in Table 134–2.[37] Of the 13,615 cases analyzed, 33.6 per cent were hospitalized, 9 per cent had pneumonia, 1.4 per cent had seizures, 0.1 per cent had encephalopathy, and 0.2 per cent died. The most severe morbidity occurred in infants younger than 6 months of age. Of this group, 71.1 per cent were hospitalized, 14.8 per cent had pneumonia, 1.9 per cent had seizures, 0.2 per cent had encephalopathy, and 0.6 per cent died.

In a study carried out in England and Wales (1977 to 1979)[257] in which there were 2295 cases, the following complications were reported: weight loss (16.8 per cent), acute bronchitis (9.8 per cent), atelectasis (0.3 per cent), bronchopneumonia (0.8 per cent), apnea (1.1 per cent), convulsions (0.6 per cent), and otitis media (7.5 per cent). Two children (0.19 per cent) had encephalitis. Other complications noted were hernia (0.19 per cent), squint (0.29 per cent), deafness (0.29 per cent), hemoptysis (0.19 per cent), subconjunctival hemorrhages (0.19 per cent), and conjunctivitis (1.39 per cent). Sixty-four children (2.89 per cent) were hospitalized; 25 (1.19 per cent) required special nursing, but none needed assisted ventilation.

The results of a study involving 94 area health authorities in Great Britain between October 1974 and March 1975 were reported in 1976.[167] In this study, the morbidity of 8092 cases of pertussis was analyzed. Fifteen per cent of the patients were infants who were younger than 1 year of age. Hospital admissions of children with pertussis (9.6 per cent of the cases) were related inversely to age. Sixty per cent of the affected infants younger than 6 months of age and 28 per cent of affected infants 6 to 11 months of age were admitted to the hospital. Of the 7317 patients treated at home, 3 per cent were described as patients with severe illness and 32

TABLE 134–2. Number of Pertussis-Related Hospitalizations, Complications, and Deaths, by Age Group (United States, 1992–1994)

		Complications									
	No. Persons with Pertussis	*Hospitalized*		*Pneumonia**		*Seizures*		*Encephalopathy*		*Deaths*	
Age Group		No.	(%)	No.	(%)	No.	(%)	No.	(%)	No.	(%)
<6 mo	4524	3217	(71.1)	671	(14.8)	87	(1.9)	11	(0.2)	25	(0.6)
6–11 mo	1094	512	(46.8)	153	(14.0)	27	(2.5)	2	(0.2)	3	(0.3)
1–4 yr	2682	580	(21.6)	248	(9.2)	45	(1.7)	3	(0.1)	1	(<0.1)
5–9 yr	1551	124	(8.0)	66	(4.3)	8	(0.5)	0		3	(0.2)
10–19 yr	2223	78	(3.5)	45	(2.0)	10	(0.4)	1	(<0.1)	0	
≥20 yr	1541	57	(3.7)	41	(2.7)	7	(0.5)	0		0	
Total	13,615†	4568‡	(33.6)	1224§	(9.0)	184	(1.4)	17	(0.1)	32	(0.2)

*Radiographically confirmed.
†Excludes 18 (0.1 per cent) persons of unknown age with pertussis.
‡Excludes six hospitalized patients of unknown age.
§Excludes one hospitalized patient of unknown age.
From Centers for Disease Control and Prevention: Pertussis: United States, January 1992–June 1995. M.M.W.R. *44*:525–529, 1995.

per cent with moderate illness by their attending general practitioners. Fifty-one per cent of children younger than 1 year of age had moderate or severe illness.

A pertussis surveillance system was introduced in conjunction with a large pertussis vaccine efficacy trial in several regions of Germany in 1990. First results of this ongoing surveillance study were published in 1993.[104] Of 601 culture-proven cases, 12.3 per cent were infants and 86.2 per cent were younger than 6 years of age. Serious complications were reported in 22 of 275 patients with follow-up. These complications included pneumonia in 5.5 per cent, apnea in 2.2 per cent, and cardiorespiratory failure in 0.4 per cent.

Season, Geography, and Sex

Pertussis occurs throughout the world.[42] Historically, there was no seasonal pattern to epidemic pertussis.[41] However, in the present vaccine era in North America, pertussis is most common in the summer and fall.[73, 88, 187] In the past, the incidence of pertussis was greater in females than males.[41] Between 1980 and 1989, this female predominance was observed again, but only in those 15 years of age or older.[73]

Transmission

Transmission is believed to occur by droplets from a coughing patient that reach the upper respiratory tract of a susceptible person. It also is possible that indirect spread occurs. The symptomatic patient could contaminate the environment with respiratory secretions. The new host-to-be has contact with the secretions and inoculates his or her own respiratory tract by the hands.[42] Attack rates in susceptible household contacts range from 70 to 100 per cent.[41, 42] Antibody studies indicate that asymptomatic infections also occur in contacts.[64, 146, 147] These asymptomatic infections are likely to be short-lived and probably are not important in regard to contagion. Transmissibility is greatest early in the illness, during the catarrhal and early paroxysmal phases.

PATHOLOGY

Inflammation of the mucosal lining of the respiratory tract may be observed.[41, 42, 142] *B. pertussis* organisms multiply only in association with ciliated epithelium, producing congestion and infiltration of the mucosa with lymphocytes and polymorphonuclear leukocytes. Inflammatory debris accumulates in the lumen of the bronchi. Peribronchial lymphoid hyperplasia occurs early in infection, followed by a necrotizing process that affects the midzonal and basilar layers of the bronchial epithelium. A bronchopneumonia may develop, with necrosis and desquamation of the superficial epithelial layer of small bronchi. Bronchiolar obstruction and atelectasis are the result of accumulation of mucous secretions.

Pathologic changes also have been described in brain and liver. Microscopic or gross cerebral hemorrhages may be noted, and cortical atrophy has been observed. These changes most likely are the result of anoxic brain damage. In some studies of pertussis encephalopathy, the findings suggested meningoencephalitis with perivascular cuffs of lymphocytes within cerebral gray matter and pleocytosis.[261] However, studies in which inflammation was demonstrated were done before the availability of modern virologic techniques. It is likely that the neurologic findings in these instances were due to interactions with neurotropic viruses or other infectious agents and were not the result of *B. pertussis* infection.[42] Fatty infiltration of the liver has been noted in patients with pertussis encephalopathy.

PATHOGENESIS AND IMMUNITY

After exposure to *B. pertussis*, the pathogenesis of infection depends on four important steps: attachment, evasion of host defenses, local damage, and systemic disease.[42, 84, 112, 184, 186, 204, 251] The biologically active antigenic components of *B. pertussis* listed in Table 134–1 have various roles in pathogenesis.

Infection is initiated in the respiratory tract by the attachment of *B. pertussis* organisms to the cilia of the ciliated epithelial cells.[251] The adhesins (FHA, PT, and pertactin) facilitate this attachment.[184, 204, 240, 251] Studies suggest that FHA and pertactin may act synergistically.[19, 132, 138] Because fimbriae of some gram-negative bacteria are important for attachment, it has been assumed that *B. pertussis* fimbriae are important in attachment. However, in one tissue culture study, fimbriae did not mediate attachment of organisms to cells.[242] However, in a more recent study, it was shown that fimbriae played a role in attachment in persistent infection.[178]

Both adenylate cyclase and PT adversely affect immune cell functions and therefore allow infection, once initiated, to continue.[42, 112, 184] PT prevents migration of lymphocytes and macrophages to areas of infection and adversely affects phagocytosis and intracellular killing. Adenylate cyclase enters phagocytic cells and catalyzes excessive production of cyclic adenosine monophosphate, which results in a decrease in phagocytosis.

Tracheal cytotoxin, heat-labile toxin, and adenylate cyclase all have been implicated as contributors to local tissue damage in the respiratory tract.[42, 84, 186] Of these toxins, tracheal cytotoxin is likely to be the most important.[84] In hamster tracheal organ cultures, tracheal cytotoxin selectively destroys ciliated cells in a manner similar to that seen in *B. pertussis* infection, and the pathologic process is similar to that noted in human pertussis autopsy studies.

Pertussis is a unique illness in that there is only one manifestation of systemic disease in uncomplicated infection: leukocytosis with lymphocytosis due to pertussis toxin.[42, 107] T and B lymphocytes increase to a similar extent in the circulation.[17] In contrast with *B. pertussis* infection, lymphocytosis is not a characteristic of *B. parapertussis* infection because this organism does not liberate PT.

The most important systemic complication of pertussis is encephalopathy, whose cause is not known. The most likely explanation is anoxia associated with coughing paroxysms.

It has been suggested that pertussis is a toxin-mediated disease due to PT.[200, 201] Although this idea still is believed by some today,[209] little evidence supports it. Undoubtedly, PT is a fascinating protein with multiple activities in experimental animals such as histamine sensitization, lymphocytosis promotion, effects upon glucose metabolism, adjuvancy, and mitogenicity.[42, 81, 184] However, in infections in humans, the only effects that appear to be due to PT are lymphocytosis and mild, compensated hyperinsulinemia. It has been suggested that PT is the cause of the prolonged cough in pertussis. But, because persistent cough is a major manifestation of *B. bronchiseptica* infection in dogs and *B. parapertussis* infection in children and both organisms do not liberate PT, this hypothesis should be refuted.[107, 195]

Cell-mediated immune function is altered by *B. pertussis* infection. In some studies, cell-mediated immunity was depressed, whereas in others it was augmented.[197]

A variety of antibodies develop after exposure of the human host to infection with *B. pertussis*. The development of agglutinins, hemagglutination-inhibiting antibodies, and bactericidal antibodies has been described.[41] ELISA techniques have demonstrated class-specific antibodies (IgA, IgE, IgG, and IgM) to many of the specific proteins of *B. pertussis*.[104, 155, 198] These antibodies develop after infection and also after immunization. Neutralizing antibody to PT toxin also occurs after both infection and immunization.[22, 99, 198] Specific IgA antibody to PT and FHA also can be demonstrated in nasopharyngeal secretions and saliva.[89, 267]

At present, it is clear that both *B. pertussis* infection and immunization with whole-cell or acellular pertussis vaccines elicit protection of varying degrees and duration against pertussis. The prevailing opinion throughout this century is that immunity after *B. pertussis* infection is lifelong, whereas vaccine-induced immunity is relatively short-lived. Although the latter clearly is true,[76] studies by members of our research group suggest that the former opinion regarding infection-induced immunity is wrong.[49, 219] Utilizing the fact that IgA antibodies to pertussis antigens (PT, FHA, and pertactin) result from infection and not vaccination, our group studied the prevalence of these antibodies in the sera of similarly aged young German and American men.[49] In Germany, routine childhood immunization was not carried out during the 1970s and 1980s and pertussis was epidemic. To our surprise, the rate and mean values of IgA antibodies in the two populations were similar, suggesting that adult infection rates were similar. In another study in Germany, we found that *B. pertussis* infections were common in adults (133 per 100,000 population) and they often occurred in those with a known history of childhood pertussis.[219]

The nature of immunity in pertussis is not known. It generally has been assumed that serum antibodies above some unknown concentrations to one or more of the pertussis antigens are responsible for protection.[64] Antibodies to PT, FHA, and pertactin have been shown to be protective in animal model systems.[19, 60, 138, 215, 220] However, at the present, no serologic correlates of immunity have been established, although several large vaccine trials were performed during the last decade.[1, 91, 96, 108, 223, 239]

In addition to humoral responses to several *B. pertussis* antigens, there is evidence that cell-mediated immune responses to PT, FHA, and pertactin also occur.[66, 77, 83, 256] Studies in a murine respiratory infection model suggest that cellular immunity plays an important role in bacterial clearance and augments antibody effects by a predominantly T–helper 1 cell stimulation.[173, 174] Studies in humans demonstrate a cellular immune response shortly after natural infection with *B. pertussis*, and this also is a preferential T–helper cell induction to PT, FHA, and pertactin.[269, 270] The role of T cells in prolonged immunity, however, needs further clarification.

Immunity after *B. pertussis* infection or pertussis vaccination does not protect against illness due to *B. parapertussis*, and, similarly, infection with *B. parapertussis* does not induce protection against disease caused by *B. pertussis*.[137, 238]

CLINICAL MANIFESTATIONS

The clinical manifestations of *B. pertussis* infection have considerable variations that depend upon age, previous immunization or infection, the presence of passively acquired antibody, and perhaps other factors, such as degree of exposure, host genetic and acquired factors, and genotype of the organism. The incubation period for pertussis varies between 6 and 20 days, with the majority of cases having their onset 7 to 10 days after exposure.

Classic Illness[42, 74, 87, 197]

Classic illness occurs as a primary infection in unimmunized children who are between 1 and 10 years of age. The illness usually lasts 6 to 8 weeks and has three stages: catarrhal, paroxysmal, and convalescent. Initial illness is characterized by rhinorrhea, lacrimation, and mild cough suggesting a common cold. The temperature usually is normal. The severity of the cough gradually increases over 1 to 2 weeks, but pertussis usually is not suspected until the cough becomes paroxysmal.

After the catarrhal period, the coughs increase in severity and number. Repetitive series of 5 to 10 or more forceful coughs during a single expiration occur. These paroxysms are followed by a sudden massive inspiratory effort, and a characteristic whoop may occur as air is inhaled forcefully through a narrowed glottis. Cyanosis, bulging eyes, protrusion of the tongue, salivation, lacrimation, and distention of neck veins occur during paroxysms. Several paroxysmal coughing episodes with their associated massive inspiratory efforts may occur sequentially until the child succeeds in dislodging the obstructing mucus. Posttussive vomiting is common. Paroxysms may occur several times per hour and occur during both day and night.

The paroxysmal episodes are exhausting, and it is not unusual for the patient to appear dazed and apathetic. Weight loss may occur due to vomiting and because eating and drinking may be resisted because they trigger attacks. Attacks also may be triggered by yawning, sneezing, or physical exertion. Between attacks, the patient may appear normal and usually is in no distress.

Common and important complications of classic pertussis include pneumonia, otitis media, seizures, and encephalopathy. Pneumonia may be due to *B. pertussis* or to secondary bacterial invaders. Atelectasis may develop secondary to mucus plugs. The forcefulness of the paroxysms can cause rupture of the alveoli, which produces interstitial or subcutaneous emphysema.

Otitis media is common and frequently is due to *Streptococcus pneumoniae*. Pertussis also has been associated with activation of latent tuberculosis. Convulsions and coma may be observed. These findings may be a reflection of cerebral hypoxia related to asphyxia. Rarely, subarachnoid and intraventricular hemorrhage may be observed. Tetanic seizures may be associated with the severe alkalosis that results from loss of gastric contents due to persistent vomiting.

Other complications that have been noted include ulcer of the frenulum of the tongue, epistaxis, melena, subconjunctival hemorrhages, subdural hematomas, spinal epidural hematoma, rupture of the diaphragm, umbilical hernia, inguinal hernia, rectal prolapse, dehydration, meningoencephalitis, syndrome of inappropriate antidiuretic hormone secretion, apnea, and nutritional disturbances.[30, 122, 159, 203, 224, 250]

The convalescent stage, which usually lasts 1 to 2 weeks, is characterized by a decreasing frequency and severity of coughing episodes, whooping, and vomiting. All cases of classic pertussis due to primary infection will have a leukocytosis due to lymphocytosis. Fever and pharyngitis are not usual manifestations in pertussis, and therefore a search for a secondary cause should be undertaken when they occur. Except for the observation of typical paroxysms, the physical examination in pertussis usually is unrewarding. Diffuse rhonchi may be noted on auscultation.

Infection with *B. parapertussis* causes an illness that is similar to that caused by *B. pertussis* but generally is less severe and of shortened duration.[107]

Mild Illness

Mild nonclassic illness due to *B. pertussis* infection is common.[106, 217] This occurs in previously vaccinated children and also as a primary infection in nonvaccinated children. We conducted a study in which we encouraged physicians to send nasopharyngeal specimens to our laboratory from children with cough illnesses whether or not the illnesses were typical of pertussis.[106] We found that of 247 culture-positive cases, 47 per cent had a total cough illness duration of 28 days or less. In 26 per cent, the duration of cough was less than 3 weeks. The vast majority of these cases occurred in unvaccinated children. In a study in which both culture and PCR were used for diagnosis of *B. pertussis* infection, we found that many mild cases were PCR-positive and culture-negative.[217] Of these cases, only 68 per cent had a cough illness of greater than or equal to 4 weeks and only 57 per cent and 32 per cent had paroxysmal cough and whoop, respectively.

Infants

Pertussis in infancy is unique. Its spectrum of clinical manifestations varies by age, immunization, and the presence or absence of transplacentally acquired antibody.[13, 37, 41, 42, 51, 73, 105, 160, 187, 192] In the United States from 1980 to 1989, the rate of hospitalization was 69 per cent, of pneumonia 22 per cent, of seizures 3 per cent, of encephalopathy 0.9 per cent, and death 0.7 per cent.[73]

B. pertussis infection in the neonate particularly is severe, with a death rate of 1.3 per cent.[13, 51, 73, 105, 160] A common presenting finding is apnea, and typical coughing is not observed. Seizures in association with apnea are not infrequent. Severe disease in young infants frequently is associated with marked leukocytosis; total white blood cell counts in the range of 30,000 to 60,000 cells/μL are seen with a lymphocytosis.

Whoop is a rare manifestation of illness in infants, and other respiratory manifestations frequently are confused with those due to respiratory viruses. [41] *B. pertussis* infection may be a cause of sudden infant death syndrome.[110, 192]

Adults

There has been an increased awareness of adult pertussis in recent years.[37, 64, 73, 175, 176, 187, 190, 203, 213, 219, 260, 266] Unrecognized pertussis cases in adults often are the source from which infants and children become infected.[13, 51, 105, 160, 187, 219] All adults previously have been exposed to *B. pertussis* antigens by immunization, infection, or both,[49, 64, 66] and this tends to modify the illness. However, in a United States study, the following cough characteristics were noted in 31 university students with laboratory-confirmed *B. pertussis* infection: the median duration was 21 days before time of evaluation, 94 per cent had one or more episodes per hour, and 90 per cent had staccato or paroxysmal quality.[175] Despite these findings, pertussis was not suspected in any of the students, and the clinical diagnoses by the primary care providers were upper respiratory tract infection (39 per cent), bronchitis (48 per cent), and other diagnoses (16 per cent). Although specific records were not available, it is likely that most of these students were vaccinated as children and had a previous, unrecognized infection.[49, 64]

In contrast with these findings in the United States, we found that adults in Germany were more likely to have typical pertussis, even though our epidemiologic data suggested that all had a previous infection and 26 per cent of 64 patients with laboratory-confirmed infection recalled having had pertussis during childhood.[49, 219] The rates of clinical manifestations in the 64 laboratory-confirmed cases were 70 per cent, paroxysms; 38 per cent, whoop; 66 per cent, posttussive phlegm; and 17 per cent, posttussive vomiting. The clinical diagnosis in 39 per cent was definite or probable pertussis; only 14 per cent were thought not to have pertussis. It should be noted that the clinical diagnosis was not made by primary physicians but by a small team of specially trained central investigators with a high awareness for pertussis.

In a German household contact study, similar findings were noted:[203] 80 per cent of 79 adults with laboratory-confirmed *B. pertussis* infections coughed for 3 or more weeks and 63 per cent had spasmodic cough for 3 or more weeks. In addition, in 53 per cent of patients, coughing was followed by choking or vomiting. However, only 8 per cent of the adults in this study had whoops. Complications that were observed included pneumonia, rib fracture, inguinal hernia, and severe weight loss.

DIAGNOSIS AND DIFFERENTIAL DIAGNOSIS

In classic disease, the clinical diagnosis of pertussis should be made without difficulty. However, the etiology of the illness could be due to *B. pertussis* or *B. parapertussis*. The history of contact with a known case (laboratory-confirmed) will help make the diagnosis in the patient with mild or atypical illness. The presence of leukocytosis with lymphocytosis in a child with a cough illness or apnea in an infant is a strong indication that the illness is due to *B. pertussis* and not *B. parapertussis*. In a matched-control comparison performed by our group, none of 11 children with culture-proven *B. parapertussis* infection compared with 7 of 22 (32 per cent) with *B. pertussis* infection had a lymphocytosis of ≥10,000 cells/μL.[107] A lymphocytosis of ≥10,000 cells/μL is observed in few other diseases.

The definitive diagnosis is made by culture or specific antibody studies. *B. pertussis* and *B. parapertussis* can be recovered from nasopharyngeal specimens and are distinguished from each other by specific agglutination reactions or by specific fluorescent antibody staining of suspicious colonies.

The routine laboratory diagnosis of *B. pertussis* infections in adults or in other atypical cases is hampered by the fact that care usually is not sought until the third or fourth week of the illness and frequently antibiotics have been administered before the possibility of pertussis was considered.[175, 219]

Serologic testing for *B. pertussis* infections in the clinical setting is neither standardized nor widely available.[42, 198] In the research setting, the use of ELISA has contributed significantly to the diagnosis of *B. pertussis* infections in many patients with negative cultures.[66, 98, 146, 147, 175, 176, 219, 266] Most useful has been the determination of IgG and IgA antibodies to PT and FHA. The most reliable proof of acute infection is the demonstration of a significant increase in antibody value between acute-phase and convalescent-phase serum specimens. Frequently, acute-phase specimen collection is delayed and therefore the acute-phase values are elevated already, so that significant increases between first and second serum specimens cannot be demonstrated. However, diagnosis frequently can be made on the basis of a high value or values on a single serum specimen.[64, 175, 219, 266]

B. parapertussis infection induces cross-reacting antibodies to *B. pertussis* FHA, so that use of this antigen alone cannot differentiate *B. pertussis* from *B. parapertussis* infections.[90]

The measurement of agglutinating antibodies also is useful for the diagnosis of *B. pertussis* infections, and because the test is simple, cheap, and accurate, it can be used in the clinical setting.[64, 109, 175, 198, 219]

Other infectious agents that cause illnesses with cough that can be confused with pertussis are *Mycoplasma pneumoniae*, *C. trachomatis*, *Chlamydia pneumoniae*, and adenoviruses and other respiratory viruses.[41, 42, 55, 57, 62, 188]

Spasmodic attacks of coughing may be observed in infants with bronchiolitis, bacterial pneumonia, cystic fibrosis, tuberculosis, and other diseases that cause lymphadenopathy with extrinsic compression of trachea and bronchi. Generally, these disorders can be differentiated from infection with *B. pertussis* by associated clinical and laboratory findings and their course. In addition, the cough associated with sinusitis can be confused with that due to *B. pertussis* infection. Airway foreign bodies on occasion can result in confusion in diagnosis. One of us has seen a child with typical pertussis in whom the head and neck surgeon performed bronchoscopy because of the concern that a foreign body was causing the problem.

TREATMENT

Several antibiotics have in vitro efficacy against *B. pertussis*.[117–119] The first choice for treatment is oral erythromycin, which will ameliorate the symptoms if given early during the course of the illness and will eliminate the organism from the nasopharynx within a few days, thereby shortening the period of contagiousness.[16] The dose for children is 50 mg/kg/day given every 6 hours for 14 days. The dose for adults is 2 g/day given every 6 hours for 14 days. Trimethoprim-sulfamethoxazole can be used as an alternative agent in those who can not tolerate erythromycin.[119] A first and so far only erythromycin-resistant strain of *B. pertussis* was isolated from a 2-month-old male infant in Yuma County, Arizona, in June 1994.[140] The isolate was highly resistant, with a minimum inhibitory concentration of >64 μg/mL (usual minimum inhibitory concentration of erythromycin, 0.02 to 0.1 μg/mL).

Supportive care includes avoidance of factors that provoke attacks of coughing and maintenance of hydration and nutrition. In the hospital, gentle suction for removal of secretions and well-humidified oxygen may be required, particularly in infants with pneumonia and significant respiratory distress. In severe infections in neonates and young infants, assisted ventilation may be necessary.

The use of corticosteroids has received attention in the treatment of pertussis. Cortisone treatment of murine pertussis increased the mortality rate.[120] In contrast, Zoumboulakis and associates[273] found that a 7-day course of steroids and erythromycin reduced the number of coughing paroxysms and episodes of vomiting significantly and the duration of symptoms was shortened. Unfortunately, this study was not controlled rigorously.

The use of salbutamol also may be of some value, but definitive studies have not established this mode of treatment.[28]

PROGNOSIS

The prognosis in pertussis is related directly to the patient's age. In older children and adults, the prognosis is good. In infants, there is a significant risk of death (0.3 to 1.3 per cent) and encephalopathy (0.5 to 1.4 per cent).[37, 73] In addition, long-term follow-up suggests that apnea or seizures at the time of disease may be associated with subsequent intellectual impairment.[235] The present availability of pediatric intensive care units and assisted ventilation has reduced the mortality in those infants who get medical care.[105] Unfortunately, many deaths occur outside of the hospital.

PREVENTION

Vaccine History and Whole-Cell Vaccines

The first pertussis vaccines were developed more than 70 years ago, and effective vaccines have enjoyed worldwide use for about 45 years. In the United States, a minimum potency standard for vaccine was established in 1949, and in 1953, a standard unit was established. Adsorbed triple vaccines (DTP) have been employed widely since originally recommended in 1947. An international standard was established in 1964, at which time it was recommended that each dose of vaccine contain at least 4 IU.[263] Potency of vaccine in international units was ascertained by the intracerebral mouse protection test, and toxicity was assessed by the mouse weight gain test. In 1962, an international opacity reference preparation was established. Ten international units of opacity indicate a concentration of approximately 10 billion organisms per milliliter.

After World War II, extensive vaccine trials were organized by the British Medical Research Council. Five British and American vaccines were evaluated in 1951 in a series of 10 field trials that involved 3801 vaccinees and 3757 children who did not receive pertussis vaccine but who did receive an anticatarrhal vaccine (controls).[162] The attack rate was 1.45 per 1000 child months in immunized children and 6.72 per 1000 child months in the control group, an overall vaccine efficacy rate of 78.4 per cent. When secondary attack rates were examined in families, an efficacy rate of 79.2 per cent was noted. The secondary attack rate in families of vaccinees was 18.2 per cent, whereas it was 87.3 per cent in the control group.

The results of 18 other trials conducted between 1948 and 1954 were published in 1956.[163] In 11 trials, various British vaccines were compared with vaccines produced in the United States. In these trials,[31] 557 children were immunized; the attack rate in vaccinees exposed at home was 14 per cent. In the other seven trials, various lots of British vaccines were compared. In 9794 immunized children, the attack rate of children exposed at home was 69 per cent. The final report of vaccine trials in Great Britain was presented in 1959.[164] Seven different vaccines were given to 13,029 children. The potency of the various vaccines, as measured by mouse protection tests, correlated well with their clinical efficacy. The secondary attack rate for vaccinated children exposed at home was 17 per cent.

The pertussis attack rate was relatively constant within the United States in the prevaccine era between 1922 and 1942 (see Fig. 134–1). From 1943 to 1976, a 150-fold reduction in attack rate was noted in association with widespread childhood pertussis immunization.

A relationship between vaccine use and disease control also was supported by data from England and Wales. The pertussis attack rate declined between 1958 and 1973 and increased dramatically between 1977 and 1983, after a marked decrease in vaccine uptake beginning in 1974.[41] The attack rate decreased with the widespread use of vaccine and increased when vaccine use decreased. Moreover, the attack rate after the decrease in vaccine use was increased most markedly in the newly susceptible cohort of children younger than 4 years of age. English children receive their pertussis immunization only in the first year of life, and protection is not long-lasting.

Improper storage, dilution, or administration of pertussis vaccine, variations in vaccine potency, variations in immunization schedules, and other factors all serve to reduce the efficacy of pertussis immunization in clinical practice, compared with the efficacy reported in clinical trials.[26, 27, 53, 123, 149, 193, 206, 207, 258]

Another measure of vaccine efficacy can be provided by comparing disease severity in unvaccinated children with that observed in vaccinated children. Such data are available from studies performed in the United Kingdom.

Vesselinova-Jenkins and associates[245] studied an outbreak of pertussis involving 229 children. When an allowance for age was made and only children 18 months of age or older were evaluated, it was reported that gasping, cyanosis, dyspnea, streaming tears, vomiting, and seizures were more common in unvaccinated children.

In another study of data from 94 health area authorities, Miller and Fletcher[167] noted that hospital admissions were more common in unimmunized children and that severity of disease in children treated at home was correlated inversely with vaccination status. Severe disease was found in only 0.9 per cent of fully immunized children, in contrast to 5 per cent of unvaccinated children. An illness of moderate severity occurred in 37 per cent of the unvaccinated group, compared with 24 per cent of the fully vaccinated individuals. In the United States, information from the Supplementary Pertussis Surveillance System revealed that pneumonia, seizures, and hospitalization were more common in unvaccinated persons than in those receiving three or more doses of vaccine.[26, 36]

The epidemics in Great Britain also made possible the study of vaccine efficacy. During the epidemic from 1977 to 1979, the attack rate in 25,780 fully immunized children in Hertfordshire was 3.6 per 1000, whereas it was 14.35 per 1000 in those partially immunized and 27.64 per 1000 in children not immunized[53]; vaccine efficacy in those fully immunized was 86.6 per cent.

Vaccine efficacy also has been studied in outbreak situations in the United States.[33–35, 64, 199] In one study from 1982 to 1983 involving 440 household contacts 6 months to 9 years of age, the secondary attack rate for unvaccinated contacts was compared with the rate in children who had received three or more DTP doses. Vaccine efficacy was found to be 91.4 per cent. A similar study during the period from 1979 to 1981 revealed an efficacy value of 82.4 per cent.

In a more recent study, Onorato and associates[199] noted that calculated efficacy varied markedly by the clinical case definition. Efficacy against any cough illness was 63 per cent, whereas it was 83 per cent if a cough duration of 21 or more days was required.

In contrast with the efficacy data determined in observational household contact studies in the United States, one of the two major U.S. vaccines showed poor efficacy in the double-blind efficacy trials carried out in Sweden and Italy.[91, 96] Specifically, the calculated efficacy after three doses in infancy was 48 per cent in Sweden and 36 per cent in Italy.

Adverse Events

Local reactions and relatively mild systemic complaints are frequent after pertussis immunization. Less commonly, severe neurologic illnesses have been noted in temporal association with DTP immunization.

The largest study in the United States designed to assess the risk of relatively common and common reactions to pertussis vaccine was performed by Baraff and associates.[8, 9, 11, 54] This study was carried out between January 1978 and December 1979. Reactions in children who received either DTP or DT immunizations were compared. A total of 15,752 DTP immunizations and 784 DT immunizations were given to children between birth and 6 years of age. These children were evaluated for reactions that occurred within 48 hours of vaccine administration. All common local and systemic reactions occurred more frequently in the DTP recipients than in the DT group. The differences between the common reactions in the two groups were all highly significant ($p < .005$).

Redness at the injection site occurred in 37.4 per cent of the DTP recipients and in 7.6 per cent of the DT vaccinees. Fever (≥38° C [100.4° F]) was noted in 46.5 per cent of DTP recipients. Temperature of 39° C (102.2° F) or higher occurred in 6.1 per cent of DTP recipients but in only 0.7 per cent of DT recipients. Drowsiness, fretfulness, vomiting, anorexia, and persistent crying were other reactions recorded in 3.1 per cent (persistent crying) to 53.4 per cent (fretfulness) of DTP recipients, compared with 0.7 per cent (persistent crying) and 22.6 per cent (fretfulness) of DT vaccinees.

In addition to these reactions, 0.1 per cent of DTP recipients in this study were reported by the parents to have a high-pitched, unusual cry; 0.6 per cent had convulsions, and 0.06 per cent had hypotonic-hyporesponsive episodes (shock, collapse). No children in the control group (DT recipients) had similar reactions; because the control group was of modest size (784 DT recipients), statistical significance could not be assigned to any of these relatively uncommon events.

Because convulsions in young children are the result of many different etiologic factors, the cause-and-effect relationship with pertussis vaccine is less clear. However, because almost half of all DTP vaccinees develop fever and febrile convulsions are not uncommon, it is reasonable to assume that many convulsions that occur in temporal association with DTP vaccination in fact are due to the immunization. Two studies have noted a significant association between pertussis immunization and febrile convulsions.[222, 247] About 1 per 1000 vaccinees older than 6 months of age will have a first febrile seizure after pertussis immunization. The concomitant use of acetaminophen (15 mg/kg/dose at the time of immunization and every 4 hours for 24 hours) and DTP vaccine has been suggested for reduction of the incidence of febrile convulsions in vaccinees.[139]

Neurologic disease and death occurring in temporal association with pertussis immunization have been of major concern throughout the vaccine era. During the last 50 years, there have been several case series and individual reports of neurologic illness after pertussis immunization; by 1979, there were more than 1000 reported cases of alleged pertussis vaccine neurologic damage.[15, 29, 39, 41, 133, 157, 259] In few of these reports was there evidence of an adequate search for other possible causes of the neurologic disease, and in none were data available for rate calculations.

Several attempts have been made to determine the frequency of neurologic disease after pertussis immunization. In 1967, Ström[234] in Sweden reported a rate of destructive encephalopathy of 1 per 170,000 children immunized. Hannik and Cohen[102] in the Netherlands reported a rate of encephalopathy temporally related to pertussis immunization of 1 per 400,000 vaccinated children.

Edsall[68] noted in 1975 that during a 12-year period in Massachusetts, not a single case of pertussis encephalopathy was brought to the attention of the Massachusetts State Laboratory, despite the immunization of approximately 1 million children with pertussis vaccine during that period. In a previous publication, however, Edsall[69] reported that one serious reaction to DTP occurred every 2 years, a rate of 1 per 180,000 children who had received pertussis vaccine.

Since 1978, the Centers for Disease Control and Prevention has maintained a monitoring system for adverse events occurring in temporal relation to immunizations.[78] Between 1978 and 1981, 139 cases of severe neurologic illness were reported; during this same period, 19.2 million children received one or more doses of pertussis vaccine. These data suggest a rate of severe events of 1 per 230,000 doses of pertussis vaccine administered. No information is available concerning residual damage in the 139 children who were reported to have had neurologic events.

In the United Kingdom, where the possible neurologic risks of pertussis immunization have received considerable attention, there have been several studies to determine incidence rates. In 1977, Stewart[228] reported a rate of one case of encephalopathy per 54,000 children. In later writings, Stewart suggested a risk rate as high as 1 per 750 children.[41] In 1981, an expert panel in Great Britain estimated a rate of brain damage from pertussis vaccination of 1 in 53,000 children.[2]

In none of the preceding rate estimates was a control group included, so that all of the estimates include children with temporally related events that were due to other causes.

A carefully designed prospective case-control study (National Childhood Encephalopathy Study [NCES]) of all hospital admissions in England, Wales, and Scotland of all children 2 to 35 months of age with acute serious neurologic disorders was undertaken between 1976 and 1979.[3, 14, 152, 168–171] The results of this study revealed for the first time an apparent statistical association between pertussis immunization and neurologic illness. It was found that a child who had received DTP vaccine within 3 and 7 days was two to five times more likely to have neurologic disease than was a child who was not immunized during the same intervals. The causal relationship between DTP immunization and neurologic illness noted in this study must be questioned, however, because both cases and controls had an equal frequency of immunization during the month preceding the index date. It is more appropriate to interpret the results as not indicating cause and effect; rather, the DTP immunization calls attention to or brings out something that is to occur anyway, but just moves it forward in time.[43]

Infantile spasms, an identifiable seizure disorder of infancy, usually has its onset in the 6-month period from 2 to 7 months of age; therefore, it is not surprising that some cases occur after DTP immunization. Simple calculations indicate that about 12 per cent of all patients destined to develop infantile spasms between 2 and 7 months of age will have the onset of illness within 7 days after DTP immunization. The temporal association between DTP immunization and infantile spasms has led many people to assume a cause-and-effect relationship. However, controlled data from the NCES in Great Britain provide strong evidence against a causative role for pertussis vaccine in infantile spasms.[14] In another study, Melchior[165] in Denmark noted that the time of onset of infantile spasms was not altered when the time of pertussis immunization was changed from 5, 6, 7, and 15 months of age to 5 weeks, 9 weeks, and 10 months of age. In both periods, 42 per cent of patients had their onset during the first 4 months of life.

Data from the NCES have been reanalyzed with exclusion of cases of infantile spasms.[168, 169] From these analyses, it has been suggested that the risk of permanent brain damage from pertussis immunization is 1 per 330,000 vaccine doses and the risk of any encephalopathy is 1 per 140,000 vaccinations. However, review of the NCES data by others indicates that both rate estimates are incorrect. Specifically, Stephenson[227] has shown that the 1 per 140,000 rate for all encephalopathy is an artifact resulting from the inclusion of nine children with febrile convulsions. Similarly, MacRae[151] has noted that the increased relative risk that was observed within 7 days of immunization (which was used to calculate the risk of brain damage of 1 per 330,000 immunizations) was offset by a decreased relative risk over the subsequent 3-week period. This, similar to the original study data and the infantile spasms data, indicates not a cause-and-effect relationship but a redistribution of events over time.[151]

In the United States, the major neurologic illness that is noted in temporal association with DTP immunization is the first seizure of what turns out to be severe epilepsy. By chance alone, this association may occur 400 times a year in the United States. Four carefully performed studies, which included about 330,000 children and 1 million immunizations, have examined the possibility that pertussis immunization is a causative factor in epilepsy; no evidence of a causative role has been found.[45, 82, 93, 222, 247]

Similar to infantile spasms, sudden infant death syndrome also occurs in early life; therefore, it is not surprising that cases are noted to occur after DTP immunization. Four sudden unexplained deaths during a 4-month period in children who had been immunized with DTP were reported on March 9, 1979, in Tennessee.[18, 31, 32] In the definitive report of this investigation, it was noted that an unusual temporal association between DTP immunization with one lot of DTP vaccine and sudden infant death syndrome had been observed. An outside panel of consultants concluded that a causal relationship could be neither established nor excluded.

Hoffman and associates[114] carried out an extensive prospective case-control study of risk factors in sudden infant death syndrome from October 1978 through December 1979. In this study with 800 cases, it was found that DTP immunization is not a risk factor in the causation of the syndrome. Other good, controlled studies have yielded similar results.[42, 92]

Schedules and Contraindications

Immunization with whole-cell vaccines generally is accomplished by providing pertussis in combination with diphtheria and tetanus toxoids (DTP adsorbed); primary immunization is initiated at 2 months of age. Additional doses of DTP are recommended at 4, 6, and 12 to 18 months of age, with a final dose between 48 and 84 months of age.[5] If pertussis is prevalent in the community, immunization can be started at 2 weeks of age, and the first three doses can be given as frequently as 4 weeks apart.

Over the years, pertussis vaccine recommendations have undergone many changes. In particular, vaccine contraindications are changing continually. It is important to note, however, that few scientific data support any of the present contraindications. The primary goal of the national immunization program is to vaccinate all infants and children. If excessive contraindications or their overinterpretation leads to a large number of unimmunized children, the program will fail and the children in the greatest need of protection will get pertussis. The most recent recommendations of the Committee on Infectious Diseases of the American Academy of Pediatrics generally should be followed. However, individual case-by-case decisions often will need to be made.

Acellular Vaccines

Research in the 1970s showed that three *B. pertussis* antigens (PT, FHA, LOS) were liberated into the medium during culture and that these antigens could be concentrated and separated by density gradient centrifugation.[42, 113] This allowed for the development and production of vaccines by six manufacturers in Japan. All six vaccines had minimal amounts or no endotoxin but different amounts of toxoided PT and FHA. In addition, it was found that some of the vaccines contained fimbriae 2 and pertactin. These new "acellular" pertussis vaccines were shown to cause a lesser frequency and severity of fever, other systemic reactions, and local side reactions than do whole-cell vaccines.[131, 194]

TABLE 134–3. Pertussis Antigens in Seven Diphtheria and Tetanus Toxoids and Acellular Pertussis Vaccines Evaluated in Recent Efficacy Trials (1990–1995)

Vaccine	Pertussis Toxin μg/Dose	Filamentous Hemagglutinin μg/Dose	Pertactin μg/Dose	Fimbriae μg/Dose
Amvax (Amvax-1)	40			
Connaught (US) Biken	23.4	23.4		
Pasteur-Merieux (PM2)	25	25		
Smith-Kline Beecham (SKB-2)	25	25		
Chiron-Biocine (CB-3)	5	2.5	2.5	
Smith-Kline Beecham (SKB-3)	25	25	8	
Connaught (Canada) (Con[Can]-5)	10	5	3	5*
Lederle Praxis/Takeda (Led/Tak-4)	3.5	3.5	2	0.8†

*Contains fimbriae 2 and 3.
†Contains fimbriae 2.

Despite limited proof of efficacy, the six vaccines were put into routine use in Japan in 1981, and they have controlled epidemic pertussis during the ensuing 16 years. However, because adequate data were not available on any single vaccine or in vaccine use in early infancy, many extensive trials subsequently have been carried out in Europe, Africa, and Japan. The findings of early trials in Sweden and Japan resulted in the licensure of two acellular vaccines for fourth and fifth doses in the United States.[1, 182]

It was noted, after extensive analyses of the data in the original efficacy trial in Sweden, that calculated efficacy varied significantly, depending upon the clinical case definition and the laboratory methods.[1, 21, 98, 230–232] Therefore, it was felt that a universal primary case definition should be developed to be used in all subsequent efficacy trials, so that different vaccines could be compared from different trials. A World Health Organization committee met in Geneva in January 1991, and a primary case definition was developed. This definition or minor variations of it have been used in the most recent efficacy trials.[264] The World Health Organization case definition is as follows: (1) an illness with 21 days or more of spasmodic cough and either culture-confirmed infection with *B. pertussis* or serologic evidence of infection with *B. pertussis* as indicated by a significant IgA or IgG antibody rise determined by ELISA against PT or FHA in paired sera or (2) contact with a case of culture-confirmed

TABLE 134–4. Vaccine Efficacy in Seven Recent Efficacy Trials

Location and Sponsor	Design	Vaccines and No. of Subjects: *Vaccine*	*No. of Subjects*	Efficacy *(%): *Schedule*	*(95% CI)*
Sweden, Stockholm; NIH-NIAID	Prospective cohort, double-blind	SKB-2	2538	3 doses (2, 4, 6 mo)	59 (51–66)
		Con(Can)-5	2551		85 (81–89)
		DTP (Con)	2001		48 (37–58)
		DT	2538		
Italy, Rome; NIH-NIAID	Prospective cohort, double-blind	SKB-3	4481	3 doses (2, 4, 6 mo)	84 (76–90)
		CB-3	4452		84 (76–90)
		DTP(Con)	4348		36 (14–52)
		DT	1470		
Sweden, Gothenburg; NIH-NIAID	Prospective cohort, double-blind	Amvax-1	1670	3 doses (3, 5, 12 mo)	71 (63–78)
		DT	1665		
Germany, Erlangen; Wyeth-Lederle	Prospective cohort, double-blind DTaP/DTP, unblinded DT	Led/Tak-4	4273	4 doses (3, 4½, 6, 15–18 mo)	82 (73–87)†
		DTP(Led)	4259		91 (85–94)†
		DT	1739		
Senegal; Pasteur-Merieux	Prospective cohort, double-blind	PM-2	1847	3 doses (2, 4, 6 mo)	86 (71–93)
		DTP(PM)	1772		96 (87–94)
	Unblinded household contact study	DTaP/DTP			
Germany, Mainz; Smith-Kline Beecham	Prospective household contact study	SKB-3	22,503	3 doses (3, 4, 5 mo)	89 (77–95)
		DTP (Behring)			97 (83–100)
		DT			
Germany, Munich; Connaught (US)	Case-control study, unblinded	Con(US)Bik-2	12,710	4 doses (2, 4, 6, 15–25 mo)	96 (78–99)
		DTP (Behring)	3200		97 (79–100)
		DT	2100		

*Using the WHO or modified WHO case definition.
†Manufacturer's determination of efficacy and not that of the study investigators.
NIH-NIAID, National Institutes of Health, National Institute for Allergy and Infectious Diseases.

pertussis in the household with onset within 28 days before or after the onset of cough in the study vaccinee. Not all members of the World Health Organization committee, including one of us (JDC), agreed with this primary case definition, because its use results in the elimination of many laboratory-confirmed cases from efficacy calculations. With this definition, vaccines that lessen the severity of disease but are poor at preventing infection will, in general, be overrated.

In 1994 and 1995, seven efficacy trials with eight candidate acellular pertussis component DTP vaccines (DTaP) in four countries were completed.[91, 96, 108, 205, 218, 239] As noted in Table 134–3, the eight vaccines are different in the number of antigens that they contain as well as the concentrations of the specific antigens. Characteristics of the studies and efficacy data are presented in Table 134–4. In all efficacy studies, confounding factors may affect results. In general, double-blind studies with placebo and whole-cell vaccine controls are ideal. However, placebo control was not ethical in countries in which DTP vaccine was recommended. Therefore, studies in Germany and Senegal used various methods to obtain efficacy data in spite of the lack of a blinded DT group. It also should be noted that observer bias can affect the results of all studies, including those with double-blind control. For example, a less efficacious vaccine that prevents typical disease but not mild disease can be determined to be more efficacious than it is if the study observers "know pertussis" and dismiss possible cases as being other respiratory illnesses and do not obtain cultures or carry out prospective follow-up.

In addition to the efficacy data presented in Table 134–4, efficacy based upon lesser cough illnesses has been presented for the two Swedish trials and the Italian trial.[91, 96, 239] The following efficacies were noted: Con(Can)-5, 78 per cent (95 per cent confidence interval [CI], 73 to 82); SKB-2, 42 per cent (95 per cent CI, 33 to 51); SKB-3, 71 per cent (95 per cent CI, 60 to 78); CB-3, 71 per cent (95 per cent CI, 61 to 79); and Amvax-1, 53 per cent (95 per cent CI, 43 to 63).

When the results of the three aforementioned double-blind studies and the original Swedish study, which also was double-blind (PT toxoid vaccine with an efficacy of 13 per cent and a PT toxoid/FHA vaccine with an efficacy of 42 per cent),[230] are analyzed, the following conclusions can be made. Monocomponent PT toxoid vaccines and two component PT toxoid/FHA vaccines are less efficacious than three or four component vaccines that contain pertactin in addition to PT toxoid and FHA. The two studies (Munich and Senegal) that suggested that PT/FHA vaccines had similar efficacy as three and four component vaccines containing pertactin were unblinded, limited by case definition, and prone to observer bias in regard to the determination of efficacy.

All eight DTaP vaccines used in the seven efficacy trials were well tolerated. In general, the DTaP vaccines caused less local reactions and systemic events than conventional DTP vaccines. High temperature, persistent crying, hypotonic-hyporesponsive episodes, and seizures did occur in recipients of DTaP vaccines, but their occurrences were significantly less frequent than in DTP vaccinees.

Because acellular vaccines are significantly less reactogenic than whole-cell vaccines, they offer the possibility of booster immunizations for adolescents and adults.[47, 48] It is our opinion that future programs with multicomponent acellular vaccines that contain pertactin and perhaps fimbriae, which include booster doses in adolescents and adults as well as universal childhood immunization, will control disease and perhaps the circulation of *B. pertussis* as well.

Isolation and Prophylactic Measures

Erythromycin in the index case shortens communicability of the organisms and thus limits spread of the disease. During the first few days of treatment, contact with susceptible persons should be avoided. In general, close contacts (household members, those in day care centers, playmates) of the index case should be protected from infection. This can be managed by the prophylactic use of erythromycin[226] for 14 days and active immunization of children younger than 7 years of age who have not completed their immunization series for pertussis.[5]

The use of erythromycin prophylactically for exposed adults frequently is recommended. In the hospital setting, this often involves many people and considerable expense. In our experience, the side effects of erythromycin are such that adult compliance is poor. Therefore, it is our opinion that erythromycin should not be used prophylactically but only for treatment at the first sign of respiratory illness in those exposed.

References

1. Ad Hoc Group for the Study of Pertussis Vaccines: Placebo-controlled trial of two acellular pertussis vaccines in Sweden: Protective efficacy and adverse events. Lancet *1*:955–960, 1988.
2. Advisory Panel of the Committee on Safety of Medicines: The collection of data relating to adverse reactions in pertussis vaccine. *In* Whooping Cough: Reports From the Committee on Safety of Medicines and the Joint Committee on Vaccination and Immunisation. London, Department of Health and Social Security, Her Majesty's Stationery Office, 1981, p. 27.
3. Alderslade, R., Bellman, M. H., Rawson, N. S. B., et al.: The National Childhood Encephalopathy Study. *In* Whooping Cough: Reports From the Committee on Safety of Medicines and the Joint Committee on Vaccination and Immunisation. London, Department of Health and Social Security, Her Majesty's Stationery Office, 1981, p. 79.
4. Amador, C., Chiner, E., Calpe, J. L., et al.: Pneumonia due to *Bordetella bronchiseptica* in a patient with AIDS. Rev. Infect. Dis. *13*:771–772, 1991.
5. American Academy of Pediatrics: Active immunization: Pertussis. *In* Peter, G. (ed.): 1994 Red Book: Report of the Committee on Infectious Diseases. 23rd ed. Elk Grove Village, American Academy of Pediatrics, 1994, pp. 7–39, 355–367.
6. Arciniega, J. L., Shahin, R. D., Burnette, W. N., et al.: Contribution of the B oligomer to the protective activity of genetically attenuated pertussis toxin. Infect. Immun. *59*:3407–3410, 1991.
7. Arico, B., and Rappuoli, R.: *Bordetella parapertussis* and *Bordetella bronchiseptica* contain transcriptionally silent pertussis toxin genes. J. Bacteriol. *169*:2847–2853, 1987.
8. Baraff, L. J., Wilkins, J., and Wehrle, P.F.: The role of antibiotics, immunizations and adenoviruses in pertussis. Pediatrics *61*:224–230, 1978.
9. Baraff, L. J., and Cherry, J. D.: Nature and rates of adverse reactions associated with pertussis immunization. *In* International Symposium on Pertussis. Bethesda, U.S. DHEW, NIH, 1979, p. 291.
10. Baraff, L. J., Manclark, C. R., Cherry, J. D., et al.: Analyses of adverse reactions to diphtheria and tetanus toxoids and pertussis vaccine by vaccine lot, endotoxin content, pertussis vaccine potency and percentage of mouse weight gain. Pediatr. Infect. Dis. J. *8*:502–507, 1989.
11. Baraff, L. J., Cody, C. L., and Cherry, J. D.: DTP-associated reactions: An analysis by injection site, manufacturer, prior reactions, and dose. Pediatrics *73*:31–36, 1984.
12. Bass, J. W., Klenk, E. L., Kotherine, J. B., et al.: Antimicrobial treatment of pertussis. J. Pediatr. *75*:768–781, 1969.
13. Beiter, A., Lewis, K., Pineda, E. F., et al.: Unrecognized maternal peripartum pertussis with subsequent fatal neonatal pertussis. Obstet. Gynecol. *82*:691–693, 1993.
14. Bellman, M. H., Ross, E. M., and Miller, D. L.: Infantile spasms and pertussis immunisation. Lancet *1*:1031–1034, 1983.
15. Berg, J. M.: Neurological complications of pertussis immunization. Br. Med. J. *2*:24, 1958.
16. Bergquist, S., Bernander, S., Dahnsjo, H., et al.: Erythromycin in the treatment of pertussis: A study of bacteriologic and clinical effects. Pediatr. Infect. Dis. J. *6*:458–461, 1987.
17. Bernales, R., Eastman, J., and Kaplan, J.: Quantitation of circulating T and B lymphocytes in children with whooping cough. Pediatr. Res. *10*:965–967, 1976.
18. Bernier, R. H., Frank, J. A., Jr., Dondero, T. J., Jr., et al.: Diphtheria-tetanus toxoids–pertussis vaccination and sudden infant deaths in Tennessee. J. Pediatr. *101*:419–421, 1982.
19. Bhargava, A., Leininger, E., Roberts, M., et al.: Filamentous hemagglutinin and the 69-kDa protein, Pertactin, promote adherence of *Bordetella pertussis* to epithelial cells and macrophages. 6th International Symposium on Pertussis. Bethesda, September 26–28, 1990, pp. 137–138.
20. Biellik, R. J., Patriarca, P. A., Mullen, J. R., et al.: Risk factors for commu-

nity- and household-acquired pertussis during a large-scale outbreak in central Wisconsin. J. Infect. Dis. *157*:1134–1141, 1988.
21. Blackwelder, W. C., Storsaeter, J., Olin, P., et al.: Acellular pertussis vaccines. Am. J. Dis. Child. *145*:1285–1289, 1991.
22. Blumberg, D. A., Mink, C. M., Cherry, J. D., et al.: Comparison of an acellular pertussis-component diphtheria-tetanus-pertussis (DTP) vaccine with a whole-cell pertussis-component DTP vaccine in 17- to 24-month-old children, with measurement of 69-kilodalton outer membrane protein antibody. J. Pediatr. *117*:46–51, 1990.
23. Bordet, J., and Gengou, O.: Le microbe de la coqueluche. Ann. Inst. Pasteur *20*:48–68, 1906.
24. Bordet, J., and Gengou, O.: L'endotoxin coquelucheuse. Ann. Inst. Pasteur. *23*:415–419, 1909.
25. Brooksaler, F., and Nelson, J. D.: Pertussis: A reappraisal and report of 190 confirmed cases. Am J. Dis. Child. *114*:389–396, 1967.
26. Broome, C. V., and Fraser, D. W.: Pertussis in the United States, 1979: A look at vaccine efficacy. J. Infect. Dis. *144*:187–190, 1981.
27. Broome, C. V., Preblud, S. R., Bruner, B., et al.: Epidemiology of pertussis, Atlanta, 1977. J. Pediatr. *98*:362–367, 1981.
28. Broomhall, J., and Herxheimer, A.: Treatment of whooping cough: The facts. Arch. Dis. Child. 59: 185–187, 1984.
29. Byers, R. K., and Moll, F. C.: Encephalopathies following prophylactic pertussis vaccine. Pediatrics *1*:437, 1948.
30. Celermajor, J. M., and Brown, J.: The neurological complications of pertussis. Med. J. Aust. *1*:1066–1069, 1966.
31. Centers for Disease Control: DTP vaccination follow-up: Tennessee. M. M. W. R. *28*:134, 1979.
32. Centers for Disease Control: DTP vaccination and sudden infant deaths: Tennessee. M. M. W. R. *28*:131, 1979.
33. Centers for Disease Control: Pertussis surveillance, 1979–1981. M. M. W. R. *31*:333, 1982.
34. Centers for Disease Control: Pertussis: Maryland, 1982. M. M. W. R. *32*:298, 1983.
35. Centers for Disease Control: Pertussis: United States, 1982 and 1983. M. M. W. R. *33*:573–576, 1984.
36. Centers for Disease Control: Pertussis surveillance: United States, 1986–88. M. M. W. R. *39*:57–66, 1990.
37. Centers for Disease Control and Prevention: Pertussis: United States, January 1992–June 1995. M. M. W. R. *44*:525–529, 1995.
38. Chaby, R., and Caroff, M.: Lipopolysaccharides of *Bordetella pertussis* endotoxin. *In* Wardlaw, A. C., and Parton, R. (eds.): Pathogenesis and Immunity in Pertussis. New York, John Wiley & Sons, 1988, pp. 247–272.
39. Chakravorty, A. P.: Blindness after use of triple antigen. Br. Med. J. *1*:105, 1963.
40. Charles, I. G., Li, J. L., Roberts, M., et al.: Identification and characterization of a protective immunodominant B cell epitope of pertactin (P.69) from *Bordetella pertussis*. Eur. J. Immunol. *21*:1147–1153, 1991.
41. Cherry, J. D.: The epidemiology of pertussis and pertussis immunization in the United Kingdom and the United States: A comparative study. Curr. Probl. Pediatr. *14*:1–78, 1984.
42. Cherry, J. D., Brunell, P. A., Golden, G. S., et al.: Report of the Task Force on Pertussis and Pertussis Immunization: 1988. Pediatrics *81* (Suppl.):939–984, 1988.
43. Cherry, J. D.: Pertussis and the vaccine controversy. *In* Root, R. K., Griffiss, J. M., Warren, K. S., et al. (eds.): Immunization. New York, Churchill Livingstone, 1989, pp. 47–63.
44. Cherry, J. D., Baraff, L. J., and Hewlett, E.: The past, present, and future of pertussis: The role of adults in epidemiology and future control. West. J. Med. *150*:319–328, 1989.
45. Cherry, J. D.: Pertussis vaccine encephalopathy: It is time to recognize it as the myth that it is. J. A. M. A. *263*:1679–1680, 1990.
46. Cherry, J. D.: Pertussis: The trials and tribulations of old and new pertussis vaccines. Vaccine *10*:1033–1038, 1992.
47. Cherry, J. D.: Acellular pertussis vaccines: A solution to the pertussis problem. J. Infect. Dis. *168*:21–24, 1993.
48. Cherry, J. D.: Strategies for diphtheria, tetanus, and pertussis (DTP) immunization. Report of the 104th Ross Conference on Pediatric Research. Columbus, Ross Products Division, Abbott Laboratories, 1994, pp. 218–225.
49. Cherry, J. D., Beer, T., Chartrand, S. A., et al.: Comparison of antibody values to *Bordetella pertussis* antigens in young German and American men. Clin. Infect. Dis. *20*:1271–1274, 1995.
50. Cherry, J. D.: Historical review of pertussis and the classical vaccine. J. Infect. Dis. *174*(Suppl.):S259–S263, 1996.
51. Christie, C. D. C., and Baltimore, R. S.: Pertussis in neonates. Am. J. Dis. Child. *143*:1199–1202, 1989.
52. Christie, C. D. C., Marx, M. L., Marchant, C. D., et al.: The 1993 epidemic of pertussis in Cincinnati: Resurgence of disease in a highly immunized population of children. N. Engl. J. Med. *331*:16–21, 1994.
53. Church, M. A.: Evidence of whooping-cough-vaccine efficacy from the 1978 whooping-cough epidemic in Hertfordshire. Lancet 2:188–190, 1979.
54. Cody, C. L., Baraff, L. J., Cherry, J. D., et al.: Nature and rates of adverse reactions associated with DTP and DT immunizations in infants and children. Pediatrics *68*:650–660, 1981.
55. Collier, A. M., Connor, J. T., and Irving, W. R., Jr.: Generalized type 5 adenovirus infection associated with the pertussis syndrome. J. Pediatr. *69*:1073–1978, 1966.
56. Cone, T. E., Jr.: Whooping cough is first described as a disease *sui generis* by Baillou in 1640. Pediatrics *46*:522, 1970.
57. Connor, J. D.: Evidence for an etiological role of adenoviral infection in pertussis syndrome. N. Engl. J. Med. *283*:390–394, 1970.
58. Conway, S. P., Balfour, A. H., and Ross, H.: Serologic diagnosis of whooping cough by enzyme-linked immunosorbent assay. Pediatr. Infect. Dis. J. *7*:570–574, 1988.
59. Cookson, B. T., Vandamme, P., Carlson, L. C., et al.: Bacteremia caused by a novel *Bordetella* species, "*B. hinzii*." J. Clin. Microbiol. *32*:2569–2571, 1994.
60. Cowell, J. L., Sato, Y., Sato, H., et al.: Separation, purification and properties of the filamentous hemagglutinin and the leukocytosis promoting factor-hemagglutinin from *Bordetella pertussis*. *In* Robbins, J. B., Hill, J. C., and Sadoff, G. (eds.): Seminars in Infectious Disease. Vol. IV. Bacterial Vaccines. International Symposium on Bacterial Vaccines. New York, Brian C. Decker Division, Thieme-Stratton, 1982, pp. 371–379.
61. Cundell, D. R., Kanthakumar, K., Taylor, G. W., et al.: Effect of tracheal cytotoxin from *Bordetella pertussis* on human neutrophil function in vitro. Infect. Immun. *62*:639–643, 1994.
62. Davis, S. F., Sutter, R. W., Strebel, P. M., et al.: Concurrent outbreaks of pertussis and *Mycoplasma pneumoniae* infection: Clinical and epidemiological characteristics of illnesses manifested by cough. Clin. Infect. Dis. *20*:621–628, 1995.
63. Decker, G. R., Lavelle, J. P., Kuman, P. N., et al.: Pneumonia due to *Bordetella bronchiseptica* in a patient with AIDS. Rev. Infect. Dis. *13*:1250–1251, 1991.
64. Deen, J. L., Mink, C. M., Cherry, J. D., et al.: A household contact study of *Bordetella pertussis* infections in adults. Clin. Infect. Dis. *21*:1211–1219, 1995.
65. DeMagistris, M. T., Romano, M., Nuti, S., et al.: Dissecting human T cell responses against *Bordetella* species. J. Exp. Med. *168*:1351–1362, 1988.
66. DeVille, J. G., Cherry, J. D., Christenson, P. D., et al.: Frequency of unrecognized *Bordetella pertussis* infections in adults. Clin. Infect. Dis. *21*:639–642, 1995.
67. Donaldson, P., and Whitaker, J. A.: Diagnosis of pertussis by fluorescent antibody staining of nasopharyngeal smears. Am. J. Dis. Child. *99*:423–427, 1960.
68. Edsall, G.: Present status of pertussis vaccination. Practitioner *215*:310–314, 1975.
69. Edsall, G.: Comment. *In* International Symposium on Pertussis, Bilthoven, 1969. Immunobiologic Standards. Vol. 13. New York, S. Karger, 1979, p. 170.
70. Eldering, G., and Kendrick, P.: A group of cultures resembling both bacillus pertussis and bacillus bronchisepticus but identical with neither. J. Bacteriol. *33*:71, 1937.
71. Eldering, G., and Kendrick, P.: *Bacillus parapertussis*: A species resembling both *Bacillus pertussis* and *Bacillus bronchiseptica* but identical with neither. J. Bacteriol. *35*:561–572, 1938.
72. Eldering, G., Hornbeck, C., and Baker, J.: Serological study of *Bordetella pertussis* and related species. J. Bacteriol. *74*:133–136, 1957.
73. Farizo, K. M., Cochi, S. L., Zell, E. R., et al.: Epidemiological features of pertussis in the United States, 1980–1989. Clin. Infect. Dis. *14*:708–719, 1992.
74. Feigin, R. D., and Cherry, J. D.: Pertussis. *In* Feigin, R. D., and Cherry, J. D. (eds.): Textbook of Pediatric Infectious Diseases. 3rd ed. Philadelphia, W. B. Saunders, 1992, pp. 1208–1218.
75. Fine, P. E. M.: Epidemiological considerations for whooping cough eradication. *In* Wardlaw, A. C., and Parton, R. (eds.): Pathogenesis and Immunity in Pertussis. New York, John Wiley & Sons, 1988, pp. 451–467.
76. Fine, P. E. M., and Clarkson, J. A.: The recurrence of whooping cough: Possible implications for assessment of vaccine efficacy. Lancet *1*:666–669, 1982.
77. Fish, F., Cowell, J. L., and Manclark, C. R.: Proliferative response of immune mouse T-lymphocytes to the lymphocytosis-promoting factor of *Bordetella pertussis*. Infect. Immun. *44*:1–6, 1984.
78. Foege, W. H.: Statement read before the Subcommittee on Investigations and General Oversight Committee on Labor and Human Resources, United States Senate, Washington, D.C., May 7, 1982.
79. Friedman, R. L.: Pertussis: The disease and new diagnostic methods. Clin. Microbiol. Rev. *1*:365–376, 1988.
80. Funke, G., Hess, T., von Graevenitz, A., et al.: Characteristics of *Bordetella hinzii* strains isolated from a cystic fibrosis patient over a 3-year period. J. Clin. Microbiol. 34:966–969, 1996.
81. Furman, B. L., Sidey, F. M., and Smith, M.: Metabolic disturbances produced by pertussis toxin. *In* Wardlaw, A. C., and Parton, R. (eds.): Pathogenesis and Immunity in Pertussis. New York, John Wiley & Sons, 1988, pp. 147–172.
82. Gale, J. L., Thapa, P. B., Wassilak, S. G. F., et al.: Risk of serious acute neurological illness after immunization with diphtheria-tetanus-pertussis vaccine: A population-based case-control study. J. A. M. A. *271*:37–41, 1994.
83. Gearing, A. J. H., Bird, C., Wadha, M., et al.: The primary and secondary

cellular immune response to whole cell *Bordetella pertussis* vaccine and its components. Clin. Exp. Immunol. *68*:275–281, 1987.
84. Goldman, W. E.: Tracheal cytotoxin of *Bordetella pertussis. In* Wardlaw, A. C., and Parton, R. (eds.): Pathogenesis and Immunity in Pertussis. New York, John Wiley & Sons, 1988, pp. 237–246.
85. Goodman, Y. E., Wort, A. J., and Jackson, F. L.: Enzyme-linked immunosorbent assay for detection of pertussis immunoglobulin A in nasopharyngeal secretions as an indicator of recent infection. J. Clin. Microbiol. *13*:286–292, 1981.
86. Goodnow, R. A.: Biology of *Bordetella bronchiseptica*. Microbiol. Rev. *44*:722–738, 1980.
87. Gordon, J. E., and Hood, R. I.: Whooping cough and its epidemiological anomalies. Am. J. Med. Sci. *222*:333–361, 1951.
88. Gordon, M., Davies, H. D., and Gold, R.: Clinical and microbiologic features of children presenting with pertussis to a Canadian pediatric hospital during an eleven-year period. Pediatr. Infect. Dis. J. *13*:617–622, 1994.
89. Granström, G., Askelof, P., and Granström, M.: Specific immunoglobulin A to *Bordetella pertussis* antigens in mucosal secretion for rapid diagnosis of whooping cough. J. Clin. Microbiol. *26*:869–874, 1988.
90. Granström, M., Lindberg, A., Askelof, P., et al.: Detection of antibodies in human serum against fimbrial haemagglutinin of *Bordetella pertussis* by enzyme-linked immunosorbent assay. J. Med. Microbiol. *15L*:85–96, 1982.
91. Greco, D., Salmaso, S., Mastrantonio, P., et al.: A controlled trial of two acellular vaccines and one whole-cell vaccine against pertussis. N. Engl. J. Med. *334*:341–348, 1996.
92. Griffin, M. R., Ray, W. A., Livengood, J. R., et al.: Risk of sudden infant death syndrome after immunization with the diphtheria-tetanus-pertussis vaccine. N. Engl. J. Med. *319*:618–623, 1988.
93. Griffin, M. R., Ray, W. A., Mortimer, E. A., et al.: Risk of seizures and encephalopathy after immunization with the diphtheria-tetanus-pertussis vaccine. J. A. M. A. *263*:1641–1645, 1990.
94. Grob, P. R., Crowder, M. J., and Robbins, J. F.: Effect of vaccination on severity and dissemination of whooping cough. Br. Med. J. *282*:1925–1928, 1981.
95. Gueirard, P., Weber, C., Coustumier, A. L., et al.: Human *Bordetella bronchiseptica* infection related to contact with infected animals: Persistence of bacteria in host. J. Clin. Microbiol. *33*:2002–2006, 1995.
96. Gustafsson, L., Hallander, H. O., Olin, P., et al.: A controlled trial of a two-component acellular, a five-component acellular, and a whole-cell pertussis vaccine. N. Engl. J. Med. *334*:349–355, 1996.
97. Hallander, H. O., Reizenstein, I., Renemar, B., et al.: Comparison of nasopharyngeal aspirates with swabs for culture of *Bordetella pertussis*. J. Clin. Microbiol. *31*:50–52, 1993.
98. Hallander, H. O., Storsaeter, J., and Mollby, R.: Evaluation of serologic and nasopharyngeal cultures for diagnosis of pertussis in a vaccine efficacy trial. J. Infect. Dis. *163*:1046–1054, 1991.
99. Halperin, S. A., Bortolussi, R., Kasina, A., et al.: Use of a Chinese hamster ovary cell cytotoxicity assay for the rapid diagnosis of pertussis. J. Clin. Microbiol. *28*:32–38, 1990.
100. Halperin, S. A., Bortolussi, R., MacLean, D., et al.: Persistence of pertussis in an immunized population: Results of the Nova Scotia Enhanced Pertussis Surveillance Program. J. Pediatr. *115*:686–693, 1989.
101. Hannah, J. H., Menozzi, F. D., Renauld, G., et al.: Sulfated glycoconjugate receptors for the *Bordetella pertussis* adhesin filamentous hemagglutinin (FHA) and mapping of the heparin-binding domain on FHA. Infect. Immun. *62*:5010–5019, 1994.
102. Hannik, C. A., and Cohen, H.: Pertussis vaccine experience in the Netherlands. *In* International Symposium on Pertussis. Bethesda, U.S. DHEW, NIH, 1979, p. 279.
103. Haward, R. A.: Scale of undernotification of infectious diseases by general practitioners. Lancet *1*:873–874, 1973.
104. Hedenskog, S., Bjorksten, B., Blennow, M., et al.: Immunoglobulin E response to pertussis toxin in whooping cough and after immunization with a whole-cell and an acellular pertussis vaccine. Int. Arch. Allergy Appl. Immunol. *89*:156–161, 1989.
105. Heininger, U., Stehr, K., and Cherry, J. D.: Serious pertussis overlooked in infants. Eur. J. Pediatr. *151*:342–343, 1992.
106. Heininger, U., Cherry, J. D., Eckhardt, T., et al.: Clinical and laboratory diagnosis of pertussis in the regions of a large vaccine efficacy trial in Germany. Pediatr. Infect. Dis. J. *12*:504–509, 1993.
107. Heininger, U., Stehr, K., Schmitt-Grohé, S., et al.: Clinical characteristics of illness caused by *Bordetella parapertussis* compared with illness caused by *Bordetella pertussis*. Pediatr. Infect. Dis. J. *13*:306–309, 1994.
108. Heininger, U.: Trial synopses: Erlangen, Germany. International Symposium on Pertussis Vaccine Trials. Rome, October 30–November 1, 1995.
109. Heininger, U., Schmitt-Grohé, S., Cherry, J. D., et al.: Der mikroagglutinationstest: Ein einfaches und sensitives verfahren zur serodiagnostik von pertussis. Klin. Pädiatr. *207*:277–280, 1995.
110. Heininger, U., Stehr, K., Schmitt-Schläpfer, G., et al.: *Bordetella pertussis* infections and sudden unexpected deaths in children. Eur. J. Pediatr. *155*:551–553, 1996.
111. Heiss, L. N., Lancaster, J. R., Corbett, J. A., et al.: Epithelial autotoxicity of nitric oxide: Role in the respiratory cytopathology of pertussis. Proc. Natl. Acad. Sci. U. S. A. *91*: 267–270, 1994.
112. Hewlett, E. L., and Gordon, V. M.: Adenylate cyclase toxin of *Bordetella pertussis. In* Wardlaw, A. C., and Parton, R. (eds.): Pathogenesis and Immunity in Pertussis. New York, John Wiley & Sons, 1988, pp. 193–209.
113. Hewlett, E. L., and Cherry, J. D.: New and improved vaccines against pertussis. *In* Woodrow, G. C., and Levine, M. M. (eds.): New Generation Vaccines. New York, Marcel Dekker, 1990, pp. 231–250.
114. Hoffman, H. J., Hunter, J. C., Damus, K., et al.: Diphtheria-tetanus-pertussis immunization and sudden infant death: Results of the National Institute of Child Health and Human Development Cooperative Epidemiological Study of Sudden Infant Death Syndrome Risk Factors. Pediatrics *79*:598–611, 1987.
115. Holmes, W. H.: Bacillary and Rickettsial Infections: Acute and Chronic: A Textbook: Black Death to White Plague. New York, Macmillan, 1940, pp. 395–414.
116. Hoppe, J. E.: Methods for isolation of *Bordetella pertussis* from patients with whooping cough. Eur. J. Clin. Microbiol. Infect. Dis. *7*:616–620, 1988.
117. Hoppe, J., and Haug, A.: Antimicrobial susceptibility of *Bordetella pertussis* (part I). Infection *16*:126–130, 1988.
118. Hoppe, J., and Eichhorn, A.: Activity of new macrolides against *Bordetella pertussis* and *Bordetella parapertussis*. Eur. J. Clin. Microbiol. Infect. Dis. *8*:653–654, 1989.
119. Hoppe, J., Halm, U., Hagedorn, H., et al.: Comparison of erythromycin ethylsuccinate and co-trimoxazole for treatment of pertussis. Infection *17*:227–231, 1989.
120. Iida, T., Kunitani, A., Komase, Y., et al.: Studies on experimental infection with *Bordetella pertussis*: Effect of cortisone on the infection and immunity in mice. Jpn. J. Exp. Med. *33*:283–295, 1983.
121. Irons, L. I., and Gorringe, A. R.: Pertussis toxin: Production, purification, molecular structure, and assay. *In* Wardlaw, A. C., and Parton, R. (eds.): Pathogenesis and Immunity in Pertussis. New York, John Wiley & Sons, 1988, pp. 95–120.
122. Jackson, F. E.: Spontaneous spinal epidural hematoma coincident with whooping cough. J. Neurosurg. *20*:715–717, 1963.
123. Jenkinson, D.: Outbreak of whooping cough in general practice. Br. Med. J. *351*:577–578, 1978.
124. Jenkinson, D.: Whooping cough: What proportion of cases is notified in an epidemic? Br. Med. J. *287*:183–185, 1983.
125. Joint Committee on Vaccination and Immunisation: The whooping cough epidemic, 1977–79. *In* Whooping Cough: Reports from the Committee on Safety in Medicine and the Joint Committee on Vaccination and Immunisation. London, Department of Health and Social Security, Her Majesty's Stationery Office, 1981, p. 170.
126. Jones, D. H., McBride, B. W., Jeffery, H., et al.: Protection of mice from *Bordetella pertussis* respiratory infection using microencapsulated pertussis fimbriae. Vaccine *13*:675–681, 1995.
127. Kendrick, P. L., Eldering, G., Dixon, M. K., et al.: Mouse protection tests in the study of pertussis vaccines. Am. J. Public Health *37*:803–810, 1947.
128. Kendrick, P. L., Eldering, G., and Eveland, W. C.: Fluorescent antibody techniques: Methods for identification of *Bordetella pertussis*. Am. J. Dis. Child. *101*:149–154, 1961.
129. Kersters, K., Hinz, K. H., Hertle, A., et al.: *Bordetella avium* sp. nov., isolated from the respiratory tracts of turkeys and other birds. Int. J. Syst. Bacteriol. *34*:56–70, 1984.
130. Khelef, N., Sakamoto, H., and Guiso, N.: Both adenylate cyclase and hemolytic activities are required by *Bordetella pertussis* to initiate infection. Microbiol. Pathog. *12*:227–235, 1992.
131. Kimura, M., and Kuno-Sakai, H.: Pertussis vaccines in Japan. Acta Paediatr. Jpn. *30*:143–153, 1988.
132. Kimura, A., Mountzouros, K. T., Relman, D. A., et al.: *Bordetella pertussis* filamentous hemagglutinin: Evaluation as a protective antigen and colonization factor in a mouse respiratory infection model. Infect. Immun. *58*:7–16, 1990.
133. Kulenkampff, M., Schwartzman, J. S., and Wilson, J.: Neurological complications of pertussis inoculation. Arch. Dis. Child. *49*:46, 1974.
134. Kurt, T. L., Yeager, A. S., Guenette, S., et al.: Spread of pertussis by hospital staff. J. A. M. A. *221*:264–267, 1972.
135. Lapin, J. H.: Whooping Cough. Springfield, IL, Charles C Thomas, 1943.
136. Lambert, H. J.: Epidemiology of a small pertussis outbreak in Kent County, Michigan. Public Health Rep. *80*:365–369, 1965.
137. Lautrop, H.: Observations on parapertussis in Denmark 1950–1957. Acta Pathol. Microbiol. Scand. *43*:255–266, 1958.
138. Leininger, E., Kenimer, J. G., and Brennan, M. J.: Surface proteins of *Bordetella pertussis*: Role in adherence. 6th International Symposium on Pertussis. Bethesda, September 26–28, 1990, pp. 25–26.
139. Lewis, K., Cherry, J. D., Sachs, M. H., et al.: The effect of prophylactic acetaminophen administration on reactions to DTP vaccination. Am. J. Dis. Child. *142*:62–65, 1988.
140. Lewis, K., Saubolle, M. A., Tenover, F. C., et al.: Pertussis caused by an erythromycin-resistant strain of *Bordetella pertussis*. Pediatr. Infect. Dis. J. *14*:388–391, 1995.
141. Lindquist, S. W., Weber, D. J., Mangum, M.E., et al.: *Bordetella holmesii* sepsis in an asplenic adolescent. Pediatr. Infect. Dis. J. *14*:813–815, 1995.
142. Linnemann, C. C., Jr.: Host-parasite interactions in pertussis. *In* Manclark, C. R., and Hill, J. C. (eds.): International Symposium on Pertussis. U.S.

Dept. of Health, Education, and Welfare. Publication No. (NIH) 79–1830. Washington, D.C., U.S. Government Printing Office, 1979, pp. 3–18.
143. Linnemann, C. C., Jr., and Nasenbeny, J.: Pertussis in the adult. Ann. Rev. Med. *28*:179–185, 1977.
144. Linnemann, C. C., Jr., Ramundo, N., Perlstein, P. H., et al.: Use of pertussis vaccine in an epidemic involving hospital staff. Lancet *2*:540–543, 1975.
145. Locht, C., Bertin, P., Menozzi, F. D., et al.: The filamentous haemagglutinin, a multifaceted adhesin produced by virulent *Bordetella* spp. Mol. Microbiol. *9*:653–660, 1993.
146. Long, S., Welkon, C., and Clark, J.: Widespread silent transmission of pertussis in families: Antibody correlates of infection and symptomatology. J. Infect. Dis. *161*:480–486, 1990.
147. Long, S., Lischner, H., Deforest, A., et al.: Serologic evidence of subclinical pertussis in immunized children. Pediatr. Infect. Dis. J. *9*: 700–705, 1990.
148. Luker, K. E., Collier, J. L., Kolodziej, E. W., et al.: *Bordetella pertussis* tracheal cytotoxin and other muramyl peptides: Distinct structure-activity relationships for respiratory epithelial cytopathology. Proc. Natl. Acad. Sci. U. S. A. *90*:2365–2369, 1993.
149. MacGregor, J. D.: Whooping-cough vaccination: A recent Shetland experience. Br. Med. J. *1*:1154, 1979.
150. MacLean, D. W.: Adults with pertussis. J. R. Coll. Gen. Pract. May:298–300, 1982.
151. MacRae, K. D.: Epidemiology, encephalopathy, and pertussis vaccine. *In* FEMS-Symposium Pertussis: Proceedings of the Conference Organized by the Society of Microbiology and Epidemiology of the GDR. Berlin, April 20–22, 1988.
152. Madge, N., Diamond, J., Miller, D., et al.: The national childhood encephalopathy study: A 10-year follow-up. Dev. Med. Child Neurol. *68* (Suppl.):1–119, 1993.
153. Madsen, T.: Whooping cough: Its bacteriology, diagnosis, prevention and treatment. Boston Med. Surg. J. *192*:50–60, 1925.
154. Makhov, A. M., Hannah, J. H., Brennan, M. J., et al: Filamentous hemagglutinin of *Bordetella pertussis*: A bacterial adhesin formed as a 50-nm monomeric rigid rod based on a 19-residue repeat motif rich in beta strains and turns. J. Mol. Biol. *241*:110–124, 1994.
155. Manclark, C. R., Meade, B. D., and Burstyn, D. G.: Serological response to *Bordetella pertussis*. *In* Rose, N. R., Friedman, H., and Fahey, J. L. (eds.): Manual of Clinical Laboratory Immunology. 3rd ed. Washington, D.C., American Society for Microbiology, 1986, pp. 388–394.
156. Mannerstedt, G.: Pertussis in adults. J. Pediatr. *5*:596–600, 1934.
157. Martin, G. I., and Weintraub, M. I.: Brachial neuritis and seventh nerve palsy: A rare hazard of DPT vaccination. Clin. Pediatr. *12*:506–507, 1973.
158. Masure, H. R.: The adenylate cyclase toxin contributes to the survival of *Bordetella pertussis* within human macrophages. Microb. Pathog. *14*:253–260, 1993.
159. Matherne, P., Matson, J., and Marks, M. I.: Pertussis complicated by the syndrome of inappropriate antidiuretic hormone secretion. Clin. Pediatr. *25*:46–48, 1986.
160. McGregor, J., Ogle, J., and Curry-Kane, G.: Perinatal pertussis. Obstet. Gynecol. *68*:582–586, 1986.
161. Meade, B. D., and Bollen, A.: Recommendations for use of the polymerase chain reaction in the diagnosis of *Bordetella pertussis* infections. J. Med. Microbiol. *41*:51–55, 1994.
162. Medical Research Council: The prevention of whooping cough by vaccination. Br. Med. J. *1*:1463–1471, 1951.
163. Medical Research Council: Vaccination against whooping cough: Relation between protection in children and results of laboratory tests. Br. Med. J. *2*:454–462, 1956.
164. Medical Research Council: Vaccination against whooping cough. Br. Med. J. *1*:994–1000, 1959.
165. Melchior, J. C.: Infantile spasms and early immunization against whooping cough: Danish survey from 1970 to 1975. Arch. Dis. Child. *52*:134, 1977.
166. Mertsola, J., Ruuskanen, O., Kuronen, T., et al.: Serologic diagnosis of pertussis: Evaluation of pertussis toxin and other antigens in enzyme-linked immunosorbent assay. J. Infect. Dis. *161*:966–971, 1990.
167. Miller, C. L., and Fletcher, W. B.: Severity of notified whooping cough. Br. Med. J. *1*:117–119, 1976.
168. Miller, D. L., Ross, E. M., Alderslade, R., et al.: Pertussis immunisation and serious acute neurological illness in children. Br. Med. J. *282*:1595–1597, 1981.
169. Miller, D., Wadsworth, J., Diamond, J., et al.: Pertussis vaccine and whooping cough as risk factors in acute neurological illness and death in young children. Dev. Biol. Stand. *61*:389–394, 1985.
170. Miller, D., Wadsworth, J., and Ross, E.: Severe neurological illness: Further analyses of the British National Childhood Encephalopathy Study. Tokai J. Exp. Clin. Med. *13*(Suppl.):145–155, 1988.
171. Miller, D., Madge, N., Diamond, J., et al.: Pertussis immunisation and serious acute neurological illnesses in children. Br. Med. J. *307*:1171–1176, 1993.
172. Miller, J. J., Jr., Silverberg, R. J., Saito, T. M., et al.: An agglutinative reaction for *Hemophilus pertussis*. II. Its relation to clinical immunity. J. Pediatr *22*:644–651, 1943.
173. Mills, K. H. G., and Redhead, K.: Cellular immunity in pertussis. J. Med. Microbiol. *39*: 163–164, 1993.
174. Mills, K. H. G., Barnard, A., Watkins, J., et al.: Cell-mediated immunity to *Bordetella pertussis*: Role of Th1 cells in bacterial clearance in a murine respiratory infection model. Infect. Immun. *61*:399–410, 1993.
175. Mink, C. A. M., Cherry, J. D., Christenson, P., et al.: A search for *Bordetella pertussis* infection in university students. Clin. Infect. Dis. *14*:464–471, 1992.
176. Mink, C., Sirota, N. M., and Nugent, S.: Outbreak of pertussis in a fully immunized adolescent and adult population. Arch. Pediatr. Adolesc. Med. *148*:153–157, 1994.
177. Mink, C. M., O'Brien, C. H., Wassilak, S., et al.: Isotype and antigen specificity of pertussis agglutinins following whole-cell pertussis vaccination and infection with *Bordetella pertussis*. Infect. Immun. *62*:1118–1120, 1994.
178. Mooi, F. A., van der Heide, H. G. J., Wellems, R., et al.: *Bordetella pertussis* fimbriae: Role in pathogenesis and mechanism of phase variation. 6th International Symposium on Pertussis. Bethesda, September 26–28, 1990, p. 63.
179. Mortimer, E. A., Jr.: Pertussis and its prevention: A family affair. J. Infect. Dis. *161*:473–479, 1990.
180. Mortimer, E. A., Jr., and Jones, P. K.: An evaluation of pertussis vaccine. Rev. Infect. Dis. *1*:927–932, 1979.
181. Mortimer, E. A., Jr., and Jones, P. K.: Pertussis vaccine in the United States: The benefit-risk ratio. *In* International Symposium on Pertussis. Bethesda, U.S. DHEW, NIH, 1979, p. 250.
182. Mortimer, E. A., Jr., Kimura, M., Cherry, J. D., et al.: Protective efficacy of the Takeda acellular pertussis vaccine combined with diphtheria and tetanus toxoids following household exposure of Japanese children. Am. J. Dis. Child. *144*:899–904, 1990.
183. Mountzouros, K. T., Kimura, A., and Cowell, J. L.: A bactericidal monoclonal antibody specific for the lipooligosaccharide of *Bordetella pertussis* reduces colonization of the respiratory tract of mice after aerosol infection with *B. pertussis*. Infect. Immun. *60*:5316–5318, 1992.
184. Munoz, J. J.: Action of pertussigen (pertussis toxin) on the host immune system. *In* Wardlaw, A. C., and Parton, R. (eds.): Pathogenesis and Immunity in Pertussis. New York, John Wiley & Sons, 1988, pp. 173–192.
185. Nagel, J., and Poot-Scholtens, E. J.: Serum IgA antibody to *Bordetella pertussis* as an indicator of infection. J. Med. Microbiol. *16*:417–426, 1983.
186. Nakase, Y., and Endoh, M.: Heat-labile toxin of *Bordetella pertussis*. *In* Wardlaw, A. C., and Parton, R. (eds.): Pathogenesis and Immunity in Pertussis. New York, John Wiley & Sons, 1988, pp. 217–229.
187. Nelson, J. D.: The changing epidemiology of pertussis in young infants: The role of adults as reservoirs of infection. Am. J. Dis. Child. *132*:371–375, 1978.
188. Nelson, K. E., Gavitt, F., Batt, M. D., et al.: The role of adenoviruses in the pertussis syndrome. J. Pediatr. *86*:335–341, 1975.
189. Nencioni, L., Pizza, M., Volpini, G., et al.: Properties of the B oligomer of pertussis toxin. Infect. Immun. *59*:4732–4734, 1991.
190. Nennig, M. E., Shinefield, H. R., Edwards, K. M., et al.: Prevalence and incidence of adult pertussis in an urban population. J. A. M. A. *275*:1672–1674, 1996.
191. Ng, V. L., Boggs, J. M., York, M. K., et al.: Recovery of *Bordetella bronchiseptica* from patients with AIDS. Clin. Infect. Dis. *15*:376–377, 1992.
192. Nicoll, A., and Gardner, A.: Whooping cough and unrecognised postperinatal mortality. Arch. Dis. Child. *63*:41–47, 1988.
193. Noah, N. D.: Attack rates of notified whooping cough in immunised and unimmunised children. Br. Med. J. *1*:128–129, 1976.
194. Noble, G. R., Bernier, R. H., Esber, E. C., et al.: Acellular and whole cell pertussis vaccines in Japan: Report of a visit by U.S. scientists. J. A. M. A. *257*:1351–1356, 1987.
195. Novotny, P.: Pathogenesis in *Bordetella* species. J. Infect. Dis. *161*:581–582, 1990.
196. Novotny, P., Chubb, A. P., Cownley, K., et al.: Biologic and protective properties of the 69-kDa outer membrane protein of *Bordetella pertussis*: A novel formulation for an acellular pertussis vaccine. J. Infect. Dis. *164*:114–122, 1991.
197. Olsen, L. C.: Pertussis. Medicine *54*:427–469, 1975.
198. Onorato, I. M., and Wassilak, S. G. F.: Laboratory diagnosis of pertussis: The state of the art. Pediatr. Infect. Dis. J. *6*:145–151, 1987.
199. Onorato, I. M., Wassilak, S. G., and Meade, B.: Efficacy of whole-cell pertussis vaccine in preschool children in the United States. J. A. M. A. *20*:2745–2749, 1992.
200. Pittman, M.: Pertussis toxin: The cause of the harmful effects and prolonged immunity of whooping cough: A hypothesis. Rev. Infect. Dis. *1*:401–412, 1979.
201. Pittman, M.: The concept of pertussis as a toxin-mediated disease. Pediatr. Infect. Dis. *3*:467–486, 1984.
202. Porter, J. F., Connor, K., and Donachie, W.: Isolation and characterization of *Bordetella parapertussis* like bacteria from ovine lungs. Microbiolology *140*:255–261, 1994.
203. Postels-Multani, S., Schmitt, H. J., Wirsing von König, C. H., et al.: Symptoms and complications of pertussis in adults. Infection *23*:139–142, 1995.
204. Preston, N. W.: Pertussis today. *In* Wardlaw, A. C., and Parton, R. (eds.): Pathogenesis and Immunity in Pertussis. New York, John Wiley & Sons, 1988, pp. 1–18.

205. Proceedings of the International Symposium on Pertussis Vaccine Trials. Rome, October 30–November 1, 1995 (in press).
206. Public Health Laboratory Service: Efficacy of whooping cough vaccines used in the United Kingdom before 1968. Br. Med. J. *4*:329–333, 1969.
207. Public Health Laboratory Service: Efficacy of pertussis vaccination in England. Br. Med. J. *285*:357, 1982.
208. Reizenstein, E., Johanson, B., Mardin, L., et al.: Diagnostic evaluation of polymerase chain reaction discriminative for *Bordetella pertussis*, *B. parapertussis*, and *B. bronchiseptica*. Diagn. Microbiol. Infect. Dis. *17*:185–191, 1993.
209. Robbins, J. B., Pittman, M., Trollfors, B., et al.: Primum non nocere: A pharmacologically inert pertussis toxoid alone should be the next pertussis vaccine. Pediatr. Infect. Dis. J. *12*:795–807, 1993.
210. Robertson, P. W., Goldberg, H., Jarvie, B. H., et al.: *Bordetella pertussis* infection: A cause of persistent cough in adults. Med. J. Aust. *146*:522–525, 1987.
211. Robinson, A., Ashworth, L. A. E., and Irons, L. I.: Serotyping *Bordetella pertussis* strains. Vaccine *7*:491–494, 1989.
212. Robinson, A., Irons, L. I., Seabrook, R. N., et al.: Structure-function studies of *Bordetella pertussis* fimbriae. *In* Manclark, C. R. (ed.): Proceedings of the Sixth International Symposium on Pertussis. Bethesda Dept. of Health and Human Services, United States Public Health Service, DHHS Publ. No. (FDA) 90, 1990, pp. 126–135.
213. Rosenthal, S., Strebel, P., Cassiday, P., et al.: Pertussis infection among adults during the 1993 outbreak in Chicago. J. Infect. Dis. *171*:1650–1652, 1995.
214. Sans, M. B., Bonal, J., Bonet, J., et al.: *Bordetella bronchiseptica* septicemia in a hemodialysis patient. Nephron *59*:676, 1991.
215. Sato, H., and Sato, Y.: *Bordetella pertussis* infection in mice: Correlation of specific antibodies against two antigens, pertussis toxin, and filamentous hemagglutinin with mouse protectivity in an intracerebral or aerosol challenge system. Infect. Immun. *46*:415–421, 1984.
216. Schläpfer, G., Senn, H. P., Berger, R., et al.: Use of the polymerase chain reaction to detect *Bordetella pertussis* in patients with mild or typical symptoms of infection. Eur. J. Clin. Microbiol. Infect. Dis. *12*:459–463, 1993.
217. Schläpfer, G., Cherry, J. D., Heininger, U., et al.: Polymerase chain reaction identification of *Bordetella pertussis* infections in vaccinees and family members in a pertussis vaccine efficacy trial in Germany. Pediatr. Infect. Dis. J. *14*:209–214, 1995.
218. Schmitt, H. J., Wirsing von König, C. H., Neiss, A., et al.: Efficacy of acellular pertussis vaccine in early childhood after household exposure. J. A. M. A. *275*:37–41, 1996.
219. Schmitt-Grohé, S., Cherry, J. D., Heininger, U., et al.: Pertussis in German adults. Clin. Infect. Dis. *21*:860–866, 1995.
220. Shahin, R. D., Brennan, M. J., Meade, B. D., et al.: Characterization of the protective capacity and immunogenicity of the 69-kD outer membrane protein of *Bordetella pertussis*. J. Exp. Med. *171*:63–73, 1990.
221. Shahin, R. D., Amsbaugh, D. F., and Leef, M. F.: Mucosal immunization with filamentous hemagglutinin protects against *Bordetella pertussis* respiratory infection. Infect. Immun. *60*:1482–1488, 1992.
222. Shields, W. D., Nielsen, C., Buch, D., et al.: Relationship of pertussis immunization to the onset of neurologic disorders: A retrospective epidemiologic study. J. Pediatr. *113*:801–805, 1988.
223. Simonond, F.: Trial synopses: Senegal. International Symposium on Pertussis Vaccine Trials. Rome, October 30–November 5, 1995.
224. Southhall, D. P., Thomas, M. G., and Lambert, H. P.: Severe hypoxaemia in pertussis. Arch. Dis. Child. *63*:598–605, 1988.
225. Steketee, R. W., Burstyn, D. G., Wassilak, S. G. F., et al.: A comparison of laboratory and clinical methods for diagnosing pertussis in an outbreak in a facility for the developmentally disabled. J. Infect. Dis. *157*:441–449, 1988.
226. Steketee, R. W., Wassilak, S. G. F., Adkins, W. N., Jr., et al.: Evidence for a high attack rate and efficacy of erythromycin prophylaxis in a pertussis outbreak in a facility for the developmentally disabled. J. Infect. Dis. *157*:434–440, 1988.
227. Stephenson, J. B. P.: A neurologist looks at neurological disease temporally related to DTP immunization. Tokai J. Exp. Clin. Med. *13*(Suppl.):157–164, 1988.
228. Stewart, G. T.: Vaccination against whooping-cough: Efficacy versus risks. Lancet *1*:234, 1977.
229. Stocks, P.: Studies in the population of England and Wales 1944–47. Studies on Medical and Population Subjects. No. 2. London, Her Majesty's Stationery Office, 1949.
230. Storsaeter, J., Hallander, H., Farrington, C. P., et al.: Secondary analyses of the efficacy of two acellular pertussis vaccines evaluated in a Swedish phase III trial. Vaccine *8*:457–461, 1990.
231. Storsaeter, J., Blackwelder, W. C., and Hallander, H. O.: Pertussis antibodies, protection, and vaccine efficacy after household exposure. Am. J. Dis. Child. *146*:167–172, 1992.
232. Storsaeter, J., and Olin, P.: Relative efficacy of two acellular pertussis vaccines during three years of passive surveillance. Vaccine *10*:142–144, 1992.
233. Strebel, P. M., Cochi, S. L., Farizo, K. M., et al.: Pertussis in Missouri: Evaluation of nasopharyngeal culture, direct fluorescent antibody testing, and clinical case definitions in the diagnosis of pertussis. Clin. Infect. Dis. *16*:276–285, 1993.
234. Ström, J.: Further experience of reactions, especially of a cerebral nature, in conjunction with triple vaccination: A study based on vaccinations in Sweden 1959–65. Br. Med. J. *4*:320, 1967.
235. Swansea Research Unit of the Royal College of General Practitioners: Study of intellectual performance of children in ordinary schools after certain serious complications of whooping cough. Br. Med. J. *295*:1044–1047, 1987.
236. Switzer, W. P., Mare, C. J., and Hubbard, E. D.: Incidence of *Bordetella bronchisepticum* in wildlife and man in Iowa. Am. J. Vet. Res. *27*:1134–1136, 1966.
237. Tamion, F., Girault, C., Chevron, V., et al.: *Bordetella bronchoseptica* pneumonia with shock in an immunocompetent patient. Scand. J. Infect. Dis. *28*:137–138, 1996.
238. Taranger, J., Trollfors, B., Lagergard, T., et al.: Parapertussis infection followed by pertussis infection. Lancet *2*:1703, 1994.
239. Trollfors, B., Taranger, J., Lagergard, T., et al.: A placebo-controlled trial of a pertussis-toxoid vaccine. N. Engl. J. Med. *333*:1045–1050, 1995.
240. Tuomanen, E.: *Bordetella pertussis* adhesins. *In* Wardlaw, A. C., and Parton, R. (eds.): Pathogenesis and Immunity in Pertussis. New York, John Wiley & Sons, 1988, pp. 75–94.
241. Ui, M.: The multiple biological activities of pertussis toxin. *In* Wardlaw, A.C., and Parton, R. (eds.): Pathogenesis and Immunity in Pertussis. New York, John Wiley & Sons, 1988, pp. 121–146.
242. Urisu, A., Cowell, J. L., and Manclark, C. R.: Filamentous hemagglutinin has a major role in mediating adherence of *Bordetella pertussis* to human WiDr cells. Infect. Immun. *52*:695–701, 1986.
243. Valenti, W. M., Pincus, P. H., and Messner, M. K.: Nosocomial pertussis: Possible spread by a hospital visitor. Am. J. Dis. Child. *134*:520–521, 1980.
244. Vancanneyt, M., Vandamme, P., and Kersters, K.: Differentiation of *Bordetella pertussis*, *B. parapertussis*, and *B. bronchiseptica* by whole-cell protein electrophoresis and fatty acid analysis. Int. J. Syst. Bacteriol. *45*:843–847, 1995.
245. Vesselinova-Jenkins, C. K., Newcombe, R. G., Gray, O. P., et al.: The effects of immunisation upon the natural history of pertussis: A family study in the Cardiff area. J. Epidemiol. Commun. Health *32*:194–199, 1978.
246. Viljanen, M. K., Ruuskanen, O., Granberg, C., et al.: Serological diagnosis of pertussis: IgM, IgA, and IgG antibodies against *Bordetella pertussis* measured by enzyme-linked immunosorbent assay (ELISA). Scand. J. Infect. Dis. *14*:117–122, 1982.
247. Walker, A. M., Jick, H., Perera, D. R., et al.: Neurologic events following diphtheria-tetanus-pertussis immunization. Pediatrics *81*:345–349, 1988.
248. Walker, K. E., and Weiss, A. A.: Characterization of the dermonecrotic toxin in members of the genus *Bordetella*. Infect. Immun. *62*:3817–3828, 1994.
249. Washburn, T. C., Medearis, D. N., and Childs, B.: Sex differences in susceptibility to infection. Pediatrics *35*:57–67, 1965.
250. Watts, E. C., and Acosta, C.: Pertussis and bilateral subdural hematomas. Am. J. Dis. Child. *118*:518–519, 1969.
251. Weiss, A. A., and Hewlett, E. L.: Virulence factors of *Bordetella pertussis*. Ann. Rev. Microbiol. *40*:661–686, 1986.
252. Weiss, A. A., and Falkow, S.: Genetic analysis of phase variation in *Bordetella pertussis*. Infect. Immun. *43*:263–269, 1984.
253. Weiss, A. A., Hewlett, E. L., Myers, G. A., et al.: Pertussis toxin and extracytoplasmic adenylate cyclase as virulence factors of *Bordetella pertussis*. J. Infect. Dis. *2*:219–222, 1984.
254. Weyant, R. S., Hollis, D. G., Weaver, R. E., et al.: *Bordetella holmesii* sp. nov., a new gram-negative species associated with septicemia. J. Clin. Microbiol. *33*:1–7, 1995.
255. Whitaker, J. A., Donaldson, P., and Nelson, J. D.: Diagnosis of pertussis by the fluorescent antibody method. N. Engl. J. Med. *263*:850–851, 1960.
256. Wiertz, E. J. H., Loggen, H. G., Walvoort, H. D., et al.: In vitro induction of antigen specific antibody synthesis and proliferation of T lymphocytes with acellular pertussis vaccines, pertussis toxin and filamentous hemagglutinin in humans. J. Biol. Stand. *17*:181–190, 1989.
257. Williams, W. O., Kwantes, W., Joynson, D. H. M., et al.: Effect of low pertussis vaccination uptake on a large community. Br. Med. J. *282*:23–26, 1981.
258. Wilson, A. T., Henderson, I. R., Moore, E. J. H., et al.: Whooping-cough: Difficulties in diagnosis and ineffectiveness of immunization. Br. Med. J. *2*:623–626, 1965.
259. Wilson, G. S.: The Hazards of Immunization. London, Althone Press, 1967.
260. Wirsing von König, C. H., Postels-Multani, S., Bock, H. L., et al.: Pertussis in adults: Frequency of transmission after household exposure. Lancet *346*:1326–1329, 1995.
261. Woolf, A. L., and Caplin, H.: Whooping cough encephalitis. Arch. Dis. Child. 3:87–91, 1956.
262. Woolfrey, B. F., and Moody, J. A.: Human infections associated with *Bordetella bronchiseptica*. Clin. Microbiol. Rev. *4*:243–255, 1991.
263. World Health Organization, Expert Committee on Biological Standardisation: Requirements for Pertussis Vaccine (Requirements for Biological Substances No. 8). 16th report (Technical report Series No. 274). Geneva, W. H. O., 1964.

264. World Health Organization meeting on case definition of pertussis. Geneva, January 10–11, 1991, MIM/EPI/PERT/9.1. Geneva, W. H. O., 1991.
265. Wortis, N., Strebel, P. M., Wharton, M., et al.: Pertussis deaths: Report of 23 cases in the United States, 1992 and 1993. Pediatrics *97*:607–612, 1996.
266. Wright, S. W., Edwards, K. M., Decker, M. D., et al.: Pertussis infections in adults with persistent cough. J. A. M. A. *273*:1044–1046, 1995.
267. Zackrisson, G., Lagergard, T., Trollfors, B., et al.: Immunoglobulin A antibodies to pertussis toxin and filamentous hemagglutinin in saliva from patients with pertussis. J. Clin. Microbiol. *28*:1502–1505, 1990.
268. Zee, A., Agterberg, C., Peeters, M., et al.: Polymerase chain reaction assay for pertussis: Simultaneous detection and discrimination of *Bordetella pertussis* and *Bordetella parapertussis*. J. Clin. Microbiol. *31*:2134–2140, 1993.
269. Zepp, F., Schmitt, H. J., Knuf, M., et al.: Specific cellular immune response after vaccination with an acellular (DTPa) pertussis vaccine and after natural disease. Abstract G73. 34th Interscience Conference on Antimicrobial Agents and Chemotherapy. Orlando, October 4–7, 1994.
270. Zepp, F., Knuf, M., Habermehl, P., et al.: Specific cell-mediated immunity after vaccination with an acellular pertussis vaccine (DTPa) in comparison to whole-pertussis vaccines (DTPw) or natural infection. Abstract G62. 35th Interscience Conference on Antimicrobial Agents and Chemotherapy. San Francisco, September 17–20, 1995.
271. Zhang, Y. L., and Sekura, R. D.: Purification and characterization of the heat-labile toxin of *Bordetella pertussis*. Infect. Immun. *59*:3754–3759, 1991.
272. Zoumboulakis, D., Anagnostakis, D., Albams, V., et al.: Steroids in treatment of pertussis: A controlled clinical trial. Arch. Dis. Child. *48*:51–54, 1973.

135

CALYMMATOBACTERIUM GRANULOMATIS

Mariam R. Chacko

Granuloma inguinale is caused by *Calymmatobacterium granulomatis*. Granuloma inguinale first was described by McLeod in 1882, and *C. granulomatis* was discovered by Donovan in 1905. This disease has been known through the years by many different names, the most common names being granuloma inguinale, Donovanosis, and granuloma venereum.[10]

THE ORGANISM

C. granulomatis is an encapsulated gram-negative rod, measuring 1.5 × 0.7 μm. Some of its characteristics resemble those of *Klebsiella*. However, the biochemical and bacteriologic characteristics of the organism have not been identified.[10]

Study of the organism reveals a complex cell envelope. In addition to having regular bacterial structures, such as mesosome, ribosomes, and nuclear material, the cytoplasm contains electron-dense polar material. The capsule contains homogeneous material of varying density and develops with maturity. Extending from the cell wall are small filamentous projections that are the size of pili. The origins of these projections are endogenous to the cell wall. The organisms are enclosed mainly in large histiocytic cells and occasionally in polymorphonuclear cells and plasma cells. They multiply intracellularly to about 30 in number and eventually cause cell rupture.[2, 10]

EPIDEMIOLOGY

Granuloma inguinale occurs predominantly in young adults and adults. It is a cause of genital ulcerative disease in tropical and subtropical regions of the world. As with all genital ulcerative diseases, granuloma inguinale has been given greater attention as a risk factor for HIV infection.[18] In South Africa, the prevalence of granuloma inguinale among patients with genital ulcer disease is reported to be approximately 10 per cent.[16]

Granuloma inguinale is rare in children. In the early 1950s, 4 per cent of 1- to 4-year-old children in a New Guinea population were found to have granuloma inguinale. The mode of transmission of the disease was thought to be from children sitting on the laps of infected adults.[10]

Granuloma inguinale has been reported since the early 1990s as endemic in South Africa, Papua New Guinea, and India and among the Aboriginal community in Australia.[23] A resurgence of the disease was reported in the late 1980s in Durban, South Africa. The Durban Health Department in South Africa identified an initial peak in males between 1969 and 1974, and a second peak of 313 cases was recorded in 1988.[20]

Granuloma inguinale is not common in the United States today. Until 1952, more than a thousand cases a year were reported to the Centers for Disease Control and Prevention. Since 1952, there has been a rapid decline in the prevalence of this disease; between 1971 and 1981, 50 to 90 cases a year were reported. Except for an isolated surge of 97 cases in 1990, fewer than 50 cases a year have been reported since 1982. In 1993, 19 cases were reported, 15 male and 4 female.[4] Granuloma inguinale was reported in a white adolescent female in California in 1985.[8] In 1991, an adult male with testicular carcinoma was diagnosed with nongenital granuloma inguinale in Texas.[14] In 1992, three unrelated cases of granuloma inguinale, seen within a period of a few weeks, were reported in Toronto; two were reported in immigrants and one in a native-born Canadian. The first patient was a recent immigrant from El Salvador, and the second patient had immigrated several years previously and had had sexual activity with a recently immigrated Jamaican. The sexual partner of the third case had come from Turkey.[9] Although the prevalence of the disease is low, it is expected to be seen in North America and Europe as a result of international travel and immigration.

Granuloma inguinale is more common in males than in females. During 1988 in Durban, the male-to-female ratio was found to be 3.2:1. However, among adolescents in the same city, the disease was more common in females than males at a ratio of 1:2. Among infected males, 22 per cent were 16 to 19 years of age, and among infected females, 44 per cent were 16 to 19 years of age. This probably is a reflection of sexual activity between adolescent females and adult males.[21]

Granuloma inguinale generally is considered a sexually transmitted disease. The risk factors and mode of transmission of the disease are not clear. In many cases, granuloma inguinale cannot be detected in sexual partners of infected persons. Nevertheless, a number of studies have reported the disease in 12 to 50 per cent of marital or steady sexual partners.[10] Anal intercourse also has been associated with rectal and penile lesions of granuloma inguinale.[12] O'Farrell and associates[19] studied the patterns of sexual behavior in men and women with genital ulcer disease and found that patients with granuloma inguinale and secondary syphilis were more likely than patients with other genital ulcer diseases to have had sexual intercourse despite the presence of ulcers. Studies reported from India and South Africa have noted a preponderance of granuloma inguinale cases among uncircumcised males with poor genital hygiene.[21]

Coexisting granuloma inguinale and other sexually transmitted diseases is common. Syphilis has been described in up to 23 per cent of patients with granuloma inguinale. In a recent report, HIV-1 antibodies were found in up to 8 per cent of males with granuloma inguinale.[21]

PATHOGENESIS AND PATHOLOGY

The primary lesion in granuloma inguinale is an indurated nodule that erodes through the skin and becomes a granulomatous heaped ulcer. Adjacent lesions form and eventually coalesce, especially in the perineal area. Secondary infection of lesions may occur, aggravating tissue destruction and scarring. *C. granulomatis* organisms invade the mononuclear endothelial cells. Extensive acanthosis and dense dermal infiltrates of mainly plasma cells and histiocytes have been observed in the indurated nodules. Polymorphonuclear cell infiltration also occurs, but lymphocytes are rare when secondary infection occurs. The pathognomonic feature of granuloma inguinale is a large, infected mononuclear cell, 25 to 90 μm in diameter, containing many intracytoplasmic cysts filled with deep-staining Donovan bodies. Metastatic spread to bones, joints, liver, and lymphatics occasionally occurs.[10]

A possible link between HLAB57 and granuloma inguinale infection may exist; class I, class II, and DQ antigens have been detected in genital ulcers of granuloma inguinale.[17] Circulating lymphocytes and tissue-level lymphocyte subpopulations in granuloma inguinale have been studied.[25, 26] T-lymphocyte and B-lymphocyte infiltrations in the tissues are almost identical, without any significant difference in ulcerogranulomatous and hypertrophic variants. Both total leukocyte and absolute lymphocyte counts are increased in the ulcerogranulomatous variant of granuloma inguinale. Total T lymphocytes; the CD4, CD8, and CD22 levels; and the CD4/CD8 ratio all are increased significantly in the ulcerogranulomatous variant. In contrast, the hypertrophic variant causes a significant elevation only in the CD4/CD8 ratio. This suggests a greater cell-mediated immune response in the ulcerogranulomatous variant of granuloma inguinale and is consistent with the paucity of Donovan bodies in smears obtained from patients with the ulcerogranulomatous variant of granuloma inguinale.[25, 26]

CLINICAL MANIFESTATIONS

The incubation period of granuloma inguinale usually is less than 2 weeks but may be as long as 3 months. The disease begins as one or more subcutaneous nodules that erode through the skin to produce clean, beefy-red, granulomatous ulcers. The lesions are defined sharply, and are painless. The ulcers feel hard when palpated. The disease is characterized by large genital ulcers that bleed easily. When left untreated at this early stage, the disease progresses, causing extensive mutilating lesions.[10] (See Chapter 49.)

The morphology of the cutaneous lesions of granuloma inguinale can vary, depending on the stage of the disease. The exuberant or hypertrophic stage appears before secondary infection develops. It consists of large, vegetating masses, with overgrowth of granulation tissue, usually in the perianal region. The ulcerative stage is accompanied by secondary infection. In this stage, large, spreading, shallow, necrotic ulcers with a foul odor may be noted. The cicatricial stage results after prolonged healing and is characterized by fibrosis, scarring, depigmentation, keloid formation, elephantiasis, and stenosis of the vagina, urethra, and anus. Among patients in Durban, ulcerogranulomatous lesions were far more common than hypertrophic and necrotic lesions. Although lymphadenopathy is unusual in granuloma inguinale, pseudobuboes and pseudoelephantiasis may be seen. Pseudobuboes are the result of deep, inguinal granulomas; pseudoelephantiasis is caused by cutaneous extension of lesions and inflammation.[6, 10, 21]

The genitalia are involved in 90 per cent of cases, the inguinal region in 10 per cent, the anal region in 5 to 10 per cent, and extragenital sites in 1 to 5 per cent. Primary lesions of the mouth, axillae, and lower abdomen have been reported.[10, 14] In males, lesions usually occur on the prepuce. They also can occur on the coronal sulcus and frenulum of the penis. As ulcers enlarge, they can be mutilating, causing urethral stenosis. The most common clinical presentation in pregnant and nonpregnant women is vulvar ulcerations. Genital tract bleeding is the next most common presentation in nonpregnant women.[1, 10, 21] Multiple sites of genital ulceration (vulva, vagina, and cervix) have been noted only in nonpregnant women.

Hematogenous spread to the head, liver, spleen, thorax, and bones can occur. These distant sites usually are associated with the primary lesions in the genital area.[10] Lesions in the oral cavity were described recently after apparently successful treatment of genital lesions.[5]

Misdiagnosis of granuloma inguinale can occur in areas where this disease is not endemic. In endemic areas, unusual presentations of granuloma inguinale may cause confusion with a wide variety of diseases. The differential diagnosis includes carcinoma, secondary syphilis, and necrotic ulcerations of amebiasis. Secondary infection can confuse the diagnosis as well.[10]

DIAGNOSIS

Successful isolation of *C. granulomatis* rarely has proved feasible. Reliable culture techniques are not yet available. Culture of the organism in the chicken embryonic yolk sac has been reported but is unsuccessful on artificial media. Isolation of the organism is hampered by the presence of innumerable bacterial contaminants and by the relatively poor characterization of *C. granulomatis*.[11]

Granuloma inguinale generally is diagnosed on clinical grounds. The accuracy of a clinical diagnosis of granuloma inguinale can be as high as 63 per cent in males and 83 per cent in females. Compared with other genital ulcers, the ulcers are larger in granuloma inguinale, are painless, bleed easily to touch, and generally are not associated with inguinal lymphadenopathy.[22]

The diagnosis of granuloma inguinale can be confirmed by identification of Donovan bodies on a stained crush specimen from the lesion (see Fig. 49–23). Appropriately stained specimens from active lesions remain the most reliable diagnostic tests. Light-microscopic examination of biopsy specimens that have been fixed in formalin and embedded in wax is less reliable. Donovan bodies rarely are seen by this method. The organisms also may be identified by electron microscopy, but the appearance of the organisms is not specific enough to allow definitive diagnosis by this method.[10, 22]

Stains used to identify Donovan bodies are Wright-Giemsa blue-black stain or Warthin-Starry silvery stain. Sections that are formalin-fixed or stained with hematoxylin and eosin are less useful for detecting Donovan bodies. The most recently described technique is a "quick" test. Specimens are obtained from friable tissue with cotton swabs, and a 1-minute rapid differentiation stain of eosin and thiazine dyes called RapiDiff stain is applied. This quick test may identify Donovan bodies in only 38 per cent of cases.[10, 11, 15]

To ensure success in identification of Donovan bodies, one must pay particular attention to the technique of obtaining a smear. A thorough search of the specimen by someone familiar with the tissue appearance of Donovan bodies is of paramount importance. Tissue for a smear or crush specimen should be obtained from the advancing edge of the ulceration using a forceps, scissors, curette, scalpel, or punch biopsy. A crush preparation minimizes the amount of debris and other organisms present on superficial layers. Preparations should be made immediately using moist tissue because drying leads to rupture of parasitized histiocytes. When *C. granulomatis* organisms are likely to be scarce or when smear or crush specimens are likely to fail, one should consider a biopsy of the lesion. Therefore, a biopsy specimen stained preferably with Giemsa or silver is recommended in very early, very sclerotic, or heavily superinfected specimens.[10, 11, 15]

Donovan bodies have been identified on Papanicolaou smears from the cervix.[3] Serologic and skin tests for granuloma inguinale are highly sensitive but not specific. More recently, a serologic test using indirect immunofluorescence technique was evaluated. The sera were tested either unabsorbed or after absorption with whole *Klebsiella pneumoniae* bacteria from patients with proven granuloma inguinale and controls. The test was found to have a sensitivity of 100 per cent, a specificity of 98 per cent, a positive predictive value of 89 per cent, and a negative predictive value of 100 per cent in diagnosing granuloma inguinale. In the absence of culture methods for *C. granulomatis*, this test may prove helpful in the diagnosis of individual cases and epidemiologic studies of granuloma inguinale in endemic areas.[7]

TREATMENT

Antibiotics with good activity against *C. granulomatis* are those effective in the therapy of gram-negative bacilli or those whose lipid solubility ensures good intracellular penetration. These include tetracyclines, erythromycin, co-trimoxazole, streptomycin, and chloramphenicol. Good results also have been reported with norfloxacin and thiamphenicol.[10, 24] In adolescents and adults, doxycycline and tetracycline are the antibiotics used most frequently. Doxycycline is provided in a dose of 100 mg twice a day, or tetracycline (500 mg orally) is provided four times a day until the lesions have healed completely (usually 3 weeks). Trimethoprim-sulfamethoxazole, 160/800 mg orally twice a day, or norfloxacin, 400 mg orally twice a day for 7 to 10 days, or erythromycin, 500 mg four times a day for 2 to 3 weeks, is an alternative treatment. Resistance to tetracycline has been encountered.[10] Children younger than 9 years of age can be treated with trimethoprim-sulfamethoxazole (10 mg/kg/day trimethoprim) or erythromycin (30 to 50 mg/kg/day).

Clinical response to antibiotics should be noted within a week of treatment; the lesions should become paler and less friable. After a week of treatment, the lesions become smaller; total healing of the area takes 3 to 5 weeks. Relapse occurs in about 10 per cent of cases, especially if the antibiotic is discontinued before the primary lesion has healed completely. Donovan bodies may reappear within 7 to 10 days.[10] Treatment can fail with coexisting HIV infection.

Merianos and associates[13] reported the possible effectiveness of ceftriaxone for chronic, recurrent granuloma inguinale. Patients in this study had been suffering from the disease for 1 to 5 years and had received 4 to 19 courses of antibiotics. A single daily, intramuscular injection of 1 g of ceftriaxone diluted in 2 mL of 1 per cent lidocaine was administered for 7 to 26 days. Clinical improvement was dramatic in most lesions, with a third of patients recovering completely without a recurrence after receiving daily doses of ceftriaxone for 7 to 10 days. Mild recurrences responded to additional ceftriaxone or short courses of oral antibiotics.[13] Vulvectomy is reserved for cases that have not responded to antibiotic treatment or for cases with severe vulvar elephantiasis.[6]

PROGNOSIS

Healing is complete in patients who seek treatment early in the course of the disease and comply with their medication and follow-up. O'Farrell[21] found complete healing of lesions in 24 per cent of patients who complied with follow-up. Complications of granuloma inguinale include pseudoelephantiasis, urethral stricture, and pelvic abscess, which may require surgery. Another complication is the acquisition of HIV infection and granuloma inguinale, especially when patients with ulcerations left untreated for a prolonged period have sexual contact with an HIV-positive partner.[10, 21]

The severe mutilating complications of granuloma inguinale primarily are a result of delayed treatment. In Durban, South Africa, almost half of the males had ulcerations for 1 to 6 months prior to presentation, and 16 per cent had ulcerations for 1 to 3 weeks. In contrast, approximately 25 per cent of females had ulcerations for 1 to 6 months and 50 per cent had ulcerations for 1 to 3 weeks.[21] Delayed medical attention may be related to limited education, ignorance of sexually transmitted diseases, absence of suitable medical facilities, or embarrassment in seeking treatment because of extensive genital lesions.

PREVENTION

Sexual partners of persons diagnosed with the disease should be traced, examined, and treated. Treatment of granuloma inguinale when the nodule first appears is associated with a benign course. Thus, community-based eradication that targets males with granuloma inguinale in endemic areas should be implemented. Programs should be aimed at identification of lesions, provision of early treatment, and prevention of severe complications. Teaching the importance of personal genital hygiene, such as instruction on simple retraction of the foreskin in the male and cleansing the penis with soap and water, also is effective.[10, 21]

References

1. Bassa, A. G., Hoosen A. A., Moodley, J., et al.: Granuloma inguinale (donovanosis) in women: An analysis of 61 cases from Durban, South Africa. Sex. Transm. Dis. *20*:164–167, 1993.
2. Chandra, M., and Jain, A. K.: Fine structure of *Calymmatous bacterium granulomatis* with particular reference to the surface structure. Ind. J. Med. Res. *93*:225–231, 1991.
3. DeBoer, A., DeBoer, F., and Van Der Merwe, J.: Cytologic identification of Donovan bodies in granuloma inguinale. Acta Cytol. *28*:126–128, 1984.
4. Division of STD/HIV Prevention: Sexually Transmitted Disease Surveillance, 1993. U.S. Department of Health and Human Services, Public Health Service. Atlanta, Centers for Disease Control and Prevention 1994, pp. 55–57.

5. Doddridge, M., and Muirhead, R.: Donovanosis of the oral cavity: Case report. Aust. Dental J. *39*:203–205, 1994.
6. Faro, S.: Lymphogranuloma venereum, chancroid, and granuloma inguinale. Obstet. Gynecol. Clin. North Am. *16*:517–530, 1989.
7. Freinkel, A. L., Dangor, Y., Koornhof, H. J., et al.: A serological test for granuloma inguinale. Genitourin. Med. *68*:269–272, 1992.
8. Growden, W. A., Lebherz, T. B., Moore, J. G., et al.: Granuloma inguinale in a white teenager: A diagnosis easily forgotten, poorly pursued. West. J. Med. *143*:105–108, 1985.
9. Hacker, P., Fisher, B. K., Dekoven, J., et al.: Granuloma inguinale: Three cases diagnosed in Toronto, Canada. Int. J. Dermatol. *31*:696–699, 1992.
10. Hart, G.: Donovanosis. *In* Holmes, K. K., Mardh, P. A., Sparling, P. E., et al. (eds.): Sexually Transmitted Disease. New York, McGraw-Hill, 1990, pp. 273–277.
11. Joseph A. K., and Rosen, T.: Laboratory techniques used in the diagnosis of chancroid, granuloma inguinale and lymphogranuloma venereum. Dermatol. Clin. *12*:1–8, 1994.
12. Marmell, M.: Donovanosis of the anus in the male: An epidemiologic consideration. Br. J. Vener. Dis. *34*:213–218, 1958.
13. Merianos, A., Gilles, M., and Chuah, J.: Ceftriaxone in the treatment of chronic donovanosis in central Australia. Genitourin. Med. *70*:84–89, 1994.
14. Morris, L. F., Cohen, P. R., and Dodd, L. G.: Nongenital granuloma inguinale in an oncology patient. Am. J. Clin. Oncol. *17*:456–460, 1994.
15. O'Farrell, N., Hoosen, A. A., Coetzee, K. D., et al.: A rapid stain for the diagnosis of granuloma inguinale. Genitourin. Med. *66*:200–201, 1990.
16. O'Farrell, N., Hoosen A. A., Coetzee, K. D., et al.: Genital ulcer disease in men in Durban, South Africa. Genitourin. Med. *67*:327–330, 1991.
17. O'Farrell, N., and Hammond, M.: HLA antigens in donovanosis (granuloma inguinale). Genitourin. Med. *67*:400–402, 1991.
18. O'Farrell, N., Windsor, I., and Becker, P.: HIV-1 infection among heterosexual attenders at a sexually transmitted diseases clinic in Durban. South Afr. J. *80*:17–20, 1991.
19. O'Farrell, N., Hoosen, A. A., Coetzee, K. D., et al.: Sexual behavior in Zulu men and women with genital ulcer disease. Genitourin. Med. *68*:245–248, 1992.
20. O'Farrell, N.: Trends in reported cases of donovanosis in Durban, South Africa. Genitourin. Med. *68*:366–369, 1992.
21. O'Farrell, N.: Clinico-epidemiological study of donovanosis in Durban, South Africa. Genitourin. Med. *69*:108–111, 1993.
22. O'Farrell, N., Hoosen, A. A., Coetzee, K. D., et al.: Genital ulcer disease: Accuracy of clinical diagnosis and strategies to improve control in Durban, South Africa. Genitourin. Med. *70*:7–11, 1994.
23. O'Farrell, N.: Global eradication of donovanosis: An opportunity for limiting the spread of HIV-1 infection. Genitourin. Med. *71*:27–31, 1995.
24. Richens, J.: The diagnosis and treatment of donovanosis (granuloma inguinale). Genitourin. Med. *67*:441–452, 1991.
25. Sehgal, V. N., Sharma, H. K., and Sharma, V. K.: Characterization of circulating lymphocytes by monoclonal antibodies in donovanosis. J. Dermatol. *18*:181–183, 1991.
26. Sehgal, V. N., Gupta, M. M., and Jain, V. K.: Tissue level lymphocyte subpopulations in donovanosis. Int. J. Dermatol. *30*:857–859, 1991.

136

CAMPYLOBACTER JEJUNI

Gloria Heresi and Thomas G. Cleary

Campylobacter jejuni is a frequent cause of enteritis and less often of extraintestinal infection in humans. Since its first recognition as a common human pathogen in the 1970s, there has been a steady increase in the appreciation of this agent's importance as a cause of disease. *C. jejuni* now is thought to be the most frequent bacterial cause of human enteritis in the United States.[4, 141]

HISTORY

The first recognition of pathologic consequences of infection with members of the group of bacteria that includes *C. jejuni* came in 1909 from studies of abortions in sheep.[92] In 1947, the sheep abortion–associated organism, *Vibrio fetus*, was isolated from a culture of blood of a pregnant woman who had an influenza-like illness and delivered a stillborn infant with a necrotic infarcted placenta.[159] In 1957, King[81, 82] hypothesized that *V. fetus*–related organisms might be associated with human enteric disease. Butzler and colleagues,[21] in 1972, showed that bacteria similar to *V. fetus* were in stools of children with diarrhea. This observation was confirmed rapidly and repeatedly.[12, 24, 48, 134, 140] Major differences in biochemical activities, growth characteristics, and DNA base nucleotide content between true vibrios and *V. fetus* led to the establishment of the new genus *Campylobacter*.[158]

THE ORGANISM

C. jejuni is a gram-negative rod that may vary in width from 0.2 to 0.9 μm and in length from 0.5 to 5.0 μm.[154] The rods may be short and S-shaped or longer spirals (Fig. 136–1). *C. jejuni* possesses a lipopolysaccharide endotoxin[121] and usually is motile due to either a single polar flagellum (monotrichous) or two flagella, one at each end of the rod (amphitrichous); nonmotile variants exist, and spores are not formed. Organisms obtained from stressed cultures may be coccoid or spherical. *C. jejuni* is a member of the family Campylobacteraceae, which contains two closely related genera, *Campylobacter* and *Arcobacter*.[153, 154] There currently are 18 species and subspecies within the genus *Campylobacter*. The species *C. jejuni* has two subspecies: *C. jejuni jejuni* and *C. jejuni doylei*. *C. jejuni doylei* can be differentiated from *C. jejuni jejuni* by the former's failure to grow at 42° C, lack of nitrate reduction,

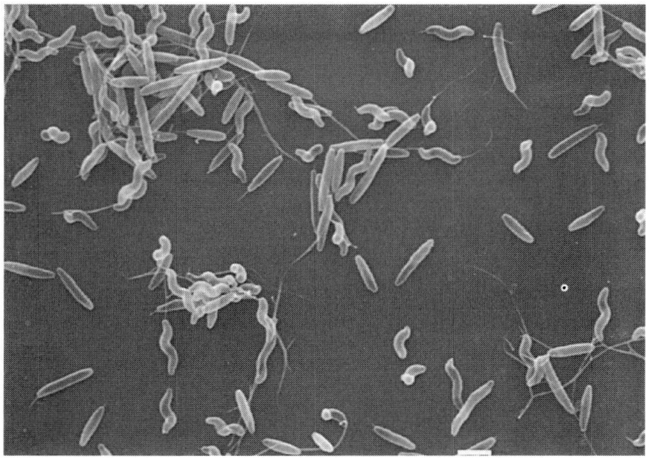

FIGURE 136–1. *Scanning electron microscopy of* Campylobacter jejuni *strain JM 001. The bar = 1 μm. (Courtesy of Dr. S. Baqar, Naval Medical Research Unit.)*

TABLE 136–1. Illustrative Studies of Isolation of *Campylobacter jejuni* from Environmental Sources

Sample		Location (Reference)	Sample Size	Positive*
Chicken	Processing plants, shops	Japan[149]	156	67.9
	Flocks on farms	England[67]	49	76.0
	Giblets	Egypt[80]	50	23.5
	Eggs from 23 farms	U.S.[8]	276	0.0
	Live birds	U.S.[8]	10	90
Duck	Giblets	Egypt[80]	50	19.0
	At reservoir	U.S.[102]	113	73.0
Goose	At reservoir	U.S.[102]	94	5.0
Turkey	Giblets	Egypt[80]	50	14.5
Squab	Giblets	Egypt[80]	50	4.0
Crane	At reservoir	U.S.[102]	91	81.0
Pig	Pork at processing plants, shops	Japan[149]	94	2.1
Cow	Beef in processing plants, shops	Japan[149]	52	0.0
	Rectal swabs	U.K.[66]	668	72.0
	Farms	Canada[160]	78	13.0
	Milk cows	U.S.[36]	78	68.0
	Milk, bulk tanks	U.S.[36]	108	0.9
Goat	Rectal swabs	Ghana[1]	72	33.3
Sheep	Rectal swabs	Ghana[1]	13	23.0
Cat	Domestic, rectal swab	U.S.[47]	430	1.0
	Zoo, rectal swab, (species-positive)	U.S.[47]	15	6.7
Monkey	Stool	U.S.[97]	50	77.0
	Stool	Indonesia[97]	50	36.0

*Per cent positive. In instances in which studies reported ranges of per cent positive, the highest rate is recorded.

and sensitivity to cephalothin. *C. jejuni* is differentiated routinely from *C. coli* by the capacity of *C. jejuni* to hydrolyze hippurate. Hippurate-negative *C. jejuni* exist,[152] but these are infrequent (5 per cent). Other pathogenic *Campylobacter*, including *C. fetus* and *C. pylori* (which has been reclassified as *Helicobacter pylori)*, are addressed in other chapters. The spectrum of disease recognized as caused by *C. jejuni*, other *Campylobacter* organisms, and related organisms is expanding.[4]

EPIDEMIOLOGY

Human infection with *C. jejuni* occurs worldwide. *C. jejuni* persists in zoonotic niches (Table 136–1), and most human infections are thought to come from these zoonotic reservoirs. *C. jejuni* is a common commensal of the gastrointestinal tract of cattle, pigs, dogs, cats, and most birds used as human food.[15, 135] *C. jejuni* infection in the United States peaks in late summer and early fall (Fig. 136–2). In subtropical areas, the peak incidence of *C. jejuni* isolation often is associated with the rainy season. In tropical climates, rates of isolation are similar year-round. Studies in volunteers have shown an incubation period of 3 days.[11] Fecal shedding of *C. jejuni* may last a median of 2 to 3 weeks, with a range of 3 days to several months.[24, 78, 103] Studies of *C. jejuni* infections in adult volunteers show the infectious dose to be as low as 500 colony-forming units.[11]

Data on the distribution of *C. jejuni* infections within populations have been interpreted as showing a linkage to the level of industrialization. In industrialized countries, *C. jejuni* infection often is found in children and adults with enteritis and seldom isolated from healthy individuals.[141] In less industrialized areas, *C. jejuni* frequently is isolated from children, even in the absence of enteritis. However, clear exam-

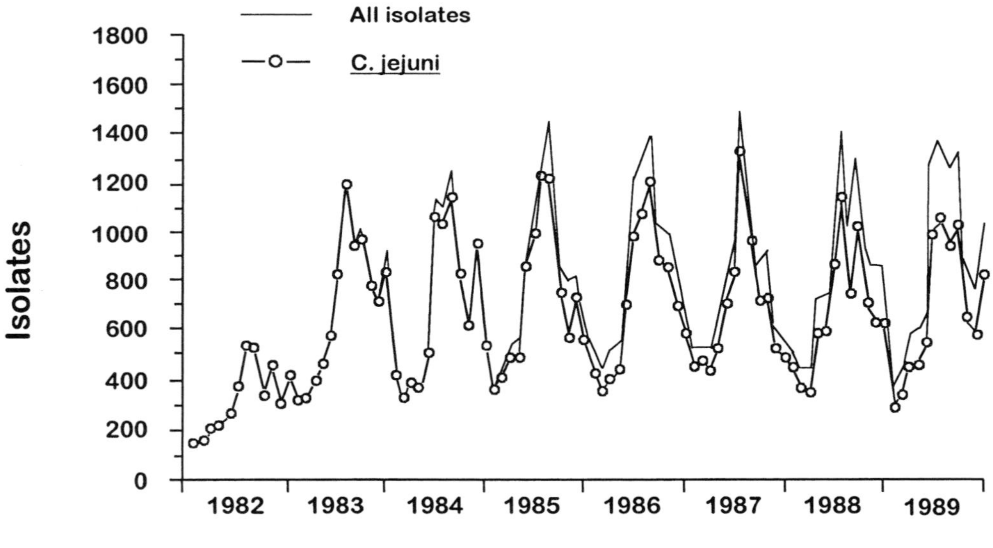

FIGURE 136–2. *Reported human* Campylobacter *isolates by month in the United States, 1982–1989. (From Tauxe, R. V.: Epidemiology of* Campylobacter jejuni *infections in the United States and other industrialized countries.* In *Nachamkin, I., Blaser, M. J., and Tompkins, L. S. (eds.):* Campylobacter jejuni: *Current Strategy and Future Trends. Washington, D.C., American Society for Microbiology, 1992, pp. 9–19.)*

TABLE 136–2. Selected Longitudinal Studies of Frequency of *Campylobacter jejuni* Infection in Children

Location (Reference)	No. of Children	Isolation of *C. jejuni* from Children*	
		With Diarrhea	*Without Diarrhea*
Guatemala[116]	321	12.1	8.1
Czechoslovakia[60]	5831	10.1	NR†
Mexico[24]	179	0.4	1.7
Thailand[144]	411	0.4	1.1

*Results are reported as per cent of stools positive.
†Not reported.

ples of "industrialized" epidemiology patterns exist in less industrialized countries and vice versa (Tables 136–2 and 136–3).

In industrialized countries, *C. jejuni* has been isolated from between 1 and 13 per cent of children with diarrhea, and the prevalence of infection in healthy individuals has been reported to be between 0 and 1.5 per cent.[12, 21, 118, 134, 141] A 5-year, laboratory-based national surveillance of *Campylobacter* species made in the United States between 1982 and 1986 showed an isolation rate of 5.5 per 100,000 person-years (with *C. jejuni* making up 99 per cent of the *Campylobacter* species isolates) (Fig. 136–3).[40] Population-based isolation rates of *Campylobacter* in the United States range from 28 to 1560 per 100,000 per year.[139, 140] Technical requirements for culturing *C. jejuni*, deficits in case reporting systems, and frequency of mild or asymptomatic *C. jejuni* infections probably combine to result in a gross underestimation of rates of infection.[4] Allos and Blaser[4] and Tauxe[141] have estimated that the actual incidence is about 1000 *C. jejuni* infections per 100,000 population per year. This rate would mean that about 1 per cent of the United States population would acquire *C. jejuni* infection per year. This rate is very close to the 1.1 per cent annual incidence of *Campylobacter* infections reported in Great Britain.[79] Population-based studies in England, the United States, and Sweden have shown a bimodal age distribution with a peak of illness in children younger than 5 years of age and a second peak in those 15 to 29 years of age.[120, 140] The highest isolation rate occurs in the first year of life (see Fig. 136–3).

In less industrialized regions, *Campylobacter* is found in association with childhood diarrhea in between 8 and 45 per cent of cases but is isolated at similar rates from healthy children[24, 28, 46]; the highest rates of *Campylobacter* isolation are in children younger than 5 years of age.[24] Cravioto and colleagues[28] showed that 75 per cent of *Campylobacter* infections occurring during the first year of life were asymptomatic.

Modes of transmission of *C. jejuni* differ between developed and developing countries. In industrialized regions, most sporadic cases occur because of handling, preparation, and consumption of contaminated raw or undercooked poultry.[12, 22, 30, 61, 129, 136, 140] Raw milk and contaminated water are less frequent sources.[63, 68, 95, 142, 161] Campylobacters are present ubiquitously in the human food chain (see Table 136–1). Poor kitchen hygiene also may play a role; the risk of infection has been shown to be associated inversely with the frequency of using soap to clean cutting boards.[140] Barbecues represent a special hazard because they permit easy transfer of bacteria from raw meats to hands and other foods and from these to the mouth.[24] Sporadic cases of *C. jejuni* infection are much more frequent than are outbreaks.

Between 1978 and 1986, 57 outbreaks of *Campylobacter* infection affecting 6441 persons were reported in the United States, including 45 food-borne outbreaks, 11 water-borne outbreaks, and 1 outbreak of unclear source in a tourist group. Of the 43 outbreaks in which a species was identified, 42 (97 per cent) were due to *C. jejuni*. A vehicle was implicated in 80 per cent of the food-borne outbreaks; 70 per cent were caused by consumption of raw milk, 8 per cent were associated with poultry, and the remaining 22 per cent were associated with other causes.[140] Most cases originating from cows appear to come from contamination of milk with bovine feces. However, direct excretion of *C. jejuni* in milk has been

TABLE 136–3. Selected Cross-Sectional Studies of Frequency of *Campylobacter jejuni* Infection in Children

Location	Frequency of Isolation of *C. jejuni* from Children [Per cent of stools with *C. jejuni* (number of children studied)]	
	With Diarrhea	*Without Diarrhea*
South Africa[18]	35.0 (78)	16.0 (63)
Zaire[32]	14.4 (416)	3.0 (200)
Rwanda[31]	9.3 (150)	0.0 (58)
Zaire[20]	8.6 (70)	0.0 (30)
Cameroon[83]	7.7 (272)	3.2 (157)
Bangladesh[56]	25.5 (102)	8.6 (93)
China[166]	18.7 (48)	8.6 (105)
China[35]	11.9 (303)	4.6 (953)
Kuwait[129]	7.0 (621)	0.0 (152)
India[99]	4.0 (607)	0.9 (529)
Saudi Arabia[26]	1.0 (7369)	0.1 (1130)
Belgium[21]	5.1 (800)	1.3 (1000)
Canada[103]	4.3 (1004)	0.0 (176)
Chile[42]	10.0 (299)	6.0 (304)

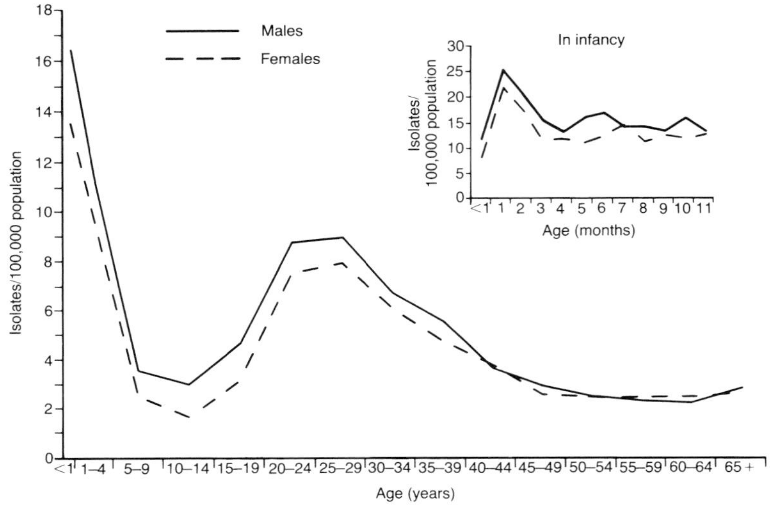

FIGURE 136–3. *Annual isolation rates of* Campylobacter, *by age and sex, United States, 1982 to 1986. (From Tauxe, R. V., Hargrett-Bean, N., Patton, C. M., et al.:* Campylobacter *isolates in the United States, 1982–1986. M. M. W. R. CDC Surveillance Summaries 37:1–13, 1988.)*

described[68, 100] and has been implicated as the source of an outbreak of disease in humans. Less frequent sources of infection include infected pets, such as cats, dogs, and birds.[132] Puppies seem a more frequent source of infection than older dogs.[150] Secondary person-to-person spread may occur where diapered children are present[109] and in the perinatal environment[157] but otherwise is infrequent. *C. jejuni* has been transmitted by transfusion.[110]

In developing countries, transmission is multifactorial. The most important are free-roaming poultry, toddlers, unsafe water supply, and lack of adequate excreta disposal. Chickens commonly are infected with *C. jejuni*[51] and often have free access to defecate in and outside the house. Toddlers have frequent contact with poultry feces, making the presence of live chickens in the house a prominent risk factor for *C. jejuni* infection. Personal and domestic hygiene education, such as penning chickens outside the house, preventing contact with their feces, and hand washing, probably would reduce transmission further.

PATHOLOGY

The majority of *C. jejuni* infections may not be associated with illness. When illness occurs, watery diarrhea, invasive enteritis, or systemic infection may result. The spectrum of pathology reflects this range of presentations. Acute watery diarrhea may occur in the absence of grossly visible pathology. Acute inflammation of the colon and rectum is the hallmark of *C. jejuni* invasive enteritis,[89] although hemorrhagic jejunitis and ileitis may occur.[39, 78, 82, 134] In those patients who have undergone proctoscopy, a normal mucosa is found in approximately 50 per cent; in the rest, mucosal edema, congestion, friability, and granularity are seen. The spectrum of histologic change ranges from minimal edema with acute and chronic inflammatory cells without vascular congestion to moderate inflammation and cryptitis to crypt abscess formation.[7] Acute appendicitis, mesenteric lymphadenitis, and ileocolitis have been reported in patients who have had appendectomies during *C. jejuni* infection.[13, 85]

PATHOGENESIS

The mechanisms by which *C. jejuni* causes diarrhea and dysentery are not well understood. Evidence consistent with the production of a heat-labile enterotoxin has been presented.[55, 71, 87, 121] However, this toxic activity is not found associated universally with isolates from individuals who have *C. jejuni* illness. Some strains produce a cytotoxin,[72, 88] but its relevance to disease is not established. Some *C. jejuni* can invade various cultured cell lines.[22, 40] Dogs,[115] rhesus monkeys,[43] rabbits,[137] mice[43] and hamsters[65] have been evaluated as models of *Campylobacter* enteritis. None faithfully reproduces the disease seen in humans. Recently, a mouse intranasal challenge model[9] has been developed for use in studies of *C. jejuni* invasiveness, and a ferret model[10] has been developed for studies of *C. jejuni*–induced diarrhea. It is not clear yet if results obtained from these newer models will yield information that correlates with disease in humans.

IMMUNITY

Evidence for protective immunity to *C. jejuni* comes mostly from studies of children in less developed countries. Such children have more frequent symptomatic infections at younger ages; with increasing age, the rate of symptomatic infection decreases.[14, 16, 17, 73–75, 90, 138, 144, 146, 162] The number of *C. jejuni* excreted per gram of stool of infected individuals also declines with increasing age,[146] as does the duration of excretion of the organism.[144] Breast feeding has been shown to protect from *C. jejuni* diarrhea.[122, 151] Further evidence of acquired immunity to *C. jejuni* comes from a study of infection in volunteers.[11] Adult volunteers who became ill after a first challenge were protected from illness after rechallenge with a homologous strain; those who were resistant to homologous rechallenge had anti–*C. jejuni* antibodies as a result of the first infection.[11] Further evidence of the importance of acquired immunity in protecting against *C. jejuni* infection is the prolonged, severe, and sometimes recurrent infections in immunodeficient patients.[91, 94, 108, 111] There is limited evidence relating the presence of specific antibodies and protection from disease. Naturally acquired *C. jejuni* infection leads to the generation of antibodies that recognize *C. jejuni* antigens, and in children in developing countries, titers of these antibodies increase with age while the rate of symptomatic infection decreases.[14, 17, 73, 90, 138, 146, 148, 162] The composite evidence convincingly argues for the existence of acquired protective immunity to *C. jejuni* disease and suggests that immunity to disease may not protect against asymptomatic colonization necessarily. The bacterial component against which the protective immune response is directed has not been proved.

Very little information is available on cellular immune responses to *C. jejuni*. Cellular responses might play important roles as helpers in antibody formation and in clearance of *C. jejuni* resident within eukaryotic cells.

A candidate oral vaccine consisting of a mixture of killed whole cells of *C. jejuni* in combination with heat-labile enterotoxin of *Escherichia coli* has been made. This vaccine was safe and induced both humoral and cellular anti–*C. jejuni* immune responses in monkeys.[9] Its efficacy remains to be determined. This prototype product is based on the successful cholera whole-cell recombinant B-subunit vaccine, which has proven efficacy in the prevention of cholera and enterotoxigenic *E. coli* disease.

CLINICAL MANIFESTATIONS

C. jejuni produces a spectrum of manifestations. The most common presentation is enteritis. Bacteremia, other systemic manifestations, and perinatal infections occur infrequently.

Enteritis

Children with *Campylobacter* enteritis may present with unformed stools, watery diarrhea, and/or inflammatory diarrhea.[12, 13, 24, 78, 103, 134] The latter can be so severe as to be misdiagnosed as inflammatory bowel disease.[134] Inflammatory diarrhea is more common in industrialized countries, and secretory watery diarrhea is more typical in underdeveloped areas.

The majority of enteric illnesses (60 to 70 per cent) subside within 7 days, although 20 to 30 per cent last for 2 weeks, and a few (5 to 10 per cent) may persist longer.[78, 103] In one-third to one-half of patients, the initial symptoms are periumbilical cramping, intense abdominal pain, malaise, myalgias, and headache. Acute abdomen or appendicitis may be suspected initially[25] because, occasionally, acute abdominal pain may be the only presenting symptom; pseudoappendicitis or mesenteric adenitis and terminal ileitis can be found.[107] The pain may be mild and intermittent for several weeks. Vomiting is common. Secretory diarrhea with 10 or more profuse watery stools per day may occur. Because this course is common in younger children, dehydration is a frequent outcome (10 per cent). Relapse of symptoms may occur.

The symptoms of inflammatory diarrhea are similar to those caused by *Shigella*, invasive *E. coli*, and *Salmonella* and are characterized by generalized malaise, fever, abdominal cramps, tenesmus, bloody stools, and the presence of fecal leukocytes on light microscopy.[89] Fever without other symptoms may occur and can be associated with febrile seizures.[165] Toxic megacolon with massive bleeding may occur.[53, 77] In neonates, blood-streaked formed stools or hematochezia may be associated with the isolation of *C. jejuni*.[53, 77] The abdomen is tender, especially in the right lower quadrant. Splenomegaly is rare.

Extraintestinal Infections

Bacteremia with *C. jejuni* is much less common than enteritis. Bacteremia was recognized first in malnourished children, patients with chronic illness or immunodeficiency, and at the extremes of age.[3, 54, 94] These findings led to the view that *C. jejuni* bacteremia was a disease of the relatively immunoincompetent. Recent data from Britain have shown that the majority of *C. jejuni* blood isolates actually are from healthy individuals who often have histories of recent gastrointestinal disease.[133] The average incidence of *Campylobacter* bacteremia for England and Wales is 1.5 per 1000 intestinal *Campylobacter* infections. The Centers for Disease Control and Prevention data report that only 0.4 per cent of *C. jejuni* isolates in the United States are from blood cultures.[140] Most *C. jejuni* strains are susceptible to killing by serum, perhaps explaining the transient nature of bacteremia and its tendency to resolve without specific therapy.

The main cause of the increased recognition of extraintestinal *Campylobacter* infections appears to be the growing application of appropriate microbiologic culture methods. It is likely that the incidence of *C. jejuni* bacteremia is underestimated. Typically, blood cultures are not taken from individuals presenting with the primary complaint of diarrhea. Rarely, cholecystitis, urinary tract infection,[29] pancreatitis,[45] and meningitis[148] are results of *Campylobacter* infection.

Perinatal Infections

Abortion or stillbirth, premature labor, neonatal sepsis, and meningitis due to *C. jejuni* rarely have been described.[113] *Campylobacter*-associated second-trimester abortion generally is preceded by a mild gastroenteritis.[98, 130] The placenta may have areas of necrosis, infarction, microabscesses, and inflammation. The most likely route of placental/fetal infection is through the blood stream, although a case with a possible ascending spread has been reported.[33] Infected infants often are premature. Illness in neonates generally is mild or asymptomatic. Symptomatic gastroenteritis and asymptomatic bloody diarrhea due to *C. jejuni* have been reported in newborn infants,[19, 103] although bacteremia and meningitis may occur.[50, 113, 148] The source of the organism in these cases generally has been the mother, who may be symptomatic or asymptomatic at the time of delivery.[19, 157]

Immunoreactive Complications

An episode of *C. jejuni* infection may be followed by immunoreactive complications, such as Guillain-Barré syndrome,[57, 58, 76, 96, 119] Reiter syndrome,[70, 112, 114] reactive arthritis,[37, 127] and erythema nodosum.

In the last decade, reports of Guillain-Barré syndrome occurring after well-documented, culture-proven *C. jejuni* infection have accumulated.[57, 58, 64, 76, 96] A preceding *C. jejuni* infection has been documented by serologic methods or stool culture in 12 to 60 per cent of Guillain-Barré cases.[58] Certain serotypes of *C. jejuni* are associated more frequently with subsequent Guillain-Barré syndrome. Kuroki and colleagues[84] studied 46 cases of Guillain-Barré in Japan with isolation of *C. jejuni* from 14, 11 of which were Penner serogroup 19[84]; the frequency of that serotype among *C. jejuni* isolates was less than 2 per cent. The possible link between preceding *C. jejuni* infection and Guillain-Barré syndrome is cross-reactivity between components shared by nerve and microbe.[57, 58] A positive correlation of serologic evidence of *C. jejuni* and the presence of antibodies to GM1 has been described[52]; lipopolysaccharide extracted from *C. jejuni* was found to have core oligosaccharide resembling human ganglioside GM1.[6]

Recent studies have shown an association of *C. jejuni* with acute motor axonal neuropathy, an illness similar to Guillain-Barré syndrome that occurs primarily in northern China[93]; 76 per cent of acute motor axonal neuropathy patients and 42 per cent of patients with acute inflammatory demyelinization polyneuropathy were positive for anti–*C. jejuni* antibodies.[59] A few cases of Miller-Fisher syndrome, a polyneuritis variant characterized by ophthalmoplegia, areflexia, and cerebellar ataxia, have been reported.[69, 167]

Reactive arthritis may be associated with *Campylobacter* enteritis, especially in adults with HLA-B27.[37, 127] Arthritis starts a few days to several weeks after the episode of diarrhea. Joint involvement can be monoarticular or multiple, as well as migratory, and it can affect large and small joints. Synovial fluid is sterile, and fever and leukocytosis are absent. Duration ranges from 1 week to several months. The course is self-limited, and the prognosis is good.

Severe, persistent, and relapsing *C. jejuni* infections have been reported in patients with immune deficiencies, including congenital and acquired hypogammaglobulinemia, and malnutrition.[3, 62, 94] In patients with AIDS, an increased frequency and severity of *C. jejuni* infection has been reported; severity correlates inversely with CD4 count.[86, 108, 111]

DIAGNOSIS

Presenting characteristics of *C. jejuni* enteritis are not sufficiently unique to allow diagnosis on clinical grounds. Differential diagnoses should include *Shigella*, *Salmonella*, invasive *E. coli*, *E. coli* O157:H7, *Yersinia enterocolitica*, *Aeromonas* species, and *Vibrio parahaemolyticus* infections and amebiasis. Consideration should be given to pseudomembranous colitis due to *Clostridium difficile* if the patient has been receiving antibiotic therapy. Fecal leukocytes are found in up to 75 per cent of cases of *Campylobacter* enteritis; gross or occult fecal blood is present in 50 per cent.[11, 12, 89] White blood cell counts usually are normal, although a shift to the left may occur. Mild elevations of alanine aminotransferase, alkaline phosphatase, and the sedimentation rate are observed in up to 25 per cent of patients.

Methods available for demonstration of *C. jejuni* include direct microscopy,[105, 106] bacteriologic culture, DNA probes,[147] polymerase chain reaction,[101] and serology.[4] DNA probes and polymerase chain reaction mainly are research tools. Serologic tests appear useful for epidemiologic investigations but are not recommended for routine diagnosis.

C. jejuni can be detected by darkfield and phase-contrast examination of fresh suspensions of stool. The distinguishing characteristic of *Campylobacter* is darting motility. Gram stain of stool showing *Vibrio* forms is said to be useful in making a presumptive diagnosis.[126] Indirect fluorescent-antibody test can be used for identification of *Campylobacter* on smears; however, standardized reagents for this procedure are not available from commercial sources.

Definitive diagnosis of *C. jejuni* infection requires the demonstration of *C. jejuni* in stool or in a tissue sample. Unfortunately, despite its frequency, not all laboratories culture for *C. jejuni*. Culture of *C. jejuni* from stool requires both special methods and special media. This can be accomplished using media that contain antibiotics,[38] (e.g., Butzler's, Skirrow's, CampyBAP), to which campylobacters are resistant. If culturing is to be done on medium free of antibiotics, diluted stool samples should be passed through a cellulose acetate membrane filter to reduce the numbers of other enteric microorganisms.[49] Inoculated plates should be incubated in 5 per cent oxygen and 10 per cent carbon dioxide at 42° C. It may take up to 72 hours for visible colonies to form. Identification of colonies as *C. jejuni/coli* is based on a Gram stain showing characteristic morphology and positive catalase and oxidase reactions. Hydrolysis of hippurate establishes an isolate as meeting the conventional inclusion criteria for *C. jejuni*. Routine media usually are adequate for isolation of *Campylobacter* from normally sterile body fluids and tissues.

TREATMENT

Most *C. jejuni* are susceptible to macrolides, quinolones, aminoglycosides, chloramphenicol, tetracycline, and clindamycin and resistant to cephalosporins, rifampin, penicillins, trimethoprim, and vancomycin.[131, 155] Patterns of antibiotic resistance in *C. jejuni* show regional differences; resistance is increasing with time (Table 136–4). Most patients with *C. jejuni* infection have mild symptoms and do not require antibiotic therapy. For these patients, oral rehydration and replacement of electrolytes are sufficient. Patients who may benefit from antibiotic therapy are those with fever, bloody stools, and symptoms of longer than a week's duration.[4] Erythromycin is considered the treatment of choice for *C. jejuni* diarrhea in those patients with proven infection who require antibiotic therapy.[5] The data on antibiotic treatment are controversial. Placebo-controlled studies of 5 days of erythromycin have shown no effect on the course of the disease.[5, 104, 163] In contrast, early erythromycin treatment of children with bloody diarrhea due to *Campylobacter* shortened both duration of diarrhea and fecal excretion of the microbe.[124]

The new macrolides, azithromycin and clarithromycin, may be as effective as erythromycin and have better tolerance. Quinolones do not modify the course of the disease but do shorten the duration of excretion of the organism. Quinolones have been advocated as a therapy for adult trav-

TABLE 136–4. Illustrative Studies of *Campylobacter jejuni* In Vitro and Antibiotic Resistance Patterns

Location	Publication Date	No. of Isolates Tested	Per cent of Isolates Resistant to				
			Erythromycin	*Ciprofloxacin*	*Tetracycline*	*Gentamicin*	*Ampicillin*
Spain[156]	1995	102	1.9	ND	22.8	0	11.0
Spain[125]	1994	230	2.3	28.5	ND	ND	ND
Nigeria[27]	1994	23	79.2	62.0	ND	0	87.5
Sweden[131]	1992	110	6.4	0.9	12.7	ND	20.9
Saudi Arabia[168]	1992	38	7.3	ND	32.7	0	ND
Spain[117]	1992	614	0.9–1.6	10.7	ND	0	ND
Japan[123]	1987	111	0	ND	55.0	0	ND
Thailand[143]	1987	43	53	ND	ND	ND	ND
Canada[145]	1986	382	0	ND	ND	0	22.0

ND, no data.

elers to regions where sulfamethoxazole-trimethoprim–resistant *Campylobacter* are prevalent because quinolones are effective in the treatment of both intestinal campylobacteriosis and shigellosis.[34] Ciprofloxacin and norfloxacin have been effective in the treatment of *Campylobacter* infection, but emergence of ciprofloxacin resistance soon after initiation of drug therapy has been reported.[2, 44, 164] In vitro studies suggest an increasing resistance to fluoroquinolones that may limit their use in the future.

All immunocompromised and bacteremic patients with *C. jejuni* infection should be treated with an appropriate antibiotic.[4] In *Campylobacter* bacteremia, gentamicin and/or imipenem therapy is recommended.[4]

References

1. Abrahams, C. A., Agbodaze, D., Nakano, T., et al.: Prevalence and antibiogram of *Campylobacter jejuni* in domestic animals in rural Ghana. Arch. Environ. Health *45*:59–62, 1990.
2. Adler-Mosca, H., Luthy-Hottenstein, J., Martinetti, L. G., et al.: Development of resistance to quinolones in five patients with campylobacteriosis treated with norfloxacin or ciprofloxacin. Eur. J. Clin. Microbiol. Infect. Dis. *10*:953, 1991.
3. Ahnen, D. J., and Brown, W. R.: *Campylobacter* enteritis in immune deficient patients. Ann. Intern. Med. *96*:187–188, 1982.
4. Allos, B. M., and Blaser, M. J.: *Campylobacter jejuni* and the expanding spectrum of related infections. Clin. Infect. Dis. *20*:1092–1099, 1995.
5. Anders, B. J., Lauer, B. A., Paisley, J. W., et al.: Double-blind placebo-controlled trial of erythromycin for treatment of *Campylobacter* enteritis. Lancet *1*:131–132, 1982.
6. Aspinall, G. O., Fujimoto, S., and McDonald, A. G.: Lipopolysaccharides from *Campylobacter jejuni* associated with Guillain-Barré syndrome patients mimic human gangliosides in structure. Infect. Immun. *62*:2122–2125, 1994.
7. Babakhani, F. K., Bradley, J. A., and Joens, L. A.: Newborn piglet model for campylobacteriosis. Infect. Immun. *61*:3466–3475, 1993.
8. Baker, R. C., Paredes, M. D., and Qureshi, R. A.: Prevalence of *Campylobacter jejuni* in eggs and poultry meat in New York State. Poultry Science *66*:766–770, 1987.
9. Baqar, S., Bourgeois, A. I., and Schultheiss, P. J., et al.: Safety and immunogenicity of a prototype oral whole-cell killed *Campylobacter* vaccine administered with a mucosal adjuvant in non-human primates. Vaccine *13*:22–28, 1995.
10. Bell, J. A., and Manning, D. D.: A domestic ferret model of immunity to *Campylobacter jejuni*-induced enteric disease. Infect. Immun. *58*:1848–1852, 1990.
11. Black, R. E., Levine, M. M., Clements, M. L., et al.: Experimental *Campylobacter jejuni* infection in humans. J. Infect. Dis. *157*:472–479, 1988.
12. Blaser, M. E., Berkowitz, I. D., LaForce, F. M., et al.: *Campylobacter* enteritis: Clinical and epidemiologic features. Ann. Intern. Med. *91*:179–185, 1979.
13. Blaser, M. J., Parsons, R. B., and Wang, W. L.: Acute colitis caused by *Campylobacter fetus* sp. *jejuni*. Gastroenterology *78*:448–453, 1980.
14. Blaser, M. J., Duncan, D. J., Osterholm, M. T., et al.: Serologic study of two clusters of infection due to *Campylobacter jejuni*. J. Infect. Dis. *147*:820–823, 1983.
15. Blaser, M. J., Taylor, D. N., and Feldman, R. A.: Epidemiology of *Campylobacter jejuni* infections. Epidemiol. Rev. *5*:157–176, 1983.
16. Blaser, M. J., and Duncan, D. J.: Human serum antibody response to *Campylobacter jejuni* infection as measured in an enzyme-linked immunosorbent assay. Infect. Immun. *44*:292–298, 1984.
17. Blaser, M. J., Taylor, D. N., and Echeverria, P.: Immune response to *Campylobacter jejuni* in a rural community in Thailand. J. Infect. Dis. *153*:249–254, 1986.
18. Bokkenheuser, V. D., Richardson, N. J., Bryner, J. H., et al.: Detection of enteric campylobacteriosis in children. J. Clin. Microbiol. *9*:227, 1979.
19. Buck, G. E., Kelly, M. T., Pichanick, A. M., et al.: *Campylobacter jejuni* in newborns: A cause of asymptomatic bloody diarrhea. Am. J. Dis. Child. *136*:744, 1982.
20. Butzler, J. P.: Related vibrios in Africa. Lancet *2*:858, 1973.
21. Butzler, J. P., Dekeyser, P., Detrain, M., et al.: Related *Vibrio* in stools. J. Pediatr. *82*:493–495, 1973.
22. Butzler, J. P., and Skirrow, M. B.: *Campylobacter* enteritis. Clin. Gastroenterol. *8*:737–765, 1979.
23. Butzler, J. P., and Oosterom, J.: *Campylobacter*: Pathogenicity and significance in foods. Int. J. Food Microbiol. *12*:1–8, 1991.
24. Calva, J. J., Ruiz-Palacios, G. M., Lopez-Vidal, A. B., et al.: Cohort study of intestinal infection with *Campylobacter* in Mexican children. Lancet *1*:503–506, 1988.
25. Chan, F. T., Stringel, G., and Mackenzie, A. M.: Isolation of *Campylobacter jejuni* from an appendix. J. Clin. Microbiol. *18*:422–424, 1983.
26. Chowdhury, M. N., and al-Eissa, Y. A.: *Campylobacter* gastroenteritis in children in Riyadh, Saudi Arabia. J. Trop. Pediatr. *38*:158–161, 1992.
27. Coker, A. O., and Adefeso, A. O.: The changing patterns of *Campylobacter jejuni/coli* in Lagos, Nigeria, after 10 years. East Afr. Med. J. *71*:437–440, 1994.
28. Cravioto, A., Reyes, R. E., Trujillo, F., et al.: Risk of diarrhea during the first year of life associated with initial and subsequent colonization by specific enteropathogens. Am. J. Epidemiol. *131*:1886–1904, 1979.
29. Davis, J. S., and Penfold, J. B.: *Campylobacter* urinary tract infection. Lancet *1*:1091–1092, 1979.
30. Deming, M. S., Tauxe, R. V., Blake, P. A., et al.: *Campylobacter* enteritis at a university: Transmission from eating chicken and from cats. Am. J. Epidemiol. *126*:526–534, 1987.
31. De Mol, P., and Bosmans, E.: *Campylobacter* enteritis in central Africa. Lancet *1*:604, 1978.
32. De Mol, P., Brasseur, D., and Lauwers, S.: *Campylobacter:* An important enteropathogen in a tropical area. Presented at the 20th Interscience Conference on Antimicrobial Agents and Chemotherapy, September 22–24, 1980, New Orleans. Washington, D.C., American Society for Microbiology, 1980.
33. Denton, K. J., and Clarke, T.: Role of *Campylobacter jejuni* as a placental pathogen. J. Clin. Pathol. *45*:171–172, 1992.
34. DuPont, H. L.: Use of quinolones in the treatment of gastrointestinal infections. Eur. J. Clin. Microbiol. Infect. Dis. *10*:325–329, 1991.
35. Desheng, L., Zhixin, C., and Boulun, W.: Age distribution of diarrhoeal and healthy children infected with *Campylobacter jejuni*. J. Trop. Med. Hyg. *95*:218–220, 1992.
36. Doyle, M. P., and Roman, D. J.: Prevalence and survival of *Campylobacter jejuni* in unpasteurized milk. Appl. Env. Microbiol. *44*:1154–1158, 1982.
37. Ebright, J. R., and Ryan, L. M.: Acute erosive reactive arthritis associated with *Campylobacter jejuni*–induced colitis. Am. J. Med. *76*:321–323, 1984.
38. Endtz, H. P., Ruijs, G. J., Zwinderman, A. H., et al.: Comparison of six media, including a semisolid agar, for the isolation of various *Campylobacter* species from stool specimens. J. Clin. Microbiol. *29*:1007–1010, 1991.
39. Evans, R. G., and Dadswell, J. V.: Human vibriosis. Br. Med. J. *3*:240, 1967.
40. Falkow, S.: Bacterial entry into eukaryotic cells. Cell *65*:1099–1102, 1991.
41. Field, L. H., Underwood, J. L., and Berry, L. J.: The role of gut flora and animal passage in the colonization of adult mice with *Campylobacter jejuni*. J. Med. Microbiol. *17*:59–66, 1984.
42. Figueroa, G., Galeno, H., Troncoso, M., et al.: Prospective study of *Campylobacter jejuni* infection in Chilean infants evaluated by culture and serology. J. Clin. Microbiol. *27*:1040–1044, 1989.
43. Fitzgeorge, R. B., Baskerville, A., and Lander, K. P.: Experimental infection of rhesus monkeys with a human strain of *Campylobacter jejuni*. J. Hyg. *86*:343–351, 1981.
44. Funke, G., Baumann, R., Penner, J. L., et al.: Development of resistance to macrolide antibiotics in an AIDS patient treated with clarithromycin for *Campylobacter jejuni* diarrhea. Eur. J. Clin. Microbiol. Infect. Dis. *13*:612, 1994.
45. Gallagher, P., Chadwick, P., Jones, D.M., et al.: Acute pancreatitis associated with *Campylobacter* infection. Br. J. Surg. *68*:383, 1981.
46. Georges-Courbot, M. C., Beraud-Cassel, A. M., Gouandjika, I., et al.: Prospective study of enteric *Campylobacter* infections in children from birth to 6 months in the Central African Republic. J. Clin. Microbiol. *25*:836–839, 1987.
47. Gifford, D. H., Shane, S. M., and Smith, R. E.: Prevalence of *Campylobacter jejuni* in *felidae* in Baton Rouge, Lousiana. Int. Zoonoses *12*:67–73, 1985.
48. Glass, R. I., Stoll, B. J., Huq, M. I., et al.: Epidemiologic and clinical features of endemic *Campylobacter jejuni* infection in Bangladesh. J. Infect. Dis. *148*:292–296, 1983.
49. Goossens, H., De Boeck, M., Coignau, H., et al.: Modified selective medium for isolation of *Campylobacter* spp. from feces: Comparison with Preston medium, a blood-free medium and a filtration system. J. Clin. Microbiol. *24*:840–843, 1986.
50. Goossens, H., Henocque, G., Kremp, L., et al.: Nosocomial outbreak of *Campylobacter jejuni* meningitis in newborn infants. Lancet *2*:146–149, 1986.
51. Grados, O., Bravo, N., Black, R. E., et al.: Paediatric *Campylobacter* diarrhea from household exposure to live chickens in Lima, Peru. Bull. World Health Org. *66*:369–374, 1988.
52. Gregson, N. A., Koblar, S., and Hughes, R. A.: Antibodies to gangliosides in Guillain-Barré syndrome: Specificity and relationship to clinical features. Q. J. Med. *86*:111–117, 1993.
53. Guandalini, S., Cucchiara, S., de Ritis, G., et al.: *Campylobacter* colitis in infants. J. Pediatr. *102*:72–74, 1983.
54. Guerrant, R. L., Lahita, R. G., Winn, W. C., Jr., et al.: Campylobacteriosis in man: Pathogenic mechanisms and review of 91 bloodstream infections. Am. J. Med. *65*:584–592, 1978.
55. Guerrant, R. L., Wanke, C. A., Pennie, R. A., et al.: Production of a unique cytotoxin by *Campylobacter jejuni*. Infect. Immun. *55*:2526–2530, 1987.
56. Haq, J. A., and Rahman, K. M.: *Campylobacter jejuni* as a cause of acute diarrhoea in children: A study at an urban hospital in Bangladesh. J. Trop. Med. Hyg. *94*:50–54, 1991.
57. Hartung, H. P., Pollard, J. D., Harvey, G. K., et al.: Immunopathogenesis

and treatment of the Guillain-Barré syndrome: Part I. Muscle Nerve *18*:137–153, 1995.
58. Hartung, H. P., Pollard, J. D., Harvey, G. K., et al.: Immunopathogenesis and treatment of the Guillain-Barré syndrome: Part II. Muscle Nerve *18*:154–164, 1995.
59. Ho, T. W., Mishu, B., Li, C. Y., et al.: Guillain-Barré syndrome in northern China: Relationship to *Campylobacter jejuni* infection and anti-glycolipid antibodies. Brain *118*:597–605, 1995.
60. Hofstetr, A., Dvorakova, A., Nikodymova, I., et al.: A 3-year follow-up study of the incidence of campylobacteriosis in a pediatric population. Ceskoslovenska Pediatrie *45*:651–654, 1990.
61. Hood, A. M., Pearson, A. D., and Shahamat, M.: The extent of surface contamination of retailed chickens with *Campylobacter jejuni* serogroups. Epidemiol. Infect. *100*:17–25, 1988.
62. Hossain, M.A., Kabir, I., Albert, M. J., et al.: *Campylobacter jejuni* bacteraemia in children with diarrhea in Bangladesh: Report of six cases. J. Diarrhoeal Dis. Res. *10*:101–104, 1992.
63. Hudson, P. J., Vogt, R. L., Brondum, B. J., et al.: Isolation of *Campylobacter jejuni* from milk during an outbreak of campylobacteriosis. J. Infect. Dis. *150*:789, 1984.
64. Hughes, R. A., and Rees, J. H.: Guillain-Barré syndrome. Curr. Opin. Neurol. *7*:386–392, 1994.
65. Humphrey, C. D., Montag, D. M., and Pittman, F. E.: Experimental infection of hamsters with *Campylobacter jejuni*. J. Infect. Dis. *151*:485–493, 1985.
66. Humphrey, T. J.: *Campylobacter jejuni* in dairy cows and raw milk. Epidemiol. Infect. *98*:263–269, 1987.
67. Humphrey, T. J., Henley, A., and Lanning, D. G.: The colonization of broiler chickens with *Campylobacter jejuni*: Some epidemiological investigations. Epidemiol. Infect. *110*:601–607, 1993.
68. Hutchinson, D. N., Bolton, F. J., Hinchliffe, P. M. et al.: Evidence of udder excretion of *Campylobacter jejuni* as the cause of milk-borne *Campylobacter* outbreak. J. Hyg. *94*:205–215, 1985.
69. Ichikawa, H., Sugita, K., Fukui, T., et al.: Fisher's syndrome following *Campylobacter jejuni* enteritis: A case report and review of the literature. Clin. Neurol. *35*:391–395, 1995.
70. Johnsen, K., Ostensen, M., Melbye, A. C., et al.: HLA-B27-negative arthritis related to *Campylobacter jejuni* enteritis in three children and two adults. Acta Med. Scand. *214*:165–168, 1983.
71. Johnson, W. M., and Lior, H.: Toxins produced by *Campylobacter jejuni* and *Campylobacter coli*. Lancet *1*:229–230, 1984.
72. Johnson, W. M., and Lior, H.: Cytotoxic and cytotonic factors produced by *Campylobacter jejuni*, *Campylobacter coli* and *Campylobacter laridis*. J. Clin. Microbiol. *24*:275–281, 1986.
73. Jones, D. M., Eldridge, J., and Dale, B.: Serological response to *Campylobacter jejuni/coli* infection. J. Clin. Pathol. *33*:767–769, 1980.
74. Jones, D. M., Robinson, D. A., and Eldridge, J.: Serological studies in two outbreaks of *Campylobacter jejuni* infection. J. Hyg. *87*:163–170, 1981.
75. Kaldor, J., Pritchard, H., Serpell, A, et al.: Serum antibodies in *Campylobacter* enteritis. J. Clin. Microbiol. *18*:1–4, 1983.
76. Kaldor, J., and Speed, B. R.: Guillain-Barré syndrome and *Campylobacter jejuni:* A serological study. Br. Med. J. Clin. Res. *288*:1867–1870, 1984.
77. Kalkay, M. N., Ayanian, Z. S., Lehaf, E. A., et al.: *Campylobacter*-induced toxic megacolon. Am. J. Gastroenterol. *78*:557–559, 1983.
78. Karmali, M. A., and Fleming, P. C.: *Campylobacter* enteritis. Can. Med. Assoc. J. *120*:1525–1532, 1979.
79. Kendall, E. J., and Tanner, E. I.: *Campylobacter* enteritis in general practice. J. Hyg. *88*:155–163, 1982.
80. Khalafalla, F. A.: *Campylobacter jejuni* in poultry giblets. Zentralbl. für Veterinarmed. *37*:31–34, 1990.
81. King, E. O.: Human infections with *Vibrio fetus* and a closely related *Vibrio*. J. Infect. Dis. *101*:119–128, 1957.
82. King, E. O.: The laboratory recognition of *Vibrio fetus* and a closely related *Vibrio* isolated from cases of human vibriosis. Ann. N. Y. Acad. Sci. *98*:700–711, 1962.
83. Koulla-Shiro, S., Loe, C., Ekoe, T.: Prevalence of *Campylobacter* enteritis in children from Yaounde (Cameroon). Central African J. Med. *41*:91–94, 1995.
84. Kuroki, S., Saida, T., Nukina, M., et al.: *Campylobacter jejuni* strains from patients with Guillain-Barré syndrome belong mostly to Penner serogroup 19 and contain beta-N-acetylglucosamine residues. Ann. Neurol. *33*:243–247, 1993.
85. Lambert, M. E., Schofield, P. F., Ironside, A. G., et al.: *Campylobacter* colitis. Br. Med. J. *1*:857–859, 1979.
86. Leyes, M., Vara, F., Reina, J., et al.: *Campylobacter* gastroenteritis in patients with human immunodeficiency virus infection. Enferm. Infecc. Microbiol. Clin. *12*:332–336, 1994.
87. Madden, J. M., McCardell, B. A., and Shah, D. B.: *Campylobacter jejuni* and *Campylobacter coli* cytotonic toxin production by members of genus *Vibrios*. Lancet *2*:1217–1218, 1984.
88. Mahajan, S., and Rodgers, F. G.: Isolation, characterization and host-cell binding properties of a cytotoxin from *Campylobacter jejuni*. J. Clin. Microbiol. *28*:1314–1320, 1990.
89. Maki, M., Maki, R., and Vesikari, T.: Fecal leukocytes in *Campylobacter*-associated diarrhea in infants. Acta Paediatr. Scand. *68*:271–272, 1979.
90. Martin, P. M., Mathiot, J., Ipero, J., et al.: Immune response to *Campylobacter jejuni* and *Campylobacter coli* in a cohort of children from birth to 2 years of age. Infect. Immun. *57*:2542–2546, 1989.
91. Martinez, R. M., Figueras, M. P., Ramos, C., et al.: *Campylobacter jejuni* and HIV infection. Enferm. Infecc. Microbiol. Clin. *12*:90–94, 1994.
92. McFadyean, F., and Stockman, S.: Report of the Departmental Committee Appointed by the Board of Agriculture and Fisheries to Inquire into Epizootic Abortion. Vol. 3. London, His Majesty's Stationery Office, 1909.
93. McKhann, G. M., Cornblath, D. R., Griffin, J. W., et al.: Acute motor axonal neuropathy: A frequent case of acute flaccid paralysis in China. Ann. Neurol. *33*:333–342, 1993.
94. Melamed, I., Bujanover, Y., Igra, Y. S., et al.: *Campylobacter* enteritis in normal and immunodeficient children. Am. J. Dis. Child. *137*:752–753, 1983.
95. Mentzing, L. O.: Waterborne outbreaks of *Campylobacter* enteritis in central Sweden. Lancet *2*:352–354, 1981.
96. Mishu, B., and Blaser, M. J.: Role of infection due to *Campylobacter jejuni* in the initiation of Guillain-Barré syndrome. Clin. Infect. Dis. *17*:104–108, 1993.
97. Morton, W. R., Bronsdon, M., Mickelson, G., et al.: Identification of *Campylobacter jejuni* in Macca fascicularis imported from Indonesia. Lab. Anim. Sci. *33*:187–188, 1983.
98. Moscuna, M., Gross, Z., Korenblum, R., et al.: Septic abortion due to *Campylobacter jejuni*. Eur. J. Clin. Microbiol. Infect. Dis. *8*:800, 1989.
99. Nath, G., Shukla, B. N., Reddy, D. C., et al.: A community study on the aetiology of childhood diarrhoea with special reference to *Campylobacter jejuni* in a semiurban slum of Varanasi, India. J. Diarrhoeal Dis. Res. *11*:165–168, 1993.
100. Orr, K. E., Lightfoot, N. F., Sisson, P. R., et al.: Direct milk excretion of *Campylobacter jejuni* in a dairy cow causing cases of human enteritis. Epidemiol. Infect. *114*:15, 1995.
101. Oyofo, B. A., Thornton, S. A., Burr, D. H., et al.: Specific detection of *Campylobacter jejuni* and *Campylobacter coli* by using polymerase chain reaction. J. Clin. Microbiol. *30*:2613–2619, 1992.
102. Pacha, R. E., Clark, G. W., Williams, E. A., et al.: Migratory birds of central Washington as reservoirs of *Campylobacter jejuni*. Can. J. Microbiol. *24*:80–82, 1988.
103. Pai, C. H., Sorger, S., Lackman, L., et al.: *Campylobacter* gastroenteritis in children. J. Pediatr. *94*:589–591, 1979.
104. Pai, C. H., Gillis, F., Toumanen, E., et al.: Erythromycin in treatment of *Campylobacter* enteritis in children. Am. J. Dis. Child. *137*:286–288, 1983.
105. Paisley, J. W., Mirret, S., Lauer, B. A., et al.: Dark-field microscopy of human feces for presumptive diagnosis of *Campylobacter fetus* subsp. *jejuni* enteritis. J. Clin. Microbiol. *15*:61–63, 1982.
106. Park, C. H., Hixon, D. L., Polhemus, A. S., et al.: A rapid diagnosis of *Campylobacter* enteritis by direct smear examination. Am. J. Clin. Pathol. *80*:388–390, 1983.
107. Perkins, D. J., and Newstead, G. L.: *Campylobacter jejuni* enterocolitis causing peritonitis, ileitis, and intestinal obstruction. Aust. N. Z. J. Surg. *64*:55–58, 1994.
108. Perlman, D. M., Ampel, N. M., Schifman, R. B., et al.: Persistent *Campylobacter jejuni* infections in patients infected with human immunodeficiency virus (HIV). Ann. Intern. Med. *108*:540–546, 1988.
109. Pearson, A. D., and Healing, T. D.: The surveillance and control of *Campylobacter* infections. Commun. Dis. Rep. R133–R139, 1992.
110. Pepersack, F., Prigogyne, T., Butzler, J. P., et al.: *Campylobacter jejuni* post-tranfusional septicaemia. Lancet *2*:911, 1979.
111. Peterson, M. C., Farr, R. W., and Castiglia, M.: Prosthetic hip infection and bacteremia due to *Campylobacter jejuni* in a patient with AIDS. Clin. Infect. Dis. *16*:439–440, 1993.
112. Peterson, M. C.: Rheumatic manifestations of *Campylobacter jejuni* and *C. fetus* infections in adults. Scand. J. Rheumatol. *23*:167–170, 1994.
113. Pickering, L. K., Guerrant, R. L., and Cleary, T. G.: Microorganisms responsible for neonatal diarrhea. In Remington, J. S., and Klein, J. O. (eds.): Infectious Diseases of the Fetus and Newborn Infant. 4th ed. Philadelphia, W. B. Saunders, 1994, pp. 1142–1222.
114. Ponka, A., Martio, J., and Kosunen, T. U.: Reiter's syndrome in association with enteritis due to *Campylobacter fetus* ssp. *jejuni*. Ann. Rheumat. Dis. *40*:414–415, 1981.
115. Prescott, J. F., Barker, I. K., Manninen, K. I., et al.: *Campylobacter jejuni* colitis in gnotobiotic dogs. Can. J. Comp. Med. *45*:377–383, 1981.
116. Ramiro-Cruz, J., Cano, F., Bartlett, A. V., et al.: Infection, diarrhea and dysentery caused by *Shigella* species and *Campylobacter jejuni* among Guatemalan rural children. Pediatr. Infect. Dis. J. *13*:216–223, 1994.
117. Reina, J., Borrel, N., and Serra, A.: Emergence of resistance to erythromycin and fluoroquinolones in thermotolerant *Campylobacter* strains isolated from feces 1987–1991. Eur. J. Clin. Microbiol. Infect. Dis. *11*:1163–1166, 1992.
118. Rettig, P. J.: *Campylobacter* infections in human beings. J. Pediatr. *94*:855–864, 1979.
119. Rhodes, K. M., and Tattersfield, A. E.: Guillain-Barré syndrome associated with *Campylobacter* infection. Br. Med. J. *285*:173–174, 1982.
120. Riley, L. W., and Finch, M. J.: Results of the first year of national surveillance of *Campylobacter* infections in the United States. J. Infect. Dis. *151*:956–959, 1985.
121. Ruiz-Palacios, G. M., Torres, J., and Escamilla, N. I.: Cholera-like entero-

toxin produced by *Campylobacter jejuni:* Characterization and clinical significance. Lancet 2:250–253, 1983.
122. Ruiz-Palacios, G. M., Calva, J. J., Pickering, L. K., et al.: Protection of breast fed infants against *Campylobacter* diarrhea by antibodies in human milk. J. Pediatr. *116*:707–713, 1990.
123. Sagara, H., Mochizuki, A., Okamura, N., et al.: Antimicrobial resistance of *Campylobacter jejuni* and *Campylobacter coli* with special reference to plasmid profiles of Japanese clinical isolates. Antimicrob. Agents Chemother. *31*:713–719, 1987.
124. Salazar-Lindo, E., Sack, B., Chea-Woo, E., et al.: Early treatment with erythromycin of *Campylobacter jejuni* associated dysentery in children. J. Pediatr. *109*:355–360, 1986.
125. Sanchez, R., Fernandez-Vaca, V., Diaz, M. D., et al.: Evolution of susceptibilities of *Campylobacter* spp to quinolones and macrolides. Antimicrob. Agents Chemother. *38*:1879–1882, 1994.
126. Sazie, E. S., and Titus, A. E.: Rapid diagnosis of *Campylobacter* enteritis. Ann. Intern. Med. *96*:62–63, 1982.
127. Schaad, U. B.: Reactive arthritis associated with *Campylobacter* enteritis. Pediatr. Infect. Dis. J. *1*:328–332, 1982.
128. Sethi, S. K., Khuffash, F. A., and al-Nakib, W.: Microbial etiology of acute gastroenteritis in hospitalized in children in Kuwait. Pediatr. Infect. Dis. J. *8*:593–597, 1989.
129. Shanker, S., Rosenfield, J. A., Davey, G. R., et al.: *Campylobacter jejuni:* Incidence in processed broilers and biotype distribution in human and broiler isolates. Appl. Environ. Microbiol. *43*:1219–1220, 1982.
130. Simor, A. E., Karmali, M. A., Jadaviji, T., et al.: Abortion and perinatal sepsis associated with *Campylobacter* infection. Rev. Infect. Dis. *8*:397–402, 1986.
131. Sjogren, E., Kaijser, B., and Werner, M.: Antimicrobial susceptibilities of *Campylobacter jejuni* and *Campylobacter coli* isolated in Sweden: A 10-year follow-up report. Antimicrob. Agents Chemother. *36*:2847–2849, 1992.
132. Skirrow, M. B.: *Campylobacter* enteritis in cats and dogs: A "new" zoonosis. Vet. Res. Commun. *5*:13–19, 1981.
133. Skirrow, M. B., Jones, D. M., Sutcliffe, E., et al.: *Campylobacter* bacteremia in England and Wales, 1981–91. Epidemiol. Infect. *110*:567–573, 1993.
134. Skirrow, M. B.: *Campylobacter* enteritis: A "new" disease. Br. Med. J. *2*:9–11, 1977.
135. Smibert, R. M.: Genus *Campylobacter. In* Krieg, N. R., and Holt, H. G. (eds.): Manual of Systematic Bacteriology. Vol. 1. Baltimore, Williams & Wilkins, 1984, p. 111.
136. Smith, M. V., and Muldoon, A. J.: *Campylobacter fetus* ssp. *jejuni (Vibrio fetus)* from commercially processed poultry. Appl. Microbiol. *27*:995, 1974.
137. Spira, W. M., Sack, R. B., and Froelich, J. L.: Simple adult rabbit model for *Vibrio cholerae* and enterotoxigenic *Escherichia coli* diarrhea. Infect. Immun. *32*:739–747, 1981.
138. Svedhem, A., Gunnarsson, H., and Kaijser, B.: Diffusion-in-gel enzyme-linked immunosorbent assay for routine detection of IgG and IgM antibodies to *Campylobacter jejuni.* J. Infect. Dis. *148*:82–92, 1983.
139. Tauxe, R. V., Deming, M. S., and Blake, P. A.: *Campylobacter jejuni* infections on college campuses: A national survey. Am. J. Public Health *75*:659–660, 1985.
140. Tauxe, R. V., Hargrett-Bean, N., Patton, C. M., et al.: *Campylobacter* isolates in the United States, 1982–1986. M. M. W. R. CDC Surveillance Summaries *37*:1–13, 1988.
141. Tauxe, R. V.: Epidemiology of *Campylobacter jejuni* infections in the United States and other industrialized countries. *In* Nachamkin, I., Blaser, M. J., and Tompkins, L. S. (eds.): *Campylobacter jejuni:* Current Strategy and Future Trends. Washington, D.C., American Society for Microbiology, 1992, pp. 9–19.
142. Taylor, D. N., McDermott, K. T., Little, J. R., et al.: *Campylobacter* enteritis from untreated water in the Rocky Mountains. Ann. Intern. Med. *99*:38–40, 1983.
143. Taylor, D. N., Blaser, M. J., Echeverria, P., et al.: Erythromycin-resistant *Campylobacter* infections in Thailand. Antimicrob. Agents Chemother. *31*:438–442, 1987.
144. Taylor, D. N., Echeverria, P., Pitarangsi, C., et al.: Influence of strain characteristics and immunity on the epidemiology of *Campylobacter* infections in Thailand. J. Clin. Microbiol. *26*:863–868, 1988.
145. Taylor, D. E., Chang, N., Garner, R. S., et al.: Incidence of antibiotic resistance and characterization of plasmids in *Campylobacter jejuni* strains isolated from clinical sources in Alberta, Canada. Can. J. Microbiol. *32*:28–32, 1986.
146. Taylor, D. N., Perlman, D. N., Echeverria, P. D., et al.: *Campylobacter* immunity and quantitative excretion rates in Thai children. J. Infect. Dis. *168*:754–758, 1993.
147. Tenover, F. C., Carlson, L., Barbagallo, S. et al.: DNA probe culture confirmation assay for identification of thermophilic *Campylobacter* species. J. Clin. Microbiol. *28*:1284–1287, 1990.
148. Thomas, K., Chan, K. N., and Riberiro, C. D.: *Campylobacter jejuni/coli* meningitis in a neonate. Br. Med. J. *280*:1301–1302, 1980.
149. Tokumaru, M., Konuma, H., and Umesako, M.: Rates of detection of *Salmonella* and *Campylobacter* in meats in response to the sample size and the infection level of each species. Int. J. Food Microbiol. *13*:41–46, 1991.
150. Torre, E., and Tello, M.: Factors influencing fecal shedding of *Campylobacter jejuni* in dogs without diarrhea. Am. J. Vet. Res. *54*:260–262, 1993.
151. Torres, O., and Cruz, J. R.: Protection against *Campylobacter* diarrhea: Role of milk IgA antibodies against bacterial surface antigens. Acta. Paediatr. *82*:835–838, 1993.
152. Totten, P. A., Patton, C. M., Tenover, F. C., et al.: Prevalence and characterization of hippurate-negative *Campylobacter jejuni* in King County, Washington. J. Clin. Microbiol. *25*:1747–1752, 1987.
153. Vandamme, P., Falsen, E., Rossau, R., et al.: Revision of *Campylobacter, Helicobacter,* and *Wolinella* taxonomy: Emendation of generic descriptions and proposal of *Arcobacter* gen. nov. Int. J. Syst. Bacteriol. *41*:81–103, 1991.
154. Vandamme, P., and De Ley, J.: Proposal for a new family, Campylobacteraceae. Int. J. Sys. Bacteriol. *41*:451–455, 1991.
155. Vanhoof, R., Gordts, B., Dierickx, R., et al.: Bacteriostatic and bactericidal activities of 24 antimicrobial agents against *Campylobacter fetus* subsp. *jejuni*. Antimicrob. Agents Chemother. *18*:118–121, 1980.
156. Velazquez, J. B., Jimenez, A., Chomon, B., et al.: Incidence and transmission of antibiotic resistance in *Campylobacter jejuni* and *Campylobacter coli.* J. Antimicrob. Chemother. *35*:173–178, 1995.
157. Vesikari, T., Huttunen, L., and Maki, R.: Perinatal *Campylobacter fetus* ssp *jejuni* enteritis. Acta Paediatr. Scand. *70*:261–263, 1981.
158. Vernon, M., and Chatelain, R.: Taxonomic study of the genus *Campylobacter* and designation of the neotype strain for the type species, *Campylobacter fetus.* Int. J. Syst. Bacteriol. *23*:122–134, 1973.
159. Vinzent, R., Dumas, J., and Picard, N.: Septicemia grave au cours de la grossesse due a vibrion: Avortement consecutif. Bull. Acad. Natl. Med. *131*:90–92, 1947.
160. Waltner-Toews, D., Martin, S. W., and Meek, A. H.: An epidemiological study of selected calf pathogens on Holstein dairy farms in southwestern Ontario. Can. J. Vet. Res. *50*:307–313, 1986.
161. Warner, D. P., Brainier, J. H., and Beran, W.: Epidemiologic study of campylobacteriosis in Iowa cattle and the possible role of unpasteurized milk as a vehicle of infection. Am. J. Vet. Res. *47*:254–258, 1986.
162. Watson, K. C., Kerr, E. J. C., and McFadzean, S. M.: Serology of human *Campylobacter* infections. J. Infect. *1*:151, 1979.
163. Williams, D., Schorling, J., Barrett, L. J., et al.: Early treatment of *Campylobacter jejuni* enteritis. Antimicrob. Agents Chemother. *33*:248–250, 1989.
164. Wretlind, B., Stromberg, A., Ostlund, L., et al.: Rapid emergence of quinolone resistance in *Campylobacter jejuni* in patients treated with norfloxacin. Scand. J. Infect. Dis. *24*:685–686, 1992.
165. Wright, E. P., and Seager, J.: Convulsions associated with *Campylobacter* enteritis. Br. Med. J. *281*:454, 1980.
166. Young, D. M., Biao, J., Zheng, Z., et al.: Isolation of *Campylobacter jejuni* in Hunan, the People's Republic of China: Epidemiology and comparison of Chinese and American methodology. Diagn. Microbiol. Infect. Dis. *5*:143–149, 1986.
167. Yuki, N., Ichikawa, H., and Doi, A.: Fisher syndrome after *Campylobacter jejuni* enteritis: Human leukocyte antigen and the bacterial serotype. J. Pediatr. *126*:55–57, 1995.
168. Zaman, R.: *Campylobacter* enteritis in Saudi Arabia. Epidemiol. Infect. *108*:51–58, 1992.

137

OTHER *CAMPYLOBACTER* SPECIES

Robert J. Leggiadro

Although they are not isolated as frequently as *Campylobacter jejuni* and *Campylobacter coli*, the "other" *Campylobacter* species are gaining recognition as human pathogens. *Campylobacter fetus*, a classic cause of perinatal infection, also is an infrequent cause of bacteremia in immunocompromised hosts. *Campylobacter upsaliensis*, *Campylobacter lari*, and *Campylobacter hyointestinalis* are associated primarily with diarrheal disease. Populations affected by these three species include normal as well as immunosuppressed hosts, especially HIV-infected persons with or without histories of animal exposure. The clinical spectrum of these organisms should be expanded as the special diagnostic tests needed to identify them become more widely available.

HISTORY

McFadyean and Stockman[41] first described the organisms now known as campylobacters in 1913. These *Vibrio*-like organisms were implicated as causes of epizootic abortion in sheep, and a few years later Smith[62] reported their association with bovine abortion as well and gave them the name *Vibrio fetus*. Although never confirmed microbiologically, it is believed that these organisms were *C. fetus*, according to current nomenclature.[33] Vinzent and associates[70] first reported *Campylobacter* infection in humans in 1947. They described a pregnant woman with *V. fetus* bacteremia who aborted subsequently at 6 months of gestation. In addition to pregnancy, gastrectomy, tooth extraction, heart disease, diabetes, and cirrhosis were predisposing conditions in King's[35] 1957 review of 15 patients with *V. fetus* bacteremia.

Many reports describing "new" *Campylobacter* species were published in the 1980s and early 1990s. *C. upsaliensis* was reported to be a pathogen in dogs and humans.[50, 57] *C. lari*, a common isolate from healthy seagulls, was found to be a cause of gastrointestinal and extraintestinal disease in humans.[3, 66] Originally identified in the intestines of swine with proliferative ileitis, *C. hyointestinalis* first was reported as a human pathogen in a homosexual man with proctitis.[20] The hydrogen-requiring campylobacters, *C. concisus*,[69] *C. rectus*,[52] and *C. curvus*, have been associated with periodontal disease. *Campylobacter sputorum* has been identified in abscesses,[45] and *Campylobacter mucosalis* was reported in two children with diarrhea.[21]

Once called *Campylobacter*-like organisms, *Helicobacter cinaedi* and *Helicobacter fenelliae* now are classified in the *Helicobacter* genus.[47] These pathogens cause enteritis and proctocolitis in homosexual men and bacteremia on occasion.[49, 68] Two former *Campylobacter* species, *Arcobacter butzleri* and *Arcobacter cryaerophilus*, are associated with abortion and enteritis in cattle and pigs, in addition to bacteremia and diarrhea in humans.[34]

MICROBIOLOGY

Campylobacter is a Greek word meaning "curved rod." Members of this genus are gram-negative, curved, S-shaped or spiral, non–spore-forming rods that are 0.2 to 0.9 μm wide and 0.5 to 5 μm long.[45] Organisms are motile by means of a single polar flagellum, but some have one flagellum at each pole.[29] They are microaerophilic and have a respiratory type of metabolism.[45] Campylobacters are oxidase-positive and reduce nitrates but do not ferment or oxidize carbohydrates.[51] Although most grow at 37° C, *C. jejuni*, the most commonly identified *Campylobacter* species in humans, grows optimally at 42° C.[1]

Most *Campylobacter* species require a microaerobic atmosphere containing approximately 5 per cent oxygen, 10 per cent carbon dioxide, and 85 per cent nitrogen for optimal recovery.[45] Some species, such as *C. sputorum*, *C. concisus*, C *mucosalis*, *C. curvus*, *C. rectus*, and *C. hyointestinalis*, may require hydrogen for primary isolation and growth. Many different selective media for *Campylobacter* isolation have been developed, but because of species differences in antibiotic resistance patterns, no single formulation isolates all species of clinical importance.[29] For example, *C. jejuni* and *C. coli* are resistant to cephalothin, whereas *C. fetus* is susceptible. A filtration method with nonselective media may be used to complement direct culture on selective media in the detection of antibiotic-susceptible *Campylobacter* species. Because of their small size and motility, *Campylobacter* may pass through filters with pores of 0.45 to 0.65 μm, whereas other enteric flora are retained.[1, 45]

Although colonies may appear on plates within 24 to 48 hours, growth of campylobacters from stool may take up to 72 to 96 hours. Primary isolation from blood may require 2 weeks.[1] Gram stain of young cultures reveals vibrioid forms, and longer incubation may yield spherical or coccoid bodies. *Campylobacter* species usually can be distinguished from one another on the basis of biochemical tests and growth characteristics (Table 137–1).

EPIDEMIOLOGY

Much needs to be learned about the epidemiology of *Campylobacter* species other than *C. jejuni* and *C. coli*, a group of organisms that made up only about 1 per cent of reported *Campylobacter* species to the Centers for Disease Control and Prevention from 1982 to 1986.[10] However, this study found that age-specific isolation rates of *C. fetus* parallel those of *C. jejuni* and *C. coli*, peaking in infancy and increasing in young adulthood, with *C. fetus* increasing substantially among the elderly. Seasonal distribution patterns of *C. jejuni*, *C. coli*, and *C. fetus* also were similar, with peaks in warm months. In this surveillance study, *C. jejuni* and *C. coli* isolate reports predominantly were from stool, whereas 54 per cent of *C. fetus* isolates with a known source were from blood.[10]

C. fetus, an important cause of sporadic abortion in cattle and sheep, may be isolated from the intestines and genital tracts of these animals.[51] It is suspected that contaminated food and water are the source of infection for sheep, cattle, and other animals, including goats, pigs, cats, dogs, hamsters, guinea pigs, antelopes, chickens, and turkeys.[24] Although the source of *C. fetus* infection in humans generally is not apparent,[30] a 1970 review of *V. fetus* infection in humans found that one-third of patients had recent contact with ani-

TABLE 137–1. Growth and Biochemical Characteristics for Species of the Genus *Campylobacter*

	Growth														Susceptibility	
Species	*25° C*	*37° C*	*42° C*	*Anaerobically*	*In CO_2 Inhibitor*	Glycine 1%	Bile 1%	Charcoal Casein Deoxycholate	Oxidase	Catalase	Urease	Hippurate	Nitrate	H_2S (TSI)	*Nalidixic Acid*	*Cephalothin*
C. lari	−	+	+	+	+	+	+	+	+	+	−	−	+	−	R	R
C. upsaliensis	−	+	+	+	+	−	+	+	+	(−)	−	−	+	−	S	S
C. fetus	+	+	(−)	−	+	+	−	−	+	+	−	−	+	−	R	S
C. hyointestinalis	(+)	+*	+	+	+	+	NA	NA	+	+	−	−	+	+	R	S
C. concisus	−	+	+	+	+	+	NA	NA	+	−	−	−	+	+	R	R
C. mucosalis	+	+	+	+	+	+	NA	NA	+	−	−	−	+	+	R	S
C. sputorum†	−	+	+	+	+	+	+	+	+	−	−	−	+	+	R	S

+, positive; −, negative; w, weak; (+), most strains positive; (−), most strains negative; S, susceptible; R, resistant; NA, data not available or found.
*Best at 35° C.
†*C. sputorum* has three biovars with different biochemical characteristics.
Adapted from Ruiz-Palacios, G., and Pickering, L. K.: *Campylobacter* and *Helicobacter* infections. *In* Feigin, R. D., and Cherry, J. D. (eds.): Textbook of Pediatric Infectious Diseases. 3rd ed. Philadelphia, W. B. Saunders, 1992, pp. 1072–2084.

mals or animal products and one-third denied such contact, with no information available for the remaining third.[7]

C. fetus bacteremia generally occurs in immunosuppressed hosts (especially elderly males), pregnant women, and neonates.[53, 67] Predisposing conditions include alcoholism or cirrhosis, diabetes mellitus, heart disease, malignancy, splenectomy, and corticosteroid or other immunosuppressive therapy.[53] *C. fetus* is not believed to be a major cause of gastroenteritis, which may be the result of its failure to grow in stool specimens evaluated by routine laboratory methods for *C. jejuni* and *C. coli*.[10, 51]

The epidemiology of human *C. fetus* infection as a foodborne, perinatal infection was reflected in Vinzent's original report, which describes a 39-year-old pregnant woman who had a history of drinking raw milk from a cow that recently had aborted a pregnancy and developed a flu-like syndrome in the sixth month of pregnancy.[70] Two blood cultures grew *C. fetus*, and, after 5 weeks of illness, a stillborn infant was delivered. In addition to raw milk,[72] *C. fetus* infection also has been associated with raw beef liver[63] and "nutritional therapy" (raw fruit, vegetable juices, and calf's liver, along with coffee enemas).[11] The latter report described nine patients with malignancy and one with systemic lupus erythematosus in whom *C. fetus* sepsis was associated with such therapy. Nine received their "nutritional therapy" in Mexico, and one died.[11]

First associated with human disease in a homosexual man with proctitis, *C. hyointestinalis* (*hyos*, hog; *intestinalis*, pertaining to the intestines) originally was isolated from the intestines of swine with proliferative ileitis.[20, 51] *C. hyointestinalis* also has been isolated from the stool of persons with nonbloody, watery diarrhea.[17] Two of these patients were homosexual men, the third an elderly woman who had been traveling in Egypt, and the fourth an infant from a large farm family who drank raw milk. These organisms are closer to *C. fetus* by DNA hybridization than any other catalase-positive *Campylobacter* species and are resistant to nalidixic acid but susceptible to cephalothin.[56]

C. lari, isolated frequently from apparently healthy sea gulls, is nalidixic acid–resistant and thermophilic.[61] The name derives from *laridis*, "of a sea bird," although sea gulls do not play a direct role in its epidemiology.[66] Epidemiologically and microbiologically similar to *C. jejuni*, *C. lari* has been reported to cause enteritis in patients with and without a history of animal exposure and bacteremia in an elderly man with multiple myeloma.[46, 59, 66]

Catalase-negative or weak *Campylobacter* species that are hippurate-negative and thermotolerant first were isolated from dogs in 1983.[57] This *C. upsaliensis* group is associated with gastroenteritis, breast abscess, and bacteremia in normal hosts, as well as with opportunistic infections in immunocompromised persons.[25, 26, 39, 50] Conditions predisposing to *C. upsaliensis* bacteremia include gallbladder surgery, ectopic pregnancy, kwashiorkor, and AIDS.[50] Routine selective media for *Campylobacter* may fail to detect this organism, which is slow-growing and cephalothin-susceptible.[27, 39, 71] Filtration methods may improve the yield from stool cultures.[26, 27]

PATHOGENESIS AND IMMUNITY

Information on the pathogenic and immune mechanisms involved in *Campylobacter* infections other than *C. jejuni* and *C. coli* is scarce. Much of what is known has been learned from animal, clinical, and epidemiologic data. The association of *Campylobacter* bacteremia with hypogammaglobulinemia, HIV infection, kwashiorkor, pregnancy, and malignancy indicates the importance of both humoral and cell-mediated immunity in host defense against this genus,[1, 39, 46, 60, 74] and the predilection of *C. fetus* for endovascular surfaces in adults and the central nervous system in neonates also is well documented.[16, 58]

In pregnant animals, *C. fetus* bacteremia occurs after ingestion of the organism, leading to infection of the placenta and fetus.[42, 48] Examination of infected animal placentas has revealed necrosis, infarction, and microabscesses, with disruption of placental circulation.[13] Placental changes similar to these have been described in humans after preterm maternal bacteremia, consistent with infection as a result of hematogenous, rather than ascending, spread.[60] Ascending infection with premature rupture of membranes and amnionitis in the absence of maternal bacteremia, resulting in stillbirth or early-onset disease, has been reported.[22, 31] Contamination of the baby at the time of vaginal delivery is important in the pathogenesis of neonatal sepsis and meningitis with *C. fetus* in liveborn infants.[40, 73]

Bacteremia may be more common with *C. fetus* than with *C. jejuni* because the former is resistant to the bactericidal effects of human serum, whereas the latter is susceptible.[4] A surface-layer protein that covers *C. fetus* functions as a capsule and appears to be an important virulence property of the organism.[5] It inhibits C3b binding, explaining both the serum resistance and the phagocytic resistance of *C. fetus*.[6]

CLINICAL MANIFESTATIONS

The clinical spectrum of non-*jejuni* or -*coli Campylobacter* infections varies with the age of the patient and the individual species involved (Table 137–2). *C. fetus* is responsible for most reported disease patterns caused by this "other *Campylobacter*" group of organisms, including prenatal, neonatal, bacteremic, and focal infections.[67] Pregnancies complicated by maternal infection with *C. fetus* may result in abortion, stillbirth, and prematurity.[12, 16, 60] Liveborn infants may suffer from sepsis and meningitis with a high case-fatality rate.

Mothers may present with fever and chills with bacteremia alone or with diarrhea. Maternal blood, placenta, cervix, vaginal, and stool cultures have yielded *C. fetus* in reported perinatal cases.[16, 40, 60, 73] Maternal outcome is excellent.

Torphy and Bond[67] reviewed eight infants, 12 hours to 22 days old, with reported *C. fetus* disease. Initial symptoms were consistent with neonatal sepsis, including fever, cough, respiratory distress, vomiting, diarrhea, cyanosis, convulsions, and jaundice. All eight developed meningitis, and six died. Four were premature, and three of these had onset of illness at 2 days of age or younger and died during the first week of life. However, a subsequent review reported three additional neonatal patients who survived *C. fetus* meningitis after presenting at 1 to 3 days of age.[73] Hemorrhagic infarction and necrosis, as well as cystic degeneration of the cerebral cortex, are the most common cerebral lesions reported in *Campylobacter* meningitis.[73]

Descriptions of *C. fetus* infection in children outside of the neonatal age group are rare.[36, 72, 74] One was a 2½-year-old child with *V. fetus* bacteremia presenting with low-grade fever for 3 weeks and a cervical mass on the day of admission who was treated successfully with penicillin.[72] Her past history included drinking raw cow's milk and untested well water. A 16-month-old girl from India whose father operated a dairy business was admitted for evaluation of fever for 10 days and seizures 5 days before admission.[36] Her provisional diagnosis was encephalitis, and a blood culture grew *V. fetus*.

TABLE 137–2. Clinical Features Associated with Infection Due to "Other" *Campylobacter*

Species	Common Clinical Features	Less Common Clinical Features	Additional Information
C. fetus	Bacteremia, sepsis, meningitis, vascular infections	Diarrhea, relapsing fevers	Not usually isolated from media containing cephalothin
C. upsaliensis	Watery diarrhea, low-grade fever, abdominal pain	Bacteremia, abscesses	Difficult to isolate because of cephalothin susceptibility
C. lari	Abdominal pain, diarrhea	Colitis, appendicitis	Seagulls frequently colonized; organism often transmitted to humans via contaminated water
C. hyointestinalis	Watery or bloody diarrhea, vomiting, abdominal pain	Bacteremia	Causes proliferative enteritis in swine
C. sputorum	Pulmonary, perianal, groin, and axillary abscesses	None described	Three clinically relevant biovars: *C. sputorum* subspecies *sputorum, C. sputorum* subspecies *bubulus,* and *Campylobacter mucosalis*
H_2-requiring campylobacters*	Periodontitis	Diarrhea, osteomyelitis, bacteremia	Uncertain role as human pathogen

*Includes *C. rectus, C. curvus,* and *C. concisus.*
Adapted from Allos, B. M., and Blaser, M. J.: *Campylobacter jejuni* and the expanding spectrum of related infections. Clin. Infect. Dis. *20*:1092–1099, 1995. University of Chicago, Publisher.

No antibiotics were administered, and the patient recovered uneventfully. The authors emphasized the undulant nature of *C. fetus* infections, similar to that of brucellosis. *C. fetus* bacteremia also was detected in a nearly 5-year-old boy with agammaglobulinemia who had a 3-week history of anorexia, lethargy, fever, and, more recently, hepatitis.[74] Blood culture grew *C. fetus,* and liver biopsy demonstrated hepatitis, with multiple areas of severe focal necrosis, bridging necrosis, and Kupffer-cell hyperplasia. He rapidly responded to ampicillin therapy.

Most reported patients with *C. fetus* infection are adult males older than 45 years of age who have bacteremia with or without focal infection.[53, 67] Most have underlying conditions, such as diabetes, malignancy, and hepatorenal or cardiovascular disease.[30] Typically, illness begins with fever, malaise, and headache. Chills and night sweats are prominent, as is weight loss in prolonged illness. Diarrhea, nausea, vomiting, and abdominal pain occur in up to 38 per cent of cases, and hepatosplenomegaly or jaundice occurs in two-thirds.[30, 74] Pulmonary involvement is rare.[7, 30]

Three patterns of invasive *C. fetus* disease have been described.[54] Clinical manifestations of the first localized infection accompanied by septicemia include meningitis,[40] endocarditis,[19] pericarditis,[44] thrombophlebitis,[9] mycotic aneurysm,[55] cellulitis,[23] gluteal abscess,[15] septic arthritis,[38] salpingitis,[8] and peritonitis.[65] The second form is transient asymptomatic bacteremia, which may be self-limited.[30, 53, 54] Prolonged and recurrent bacteremia, with waxing and waning symptoms as spontaneous relapses and remissions occur, is the third pattern of invasive *C. fetus* infection.[7, 14, 32, 54, 74]

The vascular tropism of *C. fetus,* especially in the presence of preexisting vessel damage, is well recognized.[9, 44, 74] Possible explanations for this predilection include a surface receptor on the organism with an affinity for vascular endothelium, resulting in endothelial damage and subsequent thrombus formation. In addition, the organism's microaerophilic growth requirements may be favored by venous oxygen tensions.[44] Previous valvular heart disease is common in endocarditis.[19]

A report from the Centers for Disease Control and Prevention reviewed clinical and epidemiologic information on a dozen *C. upsaliensis* isolates from 1980 to 1986.[50] Eight isolates were from blood and three from stool. Ages of the 12 patients ranged from 6 months to 83 years. Two infants with *C. upsaliensis* bacteremia that responded to amoxicillin therapy were included. One was a 10-month-old who had fever, leukocytosis, and a history of culture-negative diarrhea, bronchiolitis, and *Klebsiella* bacteremia 3 months previously. The second was a 6½-month-old with fever, respiratory distress, and erythematous tympanic membranes. A 14-month-old who lived on a farm with a private well and several household dogs and cats had a history of pica, including dirt from where chickens roamed. Stool culture obtained for evaluation of febrile, watery diarrhea yielded *C. upsaliensis,* and he recovered with erythromycin therapy.[50]

Underlying medical problems for adults with *C. upsaliensis* bacteremia included peptic ulcer disease and partial large bowel resection for a benign tumor, perforated gallbladder with peritonitis, AIDS, corticosteroid therapy, ruptured ectopic pregnancy, and cirrhosis with pancreatic insufficiency and partial gastrectomy.[50] One adult with a *C. upsaliensis* stool isolate was a 35-year-old with relapsing acute myelogenous leukemia. She was ill with fever and blood-tinged, watery diarrhea while thrombocytopenic and neutropenic. A healthy, 20-year-old student with a history of drinking raw milk and swimming in freshwater lakes and rivers was the second adult with a *C. upsaliensis* stool isolate. He had fever, severe cramping abdominal pain, and nonbloody, watery diarrhea of 3 weeks' duration, which responded to oral erythromycin.[50]

Kwashiorkor and gastroenteritis were the predominant clinical features in a retrospective series of 16 pediatric patients with *C. upsaliensis* bacteremia from South Africa.[39] The age range was 2 to 36 months, with a mean age of 15.5 months. The authors suggested that *C. upsaliensis* bacteremia was secondary to intestinal infection with the same organism, but no confirmatory stool culture data were available.[39] A gastrointestinal source also was postulated for the *C. upsaliensis* isolated from a breast abscess in a previously healthy, 46-year-old woman.[25]

C. upsaliensis was the only organism isolated in 83 patients in a large stool culture survey employing a filtration system for campylobacters in Belgium.[26] Ninety-two per cent of patients had diarrhea, which was of acute onset in most cases. Vomiting (14 per cent) and fever (7 per cent) were uncommon, and symptoms generally abated in less than a week. Gross or occult blood was identified in 25 per cent of cases, and neutrophils were seen on fecal smear in about 20 per cent. Erythromycin (11 patients) or amoxicillin (2 patients) therapy eradicated the organism, with resolution of symptoms in all 13 patients treated with antibiotics.[26]

Six clinical *C. lari* isolates were referred to the national *Campylobacter* reference laboratory at the Centers for Disease Control and Prevention in 1982 and 1983.[66] Clinical illness associated with these isolates included enteritis in four, severe crampy abdominal pain in a 7-year-old girl, and terminal bacteremia in a 71-year-old man with multiple myeloma and chronic renal failure. Ages of the four patients with enteritis were 8 months, 3 years, 22 years, and 39 years. Diarrhea was watery or mucoid, and fever was unusual. Potential exposures included consuming chicken, having contact with house pets, drinking untreated surface water, and eating raw oysters. *C. lari* colitis also developed in an HIV-infected woman.[18]

C. hyointestinalis has been isolated from stool specimens of adult and pediatric patients experiencing nonbloody, watery diarrhea[17] and from a rectal culture of a homosexual man with proctitis.[20] Clinical features of other *Campylobacter* species are displayed in Table 137–2.

DIAGNOSIS

Confirmation of *C. fetus* infection and *Campylobacter* species other than *C. jejuni* and *C. coli* is based on positive culture results from clinical specimens.[1] *C. fetus* has been isolated from blood, cerebrospinal fluid, joint effusions, bile, urine, and pleural and pericardial fluid in standard culture media.[30] Blood cultures generally are positive within 4 to 14 days. Isolation of *C. fetus* and "other" *Campylobacter* species from stool requires incubation at 37° C and media without cephalosporins. Filtration techniques also may be warranted to detect these strains in stool cultures.

TREATMENT

Gentamicin, erythromycin, and imipenem are bactericidal for *C. fetus*, as is ampicillin to a lesser extent.[19, 28, 43] Cefotaxime, ticarcillin, amikacin, chloramphenicol, clindamycin, tetracycline, and ciprofloxacin demonstrate variable activity against different *C. fetus* strains.[19] Reported synergistic antimicrobial combinations in vitro include ampicillin and gentamicin or cefazolin and imipenem with gentamicin.[19, 64]

Erythromycin continues to be the drug of choice for the majority of patients with *Campylobacter* diarrhea.[1] The newer macrolide azithromycin, which has a broader spectrum of activity than erythromycin, is effective therapy for *Campylobacter* enteritis, as well as for diarrhea caused by *Salmonella*, *Shigella*, *Vibrio cholerae*, and *Escherichia coli*, making it a useful drug in the treatment of traveler's diarrhea.[37] Increasing *Campylobacter* resistance to quinolones related to expanded use in humans and in animals used for food, especially chickens, has diminished the usefulness of quinolones, such as ciprofloxacin, in the treatment of *Campylobacter* gastroenteritis in adults.[1, 18, 37]

Gentamicin, imipenem, ampicillin, and cefotaxime are therapeutic options in *Campylobacter* bacteremia and other extraintestinal infections.[1, 2, 19, 73] Synergistic combination therapy is indicated in patients with meningitis and endocarditis, in which bactericidal activity is critical.[1, 43] Patients with *Campylobacter* in their stool who are being treated for an extraintestinal *Campylobacter* infection with gentamicin should be prescribed supplemental oral therapy, because gentamicin is ineffective against *Campylobacter* in the gut.[1]

Prolonged antimicrobial therapy and follow-up blood cultures are warranted for *C. fetus* bacteremia because of its relapsing nature.[44, 54] Chloramphenicol should be used with caution in *C. fetus* meningitis because clinical outcome and in vitro susceptibility results for this drug have been disappointing.[40, 43]

References

1. Allos, B. M., and Blaser, M. J.: *Campylobacter jejuni* and the expanding spectrum of related infections. Clin. Infect. Dis. *20*:1092–1099, 1995.
2. American Academy of Pediatrics: *Campylobacter* infections. *In* Peter, G. (ed.): 1994 Redbook: Report of the Committee on Infectious Diseases. 23rd ed. Elk Grove Village, IL, American Academy of Pediatrics, 1994, pp. 146–147.
3. Benjamin, J., Leaper, S., Owen, R. J., et al.: Description of *Campylobacter laridis*, a new species comprising the nalidixic acid resistant thermophilic *Campylobacter* (NARTC) group. Curr. Microbiol. *8*:231, 1983.
4. Blaser, M. J., Smith, P. F., and Kohler, P. A.: Susceptibility of *Campylobacter* isolates to the bactericidal activity in human serum. J. Infect. Dis. *151*:227–235, 1985.
5. Blaser, M. J., Smith, P. F., Hopkins, J. A., et al.: Pathogenesis of *Campylobacter fetus* infections: Serum resistance associated with high molecular weight surface proteins. J. Infect. Dis. *135*:696–706, 1987.
6. Blaser, M. J., Smith, P. F., Repine, J. E., et al.: Pathogenesis of *Campylobacter fetus* infections: Failure of C3b to bind explains serum and phagocytosis resistance. J. Clin. Invest. *81*:1434–1444, 1988.
7. Bokkenheuser, V.: *Vibrio fetus* infection in man. I. Ten new cases and some epidemiologic observations. Am. J. Epidemiol. *91*:400–409, 1970.
8. Brown, W. J., and Sautter, R.: *Campylobacter fetus* septicemia with concurrent salpingitis. J. Clin. Microbiol. *6*:72–75, 1977.
9. Carbone, K. M., Heinrich, M. C., and Quinn, T. C.: Thrombophlebitis and cellulitis due to *Campylobacter fetus* ssp. *fetus*: Report of four cases and a review of the literature. Medicine (Baltimore) *64*:244–250, 1985.
10. Centers for Disease Control: *Campylobacter* isolates in the United States, 1982–1986. *In* CDC Surveillance Summaries, June 1988. M. M. W. R. *37*(SS-2):1–13, 1988.
11. Centers for Disease Control: *Campylobacter* sepsis associated with "nutrition therapy." M. M. W. R. *30*:294–295, 1981.
12. Centers for Disease Control. Premature labor and neonatal sepsis caused by *Campylobacter fetus*, subsp. *fetus*: Ontario. M. M. W. R. *33*:483–484, 1984.
13. Coid, C. R., and Fox, H.: Short review: Campylobacters as placental pathogens. Placenta *4*:295–305, 1983.
14. Collins, H. S., Blevins, A., and Benter, E.: Protracted bacteremia and meningitis due to *Vibrio fetus*. Arch. Intern. Med. *113*:361, 1964.
15. de Otero, J., Pigrau, C., Buti, M., et al.: Isolation of *Campylobacter fetus* subspecies *fetus* from a gluteal abscess. Clin. Infect. Dis. *19*:557–558, 1994.
16. Eden, A. N.: Perinatal mortality caused by *Vibrio fetus*. J. Pediatr. *68*:297, 1966.
17. Edmonds, P., Patton, C. M., Griffin, P. M., et al.: *Campylobacter hyointestinalis* associated with human gastrointestinal disease in the United States. J. Clin. Microbiol. *25*:685–691, 1987.
18. Evans, T. G., and Riley, D.: *Campylobacter laridis* colitis in a human immunodeficiency virus-positive patient treated with a quinolone. Clin. Infect. Dis. *15*:172–173, 1992.
19. Farrugia, D. C., Eykyn, S. J., and Smyth, E. G.: *Campylobacter fetus* endocarditis: Two case reports and review. Clin. Infect. Dis. *18*:443–446, 1994.
20. Fennell, C. L., Rompalo, A. M., Totten, P. A., et al.: Isolation of *Campylobacter hyointestinalis* from a human. J. Clin. Microbiol. *24*:146–148, 1986.
21. Figura, N., Guglielmetti, P., Zanchi, A., et al.: Two cases of *Campylobacter mucosalis* enteritis in children. J. Clin. Microbiol. *31*:727–728, 1993.
22. Forbes, J. D., and Scheifele, D. W.: Early onset *Campylobacter* sepsis in a neonate. Pediatr. Infect. Dis. J. *6*:494, 1987.
23. Francioli, P., Hertzstein, J., Grob, J., et al.: *Campylobacter fetus* subspecies *fetus* bacteremia. Arch. Intern. Med. *145*:289–292, 1985.
24. Franklin, B., and Ulmer, D. D.: Human infection with *Vibrio fetus*. West. J. Med. *120*:200–204, 1974.
25. Gaudreau, C., and Lamothe, F.: *Campylobacter upsaliensis* isolated from a breast abscess. J. Clin. Microbiol. *30*:1354–1356, 1992.
26. Goossens, H., Vlaes, L., DeBoeck, M., et al.: Is "*Campylobacter upsaliensis*" an unrecognised cause of human diarrhoea? Lancet *335*:584–586, 1990.
27. Goossens, H., Pot, B., Vlaes, L., et al.: Characterization and description of *Campylobacter upsaliensis* isolated from human feces. J. Clin. Microbiol. *28*:1039–1046, 1990.
28. Goossens, H., Coignau, H., Vlaes, L., et al.: In vitro evaluation of antibiotic

combinations against *Campylobacter fetus*. J. Antimicrob. Chemother. *24*:195–201, 1989.
29. Griffiths, P. L., and Park, R. W. A.: Campylobacters associated with human diarrhoeal disease. J. Appl. Bacteriol. *69*:281–301, 1990.
30. Guerrant, R. L., Lahita, R. G., Winn, W. C., et al.: Campylobacteriosis in man: Pathogenic mechanisms and review of 91 bloodstream infections. Am. J. Med. *65*:584–592, 1978.
31. Hood, M., and Todd, J. M.: *Vibrio fetus*: A cause of human abortion. Am. J. Obstet. Gynecol. *80*:506, 1960.
32. Jackson, J. F., Hinton, P., and Allison, F., Jr: Human vibriosis: Report of a patient with relapsing febrile illness due to *Vibrio fetus*. Am. J. Med. *28*:986, 1960.
33. Karmali, M. A., Allen, A. K., and Fleming, P. C.: Differentiation of catalase-positive campylobacters with special reference to morphology. Int. J. System. Bacteriol. *31*:64, 1981.
34. Kiehlbauch, J. A., Brenner, D. J., Nicholson, M. A., et al.: *Campylobacter butzleri* sp. nov isolated from humans and animals with diarrheal illness. J. Clin. Microbiol. *29*:376–385, 1991.
35. King, E. O.: Human infections with *Vibrio fetus* and a closely related vibrio. J. Infect. Dis. *101*:119, 1957.
36. Koshi, G., Samuel, B. T., Malati, J., et al.: *Vibrio fetus* encephalitis with bacteremia in a child. Indian J. Med. Res. *57*:1232–1239, 1969.
37. Kuschner, R. A., Trofa, A. F., Thomas, R. J., et al.: Use of azithromycin for the treatment of *Campylobacter enteritis* in travelers to Thailand, an area where ciprofloxacin resistance is prevalent. Clin. Infect. Dis. *21*:536, 1995.
38. Kutner, L. J., and Arnold, W. D.: Septic arthritis due to *Vibrio fetus*. J. Bone Joint Surg. [Am.] *52*:161–164, 1970.
39. Lastovica, A. J., LeRoux, E., and Penner, J. L.: *Campylobacter upsaliensis* isolated from blood cultures of pediatric patients. J. Clin. Microbiol. *27*:657–659, 1989.
40. Lee, M. M., Welliver, R. C., and La Scolea, L. J.: *Campylobacter* meningitis in childhood. Pediatr. Infect. Dis. *4*:544–547, 1985.
41. McFadyean, F., and Stockman, S.: Report of the Departmental Committee Appointed by the Board of Agriculture and Fisheries to Inquire into Epizootic Abortion, London, 1909–1913. His Majesty's Stationary Office, 3:1, 1913.
42. Miller, V. A., Jensen, R., and Gilroy, J. J.: Bacteremia in pregnant sheep following oral administration of *Vibrio fetus*. Am. J. Vet. Res. *20*:677, 1959.
43. Morooka, T., Oda, T., and Shigeoka, H.: In vitro evaluation of antibiotics for treatment of meningitis caused by *Campylobacter fetus* subspecies *fetus*. Pediatr. Infect. Dis. J. *8*:653–654, 1989.
44. Morrison, V. A., Lloyd, B. D., Chia, J. K. S., et al.: Cardiovascular and bacteremic manifestations of *Campylobacter fetus* infection: Case report and review. Rev. Infect. Dis. *12*:387–392, 1990.
45. Nachamkin, I.: *Campylobacter* and *Arcobacter*. *In* Murray, P. R., Baron, E. J., Pfaller, M. A., et al. (eds.): Manual of Clinical Microbiology. 6th ed. Washington, D.C., ASM Press, 1995, pp. 483–491.
46. Nachamkin, I., Stowell, C., Skalina, D., et al.: *Campylobacter laridis* causing bacteremia in an immunosuppressed patient. Ann. Intern. Med. *101*:55–57, 1984.
47. Orlicek, S. L., Welch, D. F., and Kuhls, T. L.: Septicemia and meningitis caused by a *Helicobacter cinaedi* in a neonate. J. Clin. Microbiol. *31*:569–571, 1993.
48. Osburn, B. I., and Hoskins, R. K.: Experimentally induced *Vibrio fetus* var. *intestinalis* infection in pregnant cows. Am. J. Vet. Res. *31*:1733–1741, 1970.
49. Pasternak, J., Bolivar, R., Hopfer, R. L., et al: Bacteremia caused by *Campylobacter*-like organisms in two male homosexuals. Ann. Intern. Med. *101*:339–341, 1984.
50. Patton, C. M., Shaffer, N., Edmonds, P., et al.: Human disease associated with *Campylobacter upsaliensis* (catalase-negative or weakly positive *Campylobacter* species) in the United States. J. Clin. Microbiol. *27*:66–73, 1989.
51. Penner, J. L.: The genus *Campylobacter*: A decade of progress. Clin. Microbiol. Rev. *1*:157–172, 1988.
52. Rams, T. E., Feik, D., and Slots, J.: *Campylobacter rectus* in human periodontitis. Oral Microbiol. Immunol. *8*:230–235, 1993.
53. Rettig, P. J.: *Campylobacter* infections in human beings. J. Pediatr. *94*:855–864, 1979.
54. Righter, J., Wells, W. A., Hart, G. D., et al.: Relapsing septicemia caused by *Campylobacter fetus* subsp *fetus*. Can. Med. Assoc. J. *128*:686–689, 1983.
55. Righter, J., and Woods, J. M.: *Campylobacter* and endovascular lesions. Can. J. Surg. *28*:451–452, 1985.
56. Roop, R. M., II, Smibert, R. M., Johnson, J. L., et al.: Differential characteristics of catalase positive campylobacters correlated with DNA homology groups. Can. J. Microbiol. *30*:938–951, 1984.
57. Sanstedt, K., Ursing, J., and Walder, M.: Thermotolerant *Campylobacter* with no or weak catalase activity isolated from dogs. Curr. Microbiol. *8*:209, 1983.
58. Schmidt, U., Chmel, H., Kaminski, Z., et al.: The clinical spectrum of *Campylobacter fetus* infections: Report of five cases and review of the literature. Q. J. Med. *49*:431–432, 1980.
59. Simor, A. E., and Wilcox, L.: Enteritis associated with *Campylobacter laridis*. J. Clin. Microbiol. *25*:10–12, 1987.
60. Simor, A. E., Karmali, M. A., Jadavji, T., et al.: Abortion and perinatal sepsis associated with *Campylobacter* infection. Rev. Infect. Dis. *8*:397–402, 1986.
61. Skirrow, M. B., and Benjamin, J.: Differentiation of enteropathogenic *Campylobacter*. J. Clin. Pathol. *33*:1122, 1980.
62. Smith, T.: Spirilla associated with disease of the fetal membranes in cattle. J. Exp. Med. *28*:701, 1918.
63. Soonattrakul, W., Andersen, B. R., and Brynor, J. H.: Raw liver as a possible source of *Vibrio fetus* septicemia in man. Am. J. Med. Sci. *261*:245, 1981.
64. Spelhaug, D. R., Gilchrist, M. J. R., and Washington, J. A., II: Bactericidal activity of antibiotics against *Campylobacter fetus* subspecies *intestinalis*. J. Infect. Dis. *143*:500, 1981.
65. Targan, S. R., Chow, A. W., and Guze, L. B.: Spontaneous peritonitis of cirrhosis due to *Campylobacter fetus*. Gastroenterology *71*:311–313, 1976.
66. Tauxe, R. V., Patton, C. M., Edmonds, P., et al.: Illness associated with *Campylobacter laridis*, a newly recognized *Campylobacter* species. J. Clin. Microbiol. *21*:222–225, 1985.
67. Torphy, D. E., and Bond, W. W.: *Campylobacter fetus* infections in children. Pediatrics *64*:898–903, 1979.
68. Totten, P. A., Fennell, C. L., Tenover, F. C., et al.: *Campylobacter cinaedi* (sp. nov.) and *Campylobacter fennelliae* (sp. nov.): Two new *Campylobacter* species associated with enteric disease in homosexual men. J. Infect. Dis. *151*:131–139, 1985.
69. Vandamme, P., Falsen, E., Pot, B., et al.: Identification of EF group 22 campylobacters from gastroenteritis cases as *Campylobacter concisus*. J. Clin. Microbiol. *27*:1775–1781, 1989.
70. Vinzent, R., Dumas, J., and Picard, N.: Septicemie grave au cours de la grossesse, due à un vibrion: Avortement consecutif. Bull. Acad. Natl. Med. (Paris) *131*:90, 1947.
71. Walmsley, S. L., and Karmali, M. A.: Direct isolation of atypical thermophilic *Campylobacter* species from human feces on selective agar medium. J. Clin. Microbiol. *27*:668–670, 1989.
72. Willis, M, D., and Austin, W. J.: Human *Vibrio fetus* infection: Report of two dissimilar cases. Am. J. Dis. Child *112*:459–462, 1966.
73. Wong, S., Tam, A. Y., and Yeun, K.: *Campylobacter* infection in the neonate: Case report and review of the literature. Pediatr. Infect. Dis. J. *9*:665, 1990.
74. Wyatt, R. A., Younoszai, K., Anuras, S., et al.: *Campylobacter fetus* septicemia and hepatitis in a child with agammaglobulinemia. J. Pediatr. *91*:441–442, 1977.

138

TULAREMIA

Ching C. Lau and Ralph D. Feigin

Tularemia is an acute febrile illness caused by *Francisella tularensis*. Although it primarily is a disease of animals, humans also are highly susceptible hosts.

HISTORY

McCoy[53] published the first documented evidence of tularemia in 1911, when he described a plague-like disease in ground squirrels (*Citellus beecheyi*) that occurred in Tulare County, California. Within 2 years, McCoy and Chapin[54] isolated and characterized the organism, *Bacterium tularense*, from naturally infected ground squirrels. They also detailed the pathology produced in the ground squirrels, defined the susceptibility of other animal species to *B. tularense*, and identified fleas as vectors for the plague-like disease in 1912.

The first description of tularemia in humans may be that of Hommo-Soken, a court physician in eastern Japan.[58] In 1837, he described an illness as "hare meat poisoning." Nearly a century later, Vail[86] and Wherry and Lamb[90] independently reported the first etiologically proven case of tularemia in humans in 1914. Thereafter, knowledge of the organism, susceptible hosts, modes of transmission, and clinical manifestations of disease was acquired rapidly, and retrospective information was assessed in light of this new information. Much of the current understanding of the disease in humans originated from the work of Edward Francis,[26] a United States Public Health Service surgeon. Intrigued by the new diseases called "deer fly fever," as described by Pearse[65] in 1911, and "plague-like disease," as described by McCoy, Francis relocated to Utah in 1919 and established his laboratory in an unused coal shed.[26, 28, 29, 70] Soon thereafter, he recognized the singular cause of these two diseases and renamed them "tularemia" because of the isolation of *B. tularense* from the blood. He isolated the organism from humans and jackrabbits[25] and demonstrated the transmission of the organism by the deer fly.[28]

For a more complete historical review, the reader is referred to the classic paper of Dr. Edward Francis,[26] "A Summary of the Present Knowledge of Tularemia." Some seven decades later, this paper is accurate and contains most of the knowledge essential for understanding tularemia.

ETIOLOGY

The causative agent of tularemia, after having been placed in the genera *Bacterium, Bacillus, Brucella*, and *Pasteurella*, now is named *Francisella tularensis* in honor of Dr. Edward Francis. *F. tularensis* is a small (0.2 to 1.0 μm × 1 to 3 μm), nonmotile, non–spore-forming, highly pleomorphic, gram-negative coccobacillus.

Hesselbrock and Foshay[35] described the morphology as resembling that of the pleuropneumonia group of organisms, the usual coccoid form being a spheroidal cystic structure with a delicate, transparent cell wall. The morphology and mode of reproduction (chiefly budding) suggested relationships with fungi and the pleuropneumonia group and none with the genera *Pasteurella* and *Brucella*. Subsequent electron-microscopic studies confirmed the presence of a delicate, almost transparent cell wall, which Eigelsbach and associates[15] felt could explain the instability of lyophilized cultures.

The outstanding growth characteristic of these fastidious organisms is their requirement for cysteine or sulfhydryl compounds in amounts exceeding those usually present in nutrient media.[21] Although *F. tularensis* grows best on cysteine-glucose-blood agar and on coagulated egg yolk medium and less well in thioglycolate broth, it can be isolated in routine cultures and on enriched chocolate agar.[46, 56] Hornick[37] suggested that the addition of cycloheximide and penicillin facilitates isolation of the organism from the respiratory tract or skin ulcers.

F. tularensis is killed readily by heat. Exposure to a temperature of 56° C for 10 minutes is sufficient for killing. The organisms are not destroyed by freezing and may remain viable in frozen animal carcasses for up to 3 years. However, adequate cooking renders the meat of game birds and animals harmless. Treatment with tricresol solution (1 per cent) for 2 minutes also kills organisms in tissue; organisms from cultures are killed in 24 hours by 0.1 per cent formalin.

All strains of *F. tularensis* seem serologically identical. Individual strains may possess varying degrees of virulence. Ormsbee and associates[62] reported that the immunizing antigens seem to be concentrated in the cell wall. The purest cell-wall preparations contain at least four and possibly six different antigens, against none of which the soluble fractions seemed to provide protection when mice were immunized with these antigen preparations.

Despite serologic homogeneity, there are two distinct varieties of tularemia organisms. Those strains that are highly virulent for humans, Jellison type A (*F. tularensis* biovar *tularensis*), account for approximately 90 per cent of organisms isolated in North America and rarely are isolated elsewhere. The less virulent strains, Jellison type B (*F. tularensis* biovar *palaearctica*), are found primarily in Europe and Asia. The two strains had been found to coexist in the same ecosystem.[52]

F. tularensis does not produce any exotoxin, but pharmacologic tests indicate that the organism contains an endotoxin similar to those of gram-negative bacilli.[23]

EPIDEMIOLOGY

Tularemia is ubiquitous in the northern hemisphere between 30° and 71° north latitude.[36] It has been reported throughout the United States, in the Far East, and in Europe.[27, 59, 60, 78] *F. tularensis* has been found in Canada and Mexico but has not been reported in South America or Africa. Within the United States, the disease is most common in the South-Central region. In 1982, four states (Arkansas, Missouri, Oklahoma, and Texas) accounted for about a third of the reported cases.[9] From 1991 to 1992, 47 per cent (165 of 352) of all cases were reported from Missouri and Arkansas.[2]

Tularemia occurs year-round. However, there are peaks in summer and winter months, depending on the regions. It is more common in the central and southern states during the summer months, when ticks are more prevalent. The incidence in the northern and eastern states peaks in the winter months during the hunting season.

In the United States, the incidence of tularemia has been recorded since 1927. The number of human cases declined steadily from 1939 (2991 cases)[4] until 1975 (129 cases). Since then, the number of reported cases has increased. Since the 1980s, between 129 and 288 cases of tularemia have been reported annually. This range probably is a gross underestimate of the actual incidence. In 1968, in a serologic survey of 1936 subjects in California, approximately 1 per cent of this population had antibody against *F. tularensis*.[20] Using skin test antigens, Casper and Phillip[8] showed that 6.6 per cent of 365 persons in eastern Montana had evidence of previous infection with *F. tularensis*. Of the persons in whom skin test results were positive, 80 per cent had no previous history of the disease, indicating a high number of subclinical or self-limiting infections. The mortality rate is zero to four cases per year.

The most common sources of human infections are contact with infected animals or their carcasses and bites by ticks or tabanid flies (deer flies). Less commonly, people acquire the disease from the bite of a diseased animal or one in which the mouth has been contaminated by ingestion of a diseased animal. Numerous outbreaks of human tularemia have occurred by water transmission,[29, 42, 82, 87] the water having been contaminated by voles, beavers, and muskrats. Infection also may occur by aerosolization of the organisms, especially for laboratory workers[43, 87] and occasionally farm workers (inhalation of dust and threshings contaminated by voles and other rodents).[13, 36] Person-to-person transmission has not been documented.

Hopla,[36] in describing the ecology of tularemia, states that "rarely does one encounter a zoonotic disease of such complexity." Indeed, to understand the development of epizootics and transmission to humans, one must consider the role of numerous vertebrates (humans and other animals, both wild and domestic) and many invertebrates.

Approximately 100 species of wild mammals, 9 species of domestic animals, 25 species of birds, and several species of fish and amphibians have been found to be infected naturally,[61] but probably fewer than a dozen species of mammals are important in the transmission of *F. tularensis*.[36] Lagomorphs (rabbits and hares) and some rodents (muskrats, voles) are highly susceptible to *F. tularensis*; sheep and domestic rabbits are susceptible but have a low sensitivity to the organism; cats, cattle, dogs, and horses virtually are insusceptible to infection. Vertebrate animals are called reservoirs, but they rarely are true reservoirs because most of them become sick and either die or recover, with elimination of the organism. The varying hare (snowshoe rabbit) is less susceptible to *F. tularensis* and may serve as a reservoir because of its high natural resistance and carrier state.[24]

Humans act as terminal hosts of *F. tularensis* because they do not transmit it to other humans or to other mammals. Persons especially at risk are hunters, trappers, meat processors, cooks, sheep herders and shearers, muskrat farmers, and laboratory workers. The incidence of tularemia in children is less than that in adults because exposure is less frequent. Infection is acquired by the same routes as for adults: vector bites, animal bites, and ingestion of infected, inadequately cooked meat. In reviewing the age incidence of tularemia in Arkansas (704 cases), Washburn and Tuohy[89] found the following order of risk: agricultural workers, rural housewives, and preschool and school age children.

Many invertebrates can be infected experimentally by *F. tularensis*, but relatively few are infected naturally. In 1924, Parker and Spencer[64] first described ticks as vectors for *F. tularensis* infection in guinea pigs. However, the role of ticks in the spread of the human disease was not recognized until 1949, when Washburn and Tuohy[89] reported that 56 per cent (391 of 704) of tularemia cases in Arkansas were associated with tick exposure. To date, ticks remain the most common vectors for *F. tularensis* in the United States and can serve as reservoirs because the organism can be transmitted from generation to generation by transovarian passage.[36]

At least 13 species of ticks have been found to be infected naturally by *F. tularensis*.[36] The species involved in the transmission to humans are *Dermacentor andersoni* (wood tick), *Dermacentor variabilis* (dog tick), and *Amblyomma americanum* (Lone Star tick). A fourth tick, *Haemaphysalis leporisalustris* (rabbit tick), is important in the epidemiology of tularemia. Although this tick does not transmit tularemia directly to humans, it perpetuates the cycle of infection by acting as the sylvatic vector between rabbits.[34]

When the tick feeds on an infected animal, the organisms penetrate through the gut into the hemolymph and are disseminated throughout the body, including the salivary glands. The tick then transmits the organisms by injecting them along with saliva when it feeds on another animal. In addition, transmission by tick fecal contamination also is likely. Ticks and biting flies (i.e., deer flies) and fleas probably are responsible for the continuing endemic disease in susceptible animals and for epizootic disease. Infrequently, mosquitoes and mites mechanically may transport *F. tularensis* from animal to animal or animal to humans.[36]

There are a few reported cases of tularemia acquired by cat bite.[7, 89] Because cats rarely are infected by *F. tularensis*, such transmission probably is due to mechanical transmission from the contaminated teeth or claws of a cat that has come into contact with or has fed on an infected animal. Cat bite may be an important source of disease in children.

PATHOGENESIS

Bacterial and Host Interactions

Much of the knowledge regarding the interactions between *F. tularensis* organisms and the host was derived from experimental studies using live attenuated strains. During the second World War, live attenuated strains of *F. tularensis* were developed in the Soviet Union in an effort to produce a vaccine.[68, 84] In 1956, a mixture of attenuated strains of *F. tularensis* was transferred from the Soviet Union to the United States. From this mixture, a strain of suitable virulence was selected, tested for safety and efficacy, and designated *F. tularensis* live vaccine strain.[16, 18, 40] This strain has been used extensively in experimental studies on the development of immunity in humans.

A single *F. tularensis* organism of a virulent strain can produce fatal infection in susceptible animals, such as mice, guinea pigs, and hamsters.[92] As few as 10 organisms of a virulent strain injected intradermally or 25 organisms given by aerosol may produce systemic disease in human volunteers.[40] Tularemia is followed by effective immunospecific protection of the host; reinfection has been documented in only nine persons.[6] Studies in which the infecting bacteria were suppressed by the use of a bacteriostatic agent, such as tetracycline, show that protective immunity seems to be activated about 2 weeks after onset of the disease. When tetracycline treatment was initiated on the day of onset of tularemia and given for 10 days, early relapses were common. When tetracycline treatment was administered for 14 days, relapses were less frequent, indicating that protective immunity had begun to arise.[72]

In animals and humans, *F. tularensis* elicits both the humoral and the cell-mediated immune response. Both reach maximal levels during the second week after infection.[10] Although the presence of IgA antibodies in nasal secretions correlates with resistance to infection by aerosolized organisms, earlier works by Bellanti and associates[3] have shown that humoral immunity plays a minor role in resistance to tularemia. However, more recent animal studies showed that protection against tularemia live vaccine strain can be transferred by immune mouse serum and depends on host interferon-γ and T cells.[69] It is possible that specific antibodies are involved initially in delaying the infection, allowing time for the induction for cytokine production and specific T-cell–mediated immunity. This is consistent with the observation that although neutrophils only have a minor role in resistance to infection, mice selectively depleted of neutrophils and eosinophils by treatment with a granulocyte-specific antibody are incapable of controlling infection with a sublethal inoculum of the live vaccine strain of tularensis.[75] In addition, mice depleted of $CD4^+$ T cells, $CD8^+$ T cells, or both remained capable of controlling and partly resolving a primary sublethal *F. tularensis* infection.[11]

Because *F. tularensis* is described as a facultative intracellular parasite, it generally is believed that host immunity ultimately depends on cell-mediated immunity, just as in *Listeria monocytogenes* and *Mycobacterium tuberculosis*.[76, 91] This has been confirmed by several trials showing that vaccination with killed tularemia preparations, although it induces agglutinating serum antibodies, provides poor protection.[6, 40, 71] Numerous studies have shown that passive transfer of mononuclear leukocytes from infected animals to noninfected animals conferred resistance when the nonimmunized animals were challenged with a virulent strain.[75]

Denaturation of protein or carbohydrate of a macromolecular antigen of *F. tularensis* has shown that T-cell reactivity is associated only with protein determinants, whereas human immune serum reacts mostly with carbohydrate determinants of the organism.[1, 17, 83]

Invasion and Disease Production

The organism may gain access to the human body through the skin, conjunctiva, oropharynx, respiratory tract, or gastrointestinal tract. It spreads by the lymphatics or hematogenously, and bacteremia usually develops during the first week of infection (3 to 12 days).[43] Infection commonly involves the skin, regional lymph nodes, liver, spleen, and lungs. Rarely, the gastrointestinal tract and the central nervous system also are involved.

Histopathologic examination of mammals experimentally infected with *F. tularensis* indicates that the organism disseminates and causes cellular changes in a manner typical of intracellular parasites. After the organism is introduced into a susceptible host, multiplication occurs locally, with early spread to regional lymph nodes within 48 to 96 hours.[18] The developing cutaneous ulcer or soft tissue focus goes through a series of changes, with polymorphonuclear leukocytes being replaced by macrophages. In time, there may be necrosis, epithelioid-cell infiltrates, giant-cell formation, and true granulomas.[32, 55, 74] Organisms are difficult to demonstrate in the tissues but occasionally are found at the periphery of the lesions. In addition to the classic necrotic and granulomatous lesions, there may be degeneration of the parenchyma in the liver and spleen, as well as marked hyperplasia of the reticuloendothelial system. The pace of the illness depends on the virulence of the strain, as well as inoculum size, portal of entry, and the immune status of the host. When organisms enter the blood circulation, typical endotoxemia may ensue, sometimes in association with acute rhabdomyolysis.[41]

Autopsies in fatal cases of tularemia in humans have confirmed the findings in experimental animals.[31, 49, 67] Lymph nodes from patients with nonfatal disease have shown follicular hyperplasia with conglomerates of macrophages and caseating granulomas.[44, 49, 51, 77] These findings are similar to those seen in miliary tuberculosis. In fact, tularemia and tuberculosis may be histopathologically distinguishable only because of the difference in timing of the development of tissue changes,[44] a difference related to the more rapid replication of *F. tularensis*.

CLINICAL MANIFESTATIONS

Regardless of the portal of entry, the mode of onset of tularemia and the general features of the disease are the same. The usual incubation period of tularemia is 3 to 4 days, with a range of 1 to 21 days. The onset of symptoms is abrupt. These symptoms include fever usually higher than 39.4° C (103° F), chills, headache, myalgia, vomiting, and occasionally photophobia. Fever may be continuous or biphasic with an intermittent period of defervescence. In untreated patients, fever may persist for more than 3 weeks. Physical findings usually include lymphadenopathy, hepatosplenomegaly, pharyngitis, and skin lesions. Temperature-pulse dissociation has been described.[22] A variety of skin rashes (e.g., maculopapular, vesicular, pustular, erythema nodosum, erythema multiforme) may appear during the second week of illness,[80] and subcutaneous nodules may be present.[43]

Laboratory studies, including complete blood count, erythrocyte sedimentation rate, urinalysis, and *Proteus* OX2/OX19 titers, usually are not helpful in the diagnosis of tularemia. Interestingly, sterile pyuria has been reported in patients with tularemia, 22 per cent in one study[22] and 32 per cent in another.[66] Sterile pyuria combined with a history of fever, dysuria, or low back pain had led to an erroneous diagnosis of urinary tract infection in 11 per cent of the patients reported by Evans and associates.[22] Atypical lymphocytosis also has been reported.[30]

There are six clinical syndromes of tularemia, which can be classified by the portal of entry: ulceroglandular, glandular, oculoglandular, typhoidal, oropharyngeal, and pneumonic.

Ulceroglandular Tularemia

Ulceroglandular tularemia is the most common form of the disease, constituting greater than 75 per cent of all cases (adults and children). The organism gains access through the skin. Approximately 2 days after the onset of general symptoms, the patient complains of tender, swollen lymph nodes, most commonly in the axillary or inguinal areas. Within 24 hours, the portal of entry may become evident when a painful swollen papule develops distal to the regional node. This papule ruptures, leaving a punched-out ulcer with raised edges. The ulcer is indolent and in untreated cases may persist for longer than a month. The skin over the involved nodes may be inflamed. In untreated cases, about half of the lymph nodes suppurate and drain. In other cases, the nodes remain firm, enlarged, and tender for several months. There may be a mild, generalized lymphadenopathy and enlargement of the liver and spleen.

Glandular Tularemia

The glandular form of tularemia is almost identical to the ulceroglandular form, except that the portal of entry can not be identified. It generally is thought to be an insignificant break in the skin. Isolated cases of cervical lymphadenopathy have been related causally to *F. tularensis* infection.

Oculoglandular Tularemia

With oculoglandular tularemia, the portal of entry is the conjunctival sac, which may be inoculated by rubbing with contaminated fingers, having contact with infected water, splashing of infected liquids, or inhaling of infected aerosols. The eyelids may become edematous and the conjunctivae inflamed and painful. Numerous small, sharply defined, yellowish nodules and ulcers may be present on the palpebral conjunctivae. The regional nodes, the preauricular nodes, and the submaxillary and cervical nodes are swollen, tender, and painful. In severe cases, the axillary nodes may be involved.[26]

Typhoidal Tularemia

Typhoidal tularemia presents as a fever of unknown cause. The symptoms are those of acute septicemia with no localized skin lesions and often without lymphadenopathy. The patients are seriously ill, and shock may develop. The symptoms and signs are toxemia, continuous fever, myalgias, and severe headache. Patients may be delirious and may exhibit meningismus. Patients often complain of severe pharyngeal pain, but pharyngeal lesions may not be evident. Diarrhea occurs in this form of tularemia, in both adults and children. Sometimes, a dry cough and retrosternal pain are present. Pleuropulmonary involvement is common in adults with typhoidal tularemia.[14] In children, typhoidal tularemia can be the result of ingestion of the causative agent, and there may be necrotic lesions throughout the bowel.[14] Inhalation of aerosolized organisms is a more common mode of acquisition in adults (laboratory workers, farmers).

Oropharyngeal Tularemia

The oropharyngeal form resembles the ulceroglandular form. The infection is introduced into the oropharyngeal mucosa via infected, inadequately cooked meat. The organisms enter through abrasions, or aerosolization may occur during chewing. Local involvement consists of acute tonsillitis with cervical adenitis. The tonsils may be covered by an exudate or membrane that extends in all directions and may resemble a diphtheritic membrane. Complaints of sore throat commonly are out of proportion to the visible pathology. Ulcers sometimes are present. The cervical nodes may suppurate. Infrequently, *F. tularensis* invades the lower portions of the gastrointestinal tract, in which case vomiting, diarrhea, and abdominal pain are prominent symptoms. Awareness of the ability of *F. tularensis* to cause oropharyngeal involvement is important for the physician caring for children.[38, 48]

Pneumonic Tularemia

The pneumonic form of disease is most common in laboratory workers and is the most severe and lethal form.[40] Pneumonic tularemia may be acquired by the aerogenic route, or pulmonary disease may be associated with other forms of tularemia, particularly the typhoidal type. Dienst[14] and Miller and Bates[56] have published outstanding descriptions of pleuropulmonary tularemia. The latter stress that the symptoms and signs of pleuropulmonary tularemia are nonspecific, varying with the location and degree of pulmonary involvement. The variable radiographic features may be confused with those of tuberculosis, mycotic infections, common bacterial pneumonia, lymphoma, or carcinoma of the lung. In Miller and Bates' series of 29 patients, 6 developed pleural effusion. Because of the necrotizing nature of the pathologic process, the lung may heal, with residual fibrosis or calcification. In other instances, the disease is so fulminant that death occurs before the pathologic features can progress fully.

Additional Clinical Manifestations

In all large series of reported cases, there are patients who develop subcutaneous nodules resembling those seen in sporotrichosis. The nodules usually are distributed on the anterior or posterior surface of the arm and may extend from the primary lesion to the regional lymph nodes. Initially, they are firm and movable. Later, they become fixed to the skin and may suppurate. They vary in size from less than a centimeter to greater than several centimeters, if they become confluent. As many as 30 single nodules may be present.

Other unusual presentations of tularemia include pericarditis, appendicitis, peritonitis, liver abscess, meningitis, encephalitis, osteomyelitis, rhabdomyolysis, and venous thrombosis.

The incidence of these forms in children is somewhat different from that in adults. Although the pneumonic form previously was thought to be relatively rare in children,[48] more recent studies on the changing epidemiology and clinical manifestations of this disease have shown that pneumonic tularemia is not uncommon.[39] In a 1985 study by Jacobs and associates,[39] 14 per cent of tularemia cases in children were the pneumonic form. This contrasts with no pulmonary involvement in a series of 48 cases of tularemia in children reported by Levy and associates[48] in 1950. The distribution of these forms of tularemia also varies with geographic location. In a report of 67 children with tularemia in Finland, 79 per cent of the cases were of the ulceroglandular form, and 8 per cent were glandular.[85] This distribution is significantly different from that in the United States. In the study by Jacobs and associates,[39] who reported 28 cases of tularemia in children, 45 per cent were ulceroglandular and 25 per cent glandular.[39] The authors of the Finnish study attribute the higher proportion of the ulceroglandular form in their study to heightened awareness of the disease and early diagnosis. They believed that because tularemia is common in northern Finland, the patients usually recognize the disease and seek medical help so early that the primary ulcerations still are visible. This could explain why the glandular form was so rare in their series. In addition, the differences also could be explained by the different strains of *F. tularensis* and different vectors in the two regions.

DIAGNOSIS

The diagnosis of tularemia is established by a thorough history of possible exposure, clinical manifestations, and serial serology tests. A careful family history often is rewarding because several family members commonly are infected simultaneously. In some instances, however, a history is never elicited. Tularemia has no absolute pathognomonic features. In diagnosing tularemia, the physician must account for the endemic rate of the disease in the area, the season of the year, the clinical manifestations of the disease, and the unresponsiveness of the disease to antibiotics that are not effective against tularemia.

Diagnosis is confirmed by the standard agglutination test, which is commercially available and reliable. Unfortunately, it does not provide an early diagnosis because agglutinating antibodies usually are not detectable until the second week of illness. Occasionally, seroconversion is not confirmed until 4 to 6 weeks of illness. In rare cases, agglutinating antibody may never be detected. A fourfold increase in the convalescent titer confirms the diagnosis, but a presumptive diagnosis should be considered with acute titers greater than or equal to 1:160. This titer may indicate current or past infection, but in a clinically suspicious case, it should be considered as an indication for presumptive therapy. Patients with active disease often develop titers of greater than or equal to 1:1280 as the initial manifestation of seroconversion.

The agglutination test is specific, but cross-reaction with *Brucella* and occasionally with cholera vaccine (in recent recipients) has been reported. This can be clarified easily by simultaneous testing with the individual antigens (tularemia and brucellosis). Antibiotic therapy does not prevent the development of agglutinating antibodies.

An enzyme-linked immunosorbent assay with bacterial sonicate antigen (ELISA-S) determines the presence of IgM, IgG, and IgA antibodies to *F. tularensis*.[88] This test has the advantage of confirming the diagnosis of tularemia earlier in the illness than the agglutinating test. Like other ELISA-based methods that have been developed recently, however, the ELISA-S test is not commercially available.

Another method of early diagnosis of tularemia is the whole blood lymphocyte stimulation test.[45, 79] During an epidemic in Finland in 1983, this technique was compared with the bacterial agglutination test in the diagnosis of 200 cases. The lymphocyte stimulation test yielded positive results in 21 per cent of cases during the first week of illness and in 97 per cent during the second week. In contrast, the bacterial agglutination test detected only 2 per cent of the cases in the first week and 53 per cent in the second week.

The skin test (Foshay) is an accurate method of diagnosis[5] and is positive earlier in the illness than the agglutination test, but the skin test antigen is not commercially available.

Of the other diagnostic modalities recently evaluated, a polymerase chain reaction–based assay holds promise for early detection of *F. tularensis* infection.[50] This assay is not commercially available.

Gram-stained smears of patient specimens, such as exudate and sputum, usually do not reveal the organism. However, there is no danger in collecting the specimens, and examination of direct smears helps rule out other causative agents. Specimens should not be cultured for *F. tularensis* in the usual hospital or diagnostic laboratory because isolation of these organisms in facilities other than a level P-3 laboratory is hazardous to the laboratory personnel. If confirmation by culture is indicated, physicians should notify the laboratory of the potential for the specimen to contain *F. tularensis* so that appropriate laboratory precautions can be taken.

The differential diagnosis of tularemia depends on the clinical form of the disease. Ulceroglandular and glandular tularemia must be differentiated from disease due to ordinary bacterial pathogens, such as *Streptococcus* and *Staphylococcus*, disease due to *M. tuberculosis* and atypical mycobacteria, and cat-scratch disease. In older patients who present with inguinal lymphadenopathy, lymphogranuloma venereum, granuloma inguinale, and other sexually transmitted diseases should be considered. Occasionally, sporotrichosis and infectious mononucleosis are diagnosed in these patients. Oculoglandular fever is somewhat more distinctive, but disease due to common bacterial pathogens must be ruled out. Oropharyngeal tularemia must be differentiated from streptococcal tonsillopharyngitis and corynebacterial disease. Typhoidal tularemia can be confused with ordinary bacteremia and must be differentiated from the more common bacterial and enteric disease as well as the more classic typhoid fever. Tularemic pneumonia must be differentiated from other bacterial as well as nonbacterial pneumonia, including tuberculosis, *Mycoplasma* infection, legionnaires' disease, psittacosis, viral pneumonia, Q fever, fungal infection, and chemical pneumonitis.

TREATMENT

Streptomycin traditionally is the drug of choice for the treatment of tularemia. The recommended dose is 30 mg/kg/day to 40 mg/kg/day administered intramuscularly in two divided doses for 7 days. If a patient has mild symptoms initially or responds dramatically to therapy, it is possible to use an alternative streptomycin regimen of 30 mg/kg/day to 40 mg/kg/day for 3 days followed by 15 mg/kg/day to 20 mg/kg/day for 4 days given intramuscularly. In severe cases or if a child does not become afebrile and asymptomatic within a few days of therapy, extension of treatment beyond 7 days is indicated. Streptomycin-resistant strains of tularemia are reported, but they are rare.[63] Defervescence and alleviation of other signs and symptoms are prompt, usually occurring within several days. Response may be delayed if lymph nodes have progressed to suppuration.

Because of the recent shortage of streptomycin within the United States,* alternative antibiotic regimens must be considered. Unfortunately, because there has been a lack of controlled clinical trials of the newer antibiotics in the treatment of tularemia, experience with alternative antibiotic regimens is limited. In a review of the various treatments of tularemia reported in the literature, Enderlin and associates[19] concluded that streptomycin still is the drug of choice, with a cure rate of 97 per cent and no relapse. Gentamicin is an acceptable alternative to streptomycin, with a cure rate of 86 per cent and a relapse incidence of 6 per cent. These authors attributed some of the treatment failure with gentamicin to delay in the initiation of therapy and the short duration of therapy in some severe cases, as well as to other underlying medical problems.[19] The recommended dosage of gentamicin for tularemia is 5 mg/kg/day divided into two intramuscular doses.

Bacteriostatic agents, such as tetracycline and chloramphenicol, also have been used to treat tularemia with cure rates of 88 per cent and 77 per cent, respectively. However, these agents are considered suboptimal in the treatment of tularemia because of a high incidence of relapse after therapy is stopped (12 per cent for tetracycline and 22 per cent for chloramphenicol).[19]

Although in vitro susceptibility testing indicates that the third-generation cephalosporins may be effective against *F. tularensis*, one report showed treatment failure in eight children given ceftriaxone.[12] Treatment with other antibiotics reported sporadically in the literature include one successful case with imipenem and cilastatin,[47] six successful cases with ciprofloxacin or norfloxacin in adults,[73, 81] and four isolated cases with erythromycin.[33]

Children receiving streptomycin should be monitored for ototoxicity. Hearing screening before initiation of streptomycin or gentamicin therapy should be considered. If there is preexisting hearing loss, the alternative streptomycin regimen or gentamicin therapy with close monitoring of serum levels in severe cases can be considered. Audiologic evaluation is indicated after therapy in these cases.

Bed rest and supportive therapy are, of course, indicated. In the severely ill patient who shows signs of endotoxic shock, appropriate monitoring and intensive care unit admission are indicated, and corticosteroid therapy should be considered. Suppurative nodes may require surgical drainage.

*As of November 1995, streptomycin is available from Pfizer Streptomycin Program, Pfizer Pharmaceuticals, New York, NY (800-254-4445).

Prior to the advent of effective antimicrobial therapy, tularemia often was a protracted illness, lasting weeks or months. Then there was a long period of convalescence necessitated by debility. Antibiotics have interrupted the natural history of the disease. When the disease is diagnosed promptly, the course generally is less than a month. As a result of administering appropriate antibiotic therapy, the mortality rate has declined from 5 per cent to 30 per cent to less than 1 per cent, except in cases of fulminant pneumonic and typhoid diseases.

PREVENTION

Prevention of human tularemia depends on prevention of exposure to either the vectors or contaminated animal tissue. Children living in areas of tick endemicity should have their skin and hair checked frequently for ticks. Ticks should be removed carefully with tweezers (not with fingernails) by pulling perpendicular to the skin where they have attached.[57] Care should be taken not to squeeze the tick between the fingers. Persons living in tick-infested areas should wear clothing with tightly fitting cuffs at the wrists and ankles when staying outdoors. Tick repellents should be used on children with caution.

Children should be cautioned against handling sick or dead rodents or rabbits. Rabbits caught by household pets should be disposed of by incineration or burial. Rubber gloves should be worn for preparing game animals, and the meat should be cooked thoroughly before eating. Hunters, especially rabbit hunters, should take precautions against tularemia.

The only tularemia vaccine currently available in the United States is the *F. tularensis* live vaccine strain developed in 1960. It is unlicensed and classified as an investigational product, but it is available to laboratory personnel. This vaccine appears to have reduced significantly the incidence of typhoidal tularemia and the severity of ulceroglandular disease in laboratory personnel. The efficacy of this vaccine for prevention of naturally occurring disease in the United States is unknown.

References

1. Allen, W. P.: Immunity against tularemia: Passive protection of mice by transfer of immune tissues. J. Exp. Med. *115*:411–420, 1962.
2. Anonymous: Summary of notifiable diseases: United States, 1990. M. M. W. R. *39*:1–61, 1991.
3. Bellanti, J. A., Buescher, E. L., Brandt, W. E., et al.: Characterization of human serum and nasal hemagglutinating antibody in *Francisella tularensis*. J. Immunol. *98*:171–178, 1967.
4. Boyce, J. M.: Recent trends in the epidemiology of tularemia in the United States. J. Infect. Dis. *131*:197–199, 1914.
5. Buchanan, T. M., Brooks, G. F., and Brachman, P. S.: The tularemia skin test. Ann. Intern. Med. *74*:336–343, 1971.
6. Burke, D. S.: Immunization against tularemia: Analysis of the effectivenous of live *Francisella tularensis* vaccine in prevention of laboratory-acquired tularemia. J. Infect. Dis. *135*:55–60, 1977.
7. Callaway, G. D., Peterson, S. S., and Good, J. T.: Tularemia in southwest Missouri. Missouri Med. *51*:906–909, 1954.
8. Casper, E. A., and Phillip, R. N.: A skin test survery of tularemia in a Montana sheep-raising county. Public Health Rep. *84*:611–615, 1969.
9. Centers for Disease Control: Tularemia. M. M. W. R. Annual Summary *31*:89, 1982.
10. Claflin, J. L., and Larson, C. L.: Infection-immunity in tularemia: Specificity of cellular immunity. Infect. Immun. *5*:311–317, 1972.
11. Conlan, J. W., Sjostedt, A., and North, R. J.: $CD4^+$ and $CD8^+$ T-cell-dependent and independent host defense mechanisms can operate to control and resolve primary and secondary *Francisella tularensis* LVS infection in mice. Infect. Immun. *62*:5603–5607, 1994.
12. Cross, J. T., and Jacobs, R. F.: Tularemia: Treatment failures with outpatient use of ceftriaxone. Clin. Infect. Dis. *17*:76–80, 1993.
13. Dahlstrand, S., Ringertz, O., and Zetterberg, B.: Airborn tularemia in Sweden. Scand. J. Infect. Dis. *3*:7–16, 1971.
14. Dienst, F. T., Jr.: Tularemia: A perusal of three hundred thirty-nine cases. J. La. State Med. Soc. *115*:114–127, 1963.
15. Eigelsbach, H. T., Chambers, L. A., and Coriell, L. L.: Electron microscopy of *Bacterium tularense*. J. Bacteriol. *52*:179–185, 1946.
16. Eigelsbach, H. T., Hornick, R. B., and Tulis, J. J.: Recent studies on live tularemia vaccine. Med. Ann. D. C. *36*:282–286, 1967.
17. Eigelsbach, H. T., Hunter, D. H., Janssen, W. A., et al.: Murine model for study of cell-mediated immunity: Protection against death from fully virulent *Francisella tularensis* infection. Infect. Immun. *12*:999–1005, 1915.
18. Eigelsbach, H. T., Tulis, J. J., McGavran, M. H., et al.: Live tularemia vaccine: Host-parasite relationship in monkeys vaccinated intracutaneously or aerogemically. J. Bacteriol. *84*:1020–1027, 1962.
19. Enderlin, G., Morales, L., Jacobs, R. F., et al.: Streptomycin and alternative agents for the treatment of tularemia: Review of the literature. Clin. Infect. Dis. *19*:42–47, 1994.
20. Engelfried, J. J.: Antibodies to *Pasteurella tularensis* in a selected human population. Milit. Med. *135*:723–726, 1968.
21. Evans, M. E.: *Francisella tularensis*. Infect. Control *6*:381–383, 1985.
22. Evans, M. E., Gregary, D. W., Schaffner, W., et al.: Tularemia: A 30-year experience with 88 cases. Medicine *64*:251–269, 1985.
23. Finegold, M. J., Pulliam, J. D., Landay, M.E., et al.: Pathological changes in rabbits injected with *Pasteurella tularensis* killed by ionizing radiation. J. Infect. Dis. *119*:635–640, 1969.
24. Foshay, L.: Tularemia. Ann. Rev. Microbiol. *4*:313–330, 1950.
25. Francis, E.: A new disease of man. J. A. M. A. *78*:1015, 1922.
26. Francis, E.: A summary of the present knowledge of tularemia. Medicine *7*:411–432, 1928.
27. Francis, E.: Oculoglandular tularemia. Arch. Ophthalmol. *28*:711–741, 1942.
28. Francis, E., and Mayne, B.: Public Health Rep. *36*:1938–1946, 1921.
29. Francis, E.: Sources of infection and seasonal incidence of tularemia in man. Public Health Rep. *52*:103–113, 1937.
30. Gelfand, M. S., Mehra, N., and Simmons, B. P.: Tularemia and atypical lymphocytosis. J. Tenn. Med. Assoc. *82*:417–418, 1989.
31. Goodpasture, E. W., and House, S. J.: The pathologic anatome of tularemia in man. Am. J. Pathol. *4*:213–216, 1928.
32. Hall, W. C., Kovatch, R. M., and Schricker, R. L.: Tularemic pneumonia: Pathogenesis of the aerosol-induced disease in monkeys. J. Pathol. *110*:193–201, 1973.
33. Harrell, R. E., Jr., and Simmons, H. F.: Pleuropulmonary tularemia: Successful treatment with erythromycin. South. Med. J. *83*:1363–1364, 1990.
34. Harwood, R. F., and James, M. T. (eds.): Entomology in Human and Animal Health. New York, Macmillan, 1973, pp. 403–404.
35. Hesselbrock, W. B., and Foshay, L.: The morphology of *Bacterium tulanense*. J. Bacteriol. *49*:209–231, 1945.
36. Hopla, C. E.: The ecology of tularemia. Adv. Vet. Sci. Comp. Med. *18*:25–53, 1974.
37. Hornick, R. B.: Tularemia. *In* Hoeprich, P. D. (ed.): Infectious Diseases. New York, Harper & Row, 1972, pp. 1043–1049.
38. Hughes, W. T., Jr., and Etteldorf, J. N.: Oropharyngeal tularemia. J. Pediatr. *51*:363–372, 1957.
39. Jacobs, R. F., Condrey, Y. M., and Yamauchi, T.: Tularemia in adults and children: A changing presentation. Pediatrics *76*:818–822, 1985.
40. Jaslaw, S., Eigelsback, H. T., Prior, J. A., et al.: Tularemia vaccine study. I. Intracutaneous challenge. Arch. Intern. Med. *107*:689–701, 1961.
41. Kaiser, A. B., Rieves, O., Price, A. H., et al.: Tularemia and rhabdomyolysis. J. A. M. A. *253*:241–243, 1985.
42. Karpoff, S. P., and Antonoff, N. I.: The spread of tularemia through water, as a new factor in its epidemiology. J. Bacteriol. *32*:243–258, 1936.
43. Kavanaugh, C. N.: Tularemia: A consideration of one hundred and twenty three cases with observations at autopsy in one. Arch. Intern. Med. *55*:61–85, 1935.
44. Kitamura, S., Fukada, M., Takeda, H., et al.: Pathology of tularemia. Acta Pathol. Jpn. *6*(Suppl.):719–764, 1956.
45. Koskela, P., and Merv, E.: Cell-mediated and humoral immunity induced by a live *Francisella tularensis* vaccine. Infect. Immun. *36*:983–989, 1982.
46. Larson, B. W., and Jacobson, H. J.: Tularemia with unusual laboratory characteristics in South Dakota children. S. D. J. Med. *37*:5–10, 1984.
47. Lee, H. C., Horowitz, E., and Linder, W.: Treatment of tularemia with imipenem/cilastatin sodium. South. Med. J. *84*:1277–1278, 1991.
48. Levy, H. S., Webb, C. H., and Wilkinson, J. D.: Tularemia as a pediatric problem. Pediatrics *6*:113–122, 1950.
49. Lillie, R. D., and Francis, G.: The pathology of tularemia in man (*Homo sapiens*). *In* The Pathology of Tularemia [National Institutes of Health Bulletin 167]. Washington, D.C., Public Health Service, 1936, pp. 1–81.
50. Long, G. W., Oprandy, J. J., Narayanan, R. B., et al.: Detection of *Francisella tularensis* in blood by polymerase chain reaction. J. Clin. Microbiol. *31*:152–154, 1993.
51. Ludmerer, K. M., and Kissane, J. M. (eds.): Fever, leukopenia, acute renal failure and death in a 65-year-old man. Am. J. Med. *77*:117–124, 1984.
52. Markwitl, L. E., Hynes, N. A., de la Cruz, P., et al.: Tick-borne tularemia: An outbreak of lymphadenopathy in children. J. A. M. A. *254*:2922–2925, 1985.

53. McCoy, G. N.: A plague-like disease in rodents. Public Health Bull. *43*:53, 1911.
54. McCoy, G. N., and Chapin, C. W.: Further observations on a plague-like disease of rodents with a preliminary note on the causative agent: *Bacterium tularense*. J. Infect. Dis. *10*:61–72, 1912.
55. McGowran, M. H., White, J. D., Eigelsbach, H. T., et al.: Morphologic and immunohistochemical studies of the pathogenesis of infection and antibody formation subsequent to vaccination of macacavirus with an attenuated strain of *Pasteurella tularensis*. I. Intracutaneous vaccination. Am. J. Pathol. *41*:259–271, 1962.
56. Miller, R. P., and Bates, J. H.: Pleuropulmonary tularemia. Am. Rev. Respir. Dis. *99*:31–41, 1969.
57. Needham, G. R.: Evaluation of five popular methods for tick removal. Pediatrics *75*:997–1002, 1985.
58. Ohara, H.: Jikken Dobutsu. Exp. Amin. *11*:508–523, 1925.
59. Ohara, H.: Kensei Igaker *12*:401–410, 1926.
60. Ohara, H.: Studies on Ohare's disease. Jpn. J. Exp. Med. *24*:69–79, 1954.
61. Olsen, P. F.: Tularemia. *In* Hubbert, W. T., McCullock, W. F., and Schnurrenberger, P. R. (eds.): Diseases Transmitted from Animals to Man. Springfield, IL, Charles C Thomas, 1975, pp. 191–223.
62. Ormsbee, R. A., Bell, J. F., and Larson, C. L.: The isolation, purification and biological activity of the antigenic preparations from *Bacterium tularense*. J. Immunol. *74*:351–359, 1955.
63. Overhold, E. L., Tigertt, W. D., Kadull, P. J., et al.: Analysis of forty-two cases of laboratory acquired tularemia: Treatment with broad spectrum antibiotics. Am. J. Med. *30*:785–806, 1961.
64. Parker, R. R., and Spencer, R. R.: Public Health Rep. *39*:1057–1073, 1924.
65. Pearse, R. A.: Insect bite. Northwest Med. *3*:81, 1911.
66. Penn, R. L., and Kinasewitz, G. T.: Factors associated with a poor outcome in tularemia. Arch. Intern. Med. *147*:265–268. 1987.
67. Permar, H. H., and Maclachlan, W. W. G.: Tularemic pneumonia. Ann. Intern. Med. *5*:687–698, 1931.
68. Pollitzer, R.: History and incidence of tularemia in the Soviet Union: A review. Bronx, NY, The Institute of Contemporary Russian Studies, Fordham University, 1967.
69. Rhinehart-Jones, T. R., Fortier, A. H., and Elkins, K. L.: Transfer of immunity against lethal murine *Francisella* infection by specific antibody depends on host gamma interferon and T cells. Infect. Immun. *62*:3129–3137, 1994.
70. Rockwood, S. W.: Tularemia: What's in a name? Am. Soc. Microbiol. *49*:63–65, 1983.
71. Saslaw, S., Eigelsbach, H. T., Prior, J. A., et al.: Tularemia vaccine study. II. Respiratory challenge. Arch. Intern. Med. *107*:702–714, 1961.
72. Sawyer, W. D., Dangerfield, H. G., Hogge, A. L., et al.: Antiobiotic prophylaxis and therapy of airborne tularemia. Bacteriol. Rev. *30*:542–550, 1965.
73. Scheel, O., Reiersen, R., and Hoel, T.: Treatment of tularemia with ciprofloxacin. Eur. J. Clin. Microbiol. Infect. Dis. *11*:447–448, 1992.
74. Schricker, R. L., Eigelsbach, H. T., Mitten, J. Q., et al.: Pathogenesis of tularemia in monkeys aerogenically exposed to *Francisella tularensis* 425. Infect. Immun. *5*:734–744, 1972.
75. Sjostedt, A., Conlan, J. W., and North, R. J.: Neutrophils are critical for host defense against primary infection with the facultative intracellular bacterium *Francisella tularensis* in mice and participate in defense against reinfection. Infect. Immun. *62*:2770–2783, 1994.
76. Suter, E.: Passive transfer of acquired resistance to infection with *Mycobacterium tuberculosis* by means of cells. Am. Rev. Respir. Dis. *83*:535–543, 1961.
77. Sutinen, S., Syrjala, H., Anttila, S., et al.: Histopathology of human lymph node tularemia caused by *Francisella tularensis* var *palaearctica*. Acta Pathol. Lab. Med. *110*:42–46, 1986.
78. Suvorov, S. V., Volfertz, A. A., and Voronkova, M. M.: Vestn. Mikrobiol. *7*:293–299, 1928.
79. Syrjala, H., Herva, E., Ilonen, J., et al.: A whole blood lymphocyte stimulation test in human tularemia. J. Infect. Dis. *150*:912–915, 1984.
80. Syrjala, H., Karvonen, J., and Salminen, A.: Skin manifestations of tularemia: A study of 88 cases in northern Finland during 16 years (1967–1983). Acta Derm. Venereol. *64*:513–516, 1984.
81. Syrjala, H., Schildt, R., and Raijainen, S.: In vitro susceptibility of *Francisella tularensis* to fluoroquinolones and treatment of tularemia with norfloxacin and ciprofloxacin. Eur. J. Clin. Microbiol. Infect. Dis. *10*:68–70, 1991.
82. Tellison, W. L., Epler, D. C., Kunns, E., et al.: Tularemia in man from a domestic rural water supply. Public Health Rep. *65*:1219–1226, 1950.
83. Thorpe, B. D., and Marcus, S.: Phagocytosis and intracellular fate of *Pasteurella tularensis*. III. In vivo studies with passively transferred cells and sera. J. Immunol. *94*:578–585, 1965.
84. Tigertt, W. D.: Soviet viable *Pasteurella tularensis* vaccines: A review of selected articles. Bacteriol. Rev. *26*:254–373, 1962.
85. Uhari, M., Syrjala, H., and Salminen, A.: Tularemia in children caused by *Francisella tularensis biovar palaearctica*. Pediatr. Infect. Dis. J. *9*:80–83, 1990.
86. Vail, D. T.: Ophthalmic Res. *23*:487, 1914.
87. Van Metre, T. E., Jr., and Kadull, P. J.: Laboratory-acquired tularemia in vaccinated individuals: A report of 62 cases. Ann. Intern. Med. *50*:621–632, 1959.
88. Vilianen, M. K., Nurmi, T., and Salminen, A.: Enzyme linked immunosorbent assay (ELISA) with bacterial sonicate antigen for IgM, IgA and IgG antibodies to *Francisella tularensis*: Comparison with bacterial agglutination test and ELISA with lipopolysaccharide antigen. J. Infect. Dis. *148*:715–720, 1983.
89. Washburn, A. M., and Tuohy, J. R.: The changing picture of tularemia in Arkansas. South. Med. J. *42*:60–62, 1949.
90. Wherry, W. B., and Lamb, B. H.: Infection of man with *Bacterium tularense*. J. Infect. Dis. *15*:331–340, 1914.
91. Zinkernagel, R. M.: Restriction by H-2 gene complex of transfer of cell-mediated immunity to *Listeria monocytogenes*. Nature *251*:230–233, 1974.
92. Zinsser, H.: *Francisella*. *In* Joklich, W. K., Willett, H. P., and Amos, D. B. (eds.): Zinsser Microbiology. 18th ed. E. Norwalk, CT, Appleton-Century-Crofts, 1984, pp. 649–655.

139

HAEMOPHILUS INFLUENZAE

Joel I. Ward and Kenneth M. Zangwill

Relatively few species of the genus *Haemophilus* are pathogenic to man, and nearly all that cause human disease are either encapsulated or unencapsulated strains of *H. influenzae*. These bacteria are small gram-negative pleomorphic coccobacilli that generally are considered to be normal constituents of the microbial flora of the upper respiratory tract of man. The strains without polysaccharide capsules often cause infections of mucosal surfaces, such as otitis media, bronchitis, conjunctivitis, sinusitis, and types of pneumonia. Encapsulated strains, especially *H. influenzae* type b (Hib) strains, cause invasive diseases such as septicemia, meningitis, septic arthritis, cellulitis, epiglottitis, pneumonia, and empyema. Before Hib vaccines became widely available, *H. influenzae* was the leading cause of bacterial meningitis in the United States and in most other countries, and it also was an important cause of other bacteremic illnesses, primarily in young children. Other *Haemophilus* species, including *H. influenzae* (biogroup aegyptius), *H. ducreyi* (chancroid), *H. parainfluenzae*, *H. parahaemolyticus*, and *H. aphrophilus*, less commonly cause human infections.

The organism first was described in 1892 by Robert Pfeiffer, who isolated it from the lung and sputum of patients during the 1889–1892 pandemic of influenza. He proposed that the organism was the cause of influenza, and it initially was known as the Pfeiffer influenza bacillus.[170] The bacteria were difficult to culture on routine culture media, until it was appreciated that supplementation of X (hemin) and V (nicotinamide-adenine-dinucleotide [NAD]) factors were required for its growth. By the turn of the century, the organism had been recovered from the blood and cerebrospinal fluid (CSF) of young children with meningitis. Although doubts remained about the etiologic role of the Pfeiffer bacillus as the cause of influenza, it was not until the influenza pandemic of 1918 that its etiologic role was questioned seriously. In

1920, the organism was renamed *H. influenzae* to acknowledge its inappropriate historic association with influenza and to emphasize its requirement of blood factors for growth (from the Greek *haemophilus*, or "blood-loving").[248] In 1933, the viral etiology of influenza was discovered, which refuted any remaining confusion about the erroneous association between *H. influenzae* and influenza virus.

Key concepts relevant to the development of treatment and prevention modalities derive from the pioneering work in the early 1930s of Margaret Pittman.[173, 174] Paralleling earlier research on the pneumococcus, she defined two major categories of *H. influenzae*: encapsulated and unencapsulated strains. Among the encapsulated strains, she characterized six distinct serotypes (designated a through f), which now are known to differ biochemically in the composition of their polysaccharide capsules. She observed that Hib strains were recovered primarily from blood and CSF of young patients with meningitis, and that unencapsulated strains and other *H. influenzae* serotypes were recovered primarily from respiratory tract secretions. Furthermore, she demonstrated that antibody to Hib capsule conferred type-specific protection against lethal infection in rabbits. This observation led to the use of antiserum as the first treatment for disease, prepared by immunization with formalin-killed Hib, initially in horses and later in rabbits. Prior to this, Hib meningitis and other forms of invasive Hib disease almost always were fatal.[223] However, it was not until the late 1930s that treatment of children with meningitis using both Hib antiserum and sulfonamides substantially reduced the case fatality rate.[2, 3]

In 1933, Fothergill and Wright[72] described the age-related risk of *H. influenzae* meningitis, which affected mostly young children younger than 5 years of age. Importantly, they noted the correlation between the age-related disease risk and the absence of bactericidal antibodies. It was shown later that the major antibody contributing to the protective activity of bactericidal serum was antibody to Hib capsule.[108, 200] These observations suggested that naturally acquired type b anticapsular antibody is protective and that the early stimulation of protective immunity using vaccines might be possible.

Unfortunately, the advent of effective antimicrobial agents focused attention away from the need for primary prevention. Even with effective antimicrobial therapies and excellent hospital care, significant mortality (about 5 per cent) and neurologic morbidity (about 20 per cent) remained. Ultimately, the appreciation that the morbidity and mortality of disease could never be eliminated completely by treatment gave impetus to the development of vaccines for prevention.

In the early 1970s, investigators purified and characterized the type b capsular polysaccharide (polyribosyl-ribitol-phosphate [PRP]) and proposed it as a potential vaccine candidate. Ultimately, the protective efficacy of a PRP vaccine against invasive Hib disease was shown in older children in a 1974 field trial conducted in Finland.[166] This and other studies culminated in the licensure of PRP vaccine in the United States in 1985, thus becoming the first vaccine available for the prevention of Hib disease. Unfortunately, this vaccine induced equivocal immune responses and incomplete protection among older children and provided no protection for young infants, those at greatest disease risk.[238] Improved vaccines employed polysaccharide-protein conjugate techniques, and four such vaccines were licensed for use in children. Three of these vaccines were shown to protect young infants[18, 195] against Hib disease, and with the universal immunization of young infants, the near elimination of invasive Hib disease has been attained in many populations.[1, 19, 167]

In this chapter, reviews of the microbiology, pathogenesis, immunology, clinical spectrum, diagnosis, epidemiology, treatment and prevention of *H. influenzae* infections are presented. Brief discussions of disease caused by other *Haemophilus* species also are included.

MICROBIOLOGY

Growth

H. influenzae is a small gram-negative coccobacillus that in clinical specimens can appear to be filamentous or pleomorphic, especially when obtained from patients who have received prior antibiotics. The organism is nonmotile, non–spore-forming, and facultatively anaerobic and requires two supplemental factors for in vitro growth. The X factor (hemin) is a heat-stable, iron-containing protoporphyrin essential for activity of the electron-transport chain, which is important for aerobic growth. The heat-labile V factor is a co-enzyme, NAD. Both factors are present within erythrocytes and are released by appropriate heating or enzyme lysis of the red cells, which permit growth on chocolate agar. The requirement for these factors for growth remains the primary basis for the laboratory differentiation of *H. influenzae* from other *Haemophilus* species.[10]

The growth of *H. influenzae* is fastidious, and clinical specimens need to be inoculated promptly onto appropriate media, such as chocolate agar. The organism can be grown in most enriched liquid or solid media supplemented with X and V factors. Although not mandatory for growth, 5 to 10 per cent carbon dioxide makes some strains grow better. In blood or liquid media, *H. influenzae* may not grow to sufficient quantity to result in visual turbidity; therefore, to detect positive cultures, blood and CSF cultures should be assayed for carbon dioxide release or routinely subcultured at 24 to 48 hours. After overnight incubation on solid media, colonies appear that are 0.5 to 1.5 mm in diameter and usually are rough or granular in appearance. Encapsulated strains usually produce slightly larger colonies that are mucoid or glistening. Fermentation reactions and other metabolic activities are variable and therefore not particularly useful for identification. However, a biotyping scheme, based on the metabolism of indole, urea, and ornithine decarboxylase activity, has been used to subtype strains.

Capsular Polysaccharide

Several surface structures of *H. influenzae* appear to be important determinants of the organism's pathogenicity. Strains can have one of six serotypic polysaccharide capsules (a, b, c, d, e, f) or lack capsules (nontypable strains). The Hib capsule is of particular clinical, pathogenic, and immunologic importance because Hib accounts for 95 per cent of all strains that cause invasive disease (bacteremia or meningitis).[137] The Hib polysaccharide consists of a repeating polymer of ribosyl and ribitol phosphate (PRP) having a 1-1 linkage. The genes involved with Hib capsule production have been cloned and consist of two repeating 17-kb DNA fragments separated by a 1-kb bridge region (hex A)[101]; 98 per cent of Hib tested contain this duplication. Encapsulation often is unstable, with the loss of capsule production associated with loss of one 17-kb repeat. These strains produce type b capsule but in barely detectable amounts. Importantly, the release of Hib capsular antigen in body fluids of infected individuals can be detected by specific immunologic techniques (i.e., latex agglutination) which are useful for rapid diagnosis. The other capsular serotypes are composed of hexose rather than pentose sugars and only occasionally cause invasive disease. Types e and f less commonly cause invasive disease.

Outer-Membrane Proteins

The cell envelope of gram-negative bacteria consists of a cytoplasmic membrane, a peptidoglycan layer, and an outer membrane. The outer membrane contains protein, lipopolysaccharides, and phospholipid. Electron microscopy of encapsulated and nonencapsulated strains of *H. influenzae* demonstrate a cell envelope similar to that of other gram-negative bacteria. The importance of outer-membrane proteins (OMPs) in the pathogenesis of and immunity to *H. influenzae* disease is not clear. Some membrane proteins are involved with cell transport (porins), others are adhesins, and the functions of others remain undefined. Pili or fimbriae are protein filaments that extend from the outer-membrane and appear to mediate attachment of the organism to epithelial cells.[231] Their expression appears to be reversible, but the importance of these adhesins in the pathogenesis of disease is not well understood.

Methods have been developed for differentiating isolates of Hib by differences in electrophoretic mobility patterns of the major OMPs, and this has been useful for epidemiologic studies[85, 129] and to identify potential vaccine immunogens. Although there are two to three dozen proteins, there are four to six major proteins. To date, specific OMP patterns have not been associated clearly with virulence. However, some proteins are well conserved and can be found in essentially all *H. influenzae* strains. Specifically, proteins P1 (50,000 kDa), P2 (36,000 to 41,000 kDa), and P6 (16,600 kDa) appear to be present in all strains. They are cell surface exposed and induce bactericidal antibodies that are protective in animal challenge studies.[149, 159]

Lipopolysaccharides

The lipopolysaccharide (LPS) of encapsulated *H. influenzae* has been characterized partially. Although chemically different from the LPS of Enterobacteriaceae, the biologic activities of *H. influenzae* LPS appear similar. Hib LPS preparation produces a dermal Shwartzman reaction, is lethal to mice, causes a febrile response in rabbits, evokes polyclonal B-cell activation, and has limulus lysate activity. Human leukocytes incubated with a Hib LPS generate a potent procoagulant activity,[145] which may be relevant to the understanding of the mechanisms responsible for intravascular coagulation in severe Hib infections. LPS or endotoxin of Hib is important in the pathogenicity of the organism and appears to have little antigenic diversity,[245] although there is variability in LPS electrophoretic patterns after passage in vivo or in vitro. Consequently, electrophoretic characterization of endotoxin has not been useful as an epidemiologic tool.

Isoenzymes

Multilocus enzyme electrophoresis is a method used to characterize cytoplasmic isoenzymes of the organism. This method has been used to distinguish different Hib genotypes for epidemiologic purposes. The electrophoresis of a number of enzymes has distinguished isoenzyme differences that have been useful in genetic analyses of *H. influenzae* strains.[156] Population genetic evaluation of *H. influenzae* based on cluster analysis of multilocus enzyme electrophoretic typing has revealed that Hib strains are clonal.[155] Hib strains are distinct from nonencapsulated isolates, which are more genetically diverse.[154]

IgA Proteases

IgA proteases, bacterial enzymes whose only known substrate is human IgA-1, cleave the heavy chain at specific sites.[118–153] IgA proteases are regarded as potentially important virulence factors because mucosal defense is in part IgA mediated. *H. influenzae* produces three distinct types of IgA proteases that cleave different peptide bonds within the IgA-1 hinge region.[175]

Antibiotic Resistance

Another important microbiologic feature of *H. influenzae* has been the development of antibiotic resistance. Resistance to a wide variety of antibiotics (sulfonamides, trimethoprim-sulfamethoxazole, erythromycin, tetracycline, penicillin) has been described, but these antibiotics are not essential for therapy. Of greater importance is resistance to ampicillin, first noted in the mid-1970s,[51] because it was the primary antibiotic used for treatment of disease. Since then, ampicillin resistance has become widespread, now ranging between 5 and 40 per cent of all isolates in various parts of the world.[33, 110] The mechanism of resistance usually involves plasmid-mediated β-lactamase enzyme production, and resistant strains often are characterized by their plasmid or β-lactamase enzyme content.[110] Resistance to chloramphenicol usually is mediated by the enzyme chloramphenicol acetyltransferase.[186] Although chloramphenicol-resistant strains are rare in the United States, they are more prevalent in some areas of the world, and strains resistant to both ampicillin and chloramphenicol have been reported.[36, 225] Currently, third-generation cephalosporins are the mainstays of therapy for invasive disease; concern, however, about the potential for increasing resistance to these highly effective agents further emphasizes the need for means to prevent disease.

PATHOGENESIS

Acquisition and Carriage of Organisms

Illness caused by *H. influenzae* infection results from a series of pathogenic events, beginning with exposure to the organism, acquisition of infection, and colonization of respiratory mucosal membranes. Under natural conditions, *H. influenzae* exclusively is a pathogen of humans, and it usually is transmitted asymptomatically from person to person by transfer of respiratory secretions. The incubation period is unknown due to the fact that there may be many transmission cycles before illness occurs in a susceptible person. Furthermore, in some individuals the organism can be carried in the upper respiratory tract for many months before it causes disease.

Both typable and nontypable organisms may be part of the normal flora of the upper respiratory tract; nearly all individuals (up to 80 per cent) are colonized with nontypable strains. Hib carriage rates are lowest in adults and young infants, and highest in preschool-aged children. In a prospective longitudinal study conducted at a day care center in Dallas, Texas, where no invasive infections occurred, the average rate of colonization with Hib was 10 per cent.[150] During the 18 months of study, 71 per cent of the children 18 to 35 months of age and 48 per cent of the children 36 to 71 months of age were colonized at some time. Carriage rates can be substantially higher in households or day care centers in which there is a case. For example, the colonization prevalence rates among children in day care centers where a case of invasive disease has occurred can be as high as 58 to 91 per cent.[87, 237] Likewise, within families in which a case of invasive disease has occurred, rates of colonization of 60 to 70 per cent among siblings and 20 per cent among parents have been observed.[31, 237] It is not clear whether the high carriage rates in these exposed semi-closed populations are the cause or the result of disease.[138, 143] Close contact among exposed susceptible individuals, as occurs within families and day care centers, facilitates transmission and disease risk.

Despite a low point prevalence of Hib pharyngeal carriage (1 to 5 per cent), most young children become colonized with Hib during the first 2 to 5 years of life[138, 224] and consequently develop specific immunity.[93, 200] Hib strains may persist in the nasopharynx for months[143, 150] and often are not eliminated by treatment with antimicrobial agents that do not penetrate into respiratory secretions.[205, 206] The relationship between carriage of Hib and the subsequent development of disease and immunity is not understood. Factors that influence the efficiency of transmission and the ability of the organism to establish colonization also are poorly understood. However, two factors that likely potentiate infection and invasive disease risk are the size of the bacterial inoculum[214] and the presence of a concomitant viral infection.[120]

The inoculation of Hib organisms into the noses of infant animals results in a local infection. In the animal systems used, rhinorrhea was not noted, but nasopharyngeal washings reveal numerous polymorphonuclear leukocytes and organisms that reach a maximum density in approximately 24 hours. Shortly thereafter, bacteremia in the animals can be detected. With colonization of humans, Hib is found on the surface of the respiratory mucosa. Rarely, by electron microscopy, an organism can be seen penetrating through the nasal mucosal epithelial cell. There is an acute inflammatory response to the submucosal bacteria, but it is not marked. The exact mode of entrance of the organisms into the vascular compartment is unknown, but it is assumed that the organisms enter via lymphatics, probably carried by phagocytic cells, which are found in the submucosa. In support of this hypothesis, in four of eight rats after nasal inoculation, Rubin and Moxon[189] detected early transient bacteremia (within 30 minutes).

Presumably, bacterial cell wall components, such as pili and other adhesins, promote attachment, and capsule impedes bacterial clearance. Bacterial toxins, including LPS, impair ciliary function and damage the respiratory epithelium. *H. influenzae* also produces an IgA1 protease that degrades the predominant IgA serotype in the nasopharynx and may interfere with immunologic clearance.

Pathogenesis of Mucosal Infections

Noninvasive or mucosal infections are much more frequent than invasive bacteremic infections and cause considerable morbidity and health care cost. Mucosal infections generally are caused by nontypable *H. influenzae* strains and involve direct extension of organisms through nasal ostia to the sinuses, up the eustachian tubes to cause otitis media, and down the bronchi to cause bronchitis and pneumonia. Bacteremia rarely is involved, and such infections generally are not life-threatening. These infections appear to be enhanced by antecedent viral infection, eustachian tube malfunction, foreign bodies, or mucosal damage from smoking or other irritants.[191]

The clinical separation of invasive and noninvasive disease is not absolute, inasmuch as Hib strains can cause otitis media or sinusitis and non-Hib strains occasionally cause bacteremia or meningitis. A notable example of the latter is bacteremia and meningitis in neonates usually caused by nontypable organisms that presumably are acquired from the mother's genital tract.

Pathogenesis of Invasive Disease

Invasion occurs when there is dissemination of bacteria from the mucosa of the upper respiratory tract to the blood stream and then elsewhere in the body. The attack rate of invasive disease is a small fraction of the carrier rate. The organism appears to invade the mucosa by separating apical tight junctions of the columnar epithelium and moving intercellularly. The resulting bacteremia initially is at a low concentration but steadily increases over hours.[162] The dynamics between bacterial proliferation and clearance are influenced by antibody, complement, and phagocytes, which all influence the magnitude of the bacteremia.[92, 242] The polysaccharide capsule of Hib is antiphagocytic and a major virulence factor, and in the absence of anticapsular antibody, bacteremia increases steadily over a period of hours.[96] When the bacterial concentration exceeds 10^4 organisms/mL, metastatic seeding occurs, especially to the meninges via the choroid plexus (see later). Although meningitis constitutes most of all recognized invasive Hib disease, other potential metastatic sites include the lungs, joint synovium, pleura, peritoneum, and pericardium.

With pneumonia, cellulitis, and epiglottitis, the exact pathogenesis is less well understood, even though these invasive infections are associated with bacteremia. Presumably, pneumonia occurs following the aspiration of a critical number of virulent organisms, epiglottitis involves the focal infection of the epiglottis, and cellulitis occurs by secondary seeding of deep subcutaneous tissues via the blood stream.[81] With all forms of invasive Hib disease there is an invasion of the blood stream, either as a primary or as a secondary event.

Viral interactions enhance Hib pathogenesis.[218] It has been shown that influenza virus infection reduces neutrophil chemotaxis, bacterial killing, systemic macrophage function, numbers of circulating T cells, T-cell blastogenesis, and expression of delayed cutaneous hypersensitivity.[93] Reduced bacterial killing may be due to a defect in phagosome-lysosome fusion, a defect that is maximal at 5 to 7 days after viral infection and inoculation of Hib.

Bacteremia

During bacteremia, there is a continued clearance of organisms from the vascular compartment by antibody, complement, and the reticuloendothelial system. The balance of these processes determines the magnitude and duration of the bacteremia. If bacterial clearance is stopped by reticuloendothelial blockade, then bacterial densities increase to a maximum and death quickly occurs, presumably due to the effects of endotoxin.

Initially, bacterial concentrations are very low (about 100 organisms per milliliter of blood). They then steadily increase in density over the next 24 hours, reaching a plateau value. In young animals, this plateau level is 10^7 organisms per milliliter of blood and usually is associated with the features of human sepsis. In older animals, the plateau value is lower: about 10^4 organisms per milliliter of blood. These animals have low-grade fever but a relative paucity of symptoms. This primary bacteremia leads to seeding of serous surfaces: peritoneum, diarthrodial joints, pleura, pericardium, and meninges. Early in the infectious process, organisms can be obtained from all these surfaces but without an observable inflammatory response. As the host initiates an immunologic response, an inflammatory response ensues. In experimental animals, the first evidence of an immune response is antibody directed against somatic antigens.

Strains of Hib vary in virulence potential. Furthermore, the other five capsular types or nonencapsulated strains result in only transient, low-level, or undetectable bacteremia even with large inocula ($>10^7$ colony-forming units). Complement and the spleen are critical factors for host defense in the rat. Rats depleted of C3 that are splenectomized (or with iatrogenic splenic congestion due to hemolytic anemia) have an increased incidence and magnitude of bacteremia.[41, 251] These studies suggest the importance of the alternative pathway of complement (opsonic antibody) and of the reticuloendothelial phagocytes as determinants of intravascular clearance.

Meningitis

Bacteremia precedes the development of meningitis, except for those rare situations where there is direct extension of infection from adjacent sinuses or an ear infection. Data from experimental studies in the infant rat and the infant monkey support this hypothesis.[147] Both the magnitude and duration of bacteremia likely are the primary determinants of central nervous system (CNS) invasion. After a critical bacterial concentration is exceeded in blood, Hib appears to enter the CNS via the choroid plexus.[210] This is supported by the following data: (1) the earliest histopathologic lesion seen in the central nervous system is choroid plexitis, (2) the choroid plexus is one of the foci seeded from the blood stream, and (3) bacterial density early in the infection is greater in the lateral cerebral ventricles than in other CSF compartments.[210] Furthermore, pulse-chase experiments using tracer strains show that organisms enter the CSF through the choroid plexus and inflammation of the choroid plexus is a uniform feature of meningitis. Then, organisms infect the CSF and the arachnoid villi of the leptomeninges, causing blockage of CSF return and thereby increasing bacterial density and CSF pressure.[189] Generally, the magnitude of the CSF bacterial density correlates with the severity of clinical illness.[66, 197] Egress of CSF from the subarachnoid space is by flow through the subarachnoid villi, and bacterial density in the CSF can be increased or decreased by manipulating CSF egress, which occurs in meningitis via inflammatory responses. Choroid plexus inflammatory response is followed by pachymeningitis, which also influences CSF reabsorption and pressure. Phlebitis of the cerebral blood vessels and thrombosis can occur. All of this contributes to decreased blood flow to the cortex. The resulting increased bacterial density, inflammation, edema, cranial nerve damage, and overall increased CSF pressure cause the morbidity and mortality associated with meningitis.[65, 210] Parenchymal invasion of the brain is rare.

IMMUNOLOGY

Resistance to Hib infection depends upon the successful integration of a wide variety of host defenses, including (1) mucosal factors that prevent the organism from attaching and penetrating the respiratory epithelium; (2) activation of the alternate and classical complement pathways, which leads to killing of the organism and initiation of other inflammatory responses; (3) induction of antibody formation; (4) phagocytosis and killing by macrophages and polymorphonuclear cells in tissues, the circulation, and reticuloendothelial system; and (5) cell-mediated immunity. It is difficult to assess the role of each of these immunologic mechanisms independently or to determine which mechanisms are most important in host defense. Although antibodies are not the sole defense against bacteremia, it has been the research emphasis of vaccine development. The goal has been to induce antibodies that are bactericidal, opsonophagocytic, and ultimately protective. Although it is antibody that usually is measured in these studies, other immune factors are induced and probably play an important role in protection.

Anticapsular Antibody

Initially, antibody activity was assessed by measuring agglutinin and bactericidal titers of serum. In 1933, Fothergill and Wright[72] suggested that bactericidal activity was responsible for immunity to Hib meningitis and that acquisition of this immunity correlated with the age of the individual. Although antibodies to several surface antigens of *H. influenzae* play a role in conferring immunity, antibody to the Hib capsular polysaccharide appears to be of primary importance.[185] Newborns and young infants are at low risk of infection, presumably due to maternally acquired antibody. Young children at highest risk of disease have low or undetectable levels of antibody, whereas older children at lower risk have higher levels of antibody. By 5 years of age, most children have naturally acquired anticapsular antibody that appears to provide protection,[93, 200] although natural exposure also induces antibodies to OMPs, LPSs, and other surface antigens of the bacteria which contribute to natural immunity. The evidence that anticapsular antibodies protect humans from invasive Hib disease is considerable; they activate complement,[213, 247] are opsonophagocytic[160] and bactericidal,[72, 160] and protect animals from lethal Hib challenge.[216] Moreover, passive prophylaxis with serum preparations containing anticapsular antibody protects agammaglobulinemic patients[185] and high-risk children from invasive Hib disease.[193] Furthermore, in the preantibiotic era, immune sera was an effective therapy for Hib disease.[3, 174] Yet the most compelling evidence for the protective efficacy of PRP antibody is the clinical protection achieved in older children vaccinated with purified PRP vaccine[166] and more recently in younger infants immunized with Hib conjugate vaccines. Induction of antibody to Hib polysaccharide is the immunologic basis of all Hib vaccines.

A precise minimal level of anti-PRP antibody that is protective has not been established. Data from passive protection of agammaglobulinemic children, challenge experiments in infant rats, and studies of naturally acquired antibody levels in healthy individuals of various ages suggest that the minimum serum concentration of anti-PRP antibody that provides protection ranges from 0.05 μg/mL in animals[201] to 0.15 to 1.00 μg/mL in humans.[115, 166] Such estimates are crude and do not take into account the different functional properties of different immunoglobulins or the contribution of antibodies to other Hib antigens. Also, antibody levels decline over time, and a given peak level may not reflect levels at the time of exposure, which would predict long-term protection better.[7, 166] In a Finnish PRP vaccine trial, an antibody level of greater than 1.0 μg/mL 1 month after immunization correlated with clinical protection for a minimum of 1 year.[166] However, this antibody level might not be extrapolated readily to immunogenicity data evaluated in different studies or with different Hib conjugate vaccines.

Class and Subclass Specific Antibody

Several studies have shown variable immunoglobulin class, isotype, idiotype, and IgG subclass responses to PRP polysaccharide after natural Hib exposure, disease, and immunization.[116, 201] Most individuals respond with IgG antibodies after PRP immunization, although some children have predominantly IgA or IgM responses.[116] Schreiber and associates[201] showed that IgG antibody is bactericidal, opsonic for PMNs in the presence of complement, and protective for animals. IgM antibody equally is protective and more bactericidal than is IgG in the presence of complement, but it opsonizes poorly. IgA antibody is not bactericidal, opsonic, or protective for animals. Some have hypothesized that IgA-specific antibody blocks the activity of other more functional antibodies and thereby may depress immunity.[155, 166]

Data from experiments in mice and humans suggest that polysaccharide antigens induce restricted IgG subclass responses.[183] The findings of increased Hib disease susceptibility in IgG subclass–deficient patients (predominantly IgG2 and IgG4 deficiencies)[163, 202] and the low levels of IgG2 in children younger than 2 years of age[204] suggest that there are differences in the role of subclass-specific anticapsular antibodies. In adults, natural exposure or immunization with PRP vaccine results in a predominantly IgG2 subclass response.[113, 179] Children develop IgG1 and IgG2 antibodies after PRP immunization, but IgG1 antibodies predominate after immunization with Hib conjugate vaccines.[5, 113] Human anti-PRP antibodies express predominantly K light chains[207] and may be grouped into a few restricted clonotypes. These clonotypes and antibody specificities have been characterized by idiotype analysis[132] and amino acid sequencing of the immunoglobulin light chain.[220] Individuals of different ages produce different proportions or repertoires of antibody. Some differences in binding specificity and affinity have been described with the different anti-PRP antibodies, but it is not clear that the antibodies have different degrees of protective potency or are different substantially in proportion in individuals given different vaccines.

The role of mucosal immunity in killing Hib or inhibiting adherence or penetration of the mucosa is poorly understood, although there have been studies of secretory IgA antibody to the Hib capsule.[171, 172] Moreover, Hib strains produce an IgA protease that can inactivate mucosal antibody.[148] The recent observation of reduced carriage of Hib in children given Hib conjugate vaccines[151, 217] suggests that mucosal immunity may be important in reducing transmission of disease.

Cellular Immune Responses

Most of our understanding of the interactions of B cells, T cells, and antigen presenting cells (macrophages) derives from extensive research in mice.[56] Based upon T-cell involvement in antibody synthesis, antigens can be classified as T-dependent (thymus-dependent) or T-independent immunogens. Most protein antigens induce T-helper cell regulation of antibody synthesis and therefore are considered T-dependent. These antigens first are recognized and processed by macrophages and then presented to both T and B cells. The activated T cells induce proliferation and differentiation of specific antigen-reactive B-cell subpopulations. They also retain the memory necessary for subsequent booster responses.[14] Through the release of cytokines, T-helper cells appear to regulate (1) the magnitude of the immune response, especially in young infants, (2) the switch in immunoglobulin classes (IgM to IgG), (3) the functional activity of antibody, and (4) the capacity to elicit immunologic memory.

Polysaccharides consist of repeating oligosaccharide units and elicit weak immune responses involving minimal T-cell influences.[14] These T-independent antigens elicit antibody responses primarily by direct stimulation of B cells. In general, polysaccharide vaccines have the following T-independent immunologic characteristics: (1) delayed ontogeny of immune responsiveness in the young, (2) limited and variable quantitative immune responses, (3) restricted isotype (predominantly IgM) and IgG subclass responses, and (4) lack of booster or anamnestic response with secondary antigenic challenge.

The quest for a Hib vaccine that is immunogenic and protective for young infants has involved attempts to convert the capsular polysaccharide (PRP) antigen from a T-independent to a T-dependent antigen, employing the carrier-hapten principles first defined by Landsteiner in the first half of the twentieth century.[121] PRP can be considered a hapten and is linked covalently to a T-dependent immunogen, a carrier, to form a conjugate vaccine. The Hib conjugate vaccines, which demonstrate markedly enhanced immunogenicity, are described in a subsequent section.

Genetic Factors

Compared with protein vaccines, immune responses to most polysaccharide antigens are variable and may be influenced by genetic factors. Several studies have shown associations between immune responses to PRP vaccine and genetically determined factors, such as red cell antigens, human leukocyte antigen, or immunoglobulin allotypes.[4, 90, 203, 245] However, because many factors influence immunogenicity, it is difficult to know whether these associations have relevance, and it is difficult to control for these in studies. In addition, it is not known if the antibody differences, although statistically significant, are important clinically. No single genetic relationship regulating susceptibility or immune responses to polysaccharide antigens has been demonstrated convincingly.

Complement

The importance of complement components in host defense against Hib is evidenced by the elimination of the bactericidal activity of serum by heat, by the susceptibility of complement-depleted animals to Hib disease, and by the increased susceptibility of patients with specific congenital complement deficiencies.[53, 213, 247] Hib is capable of activating both the classical and alternate complement pathways, thereby initiating opsonophagocytosis, cell killing, and eliciting other inflammatory responses. Whereas the alternate pathway probably is most important early in the course of infection in the nonimmune host, the antibody-dependent classical complement pathway is more likely to predominate as a defense mechanism at a later stage of infection.[247] Both encapsulated and unencapsulated organisms activate complement, underscoring the importance of noncapsular antigens in host defense. Although the Hib capsule is a poor activator of the alternate complement pathway, antibody to the capsule activates both the classical and alternate pathways.[213] Other cell wall antigens activate the alternate pathway, and antibody to these antigens activates the classical pathway.[53, 213, 247] Thus, antibodies to both capsular and noncapsular antigens activate the complement system, primarily via the classical pathway. Activation of the terminal complement components mediates the bactericidal activity of serum.

Phagocytosis

Opsonization leading to phagocytosis and killing of Hib also is an important determinant of host defense. Impairment of phagocytic function or reduction in the numbers of phagocytes results in increased susceptibility to disease, as does the loss of the spleen or impairment of its function (e.g., hemoglobinopathies).[42, 177] The opsonic activity of serum is influenced greatly by the roles of complement and antibody. It appears that opsonization and phagocytosis of Hib are dependent upon (1) IgG binding, (2) antibody activation of the classical complement pathway with deposition of C3b on the bacterial surface, and (3) direct bacterial activation of the alternate complement pathway. Relatively little is known about direct cell-mediated killing of Hib.[60]

TABLE 139–1. Worldwide Incidence of Invasive *Haemophilus influenzae* Type b (Hib) Disease, Prior to the Use of Hib Vaccines, in Children Younger Than 5 Years of Age

Region	Years	Hib Meningitis*	All Hib Disease*
Australia/New Zealand	1985–1987	25–53	39–92
U.S./Canada	1959–1991	40–69	67–130
Europe	1985–1990	15–26	33–60
Israel	1985–1990	18	34
Africa	1980s	36–60	NA
South America	1989–1990	15–25	21–43
Asia	1990s	1.3–1.9	1.9–2.7

*Annual incidence per 100,000 population younger than 5 years of age.

NA, not available.

Adapted from Vadheim, C. M., and Ward, J. I.: Epidemiology in developed countries. *In* Ellis, R. W., and Granoff, D. M. (eds): Development and Clinical Uses of *Haemophilus b* Conjugate Vaccines. New York, Marcel Dekker, 1994, pp. 231–245; and Bijlmer, H. A.: Epidemiology of *Haemophilus influenzae* invasive disease in developing countries and intervention strategies. *In* Ellis, R. W., and Granoff, D. M. (eds.): Development and Clinical Uses of *Haemophilus b* Conjugate Vaccines. New York, Marcel Dekker, 1994, pp. 247–264. By courtesy of Marcel Dekker, Inc.

EPIDEMIOLOGY

Humans are the only natural host for *H. influenzae,* and asymptomatic nasopharyngeal carriage is common, usually by unencapsulated strains. Nasopharyngeal acquisition of Hib strains increases after infancy and persists for weeks to months, and most children are colonized at some time during the first 5 years of life. Colonization rates over 70 per cent occur following recent exposure in closed populations, such as among family members or day care center contacts of a patient with disease. Person-to-person transmission occurs via respiratory droplets, and fomites also may play a role. Since the asymptomatic carriage is common, the incubation period cannot be defined accurately.

The widespread use of the Hib conjugate vaccines has altered the epidemiology of invasive Hib disease dramatically. The first Hib conjugate vaccine was licensed in the United States in 1987 for use in children 18 months of age or older. Subsequently, decreases in the incidence of Hib disease were seen in older children and, unexpectedly, in unimmunized infants and children as well. This effect was attributed to a direct effect of vaccination on nasopharyngeal carriage, thus decreasing the environmental burden of Hib infection and, ultimately, transmission of disease. In late 1990, Hib conjugate vaccines were approved for use in infants beginning at 2 months of age, which heralded a dramatic decline in the incidence of invasive Hib disease in all children. In populations where immunization rates are high, the occurrence of invasive Hib disease has been eliminated almost completely.

Prior to immunization, invasive Hib disease was a leading infectious disease problem worldwide, affecting primarily young children (Table 139–1).[233, 243] Hib strains are responsible for greater than 95 per cent of invasive Hib infections in children. According to population-based studies, an estimated 20,000 to 25,000 persons developed invasive Hib disease annually in the United States, 85 per cent of which occurred in children younger than 5 years of age. The incidence of Hib meningitis and all invasive Hib disease was 40 to 69 and 67 to 130 cases per 100,000 children younger than 5 years of age, respectively. It was estimated that 1 of every 200 U.S. children developed invasive Hib disease during the first 5 years of life.[49] Hib pneumonia was estimated to cause as many as 15 per cent of ambulatory pneumonias in children under 6 years of age, but the true incidence was unknown since microbiologic diagnosis is difficult. Overall, incidence of Hib disease in the prevaccine era was similar to that for paralytic poliomyelitis during its peak epidemic years before immunization. A bimodal seasonal pattern had been observed in several studies, with one peak between September and December and a second peak between March and May.[180, 243] The attack rate of Hib was slightly higher in boys.[134]

Some population-based studies of the incidence of *H. influenzae* disease have been conducted outside the United States. Most of these studies were performed in Western Europe and show an incidence about one-third to two-thirds that in the U.S.[168, 192, 211] Incidence of Hib disease especially is high in certain ethnic groups including Aboriginal children in central Australia,[98] Navajo Native Americans, Native Alaskans, and Apache, Yakima, Athabascan, and Canadian Native Americans.[131, 144, 239, 250] *H. influenzae* appears to rank as a leading cause of bacterial meningitis in some developing countries as well.[30] As seen in the United States, substantial reduction in Hib disease has been seen with widespread vaccination programs. Studies in Asia show a disease incidence one-tenth to one-thirtieth that in the United States before vaccine introduction, but there are methodologic issues about the accuracy of these disease assessments, particularly related to antibiotic use and validity of culture results.

Children between the ages of 6 and 18 months are at highest risk of invasive Hib disease[134]; however, the age distribution of specific clinical syndromes of disease varies. The peak incidence of Hib meningitis occurs in children 6 to 9 months of age and declines markedly after 2 years of age.[75, 219] Hib cellulitis tends to occur during the first year of life, whereas epiglottitis generally occurs in children over 2 years of age. Invasive *H. influenzae* disease is much less common in adults due to the development of protective antibodies over time but occurs more frequently in immunocompromised patients. Nonetheless, Hib causes pneumonia and meningitis in adults,[80] and disease caused by other serotypes and nontypable strains are common, especially pneumonia, otitis media, bronchitis, and sinusitis, in all age groups. Most adults who develop invasive *H. influenzae* disease have an underlying condition such as chronic obstructive pulmonary disease, HIV infection, alcoholism, pregnancy, or malignancy.[27, 80]

The development of invasive Hib disease in a given individual is a consequence of a complex interaction of a variety of factors, including exposure risk, characteristics of the organism, and the host.[74] In populations with a high disease incidence, such as Native Americans, the age-specific incidence peaks in a younger age group (<6 months), presumably a result of early or intense exposure to Hib at home or in the community. Several factors that may reflect environmental exposure to the organism have been shown to be risk factors for disease, including household size,[86, 114] crowding,[226] day care,[50, 105] low family income,[73, 75] and low parental education level,[75, 114] whereas breast feeding appears to be protective.[169] Several underlying medical conditions are associated with increased risk for Hib disease, including HIV infection,[35, 198] sickle-cell anemia,[177] asplenia or splenectomy,[42] antibody[64] and complement deficiency syndromes,[69] and malignancy.[241]

Although the direct contagiousness of invasive Hib disease is limited, small outbreaks and direct secondary transmission of disease can occur. A number of studies have estimated the risk of secondary disease in household contacts in the 30 days after onset of disease in an index case. Overall, the attack rate for contacts of all ages was 0.3 per cent, representing a risk about 600-fold higher than the age-adjusted risk in the general population.[31, 236] However, attack rates varied inversely with age, with children younger than 4 years of age at greatest risk. Among household contacts, nearly two-thirds of secondary cases occurred within the first week after disease onset in the index patient.[236] Controversy exists about the degree of risk of secondary Hib disease among day care center contacts exposed to a child with invasive Hib disease. The risk of secondary disease among children younger than 2 years of age in day care centers ranges from 0 to 3.2 per cent.[12, 161] For day care center contacts older than 2 years of age, however, the risk is less than 1 per cent.

CLINICAL MANIFESTATIONS

Bacteremia

Occult bacteremia (i.e., not associated with a focus of infection) is not common in febrile children, but bacteremia does precede essentially all invasive Hib infections. In the prevaccine era, Hib was the second leading cause of occult bacteremia after *Streptococcus pneumoniae*, primarily affecting children 6 to 36 months of age. Most children present with fever and peripheral leukocytosis. Unlike *S. pneumoniae* bacteremia, the condition is not benign. Approximately 30 to 50 per cent of children with occult Hib bacteremia develop a focal infection such as meningitis, pneumonia, or cellulitis.[52, 119]

Meningitis

Meningitis is the most serious manifestation of invasive Hib disease. No clinical feature differentiates Hib meningitis from the other causes of meningitis in children. The onset of disease can be fulminant,[106] but more commonly the signs and symptoms are nonspecific (particularly in young infants) and may include irritability, fever, lethargy, poor feeding, or vomiting. Children younger than 18 months of age often do not have nuchal rigidity. Older children are more likely to present with findings of headache, photophobia, and meningismus. With fulminant Hib meningitis, very rapid neurologic deterioration may occur with increased intracranial pressure, seizures, coma, and respiratory arrest. Ten to 20 per cent of children with meningitis will have other foci of infection such as cellulitis, arthritis, or pneumonia,[11, 70] and essentially all have concomitant bacteremia.

CSF examination typically reveals a pleocytosis (mean of 4000 to 5000 white blood cells/μL) with a predominance of polymorphonuclear leukocytes. About 75 per cent of patients have hypoglycorrhachia, and about 90 per cent have an elevated CSF protein concentration. Eighty per cent of meningitis cases due to Hib will have a positive CSF Gram stain. As with other types of bacterial meningitis, however, prior antimicrobial therapy significantly decreases the concentration of Hib organisms in the CSF and decreases the sensitivity of the Gram stain.[20] Prior treatment does not affect substantially the total blood cell count and differential, glucose, or protein, thus permitting a diagnosis of meningitis. In over 90 per cent of cases, capsular antigen can be detected in CSF or serum.[240] Anemia, leukocytosis, thrombocytosis and thrombocytopenia also are observed frequently.[65]

Complications of Hib meningitis include seizures, cerebral edema, subdural effusion or empyema, inappropriate secretion of antidiuretic hormone, cortical infarction (often manifest by focal neurologic abnormalities), cerebritis, intracerebral abscess, hydrocephalus, and, rarely, cerebral herniation.[23, 65] Computed tomography and magnetic resonance imaging of the head should not be performed routinely for Hib meningitis, but they may be helpful if there are focal neurologic findings or if the clinical course becomes complicated. Small subdural effusions are common but usually are not of clinical significance.

Even with prompt intensive care, the mortality from Hib meningitis is about 5 per cent and significant long-term morbidity, including sensorineural hearing loss, delay in language acquisition, developmental delay, gross motor abnormalities, vision impairment, or behavior abnormalities, may occur in 15 to 30 per cent of survivors.[58, 59, 65, 176, 222] A substantial proportion of such abnormalities may resolve over time, emphasizing the need for long-term monitoring of these patients.[65]

Pneumonia

Hib pneumonia is indistinguishable clinically from other bacterial pneumonias. The majority of patients have a preceding upper respiratory tract infection, fever, and cough accompanied by peripheral leukocytosis with a predominance of polymorphonuclear leukocytes. Radiologically, Hib pneumonia may be segmental, lobar, interstitial, or diffuse, and over 50 per cent of cases have evidence of pleural or pericardial involvement on radiographic examination. Cavitation and pneumatoceles are rare but have been reported.[43] Computed tomography can be a useful adjunct to the evaluation of complicated disease due to Hib.[48] Blood culture, pleural fluid, tracheal aspirate, and lung aspirate cultures are positive in 75 to 90 per cent of cases. Detection of capsular polysaccharide in pleural fluid, serum, or urine can establish the diagnosis, particularly if prior antimicrobial therapy was instituted. Although fever may persist for several days while on adequate therapy, uncomplicated Hib pneumonia rarely is associated with long-term pulmonary dysfunction.

Epiglottitis (see Chapter 21)

Acute upper airway obstruction caused by Hib infection of the epiglottis and superglottic tissues occurs primarily in children 2 to 7 years of age. Onset usually is abrupt, with high fever, sore throat, dysphagia, and sepsis. Antecedent upper respiratory tract infection with cough occurs in approximately 50 per cent of patients.[26, 130] The child may drool due to an inability to swallow oropharyngeal secretions and develop progressive respiratory distress over a period of hours with tachypnea, stridor, cyanosis, and retractions. The child usually is agitated and may sit forward with the chin extended to maintain an open airway. In children younger than 2 years of age, Hib epiglottitis may present in an atypical fashion with low-grade fever and a cough suggestive of croup.[130]

The most important aspect of management of a child with epiglottitis is the maintenance of a patent airway. Nasotracheal intubation is preferable to tracheostomy because it is equally effective, is not permanent or disfiguring, and has fewer inherent risks.[16] Seventy to 90 per cent of patients with epiglottitis will have positive blood cultures; cultures from the inflamed epiglottitis should be obtained only after the airway has been secured. A lateral neck radiograph revealing dilatation of the hypopharynx and the "thumbprint" sign (swollen epiglottis)[25] can be helpful if the clinical presentation is subtle, but in most cases diagnostic studies should not delay intubation and direct inspection of the epiglottis in controlled surroundings. The mortality rate is 5 to 10 per cent, almost always related to abrupt airway obstruction.

Joint Infection

Prior to the routine use of the Hib conjugate vaccines, Hib was the leading cause of septic arthritis in children younger than 2 years of age. It affects a single large joint at the knee, ankle, elbow, or hip in over 90 per cent of cases. Contiguous osteomyelitis occurs in 10 to 20 per cent.[70, 122] No feature clearly distinguishes septic arthritis due to Hib from that due to other bacterial etiologies. Patients present with fever, and more than two-thirds present with decreased range of motion, local warmth, and swelling.[54, 70, 122] Usually, pain, swelling, and erythema of the involved joint are preceded by a nonspecific upper respiratory illness. The clinical presentation may be subtle with only decreased range of motion of the joint or abnormal gait as the presenting feature. Hib capsular antigen concentrations are very high in the infected joint fluid of children with septic arthritis, and rapid detection of antigen is useful diagnostically. Septic arthritis of the hip requires surgical drainage, and resolution generally is rapid, but long-term cartilage damage may follow Hib arthritis despite adequate therapy.[222]

Cellulitis

Cellulitis is a relatively uncommon form of Hib disease and is seen almost exclusively in children younger than 2 years of age. Most (74 per cent) is located in the cheek (buccal cellulitis), the periorbital region, and the neck[54] and rarely on the extremities. Facial cellulitis is most common in infants and presents with acute fever and a unilateral, raised, warm, tender and indurated area that may progress to a violaceous hue, although this finding is not unique to Hib disease. Aspirate cultures of the point of maximal swelling usually yield the organism, and bacteremia is usual.[71, 104] A secondary focus (including meningitis) may be present in 10 to 15 per cent of the patients.[62, 63] Orbital cellulitis usually is a complication of ethmoid sinusitis and consequently can be caused by non-Hib strains. Etiologic diagnosis can be established by blood culture or aspiration of the subcutaneous tissues. Antibiotics always are indicated, but surgical drainage depends on the degree of involvement of the tissues within the orbit.

Pericarditis

Hib pericarditis usually is a complication of adjacent pneumonia and presents with fever, ill appearance, respiratory distress, and tachycardia.[40, 182] The radiographic or clinical diagnosis can be confirmed with two-dimensional echocardiography[249] and may be suggested by finding capsular polysaccharide in the serum or pericardial fluid or in the pericardial fluid Gram stain. Cultures of pericardial fluid are positive in more than 70 per cent of cases.[54] Early drainage is an important part of the management of this illness, and early pericardectomy or pericardiostomy is preferred over repeated pericardiocentesis.[146, 182]

Neonatal Disease

H. influenzae causes 2 to 8 per cent of neonatal early-onset sepsis.[32, 234] The majority of these cases are due to nontypable strains, most of which are concordant with those isolated from the maternal genital tract. The precise pathogenesis is unknown, but neonatal disease often is associated with prematurity, low birth weight, premature rupture of membranes, and maternal chorioamnionitis, and several cases have followed cesarean delivery, suggesting in utero transmission.[190] Clinical manifestations include pneumonia, bacteremia, and conjunctivitis. More than two-thirds of neonatal *H. influenzae* disease occurs in the first day of life, with an overall mortality rate of 55 per cent.[77]

Other Invasive Infections

Other invasive Hib infections include endophthalmitis,[221] CSF shunt infections,[124, 181] necrotizing fasciitis, pyomyositis,[158] peritonitis,[45, 76] scrotal abscess,[128] brain abscesses,[68] polyserositis,[142] tenosynovitis,[157] epididymitis,[94] lung abscess,[126] periappendiceal abscess,[139] and bacterial tracheitis.[34] Invasive disease also may present with fever alone, fever with petechiae, or fever of unknown origin.[28, 232]

Nontypable Invasive Disease

Nontypable *H. influenzae* invasive disease is rare and is associated frequently with underlying medical conditions, including prematurity, malignancy, cystic fibrosis, asthma, CSF leak, CNS shunts, congenital heart disease, lymphoproliferative disorders, and immunoglobulin deficiency.[15, 46, 63, 79, 164] Reports from Africa and Papua New Guinea suggest that non-Hib strains are important causes of severe acute lower respiratory tract infections in developing countries.[95, 123]

Mucosal Infections

Unencapsulated or non-Hib strains usually cause a variety of mucosal infections, including otitis media, sinusitis, conjunctivitis, and bronchitis. *H. influenzae* is the second leading cause of acute otitis media in adults and children[21] and presents similarly to other causes of otitis, that is, with fever and symptoms referable to the upper respiratory tract with nonspecific symptoms such as irritability, vomiting, and diarrhea. Sinusitis may present with common cold symptoms that are persistent or more severe than usual. Older children and adults are more likely to complain of headache, paranasal, dental, or facial pain. Other common symptoms are a daytime cough that may worsen at night or reactive airway disease unresponsive to therapy. Rarely, chronic otitis or sinusitis may result in the development of mastoiditis or a parameningeal abscess. Conjunctivitis usually is bilateral and purulent[22] and may occur in outbreaks. Although common, these infections rarely are life-threatening and are not associated with bacteremia.

Because noninvasive infections rarely are caused by Hib, antigen detection and blood cultures rarely are of diagnostic value. The diagnosis usually is clinical, and specific etiology is not determined, but a microbiologic diagnosis can be established for lung disease by careful Gram stain and culture of sputum, for otitis media by culture of middle ear fluid obtained by tympanocentesis, for sinusitis by culture of sinus aspirate, and for conjunctivitis by Gram stain and culture of the eye discharge. Cultures of the nasopharynx to detect carriers of *H. influenzae* should not be done for the following reasons:

1. It is difficult to identify *H. influenzae* among the many bacteria colonizing the upper respiratory tract.
2. *H. influenzae* is a normal constituent of the upper airway, and its presence or absence has little diagnostic significance.

Endocarditis

H. influenzae may cause endocarditis,[55] but *H. parainfluenzae* and *H. aphrophilus* are more important causes of endocarditis, accounting for as many as 5 per cent of such cases in adults. These species are commensal organisms of the oropharynx and due to fastidious growth characteristics are included in the group of pathogens that cause "culture-negative" endocarditis known as the HACEK group.[246]

Brazilian Purpuric Fever (see Chapter 140)

Brazilian purpuric fever is a fulminant infection caused by *H. influenzae* biogroup aegyptius. Limited primarily to Brazil, the illness afflicts children younger than 10 years of age, with a median age of 30 months. Illness is characterized by a purulent conjunctivitis followed 7 to 16 days later by the acute onset of high fever, vomiting, abdominal pain, purpura, vascular collapse, and death in 70 per cent. Some children present with mild fever alone. Diagnosis is confirmed by blood culture in nearly all patients,[99] and therapy with antimicrobial agents effective against other *H. influenzae* infections is adequate.

Chancroid (see Chapter 140)

Chancroid is a sexually transmitted disease caused by *H. ducreyi*. This disease is found worldwide, especially among groups of lower socioeconomic status and the HIV-infected population.[97] The median incubation period is 5 to 7 days, after which tender papules develop in the inguinal or perirectal area. The lesions ulcerate, readily bleed, and are associated with tender lymphadenopathy in 25 to 50 per cent of patients. Because it is difficult to distinguish chancroid from other ulcerative sexually transmitted diseases, diagnosis is confirmed by culture of the ulcer or associated bubo. Testing for concomitant syphilis infection is important.[215] Oral erythromycin or parenteral ceftriaxone is the preferred treatment.

DIAGNOSIS

A high index of suspicion for the possibility of Hib disease must be maintained when evaluating children with appropriate clinical presentations and findings. The primary criterion for the diagnosis of *H. influenzae* infection is Gram stain and/or isolation of the organism from the infected focus (e.g., CSF, pleural fluid, sputum, or blood). Because most invasive Hib disease is associated with bacteremia, blood cultures should be done on any febrile child with potential Hib disease. The specimens need to be processed immediately because the organism is fastidious. Although most commercial blood culture media support the growth of *H. influenzae*, the fluid should be applied, when possible, directly to chocolate agar or a semisynthetic medium containing heme and NAD.[10] In liquid medium, growth may not be sufficient to result in turbidity; therefore for blood cultures, advanced detection systems or subcultures should be performed. Also, selective media that suppress the growth of gram-positive organisms may increase the recovery of *H. influenzae* from upper respiratory tract specimens.[38] The identification of an isolate as *H. influenzae* relies on its dependence on heme and NAD.

Other techniques that may assist in the microbiologic diagnosis include rapid antigen detection, staining techniques, and immunofluorescence. Such techniques are useful in the context of a patient whose cultures are sterile owing to prior antibiotic therapy, or they can confirm the clinical diagnosis before bacterial growth occurs. The three most commonly used techniques for antigen detection are latex particle agglutination (LPA), countercurrent immunoelectrophoresis (CIE), and coagglutination (CoA). False-positive results are rare with CSF by all three tests; however, false-positive reactions have occurred in testing of serum and urine. False-positive reactions occur due to nonspecific agglutination (i.e., rheumatoid factors) and due to antigenic cross-reactivity with *Escherichia coli, S. pneumoniae*, staphylococci, or meningococcus. Overall, the LPA appears to be more sensitive than is CoA, and LPA and CoA are more sensitive than is CIE in CSF, serum, urine, joint fluid, and pleural fluid.[111, 136, 141] False-positive results can occur in the urine of children with nasopharyngeal carriage of the organism or, more commonly, for several days after immunization with Hib conjugate vaccine.[212] Acridine orange is a fluorescent stain that binds to cellular nucleic acids and may be useful in situations in which smaller bacterial concentrations are present.[117] Immunofluorescent staining of purulent specimens from patients with partially treated disease also has been useful.[47] Several enzyme-linked immunosorbent assays for PRP detection are available. These tests generally are used in the research setting and are not of substantial clinical value.

TREATMENT

Invasive Disease

Bacteremia plays a central pathogenetic role in invasive Hib disease; therefore, occult invasion of the CNS always must be considered in the context of any manifestation of Hib infection. In addition, severe Hib disease often is fatal if not treated adequately. Therefore, cure of Hib bacteremia and its complications requires antimicrobial therapy that will (1) penetrate the blood-brain barrier to achieve bactericidal concentrations and (2) be of adequate duration to sterilize the primary and potential secondary foci. The choice of specific antibiotic therapy must take into account the local antibiotic susceptibility patterns of invasive isolates (Table 139–2). Hib resistance to several antimicrobials, including ampicillin, chloramphenicol, trimethoprim-sulfamethoxazole, rifampin, and certain second-generation cephalosporins in *H. influenzae* type b has been increasing in several areas of the world.[110]

For proven or suspected Hib meningitis, cefotaxime or ceftriaxone is recommended until the antibiotic susceptibility of the organism is known or an alternative diagnosis is established.[65] Both antibiotics have bactericidal activity against Hib, including those that produce β-lactamases, and they penetrate well into infected CSF and are well tolerated. Ceftriaxone may be useful for daily intramuscular injections, if necessary. Cefuroxime no longer appears to have a role in the treatment of *H. influenzae* meningitis in that delayed sterilization may be at least twofold more common than with standard therapy of ampicillin plus chloramphenicol or with the third-generation cephalosporins.[107, 209] Also, ampicillin, formerly a mainstay of therapy for this infection, should not be used empirically to treat infections due to Hib because up to 50 per cent of Hib isolates in the United States are resistant, usually via plasmid-mediated β-lactamase production.[110] Chloramphenicol, another medication that frequently was used to treat Hib disease, now rarely is used because safer antibiotics with greater activity are available. Although adequate bactericidal blood and CNS levels of chloramphenicol can be achieved, even with oral administration,[67, 196] its use requires monitoring of drug levels. Dose-dependent, yet reversible bone marrow toxicity may occur particularly in neonates, in patients with liver disease, or in those who require prolonged treatment. Idiosyncratic aplastic anemia, a dose-independent complication of chloramphenicol use, is extremely rare.

Cefuroxime has good activity against *H. influenzae* and is useful for empiric therapy for nonmeningitic infections such as pneumonia, periorbital cellulitis, and septic arthritis. Other parenteral agents have activity against *H. influenzae*, including imipenem-cilastatin, meropenem, ampicillin-sulbactam, aztreonam, and other third-generation cephalosporins such as ceftazidime. Imipenem-cilastatin has been associated with seizures during treatment of meningitis,[100] and its use likely will be supplanted by meropenem for situations in which resistance to third-generation cephalosporins is documented. In general, the spectrum of activity of these agents is too broad for routine use in pediatric infections in which Hib is an important pathogen.

TABLE 139–2. Selected Antimicrobial Agents for Treatment of *Haemophilus influenzae* Infections*

Antimicrobial Agent	Total Daily Dose (mg/kg)†	Dose Frequency
Parenteral		
Ampicillin	200–400	q4–6h
Cefuroxime	75–150	q8h
Cefotaxime	150–200	q6–8h
Ceftriaxone	50–100	q12–24h
Chloramphenicol	50–100	q6h
Oral		
Amoxicillin	40–60	tid
Amoxicillin-clavulanate	40–60	tid/bid
Erythromycin-sulfisoxazole	40 (erythromycin)	qid
Trimethoprim-sulfamethoxazole	8 (trimethoprim)	bid
Clarithromycin	15	bid
Azithromycin	10‡	qid
Cefuroxime axetil	30–40	bid

*The duration of therapy depends on the clinical presentation, presence of complications, and clinical response.

†The higher doses should be used for meningitis.

‡10 mg/kg is a loading dose that should be followed by 5 mg/kg daily thereafter for otitis media.

Children with occult Hib bacteremia need to be reevaluated carefully because since 30 to 50 per cent of such patients who are clinically well may develop focal disease.[52, 119] The duration of therapy is determined by the site of infection and the clinical response. Children with uncomplicated Hib meningitis can be treated for 7 to 10 days. Children with Hib cellulitis can be changed to oral therapy after several days of parenteral therapy, provided they have had a satisfactory clinical response and do not have meningitis. Patients with septic arthritis should receive at least 10 to 14 days of therapy, whereas children with pericarditis, empyema, or osteomyelitis may require longer courses of antibiotic treatment (3 to 6 weeks). These patients often can be switched to oral antibiotics after documenting susceptibility, a good therapeutic response, and adequate antimicrobial blood levels and ensuring compliance.

Equally important in the overall management of a child with invasive Hib disease is supportive care. For Hib meningitis, several studies have shown that adjunctive therapy with dexamethasone moderates the inflammatory cascade and may decrease the likelihood of hearing loss. The recommended dose is 0.6 mg/kg/day given every 6 hours for 4 days, with the first dose given just before or with the first antibiotic dose.[178] Management of the child with meningitis requires continuing careful evaluations for complications such as the development of shock, inappropriate secretion of antidiuretic hormone, seizures, subdural empyema, and secondary foci of infection. Prolonged fever is common, with about 10 per cent of children remaining febrile for at least 10 days.[65] Repeat lumbar puncture to document sterility of the CSF is not necessary in uncomplicated cases.

In children with epiglottitis, airway protection is the most important component of therapy and should be initiated even before administration of antimicrobials. Endotracheal intubation or tracheostomy is performed optimally in the operating room by personnel experienced with these procedures in children. Prior to establishing the airway, care should be taken not to precipitate laryngospasm by attempting to examine the epiglottis or by performing tests such as venipuncture. Blood cultures should be obtained and intravenous antibiotics initiated as soon as possible after the airway has been secured.

Patients with subdural empyema, pericarditis, or pleural empyema usually require percutaneous or surgical drainage. Infected joint fluid should be aspirated from the child with septic arthritis to confirm the diagnosis and to reduce pressure. Repeated aspirations or placement of a surgical drain also may be needed. Infection of the hip requires surgical incision and drainage to decompress the joint; failure to do so may result in avascular necrosis of the femoral head.

Noninvasive Disease

Noninvasive *H. influenzae* infections, usually due to nontypable strains, include otitis media, sinusitis, conjunctivitis, bronchitis, and pneumonia. Numerous orally administered antimicrobials are available to treat these infections (see Table 139–2). Despite the increasing prevalence of β-lactamase–

producing organisms, amoxicillin remains the drug of choice for empiric therapy in most areas for otitis media because of its low cost and proven safety. Several other antimicrobials with activity against *H. influenzae* are available, including amoxicillin-clavulanate, trimethoprim-sulfamethoxazole, erythromycin-sulfisoxazole, newer macrolides including clarithromycin and azithromycin, and second- and third-generation cephalosporins such as cefuroxime axetil, cefixime, cefpodoxime, and cefprozil. Cefaclor is used widely but has poor activity against β-lactamase–producing organisms and causes a serum sickness–like illness in approximately 2 per cent of recipients. The quinolone antibiotics, such as ciprofloxacin, also are active but are not licensed for use in children younger than 18 years of age because of a quinolone-induced arthropathy seen in juvenile animals. In the context of poor clinical response or isolation of β-lactamase–producing organisms, augmentin-clavulanate, cefixime, and cefpodoxime appear to be the most useful.

Most mucosal infections are treated presumptively without obtaining definitive cultures, and, consequently, the duration of therapy and the need for alternative antibiotics are based on an assessment of the clinical response. Otitis media usually is treated for 7 to 10 days, and sinusitis should be treated for at least 10 days. If resistance is suspected and leads to failure of treatment, an empiric change in antibiotics is indicated.

PREVENTION

The near elimination of invasive Hib disease in the United States and other countries is a direct result of routine use of Hib conjugate vaccines and represents a remarkable success story. Prevention with a hyperimmunoglobulin also has been shown to be effective in high-risk populations, but it is costly, of short-lived benefit, and not licensed for general use. Antimicrobial prophylaxis is effective for the prevention of secondary Hib disease, but this represents only a minor portion of the overall disease burden.

Active Immunization

The first Hib vaccine was the PRP polysaccharide vaccine, which is composed of the purified Hib capsular polysaccharide, PRP.[9, 187] In 1985, for children older than 18 months of age, this became the first vaccine to be licensed for the prevention of Hib disease. Children younger than 18 months of age had inadequate immune responses[8, 114] with PRP vaccination. PRP vaccine has immunologic properties similar to those of some other polysaccharide vaccines, which generally are considered to be T-independent immunogens. As a result, antibody responses are limited and of short duration, particularly in young children, and there is no booster response with repeated administrations of the vaccine. Furthermore, the induced antibody may have reduced functional qualities (i.e., primarily IgM, low avidity).[184, 204]

PRP vaccine was licensed based on the findings of a large, randomized clinical trial conducted in Finland in 1974[165, 166] that suggested a protective efficacy of 90 per cent for children who were immunized between 18 and 71 months of age. Subsequent to the licensure of this vaccine in the United States, it became apparent that routine use of the vaccine resulted in efficacy less than that assessed in the Finnish vaccine trial, ranging between 0 and 88 per cent.[238] This vaccine mainly is of historic significance because its role has been supplanted by the development and licensure of the PRP-protein conjugate vaccines.

Hib conjugate vaccines were developed in an effort to enhance immune responses to the PRP antigen. Basic to all conjugate vaccines is the use of a covalently linked (conjugated) immunogenic protein carrier that confers upon the PRP polysaccharide hapten recognition by T cells and macrophages and stimulation of T-dependent immunity.[121, 238] Four Hib conjugate vaccines have been developed and evaluated in infants, all of which employ PRP polysaccharide as the primary immunogen (Table 139–3): PRP-D (diphtheria toxoid), HbOC (mutant diphtheria toxin), PRP-OMP (major OMP of *Neisseria meningitidis* serogroup B), and PRP-T (tetanus toxoid). The immune response after Hib conjugate vaccination has the following general characteristics:

1. It is quantitatively enhanced, particularly in younger infants.
2. Repeat administrations of vaccine elicit booster responses.
3. There is a maturation of class-specific immunity with a predominance of IgG antibody and probably enhanced functional properties.

The first Hib conjugate vaccine licensed was PRP-D, but it was less immunogenic than the subsequent conjugate vaccines and rarely is used in the United States. In children 15 months of age or older who received PRP-D, high antibody concentrations were achieved with a single dose.[17, 102] In infants, however, fewer than half develop antibody levels greater than 1 μg/mL, even after three doses.[57, 113] A number of case-control studies have demonstrated that a single dose

TABLE 139–3. Characteristics of *Haemophilus influenzae* Type b Conjugate Vaccines

Vaccine	Polysaccharide Size (PS)	Protein Carrier	Linkage	Trade Name*
PRP-D	Medium	Diphtheria toxoid	Protein with 6-carbon spacer	ProHIBIT
HbOC	Small	CRM_{197} (mutant diphtheria toxin)	PS, no spacer	HibTITER
PRP-OMP	Medium	*Neisseria meningitidis* outer-membrane protein complex	Protein and PS with bigeneric spacer	PedvaxHIB
PRP-T	Large	Tetanus toxoid	PS with 6-carbon spacer	ActHIB

*HbOC, PRP-OMP, and PRP-T also are available in combination with diphtheria-tetanus-pertussis, diphtheria-tetanus–acellular pertussis, and hepatitis B vaccines.

HbOC, mutant diphtheria toxin; PRP-D, diphtheria toxoid; PRP-OMP, major outer-membrane protein of *Neisseria meningitidis* serogroup B; PRP-T, tetanus toxoid.

of vaccine was at least 80 per cent efficacious in preventing disease in children 18 months of age or older.[92, 244] In infants who received vaccine at 3, 4, 6, and 14 to 18 months of age, the protective efficacy after three doses was 94 per cent in Finland.[62] In contrast, a trial conducted in Native Alaskan infants found no evidence of protection in that high-risk population.[235]

A single dose of HbOC is highly immunogenic in children older than 18 months of age,[102, 133] and after three doses in infancy, high antibody levels are achieved.[57, 188] Two prospective clinical studies have shown that two or three doses of HbOC administered in the first 6 months of life provide a high degree of protective efficacy. In the Kaiser Permanente northern California region population, HbOC was 100 per cent efficacious after two doses in infancy.[18] The vaccine also was evaluated in Finland in infants who received vaccine at 4, 6, and 14 to 18 months of age,[61] and efficacy was 95 per cent after two doses. Data from a third postlicensure study in infants in Los Angeles County also suggested a protective efficacy of 89 per cent after two doses and 94 per cent after three doses.[228]

PRP-OMP induces an immune response that is less age-dependent than is the response to the other Hib conjugate vaccines. Adults and children respond to a single vaccine dose with high antibody levels.[188] In infants as young as 6 to 8 weeks of age, a single dose of PRP-OMP induces a good antibody response.[29] Also, antibody levels achieved after two doses are higher than those after two doses of any of the other conjugate vaccines,[29, 57] and a third dose does not enhance the response. PRP-OMP was evaluated in infants in a randomized, double-blind, placebo-controlled trial in a high-risk Navajo Native American population[195] who received vaccine at 2 and 4 months of age, yielding an overall efficacy of 95 per cent. Additional data from a population-based case-control study in Los Angeles County suggested a level of effectiveness similar to that seen for HbOC.[227]

PRP-T is highly immunogenic in adults and older children,[44, 199] and high concentrations of antibody are achieved in infants with a three-dose immunization series at 2, 4, and 6 months of age.[57] The protective efficacy of PRP-T was evaluated in two large prospective randomized trials that were terminated prematurely due to the licensure of other Hib conjugate vaccines for infants. More than 12,000 infants were enrolled in the studies in southern California and North Carolina, and no cases of invasive Hib disease occurred in vaccinated children compared with five cases in the control groups.[78, 229] Efficacy subsequently was shown in a study in England in which the efficacy after three doses in infancy was estimated to be 100 per cent.[24] In Finland, during the first 2 years of its general use, over 100,000 infants were immunized, and only two cases of invasive Hib disease had occurred in vaccinees, both after a single dose. No infant in any study who has received two or more doses of vaccine has developed Hib disease.[167]

HbOC, PRP-OMP, and PRP-T are licensed for use in infants at 2, 4, 6, and 12 to 15 months of age. Any Hib conjugate vaccine can be used as the booster dose or in different sequences. Several issues, however, remain regarding the use of Hib conjugate vaccines in infancy. Direct comparisons of the Hib conjugate vaccines need to be considered in the context of varying study designs, differences in vaccine lots, and different laboratory and statistical methodologies. Despite these difficulties, certain concepts are apparent:

1. All Hib conjugate vaccines are safe in infants.
2. PRP-D is the least immunogenic conjugate vaccine.
3. Only PRP-OMP induces a good immune response after one dose in young infants, but antibody levels are lower than those induced by HbOC and PRP-T after three doses.
4. PRP-OMP, HbOC, and PRP-T appear to be efficacious, but no direct comparisons of protective efficacy of these vaccines has been completed.

Also, certain mixed sequences of Hib vaccines given to infants (i.e., PRP-OMP follow by HbOC or PRP-T) may enhance the antibody response.[84, 91] In addition, the simultaneous receipt of other non-Hib vaccines and the impact of concurrent or prior receipt of the carrier protein (carrier priming)[88, 89, 127] are issues that need to be explored. Combination vaccines that include Hib (Hib-DTP, Hib-DTaP) currently are licensed, and several other combinations (Hib-hepatitis B, -IPV, -DTaP/IPV) are being evaluated in infants and children. The impact on the reactogenicity, immunogenicity, and protective efficacy of such combinations remains to be determined.

To date, essentially all *H. influenzae* vaccines are based on immunity to the Hib capsule. Antibodies to other components of the bacterium also have been shown to be bactericidal, opsonophagocytic, and protective in animal studies. Vaccines containing alternative antigens could provide supplemental protection against Hib, although this does not appear to be necessary based on the efficacy of the available Hib conjugate vaccines. More importantly, such alternative vaccines could provide immunity to non-Hib strains, which have substantial phenotypic and genetic variability[156] but are ubiquitous colonizers of the upper respiratory tract of humans and cause mucosal infections. The basic microbiologic problem hindering the development of such vaccines has been the diversity and instability of cell wall antigens between most *H. influenzae* strains. Studies have attempted to define OMPs, cell wall LPS, and fimbrial surface antigens of the organism.[13] Due to the variability of most of these antigens between heterologous strains and even among homologous strains over time, it has been difficult to find an antigen relevant to all or the majority of strains. Also, not all bacterial antigens elicit protective immunity. The focus of most investigations has been to characterize OMPs.[159] Other efforts have focused on proteins of higher molecular weight,[230] LPS, or fimbrial antigens.[112] Immunity to these other antigens has not been consistent against heterologous strains.

Passive Immunization

Although active immunization clearly is preferred for the control of Hib disease, passive immunization has potential utility in the following settings: (1) selected high-risk groups with disease risk soon after birth and too young to respond to vaccination (i.e., Eskimos or Native Americans), (2) functionally asplenic patients, (3) immunocompromised patients, and (4) for prevention of secondary disease in households, day care centers, or institutions. A human hyperimmunoglobulin from adult Hib-immunized donors called bacterial polysaccharide immunoglobulin has been prepared,[208] but it is not commercially available. Pharmacologic studies show that high levels of antibody can be achieved after intramuscular injection, and significant protective efficacy against invasive Hib disease has been demonstrated in Apache children given three doses during the first year of life.[193] Use of concurrent active immunization with bacterial polysaccharide immunoglobulin also may be an effective strategy.[125] Another possible approach in such groups would be maternal Hib immunization,[82] which induces transplacental antibody, but questions remain regarding the safety and acceptability of vaccinating pregnant women and the inability to immunize women who do not receive prenatal care.

Impact of *Haemophilus influenzae* Type b Vaccination

The impact of widespread vaccination with Hib conjugate vaccine has been dramatic and reproduced in several areas of the United States[1, 152] and many countries throughout the world.[109, 167] Exclusively using HbOC vaccine,[19] the Kaiser Permanente northern California region has eliminated Hib disease except for a rare case in an unimmunized child and just a few cases in children with incomplete immunizations. In the Kaiser Permanente southern California region,[227] PRP-D and subsequently PRP-OMP vaccines were used in older children between 1987 and 1990. Since 1990, PRP-OMP vaccine has been used almost exclusively. There were a few cases of PRP-D failure and only two cases of PRP-OMP failure; disease essentially has been eliminated. Similar control of disease has been achieved with use of PRP-OMP vaccine in Alaska and Navajo Native American populations.[194] In Los Angeles County,[227] Minnesota, Dallas,[152] and selected other U.S. sites under surveillance by the Centers for Disease Control and Prevention, similar but less complete disease eradication has been achieved. In these areas, both HbOC and PRP-OMP vaccine have been used in varying proportions over time, and complete immunization levels have not been achieved.

In general, the fall in disease incidence has exceeded expectations given the estimated proportion of the population completely immunized. In addition, in essentially all of these populations, a significant fall in disease incidence was observed among infants before the licensure and recommended use of vaccines in that age group. These findings likely are explained by reductions in Hib carriage caused by vaccination[151, 217] leading to decreased transmission from immunized children to unimmunized young children and infants.

Chemoprophylaxis

Secondary disease makes up less than 2 per cent of all cases of invasive Hib disease. Chemoprophylaxis, however, can protect susceptible persons from acquiring Hib by eliminating Hib colonization in close contacts. Children younger than 4 years of age have a 600-fold increased risk of Hib disease after household contact with a case.[236] Risk also is increased in day care center settings, but the risk is less well defined. In addition, adults and older children who are colonized can transmit Hib to susceptible children even though they are at little risk of developing invasive disease themselves.

Antimicrobial agents effective for chemoprophylaxis must achieve bactericidal levels intracellularly and in mucosal secretions. Rifampin, which achieves high concentrations in respiratory secretions,[140] is the most effective antimicrobial agent for eradicating Hib from the nasopharynx. Rifampin in a dosage of 20 mg/kg once daily (maximum daily dose, 600 mg) for 4 days eradicates Hib carriage in 95 per cent or more of household[12, 83] or day care center[87] contacts of a case. Cohort studies have shown the effectiveness of rifampin prophylaxis in preventing secondary Hib disease in household and day care center attendees.[83, 87, 135] Antimicrobials effective in treatment of Hib disease, such as ampicillin, trimethoprim-sulfamethoxazole, erythromycin-sulfisoxazole, and cefaclor, have been shown to be ineffective agents for antimicrobial prophylaxis,[103] eliminating Hib carriage in less than 70 per cent of culture-positive contacts, and, therefore, are not recommended.

Both the U.S. Public Health Service Advisory Committee on Immunization Practices[37] and the American Academy of Pediatrics Committee on Infectious Diseases[6] recommend rifampin prophylaxis for all household contacts, including adults, and for the index patient (therapeutic antibiotics do not eradicate Hib from the nasopharynx consistently) if there is a household contact younger than 4 years of age who is *not* fully immunized. Prophylaxis should be instituted as soon as possible because the risk of secondary disease is greatest during the few days after disease onset in the index patient and within 2 weeks of disease onset. In the day care center setting, there is no consensus concerning the need for chemoprophylaxis due to uncertainty about the magnitude of risk of secondary Hib disease in this setting. Some authors recommend chemoprophylaxis if there are classroom contacts younger than 2 years of age, whereas others believe that recommendations should be individualized. However, virtually all experts recommend prophylaxis if two or more cases of Hib disease have occurred among attendees within 60 days.[6, 37]

In all situations in which there is potential for secondary disease, this risk should be explained to families, emphasizing the importance of seeking prompt medical attention for febrile illnesses. Clinicians should not obtain pharyngeal cultures to determine whether or not to administer prophylaxis; this only delays prompt chemoprophylaxis.

CONCLUSION

The perspective on *Haemophilus* disease has changed dramatically in recent years. Prior to the availability of Hib conjugate vaccines, invasive Hib was one of the most important bacterial pathogens of children. It was the leading cause of bacterial meningitis and an important cause of other bacteremic illnesses. The spectrum of illness is broad, morbidity and mortality are significant, and there are subtleties to early diagnosis and appropriate management. Currently, when one considers that most antibiotic use worldwide is for upper respiratory tract infections, including otitis media, and that *H. influenzae* causes a significant proportion of these illnesses, it still can be considered an important pediatric pathogen.

Although various aspects of disease caused by *H. influenzae* have been reviewed in this chapter, it is clear that the most important aspect has been disease prevention by routine immunization of infants with polysaccharide-protein conjugate vaccines. This achievement is the culmination of more than 100 years of research on *H. influenzae.* Although historically there have been many technologic problems and misunderstandings about the organism and its pathogenesis, much has been accomplished in recent years. The impact of routine infant immunizations with Hib conjugate vaccines is relatively recent and very dramatic. The public health benefits parallel the eradication of polio and the control of other vaccine-preventable childhood diseases. Widespread Hib immunization virtually has eliminated Hib disease in the United States and in many developed countries where it is used routinely. The degree of disease control exceeds all expectations and is in excess of what known levels of immunization would have predicted. Unfortunately, Hib conjugate vaccines currently are used routinely in relatively few developing countries and electively in some additional countries, leaving most of the world without the benefit of immunization. The World Health Organization recently has taken up the challenge to expand Hib immunization worldwide.

Progress also has been achieved in the development of vaccines against other *H. influenzae* serotypes and nontypable strains. Control of infections caused by these organisms will have an important public health impact, and there may be a role for use of such vaccines in adolescents and adults. The technologies that led to the development of Hib conjugate vaccines serve as a prototype for vaccines to prevent disease caused by other encapsulated bacteria, such as the pneumococcus, meningococcus, and group B *Streptococcus*. As such, the lessons learned in the quest to eliminate Hib disease will have important implications in control of other bacterial diseases.

References

1. Adams, W. G., Deaver, K. A., Cochi, S. L., et al.: Decline of childhood *Haemophilus influenzae* type b (Hib) disease in the Hib vaccine era. J. A. M. A. *269*:221–226, 1993.
2. Alexander, H. E., Leidy, G., and MacPherson, C.: Production of types a, b, c, d, e and f *H. influenzae* antibody for diagnostic and therapeutic purposes. J. Immunol. *54*:207–211, 1946.
3. Alexander, H. E., Heidelberger, M., and Leidy, G.: The protective or curative element in type b *H. influenzae* rabbit serum. Yale J. Biol. Med. *16*:425–440, 1944.
4. Ambrosino, D. M., Schiffman, G., Gotschlich, E. C., et al.: Correlation between G2m(n) immunoglobulin allotype and human antibody response and susceptibility to polysaccharide encapsulated bacteria. J. Clin. Invest. *75*:1935–1942, 1985.
5. Ambrosino, D. M., Sood, S. K., Lee, M. C., et al.: IgG1, IgG2 and IgM responses to two *Haemophilus influenzae* type conjugate vaccines in young infants. Pediatr. Infect. Dis. J. *11*:855–859, 1992.
6. American Academy of Pediatrics: *Haemophilus influenzae* infections. *In* Peter, G (ed.): 1994 Red Book: Report of the Committee on Infectious Diseases. 23rd ed. Elk Grove Village, IL, American Academy of Pediatrics, 1994, pp. 203–216.
7. Anderson, P.: The protective level of serum antibodies to the capsular polysaccharide of *H. influenzae* type b. J. Infect. Dis. *149*:1034, 1984.
8. Anderson, P., Smith, D. H., and Ingram, D. L.: Antibody to polyribophosphate of *H. influenzae* type b in infants and children: Effect of immunization with polyribophosphate. J. Infect. Dis. *136*:S57–S62, 1977.
9. Argaman, M., Lin, T. Y., and Robbins, J. B.: Polyribitol-phosphate: An antigen of four gram-positive bacteria cross-reactive with the capsular polysaccharide of *H. influenzae* type b. J. Immunol. *112*:649–655, 1974.
10. Artman, M., Domenech, E., and Weiner, M.: Growth of *Haemophilus influenzae* in simulated blood cultures supplemented with hemin and NAD. J. Clin. Microbiol. *18*:376–379, 1983.
11. Baker, R. C., and Bausher, J. D.: Meningitis complicating acute bacteremic facial cellulitis. Pediatr. Infect. Dis. *5*:421–423, 1986.
12. Band, J. D., Fraser, D. W., and Ajello, G.: Prevention of *H. influenzae* type b disease. J. A. M. A. *251*:2381–2386, 1984.
13. Barenkamp, S. J., Granoff, D. M., and Munson, R. S., Jr.: Outer membrane protein subtypes of *Haemophilus influenzae* type b and spread of disease in day care centers. J. Infect. Dis. *144*:210–217, 1981.
14. Barrett, D. J.: Human immune responses to polysaccharide antigens: An analysis of bacterial polysaccharide vaccines in infants. *In* Barness, L. A. (ed.): Advances in Pediatrics. Chicago, Year Book Medical Publishers, 1985.
15. Bartlett, A. V., Zusman, J., and Daum, R. S.: Unusual presentations of *Haemophilus influenzae* infections in immunocompromised patients. J. Pediatr. *102*:55–58, 1983.
16. Baugh, R., and Baker, S. R.: Epiglottitis in children: Review of 24 cases. Otolaryngol. Head Neck Surg. *90*:157–162, 1982.
17. Berkowitz, C. D., Ward, J. I., Meier, K., et al.: Safety and immunogenicity of *Haemophilus influenzae* type b polysaccharide and polysaccharide diphtheria toxoid conjugate vaccines in children 15 to 24 months of age. J. Pediatr. *110*:509–514, 1987.
18. Black, S. B., Shinefield, H. R., Fireman, B., et al.: *Haemophilus influenzae* type b (HbOC) vaccine in a United States population of 61,080 children. Pediatr. Infect. Dis. J. *10*:97–104, 1991.
19. Black, S. B., and Shinefield, H. R.: Immunization with oligosaccharide conjugate *Haemophilus influenzae* type b (HbOC) vaccine on a large health maintenance organization population: Extended follow-up and impact on *Haemophilus influenzae* disease epidemiology. Pediatr. Infect. Dis. J. *11*:610–613, 1992.
20. Blazer, S., Berant, M., and Alon, U.: Bacterial meningitis: Effect of antibiotic treatment on cerebrospinal fluid. Am. J. Clin. Pathol. *80*:386–387, 1983.
21. Bluestone, C. D., Stephenson, J. S., and Martin, L. M.: Ten-year review of otitis media pathogens. Pediatr. Infect. Dis. J. *11*:S7–S11, 1992.
22. Bodor, F. F.: Conjunctivitis-otitis syndrome. Pediatrics *69*:695–698, 1982.
23. Bonadio, W. A.: Cerebral herniation syndrome as the presenting sign of *Haemophilus influenzae* meningitis. Pediatr. Emerg. Care *3*:253–255, 1987.
24. Booy, R., Moxon, E. R., MacFarlane, J. A., et al.: Efficacy of *Haemophilus influenzae* type b conjugate vaccine in Oxford region. Lancet *340*:847, 1992.
25. Bottenfield, G. W., Arcinue, E. L., Sarnaik, A., et al.: Diagnosis and management of acute epiglottitis: Report of 90 consecutive cases. Laryngoscope *90*:822–825, 1980.
26. Brilli, R. J., Benzing, G., and Cotcamp, D. H.: Epiglottitis in infants less than two years of age. Pediatr. Emerg. Care *5*:16–21, 1989.
27. Broome, C. V., and Schlech, W. F., III.: Recent developments in the epidemiology of bacterial meningitis. *In* Sande, M. A., Smith, A., and Root, R. D. (eds.): Bacterial Meningitis. Edinburgh, Churchill Livingstone, 1985, pp. 1–10.
28. Broughton, R. A., Edwards, M. S., Taber, L. H., et al.: Systemic *Haemophilus influenzae* type b infection presenting as fever of unknown origin. J. Pediatr. *98*:925–928, 1981.
29. Bulkow, L. R., Wainwright, R. B., Letson, G. W., et al.: Comparative immunogenicity of four *Haemophilus influenzae* type b conjugate vaccines in Alaska Native infants. Pediatr. Infect. Dis. J. *12*:484–492, 1993.
30. Cadoz, M., Prince-David, M., Mar, I. D., and Denis, F.: Epidemiologie et prognostic des meningites a *Haemophilus influenzae* en Afrique (901 cas). Pathol. Biol. *31*:128–133, 1983.
31. Campbell, L. R., Zedd, A. J., and Michaels, R. H.: Household spread of infection due to *H. influenzae* type b. Pediatrics *66*:115–117, 1980.
32. Campognone, P., and Singer, D. B.: Neonatal sepsis due to nontypable *Haemophilus influenzae*. Am. J. Dis. Child. *140*:117–121, 1986.
33. Campos, J., Garcia-Tornel, S., Gairi, J. M., and Fabregues, I.: Multiply resistant *H. influenzae* type b causing meningitis: Comparative clinical and laboratory study. J. Pediatr. *108*:897–902, 1986.
34. Cant, A. J., Gibson, P. J., and West, R. J.: Bacterial tracheitis in Down's syndrome. Arch. Dis. Child. *62*:962–963, 1987.
35. Casadevall, A., Dobroszycki, J., Small, C., and Pirofski, L. *Haemophilus influenzae* type b bacteremia in adults with AIDS and at risk for AIDS. Am. J. Med. *92*:587–590, 1992.
36. Centers for Disease Control: Ampicillin and chloramphenicol resistance in systemic *H. influenzae* disease. M. M. W. R. *33*:35–37, 1984.
37. Centers for Disease Control: Recommendations for use of *Haemophilus* b conjugate vaccines and a combined diphtheria, tetanus, pertussis, and *Haemophilus* b vaccine: Recommendations of the Advisory Committee on Immunization Practices (ACIP). M. M. W. R. *42*(No. RR-13):1–15, 1993.
38. Chapin, K. C., and Doern, G. V.: Selective media for recovery of *Haemophilus influenzae* from specimens contaminated with upper respiratory tract microbial flora. J. Clin. Microbiol. *17*:1163–1165, 1983.
39. Chartrand, S. A., Marks, M. I., Scribner, R. K., et al.: Moxalactam therapy of *Haemophilus influenzae* type b meningitis in children. J. Pediatr. *104*:454–459, 1984.
40. Cheatham, J. E., Jr., Grantham, R. N., Peyton, M. D., et al.: *Haemophilus influenzae* purulent pericarditis in children. J. Thorac. Cardiovasc. Surg. *79*:933–936, 1980.
41. Chen, L. T., and Moxon, E. R.: Effect of splenic congestion associated with hemolytic anemia on mortality of rats challenged with *Haemophilus influenzae* b. Am. J. Hematol. *15*:117–121, 1983.
42. Chilcote, R., Baehner, R., and Hammond, D.: Septicemia and meningitis in children splenectomized for Hodgkin's disease. N. Engl. J. Med. *295*:798–801, 1976.
43. Chitayat, D., Diamant, S. H., Lazevnick, R., et al.: *Haemophilus influenzae* b with pneumatocele formation. Pediatr. Infect. Dis. J. *5*:276, 1986.
44. Claesson, B. A., Trollfors, B., Lagergard, T., et al.: Clinical and immunologic responses to the capsular polysaccharide of *Haemophilus influenzae* type b alone or conjugated to tetanus toxoid in 18- to 23-month-old children. J. Pediatr. *112*:695–702, 1988.
45. Clark, J. H., Fitzgerald, J. F., and Kleiman, M. B.: Spontaneous bacterial peritonitis. J. Pediatr. *104*:495–500, 1984.
46. Clarke, C. W., Hannant, C. A., Scicchitano, R., et al.: Antigen of *Haemophilus influenzae* in bronchial tissue. Thorax *36*:665–668, 1981.
47. Clausen, C. R.: Detection of bacterial pathogens in purulent clinical specimens by immunofluorescence techniques. J. Clin. Microbiol. *13*:1119–1121, 1981.
48. Cleveland, R. H., and Foglia, R. P.: CT in the evaluation of pleural versus pulmonary disease in children. Pediatr. Radiol. *18*:14–19, 1988.
49. Cochi, S. L., and Broome, C. V. Vaccine prevention of *H. influenzae* type b disease: Past, present and future. Pediatr. Infect. Dis. J. *5*:12–19, 1986.
50. Cochi, S. L., Fleming, D. W., and Hightower, A. W.: Primary invasive *H. influenzae* type b disease: A population-based assessment of risk factors. J. Pediatr. *108*:887–896, 1986.
51. Committee on Infectious Diseases: Ampicillin-resistant strains of *H. influenzae* type b. Pediatrics *55*:145, 1975.
52. Cortese, M. M., Goepp, J., Almeido-Hill, J., et al.: Children with *Haemophilus influenzae* bacteremia initially treated as outpatients: Outcome in 85 American Indian children. Pediatr. Infect. Dis. J. *11*:521–525, 1992.
53. Crosson, F. J., Winkelstein, J. A., and Moxon, E. R.: Participation of complement in the nonimmune host defense against experimental *H. influenzae* type b septicemia and meningitis. Infect. Immun. *14*:882–887, 1976.
54. Dajani, A. S., Asmar, B. I., and Thirumoorthi, M. C.: Systemic *H. influenzae* disease: An overview. J. Pediatr. *94*:355–364, 1979.
55. Danford, D. A., Kugler, J. D., Cheatham, J. P., et al.: *Haemophilus influenzae* endocarditis: Successful treatment with ampicillin and early valve replacement. Nebr. Med. J. *69*:88–91, 1984.
56. Davie, J. M.: Antipolysaccharide immunity in man and animals. In Sell, S. H., and Wright, P. F. (eds.): *Haemophilus influenzae*. New York, Elsevier Science, 1982.
57. Decker, M. D., Edwards, K. M., Bradley, R., and Palmer, P.: Comparative

trial in infants of four conjugate *Haemophilus influenzae* type b vaccines. J. Pediatr. *120*:184–189, 1992.
58. Dodge, P. R., Davis, H., Feigin, R. D., et al.: Prospective evaluation of hearing impairment as a sequela of acute bacterial meningitis. N. Engl. J. Med. *311*:869–874, 1984.
59. Dodge, P. R., and Swartz, M. N.: Bacterial meningitis: A review of selected aspects. II. Special neurologic problems, post-meningitis complications and clinicopathological correlations. N. Engl. J. Med. *272*:1003–1010, 1965.
60. Drexhage, H. A., Van de Plassche, E. M., Kokje, M., et al.: Abnormalities in cell-mediated immune functions to *H. influenzae* in chronic purulent infections of the upper respiratory tract. Clin. Immunol. Immunopathol. *28*:218–228, 1983.
61. Eskola, J., Peltola, H., and Takala, A.: Protective efficacy of the *Haemophilus influenzae* type b conjugate vaccine HbOC in Finnish infants (Abstract 60). Program and Abstracts of the 30th ICAAC, Atlanta, GA, 1990.
62. Eskola, J., Kayhty, H., Takala, A. K., et al.: A randomized, prospective field trial of a conjugate vaccine in the protection of infants and young children against invasive *Haemophilus influenzae* type b disease. N. Engl. J. Med. *323*:1381–1387, 1990.
63. Falla, T. J., Dobson, S. R. M., Crook, D. W. M., et al.: Population-based study of non-typeable *Haemophilus influenzae* invasive disease in children and neonates. Lancet *341*:851–854, 1993.
64. Farrand, R. J.: Recurrent *Haemophilus* septicemia and immunoglobulin deficiency. Arch. Dis. Child. *45*:582–584, 1970.
65. Feigin, R. D., McCracken, G. H., Jr., and Klein, J. O.: Diagnosis and management of meningitis. Pediatr. Infect. Dis. J. *11*:785–814, 1992.
66. Feldman, W. E., Ginsburg, C. M., and McCracken, G. H.: Relation of concentrations of *H. influenzae* type b in cerebrospinal fluid to late sequelae of patients with meningitis. J. Pediatr. *100*:209–212, 1982.
67. Feldman, W. E., and Manning, N. S.: Effect of growth phase on the bactericidal action of chloramphenicol against *Haemophilus influenzae* type b and *Escherichia coli* K-1. Antimicrob. Agents Chemother. *23*:551–554, 1983.
68. Feldman, W. E., and Schwartz, J.: *Haemophilus influenzae* type b brain abscess complicating meningitis: Case report. Pediatrics *72*:473–475, 1983.
69. Figueroa, J. E., and Densen P.: Infectious diseases associated with complement deficiencies. Clin. Microbiol. Rev. *4*:359–395, 1991.
70. Fink, C. W., and Nelson, J. D.: Septic arthritis and osteomyelitis in children. Clin. Rheum. Dis. *12*:423–435, 1986.
71. Fleisher, G., Ludwig, S., and Campos, J.: Cellulitis: Bacterial etiology, clinical features, and laboratory findings. J. Pediatr. *97*:591–592, 1980.
72. Fothergill, L. D., and Wright, J.: Influenzal meningitis: The relation of age incidence to the bactericidal power of blood against the causal organism. J. Immunol. *24*:273–284, 1933.
73. Fraser, D. W., Geil, C. C., and Feldman, R. A.: Bacterial meningitis in Bernalillo county, New Mexico: A comparison with three other American populations. Am. J. Epidemiol. *100*:29–34, 1974.
74. Fraser, D. W.: *Haemophilus influenzae* in the community and in the home. *In* Sell, S. H., and Wright, P. F. (eds.): *Haemophilus influenzae*. Amsterdam, Elsevier, 1982, pp. 11–22.
75. Fraser, D. W., Henke, C. E., and Feldman, R. A.: Changing patterns of bacterial meningitis in Olmsted County, Minnesota. J. Infect. Dis. *238*:300–307, 1973.
76. Freij, B. J., Votteler, T. P., and McCracken, G. H.: Primary peritonitis in previously healthy children. Am. J. Dis. Child. *138*:1058–1061, 1984.
77. Friesen, C. A., and Cho, C. T.: Characteristic features of neonatal sepsis due to *Haemophilus influenzae*. Rev. Infect. Dis. *8*:777–780, 1986.
78. Fritzell, B., and Plotkin, S. A.: Efficacy and safety of a *Haemophilus influenzae* type b capsular polysaccharide-tetanus protein conjugate vaccine. J. Pediatr. *121*:355–362, 1992.
79. Gilsdorf, J. R.: *Haemophilus influenzae* non-type b infections in children. Am. J. Dis. Child. *141*:1063–1065, 1987.
80. Gilsdorf, J. R.: Bacterial meningitis in southwestern Alaska. Am. J. Epidemiol. *106*:388–391, 1977.
81. Ginsburg, C. M.: *Haemophilus influenzae* type b buccal cellulitis. J. Am. Acad. Dermatol. *4*:551–554, 1981.
82. Glezen, W. P., Englund, J. A., Siber, G. R., et al.: Maternal immunization with the capsular polysaccharide vaccine for *Haemophilus influenzae* type b. J. Infect. Dis. *165*(Suppl. 1):S134–S136, 1992.
83. Glode, M. P., Daum, R. S., Halsey, N. A., et al.: Rifampin alone and in combination with trimethoprim in chemoprophylaxis for infections due to *Haemophilus influenzae* type b. Rev. Infect. Dis. *5*(Suppl.):S549–S555, 1983.
84. Goldblatt, D., Fairley, C. K., Cartwright, K., and Miller, E.: Interchangeability of conjugated *Haemophilus influenzae* type b vaccines during primary immunisation of infants. B. M. J. *312*:817–818, 1996.
85. Granoff, D. M., Barenkamp, S. J., and Munson, R. S.: Outer membrane protein subtypes for epidemiologic investigation of *H. influenzae* type disease. *In* Sell, S. H., and Wright, P. F. (eds.): *Haemophilus influenzae*: Epidemiology, Immunology, and Prevention of Disease. New York, Elsevier Biomedical, 1982, pp. 43–55.
86. Granoff, D. M., and Basden, M.: *H. influenzae* infections in Fresno County, California: A prospective study of the effects of age, race and contact with a case on incidence of disease. J. Infect. Dis. *140*:40–46, 1980.
87. Granoff, D. M., Gilsdorf, J., and Gessert, C.: *Haemophilus influenzae* type b disease in a day care center: Eradication of carrier state by rifampin. Pediatrics *63*:397–401, 1979.
88. Granoff, D. M., Holmes, S. J., Belshe, R. B., et al.: Effect of carrier protein priming on antibody responses to *Haemophilus influenzae* type b conjugate vaccines in infants. J. A. M. A. *272*:1116–1121, 1994.
89. Granoff, D. M., Rathore, M. H., Holmes, S. J., et al.: Effect of immunity to the carrier protein on antibody responses to *Haemophilus influenzae* type b conjugate vaccines. Vaccine *11*(Suppl. 1):S46–S51, 1993.
90. Granoff, D. M., Shackelford, P. G., Pandey, J. P., et al.: Antibody responses to *H. influenzae* type b polysaccharide vaccine in relation to Km(1) and G2, (23) immunoglobulin allotypes. J. Infect. Dis. *154*:257–264, 1986.
91. Greenberg, D. P., Lieberman, J. M., Marcy, S. M., et al.: Enhanced antibody responses in infants given different sequences of heterogeneous *Haemophilus influenzae* type b conjugate vaccines. J. Pediatr. *126*:206–211, 1995.
92. Greenberg, D. P., Vadheim, C. M., Bordenave, N., et al.: Protective efficacy of *Haemophilus influenzae* type b polysaccharide and conjugate vaccines in children 18 months of age and older. J. A. M. A. *265*:987–992, 1991.
93. Greenfield, S., Peter, G., and Howie, V. M.: Acquisition of type-specific antibodies to *H. influenzae* type b. J. Pediatr. *80*:204–208, 1972.
94. Greenfield, S. P.: Type b *Haemophilus influenzae* epididymo-orchitis in the prepubertal boy. J. Urol. *136*:1311–1313, 1986.
95. Greenwood, B.: Epidemiology of acute lower respiratory tract infections, especially those due to *Haemophilus influenzae* type b, in the Gambia, West Africa. J. Infect. Dis. *165*(Suppl. 1):S26–S28, 1992.
96. Gregorius, F. K., Johnson, B. J., Stern, W. E., and Brown, W. J.: Pathogenesis of hematogenous bacterial meningitis in rabbits. J. Neurosurg. *45*:561–567, 1976.
97. Hammond, G. W., Slutchuk, M., Scatiff, J., et al.: Epidemiologic, clinical, laboratory and therapeutic features of an urban outbreak of chancroid in North America. Rev. Infect. Dis. *2*:867–869, 1980.
98. Hansman, D., Hanna, J., and Morey, F.: High prevalence of invasive *Haemophilus influenzae* disease in central Australia, 1986. Lancet *2*:927, 1986.
99. Harrison, L. H., da Silva, G. A., Pittman, M., et al.: Epidemiology and clinical spectrum of Brazilian purpuric fever. Brazilian Purpuric Fever Study Group. J. Clin. Microbiol. *27*:599–604, 1989.
100. Hellinger, W. C., and Brewer, N. S.: Imipenem. Mayo Clin. Proc. *66*:1074–1081, 1991.
101. Hoiseth, S. K., Moxon, E. A., and Silver, R. P.: Genes involved in *Haemophilus influenzae* type b expression are part of an iskilobase tandem duplication. Proc. Natl. Acad. Sci. U. S. A. *83*:1106–1110, 1986.
102. Holmes, S. J., Murphy T. V., Anderson, R. S., et al.: Immunogenicity of four *Haemophilus influenzae* type b conjugate vaccines in 17- to 19-month-old children. J. Pediatr. *118*:364–371, 1991.
103. Horner, D. B., McCracken, G. H., Ginsburg, C. M., and Zweighaft, T. C.: A comparison of three antibiotic regimens for eradication of *Haemophilus influenzae* type b from the pharynx of infants and children. Pediatrics *66*:136–138, 1980.
104. Howe, P. M., Edwardo Fajardo, J., and Orcutt, M. A.: Etiologic diagnosis of cellulitis: Comparison of aspirates obtained from the leading edge and the point of maximal inflammation. Pediatr. Infect. Dis. J. *5*:685–686, 1987.
105. Istre, G. R., Conner, J. S., and Broome, C. V.: Risk factors for primary invasive *H. influenzae* disease: Increased risk from day care attendance and school age household members. J. Pediatr. *106*:190–195, 1985.
106. Jacobs, R. F., Hsi, S., Wilson, C. B., et al.: Apparent meningococcemia: Clinical features of disease due to *Haemophilus influenzae* and *Neisseria meningitidis*. Pediatrics *72*:469–472, 1983.
107. Jacobs, R. F., Wright, M. W., Deskin, R. L., et al.: Delayed sterilization of *Haemophilus influenzae* type b meningitis with twice-daily ceftriaxone. J. A. M. A. *259*:392–394, 1988.
108. Johnston, R. B., Anderson, P., Rosen, F. S., and Smith, D. H. Characterization of human immunity to polyribophosphate, the capsular antigen of *H. influenzae* type b. Clin. Immunol. Immunopathol. *1*:234–240, 1973.
109. Jonsdottir, K. E., Steingrimsson, O., and Olafsson, O.: Immunisation of infants in Iceland against *Haemophilus influenzae* type b. Lancet *340*:252–253, 1992.
110. Jorgensen, J. H.: Update on mechanisms and prevalence of antimicrobial resistance in *Haemophilus influenzae*. Clin. Infect. Dis. *14*:1119–1123, 1992.
111. Kaplan, S. L.: Antigen detection in cerebrospinal fluid: Pros and cons. Am. J. Med. *75*(B):109–118, 1983.
112. Karasic, R. B., Beste, D. J., To, S. C., et al.: Evaluation of pilus vaccines for prevention of experimental otitis media caused by nontypable *Haemophilus influenzae*. Pediatr. Infect. Dis. J. *8*:S62–S65, 1989.
113. Kayhty, H., Eskola, J., Peltola, H., et al.: Immunogenicity in infants of a vaccine composed of a *Haemophilus influenzae* type b capsular polysaccharide mixed with DPT or conjugated to diphtheria toxoid. J. Infect. Dis. *155*:100–106, 1987.
114. Kayhty, H., Karanko, V., Peltola, H., Makela, P. H. Serum antibodies after vaccination with *H. influenzae* type b capsular polysaccharide and responses to reimmunization: No evidence of immunologic tolerance or memory. Pediatrics *74*:857–865, 1984.
115. Kayhty, H., Peltola, H., Karanko, V., et al.: The protective level of serum antibodies to the capsular polysaccharide of *H. influenzae* type b. J. Infect. Dis. *147*:1100, 1983.
116. Kayhty, H., Schneerson, R., and Sutton, A.: Class-specific antibody re-

sponse to *H. influenzae* type b capsular polysaccharide vaccine. J. Infect. Dis. *148*:767, 1983.

117. Kleiman, M. B., Reynolds, J. K., Watts, N. H., et al.: Superiority of acridine orange stain versus Gram stain in partially treated bacterial meningitis. J. Pediatr. *104*:401–404, 1984.
118. Koomey, J. M., and Falkow, S.: Nucleotide sequence homology between the immunoglobulin A1 protease genes of *Neisseria gonorrhoeae, Neisseria meningitidis,* and *Haemophilus influenzae.* Infect. Immun. *43*:101–107, 1984.
119. Korones, D. N., Marshall, G. S., and Shapiro, E. D.: Outcome of children with occult bacteremia caused by *Haemophilus influenzae* type b. Pediatr. Infect. Dis. J. *11*:516–520, 1992.
120. Krasinski, K., Nelson, J. D., Butler, S., et al.: Possible association of mycoplasma and viral respiratory infections with bacterial meningitis. Am. J. Epidemiol. *125*:499–508, 1987.
121. Landsteiner, K.: The Specificity of Serologic Reactions. Cambridge, Harvard University Press, 1945. Reprinted by Dover Publications, New York, 1962.
122. Lebel, M. H., and Nelson, J. D.: *Haemophilus influenzae* type b osteomyelitis in infants and children. Pediatr. Infect. Dis. J. *7*:250–254, 1988.
123. Lehmann, D.: Epidemiology of acute respiratory tract infections, especially those due to *Haemophilus influenzae,* in Papua New Guinean children. J. Infect. Dis. *165*(Suppl. 1):S20–S25, 1992.
124. Lerman, S. J.: *Haemophilus influenzae* infections of cerebrospinal fluid shunts. J. Neurosurg. *54*:261–263, 1981.
125. Letson, G. W., Santosham, M., Reid, R., et al.: Comparison of active and combined passive/active immunization of Navajo children against *Haemophilus influenzae* type b. Pediatr. Infect. Dis. J. *7*:747–752, 1988.
126. Lichty, E., Kleiman, M. B., Ballantine, T. V. N., et al.: Primary *Haemophilus influenzae* lung abscesses with bronchial obstruction. J. Pediatr. Surg. *17*:281–284, 1982.
127. Lieberman, J. M., Greenberg, D. P., Wong, V. K., et al. Effect of neonatal immunization with diphtheria and tetanus toxoids on antibody responses to *Haemophilus influenzae* type b conjugate vaccines. J. Pediatr. *126*:198–205, 1995.
128. Lin, Y. C., King, D. R., Birken, G. A., et al.: Acute scrotum due to *Haemophilus influenzae* type b. J. Pediatr. Surg. *23*:183–184, 1988.
129. Loeb, M. R., and Smith, D. H.: Human antibody response to individual outer membrane proteins of *Haemophilus influenzae* type b. Infect. Immun. *37*:1032–1036, 1982.
130. Losek, J. D., Dewitz-Zink, B. A., Melzer-Lange, M., et al.: Epiglottitis: Comparison of signs and symptoms in children less than 2 years old and older. Ann. Emerg. Med. *19*:55–58, 1990.
131. Losonsky, G. A., Santosham, M., Sehgal, V. M., et al.: *Haemophilus influenzae* in the White Mountain Apaches: Molecular epidemiology of a high risk population. Pediatr. Infect. Dis. J. *3*:539–547, 1984.
132. Lucas, A. H.: Expression of crossreactive idiotypes by human antibodies specific for the capsular polysaccharide of *Haemophilus influenzae* b. J. Clin. Invest. *81*:480–486, 1988.
133. Madore, D. V., Johnson, C. L., Phipps, D. C., et al.: Safety and immunogenicity of *Haemophilus influenzae* type b oligosaccharide-CRM197 conjugate vaccine in infants aged 15–23 months. Pediatrics *86*:527–534, 1990.
134. Makela, P. H., Takala, A. K., Peltola, H., and Eskola, J.: Epidemiology of invasive *Haemophilus influenzae* type b disease. J. Infect. Dis. *165*(Suppl. 1):S2–S6, 1992.
135. Makintubee, S., Istre, G. R., and Ward, J. I.: Transmission of invasive *Haemophilus influenzae* type b disease in day care settings. J. Pediatr. *111*:180–186, 1987.
136. Marcon, M. J., Hamoudi, A. C., and Cannon, J. H.: Comparative laboratory evaluation of three antigen detection methods for diagnosis of *Haemophilus influenzae* type b disease. J. Clin. Microbiol. *19*:333–337, 1984.
137. Mason, E. O., Kaplan, S. L., Lambeth, L. B., et al.: Serotype and ampicillin susceptibility of *Haemophilus influenzae* causing systemic infection in children: Three years of experience. J. Clin. Microbiol. *15*:543–546, 1982.
138. Masters, P. L., Brumfitt, W., Mendez, R. L., Likar, M.: Bacterial flora of the upper respiratory tract in Paddington families. B. M. J. *1*:1200–1205, 1958.
139. McCarthy, L. G.: *Haemophilus influenzae* associated with periappendiceal abscess. Am. J. Gastroenterol. *76*:157–159, 1981.
140. McCracken, G. H., Ginsburg, C. M., Zweighaft, T. C., and Clahsen, J.: Pharmacokinetics of rifampin in infants and children: Relevance to prophylaxis against *Haemophilus influenzae* type b disease. Pediatrics *66*:17–21, 1980.
141. McGraw, T. P., and Bruckner, D. A.: Sensitivity of commercial agglutination and counterimmunoelectrophoresis methods for the detection of *Haemophilus influenzae* type b capsular polysaccharide. Am. J. Clin. Pathol. *80*:703–706, 1983.
142. Mehl, A. L.: *Haemophilus influenzae* polyserositis. J. Pediatr. *112*:160–161, 1988.
143. Michaels, R. H., and Norden, C. W.: Pharyngeal colonization with *H. influenzae* type b: A longitudinal study of families with a child with meningitis or epiglottitis due to *H. influenzae* type b. J. Infect. Dis. *136*:222–228, 1977.
144. Michaels, R. H., and Schultz, W. F.: The frequency of *Haemophilus influenzae* infections: Analysis of racial and environmental factors. *In* Sell, S. H., and Karzon, D. T. (eds.): *Haemophilus influenzae.* Nashville, Vanderbilt University Press, 1973, pp. 243–250.
145. Miragliotta, G., Colucci, M., Semeraro, N., et al.: Platelet injury and stimulation of leukocyte procoagulant activity in vitro by a lipopolysaccharide from *Haemophilus influenzae* type b. Microbiologica *4*:173–180, 1981.
146. Morgan, R. J., Stephenson, L. W., and Woolf, P. K.: Surgical treatment of purulent pericarditis in children. J. Thorac. Cardiovasc. Surg. *85*:527–531, 1983.
147. Moxon, E. R.: Experimental studies of *H. influenzae* in a rat model. *In* Sell, S. H., and Wright, P. F. (eds.): *Haemophilus influenzae*: Epidemiology, Immunology, and Prevention of Disease. New York, Elsevier Biomedical, 1982.
148. Mulks, M. H., Kornfeld, S. J., Bragione, B., et al.: Relationship between the specificity of IgA proteases and serotypes in *H. influenzae.* J. Infect. Dis. *146*:266–274, 1982.
149. Munson, R., Jr., and Grass, S.: Purification, cloning, and sequence of outer membrane protein P1 of *Haemophilus influenzae* type b. Infect. Immun. *56*:2235–2242, 1988.
150. Murphy, T. V., Granoff, D., and Chrane, D. F.: Pharyngeal colonization with *Haemophilus influenzae* type b in children in a day care center without invasive disease. J. Pediatr. *106*:712–716, 1985.
151. Murphy, T. V., Pastor, P., Medley, F., et al.: Decreased *Haemophilus* colonization in children vaccinated with *Haemophilus influenzae* type b conjugate vaccine. J. Pediatr. *122*:517–523, 1993.
152. Murphy, T. V., White, K. E., Pastor, P., et al.: Declining incidence of *Haemophilus influenzae* type b disease since introduction of vaccination. J. A. M. A. *269*:246–248, 1993.
153. Musher, D. M., Goree, A., Baughn, R. E., et al.: Immunoglobulin A from bronchopulmonary secretions block bactericidal and opsonizing effects of antibody to nontypable *H. influenzae.* Infect. Immun. *45*:36–40, 1984.
154. Musser, J. M., Barenkamp, S. J., Granoff, D. M., et al.: Genetic relationships of serologically nontypable and serotype b strains of *Haemophilus influenzae.* Infect. Immun. *52*:183–191, 1986.
155. Musser, J. M., Kroll, J. S., Cranoff, D. M., et al.: Global genetic structure and molecular epidemiology of encapsulated *Haemophilus influenzae.* Rev. Infect. Dis. *12*:75–111, 1990.
156. Musser, J. M., Kroll, J. S., Moxon, E. R., and Selander, R. K.: Evolutionary genetics of the encapsulated strains of *Haemophilus influenzae.* Proc. Natl. Acad. Sci. U. S. A. *85*:7758–7762, 1988.
157. Mustafa, M. M., Lebel, M. H., and McCracken, G. H., Jr.: Tenosynovitis and transient arthritis associated with *Haemophilus influenzae* type b bacteremia. Pediatr. Infect. Dis. J. *7*:517–519, 1988.
158. Mustafa, M. M., Scarvey, L., Rollins, N. et al.: Primary suppurative myositis associated with *Haemophilus influenzae* type b septicemia. Pediatr. Infect. Dis. J. *7*:815–817, 1988.
159. Nelson, M. D., Murphy, T. F., van Keulen, H., et al.: Studies on P6, an important outer-membrane protein antigen of *Haemophilus influenzae.* Rev. Infect. Dis. *10*:S331–S336, 1988.
160. Newman, S. L., Waldo, B., and Johnston R. B.: Separation of serum bactericidal and opsonizing activities for *Haemophilus influenzae* type b. Infect. Immun. *8*:488–490, 1973.
161. Osterholm, M. T., Pierson, L. N., White, K. E., et al.: Risk of subsequent transmission of *Haemophilus influenzae* type b disease among children in day care. N. Engl. J. Med. *316*:1–4, 1987.
162. Ostrow, P. T., Moxon, E. R. Vernon, N., and Kapko, R.: Studies on the route of meningeal invasion following *H. influenzae* inoculation of infant rats. Lab. Invest. *40*:678–685, 1979.
163. Oxelius, V. A.: Quantitative and qualitative investigations of serum IgG subclasses in immunodeficiency diseases. Clin. Exp. Immunol. *36*:112–116, 1979.
164. Pauwels, R., Verschraegen, G., and Van Der Straeten, M.: IgE antibodies to bacteria in patients with bronchial asthma. Allergy *157*:665–669, 1980.
165. Peltola, H., Kayhty, H., and Sivonen, A.: *Haemophilus influenzae* type b capsular polysaccharide vaccine in children: A double-blind field study of 100,000 vaccinees 3 months to 5 years of age in Finland. Pediatrics *60*:730–737, 1977.
166. Peltola, H., Kayhty, H., Virtanen, M., and Makela, P. H.: Prevention of *H. influenzae* type b bacteremic infection with the capsular polysaccharide vaccine. N. Engl. J. Med. *310*:1566–1569, 1984.
167. Peltola, H., Kilpi, T., and Anttila, M.: Rapid disappearance of *Haemophilus influenzae* type b meningitis after routine childhood immunization with conjugate vaccines. Lancet *340*:592–594, 1992.
168. Peltola, H., and Virtanen, M.: Systemic *Haemophilus influenzae* infection in Finland. Clin. Pediatr. *5*:275–280, 1984.
169. Peterson, G. M., Silimperi, D. R., Chiu, C. Y., and Ward, J. I.: Effects of age, breast-feeding and household structure on *Haemophilus influenzae* type b disease risk and antibody acquisition in Alaskan Eskimos. Am. J. Epidemiol. *134*:1212–1221, 1991.
170. Pfeiffer, R.: Vorlaufige mit heilungen über die erreger der influenzae. Dtsch. Med. Wochenschr. *18*:28–34, 1892.
171. Pichichero, M. E., Hall, C. B., and Insel, R. A.: A mucosal antibody response following systemic *H. influenzae* type b infection in children. J. Clin. Invest. *67*:1482–1489, 1981.
172. Pichichero, M. E., and Insel, R. A.: Mucosal antibody response to parenteral vaccination with *H. influenzae* type b capsule. J. Allergy Clin. Immunol. *72*:481–486, 1983.

173. Pittman, M.: Variation and type specificity in the bacterial species: *H. influenzae*. J. Exp. Med. *53*:471–495, 1931.
174. Pittman, M.: The action of type-specific *H. influenzae* antiserum. J. Exp. Med. *58*:583–706, 1933.
175. Plaut, A. G.: The IgA1 proteases of pathogenic bacteria. Ann. Rev. Microbiol. *37*:603–622, 1983.
176. Pomeroy, S. L., Holmes, S. J., Dodge, P. R., and Feigin, R. D.: Seizures and other neurologic sequelae of bacterial meningitis in children. N. Engl. J. Med. *323*:1651–1657, 1990.
177. Powars, D., Overturf, G., and Turner, E.: Is there an increased risk of *H. influenzae* septicemia in children with sickle cell anemia? Pediatrics *71*:927–931, 1983.
178. Prober, C. G.: The role of steroids in the management of children with bacterial meningitis. Pediatrics *95*:29–31, 1995.
179. Ramada, K., Petersen, G. M., Heiner, D. C., et al.: Class and subclass antibodies of *H. influenzae* type capsule: Comparison of invasive disease and natural exposure. Infect. Immun. *53*:486–490, 1986.
180. Redmond, S. R., and Pichichero, M. E. *Haemophilus influenzae* type b disease: An epidemiologic study with special reference to day care centers. J. A. M. A. *252*:2581–2584, 1984.
181. Rennels, M. B., and Wald, E. R.: Treatment of *Haemophilus influenzae* type b meningitis in children with cerebrospinal fluid shunts. J. Pediatr. *97*:424–426, 1980.
182. Ricketts, R. R., Ilbawi, M. N., and Idriss, F. S.: Management of *Haemophilus influenzae* pericarditis. J. Pediatr. Surg. *17*:285–289, 1982.
183. Riesen, W. F., Skavaril, F., and Braun, D. G.: Natural infection of man with group A streptococci: Levels, restriction in class, subclass, and type, and clonal appearance of polysaccharide-group specific antibodies. Scand. J. Immunol. *5*:383–390, 1976.
184. Robbins, J. B., Park, J. C., Jr., Schneerson, R., and Whisnant, J. K.: Quantitative measurement of "natural" and immunization-induced *H. influenzae* type b capsular polysaccharide antibodies. Pediatr. Res. *7*:103–110, 1973.
185. Robbins, J. B., Schneerson, R., and Pittman, M. H.: Influenzae type b infections. *In* Germanier, R. (ed.): Bacterial Vaccines. Orlando, Academic Press, 1984, pp 290–313.
186. Roberts, M. C., Swenson, C. D., Owens, I. M., and Smith, A. L.: Characterization of chloramphenicol-resistant *H. influenzae*. Antimicrob. Agents Chemother. *18*:510–515, 1980.
187. Rodrigues, L. P., Schneerson, R., and Robbins, J. B.: Immunity to *H. influenzae* type b. I. The isolation and some physiochemical, serologic and biologic properties of the capsular polysaccharide of *H. influenzae* type b. J. Immunol. *107*:1071–1080, 1971.
188. Rowe, J. E., Messinger, I. K., Schwendeman, C. A., and Popejoy, L. A.: Three-dose vaccination of infants under 8 months of age with a conjugate *Haemophilus influenzae* type b vaccine. Mil. Med. *155*:483–486, 1990.
189. Rubin, L. G., and Moxon, E. R.: Pathogenesis of bloodstream invasion with *Haemophilus influenzae* type b. Infect. Immun. *41*:280–284, 1983.
190. Rusin, P., Adam, R. D., Petersen, E. A., et al.: *Haemophilus influenzae*: An important cause of maternal and neonatal infections. Obstet. Gynecol. *77*:92–96, 1991.
191. Saez-Llorens, X.: Pathogenesis of acute otitis media. Pediatr. Infect. Dis. J. *13*:1035–1038, 1994.
192. Salwen, K. M., Vikerfors, T., and Olcen, P.: Increased incidence of childhood bacterial meningitis: A 25-year study in a defined population in Sweden. Scand. J. Infect. Dis. *19*:1–11, 1987.
193. Santosham, M., Reid, R., and Ambrosino, D. M.: Prevention of *H. influenzae* type b (Hib) infections in high-risk infants treated with bacterial polysaccharide immune globulin. N. Engl. J. Med. *317*:923–929, 1987.
194. Santosham, M., Rivin, B., Wolff, M., et al.: Prevention of *Haemophilus influenzae* type b infections in Apache and Navajo children. J. Infect. Dis. *165*(Suppl. 1):S144–S151, 1992.
195. Santosham, M., Wolff, M., Reid, R., et al.: The efficacy in Navajo infants of a conjugate vaccine consisting of *Haemophilus influenzae* type b polysaccharide and *Neisseria meningitidis* outer-membrane protein complex. N. Engl. J. Med. *324*:1767–1772, 1991.
196. Schauf, V., Green, D. C., Van Der Stuyf, L., et al.: Chloramphenicol kills *Haemophilus influenzae* more rapidly than does ampicillin or cefamandole. Antimicrob. Agents Chemother. *23*:364–368, 1983.
197. Scheld, W. M., Parks, T. S., Winn, H. R., et al.: Clearance of bacteria from cerebrospinal fluid to blood in experimental meningitis. Infect. Immun. *24*:102–105, 1979.
198. Schlamm, H. T., and Yancovitz, S. R.: *Haemophilus influenzae* pneumonia in young adults with AIDS, ARC, or risk of AIDS. Am. J. Med. *86*:11–14, 1989.
199. Schneerson, R., Robbins, J. B., and Parke, J. C.: Quantitative and qualitative analyses of serum antibodies elicited in adults by *H. influenzae* type b and pneumococcus type 6A capsular polysaccharide-tetanus toxoid conjugates. Infect. Immun. *52*:519–528, 1986.
200. Schneerson, R., Rodrigues, L. P., Parke, J. C., and Robbins, J. B.: Immunity to disease caused by *H. influenzae* type b. II. Specificity and some biological characteristics of "natural," infection acquired and immunization induced antibody to the capsular polysaccharide. J. Immunol. *107*:1081–1089, 1971.
201. Schreiber, J. R., Barrus, V., Cates, K. L., et al.: Functional characterization of human IgG, IgM, and IgA antibody directed to the capsule of *H. influenzae* type b. J. Infect. Dis. *153*:8–16, 1986.
202. Schur, P. H., Borel, H., and Gelfand, E. W.: Selective gamma-G globulin deficiencies in patients with recurrent pyogenic infections. N. Engl. J. Med. *283*:631–634, 1970.
203. Shackelford, P. G., Granoff, D. M., and Nahm, M. H.: Relation of age, race and allotype to immunoglobulin subclass concentrations. Pediatr. Res. *19*:846–849, 1985.
204. Shackelford, P. G., Granoff, D. M., Nelson, S. J., et al.: Subclass distribution of human antibodies to *Haemophilus influenzae* type b capsular polysaccharide. J. Immunol. *138*:587–592, 1987.
205. Shapiro, E. D.: Persistent pharyngeal colonization with *H. influenzae* type b after intravenous chloramphenicol therapy. Pediatrics *67*:435–437, 1981.
206. Shapiro, E. D., and Wald, E. R.: Efficacy of rifampin in eliminating pharyngeal carriage of *H. influenzae* type b. Pediatrics *66*:5–8, 1980.
207. Siber, G. R., and Ambrosino, D. M.: Heavy and light chain restriction of human antibodies to bacterial polysaccharide antigens. *In* Morell, A., and Hydegger, U. E. (eds.): Clinical Use of Intravenous Immunoglobulins. Orlando, Academic Press, 1986, pp. 47–54.
208. Siber, G. R., Ambrosino, D. M., and McIver, J.: Preparation of human hyperimmune globulin to *Haemophilus influenzae* b, *Streptococcus pneumoniae*, and *Neisseria meningitidis*. Infect. Immun. *45*:248–254, 1984.
209. Sirinavin, S., Chiemchanya, S., Visudhipan, P., et al.: Cefuroxime treatment of bacterial meningitis in infants and children. Antimicrob. Agents Chemother. *25*:273–275, 1984.
210. Smith, A. L., Daum, R. S., Scheifele, D., et al.: Pathogenesis of *H. influenzae* meningitis. *In* Sell, S. H., and Wright, P. F. (eds.): *Haemophilus influenzae*: Epidemiology, Immunology and Prevention of Disease. New York, Elsevier Biomedical, 1982, pp. 89–109.
211. Spanjaard, L., Bol, P., Ekker, W., and Zanen, H. C.: The incidence of bacterial meningitis in The Netherlands: A comparison of three registration systems, 1977–1982. J. Infect. *11*:259–268, 1985.
212. Spinola, S. M., Sheaffer, C. I., Pholbrick, K. B., et al.: Antigenuria after *Haemophilus influenzae* type b polysaccharide immunization: A prospective study. J. Pediatr. *109*:835–838, 1986.
213. Steele, N. P., Munson, R. S., and Granoff, D. M. Antibody-dependent alternative pathway killing of *H. influenzae* type b. Infect. Immun. *44*:452, 1984.
214. Stephens, D. S., and Farley, M. M.: Pathogenic events during infections of the human nasopharynx with *Neisseria meningitidis* and *Haemophilus influenzae*. Rev. Infect. Dis. *13*:22–33, 1991.
215. Strakosch, E. A., Kendell, H. W., Craig, R. M., et al.: Clinical and laboratory investigation of 370 cases of chancroid. J. Invest. Dermatol. *6*:95–107, 1945.
216. Stull, T. L., Jacobs, R. F., and Haas, J. E.: Human serum bactericidal activity against *H. influenzae* type b. J. Clin. Microbiol. *130*:665–672, 1984.
217. Takala, A. K., Eskola, J., Leinonen, M., et al.: Reduction of oropharyngeal carriage of *Haemophilus influenzae* type b (Hib) in children immunized with an Hib conjugate vaccine. J. Infect. Dis. *164*:982–986, 1991.
218. Takala, A. K., Mourman, O., Kleemola, M., et al.: Preceding respiratory infection predisposing for primary and secondary invasive *Haemophilus influenzae* type b disease. Pediatr. Infect. Dis. J. *12*:189–195, 1993.
219. Tarr, P. I., and Peter, G.: Demographic factors in the epidemiology of *H. influenzae* meningitis in young children. J. Pediatr. *92*:884–888, 1978.
220. Tarrand, J. J., Scott, M. G., Takes, P. A., et al.: Clonal characterization of the human IgG antibody repertoire to *Haemophilus influenzae* type b polysaccharide: Demonstration of three types of V regions and their association with H and L chain isotypes. J. Immunol. *142*:2519–2526, 1989.
221. Taylor, J. R. W., Cibis, G. W., and Hamtil, L. W.: Endophthalmitis complicating *Haemophilus influenzae* type b meningitis. Arch. Ophthalmol. *98*:324–326, 1980.
222. Taylor, H. G., Mills, E. L., Ciampi, A., et al.: The sequelae of *Haemophilus influenzae* meningitis in school-age children. N. Engl. J. Med. *323*:1657–1663, 1990.
223. Todd, J. K., and Bruhn, F. W.: Severe *Haemophilus influenzae* infections: Spectrum of disease. Am. J. Dis. Child. *129*:607–611, 1975.
224. Turk, D. C.: Naso-pharyngeal carriage of *H. influenzae* type b. J. Hyg. *61*:247–256, 1963.
225. Uchiyama, N., Greene, G. R., Kitts, D. R., and Thrupp, L. D.: Meningitis due to *H. influenzae* type b resistant to ampicillin and chloramphenicol. J. Pediatr. *97*:421–424, 1980.
226. Vadheim, C. M., Greenberg, D. P., Bordenave, N., et al.: Risk factors for invasive *Haemophilus influenzae* type b in Los Angeles County children 18–60 months of age. Am. J. Epidemiol. *136*:221–235, 1992.
227. Vadheim, C. M., Greenberg, D. P., Eriksen, E., et al.: Eradication of *Haemophilus influenzae* type b disease in Southern California. Arch. Pediatr. Adolesc. Med. *148*:51–56, 1994.
228. Vadheim, C. M., Greenberg, D. P., Eriksen, E., et al.: Protection provided by *Haemophilus influenzae* type b conjugate vaccines in Los Angeles county: a case-control study. Pediatr. Infect. Dis. J. *13*:274–280, 1994.
229. Vadheim, C. M., Greenberg, D. P., Partridge, S., et al.: Effectiveness and safety of an *Haemophilus influenzae* type b conjugate vaccine (PRP-T) in young infants. Pediatrics *92*:272–279, 1993.
230. van Alphen, L., Eijk, P., Geelen-van den, B., and Dankert, J.: Immunochemical characterization of variable epitopes of outer membrane protein

P2 of nontypeable *Haemophilus influenzae*. Infect. Immun. *59*:247–252, 1991.
231. Van Ham, S. M., van Alpen, L., and Mooi, F. R.: Fimbria-mediated adherence and hemagglutination of *Haemophilus influenzae*. J. Infect. Dis. *165*(Suppl. 1):S97–S99, 1992.
232. van Nguyen, Q., Nguyen, E. A., and Weiner, L. B.: Incidence of invasive bacterial disease in children with fever and petechiae. Pediatrics *74*:77–80, 1984.
233. Wall, R. A., Corrah, P. T., Mabey, D. C. W., and Greenwood, B. M.: The etiology of lobar pneumonia in the Gambia. Bull. W. H. O. *64*:553–558, 1986.
234. Wallace, R. J., Baker, C. J., Quinones, F. J., et al.: Non-typeable *Haemophilus influenzae* (biotype 4) as a neonatal, maternal, and genital pathogen. Rev. Infect. Dis. *5*:123–136, 1983.
235. Ward, J. I., Brenneman, G., Letson, G. W., and Heyward, W. L.: The Alaska *H. influenzae* Vaccine Study Group: Limited efficacy of a *Haemophilus influenzae* type b conjugate vaccine in Alaska Native infants. N. Engl. J. Med. *323*:1393–1401, 1990.
236. Ward, J. I., Fraser, D. W., Baraff, L. J., and Plikaytis, B. D.: *H. influenzae* meningitis: A national study of secondary spread in household contacts. N. Engl. J. Med. *301*:122–126, 1979.
237. Ward, J. I., Gorman, G., and Phillips, C.: *Haemophilus influenzae* type b disease in a daycare center: Report of an outbreak. J. Pediatr. *92*:713–717, 1978.
238. Ward, J. I., Lieberman, J. M., and Cochi, S. L.: *Haemophilus influenzae* vaccines. *In* Plotkin, S. A., and Mortimer, E. A. (eds.): Vaccines. Philadelphia, W. B. Saunders, 1994, pp. 337–386.
239. Ward, J. I., Lum, M. K. W., Hall, D. B., et al.: Invasive *Haemophilus influenzae* type b disease in Alaska: Background epidemiology for a vaccine efficacy trial. J. Infect. Dis. *108*:887–896, 1986.
240. Ward, J. I., Siber, G. I., Scheifele, D. W., et al.: Rapid diagnosis of *Haemophilus influenzae* type b infections by latex particle agglutination and counterimmunoelectrophoresis. J. Pediatr. *93*:37–42, 1978.
241. Weitzman, S., and Aisenberg, A. C.: Fulminant sepsis after the successful treatment of Hodgkin's disease. Am. J. Med. *62*:47–50, 1977.
242. Weller, P. F., Smith, A. L., Smith, D. H., and Anderson, P.: Role of immunity in the clearance of bacteremia due to *H. influenzae*. J. Infect. Dis. *138*:427–436, 1978.
243. Wenger, J. D., Hightower, A. W., Facklam, R. R., et al.: Bacterial meningitis in the United States, 1986: Report of a multistate surveillance study. J. Infect. Dis. *162*:1316–1323, 1990.
244. Wenger, J. D., Pierce, R., Deaver, K. A., et al.: Efficacy of *Haemophilus influenzae* type b polysaccharide-diphtheria toxoid conjugate vaccine in US children aged 18–59 months. Lancet *338*:395–398, 1991.
245. Whisnant, J. K., Mann, D. L., Rogentine, G. N., and Robbins, J. B.: Human cell-surface structures related to *H. influenzae* type b disease. Lancet *2*:895–898, 1971.
246. Wilson, W. R., Karchmer, A. W., Dajani, A. S., et al.: Antibiotic treatment of adults with infective endocarditis due to streptococci, enterococci, staphylococci, and HACEK microorganisms. J. A. M. A. *274*:1706–1713, 1995.
247. Winkelstein, J. A., and Moxon, E. R.: The role of complement in the host's defense against *Haemophilus influenzae*. J. Infect. Dis. *165*(Suppl. 1):S62–S65, 1992.
248. Winslow, C. E., Broadhurst, J., Buchanan, R. E., et al.: The families and genera of the bacteria: Final report of the Committee of the Society of American Bacteriologists on characterization and classification of bacterial types. J. Bacteriol. *5*:191–229, 1920.
249. Wolf, W. J.: Echocardiographic features of a purulent pericardial peel. Am. Heart J. *111*:990–992, 1986.
250. Wotton, K. A., Stiver, H. G., and Hildes, J. A.: Meningitis in the central Arctic: A 4-year experience. Can. Med. Assoc. J. *124*:887–890, 1981.
251. Zwahlen, A., Winkelstein, J. A., and Moxon, E. R.: Surface determinants of *Haemophilus influenzae* pathogenicity: Comparative virulence of capsular transformants in normal and complement-depleted rats. J. Infect. Dis. *148*:385–394, 1983.

140

OTHER *HAEMOPHILUS* SPECIES

Stephen J. Barenkamp

Most serious pediatric infections caused by organisms of the *Haemophilus* genus are caused by *H. influenzae*. However, other *Haemophilus* species can cause disease occasionally. *Haemophilus* species that have been well documented as causing illness in pediatric and adolescent patients include *H. aegyptius*, *H. aphrophilus*, *H. ducreyi*, and *H. parainfluenzae*. As is discussed later, *H. aegyptius* recently has been classified as a member of the species *H. influenzae* (*H. influenzae* biogroup aegyptius), but, given the unique characteristics of this organism and the distinctive illnesses with which it is associated, it is described in this chapter. Other *Haemophilus* species, such as *H. haemolyticus* and *H. parahaemolyticus*, rarely, if ever, cause illness in the pediatric population.

Members of the *Haemophilus* genus are gram-negative coccobacillary bacteria that are facultatively anaerobic and demonstrate optimal growth when they are incubated in a humid atmosphere containing 5 to 10 per cent carbon dioxide.[19, 43, 56] Most species have fastidious nutritional requirements and require special media, supplements, or both for optimal growth.[19, 56] X factor (hemin), V factor (nicotinamide adenine dinucleotide), or both are required for in vitro growth.[78] Organisms with the "para-" prefix require V factor only. The specific nutritional requirements of *Haemophilus* isolates are one characteristic used to subclassify these organisms into the different species (Table 140–1).

HAEMOPHILUS APHROPHILUS

Bacteriology

H. aphrophilus was described first by Khairat[55] in 1940 in association with a fatal case of endocarditis. He suggested the species name *aphrophilus* because the organism required relatively high concentrations of carbon dioxide for isolation on the usual media. In earlier times, a well-known manifestation of carbon dioxide was the formation of bubbles of gas in fermenting wine (i.e., froth, or *aphros*).[8, 55] Although the organism originally was classified as a *Haemophilus* organism because of the growth requirement for X factor, more recent studies suggest that it can grow independent of this factor.[56, 76, 100] Some authors have suggested that given this X factor independence, the organism should be placed in another genus,[56, 100] but, at present, it remains in the *Haemophilus* genus.

Epidemiology and Pathogenesis

H. aphrophilus is a component of the normal oral flora. Using a selective medium, Kraut and coworkers[58] isolated the organism from gingival scrapings and interdental material of one-third of the healthy adults they examined. With respect to disease pathogenesis, it has been suggested that dental disease or manipulation predisposes to transient bacteremia, which results in seeding of distant tissue sites where localized infection subsequently develops.[8, 38, 75, 76, 88] In addition, several case reports of patients with *H. aphrophilus* disease reported an association between human infection and contact with or bites from dogs and cats.[32, 48, 75, 76, 107] However, a causal relationship has been difficult to confirm, and the mouth or respiratory tract probably is the portal of entry for the great majority of infections.

TABLE 140–1. Differential Characteristics of *Haemophilus* Species

Haemophilus Species	Factor Requirement		Hemolysis of Horse Blood	Fermentation of				Presence of Catalase	CO_2 Enhancement of Growth
	X*	V		Glucose	Sucrose	Lactose	Mannose		
H. influenzae†	+	+	−	+	−	−	−	+	+
H. haemolyticus	+	+	+	+	−	−	−	+	−
H. ducreyi	+	−	−	−	−	−	−	−	−
H. parainfluenzae	−	+	−	+	+	−	+	D	D
H. parahaemolyticus	−	+	+	+	+	−	−	+	−
H. aphrophilus	−	−	−	+	+	+	+	−	+

D, Differences encountered.
*As determined by the porphyrin test.
†Includes biogroup aegyptius.
Adapted from Campos, J. M.: *Haemophilus. In* Murray, P. R., Baron, E. J., Pfaller, M. A., et al. (eds.): Manual of Clinical Microbiology. 6th ed. Washington, D.C., American Society for Microbiology, 1995, pp. 556–565.

Clinical Manifestations

H. aphrophilus is a rare cause of infection and disease in pediatric patients, with fewer than 50 cases reported in the literature.[4, 8, 30, 32, 48, 53, 72, 112] Brain abscesses and endocarditis are the pediatric infections reported most commonly with this organism.[8, 30, 32, 48, 72, 76] Other sites of infection in children documented in the literature include the oropharynx,[8] the abdominal cavity,[8, 53] and various superficial soft tissue sites.[76, 112] Infections with *H. aphrophilus* do not appear to be associated with any distinctive clinical features compared with infection by other organisms at the same sites. However, *H. aphrophilus* infections frequently are associated with underlying conditions predisposing the host to infection, such as congenital heart disease, trauma, and immunosuppression.[8, 31, 32, 46, 72, 76, 80, 112]

Treatment

Antimicrobial susceptibility testing has not been well standardized for this organism, and disk-diffusion testing, in particular, has been found to be unreliable.[8, 27, 76, 100] Tube or agar dilution testing generally is considered to be the preferred testing method. Older reports found that *H. aphrophilus* was susceptible uniformly to a number of antibiotics, including chloramphenicol and the aminoglycosides.[8, 76, 100] Susceptibility to penicillins has been variable.

However, penicillin has been used successfully for treatment of susceptible organisms,[8, 38, 76, 107] at times in combination with aminoglycosides and other antimicrobials. Some reports document the usefulness of ceftriaxone for treatment of infection.[71, 75] A number of different antibiotics likely can treat *H. aphrophilus* infections successfully. The choice for treatment should be guided by appropriate in vitro susceptibility testing.

HAEMOPHILUS DUCREYI

Bacteriology

In 1889, Ducrey[28] originally identified *H. ducreyi* in purulent material recovered from genital ulcers of patients with soft chancre or chancroid. Although unable to culture the organism in vitro, Ducrey[28] was able to establish the specificity of the infectious agent by serial cutaneous inoculations.[73] *H. ducreyi* originally was assigned to the *Haemophilus* genus because of its requirement for hemin (X-factor) and a guanosine plus cytosine content within the expected range for *Haemophilus* species.[1, 105] However, more recent studies, including genetic transformation and DNA hybridization analyses, suggest that *H. ducreyi* is not related to the true haemophili, such as *H. influenzae,* and potentially should be placed in a separate genus.[1, 105]

Epidemiology

Chancroid is a genital ulcerative disease that is common throughout the world. It is said to be common particularly in Africa, Asia, and Latin America, where it may be a more common cause of genital ulcer disease than syphilis.[1, 73, 105] Although generally considered a relatively uncommon cause of illness in the United States, chancroid continues to be diagnosed, particularly among patients, including adolescents, who present with genital ulcer disease in large urban areas.[10, 22, 42, 93] Furthermore, more recent data suggest that chancroid may be more common in the United States than suspected previously because it can be difficult to diagnose correctly by traditional clinical and laboratory means.[22, 105] Symptomatic disease in the United States has been reported most commonly among nonwhite heterosexual males.[10, 33, 42, 73] However, symptomatic disease is not restricted to men, and female prostitutes have been implicated as important sources of infection in several of the outbreaks reported in the United States.[10, 42, 73]

H. ducreyi has been the subject of renewed medical and scientific interest since the 1980s. This interest followed from epidemiologic studies primarily from Africa that demonstrated that the presence of genital ulcer disease (much of which was chancroid) was associated strongly with an increased risk of heterosexual transmission of HIV infection.[7, 49, 59, 60, 81, 108] Mechanisms proposed to explain this enhanced transmission have included an increased shedding of HIV through the ulcers[60, 105] and perhaps an increased number of HIV-susceptible cells (e.g., CD4 T lymphocytes) in the genital ulcers of the person being infected.[105]

Pathogenesis

Relatively little is known about the pathogenesis of *H. ducreyi* infection, although some progress has been made in this area over the last few years coincident with the renewed interest in the organism.[105] Several putative virulence factors have been identified, including lipo-oligosaccharide,[18] pili,[97] a putative cytotoxin,[63, 83] a hemolysin,[77, 104] and an ability to adhere specifically to epithelial cells of genital origin.[2, 64] To date, the contribution of these proposed virulence characteristics to the pathogenesis of infection in humans has yet to be demonstrated clearly. However, several potentially useful in vivo models of *H. ducreyi* infection have been developed. These include a temperature-dependent rabbit model of dermal infection,[82] a primate model of genital chancroid infection in adult pigtailed macaques,[103] and a model of experimental human infection.[98] Additional investigations of *H. ducreyi* using these models undoubtedly will define the virulence mechanisms of the organism more clearly and should allow for evaluation of potential protective vaccines.[25, 44]

Clinical Manifestations

The incubation period of chancroid usually is between 4 and 7 days. It rarely is less than 3 days or more than 10 days.[73, 86, 87] Typically, the first lesion noted is a small inflammatory papule surrounded by a zone of erythema. Within 2 or 3 days, a pustule forms that soon ruptures, leaving a sharply circumscribed ulcer with ragged undermined edges *without* induration.[73, 87] The base of the ulcer usually has a granular appearance and always is painful. In males, the most common sites of appearance of the ulcers are on the distal prepuce, on the mucosal surface of the prepuce on the frenulum, and in the coronal sulcus. In females, most lesions are at the entrance to the vagina.[73, 87] Painful, tender, inguinal adenopathy is present in up to 50 per cent of patients and usually is unilateral. The involved lymph nodes rapidly may become fluctuant and rupture, with the formation of inguinal ulcers.[73, 87]

The combination of a painful ulcer with tender inguinal adenopathy is suggestive of chancroid and, when accompanied by suppurative inguinal adenopathy, is almost pathognomonic.[21] However, a substantial percentage of patients with *H. ducreyi* infection may have ulcers that can be confused with other genital ulcer diseases, such as herpes or syphilis.[36, 73, 87] Furthermore, as many as 10 per cent of patients with chancroid may be coinfected with *Treponema pallidum* or herpes simplex virus.[21] Thus, it becomes mandatory to establish a definitive diagnosis by laboratory means if one is to be confident about the diagnosis.

Diagnosis

As noted earlier, diagnosing chancroid on clinical grounds alone is difficult because the clinical presentation often is not classic and many clinicians do not have a great deal of experience with the disease.[21, 105] Definitive diagnosis of chancroid requires isolation of the organism from a genital ulcer or from involved lymph nodes. However, the organism is fastidious and is difficult to isolate, even under the best of circumstances.[73] To obtain specimens for culture, a swab should be used to obtain material from the purulent base of an ulcer or a fluctuant inguinal lymph node should be aspirated directly. Gram stain of purulent material may reveal gram-negative rods in the characteristic "school-of-fish" pattern, but this appearance probably is more characteristic of in vitro propagated organisms.[73] However, even with use of the selective media now recommended for isolation of *H. ducreyi*, it has been estimated that the sensitivity of culture is no higher than 80 per cent.[21]

Given the low sensitivity of culture, alternative non–culture-based diagnostic tests have been evaluated. One study examined the utility of diagnosing chancroid serologically with an enzyme-linked immunosorbent assay (ELISA) by examining the host response to either an outer-membrane protein preparation or an oligosaccharide preparation of *H. ducreyi*.[3] Although the outer-membrane protein assay was not useful because of the presence of cross-reacting antibodies in a number of the negative control sera, the oligosaccharide ELISA was found to be both sensitive and specific. Additional studies are required to confirm these initial observations and assess better the utility of the assay as a routine clinical tool.

Nucleotide-based diagnostic methods also have been described in recent years.[22, 50, 89, 105] Perhaps most promising are the polymerase chain reaction–based techniques. These assays demonstrate high sensitivity and appear to identify a number of patients with chancroid, from whom bacterial cultures for *H. ducreyi* are negative.[22, 105] Multiplex polymerase chain reaction assays that can amplify and subsequently detect DNA from *H. ducreyi*, *T. pallidum*, and herpes simplex virus from genital ulcer specimens simultaneously are undergoing field trials and have shown early promise.[22, 105]

Even if chancroid is diagnosed definitively, it is recommended that patients also be tested for HIV at the time of diagnosis. In addition, it must be remembered that up to 10 per cent of patients with chancroid may be coinfected with *T. pallidum* or herpes simplex virus.[22] Appropriate testing for these other pathogens should be considered strongly when a patient presents with any form of genital ulcer disease.

Treatment and Prevention

Successful antimicrobial treatment of genital ulcers caused by *H. ducreyi* cures infection, resolves clinical symptoms, and prevents transmission to others. However, in cases of extensive ulcerative disease, scarring may result, despite successful antimicrobial therapy.[22] The Centers for Disease Control and Prevention currently recommend one of three antibiotic regimens for treatment of chancroid in adolescents and adults.[22, 94] These are (1) azithromycin, 1 g orally in a single dose, (2) ceftriaxone, 250 mg intramuscularly in a single dose, and (3) erythromycin base, 500 mg orally four times a day for 7 days. All three regimens are effective for treatment of chancroid among patients without HIV infection.[94] Alternative antimicrobial regimens are (4) amoxicillin/clavulanic acid, 500 mg/125 mg three times daily for 1 week, and (5) ciprofloxacin, 500 mg orally twice a day for 3 days.[22, 94] The alternative regimens have not been evaluated as extensively as have the recommended regimens. A successful response to therapy usually is apparent within 48 to 72 hours, as shown by decreased ulcer tenderness and pain.[86, 94] Complete healing of ulcers may take up to 28 days but often is achieved in 7 to 14 days.[94] Healing of fluctuant adenopathy is slower than that of the ulcers and may require needle aspiration through adjacent intact skin, even during successful therapy.[22]

Patients with HIV infection must be monitored closely because they may require longer courses of antimicrobial agents than the standard regimens just outlined.[22, 94] Treatment failures have been noted with several of these regimens,[13, 94, 106] and there is some suggestion that persons who are most immunosuppressed are at the greatest risk for failure of standard regimens.[94] Some experts recommend using the erythromycin 7-day regimen for treating all HIV-infected patients because of good experience with this regimen in the HIV-infected population and limited successful experience with the alternative regimens.[94]

It is critical to identify all sexual contacts of infected persons to prevent further spread of *H. ducreyi* disease. The Centers for Disease Control and Prevention recommend that all persons who have had sexual contact with a patient with proven *H. ducreyi* infection within the 10 days before onset of the patient's symptoms be examined and treated.[22] Contacts should be examined and treated even in the absence of symptoms.

In the longer term, alternative strategies for control of chancroid should be examined. If feasible, vaccination for prevention of *H. ducreyi* infection would be a worthy goal. Data generated in animal models of infection are somewhat encouraging.[25, 44] Protective immunity to both homologous and heterologous challenge has been reported after immunization of rabbits with cell-surface extracts of *H. ducreyi*.[44] More recently, a purified pilus preparation also was reported to induce immunity in that same model.[25] Although preliminary, these data suggest that prevention of chancroid in humans by vaccination may be an achievable goal at some point in the not-too-distant future.

HAEMOPHILUS INFLUENZAE BIOGROUP AEGYPTIUS (*HAEMOPHILUS AEGYPTIUS*)

Bacteriology

H. influenzae biogroup aegyptius (*H. aegyptius*) was described originally by Koch[57] in 1883 in Egyptian patients with conjunctivitis. A more detailed description of the organism and the clinical characteristics of disease followed 3 years later in the work of Weeks.[110] The Koch-Weeks bacillus has continued to be an important cause of conjunctivitis since these initial reports. Because of several reportedly unique characteristics,[70] the Koch-Weeks bacillus originally was designated as a unique species of the *Haemophilus* genus (*H. aegyptius*) distinct from *H. influenzae*. However, more recent phenotypic and phylogenetic studies, including DNA relatedness analyses, have raised questions about the validity of this separation.[16, 101] The organism is designated currently as *H. influenzae* biogroup aegyptius, although debate continues in the literature as to the appropriateness of this designation.[66]

This organism has been the subject of intense scientific study since the 1980s as a result of its association with a newly described fulminant and often fatal disease called Brazilian purpuric fever.[14, 15] *H. influenzae* biogroup aegyptius was isolated from nine blood cultures and one hemorrhagic cerebrospinal fluid culture from 10 clinically ill children in Serrana, Sao Paulo State, Brazil.[15] The *H. influenzae* biogroup aegyptius strains causing Brazilian purpuric fever were felt initially to be members of a single virulent clone.[16, 101] This clone was characterized by the presence of several unique features, including a 24-MDa plasmid with a characteristic restriction endonuclease pattern,[16] a unique multilocus electrophoretic enzyme typing pattern,[74] one of two rRNA gene restriction fragment length polymorphisms,[16, 26, 101] a single sodium dodecyl sulfate–polyacrylamide gel electrophoresis profile using whole-cell lysates,[16] specific reactivity with monoclonal antibodies recognizing epitopes unique to Brazilian purpuric fever strains,[65, 101] and agglutination with antisera specific for the Brazilian purpuric fever clone.[16] Although most Brazilian purpuric fever–associated strains of *H. influenzae* biogroup aegyptius appear to be members of a unique clone, a few Brazilian purpuric fever–associated strains have been identified that lack some of the defining characteristics.[101, 102] Furthermore, two cases of Brazilian purpuric fever reported from Australia were associated with strains clearly distinct from the Brazilian purpuric fever clone.[66, 101]

Epidemiology

In the United States, *H. influenzae* biogroup aegyptius has remained an important cause of conjunctivitis, with disease most commonly reported from the southern states.[45] The United States has not experienced any recognized cases of Brazilian purpuric fever. In Brazil, the epidemiology of Brazilian purpuric fever has been defined more clearly over the last several years.[45] The median age of patients with Brazilian purpuric fever is from 2 to 3 years, with an overall range of ages of 3 months to 10 years.[14, 15] Brazilian purpuric fever appears to occur with the onset of warmer temperatures and is less likely during the Brazilian winter.[45] Furthermore, it appears to be more common in small agricultural towns than in larger cities.[14, 15, 45] Case-control studies attempting to identify risk factors for development of disease identified a history of preceding conjunctivitis as being associated strongly with the development of Brazilian purpuric fever[14, 15, 45] (although many of the controls also gave a history of conjunctivitis) and suggested that day care center attendance was an additional risk factor.[15]

Pathogenesis

Efforts to identify virulence factors of *H. influenzae* biogroup aegyptius responsible for the fulminant nature of Brazilian purpuric fever have been ongoing since the initial descriptions of the illness. Progress to date has been limited.[20] Brazilian purpuric fever clone strains express a number of novel or unique surface molecules or secreted proteins that theoretically could result in enhanced virulence.[16, 20, 65, 66, 90, 113] Distinctive oligosaccharide phenotypes,[20, 90] IgA proteases,[20, 66] pili,[113] and secreted proteins[20] for Brazilian purpuric fever strains have been reported. However, none has been shown to have a specific role in bacterial virulence. One study has suggested that the risk of developing Brazilian purpuric fever correlated with the lack of serum bactericidal activity against the Brazilian purpuric fever clone, but this observation needs further confirmation.[91]

Both in vitro and in vivo models have been developed for further investigating the pathogenesis of Brazilian purpuric fever.[84, 90, 111] In these model systems, Brazilian purpuric fever–associated strains demonstrated increased virulence compared with control strains not associated with Brazilian purpuric fever, but, again, the specific molecular correlates of this increased pathogenicity have yet to be identified clearly.[84, 90] It seems likely that over the next few years, the in vitro and in vivo models will prove useful in defining specific virulence factors of the Brazilian purpuric fever strain.

Clinical Manifestations

The clinical presentation of Brazilian purpuric fever is distinctive and dramatic.[14, 15, 45] The syndrome initially manifests as a purulent conjunctivitis without distinguishing characteristics. Symptoms of Brazilian purpuric fever typically appear 3 to 15 days later, after the conjunctivitis has resolved. The affected children experience the acute onset of fever, which may be associated with vomiting and abdominal pain. Death frequently ensues within 48 hours after the development of disseminated purpura, vascular collapse, and hypotensive shock. The precise pathophysiologic mechanisms responsible for progression from conjunctivitis due to the Brazilian purpuric fever clone to full-blown Brazilian purpuric fever are unknown. The overall case-fatality rate since Brazilian purpuric fever first was recognized is estimated to be 70 per cent.[45] Children may develop conjunctivitis with the Brazilian purpuric fever clone and, after recovery from the conjunctivitis, have no further problems.[45] The risk factors that predispose only some children to develop Brazilian purpuric fever are not well understood.

Treatment

Data from the limited number of Brazilian purpuric fever cases studied suggest that early antimicrobial therapy may improve survival.[15] One suggested regimen is high-dose ampicillin and chloramphenicol. The small number of patients treated to date does not permit a comparison of the efficacy of different antibiotic regimens.[15]

Most of the patients who developed Brazilian purpuric fever in the Brazilian studies were treated with topical antimicrobials for conjunctivitis, yet still developed systemic disease.[15] This suggests that local topical therapy is ineffective in eradicating the organism from the host. One study examined the relative efficacy of oral rifampin and topical chloramphenicol in eradicating conjunctival carriage of the Brazilian purpuric fever clone.[79] Although the number of patients who actually carried the Brazilian purpuric fever clone was small, rifampin was shown to be significantly better in eradicating carriage of the Brazilian purpuric fever clone than was topical chloramphenicol.

HAEMOPHILUS PARAINFLUENZAE

Bacteriology

H. parainfluenzae was identified first as a species distinct from *H. influenzae* by Rivers in 1922.[85] Both organisms are fastidious, gram-negative coccobacilli, but with in vitro culture, *H. parainfluenzae* can be propagated on nutrient agar plates with supplemental factor V alone (thus the "para" designation), rather than with both factor X and factor V, which are required by *H. influenzae* isolates (see Table 140–1). Testing for hemolysis on blood-containing media differentiates *H. parainfluenzae* from hemolysis-producing species, such as *H. haemolyticus* and *H. parahaemolyticus*.[19, 56] Recovery of *H. parainfluenzae* organisms from blood cultures is enhanced by routine subculturing of all specimens. The organisms tend to grow as small colonies along the side walls of the blood bottles or in the red cell mass, leaving the broth clear.[43] Routine subculturing to supplemented chocolate agar and incubation with supplemental carbon dioxide should allow recovery of any *H. parainfluenzae* organisms that are present.[23, 41, 43]

Epidemiology and Pathogenesis

H. parainfluenzae is found commonly in the oropharyngeal flora of normal children.[40, 62, 68] The organism can be recovered from oropharyngeal cultures of one-quarter or more of healthy children. Of children who develop serious invasive disease caused by *H. parainfluenzae*, more than one-half give histories of identifiable preceding illnesses, such as upper respiratory tract infection, otitis media, and dental infections,[5, 9, 40, 47] suggesting that local inflammation in the upper respiratory tract may predispose to transient bacteremias with this organism, which allows for seeding of other sites, such as the meninges and the heart valves. No specific virulence factors of the organism have been identified to date.

Clinical Manifestations

As was noted previously with *H. aphrophilus*, *H. parainfluenzae* remains an uncommon cause of infection in pediatric patients. However, an increasing number of cases have been reported since the 1970s.[9] The most commonly reported infection is meningitis.[5, 6, 24, 34, 35, 39, 40, 47, 54, 61, 69, 96, 109, 114] The clinical courses of the patients described with *H. parainfluenzae* meningitis are not remarkably different from those typical of acute bacterial meningitis caused by other organisms. However, the average age of the patients is 2.2 years,[9] an age significantly greater than that of the typical pediatric patient with bacterial meningitis.

The next most commonly reported infection is endocarditis.[9, 11, 12, 17, 29, 37, 67, 68, 95] *H. parainfluenzae* endocarditis has a number of unique features. The reported cases of pediatric endocarditis usually occur in adolescents and involve females more commonly than males.[9] The clinical presentation often is subacute and frequently is not associated with localizing signs on physical examination (i.e., pathologic murmurs), at least initially.[23, 67, 68] Another unique feature of *H. parainfluenzae* endocarditis is the high incidence of major arterial occlusion secondary to release of large emboli from the heart.[9, 23, 37, 67, 99] This high incidence of embolization is thought to be due to the particularly friable nature of the vegetations.[9, 37] Another characteristic feature noted by several authors is the relatively slow and variable response of endocarditis caused by this organism to antimicrobial therapy.[9, 23, 67, 68]

Other *H. parainfluenzae* infections reported in pediatric patients include brain abscesses,[40, 69] septic arthritis,[9] and urinary tract infection.[9]

Treatment

H. parainfluenzae usually is susceptible in vitro to multiple antibiotics, including chloramphenicol, aminoglycosides, trimethoprim-sulfamethoxazole, and third-generation cephalosporins.[9, 23, 51, 68] Although the majority of isolates in the past were susceptible to penicillins, more recent studies have documented an increasing incidence of β-lactamase–producing strains resistant to penicillin and ampicillin.[9, 92] For β-lactamase–negative penicillin-susceptible organisms, administration of ampicillin with an aminoglycoside has been recommended for serious *H. parainfluenzae* infections.[23, 43] Individual case reports document successful treatment with a variety of other antimicrobials, including ampicillin alone, cephalosporins, chloramphenicol, and trimethoprim-sulfamethoxazole.[17, 23, 52, 68] At present, pending results of susceptibility testing, it would be reasonable to initiate therapy for serious *H. parainfluenzae* infections with a third-generation cephalosporin, perhaps in combination with an aminoglycoside.

References

1. Albritton, W. L.: Biology of *Haemophilus ducreyi*. Microbiol. Rev. *53*:377–388, 1989.
2. Alfa, M. J., Degagne, P., and Hollyer, T.: *Haemophilus ducreyi* adheres to but does not invade cultured human foreskin cells. Infect. Immun. *61*:1735–1742, 1993.
3. Alfa, M. J., Olson, N., Degagne, P., et al.: Humoral immune response of humans to lipooligosaccharide and outer membrane proteins of *Haemophilus ducreyi*. J. Infect. Dis. *167*:1206–1210, 1993.
4. Arneborn, P., Lindquist, B. L., and Sjöberg, L.: Severe pulmonary infection by *Haemophilus aphrophilus* in a non-compromised child. Scand. J. Infect. Dis. *17*:327–329, 1985.
5. Bachman, D. S.: *Hemophilus* meningitis: Comparison of *H. influenzae* and *H. parainfluenzae*. Pediatrics *55*:526–530, 1975.
6. Barnshaw, J. A., and Phillips, C. F.: *Haemophilus parainfluenzae* meningitis in a 4-year-old boy. Pediatrics *45*:856–857, 1970.

7. Behets, F. M.-T., Liomba, G., and Lule, G.: Sexually transmitted diseases and human immunodeficiency virus control in Malawi: A field study of genital ulcer disease. J. Infect. Dis. *171*:451–455, 1995.
8. Bieger, R. C., Brewer, N. S., and Washington, J. A., II: *Haemophilus aphrophilus*: A microbiologic and clinical review and report of 42 cases. Medicine (Baltimore) *57*:345–355, 1978.
9. Black, C. T., Kupferschmid, J. P., West, K. W., et al.: *Haemophilus parainfluenzae* infections in children, with the report of a unique case. Rev. Infect. Dis. *10*:342–346, 1988.
10. Blackmore, C. A., Limpakarnjanarat, K., Rigau-Perez, J. G., et al.: An outbreak of chancroid in Orange County, California: Descriptive epidemiology and disease-control measures. J. Infect. Dis. *151*:840–844, 1985.
11. Blair, D. C., Walker, W., Sodeman, T., et al.: Bacterial endocarditis due to *Haemophilus parainfluenzae*. Chest *71*:146–149, 1977.
12. Blair, D. C., and Weiner, L. B.: Prosthetic valve endocarditis due to *Haemophilus parainfluenzae* biotype II. Am. J. Dis. Child. *133*:617–618, 1979.
13. Bogaerts, J., Kestens, L., Tello, W. M., et al.: Failure of treatment for chancroid in Rwanda is not related to human immunodeficiency virus infection: In vitro resistance of *Haemophilus ducreyi* to trimethoprim-sulfamethoxazole. Clin. Infect. Dis. *20*:924–930, 1995.
14. Brazilian Purpuric Fever Study Group: Brazilian purpuric fever: Epidemic purpura fulminans associated with antecedent purulent conjunctivitis. Lancet 2:757–761, 1987.
15. Brazilian Purpuric Fever Study Group: *Haemophilus aegyptius* bacteremia in Brazilian purpuric fever. Lancet 2:761–763, 1987.
16. Brenner, D. J., Mayer, L. W., Carlone, G. M., et al.: Biochemical, genetic, and epidemiologic characterization of *Haemophilus influenzae* biogroup aegyptius (*Haemophilus aegyptius*) strains associated with Brazilian purpuric fever. J. Clin. Microbiol. *26*:1524–1534, 1988.
17. Calio, A. J., Cusumano, S., Ullman, R. F., et al.: *Haemophilus parainfluenzae* endocarditis. Heart Lung *16*:222–223, 1987.
18. Campagnari, A. A., Wild, L. M., Griffiths, G. E., et al.: Role of lipooligosaccharides in experimental dermal lesions caused by *Haemophilus ducreyi*. Infect. Immun. *59*:2601–2608, 1991.
19. Campos, J. M.: *Haemophilus*. *In* Murray, P. R., Baron, E. J., Pfaller, M. A., et al. (eds.): Manual of Clinical Microbiology. 6th ed. Washington, D. C., American Society for Microbiology, 1995, pp. 556–565.
20. Carlone, G. M., Gorelkin, L., Gheesling, L. L., et al.: Potential virulence-associated factors in Brazilian purpuric fever. J. Clin. Microbiol. *27*:609–614, 1989.
21. Centers for Disease Control: 1993 Sexually transmitted diseases treatment guidelines. M. M. W. R. *42*(RR-14):1–102, 1993.
22. Centers for Disease Control and Prevention: Chancroid detected by polymerase chain reaction—Jackson, Mississippi, 1994–1995. M. M. W. R. *44*(30):567, 1995.
23. Chunn, C. J., Jones, S. R., McCutchan, J. A., et al.: *Haemophilus parainfluenzae* infective endocarditis. Medicine (Baltimore) *56*:99–113, 1977.
24. Davis, D. J.: *Haemophilus parainfluenzae*. Pediatr. Infect. Dis. *1*:448–449, 1982.
25. Desjardins, M., Filion, L. G., Robertson, S., et al.: Inducible immunity with a pilus preparation booster vaccination in an animal model of *Haemophilus ducreyi* infection and disease. Infect. Immun. *63*:2012–2020, 1995.
26. Dewhirst, F. E., Paster, B. J., Olsen, I., et al.: Phylogeny of 54 representative strains of species in the family *Pasteurellaceae* as determined by comparison of 16S rRNA sequences. J. Bacteriol. *174*:2002–2013, 1992.
27. Doern, G. V.: Susceptibility tests of fastidious bacteria. *In* Murray, P. R., Baron, E. J., Pfaller, M. A., et al. (eds.): Manual of Clinical Microbiology. 6th ed. Washington, D. C., American Society for Microbiology, 1995, pp. 1342–1349.
28. Ducrey, A.: Experimentelle untersuchungen über den ansteckungsstoff des weichen schankers und über die bubonen. Monatschr. Prakt. Dermatol. *9*:387, 1889.
29. Ellner, J. J., Rosenthal, M. S., Lerner, P. I., et al.: Infective endocarditis caused by slow-growing, fastidious, gram-negative bacteria. Medicine *58*:145–158, 1979.
30. Elster, S. K., Mattes, L. M., Meyers, B. R., et al.: *Haemophilus aphrophilus* endocarditis: Review of 23 cases. Am. J. Cardiol. *35*:72–79, 1975.
31. Farrington, M., Eykyn, S. J., Walker, M., et al.: Vertebral osteomyelitis due to coccobacilli of the HB group. B. M. J. *287*:1658–1660, 1983.
32. Fischbein, C. A., Beckett, K. M., and Rosenthal, A.: *Haemophilus aphrophilus* brain abscess associated with congenital heart disease. J. Pediatr. *83*:631–633, 1973.
33. Flood, J. M., Sarafian, S. K., Bolan, G. A., et al.: Multistrain outbreak of chancroid in San Francisco. 1989–1991. J. Infect. Dis. *167*:1106–1111, 1993.
34. Florman, A. L.: An acute febrile illness with rash and leucopenia due to *Haemophilus parainfluenzae*. J. Pediatr. *22*:202–204, 1943.
35. Frazier, J. P., Cleary, T. G., and Pickering, L. K.: Meningitis due to *Haemophilus parainfluenzae*: Report of three cases and review of the literature. Pediatr. Infect. Dis. *1*:117–119, 1982.
36. Gaisin, A., and Heaton, C. L.: Chancroid: Alias the soft chancre. Int. J. Dermatol. *14*:188–197, 1975.
37. Geraci, J. E., Wilkowske, C. J., Wilson, W. R., et al.: *Haemophilus* endocarditis: Report of 14 patients. Mayo Clin. Proc. *52*:209–215, 1977.
38. Gribble, M. J., and Hunter, T.: *Haemophilus aphrophilus* vertebral osteomyelitis: A case report and literature review. Diagn. Microbial. Infect. Dis. 8:189–191, 1987.
39. Gullekson, E. H., and Dumoff, M.: *Haemophilus parainfluenzae* meningitis in a newborn. J. A. M. A. *198*:1221, 1966.
40. Hable, K. A., Logan, G. B., and Washington, J. A., II: Three *Hemophilus* species: Pathogenic activity. Am. J. Dis. Child. *121*:35–37, 1971.
41. Hamed, K. A., Dormitzer, P. R., Su, C. K., et al.: *Haemophilus parainfluenzae* endocarditis: Application of a molecular approach for identification of pathogenic bacterial species. Clin. Infect. Dis. *19*:677–683, 1994.
42. Hammond, G. W., Slutchuk, M., Scatiff, J., et al.: Epidemiologic, clinical, laboratory and therapeutic features of an urban outbreak of chancroid in North America. Rev. Infect. Dis. *2*:867–879, 1980.
43. Hand, W. L.: *Haemophilus* species (including chancroid). *In* Mandell, G. L., Douglas, R. G., Jr., and Bennett, J. E. (eds.): Principles and Practice of Infectious Diseases. 4th ed. New York, Churchill Livingstone, 1994, pp. 2045–2050.
44. Hansen, E. J., Lumbley, S. R., Richardson, J. A., et al.: Induction of protective immunity to *Haemophilus ducreyi* in the temperature-dependent rabbit model of experimental chancroid. J. Immunol. *152*:184–192, 1994.
45. Harrison, L. H., daSilva, G. A., Pittman, M., et al.: Epidemiology and clinical spectrum of Brazilian purpuric fever. J. Clin. Microbiol. *27*:599–604, 1989.
46. Ho, J. L., Soukiasian, S., Oh, W. H., et al.: *Haemophilus aphrophilus* osteomyelitis. Am. J. Med. *76*:159, 1984.
47. Holt, R. N., Taylor, C. D., Schneider, H. J., et al.: Three cases of *Hemophilus parainfluenzae* meningitis. Clin. Pediatr. *13*:666–668, 1974.
48. Isom, J. B., Gordy, P. D., Selner, J. C., et al.: Brain abscess due to *Haemophilus aphrophilus*. N. Engl. J. Med. *271*:1059, 1964.
49. Jessamine, P. G., and Ronald, A. R.: Chancroid and the role of genital ulcer disease in the spread of human retrovirus. Med. Clin. North Am. *74*:1417–1431, 1990.
50. Johnson, S. R., Martin, D. H., Cammarata, C., et al.: Alterations in sample preparation increase sensitivity of PCR assay for diagnosis of chancroid. J. Clin. Microbiol. *33*:1036–1038, 1995.
51. Jorgensen, J. H., Howell, A. W., and Maher, L. A.: Antimicrobial susceptibility testing of less commonly isolated *Haemophilus* species using *Haemophilus* test medium. J. Clin. Microbiol. *28*:985–988, 1990.
52. Julander, I., Lindberg, A. A., and Svanbom, M.: *Haemophilus parainfluenzae:* An uncommon cause of septicemia and endocarditis. Scand. J. Infect. Dis. *12*:85–89, 1980.
53. Kaplan, J. M., McCracken, G. H., Jr., and Nelson, J. D.: Infections in children caused by the HB group of bacteria. J. Pediatr. *82*:398–403, 1978.
54. Kaufman, S. R., Hambly, F., Dyke, J. W., et al.: *Haemophilus parainfluenzae* meningitis: Report of two cases. Clin. Pediatr. *13*:661–663, 1974.
55. Khairat, O.: Endocarditis due to a new species of *Haemophilus*. J. Pathol. Bacteriol. *50*:497–505, 1940.
56. Kilian, M.: A taxonomic study of the genus *Haemophilus* with the proposal of a new species. J. Gen. Microbiol. *193*:9–62, 1976.
57. Koch, R.: Bericht über die tätigkeit der Deutschen Cholerakommission in Aegypten und Ostindien. Wein. Med. Wochenschr. *33*:1548, 1883.
58. Kraut, M. S., Attebery, H. R., Finegold, S. M., et al.: Detection of *Haemophilus aphrophilus* in the human oral flora with a selective medium. J. Infect. Dis. *126*:189–192, 1972.
59. Kreiss, J. K., Koech, D., Plummer, F. A., et al.: AIDS virus infections in Nairobi prostitutes: Spread of the epidemic to East Africa. N. Engl. J. Med. *314*:414–418, 1986.
60. Kreiss, J. K., Coombs, R., Plummer, F., et al.: Isolation of human immunodeficiency virus from genital ulcers in Nairobi prostitutes. J. Infect. Dis. *160*:380–384, 1989.
61. Krishnaswami, R., Schwartz, J., and Boodish, W.: Pathogenicity of *H. parainfluenza*. Pediatrics *50*:498–499, 1972.
62. Kuklinska, D., and Kilian, M.: Relative proportions of *Haemophilus* species in the throat of healthy children and adults. Eur. J. Clin. Microbiol. *3*:249–252, 1984.
63. Lagergard, T., and Purven, M.: Neutralizing antibodies to *Haemophilus ducreyi* cytotoxin. Infect. Immun. *61*:1589–1592, 1993.
64. Lammel, C. J., Dekker, N. P., Palefsky, J., et al.: In vitro model of *Haemophilus ducreyi* adherence to and entry into eukaryotic cells of genital origin. J. Infect. Dis. *167*:642–650, 1993.
65. Lesse, A. J., Gheesling, L. L., Bittner, W. E., et al.: Stable, conserved outer membrane epitope of strains of *Haemophilus influenzae* biogroup aegyptius associated with Brazilian purpuric fever. Infect. Immun. *60*:1351–1357, 1992.
66. Lomholt, H., and Kilian, M.: Distinct antigenic and genetic properties of the immunoglobulin A1 protease produced by *Haemophilus influenzae* biogroup aegyptius associated with Brazilian purpuric fever in Brazil. Infect. Immun. *63*:4389–4394, 1995
67. Lutwick, L. I., Gradon, J. D., Chapnick, E. K., et al.: *Haemophilus parainfluenzae* endocarditis treated with vegetectomy and complicated by late, fatal splenic rupture. Pediatr. Infect. Dis. J. *10*:778–781, 1991.
68. Lynn, J. D., Kane, J. G., and Parker, R. H.: *Haemophilus parainfluenzae* endocarditis: A review of forty cases. Medicine *56*:115–128, 1977.
69. Maller, R., Ånséhn, S., and Frydén, A.: *Haemophilus parainfluenzae* infection of the central nervous system: A report on two infants. Scand. J. Infect. Dis. *9*:241–242, 1977.

70. Mazloum, H. A., Kilian, M., Mohamed, Z. M., et al.: Differentiation of *Haemophilus aegyptius* and *Haemophilus influenzae*. Acta. Pathol. Microbiol. Immunol. Scand. *90*:109–112, 1982.
71. Merino, D., Saavedra, J., Pujol, E., et al.: *Haemophilus aphrophilus* as a rare cause of athritis. Clin. Infect. Dis. *19*:320–322, 1994.
72. Mesko, Z. G., Bauza, J., and Vinas, C.: Bacterial endocarditis due to *Haemophilus aphrophilus* with cerebral embolism. J. Pediatr. *89*:1031–1032, 1976.
73. Morse, S. A.: Chancroid and *Haemophilus ducreyi*. Clin. Microbiol. Rev. *2*:137–157, 1989.
74. Musser, J. M., and Selander, R. K.: Brazilian purpuric fever: Evolutionary genetic relationships of the case clone of *Haemophilus influenzae* biogroup aegyptius to encapsulated strains of *Haemophilus influenzae*. J. Infect. Dis. *161*:130–133, 1990.
75. Nahass, R. G., Cook, S., and Weinstein, M. P.: Vertebral osteomyelitis due to *Haemophilus aphrophilus*: Treatment with ceftriaxone. J. Infect. Dis. *159*:811–812, 1989.
76. Page, M. I., and King, E. O.: Infection due to *Actinobacillus actinomycetemcomitans* and *Haemophilus aphrophilus*. N. Engl. J. Med. *275*:181–188, 1966.
77. Palmer, K. L., Grass, S., and Munson, R. S., Jr.: Identification of a hemolytic activity elaborated by *Haemophilus ducreyi*. Infect. Immun. *62*:3041–3043, 1994.
78. Parker, R. H., and Hoeprich, P. D.: Disk method for rapid identification of *Hemophilus* species. Am. J. Clin. Pathol. *37*:319–327, 1962.
79. Perkins, B. A., Tondella, M. L. C., Bortolotto, I. M., et al.: Comparative efficacy of oral rifampin and topical chloramphenicol in eradicating conjunctival carriage of *Haemophilus influenzae* biogroup aegyptius. Pediatr. Infect. Dis. J. *11*:717–721, 1992.
80. Petty, B. G., Burrow, C. R., Robinson, R. A., et al.: *Haemophilus aphrophilus* meningitis followed by vertebral osteomyelitis and suppurative psoas abscess. Am. J. Med. *78*:159–162, 1985.
81. Plummer, F. A., Simonson, J. N., Cameron, D. W., et al.: Cofactors in male-female sexual transmissions of human immunodeficiency virus type 1. J. Infect. Dis. *163*:233–239, 1991.
82. Purcell, B. K., Richardson, J. A., Radoff, J. D., et al.: A temperature-dependent rabbit model for production of dermal lesions by *Haemophilus ducreyi*. J. Infect. Dis. *164*:359–367, 1991.
83. Purven, M., and Lagergard, T.: *Haemophilus ducreyi*, a cytotoxin-producing bacterium. Infect. Immun. *60*:1156–1162, 1992.
84. Quinn, F. D., Weyant, R. S., Worley, M. J., et al.: Human microvascular endothelial tissue culture cell model for studying pathogenesis of Brazilian purpuric fever. Infect. Immun. *63*:2317–2322, 1995.
85. Rivers, T. M.: Influenza-like bacilli: Growth of influenza-like bacilli on media containing only an autoclave-labile substance as an accessory food factor. Bull. Johns Hopkins Hosp. *33*:429–431, 1922.
86. Ronald, A. R., and Plummer, F. A.: Chancroid and *Haemophilus ducreyi*. Ann. Intern. Med. *102*:705–707, 1985.
87. Ronald, A. R., and Albritton, W.: Chancroid and *Haemophilus ducreyi*. *In* Holmes, K.K., Mardh, P. A., Sparling, P. F., et al. (eds): Sexually Transmitted Diseases. 2nd ed. New York, McGraw-Hill, 1990, pp. 263–271.
88. Root, T. E., Silva, E. A., Edwards, L. D., et al.: *Haemophilus aphrophilus* endocarditis with a probable primary dental focus of infection. Chest *80*:109–110, 1981.
89. Rossau, R., Duhamel, M., James, G., et al.: The development of specific rRNA-derived oligonucleotide probes for *Haemophilus ducreyi*, the causative agent of chancroid. J. Gen. Microbiol. *137*:277–285, 1991.
90. Rubin, L. G., and St. Geme, J. W., III: Role of lipooligosaccharide in virulence of the Brazilian purpuric fever clone of *Haemophilus influenzae* biogroup aegyptius for infant rats. Infect. Immun. *61*:650–655, 1993.
91. Rubin, L. G., Peters, V. B., and Ferez, M. C. C.: Bactericidal activity of human sera against a Brazilian purpuric fever (BPF) strain of *Haemophilus influenzae* biogroup aegyptius correlates with age-related occurence of BPF. J. Infect. Dis. *167*:1262–1264, 1993.
92. Scheifele, D. W., and Fussell, S. J.: Frequency of ampicillin-resistant *Haemophilus parainfluenzae* in children. J. Infect. Dis. *143*:495–498, 1981.
93. Schmid, G. P., Sanders, L. L., Jr., Blount, J. H., et al.: Chancroid in the United States: Re-establishment of an old disease. J. A. M. A. *258*:3265–3268, 1987.
94. Schulte, J. M., and Schmid, G. P.: Recommendations for treatment of chancroid, 1993. Clin. Infect. Dis. *20*(Suppl. 1):S39–S46, 1995.
95. Simon, M. W., Mitchell, B. L., O'Connor, W. N., et al.: Glomerulonephritis, pulmonary hemorrhage and coagulopathy associated with *Haemophilus parainfluenzae* endocarditis. Pediatr. Infect. Dis. *4*:183–188, 1985.
96. Smith, W. K., and Berger, H. W.: *Haemophilus parainfluenzae* meningitis: A case in an adult. Mt. Sinai J. Med. *41*:543–548, 1974.
97. Spinola, S. M., Castellazzo, A., Shero, M., et al.: Characterization of pili expressed by *Haemophilus ducreyi*. Microb. Pathol. *9*:417–426, 1990.
98. Spinola, S. M., Wild, L. M., Apicella, M. A., et al.: Experimental human infection with *Haemophilus ducreyi*. J. Infect. Dis. *169*:1146–1150, 1994.
99. Steckelberg, J. M., Murphy, J. G., Ballard, D., et al.: Emboli in infective endocarditis: The prognostic value of echocardiography. Ann. Intern. Med. *114*:635, 1978.
100. Sutter, V. L., and Finegold, S. M.: *Haemophilus aphrophilus* infections: Clinical and bacteriologic studies. Ann. N. Y. Acad. Sci. *174*:468–487, 1970.
101. Swaminathan, B., Mayer, L. W., Bibb, W. F., et al.: Microbiology of Brazilian purpuric fever and diagnostic tests. J. Clin. Microbiol. *27*:605–608, 1989.
102. Tondella, M. L. C., Quinn, F. D., and Perkins, B. A.: Brazilian purpuric fever caused by *Haemophilus influenzae* biogroup aegyptius strains lacking the 3031 plasmid. J. Infect. Dis. *171*:209–212, 1995.
103. Totten, P. A., Morton, W. R., Knitter, G. H., et al.: A primate model of chancroid. J. Infect. Dis. *169*:1284–1290, 1994.
104. Totten, P. A., Norn, D. V., and Stamm, W. E.: Characterization of the hemolytic activity of *Haemophilus ducreyi*. Infect. Immun. *63*:4409–4416, 1995.
105. Trees, D. L., and Morse, S. A.: Chancroid and *Haemophilus ducreyi*: An update. Clin. Microbiol. Rev. *8*:357–375, 1995.
106. Tyndall, M., Malisa, M., Plummer, F. A., et al.: Ceftriaxone no longer predictably cures chancroid in Kenya. J. Infect. Dis. *167*:469–471, 1993.
107. Varghese, R., Melo, J. C., Barnum, P., et al.: Endocarditis due to *Haemophilus aphrophilus*: Report of a case with possible transmission from dog to man. Chest *72*:680–682, 1977.
108. Wasserheit, J. N.: Epidemiological synergy: Interrelationships between human immunodeficiency virus infection and other sexually transmitted diseases. Sex. Transm. Dis. *19*:61–77, 1992.
109. Watson, K. C., Grimstone, J., O'Hare, A. E.: Meningitis due to *Haemophilus parainfluenzae*. J. Infect. *3*:380–384, 1981.
110. Weeks, J. E.: The bacillus of acute conjunctival catarrh, or "pink eye." Arch. Ophthalmol. *15*:441–451, 1886.
111. Weyant, R. S., Quinn, F. D., Utt, E. A., et al.: Human microvascular endothelial cell toxicity caused by Brazilian purpuric fever-associated strains of *Haemophilus influenzae* biogroup aegyptius. J. Infect. Dis. *169*:430–433, 1994.
112. White, C. B., Lampe, R. M., Copeland, R. L., et al.: Soft tissue infection associated with *Haemophilus aphrophilus*. Pediatrics *67*:434–435, 1981.
113. Whitney, A. M., and Farley, M. M.: Cloning and sequence analysis of the structural pilin gene of Brazilian purpuric fever-associated *Haemophilus influenzae* biogroup aegyptius. Infect. Immun. *61*:1559–1562, 1993.
114. Wort, A. J.: *Hemophilus parainfluenzae* meningitis. Can. Med. Assoc. J. *112*:606–607, 1975.

141

HELICOBACTER PYLORI

Mark A. Gilger

"No acid, no ulcer." Such is the dictum of modern medicine regarding peptic ulcer disease.[100] Indeed, peptic ulcers are managed successfully by acid reduction therapy. Unfortunately, the nagging problem with ulcers is their tendency to recur after treatment is completed. It now appears that most peptic ulcers have an infectious cause, thus giving a plausible explanation to the chronic, recurrent nature of this disease. The discovery of *Helicobacter pylori* in 1983 by Marshall and Warren[1] as the bacterial cause of peptic ulcer disease has stimulated worldwide interest and is revolutionizing the understanding, diagnosis, and treatment of peptic ulcer disease.

BACKGROUND

The presence of bacteria in the gastric mucosa has been known for more than 100 years. In 1874, Bottcher[13] observed bacteria in the human stomach. Bizzozero[7] described spirochetes in the stomach of dogs in 1893, and his observations were confirmed by Solomon[104] and Kasai and Kobayashi[61] in the dog, cat, rat, and monkey. Muhlens[84] and later Luger and Neuberger[71] reported spiral organisms in ulcerating carcinomas of the stomach in humans. In 1938, Doenges[25] explored the issue of gastric spirochetes and their clinical relevance. He reported a 43 per cent prevalence of spiral organisms in the human stomach in an autopsy review of 242 patients without known gastrointestinal disease. Specimen autolysis, however, made interpretation of the pathologic significance of the gastric spirochetes impossible. Freedburg and Barron[36] verified the findings of Doenges in 1940 when they identified spirochetes in the stomachs of 37 per cent of patients after partial gastric resection for carcinoma or ulcer disease. Work on the clinical significance of gastric spiral bacteria continued until a report in 1954. In an attempt to confirm the findings of spirochetes in the gastric mucosa, Palmer[89] performed an exhaustive review of gastric fundus biopsies from 1000 adult patients, 80 per cent of whom were being evaluated for upper gastrointestinal complaints and 20 per cent of whom were healthy control volunteers. Palmer noted, "None of the 1180 specimens was found to contain spirochetes or any structure which could reasonably be considered to be of spirochetal nature." He concluded that spirochetes are not part of the human gastric mucosa in health or illness. Palmer, a prominent researcher in gastritis, inadvertently may have curtailed further research into the role of gastric spiral bacteria.

In 1975, Steer,[105] using electron microscopy, noted curved bacteria in stomach biopsy specimens from patients with gastric ulcers. A few years later, Warren,[1] an Australian pathologist, noted the appearance of spiral bacteria overlaying inflamed gastric mucosa. Warren noted that this organism looked like a *Campylobacter*. He and Marshall began a series of culture experiments using *Campylobacter*-specific methods. The story culminates in 1983 and 1984, respectively, with their reports of the successful culture of the curved bacillus.[1, 78] In an attempt to fulfill the remainder of Koch's postulate, Marshall and associates[76] and Morris and Nicholson[83] independently ingested pure culture of *H. pylori*, and both developed symptomatic acute gastritis. The organism subsequently was recovered from the gastric mucosa by endoscopy and successfully cultured, thus completing Koch's postulate.

MICROBIOLOGY AND PATHOPHYSIOLOGY

H. pylori initially was named *Campylobacter pyloridis* by Marshall and Warren[1] due to its resemblance to *Campylobacter* species. Later changed to *C. pylori*, it became clear that the bacterium did not belong to any known genus. An entirely new genus—*Helicobacter*—was created, with "helico" describing the spiral shape and "pylori" denoting its typical location. *H. pylori* is a spiral-shaped, gram-negative bacteria with four to seven unipolar-sheathed flagella (Fig. 141–1).[9, 88] It is 0.5 μm wide and 3 to 5 μm long and has a smooth surface.[2, 81] It is generally S-shaped in vivo but can take on many forms, from U-shaped to cocci to rod-like.[81]

H. pylori inhabits a unique ecologic niche: the gastric submucosa. Several attributes, including adherence, shape, microaerophilism, urease production, and motility, allow adaption to the acidic gastric environment. *H. pylori* overlays the intercellular tight junctions of epithelial cells, beneath the mucous layer. Specific adhesion molecules appear to be tropic to gastric mucus-producing cells.[67] This adherence allows the organism to maintain colonization despite the rapid gastric cell turnover.[66] The spiral shape may allow the organism to

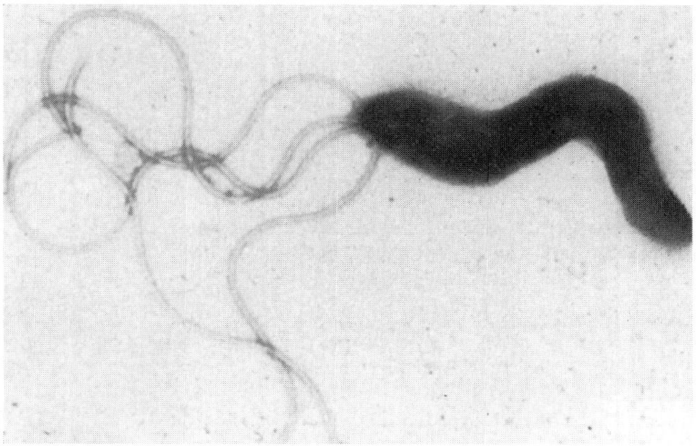

FIGURE 141–1. *Electron microscopy of* H. pylori *demonstrating the multipolar flagella and the typical spiral shape.*

corkscrew though the gastric mucus (Fig. 141–1). This spiral movement has been demonstrated in vitro using methylcellulose solutions.[66] *H. pylori* is microaerophilic and slow growing in culture media.[9, 88] One-millimeter translucent colonies grow after 5 to 7 days on blood- or serum-supplemented media with a low concentration of oxygen and carbon dioxide at a temperature of 37° C, which promotes optimal growth. This microaerophilism is well suited to the low oxygen levels of the gastric submucosa.[67] *H. pylori* is the most potent urease producer of any known microbe, surrounding itself in a cloud of ammonia.[2, 9, 88] The urea is converted to ammonium and bicarbonate.[8, 40] There is little evidence that the ammonium produced is cytoxic to gastric epithelium.[54] The bicarbonate creates an alkaline environment in the gastric submucosa. *H. pylori* produces several other enzymes, including a mucinase,[102] lipase,[99] catalase,[70] hemolysin, and cytopathic toxin.[68] The multiple, unipolar flagella (see Fig. 141–1) provide motility that may enable the organism to escape the acid lumen of the stomach[66] and evade the host immune responses.[67]

It has been suggested that *H. pylori* is more akin to normal gastrointestinal flora because the bacterium and the host can coexist for decades without apparent problems.[45] *H. pylori* infection produces inflammation, although in most cases the host is asymptomatic.[11] The inflammatory response is characterized by an infiltration of polymorphonuclear leukocytes, monocytes, lymphocytes, and plasma cells into the lamina propria (Fig. 141–2).[70] A significant immune response is produced by the host, including the production of antibodies, but it does not clear the organism in most cases.[68] *H. pylori* produces a chronic infection that persists for decades, possibly for life.[70] This lifelong colonization is accomplished by the same features that allow survival in the gastric mucosa, namely high urease production, flagellar motility, spiral shape, microaerophilism, and adherence.[70]

A number of potential virulence factors, such as urease, catalase, cytotoxin, and lipopolysaccharide, have been identified, although whether any of these actually contribute to symptomatic disease is unknown. The urease of *H. pylori* is a potent antigen, inducing elevations of antiurease IgG and IgA.[70] Interestingly, the ammonia produced by the urease does not appear to have a significant role in pathogenesis.[46] Catalase, another *H. pylori* enzyme, prevents the formation of oxygen metabolites from hydrogen peroxide in neutrophils.[32] This may provide an ability to evade host destruction. A vacuolating cytoxin has been identified in many *H. pylori*

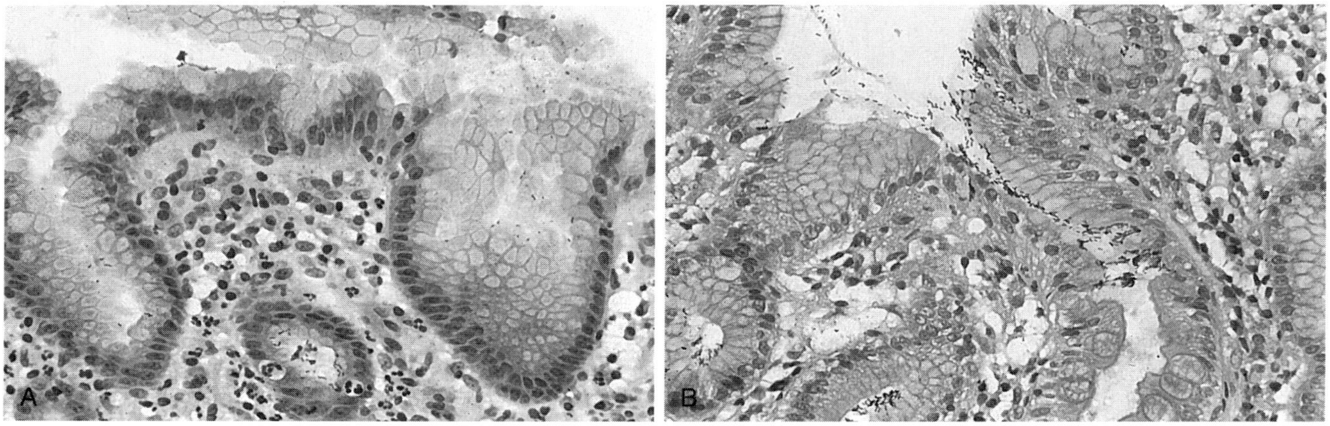

FIGURE 141–2. A, *High-power light microscopy of* H. pylori *demonstrating chronic active gastritis with small numbers of* H. pylori *seen on the epithelial surface and the mucus. An aggregate of* H. pylori *organisms is visible within the gastric pit. (Genta stain.)* B, *More* H. pylori *organisms and mild intestinal metaplasia. (*A *and* B *courtesy of Dr. Robert Genta, Baylor College of Medicine.)*

strains,[32] although it is unclear whether it is more common in patients with symptomatic disease. *H. pylori* has a peculiar lipopolysaccharide outer membrane. Unlike most gram-negative bacteria, its lipopolysaccharide coat is a significantly less potent inducer of the host complement cascade, some 1000-fold less potent than that of the Enterobacteriaceae.[70] This low biologic activity of *H. pylori's* outer membrane may be another adaptive mechanism allowing gastric colonization.[10]

EPIDEMIOLOGY

H. pylori may be the most common bacterial infection in humans, with an estimated 1 billion people in the world infected.[69] Transmission appears to be person-to-person.[65, 80, 107] The mode of transmission—whether fecal-oral, oral-oral, or other—is unknown.[106] *H. pylori* appears to be acquired in childhood,[21, 69] and humans appear to be a natural reservoir for infection.[48] There are no proven environmental sources of *H. pylori* infection, although a higher prevalence of infection has been found in Peru in families using a municipal water source versus private wells.[82]

Children appear to be important in the transmission of *H. pylori* infection, which clusters within families with children.[29, 74, 80, 87, 112] Family clustering emphasizes the role of crowding and personal hygiene in the person-to-person spread of infection. The prevalence of infection increases with age. In the United States, for example, only about 20 per cent of individuals younger than 30 years of age are infected, compared with 50 per cent of those older than 60 years of age.[75] Infection in young children is rare in the United States and developed nations.[70] The phenomenon of increasing prevalence with age most likely reflects a cohort effect, that is, the high prevalence in older persons simply reflects a higher childhood infection rate.[70] This cohort effect may be explained best by a lower standard of living during childhood of older persons. Socioeconomic status varies inversely with the prevalence of infection, with low-income individuals

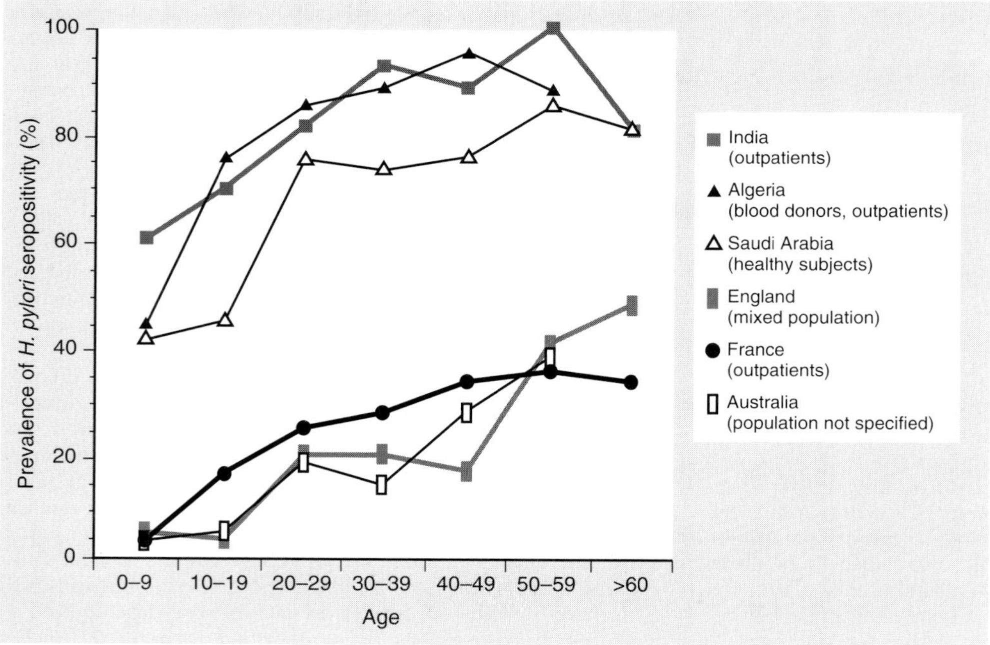

FIGURE 141–3. *Seroepidemiology of* H. pylori *infection demonstrating the difference in disease prevalence between developing and developed countries. (Data from Graham D. Y., Adam, E., Reddy, G. T. et al.: Seroepidemiology of* Helicobacter pylori *infection in India: Comparison of developing and developed countries. Dig. Dis. Sci. 36:1084–1088, 1991.)*

having the highest rates of infection.[35] There is a higher prevalence of infection in developing countries versus developed countries[80] (Fig. 141–3), and prevalence of infection varies greatly around the world. In Nigeria, for example, 58 per cent of children younger that 1 year of age were infected and 91 per cent of children older than 10 years of age were infected.[56] Such differences have been attributed to socioeconomic factors, hygiene, and the number of household occupants.[53] *H. pylori* is more prevalent in blacks and Hispanics than in whites in the United States.[103]

CLINICAL MANIFESTATIONS

There are no specific symptoms for *H. pylori* infection in children.[39, 41, 42, 51, 72, 93, 97] Symptoms such as epigastric abdominal pain, nighttime awakening with abdominal pain, hematemesis, and recurrent vomiting are suggestive, but in no way predictive, of infection.[28, 30, 62, 85] Still, these clinical symptoms are typical of peptic ulcer disease. It appears that such symptoms may be present only if *H. pylori* infection is found with a duodenal ulcer. Furthermore, the presence of *H. pylori* infection alone in both adults and children usually is asymptomatic.[24, 26, 27, 36, 43, 49, 94]

The association of *H. pylori* infection with recurrent abdominal pain of childhood remains a topic of ongoing debate. The critical issue is whether *H. pylori* antral gastritis is a source of abdominal pain. The issue remains unresolved. A logical conclusion for the pediatrician would be that a child with active upper gastrointestinal tract complaints in whom *H. pylori* infection is found deserves either treatment for the infection or diagnostic upper endoscopy to determine the presence of ulcer disease. *H. pylori* infection also has been associated with protein-losing enteropathy.[18, 55] Whether *H. pylori* infection actually causes the protein loss remains speculative.

DIAGNOSIS

The "gold standard" for diagnosis of *H. pylori* infection is culture of the organism from gastric biopsies or histologic review.[1] Upper endoscopy or other invasive means are necessary in order to obtain such biopsy specimens. In children, upper endoscopy can be quite helpful, often revealing a distinct nodularity at the antrum (Fig. 141–4), but it also may appear normal. This nodularity is found in two-thirds of infected children but only rarely in adults.[14, 52, 53] Histologically, prominent lymphoid follicles are seen. Routine hematoxylin-eosin staining may be adequate but must be performed properly to see the bacteria clearly. Alternative staining techniques, such as acridine orange, silver stains, and the "triple" stain, improve visualization.[37, 63, 73] The triple, or Genta, stain (Steiner + hematoxylin-eosin + alcian blue) may offer some distinct advantages because it is significantly more sensitive than hematoxylin-eosin staining and particularly useful for the detection of small numbers of bacteria, which often is the case in children (see Fig. 141–2). Although culture and histology require the need for endoscopy, culture may be important. In cases of recurrent *H. pylori* infection in which antibiotic resistance is suspected, culture allows in vitro antibiotic sensitivities to be determined.

Because culture requires gastric biopsy, less invasive methods have been developed (Table 141–1). These include serology, varying methods for detection of urease production, detection of salivary antibody, stool culture, polymerase chain reaction, and urine ammonia production.[92] Serology and urease activity detection by breath testing offer simple, noninvasive approaches to diagnosis and thus are attractive methods for use in children.

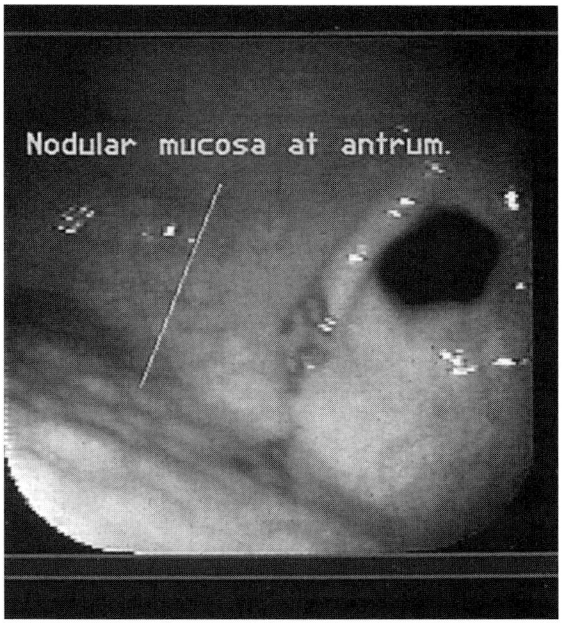

FIGURE 141–4. *Endoscopic view of the gastric antrum demonstrating the marked nodularity of the gastric surface.*

H. pylori infection induces a vigorous neutrophilic and lymphocytic (T-cell and B-cell) response that fails to clear the infection. The humoral immune response produces antibodies that can be detected in gastric secretions as well as systemically. A number of *H. pylori* antigens have been determined using bacterial cell wall sonicates, urease, or membrane extracts as the capture antigen.[19, 22, 23, 34, 101, 109] Some commercial assays have been found to have inappropriate positive and negative cut-off values for use in children.[20, 22] Care must be taken to ensure that the serologic tests employed have been verified for use in children. Although detection of IgA, polymeric IgA, and IgM antibodies against haptoglobin can be performed, they are not reproducible and thus not of any useful clinical value. Serologic diagnosis, although simple and widely available, does not indicate symptomatic disease. Because *H. pylori* can exist as an asymptomatic colonization of the gastric mucosa, significant debate exists concerning whether treatment is indicated.

H. pylori is a vigorous producer of urease. This characteristic has been used to create a variety of tests to detect the presence of urease. The urea breath test uses a labeled carbon of the urea, either radioactive carbon 14 (^{14}C)[5] or a nonradioactive, stable isotope, carbon 13 (^{13}C).[47] Patients fast 4 to 8 hours and then drink the labeled carbon accompanied by a meal to delay gastric emptying; then, the amount of labeled carbon dioxide in the breath is measured. Only those with gastric *H. pylori* present (and thus gastric urease activity to degrade the labeled urea) will be identified. Urea breath testing is useful for both the initial diagnosis and determination of successful treatment because the results return rapidly to normal after eradication. The radioactive ^{14}C method does not deserve consideration for use in children, but the stable isotope ^{13}C methodology seems highly suited as a safe, noninvasive test in children. Just as with serology, urea breath testing only indicates presence or absence of infection and does not indicate active symptomology.

The urease production of *H. pylori* can be measured directly

TABLE 141–1. Summary of Methods for Detecting *Helicobacter pylori*

Method	Sensitivity (%)	Specificity (%)	Advantages	Disadvantages
Invasive				
Histology	93–99	95–99	Widely available; detection best with special stains; can evaluate underlying mucosal damage; "gold standard"	Expensive; ≥two biopsies required; observer error; recent antibiotics or proton pump inhibitor use can lead to false-negative results
Culture of biopsy specimens	77–92	100	In vitro antibiotic susceptibility can be determined	Expensive; organism requires special transfer and culture technique; requires up to 1 week for results; recent antibiotics or proton pump inhibitor use can lead to false-negative results
Rapid urease test CLOtest hpFast PylorTek	89–98	93–98	Rapid results; easy to perform; less expensive than other invasive techniques	Formalin, simethicone, local anesthetic spray, recent antibiotics, bismuth, or proton pump inhibitor use can lead to false-negative results; poor technique or handling will affect results
Noninvasive				
Urea breath test ^{13}C ^{14}C	90–100	89–100	Inexpensive; represents entire mucosa (not subject to biopsy sampling bias)	Not currently available; antibiotics or proton pump inhibitor use can lead to false-negative results; presence of ulcer disease not determined
Serology (ELISA) HM-CAP Pylori.STAT Rapid serology FlexSure QuikVue	88–99	89–95	Inexpensive; test of choice when endoscopy is not required; good for screening or epidemiologic studies in children and adults	Possible cross-reactivity with similar bacteria; remains positive for a variable period following successful treatment; currently available rapid office-based tests require serum

ELISA, enzyme-linked immunosorbent assay
Data from Graham, D. Y.: *Helicobacter* Today. Norris Communications, Altrincham, Cheshire, United Kingdom, 1995, p. 5.

in gastric biopsy specimens using a variety of commercial assays.[79, 83] A portion of gastric biopsy specimen is placed into urea medium, and hydrolysis of urea leads to a color change in the media from tan to pink. False-negative results have been noted in children due to low numbers of organisms.[31] Such testing is useful for a rapid diagnosis during endoscopy but requires gastric biopsy. Urease activity also can be detected by measurement of another nonradioactive, stable isotope, ammonium, in the urine after oral ingestion.[60] This noninvasive test also may prove useful in children if it becomes commercially available.

H. pylori has been identified in saliva and dental plaque by culture[64] and polymerase chain reaction.[17] Others have identified salivary antibody to *H. pylori* using indirect immunofluorescence assay.[57] Viable *H. pylori* organisms have been cultured from feces in Gambian children.[108] Fecal identification of *H. pylori* would be useful for young infants but has proved to be a very difficult method with questionable reproducibility to date.

TREATMENT

Cure of *H. pylori* infection associated with peptic ulcer disease in both children and adults significantly reduces the likelihood of recurrence of ulceration.[59, 77, 95, 114] Such evidence supports a radical change in the treatment of peptic ulcer disease, from the standard acid suppression therapy to antibiotic cure of *H. pylori* infection.[79]

H. pylori infection is difficult to cure. Successful treatment usually requires two or more antibiotics,[111, 113] usually administered with an acid inhibitory agent. Confirmation of successful treatment has been defined as absence of detectable organisms by tissue biopsy or urea breath test at least 1 month after completion of treatment.[6] Because tissue biopsy is invasive, urea breath testing appears to be an excellent method for determination of successful treatment. Serologic tests are not useful for detection of cure due to the prolonged elevation of titers, which remain elevated for 6 months to 1 year or longer after treatment.

Children with recurrent abdominal pain represent a particular quandary for the pediatrician. Numerous studies of recurrent abdominal pain in children have found that *H. pylori*

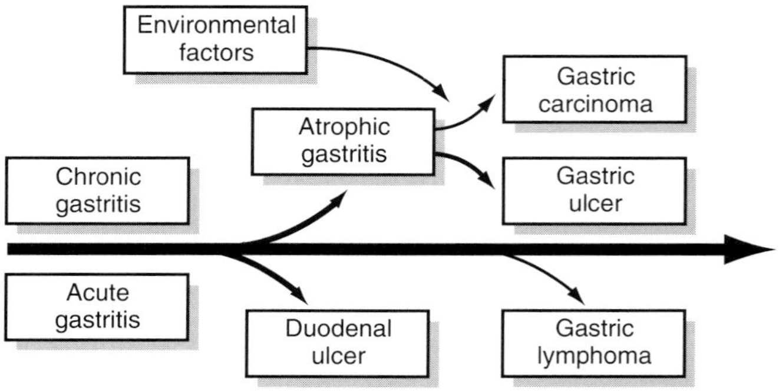

FIGURE 141–5. *Timeline of the possible outcomes of* H. pylori *infection, demonstrating the acute acquisition of infection and possible sequelae. (Data from Graham, D. Y.: Personal data.)*

infection may be a significant cause.[38, 86, 98, 107, 110] It has been argued that in any child with symptoms of ulcer disease, such as one with recurrent abdominal pain who is found to be *H. pylori*–infected, antibiotic treatment should be considered.[110]

A growing body of evidence indicates that the acquisition of *H. pylori* infection in childhood is a significant risk factor for the development of gastric cancers, such as adenocarcinoma and lymphoma (Fig. 141–5).[58, 108] Indeed, treatment of gastric lymphoma using antibiotics directed at *H. pylori* has resulted in tumor regression.[3, 113] Some argue this factor alone provides cause for the treatment of all children infected with *H. pylori*. Despite such provocative data and because most children with *H. pylori* infection have no clinical symptoms, there is no current rationale for treatment of all children.

In children, the most effective anti-*Helicobacter* treatment currently available is "triple therapy," which includes a bismuth compound (such as Pepto-Bismol), metronidazole, and amoxicillin.[75] In adults, amoxicillin is replaced by tetracycline. This therapy is given for 2 weeks, although regimens ranging from 7 to 28 days all have been reported as being successful.[75] Efficacy rates of 85 to 95 per cent have been reported for this combination. In patients allergic to penicillin, amoxicillin may be replaced with clarithromycin. Many clinicians advocate simultaneous use of an H_2-receptor antagonist, such as cimetidine or ranitidine, along with the triple therapy. This allows symptomatic relief of ulcer pain as well as a decrease in gastric acidity, which may be important. Amoxicillin and erythromycin, for example, are more active at a neutral pH.[50] Metronidazole, to which the *H. pylori* organism is highly sensitive, appears to be the mainstay of the triple therapy. Many areas outside the United States have high rates of metronidazole resistance due to overusage for other infections.[33] Unsuccessful triple therapy, even in the United States, may be due to such metronidazole resistance. No single antibiotic agent given alone is effective therapy against *H. pylori*.[77, 91, 95] Extensive study continues to determine the optimal treatment of *H. pylori*, but, to date, triple therapy remains the accepted standard.

When cure of infection has been obtained, the long-term rates of reinfection are as low as 1 per cent per year in developed countries but much higher in developing nations.[12, 91] However, reinfection may be more likely in families, especially when small children are the first infected.[4] No conclusive evidence currently exists, however, to recommend routine treatment of the entire family.[86] Until simple noninvasive tests, such as the ^{13}C urea breath test, routinely become available, reinfection rates will be difficult to determine in clinical practice.

Vaccination against *H. pylori* infection appears possible. Work in a mouse model has shown that oral immunization with a sonicate of *H. fetus* plus the adjuvant cholera toxin results in protection against an oral challenge.[15] Continued animal model investigation may yield promising direction for future vaccines.

FUTURE DIRECTIONS

Evidence continues to accumulate to confirm the role of *H. pylori* in the etiopathogenesis of peptic ulcer disease. This has caused a dramatic reappraisal of many previous notions about ulcer disease. Although the dictum "No acid, no ulcer" still holds, many other previous considerations, such as genetic predisposition, must be re-examined. Figure 141–5 demonstrates a proposed *H. pylori* timeline. It emphasizes the acquisition of an acute infection, most likely in childhood; maintenance of a chronic gastritis; and the possible progression to ulcer, atrophic gastritis, and potentially gastric carcinoma and lymphoma. Future research in children will be directed toward the epidemiology of infection because children are a natural reservoir of infection and have the potential for developing serious long-term sequelae of *H. pylori* infection.

References

1. Anonymous: Unidentified curved bacilli on gastric epithelium in active chronic gastritis. Lancet *1*:1273–1275, 1993.
2. Antonescu, C. G., and Marshall, B. J.: *Helicobacter pylori:* A potentially curable form of peptic ulcer disease. Gastroenterol. J. Club 2:3–9, 1990.
3. Ashorn, P., Lahde, P. L., Ruuska, T., et al.: Gastric lymphoma in an 11 Y/O boy: A case report. Med. Pediatr. Oncol. 22:66–67, 1994.
4. Bamford, K. B., Bickley, J., and Collins, J. S.: *Helicobacter pylori*: Comparison of DNA fingerprints provides evidence for intrafamilial infection. Gut *34*:1348–1350, 1993.
5. Bell, G. D., Weil, J., Garrison, G., et al.: ^{14}C-urea breath analysis: A noninvasive test for *Campylobacter pylori* in the stomach. Lancet *1*:1367–1368, 1987.
6. Bell, G. D.: Anti–*Helicobacter pylori* therapy: Clearance, elimination, or eradication? Lancet *337*:310–311, 1991.
7. Bizzozero, G.: Über die schlauchformigen drusen des magen darmkanals und die bezienhungen ihres epithels zu dem ober flachenepithel der schleimhaut. Arch. Mikr. Anast. *42*:82, 1893.
8. Blakeley, R. L., Hinds, J. A., Kunze, H. E., et al.: Jack bean urease (EC 3.5.1.5): Demonstration of a carbamoyl-transfer reaction and inhibitation by hydroxamic acids. Biochemistry *8*:1991–2000, 1969.
9. Blaser, M. J.: Gastric *Campylobacter*-like organisms, gastritis and pepic ulcer disease. Gastroenterology *96*:615–625, 1987.
10. Blaser, M. J.: *Helicobacter pylori*: Microbiology of a "slow" bacterial infection. Trends Microbiol. *1*:255–260, 1993.
11. Blaser, M. J.: The 10 most common questions about *Helicobacter pylori*. Infect. Dis. Clin. Pract. 2:439–440, 1993.
12. Borody, T. J., Cole, P., and Noonan, S.: Recurrence of duodenal ulcer and *Campylobacter pylori* infection after eradication. Med. J. Aust. *151*:431–435, 1989.
13. Bottcher, Dorpater Med. Z.: *5*:148, 1874.
14. Bujanover, Y., Konikoff, F., and Baratz, M.: Nodular gastritis and *Helicobacter pylori*. J. Pediatr. Gastroenterol. Nutr. *11*:41–44, 1990.
15. Chen, M., Lee, A., Haze, S, et al.: Immunization against gastric infection with *Helicobacter species*: First step in the prophylaxis of gastric cancer. Zentralbl. Bakteriol. *290*:155–165, 1993.
16. Chiba, N., Rao, B. V., and Rademaker, J. W.: Meta-analysis of the efficacy of antibiotic therapy in eradicating *Helicobacter pylori*. Am. J. Gastroenterol. *87*:1716–1720, 1992.
17. Clayton, C., Kleanthous, H., Coates, P. J., et al.: Sensitive detection of *Helicobacter pylori* by using polymerase chain reaction. J. Clin. Microbiol. *30*:192–200, 1992.
18. Cohen, H. A., Shapiro, P., Frydman, M., et al.: Childhood protein-losing enteropathy associated with *Helicobacter pylori* infection. J. Pediatr. Gastroenterol. Nutr. *13*:201–203, 1991.
19. Correa, P., Fox, J., Fontham, E., et al.: *Helicobacter pylori* and gastric carcinoma: Serum antibody prevalence in populations with contrasting cancer risks. Cancer *66*:2569–2574, 1990.
20. Crabtree, J. E., Mahoney, M. J., Taylor, J. D. et al.: Immune responses to *Helicobacter pylori* in children with recurrent abdominal pain. J. Clin. Pathol. *44*:768–773, 1991.
21. Cullen, D. J., Collins, B. J., Christiansen, K. J., et al.: When is *Helicobacter pylori* acquired? Gut *34*:1681–1682, 1993.
22. Czinn, S. J., Carr, H. S., and Speck, W. T.: Diagnosis of gastritis caused by *Helicobacter pylori* in children by means of an ELISA. Rev. Infect. Dis. *13*(Suppl. 8):S700, 1991.
23. De Giacomo, C., Lisato, L., Negrini, R., et al.: Serum antibody response to *Helicobacter pylori* in children: Epidemiologic and clinical applications. J. Pediatr. *119*:205–210, 1991.
24. Demers, B., Karmali, M., and Sherman, P.: Seroprevalence of *Helicobacter pylori* IgG antibodies in Canadian children. Ir. J. Med. Sci. *161*(Suppl. 10):78, 1992.
25. Doenges, J. L.: Spirochetes in the gastric glands of Macacus rhesus and humans without definite history of related disease. Proc. Soc. Exp. Med. Biol. *38*:536–538, 1938.
26. Dooley, C. P., Cohen, H., Fitzgibbons, P. L., et al.: Prevalence of *Helicobacter pylori* infection and histologic gastritis in asymptomatic persons. N. Engl. J. Med. *321*:1562–1566, 1989.
27. Drumm, B. *Helicobacter pylori* in the pediatric patient. Gastroenterol. Clin. North Am. *22*:169–182, 1991.
28. Drumm, B., O'Brien, A., Cutz, E., et al.: *Campylobacter pylori*–associated primary gastritis in children. Pediatrics *80*:192–195, 1987.
29. Drumm, B., Perez-Perez, G. L., Blaser, M. J., et al.: Intrafamilial clustering of *Helicobacter pylori* infection. N. Engl. J. Med. *322*:359–363, 1990.

30. Drumm, B., O'Brien, A., Cutz, E., et al.: *Campylobacter pylori*–associated primary gastritis in children. Pediatrics 80:192–195, 1987.
31. Drumm, B., Sherman, P., Cutz, E., et al.: Rapid diagnosis of *Campylobacter pylori* infection. Lancet *1*:149, 1986.
32. Dunn, B. E.: Pathogenic mechanisms of *Helicobacter pylori*. Gastroenterol. Clin. North Am. *22*:43–57, 1993.
33. European Study Group on Antibiotic Susceptibility of *Helicobacter pylori*: Results of a multicentre European survey in 1991 of metronidazole resistance in *Helicobacter pylori*. Eur. J. Clin. Microbiol. Infect. Dis. *11*:777–781; 1992.
34. Evans, D. J., Evans, D. E., Graham, D. Y., et al.: A sensitive and specific serology test for detection of *Campylobacter pylori* infection. Gastroenterology *96*:1004–1008, 1989.
35. Fiedorak, S. C., Malaty, H. M., Evans, D. L., et al.: Factors influencing the epidemiology of *Helicobacter pylori* infection in children. Pediatrics *88*:578–582, 1991.
36. Freedburg, A. S., and Barron, L. E.: The presence of spirochetes in human gastric mucosa. Am. J. Dig. Dis. *7*:443–445, 1940.
37. Genta, R. M., Robason, G. O., and Graham, D. Y.: Simultaneous visualization of *Helicobacter pylori* and gastric morphlogy: A new stain. Hum. Pathol. *25*:221–226, 1994.
38. Glassman, M. S.: *Helicobacter pylori* infection in children: A clinical overview. Clin. Pediatr. *31*(Suppl.):481–487, 1992.
39. Glassman, M., Schwartz, S., Medow, M., et al.: *Campylobacter pylori*–related gastrointestinal disease in children: Incidence and clinical findings. Dig. Dis. Sci. *34*:1501–1504, 1989.
40. Gorin, G.: On the mechanism of urease action. Biochim. Biophys. Acta *34*:268–269, 1959.
41. Gormally, S., and Drumm, B.: *Helicobacter pylori* and gastrointestinal symptoms. Arch. Dis. Child. *70*:165–166, 1994.
42. Gormally, S. M., Prakash, N., Durnin, M. T., et al.: Association of symptoms with *Helicobacter pylori* infection in children. J. Pediatr. *126*:753–756, 1995.
43. Gormally, S., Sherman, P., and Drumm, B.: Clinical syndromes of *Helicobacter pylori* infection in children. In Goodwin, C. S. (ed.): *Helicobacter pylori*: Biology and Clinical Practice. Boca Raton, FL, CRC Press, 1993, p. 85.
43a. Graham, D. Y.: *Helicobacter* today. Norris Communications, Attrincham, Cheshire, United Kingdom, 1995, p. 5.
44. Graham, D. Y., Adam, E., Reddy, G. T., et al.: Seroepidemiology of *Helicobacter Pylori* infection in India: Comparison of developing and developed countries. Dig. Dis. Sci. *36*:1084–1088, 1991.
45. Graham, D. Y., Blaser, M. J., and Soll, A. H.: *Helicobacter pylori*: Pathophysiology and epdemiology. Deerfield, IL, Discovery International, 1995, p. 9.
46. Graham, D. Y., Go, M., and Evans, D., Jr.: Urease, gastric ammonium/ammonia and *Helicobacter pylori*: The past, the present, and recommendations for future research. Aliment. Pharmacol. Ther. *6*:659–669, 1992.
47. Graham, D. Y., Klein, P. D., Evans, D. G., Jr., et al.: *Campylobacter pylori* detected noninvasively by the ^{13}C-urea breath test. Lancet *2*:1174–1177, 1987.
48. Graham, D. Y., Klein, P. D., Evans, D. G., Jr., et al.: *Helicobacter pylori*: Epidemiology, relationship to gastric cancer and the role of infants in transmission. Eur. J. Gastroenterol. Hepatol. *4*(Suppl. 1):S1–S6, 1992.
49. Graham, D. Y., Malaty, H. M., Evans, D. G., et al.: Epidemiology of *Helicobacter pylori* in an asymptomatic population in the United States: Effect of age, race and socioeconomic status. Gastroenterology *100*:1495–1501, 1991.
50. Grayson, M. L., Eliopoulos, G. M., Ferraro, M. J., et al.: Effect of varying pH on the susceptibility of *Campylobacter pylori* to antimicrobial agents. Eur. J. Clin. Microbiol. Infect. Dis. *8*:888–889, 1989.
51. Hardikar, W., Davidson, P. M., Cameron, D. J., et al.: *Helicobacter pylori* infection in children. J. Gastroenterol. Hepatol. *6*:450–454, 1991.
52. Hassell, E., and Dimmick, J. E.: Unique features of *Helicobacteri pylori* disease in children. Dig. Dis. Sci. *36*:417–423, 1991.
53. Hazell, S. L.: *H. pylori* in developing countries. *In* Hunt, R. H., and Tygat, G. N. J. (eds.): *Helicobacter pylori*: Basic Mechanisms to Clinical Cure. Dordrecht, Kluwer Academic Publishers, 1994, pp. 85–94.
54. Hazell, S. L., and Lee, A.: *Campylobacter pyloridis*, urease hydrogen ion back diffusion and gastric ulcers. Lancet *2*:15–17, 1986.
55. Hill, I. D., Sinclair-Smith, C., Lastorica, A. J., et al.: Transient protein enteropathy associated with acute gastritis and *Campylobacter pylori* gastritis. Arch Dis. Child. *62*:1215–1219, 1987.
56. Holcombe, C., Tsimuri, S., Eldridge, J., et al.: Prevalence of antibody to *Helicobacter pylori* in children in northern Nigeria. Trans. Royal Soc. Trop. Med. Hyg. *87*:19–21, 1994.
57. Husson, M. O., Gottrand, F., Truck, D. et al.: Detection of *H. pylori* in saliva using a monoclonal antibody. Zentralbl. Bakteriol. *279*:466–471, 1993.
58. Isaacson, P. G.: Gastric lymphoma and *Helicobacter pylori*. N. Engl. J. Med. *330*:1310–1311, 1994.
59. Israel, D. M., and Hassall, E.: Treatment and long-term follow up of *Helicobacter pylori*–associated duodenal ulcer disease in children. J. Pediatr. *123*:53–59, 1993.
60. Jicong, W., Guolong, L., Zhentua, Z., et al.: $^{15}NH_4+$ excretion test: A new method for detection of *Helicobacter pylori* infection. J. Clin Microbiol. *30*:181–184, 1992.
61. Kasai, K., and Kobayashi, R.: Stomach spirochetes occurring in mammals. J. Parasitol. *6*:1, 1919.
62. Kilbridge, P. M., Dahms, B. B., and Czinn, S. J.: *Campylobacter pylori*–associated gastritis and peptic ulcer disease in children. Am. J. Dis. Child. *142*:1149–1152, 1988.
63. Krajden, S., and Sherman, P.: *Helicobacter (campylobacter) pylori* and acid peptic diseases. Can. J. Gastroenterol. *4*:237–241, 1990.
64. Kradjen, S., Fuska, M., Anferson, J., et al.: Examination of human stomach biopsies, saliva and dental plaque for *Campylobacter pylori*. J. Clin. Microbiol. *27*:1397–1398, 1989.
65. Lee, A., Fox, J., and Hazell, S.: Pathology of *Helicobacter pylori*: A perspective. Infect. Immun. *61*:1601–1610, 1993.
66. Lee, A., and Mitchell, H.: Basic bacteriology of *H. pylori: H. pylori* colonization factors. *In* Hunt, R. H., and Tygat, G. N. J. (eds.): *Helicobacter pylori*: Basic Mechanisms to Clinical Cure. Dordrecht, Kluwer Academic Publishers, pp. 59–72, 1994.
67. Lee, A.: The microbiology and epidemiology of *Helicobacter pylori* infection. Scand. J. Gastroenterol. *29*(Suppl. 201):2–6, 1994.
68. Leunk, R. D., Johnson, P. T., David, B. C., et al.: Cytoxic activity in broth-culture filtrates of *Campylobacter pylori*. J. Med. Microbiol. *26*:93–99, 1988.
69. Levine, T. S., and Price, A. B.: *Helicobacter pylori*: Enough to give anyone an ulcer. Br. J. Clin. Pract. *47*:328–332, 1993.
70. Lior, H., and Johnson, W. M.: Catalase, peroxidase and superoxide dismutase activities in *Campylobacter* spp. *In* Pearson, A. D., Skirrow, M. B., Lior, H., et al. (eds.): *Campylobacter* III. London, Health Laboratory Service, 1985, pp. 226–227.
71. Luger, A., and Neuberger, H. Z.: Klin. Med. *92*:54, 1921.
72. Macarthur, C., Saunders, N., and Feldman, W.: *Helicobacter pylori*, gastroduodenal disease and recurrent abdominal pain in children. J. A. M. A. *273*:729–734, 1995.
73. Maden, E., Kemp, J., Westblom, T. U., et al.: Evaluation of staining methodologies for identifying *Campylobacter pylori*. Am. J. Clin. Pathol. *90*:450–453, 1988.
74. Malaty, H., Graham, D., Klein, P., et al.: Transmission of *Helicobacter pylori* infection: Studies in families of healthy individuals. Scand. J. Gastroenterol. *26*:927–932, 1991.
75. Marshall, B. J.: Epidemiology of *H. pylori* in Western countries. *In*: Hunt, R. H., and Tygat, G. N. J. (eds.): *Helicobacter pylori*: Basic Mechanisms to Clinical Cure. Dordrecht, Kluwer Academic Publishers, 1995, pp. 75–84.
76. Marshall, B. J., Armstrong, J. A., McGechie, D. B., et al.: Attempt to fulfill Koch's postulate for pyloric *Campylobacter*. Med. J. Aust. *125*:436–444, 1985.
77. Marshall, B. J., Goodwin, C. S., and Warren, J. R.: Prospective double-blind trial of duodenal ulcer relapse after eradication of *Campylobacter pylori*. Lancet *2*:1437–1442, 1988.
78. Marshall, B. J., Royce, H., Annear, D. I., et al.: Original isolation of *Campylobacter pyloridis* from human gastric mucosa. Microbios *25*:83–88, 1984.
79. McNutty, C. A. M., and Wise, R.: Rapid diagnosis of *Campylobacter*–associated gastritis. Lancet *1*:1443–1444, 1985.
80. Megraud, F.: Epidemiology of *Helicobacter pylori* infection. Gastroenterol. Clin. North Am. *22*:73–88, 1993.
81. Megraud, R., Bonnet, F., Garnier, M., et al.: Characterization of "*Campylobacter pyloridis*" by culture, enzymatic profile, and protein content. J. Clin. Microbiol. *22*:1007–1010, 1985.
82. Mendall, M.: Natural history and mode of transmission. *In*: Northfield, T., Mendall, M., and Goggin, P. (eds.): *Helicobacter pylori* infection: Pathophysiology, Epidemiology and Management. Boston, Kluwer Academic Publishers, 1993, 21–23.
83. Morris, A., and Nicholson, G.: Ingestion of *Campylobacter pyloridis* causes gastritis and raised fasting gastric pH. Am. J. Gastroenterol. *32*:192–199, 1987.
84. Muhlens, P. Z.: Vergleichende spirochätenstudien. Z. Hyg. Infekt. *57*:405–416, 1907.
85. Oderda, G., Dell'Olio, D., and Travassoli, K.: *Campylobacter pylori* gastritis and peptic ulcer disease in children. Am. J. Dis. Child. *143*:877, 1989.
86. Oderda, G., Vaira, D., and Ainley, C.: Eighteen-month follow-up of *Helicobacter pylori*–positive children treated with amoxicillin and tinidazaole. Gut *33*:1328–1330, 1992.
87. Oderda, G., Vaira, D., Holton, J., et al.: *Helicobacter pylori* in children with peptic ulcer and their families. Dig. Dis. Sci. *36*:572–576, 1991.
88. Ormand, J. E., and Talley, N. J.: *Helicobacter pylori*: Controversies and an approach to management. Mayo Clin. Proc. *65*:414–426, 1990.
89. Palmer, E. D.: Investigation of the gastric mucosa spirochetes of the human. Gastroenterology *27*:218–220, 1954.
90. Parsonnet, J., Friedman, G. D., and Vandersteen, D. P.: *Helicobacter pylori* infection and the risk of gastric carcinoma. N. Engl. J. Med. *325*:1127–1131, 1991.
91. Penston, J. G.: *Helicobacter pylori* eradication: Understandable caution but no excuse for inertia. Aliment. Pharmacol. Ther. *8*:369–389, 1994.
92. Pezzi, J. S., and Shiau, Y. F.: *Helicobacter pylori* and gastrointestinal disease. Am. Fam. Phys. *52*:1717–1724, 1995.
93. Prieto, G., Polanco, I., Larrauri, J., et al.: *Helicobacter pylori* infection in

children: Clinical endoscopic and histologic correlations. J. Pediatr. Gastroenterol. Nutr. *14*:420–425, 1992.
94. Peterson, W.: *Helicobacter pylori* and peptic ulcer disease. N. Engl. J. Med. *324*:1043–1048, 1991.
95. Rauws, E. A. J., and Tygat, G. N. J.: Cure of duodenal ulcer associated with eradication of *Helicobacter pylori*. Lancet *335*:1233–1239, 1990.
96. Raymond, J., Bergeret M., Benhamou, H., et al.: A two-year study of *Helicobacter pylori* in children. J. Clin. Microbiol. *32*:461–463, 1994.
97. Reifen, R., Rasooly, I., Drumm, B., et al.: *Helicobacter pylori* infection in children: Is there specific symptomatology? Dig. Dis. Sci. *39*:1488–1492, 1994.
98. Rosioru, C., Glassman, M. S., Berezin, S. H., et al.: Treatment of *Helicobacter pylori*–associated gastroduodenal disease in children: Clinical evaluation of antisecretory vs. antibacterial therapy. Dig. Dis. Sci. *38*:123–128, 1993.
99. Sarosiek, J., Slomiany, A., Van Horn, K., et al.: Lipolytic activity of *Campylobacter pylori*: Effect of sofalcone. Gastroenterology *94*:A399, 1988.
100. Schwartz, K.: Über penbtrierende magenund jejunal-geschwüre. Beltr. Ucin. Chir. *67*:96–128, 1910.
101. Sherman, P., Peptic ulcer disease in children: Diagnosis, treatment and the implication of *Helicobacter pylori*. Gastroenterol. Clin. North Am. *23*:707–725, 1994.
102. Slomiany, B. L., Bliski, J., Sarosiek, J., et al.: *Campylobacter pyloridis* degrades mucin and undermines gastric mucosal integrity. Biochem. Biophys. Res. Commun. *144*:307–314, 1987.
103. Smoak, B. L., Kelley, P. W., and Taylor D. N.: Seroprevalence of *Helicobacter pylori* infections in a cohort of U. S. Army recruits. Am. J. Epidemiol. *139*:513–519, 1994.
104. Solomon, H., Über das spirilllim des saugetiermagens und sein verhalten zu den belegzelen. Centralbl. Bakt. *19*:433, 1896.
105. Steer, H. W.: Ultrastructure of cell migration through the gastric epithelium and its relationship to bacteria. J. Clin. Pathol. *28*:639–646, 1975.
106. Talley, M. J.: Epidemiology of *Helicobacter pylori* infection. NIH Consensus Development Conference on *Helicobacter pylori* in Peptic Ulcer Disease, Bethesda, MD, February 1994, pp. 7–9.
107. Taylor, D., and Blaser, M. J.: The epidemiology of *Helicobacter pylori* infection. Epidemiol. Rev. *13*:42–59, 1991.
108. Thomas, J. E., Gibson, G. R., Darboe, M. K., et al.: Isolation of *Helicobacter pylori* from human faeces. Lancet *340*:1194–1195, 1992.
109. Thomas, J. E., Whatmore, A. M., Barer, M. R., et al.: Serodiagnosis of *Helicobacter pylori* infection in childhood. J. Clin. Microbiol. *28*:2641–2645, 1990.
110. Tolia, V.: *Helicobacter pylori* in pediatric nonulcer dyspepsia: Pathogen or commensal. Am. J. Gastroenterol. *90*:865–868, 1995.
111. Tygat, G. N. J.: Treatments that impact favorably upon the eradication of *Helicobacter pylori* and ulcer recurrence. Aliment. Pharmacol. Ther. *8*:359–368, 1994.
112. Vincent, P., Gottand, F., Pernes, P., et al.: High prevalence of *Helicobacter pylori* infection in cohabiting children: Epidemiology of a cluster with special emphasis on molecular typing. Gut *35*:313–316, 1994.
113. Wotherspoon, A. C., Doglioni, E., and Diss, T. C.: Regression of primary low-grade B-cell gastric lymphoma of mucosa-associated lymphoid tissue type after eradication of *Helicobacter pylori*. Lancet *342*:575–578, 1993.
114. Yeung, C. K., Fu, K. H., and Yeun, K. Y.: *Helicobacter pylori* and associated duodenal ulcer. Arch. Dis. Child. *65*:1212–1215, 1990.

142

KINGELLA

Thomas L. Kuhls

The genus *Kingella* comprises three species: *K. kingae, K. denitrificans,* and *K. orale*. *K. kingae* increasingly is being recognized as an important cause of invasive infections in children. With improved methods to recover this fastidious member of the family Neisseriaceae and increasing awareness that the microorganism is not a culture contaminant, *K. kingae* infections are being encountered almost annually by many pediatric infectious diseases specialists. It is assumed, however, that most *K. kingae* infections continue to be treated empirically because the organism is difficult to isolate from clinical specimens. *K. denitrificans* rarely causes endocarditis,[3, 7, 27, 32, 40, 76] empyema,[51] and chorioamnionitis[48] in adults, but it has not been reported to cause invasive disease in children. To date, *K. orale* has not been reported to cause human infections.[18]

HISTORY

During the 1950s and early 1960s, Elizabeth O. King isolated gram-negative bacilli from clinical specimens that had phenotypic and growth characteristics identical to those of *Moraxella* species, except the organisms were beta-hemolytic and did not contain catalase.[34] In honor of Dr. King, the organism initially was named *Moraxella kingii* in 1968,[34] later renamed *Moraxella kingae* in 1974,[5] and finally reclassified as *Kingella kingae* in 1976.[35] The Centers for Disease Control and Prevention received 78 *K. kingae* isolates from 1953 to 1980, of which 75 per cent were recovered from blood, bone, or joint specimens.[29] Most of the isolates were obtained from children younger than 6 years of age. During the 1980s, increasing numbers of children with *K. kingae* infections were reported because of better awareness of the microorganism and better culturing techniques of fastidious agents. It was not until the 1990s that the importance of *K. kingae* in causing invasive infections in children became apparent.

MICROBIOLOGY

Kingella species are small (0.6 to 1 μm × 1 to 3 μm), gram-negative rods that may resist Gram decolorization.[56] The organisms can appear coccoid and exist in pairs or short chains. The nonencapsulated bacilli are fastidious aerobes that grow best at 33° to 37° C in both nutrient and blood agar. At least 4 days of incubation usually is required before *Kingella* species can be detected in clinical specimens grown on agar plates, but growth can be detected earlier using radiometric detection culturing systems.[88] Two types of bacterial colonies are found on agar plates: small, smooth, and nearly translucent colonies and larger spreading colonies that appear pitted because of corrosion of the agar surface. The larger colony type, however, usually is not present after the initial colonies have been subcultured, unless the organism is cultured under anaerobic conditions. Biochemical characteristics of the genus *Kingella* include negative reactions for motility, catalase, indole, and urease and a positive reaction for oxidase. All members of the genus are able to produce trace acid from glucose.

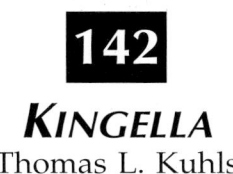

K. kingae is the only member of the genus reported to cause invasive infections in children. It can be differentiated from *K. denitrificans, K. orale,* and *Neisseria* species by a distinct narrow zone of beta-hemolysis surrounding the colonies. Unlike *K. denitrificans, K. kingae* does not reduce nitrates or nitrites and produces acid from maltose. *K. kingae* can be confused easily with isolates of *Eikenella corrodens* and *Cardio-*

bacterium hominis, both of which can cause suppurative infections in humans. Also, *K. kingae* can be misidentified as beta-hemolytic streptococci in Gram-stained specimens when decolorization is incomplete.

EPIDEMIOLOGY

Kingella species are a part of the normal oropharyngeal flora of children. In 1969, *K. kingae* was isolated from 1.1 per cent of nose and throat swabs obtained from children and adults.[33] In this study, however, the cultures only were incubated for 24 hours and selective media were not used; thus, the prevalence rate of carriage was most likely much higher. Throat and nasopharyngeal cultures were obtained from infants and children attending two day care centers in Israel.[90] Specimens were obtained every 2 weeks for a duration of 11 months and plated on selective media.[92] The monthly prevalence rates of *K. kingae* carriage ranged from 6 to 35 per cent, with the highest rates found in the months of December and April. Overall, at least one positive *K. kingae* culture was obtained in 73 per cent of the children. The rate of *K. kingae* carriage in this study was similar to previously reported rates of *Streptococcus pneumoniae* carriage in children of the same age group and much higher than the rates of *Haemophilus influenzae* type b carriage found in young children during the prevaccine era. Unlike these respiratory tract pathogens, *K. kingae* was isolated only from the tonsillar areas of the children and not from the nasopharynx. The investigators did not isolate *K. kingae* from 2- to 4-month-old infants attending a well-care clinic but did isolate the organism from 8 per cent of healthy children older than 8 years of age who were scheduled for elective surgical procedures.[90]

Osteoarticular *K. kingae* infections are most common in children 6 months to 4 years of age,[28, 41, 89] but *K. kingae* endocarditis occurs in all age groups, including adults.[12, 28, 80, 84] In southern Israel, the annual incidence of *K. kingae* invasive infections has been estimated to be 27.4 cases per 100,000 children 24 months of age or younger.[89] The rate of invasive infection was one-quarter of that found for invasive *H. influenzae* type b infections during a period when children were not receiving *H. influenzae* type b vaccine. In children with suppurative arthritis, *K. kingae* was isolated more commonly from joint aspirates that were cultured directly in BACTEC bottles than was *H. influenzae* type b.[88] Invasive *K. kingae* infections occur equally in males and females.[28, 41, 89] In two studies completed outside the United States, infections tended to occur between the months of July and December.[12, 89] Children with *K. kingae* invasive infections often have upper respiratory tract symptoms, dental procedures, or stomatitis before signs of invasive illness develop.[28, 41, 89] In Israel, 56 per cent of children with an invasive infection had evidence of a respiratory tract infection or stomatitis at the time of *K. kingae* infection.[89]

PATHOGENESIS

No studies have defined the mechanisms of pathogenesis of *Kingella* infections. *Kingella* species have type 4 pili, which may allow the organisms to adhere to the oropharyngeal epithelium.[83] It has been suggested that damage of the oropharyngeal mucosa by viruses or trauma may allow *K. kingae* to gain access to the blood stream. After a period of transient bacteremia, *K. kingae* then causes focal infection in joints, bones, disk spaces, and heart valves.

CLINICAL MANIFESTATIONS

K. kingae causes various infections in children (Table 142–1). The most common invasive *K. kingae* infection is suppurative arthritis.[28, 41, 89] Infants and young children usually present with acute monoarticular joint swelling and tenderness. To date, there have been no reported cases of polyarticular infection in children. No features of the illness distinguish it from other bacterial causes of suppurative arthritis. Patients often have symptoms of an upper respiratory tract illness or stomatitis shortly before or at the time of illness.[28, 41, 64, 89] Eighty-six per cent of children have fever higher than 38° C at presentation.[41] The knee is the joint affected most commonly.[6, 12, 13, 17, 22, 42, 57, 59, 64, 68, 75, 81, 89] However, *K. kingae* has been reported to cause infection in the hip,[4, 12, 13, 17, 89] ankle,[13, 17, 23, 43, 89] elbow,[17, 45] wrist,[24, 65, 72, 89] sternoclavicular joint,[12, 13] and shoulder.[89] Most children do not have an underlying illness that increases their susceptibility to infection, although a child undergoing therapy for acute lymphocytic leukemia did develop *K. kingae* suppurative arthritis.[64]

K. kingae osteomyelitis has a more insidious onset than suppurative arthritis, with most patients having symptoms for at least 1 week before they are diagnosed with a bone infection. Fever is present in only one-half of the children with *K. kingae* osteomyelitis.[41] The proximal femur and distal femur are the most common sites of infection,[13, 16, 23, 28, 73] which often occurs in an epiphysis.[4, 41, 46, 71, 89] Young children also develop *K. kingae* osteomyelitis of the talus[2, 12, 80] and calcaneus,[17, 28, 89, 91] although, unlike the more frequently encountered cases of osteomyelitis associated with puncture wounds, the children have relatively mild symptoms and there is no history of trauma or penetrating injury. Less commonly, *K. kingae* causes infection in the tibia,[28, 42, 71] clavicle,[66] ulna,[54] radius,[9] humerus,[89] and sternum.[16, 63] In one child with *K. kingae* osteomyelitis of the neck of the femur, the histopathologic findings of the infected bone resembled those of eosinophilic granuloma.[73]

There are numerous reports of children developing *K. kingae* spondylodiskitis.[9, 12, 13, 19, 20, 28, 41, 42, 58, 63, 85, 86] The children usually are younger than 5 years of age and have an insidious onset of back stiffness and tenderness, eventually leading to their refusal to walk. Fever was present in two-thirds of the patients, but it never was higher than 39° C.[41] Various disks from T11–12 to L5–S1 have been involved, although one patient with cervical involvement has been reported.[58]

Less than half of the reported cases of *K. kingae* endocarditis have occurred in children.[1, 4, 11, 12, 14, 15, 21, 25, 26, 28, 30, 36, 42, 43, 47, 50, 55, 61, 62, 67, 70, 80, 84, 93] Nearly three-quarters of the patients have had preexisting structural cardiac defects.[28, 84] The history and physical findings of *K. kingae* endocarditis do not differ from those seen in children with subacute endocarditis of other bacterial etiologies. At least one-third of patients with *K.*

TABLE 142–1. Infections in Children Caused by *Kingella kingae*

Suppurative arthritis
Osteomyelitis
Spondylodiskitis
Endocarditis
Transient bacteremia
Meningitis
Endophthalmitis
Pulmonary infections
Dactylitis
Subglottic and epiglottic infections
Eyelid abscesses

kingae endocarditis have oral or pharyngeal mucosal alterations prior to the development of systemic symptoms.[28, 84] Children usually present with fever, and they often have a new or changing heart murmur, splenomegaly, and petechial rashes. Patients also can present with more acute symptoms, including evidence of septic shock and cardiac failure.[12, 21, 80] *K. kingae* endocarditis occasionally has occurred in immunosuppressed persons,[12, 36, 84] including patients with AIDS.[39, 78]

Isolating *K. kingae* from the blood of a febrile infant should not suggest necessarily that the child has endocarditis. Seven children with transient *K. kingae* bacteremia during infancy who did not develop a focal infection have been identified.[87] Bacteremic children occasionally develop a rash mimicking gonococcemia[65, 70] or meningococcemia.[77] Rarer *K. kingae* infections include meningitis,[53, 77, 79, 82] endophthalmitis,[8, 28] pulmonary infections,[31, 52] dactylitis,[10, 89] subglottic[89] and epiglottic[38] infections, and an eyelid abscess.[33] A 3-year-old child with vaginitis from which *K. denitrificans* was isolated represents the only reported example of other members of the *Kingella* genus causing infection during childhood.[69]

LABORATORY FINDINGS AND DIAGNOSIS

No characteristic laboratory findings suggest the presence of an invasive *K. kingae* infection. Leukocytosis (>10,000 white blood cells/mm^3) is present in only 60 per cent of children with an invasive infection. However, the erythrocyte sedimentation rate almost always is elevated (>20 mm/hr).[41] In children with culture-proven suppurative arthritis, the leukocyte count in synovial fluid is variable (10,000 to 161,000 white blood cells/mm^3), but neutrophils usually predominate.[89] Organisms are identified by Gram stain in less than 15 per cent of clinical specimens.[28, 41] Plain radiographs demonstrate soft tissue swelling and joint effusions in one-half of the cases of suppurative arthritis, but lytic lesions or disk space narrowing develops in 95 per cent of cases of osteomyelitis or spondylodiskitis.[28] Technetium-99m bone scans help in diagnosing *K. kingae* osteomyelitis during the early course of disease when plain radiographs do not demonstrate abnormalities yet.[28] In children with *K. kingae* endocarditis, large vegetations often are demonstrated by echocardiogram, especially in children who have had symptoms for a long time, or when there is evidence of embolization.

K. kingae infection is diagnosed by isolating the organism from an appropriate clinical specimen. The organism is isolated from the blood in only 5 per cent of patients with osteoarticular *K. kingae* infections.[17] The fastidious nature of the organism, the low number of organisms found in clinical specimens, and its slow growth pattern hamper the recovery of *K. kingae*. Conventional cultures should be examined at least once per week for a total of 3 weeks to detect the organism. The recovery rate of *K. kingae* can be enhanced greatly if culture material, including purulent synovial fluid, is inoculated directly into BACTEC culture media.[88] In one study, 91 per cent of episodes of *K. kingae* suppurative arthritis would have been missed if the specimens were not cultured in BACTEC bottles.[88] Also, growth of the organism was detected within 72 hours using this culturing system. The recovery rate of *K. kingae* from clinical specimens also may be enhanced if specimens are inoculated directly into Isolator microbial tubes.[89] Once growth of the organism is detected, it is not uncommon for the clinical microbiology laboratory to have difficulty in identifying it as *K. kingae*. Clinicians should suspect that their patient has a *K. kingae* infection when slow-growing, gram-negative rods that display beta-hemolysis are isolated from a normally sterile body site.

TREATMENT AND OUTCOME

K. kingae generally is susceptible to β-lactam antibiotics.[12, 37, 60] However, two isolates have shown in vitro resistance to the antistaphylococcal β-lactams.[30, 42] A β-lactamase–positive strain of *K. kingae* was isolated from the blood of an adult patient with AIDS.[74] Similarly, a *K. denitrificans* isolate obtained from the bone marrow of a 39-year-old patient with AIDS has contained β-lactamase.[49] Isolates of *K. kingae* have been susceptible universally to second- and third-generation cephalosporins, aminoglycosides, chloramphenicol, and trimethoprim-sulfamethoxazole.[12, 37, 60] Many isolates, however, demonstrate at least partial resistance to erythromycin, clindamycin, and vancomycin.[12, 37, 60]

Children with invasive *K. kingae* infections have been treated with a variety of antibiotics, including penicillin G, ampicillin, cephalosporins, chloramphenicol, trimethoprim-sulfamethoxazole, and the antistaphylococcal β-lactams. Most infections should be treated initially with intravenous penicillin G or ampicillin because these antibiotics are relatively well tolerated and inexpensive. All *K. kingae* isolates, however, should be checked for β-lactamase activity.

The duration of antibiotic treatment for *K. kingae* osteoarticular infections has ranged from 17 days to 6 months.[41] Oral therapy with an antibiotic such as amoxicillin can be considered when gastrointestinal absorption is demonstrated and compliance can be monitored. Many clinicians use the normalization of the erythrocyte sedimentation rate as a guide to the duration of therapy. Surgical drainage of the bone, joint, or disk space usually is not required, except for infections in the hip and shoulder. The prognosis of *K. kingae* osteoarticular infections is excellent; chronic complications from initial infection have not been reported. However, persistent narrowing of the intervertebral disk space is common in cases of *K. kingae* spondylodiskitis.[41]

Patients with *K. kingae* endocarditis usually respond rapidly to antibiotic therapy and become afebrile in a few days. High-dose intravenous therapy usually is continued for 4 to 6 weeks. In cases in which prosthetic valves are infected, surgical excision of the valve usually is not needed for cure unless abscess formation occurs. Unlike osteoarticular infections, the complication rate of *K. kingae* endocarditis is high; cerebral infarction and death have been reported after embolization of vegetations.[12, 43, 44, 84]

References

1. Adachi, R., Hammerberg, O., and Richardson, H.: Infective endocarditis caused by *K. kingae*. Can. Med. Assoc. J. *128*:1087–1088, 1983.
2. Benard, M., Jean-Baptiste, A., Nelet, F., et al.: Osteomyelite a *Kingella kingae*. Arch. Fr. Pediatr. *46*:521–524, 1989.
3. Berdah, J., Feder, J. M., Bimet, F., et al.: *Kingella denitrificans* endocarditis on prosthetic aortic valve. Presse Méd. *18*:1517–1518, 1989.
4. Bosworth, D. E.: *Kingella (Moraxella) kingae* infections in children. Am. J. Dis. Child. *137*:650–653, 1983.
5. Bøvre, K., Henriksen, S. D., and Jonsson, V.: Correction of the specific epithet *kingii* in the combinations *Moraxella kingii* Henriksen and Bøvre 1968 and *Pseudomonas kingii* Jonsson 1970 to *kingae*. Int. J. Syst. Bacteriol. *24*:307, 1974.
6. Boyce, F., Cassidy, M., and Price, R.: *Kingella kingae* septic arthritis. Clin. Microbiol. Newsl. *5*:46, 1983.
7. Brown, A. M., Rothburn, M. M., Roberts, C., et al.: Septicaemia with probable endocarditis caused by *Kingella denitrificans*. J. Infect. *15*:225–228, 1987.
8. Carden, S. M., Colville, D. J., Gonis, G., et al.: *Kingella kingae* endophthalmitis in an infant. Aust. N. Z. J. Ophthalmol. *19*:217–220, 1991.

9. Chanel, C., Tiget, F., Chapvis, P., et al.: Spondylitis and osteomyelitis caused by *Kingella kingae* in children. J. Clin. Microbiol. *25*:2407–2409, 1987.
10. Chiquito, P. E., Elliott, J., and Namnyak, S. S.: *Kingella kingae* dactylitis in an infant. J. Infect. *22*:102–103, 1991.
11. Christensen, C. E., and Emmanouilides, G. C.: Bacterial endocarditis due to "*Moraxella* new species I." N. Engl. J. Med. *277*:803–804, 1967.
12. Claesson, B., Falsen, E., and Kjellman, B.: *Kingella kingae* infections: A review and a presentation of data from 10 Swedish cases. Scand. J. Infect. Dis. *17*:233–243, 1985.
13. Clement, J. L., Berard, J., Cahuzac, J. P., et al.: *Kingella kingae* osteoarthritis and osteomyelitis in children. J. Pediatr. Orthop. *8*:59–61, 1988.
14. Cohen, P. S., Maguire, J. H., and Weinstein, L.: Infective endocarditis caused by gram-negative bacteria: A review of the literature. Prog. Cardiovasc. Dis. *22*:204–242, 1980.
15. Corrigall, D., Bolen, J., Hancock, E. W., et al.: Mitral valve prolapse and infective carditis. Am. J. Med. *63*:215–222, 1977.
16. Davis, J. M., and Peel, M. M.: Osteomyelitis and septic arthritis caused by *Kingella kingae*. J. Clin. Pathol. *35*:219–222, 1982.
17. de Groot, R., Glover, D., Clausen, C., et al.: Bone and joint infections caused by *Kingella kingae*: Six cases and review of the literature. Rev. Infect. Dis. *10*:998–1004, 1988.
18. Dewhirst, F. E., Chen, C.-K. C., Paster, B. J., et al.: Phylogeny of species in the family *Neisseriaceae* isolated from human dental plaque and description of *Kingella orale* sp. nov. Int. J. Syst. Bacteriol. *43*:490–499, 1993.
19. Donnio, P. Y., Minet, J., Guerin, M. N., et al.: Spondylodiscite a *Kingella kingae* chez un enfant. Med. Mal. Infant. *12*:741–744, 1985.
20. Falsen, E., Brorson, E., and Enger, E. A.: *Moraxella kingii*: A rare cause of osteomyelitis. Z. Kinderchir. *22*:186–189, 1977.
21. Förstl, H., Ruckdeschel, G., Lang, M., et al.: Septicemia caused by *Kingella kingae*. Eur. J. Clin. Microbiol. *3*:267–269, 1984.
22. Franklin, G. W., and Shafi, N. A.: Spontaneous septic arthritis due to *Kingella kingae*. Clin. Microbiol. Newsl. *5*:53–54, 1983.
23. Gamble, J. G., and Rinsky, L. A.: *Kingella kingae* infection in healthy children. J. Pediatr. Orthop. *8*:445–449, 1988.
24. Gay, R. M., Lane, T. W., and Keller, D. C.: Septic arthritis caused by *Kingella kingae*. J. Clin. Microbiol. *17*:168–169, 1983.
25. Geraci, J. E., and Wilson, W. R.: Endocarditis due to gram-negative bacteria. Mayo Clin. Prac. *57*:145–148, 1982.
26. Giamarellou, H., and Galanakis, N.: Use of intravenous ciprofloxacin in difficult-to-treat infections. Am. J. Med. *82*(Suppl. 4A):346–351, 1987.
27. Goldman, I. S., Ellner, P. D., Francke, E. L., et al.: Infective endocarditis due to *Kingella denitrificans*. Ann. Intern. Med. *93*:152–153, 1980.
28. Goutzmanis, J. J., Gonis, G., and Gilbert, G. L.: *Kingella kingae* infection in children: Ten cases and a review of the literature. Pediatr. Infect. Dis. J. *10*:677–683, 1991.
29. Graham, D. R., Band, J. D., Thornsberry, C., et al.: Infections caused by *Moraxella, Moraxella urethralis, Moraxella*-like groups M-5 and M-6, and *Kingella kingae* in the United States, 1953–1980. Rev. Infect. Dis. *12*:423–431, 1990.
30. Grant, J. M., Bartolussi, R. A., Roy, D. L., et al.: Prosthetic valve bacterial endocarditis caused by *Kingella kingae*. Can. Med. Assoc. J. *129*:406–410, 1983.
31. Gremillion, D. H., and Crawford, G. E.: Measles pneumonia in young adults: An analysis of 106 cases. Am. J. Med. *71*:539–542, 1981.
32. Hassan, I. J., and Hayek, L.: Endocarditis caused by *Kingella denitrificans*. J. Infect. *27*:291–295, 1993.
33. Henriksen, S. D.: Corroding bacteria from the respiratory tract. Acta Pathol. Microbiol. Scand. *75*:85–90, 1969.
34. Henriksen, S. D., and Bøvre, K.: *Moraxella kingii* sp. nov., a haemolytic, saccharolytic species of the genus *Moraxella*. J. Gen. Microbiol. *51*:377–385, 1968.
35. Henriksen, S. D., and Bøvre, K.: Transfer of *Moraxella kingae* Henriksen and Bøvre to the genus *Kingella* gen. nov. in the family Neisseriaceae. Int. J. Syst. Bacteriol. *26*:447–450, 1976.
36. Huhn, P.: *Moraxella* endocarditis in a patient with systemic lupus erythematosus. W. VA Med. J. *129*:344–346, 1978.
37. Jensen, K. T., Schonheyder, H., and Thomsen, V. F.: In-vitro activity of β-lactam and other antimicrobial agents against *Kingella kingae*. J. Antimicrob. Chemother. *33*:635–640, 1994.
38. Kennedy, C. A., and Rosen, H.: *Kingella kingae* bacteremia and adult epiglottitis in a granulocytopenic host. Am. J. Med. *85*:701–702, 1988.
39. Kerlikowske, K., and Chambers, H. F.: *Kingella kingae* endocarditis in a patient with the acquired immunodeficiency syndrome. West. J. Med. *151*:558–560, 1989.
40. Khan, J. A., Sharp, S., Mann, K. R., et al.: Case report: *Kingella denitrificans* prosthetic endocarditis. Am. J. Med. Sci. *291*:187–189, 1986.
41. Lacour, M., Duarte, M., Beutler, A., et al.: Osteoarticular infections due to *Kingella kingae* in children. Eur. J. Pediatr. *150*:612–618, 1991.
42. LaSelve, H., Berard, J., Barbe, G., et al.: Osteoarthrites et osteomyelites a *Kingella kingae* chez l'enfant: A propos de 5 observations et revue de la litterature. Pediatrie *4*:294–304, 1986.
43. Le, C.T.: *Kingella (Moraxella) kingae* infections. Am. J. Dis. Child. *137*:1212–1213, 1983.
44. Lee, W. L., and Dooling, E.: Acute *Kingella kingae* endocarditis with recurrent cerebral emboli in a child with mitral prolapse. Ann. Neurol. *16*:88–89, 1984.
45. Lewis, D. A., and Settas, L.: *Kingella kingae* causing septic arthritis in Felty's syndrome. Postgrad. Med. J. *59*:525–526, 1983.
46. Lindenbaum, S., and Alexander, H.: Infections simulating bone tumours: A review of subacute osteomyelitis. Clin. Orthop. *184*:193–203, 1984.
47. Lion, C., Chatelain, R., Neimann, J. L., et al.: Endocarite a *Kingella kingae*. Med. Mal. Infect. *12*:280–284, 1982.
48. Maccato, M., McLean, W., Riddle, G., et al.: Isolation of *Kingella denitrificans* from amniotic fluid in a woman with chorioamnionitis. J. Reprod. Med. *36*:685–687, 1991.
49. Minamoto, G. Y., and Sordillo, E. M.: *Kingella denitrificans* as a cause of granulomatous disease in a patient with AIDS. Clin. Infect. Dis. *15*:1052–1053, 1992.
50. Miridjanian, A., and Berrett, M.: Infective endocarditis caused by *Moraxella kingae*. West. J. Med. *129*:344–346, 1978.
51. Molina, R., Baro, T., Torne, J., et al.: Empyema caused by *Kingella denitrificans* and *Peptostreptococcus* spp. in a patient with bronchogenic carcinoma. Eur. Respir. J. *1*:870–871, 1988.
52. Morrison, V. A., and Wagner, K. F.: Clinical manifestations of *Kingella kingae* infections: Case report and review. Rev. Infect. Dis. *11*:776–782, 1989.
53. Namnyak, S. S., Quinn, R. F. M., and Ferguson, F. D. M.: *Kingella kingae* meningitis in an infant. J. Infect. *23*:104–106, 1991.
54. Noftal, F., Mersal, A., Yaschuk, Y., et al.: Osteomyelitis due to *Kingella kingae* infection. Can. J. Surg. *31*:21–22, 1988.
55. Ødum, L., Jensen, K. T., and Slotsbjerg, T. D.: Endocarditis due to *Kingella kingae*. Eur. J. Clin. Microbiol. *3*:263–266, 1984.
56. Ødum, L., and Frederiksen, W.: Identification and characterization of *Kingella kingae*. Acta Pathol. Microbiol. Scand. *89*:311–315, 1981.
57. Patel, N. J., Moore, T. L., Wriss, T. D., et al.: *Kingella kingae* infectious arthritis: Case report and review of literature of *Kingella* and *Moraxella* infections. Arthritis Rheum. *26*:557–559, 1983.
58. Petrus, M., Rance, F., and Clément, J. L.: Cervical spondylodiscitis due to *Kingella kingae*: A case report. Ann. Pédiatr. *37*:170–172, 1990.
59. Powell, J. M., and Bass, J. W.: Septic arthritis caused by *Kingella kingae*. Am. J. Dis. Child. *137*:974–976, 1983.
60. Prère, M. F., Seguy, M., Vezard, Y., et al.: Sensibilité aux antibiotiques de *Kingella kingae*. Pathol. Biol. *34*:604–607, 1986.
61. Rabin, R. L., Wong, P., Noonan, J. A., et al.: *Kingella kingae* endocarditis in a child with a prosthetic aortic valve and bifurcation graft. Am. J. Dis. Child. *137*:403–404, 1983.
62. Ravdin, J. I., Brandstetter, R. D., Wade, M. J., et al.: Endocarditis resulting from *Kingella kingae* presenting initially as culture-negative bacterial endocarditis. Heart Lung *11*:552–554, 1982.
63. Raymond, J., Bergeret, M., Bargy, F., et al.: Isolation of two strains of *Kingella kingae* associated with septic arthritis. J. Clin. Microbiol. *24*:1100–1101, 1986.
64. Redfield, D. C., Overturf, G. D., Ewing, N. D., et al.: Bacteria, arthritis, and skin lesions due to *Kingella kingae*. Arch. Dis. Child. *55*:411, 1980.
65. Rosenbaum, J., Lieberman, D. H., and Katz, W. A.: Case report: *Moraxella* infectious arthritis: First report in an adult. Ann. Rheum. Dis. *39*:184–185, 1980.
66. Rotbart, H. A., Gelfand, W. M., and Glode, M. P.: *Kingella kingae* osteomyelitis of the clavicle. J. Pediatr. Orthop. *4*:500–502, 1984.
67. Sage, M. J., Maslowski, A. H., and MacCulloch, D.: Bacterial endocarditis due to *K. kingae*. N. Z. Med. J. *26*:795–796, 1983.
68. Salminen, I., Von Essen, R., Koota, K., et al.: A pitfall in purulent arthritis brought out in *Kingella kingae* infection of the knee. Ann. Rheum. Dis. *43*:656–657, 1984.
69. Salvo, S., Mazon, A., Kutz, M., et al.: Vaginitis por *Kingella denitrificans* en una paciente de 3 anos. Enferm. Infecc. Microbiol. Clin. *11*:395–396, 1993.
70. Shanson, D. C., and Gazzard, G. B.: *Kingella kingae* septicaemia with a clinical presentation resembling disseminated gonococcal infection. Br. Med. J. *289*:730–731, 1984.
71. Shelton, M. M., Nachtigal, M. P., Yngve, D. A., et al.: *Kingella kingae* osteomyelitis: Report of two cases involving the epiphysis. Pediatr. Infect. Dis. J. *7*:421–424, 1988.
72. Shuler, T. E., Riddle, C. D., and Potts, D.: Polymicrobic septic arthritis caused by *Kingella kingae* and enterococcus. Orthopedics *13*:254–256, 1990.
73. Skouby, S. O., and Knudsen, F. U.: *Kingella kingae* osteomyelitis mimicking an eosinophilic granuloma. Acta Paediatr. Scand. *71*:511–512, 1982.
74. Sordillo, E. M., Rendel, M., Sood, R., et al.: Septicemia due to β-lactamase–positive *Kingella kingae*. Clin. Infect. Dis. *17*:818–819, 1993.
75. Spahr, R. C.: Septic arthritis due to *Moraxella* species. J. Pediatr. *86*:310, 1975.
76. Swann, R. A., and Holmes, B.: Infective endocarditis caused by *Kingella denitrificans*. J. Clin. Pathol. *37*:1384–1387, 1984.
77. Toshniwal, R., Draghi, T. C., Kocka, F. E., et al.: Manifestations of *Kingella kingae* infections in adults: Resemblance to neisserial infections. Diagn. Microbiol. Infect. Dis. *5*:81–85, 1986.
78. Urs, S., D'Silva, B. S. V., Jeena, C. P., et al.: *Kingella kingae* septicaemia in association with HIV disease. Trop. Doc. *24*:127, 1994.
79. Van Erps, J., Schmedding, E., Naessens, A., et al.: *Kingella kingae*, a rare cause of bacterial meningitis. Clin. Neurol. Neurosurg. *94*:173–175, 1992.

80. Verbruggen, A.-M., Hauglustaine, D., Schildermans, F., et al.: Infections caused by *Kingella kingae*: Report of four cases and review. J. Infect. *13*:133–142, 1986.
81. Vincent, J., Podewell, C., Franklin, G. W., et al.: Septic arthritis due to *Kingella (Moraxella) kingii*. J. Rheumatol. *8*:501–503, 1981.
82. Walterspiel, J. N.: *Kingella kingae* meningitis with bilateral infarcts of the basal ganglia. Infection *11*:307–309, 1983.
83. Weir, S., and Marrs, C. F.: Identification of type 4 pili in *Kingella denitrificans*. Infect. Immun. *60*:3437–3441, 1992.
84. Wolff, A. H., Ullman, R. F., Strampfer, M. J., et al.: *Kingella kingae* endocarditis: Report of a case and review of the literature. Heart Lung *16*:579–583, 1987.
85. Wong, A. S., Dyke, J., Perry, D., et al.: Paraspinal mass associated with intervertebral disk infection secondary to *Moraxella kingii*. J. Pediatr. *92*:86–88, 1978.
86. Woolfrey, B. F., Lally, R. T., and Faville, R. J.: Intervertebral diskitis caused by *Kingella kingae*. Am. J. Clin. Pathol. *85*:745–749, 1986.
87. Yagupsky, P., and Dagan, R.: *Kingella kingae* bacteremia in children. Pediatr. Infect. Dis. J. *13*:1148–1149, 1994.
88. Yagupsky, P., Dagan, R., Howard, C. W., et al.: High prevalence of *Kingella kingae* in joint fluid from children with septic arthritis revealed by the BACTEC blood culture system. J. Clin. Microbiol. *30*:1278–1281, 1992.
89. Yagupsky, P., Dagan, R., Howard, C. B., et al.: Clinical features and epidemiology of invasive *Kingella kingae* infections in southern Israel. Pediatrics *92*:800–804, 1993.
90. Yagupsky, P., Dagan, R., Prajgrod, F., et al.: Respiratory carriage of *Kingella kingae* among healthy children. Pediatr. Infect. Dis. J. *14*:673–678, 1995.
91. Yagupsky, P., Howard, C. B., Einhorn, M., et al.: *Kingella kingae* osteomyelitis of the calcaneus in young children. Pediatr. Infect. Dis. J. *12*:540–541, 1993.
92. Yagupsky, P., Merires, M., Bahar, J., et al.: Evaluation of novel vancomycin-containing medium for primary isolation of *Kingella kingae* from upper respiratory tract specimens. J. Clin. Microbiol. *33*:1426–1427, 1995.
93. Zeimis, R. T., and Hanley, O. Q.: Endocarditis caused by *Kingella kingae*: Case report and review. Lab. Med. *16*:547–550, 1985.

143

LEGIONNAIRES' DISEASE, PONTIAC FEVER, AND RELATED ILLNESSES

Paul H. Edelstein

Legionnaires' disease is an acute pneumonic illness caused by gram-negative bacilli of the genus *Legionella*. Pontiac fever is a febrile, nonpneumonic, systemic illness closely associated with, if not caused by, *Legionella* species.

HISTORY

Legionnaires' disease first was recognized as a distinct clinical entity when it caused an epidemic of pneumonia at an American Legion convention in Philadelphia in 1976[55]; 221 people were affected, and 34 died. Investigators were unable to determine the exact cause of the outbreak immediately; this mystery provoked considerable fear and widespread speculation about the cause. About a half year later, two investigators at the Centers for Disease Control and Prevention, Joseph McDade and Charles Shepard,[92] announced that they had discovered the etiologic agent, a fastidious gram-negative bacillus. It was determined subsequently that both the organism and the disease had been studied previously as long ago as the 1940s but had been forgotten.[35, 44, 121] Because of the historical association with the American Legion Convention, this disease now is called legionnaires' disease, and the etiologic agents belong to the family Legionellaceae.

ETIOLOGIC AGENT

Legionella is the only genus in the family Legionellaceae. Thirty-nine species of *Legionella* and 59 serogroups within some of the species now are recognized (Table 143–1). *L. pneumophila* is the species responsible for the 1976 Philadelphia epidemic and causes the majority of cases of legionnaires' disease.[35, 38, 44, 121] Serogroup one of *L. pneumophila* is estimated to cause about 70 to 90 per cent of all cases of legionnaires' disease in previously healthy people.[39, 91] *Legionella* species and serogroups other than *L. pneumophila* serogroup 1 cause 25 to 40 per cent of nosocomial outbreaks of legionnaires' disease.[77, 91]

The Legionellaceae are obligately aerobic, mesophilic, motile, gram-negative bacilli with variable oxidase and catalase reactions.[35, 121] They do not utilize carbohydrates as a source of energy but rather metabolize amino acids. They are unique in that L-cysteine is required for growth, a characteristic shared only with *Francisella tularensis*. Also, both the cellular fatty acid and ubiquinone content differ from other mesophilic gram-negative bacilli.

The antigenic relationship among different *Legionella* species, and among serotypes of the same species is complex.[121] The serologic typing scheme is based on surface antigens (O antigens), which primarily are lipopolysaccharides. These surface antigens are shared by different species and, in rare cases, by other gram-negative bacilli, such as *Pseudomonas* species. Thus, identifying an unknown strain by use of serologic methods alone occasionally leads to a false or misleading identification. Cross-reactions also may be observed in testing for human antibodies to *Legionella*. Patients with infections caused by some *Pseudomonas* species strains, *Campylobacter jejuni*, and other gram-negative bacilli may develop antibodies to *Legionella*.[22, 32, 35, 64, 89, 121]

Because of these complexities, definite identification of *Legionella* species other than *L. pneumophila* often requires the capabilities of a research laboratory. However, isolation and presumptive identification should be within the capabilities of most clinical laboratories.[35, 121]

Legionella is ubiquitous in the aqueous environment and can be found, often in high concentrations, in lake water, ponds, bathing water, hot-water tanks, hot-water plumbing, and air-conditioning cooling towers.[121] Its optimal growth temperature ranges from about 28° to 40° C (82° to 104° F). The natural hosts and probable reservoirs of environmental *Legionella* likely are freshwater amebae, such as *Acanthamoeba* and *Hartmannella*.[53, 114, 125, 126] Factors promoting growth of *Legionella* in the environment are diverse, such as the presence of other microorganisms, use of plumbing materials that

TABLE 143–1. *Legionella* Species and Serogroups

Species	No. of Serogroups	Implicated in Human Disease
L. adelaidensis	1	No
L. anisa	1	Yes
L. birminghamensis	1	Yes
L. bozemanii	2	Yes
L. brunensis	1	No
L. cherii	1	No
L. cincinnatiensis	1	Yes
L. dumoffii	1	Yes
L. erythra	1	No
L. fairfieldensis	1	No
L. feeleii	2	Yes
L. geestiana	1	No
L. gormanii	1	Yes
L. gratiana	1	No
L. hackeliae	2	Yes
L. israelensis	1	No
L. jamestowniensis	1	No
L. jordanis	1	Yes
L. lansingensis	1	Yes
L. londinensis	1	No
L. longbeachae	2	Yes
L. maceachernii	1	Yes
L. micdadei	1	Yes
L. moravica	1	No
L. nautarum	1	No
L. oakridgensis	1	Yes
L. parisiensis	1	No
L. pneumophila	15	Yes
L. quateirensis	1	No
L. quinlivanii	1	No
L. rubrilucens	1	No
L. sainthelensi	2	Yes
L. sainticrucis	1	No
L. shakespearei	1	No
L. spiritensis	2	No
L. steigerwaltii	1	No
L. tucsonensis	1	Yes
L. wadsworthii	1	Yes
L. worsleiensis	1	No

promote bacterial growth (certain types of rubber gaskets), stagnation, and warm temperatures.[121] In the home, older municipal water distribution systems, use of electric rather than gas water heaters, and use of well water all appear to promote the presence of *Legionella* in water.[1, 106] Most newly discovered *Legionella* species have been environmental isolates not associated with clinical illness.[35, 38, 121]

Some virulence factors responsible for initiating infection have been elucidated. These include a gene that potentiates infection of macrophages (macrophage infectivity potentiator) and a gene encoding a protein that inhibits phagosomal fusion and allows intracellular growth (defect in organelle trafficking).[7–9, 30, 31, 72] Macrophage complement receptors may play a role in the uptake of the bacterium, although this is controversial.[58, 71, 102] Elegant in vitro studies have shown that *L. pneumophila,* and perhaps other species, have a unique means of evading host defenses. This evasion is by growth within alveolar macrophages, the pulmonary defense cells that ordinarily ingest and then kill invading bacteria. *L. pneumophila* is not killed actively by macrophages, which, in fact, provide sustenance for the bacterium. Poor killing of *L. pneumophila* within macrophages probably is fostered by failure of both lysophagosomal fusion and phagosomal acidification.[70] These in vitro studies have been substantiated, in part, in an animal model.[37, 97] Availability of intracellular iron appears to play a key role in the growth of intracellular *L. pneumophila.* Interferon-γ, the production of which is increased during *L. pneumophila* infection of macrophages, down-regulates the number of iron-binding receptors on macrophages. This has the effect of decreasing the availability of intracellular iron and hence limiting intracellular growth of *L. pneumophila.*[25–27]

L. pneumophila is serum-resistant.[121] High-titer antibody promotes phagocytosis but may not enhance killing. Macrophage activation factors possibly are more important than antibody in promoting phagocytosis and bacterial killing.[70]

Both exotoxins and endotoxins are produced by *L. pneumophila;* their role in the manifestations of disease or in organism invasiveness is unclear.[30, 35, 121]

EPIDEMIOLOGY

Incidence and Frequency

The incidence of pediatric legionnaires' disease has been studied only by use of serosurveys, as have most studies of the adult population.[3, 35, 54, 66, 95, 96, 100, 109, 111, 115, 121] Because of the less than absolute specificity of serologic testing, frequent failure to obtain appropriately timed paired serum samples, and almost uniform lack of culture confirmation of disease, these serosurveys can be used only as crude measurements of disease incidence.[35, 109, 121] Regardless, it appears as if pediatric legionnaires' disease rarely is the cause of pneumonia in otherwise healthy children.[2, 10, 28, 33, 57, 67, 83, 93, 105, 118] Fewer than 10 culture-confirmed cases of legionnaires' disease have been reported in otherwise normally healthy children, and fewer than 20 culture-confirmed cases have been reported in immunosuppressed children.[5, 23, 28, 33, 36, 48, 52, 75, 81, 82, 98, 103, 108, 130]

A retrospective serosurvey of 500 patients with pneumonia, 83 per cent of whom did not need hospitalization, found that only 5 of the 132 patients younger than 15 years of age (26 per cent of the total) had significant antibody titers against *L. pneumophila,* and none developed seroconversion.[54] It was estimated that the incidence of legionnaires' disease in the overall population was about 12 per 100,000 per year. In a year-long prospective study of 191 children hospitalized with pneumonia, titers rose significantly in only one child (0.92 per cent of cases with paired serum samples available).[100] In another prospective study of 52 children younger than 4 years of age with lower respiratory tract infections, no cases of legionnaires' disease were identified.[3] Four of 211 Iowa children (1 to 19 years of age) with atypical pneumonia demonstrated seroconversion to *L. pneumophila.*[111] In a retrospective Israeli serosurvey, titers rose in 2 of 37 children.[96] A 2-year prospective study in France found that only 2 of 278 children (0.7 per cent) hospitalized for pneumonia had legionnaires' disease based on seroconversion.[33] One of these two children was immunosuppressed. Using these data, one could estimate that the mean frequency of legionnaires' disease as a cause of pneumonia requiring hospitalization in the normal pediatric population is about 1 per cent. This is about the same as the 0.5 to 4 per cent frequency found in the adult population.[35, 91, 121] Legionnaires' disease is not a major cause of pneumonia in either children or adults.

The frequency of legionnaires' disease in the immunosuppressed pediatric population is unknown. Several case reports document this disease in children being treated for acute leukemia, with chronic granulomatous disease, after bone marrow or solid organ transplantation, or after being treated with steroids for other reasons.[36, 48, 63, 68, 75, 81, 82, 84, 103, 104, 115, 117, 120, 122] No large studies of this disease in the immunosuppressed pediatric population have been performed, however. One retrospective study of 55 pediatric cancer patients with atypical pneumonia found one case in which there was an antibody titer rise to *L. pneumophila.*[115] Immunosuppression in the pediatric population probably would result in a higher incidence of legionnaires' disease than that seen in the normal population; this is the case in adults.[44, 121] Nosocomial or community-acquired legionnaires' disease has been reported in several "immunologically normal" infants, who may have some degree of immunocompromise that predisposes them to this disease.[34, 51, 57, 67, 69, 77, 83, 98, 108, 130]

Whether atypical, mild, or asymptomatic *Legionella* infection occurs in children is unknown. Several cases of Pontiac fever in children were reported from a large outbreak of this disease at a recreation center in Scotland.[61] The true frequency of Pontiac fever in children is difficult to know because this diagnosis is impossible to make with certainty in the sporadic form. Several of the serosurveys already cited have found asymptomatic elevations of *L. pneumophila* antibody in widely varying frequency. Andersen and colleagues[3] found that 27 of 52 children developed an increase in antibody titer unrelated to acute illness over a period of several years; some of these children developed significantly high titers. Muldoon and colleagues[95] found that 15 per cent of 126 children sampled had antibody titers to *L. pneumophila* of 256 or greater, which was not significantly different from that seen with an adult control population. The striking thing was that the antibody titers rose with age, doubling each year until age 3 years, when the values plateaued; this finding held even when patients with pneumonia were excluded. In contrast, using a different and perhaps more specific antigen preparation, Mundel and colleagues[96] in Israel found a much lower prevalence of elevated antibody titers. That these findings may be geographic rather than methodologic is exemplified by the study of Orenstein and associates,[100] who obtained results similar to the Israeli study despite using the same type of antigen as did Andersen and colleagues.[3] The significance of these elevated titers in children without documented pneumonia is unclear and can be interpreted as cross-reactions to other colonizing or infecting bacteria, asymptomatic infection, or atypical disease.

Several investigators have examined the question of whether atypical disease caused by *Legionella* occurs in children. Unfortunately, all these studies are based exclusively on serologic testing, which, as stated before, may not be entirely specific. Italian physicians found that two children with acute, reversible cerebellar ataxia developed significant antibody titer changes to *L. pneumophila.*[99] Another Italian study found two children with pericarditis who had significant antibody changes.[119] None of 140 British infants with sudden death had measurable antibodies to *L. pneumophila,* despite suggestions that they might be linked.[127] Three studies have shown that children with cystic fibrosis have higher antibody levels to *Legionella* than do normal children, although these data especially are suspect because of known cross-reactions between *Legionella* and *Pseudomonas aeruginosa.*[32, 46, 79] Thus, despite several epidemiologic surveys, the prevalence of atypical *Legionella* infections in children is unclear.

In adults, true incidence figures are as difficult to find. Estimates based on serologic surveys range from 2 to 20 cases per 100,000 population per year.[35, 109, 121] A prospective study in Ohio found that the incidence of legionnaires' disease requiring hospitalization was about 6 per 100,000 per year, in what is felt to be a geographic region with an above-average frequency of the disease.[90, 106] Estimates of the proportion of adult pneumonias due to legionnaires' disease range from 1 to 25 per cent, with a reasonable mean of 3 per cent.[91] Mild or atypical *Legionella* infection certainly occurs in adults, although the exact incidence is unknown. This includes several outbreaks of Pontiac fever and case reports from the original Philadelphia outbreak of persons with relatively mild disease.[35, 55, 59, 60, 80, 121] Asymptomatic infection may occur in adults, based on the same types of serosurveys discussed for children. Neither oropharyngeal colonization nor a carrier state has been documented. A study of a cross-section of adults showed that about 6 per cent had oropharyngeal colonization with *L. pneumophila* on the basis of immunofluorescent studies, although none of the positive results could be confirmed by culture.[24]

Disease Outbreaks

Many epidemics of legionnaires' disease and Pontiac fever have been recognized.[23, 35, 61, 121] In the case of legionnaires' disease, most outbreaks have occurred in residents, employees, or visitors in large buildings. These include hotels, hospitals, factories, retail stores, and office buildings. Nosocomial legionnaires' disease has been reported in hospitals throughout North America and Europe. In most cases in which thorough investigations have been performed, the reservoir has been the potable water distribution system, air-conditioning cooling towers, or both.[35, 121] Outbreaks have been ended by disinfection of water and cooling tower systems by hyperchlorination or pasteurization.[35, 121] In some of these outbreaks, disease has occurred over a number of years until effective disinfection procedures were utilized. Attack rates in legionnaires' disease epidemics consistently have been less than 5 per cent overall. Incubation periods ranging from 2 to 14 days have been observed.

Pontiac fever outbreaks generally have been associated with exposure to an aerosol of warm water contaminated with *Legionella.*[60, 80, 121] Examples of this include whirlpool baths, an engine assembly plant using contaminated water to cool machine lathes, and a health department building in which condensate in the air-conditioning system was contaminated. The attack rates in Pontiac fever outbreaks have been high, in the range of 95 to 100 per cent. The incubation period is short, about 12 to 36 hours.[60]

Sporadic culture-proven cases of legionnaires' disease have been well documented. In fact, 70 to 85 per cent of cases of legionnaires' disease in the United States and elsewhere are neither nosocomial nor associated with an epidemic.[76, 77, 91] Some of these community-acquired cases represent undetected small case clusters, as has been shown for community-acquired cases in Glasgow, Scotland.[11–14] In that city, living close to a cooling tower was a risk factor for legionnaires' disease. It is likely that sporadic Pontiac fever also occurs, although this would be difficult to prove.[35, 121]

Risk factors for legionnaires' disease acquisition can be divided logically into two main categories: those that increase exposure to contaminated water and those that suppress pulmonary defense mechanisms.[35, 121] Included in the former category are occupational or residential exposure to warm or stagnant water, traveling and residence in hotels, and stays in hospitals with contaminated water distribution systems. A risk factor for residential acquisition of disease is use of well water.[106] The latter category includes general anesthesia, administration of glucocorticosteroids, cigarette smoking, chronic lung disease, and diseases or therapy that compromise the cellular immune system, including HIV infection. Males are more than twice as likely as females to develop the disease, perhaps as a result of the greater male prevalence of cigarette smoking and chronic lung disease. Middle-aged and older persons also are at higher risk than are younger persons. Other than exposure to aerosols of contaminated water, there appear to be no particular predisposing factors for the development of Pontiac fever. Exposure to patients with legionnaires' disease has not been shown to be a risk factor for disease acquisition.

PATHOLOGY, PATHOGENESIS, AND IMMUNITY

The exact mode of disease production in legionnaires' disease is unknown. Very good, but indirect, epidemiologic and pathologic evidence suggests that the initial infection results from inhalation of an aerosol rather than by the route of initial oropharyngeal colonization and subsequent aspiration.[35, 121] However, some patients undoubtedly have acquired their disease after aspiration of *Legionella*-contaminated tap water.[20, 74, 88, 124] Some investigators have speculated about the possibility of the development of a bacteremic pneumonia after ingestion and gastrointestinal tract infection, although there is little clinical, epidemiologic, or pathologic support for this hypothesis. Animal models for each of these modes of initial spread exist, and some investigators rightly argue that not enough is known about the initial event to exclude all possibilities effectively.[6, 40, 47, 65, 78, 107, 121]

L. pneumophila apparently does not adhere to ciliated columnar epithelial cells, a property that might not be important if the major mode of transmission is by aerosol.[6] Also, an exclusively environmental microorganism for which humans probably are accidental hosts may not have a selective advantage for such adherence traits.

In guinea pigs infected by the aerosol route, multiplication of *L. pneumophila* begins within 16 hours.[37] This multiplication most likely occurs within the alveolar macrophage, although some extracellular growth may occur. Several cell culture studies show that multiplication occurs only intracellularly and not in the extracellular tissue culture medium.[70] This intracellular location of bacteria protects them from serum factors such as antibody and complement as well as from the effects of those antimicrobials that are not concentrated intracellularly. Killing of *L. pneumophila* within macrophages in cell culture is limited by failure of phagolysosomal fusion.[70] Polymorphonuclear leukocytes do not ingest or kill the organism effectively in vitro, although Davis and colleagues[37] feel that they may form the bulwark of initial host defenses based on in vivo studies. Their conclusions are bolstered by the experiments of Richards and colleagues,[112] which show that polymorphonuclear leukocyte depletion in hamsters enhanced the virulence of *L. pneumophila* given intratracheally. Clinical evidence suggests that leukopenic hosts without concomitant macrophage dysfunction are not high-risk candidates for legionnaires' disease, although they may be at higher risk than the normal population.[29, 44]

The histopathologic correlate of bacterial lung invasion is intense intra-alveolar inflammation.[121] Large airways are not affected, nor are small ones to the level of the terminal bronchioles affected. Both the terminal bronchioles and alveolar ducts may be involved in the inflammatory process. The interstitial spaces generally are uninvolved, although necrosis of alveoli may bridge the interstitial spaces. The alveoli contain a variable mixture of polymorphonuclear leukocytes, alveolar macrophages, and necrotic debris. Hemorrhage is observed, as are microabscesses. Later, fibrin formation and a histiocytic predominance occur. Pleural inflammation is seen in the presence of empyema.

Gross lung changes evolve in the classic pattern of lobar pneumonia, with first red and then gray hepatization.[121] Nodes are involved occasionally. The lung segments involved often are subpleural, a finding that sometimes suggests septic or bland infarction to the clinician. The pleural space is involved variably and seemingly is more prone to infection in immunosuppressed patients. One of the most striking pulmonary findings is the usual absence of significant intrabronchial exudate.

Despite frequent signs and symptoms of extrapulmonary disease in patients with legionnaires' disease, there appear to be no specific extrapulmonary pathologic findings.[121] In fatal cases, organisms often can be recovered or detected in various reticuloendothelial organs, such as the liver or spleen; however, it is unusual to detect significant inflammation associated with this. Occasional patients have nonbacterial endocardial vegetations. Some patients have nonmassive hilar and paratracheal adenopathy, the result of bacterial adenitis. Patients may have metastatic foci with abscesses in almost any location; this includes the myocardium, pericardium, peritoneum, brain, kidney, bowel wall, perirectal region, prosthetic heart valves, and hemodialysis shunts (Table 143–2).[44, 121] Bacteremia occurs in some patients; this has been documented by positive blood cultures and is substantiated indirectly by extrapulmonary foci of infection found in some patients.[44, 121] Whether bacteremia accounts for some of the systemic clinical findings in legionnaires' disease is unproven but likely. Elaboration of toxins by *Legionella* has been postulated to account for some aspects of the systemic disease, but supporting evidence is not convincing.[121] The effect of host responses to *L. pneumophila* has not been studied as a possible explanation for these systemic manifestations. Cell culture and animal experiments show that tumor necrosis factor, interferon-γ, and other cytokines are produced during *L. pneumophila* infection, the production of which could account for some of the systemic manifestations of the infection.[15, 131]

Episodes of recurrent or relapsing legionnaires' disease in patients with elevated antibody titers support experimental evidence suggesting that the humoral immune system plays a minor role in this disease.[44] Also supporting this is the rarity of legionnaires' disease case reports in patients with hypogammaglobulinemia or other diseases in which the humoral immune system primarily is deficient. The rapidity of rise of specific antibody levels does not seem to have any clinical correlates and neither does the absolute antibody level.[44] Patients may recover from legionnaires' disease without any significant increase in antibody levels, again providing indirect evidence of the limited role of the humoral immune system.

The roles of antibody and complement in experimental models of infection vary with the model. Several studies have shown that passive or active immunization is protective against intraperitoneal and subcutaneous chamber infection in rats, mice, and guinea pigs.[4, 47, 65, 113] Preopsonization of *L. pneumophila* before intratracheal inoculation of hamsters was

TABLE 143–2. Diseases Caused by *Legionella*

Pneumonia (legionnaires' disease)	Not associated with pneumonia
Associated with pneumonia	Prosthetic heart valve endocarditis
Hemodialysis shunt infection	Sinusitis
Renal abscess	Wound infection
Brain abscess	Colitis
Myocarditis	Pleural empyema
Pericarditis	Peritonitis
Peritonitis	Pontiac fever (? toxin-mediated)
Perirectal abscess	
Pleural empyema	
Bacteremia	
Bowel wall abscess	
Myositis cellulitis	

found to be partially protective, but several investigators have shown that active immunization fails to protect against pneumonia after intratracheal, aerosol, or intranasal inoculation of large numbers of *L. pneumophila* bacteria.[6, 40, 47, 112] Protective immunity to pulmonary challenge in the guinea pig can be achieved after sublethal infection or infection with an avirulent mutant strain and by vaccination with an *L. pneumophila*–derived metalloprotease or outer-membrane protein.[16–19, 128]

Evidence for the importance of the cellular immune system in preventing infection largely is indirect and based on the greater prevalence of legionnaires' disease in immunosuppressed patients with cellular immunodeficiencies.[44, 121] Curiously, legionnaires' disease in patients with AIDS has been reported infrequently, although an epidemiologic survey showed that patients with AIDS had a disease attack rate about 40 times greater than that in the normal population.[18, 19, 91, 128] Passive transfer of spleen cells from infected animals has been shown to be protective in an intratracheal model of *L. micdadei* infection.[97] Development of cellular immunity after infection or vaccination can be demonstrated in vitro for both humans and animals; the clinical importance of this is unclear.[121]

Vaccination for prevention of legionnaires' disease may be feasible because it has been demonstrated to be effective in an animal model.[17–19, 128] Whether vaccination in susceptible host populations would be successful is unknown, even if justified economically or on epidemiologic grounds.

The pathogenesis of Pontiac fever has not been studied. No differences have been detected between an *L. pneumophila* strain isolated from an outbreak of Pontiac fever and strains isolated from outbreaks of legionnaires' disease; these studies have included examination of virulence in an animal model, toxin production, and biochemical characteristics.[121] Detailed clinical studies of patients with Pontiac fever have not been performed, which makes it difficult to know how to produce an experimental model of this disease. On the basis of its short incubation time, which can be as brief as 12 hours, it seems unlikely that this disease represents widespread bacterial multiplication within the body and more likely that it represents a toxin-induced or allergic disease. In fact, the link between *Legionella* and Pontiac fever is circumstantial; it is entirely possible that other microbes coexisting with *Legionella* may cause the disease.[60, 80] The clinical syndromes most like Pontiac fever are bath-water fever, humidifier fever, and extrinsic allergic alveolitis; it is thought that these syndromes are caused either by the direct toxic activity of inhaled endotoxin or by an allergic reaction to microorganisms, most particularly amebae such as *Naegleria*.[45, 94, 116]

CLINICAL FINDINGS OF LEGIONNAIRES' DISEASE

Signs and Symptoms

Legionnaires' disease usually presents as atypical pneumonia.[56] It is atypical in that usual pathogenic bacteria generally are not isolated from respiratory tract secretions or blood and because patients do not respond, except fortuitously, to antimicrobial agents commonly used to treat pneumonia in adults (penicillins, cephalosporins, and aminoglycosides). Beyond this, there is considerable speculation and controversy over whether there is a distinct clinical syndrome. Several prospective studies of both community-acquired and nosocomial legionnaires' disease have failed to demonstrate any clinical, radiographic, or nonspecific laboratory features that distinguish legionnaires' disease from other common causes of pneumonia.[41] The classic clinical findings are reviewed because many feel that these are distinctive for *Legionella* pneumonias. Whether legionnaires' disease in children mimics the clinical findings in adults is unknown because of the rarity of well-documented pediatric cases and the possibility of spectrum bias.

The onset of pneumonia may be either insidious or abrupt. Recurrent chills, abdominal pains, myalgia, headache, malaise, anorexia, and severe fatigue are common. Diarrhea, consisting of loose, nonbloody stools several times a day, occurs in about 30 to 40 per cent of cases. Fever may be low-grade or absent initially. Over the course of a day to several days, these nonspecific symptoms gradually worsen, often resulting in severe debilitation. Noteworthy is the frequent absence of symptoms referable to the respiratory system. Rash, splenomegaly, adenopathy, and rhinorrhea are exceptionally uncommon findings. Physical examination early in the illness generally is remarkable for a paucity of localizing findings and the frequent impression that the patient has an influenzal or typhoidal illness.

Within a day to several days after onset, the patient usually, but not always, develops high fever. Pulse-temperature dissociation occurs in about half of epidemic-associated cases. Respiratory complaints may become prominent, especially dyspnea and pleuritic chest pains. Cough is not usually a major complaint, although it is common. The sputum almost never is frankly purulent; blood-streaked sputum or frank hemoptysis is observed in 20 to 30 per cent of patients. Most patients experience confusion, cerebellar ataxia, lethargy, agitation, or some other neurologic disorder. Severe abdominal or back pain may occur, sometimes with localization. Physical examination at this time reveals a "toxic" febrile patient with apparent multisystem disease. Chest examination usually discloses findings of consolidating pneumonia, with bronchial breath sounds, increased vocal fremitus, and dullness to percussion. Depending on the stage of consolidation, rales may or may not be heard. Pleural friction rubs or signs of pleural effusion can be observed. Despite frequent symptoms of abdominal pain, it is unusual to detect signs of peritoneal irritation, such as decreased bowel sounds or rebound tenderness. Signs of meningeal irritation are rare but reported.

Most normally healthy patients recover without specific therapy, usually by day 7 to 10 of illness. Those who do not recover usually die of progressive respiratory failure, along with failure of other organ systems. Empyema, pulmonary cavitation, renal failure, memory loss, fatigue, and neurologic disorders all are potential complications and may persist for weeks to months after disease onset.

Radiographic Findings

The hallmark of legionnaires' disease on the chest radiograph is an acinar filling pattern with consolidation.[35, 44, 121] There is no distinctive predilection for any lung region; pleura-based consolidation and bilateral infiltrates may occur. Nodular infiltrates may be seen, as may cavitation in the areas of original consolidation. Purely interstitial infiltrates are distinctly uncommon in established disease but rarely occur very early in the disease process; these interstitial infiltrates rapidly progress to consolidating ones within a day or so. Pleural effusion, with or without parenchymal infiltrates, can occur. Pleural effusion has been documented as the only chest finding in patients treated early.

Laboratory Findings

General

Multiple nonspecific abnormal laboratory results can be detected in patients with legionnaires' disease.[35, 44] Hematologic abnormalities include leukocytosis or leukopenia, usually with a left shift; lymphopenia; thrombocytosis; and disseminated intravascular coagulation. Proteinuria and pyuria are common findings; myoglobinuria also may be present. Hyponatremia and hypophosphatemia commonly occur, as do elevations of aminotransferase enzymes, bilirubin, alkaline phosphatase, and creatine kinase. Severe azotemia occurs, although rarely. Arterial oxygenation usually is depressed in relation to the extent of pneumonia. Patients with severe disease also may develop severe oxygen desaturation related to either oxygen intoxication or respiratory distress syndrome. Taken together, these multiple laboratory abnormalities often suggest multisystem disease to the clinician.

Nonspecific, and occasionally confusing, laboratory abnormalities also may be seen. These include elevation of cold agglutinin titers, cold agglutinin–induced hemolytic anemia, and elevation of complement fixation titers to *Mycoplasma pneumoniae.* The elevations of *M. pneumoniae* titer probably are not due to a cross-reaction and occur in about 10 per cent of patients who develop seroconversion to *L. pneumophila*.[21, 62, 110, 129] It is possible that this represents dual infection with *M. pneumoniae* and *L. pneumophila.*

Specific

Diagnosis of legionnaires' disease is accomplished best by recovery of *Legionella* from sputum or other lower respiratory tract secretions or tissues.[44, 121] Complementary to this is detection of *Legionella* in the same materials by immunofluorescent microscopy. Other specific diagnostic methods are detection of *L. pneumophila* antigenuria and detection of *Legionella* DNA in respiratory tract specimens using the polymerase chain reaction. Serologic diagnosis is of uncertain value in children, but it is useful in adults.

Selective media and techniques now are available that facilitate the isolation of *Legionella* from sputum.[35, 121] Sputum is pretreated with an acid solution. This material, as well as a nonpretreated sample, then is plated on buffered charcoal yeast extract medium supplemented with α-ketoglutaric acid (BCYE-α) and on BCYE supplemented with antibiotics (BMPA, or PAC, and MWY, or PAV media). *Legionella* organisms grow on these media 2 to 7 days after inoculation and incubation at 35° C in air. Culture diagnosis has a higher yield than does immunofluorescent microscopy or serology and yields no false-positive results. Blood and pleural fluid cultures generally have lower yields than do respiratory tract cultures, even when plated on proper media; the low yield of blood culture may be a result of methodologic problems.

Immunofluorescent microscopy for *L. pneumophila* is a rapid and highly specific (99.9 per cent) technique for diagnosis.[35, 44] This can be performed in 1 to 2 hours after specimen receipt and, like culture, can be done with sputum. It does have several disadvantages. The test requires considerable technical expertise in reading; if it is performed by inexperienced technologists, results often are erroneous. Also, one must take scrupulous care to avoid carryover from other samples and false-positive results due to contaminated reagents. Cross-reacting organisms are rare in clinical samples; these often can be detected by experienced technologists on the basis of morphologic characteristics and staining pattern. Despite this, some cross-reacting bacteria, such as some *Pseudomonas* species strains, still cause rare false-positive results. Some strains of *Bacteroides fragilis, Streptococcus pneumoniae, Bacillus* species, and *Candida* species also can cross-react with diagnostic reagents, although cross-reactions caused by these organisms rarely, if at all, result in false-positive diagnosis of legionnaires' disease.[35, 121] Patients with tularemia may have false-positive immunofluorescent stains for *Legionella.* The most specific reagent available for immunofluorescent microscopy is a monoclonal antibody to *L. pneumophila*; this reacts with all known serogroups of the species (Genetic Systems, Seattle, Washington). Polyclonal antibodies to *L. pneumophila* serogroups 1 to 4 also are highly specific and are available from a variety of sources. However, polyclonal antibodies to other *L. pneumophila* serogroups and to other *Legionella* species give an unacceptable rate of false-positive results. A positive immunofluorescent test result not confirmed by culture, when performed, should be regarded as a possible false-positive result, and independent validating tests should be performed, if indicated. Finally, the sensitivity of the test is low, in the 25 to 80 per cent range. The reasons for low test sensitivity are that the lowest number of detectable bacteria is in the range of 10^4 cells/mL and that more antigenic types than diagnostic serum types of *Legionella* exist. A laboratory can increase the sensitivity of the test by screening for more than one antigenic type, but this increases the number of false-positive results and should be avoided in almost all situations. The best compromise is for the laboratory to screen for antigenic types common in its locale. For example, *L. pneumophila* serogroups 1 and 4 account for the vast majority of isolates in Los Angeles; in Chicago, *L. pneumophila* serogroups 1 and 6 are more common. Because of the limited sensitivity of the test, a negative result does not exclude disease.

Serologic testing is of most value in epidemiologic studies and of least value in the acute diagnosis of sporadic cases.[43] Up to 25 per cent of patients with culture-documented disease fail to undergo seroconversion against the homologous serotype; this is not related solely to early treatment or immunosuppression, although these factors may cause failure of antibody formation. Up to 3 months may be required for antibody levels to increase after onset of illness; the median time is about 2 weeks. Also, as with any other means of immunologic diagnosis of this disease, the multiplicity of antigenic types makes serologic testing extremely cumbersome. Because 5 to over 25 per cent of the normal population have elevated antibody titers to *Legionella,* only a fourfold rise in titer is considered significant. Only paired samples, drawn 3 to 6 weeks apart, should be tested. Because of day-to-day variation of test results, these samples must be tested simultaneously for optimal results. For maximum yield, samples taken as long as 9 to 12 weeks after disease onset should be tested if earlier samples reveal no changes. As with immunofluorescent detection of bacterial antigen, a negative serologic result does not exclude disease.

The specificity of serologic diagnosis is fairly high in adults, in the range of 95 to 99 per cent.[35, 121] Cross-reactive antibodies may be found in the serum of patients with leptospirosis, melioidosis, *B. fragilis* infections, *P. aeruginosa* infections, and possibly *Haemophilus influenzae* or enteric bacterial infections. However, even 99 per cent specificity is not sufficient for diagnosis of a sporadic case with certainty. If the estimated 1 per cent prevalence of legionnaires' disease in children is correct, fewer than half of all seroconversions yield truly positive results (positive predictive accuracy of 45 per cent). This, combined with the studies cited previously showing age-related elevations of anti-*Legionella* antibody in young asymptomatic children, makes serologic diagnosis of pediatric legionnaires' disease highly suspect.

Detection of soluble bacterial antigen in urine can be used to diagnose *L. pneumophila* serogroup 1 infections successfully.[35, 121] A radioimmunoassay (^{125}I) kit for this procedure is available commercially (Binax, South Portland, Maine). The major drawback of this test is that it detects only *L. pneumophila* serogroup 1 infections. Otherwise, it has an excellent sensitivity (90 to 95 per cent versus culture) and extraordinary specificity (≥99.9 per cent). In some cases, the urinary antigen test yields positive results when sputum culture for *L. pneumophila* serogroup 1 is negative. This especially is true in previously treated patients and in epidemics of legionnaires' disease.

A DNA probe test for the detection of bacterial rRNA (Gen-Probe, San Diego, California), previously available, is no longer being made. The polymerase chain reaction has been used to detect *L. pneumophila* in sputum. The polymerase chain reaction test appears both sensitive and specific, but neither is commercially available nor is validated in large studies.[73, 85–87]

None of the nonculture tests is as sensitive as is culture diagnosis under ideal circumstances. Thus, culture must be performed in every case; if desired, the other tests can be used to provide rapid answers (same day). Because none of the *Legionella*-specific tests is 100 per cent sensitive, the clinician sometimes must treat for legionnaires' disease in the absence of confirmatory laboratory tests. One or 2 days of erythromycin therapy apparently does not affect the sensitivity of the diagnostic tests, so therapy should not be withheld pending laboratory tests.

TREATMENT

No prospective clinical studies of antimicrobial therapy for legionnaires' disease have been performed. All recommendations regarding therapy, therefore, are based on retrospective and experimental studies.

Erythromycin is the drug of choice for treatment of legionnaires' disease in children. Generally, it is given intravenously in four daily divided doses of 15 mg/kg. Intravenous therapy can be changed to oral therapy (30 mg/kg/day in divided doses) once clinical improvement is evident. Therapy should be given for a minimum of 18 to 21 days and perhaps longer in cases of cavitating infiltrates and severe immunosuppression. Relapses may occur when intravenous erythromycin therapy is changed to the oral route and after too short a course of therapy. Some patients with mild illness may be treated initially with oral therapy, although generally this is not advisable.

Alternative drugs to erythromycin include tetracycline or sulfamethoxazole-trimethoprim (co-trimoxazole). Neither of these agents has been approved for this use by the Food and Drug Administration, although limited clinical and experimental data support their effectiveness. Doxycycline, because of its high lipid solubility, may be more effective than is tetracycline, although this is conjecture. The dosage of doxycycline used in adults is 4 mg/kg/day, given in one or two doses. Use of all tetracyclines is contraindicated in children younger than 9 years of age. The daily co-trimoxazole dosage is 15 to 20 mg/kg of the trimethoprim component and 75 to 100 mg/kg of the sulfamethoxazole component in three divided doses. Duration of therapy for these drugs is the same as for erythromycin.

Rifampin therapy, combined with one of the aforementioned drugs, probably is indicated for severe disease (bilateral consolidation, cavitation) and in treatment of immunosuppressed patients. The dosage is 16 to 20 mg/kg/day, given in two divided doses for the first 3 to 7 days of therapy. This drug rapidly diminishes bacterial counts in experimental disease and has been effective in combination with other drugs in patients in whom erythromycin therapy has failed. Use of this drug for treatment of legionnaires' disease is not approved by the Food and Drug Administration.

Clinical and laboratory evidence suggests that some fluoroquinolone antimicrobials (ciprofloxacin, ofloxacin, and pefloxacin) may be more effective than is erythromycin for the treatment of legionnaires' disease.[42] Use of these drugs in children is contraindicated, and their use in adults is not approved by the Food and Drug Administration for this indication. The new macrolide antimicrobial agents, such as azithromycin and clarithromycin, are more active than is erythromycin against *Legionella* in laboratory and animal studies. Both of these new macrolide antibiotics have been used to treat legionnaires' disease successfully, but whether they are more effective clinically than erythromycin is uncertain.

Treatment of extrapulmonary foci of infection does not appear to differ significantly from treatment of legionnaires' disease without extrapulmonary disease. The duration of therapy and indications for surgical drainage need to be assessed individually in these cases.

Response to Treatment

Most patients improve dramatically within a few days after initiation of specific therapy.[35, 41, 44, 121] Response has been as rapid as 6 hours after the first dose of erythromycin therapy. Patients regain their appetite, lose symptoms of myalgia and fatigue, and feel better overall. It may take as long as a week for a patient to become completely afebrile and rarely as long as a month in some severely immunosuppressed patients. The chest radiograph changes slowly and even may appear to worsen despite overall clinical improvement; progressive consolidation after 3 to 4 days of intravenous antimicrobial therapy is unusual.

The mortality rate in otherwise healthy adults who are treated promptly is about 5 per cent, whereas in treated immunosuppressed patients, it is about 20 per cent. Untreated fatality rates range from 15 to 20 per cent in normally healthy patients and upward of 80 per cent in immunosuppressed patients. Even in normally healthy patients, delayed therapy and development of respiratory failure are exceptionally poor prognostic factors.[49, 101, 123]

DIFFERENTIAL DIAGNOSIS

Other causes of atypical, or "culture-negative," pneumonia may resemble legionnaires' disease closely. *M. pneumoniae* pneumonia usually is a milder illness not requiring hospitalization. Cough is a prominent symptom in mycoplasmal pneumonia, whereas it is not in legionnaires' disease. Neither rash nor otitis is found in legionnaires' disease. Laboratory abnormalities also are more common in legionnaires' disease. Serologic testing may provide positive results for both diseases, a confusing finding that can be clarified by performing sputum cultures. Fortunately, the treatment is the same for both diseases.

Psittacosis and Q fever may resemble legionnaires' disease closely. A history of bird or cattle exposure may be helpful, but its absence does not exclude either of these zoonoses. An interstitial rather than an acinar-filling infiltrate on chest radiograph would be a point against legionnaires' disease. Pathogen-specific laboratory tests help in this differential diagnosis. A tetracycline can be used successfully for all three of these diseases.

Early in their evolution, some diseases may resemble legionnaires' disease. These include typhoid fever, acute coccidioidomycosis, influenza, the typhus or spotted fevers, and leptospirosis. It generally is easy to distinguish these diseases on the basis of their clinical evolution, the laboratory results, and the exposure or travel history.

Tularemia may pose a problem in differential diagnosis. This is because immunologic test results for legionnaires' disease can be falsely positive in tularemia and because some of the growth characteristics of *F. tularensis* closely resemble those of *Legionella*. In regions endemic for tularemia, clinicians must work closely with the laboratory to facilitate this differential diagnosis. One case record of tularemia misdiagnosed as legionnaires' disease reported that the patient responded to erythromycin therapy.

Dual infection sometimes occurs in legionnaires' disease. Coexistence of legionnaires' disease with pneumonia caused by *Mycobacterium tuberculosis*, pneumococcus, *H. influenzae*, *Neisseria meningitidis*, *Pneumocystis carinii*, *Moraxella (B.) catarrhalis*, and various viral agents has been reported. Thus, dual infection should be suspected in patients not responding to therapy for pneumonia. Pathogen-specific laboratory tests often are useful in sorting this out.

CLINICAL SYNDROMES CAUSED BY OTHER *LEGIONELLA* SPECIES

Relatively few cases have been reported of disease caused by the non–*L. pneumophila Legionella* species.[50] Of the ones described, there appear to be few differences in clinical findings, diagnostic methods, or treatment. One group contends that these infections are more difficult to treat than *L. pneumophila* infections, but it is unclear whether this represents differences in host factors or reduced susceptibility of the bacteria to antibiotic therapy.[50] It is unknown whether the lower frequency of these infections reflects decreased virulence, inadequate efforts to diagnose them, rare environmental presence, or all three. It is possible that they cause mild disease for which major diagnostic efforts are not undertaken. The mode of spread and nosocomial reservoirs of these species are not defined as well as they are for *L. pneumophila*. These infections are less likely to be diagnosed by immunologic means because fewer laboratories routinely test for all possible species. As with *L. pneumophila*, and even more so for the non–*L. pneumophila Legionella* species, treatment sometimes must be based solely on clinical suspicion without the benefit of confirmatory laboratory tests.

PONTIAC FEVER

Clinical Signs and Symptoms

Fever, myalgia, malaise, chills, and headache are the most common symptoms of Pontiac fever.[60] The symptoms may begin suddenly or have a more gradual onset over several hours. Many symptoms referable to the respiratory tract also are common, such as dry, nonproductive cough, chest pain, and pharyngitis. Nausea is common, but diarrhea and vomiting are less frequent. Neurologic symptoms such as dizziness, confusion, and poor coordination also have been reported. These symptoms usually are at their worst within a day after onset of illness and gradually resolve over a 2- to 7-day period. Physical examination shows only tachycardia and fever. Leukocytosis has been the only laboratory abnormality reported. Chest radiographs show no abnormalities. Pulmonary function testing has not been performed in patients with Pontiac fever. Rechallenge by return to the contaminated building in the original Pontiac outbreak produced only a mild illness compared with first exposure; the length of time between first and second exposure was not stated clearly.

Specific Diagnosis

The diagnosis of Pontiac fever primarily is one of exclusion.[35, 121] Significant rises in anti-*Legionella* antibody level, combined with characteristic symptoms, and isolation of *Legionella* from an aerosol source are diagnostic criteria used currently. Because of the nonspecificity of the symptoms and the ubiquitous distribution of *Legionella* in our environment, rather detailed epidemiologic and environmental studies must be performed to diagnose Pontiac fever specifically. Definitive diagnosis of sporadic cases therefore is difficult.

Treatment

Antimicrobial therapy does not appear to be effective for either the treatment or the prophylaxis of this disease. Removal of the patient from the area of the contaminated water source, while it is being disinfected, appears to be the best means of management.

References

1. Alary, M., and Joly, J. R.: Risk factors for contamination of domestic hot water systems by legionellae. Appl. Environ. Microbiol. *57*:2360, 1991.
2. Andersen, R., Bergan, T., Halvorsen, K., et al.: Legionnaires' disease combined with erythema multiforme in a 3-year-old boy. Acta Paediatr. Scand. *70*:427, 1981.
3. Andersen, R. D., Lauer, B. A., Fraser, D. W., et al.: Infections with *Legionella pneumophila* in children. J. Infect. Dis. *143*:386, 1981.
4. Arko, R. J., Wong, K. H., and Feeley, J. C.: Immunologic factors affecting the in-vivo and in-vitro survival of the Legionnaires' disease bacterium. Ann. Intern. Med. *90*:680, 1979.
5. Aubert, G., Bornstein, N., Rayet, I., et al.: Nosocomial infection with *Legionella pneumophila* serogroup 1 and 8 in a neonate. Scand. J. Infect. Dis. *22*:367, 1990.
6. Baskerville, A., Fitzgeorge, R. B., Gibson, D. H., et al.: Pathological and bacteriological findings after aerosol *Legionella pneumophila* infection of susceptible, convalescent, and antibiotic-treated animals. *In* Thornsberry, C., Balows, A., Feeley, J. C., et al. (eds.): *Legionella*. Proceedings of the 2nd International Symposium. Washington, D.C., American Society for Microbiology, 1984, pp. 131–132.
7. Berger, K. H., and Isberg, R. R.: Two distinct defects in intracellular growth complemented by a single genetic locus in *Legionella pneumophila*. Mol. Microbiol. *7*:7, 1993.
8. Berger, K. H., and Isberg, R. R.: Intracellular survival by *Legionella*. Methods Cell. Biol. *45*:247, 1994.
9. Berger, K. H., Merriam, J. J., and Isberg, R. R.: Altered intracellular targeting properties associated with mutations in the *Legionella pneumophila* dotA gene. Mol. Microbiol. *14*:809, 1994.
10. Beyer, P., Kahn, D., Horbach, J., et al.: Unusual progression of a *Legionella pneumophila* infection in a young child. Eur. J. Pediatr. *141*:173, 1984.
11. Bhopal, R.: Source of infection for sporadic Legionnaires' disease: A review. J. Infect. *30*:9, 1995.
12. Bhopal, R. S., Diggle, P., and Rowlingson, B.: Pinpointing clusters of apparently sporadic cases of Legionnaires' disease. B. M. J. *304*:1022, 1992.
13. Bhopal, R. S., and Fallon, R. J.: Variation in time and space of non-outbreak Legionnaires' disease in Scotland. Epidemiol. Infect. *106*:45, 1991.
14. Bhopal, R. S., Fallon, R. J., Buist, E. C., et al.: Proximity of the home to a cooling tower and risk of non-outbreak Legionnaires' disease. B. M. J. *302*:378, 1991.
15. Blanchard, D. K., Friedman, H., Klein, T. W., et al.: Induction of interferon-gamma and tumor necrosis factor by *Legionella pneumophila*: Augmentation of human neutrophil bactericidal activity. J. Leukoc. Biol. *45*:538, 1989.
16. Blander, S. J., Breiman, R. F., and Horwitz, M. A.: A live avirulent mutant *Legionella pneumophila* vaccine induces protective immunity against lethal aerosol challenge. J. Clin. Invest. *83*:810, 1989.
17. Blander, S. J., and Horwitz, M. A.: Vaccination with the major secretory protein of *Legionella pneumophila* induces cell-mediated and protective

immunity in a guinea pig model of Legionnaires' disease. J. Exp. Med. *169*:691, 1989.
18. Blander, S. J., and Horwitz, M. A.: Vaccination with *Legionella pneumophila* membranes induces cell-mediated and protective immunity in a guinea pig model of Legionnaires' disease: Protective immunity independent of the major secretory protein of *Legionella pneumophila*. J. Clin. Invest. *87*:1054, 1991.
19. Blander, S. J., and Horwitz, M. A.: Major cytoplasmic membrane protein of *Legionella pneumophila*, a genus common antigen and member of the hsp 60 family of heat shock proteins, induces protective immunity in a guinea pig model of Legionnaires' disease. J. Clin. Invest. *91*:717, 1993.
20. Blatt, S. P., Parkinson, M. D., Pace, E., et al.: Nosocomial Legionnaires' disease: Aspiration as a primary mode of disease acquisition. Am. J. Med. *95*:16, 1993.
21. Bornstein, N., Fleurette, J., Bosshard, S., et al.: Evaluation de la frequence des reactions serologiques croisees entre *Legionella* et mycoplasma ou chlamydia. Pathol. Biol. (Paris) *32*:165, 1984.
22. Boswell, T. C., and Kudesia, G.: Serological cross-reaction between *Legionella pneumophila* and *Campylobacter* in the indirect fluorescent antibody test. Epidemiol. Infect. *109*:291, 1992.
23. Brady, M. T.: Nosocomial legionnaires' disease in a children's hospital. J. Pediatr. *115*:46, 1989.
24. Bridge, J. A., and Edelstein, P. H.: Oropharyngeal colonization with *Legionella pneumophila*. J. Clin. Microbiol. *18*:1108, 1983.
25. Byrd, T. F., and Horwitz, M. A.: Interferon gamma-activated human monocytes downregulate transferrin receptors and inhibit the intracellular multiplication of *Legionella pneumophila* by limiting the availability of iron. J. Clin. Invest. *83*:1457, 1989.
26. Byrd, T. F., and Horwitz, M. A.: Lactoferrin inhibits or promotes *Legionella pneumophila* intracellular multiplication in nonactivated and interferon gamma-activated human monocytes depending upon its degree of iron saturation: Iron-lactoferrin and nonphysiologic iron chelates reverse monocyte activation against *Legionella pneumophila*. J. Clin. Invest. *88*:1103, 1991.
27. Byrd, T. F., and Horwitz, M. A.: Chloroquine inhibits the intracellular multiplication of *Legionella pneumophila* by limiting the availability of iron: A potential new mechanism for the therapeutic effect of chloroquine against intracellular pathogens. J. Clin. Invest. *88*:351, 1991.
28. Carlson, N. C., Kuskie, M. R., Dobyns, E. L., et al.: Legionellosis in children: An expanding spectrum. Pediatr. Infect. Dis. J. *9*:133, 1990.
29. Carratala, J., Gudiol, F., Pallares, R., et al.: Risk factors for nosocomial *Legionella pneumophila* pneumonia. Am. J. Respir. Crit. Care Med. *149*:625, 1994.
30. Cianciotto, N., Eisenstein, B. I., Engleberg, N. C., et al.: Genetics and molecular pathogenesis of *Legionella pneumophila*, an intracellular parasite of macrophages. Mol. Biol. Med. *6*:409, 1989.
31. Cianciotto, N. P., Eisenstein, B. I., Mody, C. H., et al.: A mutation in the *mip* gene results in an attenuation of *Legionella pneumophila* virulence. J. Infect. Dis. *162*:121, 1990.
32. Collins, M. T., McDonald, J., Hiby, N., et al.: Agglutinating antibody titers to members of the family Legionellaceae in cystic fibrosis patients as a result of cross-reacting antibodies to *Pseudomonas aeruginosa*. J. Clin. Microbiol. *19*:757, 1984.
33. Couvreur, J., Dournon, E., Garcia, J., et al.: La maladie des Légionnaires chez l'enfant: Enquête épidemiologique avec une nouvelle observation et revue de la littérature. Ann. Pédiatr. (Paris) *33*:379, 1986.
34. Couvreur, J., Khiati, M., Petiot, A., et al.: Pneumopathie a *Legionella pneumophila* chez un nourrisson de 4 mois et demi. Arch. Fr. Pédiatr. *40*:649, 1983.
35. Cunha, B. A., (ed.): Seminars in Respiratory Infections: Legionnaires' Disease. Vol. II. Philadelphia, Grune & Stratton, 1987.
36. Cutz, E., Thorner, P. S., Rao, C. P., et al.: Disseminated *Legionella pneumophila* infection in an infant with severe combined immunodeficiency. J. Pediatr. *100*:760, 1982.
37. Davis, G. S., Winn, W. C., Jr., Gump, D. W., et al.: The kinetics of early inflammatory events during experimental pneumonia due to *Legionella pneumophila* in guinea pigs. J. Infect. Dis. *148*:823, 1983.
38. Dennis, P. J., Brenner, D. J., Thacker, W. L., et al.: Five new *Legionella* species isolated from water. Int. J. Syst. Bacteriol. *43*:329, 1993.
39. Dournon, E., Bibb, W. F., Rajagopalan, P., et al.: Monoclonal antibody reactivity as a virulence marker for *Legionella pneumophila* serogroup 1 strains. J. Infect. Dis. *157*:496, 1988.
40. Drutz, D. J., Demarsh, P., Edelstein, P., et al.: *Legionella pneumophila* pneumonia in athymic nude mice. *In* Thornsberry, C., Balows, A., Feeley, J. C., et al. (eds.): *Legionella*. Proceedings of the 2nd International Symposium. Washington, D.C., American Society for Microbiology, 1984, pp. 134–135.
41. Edelstein, P. H.: Legionnaires' disease. Clin. Infect. Dis. *16*:741, 1993.
42. Edelstein, P. H.: Antimicrobial therapy of Legionnaires' disease: A review. Clin. Infect. Dis. *21*(Suppl. 3):S265, 1995.
43. Edelstein, P. H.: Detection of antibodies to *Legionella*. *In* Rose, N. R., de Macario, E. C., Folds, J. D., et al. (eds.): Manual of Clinical Laboratory Immunology. 5th ed. Washington, D.C., American Society for Microbiology, in press.
44. Edelstein, P. H., and Meyer, R. D.: Legionnaires' disease: A review. Chest *85*:114, 1984.
45. Edwards, J. H., Harbord, P., Skidmore, J. W. et al.: Humidifier fever. Thorax *32*:653, 1977.
46. Efthimiou, J., Hodson, M. E., Taylor, P., et al.: Importance of viruses and *Legionella pneumophila* in respiratory exacerbations of young adults with cystic fibrosis. Thorax *39*:150, 1984.
47. Eisenstein, T. K., Tamada, R., Meissler, J., et al.: Vaccination against *Legionella pneumophila*: Serum antibody correlates with protection induced by heat-killed or acetone-killed cells against intraperitoneal but not aerosol infection in guinea pigs. Infect. Immun. *45*:685, 1984.
48. Ephros, M., Engelhard, D., Maayan, S., et al.: *Legionella gormanii* pneumonia in a child with chronic granulomatous disease. Pediatr. Infect. Dis. J. *8*:726, 1989.
49. Falcó, V., Fernández de Sevilla, T., Alegre, J., et al.: *Legionella pneumophila*: A cause of severe community-acquired pneumonia. Chest *100*:1007, 1991.
50. Fang, G. D., Yu, V. L., and Vickers, R. M.: Disease due to the Legionellaceae (other than *Legionella pneumophila*): Historical, microbiological, clinical, and epidemiological review. Medicine (Baltimore) *68*:116, 1989.
51. Ferrer Marcelles, A., Garcia Hernandez, F., Elcuaz Romano, R., et al.: Neumonia por *Legionella* en un recién nacido. An. Esp. Pediatr. *30*:213, 1989.
52. Ferrer, A., Elcuaz, R. I., Giménez-Pérez, M., et al.: Legionelosis infantil. Enferm. Infecc. Microbiol. Clin. *8*:278, 1990.
53. Fields, B. S., Sanden, G. N., Barbaree, J. M., et al.: Intracellular multiplication of *Legionella pneumophila* in amoebae isolated from hospital hot water tanks. Curr. Microbiol. *18*:131, 1989.
54. Foy, H. M., Broome, C. V., Hayes, P. S., et al.: Legionnaires' disease in a prepaid medical-care group in Seattle 1963–75. Lancet *1*:767, 1979.
55. Fraser, D. W., Tsai, T. R., Orenstein, W., et al.: Legionnaires' disease: Description of an epidemic of pneumonia. N. Engl. J. Med. *297*:1189, 1977.
56. Friedman, H., Widen, R., Klein, T., et al.: *Legionella pneumophila*-induced blastogenesis of murine lymphoid cells in vitro. Infect. Immun. *43*:314, 1984.
57. Fuchs, G. J., LaRocco, M., Robinson, A., et al.: Fatal Legionnaires' disease in an infant. Pediatr. Infect. Dis. *5*:377, 1986.
58. Gibson, F. C., Tzianabos, A. O., and Rodgers, F. G.: Adherence of *Legionella pneumophila* to U-937 cells, guinea-pig alveolar macrophages, and MRC-5 cells by a novel, complement-independent binding mechanism. Can. J. Microbiol. *40*:865, 1994.
59. Girod, J. C., Reichman, R. C., Winn, W. C., Jr., et al.: Pneumonic and nonpneumonic forms of legionellosis: The result of a common-source exposure to *Legionella pneumophila*. Arch. Intern. Med. *142*:545, 1982.
60. Glick, T. H., Gregg, M. B., Berman, B., et al.: Pontiac fever: An epidemic of unknown etiology in a health department. I. Clinical and epidemiologic aspects. Am. J. Epidemiol. *107*:149, 1978.
61. Goldberg, D. J., Wrench, J. G., Collier, P. W., et al.: Lochgoilhead fever: Outbreak of non-pneumonic legionellosis due to *Legionella micdadei*. Lancet *1*:316, 1989.
62. Grady, G. F., and Gilfillan, R. F.: Relation of *Mycoplasma pneumoniae* seroreactivity, immunosuppression, and chronic disease to Legionnaires' disease: A twelve-month prospective study of sporadic cases in Massachusetts. Ann. Intern. Med. *90*:607, 1979.
63. Hartemann, E., Berthier, J. C., Barrois, S., et al.: Pnemopathie grave a legionelle chez un nourrisson immunologiquement normal. Pediatrie *38*:393, 1983.
64. Harvey, C. J., and Eykyn, S. J.: Crossreactions between *Legionella* and *Campylobacter* spp.: A clinical conundrum. J. Infect. *30*:85, 1995.
65. Hedlund, K. W., McGann, V. G., Copeland, D. S., et al.: Immunologic protection against the Legionnaires' disease bacterium in the AKR/J mouse. Ann. Intern. Med. *90*:676, 1979.
66. Helms, C. M., Viner, J. P., Renner, E. D., et al.: Legionnaires' disease among pneumonias in Iowa (FY 1972–1978). II. Epidemiologic and clinical features of 30 sporadic cases of *L. pneumophila* infection. Am. J. Med. Sci. *281*:2, 1981.
67. Hervás, J. A., Lopez, P., de la Fuente, A., et al.: Multiple organ system failure in an infant with *Legionella* infection. Pediatr. Infect. Dis. J. *7*:671, 1988.
68. Hofflin, J. M., Potasman, I., Baldwin, J. C., et al.: Infectious complications in heart transplant recipients receiving cyclosporine and corticosteroids. Ann. Intern. Med. *106*:209, 1987.
69. Horie, H., Kawakami, H., Minoshima, K., et al.: Neonatal Legionnaires' disease: Histopathological findings in an autopsied neonate. Acta Pathol. Jpn. *42*:427, 1992.
70. Horwitz, M. A.: Interactions between macrophages and *Legionella pneumophila*. Curr. Top. Microbiol. Immunol. *181*:265, 1992.
71. Husmann, L. K., and Johnson, W.: Adherence of *Legionella pneumophila* to guinea pig peritoneal macrophages, J774 mouse macrophages, and undifferentiated U937 human monocytes: Role of Fc and complement receptors. Infect. Immun. *60*:5212, 1992.
72. Isberg, R. R., Rankin, S., Roy, C. R., et al.: *Legionella pneumophila*: Factors involved in the route and response to an intracellular niche. Infect. Agents Dis. *2*:220, 1993.
73. Jaulhac, B., Nowicki, M., Bornstein, N., et al.: Detection of *Legionella* spp. in bronchoalveolar lavage fluids by DNA amplification. J. Clin. Microbiol. *30*:920, 1992.
74. Johnson, J. T., Yu, V. L., Best, M. G., et al.: Nosocomial legionellosis in

surgical patients with head-and-neck cancer: Implications for epidemiological reservoir and mode of transmission. Lancet 2:298, 1985.
75. Joly, J. R., Déry, P., Gauvreau, L., et al.: Legionnaires' disease caused by *Legionella dumoffii* in distilled water. Can. Med. Assoc. J. *135*:1274, 1986.
76. Joseph, C. A., Dedman, D., Birtles, R., et al.: Legionnaires' disease surveillance: England and Wales, 1993. Commun. Dis. Rep. C. D. R. Rev. *4*:R109, 1994.
77. Joseph, C. A., Watson, J. M., Harrison, T. G., et al.: Nosocomial Legionnaires' disease in England and Wales, 1980–92. Epidemiol. Infect. *112*:329, 1994.
78. Katz, S. M., Hammel, J. M., Matus, J. P., et al.: A self-limited febrile illness produced in guinea pigs associated with oral administration of *Legionella pneumophila*. Gastroenterology *95*:1575, 1988.
79. Katz, S. M., and Holsclaw, D. S., Jr.: Serum antibodies to *Legionella pneumophila* in patients with cystic fibrosis. J. A. M. A. *248*:2284, 1982.
80. Kaufmann, A. F., McDade, J. E., Patton, C. M. et al.: Pontiac fever: Isolation of the etiologic agent (*Legionella pneumophila*) and demonstration of its mode of transmission. Am. J. Epidemiol. *114*:337, 1981.
81. Kovatch, A. L., Jardine, D. S., Dowling, J. N., et al.: Legionellosis in children with leukemia in relapse. Pediatrics *73*:811, 1984.
82. Kugler, J. W., Armitage, J. O., Helms, C. M. et al.: Nosocomial Legionnaires' disease: Occurrence in recipients of bone marrow transplants. Am. J. Med. *74*:281, 1983.
83. Lavocat, M. P., Berthier, J. C., Rousson, A., et al.: Légionellose pulmonaire chez un enfant après noyade en eau douce. Presse Med. *16*:780, 1987.
84. Lefrancois, C., Casadevall, I., Betremieux, P., et al.: Legionellose mortelle chez un nourrisson traite par ACTH. Arch. Fr. Pédiatr. *46*:591, 1989.
85. Lindsay, D. S., Abraham, W. H., and Fallon, R. J.: Detection of mip gene by PCR for diagnosis of Legionnaires' disease. J. Clin. Microbiol. *32*:3068, 1994.
86. Maiwald, M., Kissel, K., Srimuang, S., et al.: Comparison of polymerase chain reaction and conventional culture for the detection of legionellas in hospital water samples. J. Appl. Bacteriol. *76*:216, 1994.
87. Maiwald, M., Schill, M., Stockinger, C., et al.: Detection of *Legionella* DNA in human and guinea pig urine samples by the polymerase chain reaction. Eur. J. Clin. Microbiol. Infect. Dis. *14*:25, 1995.
88. Marrie, T. J., Haldane, D., MacDonald, S., et al.: Control of endemic nosocomial legionnaires' disease by using sterile potable water for high risk patients. Epidemiol. Infect. *107*:591, 1991.
89. Marshall, L. E., Boswell, T. C., and Kudesia, G.: False positive *Legionella* serology in *Campylobacter* infection: *Campylobacter* serotypes, duration of antibody response and elimination of cross-reactions in the indirect fluorescent antibody test. Epidemiol. Infect. *112*:347, 1994.
90. Marston, B., Plouffe, J., Breiman, R., et al.: Findings of a community-based pneumonia incidence study through November 1991 [Abstract 7]. Program and Abstracts of the 1992 International Symposium on *Legionella*, January 26–29, 1992, Orlando, FL. Washington, D.C., American Society for Microbiology, 1992.
91. Marston, B. J., Lipman, H. B., and Breiman, R. F.: Surveillance for Legionnaires' disease: Risk factors for morbidity and mortality. Arch. Intern. Med. *154*:2417, 1994.
92. McDade, J. E., Shepard, C. C., Fraser, D. W., et al.: Legionnaires' disease: Isolation of a bacterium and demonstration of its role in other respiratory disease. N. Engl. J. Med. *297*:1197, 1977.
93. Millunchick, E. W., Floyd, J., and Blanks, J.: Legionnaires' disease in an immunologically normal child. Am. J. Dis. Child. *135*:1065, 1981.
94. Muittari, A., Kuusisto, P., Virtanen, P., et al.: An epidemic of extrinsic allergic alveolitis caused by tap water. Clin. Allergy *10*:77, 1980.
95. Muldoon, R. L., Jaecker, D. L., and Kiefer, H. K.: Legionnaires' disease in children. Pediatrics *67*:329, 1981.
96. Mundel, G., Goldberg, A., Boldur, I., et al.: Legionnaires' disease in Israel: Serological evidence of childhood infection. Isr. J. Med. Sci. *19*:380, 1983.
97. Myerowitz, R. L., Dowling, J. N., and Pasculle, A. W.: Immunity to Pittsburgh pneumonia agent in guinea pigs [Abstract]. 20th Interscience Conference on Antimicrobial Agents and Chemotherapy, New Orleans, 1980.
98. Nëgre, V., Chevallier, B., Dournon, E., et al.: Maladies des légionnaires noscomiale chez l'enfant: Mesures de prevention. Arch. Fr. Pédiatr. *47*:43, 1990.
99. Nigro, G., Pastoris, M. C., Fantasia, M. M., et al.: Acute cerebellar ataxia in pediatric legionellosis. Pediatrics *72*:847, 1983.
100. Orenstein, W. A., Overturf, G. D., Leedom, J. M., et al.: The frequency of *Legionella* infection prospectively determined in children hospitalized with pneumonia. J. Pediatr. *99*:403, 1981.
101. Pachon, J., Prados, M. D., Capote, F., et al.: Severe community-acquired pneumonia: Etiology, prognosis, and treatment. Am. Rev. Respir. Dis. *142*:369, 1990.
102. Payne, N. R., and Horwitz, M. A.: Phagocytosis of *Legionella pneumophila* is mediated by human monocyte complement receptors. J. Exp. Med. *166*:1377, 1987.
103. Peerless, A. G., Liebhaber, M., Anderson, S., et al.: *Legionella* pneumonia in chronic granulomatous disease. J. Pediatr. *106*:783, 1985.
104. Peeters, M., Cornu, G., and De Meyer, R.: Legionnaires' disease in an immunosuppressed child. Acta Paediatr. Belg. *33*:189, 1980.
105. Peliowski, A., and Finer, N. N.: Intractable seizures in Legionnaires disease. J. Pediatr. *109*:657, 1986.
106. Plouffe, J. F., Breiman, R. F., File, T. M., et al.: Investigation of the risk factors for sporadically occurring Legionnaires' disease, Palo Alto, Calif. Electric Power Research Institute, 1995, TR-104770s, p. i-F-2.
107. Plouffe, J. F., Para, M. F., Fuller, K. A., et al.: Oral ingestion of *Legionella pneumophila*. J. Clin. Lab. Immunol. *20*:113, 1986.
108. Quagliano, P. V., and Das Narla, L.: *Legionella* pneumonia causing multiple cavitating pulmonary nodules in a 7-month-old infant. A. J. R. *161*:367, 1993.
109. Reingold, A. L.: Role of legionellae in acute infections of the lower respiratory tract. Rev. Infect. Dis. *10*:1018, 1988.
110. Renner, E. D., Helms, C. M., Hall, N. H., et al.: Seroreactivity to *Mycoplasma pneumoniae* and *Legionella pneumophila*: Lack of a statistically significant relationship. J. Clin. Microbiol. *13*:1096, 1981.
111. Renner, E. D., Helms, C. M., Hierholzer, W. J., Jr., et al.: Legionnaires' disease in pneumonia patients in Iowa: A retrospective seroepidemiologic study, 1972–1977. Ann. Intern. Med. *90*:603, 1979.
112. Richards, S. W., Peterson, P. K., Niewoehner, D. E., et al.: *Legionella pneumophila* infection in normal and immunocompromised hamsters [Abstract]. Proceedings of the American Society Annual Meeting, 1983.
113. Rolstad, B., and Berdal, B. P.: Immune defenses against *Legionella pneumophila* in rats. Infect. Immun. *32*:805, 1981.
114. Rowbotham, T. J.: Current views on the relationships between amoebae, legionellae and man. Isr. J. Med. Sci. *22*:678, 1986.
115. Ryan, M. E., Feldman, S., Pruitt, B., et al.: Legionnaires' disease in a child with cancer. Pediatrics *64*:951, 1979.
116. Rylander, R., and Haglind, P.: Airborne endotoxins and humidifier disease. Clin. Allergy *14*:109, 1984.
117. Schmid, H., Henze, G., Schwerdtfeger, R., et al.: Fractionated total body irradiation and high-dose VP-16 with purged autologous bone marrow rescue for children with high risk relapsed acute lymphoblastic leukemia. Bone Marrow Transplant. *12*:597, 1993.
118. Simpson, R. M., Cogswell, J. J., Mitchell, E. R., et al.: Legionnaires' disease in an infant. Lancet 2:740, 1980.
119. Spanò, C., and Menozzi, M.: Legionnaire's disease in Palermo and possible involvement of *Legionella pneumophila* in cases of pericardial effusion. Infection *10*:103, 1982.
120. Sturm, R., Staneck, J. L., Myers, J. P., et al.: Pediatric Legionnaires' disease: Diagnosis by direct immunofluorescent staining of sputum. Pediatrics *68*:539, 1981.
121. Thornsberry, C., Balows, A., Feeley, J. C., et al.: *Legionella*. Proceedings of the 2nd International Symposium. Washington, D.C., American Society for Microbiology, 1984, pp. 1–371.
122. Tokunaga, Y., Concepcion, W., Berquist, W. E., et al.: Graft involvement by *Legionella* in a liver transplant recipient. Arch. Surg. *127*:475, 1992.
123. Torres, A., Serra-Batlles, J., Ferrer, A., et al.: Severe community-acquired pneumonia: Epidemiology and prognostic factors. Am. Rev. Respir. Dis. *144*:312, 1991.
124. Venezia, R. A., Agresta, M. D., Hanley, E. M., et al.: Nosocomial legionellosis associated with aspiration of nasogastric feedings diluted in tap water. Infect. Control Hosp. Epidemiol. *15*:529, 1994.
125. Wadowsky, R. M., Butler, L. J., Cook, M. K., et al.: Growth-supporting activity for *Legionella pneumophila* in tap water cultures and implication of hartmannellid amoebae as growth factors. Appl. Environ. Microbiol. *54*:2677, 1988.
126. Wadowsky, R. M., Wilson, T. M., Kapp, N. J., et al.: Multiplication of *Legionella* spp. in tap water containing *Hartmannella vermiformis*. Appl. Environ. Microbiol. *57*:1950, 1991.
127. Watson, K. C., Bain, A. D., and Bartholomew, S. E.: Legionellosis and sudden infant death syndrome. Lancet 2:1312, 1983.
128. Weeratna, R., Stamler, D. A., Edelstein, P. H., et al.: Human and guinea pig immune responses to *Legionella pneumophila* protein antigens OmpS and Hsp60. Infect. Immun. *62*:3454, 1994.
129. Wentworth, B. B., and Stiefel, H. E.: Studies of the specificity of *Legionella* serology. J. Clin. Microbiol. *15*:961, 1982.
130. Winn, W. C., Jr.: *Legionella* and the clinical microbiologist. Infect. Dis. Clin. North Am. *7*:377, 1993.
131. Yamamoto, Y., Retzlaff, C., He, P., et al.: Quantitative reverse transcription-PCR analysis of *Legionella pneumophila*-induced cytokine mRNA in different macrophage populations by high-performance liquid chromatography. Clin. Diagn. Lab. Immunol. *2*:18, 1995.

144

STREPTOBACILLUS MONILIFORMIS (RAT-BITE FEVER)

Carrie L. Byington and Robert D. Basow

Rat-bite fever is an acute febrile illness usually acquired in humans from the bite of a rat or other rodent. It is a zoonosis with worldwide distribution. *Streptobacillus moniliformis* is the leading cause of rat-bite fever in the United States, but in Asia, the illness is caused most often by a spirochete, *Spirillum minus* (see Chapter 149). Infection with *S. moniliformis* is characterized by a relapsing fever, rash, and prominent arthralgia and arthritis. Infection may be acquired after the bite of an animal, by skin or mucous membrane contact with an infected animal, or by ingestion of food or water contaminated by rats. When the organism is acquired by ingestion, the resulting illness is termed "Haverhill fever," after an outbreak that occurred in Haverhill, Massachusetts, in 1926.[31, 33]

HISTORY

The first description of rat-bite fever is found in the 2500-year-old Indian *Compendium of Medicine*, the *Susruta Samhita*.[7] In this text, a description of the illness is given that remains valid today: "The blood of any part of the human body coming in contact with the semen of rats or scratched with their nails or teeth is vitiated and gives rise to the appearance of nodes, swellings, eruptions of circular erythematous patches on skin, pustules, violent and acute erysipelas, breaking pain in the joints, extreme pain in the body, fever, anemia, aversion to food, shivering, and horripilation." The disease also was known in ancient Japan, where treatment consisted of local application of herbs and dynamite for causing an "explosion in the wound."[7]

The first modern accounts of the disease are found in a lecture by professor Eli Ives at Yale University in 1831.[17] The first case report was published in 1839.[60] In 1900, Miyake[26] gave a detailed description of the disease, which he named sodoku, from the Japanese *so* (rat) and *doku* (poison). Schottmüller[49] and Levaditi and associates[21] were the first to isolate and describe the causative agent of streptobacillary rat-bite fever in 1914 and 1925, respectively. The organism has been known as *Streptothrix muris ratti* and *Streptobacillus muris minus* but currently is referred to as *S. moniliformis*.[3]

Haverhill fever was reported first in 1926 by Place, Sutton, and Willner[33] after an outbreak of epidemic illness that was traced to contaminated milk. They called the illness erythema arthriticum epidemicum. Shortly thereafter, Parker and Hudson[31] isolated the causative organism and named it *Haverhillia multiformis*. Later, this organism was shown to be identical to *S. moniliformis*.

EPIDEMIOLOGY

There have been approximately 200 reported cases of rat-bite fever in the United States. In addition, the disease has been reported worldwide.[9, 13, 17, 21, 23, 30] *S. moniliformis* is responsible for most of the cases seen in North America, whereas the spirillary form is seen more commonly in Asia. There is only one reported case of spirillary rat-bite fever in the American literature of the last 30 years.[8] There are two reported outbreaks of Haverhill fever in the literature.[23, 31]

Rat-bite fever currently is not a reportable illness in the United States, so its true incidence is unknown. Although it is considered to be rare, it is likely that the illness is underdiagnosed. There are more than 2 million animal bites reported yearly in the United States, and rat bites account for at least 1 per cent of these.[14] De Hoff and Ross[10] reviewed animal bites in Maryland over a 3-year period and found that approximately 4.7 per cent were caused by rats or lagomorphs. Among bitten patients, the risk of rat-bite fever is significant. Richter[41] reported that in a sample of 93 persons bitten by rats in Baltimore, 10.7 per cent developed rat-bite fever. A similar study conducted in St. Louis showed an infection rate of 4 per cent.[59]

Rat-bite fever, although usually transmitted through the bite of a rat, also may be transmitted by rat scratches and has been reported after mucous membrane contact with rats. Rat-bite fever was reported following varicella in a child who handled pet rats frequently while she had open skin lesions.[35] The disease also has been transmitted to humans from mice,[39] squirrels,[25] weasels,[11] gerbils,[61] and such rat-eating carnivores as cats,[27] dogs,[32, 42] and pigs.[58] Between 10 and 100 per cent of rats, both wild and laboratory, carry *S. moniliformis* as normal nasopharyngeal flora and excrete it in their urine.[2, 56]

One-half of all reported cases of rat-bite fever in the United States over the last 25 years have involved children, usually younger than 12 years of age. Not surprisingly, children living in crowded urban centers or rural impoverished areas seem to be at greatest risk.[38] Most of the other reported cases involve laboratory personnel who handle rats.[2]

Haverhill fever is transmitted by ingestion of food or water contaminated by rats. Previous outbreaks have involved unpasteurized milk, ice cream made from raw milk, and water.[23, 33] *S. moniliformis* also can cause disease in turkeys,[28] guinea pigs,[20] and koalas,[47] and these animals could pose a potential source for infection in humans.

BACTERIOLOGY

S. moniliformis is a pleomorphic, microaerophilic, nonmotile, nonencapsulated, non–acid fast, gram-negative bacillus. It measures 1 to 5 μm in length. The organism is oxidase- and catalase-negative and will ferment glucose, maltose, fructose, galactose, and salicin.[19]

The organism is fastidious and requires special handling for isolation. Optimal growth is achieved in trypticase soy agar or broth supplemented with 20 per cent horse or rabbit serum.[31] Alternatively, brain-heart infusion broth supplemented with "Panmede" (a papain digest of ox liver) also has been shown to support the growth of *S. moniliformis*.[53] Sodium polyanethol sulfonate, which is added to most aerobic blood culture bottles at a concentration of 0.05 per cent, will inhibit the growth of *S. moniliformis* at concentrations as low as 0.0125 per cent.[52] Blood culture bottles without sodium polyanethol sulfonate added should be used for primary isolation when rat-bite fever is suspected. Sodium polyanethol sulfonate is not added to anaerobic blood culture bottles, and *S. moniliformis* may be isolated from standard anaerobic culture. Cultures should be incubated at 35° to 37° C in a humid environment with a partial pressure of carbon dioxide between 8 and 10 per cent.

The morphologic characteristics of the bacteria are dependent on its environment.[31] In favorable media, the typical appearance is that of short rods that may grow in chains. Under other conditions, the organism tends to grow in long, interwoven filaments that commonly contain beaded and fusiform swellings throughout their length. In broth culture, colonies usually appear in 2 to 10 days. The colonies are white, soft "puffballs" 1 to 2 mm in diameter. On blood agar plates, the colonies are round, gray, and glistening and measure 1 to 2 mm in diameter after 2 to 3 days of incubation.[19]

Stable L-forms of the organism develop spontaneously in vivo or in vitro. These cell-wall-deficient forms have a "fried egg" appearance with dark centers and lacy edges when grown on solid media.[19] They are resistant to penicillin and other antibiotics active against the bacterial cell wall. L-phase variants may deposit in tissues and prolong the symptoms of illness.[13]

CLINICAL MANIFESTATIONS

Streptobacillary rat-bite fever typically has an incubation period of less than 7 days, with a reported range of 1 to 22 days.[5] Young children have a predilection for shorter incubation times. The illness is characterized by the acute onset of shaking chills, fever, headache, and vomiting. Usually, the bite site is well healed, without evidence of inflammation or regional adenopathy. Within the first week of illness, more than 50 per cent of patients develop arthralgia or arthritis with or without joint effusion. The arthritis tends to be migratory, nonsymmetric, and extremely painful and involves the large joints. Within 1 to 8 days after the onset of fever, about 75 per cent of patients develop a pink-red maculopapular rash that frequently involves the palms and soles.[24] The rash, lasting up to 3 weeks, may be generalized, petechial, purpuric, or pustular, and approximately 20 per cent desquamate. With untreated infection, there may be persistent or recurrent episodes of fever and arthritis. The rash generally does not recur.

Haverhill fever is similar to streptobacillary rat-bite fever, with the abrupt onset of fever and chills (100 per cent) rash (95 per cent), and arthritis (97 per cent).[1, 24] Generally, the incubation period is 1 to 3 days. Upper respiratory and gastrointestinal complaints are common. Multiple recurrences of fever are found rarely, and the rash tends to be small and uniform in size.[23]

Complications of *S. moniliformis* infection include anemia, abscess formation, bronchopneumonia, parotitis, destructive joint disease, prostatitis, and pancreatitis.[33, 62] Unusual and potentially devastating complications include brain abscess,[12, 29] chorioamnionitis,[16] and periarteritis nodosa.[37] The most serious complication is that of bacterial endocarditis, which was uniformly fatal in the preantibiotic era.[22, 40, 46, 54] Six cases of endocarditis occurring in children younger than 18 years of age have been reported since 1934.[24, 36, 44, 50, 54, 57] Five of the six patients died during the acute illness. Four received no antibiotic treatment. In two of the cases, the patients had evidence of preexisting valvular disease, secondary to rheumatic fever. Patients present with combinations of the signs and symptoms of streptobacillary rat-bite fever and those of bacterial endocarditis, including heart murmurs, petechiae, Osler nodes, and splenomegaly. Massive pericardial effusion may complicate the endocarditis.[6]

The untreated mortality rate of *S. moniliformis* infection is 10 per cent overall.[43] The prognosis generally is excellent in patients treated with antibiotics, and the mortality rate is believed to be less than 1.5 per cent. Essentially all mortality is due to complications of endocarditis.[22]

Iron-deficiency anemia is the only complication that has been reported after Haverhill fever.[23] There have been no reported fatalities due to Haverhill fever, and the prognosis is excellent.[23]

PATHOPHYSIOLOGY AND PATHOLOGY

The factors influencing the virulence of *S. moniliformis* are not well described. The organism has an affinity for synovial tissue in both animals and humans, but the mechanisms by which *S. moniliformis* produces arthritis are unknown. Studies done in mice indicate that *S. moniliformis* is only slightly immunogenic, producing mild leukocytosis and minimal homologous antibody production. In addition, the organism is resistant to phagocytic destruction.[48] These factors may allow the development of chronic infection.

The pathologic features of streptobacillary rat-bite fever have been described in a limited number of autopsy reports. Common features include ulcerative endocarditis with secondary septic embolization in the liver and spleen, septic arthritis, and interstitial pneumonia.[3, 50] The pure interstitial pneumonia is atypical of bacterial infections. Mononuclear meningitis and erythrophagocytosis also have been reported.[50] In most reports, there is little histologic evidence of inflammation at the site of the bite.[24]

DIAGNOSIS

The correct diagnosis of rat-bite fever requires a high index of suspicion on the part of the physician. The diagnosis is suggested in a febrile patient with a history of rat exposure, but in most clinical settings, the exposure history is not elucidated until after the diagnosis is made.

Nonspecific signs include an elevation in the white blood cell count, usually in the range of 10,000 to 30,000 cells/mm^3 with a left shift, a mild anemia, and a false-positive serologic test for syphilis, which may occur in 25 per cent of patients.[43] Direct visualization of the organism on Giemsa stain of blood or joint fluid may suggest the diagnosis. Specific agglutinins appear at 10 days, reach a maximum in 1 to 3 months, and persist up to 2 years.[18] A single titer of 1:80 or greater is considered diagnostic. Fluorescent antibody and complement-fixation tests also are available at some centers.[54] An enzyme-linked immunosorbent assay has been developed, is being used to monitor infection in rodent colonies, and might be useful for human diagnosis.[4]

Ultimately, diagnosis depends on culturing the organism. The organism has been cultured from blood, joint fluid, abscesses, pericardial fluid, meninges, and tissues obtained at autopsy.[6] *S. moniliformis* possesses strict growth requirements, and choice of culture media and technique is of critical importance for optimal growth of the bacterium (see section on bacteriology). In general, routine aerobic blood cultures are not satisfactory for isolation.

If the organism is isolated, it may be identified rapidly using gas-liquid chromatography. *S. moniliformis* has a characteristic fatty acid profile, with major peaks being palmitic, linoleic, oleic, and stearic acid.[45]

The differential diagnosis for streptobacillary rat-bite fever includes illness caused by *S. minus*, which may be indistinguishable. It also includes all relapsing fevers, such as *Borrelia recurrentis*, malaria, and typhoid. Rickettsial disease, especially Rocky Mountain spotted fever, must be considered.[34] Other infectious entities include leptospirosis, Lyme disease, disseminated gonococcal infection, meningococcemia, brucellosis, syphilis, and viral infections, especially those caused by enteroviruses. Acute rheumatic fever also should be considered. Noninfectious entities include drug reactions, collagen vascular disease, and Pel-Ebstein fever.

TREATMENT AND PREVENTION

In proven cases of streptobacillary rat-bite fever, the treatment of choice is penicillin G. In adults, the dosage of penicillin should be no less than 400,000 to 600,000 IU/day continued for at least 7 days.[43] If no response is seen within 2 days, the dosage should be increased to 1.2 million IU/day. Children have been treated successfully with 20,000 to 50,000 units/kg/day of intramuscular or intravenous penicillin, up to a maximum of 1.2 million IU/day. In children who do not require hospitalization, oral penicillin V, 1 to 2 g/day in divided doses, may be given.[51] In penicillin-allergic adults, both streptomycin and tetracycline have been effective. In children, streptomycin and erythromycin have been used. Newer antibiotics, including cefuroxime, cefotaxime, gentamicin, and ciprofloxacin, have good activity against *S. moniliformis* in vitro.[15]

Endocarditis secondary to *S. moniliformis* should be treated with high-dose penicillin G in combination with streptomycin or gentamicin. In children, the dosage is 160,000 to 240,000 IU/kg/day, up to the adult maximum of 20 million IU/day.[51] Treatment should be continued for at least 4 weeks. Antibiotic susceptibility testing of the organism should be performed, and minimum inhibitory and bactericidal concentrations for several antimicrobial agents should be determined. It is desirable to have a peak serum minimum bactericidal concentration of at least 1:8. In penicillin-allergic adults or with penicillin-resistant organisms, chloramphenicol, 3 g/day for 4 weeks, has been shown to be effective.[55]

Haverhill fever is treated in much the same way, with penicillin G the current drug of choice. Most individuals can be treated as outpatients.

Rat-bite fever can be prevented by controlling rodents in urban areas, properly handling rodents, and avoiding unpasteurized milk products. If an individual is bitten by a rat, prophylactic antibiotics, such as amoxicillin or amoxicillin–clavulanic acid, probably would prevent rat-bite fever, but current data do not support the routine use of antibiotics after all rat bites.

References

1. Allbritten, F. F., Sheely, R. F., and Jeffers, W. A.: *Haverhillia multiformis* septicemia: Etiologic and clinical relationship to rat-bite fever. J. A. M. A. *114*:2360–2363, 1940.
2. Anderson, L. C., Leary, S. L., and Manning, P.: Rat-bite fever in animal laboratory personnel. Lab. Anim. Sci. *33*:292–294, 1983.
3. Blake, F.: The etiology of rat-bite fever. J. Exp. Med. *23*:39–60, 1916.
4. Boot, R., Bakker, R.H.G, Thuis, H. et al: An enzyme immunosorbent assay (ELISA) for monitoring rodent colonies for *Streptobacillus moniliformis* antibodies. Lab. Anim. *27*:350, 1993.
5. Brown, T., and Nunemaker, J.: Rat-bite fever: Review of American cases with reevaluation of its etiology and report of cases. Bull. Johns Hopkins Hosp. *70*:201–302, 1942.
6. Carbeck, R., Murphy, J., and Britt, E.: Streptobacillary rat-bite fever with massive pericardial effusion. J. A. M. A. *201*:703–704, 1967.
7. Cohen, H.: Rat-bite fever: Contributions to its history and war significance. Bull. Hist. Med. *15*:108–115, 1944.
8. Cole, J. S., Stoll, R. W., and Bulger, R. J.: Rat-bite fever: Report of three cases. Ann. Intern. Med. *71*:979–981, 1969.
9. Dalal, A.: Case of rat-bite fever treated with intravenous injection of Neosalvarsan. Practitioner *92*:449, 1914.
10. De Hoff, J. B., and Ross, L.: Animal bites. Md. State Med. J. *30*:35–45, 1981.
11. Dick, G., and Turncliff, R.: *Streptothrix* isolated from blood of a patient bitten by a weasel. J. Infect. Dis. *23*:183–187, 1918.
12. Dijkmans, B., Thomeer, R., Vielvoye, G., et al.: Brain abscess due to *Streptobacillus moniliformis* and *Actinobacterium meyerii*. Infection *12*:262–264, 1984.
13. Dolman, C.: Two cases of rat-bite fever due to *Streptobacillus moniliformis*. Can. J. Public Health *42*:228–241, 1951.
14. Edwards, M. S.: Infections due to human and animal bites. *In* Feigin, R. D., and Cherry, J. D. (eds.): Textbook of Pediatric Infectious Diseases. 3rd ed. Vol. 2. Philadelphia, W. B. Saunders, 1992, pp. 2335–2345.
15. Edwards, R., and Finch, R. G.: Characterization and antibiotic susceptibilities of *Streptobacillus moniliformis*. J. Med. Microbiol. *21*:39–42, 1986.
16. Faro, S., Walker, C., and Pierson, R.: Amnionitis with intact amniotic membranes involving *Streptobacillus moniliformis*. Obstet. Gynecol. *55*:9S–11S, 1980.
17. Francis, E.: Rat-bite fever and relapsing fever in the United States. Trans. Assoc. Am. Physicians *47*:143–151, 1932.
18. Gunning, J.: Rat-bite fever. *In* Hunter, G. W., Swartzwelder, J. C., and Clyde, D. F. (eds.): Tropical Medicine. 5th ed. Philadelphia, W. B. Saunders, 1976, pp. 245–247.
19. Holmes, B., Pickett, M. J., and Hollis, D. G.: *Streptobacillus moniliformis*. *In* Murray, P. R. (ed.): Manual of Clinical Microbiology. 6th ed. Washington, D.C., A. S. M. Press, 1995, pp. 506–507.
20. Kirchner, B. K., Lake, S. G., and Wightman, S. R.: Isolation of *Streptobacillus moniliformis* from a guinea pig with granulomatous pneumonia. Lab. Anim. Sci. *42*:519–521, 1992.
21. Levaditi, C., Nicolau, S., and Poindoux, P.: Sur le role étiologique de *Streptobacillus moniliformis* (nov. spec.) dans l'érythèma polymorphe aigu septiccemique. Compt. Rend. Acad. Sci. *180*:1188–1190, 1925.
22. McCormack, R., Kaye, D., and Hook, E.: Endocarditis due to *Streptobacillus moniliformis*: A report of two cases. J. A. M. A. *200*:77–79, 1967.
23. McEvoy, M., Noah, N., and Pilsworth, R.: Outbreak of fever caused by *Streptobacillus moniliformis*. Lancet 2:1361–1363, 1987.
24. McHugh, T., Bartlett, R., and Raymond, J.: Rat-bite fever: Report of a fatal case. Ann. Emerg. Med. *14*:119–121, 1985.
25. McMillan, B., and Boulger, L.: Squirrel-bite fever. Trans. R. Soc. Trop. Med. Hygiene *62*:567, 1968.
26. Miyake, H.: Üeber die rattenbiskrankheit. Mitt. Grenzgeb. Med. Chir. *5*:231–262, 1900.
27. Mock, H., and Morrow, A.: Rat-bite fever transmitted from a cat bite. Ill. Med. J. *61*:67–70, 1932.
28. Mohamed, Y., and Moorhead, P.: Natural *Streptobacillus moniliformis* infection in turkeys. Avian Dis. *13*:379–385, 1969.
29. Oeding, P., and Pederson, H.: Streptothrix muris ratti isolated from a brain abscess. Acta Pathol. Microbiol. Scand. *27*:436, 1950.
30. Ogata, M.: Die aetiologie der rattenbiskrankheit. Dtsch. Med. Wochenschr. *34*:1099–1102, 1908.
31. Parker, F., and Hudson, N.: The etiology of Haverhill fever (erythema arthriticum epidemicum). Am. J. Pathol. *2*:357–379, 1926.
32. Peel, M.: Dog associated bacterial infections in humans: Isolates submitted to an Australian reference laboratory. Pathology *25*:379–384, 1993.
33. Place, E., Sutton, H., and Willner, O.: Erythema arthriticum epidemicum: Preliminary report. Boston Med. Surg. J. *194*:285–287, 1926.
34. Portnoy, B. L., Satterwhite, T. K., Dyckman, J. D.: Rat-bite fever misdiagnosed as Rocky Mountain spotted fever. South. Med. J. *72*:607–609, 1979.
35. Prayer, L., and Frenk, R. W.: *Streptobacillus moniliformis* infection in a child with chickenpox. Pediatr. Infect. Dis. J. *13*:417–418, 1994.
36. Priest, W. S., Smith, J. M., and McGee, C. J.: Penicillin therapy in subacute bacterial endocarditis. Arch. Intern. Med. *79*:333–359, 1947.
37. Prouty, M., and Shater, E.: Periarteritis nodosa associated with rat-bite fever due to *Streptobacillus moniliformis* (erythema arthriticum epidemicum). J. Pediatr. *36*:605–613, 1950.
38. Raffin, B. J., and Freeman, M.: Streptobacillary rat-bite fever: A pediatric problem. Pediatrics *64*:214–217, 1979.
39. Reitzel, R., Haim, A., and Prindle, K.: Rat-bite fever from a field mouse. J. A. M. A. *106*:1090, 1936.
40. Rey, J., et al.: Les endocardites a *Streptobacillus moniliformis*. Ann. Cardiol. Angeiol. *36*:297–300, 1987.
41. Richter, C.: Incidence of rat-bites and rat-bite fever in Baltimore. J. A. M. A. *128*:324, 1945.
42. Ripley, H., and Van Sant, H.: Rat-bite fever acquired from a dog. J. A. M. A. *102*:1917, 1934.
43. Roughgarden, J.: Antimicrobial therapy of rat-bite fever. Arch. Intern. Med. *116*:39–53, 1965.
44. Roundtree, P. M., and Rohan, M.: A fatal human infection with *Streptobacillus moniliformis*. Med. J. Aust. *1*:359, 1941.
45. Rowbotham, T.: Rapid identification of *Streptobacillus moniliformis*. Lancet *2*:567, 1983.

46. Rupp, M. E.: *Streptobacillus moniliformis* endocarditis: A case report and review. Clin. Infect. Dis. *14*:769–772, 1992.
47. Russell, E. G., and Straub, E. F.: Streptobacillary pleuritis in a koala. J. Wildlife Dis. *15*:391–394, 1979.
48. Savage, N. L.: Host-parasite relationships in experimental *Streptobacillus moniliformis* arthritis in mice. Infect. Immunol. *5*:S183–S190, 1972.
49. Schottmüller, H.: Zur ätiologie und klinik der bisskrankheit. Dermatol. Wochenschr. *58*(Suppl.):77–103, 1914.
50. Sens, M. A., Brown, E. W., Wilson, L. R., et al.: Fatal *Streptobacillus moniliformis* infection in a two-month-old. Am. J. Clin. Pathol. *91*:612–616, 1989.
51. Shackelford, P. G.: Rat-bite fever. *In* Kaplan, S. L. (ed.): Current Therapy in Pediatric Infectious Disease. 3rd. ed. St. Louis, Mosby Year Book, 1993, p. 235.
52. Shanson, D. G., Gazzard, B., Midgely, J., et al.: *Streptobacillus moniliformis* isolated from blood in four cases of Haverhill fever. Lancet 2:92–94, 1983.
53. Shanson, D. G., Pratt, J., and Greene, P.: Comparison of media with and without 'Panmede' for the isolation of *Streptobacillus moniliformis* from blood culture and observation on the inhibitory effect of sodium polyanethol sulphonate. J. Med. Microbiol. *19*:181–186, 1985.
54. Simon, M., and Wilson, D.: *Streptobacillus moniliformis* endocarditis. Clin. Pediatr. *25*:110–111, 1986.
55. Stokes, J.: *Actinomycosis muris* endocarditis treated with chloramphenicol. Br. Heart J. *13*:247–251, 1951.
56. Strangeways, W.: Rats as carriers of *Streptobacillus moniliformis*. J. Pathol. Bacteriol. *37*:45–51, 1933.
57. Stuart-Harris, C. H., Wells, A. Q., Rosher, H. B., et. al.: Four cases of infective endocarditis due to organisms similar to *Haemophilus parainfluenza*, and one case due to pleomorphic *Streptobacillus*. J. Pathol. Bacteriol. *41*:407–421, 1935.
58. Washburn, R. G.: *Streptobacillus moniliformis*. *In* Mandell, G. L., Bennett, J. E., and Dolin, R. (eds.): Principles and Practice of Infectious Disease. 4th ed. New York, John Wiley & Sons, 1995, pp. 2084–2086.
59. Watkins, C.: Rat-bite fever. J. Pediatr. *28*:429–488, 1946.
60. Wilcox, W.: Violent symptoms from the bite of a rat. Am. J. Med. Sci. *26*:245–246, 1839.
61. Wilkens, E. G.: Rat-bite fever in a gerbil breeder. J. Infect. Dis. *16*:177–180, 1988.
62. Wullenweber, M.: *Streptobacillus moniliformis*, a zoonotic pathogen: Taxonomic considerations, host species, diagnosis, therapy, geographical distribution. Lab. Anim. *29*:1–15, 1995.

145

BARTONELLA (CAT-SCRATCH DISEASE)

Kenneth M. Boyer

A scratch is the beginning of what
Becomes a diagnosis that's hot.
Red, suppurating nodes
Post-skin primary bodes

"La maladie des griffes de chat."[17]

Cat-scratch disease is a subacute, regional lymphadenitis syndrome that occurs after cutaneous inoculation. Contact with cats is associated strongly with the illness, generally in the form of a scratch by claws or teeth, although cases without known cat contact have been reported. The causative agent is a newly described fastidious proteobacterium, *Bartonella henselae*. A number of complications of the disease can occur, but it generally has an indolent chronic course for 2 to 3 months, followed by spontaneous resolution.

Although cats undoubtedly have scratched children and adults for centuries, "la maladie des griffes de chat" was not described in the medical literature until 1950. Debré and associates[23] recorded the first case in a 6-year-old Parisian boy. Their description was based on clinical observations, but they also noted a positive skin test with an antigen prepared in 1946 by Hanger and Rose in New York.[9] Dr. Hanger, the owner of a "ferocious tiger cat," acquired a strong skin test reaction to this reagent after recovering from suppurative lymphadenitis. Dr. Rose had prepared the antigen from sterile pus he aspirated from his friend's affected node. This serendipitous international collaboration soon was followed by case series by Mollaret and associates[50] and Debré and colleagues[24] in France and by Daniels and MacMurray[20] in the United States that established cat-scratch disease as a distinct clinical entity and the cat-scratch skin test as the usual diagnostic confirmation.

ETIOLOGY

Elucidation of the cause of cat-scratch disease and its transmission mechanism over the past 15 years is one of the fascinating stories in the field of infectious diseases.[2, 57] The first clue was the visualization by Wear and associates,[47, 71, 72] in 1983, of small, pleomorphic, gram-negative bacilli in biopsy materials from nodes and primary granulomas stained by the Warthin-Starry silver impregnation technique. In lymph nodes, the bacilli were seen intracellularly in capillaries and in macrophages lining sinuses in or near the germinal centers. In primary skin granulomas, bacilli were seen in clumps in collagen bundles, aligned along the axis of collagen fibers. They were identified more readily in developing lesions than in suppurative nodes. Electron-microscopic examination of the bacilli revealed a trilaminar membrane structure (an outer membrane, a central peptidoglycan-like layer, and an inner plasma membrane).

An organism was cultured by English and colleagues[29] from an affected lymph node using biphasic brain-heart media. This organism, named *Afipia felis*, was presumed to be the bacterium visualized by Wear. Disconcerting, however, was the fact that patients recovering from cat-scratch disease seldom developed a serologic response to this organism.[26, 65] Further study now has discredited *A. felis* as the etiology of most cases.

A second breakthrough was the use of polymerase chain reaction (PCR) amplification of ribosomal DNA to identify another previously undescribed organism, *Rochalimaea henselae*. This bacterium first was detected in the skin and liver, respectively, of HIV-infected adults with bacillary angiomatosis and bacillary peliosis hepatitis.[53, 58, 59] Because silver staining and electron microscopy of tissue sections revealed bacillary organisms indistinguishable from those seen in cat-scratch disease, several authors hypothesized that these conditions might represent disseminated cat-scratch disease in the compromised host.[35, 39] Successful cultivation of the same organism from the blood of a group of immunocompromised patients with prolonged fever[54, 62, 73] and from the skin lesions of patients with bacillary angiomatosis[36] made possible definitive taxonomic classification. It also permitted the development of serologic tests and more reliable culture techniques. As a result, *R. henselae* now is reclassified as *B. henselae*, based on its strong nucleic acid homology to the other medically important *Bartonella* species, *B. bacilliformis* and *B. quintana*.[7]

That *B. henselae* is the cause of cat-scratch disease now has been established beyond doubt. Indirect immunofluorescence[26, 56, 57, 75] and enzyme immunoassay serologic tests[65] have been positive in 84 to 100 per cent of cases in several prospective studies, whereas the prevalence of antibody in controls generally is less than 5 per cent. *B. henselae* has been cultured from affected nodes[27] and detected by PCR in 21 of 25 samples of lymph node tissues.[4] A strong confirmatory observation has been the detection of *B. henselae* nucleic acid sequences in a number of lots of cat-scratch skin test antigen.[3] None of these studies has been supportive of *A. felis* as the etiology of even a small minority of cases.

TRANSMISSION

Cat-scratch disease is transmitted by cutaneous inoculation, frequently recognized in retrospect by the patient. In four large case series,[12, 21, 46, 63] 87 to 99 per cent of patients had contact with cats; 57 to 73 per cent had a definite cat scratch or bite. Isolated cases without known cat contact have been ascribed to minor skin trauma by dog scratches, wood splinters, pins, fish hooks, cactus spines, and porcupine quills.[68] In most cases in which a history of cat scratch can be elicited, the animal is a kitten younger than 6 months of age.[76]

Isolation of *B. henselae* from the blood of naturally infected cats and the demonstration that cats remain highly bacteremic ($>10^3$ colony forming units/mL of blood) for several months have implicated cats as the zoonotic reservoir for the organism.[34, 38, 55] In California, the number of infected cats is substantial. In one study, *B. henselae* strains were isolated from the blood of 25 of 61 (41 per cent) apparently healthy impounded or pet cats![34] In another, antibodies were demonstrated in 81 per cent of 205 cats.[15] Kittens are bacteremic more frequently than are adult cats.[26]

Although transmission from cats to humans is by means of a scratch or bite, transmission between cats has been shown to be arthropod-borne. The vector is the cat flea, *Ctenocephalides felis*. *B. henselae* has been isolated from surface-sterilized fleas infesting bacteremic cats.[34] Seroprevalence studies of pet cats from geographically diverse regions of the United States have revealed higher prevalences of *B. henselae* antibodies in warm, humid climates, where fleas are more common.[32] In an elegant series of transmission studies, Chomel and associates[16] have demonstrated that *B. henselae* can be transmitted from bacteremic to specific-pathogen–free kittens by transfer of fleas from one group of animals to the other. Housing bacteremic cats with specific-pathogen–free animals in the absence of fleas, however, did not result in transmission.

The precise mechanism of cat to human transmission remains somewhat unclear. In one study, multiple attempts to amplify *B. henselae* DNA from the nail clippings of flea-infested bacteremic kittens were unsuccessful.[26]

EPIDEMIOLOGY

Seasonality has been noted in most case series of cat-scratch disease. In temperate zones, the disease occurs predominantly in the fall and winter. Of 459 cases in which date of onset was reported, 88 per cent occurred in the months of September through March.[68] Marked seasonal fluctuations have been interpreted in several instances as community epidemics.[69] For example, there is a report of an August–September case cluster of cat-scratch encephalopathy cases in Florida.[51] There is some seasonality in the breeding of house cats, with most litters born in summer months. Thus, it may be that seasonal variation in incidence simply reflects seasonal variation in acquiring new family pets. In tropical climates, however, seasonal variation is not observed.

Large case series amassed in Paris,[21] Toronto,[63] Washington, D.C.,[21, 45, 46] Minneapolis,[68] and Jacksonville[11, 12] attest to the frequency of cat-scratch disease as a cause of chronic lymphadenitis. One report estimates an incidence in ambulatory patients in the United States of 9.3 per 100,000 population (22,000 cases) per year.[31] Individual case reports from numerous countries indicate a worldwide distribution.[68]

Cat-scratch disease is more common in children than adults, with the peak in case numbers falling between 2 and 14 years of age.[11, 22] Clustering of cases within families has been noted frequently, generally in association with acquiring new pets.[70] Veterinarians as an occupational group appear to have greater likelihood of exposure to the disease.[30, 33] Increased prevalences of skin test reactivity among veterinarians and asymptomatic relatives within family case clusters[70] indicate that some infections may be subclinical. Use of serologic tests for *B. henselae* can be expected further to clarify this issue.

PATHOLOGY

The pathology of the primary inoculation site and that of the affected lymph nodes are similar.[8, 75] Both show a characteristic central avascular necrotic area surrounded by lymphocytes, with some giant cells and histiocytes. Three evolutionary stages are recognized within affected lymph nodes; all may coexist in the same node. Initially, there is generalized enlargement of the node with thickening of the cortex and hypertrophy of the germinal centers. Lymphocytes are the predominant cell type, and epithelioid granulomas containing Langhans giant cells may be scattered throughout the node. In the middle stage, granulomas become distributed more densely, fuse, and become infiltrated with polymorphonuclear leukocytes. Central necrosis of the epithelioid granulomas begins at this stage. Progression of the process leads to formation of large pus-filled sinuses, the chief late feature. The capsule of the node may rupture, with drainage of pus into surrounding tissues, resulting in a fibrotic inflammatory reaction and binding of the node to adjacent structures. The early stage of the lesion may resemble lymphoma or sarcoidosis; in later stages, the histopathologic features resemble those of tularemia, lymphogranuloma venereum, brucellosis, and mycobacterial infection.[14]

CLINICAL MANIFESTATIONS

After an incubation period ranging from 3 to 30 days, usually between 7 and 12 days, one or more red papules measuring 2 to 5 mm in diameter develop at the site of cutaneous inoculation, often within the line of a previous cat scratch (Fig. 145–1). Although often overlooked, such primary lesions were found with careful search in 93 per cent of affected patients in one series.[12] The lesions persist until the development of lymphadenopathy, generally a period of 1 to 4 weeks.

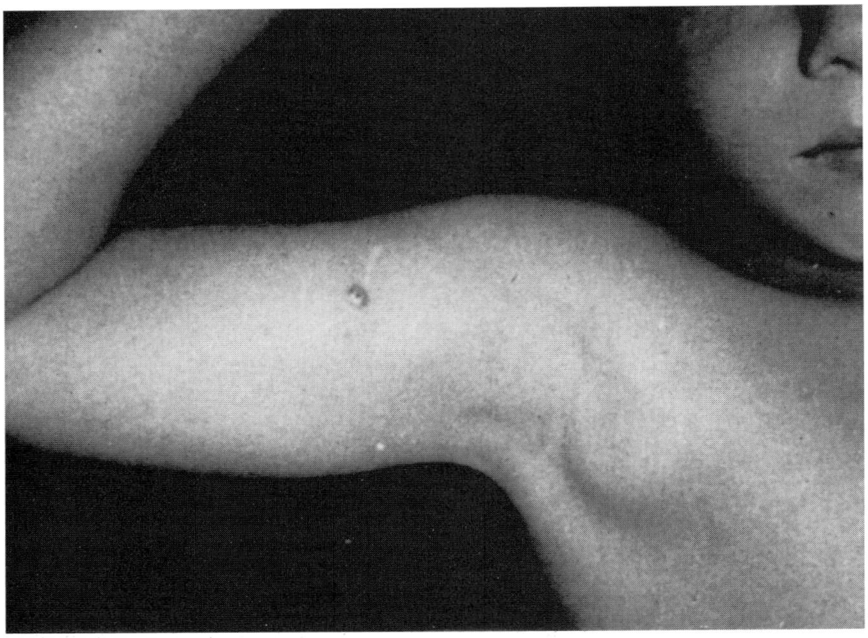

FIGURE 145–1. *Cat-scratch disease involving an axillary lymph node with primary granuloma of the upper arm. Note that the primary lesion is within the line of a healed cat scratch. (Courtesy of Hugh A. Carithers, M.D.)*

Chronic lymphadenitis is the hallmark of cat-scratch disease (see Fig. 145–1), most frequently affecting the first or second sets of nodes draining the site of inoculation. Intervening lymphangitis does not occur. The sites affected most frequently, in decreasing order, are the axillary, cervical, submandibular, preauricular, epitrochlear, femoral, and inguinal lymph node groups.[11, 28, 46] Involvement of more than one lymph node group, either within the same regional drainage or at an unrelated site, is present in 10 to 20 per cent of cases.[46, 63] At a given site, about one half of cases will involve a single node and the other half, multiple nodes.[46]

Affected nodes usually are tender, and the overlying skin becomes warm, red, and indurated. Between 10 and 40 per cent of them eventually suppurate, occasionally with formation of a sinus tract to the skin surface.[12, 45] The duration of lymph node enlargement is 4 to 6 weeks, with persistence for up to 12 months in exceptional cases. Nodes that have drained to the skin surface frequently produce some residual scarring.

Despite the common appellation *cat-scratch fever,* the majority of patients lack constitutional symptoms.[46] Elevated temperatures are documented in about 30 per cent of patients and, when present, generally are in the range of 38° to 39° C. Other nonspecific symptoms may include malaise, anorexia, fatigue, and headache.

A distinctive manifestation of cat-scratch disease is Parinaud oculoglandular syndrome (Figs. 145–2 and 145–3).[10, 44, 72] The site of primary inoculation is the conjunctiva of one eye or the eyelid. Mild to moderate conjunctivitis accompanies the primary lesion. Preauricular lymph nodes are the corresponding regional site of adenopathy. The involved preauricular nodes may be within the substance of the parotid gland, but exocrine tissue typically is not involved.[21] Although the oculoglandular syndrome may be induced by other agents, notably *Francisella tularensis,* the most common cause appears to be cat-scratch disease.

The most serious complication of cat-scratch disease is involvement of the central nervous system, chiefly in the form of encephalopathy or encephalitis.[13, 14, 41, 51, 52, 54, 61] High fever and convulsions develop within 6 weeks of the onset of lymphadenopathy, followed by alteration in the level of consciousness, headache, and muscle weakness. The cerebrospinal fluid is normal or shows minimal pleocytosis or elevation of protein. Electroencephalograms show diffuse slowing or focal abnormalities in most patients. Recovery has occurred without residua in nearly all of the well-documented cases in the literature. A few patients had prolonged convalescence and required anticonvulsant therapy for persistent seizure foci. The incidence of encephalopathy is low, but it can be the presenting manifestation of cat-scratch disease.[13]

A variety of exanthems have been reported to occur in cat-scratch disease, most frequently an evanescent maculopapular rash that occurs in about 7 per cent of patients early in the course of the disease.[12] Erythema nodosum has been noted in a number of reports but appears to be a less common manifestation.[22, 77] Thrombocytopenic purpura is quite rare but potentially serious. All reported cases have proved

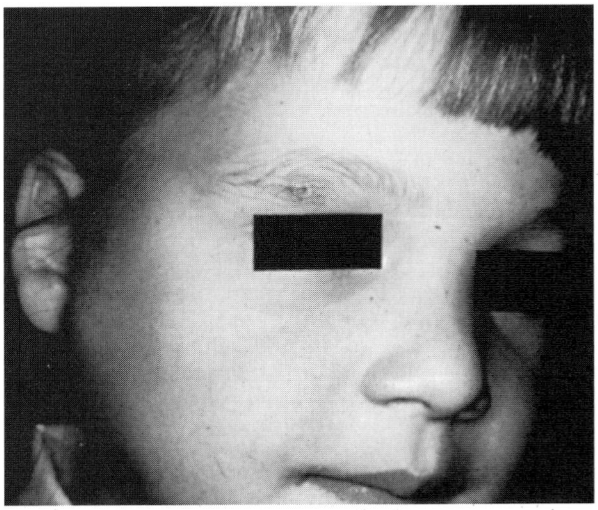

FIGURE 145–2. *Child with oculoglandular syndrome of Parinaud as a manifestation of cat-scratch disease. Note the parotid swelling and the primary site in the right eyebrow. (Courtesy of James D. Cherry, M.D.)*

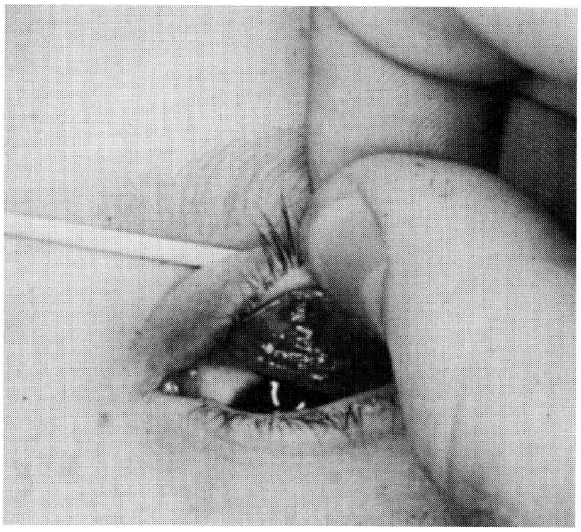

FIGURE 145–3. *Sibling of the patient in Figure 145–2. This child also has the oculoglandular syndrome. Note the primary site on the left palpebral conjunctival surface. (Courtesy of James D. Cherry, M.D.)*

to be transient. Increased marrow megakaryocytes in several cases suggest an immunopathologic mechanism.[5, 12]

Osteolytic bone lesions have been noted in several well-documented cases.[1, 12, 19] In one affected patient, biopsy of the lesion in the ilium revealed a granulomatous reaction typical of cat-scratch disease. In all of the reported cases, the involved bone site has been anatomically remote from the site of primary inoculation, which suggests the likelihood of hematogenous spread.

Granulomatous hepatitis is a newly recognized "systemic" manifestation of cat-scratch disease and may present as fever of unknown origin with or without lymphadenopathy.[6, 25, 40, 43, 60] The reported cases have shown characteristic multiple hypodense lesions in the liver on computed tomography scan, in some instances with similar lesions in the spleen. Confirmation of the diagnosis in these cases has been based on characteristic histopathology, visualization of organisms with Warthin-Starry staining, and positive skin tests.

Other rare complications that have been ascribed to cat-scratch disease include mesenteric lymphadenitis, pneumonia, arthralgia, subacute iritis, chorioretinitis, optic neuritis, urethritis, lymphedema, and thyroiditis.[48, 67, 68] Newer diagnostic techniques undoubtedly will clarify the spectrum and incidence of complications of cat-scratch disease in normal and immunocompromised children.

DIAGNOSIS AND DIFFERENTIAL DIAGNOSIS

Before its etiology was established, a number of criteria for the diagnosis of cat-scratch disease were proposed.[12, 45, 46, 68] A current version is based on the Carithers "rule of five."[42] Subacute or chronic regional lymphadenopathy is assigned one point, and two each are assigned for cat contact, an inoculation site on physical examination, and a positive serology or cat-scratch (Hanger-Rose) skin test. A total of five points is considered strongly suggestive of the diagnosis, and seven points is definitive. The cat-scratch skin test, however, now should be considered obsolete. Reagents are unstandardized, have the potential for transmission of known and unknown pathogens, and appear to yield results that have less sensitivity than serologic studies.[26, 65] Although not available in most hospitals, indirect immunofluorescence and enzyme immunoassay serologic tests for *B. henselae* now are performed by a number of commercial and reference laboratories.

Cultivation of *B. henselae* from a suppurative lymph node is difficult.[74] Even under optimal circumstances in prospective studies, most cultures are negative, perhaps reflecting a decline in organism viability and numbers at the stage when specimens are obtained most easily by needle aspiration.[26] Histopathologic studies at the inoculation site or of a surgically excised lymph node, using hematoxylin-eosin as well as Warthin-Starry silver impregnation staining, may be strongly supportive of the diagnosis.[14] Detection of *B. henselae* nucleic acid by PCR amplification of lymph node materials appears to be highly sensitive and specific but as yet is available only in research laboratories.[4]

The differential diagnosis of cat-scratch disease can include virtually all known causes of lymphadenopathy.[14] As a general rule, the diagnosis is favored by chronicity, unilaterality, tenderness, and characteristic sites of involvement, such as axillary, epitrochlear, and preauricular nodes. Cervical, femoral, inguinal, and generalized lymph node involvement is less typical for cat-scratch disease and necessitates more care in differential diagnosis.

The major differential considerations are listed in Table 145–1. The most common diagnoses in 85 patients with adenopathy and negative cat-scratch skin tests in one series were pyogenic lymphadenitis and/or abscess (29 patients), benign or malignant neoplasm (12 patients), and mycobacterial cervical adenitis (10 patients).[45] Other lymphadenopathic conditions, particularly tularemia, toxoplasmosis, plague, rat-bite fever, fungal infections, and Kawasaki disease, must be considered because of the need for specific therapy.

TREATMENT AND PROGNOSIS

Management of affected patients generally is considered to be expectant. No controlled trials of antimicrobial treatment for cat-scratch disease have been performed.[11, 48] Indeed, the

TABLE 145–1. Differential Diagnosis of Cat-Scratch Disease

Infections	Other Conditions
Pyogenic lymphadenitis/ abscess	Hodgkin disease
Atypical mycobacterial lymphadenitis	Non-Hodgkin lymphoma
Lymphogranuloma venereum	Langerhans cell histiocytosis
Infectious mononucleosis	Thyroglossal duct cyst
Tuberculosis	Cystic hygroma
Tularemia*	Dermoid cyst
Toxoplasmosis*	Branchial cleft cyst
Plague*	Sarcoidosis
Rat-bite fever	Kawasaki disease
Sporotrichosis*	Kikuchi-Fujimoto disease
Blastomycosis	Rosai-Dorfman disease
Histoplasmosis	Systemic lupus erythematosus
Nocardiosis	
Syphilis	
Symptomatic HIV infection	

*Known to be transmitted by cats.

diagnosis is considered most often in the context of failure to respond to empiric treatment of presumed staphylococcal lymphadenitis with dicloxacillin or a first-generation cephalosporin. Anecdotal experience, however, has suggested accelerated resolution of affected nodes after treatment with gentamicin[6] and trimethoprim-sulfamethoxazole.[18] Adult patients with bacillary angiomatosis, peliosis hepatitis, and *B. henselae* bacteremia have been treated successfully with long-term erythromycin and tetracycline.[37] Agar dilation susceptibility testing of three reference strains of *B. henselae* revealed inhibition by low concentrations of penicillin G, amoxicillin, gentamicin, rifampin, erythromycin, clarithromycin, and azithromycin (the lowest minimum inhibitory concentration of all tested drugs).[49] Relatively high minimum inhibitory concentrations were seen with oxacillin, cephalothin, clindamycin, and ciprofloxacin. These data suggest that it now is reasonable to consider a trial of macrolide therapy for a child with suspected or proven cat-scratch disease.

Suppurative nodes are treated best by needle aspiration, repeated if necessary. The needle track for aspiration should course through normal skin adjacent to the node, so that the risk of forming a draining sinus is minimized. Aspirated pus should be cultured, with an emphasis on recovery of pyogenic organisms, fungi, and mycobacteria. Surgical excision of affected nodes generally is unnecessary but is indicated when there is uncertainty about the diagnosis or an atypical or prolonged course. Incision and drainage should not be done because this leads to prolonged drainage and scar formation.

Most patients with cat-scratch disease have a benign course. Systemic symptoms usually last less than 2 weeks. Affected nodes may be painful for several weeks and remain enlarged for a number of months. Cases with such complications as encephalopathy, thrombocytopenic purpura, granulomatous hepatitis, chorioretinitis or bone lesions generally have a more prolonged course but also have a good long-term prognosis. Reinfection appears to be an extremely rare occurrence.[26, 66]

PREVENTION

The ideal preventive approach probably is to avoid cats, particularly aggressive play with young kittens. Destroying a family pet to which cases of cat-scratch disease have been attributed seems rather drastic because the capacity for disease transmission appears to be transient and cat-scratch disease is a rare and relatively late complication of a scratch. However, declawing such a pet might be considered. Perhaps more important, control of flea infestation has the potential for limiting transmission between cats and therefore is a practical preventive measure. In any case, if the owners of the 57 million cats in the United States are to be believed, the benefits of cat ownership appear to outweigh the risks!

References

1. Adams, W. C., and Hindman, S. M.: Cat-scratch disease associated with an osteolytic lesion. J. Pediatr. *44*:665–669, 1954.
2. Adal, K. A., Cockerell, C. J., and Petri, W. A.: Cat scratch disease, bacillary angiomatosis, and other infections due to *Rochalimaea*. N. Engl. J. Med. *330*:1509–1515, 1994.
3. Anderson, B., Kelley, C., Threlkel, R., et al.: Detection of *Rochalimaea henselae* in cat scratch disease skin test antigens. J. Infect. Dis. *168*:1034–1036, 1993.
4. Anderson, B., Sims K., Regnery, R., et al.: Detection of *Rochalimaea henselae* DNA in specimens from cat scratch disease patients by PCR. J. Clin. Microbiol. *32*:942–948, 1994.
5. Billo, O. E., and Wolff, J. A.: Thrombocytopenic purpura due to cat-scratch disease. J. A. M. A. *174*:1824–1826, 1960.
6. Bogue, C. W., Wise, J. D., Gray, G. F., et al.: Antibiotic therapy for cat-scratch disease. J. A. M. A. *262*:813–816, 1989.
7. Brenner, D. J., O'Connor, S. P., Winkler, H. H., et al.: Proposals to unify the genera *Bartonella* and *Rochalimaea*, with descriptions of *Bartonella quintana* comb. nov., *Bartonella vinsonii* comb. nov., *Bartonella henselae* comb. nov., and *Bartonella elizabethae* comb. nov., and to remove the family Bartonellaceae from the order Rickettsiales. Int. J. Syst. Bacteriol. *43*:777–786, 1993.
8. Campbell, J. A. H.: Cat scratch disease. Pathol. Ann. *12*:277–292, 1977.
9. Carithers, H. A.: Cat-scratch disease: Notes on its history. Am. J. Dis. Child. *119*:200–203, 1970.
10. Carithers, H. A.: Oculoglandular disease of Parinaud: A manifestation of cat scratch disease. Am. J. Dis. Child. *132*:1195–1200, 1978.
11. Carithers, H. A.: Cat-scratch disease: An overview based on a study of 1,200 patients. Am. J. Dis. Child. *139*:1124–1133, 1985.
12. Carithers, H. A., Carithers, C. M., and Edward, R. O., Jr.: Cat-scratch disease: Its natural history. J. A. M. A. *207*:312–316, 1969.
13. Carithers, H. A., Margileth, A. M.: Cat-scratch disease: Acute encephalopathy and other neurological manifestations. Am. J. Dis. Child. *145*:98–101, 1991.
14. Case Records of the Massachusetts General Hospital: Case 22-1992: A 6½-year-old girl with status epilepticus, cervical lymphadenopathy, pleural effusions, and respiratory distress. N. Engl. J. Med. *326*:1480–1489, 1992.
15. Chomel, B. B., Abbott, R. G., Kasten, R. W., et al.: *Bartonella henselae* prevalence in domestic cats in California: Risk factors and association between bacteremia and antibody titers. J. Clin. Microbiol. *33*:2445–2450, 1995.
16. Chomel, B. B., Kasten, R. W., Floyd-Hawkins, K., et al.: Experimental transmission of *Bartonella henselae* by the cat flea. J. Clin. Microbiol. *34*:1952–1956, 1996.
17. Clyde, W. A., Jr.: On cat-scratch disease. Pediatr. Infect. Dis. *2*:405, 1983.
18. Collipp, P. J.: Cat-scratch disease therapy. Am. J. Dis. Child. *143*:1261, 1989.
19. Collipp, P. J., and Koch, R.: Cat-scratch fever associated with an osteolytic lesion. N. Engl. J. Med. *260*:278–280, 1959.
20. Daniels, W. B., and MacMurray, F. G.: Cat-scratch disease: Nonbacterial regional lymphadenitis. Arch. Intern. Med. *88*:736–751, 1951.
21. Daniels, W. B., and MacMurray, F. G.: Cat-scratch disease: Report of one hundred sixty cases. J. A. M. A. *154*:1247–1251, 1954.
22. Debré, R., and Job, J. C.: La maladie des griffes de chat. Acta. Pediatr. Scand. *43* (Suppl.):1–86, 1954.
23. Debré, R., Lamy, M., Jammett, M. L., et al.: La maladie des griffes de chat. Bull. Mem. Soc. Med. Hôp. Paris *66*:76–79, 1950.
24. Debré, R., Lamy, M., Jammett, M. L., et al.: La maladie des griffes de chat. Semaine Hôp. Paris *26*:1895–1904, 1950.
25. Delahoussey, P. M., and Osborne, B. M.: Cat-scratch disease presenting as abdominal visceral granulomas. J. Infect. Dis. *161*:71–78, 1990.
26. Demers, D. M., Bass, J. W., Vincent, J. M., et al.: Cat-scratch disease in Hawaii: Etiology and seroepidemiology. J. Pediatr. *127*:23–26, 1995.
27. Dolan, M. J., Wong, M. T., Regnery, R. L., et al.: Syndrome of *Rochalimaea henselae* adenitis suggesting cat scratch disease. Ann. Intern. Med. *118*:331–336, 1993.
28. Earle, A. S., and Wolinsky, E.: Cat scratch disease with involvement of intra-parotid lymph nodes. Plast. Reconstruct. Surg. *61*:917–919, 1978.
29. English, C. K., Wear, D. J., Margileth, A. M., et al.: Cat-scratch disease: Isolation and culture of the bacterial agent. J. A. M. A. *259*:1347–1352, 1988.
30. Gifford, H.: Skin-test reactions to cat-scratch disease among veterinarians. Arch. Intern. Med. *95*:828–833, 1955.
31. Jackson, L. A., Perkins, B. A., and Wenger, J. D.: Cat scratch disease in the United States: An analysis of three national data bases. Am. J. Public Health *83*:1707–1711, 1993.
32. Jameson, P., Greene, C., Regnery, R., et al.: Prevalence of *Bartonella henselae* in pet cats throughout regions of North America. J. Infect. Dis. *172*:1145–1149, 1995.
33. Kalter, S. S.: A survey of cat scratch disease among veterinarians. J. Am. Vet. Med. Assoc. *144*:1281–1282, 1964.
34. Koehler, J. E., Glaser, C. A., and Tuppero, J. W.: *Rochalemaea henselae* infection: A new zoonosis with the domestic cat as the reservoir. J. A. M. A. *271*:531–535, 1994.
35. Koehler, J. E., LeBoit, P. E., Egbert, B. M., et al.: Cutaneous vascular lesions and disseminated cat-scratch disease in patients with the acquired immunodeficiency syndrome (AIDS) and AIDS-related complex. Ann. Intern. Med. *109*:449–455, 1988.
36. Koehler, J. E., Quinn, F. D., Berger, T. G., et al.: Isolation of *Rochalimaea* species from cutaneous and osseous lesions of bacillary angiomatosis. N. Engl. J. Med. *327*:1625–1631, 1992.
37. Koehler, J. E., Tappero, J. W.: Bacillary angiomatosis and bacillary peliosis in patients infected with human immunodeficiency virus. Clin. Infect. Dis. *17*:612–624, 1993.
38. Kordick, D. L., Wilson, K. H., Sexton, D. J., et al.: Prolonged *Bartonella* bacteremia in cats associated with cat-scratch disease patients. J. Clin. Microbiol. *33*:3245–3251, 1995.
39. LeBoit, P. E., Berger, T. G., Egbert, B. M., et al.: Bacillary angiomatosis: The histopathology and differential diagnosis of a pseudoneoplastic infection in patients with human immunodeficiency virus disease. Am. J. Surg. Pathol. *13*:909–920, 1989.

40. Lenoir, A. A., Storch, G. A., DeSchryver-Kecskemeti, K., et al.: Granulomatous hepatitis associated with cat scratch disease. Lancet *1*:1132–1136, 1988.
41. Lewis, D. W., and Tucker, S. H.: Central nervous system involvement in cat scratch disease. Pediatrics *77*:714–721, 1986.
42. Malatack, J. J.: Cat-scratch disease. *In* Burg, F. D., Ingelfinger, J. R., Wald, E. R., et al. (eds.): Current Pediatric Therapy. Philadelphia, W. B. Saunders, 1996, pp. 593–594.
43. Malatack, J. J., Altman, H. A., Nard, J. A., et al.: Cat-scratch disease without adenopathy. J. Pediatr. *114*:101–104, 1989.
44. Margileth, A. M.: Cat scratch disease as a cause of the oculoglandular syndrome of Parinaud. Pediatrics *20*:1000–1005, 1957.
45. Margileth, A. M.: Cat scratch disease: Nonbacterial regional lymphadenitis. Pediatrics *42*:803–818, 1968.
46. Margileth, A. M.: Cat scratch disease. Adv. Pediatr. Infect. Dis. *8*:1–21, 1993.
47. Margileth, A. M., Wear, D. J., Hadfield, T. L., et al.: Cat scratch disease: Bacteria in skin at the primary inoculation site. J. A. M. A. *252*:928–931, 1984.
48. Margileth, A. M., Wear, D. J., and English, C. K.: Systemic cat scratch disease: Report of 23 patients with prolonged or recurrent severe bacterial infection. J. Infect. Dis. *155*:390–402, 1987.
49. Maurin, M., Gusquet, S., Ducco, C., et al.: MIC's of 28 antibiotic compounds for 14 *Bartonella* (formerly *Rochalimaea)* isolates. Antimicrob. Agents Chemother. *39*:2387–2391, 1995.
50. Mollaret, P., Reilly, J., Bastin, R., et al.: Sur un adénopathie régionale subaiguë et spontanément curable, avec intradermo-réaction et lésions ganglionnaires particulières. Bull Mem. Soc. Méd. Hôp. Paris *66*:424–449, 1950.
51. Noah, D. L., Breese, J. S., Gorensek, M. J., et al.: Cluster of five children with acute encephalopathy associated with cat-scratch disease in south Florida. Pediatr. Infect. Dis. J. *14*:866–869, 1995.
52. Paxson, E. M., and McKay, R. J.: Neurologic symptoms associated with cat scratch disease. Pediatrics *20*:18–22, 1957.
53. Perkocha, L. A., Geaghan, S. M., Yen, T. S. B., et al.: Clinical and pathological features of bacillary peliosis hepatitis in association with human immunodeficiency virus infection. N. Engl. J. Med. *323*:1581–1586, 1990.
54. Regnery, R. L., Anderson, B. E., Clarridge, J. E., III, et al.: Characterization of a novel *Rochalimaea* species, *R. henselae* sp. nov., isolated from blood of a febrile, HIV-positive patient. J. Clin. Microbiol. *30*:265–274, 1992.
55. Regnery, R. L., Martin, M., and Olson, J. G.: Naturally occurring *Rochalimaea hemselae* infection in domestic cats. Lancet *340*:557–558, 1992.
56. Regnery, R., Olson, J. G., Perkins, B. A., et al.: Serological response to "*Rochalimaea hemselae*" antigen in suspected cat scratch disease. Lancet *339*:1443–1445, 1992.
57. Regnery, R., and Tappero, J.: Unraveling mysteries associated with cat-scratch disease, bacillary angiomatosis, and related syndromes. Emerg. Infect. Dis. *1*:16–21, 1995.
58. Relman, D. A., Falkow, S., LeBoit, P. E., et al.: The organism causing bacillary angiomatosis, peliosis hepatitis, and fever and bacteremia in immunocompromised patients. N. Engl. J. Med. *324*:1514, 1991.
59. Relman, D. A., Loutit, J. S., Schmidt, T. M., et al.: The agent of bacillary angiomatosis: An approach to the identification of uncultured pathogens. N. Engl. J. Med. *323*:1573–1580, 1990.
60. Rizkallah, M. F., Meyer, L., and Ayoub, E. M.: Hepatic and splenic abscesses in cat-scratch disease. Pediatr. Infect. Dis. J. *7*:191–195, 1988.
61. Selby, G., and Grant, L. W.: Cerebral arteritis in cat-scratch disease. Neurology *29*:1413–1418, 1979.
62. Slater, L. N., Welch, D. F., Hensel, D., et al.: A newly recognized fastidious gram-negative pathogen as a cause of fever and bacteremia. N. Engl. J. Med. *323*:1587–1593, 1990.
63. Spaulding, W. B., and Hennessy, J. N.: Cat scratch disease: A study of eighty-three cases. Am. J. Med. *28*:504–509, 1960.
64. Steiner, M. M., Vuckovitch, D., and Hadawi, S. A.: Cat-scratch disease with encephalopathy. J. Pediatr. *62*:514–520, 1963.
65. Szelc-Kelly, C. M., Goral, S., Perez-Perez, G. I., et al.: Serologic responses to *Bartonella* and *Afipia* antigens in patients with cat scratch disease. Pediatrics *96*:1137–1142, 1995.
66. Townsend, E. H., Jr., and Cravitz, L.: Cat-scratch disease: Recurrence after three years. Am. J. Dis. Child. *110*:213–214, 1965.
67. Ulrich, G. G., Waecker, N. J., Meister, S. J., et al.: Cat scratch disease associated with neuroretinitis in a six-year-old girl. Ophthalmology *99*:246–249, 1992.
68. Warwick, W. J.: The cat-scratch syndrome, many diseases or one disease? Progr. Med. Virol. *9*:256–301, 1967.
69. Warwick, W. J., and Good, R. A.: Cat-scratch disease in Minnesota. I. Evidence for its epidemic occurrence. Am. J. Dis. Child. *100*:228–235, 1960.
70. Warwick, W. J., and Good, R. A.: Cat-scratch disease in Minnesota. II. The family epidemics. Am. J. Dis. Child. *100*:236–240, 1960.
71. Wear, D. J., Margileth, A. M., Hadfield, T. L., et al.: Cat scratch disease: A bacterial infection. Science *221*:1403–1405, 1983.
72. Wear, D. J., Malaty, R. H., Zimmerman, L. E., et al.: Cat scratch disease bacilli in the conjunctiva of patients with Parinaud's oculoglandular syndrome. Ophthalmology *92*:1282–1287, 1985.
73. Welch, D. F., Pickett, D. A., Slater, L. N., et al.: *Rochalimaea henselae* sp. nov., a cause of septicemia, bacillary angiomatosis, and parenchymal bacillary peliosis. J. Clin. Microbiol. *30*:275–280, 1992.
74. Welch, D. F., and Slater, L. N.: Bartonella. *In* Murray, P. R., Baron, E. J., Pfaller, M. A., et al. (eds.): Manual of Clinical Microbiology. Washington, D.C., American Society for Microbiology, 1995, pp. 690–695.
75. Winship, T.: Pathologic changes in so-called cat-scratch fever. Am. J. Clin. Pathol. *23*:1012–1018, 1953.
76. Zangwill, K. M., Hamilton, D. H., Perkins, B. A., et al: Cat scratch disease in Connecticut: Epidemiology, risk factors, and evaluation of a new diagnostic test. N. Engl. J. Med. 329:8–13, 1993.
77. Zeigler, L. K.: A case of cat-scratch disease complicated by erythema nodosum. Clin. Proc. Child. Hosp. D. C. *15*:71–74, 1959.

SUBSECTION SIX

TREPONEMATACEAE

146

BORRELIA (RELAPSING FEVER)

Kenneth M. Boyer

Relapsing fever is a vector-borne bacterial infection. It is characterized by recurring febrile attacks separated by periods of relative well-being. Spirochetes of the genus *Borrelia* cause the disease. It may be transmitted by lice (epidemic relapsing fever) or ticks (endemic relapsing fever).

Relapsing fever first was differentiated from other intermittently febrile conditions in 1868 by Obermeir,[5] who noted the presence of "myriads of living and actively motile spirilla in the blood of relapsing fever patients during the febrile attack." At the turn of the century, Mackie, in India, and Nicolle, in Tunisia, elucidated transmission of the epidemic disease by the human body louse. Concurrently, in equatorial Africa, Dutton and Todd discovered that sporadic cases could be transmitted by argasid (soft) ticks.

Massive outbreaks of louse-borne relapsing fever accompanied social and hygienic disruption in Europe and North Africa in the wake of both World Wars. At present, louse-borne disease is reported in appreciable numbers only from Ethiopia and Sudan. Tick-borne relapsing fever persists as an uncommon but widely dispersed infection in many countries, including the western United States.

THE ORGANISM

The borreliae that cause relapsing fever differ from other pathogenic spirochetes (such as *Leptospira* and *Treponema*) in their loose-coiled morphology and ready staining by Wright or Giemsa stain. These two characteristics permit identification of the organisms in blood smears, a diagnostic finding that is unique among bacterial diseases (Fig. 146–1). *B. burg-*

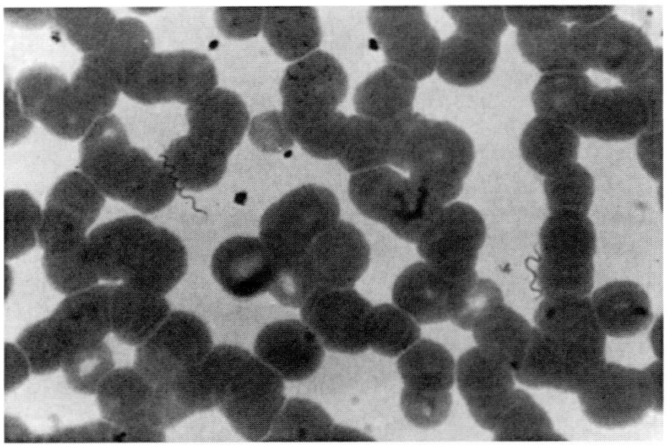

FIGURE 146–1. Borrelia hermsii *spirochetes in the peripheral blood smear of a 20-year-old patient with tick-borne relapsing fever. (Wright stain × 1000.) (From Boyer, K. M., Munford, R. S., Maupin, G. O., et al.: Tick-borne relapsing fever: An interstate outbreak originating at Grand Canyon National Park. Am. J. Epidemiol. 105:469–479, 1977.)*

dorferi, the cause of Lyme disease, is not seen in peripheral smears, an important point in differential diagnosis.

Borrelia microorganisms are extremely fastidious in cultivation, and taxonomic classification has depended on the specificity of strain-vector relationships.[11, 20] *B. recurrentis* is transmitted by the human body louse *(Pediculus humanus humanus)*. The other species that cause relapsing fever are transmitted by ticks of the genus *Ornithodoros* (Table 146–1).

Propagation of *B. recurrentis, B. hispanica, B. hermsii,* and *B. turicatae* in complex artificial media has been accomplished.[28] In common with other pathogenic spirochetes, borreliae require long-chain fatty acids for growth. They are microaerophilic and metabolize glucose by glycolysis, with resulting accumulation of lactic acid. Further study of metabolism and DNA homology eventually may simplify their taxonomy. The guanine and cytosine content in the multiple copies of borrelial genomic DNA is an exceptionally low 27 to 32 per cent.[3] *B. burgdorferi* has a 30 to 44 per cent DNA homology to *B. hermsii*.[25] It is clearly a distinct species and perhaps a distinct genus. The 86 per cent DNA homology between *B. turicatae* and *B. hermsii*, however, suggests a much closer taxonomic and evolutionary relationship.[3]

TRANSMISSION

Body lice that transmit relapsing fever become infected by feeding on a spirochetemic patient. Ingested spirochetes enter the hemolymph through the gut epithelium and multiply there. Except for the central ganglion, other tissues such as salivary glands and genital organs are not invaded. Once infected, lice remain so for their entire life but do not transmit the organisms to their progeny. Transmission to humans takes place by contamination of the bite wound with infectious hemolymph, when lice are crushed or wounded by scratching. Intermediate hosts for *B. recurrentis* other than humans are not known.[21]

The development of borreliae in *Ornithodoros* ticks differs from that in body lice. After the tick engorges on an infected host, spirochetes invade all tissues, including the salivary glands, and, in most instances, the female genital tract. The latter phenomenon results in transovarial infection of progeny, an important survival mechanism. Once infected, ticks remain capable of transmitting infection for years via secretions of infectious saliva or coxal fluid. *Ornithodoros* ticks typically are night feeders and take blood meals lasting an average of 15 minutes, after which they detach themselves. Their bites usually are painless and are noted infrequently. With the exception of *O. moubata*, ticks that transmit relapsing fever are maintained in nature by intermediate hosts. Rodents and other small mammals are the major reservoirs of both ticks and tick-borne borreliae.[10, 20, 21, 50]

EPIDEMIOLOGY

The epidemiology of relapsing fever is determined by the habits of its vectors. Acquisition of louse-borne relapsing fever occurs under conditions of crowding, cold weather, and poor hygiene, which favor the spread of lice. Thus, epidemics have occurred in the setting of wars, earthquakes, famines, and floods, often in association with epidemic typhus. In Addis Ababa, Ethiopia, where an estimated 1000 cases of louse-borne relapsing fever occur each year, nomadic tribesmen and seasonal laborers living under conditions of extreme poverty are at risk.[9]

Most foci of tick-borne relapsing fever exist in nature in rather closed environments, such as rodent burrows, nests, or caves. In Africa, Asia, and South America, primitive dwellings with dirt floors, thatched roofs, and rodent nests often harbor endemic species of *Ornithodoros*. In more sophisticated societies, people become part of these ecologic systems only when "roughing it." In the western United States, for example, where *O. hermsi* transmits most cases, a history of sleeping in old summer cabins in forested mountain areas is the rule.[18, 24, 50] In well-studied outbreaks occurring at Browne Mountain, Spokane County, Washington[48]; Big Bear Lake,

TABLE 146–1. Important Borreliae Causing Relapsing Fever, Their Vectors, and Their Current Geographic Distribution

Borrelia Species	Vector	Geographic Distribution
B. recurrentis	*Pediculus humanus humanus*	Ethiopia, Sudan
B. caucasica	*Ornithodoros verrucosus*	Iraq, southwestern former U.S.S.R.
B. crocidurae	*O. erraticus* (small variant)	North Africa, Middle East
B. duttonii	*O. moubata*	East and Central Africa
B. hermsii	*O. hermsi*	Western U.S. and Canada
B. hispanica	*O. erraticus* (large variant)	Spain, western North Africa
B. latyschewii	*O. tartakowskyi*	Iran, central Asia
B. mazzottii	*O. talaje*	Mexico, Central America
B. parkeri	*O. parkeri*	Western U.S.
B. persica	*O. tholozani*	Middle East, western Asia
B. turicatae	*O. turicata*	Southwestern U.S., Mexico
B. venezuelensis	*O. rudis*	Northern South America

Data from references 3, 10, 11, and 20.

San Bernardino County, California[16]; and North Rim, Grand Canyon National Park, Arizona,[6, 17] cabins that were the sources of cases were found to contain large rodent nests from which infective ticks were recovered.

PATHOGENESIS AND PATHOLOGY

Borreliae undergo spontaneous antigenic variation both in vivo and in vitro.[46] Repeated episodes of dense spirochetemia (10^5 to 10^8 organisms/mL), each involving a different antigenic variant, account for the cyclic nature of relapsing fever.[31] In relapsing fever borreliae, the immunodominant surface protein is called variable major protein (VMP). In serial passage in mice, progeny of a single organism can give rise to as many as 40 antigenically distinctive VMPs.[1, 27, 40] Different VMPs have some sequence homology but generally differ by considerably more than a single point mutation.[3, 37] The VMP genes of *B. hermsii* are located on multiple copies of linear plasmids. Antigenic variation can be conferred by interplasmidic and intraplasmidic recombination events as well as by point mutations in the VMP gene. The mechanisms are reminiscent of those employed in B cells to generate antibody diversity.[2, 29, 37, 40] With each remission of the disease, antibodies produced against the variant strain result in immobilization, opsonization, and agglutination.[13, 15, 31] Agglutinated organisms are phagocytosed and cleared from the circulation. Experimental animal studies indicate that during remissions, borreliae persist in the central nervous system, bone marrow, spleen, and liver.[21]

Major pathologic findings in fatal cases include widespread petechial hemorrhages of visceral surfaces, splenomegaly and hepatomegaly, often with multiple necrotic foci, and a diffuse histiocytic interstitial myocarditis.[21, 26] Other features of cases with fatal outcome include intercurrent infections, such as pneumonia, salmonellosis, or reactivated malaria; hemorrhages of the central nervous system; meningitis; disseminated intravascular coagulation; splenic rupture; hepatic coma; and cardiac arrhythmia.[21, 26] Borreliae cross the placenta, and infection during pregnancy results in abortion or severe infection of full-term neonates.[22, 45]

CLINICAL MANIFESTATIONS

After an incubation period of 5 to 11 days, relapsing fever has a sudden onset with high fever (39° to 41° C [102.2° to 105.8° F]), chills, headache, and myalgia. An initial illness of 3 to 6 days' duration will be followed by about a week during which the patient is afebrile and feels weak but improved. Relapse occurs with "flu-like" symptoms similar to the initial episode. As many as 10 febrile attacks have been recorded in untreated tick-borne cases. Four episodes is the usual maximum in louse-borne disease. Resolution of febrile attacks, either spontaneously or after antibiotic administration, is by crisis. Relapses become progressively shorter and milder as the afebrile intervals lengthen (Fig. 146–2).[7]

Other clinical features are inconstant and reflect the nature of the infecting organism and the condition of the host. *B. recurrentis* and *B. duttonii* infections are uniformly severe; infections by other species tend to be somewhat milder. Splenomegaly and hepatomegaly, often with associated tenderness, are characteristic. A fleeting macular rash of the trunk, which may become generalized or petechial, is common. Meningeal irritation, iridocyclitis, epistaxis, and myocarditis are more variable in their incidence but may be prominent features.[26, 44] Inflammation at the site of inoculation and regional lymphadenopathy are not seen. Thrombocytopenia, hyperbilirubinemia, and elevated liver enzymes are frequent laboratory abnormalities.

DIAGNOSIS AND DIFFERENTIAL DIAGNOSIS

Although an appropriate history of exposure is by far the most helpful clue to the diagnosis of relapsing fever,[30] physicians caring for patients who have vacationed in distant endemic areas may not consider the possibility. Often it is an alert hematology technician who first makes the diagnosis by recognizing loosely coiled spirochetes in a Wright-stained smear of the patient's peripheral blood. Although routine smears usually are positive while the patient has fever, increased sensitivity is obtained by examination of dehemo-

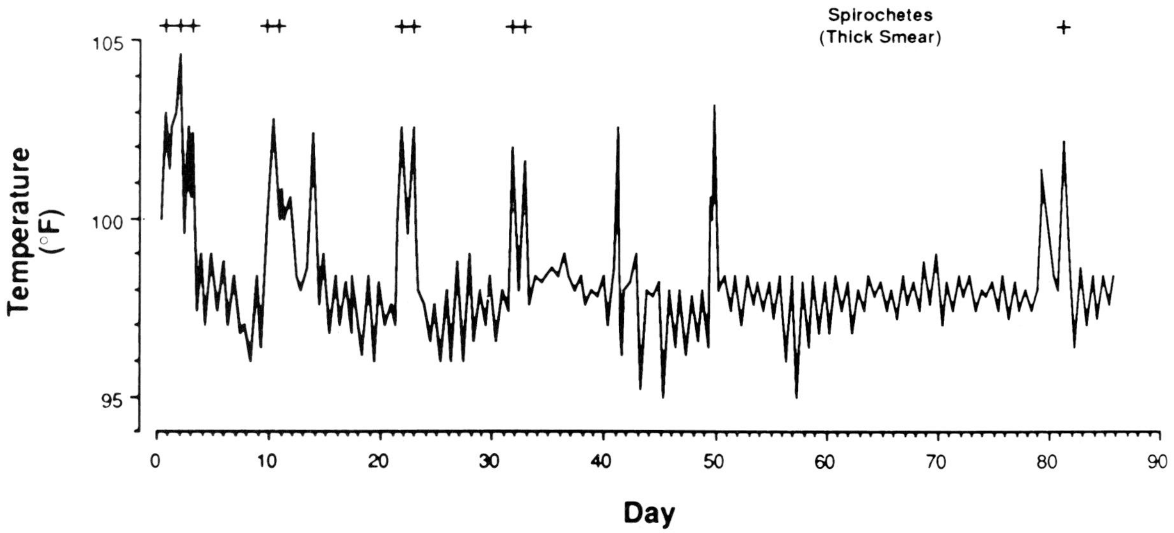

FIGURE 146–2. *Febrile course of untreated tick-borne relapsing fever caused by* Borrelia duttonii. *Thick blood smears were examined for spirochetes on each day of illness, with positive results indicated by a plus sign (+). (Adapted from Breinl, A., Dutton, J. E., Kinghorn, A., et al.: An experimental study of the parasite of the African tick fever. Memoir XXI of the Liverpool School of Tropical Medicine. London, Williams & Norgate, 1906.)*

globinized thick smears or buffy coat preparations stained with Giemsa[23] or acridine orange.[43] Species-specific fluoresceinated monoclonal antibodies further can enhance detection of borreliae in blood smears.[42] Immature laboratory mice, which readily develop spirochetemia after intraperitoneal inoculation with infected blood, provide the most sensitive system for specific diagnosis during the late relapses or remission periods.[20] Because of the fastidiousness of *Borrelia*, routine blood cultures are helpful only in excluding other causes of bacteremia.

Weil-Felix agglutination of *Proteus* OX-K provides supportive evidence of the diagnosis.[51] Indirect fluorescent antibody tests are more sensitive but are limited by species and relapse variations in antigenic content. Moreover, they may yield false-positive results in Lyme disease and other spirochetal infections.[27] Conversely, enzyme-linked immunosorbent assays and immunoblot serologic tests for Lyme disease may yield false-positive results in patients with relapsing fever.[39]

Because of its nonspecific presenting symptoms and spontaneous remissions, relapsing fever may be misdiagnosed as influenza or enteroviral infection. The "saddle back" fever pattern of Colorado tick fever may resemble relapsing fever, but this condition may be recognized by its characteristic leukopenia. Other tick-transmitted illnesses, such as Lyme borreliosis, tularemia, Rocky Mountain spotted fever, and human erlichiosis, may be suggested by a history of tick exposure. In developing countries, malaria, typhoid fever, and rickettsial diseases may show similar clinical findings and are important to differentiate. The microgametocytes of *Plasmodium virax* may look similar to borreliae in a peripheral blood smear.[17a] The periodic fevers, such as familial Mediterranean fever, hyperimmunoglobulin D syndrome, and the "FAPA" syndrome (fever, aphthous stomatitis, pharyngitis, and adenitis) may resemble relapsing fever but generally have longer intervals between febrile episodes.[32] Empiric treatment with broad-spectrum antibiotics may modify the characteristic fever pattern of relapsing fever or cure it before a diagnosis is made.

TREATMENT

Because of difficulties in cultivation, no in vitro data are available to compare the efficacy of antimicrobial agents against relapsing fever borreliae. Oral or parenteral tetracycline, erythromycin, and chloramphenicol are clinically effective, whereas intramuscular procaine penicillin G and oral ampicillin result in relapse rates of about 5 per cent and 30 per cent, respectively. Ceftriaxone and amoxicillin probably also are effective drugs, as indicated by anecdotal experience[33] and by analogy to their efficacy in Lyme disease. The newer macrolides clarithromycin and azithromycin also may have efficacy. Doxycycline (100 mg orally), tetracycline (250 mg intravenously or 500 mg orally), and erythromycin (250 mg intravenously or 500 mg orally) have been used successfully as single-dose regimens for the treatment of adults with louse-borne relapsing fever in Ethiopia.[14, 35, 36] Such regimens have the advantages of low cost and at least partial efficacy against other louse-borne diseases, such as typhus.

Erythromycin is considered the drug of choice for children younger than 8 years of age; tetracycline is considered the drug of choice for older patients. For a febrile patient, however, oral phenoxymethyl penicillin (a single dose of 7.5 mg/kg) or intravenous penicillin G (10,000 units/kg infused over 30 minutes) is recommended as initial therapy. Either should lead to gradual clearance of circulating spirochetes and defervescence. Thereafter, a 10-day course of oral erythromycin or tetracycline (40 mg/kg/day divided every 6 hours) will eradicate tissue spirochetes and prevent relapse.[36] For the afebrile child between relapses, erythromycin or tetracycline may be given alone without initial penicillin therapy.

Other than the choice of antimicrobial therapy, the major concern in treating relapsing fever is the frequent occurrence of the Jarisch-Herxheimer reaction in the first hours after initiating therapy. This response, an exaggeration of the crisis that normally terminates febrile attacks, is characterized by rigors and hyperthermia followed by drenching sweats, hypotension, and prostration.[8] It may be fatal in louse-borne disease but generally is less severe in tick-borne cases. Rapid clearance of blood stream spirochetes initiates the process.[8, 14, 47, 49] Release of inflammatory mediators, such as tumor necrosis factor, interleukin-6, and interleukin-8, after bacterial lysis or phagocytosis probably is the major pathophysiologic mechanism.[4, 12, 13, 15, 34, 38] Three approaches to controlling this response have been tried—supportive measures, gradual killing of spirochetes, and pharmacologic blockade. The usual supportive measures involve volume expansion and antipyretics. Penicillins result in slower elimination of circulating borreliae and yield a more prolonged but less severe reaction than tetracycline or erythromycin.[41, 49] Steroids (e.g., hydrocortisone) and pure opioid antagonists (e.g., naloxone) do not block the reaction. The opioid antagonist and partial agonist meptazinol (available in Great Britain; not licensed in the United States) effectively blocks the reaction.[47] Fekade and colleagues[19] have demonstrated that pretreatment with sheep anti–tumor necrosis factor–α Fab antibody fragments suppresses Jarisch-Herxheimer reactions and reduces the associated increases in plasma concentrations of interleukin-6 and interleukin-8.

At present, the most reasonable approach to limiting Jarisch-Herxheimer reactions is to provide close nursing supervision (either in hospital or in an office or emergency treatment room) during the first 12 hours after therapy. During this period, an intravenous line should be in place. The use of oral penicillin as initial therapy is recommended. Positioning, volume expansion, sponging, and antipyretics should be used as is necessary to control changes in blood pressure, pulse, and temperature.

PROGNOSIS

With current therapy, case fatality rates from relapsing fever are less than 5 per cent.[44] Without treatment, louse-borne disease, in particular, carries a much higher risk of fatality. Late relapses may occur, particularly in cases with an incompletely treated central nervous system "sanctuary."[33] Permanent sequelae are rare. In untreated cases, immunity persists for several years. In treated cases, the duration of immunity is unknown.

PREVENTION

Louse-borne relapsing fever is internationally notifiable to the World Health Organization. Tick-borne relapsing fever is reportable to state health authorities in the United States only in California, but its occurrence in national parks and other public recreational settings makes optional reporting desirable.

Prevention of relapsing fever largely is a problem of avoiding its vectors. In outbreaks of louse-borne disease, time-honored measures, such as environmental dusting with insecticide, cutting hair short, laundering at 49° C (120° F), and applying residual insecticides to clothing and bedding, have been effective.[4a] In individual cases of louse-borne disease, eradication of pediculosis with 5 per cent permethrin or 1 per cent lindane is an essential adjunct to specific therapy.

In endemic foci of tick-borne disease, the habits of *Ornithodoros* and of humans determine the environmental and personal measures necessary.[6, 16, 17] In the United States, increasing utilization of wilderness recreational areas by the public calls for an increased awareness of relapsing fever and its potential transmission. Dwellings in endemic areas should employ "rodent-proof" construction of foundations and soffits. In unsatisfactory buildings, removal of rodent nesting materials and liberal spraying of walls, floors, ceilings, and crawl spaces with 1.1 per cent *o*-isopropoxyphenyl *N*-methylcarbamate (Baygon) or a similar residual insecticide are proven preventive measures.[6] Use of insect repellents has been recommended in some instances, but their effectiveness is not established.

References

1. Barbour, A. G., Barrera, O., and Judd, R. C.: Structural analysis of the variable major proteins of *Borrelia hermsii*. J. Exp. Med. *158*:2127–2140, 1983.
2. Barbour, A. G., Carter, C. J., Burman, N., et al.: Tandem insertion sequence-like elements define the expression site for variable antigen genes of *Borrelia hermsii*. Infect. Immun. *59*:390–397, 1991.
3. Barbour, A. G., and Hayes, S. F.: Biology of *Borrelia* species. Microbiol. Rev. *50*:381–400, 1986.
4. Barbour, A. G., Todd, W. J., and Stoenner, H. G.: Action of penicillin on *Borrelia hermsii*. Antimicrob. Agents Chemother. *21*:823–829, 1982.

4a. Benenson, A. S.: Control of Communicable Diseases Manual: An Official Report of the American Public Health Association. Washington, D. C., The Association, 1995, pp. 345–347, 392–395.

5. Birkhaug, K.: Otto H. F. Obermeier. *In* Moulton, F. R. (ed.): A Symposium on Relapsing Fever in the Americas. Washington, D.C., American Association for the Advancement of Science, 1942, pp. 7–14.
6. Boyer, K. M., Munford, R. S., Maupin, G. O., et al.: Tick-borne relapsing fever: An interstate outbreak originating at Grand Canyon National Park. Am. J. Epidemiol. *105*:469–479, 1977.
7. Breinl, A., Dutton, J. E., Kinghorn, A., et al.: An experimental study of the parasite of the African tick fever. Memoir XXI of the Liverpool School of Tropical Medicine. London, Williams & Norgate, 1906.
8. Bryceson, A. D. M.: Clinical pathology of the Jarisch-Herxheimer reaction. J. Infect. Dis. *133*:696–704, 1976.
9. Bryceson, A. D. M., Parry, E. H. O., Perine, P. L., et al.: Louse-borne relapsing fever. Q. J. Med. *39*:129–170, 1970.
10. Burgdorfer, W.: Epidemiology of the relapsing fevers. *In* Johnson, R. C. (ed.): The Biology of Parasitic Spirochetes. New York, Academic Press, 1976, pp. 191–200.
11. Burgdorfer, W., Rosa, P. A., and Schwan, T. G.: *Borrelia*. *In* Murray, P. R., Barou, E. J., Pfaller, M. A., et al. (eds.): Manual of Clinical Microbiology. Washington, D.C., American Society for Microbiology, 1995, pp. 626–635.
12. Butler, T.: Relapsing fever: New lessons about antibiotic action. Ann. Intern. Med. *102*:397–399, 1985.
13. Butler, T., Aikawa, M., Habte-Michael, A., et al.: Phagocytosis of *Borrelia recurrentis* by blood polymorphonuclear leukocytes is enhanced by antibiotic treatment. Infect. Immun. *28*:1009–1013, 1980.
14. Butler, T., Jones, P. K., and Wallace, C. K.: *Borrelia recurrentis* infection: Single-dose antibiotic regimens and management of the Jarisch-Herxheimer reaction. J. Infect. Dis. *137*:573–577, 1978.
15. Butler, T., Spagnuolo, P. J., Goldsmith, G. H., et al.: Interaction of *Borrelia* spirochetes with human mononuclear leukocytes causes production of leukocytic pyrogen and thromboplastin. J. Lab. Clin. Med. *99*:709–721, 1982.
16. Centers for Disease Control: Common source outbreak of relapsing fever: California. M. M. W. R. *39*:579–586, 1990.
17. Centers for Disease Control: Outbreak of relapsing fever: Grand Canyon National Park, Arizona, 1991. M. M. W. R. *40*:296–303, 1991.

17a. Dworkin, M. S., Anderson, D. E., Thompson, E., et al.: Photo quiz: Relapse of *Plasmodium virax* malaria with the presence of microgametes. Clin. Infect. Dis. *24*:447–448, 1997.

18. Edall, T. A., Emerson, J. K., Maupin, G. O., et al.: Tick-borne relapsing fever in Colorado: Historical review and report of cases. J. A. M. A. *241*:2279–2282, 1979.
19. Fekade, D., Knox, K., Hussein K., et al.: Prevention of Jarisch-Herxheimer reactions by treatment with antibodies against tumor necrosis factor α. N. Engl. J. Med. 335:311–315, 1996.
20. Felsenfeld, O.: *Borrelia*, human relapsing fever, and parasite-vector-host relationships. Bacteriol. Rev. *29*:46–74, 1965.
21. Felsenfeld, O.: *Borrelia*: Strains, Vectors, Human and Animal Borreliosis. St. Louis, Warren H. Green, 1971.
22. Fuchs, P. C., and Oyama, A. A.: Neonatal relapsing fever due to transplacental transmission of *Borrelia*. J. A. M. A. *208*:690–692, 1969.
23. Goldsmid, J. M., and Mahomed, K.: The use of the microhematocrit for the recovery of *Borrelia duttonii* from the blood. Am. J. Clin. Pathol. *58*:165–169, 1972.
24. Horton, J. M., and Blaser, M. J.: The spectrum of relapsing fever in the Rocky Mountains. Arch. Intern. Med. *145*:871–875, 1985.
25. Hyde, F. W., and Johnson, R. C.: Genetic relationship of Lyme disease spirochetes to *Borrelia, Treponema*, and *Leptospira* spp. J. Clin. Microbiol. *20*:151–154, 1984.
26. Judge, D. M., Samuel, I., Perine, P. L., et al.: Louse-borne relapsing fever in man. Arch. Pathol. *97*:136–140, 1974.
27. Kehl, K. S.: Relapsing fever: Role of borrelial antigens. Clin. Microbiol. Newsl. *7*:25–27, 1985.
28. Kelly, R. T.: Cultivation of *Borrelia hermsii*. Science *173*:443–444, 1971.
29. Kitten, T., and Barbour, A. G.: Juxtaposition of expressed variable antigen genes with a conserved telomere in the bacterium *Borrelia hermsii*. Proc. Natl. Acad. Sci. U. S. A. *87*:6077–6081, 1990.
30. Le, C. T.: Tick-borne relapsing fever in children. Pediatrics *66*:963–966, 1980.
31. Meleney, H. E.: Relapse phenomena of *Spironema recurrentis*. J. Exp. Med. *48*:65–82, 1928.
32. Miller, L. C., Sisson, B. A., Tucker, L. B., et al.: Prolonged fevers of unknown origin in children: Patterns of presentation and outcome. J. Pediatr. *129*:419–423, 1996.
33. Nassif, X., Dupont, B., Fleury, J., et al.: Ceftriaxone in relapsing fever. Lancet *2*:394, 1988.
34. Negussie, Y., Remick, D. G., DeForge, L. E., et al.: Detection of plasma tumor necrosis factor, interleukins 6 and 8 during the Jarisch-Herxheimer reaction of relapsing fever. J. Exp. Med. *175*:1207–1212, 1992.
35. Perine, P. L., Krause, D. W., Awoke, S., et al.: Single-dose doxycycline treatment of louse-borne relapsing fever and endemic typhus. Lancet *2*:742–744, 1974.
36. Perine, P. L., and Tekly, B.: Antibiotic treatment of louse-borne relapsing fever in Ethiopia: A report of 377 cases. Am. J. Trop. Med. Hyg. *32*:1096–1100, 1983.
37. Plasterk, R. H. A., Simon, M. I., and Barbour, A. G.: Transposition of structural genes to an expression sequence on a linear plasmid causes antigenic variation in the bacterium *Borrelia hermsii*. Nature *318*:257–263, 1985.
38. Randolph, J. D., Norgard, M. V., Brandt, M. E., et al.: Lipoproteins of *Borrelia burgdorferi* and *Treponema pallidum* activate cachectin/tumor necrosis factor synthesis: Analysis using a CAT reporter construct. J. Immunol. *147*:1968–1974, 1991.
39. Rath, P. U., Ragler, G., Schonberg, A., et al.: Relapsing fever and its serological discrimination from Lyme borreliosis. Infection *20*:283–286, 1992.
40. Restrepo, B. I., and Barbour, A. G.: Antigenic diversity in the bacterium *B. hermsii* through "somatic mutations" in rearranged *vmp* genes. Cell *78*:867–876, 1994.
41. Salih, S. Y., and Mustafa, D.: Louse-borne relapsing fever. II. Combined penicillin and tetracycline therapy in 160 Sudanese patients. Trans. R. Soc. Trop. Med. Hyg. *71*:49–51, 1977.
42. Schwan, T. G., Gage, K. L., Karstens, R. L., et al.: Identification of the tick-borne relapsing fever spirochete *Borrelia hermsii* by using a species-specific monoclonal antibody. J. Clin. Microbiol. *30*:790–795, 1992.
43. Sciotto, C. G., Lauer, B. A., White, W. L., et al.: Detection of *Borrelia* in acridine orange-stained blood smears by fluorescence microscopy. Arch. Pathol. Lab. Med. *107*:384–386, 1983.
44. Southern, P. M., and Sanford, J. P.: Relapsing fever: A clinical and microbiological review. Medicine *48*:129–149, 1969.
45. Steenbarger, J. R.: Congenital tick-borne relapsing fever: Report of a case with first documentation of transplacental transmission. Birth Defects *18*:39–45, 1982.
46. Stoenner, H. G., Dodd, T., and Larsen, C.: Antigenic variation of *Borrelia hermsii*. J. Exp. Med. *156*:1297–1311, 1982.
47. Teklu, B., Habte-Michael, A., Warrell, D. A., et al.: Meptazinol diminishes the Jarisch-Herxheimer reaction of relapsing fever. Lancet *1*:835–839, 1983.
48. Thompson, R. S., Burgdorfer, W., Russell, R., et al.: Outbreak of tick-borne relapsing fever in Spokane County, Washington. J. A. M. A. *310*:1045–1050, 1969.
49. Warrell, D. A., Perine, P. L., Krause, D. W., et al.: Pathophysiology and immunology of the Jarisch-Herxheimer reaction in louse-borne relapsing fever: Comparison of tetracycline and slow release penicillin. J. Infect. Dis. *147*:898–909, 1983.
50. Wynns, H. L.: The epidemiology of relapsing fever. *In* Moulton, F. R. (ed.): A Symposium on Relapsing Fever in the Americas. Washington, D.C., American Association for the Advancement of Science, 1942, pp. 100–105.
51. Zarafonetis, C. J. D., Ingraham, H. S., and Berry, J. F.: Weil-Felix and typhus complement-fixation tests in relapsing fever, with special reference to *B. proteus* OX-K agglutination. J. Immunol. *52*:189–199, 1946.

147

BORRELIA (LYME DISEASE)

Barbara W. Stechenberg

Lyme disease, recognized initially in 1975, first was brought to medical attention through the concern of two mothers from Lyme, Connecticut; one contacted the Connecticut State Health Department, and the other contacted physicians at Yale about the unusual illness spreading through their community, a small town about 15 km north of Long Island Sound near the mouth of the Connecticut River. Their inquiries sparked an intensive clinical and epidemiologic investigation that has yielded much of the information about this disorder—its wide spectrum of clinical manifestations, etiology, pathogenesis, and treatment.

From these investigations, a distinct pattern of signs and symptoms emerged as a newly described disorder. Actually, the characteristic skin lesions soon were recognized as erythema (chronicum) migrans, a skin lesion that had been associated with a similar, but more limited, illness in Europe since the early 1920s.

THE ORGANISM

Because of certain epidemiologic characteristics, particularly the geographic and seasonal clustering of cases, an infectious etiology, particularly associated with an arthropod or other vector, was sought. Early speculation that Lyme disease might be caused by a virus diminished with the report of rapid resolution of erythema migrans and other symptoms with early treatment with penicillin or tetracycline.[87]

In 1982, Burgdorfer and associates[17] isolated a *Treponema*-like spirochete from the midgut of the tick *Ixodes dammini*. The spirochete has irregular coils ranging in size from 10 to 30 μm in length and from 0.18 to 0.25 μm in diameter. Electron microscopy demonstrates their close association with the microvillar brush border of intestinal epithelium.

When infected *I. dammini* ticks were allowed to feed on New Zealand white rabbits, there was no immediate adverse effect. However, 10 to 12 weeks after tick engorgement, small skin lesions developed that progressed into typical erythema migrans. The sera of all exposed rabbits yielded high titers of antibody to the spirochetes by indirect immunofluorescence. Sera from nine patients with clinically diagnosed Lyme disease also demonstrated positive reactions.[17]

The etiologic role of these spirochetes has been defined further. Steere and associates[85] isolated the spirochete from blood, skin, and cerebrospinal fluid of 3 of 56 patients with Lyme disease and from 21 of 110 *I. dammini* ticks studied. More than 90 per cent of the patients had a characteristic IgM and IgG antibody response; IgM antibody titers reached a peak between the third and sixth weeks after onset, and IgG antibodies rose slowly to reach a peak when arthritis was present. Benach and associates[12] isolated the same spirochete from 2 of 36 patients with Lyme disease in New York. These patients also had a similar rise in antispirochetal antibodies. Berger and his group[15] demonstrated the spirochete in 6 of 14 patients in whom the cutaneous lesions of erythema migrans were studied; 4 of these 6 positive specimens were obtained from the peripheries of lesions. Berger was able to demonstrate the organisms in secondary lesions.[15]

Although morphologically similar to known pathogenic *Treponema* organisms, the *I. dammini* spirochete is distinctive because it grows on artificial media. Growth of this fastidious, microaerophilic organism occurs best at 33° C in a complex liquid medium called Barbour-Stoenner-Kelly medium.[7] The organism has an apparent slime layer, an outer membrane that is associated loosely with the underlying structures, flagella (7 to 11), a cell wall, and cytoplasmic constituents.[85] It is coiled more loosely and is longer than other spirochetes. It resembles borreliae most closely and has been designated *Borrelia burgdorferi*.

B. burgdorferi contains many different proteins. Six outer-membrane proteins have been identified—outer-surface protein A (OspA) (molecular weight 30 to 32 kDa), outer-surface protein B (OspB) (34 kDa), outer-surface protein C (OspC) (22 to 25 kDa), outer-surface protein D (OspD) (28 to 30 kDa), outer-surface protein E (OspE) (19 kDa), and outer-surface protein F (OspF (26 kDa)—that act as surface antigens. Other polypeptides include the 41-kDa flagellar antigen, several heat shock proteins, and a 93-kDa antigen that is part of the protoplasmic cylinder. A 49-kilobase linear plasmid contains genes that encode for the two major outer surface proteins, OspA and OspB.[8] In fact, all isolates of *B. burgdorferi* examined have had four to nine pieces of extrachromosomal plasmid DNA, both supercoiled and linear.[9]

Strain differences in DNA and plasmid composition,[52] ultrastructure, and outer-surface proteins have been identified between American and European strains, with the European strains generally being more diverse. Three genomic groups of the *B. burgdorferi* sensu lato complex now have been identified using several methods. To date, all North American strains have belonged to group *B. burgdorferi* sensu stricto. All three groups have been found in Europe, but group 2, *B. garinii*, and group 3, *B. afzelii*, are more common.[6, 18] These differences may account for variability in clinical expression.

EPIDEMIOLOGY

Evidence for the tick vector had accumulated early in the investigations. During 1977, the incidence of Lyme disease was 30 times greater on the eastern bank of the Connecticut River than on the western shore.[81, 92] Case-control studies of patients, mainly children and young adults, and their neighbors revealed that patients did not participate in more outdoor activities but were more likely to have a cat or farm animal, a pet with ticks, or a tick bite in the year of the study. Ixodid ticks were identified as the likely vector. These ticks have a complex life cycle that spans 2 years, during which they feed once during each of their three stages. In the United States, the white-footed mouse is the preferred host for both the larval and the nymph stages. The larvae feed in late summer, the nymphs in spring or early summer. It is important that this animal is the host for both of these stages and that it is tolerant to infection. It is the host-seeking behavior of the nymphs in late May that initiates the Lyme disease season each year. Although the prevalence of spirochetes in this stage (20 to 25 per cent) is approximately half that found in the adult, nymphs are responsible for nearly

90 per cent of Lyme disease cases.[34] This may be related to their smaller size, their greater abundance, and the coincidence of their peak feeding activity with human outdoor activity. The white-tailed deer is the preferred host for the adult stages and acts as the reservoir over winter months. The adult tick feeds in the fall or winter.

Since the association of the *Ixodes* genus of tick with a large number of cases reported from the Lyme, Connecticut, area, Lyme disease has been reported in at least 46 states and now is the most common vector-borne disease in the United States. The major geographic areas with clusters of cases include the eastern seaboard (particularly from Massachusetts to Maryland), the upper Midwest (Wisconsin and Minnesota), and the West (California, Nevada, Utah, and Oregon). Massachusetts, Rhode Island, Connecticut, New York, New Jersey, Wisconsin, and Minnesota account for 90 per cent of cases. In the East, the tick associated with disease is the *I. dammini* or *scapularis* tick; in the West, it is *I. pacificus*.

In Europe, cases of erythema migrans with and without meningopolyneuritis have occurred within the range of the *I. ricinus* tick, although one case described outside the range of this vector has been ascribed to mosquito bites.[72] Isolated cases over a wide distribution, including Australia, where none of the vectors recognized currently are known to exist, suggest that the disease may be more widespread than first realized and may have a broader range of potential vectors. In fact, there is evidence that *Amblyomma americanum* (lone star) ticks also harbor the organism.[73] This particularly is important because of its large range. Mosquitoes and deer flies may become infected with the organism but do not appear to be able to transmit the organism to humans.[55]

B. burgdorferi is widespread in the animal kingdom. Virtually any feral or domestic animal can act as an intermediate host. Birds frequently are carriers and may account for the unusual dispersal pattern of Lyme disease.[3] The greatest reservoir continues to be white-footed mice and deer. Wild animals do not develop illness; however, clinical Lyme disease may occur in domestic animals, such as dogs and horses.

As expected with this vector, the disease has a high occurrence in the summer and early fall, with clustering of patients in wooded and sparsely settled areas. The age range of reported cases has been from 2 to 88 years, with a slight male predominance.

PATHOGENESIS

Lyme disease appears to result from direct infection by and the immune response of the host to *B. burgdorferi*. The spirochete is injected into the blood stream through the saliva of the tick or deposited on the skin in fecal material.[13] After an incubation period of from 3 to 32 days, the spirochete may invade or migrate to the skin, causing erythema migrans, or enter the blood stream, migrating to distant sites. The organism has shown in vitro resistance to elimination by phagocytic cells, thereby increasing infectivity of the spirochete.[36] It has been isolated from cerebrospinal fluid in patients with neurologic symptoms up to 10 weeks after the initial tick bite. Success with antibiotic treatment provides evidence that the spirochete still is alive when arthritis is present.[84] The late complications probably are caused by a direct effect of infection with viable organisms and the immunologic response to them. The spirochete can adhere to many different types of mammalian cells and is a potent inducer of tumor necrosis factor and interleukin-1β and interleukin-6.[42] In a rat model, permeability changes in the blood-brain barrier begin within 12 hours of inoculation of the organism, and the spirochete can be cultured from cerebrospinal fluid within 24 hours.[35]

Initially, the immune response seems to be suppressed, which may aid dissemination. The specific IgM response peaks between the third and sixth weeks of infection. It often is associated with polyclonal activation of B cells, causing elevated total serum IgM levels, circulating immune complexes, and cryoglobulins.[45] The specific IgG response develops initially over the first 6 to 8 weeks but then matures over months with the development of a wide array of antibodies to both protein and nonprotein antigens. The unusual persistence of the IgM response in patients with severe disease suggests that such patients have a defect in their helper T-cell function necessary to switch from IgM to IgG production.[85] Patients with severe and prolonged illness, particularly arthritis or neurologic disease, often have the B-cell alloantigen HLA-DR4.[83]

Histologically, all affected tissues show infiltration of lymphocytes and plasma cells. Some degree of vascular damage may be seen in many sites, suggesting that the organism may have been in or around the vessels. *B. burgdorferi* seems to survive for long periods in certain areas, particularly the skin, nervous system, and joints. How it does this is an area of intense research.

CLINICAL MANIFESTATIONS

The clinical findings in Lyme disease can be divided into three stages on the basis of chronologic relationship to the original bite. In the first stage, the skin lesions are most prominent; in the second stage, cardiac and neurologic findings predominate; and in the third stage, arthritis is most common. Any of these findings may occur in isolation or recurrently. Asbrink and Hovmark[4] have proposed a clinical classification analogous to that of syphilis, with early infection divided into stage 1 (localized erythema migrans), followed days to weeks later by stage 2 (early disseminated infection), with late or persistent infection as stage 3.

The most common of the clinical manifestations is the skin rash, erythema migrans (Fig. 147–1). This rash usually begins 3 to 30 days after a tick bite, although only about one-third of patients give a specific history of a bite. This may relate to the small size of the tick. An erythematous macule or papule forms at the site of the bite. This gradually enlarges to form a large, plaque-like, erythematous annular lesion. The median diameter is 16 cm, but it may reach 68 cm.[16] The outer border usually is erythematous and flat, although it may be indurated. The middle area may show clearing, but the center sometimes is indurated or erythematous or may have vesicles. The lesions often are hot to touch and otherwise asymptomatic but may burn, prickle, or itch. They may occur on any area of the body; usual sites include the thigh, buttocks, and axillae; intertriginous areas; or places where underwear may be tight. Mucosal lesions do not occur. Multiple secondary annular lesions occur in 20 to 50 per cent of the patients, usually within a few days of the primary lesion. These secondary lesions are evidence of dissemination (stage 2).

The average duration of the initial skin lesion is about 3 weeks. It gradually resolves, sometimes with a bluish hue as it fades. Lesions can recur for up to a year or more, often coincident with subsequent attacks of arthritis. Among patients treated with appropriate antibiotics, the lesions usually resolve within several days.

The skin lesions often are associated with systemic symptoms, most commonly malaise, fatigue, headache, stiff neck, and arthralgias; additionally, there may be backache, myal-

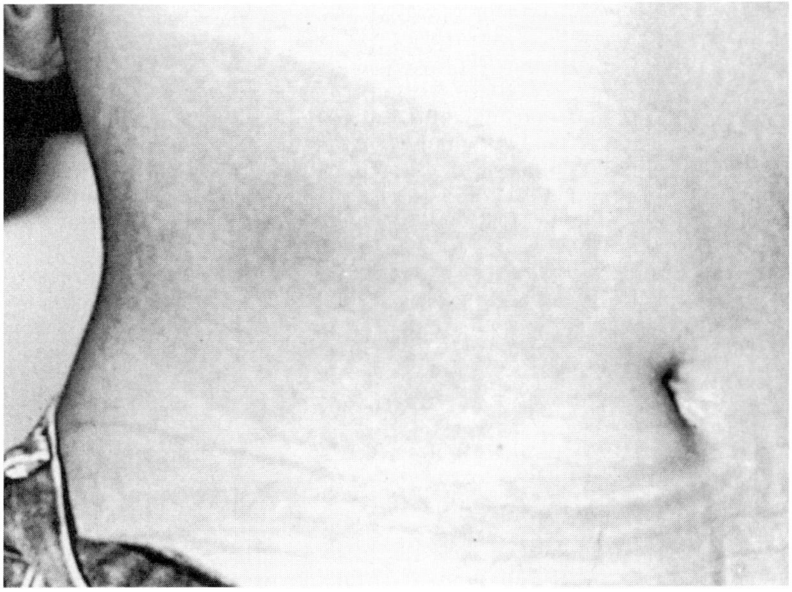

FIGURE 147–1. *The typical skin lesion of Lyme disease, erythema (chronicum) migrans. The lesion had progressed from about 3 cm to this size within a week. (Courtesy of Drs. Jane Grant-Kels and Nadine Wenner.)*

gias, nausea, vomiting, and sore throat. Fever usually is low-grade but can be as high as 40° C with chills. Fever is more common in children than adults.[94] Lymphadenopathy, usually regional and associated with erythema migrans but occasionally generalized, may occur. Occasionally, a malar rash, conjunctivitis, or pharyngitis is present. In about 10 per cent of patients, signs and symptoms consistent with anicteric hepatitis, including hepatomegaly and right upper quadrant tenderness, are present. Most symptoms resolve over a few days, but some patients experience intermittent and fluctuating symptoms over a period of several weeks. Feder and associates[32] described a group of five children who presented with a flu-like illness without erythema migrans that was documented serologically as Lyme disease.

Another skin lesion seen in early disseminated disease is *Borrelia* lymphocytoma. Seen in Europe in about 1 per cent of cases of Lyme disease, it usually presents as a firm, red, red-brown, or red-purple nodule or papule, seen principally on the pinna of the ear in children or on the nipple or areola on adults.[56]

The late skin manifestation is acrodermatitis chronica atrophicans, a progressive dermatologic condition that develops slowly with increasing erythema and pigmentation changes of the skin of an extremity, which spreads over its extensor surface. After initial hyperpigmentation, hypopigmented areas develop, and eventually the skin becomes frail. It is seen primarily in European cases. This condition has been associated with elevated antibodies to *B. burgdorferi* and response to antibiotic therapy.[59] Other associated lesions are fibrotic nodules, other sclerotic and atrophic lesions, and, rarely, eosinophilic fasciitis and progressive facial hemiatrophy.[40, 56]

Although early Lyme disease can cause symptoms of meningeal irritation and headache, they usually are benign and self-limited. Neurologic abnormalities occur roughly within 4 weeks (range, 2 to 11 weeks but can be up to months) after the tick bite. The spectrum of involvement is wide, including aseptic meningitis, meningoencephalitis, chorea, cerebellar ataxia, cranial neuritis, radiculopathies, mononeuritis multiplex, and myelitis.[24, 43, 65] The most common is aseptic meningitis, presenting with headache and stiff neck, often associated with nausea and vomiting, sensory disturbance, photophobia, and irritability. Cerebrospinal fluid findings are similar to those seen in patients with viral meningitis. The symptoms may occur intermittently for weeks, with mild headache persisting between attacks until spontaneous remission occurs. Up to two-thirds of adult patients exhibit subtle findings of parenchymal abnormality or encephalitis[33] with somnolence, emotional lability, memory loss, poor concentration, or behavioral changes. In a series of children with neurologic manifestations, behavior changes that did not predate the Lyme disease were rare, as were meningoradiculitis and peripheral neuropathy syndromes.[11]

The seventh cranial nerve is involved most frequently in Lyme disease; unilateral or bilateral facial palsies occur in up to 11 per cent of patients.[20] Seventh nerve palsy is seen in about 50 per cent of patients with meningitis; it also can occur alone. Other cranial nerves, particularly III and IV, are involved less frequently. Several children with pseudotumor cerebri in association with Lyme disease have been reported.[11, 40, 64]

It has become clear that neurologic involvement can occur in the third stage of illness months to years after the initial infection. These patients present with neuropsychiatric symptoms, focal central nervous system disease, or, rarely, severe incapacitating fatigue.[43, 61] These findings are extremely rare in children.[11, 75]

Conjunctivitis is an infrequent early ophthalmologic manifestation that usually is transient.[78] A case has been described of iritis progressing to panophthalmitis and unilateral blindness.[82] Spirochetes consistent with *B. burgdorferi* were found in vitreous debris. Other eye manifestations include optic neuritis, iritis, and keratitis.[10]

Cardiac abnormalities occur in about 10 per cent of patients, usually within several weeks (average, 5 weeks; range, 3 to 21 weeks after the bite). Seen most commonly in young adult males, they range from fluctuating degrees of atrioventricular block to myopericarditis and left ventricular dysfunction.[58, 79] Cardiac involvement usually is brief (3 days to 6 weeks). Patients with cardiac involvement usually have other evidence of more severe systemic disease, such as fever, rash, arthritis, or neurologic findings. Although described in children, these cardiac findings are uncommon among pediatric patients.

The second most common manifestation of Lyme disease after erythema migrans is arthritis, which occurs in approximately half of the patients without treatment.[25, 88] It begins typically 4 weeks after the skin lesion (5 to 6 weeks after the bite), although the time span can vary from less than 1 week to many months, and a small percentage of patients do not recall any skin lesions. The arthritis usually is of sudden onset, monoarticular or oligoarticular, and occasionally migratory. Large joints, often those closest to the initial rash, are affected most commonly. The knee is by far the joint involved most frequently, followed by the shoulder, elbow, temporomandibular joint, ankle, wrist, and hip.[28] They become swollen, warm, and painful but rarely red. The usual duration of the first episode is about 1 week, but sometimes the episode persists for several months.

Recurrent attacks of arthritis are common. Among the initial 51 patients studied, 35 (69 per cent) had recurrent attacks.[78, 88] The median number of recurrent attacks was three. During recurrences, usually more joints are involved than in the initial episode. These attacks last about 1 week, with intervals of 1 week to 2 years between attacks. Children experience complete remissions between attacks; however, adults often have persistent asymptomatic joint effusions or mild morning stiffness. Approximately 10 per cent of all patients with Lyme disease develop a severe chronic erosive arthritis; this occurs about 1 year after the initial manifestations and often is associated with HLA-DR4.[83] A rare, unusual complication is rupture of a Baker cyst, which causes a pseudothrombophlebitis.

Other unusual manifestations of Lyme disease include recurrent hepatitis,[39] myositis,[5] eosinophilic lymphadenitis,[63] and adult respiratory distress syndrome.[51]

Maternal-fetal transmission of *B. burgdorferi* has been documented in two infants, one with congenital heart disease,[71] the other with encephalitis.[93] Neither case had evidence of tissue inflammation. A stillbirth after maternal Lyme disease also has been reported.[54] An analysis of 19 cases of Lyme disease during pregnancy revealed five pregnancies (26 per cent) with adverse outcomes. These occurred in all three trimesters, and no two were the same.[57] In a study of 463 infants, no association between congenital malformations and the presence of antibody to *B. burgdorferi* in cord blood or IgM antibody could be established.[95]

Strobino and associates,[90] in a prospective study of approximately 2000 pregnant women in an endemic area, found no evidence of fetal wasting, prematurity, or congenital malformations attributable to Lyme disease. Gerber and Zalneraitis[38] surveyed pediatric neurologists in a large endemic area to determine the prevalence of clinically significant nervous system disease that might be attributable to transplacental transmission; they found no cases that met their case definition.

The association of Lyme disease with adverse fetal outcomes appears to be unusual; however, continued surveillance of pregnant women as well as prompt diagnosis and treatment should be emphasized.

DIFFERENTIAL DIAGNOSIS

When the characteristic erythema migrans rash is present and recognized, there should be little problem identifying the etiology of subsequent symptoms. However, particularly when the presentation is atypical, the differential diagnosis is broad.

If the rash is not recognized as erythema migrans, it may be confused with streptococcal cellulitis. Erythema multiforme might be a consideration, but the lesions in that disorder often are smaller and urticarial or vesicular, are seen on mucosal surfaces, and are associated often with drug exposure. Erythema marginatum usually is smaller and less annular. If there is a necrotic or vesicular center in the erythema migrans lesion, it may resemble the lesion of tularemia, but the latter is not expansive and not associated with similar complications. Occasionally, a superficial reaction to a tick bite proves confusing, but usually the time course helps. There should be a hiatus of at least 3 days between the bite and erythema migrans.

It particularly is important to distinguish Lyme disease from acute rheumatic fever. If the skin lesion is misdiagnosed and migratory arthritis is noted in association with nonspecific electrocardiographic changes, such as prolonged PR interval, one erroneously may assume that the modified Jones criteria have been fulfilled. Fortunately, in Lyme disease, there usually is no evidence of antecedent streptococcal infection, and the specific natures of rheumatologic and cardiac involvement are different.

Other forms of arthritis that may be confused with Lyme disease include (1) pauciarticular juvenile rheumatoid arthritis, (2) psoriatic arthritis, (3) reactive arthritis associated with *Salmonella, Shigella,* or *Yersinia* infections, (4) Reiter syndrome, and (5) postinfectious or infectious arthritis, such as that associated with rubella, hepatitis B, or echoviruses. Several distinctive features usually allow prompt differentiation from Lyme disease.

The major neurologic manifestation of aseptic meningitis may be confused with enteroviral, leptospiral, or early tuberculous meningitis. When it becomes more chronic and relapsing, one must consider sarcoidosis, Mollaret meningitis, Behçet disease, and multiple sclerosis.

SPECIFIC DIAGNOSIS

The diagnosis of Lyme disease is made best on clinical and epidemiologic grounds and often can be established early in the course of illness from the gross appearance of erythema migrans.

Routine laboratory testing usually is nonspecific and not helpful. The sedimentation rate often is elevated. Leukocyte counts commonly are normal. Serum glutamic-oxaloacetic transaminase and serum glutamic-pyruvic transaminase levels may be elevated mildly early in the disease. Complement studies may be normal, low, or high. Serum IgG and IgA usually are normal; however, IgM and cryoglobulin IgM often are elevated, particularly in those patients with severe disease or those patients who later develop neurologic complications or arthritis. Immune complexes as measured by Clq binding (or other methods) may be found in patients with Lyme disease and may be involved in the pathogenesis. They may be present at the time of diagnosis and then clear in those patients without neurologic or cardiac involvement or localize to the synovium in those with arthritis.[45]

Examination of the synovial fluid in patients with arthritis demonstrates elevated leukocyte counts from 500 to 98,000 cells/mm^3 with a predominance of polymorphonuclear leukocytes. Total protein usually is between 3 and 8 g/dL.

Patients with aseptic meningitis often have cerebrospinal fluid pleocytosis, with counts ranging from 25 to 450 cells/mm^3, usually with a lymphocytic predominance. Total protein may be elevated mildly, and glucose levels (cerebrospinal fluid/blood ratio) usually are normal.

The yield from cultures and direct visualization techniques is too low to make them practical for diagnosis. Therefore, serology currently is the only practical laboratory technique for diagnosis. Although indirect immunofluorescence first was used to evaluate the immune response to *B. burgdorferi*, the enzyme-linked immunosorbent assay appears to be more sensitive and specific.[22, 69] However, there is no standardization of testing, and interlaboratory variation in results may be marked.[46] Any serologic results must be interpreted with care. Serologic testing only should be undertaken when the clinical and epidemiologic investigation suggests Lyme disease as the diagnosis.

False-negative results are common early in the infection.[77] However, Berardi and associates[14] have developed a sensitive capture IgM enzyme-linked immunosorbent assay that demonstrates an IgM response in up to 90 per cent of patients with early disease. Some patients treated with antibiotics early in the disease may not show an antibody response. In one study, 17 patients with a variety of symptoms were found to be seronegative but to have mononuclear cells with a proliferative response to *B. burgdorferi*.[26] The significance of such responses remains to be seen, but this finding should be considered extremely uncommon.

New techniques to increase sensitivity, specificity, or both include enzyme-linked immunosorbent assay using flagellar antigen,[44] immunoblotting,[41] and polymerase chain reaction.[60] Immunoblotting, particularly, may be used to identify false-positive results.[68] The Western blot or immunoblotting separates surface and subsurface proteins of *B. burgdorferi* by polyacrylamide gel electrophoresis, which then are reacted with patients' sera. This technique is more specific than enzyme-linked immunosorbent or immunofluorescent assay and particularly is useful to identify false-positive results.[37, 41, 68]

The Centers for Disease Control and Prevention, as a result of a national conference on serologic diagnosis of Lyme disease, recommends a two-test approach for active disease and for previous infection using a sensitive enzyme immunoassay or immunofluorescent assay followed by a Western blot if the initial test is positive or equivocal.[19] Negative results need not be validated. For Western blot in the first 4 weeks of disease, both IgM and IgG procedures should be performed. A positive IgM test result alone is not recommended for use for determining active disease in persons with illnesses of greater than 1 month's duration because of a high false-positive rate for current infection. If serologic results in a patient with suspected early Lyme disease are negative, paired acute and convalescent specimens should be obtained. Serum samples from persons with disseminated or late-stage disease almost always have a strong IgG response to *B. burgdorferi* antigens. It is recommended that an IgM immunoblot result be considered positive if two of the following three bands are present: 24 kDa (OspC), 39 kDa (BmpA), and 41 kDa (Fla).[31] An IgG immunoblot result is considered positive if 5 of the following 10 bands are present: 18 kDa, 21 kDa (OspC), 28 kDa, 30 kDa, 39 kDa (BmpA0), 41 kDa (Fla), 45 kDa, 58 kDa, 66 kDa, and 93 kDa.[29]

In addition to false-positive results, 5 to 10 per cent of patients in the United States have asymptomatic *B. burgdorferi* infection; these serologic results may interfere with the diagnosis of another significant illness.

Polymerase chain reaction has been used to amplify and detect *B. burgdorferi* DNA in cultured spirochetes, infected animals, and patients with Lyme disease.[60, 66, 74] DNA sequences can be detected in blood, urine, cerebrospinal fluid, skin, and synovial fluid. *B. burgdorferi* DNA was detected in 75 of 88 synovial fluid samples from patients with Lyme disease.[60] The usefulness of polymerase chain reaction in clinical situations is an area of active research, but its use may be limited by problems with sensitivity and specificity.[60, 66, 74]

The diagnosis of neurologic manifestations of Lyme disease particularly is difficult. Comparing intrathecal antibody assay results with serum results may be helpful.[80]

Because of the delay in specific antibody response and the possible ablation of this response in patients with localized disease who are treated early, recognition of the clinical picture—erythema migrans, a "flu-like" or "meningitis-like" illness in the summer, or both—is essential for prompt diagnosis and treatment.

TREATMENT

Even before the spirochete was identified as the causative agent of Lyme disease, antibiotic treatment of adults with penicillin or tetracycline was associated with more rapid resolution of the rash and its associated symptoms.[87] Subsequent studies have confirmed that impression; tetracycline may be more effective in preventing late complications (meningoencephalitis, myocarditis, and arthritis) of the disease.[86] None of 88 patients treated with tetracycline developed such complications, compared with 7.5 per cent (3 of 40) of a group of patients treated with penicillin. However, nearly half of all treated patients still had minor late symptoms, such as headache, musculoskeletal pain, and lethargy. These complications correlated significantly with the initial severity of illness.

Antibiotic sensitivities to *B. burgdorferi* have been determined in vitro and in experimental animals.[47, 49] Although the methods are not standardized, there is general agreement that the organism is highly sensitive to tetracycline. It also is susceptible to ampicillin, ceftriaxone, and imipenem. Unlike *Treponema pallidum*, *B. burgdorferi* is only moderately sensitive to penicillin. Aminoglycosides and rifampin have no activity, whereas oxacillin and chloramphenicol are only moderately active. Erythromycin appears active in vitro but may be less so in vivo.

In fact, azithromycin and clarithromycin both are more active, although the clinical efficacy of either is controversial.[27] Newer oral cephalosporins, particularly cefixime and cefuroxime axetil, hold promise.[2, 48] Cefuroxime axetil was comparable with doxycycline in a clinical trial in patients with early Lyme disease.[53]

Recommendations for treatment continue to evolve. For early Lyme disease, oral tetracycline, 250 mg orally four times a day, or doxycycline, 100 mg twice a day for 10 to 30 days, is effective for adults and children older than 8 years of age. In younger children, amoxicillin, 30 to 50 mg/kg/day in three divided doses, for the same duration appears to be the best choice, with cefuroxime axetil, 30 to 40 mg/kg/day in two divided doses, as an alternative. For penicillin-allergic children who cannot tolerate a cephalosporin, erythromycin, 30 to 50 mg/kg/day in four divided doses, for the same period may be used, although its efficacy is less clear. The duration of treatment is based on clinical response.

Patients with isolated seventh nerve palsy should be treated with oral regimens to prevent further complications. If the palsy is associated with other neurologic complications, parenteral therapy should be initiated.

Adults with neurologic complications, particularly Lyme meningitis, have been treated successfully with large doses of penicillin G (20 million IU/day).[89] No large trials have been reported in children; however, penicillin, 300,000 IU/kg/day, appeared to be beneficial in two cases of pseudotumor cerebri.[64]

Patients with established Lyme arthritis also have been treated successfully with high-dose penicillin but without universal efficacy.[84] In an uncontrolled study of 33 children with arthritis, 31 were treated with oral therapy alone for 3 to 4 weeks, with elimination of synovitis and recurrent attacks.[23, 30] This approach can be considered for arthritis in children, although parenteral therapy may be necessary.

The exquisite sensitivity of the organism to ceftriaxone makes it an attractive alternative for parenteral therapy, and it has become the drug of choice. The dose of ceftriaxone is 75 to 100 mg/kg/day up to 2 g a day. In a study of 23 patients with late Lyme disease, Dattwyler and associates[25] reported superior efficacy of ceftriaxone over penicillin. Cefotaxime is a reasonable alternative. The duration of parenteral therapy for neurologic or rheumatologic disease is not clear but should be a minimum of 14 days.

The self-limited nature of the acute arthritis obviates the need for any analgesics other than acetaminophen or nonsteroidal anti-inflammatory agents. Patients with chronic arthritis usually have been treated with the nonsteroidal anti-inflammatory agents.

Patients with cardiac complications usually do not require specific treatment other than an oral antibiotic regimen, although those with heart block may require temporary pacing.[79]

PROGNOSIS AND PREVENTION

Most patients with Lyme disease, particularly those treated promptly with an appropriate antibiotic, have an uncomplicated course. Series in children point to an excellent prognosis in most cases. A review of 65 children treated for erythema migrans and followed for a mean of more than 3 years found them all to be well and without findings of late Lyme disease.[70] Another prospective study of children with newly diagnosed disease of any stage found that all the children were cured.[75] Rose and associates[67] described 44 children with arthritis who all had an excellent prognosis. A study of cognitive sequelae in children treated for Lyme disease showed no differences between the Lyme disease and control groups.[1] In fact, a study of children with arthritis who initially were untreated for at least 4 years found few children with late or chronic problems.[91]

For the small percentage with chronic arthritis, the course may be variable, although the illness may resolve after 12 to 16 months. With earlier treatment, this group should be held to a minimum.

The prompt recognition of this disease with its diverse manifestations should lead to early treatment and resolution. The only prevention is avoidance of contact with the tick vector.

Even in endemic areas where a large percentage of the ticks are infected, the chance of acquiring disease is not great and depends in part on the duration of attachment of the tick. Attachment for more than 24 hours may be required.[62] A small study of prophylactic antibiotics for tick bites showed a low risk of acquiring disease that was similar to the risk of adverse reaction to penicillin.[21] In a study of prophylaxis after tick bites in a highly endemic area, the risk of infection in the placebo-treated group was only 1.2 per cent. The authors concluded that, even in an endemic area, the use of routine prophylactic antibiotics is not indicated.[76] However, there may be situations such as a highly engorged tick on a pregnant woman, in which prophylaxis might be considered. Ten days of oral therapy should be adequate.

Important preventive measures include (1) avoiding high-risk areas, particularly wooded, grassy areas, (2) when walking in such areas, wearing light-colored, long pants tucked into socks, sneakers, and long-sleeved shirts, (3) using insect repellents such as DEET (for skin) and permethrin (for clothing), (4) most important, conducting careful "tick patrols" every day or after every potential exposure to look carefully for the ticks, and (5) removing ticks by pulling them straight out with tweezers or protected fingers.

Active immunization against *B. burgdorferi* actively is being pursued. A phase I trial of a recombinant OspA vaccine showed it to be safe and immunogenic.[50]

References

1. Adams, W. V., Rose, C. D., Eppes, S. C., et al.: Cognitive effects of Lyme disease in children. Pediatrics *94*:185–189, 1994.
2. Agger, W. A., Callister, S. M., and Jobe, D. A.: In vitro susceptibles of *Borrelia burgdorferi* to five oral cephalosporins and ceftriaxone. Antimicrob. Agents Chemother. *36*:1788–1790, 1995.
3. Anderson, J. F., and Magnarelli, L. A.: Avian and mammalian hosts for spirochete-infected ticks and insects in a Lyme disease focus in Connecticut. Yale J. Biol. Med. *57*:627–641, 1984.
4. Asbrink, E., and Hovmark, A.: Early and late cutaneous manifestations of Ixodes-borne borreliosis (erythema migrans borreliosis, Lyme borreliosis). Ann. N. Y. Acad. Sci. *539*:4–15, 1988.
5. Atlas, E., Novak, S. N., Duray, P. H., et al.: Lyme myositis: Muscle invasion by *Borrelia burgdorferi*. Ann. Intern. Med. *109*:245–246, 1988.
6. Baranton, G, Postic, D. Saint-Girons, I., et al.: Delineation of *Borrelia Burgdorferi* sensu stricto, *Borrelia garinii* sp. nov. and group VS461 associated with Lyme borreliosis. Int. Syst. Bacteriol. *42*:378–383, 1992.
7. Barbour, A. G.: Isolation and cultivation of Lyme disease spirochetes. Yale J. Biol. Med. *57*:521–525, 1984.
8. Barbour, A. G.: The molecular biology of Borrelia. Rev. Infect. Dis. *11*:S1470–S1474, 1989.
9. Barbour, A. G.: Plasmid analysis of *Borrelia burgdorferi*, the Lyme disease agent. J. Clin. Microbiol. *26*:475–478, 1988.
10. Baum, J., Barza, M., Weinstein, P., et al.: Bilateral keratitis as a manifestation of Lyme disease. Am. J. Ophthalmol. *105*:75–77, 1988.
11. Belman, A. L., Iyer, M. Coyle, P. K., et al.: Neurologic manifestations in children with North American Lyme disease. Neurology *43*:2609–2614, 1994.
12. Benach, J. L., Bosler, E. M., Hanrahan, J. P., et al.: Spirochetes isolated from the blood of two patients with Lyme disease. N. Engl. J. Med. *308*:740–742, 1983.
13. Benach, J. L., Coleman, J. L., Skinner, R. A., et al.: Adult *Ixodes dammini* on rabbits: A hypothesis for the development and transmission of *Borrelia burgdorferi*. J. Infect. Dis. *155*:1300–1306, 1987.
14. Berardi, V. P., Weeks, K. E., and Steere, A. C.: Serodiagnosis of early Lyme disease: Analysis of IgM and IgG antibody responses by using an antibody capture enzyme immunoassay. J. Infect. Dis. *158*:754–760, 1988.
15. Berger, B. W., Clemmensen, O. J., and Ackerman, A. B.: Lyme disease is a spirochetosis: A review of the disease and evidence for its cause. Am. J. Dermatopathol. *5*:111–124, 1983.
16. Bruhn, F. W.: Lyme disease. Am. J. Dis. Child. *138*:467–470, 1984.
17. Burgdorfer, W., Barbour, A. G., Hayes, S. F., et al.: Lyme disease: A tick-borne spirochetosis? Science *216*:1317–1319, 1982.
18. Canica, M. M., Nato, F., duMerle, L., et al.: Monoclonal antibodies for identification of *B. burgdorferi*. sp. nov. associated with late cutaneous manifestations of Lyme borreliosis. Scand. J. Infect. Dis. *25*:441–448, 1993.
19. Centers for Disease Control and Prevention: Recommendations for test performance and interpretation from the second national conference on serologic diagnosis of Lyme disease. M. M. W. R. *44*:590–591, 1995.
20. Clark, J. R., Carlson, R. D., Sasaki, C. T., et al.: Facial paralysis in Lyme disease. Laryngoscope *95*:1341–1345, 1985.
21. Costello, C. M., Steere, A. C., Pinkerton, R. E., et al.: Prospective study of tick bites in an endemic area for Lyme disease. J. Infect. Dis. *159*:136–139, 1989.
22. Craft, J. E., Grodzicki, R. L., and Steere, A. C.: Antibody response in Lyme disease: Evaluation of diagnostic tests. J. Infect. Dis. *149*:789–795, 1984.
23. Culp, R. W., Eichenfield, A. H., Davidson, R. S., et al.: Lyme arthritis in children. J. Bone Joint Surg. [Am.] *69*:96–99, 1987.
24. Darras, B. T., Annunziato, D., and Leggiadro, R. J.: Lyme disease with neurologic abnormalities. Pediatr. Infect. Dis. *2*:47–49, 1982.
25. Dattwyler, R. J., Halperin, J. J., Volkman, D. J., et al.: Treatment of late Lyme borreliosis: Randomized comparison of ceftriaxone and penicillin. Lancet *1*:1191–1194, 1988.
26. Dattwyler, R. J., Volkman, D. J., Luft, B. J., et al.: Seronegative Lyme disease: Dissociation of specific T- and B-lymphocyte responses to *Borrelia burgdorferi*. N. Engl. J. Med. *319*:1441–1446, 1988.
27. Dever, L. L., Jogensen, J. H., and Barbour, A. G.: Comparative in vitro activities of clarithromycin, azithromycin, and erythromycin against *Borrelia burgdorferi*. Antimicrob. Agents Chemother. *37*:1704–1706, 1993.
28. Doughty, R. A.: Lyme disease. Pediatr. Rev. *6*:20–25, 1984.
29. Dressler, F., Whalen, J. A., Reinhardt, B. N., et al.: Western blotting in the serodiagnosis of Lyme disease. J. Infect. *167*:392–400, 1993.
30. Eichenfield, A. H., Goldsmith, D. P., Benach, J. L., et al.: Childhood Lyme arthritis: Experience in an endemic area. J. Pediatr. *109*:753–758, 1986.
31. Engstrom, S. M., Snoop, E., and Johnson, R. C.: Immunoblot interpretation

criteria for serodiagnosis of early Lyme disease. J. Clin. Microbiol. *33*:419–427, 1995.
32. Feder, H. M., Gerber, M. A., Drause, P. J., et al.: Early Lyme disease: A flu-like illness without erythema migrans. Pediatrics *91*:456–459, 1993.
33. Feder, H. M., Zalneraitis, E. L., and Reik, L.: Lyme disease: Acute focal meningoencephalitis in a child. Pediatrics *82*:931–934, 1988.
34. Fish, D.: Environmental risk and prevention of Lyme disease. Am. J. Med. *98*(Suppl. 4A):2S–7S, 1995.
35. Garcia-Monco, J. C., Villar, B. F., Alen, J. C., et al.: *Borrelia burgdorferi* in the central nervous system: Experimental and clinical evidence of early invasion. J. Infect. Dis. *161*:1187–1193, 1990.
36. Georgilis, K., Steere, A. C., and Klempner, M. S.: Infectivity of *Borrelia burgdorferi* correlates with resistance to elimination by phagocytic cells. J. Infect. Dis. *163*:150–155, 1991.
37. Gerber, M. D., and Shapiro, E. D.: Diagnosis of Lyme disease in children. J. Pediatr. *121*:157–162, 1992.
38. Gerber, M. D., and Zalneraitis, E. L.: Childhood neurologic disorders and Lyme disease during pregnancy. Pediatr. Neurol. *11*:41–43, 1994.
39. Goellner, M. H., Agger, W. A., Burgess, J. H., et al.: Hepatitis due to recurrent Lyme disease. Ann. Intern. Med. *108*:707–708, 1988.
40. Granter, S. R, Barnhill, R. L., Hewins, M. E., et al.: Identification of *Borrelia burgdorferi* in diffuse fasciitis with peripheral eosinophilia: *Borrelia fasciitis*. J. A. M. A. *272*:1283–1285, 1994.
41. Grodzicki, R. L., and Steere, A. C.: Comparison of immunoblotting and indirect enzyme-linked immunosorbent assay using different antigen preparations for diagnosing early Lyme disease. J. Infect. Dis. *157*:790–797, 1988.
42. Habicht, G. S., Katona, L. I., and Benach, J. L.: Cytokines and the pathogenesis of neuroborreliosis: *B. burgdorferi* induces glioma cells to secrete interleukin-6. J. Infect. Dis. *164*:568–574, 1991.
43. Halperin, J. J., Luft, B. J., Anand, A. K., et al.: Lyme neuroborreliosis: Central nervous system manifestations. Neurology *39*:753–759, 1989.
44. Hansen, K., and Asbrink, E.: Serodiagnosis of erythema migrans and acrodermatitis chronica atrophicans by the *Borrelia burgdorferi* flagellum enzyme-linked immunosorbent assay. J. Clin. Microbiol. *27*:545–551, 1989.
45. Hardin, J. A., Steere, A. C., and Malawista, S. E.: Immune complexes and the evolution of Lyme arthritis. N. Engl. J. Med. *301*:1358, 1979.
46. Hedberg, C. W., Osterholm, M. T., MacDonald, K. L., et al.: An interlaboratory study of antibody to *Borrelia burgdorferi*. J. Infect. Dis. *6*:1325–1327, 1987.
47. Johnson, R. C., Klein, G. C., Schmid, G. P., et al.: Susceptibility of the Lyme disease spirochete to seven antimicrobial agents. Yale J. Biol. Med. *57*:549–553, 1984.
48. Johnson, R. C., Kodner, C. B., Jurkovich, P. J., et al.: Comparative in vitro and in vivo susceptibilities of the Lyme disease spirochete *Borrelia burgdorferi* to cefuroxime and other antimicrobial agents. Antimicrob. Agents Chemother. *34*:2133–2136, 1990.
49. Johnson, R. C., Kodner, C., and Russel, M.: In vitro and in vivo susceptibility of the Lyme disease spirochete, *Borrelia burgdorferi* to four antimicrobial agents. Antimicrob. Agents Chemother. *31*:164–167, 1987.
50. Keller, D., Koster, F. T., Marks, D. H., et al.: Safety and immunogenicity of a recombinant outer surface protein A Lyme vaccine. J. A. M. A. *27*:1764–1768, 1994.
51. Kirsch, M., Ruben, F. L., Steere, A. C., et al.: Fatal adult respiratory distress syndrome in a patient with Lyme disease. J. A. M. A. *259*:2737–2739, 1988.
52. LeFebvre, R. B., Perng, G. C., and Johnson, R. C.: Characterization of *Borrelia burgdorferi* isolates by restriction endonuclease analysis and DNA hybridization. J. Clin. Microbiol. *27*:636–639, 1989.
53. Luger, S. W., Paparone, P., Wormser, G. P., et al.: Comparison of cefuroxime axetil and doxycycline in treatment of patients with early Lyme disease associated with erythema migrans. Antimicrob. Agents Chemother. *39*:661–667, 1995.
54. MacDonald, A. B., Benach, J. L., and Burgdorfer, W.: Still birth following maternal Lyme disease. N. Y. State J. Med. *87*:615–616, 1987.
55. Magnarelli, L. A., and Anderson, J. F.: Ticks and biting insects infected with the etiologic agent of Lyme disease, *Borrelia burgdorferi*. J. Clin. Microbiol. *26*:1482–1486, 1988.
56. Malane, M. S., Grant-Kels, J. M., Feder, H. M., et al.: Diagnosis of Lyme disease based on dermatologic manifestations. Ann. Intern. Med. *114*:490–498, 1991.
57. Markowitz, L. E., Steere, A. C., Benach, J. L., et al.: Lyme disease during pregnancy. J. A. M. A. *255*:3394–3396, 1986.
58. McAlister, H. F., Klementowicz, P. T., Andrews, C., et al.: Lyme carditis: An important cause of reversible heart block. Ann. Intern. Med. *110*:339–345, 1989.
59. Nadal, D., Gundelfinger, R., Flueler, U., et al.: Acrodermatitis chronica atrophicans. Arch. Dis. Child. *63*:72–74, 1988.
60. Nocton, J. J., Dressler, F., Rutledge, B. J., et al.: Detection of *Borrelia burgdorferi* DNA by polymerase chain reaction in synovial fluid from patients with Lyme arthritis. N. Engl. J. Med. *330*:329–234, 1994.
61. Pachner, A. R., Duray, P., and Steere, A. C.: Central nervous system manifestations of Lyme disease. Arch. Neurol. *46*:790–795, 1989.
62. Piesman, J., Mather, T. N., Sinsky, R. J., et al.: Duration of tick attachment and *Borrelia burgdorferi* transmission. J. Clin. Microbiol. *25*:557–558, 1987.
63. Ramakrishnan, T., Gloster, E., Bonagura, V. R., et al.: Eosinophilic lymphadenitis in Lyme disease. Pediatr. Infect. Dis. *8*:180–181, 1989.
64. Raucher, H. S., Kaufman, D. M., Goldfarb, J., et al.: Pseudotumor cerebri and Lyme disease: A new association. J. Pediatr. *107*:931–933, 1985.
65. Reik, L., Steere, A. C., Bartenhagen, N. H., et al.: Neurologic abnormalities of Lyme disease. Medicine *58*:281–294, 1979.
66. Rosa, P. A., and Schwan, T. G.: A specific and sensitive assay for the Lyme disease spirochete *Borrelia burgdorferi* using the polymerase chain reaction. J. Infect. Dis. *160*:1018–1029, 1989.
67. Rose, C. D., Fawcett, P. T., Epps, S. C., et al.: Pediatric Lyme arthritis: Clinical spectrum and outcome. J. Pediatr. Orthop. *14*:238–241, 1994.
68. Rose, C. D., Fawcett, P. T., Singsen, B. H., et al.: Use of Western blot and enzyme-linked immunosorbent assays to assist in the diagnosis of Lyme disease. Pediatrics *88*:465–470, 1991.
69. Russell, H., Sampson, J. S., Schmid, G. P., et al.: Enzyme-linked immunoabsorbent assay and indirect immunofluorescence assay for Lyme disease. J. Infect. Dis. *149*:465–470, 1984.
70. Salazar, J. C., Gerber, M. A., and Goff, C. W.: Longterm outcome of Lyme disease in children given early treatment. J. Pediatr. *122*:591–593, 1993.
71. Schlesinger, P. A., Duray, P. H., Durk, B. A., et al.: Maternal-fetal transmission of the Lyme disease spirochete, *Borrelia burgdorferi*. Ann. Intern. Med. *103*:67–68, 1985.
72. Schmid, G. P.: The global distribution of Lyme disease. Rev. Infect. Dis. *7*:41–50, 1985.
73. Schulze, T., Bowen, G. S., Bosler, E. M., et al.: *Ambylomma americanum*: A potential vector of Lyme disease in New Jersey. Science *224*:601–603, 1984.
74. Schwartz, I., Wormser, G. P., Schwartz, J. J., et al.: Diagnosis of early Lyme disease by polymerase chain reaction amplification and culture of skin biopsies from erythema migrans lesions. J. Clin. Microbiol. *30*:3082–3088, 1992.
75. Shapiro, E. D.: Lyme disease in children. Am. J. Med. *98*(Suppl. 4A):69S–73S, 1995.
76. Shapiro, E. D., Gerber, M. A., Holabird, N. B., et al.: A controlled trial of antimicrobial prophylaxis for Lyme disease after deer-tick bites. N. Engl. J. Med. *327*:1769–1773, 1992.
77. Shrestha, M., Grodzicki, R. L., and Steere, A. C.: Diagnosing early Lyme disease. Am. J. Med. *78*:235–240, 1985.
78. Steere, A. C., Bartenhagen, N. H., Craft, J. E., et al.: The early clinical manifestations of Lyme disease. Ann. Intern. Med. *99*:22–26, 1983.
79. Steere, A. C., Batsford, W. P., Weinberg, M., et al.: Lyme carditis: Cardiac abnormalities of Lyme disease. Ann. Intern. Med. *93*:8–16, 1980.
80. Steere, A. C., Berardi, V. P., Weeks, K. E., et al.: Evaluation of the intrathecal antibody response to *Borrelia burgdorferi* as a diagnostic test for Lyme neuroborreliosis. J. Infect. Dis. *161*:1203–1209, 1990.
81. Steere, A. C., Broderick, T. F., and Malawista, S. E.: Erythema chronicum migrans and Lyme arthritis: Epidemiologic evidence for a tick vector. Am. J. Epidemiol. *108*:312–321, 1978.
82. Steere, A. C., Duray, P. H., Kauffmann, D. J. H., et al.: Unilateral blindness caused by infection with the Lyme disease spirochete, *Borrelia burgdorferi*. Ann. Intern. Med. *103*:382–384, 1985.
83. Steere, A. C., Dwyer, E., and Winchester, R.: Association of chronic Lyme arthritis with HLA-DR4 and HLA-DR2 alleles. N. Engl. J. Med. *323*:219–223, 1990.
84. Steere, A. C., Green, J., Schoen, R. T., et al.: Successful parenteral penicillin therapy of established Lyme arthritis. N. Engl. J. Med. *312*:869–874, 1985.
85. Steere, A. C., Grodzicki, R. L., Kernblatt, A. N., et al.: The spirochetal etiology of Lyme disease. N. Engl. J. Med. *308*:733–740, 1983.
86. Steere, A. C., Hutchinson, G. J., Rahn, D. W., et al.: Treatment of the early manifestations of Lyme disease. Ann. Intern. Med. *99*:22–26, 1983.
87. Steere, A. C., Malawista, S. E., Newman, J. H., et al.: Antibiotic therapy in Lyme disease. Ann. Intern. Med. *93*:1–8, 1980.
88. Steere, A. C., Malawista, S. E., Snydman, D. R., et al.: Lyme arthritis. Arthritis Rheum. *20*:7–17, 1977.
89. Steere, A. C., Pachner, A. R., and Malawista, S. E.: Neurologic abnormalities of Lyme disease: Successful treatment with high-dose intravenous penicillin. Ann. Intern. Med. *99*:767–772, 1983.
90. Strobino, B. A., Williams, C. L., Abid, S., et al.: Lyme disease and pregnancy outcome: A prospective study of two thousand prenatal patients. Am. J. Obstet. Gynecol. *169*:367–374, 1993.
91. Szer, I. S., Taylor, E., and Steere, A. C.: The long-term course of Lyme arthritis in children. N. Engl. J. Med. *325*:159–163, 1991.
92. Wallis, R. C., Brown, S. E., Kloter, K. O., et al.: Erythema chronicum migrans and Lyme arthritis: Field study of ticks. Am. J. Epidemiol. *105*:322–327, 1978.
93. Weber, K., Bratzke, H. J., Neubert, U., et al.: *Borrelia burgdorferi* in a newborn despite oral penicillin for Lyme borreliosis during pregnancy. Pediatr. Infect. Dis. *7*:286–289, 1988.
94. Williams, C. L., Strobino, B., Lee, A., et al.: Lyme disease in childhood: Clinical and epidemiologic features of ninety cases. Pediatr. Infect. Dis. *9*:10–14, 1990.
95. Williams, C. L., Benach, J. L., Curran, A. S., et al.: Lyme disease during pregnancy: A cord blood serosurvey. Ann. N. Y. Acad. Sci. *539*:504–506, 1988.

148

Leptospirosis

Ralph D. Feigin and Donald C. Anderson

HISTORY

Weil[166] is credited with the first description of leptospirosis in 1886. It was not until 1915, however, that the causal agent, "spirochaeta icterohaemorrhagiae," was identified by Inada and associates.[82] Two years earlier, Stimson[139] unknowingly had identified the same organism within sections of kidney obtained from a patient who had been diagnosed incorrectly as having yellow fever.

Noguchi[108] first recovered this organism from a Norway rat in 1917; in 1922, the first case of Weil disease in a person associated with rat exposure was identified.[161] For many years, the rat was considered the only animal host of *Leptospira icterohaemorrhagiae.* In 1944, Randall and associates[115] isolated this agent from a naturally infected dog, and *L. icterohaemorrhagiae* subsequently has been associated with many animal hosts, including goats, swine, cattle, and hamsters.

In 1938 and 1939, Meyer and associates[99] popularized the concept that infection with *Leptospira canicola* caused disease in dogs and humans in the United States. "Canicola fever" first was reported in Great Britain in 1946,[13] and in 1951, it was noted that 40 per cent of the dogs in Great Britain were seropositive.[31] Surveys have confirmed the presence of *L. canicola* infection in species other than dogs.[124, 158]

In 1950, Gochenour and colleagues[69] identified *Leptospira pomona* as the agent responsible for leptospirosis in cows. Widespread *L. pomona* infection among cattle in the United States was recognized quickly, and, in time, this stimulated extensive epidemiologic investigations in livestock. Infection of cattle with *Leptospira hebdomidis* and *Leptospira grippotyphosa* was identified, and, concomitantly, infection of swine and horses with *L. pomona* was documented.[77] In Europe, *L. pomona* was identified as the agent responsible for "swineherd disease," and it was recovered from other domestic animals as well. In 1951, the first human cases of *L. pomona* infection were identified.

Recognition of many new serotypes of leptospires followed the establishment in the early 1950s of serologic diagnostic services for leptospires by the Centers for Disease Control and Prevention and the Walter Reed Army Institute of Research. Along with the identification of additional leptospiral serotypes, the clinical disease spectrum associated with infection by leptospires was elucidated. Patients with autumnal fever (a disease in Japanese peasants and potters) and Fort Bragg fever (a febrile illness associated with pretibial eruptions described in army recruits) were shown to suffer from leptospirosis caused by *Leptospira autumnalis.*[121] "Mud fever," "pea-pickers disease," and "European swamp fever," terms that were used to describe a disease of undetermined etiology in East Germany, the Far East, and western Poland, were shown to be examples of leptospirosis caused by *L. grippotyphosa.*[36, 68] Seven-day fever in Japan, Wycon fever and Bushy Creek fever in the United States, canefield fever in Australia, and swineherd disease in Europe were identified as examples of infection caused by *L. hebdomidis, L. canicola, L. pomona, Leptospira australis,* and *L. pomona,* respectively.[17, 22, 27, 42, 77]

It now is apparent that leptospirosis is a disease caused by a single family of organisms, of which there are multiple serogroups and serotypes,[2] and that it is characterized by a broad spectrum of clinical findings.[112] In the *Leptospira* genus, the species *Leptospira interrogans* is pathogenic for animals and humans.[12] There are at least 180 strains called serovars (serotypes), which are divided into serogroups on the basis of common antigens.

EPIDEMIOLOGY

Animal Reservoirs

Among mammals, rodents are the most important reservoir of leptospires, but nearly all mammals may be infected and can transmit the disease. In various parts of the world, rats, field mice, moles, gerbils, coypus, hedgehogs, shrews, dogs, foxes, jackals, mongooses, civets, skunks, raccoons, bandicoots, opossums, and cattle have been implicated as sources of human infection.[14, 48, 52, 55, 75, 121, 149, 152, 155, 156] Leptospires also have been isolated in reptiles and birds, but the epidemiologic significance of these animals in terms of maintenance of the organism in nature or transmission of disease to humans is not clear. For many species, infectivity rates of 10 to 50 per cent have been reported frequently.[77] During epizootics, the circulation of leptospires among many species of animals living within a given biocenosis has been well recognized.[47]

A biologic equilibrium exists between some strains of leptospires and a number of species of animals, whereby these organisms remain within the convoluted tubules of the kidneys of the host without producing any pathogenic effect on the tubular epithelium. When this equilibrium is not established, the animal may become ill or may die.[14, 55] Studies performed in skunks suggest that local resistance appears soon after infection. The failure of leptospires to elicit a significant systemic antibody response in certain animal species may be due to development of this local immunity.[144] Some animals fail to develop homologous antibody titers but harbor leptospires in the kidneys for extended periods.[144] Thus, lack of a positive titer to leptospires, as determined during the course of serologic surveys of animal populations, does not indicate absence of infection. For this reason, serologic surveys of animal populations cannot reflect accurately the true incidence of leptospiral infection.

It now is well established that a particular host species may serve as a reservoir for one or more serotypes of leptospires and that a particular serotype may be hosted by many different animal species. Turner[152, 155] stressed that a particular animal species serves commonly as a reservoir for selected serotypes but temporarily may be infected and serve as an incidental host for other serotypes with which it usually is not infected. Two or more animal hosts for the same serotype may be present in the same geographic area. These newer insights have replaced earlier epidemiologic concepts of leptospirosis concerning a "host of election." Although any animal susceptible to infection by leptospires may become a urinary "shedder" of the organisms temporarily, only selected animal species with "biologic sympathy" for a particular strain of leptospires can become a principal or maintenance host of the serotype.[14]

Transmission of Leptospires to Humans

Transmission of leptospires to humans occurs after either contact with blood, urine, tissues, or organs of infected animals or exposure to an environment that has been contaminated by leptospires. Humans usually represent a dead end in the chain of infection, for although it is possible theoretically, person-to-person transmission is rare. Upon direct exposure of humans to infected animals, leptospires may enter breaks in the skin or may penetrate the mucous membranes, including the conjunctiva, nasopharynx, and vagina.[17, 48, 120, 152] Human-to-human transmission has been reported via human milk obtained by a breast-fed infant from a lactating mother who was infected with *L. interrogans*.[26]

Indirect transmission of leptospires to humans (from soil or water) depends on the presence of an environment that favors the survival of leptospires outside the animal host. A warm climate (25° C [77° F]), the presence of moisture, and pH values of soil or surface water between 6.2 and 8 are optimal for survival of leptospires. These conditions prevail in many tropical regions throughout the year and in temperate climates during the late spring, summer, and autumn months. Conversely, survival of leptospires outside the animal host is impeded by chemical pollution, salinity, and various absorptive properties of clay in the soil.[48, 152]

Smith and Self[132] demonstrated survival of leptospires in cultures of infected soil for 43 days. *L. icterohaemorrhagiae* recovered from the soil of lawns in suburban communities has been indicted in an epidemic of leptospirosis in Missouri,[37] and a case of human leptospirosis has been reported in a soil scientist who became infected after handling a soil sample that had been collected in North Queensland, Australia, and transported 1100 miles during a period of 48 hours.[148]

Fresh water, particularly that contaminated by rat urine, has been recognized as an important vehicle for transmission of leptospiral infection.[67, 152] Drinking water from a fountain also has been associated with an outbreak of leptospirosis.[33] The urine of infected cows may contain up to 100 million leptospires per milliliter. If conditions are favorable, surface water contaminated by the urine of infected cattle may remain infectious for several weeks.[34]

Venereal transmission of leptospirosis is important in rodents and can occur in livestock. Leptospires have been recovered from the semen of bulls and have been transmitted by artificial insemination and by coitus. The possibility of seminal transmission in humans remains speculative.[39] Transplacental infection of the fetus in utero is well documented in livestock and other animals and may occur in humans.[43, 48, 152, 154]

The importance of occupation as related to the risk of leptospirosis was emphasized in 1965.[77] Disease appeared to be most frequent in persons with occupations that required exposure to cattle or swine or to water contaminated by rat urine. During the past several decades, the number of cases acquired during outdoor recreation has increased. In rural areas, the U.S. Department of Agriculture promoted and aided in the development of farm ponds. These ponds, along with streams and rivers, are used widely for recreation and as a water supply for livestock and wild animals.[111] It is not surprising that many outbreaks of human leptospirosis have been attributed to water used for dual purposes.[22, 64, 117, 121]

More recently, leptospirosis has become more prevalent in children, students, and housewives than in adults with occupational exposure; cases from urban and suburban communities have been reported more frequently than cases from rural areas.[37] The dog has been incriminated increasingly as an important vector and as a reservoir of this disease. Although immunization of dogs against leptospirosis is possible, it is important to remember that (1) the immunization may not prevent the dog from renal carriage and excretion of the organism, (2) canine immunity after immunization may persist for but 1 year, and (3) immunity, when established, is effective only for those serotypes found in the canine vaccine.[14] The immunized pet dog has been identified as a previously unrecognized threat to people.[14] The exact prevalence in each community of immunized dogs that excrete leptospires is unknown. In one survey of suburban and urban areas, however, between 15 and 40 per cent of dogs were found to be infected.[21] These data are consistent with reports from the Centers for Disease Control and Prevention; dogs were implicated in 58 per cent of the 820 known cases of leptospirosis reported between 1962 and 1971.[37]

In a study performed in Detroit, 90 per cent of rats carried *L. icterohemorrhagiae*.[51] Strain-specific tests were performed, comparing antibody titers in the sera of inner-city and suburban children. Thirty-one per cent of inner-city children had antibodies against *L. icterohaemorrhagiae;* 10 per cent of suburban children also had antibodies to this organism.

PATHOPHYSIOLOGY

After penetration of the skin or mucous membranes, leptospires invade the blood stream and spread throughout the body to produce the protean manifestation of the disease.[56, 57, 136] Stavitsky[136] has suggested that the speed with which the leptospire revolves in a corkscrew fashion enables it to bore through connective tissue. This suggestion correlates with observations in humans, which show that leptospires regularly invade the anterior chamber of the eye and the subarachnoid space without eliciting a significant inflammatory response.[74] Volland and Brede[160] detected hyaluronidase in fluid filtered from leptospiral cultures and cited this as a reason for the unusual invasive property of leptospires.

Specific factors responsible for the virulence of leptospires remain unknown. The possible role played by animal hosts in determining the virulence of leptospires for humans remains speculative. Faine[56] compared the fate of virulent and nonvirulent strains of *L. icterohaemorrhagiae* in guinea pigs. Both strains behaved similarly after intraperitoneal infection, but virulent organisms survived and multiplied whereas avirulent strains did not. Both virulent and avirulent strains were taken up by fixed phagocytes in reticuloendothelial tissues in vivo. Phagocytosis or chemotaxis was not noted with either strain in vitro or in vivo. Virulent and avirulent strains appeared to be identical serologically. Faine[57] also showed that the severity of lesions correlated positively with the number of organisms present and that a discrete number of organisms were required to cause death. The logarithm of the dose for strains of a given virulence was related constantly to survival time after ingestion. This relationship was correlated with growth rate in vivo. Faine[56] also suggested that the low proportion of virulent organisms within avirulent strains permitted modification of the disease process by antibodies that have sufficient time to develop before the disease process becomes irreversible. He hypothesized that virulence results from the selective multiplication of virulent leptospires in vivo. This hypothesis was supported by the fact that maximum virulence can be regained after a single animal passage that follows isolation in culture. Virulence may be lost in culture by mutation to nonvirulent forms.

Nonspecific resistance to leptospirosis is not mediated by differences in phagocytosis of leptospires among animals. Specific resistance, however, apparently is mediated by antibody. Antibody increases the efficacy of clearance of leptospires from the blood stream by enhancing opsonization and hence improving phagocytosis.[42] Wang and associates[162] demonstrated that polymorphonuclear leukocytes are not an efficient defense factor for pathogenic leptospires in nonimmune hosts. Virulence of leptospires appears to be related to their ability to resist killing both by serum and by neutrophils.

Clinical and histologic findings in human and animal leptospirosis have suggested that the pathogenicity of leptospirosis may, in part, be the result of enzyme, toxin, or other metabolites that are elaborated by or released from lysed leptospires.[1, 7, 8, 10, 20, 56, 63, 71, 73, 78, 114, 146] Imamura and associates[81] demonstrated the presence of a thermostable dermal necrotizing toxin in extracts of suspension of *L. icterohaemorrhagiae* by noting the necrotizing effects that followed intradermal injection into guinea pigs or rabbits. The skin-necrotizing effect was attributed to the presence of insoluble particles of leptospires in the sonification supernatant.[54]

Clinical and histologic findings observed in leptospirosis are similar to those noted in animals given endotoxin, which suggests that the endotoxin may, in part, be responsible for the pathogenic action of leptospires.[145] Arean and associates[10] were unable to demonstrate the presence of endotoxin in extracts of leptospires and concluded that *L. icterohaemorrhagiae* contained either no endotoxin or one that was labile and readily destroyed by chemical agents in the process of infection. Further study by the same investigators, however, suggested the elaboration of some other undefined toxins that may play a role in the pathogenic action of leptospires.[9] The inoculation of rabbits by Gourley and Low[72] intravenously with disintegrated cells or extracts of cells of *L. canicola* and *L. icterohaemorrhagiae* has been followed by fever, leukopenia, thrombocytopenia, and, later, leukocytosis. Their findings suggested the presence of endotoxin in these serotypes. Finco and Low,[60] utilizing preparations *of L. canicola* organisms and several bioassay procedures, showed that *L. canicola* had little ability to elicit biologic responses characteristic of endotoxins. One thousand to 1 million more *L. canicola* organisms (on the basis of dry weight) were required to produce a febrile response in rabbits of a magnitude similar to that elicited by *Escherichia coli.* The results suggest that *L. canicola* contains material with weak endotoxin activity. Massive quantities of *L. canicola* would be required to produce endotoxin-related disease. Finco and Low[60] concluded that (1) other factors related to leptospiral infection may increase the susceptibility of the host to endotoxin during leptospirosis, or (2) endotoxin from the intestinal lumen may gain access to the blood stream during the course of leptospirosis.

The development of hemolytic anemia and jaundice in patients with leptospirosis has suggested a role for hemolysis in the pathogenesis of this disease. Alexander and associates[4] reported the presence of a heat-labile, oxygen-stable, nondialyzable hemolysin in the supernate of leptospiral cultures; subsequently, Russell[118] noted that this hemolysin could be inhibited by leptospiral antiserum. Hemolysis may persist during leptospirosis, despite the development of serum antibodies, which suggests that circulating hemolysin is adsorbed by erythrocytes early during the course of leptospirosis and that the erythrocytes lyse subsequently,[20, 104] despite the presence of circulating antibody. The hemolysin is thermolabile and can be inactivated by trypsin and precipitated by ammonium sulfates, which suggests that it is, in part, a protein moiety.[4, 7] To date, attempts to isolate hemolysins from strains of *L. icterohaemorrhagiae* have failed. The precise role of hemolysins in human disease remains unclear.

A toxic and pathogenic potential in vivo for lipid products of leptospiral metabolism has been suggested.[1] The cell wall of the leptospire is high in lipid content; component fatty acids vary among leptospiral strains. Lipids are utilized as a source of energy by the leptospires.[1] Saprophytic leptospires invariably possess lipase activity, whereas pathogenic leptospires may be lipase-positive or lipase-negative.[1] Kasarov and Addamiano[88] investigated the lipolytic activity of leptospires on serum lipoproteins. On the basis of their ability to attack these lipoproteins, leptospires can be divided into three groups: (1) strains that degrade lecithin and sphingomyelin, (2) strains that degrade neither lecithin nor sphingomyelin, and (3) strains degrading lecithin but not sphingomyelin. Virulent leptospires behaved as group 1 and 2 strains, whereas saprophytic leptospires behaved as a group 3 strain.

A prominent feature of experimental leptospirosis is hemorrhagic diathesis that increases in severity before death.[8] Many investigators have attributed bleeding to depletion of serum prothrombin, to thrombocytopenia, or to both.[41, 74, 114] Prothrombin activity, however, can be corrected in children and adults with leptospirosis by the administration of vitamin K without otherwise altering the severity of the hemorrhagic diathesis.[8, 66, 139] Moreover, thrombocytopenia is not a consistent concomitant in patients who bleed during the course of leptospirosis. For these reasons, the hemorrhagic diathesis most likely reflects widespread damage to the capillary endothelium.[10, 36, 52, 162] The precise mechanism of capillary injury is uncertain, but it has been suggested that the damage was induced by toxin.[8] Generally, hemorrhage is restricted to the skin or mucosal surfaces, but, rarely, death may follow a massive gastrointestinal hemorrhage or bleeding into a vital organ.[74]

In humans, profound derangement in hepatic function has been demonstrated. Liver cell necrosis, however, is infrequent, and thus the activity of aspartate aminotransferase and alanine aminotransferase generally is elevated only slightly.

The most striking clinical manifestation of hepatic dysfunction is jaundice. Laboratory evidence of hepatic involvement in human leptospirosis includes the following: impaired bromsulfophthalein excretion, positive cephalin flocculation reactions, reduced esterification of cholesterol, abnormal galactose tolerance tests, impaired production of the clotting factors dependent on vitamin K, decreased serum albumin, and increased serum globulins. These abnormalities have been noted in icteric and anicteric patients with leptospirosis.

Several theories attempt to explain the jaundice of leptospirosis. Early investigation suggested that hyperbilirubinemia was the result of a hemolytic anemia.[19] Considerable evidence does not support the hemolytic theory; attempts to demonstrate hemolysin elaboration by *L. icterohaemorrhagiae,* a serotype associated frequently with hyperbilirubinemia in humans, have failed repeatedly.[8] Variability in the presence of anemia, the poor temporal association between anemia (when present) and the development of icterus, the absence of hemoglobinuria and reticulocytosis, and generally normal fecal urobilinogen values provide evidence that hemolysis is not the cause of jaundice in many patients with leptospirosis.[114]

On the other hand, a significant hemolytic process can be documented in selected persons.[146] Hemoglobinuria has been documented early in the course of leptospirosis, even before the development of jaundice.[6, 84] It has been recognized that significant anemia is a feature only of icteric cases of leptospirosis. It seems most likely that hemolysis occurs in selected cases of severe leptospirosis in humans and that it may contribute to the development of jaundice in some cases.[52, 146]

One must conclude that the hepatic manifestations of leptospirosis, including jaundice, are most likely the result of hepatocellular injury because hemolysis is not a consistent finding and neither intrahepatic nor extrahepatic biliary stasis has been observed morphologically or clinically.[8, 114, 161] Although hepatocellular injury occurs, hepatocellular destruction is not significant, as reflected by the complete recovery without residual hepatic dysfunction, even in survivors of severe icteric leptospirosis. Histologic changes that have been observed consistently include disorganization of liver cell plates; variation in the shape and size of parenchymal cells; large numbers of bi-, tri-, and multinucleated cells with bizarre nuclei; proliferation of Kupffer cells with erythrophagocytosis; and cholestasis associated with scant infiltrates of round cells in the periportal spaces.[7, 24, 52] These changes also have been observed in anicteric patients.[24] Electron microscopy has demonstrated alterations in cell membranes, alteration or destruction of mitochondria, and a predominance of smooth over rough endoplasmic reticulum in hepatocytes, reflecting an altered protein turnover.[50]

Additional evidence of hepatocellular damage is provided by the histochemical demonstration of reduced activity of succinic, isocitric, glutamic, and lactate dehydrogenases concomitant with functional alteration,[9] findings suggesting that the fundamental hepatic lesion is subcellular and that critical cellular enzyme systems somehow are affected. Presumably, hepatocellular damage is not caused by the direct action of leptospiral organisms because the most severe pathologic changes are noted at a time when leptospires are difficult to demonstrate in tissue section.[71] Moreover, leptospires rarely have been identified in sections of hepatic tissue. The elaboration of one or more toxins by leptospires or the release of various products after lysis, which may be injurious to hepatocytes, is the most plausible explanation for hepatic injury at this time.

Renal failure is an important cause of death in patients with leptospirosis. In patients who have died during the first week of disease, renal changes included cloudy swelling or isolated tubular epithelial cell necrosis previously involving the distal convoluted tubule and the ascending loop of Henle, isolated foci of acute vasculitis, segmental thickening of the basement membrane, and isolated areas of mild interstitial edema with lymphocytic infiltrates. In patients who have died during the second week of the illness, numerous foci of tubular epithelial necrosis have been apparent. Interstitial edema and infiltrates of lymphocytes, monocytes, plasma cells, and neutrophils are more prominent. When patients die after the twelfth day of illness, the inflammatory infiltrate is widespread and involves the medulla as well as the cortex. Foci of tubular necrosis and interstitial inflammation are large, irregular, and packed densely with plasma cells, monocytes, lymphocytes, and neutrophils. Cells lining the lumen of the renal tubules are distended and disorganized and contain hyaline, granular, epithelial, and even bile casts. The glomeruli show mesangial hyperplasia, focal fusion of foot processes, moderate cloudy swelling of the epithelium in the Bowman capsule, and basement membrane thickening.[7, 9, 45, 50, 80, 91, 131, 167] The changes observed in epithelial cells may be responsible for the protein leak observed clinically as proteinuria.[40] Leptospires have been demonstrated in the liver or renal tubules and less frequently in the interstices of the renal cortex.[7, 52, 91]

Although some investigators[80] have emphasized that interstitial nephritis is the fundamental lesion of leptospirosis, renal failure primarily is the result of tubular damage. Interstitial nephritis occurs primarily in persons who have survived until inflammation has had an opportunity to develop. Interstitial nephritis frequently is absent in patients with fulminant disease.[7]

Hypoxia may contribute significantly to the pathogenesis of renal dysfunction in leptospirosis. The focal distribution of the lesions suggests a relationship to impaired renal blood flow. Even in relatively mild cases of leptospirosis in which glomerular function remains unaffected, tubular function as measured by the excretion of para-aminohippurate is reduced markedly.[12, 45] In severe cases, the tubular maximum for para-aminohippurate becomes negligible, and glomerular filtration drops precipitously. On the basis of observations of this type, it has been concluded that impaired renal blood flow is the fundamental alteration of the nephropathy of leptospirosis. Histochemical and enzymatic studies also demonstrate hypoxic damage and suggest renal ischemia.[9] Diminution in renal perfusion in leptospirosis also is suggested by the clinical occurrence of hypovolemia, hypotension, and circulatory collapse.[24, 54, 64, 92] The reversible oliguria frequently observed during the course of leptospirosis has been attributed to reduced renal blood flow resulting from hypotension, a deficit of extracellular fluid, or both.[52] During periods of oliguria, decreased glomerular filtration rates have been noted. Renal function recovers first by restitution of glomerular function; subsequently, and more slowly, renal tubular function improves.[8]

Hypovolemia or hypotension in patients with leptospirosis may reflect dehydration secondary to vomiting, increased insensible water loss, diminished intake of fluid, and, rarely, massive gastrointestinal hemorrhage.[52, 61] A decrease in intravascular volume due to a shift of fluid from the intravascular to the extracellular spaces as a result of severe endothelial injury also may occur.

Rarely, during human leptospirosis, adrenal insufficiency follows hemorrhagic infarction of the adrenal glands.[133] Vascular collapse observed terminally in fatal cases may, in part, reflect adrenal insufficiency secondary to hemorrhage. However, this cannot be the cause of the reversible state of shock that is noted early during the course of leptospirosis.

Cardiac dysfunction also may lead to hypoperfusion in severe leptospirosis. Focal hemorrhagic myocarditis, acute coronary arteritis, pericarditis, aortitis, and cardiac arrhythmias also have been well documented. Rarely, sudden death results from congestive heart failure or arrhythmias.[7, 49, 126, 133, 143] Cardiac malfunction also may develop secondary to hypertension, hypovolemia, electrolyte imbalance, or uremia. Peripheral vascular collapse in leptospirosis most often occurs regardless of any cardiac involvement, obvious dehydration, or massive hemorrhage. Regardless of the etiologic factor, shock is common in the course of severe leptospirosis.

Pulmonary lesions in leptospirosis generally are the result of hemorrhage rather than of acute inflammation. In selected cases, acute inflammation is noted but generally reflects a secondary pyogenic infection. Localized or confluent hemorrhagic pneumonitis may be noted, and petechial and ecchymotic hemorrhages are noted throughout the lungs, pleura, and tracheobronchial tree.[128] Acute hemorrhagic lobar pneumonia and massive hemoptysis have been observed in fatal cases.[11] Silverstein[128] suggested that pulmonary capillary damage was the result of a toxin because leptospires have not been demonstrated in the lungs.

Central or peripheral nervous system involvement may be striking. Most investigators agree that signs of meningeal inflammation cannot be attributed to invasion of the meninges by leptospires. Leptospires frequently are isolated from cerebrospinal fluid that otherwise is normal; thus, there appears to be minimal reaction to the presence of leptospires in the meninges. The leptospires disappear rapidly after onset of meningeal signs, usually during the second week of disease. Because meningeal reaction occurs only after the development of antibody, it has been suggested that leptospiral meningitis is a reflection of an antigen-antibody reaction.[14, 74] Meningitis as a result of hypersensitivity may explain the absence of pleocytosis in the early stages of meningeal involvement, the abrupt onset of meningitis at the end of the first week of leptospiral disease, and the good prognosis of patients with leptospirosis who have central nervous system involvement.

Pathologic examination of the meninges may reveal nothing[7] or may show thickening of the meninges, a slight increase in the number of arachnoid cells, and a predominance of mononuclear cells in the exudate.[11]

Uncommon features of leptospirosis include encephalitis, myelitis, radiculitis, and peripheral neuritis. When present, they occur during the second week of illness.[52] These neurologic findings also may be the result of hypersensitivity reactions similar to those seen in other postinfectious encephalitis syndromes.[100, 101] Koppisch and Bond,[91] however, demonstrated perivascular infiltration of blood vessels in the spinal cord, basal ganglia, hippocampus, and white matter of the cerebellum and in the subcortical areas of the cerebrum; these changes are not pathologic features of postinfectious viral encephalitis.[7, 70] In certain cases, neurologic manifestations have been attributed to subarachnoid, peripapillary, and subdural hemorrhages.[32, 34]

The aqueous humor provides a protective environment for leptospires; despite the development of high antibody titers in serum, leptospires may remain viable in the anterior chamber of the eye for many months.[3] Persistence of leptospires in the aqueous humor may be responsible for the recurrent, chronic, or latent uveitis syndromes that have been seen in patients with leptospirosis. The acute ocular inflammatory response seen during the leptospirotic phase of the disease generally disappears without complications and with little or no opacification of the vitreous. Chronic ocular involvement is less common but is more significant because anterior uveal inflammation and vitreous opacification may occur. Development of a hypopyon during the course of leptospirosis may be followed by loss of vision. Pathologic descriptions of ocular tissue from patients with leptospirosis are limited, which precludes a better understanding of the pathogenesis of the ocular involvement.

The myalgia reported so frequently in patients with leptospirosis most likely relates to the pathologic process that has been noted.[92] Biopsy specimens obtained early in the course of leptospirosis have vacuoles within the cytoplasm of the myofibril. Subsequent focal cytoplasmic changes include fragmentation and loss of cellular detail, which results in homogeneous or irregular acidophilic masses. Polymorphonuclear infiltrates that may be noted in affected areas are minimal, even in muscle fibers that are affected severely. Infiltration by sarcoblasts, with new myofibril formation, leads ultimately to healing without significant fibrosis.[25, 84] Histologic changes in the muscles of patients with mild infection usually are minimal.[52] Pathologic evidence of myopathy resolves completely and promptly in most cases; pathologic changes usually are absent in the muscles of patients dying in the second week of disease.[146]

The selective involvement of certain muscle groups in some patients with leptospirosis is not explained. Any or all muscles may be affected; generalized myalgia is common. Myalgia is an early clinical feature concurrent with leptospirosis, and these clinical findings are correlated with the timing of the histologic changes in muscle. Generally, muscle pain subsides promptly as leptospiral agglutinin titers develop and the septicemic stage of leptospirosis ends. These observations are consistent with active invasion of skeletal muscle by leptospires, rather than from a toxin-related effect.[92, 134] Antigens of leptospires have been demonstrated by fluorescent antibody techniques in patients infected with *L. icterohemorrhagiae*.[127]

The epicardium, endocardium, and myocardium all may be involved during leptospirosis. Arean[7] described focal or diffuse epicardial hemorrhages with or without lymphocytic and monocytic infiltrates in 10 fatal cases. In four patients, mesothelial desquamation and fibrin formation in the pericardial cavity also were noted. Myocardial changes included focal or diffuse lesions characterized by interstitial edema with fragmented fibers and infiltrates of monocytes, lymphocytes, and plasma cells. Neutrophilic infiltrates also were seen in most necrotic foci. Aortic insufficiency due to focal endocarditis involving the aortic valves also was noted.[7] Patchy interstitial edema, cellular infiltrates, necrosis, and focal hemorrhagic lesions have been noted in other patients.[70, 146] In most cases, these findings are not mirrored by clinical findings. Rarely, leptospires have been demonstrated in myocardium.[52]

Except for focal hemorrhages, no characteristic lesions have been noted in adrenal glands, lymph nodes, spleen, gastrointestinal tract, pancreas, ureter, or bladder. Interstitial edema with monocytic and lymphocytic infiltrates has been found in testicular tissue associated with impaired spermatogenesis.[70] Bone involvement in leptospirosis is not a significant feature clinically or pathologically, and there is no explanation for the apparent failure of leptospires to proliferate in bone.[83]

CLINICAL MANIFESTATIONS

Leptospirosis is an acute systemic infection characterized by extensive vasculitis. Serologic surveys in human populations indicate that a large number of subclinical infections also occur. Surveys of veterinarians and packing house and abattoir workers reveal positive leptospiral titers in 5 to 16 per cent of persons tested.[85, 102, 103, 147]

A low index of suspicion of this disorder in physicians, coupled with the diversity and nonspecificity of its presentation, accounts for the significant number of cases that go unrecognized. In one series of 483 proven cases, only 17 per cent were diagnosed initially as leptospirosis.[22]

The incubation period generally is 7 to 12 days, but a range of 2 to 20 days has been noted.[123, 136, 156] The incubation period does not vary significantly among serotypes and is not of prognostic significance. Variability in incubation period may be attributed to the dose of virulent organisms to which the host is exposed and to the portal of entry of the organism.[123, 136, 156]

The clinical course of leptospirosis varies, but it is generally predictable: both anicteric and icteric leptospirosis follow a biphasic course (Fig. 148–1).

The first stage (septicemic phase) is characterized by acute systemic infection. The onset of symptoms is abrupt. This phase terminates after 4 to 7 days; symptomatic improvement and defervescence of fever coincide with disappearance of leptospires from the blood, cerebrospinal fluid, and all other tissues, with the exception of the aqueous humor and renal parenchyma. Antibody titers to leptospires develop rapidly; this immune response heralds the second or "immune" stage of the illness.

The immune or second stage lasts 4 to 30 days. Leptospiruria is prevalent and continues for 1 week to 1 month; generally, it is unaffected by antibiotic therapy. Meningitis or hepatic or renal manifestations, when present, reach peak intensity during this stage of the disease.

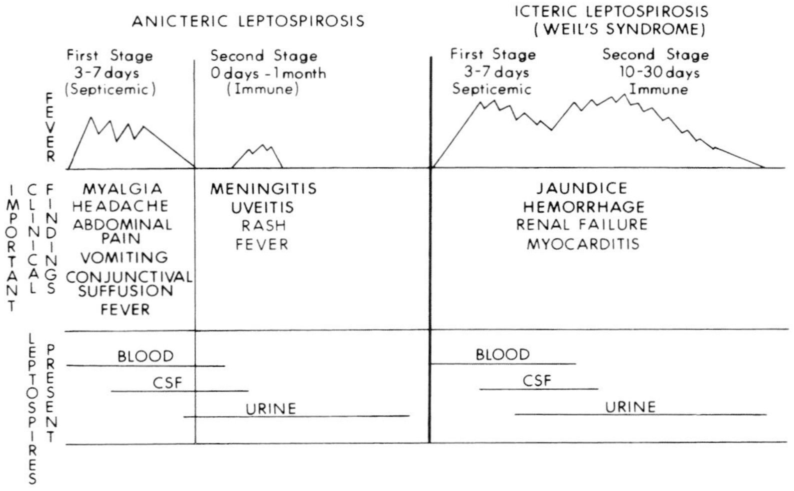

FIGURE 148–1. *The clinical course of leptospirosis: anicteric and icteric disease.*

Anicteric Leptospirosis

Ninety per cent or more of all leptospirosis patients are anicteric. They frequently escape definitive diagnosis because jaundice and azotemia are absent. The onset of the septicemic phase of anicteric leptospirosis is abrupt[53] and is heralded by fever, malaise, headache, myalgia, and, occasionally, prostration and circulatory collapse.[95] Chills, remittent fever, headaches, severe myalgia, and abdominal pain are prominent for 4 to 7 days. Fever defervesces by lysis, and other symptoms resolve. Death is extraordinarily rare in the first stage of anicteric illness. Some patients with anicteric leptospirosis do not experience a biphasic illness and remain asymptomatic after the first week.[53]

The second phase of anicteric disease may be characterized by fever, uveitis, rash, headache, and meningitis. If present, fever usually is brief and has a lower peak than that of the septicemic phase.[52, 53, 77] Maximum temperatures range from 38.2° to 40.6° C (100° to 105° F) with one or more daily peaks. Recurrence of fever 2 or 3 weeks after leptospirosis resolves is not unusual, but there are no reports of the isolation of leptospires from blood to document relapse on these occasions. Relapse occurs generally when the immune response of the host is peaking and at a time of maximal leptospiruria, which suggests an allergic or immune basis for the febrile episodes.[24] Headache may be intense and generally is not controlled well by analgesics. Generally, it is frontal in distribution and characterized as bitemporal or occipital. It may be associated with retrobulbar pain.[44, 52, 53] Persistence or recurrence of headache after termination of the septicemic phase of disease usually indicates the onset of meningitis. The factors responsible for headache in the septicemic phase of leptospirosis are unknown.

Restlessness, nocturnal confusion, mood disturbances, and mild alterations in consciousness usually are brief and common to both stages of leptospirosis.[52, 77] Delirium, hallucinations, psychotic behavior, and suicidal tendencies have been reported.[52, 77]

Anorexia, nausea, vomiting, and abdominal pain may be reported in both stages of anicteric disease. Constipation, diarrhea, and gastrointestinal hemorrhage also have been documented.[52, 95, 108] Generally, hemorrhagic complications are associated exclusively with icteric disease.

Physical examination during the septicemic stage may reveal dehydration, muscle tenderness, conjunctival suffusion, generalized lymphadenopathy, hepatosplenomegaly, and skin rashes that may be macular, maculopapular, erythematous, urticarial, petechial, purpuric, hemorrhagic, or desquamating. Skin lesions are most prominent over the trunk, but any area of the body may be affected. Pretibial eruptions have been noted in patients with infection due to *L. autumnalis*, but other serotypes also may cause disease with pretibial eruptions. Recurrent, transient, urticarial eruptions have appeared for many days after resolution of other manifestations of leptospirosis. Pharyngitis, rales, arthritis, and nonpitting edema are less common.[5, 7, 23, 44, 53, 77, 84, 95, 119, 151, 156] Tachycardia is common, and cardiac arrhythmias occur occasionally.[110, 133] Hypotension is rare in anicteric leptospirosis.[53]

Muscle pain and tenderness may be generalized, but the muscles of the calf, lumbosacral spine, and abdomen are affected most frequently. Tenderness and rigidity of the abdominal wall may suggest the possibility of an acute surgical abdomen. Tenderness of the muscles adjacent to the cervical spine often causes nuchal rigidity in patients without meningeal involvement. Muscle tenderness usually subsides with termination of the septicemic stage of the disease.

Conjunctival suffusion, photophobia, ocular pain, and conjunctival hemorrhage are more specifically helpful diagnostic signs. Chemosis and inflammatory exudates generally are absent, despite marked conjunctival infection. In anicteric disease, conjunctival infection primarily involves the bulbar conjunctiva only. It appears by the third day of illness and disappears 3 days to 3 weeks later.

Abdominal pain and tenderness, when associated with vomiting and hypoactive bowel sounds, clearly suggest the possibility of a surgical abdomen and present a challenging diagnostic problem because acute intra-abdominal catastrophes may complicate the natural history of this disease. Nonobstructive, toxic dilation of the gallbladder requiring cholecystotomy has been noted repeatedly in children with leptospirosis (Fig. 148–2). Pain of this type must be differentiated from myositis, subperitoneal or subserosal hemorrhages, abdominal wall causalgia, or pancreatitis, all of which may occur in some children with anicteric or icteric disease.

Pulmonary involvement may be observed in anicteric patients, generally during the septicemic phase, and usually is manifested by a dry, hacking cough, occasionally productive of blood-stained sputum, or by the finding of infiltrates on a chest radiograph.[23, 113, 128] Hemoptysis, chest pain, respiratory distress, and cyanosis appear rarely during anicteric disease.[113] Hemoptysis, when present, clears in 3 to 5 days. Physical examination of the chest may reveal rales, evidence of consolidation, or pleural or pericardial friction rub.

Chest radiographs may show (1) confluent infiltrates or massive consolidation representing larger areas of pulmonary hemorrhage, (2) small, patchy, snowflake-like lesions in the periphery of the lung fields that are restricted to a few intercostal spaces or disseminated widely, and (3) solitary, patchy lesions with ill-defined margins.[113, 163] Of these radiographic appearances, the second is most common. Small pleural effusions are rare in anicteric disease,[163] and hilar adenopathy has not been described. Although the chest radiograph may help delineate the extent of pulmonary disease, it does not provide information that could be considered pathognomonic of leptospirosis.

Other signs and symptoms of the septicemic phase of anicteric leptospirosis that have been reported include parotitis,[19] orchitis,[140] epididymitis,[77] prostatitis,[77] otitis media,[23] arthralgia,[23, 52, 77] and monoarticular or polyarticular arthritis.[52]

The hallmark of the immune phase of anicteric leptospirosis is meningitis, and it is reflected by cerebrospinal fluid pleocytosis with or without meningeal symptoms or signs. During the leptospirotic phase, leptospires may be found in the subarachnoid space unassociated with the presence of inflammatory cells. As an antibody titer develops, leptospires are cleared rapidly from the cerebrospinal fluid, and an inflammatory response develops.[52] If the cerebrospinal fluid is examined during the second week of illness in all patients with anicteric leptospirosis, a meningeal reaction can be demonstrated in more than 80 per cent, but only 50 per cent of these patients have clinical signs and symptoms of meningitis.[35, 52] The severity of meningitis varies and does not correlate with the severity of other clinical manifestations of leptospirosis. Symptoms referable to the nervous system usually subside within 1 or 2 days but rarely persist for 2 or 3 weeks. The cerebrospinal fluid pleocytosis may persist for 2 to 3 months but generally disappears within 7 to 21 days.[52] In some cases, patients are asymptomatic during the septicemic phase of leptospirosis but seek medical attention during the immune phase because of headache, vomiting, and nuchal rigidity. Papilledema has been observed in patients with leptospirosis but is rare.[32]

Lumbar puncture may reveal cerebrospinal fluid pressures varying from normal to 350 mm H_2O. Mean values generally are less than 200 mm H_2O.[79] Cell counts within cerebrospinal fluid vary from normal to more than 500 cells/mm^3; generally, fewer than 500 cells have been reported.[52, 77] Polymorphonuclear leukocytes predominate early during the immune phase, but mononuclear cells subsequently predominate. Protein concentrations within the cerebrospinal fluid range from normal to 300 mg/dL. In some cases, protein values have been elevated in the absence of pleocytosis. Abnormal values may persist for several weeks after clinical symptoms resolve.[23, 35, 77, 96, 97] Glucose concentrations within the cerebrospinal fluid generally are normal.[35, 53, 96]

Encephalitis, focal weakness, spasticity, paralysis, nystagmus, peripheral neuritis, cranial nerve paralysis, seizures, radiculitis, visual disturbances, myelitis, or Guillain-Barré syndrome may appear with or subsequent to the immune stage of anicteric disease.[52, 54, 77, 96, 100, 117, 159] Generally, these symptoms resolve, but complete resolution may require several weeks to months. Neurologic sequelae secondary to central nervous system hemolysis may occur.[32, 34]

The anterior uveal tract may be affected as early as the third week of illness, but symptoms may be found up to 1 year after the onset of leptospirosis. The conjunctival suffusion (characteristic during the septicemic phase) is not found in the immune stage of the disease. Rather, iritis, iridocyclitis, and, occasionally, chorioretinitis are noted.[22, 52, 53, 77] Uveal involvement may be unilateral or bilateral and may occur as a single, self-limited episode, as recurrent episodes, or as a chronic unrelenting process.[29, 52] The severity of the uveitis does not correlate with the severity of other clinical manifestations. When uveitis is transient or self-limited, complete

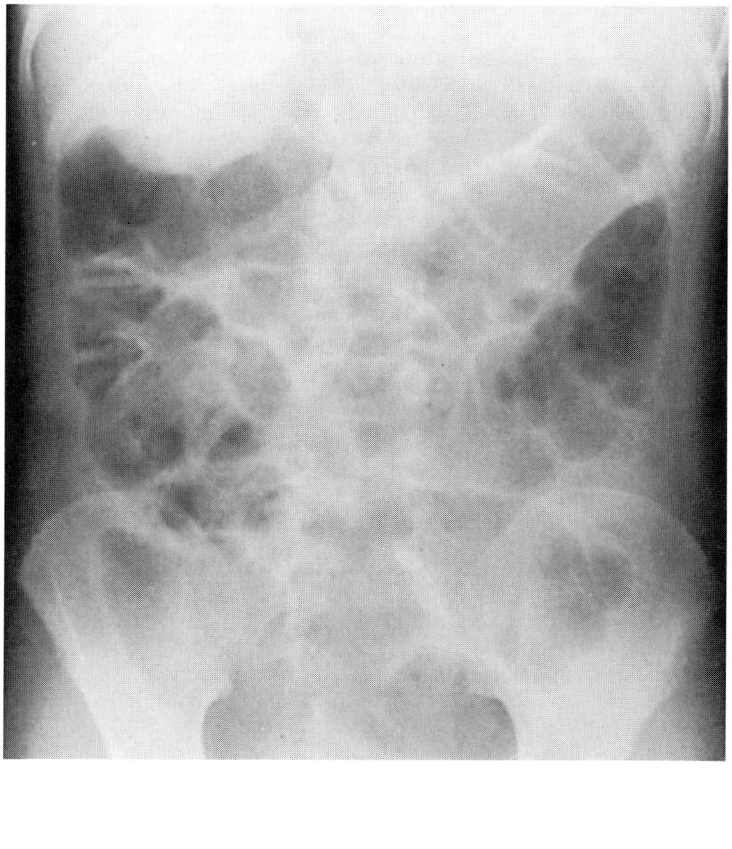

FIGURE 148–2. *Radiograph demonstrating a dilated, opaque gallbladder protruding from the inferior margin of the liver, presenting nonobstructed toxic dilation of the gallbladder in a child with leptospirosis.*

healing is the rule, but, in some cases, blindness and cataract formation are noted.

The precise incidence of involvement of the uveal tract is unclear because symptoms may be minimal or may not appear until after other clinical manifestations have resolved completely. The generally benign course of uveitis may be attributable to the capacity of leptospires to survive in the aqueous humor without eliciting an intense inflammatory response.[53] Despite the presence of high titers of specific antibodies to leptospires in the serum, antibodies to leptospires are absent or found in low titer in the aqueous humor.

Leptospiruria is the rule during the immune stage of anicteric leptospirosis, and it is not associated with impaired renal function. In contrast with many animal species, humans do not serve as a reservoir for leptospires; leptospiruria is transient. In anicteric patients, proteinuria, pyuria, microscopic hematuria, and mild to moderate azotemia may be observed.[23]

The white blood cell count may be low, normal, or elevated. Neutrophilia is the rule, regardless of the total white blood cell count. Leukocytosis generally is associated with hepatic involvement. Anemia is an inconsistent finding; when present, it may be attributable to blood loss, vascular damage, or hemolysis. In the absence of blood loss, significant anemia is not a manifestation of anicteric cases. The sedimentation rate consistently is elevated.

Icteric Leptospirosis (Weil Syndrome)

The term "Weil syndrome" should be applied to define a form of leptospirosis that is distinctive in clinical expression but nonspecific with respect to serotypic etiologic agents. In addition to the symptoms and signs of anicteric leptospirosis, Weil syndrome is set apart by the presence of impaired hepatic and renal function, vascular collapse, hemorrhage, severe alterations in consciousness, and a high mortality rate.

Weil syndrome may be heterogeneous in presentation, and the course may be dominated by symptoms of renal, hepatic, or vascular dysfunction. Jaundice and azotemia may be so severe that the biphasic course of illness is not observed. Fever may persist without defervescence between the septicemic and immune stages and is more prominent and of longer duration during the immune stage than in anicteric cases. The mortality rate, despite adequate supportive care, is between 5 and 10 per cent.

Jaundice remains the hallmark of Weil syndrome. The intensity of jaundice varies; maximum total serum bilirubin concentration in the range of 60 to 80 mg/dL has been reported.[96] Usually, the bilirubin concentration is less than 20 mg/dL. Both direct- and indirect-reacting bilirubin increase, but an increase in the direct fraction usually accounts for most of the bilirubin elevation.[137] Jaundice may appear as early as the third day of illness or may not appear until the second week.[11, 53] The concentration of serum bilirubin peaks within the first 7 days after onset of jaundice in 85 per cent of cases.[114]

Modest elevations of serum alkaline phosphatase and depressed activity of plasma prothrombin are noted occasionally.[114] Hypoprothrombinemia responds uniformly to parenteral administration of vitamin K. Serum albumin may be depressed; concentrations of 2 to 2.5 g are not unexpected.[137] Aspartate aminotransferase and alanine aminotransferase are elevated minimally; these values rarely exceed 100 and 200 U. Abnormal cephalothin flocculation and thymic turbidity values are noted generally, and the urine may contain bilirubin and urobilinogen.

Hepatomegaly is found in about 24 per cent of patients, a frequency that is no greater than in anicteric cases.[52] Transient biliary obstruction, probably intrahepatic, may occur, but there is no evidence that obstructive phenomena are the primary mechanism of impaired hepatic function. Even in severely icteric cases, acholic stools generally are not observed.[52, 77] Pruritus has been reported rarely in patients with leptospirosis.[52] The presence of abnormal urinary urobilinogen values in the absence of acholic stools suggests the patency of the biliary tract in most cases.[114]

In some reports of children with leptospirosis, acalculous cholecystitis has been seen in 55 per cent of cases.[138] In these cases, right upper quadrant pain, tenderness, and a palpable mass were present. Abdominal radiographs confirmed the presence of a mass in the region of the gallbladder. When cholecystotomy was performed, a massively distended gallbladder containing colorless bile was noted. Routine aerobic and anaerobic cultures of bile were negative, but cultures for leptospires were positive.

Hepatic dysfunction is not an important cause of death in patients with leptospirosis. It is present, however, in most patients who die of this disease, and, conversely, a fatal outcome is extremely rare in the absence of hepatic dysfunction.[23] Renal dysfunction, cardiovascular collapse, and hemorrhagic complications occur most often in patients whose icterus is most prominent.

Renal dysfunction may be observed in all forms of leptospirosis, regardless of the severity of disease or of the serotype causing infection.[23, 52, 77] Symptoms attributable to functional renal impairment generally are observed only during icteric leptospirosis.[11, 23, 52, 53, 156] During the leptospirotic phase, abnormal urinalysis results are noted in up to 80 per cent of cases.[23, 52, 138] Proteinuria is the most frequent abnormality and generally is mild. Hyaline or granular casts and cellular elements (red and white blood cells) may be found in the urinary sediment. Microscopic or gross hematuria is noted in many patients and most likely reflects the presence of a hemorrhagic diathesis rather than glomerular injury.[159]

Fatal cases of icteric leptospirosis have been reported in which urinalysis results were normal.[11] Abnormalities of urinary sediment and proteinuria may persist for weeks in patients without significant azotemia.[18]

Oliguria or anuria may be noted as early as the third day of illness but is more common after the first week. Generally, blood urea nitrogen values remain below 100 mg/dL, but values may exceed 300 mg/dL in some cases.[77, 109] The height of the blood urea nitrogen value is not of prognostic value in individual cases, but in groups of patients, it correlates well with outcome.[146]

Azotemic patients with leptospirosis can be divided into two groups: (1) those with decreased renal perfusion (urine osmolality/plasma osmolality ratio [Uosm:Posm] of about 2:1) and a good response to fluid administration and (2) those with a Uosm:Posm ratio close to 1:1, with impaired resorption of sodium and water from the renal tubules and no response to fluid administration. The manifestations of the second group of patients are those of acute tubular necrosis. The factors responsible for oliguria in the first group of patients (those with prerenal azotemia), including hypotension, shock, and volume depletion, if uncorrected, ultimately may progress to acute tubular necrosis as well.

Anuria is an ominous sign, and diuresis is a good prognostic omen.[11] Impairment in renal function may persist, and fatalities have been recorded after the onset of diuresis.[109] Hyposthenuria can persist for months in some cases.[53] Some evidence of renal disease has been demonstrated by renal function tests and renal biopsies for as long as 6 months after the onset of leptospirosis.[16] Renal failure is the principal cause of death in patients with leptospirosis, but it generally is reversible in time.

Cardiac involvement is relatively infrequent, but when it is present, congestive heart failure and cardiovascular collapse may occur.[53, 84] Electrocardiographic changes are seen in all forms of leptospirosis.[110] In one series of patients, electrocardiograms obtained during the first week of illness were abnormal in 90 per cent of patients at a time when none had signs or symptoms of congestive failure, pericarditis, or hypotension.[110] The electrocardiographic abnormalities disappeared by 10 days in most cases. The electrocardiographic changes that have been described are nonspecific findings common to many infectious diseases or attributable to fever alone.[110]

Cerebrovascular accidents may be noted in patients with leptospirosis.[94] In one study of 21 cases in which postmortem examination was performed, subarachnoid hemorrhage was described in one case, cerebral hemorrhage in two, and recent cerebral infarction in one.

Hyponatremia is a rather consistent finding in patients with severe icteric leptospirosis. The hyponatremia appears to be the result of (1) failure of the sodium pump, which causes sodium to move intracellularly in exchange for potassium, and (2) a redistribution of fluid such that the extracellular fluid space is expanded at the expense of the intracellular space. Hyponatremia in these patients may be unresponsive to either sodium replacement or fluid restriction. It is treated best by fluid restriction, which can be continued unless systemic blood pressure falls. Clinical improvement in the patient generally follows a spontaneous increase in serum sodium, and this may occur before any other evidence of clinical improvement is noted.

LABORATORY DIAGNOSIS

Whenever possible, the physician should utilize laboratory facilities in which cultural and serologic tests for leptospirosis are routine. The authors recommend that specimens be sent to the standard reference laboratory, the National Leptospirosis Laboratory at the Centers for Disease Control and Prevention in Atlanta. Despite proper collection and handling of specimens, laboratory confirmation of cases of leptospirosis may be difficult, even for facilities with skill in this area.

A confirmed case of leptospirosis, as defined by the U.S. Department of Health and Human Services, fulfills one of the following criteria: (1) clinical specimens that are culture-positive for leptospires or (2) clinical symptoms compatible with leptospirosis and either a seroconversion or a fourfold or greater rise in the microscopic agglutination titer between acute and convalescent sera specimens obtained 2 or more weeks apart and studied at the same laboratory.

Presumptive leptospirosis is defined as the presentation of clinical symptoms that are compatible with leptospirosis and a microscopic agglutination titer of 1:100 or greater, a positive macroscopic agglutination slide test reaction on a single serum specimen obtained after the onset of symptoms, or a stable microscopic agglutination titer of 1:100 or greater in two or more serum specimens obtained after the onset of symptoms.

Identification by Culture

Leptospires can be recovered from blood or cerebrospinal fluid obtained from patients during the septicemic stage of illness or from urine during the immune stage. Other than these body fluids, only tissue sections obtained by biopsy or at necropsy are sources from which organisms can be recovered. Rarely, organisms are isolated from intraocular fluid during convalescence.[3]

Media for the cultivation of leptospires generally contain a buffered solution, with or without peptone and with or without 0.1 to 0.2 per cent agar to which rabbit serum has been added to provide a final concentration in the medium of 5 to 10 per cent. In addition, a pH between 7.2 and 7.8 appears to be essential. Clinical materials obtained for culture frequently are contaminated; antimicrobial agents, including neomycin, vancomycin, or bacitracin, added to leptospiral media in low concentration have been found to be effective in reducing contamination and exert little if any effect on leptospires.

For routine use, Fletcher semisolid medium[62] or EMJH semisolid medium[86, 136] is recommended. Stuart medium[141] has been used to prepare and maintain antigens for serologic tests. Tween 80-albumin medium (OAC) was developed not long ago and is commercially available. This medium appears to be superior for primary isolation of leptospires.

Several solid media are available but appear to be most useful for the isolation and purification of leptospires from contaminated natural materials, such as water.[142, 154] The preparation, use, and maintenance of these solid media and other media are described in other works.[98, 142, 154]

Multiple cultures should be obtained from patients with leptospirosis because the concentration of organisms in blood at any point in time is low.[86] Freshly drawn blood is most desirable, but leptospires may remain viable in anticoagulated blood for up to 11 days.[141] Blood should be inoculated into several tubes of semisolid media. The number of drops of blood placed into each tube should be varied (one to four drops). Excessive amounts of blood inhibit the growth of leptospires, so a small inoculum gives the best results.[62] Cultures are incubated at 28° to 30° C (82.4° to 86° F) in the dark for 6 weeks or longer.

In semisolid media, leptospires grow in a concentrated ring about 0.5 to 1 cm below the surface. Growth may not be detected in Fletcher semisolid media for several weeks but may occur earlier in polysorbate medium.

Contaminated specimens or suspensions of primary cultures in which contamination is suspected may be inoculated into hamsters. Upon death of any animal, phlebotomy or necropsy is performed, and sections of liver, kidney, and brain then are recultured in appropriate semisolid media.

If collected during the septicemic phase, cerebrospinal fluid may be cultured in the same manner as blood is.

Urine serves as the main source from which leptospires can be isolated during the immune and convalescent phases of leptospirosis. A clean-voided urine may be inoculated directly into an appropriate semisolid medium. Urine specimens must be diluted with sterile, buffered saline solution to ensure growth.[146] Best results are obtained by adding 0.1 mL of urine to 0.9 mL of buffered saline before inoculation into 5 mL of semisolid medium. This procedure can be continued with four additional dilutions. Other bacterial contaminants that may be present in undiluted urine cultures generally do not survive in these cultures after dilution.[142]

Identification by Means Other Than Culture

The morphologic appearances of all members of the genus *Leptospira* are similar. They are slender, thread-like organisms about 0.1 μm in diameter and 6 to 12 μm in length, tightly coiled on their long axis. Like other spirochetes, they cannot be seen in wet preparations by lightfield microscopy, but, on darkfield examination, they may be observed readily. For the detection of one leptospire per high-power field by darkfield examination, a concentration of 10,000 to 20,000 leptospires per milliliter of fluid is needed.[154] At best, darkfield examination should be considered an aid that may suggest but not establish a diagnosis of leptospirosis.

Leptospires can be stained by several silver impregnation techniques.[30, 89, 98, 142, 154] The modified method of Van Orden has been used at the Centers for Disease Control and Prevention for demonstrating organisms in tissue sections of liver, kidney, or other tissues. Infecting serotypes cannot be differentiated by silver impregnation techniques. Leptospiral antigen also has been detected by the use of an immunoperoxidase staining procedure.[59]

Fluorescent-antibody techniques may be applied successfully to the detection of leptospires in urine or tissue.[105, 106, 142, 154] This test is based on specific antigen-antibody reactions utilizing fluorescence-tagged antisera. In theory, the fluorescent-antibody reaction should demonstrate distorted and fragmented as well as whole organisms, but caution is required. Control specimens that have been treated with unlabeled antiserum before addition of fluorescein-labeled antiserum should be employed.[98] The control specimen should not fluoresce. The fluorescent-antibody technique may provide the physician with useful information in the course of the disease in some patients. Positive results, however, are considered only as presumptive evidence of infection.

In addition to this technique, DNA hybridization techniques or nucleic acid amplification procedures, including polymerase chain reaction protocols using leptospiral-specific cDNA probes or oligonucleotide primers, can be used to detect the presence of leptospires in body fluids or culture supernatants. These techniques currently are under development in the laboratories of the Leptospirosis Branch at the Centers for Disease Control and Prevention, but proof of their superiority in terms of sensitivity or specificity in detecting leptospiral organisms in body fluids or other clinical samples has not been established yet.

Serologic Tests

Evaluating serologic findings to supplement clinical and epidemiologic information generally is recommended as a first step in establishing a diagnosis of leptospirosis. The most widely used specific serologic test for leptospirosis is the microscopic agglutination test (MAT), in which live antigen is utilized. This test is time-consuming and potentially hazardous to the technician but is considered the reference test against which all other tests are evaluated. Formalinized antigens can be used for the MAT, and these are preferred in some laboratories, but the titers obtained are lower than those obtained with live antigens, and more cross-reactions with heterologous serotypes occur. Generally, serum is used for the MAT or other agglutination tests, but cerebrospinal fluid, urine, bile, or aqueous humor may be employed.[98]

In the United States, 20 leptospiral strains representative of the serogroups known to be present in this country currently are used to prepare antigens for MATs performed at the Centers for Disease Control and Prevention. Serotypes representative of serogroups in other countries can be added to the battery, and others may be deleted, if desired. Killed antigens remain stable for at least 12 months and are commercially available either individually or in pools. Sulzer and associates[142] have provided detailed descriptions of the methods for performance of the MAT. Modifications of the MAT have been developed and include the semimicro method and microtiter techniques.[65]

A newer serologic test diffusion in gel, the enzyme-linked immunosorbent assay (ELISA), has been compared with MAT for the serologic diagnosis of leptospirosis.[47] The results suggest that this test is a viable alternative to the MAT because of its sensitivity, potential for standardization, and simplicity. Variations of this test have been developed; rapid serodiagnosis of leptospirosis with the use of an IgM-specific dot ELISA has proved to be as sensitive and specific as MATs.[164] The dot ELISAs are inexpensive and simple to perform, and they utilize minute volumes of leptospiral antigens.

Other tests that may be used for the serologic diagnosis of leptospirosis include a complement-fixation assay,[38] a hemolytic test,[38] an indirect immunofluorescent test,[150] an erythrocyte-sensitizing substance test,[38] and countercurrent immunoelectrophoresis.[107] These tests are genus-specific and may yield positive results earlier in the course of leptospirosis than do the agglutination tests. Their results also revert to negative earlier, so these tests are of little value for serologic surveys. They may be of value in distinguishing current from past infections when agglutination test results are equivocal.[141, 142] Other works[38, 46, 116, 150, 154] provide specific details concerning the use of these techniques.

An indirect hemagglutination test offers the advantage of detecting antibodies as early as the fourth day after the onset of illness. It is genus-specific, is less time-consuming, and requires but one antigen in the test system. It has an excellent sensitivity and specificity and may replace the MAT as the screening test of choice.[142]

Agglutination tests have been considered to be serotype-specific. Because of the antigenic complexity of leptospires, however, cross-agglutination reactions occur; serotypes that belong to the same serogroup cross-react at high titers. Early in the course of leptospirosis, heterologous reactions may be stronger than homologous reactions. Because of these paradoxic cross-reactions, one should not depend on serologic determination alone to define the infecting serotype. When agglutination tests are performed on serial specimens over time, the homologous reaction becomes the dominant one in most cases. Agglutination absorption studies may be necessary to define the infecting serotype in some cases. The antigen (serotype) that absorbs out agglutinin to all the serotypes in a serogroup is most likely the infecting serotype.[98, 137, 153]

A passive microcapsule agglutination test has been developed that utilizes chemically stable microcapsules instead of sheep erythrocytes.[11] Compared with the MAT, the passive microcapsule agglutination test showed a relatively greater degree of genus specificity and 4- to 32-fold higher titers. The sensitized microcapsules were stable for at least 1 year. This test is simple and reproducible and can be employed readily in the routine laboratory. Moreover, the test appears to be more sensitive than is the MAT in the early stages of leptospirosis.[125]

A positive leptospiral agglutination reaction generally is not found until the sixth to twelfth day of illness, and maximal levels are reached at between 21 and 28 days. After recovery, low titers may persist for many years. One blood sample should be obtained early in the course of illness, and a second should be obtained at the end of 1 month. Negative reactions in serial samples do not exclude the possibility of leptospirosis because patients may be infected with a serotype not included in the battery of test antigens or with a previously unrecognized serotype. Moreover, the titer may have peaked before the collection of an acute-phase specimen. Antibiotic therapy also may suppress the development of positive titers or delay their appearance.[75, 98] Peak microscopic agglutination titers of 1:3000 to 1:100,000 usually are reached during the third week of illness.[52, 153] An unchanging titer of 1:100 on two successive serum specimens has been defined as sufficient for making a presumptive diagnosis of leptospirosis. A fourfold increase in titers between acute and convalescent sera is indisputable evidence of active leptospirosis.

TREATMENT

To be of maximum therapeutic benefit, an antimicrobial agent would have to be administered before invading organisms damage the endothelium of blood vessels and various organs or tissues. One of the problems in evaluating the efficacy of treatment is the fact that, generally, leptospirosis is a self-limited disease with a favorable prognosis. Even patients with severe icteric leptospirosis may recover without specific treatment.

Most claims of the beneficial value of antimicrobial agents in human leptospirosis are based on the response of individual patients rather than on controlled studies. Hall and associates[76] compared the effects of penicillin, chloramphenicol, chlortetracycline (Aureomycin), and Terramycin with placebo in 67 confirmed cases of leptospirosis. No appreciable effect of antibiotics could be demonstrated on the duration or severity of illness or on the prevention or amelioration of central nervous system, hepatic, renal, or hemorrhagic complications of this disease. Moreover, the duration of leptospiremia and the persistence of organisms in cerebrospinal fluid were not altered by treatment. Kocen[90] compared the effects of penicillin given on the fourth day of illness in 28 patients with a control group of 33 who were given only supportive care and reported that the duration of fever was shorter and the incidence of jaundice, meningismus, renal involvement, and hemorrhagic manifestations was diminished in the treated group.[90] None of these controlled studies was entirely satisfactory with respect to randomization of patients.

McClain and associates[94a] studied the therapeutic efficacy of doxycycline in military recruits contracting leptospirosis while training at the Jungle Operations Training Center in Panama. Twenty-nine patients with anicteric disease were treated in a randomized, double-blinded fashion with doxycycline, 100 mg orally twice a day, or with placebo. Therapy was administered for 7 days in the hospital, after which patients were followed for 3 weeks. The duration of illness before therapy and the severity of illness were similar in both study groups. Doxycycline reduced the duration of illness by 2 days and favorably influenced fever, malaise, headache, and myalgias. Treatment also prevented leptospiruria, and no significant adverse effects of doxycycline administration were observed.

In another randomized, double-blinded, placebo-controlled field trial at the same military training site, Takafuji and associates[144a] demonstrated that doxycycline (200-mg oral dose) given weekly or at the completion of jungle training was highly effective in preventing the onset of clinical leptospirosis. Twenty cases of disease were documented in the placebo group (attack rate = 4.2 per cent), compared with only one case in the treatment group (attack rate = 0.2 per cent), findings supporting the prophylactic utility of doxycycline in this setting.

Watt and associates[165] reported the results of a trial in which a 7-day course of large intravenous doses of penicillin (4 million U/m^2/day) was compared with placebo in a randomized, double-blind trial involving 42 patients. All of the patients had severe, advanced disease. Every measurable aspect of the disease was affected favorably by penicillin. The duration of fever was shortened significantly ($p < .005$) in the group receiving penicillin. Penicillin therapy decreased the number of days of hospitalization and prevented leptospiruria. These investigators concluded that intravenous penicillin should be given to patients with severe leptospirosis, even if therapy can be initiated only late in the course of their disease.

Treatment with penicillin or tetracycline (to be avoided in children younger than 9 years of age) should be initiated if the diagnosis of leptospirosis is suspected early in the course of the disease. Parenteral aqueous penicillin G, 6 to 8 million U/m^2/day in six divided doses, should provide optimal blood and tissue concentration of penicillin. For patients sensitive to penicillin, tetracycline, 10 to 20 mg/kg/day intravenously, or 25 to 50 mg/kg/day orally in four divided doses for 1 week, should be provided.

The management of leptospirosis requires careful attention to supportive care. Fluid and electrolyte balance requires meticulous attention. Dehydration, cardiovascular collapse, and acute renal failure may require prompt and specific treatment. In some cases, acute renal failure may be prevented by ensuring adequate renal perfusion and appropriate fluid administration early in the course of disease, when prerenal azotemia and shock may be seen.[18, 129] If prerenal azotemia is suspected, diuresis should be attempted promptly with administration of a fluid or colloid load designed to expand extracellular volume and replace extracellular fluid deficits.[18] In patients who do not respond to such therapy, acute tubular necrosis may be suspected and appropriate fluid restriction should be initiated. If azotemia is severe or prolonged, peritoneal dialysis or hemodialysis should be instituted.[58, 157] The use of exchange transfusion has been suggested in patients with marked hyperbilirubinemia.[106, 109, 130]

The use of corticosteroids in the treatment of severe cases has not been evaluated critically, but their use has been suggested in patients with impending hepatic coma.[53] Anecdotal reports also suggest that corticosteroids may be of value in patients with profound hypotension or shock.

PREVENTION

Benches in rat-infested, fish-gutting sheds and sewers may be decontaminated. Hygienic conditions should be encouraged in slaughterhouses, farmyard buildings, and bathing pools. In addition to hygiene, prevention of leptospirosis primarily depends on immunization of animals. Immunization of workers at high risk for leptospirosis has been used successfully in mines in Japan and Poland and in rice fields in Italy and Spain.[152]

Leptospire bacterins are commercially available and have been evaluated for safety and efficacy in laboratory animals and in domestic livestock.[28, 87, 122, 135] The degree of protection that is attained depends largely on the antigenic potential of the immunizing agent. Requirements for *L. pomona* vaccine used in cattle are such that not more than $\frac{1}{800}$ of the dose recommended for cattle must protect 80 per cent of hamsters challenged intraperitoneally 14 to 18 days postvaccination with a dose of 100 hamster LD_{50}s. In contrast, most dogs are immunized with a vaccine that is but one-tenth the potency of that used for cattle. The majority of dogs so immunized has been protected against disease but not necessarily from carrying and excreting leptospires in their urine. Trends documenting that many cases of leptospirosis in children have been associated with dog contact suggest more stringent requirements for the immunization of pet dogs.

References

1. Abdussalam, M., Alexander, A. D., Babudieri, B., et al.: Research needs in leptospirosis. Bull. W. H. O. *47*:113–122, 1971–1972.
2. Addamiano, L.: Classificazione serologica di alcuniceppi di leptospire provenienti dall Indonesia [Serological classification of strains of Leptospira from Indonesia]. Rend. 1st Super. Sanita. *22*:5–12, 1959.
3. Alexander, A., Baer, A., Fair, J. P., et al.: Leptospiral uveitis: Report of bacteriologically verified cases. Arch. Ophthalmol. *48*:292–297, 1952.
4. Alexander, A. D., Smith, O. H., Hiatt, C. W., et al.: Presence of hemolysin in cultures of pathogenic leptospires. Proc. Soc. Exp. Biol. Med. *91*:205–211, 1956.
5. Allen, G. L., Weber, D. R., and Russell, P. K.: The clinical picture of leptospirosis in American soldiers in Vietnam. Milit. Med. *133*:275–280, 1968.
6. Alston, J. M., and Broom, J. C.: Leptospirosis in Man and Animals. Edinburgh and London, E. & S. Livingston, 1958.
7. Arean, V. M.: The pathologic anatomy and pathogenesis of fatal human leptospirosis (Weil's disease). Am. J. Pathol. *40*:393–414, 1962.
8. Arean, V. M.: Studies on the pathogenesis of leptospirosis. II. A clinicopathologic evaluation of hepatic and renal function in experimental leptospiral infections. Lab. Invest. *11*:273–288, 1962.
9. Arean, V. M., and Henry, J. B.: Studies on the pathogenesis of leptospirosis. IV. The behavior of transaminases and oxidative enzymes in experimental leptospirosis: A histochemical and biochemical assay. Am. J. Trop. Med. Hyg. *13*:430–442, 1964.
10. Arean, V. M., Sarasin, G., and Green, J. H.: The pathogenesis of leptospirosis: Toxin production by *Leptospira icterohemorrhagiae.* Am. J. Vet. Res. *25*:836–842, 1964.
11. Arimitsu, Y., Kobayashi, S., Akama, K., et al.: Development of a simple serological method for diagnosing leptospirosis: A microcapsule agglutination test. J. Clin. Microbiol. *15*:835–841, 1982.
12. Austoni, M., and Cora, D.: Data on the pathogenesis and therapy of acute renal insufficiency in leptospirosis. Clin. Ter. *18*:233–243, 1960.
13. Baber, M. D., and Stuart, R. D.: Leptospirosis canicola: Case treated with penicillin. Lancet *2*:594–596, 1946.
14. Babudieri, B.: Animal reservoirs of leptospires. Ann. N. Y. Acad. Sci. *70*:393–413, 1958.
15. Babudieri, B.: Laboratory diagnosis of leptospirosis. Bull. W. H. O. *24*:45–58, 1961.
16. Bain, B. J., Ribush, N. T., Nicoll, P., et al.: Renal failure and transient paraproteinemia due to *Leptospira pomona.* Arch. Intern. Med. *131*:740–745, 1973.
17. Barciscewski, M., and Domanski, E.: Przypadek zakazenia choroba Weila w pracowni [Case of Weil's disease acquired in a laboratory]. Pol. Typ. Lek. *6*:1550–1551, 1951.
18. Barrett-Connor, E., Child, C. M., and Carter, M. J.: Renal failure in leptospirosis. South. Med. J. *63*:580–583, 1970.
19. Basile, C.: Pathology and pathogenesis of spirochetosis icterohemorrhagiae. J. Pathol. Bacteriol. *24*:277–285, 1921.
20. Bauer, D. C., Eames, L. N., Sleight, S. D., et al.: The significance of leptospiral hemolysin in the pathogenesis of *Leptospira pomona* infections. J. Infect. Dis. *108*:229–236, 1961.
21. Beck, A., and Barbehenn, K. R.: The Status of Leptospirosis in the St. Louis Area: Final Report to the Commissioners of Health. St. Louis City and University City, Missouri, 1974.
22. Beeson, P. B., Hankey, D. D., and Cooper, C. F., Jr.: Leptospiral iridocyclitis: Evidence of human infection with *Leptospira pomona* in the United States. J. A. M. A. *145*:229–230, 1951.
23. Berman, S. J., Tsai, C., Holmes, K., et al.: Sporadic anicteric leptospirosis in South Vietnam: A study in 150 patients. Ann. Intern. Med. *79*:167–173, 1973.
24. Bhamarapravati, N., Boonyapaknavig, V., Viranuvatti, V., et al.: Liver changes in leptospirosis: A study of needle biopsies in twenty-two cases. Am. J. Proctol. *17*:480–487, 1966.
25. Blake, F. G.: Weil's disease in the United States: Report of a case in Connecticut. N. Engl. J. Med. *223*:5561–5565, 1940.
26. Bolin, C. A., and Koellner, P.: Human-to-human transmission of *Leptospira interrogans* by milk. J. Infect. Dis. *158*:246–247, 1988.
27. Bowdoin, C. D.: New disease entity. J. Med. Assoc. Ga. *31*:437, 1942.
28. Bramel, R. G., and Scheidy, S. F.: The effect of revaccination of horses and cattle with *Leptospira pomona* bacterin. J. Am. Vet. Med. Assoc. *128*:399–400, 1956.
29. Brand, N., and Moshe, H. B.: Human leptospirosis associated with eye complications. Isr. Med. J. *22*:182–184, 1963.
30. Bridges, C. H., and Luna, L.: Kerr's improved Warthin-Starry technic. Lab. Invest. *6*:357–367, 1957.
31. Broom, J. C.: Canicola fever in Great Britain. Monthly Bull. Ministry Health *10*:258–265, 1951.
32. Buzzard, E. M., and Wylie, J. A. H.: Meningitis leptospirosa. Lancet *2*:417–420, 1947.
33. Cacciapuoti, B., Ciceroni, L., Maffei, C., et al.: A waterborne outbreak of leptospirosis. Am. J. Epidemiol. *126*:535–545, 1987.
34. Carayon, A., and Fouin, G.: Encephalite pseudotumorale et leptomeningite hemorragique en "plaques" sousdurales, complication tardive d'une leptospirose icterohemorrhagique en Extreme-Orient. Med. Trop. *13*:698–702, 1953; Bull. Hyg. *29*:1226–1227, 1954.
35. Cargill, W. H., Jr., and Beeson, P. B.: The value of spinal fluid examination as a diagnostic procedure in Weil's disease. Ann. Intern. Med. *27*:396–400, 1947.
36. Carrasco, E. D., and Dunkelberg, W. E.: European swamp fever: Leptospirosis due to leptospiral grippotyphosa. A case report. Milit. Med. *127*:569–570, 1962.
37. Centers for Disease Control: Annual Summary of Leptospirosis for 1972. Atlanta, 1974.
38. Chang, R. S., Smith, O. J. W., McComb, D. C., et al.: The use of erythrocyte-sensitizing substance in the diagnosis of leptospirosis. Am. J. Trop. Med. Hyg. *6*:101–107, 1957.
39. Chung, H. L., Ts'ao, W. C., Mo, P. S., et al.: Transplacental or congenital infection of leptospirosis: Clinical and experimental observations. Chin. Med. J. (Peking) *82*:777–782, 1963.
40. Chung, J.: Electron microscopic aspects of renal pathology. *In* Becker, E. L. (ed.): Structural Basis of Renal Disease. New York, Harper & Row, 1968, pp. 132–196.
41. Clapper, M., and Myers, G. B.: Clinical manifestations of Weil's disease with particular reference to meningitis. Arch. Intern. Med. *72*:18–30, 1943.
42. Cockburn, T. A., Vavra, J. D., Spencer, S. S., et al.: Human leptospirosis associated with a swimming pool, diagnosed after eleven years. Am. J. Hyg. *60*:1–7, 1954.
43. Coghlan, J. D., and Norval, J.: Canicola fever in man from contact with infected pigs: Further observations. Br. Med. J. *1*:1711–1713, 1960.
44. Cohn, A. P., and Howard, A. A.: Common characteristics of leptospirosis: A report of 11 cases. Ann. Intern. Med. *54*:57–65, 1961.
45. Cora, D.: La funzionalita renale nel morbo di Weil. G. Clin. Med. *37*:1295, 1956.
46. Cox, D. C.: Hemolysis of sheep erythrocytes sensitized with leptospiral extracts. Proc. Soc. Exp. Biol. Med. *90*:610–615, 1955.
47. Cursons, R., and Pyke, P.: Diffusion in gel-enzyme-linked immunosorbent assay: A new serological test for leptospirosis. J. Clin. Pathol. *34*:1128–1131, 1981.
48. Daniels, W. B., and Grennan, H. A.: Pretibial fever, an obscure disease. J. A. M. A. *122*:361–365, 1943.
49. de Brito, T., Morais, C. F., Yasuda, P. H., et al.: Cardiovascular involvement in human and experimental leptospirosis: Pathologic findings and immunohistochemical detection of leptospiral antigen. Ann. Trop. Med. Parasitol. *81*:207–214, 1987.
50. de Brito, T., Penna, D. O., Pereira, V. C., et al.: Kidney biopsies in human leptospirosis: A biochemical and electron microscopy study. Virchows Arch. [A] *343*:124–135, 1967.
51. Demers, R. Y., Thiermann, A., Demers, P., et al.: Exposure to *Leptospira icterohaemorrhagiae* in inner city and suburban children: A serologic comparison. J. Fam. Pract. *17*:1007–1011, 1983.
52. Edwards, G. A., and Domm, B. M.: Human leptospirosis. Medicine (Baltimore) *39*:117–156, 1960.
53. Edwards, G. A., and Domm, B. M.: Leptospirosis. II. Med. Times *94*:1086–1095, 1966.
54. Elian, M., Tamir, M., and Bornstein, B.: Unusual case of brachial plexitis in relation to leptospires and Coxsackie virus. Confin. Neurol. *26*:1–6, 1965.
55. Emanuel, M. L., Mackerras, I. M., and Smith, D. J.: The epidemiology of leptospirosis in North Queensland. I. General surgery of animal hosts. J. Hyg. (Camb.) *62*:451–484, 1964.
56. Faine, S.: Virulence in *Leptospira.* I. Reactions of guineapigs to experimental infection with *Leptospira icterohemorrhagiae.* Br. J. Exp. Pathol. *38*:1–8, 1957.
57. Faine, S.: Virulence in *Leptospira.* II. The growth in vivo of virulent *Leptospira icterohemorrhagiae.* Br. J. Exp. Pathol. *38*:8–14, 1957.
58. Feigin, R. D., Lobes, L. A., Anderson, D. C., et al.: Human leptospirosis from immunized dogs. Ann. Intern. Med. *79*:777–785, 1973.
59. Ferreira Alvas, V. A., Vianna, M. R., Yasuda, P. H., et al.: Detection of leptospiral antigens in the human liver and kidney using an immunoperoxidase staining procedure. J. Pathol. *115*:125–131, 1987.
60. Finco, D. R., and Low, D. G.: Endotoxin properties of *Leptospira canicola.* Am. J. Vet. Res. *28*:1863–1872, 1967.
61. Finco, D. R., and Low, D. G.: Water, electrolyte, and acid-base alterations in experimental canine leptospirosis. Am. J. Vet. Res. *29*:1799–1807, 1968.
62. Fletcher, W.: Recent work on leptospirosis, tsutsugamushi disease and tropical typhus in the Federated Malay States. Trans. R. Soc. Trop. Med. Hyg. *21*:265–288, 1928.
63. Fukushima, B., and Hosoya, S.: Sci. Rep. Govt. Inst. Infect. Dis., Tokyo Imperial University *5*:151–169, 1926.
64. Galton, M. M., Menges, R. W., Shotts, E. B., Jr., et al.: Leptospirosis. PHS Publication No. 951. Washington, D.C., U.S. Government Printing Office, 1962.
65. Galton, M. M., Sulzer, C. R., Santa Rosa, A., et al.: Application of a

microtechnique to the agglutination test for leptospiral antibodies. Appl. Microbiol. *13*:81–85, 1965.
66. Geszti, O., Chung, H. L., and Ts'ao, W. C.: Studies on blood coagulation disorders in experimental leptospirosis. Chin. Med. J. *75*:603–615, 1957.
67. Gillespie, R. W., and Ryn, J.: Epidemiology of leptospirosis. Am. J. Public Health *53*:950–955, 1963.
68. Gochenour, W. S., Jr., Smadel, J. E., Jackson, E. B., et al.: Leptospiral etiology of Fort Bragg fever. Public Health Rep. *67*:811–813, 1952.
69. Gochenour, W. S., Jr., Yager, R. H., and Wetmore, P. W.: Antigenic similarity of bovine strains of leptospira (United States) and *Leptospira pomona*. Proc. Soc. Exp. Biol. Med. *74*:199–202, 1950.
70. Goebel, A., and Koburg, E.: Experimentelle untersuchungen zur frage der nierenveranderungen bei respirattorescher insuffizienz [Experimental studies on the problem of kidney changes in respiratory insufficiency]. Beitr. Pathol. Anat. *120*:111–124, 1959.
71. Gourley, I. M.: Studies of Experimental Canine Leptospirosis. Thesis, University of Minnesota Graduate School, Minneapolis, 1962.
72. Gourley, I. M., and Low, D. G.: In vitro aggregation of canine blood platelets and liquefaction of blood clots by leptospires. Am. J. Vet. Res. *23*:1252–1256, 1962.
73. Green, J. H., and Arean, V. M.: Virulence and distribution of *Leptospira icterohemorrhagiae* in experimental guinea pig infections. Am. J. Vet. Res. *25*:264–267, 1964.
74. Gsell, O.: Leptospirosis. Bern, Hans Huber Verlag, 1952.
75. Gsell, O.: Epidemiology of the leptospiroses. *In* Symposium of the Leptospiroses, December 11–12, 1952. Medical Science Publication No. 1. Washington, D.C., U.S. Government Printing Office, 1953, pp. 4–23.
76. Hall, H. E., Hightower, J. A., Rivera, R. D., et al.: Evaluation of antibiotic therapy in human leptospirosis. Ann. Intern. Med. *35*:981–998, 1951.
77. Heath, C. W., Jr., Alexander, A. D., and Galton, M. M.: Leptospirosis in the United States. N. Engl. J. Med. *273*:857–922, 1965.
78. Hubbart, W. R.: Immunologic Studies on Leptospirosis. Thesis, University of California Graduate School, Los Angeles, 1964.
79. Hubbert, W. T., and Humphrey, G. L.: Epidemiology of leptospirosis in California: A cause of aseptic meningitis. Calif. Med. *108*:113–116, 1968.
80. Hutchison, J. H., Poppard, J. S., White, M. H. G., et al.: Outbreak of Weil's disease in the British army in Italy; clinical study; post-mortem and histological findings. Br. Med. J. *1*:81–83, 1946.
81. Imamura, S., Kuribayashi, K., and Kameta, M.: Studies on toxins of pathogenic *Leptospira*. Jpn. J. Microbiol. *1*:43–47, 1957.
82. Inada, R., Ido, Y., Hoki, R., et al.: The etiology, mode of infection and specific therapy of Weil's disease (spirochaetosis icterohaemorrhagica). J. Exp. Med. *23*:377–402, 1916.
83. Jacobs, J. H.: Spondylitis following Weil's disease. Ann. Rheum. Dis. *10*:61–63, 1951.
84. Jeghers, H. J., Houghton, J. D., and Foley, J. A.: Weil's disease: Report of case with postmortem observations and review of recent literature. Arch. Pathol. *20*:447–476, 1935.
85. Johnson, D. W.: The Australian leptospiroses. Med. J. Aust. *2*:724–731, 1950.
86. Johnson, R. C., and Harris, V. G.: Differentiation of pathogenic and saprophytic leptospires. I. Growth at low temperatures. J. Bacteriol. *94*:27–31, 1967.
87. Kahrs, R. F., and Baker, J. A.: Combined vaccines for dairy cattle. U.S. Livestock Sanitary Association, Proceedings of 69th Annual Meeting, 1966, p. 177.
88. Kasarov, L. B., and Addamiano, L.: Metabolism of the lipoproteins of serum by leptospires: Degradation of the triglycerides. J. Med. Microbiol. *2*:165–168, 1969.
89. Kerr, D. A.: Improved Warthin-Starry technique of staining spirochetes in tissue section. Am. J. Clin. Pathol. *2*(Tech. Suppl.):63–67, 1938.
90. Kocen, R. S.: Leptospirosis, a comparison of symptomatic and penicillin therapy. Br. Med. J. *1*:1181–1183, 1962.
91. Koppisch, E., and Bond, W. M.: The morbid anatomy of human leptospirosis: A report on thirteen fatal cases. *In* Symposium on the Leptospiroses, December 11–12, 1952. Medical Science Publication No. 1. Washington, D.C., U.S. Government Printing Office, 1953, pp. 83–105.
92. Laurain, A. R.: Lesions of skeletal muscle in leptospirosis: Review of reports and an experimental study. Am. J. Pathol. *31*:501–514, 1955.
93. Lawson, J. H.: Leptospirosis in the west of Scotland. Scott. Med. J. *1*:220–224, 1972.
94. Lessa, I., and Cortes, E.: Cerebrovascular accident as a complication of leptospirosis. Lancet 2:1113, 1981.
94a. McClain, J. B., Ballou, W. R., Harrison, S. M., et al.: Doxycycline therapy for leptospirosis. Ann. Intern. Med. *100*:696–698, 1984.
95. McCrumb, F. R., Jr., Stockard, J. L., Robinson, C. R., et al.: Leptospirosis in Malaya. I. Sporadic cases among military and civilian personnel. Am. J. Trop. Med. Hyg. *6*:238–256, 1952.
96. McCulloch, W. F., Braun, J. L., and Robinson, R. G.: Leptospiral meningitis. J. Iowa Med. Soc. *52*:728–731, 1962.
97. McNee, J. W.: Spirochaetal jaundice: The morbid anatomy and mechanism of production of the icterus. J. Pathol. Bacteriol. *23*:342–349, 1919.
98. Menges, R. W., Galton, M. M., and Hall, A. D.: Diagnosis of leptospirosis from urine specimens by direct culture following bladder tapping. J. Am. Vet. Med. Assoc. *132*:58–60, 1958.
99. Meyer, K. F., Anderson-Stewart, B., and Eddie, B.: Canine leptospirosis in the United States. J. Am. Vet. Med. Assoc. *95*:710–729, 1939.
100. Middleton, J. E.: Canicola fever with neurological complications. Br. Med. J. *2*:25–26, 1955.
101. Miller, H. G., Stanton, J. B., and Gibbons, J. L.: Parainfectious encephalomyelitis and related syndromes: A critical review of the neurological complication of certain specific fevers. Q. J. Med. *25*:427, 1956.
102. Miller, N. G., and Wilson, R. B.: In vivo and in vitro observations of *Leptospira pomona* by electron microscopy. J. Bacteriol. *84*:569–576, 1962.
103. Morse, E. V., Allen, V., and Worley, G., Jr.: Brucellosis and leptospirosis serological test results on serums of Wisconsin veterinarians. J. Am. Vet. Med. Assoc. *126*:59, 1955.
104. Morse, E. V., Morter, R. L., Langham, R. F., et al.: Experimental bovine leptospirosis, *Leptospira pomona* infection. J. Infect. Dis. *101*:129–136, 1957.
105. Moulton, J. E., and Howarth, J. A.: The demonstration of *Leptospira canicola* in hamster kidneys by means of fluorescent antibody. Cornell Vet. *47*:524–532, 1957.
106. Murphy, K. J.: Exchange transfusion and albumin infusion for severe leptospiral jaundice. Med. J. Aust. *1*:1299–1300, 1969.
107. Myers, D. M.: Serodiagnosis of human leptospirosis by countercurrent immunoelectrophoresis. J. Clin. Microbiol. *25*:897–899, 1987.
108. Noguchi, H.: *Spirochaeta icterohaemorrhagiae* in American wild rats and its relation to the Japanese and European strains. J. Exp. Med. *25*:755–763, 1917.
109. Ooi, B. S., Chen, B. T. M., Tan, K. K., et al.: Human renal leptospirosis. Am. J. Trop. Med. Hyg. *21*:336–341, 1972.
110. Parsons, M.: Electrocardiographic changes in leptospirosis. Br. Med. J. *2*:201–203, 1965.
111. Pertzelan, A., and Pruzanski, W.: *Leptospira canicola* infection: Report of 81 cases and review of the literature. Am. J. Trop. Med. Hyg. *12*:75–81, 1963.
112. Peter, G.: Leptospirosis: A zoonosis of protean manifestations. Pediatr. Infect. Dis. *1*:282–288, 1982.
113. Poh, S. C., and Soh, C. S.: Lung manifestations in leptospirosis. Thorax *25*:751–755, 1970.
114. Ramos-Morales, F., Diaz-Rivera, R. S., Cintron-Rivera, A. A., et al.: The pathogenesis of leptospiral jaundice. Ann. Intern. Med. *51*:861–878, 1959.
115. Randall, R., and Cooper, H. R.: Golden hamster *(Cricetus auratus)* as test animal for diagnosis of leptospirosis. Science *100*:133–134, 1944.
116. Randall, R., Wetmore, P. W., and Warner, A. R.: Sonic-vibrated leptospirae as antigens in complement fixation test for diagnosis of leptospirosis. J. Lab. Clin. Med. *34*:1411–1415, 1949.
117. Rimpan, W.: Die Leptospirose. Munich, Urban & Schwarzenberg, 1950.
118. Russell, C. M.: A hemolysin associated with leptospirae. J. Immunol. *77*:405–409, 1956.
119. Russell, R. W. R.: Clinical features of tropical leptospirosis. Ann. Trop. Med. Parasitol. *53*:416–420, 1959.
120. Sarasin, G., Tucker, D. N., and Arean, V. M.: Accidental laboratory infection caused by *Leptospira icterohaemorrhagiae:* Report of a case. Am. J. Clin. Pathol. *40*:146–150, 1963.
121. Schaeffer, M.: Leptospiral meningitis: Investigation of a water-borne epidemic due to *L. pomona*. J. Clin. Invest. *30*:670–671, 1951.
122. Scheidy, S. F.: Leptospirosis vaccination studies in cattle, swine, sheep, and horses. J. Am. Vet. Med. Assoc. *131*:366–368, 1957.
123. Schuffner, W.: Recent work on leptospirosis. Trans. R. Soc. Trop. Med. Hyg. *28*:7–37, 1934.
124. Seiler, H. E., Noval, J., and Coghlan, J. D.: Leptospirosis in piggery workers. Nature *177*:1042, 1956.
125. Seki, M., Sato, T., Arimitsu, Y., et al.: One-point method for serological diagnosis of leptospirosis: A microcapsule agglutination test. Epidemiol. Infect. *99*:399–405, 1987.
126. Senekjie, H. A.: The clinical manifestations of leptospirosis in Louisiana. J. A. M. A. *126*:5–10, 1944.
127. Sheldon, W. H.: Lesions of muscle in spirochetal jaundice (Weil's disease; spirochetoses icterohemorrhagica). Arch. Intern. Med. *75*:119–124, 1945.
128. Silverstein, C. M.: Pulmonary manifestations of leptospirosis. Radiology *61*:327–334, 1953.
129. Sitprija, V.: Renal involvement in human leptospirosis. Br. Med. J. *2*:656–658, 1968.
130. Sitprija, V., and Chusilp, S.: Renal failure and hyperbilirubinemia in leptospirosis: Treatment with exchange transfusion. Med. J. Aust. *1*:171–173, 1973.
131. Sitprija, V., and Evans, H.: The kidney in human leptospirosis. Am. J. Med. *49*:780–788, 1970.
132. Smith, D. J. W., and Self, H. R.: Observations on the survival of *Leptospira australis* A in soil and water. J. Hyg. (Lond.) *53*:436–444, 1955.
133. Sodeman, W. A., and Kilough, J. H.: Cardiac manifestations of Weil's disease. Am. J. Trop. Med. *31*:479–488, 1951.
134. Solbrig, A. U., Sher, J. H., and Kula, R. W.: Rhabdomyolysis in leptospirosis (Weil's disease). J. Infect. Dis. *156*:692–693, 1987.
135. Stalheim, O. H., and Wilson, J. B.: Antigenicity and immunogenicity of leptospires grown in chemically characterized medium. Am. J. Vet. Res. *25*:1277–1280, 1964.
136. Stavitsky, A. B.: Studies on the pathogenesis of leptospirosis. J. Infect. Dis. *76*:179–192, 1945.

137. Sterling, K.: Hepatic function in Weil's disease. Gastroenterology *15*:52–58, 1950.
138. Stiles, W. W., Goldstein, J. D., and McCann, W. S.: Leptospiral nephritis. J. A. M. A. *131*:1271–1274, 1946.
139. Stimson, A. M.: Note on an organism found in yellow-fever tissue. Public Health Rep. *22*:541, 1907.
140. Stoenner, H. G., and Marlean, D.: Leptospirosis ballum contracted from Swiss albino mice. Arch. Intern. Med. *101*:606–610, 1958.
141. Stuart, R. D.: Transport problems in public health bacteriology: The use of transport media and other devices to maintain the viability of bacteria in specimens. Can. J. Public Health *47*:115–122, 1956.
142. Sulzer, C. R., Glosser, J. W., Rogers, F., et al.: Evaluation of an indirect hemagglutination test for the diagnosis of human leptospirosis. J. Clin. Microbiol. *2*:218–221, 1975.
143. Sutliff, W. D., Shepard, R., and Dunham, W. B.: Acute *Leptospira pomona* arthritis and myocarditis. Ann. Intern. Med. *39*:134–140, 1953.
144. Tabel, H., and Karstad, L.: The renal carrier state of experimental *Leptospira pomona* infections in skunks *(Mephitis mephitis)*. Am. J. Epidemiol. *85*:9–15, 1967.
144a. Takafuji, E. T., Kirkpatrick, J. W., Miller, R. N., et al.: An efficacy trial of doxycycline chemoprophylaxis against leptospirosis. N. Engl. J. Med. *310*:497–500, 1984.
145. Thomas, L.: Physiological disturbances produced by endotoxins. Annu. Rev. Physiol. *16*:467–490, 1954.
146. Thomson, J. G.: Fatal Weil's disease with myocarditis in South Africa. S. Afr. Med. J. *38*:696–700, 1964.
147. Tobie, J. E., and McCullough, N. B.: Serologic evidence of *Leptospira pomona* infections in meat inspectors. J. Am. Vet. Med. Assoc. *138*:434–436, 1961.
148. Tonge, J. I., and Smith, D. J.: Leptospirosis acquired from soil. Med. J. Aust. *48*:711–712, 1961.
149. Torten, M., Birnbaum, S., Klingberg, M. A., et al.: Epidemiologic investigation of an outbreak of leptospirosis in the Upper Galilee, Israel. Am. J. Epidemiol. *91*:52–58, 1970.
150. Torten, M., Shenberg, E., and van der Hoeden, J.: The use of immunofluorescence in the diagnosis of human leptospirosis by a genus-specific antigen. J. Infect. Dis. *116*:537–543, 1966.
151. Trimble, A. P.: Clinical aspects of leptospirosis in Malaya. Proc. R. Soc. Med. *50*:125–128, 1957.
152. Turner, L. H.: Leptospirosis. I. Trans. R. Soc. Trop. Med. Hyg. *61*:842–855, 1967.
153. Turner, L. H.: Leptospirosis. II. Trans. R. Soc. Trop. Med. Hyg. *62*:880–899, 1968.
154. Turner, L. H.: Leptospirosis. III. Maintenance, isolation and demonstration of leptospires. Trans. R. Soc. Trop. Med. Hyg. *64*:623–646, 1970.
155. Turner, L. H.: Leptospirosis. Br. Med. J. *1*:231–235, 1969.
156. Turner, L. H.: Leptospirosis. Br. Med. J. *1*:537–540, 1973.
157. Valek, K., Neuwirtova, R., and Chytil, M.: Treatment of acute renal failure in the course of Weil's disease by the artificial kidney. Rev. Czech. Med. *5*:32–39, 1959.
158. van der Hoeden, J., Shenberg, E., and Torten, M.: The epidemiological complexity of *Leptospira canicola* infection of man and animals in Israel. Isr. J. Med. Sci. *3*:880–884, 1967.
159. Van Thiele, P. H.: The Leptospiroses. Leiden, Universitaire Pers Leiden, 1948.
160. Volland, W., and Brede, H. D.: Zur frage der hyaluronidasebildung durch Leptospiren: Ein beitrag zum problem der meningitisentstehung und der blut-gehirnschranke [On the production of hyaluronidase by leptospires with reference to meningitis and the hemoencephalic barrier]. Med. Monatsschr. *5*:698, 1951; Bull. Hyg. (Lond.) *27*:251–252, 1952.
161. Wadsworth, A., Langworthy, H. V., Stewart, F. O., et al.: Infectious jaundice occurring in New York State: Preliminary report of an investigation, with report of a case of accidental infection of the human subject with *Leptospira icterohaemorrhagiae* from the rat. J. A. M. A. *78*:1120, 1922.
162. Wang, B., Sullivan, J., Sullivan, G. W., et al.: Interaction of leptospires with human polymorphonuclear neutrophils. Infect. Immun. *44*:459–464, 1984.
163. Wang, C. P., Chi, C. W., and Lu, F. L.: Studies on anicteric leptospirosis. III. Roentgenologic observations of pulmonary changes. Chin. Med. J. (Peking) *84*:298–306, 1965.
164. Watt, G., Alquiza, L. M., Padre, L. P., et al.: The rapid diagnosis of leptospirosis: A prospective comparison of the DOT enzyme-linked immunosorbent assay and the genus-specific microscopic agglutination test at different stages of illness. J. Infect. Dis. *157*:840–842, 1988.
165. Watt, G., Padre, L. P., Tuazon, M. L., et al.: Placebo-controlled trial of intravenous penicillin for severe and late leptospirosis. Lancet *1*:433–435, 1988.
166. Weil, A.: Ueber eine eigenthumliche, mit milztumor, icterus und nephritis einhergehende, acute infectionskrankheit. Dtsch. Arch. Klin. Med. *39*:209–232, 1886.
167. Wylie, J. A. H.: Relative importance of renal and hepatic lesions in experimental leptospirosis icterohemorrhagiae. J. Pathol. Bacteriol. *58*:351–358, 1946.

149

SPIRILLUM MINUS (RAT-BITE FEVER)

Carrie L. Byington and Robert D. Basow

Spirillum minus is one of the causative agents of rat-bite fever, or sodoku. Rat-bite fever also may be caused by *Streptobacillus moniliformis* (see Chapter 144). *S. minus* is a spirochete that was isolated first by Futaki and associates in 1917.[3] The original name for the organism was *Spirochaeta morsus muris*. *S. minus* is the most frequent cause of rat-bite fever in Asia. There has been only one reported case of spirillary rat-bite fever in the American literature of the last 30 years.[2]

BACTERIOLOGY

S. minus is a short, rigid, aerobic, gram-negative, flagellated spirochete measuring 2 to 5 μm in length. The organism is thicker than *Treponema pallidum* and usually contains two to five regular sharp turns along its length. On darkfield microscopy, the organism moves quickly, using the terminal flagellum.[3] In general, it is thought that *S. minus*, like other spirochetes, does not grow on artificial media and requires animal inoculation for successful isolation.[10] There are, however, two reports in the literature from Mt. Sinai Hospital reporting the isolation of *S. minus* in broth.[5, 9] The cases, however, may have represented other infectious illnesses.

EPIDEMIOLOGY AND PATHOLOGY

The epidemiology of spirillary rat-bite fever is similar to that of the streptobacillary form. Disease appears to be transmitted primarily through rat bites. Approximately 25 per cent of rats are carriers of *S. minus* in the nasopharynx, and rats with conjunctivitis have been shown to have *S. minus* in the eye discharges that drain into their mouths.[6] Disease has not been reported after oral ingestion of the organism. Human-to-human transmission has not been reported but conceivably could occur during blood transfusions.

Gunning[4] has given an excellent description of the pathologic changes of *S. minus* infection. The infection provokes edema, mononuclear leukocyte infiltration, and necrosis at the site of inoculation. Regional lymph nodes are hyperplastic. The relapsing symptoms are associated with invasion of the blood by spirilla. There may be toxic, hemorrhagic, or necrotic changes in the liver and kidney.

CLINICAL MANIFESTATIONS

The incubation period of spirillary rat-bite fever typically is longer than that of the streptobacillary form, averaging 14 to 18 days, with a range of 1 to 36 days.[1] The disease is heralded by the appearance of an indurated lesion at the site of the initially healed bite, which coincides with the onset of fever and chills. There may be chancre formation or ulceration at the site, and regional lymphadenopathy is common. The temperature may reach 41° C in a stepwise fashion over 2 to 4 days and fall abruptly.[4] There may be six to eight regularly occurring relapses of fever separated by afebrile periods lasting 3 to 7 days. During febrile periods, the patient also may experience myalgia, headache, and vomiting. Approximately 50 per cent of patients develop a purple to red-brown rash consisting of large macules with occasional indurated erythematous plaques or urticarial lesions.[10] As opposed to streptobacillary rat-bite fever, joint manifestations are rare. In untreated cases, the illness may persist for 3 to 8 weeks, but relapses have occurred after months or years.[8]

Spontaneous cures are the general rule, but several untreated cases have persisted for more than 1 year.[10] The untreated mortality rate is reported to be 6.5 per cent.[1] In protracted, untreated cases, severe complications include endocarditis, meningitis, myocarditis, hepatitis, and nephritis.[4] Anemia, weight loss, and severe diarrhea are common complications in infants and children. Epididymitis, nuchal rigidity, headache, pleurisy, pleural effusion, and splenomegaly also have been reported.[7]

The differential diagnosis includes streptobacillary rat-bite fever, as well as many other infectious and noninfectious diseases (see Chapter 144 for details).

DIAGNOSIS

Definitive diagnosis requires isolation and identification of the spirochete, which is difficult. Although the organism rarely may be seen on peripheral blood smear, animal inoculation usually is required for isolation. Blood or wound aspirates are injected intraperitoneally into guinea pigs or mice. The spirochetes then may be recovered in 5 to 15 days from the animals' blood, which is examined under darkfield microscopy. This process is time-consuming and may not be available in most centers. In addition, the inoculated animals must be screened carefully for prior *Spirillum* carriage.

Nonspecific diagnostic criteria include a false-positive test for syphilis in 50 per cent of patients, white blood cell count between 10,000 and 20,000 cells/mm^3, and a moderate anemia.[1, 10] There are no specific serologic tests for *S. minus*.

TREATMENT

S. minus is considerably more sensitive to penicillin than is *S. moniliformis*. In one study, a dosage as low as 24,000 units/day for 5 days was shown to be effective.[8] However, because it is difficult to distinguish spirillary disease from streptobacillary disease and the two may coexist, it is important in the acute stage to treat with dosages effective against *S. moniliformis* (see Chapter 144 for further details).

References

1. Brown, T., and Nunemaker, J.: Rat-bite fever: Review of American cases with reevaluation of its etiology and report of cases. Bull. Johns Hopkins Hosp. *70*:201–302, 1942.
2. Cole, J. S., Stoll, R. W., and Bulger, R. J.: Rat-bite fever: Report of three cases. Ann. Intern. Med. *71*:979–81, 1969.
3. Futaki, K., Takaki, I., and Taniguchi, T.: *Spirochaeta morsus muris* n. sp.: The cause of rat-bite fever. J. Exp. Med. *25*:33–44, 1917.
4. Gunning, J.: Rat-bite fever. *In* Hunter, G. W., Swartzwelder, J. C., and Clyde, D. F. (eds.): Tropical Medicine. 5th ed. Philadelphia, W. B. Saunders, 1976, pp. 245–247.
5. Hitzig, W. M., and Liebman, A.: Subacute endocarditis associated with a spirillum: Report of a case with repeated isolation of the organism from the blood. Arch. Int. Med. *73*:415, 1944.
6. McDermott, E.: Rat-bite fever: Study of experimental disease with critical review of literature. Q. J. Med. *21*:433–458, 1928.
7. Robertson, A.: *Spirillum minus*: Etiological agent of rat-bite fever. Ann. Trop. Med. *24*:367, 1930.
8. Roughgarden, J.: Antimicrobial therapy of rat-bite fever. Arch. Intern. Med. *116*:39–53, 1965.
9. Shwartzman, G., Florman, A. L., Bass, M. H., et al.: Repeated recovery of a spirillum by blood culture from two children with prolonged and recurrent fevers. Pediatrics *8*:227, 1951.
10. Taber, L., and Feigin, R. D.: Spirochetal infections. Pediatr. Clin. North Am. *26*:377–413, 1979.

150

SYPHILIS

Laura T. Gutman

Syphilis first was recognized in Europe at the end of the fifteenth century. It appeared first in the Mediterranean area, from which it spread and rapidly reached epidemic proportions. Although the European origin of the disease is unknown, the possibility that the disease was introduced from the West Indies by Columbus's crew has been considered. Alternatively, endemic African disease may have been imported by travelers. Some also consider it probable that the endemic yaws and bejel of African peoples appeared as virulent syphilis in a susceptible European population.

Syphilis initially was called the "Italian disease," the "French disease," and the "great pox" (as distinguished from smallpox). Its venereal transmission was not recognized until the eighteenth century. Delineation of characteristics of syphilis was hindered by the confusion of its symptoms with those of gonorrhea. In 1767, John Hunter, a great English experimental biologist and physician, inoculated himself with urethral exudate from a patient with gonorrhea. Unfortunately, the patient also had syphilis, and the subsequent symptoms experienced by Hunter convinced two generations of physicians of the unity of gonorrhea and syphilis. The separate nature of gonorrhea and syphilis was demonstrated in 1838 by Ricord, who reported his observations on more than 2500 human inoculations. Recognition of the stages of syphilis followed, and in 1905, Schaudinn and Hoffman discovered the causative agent. The following year Wassermann introduced the diagnostic blood test that bears his name.

THE ORGANISM

Morphologic characteristics are the primary features by which members of the family Spirochaetaceae are placed into a single taxon. Spirochetes are helix-shaped, heterotrophic bacteria. These organisms are slender, coiled, and flexible, with one or more complete turns in the helix. Spirochetes are motile, their motility resulting from the action of axial fibrils rather than flagella. There are five genera in the family Spirochaetaceae, of which only *Treponema, Borrelia,* and *Leptospira* species cause major human illnesses. Differentiation among genera of the family Spirochaetaceae is based primarily on the morphology of the organism.

The name *Treponema* is derived from the Greek words meaning "turning thread." Individual organisms are 5 to 20 μm in length and 0.092 to 0.5 μm in diameter and have finely tapered ends. Whole cells appear to have a flat wave with one or more planes per cell, giving the appearance of a helical coil. There are 8 to 14 waves per cell, distributed evenly. They exhibit a sluggish mobility, with drifting motion and graceful flexuous movements. These organisms rarely rotate but are motile in liquid and solid media.

The internal structure of *Treponema pallidum* is in general similar to that of other spirochetes. An outermost thin, three-layered membrane surrounds the protoplasmic cylinder of the cell. Intracytoplasmic microtubules have been described, and such structures may be specific for *Treponema* species.

The six axial fibrils are long, flagella-like, intracellular organelles that originate at either end of the cell from knoblike structures and extend toward the other end. Axial fibrils are variable in length but overlap one another near the middle of the cell. These fibrils are thought to determine the spiral shape of the cells and are responsible for the characteristic motility exhibited by members of Spirochaetaceae.

Virulent strains of *T. pallidum* are propagated only by intratesticular inoculation of rabbits, and the inability to propagate the organisms in vitro has hampered study of these microorganisms. Division time of the organism in rabbits is about 30 hours. Velocity sedimentation employing discontinuous gradients of Hypaque successfully has purified and concentrated treponemes extracted from infected rabbit testes. These organisms retain the antigens for the fluorescence test, although motility is lost.

Limited cultivation of *T. pallidum* on monolayers of baby hamster kidney cells in 7 per cent carbon dioxide has been reported recently. Research with in vitro characteristics of these organisms also has resulted in the description of adherence of virulent *T. pallidum* to primary cell cultures of rabbit testicular cells and to an established continuous line of human epithelial cells (HEp-2). To date, however, direct in vitro culture for diagnosis of *T. pallidum* disease has not been possible.

TRANSMISSION

Acquired Syphilis

Syphilis is not a highly contagious disease. A person who has had sexual contact with an infected partner has approximately 1 chance in 10 of acquiring disease. The ID_{50} to humans experimentally has been estimated to be 57 organisms. *T. pallidum* has the capability to invade the intact mucous membrane or the skin in areas of abrasion. Direct inoculation from contact with an infected person is necessary for infection because survival of the organism outside the host is very limited. Sexual contact is the common method of transmission of acquired disease, and the site of inoculation usually is on the genital organs: the vagina or cervix in females and the penis in males. Other sites include lips and abraded areas of the skin. Examining physicians and pathologists may be infected by contact if appropriate barrier protection is not provided.

Congenital Syphilis

Congenital syphilis usually results from transplacental infection of the developing fetus, but a newborn occasionally may be infected by contact at delivery with a chancre of the birth canal. Hematogenous infection of the infant can occur throughout pregnancy. Occasional reports in the literature describing treponemes in fetal tissue or placentas prior to the fifth month of gestation were disputed for decades, but recent reports describe the results of examination of tissues from therapeutic abortions accomplished prior to 12 weeks of gestation.[22, 31] In two fetuses, treponemal organisms were visualized by Warthin-Starry silver stain and immunofluorescence of the fetal tissues at gestational ages of 9 to 10 weeks. The expected inflammatory response was not observed in these two fetuses but was found in infected fetuses after the fifteenth week of pregnancy. These investigators noted that investigators in the older literature describing syphilitic fetuses or placentas worked with the products of spontaneous abortions. Such fetal loss due to syphilis occurred only after 18 weeks of gestation, implying that the fetal loss was a reflection of damage incurred as a result of the host response to the organism. The observation of sequential acquisition by the fetus of the ability to respond to a variety of antigens suggests that inflammation can be present only after the fetus acquires the immunologic ability to recognize the treponeme.[71] It also is true that the layer of Langhans cells in the placenta is intact until the sixteenth week of gestation, but this does not appear to be a barrier to invasion of the fetus by *T. pallidum*.

EPIDEMIOLOGY

Since the latter part of the 1980s, there has been a rapid increase in the rate and numbers of cases of primary and secondary syphilis, and with the increases in disease of adults has been an increase in rates of congenital syphilis. Rates have been greatest in urban centers, and the disease has been centered in populations in which substance abuse is common and in which prostitution is practiced. One of the cycles of infection is in groups in which sex is exchanged for drugs. An earlier rise in incidence in male homosexuals appears to have leveled or decreased.

Syphilis is one of the ulcer-causing diseases that are associated with increased transmission of HIV. In this regard, increasing proportions of newborns who are infected with congenital syphilis also are born to mothers with HIV, and vice versa. In 1987, the reported rate of congenital syphilis was 10.5 cases/100,000 live births. By 1991, there were 4398 cases of congenital syphilis (107/100,00 live births). These rates reflect a reporting case definition that was changed in 1988 and undoubtedly also reflect substantial underreporting of actual disease[79] (see section on diagnosis). However, there

TABLE 150–1. Prenatal Care and the Occurrence* of Congenital Syphilis in Infants

Care	Study: *Mascola et al., 1984*[49] *(n = 50)*	Study: *Coles et al., 1995*[16] *(n = 318)*
No prenatal care	56	46
First prenatal test negative; testing not repeated in late pregnancy	6	14
Medical mismanagement	6	10
Failure of conventional prenatal syphilis treatment of mother	8	5
Negative maternal syphilis test at delivery	14	—
Infection late in pregnancy or no prenatal care until late in pregnancy	—	20
Mother not tested	8	3
Laboratory error	2	—

*Numbers represent percentage of total cases in study.
Adapted from Gutman, L. T.: Congenital syphilis. *In* Mandell, G. L. (ed.): Atlas of Infectious Disease. Volume 5: Sexually Transmitted Diseases. Philadelphia, Current Medicine, 1996.

also was a genuine increase in case rates.[40] Case rates of congenital syphilis were greatest in the Northeast (186.2 cases/100,000) and lowest in the Midwest (54.8/100,000).[23]

Strenuous attempts have been made in the United States to control syphilis, primarily by early treatment of contact cases. Persons who acquire syphilis characteristically are young and often promiscuous, having had contact with an average of five persons during the incubation period. Because there is a high rate of dual infection (8 per cent), some persons identified and treated for gonorrhea also will be treated for syphilis while in the preprimary stage of disease.

Factors contributing to the increased rates of syphilis in recent years have included HIV infection, scarce and overwhelmed public health resources, and failure to implement safer sexual practices, especially among adolescents and young adults.

Congenital syphilis is a disease that should be amenable almost fully to eradication if currently available prenatal health measures were implemented completely. Table 150–1 presents two studies of prenatal care of women who delivered infants with congential syphilis and indicates the hurdles that control of the disease will have to overcome.

There is little doubt that penicillin was a major reason for the decline of the treponematoses seen in the early 1950s.[24] Other factors must be considered in the attempted eradication of these infections. For example, nonvenereal endemic treponemal infections (endemic syphilis, bejel, yaws, pinta) have continued to flourish in underdeveloped areas of the world where hygiene is poor, despite the introduction of penicillin. Progress in control of these diseases requires that mass treatment programs be coupled with efforts to improve local living conditions. In areas where this could be accomplished, a resulting decline in endemic treponematoses occurred.

PATHOLOGY

Syphilis often is a lifelong infection that progresses in three clear characteristic stages (Fig. 150–1). After initial invasion through mucous membranes or skin, the organism undergoes rapid multiplication and is disseminated widely. Spread through the perivascular lymphatics and then through the systemic circulation occurs before the clinical development of the primary lesion. Ten to 90 days later, usually within 3 to 4 weeks, the patient manifests an inflammatory response to the infection at the site of the inoculation. The resulting lesion, the chancre, is characterized by the profuse discharge of spirochetes; accumulation of mononuclear leukocytes, lymphocytes, and plasma cells; and the swelling of capillary endothelia. The regional lymph nodes are enlarged, and the cellular infiltrate resembles that of the primary lesions. Resolution of the primary lesion is by fibrosis.

Secondary lesions develop when tissues of ectodermal origin, such as skin, mucous membranes, and central nervous system, participate in an inflammatory response. Mucous patches in the mouth are caused by local vasculitis. The cellular infiltrate resembles that of the primary lesion, with the predominance of plasma cells. There is little or no necrosis, and healing is without scarring but may include pigmentary changes.

Tertiary syphilis may involve any organ system and often is asymmetric. Gummata are lesions typified by extensive necrosis, a few giant cells, and a paucity of organisms. They

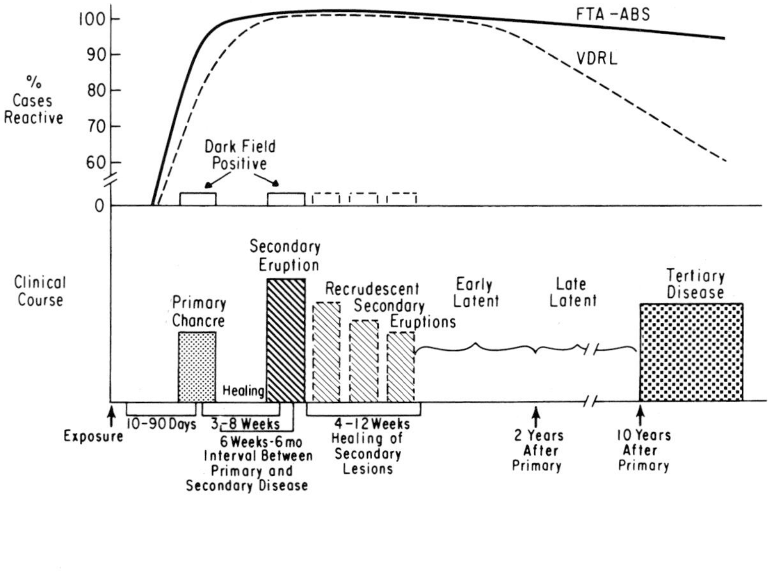

FIGURE 150–1. *The course of untreated syphilis.*

commonly occur in internal organs, bone, and skin. The other major form of tertiary lesion is a diffuse chronic inflammation, with plasma cells and lymphocytes but without caseation, that may result in an aneurysm of the aorta, paralytic dementia, or tabes dorsalis. Chronic swelling of the capillary endothelium and fibrosis result in the characteristic tissue changes.

Congenital syphilis is a result of hematogenous infection and the disseminated involvement of almost all viscera. The intense inflammatory response occurs in the perivascular framework and interstitial stroma rather than the parenchyma.[54] Bone, liver, pancreas, intestine, kidney, and spleen are tissues that are involved most reproducibly and severely. Other tissues, such as the brain, lymph nodes, and lungs, may be infected as well. The gastrointestinal tract shows a pattern of mononuclear cell infiltration in the mucosa and submucosa, with subsequent widening of the submucosa by the ensuing fibrosis. This is most prominent in the small bowel. In the kidney, a perivascular inflammation, particularly in the juxtamedullary region, is evident. The basic architecture of the tissue influences the ultimate pattern of involvement. For example, the deposition of collagen around arteries of the spleen produces a typical onion-skin appearance. Periosteum and epiphyses are the most affected portions of bone, and syphilitic granulation tissue may interfere with bone formation. Pancreatitis also is observed, with typical inflammation and fibrosis. The fetus or newborn shows diffuse extramedullary hematopoiesis in many tissues. There are several histopathologic features of placentas of infants with congenital syphilis. Three features commonly are seen: enlarged and hypercellular villi, proliferative fetal vascular changes, and both acute and chronic inflammation of the villi.[28a] Spirochetes may be identified in placental tissue using conventional staining, although they may be difficult to visualize. Nucleac acid amplification methods also have been used to identify *T. pallidum* genome in involved placental specimens.[28a]

PATHOGENESIS AND IMMUNE RESPONSE

The pathogenesis of syphilis will not be understood until we can understand why on the one hand there is a vigorous host immune response to infection, but on the other hand the infection may persist for life in the presence of this response. In addition, prior infection does not confer resistance to reinfection. Information concerning host and bacterial interactions that may pertain to these questions is described briefly.

Treponemal Virulence-Associated Factors

Virulent *T. pallidum* attach to host cells during parasitism and are oriented by the proximal hook to the host cell surface. There appears to be a ligand-receptor adherence mechanism involving the treponemal outer-membrane proteins. Virulent strains attach to metabolically active mammalian cells, and treponemes are capable of multiplication only during attachment. Fetal and infant cells appear to support treponemal growth maximally, and capillary cells are the prime target of parasitism. Virulent treponemal strains produce hyaluronidase, which may facilitate the perivascular infiltration that is apparent by histopathologic study. These strains also may invade the ground substance that joins capillary endothelial cells.

Virulent *T. pallidum* is coated with fibronectin of host origin. This coating appears to protect the organism from antibody-mediated phagocytosis; allows the organism to adhere to the surface of host phagocytes with only limited ingestion of the organisms; may block complement-mediated lysis of the coated treponemes; and, finally, may allow the treponemes additionally to acquire physiologically active host proteins, such as ceruloplasmin and transferrin, on which they are dependent.[58]

Host Response

Treponemes appear to persist in extracellular loci with little or no inflammatory response elicited. It is known that polymorphonuclear leukocytes ingest virulent treponemes, incorporate them into phagocytic vacuoles, degranulate, and digest *T. pallidum*. In addition, phagocytosis occurs relatively slowly and is facilitated by the presence of immune serum.[2] However, relatively large numbers of treponemes are needed in order to elicit this response, and small numbers may escape recognition.[52]

Alterations in host cell-mediated immunity occur during primary and secondary stages of syphilis. During early stages of disease, all aspects of cell-mediated immunity are suppressed, including responses to nonspecific T-cell mitogens. Blastogenesis to treponemal antigens is not demonstrable until late in secondary disease. Natural killer cell activity is increased in early primary syphilis and depressed in secondary and latent syphilis.[37] There is some evidence to support the idea that lymphocytes from previously infected animals confer moderate protection to nonimmune animals. However, the extent to which these alterations in cellular function during infection affect the outcome or progression of disease remains uncertain.

During the initial infection with *T. pallidum*, humoral IgG and IgM antibodies are detectable by the time the chancre appears. In primary syphilis, the main IgG subclass is IgG1, whereas in secondary syphilis, IgG1 and IgG3 predominate.[6] If the patient is treated adequately, IgM antibody declines during the next 1 to 2 years, but IgG antibody usually persists through the lifetime of the patient. The stages of syphilis evolve, in spite of humoral antibody response.

Persons with untreated syphilis have only a relative resistance to reinfection, so that the development of a chancre with reinfection is unusual and probably depends on the challenge inoculum. After re-exposure, untreated persons may develop an increased humoral antibody level.

In persons who have been treated for syphilis, especially if treatment was given during the secondary or earlier stages, the protective effect of prior disease is minor, and active disease after reinfection is common. This applies to persons who maintain a reactive nontreponemal antibody test (Serofast), as well as to those who are serononreactive. Patients who have been treated for congenital syphilis also may acquire symptomatic disease.[25, 56] In summary, although active or prior syphilis modifies the response of the patient to subsequent reinfection, protection is only relative and is unreliable.

Secondary syphilis and congenital infection may be accompanied by the nephrotic syndrome. The nephrosis characteristically responds rapidly to penicillin, and light microscopy reveals membranous glomerulonephritis with glomerular mesangial cell proliferation. The subendothelial basement membrane deposits contain IgG and C3 or only globulin. Acute syphilitic glomerulonephritis appears to be an immune complex disease.[9, 27, 38] In infants with congenital syphilis, analysis of circulating immune complexes using immunoblotting methods demonstrated the presence of an 83-kDa

T. pallidum antigen.[20] Similiar findings have been made with secondary syphilis.

CLINICAL MANIFESTATIONS

It is characteristic for the course of untreated syphilis to progress through three or four stages over a period of many years. Information on the natural history of untreated syphilis primarily comes from follow-up studies of almost 2000 untreated syphilitic patients who were seen initially between 1891 and 1910 in the clinic of Dr. Boeck. The subsequent studies of these patients by Dr. Bruusgaard and by other epidemiologists later provided the basis for most of our concepts of the consequences of this disease. A summary of some of these studies has been done by Clark and Danbolt.[14] Figure 150–1 depicts some of the characteristics of an untreated course of disease.

Acquired Syphilis

Most recognized syphilitic disease in children is congenital. Acquired syphilis in prepubertal children seldom is reported and is assumed to resemble the clinical course of acquired syphilis in adulthood. Children with acquired syphilis should be assumed to have been infected through contact during child sexual abuse, unless another method of transmission is identified. Although acquired syphilis during sexual abuse seems to be a relatively rare event, the author has treated two children who acquired syphilis through abuse; one had progressed to general paresis, and the other presented with primary and secondary disease.

The decision to screen for syphilis during the medical evaluation of a child who is suspected of having been abused should be decided on an individual basis, in part because a difficult aspect of the follow-up is the requirement of repeat serologic assays in 3 to 6 months. Children who should be considered for this evaluation include those who are infected with another sexually transmitted disease, who have physical signs of sexual abuse, who are in a social setting in which the adults are at high risk for syphilis, or who have any finding suggestive of syphilis.[7, 42, 69, 70] In addition, children who may have acquired HIV through sexual abuse should be evaluated for syphilis.

Primary Disease

The chancre of primary syphilis typically is a single lesion, nontender and firm, with a clean surface, raised border, and reddish color. It may be overlooked by women, in whom it frequently is situated on the cervix or vaginal wall. Systemic signs or symptoms are absent, but adjacent lymph nodes frequently are enlarged and nontender. (See reference 30 for depictions of childen with acquired primary syphilis.)

Secondary Disease

Two to 10 weeks after the primary lesions, the patient may experience secondary disease. Prominent findings include fever, sore throat, generalized lymphadenopathy, headache, and rash. Involvement of the palms and soles is common, in contradistinction to many other dermatologic conditions. On mucous membranes, the lesions may appear as white mucous patches. Condylomata lata occur around moist areas, such as the anus and vagina. All secondary lesions of the skin and mucous membranes are highly infectious. Acquired syphilis in early childhood may reveal minimal dermal findings.[1]

After the late episode of secondary disease, the patient enters the stage of latent disease; the first 4 years are considered early latent, and the subsequent period is late latent. Persons in the late latent stage of disease have no signs or symptoms of active syphilis but remain seroreactive. If therapy for syphilis is given first during this stage, the patient is unlikely to show regression of nontreponemal antibody determinations. Approximately 60 per cent of untreated patients in the late latent stages continue to have an asymptomatic course, whereas 40 per cent develop symptoms of late or tertiary disease. Progress of disease from late latent to late symptomatic syphilis usually is prevented if appropriate antimicrobial therapy is given at this stage. (See reference 30 for depictions of children with acquired secondary syphilis.)

Tertiary Disease

Three to 10 years after the last evidence of secondary disease, the patient may develop nonprogressive, localized lesions of the dermal elements or supporting structures of the body, called gummata. Because these lesions are relatively quiescent, the term benign tertiary syphilis often is used. Spirochetes are extremely sparse or absent. The gummatous reaction primarily is a pronounced immunologic reaction of the host.

Neurosyphilis

During the early stage of syphilis, approximately one-third of all patients have involvement of the central nervous system. If untreated, only half of these patients develop late neurosyphilis. The interval between primary disease and late neurosyphilis usually is more than 5 years. However, several of the few children recognized to have acquired (vs. congenital) late neurosyphilis have developed symptomatic disease at a very early age. It is possible that the disease progresses more rapidly in children than in adults.

Late neurosyphilis may be asymptomatic or, if symptomatic, may occur in a variety of ways. Classic presentations include paralytic dementia, tabes dorsalis, amyotrophic lateral sclerosis, meningovascular syphilis, seizures, optic atrophy, and gummatous changes of the cord. Neurosyphilis may resemble virtually any other neurologic disease.

Cardiovascular Syphilis

Approximately 10 to 40 years after primary syphilis, the untreated patient may develop signs of cardiovascular involvement. Most commonly involved are the great vessels of the heart, where syphilitic aortic and pulmonary arteritis develop. The inflammatory reaction also may cause stenosis, with resulting angina, myocardial insufficiency, and death.

Congenital Syphilis

Syphilitic pregnant women who have not received therapy or have received inadequate therapy may transmit the infection to their fetuses at any clinical stage of their disease. Seventy to 100 per cent of all pregnant women with untreated primary syphilis, 90 per cent of women with secondary syphilis, and approximately 30 per cent of women with latent syphilis may transmit the infection to their fetuses. In general, the greater the time that has elapsed since the woman's primary or secondary infection, the less likely she is to transmit disease to the fetus. From 1988 to 1991, approximately 10 to 50 cases of congenital syphilis were reported to occur per 100 cases of primary or secondary syphilis in women of child-bearing age.[23] In 1994, there were 56 cases of congenital syphilis per 100,000 live births.

At the onset of congenital syphilis, *T. pallidum* is liberated directly into the circulation of the fetus, resulting in spirochetemia with widespread dissemination.

The outcome of untreated fetal infection is variable. Intrauterine death occurs in an estimated 25 per cent of infections, with abortion usually occurring after the first trimester. Perinatal death may occur in another 25 to 30 per cent of untreated infected babies.[54] In a study of the perinatal outcome of congenital syphilis, the fatality rate for the infant was 464 per 1000 infected births. Of the fatalities, 27 per cent were neonatal deaths, and 73 per cent were stillbirths.[64] Those infants who survive delivery have a broad spectrum of manifestations.

The signs and symptoms of congenital syphilis are divided arbitrarily into early manifestations, which appear in the first 2 years of life, and late manifestations, which emerge anytime thereafter.

Early Congenital Syphilis

The abnormal physical and laboratory findings in early congenital syphilis are varied and unpredictable. Table 150–2 lists the major physical and laboratory findings from 310 reported cases of early congenital syphilis. These undoubtedly are minimal rates for each finding. The onset is between birth and about 3 months of age, with most cases occurring within the first 5 weeks of age. If the infection is transmitted at or close to the time of delivery, which is a common occurrence, the baby with congenital syphilis may appear perfectly normal at birth, only to appear later in the newborn period with "septic" syphilis characterized by multiorgan involvement. The neonate in the immediate newborn period may have only hepatosplenomegaly with or without jaundice.

SKELETAL SYSTEM. Because of their frequency and early appearance, the roentgenographic changes in the bones are of diagnostic value. The femur and humerus are involved most often. Roentgenographically, accumulating calcified matrix is seen at the epiphyseal margin, which may be smooth or serrated. The serrated appearance is known as Wegner sign and represents points of calcified cartilage along the nutrient cartilage canal. A zone of rarefaction at the epiphyseal line may be seen, which represents syphilitic granulation tissue containing a few scattered calcified remnants and a mass of connective tissue containing areas of perivascular infiltration of small round cells. Irregular areas of increased density and rarefaction produce the moth-eaten appearance of the roentgenogram. Epiphyseal separation may occur as a result of a fracture of the brittle layer of calcified cartilage. Irregular periosteal thickening also is common. The changes usually are present at birth but may appear in the first few weeks of life. The bony changes, osteochondritis and periostitis, are self-limited and usually are healed in the first 6 months, even in the absence of specific therapy. These are painful lesions, and pain on motion often leads an affected infant to appear to have a limb paralysis.

TABLE 150–2. Findings in 310 Cases of Early Congenital Syphilis

Findings	Number of Patients
Hepatomegaly	100
Skeletal abnormalities	91
Birth weight <2500 g	51
Skin lesions	45
Hyperbilirubinemia	40
Pneumonia	51
Splenomegaly	56
Severe anemia, hydrops, edema	50
Snuffles, nasal discharge	27
Painful limbs	22
Pancreatitis	14
Cerebrospinal fluid abnormalities	21
Nephritis	11
Failure to thrive	10
Testicular mass	1
Chorioretinitis	1
Hypoglobulinemia	1

Data from references 11, 17, 38, 44, 55, 64, 75, and 76.

RHINITIS. Rhinitis, coryza, or snuffles are likely to mark the onset of congenital syphilis. Usually, it appears in the first week of life and seldom later than the third month. The snuffles are more severe and persist longer than the common cold, often are bloody, and frequently are associated with laryngitis.

RASH. The syphilitic rash usually appears 1 to 2 weeks after the rhinitis. The typical eruption is maculopapular and consists of small spots that are dark red-copper. If the rash is present at birth, it often is bullous. The rash is most severe on the hands and feet. The rash comes out slowly, taking 1 to 3 weeks, and is followed by desquamation. As the rash fades, the lesions become coppery or dusky red, and pigmentation may persist. (See reference 30 for depictions of a variety of cutaneous manifestations of early congenital syphilis.)

FISSURES AND MUCOUS PATCHES. Fissures and mucous patches are not seen often but are highly characteristic features of congenital syphilis. The fissures develop about the lips, nares, and anus. They bleed readily and heal with scarring. A cluster of scars radiating around the mouth is named rhagades. Mucous patches may be found on any of the mucous membranes, especially in the mouth and genitalia. Condylomata are raised, moist lesions appearing on areas of the skin where there is moisture or friction. They are highly infectious.

HEMATOLOGIC FINDINGS. Anemia, thrombocytopenia, hemolytic processes, and both leukopenia and leukocytosis characterize congenital syphilis. The hemolytic process is Coombs test–negative and often accompanied by cryoglobulinemia, immune complex formation, and macroglobulinemia. The hemolysis, like the liver disease, is refractory to therapy and may persist for weeks. Paroxysmal nocturnal hemoglobinuria is a late manifestation of congenital syphilis.

CENTRAL NERVOUS SYSTEM INVOLVEMENT. Because of the wide range of normal values for cerebrospinal fluid protein, red blood cells, and white blood cells in the perinatal period, it has been difficult to define the proportion of infants with congenital syphilis who have abnormalities of those laboratory values. Current consensus identifies an abnormal cerebrospinal fluid white blood cell count in infants being evaluated for possible congenital syphilis as >25 cells/mm^3 and protein as >150/dL. In the era prior to penicillin therapy, approximately 15 per cent of infants with congenital syphilis developed findings of meningovascular disease. These findings included meningitis, meningeal irritation, bulging fontanelle, and seizures.

The only specific diagnosis for central nervous system disease in congenital syphilis is the presence of a reactive Venereal Disease Research Laboratory (VDRL) test from the cerebrospinal fluid. However, children may fail to have a reactive VDRL test on initial examination and still develop later signs of neurosyphilis. Therefore, it is recommended that all children with the diagnosis of congenital syphilis receive therapy that is adequate for the care of neurosyphilis, regardless of cerebrospinal fluid findings.

PNEUMONIA. Syphilitic pneumonia is a common finding in congenital syphilis and causes a fluffy, diffuse infiltrate involving all lung areas. It is termed pneumonia alba. Follow-up evaluation of children who have recovered from congenital syphilis has shown that at least 10 per cent have chronic pulmonary disease.

HEPATOSPLENOMEGALY. Neonatal syphilitic hepatitis is associated with visible *Treponema* on biopsy of liver tissue, hepatomegaly, and cholestasis. Aspartate aminotransferase, alkaline phosphatase, and alanine aminotransferase determinations often are elevated, and prothrombin time may be delayed. The liver disease often resolves slowly, even after apparently adequate therapy.[67] Other gastrointestinal presentations of congenital syphilis include necrotizing enterocolitis.

ECTODERMAL CHANGES. Ectodermal changes in syphilitic infants include suppuration and exfoliation of the nails, loss of hair and eyebrows, choroiditis, and iritis.

Neonates and infants with congenital syphilis may resemble babies with other illnesses peculiar to newborns, including toxoplasmosis, rubella, cytomegalovirus infection, herpes simplex virus infection, "sepsis" of the newborn, blood group incompatibilities, battered child syndrome, "periostitis" of prematurity, neonatal hepatitis, and osteomyelitis.

Late Congenital Syphilis

Late manifestations of congenital syphilis are the result of scarring from the early systemic disease and include involvement of the teeth, bones, eyes, and eighth nerve; gummata in the viscera, skin, or mucous membranes; and neurosyphilis (Table 150–3). Approximately 40 per cent of surviving and untreated infected infants, as reported in the early literature, develop late manifestations of infection. Some of these changes can be prevented by treatment of the mother during pregnancy or of the infant prior to 3 months of age. In contrast, treatment of 15 children at 4 months of age or later showed 7 with dental changes.[60] Other stigmata (e.g., keratitis saber skin) may occur or progress, despite appropriate therapy.

TABLE 150–3. Stigmata of Late Congenital Syphilis*

Stigmata	Per Cent of Total Patients
Frontal boss of Parrott	87
Short maxilla	84
High palatal arch	76
Hutchinson triad	75
Hutchinson teeth	63
Interstitial keratitis	9
Eighth nerve deafness	3
Saddle nose	73
Mulberry molars	65
Higouménakis sign	39
Relative protuberance of mandible	26
Rhagades	7
Saber shin	4
Scaphoid scapulae	0.7
Clutton joint	0.3

*An analysis of 271 patients.

Adapted from Fiumara, N. J., and Lessell, S.: Manifestations of late congenital syphilis. Arch. Dermatol. *102*:78–83, 1970. Copyright 1970, American Medical Association.

TEETH. Characteristic changes are found in the permanent upper central incisors, which present a notched appearance of the biting edges; x-ray study leads to diagnosis, even while deciduous teeth are in place. These are Hutchinson teeth. If first molars show maldevelopment of the cusps, the finding is called mulberry or moon molars.

INTERSTITIAL KERATITIS. Interstitial keratitis is the most common late lesion. It may appear at any age between 4 and 30 years or later but characteristically appears when the patient is close to puberty. A ground-glass appearance may develop in the cornea, accompanied by vascularization of the adjacent sclera. These changes become bilateral and usually lead to blindness.

NEUROSYPHILIS. The same manifestations of neurosyphilis seen in acquired syphilis may occur in congenital syphilis. Paresis is seen more frequently and tabes dorsalis less frequently in the congenital form than in the acquired form of the disease.

EIGHTH NERVE DEAFNESS. Hearing loss usually is sudden and appears around 8 to 10 years of age. It often accompanies interstitial keratitis. The constellation of eighth nerve deafness, interstitial keratitis, and Hutchinson teeth is called the Hutchinson triad.

BONE CHANGES. Bone changes include the sclerosing lesions, saber shin and frontal bossing, and the gummatous or destructive lesion of saddle nose. Perforation of the hard palate almost is pathognomonic of congenital syphilis.

CLUTTON JOINT. This is painless arthritis of the knees and, rarely, other joints.

CUTANEOUS LESIONS. Rhagades represent scars resulting from persistent rhinitis during infancy and rarely are seen today.

Nonspecific sequelae of congenital syphilis have not been described well because follow-up studies of children with congenital syphilis are minimal. Other findings that have been reported include failure to thrive in 41 per cent, chronic lung disease in 10 per cent, and necrotizing enterocolitis in 3 per cent.[64] Numerous children with symptomatic congenital syphilis also present with sepsis due to other bacteria, including *Escherichia coli*, group B streptococci, and *Yersinia* species.

Syphilis in Pregnancy

The investigations of Taber and Huber[75] illustrate the importance of recognition and appropriate therapy of syphilis in pregnant women. In this study, 22 women with syphilis were undiagnosed during pregnancy and therefore did not receive prenatal therapy. Eleven infants were followed without initial therapy. At delivery, all were asymptomatic clinically, four had a reactive VDRL test, five had a nonreactive VDRL test, and two were not tested. All these infants were readmitted with obvious disease involving multisystem infection, three with proven spirochetal hepatitis, two with nephrotic syndrome, and three with central nervous system involvement. This experience again emphasizes the importance of transmission of infection late in gestation, leading to delivery of infants who are well clinically but whose disease emerges in the weeks after delivery if untreated.[21]

DIAGNOSIS

Efforts to diagnose infectious syphilis suffer from the lack of a method to culture the organisms on laboratory media. Four methods are useful in the diagnosis of syphilis: (1) direct visualization of the organism by darkfield microscopy, fluorescent antibody technique, or special stains of infected tissue; (2) animal inoculation; (3) demonstration of serologic reactions typical of syphilis; (4) demonstration of the organism by histopathology; and (5) demonstration of exposure of an infant to a mother whose disease was untreated or treated inadequately.

Patients with a primary chancre as well as with active secondary lesions may be diagnosed by darkfield microscopy. Because this depends on direct visualization of motile spirochetes, the organisms must be active and viable. Prior use of many antibiotics rapidly destroys the motility of the organisms, as do many topical disinfectants. Serous fluid from the base of the lesion should be collected for darkfield examination. Syphilitic lesions of the mouth may harbor indigenous treponemes, of which the morphologic similarity to pathogenic species can confuse the interpretation of findings. Direct darkfield examination is, however, particularly helpful in making a diagnosis early in the disease, prior to the development of seroreactivity. If a darkfield microscope is unavailable, a direct fluorescent antibody stain for *T. pallidum* may be made. Exudate is collected in capillary tubes or slides and stained with specific antibody. Amniotic fluid may be examined for the presence of spirochetes using darkfield microscopy, fluorescent antitreponemal staining, and amniotic fluid VDRL test.[29, 78]

Most patients with syphilis that has progressed beyond the primary stage are diagnosed by serologic methods.

Serologic Tests

The two types of serologic tests for syphilis are the nontreponemal antigen tests and the treponemal antigen tests (Table 150–4). Although the latter tests indicate experience with a treponemal infection, they cross-react with the antigen of other treponemal diseases, such as those causing yaws and pinta. Therefore, no test is specific for syphilis, and no test is completely sensitive. Efforts to produce a more sensitive and more specific test are continuous. A promising approach is the use of recombinant clones expressing immunogenic proteins of *T. pallidum* to investigate pathogen-specific antigens.[35] Some of these products are under investigation for use as diagnostic material.[67a]

NONTREPONEMAL TESTS. The original test for syphilis, as described by Wassermann, used syphilitic tissue as complement-fixing antigen to detect the presence of antibody (reagin) that is induced by *T. pallidum*. Extracts of other normal tissue, such as beef heart, had similar properties, and

TABLE 150–4. Standard Serologic Tests for Syphilis

			Per Cent Reactivity During		
Antigen	**Antigen Source**	**Test**	***Primary Stage***	***Secondary Stage***	***Tertiary Stage***
Nontreponemal reagin	Extracts of tissue (cardiolipin-lecithin-cholesterol)	VDRL	78	95	71
		RPR	86	98	73
Treponemal	*Treponema pallidum*	MHA-TP	76	100	94
		FTA-ABS	84	100	97

FTA-ABS, fluorescent treponemal antibody absorption; MHA-TP, microhemagglutination–*Treponema pallidum;* RPR, rapid plasma reagin; VDRL, Venereal Disease Research Laboratory.

purification and standardization of these materials led to the use as antigen of a preparation containing cardiolipin and lecithin in cholesterol.

Two tests currently using cardiolipin, lecithin, and cholesterol are the VDRL and rapid plasma reagin tests. These tests measure IgM and IgG antibiodies nondescriminatively. The tests provide similar clinical information and have similar advantages. They are inexpensive to perform and demonstrate rising and falling antibody titers that often correlate with adequacy of therapy and the clinical status of a patient. Disadvantages include a relatively high proportion of biologic acute and chronic false-positive reactors and an increasing proportion of false-negative reactions in the later stages of untreated syphilis. The technical difficulties include a negative reaction due to the prozone phenomenon when only undiluted serum is tested.

The VDRL test is used commonly to screen newborn infants for possible infection with *T. pallidum*. Transplacental passage of IgG antibodies to the infant means that mothers with positive VDRL tests usually will transmit these antibodies to their infants. Review of the relationship of maternal to newborn VDRL tests was included in the study by Taber and Huber[75] of mothers who were undiagnosed and untreated. Although 12 of 22 mothers had VDRL test results two to four times that of their babies, 6 of these women and their babies had nonreactive serology at the time of delivery. These and other data have shown that it was unusual for the infant to have a VDRL test of greater titer than its mother's, even if the infant was incubating congenital syphilis.[73]

TREPONEMAL TESTS. The most significant development of the past three decades in the serologic study of syphilis was the detection of treponemal antibody by fluorescein-labeled antihuman antibody. These tests are used to confirm the validity of a positive nontreponemal test, to diagnose congenital syphilis, and to diagnose late stages of syphilis. The tests are both sensitive and reliable.

Fluorescent treponemal antibody absorption (FTA-ABS) tests use lyophilized Nichols strain organisms as antigen and are tests that measure both IgG and IgM. Antigen is fixed to a slide, and the test serum is applied, allowing reaction of antitreponemal antibody with antigen. The slide is layered with fluorescein isothiocyanate-labeled antihuman gamma globulin, and the presence or absence of antibody is determined by fluorescent microscopy.

Test sera are preabsorbed with sorbent to eliminate group-reactive antibody. Thus, the test is rendered relatively specific for disease with virulent treponemal species, usually *T. pallidum*. However, the FTA-ABS test is expensive and time consuming. It is, therefore, recommended not for general screening but for confirmation of positive nontreponemal tests and diagnosis of later stages of syphilis in which the results of nontreponemal tests may be falsely negative.

Microhemagglutination–*T. pallidum* tests depend on the passive hemaggutination of erythrocytes that have been sensitized with Nichols strain *T. pallidum*. The test has been automated and is both easy to perform technically and inexpensive. It is as sensitive as the FTA-ABS tests, except in primary syphilis, and is highly specific. Like the FTA-ABS test, it is unlikely to revert to a nonreactive state after treatment of the patient and unless treatment is given very early.

PROVISIONAL TESTS. Several tests are in development and are recognized to be likely to progress to a standardized test if further studies confirm initial results. One of these that tests for IgM antibody is the Capita syphilis M test.[45] These studies provide some hope that a reliable assay for IgM antibody in infancy eventually may assist in the diagnosis or ruling out of congenital syphilis in exposed but asymptomatic infants.[10, 73] More studies are needed before this test or other IgM tests will be accepted as a standard assay.

In the diagnosis of congenital syphilis, it would be most helpful if there were a means to differentiate between passive transplacental transfer of maternal antibody to the fetus and production by the fetus of endogenous antitreponemal antibody. Because antibodies of the IgM class do not cross the placenta, detection of IgM antibody in the fetal circulation usually indicates antibody production by the fetus because of active fetal infection. The development of a fluorescent antihuman antibody that is specific for IgM-class antitreponemal antibody is the IgM–FTA-ABS test. A reactive test with infant blood is strong evidence of active congenital disease.[3, 39, 66] However, a negative test does not eliminate the possibility of congenital syphilis. The test is insensitive when the onset of disease is delayed. Occasional false-positive IgM–FTA-ABS tests occur because of the presence of an IgM anti-IgG antibody. For these reasons, the Centers for Disease Control and Prevention have recommended that the IgM–FTA-ABS test be suspended for diagnostic testing of newborns, and the test is available only as a provisional test.

Efforts to develop a sensitive and specific serologic test for congenital syphilis have led to the identification of antigenic components of *T. pallidum* that are epitopes for the immune response. A 37-kDa membrane protein is a dipoprotein[74] and the target of IgM antibody formation in the sera of congenitally infected infants.[19] Another protein that is recognized by infected infants, using an immunoblot technique, is a 47-kDa protein. Efforts to develop diagnostic tests based on these findings are active.[43, 67]

False-Positive Reactions

All of the available serologic tests for syphilis produce occasional reactive results in patients for whom there is no other evidence of syphilitic infection. These reactions usually are called biologic false-positive (BFP), as distinct from positive reactions due to technical errors. The majority of BFP reactions occur with nontreponemal tests; approximately 1 per cent of normal adults will have a BFP reaction by nontreponemal antigen tests. These reactions probably are not more common in pregnancy than in the general population. Reaginic antibody is reactive with at least 200 antigens other than those of *T. pallidum*, and although the specific stimulus for this antibody in syphilis as well as other diseases is unknown, it may represent antibody to cellular lipoidal antigens of the host that are liberated during various diseases. For clinical purposes, BFP reactions may be classified as acute, in which the reactivity resolves within 6 months, or chronic, in which reactivity is persistent.

ACUTE BIOLOGIC FALSE-POSITIVE REACTIONS. Most BFP reactions are detected by nontreponemal tests and occur in patients with other acute illnesses, especially pneumonia, hepatitis, and viral exanthematous disease, or after vaccinations. The prognosis for the patient's health is not affected by the finding. The titer of antibody usually is low, less than 1:8, and in most instances the FTS-ABS is nonreactive. Approximately two-thirds of patients with BFP reactions have acute reactions, and reactivity subsides in 6 months or less.

CHRONIC BIOLOGIC FALSE-POSITIVE REACTIONS. Many patients with chronic BFP reactions have or develop systemic disease. Drug addiction, chronic hepatitis, old age, leprosy, and collagen vascular disease are associated highly with chronic BFP reactions. There may be a familial predisposition to this finding. The antibody detected by the VDRL test in chronic BFP reactions predominantly is IgM, whereas in syphilis it mainly is IgG. Patients with chronic BFP reactions and systemic lupus erythematosus commonly also have a reactive FTA-ABS test.[46] The triosephosphate isomerase test may be helpful in the differential diagnosis in these instances. A particularly concerning finding has been that there appears to be a relative increase in both acute and chronic BFP reactions in women who are infected with HIV.[5]

TABLE 150–5. Case Definitions for Confirmed or Presumptive Congenital Syphilis

Confirmed

Treponema pallidum identified from lesions, placenta, umbilical cord, or autopsy

Presumptive

Infant's mother had evidence of syphilis and was untreated or inadequately treated

or

Infant had a positive serologic test for syphilis and any of the following:
- Positive physical findings
- Positive cerebrospinal fluid Venereal Disease Research Laboratory test
- Cerebrospinal fluid cells or protein is abnormal
- Osteitis appears on long-bone radiograph
- Infant's serologic test for syphilis is 4 × that of the mother's
- Fluorescent treponemal antibody absorption 19S is IgM-positive
- Placentitis or funicitis

or

The infant's mother had contact within 90 days prior to delivery with a person with primary or secondary syphilis and the mother had been untreated

Criteria for Diagnosis of Early Congenital Syphilis

The diagnosis of early congenital syphilis is based upon clinical, serologic, and epidemiologic considerations. Case definitions for the diagnosis of congenital syphilis are found in Table 150–5. The evaluation includes an assessment of the mother for general risk factors for increased rates of syphilis (Table 150–6), followed by an evaluation of the mother's current known serologic status (Table 150–7). If the mother has been treated, the clinician must assess the adequacy of therapy (Table 150–8).

If the mother's serologic assays have been positive, the infant also must be assessed for clinically apparent disease (Table 150–9). It should be noted that patients with early

TABLE 150–6. General Maternal Risk Factors Associated with Increased Rates of Early Syphilis in Pregnancy

Infection with HIV
Adolescent or unmarried status
History of sexually transmitted disease
Substance abuse, especially cocaine
Inadequate or absent prenatal care
Prostitution or promiscuity
Localized populations or geographic areas
Treatment of gonorrhea with ciprofloxacin or spectinomycin
Poor communication among medical personnel regarding maternal/infant status

Data from references 18, 41, 57, 63, and 77.

TABLE 150–7. Components of the Epidemiologic Evaluation of an Infant's Mother for Presumptive Congenital Syphilis of the Infant

- Evaluate mother for prior history of syphilis or major risk factors for syphilis
- If mother received treatment for syphilis, evaluate course of therapy for adequacy in the eradication of congenital syphilis (see Table 150–8)
- Evaluate current maternal status with a nontreponemal test (e.g., Venereal Disease Research Laboratory, rapid plasma reagin) or a treponemal test (e.g., fluorescent treponemal antibody absorption, microhemagglutination–*Treponema pallidum*)
- If mother is identified clinically or through contact tracing as having early syphilis during the 3 months after delivery, reevaluate the child and consider therapy at that time
- Note that higher maternal titers to nontreponemal tests are associated with failure of maternal therapy to prevent congenital disease[47]
- Note that unknown duration of maternal syphilis is associated with failure of maternal therapy to prevent congenital disease[47]

congenital syphilis have a significant incidence of other infections, including cytomegalovirus infection, toxoplasmosis, other sexually transmitted diseases, and bacteremia. The diagnosis of congenital syphilis particularly may be difficult when another infection is present. Both VDRL and FTA-ABS measure IgG antibody and therefore do not distinguish disease of the infant from maternally derived antibody. Many infants are born to women who have had syphilis in the past, received therapy, and remained seroreactive. Their infants also will be seroreactive. Assuring that the infant does not have congenital disease in the immediate newborn period may not be possible.

The limitations of interpretation of the infant's serologic results are seen in Figure 150–2. At any given time, the clinician may not know if an asymptomatic infant is or is not infected and is or is not reflecting maternal antibody. Figure 150–2 depicts the four major patterns of VDRL results from infants who initially were well clinically and were not treated in the perinatal period. Pattern *A* describes children who receive passive transfer of maternal antibody, do not have disease, have progressive decrease of titer of antibody to a nondetectable level, and have a nondetectable reaction at 2 to 3 months of age. These children need not receive therapy.

Pattern *B* depicts infants to whom disease is transmitted

TABLE 150–8. Circumstances in Which Maternal Therapy for Syphilis May Be Presumed to Be Subtherapeutic

- Treatment with a nonpenicillin regimen
- History of maternal treatment was not documented fully or verifiable
- Treatment during the month prior to delivery
- Treatment in HIV-infected women with a regimen that is not standard for neurosyphilis
- Serial posttherapy assays of maternal nontreponemal antibody titers were not performed
- Serial posttherapy assays of maternal nontreponemal antibody titers did not show fourfold decline in titers, thus suggesting failure to eradicate infection or relapse or reinfection

TABLE 150–9. Components of the Medical Evaluation of an Infant for Suspected Congenital Syphilis

- A thorough physical examination for physical evidence of congenital syphilis
- A quantitative nontreponemal serologic test for syphilis performed on the infant's peripheral sera
- Cerebrospinal fluid analysis for cells, protein, and Venereal Disease Research Laboratory test
- Long bone roentgenography
- Chest roentgenography
- Complete blood cell count
- Liver function tests
- Where available, determination of the presence of antitreponemal immunoglobulin antibody
- Pathologic examination of the placenta or amniotic cord using specific fluorescent antitreponemal antibody staining
- If any other signs of disease occur, complete an ophthalmic examination
- Auditory brain stem response

at delivery and who are well clinically at delivery. In this group, the mothers are seroreactive and the infant receives maternal antibody, which is catabolized and decreases for a few weeks. However, the infant begins to produce antibody at about 3 to 4 weeks of age and if untreated may present with congenital syphilis at about 3 to 6 weeks of age.

Pattern *C* is difficult to interpret. These children often have a relatively low titer of antibody at birth, but the antibody does not decrease to nonreactive, and at 6 weeks to 3 months of age, the children still are seroreactive. Although these children may or may not have active disease, the author recommends that they receive a full course of therapy.

Pattern *D* depicts infants whose mothers have acquired syphilis very near to the time of delivery and the infant therefore is well clinically, receives no maternal antibody, and is seronegative. In these instances, the infection is transmitted to the infant at delivery, and if left untreated, the child usually will present with disease at about 3 to 6 weeks of age. Congenital disease in these children will be recognized prior to development of symptomatic illness only if the mother's illness is recognized (a chancre or early secondary eruption) or she is identified as a contact. Table 150–9 lists

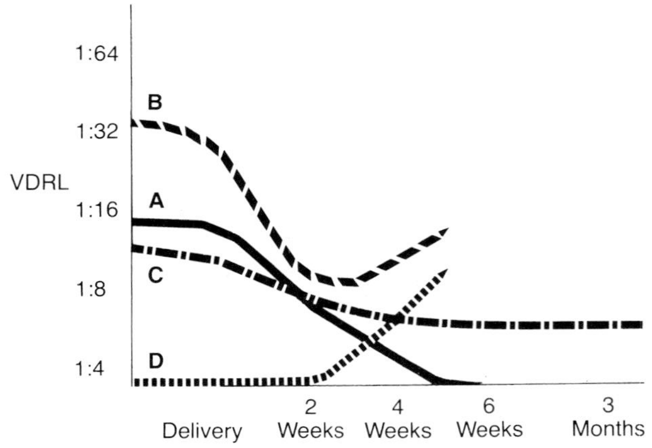

FIGURE 150–2. *Patterns of serologic findings in infants with congenital syphilis or passive transfer of maternal antibody.* A, *Passive transfer of maternal antibody: no disease.* B, *Passive transfer of maternal antibody: later onset of disease.* C, *Passive transfer of maternal antibody: indeterminate status for the infant.* D, *Perinatal infection of mother and infant: later onset of disease.*

TABLE 150–10. Clinical Findings of 148 Infants Whose Mothers Had Syphilis and Whose Treatment Was Adequate, Inadequate, or Not Provided

	Maternal Treatment		
Infant Findings	*None* (n = *72*)	*Inadequate* (n = *31*)	*Adequate* (n = *45*)
Clinical disease	3	0	0
Positive CSF-VDRL test	7	4	0
Abnormal bone radiograph	6	0	0
Stillbirth	6	0	0
Total (any abnormality)	22 (31%)	4 (13%)	0

CSF, cerebrospinal fluid; VDRL, Venereal Disease Research Laboratory.

From Reyes, M. P., Hunt, N., Ostrea, E. M., et al.: Maternal/congenital syphilis in a large tertiary care urban hospital. Clin. Infect. Dis. *17:*1041–1046, 1993. University of Chicago, publisher.

the major components of the medical evaluation of an infant for suspected congenital syphilis.

In 1988, it was recognized that prior definitions of congenital syphilis that had been used for surveillance and for treatment decisions had been difficult to apply to the clinical setting because they required a diagnosis that often could be made only over a period of weeks or months. During that period, many children were lost to follow-up and therefore were neither treated nor reported.[15] Because of the high incidence of congenital disease in infants born to inadequately treated mothers, current definitions of congenital syphilis for a presumptive case (which should be reported and treated) require only (1) that the infant be born to a mother with untreated or inadequately treated syphilis or (2) that the child have physical or laboratory signs of congenital syphilis. A summary of the surveillance case definition used since 1988 is seen in Table 150–5. There are minor differences among case definitions of congenital syphilis as formulated by several agencies and experts.[64a] Note the following two points:

1. The newborn who is well clinically but was born to a mother who had contact within 90 days before delivery with a person with primary or secondary syphilis and who had not been treated or had been treated inadequately is a presumptive case. This includes infants of mothers with nonreactive serology.
2. Although recommendations for therapy commonly have assumed that adequate therapy of a mother with primary or secondary syphilis during pregnancy will prevent congenital syphilis with a high degree of reliability, reasons to doubt this premise have emerged.[49, 79] In particular, treatment failures in which the infant developed syphilis despite maternal therapy have been reported when the mother first was treated within 30 days of delivery.[8, 50, 51, 64] Therefore, infants born to mothers who were treated within 30 days of delivery are considered to have been treated inadequately, and the baby should receive a full course of therapy.

A listing of the various circumstances in which maternal therapy may be presumed to be subtherapeutic is given in Table 150–8. The consequences of inadequate therapy of the mother are shown in data on Table 150–10. In that experience, 13 per cent of children born to inadequately treated mothers had congenital syphilis, all of which was neurosyphilis.[63]

TREATMENT

T. pallidum is extremely sensitive to penicillin, as defined by experimental animal work. The minimal inhibitory concentration of penicillin is approximately 0.004 U (or 0.0025 μg/mL). There is no evidence of increasing resistance to penicillin by the spirochetes, but such evidence would come only from the recognition of therapeutic failures. Effective treatment of syphilis must maintain a minimal inhibitory concentration of 0.03 U/mL of penicillin in serum (or cerebrospinal fluid) for 7 to 10 days. Therapy is designed to achieve and maintain several times the necessary inhibiting levels and to avoid penicillin-free intervals during therapy. Penicillin remains the drug of first choice because of its established efficacy and minimal toxicity. Penicillin regimens for treatment of gonorrhea are sufficient to treat preprimary syphilis.

Syphilis in Pregnancy

All pregnant women should have a nontreponemal serologic test for syphilis at the first prenatal visit. A second test should be done during the third trimester, especially in those at increased risk of contracting disease. Seropositivity with a nontreponemal test requires complete evaluation, including quantitative nontreponemal serology and confirmatory treponemal serology. In the absence of clinical symptoms or proven exposure to an active case and with a negative treponemal test, treatment may be withheld and studies repeated in 4 weeks. When epidemiologic, clinical, or serologic evidence of infection is present or the diagnosis can not be excluded, treatment should be instituted. Patients who have been treated adequately in the past do not require additional therapy unless quantitative serology shows persisting high titer, fourfold increase, or other evidence of reinfection. The clinician should err on the side of more complete therapy if in doubt.

It is a policy statement of the Centers of Disease Control and Prevention that no infant should leave the hospital without the serologic status of the infant's mother having been documented at least once during pregnancy. Serologic testing also should be performed at delivery in communities and populations at risk of acquiring congenital syphilis.[4, 12] In this era of early and very early discharge from the hospital after deliveries, fulfilling the policy goal may require careful planning and advocacy by the clinician (Table 150–11).

Acquired Syphilis

Early syphilis may be treated with benzathine penicillin G, 2.4 million units intramuscularly in a single dose. It is recommended by some experts that the dose be repeated in 1 week.

Syphilis of more than 1 year's duration requires benzathine penicillin G, 7.2 million units administered as 2.4 million units weekly for 3 weeks.

Because neurosyphilis may be asymptomatic and can be

TABLE 150–11. Comparison of Yield of Positive Assays from Clinical Specimens for Screening of Congenital Syphilis at Delivery (n = 3306 liveborns)

Total positive assays	= 73 (2.2%)
Maternal sera positive	= 68/72 (94%)
Neonatal venopuncture sera positive	= 43/68 (63%)
Cord sera positive	= 30/60 (50%)

Data from Chabra, R. S., Brion, L. P., Castro, M., et al.: Comparison of maternal sera, cord blood and neonatal sera for detecting presumptive congenital syphilis: Relationship with maternal treatment. Pediatrics *91:*88–91, 1993.

defined accurately only by examination of cerebrospinal fluid, a lumbar puncture is recommended for patients with disease of more than 1 year's duration. Benzathine penicillin does not produce inhibitory cerebrospinal fluid levels of penicillin reliably.[72] Therefore, shorter-acting penicillins must be employed for neurosyphilis. In evaluating a patient for neurosyphilis, a cerebrospinal fluid specimen without contamination by peripheral blood is needed.[36] Recommended therapy is aqueous crystalline penicillin G, 12 to 24 million units, administered 2 to 4 million units every 4 hours intravenously for 10 to 14 days, *or* procaine penicillin, 2 to 4 million units intramuscularly daily plus probenecid, 500 mg orally four times per day, both for 10 to 14 days.

Any history of penicillin allergy should be documented clearly, and, if necessary, patients should receive skin testing, desensitization, and therapy with penicillin; other regimens confer a high risk that the fetus will not be treated adequately.[24, 59]

Pregnant Women Infected with HIV

Women who are HIV-infected and who have evidence of syphilis should receive treatment regimens that are recommended for persons with neurosyphilis (see earlier).

The follow-up on treated HIV-infected women must be thorough and frequent. The efficacy of therapy for syphilis in eradicating infection from HIV-infected women appears to be less secure than that in HIV-noninfected women and may require additional courses of therapy.[32, 53]

Follow-up of all pregnant women treated for syphilis requires quantitative serology at monthly intervals throughout pregnancy.

Normally, there is a fourfold or greater decline in nontreponemal assay titer during the 6 months after therapy for primary or secondary disease.[65] Subsequent follow-up with quantitative serology at 3, 6, and 12 months is necessary for early syphilis and is extended to 24 months for syphilis of longer duration. Patients with neurosyphilis require examinations and repeat cerebrospinal fluid examinations at 3-year intervals, especially if a drug other than penicillin was employed.

Retreatment for syphilis is considered when clinical signs or symptoms persist or recur, if there is a sustained fourfold increase in titer of a nontreponemal serologic test, or if therapy fails to produce a fourfold fall in originally high titers.

Patients who received therapy for gonorrhea with ceftriaxone have a high rate of cure of preprimary syphilis, but failures have occurred, and efficacy in pregnancy is not well studied.[33] This regimen therefore can not be assumed to have provided adequate therapy for syphilis in pregnancy.

Congenital Syphilis

All infants born to women with reactive serologic tests for syphilis should have a thorough physical examination that focuses on finding evidence of congenital syphilis. Pathologic examination of the placenta or umbilical cord using specific fluorescent antitreponemal antibody staining is recommended[28a, 60a] (Table 150–9).

Symptomatic infants include those with physical evidence of active disease, x-ray evidence of disease, a reactive cerebrospinal fluid VDRL test, elevated cerebrospinal fluid white blood cell count (>25 white blood cells/mm^3) and/or protein (>150 mg/dL), a quantitative nontreponemal serologic titer that is at least fourfold greater than the mother's titer, or placentitis or funicitis.

The recommended treatment regimens are aqueous crystalline penicillin G, 50,000 units/kg/dose intravenously every 12 hours during the first 7 days of life and every 8 hours thereafter for 10 days, or procaine penicillin G, 50,000 units/kg/dose intramuscularly in a single daily dose for 10 days.

The decision that an apparently well or ill infant does or does not require therapy for congenital syphilis must rest upon the physical examination, history of disease and treatment of the mother, results of a lumbar puncture, and serologic study.

Asymptomatic infants include those with a normal physical examination and serum quantitiative nontreponemal serologic titer the same or less than that of the mother. In these instances, treatment of the infant is dependent on the maternal treatment history and stage of infection.

If the maternal treatment was adequate and occurred before pregnancy and the mother maintained a stable low titer during pergnancy and at delivery, the infant does not require further evaluation and does not require treatment. If the maternal treatment was adequate, was given during pregnancy, and was given more than 4 weeks prior to delivery, the infant does not require cerebrospinal fluid evaluation or radiologic evaluation. In this instance, however, it is recommended that the infant receive a single dose of benzathine penicillin G, 50,000 units/kg intramuscularly.

Recent studies have re-evaluated the efficacy of treatment regimens for asymptomatic children who are born to mothers in whom the treatment for possible syphilis was suboptimal. Paryani and colleagues[55a] randomized 152 infants to receive either one injection of bicillin or a 10-day course of parenteral procaine penicillin. All study infants were asymptomatic on physical examination and had normal cerebrospinal fluid evaluation, normal x-ray studies of long bones, and no visceral abnormalities. The results of both forms of therapy were excellent, with no treatment failures. This study indicates that single-dose therapy may have a high rate of success when the child has negative studies and is asymptomatic. Failures of such therapy have been reported, but the frequency is unknown and appears to be low.[8, 79] These considerations are incorporated into treatment recommendations.

If the mother's treatment was inadequate, undocumented, or nonpenicillin or was administered less than 4 weeks prior to delivery, the infant may receive the following evaluations and regimens: aqueous penicillin G or procaine penicillin G (see earlier) for 10 days or benzathine penicillin G, 50,000 units/kg as a single dose, if the infant's evaluation (including cerebrospinal fluid examination, long-bone radiographs, and complete blood count) was normal and follow-up is certain.

Among asymptomatic infants, the yield of abnormal findings from examination of the cerebrospinal fluid has been very low in some experiences and appreciable in others.[7a, 63] A primary benefit of obtaining cerebrospinal fluid studies from infants who are receiving a 10-day parenteral course of aqueous or procaine penicillin therapy is identification of infants for whom follow-up of abnormal cerebrospinal fluid results should be accomplished. Benzathine penicillin regimens should be restricted to infants known to have a normal cerebrospinal fluid evaluation.

After the newborn period, children discovered to have syphilis should have a cerebrospinal fluid examination to rule out existing neurosyphilis. Children with late congenital syphilis or neurosyphilis should be treated with 200,000 to 300,000 U/kg/day of aqueous crystalline penicillin G, given as 50,000 U/kg every 4 to 6 hours for a minimum of 10 to 14 days. Older children with definite acquired syphilis and a normal neurologic examination may be treated with benzathine penicillin G, 50,000 U/kg intramuscularly to a maximal dose of 2.4 million units.

TABLE 150–12. Recommended Follow-Up of Infants with Congenital Syphilis or Seroreactive Status

Children with Congenital Syphilis

Repeat serologic assays at 1, 2, 4, 6, and 12 months of age
Nontreponemal assay should be nonreactive by 6 months
Repeat cerebrospinal fluid Venereal Disease Research Laboratory test at 6 months of age. If positive, re-treat infant
Monitor yearly for neurologic, hearing, and ophthalmic disorders
Perform yearly developmental evaluation

Children with Reactive Serologic Assays Who Were Not Treated Post Delivery

Repeat serologic assays at 1, 2, 4, 6, and 12 months of age
Nontreponemal assay should be nonreactive by 6 months
If nontreponemal assay is reactive at 6 months, reevaluate child (including cerebrospinal fluid test) and treat

Data from Ikeda, M. K., and Jenson, H. B.: Evaluation and treatment of congenital syphilis. J. Pediatr. *117*:843–852, 1990; and Rathbun, K. C.: Congenital syphilis: A proposal for improved surveillance, diagnosis and treatment. Sex. Transm. Dis. *10*:102–107, 1983.

Table 150–12 summarizes recommendations concerning follow-up of infants after treatment for congenital syphilis, as well as of seroreactive infants who were not treated because of the presumed adequacy of the management of the mother's serologic status.[34, 61]

Untreated infants should be seen at 1, 2, 4, 6, and 12 months of age and serologic tests repeated until two negative assays are obtained. If the child is not seronegative by 6 months of age, the child should be re-evaluated clinically and treated. The patient should be evaluated thoroughly for the extent of disease if there is serologic evidence of failure of treatment or of recurrent disease.

Two to 12 hours after the treatment of syphilis, a variable proportion of patients develop an acute systemic (Jarisch-Herxheimer) reaction usually consisting of headache, malaise, temperature to 38° C or higher, and resolution within a day. The reaction is observed most commonly in the early stages of syphilis,[3] probably represents a reaction to liberated endotoxin,[28] and does not affect the course of recovery. In the later stages of syphilis, fewer than one in four patients develop the reaction. Most reactions in late syphilis clinically are insignificant, but an occasional reaction may produce damage to the central nervous system or cardiovascular system.

In most patients receiving appropriate therapy during the primary or secondary stages, active disease totally and permanently is arrested. Persistent seroreactivity as measured by the FTA-ABS test may be avoided if treatment is given during the preprimary stage, but seldom thereafter. Nevertheless, progression to tertiary disease seldom, if ever, occurs. Similarly, therapy during early or late latent syphilis averts the development of symptomatic tertiary disease. Antimicrobial therapy for symptomatic neurosyphilis, optic neuritis, and cardiovascular syphilis may not be followed by significant clinical improvement, and established damage to vital organs may fail to resolve.

PREVENTION

Methods to control the spread of syphilis have relied extensively on treatment of case contacts. Persons with active syphilis are interviewed to identify all sexual contacts that may have occurred during the incubation period. The contacts are examined, and, if they are not infectious, they receive treatment appropriate for primary syphilis. Thus, advantage is taken of the long incubation period of syphilis by preventing disease in contacts before they themselves can transmit infection.

Prevention of congenital syphilis is based on serologic examination of women in early and late pregnancy. Because women may acquire syphilis during pregnancy, repeat serology should be performed in late pregnancy even when early assays were nonreactive.[4] Many states require examination of mother and/or infant blood samples at the time of delivery.

References

1. Ackerman, A. B., Goldfaden, G., and Cosmides, J. C.: Acquired syphilis in early childhood. Arch. Dermatol. *106*:92, 1972.
2. Alder, J. D., Friess, L., Tengowski, M., et al.: Phagocytosis of opsonized *Treponema pallidum* subsp. *pallidum* proceeds slowly. Infect. Immun. *58*:1167–1173, 1990.
3. Alford, C. A., Jr., Polt, S. S., Cassady, G. E., et al.: γ-M-fluorescent treponemal antibody in the diagnosis of congenital syphilis. N. Engl. J. Med. *280*:1086–1091, 1969.
4. Al-Salihi, F. L., Curran, J. P., and Shteir, O. A.: Occurrence of fetal syphilis after a nonreactive early gestational serologic test. J. Pediatr. *78*:121–123, 1971.
5. Augenbraun, M. H., DeHovitz, J. A., Feldman, J., et al.: Biological false-positive syphilis test results for women infected with human immunodeficiency virus. Clin. Infect. Dis. *19*:1040–1044, 1994.
6. Baughn, R. E., Jorizzo, J. L., Adams, C. B., et al.: Ig class and IgG subclass responses to *Treponema pallidum* in patients with syphilis. J. Clin. Immunol. *8*:128–139, 1988.
7. Bays, J., and Chadwick, D.: The serologic test for syphilis in sexually abused children and adolescents. Adolesc. Pediatr. Gynecol. *4*:148–151, 1991.
8. Beck-Sague, C., and Alexander, R.: Failure of benzathine penicillin and treatment in early congenital syphilis. Pediatr. Infect. Dis. *6*:1061–1064, 1987.

8a. Beeram, M. R., Chopde, N., Dawood, Y., et al: Lumbar puncture in the evaluation of possible asymptomatic congenital syphilis in neonates. J. Pediatr. *128*:125–129, 1996.

9. Braunstein, G. D., Lewis, E. J., Galvanek, E. G., et al.: The nephrotic syndrome associated with secondary syphilis. Am. J. Med. *48*:643–648, 1970.
10. Bromberg, K., Rawstron, S., and Tannis, G.: Diagnosis of congenital syphilis by combining *Treponema pallidum*–specific IgM detection with immunofluorescent antigen detection of *T. pallidum*. J. Infect. Dis. *168*:238, 1993.
11. Bulova, S. I., Schwartz, E., and Harrer, W. V.: Hydrops fetalis and congenital syphilis. Pediatrics *49*:285–287, 1972.
12. Centers for Disease Control and Prevention: 1993 sexually transmitted diseases treatment guidelines. M. M. W. R. *42*:1–102, 1993.
13. Chabra, R. S., Brion, L. P., Castro, M., et al.: Comparison of maternal sera, cord blood and neonatal sera for detecting presumptive congenital syphilis: Relationship with maternal treatment. Pediatrics *91*:88–91, 1993.
14. Clark, E. G., and Danbolt, N.: The Oslo study of the natural course of untreated syphilis: An epidemiologic investigation based on a re-study of the Boeck-Bruusgaard material. Med. Clin. North Am. *48*:613–623, 1964.
15. Cohen, D. A., Boyd, D., Pabhudas, I., et al.: The effects of case definition, maternal screening, and reporting criteria on rates of congenital syphilis. Am. J. Public Health *80*:316–317, 1990.
16. Coles, F. B., Hipp, S. S., Siberstein, G. S., et al.: Congenital syphilis surveillance in upstate New York, 1989–1992: Implications for prevention and clinical management. J. Infect. Dis. *171*:732–735, 1995.
17. Cremin, B. J., and Fisher, R. M.: The lesions of congenital syphilis. Br. J. Radiol. *43*:333–341, 1970.
18. Desenclos, J.-C. A., Scaggs, M., and Wroten, J. E.: Characteristics of mothers of live infants with congenital syphilis in Florida, 1987–1989. Am. J. Epidemiol. *136*:657–661, 1992.
19. Dobson, S. R. M., Taber, L. H., and Baughn, R. E.: Recognition of *Treponema pallidum* antigens by IgM and IgG antibodies in congenitally infected newborns and their mothers. J. Infect. Dis. *157*:903–910, 1988.
20. Dobson, S. R. M., Taber, L. H., and Baughn, R. E.: Characterization of the components in circulating immune complexes from infants with congenital syphilis. J. Infect. Dis. *158*:940–947, 1988.
21. Dorfman, D. H., and Glaser, J. H.: Congenital syphilis presenting in infants after the newborn period. N. Engl. J. Med. *323*:1299–1302, 1990.
22. Dorman, H. G., and Sahyun, B. F.: Identification and significance of spirochetes in placenta: Report of 105 cases with positive findings. Am. J. Obstet. Gynecol. *33*:954–967, 1937.
23. Dunn, R. A., Webster, L. A., and Nakashima, A. K.: Surveillance for

geographic and secular trends in congenital syphilis: United States, 1983–1991. M. M. W. R. *42*:59–71, 1993.

24. Fenton, L. J., and Light, I. J.: Congenital syphilis after maternal treatment with erythromycin. Obstet. Gynecol. *47*:492–494, 1976.
25. Fiumara, N. J.: Acquired syphilis in three patients with congenital syphilis. N. Engl. J. Med. *290*:1110–1120, 1974.
26. Fiumara, N. J., and Lessell, S.: Manifestations of late congenital syphilis. Arch. Dermatol. *102*:78–83, 1970.
27. Gamble, C. N., and Reardan, J. B.: Immunopathogenesis of syphilitic glomerulonephritis. N. Engl. J. Med. *292*:449–454, 1975.
28. Gelfand, J. A., Elin, R. J., Berry, F. W., Jr., et al.: Endotoxemia associated with the Jarisch-Herxheimer reaction. N. Engl. J. Med. *295*:211–213, 1976.

28a. Genest, D. R., Choi-Hong, S. R., Tate, J. E., et al: Diagnosis of congenital syphilis from placental examination: Comparison of histopathology, Steiner stain, and polymerase chain reaction for *Treponema pallidum* DNA. Hum. Pathol. *27*:366–372, 1996.

29. Glover, D. D., Winter, C. A., Charles, D., et al.: Diagnostic considerations in intra-amniotic syphilis. Sex. Transm. Dis. *12*:145–149, 1985.
30. Gutman, L. T.: Congenital syphilis. *In* Mandell, G. L. (ed.): Atlas of Infectious Disease. Volume 5: Sexually Transmitted Diseases. Philadelphia, Current Medicine, 1996.
31. Harter, C. A., and Benirschke, K.: Fetal syphilis in the first trimester. Am. J. Obstet. Gynecol. *124*:705–711, 1976.
32. Haas, J. S., Bolan, G., Larsen, S. A., et al.: Sensitivity of treponemal tests for detecting prior treated syphilis during human immunodeficiency virus infection. J. Infect. Dis. *162*:862–866, 1990.
33. Hook, E. W., Roddy, R. E., and Hardsfield, H. H.: Ceftriaxone therapy for incubating and early syphilis. J. Infect. Dis. *158*:881–884, 1988.
34. Ikeda, M. K., and Jenson, H. B.: Evaluation and treatment of congenital syphilis. J. Pediatr. *117*:843–852, 1990.
35. Isaacs, R. D., and Radolf, J. D.: Molecular approaches to improved syphilis serodiagnosis. Serodiagn. Immunother. Infect. Dis. *3*:299–306, 1989.
36. Izzat, N. N., Bartruff, J. K., Glicksman, J. M., et al.: Validity of the VDRL test on cerebrospinal fluid contaminated by blood. Br. J. Vener. Dis. *47*:162–164, 1971.
37. Jensen, J. R., Thestrup-Pedersen, K., and From, E.: Fluctuations in natural killer cell activity in early syphilis. Br. J. Vener. Dis. *59*:30–32, 1983.
38. Kaplan, B. S., Wiglesworth, F. W., Marks, M. I., et al.: The glomerulopathy of congenital syphilis: An immune deposit disease. J. Pediatr. *81*:1154–1156, 1972.
39. Kaufman, R. E., Olansky, D. C., and Wiesner, P. J.: The FTA-ABS (IgM) test for neonatal congenital syphilis: A critical review. J. Am. Vener. Dis. Assoc. *1*:78–84, 1974.
40. Klass, P. E., Brown, E. R., and Pelton, S. I.: The incidence of prenatal syphilis at the Boston City Hospital: A comparison across four decades. Pediatrics *94*:24–28, 1994.
41. Knight, J., Richardson, A. C., and White, K. C.: The role of syphilis serology in the evaluation of suspected sexual abuse. Pediatr. Infect. Dis. J. *11*:125–127, 1992.
42. Lande, M. B., Richardson, A. C., and White, K. C.: The role of syphilis in the evaluation of suspected sexual abuse. Pediatr. Infect. Dis. J. *11*:125–127, 1992.
43. Larsen, S. A., Steiner, B. M., and Rudolph, A. H.: Laboratory diagnosis and intrepretation of tests for syphilis. Clin. Microbiol. Rev. *8*:1–21, 1995.
44. Lascari, A. D., Diamond, J., and Nolan, B. E.: Anemia as the only presenting manifestation of congenital syphilis. Clin. Pediatr. *15*:90–91, 1976.
45. Lefevre, J. C., Betrand, M. A., and Bauriaud, R.: Evaluation of the Capita enzyme immunoassays for detection of immunoglobulins G and M to *Treponema pallidum* in syphilis. J. Clin. Microbiol. *28*:1704–1707, 1990.
46. Lesser, R. P., and O'Connell, E. J.: Positive fluorescent treponemal antibody test in systemic lupus erythematosus in childhood: Report of a case. J. Pediatr. *79*:1006–1008, 1971.
47. McFarlin, B. L., Bottoms, S. F., Dock, B. S., et al.: Epidemic syphilis: Maternal factors associated with congenital infection. Am. J. Obstret. Gynecol. *170*:535–540, 1994.
48. Macias, E. G., Eller, J. J., Huber, T. W., et al.: Immunofluorescence of tracheal secretions in neonatal syphilis. Pediatrics *53*:947–949, 1974.
49. Mascola, L., Pelosi, R., Blount, J. H., et al.: Congenital syphilis: Why is it still occurring? J. A. M. A. *252*:1719–1722, 1984.
50. Mascola, L., Pelosi, R., and Alexander, C. E.: Inadequate treatment of syphilis in pregnancy. Am. J. Obstet. Gynecol. *150*:945–947, 1984.
51. Mascola, L., Pelosi, R., Blount, J. A., et al.: Congenital syphilis revisited. Am. J. Dis. Child. *139*:575–580, 1985.
52. Musher, D. M., Hague-Park, M., Gyorkey, F., et al.: The interaction between *Treponema pallidum* and human polymorphonuclear leukocytes. J. Infect. Dis. *147*:77–86, 1983.
53. Musher, D. M., Hamill, R. J., and Baughn, R. E.: Effect of human immunodeficiency virus (HIV) infection on the course of syphilis and on the response to treatment. Ann. Intern. Med. *113*:872–881, 1990.
54. Nabarro, J. N. D.: Congenital Syphilis. Baltimore, Williams & Wilkins, 1954.
55. Oppenheimer, E. H., and Hardy, J. B.: Congenital syphilis in the newborn infant: Clinical and pathological observations in recent cases. Johns Hopkins Med. J. *129*:63–82, 1971.

55a. Paryani, S. G., Vaugh, A. J., Crosby, M., et al: Treatment of asymptomatic congenital syphilis benzathine versus procaine penicillin G therapy. J. Pediatr. *125*:471–475, 1994.

56. Pavithran, K.: Acquired syphilis in a patient with late congenital syphilis. Sex. Transm. Dis. *14*:119–121, 1987.
57. Peterman, T. A., Zaidi, A. A., Lieb, S., et al.: Incubating syphilis in patients treated for gonorrhea: A comparison of treatment regimens. J. Infect. Dis. *170*:689–692, 1994.
58. Peterson, K., Baseman, J. B., and Alderete, J. F.: *Treponema pallidum* receptor binding proteins interact with fibronectin. J. Exp. Med. *157*:1958–1970, 1983.
59. Philipson, A., Sabeth, L. D., and Charles, D.: Transplacental passage of erythromycin and clindamycin. N. Engl. J. Med. *288*:1219–1221, 1973.
60. Putkonen, T.: Does early treatment prevent dental changes in congenital syphilis? Acta Derm. Venerol. *43*:240–249, 1963.

60a. Qureshi, F., Jacques, S. M., and Reyes, M. P.: Placental histopathology in syphilis. Hum. Pathol. *24*:779–784, 1993.

60b. Rathbun, K. C.: Congenital syphilis. Sex. Transm. Dis. *10*:93–99, 1983.

61. Rathbun, K. C.: Congenital syphilis: A proposal for improved surveillance, diagnosis and treatment. Sex. Transm. Dis. *10*:102–107, 1983.
62. Rawston, S. A., and Bromberg, K.: Comparison of maternal and newborn serologic tests for syphilis. Am. J. Dis. Child. *145*:1383–1388, 1991.
63. Reyes, M. P., Hunt, N., Ostrea, E. M., et al.: Maternal/congenital syphilis in a large tertiary care urban hospital. Clin. Infect. Dis. *17*:1041–1046, 1993.
64. Ricci, J. M., Fojaco, R. M., and O'Sullivan, M. J.: Congenital syphilis: The University of Miami/Jackson Memorial Medical Center experience, 1986–1988. Obstet. Gynecol. *74*:687–693, 1989.

64a. Risser, W. L., and Hwang, L.-Y.: Problems in the current case definitions of congenital syphilis. J. Pediatr. *129*:499–505, 1996.

65. Romanowski, B., Sutherland, R., and Fick, G. H.: Serologic response to treatment of infectious syphilis. Ann. Intern. Med. *114*:1005–1009, 1991.
66. Rosen, E. U., and Richardson, N. J.: A reappraisal of the value of the IgM fluorescent treponemal antibody absorption test in the diagnosis of congenital syphilis. J. Pediatr. *87*:38–42, 1975.
67. Sanchez, P. J., McCracken, G. H., Wendel, G. D., et al.: Molecular analysis of the fetal IgM response to *Treponema pallidum* antigens: Implications for improved serodiagnosis of congenital syphilis. J. Infect. Dis. *159*:508–517, 1989.

67a. Sanchez, P. J., Wendel, G. D., Grimpel, E., et al.: Evaluation of molecular methodologies and rabbit infectivity testing for the diagnosis of congenital syphilis and central nervous system invasion by *Treponema pallidum*. J. Infect. Dis. *167*:148–157, 1993.

68. Shah, M. C., and Barton, L. L.: Congenital syphilitic hepatitis. Pediatr. Infect. Dis. *8*:891–892, 1989.
69. Shew, M. L., and Fortenberry, J. D.: Syphilis screening in adolescents. J. Adolesc. Health *13*:303–305, 1992.
70. Silber, T. J., and Milard, M. F.: The clinical spectrum of syphilis in adolescence. Adolesc. Health Care *5*:112–116, 1984.
71. Silverstein, A. M.: Congenital syphilis and the timing of immunogenesis in the human fetus. Nature *194*:196–197, 1962.
72. Speer, M. E., Taber, L. H., Clark, D. B., et al.: Cerebrospinal fluid levels of benzathine penicillin in the neonate. J. Pediatr. *91*:996–997, 1977.
73. Stoll, B. J., Lee, F. K., Larsen, S., et al:. Clinical and serologic evaluation of neonates for congenital syphilis: A continuing diagnostic dilemma. J. Infect. Dis. *167*:415–422, 1993.
74. Swancott, M. A., Radolf, J. D., and Norgard, M. V.: The 34-kilodalton membrane immunogen of *Treponema pallidum* is a lipoprotein. Infect. Immun. *58*:384–392, 1990.
75. Taber, L. H., and Huber, T. W.: Congenital syphilis. Prog. Clin. Biol. Res. *3*:183–190, 1975.
76. Tan, K. L.: The re-emergence of early congenital syphilis. Acta Pediatr. Scand. *62*:601–607, 1973.
77. Webber, M. P., Lambert, G., Bateman, D. A., et al.: Maternal risk factors for congenital syphilis: A case-control study. Am. J. Epidemiol. *137*:415–422, 1993.
78. Wendel, G. D., Maberry, M. C., Christmas, J. T., et al.: Examination of amniotic fluid in diagnosing congenital syphilis with fetal death. Obstet. Gynecol. *74*:967–970, 1989.
79. Woolf, A., Wilfert, C. M., Kelsey, D. B., et al.: Childhood syphilis in North Carolina. N. C. Med. J. *41*:443–449, 1980.
80. Zenker, P. N., and Berman, S. M.: Congenital syphilis: Reporting and reality. Am. J. Public Health *80*:271–272, 1990.

151

NONVENEREAL TREPONEMATOSES

James N. Miller and Craig W. Beachler

Pinta, yaws, and endemic syphilis are the three chronic granulomatous diseases that constitute the pathogenic nonvenereal treponematoses of humans. These diseases are caused by morphologically indistinguishable treponemes found almost exclusively in underdeveloped populations of the tropical and bordering arid areas of the world. On the basis of 100 per cent DNA sequence homology for the etiologic agents of syphilis and yaws[35] and the consideration by most investigators that the etiologic agent of endemic syphilis is a variant of *Treponema pallidum*,[27] the pathogenic treponemes have been given subspecies designations as follows: syphilis, *T. pallidum* subspecies *pallidum* (*T. pallidum*); yaws, *T. pallidum* subspecies *pertenue* (*T. pertenue*); endemic syphilis, *T. pallidum* subspecies *endemicum* (*T. pallidum*). The designation for the causative agent of pinta remains *T. carateum* (*T. herrejoni*).

Agents responsible for the nonvenereal treponematoses are transmitted from person to person by means of skin or mucous membrane contact. Close contact with children or young adults, traumatized areas of skin, lack of clothing, and personal hygiene are important factors in transmission of these diseases. All three nonvenereal treponematoses are potentially debilitating diseases that have enormous social and economic implications within endemic areas. Although their worldwide prevalence in general has been reduced considerably by means of seroepidemiologic and mass treatment campaigns sponsored by the World Health Organization (WHO) and UNICEF, they still remain a public health problem in several areas of the world where sporadic outbreaks continue to occur.[39, 53]

These diseases have existed for centuries. In theory, they appear to have originated from mutant forms of ancient treponemes, commencing with the human acquisition of pinta from an animal infection in the Euro-Afro-Asian land mass sometime before 20,000 B.C. Pinta presumably spread throughout the world by 15,000 B.C. and became isolated in the Americas by shifting continents. By 10,000 B.C., climate-induced mutations gave rise to yaws in the tropical areas of Asia and Africa as the benign pinta-producing treponemes became more invasive and destructive. The emergence of the Bering Strait isolated the Americas. Finally, in the arid lands bordering the tropical zones, yaws-producing treponemes again mutated by 7000 B.C. Natural selection within populations more fully clothed gave rise to treponemes that spread not by skin contact but by mucous membrane contact, namely, the etiologic agent of bejel or endemic syphilis.[18]

On morphologic examination, the treponemes are thin, tightly coiled organisms that do not stain or stain poorly with the usual aniline dyes. They contain 4 to 14 spirals and are actively motile by virtue of periplasmic flagella. The organisms are quite fragile and sensitive to drying, atmospheric oxygen, and temperatures above 35° C (95° F). Although limited multiplication of *T. pallidum* subspecies *pallidum* has been achieved in a tissue-culture system,[10] this has not been accomplished as yet with the nonvenereal pathogenic treponemes. Furthermore, none of the human pathogenic treponemes has been cultured in or on artificial media. They can, however, be identified in infected skin or mucous membrane lesions by darkfield microscopy.

Material should be removed aseptically and immediately examined unstained. In tissue from biopsy material, silver impregnation methods can be used to identify organisms,[25] but care must be taken to distinguish them from morphologically similar tissue artifacts. Little can be done to distinguish the various species of pathogenic treponemes. Clinical and epidemiologic features of each disease state from which the treponeme is recovered constitute the primary method of differentiation. Despite differences in methods of transmission, clinical disease, and geographic distribution, all human treponemes remain sensitive to penicillin.[51] Although not practical, further differentiation is based on the response of animal models to experimental infection.[22, 28, 40, 44, 45] Each of the pathogenic treponemes stimulates cross-reactive antibodies assayed in the serologic diagnosis of the human diseases by nontreponemal (VDRL, RPR Circle Card) and treponemal (FTA-ABS, MHA-TP, and TPI) tests. Furthermore, varying degrees of homologous resistance and cross-immunity exist after infection with any of these spirochetes.[22, 23, 31, 33, 44, 49]

PINTA

Pinta (mal del pinto, carate) is a chronic, contagious, nonvenereally transmitted treponemal disease presumed to be the most primitive of the human treponematoses. It can affect children and adults of all age groups, producing dyschromic skin lesions without pathogenic involvement of deeper organ structures. Pinta is not a fatal disease but a disfiguring one, which results in social ostracism and an inability to adjust to an urban society.

Biology and Immunology

Pinta is caused by *T. carateum*, which is morphologically indistinguishable from the other pathogenic treponemes. The organism is characterized mainly by its isolation from patients with clinically apparent pinta and by its lack of pathogenicity for small laboratory animals. Only the chimpanzee has been shown to be susceptible to experimental infection.[28, 29] Human studies by Medina[33] suggest that *T. carateum* induces significant protection against homologous reinfection as well as cross-immunity against the treponemes of yaws and syphilis; however, these two subspecies of *T. pallidum* fail to confer cross-protection against *T. carateum*.[33]

Epidemiology

Pinta is found primarily among the primitive, underprivileged Indians of tropical Central and South America. It occurs in major river basins of Mexico, Venezuela, Colombia, Brazil, Peru, and Ecuador. Cases also have been reported in Argentina, Chile, Haiti, Guatemala, Dominican Republic, Honduras, Nicaragua, and Bolivia. Pinta rarely occurs at higher elevations in the mountain regions of these countries. Coastal areas surprisingly are devoid of the disease. In the early 1920s, there were approximately 500,000 cases throughout Latin America; however, today, as a result of the seroepidemiologic and mass treatment campaigns, few cases have been reported.

The disease is found where poor hygienic and crowded conditions exist. Although endemic areas basically are rural, tribal tradition allows very close contact among its members. These tropical societies, with their absence of shoes and clothes, continually subject exposed skin to trauma and to contact with infectious lesions. Transmission of *T. carateum* occurs primarily by intimate skin-to-skin contact; a break in the skin is required for invasion of the treponeme. Pinta is not acquired congenitally or by blood transfusion. The proposed transmission of the disease by insect vectors has been disproved[33]; insects probably initiate disease by producing the necessary breaks in the skin.[9] Pinta is distributed equally between males and females and among all races in endemic areas. Furthermore, it is acquired primarily by young adults aged 15 to 20 years,[39] frequently spreading to family members because of crowded living conditions.

Pathogenesis and Pathology

T. carateum penetrates skin through breaks in the epidermis, with resultant damage restricted to the dermal and epidermal tissues. The organisms multiply in these layers, eliciting cellular proliferation as well as a plasma cell, lymphocyte, and macrophage infiltration. The resulting primary lesion may appear on any area of exposed skin but most often occurs on the legs, the dorsum of the foot, the forearm, or the back of the hands.[39] The lesion enlarges as a result of continual progression and direct extension or by coalescing with adjacent primary lesions; occasionally, a regional lymphadenopathy develops. Secondary lesions, known as pintids, result from treponemal dissemination and exhibit a cellular proliferation and infiltration similar to that of the primary lesion. In contrast to venereal syphilis, blood vessels remain intact and do not show proliferation. The dyschromic or multicolored nature of the primary and secondary lesions is more characteristic of older rather than of younger lesions, in which pigmentary changes usually are minimal. The variously pigmented older lesions may show hyperkeratosis or parakeratosis. Large numbers of treponemes can be found throughout the dermis and epidermis in the highly contagious primary and secondary lesions.

Late pinta is characterized by pigmentary changes, from dyschromic treponeme-containing lesions to achromic treponeme-free lesions.[39] This depigmentation process occurs at different rates even within the same lesion, which gives rise to different degrees of hypochromia and atrophy around dyschromic and achromic lesions.[39] There may be a concomitant lack of hair follicles and sebaceous glands.[7]

Clinical Manifestations

Pinta is characterized by a continuing production of early infectious lesions from either direct extension or dissemination and by the concomitant presence of lesions in various stages of dyschromia and achromia. The lesions are not well delineated, often merge, and may be accompanied by regional lymphadenopathy. Primary, secondary, and tertiary stages may or may not occur simultaneously.

The early stage of pinta includes the initial lesions, occasional regional lymphadenopathy, and secondary lesions resulting from treponemal dissemination. A primary lesion (not always evident) develops after an incubation period of 3 days to 2 months, usually 2 to 3 weeks. The primary lesion begins as one or more small erythematous papules that may appear scaly and indurated. The papules progressively enlarge over 1 to 3 months, often coalescing, becoming pigmented and more scaly and erythematous, and developing heaped-up margins. Occasionally, there is an accompanying regional lymphadenopathy. The lesion may disappear in several months or may continue to enlarge for several years, forming larger psoriasiform plaques that coalesce further.

The primary lesions of pinta generally overlap development of the secondary lesions or pintids, which appear 3 to 9 months after infection. This is the stage of dissemination, and almost any area of the skin can be involved. They occur typically on exposed areas of skin and are variously pigmented. The degree of pigmentation is related to the state of lesion development, the age of the lesion, the degree of sun exposure, and the host's natural pigmentation. Pintids begin as small, scaly papules that gradually enlarge and coalesce. Several colors may exist within the same lesion. Initially, pintids usually are red to violaceous; later, they become slate-blue, gray, or black as a result of photosensitization. Lesions on the legs typically are yellow-brown or dark-brown.

Serologic surveys suggest that a latent form of pinta exists, although this has not been established clearly.[8]

The late stage of pinta is characterized by the development of depigmented lesions. Achromia usually begins several years after the onset of the disease but may appear as early as 3 months. Areas of depigmentation spread slowly, leaving large achromic lesions as the end result. Early achromia tends to be asymmetric, whereas later depigmented lesions are symmetric. Characteristic of the Cuban form of pinta is the development of hyperkeratosis of the palms and soles.

Diagnosis

A presumptive diagnosis of pinta is based on the typical clinical presentation of a patient from a known endemic area. Laboratory tests are essential in characterizing pinta as a treponemal disease and include darkfield examination of early lesions and serologic tests for syphilis.

Darkfield examination of fluid obtained from the initial lesion or from pintids generally will reveal the presence of treponemes. As the lesions become achromic, treponemes are more difficult to find. For all practical purposes, achromic lesions are devoid of organisms. Silver impregnation of biopsy material from skin lesions or lymph nodes may reveal the organisms, but care must be taken in differentiating treponemes from tissue artifact. Both the nontreponemal (VDRL and RPR Circle Card) and treponemal (FTA-ABS, MHA-TP, and TPI) tests, originally designed for use in venereal syphilis, may not become reactive for as late as 4 months after the development of the initial lesion. Reactivity with these assays points to the antigenic cross-reactivity among the pathogenic treponemes and the inability to differentiate among the treponematoses solely on this basis.[39] Furthermore, it is important to note that the nontreponemal tests are, at best, screening procedures; false-positive reactions due to a variety of conditions and nontreponemal diseases can occur.[36] Many chronic dermatologic entities characterized by scaly, psoriasiform lesions or by dyschromia or depigmentation can be confused with pinta in endemic areas. Maculopapulosquamous diseases, including psoriasis, parapsoriasis, and lichen planus, as well as such dyschromic dermatologic diseases as vitiligo, ochronosis, and argyria, must be taken into consideration. Combined nontreponemal and treponemal tests will aid greatly in the differentiation.

Prognosis

Pinta is not a fatal disease; it produces changes related only to the skin. Untreated, the patient frequently develops large achromic cutaneous blemishes. The major resulting problem is one of social ostracism from the community. These infected members are removed from the urban society and find refuge in the rural areas. This further separates the patient from the principal sources of medical therapy.

Treatment and Prevention

The treatment of choice is benzathine penicillin G; those older than 10 years of age with clinical disease, in a period of latency, or in the incubatory stage and contacts of cases should receive 1.2 million units of benzathine penicillin G intramuscularly in a single dose; children younger than 10 years of age should receive 600,000 units in a single dose by the same route.[39, 53] Tetracycline is the antibiotic of choice for penicillin-allergic patients older than 8 years of age and not pregnant. The recommended dose is 500 mg by mouth four times daily for 15 days (total dose of 30 g)[39]; children between 8 and 15 years of age may be given half the dose.[39] Studies to determine the effectiveness of erythromycin have not been reported, although the same dosage and route as recommended for tetracycline probably are effective for those 8 years of age or older[39]; those younger than 8 years of age should be given doses adjusted for their body weight.[39]

The clinical response to therapy is remarkably slow in pinta. Primary and early secondary lesions take 4 to 6 months to disappear, whereas late secondary lesions require 6 to 12 months for complete healing to occur.[41] Hyperchromic lesions heal without residua, and hypochromic lesions often result in depigmented areas. Old achromic lesions usually remain intact without repigmentation. In general, the serologic response to therapy is absent or slow in pinta. Treponemal tests tend to remain reactive for life; nontreponemal tests may take years to decline after adequate therapy.[34]

Early campaigns to eradicate pinta proved that the prevalence of the disease could be reduced significantly by improving personal hygiene, by mass treatment of patients and contacts with penicillin, and by seroepidemiologic campaigns.

YAWS

Yaws (framboesia, pian, buba, bouba) is a communicable, nonvenereally transmitted treponematosis of the tropical zones. The disease is characterized by its early acquisition (usually before puberty) and its chronic, relapsing pattern of early benign lesions separated by periods of latency that terminate with late destructive lesions of skin, bones, and cartilaginous tissues.

Historically, yaws is another ancient treponematosis that, in theory, arose around 10,000 B.C. in Africa and Asia from a mutant form of pinta more suitable to tropical climates. From here, the disease was brought to the Americas by African slaves and remains today almost exclusively among their descendants. The interesting distribution of yaws in South America, for example, corresponds to the distribution of persons of African descent.[18] A very prevalent disease in the early part of this century, yaws was estimated to have affected more than 50 million people. Although seroepidemiologic and mass treatment campaigns sponsored by the WHO and UNICEF have reduced its overall prevalence drastically,[16] endemic areas of concern continue to exist.[39, 53]

Biology and Immunology

T. pallidum subspecies *pertenue*, the etiologic agent of yaws, is morphologically identical to other pathogenic treponemes. The organisms can be stored either in 15 per cent glycerol at –70° C (–94° F) or in liquid nitrogen and still retain their virulence for long periods.[25, 48] Rabbits experimentally infected by both the intratesticular and intradermal routes produce visible lesions and regional lymphadenopathy.[22, 48] However, four features commonly observed in experimental yaws infection differentiate it from experimental syphilis in the rabbit: (1) the relative absence of induration in the initial testicular lesions; (2) small focal lesions in or immediately beneath the visceral tunic of the testis, which give rise to a granular periorchitis; (3) the relative absence of induration in initial skin lesions; and (4) the relative scarcity of generalized (metastatic) lesions.[48] Both outbred and inbred hamsters can be infected experimentally with yaws treponeme strains by the intradermal route in the groin, with the production of chronic, ulcerative skin lesions, and, in most cases, generalized lymphadenopathy.[22, 44, 48] In contrast, intradermal groin infection of hamsters with *T. pallidum* subspecies *pallidum* rarely produces skin lesions but consistently results in generalized lymphadenopathy with larger numbers of treponemes within the nodes.[22, 45, 48]

On the basis of human and experimental studies, the organism stimulates a significant degree of homologous resistance to reinfection and superinfection as well as cross-immunity to *T. pallidum* subspecies *pallidum* and *endemicum*.[22, 26, 32, 44, 48]

Epidemiology

Yaws is a disease of tropical countries found primarily among the rural populations. It exists in the warm, moist, endemic areas of rural Africa, Southeast Asia, the Caribbean, and central and southern Africa. As indicated, seroepidemiologic and mass treatment campaigns have resulted in a significant reduction in prevalence of the disease in most of these areas. However, the failure of many countries to integrate active control measures into the functions of local health services has led to a gradual build-up and extension of yaws reservoirs, with the emergence of significant numbers of new, active cases since 1974 in Ghana, Togo Benin, Indonesia, and the Ivory Coast.[53] In a WHO survey in the Central African Republic, Congo, and Gabori, clinical yaws was detected in more than 20 per cent of the Pygmy population and reactive serologic tests were obtained in 80 per cent.[53]

Poor hygiene, close crowding among children (especially in sleeping areas), and lack of protective clothing facilitate transmission of the disease by direct skin-to-skin contact, whereby *T. pallidum* subspecies *pertenue* enters traumatized exposed areas from an infected lesion. The usual portals of entry are the lower extremities, head, face, and mouth. The presence of treponemal antibodies and isolation of treponemes (most probably *T. pallidum* subspecies *pertenue* from West African monkeys[2, 11]) suggest the possibility that primates in this area may act as a reservoir for spread of the disease.

Yaws usually is acquired before puberty and therefore is most prevalent among children. Inasmuch as such a large percentage of the population contracts the disease in infancy, young children represent the primary reservoir. Older children and adults generally are not infectious; therefore, congenital and sexual transmission does not occur. Both males and females are affected equally.

Pathogenesis and Pathology

T. pallidum subspecies *pertenue* enters the host through abraded skin and, most frequently, below the knees. The organisms multiply locally and in the regional lymph nodes; epithelial hyperplasia and plasma cell, lymphocytic, and macrophage infiltration are elicited. The end result is the formation of a primary lesion and lymphadenopathy containing numerous treponemes. Shortly after their introduction into the host, organisms are carried to skin, bone, and cartilage via the circulation. Disseminated treponemes in these tissues multiply, elicit a chronic inflammatory response similar to that seen in the primary lesion, and produce distant papillomas, lymphadenopathy, hyperkeratosis, and bone involvement that develop uninterruptedly until they are reversed by either immune mechanisms or treatment. In contrast to those associated with venereal syphilis, vascular changes are discrete or do not occur in cutaneous yaws.

The untreated primary and secondary cutaneous lesions generally heal with only minimal scarring unless they are complicated by secondary bacterial infection. The healing process and maintenance of latency appear to involve both humoral and cellular mechanisms of immunity.[43] Relapses may occur during latency and, together with late disease, may be due to a breakdown in the immune state, the development of antigenic variation by the treponeme, or both.

The late gummatous lesions are thought to be due to a hypersensitivity-induced mechanism similar to that postulated for the syphilitic gumma. Bone changes in late yaws most often involve the long bones and manifest as hypertrophic periostitis, gummatous periostitis, osteitis, and nodular or generalized osteomyelitis.[19] Juxta-articular nodules occur near major joints and are characterized as nonspecific granulomas.[6]

Clinical Manifestations

Yaws is a chronic, debilitating disease characterized by early infectious lesions; periods of latency and relapse; and late destructive lesions of cutaneous, subcutaneous, cartilaginous, and bony tissue. After an incubation period of 9 to 90 days (usually about 3 weeks), the primary lesion forms at the site of inoculation and is accompanied by regional lymphadenopathy. The lesion typically appears as a raised papule that enlarges to become a hyperkeratotic papilloma measuring 2 to 5 cm in diameter, referred to as a mother yaw. It undergoes shallow ulceration and persists from a few months to as long as 3 years, at which time healing occurs with a resultant hypopigmented scar.[6] Before or weeks to months after healing of the mother yaw, crops of secondary, generalized, nondestructive papular lesions appear together with lymphadenopathy and malaise. Some papules fade, whereas others enlarge to become papillomatous lesions referred to as satellite secondaries or daughter yaws. The multiple papillomas are circular, raised, red-yellow lesions with a granular, lobulated, and verrucous surface. They contain numerous treponemes, usually measure 1 to 3 cm in diameter, and produce a yellow discharge that dries to form a black scab. Hyperkeratotic involvement of the palms and soles is common. Painful fissuring of the soles may cause the patient to walk on the sides of the feet, thus producing the characteristic gait of crab yaws.[6] Bone pain may be severe, and nondestructive long bone lesions, including periostitis, osteitis, and osteomyelitis, may occur.[6, 17] Untreated secondary lesions may persist for more than 6 months, at which time, owing to the development of host immune mechanisms, they usually heal without scarring or residual defects unless ulceration due to secondary bacterial infection occurs. It should be noted that during the dry season, early yaws lesions often are atypical, tending to be macular and fewer in number; papillomas, which are small, scanty, dry, flat, and grayish in appearance and of short duration (approximately 1 month), are confined mainly to the hidden, protected, moist skin folds.[37, 39, 50]

Despite healing, some treponemes evade the immune process and persist in the affected tissues (latency). Latency frequently is interrupted by relapses, which tend to occur several times over a 3- to 5-year period. Fewer lesions are produced with each relapse, and they tend to be localized to the periaxillary, perianal, or circumoral area.[39] After cessation of the relapses and usually after a latent period of 3 to several years, tertiary lesions occur in up to 10 per cent of patients[39]; the latent state persists in the remaining patients for their lifetime.

The tertiary lesions characteristically are solitary and destructive; they involve skin, subcutaneous tissue, bone, and/or cartilage and most commonly occur after the onset of puberty. Painful hyperkeratosis of the palms and soles similar to that seen in early yaws is common. Other lesions develop as ulcerating, subcutaneous nodules and may heal spontaneously to form scars or extend widely from their margins. The scarring results in depigmentation and, at times, contractions. Bone deformities of late yaws include chronic hypertrophic periostitis, osteitis, gummatous periostitis, and osteomyelitis, each of which may ulcerate through the skin.[19] Gangosa, or rhinopharyngitis mutilans, the destructive gummatous ulceration of the skin and bones of the central face, as well as juxta-articular nodules, ganglions of tendon sheaths, and sabre tibiae, also may occur as manifestations of the late disease.[19] Gondou, a hypertrophic osteitis of the frontal processes of the maxillae once commonly seen among western Africans with yaws, is not a proven manifestation of the disease.[6]

Diagnosis

As with the other nonvenereal treponematoses, a presumptive diagnosis is based largely on clinical presentation of the disease in an endemic area. The diagnosis of yaws in nonendemic areas or during periods of latency is difficult. Although darkfield examination of early lesions and lymph nodes permits visualization of treponemes, late lesions usually contain few, if any, organisms. Silver impregnation of biopsy material from late lesions or lymph nodes may reveal treponemes, but again, care must be taken in differentiating the organisms from tissue artifact.

Nontreponemal and treponemal tests for syphilis become reactive during the first few weeks of illness, a reflection, again, of the shared antigens of pathogenic treponemes. As previously indicated, care must be taken in the utilization of only nontreponemal tests in diagnosis because of the possibility of false-positive reactions among patients with nontreponemal diseases or conditions.[36] Furthermore, the differentiation of the treponematoses from one another solely on the basis of serologic testing is not possible because of shared antigens.[12, 39] The coexistence of yaws and endemic syphilis in certain geographic locations, together with their often identical clinical manifestations, renders both darkfield and serologic assays useless for differentiating these diseases in such areas.[39] Similar limitations are applicable in differentiating venereal syphilis from yaws or endemic syphilis in nonendemic areas.[39] Under these circumstances, the diagnosis can be based only on a careful history and epidemiologic data.[39] In tropical areas, numerous other diseases may be confused with yaws.[21, 39] Impetigo and chronic tropical ulcers are found frequently and usually respond to penicillin therapy. Ecthyma may produce ulcers that occasionally are similar to the ulcerative papillomas of yaws. Other diseases that must be differentiated from yaws skin lesions include vitamin deficiencies, early leprosy, venereal syphilis, tinea versicolor, molluscum contagiosum, scabies, lichen planus, plantar warts, tungiasis, psoriasis, and cutaneous leishmaniasis. Sickle-cell disease, tuberculosis, and bacterial osteomyelitis may produce clinical manifestations that mimic the bone lesions of yaws. Combined nontreponemal and treponemal tests will aid greatly in the differentiation.

Prognosis

Yaws is not a benign disease. If left untreated, it can produce destructive, disfiguring lesions of the face, feet, and hands, as well as disabling and painful lesions of the fingers and long bones. Ulcers near joints may result in crippling contractures. Secondary bacterial infection of ulcers and of protruding bone lesions can result in further permanent damage to skin and bone tissues. Fractures generally are not a problem.

Treatment and Prevention

As with pinta, the treatment of choice is benzathine penicillin G; those older than 10 years of age with clinical disease, in a period of latency, or in the incubatory stages and contacts of cases should receive 1.2 million units of benzathine penicillin G intramuscularly in a single dose; children younger than 10 years of age should receive 600,000 units in a single dose by the same route.[39, 53] Tetracycline is the antibiotic of choice for penicillin-allergic patients older than 8 years of age and not pregnant. The recommended dosage is 500 mg by mouth four times daily for 15 days (total dose of 30 g)[39]; children between 8 and 15 years of age may be given half the dose.[39] Studies to determine the efficacy of erythromycin have not been reported, although the same dosage and route as recommended for tetracycline probably are effective for those 8 years of age or older[39]; those younger than 8 years of age should be given doses adjusted for their body weight.[39]

Therapy renders early lesions noninfectious in a few days, with complete healing in 7 to 10 days. Recurrences after treatment may occur as a result of reinfection.[20] Late lesions heal more slowly after therapy and may require surgery. Nontreponemal test titers may revert to nonreactive if the patient is treated early in the course of the disease. However, the longer the patient remains untreated, the more slowly will conversion to seronegativity occur.[5] As with each of the treponemal diseases, treponemal tests remain reactive for life after adequate therapy.

Improvement of living conditions and the general hygiene of the community, mass treatment of patients and contacts, and seroepidemiologic campaigns contribute significantly to the prevention of yaws.

ENDEMIC SYPHILIS

Endemic syphilis (bejel, njovera, siti, dichuchwa) is a chronic, nonvenereally transmitted disease of prepubescent children. It occurs in the warm, dry, arid regions of the world[39]; lesions are confined to the skin, bone, and cartilage. The disease, known to exist for centuries in Africa, has been recorded in epidemic proportions in areas where conditions among children allow transmission. As with yaws, although seroepidemiologic and mass treatment campaigns have reduced its overall prevalence drastically,[16, 39] endemic areas of concern continue to exist.[38, 39, 53]

Biology and Immunology

T. pallidum subspecies *endemicum*, the etiologic agent of endemic syphilis, morphologically is identical to the other pathogenic treponemes. Like *T. pallidum* subspecies *pallidum* and *pertenue*, the organisms can be stored in 15 per cent glycerol at –70° C (–94° F) or in liquid nitrogen and still retain their virulence for long periods.[25, 48] *T. pallidum* subspecies *endemicum* exhibits further similarity to these treponemes by producing visible lesions and generalized lymphadenopathy in rabbits experimentally infected by the intratesticular and intradermal routes.[22, 48] However, the degree of lesion induration generally is less than that observed in *T. pallidum* subspecies *pallidum* infection, whereas the frequency of granular periorchitis is intermediate between that seen with strains of yaws and venereal syphilis treponemes.[22, 48] As with *T. pallidum* subspecies *pertenue* infection, but in contrast to infection with *T. pallidum* subspecies *pallidum*, generalized (metastatic) lesions have not been observed in the rabbit.[22] Further similarities to the yaws treponeme are evidenced by the response of hamsters to infection. Both outbred and inbred hamsters can be infected experimentally by the intradermal route in the groin, with the production of chronic, ulcerative skin lesions and generalized lymphadenopathy.[22, 45, 48] However, as indicated earlier, infection of hamsters with *T. pallidum* subspecies *pallidum* by the same route rarely produces skin lesions but consistently results in generalized lymphadenopathy with large numbers of treponemes in the nodes.[22, 45, 48]

On the basis of experimental studies in inbred hamsters, *T. pallidum* subspecies *endemicum* stimulates a high degree of homologous resistance to reinfection as well as cross-immunity to *T. pallidum* subspecies *pallidum* and *pertenue*.[45]

Epidemiology

Endemic syphilis continues to persist in the warm, drier desert areas bordering the tropical belt. It is prevalent primarily among the seminomadic rural populations in the Arabian peninsula and along the southern border of the Sahara desert in Africa known as the "Sahel region"[38, 39]; a significant resurgence occurred in Mali, Mauritania, Niger, and the upper Volta during the 1970s.[39, 53] Although scattered endemic foci did exist in central Asia, Australia, the former Yugoslavia, and India, they now virtually have been eliminated from these areas by mass treatment campaigns.[38, 39]

As with pinta and yaws, endemic syphilis propagates under conditions of poor hygiene, crowding, and little or no clothing. Oral mucous membrane transmission is favored through contaminated objects, such as drinking vessels and kitchen utensils, as well as through contact with saliva-contaminated fingers and mouth-to-mouth contact.[4, 24] Transmission may occur via direct oral lesion-to-skin contact.[39] Occasionally, a previously uninfected nursing mother will develop a primary lesion on or near the nipple after the transfer of treponemes from her infected infant.[14, 52] Congenital transmission does not occur, and the role of insect vectors, such as flies, is uncertain.

Endemic syphilis occurs predominantly among children, with onset usually in those younger than 15 years of age[4] and with equal sex distribution. Spread occurs most commonly within the family, and active disease can be present in more than one family member at any given time.

Pathogenesis and Pathology

T. pallidum subspecies *endemicum* enters the host most often through the oral mucosa. The relatively small number of treponemes introduced into a susceptible host usually precludes the local multiplication and host inflammatory response required to produce a visible primary buccal lesion.[14] When a primary lesion does occur, it appears as a papule or ulcer resulting from a chronic inflammatory response to the proliferating organisms consisting of a plasma cell, lymphocytic, and macrophage infiltration. Endothelial cell swelling of small blood vessels also is evident.

The organisms are carried to the regional lymph nodes within a few hours of entry, commonly into the oral mucosa portal entry. They multiply and elicit epithelial hyperplasia as well as plasma cell, lymphocytic, and macrophage infiltration, with resultant lymphadenopathy. Dissemination occurs via the circulation, and the organisms are carried to the skin, bone, oral mucosa, axillae, and anogenital regions, where they multiply and elicit a chronic inflammatory response characterized by a cellular infiltration, as seen in the lymph nodes. Vascular changes and perivascular cuffing are prominent.

The untreated early lesions heal owing to mechanisms thought to involve both humoral and cellular immune responses by the host,[42] and the patient enters into a state of latency. Maintenance of latency is thought to involve similar mechanisms. The occurrence of infectious relapses during the latent period still is uncertain.

The late lesions of endemic syphilis are strikingly similar to those of late yaws. Both late disease and relapses (if they occur) may be due to a hypersensitivity-induced mechanism similar to that postulated for the syphilitic gumma.[14, 15] Juxta-articular nodules may occur and represent a nonspecific granulomatous response occurring near major joints.[6] It has been proposed that the rarity of cardiovascular and neurologic manifestations may be due to the slow acquisition of small numbers of organisms over a long period, which results in the immunologic protection of the heart and nervous system.[14, 30]

Clinical Manifestations

Endemic syphilis is a chronic, often debilitating disease characterized by early infectious secondary lesions, variable periods of latency, and late destructive lesions of cutaneous, subcutaneous, and bone tissues. As indicated, primary lesions are rare. They appear usually on the breast or nipple as a papule or shallow ulcer similar to that seen in primary venereal syphilis after an approximate 3-week incubation period[1]; they may persist for years before healing.[24]

Even without the appearance of a primary lesion, generalized infection occurs as a result of early dissemination. The onset begins after an incubation period thought to approximate that of secondary venereal syphilis and is characterized by the presence of highly infectious, relatively painless, ulcerative mucous patches on the oropharyngeal mucosa, including the tongue, lips, palate, tonsils, and larynx, with accompanying regional lymphadenopathy. Involvement of the larynx usually results in hoarseness.[6] Split papules or angular stomatitis occurs at the angles of the mouth. Osteoperiostitis of the long bones of the lower extremities, similar to that seen in yaws, is a common early manifestation causing nocturnal leg pains.[6] Occasionally, axillary and anogenital "secondary-type" lesions result, which consist of condylomata similar to yaws or dry papilloma annular patches, with accompanying axillary and inguinal lymphadenopathy. Disseminated papules that are indistinguishable from those seen in secondary venereal syphilis may occur. Other forms of cutaneous lesions can occur but are rare.

Untreated secondary lesions may persist for 6 to 9 months, at which time healing occurs because of the development of host immunity. This period of latency is variable and, like yaws, may last for 3 to several years.

Most patients develop tertiary manifestations. Late lesions generally occur during adolescence or adult life and may resemble those seen in either late yaws or late venereal syphilis. Gummata may affect any part of the body but commonly occur in the nasopharynx, skin, and bone, which results in destructive, disfiguring, chronic ulcerations characteristic of gangosa or gangosa-like lesions. Late gummatous lesions can occur during childhood, possibly as a result of superinfection in an already infected host.[13] Bone involvement also is common and results in painful lesions. This involves osteitis with gumma formation and, like yaws, periostitis affecting most frequently the long bones of the lower extremities. Bilateral synovitis, especially of the knees, occasionally may occur with concomitant juxta-articular nodules.[13] The cardiovascular and neurologic findings common to venereal syphilis are rare in endemic syphilis; when clinical manifestations occur, they usually are atypical and very mild.[3]

Endemic syphilis appears to have become "clinically attenuated" in Saudi Arabia.[38] Once florid, the classic disease seems to have been replaced by a milder form in which the number, severity, and duration of both early and late lesions are reduced and seroreactive latent infection is increased.[38] The most common late manifestation observed in this study was painful osteoperiostitis of the legs affecting mainly the tibia and fibula. It has been postulated that attenuation has occurred due to improvement in hygienic conditions, with resultant lesser re-exposure to potential superinfection.[38]

Diagnosis

Endemic syphilis, like pinta and yaws, is diagnosed presumptively from the typical clinical presentation of patients living in known endemic areas. The diagnosis of the disease as a treponemal infection can be confirmed by the darkfield examination of serous exudate from mucous membrane or cutaneous lesions and by the use of both nontreponemal and treponemal serologic tests. Seroreactivity approaches 100 per cent in patients presenting with clinical manifestations characteristic of early secondary endemic syphilis. It bears repeating, however, that the coexistence of yaws and endemic syphilis in certain geographic locations, together with their often indistinguishable clinical manifestations, renders both darkfield and serologic assays useless for differentiating these diseases in such areas.[39] Similarly, in nonendemic areas, venereal syphilis may not be distinguishable from yaws or endemic syphilis by the use of these laboratory procedures. Under these circumstances, the diagnosis can be based only on a careful case history and epidemiologic data.[39] The same nontreponemal diseases that can simulate the clinical manifestations of yaws and venereal syphilis also can confuse the diagnosis of endemic syphilis, which again stresses the importance of utilizing both nontreponemal and treponemal serologic tests in the differential diagnosis.

Prognosis

The main complication of endemic syphilis is the destructive gummatous lesions of the face and bones. Severely disfiguring and disabling, these lesions prevent the patient from working effectively in the community. Many of the bone lesions are extremely painful and incapacitating. The prognosis for the rare cardiovascular and neurologic manifestations is unknown.

Treatment and Prevention

Like the other pathogenic human treponemes, *T. pallidum* subspecies *endemicum* is highly susceptible to penicillin G. It should be administered to those older than 10 years of age with clinical disease, in a period of latency, or in the incubatory stage and to contacts of cases as the long-acting benzathine penicillin G in a single intramuscular dose of 1.2 million units; children younger than 10 years of age should be given 600,000 units in a single dose by the same route.[39, 53] In the penicillin-allergic patient older than 8 years of age and not pregnant, tetracycline is the antibiotic of choice. The recommended dose is 500 mg by mouth, four times daily for 15 days (total dose of 30 g)[39]; children between 8 and 15 years of age may be given half the dose.[39] Studies to determine the efficacy of erythromycin have not been reported, although the same dosage and route as recommended for tetracycline probably are effective for those 8 years of age or older[39]; those younger than 8 years of age should be given doses adjusted for their body weight.[39]

Infectious lesions rapidly disappear, and relapses usually are prevented after therapy. As in yaws, nontreponemal test titers may revert to nonreactive if the patient is treated early in the course of the disease. However, treatment during the later stages may result in the persistence of relatively high titers.[5] As with each of the treponemal diseases, treponemal tests remain reactive for life after adequate therapy.

Control of the disease in endemic areas requires mass treatment and seroepidemiologic campaigns coupled with an improvement in the hygiene of the community.

References

1. Akrawi, F.: Is bejel syphilis? Br. J. Vener. Dis. *25*:115–123, 1949.
2. Baylet, R., Thivolet, J., Sepetjian, M., et al.: La treponematose naturelle ouverte du singe *Papio papio* en Casamance. Bull. Soc. Pathol. Exot. *64*:842–846, 1971.
3. Csonka, G. W.: Clinical aspects of bejel. Br. J. Vener. Dis. *29*:95–103, 1953.
4. Cutler, J. C.: Endemic syphilis, yaws, and pinta. *In* Johnson, R. C. (ed.): The Biology of Parasitic Spirochetes. New York, Academic Press, 1976, pp. 365–373.
5. Demis, D. J.: Nonsyphilitic treponematoses. *In* Hoeprich, P. D. (ed.): Infectious Diseases. New York, Harper & Row, 1977, pp. 823–835.
6. Dooley, J. R., and Binford, C. H.: Treponematoses. *In* Binford, C. H., and Connor, D. H. (eds.): Pathology of Tropical and Extraordinary Diseases. Vol. 1. Washington, D.C., Armed Forces Institute of Pathology, 1976, pp. 10–117.
7. Edmundson, W. F.: Pinta. *In* Demis, D. J., Dobson, R. C., and McGuire, J. (eds.): Clinical Dermatology. Vol. 3. New York, Harper & Row, 1976, pp. 1–12.
8. Edmundson, W. F., Demis, D. J., and Bejarino, G.: A clinico-serologic study of pinta in the Alto Beni Region, Bolivia. Dermatol. Int. *6*:64–76, 1967.
9. Edmundson, W. F., Lopez Rico, A., and Olansky, S.: A study of pinta in the Tepalcatepec Basin, Michoacan, Mexico. Am. J. Syph. *37*:201–225, 1953.
10. Fieldsteel, A. H., Cox, D. L., and Moeckli, R. A.: Cultivation of virulent *Treponema pallidum* in tissue culture. Infect. Immun. *32*:908–915, 1981.
11. Fribourg-Blanc, A., Niel, G., and Mollaret, H. H.: Note sur quelques aspects immunologiques du cynocephale african. Bull. Soc. Pathol. Exot. *56*:474–485, 1963.
12. Garner, M. F., Backhouse, J. L., Cook, C. A., et al.: Fluorescent treponemal antibody absorption (FTA-ABS) test in yaws. Br. J. Vener. Dis. *46*:284–286, 1970.
13. Grin, E. I.: Endemic syphilis (bejel). *In* Demis, D. J., Dobson, R. C., and McGuire, J. (eds.): Clinical Dermatology. Vol. 3. New York, Harper & Row, 1976, pp. 1–7.
14. Grin, E. I.: Epidemiology and control of endemic syphilis. W. H. O. Monogr. Ser. *11*, 1953.
15. Guthe, T., and Luger, A.: Epidemiologic aspects of nonvenereal endemic syphilis. Dermatologica *115*:248–272, 1957.
16. Guthe, T., and Wilcox, R. R.: Changing concepts in the epidemiology and control of the treponematoses. Chron. W. H. O., Special Number *8*:33–69, 1954.
17. Hackett, C. J.: Bone Lesions of Yaws in Uganda. Oxford, Blackwell Scientific Publications, 1951.
18. Hackett, C. J.: On the origin of the human treponematoses. Bull. W. H. O. *29*:7–41, 1963.
19. Hackett, C. J.: Yaws. *In* Demis, D. J., Dobson, R. C., and McGuire, J. (eds.): Clinical Dermatology. Vol. 3. New York, Harper & Row, 1976, pp. 1–19.
20. Hackett, C. J., and Guthe, T.: Some important aspects of yaws eradication. Bull. W. H. O. *15*:869–896, 1956.
21. Hackett, C. J., and Loewenthal, L. J. A.: Differential diagnosis of yaws. W. H. O. Monogr. Ser. *45*:1–88, 1960.
22. Hardy, P. H.: Pathogenic treponemes. *In* Johnson, R. C. (ed.): The Biology of Parasitic Spirochetes. New York, Academic Press, 1976, pp. 107–119.
23. Hill, K. R.: Non-specific factors in the epidemiology of yaws. Bull. W. H. O. *8*:17–47, 1953.
24. Hudson, E. H.: Non-venereal Syphilis. Edinburgh, E. & S. Livingstone, Ltd., 1958.
25. Kelly, R. T.: Treponema. *In* Lennette, E. H., Spaulding, E. H., and Truant, J. P. (eds.): Manual of Clinical Microbiology. Washington, D.C., American Society for Microbiology, 1975, pp. 358–360.
26. Knox, J. M., Musher, D., and Guzick, N. D.: The pathogenesis of syphilis and the related treponematoses. *In* Johnson, R. C. (ed.): The Biology of Parasitic Spirochetes. New York, Academic Press, 1976, pp. 249–259.
27. Krieg, N. R., and Holt, J. G. (eds.): Bergey's Manual of Systematic Bacteriology. Vol. 1. Baltimore/London, Williams & Wilkins, 1984, p. 50.
28. Kuhn, U. S. G., III, Medina, R., Cohen, P. G., et al.: Inoculation pinta in chimpanzees. Br. J. Vener. Dis. *46*:311–312, 1970.
29. Kuhn, U. S. G., III, Varela, G., Chandler, Jr., F. W., et al.: Experimental pinta in the chimpanzee. J. A. M. A. *206*:829, 1968.
30. Luger, A., and Schmid, E. E.: Immunity of the central nervous system in endemic syphilis. Dermatol. Wochenschr. *143*:617–637, 1961.
31. Magnuson, H. J., Thomas, E. W., Olansky, M. D., et al.: Inoculation syphilis in human volunteers. Medicine *35*:33–82, 1956.
32. McLeod, C. P., and Magnuson, H. J.: Study of cross-immunity between syphilis and yaws in treated rabbits. J. Vener. Dis. Infect. *32*:305–309, 1951.
33. Medina, R.: Pinta in South America. *In* Fogarty International Center Symposium Documents: Yaws and Other Endemic Treponematoses. April 16–18, 1984.
34. Mesa, J., Restrepo, A., and Cortes, A.: A study of fluorescent treponemal antibody absorption (FTA-ABS) and VDRL tests in pinta. Int. J. Dermatol. *12*:135–138, 1973.
35. Miao, R. M., and Fieldsteel, A. H.: Genetic relationship between *Treponema pallidum* and *Treponema pertenue*, two noncultivable human pathogens. J. Bacteriol. *141*:427–429, 1980.
36. Miller, J. N.: Value and limitations of nontreponemal and treponemal tests in the laboratory diagnosis of syphilis. Clin. Obstet. Gynecol. *18*:191–203, 1975.
37. Niemal, P. L. A., Brunings, E. A., and Menke, H. E.: Attenuated yaws in Surinam. Br. J. Vener. Dis. *55*:99–101, 1979.
38. Pace, J. L., and Csonka, G. W.: Endemic non-venereal syphilis (bejel) in Saudi Arabia. Br. J. Vener. Dis. *60*:293–297, 1984.
39. Perine, P. L., Hopkins, D. R., Niemel, P. L. A., et al.: Handbook of Endemic Treponematoses. Geneva, World Health Organization, 1984.
40. Pierce, C. S., Wicher, K., and Nakeeb, S.: Experimental syphilis: Guinea pig model. Br. J. Vener. Dis. *59*:157–168, 1983.
41. Rein, C. R.: Bacteriologic and serologic aspects of pinta. Am. J. Syph. *38*:336–340, 1954.
42. Schell, R. F., Chan, J. K., and LeFrock, J. L.: Endemic syphilis: Passive transfer of resistance with serum and cells in hamsters. J. Infect. Dis. *140*:378–383, 1979.
43. Schell, R. F., LeFrock, J. L., and Babu, J. P.: Passive transfer of resistance to frambesial infection in hamsters. Infect. Immun. *21*:430–435, 1978.
44. Schell, R. F., LeFrock, J. L., Babu, J. P., et al.: Use of CB hamster in the study of *Treponema pertenue*. Br. J. Vener. Dis. *55*:316–319, 1979.
45. Schell, R. F., LeFrock, J. L., Chan, J. K., et al.: LSH hamster model of syphilitic infection. Infect. Immun. *28*:909–913, 1980.
46. Schöbl, O., and Miyao, I.: Immunologic relation between yaws and syphilis. Philipp. J. Sci. *40*:91–109, 1929.
47. Turner, T. B.: The resistance of yaws and syphilis patients to reinoculation with yaws spirochetes. Am. J. Hyg. *23*:431–448, 1936.
48. Turner, T. B., and Hollander, D. H.: Biology of the Treponematoses. Geneva, World Health Organization, 1957.
49. Turner, T. B., McLeod, C. P., and Updyke, E. L.: Crossimmunity in experimental syphilis, yaws, and venereal spirochetosis of rabbits. Am. J. Hyg. *46*:287–295, 1947.
50. Vorst, F. A.: Attenuating endemic treponematoses. Thesis, University of Amsterdam, 1974.
51. Wilcox, R. R.: Changing patterns of treponemal disease. Br. J. Vener. Dis. *50*:169–178, 1974.
52. Wilcox, R. R.: Endemic syphilis in Africa. S. Afr. Med. J. *25*:501–504, 1951.
53. WHO Technical Report Series No. 674: Treponemal Infections. Geneva, World Health Organization, 1982.

❑ ❑ ❑

SUBSECTION SEVEN

ANAEROBIC BACTERIA

152

CLOSTRIDIAL INTOXICATION AND INFECTION

W. Lance George

BOTULISM

Botulism is an acute descending flaccid paralysis that results when the neurotoxin of *Clostridium botulinum* blocks neuromuscular transmission. Three forms of botulism exist: infant (the most common), food-borne, and wound. A fourth category, "unclassified," was created by the Centers for Disease Control and Prevention (CDC) for those adult patients who lack an apparent food or wound source of botulinus toxin and whose cases, it was hypothesized, might have an infant-type pathogenesis.[6] Infant botulism is discussed in Chapter 153.

Epidemiology and Etiology

There are seven antigenically distinct types of botulinus toxin, designated by the letters A through G. Disease in humans is caused by toxin types A, B, E, F (rarely), and possibly G.[1, 3, 5, 6, 8, 9, 12, 14, 15] Types C and D cause botulism in animals.[5, 14] The toxin type has been determined in one-third of the food-borne botulism outbreaks in the United States. About one-fourth of all outbreaks involve type A; 8 per cent, type B; 4 per cent, type E; and 0.1 per cent, type F. Type A is seen primarily in the western states; type B is more common in the eastern states. Type E predominates in Alaska and the Great Lakes region, and type F has been reported only in California.

Botulinus toxin probably is the most lethal of all naturally occurring compounds. It is heat-labile; 5 minutes of boiling destroys the toxin, and little remains after 30 minutes of exposure at 80° C. Toxin is produced by *C. botulinum* at all temperatures at which growth occurs (3° to 48° C). Toxin also is formed at all pH values at which growth occurs (pH 4.8 to 8.5), but the toxin is unstable at pH values greater than 7. The presence of organisms in improperly processed acidic food, however, can allow toxin production.[5, 6, 14] Type E toxin may be produced quickly in small fragments of fish exposed to air and at lower pH values and cooler temperatures than is true for other toxin types.[5]

The majority of outbreaks of botulism in the United States are traceable to home-processed foods; an increase in the number of cases of botulism may reflect increased home canning activity in recent years. The most important food vehicles are vegetables, fish, fruits, and condiments. Type E botulism almost always is traceable to fish and fish products, but types A and B also may be involved in outbreaks related to this type of food. Recent outbreaks have been traced to unusual foods, for example, potato salad and sautéed onions served by restaurants, and to commercial frozen pot pies mishandled at home.

Wound botulism results from infection of traumatized tissue by *C. botulinum*, type A or B, and subsequent toxin production.[12] Although infrequently reported (<50 cases worldwide as of 1985), it is a disease of pediatric concern: about half of the cases in the United States have occurred in children and teenagers, most of whom were boys with compound extremity fractures. In recent years, the disease also has been recognized in Australia, China, France, and Italy.

Pathophysiology

Botulinus toxin is absorbed from the proximal intestine or an infected wound into the lymphatics and then distributed hematogenously to peripheral cholinergic nerve synapses, most notably the neuromuscular junction. The toxin does not cross the blood-brain barrier. The nerve endings take up the toxin, which then irreversibly blocks acetylcholine release and results clinically in flaccid paralysis.[5, 6, 14] The cranial nerves are affected earliest and often most severely. Death occurs mainly from respiratory muscle paralysis (asphyxia) or its complications, such as cardiac arrhythmia, aspiration, and pneumonia. Recovery occurs by regeneration of terminal motor neurons and formation of new motor endplates.

Clinical Manifestations

The illness begins as a descending symmetric motor paralysis first affecting muscles supplied by the cranial nerves.[5] There is no sensory disturbance, but vision may be impaired and hearing distorted because of cranial nerve involvement. Mental processes remain clear, but there may be anxiety and agitation. Fever is absent unless a secondary bacterial infection occurs. The triad of bulbar palsies (including sluggish or absent pupillary response to light), lucid sensorium, and absent fever always should bring botulism to mind.

Common symptoms include diplopia, dysarthria, and dysphagia. The degree of ocular involvement is quite variable; in severe cases, the pupils may become fixed and dilated. The mucous membranes of the mouth, tongue, and pharynx may be so dry that pain results, which may lead to the mistaken diagnosis of pharyngitis. Dizziness or vertigo may occur. Urinary retention, occasionally with stress incontinence, may be seen.

Two-thirds of patients have no gastrointestinal symptoms. In those who do, with type A or type B botulism, the gastrointestinal manifestations primarily are abdominal pain, cramps, fullness, and diarrhea. However, after an initial period of diarrhea, constipation or obstipation may be noted and indeed is more typical of the disease. In contrast to the other types, most patients with type E botulism first have gastrointestinal symptoms. Included are nausea, vomiting, substernal burning or pain, abdominal distention, and decreased bowel sounds. The most common signs encountered in botulism are respiratory impairment; specific muscle weakness or paralysis; eye muscle involvement, including ptosis; dry throat, mouth, or tongue; dilated fixed pupils; and ataxia. Respiratory involvement, even aside from aspiration pneumonia, is fairly common. Vital capacity is a more sensitive indicator of respiratory compromise than blood gas measurement. Postural hypotension, nystagmus, and somnolence may be noted.

The usual interval between food ingestion and onset of symptoms is 18 to 36 hours, but it may be as short as a few hours or as long as 8 days. In general, the patients with the shorter incubation periods are affected more severely and have a poorer prognosis. The shortness of the incubation period and the severity of illness correlate with the amount of toxin ingested.

The symptoms of wound botulism are similar to those of food botulism, but there may be some important differences.[12] Fever may or may not be present. Constipation occurs, but nausea and vomiting do not. Unilateral sensory changes in association with the trauma or infection may occur. There may be grossly purulent drainage in the wound itself, but sometimes the wounds show no evidence of infection. The incubation period of wound botulism usually is 4 to 14 days.

Differential Diagnosis

The differential diagnosis of botulism includes myasthenia gravis, cerebral vascular accidents, Guillain-Barré syndrome (particularly the Miller-Fisher variant), tick paralysis, chemical intoxication, diphtheritic polyneuritis, psychiatric disease, and the Eaton-Lambert syndrome.[5, 14]

Ordinary bacterial food poisonings usually are not a problem in differential diagnosis because of the absence of cranial nerve involvement. Chemical food poisoning may cause neurologic manifestations, but the signs of this almost always appear within minutes or at most hours after consumption of contaminated food. Atropine poisoning has a very rapid onset and is distinctive because of facial flushing and hallucinations. Shellfish and fish poisoning has a rapid onset and often causes characteristic paresthesias, tremors, and other signs. Mushroom poisoning causes severe abdominal pain, violent vomiting, diarrhea, and coma.

Myasthenia gravis usually spares pupillary oculomotor function. An edrophonium (Tensilon) test should be performed. Guillain-Barré syndrome can mimic botulism but usually shows ascending peripheral paralysis and, later, cranial nerve involvement. Muscle cramps, paresthesias, and elevated protein content in the cerebrospinal fluid in the absence of cells help distinguish this disease. Electromyography may be extremely helpful in differentiating botulism from atypical cases of Guillain-Barré syndrome.

The problem of identifying a case is complicated by reports of patients with features not characteristic of either botulism or the action of botulinus toxin, such as paresthesias, asymmetric weakness of extremities, asymmetric ptosis, slightly elevated cerebrospinal fluid protein, and a "positive" response to edrophonium. Some of these symptoms may be a consequence of the high anxiety that prevails among persons who know they have eaten a food that contains botulinus toxin.

Specific Diagnosis

Confirmation of the diagnosis of botulism depends primarily on detection of the toxin or the organism in the patient or in the implicated food or wound.[2, 5, 14] Specimens to be examined for botulinus toxin include serum, gastric contents or vomitus, feces (at least 50 g when possible), and exudates from wounds and tissues. These should be obtained as soon as possible and before antitoxin is given. This particularly is important for blood specimens. When feasible, 30 mL of blood should be obtained in a large vacuum tube and sent without separation of the serum to the nearest laboratory capable of carrying out the mouse neutralization test and other tests for toxin. State health departments or the CDC can provide advice regarding specimen collection and handling and laboratories to which samples can be sent (see later).

Specimens should be refrigerated and examined as quickly as possible after collection. Whenever possible, suspect food should be kept sealed in the original container. Sterile unbreakable containers should be used for other food samples. Specimens to be shipped to laboratories must be placed in leak-proof containers, packed with ice in a second leak-proof, insulated container, and marked "Danger, hazardous material." Extreme caution should be used in handling materials that may contain botulinus toxin because even minute quantities of toxin acquired by ingestion, inhalation, or absorption through the eye or a break in the skin may cause profound intoxication and death.

Laboratory confirmation of suspected botulism should be attempted, even late in the clinical course. Detection of the organism itself may be done by culture (preferably by means of spore selection procedures and a selective medium), by fluorescent antibody technique, and, in a presumptive manner, by gas chromatography.

The CDC found botulinus toxin in the stools of 19 of 56 patients and in the sera of 20 of 60 patients with clinical botulism. Toxin was not detected in specimens from 246 persons with an illness other than botulism or no illness at all. *C. botulinum* was identified in stools of 36 of 60 clinical botulism patients and in 4 of 27 asymptomatic contacts of such patients but not in the stools of 65 persons not associated with confirmed botulism. When stool and serum samples were examined, confirmatory evidence was obtained for more than 70 per cent of botulism cases. Thus, the detection of *C. botulinum* toxin or organisms in the stool of a symptomatic person should be considered diagnostic.

Treatment

The mainstay of therapy in all forms of botulism is meticulous supportive care, with particular attention to the respiratory and nutritional needs of the patient and to anticipation of potential complications for the purpose of preventing them.[5, 6] Symptomatic persons known to have ingested toxin-containing food should be hospitalized, with careful monitoring of respiratory and cardiac function. Measurement of vital capacity is a useful index of clinical status.

In food-borne botulism, if the patient is seen early, emetics and gastric lavage should be used for reducing the amount of unabsorbed toxin. Trivalent (ABE) botulinus antitoxin, a horse serum product, is considered a routine part of the therapy of food-borne botulism, although conclusive evidence of its efficacy is lacking.[5, 15] The antitoxin is used to neutralize circulating botulinus toxin that is found in about 30 per cent of patients with food-borne botulism. Low-dose, subcutaneous heparin should be considered for patients with severe paralysis and an anticipated long hospitalization. Treatment of a single patient with suspected or proven food-borne botulism requires immediate notification of state and federal (CDC) health officials, who also are the antitoxin source, because the food responsible for the index patient's illness still may be available to other persons. The appropriate initial contact is via the state health department. If they can not be reached, then the CDC should be contacted immediately (CDC telephone: 404-639-2206, days, or 404-639-2888, nights).

A commonly encountered problem is the management of the "possible outbreak" of food-borne botulism that comes to attention once someone has sampled a food of dubious color, odor, or taste, often obtained from an obviously swollen or damaged can. The patient may or may not already have gastrointestinal signs and symptoms. The physician's dilemmas are whether or not to admit the patient for further observation and whether or not to administer botulinus antitoxin. Almost all of these situations eventually are found not to represent an exposure to botulinus toxin, and as a consequence, the following procedure generally is practiced.

Locate all persons who ate the suspect food and determine whether any have symptoms or signs of botulism.[5] If the patients are seen soon after the suspect meal, use of gastric lavage, emetics, and cathartics deserves consideration. Arrange to have antitoxin easily available. Collect and refrigerate any samples of the suspect food that may remain. The health authorities should assist the clinician with these tasks. Obtain the fecal and serum specimens needed to establish the diagnosis. If neurologic signs are present, try to identify defective neuromuscular transmission by electromyelography. If neurologic signs are absent, the patient(s) and the family should be told the early signs of botulinus intoxication and should be instructed to return at the first manifestation of ptosis, diplopia, blurred vision, dysphonia, dysarthria, or dysphagia. Because of the serious side effects of equine botulinus antitoxin, its administration before the development of signs of illness or before the laboratory identification of botulinus toxin in the suspect food generally is not recommended or practiced. An exception is made when the epidemiologic setting or the clinical findings are so compelling that only food-borne botulism can explain the illness.

When wound botulism is suspected, exploration and débridement of the site must be undertaken, ideally after antitoxin administration has begun. Arrangements should be made to obtain anaerobic cultures in the operating room and to begin antibiotic therapy there. Penicillin (10 to 12 million units per day for adult-size patients for 10 to 14 days) is the drug of choice. To ensure that all circulating toxin has been neutralized, a serum specimen should be obtained after antitoxin administration. Guanidine has been used to treat some cases of food-borne and wound botulism, but convincing evidence of efficacy is lacking.

Prognosis

The mortality with botulism usually is 20 to 25 per cent. It is lower with type B disease (10 per cent) than with type A or E disease.[5, 14] The mortality rate is lower in individuals younger than 20 years of age (10 per cent). An important factor, as noted, is the dose of toxin ingested as reflected by the length of the incubation period. The longer the incubation period, the better the prognosis. If the index case in an outbreak can be detected early, other patients exposed to the same food will have a much better prognosis. Recovery may be prolonged, and some symptoms (e.g., fatigability) may persist for as long as 1 year. Most patients recover entirely.

Prevention

Local and state health authorities and the CDC should be notified immediately of all suspected cases of botulism so that appropriate investigations can be undertaken. Although commercial products still occasionally are responsible for botulism, control measures taken by the industry have done a great deal to prevent botulism from this source. The need continues to instruct home canners on appropriate means for sterilizing containers and food before preserving and about adequate cooking of foods before serving.[5, 14] In canning, a pressure cooker must be used to obtain temperatures well above boiling in order to destroy the spores of *C. botulinum* types A and B. For certain foods, a temperature of 116° C is recommended. Spores of *C. botulinum* are destroyed at 120° C after 30 minutes. Pressure cookers set at 15 pounds will achieve this temperature. Corrections for higher altitudes must be made. Home-canned foods should be boiled for 10 minutes before serving.

CLOSTRIDIAL INFECTIONS

Clostridia are encountered less commonly than non–spore-forming anaerobic bacteria in infection, but these spore formers, rarely, may produce devastating disease. Overall, clostridia are encountered in 5 to 10 per cent of anaerobic or mixed anaerobic infections.[1, 4–6, 16] *C. perfringens* is the species encountered most commonly. It may be isolated in pure culture but more commonly is part of a mixed flora involving other anaerobes and nonanaerobes at times as well. Other species that are important clinically and/or encountered commonly include *C. novyi, C. septicum, C. bifermentans, C. histolyticum,* and *C. sordellii* (together with *C. perfringens,* these are the "gas gangrene group"); *C. tetani* (see Chapter 154); *C. difficile,* a major pathogen in pseudomembranous colitis; and a group of clostridia important in infections other than gas gangrene or myonecrosis (wound infection, abscesses, bacteremia, etc.)—*C. perfringens, C. ramosum, C. bifermentans, C. sphenoides, C. sporogenes,* and others.

Clostridia may be involved in a wide variety of infections throughout the body. Certain of these infections have a distinctive clinical picture; these will be discussed in this chapter. A number of other infections are not distinctive and will not be discussed specifically here, including peritonitis, intra-abdominal infection, wound infections, soft tissue infections, and occasionally pleuropulmonary infection, central nervous system infection, and urinary tract infection. Emphysematous cholecystitis involving *C. perfringens* has distinctive features, but it is not encountered in the pediatric age group and so will not be discussed. Bacteremia involving *C. perfringens* may or may not have distinctive features. The distinctive intravascular hemolysis that may occur with *C. perfringens* bacteremia will be discussed in connection with female genital tract infections due to this organism.

Epidemiology

The vast majority of clostridial infections are of endogenous origin. Even those secondary to trauma and contamination of a wound with foreign bodies usually involve *C. perfringens* or other clostridia from the host's flora, chiefly the intestinal tract.

Pathophysiology

The chief sites of normal carriage of *C. perfringens* in humans are the colon and the vagina.[5, 6] Many other clostridial species are found in the bowel. These organisms may gain access to tissues through wounds (surgical or traumatic), by virtue of perforation of abdominal viscera, or because of local disease, such as tumor. The organism then may grow in the tissues if the oxidation-reduction potential is low or host defense mechanisms are impaired or both. Factors favoring anaerobic growth include necrotic tissue, poor blood supply, the presence of foreign bodies, or previous multiplication of other bacteria in the wound, leading to a lowered oxidation-reduction potential.

C. perfringens produces at least a dozen different extracellular toxins or other factors that account for its pathogenicity.[5] The most important of these is the alpha-toxin, a lecithinase, the main one accounting for destruction of tissue, hemolysis, and death. Other important factors include collagenase, hyaluronidase, leukocidin, deoxyribonuclease, and fibrinolysin. The enterotoxins produced by some strains of *C. perfringens* and of *C. difficile* are important in the pathogenesis of certain gastrointestinal diseases, which will be discussed. Gas gangrene, or clostridial myonecrosis, is characterized by profound toxicity, necrosis of muscle, edema, thrombosis of small vessels, gas bubbles in the tissues, and minimal infiltration of leukocytes (probably due to destruction of leukocytes at the site).

Clinical Manifestations

Gas Gangrene or Myonecrosis

Although other clostridia also are involved in gas gangrene, *C. perfringens* is the causative species in approximately 90 to 95 per cent of cases. Clostridial myonecrosis may occur in the absence of a traumatic wound. This disease is referred to as spontaneous myonecrosis and is due to bacteremic seeding of muscle with either *C. perfringens* or *C. septicum.* The usual source of the organism is the bowel, and the usual predisposing factors are mucosal tumors of the bowel or ulcerations produced by cytotoxic chemotherapy.[6] The typical case of clostridial myonecrosis manifests with sudden appearance of pain in the region of a wound.[5] The pain increases in severity but remains localized to the infected area. Next there is local swelling and edema, and a thin hemorrhagic exudate appears. The pulse is very rapid, out of proportion to the mild temperature elevation. Initially, the skin is tense, white, somewhat colder than normal, and very tender. Bronze discoloration appears and increases with time. The process extends and becomes more severe, and the patient becomes toxemic. The skin becomes dusky or bronzed, and bullae filled with dark-red or purple fluid appear. Crepitus due to gas may be noted, but the amount of gas produced generally is small. A peculiar sweet smell may be noted in some cases. Occasionally, there may be a fetid odor that probably reflects the presence of a *Clostridium* organism other than *C. perfringens.*[6] There may be toxic delirium and later overwhelming prostration and toxemia. Some patients are alert and apprehensive, and others are apathetic. Later in the course of the disease, shock supervenes. At operation, early changes in the muscle consist primarily of edema and pallor, but later there is increased reddening with mottled purple. The consistency of the muscle may be pasty or mucoid, and contractility disappears. Eventually, the muscle becomes diffusely gangrenous, dark greenish-purple or black, friable, and even liquefied.

Soft Tissue Infection

C. perfringens and other clostridia also may be involved in less dramatic and less serious infections ranging from minor superficial infections to anaerobic cellulitis and necrotizing fasciitis.[6] The clinical picture in these various infections is no different from that noted with other types of organisms and thus is not discussed further here. It is interesting to note that *C. perfringens* has been isolated from bullous impetigo.

Septic Abortion and Puerperal Sepsis

C. perfringens infections of the uterus usually occur after incomplete abortions induced under nonsterile conditions.[5] Occasionally, this type of infection will occur after spontaneous abortion, prolonged labor, ruptured membranes, or operative interference with pregnancy. Early symptoms include uterine bleeding, suprapubic and back pain, chills, and fever.[5, 6] The incubation period after the precipitating event usually is several days, but it may be less than 24 hours. In addition to vaginal bleeding, there often is a foul-smelling, brown vaginal discharge containing necrotic tissue. The uterus is tender, and the lower abdominal wall may be tense. Nausea, vomiting, and diarrhea may occur. Generalized peritonitis may complicate the picture. The most striking systemic manifestation of the disease, however, is massive intravascular hemolysis with hemoglobinemia, hemoglobinuria, and jaundice. Shock and acute renal failure may complicate the picture. Intrauterine gas formation may be detected.

Pseudomembranous Colitis

Pseudomembranous colitis, generally characterized by profuse watery diarrhea, abdominal cramps, fever, leukocytosis, and small (2 to 5 mm) raised, yellowish plaques on the colonic mucosa, represents the most severe end of a disease spectrum that the toxins of *C. difficile* can produce.[6, 7, 13] At the other end of the spectrum are found asymptomatic carriage and mild diarrhea.[13] *C. difficile* diarrhea and colitis almost invariably follow antimicrobial treatment, the most common precipitants being ampicillin, clindamycin, and cephalosporins.[6, 13] However, almost any antibacterial agent can set off the illness. Sporadic, non–antibiotic-associated cases have been recognized. The spectrum of *C. difficile*–associated diarrhea ranges from a trivial, self-limited disease to that of a severe illness that simulates an intra-abdominal catastrophe. Fever to 104° C, leukocytosis to 25,000 cells/mm^3, and hypoalbuminemia occur in approximately one-quarter of patients. Stools range from 3 or 4 to 20 per day and may be loose, watery, or bloody with mucus; associated abdominal cramping is relatively common.[6] Occasionally, pseudomembranous colitis may be caused by *Staphylococcus aureus* or by clostridia other than *C. difficile* (e.g., *C. perfringens* type C).

Many determinants of the illness remain to be clarified. Toddlers, and particularly infants, may harbor the bacterium and its toxins asymptomatically within the intestinal flora, whereas in healthy older children and adults, *C. difficile* is found infrequently (approximately 2 per cent intestinal carriage rate).[10, 13, 17] Recently developed typing systems may help distinguish pathogenic from nonpathogenic strains of *C. difficile.*

Other Enteric Infections

A mild and self-limited but very common form of food poisoning may be caused by *C. perfringens,* meat and meat products being the major vehicles for such outbreaks.[5, 6] The incubation period after ingestion of the contaminated food varies from 6 to 24 hours but usually is 8 to 12 hours. The major symptoms are crampy abdominal pain and diarrhea. The stools are liquid but do not contain blood or mucus. Nausea may be present on occasion, but vomiting is rare. The illness usually lasts less than 24 hours.

Rarely, *C. perfringens* also may produce a very severe type of necrotizing enteritis. Although food poisoning is produced by *C. perfringens* type A, the necrotizing enteritis involves *C. perfringens* type C.[11] Consumption of excessive amounts of rich food by people normally on a low-protein diet and with decreased levels of digestive proteases seems to be an important background factor. Additionally, proteases may be blocked by ingestion of trypsin inhibitors found in sweet potatoes. In some cases, consumption of contaminated canned meat is involved. In New Guinea, the disease is associated with traditional pig-feasting activities in which large quantities of pork are consumed. The disease is characterized by abdominal cramps, vomiting, shock, diarrhea (sometimes bloody), and acute inflammation of the small intestine with areas of necrosis and gangrene, particularly in the jejunum.

Miscellaneous Infections Due to Clostridia

Panophthalmitis involving *C. perfringens* or, occasionally, other clostridia is secondary to injury, usually with retention of a foreign body.[5] Gas gangrene panophthalmitis occurs after a perforating wound of the globe. Pain and loss of vision occur within 12 hours after the injury. By 18 hours, there is evidence of a fulminating panophthalmitis with chemosis and brawny swelling of the lids, proptosis, hypopyon, increased intraocular tension, gas bubbles in the anterior chamber, and necrosis of the wound margins.

Pneumatosis cystoides intestinalis can be produced in animals with *C. perfringens,* and this organism has been recovered from this process in humans.[5, 6] Pneumatosis cystoides intestinalis may be found in conjunction with toxic megacolon and neonatal necrotizing enterocolitis and as a complication of ileal bypass for obesity.

Specific Diagnosis

The diagnosis of gas gangrene must be made on clinical grounds. The presence of a gas-forming infection and recovery of *C. perfringens* from the wound do not establish the diagnosis of gas gangrene. The key to this diagnosis is demonstration of myonecrosis. Clostridial myonecrosis must be differentiated from other gas-forming, soft tissue infections, which may or may not involve *C. perfringens,* and from other causes of myonecrosis. The sudden onset, extreme toxemia, and severe pain that are noted in clostridial myonecrosis represent important differential features. Entities such as anaerobic cellulitis and streptococcal myonecrosis have a gradual onset, slight toxemia, and less pain in comparison with clostridial myonecrosis. Synergistic nonclostridial anaerobic myonecrosis is a severe infection characterized by discrete areas of blue-gray necrosis of skin, with extensive involvement of underlying soft tissue and muscle and foul "dishwater" pus. Anaerobic cellulitis typically has much more gas and does not involve muscle.

In streptococcal myonecrosis, initially there is edema of the muscle, and then the muscle has a hemorrhagic appearance.[5] Specimens for Gram staining and culture should be obtained from the involved muscle rather than from the wound surface. Large gram-positive rods will be demonstrated on Gram stain in clostridial myonecrosis; no white blood cells may be demonstrable, or the white blood cells present may be distorted significantly as a function of the toxin of *C. perfringens* acting on them. Anaerobic cellulitis typically shows a mixture of organisms, which may include *C. perfringens.* Streptococcal myonecrosis reveals anaerobic streptococci, sometimes along with group A streptococci, *S. aureus,* and other organisms.[5] In synergistic nonclostridial anaerobic myonecrosis, *Bacteroides* organisms seem to be key pathogens, along with anaerobic cocci and nonanaerobic gram-negative bacilli.[6] It is important in obtaining material for culture to place this under anaerobic conditions promptly for transport to the laboratory. Anaerobic blood cultures also should be obtained.

Uterine infection due to *C. perfringens* varies in severity from secondary invasion of necrotic material in the uterus or a dead fetus to invasion of intact uterine muscle producing myonecrosis and physometra.[5] Although bacteremia is relatively uncommon in gas gangrene, uterine infection with *C. perfringens* frequently is accompanied by sepsis, leading to the dramatic picture of intravascular hemolysis described earlier. Demonstration of a severe hemolytic anemia in association with uterine infection essentially is diagnostic. Anaerobic blood cultures should be obtained.

Clostridia, particularly *C. perfringens,* occasionally are isolated from the blood of a patient with a clinically benign course. The usual scenario is that a hospitalized patient has a single fever spike of unclear etiology, and blood cultures are done as part of the evaluation; by the time the culture becomes positive, there is no evidence of an infectious process. This transient and benign bacteremia probably originates from the colonic flora.[6]

C. perfringens food poisoning usually is seen in a setting of a sizable outbreak.[6] The organism grows to high counts in the responsible food and then sets up an infection in the host with production of enterotoxin in the colon of patients. Demonstration of large numbers of *C. perfringens* ($>10^6$/g) in the implicated food and demonstration of the same serotype of *C. perfringens* from the stools of affected individuals and from the food are important in documenting the nature of the food poisoning. Enterotoxin also may be demonstrated in the stools of affected individuals, and the *C. perfringens* recovered from the stool or food can be demonstrated to produce enterotoxin in vitro. Necrotizing enteritis due to *C. perfringens* may be suspected by virtue of the dramatic clinical picture and confirmed by demonstration of *C. perfringens* type C in the stool or suspect food or serum antibody to the beta-toxin of the organism.

C. difficile is isolated conveniently by use of a selective medium, cycloserine-cefoxitin-fructose agar. Its toxin B (cytotoxin) is identified most easily by tissue culture assay, which is the gold standard for diagnosis of antibiotic-associated diarrhea.[6] A simple latex particle agglutination test for detection of *C. difficile* is available and is used in some laboratories as a screening test. Other tests for toxins A and B have been developed; these may be performed more rapidly than the tissue culture assay, but they lack sensitivity, specificity, or both. Sigmoidoscopy or colonoscopy is needed to identify the characteristic mucosal plaques of pseudomembranous colitis that are diagnostic of the disease.

Interpreting the significance of finding *C. difficile* or its toxins in very young patients with diarrhea is difficult because infants and toddlers have such a high rate of asymptomatic carriage.[10, 13, 17] Quantitation of toxin or organisms has not correlated with presence or absence of symptoms. Consequently, once the possible presence of other diarrhea-producing pathogens (e.g., rotavirus, *Salmonella*) has been excluded, an effort should be made to stop the presumptive precipitating antibacterial agent. If diarrhea with mucus or blood persists, endoscopy should be considered and specific therapy begun.

Treatment

The most important aspect of treating clostridial myonecrosis is immediate surgical intervention with radical débridement and drainage and decompression of fascial compartments.[5, 6] The wound should not be closed after this surgery. It is crucial that all bits of necrotic muscle and other tissue be removed. Polyvalent gas gangrene antitoxin was never established firmly as beneficial in the context of modern therapy, although some authorities still favored its use. However, this product no longer is being produced. Hyperbaric oxygen is recommended enthusiastically by some, but there is no definitive evidence that its use reduces mortality. It does facilitate demarcation of a limb with impaired vascular supply, and it appears to slow down or arrest local spread of the gangrenous infection. Clearly, however, hyperbaric oxygen must not be used as a substitute for any of the important principles of surgical management. Antimicrobial therapy also is important as an adjunct, with penicillin G the drug of choice.[5, 6] In individuals who are allergic to penicillin G, cephalosporins may be used. Chloramphenicol is active routinely against all clostridia. Clindamycin is very active against *C. perfringens,* but 20 to 30 per cent of strains of other species of *Clostridium* that may accompany *C. perfringens* may be resistant.[5, 6]

Clostridial cellulitis is treated by incision and drainage and antimicrobial therapy. Radical débridement is not necessary, but it is important to lay the tissues open to effect proper drainage and to permit removal of all necrotic tissue.[5, 6]

Uterine curettage should be performed for diagnosis and treatment of postabortal or puerperal clostridial infections.[5] Hysterectomy may be required if there is involvement of the myometrium and if the patient's condition is deteriorating. At times, perforation of the uterus may be present without typical clinical findings. Exchange transfusion has been recommended in sepsis due to *C. perfringens* when there is significant intravascular hemolysis.

Food poisoning due to *C. perfringens* is self-limited and requires no therapy. Antitoxin to the beta-toxin produced by *C. perfringens* type C has been of considerable benefit in the treatment of necrotizing enteritis due to this organism.

In any serious infection due to *C. perfringens* or other clostridia, the usual support measures for shock, dehydration, anemia, and renal insufficiency are utilized as indicated.

With the recent and rapid increase in the recovery of vancomycin-resistant enterococci (as many as 20 per cent of enterococcal isolates in some intensive care units), many experts and the CDC have suggested that vancomycin should be used only to treat *C. difficile*–induced diarrhea (presumably referring to adults) as a last resort. The rationale is that a major reservoir for enterococci is the human gastrointestinal tract, and vancomycin, when administered orally, achieves exceedingly high gut levels; this would seem to be an ideal means to promote an ever-increasing prevalence of vancomycin-resistant enterococci. Keeping the aforementioned codicil in mind, if treatment of *C. difficile* diarrhea is needed, it should be either with oral vancomycin or with oral metronidazole (30 mg/kg/day divided every 6 hours). Orally administered bacitracin also may be useful, although some experts believe that it may be less effective than metronidazole or vancomycin. In the child older than 2 years of age, the detection of *C. difficile* cytotoxin in the appropriate clinical setting virtually is diagnostic for *C. difficile*–induced disease and therefore should be acted upon accordingly. The usually recommended pediatric dose of oral vancomycin is 50 mg/kg/day, divided every 6 hours, for 7 to 14 days. If one can judge from extensive experience in adults, it is probable that a lower dose (10 to 30 mg/kg/day) would be sufficient in children. Improvement should occur within 3 to 5 days.[13]

Treatment of pseudomembranous colitis due to *C. difficile* involves discontinuation of the offending drug, when feasible, and use of oral metronidazole or vancomycin as noted earlier.[6]

Prognosis

The mortality in gas gangrene varies between 15 and 35 per cent and is worse when large muscle groups, such as those of the buttock, thigh, leg, and shoulder, are involved or when areas that are difficult to débride, such as the viscera and pelvis, are involved with disease. Clostridial cellulitis has a much better prognosis, but aggressive therapy still is important in minimizing mortality. The mortality in postabortal clostridial sepsis still is 50 to 85 per cent. *C. perfringens* food poisoning has an excellent prognosis, but mortality is significant in necrotizing enteritis due to *C. perfringens* type C.

Prevention

Wounds involving areas with large muscle masses particularly are prone to gas gangrene, as are compound fractures, severe crushing injuries, and injuries secondary to high-velocity missiles. Extensive laceration or devitalization of muscle tissue, impairment of the main blood supply to a limb or large muscle group, and contamination by dirt and particularly by bowel contents all predispose to clostridial myonecrosis. The most important aspect of prophylaxis by far is early and adequate surgical management.[5, 6] All devitalized tissue must be débrided; meticulous hemostasis is very important. Primary closure and tight packing of the wound should be avoided. All aspects of the wound must be drained adequately. If a cast must be applied, it should be bivalved from the outset. Hyperbaric oxygen is not indicated prophylactically. Antimicrobial prophylaxis, however, definitely is indicated. Penicillin is the drug of choice and should be given as early as possible after injury. It must be emphasized that antimicrobial prophylaxis is strictly adjunctive and far from adequate by itself. It has been shown that bathing, particularly showering, and application of a compress wet with an iodophor for 15 minutes reduce the skin count of *C. perfringens* significantly and minimize the likelihood of postoperative gas gangrene. This type of decontamination, of course, also may be useful in the management of traumatic wounds.

Prevention of clostridial uterine infection involves being certain that all products of conception are removed during abortion and that retained portions of the placenta are removed immediately after the third stage of labor. Prolonged labor should be anticipated when possible and analgesics employed judiciously. During labor, particularly with ruptured membranes, pelvic and rectal examinations should be kept to a minimum. During delivery, trauma should be minimized and lacerations repaired according to accepted surgical principles.

Proper sanitation in food-preparing facilities and adequate refrigeration are important safeguards against *C. perfringens* food poisoning. In areas where necrotizing enteritis due to *C. perfringens* type C is found with some frequency (such as New Guinea), a *C. perfringens* type C toxoid has been given with encouraging results. Much remains to be learned about precipitating and host factors in *C. difficile* colitis. The hospital environment has been shown to be a reservoir of this spore-forming bacterium. In infants, *C. difficile* is found more frequently in formula-fed than in breast-fed babies. One-third to one-half of women have antibody in their milk that neutralizes *C. difficile* cytotoxin; as a consequence, breast feeding may help protect some infants against illness.[13]

References

1. Brook, I.: Anaerobic Infections in Childhood. Boston, G. K. Hall Medical Publishers, 1983.
2. Centers for Disease Control: Botulism in the United States, 1899–1977. Handbook for Epidemiologists, Clinicians and Laboratory Workers. At-

lanta, Centers for Disease Control, U.S. Department of Health, Education and Welfare, May 1979.
3. Dowell, V. R., Jr.: Botulism and tetanus: Selected epidemiologic and microbiologic aspects. Rev. Infect. Dis. 6(Suppl. 1):S202–S207, 1984.
4. Dunkle, L. M., Brotherton, T. J., and Feigen, R. D.: Anaerobic infections in children: A prospective study. Pediatrics 57:311–320, 1976.
5. Finegold, S. M.: Anaerobic Bacteria in Human Disease. New York, Academic Press, 1977.
6. Finegold, S. M., and George, W. L. (eds.): Anaerobic Infections in Humans. San Diego, Academic Press, 1989.
7. George, W. L.: Antimicrobial agent-associated colitis and diarrhea: Historical background and clinical aspects. Rev. Infect. Dis. 6(Suppl. 1):S208–S213, 1984.
8. Horowitz, M. A., Hughes, J. M., Merson, M. H., et al.: Food-borne botulism in the United States, 1970–1975. J. Infect. Dis. 136:153–159, 1977.
9. Hughes, L. M., Blumenthal, J. R., Merson, M. H., et al.: Clinical features of types A and B food-borne botulism. Ann. Intern. Med. 95:442–445, 1981.
10. Jarvis, W. R., and Feldman, R. A.: *Clostridium difficile* and gastroenteritis: How strong is the association in children? Pediatr. Infect. Dis. 3:4–6, 1984.
11. Lawrence, G., and Walker, P. D.: Pathogenesis of enteritis necroticans in Papua, New Guinea. Lancet 1:125–126, 1976.
12. Merson, M. H., and Dowell, Jr., V. R.: Epidemiologic, clinical and laboratory aspects of wound botulism. N. Engl. J. Med. 289:1005–1010, 1973.
13. Rolfe, R. D., and Finegold, S. M. (eds.): *Clostridium difficile:* Its Role in Intestinal Disease. San Diego, Academic Press, 1988.
14. Smith, L., and Sugiyama, H.: Botulism: The Organism, Its Toxins, the Disease. 2nd ed. Springfield, Charles C Thomas, 1977.
15. Tacket, C. O., Shandera, W. X., Mann, J. M., et al.: Equine antitoxin use and other factors that predict outcome in type A food-borne botulism. Am. J. Med. 76:794–798, 1984.
16. Thirumoorthia, M. C., Keen, B. M., and Djani, A. S.: Anaerobic infections in children: A prospective study. J. Clin. Microbiol. 3:318–323, 1976.
17. Welch, D. F., and Marks, M. I.: Is *Clostridium difficile* pathogenic in infants? J. Pediatr. 100:393–395, 1982.

153

INFANT BOTULISM

Stephen S. Arnon

Of the three forms of human botulism (food-borne, wound, and infant), infant botulism is the most recently recognized (1976) and in the United States the most common. Now recognized globally, infant botulism results from a unique pathogenesis. Ingested spores of *Clostridium botulinum* germinate, colonize the infant colon, and in it produce botulinum neurotoxin. The toxin then is absorbed, binds to peripheral cholinergic synapses, and causes flaccid paralysis. Knowledge of this intestinal pathogenesis resulted in the discovery of novel pathogenic strains of *Clostridium baratii* and *Clostridium butyricum*, each of which can make a botulinum-like neurotoxin and cause the clinical picture of infant botulism. Discovery of these strains enlarged the number of organisms known to cause the "intestinal toxemias of infancy," of which infant botulism is the prototype.[5] Parenthetically, adults and older children rarely may become susceptible to infant-type botulism after broad-spectrum antibiotic treatment and intestinal surgery, inflammatory bowel disease,[1, 18, 23, 42] or procedures associated with bone marrow transplantation.[60]

HISTORY

Infant botulism is not a new disease; rather, it is a newly recognized one. The first laboratory-proven case of human infant botulism occurred in California in 1931, although it was misdiagnosed at the time.[10] Decades later and well before the etiology of the disease was apparent, the characteristic clinical features of infant botulism had become evident to discerning observers. In 1974, Grover and associates[27] described nine patients from Pennsylvania with a neurologic syndrome of undetermined cause that from today's perspective almost certainly was infant botulism. The same idiopathic syndrome was recognized in southern California and was reported by Ramseyer and colleagues[57] in 1976 to have a characteristic electromyographic pattern. In 1977, Clay and associates[19] linked their eight patients to infant botulism.

The first report of frank botulism in infancy was by Pickett and colleagues[56] in 1976. Although the source of botulinum neurotoxin for their two patients was undetermined, the possibility of its in vivo production was suggested.[44, 56] The diagnosis of botulism in these and other California patients was established by identification of *C. botulinum* toxin and organisms in the infants' feces.[44] Evidence also was obtained that ingested spores of *C. botulinum* had produced the toxin in the infants' intestinal tract.[8, 44, 78]

In subsequent years, the clinical spectrum of infant botulism was found to include mild, outpatient cases and sudden unexpected death indistinguishable from typical sudden infant death syndrome.[9, 55, 63, 74] In 1985, a *C. baratii* strain that produced a type F–like botulinum neurotoxin was recognized belatedly as the true cause of a case of infant botulism that occurred in New Mexico in 1979,[28, 31] and, in 1986, a *C. butyricum* strain that produced a type E–like botulinum neurotoxin was recognized as the cause of two cases of infant botulism in Rome, Italy.[12] These latter two novel clostridia were discovered only because they caused human infant botulism; their existence suggests that others like them await discovery.

ETIOLOGIC AGENT

C. botulinum is a gram-positive, spore-forming, obligate anaerobe whose natural habitat worldwide is the soil. Consequently, *C. botulinum* is as ubiquitous as the dust on which it may travel, and, hence, its spores commonly are present on fresh fruits, vegetables, and other agricultural products, such as honey. The members of the *C. botulinum* species are so diverse in their biochemical capabilities that they would not be grouped as a single species except for the similar neurotoxin molecule that each strain produces[62]; at present, the *C. botulinum* species is subdivided into six groups based on metabolic characteristics.[12] Almost all cases of infant botulism in the United States have been caused by group I proteolytic type A or type B strains. Unusual strains of *C. baratii* and *C. butyricum* that make botulinum-like toxins E and F also cause infant botulism.[12, 28, 67, 52, 77]

In general, each vegetative cell of *C. botulinum* produces just one of seven serologically distinguishable toxins, which arbitrarily have been assigned the letters A to G. Antitoxin raised against one toxin type does not protect against any of the other six toxin types. The different toxin types serve as convenient epidemiologic and clinical markers. Each toxin molecule is a simple protein consisting of two polypeptide chains of approximately 100,000 (heavy chain) and 50,000 (light chain) daltons joined by a disulfide bond. Botulinum toxin is the most poisonous substance known.[24] By extrapolation from studies with adult primates, the lethal dose in the blood stream of man is approximately 1 nanogram/kg body weight.[24] Its potency for infants may be even higher because of the narrowness of their pharyngeal airway.[74]

After centuries of awe and mystery, the basis of the phenomenal potency of the botulinum (and tetanus) toxins recently was shown to be enzymatic. The light chain of each neurotoxin is a Zn^{++}-containing protease that hydrolyzes one of three intracellular proteins needed for vesicle fusion and acetylcholine release into the synaptic cleft.[48, 51]

PATHOGENESIS

Infant botulism results from a unique infectious disease pathway. Ingested spores of *C. botulinum* germinate, colonize the infant colon, and produce botulinum neurotoxin in it.[8, 29, 46, 53, 54, 78] The toxin subsequently is absorbed and carried by the blood stream to peripheral cholinergic synapses, where it binds irreversibly. The light chain then is taken into the cytosol of the neuron, where it blocks the release of acetylcholine by enzymatic cleavage of "fusion complex" proteins.[48, 51] Clinically, the most important of the peripheral cholinergic synapses is the neuromuscular junction; the toxin's action results in flaccid paralysis and hypotonia. Preganglionic cholinergic synapses in the autonomic nervous system also may be affected.[41, 59]

By use of a mouse model system of intestinal colonization (in which the animals paradoxically remained symptom-free), Sugiyama and colleagues[14, 47, 68] have demonstrated that the intestinal microflora of adult animals ordinarily prevent colonization of the gut by *C. botulinum*. Administration of 10^6 type A spores failed to colonize the intestine of normal adult mice, whereas after treatment for $2\frac{1}{2}$ days with a combination of oral erythromycin and kanamycin, half the mice could be colonized by just 2×10^4 spores. When the antibiotic-treated mice were placed in cages with normal mice, they lost their susceptibility to intestinal colonization after 3 days.[14] (Mice normally are coprophagic.) In addition, adult germ-free mice could be colonized intestinally by just 10 *C. botulinum* type A spores. When the germ-free adult animals were placed in a room with conventional mice, in 3 days the formerly germ-free animals became resistant to colonization by 10^5 spores.[47]

In contrast to the experimental work with adult mice, normal infant mice were susceptible to intestinal colonization by *C. botulinum* spores.[68] Like human infants, the normal infant mice were susceptible to colonization only for a limited period (7 to 13 days of age). Susceptibility of the infant mice peaked between days 8 and 11 in a pattern reminiscent of the peaking of susceptibility seen between 2 and 4 months of age in human infant botulism (Fig. 153–1).[6, 68] The infective dose of spores for infant mice was much smaller than that of their antibiotic-treated adult counterparts; the 50 per cent infective dose for normal infants was only 700 spores. In one

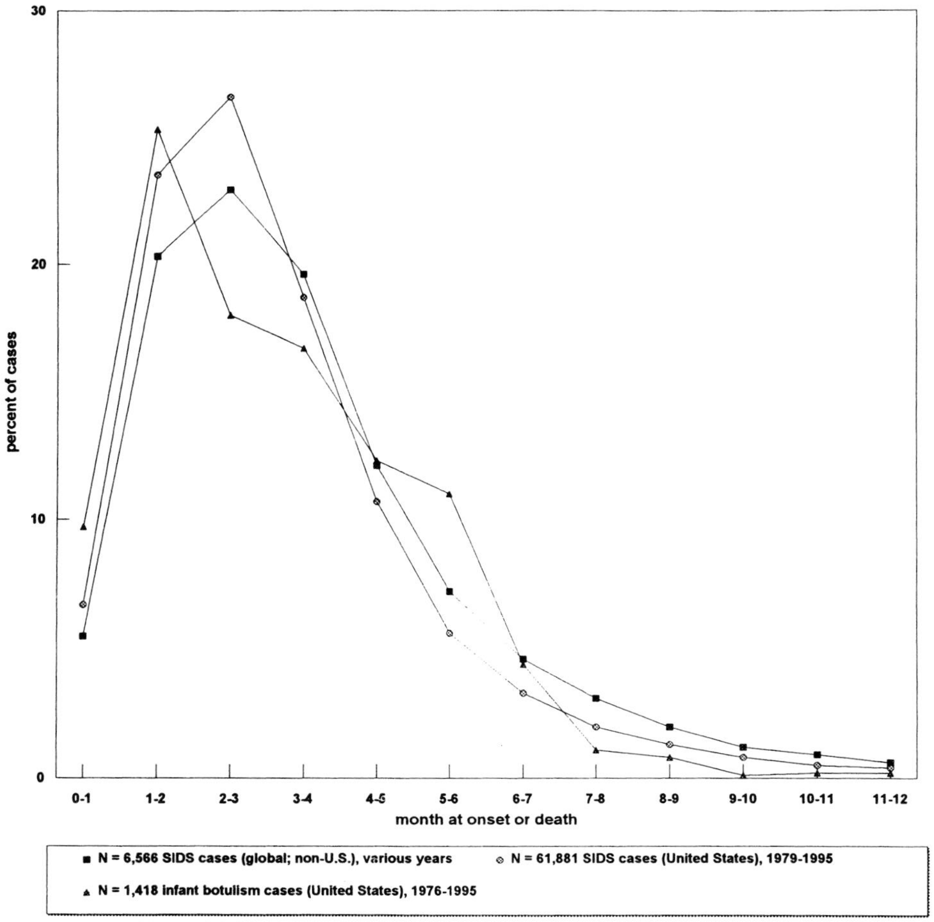

FIGURE 153–1. *The age distributions of infant botulism and sudden infant death syndrome (SIDS).*

experiment, just 10 spores colonized an infant mouse.[68] The minimum infective dose of *C. botulinum* spores for human infants is not known, but from exposure to spore-containing honeys, it has been estimated to be as low as 10 to 100.[9]

Recognition of the central role of the host intestinal microflora in determining susceptibility or resistance to colonization by *C. botulinum* has directed attention to those factors that may influence the composition of the normal microflora. Diet may be the most important of these factors. In comparison with the adult-type flora, the infant flora is simpler, with fewer genera and species. The dominant members vary, depending in part on whether the infant is fed only breast milk, only formula milk, or a mixture of the two.[66] Also, the composition of the intestinal flora is changed if solid foods, such as cereals, become part of the infant's diet. The normal human infant microflora contain several bacterial species, mainly *Bifidobacterium* and *Bacteroides*, that in vitro can inhibit the multiplication of *C. botulinum*.[70]

Onset of infant botulism occurs at a significantly younger age in formula-fed infants (7.6 weeks) than in breast-fed infants (13.7 weeks),[7] perhaps reflecting the earlier availability in formula-fed infants of suitable ecologic niches[7, 41, 65, 66] and the formula-fed infants' lack of the immune factors (e.g., sIgA, lactoferrin) contained in human milk.[2, 4, 26] In addition, introduction of solid foods may "perturb" the intestinal microflora[66] and thereby aid *C. botulinum* colonization.[4, 6, 41, 64]

An additional physiologic risk factor for infant botulism is a slower gut motility, as measured by frequency of defecation before onset of illness.[64] Less than one bowel movement per day is a risk factor for both breast-fed and formula-fed infants, but this occurred in just 50 per cent of the cases.[59a]

EPIDEMIOLOGY

Any discussion of the epidemiology of infant botulism should be prefaced by the caveat that almost all presently available information is derived from study of only part of the clinical spectrum, namely, the hospitalized patients. Accordingly, current perspectives may need to be modified as the outpatient and sudden-death portions of the clinical spectrum become defined more fully. Also, the perceived incidence remains more a reflection of physician awareness and access to diagnostic testing than of actual disease occurrence. About half (48 per cent) of U.S. cases have been reported from California, which has the largest number of births of any state. However, California does not have the highest incidence of infant botulism once adjustment is made for differences in annual births (Table 153–1). Notably, 8 of the 10 highest incidence states are located west of the Rocky Mountains.

TABLE 153–1. Cases and Incidence of Infant Botulism, Top 10 Incidence States, United States, 1977–1995

State	Cases	Incidence*
Delaware	20	11.0
Hawaii	35	10.3
Utah	58	8.3
California	631	7.1
Pennsylvania	153	5.2
Oregon	28	3.7
Washington	45	3.6
Idaho	11	3.5
New Mexico	16	3.3
Arizona	25	2.4

*Per 100,000 live births per year.

A unique epidemiologic feature of infant botulism is its age distribution, which, perhaps coincidentally, virtually is identical to the age distribution of sudden infant death syndrome (see Fig. 153–1).[6, 9, 17, 64] All cases of infant botulism reported to date have occurred in children younger than 1 year of age. Some 95 per cent of cases occur in the first 6 months of life; the remaining 5 per cent are distributed over the subsequent 6 months. The youngest known patient was 6 days old at onset,[34, 73] and the oldest was 351 days.[32] The illness has occurred in all major racial and ethnic groups and in approximately equal proportions in males and females. A national seasonality is not evident.

Infant botulism now has been reported from all inhabited continents except Africa. In the United States, with four exceptions, all hospitalized cases known as of December 1996 were caused either by *C. botulinum* type A or type B (or, in one case, both). Forty-three of the 50 states, representing all regions of the country and including Alaska and Hawaii, now have reported infant botulism. In general, the distribution of cases by toxin type has paralleled the distribution of toxin types in U.S. soils,[61] type B cases predominating from the great plains eastward and type A cases predominating from the Rocky Mountains westward. Of the four exceptional toxin types, two cases in New Mexico and Oregon resulted from a type F–like toxin produced by *C. baratii* strains,[28, 31, 52] and the other two cases were caused by a *C. botulinum* strain that produced mostly type B and some type F toxin (designated type B_f). One patient with B_f illness lived in New Mexico, and the other patient had traveled there immediately before onset of illness.

Geographic clustering has been noted. In Pennsylvania, 43 of 53 cases in the period 1977 to 1983 occurred in four suburban counties that form an arc bordering the city of Philadelphia.[40] In Colorado, three type A cases occurred in three separate families in a small town with approximately 300 annual births. Two of the infants had used the same crib sequentially; environmental samples, including the crib, soils, and household dust, yielded *C. botulinum* type A.[35] In California, two type A cases occurred 5 years apart in the children of two families who lived one house apart. In another California family, two successive infants each acquired type A infant botulism, but the third child born in sequence did not. Soil and dust specimens from the house contained *C. botulinum* type A.

The role of breast feeding and formula feeding as factors possibly predisposing to illness remains unsettled. All studies to date have identified an association between being breast-fed and being hospitalized for infant botulism.[2, 7, 40, 41, 49, 64, 74] This finding has resulted in one perspective that holds that breast feeding predisposes to illness,[40, 41, 64] whereas the other perspective holds that breast feeding slows onset sufficiently to permit hospitalization to occur.[2, 4, 6, 7] However, among hospitalized patients, the mean age at onset of formula-fed infants (7.6 weeks) was significantly younger and about half that of breast-fed infants (13.8 weeks). In addition, the fulminant-onset infant botulism patients who stopped breathing and died at home all were formula-fed.[7] It appears that the relative susceptibilities of formula-fed and breast-fed infants to infant botulism and the resultant severity of their disease may reflect differences in the availability of suitable ecologic niches in the intestinal flora for *C. botulinum*, differences in the availability of immune factors (such as lactoferrin and secretory IgA) are contained in human milk but not in formula milk,[26] or other differences not identified yet.

Honey is the one dietary reservoir of *C. botulinum* spores thus far definitively linked to infant botulism by both laboratory and epidemiologic evidence.[6, 10, 30, 33, 37, 43, 45, 58, 69] To date, 32 instances worldwide are known in which *C. botulinum* spores have been found in the actual honey fed to the affected infant before the onset of illness. In each instance, the toxin type (A or B) of the spores in the honey matched the toxin type (A or B) of the *C. botulinum* that caused the infant's illness; the probability that such perfect concordance occurred by chance is less than 1 in 1 billion. *C. botulinum* spores have been found in honeys originating in the United States, Canada, Australia, China (Taiwan), Japan, and Central America[30, 33, 37, 43, 45, 58, 69] but not in honeys from the United Kingdom.[13] For these reasons and because honey is nutritionally nonessential, all major pediatric, public health, and honey industry agencies in the United States have joined in the recommendation that honey not be fed to infants (see references in Arnon and colleagues' study[6]).

Discussion of the possible role of corn syrups in infant botulism is necessitated by two reports. In 1982, the U.S. Food and Drug Administration found *C. botulinum* type B spores in approximately 0.5 per cent (5 of 961) of previously unopened retail samples of light and dark corn syrups[37]; the manufacturer then made changes in the production process. In 1989, the federal Centers for Disease Control and Prevention reported a 2-year epidemiologic study of U.S. cases from all states except California.[64] By subgrouping patients by age and using logistic regression modeling techniques, it was possible to obtain a statistical association between the triad of corn syrup exposure, breast feeding, and an age at onset of 2 months or older.

In contrast to these reports, a 1988 Canadian survey found no *C. botulinum* spores in 43 corn syrup samples.[30] A 1991 Food and Drug Administration market survey of 783 syrups (354 of which were light corn syrup and 271 dark corn syrup) concluded that none contained *C. botulinum* spores.[39] A California study (unpublished) of 103 corn syrups, 72 of which had been fed to infants who subsequently became ill with infant botulism, did not find *C. botulinum* in any sample. Also, a 1979 epidemiologic study that simply compared corn syrup exposure rates in 41 cases and 107 control infants identified corn syrup feeding as a significant protective factor against type A infant botulism.[10] The explanation offered for the latter observation was that if a parent chose corn syrup as a sweetener for the infant, he or she was unlikely to have fed the child honey as a second sweetener. Thus, on the basis of presently available evidence, it appears that corn syrups do not constitute a source of *C. botulinum* spores or a risk factor for infant botulism. In addition to specific testing of honeys and syrups, hundreds of traditional and nontraditional infant food items, including formula milk, have been examined and found not to contain *C. botulinum*.[43]

Besides honey, potential environmental sources of *C. botulinum* spores have been identified in many locales. In Pennsylvania, the soil;[41] in Australia, the soil and cistern water;[50] and in California, the soil and vacuum cleaner dust[6] obtained from case homes were found to contain *C. botulinum*, whose toxin type (A or B) in each instance matched that of the ill infant. However, despite the foregoing, it deserves emphasis that for the majority of cases of infant botulism, no source of *C. botulinum* spores is ever identified, even circumstantially. In these cases, it is likely that illness was acquired by swallowing spores adherent to airborne microscopic (invisible) dust.

CLINICAL MANIFESTATIONS

Like other infectious diseases, infant botulism displays a spectrum in its clinical severity.[4, 6–9, 41, 55, 59, 63, 74] To date, almost all recognized cases sufficiently have been hypotonic and weak to need hospitalization. Consequently, it is from the hospitalized patient that the present picture of infant botulism is derived. However, outpatient cases that displayed only a few days of lethargy, poor feeding, and some decrease in bowel movement frequency have been detected by alert physicians familiar with the more "classic" illness. At the opposite end of the clinical spectrum are those few cases whose history and presentation were indistinguishable from those of typical cases of sudden infant death syndrome (crib death),[9, 55, 63, 74] about 1 in 20 of which (in California) appears to result from fulminant infant botulism.[6, 9]

The onset of infant botulism ranges from the insidious to the abrupt. At one extreme are patients who were nursing normally 6 hours before becoming so floppy that acute meningitis was the diagnosis at presentation, and at the other extreme are patients who returned to their physicians four times in a week as the signs of illness gradually became manifest.

In the "classic" case, the first sign of illness almost always is constipation (defined as 3 or more days without defecation in a previously regular infant), yet the constipation often is overlooked. A few patients (<5%) will present without a history of constipation. Usually, a mother first notices listlessness, lethargy, and poor feeding, together with breast engorgement if the infant had been nursing. The increasing weakness over the ensuing 1 to 4 days usually brings the baby to medical attention.

Botulism is manifested clinically as a symmetric, descending paralysis. Early on, weakness and hypotonia characterize the illness, and the remainder of the physical examination not involving the neuromuscular system is normal. The first signs of illness are found in the cranial nerves; *it is not possible to have infant botulism without having bulbar palsies*. The typical patient has an expressionless face, a feeble cry, ptosis (evident when the eyelids must work against gravity), poor head control, and generalized weakness and hypotonia (Fig. 153–2). Eye muscle paralysis varies, and the pupils often are midposition and initially briskly reactive (Table 153–2). The gag, suck, and swallow reflexes are impaired, as well as the corneal reflex if it is tested repetitively. Deep tendon reflexes often are normal at presentation and diminish subsequently as the paralysis extends and increases. The "frog's legs" sign often is seen. Patients are afebrile unless a secondary infection (e.g., aspiration pneumonia) is present.

The results of most laboratory and clinical studies are normal. At admission, there may be evidence of mild dehydration and of fat mobilization because of diminished oral intake. Occasionally at admission, the cerebrospinal fluid protein concentration becomes elevated because of the mild dehydration. If infant botulism is suspected soon after admission, electroencephalography, computed tomography, and magnetic resonance imaging seldom are required; but if done, these examinations yield nonspecific or normal results. Electromyography offers rapid bedside confirmation of the clinical diagnosis (see Differential Diagnosis and Diagnosis).[20, 22]

It sometimes is possible to identify small amounts (<5 mouse LD_{50}/mL) of botulinum toxin in serum specimens if these are collected early in the illness.[12, 29, 54, 72, 76] In one report, almost one patient in eight had toxin demonstrable in serum.[29] The definitively diagnostic laboratory study is the examination of feces for the presence of *C. botulinum* organisms and toxin, which is the only way to identify the neurotoxin type (A, B, or other) responsible for the illness. Clinically suspected cases that lack an identified toxin type will not be included in official tallies of infant botulism.[16]

The usual hospital course of infant botulism has certain

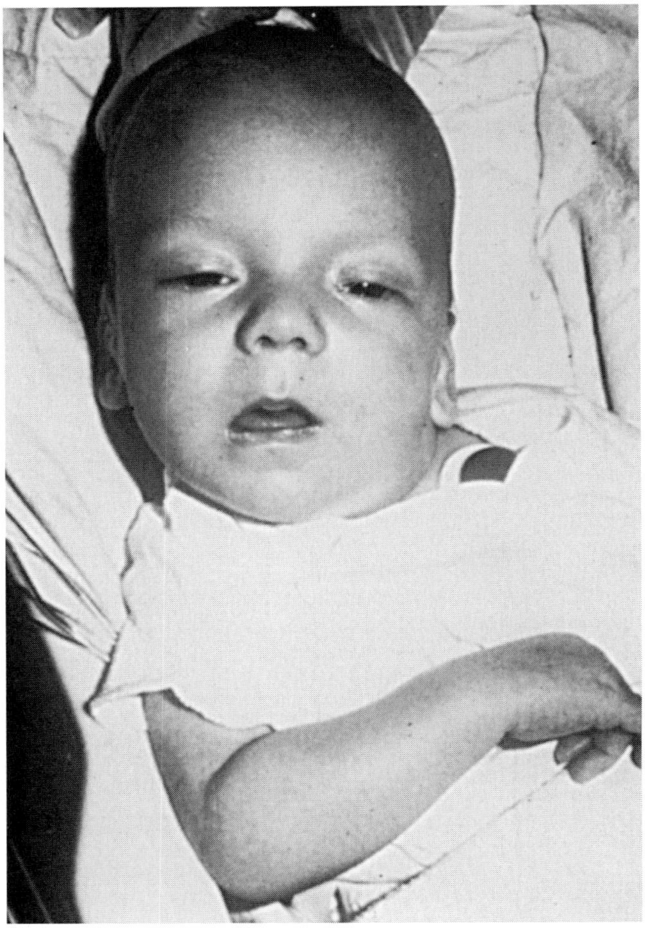

FIGURE 153–2. *Mildly affected, 7-week-old infant with botulism. Note the minimal signs, including ptosis, mildly disconjugate gaze, expressionless face, slack jaw, and neck and arm hypotonia.*

general features.[36, 41, 59] After the increasing weakness has necessitated admission, the weakness and hypotonia continue to progress and usually become generalized. The deep tendon reflexes, which may be normal at admission, may diminish or disappear temporarily. The nadir of paresis and paralysis usually occurs within 1 to 2 weeks after admission. Patients often remain at their nadir for as long as 1 to 3 weeks before showing signs of improvement. However, once strength and tone begin to return, the improvement continues steadily and gradually over the ensuing weeks in the absence of complications (Table 153–3).

In the California experience, infant botulism does not have a relapsing course, and perceived "relapses" have been found to be, in retrospect, an indication either of the onset of a complication (see Table 153–3) or of a premature discharge. However, the clinical experience elsewhere with regard to relapses has been different.[25, 59] The patient is ready for discharge when gag, suck, and swallow sufficiently are strong both to protect the airway against accidental aspiration and to ensure adequacy of oral intake. Parents also may be taught to feed by gavage at home. In either situation, discharge may occur safely while head-lag and constipation still are present.

DIFFERENTIAL DIAGNOSIS AND DIAGNOSIS

When initially brought to medical attention, patients with infant botulism often are so mildly weak and hypotonic that the illness is not suspected. Even today, more than 20 years after the first recognition of the disease, suspected sepsis remains the most common admission diagnosis for patients with infant botulism. A careful history (constipation commonly is overlooked) and physical examination (especially cranial nerve function) usually can identify infant botulism patients correctly and render unnecessary most additional testing for the other entities typically suspected (Table 153–4).

The diagnosis of infant botulism is established by identification of *C. botulinum* organisms in the feces of an infant with clinical signs consistent with the paralyzing action of botulinum toxin.[36, 44] Extensive studies have demonstrated that *C. botulinum* is not part of the normal resident flora of infants or adults.[6, 29, 65, 66] If the fecal specimen is obtained early enough in illness, it also will contain botulinum toxin. Because of the patient's constipation, an enema with sterile, nonbacteriostatic water (not saline) commonly is needed for obtaining a fecal specimen for diagnostic examination. A

TABLE 153–2. Neurologic Signs Helpful in the Diagnosis of Infant Botulism

Test	Findings
1. Take the patient to a dark room. Shine a bright light into the eye; note the quickness of pupillary constriction. Remove the light when the constriction is maximal; let the pupil dilate again. Then immediately repeat the light, continuing thus for 1 to 3 minutes.	The initially brisk pupillary response may become sluggish and the pupil unable to constrict maximally. (Fatigability with repetitive muscle contraction is the clinical hallmark of botulism.)
2. Shine a bright light onto the fovea, keeping it there for 1 to 3 minutes, even if the infant tries to deviate his eyes.	Latent ophthalmoplegia may be elicited, and/or purposeful efforts to avoid the light may diminish.
3. Place a clean fifth finger in the infant's mouth, taking care not to obstruct the airway. Note the strength and duration of the reflex sucking.	The suck is weak and poorly sustained.

Adapted from Arnon, S. S.: Infant botulism. Annu. Rev. Med. *31*:541–560, 1980. (Reproduced with permission by Annual Reviews, Inc.)

TABLE 153–3. Complications of Infant Botulism

Adult respiratory distress syndrome
Aspiration
Clostridium difficile colitis
Fracture of the femur (nosocomial)
Inappropriate antidiuretic hormone secretion
Misplaced or plugged endotracheal tube
Necrotizing enterocolitis
Otitis media
Pneumonia
Recurrent atelectasis
Seizures secondary to hyponatremia
Sepsis
Tension pneumothorax
Transfusion reaction
Urinary tract infection
Subglottic stenosis
Tracheal granuloma
Tracheitis
Tracheomalacia

TABLE 153–4. Working Differential Diagnosis of Infant Botulism

Admission Diagnoses	Subsequent Working Diagnoses
R/O sepsis	Hypothyroidism
Dehydration	Metabolic encephalopathy
Viral syndrome	Amino acid metabolic disorder
Pneumonia	Heavy metal poisoning (Pb, Mg, As)
Idiopathic hypotonia	Drug ingestion
Failure to thrive	Poliomyelitis
	Brain stem encephalitis
	Myasthenia gravis
	Viral polyneuritis
	Guillain-Barré syndrome
	Hirschsprung disease
	Werdnig-Hoffmann disease

mouse neutralization test remains the most sensitive and specific assay for botulinum toxin.[16] Laboratory diagnosis that identifies the toxin type responsible for illness is essential for the case to be registered as infant botulism and is important to prognosis; mean hospital stay is significantly longer in type A cases (see Treatment).[16] Physicians are reminded that in most states, botulism or suspected botulism (all types) is an immediately reportable illness.

At the bedside, electromyography can be helpful in ambiguous situations, in that when a clinically weak muscle is tested, the electromyography often discloses a pattern known by the acronym BSAP (brief, small, abundant motor-unit potentials).[8, 19, 20, 22, 57, 59] The edrophonium (Tensilon) test is unnecessary in that congenital myasthenia gravis can be excluded by history, and de novo myasthenia does not occur at this age because of the immaturity of an infant's immune system. Likewise, Guillain-Barré syndrome that is well documented by finding a consistently elevated protein concentration in the cerebrospinal fluid is of negligible occurrence in infancy. In infant botulism, the cerebrospinal fluid protein concentration is normal, an occasional exception being that of the specimen collected while the child is mildly dehydrated.

TREATMENT

Specific treatment for infant botulism is now available. In California, a recently completed 5-year, randomized, double-blinded, placebo-controlled treatment trial demonstrated the safety and efficacy of human-derived botulinum antitoxin, formally known as botulism immune globulin (BIG).[24, 39] Use of BIG reduced mean hospital stay per case from approximately 5.5 weeks to approximately 2.5 weeks ($p < .001$) and reduced mean hospitalization cost per case by approximately \$70,000 ($p < .001$). Treatment with BIG should be started as early in the illness as possible. In the United States, BIG may be obtained from the California Department of Health Services (24-hour telephone: 510-540-2646) under a U.S. Food and Drug Administration–approved Treatment Investigational New Drug (IND) protocol.

Successful management of infant botulism also depends on meticulous supportive care and the anticipation and avoidance of potentially fatal complications (see Table 153–3). Feeding and breathing generally require the most attention. At admission, patients should receive cardiac, respiratory, and transcutaneous blood gas monitoring (especially carbon dioxide pressure) until it is clear that the paralysis no longer is progressing. An endotracheal tube often is necessary to maintain and protect the airway, even in the absence of a need for mechanical ventilation.

A third cornerstone of management is forbearance. Antibiotics should be reserved to treat the principal secondary infections (pneumonia, urinary tract infection, otitis media) because their use may result in lysis of intraintestinal *C. botulinum* with liberation of intracellular neurotoxin into the gut lumen. This potential problem may be avoided by use of nalidixic acid or the combination trimethoprim-sulfamethoxazole, antibiotics to which *C. botulinum* is known to be resistant.[71]

Surprisingly, the use of tracheostomy varies geographically, from a high of 32 per cent of 57 patients in one East Coast U.S. hospital[59] to a low of less than 1 per cent of 690 California patients. The California experience suggests that tracheostomy can be avoided for most patients if two simple positioning measures are used. First, for expansion of the thoracic cage and assistance in diaphragmatic function, patients should be placed in an older-style crib, the rigid bottom mattress of which can be lifted to elevate the entire body to a 30-degree angle. Second, for tipping the head back and to maintain normal curvature of neck and airway, a soft cloth should be rolled to the thickness of about three fingers and placed under just the child's neck. This maneuver allows oral secretions to drain away from the trachea and into the true posterior pharynx, where they are swallowed most easily.

Use of intravenous feeding (hyperalimentation) is discouraged because of its potential for secondary infection and because of the success obtained with nasogastric or nasojejunal tube feeding. Mother's milk is the nutritional fluid of choice. Isolation measures or "enteric precautions" are not required, but meticulous hand washing is. Soiled diapers should be autoclaved because they can be expected to contain botulinum neurotoxin as well as viable spores and vegetative cells of *C. botulinum*. For this reason, staff with open lesions on their hands should not handle the diapers.

Hospital stay of all 508 California patients hospitalized 1976–1991 averaged just over 1 month (4.9 weeks). However, the mean length of stay differed significantly ($p < .0001$) between the 307 type A cases (5.7 weeks) and the 201 type B cases (3.6 weeks), in large part because the major complications and multimonth hospitalizations occurred mainly in type A cases. Thus, illness caused by type A toxin appears to be potentially, but not invariably, more severe than that caused by type B toxin.

OUTCOME AND PROGNOSIS

Recovery from infant botulism occurs through regeneration of the poisoned terminal unmyelinated nerve endings. The newly synthesized nerve twigs then induce formation of new motor endplates that are indistinguishable functionally and morphologically from the original ones.[21] In experimental animals and in humans, completion of this process takes several weeks.[21] Consequently, in the absence of hypoxic cerebral complications, full and complete recovery of strength and tone is the expected outcome of infant botulism. In addition, because botulinum toxin does not cross the blood-brain barrier to any functional degree, the child's intelligence and personality remain as originally endowed. Parents often need reassurance on this latter point. Reinfection with the same or a different toxin type of *C. botulinum* has not occurred. In the United States, in hospitalized patients, the case-fatality ratio is less than 1 per cent, a reflection of and tribute to the high quality of intensive care given to these critically ill infants. In other countries, the experience has not been so fortunate.

PREVENTION

At present, the one known way to prevent infant botulism is not to feed honey to infants, and all major pediatric and public health agencies have endorsed this recommendation.

Breast feeding may help moderate the rapidity of onset and the severity of illness. Persuasive evidence that links infant botulism to ingestion of corn or other syrups is lacking. Mean hospital costs in California (1984–1991) exceeded $88,000 per case (1996 dollars; data collection began in 1984), and the patient with the most protracted illness was hospitalized for 10 months in 1988 at a cost of over $960,000 (1996 dollars). These economic facts combine with humanitarian considerations to make a compelling case for the prevention of infant botulism.

Suggested Readings

Smith, L. D. S., and Sugiyama, H. (eds.): Botulism: The Organism, Its Toxins, the Disease. 2nd ed. Springfield, IL, Charles C Thomas, 1988.

Montecucco, C. (ed.): Clostridial Neurotoxins: The Molecular Pathogenesis of Tetanus and Botulism. New York, Springer, 1995.

References

1. Arnon, S. S.: Botulism as an intestinal toxemia. *In* Blaser, M. J., Smith, P. D., Ravdin, J. I., et al. (eds.): Infections of the Gastrointestinal Tract. New York, Raven Press, 1995, pp. 257–271.
2. Arnon, S. S.: Breast feeding and toxigenic intestinal infections: Missing links in crib death? Rev. Infect. Dis. *6*:S193–S201, 1984.
3. Arnon, S. S.: Clinical trial of human botulism immune globulin. *In* Das Gupta, B. R. (ed.): Botulinum and Tetanus Neurotoxins: Neurotransmission and Biomedical Aspects. New York, Plenum Press, 1993, pp. 477–482.
4. Arnon, S. S.: Infant botulism. Annu. Rev. Med. *31*:541–560, 1980.
5. Arnon, S. S.: Infant botulism: Anticipating the second decade. J. Infect. Dis. *154*:201–206, 1986.
6. Arnon, S. S., Damus, K., and Chin, J.: Infant botulism: Epidemiology and relation to sudden infant death syndrome. Epidemiol. Rev. *3*:45–66, 1981.
7. Arnon, S. S., Damus, K., Thompson, B., et al.: Protective role of human milk against sudden death from infant botulism. J. Pediatr. *100*:568–573, 1982.
8. Arnon, S. S., Midura, T. F., Clay, S. A., et al.: Infant botulism: Epidemiological, clinical, and laboratory aspects. J. A. M. A. *237*:1946–1951, 1977.
9. Arnon, S. S., Midura, T. F., Damus, K., et al.: Intestinal infection and toxin production by *Clostridium botulinum* as one cause of sudden infant death syndrome. Lancet *1*:1273–1277, 1978.
10. Arnon, S. S., Midura, T. F., Damus, K., et al.: Honey and other environmental risk factors for infant botulism. J. Pediatr. *94*:331–336, 1979.
11. Arnon, S. S., Werner, S. B., Faber, H. K., et al.: Infant botulism in 1931: Discovery of a misclassified case. Am. J. Dis. Child. *133*:580–582, 1979.
12. Aureli, P., Fenicia, L., Pasolini, B., et al.: Two cases of type E infant botulism in Italy caused by neurotoxigenic *Clostridium butyricum*. J. Infect. Dis. *54*:207–211, 1986.
13. Berry, P. R., Gilbert, R. J., Oliver, R. W. A., et al.: Some preliminary studies on the low incidence of infant botulism in the United Kingdom. Corres. J. Clin. Pathol. *40*:121, 1987.
14. Burr, D. H., Sugiyama, H., and Jarvis, G.: Susceptibility to enteric botulinum colonization of antibiotic-treated adult mice. Infect. Immun. *36*:103–106, 1982.
15. Centers for Disease Control: Botulism in the United States, 1899–1977. Handbook for Epidemiologists, Clinicians, and Laboratory Workers. Atlanta, Centers for Disease Control, May 1979.
16. Centers for Disease Control: Case definitions for public health surveillance. M. M. W. R. *39*(RR-13):6–7, 1990.
17. Centers for Disease Control and Prevention: Sudden infant death syndrome: United States, 1983–1994. M. M. W. R. *45*:859–863, 1996.
18. Chia, J. K., Clark, J. B., Ryan, C. A., et al.: Botulism in an adult associated with food-borne intestinal infection with *Clostridium botulinum*. N. Engl. J. Med. *315*:239–240, 1986.
19. Clay, S. A., Ramseyer, J. C., Fishman, L. S., et al.: Acute infantile motor unit disorder: Infantile botulism? Arch. Neurol. *345*:236–243, 1977.
20. Cornblath, D. R., Sladky, J. T., and Sumner, A. J.: Clinical electrophysiology of infantile botulism. Muscle Nerve *6*:448–452, 1983.
21. Duchen, L. W.: Motor nerve growth induced by botulinum toxin as a regenerative phenomenon. Proc. R. Soc. Med. *65*:196–197, 1972.
22. Engel, W. K.: Brief, small, abundant motor-unit action potentials: A further critique of electromyographic interpretation. Neurology *25*:173–176, 1975.
23. Freedman, M., Armstrong, R. M., Killian, J. M., et al.: Botulism in a patient with jejunoileal bypass. Ann. Neurol. *20*:641–643, 1986.
24. Gill, D. M.: Bacterial toxins: A table of lethal amounts. Microbiol. Rev. *46*:86–94, 1982.
25. Glauser, T. A., Maguire, H. C., and Sladky, J. T.: Relapse of infant botulism. Ann. Neurol. *28*:187–189, 1990.
26. Goldman, A. S., and Goldblum, R. M.: Immunologic system in human milk: Characteristics and effects. *In* Lebenthal, E. (ed.): Textbook of Gastroenterology and Nutrition in Infancy. 2nd ed. New York, Raven Press, 1989, pp. 135–142.
27. Grover, W. D., Peckham, G. J., and Berman, P. H.: Recovery following cranial nerve dysfunction and muscle weakness in infancy. Dev. Med. Child. Neurol. *16*:163–171, 1974.
28. Hall, J. D., McCroskey, L. M., Pincomb, B. J., et al.: Isolation of an organism resembling *Clostridium barati* which produces type F botulinal toxin from an infant with botulism. J. Clin. Microbiol. *21*:654–655, 1985.
29. Hatheway, C. L., and McCroskey, L. M.: Examination of feces and serum for diagnosis of infant botulism in 336 patients. J. Clin. Microbiol. *25*:2334–2338, 1987.
30. Hauschild, A. H. W., Hilsheimer, R., Weiss, K. F., et al.: *Clostridium botulinum* in honey, syrups and dry infant cereals. J. Food Protect. *51*:892–894, 1988.
31. Hoffman, R. E., Pincomb, B. J., Skeels, M. R., et al.: Type F infant botulism. Am. J. Dis. Child. *136*:270–271, 1982.
32. Hubert, P., Roy, C., and Caille, B.: Un cas de botulisme chez un nourrisson de 11 mois. Arch. Fr. Pediatr. *44*:129–130, 1987.
33. Huhtanen, C. N., Knox, D., and Shimanuki, H.: Incidence and origin of *Clostridium botulinum* spores in honey. J. Food Protect. *44*:812–815, 1981.
34. Hurst, D. L., and Marsh, W. W.: Early severe infantile botulism. J. Pediatr. *122*:909–911, 1993.
35. Istre, G. R., Compton, R., Novotny, T., et al.: Infant botulism: Three cases in a small town. Am. J. Dis. Child. *140*:1013–1014, 1986.
36. Johnson, R. O., Clay, S. A., and Arnon, S. S.: Diagnosis and management of infant botulism. Am. J. Dis. Child. *133*:586–593, 1979.
37. Kautter, D. A., Lilly, T., Jr., Solomon, H. M., et al.: *Clostridium botulinum* spores in infant foods: A survey. J. Food Protect. *45*:1028–1029, 1982.
38. Lewis, G. E., Jr.: Approaches to the prophylaxis, immunotherapy, and chemotherapy of botulism. *In* Lewis, G. E., Jr. (ed.): Biomedical Aspects of Botulism. New York, Academic Press, 1981, pp. 261–270.
39. Lilly, T., Jr., Rhodehamel, E. J., Kautter, D. A., et al.: Incidence of *Clostridium botulinum* spores in corn syrup and other syrups. J. Food Protect. *54*:585–587, 1991.
40. Long, S. S.: Epidemiologic study of infant botulism in Pennsylvania: Report of the infant botulism study group. J. Pediatr. *75*:928–934, 1985.
41. Long, S. S., Gajewski, J. L., Brown, L. W., et al.: Clinical, laboratory, and environmental features of infant botulism in southeastern Pennsylvania. Pediatrics *75*:935–941, 1985.
42. McCroskey, L. M., and Hatheway, C. L.: Laboratory findings in four cases of adult botulism suggest colonization of the intestinal tract. J. Clin. Microbiol. *26*:1052–1054, 1988.
43. Midura, T. F.: Laboratory aspects of infant botulism in California. Rev. Infect. Dis. *1*:652–654, 1979.
44. Midura, T. F., and Arnon, S. S.: Infant botulism: Identification of *Clostridium botulinum* and its toxins in faeces. Lancet *2*:934–936, 1976.
45. Midura, T. F., Snowden, S., Wood, R. M., et al.: Isolation of *Clostridium botulinum* from honey. J. Clin. Microbiol. *9*:282–283, 1979.
46. Mills, D. C., and Arnon, S. S.: The large intestine as the site of *Clostridium botulinum* colonization in human infant botulism. J. Infect. Dis. *156*:997–998, 1987.
47. Moberg, L. J., and Sugiyama, H.: Microbial ecologic basis of infant botulism as studied with germfree mice. Infect. Immun. *25*:653–657, 1979.
48. Montecucco, C., and Schiavo, G.: Tetanus and botulism neurotoxins: A new group of zinc proteases. Trends Biochem. Sci. *18*:324–327, 1993.
49. Morris, J. G., Jr., Snyder, J. D., Wilson, R., et al.: Infant botulism in the United States: An epidemiologic study of cases occurring outside of California. Am. J. Public Health *73*:1385–1388, 1983.
50. Murrell, W. G., and Stewart, B. J.: Botulism in New South Wales, 1980–1981. Med. J. Austr. *1*:13–17, 1983.
51. Niemann, H., Blasi, J., and Jahn, R.: Clostridial neurotoxins: New tools for dissecting exocytosis. Trends Cell. Biol. *4*:179–185, 1994.
52. Paisley, J. W., Lauer, B. A., and Arnon, S. S.: A second case of infant botulism type F caused by *Clostridium baratii*. Pediatr. Infect. Dis. J. *14*:912–914, 1995.
53. Paton, J. C., Lawrence, A. J., and Manson, J. I.: Quantitation of *Clostridium botulinum* organisms and toxin in the feces of an infant with botulism. J. Clin. Microbiol. *15*:1–4, 1982.
54. Paton, J. C., Lawrence, A. J., and Steven, I. M.: Quantities of *Clostridium botulinum* organisms and toxin in feces and presence of *Clostridium botulinum* toxin in the serum of an infant with botulism. J. Clin. Microbiol. *17*:13–15, 1983.
55. Peterson, D. R., Eklund, M. W., and Chinn, N. M.: The sudden infant death syndrome and infant botulism. Rev. Infect. Dis. *1*:S630–S634, 1979.
56. Pickett, J., Berg, B., Chaplin, E., et al.: Syndrome of botulism in infancy: Clinical and electrophysiologic study. N. Engl. J. Med. *295*:770–772, 1976.
57. Ramseyer, J. C., Clay, S. A., and Fishman, L. S.: Electromyographic studies in acute infantile polyneuropathy. Neurology *26*:364, 1976.
58. Sakaguchi, G., Sakaguchi, S., Kamata, Y., et al.: Distinct characteristics of *Clostridium botulinum* type A strains and their toxin associated with infant botulism in Japan. Int. J. Food Microbiol. *11*:231–242, 1990.
59. Schreiner, M. S., Field, E., and Ruddy, R.: Infant botulism: A review of 12 years' experience at the Children's Hospital of Philadelphia. Pediatrics *87*:159–165, 1991.

59a. Schwarz, D. J., Arnon, J. M., and Arnon, S. S.: Epidemiological aspects of

infant botulism in California, 1976–1991. *In* DasGupta, B. R. (ed.): Botulinum and Tetanus Neurotoxins: Neurotransmission and Biomedical Aspects. New York, Plenum Press, 1993.
60. Shen, W-P. V., Felsing, N., Lang, D., et al.: Development of infant botulism in a 3-year-old female with neuroblastoma following autologous bone marrow transplantation: Potential use of human botulism immune globulin. Bone Marrow Transpl. *13*:345–347, 1994.
61. Smith, L. D. S.: The occurrence of *Clostridium botulinum* and *Clostridium tetani* in the soil of the United States. Health Lab. Sci. *15*:74–80, 1978.
62. Smith, L. D. S., and Sugiyama, H. (eds.): Botulism: The Organism, Its Toxins, the Disease. 2nd ed. Springfield, IL, Charles C Thomas, 1988.
63. Sonnabend, O. A. R., Sonnabend, W. F. F., Krech, U., et al.: Continuous microbiological and pathological study of 70 sudden and unexpected deaths: Toxigenic intestinal *Clostridium botulinum* infection in 9 cases of sudden infant death syndrome. Lancet *1*:237–240, 1985.
64. Spika, J. S., Shaffer, N., Hargrett-Bean, N., et al.: Risk factors for infant botulism in the United States. Am. J. Dis. Child. *143*:828–832, 1989.
65. Stark, P. L., and Lee, A.: Clostridia isolated from the feces of infants during the first year of life. J. Pediatr. *100*:362–365, 1982.
66. Stark, P. L., and Lee, A.: The microbial ecology of the large bowel of breast-fed and formula-fed infants during the first year of life. J. Med. Microbiol. *15*:189–203, 1982.
67. Suen, J. C., Hatheway, C. L., Steigerwalt, A. G., et al.: Genetic confirmation of identities of neurotoxigenic *Clostridium barati* and *Clostridium butyricum* implicated as agents of infant botulism. J. Clin. Microbiol. *26*:2191–2192, 1988.
68. Sugiyama, H., and Mills, D. C.: Intraintestinal toxin in infant mice challenged intragastrically with *Clostridium botulinum* spores. Infect. Immun. *21*:59–63, 1978.
69. Sugiyama, H., Mills, D. C., and Kuo, L.-J. C.: Number of *Clostridium botulinum* spores in honey. J. Food Protect. *41*:848–850, 1978.
70. Sullivan, N. M., Mills, D. C., Riemann, H. P., et al.: Inhibition of growth of *Clostridium botulinum* by intestinal microflora isolated from healthy infants. Microbial. Ecol. Health Dis. *1*:179–192, 1988.
71. Swenson, J. M., Thornsberry, C., McCroskey, L. M., et al.: Susceptibility of *Clostridium botulinum* to thirteen antimicrobial agents. Antimicrob. Agents Chemother. *18*:13–19, 1980.
72. Takahashi, M., Noda, H., Takeshita, S. et al.: Attempts to quantify *Clostridium botulinum* type A toxin and antitoxin in serum of two cases of infant botulism in Japan. Jpn. J. Med. Sci. Biol. *43*:233–237, 1990.
73. Thilo, E. H., and Townsend, S. F.: Infant botulism at 1 week of age: Report of two cases. Pediatrics *92*:151–153, 1993.
74. Thompson, J. A., Glasgow, L. A., Warpinski, J. R., et al.: Infant botulism: Clinical spectrum and epidemiology. Pediatrics *66*:936–942, 1980.
75. Tonkin, S.: Sudden infant death syndrome: Hypothesis of causation. Pediatrics *55*:650–661, 1975.
76. Toyoguchi, S., Tsugu, H. Nariai, A., et al.: Infant botulism with Down syndrome. Acta Pediatr. Jpn. *33*:394–397, 1991.
77. Trethon, A., Budai, J., Herendi, A., et al.: Infant botulism. Orv. Hetil. *28*:1497–1499, 1995.
78. Wilcke, B. W., Jr., Midura, T. F., and Arnon, S. S.: Quantitative evidence of intestinal colonization by *Clostridium botulinum* in four cases of infant botulism. J. Infect. Dis. *141*:419–423, 1980.

154

TETANUS

Louis L. Weinstein, Rick E. Harrison, and James D. Cherry

Tetanus is caused by the anaerobic, spore-forming bacillus *Clostridium tetani*, an organism present in soil and human and animal feces. The clinical symptoms are not due to infection but result from a specific toxin, tetanospasmin, that is produced at the site of injury and acts primarily on the spinal cord but also on brain, motor endplates, and autonomic nerves. The disease may appear as a local form or a more generalized syndrome. It is characterized by tonic spasms of skeletal muscles, little or no fever, and occasional spasms of the glottis and larynx. Bilateral trismus is the most common sign. Active immunization is highly protective. Although tetanus is well controlled today in developed countries throughout the world, it still is a major cause of death in developing countries.[22] In 1993, an estimated 515,000 deaths were caused by neonatal tetanus.

HISTORY

The first description of tetanus in recorded medical history probably was written by Hippocrates.[47] A vivid picture of the clinical course of the disease was recorded by Aretaeus the Cappadocian in the second century.[6] Very little of importance was added to this during the following 18 centuries. The transmissibility of tetanus was demonstrated by Carle and Rattone[19] in 1884. They reported that when the sciatic nerves of rabbits were injected with the contents of a human "pustule," the animals developed the characteristic disease in 2 to 3 days; inoculation of tissue obtained from their nervous systems into healthy rabbits produced a similar syndrome. The role of soil in the pathogenesis of tetanus was demonstrated by Nicolaier[71] in 1885; although he saw the organism, he was unable to recover it.

The bacterium responsible for the disease first was identified by Rosenbach,[83] who described a bacillus containing a round terminal spore in pus obtained from a human case; tetanus developed when the purulent exudate was injected into animals. *C. tetani* was isolated by Kitasato,[53] who fulfilled Koch's postulate with it in 1889. One year later, von Behring and Kitasato[100] reported the appearance of specific antitoxin in the serum of animals given injections of the tetanus toxin produced by the organism. This was followed, in 1926, by the development of toxoid, injections of which produced immunity.

MICROBIOLOGY

The vegetative form of *C. tetani* is a gram-positive, spore-forming, motile, anaerobic bacillus that measures 0.3 to 0.5 μm in width and 2.0 to 2.5 μm in length; in culture, long filament-like cells develop.[9, 16, 101, 104] *C. tetani* is a strict anaerobe that grows best at 33° to 37° C; it can be cultured in a number of different routine media used for anaerobic organisms, such as thioglycolate, casein hydrolysate, and cooked meat. Enhanced growth occurs in medium supplemented with reducing substances and maintained at a neutral or alkaline pH. With growth, gas with a fetid odor usually is produced.

The first step in the process of formation of spores is the development of a bulge at one end of the organism; this contains the spore and is responsible for the characteristic drumstick or tennis racquet appearance. As sporulation progresses, the organism is decreased in length and the spores are extruded. They stain poorly by the Gram method. Sporulation occurs in tissues as well as in vitro. Sporulation is dependent upon the composition of the medium and the temperature of the culture. Enhanced sporulation occurs in the presence of oleic acid, phosphates, 1 to 2 per cent sodium chloride, and manganese salts.[9, 16, 101] In vivo sporulation is enhanced by lactic acid and other substances toxic to cells. Sporulation is inhibited by high and low temperatures (>41° C and <25° C), glucose, fatty acids, and potassium salts. The metabolic activity of *C. tetani* is limited; carbohydrates and proteins are digested poorly; the vegetative, nonsporulated forms are killed easily by heat and a number of disinfecting agents. In contrast, the spores are resistant to boiling and phenol, cresol, 1:1000 bichloride of mercury, and other disinfectants; however, they are destroyed by heating at 120° C for 15 to 20 minutes. If not exposed to sunlight, the spores may survive in soil for months to years. They also may constitute part of the normal intestinal microflora of some horses, cows, guinea pigs, sheep, dogs, cats, rats, chickens, and humans.

Three nonpathogenic clostridia are present in soil and in human and animal feces: *Clostridium tetanomorphum, Clostridium tertium,* and *Clostridium tetanoides.* This may cause diagnostic confusion because they are similar morphologically to the organism responsible for tetanus. *C. tetani* is recovered much more commonly from cultivated than from virgin or uncultivated soil. Rural dwellers and people engaged in agricultural occupations have a higher rate of intestinal, skin, and oral carriage of the organism than have city dwellers. Dust and dirt from houses, streets, and operating rooms, as well as solutions of heroin, have been found contaminated with the organism.

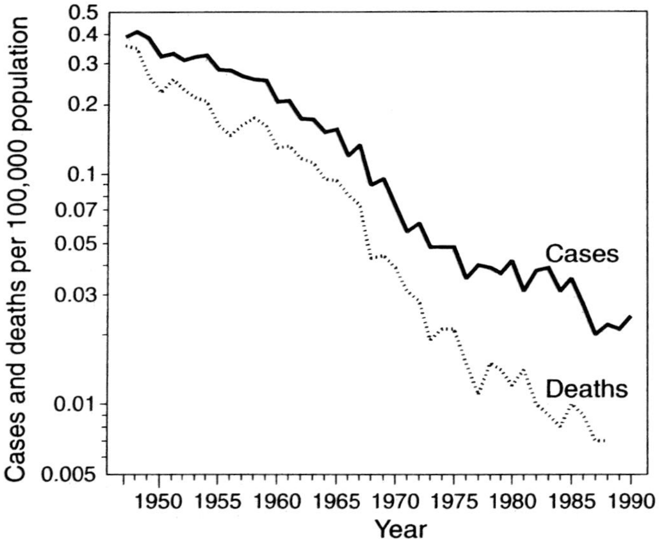

FIGURE 154–1. *The reported incidence of tetanus and tetanus-related deaths in the United States from 1947 to 1990. (From Centers for Disease Control and Prevention: Tetanus surveillance: United States, 1989–1990. M. M. W. R. 41[No. SS-8]:1–9, 1992.)*

EPIDEMIOLOGY

Source of Exposure

The predominant reservoir of *C. tetani* is the soil; *C. tetani* also is part of the normal flora of the intestinal tracts of animals, both herbivores and omnivores.[101] Intestinal spores and bacilli are shed in the feces of animals and contribute to the soil reservoir.

The worldwide morbidity and mortality due to tetanus is related inversely to adequate immunization with tetanus toxoid and directly related to suboptimal hygiene and childbirth practices and wound care.[101] Throughout the world, tetanus has a seasonal trend; more cases occur in the summer or in "wet" seasons. Rates of illness are highest in countries near the equator with fertile soil.

Acute wounds, including relatively minor wounds, are the site of most *C. tetani* infections leading to tetanus. Infection also is related to parenteral drug use and surgical procedures. In many cases, the source of exposure is unknown. The source of infection in neonatal tetanus is the umbilical cord or stump due to unsterile delivery conditions and unhygienic cultural rituals involving the umbilical stump.[48, 55]

Incidence

The reported incidence of tetanus and tetanus-related deaths in the United States from 1947 to 1990 is presented in Figure 154–1, and the reported cases and their incidence are presented by age group for 1989 and 1990 in Figure 154–2.[21] From 1947 through 1976, the incidence of tetanus fell 10-fold; since 1976, the continued fall in incidence has been less than twofold. During the same period, mortality fell from 91 per cent in 1947 to 44 per cent in 1976 to 24 per cent in 1989 and 1990.

As noted in Figure 154–2, 58 per cent of the cases in 1989 and 1990 were 60 years of age or older and only 6 per cent were children or adolescents. Of the 110 cases of tetanus in 1989 and 1990, the immunization status was known in 57 (52 per cent). Of this group, 65 per cent were unimmunized and 79 per cent had two or fewer doses of vaccine. Twelve patients had received three or more doses of vaccine and of these, the last dose was received more than 10 years before the illness in eight (67 per cent). Fifty-two per cent of the cases in 1989 and 1990 occurred in females.

PATHOGENESIS

Tetanus is, by strictest definition, not a true infection. Spores introduced at a site of injury remain harmless until, stimulated by a variety of factors, they are converted to vegetative forms that multiply but do not produce injury to tissue or provoke an inflammatory response. The clinical syndrome is caused entirely by toxin elaborated in the area where the vegetative cells are growing. *C. tetani* produces two exotoxins: tetanolysin and tetanospasmin. Tetanolysin

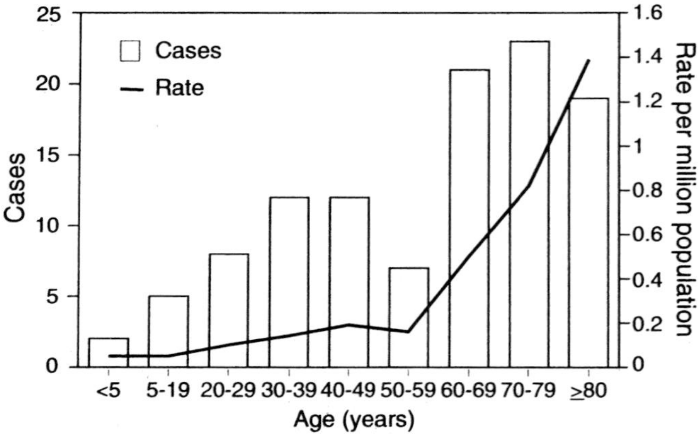

FIGURE 154–2. *The reported tetanus cases and incidence rates by age group in the United States in 1989 and 1990. (From Centers for Disease Control: Tetanus surveillance: United States, 1989–1990. M. M. W. R. 41[No. SS-8]:1–9, 1992.)*

produces hemolysis but plays no role in the disease. The activity of tetanospasmin is responsible for all the clinical features of the disease. Purified tetanospasmin is a protein, with a molecular weight of about 67,000 daltons.[75] One milligram contains 6,400,000 lethal doses for mice; 0.00001 mg may kill a 20-gram mouse in 2 hours. With the exception of the toxin produced by *Clostridium botulinum*, tetanospasmin currently is the most potent known poison. Humans are most susceptible to this agent, requiring 1/2500 and 1/350,000 of the dose fatal for cats and chickens, respectively.

C. tetani is introduced into an area of injury as the spore, the form usually present in soil and intestinal contents. Disease does not develop until the spores are converted to the toxin-elaborating bacillus. This does not follow simple inoculation of spores. When these are injected into animals with very sharp needles so that tissue is not injured but merely separated, tetanus does not develop. However, the addition of a small quantity of calcium chloride to a suspension of spores before injection leads to the development of the typical disease. This is not due to a specific effect of the cation on conversion of the spore to the vegetative form of the organism but is related to the necrosis of tissue produced by it, which leads to a reduction in oxidation reduction potential and oxygen tension, factors involved in vegetation of the spore; the same effects are produced by the presence of a foreign body, trauma, or a localized suppurative process.

The pathway by which toxin elaborated at the site at which *C. tetani* is multiplying reaches the central nervous system has been a matter of controversy. It first was thought that tetanospasmin was absorbed chiefly by motor nerve endings and then traveled along axis cylinders to the anterior horn cells.[82] Symptoms of the disease were thought to appear only after the toxin had reached the nervous system, with the initial tetanic contractions occurring first in the injured extremity, then in the opposite limb, and finally as the toxin diffused through the spinal cord in all the muscles. It was suggested that a small amount of toxin was absorbed into the lymph and carried to the blood stream, from which it was taken up by motor nerve endings in various parts of the body.[65]

Abel and associates[1] postulated that toxin reached the nervous system via the arterial circulation and suggested the following series of events. Some of the toxin diffuses from the local site of injury into adjacent skeletal muscle and acts on the neuromuscular organs to produce a state of maintained contraction: *local tetanus*. Some also enters the lymphatics and blood stream, from which it is taken up by specifically reactive cells in the spinal cord, medulla, and the motor end-organs of muscle.

Friedemann and his colleagues[40] noted that tetanus toxin did not penetrate the blood-brain barrier and therefore questioned hematogenous transmission. This led attention to be focused on transport of tetanospasmin in nerves. Wright and his coworkers[107] observed that direct injection of toxin into the vagal, facial, or hypoglossal nerves of rabbits led, within 24 hours, to the development of a syndrome characteristic of involvement of the brain stem, as indicated by the appearance of strabismus, immobility of the hairs in the nasal cavity, salivation, bradycardia, and torticollis.[107] Inoculation of the vagus resulted in the successive development of these manifestations; those dependent on innervation from motor nuclei in close proximity to the nerve tended to appear early. This hypothesis is supported by observations indicating that a variety of substances, including India ink and radioactive compounds, migrate along peripheral nerves to the central nervous system after intraneural injection.[37] This, together with the demonstration by numerous investigators that toxin is present in the peripheral nerves closest to the site of inoculation, supports the concept of transport of tetanospasmin in the tissues of the nervous system.

Knowledge of the specific mechanisms involved in the absorption of tetanus toxin and of its mechanisms of action on body cells is incomplete. Most of the presently available evidence indicates that some element of the peripheral nerve is involved. Whether transport occurs in the axis cylinder, the perineural space, or lymphatics still is unsettled. Tetanus toxin is carried to the neurons of the sciatic nerve via the neurofibrillae in axis cylinders at a rate of about 3.35 mm per hour.[82]

PATHOPHYSIOLOGY

Tetanospasmin exerts its effects in four areas of the nervous system: (1) the motor end-plates in skeletal muscle, (2) the spinal cord, (3) the brain, and (4) (in some cases) the sympathetic nervous system.[12, 14, 15, 18, 29, 50, 51, 89, 98, 109]

Motor End-Plates in Skeletal Muscle

Tetanus toxin has been noted to interfere with neuromuscular transmission. Release of acetylcholine from the nerve terminals in muscle is inhibited. The presence of tetanospasmin in the transverse and terminal sacs of the longitudinal elements of the sarcotubular system of the skeletal muscles suggests that it acts by interfering with contraction coupling or with the mechanisms involved in contraction and relaxation. These phenomena probably are involved in the pathogenesis of local tetanus.

Spinal Cord

The effects of the toxin on the spinal cord practically are identical to those produced by strychnine. It does not act on reflex arcs that include only sensory and motor neurons (two-neuron or monosynaptic reflexes). However, the toxin profoundly alters the activity of the more complex polysynaptic reflexes involving interneurons. This leads to the inhibition of antagonists. Hyperpolarization of the membranes of neurons, a mechanism normally operating when direct inhibitory pathways are stimulated, is suppressed. Depolarization associated with excitation is not affected. Whether tetanospasmin blocks inhibitory synapses by preventing release of the inhibitory transmitter substance or by suppressing the action of this substance on the membrane of motor neurons is unknown presently. Selective blocking of inhibitory synapses in the central nervous system appears adequate to account for the primary phenomena of tetanus. Unchecked and uncoordinated excitatory impulses multiply and traverse reflex pathways to produce the characteristic tetanic spasms of muscles.

Brain

It has been suggested that the action of tetanospasmin on brain may be responsible for the typical seizures of tetanus.[12] This is supported, in part, by the observation that the cerebral gangliosides fix the toxin. The antidromic inhibition of evoked cortical activity is decreased. The effects of tetanospasmin on brain are the same as those on the spinal cord, as well as those that follow exposure to strychnine.

Sympathetic Nervous System

Manifestations indicating dysfunction of the sympathetic nervous system have been observed in some patients with tetanus. Among these are profuse sweating, peripheral vasoconstriction, labile hypertension, cardiac arrhythmias, tachycardia, increased output of carbon dioxide, elevated urinary concentrations of catecholamines, and hypotension late in the course of the disease.

CLINICAL MANIFESTATIONS

Although it may be as short as 1 day or as long as several months, the incubation period of tetanus usually is 3 to 21 days. There may be a direct relation between the distance of the site of invasion by *C. tetani* from the central nervous system and the length of the interval between injury and onset of disease; the greater the distance between the local area and the central nervous system, the longer, in general, the incubation period. Sustained or separated repeated tonic spasms of isolated or multiple muscles are the characteristic clinical feature of the disease. Tetanus may appear in two forms: generalized and local.

Local Tetanus

This presentation probably is more common than recognized. Although it is thought to be infrequent, this probably is so because it may be uncommon as an isolated syndrome or because by the time diffuse involvement has occurred, the spasms in the muscles in the area of the site of entry of the organisms cannot be separated from the generalized ones. Local manifestations frequently precede the generalized disorder. The characteristic abnormality in local tetanus is unyielding, persistent, painful rigidity of the group of muscles that lies in close proximity to the site at which *C. tetani* was introduced. It often is present when a dose of antitoxin adequate to inactivate circulating toxin but insufficient to neutralize that which has accumulated at the site of injury has been given. Symptoms may persist for several weeks or months and finally disappear without leaving any residua.[66] Local tetanus may be the only manifestation, usually is mild, and has a fatality rate of about 1 per cent.

Cephalic Tetanus

This is a variant of local tetanus. It usually follows the introduction of *C. tetani* in the course of injuries to the scalp, eye, face, ear, or neck; chronic otitis media; and, rarely, tonsillectomy.[7] Insect bites of the face or head, especially if secondarily infected by pyogenic organisms, also may serve as portals of entry for the organism. The incubation period of this syndrome is short, frequently no more than 1 to 2 days. The outstanding clinical features are palsies of cranial nerves III, IV, VII, IX, X, and XII; these may be involved singly or in any combination. Dysfunction may persist for days or many months. In general, the prognosis for survival is poor. However, if death does not intervene, complete recovery, without residual neurologic dysfunction, is the rule. In some, but not all, instances, generalized tetanus may develop during the course of the cephalic form of the disease.

Generalized Tetanus

This is the most common presentation of the disease.[81] Despite the general impression that inoculation of the organism is associated most frequently with deep penetrating injury, the portal of entry in about 80 per cent of cases is an insignificant wound.[76] Burns, injuries induced by blank cartridges, deep punctures, furunculosis, dental extraction, embedded splinters, decubitus ulcers, hypodermic injections, and compound fractures complicated by chronic active osteomyelitis are typical situations in which tetanus may develop because the environment in the tissues is optimal (reduction in oxidation reduction potential and tension of oxygen) for conversion of spores to the toxin-producing vegetative organisms. Iatrogenic disease has followed the use of smallpox vaccine and surgical sutures contaminated by the spores of *C. tetani*. It also has occurred as a postoperative complication in patients exposed to the organisms present in the dust of operating rooms.[80, 88] Very *minor* injuries, such as penetration by "clean" sewing needles and bites by chiggers, bees, and scorpions, have been recorded as portals of entry. Tetanus also has followed induced abortions, usually carried out under poor asepsis.

The presenting manifestation in more than 50 per cent of cases of generalized tetanus is trismus; it may be unilateral early in the disease but becomes bilateral within a short time. In some cases, it may be absent during the entire course of the illness or appear only after other abnormalities have become apparent. In some instances, the only symptoms and signs may be irritability, restlessness, stiffness of the neck, difficulty in swallowing, and rigidity of the abdominal or thoracic muscles; these may be present singly or in various combinations. The diagnostic importance of trismus cannot be overemphasized, despite the fact that it may be associated with a number of disorders unrelated to tetanus. Among these are postmeasles encephalitis; trichinosis; suppurative and other types of parotitis; tender cervical lymphadenopathy; infected, impacted upper molar teeth; and exposure to phenothiazine drugs.

As activity of tetanospasmin persists, groups of muscles other than the masseters may become involved, featured by tonic spasms of the jaw, neck, back, and abdomen. Unrelenting trismus leads to the development of a characteristic facial expression, the sardonic smile (risus sardonicus). The abdominal and spinal muscles may become rigid. Intense and sustained contraction of the muscles of the chest and back results in persistent opisthotonos; in young children, this may be so severe that the youngster lies on one side with the soles of the feet resting on the top of the head.

Generalized seizures, tetanospasms, are unique in their appearance and peculiar to this disease. Characteristically, there is a sudden burst of tonic contraction of all groups of muscles that leads to the development of opisthotonus, flexion and abduction of the arms, clenching of the fists on the chest, and extension of the legs. Pain in the spastic muscles usually is severe. In some patients, glottal and laryngeal spasm, with the chest in the position of full inspiration, may develop. During such an episode, the face becomes florid, the neck veins are distended markedly, and cyanosis develops. All of the features of this syndrome are consistent with an intense and sustained Valsalva maneuver; unless the tonic contraction of the glottis and larynx subsides or tracheostomy is carried out, death results. Dysphagia and hydrophobia may develop as isolated phenomena in the absence of a generalized tetanospasm. Dysuria or urinary retention also may occur.

Electroencephalographic studies of patients have indicated involvement of the brain. Of 106 patients studied by Luisto,[59] 76 per cent were found to have an abnormal electroencephalogram. When patients of the same age and sex who had not had tetanus were compared with 40 individuals who had had the disease 7 years earlier, it was noted that the latter had more muscle fatigue and cramps; difficulty in speech, balance, and memory; and more peripheral paresis, muscular atrophy, decreased or absent tendon reflexes, and impaired mental capacity.[58]

The generalized seizures of tetanus often are triggered by very slight external stimuli, such as a light breeze, talking, a bump on the bed, or slight touching of the patient. The intense work generated by sustained or frequently repeated tetanospasms often leads to increases of body temperature of 2° to 5° F or more.

The intense suffering of patients with the generalized tonic seizures of tetanus and the total frustration of the physician, who in ancient times had to stand by helpless, unable to alter the course of the disease, were described best by Aretaeus[6] in the second century B.C.; no better description has ever appeared:

> An inhuman calamity! An unseemly sight! A spectacle painful even to the beholder, an incurable malady! Owing to the distortion, not to be recognized by the dearest friends; and hence the prayers of the spectators, which formerly would have been reckoned not pious, now becomes good, that the patient may depart from life, or being a deliverance from the pains and unseemly evils attendant on it. But neither can the physician, though present and looking on, furnish any assistance, as regards life, relief from pain or from deformity. For if he should wish to straighten the limbs, he can do so only by cutting and breaking those of a living man. With them, then, who are overpowered by this disease, he can merely sympathize. This is the great misfortune of the physician.

Heroin Addicts

When persons addicted to heroin develop generalized tetanus, a number of clinical features differ from those present in people who do not use drugs. Among these are much higher levels of fever; absence of trismus at onset and throughout the course of the disease or its appearance sometime after other manifestations have been present; marked stiffness of the neck and back, which in the absence of trismus may be confused with meningitis (the normal cerebrospinal fluid of tetanus excludes this possibility); and early onset of coma. Prophylaxis is less effective in addicted than in nonaddicted persons. The fatality rate approaches 100 per cent.

Neonatal Tetanus

Although neonatal tetanus is of very minor importance in the developed areas of the world, it has been a major cause of death in infants in the developing countries.[22, 23, 55, 61, 93, 101] In 1993, it was estimated that there were 515,000 deaths due to neonatal tetanus worldwide.[22] These deaths predominantly occurred in Southeast Asia (34.2 per cent), Africa (28.2 per cent), the Western Pacific, including China (21.4 per cent), and the eastern Mediterranean region (15.7 per cent). The global mortality rate in 1993 was estimated to be 4.1 per 1000 live births. The very high frequency of neonatal tetanus in these areas probably is related to the conditions surrounding the birth of infants. Most babies are born in very unhygienic environments; delivery rarely takes place in a good hospital. In addition, unclean instruments are used to sever the umbilical cord, rags often contaminated with soil or feces are used as dressings, and mud and manure are applied directly to the umbilical stump. In a recent study in Senegal that examined risk factors of neonatal tetanus, it was found that the major source of *C. tetani* was the hands of the birth attendant and the mode of contamination of the infant related to the method that the birth attendant and the mother used to dress the umbilical cord stump.[55]

Neonatal tetanus usually begins 3 to 14 days after birth with poor sucking and excessive crying.[102] Manifestations include trismus, difficulty swallowing, other tetanic spasms, and frequently marked opisthotonos.

A study of the causes of death in patients with neonatal tetanus by Salimpour[85] indicated pulmonary disease to be most common. Bronchopneumonia and/or hemorrhage in the lungs was the most frequent finding at autopsy. Among the nonpulmonary disorders responsible for a fatal outcome were hepatitis, omphalitis, cerebral hemorrhage, thrombosis, and rupture of the renal vein. As has been noted not only in infants but also in older children and adults with tetanus, it is very uncommon to find any gross or histologic abnormalities. The complications described by Salimpour,[85] especially those involving the lungs, probably are related to aspiration associated with the laryngoglottal spasm characteristic of the disease. Indicators of poor prognosis in neonates include younger than 10 days of age when admitted to the hospital, symptoms of less than 5 days' duration, presence of risus sardonicus, and fever.[45]

DIAGNOSIS

Differential Diagnosis

The differential diagnosis is affected by the major clinical manifestations of the illness.[101] Cephalic tetanus may be confused with Bell palsy, trigeminal neuritis, and encephalitis, whereas generalized tetanus can be confused with rabies, strychnine poisoning, and phenothiazine reactions. Trismus can result from dental problems, tonsillitis, peritonsillar abscess, temporomandibular joint dysfunction, and parotitis. Tetany due to hypocalcemia or hyperventilation also should be considered.

Specific Diagnosis

The diagnosis of tetanus is established on the basis of the history of an injury, particularly one in which either soil or fecal material has been introduced. In a small number of cases, especially those in which there has been a relatively long incubation period, the site of entry of the organism may be healed and undetectable. Laboratory studies are of little help. Peripheral leukocytosis may or may not be present. The characteristic gram-positive rods, some of which may contain subterminal spores, may be seen occasionally in stained material obtained from the wound that has served as the portal of entry. Anaerobic cultures of exudate or necrotic tissue may grow typical sporulated rods and vegetative forms; the yield of positive findings tends to be low.[25]

Low or undetectable levels of serum antitoxin at the time of illness onset is supportive of the diagnosis, but occasionally serum antitoxin is present.[101] Rises in antitoxin titers after infections are uncommon, so paired sera study for the retrospective diagnosis usually is not helpful; in addition, this form of serologic diagnosis is not possible when therapy included active immunization. In selected cases, electrophysiologic studies of the masseter muscle may be helpful.[8] There is a characteristic absence or shortening of the silent period due to the failure of Renshaw cell inhibition; exaggerated f-responses indicating hyperexcitability also may be noted.

TREATMENT

Management of generalized tetanus is directed to the following goals:

1. Neutralization of toxin still present in the blood before it comes in contact with the nervous system. This is accomplished by the administration of antitoxin as soon as the possibility of the disease is suspected or confirmed.[12] There is, however, no acceptable evidence that toxin, once fixed to tissues, can be inactivated by antitoxin. In fact, the effectiveness of even large doses of antitoxin in reducing the fatality rate has been questioned.

2. Surgical removal of the site of entry of the organism, when possible. This eliminates the "factory" in which tetanospasmin is being produced. Omphalectomy has been performed with good results in children with neonatal tetanus.[30] Hysterectomy has been recommended when the disease has complicated induced and often septic abortions; however, patients whose infected uterus is not removed occasionally may survive. When the surgical procedure may be mutilating, as is the case with lesions on the face, it should not be carried out.

3. Constant and meticulous nursing care.

4. Close monitoring of fluid, electrolyte, and caloric balance because it frequently is abnormal, especially in patients with high temperature and repeated seizures, as well as in those unable to take food or liquids because of severe trismus, dysphagia, or hydrophobia.

The slightest external stimulus may precipitate potentially lethal seizures in persons with diffuse disease. For this reason, it is imperative that all therapeutic and other manipulations be well coordinated and carefully scheduled, so that the risk of tetanospasms is reduced to a minimum. All maneuvers are performed best after patients have received optimal sedation and relaxation. A quiet, darkened room in which the light is subdued and the doors padded, removed as far as possible from the mainstream of hospital traffic, is ideal, but at the same time the patient requires constant monitoring and observation in an intensive care environment.

The antitoxin of choice for the treatment of tetanus is human tetanus immunoglobulin (TIG); the dose is 3000 to 6000 units, intramuscularly. A second dose does not appear to be necessary. When tetanus immunoglobulin is not available, equine antitoxin (EA) may be used; it should be avoided, however, if at all possible. The dose is 100,000 units; half is injected intramuscularly, after appropriate tests to rule out sensitivity to horse serum have been carried out. If this is well tolerated, the rest is given intravenously *slowly*. Patients sensitized to horse serum must be desensitized. An intramuscular injection of 80,000 units of equine antitoxin produces maximal concentrations of antibody in the blood in 48 to 72 hours; very good levels may be maintained for 7 days.[96, 97] Intravenous administration of the same dose yields concentrations of 40 or more units of antitoxin per milliliter of serum after 6 hours; this may persist for about 48 hours. There essentially is no difference in the circulating quantities of antitoxin 7 days after it is given by either route. Local instillation of antitoxin around the known or suspected wound may be of value if excision is not possible; it also has been recommended prior to surgical removal of the injured area.

Penicillin kills the vegetative forms of *C. tetani*. Parenteral administration of penicillin G, 100,000 units/kg/day intravenously every 6 hours for 10 days, until recently has been recommended in all cases of tetanus. It has been suggested that penicillin may act as an agonist to tetanospasmin by inhibiting the release of gamma-aminobutyric acid.[101] Because of this and the results of a controlled study in Indonesia, metronidazole has become the antimicrobial treatment of choice in many centers.[3] Metronidazole dosage is 30 mg/kg/day intravenously given every 6 hours after an initial dose of 15 mg/kg. The usual duration of therapy is 7 to 10 days.

The spasticity and seizures of tetanus are due to exaggerated reflex responses to afferent stimuli as a result of suppression of balancing central inhibition. Several classes of drugs that act at different sites along the reflex pathway are useful for the control of these manifestations. Among these are hypnotics and sedatives, which reduce sensory input and generalized excitability; general anesthetics, which produce broad depression of the central nervous system; centrally acting muscle relaxants or spinal depressants, which lower reflex activity and decrease motor output from the spinal cord; and neuromuscular blocking agents, which inhibit transmission of excess motor nerve activity to effector muscles.

The ideal drug for the treatment of tetanus must control seizures and decrease spasticity, without impairing respiration, voluntary movement, or consciousness. The activity of an agent in inhibiting the convulsions induced by strychnine usually has been a reliable guide for the prediction of effectiveness in the management of tetanus. However, this may not be reliable always. For example, although the phenothiazines act as anticonvulsants in both naturally occurring and experimentally produced tetanus, they fail to control the seizure induced by strychnine. Creech and associates[28] point out, "It may be concluded that any type of sedative or hypnotic agent, when properly administered so as to avoid respiratory depression, has the same effect or lack of effect upon the outcome of tetanus."

Historically, many different drugs have been utilized for the patient with tetanus. Secobarbital sodium (Seconal) and pentobarbital (Nembutal) have been favored for their relatively short half-life.[50, 67] The barbiturates, however, may have deleterious effects on both the respiratory and cardiovascular systems. The patient heavily sedated with barbiturates often will have a rise in carbon dioxide pressure and a fall in oxygen pressure as well as hypotension and a fall in cardiac output. Additionally, the barbiturates have a lower therapeutic index than do the benzodiazepines.[77] Chlorpromazine (Thorazine) also has been utilized to control the muscle spasms of tetanus but also has some drawbacks.[26] Chlorpromazine actually may lower the seizure threshold and should be utilized, if at all, only with concomitant anticonvulsant therapy. The acute dystonic reactions occasionally seen with chlorpromazine can confuse markedly the picture in a patient having tetanic spasms and rigidity. Akathisia, the need of the patient to be in constant movement, is another extrapyramidal effect occasionally seen with the phenothiazines and would be undesirable in the patient susceptible to tetanic spasms. Meprobamate historically was used to control the tonic spasms of tetanus.[74] It is relatively ineffective when given orally or intramuscularly (dissolved in propylene glycol).[67]

The barbiturates, phenothiazines, and meprobamate no longer are first-line antispasmodic drugs; the benzodiazepines are the preferred drugs for the spasms and rigidity associated with tetanus.[27] They also have the advantage of being potent anticonvulsants as well as sedative hypnotic agents. Additionally, they are gamma-aminobutyric acid agonists, perhaps partially overcoming the effect of tetanospasmin interfering with the normally inhibitory effect of gamma-aminobutyric acid.[95] Diazepam (Valium) and lorazepam (Ativan) have been the most frequently utilized benzodiazepines for tetanus. Lorazepam has a somewhat longer half-life and may be preferred for this reason. Very large total daily doses of diazepam (500 mg) or lorazepam (200 mg) may be required.[99] Both drugs are in propylene glycol solution for intravenous dosage, and the large doses required may result in significant propylene glycol toxicity, including a metabolic acidosis. For this reason, the enteral preparation that is free of propylene glycol should be given enterally if at all possible.[10]

Midazolam (Versed) is a short-acting benzodiazepine soluble in water and thus does not include propylene glycol in the parenteral formulation. Because of its short half-life, it should be administered as a continuous infusion and may require an initial infusion dose of 0.1 to 0.3 mg/kg/hour. The benzodiazepines all induce tachyphylaxis and will require escalation of dosage with time. Dosage should be titrated to prevent tetanic spasms and provide adequate sedation instead of relying on a specified dose. To avoid withdrawal symptoms after long-term use, the benzodiazepines should be tapered off over several weeks.

When the benzodiazepines are unable to control the spasms and rigidity associated with tetanus, neuromuscular blockage is indicated. Although succinylcholine has been utilized in the past,[39] newer agents have supplanted its use. Additionally, there are theoretical reasons to avoid the use of succinylcholine. With functional denervation of the motor end-plate in those neuromuscular junctions directly affected by tetanospasmin, succinylcholine may result in exaggerated potassium release and hyperkalemia. This has been associated with cardiac dysrhythmias and death in other denervating conditions. For this reason, nondepolarizing agents should be utilized. Potential agents would include pancuronium, vecuronium, atracurium, and rocuronium.

Pancuronium can cause tachycardia via a blockade of cardiac muscarinic receptors and would be relatively contraindicated in patients with autonomic instability. Atracurium has a metabolite, laudanosine, which has been shown to have cerebral excitatory effects in animals, including seizures. Atracurium also may cause histamine release with resultant pruritus and a decrease in blood pressure. Vecuromium and rocuronium cause only rare histamine release and have no effect on either autonomic ganglia or cardiac muscarinic receptors, making them the preferred neuromuscular blocking agents in tetanus.[49]

The neuromuscular blocking drugs should be utilized only by physicians experienced in their use, typically anesthesiologists or intensivists, in a critical care environment.[54] Although the neuromuscular blockers formerly were used at low doses to preserve diaphragmatic function and spontaneous respirations, current thought is that they should be utilized in conjunction with endotracheal intubation and ventilatory support. It is critical to remember that the neuromuscular blocking drugs have no effect on cortical function and have no sedative effect. The benzodiazepines are good sedatives and have significant amnestic effect. They are not, however, analgesics, and if pain is present (such as from previous muscle spasms), morphine sulfate is an effective analgesic. It also may be helpful in treating sympathetic hyperactivity. If sympathetic overactivity remains problematic, a combined alpha- and beta-receptor blocker, such as labetolol, should be utilized. A beta blocker such as propranolol alone should be avoided because the unopposed alpha-mediated vasoconstriction could lead to significant hypertension. Clonidine and epidural anesthesia are alternative therapies for increased sympathetic discharge.

The management approach to the patient with tetanus spasms or rigidity should be one of escalation of therapy based on need. Benzodiazepines should be utilized initially, often requiring high doses. If this results in compromise of the airway or inadequate ventilation, endotracheal intubation should be performed with a nondepolarizing neuromuscular blocking agent. Intubation also should be performed if spasms result in airway obstruction. It has been advocated that heroin addicts with tetanus have an airway established because of the fulminant course of the disease.[74]

Sixty-six per cent of 103 children 1 to 12 years of age with severe tetanus studied by Wesley and Pathes[103] required management with total muscle paralysis and intermittent positive pressure ventilation. The death rate in this group was 14.5 per cent.

Although it has been reported[70] that the intrathecal administration of antitetanus serum did not improve the rate of survival in neonatal tetanus, results of a study by Mongi and colleagues[68] led them to recommend this form of therapy. They found that intrathecal serotherapy may be of great value in the management of tetanus. Their experience indicated that the death rate from this disease in patients given intrathecal therapy was 45 per cent, whereas in those who did not receive this agent it was 82 per cent. However, the results of a recent meta-analysis led Abrutyn and Berlin[2] to conclude that intrathecal therapy with either equine antitoxin or tetanus immunoglobulin is not of proven benefit and therefore only should be given during well-designed, controlled therapeutic trials.

Very careful attention must be paid to care of the skin, bladder, mouth, and bowel of patients with tetanus. Adequate fluid and electrolyte balance must be maintained. Feeding by gavage in those unable to eat because of severe trismus, dysphagia, or hydrophobia has been suggested to ensure an optimal caloric intake. Gastric emptying may be impaired, and a transpyloric feeding tube will facilitate adequate nutritional support with a continuous infusion of age-appropriate enteral formula. The transpyloric placement of the feeding tube also may decrease the risk of aspiration.

The use of dantrolene with conservative treatment has been reported to reduce significantly the fatality rate associated with tetanus.[5] It has been suggested that both sympathetic and parasympathetic nervous systems need to be blocked in order to stabilize hemodynamics. This may be produced by spinal anesthesia.[90] Patients with tetanus treated with metronidazole have been found to have a lower fatality rate, a shorter stay in the hospital, and an improved response to treatment.[3] The intravenous administration of morphine to patients with tetanus has been noted to reduce arterial blood pressure and systemic vascular resistance.[81]

Patients who have survived an episode of tetanus must be immunized actively after recovery because antitoxin usually is not detectable in the serum for as long as 3 months after recovery.[96] Recurrent attacks of the disease are rare.[17]

Studies in mice have shown that adrenocortical steroids are without effect in altering the course of tetanus. The administration of cortisone after a significant delay between the injection of toxin and antitoxin or after clinical manifestations had appeared was found not only to be without benefit but also to decrease the effectiveness of the antitoxin.[24] Other studies also have indicated a lack of therapeutic effect[44, 97] but have not demonstrated deleterious effects. Critically evaluated clinical experiences have confirmed this finding.[57]

PROGNOSIS

The average fatality rate associated with tetanus ranges from 25 to 70 per cent. Mortality can be reduced to 10 to 20 per cent with modern intensive care.[101] The risk of death in patients with tetanus neonatorum is particularly high; it was reported to be 99.5 per cent in a group of 5794 cases reported in 1930.[46] With modern treatment and high-intensity supportive care, mortality in neonatal tetanus can be reduced to about 25 per cent.[101] Heroin addicts are highly susceptible to the development of very severe disease and are likely to die.[52]

A variety of other factors play important roles in determining the outcome of tetanus. Patients in the second and third decade of life have a higher rate of recovery than do those who are elderly. There is an inverse relationship between the length of the incubation period and the risk, first pointed out by Hippocrates. It has been noted that the risk of death is about 58 per cent when the interval between injury and onset of tetanus is 2 to 10 days. When the interval is 11 to 22 days or longer, fatality rates have been 35 to 17 per cent, respectively. There also appears to be a relation between the period elapsing from the time of appearance of the first signs of tetanus and the development of the first seizure or maximal intensity of the disease; the shorter this interval, the poorer the prognosis.[25]

The clinical form of tetanus also influences the outcome. Cephalic tetanus and tetanus neonatorum are associated with the highest incidence of death. In contrast, local tetanus, unless complicated by the development of the generalized syndrome, has an excellent prognosis. The early prophylactic administration of antitoxin markedly increases the frequency of survival, even when tetanus develops.

CAUSE OF DEATH

Because the clinical course of tetanus may be prolonged and the therapy employed complex and potentially dangerous, the cause of death often is not clear. Animals may die after injection of toxin without developing recognizable signs of the disease.[38] Studies in parabiotic rats have suggested that tetanospasmin exerts a lethal effect on the respiratory center.[87] Involvement of the medulla has been observed in experimental animals and humans in whom episodes of respiratory failure, often in the absence of seizures, have been described.[54, 107] The action of the toxin on brain has been postulated as the cause of hyperpyrexia, tachycardia, hypotension, bulbar palsy, and cardiac arrest.[69] Myocardial damage also may occur; both histologic and electrocardiographic abnormalities have been described.[73]

Death may occur during a convulsion; the specific mechanisms involved are not always clear. Laryngospasm and disturbances of balance of electrolytes may play important roles. Pneumonia complicating aspiration, induced by inability to swallow and oversedation, is common. It directly may be responsible for death or may contribute to a fatal outcome by increasing the degree of anoxia of the respiratory center.

PREVENTION

As noted in Figure 154–1, tetanus in the United States has decreased dramatically, and this decline can be attributed to routine universal use of tetanus toxoid and improved wound management, including use of tetanus prophylaxis in emergency rooms.

Active Immunization

For complete information regarding tetanus immunization, the reader is referred to the most recent recommendations of the Advisory Committee on Immunization Practices of the U.S. Public Health Service,[20] the recommendations of the Committee on Infectious Diseases of the American Academy of Pediatrics,[4] and product information from vaccine manufacturers.

In the United States, primary immunization against tetanus is performed in conjunction with immunization against diphtheria and pertussis with diphtheria and tetanus toxoids and pertussis vaccine adsorbed (DTP). The schedule involves an initial series of three doses of vaccine at 2, 4, and 6 months of age, a reinforcing dose at 12 to 18 months of age, and a booster dose at 4 to 6 years of age. After the initial series, additional booster doses of adult-type diphtheria and tetanus toxoids adsorbed (Td) are recommended at 10-year intervals. The minimal serum level of antitoxin needed for protection is 0.01 IU/mL.[33, 60, 63, 91] After the initial three-dose series, the reinforcing dose, and the booster dose in the schedule just described, levels of antitoxin 100- to 1000-fold higher than 0.01 IU/mL are attained and levels higher than 0.01 IU/mL persist in nearly all vaccinees until the scheduled subsequent dose.

Side effects of DTP immunization mainly are due to the pertussis component and are discussed in Chapter 134. A fluid tetanus toxoid also is available for booster doses, but it has limited use.

Tetanus Prophylaxis in Wound Management[20]

Antimicrobial prophylaxis against tetanus is neither practical nor useful in managing wounds. Wound cleaning, débridement when indicated, and proper immunization are important. The need for tetanus toxoid (active immunization), with or without tetanus immunoglobulin (passive immunization), depends on both the condition of the wound and the patient's vaccination history (Table 154–1). Rarely has tetanus occurred among persons with documentation of having received a primary series of toxoid injections.

A thorough attempt must be made to determine whether a patient has completed primary vaccination. Patients with unknown or uncertain previous vaccination histories should be considered to have had no previous tetanus toxoid doses. Persons who had military service since 1941 can be considered to have received at least one dose. Although most people in the military since 1941 may have completed a primary series of tetanus toxoid, this cannot be assumed for each individual. Patients who have not completed a primary series

TABLE 154–1. Summary Guide to Tetanus Prophylaxis in Routine Wound Management, 1991

History of Adsorbed Tetanus Toxoid (doses)	Clean, Minor Wounds		All Other Wounds*	
	Td†	*TIG*	*Td*†	*TIG*
Unknown or <three	Yes	No	Yes	Yes
≥Three‡	No§	No	No‖	No

*Such as, but not limited to, wounds contaminated with dirt, feces, soil, and saliva; puncture wounds; avulsions; and wounds resulting from missiles, crushing, burns, and frostbite.

†For children younger than 7 years of age, diphtheria-tetanus-pertussis vaccine (diphtheria-tetanus if pertussis vaccine is contraindicated) is preferred to tetanus toxoid alone. For persons 7 years of age or older, Td is preferred to tetanus toxoid alone.

‡If only three doses of fluid toxoid have been received, a fourth dose of toxoid, preferably an adsorbed toxoid, should be given.

§Yes, if >10 years since last dose.

‖Yes, if >5 years since last dose (more frequent boosters are not needed and can accentuate side effects).

Td, adult-type diphtheria and tetanus toxoids; TIG, tetanus immunoglobulin.

From Centers for Disease Control: Diphtheria, tetanus and pertussis: Recommendations for vaccine use and other preventive measures; recommendations of the Immunization Practices Advisory Committee (ACIP). M. M. W. R. *40*(No. RR-10):2–28, 1991.

may require tetanus toxoid and passive immunization at the time of wound cleaning and débridement (see Table 154–1).

Available evidence indicates that complete primary vaccination with tetanus toxoid provides long-lasting protection 10 or more years for most recipients. Consequently, after complete primary tetanus vaccination, boosters—even for wound management—need be given only every 10 years when wounds are minor and uncontaminated. For other wounds, a booster is appropriate if the patient has not received tetanus toxoid within the preceding 5 years. Persons who have received at least two doses of tetanus toxoid rapidly develop antitoxin antibodies.

Td is the preferred preparation for active tetanus immunization in wound management of patients 7 years of age or older. Because a large proportion of adults are susceptible, this plan enhances diphtheria protection. Thus, by taking advantage of acute health care visits, such as for wound management, some patients can be protected who otherwise would remain susceptible. For routine wound management among children younger than 7 years of age who are not vaccinated adequately, DTP should be used instead of single-antigen tetanus toxoid. Td may be used if pertussis vaccine is contraindicated or individual circumstances are such that potential febrile reactions after DTP administration might confound the management of the patient. For inadequately vaccinated patients of all ages, completion of primary vaccination at the time of discharge or at follow-up visits should be ensured.

If passive immunization is needed, human tetanus immunoglobulin is the product of choice. It provides protection longer than antitoxin of animal origin does and causes few adverse reactions. The tetanus immunoglobulin prophylactic dose that currently is recommended for wounds of average severity is 250 units intramuscularly. When tetanus toxoid and tetanus immunoglobulin are given concurrently, separate syringes and separate sites should be used. The Advisory Committee on Immunization Practices recommends the use of only adsorbed toxoid in this situation.

Neonatal Tetanus

Several approaches have been made to reduce the incidence and fatality rate of neonatal tetanus in the developing areas of the world. Among these are (1) educating pregnant women concerning the danger of using contaminated materials for cutting the umbilical cord and covering the stump; (2) training midwives in the application of modern techniques of obstetric asepsis; (3) developing hospitals in which babies are born under strict asepsis; and (4) immunizing of all women of child-bearing age or, if this cannot be done, all who are pregnant. It is clear, however, that it may not be feasible to immunize all individuals in all of the developing areas. If universal immunization is not possible, emphasis should be placed upon immunizing women of child-bearing age. Studies carried out by the World Health Organization have demonstrated that this is practical and leads to an appreciable reduction in the incidence of neonatal tetanus.[34–36, 93] Babies born to mothers who have been immunized during pregnancy not only have adequate levels of circulating antibody but also are protected against acquiring the disease. It has been noted that the level of protective antibody in newborns and the magnitude of the transfer rate of passive immunity to tetanus depend directly on the level of tetanus antitoxin in maternal serum. Mothers who had tetanus antitoxin of 1.28 IU/mL or more could transfer protection to almost all of the newborns (97 to 100 per cent), irrespective of the doses of tetanus toxoid administered. However, mothers who had received two doses of tetanus toxoid during pregnancy not only conferred good protection but also transferred high antitoxin levels to their newborns.[86]

In 1989, the World Health Organization adopted a resolution to eliminate neonatal tetanus worldwide,[105] and in 1990, the World Summit for Children issued a declaration for global elimination of neonatal tetanus by the end of 1995.[22, 106] In 1993, the World Health Organization's goal was defined as the elimination of neonatal tetanus as a public health problem by reducing its incidence to less than one case per 1000 live births for all health districts.[42]

From 1989 to 1993, vaccination coverage with two or more doses of tetanus toxoid among pregnant women in risk areas increased from 27 to 45 per cent. To achieve and maintain neonatal tetanus elimination, 80 per cent or more of infants need to be protected at birth through vaccination of their mothers with at least two doses of tetanus toxoid or through clean delivery and cord care practices.[42]

References

1. Abel, J. J., Firor, W. M., and Chalain, W.: Researches on tetanus. IX. Further evidence to show that tetanus toxin is not carried to central neurons by way of the axis cylinders of motor nerves. Bull. Johns Hopkins Hosp. *63*:373–403, 1938.
2. Abrutyn, E., and Berlin, J. A.: Intrathecal therapy in tetanus: A meta-analysis. J. A. M. A. *266*:2262–2267, 1991.
3. Ahmadsyah, I., and Salim, A.: Treatment of tetanus: An open study to compare the efficacy of procaine penicillin with metronidazole in the treatment of moderate tetanus. Br. Med. J. *29*:640–650, 1985.
4. American Academy of Pediatrics: Active and passive immunization. *In* Peter, G. (ed.): 1994 Red Book: Report of the Committee on Infectious Diseases. 23rd ed. Elk Grove Village, IL, American Academy of Pediatrics, 1994, pp. 7–71.
5. Aguilar Bernal, O. R., Bender, M. A., and Lacy, M. E.: Efficacy of dantrolene sodium in management of tetanus in children. J. R. Soc. Med. *79*:277–281, 1986.
6. Aretaeus: Tetanus. *In* Major, R. H.: Classic Descriptions of Disease. 2nd ed. Springfield, IL, Charles C Thomas, 1939, pp. 148–149.
7. Bagratuni, L.: Cephalic tetanus. Br. Med. J. *1*:461–463, 1952.
8. Bartlett, J. G.: *Clostridium tetani*. *In* Gorbac, S. L., Bartlett, J. G., and Blacklow, N. R. (eds.): Infectious Diseases. Philadelphia, W. B. Saunders, 1992, pp. 1580–1583.
9. Bizzini, B.: Tetanus. *In* Germanier, R. (ed.): Bacterial Vaccines. Orlando, Academic Press, 1984, pp. 38–68.
10. Bleck, T. P.: Tetanus: Pathophysiology, management and prophylaxis. Dis. Mon. *37*:545–603, 1991.
11. Botticelli, J. T., and Waisbren, B. A.: Tetanus in an urban community. Am. J. Med. Sci. *242*:44–50, 1961.
12. Bradley, K., Easton, D. M., and Eccles, J. C.: Investigation of primary or direct inhibition. J. Physiol. *122*:474–478, 1953.
13. Brand, D. A., Acampora, D., Gottlieb, L. D., et al.: Adequacy of antitetanus prophylaxis in six hospital emergency rooms. N. Engl. J. Med. *308*:630–640, 1983.
14. Brooks, V. B., Curtis, D. R., and Eccles, J. C.: Mode of action of tetanus toxin. Nature *175*:120–121, 1955.
15. Brooks, V. B., and Asanuma, H.: Action of tetanus toxin in the cerebral cortex. Science *137*:674–676, 1962.
16. Bytchenko, B. Microbiology of tetanus. *In* Veronesi, R. (ed.): Tetanus: Important New Concepts. Amsterdam, Excerpta Medica, 1981, pp. 28–39.
17. Cain, H. O., and Falco, F. G.: Recurrent tetanus. Calif. Med. *97*:31–33, 1962.
18. Carrea, R., and Lanari, A.: Chronic effect of tetanus toxin applied locally to the cerebral cortex of the dog. Science *137*:342–343, 1962.
19. Carle and Rattone: Studio esperimentale sull'eziologia del tetano. G. Acad. Med. Torino *32*:174–180, 1884.
20. Centers for Disease Control: Diphtheria, tetanus and pertussis: Recommendations for vaccine use and other preventive measures; recommendations of the Immunization Practices Advisory Committee (ACIP). M. M. W. R. *40*(No. RR-10):2–28, 1991.
21. Centers for Disease Control and Prevention: Tetanus surveillance: United States, 1989–1990. M. M. W. R. *41*(No. SS-8): 1–9, 1992.
22. Centers for Disease Control and Prevention: Progress toward the global elimination of neonatal tetanus. M. M. W. R. *43*(No. 48):S89–S94, 1994.
23. Centers for Disease Control and Prevention: Progress toward elimination of neonatal tetanus: Egypt, 1988–1994. M. M. W. R. *45*(No. 4):89–92, 1996.
24. Chang, T. W., and Weinstein, L.: Effect of cortisone on treatment of tetanus with antitoxin. Proc. Soc. Exp. Biol. Med. *94*:431–433, 1957.

25. Christensen, N. A., and Thurber, D. L.: Clinical experience with tetanus: 91 cases. Staff Meetings Mayo Clin. *32*:146–157, 1957.
26. Cole, A. C. E., and Robertson, D. H. H.: Chlorpromazine in the management of tetanus. Lancet *2*:1063–1064, 1955.
27. Cordova, A. B.: Control of the spasms of tetanus with diazepam (Valium). Clin. Pediatr. *8*:712–716, 1969.
28. Creech, O., Glover, A., and Ochsner, A.: Tetanus: Evaluation of treatment at Charity Hospital, New Orleans, Louisiana. Ann. Surg. *146*:369, 1957.
29. Davies, J. R., Morgan, R. S., Wright, E. A., et al.: The effect of local tetanus intoxication of the hind limb reflexes of the rabbit. Arch. Int. Physiol. *62*:248–263, 1954.
30. Dietrich, H. F.: Tetanus neonatorum. J. A. M. A. *147*:1038–1040, 1951.
31. Edsall, G.: Specific prophylaxis of tetanus. J. A. M. A. *171*:417–427, 1959.
32. Edsall, G., Elliott, M. W., Peebles, T. C., et al.: Excessive use of tetanus boosters. J. A. M. A. *202*:17–19, 1967.
33. Edsall, G.: Problems in the immunology and control of tetanus. Med. J. Aust. *2*:216–220, 1976.
34. Expanded Programme on Immunization: Reduction of neonatal deaths by immunizing women against tetanus: Weekly epidemiological record. Bull. W. H. O. *56*:185–186, 1981.
35. Expanded Programme on Immunization: Prevention of neonatal tetanus: Weekly epidemiological record. Bull. W. H. O. *57*:137–142, 1982.
36. Expanded Programme on Immunization: Global Advisory Group Meeting. Weekly Advisory Group Meeting. Weekly epidemiological record. Bull. W. H. O. *58*:15–18, 1983.
37. Fedinec, A. A., and Matzke, H. A.: The role of tissue spaces and nerve fibers in the spread of tetanus toxin in the rat. Univ. Kansas Sci. Bull. *38*:1439–1498, 1958.
38. Firor, W. M., Lamont, A., and Shumacker, H. B.: Studies on the cause of death in tetanus. Ann. Surg. *111*:246, 1940.
39. Forrester, A. T. T.: Treatment of tetanus with succinylcholine. Br. Med. J. *2*:342–344, 1954.
40. Friedemann, U., Zuger, B., and Hollander, A.: Investigations on the pathogenesis of tetanus, I and II. J. Immunol. *36*:473–484, 485–488, 1939.
41. Friedlander, F. C.: Tetanus neonatorum. J. Pediatr. *39*:448–454, 1951.
42. Global Advisory Group: Expanded Program on Immunization. World Health Organization. Achieving the major disease control goals. Wkly. Epidemiol. Rec. *69*:29–31, 34–35, 1994.
43. Godfrey, M. P., Parsons, V., and Rawstron, J. R.: Rapid destruction of antitetanus serum in a patient previously sensitized to horse serum. Lancet *2*:1229–1230, 1960.
44. Green, A. E., Ambrus, J. L., and Gershenfeld, L.: Effect of cortisone and desoxycorticosterone on infection with tetanus spores and on toxicity of tetanus toxin. Antibiot. Chemother. *3*:1221, 1953.
45. Gurses, N., and Aydin, M.: Factors affecting prognosis of neonatal tetanus. Scand. J. Infect. Dis. *25*:353–355, 1993.
46. Hines, E. A., Jr.: Tetanus neonatorum: Report of a case with recovery. Am. J. Dis. Child. *39*:560–572, 1930.
47. Hippocrates: Tetanus. *In* Major, H. H. (ed.): Classic Descriptions of Disease. 2nd ed. Springfield, IL, Charles C Thomas, 1939, pp. 148–149.
48. Hlady, W. G., Bennett, J. V., Samadi, A. R., et al.: Neonatal tetanus in rural Bangladesh: Risk factors and toxoid efficacy. Am. J. Public Health *82*:1365–1369, 1992.
49. Howder, C. L.: Cardiopulmonary Pharmacology. Baltimore, Williams & Wilkins, 1996, p. 316.
50. Jenkins, M. T., and Luhn, N. R.: Active management of tetanus. Anaesthesiology *23*:690–709, 1962.
51. Kaeser, H. E., and Saner, A.: Tetanus toxin, a neuromuscular blocking agent. Nature (Lond.) *223*:842, 1969.
52. Kerr, J. H., Corbett, J. L., Prys-Roberts, C., et al.: Involvement of the sympathetic nervous system in tetanus. Lancet *2*:236–241, 1968.
53. Kitasato, S.: Ueber den tetanus bacillus. Z. Hyg. Infektkr. *7*:225–234, 1889.
54. Laurence, D. R., and Webster, R. A.: Pathologic physiology, pharmacology and therapeutics of tetanus. Clin. Pharmacol. Therap. *4*:36–72, 1963.
55. Leroy, O., and Garenne, M.: Risk factors of neonatal tetanus in Senegal. Int. J. Epidemiol. *20*:521–526, 1991.
56. Levinson, A., Marska, R. L., and Shein, M. K.: Tetanus in heroin addicts. J. A. M. A. *157*:658–660, 1955.
57. Lewis, R. A., Satoskar, R. S., Joag, C. G., et al.: Cortisone and hydrocortisone given parenterally and orally in severe tetanus. J. A. M. A. *156*:479, 1954.
58. Luisto, M.: Outcome and neurological sequelae of patients after tetanus. Acta. Neurol. Scand. *80*:504–511, 1989.
59. Luisto, M.: Tetanus in Finland: Diagnostic problems and complications. Ann. Med. *22*:15–19, 1990.
60. MacLennan, R., Schofield, F. D., Pitman, M., et al.: Immunization against neonatal tetanus in New Guinea: Antitoxin response of pregnant women to adjuvant and plain toxoids. Bull. W. H. O. *32*:683–697, 1965.
61. Malgaard, B., Mutie, D. M., and Kimani, G.: A cluster survey of mortality due to neonatal tetanus in Kenya. Int. J. Epidemiol. *12*:124–127, 1988.
62. McComb, J. A., and Dwyer, R. C.: Passive-active immunization with tetanus immune globulin (human). N. Engl. J. Med. *268*:857–862, 1963.
63. McComb, J. A.: The prophylactic dose of homologous tetanus antitoxin. N. Engl. J. Med. *270*:175–178, 1964.
64. Mellanby, J., Van Heyningen, W. E., and Whitaker, V. P.: Fixation of tetanus toxin by subcellular fractions of brain. J. Neurochem. *12*:77–79, 1965.
65. Meyer, H., and Ransom, F.: Untersuchungen ueber den tetanus. Arch. Exp. Pathol. Pharmakol. *49*:369–416, 1903.
66. Millard, A. H.: Local tetanus. Lancet *2*:844–846, 1954.
67. Miller, C. L., and Stoelting, V. K.: Recent evaluation of the treatment of tetanus. J. A. M. A. *168*:393–394, 1958.
68. Mongi, P. S., Moise, R. L., Msengi, A. E., et al.: Tetanus neonatorum experience with intrathecal serotherapy at Muhumbili Medical Center. Am. Trop. Med. *7*:27–31, 1987.
69. Montgomery, R. D.: The cause of death in tetanus. West Indian Med. J. *10*:84, 1961.
70. Nesquay, E., and Nkrumah, F. K.: Failure of intrathecal antitetanus serum to improve survival in neonatal tetanus. Arch. Dis. Child. *58*:276–278, 1983.
71. Nicolaier, A.: Ueber infectiosen tetanus. Dtsch. Med. Wochenschr. *10*:842–884, 1884.
72. Peebles, T. C., Levine, L., Eldred, M. C., et al.: Tetanus-toxoid emergency boosters. N. Engl. J. Med. *280*:575–581, 1969.
73. Perez, L. R.: The electrocardiogram in tetanus. Rev. Clin. Espann. *75*:20, 1959.
74. Perlstein, M. A., Stein, M. D., and Elam, H.: Routine treatment of tetanus. J. A. M. A. *173*:1536–1541, 1960.
75. Pillemer, L., Wittler, R. G., and Grossberg, D. B.: The isolation and crystallization of tetanal toxin. Science *103*:615–616, 1946.
76. Pratt, E. L.: Clinical tetanus: A study of 56 cases, with special reference to methods of prevention and a plan for evaluating treatment. J. A. M. A. *129*:1243–1247, 1945.
77. Rall, T. W.: Hypnotics and sedatives. *In* Goodman and Gilman's The Pharmacologic Basis of Therapeutics. Section III. Drugs Acting on the Central Nervous System. New York, Pergamon Press, 1990, pp. 345–382.
78. Ramon, G., and Zoeller, C.: L'immunite antitetanique par l'anatoxine chez l'homme. Presse Med. *34*:485, 1926.
79. Risk, W. S., Bosch, E. P., Kimura, J., et al.: Chronic tetanus: Clinical report and histochemistry of muscle. Muscle Nerve *4*:363–366, 1981.
80. Robinson, D. T., McLeod, J. S., and Downie, A. W.: Dust in surgical theatres. Lancet *1*:152–154, 1946.
81. Rock, D. A., Wesley, A. G., Pather, M., et al.: Morphine in tetanus: The management of sympathetic nervous system overactivity. S. Afr. Med. *20*:666–668, 1986.
82. Roofe, P. G.: Role of the axis cylinder in transport of tetanus toxin. Science *105*:180–181, 1947.
83. Rosenbach: Arch. Klin. Chir. *34*:306, 1887.
84. Rubbo, S. D., and Suri, J. C.: Passive immunization against tetanus with human immune globulin. Br. Med. J. *2*:79–81, 1962.
85. Salimpour, R.: Cause of death in tetanus neonatorum. Arch. Dis. Child. *32*:587–589, 1977.
86. Sangpetchsong, V., Vichaikummart, S., Vichitnant, A., et al.: Transfer of transplacental immunity from unimmunized and immunized mothers. Southeast Asian J. Trop. Med. Public Health *15*:275–280, 1984.
87. Schellenberg, D. B., and Matzke, H. A.: The development of tetanus in parabiotic rats. J. Immunol. *80*:367, 1958.
88. Sevitt, S.: Source of two hospital-infected cases of tetanus. Lancet *2*:1075–1078, 1949.
89. Sherrington, C. S.: The Integrative Action of the Nervous System. New York, Yale University Press, 1906, pp. 303, 112.
90. Shibuya, M., Sugimoto, H., Sugimoto, T., et al.: The use of spinal anesthesia in severe tetanus with autonomic disturbances. J. Trauma *29*:1423–1429, 1989.
91. Smith, J. W. G.: Diphtheria and tetanus toxoids. Br. Med. Bull. *25*:177–182, 1969.
92. Smolens, J., Vogt, A. B., Crawford, M. N., et al.: The persistence in the human circulation of horse and human tetanus antitoxins. J. Pediatr. *59*:899–902, 1961.
93. Stanfield, J. P., and Galazaka, A.: Neonatal tetanus in the world today. Bull. W. H. O. *62*:647–669, 1984.
94. Talmage, D. W., Dixon, F. J., Bukantz, S. C., et al.: Antigen elimination from the blood as an early manifestation of the immune response. J. Immunol. *67*:243–255, 1951.
95. Tallman, J. F., Gallagher, D. W.: The GABAergic system: A locus of benzodiazepine action. Ann. Rev. Neurosci. *8*:21–44, 1985.
96. Turner, T. B., Stafford, E. S., and Goldman, L.: Studies on the duration of protection afforded by active immunization against tetanus. Bull. Johns Hopkins Hosp. *94*:204–217, 1954.
97. Turner, T. B., Velasco-Joven, E. A., and Prudovsky, S.: Studies on the prophylaxis and treatment of tetanus. Bull. Johns Hopkins Hosp. *102*:71–84, 1958.
98. Van Heyningen, W. E., and Miller, P. A.: The fixation of tetanus toxin by ganglioside. J. Gen. Microbiol. *24*:107–119, 1961.
99. Vassa, T., Yahnik, V. H., Joshi, K. R., et al.: Comparative clinical trial of diazepam with other conventional drugs in tetanus. Postgrad. Med. J. *50*:755–758, 1974.
100. Von Behring, E., and Kitasato, S.: Ueber des zustandekommen der diph-

terie-immunitat und der tetanus-immunitat bei tieren. Dtsch. Med. Wochenschr. *16*:1113–1114, 1890.
101. Wassilak, S. G. F., Orenstein, W. A., and Sutter, R. W.: Tetanus toxoid. *In* Plotkin, S. A., and Mortimer, E. A. (eds.): Vaccines. 2nd ed. Philadelphia, W. B. Saunders, 1994, pp. 57–90.
102. Weinstein, L.: Tetanus. N. Engl. J. Med. *289*:1293–1296, 1973.
103. Wesley, A. G., and Pathes, M.: Tetanus in children: An 11 year review. Ann. Trop. Med. Paediatr. *7*:32–37, 1987.
104. Willis, A. T.: *Clostridium*: The spore-bearing anaerobes. *In* Wilson, G., Miles, A., and Parker, M. T. (eds.): Topley and Wilson's Principles of Bacteriology, Virology and Immunity. Vol. 2. Baltimore, Williams & Wilkins, 1983, pp. 442–475.
105. World Health Assembly: Expanded Program on Immunization. Geneva, World Health Organization, May 19, 1989 (Resolution WHA42.32).
106. World Health Organization: Revised plan of action for neonatal tetanus elimination. Geneva, World Health Organization, Expanded Program on Immunization, 1993. Publication no. WHO/EPI/GEN/93.13.
107. Wright, E. A., Morgan, R. S., and Wright, G. P.: Tetanus intoxication of the brain stem in rabbits. J. Pathol. Bacteriol. *62*:569–583, 1950.
108. Young, L. S., LaForce, F. M., and Bennett, J. V.: An evaluation of serologic and antimicrobial therapy in the treatment of tetanus in the United States. J. Infect. Dis. *120*:153–159, 1969.
109. Zacks, S. I., and Shef, M. F.: Tetanus toxin: Fine structure localization of binding sites in striated muscle. Science *159*:643–644, 1968.

155

ACTINOMYCOSIS

Suzanne Maxson and Richard F. Jacobs

Human actinomycosis is a clinical illness with a typical histologic presentation that is due to a variety of pathogens. It often is polymicrobial, and *Actinobacillus actinomycetemcomitans* frequently is a copathogen. It is endogenous worldwide, with sporadic cases reported annually. Occurrence of the disease is unrelated to age, sex, season, or occupation, although it decidedly is uncommon in the pediatric population. These organisms have the ability to spread locally without regard to fascial planes or other anatomic barriers. Actinomycosis is characterized by localized swelling with suppuration, abscess formation, and draining sinuses. The abscesses have fibrous walls and are filled with pus and characteristic sulfur granules. The three most common types of actinomycosis are oral and cervical-facial, thoracic, and abdominal. However, involvement of the liver, female reproductive tract, and brain have been described. Definitive diagnosis of the infection rests upon isolation of the organism from pus or identification of sulfur granules on histopathologic sections of biopsy material. Adequate treatment generally consists of surgical removal of the lesion and/or prolonged antibiotic therapy.

MICROBIOLOGY

The clinical entity of actinomycosis is caused by species of the genera *Actinomyces* and *Propionibacterium*. Human actinomycosis most often is caused by *Actinomyces israelii,* although *A. naeslundii, A. viscosus, A. odontolyticus, A. meyeri*, and *A. pyogenes* also are causes of human illness. *A. bovis, A. denticolens, A. howellii, A. hordeovulneris*, and *A. slackii* primarily are animal pathogens. *Propionibacterium propionica* is the only species in the *Propionibacterium* genus, and it also is a cause of human actinomycosis.

These bacterial organisms are irregular, non–spore-forming, non–acid-fast, nonmotile, gram-positive rods. They grow well in most rich culture media and have varying oxygen requirements. For example, *A. israelii* requires anaerobic conditions for growth. *A. viscosus*, however, grows in an aerobic environment with carbon dioxide. These species ferment carbohydrates as their source of energy for growth.[5] They originally were thought to be fungi because of the mycelial appearance of the organisms in sulfur granules and because of their branching morphology. However, neither genus contains chitin or glucans, which are characteristic macromolecules of fungi. These organisms are members of the endogenous flora of mucous membranes. *A. israelii* always is found in the oral cavity when the appropriate anaerobic culture technique is used. It also has been found in the gastrointestinal tract, bronchi, and female genital tract.[13]

A. actinomycetemcomitans is a fastidious, gram-negative rod that frequently complicates actinomycosis caused by *A. israelii* (see Chapter 131). In addition to being associated with actinomycosis, it has been implicated as a pathogen in periodontal disease and is part of the oral flora. This organism is characterized by slow growth in culture and the need for incubation in an atmosphere enhanced with carbon dioxide.[7] Other bacterial species isolated concomitantly in human actinomycosis are *Eikenella corrodens, Fusobacterium, Bacteroides, Capnocytophaga, Staphylococcus, Streptococcus*, and Enterobacteriaceae.

PATHOGENESIS

The organisms that cause actinomycosis normally are found in the oral flora. Disruption of this mucous membrane likely is the initiating event for oral and cervical-facial disease. The organisms then invade locally and spread without regard to fascial planes. The exact mechanism for this spread is unknown but may be related to the ability of these organisms to suppress part of the host immune system. Organisms of the *Actinomyces* genus have been shown to be chemotactic, to activate lymphocyte blastogenesis, and to stimulate the release of lysosomal enzymes from polymorphonuclear leukocytes and macrophages.[5] In addition, the copathogens involved in this infection may reduce local oxygen tension. Dental extractions are associated with mucosal breaks and tissue necrosis and may predispose to oral or cervical-facial actinomycosis.[12] Hematogenous dissemination eventually can occur but is uncommon. Gastrointestinal disease probably is associated with the disruption of the mucosal barrier similar to oral and cervical-facial disease.[13] Organisms causing pulmonary actinomycosis likely reach the lungs through aspiration. Numerous reports exist in the literature associating actinomycosis with intrauterine contraceptive devices (IUCDs), and there is some question regarding the association of foreign bodies with actinomycosis.[2]

PATHOLOGY

Actinomycosis most commonly presents as a chronic infection with single or multiple indurated swellings. These lesions eventually soften, become fluctuant, and suppurate. The walls are fibrous and firm and often described as wooden, which frequently results in their confusion with neoplasms. Over time, sinus tracts form and extend through the overlying skin or to adjacent bones or tissues. The overlying skin may have a bluish hue.[13]

Histologically, a typical lesion has a central purulent area containing neutrophils and sulfur granules, surrounded by an outer zone of granulation with collagen fibers and fibroblasts. Sulfur granules are firm, yellowish granules containing the organisms and virtually are diagnostic of actinomycosis. In addition to neutrophils, lymphocytes and plasma cells frequently are seen in the lesions; eosinophils and multinucleated giant cells occasionally are seen.[13]

CLINICAL MANIFESTATIONS

There are three important sites of actinomycotic infection. The order of frequency of occurrence is oral and cervical-facial, abdominal, and thoracic. Actinomycosis resembles several other chronic inflammatory diseases and must be differentiated from mycotic infections, tuberculosis, appendicitis, *Yersinia enterocolitica* pseudoappendicitis, osteomyelitis, amebiasis, hepatic abscess, and other chronic bacterial infections, including nocardiosis.

Because oral and cervical-facial actinomycosis occurs after disruption of the mucous membranes in the mouth or oropharynx, patients who have this type of actinomycosis may have a history of oral surgery, dental procedures, or trauma to the mouth. They may present clinically with pain, trismus, firm swelling, and fistulas with drainage that contains the characteristic sulfur granules (Figs. 155–1 and 155–2). Patients most commonly have a chronic disease course but may present acutely with cellulitis. Infection may spread via sinus tracts to the cranial bones, which gives rise to meningitis. Bone is not involved early in the disease, but later a periostitis may develop. The marked ability of the organisms in the disease to burrow through tissue planes and even bone differentiates actinomycosis from nocardiosis and is an important characteristic of this infection. The cervical-facial type of actinomycosis, or "lumpy jaw," has the best prognosis.

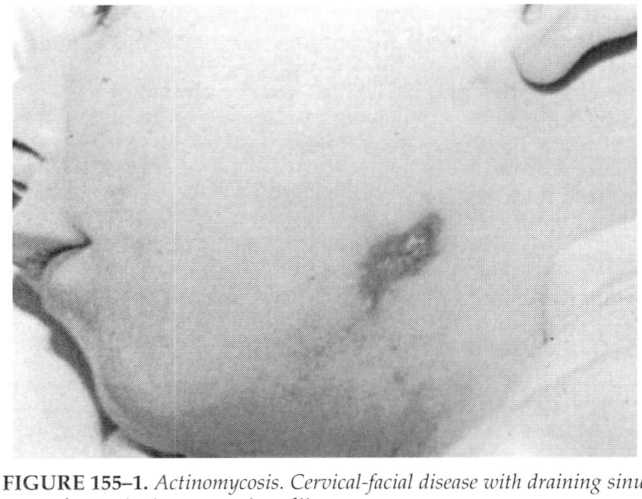

FIGURE 155–1. *Actinomycosis. Cervical-facial disease with draining sinus tracts due to* Actinomyces israelii.

With surgical débridement and excision as an adjunct to proper antibiotic therapy, the disease usually is cured.

Because abdominal actinomycosis also is the result of disruption of the mucosa of the gastrointestinal tract, patients may present with a history of gastrointestinal surgery, diverticulitis, or appendicitis. There also may be a history of trauma to the abdomen. Patients may have chills, fever, night sweats, and weight loss. The course is indolent and similar to that of tuberculous peritonitis. Because appendicitis is the most common predisposing event, on physical examination the patients may have a hard, irregular mass in the ileocecal area that softens and then drains to the outside. Extension from such foci usually is by direct continuity (or, rarely, is hematogenous) and involves any tissue or organ, including muscle, liver, spleen, kidney, fallopian tubes, ovaries, uterus, testes, bladder, or rectum. A delayed diagnosis of actinomycosis involving the abdomen or pelvis is typical.

The diagnosis of pulmonary actinomycosis depends on a high index of suspicion, because neither the clinical nor radiographic presentation is specific. Patients may have a history of, or risk factors for, aspiration. This type of actinomycosis also occurs after introduction of a colonized foreign body. Patients with oral or cervical-facial or abdominal actinomycotic infections are at risk for pulmonary infection from direct or hematogenous spread. A history of these preexisting infections should heighten the index of suspicion. The principal symptoms include chest pain, fever, productive cough, and weight loss. The infection frequently dissects along tissue planes and may extend through the chest wall or diaphragm, producing multiple sinuses. These characteristic sinus tracts contain small abscesses and purulent drainage. Adults with thoracic actinomycosis usually have abnormal local defenses, such as chronic bronchitis, bronchiectasis, or emphysema. However, pediatric patients have been shown to have predisposing factors less often.[17] The differential diagnosis of pulmonary actinomycosis includes tuberculosis and lung abscess.

Women wearing IUCDs are at risk for the development of pelvic actinomycosis. These patients may present with vaginal discharge, pelvic pain, abdominal pain, menorrhagia, fever, pelvic mass, a history of pelvic inflammatory disease, and/or a history of prolonged IUCD use. The risk is more significant if the IUCD has been in place for longer than 2 to 3 years. It is thought that these devices cause an inflammatory response in the endometrium with focal necrosis. This anaerobic environment encourages the growth of *A. israelii.* In these patients, removal of the IUCD and treatment with antibiotics are necessary.[2]

Hepatic involvement occurs in approximately 15 per cent of cases of abdominal actinomycosis. Involvement of the liver can occur through direct extension from a subdiaphragmatic or subhepatic abscess. It also is common in disseminated actinomycosis.[13] Occult disruption of the gastrointestinal mucosa may provide a portal of entry for the organisms in cases of primary or isolated hepatic disease. Presenting symptoms may include fever, abdominal pain, anorexia, weight loss, nausea, vomiting, shoulder pain, back pain, or diarrhea. The presentation usually is indolent, with 1 to 6 months of symptoms. On physical examination, the patient commonly will have fever, abdominal tenderness, and hepatomegaly. There may be a palpable abdominal mass, jaundice, or draining sinuses. Hepatic actinomycosis has been reported to occur in children after an appendectomy.[8] Other causes of liver masses included in the differential diagnosis are pyogenic abscess, amebiasis, and malignancy.

Laryngeal actinomycosis rarely has been reported in older teenagers.[10] Colonization of the oropharynx with these organisms may be involved in the development of obstructive tonsillar hypertrophy.[12] There are several adult cases of pericardial actinomycosis in the literature.[3] Actinomycetes have been isolated from nearly every organ in the body, including the kidneys, brain, breasts, mastoids, male genitourinary tract, and eyes. *A. pyogenes* only rarely has been implicated as a cause of human infection, but there are reported cases of septicemia, endocarditis, meningitis, arthritis, empyema, pneumonia, otitis media, cystitis, mastoiditis, appendicitis, and cutaneous infection.[1, 4]

A. actinomycetemcomitans is a pathogen in at least 30 per cent of actinomycotic infections.[7] Failure to recognize this organism and treat it adequately has resulted in clinical relapse and deterioration in infected patients with actinomycosis.[9, 18] Severe forms of periodontitis, particularly localized juvenile periodontitis, also are associated with this pathogen, and studies have shown that it strongly is related to children in the 10- to 19-year-old age group.[15] Additionally, it is one of the HACEK (HACEK also includes *Haemophilus aphrophilus, Cardiobacterium hominis, Eikenella corrodens*, and *Kingella kingae*) organisms that has a propensity for infecting heart valves. Endocarditis caused by this organism usually is insidious, with fever occurring in less than 50 per cent of cases.[7] This organism also has been reported to cause pericarditis, meningitis, brain abscess, parotitis, synovitis, osteomyelitis, urinary tract infection, pneumonia, and empyema.[7]

DIAGNOSIS

To make a definitive diagnosis of actinomycosis, the clinician must isolate the causative organism from tissue or pus from a normally sterile body site, such as the lungs. Isolation of the organism from the oral cavity or the female genital tract without clinical evidence of disease is, therefore, not diagnostic. Because the organisms that cause actinomycosis are exquisitely sensitive to antibiotics, it is important that clinical specimens be obtained prior to their use. They should be processed carefully to maintain anaerobic conditions. The specimens should undergo routine Gram stain, which will reveal gram-positive rods that are non–acid-fast and appear in diphtheroidal arrangements with or without branching.[5] The Gram stain is more sensitive than culture, particularly if the patient has been given antibiotics. Immunofluorescence is available for confirmation of organisms in biopsy specimens with suggestive Gram stains. Growth on media usually appears within 5 to 7 days but may take 2 to 4 weeks.[13]

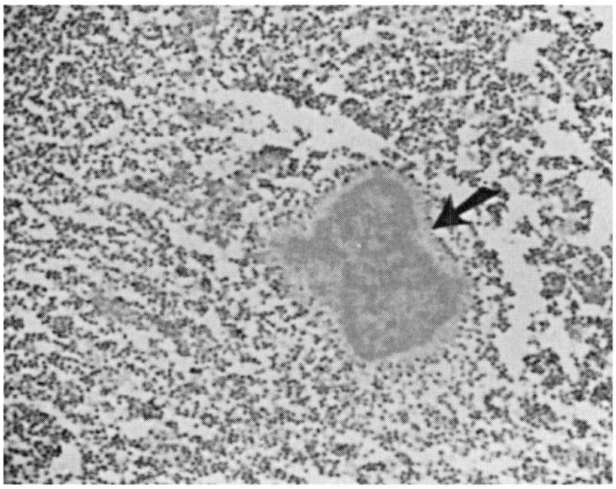

FIGURE 155–2. *Abcess containing actinomycotic granule surrounded by purulent exudate. The peripheral clubbing (arrow) is stained by eosin. (H and E × 52.)*

True microbiologic identification of these organisms is uncommon, and diagnosis most often rests on the clinical picture, with identification of the characteristic sulfur granules. The sulfur granules may be found by drawing pus from a lesion, on the bandage covering the lesion, or in surgical specimens (Fig. 155–2). Pus that is poured down the side of a glass will leave sulfur granules adherent to the sides so that the granules will be identified more easily. On hematoxylin and eosin stain, the granules are eosinophilic or variably surrounded by a radiating fringe of eosinophilic clubs. Washed, crushed granules or well-mixed pus in the absence of granules is cultured on a rich medium, such as brain-heart infusion blood agar, and incubated anaerobically and aerobically with added carbon dioxide. Plates can be examined at 24 hours and after 5 to 7 days for the characteristic colonies of *Actinomyces*.[5]

Various imaging modalities have been useful in diagnosing and characterizing actinomycosis. Computed tomography has been shown to help differentiate between inflammatory masses and tumors. Additionally, the location, extension, and relation between the mass and surrounding structures can be defined better. Ultrasonography has been shown in one report to reveal a mass with an ill-defined margin that was hypoechoic with intrinsic hyperechoic spots.[14] There currently are no skin tests available for screening purposes and no useful serologic tests for actinomycosis.[3]

A. actinomycetemcomitans can be cultured on blood and chocolate agar but grows poorly on MacConkey agar. The cultures require incubation in an enhanced carbon dioxide atmosphere. Growth of the organism in a blood culture may take up to 9 days in patients with endocarditis, and thus the cultures should be held longer. The organism on Gram stain appears coccoid to coccobacillary.[7] A rapid latex agglutination test and a polymerase chain reaction test are being developed for diagnosis of this organism.[6, 11] Because of the frequency of coinfection with this organism in cases of actinomycosis, attempts always should be made to isolate this organism in these patients.

TREATMENT

The mainstays of therapy for actinomycosis remain surgical débridement or removal of the lesion and prolonged antimicrobial therapy. Most experts still recommend drainage of abscesses, fistulotomy, sinus tract excision, and debulking of large masses, although there are numerous successful outcomes reported in the literature with antimicrobial therapy alone.[8, 13] The option to treat medically and observe for clinical response seems reasonable in the stable, noncritical patient. The antibiotic of choice is penicillin. The total duration of therapy recommended ranges from 6 to 12 months. For persons who are allergic to penicillin, tetracycline or erythromycin is acceptable. Other alternatives are clindamycin, chloramphenicol, and the third-generation cephalosporins. Three weeks of daily ceftriaxone followed by prolonged ampicillin was effective treatment in one case.[17] Because this is an uncommon disease in children with no significant randomized prospective treatment trials, most authors still recommend 4 to 6 weeks of intravenous therapy followed by oral therapy for a prolonged period. The duration of total therapy is based upon clinical and radiographic follow-up. Thoracic actinomycosis has been treated successfully with a total duration of therapy of only 4 months.[16]

Because co-infection with *A. actinomycetemcomitans* occurs regularly, it is important to consider covering this organism empirically, especially in the critically ill patient. It is susceptible to newer cephalosporins, rifampin, trimethoprim-sulfamethoxazole, aminoglycosides, ciprofloxacin, tetracycline, azithromycin, and chloramphenicol. It is susceptible to penicillin and ampicillin in vitro, but test results do not correlate necessarily with clinical outcome. Vancomycin, erythromycin, and clindamycin have very little activity against this organism.[7] In some patients with periodontitis associated with this organism, a combination of mechanical periodontal treatment with metronidazole plus amoxicillin is effective for subgingival suppression.

References

1. Drancourt, M.: Two cases of *Actinomyces pyogenes* infection in humans. Eur. J. Microbiol. Infect. Dis. *12*:55–57, 1993.
2. Evans, D. P. T.: *Actinomyces israelii* in the female genital tract: A review. Genitourin. Med. *69*:54–59,1993.
3. Fife, T. D., Finegold S. M., and Grennan T.: Pericardial actinomycosis: Case report and review. Rev. Infect. Dis. *13*:120–126, 1991.
4. Gahrn-Hansen, B., and Frederiksen W.: Human infections with *Actinomyces pyogenes (Corynebacterium pyogenes)*. Diag. Microbiol. Infect. Dis. *15*:349–354, 1992.
5. Gerencser, M. A.: *Actinomyces, Arachnia,* and *Streptomyces. In* Baron, S. (ed.): Medical Microbiology. 3rd ed. New York, Churchill Livingstone, 1991, pp. 469–477.
6. Leys J. E., Griffen, A. L., Strong, S. J., et al.: Detection and strain identification of *Actinobacillus actinomycetemcomitans* by nested PCR. J. Clin. Microbiol. *32*:1288–1294, 1994.
7. McGowan J. E., and Steinberg J. P.: Other gram-negative bacilli. *In* Mandell, G. L., Bennett, J. E., and Dolin, R. (eds.): Principles and Practices of Infectious Disease, New York, Churchill Livingstone, 1995, pp. 2106–2107.
8. Miyamoto, M. I., and Fang, F. C.: Pyogenic liver abscess involving *Actinomyces*: Case report and review. Clin. Infect. Dis. *16*:303–309, 1993.
9. Morris, J. F., and Sewell, D. L.: Necrotizing pneumonia caused by mixed infection with *Actinobacillus actinomycetemcomitans* and *Actinomyces israelii:* Case report and review. Clin. Infect. Dis. *18*:450–452, 1994.
10. Nelson, E. G., and Tybor, A. G.: Actinomycosis of the larynx. Ear Nose Throat J. *71*:356–358, 1992.
11. Nisengard, R. J., Mikulski, L., McDuffie, D., et al.: Development of a rapid latex agglutination test for periodontal pathogens. J. Periodontol. *63*:611–617, 1992.
12. Pransky, M., Feldman, J. I., Kearns, D. B., et al.: Actinomycosis in obstructive tonsillar hypertrophy and recurrent tonsillitis. Arch. Otolaryngol. *117*:883–885, 1991.
13. Russo, T. A.: Agents of actinomycosis. *In* Mandell, G. L., Bennett, J. E., and Dolin, R. (eds.): Principles and Practices of Infectious Diseases. New York, Churchill Livingstone, 1995, pp. 2280–2288.
14. Sa'do, B., Kazunori, Y., Yuasa, K., et al.: Multimodality imaging of cervicofacial actinomycosis. Oral Surg. Oral Med. Oral Pathol. *76*:772–778, 1993.
15. Savitt, E. D., and Kent, R. L.: Distribution of *Actinobacillus actinomycetemcomitans* and *Porphyromonas gingivalis*. J. Periodontol. *62*:490–494, 1991.
16. Skoutelis, A., Petrochilow, J., and Bassaris, H.: Successful treatment of thoracic actinomycosis with ceftriaxone. Clin. Infect. Dis. *19*:161–162, 1994.
17. Snape, P. S.: Thoracic actinomycosis: An unusual childhood infection. South. Med. J. *86*:222–224, 1993.
18. Tyrrell, J., Noone, P., and Prichard, J. S.: Thoracic actinomycosis complicated by *Actinobacillus actinomycetemcomitans:* Case report and review of literature. Respir. Med. *86*:341–343, 1992.

156

OTHER ANAEROBIC INFECTIONS

Lisa M. Dunkle and Mark S. Munsey

The existence of bacteria requiring an environment without oxygen for growth and replication has been known since Leeuwenhoek's observations in the seventeenth century. Pasteur noted bacterial fermentation in 1861 and introduced the term *anaerobies*, and Welch described what now is recognized as *Clostridium perfringens* in 1896. Numerous studies documenting the importance of anaerobic organisms in abdominal and gynecologic infections were published during the first half of the twentieth century but largely went unnoticed. The significance of these organisms in clinical infection has become appreciated widely only since relatively simple anaerobic culture techniques have been devised.

The frequency of anaerobic infection has been dealt with most extensively in adults, but several studies have documented the occurrence and importance of anaerobic infection in infants and children. Anaerobic organisms, when sought, have been found to cause 5 to 10 per cent of all clinically significant bacteremic episodes in infants and children. Other infections, such as peritonitis, abscesses, and a variety of soft tissue infections, also are caused by anaerobes in varying frequency. Most investigators agree that anaerobic infections are less frequent in children than in adults but that they should be considered and sought in high-risk situations or in cases of unexplained clinical sepsis.[9–11, 13–17, 23, 24, 26, 27, 29, 30, 32, 35, 42, 51]

BACTERIOLOGY

The organisms commonly involved in clinical anaerobic infection are a small portion of the vast taxonomy of anaerobic bacteria and represent a minority even of those organisms existing as normal flora of skin and mucous membranes. In general, they can be categorized according to their morphologic characteristics and Gram-staining properties and are listed in Table 156–1. Reflected in the table are the adopted taxonomic changes that resulted in the assignment of several *Bacteroides* species to the *Prevotella* and *Porphyromonas* genera[89, 98] and the designation of all of the clinically significant *Peptococcus* species (except *P. niger*) as *Peptostreptococcus* species.[22, 98]

The primary characteristic that differentiates these organisms from aerobic bacteria is the requirement of an anaerobic environment for viability and growth. Anaerobic metabolism

TABLE 156–1. Anaerobic Bacteria Responsible for Clinical Infection

Gram-Positive	Gram-Negative
Cocci	Cocci
Peptostreptococcus	*Veillonella*
Microaerophilic *Streptococcus*	Bacilli
Bacilli	*Bacteroides fragilis*
Clostridium species	*Prevotella melaninogenica* and related species
Eubacterium	*Prevotella oralis* and related species
Propionibacterium	*Porphyromonas* species
	Fusobacterium species

is more primitive than aerobic in that oxygen is not used as the final electron acceptor, and, thus, less energy is produced from equivalent quantities of substrate. Nonetheless, anaerobic metabolism may be more widespread and flexible than aerobic because it may proceed so long as any fermentable substrate is available and need not rely on the presence of oxygen. The limiting factor in the cultivation of anaerobes appears to be their aerointolerance; that is, oxygen is actively toxic to anaerobic organisms.[75]

The reason for the toxicity of oxygen is not clear, but it appears to be related to several chemical processes.[57, 74, 77] The absence of the enzyme catalase in some anaerobic organisms leads to their self-destruction by hydrogen peroxide when it is generated in the presence of oxygen. This mechanism appears operative in some strains of *Bifidobacterium* and *Clostridium*. Other species, including *Peptostreptococcus, Prevotella,* and *Bacteroides,* are aerointolerant, despite the production of measurable quantities of catalase. Bubbling oxygen through cultures of a number of anaerobic organisms inhibits growth without a demonstrable accumulation of hydrogen peroxide, and the addition of catalase to culture medium does not allow growth reliably in an oxygen-containing atmosphere. Thus, absence of catalase cannot explain fully the susceptibility to toxicity of oxygen. Similarly, a deficiency of superoxide dismutase has been detected in some anaerobic organisms, leading to susceptibility to the highly toxic intermediary superoxide anion (O^-_2), which results from oxygen reduction. Other strains do, however, produce superoxide dismutase, yet remain strictly anaerobic.

The effect of oxygen on the oxidation-reduction (redox) potential of an organism's environment probably is the major reason for the aerointolerance of anaerobic microorganisms. The redox potential (Eh) of a system, measured in millivolts (mV) against a standard hydrogen half-cell with an Eh of 0 mV at pH 0 and an Eh of -420 mV at pH 7.0, is a measure of its tendency to accept electrons. It is clear from numerous studies that there is a maximal redox potential at pH 7.0, above which most anaerobic organisms cannot grow. This value varies among strains and may be altered by changes in pH or gaseous atmosphere.

The reason that a higher Eh may be growth-limiting for anaerobes is not entirely clear but probably is related to the inability of the organisms in higher redox environments to maintain critical enzymes in the reduced state that is necessary for metabolism.

Growth of anaerobic organisms in vivo rarely is hampered by the requirement of a reduced atmosphere because reduced substances are the natural products of metabolism in most living tissues. In vitro cultivation of anaerobic organisms, however, depends to a large extent upon the creation of a sufficiently reduced and/or oxygen-free atmosphere to allow growth. Methods used in the laboratory to ensure growth of anaerobes include the addition to media of reducing substances, such as thioglycolate, dithiothreitol, cysteine, iron shavings, or chopped meat, and the processing of cultures in an oxygen-free atmosphere. Although broth medium with added reducing substances may support some anaerobic growth with incubation under aerobic conditions, solid media on which organisms may be isolated and identified must be processed and incubated in an oxygen-free atmosphere.[61]

There are two methods available for general use in clinical laboratories that fulfill this requirement. The systems used most widely are those utilizing a jar or bag in which inoculated plates are placed and an anaerobic atmosphere is generated by the elaboration of hydrogen and carbon dioxide in the presence of a palladinized alumina catalyst. In the hands of experienced personnel who take considerable care in the preparation and inoculation of solid media, this system is satisfactory for the recovery of even quite oxygen-sensitive microbes. A more extensive system for processing cultures is the anaerobic glove box, which is a flexible chamber with gloves attached for manipulation of the culture materials inside. Incubators and all necessary equipment are kept inside the chamber, and access is via a double-seal system, which maintains the oxygen-free gas mixture within. The commercial systems allowing generation of an anaerobic atmosphere in bags or individual culture plates are simple and attractive for the processing of anaerobic organisms, even in smaller clinical laboratories.[4, 52, 102]

Whatever system is used for the cultivation of anaerobes, it is critical that culture material obtained from patients be handled with care and dispatched so that organisms are not exposed to air prior to inoculation on reduced medium. Ideally, material should be inoculated at the bedside into a prereduced broth containing substrate, usually glucose, and chopped meat. This serves as the initial culture medium, and organisms may be subcultured and isolated from it. Somewhat less desirable, but still satisfactory, methods of handling cultures use anaerobic transport media containing reducing agents that maintain, but do not nourish, organisms prior to inoculation into culture medium in the laboratory. All of these methods of handling cultures require the rapid transport of material to the laboratory to be placed in an oxygen-free atmosphere.[36, 37] Once in the laboratory, the cultures may be processed using numerous systems of plating media. Most systems include selective media containing antibiotics that suppress the growth of facultative organisms, which otherwise might overgrow the anaerobic organisms. All media should be prereduced and sterilized anaerobically. More specific information regarding the cultivation of anaerobic organisms is available in several standard guides and textbooks.[59, 73, 98]

Identification of anaerobic strains can be achieved by using selective fermentative substrates and a variety of biochemical reactions, but it is facilitated greatly by gas-liquid chromatographic analysis of volatile and nonvolatile acids produced by the organisms in culture. Systems of identification of anaerobic microorganisms are described in several publications; the most widely used is that devised by the Anaerobe Laboratory at the Virginia Polytechnic Institute (VPI).[59, 73] Again, numerous commercial kits have been introduced that offer simplified batteries of biochemical tests for metabolic products or enzymes produced by the anaerobic organisms. These "mini-systems" are compared routinely with the VPI system and generally demonstrate good reliability and accuracy in the hands of those familiar with traditional biochemical identification of anaerobic organisms.

ETIOLOGY

The organisms most commonly involved in clinical infections are described briefly in Table 156–2. More complete bacteriologic information is available in the standard texts of anaerobic microbiology.[59, 73, 98]

Infection by anaerobic organisms most frequently involves endogenous flora. Thus, most anaerobic infection follows some alteration in the physical barrier to endogenous microbes and further compromise in the viability of infected tissues. Devitalized tissue provides the necessary low Eh and oxygen-free environment for the growth of anaerobic organisms. Reduction in the Eh also is achieved by concomitant inoculation with several microbes, resulting in a symbiotic infection involving organisms generally considered nonpathogenic, as well as recognized pathogens. Introduction of organisms into host tissues may occur through physical

TABLE 156–2. Characteristics of Anaerobic Bacteria Responsible for Clinical Infections

Organism	Colonial and Microscopic Morphologic Characteristics	Growth Characteristics	Extracellular Products and Toxins	Serotypes
Bacteroides fragilis	Convex, white-gray, glistening colony; foul odor. Size = 0.5–0.8 μ × 1.5–4.5 μ. Pleomorphic gram-negative bacillus with rounded end; vacuoles variably present.	Not inhibited by bile; indole and catalase variable; resistant to penicillin, kanamycin, vancomycin. Fermentation products: acetic, succinic, formic, isovaleric, lactic, propionic acids.	Heparinase; endotoxin. Many strains beta-lactamase–positive.	Major virulence factor is capsular polysaccharide.
Clostridium perfringens	Convex, gray, opaque colony with wide, double zone of hemolysis. Size = 0.8–1.5 μ × 2–4 μ. Gram-positive bacilli. No spores in infected tissue.	Optimum temp. 45° C with gas production. Grows rapidly in basic protein broth, e.g., TSB in anaerobic atmosphere. Ferments dextrose, lactose, sucrose. Reduces nitrate; liquefies gelatin. Produces lecithinase. Fermentation products: acetic, butyric acids.	Twelve toxins, alpha to nu. Major lethal: alpha, beta, epsilon, iota.	A–E based on toxin production. Types A and C most common human pathogens.
Peptostreptococcus	Convex, opaque, gray-white, smooth or matte colonies; rarely hemolytic. Size = 0.6–1 μ. Gram-positive cocci in chains.	Five species according to VPI classification. Differentiated by fermentation of maltose, cellobiose, sorbose and by size. Fermentation products: primarily acetic or lactic acids.	None known.	None differentiated. Few strains of *P. anaerobius* are Lancefield group D.
Fusobacterium	Flat-coned, opaque centers with translucent borders; non- or minimally hemolytic; flecked centers seen with *F. nucleatum*. Size = 0.6 μ × 5–10 μ. Slender, gram-negative bacilli with tapered ends. May show pleomorphism.	Tolerant of higher redox potential. Six commonly pathogenic species. Differentiated by a variety of biochemical reactions. All produce butyric acid.	*Necrophorum* produces leukocidin and hemolysin, both antiphagocytic. Nucleatum beta-lactamase–positive.	Type-specific polysaccharide antigens. Single-protein antigen stimulates antibody in most humans.
Prevotella melaninogenica	There are 0.5–2.0-mm convex colonies; light-gray, young colonies; black-pigmented colonies after 5–7 days. Fluoresce red. Size = 0.3 μ × 0.6 μ. Gram-negative bacilli, uniform in size and staining. Related species: *P. denticola, P. loeschii, P. intermedia.*	Inhibited by bile. Hydrolyzes starch; ferments sucrose, lactose, mannose.	Collagenase produced at optimum pH 6.8–7.3. Requires Ca^{++} for activity. Endotoxin, protease, phospholipase. Many strains beta-lactamase–positive.	Major virulence factor is capsule polysaccharide.
Prevotella oralis	Yellow, translucent, smooth, 1–2-mm convex colonies. Nonhemolytic. Gram-negative nonmotile bacilli. *Ovalis* form, 0.5–1 μ wide, 1–4 μ long; *elongatus* form, 3–8 μ long. Related species: *P. oris. P. baccae.*	Hydrolyzes starch; ferments sucrose, lactose, cellobiose, mannose; hydrolyzes esculin. Inhibited by 10 per cent bile.	Many strains beta-lactamase–positive	None described.

TABLE 156–2. Characteristics of Anaerobic Bacteria Responsible for Clinical Infections *Continued*

Organism	Colonial and Microscopic Morphologic Characteristics	Growth Characteristics	Extracellular Products and Toxins	Serotypes
Clostridium septicum	Semitranslucent, gray, glossy, 2–5-mm raised colonies with irregular margins. Wide zone of hemolysis. May be swarming. Size = 0.8 μ × 3–5 μ. Pleomorphic gram-positive bacilli with small, subterminal spores. Motile.	Optimum growth at 40° C. Moderately aerotolerant. Liquefies gelatin; hydrolyzes casein. Fermentation products: predominantly acetic, butyric acids.	Four toxins (alpha to delta). Most clinically significant is alpha toxin, a lethal, necrotizing, hemolytic toxin. Others are a deoxyribonuclease, a hyaluronidase, an oxygen-labile lysin.	Six serotypes based on either of two somatic and one or two of five flagellar antigens. All strains share common spore antigen A.
Clostridium difficile	Spreading 2–4-mm yellow colonies with irregular margins and dense centers. Size = 3–5 μ. Gram-positive bacilli with subterminal spores. Nonhemolytic.	Hydrolyzes esculin; liquefies gelatin; ferments glucose, fructose, mannose, cellobiose; produces acetic, butyric, isocaproic acids from glucose.	D-1 and D-2, both heat labile, immunologically distinct enterotoxins.	None described.
Eubacterium	Colonies are 1 mm with low convexity, translucent or semiopaque. Nonhemolytic. *E. lentum* is 0.6 μ × 2–3 μ, gram-positive. *E. limosum* is 1–15 μ × 4–6 μ, moderately pleomorphic.	*E. lentum* is relatively inactive but does reduce nitrate. *E. limosum* ferments some carbohydrates and hydrolyzes esculin. Fermentation products: acetic, lactic acids.	None described.	None described.
Propionibacterium acnes	Convex, shiny, opaque, 1–2-mm colonies with narrow zone of hemolysis. Size = 0.3–1.3 μ × 1–10 μ. Gram-positive bacilli with pleomorphism.	Ferments only monosaccharides; hydrolyzes gelatin; digests casein; reduces nitrate; indole-positive. Fermentation products: acetic, propionic acids.	Several exoenzymes, including hyaluronidase, chondroitin sulfatase, lipase.	Two serotypes without clinical significance.
Veillonella	Convex, glistening, nonhemolytic colonies. Size = 0.2 μ. Gram-negative cocci in pairs, chains, clumps.	Relatively inactive but does reduce nitrate. Ferments lactate; produces acetate, propionate, hydrogen. *V. alcalescens* produces pseudocatalase.	Endotoxin.	None described.

TSB, trypticase soy broth; VPI, Virginia Polytechnic Institute.

breaks in mucosal integrity or may result from invasion by organisms with increased potential for adherence to host cells, possibly in the absence of specific surface immunoglobulins. Whatever the mechanism of initiation, polymicrobial infection with endogenous flora results frequently.

Other deficiencies in host defense mechanisms, such as concurrent malignancy, premature birth, or immune suppression by drugs or disease, are associated with increased frequency of serious anaerobic infection. Compromise of tissues in the otherwise normal host by surgery, injury, or vascular embarrassment also predisposes to anaerobic infection.

Because most anaerobic infections are endogenous in etiology, transmission among patients is unlikely and specific isolation measures are not warranted. Patients with draining wounds that may contain aerobic pathogens may require isolation. Most authorities recommend enteric isolation for patients with *C. difficile*, antibiotic-associated colitis, but this has not been shown clearly to block transmission in the hospital setting.

EPIDEMIOLOGY

The epidemiology of anaerobic infections in infants and children has been documented in prospective series as well as in many isolated reports. The frequency of anaerobic infections in general appears to be somewhat lower in children than in adults. This perhaps is because of the lower incidence in children of debilitating disease and certain types of infection, such as lung abscess, empyema, liver abscess, peritoneal abscess, and all forms of obstetric and gynecologic infections, all of which involve anaerobes in up to 90 per cent of cases in adults.[27] Anaerobic septicemia also is somewhat less common in children, constituting only 5 to 8 per cent of all clinically significant episodes of bacteremia.[35, 42, 53]

Anaerobic bacteria are isolated most frequently from children with peritonitis caused by appendicitis or gastrointestinal perforation. The organisms recovered represent fecal flora, with *Bacteroides fragilis* being the most common isolate. In the majority of children with peritonitis, the infection is polymicrobial and *Escherichia coli* frequently is isolated concurrently. Virtually all cases of secondary peritonitis and associated wound infections yield anaerobic organisms when these are sought.[13, 70] Anaerobic bacteremia in children is seen in several clinical situations. It may result from dissemination from a focus of infection, commonly of gastrointestinal location, including the oral cavity. Alternatively, bacteremia occurs in patients with chronic disease or compromised host defenses. The single underlying disease most commonly associated with anaerobic septicemia in one series was leukemia.[42] The organisms recovered from patients with septicemia are the gram-negative, non–spore-forming bacilli *Bacteroides* and *Fusobacterium*, *Clostridium*, and the gram-positive cocci and *Peptostreptococcus*. Osteomyelitis and septic arthritis occasionally complicate anaerobic bacteremia. The clinical manifestations do not differ from those of bone and joint infections due to more common aerobic pathogens. Thus, appropriate specimens should be obtained for anaerobic culture whenever drainage or biopsy procedures are performed, and anaerobic infections seriously should be considered in osteomyelitis of unclear etiology.[78, 83]

Brain abscesses almost invariably yield anaerobic organisms in children, as in adults. These uncommon infections usually occur in the setting of patients with chronic otitis, mastoiditis, or sinusitis or in children with cyanotic congenital heart disease. Other forms of anaerobic central nervous system infection are rare and have been reported usually as a complication of surgery or foreign body implantation.[16, 71]

Cutaneous abscesses and wounds in children commonly may yield anaerobic organisms if cultures are obtained properly. The infections usually are polymicrobial, involve both anaerobic and facultative organisms, and are found in sites related to the gastrointestinal and genitourinary tracts.[15, 26] Chronic or acute infections of mastoids, paranasal sinuses, and middle ear may be caused by anaerobes.[10, 14, 17, 23, 29, 32, 34, 97] Animal or human bites typically are polymicrobial, involving the aerobic and anaerobic flora of the skin and mouth.[21, 47, 49]

The role of anaerobic organisms, particularly beta-lactamase producers, in acute or chronic tonsillopharyngitis is strongly suggested. Considerable data suggest that these strains are present in substantial numbers in crypt abscesses, deep within chronically inflamed tonsils, and in parapharyngeal abscesses.[11, 33] Data from in vitro and in vivo studies have demonstrated that beta-lactamase from one species in a polymicrobial infection can protect another species that does not produce the enzyme.[18, 19] Thus, it seems prudent to consider penicillin-resistant anaerobes as potential etiologic agents in serious parapharyngeal infections.[25, 56]

In addition to those sites that prominently are associated with anaerobic infection, virtually any form of local infection may in occasional cases yield anaerobes; specific cultures for these organisms should be performed in all cases of deep-seated infection. This particularly is true in patients with underlying diseases that predispose to opportunistic infection and in sites of infection involving devitalized tissue.[9, 87]

PATHOGENESIS

The pathogenesis of anaerobic infections reflects the complex interaction of host defense mechanisms, including tissue blood supply and viability, and the virulence factors peculiar to each organism. Considerable data have been gathered from specific situations, furthering our understanding of the development of these infections.

There is an appreciation for the role of bacterial adherence factors in the initiation of infection. Some strains of *Prevotella melaninogenica* (formerly *B. melaninogenicus*) and *Fusobacterium nucleatum* have been shown to adhere preferentially to epithelial cells of the crevices of the oral cavity.[58, 67, 79] The pili they possess enable them to adhere to mucosal membranes,[78, 93] and the possession of a capsule provides protection against opsonophagocytosis.[86, 92] Brook and associates[31] reported that capsules were possessed by 83 per cent of anaerobic species isolated from the blood of bacteremic patients and by 78 per cent of anaerobes isolated from abscesses (*B. fragilis* and *P. melaninogenica* groups). Pili, on the other hand, were found in only 6 per cent of anaerobic blood isolates but in 75 to 92 per cent of abscess isolates.[20] In comparison, only 10 per cent of control isolates were encapsulated and 69 to 81 per cent were piliated. These results suggest that these morphologic characteristics, particularly encapsulation, may play an important role in the pathophysiology of invasive infection, as has been demonstrated for aerobic pathogens.

The multiple proteolytic exotoxins and enzymes elaborated by many of the anaerobic organisms shown in Table 156–2 likely are responsible for the necrotizing nature of many anaerobic infections, such as pneumonia and cellulitis. The kappa-toxin of *C. perfringens*, for example, has been shown after intramuscular injection to cause collagen degradation, necrosis, and extravasation of blood similar to that seen in gas gangrene.[94] Further, these toxins may contribute to the pathogenesis of the synergistic infections common to anaerobes, in which several relatively nonpathogenic organisms contribute to each other's virulence.[38] An example is invasive infection due to *P. melaninogenica* made possible by the vitamin K elaborated by facultative organisms, such as diphtheroids or *E. coli* present concomitantly. Bacterial synergism also contributes to the reduction in Eh, which is necessary for anaerobic infection.[80]

Some cell-wall virulence factors also have been shown to have a direct role in the pathogenesis of some clinical manifestations, such as the activation of Hageman factor (clotting factor XII) by the lipopolysaccharide of several *Bacteroides* species, which contributes to the thrombophlebitis commonly associated with these infections.[8] The extensively studied animal model of peritoneal infection after gastrointestinal perforation has shown that the capsular polysaccharide of *B. fragilis* solely is responsible for the promotion of abscess formation, in contrast to the aerobic pathogens that predominate in generalized peritonitis.[64, 81, 82, 91] In addition, metabolic products of these organisms, such as the high levels of ammonia produced by some strains such as *P. melaninogenica*, also may be capable of damaging host tissues.

Interaction with host defenses also contributes to pathogenesis but is, as yet, incompletely understood. Certain strains of *Bacteroides*, *Fusobacterium*, and *Prevotella* have been shown to activate complement by both classic and alternate pathways, resulting in generation of chemotactic factors and leading to local accumulation of leukocytes.[65] Capsular polysaccharides then protect against phagocytosis, although the mechanism of the protection is unknown.[7] An effect of T lymphocytes on both the development of and protection from abscess formation has been demonstrated.[90] Certain suppressor T cells appear to contribute to abscess formation, perhaps through the elaboration of chemoattractants of polymorphonuclear leukocytes. A second suppressor T cell appears to play a role in the protection against abscess formation in the animal model, perhaps through the elaboration of a lymphokine that binds the capsular polysaccharide responsible for abscess formation.[90] The interaction between these two processes is not understood fully.

IMMUNOLOGY

The immune mechanisms involved in anaerobic infections are poorly understood. The toxin-produced diseases of tetanus and botulism are known to be prevented or modified by specific antibody, and the role of protective immunity has been documented clearly. In animal studies, inoculation with the capsular polysaccharide of *B. fragilis* provided protection against abscess formation on subsequent challenge.[39, 63] This effect was shown to be T-cell mediated, whereas humoral immune responses affected the clearance of bacteria in the bacteremic phase of the infection. No data in this regard are available from humans. Opsonophagocytosis and intracellular killing of several *Bacteroides* species have been shown to be facilitated by IgM antibodies but not by IgG or IgA in normal human sera.[7] The alternate pathway of complement also is required in this process.[6] Definitive data from humans regarding the development of specific immunity after infection or protection from subsequent infection are not available.[69]

CLINICAL MANIFESTATIONS

The common clinical syndromes in children that may be caused by anaerobic organisms are listed in Table 156–3. Tetanus, botulism, and actinomycosis are discussed in other chapters.

In general, the clinical appearance of these infections is not different from that of similar infections caused by facultative organisms. Gas formation may be seen with facultative organisms as well as *Clostridium* and other anaerobes. The major clinical distinction, when present, is the foul odor associated with anaerobic infection.

Anaerobic organisms may cause infection in most of the same sites seen in adults, although pleuropulmonary and pelvic anaerobic infections are unusual in children. Occasionally, children are seen with anaerobic osteomyelitis, soft tissue cellulitis and abscesses, and perinephric and scrotal abscesses. Meningitis caused by anaerobic organisms is reported only rarely in children.

TABLE 156–3. Clinical Infections Caused by Anaerobes in Children

Peritonitis and peritoneal abscess
Wound infection after abdominal surgery
Bacteremia associated with gastrointestinal disease
Septicemia in immunocompromised host
Abscesses and cellulitis associated with oropharyngeal disease
Cervical adenitis
Otitis media
Dental abscess; periodontitis
Peritonsillar abscess
Branchial cleft cyst infection
Paranasal sinusitis
Ludwig angina
Human and animal bites
Soft tissue cellulitis, including paronychia
Cholangitis associated with Kasai procedure for biliary hypoplasia
Brain abscess

Because of the toxins produced, significant systemic disease may accompany local anaerobic infections. Endotoxin is elaborated by gram-negative anaerobes, and typical endotoxin shock may occur with serious anaerobic infections. In addition, hemolysis, vascular collapse, jaundice, and severe toxigenic diarrhea may result from toxins elaborated by *Clostridium* and *Fusobacterium*.[2, 8, 38]

The classic syndromes of gas gangrene, progressive synergistic gangrene, synergistic necrotizing cellulitis, nonclostridial crepitant cellulitis, chronic burrowing ulcer, and necrotizing fasciitis are manifestations of anaerobic or mixed soft tissue infections, and all are rare in children. This probably results from the generally healthy vascular supply to children's tissues. When a compromised blood supply is present, these characteristic infections may occur just as they do in adults.[100]

The specific anaerobic strains isolated from anaerobic infections usually are those endogenous flora common to the anatomic site involved. Abdominal infections and associated septicemia commonly are caused by *B. fragilis, Fusobacterium,* and *Clostridium*.[13, 70] Primary anaerobic septicemia in immune-compromised children also is caused most frequently by these organisms and therefore is believed to be due to invasion by gastrointestinal microbes. Ascending cholangitis in infants who have undergone surgical palliation for biliary atresia is a complication that may involve anaerobic as well as aerobic gastrointestinal organisms.

Deep cellulitis and abscess formation around the oropharynx, including peritonsillar abscess, periodontitis, dental abscess, and secondary facial cellulitis, most commonly involve *P. melaninogenica, Porphyromonas asaccharolytica, Fusobacterium, Peptostreptococcus,* and, occasionally, *B. fragilis* or other *Bacteroides* species.[30, 77] Aerobes commonly are isolated concomitantly. The syndrome of Ludwig angina has a characteristic clinical picture of rapidly progressive, submental, spreading cellulitis, which elevates the tongue from the floor of the mouth and may encroach on the airway. Systemic toxicity usually is severe. The organisms involved usually are *Fusobacterium* and anaerobic cocci. Spirochetes may be seen in aspirated material.[72] Soft tissue infections after contamination of wounds may be caused by *Clostridium,* anaerobic gram-positive cocci, or these organisms in combination with aerobic streptococci or staphylococci. Gram-negative aerobic or anaerobic organisms may be involved as well. Wound infections of human or animal bites typically involve anaerobes among their polymicrobial flora.[21, 47, 49]

The clinical manifestations of brain abscess due to anaerobic organisms are indistinguishable from those involving only aerobes. The predominant anaerobes in these abscesses include *Peptostreptococcus, B. fragilis, Veillonella,* and *Fusobacterium*.[16, 71]

DIAGNOSIS

The diagnosis of anaerobic infection requires a high index of suspicion and Gram stain and culture of material collected in the appropriate manner. Culture of the organisms is the only method of confirming clinical suspicion. In obtaining material to be cultured, care must be taken to aspirate the infected site directly without contamination by endogenous flora of mucous membranes. Purulent material obtained after incision of abscesses may yield unreliable results. Similarly, expectorated sputum or drainage from mastoids and sinuses may be contaminated by mucosal flora, and the culture may be rendered unreliable. These materials should be obtained by aspiration, bypassing the oropharyngeal mucosa.[27, 33] Gram-stained smears of all aspirated material should be examined for characteristic forms as described in Table 156–2 and used to complement culture results, which may be compromised by the fastidious nature of many anaerobic pathogens. Direct immunofluorescence of these materials using specific antibodies for a variety of organisms, most specifically *B. fragilis* and *P. melaninogenica*, has been useful in some instances for rapid diagnosis, although nonspecific reactions do occur.[101] Culture material must be handled with care and dispatch, as described previously, to ensure recovery of organisms. Radiographs demonstrating gas in infected tissues may be helpful but are nonspecific. Enzyme immunoassay kits for the rapid detection of *C. difficile* toxins in stool are commercially available. Sensitivities between 93 per cent and 100 per cent have been reported.[1]

Other modes of more rapid diagnosis, including immunologic detection of anaerobic bacterial antigens in body fluids and gas-liquid chromatography analysis of infected fluids, have not been perfected. Lack of specificity remains a problem with the use of gas-liquid chromatography on clinical specimens, and latex particle agglutination and enzyme-linked immunosorbent assay[55, 76] have not reached the level of reliability achieved by systems in use for diagnosis of aerobic infections. Nucleic acid hybridization techniques are not yet sufficiently reliable or practical for adoption in the clinical laboratory.[66] Antibodies to certain anaerobic toxins are detectable in human sera, but these have not become clinically useful except in the case of tetanus or botulism.

TREATMENT

The treatment of anaerobic infection usually involves appropriate débridement and antibiotic therapy. Other therapeutic modalities have been proposed and used in certain instances, but experience in children generally is limited, and clear-cut recommendations are not available.

As in the case of aerobic abscess formation, anaerobic abscesses usually require incision and drainage. Deep abscesses in the abdominal cavity should be opened and drained and the area irrigated with physiologic saline, if possible, to increase the local Eh and minimize recurrent growth of anaerobes. Generalized peritonitis may respond best to this therapy as well. Anaerobic lung abscess and empyema, which are rare in children, require drainage, but irrigation rarely is indicated. As an alternative to surgical incision and drainage, percutaneous drainage guided by any of several different imaging techniques has been utilized successfully in the treatment of a variety of different abscesses.[28, 44, 54]

Anaerobic abscesses associated with the oropharynx usually respond to incision and drainage without irrigation, although excision of such malformations as branchial cleft cyst should be performed. Brain abscesses of sufficient size generally respond best to drainage, although computed tomography has documented the resolution of even some large abscesses with prolonged medical therapy alone. The occurrence of multiple or loculated abscesses may make surgical drainage impractical. Most authorities agree, however, that the outcome for abscesses larger than 2 cm in diameter is improved by drainage and that excision remains the management of choice for well-encapsulated lesions. Smaller lesions and those documented prior to encapsulation commonly respond to prolonged medical therapy alone.[3, 5, 71]

Surgical management of anaerobic cellulitis usually requires prompt and extensive débridement in addition to antibiotic therapy to prevent spread and more extensive tissue loss. This particularly is true of clostridial gas gangrene, but it also is necessary in progressive synergistic gangrene, necrotizing fasciitis, and anaerobic myositis. In contrast to aerobic soft tissue infections, severe anaerobic cellulitis frequently does not respond to antibiotics alone.[61, 95, 100] This may be due to the fact that most antibiotics function poorly in the markedly reduced Eh of anaerobic infections.

The choice of antibiotics for the management of anaerobic infection in general must be based on a recognition of the organisms likely to be involved in various anatomic sites and on published studies of susceptibilities. Antibiotic susceptibility studies should be obtained on pathogens isolated in order to guide the choice of the most effective and least toxic agents. Media and equipment now are commercially available, and, given the variability in susceptibility patterns observed nationwide, such testing is important in determining optimal therapy.[40, 43, 85]

Most gram-positive anaerobes, *Veillonella*, and *Fusobacterium* species (except *F. nucleatum*) are, to date, sensitive to clinically achievable levels of penicillin. Semisynthetic penicillin derivatives, such as ampicillin, methicillin, oxacillin, and nafcillin, are less active than the parent compound, but the very high levels of these drugs achieved with the parenteral administration of large doses appear to be adequate in some cases. Nonetheless, when infection due to anaerobes expected to be sensitive to penicillin is suspected, penicillin G should be used. Penicillin V is less effective. Penicillin G should be administered in doses of 100,000 to 200,000 U/kg/day. Intravenous ampicillin, oxacillin, and methicillin, if used, should be given in divided doses of 200 mg/kg/day. Oral penicillin G may be used in similar doses in patients who do not require intensive intravenous therapy.

Agents effective against penicillin-resistant anaerobic strains have been sought for a number of years. The organism that most commonly presents this problem is *B. fragilis*, although a growing proportion of other *Bacteroides* species, *P. melaninogenica*, *Porphyromonas* species, *F. nucleatum*, and occasional *Clostridium* species now demonstrate resistance.

In general, clindamycin is the drug of choice for suspected serious penicillin-resistant infections in children because of its overall efficacy and low potential for toxicity. Pseudomembranous enterocolitis occurs rarely in children and more frequently is associated with other antimicrobial agents.[99] A growing proportion of *Bacteroides* species demonstrate in vitro resistance to clindamycin, whereas they remain sensitive to imipenem-cilastatin and to metronidazole. Penicillins in combination with beta-lactamase inhibitors (clavulanic acid, sulbactam, and tazobactam) also have demonstrated good activity against penicillin-resistant bacteria.[12, 18, 88, 96] For superficial infections, such as cellulitis and bite wound infections, amoxicillin–clavulanate potassium has become the drug of choice.

Chloramphenicol remains the drug of choice for penicillin-resistant central nervous system infections because of its excellent penetration of the central nervous system, whereas clindamycin does not cross the blood-brain barrier. Metronidazole is being used increasingly for anaerobic infections, including brain abscess, with apparently good results.[60, 68] Comparative clinical trials in children are not available, but its excellent bactericidal activity against the penicillin-resistant anaerobes makes metronidazole an attractive drug for these serious infections. It should be combined with penicillin or an aminoglycoside because concomitant aerobic infection usually is present.[88]

The extended-generation cephalosporins on the market and in development exhibit variable efficacy against all groups of anaerobes and should not be relied upon without culture results demonstrating susceptibility to these agents.[48, 50, 84] The ureido penicillins demonstrate broader activity than the cephalosporins, but their inhibitory concentrations are significantly higher than those of any of the "first-line" drugs.[45, 46] Older first-generation cephalosporins and aminoglycosides, frequently used for aerobic gram-negative infections, have no activity against *B. fragilis*.

The dose of clindamycin is 20 to 40 mg/kg/day in three or four divided intravenous doses, with the higher dose being administered in severe illnesses. Similar doses of clindamycin can be administered orally when the clinical response and condition of the patient warrant. Imipenem, with which there is relatively little pediatric experience and no label indication, generally is used in doses of 60 to 100 mg/kg/day divided every 6 hours. Dose adjustment must be made for patients with significant renal impairment. Metronidazole has been used in the same doses administered to adults, although safety and efficacy have not been determined. The dose is 15 mg/kg as an intravenous loading dose and a maintenance dose of 30 mg/kg/day in four divided doses. Accumulation of drug has been demonstrated in patients with significant hepatic dysfunction.

Amoxicillin–clavulanate potassium is administered at 20 mg/kg/day (amoxicillin component) in three divided doses for children weighing less than 40 kg, but for treatment of otitis media, sinusitis, lower respiratory tract infections, and serious infections, the dose is 40 mg/kg/day. Adult dose levels are used for children weighing more than 40 kg (500-mg tablets for respiratory tract infections and serious infections, 250-mg tablets for other infections). Piperacillin-tazobactam and ampicillin-sulbactam, neither of which has a label indication or significant reported pediatric experience, are dosed at 200 to 300 mg/kg/day (penicillin component) in four divided doses; the higher dose should be used for more serious infections. Amoxicillin-clavulanate and piperacillin-tazobactam both are associated with a significant incidence of gastrointestinal side effects, whereas ampicillin-sulbactam appears to be free of this complication. Only amoxicillin-clavulanate is available in oral dosage forms, whereas the other agents require parenteral administration.

Chloramphenicol succinate is administered to children with normal hepatic function and infants older than 3 months of age in a dose of 100 mg/kg/day in four divided intravenous doses. Younger infants and children with hepatic dysfunction should receive 25 to 50 mg/kg/day in two or four divided intravenous infusions, the lower dose being administered to premature infants and those younger than 2 weeks of age. It is imperative that serum levels of chloramphenicol be monitored in young infants receiving the drug in order to maintain therapeutic and nontoxic levels. Serum levels between 15 and 30 μg/mL meet this requirement. Concurrent concentrations of chloramphenicol in the cerebrospinal fluid are 40 to 60 per cent of blood levels.[41] Assessment of bone marrow function by complete blood count, reticulocyte count, and platelet count should be performed frequently during chloramphenicol therapy. An absolute neutrophil count of less than 1000 is an indication to interrupt administration of the drug.

The duration of antimicrobial therapy for anaerobic infections does not differ from that recommended for the same infections of aerobic etiology. Minor soft tissue infections generally are treated for 10 to 14 days, septicemia for 10 days to 3 weeks, bone and joint infections for 6 weeks or more, and brain abscesses for 6 to 8 weeks or more.

Hyperbaric oxygen has been used and recommended by some for the treatment of rapidly progressive anaerobic infections, particularly the soft tissue infections of gas gangrene and necrotizing fasciitis. This mode of therapy may reduce the systemic toxicity of these diseases and may prevent the spread of infection with its attendant need for further surgical débridement. The potential toxicity of this therapy is significant and its value in children uncertain; it should be administered only by experienced physicians in adequate facilities. Hyperbaric oxygen does not obviate the need for standard therapy with surgery and antibiotics.[62, 100]

Antitoxin should be administered to patients with tetanus, and polyvalent clostridial antitoxin has been helpful in lowering the mortality associated with gas gangrene in patients with war wounds. Little experience with this latter material is available in civilian patients or, more particularly, in children. Recommendations for this mode of therapy are presented in other chapters.

PROGNOSIS

The outcome for patients with severe anaerobic infections generally is related to the severity of underlying disease and to the rapidity with which the infection is recognized and treated effectively with surgery or appropriate antibiotics. Peritonitis, peritoneal abscess, and abdominal wound infection in otherwise normal hosts carry a good prognosis when their anaerobic etiology is recognized, surgical drainage and débridement are carried out, and an antibiotic effective against *B. fragilis* is administered. This also is true of secondary septicemia associated with intra-abdominal anaerobic infection. When endotoxic shock, disseminated intravascular coagulopathy, or metastatic foci of infection supervene, the prognosis for favorable outcome diminishes and reflects the effectiveness of treatment for these complications. Anaerobic septicemia in patients with malignancy or other compromise of immunity carries a poor prognosis, as does generalized bacterial infection of any etiology.

Data regarding the prognosis of anaerobic bacteremia in infants are conflicting and probably reflect differing circumstances under which cultures are obtained. Transient anaerobic bacteremia in newborn infants occurs approximately one tenth as frequently as aerobic bacteremia and appears to cause little or no morbidity and a reported mortality rate of 4 per cent. When anaerobic bacteremia produced clinical disease in a prospective series of patients, the mortality rate was 37.5 per cent and probably reflected the severity of underlying disease, such as necrotizing enterocolitis, which accompanied or preceded the infection.[42, 53]

Abscesses and cellulitis surrounding the oropharynx have an almost uniformly good prognosis with adequate drainage and antimicrobial therapy. The complications of airway compromise, spontaneous rupture into pharynx or trachea, carotid artery invasion, jugular venous thrombosis, and dissection into the neck or mediastinum are rare. Cavernous sinus thrombosis is a potentially fatal complication of sinusitis. All these complications are exceedingly rare, probably because most children with suppurative infections of this nature receive some form of penicillin to which anaerobes are sensitive, even when anaerobic infection is not suspected.

Superficial anaerobic cellulitis and abscesses respond well to débridement and appropriate antibiotics. Progressive soft tissue infections caused by toxin-producing anaerobes, such as *Clostridium*, however, carry a very poor prognosis for saving the affected limb, and death may occur in as many as 15 per cent of cases, despite vigorous therapy.[100]

Anaerobic cholangitis in patients who have undergone the Kasai procedure is difficult to eradicate, primarily because of the underlying biliary pathology. The poor prognosis of this disease reflects this problem.

The prognosis in patients with brain abscess relates almost entirely to the neuroanatomic location of the abscess, the ease with which it can be drained surgically, and the degree to which the mass effect of the abscess and surrounding edema compromises the intracranial contents. The mortality rate overall approaches 20 per cent, although lesions located in the cerebral hemispheres carry a significantly better prognosis than those in the cerebellum or brain stem structures. Death commonly occurs after rupture of the abscess into the ventricular system, brain stem herniation, or iatrogenic intracranial hemorrhage. Of importance, such hemorrhage has been observed in approximately 10 per cent of patients undergoing needle aspiration of abscesses. Patients who present with severely altered mental status have a very poor prognosis.[71]

PREVENTION

Because the majority of anaerobic infections are caused by endogenous flora, prevention through isolation techniques or immunization generally is not possible. Severe anaerobic infections caused by bowel flora after gastrointestinal compromise or perforation frequently can be prevented by early and judicious surgery combined with appropriate antibiotic coverage for *B. fragilis* in addition to aerobic pathogens involved. This therapy really constitutes early treatment for infection rather than prophylaxis. Similar management of other potentially contaminated sites may prevent the development of severe infection.

Superficial wounds that are expected to be contaminated by anaerobes should be irrigated copiously and allowed to heal by secondary intention, if possible. This particularly is true of the ragged lacerations caused by animal or human bites. Appropriate antibiotics may help to prevent severe infection.

The only disease caused by anaerobes for which active immunization is possible is tetanus, which is described in another chapter. Passive immunity to tetanus in the form of human hyperimmune antiserum should be given to patients with severe, contaminated wounds.

References

1. Altaie, S. S., Meyer, P., and Dryja, D.: Comparison of two commercially available enzyme immunoassays for detection of *Clostridium difficile* in stool specimens. J. Clin. Microbiol. *32*:51–53, 1994.
2. Banno, Y., Kobayashi, T., Kono, H., et al.: Biochemical characterization and biologic actions of two toxins (D-1 and D-2) from *Clostridium difficile*. Rev. Infect. Dis. *6*:S11–24, 1984.
3. Barsoum, A. H., Lewis, H. C., and Cannillo, K. L.: Nonoperative treatment of multiple brain abscesses. Surg. Neurol. *16*:283–287, 1981.
4. Beaucage, C. M., and Onderdonk, A. B.: Evaluation of a pre-reduced anaerobically sterilized medium (PRAS II) system for identification of anaerobic organisms. J. Clin. Microbiol. *16*:570–572, 1982.
5. Berg, B., Franklin, G., Cuneo, R., et al.: Nonsurgical cure of brain abscess: Early diagnosis and follow-up with computerized tomography. Ann. Neurol. *3*:474–478, 1978.
6. Bjornson, A. B.: Role of complement in host resistance against members of the *Bacteroidaceae*. Rev. Infect. Dis. *6*:S34–39, 1984.
7. Bjornson, A. B., Bjornson, H. S., and Kitko, B. P.: Participation of normal human immunoglobulins M, G, and A in opsonophagocytosis and intracellular killing of *B. fragilis* and *B. thetaiotaomicron* by human polymorphonuclear leukocytes. Infect. Immun. *28*:633–637, 1980.
8. Bjornson, H. S.: Activation of Hageman factor by lipopolysaccharides of *B. fragilis*, *B. vulgatus* and *Fusobacterium mortiferum*. Rev. Infect. Dis. *6*:S30–33, 1984.
9. Brook, I.: Aerobic and anaerobic bacteriology of cervical adenitis in children. Clin. Pediatr. (Phila.) *19*:693–696, 1980.
10. Brook, I.: Aerobic and anaerobic bacteriology of chronic mastoiditis in children. Am. J. Dis. Child. *135*:478–479, 1981.
11. Brook, I.: Aerobic and anaerobic bacteriology of peritonsillar abscess in children. Acta Paediatr. Scand. *70*:831–835, 1981.
12. Brook, I.: Anaerobic infections in children with neurological impairments. Am. J. Ment. Ret. *99*:579–594, 1995.
13. Brook, I.: Bacterial studies of peritoneal cavity and postoperative surgical wound drainage following perforated appendix in children. Ann. Surg. *192*:208–212, 1980.
14. Brook, I.: Bacteriologic features of chronic sinusitis in children. J. A. M. A. *246*:967–969, 1981.
15. Brook, I.: Bacteriologic study of paronychia in children. Am. J. Surg. *141*:703–705, 1981.
16. Brook, I.: Bacteriology of intracranial abscess in children. J. Neurosurg. *54*:484–488, 1981.
17. Brook, I.: Chronic otitis media in children: Microbiological studies. Am. J. Dis. Child. *134*:564–566, 1980.
18. Brook, I.: Controversies in anaerobic infections in childhood. Curr. Probl. Pediatr. *17*:557–660, 1987.
19. Brook, I.: Direct and indirect pathogenicity of anaerobic bacteria in respiratory tract infections in children. Adv. Pediatr. *34*:357–378, 1987.
20. Brook, I.: Intra-abdominal infections in children. Drugs *46*:53–62, 1993.
21. Brook, I.: Microbiology of human and animal bite wounds in children. Pediatr. Infect. Dis. J. *6*:29–32, 1987.
22. Brook, I.: Peptostreptococcal infection in children. Scand. J. Infect. Dis. *26*:503–510, 1994.
23. Brook, I.: Microbiology of chronic otitis media with perforation in children. Microbiologic studies. Am. J. Dis. Child. *134*:564–566, 1980.
24. Brook, I.: The role of anaerobic bacteria in pediatric infections. Adv. Pediatr. *27*:163–197, 1980.
25. Brook, I., Calhoun, L. and Yocum, P.: Beta-lactamase–producing isolates of *Bacteroides* species from children. Antimicrob. Agents Chemother. *18*:164–166, 1980.
26. Brook, I., and Finegold, S. M.: Aerobic and anaerobic bacteriology of cutaneous abscesses in children. Pediatrics *67*:891–895, 1981.
27. Brook, I., and Finegold, S. M.: Bacteriology and therapy of lung abscess in children. J. Pediatr. *94*:10–12, 1979.
28. Brook, I., and Fraizer, E. H.: Role of anaerobic bacteria in liver abscesses in children. Pediatr. Infect. Dis. J. *12*:743–746, 1993.
29. Brook, I., Friedman, E., Rodriguez, W. J., et al.: Complications of sinusitis in children. Pediatrics *66*:568–572, 1980.
30. Brook, I., Grimm, S., and Kielich, R. B.: Bacteriology of acute periapical abscess in children. J. Endodontics *7*:378–380, 1981.
31. Brook, I., Myhal, L. A., and Dorsey, C. H.: Encapsulation and pilus formation of *Bacteroides* spp. in normal flora, abscesses and blood. J. Infect. *25*:251–257, 1992.
32. Brook, I., and Schwartz, R.: Anaerobic bacteria in acute otitis media. Acta Otolaryngol. *91*:111–114, 1981.
33. Brook, I., Yocum, P., and Shah, K.: Surface vs. core-tonsillar aerobic and anaerobic flora in recurrent tonsillitis. J. A. M. A. *244*:1696–1698, 1980.
34. Busch, D. F.: Anaerobes in infection of the head and neck and ear, nose and throat. Rev. Infect. Dis. *6*:S115–122, 1984.
35. Chow, A. W., Leake, R. D., Yamauchi, T., et al.: The significance of anaerobes in neonatal bacteremia: Analysis of 23 cases and review of the literature. Pediatrics *54*:736–745, 1974.
36. Citron, D. M.: Specimen collection and transport, anaerobic culture techniques and identification of anaerobes. Rev. Infect. Dis. *6*:S51–58, 1984.
37. Collee, J. G.: Factors contributing to loss of anaerobic bacteria in transit from the patient to the laboratory. Infection *8*:S145–147, 1980.
38. Coyle-Dennis, J. E., and Lauerman, L. H.: Correlations between leukocidin production and virulence of two isolates of *Fusobacterium necrophorum*. Am. J. Vet. Res. *40*:274–276, 1979.
39. Crabb, J. H., Finberg, R., Onderdonk, A. B., et al.: T cell regulation of *Bacteroides fragilis*–induced intraabdominal abscesses. Rev. Infect. Dis. *12*(Suppl. 2):S178–184, 1990.
40. Cuchural, G., Jacobus, N., Gorbach, S. L., et al.: A survey of *Bacteroides* susceptibility in the United States. J. Antimicrob. Chemother. *8*:27–31, 1981.
41. Dunkle, L. M.: Central nervous system chloramphenicol concentration in premature infants. Antimicrob. Agents Chemother. *13*:427–429, 1978.
42. Dunkle, L. M., Brotherton, T. J., and Feigin, R. D.: Anaerobic infections in children: A prospective survey. Pediatrics *57*:311–320, 1976.
43. Edson, R. S., Rosenblatt, J. E., Lee, D. T., et al.: Recent experience with antimicrobial susceptibility of anaerobic bacteria. Mayo Clin. Proc. *57*:734–741, 1982.
44. Finegold, S. M.: Future aspects of the treatment and prophylaxis of anaerobic infections. Drugs Exp. Clin. Res. *X*(3):179–185, 1984.
45. Fu, K. P., and Neu, H. C.: Azlocillin and mezlocillin: New ureido penicillins. Antimicrob. Agents Chemother. *13*:930–938, 1978.
46. Fu, K. P., and Neu, H. C.: Piperacillin, a new penicillin active against many bacteria resistant to other penicillins. Antimicrob. Agents Chemother. *13*:358–367, 1978.
47. Goldstein, E. J. C.: Bite wounds and infection. Clin. Infect. Dis. *14*:633–640, 1992.
48. Goldstein, E. J. C.: Selected nonsurgical anaerobic infections: Therapeutic choices and the effective armamentarium. Clin. Infect. Dis. *18*(Suppl. 4):S273–S279, 1994.
49. Goldstein, E. J. C., and Richwald, G. A.: Human and animal bite wounds. Am. Fam. Phys. (U. S.) *36*:101–109, 1987.
50. Gorbach, S. L.: Antibiotic treatment of anaerobic infections. Clin. Infect. Dis. *18*(Suppl.4):S305–S310, 1994.

51. Gorbach, S. L., and Bartlett, J. G.: Anaerobic infections. N. Engl. J. Med. *290*:1177–1184, 1237–1245, 1289–1294, 1974.
52. Hansen, S. L., and Stewart, B. J.: Comparison of API and Minitek to CDC methods for the biochemical characterization of anaerobes. J. Clin. Microbiol. *4*:227–231, 1976.
53. Harrod, J. R., and Stevens, D. A.: Anaerobic infections in the newborn infant. J. Pediatr. *85*:399–402, 1974.
54. Hasdemir, M. G., and Ebeling, U.: CT-guided stereotactic aspiration and treatment of brain abscesses. Acta Neurochir. (Wien) *125*:58–63, 1993.
55. Hazenberg, M. P., van de Merwe, J. P., Pēna, A. S., et al.: Antibodies to *Coprococcus comes* in sera of patients with Crohn's disease: Isolation and purification of the agglutinating antigen tested with an ELISA technique. J. Clin. Lab. Immunol. *23*:143–148, 1987.
56. Heimdahl, A., Vonkonow, L., and Nord, C. E.: Isolation of beta-lactamase–producing *Bacteroides* strains associated with clinical failures with penicillin treatment of human orofacial infection. Arch. Oral Biol. *25*:689–692, 1980.
57. Hewitt, L. F.: Influence of hydrogen ion concentration and oxidation-reduction conditions on bacterial behavior. Symposia Soc. Gen. Microbiol. *7*:42, 1957.
58. Hofstad, T.: Pathogenicity of anaerobic gram negative rods: Possible mechanisms. Rev. Infect. Dis. *6*:189–199, 1984.
59. Holdeman, L. V., Cato, E. P., and Moore, W. E. C. (eds.): Anaerobic Laboratory Manual. Blacksburg, Anaerobe Laboratory, Virginia Polytechnic Institute and State University, 1977.
60. Jacobs, J. A., Hendriks, J. J. E., Verschure, P. D. M., et al.: Meningitis due to *Fusobacterium necrophorum* subspecies *necrophorum:* Case report and review of the literature. Infection *21*:57–60, 1993.
61. Jonsimies-Somer, H. R., and Finegold, S. M.: Problems encountered in clinical anaerobic bacteriology. Rev. Infect. Dis. *6*:S45–S50, 1984.
62. Kaiser, R. E., and Cerra, F. B.: Progressive necrotizing surgical infections: A unified approach. J. Trauma *21*:349–353, 1981.
63. Kasper, D. L., Finberg, R. F., Crabb, J., et al.: Immune mechanisms in the prevention of intra-abdominal abscess formation. Scand. J. Infect. Dis. *62*(Suppl.):29–34, 1989.
64. Kasper, D. L., Lindberg, A. A., Weintraub, A., et al.: Capsular polysaccharides and lipopolysaccharides from two strains of *Bacteroides fragilis.* Rev. Infect. Dis. *6*:S25–S29, 1984.
65. Klempner, M. S.: Interactions of polymorphonuclear leukocytes with anaerobic bacteria. Rev. Infect. Dis. *6*:S40–S43, 1984.
66. Kuritza, A. P., Getty, C. E., Shaughnessy, P., et al.: DNA probes for identification of clinically important *Bacteroides* species. J. Clin. Microbiol. *23*:343–349, 1986.
67. Lee, S. W., Alexander, B., and McGowan, B.: Purification, characterization and serologic characteristics of *Bacteroides nodosus* pili and use of a purified pili vaccine in sheep. Am. J. Vet. Res. *44*:1676–1681, 1983.
68. Lerner, D. N., Choi, S. S., Zalzal, G. H., et al.: Intracranial complications of sinusitis in childhood. Ann. Otol. Rhinol. Laryngol. *104*:288–293, 1995.
69. Lindberg, A. A., Weintraub, A., and Nord, C. E.: The humeral antibody response to *Bacteroides fragilis* infections in humans. Scand. Infect. Dis. *19*:46–51, 1979.
70. Marchildon, M. B., and Dudgeon, D. L.: Perforated appendicitis: Current experience in a children's hospital. Ann. Surg. *185*:84–87, 1977.
71. Mathiesen, G. E., Meyer, R. D., George, W. L., et al.: Brain abscess and cerebritis. Rev. Infect. Dis. *6*:S101–S106, 1984.
72. Meyers, B. R., Lawson, W., and Hirschman, S. Z.: Ludwig's angina: Case report with review of bacteriology and current therapy. Am. J. Med. *53*:257–260, 1972.
73. Moore, L. V. H., and Moore, W. E. C.: Anaerobe Lab Manual Update, Virginia Polytechnic Institute and State University, 1991.
74. Morris, J. G.: The biochemical basis of oxygen sensitivity. J. Gen. Microbiol. *60*:111, 1970.
75. Morris, J. G.: Oxygen tolerance/intolerance of anaerobic bacteria. *In* Gottschalk, G., Pennig, N., and Werner, H. (eds.): Anaerobes and Anaerobic Infections. Stuttgart, Gustav Fischer Verlag, 1980.
76. Nagahama, M., Kobayashi, K., Ochi, S., et al.: Enzyme-linked immunosorbent assay for rapid detection of toxins from *Clostridium perfringens.* FEMS Microbiol. Lett. *84*:41–44, 1991.
77. Newman, M. G.: Anaerobic oral and dental infection. Rev. Infect. Dis. *6*:S107–S114, 1984.
78. Ogden, J. A., and Light, T. R.: Pediatric osteomyelitis. III. Anaerobic microorganisms. Clin. Orthop. *145*:230–236, 1979.
79. Okuda, K., Slots, J., and Genco, R. J.: *Bacteroides gingivalis*, *Bacteroides asaccharolyticus*, and *Bacteroides melaninogenicus* subspecies: Cell surface morphology and adherence to erythrocytes and human buccal epithelial cells. Curr. Microbiol. *6*:7–12, 1981.
80. Onderdonk, A. B., Bartlett, J. G., Louie, T., et al.: Microbial synergy in experimental intra-abdominal abscess. Infect. Immun. *13*:22–26, 1976.
81. Onderdonk, A. B., Kasper, D. L., Cisneros, R. L., et al.: The capsular polysaccharide of *Bacteroides fragilis* as a virulence factor. J. Infect. Dis. *136*:82–89, 1977.
82. Onderdonk, A. B., Shapiro, M. E., Finberg, R. W., et al.: Use of a model of intra-abdominal sepsis for studies of the pathogenicity of *B. fragilis.* Rev. Infect. Dis. *6*:S91–S95, 1984.
83. Raff, M. J., and Melo, J. C.: Anaerobic osteomyelitis. Medicine *57*:83–103, 1978.
84. Rolfe, R. D., and Finegold, S. M.: Comparative in vitro activity of new beta-lactam antibiotics against anaerobic bacteria. Antimicrob. Agents Chemother. *20*:600–609, 1981.
85. Rosenblatt, J. E.: Antimicrobial susceptibility testing of anaerobic bacteria. Rev. Infect. Dis. *6*:S242–S248, 1984.
86. Rotstein, O. D.: Interactions between leukocytes and anaerobic bacteria in polymicrobial surgical infections. Clin. Infect. Dis. *16*(Suppl. 4):S190–S194, 1993.
87. Sabbaj, J.: Anaerobes in liver abscess. Rev. Infect. Dis. *6*:S152–S156, 1984.
88. Sanders, C. V., and Aldridge, K. E.: Antimicrobial therapy of anaerobic infections, 1991. Pharmacotherapy *11*(Pt. 2):72S–79S, 1991.
89. Shah, H. N., and Collins, D. M.: *Prevotella*, a new genus to include *Bacteroides melaninogenicus* and related species formerly classified in the genus *Bacteroides.* Int. J. Syst. Bacteriol. 205–208, April 1990.
90. Shapiro, M. E., Kasper, D. L., Zaleznik, D. F., et al.: Cellular control of abscess formation: Role of T cells in the regulation of abscesses formed in response to *Bacteroides fragilis.* J. Immunol. *137*:341–346, 1986.
91. Shapiro, M. E., Onderdonk, A. B., Kasper, D. L., et al.: Cellular immunity to *Bacteroides fragilis* capsular polysaccharide. J. Exp. Med. *155*:1188–1197, 1982.
92. Simon, G. L., Klempner, M. S., Kasper, D. L., et al.: Alterations in opsonophagocytic killing by neutrophils of *Bacteroides fragilis* associated with animal and laboratory passage: Effect of capsular polysaccharide. J. Infect. Dis. *145*:72–77, 1982.
93. Slots, J., and Gibbons, R. J.: Attachment of *Bacteroides melaninogenicus* subsp. *asaccharolyticus* to oral surfaces and its possible role in colonization of the mouth of periodontal pockets. Infect. Immun. *19*:254–264, 1978.
94. Smith, L. D.: Virulence factors of *C. perfringens.* Rev. Infect. Dis. *1*:254–260, 1979.
95. Stamenkovic, I., and Lew, P. D.: Early recognition of potentially fatal necrotizing fasciitis. N. Engl. J. Med. *310*:1689–1693, 1984.
96. Styrt, B., and Gorbach, S. L.: Recent developments in the understanding of the pathogenesis and treatment of anaerobic infections (second of two parts). N. Engl. J. Med. *321*:298–302, 1989.
97. Sugita, R., Kawamura, S., and Ichikawa, G.: Studies on anaerobic bacteria in chronic otitis media. Laryngoscope *91*:816–821, 1981.
98. Summanen, P., Baron, E. J., Citron, D. M., et al.: Wadsworth Anaerobic Bacteriology Manual. 5th ed. Belmont, CA, Star Publishing Co., 1993.
99. Viscidi, R. P., and Bartlett, J. G.: Antibiotic-associated pseudomembranous colitis in children. Pediatrics *67*:381–386, 1981.
100. Weinstein, L., and Barza, M. A.: Gas gangrene. N. Engl. J. Med. *289*:1129–1131, 1973.
101. Weissfeld, A. S., and Sonnenwirth, A. C.: Rapid detection and identification of *B. fragilis* and *B. melaninogenicus* by immunofluorescence. J. Clin. Microbiol. *13*:798–800, 1981.
102. Wren, M. W. D.: Multiple selective media for the isolation of anaerobic bacteria from clinical specimens. J. Clin. Pathol. *33*:61–65, 1980.

SECTION SEVENTEEN

VIRAL INFECTIONS

❏ ❏ ❏

157

NOMENCLATURE AND CLASSIFICATION OF VIRUSES

Joseph L. Melnick

HISTORY

Virology developed from pathology. Consequently, until the middle of the twentieth century, viruses were classified according to the diseases they caused rather than according to the properties of the virus particle. An explosive period of discovery and characterization of animal viruses then took place. Knowledge that has been gained about the viruses themselves has allowed establishment of taxonomic groupings for these agents. It appears that most of the major groups of viruses that infect vertebrates—at least those of human beings and of the animals important to humans—have been recognized and described. Many of the groupings, initially established on tentative and provisional bases, now appear to form real families and genera in which the members are related in fundamental ways. For example, the validity of the original classification of the enteroviruses together, on the basis of an enteric habitat and small size, is being borne out by x-ray crystallography and by sophisticated techniques of molecular virology, such as sequence homology, that compare the genetic makeup of different members of the group and their mode of replication. The change has been reflected in the name of the committee responsible for such matters. The original name, International Committee on Nomenclature of Viruses (ICNV), was changed in 1974 to International Committee on Taxonomy of Viruses (ICTV).

The ICNV was established in 1966 at a historic international meeting in Moscow, the capital of the country in which viruses first had been discovered 75 years earlier by Ivanovski. Several reports of the ICNV/ICTV have been published,[12, 23, 25a, 43, 44, 72] dealing with viruses of humans, lower animals, insects, plants, and bacteria, as well as viruses of fungi and even mycoplasma; summaries of the properties of these groups of viruses as related to their taxonomic placement also have been included. Specialized study groups and subcommittees make recommendations to the ICTV regarding particular groupings or aspects of viral taxonomy. Reports on this work appeared regularly in *Intervirology* and now in *Archives of Virology*, the journal of the Virology Section of the IUMS (International Union of Microbiological Societies). Other reviews also are available on virus taxonomy and its historical development[11, 45] and on the taxonomy of vertebrate viruses.[2, 48, 49]

Figures 157–1 and 157–2 provide reference points for the discussion of classification that follows. Comparison of these figures also illustrates the patterns of development in knowledge of virus composition and structure. Figure 157–1 is taken from a text first published in 1967[18]; it remains fundamentally applicable in present-day virology. Figure 157–2 not only includes additional knowledge gained but also illustrates the variety of size and structure found among the viruses of vertebrates.[44]

Viruses now are separated into families on the basis of type and form of the nucleic acid genome and the size, shape, substructure, and mode of replication of the virus particle. Within each family, classifications of genera and species are based on antigenicity in addition to other properties. In some families, subfamilies and subgenera also have been set apart.

Figures 157–3 to 157–7 are schematic diagrams illustrating separation of viruses of vertebrates into 21 families. Figure 157–3 includes vertebrate viruses that have a DNA genome, cubic capsid symmetry, and a naked, unenveloped nucleocapsid. Figure 157–4 depicts DNA-containing viruses that have envelopes or complex coats. RNA-containing viruses are presented in three figures: Figure 157–5, those with cubic capsid symmetry; Figure 157–6, those with capsids having helical symmetry; and Figure 157–7, those with either asymmetric or unknown capsid architecture. Comments follow concerning these virus families and some emerging challenges for viral taxonomists.

The members of virus families and the genera to which they belong are given in Table 157–1.

ARBOVIRUSES

More than 350 agents are known as the arbovirus group.[6] These arthropod-borne viruses survive in nature through a complex cycle involving vertebrate hosts and arthropods. The latter serve as vectors transmitting the viruses by their bites. This ecologic grouping of the arboviruses, based on transmission, remains very useful epidemiologically despite the wide diversity of its members with regard to properties of the virion. Most arboviruses now have been characterized sufficiently well to permit their taxonomic placement into virus families. Their classic serologic interrelationships previously delineated by arbovirologists have been found to be paralleled by morphologic similarities. Arboviruses now are included in a number of families, chiefly **Togaviridae, Flaviviridae, Bunyaviridae, Rhabdoviridae, Arenaviridae,** and **Reoviridae.**

THE HEPATITIS VIRUSES

At least five viruses belonging to different families now are recognized as pathogens causing inflammation and necrosis of the liver (Table 157–2).[30]

Hepatitis A Virus (HAV)

This virus originally was classified as enterovirus 72, within the family **Picornaviridae.** It now is clear, however,

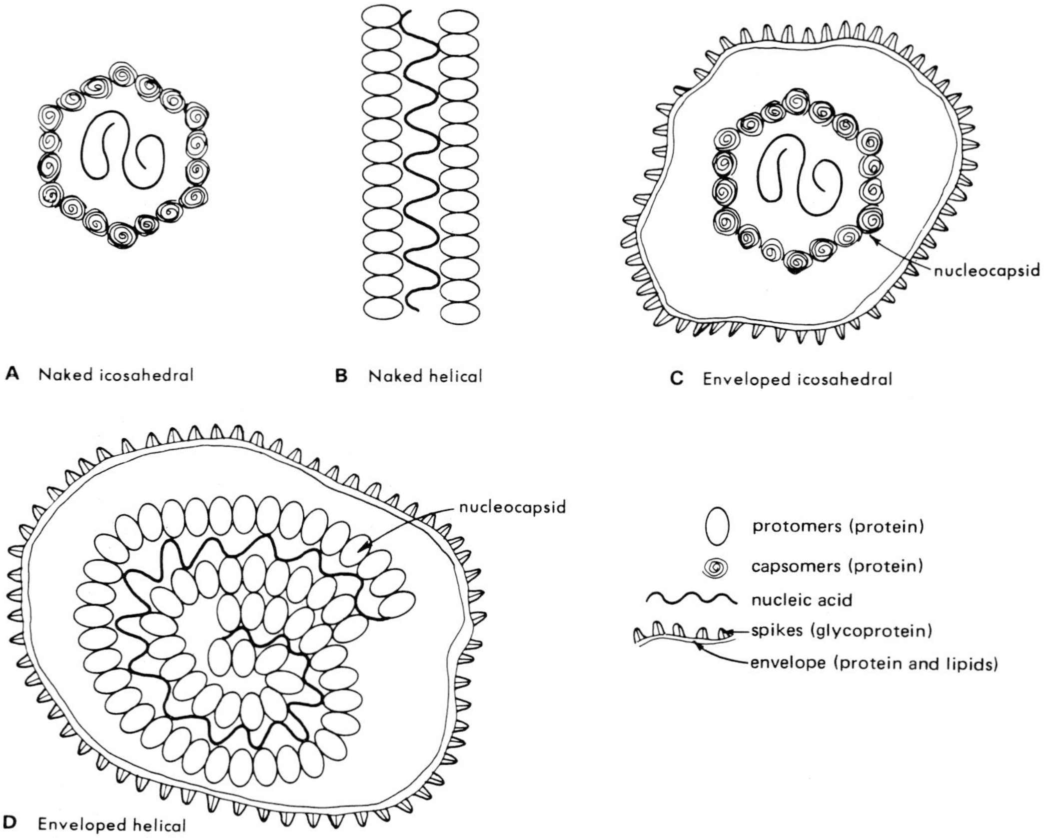

FIGURE 157–1. *Schematic diagram of simple forms of virions and their components. The naked icosahedral virions resemble small crystals; the naked helical virions resemble rods with a fine regular helical pattern in their surface. The enveloped icosahedral virions are made up of icosahedral nucleocapsids surrounded by the envelope; the enveloped helical virions are helical nucleocapsids bent to form a coarse, often irregular, coil within the envelope. (From Davis, B. D., Dulbecco, R., Eisen, H. N., et al.: Microbiology. 4th ed. Philadelphia, J. B. Lippincott, 1990, p. 772.)*

that HAV is sufficiently different from other members of **Picornaviridae** to warrant the establishment of a fifth genus, *Heparnavirus* (hepa-RNA-virus), denoting the hepatotropism of this RNA-containing virus. HAV is heat-stable and is resistant to both guanidine and disoxanil. The structural protein VP4 is very small, and the size order of proteins VP2 and VP3 is reversed.

Hepatitis B Virus (HBV)

As described in the discussion of taxonomic families later in this chapter, the family **Hepadnaviridae** (hepa-DNA-virus) has been established in recognition of the unique properties of these viruses. At present, five hepadnaviruses are recognized; all require a reverse transcription step in genome replication that is accompanied by secretion of large amounts of particulate envelope antigen into the circulation of the infected host. All hepadnaviruses have the capacity to induce persistent infections in their natural hosts and frequently are associated with hepatocellular carcinoma.

Hepatitis C Virus (HCV)

The first descriptions of this parenterally transmitted agent of non-A, non-B hepatitis showed that transmission to susceptible chimpanzees was abolished by prior exposure of the virus to chloroform but that infectivity was not lost on passage through filters with a small pore size (less than 80 nm). Taken together with an estimated sedimentation coefficient in excess of 150, these data at first suggested HCV to be a togavirus or a flavivirus. However, the entire genomic sequence of hepa-C-virus has been elucidated. The genome is similar to that of a flavivirus, although homology studies show similarities to members of the *Pestivirus* genus within the family **Togaviridae**, a genus that includes bovine virus diarrhea virus and hog cholera virus, often referred to as the mucosal disease viruses.

No full-length cDNA clone has been shown to be infectious. The 5′ noncoding region of the virus is the most highly conserved region of the virus genome. The genomes of different isolates are closely related yet heterogenous sequences (quasi-species) centered around one dominant sequence (the master sequence). Quasi-species are believed to lead to chronic infection (escape from neutralizing antibody) or vaccine failure.[14a]

Hepatitis Delta Virus (HDV)

This virus is defective. In order to replicate, helper functions coded for by HBV are required. HDV in many respects closely resembles certain infectious subviral RNA agents found in plants and animals such as viroids and satellite viruses. However, the translation of HDV RNA and its helper

Text continued on page 1610

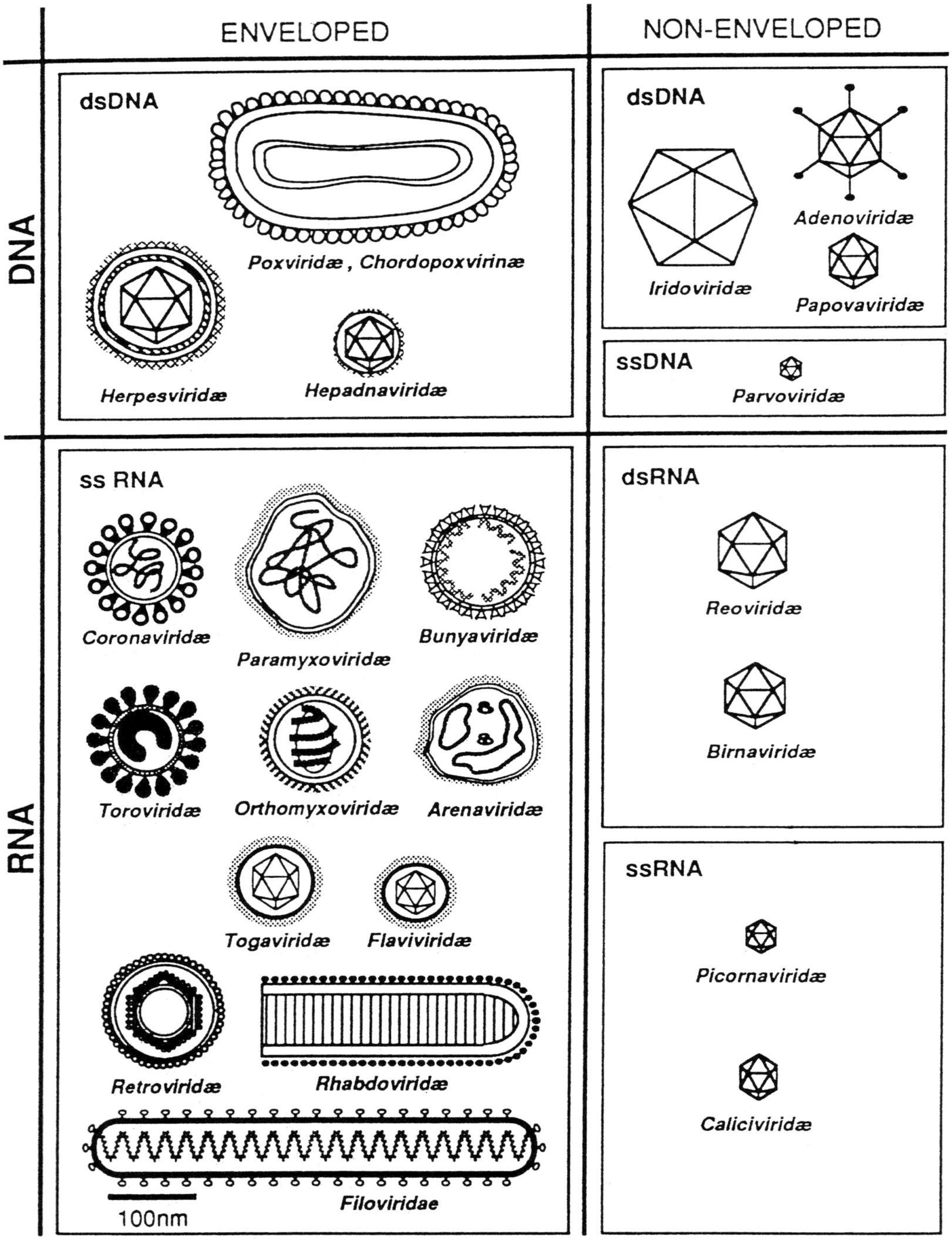

FIGURE 157–2. *Diagram illustrating the shapes and relative sizes of animal viruses of the major families (bar = 100 nm). Representative members that infect humans are listed in parentheses. (From Francki, R. I. B., Fauquet, C. M., Knudson, D. L., et al. (eds.): 5th Report of the International Committee on Taxonomy of Viruses. Arch. Virol. 2(Suppl.):1–450, 1991.)*

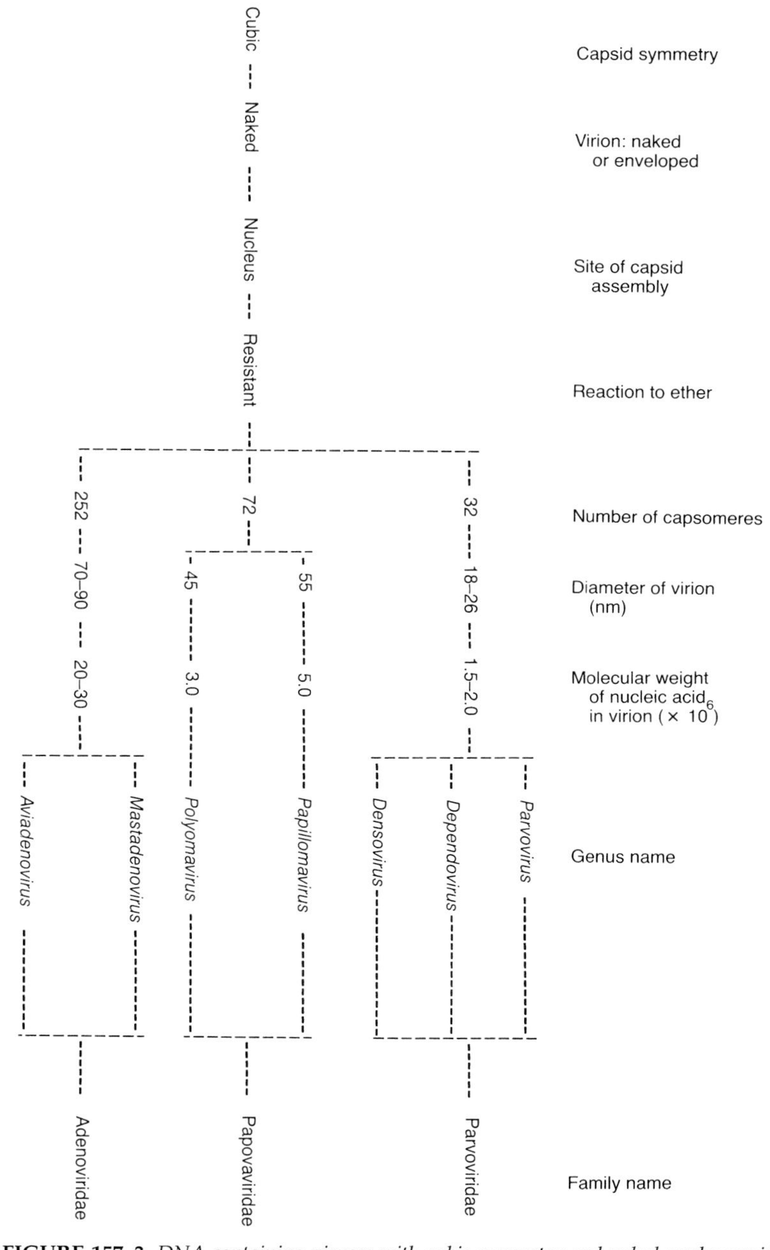

FIGURE 157–3. *DNA-containing viruses with cubic symmetry and naked nucleocapsid.*

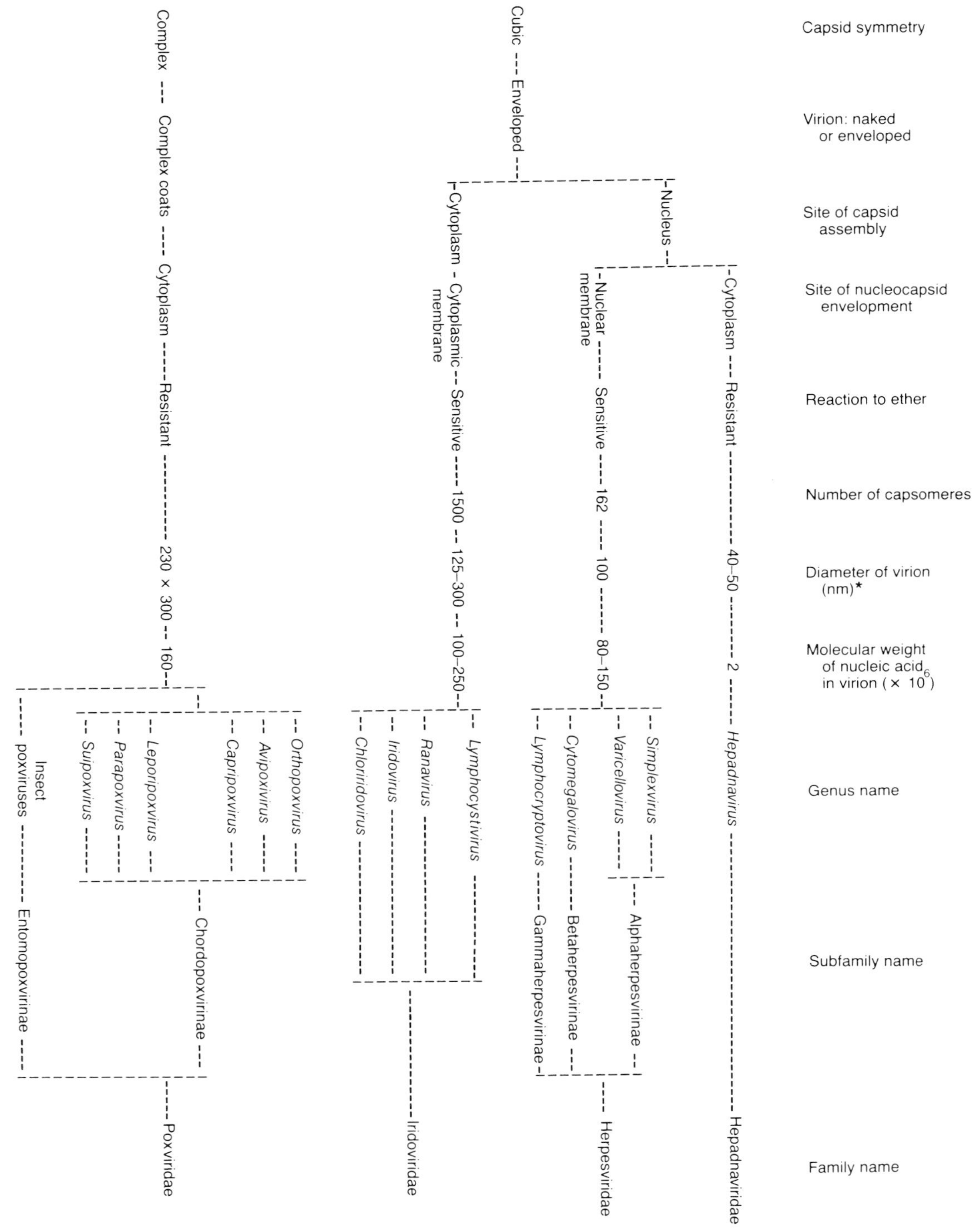

FIGURE 157–4. *DNA-containing viruses with envelopes or complex coats. (*Diameter, or diameter times length.)*

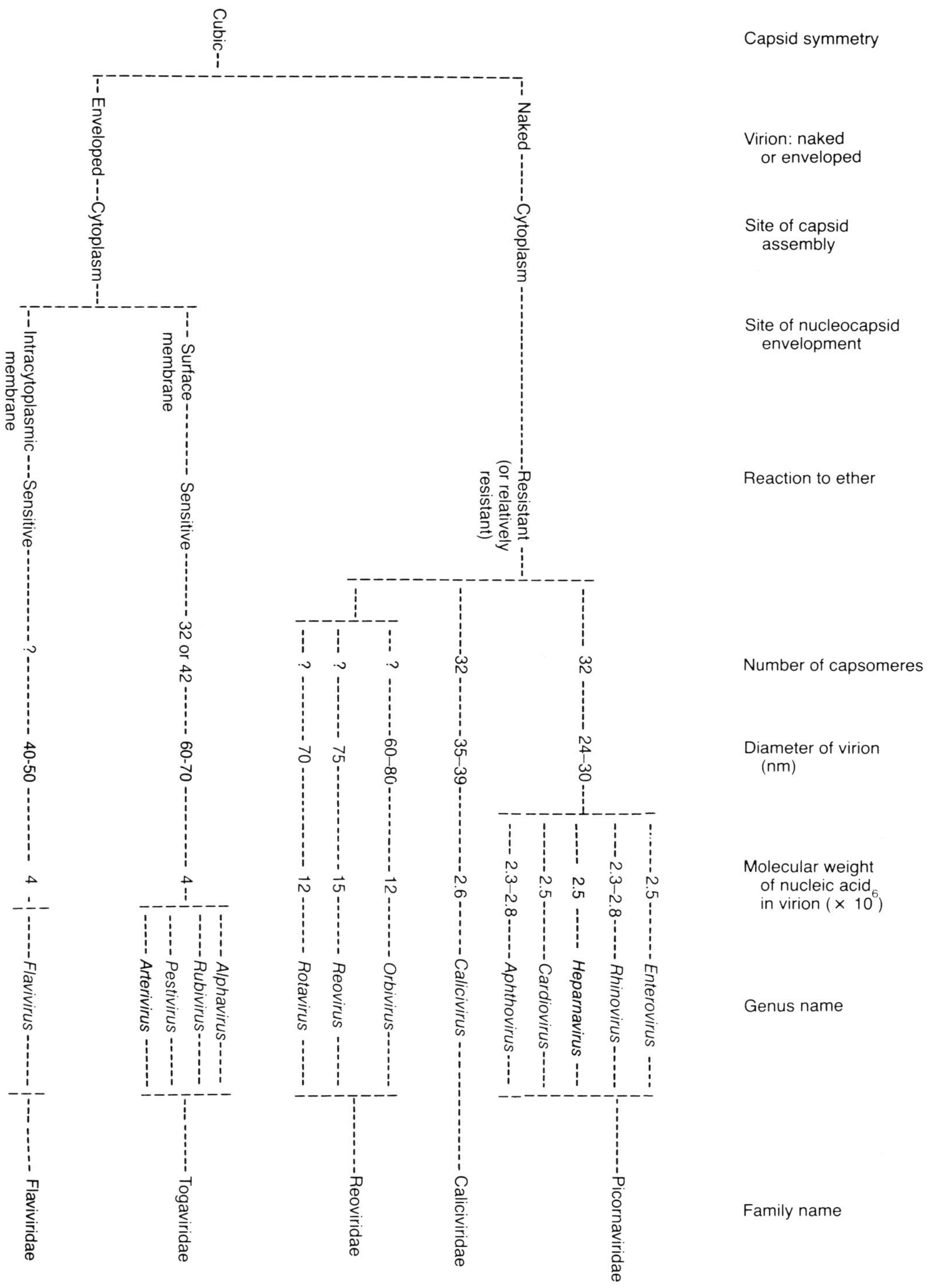

FIGURE 157–5. *RNA-containing viruses with cubic capsid symmetry. Members of the family Reoviridae possess a double protein capsid shell in which the exact number and spatial arrangements of capsomeres are difficult to determine.*

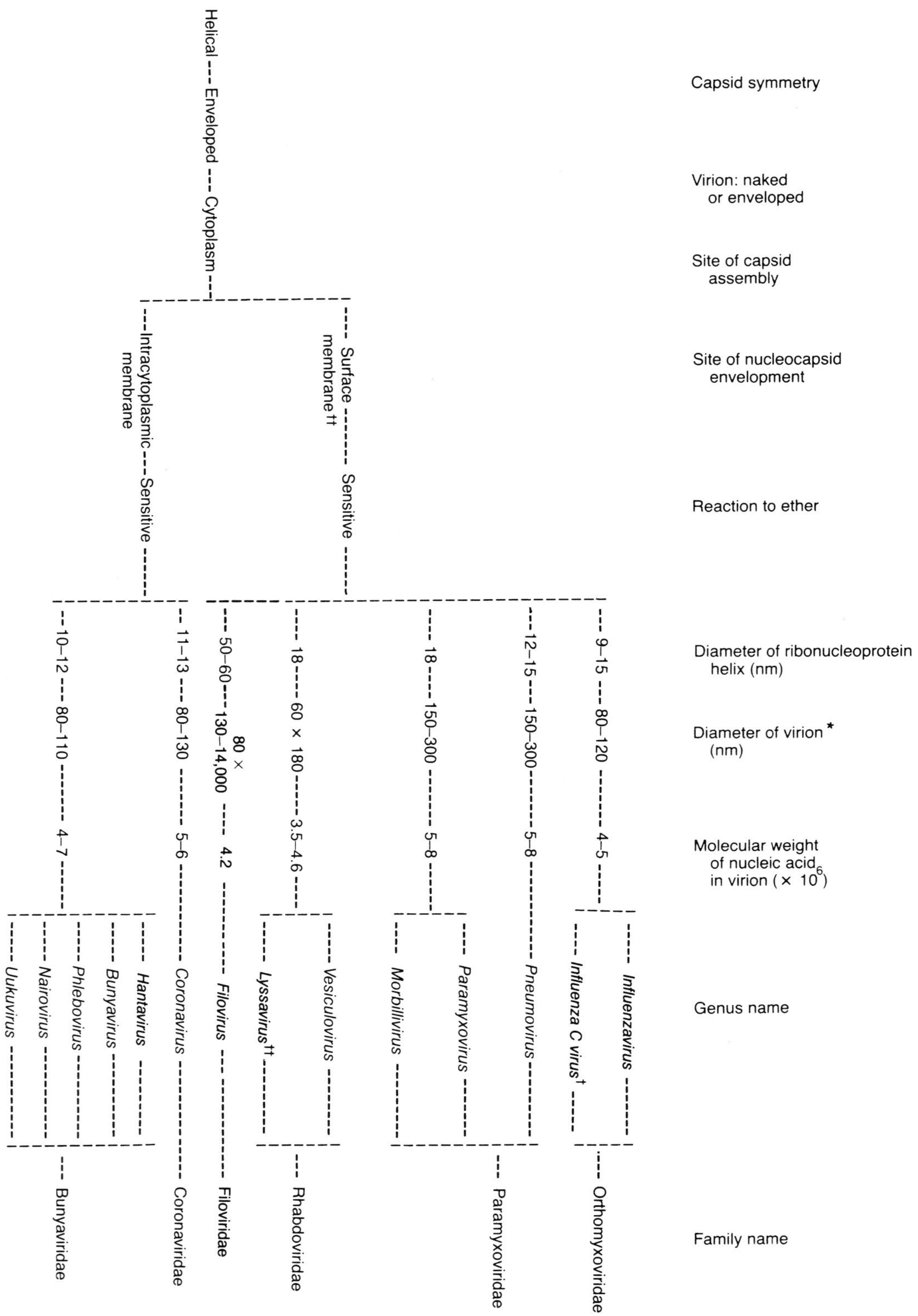

FIGURE 157–6. *RNA-containing viruses with helical symmetry. (*Diameter, or diameter times length. †Influenza virus type C is a separate genus but has not been given an official genus name. ‡Rabies virus buds predominantly from intracytoplasmic membranes.)*

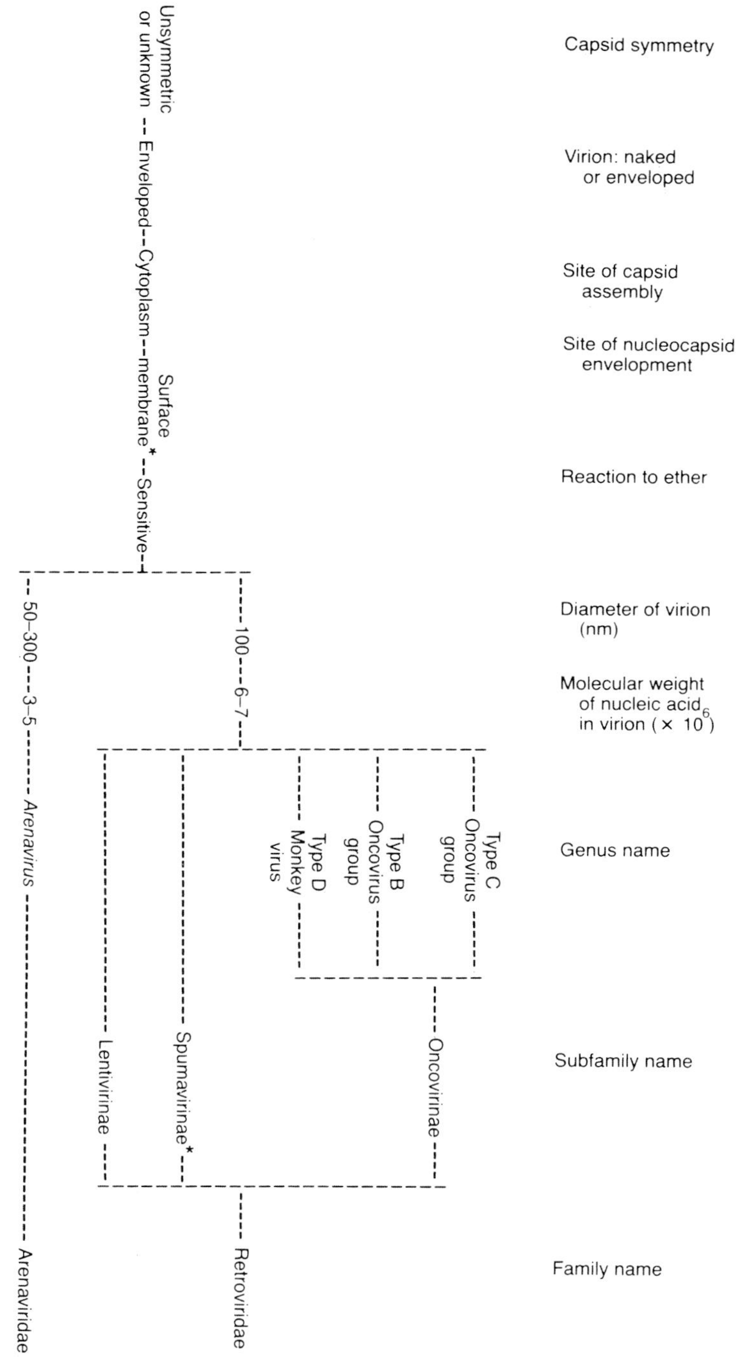

FIGURE 157–7. *RNA-containing viruses with unusually complex architecture. (*Members of Spumavirinae bud into intracytoplasmic vacuoles.)*

TABLE 157–1. Members of Virus Families, with Emphasis on Viruses that Infect Humans

Family	Genus	Common Species	No. of Members
Picornaviridae	*Enterovirus*	Polioviruses	3
		Coxsackieviruses, group A	23
		Coxsackieviruses, group B	6
		Echoviruses	31
		Enteroviruses 68 through 71	4
		Viruses of other vertebrates	>34
	Heparnavirus	Hepatitis A virus	1
		Hepatitis A virus of monkeys	>2
	Cardiovirus	Encephalomyocarditis virus and mengovirus; mouse encephalomyelitis virus	3
	Rhinovirus	Virus types infecting humans	>115
		Viruses of cattle	2
	Aphthovirus	Foot-and-mouth disease viruses of cattle and other cloven-hoofed animals	7
Caliciviridae	*Calicivirus*	Vesicular exanthema of swine virus	13
		Viruses of cats and sea lions (possible member: Norwalk gastroenteritis virus of humans)	Many
Reoviridae	*Reovirus*	Viruses of humans, monkeys, and lower vertebrates	3
		Viruses of birds	>5
	Orbivirus	17 subgroups, including Colorado tick fever and Kemerovo viruses of humans; also bluetongue virus of sheep and African horse sickness virus	>90
	Rotavirus	Human rotaviruses	>6
		Rotaviruses of many mammals, including SA-11 virus of monkeys and Nebraska calf diarrhea virus	Many
Birnaviridae	*Birnavirus*	Infectious pancreatic necrosis virus of fish; infectious bursal disease virus of chickens	2
Togaviridae	*Alphavirus*	Sindbis virus and many other mosquito-borne viruses, including viruses of eastern equine, Venezuelan, and western equine encephalitis and Semliki Forest virus	23
	Rubivirus	Rubella virus	1
	Pestivirus	Viruses of cattle and pigs	>3
Flaviviridae	*Flavivirus*	Yellow fever virus and other mosquito-borne viruses, including viruses of dengue; of Japanese, Murray Valley, and St. Louis encephalitis; and of West Nile fever	26
		Tick-borne viruses, including viruses of Kyasanur Forest disease, Omsk hemorrhagic fever, European and Far Eastern tick-borne encephalitis of humans, and louping ill of sheep	11
		Viruses whose vectors are unknown	17
		Hepatitis C virus	1
Orthomyxoviridae	*Influenzavirus*	Influenza virus type A	Many
		Influenza virus type B	Several
		Influenza virus type C	1
Paramyxoviridae	*Paramyxovirus*	Human parainfluenza viruses, including Sendai virus	4
		Mumps virus	1
		Newcastle disease virus of fowl; viruses of other diseases of birds and mammals	>6
	Morbillivirus	Measles virus	1
		Rinderpest virus of cattle	1
		Distemper virus of dogs	1
		Peste-des-petits-ruminants virus of sheep and goats	1
	Pneumovirus	Human respiratory syncytial virus	1
		Respiratory disease viruses of cattle and mice	?
Rhabdoviridae	*Vesiculovirus*	Vesicular stomatitis virus of horses, cattle, and pigs	Several
	Lyssavirus	Rabies virus	1
		Lagos bat virus and others	>5
Filoviridae	*Filovirus*	Marburg virus	1
		Ebola virus	2
Coronaviridae	*Coronavirus*	Human coronavirus	2
		Mouse hepatitis virus, infectious bronchitis virus of fowl, and other agents infecting pigs and other vertebrates	>4
Bunyaviridae	*Bunyavirus*	Bunyamwera virus	>145
		California encephalitis viruses	
		LaCrosse virus, other serologically cross-related groups, and several ungrouped viruses	
	Phlebovirus	Sandfly fever viruses	>30
		Other viruses of humans and lower animals, including Rift Valley fever virus of sheep and other ruminants, which may cause human disease	

TABLE 157–1. Members of Virus Families, with Emphasis on Viruses that Infect Humans *Continued*

Family	Genus	Common Species	No. of Members
Bunyaviridae	*Nairovirus*	Crimean-Congo hemorrhagic fever virus	
Continued		Viruses of five other serogroups, including the virus of Nairobi sheep disease	>27
	Uukuvirus	Uukuniemi virus and six other agents, all belonging to the same serogroup (infect rodents and ticks)	7
	Hantavirus	Hantaan virus of hemorrhagic fever with renal syndrome	Many
Retroviridae			
Oncovirinae	Type C oncovirus group	Sarcoma and leukemia viruses of mice, cats, cattle, birds, snakes, and primates	>15
	HTLV-BLV group	Human T-cell lymphotropic virus types 1 and 2	4
	Type B oncovirus group	Mammary tumor virus of mice (and humans?)	?
	Type D oncovirus group	Monkey (mammary tumor?) virus (Mason-Pfizer monkey virus)	?
Spumavirinae	*Spumavirus*	Syncytial and foamy viruses of humans, monkeys, cattle, and cats	>4
Lentivirinae	*Lentivirus*	HIV	2
		Visna, maedi, and progressive pneumonia viruses of sheep	?
Avenaviridae	*Arenavirus*	Lymphocytic choriomeningitis virus of mice	
		Lassa fever virus	1
		Viruses of Tacaribe complex, including Junin and Machupo	1
		viruses of South Amerian hemorrhagic fevers	>8
Parvoviridae	*Parvovirus*	Human parvovirus B19	
		Aleutian mink disease virus; viruses of rodents, pigs, cattle, cats	>1
		and dogs	Many
	Dependovirus	Adeno-associated virus (adeno-satellite virus): human (types 1 through 5); monkey (type 4); also of cattle, dogs, and birds	>8
Papovaviridae	*Papillomavirus*	Human papillomaviruses (warts)	Many
		Rabbit (Shope) papillomavirus	1
		Papillomaviruses of other mammals	Many
	Polyomavirus	Polyomavirus of mice	1
		JC and BK viruses of humans	2
		Simian virus 40 of rhesus monkeys	1
		Lymphotropic virus of African green monkeys	1
		Viruses of mice, rabbits, and baboons	>5
Adenoviridae	*Mastadenovirus*	Human adenoviruses	>36
		Viruses of other mammals	>45
	Aviadenovirus	Viruses of birds	>13
Hepadnaviridae	*Hepadnavirus*	Human hepatitis B virus	1
		Hepatitis B viruses of woodchucks, ground squirrels, and ducks	>3
Herpesviridae			
Alphaherpesvirinae	*Simplexvirus*	Human herpes simplex virus types 1 and 2	2
		Bovine mammillitis virus	1
	Varicellovirus	Varicella-zoster virus (herpesvirus 3)	1
		Herpes B virus of monkeys	1
		Pseudorabies virus	1
		Equine rhinopneumonitis virus	1
Betaherpesvirinae	*Cytomegalovirus*	Human cytomegalovirus (herpesvirus 5)	1
	Muromegalovirus	Mouse cytomegalovirus	1
Gammaherpesvirinae	*Lymphocryptovirus*	Epstein-Barr virus (herpesvirus 4)	1
	Thetalymphocryptovirus	Marek disease herpesvirus of fowl	1
	Rhadinovirus	Herpesvirus saimiri and others	>2
Iridoviridae	*Iridovirus*	Iridescent insect viruses	Several
		African swine fever virus (?)	1
	Ranavirus	Frog viruses	>30
	Piscinivirus	Fish viruses	Several
Poxviridae			
Chordopoxvirinae	*Orthopoxvirus*	Vaccinia virus	
(poxviruses of			
vertebrates)			1
		Smallpox virus (variola)	1
		Poxviruses of lower animals	>6
	Parapoxvirus	Orf virus and other viruses of ungulates	?
		Virus of milker's nodule	1
	Avipoxvirus	Fowlpox virus and other viruses of birds	
	Capripoxvirus	Viruses of sheep and goats	8
	Leporipoxvirus	Myxoma virus of hares	3
		Fibroma viruses of rabbits and squirrels	4
	Suipoxvirus	Swinepox virus	1
	Yatapoxvirus	Yabapox and tanapox viruses	2
	Molluscipoxvirus	Molluscum contagiosum virus	1
Entomopoxvirinae		Poxviruses of insects	>24

TABLE 157–2. General Characteristics of Hepatitis Viruses

Virus*	Hepatitis A	Hepatitis B	Hepatitis C	Hepatitis D	Hepatitis E
Family	Picornaviridae	Hepadnaviridae	Flaviviridae	Unclassified	(Caliciviridae)
Genus	*Heparnavirus*	*Hepadnavirus*	*Hepa-C-virus*	*Deltavirus*	*Hepevirus*
Genome	s-s RNA	d-s DNA	s-s RNA	s-s RNA	s-s RNA
Virion	27 nm Icosahedral	42 nm Spherical	30 to 60 nm particle	35 nm Spherical	27 to 34 nm Icosahedral
Envelope	No	Yes (HBsAg)	Yes	Yes (HBsAg)	No
Stability	Heat- and acid-stable	Acid-sensitive	Ether-sensitive	Acid-sensitive	Heat-stable
Replication	(+) strand RNA	(+) strand RNA intermediate	(+) strand RNA	Requires HBV helper function	(+) strand RNA
Host range	Human Chimpanzee Marmoset	Human Chimpanzee Gibbon Woodchuck Pekin duck	Human Chimpanzee	Human Chimpanzee Woodchuck Pekin duck	Human Chimpanzee Monkey

*Hepatitis F and G have been reported, but not enough is known to permit their classification.
HBV, hepatitis B virus.

dependency on HBV for the formation of new particles is distinct from the behavior of plant viroids.

Hepatitis E Virus (HEV)

This virus is the agent of enterically transmitted non-A, non-B hepatitis. Hepevirus (hep-E-virus) has a diameter of 32 to 34 nm, with a morphology resembling that of the caliciviruses.

VERTEBRATE VIRUSES WITH A DNA GENOME

Parvoviridae

Originally named picodnaviruses to reflect their small size and DNA-containing genome,[46] the family **Parvoviridae**[3, 63] now includes three named genera: *Parvovirus, Densovirus,* and *Dependovirus.* A member prevalent in children is adeno-associated satellite virus, which exists as several serotypes. Reading from the left-hand side of Figure 157–3, these DNA-containing viruses have cubic symmetry and a naked (unenveloped) nucleocapsid; during replication, capsid assembly takes place in the nucleus of the host cell.* Infectivity is resistant not only to ether and other lipid solvents but also to heat (56° C for 60 minutes). The virus particle is 18 to 26 nm in diameter, and the molecular weight of the nucleic acid in the virion is 1.5 to 2.0 $\times$ 10^6 (as compared, for example, with 160 $\times$ 10^6 for the DNA of poxviruses). There are 32 capsomeres that form the outer layers of the nucleocapsid, each 2 to 4 nm in diameter.

The genus *Parvovirus* constitutes autonomously replicating viruses of several vertebrate species. These include parvoviruses of humans, as well as the prototype for the genus, Kilham's rat virus, the virus of Aleutian disease of mink, and others (of cat, cow, dog, goose, mouse, pig, rabbit). A host range mutant of feline panleukopenia virus has become widely known as a serious pathogen of dogs. This virus induces acute enteritis with leukopenia in young and adult dogs as well as myocarditis in puppies. Infections with this virus have reached enzootic proportions around the world.

Members of the *Densovirus* genus also replicate autonomously; they are viruses of insects but also can produce cytopathic effects in cultures of certain vertebrate cells (L cells).

In contrast, members of the *Dependovirus* genus (adeno-satellite viruses) are defective; that is, they cannot multiply in the absence of a coinfecting adenovirus or herpesvirus as a "helper virus." Satellite viruses occur in cow, chicken, dog, horse, human, and monkey hosts.

Parvoviruses are the only DNA-containing viruses of vertebrates whose DNA genome is single-stranded within the virion; all the others (Figs. 157–3 and 157–4) have double-stranded DNA. In the case of dependoviruses and densoviruses, separate virions contain single strands of positive-sense or negative-sense DNA; these strands are complementary, and when isolated from the virion shells, they come together to form a double strand. Members of the genus *Parvovirus* preferentially encapsidate single-stranded DNA of negative polarity. For some members of the genus *Parvovirus,* the DNA in the virion is a negative strand only. This initially was believed to be true of all members of this genus, but further study has indicated considerable variation. In other members of the genus, plus-strand DNA also is incorporated. The percentage of particles that also contain a strand of DNA of positive polarity may vary from 1 to 50; the reasons for the variations have not yet been defined.

Members of the *Parvovirus* genus show marked preference for actively dividing cells, have been shown to be transmissible transplacentally, and have received attention for their special disease potential in fetuses and neonates.[35, 42]

Disease in human beings is associated with several members of **Parvoviridae.** Within the genus *Parvovirus,* strain B19 has been shown to cause a transient shutdown of red blood cell production by killing the late erythroid progenitor cells.[1] This shutdown presents particular problems for individuals already suffering from hemolytic anemias, such as sickle-cell anemia, causing aplastic crises. A virus named RA-1, which is associated with rheumatoid arthritis, is another member of the genus that infects humans.[64] Parvovirus B19 in normal persons may cause erythema infectiosum, or "fifth disease," of childhood.[1, 63] Maternal infection with a parvovirus has been documented in temporal association with a generalized fetal infection and hydrops fetalis.[14]

*For the DNA viruses whose capsid assembly takes place in the nucleus (not only parvoviruses but also papovaviruses, adenoviruses, and herpesviruses), a phase of replication—that is, viral protein synthesis—occurs in the cytoplasm. Messenger RNA of these viruses is associated with polyribosomes.

Papovaviridae

The members of **Papovaviridae**[15, 44, 47, 51] are relatively small, ether-resistant viruses that contain a single molecule of double-stranded DNA in circular form. Many are unusually heat-stable, surviving temperatures that inactivate most viruses. Other properties are shown in Figure 157–3. The representatives that infect human beings are the papilloma, or wart, viruses and the JC and BK viruses; these latter viruses were isolated from the brain tissue of patients with progressive multifocal leukoencephalopathy (PML) and from the urine of immunosuppressed renal transplant recipients, respectively. In addition, several isolates that appear to be identical to simian virus 40 (SV40) of monkeys also have been isolated from patients with PML. Papovaviruses produce latent and chronic infections in their natural hosts. Many of them produce tumors, particularly in experimentally infected rodents, thus serving as models for studying viral carcinogenesis. The viral DNA integrates into cellular chromosomes of transformed cells.

Two genera have been established: *Papillomavirus* and *Polyomavirus*. The genus *Papillomavirus* has as its type species the well-known rabbit (Shope) papillomavirus. Other members are known for humans (several types) and other vertebrate species. Each virus species contains a distinct surface antigen, but all members of a genus share a common antigen revealed by disrupting the virions. Thus far, papillomaviruses have not been cultivated successfully in tissue culture. Some investigations[38, 73] suggest that human genital infection by papillomaviruses may be at least a cofactor in the development of cancer of the uterine cervix.

The term polyomavirus for the human viruses of this genus is an unfortunate choice because these viruses of humans, such as JC and BK, have not been shown to be "polyoma" in character; that is, they do not "produce many types of tumors in the natural host." For example, although antibodies against BK virus are widespread in the population, human tumors and human malignant cell lines have been negative when analyzed for BK virus–specific DNA sequences. Because the probes used would have been able to detect one copy of BK virus DNA if only 10 per cent of the cells were tumor cells, the results are very strong evidence that the tumors analyzed did not have a BK virus etiology. The tumors tested represent about 50 per cent of all types of cancers in the United States; thus, there is no evidence that this "polyomavirus" is involved in production of these tumors in the human host.

Adenoviridae

The adenovirus virion[12, 44, 71] is a nonenveloped isometric particle with icosahedral symmetry. The particles are 70 to 90 nm in diameter, with 252 capsomeres, each 7 to 9 nm in diameter; 240 are hexons; and there are 12 vertex capsomeres (or penton bases), which antigenically are distinct from the hexons and carry one or two filamentous projections. The adenovirus genome is a single linear molecule of double-stranded DNA with a molecular weight of 20 to 30 $\times 10^6$. At least 36 serotypes infect humans, and there are distinct serotypes for a number of other species. Adenoviruses have a predilection for mucous membranes and may persist for years in lymphoid tissue. Some cause acute respiratory diseases, febrile catarrhs, pharyngitis, and conjunctivitis. Human adenoviruses rarely cause disease in laboratory animals, but certain serotypes do produce tumors in newborn hamsters. All mammalian adenoviruses (genus *Mastadenovirus*) share common antigens; these antigens are different from the corresponding antigens of members of the genus *Aviadenovirus*, whose members infect birds.

Human adenovirus species are designated by the letter h followed by the present Arabic number series (for example, *Mastadenovirus* h 1). Adenoviruses of domestic animals are designated by a three-letter code based on the genus of the respective host animal (for example, *Mastadenovirus* bos 1). Thus, for the adenoviruses of humans, the species are h 1 to h 42; for those of cattle, bos 1 to bos 9; for those of pig, sus 1 to sus 4. Species of aviadenoviruses are named in the same way: for the adenoviruses of fowl, gal 1 to gal 9; of turkeys, mel 1 to mel 2; and so on.

Hepadnaviridae

Among the various hepatitis viruses (Table 157–1), a new family, **Hepadnaviridae,**[12, 56] has been recognized (Fig. 157–4). The proposed name is appropriate, reflecting the DNA-containing genomes of its members and their replication within hepatocytes.[56] So far the evidence supports one genus that includes several species.

HBV of humans and three similar viruses found in woodchucks *(Marmota monax)*, Beechey ground squirrels *(Spermophilus beecheyi)*, and Pekin ducks *(Anas domesticus)* share many features. All members of the family share some antigens as well as similar morphologic characteristics and behavior in the infected host: formation of large amounts of excess viral coat protein in the form of small spherical and tubular particles. The viruses replicate in the liver and are associated with acute and chronic hepatitis. More than 200 million persons are persistent carriers of the human virus and are at very high risk of developing liver cancer. The woodchuck HBV also causes liver cancer in its natural host. Fragments of viral DNA may be found in the liver cancer cells of both species.

Further details[56] on the properties shared by hepadnaviruses include (1) characteristic ultrastructure of the virion: a double-shelled particle 40 to 50 nm in diameter with a core 27 nm in diameter and incomplete forms (22-nm spheres and filaments); (2) circular viral DNA with length corresponding to DNA of 3200 base pairs and containing a single-stranded region; (3) virion DNA polymerase that repairs the single-stranded region in the viral DNA; (4) polypeptide covalently attached to the 5′ end of the long DNA strand; (5) characteristic surface, core, and "e" antigens in the virion; (6) characteristic virion polypeptides; (7) sharing of some DNA and virion polypeptide homology; (8) protein kinase activity in the virion core; (9) liver tropism; (10) persistent infection with large amounts of incomplete viral forms continuously in the blood; and (11) infection associated with hepatitis, hepatocellular carcinoma, and immune-complex–mediated extrahepatic tissue injury.

Herpesviridae

The herpesvirus family, **Herpesviridae,**[12, 44, 57] is a diverse group of viruses identified by their structure. As indicated in Figure 157–4, the virus particle consists of a DNA-containing core enclosed by an icosahedral capsid with 162 hollow cylindric capsomeres. The enveloped virion is 120 to 200 nm in diameter and consists of four structural components. The core consists of a fibrillar spool on which the DNA is wrapped. The ends of the fibers are anchored to the underside of the capsid shell. The capsid (100 to 110 nm in diameter) is an icosahedron with 5 capsomeres on each edge; it contains 150 hexameric and 12 pentameric capsomeres. Surrounding the capsid is a tegument consisting of globular material, and surrounding the tegument is the envelope, a bilayered, lipid- and protein-containing membrane.

The double-stranded DNA of various herpesviruses differs considerably in size (molecular weight, 80 to 150 × 10^6), cytosine and guanosine content (35 to 75 per cent), and structural complexity. The prototype, human herpes simplex virus, has a complex structural organization; included in the genome are a terminally redundant section and internal inverted repetition of sequences present at both ends of the DNA molecule, with a long and short unique sequence region. For other members of the family, the genome may have a simpler structural organization. The DNA of herpesviruses is sufficiently large to carry the genetic code for 80 to 100 proteins, of which about 50 have been observed. Of these, as many as 30 may be structural proteins of the virion, whereas others may be virus-induced enzymes, including thymidine kinase, DNA polymerase, and DNase. Neutralizing antibody reacts with major viral glycoproteins located in the viral envelope.

Herpesviruses are noted for their ability to establish latent or persistent infections, or both; these may last for the lifetime of the host, even in the presence of circulating antibodies. Particular interest has been generated by the association of Epstein-Barr herpesvirus with human Burkitt lymphoma and nasopharyngeal carcinoma and by the possible role of the genital herpesvirus (herpes simplex virus type 2) in cancer of the uterine cervix and the vulva. Several simian herpesviruses have been shown to be oncogenic in experimentally infected animals. Infections of heterologous species are in many cases very serious; examples are the fatal meningoencephalitis of humans caused by a simian herpesvirus, the so-called B virus, and fatal encephalitis of cattle caused by swine pseudorabies virus. Human diseases caused by herpesviruses include oral and genital herpes lesions, chickenpox and shingles due to varicella-zoster virus, cytomegalic inclusion disease, and infectious mononucleosis.

Subfamilies have been established within **Herpesviridae,** based chiefly on host range, duration of reproductive cycle, cytopathology, and characteristics of latent infections. Alphaherpesvirinae are rapidly growing, highly cytolytic viruses that are characterized by a variable host range and a short reproductive cycle with rapid spread of infection in cell culture, resulting in mass destruction of susceptible cells. The establishment of carrier cultures of susceptible cells harboring nondefective genomes is difficult to accomplish. Latent infections are seen frequently, but not exclusively, in ganglia. Three genera have been proposed for viruses in this subfamily. They are *Simplexvirus,* to include herpes simplex viruses and similar agents; *Poikilovirus,* to include pseudorabies-like viruses; and *Varicellavirus,* thus far including only the varicella-zoster virus (species designation, human herpesvirus 3 [HHV-3] or human alphaherpesvirus 3). The second species label illustrates an alternative designation for individual herpesviruses to show clearly their subfamily affiliation, for example, human alphaherpesvirus 1, murid betaherpesvirus 1, and gallid gammaherpesvirus 2.

Betaherpesvirinae (slow-growing, cytomegalic viruses) are characterized by a narrow host range in vivo, a relatively long reproductive cycle, and slowly progressing lytic foci in cell culture. Infected cells frequently become enlarged (cytomegalia) both in vitro and in vivo. Inclusions containing DNA frequently are present in both the nucleus and the cytoplasm. Carrier cultures are established easily. Latent infections may be established in secretory glands, lymphoreticular cells, kidneys, and other tissues. Genera within the Betaherpesvirinae include *Cytomegalovirus,* containing the human cytomegaloviruses (species designation, HHV-5), and *Muromegalovirus,* cytomegaloviruses of mice (species, murid herpesvirus 1). One herpesvirus, isolated from leukocytes and capable of infecting both T cells and B cells in vitro, has been designated lymphotropic human herpesvirus or HHV-6.[21] The genome of the virus exhibits marked cross-hybridization with human cytomegalovirus and therefore provisionally is classified as a member of the Betaherpesvirinae.

HHV-6 has been shown to be an etiologic agent of exanthem subitum.[72a] The HHV-6 isolates are classified into two distinct groups according to genetic, antigenic, and other markers. Another herpesvirus, HHV-7, was isolated first in 1990 in $CD4^+$ T cells from a healthy person. It is different from but close to HHV-6. HHV-7 now is recognized as another causal agent of exanthem subitum.[66a] Most children have antibodies by the time they are 4 years old. Both viruses exist in the cervixes of infected women in late pregnancy and may cause perinatal infection.[54a]

For the Gammaherpesvirinae, the host range in vivo usually is limited to the same family or order as the host that it naturally infects. In vitro, all members of Gammaherpesvirinae replicate in lymphoblastoid cells; some also cause lytic infections in some types of epithelioid and fibroblastoid cells. Viruses in this group are specific for either B or T lymphocytes. The genera proposed for this subfamily are *Lymphocryptovirus,* which includes Epstein-Barr virus (HHV-4) and Epstein-Barr–like viruses of baboon and of chimpanzee (cercopithecine herpesvirus 12 and pongine herpesvirus 1, respectively); *Thetalymphocryptovirus,* Marek disease herpesvirus (gallid herpesvirus 2) and related viruses; and *Rhadinovirus,* to include herpesvirus ateles, herpesvirus saimiri, and similar agents (ateline herpesviruses 2 and 3; saimiriine herpesvirus 2).

Iridoviridae

The best-known members of the family **Iridoviridae**[5, 12] are the small, iridescent viruses of insects (for example, *Tipula* iridescent virus), now placed in the genus *Iridovirus,* and the large iridescent viruses of insects (genus *Chloriridovirus*). However, other members of this family are important pathogens of vertebrates, particularly of frogs and fish. No iridovirus of humans is known. Vertebrate iridoviruses are enveloped; iridoviruses that infect insects contain a lipid fraction in the virion as an integral part of the icosahedral shell but do not have envelopes as such. The genome is a single large molecule of linear double-stranded DNA, possibly two molecules in some viruses.

Poxviridae

Poxviruses[12, 24, 44] are large viruses that are brick-shaped or ovoid in form. The virion structure is complex: an external coat contains lipid and tubular or globular protein structures; the coat encloses one or two lateral bodies and an internal body (core) that contains the genome. In the virion are more than 30 structural proteins and several viral enzymes, including a DNA-dependent RNA polymerase. The genome is a single molecule of double-stranded DNA. This is the major family of DNA-containing viruses whose members replicate entirely within the cytoplasm; a number of them produce intracytoplasmic inclusion bodies (type B, viral factory; and type A, cytoplasmic accumulation). The genus *Orthopoxvirus* includes smallpox (variola) virus as well as vaccinia virus and other poxviruses of vertebrates. Orthopoxviruses produce a hemagglutinin separate from the virion; the hemagglutinin is serologically specific and is a lipid-rich pleomorphic particle 50 to 65 nm in diameter. As a result of the vaccination program of the World Health Organization, smallpox virus seems to have been eradicated from the world.[25]

Most poxviruses of vertebrates share at least one antigen; members of each genus of vertebrate poxviruses have additional antigens in common. Genetic recombination occurs within genera; nongenetic reactivation occurs both within and between genera of the poxviruses that infect vertebrates. Some of the animal poxviruses (for example, monkeypox virus) can infect humans, and with the eradication of smallpox from the world, human infections by these agents might be detected more frequently.

Two subfamilies have now been defined: Chordopoxvirinae, which includes the poxviruses that infect vertebrates (genera *Orthopoxvirus, Avipoxvirus, Capripoxvirus, Leporipoxvirus, Parapoxvirus,* and *Suipoxvirus*), and Entomopoxvirinae, which includes the poxviruses that infect insects.

VERTEBRATE VIRUSES WITH AN RNA GENOME

Picornaviridae

Picornaviridae[16, 44, 50, 58] is represented at the top of Figure 157–5. These agents—the smallest of the vertebrate viruses with RNA genomes—have been classed in four genera and several hundred species.

More than 70 members of the genus *Enterovirus* are known to infect humans; these include polioviruses, coxsackieviruses of the A and B groups, echoviruses, and enterovirus serotypes that have been assigned sequential numbers (to date, enterovirus 68 to 72) rather than being placed in the echovirus or coxsackievirus subgroups (since the distinctions among these groups have been found to be less sharp than was recognized when these subdivisions initially were established).

More than 100 viruses infecting humans belong to the genus *Rhinovirus.* Numerous enteroviruses and rhinoviruses also exist for other host species. A third genus in the family, *Cardiovirus,* is typified by encephalomyocarditis virus of mice that also may (rarely) infect humans. The fourth genus, *Aphthovirus,* includes the economically important foot-and-mouth-disease viruses of cattle.

The picornavirus genome is one piece of linear, single-stranded positive-sense RNA of low molecular weight (about 2.5×10^6). The RNA is infectious and serves as its own messenger for protein translation. The virion is about 27 nm in diameter; it contains 60 copies of each of the four major polypeptides (molecular weights, 33,000, 27,000, 23,000, and 6000). The enteroviruses and cardioviruses are acid-stable and have a buoyant density in CsCl of about 1.34 g/cm^3; in contrast, the rhinoviruses and aphthoviruses are acid-labile and have a higher buoyant density, about 1.4 g/cm^3.

After decades of investigation, hepatitis A virus (HAV) has been classified as a picornavirus. Although it resembles enteroviruses in many respects,[28, 29] it differs in gene and amino acid sequences and also in its resistance to thermal inactivation. In comparative studies, 50 per cent of the particles in a poliovirus type 2 preparation disintegrate during heating at pH 7 for 10 minutes at 43° C, whereas under the same conditions, 61° C is required to produce disintegration of 50 per cent of the HAV particles. However, HAV, like the enteroviruses, is stabilized by $MgCl_2$ against thermal inactivation. In the presence of 1 mol/L $MgCl_2$, the temperatures required to produce 50 per cent destruction of the particles are shifted to 61° C for poliovirus type 1 and to 81° C for HAV.

The diseases caused by picornaviruses range from paralytic poliomyelitis to aseptic meningitis, hepatitis, pleurodynia, myocarditis, skin rashes, and common colds; inapparent infection is very common. Different viruses may produce the same syndrome; on the other hand, the same picornavirus may cause more than a single syndrome.

Strain differentiation among the polioviruses is of direct concern in public health and medical virology. In the years since 1951 (when the existence of three poliovirus serotypes was established), differences within serotypes have been demonstrated in the genomic RNA by nucleotide mapping and in the protein coat by the use of highly strain-specific monoclonal antibody. Poliovirus isolates are identified by type, country (or city), strain number, and year of isolation. Thus, P1/England/119/65 designates a type 1 poliovirus strain, number 119, that was isolated in England in 1965.

The situation with regard to acute hemorrhagic conjunctivitis (AHC) is pertinent. The first epidemic occurred in West Africa in 1969, the second in Southeast Asia in 1970. A variant of coxsackievirus A24 was isolated in Singapore in 1970 and in subsequent AHC epidemics in Hong Kong and India, but there was no spread to other parts of the world. The first epidemic swept along the coastal areas of West, East, and North Africa, reaching India, Japan, and Southeast Asia in 1971. Tens of millions were affected. This large pandemic yielded a new virus, enterovirus 70 (EV70). EV70 continues to be the agent most often associated with AHC.[31a]

The disease, generally localized to the eye, is characterized by subconjunctival hemorrhage. EV70 is highly contagious, spreading rapidly under crowded and unhygienic conditions; warm, humid, coastal climates seem to be particularly favorable for its transmission. Intrafamilial spread is common. Some localized outbreaks, especially in developed countries, have centered around eye clinics.

Serologic surveys in Japan, Ghana, and Indonesia have confirmed that the virus was not prevalent before the pandemic and that after the outbreak antibodies appeared in the populations involved. Multiple epidemics have occurred within a 5-year period in the same regions, particularly in Southeast Asia, suggesting that immunity may be short lived.

Until 1981, virtually no infection or disease caused by EV70 had been reported in Australia and the Americas. Among more than 1000 serum samples collected between 1971 and 1974 from residents of the United States, only 3 contained antibodies to the virus. Nevertheless, when the virus was introduced into the United States in 1980, a secondary spread did not take place. However, this situation changed in 1981. Early in 1981, AHC reappeared in some of the countries from which it had been absent for a number of years. The disease spread widely in Africa and Asia, and this time it also spread extensively in the Caribbean area, in northern South America, and in Central America during the spring and summer of 1981. In the early autumn, an explosive outbreak occurred in Miami, Florida, involving thousands of cases. The diagnosis and study of AHC caused by EV70 have been complicated by the difficulty of isolating the virus. Most of the recent outbreaks have been identified solely by serologic means.

EV70 isolates obtained from widely separated locales (Asia and the Americas) during the same pandemic period, 1980 to 1981, were found to be closely related by ribonuclease T1-resistant oligonucleotide mapping. The similarities among contemporaneous strains from distant regions suggest that only one basic genotype of this virus appears to be in circulation worldwide at any one time. It appears that AHC started from a single focus in West Africa, very likely Ghana, and that the etiologic agent, EV70, is an enterovirus that newly has appeared and has been undergoing a continuing evolution at a constant rate in many parts of the world during recent years. At about the same time, a variant of coxsackievirus A24 evolved independently in Southeast Asia.[31a]

Caliciviridae

Caliciviruses[32, 33, 59] contain a single molecule of linear, infectious, single-stranded, positive-sense RNA, with a molecular weight of 2.6 to 2.8. The virion is 36 to 39 nm in diameter, with 32 cup-shaped surface depressions arranged in icosahedral symmetry. There is no lipid and no envelope, and there is a single major structural polypeptide (molecular weight about 70×10^3) that is present in 180 copies.

Calicivirus is the only genus known; the type species is vesicular exanthema of swine virus. A number of other serotypes infect cats and sea lions.

There seem to be at least five types of human caliciviruses that have been observed in human feces in association with gastroenteric disease. They have failed to show relationship to the animal caliciviruses. The possible relationships of these agents to the virus of Norwalk gastroenteritis also remain to be resolved. The Norwalk virus, a widespread human agent causing acute epidemic gastroenteritis, has a virion protein structure similar to that of the caliciviruses; however, the size of its RNA genome and the diameter of the virion suggest similarity to enteroviruses.[32]

Reoviridae

For members of **Reoviridae** (Fig. 157–5),[44, 60, 67] the virion has an isometric nucleocapsid 60 to 80 nm in diameter. The genome consists of 10 to 12 pieces of linear double-stranded RNA with a total molecular weight of 12 to 20×10^6. The nucleocapsid has a double shell; the particle with the outer coat removed is called the core. There is no lipid envelope. The structure of the outer capsid layer is indistinct, but icosahedral symmetry has been demonstrated in the inner capsid layers of all three recognized groups of reoviruses that infect vertebrates, that is, the genera *Reovirus, Orbivirus,* and *Rotavirus.*

The members of the genus *Reovirus* that infect human beings are found in the enteric tract, but their association with disease is not always clear; members of this genus recovered from lower animals are similar to those infecting humans. The genus *Orbivirus* includes numerous viruses that infect both vertebrates and invertebrates; some have been considered to be arboviruses, and several have been recovered only from insects. The diseases caused by orbiviruses include blue-tongue, African horse sickness, Colorado tick fever of humans, and epizootic hemorrhagic disease of deer.

The members of the *Rotavirus* genus[22] that infect human beings have been recognized as major pathogens of nonbacterial infantile diarrhea. The gastroenteritis syndrome is clinically more severe and of longer duration than the illness caused by the calicivirus-like "Norwalk virus"; it occurs in sporadic outbreaks rather than epidemic form. Rotavirus infection is one of the most common childhood illnesses throughout the world and is a leading cause of death among children in developing countries. Other members of this antigenically interrelated rotavirus group include calf diarrhea virus, the virus of epizootic diarrhea of infant mice, SA11 rotavirus of monkeys, and similar viruses from swine and other species. For the human rotaviruses, two subgroups and at least six serotypes are known. The subgroup antigen, VP6, coded for by the sixth genomic segment, is located in the major inner capsid protein. Serotype antigens coded for by the fourth and ninth genomic segments, VP4 and VP9, are located in the major outer capsid protein. Antibodies directed against the serotype antigens neutralize the infectivity of the virion.[22]

Togaviridae[6, 12, 69]

Members of this family include most arboviruses of antigenic group A, now classed as the genus *Alphavirus,* as well as genera that include nonarthropod-borne togaviruses—rubella *(Rubivirus)*; the mucosal disease virus group *(Pestivirus)*; and a newly designated genus, *Arterivirus* (equine arteritis virus)—for which the avenues of transmission are not known. The genus *Flavivirus* has been removed from **Togaviridae** and elevated to the status of a separate family, **Flaviviridae.**

Virions of **Togaviridae** are spherical, 60 to 70 nm in diameter. A lipoprotein envelope with lipid and virus-specified glycopeptides (usually two) is tightly bound to a nucleocapsid 25 to 35 nm in diameter, with proven or presumed icosahedral symmetry. Surface projections protrude from the envelope. The genome is a single linear molecule of single-stranded positive-sense RNA of molecular weight 4×10^6, which is infectious. The 5′ end is capped, and the 3′ end is polyadenylated. Full-length and subgenomic messenger RNAs have been demonstrated, and posttranslational cleavage of polyproteins occurs during RNA replication. Togaviruses replicate within the cytoplasm, mature at the plasma membrane, and assemble by budding.

The alphaviruses include many of the major human arboviral pathogens: the viruses of Venezuelan, eastern, and western equine encephalitis and a number of other viruses. Rubella virus thus far is the only member of the genus *Rubivirus.* Members of the *Pestivirus* genus include bovine virus diarrhea (mucosal disease complex) virus, hog cholera (European swine fever) virus, and border disease virus. The only member of the genus *Arterivirus* is equine arteritis virus. Lactic dehydrogenase virus of mice is considered a possible member of the togavirus family.

Flaviviridae[12, 61, 70]

Members of this newly established family include the members of the genus *Flavivirus,* which previously had been included in **Togaviridae.** Its members differ from the genus *Alphavirus* of **Togaviridae** in the molecular structure of the virion, the gene sequence and replication strategy, and their mode of morphogenesis.

This family includes a number of serious human pathogens. Among them are the mosquito-borne viruses of yellow fever, West Nile fever, Japanese encephalitis, St. Louis encephalitis, Murray Valley encephalitis, and dengue, as well as the tick-borne agents of Omsk hemorrhagic fever and Russian spring-summer encephalitis.

The flavivirus virion, 40 to 50 nm in diameter, is slightly smaller than that of togaviruses, and in contrast to the icosahedral symmetry of the alphavirus nucleocapsid, the symmetry of the flavivirus nucleocapsid has not been defined fully. Whereas the togavirus envelope usually contains two species of glycoprotein, that of flaviviruses contains only one. As with the togaviruses, the flavivirus genome is a single linear molecule of single-stranded positive-sense RNA of molecular weight 4×10^6, which is infectious. The 5′ end is capped, but—unlike that of togaviruses—the 3′ end is not polyadenylated. As yet, no subgenomic messenger RNA or polyprotein precursors have been detected for flaviviruses. In contrast to the alphaviruses, which mature at the plasma membrane, virions of **Flaviviridae** mature within cisternae, and their morphogenesis is not defined clearly.

Orthomyxoviridae

All orthomyxoviruses[20, 36, 44] recognized to date are influenza viruses. The ribonucleoprotein capsid is helically symmetrical and 9 to 15 nm in diameter (Figure 157–6). The genome is linear, single-stranded negative-sense RNA in eight segments, with a total molecular weight of about 5×10^6. The virions may be spherical, elongated, or filamentous; they are 80 to 120 nm in diameter. For most members of the family, "spikes" project from the surface of the envelope; these are glycosylated protein peplomers 10 to 14 nm long and 4 nm in diameter, consisting of two types: the hemagglutinin and the neuraminidase. In the nomenclature of variants of influenza type A that frequently arise either as minor variants or as major new strains, these two antigens are designated, for example, H1N1 and H3N2.

Reassortment of genes between viruses of the same type readily occurs in mixed infections, producing new genetic combinations. This frequency of recombination, particularly among members of type A, is a factor in the occurrence of periodic epidemics and pandemics of influenza. The genus *Influenzavirus* includes viruses of type A and type B. Type C may prove to be a separate genus. In type A are included the agents of human, equine, and swine influenza, and of fowl plague. For types B and C, only human strains are known.

Identification and clear description of influenza subtypes, particularly within type A, long have been recognized as essential for dealing with the antigenic variability of these viruses and the periodic emergence of new strains against which population immunity is low or absent. The recommended nomenclature includes a type and strain designation and a description of the antigenic specificity of the surface antigens, the hemagglutinin (H) and the neuraminidase (N). For all three types, the strain designation includes information on the antigenic type of the virus (based on the antigenic specificity of the nucleoprotein) as A, B, or C; the host of origin (for strains isolated from nonhuman species); geographic origin; strain number; and year of isolation. For viruses of type A, this strain designation is followed by a second part, in parentheses, indicating the antigenic subtype of the H and of the N antigens. For influenza A viruses from all species, the H antigens are grouped into 12 subtypes, H1 to H12; the N antigens are grouped into 9 subtypes, N1 to N9. Although it is recognized that antigenic variation also occurs among influenza B strains, division into subtypes is not recommended. Table 157–3 contains examples of reference strains from humans, swine, and horses, using this nomenclature. (See Figure 157–6 for these viruses and those that follow.)

TABLE 157–3. Examples of Reference Strains for Subtypes of Hemagglutinin and Neuraminidase Antigens of Influenza A Viruses Isolated from Humans, Swine, and Horses

H and N Subtypes	Reference Strains
H1N1	A/PR/8/34 (H1N1)
	A/New Jersey/8/76 (H1N1)
H2N2	A/Singapore/1/57 (H2N2)
H3N2	A/Texas/1/77 (H3N2)
H1N1	A/swine/Wisconsin/67 (H1N1)
H3N2	A/swine/Taiwan/1/70 (H3N2)
H7N7	A/equine/Prague/1/56 (H7N7)
H3N8	A/equine/Miami/1/63 (H3N8)

Paramyxoviridae

For members of the family **Paramyxoviridae**,[37, 44] the virions usually are pleomorphic but roughly spherical and 150 to 300 nm in diameter; there also may be filamentous forms several micrometers long. On the lipid bilayer envelope are surface projections. The genome consists of single-stranded, negative-sense RNA in unsegmented, linear form. The helical nucleocapsid is 12 to 18 nm in diameter. Virions are formed in the cytoplasm by budding from the plasma membrane. Infectivity is sensitive to ether, acid, and heat, but paramyxoviruses (unlike orthomyxoviruses) are resistant to dactinomycin.

The genera include *Paramyxovirus* (parainfluenza viruses of humans and of several animal species; mumps virus; Newcastle disease virus; and Yucaipa and other avian paramyxoviruses); *Morbillivirus* (the viruses of measles, canine distemper, rinderpest, and peste de petits ruminants); and *Pneumovirus* (respiratory syncytial viruses of human beings and of cattle and pneumonia virus of mice). Members of the genus *Paramyxovirus* have both hemagglutinin and neuraminidase in the virion. *Morbillivirus* members have hemagglutinin in the viral envelope but not neuraminidase, whereas virions of viruses of the genus *Pneumovirus* contain neither hemagglutinin nor neuraminidase but may contain fusion glycoprotein. Paramyxoviruses are genetically stable, and genetic recombination does not occur.

Rhabdoviridae

Virions of **Rhabdoviridae**[13, 68] are enveloped with surface projections and rod shaped, resembling a bullet (with one end rounded and the other flattened) or are bacilliform. Within the lipoprotein envelope and membrane protein is enclosed the long tubular nucleocapsid, about 50 nm in diameter, which is helically symmetric. The nucleocapsid contains a transcriptase and is infectious. The genome of single-stranded, negative-sense RNA is in unsegmented, linear form.

Some rhabdoviruses multiply in arthropods as well as in vertebrates or higher plants; some of these are typical arboviruses, for which arthropods act as true vectors of virus transmission; others multiply only in insects. Infectivity is sensitive to ether, acid, and heat.

The genera that include agents infecting vertebrates are *Lyssavirus* (rabies virus and several other viruses that infect humans, as well as some agents thus far isolated only from insects) and *Vesiculovirus* (vesicular stomatitis virus and antigenically interrelated viruses from various animal species). Among the vesiculoviruses are Chandipura virus (from humans).

Filoviridae[12, 34, 53]

Marburg virus is a simian virus highly pathogenic for man, producing a severe hemorrhagic fever syndrome, and Ebola virus is a newly recognized agent of outbreaks of hemorrhagic fever in Africa. Both of these agents are considered dangerous pathogens that should be studied in the laboratory only under maximum containment.

These viruses resemble rhabdoviruses in some respects and

were at first considered for inclusion in that family. However, it has become clear that they are significantly different from any other known vertebrate viruses, and they are established as a separate family.

By electron microscopy, the virus particles are pleomorphic, often appearing as exceedingly long filamentous forms (the basis for the name), sometimes branching extensively, sometimes appearing as U-shaped or circular forms or in the shape of the numeral 6. The diameter of the virions is 80 nm, but their length may range from 130 to 14,000 nm. In terms of infectivity, the infectious unit is 790 nm (Marburg) or 970 nm (Ebola). The virion has a lipid-containing envelope with surface projections. The nucleocapsid consists of a central axis 20 to 30 nm in diameter, surrounded by a helically wound capsid of 50 to 60 nm, and the genome is a single molecule of negative single-stranded RNA of molecular weight 4.2×10^6. The virion contains at least five major polypeptides. In replication, viral proteins accumulate in cytoplasm and plasma membranes, the nucleocapsid is assembled in the cytoplasm, and the virus matures by budding.

Coronaviridae

Coronaviridae[44, 62] is named for unique petal-shaped or club-shaped peplomers (about 20 nm long) that project from the envelope; in negatively stained electron micrographs, these projections form a fringe resembling the solar corona. The particles are pleomorphic. The internal ribonucleoprotein is seen as a loosely wound helical structure with a diameter of 10 to 20 nm (or a long strand 1 or 2 nm in diameter). The genome consists of one large molecule of single-stranded, positive-sense RNA. Nucleocapsids develop in the cytoplasm and mature by budding through intracytoplasmic membranes into cisternae. Infectivity is sensitive to ether, acid, and heat.

A single genus, *Coronavirus,* has been designated. Several serotypes of human coronaviruses have been isolated from patients with acute upper respiratory tract illnesses. The best-known of these human isolates are 229E and OC43; successful isolations have depended chiefly on the use of human embryonic tracheal and nasal organ cultures. There are distinct coronaviruses that infect a number of other vertebrate species: avian infectious bronchitis virus, mouse hepatitis virus, porcine transmissible gastroenteritis virus, and porcine hemagglutinating encephalitis virus. Probable members include canine coronavirus, the coronavirus of turkey bluecomb disease, neonatal calf diarrhea coronavirus, and at least two viruses infecting rats.

Two antigenic groups of mammalian coronaviruses and two antigenic groups of avian coronaviruses have been recognized. Human coronavirus 229E and other isolates belong to one of these groups, and human coronavirus OC43 and other human agents belong to the other.

Coronaviruses readily establish persistent infection in animals, often leading to subacute or chronic diseases. They provide a model for the study of persistent viral infections.

Bunyaviridae

Bunyaviridae[7, 12, 44] is the largest taxonomic grouping assigned to include an antigenically interrelated set of arboviruses. It includes at least 225 viruses (serotypes, subtypes, and varieties) that infect vertebrates and/or invertebrates. They are spherical virions, 80 to 110 nm in diameter, with a lipid-containing unit membrane envelope from which protrude polypeptide spikes 5 to 10 nm long. The virions develop in the cytoplasm and mature by budding through intracytoplasmic membranes into smooth-surfaced vesicles in or near the Golgi region of the cell. Infectivity is sensitive to ether, acid, and heat. Virus particles hemagglutinate.

The nucleic acid consists of three molecules of negative-sense, single-stranded RNA; the three ribonucleocapsids are composed of long, circular helical strands, 2.0 to 2.5 nm in diameter, sometimes supercoiled, with lengths of 0.2 to 3.0 μm.

Subdivision of the family **Bunyaviridae** into genera reflects both antigenic supergroup relationships and molecular similarities and differences. Most of the 124 or more members of the genus *Bunyavirus* belong to 13 serologically cross-related groups; several ungrouped arboviruses also are included; most are transmitted by mosquitoes. Among the members are the virus of California encephalitis and also the La Crosse virus, which causes human encephalitis with occasional fatal outcome, as well as other viruses that cause febrile diseases in human beings. Other bunyaviruses cause disease in some ruminants.

The genus *Phlebovirus* includes the virus of phlebotomus (sandfly) fever of humans, Rift Valley fever virus, and at least 28 other viruses. The agents predominantly are transmitted by sandfly, but some have been recovered from mosquitoes. A wide variety of vertebrates, especially rodents, may be infected. Rift Valley fever virus, a serious pathogen of sheep, has caused large epidemics among humans in Africa.

The genus *Nairovirus,* named from the virus of Nairobi sheep disease, has as its prototype the more intensively studied Crimean-Congo hemorrhagic fever virus of humans. Nairoviruses are transmitted predominantly by ticks. At least 19 serotypes belong to this genus.

Members of the genus *Uukuvirus* also are transmitted by ticks. The genus includes the type species, Uukuniemi virus, and six other viruses. They have been isolated in nature but have no known pathogenicity for humans.

Another important set of human pathogens has been shown to belong to the family **Bunyaviridae.** They are antigenically related to each other but not to other members of the family, and they apparently are not transmitted via arthropods. Human illness caused by Hantaan virus—the prototype strain—has been recognized in the Far East as Korean hemorrhagic fever, and a variant is known in Scandinavian and Eastern European countries as epidemic nephropathy.[39] There have been several instances of infection among staff members handling laboratory rats infected with the virus, both in the Far East and in Europe. In Belgium, there also have been sporadic cases with no apparent link to an outbreak or to each other.

These agents have been proposed to constitute a separate genus, *Hantavirus.* Besides the fundamental properties of **Bunyaviridae,** the hantaviruses that have been studied share a unique nucleotide sequence at the 3′ end of each of their three RNA segments—differing from the corresponding sequences of the other genera.

The illnesses caused by these viruses have been given a variety of names, the most common being hemorrhagic fever with renal syndrome, or HFRS, and muroid virus nephropathy. However, hemorrhagic symptoms are not present regularly.

In 1993, an epidemic caused by Hantavirus occurred in the southwestern United States and then spread. More than 100 cases of hantavirus pulmonary syndrome were reported in 21 states, including New York. In addition, seven cases were diagnosed in Canada and four in Brazil. About 40 per cent of the cases were fatal. In the United States, the virus is spread by deer mice, white-footed mice, and cotton rats. A vaccine has been made by inserting hantavirus gene into vaccine virus, but it has not had wide use.

Retroviridae[9, 17, 27, 31, 52]

The viruses in this family (Fig. 157–7) include not only the RNA tumor viruses (oncornaviruses, leukoviruses) that are assigned to a subfamily, Oncovirinae, but also the slow viruses of the maedi/visna group (the subfamily Lentivirinae) and the foamy virus group of agents that form syncytia in cell cultures (assigned to the subfamily Spumavirinae [Fig. 157–7]). The HIVs associated with AIDS are members of Lentivirinae.[54]

Retroviruses characteristically have a reverse transcriptase (RNA-dependent DNA polymerase) within the virion. The spherical virions, 80 to 100 nm in diameter, have glycoprotein surface projections approximately 8 nm in diameter. Within the envelope is an inner shell or capsid, probably icosahedral, containing ribonucleoprotein that possibly is helical. The genome is an inverted dimer of linear, single-stranded, positive RNA that dissociates readily into two or three pieces. Replication of the viral RNA involves a DNA provirus that is integrated into host cellular DNA.

Endogenous members of Oncovirinae may be part of the germ line of vertebrate hosts, being inherited as mendelian genes. The oncovirus genes may not be expressed but can be activated by physical and chemical agents, by superinfection with other oncoviruses, and even by herpesviruses. It was through studies of oncoviruses that the cellular "oncogenes" became recognized.[9]

The subfamily Oncovirinae has been divided into types A, B, C, and a possible type D, according to morphologic, antigenic, and enzymatic differences. Two of these groups have been designated formally as genus-level, and a third genus-level group (type D) tentatively has been defined. The type C oncovirus group includes mammalian, avian, and reptilian subgenus groupings, as well as a number of ungrouped species. Two members of Oncovirinae type C that infect humans, HTLV-I and HTLV-II, have been recognized; they are associated with human T-cell leukemias.[31] The type B oncovirus group includes the mouse mammary tumor virus and probably similar viruses from guinea pigs and perhaps other species. Type D includes viruses of monkeys. Special features observed in thin-section electron microscopy include an outer envelope, an inner membrane or shell, and a central nucleoid.

The members of the subfamily Spumavirinae, "foamy viruses," do not induce tumors or cellular transformation but cause persistent asymptomatic infections in natural and experimental host animals. They perhaps have been best known because they induce syncytia in cell cultures being prepared for cultivation of other viruses. Foamy or syncytial viruses are known for a number of mammalian species, including man.

The slow viruses of the maedi/visna group that have been placed in the subfamily Lentivirinae are morphologically and chemically like other members of **Retroviridae** but do not induce tumors.[54] Visna virus resembles type C oncoviruses in morphology, physical properties, and chemical composition. Synthesis of viral DNA continues throughout the infectious cycle under permissive conditions. Most of the DNA is extrachromosomal, but integrated DNA is present. It is not clear whether the integration is required for replication. Natural visna infections are known only in sheep, in which the virus causes panleukoencephalitis and infects all the organs of the animal. Pathologic changes, however, are confined chiefly to the brain, lungs, and reticuloendothelial system. The incubation period is long, and virus can be recovered from the animal as long as 4 years after inoculation. Serologically related viruses (variously designated in different countries as maedi or progressive pneumonia viruses) cause interstitial pneumonia.

The most widespread and severe human disease caused by members of **Retroviridae** is AIDS.[27, 31, 52] This immunoregulatory disorder often is fatal because it predisposes the infected individual to severe opportunistic infections and cancers. Susceptibility results from the depletion of helper T lymphocytes by HIV. In initial studies, the virus was called human T-lymphotropic virus type III, lymphadenopathy-associated virus, and AIDS-related virus.

HIV strains possess the physicochemical properties typical of **Retroviridae.** Two types have been recognized. Type 1 is more widespread and more virulent. Their unique morphologic characteristic is a cylindrical nucleoid in the mature virion. The genome of HIV-1 is known to encode at least seven genes, including the three structural genes *(gag, pol,* and *env)* and two transactivating genes *(tat)*.[66]

HIV is T-lymphotropic, especially for a particular group of helper T cells—those identified by monoclonal antibody OKT4 (Leu-3). Cell infection produces a pronounced cytopathic effect, including the formation of multinucleated giant cells, and cell death follows. The depletion of this CD4 subset of lymphocytes is a hallmark of AIDS. In contrast to the effect of other retrovirus pathogens of humans (HTLV-I and HTLV-II), the target cells are killed, not transformed. HIV also may infect other cell types, particularly macrophages that do not carry the CD4 antigen.

No animal model has been developed for AIDS. Although chimpanzees can be infected by HIV and develop antibodies and transient changes in T-cell ratios, they do not develop clinical signs of AIDS.

HIV is a completely exogenous virus, in contrast to the transforming retroviruses in which the viral genome is part of the conserved cellular genes. Individuals become infected by the introduction of HIV from outside sources and not by activation of silent viral sequences contained in cellular DNA. After an individual is exposed to HIV, proviral DNA is integrated into the cellular DNA of infected cells.

Isolates of HIV usually exhibit considerable divergence, particularly in the gene that codes for viral envelope proteins. This is in keeping with the behavior of visna virus, the *Lentivirus* prototype, which undergoes progressive antigenic variation in reaction to the host's immune response during persistent infection. This property of HIV may complicate efforts in vaccine development.

Arenaviridae

Members of the family **Arenaviridae**[8, 40, 44] have spherical or pleomorphic virions, ranging from 50 to 300 nm in diameter. The envelope, a dense lipid bilayer membrane, bears club-shaped surface projections 10 nm long. Within the virion core are electron-dense RNA-containing granules, about 20 to 25 nm in diameter, that resemble ribosomes in size, shape, and density. The genome is single-stranded, negative-sense RNA. Most member viruses have a single restricted rodent host in which persistent infection occurs, accompanied by viremia, viruria, or both. Spread to other mammals, including humans, can occur but is unusual.

A single genus has been established: *Arenavirus.* The type species is lymphocytic choriomeningitis virus, which can establish persistent infection causing immune complex disease in congenitally or neonatally infected mice; occasionally it can infect humans, causing aseptic meningitis. The family also includes Lassa virus which, when it spreads to humans, causes a severe febrile illness with a high mortality rate. Other arenaviruses are members of the Tacaribe complex of antigenically interrelated arboviruses: Pichinde virus, the Junin and Machupo viruses of South American hemorrhagic fevers, and several other arthropod-borne viruses.

EMERGING PROBLEMS IN VIRUS CLASSIFICATION

In addition to certain unclassified but known viral agents, some of the current and developing problems that viral taxonomists need to address are those presented by recently discovered forms of life that have properties differing from those of any other known biologic entities, such as the forms termed viroids and prions. Another kind of problem is presented by viral hybrids (between unrelated viruses), pseudotypes, pseudovirions, and recombinant DNA.

Viroids

Viroids,[19] which constitute a class of infectious agents smaller than viruses, are known to cause several diseases of plants (e.g., potato spindle tuber disease). Ultimately they may be found to cause disease in humans and animals, but their mechanisms of pathogenicity as yet are unknown. Viroids exhibit the properties of nucleic acids in crude extracts; that is, they are not sensitive to heat and organic solvents but are sensitive to nucleases, and they do not appear to have a protein coat.

Plant viroids are single-stranded, covalently closed, circular RNA molecules (molecular weights, 70,000 to 120,000) consisting of about 360 nucleotides and comprising a highly base-paired rodlike structure with unique properties. Each is arranged into 26 double-stranded regions separated by 25 regions of unpaired bases embodied in single-stranded internal loops; there is a loop at each end of the rodlike molecule. These features endow the viroid RNA molecule with structural, thermodynamic, and kinetic properties very similar to those of a double-stranded DNA molecule of the same molecular weight and G + C (guanine plus cytosine) content.

Viroids replicate by an entirely novel mechanism in which infecting viroid RNA molecules are copied by the host enzyme normally responsible for synthesis of nuclear precursors to messenger RNA. Thus, DNA-dependent RNA polymerase purified from healthy plant tissue is capable of synthesizing linear viroid RNA copies of full length from viroid RNA templates in vitro.

Comparative sequence analysis of a major group of plant viroids reveals striking similarities with the ends of transposable genetic elements. These similarities have led to speculation that viroids may have originated from transposable elements or retroviral proviruses by deletion of interior portions of the viral DNA.

Prions[4, 55]

Unusual kinds of infectious agents that may be similar to viroids have been implicated in degenerative brain diseases such as scrapie in sheep and Creutzfeldt-Jakob disease, a rare form of early senile dementia in humans.[26, 41] The scrapie agent has been considered to be an infectious DNA molecule with a molecular weight of 70,000 to 100,000, similar in size to plant RNA viroids. However, a new concept has been proposed as to the nature of the scrapie agent. The agent may be a small *pro*teinaceous *in*fectious particle, the *prion*. The prion protein, PrP 27-30, has a molecular weight of 27,000 to 30,000. PrP 27-30 co-purifies with scrapie infectivity, aggregates, and behaves like amyloid. Preparations containing only PrP and no detectable nucleic acid have been found in many normal brains, but PrP has been reported to accumulate in infected brains.[10, 41, 55]

A number of lines of evidence are set forth for consideration, including the marked resistance of the scrapie agent to procedures that attack most nucleic acids, its inactivation by procedures directed against proteins, its heterogeneity of size, and other novel properties. The evidence assembled is not claimed to rule out the possibility that a very small nucleic acid may be present, buried within a tightly packed protein shell; neither does it rule out the possible presence of a highly unusual nucleic acid, whose coat or chemical structure protects it from most procedures that inactivate nucleic acids.

If prions are devoid of nucleic acid, they are unique among microorganisms. If such is proved true, many new questions will be raised, including that of the mode whereby an infectious protein could replicate.

Virus Hybrids

The fact that hybrids[15] of unrelated viruses exist in nature should be recognized more widely. If the simian papovavirus SV40 had not been known already as a virus before the discovery of SV40-adenovirus hybrid particles, these particles would have presented viral taxonomists with a very confusing puzzle. In these hybrid particles, portions of the SV40 genome are linked covalently to adenovirus genetic material encased within an adenovirus coat. They would have seemed to be virions of a new and strange virus that reached antigenically as an adenovirus but that had many properties unlike those of an adenovirus when grown in culture.

A similar problem of identification and classification exists with regard to another type of particle found in some human adenovirus populations. That particle, termed MAC (monkey-adapting component), behaves somewhat like the SV40-adenovirus particle, permitting the true human adenovirus to replicate in monkey cell cultures. The particle, with a MAC genome and an adenovirus coat, does not contain any SV40 nucleic acid fragments, and its origin remains unknown.

Virus hybrids now can be produced in the laboratory by recombinant DNA methods.

Pseudovirions

Another virus form that is difficult to classify is the pseudovirion. During virus replication, the capsid sometimes encloses host nucleic acid rather than viral nucleic acid. When observed by electron microscopy, such particles look like ordinary virus particles, but they do not replicate. Pseudovirions contain the "wrong" nucleic acid. For example, fragments of host-cell DNA (instead of viral DNA) may be incorporated into papovavirus capsids, forming pseudovirion particles. This situation resembles the phenomenon of generalized transduction by bacteriophages (i.e., transfer of random portions of nucleic acid from donor to recipient bacterial cells).

Hybridization studies also indicate the occurrence of covalent linkage of cell DNA segments into the circular DNA of papovaviruses during replication in cells infected at high multiplicity. This phenomenon is analogous to specialized transduction by bacteriophages (i.e., transfer by virus of a specific segment of donor bacterial cell DNA). Furthermore, a DNA segment containing functional genes of a lambda bacteriophage has been incorporated into the circular DNA of papovavirus SV40. These findings open avenues for the study of possible transducing events in eukaryotic cells whereby functionally defined segments of genetic information might be transmitted from cell to cell. Pseudovirions present the taxonomist with problems based on natural events, and future laboratory manipulations probably will add to these problems of classification.

Recombinant DNA

Recently developed techniques allow DNA to be cleaved into specific pieces by use of restriction endonucleases from bacteria. The distinct fragments can be recombined and replicated. The genomic materials from two distinct viruses multiply together, and these new forms pose many new problems for classification.[65] Already available are vaccinia viruses that contain genes of HIV, HBV, influenza virus, and herpes simplex virus. Such recombinants grow in all hosts in which native vaccinia virus can replicate. Other virus vectors that have been developed include attenuated poliovirus and adenovirus vaccines, which can carry genes of HIV and HBV and can infect hosts by the oral route.

References

1. Anderson, M. J.: Parvoviruses as agents of human disease. Prog. Med. Virol. *34*:55–69, 1987.
2. Andrewes, D., Pereira, H. G., and Wildy, P.: Viruses of Vertebrates. 4th ed. New York, Macmillan, 1978.
3. Bachmann, P. A., Hoggan, M. D., Kurstak, E., et al.: *Parvoviridae:* Second report. Intervirology *11*:248–254, 1979.
4. Barry, R. A., Kent, S. B. H., McKinley, M. P., et al.: Scrapie and cellular prion proteins share polypeptide epitopes. J. Infect. Dis. *153*:848–854, 1986.
5. Bellett, A. J. D.: The iridescent virus group. Adv. Virus Res. *13*:225–246, 1968.
6. Berge, T. O.: International Catalogue of Arboviruses Including Certain Other Viruses of Vertebrates. DHEW Pub. No. (CDC) 75–8301, U. S. Dept. of Health, Education, and Welfare, 1975.
7. Bishop, D. H. L.: *Bunyaviridae. In* Fields, B. N., Knipe, D. M., Chanock, R. M., et al.: (eds.): Virology. 2nd ed. Vol. 1. New York, Raven Press, 1990, pp. 1155–1173.
8. Bishop, D. H. L.: *Arenaviridae* and their replication. *In* Fields, B. N., Knipe, D. M., Chanock, R. M., et al. (eds.): Virology. 2nd ed. Vol. 1. New York, Raven Press, 1990, pp. 1231–1243.
9. Bishop, J. M.: Exploring carcinogenesis with retroviral and cellular oncogenes. Prog. Med. Virol. *32*:5–14, 1985.
10. Bockman, J. M., Kingsbury, D. T., McKinley, M. P., et al.: Creutzfeldt-Jakob disease prion proteins in human brains. N. Engl. J. Med. *312*:73–78, 1985.
11. Brown, F.: Classification of viruses. *In* Brown, F., and Wilson, G. (eds.): Topley and Wilson's Principles of Bacteriology, Virology and Immunity. 7th ed., Vol. 4. Baltimore, Williams & Wilkins, 1984, pp. 1–13.
12. Brown, F.: Classification and nomenclature of viruses. Intervirology *25*:141–143, 1986; *30*:181–186, 1989.
13. Brown, F., Bishop, D. H. L., Crick, J., et al.: *Rhabdoviridae.* Intervirology *12*:1–7, 1979.
14. Brown, T., Anand, A., Ritchie, L. D., et al.: Intrauterine parvovirus infection associated with hydrops fetalis. Lancet *ii*:1033–1034, 1984.
14a. Bukh, J., Miller, R. H., and Purcell, R. H.: Genetic heterogeneity of hepatitis C virus: Quasi-species and genotypes. Semin. Liver Dis. *15*:41–63, 1995.
15. Butel, J. S., and Melnick, J. L.: Recent advances in molecular pathology. The state of the viral genome in cells transformed by simian virus 40: A review. Exp. Mol. Pathol. *17*:103–119, 1972.
16. Cooper, P. D., Agol, V. I., Bachrach, H. L., et al.: *Picornaviridae:* Second report. Intervirology *10*:165–180, 1978.
17. Dalton, A. G., Melnick, J. L., Bauer, H., et al.: The case for a family of reverse transcriptase viruses: *Retraviridae.* Intervirology *4*:201–206, 1974.
18. Davis, B. D., Dulbecco, R., Eisen, H. N., et al.: Microbiology. 4th ed. Philadelphia, J. B. Lippincott, 1990.
19. Diener, T. O.: Portraits of viruses: Portrait of the viroid. Intervirology *22*:1–16, 1984.
20. Dowdle, W. R., Davenport, F. M., Fukumi, H., et al.: *Orthomyxoviridae.* Intervirology *5*:245–251, 1975.
21. Efstathiou, S., Compels, U. A., Craxton, M. A., et al.: DNA homology between a novel human herpesvirus (HHV-6) and human cytomegalovirus. Lancet *1*:63–64, 1988.
22. Estes, M. K.: Rotaviruses and their replication. *In* Fields, B. N., Knipe, D. M., Chanock, R. M., et al. (eds.): Virology. 2nd ed., Vol. 2. New York, Raven Press, 1990, pp. 1329–1352.
23. Fenner, F.: Classification and nomenclature of viruses: Second report of the International Committee on Taxonomy of Viruses. Intervirology *7*:1–116, 1976.
24. Fenner, F.: Portraits of viruses: The poxviruses. Intervirology *11*:137–157, 1979.
25. Fenner, F.: Poxviruses. *In* Fields, B. N., Knipe, D. M., Chanock, R. M., et al. (eds.): Virology. 2nd ed., Vol. 2. New York, Raven Press, 1990, pp. 2113–2133.
25a. Francki, R. I. B., Fauquet, C. M., Knudson, D. L., et al. (eds.): Classification and Nomenclature of Viruses. 5th Report of the International Committee on Taxonomy of Viruses. Arch. Virol. 2(Suppl.):1–450, 1991.
26. Gajdusek, D. C.: Subacute spongiform encephalopathies: Transmissible cerebral amyloidoses caused by unconventional viruses. *In* Fields, B. N., Knipe, D. M., Chanock, R. M., et al. (eds.): Virology. 2nd ed., Vol. 2. New York, Raven Press, 1990, pp. 2289–2324.
27. Gallo, R. C., Essex, M., and Gross, L. (eds.): Human T-Cell Leukemia Viruses. Cold Spring Harbor, N.Y., Cold Spring Harbor Press, 1984.
28. Gust, I. D., Coulepis, A. G., Feinstone, S. M., et al.: Taxonomic classification of hepatitis A virus. Intervirology *20*:1–7, 1983.
29. Hollinger, F. B., and Ticehurst, J.: Hepatitis A virus. *In* Fields, B. N., Knipe, D. M., Chanock, R. M., et al. (eds.): Virology. 2nd ed., Vol. 1. New York, Raven Press, 1990, pp. 631–670.
30. Howard, C. R., and Melnick, J. L.: The classification and taxonomy of hepatitis viruses. *In* Hollinger, F. B., Lemon, S. M., and Margolis, H. (eds.): Viral Hepatitis and Liver Disease: Proceedings of the 1990 International Symposium on Viral Hepatitis (7th Triennial Congress on Viral Hepatitis). Baltimore, Williams & Wilkins, 1991, pp. 890–892.
31. Human Retrovirus Subcommittee, International Committee on Taxonomy of Viruses: Human immunodeficiency viruses. Science *232*:697, 1986.
31a. Ishii, K., Uchida, Y., Miyamura, K., et al. (eds.): Acute Hemorrhagic Conjunctivititis. Tokyo, University of Tokyo Press, 1989, pp. 1–429.
32. Jiang, X., Graham, D. Y., Wang, K., et al.: Norwalk virus genome cloning and characterization. Science *250*:1580–1583, 1990.
33. Kapikian, A. Z., and Chanock, R. M.: Norwalk group of viruses. *In* Fields, B. N., Knipe, D. M., Chanock, R. M., et al. (eds.): Virology. 2nd ed., Vol. 1. New York, Raven Press, 1990, pp. 671–693.
34. Kiley, M. P., Bowen, E. T. W., Eddy, G. A., et al.: *Filoviridae:* A taxonomic home for Marburg and Ebola viruses? Intervirology *18*:24–32, 1982.
35. Kilham, L., and Margolis, G.: Problems of human concern arising from animal models of intrauterine and neonatal infections due to viruses: A review. I. Introduction and virologic studies. Prog. Med. Virol. *20*:131–143, 1975.
36. Kingsbury, D. W.: *Orthomyxoviridae* and their replication. *In* Fields, B. N., Knipe, D. M., Chanock, R. M., et al. (eds.): Virology. 2nd ed., Vol. 1. New York, Raven Press, 1990, pp. 1075–1089.
37. Kingsbury, D. W.: *Paramyxoviridae* and their replication. *In* Fields, B. N., Knipe, D. M., Chanock, R. M., et al. (eds.): Virology. 2nd ed., Vol. 1. New York, Raven Press, 1990, pp. 945–962.
38. Lancaster, W. D., Kurman, R. J., Sanz, L. E., et al.: Human papillomavirus: Detection of viral DNA sequences and evidence for molecular heterogeneity in metaplasias and dysplasias of the uterine cervix. Intervirology *20*:202–212, 1983.
39. Lee, H. W., and van der Groen, G.: Hemorrhagic fever with renal syndrome. Prog. Med. Virol. *36*:62–102, 1989.
40. Lehmann-Grube, F.: Portraits of viruses: Arenaviruses. Intervirology *22*:121–145, 1984.
41. Manuelidis, L., and Manuelidis, E. E.: Recent developments in scrapie and Creutzfeldt-Jakob disease. Prog. Med. Virol. *33*:78–98, 1986.
42. Margolis, G., and Kilham, L.: Problems of human concern arising from animal models of intrauterine and neonatal infections due to viruses: A review. II. Pathologic studies. Prog. Med. Virol. *20*:144–179, 1975.
43. Matthews, R. E. F.: Classification and nomenclature of viruses: Third report of the International Committee on Taxonomy of Viruses. Intervirology *12*:129–296, 1979.
44. Matthews, R. E. F.: Classification and nomenclature of viruses: Fourth report of the International Committee on Taxonomy of Viruses. Intervirology *17*:1–199, 1982.
45. Matthews, R. E. F. (ed.): A Critical Appraisal of Viral Taxonomy. Boca Raton, FL, CRC Press, 1983.
46. Mayor, H. D., and Melnick, J. L.: Small deoxyribonucleic acid-containing viruses (picodnavirus group). Nature *210*:331–332, 1966.
47. Melnick, J. L.: Papovavirus group. Science *135*:1128–1130, 1962.
48. Melnick, J. L.: Taxonomy and nomenclature of viruses, 1982. Prog. Med. Virol. *28*:208–221, 1982.
49. Melnick, J. L.: Taxonomy of viruses. *In* Manual of Clinical Microbiology. 5th ed. Washington, D.C., American Society for Microbiology, 1991, pp. 811–817.
50. Melnick, J. L., Agol, V. I., Bachrach, H. L., et al.: *Picornaviridae.* Intervirology *4*:303–316, 1974.

51. Melnick, J. L., Allison, A. C., Butel, J. S., et al.: *Papovaviridae.* Intervirology 3:106–120, 1974.
52. Montagnier, L., and Alizon, M.: The human immune deficiency virus (HIV): An update. Ann. Inst. Pasteur Virol. *138*:1–11, 1987.
53. Murphy, F. A., Kiley, M. P., and Fisher-Hoch, S. P.: Marburg and Ebola viruses. *In* Fields, B. N., Knipe, D. M., Chanock, R. M., et al. (eds.): Virology. 2nd ed., Vol. 1. New York, Raven Press, 1990, pp. 933–942.
54. Narayan, O., and Clements, J. E.: Lentiviruses. *In* Fields, B. N., Knipe, D. M., Chanock, R. M., et al. (eds.): Virology. 2nd ed., Vol. 2. New York, Raven Press, 1990, pp. 1571–1589.
54a. Okuno, T., Oishi, H., Hayashi, K., et al.: Human herpesviruses 6 and 7 in cervixes of pregnant women. J. Clin. Microbiol. *33*:1968–1970, 1995.
55. Prusiner, S. B.: Prions: Novel infectious pathogens. Adv. Virus Res. *29*:1–56, 1984.
56. Robinson, W. S.: *Hepadnaviridae* and their replication. *In* Fields, B. N., Knipe, D. M., Chanock, R. M., et al. (eds.): Virology. 2nd ed., Vol. 2. New York, Raven Press, 1990, pp. 2137–2169.
57. Roizman, B., Carmichael, L. E., Deinhardt, F., et al.: *Herpesviridae:* Definition, provisional nomenclature, and taxonomy. Intervirology *16*:201–217, 1981.
58. Rueckert, R. R.: *Picornaviridae* and their replication. *In* Fields, B. N., Knipe, D. M., Chanock, R. M., et al. (eds.): Virology. 2nd ed., Vol. 1. New York, Raven Press, 1990, pp. 507–548.
59. Schaffer, F. L., Bachrach, H. L., Brown, F., et al.: *Caliciviridae.* Intervirology *14*:1–6, 1980.
60. Schiff, L. A., and Fields, B. N.: Reoviruses and their replication. *In* Fields, B. N., Knipe, D. M., Chanock, R. M., et al. (eds.): Virology. 2nd ed., Vol. 2. New York, Raven Press, 1990, pp. 1275–1306.
61. Schlesinger, A., and Schlesinger, M. J.: Replication of *Togaviridae* and *Flaviviridae. In* Fields, B. N., Knipe, D. M., Chanock, R. M., et al. (eds.): Virology. 2nd ed., Vol. 1. New York, Raven Press, 1990, pp. 697–711.
62. Siddell, S. G., Anderson, R., Cavanagh, D., et al.: *Coronaviridae.* Intervirology *20*:181–189, 1983.
63. Siegl, S., Bates, R. C., Berns, K. I., et al.: Characteristics and taxonomy of *Parvoviridae.* Intervirology *23*:61–73, 1985.
64. Simpson, R. A., McGinty, L., Simon, L., et al.: Association of parvoviruses with rheumatoid arthritis in humans. Science *223*:1425–1428, 1984.
65. Smith, G. L., Mackett, M., and Moss, B.: Infectious vaccinia virus recombinants that express hepatitis B virus surface antigen. Nature *302*:490–495, 1983.
66. Sodroski, J., Rosen, C., Wong-Staal, F., et al.: *Trans*-acting transcriptional regulation of human T-cell leukemia virus type III long terminal repeat. Science *227*:171–173, 1985.
66a. Tanaka, K., Kondo, T., Torigoe, S., et al.: Human herpesvirus 7: Another causal agent for roseola. J. Pediatr. *125*:105, 1994.
67. Tyler, K. L., and Fields, B. N.: Reoviruses. *In* Fields, B. N., Knipe, D. M., Chanock, R. M., et al. (eds.): Virology. 2nd ed., Vol. 2. New York, Raven Press, 1990, pp. 1307–1328.
68. Wagner, R. R.: *Rhabdoviridae* and their replication. *In* Fields, B. N., Knipe, D. M., Chanock, R. M., et al. (eds.): Virology. 2nd ed., Vol. 2. New York, Raven Press, 1990, pp. 867–881.
69. Westaway, E. G., Brinton, M. A., Gaidamovich, S. Y., et al.: *Togaviridae.* Intervirology *24*:125–139, 1985.
70. Westaway, E. G., Brinton, M. A., Gaidamovich, S. Y., et al.: *Flaviviridae.* Intervirology *24*:183–192, 1985.
71. Wigand, R., Bartha, A., Dreizin, R. S., et al.: *Adenoviridae*: Second report. Intervirology *18*:169–176, 1982.
72. Wildy, P.: Classification and Nomenclature of Viruses: First Report of the International Committee on Nomenclature of Viruses. Monographs in Virology. Vol. 5. Basel, S. Karger, 1971.
72a. Yamanishi, K., Okuno, T., Shiraki, M., et al.: Identification of human herpesvirus 6 as a causal agent for exanthem subitum. Lancet *i*:1065–1067, 1988.
73. zur Hausen, H.: Genital papillomavirus infections. *In* Melnick, J. L., Ochoa, S., and Oro, J. (eds.): Viruses, Oncogenes, and Cancer (Based on the 1983 Duran-Reynals International Symposium). Prog. Med. Virol. *32*:15–21, 1985.

DNA VIRUSES

❑ ❑ ❑

SUBSECTION ONE
PARVOVIRIDAE

158

PARVOVIRUSES

James D. Cherry

Parvoviruses infect a great variety of species in nature. The family *Parvoviridae* includes two subfamilies: *Parvovirinae* and *Densovirinae*.[96] The subfamily *Parvovirinae* has three genera: *Erythrovirus*, *Parvovirus*, and *Dependovirus*; the subfamily *Densovirinae* also has three genera: *Densovirus*, *Iteravirus*, and *Centravirus*. Densonucleosis viruses (*Densovirus* species) infect insect hosts and have not been found in humans or mammals.[22, 153] Human parvovirus B19 is the only member of the recently created genus *Erythrovirus*, and until recently it was classified in the genus *Parvovirus*. Parvovirus B19 is autonomous and does not require the presence of a helper virus.

Erythema infectiosum is the common clinical manifestation of parvovirus B19 infection. Other clinical manifestations include arthralgia and arthritis, aplastic crisis in patients with red blood cell defects, chronic anemia in immunocompromised patients, fetal hydrops, neurologic disease, and possibly other significant illnesses.

HISTORY

The first parvoviruses to be discovered infecting humans were found in stool specimens by electron microscopy.[154] These fecal parvoviruses have been linked with gastrointestinal symptoms, often in outbreaks associated with the consumption of shellfish.[63, 204] Their precise pathogenic role remains unclear because these viruses also may be found in the feces of asymptomatic individuals.[154]

In 1974, a second type of parvovirus was discovered in the serum of asymptomatic blood donors.[56] Discovered by chance as an agent responsible for false-positive results in the counterimmunoelectrophoresis tests then in use for the detection of hepatitis B virus surface antigen, they were revealed by electron microscopy to be uniform icosahedral particles with a mean diameter of 23 nm.

Preliminary studies of the physicochemical nature of this agent suggested its probable identity as a member of the family *Parvoviridae*.[56] In the following years, reports concerning this virus named it variously as human parvovirus-like agent, serum parvovirus-like virus,[51] and B19[190] after one of the original isolates. After the elucidation of its chemical properties in 1983,[49, 198] the virus was referred to as human parvovirus, or human serum parvovirus to denote that it is distinct from the fecal particles. Today the virus most commonly is called human parvovirus B19 or just B19 virus.[4, 53, 99]

For a number of years after its discovery, B19 virus infection appeared to be either asymptomatic or associated with a nonspecific febrile illness.[190] However, in the early 1980s, the central role of B19 virus in the etiology of aplastic crisis in chronic hemolytic anemias was identified.[62, 97, 166, 187] Soon thereafter came the appreciation that erythema infectiosum (fifth disease) is the common manifestation of B19 virus infection.[11] Ten years ago, the association between B19 virus infection in pregnancy and fetal death was observed, and during the last decade, the clinical spectrum of B19 virus infection has broadened considerably.[3, 88, 99, 218]

Although human parvovirus B19 was not discovered until 1974, its most common clinical disease (erythema infectiosum) was described almost 200 years ago.[25]

Tschamer's report in 1889[203] was considered by most reviewers to be the first description of erythema infectiosum. However, Boysen[25] noted that an English dermatologist, Robert Willan, had reported the illness first in 1799 and then more completely in 1840.

After Tschamer's report came a succession of Austrian and German reports of the illness.[25] Tschamer thought that erythema infectiosum was a manifestation of rubella, but a few years later, Escherich[67] suggested that it was a specific disease. Stricker[197] in 1899 gave the name erythema infectiosum to the clinical entity.

In 1905, Shaw,[189] having observed cases of erythema infectiosum in Austria, published the first account in the American literature. Herrick[90] was the first to document in detail an outbreak in the United States; however, cases of erythema infectiosum had been observed previously in St. Louis[224] and in Hamburg, New York.[90] Over the last 65 years, numerous outbreaks and epidemics have been described in North America.[2, 13, 16, 18, 20, 27, 39, 43, 47, 50, 54, 64, 71, 73, 75, 79, 100, 115, 116, 120, 130, 139, 158, 159, 168, 192, 208, 209, 215, 216, 227] Erythema infectiosum frequently is referred to as fifth disease and in the past also was called ring rubella, large-spotted disease, and epidemic megaloerythema.

PROPERTIES OF THE VIRUS

Human parvovirus B19 is a naked icosahedral virus with a mean diameter of 23 nm and a mean buoyant density in cesium chloride of 1.43 g/dL.[56] The capsid is formed from two major structural proteins (VP1 and VP2) discernible by sodium dodecyl sulfate polyacrylamide gel electrophoresis.[49] VP2 is the major structural protein with a molecular weight of 58 kDa; VP1 has a molecular weight of 84 kDa. Ninety-six per cent of the capsid is in VP2 and 4 per cent is in VP1. The major nonstructural protein (NS1) has a molecular weight of 77 kDa. The genome consists of a single molecule of single-stranded DNA approximately 5.6 kb in length.[60] The DNA in B19 virus occurs as both plus and minus strands in approximately equal numbers.[99] When virions are disrupted with protease, the two complementary strands anneal to form a stable duplex.[198] At each end of the molecule are palindromic sequences forming "hairpin" loops. The hairpin at the 3′ end of the genome serves as a primer for DNA polymerases. The hairpin duplex at the 5′ end of the molecule comprises sequences that are neither complementary to those at the 3′ end, as is found in dependoviruses, nor as highly complementary within this 5′ end as are those at the 3′ end.[57]

Parvovirus infectivity is relatively heat-stable, tolerant of a wide range of pH, and resistant to ether.[12] Successful replication of parvoviruses can be accomplished only in a dividing cell because of the absolute requirement for host cell function(s) found in late S phase.[87] Human parvovirus B19 can be propagated only in human erythropoietic cells from the bone marrow and in primary fetal liver culture.[29, 152, 195, 196, 201]

The cellular receptor for B19 virus infection is the blood group P antigen.[30] This antigen is found on erythroblasts, megakaryoblasts, and endothelial cells. People who lack the P protein are resistant to infection with B19 virus.[32]

Antigenically, this human parvovirus seems distinct from the parvovirus-like particles found in feces,[155] as well as from the human dependoviruses and autonomous animal parvoviruses.[56] However, the nucleotide sequence and hybridization results reported by Turton and associates[204] suggest that the viruses from gastroenteritis cases in 1977 and 1986 are similar to B19. In contrast to animal parvoviruses, no hemagglutinin has been demonstrated.

The degree to which B19 virus is related to other mammalian parvovirus types has been investigated by the technique of DNA:DNA hybridization. Although no relationship is discernible with the human dependoviruses, a distant evolutionary relationship to the genomes of autonomous parvoviruses of rodents is apparent. Interestingly, this relationship is closer than that between B19 virus and the parvoviruses infecting domestic animals (bovine, feline, and canine parvoviruses).[57]

Parvovirus B19 does not grow in routine tissue cultures. It will grow in erythroid progenitor cells from human bone marrow, fetal liver, erythroid cells from a patient with erythroleukemia, and human umbilical cord and peripheral blood.[99] It only grows in dividing cells, and therefore all of the aforementioned tissue culture systems require the addition of erythropoietin. Parvovirus B19 also has been propagated in megakaryoblastoid cell lines.

EPIDEMIOLOGY

Outbreaks of erythema infectiosum have been observed throughout the world, but most reports have come from nontropical regions. The epidemic pattern of erythema infectiosum surprisingly is similar to that of rubella. Community epidemics are most prevalent in the winter and spring, and they usually last for 3 to 6 months. In a review of 30 well-described epidemics,[2, 6, 13, 18, 25, 27, 43, 47, 50, 54, 64, 71, 79, 90, 100, 115, 116, 120, 139, 159, 168, 192, 208, 214, 216, 227] 26 had their onset in the period from December through May and 23 of the 30 peaked in March, April, or May. When the North American literature for the last 50 years is examined, a cyclic pattern appears with peaks in disease activity about every 6 years. The peak periods last for an average of 3 years. A longitudinal study of aplastic crisis among persons with sickle-cell anemia in Jamaica suggested peaks of incidence every 2 to 3 years in this island population.[187]

The case-to-case interval of erythema infectiosum is reported to be between 4 and 14 days.[2, 11, 64, 79, 162, 208, 216] In an elementary school epidemic, Greenwald and Bashe[79] noted that the mean case-to-case interval was 8.7 days. Ager and associates[2] in their studies noted clustering of intervals between cases of 7 to 11 days. Edelson and Altman[64] noted in a student who had been out of the country the occurrence of illness 4 days after his return. The data of Wilcox and Evans[216] on multiple cases in households suggest that the case-to-case interval usually is closer to 12 to 14 days. In a volunteer study in which adults were inoculated intranasally, the incubation time to the onset of the rash was 17 to 18 days.[8] From this study, the case-to-case interval in the community would be expected to be between 6 and 12 days. This prediction accords well with the intervals in the studies noted earlier, as well as the intervals observed in patients with hematologic diseases and aplastic crisis.[133]

In epidemics, the attack rate is high. Lauer and colleagues[115] noted an overall attack rate of 24.3 per cent in schoolchildren in grades kindergarten through eight. Similar attack rates were noted in two other school-related outbreaks.[64, 79] In the community as a whole, the attack rate is highest in children 5 to 14 years of age,[1, 2] but secondary cases occur in preschool children, teachers, and parents. In the home, secondary cases are reported more commonly in mothers than in fathers.[2] In school epidemics, the attack rate is considerably higher in girls than in boys.[2, 64, 115] Prevalence studies of serum IgG antibody to B19 virus have noted that 40 to 60 per cent of adults are seropositive and 2 to 21 per cent of children younger than 11 years of age are seropositive.[4–6, 51] Nosocomial infections occur; most often, the index case is an unrecognized chronically infected patient.[1, 110, 161] During community outbreaks, the risk in hospital workers is no greater than it is in other community residents.

Although erythema infectiosum long had been postulated to be transmitted by droplet via the respiratory tract,[2] proof of this was not obtained until a group of volunteers were infected successfully with B19 virus after intranasal inoculation. One week after inoculation, virus was excreted from the respiratory tract for 6 days.[8]

Parvovirus B19 infection also can be transmitted by blood transfusion and clotting factor concentrates but not by immunoglobulin preparations.[127, 134, 220]

PATHOGENESIS AND PATHOLOGY

The pathogenesis of parvovirus disease involves two quite separate components. The first is due to the lytic infection of susceptible dividing cells and the second to interaction with the products of the immune response.

As stated earlier, parvoviruses only replicate in dividing cells. Thus, infection of an organ or tissue in which a significant proportion of the cells are dividing may give rise to organ-specific disease. This is seen clearly in canine and feline parvovirus infections, in which virus replication in the crypt cells of the intestine gives rise to a severe and often fatal enteritis.[85, 122]

Parvovirus B19 is believed not to infect cells of the gastrointestinal tract; virus could not be detected in feces of volunteers,[8] nor have viruses of this type been found in stool specimens.

Gaining entry via the respiratory tract, the virus sets up a systemic infection with copious viremia (Fig. 158–1), in which 10^{10} or 10^{11} virus particles per milliliter of blood is not an uncommon finding.[8, 163]

Parvovirus infection results in profound reticulocytopenia for some 7 to 10 days commencing during viremia.[8] In vitro studies on cultured bone marrow and peripheral blood have shown that B19 virus inhibits the formation of blast-forming unit erythroid colonies, suggesting that an early erythrocyte precursor cell is susceptible to virus infection. Granulocytes and megakaryocytes are unaffected by virus in these in vitro systems. However, during B19 virus infection in the normal host, a clinically insignificant lymphopenia and neutropenia as well as a drop in platelet numbers occur.[8, 162] The mechanisms of the loss of these cells from the peripheral blood remain to be determined. Srivastava and associates[195] noted that B19 virus infection of bone marrow cells in culture results in suppression of megakaryocyte colony formation. In this study, there appeared to be tropism of B19 virus for cells other than the erythroid progenitor cell, although viral DNA replication did not occur in the megakaryocyte-enriched fractions. They suggested that the virus might be toxic to cell populations that are nonpermissive for viral DNA replication.

As noted in Figure 158–1, viremia ends at the time of

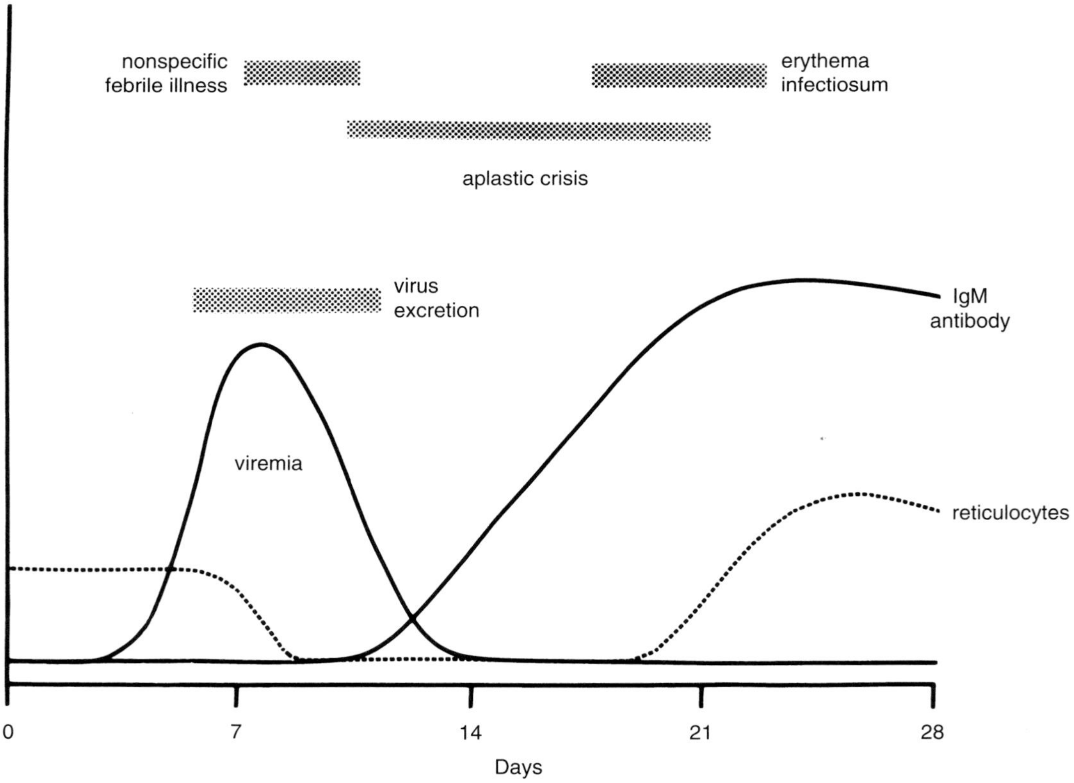

FIGURE 158–1. *Selected virologic, immunologic, hematologic, and clinical events in parvovirus B19 virus infections.*

appearance of specific IgM antibody. In addition, it has been found that the appearance of antibody neutralizes the inhibitory effect of B19 virus on erythrocyte colony formation in vitro.[223] These findings plus the fact that a cellular (T-cell) response to B19 virus has not been demonstrated suggest that the humoral response is the crucial factor in recovery from disease.[113] The early IgM response almost entirely is VP2-specific. IgG antibody first appears about 2 weeks after exposure and later becomes the major antibody subclass; in contrast with the initial IgM response, the IgG response is directed at VP1 rather than VP2.

The most common result of infection with B19 virus is erythema infectiosum. Figure 158–1 shows that the symptoms of this disease begin 17 or 18 days after inoculation and about 1 week after virus can be detected in either throat swabs or blood. Skin biopsy results have been reported in three studies.[20, 80, 93] In three skin biopsies from regions of reticulated eruption, Bard and Perry[20] noted either normal skin or very mild inflammatory changes. Hoffman[93] described edema in the epidermis and perivascular infiltration with mononuclear cells; he also noted swelling of the endothelium of the superficial vessels and cleavage spaces between the epidermis and dermis. The histopathology was investigated in 10 cases by Grimmer and Joseph[80]; they reported dilation of blood vessels with lymphocytic and occasional plasma cell perivascular infiltration. However, the clinical manifestations of many of the cases in the epidemic that Grimmer and Joseph[80] studied were quite atypical.

Virus-specific IgM is present at the time of the onset of the rash in erythema infectiosum, so that although the mechanisms of production of the rash (and arthralgia) of erythema infectiosum remain to be elucidated, it is not unreasonable to postulate an immune-mediated pathogenesis. The perivascular infiltrations noted by Hoffman[93] would support this suggestion. However, Schwarz and colleagues[185] have found both viral capsid proteins and viral DNA in a skin biopsy of the rash in a patient with erythema infectiosum. They therefore suggest that the rash may be a direct effect of the virus rather than being immune complex–mediated.

Intrauterine infection results in infection of the fetus and frequently abortion.[3, 4, 39, 42, 75, 102, 165, 171, 183, 218, 222] The main finding in the infected fetuses is hydrops fetalis, which results from the anemia due to the infection of the erythrocyte precursor cells. Intranuclear inclusions are seen in nucleated red blood cells, and viral particles are identified in the same cells by electron microscopy.[42]

In immunocompromised patients, persistent infection with B19 virus often occurs.[113] This is due to the failure to produce effective neutralizing antibodies.

CLINICAL MANIFESTATIONS

Infection with human parvovirus B19 results in a spectrum of clinical manifestations; classic cases of erythema infectiosum occupy a central position in this spectrum. Other major manifestations include arthritis and arthralgia, intrauterine infection and hydrops fetalis, transient aplastic crisis in patients with a variety of underlying hemolytic illnesses, and persistent infection with chronic anemia in patients with immunodeficiencies. In addition, subclinical, nonexanthematous infection occurs and especially is common among children.[8, 162]

Other less common illnesses include myocarditis, vasculitis, glomerulonephritis, and neurologic disease. Finally, associations between B19 virus infection and Kawasaki disease, chronic fatigue syndrome, systemic lupus erythematosus, Kikuchi disease, hepatic dysfunction, and Wegener granulomatosis have been noted, but causality has not been established.

Erythema Infectiosum

Although a search of the literature relating to erythema infectiosum outbreaks reveals a conspicuous absence of prodromal symptoms in cases, infected volunteers have had febrile episodes with nonspecific symptoms of headache, chills, myalgia, and malaise accompanying the viremic phase of the B19 virus infection (see Fig. 158–1).[8] These symptoms last for 2 to 3 days and coincide with excretion of virus from the pharynx. There then is a period of 7 days during which individuals are free of symptoms before the onset of the second, exanthematous phase of illness. It is likely that the relatively long period between the symptoms in this biphasic illness has prevented the recognition of the link between these nonspecific prodromal symptoms and erythema infectiosum.

The exanthem in classic cases of erythema infectiosum occurs in three stages.[2, 16, 27, 43, 45, 47, 79, 189, 208–210] The first stage begins 18 days after the acquisition of infection and is characterized by a fiery red rash on the cheeks (see Fig. 67–6) (slapped-cheek appearance). The edges of the involved areas may be raised slightly, and there is relative circumoral pallor. At this stage, the appearance may be suggestive of scarlet fever, drug sensitivity or other allergic reaction, or collagen vascular disease. The facial exanthem is aggravated by the transition from outdoors to a warm room.

The second stage of the exanthem occurs 1 to 4 days after the onset of facial involvement, with the appearance of an erythematous, maculopapular rash on the trunk and limbs. This rash is discrete initially but spreads to involve large areas. Toward the end of this stage, there is central clearing of the rash from these areas to give the characteristic lacy or reticular pattern (see Fig. 67–7).

The third stage of the exanthem is highly variable in duration, lasting from 1 to 3 or more weeks, and is characterized by marked changes in the intensity of the rash with periodic complete evanescence and recrudescence. These fluctuations are related to environmental factors such as exposure to sunlight and temperature (a hot bath may result in recrudescence in an apparently recovered child).

The rash often is pruritic, especially in adults, and generally is more prominent on the extensor surfaces; the palms and soles rarely are affected. Slight desquamation has been noted in a small number of patients in most reviews.

Although classic cases of erythema infectiosum are easy to recognize clinically, especially during outbreaks, there is a wide variation in the form of the exanthem from a very faint, fleeting rash to a florid exanthem, confluent over large areas (see Fig. 67–8). In many cases, the illness may be indistinguishable from rubella.

The overwhelming majority of cases of erythema infectiosum have no enanthem. Kerr and Marsh[100] and Condon[54] noted a few children with pharyngitis.

Other symptoms and signs are uncommon in erythema infectiosum (Table 158–1). In general, complaints are more frequent in adults than children. Headache is noted in about one-fifth of childhood cases and about half of the afflicted adults. Joint pain and swelling and myalgia particularly are troublesome in adults.

Routine laboratory studies are of little use in erythema infectiosum. The leukocyte count usually is normal, although a mild eosinophilia is noted occasionally.[16, 25, 209, 210]

The most common complication of erythema infectiosum is joint involvement; this is relatively rare in children (<10 per cent of cases), but in adults it is the norm, occurring in 80 per cent or more of the cases.[4, 10, 11, 16, 88, 140, 169, 170, 211, 215] There is a range of severity, from mild arthralgia to frank arthritis. The joints most commonly involved are the knees, ankles,

TABLE 158–1. Frequency of Symptoms and Signs in Erythema Infectiosum

Sign or Symptom	Per Cent Occurrence	
	Children	*Adults*
Rash	100	100
Pruritus	15	50
Headache	20	50
Fever	15	25
Sore throat	15	15
Coryza	10	15
Cough	8	8
Sore eyes	10	10
Anorexia	15	22
Nausea	7	26
Vomiting	4	7
Diarrhea	4	12
Abdominal pain	10	15
Joint pain	10	70
Joint swelling	5	60
Myalgia	4	50

Data from references 2, 64, 79, 209.

and proximal interphalangeal; symptoms usually are bilateral. Joint involvement usually is transient, lasting only a few days. In some individuals, symptoms may persist for some weeks or, rarely, months. Where joint involvement follows an exanthem, diagnosis may be adduced, but this is not invariably the case. As with rubella, the frequency of arthralgia and arthritis is higher in women than men.

Other complications of erythema infectiosum include cases of transient hemolytic anemia, encephalitis with recovery without residua, encephalopathy in a 9-month-old boy resulting in permanent sequelae, thrombocytopenic purpura, Henoch-Schönlein purpura, myocarditis, and pseudoappendicitis.[17, 69, 84, 95, 117, 118, 132, 176, 211]

Other Exanthems

Grimmer and Joseph[80] described cases in which the rashes were morbilliform, hemorrhagic, urticarial, vesicular, and erythema multiforme–like. Their studies were conducted during an epidemic of erythema infectiosum in Berlin, Germany, in which it was estimated that 50,000 persons were affected. It is quite possible that the cases with markedly unusual manifestations were not of the same etiology as the typical cases. However, other authors also have noted papular, purpuric, vesicular, urticarial, and morbilliform eruptions.[43, 54, 55, 119, 124, 141, 159]

García-Tapia and associates[74] described a 5-year-old girl with erythema multiforme bullosum without other systemic manifestations; the patient's serum had B19 virus–specific IgM antibody. Several adults with a papular-purpuric or petechial "glove and sock" syndrome have been described.[15, 23, 83]

Grimmer and Joseph[80] stated that the majority of their cases in the Berlin epidemic had dark red spots of the pharynx, gums, soft palate, and uvula. These cases, again, must be regarded with some suspicion because the investigators also noted genital lesions and conjunctivitis in a few patients.

Aplastic Crisis

In individuals with chronic hemolytic anemia, the profound reticulocytopenia of human parvovirus B19 infection results in the depression of hemoglobin concentrations to critical levels.[4, 7, 39, 62, 76, 77, 86, 97, 119, 133, 150, 166, 174, 187, 198, 222, 223] With the resolution of infection, reticulocytes reappear in the peripheral blood and hemoglobin concentrations return to the normal steady state values for these patients. This transient arrest of erythrocyte production is termed aplastic crisis and may occur in any individual whose erythrocytes have a short life span. Examples of such conditions include sickle-cell anemia,[77, 187] hereditary spherocytosis,[66, 86, 97, 150] thalassemia,[119, 166] glucose-6-phosphate dehydrogenase deficiency,[76] and pyruvate kinase deficiency.[62]

Serjeant and coworkers[188] studied the epidemiology of B19 virus infection over time in 308 children with homozygous sickle-cell disease and in 239 controls with normal hemoglobin. B19 virus infection accounted for all 91 aplastic crises that occurred. Twenty-three additional patients with sickle-cell disease had B19 virus infections; of these, 10 had mild hematologic changes and 13 had no changes. By 15 years of age, about 40 per cent of the sickle-cell group and the control group had IgG antibody to B19 virus, indicating equal infection rates in the two groups. No patient or control had two infections due to B19 virus.

Rao and colleagues[167] found that 70 per cent of patients with transient aplastic crisis admitted to their hospitals during a 7-year period had B19 viral infections. No patients had chronic or recurrent infections. In the study of 48 patients with aplastic crises, Mallouh and Qudah[125] found B19 virus infection in 91 per cent. In addition to the anemia, 21 per cent of the patients had leukopenia, 27 per cent had neutropenia, and 42 per cent had thrombocytopenia. The same investigators noted acute splenic sequestration together with aplastic crisis in three patients with sickle-cell disease and B19 virus infection.[124] Lowenthal and associates[121] noted three young adults with sickle-cell acute chest syndrome associated with B19 virus infection.

Interestingly, reports of exanthematous illness occurring after aplastic crisis are rare. However, cases of aplastic crisis require transfusion with packed cells, and it is possible that rashes occurring after such treatment would be regarded as transfusion reactions. Joint symptoms are fairly frequent in cases such as sickle-cell anemia, so that although they may occur as a result of B19 infection, they may be diagnosed as "painful crises."

As noted earlier, human parvovirus B19 infection does not result invariably in aplastic crisis in the chronic hemolytic anemic patient. Some individuals escape this complication if they have been transfused recently,[7] possibly because of a protective effect of transfused antibody (more than 60 per cent of donors are immune), the substitution of longer-lived, donated erythrocytes for the patients' own fragile ones, or a combination of these two. Certainly among individuals suffering the more severe form of beta-thalassemia, aplastic crisis is a rare complication; in such cases, the anemia is so severe that the patient is maintained by regular, frequent transfusions.

Among populations in which aplastic crisis does occur, the severity of the episode varies between individuals. This may reflect the variation in erythrocyte life span between these patients.[7]

Arthritis and Arthralgia

As noted earlier, acute arthritis and arthralgia are common occurrences in erythema infectiosum. In most instances, the joint symptoms subside within a few weeks, but arthralgia and arthritis persist occasionally. It also has been observed that joint manifestations due to B19 virus infections can occur without any exanthem or with an exanthem not typical of erythema infectiosum. These findings have led to investigations relating to the role of B19 virus in rheumatoid arthritis.[70, 82, 88, 99, 129, 146, 148, 164]

Nocton and coworkers[148] studied 22 patients seen in their rheumatology clinic who had serologic or clinical evidence of B19 virus infection. Of this group, six children had persistent arthritis that would fulfill criteria for the diagnosis of junvenile rheumatoid arthritis. Mimori and associates[129] found that patients with refractory polyarticular juvenile rheumatoid arthritis had a higher frequency of IgG antibody to B19 virus (5 of 7) than age-matched controls (5 of 60). However, on examining these data, it is clear that the antibody prevalence in the controls is lower than should be expected. Nikkari and associates[146, 147] in Finland have done extensive studies and note that chronic rheumatoid-like arthropathies triggered by B19 virus occasionally occur. However, their data do not support a general role for B19 virus in the etiology or pathogenesis of rheumatoid arthritis.

Tyndall and colleagues[205] noted an adult woman with erosive polyarthritis associated with a B19 virus infection, and Samii and coworkers[179] reported two adults with bilateral carpal tunnel syndrome associated with B19 virus infections. Berg and associates[21] could find no association with either IgG or IgM antibody to B19 virus and fibromyalgia in a study of 26 adult women and matched controls.

Infection in Immunocompromised Patients

Some immunodeficient patients suffer chronic B19 virus infections.[4, 34, 44, 58, 81, 88, 99, 106, 111, 123, 137, 145, 149, 160, 221, 222] These patients have persistent anemia due to a continuous lysis of red cell precursors. This problem has been noted most commonly in children with acute lymphocytic leukemia.[38, 58, 106, 111]

It also occurs in other acquired and congenital immunodeficiency states. Viremia and anemia may, if untreated, persist for years. Fatigue and pallor are the most common clinical findings, and other findings of B19 virus infections, such as exanthem and arthralgia, are rare. Because of immunodeficiency, IgM antibody studies usually are not useful in diagnosis. Therefore, diagnosis of persistent B19 virus infection depends upon demonstration of specific B19 antigen or DNA in the blood.

Intrauterine Infection

Although a large epidemiologic study of an outbreak of erythema infectiosum more than 30 years ago failed to reveal evidence of teratogenicity, virologic and serologic studies during the last decade indicate that B19 virus crosses the placenta and causes infection in the fetus.[2–4, 26, 33, 34, 39, 61, 75, 78, 88, 99, 102, 103, 105, 107, 157, 165, 171–173, 178, 193, 202, 206, 217–219, 222, 225] Infection in pregnancy results in fetal hydrops, fetal death, and miscarriage. To determine the rate and outcome of fetal infection after infection in pregnant women, a large prospective study was carried out in England during a $3\frac{1}{2}$-year period from January 1985 to June 1988.[165] Of 186 pregnancies, 156 (84 per cent) resulted in the birth of normal babies. At 1-year follow-up, all 114 of those with available clinical information had no appreciable abnormalities; 27 of these infants had serologic evidence of intrauterine infection. The overall fetal loss rate was 16 per cent, with an excess occurring during the second trimester. Virologic study indicated that the risk of fetal death due to B19 virus infection during pregnancy was 9 per cent and the transplacental transmission rate was 33 per cent.

In a study in Connecticut related to a large outbreak of erythema infectiosum in which 39 infected pregnant women were monitored, it was found that two miscarriages occurred.[172] Fetal loss due to B19 virus infection was estimated to be 5 per cent. In another study in Spain, fetal loss occurred in only 1 of 60 women with B19 virus infections during pregnancy.[78]

Koch and colleagues[107] performed follow-up examinations on 19 infants born to mothers who had serologically confirmed B19 virus infections between the fourth and thirty-eighth week of gestation. None of these infants developed hydrops during pregnancy, and all were normal after birth. One child, whose mother had erythema infectiosum at approximately the twentieth week of gestation, had a persistent asymptomatic infection for at least the first 7 months of life. Donders and coworkers[61] noted a child in whom a sonogram revealed fetal hydrops at 30 weeks' gestation. A cordocentesis revealed a hemoglobin concentration of 2.4 g/dL. One week later, a hydropic 1550-g infant was delivered by cesarean section. The baby's bone marrow showed an arrest in erythropoiesis with giant pronormoblasts. The baby received multiple transfusions for the first 4 months of life, and B19 viral DNA was identified in the blood at 19 weeks of age. At 2 years of age, this child was found to be clinically, hematologically, and immunologically normal.

In contrast with the case just noted, Brown and associates[33] noted a baby with a similar exposure and delivery history who had persistent anemia and in spite of therapy was transfusion-dependent at 4 years of age. In addition, Brown and associates reported two other infants who had received intrauterine transfusions for fetal hydrops and who had persistent anemias after birth.

At the present, a large number of babies who were exposed to B19 virus in utero have been studied, and there is no convincing evidence of specific congenital malformations.[102, 135, 165, 171, 172, 218] However, van Elsacker-Niele and associates[206] noted B19 virus infection in cells other than those of the erythroid series in two aborted fetuses. Ocular malformation was noted in one, and evidence of extensive inflammatory reactions in all fetal and placental tissues was noted in both.

Tiesson and colleagues[202] noted an aborted fetus with a bilateral cleft lip, alveolus, and palate; micrognathia; and webbed joints. In another aborted fetus, ocular abnormalities similar to those seen in congenital rubella were noted.[213] A newborn with anemia, blueberry-muffin rash, and hepatomegaly from whom parvovirus B19 virus gene sequences were found in the liver and placenta has been reported.[191]

Neurologic Illness

Suzuki and associates[199] reported a 20-day-old infant with fever (temperature, 39.8° C) and aseptic meningitis with B19 virus–specific IgM antibody in the blood. The child's temperature returned to normal on the fourth hospital day, but her hemoglobin decreased from 11.7 g/100 mL to 9 g/100 mL on day 36. Occasional other cases of aseptic meningitis and encephalitis have been reported.[40, 88, 99, 109, 151]

Other Illnesses

One adult patient had chronic red cell aplasia for a 10-year period, which was treated with regular blood transfusions.[112] After diagnosis of persistent B19 virus infection, the patient was treated with intravenous immunoglobulin, which resulted in an apparent cure. A presumably immunologically normal woman had recurrent episodes of paresthesia over a 4-year period in conjunction with persistent B19 virus DNA in her blood.[68] Evidence of persistent infection in immunologically normal patients has been noted in other studies.[98, 138]

McClain and coworkers[126] studied 19 children with primary neutropenia; parvovirus B19 DNA was found in the bone marrow of 15. A 12-year-old boy with hemophagocytic syndrome associated with B19 virus infection has been reported.[24] This child recovered after splenectomy.

B19 virus–associated hemophagocytic syndrome also has been noted in two patients with hereditary spherocytosis.[136] Recently, Heegaard and colleagues[89] found B19 virus DNA in 3 of 11 bone marrow smears from children with Diamond-Blackfan syndrome. The three B19 virus–positive patients experienced remission after steroid therapy, whereas the seven patients without evidence of B19 virus infection have required continued steroid treatment.

An association between parvovirus B19 infection and Kawasaki disease has been observed recently.[94, 144] Nigro and associates[144] found that 10 of 15 patients with Kawasaki disease had evidence of active or recent infection with B19 virus.

Langnas and colleagues[114] noted an association between B19 virus infection and fulminant liver failure and associated aplastic anemia. However, this study is troubling because B19 virus DNA also was found in liver specimens of 5 (15 per cent) of the controls. A 7-month-old infant with myocarditis associated with B19 virus infection has been described,[156] and a 12-year-old boy with Wegener granulomatosis and persistent B19 infection has been reported.[144]

DIAGNOSIS

Differential Diagnosis

Because the exanthem of erythema infectiosum is truly unique, its diagnosis should be easy. During epidemics, no difficulties should arise, but sporadic cases can be a problem. In the differential diagnosis, rubella and scarlet fever are of most concern. Because rubella virus has been recovered from some patients with illness thought to be erythema infectiosum[18] and because an erythema infectiosum–like illness was observed in volunteers who received intranasal administration of a rubella virus strain recovered from a patient with erythema infectiosum–like illness,[180] this diagnostic possibility always should be considered. When the risk of congenital rubella is a possibility, rubella-specific diagnostic tests should be performed (see Chapter 177).

Erythema infectiosum can be differentiated from scarlet fever by the usual lack of pharyngitis in the former and a positive culture for *Streptococcus pyogenes* in the latter. Other differential diagnostic considerations are other infectious exanthems (see Chapter 67), collagen vascular diseases, drug reactions, and allergic responses to environmental substances. Although a presumptive diagnosis of erythema infectiosum may be made by exclusion of other etiologic possibilities, definitive diagnosis only may be made by specific serologic tests or the identification of B19 antigens or DNA in blood or tissue specimens.

Aplastic crisis in a patient with a chronic hemolytic anemia may be diagnosed by finding a hemoglobin concentration 2 or more g/dL below the steady state value for that patient together with a reticulocyte count either less than 0.2 per cent of the steady state value or elevated above the steady state value (indicative of hyperplasia of erythrocyte precursors in the recovery phase). Although B19 virus infection is the most common cause of aplastic crisis, moderate to severe degrees of hypoplasia may be associated with systemic bacterial infections (e.g., *Salmonella*, pneumococcal) or marrow-suppressive drugs (e.g., chloramphenicol).[128, 187]

Specific Diagnosis

Several tests have been developed and refined that allow the reliable serologic diagnosis of acute and past B19 virus infection and the demonstration of B19 virus in blood and tissues.[4, 9, 14, 28, 35, 36, 41, 48, 52, 59, 65, 72, 91, 101, 104, 108, 131, 143, 177, 181, 184, 200, 212, 226] IgM and IgG antibody can be detected by enzyme immunoassay, hemadherence, radioimmunoassay, or immunofluorescence; antigen can be detected by DNA hybridization, polymerase chain reaction, or electron microscopy.

In the normal host, acute or recent infection is determined best by the demonstration of specific IgM antibody. In immunocompromised patients with suspected acute or chronic infections, diagnosis is accomplished by detection of antigen in the blood. Similarly, antigen detection also can be used early in aplastic crisis and to study aborted fetal tissues.

Past infection and immunity to B19 virus are determined by the demonstration of specific serum IgG antibody.

Some caution should be observed in accepting results of IgM serology and antigen detection in unusual clinical circumstances. The sensitivity and specificity of the various serologic tests vary, and additional false-positive and -negative results can be expected based upon the skill of workers in individual laboratories.[35, 52] Antigen detection systems can be contaminated, and this contamination may not be discernable by conventional controls. When the results of tests on specimens from patients with unusual illnesses are positive, repeating the tests in a different laboratory is worthwhile.

Söderlund and associates[194] recently reported an IgG avidity assay that is highly sensitive and specific for the identification of recent primary infections with parvovirus B19. Persistent infection may be determined by the presence of IgG antibody to NS1.[207]

TREATMENT, PROGNOSIS, AND PREVENTION

There is no specific treatment for B19 virus infection. Symptomatic therapy for erythema infectiosum rarely is necessary, especially among children. Starch baths may be helpful in reducing pruritus. Arthralgia or arthritis may be troublesome and may be treated with analgesics.

Cases of aplastic crisis may require transfusion of erythrocytes to raise the peripheral hemoglobin concentration.

The outlook in virtually all cases of erythema infectiosum is excellent. If patients with aplastic crisis receive transfusion with packed erythrocytes when necessary, the prognosis for these patients also is excellent. If B19 virus infection occurs during pregnancy, the pregnancy should be monitored carefully. At delivery, examination of cord blood or blood from the neonate for virus and IgM antibody will reveal whether or not the virus has crossed the placenta and infected the fetus. When this has occurred, the child should be examined carefully for any defect and followed up for some years to exclude the possibility of delayed sequelae.

It has been suggested that pregnant women with symptomatic B19 virus infections be monitored for fetal aplastic crisis by monitoring maternal serum for elevated levels of alpha-fetoprotein.[37] If elevated levels are found, then serial ultrasonography can be performed to detect hydrops fetalis. Fetal hydrops can be treated with in utero transfusions.[175] However, this approach is considered risky because of the demonstration of extensive infection in aborted fetuses and the potential for congenital malformation.

Therapeutic abortion is not indicated in pregnant women with documented B19 virus infections.

The virus is spread via the respiratory route, but cases of erythema infectiosum no longer are infectious, so that isolation of exanthematous patients serves no useful role. Patients with aplastic crisis may be excreting virus at presentation; therefore, they should be isolated from patients susceptible to this more severe manifestation of infection (patients with seronegative chronic hemolytic anemia, immunocompromised patients, and pregnant women). In immunocompromised patients with chronic B19 virus infections and in patients with persistent anemia, intravenous immunoglobulin therapy should be considered.[106]

Candidate recombinant vaccines containing B19 virus–empty capsids are being developed, and some are immunogenic in animals.[19]

References

1. Adler, S. P., Manganello, A. M. A., Koch, W. C., et al.: Risk of human parvovirus B19 infections among school and hospital employees during endemic periods. J. Infect. Dis. *168*:361–368, 1993.
2. Ager, E. A., Chin, T. D. Y., and Poland, J. D.: Epidemic erythema infectiosum. N. Engl. J. Med. *275*:1326–1331, 1966.
3. Anand, A., Gray, E. S., Brown, T., et al.: Human parvovirus infection in pregnancy and hydrops fetalis. N. Engl. J. Med. *316*:183–186, 1987.
4. Anderson, L. J.: Human parvoviruses. J. Infect. Dis. *161*:603–608, 1990.
5. Anderson, L. J., Tsou, C., Parker, R. A., et al.: Detection of antibodies and antigens of human parvovirus B19 by enzyme-linked immunosorbent assay. J. Clin. Microbiol. *24*:522–526, 1986.
6. Anderson, M. J., and Cohen, B. J.: Human parvovirus B19 infections in United Kingdom 1984–86. Lancet *1*:738–739, 1987.
7. Anderson, M. J., Davis, L. R., Hodgson, J., et al.: Occurrence of infection with a parvovirus-like agent in children with sickle cell anemia during a two-year period. J. Clin. Pathol. *35*:744–749, 1982.
8. Anderson, M. J., Higgins, P. G., Davis, L. R., et al.: Experimental parvovirus infection in man. J. Infect. Dis. *152*:257–265, 1985.
9. Anderson, M. J., Jones, S. E., and Minson, A. C.: Diagnosis of human parvovirus infection by dot-blot hybridization using cloned viral DNA. J. Med. Virol. *15*:163–172, 1985.
10. Anderson, M. J., Kidd, I. M., and Morgan-Capner, P.: Human parvovirus and rubella-like illness. Lancet *2*:663, 1985.
11. Anderson, M. J., Lewis, E., Kidd, I. M., et al.: An outbreak of erythema infectiosum associated with human parvovirus infection. J. Hyg. *93*:85–93, 1984.
12. Andrewes, C. H., Pereira, H. G., and Wildy, P.: *Parvoviridae*. *In* Andrewes, C. H., Pereira, H. G., and Wildy, D. (eds.): Viruses of Vertebrates. London, Bailliere Tindall, 1978, pp. 255–271.
13. Auriemma, P. R.: Erythema infectiosum: Report on a familial outbreak. Am. J. Public Health *44*:1450–1454, 1954.
14. Azzi, A., Zakrzewska, K., Gentilomi, G., et al.: Detection of B19 parvovirus infections by a dot-blot hybridization assay using a digoxigenin-labelled probe. J. Virol. Methods *27*:125–134, 1990.
15. Bagot, M., and Revuz, J.: Papular-purpuric "gloves and socks" syndrome: Primary infection with parvovirus B19? J. Am. Acad. Dermatol. *25*:341–342, 1991.
16. Balfour, H. H., Jr.: Erythema infectiosum (fifth disease): Clinical review and description of 91 cases seen in an epidemic. Clin. Pediatr. *8*:721–727, 1969.
17. Balfour, H. H., Jr., Schiff, G. M., and Bloom, J. E.: Encephalitis associated with erythema infectiosum. J. Pediatr. *77*:133–136, 1970.
18. Balfour, H. H., Jr., May, D. B., Rotte, T. C., et al.: A study of erythema infectiosum: Recovery of rubella virus and echovirus-12. Pediatrics *50*:285–290, 1972.
19. Bansal, G. P., Hatfield, J. A., Dunn, F. E., et al.: Candidate recombinant vaccine for human B19 parvovirus. J. Infect. Dis. *167*:1034–1044, 1993.
20. Bard, J. W., and Perry, H. O.: Erythema infectiosum. Arch. Dermatol. *93*:49–53, 1966.
21. Berg, A. M., Naides, S. J., and Simms, R. W.: Established fibromyalgia syndrome and parvovirus B19 infection. J. Rheumatol. *20*:1941–1943, 1993.
22. Berns, K. I.: *Parvoviridae* and their replication. *In* Fields, B. N., and Knipe, D. M. (eds.): Virology. Vol. 2. 2nd ed. New York, Raven Press, 1990, pp. 1743–1764.
23. Bessis, D., Lamaury, I., Jonquet, O., et al.: Human parvovirus B19 induced papular-purpuric "gloves and socks" syndrome. Eur. J. Dermatol. *4*:133–134, 1994.
24. Boruchoff, S. E., Woda, B. A., Pihan, G. A., et al.: Parvovirus B19–associated hemophagocytic syndrome. Arch. Intern. Med. *150*:897–899, 1990.
25. Boysen, G.: Erythema infectiosum. Acta Paediatr. *31*:211–224, 1944.
26. Brandenburg, H., Los, F. J., and Cohen-Overbeek, T. E.: A case of early intrauterine parvovirus B19 infection. Prenatal Diagn. *16*:75–77, 1996.
27. Brass, C., Elliott, L. M., and Stevens, D. A.: Academy rash: A probable epidemic of erythema infectiosum (fifth disease). J. A. M. A. *248*:568–572, 1982.
28. Brown, C. S., van Bussel, M., Wassenaar, A. L. M., et al.: An immunofluorescence assay for the detection of parvovirus B19 IgG and IgM antibodies based on recombinant viral antigen. J. Virol. Methods *29*:53–62, 1990.
29. Brown, K. E., Mori, J., Cohen, B. J., et al.: In vitro propagation of parvovirus B19 in primary foetal liver culture. J. Gen. Virol. *72*:741–745, 1991.
30. Brown, K. E., Anderson, S. M., and Young, N. S.: Erythrocyte P antigen: Cellular receptor for B19 parvovirus. Science *262*:114–117, 1993.
31. Brown, K. E., Young, N. S., and Liu, J. M.: Molecular, cellular and clinical aspects of parvovirus B19 infection. Crit. Rev. Oncol. Hematol. *16*:1–31, 1994.
32. Brown, K. E., Hibbs, J. R., Gallinella, G., et al.: Resistance to parvovirus B19 infection due to lack of virus receptor (erythrocyte P antigen). N. Engl. J. Med. *330*:1192–1196, 1994.
33. Brown, K. E., Green, S. W., de Mayolo, J. A., et al.: Congenital anaemia after transplacental B19 parvovirus infection. Lancet *343*:895–896, 1994.
34. Brown, T., Anand, A., Ritchie, L. D., et al.: Intrauterine human parvovirus infection and hydrops fetalis. Lancet *2*:1033–1034, 1984.
35. Bruu, A. L., and Nordb, S. A.: Evaluation of five commercial tests for detection of immunoglobulin M antibodies to human parvovirus B19. J. Clin. Microbiol. *33*:1363–1365, 1995.
36. Carrière, C., Boulanger, P., and Delsert, C.: Rapid and sensitive method for the detection of B19 virus DNA using the polymerase chain reaction with nested primers. J. Virol. Methods *44*:221–234, 1993.
37. Carrington, D., Whittle, M. J., Gibson, A. A. M., et al.: Maternal serum alpha fetoprotein: A marker of fetal aplastic crisis during intrauterine human parvovirus infection. Lancet *1*:433–435, 1987.
38. Carstensen, H., Ornvold, K., and Cohen, B. J.: Human parvovirus B19 infection associated with prolonged erythroblastopenia in a leukemic child. Pediatr. Infect. Dis. *8*:56, 1989.
39. Cartter, M. L., Farley, T. A., Rosengren, S., et al.: Occupational risk factors for infection with parvovirus B19 among pregnant women. J. Infect. Dis. *163*:282–285, 1991.
40. Cassinotti, P., Schultze, D., Schlageter, P., et al.: Persistent human parvovirus B19 infection following an acute infection with meningitis in an immunocompetent patient. Eur. J. Clin. Microbiol. Infect. Dis. *12*:701–704, 1993.
41. Cassinotti, P., Weitz, M., and Siegl, G.: Human parvovirus B19 infections: Routine diagnosis by a new nested polymerase chain reaction assay. J. Med. Virol. *40*:228–234, 1993.
42. Caul, E. O., Usher, M. J., and Burton, P. A.: Intrauterine infection with human parvovirus B19: A light and electron microscopy study. J. Med. Virol. *24*:55–66, 1988.
43. Chargin, L., Sobel, N., and Goldstein, H.: Erythema infectiosum: Report of an extensive epidemic. Arch. Dermatol. Syph. *47*:467–477, 1942.
44. Chernak, E., Dubin, G., Henry, D., et al.: Infection due to parvovirus B19 in patients infected with human immunodeficiency virus. Clin. Infect. Dis. *20*:170–173, 1995.
45. Cherry, J. D.: Newer viral exanthems. Adv. Pediatr. *16*:233–286, 1969.
46. Chorba, T., Coccia, P., Holman, R. C., et al.: The role of parvovirus B19 in aplastic crisis and erythema infectiosum (fifth disease). J. Infect. Dis. *154*:383–393, 1986.
47. Clarke, H. C.: Erythema infectiosum: An epidemic with a probable post-erythema phase. Can. Med. Assoc. J. *130*:603–604, 1984.
48. Clewley, J. P., Cohen, B. J., and Field, A. M.: Detection of parvovirus B19 DNA, antigen, and particles in the human fetus. J. Med. Virol. *23*:367–376, 1987.
49. Clewley, J. P.: Biochemical characterization of a human parvovirus. J. Gen. Virol. *65*:241–244, 1984.
50. Coe, H. C., and Kelly, F. L.: Erythema infectiosum. Calif. West. Med. *36*:39–40, 1932.
51. Cohen, B. J., Mortimer, P. P., and Pereira, M. S.: Diagnostic assays with monoclonal antibodies for the human serum parvovirus-like virus (SPLV). J. Hyg. (Camb.) *91*:113–130, 1983.
52. Cohen, B. J., and Bates, C. M.: Evaluation of 4 commercial test kits for parvovirus B19-specific IgM. J. Virol. Methods *55*:11–25, 1995.
53. Collett, M. S., and Young, N. S.: Prospects for a human B19 parvovirus vaccine. Rev. Med. Virol. *4*:91–103, 1994.
54. Condon, F. J.: Erythema infectiosum: Report of an areawide outbreak. Am. J. Public Health *49*:528–535, 1959.
55. Conway, S. P., Cohen, B. J., Field, A. M., et al.: A family outbreak of parvovirus B19 infection with petechial rash in a 7-year-old boy. J. Infect. *15*:110–112, 1987.
56. Cossart, Y. E., Field, A. M., Cant, B., et al.: Parvovirus-like particles in human sera. Lancet *1*:72–73, 1975.
57. Cotmore, S., and Tattersall, P.: Characterization and molecular cloning of a human parvovirus genome. Science *226*:1161–1165, 1984.
58. Coulombel, L., Morinet, F., Mielot, F., et al.: Parvovirus infection, leukemia, and immunodeficiency. Lancet *1*:101–102, 1989.
59. Cubel, R. C. N., Oliveira, S. A., Brown, D. W. G., et al.: Diagnosis of parvovirus B19 infection by detection of specific immunoglobulin M antibody in saliva. J. Clin. Microbiol. *34*:205–207, 1996.
60. Deiss, V., Tratschin, J. D., Weitz, M., et al.: Cloning of the human parvovi-

rus B19 genome and structural analysis of its palindromic termini. Virology *175*:247–254, 1990.
61. Donders, G. G. G., Van Lierde, S., Van Elsacker-Niele, A. M. W., et al.: Survival after intrauterine parvovirus B19 infection with persistence in early infancy: A two-year follow-up. Pediatr. Infect. Dis. J. *13*:234–236, 1994.
62. Duncan, J. R., Capellini, M. D., Anderson, M. J., et al.: Aplastic crisis due to parvovirus infection in pyruvate kinase deficiency. Lancet 2:14–16, 1983.
63. Dunnet, W. N., Thorm, B. T., and Ayling, R. G.: Food poisoning from oysters. C. D. R. *36*:3, 1984.
64. Edelson, R. N., and Altman, R.: Erythema infectiosum: A statewide outbreak. J. Med. Soc. New Jersey *67*:805–809, 1970.
65. Erdman, D. D., Durigon, E. L., and Holloway, B. P.: Detection of human parvovirus B19 DNA PCR products by RNA probe hybridization enzyme immunoassay. J. Clin. Microbiol. *32*:2295–2298, 1994.
66. Eriksson, B. M., Stromberg, A., and Kreuger, A.: Human parvovirus B19 infection with severe anemia affecting mother and son. Scand. J. Infect. Dis. *20*:335–337, 1988.
67. Escherich, T.: Discussion. Comptes-rendus du XII Congres International de Medecin. Moscow, S. P. Yakovlev, *3*:133, 1898.
68. Faden, H., Gary, G. W., and Anderson, L. J.: Chronic parvovirus infection in a presumably immunologically healthy woman. Clin. Infect. Dis. *15*:595–597, 1992.
69. Foreman, N. K., Oakhill, A., and Caul, E. O.: Parvovirus-associated thrombocytopenic purpura. Lancet 2:1426–1427, 1988.
70. Foto, F., Saag, K. G., Scharosch, L. L., et al.: Parvovirus B19–specific DNA in bone marrow from B19 arthropathy patients: Evidence for B19 virus persistence. J. Infect. Dis. *167*:744–748, 1993.
71. Fox, M. J., and Clark, J. M.: Erythema infectiosum. Am. J. Dis. Child. *73*:453–457, 1947.
72. Fridell, E., Trojnar, J., and Wahren, B.: A new peptide for human parvovirus B19 antibody detection. Scand. J. Infect. Dis. *21*:597–603, 1989.
73. Fried, R. I.: Erythema infectiosum: Fifth disease, a clinical note. Ohio St. Med. J. *47*:1027–1028, 1951.
74. García-Tapia, A. M., del Alamo, C. F. G., Girón, J. A., et al.: Spectrum of parvovirus B19 infection: Analysis of an outbreak of 43 cases in Cadiz, Spain. Clin. Infect. Dis. *21*:1424–1430, 1995.
75. Gillespie, S. M., Cartter, M. L., Asch, S., et al.: Occupational risk of human parvovirus B19 infection for school and day-care personnel during an outbreak of erythema infectiosum. J. A. M. A. *263*:2061–2065, 1990.
76. Goldman, F., Rotbart, H., Gutierrez, K., et al.: Parvovirus-associated aplastic crisis in a patient with red blood cell glucose-6-phosphate dehydrogenase deficiency. Pediatr. Infect. Dis. *9*:593–594, 1990.
77. Gowda, N., Rao, S. P., Cohen, B., et al.: Human parvovirus infection in patients with sickle cell disease with and without hypoplastic crisis. J. Pediatr. *110*:81–84, 1987.
78. Gratacós, E., Torres, P. J., Vidal, J., et al.: The incidence of human parvovirus B19 infection during pregnancy and its impact on perinatal outcome. J. Infect. Dis. *171*:1360–1363, 1995.
79. Greenwald, P., and Bashe, W. J., Jr.: An epidemic of erythema infectiosum. Am. J. Dis. Child. *107*:30–34, 1964.
80. Grimmer, H., and Joseph, A.: An epidemic of infectious erythema in Germany. Arch. Dermatol. *80*:283–285, 1959.
81. Gyllensten, K., Sönnerborg, A., Jorup-Rönström, C. J., et al.: Parvovirus B19 infection in HIV-1 infected patients with anemia. Infection *22*:356–358, 1994.
82. Hajeer, A. H., MacGregor, A. J., Rigby, A. S., et al.: Influence of previous exposure to human parvovirus B19 infection in explaining susceptibility to rheumatoid arthritis: An analysis of disease discordant twin pairs. J. Rheum. Dis. *53*:137–139, 1994.
83. Halasz, C. L. G., Cormier, D., and Den, M.: Petechial glove and sock syndrome caused by parvovirus B19. J. Am. Acad. Dermatol. *27*:835–838, 1992.
84. Hall, C. B., and Horner, F. A.: Encephalopathy with erythema infectiosum. Am. J. Dis. Child. *131*:65–67, 1977.
85. Hammon, W. D., and Enders, J. F.: A virus disease of cats, principally characterized by aleucocytosis, enteric lesions and the presence of intranuclear inclusion bodies. J. Exp. Med. *69*:327–352, 1939.
86. Hanada, T., Koike, K., Takeya, T., et al.: Human parvovirus B19–induced transient pancytopenia in a child with hereditary spherocytosis. Br. J. Haematol. *70*:113–115, 1988.
87. Hauswirth, W. W.: Autonomous parvovirus DNA structure and replication. *In* Berns, K. I. (ed.): The Parvoviruses. London, Plenum Press, 1983, pp. 129–152.
88. Heegaard, E. D., and Hornsleth, A.: Parvovirus: The expanding spectrum of disease. Acta Paediatr. *84*:109–117, 1995.
89. Heegaard, E. D., Hasle, H., Clausen, N., et al.: Parvovirus B19 infection and Diamond-Blackfan anaemia. Acta Paediatr. *85*:299–302, 1996.
90. Herrick, T. P.: Erythema infectiosum: A clinical report of 74 cases. Am. J. Dis. Child. *31*:486–495, 1926.
91. Hicks, K. E., Beard, S., Cohen, B. J., et al.: A simple and sensitive DNA hybridization assay used for the routine diagnosis of human parvovirus B19 infection. J. Clin. Microbiol. *33*:2473–2475, 1995.
92. Higgins, C. S., and Anderson, M. J.: Acute parvovirus infection associated with chronic arthritis. Unpublished data.
93. Hoffman, E.: Erythema infectiosum (groszflecken oder ringelroteln). Dtsch. Med. Wochenschr. *1*:777–779, 1916.
94. Holm, J. M., Hansen, L. K., and Oxhøj, H.: Kawasaki disease associated with parvovirus B19 infection. Eur. J. Paediatr. *154*:633–634, 1995.
95. Inoue, S., Kinra, N. K., Mukkamala, S., et al.: Parvovirus B19 infection: Aplastic crisis, erythema infectiosum and idiopathic thrombocytopenic purpura. Pediatr. Infect. Dis. *10*:251–253, 1991.
96. International Committee on Taxonomy of Viruses: Virus taxonomy update. Arch. Virol. *133*:491–495, 1993.
97. Kelleher, J. H., Luban, N. L. C., Mortimer, P. P., et al.: The human serum "parvovirus": A specific cause of aplastic crisis in hereditary spherocytosis. J. Pediatr. *102*:720–722, 1983.
98. Kerr, J. R., Curran, M. D., Moore, J. E., et al.: Persistent parvovirus B19 infection. Lancet *345*:1118, 1995.
99. Kerr, J. R.: Parvovirus B19 infection. Eur. J. Clin. Microbiol. Infect. Dis. *15*:10–29, 1996.
100. Kerr, P. S., and Marsh, E. H.: Outbreak of erythema infectiosum in Elmsford, N.Y. Am. J. Public Health *23*:1271–1274, 1933.
101. Kim, E. C., Durigon, E. L., Erdman, D. D., et al.: Chemiluminescent microwell hybridization assay for direct detection of human parvovirus B19 DNA. J. Virol. Methods *50*:349–354, 1994.
102. Kinney, J. S., Anderson, L. J., Farrar, J., et al.: Risk of adverse outcomes of pregnancy after human parvovirus B19 infection. J. Infect. Dis. *157*:663–667, 1988.
103. Knott, P. D., Welply, G. A. C., and Anderson, M. J.: Serologically proven intrauterine infection with parvovirus. Br. Med. J. *289*:1660, 1984.
104. Koch, W. C., and Adler, S. P.: Detection of human parvovirus B19 DNA by using the polymerase chain reaction. J. Clin. Microbiol. *28*:65–69, 1990.
105. Koch, W. C., and Adler, S. P.: Human parvovirus B19 infections in women of childbearing age and within families. Pediatr. Infect. Dis. *8*:83–87, 1989.
106. Koch, W. C., Massey, G., Russell, C. E., et al.: Manifestations and treatment of human parvovirus B19 infection in immunocompromised patients. J. Pediatr. *116*:355–359, 1990.
107. Koch, W. C., Adler, S. P., and Harger, J.: Intrauterine parvovirus B19 infection may cause an asymptomatic or recurrent postnatal infection. Pediatr. Infect. Dis. J. *12*:747–750, 1993.
108. Koch, W. C.: A synthetic parvovirus B19 capsid protein can replace viral antigen in antibody-capture enzyme immunoassays. J. Virol. Methods *55*:67–82, 1995.
109. Koduri, P. R., and Naides, S. J.: Aseptic meningitis caused by parvovirus B19. Clin. Infect. Dis. *21*:1053, 1995.
110. Koziol, D. E., Kurtzman, G., Ayub, J., et al.: Nosocomial human parvovirus B19 infection: Lack of transmission from a chronically infected patient to hospital staff. Infect. Control Hosp. Epidemiol. *13*:343–348, 1992.
111. Kurtzman, G. J., Cohen, B., Meyers, P., et al.: Persistent B19 parvovirus infection as a cause of severe chronic anaemia in children with acute lymphocytic leukaemia. Lancet 2:1159–1162, 1988.
112. Kurtzman, G., Frickhofen, N., Kimball, J., et al.: Pure red-cell aplasia of ten years' duration due to persistent parvovirus B19 infection and its cure with immunoglobulin therapy. N. Engl. J. Med. *321*:519–523, 1989.
113. Kurtzman, G. J., Cohen, B. J., Field, A. M., et al.: Immune response to B19 parvovirus and an antibody defect in persistent viral infection. J. Clin. Invest. *84*:1114–1123, 1989.
114. Langnas, A. N., Markin, R. S., Cattral, M. S., et al.: Parvovirus B19 as a possible causative agent of fulminant liver failure and associated aplastic anemia. Hepatology *22*:1661–1665, 1995.
115. Lauer, B. A., MacCormack, J. N., and Wilfert, C.: Erythema infectiosum: An elementary school outbreak. Am. J. Dis. Child. *130*:252–254, 1976.
116. Lawton, A. L., and Smith, R. E.: Erythema infectiosum: A clinical study of an epidemic in Branford, Conn. Arch. Intern. Med. *47*:28–41, 1931.
117. Lefrère, J. J., Courouće, A. M., Girot, R., et al.: Human parvovirus and thalassaemia. J. Infect. *13*:45–49, 1986.
118. Lefrère, J. J., Courouće, A. M., and Kaplan, C.: Parvovirus and idiopathic thrombocytopenic purpura. Lancet *1*:279, 1989.
119. Lefrère, J. J., Courouće, A. M., Muller, J. Y., et al.: Human parvovirus and purpura. Lancet *2*:730, 1985.
120. Lies, W., III, and Morgan, S. K.: Erythema infectiosum (fifth disease): Report of an outbreak. J. Med. Assoc. Ala. *32*:331–332, 1963.
121. Lowenthal, E. A., Wells, A., Emanuel, P. D., et al.: Sickle cell acute chest syndrome associated with parvovirus B19 infection: Case series and review. Am. J. Hematol. *51*:207–213, 1996.
122. Macartney, L., McCandlish, I. A. P., Thompson, H., et al.: Canine parvovirus enteritis 2: Pathogenesis. Vet. Rec. *115*:453–460, 1984.
123. Malarme, M., Vandervelde, D., and Brasseur, M.: Parvovirus infection, leukemia and immunodeficiency. Lancet *1*:1457, 1989.
124. Mallouh, A. A., and Qudah, A.: Acute splenic sequestration together with aplastic crisis caused by human parvovirus B19 in patients with sickle cell disease. J. Pediatr. *122*:593–595, 1993.
125. Mallouh, A. A., and Qudah, A.: An epidemic of aplastic crisis caused by human parvovirus B19. Pediatr. Infect. Dis. J. *14*:31–34, 1995.
126. McClain, K., Estrov, Z., Chen, H., et al.: Chronic neutropenia of childhood: Frequent association with parvovirus infection and correlations with bone marrow culture studies. Br. J. Hematol. *85*:57–62, 1993.

127. McOmish, F., Yap, P. L., Jordan, A., et al.: Detection of parvovirus B19 in donated blood: A model system for screening by polymerase chain reaction. J. Clin. Microbiol. *321*:323–328, 1993.
128. Megas, H., Papidiki, E., and Constantinides, B.: *Salmonella* septicemia and aplastic crisis in a patient with sickle cell anemia. Acta. Paediatr. *50*:517–521, 1961.
129. Mimori, A., Misaki, Y., Hachiya, T., et al.: Prevalence of antihuman parvovirus B19 IgG antibodies in patients with refractory rheumatoid arthritis and polyarticular juvenile rheumatoid arthritis. Rheumatol. Int. *14*:87–90, 1994.
130. Moore, W. F.: Erythema infectiosum: Review, and report of two cases. Hawaii Med. J. *16*:35–36, 1956.
131. Mori, J., Field, A. M., Clewley, J. P., et al.: Dot blot hybridization assay of B19 virus DNA in clinical specimens. J. Clin. Microbiol. *27*:459–464, 1989.
132. Morinet, F., Monsuez, J. J., Roger, P., et al.: Parvovirus B19 associated with pseudoappendicitis. Lancet 2:1466, 1987.
133. Mortimer, P. P.: Hypothesis: The aplastic crisis of hereditary spherocytosis is due to a single transmissible agent. J. Clin. Pathol. *36*:445–448, 1983.
134. Mortimer, P. P., Luban, N. L. C., Kelleher, J. F., et al.: Transmission of serum parvovirus like virus by clotting factor concentrates. Lancet *ii*:482–484, 1983.
135. Mortimer, P. P., Cohen, B. J., Buckley, M. M., et al.: Human parvovirus and the fetus. Lancet *2*:1012, 1985.
136. Muir, K., Todd, W. T. A., Watson, W. H., et al.: Viral-associated haemophagocytosis with parvovirus B19–related pancytopenia. Lancet *339*:1139–1140, 1992.
137. Musiani, M., Zerbini, M., Gentilomi, G., et al.: Persistent B19 parvovirus infections in haemophilic HIV-1 infected patients. J. Med. Virol. *46*:103–108, 1995.
138. Musiani, M., Zerbini, M., Gentilomi, G., et al.: Parvovirus B19 clearance from peripheral blood after acute infection. J. Infect. Dis. *172*:1360–1363, 1995.
139. Naides, S. J.: Erythema infectiosum (fifth disease) occurrence in Iowa. Am. J. Public Health *78*:1230–1231, 1988.
140. Naides, S. J., and Field, E. H.: Transient rheumatoid factor positivity in acute human parvovirus B19 infection. Arch. Intern. Med. *148*:2587–2589, 1988.
141. Naides, S. J., Piette, W., Veach, L. A., et al.: Human parvovirus B19 induced vesiculopustular skin eruption. Am. J. Med. *84*:968–972, 1988.
142. Naides, S. J., Howard, E. J., Swack, N. S., et al.: Parvovirus B19 infection inhuman immunodeficiency virus type 1–infected persons failing or intolerant to zidovudine therapy. J. Infect. Dis. *168*:101–105, 1993.
143. Nascimento, J. P., Hallam, N. F., Mori, J., et al.: Detection of B19 parvovirus in human fetal tissues by in situ hybridisation. J. Med. Virol. *33*:77–82, 1991.
144. Nigro, G., Zerbini, M., Krysztofiak, A., et al.: Active or recent parvovirus B19 infection in children with Kawasaki disease. Lancet *343*:1260–1261, 1994.
145. Nikkari, S., Mertsola, J., Korvenranta, H., et al.: Wegener's granulomatosis and parvovirus B19 infection. Arthritis Rheum. *37*:1707–1708, 1994.
146. Nikkari, S., Luukkainen, R., Möttönen, T., et al.: Does parvovirus B19 have a role in rheumatoid arthritis? Ann. Rheum. Dis. *53*:106–111, 1994.
147. Nikkari, S., Roivainen, A., Hannonen, P., et al.: Persistence of parvovirus B19 in synovial fluid and bone marrow. Ann. Rheum. Dis. *54*:597–600, 1995.
148. Nocton, J. J., Miller, L. C., Tucker, L. B., et al.: Human parvovirus B19–associated arthritis in children. J. Pediatr. *122*:186–190, 1993.
149. Nour, B., Green, M., Michaels, M., et al.: Parvovirus B19 infection in pediatric transplant patients. Transplantation *56*:835–838, 1993.
150. Nunoue, T., Koike, T., Koike, R., et al.: Infection with human parvovirus B19 aplasia of the bone marrow and a rash in hereditary spherocytosis. J. Infect. *14*:67–70, 1987.
151. Okumura, A., and Ichikawa, T.: Aseptic meningitis caused by human parvovirus B19. Arch. Dis. Child. *68*:784–785, 1993.
152. Ozawa, K., Kurtzman, G., and Young, N.: Replication of the B19 parvovirus in human bone marrow cell cultures. Science *233*:883–886, 1986.
153. Pattison, J. R.: Parvoviruses: Medical and biological aspects. *In* Fields, B. N., and Knipe, D. M. (eds.): Virology. Vol. 2. 2nd ed. New York, Raven Press, 1990, pp. 1765–1782.
154. Paver, W. K., Caul, E. O., Ashley, C. R., et al.: A small virus in human feces. Lancet *1*:664–665, 1973.
155. Paver, W. K., and Clarke, S. K. R.: Comparison of human fecal and serum parvovirus-like viruses. J. Clin. Microbiol. *4*:67–70, 1976.
156. Peschgens, T., Merz, U., Steidel, K., et al.: Parvovirus B19–assoziierte myokarditis bei einem 7-monate-alten kind. Pädiatr. Grenzgeb. *32*:527–530, 1994.
157. Petrikovsky, B. M., Baker, D., and Schneider, E.: Fetal hydrops secondary to human parvovirus infection in early pregnancy. Prenatal Diagn. *16*:342–344, 1996.
158. Phillips, I. E.: Erythema infectiosum: Outbreak in Bristol, Tennessee-Virginia area. Arch. Dermatol. Syph. *67*:628–629, 1953.
159. Phillips, I. E.: Erythema infectiosum: Clinical and epidemiological observations. South. Med. J. *47*:253–257, 1954.
160. Pillay, D., Patou, G., Griffiths, P. D., et al.: Secondary parvovirus B19 infection in an immunocompromised child. Pediatr. Infect. Dis. J. *10*:623–624, 1991.
161. Pillay, D., Patou, G., Hurt, S., et al.: Parvovirus B19 outbreak in a children's ward. Lancet *339*:107–109, 1992.
162. Plummer, F. A., Hammond, G. W., Forward, K., et al.: An erythema infectiosum–like illness caused by human parvovirus infection. N. Engl. J. Med. *313*:74–79, 1985.
163. Potter, C. G., Potter, A. C., Hatton, C. S. R., et al.: Variation of erythroid and myeloid precursors in the marrow and peripheral blood of volunteer subjects infected with human parvovirus (B19). J. Clin. Invest. *79*:1486–1492, 1987.
164. Pouchot, J., Ouakil, H., Debin, M. L., et al.: Adult Still's disease associated with acute human parvovirus B19 infection. Lancet *341*:1280–1281, 1993.
165. Public Health Laboratory Service Working Party on Fifth Disease: Prospective study of human parvovirus (B19) infection in pregnancy. Br. Med. J. *300*:1166–1170, 1990.
166. Rao, K. R. P., Patel, A. R., Anderson, M. J., et al.: Infection with a parvovirus-like virus and aplastic crisis in chronic hemolytic anemia. Ann. Intern. Med. *98*:930–932, 1983.
167. Rao, S. P., Miller, S. T., and Cohen, B. J.: Transient aplastic crisis in patients with sickle cell disease. Am. J. Dis. Child. *146*:1328–1330, 1992.
168. Rector, J. M.: Erythema infectiosum: Clinical observations during an epidemic. J. Pediatr. *15*:540–545, 1939.
169. Reid, D. M., Reid, T. M. S., Brown, T., et al.: Human parvovirus-associated arthritis: A clinical and laboratory description. Lancet *2*:422–425, 1985.
170. Rivier, G., Gerster, J. C., Terrier, P., et al.: Parvovirus B19–associated monoarthritis in a 5-year-old boy. J. Rheumatol. *22*:766–767, 1995.
171. Rodis, J. F., Hovick, T. J., Jr., Quinn, D. L., et al.: Human parvovirus infection in pregnancy. Obstet. Gynecol. *72*:733–738, 1988.
172. Rodis, J. F., Quinn, D. L., Gary, G. W., Jr., et al.: Management and outcomes of pregnancies complicated by human B19 parvovirus infection: A prospective study. Am. J. Obstet. Gynecol. *163*:1168–1171, 1990.
173. Rogers, B. B., Singer, D. B., Mak, S. K., et al.: Detection of human parvovirus B19 in early spontaneous abortuses using serology, histology, electron microscopy, in situ hybridization, and the polymerase chain reaction. Obstet. Gynecol. *81*:402–408, 1993.
174. Saarinen, U. M., Chorba, T. L., Tattersall, P., et al.: Human parvovirus B19–induced epidemic acute red cell aplasia in patients with hereditary hemolytic anemia. Blood *67*:1411–1417, 1986.
175. Sahakian, V., Weiner, C. P., Naides, S. J., et al.: Intrauterine transfusion treatment of nonimmune hydrops fetalis secondary to human parvovirus B19 infection. Am. J. Obstet. Gynecol. *164*:1090–1091, 1991.
176. Saint-Martin, J., Choulot, J. J., Bonnaud, E., et al.: Myocarditis caused by parvovirus. J. Pediatr. *116*:1007–1008, 1990.
177. Salimans, M. M. M., Holsappel, S., van de Rijke, F. M., et al.: Rapid detection of human parvovirus B19 DNA by dot-hybridization and the polymerase chain reaction. J. Virol. Methods *23*:19–28, 1989.
178. Saller, D. N., Rogers, B. B., and Canick, J. A.: Maternal serum biochemical markers in pregnancies with fetal parvovirus B19 infection. Prenatal Diagn. *13*:467–471, 1993.
179. Samii, K., Cassinotti, P., de Freudenreich, J., et al.: Acute bilateral carpal tunnel syndrome associated with human parvovirus B19 infection. Clin. Infect. Dis. *22*:162–164, 1996.
180. Schiff, G., Linnemann, C., Balfour, H., et al.: Challenge study with rubella virus isolated from a patient with erythema infectiosum. Clin. Res. *19*:675, 1971.
181. Schwarz, T. F., Roggendorf, M., and Deinhardt, F.: Human parvovirus B19: ELISA and immunoblot assays. J. Virol. Methods *20*:155–168, 1988.
182. Schwarz, T. F., Bruns, R., Schröder, C., et al.: Human parvovirus B19 infection associated with vascular purpura and vasculitis. Infection *17*:170–171, 1989.
183. Schwarz, T. F., Nerlich, A., Hottenträger, B., et al.: Parvovirus B19 infection of the fetus: Histology and in situ hybridization. Am. J. Clin. Pathol. *96*:121–126, 1991.
184. Schwarz, T. F., Jäger, G., Holzgreve, W., et al.: Diagnosis of human parvovirus B19 infections by polymerase chain reaction. Scand. J. Infect. Dis. *24*:691–696, 1992.
185. Schwarz, T. F., Wiersbitzky, S., and Pambor, M.: Case report: Detection of parvovirus B19 in a skin biopsy of a patient with erythema infectiosum. J. Med. Virol. *43*:171–174, 1994.
186. Semble, E. L., Agudelo, C. A., and Pegram, P. S.: Human parvovirus B19 arthropathy in two adults after contact with childhood erythema infectiosum. Am. J. Med. *83*:560–562, 1987.
187. Serjeant, G. R., Mason, J., Topley, J. M., et al.: Outbreak of aplastic crisis in sickle cell anemia associated with parvovirus-like agent. Lancet *2*:595–597, 1981.
188. Serjeant, G. R., Serjeant, B. E., Thomas, P. W., et al.: Human parvovirus infection in homozygous sickle cell disease. Lancet *341*:1237–1240, 1993.
189. Shaw, H. L. K.: Erythema infectiosum. Am. J. Med. Sci. *129*:16–22, 1905.
190. Shneerson, J. M., Mortimer, P. P., and Vandervelde, E. M.: Febrile illness due to a parvovirus. Br. Med. J. *2*:1580, 1980.
191. Silver, M. M., Hellmann, J., Zielenska, M., et al.: Anemia, blueberry-muffin rash, and hepatomegaly in a newborn infant. J. Pediatr. *128*:579–586, 1996.

192. Smith, E. H.: An epidemic of erythema infectiosum, "the fifth disease." Arch. Pediatr. *46*:456–458, 1929.
193. Smoleniec, J. S., Pillal, M., Caul, E. O., et al.: Subclinical transplacental parvovirus B19 infection: An increased fetal risk? Lancet *343*:1100–1101, 1994.
194. Söderlund, M., Brown, C. S., Cohen, B. J., et al.: Accurate serodiagnosis of B19 parvovirus infections by measurement of IgG avidity. J. Infect. Dis. *171*:710–713, 1995.
195. Srivastava, A., Bruno, E., Briddell, R., et al.: Parvovirus B19–induced perturbation of human megakaryocytopoiesis in vitro. Blood *76*:1997–2004, 1990.
196. Srivastava, A., and Lu, L.: Replication of B19 parvovirus in highly enriched hematopoietic progenitor cells from normal human bone marrow. J. Virol. *62*:3059–3063, 1988.
197. Stricker, G.: Die neue kindersenche in der umgebung von giessen (erythema infectiosum). Z. Prakt. Aerzte *40*:121, 1899.
198. Summers, J., Jones, S. E., and Anderson, M. J.: Characterization of the agent of erythrocyte aplasia as a human parvovirus. J. Gen. Virol. *64*:2527–2532, 1983.
199. Suzuki, N., Terada, S., and Inoue, M.: Neonatal meningitis with human parvovirus B19 infection. Arch. Dis. Child. *73*:196–197, 1995.
200. Tabrizi, S. N., Chen, S., Borg, A. J., et al.: Use of polymerase chain reaction for detection of human parvovirus B19. J. Infect. Dis. *170*:1047–1048, 1994.
201. Takahashi, T., Ozawa, K., Takahashi, K., et al.: Susceptibility of human erythropoietic cells to B19 parvovirus in vitro increases with differentiation. Blood *75*:603–610, 1990.
202. Tiessen, R. G., van Elsacker-Niele, A. M. W., Vermeij-Keers, C., et al.: A fetus with a parvovirus B19 infection and congenital anomalies. Prenatal Diagn. *14*:173–176, 1994.
203. Tschamer, A.: Ueber ortliche rotheln. Jahrb. Kinderheilk. *29*:372–374, 1889.
204. Turton, J., Appleton, H., and Clewley, J. P.: Similarities in nucleotide sequence between serum and faecal human parvovirus DNA. Epidemiol. Infect. *105*:197–201, 1990.
205. Tyndall, A., Jelk, W., and Hirsch, H. H.: Parvovirus B19 and erosive polyarthritis. Lancet *343*:480–481, 1994.
206. van Elsacker-Niele, A. M. W., Salimans, M. M. M., Weiland, H. T., et al.: Fetal pathology in human parvovirus B19 infection. Br. J. Obstet. Gynaecol. *96*:768–775, 1989.
207. Von Poblotzki, A., Hemauer, A., Gigler, A., et al.: Antibodies to the nonstructural protein of parvovirus B19 in persistently infected patients: Implications for pathogenesis. J. Infect. Dis. *172*:1356–1359, 1995.
208. Wadlington, W. B.: Erythema infectiosum: Report of an epidemic. J. Tenn. St. Med. Assoc. *50*:1–5, 1957.
209. Wadlington, W. B.: Erythema infectiosum. J. A. M. A. *192*:58–60, 1965.
210. Wadlington, W. B.: Erythema infectiosum (fifth disease). Am. J. Dis. Child. *110*:443–444, 1965.
211. Wadlington, W. B., and Riley, H. D., Jr.: Arthritis and hemolytic anemia following erythema infectiosum. J. A. M. A. *203*:473–475, 1968.
212. Wang, Q. Y., and Erdman, D. D.: Development and evaluation of capture immunoglobulin G and M hemadherence assays by using human type O erythrocytes and recombinant parvovirus B19 antigen. J. Clin. Microbiol. *33*:2466–2467, 1995.
213. Weiland, H. T., Vermey-Keers, C., Salimans, M. M. M., et al.: Parvovirus B19 associated with fetal abnormality. Lancet *1*:682–683, 1987.
214. Werner, G. H., Brachman, P. S., Ketler, A., et al.: A new viral agent associated with erythema infectiosum. Ann. N.Y. Acad. Sci. *67*:338–345, 1956–57.
215. White, D. G., Woolf, A. D., Mortimer, P. P., et al.: Human parvovirus arthropathy. Lancet *2*:419–421, 1985.
216. Wilcox, K. R., and Evans, A. S.: Erythema infectiosum: Report of an outbreak in Marshfield, Wisconsin. Wis. Med. J., March 1958.
217. Willekes, C., Roumen, F. J. M. E., Van Elsacker-Niele, A. M. W., et al.: Human parvovirus B19 infection and unbalanced translocation in a case of hydrops fetalis. Prenatal Diagn. *14*:181–185, 1994.
218. Woernle, C. H., Anderson, L. J., Tattersall, P., et al.: Human parvovirus B19 infection during pregnancy. J. Infect. Dis. *156*:17–20, 1987.
219. Yaegashi, N., Okamura, K., Tsunoda, A., et al.: A study by means of a new assay of the relationship between an outbreak of erythema infectiosum and non-immune hydrops fetalis caused by human parvovirus B19. J. Infect. *31*:195–200, 1995.
220. Yee, T. T., Cohen, B. J., Pasi, K. J., et al.: Transmission of symptomatic parvovirus B19 infection by clotting factor concentrate. Br. J. Haematol. *93*:457–459, 1996.
221. Yoto, Y., Kudoh, T., Suzuki, N., et al.: Retrospective study on the influence of human parvovirus B19 infection among children with malignant diseases. Acta Haematol. *90*:8–12, 1993.
222. Young, N.: Hematologic and hematopoietic consequences of B19 parvovirus infection. Semin. Hematol. *25*:159–172, 1988.
223. Young, N. S., Mortimer, P. P., Moore, J. G., et al.: Characterization of a virus that causes transient aplastic crisis. J. Clin. Invest. *73*:224–230, 1984.
224. Zahorsky, J.: An epidemic of erythema infectiosum. Am. J. Dis. Child. *28*:261–262, 1924.
225. Zerbini, M., Musiani, M., Gentilomi, G., et al.: Symptomatic parvovirus B19 infection of one fetus in a twin pregnancy. Clin. Infect. Dis. *17*:262–263, 1993.
226. Zerbini, M., Gibellini, D., Musiani, M., et al.: Automated detection of digoxigenin-labelled B19 parvovirus amplicons by a capture hybridization assay. J. Virol. Methods *55*:1–9, 1995.
227. Zuckerman, S. N.: Erythema infectiosum, with report of an epidemic in San Francisco. Arch. Pediatr. *57*:168–176, 1940.

❑ ❑ ❑

SUBSECTION TWO
PAPILLOVIRIDAE

159

HUMAN PAPILLOMAVIRUSES

Gail J. Demmler

The human papillomaviruses (HPVs) are responsible for a variety of benign yet bothersome cutaneous proliferations, including common skin warts. However, HPVs also have been associated with serious, even life-threatening, illnesses, including genitourinary cancers and respiratory papillomatosis. Our current understanding of the complex role these viruses play in these diverse clinical presentations remains incomplete, and management of these diseases remains an ongoing challenge.

HISTORY

Warts or papillomas have been recognized for centuries to occur at a variety of different body sites, including the skin, genital tract, oral cavity, conjunctiva, and respiratory tract. Their infectious nature has been suspected by clinicians for many decades and has been the product of much folklore. The viral etiology of warts was discovered scientifically, however, in 1907, when human volunteers were inoculated experimentally with a cell-free extract prepared from wart tissue.[35] These early experiments also suggested that warts could be transmitted from person to person. When electron microscopy became available in the 1940s, virus particles were visualized within many of these clinical sites, initially in skin warts and subsequently in genital warts, confirming the viral etiology of these lesions. However, despite the abundance of virus particles seen in some lesions, such as skin warts, virologic investigation of the disease processes was hampered by the inability to propagate the papillomaviruses in cell culture or laboratory animals. The limited amount of information available from the study of virus particles obtained directly from wart tissue led to speculation, in the 1960s, that HPVs were composed of a single virus type. Scientists further theorized that the specific body site and epithelium involved, rather than the virus type, were responsible for each characteristic morphology and disease process.[155] With the advent of molecular biology techniques in the 1970s, however, more than 70 different types of HPVs were recognized, and it quickly became clear that specific clinical diseases were associated with infection with specific HPV types. Most recently, HPV infection of the genital tract has emerged as one of the most prevalent sexually transmitted infections, and the link to some squamous cell carcinomas of the cervix has been strengthened. In addition, at least two mucosal HPV types appear to produce respiratory papillomatosis in pediatric patients. Finally, the role of some cutaneous HPV types in the evolution of squamous cell carcinoma from wart lesions in patients with epidermodysplasia verruciformis (EV) recently has been elucidated. The challenges for the future revolve around effective treatment strategies because current measures are palliative, at best, and most lesions recur. New antiviral chemotherapeutic agents are being developed, and immunomodulators, such as interferon, provide promise for therapy of serious disease due to HPVs.

VIROLOGY

The papillomaviruses are members of the family *Papovaviridae*, which contains two genera, *Papillomavirus*, which contains many types of both animal and HPVs, and *Polyomavirus*, which contains BK virus, JC virus, and simian virus 40.

The HPVs are small, nonenveloped viruses with a diameter of about 55 nm. They have a capsid composed of 72 capsomers arranged in icosahedral symmetry and a genome composed of double-stranded circular DNA that is approximately 8 kb in length. The complete nucleotide sequence is available for some HPVs, and partial information is available for all HPV types. The genome is divided into three regions, early, late, and regulatory, and many nucleotide sequences are shared between types. The early region is approximately 4.5 kb in length, contains eight open reading frames (E1 to E8), and encodes genes that produce proteins required for viral DNA replication and cellular transformation (Table 159–1). The late region is approximately 2.5 kb in length, contains two open reading frames (L1 and L2), and codes for major and minor capsid structural proteins. The regulatory or long control region is located between the early and late regions. It is about 1 kb in length and contains the origin of replication and many control elements for viral transcription and replication.[140] The virus appears to replicate solely in the nucleus of the cell, in association with low-molecular-weight histones. Because the HPV genome codes for only 10 proteins, it does not have a viral protease, DNA polymerase, or other enzymes involved in nucleotide metabolism and, therefore, requires many host cell enzymes and cellular differentiation to complete its viral replicative life cycle.

The life cycle of HPVs is integrated intimately with the life cycle and maturation of epithelial cells. Initial virus infection probably occurs in the basal keratinocyte, with early transcription of the viral genome regulated by the E2 protein. Cellular proliferation and perturbation of the keratinocyte differentiation then are induced by the E6 and E7 proteins. The cells are stimulated in the S phase of the cell cycle, and the host enzymes for DNA synthesis are used by the virus to complete viral DNA replication. After double-stranded DNA is produced, L1 and L2, the major and minor capsid proteins, and E4, a late-associated structural protein whose gene is located in the early region of the genome, are synthesized. During the final stages of cellular keratinocyte differentiation, the final stages of virus production also occur with assembly of complete viral particles. However, progeny viruses are not released until dead keratinocytes are sloughed from the surface of the epithelium.

TABLE 159–1. Major Human Papillomavirus Genes

Gene	Protein Products and Function
Early (E) Region	
E1	Viral regulatory protein that initiates viral DNA replication
E2	Viral regulatory protein that controls replication and inhibits or activates early transcription of the viral genome
E3	Unknown
E4	A late viral protein that controls viral maturation; expressed in terminally differentiated keratinocytes
E5	Major transforming protein; causes cellular proliferation
E6	Major transforming oncoprotein; associates with the cellular target, p53, a tumor suppressor protein, and promotes its proteolytic degradation; causes cellular proliferation and perturbation of keratinocyte differentiation
E7	Major transforming protein; associates with the cellular target, pRB, and inactivates its cell cycle restriction function; causes cellular proliferation and perturbation of keratinocyte differentiation
E8	Unknown; ? regulates viral DNA replication
Late (L) Region	
L1	Major structural viral capsid protein
L2	Minor structural viral capsid protein

Papillomaviruses display a high degree of species, tissue, and cellular specificity. HPVs appear to infect only humans, and most animal papillomaviruses also do not infect other species. They also primarily infect the surface squamous epithelium of the skin or mucosa, and specific viral types appear to have a preference for either skin or mucosa, as well as for specific body sites. However, some HPV types recently have been detected in transitional and cuboidal epithelium in the anogenital tract. At least 70 types of HPVs have been recognized, according to DNA homology studies, and they fall naturally into two main groups: cutaneous and mucosal (Table 159–2). The cutaneous HPVs contain types from a variety of benign skin warts, as well as more than 15 types recovered from a small group of patients with a rare dermatologic disorder: EV. The mucosal HPVs occur mainly in the genital tract but also infect and produce disease at other mucosal sites, such as the respiratory tract, the oral

TABLE 159–2. Human Papillomavirus (HPV) Types and Associated Clinical Conditions

Condition	Usual Location	Morphology	HPV Type
Cutaneous (Skin) Warts			
Common (verrucae vulgares)	Hands, lips, extremities	Multiple, dome-shaped	2, 4
Plantar (verrucae plantares)	Bottom of feet	Single, painful	1
Flat (verrucae planae)	Arms, face, knees	Multiple	3, 10, 28, 41
Filiform	Face, neck	Multiple, thread-like	2, 4
Mosaic	Feet, hands	Multiple, superficial	7
Butcher's	Hands	Multiple, dome-shaped	7
Epidermodysplasia verruciformis	Face, trunk, extremities	Multiple flat warts or reddish-brown plaques	5, 8, 9, 12, 14, 15, 17, 19–25, 36–38, 47, 49
Immunosuppressed patients	Face, trunk, extremities	Dome or epidermodysplasia verruciformis–like plaques; may be persistent or progressive	1–5, 8, 10, 20, 23, 28, 49
Muscosal (Anogenital) Warts			
Subclinical	Cervix	Asymptomatic	6, 11, 13, 16, 18, 30–35, 39, 40, 42–45, 51–59
Condylomata acuminata	Cervix, vulva, urethra, anus, penis, scrotum	Multiple exophytic, pink, gray	6, 11, 16
Flat condylomata	Cervix	Asymptomatic, flat plaques	6, 11, 16, 18, 31
Giant condylomata acuminata (Buschke-Löwenstein tumors)	Perirectal area	Large, tumor-like	6, 11
Bowenoid papulosis	Penis, vulva, perirectal area	Multiple, large	16
Cervical cancer	Cervix	Asymptomatic; pigmented papillomas; erythematous or white plaques; ulcerations; mass lesion	Strong association: 16, 18, 31, 45 Moderate association: 30, 33, 35, 39, 51, 52, 56, 58, 59, 68 Weak association: 6, 11, 26, 43, 44, 34, 40, 53–55, 57, 62, 66
Vulvar cancer	Vulva	Asymptomatic; pigmented papillomas; erythematous or white plaques; ulcerations; mass lesion	16
Penile cancer	Penis	Painless, ulcerative mass lesion	16
Anal cancer	Perianal area	Asymptomatic; pigmented papillomas; erythematous or white plaques; ulcerations; mass lesion	16, 18, 31
Ovarian cancer	Ovaries	Unknown	6?, 16?, 18?
Mucosal (Other) Warts			
Respiratory papillomatosis	Larynx, trachea, bronchi, lungs	Multiple papillomas	6, 11
Nasal and paranasal papillomas	Nose, paranasal sinuses	Single or multiple papillomas	6, 11, 57, 57b
Focal epithelial hyperplasia (Heck disease)	Oral cavity	Discrete, multiple nodules	13, 32
Oral cavity papillomas	Gums, buccal mucosa, soft palate, tonsils	Single or multiple papillomas	6, 11, 16
Conjunctival papillomas	Conjunctivae	Single or multiple papillomas	6, 11, 16
Giant cell hepatitis	Liver	Unknown	6?

cavity, and the conjunctiva. The mucosal HPVs also can be subgrouped into low, high, and intermediate or moderate risk types, depending on the frequency they are found in invasive cancers.[13, 101, 180, 190]

It has not been possible to propagate HPVs in monolayer cell culture to yield full viral particles yet, probably because full epithelial cell differentiation and keratinization of squamous epithelial cells are required for the virus to replicate completely, and this differentiation is not achieved in conventional cell culture. Therefore, other methods have been developed to study the biology of HPVs. For example, research laboratories successfully have propagated a few papillomaviruses by inoculating virion extracts into susceptible tissue and transplanting this tissue into athymic nude mice.[88] Molecular assays of viral transformation with cloned HPV DNA have been used to define the viral genes involved in the induction of cellular proliferation and transformation. Also, rabbit papillomavirus animal models have been used to study the function of the E5 protein. In addition, the three-dimensional structure of the important viral proteins, such as E2 and potentially E6 and E7, have been determined by x-ray crystallography and multidimensional nuclear magnetic resonance spectroscopy.

Induction of cellular proliferation is the hallmark of infection with the papillomaviruses. Warts, for example, arise when a cell or small group of cells in the basal cell layer of the epithelium is infected with an HPV type. The viral DNA replicates in an episomal or small circular form and stimulates the cells to proliferate and produce a self-limited tumor, also called a papilloma, or wart. In the wart, all layers of the normal epithelium are present, but there is a hyperplasia of the prickle cell layer, called acanthosis. Hyperkeratosis is common in cutaneous warts but usually is absent in mucosal warts. Viral particles are produced in the differentiated, uppermost granular layers of the epithelium, and it is here where the viral cytopathic effect (koilocytosis), characteristic of HPVs, is displayed. Benign lesions express both early and late genes, but if the lesion progresses toward malignancy, the expression of the capsid antigens and production of viral particles are inhibited and only early region transcripts and proteins are detectable. When invasive cancer occurs, the viral DNA usually is integrated into the cellular genome. Another unique characteristic of the HPVs is the presence of latent or persistent viral genome in apparently normal cells. This persistence probably accounts for the recurrence of both genital and laryngeal papillomas, even after apparently successful treatment and prolonged disease-free periods.[55, 179]

EPIDEMIOLOGY

Epidemiologic information on the HPVs is scant, primarily because HPV infection is not a reportable disease and routine serologic tools to study large populations are unavailable. Most of the early epidemiologic studies on HPVs based their incidence and prevalence on physical examination that detected clinical lesions, such as warts, that were characteristic of HPV infection. Seroepidemiologic studies of HPV infection largely are unavailable because the inability to grow large quantities of the virus in cell culture has hampered the production of large quantities of antigens needed to develop serologic tests. In addition, because HPV infection and disease are localized in the epithelium, a systemic humoral immune response may be difficult to detect. Recent epidemiologic studies have focused on the prevalence of HPV infection in certain groups by detection of viral DNA in tissue. However, interpretation and comparison of the results of various studies are complicated by the variable sensitivity and specificity of the molecular methods used in each study.

The papillomaviruses are widespread in nature, and infection with HPVs occurs in people of all ages from all parts of the world. These viruses infect squamous epithelium at several body sites, and individual HPV types display marked specificity for a particular site. Infection appears to be transmitted through fomites, moisture, and minor skin trauma in cutaneous warts; by sexual intercourse in genital warts and condyloma; and during birth through an infected maternal birth canal in patients with juvenile-onset respiratory papillomatosis. In addition, HPV DNA has been detected in the aerosolized smoke and vapor from laser and electrocautery treatment of patients with cutaneous and genital warts and laryngeal papillomatosis, and anecdotal reports of possible transmission from the patient to the surgeon exist.[1, 53, 62, 160, 161] The incubation period for most infections varies from 3 weeks to as long as 8 months, with an average of about 3 months. In respiratory papillomatosis, the incubation period may be 5 years or longer and with cervical cancer 10 years or longer. Infection with HPVs may be asymptomatic; some may produce benign, barely noticeable warts; others may produce recurrent or growing lesions that are life-threatening and resistant to treatment; and a few infections may progress to invasive, even fatal, cancer. The outcome of an infection with HPV is influenced by several factors, including virus type, location of the lesion, immunologic status of the host, environmental and infectious cofactors, and the nature of the epithelium that has been infected.

Cutaneous warts are rare in children younger than 5 years of age but are relatively common in older children, adolescents, and young adults. In fact, as many as 10 per cent of school age children may have warts at some site on their body at any given time, and up to 50 per cent of individuals may have had cutaneous warts at some time during their life. Certain activities, such as use of public swimming pools and tattooing, or occupations, such as butchers, handlers of meat, poultry, and fish, and workers in slaughterhouses, appear to carry an increased risk of acquiring cutaneous warts.[41, 81, 100, 157, 186] Most warts regress within 2 years, presumably because the host mounts a cell-mediated immune response. Warts may increase in number and size, however, if the individual is immunocompromised, is pregnant, or has the rare familial disorder EV. The genotypes of HPV recovered from skin warts correlate, although not absolutely, with the morphology and body site of the wart. For example, HPV-1 is associated with deep plantar warts, HPV-2 with common skin warts, HPV-3 and HPV-10 with flat skin warts, and HPV-7 with butcher's warts, whereas a large number of different HPV types can be recovered from patients with EV (see Table 159–2).

Infection of the genital tract with HPVs also appears to be common, but the prevalence varies widely, according to the population studied and the criteria used to define infection. For example, it is estimated that 1 to 2 per cent of sexually active individuals have external anogenital warts, or condyloma acuminatum. However, when cytologic methods to detect subclinical disease are used, up to 10 per cent of sexually active women have been shown to have HPV-related disease of the cervix. Even higher prevalence rates have been observed when highly sensitive molecular techniques that detect both asymptomatic infection and disease are used. For example, one study of young university women found that 46 per cent were positive for at least one HPV type when extremely sensitive polymerase chain reaction (PCR)–based methods were employed.[9] Furthermore, recent studies suggest that up to 75 per cent of women have been infected with HPV at some time during their life.[165, 184] In contrast, older women appear to have a lower prevalence of HPV infection than younger women, even when sensitive molecular methods are used.[118, 162] Not all genital infections with HPVs may be transmitted sexually, however, because HPV DNA also has been detected on medical instruments and on the underwear of patients with genital HPV disease, suggesting that genital tract HPVs in certain circumstances may be transmitted by fomites, similar to cutaneous warts.[14, 53]

Most epidemiologic studies suggest that HPV infection of the genital tract is a sexually transmitted disease and that age and number of lifetime sexual partners are both independent risk factors for infection.[120] Of particular concern is the high and apparently increasing prevalence of cervical HPV infection in adolescents. In fact, recent epidemiologic evidence suggests that infection with HPV is the most common sexually transmitted disease in adolescent women. For example, in one recent study conducted in more than 600 adolescents who attended three urban clinics in Colorado, 24 per cent of the patients had evidence of HPV infection (15 per cent with clinically apparent genital warts, 36 per cent with subclinical HPV infection detected cytologically, and 49 per cent with subclinical infection detected by the presence of HPV DNA in cervical tissue).[78] In another study of sexually active adolescents, an incidence rate of 29 per cent was observed during a 13.3-month study period.[154] Whether this high prevalence of HPV infection represents persistent infection with the same HPV genotype or reinfection with a new HPV genotype remains controversial. For example, one study in Panama showed that the proportion of women with HPV infection increased according to the number of consecutive specimens tested (21 per cent to 82 per cent in a cohort of high-risk subjects sampled monthly for at least six visits) and suggested that persistent HPV infection with periodic viral shedding was the most likely explanation.[148] In contrast, other studies have shown that detection of the same HPV DNA genotype on second examination is unusual and suggested that spontaneous regression or resolution, followed by reinfection with a new type of HPV, occurred.[128, 154]

Epidemiologic observations show a strong link between HPV infection and cervical cancer because they both have characteristics of a sexually transmitted disease. For example, number of lifetime sexual partners is a risk factor for both HPV infection and cervical cancer. Furthermore, women with a history of genital warts are more likely to develop cervical carcinoma than are women with a negative history, and women married to men who develop cancer of the penis are significantly more likely to develop cervical cancer.[57, 66] There also are associations between specific genotypes of HPV infection and the presence of invasive cervical cancer. HPV-16, -18, -31, and -45 are associated strongly with cervical cancer; HPV-33, -35, -39, -51, -52, -56, -58, -59, and -68 have a moderate association with cervical cancer; and HPV-6, -11, -26, -42, -43, -44, -53, -54, -55, -62, and -66 rarely have been seen in cancerous lesions of the cervix.[169] In addition, cohort studies showed that presence of HPV DNA precedes the development of preinvasive cervical lesions.[146] However, despite strong circumstantial evidence and compelling laboratory documentation of the role HPV plays in cervical cancer, it appears that HPV infection alone is neither sufficient nor necessary for cervical cancer to develop. The disease still may be multifactorial in etiology, involving cofactors such as demography, genetics, socioeconomic status, race and ethnicity, age, nutrition and other dietary factors, pregnancy and parity, hormonal exposure, use of oral contraceptives, smoking, immune status, and the presence of other sexually transmitted infections and diseases.[30, 120, 146, 169]

Another potential consequence of genital infection with HPV is perinatal transmission of the virus from mother to infant. Genital HPVs, including high-risk genotypes 16 and 18 and lower risk genotypes 6 and 11, may be transmitted from mother to infant, presumably by passage through an infected birth canal, although ascending infection and postnatal acquisition also are possibilities.[26, 135] HPV DNA has been detected in buccal and genital cells obtained from infants born to mothers infected with HPV-16 and -18, and pregnant women with a high viral load of HPV DNA in cervical cells are more likely to transmit HPV infection to their newborn infants than are those mothers with a low viral load.[83] Furthermore, a recent study has demonstrated that HPV DNA may persist for at least 6 months in perinatally infected infants.[26] In fact, infection of the oral mucosa appears to be a common event in healthy adults and children. In adults, DNA from HPV-6 and -16 has been detected by PCR in 17 and 23 per cent of oral mucosa samples, and in preschool children, 24 and 19 per cent of oral samples, respectively.[79] The consequences of infection of the oral mucosa with genital-type and other HPVs range from asymptomatic infection to a variety of oral, respiratory, and ocular lesions. For example, HPV-6, -11, -16, and -18 have been seen in leukoplakia, lichen planus, oral papillomas, squamous cell carcinoma of the tongue, and verrucous carcinoma of the larynx.[23, 42, 106] Dysplastic and malignant lesions of the ocular conjunctiva and cornea also have been associated with HPV-16.[115] HPV-6 and -11 have been associated with juvenile and adult-onset laryngeal papillomatosis.[124] Circumstantial evidence implicating perinatal transmission of HPV as a cause of respiratory papillomatosis includes retrospective analyses that have shown an association between juvenile laryngeal papillomatosis and genital warts in the mother at the time of delivery.[11, 38, 145] Juvenile laryngeal papillomatosis also appears uncommon in children delivered by cesarean section.[170] It also must be noted, however, that this disease has a bimodal age distribution. Although the peak incidence of the disease occurs between birth and 5 years of age, almost one-half of patients with HPV-associated laryngeal papillomatosis present for the first time in adulthood.[37]

CLINICAL MANIFESTATIONS

Cutaneous Warts

Common cutaneous skin warts, or verrucae, have variable morphology and may appear at any location on the skin.[29, 169] Common skin warts, or verrucae vulgares, usually are well-demarcated, dome-shaped papules with multiple conical projections (papillomatosis) that give the surface of the wart a rough appearance and texture. Common warts usually occur on the hands, especially the dorsum, but also frequently are seen between the fingers, periungually, and on the palms and soles. They occasionally may be mosaic and spread superficially over the skin, or they may be filiform in morphology and appear as thread-like warts on the face and neck. They most commonly are associated with HPV-2 and -4. Butcher's warts, a form of cutaneous wart seen in meat and poultry handlers who suffer repeated minor trauma to the hands, is associated with HPV-7. Plantar warts, also called verrucae plantares, are most common in adolescents and young adults. They usually are single lesions and have a highly thickened corneal layer or hyperkeratosis, with areas of punctate bleeding. They also are painful because they usually are found on pressure-bearing points on the plantar surface of the foot or the palms of the hand. They usually are associated with HPV-1. Flat warts, or verrucae planae, in contrast, do not have papillomatosis or hyperkatosis, and they often are multiple. These warts are more common in young children and occur most frequently on the arms, face, and knees. HPV-3, -10, -28, and -41 have been associated with flat warts.[29, 169] Although the clinical appearance of cutaneous warts almost always is diagnostic, the differential diagnosis includes other viral skin disorders, such as molluscum contagiosum, and other infectious diseases, such as actinomycosis, blastomycosis, sporotrichosis, leishmaniasis, chronic vegetating pyoderma, atypical mycobacterial infection (e.g., swimming pool granuloma), and tuberculosis verrucosa cutis (warty tuberculosis). Giant verrucae or warts also must be differentiated from squamous cell carcinoma.

Epidermodysplasia Verruciformis

EV, a rare skin disorder that presents in infancy or early childhood, is characterized by the inability to resolve HPV-induced, cutaneous wart–like lesions.[107] Seen worldwide, this disease is familial, and there is a history of parental consanguinity in approximately 10 per cent of reported cases, implying a genetic basis for the disease. Although both autosomal recessive and X-linked recessive forms of inheritance have been observed, the precise genetic defect or mode of inheritance remains elusive.[4, 43, 107, 169] Patients with EV also have both nonspecific and HPV-specific defects in cell-mediated immunity, especially T-cell defects, and some patients will have developmental disabilities.[39, 65, 77, 108–110] Although the lesions seen with EV are polymorphic, two clinical types of warts primarily are seen in these patients: flat warts and red or reddish-brown macular plaques. Both the flat warts and plaques appear first on the face, trunk, and extremities. They slowly will become confluent and then appear to disseminate. Occasionally, the plaques may be achromatic with pigmented borders and resemble pityriasis versicolor.

Malignant transformation occurs in 30 to 50 per cent of patients with EV and occurs during adulthood, usually decades after the initial presentation in childhood. Therefore, long-term, careful clinical follow-up of children diagnosed with EV is important. The malignant transformation occurs in multiple foci in the reddish-brown plaque lesions, especially on areas such as the forehead that are exposed frequently to sunlight or other ultraviolet light. It also is more likely to occur if the patient is infected with highly oncogenic HPV-5, -8, or -47. The tumors that result usually are slow-growing yet locally destructive. Histopathologically, they may appear as an in situ or invasive carcinoma.[77] They generally do not metastasize unless exposed to cocarcinogens, such as x-ray irradiation.[134] The skin cancers in EV patients, although a serious and challenging clinical entity, also provide an excellent example and scientific model to study host factors, such as genetic defects; infecting virus type of HPV; and environmental factors, such as ultraviolet light, in the genesis of malignant transformation and the development of cancer.[169]

Patients with EV may be infected with multiple types of HPVs, including HPV-3 and -10 that are associated with flat warts in healthy individuals.[107, 169] The HPV types most commonly associated with lesions in EV patients, however, are 5, 8, 17, and 20, which usually are not seen in the general population. Other HPV types associated with this disorder are 9, 12, 14, 15, 19–25, 36–38, 47, and 49. The EV-associated HPV types that have a high oncogenic potential are 5, 8, and 47 because they appear in more than 90 per cent of skin carcinomas in EV patients, whereas HPV-14, -20, -21, and -25 appear to have a low oncogenic potential because they usually are detected only in benign skin lesions of patients with EV. It is likely that healthy individuals are infected asymptomatically with many of the HPV types seen in the lesions of patients with EV and that an immunologic defect allows the HPV infection to produce a chronic disease process. For example, HPV-8 antibodies have been found in healthy individuals, and HPV-5 and -8 DNA has been found in refractory warts and skin carcinoma of immunocompromised patients, such as renal allograft recipients.[68, 103, 141, 178]

The appearance of EV-like skin lesions also may be seen in individuals who are immunocompromised from HIV infection, as well as in transplant recipients, those receiving cancer chemotherapy, and other immunosuppressed patients.[12, 24, 48, 144, 158, 159, 172, 176, 187, 191] These lesions may appear as brownish plaques, like typical EV lesions, or they also may be morphologically similar to flat or common cutaneous warts. Skin warts in immunocompromised patients may be single or multiple, and they may persist or progress. These patients also have a high risk of squamous cell carcinomas, with the risk increasing with exposure to sunlight or ultraviolet light, as well as long duration of immunosuppression.[130, 191] A variety of HPV types have been identified in patients who are immunosuppressed. For example, all the main types of HPVs (1–4, 28) associated with skin warts in the general population have been detected in immunosuppressed patients. Also, HPV-5, -8, -10, -20, -23, -28, and -49 that are associated primarily with EV have been detected, either alone or in combinations, in immunosuppressed patients, especially renal transplant recipients.[107]

Infections of the Genital Tract

Genital tract infection with the mucosal HPVs probably is the most prevalent sexually transmitted infection due to a viral pathogen and, because of its link to cervical cancer, most likely imposes a far greater morbidity on the general population than does cutaneous infection with HPVs. Genital tract infection with HPVs may be latent, active yet asymptomatic, manifest as genital warts or condyloma, or associated with various stages of cervical cytologic and histologic abnormalities, including low- and high-grade squamous intraepithelial lesions, carcinoma in situ, and invasive carcinoma of the cervix. Pregnancy and immunosuppression have been associated with an increased prevalence of HPV infection and disease.

Asymptomatic or subclinical infection occurs in up to 10 per cent of women older than 15 years of age and may be as high as 30 per cent in some sexually active adolescent populations. It involves all genital HPVs (types 6, 11, 13, 16, 18, 30 to 35, 39, 40, 42 to 45, and 51 to 59).[169, 198] The outcome of infection with a genital HPV is variable and includes resolution of the infection and elimination of viral DNA, viral persistence with no cytologic abnormalities of the cervix, transient cytologic abnormalities that resolve completely in a few months, cytologic abnormalities that persist, and cytologic abnormalities that progress to in situ or invasive cervical cancer. Although the frequencies of these different outcomes of genital HPV infection are not known precisely, it appears that complete resolution of the infection is the most frequent occurrence, whereas invasive cancer is the rarest outcome. It is unknown if reinfection with the same strain of HPV can occur. However, viral persistence appears to be likely in HPV infections with cancer-related HPVs, especially types 16, 18, and 33, and in older women.[75, 169] Subclinical HPV infections do not cause symptoms and may be detectable only using sensitive molecular techniques that detect HPV DNA in cervical tissue. Subclinical HPV infection also may produce subtle flat lesions that only can be detected using acetic acid treatment followed by colposcopy.

The most common clinical manifestation of HPV infection of the genital tract is condyloma acuminatum, or genital warts. These warts usually are caused by infection with HPV-6 and -11 and occasionally -16. They usually are multiple; exophytic; pink, purplish, or gray; and papular or pedunculated lesions composed of short or long fronds of connective tissue covered by acanthotic squamous epithelium. In females, they involve the vaginal introitus, vulva, perineum, cervix, urethra, and anus. The lesions usually are asymptomatic but may cause itching, burning, or pain. During pregnancy, genital warts may increase in number and size and regress after delivery. In males, genital warts occur on the penis, scrotum, perineum, and anus. They usually are asymptomatic but may cause itching, burning, and dyspareunia. Adult and adolescent women and men, as well as children, with external anogenital warts also may have HPV infection at internal cervical-vaginal or intra-anal mucosal sites.[70, 76, 85, 86] In addition to typical papillary warts, flat condylomata may occur, especially in the cervix. These flat warts are difficult to visualize with the naked eye, and their detection may be aided by colposcopy. Flat condylomata usually are caused by HPV-6, -11, -16, -18, and -31 and may progress to low- and high-grade cervical intraepithelial lesions.[169] Infection with HIV increases the risk for HPV infection and HPV-associated genital lesions and neoplasias in adult men and women, and therefore these patients should be examined carefully for these conditions.[36, 192] Whether HIV infection increases the risk for HPV infection or disease in adolescents and children also is a concern but is unclear at this time.[156, 175] Immunosuppression from chemotherapy and transplantation also is associated with increased risk for HPV-associated genital infection, disease, and malignant transformation. In adolescents, anogenital warts may develop within 1 to 2 months after consensual sexual activity, as well as after sexual assault.[84] Infants and children also may have anogenital warts, which may result from sexual abuse or from perinatal transmission.[40, 70, 71] The risk for a sexually abused child to develop genital warts is not identified clearly; however, it is known that approximately half of the cases of genital warts in children reported in the literature appear to be related to sexual abuse. In addition, molecular techniques have shown that anogenital warts in children contain HPV DNA from types 6, 11, or 16, the same types responsible for genital warts in adults, whereas HPV DNA from types 1, 2, and 4 that cause common cutaneous warts has not been found in anogenital warts in children.[40] Anogenital warts in children are more likely to be acquired by sexual abuse than by perinatal transmission if the child is older than 2 years of age because this period is outside the plausible incubation period of perinatal transmission of HPV. The differential diagnosis of anogenital warts includes other infectious diseases, such as condyloma lata associated with secondary syphilis and molluscum contagiosum, as well as noninfectious disorders, such as epithelial papillae, enlarged sebaceous glands or sebaceous cysts, seborrheic keratosis, lentigo, pigmented nevi, skin tags, hemorrhoids, Crohn disease, and carcinoma.

Giant condylomata acuminata may occur on the penis, vulva, or perirectal area. These giant tumor-like lesions also are called Buschke-Löwenstein tumors and condylomatous carcinomas and were reported first by Buschke in Germany in 1896. The growth of these lesions is indolent and rarely may cause inguinal lymphadenopthy, fistulous tracts, inflammation, fibrosis, and hemorrhage of the surrounding tissues. Histologically, these lesions are benign and appear similar to typical anogenital warts. However, progression to dysplasia and carcinoma has been documented. Buschke-Löwenstein tumors are associated with HPV-6 and -11, in contrast to invasive genital carcinomas, which most commonly are associated with HPV-16 and -18.[127]

Progression of HPV-induced anogenital condylomatous lesions to dysplasia or invasive carcinomas is well documented but unusual.[92, 146, 195] Most anogenital carcinomas probably arise from infection with high-risk HPV-16 and -18, because worldwide more than 70 per cent of human cervical cancers contain DNA from HPV-16 or -18.[92, 147] This epidemiologic observation complements in vitro studies that document the transforming properties of these viral types.[169, 197] Other risks and cofactors for cervical cancer also have been identified, and it is likely that the progression from subclinical infection to carcinoma is multifactorial.[169] Invasive cervical cancer appears to evolve in a progressive cascade of cervical epithelial abnormalities that recently have been reclassified. These abnormalities currently are referred to as low-grade and high-grade squamous intraepithelial lesions. The category low-grade squamous intraepithelial lesions includes subclinical HPV infection, condyloma, and what was known formerly as grade 1 cervical intraepithelial neoplasia, or mild dysplasia. In the high-grade squamous intraepithelial lesions category, most or all of the thickness of the cervical epithelium is replaced by abnormal cells or microinvasive carcinoma. It includes what previously was referred to as grades 2 and 3 cervical intraepithelial neoplasia, or moderate to severe dysplasia, and carcinoma in situ. If not detected and treated, high-grade squamous intraepithelial lesions may evolve into invasive carcinoma, breach the basement membrane, and metastasize to regional lymph nodes and other parts of the body. The HPV types that have a strong association with invasive cervical cancer are 16, 18, 31, and 45, whereas types 33, 35, 39, 51, 52, 56, 58, 59, and 68 only moderately are associated with cervical cancer. The remaining types (6, 11, 26, 43, 44, 53–55, 62, and 66) rarely have been associated with cancer. Cervical cancer usually is asymptomatic and detected by cytologic screen. However, patients with advanced invasive cervical cancer may have abnormal menstrual bleeding or pain. The lesions also may be visible by direct visual inspection and appear as pigmented papillomas, erythematous plaques, or leukoplakic lesions or, if further advanced, as ulcerations or large masses. Squamous carcinoma of the penis is quite rare, especially in countries that practice routine newborn circumcision. However, when penile cancer does occur, it usually presents as a painless, slowly enlarging ulcerative mass.

Bowenoid papulosis is another manifestation of HPV infection of the anogenital tract. It usually occurs in young adults younger than 40 years of age and is characterized by multiple, large maculopapular lesions that are erythematous and reddish, purplish, or brownish, with a smooth, velvety surface. These lesions may regress spontaneously or persist. Bowenoid papulosis is associated with HPV-16 and histologically appears to be high-grade squamous intraepithelial lesions or squamous cell carcinoma in situ. Bowen disease, on the other hand, is seen in patients older than 40 years of age and causes single, reddish, scaling or crusting lesions that histologically also appear to be high-grade squamous intraepithelial lesions.[195]

Traditionally, cervical dysplasia and carcinomas have been considered disorders of middle-aged and older women. However, over the past 10 to 20 years, the prevalence of HPV infection and abnormal cervical cytology in young women and adolescents has increased. For example, recent studies suggest 18 to 53 per cent prevalence rates for HPV infection in sexually active adolescents, with high-risk HPV-16 and -18 being the most common types detected.[78] The prevalence of cervical low- and high-grade squamous intraepithelial lesions detected by Papanicolaou smears from adolescents also appears to have increased from 3 per cent in the 1970s to 18 per cent in the 1990s.[156] These alarming observations should alert physicians who care for adolescents and suggest that an epidemic of cervical cancer may occur in the near future.

Recurrent Respiratory Papillomatosis

Recurrent respiratory papillomatosis (RRP) is a rare, histologically benign, yet paradoxically life-threatening, condition caused by HPV-6 and -11. Worldwide, it probably is the most common tumor of the larynx in children, with incidences between 0.1 to 2.8 per 100,000 observed.[173, 189] In the United States, the estimated incidence in children is 0.6 per 100,000, with an estimated 1500 patients newly diagnosed each year.[123, 189] The disease may be seen in both children and adults. Approximately two-thirds of cases of RRP are seen in children and also may be called juvenile respiratory papillomatosis. Approximately one-fourth of the cases in children will present before 1 year of age, half by 5 years of age, and the remaining by 10 years of age. Adult-onset RRP usually manifests between 20 and 40 years of age.[169]

Circumstantial evidence suggests that infants and children with RRP most likely acquire HPV perinatally during passage through an HPV-infected birth canal. For example, 30 to 60 per cent of mothers of children with RRP have a history of genital warts, compared with less than 5 per cent of mothers of children who do not have RRP.[137, 145] Furthermore, children with RRP rarely are born by cesarean section. HPV-6 and -11, most commonly associated with RRP, also are responsible for most of the genital warts seen in women.[52, 169] HPV DNA also has been detected in the oropharynx of infants born to mothers with genital HPV infection.[169] However, only a small proportion of infants born to mothers with genital warts or subclinical HPV infection develop RRP. The mode of transmission of HPV-6 and -11 in adult-onset RRP is unknown. The most common presenting symptom of RRP is hoarseness or a change in voice. Infants and toddlers may have a hoarse cry, stridor, airway obstruction, respiratory distress, or difficulty in phonation. They also may present with a croup-like illness. The most common site for RRP is the true vocal cord of the larynx. Supra- and subglottic extension of the lesions also may occur. The disease also may involve the trachea, bronchi, palate, nasopharynx, paranasal sinuses, and lungs. When the lungs are involved, pulmonary nodules, atelectasis, and secondary bacterial pneumonia may occur (Fig. 159–1). The disease also may produce permanent lung damage with bronchiectasis and cavitations (Fig. 159–2). In approximately 2 to 3 per cent of patients, progression to invasive squamous papillomatosis and even malignant transformation to a squamous cell carcinoma will occur, with invasion of the soft tissues of the neck, esophagus, and lung parenchyma (Fig. 159–3). This incidence increases to 14 per cent in patients who received radiation therapy that commonly was used up to 1970 to treat RRP.[63, 111, 164] Smoking and severe, recurrent disease also appear to increase the risk for malignant transformation in adolescents and adults. In addition, sudden and unexpected death may occur from airway obstruction if the lesions obstruct the laryngeal lumen.[174] The clinical course of RRP is highly variable, characterized by common and unpredictable remissions and exacerbations, even despite apparently successful removal of the lesions.

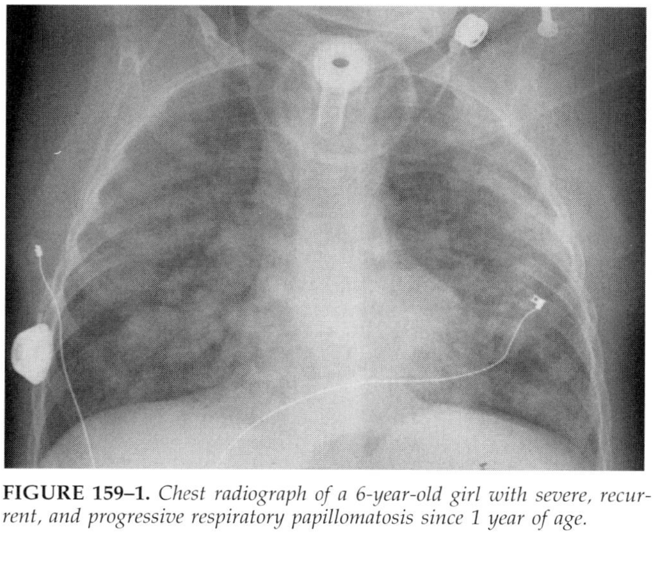

FIGURE 159–1. *Chest radiograph of a 6-year-old girl with severe, recurrent, and progressive respiratory papillomatosis since 1 year of age.*

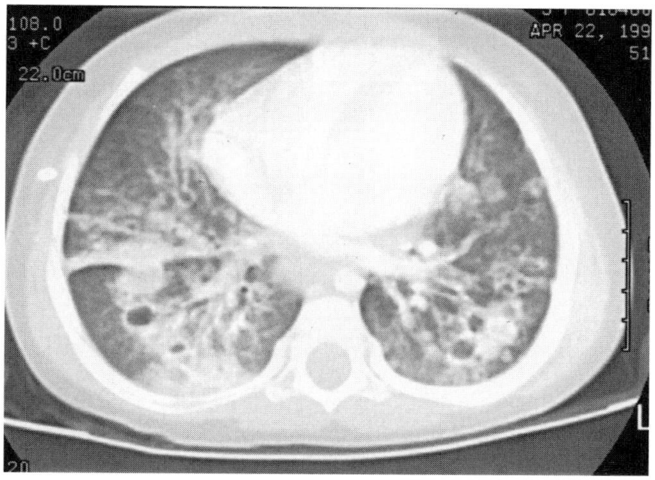

FIGURE 159–2. *Chest computed tomograph of a 6-year-old girl with severe, recurrent, and progressive respiratory papillomatosis showing pulmonary nodules, bronchiectasis, and cavitations.*

Nasal and Paranasal Papillomas

Nasal papillomas or warts are rare tumors that may occur at any age, including childhood, and may present as solitary lesions or in combination with papillomas elsewhere in the respiratory tract.[22, 152] Histologically, they usually resemble laryngeal papillomas seen in RRP. They most commonly are caused by HPV-6 and -11, although HPV-16, -57, and -57b also have been detected in nasal papillomas. Cocaine snorting is one risk factor for development of nasal papillomas.[167] Papillomas also may involve the paranasal sinuses.[22, 152]

Papillomas of the Oral Cavity

Papillomas or warts in the oral cavity are heterogeneous etiologically and may be caused by cutaneous HPV types that are associated with warts on the skin, as well as mucosal HPV types that are associated with genital warts. For example, focal epithelial hyperplasia, also called Heck disease, is a rare, yet well-defined clinical condition of the oral mucosa associated with HPV-13 and -32, which only infect the oral cavity.[169, 183] It occurs worldwide but is most prevalent in Central and South America, Alaska, and Greenland. Focal epithelial hyperplasia may occur in children or adults and often clusters in families or geographic regions.[132] The lesions are discrete, multiple, elevated nodules readily visible on the oral mucosa. They may persist for years or resolve spontaneously. They do not, however, appear to undergo malignant transformation, nor do they appear to metastasize to other parts of the body. Warts due to HPV-2, the same type associated with verrucae vulgares or common cutaneous warts of the skin, may occur on the lips and on the mucosa of the oral cavity.[49] Oral papillomas involving the gums, buccal mucosa, soft palate, and tonsils also may be caused by HPV-6, -11, and -16, which primarily are associated with genital warts, or condylomata acuminata.[125, 169]

Conjunctival Papillomas

Conjunctival papillomas occur in all age groups but are exceedingly rare. They may be asymptomatic initially, then cause a constant foreign body sensation or chronic conjunctivitis. When large, they appear as pink mulberry- or

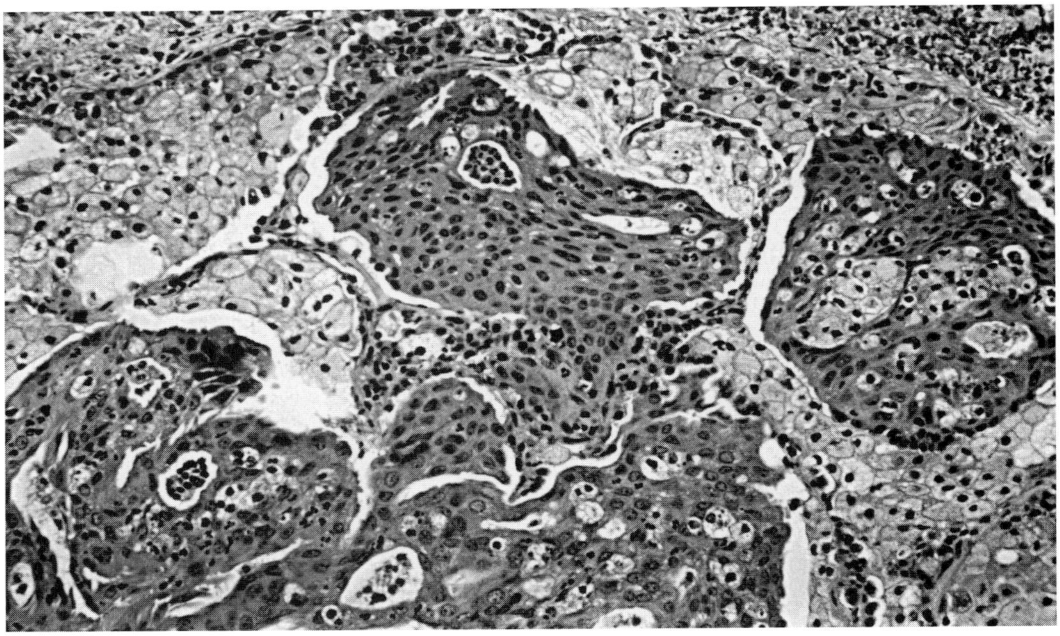

FIGURE 159–3. *Lung biopsy tissue (hematoxylin and eosin stain, 50 × original magnification, light microscopy) from a 6-year-old girl with severe, progressive, recurrent, respiratory papillomatosis. This tissue shows invasive squamous papillomatosis. The squamous cells are growing along preformed pulmonary structures, but there is no evidence of malignancy, at this time, because there is no invasion of the lung tissue. (Courtesy of Dr. Claire Langston, Department of Pathology, Baylor College of Medicine and Texas Children's Hospital, Houston, TX.)*

cauliflower-like growths that may cause pain or interfere with lid closure. In most children and some adults, they appear to be caused by HPV-6 and -11, which characteristically infect the genital tract, and therefore may be transmitted during birth, similar to RRP.[93, 116] HPV-16, another HPV that commonly infects the genital tract, also has been associated with conjunctival and lacrimal sac carcinomas in adults.[105, 115]

Gastrointestinal Papillomas and Cancer

Esophageal infection with HPV may be asymptomatic or produce papillomas that cause dysphagia.[6] HPVs also, along with a variety of cofactors, may be involved in the genesis of esophageal carcinoma.[28] Similarly, HPV DNA has been detected in tissue samples from patients with colon cancer but with unclear implications as to their role.[169] The association of HPVs with anal warts, anal squamous intraepithelial lesions, and anal cancer, however, appears strong. Infection with HPV-16, -18, and -31 most commonly occurs, but mere infection with these specific HPV types does not appear sufficient for the development of cancer. Similar to cervical cancer, it also appears that cofactors such as other sexually transmitted diseases or chemical carcinogens (e.g., tobacco) may be involved in the pathogenesis of anal cancer.[91, 127]

Liver Disease

Recent reports also have suggested that HPVs may play a role in liver disease. For example, HPV DNA, especially HPV-6, has been detected using sensitive molecular techniques in the liver of patients with neonatal giant cell hepatitis, postinfantile giant cell hepatitis, post–liver transplantation giant cell hepatitis, and primary hepatocellular carcinoma.[45, 136, 168] However, the pathogenic role of HPV in these diseases, although an intriguing possibility, remains unproven at this time.

Other Cancers

The potential role of HPVs in the pathogenesis of a variety of unusual cancers has been explored by a variety of investigators, using different approaches, with conflicting results. Therefore, the role of HPVs in these cancers remains unproven at this time. For example, HPV DNA from types 6, 16, and 18 has been detected in the tissue from some but not all patients with ovarian carcinoma.[169, 188] HPVs also have been detected in tissue from patients with cancer of the endometrium, urethra, urinary bladder, and prostate, with unclear pathogenic implications.[169]

LABORATORY DIAGNOSIS

The typical appearance of verrucae vulgares on the skin and condylomata acuminata in the anogenital area in otherwise healthy individuals usually is sufficient to make the clinical diagnosis of these HPV-associated illnesses. However, laboratory confirmation of HPV-associated lesions may be necessary in unusual presentations in healthy individuals, in immunocompromised patients, and in patients with suspected malignant lesions. Methods commonly and traditionally used in viral diagnosis, such as cell culture, serology, and electron microscopy, have limited clinical utility in detecting HPV infection, whereas a variety of molecular methods, used alone or in combination, have proved quite useful in research and clinical settings. Cytologic and histologic approaches also are useful in diagnosing HPV-associated cancers.

Electron Microscopy

Virions with typical papillomavirus morphology can be detected in abundance in cutaneous warts but are difficult to detect in tissue from patients with RRP, genital warts, or histologically diagnosed cancers.

Cell Culture

None of the papillomaviruses have been propagated in cell culture monolayer. Therefore, routine viral cultures available in most diagnostic virology laboratories will not detect the presence of HPVs. Research laboratories have shown that HPV-1, when inoculated into skin keratinocytes or respiratory tract–derived epithelial cells, will replicate its DNA transiently in an episomal form over several serial passages. However, viral capsid proteins and intact viral particles are not produced.[34] Other research laboratories have inoculated cervical tissue with extracts of HPV-11 virions obtained from condyloma acuminatum lesions and later transplanted the tissue beneath the renal capsule of athymic nude mice.[88] After several months, viral cytopathic effects have been seen and viral capsid antigen and complete viral particles were produced. Clearly, these research methods need refinement before the routine cultivation of HPVs becomes available to the clinician.

Serology

The inability to cultivate the papillomaviruses routinely has hampered the development of serologic tests to detect and study the humoral responses to infection with HPVs significantly. Therefore, routine serologic assays to detect group- and type-specific antibody to HPVs are not available to the clinician currently. However, research laboratories continue to study the humoral response to HPV by a variety of methods. For example, serologic studies using purified virions of HPV-1 from plantar warts and HPV-11 obtained from mouse xenograft systems have revealed associations between seropositivity and clinical symptoms of infection with these HPV types.[19–22, 33, 89, 142, 177, 193] Other studies of serologic response to HPV have employed recombinant DNA methods to clone and express late region L1 and L2 proteins with bacterial fusion proteins.[56, 64, 80, 201, 202] Most recently, investigators have used vaccinia virus or baculovirus expression systems to produce virion-like particles composed primarily of viral capsids of HPV-1, -6, -11, and -16.[25, 67, 94, 126, 153, 182] However, it appears that these serologic assays using intact virions or virion-like particles, although technically the most successful to date, still have problems with sensitivity and specificity. Persistent, high-titer humoral responses are not detected in HPV infections, and, in contrast to other sexually transmitted viral infections (e.g., herpes simplex virus, HIV, hepatitis B virus infections), seroconversion does not appear to be a clearly defined marker for primary HPV infection. Cross-reactivity between HPV types also appears to occur, which limits the specificity of current assays. In addition to efforts to delineate the virus-specific humoral responses to HPV infection and HPV-associated cancers by measuring antibodies to HPV capsid proteins and HPV transforming proteins, studies evaluating serologic markers as predictors of invasive genital tract disease and ultimate survival also are being conducted.[182]

Colposcopy

Colposcopy is an important procedure to perform in women with abnormal Papanicolaou smears or external anogenital warts. It also may be used to diagnose asymptomatic, flat cervical warts in women whose sexual partners have external anogenital warts or to follow women who are considered to be at high risk for genital HPV infection for other reasons. The urethral meatus, penis, scrotum, and anus of males also may be inspected with a colposcope. The procedure usually is performed by gynecologists, urologists, and family practitioners, as well as pediatricians who are specialists in adolescent medicine. Briefly, the cervix and vulva in females or urethral meatus, penis, scrotum, and anus in males are visualized under magnification with a colposcope to identify lesions, with special attention to their topography, presence of abnormal whitening, and vascular architecture. The area then is soaked in dilute acetic acid (3 to 5 per cent) and visualized again for the presence of previously undetected lesions that appear as whitened plaques. Whitening after acetic acid application, however, is not specific for HPV infection or disease, and biopsy is required for definitive diagnosis. Colposcopic examination of the cervix not only gives a more accurate assessment of the anatomic extent of suspicious lesions or neoplasia but also allows the colposcopist to direct biopsies of suspicious areas accurately. Tissue biopsies then may be sent for histologic examination and detection of HPV DNA by molecular techniques.

Cytology

Obtaining exfoliated cervical cells and staining them by the Papanicolaou method is a routine procedure that detects the majority of HPV infections and dramatically has reduced the incidence of invasive squamous cell carcinoma of the cervix. It should be performed routinely in all sexually active females, including adolescents. It also has been evaluated as a screening examination of exfoliated urethral cells from males and in the urine from both men and women, with less success and acceptance than cervical cell screening.[126] Papanicolaou smear screening, however, is limited by the expertise of the physician who obtains the specimen and the pathologist who performs the cytologic analysis.[122] For example, because most cervical neoplasia arises at the junction of the squamous and columnar epithelium of the cervix (transformation zone), care must be taken to obtain cells from this region. Interobserver variability also exists among pathologists who read Papanicolaou smears. Furthermore, Papanicolaou smears are not as sensitive as colposcopy for detecting cervical cancer, and a negative Papanicolaou smear does not eliminate the diagnosis in women at high risk for cervical cancer. Therefore, women with anogenital warts and those who are immunosuppressed should have colposcopic examination to detect subclinical cervical lesions and not just a Papanicolaou smear.

The cytologic abnormality that is specific and characteristic of HPV infection is the presence of koilocytosis (derived from the Greek word *koilos*, which means "hollow" or "cavity") or koilocytotic cells that display fat, swollen, wrinkled, or raisinoid nuclei surrounded by a halo. Other abnormalities, including dyskeratosis, parakeratosis, and hyperkeratosis, may occur but are considered secondary or nonspecific. The prevalence of cytologic abnormalities in women screened by Papanicolaou smears consistently has been estimated at 2 to 3 per cent. Most abnormalities, however, resolve spontaneously in 3 to 6 months, but some persist and rarely may progress to cervical squamous cell carcinoma. If the infection progresses to disease, the koilocytosis characteristic of viral expression diminishes and the cells begin to display dysplastic changes and nuclear abnormalities. These abnormalities currently are graded into two categories: (1) low-grade squamous intraepithelial lesions, which include very mild dysplasia and the former grade 1 cervical intraepithelial neoplasia, and (2) high-grade squamous intraepithelial lesions, which include moderate to severe dysplasia and carcinoma in situ and the former grades 2 and 3 cervical intraepithelial neoplasia.[5]

Histology

HPV infection may occur in histologically normal tissue and be detected only by molecular methods that detect viral DNA. Benign and asymptomatic HPV infection also may cause koilocytosis, the typical histologic feature of HPV infection, which has specific nuclear and cytoplasmic characteristics. Condyloma acuminatum lesions display not only koilocytosis but also other histopathologic characteristics of active HPV infection, such as hyperkeratosis, parakeratosis, acanthosis, and lengthening of the rete pegs. Atypical features, such as mitotic figures above the basal layer, dysplastic cells, and single-cell keratinization, suggest dysplasia, such as bowenoid papulosis. Precancerous and cancerous lesions of the cervix and penis also may be graded as low-grade or high-grade squamous intraepithelial lesions and invasive squamous cell carcinoma.

The histologic examination of tissue for the presence of HPV-associated disease may be augmented in certain circumstances by the detection of shared, genus-specific HPV capsid antigens that may be identified by immunohistochemistry using immunoperoxidase-labeled antibodies raised to bovine papillomavirus capsid antigen. This procedure usually is successful in identifying HPV antigens in low-grade squamous intraepithelial lesions but rarely detects antigen in high-grade squamous intraepithelial lesions because of the biology of HPV expression in these cancerous cells. Similarly, it is unusual to detect HPV antigens by this method in cutaneous or anogenital warts or other HPV-associated cancers. In addition, the utility of this method to type the HPV infection currently is limited because unique, type-specific HPV capsid antigens are available only in research laboratories.[200]

Molecular Methods That Detect Human Papillomavirus DNA

HPV DNA may be detected in tissue by several methods, including dot-blot, slot-blot, Southern blot, and in situ hybridization assays, and amplification procedures, such as PCR. HPV DNA has been detected by these methods in the majority of HPV-associated neoplasias but also in a significant proportion of asymptomatic individuals, including women with normal Papanicolaou smears. The variability of HPV DNA detection between studies is great and appears to be influenced by the population studied, the frequency and type of sampling, and the sensitivity and specificity of the molecular methods used. Because type-specific antisera are not available for HPVs, the diagnosis of type-specific HPV infection or disease requires molecular DNA methods.

Southern Blot Hybridization

Southern blot hybridization is considered the reference standard for detection of HPV DNA in clinical samples. In this assay, nucleic acid is extracted from the sample, which usually is fresh tissue or exfoliated cervical cells, and digested or cleaved into smaller fragments with restriction enzymes. These fragments then are separated by gel electrophoresis and transferred onto special filter papers. Hybridization with radio-labeled probes directed against specific HPV DNA sequences then is performed. The advantages of Southern blot hybridization include good sensitivity (approximately 10^5 DNA copies) and specificity and the ability to distinguish HPV types easily. Disadvantages of this method include the need for special equipment and expertise. It also is technically expensive and time-consuming and requires a large sample of tissue that is destroyed during the DNA isolation procedure.

Dot- and Slot-Blot Hybridization

Dot- and slot-blot hybridization apply extracted DNA from a sample directly to a specific area (dot or slot) of a filter paper, bypassing the gel electrophoresis and transfer steps of Southern hybridization. The filters are incubated with a solution containing a complementary probe, followed by stringency washes to remove an unhybridized probe.[9, 200] Detection of successful hybridization is by autoradiography if a ^{32}P-labeled probe is employed or by colorimetric reaction if an enzyme-labeled probe is used. The advantages of dot-blot hybridization include commercial availability of some assays, ease of performance, rapid turn-around time, and low cost. Sensitivity and specificity generally are slightly below those of Southern blot analysis, but the method sufficiently is sensitive to detect HPV DNA in cytologically normal, as well as abnormal, cervical samples, and its use, in combination with the Papanicolaou smear, has been advocated to improve identification of women at high risk for cervical cancer.[69, 121] Dot-blot hybridization may be performed on tissue samples or cervical swabs collected in a special sample transport media or buffer, and its utility in screening urine for HPV DNA also has been explored.[126] Typing of HPV DNA also may be performed by dot-blot hybridization methods. For example, one commercial kit, by using a combination of radio-labeled probe mixtures, delineates up to seven types of HPV by category group: types 6/11, types 16/18, and types 31/33/35.[69, 121, 194] In addition, probes to detect almost all HPV types have been developed in a variety of research laboratories.

A novel, nonradioactive, chemiluminescent liquid hybridization assay (hybrid capture assay) is commercially available and detects up to 14 HPV types, divided into high-risk (types 16, 18, 31, 33, 35, 45, 51, 52, 56) and low-risk (types 6, 11, 42, 43, 44) groups, based on association with cervical cancer.[163] This DNA hybrid capture assay is relatively rapid and simple to perform and is unique because it provides quantitative data that reflect viral concentration.

In Situ Hybridization

In situ tissue hybridization assays are performed directly on fresh or fixed tissue sections or on cytologic specimens and have the unique advantage of allowing the examiner to correlate histopathologic abnormalities with the location of HPV DNA. They may be performed with radioactive probes or enzyme-labeled probes. The sensitivity of many in situ hybridization assays is less than that of Southern blot assays, especially if enzyme-labeled probes are employed.[27, 129, 185, 200] Commercial reagents and kits are available. However, this methodology remains technically challenging.

DNA Amplification Assays

DNA amplification systems, primarily PCR-based, recently have been applied to detect HPV DNA in clinical samples. Current PCR methodology uses oligonucleotide primers and a thermostable DNA polymerase, known as *Taq* polymerase, to drive a reaction that allows the exponential production of copies of a target piece of DNA. This target DNA is detected preliminarily using gel electrophoresis and confirmed using a complementary radioactive or enzyme-labeled probe. Numerous strategies have been explored. However, many laboratories now use PCR amplification with degenerate or consensus primers that are capable of recognizing a portion of one of the late genes from a broad spectrum of papillomaviruses. The popular MY09 (primer for the negative strand)/MY11 (primer for the positive strand) primer system amplifies a 450–base pair target region located in the HPV L1 open-reading frame that contains both conserved regions that are common to most or all papillomaviruses and divergent regions that appear to be unique for each HPV DNA type.[112] Amplification and detection by the MY9/MY11 primers in a PCR assay identify HPV DNA, which can be confirmed using "generic" HPV probe mixes. Typing of known HPV types then can be performed using type-specific HPV probes that are labeled oligonucleotides composed of sequences complementary to each viral type. Alternatively, restriction fragment length polymorphism or sequence analysis can be performed on the PCR product to identify new HPV types that are unable to be typed using available type-specific probes.[16, 131, 138, 139]

HPV DNA detection by PCR-based methods can be performed on a variety of specimens, including fresh or fixed tissue, exfoliated urethral and cervical cells, and urine, and the machinery and reagents to perform the testing readily are available.[196] However, a well-designed laboratory facility and technical personnel experienced in PCR-based diagnostics who rigidly adhere to carryover precautions are necessary to perform the tests properly and avoid the pitfalls of false-positive reactions due to contamination of specimens. In addition, internal reaction controls must be employed to evaluate sample processing amplification and control for false-negative reactions caused by inadequate DNA recovery and PCR reaction failures. Variations on the traditional PCR methodology to detect HPV DNA also have been reported. For example, single- and double-tube nested PCR tests, extremely sensitive methods that detect very low–copy number levels of DNA, have detected and typed EV-associated HPVs in cutaneous cancers from renal transplant recipients and have been used to study HPVs associated with genital infection and cancer.[15, 203]

Both the major advantage and the major disadvantage of detection of HPV DNA by PCR-based methods is extreme sensitivity, which theoretically is estimated to be one DNA copy but practically has been observed to be between 10 and 100 DNA copies. Although useful as a research tool to study the epidemiology of HPV infection, the clinical application of this and other DNA detection methods for HPV infection and disease currently is evolving. For example, using traditional methods of Papanicolaou smear screening, colposcopy, and biopsy, the prevalence of cytologic, colposcopic, and histologic abnormalities of the cervix in the general population consistently has been estimated to be between 2 and 3 per cent.[200] However, wide ranges of prevalence between 7 and 82 per cent for HPV infection detected by molecular methods have been reported and vary according to the population studied and the methodology used, with PCR-based methods in high-risk groups having the highest prevalence rates.[9, 85, 102, 148, 199, 204] The recognition that HPVs, especially high-risk types 16 and 18, are associated with cervical and other cancers, suggests that the detection of HPV DNA may be used as an adjunct to cytologic screening by Papanicolaou smear and offers the potential opportunity to identify women with cervical neoplasia who have false-negative Papanicolaou smears. On the other hand, the significance of the presence of HPV DNA, even if it is from a high-risk type, in histologically normal tissue is unclear, and the presence of HPV DNA, no matter what type, in histologically abnormal tissue does not influence management at this time. Further studies are needed to explore and resolve the clinical role of DNA-based diagnostics in the management of HPV infections.

TREATMENT

Most cutaneous and mucosal HPV-associated warts and lesions in healthy individuals will regress spontaneously in 1 to 2 years. Treatment may be desirable if the lesions are large, multiple, or recurrent; if they cause pain or discomfort; or if they are undesirable cosmetically. Treatment is mandatory if the lesions are life-threatening, such as laryngeal papillomas that obstruct the airway and cervical cancer. A variety of treatment strategies are available, but none produces a universally effective or permanent cure. Rather, current approaches focus on reduction of the clinically apparent lesion, and most require repetitive application. Clinically significant HPV-associated lesions also usually require the additional expertise of a specialist. For example, a dermatologist should be consulted to assist in the management of a patient with severe recalcitrant cutaneous warts, a gynecologist and oncologist for patients with cervical cancer, an ophthalmologist for a patient with conjunctival papillomas, and an otolaryngologist and pulmonologist for children and adults with severe RRP. These specialists are likely to know the currently available treatment regimens most effective for each patient's HPV clinical manifestation. The role of the infectious diseases specialist in the management of HPV-associated disease is evolving and may become more prominent as HPV-specific antiviral chemotherapy becomes available for clinical trials and eventually for routine clinical use in patients. Current standard therapies focus on the physical, surgical, or chemical destruction of the clinical manifestation of the HPV infection, such as the wart or papilloma.

Surgical techniques to treat papillomas include traditional local excision by knife, cryotherapy with liquid nitrogen or dry ice, electrocautery and curettage, and ultrasonication.[8, 17, 18, 82, 113, 171] Newer ablative surgical techniques that use carbon dioxide laser vaporization and flash-lamp pulsed dye laser therapy allow more precise and complete removal of visible papillomas and are becoming widely used to treat genital and laryngeal papillomas.[54, 150, 181] Surgical excision by knife remains the initial mainstay of many HPV diseases, however, because it provides tissue for a histopathologic diagnosis as well as removal or debulking of large lesions. Ablation by cryotherapy using liquid nitrogen, electrocautery, or laser vaporization may be used to remove small, single, or multiple lesions or be used in combination with surgery in large or difficult lesions.[119] These surgical therapies also may release viral antigens and produce local and systemic immunologic stimulation that may assist in eradicating the lesions. The disadvantages of these physical methods of wart and papilloma removal include pain, scarring, and disfigurement. They also are relatively invasive and impractical for patients with disseminated disease. Furthermore, recurrent treatments usually are necessary. In addition, laser vapors contain HPV DNA and may be a vehicle for spreading the infection in the patient or to the treating physician or surgeon, and the vapors or smoke plume should be contained.[62] Recurrence of lesions after treatment is common and most likely is due to the presence of HPV DNA sequences in clinically and histologically normal epithelium adjacent to and beyond the treatment area.[55]

Warts and papillomas also may be disrupted physically and removed by using chemical ablatives that are applied topically to the lesion. Simple organic acids, such as bi- and tri-chloracetic acid or salicylic acids applied twice daily for several days, have shown some success in localized treatment of skin and genital warts.[59] They are caustic substances that produce a white slough that peels off, and they can be applied weekly until the lesion is destroyed.[59] Antimiotic agents, such as the traditional podophyllin or the newer preparation podophyllotoxin, can be applied twice daily for several weeks. Antimetabolites, such as bleomycin, cantharidine, and 5-fluorouracil, also have shown efficacy when administered locally once or twice a week because they inhibit the cellular proliferation induced by HPV infection.[87, 143] These topical chemicals usually are easy to apply to skin and genital warts, but they also may cause local pain, redness, swelling, irritation, blisters, and scarring.[87] They also are not virus-specific, and recurrences are common. They also are impractical for extensive lesions and may be toxic if used in certain circumstances. For example, they may damage the cornea if used to treat conjunctival papillomas, and they should not be used in pregnant women.[119] The systemically administered antitumor agent methotrexate also has been administered to individual patients with disseminated HPV disease with variable success.

Immunomodulation is another treatment strategy for HPV-associated disease. A systemic immunologic response likely is responsible for the spontaneous regression frequently observed in cutaneous and mucosal warts. Therefore, stimulation of the immune system using immunomodulators also may produce remission in patients with HPV-associated disease. Interferons have antiviral, antiproliferative, and immunomodulating properties. There are more than 10 years of clinical research experience treating HPV-associated disease with interferon administered topically, intralesionally, or systemically by subcutaneous injection. Both lymphoblastoid (alpha) and fibroblast (beta) interferon have been used with some success to treat patients with genital warts and respiratory papillomatosis topically, locally, and systemically.[47, 58, 60, 149, 166, 169] However, gamma interferon has not been shown to be beneficial. Both recombinant and natural source alpha interferon preparations have been shown in placebo-controlled trials to be effective and are approved by the U.S. Food and Drug Administration for the intralesional treatment of genital warts.[47, 58] A 25- to 30-gauge needle is used to inject approximately 0.1 mL (1×10^6 units) at the base of up to five warts at a time for a total dose of 5×10^6 units at each visit. This dose is repeated two to three times weekly for 3 weeks. Maximum effect usually is seen within 4 to 8 weeks. Repeat injections also may be given if warts are persistent or recurrent. Interferon therapy also may be effective if used alone or in combination with laser surgery to treat patients with RRP.[73, 74, 95, 96, 104] Fever, headache, chills, and myalgias frequently occur with local and systemic interferon treatment. Severe and persistent fatigue, nausea, and leukopenia also are fairly common adverse reactions, especially with systemically administered interferon. Systemic natural leukocyte interferon also causes regression of warts and reduction of virus load in tissues in patients with EV.[2] Cimetidine, an immunomodulator that alters lymphocyte function, has been used in an attempt to treat children with recalcitrant cutaneous warts.[133] Contact and systemic immunotherapy with diphenylcyclapropenone also has been tried as an alternative treatment for HPV-associated disease but with little success.[169]

Retinoids and retinoic acid, which are analogs of vitamin A, can regulate growth and differentiation of malignant, premalignant, and even normal cells.[151] Clinically, they have a documented effect against squamous cell carcinomas.[98, 99] For these reasons, anecdotal reports and small series of patients have emerged reporting the use of retinoic acid to treat HPV-associated disease, especially RRP. In these reports, retinoids have been used with varying success, primarily as adjuvant agents with surgical therapy, to treat adult patients with severe, refractory RRP.[3, 10, 46] The combination of interferon and retinoic acid has been shown to be synergistic against breast cancer cells in vitro and potentially may be useful in refractory cases of RRP.[114]

Specific HPV antiviral chemotherapy is a promising direction for the future. The ideal anti-HPV drug would eliminate existing lesions swiftly and safely, eradicate latent HPV DNA to prevent recurrences, and permit the host to develop natural immunity against future reinfection and disease. Unique aspects of HPV infection and disease, however, make designing specific antiviral therapies a challenge. For example, HPV disease usually is focal, the virus intricately is involved in the cell's life cycle, and there is great diversity of more than 70 genotypes. The inability to grow HPVs readily in cell culture also hampers the ability to study the antiviral properties and cellular toxicities of candidate compounds. Molecular assays that isolate individual viral functions therefore have been used to evaluate the ability of antiviral compounds to inhibit each individual step in the virus life cycle. Furthermore, animal models for HPV-associated disease are lacking. Despite these challenges, the in vitro, antiviral activity and clinical efficacy of a variety of compounds have been studied. For example, ribavirin, a nucleoside analog with a broad antiviral spectrum, has been used in clinical trials for the treatment of laryngeal papillomatosis.[117] Cidofovir, a newly licensed antiviral compound to treat serious disease due to cytomegalovirus, also is being studied in patients with HPV-associated genital papillomas and RRP. In addition, novel strategies such as antisense oligonucleotides and therapeutic DNA vaccines may be investigated in the near future.

PREVENTION

Prevention of HPV infection and disease involves two potential approaches: behavioral strategies and vaccines. Prevention of genital HPV infection includes the use of barrier methods, such as condoms, to reduce transmission between sexual partners. Hospital infection control policies should address the potential transmissibility of HPV from patient to health care workers during laser vaporization and electrocautery therapy. Care should be taken to wear protective mask and eye wear and to use appropriate and well-functioning suction devices during these procedures.

There appears to be substantial medical and industry interest in the development of prophylactic vaccines to prevent HPV infection and therapeutic vaccines to treat HPV-associated disease; however, several challenges for the design of HPV vaccines exist. For example, a successful vaccine probably would need to induce broad-spectrum immunity that covers all HPV types. Studies of the immunogenicity and efficacy of new HPV vaccines should appraise whether natural HPV infection induces strong and lasting systemic or local immunity to reinfection. There also are few suitable animal models for HPV vaccine studies and none for cervical cancer, which is the main impetus for vaccine development. Finally, HPV infection and disease primarily are confined to the epithelial surface. Therefore, a successful vaccine probably should be able to induce protective secretory IgA, especially in the genital tract.

Despite these challenges, vaccines suitable for prophylaxis are in the research and developmental stages. Most efforts to produce an HPV vaccine have focused on L1, the major capsid protein and primary constituent of the surface of the mature HPV particle.[61] Large quantities of conformationally correct viral capsid proteins L1 and L2 have been produced as noninfectious, "virus-like" particles in the baculovirus and vaccinia virus expression systems, and some forms have been shown to induce neutralizing antibodies in animal model systems.[31, 72, 97] Most recently, a novel polynucleotide DNA vaccine that contains DNA encoding the major capsid protein L1 has been developed. It also appears to be a promising vaccine that could protect humans against HPV infection and simplify production of a multivalent vaccine by combining plasmids that encode the capsid proteins of different HPV types.[44] Therapeutic vaccines most likely would need to induce cytotoxic T-cell responses against viral antigens such as the major capsid protein L1 and E6 and E7, the major transforming proteins. These vaccines may be possible in the near future if research and development continue.

References

1. Abramson, A., DiLoreno, T. P., and Steinberg, B.: Is papillomavirus detectable in the plume of laser-treated laryngeal papilloma? Arch. Otolaryngol. Head. Neck. Surg. *116*:604–607, 1990.
2. Adrophy, E.: Papillomaviruses and interferon. Ciba Found. Symp.*120*:221–229, 1986.
3. Alberts, D., Coulthard, S., Meys Kens, F., et al.: Regression of aggressive laryngeal papillomatosis with 13-cis-retinoic acid (Accutane). J. Biol. Response Med. *5*:124–128, 1986.
4. Androphy, E., Dvoretzky, I., and Lowy, D.: X-linked inheritance of epidermodysplasia verruciformis: Genetic and virologic studies of a kindred. Arch. Dermatol. *121*:864–868, 1985.
5. Anonymous: National Cancer Institute Workshop. The 1988 Bethesda System for Reporting Cervical/Vaginal Cytologic Diagnoses: J. A. M. A. *262*:931–940, 1998.
6. Baehr, P., and McDonald, G.: Infections of the esophagus. *In* Surawicz, C., and Owen, R. (eds.): Gastrointestinal and Hepatic Infections. Philadelphia, W. B. Saunders, 1995, pp. 3–33.
7. Barr, B., Benton, C., McLaren, K., et al.: Human papillomavirus infection and skin cancer in renal allograft recipients. Lancet *i*:124–129, 1989.
8. Bashi, S.: Cryotherapy versus podophyllin in the treatment of genital warts. Int. J. Dermatol. *24*:535–536, 1985.
9. Bauer, H., Ting, Y., Greer, C., et al.: Genital human papillomavirus infection in female university students as determined by a PCR-based method. J. A. M. A. *265*:472–477, 1991.
10. Bell, R., Hong, W., Itri, L., et al.: The use of *cis*-retinoic acid in recurrent respiratory papillomatosis of the larynx: A randomized pilot study. Am. J. Otolaryngol. *9*:161–164, 1988.
11. Bennett, R., and Powell, K.: Human papillomaviruses: Associations between laryngeal papillomas and genital warts. Pediatr. Infect. Dis. J. *6*:229–232, 1987.
12. Berger, T., Sawchuk, W., Leonardi, C., et al.: Epidermodysplasia verruciformis associated with human immunodeficiency virus disease. Br. J. Dermatol. *124*:79–83, 1991.
13 Bergeron, C., Barrasso, R., Beaudenon, S., et al.: Human papillomaviruses associated with cervical intraepithelial neoplasia: Great diversity and distinct distribution in low- and high-grade lesions. Am. J. Surg. Pathol. *16*:641–649, 1992.
14. Bergeron, C., Ferenczy, A., and Richart, R.: Underwear: Contamination by human papillomaviruses. Am. J. Obstet. Gynecol. *162*:25–29, 1990.
15. Berkhout, R., Tieben, L., Smits, H., et al.: Nested PCR approach for detection and typing of epidermodysplasia verruciformis–associated human papillomavirus types in cutaneous cancers from renal transplant recipients. J. Clin. Microbiol. *33*:690–695, 1995.
16. Bernard, H., Chan, S., Manos, M., et al.: Identification and assessment of known and novel human papillomaviruses by polymerase chain reaction amplification, restriction fragment length polymorphisms, nucleotide sequence, and phylogenetic algorithms. J. Infect. Dis. *170*:1077–1085, 1994.
17. Billingham, R., and Lewis, F.: Laser versus electrical cautery in the treatment of condylomata acuminata of the anus. Surg. Gynecol. Obstet. *155*:865–867, 1982.
18. Birch, H., and Mankart, H.: Ultrasound for juvenile laryngeal papillomas. Arch. Otolaryngol. *77*:603–608, 1963.
19. Bonnez, W., Da Rin, C., Rose, R., et al.: Evolution of the antibody response to human papillomavirus type 11 (HPV-11) in patients with condyloma acuminatum according to treatment response. J. Med. Virol. *39*:340–344, 1993.
20. Bonnez, W., Da Rin, C., Rose, R., et al.: Use of human papillomavirus type 11 virions in an ELISA to detect specific antibodies in humans with condylomata acuminata. J. Gen. Virol. *72*:1343–1347, 1991.
21. Bonnez, W., Kashima, H., Leventhal, B., et al.: Antibody response to human papillomavirus (HPV) type 11 in children with juvenile-onset recurrent respiratory papillomatosis (RRP). Virology *188*:384–387, 1992.
22. Brandsma, J., Abramson, A., Sciubba, J., et al.: Papillomavirus infection of the nose. *In* Steinberg, B., Brandsma, J., and Taichman, L. (eds.): Papillomaviruses and Cancer Cells. Vol. 5. New York, Cold Spring Harbor Laboratory, 1987, pp. 301–308.
23. Brandsma, J., Steinberg, B., Abramson, A., et al.: Presence of human papillomavirus type 16 related sequences in verrucous carcinoma of the larynx. Cancer Res. *46*:2185–2188, 1986.
24. Bunney, M., Barr, B., McLoren, K., et al.: Human papillomavirus type 5 and skin cancer in renal allograft recipients. Lancet *ii*:151–152, 1987.
25. Carter, J., Hagenensee, M., Taflin, M., et al.: HPV-1 capsids expressed in vitro detect human serum antibodies associated with foot warts. Virology *195*:456–462, 1993.
26. Cason, J., Kaye, J., Jewers, R., et al.: Perinatal infection and persistence of human papillomavirus types 16 and 18 in infants. J. Med. Virol. *47*:209–218, 1995.
27. Caussy, D., Orr, W., Daya, A., et al.: Evaluation of methods for detecting human papillomavirus deoxyribonucleotide sequences in clinical specimens. J. Clin. Microbiol. *26*:236–243, 1988.
28. Chang, F., Syrjanen, S., Wang, L., et al.: Infectious agents in the etiology of esophageal cancer. Gastroenterology *103*:1336–1348, 1992.
29. Chen, S., Tsao, Y., Lee, J., et al.: Characterization and analysis of human papillomaviruses of skin warts. Arch. Dermatol. Res. *285*:460–465, 1993.
30. Chen-Yang, S., Ho, M., Chang, S., et al.: High rate of concurrent genital infections with human cytomegalovirus and human papillomaviruses in cervical cancer patients. J. Infect. Dis. *168*:449–452, 1993.
31. Christensen, N., Hopful, R., DiAngelo, S., et al.: Assembled baculovirus-expressed human papillomavirus type 11 L1 capsid protein virus-like particles are recognized by neutralizing monoclonal antibodies and induce high titers of neutralizing antibodies. J. Gen. Virol. *75*:2271–2276, 1994.
32. Christensen, N., Krieder, J., Cladel, N., et al.: Immunological cross-reactivity to laboratory-produced HPV-11 virions of polysera raised against bacterially derived fusion proteins and synthetic peptides of HPV-6b and HPV-16 capsid proteins. Virology *175*:1–9, 1990.
33. Christensen, N., Kreider, J., Shah, K., et al.: Detection of human serum antibodies that neutralize infectious human papillomavirus type 11 virions. J. Gen. Virol. *73*:1261–1267, 1992.
34. Christian, C., Reddel, R., Gerwin, B., et al.: Infection of cultured human cells of respiratory tract origin with human papillomavirus type 1. *In* Steinberg, B., Brandsma, J., and Taichman, L. (eds.): Papillomaviruses and Cancer Cells. Vol. 5. New York, Cold Spring Harbor Laboratory, 1987, pp. 165–179.
35. Ciuffo, G.: Innesto positivo con filtrato di verruca vulgare. G. Ital. Mal. Venereol. *48*:12–17, 1907.
36. Clark, R., Brandon, W., Dumestre, J., et al.: Clinical manifestations of infection with the human immunodeficiency virus in women in Louisiana. Clin. Infect. Dis. *17*:165–172, 1993.
37. Cohen, S., Seltzer, S., Geller, K., et al.: Papilloma of the larynx and tracheobronchial tree in children: A retrospective study. Ann. Otol. Rhinol. Laryngol. *89*:497–503, 1980.
38. Cook, T., Cohn, A., Brunschwig, J., et al.: Laryngeal papilloma: Etiologic and therapeutic considerations. Ann. Otol. Rhinol. Laryngol. *82*:649–655, 1973.
39. Cooper, K., Androphy, E., Lowy, D., et al.: Antigen presentation and T-cell activation in epidermodysplasia verruciformis. J. Invest. Dermatol. *94*:769–776, 1990.
40. Davis, A., and Emans, S.: Human papillomavirus infection in the pediatric and adolescent patient. J. Pediatr. *115*:1–9, 1989.
41. de Peuter, M., De Clercq, B., Minette, A., et al.: An epidemiologic survey of virus warts of the hands among butchers. Br. J. Dermatol. *96*:427–431, 1977.
42. de Villiers, E., Weidauer, H., Otto, H., et al.: Papillomavirus DNA in human carcinomas. Int. J. Cancer *36*:575–578, 1985.
43. Deau, M., Favre, M., and Orth, G.: Genetic heterogeneity among papillomaviruses (HPV) associated with epidermodysplasia verruciformis: Evidence for multiple allelic forms of HPV 5 and HPV 8 E6 genes. Virology *184*:492–503, 1991.
44. Donelly, J., Martinez, D., Jansen, K., et al.: Protection against papillomavirus with a polynucleotide vaccine. J. Infect. Dis. *713*:314–320, 1996.
45. Drut, R., Gomez, M. A., Drut, R. M., et al.: Human papillomavirus (HPV)-associated neonatal giant cell hepatitis (NGCH). Pediatr. Pathol. Lab. Med. *16*:403–412, 1996.
46. Eicher, S., Taylor-Cooley, L., and Donovan, D.: Isotretinoid therapy for recurrent respiratory papillomatosis. Arch. Otolaryngol. Head Neck Surg. *120*:405–409, 1994.
47. Eron, J., Judson, F., Tucker, S., et al.: Interferon therapy for condyloma acuminatum. N. Engl. J. Med. *315*:1059–1064, 1986.
48. Euvrard, S., Chardonnet, Y., Pouteil-Noble, C., et al.: Association of skin malignancies with various and multiple carcinogenic and noncarcino-

genic human papillomaviruses in renal transplant recipients. Cancer *72*:2198–2206, 1993.
49. Eversole, L., Laipis, P., and Green, T.: Human papillomavirus type 2 DNA in oral and labial verruca vulgaris. J. Cutan. Pathol. *14*:319–325, 1987.
50. Favre, M., Obalek, S., Jablonska, S., et al.: Human papillomavirus type 49: A type isolated from flat warts of renal transplant patients. J. Virol. *63*:4909–4914, 1989.
51. Ferenczy, A.: Comparison of 5-fluorouracil and CO_2 laser for treatment of vaginal condylomata. Obstet. Gynecol. *64*:773–778, 1984.
52. Ferenczy, A.: HPV-associated lesions in pregnancy and their clinical implications. Clin. Obstet. Gynecol. *32*:191–199, 1989.
53. Ferenczy, A., Bergeron, C., and Richard, R.: Human papillomavirus DNA in CO_2-laser-generated plume of smoke and its consequences to surgeon. Obstet. Gynecol. *75*:114–118, 1990.
54. Ferenczy, A., Bergeron, C., and Richard, R.: Human papillomavirus DNA in fomites on objects used for the management of patients with genital human papillomavirus infections. Obstet. Gynecol. *74*:950–954, 1989.
55. Ferenczy, A., Mitae, M., Nagai, N., et al.: Latent papillomavirus and recurring genital warts. N. Engl. J. Med. *313*:784–788, 1985.
56. Firzlaff, J., Kiviat, N., Beckman, A., et al.: Detection of human papillomavirus capsid antigens in various squamous epithelial lesions using antibodies directed against the L1 and L2 open reading frames. Virology *164*:476–477, 1988.
57. Franchesci, S., Doll, R., Gallwey, J., et al.: Genital warts and cervical neoplasm: An epidemiological study. Br. J. Cancer *48*:621–628, 1983.
58. Friedman-Kien, A., Eron, L., Conant, M., et al.: Natural interferon alfa for treatment of condyloma acuminatum. J. A. M. A. *259*:533–538, 1988.
59. Gabriel, C., and Thin, R.: Treatment of anogenital warts: Comparison of trichloracetic acid and podophyllin versus podophyllin alone. Br. J. Vener. Dis. *59*:124–126, 1983.
60. Gall, S., Hughes, C., and Trofatter, K.: Interferon for the therapy of condyloma acuminatum. Am. J. Obstet. Gynecol. *153*:157–163, 1985.
61. Galloway, D.: Human papillomavirus vaccines: A warty problem. Infect. Agents Dis. *3*:187–193, 1994.
62. Garden, J., Banion, M., Schelnitz, L., et al.: Papillomavirus in the vapor of carbon dioxide laser-treated verrucae. J. A. M. A. *259*:1199–1202, 1988.
63. Gaylis, B., and Hayden, R.: Recurrent respiratory papillomatosis: Progression to invasion and malignancy. Am. J. Otolaryngol. *12*:104–112, 1991.
64. Ghim, S., Jenson, A., and Schlegel, R.: HPV-1 L1 protein expressed in cos cells displays conformational epitopes found on intact virions. Virology *190*:548–552, 1992.
65. Glinski, W., Obalek, S., Jablonska, S., et al.: T cell defect in patients with epidermodysplasia verruciformis due to human papillomavirus type 3 and 5. Dermatologica *162*:141–147, 1981.
66. Graham, S., Priore, R., Graham, M., et al.: Genital cancer in wives of penile cancer patients. Cancer *44*:1870–1874, 1979.
67. Greer, C., Wheeler, C., Ladner, M., et al.: Human papillomavirus (HPV) type distribution and serological response to HPV type 6 virus-like particles in patients with genital warts. J. Clin. Microbiol. *33*:2058–2063, 1995.
68. Gross, G., Ellinger, K., Roussaki, A., et al.: Epidermodysplasia verruciformis in a patient with Hodgkin's disease: Characterization of a new papillomavirus type and interferon treatment. J. Invest. Dermatol. *91*:43–48, 1988.
69. Guerrero, E., Daniel, R., Bosch, F., et al.: Comparison of ViraPap, Southern hybridization, and polymerase chain reaction methods for human papillomavirus identification in an epidemiological investigation of cervical cancer. J. Clin. Microbiol. *30*:2951–2959, 1992.
70. Gutman, L., St. Claire, K., Everett, V., et al.: Cervical-vaginal and intraanal human papillomavirus infection of young girls with external genital warts. J. Infect. Dis. *170*:339–344, 1994.
71. Gutman, L., St. Claire, K., Herman-Giddens, M., et al.: Evaluation of sexually abused and nonabused young girls for intravaginal human papillomavirus infection. Am. J. Dis. Child. *146*:694–699, 1992.
72. Hagensee, M., Olson, N., Baker, T., et al.: Three-dimensional structure of vaccinia-virus–produced human papillomavirus type 1 capsids. J. Virol. *68*:4503–4505, 1994.
73. Haglund, S., Lundquist, P., Cantell, K., et al.: Interferon therapy in juvenile laryngeal papillomatosis. Arch. Otolaryngol. Head Neck Surg. *107*:327–332, 1981.
74. Healy, G., Gelber, R., Trowbridge, A., et al.: Treatment of recurrent respiratory papillomatosis with human leukocyte interferon. N. Engl. J. Med. *319*:401–407, 1988.
75. Hildesheim, A., Schiffman, M., Gravitt, P., et al.: Persistence of type-specific human papillomavirus infection among cytologically normal women in Portland, Oregon. J. Infect. Dis. *169*:235–240, 1994.
76. Horn, J., McQuillan, G., Shah, K., et al.: Genital human papillomavirus infections in patients attending an inner-city STD clinic. Sex. Transm. Dis. *18*:183–187, 1991.
77. Jablonska, S., Biczysko, W., Jakubowicz, K., et al.: The ultrastructure of transitional status to Bowen's disease and invasive Bowen's carcinoma in epidermodysplasia verruciformis. Dermatologica *140*:186–194, 1970.
78. Jamison, J., Kaplan, D., Hamman, R., et al.: Spectrum of genital human papillomavirus infection in a female adolescent population. Sex. Transm. Dis. *22*:236–243, 1995.
79. Jenison, S., Xiu-ping, Y., Valentine, J., et al.: Evidence of prevalent genital-type human papillomavirus infections in adults and children. J. Infect. Dis. *162*:60–69, 1990.
80. Jenison, S., Yu, X., Valentin, J., et al.: Human antibodies react with an epitope of the human papillomavirus type 6b L1 open reading frame which is distinct from the type-common epitope. J. Virol. *63*:809–818, 1989.
81. Jennings, L., Ross, A., and Faoagali, J.: The prevalence of warts on the hands of workers in a New Zealand slaughterhouse. N. Z. Med. J. *97*:473–476, 1984.
82. Jensen, S.: Comparison of podophyllin application with simple surgical excision in clearance and recurrence of perianal condylomata acuminata. Lancet *2*:1146–1148, 1985.
83. Kaye, J., Cason, J., Pakarian, F., et al.: Viral load as a determinant for transmission of human papillomavirus type 16 from mother to infant. J. Med. Virol. *44*:415–421, 1994.
84. Kellogg, N., and Parra, J.: The progression of human papillomavirus lesions in sexual assault victims. Pediatrics *96*:1163–1167, 1995.
85. Kiviat, N., Koutsky, L., Paavonen, J., et al.: Prevalence of genital papillomavirus infection among women attending a college student health clinic or a sexually transmitted disease clinic. J. Infect. Dis. *159*:293–302, 1989.
86. Kjaer, S., Dahl, C., Engholm, G., et al.: Case-control study of risk factors for cervical neoplasia in Denmark: Role of sexual activity, reproductive factors, and venereal infections. Cancer Causes Control *3*:339–348, 1992.
87. Krebs, H. B.: Treatment of vaginal condylomata acuminata by weekly topical application of 5-fluorouracil. Obstet. Gynecol. *70*:68–71, 1987.
88. Kreider, J. W., Howett, M. K., Gill, N. L., et al.: In vivo transformation of human skin with human papillomavirus type 11 from condylomata acuminata. J. Virol. *59*:369, 1986.
89. Kreider, J., Howett, M., Leure-Dupree, A., et al.: Laboratory production in vivo of infectious human papillomavirus type 11. J. Virol. *61*:590–593, 1987.
90. Krogh, G.: Genitoanal papillomavirus infection: Diagnostic and therapeutic objectives in the light of current epidemiological observations. Int. J. STD AIDS *2*:391–404, 1991.
91. Kuypers, J., and Kiviat, N.: Anal papillomavirus infections. *In* Surawicz, C., and Owen, R. (eds.): Gastrointestinal and Hepatic Infections. Philadelphia, W. B. Saunders, 1995, pp. 279–285.
92. Labropoulou, V., Diakomanolis, E., Dailianas, S., et al.: Genital papillomavirus in Greek women with high-grade cervical intraepithelial neoplasia and cervical carcinoma. J. Med. Virol. *48*:80–87, 1996.
93. Lass, J., Grove, A., Papale, J., et al.: Detection of human papillomavirus DNA sequences in conjunctival papilloma. Am. J. Ophthalmol. *96*:670–674, 1983.
94. Le Cann, P., Touze, A., Enogat, N., et al.: Detection of antibodies against human papillomavirus (HPV) type 16 virions by enzyme-linked immunosorbent assay using recombinant HPV L1 capsids produced by recombinant baculovirus. J. Clin. Microbiol. *33*:1380–1382, 1995.
95. Leventhal, B., Kashima, H., Mounts, P., et al.: Long-term response of recurrent respiratory papillomatosis to treatment with lymphoblastoid interferon alfa-n1. N. Engl. J. Med. *325*:613–617, 1991.
96. Leventhal, B., Kashima, H., Weck, P., et al.: Randomized surgical adjuvant trial of alfa-n1 in recurrent papillomatosis. Arch. Otolaryngol. Head Neck Surg. *114*:1163–1169, 1988.
97. Lin, Y., Borenstein, L., Ahmed, R., et al.: Cottontail rabbit papillomavirus L1 protein-based vaccines: Protection is achieved only with a full-length, nondenatured product. J. Virol. *678*:4154–4162, 1993.
98. Lippman, S., and Meyskens, F.: Treatment of advanced squamous cell carcinoma of the skin with isotretinoin. Ann. Intern. Med. *107*:499–501, 1987.
99. Lippman, S., Kessler, J., Al-Sarraf, M., et al.: Treatment of advanced squamous cell carcinoma of the head and neck with isotretinoin: A phase II randomized trial. Invest. New Drugs *6*:51–56, 1988.
100. Long, G., and Rickman, L.: Infectious complications of tattoos. Clin. Infect. Dis. *18*:610–619, 1994.
101. Lorincz, A. T., Reid, R., Jenson, B., et al.: Human papillomavirus infection of the cervix: Relative risk associations of 15 common anogenital types. Obstet. Gynecol. *79*:328–337, 1992.
102. Lorincz, A., Schiffman, M., Jaffurs, W., et al.: Temporal associations of human papillomavirus infection with cervical cytological abnormalities. Am. J. Obstet. Gynecol. *162*:645–651, 1990.
103. Lutzner, M., Orth, G., Dutranquay, V., et al.: Detection of human papillomavirus type 5 DNA in skin cancers of an immunosuppressed renal allograft recipient. Lancet *ii*:422–424, 1983.
104. Lyons, G., Schlosser, J., Lousteau, R., et al.: Laser surgery and immunotherapy in the management of laryngeal papilloma. Laryngoscope *88*:1586–1588, 1978.
105. Madreperla, S., Green, W., Daniel, R., et al.: Human papillomavirus in primary epithelial tumors of the lacrimal sac. Ophthalmology *100*:569–573, 1993.
106. Maitland, N., Cox, M., Lynas, C., et al.: Detection of human papillomavirus DNA in biopsies of human oral tissue. Br. J. Cancer *56*:245–250, 1987.
107. Majewski, S., and Jabloska, S.: Epidermodysplasia verruciformis as a model of human papillomavirus-induced genetic cancer of the skin. Arch. Dermatol. *131*:1312–1318, 1995.
108. Majewski, S., and Jablonska, S.: Epidermodysplasia verruciformis: Immu-

nological and clinical aspects. Curr. Topics Microbiol. Immunol. *186*:157–175, 1994.
109. Majewski, S., Malejczyk, J., Jablonska, S., et al.: Natural cell-mediated cytotoxicity against various target cells in patients with epidermodysplasia verruciformis. J. Am. Acad. Dermatol. *22*:423–427, 1990.
110. Majewski, S., Skopinska-Rozewska, E., Jablonska, S., et al.: Partial detects of cell-mediated immunity in patients with epidermodysplasia verruciformis. J. Am. Acad. Dermatol. *15*:966–973, 1986.
111. Majoros, M., Parkhill, E., and Devine, K.: Papillomas of the larynx in children: A clinicopathologic study. Am. J. Surg. *108*:470–475, 1964.
112. Manos, M., Ting, Y., Wright, D., et al.: The use of polymerase chain reaction amplification for the detection of genital human papillomaviruses. Cancer Cells *7*:209–214, 1989.
113. Marres, E., Wentges, R., and Brinkman, W.: Cryosurgical treatment of juvenile laryngeal papillomatosis. Laryngoscope *76*:1979–1983, 1966.
114. Marth, C., Daxenbichler, G., and Dapunt, O.: Synergistic antiproliferative effect of human recombinant interferons and retinoic acid in cultured breast cancer cells. J. Natl. Cancer Inst. *77*:1197–1202, 1986.
115. McDonnell, J., Mayr, A., and Martin, W.: DNA of human papillomavirus type 16 in dysplastic and malignant lesions of the conjunctiva and cornea. N. Engl. J. Med. *320*:1442–1446, 1989.
116. McDonnell, P., McDonnell, J., Kessis, T., et al.: Detection of human papillomavirus type 6/11 DNA in conjunctival papillomas by in situ hybridization with radioactive probes. Hum. Pathol. *18*:1115–1119, 1987.
117. McGlennen, R., Adams, G., Lewis, C., et al.: Pilot trial of ribavirin for the treatment of laryngeal papillomatosis. Head Neck *15*:504–513, 1993.
118. Melkert, P., Hopman, E., van der Brule, A., et al.: Prevalence of HPV in cytomorphologically normal cervical smears, as determined by the polymerase chain reaction, is age-dependent. Int. J. Cancer. *53*:919–923, 1993.
119. Miller, D., Brodell, R., and Levine, M.: The conjunctival wart: Report of a case and review of treatment options. Ophthal Surg. *25*:545–548, 1994.
120. Morrison, E.: Natural history of cervical infection with human papillomaviruses. Clin. Infect. Dis. *18*:172–180, 1994.
121. Moscicki, A., Palefsky, J., Gonzales, J., et al.: The association between human papillomavirus deoxyribonucleic acid status and the results of cytologic rescreening tests in young, sexually active women. Am. J. Obstet. Gynecol. *165*:67–71, 1991.
122. Moscicki, A., Palesfsky, J., Smith, G., et al.: Colposcopic and histologic findings and human papillomavirus (HPV) DNA test variability in young women positive for HPV DNA. J. Infect. Dis. *166*:951–957, 1992.
123. Mounts, P., and Kashima, H.: Associated of human papillomavirus subtype and clinical course in respiratory papillomatosis. Laryngoscope *94*:28–33, 1984.
124. Mounts, P., Sha, K. V., and Kashima, H.: Viral etiology of juvenile- and adult-onset squamous papilloma of the larynx. Proc. Natl. Acad. Sci. U. S. A. *79*:5425–5429, 1982.
125. Naghashfar, Z., Sawada, E., Kutcher, M., et al.: Identification of genital tract papillomaviruses HPV-6 and HPV-16 in warts of the oral cavity. J. Med. Virol. *17*:313–324, 1985.
126. Nahhas, W., Marshall, M., Ponziani, J., et al.: Evaluation of urinary cytology of male sexual partners of women with cervical intraepithelial neoplasia and human papillomavirus infection. Gynecol. Oncol. *24*:279, 1985.
127. Noffsinger, A., Witte, D., and Fenoglio-Preiser, C. M.: The relationship of human papillomaviruses to anorectal neoplasia. Cancer *70*:1276–1287, 1992.
128. Nuovo, G., and Pedemonte, B.: Human papillomavirus types and recurrent cervical warts. J. A. M. A.. *263*:1223–1226, 1990.
129. Nuovo, G., and Richart, R.: A comparison of slot blot, Southern blot, and in situ hybridization analyses for human papillomavirus DNA in genital tract lesions. Obstet. Gynecol. *74*:673–678, 1989.
130. Obalek, S., Favre, M., Szymanczyk, J., et al.: Human papillomavirus (HPV) types specific of epidermolysis verruciformis detected in warts induced by HPV3 or HPV3-related types in immunosuppressed patients. J. Invest. Dermatol. *98*:936–941, 1992.
131. Ong, C., Bernard, H., and Villa, L.: Identification and genomic sequences of three novel human papillomavirus sequences in cervical smears of Amazonian Indians. J. Infect. Dis. *170*:1086–1088, 1994.
132. Oraetiruys-Clausen, F.: Rare oral viral disorder (molluscum contagiosum, localized keratoacanthoma, verrucae, condyloma acuminatum, and focal epithelial hyperplasia). Oral Surg. Oral Med. Oral Pathol. *34*:604–618, 1972.
133. Orlow, S. J., and Paller, A.: Cimetidine therapy for multiple viral warts in children. J. Am. Acad. Dermatol. *28*:794–796, 1993.
134. Ostrow, R., Bender, M., Nhmura, M., et al.: Human papillomavirus DNA in cutaneous primary and metastasized squamous cell carcinomas from patients with epidermodysplasia verruciformis. Proc. Natl. Acad. Sci. U. S. A. *87*:8170–8174, 1990.
135. Pakarian, F., Kaye, J., Cason, J., et al.: Cancer associated human papillomaviruses: Perinatal transmission and persistence. Br. J. Obstet. Gynaecol. *101*:514–517, 1994.
136. Pappo, O., Yunis, E., Jordan, J., et al.: Recurrent and de novo giant cell hepatitis after orthotopic liver transplantation. Am. J. Surg. Pathol. *18*:804–813, 1994.
137. Pastner, B., Baker, D., and Jackman, E.: Human papillomavirus. *In* Gonik, B. (ed.): Viral Diseases in Pregnancy. New York, Springer-Verlag, 1994, pp. 185–195.
138. Peyton, C., Jansen, A., Wheeler, C., et al.: A novel human papillomavirus sequence from an international cervical cancer study. J. Infect. Dis. *170*:1093–1095, 1994.
139. Peyton, C., and Wheeler, C.: Identification of five novel human papillomavirus sequences in the New Mexico triethnic population. J. Infect. Dis. *170*:1089–1092, 1994.
140. Pfister, H.: Biology and biochemistry of papillomaviruses. Rev. Physiol. Biochem. Pharmacol. *99*:111–181, 1984.
141. Pfister, H., Iftner, T., and Fuchs, P.: Papillomaviruses from epidermodysplasia verruciformis patients and renal allograft recipients. *In* Howley, P. M., and Broker, T. R. (eds.): Papillomaviruses: Molecular and Clinical Aspects. Proceedings of the Burroughs-Wellcome-UCLA Symposium held in Steamboat Springs, Colorado, April 8–14, 1985. New York, Liss, 1985, pp. 85–100.
142. Pfister, H., and zur Hausen, H.: Seroepidemiological studies of human papillomavirus (HPV-1) infections. Int. J. Cancer *21*:161–165, 1978.
143. Phelps, W., and Alexander, K.: Antiviral therapy for human papillomaviruses: Rationale and prospects. Ann. Intern. Med. *123*:368–382, 1995.
144. Prose, N., von Knegel-Doeberitz, C., Miller, S., et al.: Widespread flat warts associated with human papillomavirus type 5: A cutaneous manifestation of human immunodeficiency virus infection. J. Am. Acad. Dermatol. *23*:978–981, 1990.
145. Quick, C., Watts, S., Krzyzek, R., et al.: Relationship between condylomata and laryngeal papillomata: Clinical and molecular virological evidence. Ann. Otol. Rhinol. Laryngol. *89*:467–471, 1980.
146. Reeves, W., Rawls, W., and Brinton, L.: Epidemiology of genital papillomaviruses and cervical cancer. Rev. Infect. Dis. *11*:426–439, 1989.
147. Reeves, W., Brinton, L., Garcia, M., et al.: Human papillomavirus infection and cervical cancer in Latin America. N. Engl. J. Med. *320*:1437–1441, 1989.
148. Reeves, W., Arosemena, J., Garcia, M., et al.: Genital human papillomavirus infection in Panama City prostitutes. J. Infect. Dis. *160*:599–603, 1989.
149. Reichman, R., Oakes, D., Bonnez, W., et al.: Treatment of condyloma acuminatum with three different interferons administered intralesionally: A double-blind, placebo-controlled trial. Ann. Intern. Med. *108*:675–679, 1988.
150. Reid, R.: Superficial laser vulvectomy. I. The efficacy of extended superficial ablation for refractory and very extensive condylomas. Am. J. Obstet. Gynecol. *151*:1047–1052, 1985.
151. Repucci, A., DiLorenzo, T., Abramson, A., et al.: In vitro modulation of human laryngeal papilloma cell differentiated by retinoic acid. Otolaryngol. Head Neck Surg. *105*:528–532, 1991.
152. Respler, D. A., Jahn, A., Pater, A., et al.: Isolation and characterization of papillomavirus DNA from nasal inverting papilloma. Ann. Otol. Rhinol. Laryngol. *96*:107–173, 1987.
153. Rose, R., Bonnez, W., Reichman, R., et al.: Expression of human papillomavirus type 11 L1 protein in insect cells: In vivo and in vitro assembly of virus-like particles. J. Virol. *67*:1936–1944, 1993.
154. Rosenfeld, W., Rose, E., Vermund, S., et al.: Follow-up evaluation of cervicovaginal human papillomavirus infection in adolescents. J. Pediatr. *121*:307–311, 1992.
155. Rowson, K., and Mahy, B.: Human papova (wart) virus. Bacteriol. Rev. *31*:110–131, 1967.
156. Roye, C.: Abnormal cervical cytology in adolescents: A literature review. J. Adolesc. Health *13*:643–650, 1992.
157. Rudlinger, R., Bunney, M., Grob, R., et al.: Warts in fish handlers. Br. J. Dermatol. *120*:375–380, 1989.
158. Rudinger, R., and Grob, R.: Papillomavirus infection and skin cancer in renal allograft recipients. Lancet *ii*:1132–1133, 1989.
159. Rudinger, R., Smith, J., Bunney, M., et al.: Human papillomavirus infections in a group of renal transplant recipients. Br. J. Dermatol. *115*:681–692, 1986.
160. Sawchuk, W., Weber, P., Lowy, D., et al.: Infectious papillomavirus in the vapor of warts treated with carbon dioxide laser or electrocoagulation: Detection and protection. J. Am. Acad. Dermatol. *21*:41–29, 1989.
161. Sawchuk, W., and Felton, R.: Infectious potential of aerosolized particles. Arch. Dermatol. *125*:1689–1692, 1989.
162. Schiffman, M.: Recent progress in defining the epidemiology of human papillomavirus infection and cervical neoplasia. J. Natl. Cancer. Inst. *84*:394–398, 1992.
163. Schiffman, M., Kiviat, N., Burk, R., et al.: Accuracy and interlaboratory reliability of human papillomavirus DNA testing for hybrid capture. J. Clin. Microbiol. *33*:545–550, 1995.
164. Schnadig, V., Clark, W., Clegg, T., et al.: Invasive papillomatosis and squamous carcinoma complicating juvenile laryngeal papillomatosis. Arch. Otolaryngol. Head Neck Surg. *112*:966–971, 1986.
165. Schneider, A., Kirchoff, T., Meinhardt, G., et al.: Repeated evaluation of human papillomavirus 16 status in cervical swabs of young women with a history of normal papanicolaou smears. Obstet. Gynecol. *79*:683–693, 1992.
166. Schonfeld, A., Nitke, S., Schattner, A., et al.: Intramuscular human interferon-beta injections in treatment of condylomata acuminata. Lancet *1*:1038–1042, 1984.

167. Schuster, D.: Snorter's warts. Arch. Dermatol. *132*:571, 1987.
168. Scinicariello, F., Sato, T., Lee, C. S., et al.: Detection of human papillomavirus in primary hepatocellular carcinoma. Anticancer Res. *16*:763–766, 1992.
169. Shah, K., and Howley, P.: Papillomaviruses. *In* Fields, B., Knipe, D., and Howley, P. (eds.): Virology. Philadelphia, Lippincott-Raven, 1996, pp. 2077–2109.
170. Shah, K., Kashima, H., Polk, B., et al.: Rarity of cesarean delivery in cases of juvenile-onset respiratory papillomatosis. Obstet. Gynecol. *68*:795–799, 1986.
171. Singleton, G., and Adkins, W.: Cryosurgical treatment of juvenile laryngeal papillomatosis: An eight-year experience. Ann. Otol. Rhinol. Laryngol. *81*:784–790, 1972.
172. Slawsky, L., Gilson, R., Hockley, A., et al.: Epidermodysplasia verruciformis associated with severe immunodeficiency, lymphoma, and disseminated molluscum contagiosum. J. Am. Acad. Dermatol. *27*:448–450, 1992.
173. Solomon, D., Smith, R., Kashima, H., et al.: Malignant transformation in non-irradiated recurrent respiratory papillomatosis. Laryngoscope *95*:900–904, 1985.
174. Sperry, K.: Lethal asphyxiating juvenile laryngeal papillomatosis. Am. J. Foren. Med. Pathol. *15*:146–150, 1994.
175. St. Louis, M., Icenogle, J., Manzila, T., et al.: Genital types of papillomavirus in children of women with HIV-1 infection in Kinshasa, Zaire. Int. J. Cancer *54*:181–184, 1993.
176. Stark, L., Arends, M., McLaren, K., et al.: Prevalence of human papillomavirus DNA in cutaneous neoplasms from renal allograft recipients supports a possible viral role in tumour promotion. Br. J. Dermatol. *69*:222–229, 1994.
177. Steele, J., and Gallimore, P.: Humoral assays of human sera to disrupted and nondisrupted epitopes of human papillomavirus type 1. Virology *174*:388–398, 1990.
178. Steger, G., Olszewsky, M., Stockfleth, E., et al.: Prevalence of antibodies to human papillomavirus type 8 in human sera. J. Virol. *64*:4399–4405, 1990.
179. Steinberg, B., Topp, W., Schneider, P. S., et al.: Laryngeal papillomavirus infection during clinical remission. N. Engl. J. Med. *308*:1261–1264, 1983.
180. Stellato, G., Nieminen, P., Aho, H., et al.: Human papillomavirus infection of the female genital tract: Correlation of HPV DNA with cytologic, colposcopic, and natural history findings. Eur. J. Gynaecol. Oncol. *13*:262–267, 1994.
181. Strong, M., Vaughan, C., Cooperband, S., et al.: Recurrent respiratory papillomatosis: Management with the CO_2 laser. Ann. Otol. Rhinol. Laryngol. *85*:508–516, 1976.
182. Sun, Y., Eluf-Neto, J., Bosch, F., et al.: Human papillomavirus (HPV)-related serologic markers of invasive cervical carcinoma in Brazil. Cancer Epidemiol. Biomarkers Pres. *3*:341–374, 1994.
183. Syrjanen, S.: Human papillomavirus infections in the oral cavity. *In* Syrjanen, K., Gissmann, L., and Koss, L. (eds.): Papillomaviruses and Human Disease. New York, Springer-Verlag, 1987, pp. 104–137.
184. Syrjanen, K., Hakama, M., Saarikoski, S., et al.: Prevalence, incidence, and estimated life-time risk of cervical human papillomavirus infections in a nonselected Finnish female population. Sex. Transm. Dis. *17*:15–32, 1990.
185. Syrjanen, S., Paranen, P., Mantyjarvi, R., et al.: Sensitivity of in situ hybridization techniques using biotin- and ^{35}S-labeled human papillomavirus (HPV) DNA probes. J. Virol. Methods *19*:225–238, 1988.
186. Taylor, S.: A prevalence study of warts on the hands in a poultry processing and packing station. J. Soc. Occup. Med. *30*:20–23, 1980.
187. Tieben, L., Berkhout, R., Smits, H., et al.: Detection of epidermodysplasia verruciformis-like human papillomavirus types in malignant and premalignant skin lesions of renal transplant recipients. Br. J. Dermatol. *131*:226–230, 1994.
188. Trottier, A., Provencher, D., Mes-Masson, A., et al.: Absence of human papillomavirus sequences in ovarian pathologies. J. Clin. Microbiol. *33*:1011–1013, 1995.
189. Ushikai, M., Fujiyoshi, T., Kono, M., et al.: Detection and cloning of human papillomavirus DNA associated with recurrent respiratory papillomatosis in Thailand. Jpn. J. Cancer Res. *85*:699–703, 1994.
190. van den Brule, A., Walboomers, J., du Maine, M., et al.: Difference in prevalence of human papillomavirus genotypes in cytomorphologically normal cervical smears is associated with a history of cervical intraepithelial neoplasia. Int. J. Cancer *48*:404–408, 1991.
191. Van der Leest, R., Zachow, K., Ostrow, R., et al.: Human papillomavirus heterogeneity in 36 renal transplant recipients. Arch. Dermatol. *123*:354–357, 1987.
192. Vernon, S., Holmes, K., and Reeves, W.: Human papillomavirus infection and associated disease in persons infected with human immunodeficiency virus. Clin. Infect. Dis. *21*:S121–S124, 1995.
193. Viac, J., Chomel, J., Chardonnet, Y., et al.: Incidence of antibodies to human papillomavirus type 1 in patients with cutaneous and mucosal papillomas. J. Med. Virol. *31*:18–21, 1990.
194. ViraPap and ViraType HPV DNA typing kit manuals and product information. Gaithersburg, Life Technologies, Bethesda Research Laboratories, 1989.
195. von Krogh, G.: Clinical relevance and evaluation of genitoanal papilloma virus infection in the male. Semin. Dermatol. *11*:229–240, 1992.
196. Vossler, J., Forbes, B., and Adelson, M.: Evaluation of the polymerase chain reaction for the detection of human papillomavirus from urine. J. Med. Virol. *45*:354–360, 1995.
197. Vousden, K.: Mechanisms of transformation by HPV. *In* Stern, P., and Stanley, M. (eds.): Human Papillomaviruses and Cervical Cancer: Biology and Immunology. Oxford, Oxford University Press, 1994, pp. 92–116.
198. Walboomers, J., Husman, A., van den Brule, A., et al.: Detection of genital human papillomavirus infections: Critical review of methods and prevalence studies in relation to cervical cancer. *In* Stern, P., and Stanley, M. (eds.): Human Papillomaviruses and Cervical Cancer: Biology and Immunology. Oxford, Oxford University Press, 1994, pp. 41–71.
199. Ward, P., Parry, G., Yule, R., et al.: Human papillomavirus subtype 16a. Lancet *1*:170, 1989.
200. Wilbur, D., and Stoler, M.: Testing for human papillomavirus: Basic pathobiology of infection, methodologies, and implications for clinical use. Yale J. Biol. Med. *64*:113–125, 1991.
201. Yaegashi, N., Jenison, S., Batra, M., et al.: Human antibodies recognize multiple distinct type-specific and cross-reactive regions of the minor capsid proteins of human papillomavirus types 6 and 11. J. Virol. *66*:2008–2119, 1992.
202. Yaegashi, N., Jenison, S., Valentine, J., et al.: Characterization of murine polyclonal antisera and monoclonal antibodies generated against intact and denatured human papillomavirus type 2 virions. J. Virol. *65*:1578–1583, 1991.
203. Ylitalo, N., Bergstrom, T., and Gyllensten, U.: Detection of genital human papillomavirus by single-tube nested PCR and type-specific oligonucleotide hybridization. J. Clin. Microbiol. *33*:1822–1828, 1995.
204. Young, L., Bevan, I., Johnson, M., et al.: The polymerase chain reaction: A new epidemiological tool for investigating cervical human papillomavirus infection. Br. Med. J. *298*:14–18, 1989.

160

SLOW VIRUSES

William J. Britt

Transmissible diseases with unusually long incubation periods and protracted clinical courses were recognized in domestic animals long before similar diseases were shown to exist in humans. Although the etiologic agents responsible for these uncommon diseases were unknown, many early investigators suspected that conventional infectious agents were inducing the unconventional clinical features unique to these diseases. In 1954, Bjorn Sigurdsson,[313] a veterinary pathologist with a long interest in diseases of sheep, put forth the term *slow viral diseases* and suggested criteria for such diseases: (1) a long initial period of latency measured in months to years, (2) a protracted and progressive clinical course beginning after the onset of clinical symptoms, and (3) limitation of the infection to a single organ system. Other general terms for these diseases have included *transmissible diseases caused by unconventional agents*; however, for purposes of this discussion, we will continue to use the term *slow viral diseases* because this terminology is consistent with the progressive, subacute clinical manifestation of these infections.

Initially, Sigurdsson included only animal diseases, such as scrapie and maedi of sheep and a variety of retrovirus-induced tumors in mice and chicken. Slow viral diseases thus represented a curious group of diseases limited to livestock that held little interest for most physicians. However, in 1959, William Hadlow,[137] a perceptive veterinary pathologist, noted the striking similarity between the clinical and pathologic findings of scrapie in sheep and the degenerative disease of the central nervous system (CNS) of the Fore people in New Guinea known as kuru. Subsequent studies demonstrated the transmissible nature of this disease. Since these early observations, interest in human slow virus diseases has increased greatly, and, in 1976, D. Carleton Gajdusek was awarded the Nobel Prize in Medicine for his pioneering studies in this group of diseases. Research into the pathogenesis of these diseases has continued, with major advances in the etiology of transmissible spongiform encephalopathies being reported in the last several years. Furthermore, previously rare diseases, such as progressive multifocal leukoencephalopathy, have become significantly more frequent with the emergence of AIDS in the developed world. Other slow viral diseases, such as subacute sclerosing panencephalitis (SSPE), continue to represent a major cause of progressive brain disease in developing nations. Thus, this group of unique infectious diseases continues to hold great interest for both the investigator and practitioner.

Many different viruses have been shown to induce persistent infection in humans (Table 160–1). The pathways leading to persistent viral infection are diverse but in general can result from a latent infection with periodic reactivations or can be a chronic, continuously productive infection. Latency can be defined as the maintenance of viral genetic material within viable cells that can reactivate and result in productive replication of virus. The herpesviruses perhaps are the most widely studied viral pathogens that routinely induce latent infections in humans. Detailed studies of herpes simplex virus (HSV) and Epstein-Barr virus clearly have demonstrated that viral genetic material can be maintained for extended periods in vivo and then reactivated after perturbation with pharmacologic or physical agents. The mechanisms associated with the establishment, maintenance, and reactivation of latent infections only are beginning to be unraveled. Most studies suggest a complex interplay between the host cell and the virus, in which host cellular functions limit viral transcription. Expression of latency-associated transcripts in HSV-infected cervical ganglia has been suggested to play a role in the maintenance of latency by repressing expression of essential replicative functions of the virus; however, several studies have failed to demonstrate a direct role of latency-associated transcripts in the maintenance of HSV latency.[296] It is unlikely that herpesvirus DNA integration into the host DNA plays an important role in herpesvirus latency. In contrast, retroviruses insert viral nucleic acid into host DNA as part of their replicative cycle and therefore can link their expression and replication to expression of host genes. Hepatitis B virus also can integrate its DNA into the host-cell genetic material, perhaps contributing to viral persistence after infection with this agent.[40, 308] Although detailed mechanisms associated with most latent viral infections are unknown, it can be argued that latency is advantageous for survival of a virus within an animal species. Latency provides an important means of escape from host immunity by shielding virus-infected cells from the acute phase of antiviral immune responses. Latent infection also permits amplification and repeated spread of infectious virus to adjacent cells during periods of reactivation. Finally, by effectively prolonging the duration of viral shedding, latent infection increases the potential for virus spread within a population.

Chronic productive infection represents a second pathway leading to persistent infection in humans. As with latent infections, a large number of viruses have been shown to induce chronic productive infection (see Table 160–1). Productive infection can persist as the result of failure of the immune system to eliminate the infectious agent, from viral mutations resulting in the loss of antigenicity or decreased virus or viral antigen production, or from host-cell restriction of viral expression. Examples of the inability of the host immune system to eliminate infectious virus include enterovirus infections in children with inherited immunodeficiencies,[80] herpesvirus infection during pharmacologic immunosuppression associated with allograft transplantation,[150] and certain congenital infections.[2] Virus mutations may result in the production of progeny virus that escapes the immune response, such as observed in primate lentivirus infec-

TABLE 160–1. Some Human Viruses Associated with Persistent Infections

Family	Genus	Virus	Persistent Infection in Humans
Papovaviridae	*Polyomavirus*	Simian vacuolating agent (SV40), JC virus	Progressive multifocal leukoencephalopathy
Herpesviridae	*Alphaherpesviridae*	Herpes simplex I, herpes simplex II, varicella-zoster virus	Recurrent oral, genital, and skin eruptions
	Betaherpesviridae	Cytomegalovirus, human herpesvirus 6, human herpesvirus 7	Persistent oral, genital, and urinary tract shedding; congenital infection
	Gammaherpesviridae	Epstein-Barr virus	Persistent nasopharyngeal shedding; persistent infection of B lymphocytes
Togaviridae	*Rubivirus*	Rubella virus	Progressive rubella panencephalitis; congenital rubella syndrome
Paramyxoviridae	*Morbilivirus*	Measles virus	Subacute sclerosing panencephalitis
Rhabdoviridae	*Lyssavirus*	Rabies virus	Encephalitis
Hepadnaviridae		Hepatitis B virus	Hepatitis
Retroviridae	*Lentivirinae*	Human T-cell leukemia virus (1–11); HIV-1, HIV-2	Leukemia; AIDS
Picornaviridae	*Enterovirus*	Poliovirus, echovirus	Chronic meningoencephalitis in immunodeficient children
Flaviridae	*Hepatitis C*	Hepatitis C	Chronic hepatitis

Adapted from Vilcek, J., and Sreevalsan, T.: Fundamentals of virus structure and replication. *In* Galasso, G. J., Merigan, T. C., and Buchanan, R. A. (eds.): Antiviral Agents and Viral Diseases of Man. New York, Raven Press, 1984, pp. 10–11.

tions.[250, 301] The production of defective viral particles may limit the immune clearance of infectious particles or directly inhibit virus production.[92, 164] This latter pathway can predispose to chronic productive infection by providing subthreshold amounts of viral antigen for induction of an immune response. Lastly, alterations in the host-cell response after virus infection through either mutation or differentiation may lead to depressed or restricted virus replication. Restricted viral replication can result in subthreshold levels of viral antigen expression and provide an inadequate stimulus to the immune response. As could be expected, each of these mechanisms of persistent infection offers distinct advantages for continued survival of a virus in the face of host-derived antiviral immune responses. The division of persistent infections into categories of latent and chronic productive is arbitrary; in many cases, viruses utilize both pathways to establish persistent infections.

A characteristic finding of infections resulting from agents associated with slow viral diseases is the restriction of clinical disease and, in most cases, pathologic changes to the CNS. Several characteristics of the CNS appear to predispose it to persistent viral infection. The CNS is a relatively immunologically privileged site, and it is devoid of a functional lymphatic system for removal of antigens and presentation to the systemic immune system. In addition, the blood-brain barrier provided by the tight junctions of the vasculature in the CNS limits the passage of soluble molecules, such as immunoglobulins, as well as lymphoid cells from the systemic immune system into the CNS. Finally, cells of the CNS constitutively express low levels of class I and II major histocompatibility antigens, cell-surface proteins that play a fundamental role in the induction and regulation of immune responses.[12, 96, 150, 203, 225] Although de novo immune responses by resident cells of the CNS appear to be limited, infiltration of lymphoid cells from the peripheral blood can induce significant inflammatory responses within the CNS. Many of these responses develop as a result of the pleiotropic effects of potent cytokines and lymphokines on glial cells.[23] Documented responses include increased expression of class I and II major histocompatibility antigens on glial cells and induction of interleukin-1 (IL-1) secretion by astrocytes and microglial cells.[23] Likewise, exposure of vascular endothelial cells to such cytokines as IL-1 can result in increased expression of adhesion molecules and further recruitment of inflammatory cells to the site. This cascade, however, almost entirely is dependent on the presence of lymphoid cells of the peripheral blood within the CNS. Slowly progressive infections, such as those associated with slow viral diseases, may fall below the threshold required for induction of an immune response in the systemic immune system. More recent reviews in this active area of research are provided for the interested reader.[23, 286]

The myriad of cell types within the CNS and its supporting vascular supply provide infecting viruses with targets of differing permissivity to infection and viral replication. Furthermore, the characteristics of the viral infection can be expected to differ depending on the type of infected cell. For example, human papovavirus infection of the CNS leading to the clinical findings of progressive multifocal leukoencephalopathy (PML) is characterized by very different phenotypic alterations in different cell types within the CNS. If infected, neurons appear unchanged, infected oligodendrocytes often exhibit cytopathic changes, and astrocytes undergo what appears to be virus-induced transformation.[370] The complex developmental program of the CNS, which may continue after birth, ensures that cells at varying stages of differentiation will be exposed to infecting viruses. Thus, cell types not permissive to viral infection in their fully differentiated phenotype could be infected early in their developmental program. These, in turn, could act as a reservoir and as a result facilitate infection of the remainder of cells in the CNS.

Finally, the limited self-renewal capacity of many of the cellular components of the CNS as well as the complex interplay between cells of the CNS increases the likelihood of clinical disease early in the course of even slowly progressive infections. In some cases, chronic infection may not result in obvious cytopathology but yet interfere with normal functions of the CNS, as originally proposed by Oldstone and colleagues.[258] Persistent infection with hepatitis B virus in an organ with extensive self-renewal capacity, such as the liver, may be well tolerated by the host, whereas a similar persistent infection of the CNS with its limited capacity to regenerate often leads to clinically apparent, progressive disease. Thus, several characteristics of the CNS not only contribute to the likelihood of establishing a persistent infection, but also lead to the progressive nature of CNS dysfunction associated with these infections. Perhaps the clinical findings that have been associated previously with the group of diseases classified as slow viral diseases or diseases caused by unconventional agents merely reflect the natural history of chronic, subacute infections of the parenchyma of the CNS.

SUBACUTE SCLEROSING PANENCEPHALITIS

SSPE is an uncommon, slowly progressive disease of the CNS with an almost invariably fatal outcome. The disease was recognized by a number of investigators early in the twentieth century.[32, 81, 300, 343] In 1950, Greenfield[134] presented evidence that many of these reports actually described similar diseases and proposed that these diseases be unified under a single term. Several early accounts, especially those published by Dawson in 1933,[81] suggested a viral etiology of this disease; however, it was not until the mid-1960s that measles virus clearly was demonstrated to be the causative agent.[36, 73, 159, 268, 336] Interestingly, it has been suggested that several inflammatory diseases of the CNS, including progressive rubella encephalopathy, HIV encephalomyelitis, tropical spastic paraparesis, postinfectious encephalomyelitis, and SSPE, all may have a final common pathway of immune-mediated white matter destruction.[273]

Epidemiology

SSPE is a rare disease with an annual incidence of approximately 1 case per 1,000,000 population in most of the developed world, including the United States. The incidence after wild-type measles virus infection is about 1 case per 100,000 population. As will be discussed later, the introduction of universal measles immunization in many countries in Western Europe and North America has resulted in a dramatic decrease in the incidence of measles and SSPE. An example of the impact of universal measles immunization on the incidence of SSPE is illustrated by the experience in the Netherlands, where the incidence of SSPE has fallen from $1/10^6$ between 1976 and 1979 to $1/10^7$ between 1987 and 1990 and appears directly related to the incorporation of measles into national childhood vaccines policies in 1976.[20] The incidence of SSPE in some underdeveloped nations greatly exceeds that of developed nations. In southern India, the incidence of SSPE may be as high as $21/10^6$ population,[303] and in Pakistan, the rate has been estimated to be $100/10^6$.[196] A report from New Guinea has suggested a similarly high incidence of SSPE.[214] Several characteristics of natural measles virus infection in developing countries have been associated with the development of SSPE, including the high incidence of measles and the frequent occurrence of measles in children younger than 2 years of age. Both of these risk factors for SSPE are modifiable, if not preventable, by vaccination.

The disease has been reported in all countries of the world, and, although no outbreaks have been reported, clustering of cases has prompted suggestions that environmental factors or unique strains of viruses may contribute to the development of SSPE after measles. The epidemiologic study of SSPE in the Netherlands described 4 cases of SSPE in 1 year in one city of 120,000 people, which calculated to 4 cases of SSPE per 6000 cases of measles, a rate 10-fold greater than that for the rest of the country.[20] The incidence of SSPE has been reported to be about five times higher in the southeastern United States than that in other regions of the country,[142, 172, 239] also suggesting the possibility of environmental cofactors. In addition, there has been a preponderance of SSPE cases in the United States, as well as in other developed and underdeveloped countries in children from rural areas, independent of the incidence of measles in these areas.[52, 53, 142, 216, 238, 239] There appears to be no racial predilection, although whites represent the largest number of cases.[172, 239] Studies have suggested a remarkable increase in the representation of Hispanic children with SSPE.[101] The incidence of SSPE consistently is two to three times more common in males than females.[20, 172, 257] To date, no relationship between any human leukocyte antigen genotype and the development of SSPE has been demonstrated, and cases of SSPE in only one member of identical twins have been reported.[70, 86, 160] The usual age of presentation in the prevaccine era was between 6 and 10 years, with ranges of 2 to 35 years being reported.[20, 113, 114, 142, 257] The youngest case reported was a 10-month-old child and the oldest, a 52-year-old man with depressed cellular immunity.[30, 330] In most cases, symptoms attributable to SSPE begin some 4 to 8 years after measles virus infection; however, in some series, older patients (older than 10 years of age) appeared to have experienced a prolonged period between measles virus infection and the development of SSPE.[20, 172, 239]

Although several risk factors for the development of SSPE have been demonstrated repeatedly, the most consistent is the acquisition of measles before the second birthday.[20, 85, 142, 239, 257, 303] It has been estimated that at least 50 per cent of those with SSPE have had early measles.[142] In India, it is estimated that 60 per cent of measles infections occur before 2 years of age, possibly contributing to the high incidence of SSPE in this country.[303] Other risk factors have included exposure to animals.[142]

The decreased incidence of SSPE after institution of an effective measles vaccine program has been demonstrated in several countries.[20, 145, 213, 257] As noted earlier, the incidence of SSPE in the Netherlands has fallen 10-fold since universal vaccination.[20] The incidence in Japan also has fallen at least 10-fold and possibly more.[257] Poor compliance of measles vaccination in Great Britain and France in the 1980s was thought to be an explanation for the unchanging incidence of SSPE in these countries.[237, 292, 326] Development of SSPE after measles vaccination apparently occurs. In a case-control study of SSPE patients in the United States, 17 of 52 (32.7 per cent) SSPE patients had received measles vaccine prior to the development of disease.[142] Similarly, SSPE after measles immunization has been suggested by studies from the Netherlands, but the incidence of vaccine-related SSPE is estimated to be less than 1 case per 2.5 million immunizations.[20] In Japan, the estimated incidence of measles vaccine–related SSPE is 0.9 cases per million doses of vaccine.[257] An inherent problem common to all of these studies is the inability to identify patients with subclinical, wild-type measles virus infection prior to vaccination. Subclinical measles virus infections are thought to be common in underdeveloped countries, as illustrated by studies from India that suggest that up to 20 to 40 per cent of patients with measles may have a subclinical infection.[303] Because maternally derived measles antibody could modify the course of measles virus infection, it is likely that measles acquisition in early infancy could present with minimal findings.[287] Overall, the current analysis of the effect of measles immunization programs on the incidence of SSPE reveals a marked benefit.

Clinical Manifestations

The clinical course of SSPE has been described by a number of investigators, and several different clinical staging systems have been developed. The staging system of Jabbour seems to be the most straightforward and is used widely in the literature (Table 160–2). The interested reader is referred to a detailed description of five cases of SSPE, which probably represent the most thorough clinical description of the disease thus far published.[109]

The initial stage of the disease can be described best as a period of progressive psychointellectual disturbances.[294] These disturbances can include lability of mood, deterioration of school performance, hyperactivity or lethargy, depression, and occasionally altered states of consciousness. Although retrospective analysis often allows precise definition of the onset of SSPE, many of these disturbances are so subtle that they escape parental or physician detection. Physical findings vary and often are nonspecific. A peculiar pigmented retinopathy has been observed in a small number of patients.[149, 304, 375] The duration in stage I varies, depending on the clinical staging system, but in larger series, this stage is

TABLE 160–2. Clinical Stages of Subacute Sclerosing Panencephalitis

Stage I: Cerebral Signs (Psychointellectual Dysfunction)
Mood changes
Anxiety, depression
Intellectual deterioration
Memory loss
Lethargy
Stage II: Convulsive and Motor Signs
Myoclonus
Incoordination
Tremors
Choreoathetoid movements
Stage III: Coma and Opisthotonus
Spasticity
Rigidity
Unresponsive to stimulus
Wandering eyes, pathologic laughter
Stage IV: Mutism, Loss of Cortical Function, and Autonomic Dysfunction
Hyperpyrexia
Diaphoresis
Hypotonia
Heightened startle reflex

Adapted from Jabbour, J. T., Duenas, D. A., Sever, J. L., et al.: Epidemiology of SSPE: A report from the SSPE registry. J. A. M. A. *220*:959–962, 1972. Copyright 1972, American Medical Association.

relatively short, usually lasting less than 6 months.[294] Interestingly, the duration in stage I appeared to be prolonged in older patients, compared with patients younger than 10 years of age in the series from the Netherlands.[20] Accelerated progression to stage II has been reported.[294]

Stage II is characterized best by a variety of convulsive and motor disorders. The motor disorders are striking, ranging from akinetic drop attacks to violent myoclonic jerks. The motor disturbances have been described consistently as stereotypic and rhythmic. Rigidity and/or spasticity may be present in the later part of this stage.[109, 112, 294, 295] Extrapyramidal findings, such as choreoathetotic and ballismic movements as well as parkinsonism with abnormalities in the basal ganglia, have been reported.[112, 295, 373] Intellectual functions continue to deteriorate, but patients may retain receptive function during this stage. In one series of patients, up to 50 per cent with stage II disease had abnormal retinal findings, including optic atrophy.[295] The duration of this stage is quite protracted, with as many as 50 per cent of patients remaining in this stage for longer than 6 months and as many as 20 per cent remaining longer than 1 year.[294]

Progression to stage III is suggested by increased frequency of myoclonic jerks, development of spasticity or rigidity, and decerebrate and decorticate posturing. Hypothalamic dysfunction becomes prominent, with hyperpyrexia, diaphoresis, and periods of pallor and flushing.[294] Cortical activity rapidly decreases, and patients usually become comatose in this preterminal stage of disease. Duration of this stage is relatively short, lasting less than 6 months in most cases.[112, 294] Death usually is associated with complications that accompany the vegetative state, although destruction of essential structures within the brain stem and/or hypothalamus may result in death.[294]

The previous descriptions account for the vast majority of patients with SSPE; however, a significant number may exhibit a less predictable course. Some 5 to 10 per cent of patients can be expected to have a prolonged survival measured in years.[175, 294] These patients may progress to stage II or III and then remain static without relapse, or they can experience a periodic and sometimes fatal relapse of disease.[72, 294, 295] Conversely, some 10 per cent of patients may have a fulminant, rapidly progressive course lasting less than 3 months.[13, 129, 314, 327, 329]

Laboratory Findings

The definitive diagnosis of SSPE relies on a combination of laboratory findings and a compatible clinical course. Prior to association between measles and SSPE, the electroencephalogram (EEG) was extremely helpful in making the diagnosis.[112, 222, 294] The classic pattern of the EEG in SSPE is described as periodic, synchronous, bilateral discharges with a frequency of 3 to 20 seconds.[71, 109] The discharge contains high-amplitude polyphasic slow wave complexes, often consisting of two or more delta waves.[222] Frequently, the background of the EEG is suppressed, thus creating the familiar burst suppression pattern. The EEG provides little help in predicting progression of SSPE. It also should be noted that the absence of the classic EEG findings as well as other EEG abnormalities has been reported in patients with SSPE.[112, 169, 175, 311] Alternatively, the finding of periodic generalized bursts of fast waves should prompt consideration of SSPE.[223]

Recent advances in imaging technology have aided greatly in the diagnosis of SSPE. Computed tomographic (CT) scans are abnormal in more than 50 per cent of patients with SSPE, but the findings often are nonspecific.[83, 97, 198, 253, 269] In the later stages of the disease, cortical atrophy often is a prominent finding on CT scan. Magnetic resonance imaging (MRI) of patients with SSPE has revealed the presence of focal lesions consistent with inflammation, often in the white matter, in multiple areas of the brain.[83] In some cases, the location of abnormalities detected by MRI closely reflects the clinical symptomatology of the patient, whereas in others, the MRI findings have not correlated with clinical findings.[365] Finally, brain biopsy has been used as an important means of diagnosis in the past and still is of considerable value in atypical cases.

Perhaps the most useful laboratory examination of the patient with suspected SSPE is the examination of the cerebrospinal fluid (CSF). Normal to slightly increased levels of protein with an absolute increase in the gamma globulin fraction are a consistent finding in patients with SSPE.[175] Furthermore, the increase in the gamma globulin fraction is due almost exclusively to elevation of immunoglobulin.[312, 352] Additional studies have shown that 20 to 40 per cent of the CSF IgG was oligoclonal[312, 352] and that the oligoclonal fraction contained antimeasles antibodies.[346, 347] This finding almost is pathognomonic for SSPE in patients with compatible clinical presentations. All isotypes of antibodies have been found in the CSF, although the finding of IgM antimeasles antibody remains controversial.[103, 183, 226, 267, 377] Because the levels of antimeasles antibodies within the CSF are elevated as well as oligoclonal, most investigators believe that these antibodies are produced locally within the CNS, apparently in response to ongoing measles virus replication.[74] Other CSF findings include normal levels of glucose and slight pleocytosis consisting primarily of lymphocytes. Patients with SSPE have normal to elevated levels of circulating antimeasles antibody; in some cases, this antibody response also appears clonally restricted.[233, 345]

Pathogenesis and Pathology

Autopsy specimens from patients who died of SSPE reveal mild to striking changes in the gross appearance of the cerebral cortex, with ventriculomegaly in some cases. Histopathologic changes included minimal meningeal cellular infiltrate, with a perivascular accumulation of lymphocytes and plasma cells. Within involved areas of the brain, dense infiltrates of T lymphocytes and marked cellular expression of class II major histocompatibility antigens have been described.[104, 199, 248, 249] A prominent microglial and astrocytic hyperplasia often was present. Several investigators have disagreed on the relative involvement of the white and gray matter, but this issue appears to have been resolved by adaptation of Greenfield's terminology of panencephalitis.[134] One of the characteristics of SSPE was the presence of intranuclear and cytoplasmic inclusion bodies. It was the study of these structures by electron microscopy in 1965 that led to the finding of paramyxovirus-like particles in autopsy material.[36, 336] Subsequently, Connolly and colleagues[73] described the presence of measles virus antibody in the CSF of patients with SSPE as well as the presence of measles virus antigens in brain tissue from autopsy specimens of SSPE patients. Shortly thereafter, several laboratories reported the recovery of defective measles virus in specimens of brain from patients with SSPE.[159, 268] Virus was isolated only by cocultivation and not as cell-free material. Together these findings suggested that SSPE was caused by a persistent infection of the brain by measles virus.

The suggestion that a chronic measles virus infection was the etiology of SSPE raised many more questions about the pathogenesis of this disease than it answered. Several mechanisms, such as an abnormal host immune response to a common infection or a mutant virus, have elicited the most interest. Available data suggest that it may be a combination of these two possibilities. Several observations of the natural history of SSPE are consistent with an abnormal host immune response to a primary measles infection. These include (1) the chronicity of measles virus infection in children with SSPE indicated a failure to eliminate the agent; (2) the importance of early acquisition of measles virus in the development of SSPE suggested that the immature immune system may predispose the host to a persistent infection; and (3) the onset of clinical disease long after a primary infection also suggested a failure of a previously protective immune response. Early on it was thought that patients with SSPE had subtle defects in cellular immune responses as measured by decreased cutaneous reactivity to common skin test antigens, decreased lymphocyte proliferative responses to mitogens and measles virus antigens, and reduced production of cytokines.[126] Subsequent studies failed to confirm these conclusions, and most investigators now believe that patients with SSPE can generate vigorous cellular immune responses after exposure to mitogen and measles-specific antigens.[39, 89, 152] More recent studies have demonstrated the presence of several cytokines in brain lesions from SSPE patients, including IL-1b, IL-2, IL-6, tumor necrosis factor, heat-labile toxin, and interferon-γ, as well as other markers of immune activation.[234, 249] Still, there continues to be some debate about the immunocompetence of patients with SSPE.[87] Finally, measles virus is associated with a chronic progressive encephalitis in immunocompromised patients (measles inclusion body encephalitis); however, the clinical course and histologic findings of this disease clearly are different than those of SSPE.[247]

In contrast to the questions that surround the cellular response to measles virus in patients with SSPE, antibody responses to measles virus–encoded proteins are well preserved. As noted earlier, antibodies of all isotypes are produced peripherally and within the CNS. Antibodies against all of the proteins encoded by measles, including the M (matrix) protein, have been detected in the sera from patients with SSPE.[88, 141, 144] The paradox of elevated levels of circulating antimeasles antibody as well as CSF antimeasles antibody in the face of persistent infection suggested a possible immune-mediated etiology of this disease. Evidence has been presented that antimeasles antibody could interfere with virus spread and syncytial formation.[300] Fujinami and colleagues[113] demonstrated that antimeasles antibody reversibly could modulate the intracellular expression of measles virus–encoded proteins, therefore providing a mechanism by which antiviral antibody could convert an acute productive infection into a chronic persistent infection. This decrease in measles antigen expression also could shelter virus-infected cells from immunologic recognition.[259] This hypothesis also is supported by observations suggesting that early measles acquisition predisposes to the development of SSPE in that the limited quantity of passively acquired maternal antimeasles antibody may be insufficient to prevent infection and dissemination of measles virus but adequate to modulate measles virus expression. This series of events then would predispose to the development of a chronic persistent infection. Animal models consistent with this disease mechanism have been described.[176, 288, 338]

The second general mechanism for the development of SSPE is the generation of viral mutants during acute infection that then can establish a persistent infection. Persistence may result from antigenic variability or a viral mutation leading to decreased production of viral proteins below a level recognizable by the immune system and/or an extension of cell tropism. It is well documented that measles viruses from the CNS of SSPE patients are replication-defective. Analysis of these isolates does not define a virulence feature of SSPE strains but does suggest several mechanisms that could account for the generation of viral mutants. A great deal of interest has been focused on the decreased expression of the M protein in explants of brain tissue from patients with SSPE.[139, 140, 210] This viral phenotype also was consistent with the decreased production of anti-M antibody in patients with SSPE, suggesting the possibility of subthreshold production of antigen in these patients.[56, 141, 354, 372] Although the decreased expression of M protein was proposed originally as the mechanism for the persistence of mutant measles virus in patients with SSPE, subsequent studies have shown that this is only one of many mutant phenotypes in strains of measles virus associated with SSPE.

More recent studies of the replication of measles virus have revealed several mechanisms that favor the production of mutant viruses. The RNA polymerase of measles viruses, like that of other RNA viruses, does not have proofreading functions and therefore frequently misincorporates nucleotides.[55, 153] Thus, mutant progeny virus arises regularly and can be selected either by host immune responses or because of its extended host-cell tropism. In addition to this general mechanism of genetic diversity in RNA viruses, measles virus also exhibits what has been described originally as biased hypermutation and more recently as A/I hypermutation.[56, 57] This mutational event results in clusters of U (uridine) to C (cytidine) or A (adenosine) to G (guanosine) transitions, possibly as the result of novel host-derived enzymatic activity referred to double-stranded RNA unwindase.[16, 17] This activity results in the replacement of A residues with inosines in duplex RNA molecules formed between genomic RNA and mRNA. Replication of the inosine-modified genomic strand then results in the replacement of U by C. Evidence of this proposed mutational event has been found in the genomes of measles viruses from the brains of patients with SSPE, in which up to 132 of a possible 266 U residues in the M coding sequence were converted to C.[55]

Studies clearly have demonstrated that the M gene is the most heavily mutated of measles virus genes, often with early stop codons. It has been stressed that this mechanism of genetic change is operative during lytic as well as persistent infection, and mutants that persist must do so as the result of growth advantage, such as evasion of the host immune response. The frequent mutations in the M gene suggest that the measles virus can tolerate extensive genetic change in the M protein yet still replicate within cells of the CNS. The finding of clonal spread of a hypermutated measles virus genome within the brain of a patient with SSPE is consistent with this hypothesis.[11] Other genes of the measles virus also exhibit mutations that alter function, including the gene encoding the hemagglutinin (H) protein. Interestingly, mutations of this protein have been shown to limit cell surface expression but not the function of hemagglutinin in the replicative cycle of measles virus.[31] Cells infected with this phenotype likely are poorly recognized by the immune system because of the limited cell-surface expression of the H protein, yet enough functional activity remains to allow spread of the mutant virus within the CNS by a mechanism of cell-to-cell fusion. Thus, the generation of measles viruses that can induce disease and establish persistent infections results from viral strategies of genetic diversity coupled with selective pressure of the host immune response.

Treatment

The treatment of SSPE remains controversial, and as yet no antiviral agent has been efficacious consistently. In the past, 5-bromo-2-deoxyuridine,[112] transfer factor,[180] ribavirin,[256] and amantadine[174] have proved to be of little value. In the 1970s, an antiviral agent, isoprinosine (Inosiplex), was introduced and thought to have antiviral activity in vivo and in vitro, although this claim remains controversial. Some studies have suggested that isoprinosine treatment may result in stabilization, prolongation of survival, or actual clinical improvement in up to 50 to 60 per cent of patients.[167, 325] In a larger study, 98 patients with SSPE were treated continuously, and their actuarial survival was compared with that of 500 historical controls.[179] The results of this study showed that median survival for the treated patients was 3.2 years, compared with 1.2 years for the historical controls. The use of historical controls, however, raised a number of questions about the validity of the results.[64] The results of this trial also suggested a greater benefit of isoprinosine in patients with more slowly progressive SSPE.[99, 100] Other studies have not demonstrated any efficacy of isoprinosine.[136, 316] One study suggested that a combination of intrathecal interferon-α and oral isoprinosine gave a response rate of approximately 50 per cent in a series of patients with SSPE.[374] The combination of interferon and isoprinosine may warrant further evaluation, but at this time there appears to be no effective therapy for SSPE. The obvious approach is to limit the number of children infected with wild-type measles virus through continued immunization programs.

PROGRESSIVE RUBELLA PANENCEPHALITIS

Progressive rubella panencephalitis (PRP) is an extremely rare degenerative disease of the CNS. The disease continues to remain a medical curiosity, with only 10 cases reported in the medical literature.[177] The initial case report occurred in a 14-year-old boy in France with a progressive encephalitis and elevated titers of antirubella antibody in his serum and CSF.[207] Shortly thereafter, four cases of a similar progressive encephalitis in children with previously stable congenital rubella syndrome were described.[339, 355] In one of these patients, rubella virus was isolated from the brain.[355] Additional case reports suggest that PRP can occur either in children with stigmata of congenital rubella syndrome or in children acquiring rubella virus infection in childhood.[173, 340, 368]

Epidemiology

All cases of PRP thus far reported have occurred in males. In children with congenital rubella syndrome, the development of PRP occurred some 12 years after birth. In each of these cases, the neurologic abnormalities associated with congenital rubella were stable and had shown no evidence of progression. Likewise, in the few cases that have occurred after acute rubella virus infection, neurologic findings developed 8 to 12 years later. The rubella pandemic of 1964 was not associated with an increase in PRP, nor have cases been reported in Great Britain, a country with a significant incidence of congenital rubella syndrome secondary to an inconsistent immunization program. None of the reported cases has occurred after live rubella vaccination.

Clinical Manifestations

Although many of the cases of PRP exhibited signs of static congenital rubella syndrome, all patients presented with obvious neurologic deterioration. Much like the presentation of SSPE, patients with PRP initially may exhibit subtle intellectual dysfunction leading to poor school performance or behavioral changes. In reported cases, the initial clinical findings included ataxia, seizures, global dementia, and pyramidal tract findings.[339, 355] There were no findings of acute CNS inflammation, such as fever, meningismus, or headache.[84, 339, 355, 368] The course of disease is described best as slowly progressive with periods of remission and relapse. Survival with devastating CNS damage has exceeded 2 years.

Laboratory Findings

Routine laboratory testing is not helpful. Nonspecific changes in the EEG may be present but are of little diagnostic aid. Imaging studies are consistent with cortical atrophy. The examination of the CSF is essential for diagnosis of PRP. A pleocytosis consisting of mononuclear cells with normal glucose values is present in most patients. The CSF protein markedly is elevated secondary to the presence of oligoclonal IgG specific for rubella structural proteins.[173, 235, 339, 340]

Pathogenesis and Pathology

Invasive procedures, such as brain biopsy, can provide a definitive diagnosis in suspected cases of PRP. The histopathologic findings of brain from patients with PRP include demyelination, fragmentation of axons, astrocytosis, and extensive perivascular cuffing of vessels with lymphocytes and plasma cells.[340, 341, 371] Periodic acid–Schiff–positive material, as well as mineralization of vessels, has been demonstrated, suggesting the presence of endothelial damage.[340, 341, 371] Frank vasculitis is not present. Electron microscopic analysis of biopsy material has not been helpful. Rubella virus has been isolated successfully using cocultivation techniques in one case.[355] Attempts to document rubella virus–encoded antigens in involved areas of brain have been unsuccessful.[340] Immunofluorescent methodologies have demonstrated both immunoglobulins and complement deposits in vessels within affected areas, indicating the presence of immune complexes.[340]

The pathogenesis of PRP is poorly understood. Studies of children with the congenital rubella syndrome have shown that rubella virus can replicate for extended periods within the CNS.[84, 241] The virus has been isolated from nervous tissue of children up to 3 years of age with congenital rubella.[235] Long-term follow-up of these children has provided no evidence of chronic productive infection.[3] Levels of antibody to rubella often wane in the majority of patients, and many of these patients will exhibit a boost in antibody titer after exposure to wild-type rubella or vaccination with live virus.[3] Clinical follow-up also indicates that children with congenital rubella have static neurologic abnormalities and that progressive neurologic deterioration is extremely uncommon.[3] The persistence of rubella in the CNS in patients with rubella virus infection acquired later in life is even more unlikely because these patients quickly clear their infection. Thus, there is no common biologic precedence for a persistent productive rubella infection of 8 to 12 years' duration, as is seen in patients with PRP.

Patients with PRP apparently have no obvious deficits in immune responsiveness. Because many of these studies were done without the availability of more sophisticated methodologies, it is quite conceivable that subtle defects in immune responses have been overlooked. An extensive study of two cases of PRP revealed normal levels of T and B lymphocytes, cutaneous reactivity to skin test antigens, and in vitro lymphocyte responses to mitogens.[369] However, in one of the patients, a decreased response to rubella antigens was demonstrated in in vitro lymphocyte proliferation assays.[369] Levels of antirubella antibodies were elevated in these patients, and rubella-specific antibodies were found in the CSF.[369] Thus, a defect in the immune response to rubella is not a consistent finding in these patients and does not explain the persistence of rubella virus infection in this group of patients.

The emergence of a viral mutant and subsequent persistence in the CNS of PRP patients are not well supported by the limited virologic findings. Rubella virus has been isolated from only one patient with PRP, and this isolate has been shown to be similar biochemically and biologically to wild-type virus.[76, 355] Alternatively, it could be argued that the failure to isolate replicating rubella virus from patients with PRP still is compatible with a persistently replicating mutant virus that can not be cultivated in vitro. In the absence of more patients with this disease, it is unlikely that this issue will be explored adequately.

Another possible explanation for the pathogenesis of PRP is the deposition of immune complexes within vessel walls leading to tissue infarction and disease. Circulating immune complexes have been demonstrated in PRP, and rubella virus antigens have been detected within these complexes.[75, 356] IgG has been demonstrated in the vessel walls in affected brain along with lymphocytes and plasma cells.[340] Thus, one could propose a chronic, subacute vasculitis initiated by persistent rubella virus infection leading to tissue infarction. Similar vascular changes have been seen in patients with congenital rubella syndrome.[3] This mechanism does not require the persistence of rubella virus in the CNS because a peripheral site of virus replication still could produce circulating immune complexes. However, the selective involvement of the CNS and the local production of anti–rubella virus antibody argue for persistence of this virus in the CNS.

Treatment

At present, there is no treatment for this disease. One patient was treated with isoprinosine without demonstrable benefit.[369]

PROGRESSIVE MULTIFOCAL LEUKOENCEPHALOPATHY

PML is an uncommon, demyelinating, degenerative disease of the CNS caused by human papovaviruses. PML was a rare disease prior to the emergence of AIDS as an epidemic illness. A review of the literature in the early 1980s indicated that only 150 to 200 cases had been reported.[351] In most of the original reports, PML was confined to allograft recipients, individuals with lymphoproliferative disorders, and children with congenital immunodeficiencies; however, AIDS now is the most common underlying disease associated with PML.[24, 154, 363] PML first was described in 1958 by Åstrom and associates[8] in a group of patients with lymphoproliferative diseases. Although a viral etiology was suspected, it was not until 1964, when electron microscopy of involved brain revealed a crystalline array of papovavirus-like particles, that the search for a causative virus began.[317, 380] In 1971, investigators at the University of Wisconsin isolated a novel papovavirus, JC virus, which subsequently has been associated with the vast majority of cases of PML.[265] Weiner and colleagues[357] at Johns Hopkins University isolated a similar papovavirus, simian vacuolating agent 40 (SV40), from two different patients. The isolation of SV40 was disturbing because 10 to 40 million Americans had been inoculated between 1955 and 1971 with SV40-contaminated, killed poliovirus vaccine.[309] Fortunately, there have been very few cases of PML that have been associated with SV40. In addition, a case of SV40-associated PML has been reexamined and found to be associated with JC virus.[102] Investigators in Great Britain isolated a third type of papovavirus, BK, from the urine of a renal transplant patient, but this virus has not been associated with documented cases of PML.[125]

Epidemiology

Antibody reactivity to JC virus is present in 30 per cent of children by 4 years of age, 50 per cent by 6 years of age, and 80 to 90 per cent by adulthood.[63, 310, 351] These data indicate that infection with JC virus nearly is universal in most populations. In addition, JC virus has been detected in autopsy specimens from normal individuals without PML, suggesting that this virus can infect the CNS and not result in disease.[245, 360] Cases of PML have been reported from all regions of the world, as could be expected because of the worldwide prevalence of JC virus.[351] Prior to the AIDS epidemic, most cases of PML were reported in middle-aged individuals, although a case of PML occurred in a 5-year-old child with a congenital immunodeficiency.[276, 324, 351]

Because PML now most commonly is associated with AIDS, its epidemiology follows that of infections with HIV. The incidence of PML in the United States in 1987 was calculated to be approximately 5.7 cases per 10,000,000 population and in males, 9.4 cases per 10,000,000 population.[154] Between 1981 and 1990, there were 971 documented cases of PML reported to the Centers for Disease Control and Prevention.[154] Estimates of the incidence of PML in AIDS patients have ranged from 1 to 4 per cent.[24, 25, 130, 201] Cases of PML developing in pediatric AIDS patients have been reported.[27, 344] PML has been associated with a variety of lymphoproliferative diseases, aggressively treated connective tissue diseases, allotransplantation, and infectious syndromes, such as sarcoidosis.[8, 108, 188, 264, 290, 298, 321] An extremely rare subset of patients without apparent underlying abnormality in immunologic reactivity have developed PML.[349]

Clinical Manifestations

Most individual case reports have described an insidious onset of a variety of neurologic abnormalities in patients with significant underlying immunosuppression. Simultaneous changes in motor, sensory, and higher intellectual functions may be present. In a group of adult patients with AIDS and PML, about 50 per cent presented with weakness as the initial presenting complaint.[24] Nearly the same number of patients had cognitive dysfunction or disturbances in speech or language.[24] The presentation of PML in children with AIDS has been similar, with weakness, hemiparesis, and changes in mentation.[24, 344] Other presentations more commonly reported in older studies include ataxia and symptoms consistent with an intracranial mass.[178, 211, 266, 276, 348] Fever is not a component of PML, and its presence should alert physicians to other infectious causes of neurologic disease. Death usually occurs after the development of coma.

The disease is slowly but relentlessly progressive. Early reports indicated that the course of the disease from onset until death was in the range of 3 to 6 months.[379] More recent reports suggest a more variable course, ranging from weeks to years, depending on the course of the patient's underlying immunodeficiency.[24, 26, 130, 306, 363] The clinical course of PML in patients with AIDS can be altered indirectly by successful antiretroviral therapy.[318]

Laboratory Findings

The presence of slowly evolving neurologic abnormalities in an immunocompromised host should suggest the diagnosis of PML. Until recently, noninvasive diagnostic approaches have been unreliable. Serologic studies are of little use because all patients have had previous exposure to the JC virus. Furthermore, in most patient populations in which PML develops, individual patients are severely immunocompromised. Thus, the presence or absence of JC virus–specific antibody is of little value. Examination of the CSF with routine methodologies generally reveals no significant abnormalities. Evidence of inflammation is not present in most cases, with the exception of mildly elevated CSF protein. An early report suggested that papovavirus antigen could be detected in the CSF of patients with PML[270]; however, this assay has not become routine in most centers. The EEG shows a variety of nonspecific changes, most commonly generalized slowing.[106] Neuroimaging studies reveal a variety of findings. CT scans have been shown to be of value in making a presumptive diagnosis.[165, 246, 274, 275] Characteristic findings include multiple radiolucent areas within the white matter. MRI has proved to be of even greater value in the diagnosis of PML.[135, 146, 221, 252, 275, 361] In contrast to CT findings, MRI findings often define unsuspected abnormalities within areas of the brain, such as the basal ganglia and brain stem.

With the advent of polymerase chain reaction (PCR) as an important tool of the diagnostic microbiology laboratory, several studies have verified its use in the diagnosis of PML. Multiple studies have demonstrated that PCR of CSF from patients with PML can detect JC virus sequences with a high level of sensitivity (>80–90%) and specificity (>90%).[110, 230, 244, 353] The predictive value of the CSF PCR for JC virus with patients with suspected PML is such that many investigators have suggested that CSF PCR should replace brain biopsy for the diagnosis of PML. Many investigators likely would agree with this approach only if a finite number of pathogens could cause disease in immunocompromised hosts; however, the differential diagnosis for CNS dysfunction in patients with diseases such as AIDS is large and complex. This fact makes the argument promoting PCR as a replacement for brain biopsy untenable because brain biopsy often uncovers unsuspected disease in patients with preoperative diagnosis of PML.

Biopsy of diseased brain, especially CT-aided stereotaxic biopsy, provides a straightforward approach for the diagnosis of PML.[65, 107, 168, 208] Once localized by CT scan, stereotaxic biopsy can provide sufficient tissue for routine histology and electron microscopy as well as in situ hybridization, PCR, and immunocytochemical assays.[1, 138, 151, 170, 315, 323] Perhaps the most important information obtained from a brain biopsy in this setting is the diagnosis of potentially treatable diseases, such as toxoplasmosis.

Pathogenesis and Pathology

The histologic findings of diseased tissue from PML cases illustrate the pleiotropic effects of the JC virus on cells of the CNS. Microscopic examination of involved tissue reveals characteristic alteration in the appearance and distribution of oligodendrocytes. They have greatly enlarged, deeply basophilic nuclei, and, occasionally, an internuclear inclusion body can be seen. The abnormal oligodendrocytes are found on the advancing edge of the enlarging focus, whereas in the demyelinated center of the focal infection, few if any oligodendrocytes are present.[33, 138, 151, 351] Enlarged and reactive-appearing astrocytes with pleomorphic, hyperchromic nuclei are present within the center of the demyelinated focus. These giant astrocytes are said to resemble the malignant astrocyte of glioblastomas.[151, 351] The lesions do not contain well-organized inflammatory cell infiltrates, but, occasionally, phagocytic cells of the peripheral immune system can be seen infiltrating the lesions.

The pathogenesis of PML is presumed to be a persistent, lytic infection of the CNS by JC virus. The loss of oligodendrocytes and demyelinization results in many of the clinical findings associated with PML. The presence of multiple foci suggest a hematogenous spread of the virus. Consistent with this proposed route of spread has been the finding of JC virus in peripheral blood monocytes.[95] Because the foci often are of similar size, it was assumed that this spread occurred shortly before the onset of disease; however, recent data suggest that JC virus is in the brain of normal, nondiseased hosts.[95] Thus, PML may be the result of local reactivation of JC virus and not secondary to viremic spread to the CNS shortly before onset of the clinical symptoms. Although the timing of CNS seeding is unknown, existing data have shown that in the absence of normal immunity, the JC virus can continue productive, lytic infection of the human nervous system. Lastly, two strains of JC virus have been identified in patients with PML.[10] They appear to be derived from a single ancestral virus, and no evidence has been presented suggesting the presence of specific CNS tropism or virulence characteristics associated with one or the other type.

Treatment

The treatment of PML generally has been unrewarding. Reports from the older literature describe the use of a variety of antiviral agents, including adenine arabinoside, interferon, idoxuridine, and cytosine arabinoside.[157, 289, 331, 351, 362] With the exception of cytosine arabinoside, none of these agents has produced responses in a significant number of patients. The clinical responses to cytosine arabinoside have been extremely variable but in general are disappointing.[7, 148] Discontinuing all immunosuppression in a few renal transplant patients with PML has resulted in stabilization of the disease and possibly return of some neurologic function.[350] This approach obviously is of value only in patients whose immunosuppression can be reversed safely. Furthermore, this approach requires a high index of suspicion and a rapid, aggressive approach to the diagnosis because the structural damage caused by this persistent virus infection can not be reversed.

TRANSMISSIBLE SPONGIFORM ENCEPHALOPATHIES (CREUTZFELDT-JAKOB DISEASE, KURU, GERSTMANN-STRAUSSLER-SCHEINKER DISEASE, FATAL FAMILIAL INSOMNIA, SPASTIC PARAPARESIS WITH DEMENTIA)

The general category of transmissible spongiform encephalopathies, more recently termed *transmissible cerebral amyloidoses*, includes at least five distinct human diseases, as well as similar transmissible diseases of animals (Table 160–3). The most recently described member of this group of diseases was discovered after an outbreak of a spongiform encepha-

TABLE 160–3. Naturally Occurring Transmissible Spongiform Encephalopathies

Host	Disease
Human	Kuru
	Creutzfeldt-Jakob disease
	Sporadic
	Familial
	Gerstmann-Straussler-Scheinker syndrome
	Fatal familial insomnia
Sheep, goats	Scrapie
Mink	Transmissible mink encephalopathy
Deer	Chronic wasting disease
Cattle	Bovine spongiform encephalopathy
Cat	Feline spongiform encephalopathy

lopathy of cattle in Great Britain in the mid-1980s. This disease of domestic cattle initially was termed *mad cow disease*. Subsequently, this disease was shown to be transmissible.[38] Mad cow disease has been renamed *bovine spongiform encephalopathy*.[155, 156, 229, 366] Although bovine spongiform encephalopathy appeared to be a new disease of cattle because no cases were identified prior to 1985, it was shown to be endemic in 1 to 5 per cent of dairy herds in Great Britain.[37, 38] More recently, it has been demonstrated that bovine spongiform encephalopathy was transmitted through the meat and bone meal fed to dairy cattle as a nutritional supplement. Concern was raised about the potential transmission of this disease to humans after consumption of contaminated beef, but to date no human cases of spongiform encephalopathy have been linked directly to consumption of contaminated beef.

This group of degenerative diseases of the CNS clearly fits Sigurdsson's original criteria for a slow viral disease. Each disease is characterized by a prolonged incubation or latent period and a relentlessly progressive clinical course after onset of clinical symptoms, and in nature each disease appears to be limited to a single species. The diseases induce many of the same histopathologic findings in the CNS of their respective hosts, suggesting a common, albeit incompletely characterized and unconventional, agent. Common to these diseases are amyloid fibrils and amyloid plaques in involved areas of the CNS. This characteristic has prompted some investigators to reclassify these diseases as transmissible cerebral amyloidosis.[93, 120–122, 367] Another common feature of these diseases, and perhaps the most intriguing, is the unique set of chemical and biologic characteristics of the agents that are thought to induce these diseases. It appears that agents associated with transmissible spongiform encephalopathies are similar, if not identical, in size, chemical composition, and biologic activity in the diverse diseases of humans and animals. In contrast to Sigurdsson's original criteria for slow viral diseases, the agents inducing human diseases have been transmitted and propagated in nonhuman primates, goats, guinea pigs, mice, and hamsters.[120]

The study of spongiform encephalopathies began with the investigations into the cause of scrapie, a degenerative disease of the CNS of sheep. Although this disease has been recognized for more than 250 years, it was not until 1936 that it was shown to be transmissible.[78] The recognition of the similarities between a newly described human disease, kuru, and scrapie set the stage for the experimental verification that kuru and Creutzfeldt-Jakob disease (CJD) were transmissible encephalopathies.[137] The proposal of Prusiner that an infectious proteinaceous particle without DNA or RNA was the transmissible agent responsible for these diseases continues to invoke considerable skepticism, in spite of extensive supporting evidence.[277, 278, 280] Brief descriptions of human spongiform encephalopathies are provided later. More definitive works are available.[21, 82, 123, 186]

Epidemiology

The discussion of the natural history of kuru is one of the most interesting studies in medical epidemiology. Although the disease no longer occurs in the Fore people of New Guinea, a brief description of the disease is informative for understanding the epidemiologic features of other spongiform encephalopathies. The disease was noted first in 1955 by Vincent Zigas, an Australian medical officer stationed in New Guinea.[376] Zigas became aware of an endemic, fatal, subacute neurodegenerative disease limited to one linguistic group of highland natives. In addition to their primitive lifestyle, these people also practiced ritual endocannibalism, that is, eating dead members of the tribe. Gajdusek and Zigas eventually showed that the disease was limited to the Fore linguistic group and that kuru occurred only in non-Fore people as the result of intermarriage.[4] In the initial reports, the incidence of kuru was extremely high, occurring in 1 per cent of the population and accounting for 50 per cent of all deaths in the tribe.[4] The disease predominantly affected females, with a female:male ratio of 2.4:1.[4] Analysis of the mortality rates also revealed a striking difference between the age of death in men and women. Women exhibited a bimodal death curve, with a peak in adolescence and the second peak between 30 and 39 years of age.[4] Men, on the other hand, died in adolescence. Because kuru results in death within 12 months after clinical onset, it appeared as though women were acquiring the disease during childhood and adolescence. Additional epidemiologic data suggested that the cannibalism practiced by this tribe was of critical importance to the development of the disease. The ritual of endocannibalism of this tribe was practiced primarily by the women who prepared and ingested the brains of dead relatives, many of whom had died of kuru.[127] After barehanded preparation of the brain in bamboo cylinders, the Fore women would wipe the kuru-contaminated material over their bodies and hair. Subsequent transmission studies in nonhuman primates revealed that kuru was associated with contact with infected brain and that the incubation period may be as long as 20 years.[118, 284] Early titration of brain from a kuru victim revealed that the infectivity of this material was on the order of 10^8 infectious particles per gram of tissue.[118] Thus, it initially was assumed that kuru was transmitted by ingestion of infected brain. When numerous attempts to transmit kuru failed, most investigators proposed that kuru was transmitted to women during the handling of infected brain through open sores, possibly caused by endemic scabies.[127] More recent experiments have shown that kuru (and CJD) can be transmitted orally, although at a much reduced efficiency.[127] Either mode of transmission would explain the bimodal distribution of mortality of kuru in women and the high incidence of kuru deaths in adolescent boys, because both males and females would be exposed to infected brain early in infancy when they were in close physical contact with their mothers and the handling of infected brains. Females would have an additional exposure in adolescence when they participated in ritual cannibalism. Because cannibalism no longer is practiced by this tribe, the incidence of kuru has fallen dramatically and disappeared in some villages.[4] By 1985, there were no cases of kuru in individuals younger than 30 years of age. The origin of kuru in the Fore people is unknown, but a likely explanation would be that a sporadic case of CJD could have occurred in the Fore population, with resulting spread secondary to their practice of cannibalism.[117, 118]

Although the nature of the kuru agent remains a contentious issue, the natural history of the disease is well defined. Unfortunately, neither the agent nor the natural history of CJD is well-defined. CJD occurs worldwide, with an annual incidence of 1 case per 1,000,000 population.[45, 46, 143, 197, 364] Genetic factors are important because 5 to 10 per cent of cases are familial, possibly associated with mutations in the cellular prion protein (PrP), which has been suggested to be causative of CJD.[15, 46, 54, 116, 143, 227] In addition, variants of CJD, such as Gerstmann-Straussler-Scheinker (GSS) syndrome, clearly are familial in their mode of transmission.[161, 200] The incidence of CJD also markedly is increased in some ethnic groups, such as Libyan-born Jews, who have an annual incidence of CJD as high as 40 cases per 1,000,000 population.[132, 254] Initial epidemiologic studies implicated the ingestion of lightly cooked sheep brain and sheep eyeballs by this ethnic group as the likely etiology for the increased incidence of CJD; however, recent studies have demonstrated a mutation in the cellular PrP gene in Libyan-born Jews with CJD, suggesting the genetic basis for this disease.[5, 162] The familial forms of CJD exhibit an autosomal dominant mode of inheritance. Another feature of the epidemiology of nonfamilial CJD is the lack of evidence of transmission to spouses of sporadic cases, suggesting that CJD is not maintained in the population by a case-to-case contact.[46, 364] There is no evidence of vertical transmission in sporadic cases of CJD.[46] Finally, there is little evidence that an environmental factor or dietary practices are associated with sporadic CJD.[46] An extensive review of 300 cases of experimentally verified transmissible spongiform encephalopathies collected by investigators at the National Institutes of Health has been published recently.[48]

CJD is a disease primarily of middle-aged people, with a mean age of onset of 55 to 60 years and a range of 20 to 84 years.[44] CJD has been reported in a 17-year-old boy and in a 20-year-old woman.[242, 263] Similar clinical diseases and compatible pathologic findings have been seen in children with progressive CNS degenerative diseases, and transmissibility studies suggest that some of these diseases could be CJD-like.[215, 220] The incubation period of naturally occurring CJD is unknown, but inoculation of the CNS in three individuals with contaminated material resulted in disease within 15 to 30 months.[98, 215, 228] Death usually occurs within 12 months of the onset of clinical symptoms.[47, 217, 228] A variety of epidemiologically defined risk factors have been associated with the development of CJD, including previous neurosurgical procedures, CNS trauma, ingestion of CNS tissue from animals, and ingestion of lamb.[98, 181, 195] Other studies do not support these associations.[46, 66] Eight patients have developed CJD after treatment with human cadaveric–derived growth hormone.[41, 42, 77, 224, 251, 293] Additional cases of CJD have occurred as a result of cadaveric dural grafts.[206, 337] An especially disturbing report documented the transmission of CJD to a chimpanzee by stereotactic electrodes initially used in a patient with CJD. The electrodes were sterilized with both ethanol and formalin and stored for 2 years prior to their use in this experiment.[128] Scrapie has been transmitted in mice by conjunctival inoculation.[307] There have been no cases of CJD or other spongiform diseases related to the transfusion of blood products.[120, 131] At present, the mode of transmission of naturally acquired CJD, the incubation period, the susceptibility, and the possibility of subclinical infections remain inadequately defined.

Clinical Manifestations

The clinical course of kuru is described because it will offer an interesting comparison to that of CJD. Those interested in a more detailed discussion of this disease are referred to a more comprehensive work.[105] Kuru presents initially with loss of coordination, usually exacerbated by stress or fatigue. These early symptoms progress rapidly to loss of balance, inability to maintain posture, clumsiness in gait, and slurred speech. The disease then progresses to severe ataxia, inability to remain upright, exaggerated muscle contractions, and inability to chew food and swallow. Death follows, usually from aspiration, infection, or starvation. In contrast to CJD, dementia is not a prominent finding in kuru. Juvenile kuru resembles the adult form of the disease; however, abnormal eye findings, including strabismus, diplopia, nystagmus, and ptosis, are quite common. In addition, the juvenile form is more rapidly progressive, with death occurring in less than 6 months.[158] Although the incubation period of kuru can be as long as 22 years, once clinical symptoms appear, the disease follows a consistent and predictable course.

The early stages and symptoms of CJD are somewhat more subtle and complex than those described for kuru. The initial stages of the disease are characterized by symptoms of motor and sensory dysfunction, including disturbances of gait, visual abnormalities, headaches, dizziness, and paresthesias.[297] Psychointellectual dysfunction, including loss of memory, speech abnormalities, anxiety, and depression, also is a common finding.[218] Fever is not a finding in the early stages of CJD. In the second stage, patients develop objective evidence of motor, sensory, and intellectual impairment. The terminal phase is characterized by progressive motor, sensory, and intellectual deterioration. Additional findings include spasticity or rigidity, cerebellar dysfunction, myoclonus, seizures, and profound dementia. Death usually is secondary to infection, and more than 90 per cent of patients in one reported series died in an akinetic rigid state, occasionally with decerebrate or decorticate posturing.[44, 297]

Other variants of spongiform encephalopathies include spastic paraparesis with dementia and fatal familial insomnia.[124, 191, 232, 240, 243] The interesting syndrome of fatal familial insomnia now can be classified formally as a transmissible spongiform encephalopathy because the disease has been transmitted to experimental animals.[333] Clinical characteristics of this familial disease include a mean age of onset of 51 years (range, 20 to 71 years), with a duration of disease of 14 months.[124] Late in the disease, several neuroendocrine systems can be involved, leading to multiple clinical signs and symptoms. Disease presentation can include progressive insomnia that is resistant to diazepam and barbiturates.[124] Other presenting signs include impairment of cognitive functions, such as loss of memory and deficits in attention. Abnormal circadian rhythms of growth hormone, prolactin, and melatonin secretion have been described.[271, 272] In the later stages of the disease, progressive motor system involvement is manifested by dysarthria, dysphagia, ataxia, and myoclonus.[124]

Laboratory Findings

The routine laboratory findings in cases of human spongiform encephalopathies are nonspecific and in most cases nondiagnostic. This discussion will be limited to the diagnosis of CJD; variants such as GSS syndrome and fatal familial insomnia have similar findings, especially histopathologic findings. Serologic studies are of no value because naturally occurring antibody responses to the proposed etiologic agents of spongiform encephalopathies have not been demonstrated. There is no evidence of systemic or CNS inflammation. The CSF exhibits no specific abnormalities.[260] Noninvasive imaging studies are of some value in excluding other diseases that may present with signs and symptoms of CJD. Imaging studies of the brain have revealed findings consistent with cortical atrophy in the late stages of the diseases; however, their use during initial presentation is limited. In reported cases, both MRI and CT findings were nonspecific.[90, 147, 171, 190, 261, 332, 342] A review of the MRI findings of four confirmed cases of CJD suggested that increased signals in T2-weighted images of the basal ganglia possibly were a relatively specific sign for CJD.[14] The EEG has been thought to be useful in the diagnosis of CJD and its variants because abnormalities in the tracing are thought to be characteristic.[9, 35, 69, 209, 305, 378] In the early phases of the disease, the EEG may show only nonspecific slow-wave activity or mild background disorganization. With progression, the EEG evolves into semiperiodic slow-wave patterns. The most characteristic pattern is that of one- to two-cycle-per-second triphasic sharp-wave activity superimposed on diminished background activity.[35, 43] Serial EEG tracings are of much greater diagnostic aid than a single recording. Finally, the EEG findings are not diagnostic in themselves and must be correlated with other clinical and laboratory findings.

Definitive diagnosis of CJD requires the use of brain biopsy, followed by histologic examination by an experienced pathologist. Because the pathologic abnormalities are not distributed homogeneously throughout the brain, this procedure often fails to provide a definitive diagnosis. The classic triad of microscopic changes consisting of neuronal loss, status spongiosis, and proliferation of hypertrophic astrocytes with or without microgliosis is found within involved areas.[19] Amyloid plaque formation also can be found in biopsy specimens from some patients.[19, 21, 192–194, 204, 205] Status spongiosis, although not limited to the transmissible spongiform encephalopathies, nonetheless is characteristic of the disease.[21, 202] The term is used to describe the vacuolation of the neuropil caused by degenerating neurons and collapse of the cortical cytoarchitecture.[21] In some cases, the distribution of pathologic findings appears to correlate with specific spongiform encephalopathies. For instance, the observation of spongiform changes in fatal familial insomnia has been noted predominantly in the thalamus.[21, 232] Whether the distribution of spongiform lesions is related to the pathogenesis of these disorders or merely reflects the duration of disease prior to onset of clinical symptomatology is unclear.

Current thinking in this field of study is that an abnormal isoform of a normal cellular protein may be the common final pathway of this group of diseases. This proposed mechanism of disease induction has prompted several laboratories to develop immunocytochemical methods for detection of mutant forms of these cellular proteins. Biopsy specimens that demonstrate the accumulation of these proteins or the presence of mutant forms of this protein can suggest the diagnosis of a transmissible spongiform disease or, perhaps more commonly termed, a prion-associated disease (see following section). The availability of antisera and monoclonal antibodies to PrP and mutant forms of this protein has permitted the development of reliable assays for immunocytochemical analysis of suspected cases of spongiform encephalopathies. Although the specificity and sensitivity of these assays now are being defined, early reports suggest more widespread prion deposition in the brain than previously thought.[21, 205, 334] As more laboratories become experienced with this technology, it no doubt will enhance laboratory diagnosis of this group of diseases. PCR analysis of mutations within the cellular prion coding sequence has been useful for defining inherited forms of spongiform encephalopathies and should be included in the laboratory evaluation of patients with sporadically occurring forms of these diseases.[334]

Pathogenesis and Pathology

The pathogenesis of the human spongiform encephalopathies is unknown. Animal models of these diseases have provided most of our current understanding of the possible etiology of these rare diseases. Although the natural route of transmission of transmissible spongiform encephalopathies in humans is unknown, the agent(s) can be transmitted to experimental animals by a variety of parenteral routes. Regardless of inoculation site, the agent initially replicates in the spleen and liver and then likely spreads to the CNS.[219] In some animal models, such as scrapie in mice, the agent can be transmitted orally, although the oral route requires 10^9 more infectious particles than does intracerebral route.[277] Neither vertical transmission nor transmission from placental tissue has been documented.[6] Familial forms have been documented, and, as noted previously, inheritance is that of an autosomal dominant trait.

The immune system appears to have little influence on the development or course of transmissible spongiform encephalopathy. Vaccination with inactivated material has failed to prevent disease induction upon challenge.[322] In tissue specimens, no evidence of inflammatory cells is present. Immunosuppressive agents do not shorten the incubation period of scrapie in laboratory animals. Strong serologic responses to neurofilament proteins have been reported in patients with CJD and kuru.[12] Whether this represents a specific immune response or an epiphenomenon similar to the findings of anti–smooth muscle antibodies in chronic active hepatitis is not known. To date, it would appear that the degenerative changes associated with transmissible spongiform encephalopathy result from cytopathic effects of the agent(s) and are secondary to immunologic attack.

The most intriguing and recently the most revealing aspect of these diseases is the nature of the putative etiologic agent. Intense research has defined an entirely new strategy of disease induction and self-replication for an agent that may not harbor nucleic acid. Although the majority of the following discussion will be limited to experimental results obtained with the scrapie agent, overwhelming evidence indicates that agents ultimately responsible for induction of CJD, GSS syndrome, fatal familial insomnia, and kuru have the same properties.

The infectious agent associated with scrapie is extremely small. Its estimated size is less than 50 nm.[166] As shown in Table 160–4, the agent is resistant to a wide variety of chemical agents that normally inactivate viruses. Numerous experimental systems have shown repeatedly that the scrapie agent does not contain nucleic acid of sufficient size to encode any self-replicative functions (see Table 160–4). Furthermore and of noted concern to pathologists, the agent is incredibly resistant to most conventional decontamination techniques.[21] In fact, heating the agent to 360° C resulted in only about a 90 per cent reduction in infectivity.[119]

In 1982, Prusiner[277] introduced the term *prion* to describe the small proteinaceous particles isolated from the brains of scrapie-infected hamsters. Scrapie infectivity was shown to purify with the particles. In addition, the particles were shown to have many of the same biochemical characteristics as the scrapie agent, most notably resistance to conventional methods of eliminating infectivity of known viruses. Antisera prepared against these particles detected similar structures in amyloid plaques of brain tissue from CJD patients and from animals given homogenized brain from CJD patients.[182, 192–194, 299] At this time, three possible structures were proposed for the scrapie particle: (1) protein surrounding nucleic acid, (2) protein surrounding a small noncoding polynucleotide, and (3) an infectious protein without accompanying nucleic

TABLE 160–4. Chemical Properties of the Scrapie Agent

Treatment	Resistant	Sensitive
Agents Modifying Proteins		
Proteases		Proteinase K, trypsin
Chemical modification	Formaldehyde	Diethylpyrocarbonate
Detergent	Triton X-100, NP40, Sarkosyl	Sodium dodecyl sulfate
Ions	Na^+, K^+, ethylenediamine-tetraacetic acid	Thiocyanate, trichloroacetic acid
Organic solvents	Methanol, ethanol, chloroform, ether	Phenol
Heat	100° F for 1 hour	Sodium hydroxide, hypochlorite (bleach)
Agents Modifying Nucleic Agents		
Nucleases	Ribonucleases, deoxyribonucleases	
Ultraviolet irradiation (254 nm)	Stable up to 42 kJ/m^2	
Psoralen photoreaction	Stable	
Chemical	Zinc hydrolysis, hydroxylamine	

Modfied from Prusiner, S. B.: Novel proteinaceous infectious particles cause scrapie. Science *216*:136–144, 1982. Copyright 1982 by the American Association for the Advancement of Science.

acid.[280] The particle was purified further and shown to consist of a single protein, PrP, a 27,000- to 30,000-dalton glycoprotein that is highly insoluble and aggregates during purification. Interestingly, antisera raised against PrP detected a 33,000- to 35,000-dalton protein in the brains of both diseased and normal animals, which suggested that PrP was encoded by a host gene.[280] This suggestion was confirmed by the detection of PrP-specific messenger RNA in both scrapie-infected and normal brain tissue.[68, 212] Initial experiments failed to transmit scrapie with recombinant PrP, leading investigators to propose that PrP was a cellular protein associated with the as yet unidentified infectious agent.[60, 61] These experimental results were clouded by the fact that in vitro–derived PrP failed to aggregate into scrapie-associated fibrils and remained sensitive to the protease proteinase K, both characteristic of scrapie-associated PrP.[22, 51, 59, 62, 231, 236, 279, 300, 320] Further investigations have shown that PrP from normal brain and that found in brain from transmissible encephalopathies physically and chemically are distinct as well as exhibit different subcellular locations.[22, 34, 62, 285, 302, 319, 328] Most notably, scrapie-associated PrP exists as an aggregate after detergent extraction and, upon treatment with proteinase K, remains as a 27,000- to 30,000-dalton protein as the result of cleavage of its N-terminal 67 amino acids.[231, 236, 359] Forms similar to the PrP 27-30 can be found in the brains of patients with all transmissible spongiform encephalopathies, including patients with CJD, GSS syndrome, and kuru.[359] Both normal cellular and scrapie-associated PrP are glycosylated membrane proteins, but only the normal cellular form can be released by treatment with phospholipase activity directed at a membrane phosphatidylinositol linkage. Additional experiments have provided evidence for altered cellular compartmentalization of the scrapie-associated PrP.[22, 34, 62, 194, 285, 302, 319]

The finding of a cellular gene encoding an apparently disease-producing protein has been of great interest. Mapping of the gene demonstrated that it was on chromosome 20.[255, 262] Subsequent studies with familial forms of transmissible spongiform encephalopathies, such as GSS syndrome, documented mutations in the cellular gene encoding PrP.[94, 133, 163] The PrP gene in patients with GSS syndrome, an autosomal dominant disorder, has been shown to contain C to T changes in codon 102, which produces an amino acid change of proline to leucine at position 102.[161, 163] The change in the primary sequence of PrP in GSS syndrome patients is associated with the pathologic changes seen in other transmissible spongiform encephalopathies. This phenotype associated with the mutant PrP can be transmitted to experimental animals.[291] Several other PrP mutant genotypes have been described (Table 160–5). These observations also provide an explanation for the sporadic cases of CJD. Somatic mutations in the PrP gene or error in transcription/translation could give rise to a mutant and pathogenetic PrP and lead to CJD.

The proposal that a nonnucleic acid–containing protein agent could transmit disease has not been met with universal acceptance. Several investigators have suggested that PrP may be the structural component of a more complex infectious agent. Implicit in this argument is that the agent con-

TABLE 160–5. Mutations in Prion Protein (PrP) c Associated with Human Disease

Mutation	PrP Genotype	Clinical Findings
Insertions*	120 bp	Dementia, myoclonus
	144 bp	Dementia, ataxia
	168 bp	Dementia
	196 bp	Ataxia, myoclonus
	216 bp	Ataxia, dementia
Point mutations	102 *(leu)*	Gerstmann-Straussler-Scheinkler syndrome
	117 *(val)*	Dementia, extra pyramidal tract findings
	198 *(ser)*	Gerstmann-Straussler-Scheinker syndrome subtype
	217 *(arg)*	Ataxia, dementia
	200 *(lys)*	Similar to Creutzfeldt-Jakob disease
	178 *(asn)*	Dementia, ataxia, extrapyramidal tract signs
	129 *(val)*	Dementia, ataxia
	178 *(asn)* and 129 *(met)*	Sleep disorders, ataxia, extrapyramidal tract findings

*Octameric insertion into coding sequence of PrP c.
bp, base pairs.
Adapted from Gambetti, P., Petersen, R., Monari, L., et al.: Fatal familial insomnia and the widening spectrum of prion diseases. Br. Med. Bull. *49*:980–994, 1993.

tains nucleic acid, which allows replication of the agent and thus conservation of its phenotype as the result of genetic information. The most consistent argument for the presence of genetic material has been the discovery of strains of scrapie and other agents inducing spongiform changes that retain their phenotypic behavior in vivo.[49, 91, 111, 182, 184, 185, 189] Furthermore, there is a well-characterized species barrier, such that transmission results in spongiform changes associated with the host animal PrP and not that of the exogenous PrP. Ultraviolet inactivation of PrP has suggested that if nucleic acid is present, it must be less than 30 base pairs in length, a size too small to encode a conventional infectious agent.

The synthesis of experimental data has allowed the description of a novel mode of transmission of this group of diseases. PrP is proposed to act as a nucleation center in the brain and induce the formation of amyloid plaques characteristic of transmissible spongiform encephalopathies.[79, 93, 281, 358] Thus, much like crystallization in vitro, exogenous PrP could lead to the formation of crystalline arrays of amyloid material in the CNS, leading to cell death, release of additional PrP, and generation of more nucleation centers, eventually leading to disease. How does this theory explain the strain-dependent phenotypes of different scrapie isolates? This question was addressed in a landmark observation.[29] The PrP phenotype of different isolates of PrP from transmissible mink encephalopathy was shown to be transmissible in a cell-free system, demonstrating for the first time that the conformation of disease-associated protein could modify a host-cell–derived protein in such a manner as to propagate the specific conformation of the disease-associated protein.[29] Thus, infectivity of the PrP would fulfill the conventional paradigms of information transfer associated with nucleic acids within an infectious agent yet rely on the chemical consistency of protein folding to reproduce faithfully the disease-producing phenotype.[82, 282, 283]

Treatment

Treatment of transmissible spongiform encephalopathies has included both interferon and adenine arabinoside.[115, 197] It is impossible to discern if either agent provided any clinical benefit to the small number of patients in these reports. Caughey[58] has shown that sulphated glycans, such as the dye congo red, can inhibit the formation of misfolded and aggregated cellular PrP in vitro. This finding raises the possibility that therapeutic agents with similar activities could be used to limit cerebral amyloid formation associated with diseases such as CJD.

Perhaps of greater immediate importance is the prevention of medically transmitted spongiform encephalopathies.[18, 28, 50, 67, 173, 187, 335] Several studies have shown that sodium hypochlorite solutions can eliminate infectivity effectively.[335] A thorough discussion of safe handling of contaminated material has been presented.[21] There still remains considerable debate about the proper decontamination of neurosurgical instruments.[21]

References

1. Aksamit, A. J.: Nonradioactive in situ hybridization in progressive multifocal leukoencephalopathy. Mayo Clin. Proc. *68*:899–910, 1993.
2. Alford, C. A.: Chronic intrauterine and perinatal infections. *In* Galasso, G. J., Merigan, T. C., and Buchanan, R. A. (eds.): Antiviral Agents and Viral Diseases of Man. 2nd ed. New York, Raven Press, 1984, pp. 433–486.
3. Alford, C. A., and Griffiths, P. D.: Rubella. *In* Remington, J. S., and Klein, J. O. (eds.): Infectious Diseases of the Fetus and Newborn Infant. Philadelphia, W. B. Saunders, 1983, pp. 69–103.
4. Alpers, M. P.: Epidemiology and ecology of kuru. *In* Prusiner, S. B., and Hadlow, W. J. (eds.): Slow Transmissible Diseases of the Nervous System. New York, Academic Press, 1979, pp. 67–90.
5. Alter, M.: Creutzfeldt-Jakob disease: Hypothesis for high incidence in Libyan Jews in Israel. Science *186*:848, 1974.
6. Amyx, H. L., Gibbs, C. J., Gajdusek, D. C., et al.: Absence of vertical transmission of subacute spongiform viral encephalopathies in experimental primates. Proc. Soc. Exp. Biol. Med. *166*:469–471, 1981.
7. Antinori, A., De Luca, A., Ammassari, A., et al.: Failure of cytarabine and increased JC virus-DNA burden in the cerebrospinal fluid of patients with AIDS-related progressive multifocal leucoencephalopathy. AIDS *8*:1022–1024, 1994.
8. Åstrom, K. E., Mancall, E. L., and Richardson, E. P.: Progressive multifocal leukoencephalopathy. Brain *81*:93–111, 1958.
9. Au, W. J., Gabor, A. J., Vijayan, N., et al.: Periodic lateralized epileptiform complexes (PLEDs) in Creutzfeldt-Jakob disease. Neurology *30*:611–617, 1980.
10. Ault, G. S., and Stoner, G. L.: Two major types of JC virus defined in progressive multifocal leukoencephalopathy brain by early and late coding region DNA sequences. J. Gen. Virol. *73*:2669–2678, 1992.
11. Baczko, K., Pardowitz, J., Rima, B. K., et al.: Constant and variable regions of measles virus proteins encoded by the nucleocapsid and phosphoprotein genes derived from lytic and persistent viruses. Virology *190*:469–474, 1992.
12. Bahmanyar, S., Moreau-Dubois, M. C., Brown, P., et al.: Serum antibodies to neurofilament antigens in patients with neurological and other diseases and in healthy controls. J. Neuroimmunol. *5*:191–196, 1983.
13. Baram, T. Z., Gonzalez, G. I., Xie, Z. D., et al.: Subacute sclerosing panencephalitis in an infant: Diagnostic role of viral genome analysis. Ann. Neurol. *36*:103–108, 1994.
14. Barboriak, D. P., Provenzale, J. M., and Boyko, O. B.: MR diagnosis of Creutzfeldt-Jakob disease: Significance of high signal intensity of the basal ganglia. Am. J. Radiol. *162*:137–140, 1994.
15. Baron, H., Cathala, F., Brown, P., et al.: Familial Creutzfeldt-Jakob disease in France: Epidemiological implications. Eur. J. Epidemiol. *2*:252–264, 1986.
16. Bass, B. L., and Weintraub, H.: An unwinding activity that covalently modifies its double-stranded RNA substrate. Cell *55*:1089–1098, 1988.
17. Bass, B. L., Weintraub, H., Cattaneo, R., et al.: Biased hypermutation of viral RNA genomes could be due to unwinding/modification of double-stranded RNA. Cell *56*:331, 1989.
18. Bastian, F. O., and Jennings, R. A.: Creutzfeldt-Jakob disease: Procedures for handling diagnostic and research materials. Infect. Control *5*:48–50, 1984.
19. Beck, E., and Daniel, P. M.: Kuru and Creutzfeldt-Jakob disease: Neuropathological lesions and their significance. *In* Prusiner, S. B., and Hadlow, W. J. (eds.): Slow Transmissible Diseases of the Nervous System. New York, Academic Press, 1979, pp. 253–270.
20. Beersma, M. F., Galama, J. M., Van Druten, H. A., et al.: Subacute sclerosing panencephalitis in the Netherlands: 1976–1990. Int. J. Epidemiol. *21*:583–588, 1992.
21. Bell, J. E., and Ironside, J. W.: Neuropathology of spongiform encephalopathies in humans. Br. Med. Bull. *49*:738–777, 1993.
22. Bendheim, P. E., Potempska, A., Kascsak, R. J., et al.: Purification and partial characterization of the normal cellular homologue of the scrapie agent protein. J. Infect. Dis. *158*:1198–1208, 1988.
23. Benveniste, E. N.: Role of cytokines in multiple sclerosis, autoimmune encephalitis, and other neurological disorders. *In* Aggarawal, B., and Puri, R. (eds.): Human Cytokines: Their Role in Disease and Therapy. Boston, Blackwell Scientific, 1994, pp. 195–215.
24. Berger, J. R., Kaszovitz, B., Post, M. J., et al.: Progressive multifocal leukoencephalopathy associated with human immunodeficiency virus infection: A review of the literature with a report of sixteen cases. Ann. Intern. Med. *107*:78–87, 1987.
25. Berger, J. R., Moskowitz, L., Fischl, M., et al.: Neurological complications in the acquired immune deficiency syndrome: Often the initial manifestation. Neurology *34*:134–135, 1984.
26. Berger, J. R., and Mucke, L.: Prolonged survival and partial recovery in AIDS-associated progressive multifocal leukoencephalopathy. Neurology *38*:1060–1065, 1988.
27. Berger, J. R., Scott, G., Albrecht, J., et al.: Progressive multifocal leukoencephalopathy in HIV-1–infected children. AIDS *6*:837–841, 1992.
28. Bernoulli, C., Siegfried, J., and Baumgartner, G.: Danger of accidental person-to-person transmission of Creutzfeldt-Jakob disease by surgery. Lancet *1*:478–479, 1977.
29. Bessen, R. A., Kocisko, D. A., Raymond, G. J., et al.: Non-genetic propagation of strain-specific properties of scrapie prion protein. Nature *375*:698–700, 1995.
30. Bhettay, M. A., Kipps, A., and McDonald, R.: Early onset of subacute sclerosing panencephalitis. J. Pediatr. *89*:271–272, 1976.
31. Billeter, M. A., Cattaneo, R., Spielhofer, P., et al.: Generation and properties of measles virus mutations typically associated with subacute sclerosing panencephalitis. Ann. N.Y. Acad. Sci. *724*:367–377, 1994.
32. Bodechtel, G., and Guttmann, E.: Diffuse encephalitis mit sklerosierender

entzurdurg des hemispharemarkes. Z. Gesamte Neurol. Psychiatrie *133*:601–610, 1931.
33. Boldorini, R., Cristina, S., Vago, L., et al.: Ultrastructural studies in the lytic phase of progressive multifocal leukoencephalopathy in AIDS patients. Ultrastruc. Pathol. *17*:599–609, 1993.
34. Borchelt, D. R., Scott, M., Taraboulos, A., et al.: Scrapie and cellular prion proteins differ in their kinetics of synthesis and topology in cultured cells. J. Cell. Biol. *110*:743–752, 1990.
35. Bortone, E., Bettoni, L., Giorgi, C., et al.: Reliability of EEG in the diagnosis of Creutzfeldt-Jakob disease. Electroencephalogr. Clin. Neurophysiol. *90*:323–330, 1994.
36. Bouteille, M., Fontaine, C., and Vedrenne, C., et al.: Sur un cas d'encephalite subaigue à l'inclusions étude anatomoclinique et ultrastructurale. Rev. Neurol. (Paris) *113*:454–474, 1965.
37. Bradley, R.: Bovine spongiform encephalopathy (BSE): The current situation and research. Eur. J. Epidemiol. *7*:532–544, 1991.
38. Bradley, R., and Wilesmith, J. W.: Epidemiology and control of bovine spongiform encephalopathy (BSE). Br. Med. Bull. *49*:932–959, 1993.
39. Brajczewska, F. W., Iwinska, B., Kruszewska, J., et al.: Interleukin 1 and 2 production by peripheral blood mononuclear cells in subacute sclerosing panencephalitis and exacerbation of multiple sclerosis. Acta Neurol. Scand. *80*:390–393, 1989.
40. Brechot, C., Pourcel, C., Louise, A., et al.: Presence of integrated hepatitis B virus DNA sequences in cellular DNA in human hepatocellular carcinoma. Nature *286*:533–535, 1980.
41. Brown, P.: The decline and fall of Creutzfeldt-Jakob disease associated with human growth hormone therapy. Neurology *38*:1135–1137, 1988.
42. Brown, P.: Human growth hormone therapy and Creutzfeldt-Jakob disease: A drama in three acts. Pediatrics *81*:85–92, 1988.
43. Brown, P.: EEG findings in Creutzfeldt-Jakob disease. J. A. M. A. *269*:3168, 1993.
44. Brown, P., Cathala, F., Castaigne, P., et al.: Creutzfeldt-Jakob disease: Clinical analysis of a consecutive series of 230 neuropathologically verified cases. Ann. Neurol. *20*:597–602, 1986.
45. Brown, P., Cathala, F., and Gajdusek, D. C.: Creutzfeldt-Jakob disease decade 1968–1977. Ann. Neurol. *6*:438–446, 1978.
46. Brown, P., Cathala, F., Raubertas, R. F., et al.: The epidemiology of Creutzfeldt-Jakob disease: Conclusion of a 15-year investigation in France and review of the world literature. Neurology *37*:895–904, 1987.
47. Brown, P., Cathala, F., Sadowsky, D., et al.: Creutzfeldt-Jakob disease in France. II. Clinical characteristics of 124 consecutive verified cases during the decade 1968–1977. Ann. Neurol. *6*:430–437, 1979.
48. Brown, P., Gibbs, C. J., Jr., Rodgers-Johnson, P., et al.: Human spongiform encephalopathy: The National Institutes of Health series of 300 cases of experimentally transmitted disease. Ann. Neurol. *35*:513–529, 1994.
49. Bruce, M. E., and Dickinson, A. G.: Biological evidence that scrapie agent has an independent genome. J. Gen. Virol. *68*:79–89, 1987.
50. Brumback, R. A.: Routine use of phenolized formalin in fixation of autopsy brain tissue to reduce risk of inadvertent transmission of Creutzfeldt-Jakob disease. N. Engl. J. Med. *319*:654, 1988.
51. Butler, D. A., Scott, M. R., Bockman, J. M., et al.: Scrapie-infected murine neuroblastoma cells produce protease-resistant prion proteins. J. Virol. *62*:1558–1564, 1988.
52. Canal, N., and Torck, P.: An epidemiologic study of subacute sclerosing leucoencephalitis in Belgium. J. Neurol. Sci. *1*:380–389, 1964.
53. Canelas, H. M., Juliano, O. F., Lefevre, A. B., et al.: Subacute sclerosing leucoencephalitis: An epidemiological, clinical, and biochemical study of 31 cases. Arg. Neuropsiquiatr. *25*:255–268, 1967.
54. Cathala, F., Chatelain, J., Brown, P., et al.: Familial Cretuzfeldt-Jakob disease: Autosomal dominance in 14 members over three generations. J. Neurol. Sci. *47*:343–351, 1980.
55. Cattaneo, R., and Billeter, M. A.: Mutations and A/I hypermutations in measles virus persistent infections. Curr. Top. Microbiol. Immunol. *176*:63–74, 1992.
56. Cattaneo, R., Schmid, A., Billeter, M. A., et al.: Multiple viral mutations rather than host factors cause defective measles virus gene expression in subacute sclerosing panencephalitis cell line. J. Virol. *62*:1388–1397, 1988.
57. Cattaneo, R., Schmid, A., Eschle, D., et al.: Biased hypermutation and other genetic changes in defective measles viruses in human brain infections. Cell *55*:255–265, 1988.
58. Caughey, B.: Scrapie associated PrP accumulation and its prevention: Insights from cell culture. Br. Med. Bull. *49*:860–872, 1993.
59. Caughey, B., Neary, K., Buller, R., et al.: Normal and scrapie-associated forms of prion protein differ in their sensitivities to phospholipse and proteases in intact neuroblastoma cells. J. Virol. *64*:1093–1101, 1990.
60. Caughey, B., Race, R., Vogel, M., et al.: In vitro expression of cloned PrP cDNA derived from scrapie-infected mouse brain: Lack of transmission of scrapie infectivity. Ciba Found. Symp. *135*:197–208, 1988.
61. Caughey, B., Race, R. E., Vogel, M., et al.: In vitro expression in eukaryotic cells of a prion protein gene cloned from scrapie-infected mouse brain. Proc. Natl. Acad. Sci. U. S. A. *85*:4657–4661, 1988.
62. Caughey, B., Race, R., Vogel, M., et al.: Prion protein biosynthesis in scrapie-infected and uninfected neuroblastoma cells. J. Virol. *63*:175–181, 1989.
63. Chaisson, R. E., and Griffin, D. E.: Progressive multifocal leukoencephalopathy in AIDS. J. A. M. A. *264*:79–82, 1990.
64. Chalmers, T. C., and Smith, H.: Inosiplex and SSPE. Lancet *1*:1475, 1982.
65. Chappell, E. T., Guthrie, B. L., and Orenstein, J.: The role of stereotactic biopsy in the management of HIV-related focal brain lesions. Neurosurgery *30*:825–829, 1992.
66. Chatelain, J., Cathala, J., Brown, P., et al.: Epidemiological comparisons between Creutzfeldt-Jakob disease and scrapie in France during a 12-year period, 1968–1979. J. Neurol. Sci. *51*:329–337, 1981.
67. Chatiguy, M. A., and Prusiner, S. B.: Biohazards of investigations on the transmissible spongiform encephalopathies. Rev. Infect. Dis. *2*:713–724, 1980.
68. Chesebro, B., Race, R., Wehrly, K., et al.: Identification of scrapie PRION protein-specific mRNA in scrapie-infected and uninfected brain. Nature *315*:331–333, 1985.
69. Chiofalo, N., Fuentes, A. L., and G'Alvez, S.: Serial EEG findings in 27 cases of Creutzfeldt-Jakob disease. Arch. Neurol. *37*:143–145, 1980.
70. Cianchetti, C., Marrosu, M. G., Manconi, P. E., et al.: Subacute sclerosing panencephalitis in only one of identical twins: Case report with study of cell-mediated immunity. Eur. Neurol. *22*:428–432, 1983.
71. Cobb, W., and Hill, D.: EEG in subacute progressive encephalitis. Brain *73*:392–404, 1950.
72. Cobb, W. A., Marshall, J., and Scarrvilli, F.: Long survival in subacute sclerosing panencephalitis. J. Neurol. Neurosurg. Psychiatr. *47*:176–183, 1984.
73. Connolly, J. H., Allen, I. V., Hurwitz, L. J., et al.: Measles-virus antibody and antigen in subacute sclerosing panencephalitis. Lancet *1*:542–544, 1967.
74. Conrad, A. J., Chiang, E. Y., Andeen, L. E., et al.: Quantitation of intrathecal measles virus IgG antibody synthesis rate: Subacute sclerosing panencephalitis and multiple sclerosis. J. Neuroimmunol. *54*:99–108, 1994.
75. Coyle, P. K., and Wolinsky, J. S.: Characterization of immune complexes in progressive rubella panencephalitis. Ann. Neurol. *9*:557–562, 1981.
76. Cremer, N. E., Oshiro, L. S., Weil, M. L., et al.: Isolation of rubella virus from brain in chronic progressive panencephalitis. J. Gen. Virol. *29*:143–153, 1975.
77. Croxson, M., Brown, P., Synek, B., et al.: A new case of Creutzfeldt-Jakob disease associated with human growth hormone therapy in New Zealand. Neurology *38*:1128–1130, 1988.
78. Cuille, J., and Chelle, P. L.: Pathologie animale la maladie dile tremblante du mouton est-elle inoculable. C. R. Acad. Sci. *203*:1552–1554, 1936.
79. Czub, M., Braig, H. R., and Diringer, H.: Replication of the scrapie agent in hamsters infected intracerebrally confirms the pathogenesis of an amyloid-inducing virosis. J. Gen. Virol. *69*:1753–1756, 1988.
80. Davis, L. E., Bodian, D., Price, D., et al.: Chronic progressive poliomyelitis secondary to vaccination of an immunodeficient child. N. Engl. J. Med. *297*:241–245, 1977.
81. Dawson, J. R.: Cellular inclusions in cerebral lesions of lethargic encephalitis. Am. J. Pathol. *9*:7–15, 1933.
82. DeArmond, S. J.: Overview of the transmissible spongiform encephalopathies: Prion protein disorders. Br. Med. Bull. *49*:725–737, 1993.
83. Defanti, C. A., Franza, A., D'Angelo, et al.: SSPE: Clinical, EEG and neuroradiological findings in a series of 69 cases. *In* Bergamini, F., Defanti, C. A., and Ferrante, P. (eds.): Subacute Sclerosing Panencephalitis: A Reappraisal. Amsterdam, Elsevier, 1986, pp. 121–131.
84. Desmond, M. M., Fisher, E. S., Vorderman, A. L., et al.: The longitudinal course of congenital rubella encephalitis in nonretarded children. J. Pediatr. *93*:584–591, 1978.
85. Detels, R., Brody, J. A., McNew, J., et al.: Further epidemiologic studies of subacute sclerosing panencephalitis. Lancet *2*:11–14, 1973.
86. Dhib-Jalbut, S., and Haddad, F. S.: Subacute sclerosing panencephalitis in one member of identical twins. Neuropediatrics *15*:49–51, 1984.
87. Dhib-Jalbut, S., Jacobson, S., McFarlin, D. E., et al.: Impaired human leukocyte antigen–restricted measles virus–specific cytotoxic T-cell response in subacute sclerosing panencephalitis. Ann. Neurol. *25*:272–280, 1989.
88. Dhib-Jalbut, S., McFarland, H. F., Mingioli, E. S., et al.: Humoral and cellular immune responses to matrix protein of measles virus in subacute sclerosing panencephalitis. J. Virol. *62*:2483–2489, 1988.
89. Dhib-Jalbut, S. S., Abdelnoor, A. M., and Haddad, F. S.: Cellular and humoral immunity in subacute sclerosing panencephalitis. Infect. Immun. *33*:34–42, 1981.
90. Di Rocco, A., Molinari, S., Stollman, A. L., et al.: MRI abnormalities in Creutzfeldt-Jakob disease. Neuroradiology *35*:584–585, 1993.
91. Dickenson, A. G., Fraser, H., McConnell, I., et al.: Extraneural competition between different scrapie agents leading to loss of infectivity. Nature *253*:556, 1975.
92. Dimmock, N. J., and Barrett, A. D.: Defective viruses in diseases. Curr. Top. Microbiol. Immunol. *128*:55–84, 1986.
93. Diringer, H., Braig, H. R., and Czub, M.: Scrapie: A virus-induced amyloidosis of the brain. Ciba Found. Symp. *135*:135–145, 1988.
94. Doh-ura, K., Tateishi, J., Kitamoto, T., et al.: Creutzfeldt-Jakob disease patients with congophilic kuru plaques have the missense variant prion protein common to Gerstmann-Straussler syndrome. Ann. Neurol. *27*:121–126, 1990.

95. Dorries, K., Vogel, E., Gunther, S., et al.: Infection of human polyomaviruses JC and BK in peripheral blood leukocytes from immunocompetent individuals. Virology *198*:59–70, 1994.
96. Drew, P., Lonergan, M., Goldstein, M., et al.: Regulation of MHC class I and §-microglobulin gene expression in human neuronal cells. J. Immunol. *150*:3300–3310, 1993.
97. Duda, E. E., Huttenlocher, P. R., and Patronas, N. J.: CT of subacute sclerosing panencephalitis. Am. J. Neuroradiol. *1*:35–38, 1980.
98. Duffy, P., Wolf, J., Collins, G., et al.: Possible person-to-person transmission of Creutzfeldt-Jakob disease. N. Engl. J. Med. *290*:692–693, 1974.
99. Durant, R. H., and Dyken, P. R.: The effect of Inosiplex on the survival of subacute sclerosing panencephalitis. Neurology *33*:1053–1055, 1983.
100. Durant, R. H., Dyken, P. R., and Swift, A. V.: The influence of Inosiplex treatment on the neurological disability of patients with subacute sclerosing panencephalitis. J. Pediatr. *101*:1982.
101. Dyken, P. R., Cunningham, S. C., and Ward, L. C.: Changing character of subacute sclerosing panencephalitis in the United States. Pediatr. Neurol. *5*:339–341, 1989.
102. Eizuru, Y., Sakihama, K., Minamishima, Y., et al.: Re-evaluation of a case of progressive multifocal leukoencephalopathy previously diagnosed as simian virus 40 (SV40) etiology [published erratum appears in Acta Pathol. Jpn. *43*:535, 1993]. Acta Pathol. Jpn. *43*:327–332, 1993.
103. Esiri, M. M., Oppenheimer, D. R., Brownell, B., et al.: Distribution of measles antigen and immunoglobulin-containing cells in the CNS in subacute sclerosing panencephalitis (SSPE) and atypical measles encephalitis. J. Neurol. Sci. *53*:29–43, 1982.
104. Esiri, M. M., Reading, M. C., Squier, M. V., et al.: Immunocytochemical characterization of the macrophage and lymphocyte infiltrate in the brain in six cases of human encephalitis of varied aetiology. Neuropathol. Appl. Neurobiol. *15*:289–305, 1989.
105. Farguhan, J., and Gajdusek, D. C.: Kuru: Correspondence on the Discovery and Original Investigation. New York, Raven Press, 1979.
106. Farrell, O. F.: The EEG in progressive multifocal leukoencephalopathy. Electroencephalogr. Clin. Neurophysiol. *26*:200–205, 1969.
107. Feiden, W., Bise, K., Steude, U., et al.: The stereotactic biopsy diagnosis of focal intracerebral lesions in AIDS patients. Acta Neurol. Scand. *87*:228–233, 1993.
108. Flomenbaum, M. A., Jarcho, J. A., and Schoen, F. J.: Progressive multifocal leukoencephalopathy fifty-seven months after heart transplantation. J. Heart Lung Transplant. *10*:888–893, 1991.
109. Foley, J., and William, D.: Inclusion encephalitis and its relation to subacute sclerosing panencephalitis. Q. J. Med. *22*:157–194, 1953.
110. Fong, I. W., Britton, C. B., Luinstra, K. E., et al.: Diagnostic value of detecting JC virus DNA in cerebrospinal fluid of patients with progressive multifocal leukoencephalopathy. J. Clin. Microbiol. *33*:484–486, 1995.
111. Fraser, H., and Dickinson, A. G.: Scrapie in mice: Agent-strain differences in the distribution and intensity of grey matter vacuolation. J. Comp. Pathol. *82*:29–40, 1973.
112. Freeman, J. M.: The clinical spectrum and early diagnosis of Dawson's encephalitis. J. Pediatr. *75*:590–603, 1969.
113. Fujinami, R. S., and Oldstone, M. B. A.: Alterations in expression of measles virus polypeptides by antibody in molecular events in antibody-induced antigenic modulation. J. Immunol. *125*:78–85, 1980.
114. Fukuyama, Y., Nihei, Y., Matsumoto, S., et al.: Clinical effects of MND-19 (Inosiplex) on subacute sclerosing panencephalitis: A multi-institutional collaborative study: The Inosiplex-SSPE Research Committee. Brain Dev. *9*:270–282, 1987.
115. Furlow, T. W., Whitley, R. J., and Wilmes, F.: Repeated suppression of Creutzfeldt-Jakob disease with vidarabine. Lancet *2*:564–565, 1982.
116. G'Alvez, S., Cartier, L., Monari, M., et al.: Familial Creutzfeldt-Jakob disease in Chile. J. Neurol. Sci. *59*:139–147, 1983.
117. Gajdusek, D. C.: Journals 1959–1983. 34 volumes, published in limited edition.
118. Gajdusek, D. C.: Unconventional viruses and the origin and disappearance of kuru. Science *197*:943–960, 1977.
119. Gajdusek, D. C.: Mudd Award Lecture. VIIIth International Congress of Virology, Berlin. August 26–31, 1990.
120. Gajdusek, D. C.: Subacute spongiform encephalopathies: Transmissible cerebral amyloidoses caused by unconventional viruses. *In* Fields, B. N., Knipe, D. M., Chanock, R. M., et al. (eds.): Virology. 2nd ed. New York, Raven Press, 1990, pp. 2289–2334.
121. Gajdusek, D. C.: Nucleation of amyloidogenesis in infectious and noninfectious amyloidoses of brain. Ann. N. Y. Acad. Sci. *724*:173–190, 1994.
122. Gajdusek, D. C.: Spontaneous generation of infectious nucleating amyloids in the transmissible and nontransmissible cerebral amyloidoses. Mol. Neurobiol. *8*:1–13, 1994.
123. Gajdusek, D. C.: Infectious amyloids: Subacute spongiform encephalopathies as transmissible cerebral amyloidoses. *In* Fields, B. N., Knipe, D. M., Howley, P. M., et al. (eds.): Virology. 3rd ed. Philadelphia, Lippincott-Raven, 1996, pp. 2851–2900.
124. Gambetti, P., Petersen, R., Monari, L., et al.: Fatal familial insomnia and the widening spectrum of prion diseases. Br. Med. Bull. *49*:980–994, 1993.
125. Gardner, S. D., Field, A. M., Coleman, D. V., et al.: New human papovavirus (BK) isolated from urine after renal transplantation. Lancet *1*:1253–1257, 1971.
126. Gerson, K. L., and Haslam, R. H. A.: Subtle immunologic abnormalities in four boys with subacute sclerosing panencephalitis. N. Engl. J. Med. *285*:78–82, 1971.
127. Gibbs, C. J.: Virus-induced subacute degenerative diseases of the central nervous system. Ophthalmology *87*:1208–1218, 1980.
128. Gibbs, C. J., Asher, D. M., Kobrine, A., et al.: Transmission of Creutzfeldt-Jakob disease to a chimpanzee by electrodes contaminated during neurosurgery. J. Neurol. Neurosurg. Psych. *57*:757–758, 1994.
129. Gilden, D. H., Rorke, L. B., and Tanaka, R.: Acute SSPE. Arch. Neurol. *32*:644–646, 1975.
130. Gillespie, S. M., Chang, Y., Lemp, G., et al.: Progressive multifocal leukoencephalopathy in persons infected with human immunodeficiency virus, San Francisco, 1981–1989. Ann. Neurol. *30*:597–604, 1991.
131. Godec, M. S., Asher, D. M., Kozachuk, W. E., et al.: Blood buffy coat from Alzheimer's disease patients and their relatives does not transmit spongiform encephalopathy to hamsters. Neurology *44*:1111–1115, 1994.
132. Goldberg, H., Alter, M., and Kahana, E.: The Libyan Jewish focus of Creutzfeldt-Jakob disease: A search for the modes of natural transmission. *In* Prusiner, S. B., and Hadlow, W. J. (eds.): Slow Transmissible Diseases of the Nervous System. New York, Academic Press, 1979, pp. 451–460.
133. Goldgaber, D., Goldfarb, L. G., Brown, P., et al.: Mutations in familial Creutzfeldt-Jakob disease and Gerstmann-Straussler-Scheinker's syndrome. Exp. Neurol. *106*:204–206, 1989.
134. Greenfield, J. G.: Encephalitis and encephalomyelitis in England and Wales during the last decade. Brain *73*:141–166, 1950.
135. Guilleux, M. H., Steiner, R. E., and Young, I. R.: MR imaging in progressive multifocal leukoencephalopathy. Am. J. Neuroradiol. *7*:1033–1035, 1986.
136. Haddad, F. S., and Risk, W. S.: Isoprinosine treatment in 18 patients with subacute sclerosing panencephalitis: A controlled study. Ann. Neurol. *7*:185–188, 1980.
137. Hadlow, W. J.: Scrapie and kuru. Lancet *2*:289, 1959.
138. Hair, L. S., Nuovo, G., Powers, J. M., et al.: Progressive multifocal leukoencephalopathy in patients with human immunodeficiency virus. Hum. Pathol. *23*:663–667, 1992.
139. Hall, W. W., and Chopin, P. W.: Evidence for lack of synthesis of the M polypeptide of measles virus in brain cells in subacute sclerosing panencephalitis. Virology *99*:443–447, 1979.
140. Hall, W. W., and Chopin, P. W.: Measles virus proteins in the brain tissue of patients with subacute sclerosing panencephalitis: Absence of the M proteins. N. Engl. J. Med. *304*:1152–1155, 1981.
141. Hall, W. W., Lamb, R. A., and Choppin, P. W.: Measles and subacute sclerosing panencephalitis virus proteins: Lack of antibodies to the M protein in patients with subacute sclerosing panencephalitis. Proc. Natl. Acad. Sci. U. S. A. *76*:2047–2051, 1979.
142. Halsey, N. A., Modlin, J. F., Jabbour, J. T., et al.: Risk factors in subacute sclerosing panencephalitis: A case control study. Am. J. Epidemiol. *111*:415–424, 1980.
143. Haltia, M., Kovanen, J., Van Crevel, H., et al.: Familial Creutzfeldt-Jakob disease. J. Neurol. Sci. *42*:381–389, 1979.
144. Handzel, Z. T., Gadoth, N., Idar, D., et al.: Cell mediated immunity and effects of thymic humoral factor in 15 patients with SSPE. Brain Dev. *5*:29–35, 1983.
145. Haraguchi, T., Fisher, S., Olofsson, S., et al.: Asparagine-linked glycosylation of the scrapie and cellular prion proteins. Arch. Biochem. Biophys. *274*:1–13, 1989.
146. Hawkins, C. P., McLaughlin, J. E., Kendall, B. E., et al.: Pathological findings correlated with MRI in HIV infection. Neuroradiology *35*:264–268, 1993.
147. Hayashi, R., Hanyu, N., Kuwabara, T., et al.: Serial computed tomographic and electroencephalographic studies in Creutzfeldt-Jakob disease. Acta Neurol. Scand. *85*:161–165, 1992.
148. Heide, W., Kompf, D., Reusche, E., et al.: Failure of cytarabine/interferon therapy in progressive multifocal leukoencephalopathy. Ann. Neurol. *37*:412–413, 1995.
149. Hiatt, R. L., Grizzard, H. T., McNeer, P., et al.: Ophthalmologic manifestations of SSPE. Trans. Am. Acad. Ophthalmol. Otolaryngol. *75*:344–350, 1971.
150. Hirsch, M. S.: Herpes group virus infections in the compromised host. *In* Rubin, R. H., and Young, L. (eds.): Clinical Approach to Infection in the Immunocompromised Host. New York, Plenum Press, 1988, pp. 389–415.
151. Ho, K., Garancis, J. C., Paegle, R. D., et al.: Progressive multifocal leukoencephalopathy and malignant lymphoma of the brain in a patient with immunosuppressive therapy. Acta Neuropathol. *52*:81–83, 1980.
152. Hofman, F. M., Hinton, D. R., Baemayr, J., et al.: Lymphokines and immunoregulatory molecules in subacute sclerosing panencephalitis. Clin. Immunol. Immunopathol. *58*:331–342, 1991.
153. Holland, J., Spindler, K., Horodyski, F., et al.: Rapid evolution of RNA genomes. Science *215*:1577–1585, 1982.
154. Holman, R. C., Janssen, R. S., Buehler, J. W., et al.: Epidemiology of progressive multifocal leukoencephalopathy in the United States: Analysis of national mortality and AIDS surveillance data. Neurology *41*:1733–1736, 1991.
155. Hope, J., Reekie, L. J. D., Hunter, N., et al.: Fibrils from brains of cows

with new cattle disease contain scrapie-associated protein. Nature *366*:390–392, 1988.
156. Hope, J., Ritchie, L., Farquhar, C., et al.: Bovine spongiform encephalopathy: A scrapie-like disease of British cattle. Prog. Clin. Biol. Res. *317*:659–667, 1989.
157. Horn, G. V., Bastian, F. O., and Moake, J. L.: Progressive multifocal leukoencephalopathy: Failure of response to transfer factor and cytarabine. Neurology *28*:794–797, 1978.
158. Hornabrook, R. W.: Kuru and clinical neurology. *In* Prusiner, S. B., and Hadlow, W. J. (eds.): Slow Transmissible Diseases of the Nervous System. New York, Academic Press, 1979, pp. 37–66.
159. Horta-Barbosa, L., Fuccillo, D. A., Sever, J. L., et al.: Subacute sclerosing panencephalitis: Isolation of measles virus from a brain biopsy. Nature *221*:974, 1969.
160. Houff, S. A., Madden, D. L., and Sever, J. L.: Subacute sclerosing panencephalitis in only one of identical twins: A seven year follow-up. Arch. Neurol. *36*:854–856, 1979.
161. Hsiao, K., Baker, H. F., Crow, T. J., et al.: Linkage of a prion protein missense variant to Gerstmann-Straussler syndrome. Nature *338*:342–345, 1989.
162. Hsiao, K., Meiner, Z., Kahana, E., et al.: Mutation of the prion protein in Libyan Jews with Creutzfeldt-Jakob disease. N. Engl. J. Med. *324*:1091–1097, 1991.
163. Hsiao, K. K., Westaway, D. A., and Prusiner, S. B.: An amino acid substitution in the prion protein of ataxic Gerstmann-Straussler syndrome. Am. J. Hum. Genet. *43*:A87, 1988.
164. Huang, A. S.: Modulation of viral disease processes by defective interfering particles. *In* Domingo, E., Holland, J. J., and Ahlquist, P. (eds.): RNA Genetics. Vol. III. Boca Raton, CRC Press, 1988, pp. 195–208.
165. Huckman, M. S.: Computed tomography in the diagnosis of degenerative brain disease. Radiol. Clin. North Am. *20*:169–183, 1982.
166. Hunter, G. D.: The enigma of the scrapie agent: Biochemical approaches and the involvement of membranes and nucleic acids. *In* Prusiner, S. B., and Hadlow, W. J. (eds.): Slow Transmissible Diseases of the Nervous System. New York, Academic Press, 1979, pp. 365–385.
167. Huttenlocker, P. R., and Mattson, R. H.: Isoprinosine in subacute sclerosing panencephalitis. Neurology *29*:763–771, 1979.
168. Iacoangeli, M., Roselli, R., Antinori, A., et al.: Experience with brain biopsy in acquired immune deficiency syndrome-related focal lesions of the central nervous system. Br. J. Surg. *81*:1508–1511, 1994.
169. Ibrahim, M. M., and Jetuons, P. M.: The value of electroencephalography in the diagnosis of subacute sclerosing panencephalitis. Dev. Med. Child. Neurol. *16*:295–307, 1974.
170. Ironside, J. W., Lewis, F. A., Blythe, D., et al.: The identification of cells containing JC papovavirus DNA in progressive multifocal leukoencephalopathy by combined in situ hybridization and immunocytochemistry. J. Pathol. *157*:291–297, 1989.
171. Iwasaki, Y., Ikeda, K., Tagaya, N., et al.: Magnetic resonance imaging and neuropathological findings in two patients with Creutzfeldt-Jakob disease. J. Neurol. Sci. *126*:228–231, 1994.
172. Jabbour, J. T., Duenas, D. A., Sever, J. L., et al.: Epidemiology of SSPE, a report of the SSPE registry. J. A. M. A. *220*:959–962, 1972.
173. Jan, J. E., Tingle, A. J., Donald, G., et al.: Progressive rubella panencephalitis: Clinical course and response to isoprinosine. Dev. Med. Child. Neurol. *21*:648–652, 1979.
174. Jayakumar, P. N., Taly, A. B., Arya, B. Y., et al.: Computed tomography in subacute sclerosing panencephalitis: Report of 15 cases. Acta Neurol. Scand. *4*:328–330, 1988.
175. Johannes, R. S., and Sever, J. L.: Subacute sclerosing panencephalitis. Annu. Rev. Med. *26*:589–601, 1975.
176. Johnson, K. P., Norrby, E., Swoveland, P., et al.: Experimental subacute sclerosing panencephalitis: Selective disappearance of measles virus matrix protein from the central nervous system. J. Infect. Dis. *144*:161–169, 1981.
177. Johnson, R. T.: Chronic inflammatory and demyelinating diseases. *In* Johnson, R. T. (ed.): Viral Infections of the Nervous System. New York, Raven Press, 1982, pp. 237–270.
178. Johnson, R. T.: Viral Infections of the Nervous System. New York, Raven Press, 1982.
179. Jones, C. E., Dyken, P. R., Huttenlocker, P. R., et al.: Inosiplex therapy in subacute sclerosing panencephalitis: A multicenter non-randomized study in 98 patients. Lancet *1*:1034–1037, 1982.
180. Kackell, Y. M., Grob, P. J., Kreth, W. H., et al.: Transfer factor therapy in patients with subacute sclerosing panencephalitis. J. Neurol. *211*:39–49, 1975.
181. Kamin, M., and Patten, B. M.: Creutzfeldt-Jakob disease: Possible transmission to humans by consumption of wild animal brains. Am. J. Med. *76*:142–145, 1984.
182. Kascsak, R. J., Rubenstein, R., Merz, P. A., et al.: Immunological comparison of scrapie-associated fibrils isolated from animals infected with four different scrapie strains. J. Virol. *59*:676–683, 1986.
183. Kiessling, W. R., Hall, W. W., Yung, L. L., et al.: Measles specific immunoglobulin-M response in subacute sclerosing panencephalitis. Lancet *1*:324–327, 1977.
184. Kimberlin, R. H., and Walker, C. A.: Characteristics of a short incubation model of scrapie in the golden hamster. J. Gen. Virol. *34*:295–304, 1977.
185. Kimberlin, R. H., and Walker, C. A.: Evidence that the transmission of one source of scrapie agent to hamsters involves separation of agent strains from a mixture. J. Gen. Virol. *39*:487–496, 1978.
186. Kimberlin, R. H., and Walker, C. A.: Pathogenesis of experimental scrapie. Ciba Found. Symp. *135*:37–62, 1988.
187. Kimberlin, R. H., Walker, C. A., Millson, C. G., et al.: Disinfection studies with two strains of mouse passaged scrapie agent: Guidelines for Creutzfeldt-Jakob and related agents. J. Neurol. Sci. *59*:355–369, 1983.
188. King, J. O., Hart, D. H., Sullivan, J. R., et al.: Progressive multifocal leukoencephalopathy. Clin. Exp. Neurol. *17*:125–134, 1981.
189. Kingsbury, D. T., Kasper, K. C., Stites, D. P., et al.: Genetic control of scrapie and Creutzfeldt-Jakob disease in mice. J. Immunol. *131*:491–496, 1983.
190. Kirk, A., and Ang, L. C.: Unilateral Creutzfeldt-Jakob disease presenting as rapidly progressive aphasia. Can. J. Neurol. Sci. *21*:350–352, 1994.
191. Kitamoto, T., Amano, N., Terao, Y., et al.: A new inherited prion disease (PrP-P105L mutation) showing spastic paraparesis. Ann. Neurol. *34*:808–813, 1993.
192. Kitamoto, T., Tateishi, J., and Sato, Y.: Immunohistochemical verification of senile and kuru plaques in Creutzfeldt-Jakob disease and the allied disease. Ann. Neurol. *24*:537–542, 1988.
193. Kitamoto, T., Tateishi, J., Sawa, H., et al.: Positive transmission of Creutzfeldt-Jakob disease verified by murine kuru plaques. Lab. Invest. *60*:507–512, 1989.
194. Kitamoto, T., Tateishi, J., Tashima, T., et al.: Amyloid plaques in Creutzfeldt-Jakob disease stain with prion protein antibodies. Ann. Neurol. *20*:204–208, 1986.
195. Kondo, K., and Kuroiua, Y.: A case control study of Creutzfeldt-Jakob disease: association with physical injuries. Ann. Neurol. *11*:377–381, 1982.
196. Kondo, K., Takasu, T., and Ahmed, A.: Neurological diseases in Karachi, Pakistan: Elevated occurrence of subacute sclerosing panencephalitis. Neuroepidemiology *7*:66–80, 1988.
197. Kovanen, J., and Haltia, M.: Descriptive epidemiology of Creutzfeldt-Jakob disease in Finland. Acta Neurol. Scand. *77*:474–480, 1988.
198. Krawiecke, N. S., Dyken, P. R., El Gammal, T., et al.: Computed tomography of the brain in subacute sclerosing panencephalitis. Ann. Neurol. *15*:489–493, 1984.
199. Kreth, H. W., Dunker, R., Rodt, M., et al.: Immunohistochemical identification of T-lymphocytes in the central nervous system of patients with multiple sclerosis and subacute sclerosing panencephalitis. J. Neuroimmunol. 2:177–183, 1982.
200. Kretzschmar, H. A., Honold, A. G., Seitelberger, F., et al.: Prion protein mutation in family first reported by Gerstmann, Straussler, and Scheinker. Lancet *337*:1160, 1991.
201. Krupp, L. B., Lipton, R. B., Swerdlow, M. L., et al.: Progressive multifocal leukoencephalopathy: Clinical and radiographic features. Ann. Neurol. *17*:344–349, 1985.
202. Kuroiwa, Y., Celesia, G. C., and Chung, H. D.: Periodic EEG discharges and status spongiosus of the cerebral cortex in anoxic encephalopathy: A necropsy case report. J. Neurol. Neurosurg. Psychiatry *45*:740–742, 1982.
203. Lampson, L.: Molecular basis of the immune response to neural antigens. Trends Neurosci. *10*:211–216, 1987.
204. Lantos, P. L.: From slow virus to prion: A review of transmissible spongiform encephalopathies. Histopathology *20*:1–11, 1992.
205. Lantos, P. L., McGill, I. S., Janota, I., et al.: Prion protein immunocytochemistry helps to establish the true incidence of prion diseases. Neurosci. Lett. *147*:67–71, 1992.
206. Leads from the MMWR: Creutzfeldt-Jakob disease in a second patient who received a cadaveric dura mater graft. J. A. M. A. *261*:1118, 1989.
207. Lebon, P., and Lyon, G.: Non-congenital rubella encephalitis. Lancet *2*:468, 1974.
208. Levy, R. M., Russell, E., Yungbluth, M., et al.: The efficacy of image-guided stereotactic brain biopsy in neurologically symptomatic acquired immunodeficiency syndrome patients. Neurosurgery *30*:186–189, 1992.
209. Levy, S. R., Chiappa, K. H., Burke, C. J., et al.: Early evolution and incidence of electroencephalographic abnormalities in Creutzfeldt-Jakob disease. J. Clin. Neurophysiol. *3*:1–21, 1986.
210. Lin, F. H., and Thormar, H.: Absence of M protein in a cell-associated subacute sclerosing panencephalitis virus. Nature *285*:490–492, 1980.
211. Lipton, R. B., Krupp, L., Houroupian, D., et al.: Progressive multifocal leukoencephalopathy of the posterior fossa in an AIDS patient: Clinical, radiographic and evoked potential findings. Eur. Neurol. *28*:258–261, 1988.
212. Locht, C., Chesebro, B., Race, R., et al.: Molecular cloning and complete sequence of prion protein cDNA from mouse brain infected with the scrapie agent. Proc. Natl. Acad. Sci. U. S. A. *83*:6372–6376, 1986.
213. Loeber, G., and Dorries, K.: DNA rearrangements in organ-specific variants of polyomavirus JC strain GS. J. Virol. *62*:1730–1735, 1988.
214. Lucas, K. M., Sanders, R. C., Rongap, A., et al.: Subacute sclerosing panencephalitis (SSPE) in Papua New Guinea: A high incidence in young children. Epidemiol. Infect. *108*:547–53, 1992.
215. Luo, Y., and Huang, K.: Spongy degeneration of the CNS in infancy. Arch. Neurol. *41*:164–170, 1984.

216. Makenzie, D. J. M., Kipps, A., and McDonald, R.: Subacute sclerosing panencephalitis in southern Africa. S. Afr. Med. J. *49*:2083–2086, 1975.
217. Malmgren, R., Kurland, L., Mokri, B., et al.: The epidemiology of Creutzfeldt-Jakob disease. *In* Prusiner, S. B., and Hadlow, W. J. (eds.): Slow Transmissible Diseases of the Nervous System. New York, Academic Press, 1979, pp. 93–113.
218. Mandell, A. M., Alexander, M. P., and Carpenter, S.: Creutzfeldt-Jakob disease presenting as isolated aphasia. Neurology *39*:55–58, 1989.
219. Manuelidis, E. E., Gorgacs, E. J., and Manuelidis, L.: Viremia in experimental Creutzfeldt-Jakob disease. Science *200*:1069–1071, 1978.
220. Manuelidis, E. E., and Rorke, L. B.: Transmission of Alpers' disease (chronic progressive encephalopathy) produces experimental Creutzfeldt-Jakob disease in hamsters. Neurology *39*:615–621, 1989.
221. Mark, A. S., and Atlas, S. W.: Progressive multifocal leukoencephalopathy in patients with AIDS: Appearance on MR images. Radiology *173*:517–520, 1989.
222. Markard, O. N., and Panszi, J. G.: The electroencephalogram in subacute sclerosing panencephalitis. Arch. Neurol. *32*:719–726, 1975.
223. Martinovic, Z.: Periodic generalized bursts of fast waves in subacute sclerosing panencephalitis. Electroencephalogr. Clin. Neurophysiol. *63*:236–238, 1986.
224. Marzewski, D. J., Towfighi, J., Harrington, M. G., et al.: Creutzfeldt-Jakob disease following pituitary-derived human growth hormone therapy: A new American case. Neurology *38*:1131–1133, 1988.
225. Massa, P. T., Ozato, K., and McFarlin, D. E.: Cell type–specific regulation of major histocompatibility complex (MHC) class I gene expression in astrocytes, oligodendrocytes and neurons. Glia *8*:201–207, 1993.
226. Massaro, A. R., Agliano, A. M., and Grillo, R.: Immunoglobulin M specific for measles in serum and cerebrospinal fluid of patients with multiple sclerosis and other neurological diseases. J. Neurol. *217*:191–194, 1978.
227. Masters, C. L., Gajdusek, D. C., and Gibbs, C. J.: The familial occurrence of Creutzfeldt-Jakob disease and Alzheimer's disease. Brain *104*:535–558, 1981.
228. Masters, C. L., Harris, J. O., Gajdusek, D. C., et al.: Creutzfeldt-Jakob disease: Patterns of worldwide occurrence and the significance of familial and sporadic clustering. Ann. Neurol. *5*:177–188, 1979.
229. Matthews, W. B.: Bovine spongiform encephalopathy. Br. Med. J. *300*:412–413, 1990.
230. McGuire, D., Barhite, S., Hollander, H., et al.: JC virus DNA in cerebrospinal fluid of human immunodeficiency virus-infected patients: Predictive value for progressive multifocal leukoencephalopathy. Ann. Neurol. *37*:395–399, 1995.
231. McKinley, M. P., Bolton, D. C., and Prusiner, S. B.: A protease-resistant protein is a structural comnponent of the scrapie prion. Cell *35*:57–62, 1983.
232. Medori, R., Tritschler, H. J., LeBlanc, A., et al.: Fatal familial insomnia: A prion disease with a mutation at codon 178 of the prion protein gene. N. Engl. J. Med. *326*:444–449, 1992.
233. Mehta, P. D., Patrick, B. A., and Thormal, H.: Measles-specific IgG in CSF and serum from patients with subacute sclerosing panencephalitis. Immunology *46*:423–428, 1982.
234. Mehta, P. D., Thormar, H., Kulczycki, J., et al.: Immune response in subacute sclerosing panencephalitis. Ann. N. Y. Acad. Sci. *724*:378–384, 1994.
235. Menser, M. A., Harley, J. D., and Herzberg, R.: Persistence of virus in lens for three years after prenatal rubella. Lancet *2*:387–388, 1967.
236. Meyer, R. K., McKinley, M. P., Bowman, K. A., et al.: Separation and properties of cellular and scrapie prion proteins. Proc. Natl. Acad. Sci. U. S. A. *83*:2310–2314, 1986.
237. Miller, C. L.: Current impact of measles in the United Kingdom. Rev. Infect. Dis. *5*:427–432, 1983.
238. Modlin, J. F., Halsey, N. A., Conrad, J. L., et al.: Subacute sclerosing panencephalitis: A report of the National Registry. J. Pediatr. *94*:231–236, 1979.
239. Modlin, J. F., Halsey, N. A., Eddins, D. L., et al.: Epidemiology of subacute sclerosing panencephalitis. J. Pediatr. *94*:231–236, 1979.
240. Monari, L., Chen, S. G., Brown, P., et al.: Fatal familial insomnia and familial Creutzfeldt-Jakob disease: Different prion proteins determined by a DNA polymorphism. Proc. Natl. Acad. Sci. U. S. A. *91*:2839–2842, 1994.
241. Monef, G. R. G., and Sever, J. L.: Chronic infection of the central nervous system with rubella virus. Neurology *16*:111–116, 1966.
242. Monreal, J., Collins, G. H., Masters, C. L., et al.: Creutzfeldt-Jakob disease in an adolescent. J. Neurol. Sci. *52*:341–350, 1981.
243. Montagna, P., Cortelli, P., Gambetti, P., et al.: Fatal familial insomnia: Sleep, neuroendocrine and vegetative alterations. Adv. Neuroimmunol. *5*:13–21, 1995.
244. Moret, H., Guichard, M., Matheron, S., et al.: Virological diagnosis of progressive multifocal leukoencephalopathy: Detection of JC virus DNA in cerebrospinal fluid and brain tissue of AIDS patients. J. Clin. Microbiol. *31*:3310–3313, 1993.
245. Mori, M., Aoki, N., Shimada, H., et al.: Detection of JC virus in the brains of aged patients without progressive multifocal leukoencephalopathy by the polymerase chain reaction and southern hybridization analysis. Neurosci. Lett. *141*:151–155, 1992.
246. Mundinger, A., Adam, T., Ott, D., et al.: CT and MRI: Prognostic tools in patients with AIDS and neurological deficits. Neuroradiology *35*:75–78, 1992.
247. Mustafa, M. M., Weitman, S. D., Winick, N. J., et al.: Subacute measles encephalitis in the young immunocompromised host: Report of two cases diagnosed by polymerase chain reaction and treated with ribavirin and review of the literature. Clin. Infect. Dis. *16*:654–660, 1993.
248. Nagano, I., Nakamura, S., Yoshioka, M., et al.: Immunocytochemical analysis of the cellular infiltrate in brain lesions in subacute sclerosing panencephalitis. Neurology *41*:1639–42, 1991.
249. Nagano, I., Nakamura, S., Yoshioka, M., et al.: Expression of cytokines in brain lesions in subacute sclerosing panencephalitis. Neurology *44*:710–715, 1994.
250. Narayan, O., and Clements, J. E.: Biology and pathogenesis of lentiviruses of ruminant animals. *In* Wong-Staal, F., and Gallo, R. C. (eds.): Retrovirus Biology: An Emerging Role in Human Biology. New York, Marcel Dekker, 1988, pp. 117–147.
251. New, M. I., Brown, P., Temeck, J. W., et al.: Preclinical Creutzfeldt-Jakob disease discovered at autopsy in a human growth hormone recipient. Neurology *38*:1133–1134, 1988.
252. Newton, H. B., Makley, M., Slivka, A. P., et al.: Progressive multifocal leukoencephalopathy presenting as multiple enhancing lesions on MRI: Case report and literature review. J. Neuroimaging *5*:125–128, 1995.
253. Noetzel, M. J., and Dodson, W. E.: Progressive CT abnormalities desite clinical improvement in SSPE treated with Inosiplex. Ann. Neurol. *13*:457–460, 1983.
254. Oesch, B., Groth, D. F., Prusiner, S. B., et al.: Search for a scrapie-specific nucleic acid: A progress report. Ciba Found. Symp. *135*:209–223, 1988.
255. Oesch, B., Westaway, D., Walchli, M., et al.: A cellular gene encodes scrapie PrP 27-30 protein. Cell *40*:735–746, 1985.
256. Ogle, J. W., Toltzis, P., Parker, W. D., et al.: Oral ribavirin therapy for subacute sclerosing panencephalitis. J. Infect. Dis. *159*:748–750, 1989.
257. Okuno, Y., Nakao, T., Ishida, N., et al.: Incidence of subacute sclerosing panencephalitis following measels and measles vaccine in Japan. Int. J. Epidemiol. *18*:684–689, 1989.
258. Oldstone, M. B. A., Holmstoen, J., and Welsh, R. M.: Alterations of acetylcholine enzymes in neuroblastoma cells persistently infected with lymphocytic choriomeningitis virus. J. Cell. Physiol. *91*:459–472, 1977.
259. Oldstone, M. B. A., and Tishon, A.: Immunologic injury in measles virus infection. IV. Antigenic modulation and abrogation of lymphocyte lysis of virus-infected cells. Clin. Immunol. Immunopathol. *9*:55–62, 1978.
260. Olsson, J. E.: Brain and CSF proteins in Creutzfeldt-Jakob disease. Eur. Neurol. *19*:85–90, 1980.
261. Onofrj, M., Fulgente, T., Gambi, D., et al.: Early MRI findings in Creutzfeldt-Jakob disease. J. Neurol. *240*:423–426, 1993.
262. Owen, F., Poulter, M., Lofthouse, R., et al.: Insertion in prion protein gene in familial Creutzfeldt-Jakob disease. Lancet *1*:51–52, 1989.
263. Packer, R. J., Cornblath, D. R., Gonatas, N. K., et al.: Creutzfeldt-Jakob disease in a 20-year-old woman. Neurology *30*:492–496, 1980.
264. Padgett, B. L., and Walker, D. L.: Virologic and serologic studies of progressive multifocal leukoencephalopathy. Prog. Clin. Biol. Res. *105*:107–117, 1983.
265. Padgett, B. L., Walker, D. L., and Zurhein, G. M.: Cultivation of papova-like virus from human brain with progressive multifocal leukoencephalopathy. Lancet *1*:1257–1259, 1971.
266. Parr, J., Horoupian, D. S., and Winkelman, A. C.: Cerebellar form of progressive multifocal leukoencephalopathy (PML). Can. J. Neurol. Sci. *6*:123–128, 1979.
267. Patrick, B. A., Mehta, P. D., and Sobczyk, W.: Measles-virus specific immunoglobulin D antibody in cerebrospinal fluid and serum from patients with subacute sclerosing panencephalitis and multiple sclerosis. J. Neurol. Immunol. *26*:69–74, 1990.
268. Payne, F. E., Baublis, J. V., and Itabashi, H. H.: Isolation of measles virus from cell cultures of brain from a patient with subacute sclerosing panencephalitis. N. Engl. J. Med. *281*:585–587, 1969.
269. Pedersen, H., and Wulff, C. H.: Computed tomographic findings of early subacute sclerosing panencephalitis. Neuroradiology *23*:31–32, 1982.
270. Peters, A. C., Versteeg, J., Bots, G. T., et al.: Progressive multifocal leukoencephalopathy: Immunofluorescent demonstration of simian virus 40 antigen in CSF cells and response to cytarabine therapy. Arch. Neurol. *37*:497–501, 1980.
271. Portaluppi, F., Cortelli, P., Avoni, P., et al.: Diurnal blood pressure variation and hormonal correlates in fatal familial insomnia. Hypertension *23*:569–576, 1994.
272. Portaluppi, F., Cortelli, P., Avoni, P., et al.: Progressive disruption of the circadian rhythm of melatonin in fatal familial insomnia. J. Clin. Endocrinol. Metab. *78*:1075–1078, 1994.
273. Posner, C. M.: Notes on the pathogenesis of subacute sclerosing panencephalitis. J. Neurol. Sci. *95*:219–224, 1990.
274. Post, M. J., Kursunoglu, S. J., Hensley, G. T., et al.: Cranial CT in acquired immunodeficiency syndrome: Spectrum of diseases and optimal contrast enhancement technique. Am. J. Radiol. *145*:929–940, 1985.
275. Post, M. J., Sheldon, J. J., Hensley, G. T., et al.: Central nervous system disease in acquired immunodeficiency syndrome: Prospective correlation using CT, MR imaging, and pathologic studies. Radiology *158*:141–148, 1986.

276. Preskorn, S. H., and Watanabe, I.: Progressive multifocal leukoencephalopathy: Cerebral mass lesions. Surg. Neurol. *12*:231–234, 1979.
277. Prusiner, S. B.: Novel proteinaceous infectious particles cause scrapie. Science *216*:136–144, 1982.
278. Prusiner, S. B.: Prions and neurodegenerative disease. N. Engl. J. Med. *317*:1571–1581, 1987.
279. Prusiner, S. B.: Creutzfeldt-Jakob disease and scrapie prions. Alzheimer Dis. Assoc. Disord. *3*:52–78, 1989.
280. Prusiner, S. B.: Scrapie prions. Annu. Rev. Microbiol. *43*:345–374, 1989.
281. Prusiner, S. B.: Transgenetics and cell biology of prion diseases: Investigations of PrPSc synthesis and diversity. Br. Med. Bull. *49*:873–912, 1993.
282. Prusiner, S. B.: Biology and genetics of prion diseases. Annu. Rev. Microbiol. *48*:655–686, 1994.
283. Prusiner, S. B., and DeArmond, S. J.: Molecular biology and pathology of scrapie and the prion diseases of humans. Brain Pathol. *1*:297–310, 1991.
284. Prusiner, S. B., Gajdusek, D. C., and Alpers, M. P.: Kuru with incubation periods extending two decades. Ann. Neurol. *12*:1–9, 1982.
285. Race, R. E., Caughey, B., Graham, K., et al.: Analyses of frequency of infection, specific infectivity, and prion protein biosynthesis in scrapie-infected neuroblastoma cell clones. J. Virol. *62*:2845–2849, 1988.
286. Rall, G. F., Mucke, L., and Oldstone, M. B. A.: Consequences of cytotoxic T lymphocyte interaction with major histocompatibility complex class I expression neurons in vivo. J. Exp. Med. *182*:1201–1212, 1995.
287. Rammohan, K. W., McFarland, H. F., Bellini, W. J., et al.: Antibody-mediated modification of encephalitis induced by hamster neurotropic measles virus. J. Infect. Dis. *147*:546–550, 1983.
288. Rammohan, K. W., McFarland, H. F., and McFarlin, D. E.: Subacute sclerosing panencephalitis after passive immunization and natural measles infection: Role of antibody in persistence of measles virus. Neurology *32*:390–394, 1982.
289. Rand, K. H., Johnson, K. P., Rubinstein, L. J., et al.: Adenine arabinoside in the treatment of progressive multifocal leukoencephalopathy: Use of virus-containing cells in the urine to assess response to therapy. Ann. Neurol. *1*:458–462, 1977.
290. Rankin, E., and Scaravilli, F.: Progressive multifocal leukoencephalopathy in a patient with rheumatoid arthritis and polymyositis. J. Rheumatol. *22*:777–779, 1995.
291. Rao, C. V., Brennan, T. G., and Garcia, J. H.: Computed tomography in the diagnosis of Creutzfeldt-Jakob disease. J. Comput. Assist. Tomogr. *1*:211–215, 1977.
292. Rey, M., Celers, J., Mouton, Y., et al.: Impact of measles in France. Rev. Infect. Dis. *5*:433–438, 1983.
293. Richard, P., Renault, F., Ostre, C., et al.: Neurophysiological follow-up in two children with Creutzfeldt-Jakob disease after human growth hormone treatment. Electroencephalogr. Clin. Neurophysiol. *91*:100–107, 1994.
294. Risk, W., and Haddad, F. S.: The variable natural history of subacute sclerosing panencephalitis. Arch. Neurol. *36*:610–615, 1979.
295. Robertson, W. C., Clark, D. B., and Markesber, W. R.: Review of 38 cases of subacute sclerosing panencephalitis: Effect of amantadine on natural course of the disease. Ann. Neurol. *8*:422–425, 1980.
296. Roizman, B., and Sears, A. E.: Herpes simplex viruses and their replication. *In* Fields, B. N., Knipe, D. M., Howley, P. M., et al. (eds.): Virology. 3rd ed. Philadelphia, Lippincott-Raven, 1996, pp. 2231–2293.
297. Roose, R., Gajdusek, D. C., and Gibbs, C. J.: The clinical characteristics of transmissible Creutzfeldt-Jakob disease. Brain *96*:1–20, 1973.
298. Rosenbloom, M. A., and Uphoff, D. F.: The association of progressive multifocal leukoencephalopathy and sarcoidosis. Chest *83*:572–575, 1983.
299. Rubenstein, R., Merz, P. A., Kascsak, R. J., et al.: Detection of scrapie-associated fibrils (SAF) and SAF proteins from scrapie-affected sheep. J. Infect. Dis. *156*:36–42, 1987.
300. Rustigan, R.: Persistent infection of cells in culture by measles virus. I. Development and characteristics of HeLa sublines persistently infected with complete virus. J. Bacteriol. *92*:1792–1804, 1966.
301. Rwambo, P. M., Issel, C. J., Adams, W. V. J., et al.: Equine infectious anemia virus (EIAV) humoral responses of recipient ponies and antigenic variation during persistent infection. Arch. Virol. *111*:199–212, 1990.
302. Safar, J., Ceroni, M., Piccardo, P., et al.: Subcellular distribution and physiochemical properties of scrapie-associated precursor protein and relationship with scrapie agent. Neurology *40*:503–508, 1990.
303. Saha, V., John, T. J., Mukundan, P., et al.: High incidence of subacute sclerosing panencephalitis in south India. Epidemiol. Infect. *104*:151–156, 1990.
304. Salmon, J. F., Pan, E. L., and Murray, A. D.: Visual loss with dancing extremities and mental disturbances. Survey Ophthalmol. *35*:299–306, 1991.
305. Schlenska, G. K., and Walter, G. F.: Temporal evolution of electroencephalographic abnormalities in Creutzfeldt-Jakob disease. J. Neurol. *236*:456–460, 1989.
306. Schlitt, M., Morawetz, R. B., Bonnin, J., et al.: Progressive multifocal leukoencephalopathy: Three patients diagnosed by brain biopsy, with prolonged survival in two. Neurosurgery *18*:407–414, 1986.
307. Scott, J. R., Foster, J. D., and Fraser, H.: Conjunctival instillation of scrapie in mice can produce disease. Vet. Microbiol. *34*:305–309, 1993.
308. Shafritz, D., Shouval, D., Sherman, H., et al.: Integration of hepatitis B virus DNA into the genome of liver cell in chronic liver disease and hepatocellular carcinoma. N. Engl. J. Med. *305*:1067–1073, 1981.
309. Shah, K., and Nathanson, N.: Human exposure to SV40: Review and comment. Am. J. Epidemiol. *103*:1–12, 1976.
310. Shah, K. V.: Polyomaviruses. *In* Fields, B. N., Knipe, D. M., Chanock, R. M., et al. (eds.): Virology. 2nd ed. New York, Raven Press, 1990, pp. 1609–1623.
311. Sharp, G. B., Laney, S. M., Westmoreland, B. F., et al.: Atypical electroencephalographic pattern in a patient with subacute sclerosing panencephalitis. Electroencephalogr. Clin. Neurophysiol. *78*:311–313, 1991.
312. Siemes, H., Siegert, M., Hanefeld, F., et al.: Oligoclonal gamma-globulin banding of cerebrospinal fluid in patients with subacute sclerosing panencephalitis: Comparison of the electrophoretic pattern with that in multiple sclerosis and congenital infection. J. Neurol. Sci. *32*:395–409, 1977.
313. Sigurdsson, B.: Rida, a chronic encephalitis of sheep, with general remarks on infections which develop slowly and some of their special characteristics. Br. Vet. J. *110*:341–354, 1954.
314. Silva, C. A., Paula-Barbosa, M. M., Pereira, S., et al.: Two cases of rapidly progressive subacute sclerosing panencephalitis: Neuropathological findings. Arch. Neurol. *38*:109–113, 1981.
315. Silver, S. A., Arthur, R. R., Erozan, Y. S., et al.: Diagnosis of progressive multifocal leukoencephalopathy by stereotactic brain biopsy utilizing immunohistochemistry and the polymerase chain reaction. Acta Cytol. *39*:35–44, 1995.
316. Silverberg, R., Brenner, T., and Abramsky, O.: Inosiplex in the treatment of subacute sclerosing panencephalitis. Arch. Neurol. *36*:374–375, 1979.
317. Silverman, L., and Rubinstein, L. J.: Electron microscopic observations on a case of progressive multifocal luekoencephalopathy. Acta Neuropathol. *5*:215–224, 1965.
318. Singer, E. J., Stoner, G. L., Singer, P., et al.: AIDS presenting as progressive multifocal leukoencephalopathy with clinical response to zidovudine. Acta Neurol. Scand. *90*:443–447, 1994.
319. Somerville, R. A., and Ritchie, L. A.: Differential glycosylation of the protein (PrP) forming scrapie-associated fibrils. J. Gen. Virol. *71*:833–839, 1990.
320. Somerville, R. A., Ritchie, L. A., and Gibson, P. H.: Structural and biochemical evidence that scrapie-associated fibrils assemble in vivo. J. Gen. Virol. *70*:25–35, 1989.
321. Sponzilli, E. E., Smith, J. K., Malamud, M., et al.: Progressive multifocal leukoencephalopathy: A complication of immunosuppressive treatment. Neurology *32*:200–203, 1975.
322. Stites, D. P.: The immunology of scrapie. *In* Prusiner, S. B., and Hadlow, W. J. (eds.): Slow Transmissible Diseases of the Nervous System. New York, Academic Press, 1979, pp. 211–221.
323. Stoner, G. L., Soffer, D., Ryschkewitsch, C. F., et al.: A double-label method detects both early (T-antigen) and late (capsid) proteins of JC virus in progressive multifocal leukoencephalopathy brain tissue from AIDS and non-AIDS patients. J. Neuroimmunol. *19*:223–236, 1988.
324. Stoner, G. L., Walker, D. L., and Webster, H. D.: Age distribution of progressive multifocal leukoencephalopathy. Acta Neurol. Scand. *78*:307–312, 1988.
325. Streletz, L. J., and Cracco, J.: The effect of isoprinosine in subacute sclerosing panencephalitis (SSPE). Ann. Neurol. *1*:183–184, 1977.
326. Sussman, J., and Compston, D. A.: Subacute sclerosing panencephalitis in Wales. Q. J. Med. *87*:23–34, 1994.
327. Takayama, S., Iwasaki, Y., Yamanouchi, H., et al.: Characteristic clinical features in a case of fulminant subacute sclerosing panencephalitis. Brain Dev. *16*:132–135, 1994.
328. Tamai, Y., Kojima, H., Ohtani, Y., et al.: Subcellular distribution of the transmissible agent in Creutzfeldt-Jakob disease mouse brain. Microbiol. Immunol. *33*:35–42, 1989.
329. Tamari, H., Matsukura, M., Matsuda, I., et al.: An acute variant of subacute sclerosing panencephalitis: An autopsy case report. Brain Dev. *3*:87–91, 1981.
330. Tanaka, J., Nakamura, H., and Fukada, T.: Adult-onset subacute sclerosing panencephalitis: Immunocytochemical and electron microscopic demonstration of the viral antigen. Clin. Neuropathol. *6*:30–37, 1987.
331. Tarsy, D., Holden, E. M., Segarra, J. M., et al.: 5-Iodo-2-deoxyuridine (IUDR; NSC-39661) given intraventricularly in the treatment of progressive multifocal leukoencephalopathy. Cancer Chemother. Rep. *57*:73–78, 1973.
332. Tartaro, A., Fulgente, T., Delli Pizzi, C., et al.: MRI alterations as an early finding in Creutzfeldt-Jakob disease. Eur. J. Radiol. *17*:155–158, 1993.
333. Tateishi, J., Brown, P., Kitamoto, T., et al.: First experimental transmission of fatal familial insomnia. Nature *376*:434–435, 1995.
334. Tateishi, J., and Kitamoto, T.: Developments in diagnosis for prion diseases. Br. Med. Bull. *49*:971–979, 1993.
335. Taylor, D. M.: Scrapie agent decontamination: Implications for bovine spongiform encephalopathy. Vet. Rec. *124*:291–292, 1989.
336. Tellez-Nagel, J., and Harler, D. H.: Subacute sclerosing leukoencephalitis. I. Clinicopathological, electron microscopic and virological observations. J. Neuropathol. Exp. Neurol. *25*:560, 1966.
337. Thadani, V., Penar, P. L., Partington, J., et al.: Creutzfeldt-Jakob disease

probably acquired from a cadaveric dura mater graft: Case report. J. Neurosurg. *69*:766–769, 1988.

338. Thormar, H., Mehta, P. D., Lin, F. H., et al.: Presence of oligoclonal immunoglobulin G bands and lack of matrix protein antibodies in cerebrospinal fluids and sera of ferrets with measles virus encelphalitis. Infect. Immun. *41*:1205–1211, 1983.
339. Townsend, J. J., Baringer, J. R., Wolinsky, J. S., et al.: Progressive rubella panencephalitis: Late onset after congenital rubella. N. Engl. J. Med. *292*:990–993, 1975.
340. Townsend, J. J., Stroop, W. G., Baringer, J. R., et al.: Neuropathology of progressive rubella panencephalitis after childhood rubella. Neurology *32*:185–190, 1982.
341. Townsend, J. J., Wolinsky, J. S., and Baringer, J. R.: The neuropathology of progressive rubella panencephalitis of late onset. Brain *99*:81–90, 1979.
342. Uchino, A., Yoshinaga, M., Shiokawa, O., et al.: Serial MR imaging in Creutzfeldt-Jakob disease. Neuroradiolgy *33*:364–367, 1991.
343. Van Bogaert, L., et al.: Sur la sclerose inflammatorie de la substance blanche des hemispheres (Spielmeyer). Rev. Neurol. *71*:679, 1939.
344. Vandersteenhoven, J. J., Dbaibo, G., Boyko, O. B., et al.: Progressive multifocal leukoencephalopathy in pediatric acquired immunodeficiency syndrome. Pediatr. Infect. Dis. J. *11*:232–237, 1992.
345. Vandvik, B.: Oligoclonal measles virus specific IgG antibodies isolated from sera of patients with subacute sclerosing panencephalitis. Scand. J. Immunol. *6*:641–649, 1977.
346. Vandvik, B., and Norrby, E.: Oligoclonal IgG antibody response in the central nervous system to different measles virus antigen in subacute sclerosing panencephalitis. Proc. Natl. Acad. Sci. U. S. A. *70*:1600–1604, 1973.
347. Vandvik, B., Norrby, E., Nordal, H. J., et al.: Oligoclonal measles-virus specific IgG antibodies isolated from cerebrospinal fluids, brain extracts, and sera from patients with subacute sclerosing panencephalitis and multiple sclerosis. Scand. J. Immunol. *5*:979–992, 1976.
348. Vanneste, J. A., Bellot, S. M., and Stam, F. C.: Progressive multifocal leukoencephalopathy presenting as a single mass lesion. Eur. Neurol. *23*:113–118, 1984.
349. Walker, D. L.: Progressive multifocal leukoencephalopathy: An opportunistic viral infection of the central nervous system. *In* Vinken, P. J., and Gruyn, G. W. (eds.): Handbook of Clinical Neurology. Vol. 34. Infections of the Central Nervous System. Amsterdam, North-Holland, 1978, pp. 307–329.
350. Walker, D. L.: Personal communication, 1985.
351. Walker, D. L., and Padgett, B. L.: Progressive multifocal leukoencephalopathy. *In* Fraenkel-Conrat, H., and Wagner, R. R. (eds.): Comprehensive Virology. Vol. 18. New York, Plenum Press, 1983, pp. 161–193.
352. Walker, R. W., and Thompson, E. J.: The cerebrospinal fluid in subacute sclerosing panencephalitis and multiple sclerosis. Prog. Brain Res. *59*:375–390, 1983.
353. Weber, T., Turner, R. W., Frye, S., et al.: Specific diagnosis of progressive multifocal leukoencephalopathy by polymerase chain reaction. J. Infect. Dis. *169*:1138–1141, 1994.
354. Wechsler, S. L., Weiner, H. L., and Fields, B. N.: Immune response in subacute sclerosing panencephalitis: Reduced antibody response to the matrix protein of measles virus. J. Immunol. *123*:884–889, 1979.
355. Weil, M. L., Itabashi, H. H., Cremer, N. E., et al.: Chronic progressive panencephalitis due to rubella virus simulating subacute sclerosing panencephalitis. N. Engl. J. Med. *292*:994–998, 1975.
356. Weil, M. L., Perrin, L., Buimovici-Klein, E., et al.: Immunological abnormalities associated with chronic progressive panencephalitis due to congenital infection with rubella virus. Clin. Res. *24*:185, 1976.
357. Weiner, L. P., Herndon, R. M., Narayan, O., et al.: Isolation of virus related to SV40 from patients with progressive multifocal leukoencephalopathy. N. Engl. J. Med. *286*:385–390, 1972.
358. Weissmann, C.: Prion diseases: Yielding under the strain. Nature *375*:628–629, 1995.
359. Westaway, D., Goodman, P. A., Mirenda, C. A., et al.: Distinct prion proteins in short and long scrapie incubation period mice. Cell *51*:651–662, 1987.
360. White, F., Ishaq, M., Stoner, G. L., et al.: JC virus DNA is present in many human brain samples from patients without progressive multifocal leukoencephalopathy. J. Virol. *66*:5726–5734, 1992.
361. Whiteman, M. L., Post, M. J., Berger, J. R., et al.: Progressive multifocal leukoencephalopathy in 47 HIV-seropositive patients: Neuroimaging with clinical and pathologic correlation. Radiology *187*:233–240, 1993.
362. Whitley, R. J.: Personal communication, 1985.
363. Wiley, C. A., Grafe, M., Kennedy, C., et al.: Human immunodeficiency virus (HIV) and JC virus in acquired immune deficiency syndrome (AIDS) patients with progressive multifocal leukoencephalopathy. Acta Neuropathol. *76*:338–346, 1988.
364. Will, R. G.: Epidemiology of Creutzfeldt-Jakob disease. Br. Med. Bull. *49*:960–970, 1993.
365. Winer, J. B., Pires, M., Kermode, A., et al.: Resolving MRI abnormalities with progression of subacute sclerosing panencephalitis. Neuroradiology *33*:178–80, 1991.
366. Winter, M. H., Aldridge, B. M., Scott, P. R., et al.: Occurrence of 14 cases of bovine spongiform encephalopathy in a closed dairy herd. Br. Vet. J. *145*:191–194, 1989.
367. Wisniewski, H. M., and Wrzolek, M.: Pathogenesis of amyloid formation in Alzheimer's disease, Down's syndrome and scrapie. Ciba Found. Symp. *135*:224–238, 1988.
368. Wolinsky, J. S., Berg, B. O., and Maitland, C. T.: Progressive rubella panencephalitis. Arch. Neurol. *33*:722–723, 1976.
369. Wolinsky, J. S., Dau, P. C., Buimovici-Klein, E., et al.: Progressive rubella panencephalitis: Immunovirological studies and results of isoprinosine therapy. Clin. Exp. Immunol *35*:397–404, 1979.
370. Wolinsky, J. S., and Johnson, R. T.: Role of viruses in chronic neurological diseases. *In* Fraenkel-Conrat, H., and Wagner, R. R. (eds.): Comprehensive Virology. Vol. 16. New York, Plenum Press, 1980, pp. 257–291.
371. Wolinsky, J. S., Waxham, M. N., Hess, J. L., et al.: Immunochemical features of a case of progressive rubella panencephalitis. Clin. Exp. Immunol. *48*:359–366, 1982.
372. Wong, T. C., Ayata, M., Hirano, A., et al.: Generalized and localized biased hypermutation affecting the matrix gene of a measles virus strain that causes subacute sclerosing panencephalitis. J. Virol. *63*:5464–5468, 1989.
373. Woodward, K. G., Weinberg, P. E., and Lipton, H. L.: Basal ganglia involvement in subacute sclerosing panencephalitis: CT and MR demonstration. J. Comput. Assist. Tomogr. *12*:489–491, 1988.
374. Yalaz, K., Anlar, B., Oktem, F., et al.: Intraventricular interferon and oral inosiplex in the treatment of subacute sclerosing panencephalitis. Neurology *42*:488–491, 1992.
375. Zagami, A. S., and Lethlean, A. K.: Chorioretinitis as a possible very early manifestation of subacute sclerosing panencephalitis. Aust. N. Z. J. Med. *21*:350–352, 1991.
376. Zigas, V., and Gajdusek, D. C.: Kuru: Clinical study of a new syndrome resembling paralysis agitans in natives of the eastern highlands of Australian New Guinea. Med. J. Aust. *2*:745–754, 1957.
377. Ziola, B., Salmi, A., Panelius, M., et al.: Measles-virus specific IgM antibodies and IgM-class rheumatoid factor in serum and cerebrospinal fluid of subacute sclerosing panencephalitis patients. Clin. Immunol. Immunopathol. *13*:462–474, 1979.
378. Zochodne, D. W., Young, G. B., McLachlan, R. S., et al.: Creutzfeldt-Jakob disease without periodic sharp wave complexes: A clinical, electroencephalographic, and pathologic study. Neurology *38*:1056–1060, 1988.
379. Zurhein, G. M.: Virions in progressive multifocal leukoencephalopathy. *In* Minckler, J. (ed.): Pathology of the Nervous System. Vol. 3. New York, McGraw-Hill, 1968, pp. 2893–2912.
380. Zurhein, G. M., and Chou, S. M.: Particles resembling papova viruses in human cerebral demyelination disease. Science *148*:1477–1479, 1965.

❑ ❑ ❑

SUBSECTION THREE

ADENOVIRIDAE

161

ADENOVIRUSES

James D. Cherry

Adenoviruses are responsible for a varied array of illnesses in children.[1, 34, 36, 55, 99, 122, 331, 350, 384] Most commonly, they are associated with respiratory illness and gastroenteritis, but cardiac, neurologic, cutaneous, urinary, and lymphatic manifestations also occur frequently. Although many of the clinical presentations of adenoviral infections are distinctive, the specific viral etiologic agent rarely is recognized by physicians.

Adenoviruses first were noted in explant cultures of human adenoid tissue; this finding, plus the observation of their apparent general affinity for lymphatic tissue, led to their name.[101, 105, 122, 327]

HISTORY

The first adenoviral strains were not isolated until 1953, when tissue culture techniques became available, although epidemic disease due to adenoviruses had been observed throughout the first half of the century. Epidemic keratoconjunctivitis first was noted and reported in Austria by several physicians in 1889.[2, 124, 317, 337, 357] Major outbreaks of epidemic keratoconjunctivitis were reported in Bombay in 1901, in Madras in 1920 and 1928, in Hawaii in 1941, and on the West Coast of the United States in 1942.[162, 176, 177, 216, 413]

Epidemics of illness such as pharyngoconjunctival fever have been observed throughout this century. Béal[13] in 1907 was the first to report the syndrome; in the 1920s, epidemics associated with swimming in public pools and in lakes were noted in Germany and the United States.[11, 291] Initial studies by Rowe and colleagues[327] revealed cytopathic changes in explant tissue cultures of surgically removed human adenoids. Fluids from these cultures caused distinctive cytopathologic changes in other tissue cultures, and antiserum prepared in hyperimmunized rabbits neutralized the effect. In 1954, Hilleman and Werner[172] isolated similar cytopathic agents from throat washings of military recruits with febrile acute respiratory disease. Shortly thereafter, epidemic keratoconjunctivitis and pharyngoconjunctival fever were seen to be illnesses of adenoviral etiologies.[80, 83–85, 195]

Initially, adenoviruses were known by the following names: adenoid degeneration (AD) agent because of its recovery in human adenoid tissue explants[327]; respiratory illness patient number 67 (RI-67) agent, which was recovered from a military recruit with primary atypical pneumonia during an epidemic of acute respiratory disease[172, 173]; adenoidal-pharyngeal-conjunctival (APC) agent[183]; and acute respiratory disease (ARD) agent.[65] In 1956, the early investigators in the field selected the term *adenovirus* for the new group of viruses. The name suggested the characteristic involvement of lymphadenoid tissue as well as the tissue of the first reported isolation.[101]

Because of considerable morbidity and major economic considerations relating to adenoviral epidemic respiratory disease in military recruits, the development of vaccines received attention early. Initially, inactivated vaccines were produced; these achieved some degree of success.[149, 174, 230] Later, live viral preparations grown in diploid human fibroblast tissue cultures became available and have proved quite successful in the control of specific adenoviral infections in the military services.[93, 94, 142, 230, 324, 349, 373–376]

In 1975, the enteric adenoviruses (adenovirus types 40 and 41) first were reported.[112, 339, 401] These were demonstrated by electron microscopy, and subsequently they were shown to be a significant cause of diarrhea in children.[36, 61, 222, 258, 308, 371, 382, 384]

PROPERTIES OF THE VIRUS

Classification

Adenoviruses that infect humans are placed in the family *Adenoviridae* and the genus *Mastadenovirus*.[109, 181, 252] At present, 49 immunologically distinct adenoviral types have been recovered from humans.[87, 88, 109, 166–171, 182, 212, 338, 395, 396, 405] Additional adenoviral types have been isolated from monkeys, cattle, dogs, mice, and chickens.[164, 167–169] Mammalian adenoviruses have a common generic antigen, which can be identified by complement fixation and enzyme-linked immunosorbent assay (ELISA).[197, 299, 321, 404] Individual serotypes are identified by neutralization.[167, 168, 232]

Adenoviruses originally were subclassified on the basis of four hemagglutination patterns with rat and rhesus monkey red blood cells.[325] This subclassification is updated in Table 161–1. In 1962, it was found that adenovirus type 12 could cause tumors in hamsters, and soon thereafter it was realized

TABLE 161–1. Separation of Human Adenoviruses into Subgroups by Ability to Agglutinate Rhesus Monkey and Rat Erythrocytes

Subgroups	Characteristics	Types
I	Complete agglutination of monkey erythrocytes	3, 7, 11, 14, 16, 21, 34, 35
II	Complete agglutination of rat erythrocytes	8–10, 13, 15, 17, 19, 20, 22–30, 32, 33, 36–39, 42–49
III	Partial agglutination of rat erythrocytes	1, 2, 4–6, 40, 41
IV	No or little agglutination of monkey or rat erythrocytes	12, 18, 31

Data from references 164, 171, 181, 182, 204, 212, 230, 280, 281, 338, 403.

that adenoviruses also could be classified by their oncogenic potential in rodents.[185, 378] Grouping by oncogenic potential was similar, with few exceptions, to hemagglutination properties: hemagglutination group I organisms had moderate oncogenic potential, group II and group III organisms had low or no potential, and group IV organisms had high oncogenic potential.[135, 181, 189]

Adenoviruses also have been subclassified (A to F) on the basis of the percentage of guanine plus cytosine in their DNA and other biochemical and biophysical criteria[171, 212, 305, 338, 396–398] (Table 161–2). In general, subgroup A organisms are the same as hemagglutination group IV; subgroup B, the same as hemagglutination group I; subgroup C, E, and F, the same as hemagglutination group III; and subgroup D, the same as hemagglutination group II.

Physical Properties

Adenoviruses are nonenveloped DNA viruses that are 65 to 80 nm in diameter.[109, 135, 180, 181, 189, 219, 252] The virion is composed of a protein capsid made up of 252 capsomeres and a nucleoprotein core that contains the DNA viral genome and two to four internal proteins.[311] The virion is roughly spherical in the form of an icosahedron; each of the 20 sides is an equilateral triangle with the vertices of each converging in groups of five, resulting in 12 pentagonal vertices.[36, 122, 180] Each vertex capsomere contacts five other capsomeres and is designated a penton. Each penton contains a base plate and a rod-like projection, the fiber. There are 240 nonvertex capsomeres, which occur in groups of six and are known as hexons.[219, 281, 383] The hexons contain the generic complement-fixing antigen.[122] Each capsomere has a diameter of 8 nm and a central hole 2 to 3 nm in diameter.[408] The capsomeres constitute 87 per cent of the dry weight of the virion.

TABLE 161–2. Grouping of Human Adenoviral Serotypes Based upon Biochemical and Biophysical Criteria

Subgroup	Adenovirus Types	Location and Manifestations of Infection
A	12, 18, 31	Gastrointestinal; may cause disease in children
B:1	3, 7, 16, 21	Respiratory, eye, and gastrointestinal symptomatic infections
B:2	11, 14, 34, 35	Urinary and respiratory; symptomatic urinary tract infections (particularly in immunosuppressed patients) and symptomatic respiratory infections
C	1, 2, 5, 6	Respiratory and gastrointestinal; symptomatic respiratory and hepatitis in immunosuppressed patients
D	8–10, 13, 15, 17, 19, 20, 22–30, 32, 33, 36–39, 42–49	Eye and gastrointestinal; symptomatic eye infections, gastrointestinal infections in HIV-infected patients
E	4	Symptomatic eye and respiratory infections
F	40, 41	Symptomatic gastrointestinal infections

Data from references 171, 181, 212, 230, 305, 338, 372, 396.

The central core of the virion, which constitutes 12 to 14 per cent of its dry weight, is composed of linear double-stranded DNA (molecular weight, 23.85×10^6 daltons for adenovirus type 2) and two to four basic proteins.[125, 181, 408]

Adenoviruses are highly stable in general.[91, 122, 133, 189, 232] They are resistant to lipid solvents and retain activity at pH ranges from 2 to 10.

At 24° C, maximal infectivity is maintained between pH 6 and 9.5. Adenoviruses are stable at room temperature for 2 weeks, at 36° C for 7 days, and for at least 70 days at 4° C. Infectivity is destroyed by heating to 56° C for 30 minutes. Sodium dodecyl sulfate (0.25 per cent) inactivates virus by the disruption of the capsid.[219]

Antigenic Composition

The antigenic determinants of adenoviruses are contained on the protein structural subunits (hexons, pentons, and fibers).[383] The hexon antigen (alpha component) carries the generic antigenic component that is common to all mammalian adenoviruses and is measured by complement fixation or ELISA. Another hexon antigen (epsilon component) reacts with neutralizing antibodies lacking hemagglutination-inhibiting activity. The antigen related to viral fiber also induces type-specific neutralizing antibody for some adenoviral types. Minor antigens are related to the pentons. One of these (the cell-detaching factor) causes the rounding and clumping of tissue culture cells.

Gerna and associates,[131] using the immunoperoxidase antibody technique, found that the early antigens of all serotypes belonging to one group (see Table 161–1) reacted strongly with all type-specific immune sera of the same group.

Tissue Culture Growth

Although adenoviruses can be grown in a wide variety of cells of human epithelial origin, primary or diploid cultures of human embryonic kidney are preferable for the recovery of agents from clinical specimens.[232] Continuous cell lines such as HeLa and HEp-2 also are quite sensitive.[161, 189, 328] Adenoviruses also will grow in monkey kidney tissue culture, but the evolution of the cytopathic effect is considerably slower than that occurring in cells of human origin. In addition, the cytopathic effect is more variable in monkey kidney tissue culture, and many isolates will be missed.

Enteric adenoviruses have been identified in human feces by electron microscopy.[36, 73, 87, 197, 211, 316, 320, 382, 396, 404] These enteric adenoviruses, identified as type 40 and type 41, usually do not grow in standard tissue culture systems. Both viral types will grow in Graham 293 cells (a human embryonic kidney cell line transformed by adenovirus type 5); type 40 also will grow in tertiary monkey kidney cells, and some strains of type 41 will grow in HEp-2, Chang conjunctiva cells, and tertiary cynomolgus cells.[366, 395] More recently, Grabow and associates[143] noted that the PLC/PRG/5 cell line was 100 times more sensitive to a laboratory strain of adenovirus type 41 and 10 times more sensitive to a laboratory strain of adenovirus type 40 than Graham 293 cells were.

Specimens for viral culture may be obtained from eye, pharynx, blood, lungs, pleural and pericardial fluids, liver, stool, intestinal epithelium, lymph nodes, cerebrospinal fluid, brain, urine, and renal tissue. For best isolation rates, clinical specimens should be inoculated in cell cultures within 6 hours of collection. Tissue culture tubes are incubated best at 37° C, and rolling offers no advantage over stationary incubation.[232] Although there is considerable variability in the cytopathic effect, the most consistent finding is marked rounding and clumping of cells, often in grape-like clusters.[311, 314] Cytopathic effect may be noted as early as 1 to 2 days after inoculation, but it may be delayed as long as 4 weeks. The use of the shell viral technique in which infected cells in a specimen are centrifuged onto HEp-2 tissue culture cells yields positive cultures in 1 to 2 days.[102] The cytopathic effect characteristically is followed by detachment of the entire cell sheet from the glass of the tissue culture tube within 2 to 4 days.[145, 162, 300, 328, 330]

Virus Multiplication

Initial attachment of adenoviruses to cells is relatively slow, requiring up to 6 hours.[81, 134, 189] Penetration into the host cell occurs rapidly, either by phagocytosis or by direct entry through the plasma membrane.[189, 239] The eclipse period with adenoviruses varies from 11 to 21 hours, depending on serotype.[134, 189] During eclipse, viral DNA uncoating requires approximately 2 hours when it is determined biochemically.[189] After uncoating, the viral DNA rapidly enters the nucleus of the cell and disassociates from its internal protein.[81, 135, 239] After the eclipse period, there is an accumulation of viral DNA, which often doubles the content of the infected cell and becomes a part of the typical inclusion bodies of the infected cells.[135]

Characteristic cytopathic changes in tissue culture, as demonstrated by light microscopy of hematoxylin and eosin–stained material or by electron microscopy, appear as early as 8 to 24 hours after infection.[31, 32, 153] Two types of intranuclear alterations may be seen. In the first, early, small, discrete, eosinophilic inclusions are observed. These gradually enlarge, become more prominent, and then form a large crystalline central mass surrounded by a clear zone or halo.[32, 140] This type of early cytopathic effect appears to occur in cells that contain only small amounts of infectious virus.[33] The second type of intranuclear alteration, which generally is a later occurrence, consists of large, basophilic, intranuclear inclusions.[32] Occasionally, giant forms measuring greater than 14 μm are noted.[33] These mature inclusions may expand greatly the nucleus of the cell and have a DNA content 10 times greater than that of an uninfected cell. They contain a large amount of viral antigen and infective virus. Cytopathic changes vary considerably with the different adenoviral serotypes.[31, 219]

In general, virus remains within the nucleus of intact, infected cells, so that less than 1 per cent of the total virus content of a culture is free within the extracellular fluid at any one time.[219]

Animal Susceptibility

Human adenoviruses usually do not produce clinical illness in laboratory animals, although infections with several different serotypes have occurred in selected animals.[189] When adenoviral strains were administered intranasally to young, "pathogen-free," colostrum-deprived pigs or 1-month-old cotton rats, the animals developed pneumonia, and intranuclear inclusions were observed microscopically in the lungs.[189, 289] An adenovirus type 5 strain was given intravenously to a rabbit, and the virus was recovered from the animal's spleen when it was removed 2 months later. Many adenoviral strains will propagate in many different animal tissue cultures. In addition, in some cultures, marked cytopathic effects are observed, but little infectious virus is produced.

Adeno-Associated Viruses

Adeno-associated viruses are a group of small, defective, single-stranded, DNA-containing, virus-like particles that replicate in tissue culture only in the presence of adenoviruses.[26, 81, 122, 189, 210, 350] Four serologic types have been identified; however, only types 2 and 3 have been recovered in humans.[122, 219] These agents have been isolated from throat and anal swab specimens of children from whom adenoviral strains also were isolated.[26] About 30 per cent of children have complement-fixing antibody to adeno-associated virus types 2 and 3; most of these children have had evidence of adenoviral infection as well.[27] Neutralizing antibody to adeno-associated virus types 2 and 3 is noted in the sera of 60 to 80 per cent of children 8 to 14 years of age.[294] The specific relevance of adeno-associated viruses currently is unknown.

EPIDEMIOLOGY

General Prevalence

Adenoviral infections account for 2 to 5 per cent of total respiratory illnesses.[62, 68, 118, 119, 302] Respiratory viral illness in children that is due to adenoviruses has been estimated to be from 2 to 24 per cent.[34, 49, 51, 179, 237, 246] Adenoviruses are implicated in the clinical illnesses of children in these percentages: 5 to 11 per cent of upper respiratory tract infection, 4 to 10 per cent of pharyngitis, 3 to 9 per cent of croup, 5 to 11 per cent of bronchitis, 2 to 10 per cent of bronchiolitis, and 4 to 10 per cent of pneumonia.[34, 49–51, 120, 266, 297] Enteric adenoviral infections are the cause of 5 to 15 per cent of acute diarrheal illnesses in children.[61, 73, 235, 258, 308, 316, 382, 384] Specific categories of illness with adenoviruses vary in respect to viral serotypes, patient age, socioeconomic status, and environmental conditions.[47, 151, 160, 198, 416] Adenoviruses have a predilection for infants and children younger than 5 years of age who spend portions of their days in closed environments, such as day care centers, orphanages, and other institutions.[17, 18, 47, 155, 238, 394] Epidemics of disease due to adenoviral infections have been associated with swimming pools, day care centers, resident schools, certain industries, hospitals, physician's offices, and young recruits in early basic military training.[57, 76, 195, 196, 218, 233, 247, 290, 295, 306, 319, 347, 381, 417] Adenoviruses are recovered commonly from children in tropical countries and where there is crowding, such as in lower socioeconomic settings.[47, 49, 63, 198, 416]

Age Incidence and Prevalence

Although adenoviral infections occur in all age groups, the incidence of infection generally is related inversely to age.[219] More than 90 per cent of newborn infants have demonstrable transplacentally acquired complement-fixing adenoviral serum antibody.[272, 359] Most infants have neutralizing antibody to one or more of the common adenoviral types, and this appears to be protective during the first 6 months of life. When adenoviral infection does occur in the neonate, it often is severe and occasionally fatal.[7, 421] By the sixth month of life, adenoviral complement-fixing antibody can be demonstrated in only 14 per cent of infants. By 1 year of age, complement-fixing adenoviral antibody is observed in 44 to 50 per cent of the serums tested.[183, 275]

The incidence of adenoviral infection peaks in infants and children between 6 months and 5 years of age.[257, 302] By 5 years of age, 70 to 80 per cent of children have neutralizing antibody to adenovirus types 1 and 2, and 50 per cent have antibody to adenovirus type 5.[90, 118, 183, 192, 296, 302, 389]

Adenoviral infections also are common in grade school and junior high school children, but the incidence diminishes in high school adolescents. Adenoviral infections occur in only 1 to 2 per cent of college students, and they are noted infrequently in civilian adults.[103, 104, 106, 146, 360] About 1 per cent of adults with respiratory infectious illness will have adenoviral infection; in hospitalized adults, the incidence is about 4 per cent.[146] The most common adenoviral respiratory infections in children are due to types 1, 2, 3, and 5.[17, 389, 392, 394] Types 6 and 7 are the next most frequent isolates associated with childhood respiratory infection. Adenovirus types 40 and 41 are the most common causes of diarrhea.[61, 221, 235]

Military Recruits

Epidemic adenoviral disease is common in military recruits, with virtually all illness occurring during the first 8 weeks of basic training.[116, 251, 385, 391] The attack rate has varied between 40 and 90 per cent.[116, 145, 245, 388] Adenoviruses account for 30 to 70 per cent of acute respiratory disease, 67 per cent of common cold–like illnesses, 62 to 77 per cent of acute febrile pharyngitis and tonsillitis, 67 per cent of bronchitis, and 24 per cent of pneumonia.[22, 117] Some adenoviral infections are associated with minimal or no symptoms.[117, 145]

Geographic Distribution

Adenoviral infections have been noted throughout the world.[51, 53, 75, 107, 115, 122, 123, 125, 141, 160, 165, 175, 188, 192, 194, 198, 205, 210, 217–219, 223, 226, 261, 262, 293, 342, 344, 353, 357, 359, 362, 368, 381, 385–389, 408, 415, 416] Epidemic, endemic, and sporadic infections all occur.

Seasonal Patterns

Sporadic infections with adenoviruses occur throughout the year.[118, 121, 139, 175, 184, 237, 246, 261, 266] Epidemic adenoviral respiratory disease is most common in the winter, spring, and early summer.[28, 35, 122, 155, 178, 192, 223, 293, 310, 389, 391] Seasonal patterns depend on serotypes, population groups, and exposure. Epidemics of disease in military recruits commonly associated with adenovirus types 4 and 7 are most common in the winter and spring.[28, 116, 117, 174] Pharyngoconjunctival fever epidemics have been noted most commonly in the summer months in school-age children in association with summer camps or swimming pools.[247, 387, 408] No seasonal pattern has been identified in adenoviral gastroenteritis.[73, 211, 320, 382]

Host and Social Factors

No difference is apparent between males and females in the incidence of adenoviral infections, although a higher illness rate has been reported occasionally in males.[162]

Susceptibility to adenoviral infection apparently does not vary by race. More severe disease has been noted in infants of native and Indian populations in New Zealand and Canada.[15, 141] However, the relationship of these findings to socioeconomic conditions was not identified initially.

The incidence of adenoviral infections is greatest in lower socioeconomic population groups.[198] Spread of infection has been observed in day care centers, schools, children's homes, hospitals, clinics, physician's offices, and certain industrial settings.[17, 18, 21, 57, 151, 153, 196, 290, 295, 308, 347, 384, 417] Severe, overwhelming illness, including bronchiolitis and pneumonia with severe pulmonary residua, has been reported in neonates, small infants, and, occasionally, adults.[7, 160, 234] Adenoviral infections are a significant problem in the immunocompromised host, and when they occur, they frequently are severe and occasionally are fatal.[45, 46, 77, 82, 113, 147, 240, 255, 285, 351, 421]

Spread of Infection

Adenoviruses are isolated commonly from the conjunctiva, throat, and stool. Despite the ease of virus isolation, the effectiveness of spread of infection in the general population varies considerably.[49] Adenovirus types 1, 2, 3, 5, and 7 are effective spreaders; however, they are not as highly contagious as varicella, measles, and influenza viruses.[49, 50] Close contact appears to be necessary for infection to spread from one person to another.[359] Illness does not spread rapidly in the usual school environment but does spread dramatically in closed environments.[18, 50, 155, 184] Although adenovirus type 4 spreads less effectively in the general population, spread is rapid in nonimmune military recruits who live in close contact with each other.[58] In an outbreak of adenovirus type 7 in a children's home, 84 per cent of the residents were shown to be infected.

Transmission of virus is by aerosolized droplets reaching the conjunctiva, nose, or throat or, alternatively, by the fecal-oral route. In volunteer studies, adenoviruses have been shown to spread by small droplet aerosols and to a lesser degree by large droplets.[8, 69, 70] Adenovirus type 4 has been recovered from room air and cough samples of patients with the virus in their throats.[9]

In epidemics of pharyngoconjunctival fever, the virus appears to spread from contaminated swimming pool water to the eyes of the recipients. Epidemics of keratoconjunctivitis have occurred because of contact with contaminated ophthalmic instruments and contaminated fingers.[12, 83, 173, 195, 196, 205, 218, 261, 352] In day care centers, orphanages, and the military, transmission probably most commonly is through small droplet aerosols in crowded quarters.[306] An alternative in children is the fecal-oral route. The enteric adenoviruses have been identified in fecal specimens for about 8 days after the onset of gastroenteritis.[211]

Family members may excrete adenoviruses in their feces intermittently for prolonged periods after initial infection.[34, 118] In one study, 20 per cent of persons excreted adenoviruses in the stool for more than 3 months. Intrahousehold spread appears to continue as long as there are susceptible family members.[118] Infants born into households in which household members are adenoviral fecal excretors often become infected, presumably through the fecal-oral route. In general, 50 per cent of susceptible household members will experience infection, although the rate varies inversely with age and also depends on the serotype of adenovirus. Reinfection with specific adenoviral serotypes occurs, but most are asymptomatic or associated with only minimal illness.

Nosocomial spread of both respiratory and enteric adenoviruses is common and has been the cause of fatal illnesses in infants and immunocompromised patients.[3, 89, 111, 220, 347, 421]

PATHOGENESIS AND PATHOLOGY

Adenoviral infections usually are acute and self-limited, and therefore the opportunity to study the pathogenesis and pathologic process has been infrequent. The study of pathologic mechanisms has been carried out in human volunteers, tissue and organ culture systems, and recent murine model systems and by the examination of specimens from persons dying of adenoviral disease.

Viral Infection

In general, the characteristics of adenoviral infection depend on the host and the serotype of the agent.[21, 34, 40, 64, 136–138, 272, 307, 354, 401, 412] In most respiratory illnesses, initial viral infection occurs in the respiratory tract and involves the mucous membranes of the nose, oropharynx, and conjunctiva. Adenoviral agents have been isolated from sputum and oral secretions from 2 days before the onset of clinical illness up to 8 days after the onset of symptoms. Deeper respiratory involvement of the trachea, pleurae, and lung may result from progression of local infection or perhaps be a result of viremia. Gastrointestinal infection in conjunction with respiratory infection also occurs early and probably is the result of swallowed virus. Stool isolates of respiratory viral types frequently are noted concomitantly with respiratory tract infection. However, in contrast to the upper respiratory infection, the virus may persist for a long period in the lower gastrointestinal tract. Infection with enteric adenoviral types is presumed to involve intestinal epithelial cells. In one fatal infection, adenoviral antigen was demonstrated in jejunal cells.[316, 402]

In experimental studies with aerosolized adenovirus type 4, recovery of virus from throat specimens occurred on day 5 or 6, progressed to a maximum concentration at day 11 or 12, and was uncommon after day 20. Maximal recovery of adenovirus type 4 from anal specimens occurred on day 13 and continued for more than 3 weeks. Adenovirus types 26 and 27 inoculated into the conjunctiva resulted in short-term isolation of virus from the eyes on days 3 to 7 and, less frequently, from the throat on day 4.[203] Viral isolation from the rectum was common beginning at the end of the first week. Maximal fecal shedding occurred during the second and third week.

Adenoviruses may invade the blood stream early in disease, as evidenced by the occurrence of maculopapular, morbilliform, and/or petechial exanthems and also the recovery of virus from multiple organs, such as the brain, kidney, urinary bladder, lymphoid tissue, and liver, and at postmortem examination.[6, 7, 21, 29, 40, 52, 141, 148, 150, 241, 248] The virus has been cultured from the mononuclear cells of heparinized blood.[6]

Pathology

Early pathologic changes are observed in the epithelium of the respiratory tract. Severity of adenoviral involvement varies with the different serotypes. In tracheal organ cultures, the growth of adenovirus type 7 was characterized by an initial focal cytopathologic effect at 100 hours that quickly progressed to involve the whole epithelium.[71] Frequently, the cilia of incision-bearing cells were noted to be intact. In contrast to the findings with adenovirus type 7, a type 12 strain resulted in only a mild cytopathologic effect on the organ culture system.[71]

Microscopic examination of autopsy material in patients dying of adenoviral pneumonia revealed a loss of cilia in the tracheal epithelium, a proliferation of other respiratory epithelial cells, and the presence of intranuclear inclusions.[14, 21, 40, 52, 123, 406, 409, 411, 422] In severe pneumonia, total destruction with necrotizing bronchitis, bronchiolitis, and pneumonia is observed (Fig. 161–1). A mononuclear cellular infiltration is seen; hyaline membranes and necrosis are present. Cilia and goblet cells are absent, and muscle fiber bundles and elastic fibers are dispersed. Frequently, epithelial cells have a characteristic appearance with adenoviral infection. These infected cells grossly are enlarged and lose nuclear membranes; the nuclear material has migrated into the cytoplasm.[307] Blood vessels show edema, filament separation of their walls, and, occasionally, thrombosis.[422]

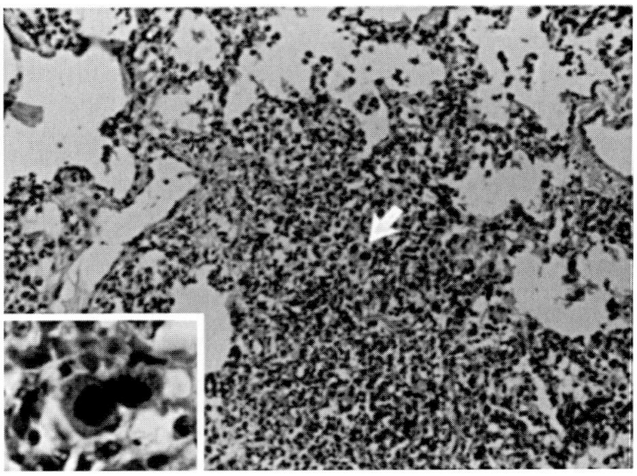

FIGURE 161–1. *The lung of a 17-month-old infant with adenoviral pneumonia. The infant died 10 days after the onset of illness, and there was no other contributing disease. The adenovirus isolated was not typed. A patchy pneumonia is present, and the arrow indicates two cells with nuclear inclusions.* Inset, *two similar cells with typical adenoviral nuclear inclusions at a higher magnification. (H and E × 190; inset × 770.) (Courtesy of Dr. David D. Porter, Department of Pathology, UCLA School of Medicine.)*

On histologic examination, adenoviral inclusions are characterized by small eosinophilic and larger basophilic intranuclear bodies.[14, 123, 272, 354]

Hepatic involvement in adenoviral infection has been reported frequently.[2, 9, 21, 46, 123, 307, 351] In addition to the isolation of virus from the liver, focal areas of liver necrosis accompanied by characteristic hepatic intranuclear inclusions have been demonstrated.[2, 46, 421] Electron microscopic examination has revealed adenoviral particles within the intranuclear inclusions.[2, 21, 307, 406, 421] Hematogenous spread to the central nervous system has been observed.[344] In most instances of adenoviral central nervous system infection, there has been an associated pneumonia.[72, 344] In central nervous system disease, the brain is edematous and congested. On microscopic examination, a perivascular accumulation of lymphocytes is noted, along with gigantic nuclear inclusions in the cortical neurons. Viral particles within these nuclear inclusions have been observed by electron microscopy.[60]

In epidemic keratoconjunctivitis due to adenovirus type 8, the walls of the conjunctival vessels are damaged, and aneurysms are present. The surrounding conjunctival connective tissue is edematous. It has been suggested that the virus penetrates the cornea along the nerves deep into the epithelial layers in a manner similar to that occurring in herpes simplex virus infection.[393]

Adenoviral strains have been isolated from and intranuclear inclusions have been demonstrated in renal tubular epithelium, lymph nodes, muscle, and gastrointestinal epithelium.[19, 46, 402, 419–421]

Immunologic Events

The local responses in adenoviral infections depend on the site of viral inoculation, the method of transmission, the viral serotype, the concentration of the inoculum, and the antibody status of the host. Three days after infection, when virus can be recovered from the nasopharynx, marked transudation of proteins from the serum into the respiratory tract occurs, along with production of secretory IgA antibody.[250] About 7 days after the onset of illness, serum-neutralizing, hemagglutination-inhibiting, and complement-fixing antibodies appear.[81, 231] At the same time, the nasal secretions contain specific IgA and IgG antibody.[20] In general, neutralizing antibody is the most sensitive indicator of adenoviral infection, hemagglutination-inhibiting antibody is less sensitive, and complement-fixing antibody is the least sensitive.[218, 308] Antibody titers peak in 2 to 3 weeks; complement-fixing antibody declines in 2 to 3 months but may persist for up to a year.[81] Neutralizing antibody persists for a longer period and is measurable in many instances for periods of up to 10 years. Reinfection with the same adenoviral serotype is rare because there is type-specific immunity.[16, 329]

Although alterations in leukocytes are not common, a decrease in lymphocytes before or at the onset of clinical illness and an increase in neutrophils early in the disease, followed by a decrease later, have been observed. Neutropenia may occur in severe disseminated illness. This is attributed to a direct toxic effect of virus on leukocytes, marrow reserves, or both.[92] The erythrocyte sedimentation rates of children have been normal or elevated to 55 mm/hour.[357, 359]

Recent studies by Ginsberg and associates[136–138] in murine adenovirus pneumonia model systems noted that tumor necrosis factor–α, interleukin-1, and interleukin-6 were elaborated during the first 2 to 3 days of infection. However, only tumor necrosis factor–α played an early role in the early phase of pathogenesis. The second phase of the inflammatory response is due to the infiltration of cytotoxic T cells.

Mistchenko and colleagues[259] studied cytokines and adenovirus-specific circulating immune complexes in 38 children with adenoviral infections. They placed the patients into three groups based upon the severity of their respiratory illnesses: moderate illness, severe illness, and fatal illness. Serum interleukin-1 was not detected in those children with moderate illness but was found in 7 of 12 of those with severe illness and in 13 of 16 of the children who died. Tumor necrosis factor–α frequently was present in the sera of fatal cases, but it was not present in sera of moderately ill children, and it was present in the sera of only 2 of 12 patients with severe but nonfatal illnesses. Interleukin-8 was noted in all sera, but values were the highest in children with fatal illnesses. Serum immune complexes (IgG-containing) were found in 7 of 16 of the children who died. Finally, patients with increased concentrations of interleukin-6, interleukin-8, and tumor necrosis factor–α were those with hypoperfusion, febrile peaks, seizures, and a manifestation of septic shock. Five of 10 children with severe or fatal illnesses had serum autoantibodies specific for smooth muscle.

CLINICAL MANIFESTATIONS

Adenoviral infections are exceedingly common, and the spectrum of disease is quite broad (Table 161–3). As noted in Table 161–3, there are some specific adenoviral diseases; however, the overall majority of infections involve a variety of anatomically associated illnesses. In many instances, similar illnesses are caused by other respiratory viruses, and the clinical spectrums of the various adenoviral serotypes frequently overlap. Certain specific adenoviral types do have clinical characteristics that facilitate etiologic diagnosis, however.

Respiratory Tract

Common Cold

Although adenoviruses frequently receive etiologic consideration in colds, they, in fact, only rarely are associated with this illness.[199] One report associated adenovirus with 3 per cent of common colds in children,[302] and in another study, 6.4 per cent of children with coryza had adenoviral isolates.[99] Respiratory tract infections with adenoviruses usually are associated with fever and, frequently, with some degree of pharyngitis; therefore, when strict clinical criteria are applied, they do not qualify as colds.[184, 360] Occasionally, adenoviruses, particularly types 1, 2, 3, 5, and 7, have been recovered from patients with typical colds.

Nasopharyngitis, Pharyngitis, and Tonsillitis

Adenoviral pharyngitis is an acute illness characterized by fever, sore throat, extensive exudative tonsillitis, and, often, cervical adenopathy.[99, 199, 262, 350] In two studies involving 74 children with adenoviral pharyngitis, Ruuskanen and associates[331, 332] described the pharyngeal findings. Most commonly, only mild inflammation and redness were observed. When exudates were present, they found them to be thick and membranous, thin and follicular, or thin and spotty; most typical were follicular and spotty exudates. Associated symptoms include malaise, headache, myalgia, chills, and cough. In infants and preschool children, nasal congestion and discharge are noticeable and abdominal pain is a common complaint.[389] Children with adenoviral acute febrile pharyngitis also frequently have laryngotracheitis, bronchitis, or pneumonia.[416] The usual duration of illness varies from 5 to 7 days, although occasionally symptoms persist well into the second week.[331]

Acute febrile pharyngitis is the most common adenoviral illness in children and particularly is important as an epidemic illness in closed environments.[18, 350, 359, 415] For example, in an epidemic in a children's home, 63 per cent of the residents were infected with adenovirus type 7a.[155] Moffet and colleagues[262] noted that adenoviruses were the most common etiologic agents recovered from hospitalized preschool children with febrile exudative pharyngitis; 23 per cent of the children they studied had adenoviral infections. In a university student health service study, 2.4 per cent of illnesses with acute febrile pharyngitis were due to adenoviruses.[271] Adenoviruses account for 37 to 75 per cent of nonstreptococcal pharyngitis in military recruits.

In children, 86 per cent of febrile pharyngitis is associated with adenovirus types 1, 2, 3, 5, and 7.[155, 184, 262]

On occasion, adenovirus types 7a, 9, 14, 15, and the intermediate strain 21/H21 + 35[170, 350, 359] also have been noted in association with pharyngitis. In military recruits, adenovirus types 4 and 7 are the main etiologic agents.

Acute Respiratory Disease

Acute respiratory disease is an epidemic disease that occurs predominantly in military recruit populations. This illness was studied extensively during World War II by the Commission on Acute Respiratory Diseases, and although individual cases were quite undifferentiated, the epidemiologic aspects of the outbreaks clearly indicated a specific etiologic agent.[65, 132, 350, 361, 381, 386] The disease is an acute, febrile, respiratory illness of short duration with constitutional and localized respiratory symptoms.[129] After an incubation period of 5 to 7 days, a patient develops fever (mean, 39.5° C), pharyngitis, laryngitis, tracheitis, and nonproductive cough.[25, 79, 132, 296] The initial dry, hacking cough may progress to paroxysms. Malaise, myalgia, chills, headache, dizziness, rhinitis, conjunctivitis, abdominal pain, and local cervical lymphadenopathy are common complaints.[79] The inflammatory process may spread to the bronchi, the bronchioles, and the parenchyma of the lungs. In epidemics, as many as 67 per cent of

TABLE 161–3. Clinical Spectrum of Adenoviral Infections

System	Illness Category	Epidemic Occurrence	Frequency	Adenoviral Types
Respiratory	Common cold	No	Rare	1, 2, 3, 5, 7
	Nasopharyngitis, pharyngitis, and tonsillitis	Yes	Common	1,* 2,* 3,* 4, 5,* 7,* 7a, 14, 15, (21/H21 + 35)†
	Acute respiratory disease	Yes (in military recruits)	Very common	2, 3, 4,* 5, 7,* 8, 11, 14, 21
	Acute laryngotracheitis	No	Occasional	1, 2, 3, 5, 6, 7
	Acute bronchiolitis	No	Occasional	3, 7, 21
	Pneumonia (civilian population)	Yes	Common	1, 2, 3,* 4, 5, 7,* 7a,* 8, 11, 21,* (21/H21 + 35),† 35
	Atypical pneumonia in military recruits	Yes	Common	4,* 7,* 21
	Pertussis-like syndrome	No	Rare	1, 2, 3, 5, 12, 19
	Bronchiolitis obliterans	No	Rare	7, 21
	Unilateral hyperlucent lung	No	Rare	7, 21
Eye	Acute follicular conjunctivitis	Yes	Common	1, 2, 3, 4, 6, 7, 9, 10, 11, 15, 16, 17, 19, 20, 22, 37
	Pharyngoconjunctival fever	Yes	Common	1, 2,* 3,* 4,* 5, 6, 7,* 7a,* 8, 14,* 37
	Epidemic keratoconjunctivitis	Yes	Occasional	2, 3, 4, 5, 7, 8,* 10, 11, 13, 14, 15, 16, 17, 19, 23, 29, 37
Skin	Morbilliform and rubelliform exanthem	Rare	Occasional	3, 4, 7, 7a
	Roseola-like	No	Occasional	1, 2
	Stevens-Johnson syndrome	No	Rare	7
	Petechial exanthem	No	Rare	7
Genitourinary	Acute hemorrhagic cystitis	No	Rare	7, 11, 21
	Nephritis	No	Rare	3, 4, 7a
	Orchitis	No	Rare	Unknown
	Oculogenital syndrome	Yes	Rare	19, 37
Gastrointestinal	Gastroenteritis	Yes	Common	1, 2, 3,* 5, 7,* 11, 12, 15, 17, 31,* 32, 33, 40,* 41*
	Mesenteric lymphadenitis	No	Rare	1, 2, 3, 5, 7
	Intussusception	No	Rare	1, 2, 3, 5, 6, 7
	Appendicitis	No	Rare	1, 2, 7
	Hepatitis	No	Rare	1, 2, 3, 5,* 7, (11 + 35/H11 + 35)†
Heart	Myocarditis	No	Rare	7, 7a, 21
	Pericarditis	No	Rare	7
Neurologic	Encephalitis and meningitis	No	Rare	1, 2, 3, 5, 6, 7, 11, 12, 32
Joint	Arthritis	No	Rare	7
Auditory	Deafness	No	Rare	3
Endocrine	Thyroiditis	No	Rare	Unknown

*Most common.
†Intermediate strain.

those affected wheeze and have other evidence of small airway obstruction; pneumonia occurs in 10 to 20 per cent.[174, 234, 265] The illness gradually resolves over an 8- to 36-day period.[122] Early in the illness, the total white blood cell count may be slightly elevated, with a slight increase in the percentage of polymorphonuclear leukocytes.

In experimental aerosol-induced acute respiratory disease, the incubation period ranged between 6 and 13 days.[70] Typical illness included fever to 39° C, rhinitis, prostration, malaise, myalgia, and headache. Pneumonia occurred occasionally. The virus was recovered from throat culture specimens 5 days after inoculation, from the nose at 6 days, and after 9 days in fecal specimens. Serum-neutralizing antibody responses occurred between the third and fourth weeks. All ill volunteers demonstrated a leukopenia and an elevated erythrocyte sedimentation rate during illness.

The syndrome is most common in military recruits early in basic training; illness has been documented in up to 90 per cent of new trainees within the first 8 weeks of arrival at a training site.[174] The usual etiologic agents are adenovirus types 4 and 7. Occasionally, epidemics have been associated with adenovirus types 3, 11, 14, and 21.[122] Sporadic cases have been noted in association with adenovirus types 2, 5, and 8.[174, 296] The peak seasons of illness are winter and spring.[174] Although illness may occur in civilian adults, it is uncommon and not epidemic. In volunteer studies, subjects with serum antibody to a particular adenoviral type are protected against disease with that type upon intranasal inoculation.[16, 70]

In children, epidemic acute respiratory disease has not been described. However, sporadic comparative illness, usually clinically identified as acute bronchitis, commonly is the result of adenoviral infection.[416] Adenovirus type 7 is the most common etiologic agent in these cases.

Acute Laryngotracheitis

Adenoviruses on occasion have been implicated in the causation of acute laryngotracheitis. In general, croup due to adenoviruses is not severe and frequently manifests only as a barking, brassy cough. Laryngotracheitis often is seen in association with febrile pharyngitis, bronchiolitis, and pneumonia.[416] Epidemics have not been observed. Adenovirus types 1, 2, 3, 5, 6, and 7 have been implicated as etiologic agents.

Acute Bronchiolitis

Adenoviruses account for approximately 5 per cent of the cases of bronchiolitis in infants.[409] Bronchiolitis due to adenoviral infection is sporadic and usually similar to illness associated with other viral agents. Adenoviral bronchiolitis occurring early in infancy on occasion has been fatal or associated with serious residual lung damage and chronic disease.[400] This severe illness has been associated with serotypes 3, 7, and 21.

Pneumonia

YOUNG CHILDREN. Adenoviruses are common isolates in children with pneumonia. Their overall frequency in the causation of nonbacterial pneumonia in children is less than that of respiratory syncytial virus and parainfluenza virus type 3, but an alarming number of fatal illnesses have been noted. Severe and fatal illnesses in infants and young children have been noted in association with adenovirus types 1, 2, 3, 4, 5, 7, 7a, 8, 19, 21, 35, and the intermediate strain 21/H21 + 35.[6, 14, 15, 21, 39, 40, 52, 58, 89, 127, 141, 172, 191, 200, 201, 213–215, 223, 241, 248, 284, 293, 304, 318, 344, 345, 354, 357, 411] The more severe cases of pneumonias have been associated with types 3, 7, and 21.[345, 411] Adenoviral pneumonia has been epidemic and sporadic.[52, 58]

Severe pneumonia is most common in neonates and young children 3 to 18 months of age.[14, 15, 21, 39, 40, 67, 89, 141, 200, 215, 226, 248, 304, 318] The onset of illness is acute, with persistent cough and fever (>39° C). On physical examination, moderate to severe dyspnea is apparent, as is the associated tachypnea. Inspiratory and expiratory wheezes and rales on auscultation are heard. Other signs and symptoms include lethargy, diarrhea and vomiting, pharyngitis, and, occasionally, conjunctivitis. Extrapulmonary complications are common: meningitis, encephalitis, seizures, splenomegaly, hepatomegaly and hepatitis, myocarditis, nephritis, bleeding tendency, and exanthems.[21, 40, 52, 67, 226, 344, 345, 354, 357] Chest radiographs reveal diffuse infiltrates, which usually are bilateral and bronchial, peribronchial, or interstitial.[14, 226, 407] Hyperinflation and lobar collapse are frequent.[141] Rarely, pleural effusions or mediastinal lymphadenopathy has been described.[226] In surviving infants, symptoms persist for 2 to 4 weeks, and radiographic changes resolve slowly, frequently being present at the 3-week follow-up examination.[52, 58, 345] Recovery often is gradual, and exacerbations are common.[191, 293]

Serious sequelae often result from adenoviral lower respiratory disease, particularly in association with adenovirus types 3, 7, 7a, and 21.[10, 15, 141, 191, 226, 345] These include bronchiectasis, bronchiolitis obliterans, and unilateral hyperlucent lung.[10, 15, 226, 243, 345, 409] It has been estimated that 14 to 60 per cent of children with documented adenoviral lower respiratory tract disease have some degree of permanent pulmonary sequelae.[141, 226, 345, 346] In a study of 27 children 10 years after documented adenoviral type 7 pneumonia, 12 children had radiographic evidence of bronchiectasis or residual pulmonary changes; 16 children had abnormal pulmonary function studies.[346]

Maček and associates[242] have suggested that persistent adenoviral infections may be the cause of chronic airway obstructive disease in children. They noted adenoviral antigen in bronchoalveolar lavage specimens from 31 of 34 patients with chronic disease but from no bronchoalveolar lavage specimens from a control group.

On occasion, severe and fatal adenoviral pneumonia has been related to malnutrition, environmental crowding, or a preceding severe viral disease, such as measles.[10, 14, 15, 141, 223, 272, 345]

Severe adenoviral pneumonia associated with adenovirus types 3 and 7 also has been reported occasionally in previously healthy adults.[298, 306, 348] One adult had severe pneumonia due to adenovirus type 21, which was associated with myalgia, rhabdomyolysis, and myoglobinuria.[412]

ATYPICAL PNEUMONIA IN MILITARY RECRUITS. About 7 to 20 per cent of cases of pneumonia in military recruits are associated with adenoviral infection.[42, 117, 130] Adenoviral primary atypical pneumonia commonly occurs in the winter months and usually is associated with adenovirus types 4, 7, and 21.[117] The illness is associated with fever, cough, sore throat, rhinorrhea, and chest pain. Other common symptoms include nausea, vomiting, myalgia, headache, and diarrhea. On physical examination, rales and pharyngitis are noted in almost all cases. Rhinitis and generalized lymphadenopathy are observed in about half of those afflicted, and occasionally conjunctivitis is noted. Chest radiographs reveal a bilaterally mottled appearance, most prominent in the lower lobes; these remain abnormal from 4 to 36 days.[42] Although serum cold agglutinins are observed, titers of 1:32 or higher are noted in only 18 per cent of patients.[42, 130]

Fatal pneumonia, absolute leukopenia, and disseminated disease have been reported in four previously healthy military trainees. Adenovirus type 7 was the etiologic agent in three of these cases, and the fourth illness was due to adenovirus type 4.[95, 234]

PERTUSSIS-LIKE SYNDROME. A pertussis-like illness has been noted in association with several adenoviruses, including types 1, 2, 3, 5, 12, and 19.[64, 66, 155, 274, 287] The illness is most common in infants younger than 36 months of age. The onset of illness is insidious and initially suggestive of a cold. Cough becomes progressively worse and by 1 to 2 weeks is paroxysmal. Severe recurrent episodes of paroxysms result in the production of mucus, posttussive fatigue, and vomiting.[66] About 50 per cent of children have a typical whoop, and cyanosis occurs with paroxysms. Peripheral leukocytosis, ranging from 25,000 to 125,000 cells/mm^3, with lymphocytosis and thrombocytosis, is the usual finding.[64, 287] Recovery time ranges from 4 to 10 weeks from onset of illness.[66] Radiologic evidence of bronchiolitis is present in most children; interstitial pneumonia occurs occasionally. In my opinion, most and probably all of these pertussis-like illnesses are indeed *Bordetella pertussis* infections in which the adenovirus is a coinfecting agent.

BRONCHIOLITIS OBLITERANS. Bronchiolitis obliterans is a chronic bronchiolitis that initially was described in 1901 by Lange.[227] It has been noted to occur after measles, influenza, and pertussis and after the inhalation of toxic substances.[10, 15, 409] Adenovirus types 7 and 21 have resulted in a bronchiolitis obliterans–type chronic illness. With adenoviruses, a severe necrotizing bronchiolitis occurs that heals with fibrosis and predominantly obliterates small airways.[15] The onset of disease occurs with acute febrile illness, cough, and respiratory distress. Disease may wax and wane for several weeks or months and is associated with recurrent episodes of atelectasis, pneumonia, and wheezing. Although some children recover from these episodes, the remainder have chronic pulmonary disease, including irreversible atelectasis, bronchiectasis, or hyperlucent lung syndrome.[15, 400, 409]

UNILATERAL HYPERLUCENT LUNG. Unilateral hyperlucent lung is a well-defined syndrome characterized by increased translucency of all or part of one lung, with reduction in lung size.[74, 243] The unilateral hyperlucency is associated with a decrease in the size and number of pulmonary vessels, as observed on pulmonary angiograms, and an absence of peripheral filling at bronchography.[243] Although the disease may be secondary to a number of causes, including pneumonia due to other viruses, it has been noted to occur after severe necrotizing bronchiolitis and pneumonia due to adenovirus types 7 and 21.[243, 409]

CONGENITAL PLEURAL EFFUSION. An infant with a congenital pleural effusion from which an adenovirus type 3 was recovered has been reported.[254]

Eye

Acute Follicular Conjunctivitis

Acute follicular conjunctivitis is the most common and benign of the adenoviral infections of the eye. The infection in this disease is confined to the eye, usually is unilateral, and is manifest by follicular lesions on the conjunctival surface. Symptoms occur after an incubation period of 5 to 7 days and include lacrimation, itching, burning, foreign body sensation, and conjunctival erythema.[90] Examination shows erythema and lymphoid follicular hyperplasia in the conjunctiva in association with serous drainage and increased lacrimation. Occasionally, adenopathy of the preauricular lymph nodes is seen. Symptoms resolve in 10 days to 3 weeks, with recovery usually complete.[69, 90] Adenovirus types 1, 2, 3, 4, 6, 7, 9, 10, 11, 15, 16, 17, 19, 20, 22, and 37 have been isolated from the eyes of afflicted patients.[30, 67, 90, 336, 341]

Pharyngoconjunctival Fever

Pharyngoconjunctival fever is presented in detail in Chapter 12.

Epidemic Keratoconjunctivitis

Epidemic keratoconjunctivitis is caused most commonly by adenovirus type 8, but it also has resulted from infection with adenovirus types 2, 3, 4, 5, 7, 10, 11, 13, 14, 15, 16, 17, 19, 22, 23, 29, and 37.[12, 30, 44, 70, 78, 80, 83, 85, 86, 107, 151, 152, 156, 195, 196, 205, 206, 209, 261, 263, 277, 279, 336, 352, 369, 415] Currently, adenovirus type 37 is the most common virus recovered from patients with epidemic keratoconjunctivitis in the United States and Europe. The most severe disease is associated with adenovirus types 5, 8, and 19.[78]

The illness is most common in adults, but there are a few reports of disease in children.[156, 261, 368] There is no seasonal pattern. Although transmission of the viral agent from the respiratory tract to the eye occurs in sporadic cases, the usual method of viral spread is by contaminated ophthalmic instruments and eye solutions, hand-to-eye contact by medical personnel and others, swimming pools, or hands or fomites in close contact situations, such as in families and in industry.[12, 44, 78, 80, 83, 114, 195, 218, 247, 261, 263, 368, 399] The incubation period usually is 5 to 10 days but ranges from as short a period as 2 days to as long as 2 weeks.[80, 218] The initial symptom usually is unilateral, acute, follicular conjunctivitis that suggests a foreign body. Photophobia, lacrimation, discharge, hyperemia, and edema of the conjunctiva are notable. Preauricular adenopathy occurs in up to 90 per cent of patients, and 50 per cent of those afflicted have pharyngitis and rhinitis. Spread to the other eye may occur in 2 to 7 days. Seven to 10 days after the onset of disease, the conjunctivitis resolves and painful, superficial, punctate, epithelial opacities appear in the center of the cornea. These lesions frequently extend subepithelially and then heal, leaving subepithelial infiltrates that may persist for months. In severe cases, hazy vision may persist for several years.[12]

An infantile form of epidemic keratoconjunctivitis, usually affecting infants younger than 2 years of age, has been described. This pseudomembranous or membranous conjunctivitis usually is accompanied by high fever, pharyngitis, otitis media, diarrhea, and vomiting. Preauricular lymphadenopathy usually is absent.[368]

Virus can be recovered from the eye for a usual period of approximately 2 weeks but has been cultured for 2 to 3 years in patients with chronic papillary conjunctivitis.[78, 303] In acute illness, conjunctival scrapings obtained during the first 10 days of infection reveal characteristic inclusion bodies when they are Giemsa-stained.[188] Virus-specific fluorescent antibody staining is diagnostic in epidemic keratoconjunctivitis.[340] Preparations of corneal and conjunctival epithelia reveal adenoviral particles when they are examined with the electron microscope.[85]

Skin

Adenovirus types 1, 2, 3, 4, 7, and 7a, plus several unknown types, have been noted in association with exanthematous disease.[54] The most common cutaneous manifestation associated with adenoviral infection is an erythematous maculopapular rash that appears while the child is febrile. In many instances, children with this illness have been thought to have either measles or rubella.[223] In the majority of adenoviral infections with exanthems, other clinical findings more characteristic of adenoviruses, such as conjunctivitis, rhinitis, pharyngitis, and lymphadenopathy, also are present. In some instances, the exanthem truly is morbilliform with characteristic confluence, but Koplik spots do not occur.

A widespread erythematous rash often is present early in the course of severe pneumonia in infants.[141] Chany and colleagues[52] noted a measles-like rash in five patients who died of adenoviral type 7a pneumonia. One report notes a child with an adenoviral type 7 infection and illness suggestive of meningococcemia.[333] This patient had fever, vomiting, diarrhea, and a petechial exanthem.

On several occasions, illness characterized by fever and defervescence and then the appearance of a maculopapular rash suggesting the diagnosis of roseola infantum has been observed.[115, 125, 193, 194, 276] Adenoviral infections also are confused with rubella. However, the respiratory symptoms and the degree of fever associated with adenoviral infections should clarify the diagnosis. With rubella, respiratory complaints and fever are minimal. On occasion, severe disease with Stevens-Johnson syndrome has been noted. In these cases, pneumonia frequently is noted, and the illness is quite similar to that caused by *Mycoplasma pneumoniae* infection.

Lähdeaho and associates[225] have noted that serum antibodies to the E1b protein-derived peptides of the enteric adenovirus type 40 are associated with dermatitis herpetiformis.

Genitourinary Tract

Acute Hemorrhagic Cystitis

Acute hemorrhagic cystitis is an uncommon manifestation of adenoviral infection characterized by the sudden onset of dysuria and frequency, with hematuria 12 to 24 hours later.[228, 267–269, 283] Occasionally, fever, suprapubic pain, and enuresis occur. Antecedent upper respiratory infection is noted in some children. Symptoms persist for a few days to 2 weeks. The usual duration is about 5 days. The disease has been reported in both the United States and Japan. It occurs primarily in children, most often boys, and usually is associated with adenovirus type 11. Occasionally, adenovirus types 7 and 21 have been implicated. Adenoviral antigen has been identified by immunofluorescence in exfoliated bladder cells. Although there have been no known sequelae, the long-term prognosis is unknown.[269]

Nephritis

Hematuria occasionally has been noted in infants with severe pneumonia and disseminated adenoviral infection. Red blood cells and occasionally red blood cell casts in the urine also have been noted in some children with upper respiratory illnesses due to adenoviruses and specifically in patients with pharyngoconjunctival fever associated with adenovirus types 3, 4, and 7a.[350, 355, 387, 389] In one instance, a young boy had a maculopapular and petechial exanthem and thrombocytopenia associated with adenovirus type 7 infection. Hematuria also was noted.

Orchitis

Orchitis was noted in one child who had a 5-day history of pain and fever, erythema, and swelling of the right testicle.[273] The testicular involvement resolved in several days, and the illness was associated with a 16-fold adenoviral complement-fixation antibody titer rise.

Oculogenital Syndrome

In 1976, Laverty and associates[228] reported a woman who, in addition to pharyngoconjunctival fever, had cervicitis and paresthesia of the legs; an adenovirus type 19 was recovered from this woman's cervix. In Perth, Australia, adenovirus type 19 was recovered from the genital tracts of 59 men and women being examined for genital herpes simplex virus infection in a sexually transmitted diseases clinic.[188] Several of the patients also had conjunctivitis, and, in two, adenovirus type 19 also was isolated from conjunctival specimens. Similar oculogenital illnesses have been noted in association with adenoviral types 2, 8, and 37.[48, 336, 364]

Hemolytic-Uremic Syndrome

Two 2-year-old children with hemolytic-uremic syndrome in association with adenoviral infections have been described.[24]

Gastrointestinal Tract

Gastroenteritis

Infantile diarrhea has been associated with epidemic and sporadic adenoviral diseases such as acute upper respiratory infections, severe pneumonia, and pharyngoconjunctival fever.[115, 226, 350, 358, 402] Outbreaks of diarrhea, characterized by acute abdominal pain followed by diarrhea, nausea and vomiting, fever, headache, and pharyngitis, have been associated with infections with adenovirus types 3 and 7.[128, 359] Other symptoms occurring in patients with diarrhea include conjunctivitis, rhinitis, pharyngotonsillitis, hepatomegaly, and cervical adenitis.[358] In two patients who had diarrhea and upper respiratory illness in association with adenoviral type 15 infection, viral particles were visualized at autopsy by electron microscopy within the nuclei of mucosal cells.[97]

The widespread use of electron microscopy for the study of rotavirus diarrhea led to the finding of previously unrecognized adenoviruses that were fastidious and could not be grown in routine cell cultures.[112, 339] These adenoviruses, now identified as type 40 and type 41, have been shown subsequently to be important causes of gastroenteritis in children.[36, 38, 61, 221, 222, 258, 286, 308, 320, 371, 382, 384] In enteric adenoviral infections, diarrhea is the most prominent symptom.[382] In children with adenovirus type 40 infections, Uhnoo and colleagues[382] found that the mean duration was 8.6 days, whereas it was 12.2 days in those infected with adenovirus type 41. Most illnesses occur in children younger than 3 years of age; the mean age for adenoviral type 40 diarrhea was 15.2 months, whereas it was 28.3 months in type 41 illnesses. Most patients had mild vomiting, which lasted about 2 days. When compared with illnesses due to established respiratory adenoviruses, fever was less common, less severe, and of less duration in enteric adenoviral infections. Upper respiratory symptoms and signs, such as pharyngitis, coryza, cough, and otitis media, were noted in 21 per cent of the children with enteric adenoviral infections. Brandt and colleagues[37] have noted that dual infections with respiratory viruses (such as respiratory syncytial virus and enteric adenoviruses) are common, so that caution should be observed in attributing respiratory symptoms to enteric adenoviruses.

Yolken and Franklin[418] found that enteric adenoviruses were an important cause of nosocomial diarrhea in infants who had prior gastrointestinal surgery for necrotizing enterocolitis.

Mesenteric Lymphadenitis

Adenoviral serotypes 1, 2, 3, 5, and 7 have been recovered from lymph nodes and appendix in cases of mesenteric lymphadenitis.[19, 29, 217] Patients with mesenteric lymphadenitis frequently have abdominal pain and other symptoms similar to acute appendicitis. Pharyngitis is a frequent associated finding. Mesenteric adenitis often is associated with concurrent or recent adenoviral illness.[67, 312] Often, the peak incidence of mesenteric lymphadenitis occurs when adenoviral illness is common in the community.

Intussusception

The suggestion that adenoviruses could be an etiologic factor in intussusception arose because these agents frequently can be recovered from throat, stool, and mesenteric lymph node specimens obtained from children operated on for intussusception.[19, 23, 63, 129, 282, 306, 326, 419, 420] Most children with intussusception were younger than 2 years of age; some had preceding respiratory symptoms.[326, 420] Adenovirus serotypes 1, 2, 3, 5, 6, and 7 have been implicated. Typical adenoviral intranuclear inclusions have been demonstrated by electron microscopy in cells in stool, intestinal epithelia (ileum), and the appendix.[282, 419, 420] Mesenteric lymph nodes often are enlarged at surgery.[419] Antibody titer rises to adenoviruses have been noted in children after intussusception. It has been suggested that bowel wall hypermotility due to direct viral involvement or the hypertrophy of lymphatic tissue is the lead point for the intussusception.[19, 63, 129, 282, 310, 326, 419, 420]

Appendicitis

Adenoviruses have been associated with both acute and chronic appendicitis.[29] Right iliac fossa abdominal pain associated with sore throat is a common finding. The virus has been isolated from the appendix and mesenteric lymph nodes at surgery. During acute infection, lymphoid follicles of the ileum, appendix, and mesenteric lymph nodes are infected with virus. In chronic infection, adenovirus remains in cells; on microscopic examination, slight inflammation is seen in the appendix.

Hepatitis

Hepatitis in association with adenoviral infection has been reported many times in small infants, in children with overwhelming disseminated diseases, and in immunocompromised patients.[2, 9, 21, 40, 46, 214, 421] In one study, 27 of 30 persons thought to have sporadic infectious hepatitis were found to be infected with adenovirus type 5.[157] Adenovirus types 1, 2, and 3 were isolated from stool specimens of 12 children younger than 3 years of age in an outbreak of infectious hepatitis on a Native American reservation in Arizona.[158]

In one report, three children with severe, fatal adenoviral type 7 pneumonia had associated findings that simulated Reye syndrome: lethargy, diarrhea, seizures, elevated cerebrospinal fluid pressure, myocarditis, hepatitis, and disseminated intravascular coagulation.[224] Edwards and colleagues[100] reported three children with Reye syndrome and adenoviral infections. They suggested that adenoviruses might be an important agent in initiating the syndrome.

Heart

Myocarditis

In children, myocarditis has been noted in association with severe pneumonia and disseminated disease due to adenovirus types 7, 7a, and 21.[159] Similar cardiac involvement has been noted in military recruits with severe acute respiratory disease.[52, 58, 159, 350]

Pericarditis

Pericarditis has been associated with severe adenoviral pneumonia. In a patient with adenoviral type 7 pneumonia, electrocardiographic changes consistent with pericarditis were demonstrated, and the virus was isolated in high titer from pericardial fluid at postmortem examination.[272] Recently, Mistchenko and coworkers[260] reported a 10-month-old boy with fatal pericarditis due to adenovirus type 7. In serum and pericardial fluid from this child, interleukin-6, tumor necrosis factor–α, and adenovirus-specific immune complexes were identified.

Neurologic

Although central nervous system disease in adenoviral infection is uncommon, a variety of clinical manifestations have been observed. Both meningitis and encephalitis have been noted as the major manifestations of adenoviral infections or in association with severe disease at other body sites.[306, 310] Adenovirus types 1, 2, 3, 5, 6, 7, 12, and 32, in isolated instances, have been recovered from both brain and cerebrospinal fluid.[67, 72, 108, 126, 208, 301, 323, 344, 357, 362] In two children with respiratory and central nervous system symptoms, adenoviruses were recovered from the spinal fluid.[108] One child was convalescing from herpes zoster and the other from varicella. Adenovirus type 7 was recovered from tissue cultures of brain from an elderly patient with chronic schizophrenia.[241] In another instance, an adenovirus type 32 was recovered from the brain of a man with lymphosarcoma and subacute encephalitis.[60, 323] In an epidemic of adenoviral infection due to type 7, 25 per cent of the hospitalized patients had symptoms referable to the central nervous system.[344, 345] Many of the patients died; those who survived had little residual. Too few cases are reported in the literature to predict accurately the prognosis of central nervous system disease in children.

Other Manifestations

Arthritis

Arthritis has been noted in association with adenoviral type 7 infection.[292] The illness was characterized by fever, acute respiratory symptoms, erythematous macular rash, aseptic meningitis, and inflammatory arthritis of both knees.

Thyroiditis

In 1964, Swann[363] reported five patients with acute thyroiditis and thyroid enlargement in whom serologic study revealed greater than fourfold titer rises in adenoviral complement-fixing antibody.

Deafness

Deafness of sudden onset was reported in an adult with a 2-day history of sore throat, low-grade fever, rhinorrhea, and cough. Adenovirus type 3 was isolated from the patient's throat, and a greater than fourfold neutralizing antibody titer rise to this virus was observed.[190]

Infection in the Immunocompromised Host

Adenovirus types 1, 2, 4, 5, 6, 7, 7a, 11, 29, 31, 32, 34, and 35 have been recovered from children and adults who were immunocompromised by immunodeficiency diseases, malignancies, steroid therapy, immunosuppressive therapy, radiation therapy, and transplantation procedures.[2, 45, 46, 60, 77, 82, 113, 147, 166, 207, 240, 271, 278, 285, 323, 342, 343, 351, 379, 406, 421] Although there are few data relating to morbidity and mortality from adenoviral infections in patients who are immunocompromised, recent evidence suggests a generally greater severity of illness. Scattered reports have noted an association between adenoviral infections and viruria and hemorrhagic cystitis in renal transplant patients.[110, 227] A fatal case of subacute meningoencephalitis due to an adenovirus in a bone marrow transplant patient has been described.[82]

In many instances, a fulminant, bacterial, sepsis-like picture with high fever, cough, and lethargy is associated with adenoviral infections in compromised patients.[421] Severe pneumonia often is demonstrated, both clinically and radiologically, and hepatic involvement with disseminated intravascular coagulation also is frequent. Fatalities are reported, and recovery often is slow.

Congenital and Neonatal Infections

Neonatal and congenital adenoviral infections reflect disseminated infection with the involvement of multiple organs.[1, 39, 59, 215, 288, 357] Major manifestations include hepatosplenomegaly, progressive pneumonia, hepatitis, and thrombocytopenia. Towbin and colleagues[377] noted intrauterine adenoviral myocarditis that presented as nonimmune hydrops fetalis. Illnesses frequently present as an early-onset sepsis syndrome.

DIAGNOSIS

Differential Diagnosis

The differential diagnosis of adenoviral infection must be subcategorized on the basis of the major clinical manifestations. In many instances, because of specific clinical symptoms, such as pharyngoconjunctival fever or epidemic keratoconjunctivitis, the adenoviral etiology strongly can be suspected. In other, more general respiratory diseases, such as pharyngitis, bronchitis, croup, bronchiolitis, and pneumonia, the adenoviral etiology can not be established on clinical grounds. Fever in adenoviral respiratory infections tends to be higher than that occurring in parainfluenza and respiratory syncytial viral infections but similar to that occurring in influenza A and B virus infections.[313] High and prolonged fever is as common in adenoviral infections as it is in bacterial respiratory infections.

In pharyngitis, adenoviral infection must be differentiated both from other viral diseases, such as those due to Epstein-Barr, parainfluenza, and influenza viruses and enteroviruses, and from streptococcal disease. In the young child, follicular pharyngitis is more likely to be due to adenoviral than to streptococcal infection.

Adenoviral pneumonia in young children frequently is not distinguishable on clinical grounds from that caused by bacteria. In older children and adolescents in particular, adenoviral pneumonia frequently can be differentiated from bacterial disease by its bilateral nature. The differentiation of adenoviral illness from disease due to *M. pneumoniae* is more difficult; however, cold agglutinin titers generally are higher and more persistently positive in mycoplasmal disease.

Adenoviral eye disease must be differentiated from that due to viruses of the herpes group, *Chlamydia* species, and bacteria, including *Neisseria gonorrhoeae.*

Diarrhea due to enteric adenoviruses can be differentiated from other viral diarrheas by electron microscopy, specific culture or identification by ELISA, and specific culture of the enteric agents in 293 cell culture. Enteric bacterial and parasitic agents also must be considered in the differential diagnosis.

Because of high relatively prolonged fever in association with lymphadenopathy, exanthem, and enanthem, adenoviral infections often are confused with Kawasaki disease.[56] Because it is important to treat Kawasaki disease early with intravenous immunoglobulin, adenoviral infections should be considered early and appropriate studies performed.

Specific Diagnosis

Adenoviral infection can be diagnosed specifically by viral isolation in an appropriate tissue culture system or by a direct antigen detection assay. Most adenoviral types can be recovered from clinical specimens in primary or diploid cultures of human embryonic kidney.[232] The enteric viral types 40 and 41 can be grown in 293 cells.[366, 395] The rapidity of detection of adenoviruses by culture is enhanced by the use of centrifugation of specimens in shell vials or plastic-welled plates.[98, 102, 244]

The direct identification of adenoviruses in respiratory secretions by radioimmunoassay, immunofluorescence, and ELISA is now done widely.[41, 244, 253, 315, 331, 332, 334, 370] However, in general, the sensitivity, compared with that of virus isolation, is relatively low; on the other hand, the specificity is high (>95 per cent). Rapid techniques for the identification of enteric adenoviruses in general have been sensitive and specific.[4, 144, 163, 335, 382, 410] However, in newborns, false-positive results with a latex agglutination test have been reported.[187] Several techniques using DNA probes have been studied and show promise for the rapid identification of both respiratory and enteric adenoviral infections.[43, 186, 367] Polymerase chain reaction (PCR) also shows promise for the rapid detection of adenoviral infections but at present lacks the sensitivity of culture.[5, 264] PCR also can be used for the identification of adenovirus DNA in formalin-fixed, paraffin-embedded tissues.[380]

Acute infection also can be demonstrated serologically by the demonstration of specific IgM serum antibody.[253] Infection can be confirmed serologically by the demonstration of an antibody titer rise in two sequential serum samples. Antibody response to the adenovirus group antigen can be detected by complement fixation or ELISA. Type-specific antibodies can be determined by neutralization, ELISA, or hemagglutination inhibition.

TREATMENT

During the febrile period of illness, adequate hydration should be maintained and excessive activity should be discouraged. The fever may be controlled with acetaminophen. In children with eye involvement, careful attention should be paid to the possibility of secondary bacterial infection. If local purulence develops, cultures should be taken and topical antimicrobial therapy started. Steroid-containing ophthalmic ointments should be avoided.

In a number of instances, immunocompromised patients with disseminated adenoviral infections have been treated with ribavirin administered intravenously and successful outcomes have been reported.[202, 236, 249, 270, 414] In one instance, a loading dose of 30 mg/kg/day in three doses was followed by maintenance therapy with 15 mg/kg/day.[249]

Human fibroblast-derived interferon, applied topically, was used to treat epidemic adenovirus keratoconjunctivitis in a comparative trial.[322] The duration of illness was reduced in the interferon-treated patients, but many of the control patients received dexamethasone. A child with combined immunodeficiency and a severe diffuse adenovirus type 7a pneumonia improved dramatically after a large dose of high-titered adenovirus type 7a immune serum globulin.[77]

PREVENTION

Serious incapacitating epidemics in military recruits in basic training caused by adenoviruses led to the development of adenoviral vaccines.[7, 230] Initial vaccines were formalin-inactivated preparations of monkey kidney tissue culture-grown virus, which were administered parenterally.[6, 149, 174] These vaccines achieved only limited success because of variable degrees of potency in different vaccine lots.[15] An inactivated adenoviral vaccine that contained types 3, 4, and 7 was prepared in monkey tissue culture for trial in children.[390] Three doses of this vaccine resulted in high levels of neutralizing antibody to the three viral types, and this antibody persisted in the majority of infants for at least 1 year. Many of the initial lots of inactivated adenoviral vaccine were found to contain live simian adenoviruses that were capable of producing neoplasms in suckling hamsters. Because of this, inactivated vaccine trials were discontinued. Next, a live attenuated adenovirus type 4 vaccine that was cultivated in human diploid tissue culture was developed and administered orally by enteric-coated capsule to volunteers.[149] Asymptomatic gastrointestinal infection occurred, and a good serum-neutralizing antibody response was elicited.[149, 349, 353] Most recipients of live oral vaccine excrete virus in the stool for several days to a month after vaccination. With military use of the vaccine, stool shedding was not associated with transmission of virus to nonimmune contacts.[265] In other studies, of married couples and families with children, virus was transmitted to nonimmune contacts.[265, 353] Transmission usually occurred without illness.[265]

The administration of live enteric-coated adenovirus types 4 and 7 vaccine resulted in a significant decrease in the incidence of acute respiratory disease in military recruits.[96, 142, 365] With use of this vaccine, acute respiratory disease caused by other serotypes, including adenovirus type 21, became more prevalent, however.[388] There have been few attempts to protect children with live adenoviral vaccines. In one study, live enteric-coated adenovirus type 4 vaccine was given to children 5 to 11 years of age. Asymptomatic gastrointestinal infection resulted from vaccine administration.

PROGNOSIS

The overall prognosis in adenoviral infections generally is excellent. Secondary bacterial complications, if untreated, can result in the prolongation of illness and permanent sequelae in some instances. The prognosis in adenoviral infection in the very young and in immunocompromised patients must be guarded.

References

1. Abzug, M. J., and Levin, M. J.: Neonatal adenovirus infection: Four patients and review of the literature. Pediatrics *87*:890–896, 1991.
2. Adler, H.: Keratitis sub-epithelialis. Centralbl. Prakt. Augenh. *13*:289–295, 1889.
3. Adrian, T., Wigans, R., and Richter, J.: Gastroenteritis in infants, associated with a genome type of adenovirus 31 and with combined rotavirus and adenovirus 31 infection. Eur. J. Pediatr. *146*:38–40, 1987.
4. Ahluwalia, G. S., Scott-Taylor, T. H., Klisko, B., et al.: Comparison of detection methods for adenovirus from enteric clinical specimens. Diagn. Microbiol. Infect. Dis. *18*:161–166, 1994.
5. Allard, A., Girones, R., Juto, P., et al.: Polymerase chain reaction for detection of adenoviruses in stool samples. J. Clin. Microbiol. *28*:2659–2667, 1990.
6. Andiman, W. A., Jacobson, R. I., and Tucker, G.: Leukocyte-associated viremia with adenovirus type 2 in an infant with lower-respiratory-tract disease. N. Engl. J. Med. *297*:100–101, 1977.
7. Angella, J. J., and Connor, J. D.: Neonatal infection caused by adenovirus type 7. J. Pediatr. *72*:474–478, 1968.
8. Artenstein, M. S., Miller, W. S., Lamson, T. H., et al.: Large-volume air sampling for meningococci and adenoviruses. Am. J. Epidemiol. *87*:567–577, 1968.
9. Aterman, K., Embil, J., Easterbrook, K. B., et al.: Liver necrosis, adenovirus type 2 and thymic dysplasia. Virchows Arch. (Pathol. Anat.) *360*:155–171, 1973.
10. Azizirad, H., Polgar, G., Borns, P. F., et al.: Bronchiolitis obliterans. Clin. Pediatr. *14*:572–584, 1975.
11. Bahn, C. A.: Swimming bath conjunctivitis. New Orleans Med. Surg. J. *79*:586–590, 1927.
12. Barnard, D. L., Hart, J. C. D., Marmion, V. J., et al.: Outbreak in Bristol of conjunctivitis caused by adenovirus type 8, and its epidemiology and control. Br. Med. J. *2*:165–169, 1973.
13. Béal, R.: Sur une forme particulière de conjonctivite aigue avec follicules. Annales D'Oculistique, Jan. 1907, pp. 1–33.
14. Becroft, D. M. O.: Histopathology of fatal adenovirus infection of the respiratory tract in young children. J. Clin. Pathol. *20*:561–569, 1967.
15. Becroft, D. M. O.: Bronchiolitis obliterans, bronchiectasis, and other sequelae of adenovirus type 21 infection in young children. J. Clin. Pathol. *24*:72–82, 1971.
16. Bell, J. A., Ward, T. G., Huebner, R. J., et al.: Studies of adenoviruses (APC) in volunteers. Am. J. Public Health *46*:1130–1146, 1956.
17. Bell, J. A., Huebner, R. J., Rosen, L., et al.: Illness and microbial experiences of nursery children at junior village. Am. J. Hyg. *74*:267–292, 1961.
18. Bell, T. M., Turner, G., Macdonald, A., et al.: Type-3 adenovirus infection. Lancet *2*:1327–1329, 1960.
19. Bell, T. M., and Steyn, J. H.: Viruses in lymph nodes of children with mesenteric adenitis and intussusception. Br. Med. J. *5306*:700–702, 1962.
20. Bellanti, J. A., Artenstein, M. S., Brandt, B. L., et al.: Immunoglobulin responses in serum and nasal secretions after natural adenovirus infections. J. Immunol. *103*:891–898, 1969.
21. Benyesh-Melnick, M., and Rosenberg, H. S.: The isolation of adenovirus type 7 from a fatal case of pneumonia and disseminated disease. J. Pediatr. *64*:83–87, 1964.
22. Berge, T. O., England, B., Mauris, C., et al.: Etiology of acute respiratory disease among service personnel at Fort Ord, California. Am. J. Hyg. *62*:283–294, 1955.
23. Bhisitkul, D. M., Todd, K. M., and Listernick, R.: Adenovirus infection and childhood intussusception. Am. J. Dis. Child. *146*:1331–1333, 1992.
24. Blachar, Y., Leibovitz, E., and Levin, S.: The interferon system in two patients with hemolytic uremic syndrome associated with adenovirus infection. Acta Paediatr. Scand. *79*:108–109, 1990.
25. Blacklock, J. W. S.: Section of pathology with section of epidemiology and preventive medicine: Discussion on adenovirus infections. Proc. R. Soc. Med. *50*:753–755, 1957.
26. Blacklow, N. R., Hoggan, M. D., Kapikian, A. Z., et al.: Epidemiology of adenovirus-associated virus infection in a nursery population. Am. J. Epidemiol. *88*:368–378, 1968.
27. Blacklow, N. R., Hoggan, M. D., Sereno, M. S., et al.: A seroepidemiologic study of adenovirus-associated virus infection in infants and children. Am. J. Epidemiol. *94*:359–366, 1971.
28. Bloom, H. H., Forsyth, B. R., Johnson, K. M., et al.: Patterns of adenovirus infections in Marine Corps personnel. I. A 42-month survey in recruit and nonrecruit populations. Am. J. Hyg. *80*:328–342, 1964.
29. Bonard, E. C., and Paccaud, M. F.: Abdominal adenovirosis and appendicitis. Helv. Med. Acta *33*:164–171, 1966.
30. Boniuk, M., Phillips, C. A., and Friedman, J. B.: Chronic adenovirus type 2 keratitis in man. N. Engl. J. Med. *273*:924–925, 1965.
31. Boyer, G. S., Leuchtenberger, C., and Ginsberg, H. S.: Cytological and cytochemical studies of HeLa cells infected with adenoviruses. J. Exp. Med. *105*:195–214, 1957.
32. Boyer, G. S., Denny, F. W., Jr., and Ginsberg, H. S.: Sequential cellular changes produced by types 5 and 7 adenoviruses in HeLa cells and in human amniotic cells: Cytological studies aided by fluorescein-labelled antibody. J. Exp. Med. *110*:827–843, 1959.
33. Boyer, G. S., Denny, F. W., Jr., Miller, I., et al.: Correlation of production of infectious virus with sequential stages of cytologic alteration in HeLa cells infected with adenoviruses types 5 and 7. J. Exp. Med. *112*:865–882, 1960.
34. Brandt, C. D., Kim, H. W., Vargosko, A. J., et al.: Infections in 18,000 infants and children in a controlled study of respiratory tract disease. I. Adenovirus pathogenicity in relation to serologic type and illness syndrome. Am. J. Epidemiol. *90*:484–500, 1969.
35. Brandt, C. D., Kim, H. W., Jeffries, B. C., et al.: Infections in 18,000 infants and children in a controlled study of respiratory tract disease. II. Variation in adenovirus infections by year and season. Am. J. Epidemiol. *95*:218–227, 1972.
36. Brandt, C. D., Kim, H. W., Rodriguez, W. J., et al.: Adenoviruses and pediatric gastroenteritis. J. Infect. Dis. *151*:437–443, 1985.
37. Brandt, C. D., Kim, H. W., Rodriguez, W. J., et al.: Simultaneous infections with different enteric and respiratory tract viruses. J. Clin. Microbiol. *23*:177–179, 1986.
38. Brown, M.: Laboratory identification of adenoviruses associated with gastroenteritis in Canada from 1983 to 1986. J. Clin. Microbiol. *28*:1525–1529, 1990.
39. Brown, M., Rossier, E., Carpenter, B., et al.: Fatal adenovirus type 35 infection in newborns. Pediatr. Infect. Dis. J. *10*:955–956, 1991.
40. Brown, R. S., Nogrady, B., Spence, L., et al.: An outbreak of adenovirus type 7 infection in children in Montreal. Can. Med. Assoc. J. *108*:434–439, 1973.
41. Bruckova, M., Grandien, M., Pettersson, C. A., et al.: Use of nasal and pharyngeal swabs for rapid detection of respiratory syncytial virus and adenovirus antigens by enzyme-linked immunosorbent assay. J. Clin. Microbiol. *27*:1867–1869, 1989.
42. Bryant, R. E., and Rhoades, E. R.: Clinical features of adenoviral pneumonia in Air Force recruits. Am. Rev. Respir. Dis. *96*:717–723, 1967.
43. Buitenwerf, J., Louwerens, J. J., and DeJong, J. C.: A simple and rapid method for typing adenoviruses 40 and 41 without cultivation. J. Virol. Methods *10*:39–44, 1985.
44. Burns, R. P., and Potter, M. H.: Epidemic keratoconjunctivitis due to adenovirus type 19. Am. J. Ophthalmol. *81*:27–29, 1976.
45. Cames, B., Rahler, J., Burtomboy, G., et al.: Acute adenovirus hepatitis in liver transplant recipients. J. Pediatr. *120*:33–37, 1992.
46. Carmichael, G. P., Jr., Zahradnik, J. M., Moyer, G. H., et al.: Adenovirus hepatitis in an immunosuppressed adult patient. Am. J. Clin. Pathol. *71*:352–355, 1979.
47. Cesario, T. C., Kriel, R. L., Caldwell, G. G., et al.: Epidemiologic observations of virus infections in a closed population of young children. Am. J. Epidemiol. *94*:457–466, 1971.
48. Cevenini, R., Donati, M., Landini, M. P., et al.: Adenovirus associated with an oculo-genital infection. Microbiologica *2*:425–427, 1979.
49. Chanock, R. M., and Parrott, R. H.: Acute respiratory disease in infancy and childhood: Present understanding and prospects for prevention. Pediatrics *36*:21–39, 1965.

50. Chanock, R. M., Mufson, M. A., and Johnson, K. M.: Comparative biology and ecology of human virus and mycoplasma respiratory pathogens. Prog. Med. Virol. *7*:208–252, 1965.
51. Chanock, R. M., Chambon, L., Chang, W., et al.: WHO respiratory disease survey in children: A serological study. Bull. W. H. O. *37*:363–369, 1967.
52. Chany, C., Lepine, P., Lelong, M., et al.: Severe and fatal pneumonia in infants and young children associated with adenovirus infections. Am. J. Hyg. *67*:367–378, 1958.
53. Chapple, P. J.: A survey of antibodies to adenovirus 8 and coxsackievirus A21 in human sera. Bull. W. H. O. *34*:243–248, 1966.
54. Cherry, J. D.: Newer viral exanthems. *In* Schulman, I. (ed.): Advances in Pediatrics. Vol. 16. Chicago, Year Book Medical Publishers, 1969, pp. 233–286.
55. Cherry, J. D.: Newer respiratory viruses. Their role in respiratory illnesses of children. *In* Schulman, I. (ed.): Advances in Pediatrics. Vol. 20. Chicago, Year Book Medical Publishers, 1973, pp. 225–290.
56. Cherry, J. D.: Unpublished observation.
57. Chiba, S., Nakata, S., Nakamura, I., et al.: Outbreak of infantile gastroenteritis due to type 40 adenovirus. Lancet *2*:954–957, 1983.
58. Chin-Hsien, T.: Adenovirus pneumonia epidemic among Peking infants and preschool children in 1958. Chinese Med. J. *80*:331–339, 1960.
59. Chiou, C. C., Soong, W. J., Hwang, B., et al.: Congenital adenoviral infection. Pediatr. Infect. Dis. J. *13*:664–665, 1994.
60. Chou, S. M., Roos, R., Burrell, R., et al.: Subacute focal adenovirus encephalitis. J. Neuropathol. Exp. Neurol. *32*:34–50, 1973.
61. Christensen, M. L.: Human viral gastroenteritis. Clin. Microbiol. Rev. *2*:51–89, 1989.
62. Claesson, B. A., Trollfors, B., Brolin, I., et al.: Etiology of community-acquired pneumonia in children based on antibody responses to bacterial and viral antigens. Pediatr. Infect. Dis. J. *8*:856–861, 1989.
63. Clarke, E. J., Phillips, I. A., and Alexander, E. R.: Adenovirus infection in intussusception in children in Taiwan. J. A. M. A. *208*:1671–1674, 1969.
64. Collier, A. M., Connor, J. D., and Irving, W. R., Jr.: Generalized type 5 adenovirus infection associated with the pertussis syndrome. J. Pediatr. *69*:1073–1078, 1966.
65. Commission on Acute Respiratory Diseases: Acute respiratory disease among new recruits. Am. J. Public Health *36*:439–450, 1946.
66. Connor, J. D.: Evidence for an etiologic role of adenoviral infection in pertussis syndrome. N. Engl. J. Med. *283*:390–394, 1970.
67. Connor, J. D., Buchta, R. M., DeGenaro, F., Jr., et al.: Potpourri of adenoviral infections. West. J. Med. *120*:55–61, 1974.
68. Cooney, M. K., Hall, C. E., and Fox, J. P.: The Seattle virus watch. III. Evaluation of isolation methods and summary of infections detected by virus isolations. Am. J. Epidemiol. *96*:286–305, 1972.
69. Couch, R. B., Cate, T. R., Douglas, R. G., Jr., et al.: Effect of route of inoculation on experimental respiratory viral disease in volunteers and evidence for airborne transmission. Bacteriol. Rev. *30*:517–529, 1966.
70. Couch, R. B., Cate, T. R., Fleet, W. F., et al.: Aerosol-induced adenoviral illness resembling the naturally occurring illness in military recruits. Am. Rev. Respir. Dis. *93*:529–535, 1965.
71. Craighead, J. E.: Cytopathology of adenoviruses types 7 and 12 in human respiratory epithelium. Lab. Invest. *22*:553–557, 1970.
72. Crandell, R. A., Dowdle, W. R., Holcomb, T. M., et al.: A fatal illness associated with two viruses: An intermediate adenovirus type (21–26) and influenza A2. J. Pediatr. *72*:467–473, 1968.
73. Cukor, G., and Blacklow, N. R.: Human viral gastroenteritis. Microbiol. Rev. *48*:157–179, 1984.
74. Cumming, G. R., Macpherson, R. I., and Chernick, V.: Unilateral hyperlucent lung syndrome in children. J. Pediatr. *78*:250–260, 1971.
75. D'Ambrosio, E., Del Grosso, N., Chicca, A., et al.: Neutralizing antibodies against 33 human adenoviruses in normal children in Rome. J. Hyg. (Camb.) *89*:155–161, 1982.
76. D'Angelo, L. J., Hierholzer, J. C., Keenlyside, R. A., et al.: Pharyngoconjunctival fever caused by adenovirus type 4: Report of a swimming pool–related outbreak with recovery of virus from pool water. J. Infect. Dis. *140*:42–47, 1979.
77. Dagan, R., Schwartz, R. H., Insel, R. A., et al.: Severe diffuse adenovirus 7a pneumonia in a child with combined immunodeficiency: Possible therapeutic effect of human immune serum globulin containing specific neutralizing antibody. Pediatr. Infect. Dis. *3*:246–250, 1984.
78. Darougar, S., Quinlan, M. P., Gibson, J. A., et al.: Epidemic keratoconjunctivitis and chronic papillary conjunctivitis in London due to adenovirus type 19. Br. J. Ophthalmol. *61*:76–85, 1977.
79. Dascomb, H. E., and Hilleman, M. R.: Clinical and laboratory studies in patients with respiratory disease caused by adenoviruses (RI-APC-ARD agents). Am. J. Med. *21*:161–174, 1956.
80. Davidson, S.I.: Epidemic kerato-conjunctivitis: Report of an outbreak which resulted in ward cross-infection. Br. J. Ophthalmol. *48*:573–580, 1964.
81. Davis, B. D., Dulbecco, R., Eisen, H. N., et al.: Microbiology. Hagerstown, Harper & Row, 1973, pp. 1222–1236.
82. Davis, D., Henslee, P. J., and Markesbery, W. R.: Fatal adenovirus meningoencephalitis in a bone marrow transplant patient. Ann. Neurol. *23*:385–389, 1988.
83. Dawson, C., and Darrell, R.: Infections due to adenovirus type 8 in the United States. I. An outbreak of epidemic keratoconjunctivitis originating in a physician's office. N. Engl. J. Med. *268*:1031–1033, 1963.
84. Dawson, C., Darrell, R., Hanna, L., et al.: Infections due to adenovirus type 8 in the United States. II. Community-wide infection with adenovirus type 8. N. Engl. J. Med. *268*:1034–1037, 1963.
85. Dawson, C. R., Hanna, L., and Togni, B.: Adenovirus type 8 infections in the United States. IV. Observations on the pathogenesis of lesions in severe eye disease. Arch. Ophthalmol. *87*:258–268, 1972.
86. Dawson, C. R., O'Day, D., and Vastine, D.: Adenovirus 19, a cause of epidemic keratoconjunctivitis, not acute hemorrhagic conjunctivitis. N. Engl. J. Med. *293*:45–46, 1975.
87. de Jong, J. C., Wigand, R., Kidd, A. H., et al.: Candidate adenoviruses 40 and 41: Fastidious adenoviruses from human infant stool. J. Med. Virol. *11*:215–231, 1983.
88. de Jong, J. C., Wigand, R., Wadell, G., et al.: Adenovirus 37: Identification and characterization of a medically important new adenovirus type of subgroup D. J. Med. Virol. *7*:105–118, 1981.
89. deSilva, L. M., Colditz, P., and Wadell, G.: Adenovirus type 7 infections in children in New South Wales, Australia. J. Med. Virol. *29*:28–32, 1989.
90. Denny, F. W., Jr.: Viruses newly isolated from the upper respiratory tract. Pediatr. Clin. North Am. *7*:295–314, 1960.
91. Denny, F. W., Jr., and Ginsberg, H. S.: Certain biological characteristics of adenovirus types 5, 6, 7, and 14. J. Immunol. *86*:567–574, 1961.
92. Douglas, R. G., Jr., Alford, R. H., Cate, T. R., et al.: The leukocyte response during viral respiratory illness in man. Ann. Intern. Med. *64*:521–530, 1966.
93. Dudding, B. A., Bartelloni, P. J., Scott, R. M., et al.: Enteric immunization with live adenovirus type 21 vaccine. Infect. Immun. *5*:295–299, 1972.
94. Dudding, B. A., Top, F. H., Jr., Scott, R. M., et al.: An analysis of hospitalizations for acute respiratory disease in recruits immunized with adenovirus type 4 and type 7 vaccines. Am. J. Epidemiol. *95*:141–147, 1972.
95. Dudding, B. A., Wagner, S. C., Zeller, J. A., et al.: Fatal pneumonia associated with adenovirus type 7 in three military trainees. N. Engl. J. Med. *286*:1289–1292, 1972.
96. Dudding, B. A., Top, F. H., Jr., Winter, P. E., et al.: Acute respiratory disease in military trainees: The adenovirus surveillance program, 1966–1971. Am. J. Epidemiol. *97*:187–198, 1973.
97. Duncan, I. B. R.: Adenovirus type 15 and human thyroid tissue-culture. Lancet *1*:829–830, 1960.
98. Durepaire, N., Ranger-Rogez, S., and Denis, F.: Evaluation of rapid culture centrifugation method for adenovirus detection in stools. Diagn. Microbiol. Infect. Dis. *24*:25–29, 1996.
99. Edwards, K. M., Thompson, J., Paolini, J., et al.: Adenovirus infections in young children. Pediatrics *76*:420–424, 1985.
100. Edwards, K. M., Bennett, S. R., Garner, W. L., et al.: Reye's syndrome associated with adenovirus infections in infants. Am. J. Dis. Child. *139*:343–346, 1985.
101. Enders, J. F., Bell, J. A., Dingle, J. H., et al.: "Adenoviruses": Group name proposed for new respiratory-tract viruses. Science *124*:119–120, 1956.
102. Espy, M. J., Hierholzer, J. C., and Smith, T. F.: The effect of centrifugation on the rapid detection of adenovirus in shell vials. Am. J. Clin. Pathol. *88*:358–360, 1987.
103. Evans, A. S.: Acute respiratory disease in University of Wisconsin students. N. Engl. J. Med. *256*:377–384, 1957.
104. Evans, A. S.: Adenovirus infections in children and young adults: With comments on vaccination. N. Engl. J. Med. *259*:464–468, 1958.
105. Evans, A. S.: Latent adenovirus infections of the human respiratory tract. Am. J. Hyg. *67*:256–266, 1958.
106. Evans, A. S., and Dick, E. C.: Acute pharyngitis and tonsillitis in University of Wisconsin students. J. A. M. A. *190*:699–708, 1964.
107. Farkas, E., Jancso, A., and Radnot, M.: Clinical and virologic studies: On the first widespread outbreak of epidemic keratoconjunctivitis in Hungary. Am. J. Ophthalmol. *60*:78–82, 1965.
108. Faulkner, R., and Van Rooyen, C. E.: Adenoviruses types 3 and 5 isolated from the cerebrospinal fluid of children. Can. Med. Assoc. J. *87*:1123–1125, 1962.
109. Fenner, F.: Classification and nomenclature of viruses. Intervirology *7*:1–115, 1976.
110. Fiala, M., Payne, J. E., Berne, T. V., et al.: Role of adenovirus type 11 in hemorrhagic cystitis secondary to immunosuppression. J. Urol. *112*:595–597, 1974.
111. Finn, A., Anday, E., and Talbot, G. H.: An epidemic of adenovirus 7a infection in a neonatal nursery: Course, morbidity, and management. Infect. Control Hosp. Epidemiol. *9*:398–404, 1988.
112. Flewett, T. H., Bryden, A. S., Davies, H., et al.: Epidemic viral enteritis in a long-stay children's ward. Lancet *1*:4–5, 1975.
113. Flomenberg, P., Babbitt, J., Drobyski, W. R., et al.: Increasing incidence of adenovirus disease in bone marrow transplant recipients. J. Infect. Dis. *169*:775–781, 1994.
114. Ford, E., Nelson, K. E., and Warren, D.: Epidemiology of epidemic keratoconjunctivitis. Epidemiol. Rev. *9*:244–261, 1987.
115. Forssell, P., Halonen, H., Stenstrom, R., et al.: An adenovirus epidemic due to types 1 and 2. Ann. Pediatr. Fenn. *8*:35–44, 1962.
116. Forsyth, B. R., Bloom, H. H., Johnson, K. M., et al.: Patterns of adenovirus

infections in Marine Corps personnel. II. Longitudinal study of successive advanced recruit training companies. Am. J. Hyg. *80*:343–355, 1964.
117. Forsyth, B. R., Bloom, H. H., Johnson, K. M., et al.: Etiology of primary atypical pneumonia in a military population. J. A. M. A. *191*:92–96, 1965.
118. Fox, J. P., Brandt, C. D., Wassermann, F. E., et al.: The virus watch program: A continuing surveillance of viral infections in metropolitan New York families. VI. Observations of adenovirus infections: Virus excretion patterns, antibody response, efficiency of surveillance, patterns of infection, and relation to illness. Am. J. Epidemiol. *89*:25–50, 1969.
119. Fox, J. P., Hall, C. E., and Cooney, M. K.: The Seattle virus watch. VII. Observations of adenovirus infections. Am. J. Epidemiol. *105*:362–386, 1977.
120. Foy, H. M., Cooney, M. K., Maletzky, A. J., et al.: Incidence and etiology of pneumonia, croup and bronchiolitis in preschool children belonging to a prepaid medical care group over a four-year period. Am. J. Epidemiol. *97*:80–92, 1973.
121. Foy, H. M., Cooney, M. K., McMahan, R., et al.: Viral and mycoplasmal pneumonia in a prepaid medical care group during an eight-year period. Am. J. Epidemiol. *97*:93–102, 1973.
122. Foy, H. M.: Adenoviruses. *In* Evans, A. S. (ed.): Viral Infections of Humans: Epidemiology and Control. 3rd ed. New York, Plenum, 1989, pp. 77–94.
123. Freiman, I., Super, M., Joosting, A. C. C., et al.: An epidemic of adenovirus type 7 bronchopneumonia in Bantu children. Afr. Med. J. *45*:107–109, 1971.
124. Fuchs, E.: Keratitis punctata superficialis. Wien. Klin. Wochenschr. *2*:837–841, 1889.
125. Fukumi, H., Nishikawa, F., Kokuku, Y., et al.: Isolation of adenovirus from an exanthematous infection resembling roseola infantum. Jpn. J. Med. Sci. Biol. *10*:87–91, 1957.
126. Gabrielson, M. O., Joseph, C., and Hsiung, G. D.: Encephalitis associated with adenovirus type 7 occurring in a family outbreak. J. Pediatr. *68*:142–144, 1966.
127. Garcia, A. G. P., Fonseca, M. E. F., DeBonis, M., et al.: Morphological and virological studies in six autopsies of children with adenovirus pneumonia. Mem. Inst. Oswaldo Cruz, Rio de Janeiro, *88*:141–147, 1993.
128. Gardner, P. S., McGregor, C. B., and Dick, K.: Association between diarrhoea and adenovirus type 7. Br. Med. J. *1*:91–93, 1960.
129. Gardner, P. S., Knox, E. G., Court, S. D. M., et al.: Virus infection and intussusception in childhood. Br. Med. J. *2*:697–700, 1962.
130. George, R. B., Ziskind, M. M., Rasch, J. R., et al.: *Mycoplasma* and adenovirus pneumonias: Comparison with other atypical pneumonias in a military population. Ann. Intern. Med. *65*:931–942, 1966.
131. Gerna, G., Cattaneo, E., Revello, M. G., et al.: Grouping of human adenoviruses by early antigen reactivity. J. Infect. Dis. *145*:678–682, 1982.
132. Ginsberg, H. S., Gold, E., Jordan, W. S., Jr., et al.: Relation of the new respiratory agents to acute respiratory diseases. Am. J. Public Health *45*:915–922, 1955.
133. Ginsberg, H. S.: Characteristics of the new respiratory viruses (adenoviruses). II. Stability to temperature and pH alterations. Proc. Soc. Exp. Biol. Med. *93*:48–52, 1956.
134. Ginsberg, H. S.: Characteristics of the adenoviruses. III. Reproductive cycle of types 1 to 4. J. Exp. Med. *107*:133–152, 1958.
135. Ginsberg, H. S.: Adenoviruses. Am. J. Clin. Pathol. *57*:771–776, 1972.
136. Ginsberg, H. S., Horswood, R. L., Chanock, R. M., et al.: Role of early genes in pathogenesis of adenovirus pneumonia. Proc. Natl. Acad. Sci. U. S. A. *87*:6191–6195, 1990.
137. Ginsberg, H. S., Moldawer, L. L., Sehgal, P. B., et al.: A mouse model for investigating the molecular pathogenesis of adenovirus pneumonia. Proc. Natl. Acad. Sci. U. S. A. *88*:1651–1655, 1991.
138. Ginsberg, H. S., and Prince, G. A.: The molecular basis of adenovirus pathogenesis. Infect. Agents Dis. *3*:1–8, 1994.
139. Glezen, W. P., Loda, F. A., Clyde, W. A., Jr., et al.: Epidemiologic patterns of acute lower respiratory disease of children in a pediatric group practice. J. Pediatr. *78*:397–406, 1971.
140. Godman, G. C., Morgan, C., Brietenfeld, P. M., et al.: A correlative study by electron and light microscopy of the development of type 5 adenovirus. II. Light microscopy. J. Exp. Med. *112*:383–401, 1960.
141. Gold, R., Wilt, J. C., Adhikari, P. K., et al.: Adenoviral pneumonia and its complications in infancy and childhood. J. Can. Assoc. Radiol. *20*:218–224, 1969.
142. Gooch, W. M., and Mogabgab, W. J.: Simultaneous oral administration of live adenovirus 4 and 7 vaccines: Protection and lack of emergency of other types. Arch. Environ. Health *25*:388–394, 1972.
143. Grabow, W. O. K., Puttergill, D. L., and Bosch, A.: Propagation of adenovirus types 40 and 41 in the PLC/PRF/5 primary liver carcinoma cell line. J. Virol. Methods *37*:201–208, 1992.
144. Grandien, M., Pettersson, C. A., Svensson, L., et al.: Latex agglutination test for adenovirus diagnosis in diarrheal disease. J. Med. Virol. *23*:311–316, 1987.
145. Grayston, J. T., Woolridge, R. L., Loosli, C. G., et al.: Adenovirus infections in naval recruits. J. Infect. Dis. *104*:61–70, 1957.
146. Grayston, J. T., Lashof, J. C., Loosli, C. G., et al.: Adenoviruses. III. Their etiological role in acute respiratory diseases in civilian adults. J. Infect. Dis. *103*:93–101, 1958.
147. Green, W. R., Greaves, W. L., Frederick, W. R., et al.: Renal infection due to adenovirus in a patient with human immunodeficiency virus infection. Clin. Infect. Dis. *18*:989–991, 1994.
148. Gresser, I., and Kibrick, S.: Isolation of vaccinia virus and type 1 adenovirus from urine. N. Engl. J. Med. *265*:743–744, 1961.
149. Griffin, J. P., and Greenberg, B. H.: Live and inactivated adenovirus vaccines: Clinical evaluation of efficacy in prevention of acute respiratory disease. Arch. Intern. Med. *125*:981–986, 1970.
150. Gutekunst, R. R., and Heggie, A. D.: Viremia and viruria in adenovirus infections: Detection in patients with rubella or rubelliform illness. N. Engl. J. Med. *264*:374–378, 1961.
151. Guyer, B., O'Day, D. M., Hierholzer, J. C., et al.: Epidemic keratoconjunctivitis: A community outbreak of mixed adenovirus type 8 and type 19 infection. J. Infect. Dis. *132*:142–150, 1975.
152. Hara, J., Ishibashi, T., Fujimoto, F., et al.: Adenovirus type 10 keratoconjunctivitis with increased intraocular pressure. Am. J. Ophthalmol. *90*:481–484, 1980.
153. Harford, C. G., Hamlin, A., Parker, E., et al.: Electron microscopy of HeLa cells infected with adenoviruses. J. Exp. Med. *104*:443–453, 1956.
154. Harnett, G. B., and Newnham, W. A.: Isolation of adenovirus type 19 from the male and female genital tracts. Br. J. Vener. Dis. *57*:55–57, 1981.
155. Harris, D. J., Wulff, H., Ray, C. G., et al.: Viruses and disease. III. An outbreak of adenovirus type 7a in a children's home. Am. J. Epidemiol. *93*:399–402, 1971.
156. Harrison, H. R., Howe, P., Minnich, L., et al.: A cluster of adenovirus 19 infections with multiple clinical manifestations. J. Pediatr. *94*:917–919, 1979.
157. Hartwell, W. V., Love, G. J., and Eidenbock, M. P.: Adenovirus in blood clots from cases of infectious hepatitis. Science *152*:1390, 1966.
158. Hatch, M. H., and Siem, R. A.: Viruses isolated from children with infectious hepatitis. Am. J. Epidemiol. *84*:495–509, 1966.
159. Henson, D., and Mufson, M. A.: Myocarditis and pneumonitis with type 21 adenovirus infection: Association with fatal myocarditis and pneumonitis. Am. J. Dis. Child. *121*:334–339, 1971.
160. Herbert, F. A., Wilkinson, D., Burchak, E., et al.: Adenovirus type 3 pneumonia causing lung damage in childhood. Can. Med. Assoc. J. *116*:274–276, 1977.
161. Herbert, H.: Superficial punctate keratitis associated with an encapsulated bacillus. Ophthalmol. Rev. *20*:339–345, 1901.
162. Herrmann, E. C., Jr.: Experiences in laboratory diagnosis of adenovirus infections in routine medical practice. Mayo Clin. Proc. *43*:635–644, 1968.
163. Herrmann, J. E., Perron-Henry, D. M., and Blacklow, N. R.: Antigen detection with monoclonal antibodies for the diagnosis of adenovirus gastroenteritis. J. Infect. Dis. *155*:1167–1171, 1987.
164. Hierholzer, J. C.: Further subgrouping of the human adenoviruses by differential hemagglutination. J. Infect. Dis. *128*:541–550, 1973.
165. Hierholzer, J. C., Pumarola, A., Rodriguez-Torres, A., et al.: Occurrence of respiratory illness due to an atypical strain of adenovirus type 11 during a large outbreak in Spanish military recruits. Am. J. Epidemiol. *99*:434–442, 1974.
166. Hierholzer, J. C., Atuk, N. O., and Gwaltney, J. M., Jr.: New human adenovirus isolated from a renal transplant recipient: Description and characterization of candidate adenovirus type 34. J. Clin. Microbiol. *1*:366–376, 1975.
167. Hierholzer, J. C., Gamble, W. C., and Dowdle, W. R.: Reference equine antisera to 33 human adenovirus types: Homologous and heterologous titers. J. Clin. Microbiol. *1*:65–74, 1975.
168. Hierholzer, J. C., and Bingham, P. G.: Vero microcultures for adenovirus neutralization tests. J. Clin. Microbiol. *7*:499–506, 1978.
169. Hierholzer, J. C., Kemp, M. C., Gary, G. W., Jr., et al.: New human adenovirus associated with respiratory illness: Candidate adenovirus type 39. J. Clin. Microbiol. *16*:15–21, 1982.
170. Hierholzer, J. C., Torrence, A. E., and Wright, P. F.: Generalized viral illness caused by an intermediate strain of adenovirus (21/H21+35). J. Infect. Dis. *141*:281–288, 1980.
171. Hierholzer, J. C., Stone, Y. O., and Broderson, J. R.: Antigenic relationships among the 47 human adenoviruses determined in reference horse antisera. Arch. Virol. *121*:179–197, 1991.
172. Hilleman, M. R., and Werner, J. H.: Recovery of new agent from patients with acute respiratory illness. Proc. Soc. Exp. Biol. Med. *85*:183–188, 1954.
173. Hilleman, M. R., Tousimis, A. J., and Werner, J. H.: Biophysical characterization of the RI (RI-67) viruses. Proc. Soc. Exp. Biol. Med. *89*:587–593, 1955.
174. Hilleman, M. R.: Epidemiology of adenovirus respiratory infections in military recruit populations. Ann. N. Y. Acad. Sci. *67*:262–272, 1957.
175. Hillis, W. D., Cooper, M. R., and Bang, F. B.: Adenovirus infections in West Bengal. I. Persistence of viruses in infants and young children. Indian J. Med. Res. *61*:1–9, 1973.
176. Hogan, M. J., and Crawford, J. W.: Epidemic keratoconjunctivitis (superficial punctate keratitis, keratitis subepithelialis, keratitis maculosa, keratitis nummularis): With a review of the literature and a report of 125 cases. Am. J. Ophthalmol. *25*:1059–1078, 1942.
177. Holmes, W. J.: Epidemic infectious conjunctivitis. Hawaiian Med. J. *1*:11–12, 1941.
178. Holzel, A., Parker, L., Patterson, W. H., et al.: Virus isolations from throats

of children admitted to hospital with respiratory and other diseases: Manchester 1962–1964. Br. Med. J. *1*:614–619, 1965.
179. Horn, M. E. C., Brain, E., Gregg, I., et al.: Respiratory viral infection in childhood: A survey in general practice, Roehampton 1967–1972. J. Hyg. (Camb.) *74*:157–168, 1975.
180. Horne, R. W., Brenner, S., Waterson, A. P., et al.: The icosahedral form of an adenovirus. J. Mol. Biol. *1*:84–86, 1959.
181. Horwitz, M. S.: *Adenoviridae* and their replication. *In* Fields, B. N., Knipe, D. M., Chanock, R. M., et al.: Virology. 2nd ed. New York, Raven Press, 1990, pp. 1679–1721.
182. Horwitz, M. S.: Adenoviruses. *In* Fields, B. N., Knipe, D. M., Chanock, R. M., et al.: Virology. 2nd ed. New York, Raven Press, 1990, pp. 1723–1739.
183. Huebner, R. J., Rowe, W. P., Ward, T. G., et al.: Adenoidal-pharyngeal-conjunctival agents: A newly recognized group of common viruses of the respiratory system. N. Engl. J. Med. *251*:1077–1086, 1954.
184. Huebner, R. J., Rowe, W. P., and Chanock, R. M.: Newly recognized respiratory tract viruses. Ann. Rev. Microbiol. *12*:49–76, 1958.
185. Huebner, R. J., Casey, M. J., Chanock, R. M., et al.: Tumors induced in hamsters by a strain of adenovirus type 3: Sharing of tumor antigens and neoantigens with those produced by adenovirus type 7 tumors. Proc. Natl. Acad. Sci. U. S. A. *54*:381–388, 1965.
186. Hypia, T.: Detection of adenovirus in nasopharyngeal specimens by radioactive and nonradioactive DNA probes. J. Clin. Microbiol. *21*:730–733, 1985.
187. Ieven, M., Van Reempts, P., Overmeier, B. V., et al.: A pseudoepidemic of adenoviruses in a neonatal care unit. Diagn. Microbiol. Infect. Dis. *18*:157–159, 1994.
188. Imre, G., Korchmaros, I., Geck, P., et al.: Antigenic specificity of inclusion bodies in epidemic keratoconjunctivitis. Ophthalmologica *148*:7–12, 1964.
189. Jackson, G. G., and Muldoon, R. L.: Viruses causing common respiratory infection in man. IV. Reoviruses and adenoviruses. J. Infect. Dis. *128*:811–866, 1973.
190. Jaffe, B. F., and Maassab, H. F.: Sudden deafness associated with adenovirus infection. N. Engl. J. Med. *276*:1406–1408, 1967.
191. James, A. G., Lang, W. R., Liang, A. Y., et al.: Adenovirus type 21 bronchopneumonia in infants and young children. J. Pediatr. *95*:530–533, 1979.
192. Jansson, E., and Wager, O.: Adenovirus antibodies in patients with respiratory infection. Ann. Med. Intern. Fenn. *50*:221–227, 1961.
193. Jansson, E., Wager, O., Forssell, P., et al.: An exanthema subitum-like rash in patients with adenovirus infection. Ann. Paediatr. Fenn. *7*:3–11, 1961.
194. Jansson, E., Wager, O., Forssell, P., et al.: Epidemic occurrence of adenovirus type 7 infection in Helsinki. Ann. Paediatr. Fenn. *8*:24–34, 1962.
195. Jawetz, E.: The story of shipyard eye. Br. Med. J. *1*:873–876, 1959.
196. Jernigan, J. A., Lowry, B. S., Hayden, F. G., et al.: Adenovirus type 8 epidemic keratoconjunctivitis in an eye clinic: Risk factors and control. J. Infect. Dis. *167*:307–313, 1993.
197. Johansson, M. E., Uhnoo, I., Kidd, A. H., et al.: Direct identification of enteric adenovirus, a candidate new serotype, associated with infantile gastroenteritis. J. Clin. Microbiol. *12*:95–100, 1980.
198. Joncas, J., Moisan, A., and Pavilanis, V.: Incidence of adenovirus infection: A family study. Can. Med. Assoc. J. *87*:52–58, 1962.
199. Jordan, W. S., Jr., Badger, G. F., Curtiss, C., et al.: A study of illness in a group of Cleveland families. X. The occurrence of adenovirus infections. Am. J. Hyg. *64*:336–348, 1956.
200. Kajon, A. E., Murtagh, P., Franco, S. G., et al.: A new genome type of adenovirus 3 associated with severe lower acute respiratory infection in children. J. Med. Virol. *30*:73–76, 1990.
201. Kajon, A. E., and Wadell, G.: Molecular epidemiology of adenoviruses associated with acute lower respiratory disease of children in Buenos Aires, Argentina (1984–1988). J. Med. Virol. *36*:292–297, 1992.
202. Kapelushnik, J., Or, R., Delukina, M., et al.: Intravenous ribavirin therapy for adenovirus gastroenteritis after bone marrow transplantation. J. Pediatr. Gastroenterol. Nutr. *21*:110–112, 1995.
203. Kasel, J. A., Evans, H. E., Spickard, A., et al.: Conjunctivitis and enteric infection with adenovirus types 26 and 27: Responses to primary, secondary and reciprocal cross-challenges. Am. J. Hyg. *77*:265–282, 1963.
204. Kasel, J. A., Banks, P. A., Wigand, R., et al.: An immunologic classification of heterotypic antibody responses to adenoviruses in man. Proc. Soc. Exp. Biol. Med. *119*:1162–1165, 1965.
205. Kasova, V., Brackova, M., Kotelensky, F., et al.: Isolation of adenovirus type 29 from an outbreak of epidemic keratoconjunctivitis. Acta Virol. *21*:173, 1977.
206. Keenlyside, R. A., Hierholzer, J. C., and D'Angelo, L. J.: Keratoconjunctivitis associated with adenovirus type 37: An extended outbreak in an ophthalmologist's office. J. Infect. Dis. *147*:191–198, 1983.
207. Keller, E. W., Rubin, R. H., Black, P. H., et al.: Isolation of adenovirus type 34 from a renal transplant recipient with interstitial pneumonia. Transplantation *23*:188–191, 1977.
208. Kelsey, D. S.: Adenovirus meningoencephalitis. Pediatrics *61*:291–293, 1978.
209. Kemp, M. C., Hierholzer, J. C., Cabradilla, C. P., et al.: The changing etiology of epidemic keratoconjunctivitis: Antigenic and restriction enzyme analyses of adenovirus types 19 and 37 isolated over a 10-year period. J. Infect. Dis. *148*:24–33, 1983.
210. Kendall, E. J. C., Cook, G. T., and Stone, D. M.: Acute respiratory infections in children: Isolation of coxsackie B virus and adenovirus during a survey in a general practice. Br. Med. J. *2*:1180–1184, 1960.
211. Kidd, A. H., Cosgrove, B. P., Brown, R. A., et al.: Faecal adenoviruses from Glasgow babies: Studies on culture and identity. J. Hyg. (Camb.) *88*:463–474, 1982.
212. Kidd, A. H., Jonsson, M., Garwicz, D., et al.: Rapid subgenus identification of human adenovirus isolates by a general PCR. J. Clin. Microbiol. *34*:622–627, 1996.
213. Kim, K. S.: Fatal pneumonia caused by adenovirus type 35. Am. J. Dis. Child. *135*:473–475, 1981.
214. Kim, Y. J., Schmidt, N. J., and Mirkovic, R. R.: Isolation of an intermediate type of adenovirus from a child with fulminant hepatitis. J. Infect. Dis. *152*:844, 1985.
215. Kinney, J. S., Hierholzer, J. C., and Thibeault, D. W.: Neonatal pulmonary insufficiency caused by adenovirus infection successfully treated with extracorporeal membrane oxygenation. J. Pediatr. *125*:110–112, 1994.
216. Kirkpatrick, H.: An epidemic of macular keratitis. Br. J. Ophthalmol. *4*:16–20, 1920.
217. Kjellen, L., Sterner, G., and Svedmyr, A.: On the occurrence of adenoviruses in Sweden. Acta Paediatr. *46*:164–176, 1957.
218. Kjer, P., and Mordhorst, C. H.: Studies on an epidemic of keratoconjunctivitis caused by adenovirus type 8. II. Clinical and epidemiological aspects. Acta Ophthalmol. *39*:984–992, 1961.
219. Knight, V., and Kasel, J. A.: Adenoviruses. *In* Knight, V. (ed.): Viral and Mycoplasmal Infections of the Respiratory Tract. Philadelphia, Lea & Febiger, 1973, pp. 65–86.
220. Koneru, B., Jaffe, R., Esquivel, C. O., et al.: Adenoviral infections in pediatric liver transplant recipients. J. A. M. A. *258*:489–492, 1987.
221. Kotloff, K. L., Losonsky, G. A., Morris, J. G., Jr., et al.: Enteric adenovirus infection and childhood diarrhea: An epidemiologic study in three clinical settings. Pediatrics *84*:219–225, 1989.
222. Krajden, M., Brown, M., Petrasek, A., et al.: Clinical features of adenovirus enteritis: A review of 127 cases. Pediatr. Infect. Dis. J. *9*:636–641, 1990.
223. Kuei-Fang, J., Ying, T., Yu-Ch'un, L., et al.: The role of adenovirus in the etiology of infantile pneumonia and pneumonia complicating measles. Chin. Med. J. *81*:141–146, 1962.
224. Ladisch, S., Lovejoy, F. H., Hierholzer, J. C., et al.: Extrapulmonary manifestations of adenovirus type 7 pneumonia simulating Reye syndrome and the possible role of an adenovirus toxin. J. Pediatr. *95*:348–355, 1979.
225. Lähdeaho, M. L., Parkkonen, P., Reunala, T., et al.: Antibodies to E1b protein-derived peptides of enteric adenovirus type 40 are associated with celiac disease and dermatitis herpetiformis. Clin. Immunol. Immunopathol. *69*:300–305, 1993.
226. Lang, W. R., Howden, C. W., Laws, J., et al.: Bronchopneumonia with serious sequelae in children with evidence of adenovirus type 21 infection. Br. Med. J. *1*:73–79, 1969.
227. Lange, W.: Über eine eigentumliche erkrankung der kleinen bronchien und bronchiolen. Dtsch. Arch. Klin. Med. *70*:342, 1901.
228. Laverty, C. R., Russell, P., Black, J., et al.: Adenovirus infection of the cervix. Acta Cytol. (Baltimore) *21*:114–117, 1977.
229. Lee, H. J., Pyo, J. W., Choi, E. H., et al.: Isolation of adenovirus type 7 from the urine of children with acute hemorrhagic cystitis. Pediatr. Infect. Dis. J. *15*:633–634, 1996.
230. Lee, S. G., and Hung, P. P.: Vaccines for control of respiratory disease caused by adenoviruses. Rev. Med. Virol. *3*:209–216, 1993.
231. Lehrich, J. R., Kasel, J. A., and Rossen, R. D.: Immunoglobulin classes of neutralizing antibody formed after human inoculation with soluble adenoviral antigens. J. Immunol. *97*:654–662, 1966.
232. Lennette, E. H., and Schmidt, N. J. (eds.): Diagnostic Procedures for Viral and Rickettsial Infections. 4th ed. New York, American Public Health Association, 1969, pp. 205–225.
233. Levandowski, R. A., and Rubenis, M.: Nosocomial conjunctivitis caused by adenovirus type 4. J. Infect. Dis. *143*:28–31, 1981.
234. Levin, S., Dietrich, J., and Guillory, J.: Fatal nonbacterial pneumonia associated with adenovirus type 4: Occurrence in an adult. J. A. M. A. *201*:155–157, 1967.
235. Lew, J. F., Glass, R. I., Petric, M., et al.: Six-year retrospective surveillance of gastroenteritis viruses identified at 10 electron microscopy centers in the United States and Canada. Pediatr. Infect. Dis. J. *9*:709–714, 1990.
236. Liles, W. C., Cushing, H., Holt, S., et al.: Severe adenoviral nephritis following bone marrow transplantation. Bone Marrow Transplant. *12*:409–412, 1993.
237. Loda, F. A., Clyde, W. A., Jr., Glezen, W. P., et al.: Studies on the role of viruses, bacteria, and *M. pneumoniae* as causes of lower respiratory tract infections in children. J. Pediatr. *72*:161–176, 1968.
238. Loda, F. A., Glezen, W. P., and Clyde, W. A., Jr.: Respiratory disease in group day care. Pediatrics *49*:428–437, 1972.
239. Lonberg-Holm, K., and Philipson, L.: Early events of virus-cell interaction in an adenovirus system. J. Virol. *4*:323–338, 1969.
240. Londergan, T. A., and Walzak, M. P.: Hemorrhagic cystitis due to adenovirus infection following bone marrow transplantation. J. Urol. *151*:1013–1014, 1994.
241. Lord, A., Sutton, R. N. P., and Corsellis, J. A. N.: Recovery of adenovirus

type 7 from human brain cell cultures. J. Neurol. Neurosurg. Psychiatry *38*:710–712, 1975.

242. Maček, V., Sorli, J., Kopriva, S., et al.: Persistent adenoviral infection and chronic airway obstruction in children. Am. J. Respir. Crit. Care Med. *150*:7–10, 1994.
243. Macpherson, R. I., Cumming, G. R., and Chernick, V.: Unilateral hyperlucent lung: A complication of viral pneumonia. J. Can. Assoc. Radiol. *20*:225–231, 1969.
244. Mahafzah, A. M., and Landry, M. L.: Evaluation of immunofluorescent reagents, centrifugation, and conventional cultures for the diagnosis of adenovirus infection. Diagn. Microbiol. Infect. Dis. *12*:407–411, 1989.
245. Maisel, J. C., Pierce, W. E., Crawford, Y. E., et al.: Virus pneumonia and adenovirus infection: A reappraisal. Am. J. Hyg. *75*:56–68, 1962.
246. Maletzky, A. J., Cooney, M. K., Luce, R., et al.: Epidemiology of viral and mycoplasmal agents associated with childhood lower respiratory illness in a civilian population. J. Pediatr. *78*:407–414, 1971.
247. Martone, W. J., Hierholzer, J. C., Keenlyside, R. A., et al.: An outbreak of adenovirus type 3 disease at a private recreation center swimming pool. Am. J. Epidemiol. *111*:229–237, 1980.
248. Matsuoka, T., Naito, T., Kubota, Y., et al.: Disseminated adenovirus (type 19) infection in a neonate: Rapid detection of the infection by immunofluorescence. Acta Paediatr. Scand. *79*:568–571, 1990.
249. McCarthy, A. J., Bergin, M., DeSilva, L. M., et al.: Intravenous ribavirin therapy for disseminated adenovirus infection. Pediatr. Infect. Dis. J. *14*:1003–1004, 1995.
250. McCormick, D. P., Wenzel, R. P., Davies, J. A., et al.: Nasal secretion protein responses in patients with wild-type adenovirus disease. Infect. Immun. *6*:282–288, 1972.
251. McNamara, M. J., Pierce, W. E., Crawford, Y. E., et al.: Patterns of adenovirus infection in the respiratory diseases of naval recruits: A longitudinal study of two companies of naval recruits. Am. Rev. Respir. Dis. *86*:485–494, 1962.
252. Melnick, J. L.: Taxonomy of viruses, 1976. Prog. Med. Virol. *22*:211–221, 1976.
253. Meurman, O., Ruuskanen, O., and Sarkkinen, H.: Immunoassay diagnosis of adenovirus infections in children. J. Clin. Microbiol. *18*:1190–1195, 1983.
254. Meyer, K., Girgis, N., and McGravey, V.: Adenovirus associated with congenital pleural effusion. J. Pediatr. *107*:433–435, 1985.
255. Michaels, M. G., Green, M., Wald, E. R., et al.: Adenovirus infection in pediatric liver transplant recipients. J. Infect. Dis. *165*:170–174, 1992.
256. Mikol, J., Felten-Papaiconomou, A., Ferchal, F., et al.: Inclusion-body myositis: Clinicopathological studies and isolation of an adenovirus type 2 from muscle biopsy specimen. Ann. Neurol. *11*:576–581, 1982.
257. Miller, D. G., Gabrielson, M. O., and Horstmann, D. M.: Clinical virology and viral surveillance in a pediatric group practice: The use of double-seeded tissue culture tubes for primary virus isolation. Am. J. Epidemiol. *88*:245–256, 1968.
258. Mistchenko, A. S., Huberman, K. H., Gomez, J. A., et al.: Epidemiology of enteric adenovirus infection in prospectively monitored Argentine families. Epidemiol. Infect. *109*:539–546, 1992.
259. Mistchenko, A. S., Diez, R. A., Mariani, A. L., et al.: Cytokines in adenoviral disease in children: Association of interleukin-6, interleukin-8, and tumor necrosis factor alpha levels with clinical outcome. J. Pediatr. *124*:714–720, 1994.
260. Mistchenko, A. S., Maffey, A. F., Casal, G., et al.: Adenoviral pericarditis: High levels of interleukin-6 in pericardial fluid. Pediatr. Infect. Dis. J. *14*:1007–1009, 1995.
261. Mitsui, Y., Hanna, L., Hanabusa, J., et al.: Association of adenovirus type 8 with epidemic keratoconjunctivitis. Arch. Ophthalmol. *61*:891–898, 1959.
262. Moffet, H. L., Siegel, A. C., and Doyle, H. K.: Nonstreptococcal pharyngitis. J. Pediatr. *73*:51–60, 1968.
263. Mordhorst, C. H., and Kjer, P.: Studies on an epidemic of keratoconjunctivitis caused by adenovirus type 8. I. Virus isolation in human amniotic cells, and serological observations. Acta Ophthalmol. *39*:974–983, 1961.
264. Morris, D. J., Cooper, R. J., Barr, T., et al.: Polymerase chain reaction for rapid diagnosis of respiratory adenovirus infection. J. Infect. *32*:113–117, 1996.
265. Mueller, R. E., Muldoon, R. L., and Jackson, G. G.: Communicability of enteric live adenovirus type 4 vaccine in families. J. Infect. Dis. *119*:60–66, 1969.
266. Mufson, M. A., Krause, H. E., Mocega, H. E., et al.: Viruses, *Mycoplasma pneumoniae* and bacteria associated with lower respiratory tract disease among infants. Am. J. Epidemiol. *91*:192–202, 1970.
267. Mufson, M. A., Zollar, L. M., Mankad, V. N., et al.: Adenovirus infection in acute hemorrhagic cystitis. Am. J. Dis. Child. *121*:281–285, 1971.
268. Mufson, M. A., Belshe, R. B., Horrigan, T. J., et al.: Cause of acute hemorrhagic cystitis in children. Am. J. Dis. Child. *126*:605–609, 1973.
269. Mufson, M. A., and Belshe, R. B.: A review of adenoviruses in the etiology of acute hemorrhagic cystitis. J. Urol. *115*:191–194, 1976.
270. Murphy, G. F., Wood, D. P., Jr., McRoberts, J. W., et al: Adenovirus associated haemorrhagic cystitis treated with intravenous ribavirin. J. Urol. *149*:565–566, 1993.
271. Myerowitz, R. L., Stalder, H., Oxman, M. N., et al.: Fatal disseminated adenovirus infection in a renal transplant recipient. Am. J. Med. *59*:591–598, 1975.
272. Nahmias, A. J., Griffith, D., and Snitzer, J.: Fatal pneumonia associated with adenovirus type 7. Am. J. Dis. Child. *114*:36–41, 1967.
273. Naveh, Y., and Friedman, A.: Orchitis associated with adenoviral infection. Am. J. Dis. Child. *129*:257–258, 1975.
274. Nelson, K. E., Gavitt, F., Batt, M. D., et al.: The role of adenoviruses in the pertussis syndrome. J. Pediatr. *86*:335–341, 1975.
275. Nemir, R. L., O'Hare, D., Goldstein, S., et al.: Adenovirus complement-fixing antibody titers from birth through the first year of life: A longitudinal study. Pediatrics *32*:497–500, 1963.
276. Neva, F. A., and Enders, J. F.: Isolation of a cytopathogenic agent from an infant with a disease in certain respects resembling roseola infantum. J. Immunol. *72*:315–321, 1954.
277. Newland, J. C., and Cooney, M. K.: Characteristics of an adenovirus type 19 conjunctivitis isolate and evidence for a subgroup associated with epidemic conjunctivitis. Infect. Immun. *21*:303–309, 1978.
278. Niemann, T. H., Trigg, M. E., Winick, N., et al.: Disseminated adenoviral infection presenting as acute pancreatitis. Hum. Pathol. *24*:1145–1148, 1993.
279. Noda, M., Miyamoto, Y., Ikeda, Y., et al.: Intermediate human adenovirus type 22/H10, 19, 37 as a new etiological agent of conjunctivitis. J. Clin. Microbiol. *29*:1286–1289, 1991.
280. Norrby, E.: Biological significance of structural adenovirus components. Curr. Top. Microbiol. *43*:1–43, 1968.
281. Norrby, E.: The structural and functional diversity of adenovirus capsid components. J. Gen. Virol. *5*:221–236, 1969.
282. Numazaki, Y., Yano, N., Ikeda, M., et al.: Adenovirus infection in intussusception of Japanese infants. Jpn. J. Microbiol. *17*:87–89, 1973.
283. Numazaki, Y., Kumasaka, T., Yano, N., et al.: Further study on acute hemorrhagic cystitis due to adenovirus type 11. N. Engl. J. Med. *289*:344–347, 1973.
284. Odio, C., McCracken, G. H., Jr., and Nelson, J. D.: Disseminated adenovirus infection: A case report and review of literature. Pediatr. Infect. Dis. *2*:46–48, 1984.
285. Ohori, N. P., Michaels, M. G., Jaffe, R., et al.: Adenovirus pneumonia in lung transplant recipients. Hum. Pathol. *26*:1073–1079, 1995.
286. Oishi, I., Yamazaki, K., Minekawa, Y., et al.: Three-year survey of the epidemiology of rotavirus, enteric adenovirus, and some small spherical viruses including "Osaka-agent" associated with infantile diarrhea. Biken J. *28*:9–19, 1985.
287. Olson, L. C., Miller, G., and Hanshaw, J. B.: Acute infectious lymphocytosis presenting as a pertussis-like illness: Its association with adenovirus type 12. Lancet *1*:200–201, 1964.
288. Osamura, T., Mizuta, R., Yoshioka, H., et al.: Isolation of adenovirus type 11 from the brain of a neonate with pneumonia and encephalitis. Eur. J. Pediatr. *152*:496–499, 1993.
289. Pacini, D. L., Dubovi, E. J., and Clyde, W. A., Jr.: A new animal model for human respiratory tract disease due to adenovirus. J. Infect. Dis. *150*:92–97, 1984.
290. Pacini, D. L., Collier, A. M., and Henderson, F. W.: Adenovirus infections and respiratory illnesses in children in group day care. J. Infect. Dis. *156*:920–927, 1987.
291. Paderstein, R.: Was ist schwimmbad-konjunktivitis? Klin. Monat. Augenheilk. *74*:634–642, 1925.
292. Panush, R. S.: Adenovirus arthritis. Arthritis Rheum. *17*:534–536, 1974.
293. Parker, W. L., Wilt, J. C., and Stakiw, W.: Adenovirus infections. Can. J. Public Health *52*:246–251, 1961.
294. Parks, W. P., Boucher, D. W., Milnick, J. L., et al.: Seroepidemiological and ecological studies of the adenovirus-associated satellite viruses. Infect. Immun. *2*:716–722, 1970.
295. Parrott, R. H., Rowe, W. P., Huebner, R. J., et al.: Outbreak of febrile pharyngitis and conjunctivitis associated with type 3 adenoidal-pharyngeal-conjunctival virus infection. N. Engl. J. Med. *251*:1087–1090, 1954.
296. Parrott, R, H.: Newly isolated viruses in respiratory disease. Pediatrics *20*:1066–1083, 1957.
297. Parrott, R. H.: Viral respiratory tract illnesses in children. Bull. N. Y. Acad. Med. *39*:629–648, 1963.
298. Pearson, R. D., Hall, W. J., Menegus, M. A., et al.: Diffuse pneumonitis due to adenovirus type 21 in a civilian. Chest *78*:107–109, 1980.
299. Pereira, H. G.: Typing of adenoidal-pharyngeal-conjunctival (APC) viruses by complement-fixation. J. Pathol. Bacteriol. *72*:105–109, 1956.
300. Pereira, H. G.: A protein factor responsible for the early cytopathic effect of adenoviruses. Microbiology *6*:601–611, 1958.
301. Pereira, M. S., and MacCallum, F. O.: Infection with adenovirus type 12. Lancet *1*:198–199, 1964.
302. Pereira, M. S.: Adenovirus infections. Postgrad. Med. J. *49*:798–801, 1973.
303. Pettit, T. H., and Holland, G. N.: Chronic keratoconjunctivitis associated with ocular adenovirus infection. Am. J. Ophthalmol. *88*:748–751, 1979.
304. Piedra, P. A., Kasel, J. A., Norton, H. J., et al.: Description of an adenovirus type 8 outbreak in hospitalized neonates born prematurely. Pediatr. Infect. Dis. J. *11*:460–465, 1992.
305. Piña, M., and Green, M.: Biochemical studies on adenovirus multiplication. IX. Chemical and base composition analysis of 28 human adenoviruses. Proc. Natl. Acad. Sci. U. S. A. *54*:547–551, 1965.

306. Pingleton, S. K., Pingleton, W. W., Hill, R. H., et al.: Type 3 adenoviral pneumonia occurring in a respiratory intensive care unit. Chest *73*:554–555, 1978.
307. Pinkerton, H., and Carroll, S.: Fatal adenovirus pneumonia in infants: Correlation of histologic and electron microscopic observations. Am. J. Pathol. *65*:543–548, 1971.
308. Poerregaard, A., Hjelt, K., Genner, J., et al.: Role of enteric adenoviruses in acute gastroenteritis in children attending day-care centres. Acta Paediatr. Scand. *79*:370–371, 1990.
309. Portnoy, B., Salvatore, M. A., Hanes, B., et al.: The sensitivity of the complement fixation test for the detection of adenovirus infections in infants and children with lower respiratory disease. Am. J. Epidemiol. *86*:362–372, 1967.
310. Potter, C. W.: Adenovirus infection as an aetiological factor in intussusception of infants and young children. J. Pathol. Bacteriol. *88*:263–274, 1964.
311. Prage, L., Pettersson, U., and Philipson, L.: Internal basic proteins in adenovirus. Virology *36*:508–511, 1968.
312. Prince, R. L.: Evidence for an aetiological role for adenovirus type 7 in the mesenteric adenitis syndrome. Med. J. Aust. *2*:56–57, 1979.
313. Putto, A., Ruuskanen, O., and Meurman, O.: Fever in respiratory virus infections. Am. J. Dis. Child. *140*:1159–1163, 1986.
314. Rafajko, R. R.: Differences in cytopathic effects of adenovirus in monkey kidney tissue culture. Proc. Soc. Exp. Biol. Med. *119*:975–982, 1965.
315. Ray, C. G., and Minnich, L. L.: Efficiency of immunofluorescence for rapid detection of common respiratory viruses. J. Clin. Microbiol. *25*:355–357, 1987.
316. Retter, M., Middleton, P. J., Tam, J. S., et al.: Enteric adenoviruses: Detection, replication, and significance. J. Clin. Microbiol. *10*:574–578, 1979.
317. Reuss, V. A.: Keratitis maculosa. Wien. Klin. Wochenschr. *2*:665–666, 1889.
318. Reynolds, M. A., Hart, C. A., Sills, J. A., et al.: Two cases of adenovirus type 1 pneumonia: Diagnosis by direct electron microscopy and culture. Pediatr. Infect. Dis. *5*:105–107, 1986.
319. Richmond, S. J., Caul, E. O., Dunn, S. M., et al.: An outbreak of gastroenteritis in young children caused by adenoviruses. Lancet *1*:1178–1180, 1979.
320. Rodriguez, W. J., Kim, H. W., Brandt, C. D., et al.: Fecal adenoviruses from a longitudinal study of families in metropolitan Washington, D. C.: Laboratory, clinical, and epidemiologic observations. J. Pediatr. *107*:514–520, 1985.
321. Roggendorf, M., Wigand, R., Deinhardt, F., et al.: Enzyme-linked immunosorbent assay for acute adenovirus infection. J. Virol. Methods *4*:27–35, 1982.
322. Romano, A., Revel, M., Guarari-Rotman, D., et al.: Use of human fibroblast-derived (beta) interferon in the treatment of epidemic adenovirus keratoconjunctivitis. J. Interferon Res. *1*:95–100, 1980.
323. Roos, R., Chou, S. M., Basnight, M., et al.: Isolation of an adenovirus 32 strain from human brain in a case of subacute encephalitis. Proc. Soc. Exp. Biol. Med. *139*:636–640, 1972.
324. Rose, H. M., Lamson, R. H., and Buescher, E. L.: Adenoviral infection in military recruits: Emergence of type 7 and 21 infections in recruits immunized with type 4 oral vaccine. Arch. Environ. Health *21*:356–361, 1970.
325. Rosen, L.: A hemagglutination-inhibition technique for typing adenoviruses. Am. J. Hyg. *71*:120–128, 1959.
326. Ross, J. G., Potter, C. W., and Zachary, R. B.: Adenovirus infection in association with intussusception in infancy. Lancet *2*:221–223, 1962.
327. Rowe, W. P., Huebner, R. J., Gilmore, L. K., et al.: Isolation of a cytopathogenic agent from human adenoids undergoing spontaneous degeneration in tissue culture. Proc. Soc. Exp. Biol. Med. *84*:570–573, 1955.
328. Rowe, W. P., Huebner, R. J., Hartley, J. W., et al.: Studies of the adenoidal-pharyngeal-conjunctival (APC) group of viruses. Am. J. Hyg. *61*:197–218, 1955.
329. Rowe, W. P., and Huebner, R. J.: Present knowledge of the clinical significance of the adenoidal-pharyngeal-conjunctival group of viruses. Am. J. Trop. Med. Hyg. *5*:453–460, 1956.
330. Rowe, W. P., Hartley, J. W., Roizman, B., et al.: Characterization of a factor formed in the course of adenovirus infection of tissue cultures causing detachment of cells from glass. J. Exp. Med. *108*:713–729, 1958.
331. Ruuskanen, O., Meurman, O., and Sarkkinen, J.: Adenoviral diseases in children: A study of 105 hospital cases. Pediatrics *76*:79–83, 1985.
332. Ruuskanen, O., Sarkkinen, H., Meurman, O., et al.: Rapid diagnosis of adenoviral tonsillitis: A prospective clinical study. J. Pediatr. *104*:725–728, 1984.
333. Sahler, O. J. Z., and Wilfert, C. M.: Fever and petechiae with adenovirus type 7 infection. Pediatrics *53*:233–235, 1974.
334. Salomón, H. E., Grandien, M., Avila, M. M., et al.: Comparison of three techniques for detection of respiratory viruses in nasopharyngeal aspirates from children with lower acute respiratory infections. J. Med. Virol. *28*:159–162, 1989.
335. Sanekata, T., Taniguchi, K., Demura, M., et al.: Detection of adenovirus type 41 in stool samples by a latex agglutination method. J. Immunol. Methods *127*:235–239, 1990.
336. Schaap, G. J. P., de Jong, J. C., van Bijsterveld, O. P., et al.: A new intermediate adenovirus type causing conjunctivitis. Arch. Ophthalmol. *97*:2336–2338, 1979.
337. Schloesser, C.: Comments on keratitis punctata. Centralbl. Prakt. Augenh. *13*:360, 1889.
338. Schnurr, D., and Dondero, M. E.: Two new candidate adenovirus serotypes. Intervirology *36*:79–83, 1993.
339. Schoub, B. D., Koornhof, H. L., Lecatsas, G., et al.: Virus in acute summer gastroenteritis in black infants. Lancet *1*:1093–1094, 1975.
340. Schwartz, H. S., Vastine, D. W., Yamashiroya, H., et al.: Immunofluorescent detection of adenovirus antigen in epidemic keratoconjunctivitis. Invest. Ophthalmol. *15*:199–207, 1976.
341. Severe, J. L., and Traub, R. G.: Conjunctivitis with follicles associated with adenovirus type 22. N. Engl. J. Med. *266*:1375–1376, 1962.
342. Shields, A. F., Hackman, R. C., Fife, K. H., et al.: Adenovirus infections in patients undergoing bone-marrow transplantation. N. Engl. J. Med. *312*:529–533, 1985.
343. Siegal, F. P., Dikman, S. H., Arayata, R. B., et al.: Fatal disseminated adenovirus 11 pneumonia in an agammaglobulinemic patient. Am. J. Med. *71*:1062–1067, 1981.
344. Simila, S., Jouppila, R., Salmi, A., et al.: Encephalomeningitis in children associated with an adenovirus type 7 epidemic. Acta Paediatr. Scand. *59*:310–316, 1970.
345. Simila, S., Ylikorkala, O., and Wasz-Hockert, O.: Type 7 adenovirus pneumonia. J. Pediatr. *79*:605–611, 1971.
346. Simila, S., Linna, O., Lanning, P., et al.: Chronic lung damage caused by adenovirus type 7: A ten-year follow-up study. Chest *80*:127–131, 1981.
347. Singh-Naz, N., Brown, M., and Ganeshananthan, M.: Nosocomial adenovirus infection: Molecular epidemiology of an outbreak. Pediatr. Infect. Dis. J. *12*:922–925, 1993.
348. Smith, R. H.: Fatal adenovirus infection with misleading positive serology for infectious mononucleosis. Lancet *1*:299–300, 1979.
349. Smith, T. J., Buescher, E. L., Top, F. H., Jr., et al.: Experimental respiratory infection with type 4 adenovirus vaccine in volunteers: Clinical and immunological responses. J. Infect. Dis. *122*:239–248, 1970.
350. Sohier, R., Chardonnet, Y., and Prunieras, M.: Adenoviruses: Status of current knowledge. Prog. Med. Virol. *7*:253–325, 1965.
351. South, M. A., Dolen, J., Beach, D. K., et al.: Fatal adenovirus hepatic necrosis in severe combined immune deficiency. Pediatr. Infect. Dis. *1*:416–419, 1982.
352. Sprague, J. B., Hierholzer, J. C., Currier, R. W., II, et al.: Epidemic keratoconjunctivitis: A severe industrial outbreak due to adenovirus type 8. N. Engl. J. Med. *289*:1341–1346, 1973.
353. Stanley, E. D., and Jackson, G. G.: Spread of enteric live adenovirus type 4 vaccine in married couples. J. Infect. Dis. *119*:51–59, 1969.
354. Steen-Johnsen, J., Orstavik, I., and Attramadal, A.: Severe illnesses due to adenovirus type 7 in children. Acta Paediatr. Scand. *58*:157–163, 1969.
355. Steigbigel, R. T., LaScolea, L. J., Jr., and Marx, G.: Renal hematuria associated with adenovirus 7a infection. Am. J. Dis. Child. *132*:208–210, 1978.
356. Stellwag, V. K.: A peculiar form of corneal inflammation. Wien. Klin. Wochenschr. *August*:613–614, 1889.
357. Sterner, G.: Infections with adenovirus type 7 in children and their relationship to acute respiratory disease. Acta Paediatr. *48*:287–298, 1959.
358. Sterner, G., Gerzen, P., Ohlson, M., et al.: Acute respiratory illness and gastroenteritis in association with adenovirus type 7 infections. Acta Paediatr. *50*:457–468, 1961.
359. Sterner, G.: Adenovirus infection in childhood: An epidemiological and clinical survey among Swedish children. Acta Paediatr. *142*:5–30, 1962.
360. Stovin, S.: Sporadic acute respiratory infections in adults with special reference to adenovirus infections. J. Hyg. *56*:404–414, 1958.
361. Stuart-Harris, C. H.: The adenoviruses and respiratory disease in man. Lectures on the Scientific Basis of Medicine *8*:148–164, 1958–59.
362. Sutton, R. N. P., Pullen, H. J. M., Blackledge, P., et al.: Adenovirus type 7: 1971–74. Lancet *2*:987–991, 1976.
363. Swann, N. H.: Acute thyroiditis: Five cases associated with adenovirus infection. Metabolism *13*:908–910, 1964.
364. Swenson, P. D., Lowens, M. S., Celum, C. L., et al.: Adenovirus types 2, 8 and 37 associated with genital infections in patients attending a sexually transmitted disease clinic. J. Clin. Microbiol. *33*:2728–2731, 1995.
365. Takafuji, E. T., Gaydos, J. C., Allen, R. G., et al.: Simultaneous administration of live, enteric-coated adenovirus types 4, 7, and 21 vaccines: Safety and immunogenicity. J. Infect. Dis. *140*:48–53, 1979.
366. Takiff, H. E., Straus, S. E., and Garon, C. F.: Propagation and in vitro studies of previously non-cultivable enteral adenoviruses in 293 cells. Lancet *2*:832–834, 1981.
367. Takiff, H. E., Seidlin, M., Krause, P., et al.: Detection of enteric adenoviruses by dot-blot hybridization using a molecularly cloned viral DNA probe. J. Med. Virol. *16*:107–118, 1985.
368. Tanaka, C.: Epidemic keratoconjunctivitis in Japan and the Orient. Am. J. Ophthalmol. *43*:46–50, 1957.
369. Tanaka, C.: A study of the relationship between adenovirus and epidemic keratoconjunctivitis. Arch. Ophthalmol. *59*:49–54, 1958.
370. Thiele, G. M., Okano, M., and Purtilo, D. T.: Enzyme-linked immunosorbent assay (ELISA) for detecting antibodies in sera of patients with adenovirus infection. J. Virol. Methods *23*:321–332, 1989.
371. Tiemessen, C. T., Wegerhoff, F. O., Erasmus, M. J., et al.: Infection by enteric adenoviruses, rotaviruses, and other agents in a rural African environment. J. Med. Virol. *28*:176–182, 1989.

372. Tiemessen, C. T., and Kidd, A. H.: The subgroup F adenoviruses. J. Gen. Virol. 76:481–497, 1995.
373. Top, F. H., Jr., Dudding, B. A., Russell, P. K., et al.: Control of respiratory disease in recruits with types 4 and 7 adenovirus vaccines. Am. J. Epidemiol. 94:142–146, 1971.
374. Top, F. H., Jr., Grossman, R. A., Bartelloni, P. J., et al.: Immunization with live types 7 and 4 adenovirus vaccines. I. Safety, infectivity, and potency of adenovirus type 7 vaccine in humans. J. Infect. Dis. 124:148–154, 1971.
375. Top, F. H., Jr., Buescher, E. L., Bancroft, W. H., et al.: Immunization with live types 7 and 4 adenovirus vaccines. II. Antibody response and protective effect against acute respiratory disease due to adenovirus type 7. J. Infect. Dis. 124:155–160, 1971.
376. Top, F. H., Jr.: Control of adenovirus acute respiratory disease in U. S. Army trainees. Yale J. Biol. Med. 48:185–195, 1975.
377. Towbin, J. A., Griffin, L. D., Martin, A. B., et al: Intrauterine adenoviral myocarditis presenting as nonimmune hydrops fetalis: Diagnosis by polymerase chain reaction. Pediatr. Infect. Dis. J. 13:144–150, 1994.
378. Trentin, J. J., Yabe, Y., and Taylor, G.: The quest for human cancer viruses. Science 137:835–849, 1962.
379. Trifajova, J., Bruckova, M., Ryc, M., et al.: Type 5 adenovirus isolated from urine of patient with Hodgkin's disease. J. Hyg. Epidemiol. Microbiol. Immunol. 25:321–323, 1981.
380. Turner, P. C., Bailey, A. S., Cooper, R. J., et al.: The polymerase chain reaction for detecting adenovirus DNA in formalin-fixed, paraffin-embeddded tissue obtained post mortem. J. Infect. 27:43–46, 1993.
381. Tyrrell, D. A. J., Balducci, D., and Zaiman, T. E.: Acute infections of the respiratory tract and the adenoviruses. Lancet 2:1326–1330, 1956.
382. Uhnoo, I., Wadell, G., Svensson, L., et al.: Importance of enteric adenoviruses 40 and 41 in acute gastroenteritis in infants and young children. J. Clin. Microbiol. 20:365–372, 1984.
383. Valentine, R. C., and Pereira, H. G.: Antigens and structure of the adenovirus. J. Mol. Biol. 13:13–20, 1965.
384. Van, R., Wun, C. C., O'Ryan, M. L., et al.: Outbreaks of human enteric adenovirus types 40 and 41 in Houston day care centers. J. Pediatr. 120:516–520, 1992.
385. Van Der Veen, J., and Kok, G.: Isolation and typing of adenoviruses recovered from military recruits with acute respiratory disease in the Netherlands. Am. J. Hyg. 65:119–129, 1957.
386. Van Der Veen, J.: Infections with adenovirus in Europe. Soc. Belge Med. Trop. Ann. 38:891–904, 1958.
387. Van Der Veen, J., and Ven Der Ploeg, G.: An outbreak of pharyngoconjunctival fever caused by types 3 and 4 adenovirus at Waalwijk, the Netherlands. Am. J. Hyg. 68:95–105, 1958.
388. Van Der Veen, J., and Dijkman, J. H.: Association of type 21 adenovirus with acute respiratory illness in military recruits. Am. J. Hyg. 76:149–159, 1962.
389. Van Der Veen, J.: The role of adenoviruses in respiratory disease. Am. Rev. Respir. Dis. 88:167–180, 1963.
390. Van Der Veen, J., Van Zaane, D. J., Sprangers, M. A., et al.: Homotypic and heterotypic antibody response in infants to adenovirus vaccine. Arch. Gesamte. Virusforsch. 21:320–333, 1967.
391. Van Der Veen, J., Oei, K. G., and Arbarbanal, M. F. W.: Patterns of infections with adenovirus types 4, 7, and 21 in military recruits during a 9-year survey. J. Hyg. (Camb.) 67:255–268, 1969.
392. Vargosko, A. J., Kim, H. W., Parrott, R. H., et al.: Recovery and identification of adenovirus in infections of infants and children. Bacteriol. Rev. 29:487–495, 1965.
393. Vass, Z.: Histological findings in epidemic keratoconjunctivitis. Acta Ophthalmol. 42:119–121, 1964.
394. Vihma, L.: Surveillance of acute viral respiratory diseases in children. Acta Paediatr. Scand. 192:27–41, 1969.
395. Wadell, G., Sundell, G., and de Jong, J. C.: Characterization of candidate adenovirus 37 by SDS-polyacrylamide gel electrophoresis of virion polypeptides and DNA restriction site mapping. J. Med. Virol. 7:119–125, 1981.
396. Wadell, G.: Molecular epidemiology of human adenoviruses. Curr. Top. Microbiol. Immunol. 110:191–220, 1984.
397. Wadell, G.: Classification of human adenoviruses by SDS polyacrylamide gel electrophoresis of structural polypeptides. Intervirology 11:47–57, 1979.
398. Wadell, G., Hammarskhold, M. L., Winberg, G., et al.: Genetic variability of adenoviruses. Ann. N. Y. Acad. Sci. 354:16–42, 1980.
399. Warren, D., Nelson, K. E., Farrar, J. A., et al.: A large outbreak of epidemic keratoconjunctivitis: Problems in controlling nosocomial spread. J. Infect. Dis. 160:938–943, 1989.
400. Wenman, W. M., Pagtakhan, R. D., Reed, M. H., et al.: Adenovirus bronchiolitis in Manitoba: Epidemiologic, clinical, and radiologic features. Chest 81:605–609, 1982.
401. White, G. P. B., and Stancliffe, D.: Viruses and gastroenteritis. Lancet 2:703, 1975.
402. Whitelaw, A., Davies, H., and Parry, J.: Electron microscopy of fatal adenovirus gastroenteritis. Lancet 1:361, 1977.
403. Wigand, R., and Keller, D.: Relationship of human adenoviruses 12, 18 and 31 as determined by hemagglutination inhibition. J. Med. Virol. 2:137–142, 1978.
404. Wigand, R., Baumeister, H. G., Maass, G., et al.: Isolation and identification of enteric adenoviruses. J. Med. Virol. 11:233–240, 1983.
405. Wigand, R., Gelderblom, H., and Wadell, G.: New human adenovirus (candidate adenovirus 36), a novel member of subgroup D. Arch. Virol. 64:225–233, 1980.
406. Wigger, H. J., and Blanc, W. A.: Fatal hepatic and bronchial necrosis in adenovirus infection with thymic alymphoplasia. N. Engl. J. Med. 275:870–874, 1966.
407. Wildin, S. R., Chonmaitree, T., and Swischuk, L. E.: Roentgenographic features of common pediatric viral respiratory tract infections. Am. J. Dis. Child. 142:43–46, 1988.
408. Wilt, J. C., and Stackiw, W.: Adenovirus infections in Manitoba. Can. Med. Assoc. J. 102:269–272, 1970.
409. Wohl, M. E. B., and Chernick, V.: Bronchiolitis. Am. Rev. Respir. Dis. 118:759–781, 1978.
410. Wood, D. J., Bijlsma, K., de Jong, J. C., et al.: Evaluation of a commercial monoclonal antibody-based enzyme immunoassay for detection of adenovirus types 40 and 41 in stool specimens. J. Clin. Microbiol. 27:1155–1158, 1989.
411. Wright, H. T., Beckwith, J. B., and Gwinn, J. L.: A fatal case of inclusion body pneumonia in an infant infected with adenovirus type 3. J. Pediatr. 64:528–533, 1964.
412. Wright, J., Couchonnal, G., and Hodges, G. R.: Adenovirus type 21 infection: Occurrence with pneumonia, rhabdomyolysis, and myoglobinuria in an adult. J. A. M. A. 241:2420–2421, 1979.
413. Wright, R. E.: Superficial punctate keratitis. Br. J. Ophthalmol. 14:257–291, 1930.
414. Wulffraat, N., Geelan, S., van Dijken, P., et al.: Recovery from adenovirus pneumonia in a severe combined immunodeficiency patient treated with intravenous ribavirin. Transplantation 59:927, 1995.
415. Yin-Coggrave, M.: Isolation of adenoviruses from cases of epidemic keratoconjunctivitis in Singapore. Am. J. Ophthalmol. 55:575–583, 1963.
416. Yodfat, Y., and Nishmi, M.: Successive overlapping outbreaks of febrile pharyngitis and pharyngoconjunctival fever, associated with adenovirus types 2 and 7, in a kibbutz. Isr. J. Med. Sci. 10:1505–1509, 1974.
417. Yolken, R. H., Lawrence, F., Leister, F., et al.: Gastroenteritis associated with enteric type adenovirus in hospitalized infants. J. Pediatr. 101:21–26, 1982.
418. Yolken, R. H., and Franklin, C. C.: Gastrointestinal adenovirus: An important cause of morbidity in patients with necrotizing enterocolitis and gastrointestinal surgery. Pediatr. Infect. Dis. 4:42–47, 1985.
419. Yunis, E. J., and Hashida, Y.: Electron microscopic demonstration of adenovirus in appendix vermiformis in a case of ileocecal intussusception. Pediatrics 51:566–570, 1973.
420. Yunis, E. J., Atchison, R. W., Michaels, R. H., et al.: Adenovirus and ileocecal intussusception. Lab. Invest. 33:347–351, 1975.
421. Zahradnik, J. M., Spencer, M. J., and Porter, D. D.: Adenovirus infection in the immunocompromised patient. Am. J. Med. 68:725–732, 1980.
422. Zinserling, A.: Peculiarities of lesions in viral and mycoplasmal infections of the respiratory tract. Virchows Arch. (Pathol. Anat.) 356:259–273, 1972.

❑ ❑ ❑

SUBSECTION FOUR

HEPATOVIRIDAE

162

HEPATITIS B AND D VIRUSES

James D. Cherry, Karin Nielsen, and Jorge Vargas

Hepatitis B Virus

(see also Chapter 55)

Hepatitis B virus (HBV) is the single human agent in the family *Hepadnaviridae*.[63] It causes a wide spectrum of clinical manifestations ranging from asymptomatic infection to fulminant fatal hepatitis.[7, 81, 106, 107, 189] HBV infection is a major cause of acute hepatitis throughout the world, and a substantial number of infections become chronic. Chronically infected children develop chronic liver disease (cirrhosis, chronic active hepatitis, chronic persistent hepatitis) or primary hepatocellular carcinoma in later life.

Each year, an estimated 300,000 persons in the United States, primarily young adults, are infected with HBV.[39] One-quarter become ill with jaundice, more than 10,000 patients require hospitalization, and an average of 250 die of fulminant disease. The United States currently contains an estimated pool of 750,000 to 1,000,000 infectious carriers. Approximately 25 per cent of carriers develop chronic active hepatitis, which often progresses to cirrhosis. Furthermore, HBV carriers have a risk of developing primary liver cancer that is 12 to 300 times higher than that of other persons. An estimated 4000 persons die each year from hepatitis B–related cirrhosis, and more than 800 die from hepatitis B–related liver cancer.

HBV nomenclature is presented in Table 162–1.

HISTORY

Although endemic and epidemic illnesses with jaundice were noted in the Babylonian Talmud and the writings of Hippocrates more than 2000 years ago, it was not until 1885 that a parenterally transmitted illness consistent with HBV infection was observed.[120] Lurman[120] noted that 15 per cent of 1289 shipyard workers in Bremen, Germany, developed jaundice 2 to 8 months after they had received a smallpox vaccine prepared from human "lymph." Over the ensuing 50 years, other cases, as well as minor and major outbreaks of hepatitis, were associated with exposure to or injection with products containing human blood.[81] In 1943, cases of hepatitis after exposure to human blood products were grouped together and called homologous serum jaundice.[128]

In 1937, Findlay and MacCallum[58] noted that hepatitis occurred in volunteers who had received an attenuated yellow fever vaccine that contained human serum for stabilization. The use of this same type of yellow fever vaccine in United States military troops early in 1942 resulted in a significant epidemic of hepatitis[52, 156]; 28,000 cases and 62 deaths occurred. Later serologic studies confirmed that this military epidemic was due to HBV.[158]

After the realization of two epidemiologically distinct forms of hepatitis, the terms hepatitis A (infectious hepatitis) and hepatitis B (homologous serum jaundice) were suggested by MacCallum[121] in 1947. Subsequent studies by Krugman and associates[106–108] during the late 1950s through the early 1970s at the Willowbrook State School for the Mentally Handicapped contributed significantly to the understanding of hepatitis A and hepatitis B.

HBV was discovered by accident. In a study in which inherited polymorphic traits were looked for, the sera from multiply transfused hemophilia patients from throughout the world were examined.[23, 81] A unique antigen was noted in the serum of an Australian aborigine. This antigen (Australia

TABLE 162–1. Hepatitis B Virus Nomenclature

Abbreviation	Term	Definition/Comments
HBV	Hepatitis B virus	Etiologic agent of "serum" hepatitis; also known as Dane particle
HBsAg	Hepatitis B surface antigen	Surface antigen(s) of HBV detectable in large quantity in serum; several subtypes identified
HBeAg	Hepatitis B e antigen	Soluble antigen; correlates with HBV replication, high-titer HBV in serum, and infectivity of serum
HBcAg	Hepatitis B core antigen	No commercial test available
Anti-HBs	Antibody to HBsAg	Indicates past infection with and immunity to HBV, passive antibody from HBIG, or immune response from hepatitis B vaccine
Anti-HBe	Antibody to HBeAg	Presence in serum of HBsAg carrier indicates lower titer of HBV
Anti-HBc	Antibody to HBcAg	Indicates prior infection with HBV at some undefined time
IgM anti-HBc	IgM class antibody to HBcAg	Indicates recent infection with HBV; detectable for 4 to 6 months after infection
HBIG	Hepatitis B immunoglobulin	Contains high-titer antibodies to HBV

[Au] antigen) is known now to be the HBV surface antigen (HBsAg). In 1970, HBV was detected, and shortly thereafter the hepatitis B core antigen (HBcAg), the viral DNA, and the hepatitis B e antigen (HBeAg) were described.

Because HBV could not be grown in tissue culture systems, original vaccine studies used plasma-derived, highly purified HBsAg particles.[106] These trials were successful because antibody to HBsAg neutralized HBV. Subsequently, genetically engineered HBsAg vaccines replaced plasma-derived products. A plasma-derived vaccine was licensed in the United States in 1981, and recombinant vaccines have been available since July 1986.

THE VIRUS

Structure of the Virion

(see Fig. 55–3)

HBV belongs to the family of DNA viruses named *Hepadnaviridae*.[63] These viruses also are found in other mammalian (squirrels and woodchucks) and avian (Peking ducks) species. Hepadnaviruses all have common features, including virion size and structure, antigenic composition, DNA size, and pattern of viral replication. Cells infected with HBV produce many types of virus-related particles.[49, 66, 144] Via electron microscopy, sera of infected persons have been shown to harbor three types of particles. All three particles share a common surface antigen known as HBsAg, which is present at high concentrations in the sera of infected persons. The first group, identified by Dane in 1970,[49] is composed of 42- to 47-nm, double-shelled particles. These particles, known as Dane particles, are the infectious virions of HBV. Infected persons may harbor as many as 10^{10} infectious virions/mL of serum.[168]

The Dane particle contains an outer shell with a lipoprotein envelope harboring viral glycoproteins, which are identified serologically as HBsAg.[24] Antibody directed against HBsAg has neutralizing potential.[24] In addition, the particle contains an inner core or nucleocapsid of 25 to 27 nm that harbors a structural protein identified as the C protein, serologically identified as HBcAg.[8, 84, 87] The core contains the viral DNA[167] and polymerase[99, 145] activity that is involved in viral genomic replication. The core also has protein kinase activity, although its biologic role is uncertain.[5, 122, 149] HBV also contains 17- to 25-nm spherical particles that have no nucleic acid (hence are noninfectious) and are numerous (present in numbers 10^4 to 10^6 times that of the Dane particles). The third type of particles are 20-nm diameter, filamentous particles present in smaller amounts. Both types of particles are composed of HBsAg and host-derived lipids.[3, 65, 138] All three particles highly are immunogenic and induce an HBsAg-neutralizing antibody response.[103]

The HBsAg contains a heterogeneous group of antigens, which makes subtyping of the virus possible.[141] One antigen—a—is common to all viral strains. In addition, there are two pairs of subtype-specific determinants per virus. The pairs are d or y and w or r. Thus, there are four major HBsAg subtypes: HBsAg/adw, HBsAg/ayw, HBsAg/adr, and HBsAg/ayr. Subtyping with monospecific antisera can be performed by immunodiffusion or other immunologic methods (see Fig. 55–5).

Viral Genome

(see Fig. 55–4)

The DNA of the hepatitis B virion is a circular, partially duplex molecule with a structure of not completely symmetric DNA strains.[2] The viral minus strand is unit length and has protein covalently linked to its 5′ end,[67] whereas the plus strand is less than unit length and has capped oligoribonucleotide at its 5′ end.[116, 159] Therefore, the virion DNA has a single-stranded region (or gap) of fixed polarity but variable length. The virion has a polymerase, however, which is capable of repairing the gap in the template. By molecular cloning, it has been noted that the coding organization of HBV DNA is highly compact, with every nucleotide in the genome being within a coding region and more than half of the sequence being translated in more than one frame.[61, 176] There are four open-reading frames (ORFs) present in the DNA: ORF *P*, ORF *C*, ORF *S*/pre-*S*, and ORF *X*. The *P* gene encodes for the viral polymerase, which is crucial for viral replication.[2] ORF *P* encodes the terminal protein found on minus-strand DNA,[25] ORF *C* encodes the structural protein of the nucleocapsid,[136] ORF *S*/ pre-*S* encodes the viral surface glycoproteins,[177] and ORF *X* encodes a regulatory protein whose function is not yet well understood.[151]

HBV is similar to the other hepadnaviruses so far described (woodchuck hepatitis virus [WHV], ground squirrel hepatitis virus [GSHV], duck hepatitis virus [DHV]).[63] All have enveloped virions with relaxed, circular, partially duplex DNA, virion polymerases, subviral particles, narrow host range, and hepatotropism.[2]

Viral Life Cycle Overview

HBV flow of genetic information is from DNA to RNA to DNA. Unlike other DNA viruses, viral DNA replication does not occur by semiconservative DNA synthesis but by reverse transcription of an RNA intermediate.[166] After binding of the virus to receptors on the cell surface, virion nucleocapsids are delivered to the cytoplasm, where they translocate to the nucleus. There they mature their genomic DNA to the cccDNA form (a nuclear pool of viral covalently closed circular DNA that serves as a template for reverse transcription). This form of DNA then is transcribed by host RNA polymerase II, and the resulting RNAs are translated to originate the *P*, *C*, *S*/pre-*S*, and *X* gene products.[2] These viral pregenomic RNAs then are encapsidated into the cytoplasm with the *P* gene product.[166] DNA synthesis then is initiated, and the RNA template is degradated. After minus-strand synthesis and sequential plus-strand synthesis are completed, the progeny cores then bud into intracellular membranes and acquire their glycoprotein envelope.[97] The enveloped virions are secreted by vesicular transport.[100]

Recently, novel cell culture lines have been developed that permit further evaluation of the replicative cycle of hepadnaviruses.[2] Fresh primary duck hepatocytes support infection with DHV, but these cells do not have much cell division and cannot undergo passage.[62, 140, 174] Immortalized hepatoma cell lines, such as HepG2, HuH7, and chick LMH, can support viral replication and release if transfected with cloned HBV DNA.[63, 85] However, there still is no efficient tissue culture technique that supports HBV infection. In the cell culture systems presently available, it has been noted that the viral replicative cycle is not cytopathic. Infected hepatocytes are normal morphologically and display growth rates identical to those of uninfected controls.[63]

Viral Attachment and Entry

Studies of the early phases of the viral life cycle have been conducted primarily using DHV as a prototype for *Hepadnaviridae*.[2] There are two components to the bindings reaction: one is of low affinity and is nonsaturable, and the second is of high affinity and saturable.[101] At 37° C, entry and viral infection occur. After binding takes place, the virus must fuse with the host cell membrane. It appears that this phenomenon occurs by a pH-independent mechanism.[143] Experiments have shown that the binding and entry processes are slow, with maximal infection occurring after 16 hours of cell exposure to the inoculum.[140] The viral envelope components that appear to be involved primarily in the cell fusion interactions are the pre-S proteins.[101] Studies demonstrate that monoclonal antibodies to these proteins prevent infection of primary duck hepatocytes.[101] The pre-S proteins also appear to determine the narrow spectrum of the viral host determination (i.e., if the virus entry process is bypassed by transfection into heterologous cells, viral replication of heron HBV [HHBV] is able to replicate normally in duck cells, which normally are not infectible by this virus).[2, 162]

With regard to the cellular receptors for the hepadnaviruses, studies still are ongoing. Many proteins bind to the HBV envelope glycoproteins, such as apolipoprotein H[38] and endonexin 2 (a phospholipid binding protein),[77] which bind to HBV S particles. Receptors for pre-S proteins still have not been identified, and the biologic significance of these findings are yet to be determined. The mechanisms by which viral DNA is delivered to the nucleus following entry still are unclear as well. In the nucleus, viral DNA is transformed to the cccDNA form, which entails repair of the single-stranded gap, removal of the 5′ terminal structures, and covalent ligation of the strands.[2] It appears that host mechanisms contribute highly to this process.[102]

Viral Transcription

Several viral transcripts have been identified for HBV, but their function in the viral life cycle still is uncertain. These transcripts are either genomic or subgenomic and are able to translate specific viral gene products.[2] Genomic RNAs can serve as templates for viral DNA synthesis and as messages for ORF *pre-C*, *C*, and *P* translation.[2] Subgenomic RNAs function as messenger RNAs for the translation of the envelope and X proteins. Several viral promoters originate the viral transcripts. They are the genomic RNAs,[82] the L protein mRNA (pre-*S1* promoter),[42] the M and S protein mRNAs (*S* promoter),[42] and the X protein mRNA (*X* promoter).[161] Two genomic regions appear to function as enhancer elements of the viral promoters: enhancer I (*EnI*) and enhancer II (*EnII*).[43, 44] *EnI* is located between the *S* and *X* coding regions, and it up-regulates all viral promoters.[91] *EnII* has been shown so far to up-regulate the *S* promoter.[119] Deletion of any of the enhancers decreases viral transcription significantly.

Genomic Replication

The ORF *P* region of hepadnaviruses encodes for the viral polymerases. There are considerable similarities between this region and the coding regions for retroviral reverse transcriptases.[170] Changes in ORF *P* inactivate viral DNA synthesis.[13] However, unlike retroviruses, hepadnaviruses do not have integrases; therefore, there are no homologies between ORF *P* and reverse transcribing regions for integrases (and for proteases as well).[132] The first step in HBV genomic replication is the encapsidation of the genomic RNA template.[166] The pregenomic RNA is encapsidated into the core particle.[55] In order to package this small RNA portion into the capsid, both C protein and *P* gene products are required.[79] Encapsidation of polymerase occurs by binding of the P protein to the RNA that will be packaged.[12] Single-stranded pregenomic RNA is converted to partially duplex virion DNA through reverse transcription. The P protein interacts with the 5′ end of the pregenomic RNA.

Reverse transcription then is initiated by P at the 5′ stem-loop, with minus-strand DNA being extended by three to four nucleotides. P then is attached covalently to the new DNA, and both are transferred to the 3′ copy of the direct repeat 1 (DR1), with the DNA being extended. While the minus strand is being elongated, pregenomic RNA is degraded by the RNaseH of P. P then reaches the 5′ end of the template, where an RNA oligomer is formed. This oligomer translocates and anneals to direct repeat 2 (DR2), where it serves as a primer for plus-strand DNA synthesis. The plus strand is elongated to the 5′ end of the minus-strand DNA template. A second template transfer then occurs, with complementary sequences at the 3′ end of the minus-strand DNA enabling the genome to become circular.[169]

Viral Assembly and Release

The 20-nm subviral particles are assembled between the endoplasmic reticulum and the Golgi apparatus.[92] These 20-nm particles contain predominantly S proteins, which are synthesized in the endoplasmic reticulum.[71] In addition, these particles may contain M subunits but generally do not have L proteins.[75] The assembly process is encoded totally in the S domain.[112] Assembled particles are transported via the secretory pathway and transverse the Golgi complex.[100, 165] The S protein carries out the entire assembly process without the involvement of other viral proteins.[2] Therefore, subviral particles containing only envelope proteins are released. In vitro studies have shown that overexpression of L proteins gives rise to filamentous viral particles in the endoplasmic reticulum.[46] It appears that the overabundance of L, M, and S aggregates is cytopathic to hepatocytes in vitro. Similar cytopathic features have been seen in human infections with HBV, yet the role of envelope protein expression in hepatocyte injury remains to be determined.[2]

The assembly of the Dane particle differs from the assembly of the 20-nm particles in that all three proteins—L, M, and S—are present.[75] Studies of HepG2 cell lines transfected with HBV mutants missing L, M, or S proteins have shown that no virus budding occurs if the envelope proteins are not present (mutations in S) and that for virion formation and release, both L and S proteins are needed.[29] It appears that M proteins are not necessary for viral assembly.

Viral Persistence

Nuclear cccDNA appears to be crucial to viral persistence. Hepatocytes that harbor this form of viral genome are the only ones that produce virus.[2] As mentioned earlier, the replicative cycle of HBV is not cytopathic to hepatocytes, and therefore cells multiply normally. The cytoplasmic mechanism of reverse transcription, which delivers all cccDNA, and consequent delivery of this product to the nucleus hence must be passed on to progeny cells. The mechanisms by which this process unfolds still are under investigation.[63]

EPIDEMIOLOGY

Incidence and Prevalence

The prevalence of hepatitis B serologic markers (HBsAg and antibody to HBsAg) vary markedly throughout the world.[50, 81] Patterns of this serologic prevalence are presented

TABLE 162–2. Geographic Patterns of Hepatitis B Virus Serologic Prevalence and Occurrence of Neonatal and Childhood Infections

Prevalence	HBsAg	Anti-HBs	Neonatal/ Childhood Infection	Geography
Low	0.1–0.5%	4–6%	Rare	North America, Western Europe, Australia
Intermediate	2–7%	20–55%	Uncommon	Eastern Europe, Mediterranean, South America, Middle East, Russia, Japan
High	8–20%	70–95%	Common	China, Southeast Asia, tropical Africa, Pacific Islands, Middle East, South America

Data from Deinhart, F., Gust, I. D., on behalf of the participants in an informal WHO meeting: Viral hepatitis. Bull. W. H. O. *60*:661–691, 1982; and Hollinger, F. B.: Hepatitis B virus. *In* Fields, B. N., Knipe, D. M., Howley, P. M., et al. (eds.): Fields Virology. 3rd ed. Philadelphia, Lippincott-Raven, 1996, pp. 2739–2807.
HBsAg, hepatitis B surface antigen; anti-HBs, antibody to HBsAg.

in Table 162–2. The prevalence of hepatitis B serologic markers in the United States by various population groups in 1990 is presented in Table 162–3. Note the marked difference in HBsAg prevalence and other markers of past infection in the high-risk categories compared with the general population.

Reported cases of hepatitis B per 100,000 population in the United States from 1966 to 1994 are presented in Figure 162–1. Some of the increase in hepatitis B incidence during 1966 to 1985 can be attributed to improvements in serologic diagnosis, and some of the decline since 1985 may be due to changes in state reporting practices.[35] There were 26,654 cases (rate 11.5/100,000) in 1985 and 12,517 cases (rate 4.8/100,000) in 1994.[35, 36] A summary of reported cases by age group in the United States in 1994 is presented in Table 162–4. Of the total cases, only 3 per cent occurred in children and 6.45 per cent occurred in adolescents.[36] Of the 12,517 cases, race data were available for 8891 (71 per cent); 1.14 per cent were Native American or Alaskan Natives, 9.41 per cent were Asian or Pacific Islanders, 30.87 per cent were black, 58.01 per cent were white, and 0.56 per cent were classified as other.

TABLE 162–3. Prevalence of Hepatitis B Virus (HBV) Serologic Markers in Various Population Groups in the United States

	Prevalence of Serologic Markers of HBV Infection	
Population Group	***Hepatitis B Surface Antigen (%)***	***Any Marker (%)***
Immigrants/refugees from areas of high HBV endemicity	13	70–85
Alaskan Natives/Pacific Islanders	5–15	40–70
Clients in institutions for the developmentally disabled	10–20	35–80
Users of illicit parenteral drugs	7	60–80
Sexually active homosexual men	6	35–80
Household contacts of HBV carriers	3–6	30–60
Patients of hemodialysis units	3–10	20–80
Health care workers (frequent)	1–2	15–30
Prisoners (male)	1–8	10–80
Staff of institutions for the developmentally disabled	1	10–25
Heterosexuals with multiple partners	0.5	5–20
Health care workers (no or infrequent blood contact)	0.3	3–10
General population (NHANES II)*		
Blacks	0.9	14
Whites	0.2	3

* Second National Health and Nutrition Examination Survey.
Data from Centers for Disease Control: Protection against viral hepatitis: Recommendations of the Immunization Practices Advisory Committee (ACIP). M. M. W. R. *39*:1–23, 1990.

Transmission and Risk Factors

HBV infection occurs when the blood or other body fluids (containing the virus) of an infected person enter the blood of an uninfected person. This can occur directly, such as by blood transfusion, or less directly by breaks in the skin and mucous membrane barriers of the contact becoming exposed to blood or other body fluids of an infected person.

The incubation period of HBV infection is long (45 to 160 days; average = 120 days), and the onset of acute disease generally is insidious.[39] A variable proportion of persons infected with HBV become chronically infected with the virus. The HBV carrier is central to the epidemiology of HBV transmission. A carrier is defined as a person who is either HBsAg-positive on at least two occasions (at least 6 months apart) or who is HBsAg-positive and IgM anti-HBc–negative when a single serum specimen is tested. Although the degree of infectivity is correlated best with HBeAg positivity, any person positive for HBsAg potentially is infectious. The likelihood of becoming chronically infected with HBV varies inversely with the age at which infection occurs. HBV transmitted from HBsAg-positive mothers to their newborns results in HBV carriage for up to 90 per cent of infants. Between 25 and 50 per cent of children infected before 5 years of age become carriers, whereas only 6 to 10 per cent of acutely infected adults become carriers.

Carriers and persons with acute infection have the highest concentrations of HBV in blood and serous fluids.[39] A lower concentration is present in other body fluids, such as saliva and semen. Transmission occurs via percutaneous or permucosal routes, and infective blood or body fluids can be introduced at birth, through sexual contact, or by contaminated needles. Infection also can occur in settings of continuous close personal contact (such as in households or among children in institutions for the developmentally disabled), pre-

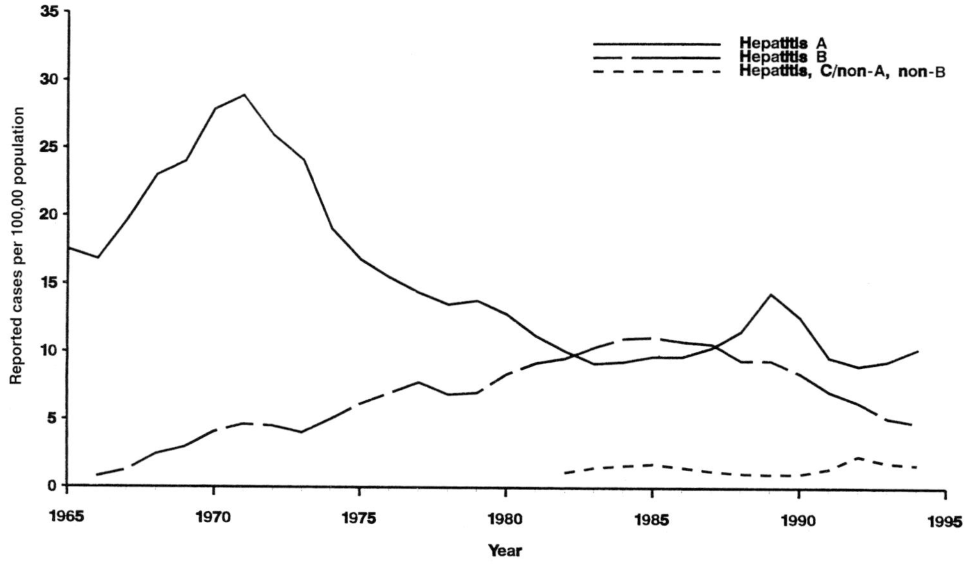

FIGURE 162–1. *Reported rates of hepatitis A, B, and non-A, non-B (C) by year in the United States. (From Centers for Disease Control and Prevention: Update: Recommendations to prevent hepatitis B virus transmission: United States. M. M. W. R. 44:574–575, 1995.)*

sumably via inapparent or unnoticed contact of infective secretions with skin lesions or mucosal surfaces. Transmission of infection by transfusion of blood or blood products is rare because of routine screening of blood for HBsAg and because of current donor selection procedures. Transmission of HBV from infected health care workers to patients is uncommon but has been documented during types of invasive procedures (e.g., oral, gynecologic, and thoracic surgery).[74, 98, 117] Adherence to aseptic techniques minimizes the risk of transmission. HBV is not transmitted via the fecal-oral route.

Worldwide, HBV infection is a major cause of acute and chronic hepatitis, cirrhosis, and primary hepatocellular carcinoma.[39] The frequency of HBV infection and patterns of transmission vary markedly in different parts of the world (see Table 162–2). In the United States, Western Europe, and Australia, it is a disease of low endemicity, with infection occurring primarily during adulthood and with only 0.2 to 0.9 per cent of the population being infected chronically. In contrast, HBV infection is highly endemic in China and Southeast Asia, most of Africa, most Pacific Islands, parts of the Middle East, and in the Amazon Basin. In these areas, most persons acquire infection at birth or during childhood, and 8 to 15 per cent of the population are infected chronically with HBV. In other parts of the world, HBV infection is moderately endemic, with 2 to 7 per cent of the population being HBV carriers.

Serologic surveys in the United States demonstrate that although HBV infection is uncommon among adults in the general population, it is highly prevalent in certain groups.[39] Those at risk, based on the prevalence of serologic markers of infection, are described in Table 162–3. Persons born in areas of high HBV endemicity and their descendants remain at high risk of infection, as do certain populations in which HBV is highly endemic (Alaskan Natives and Pacific Islanders). Certain lifestyles (e.g., homosexual activity, intravenous drug abuse) result in early acquisition of HBV infection and high rates of infection. Persons who have heterosexual activity with multiple partners are at significant risk of infection. Inmates of prisons have a high prevalence of HBV markers, usually because of parenteral drug abuse before or during imprisonment. Patients in custodial institutions for the developmentally disabled also are at increased risk of HBV infection. Household contacts and sexual partners of HBV carriers are at increased risk, as are hemodialysis patients and recipients of certain plasma-derived products that have not been inactivated (e.g., anti-hemophilic factor).

Those at occupational risk of HBV infection include medical and dental workers, related laboratory and support personnel, and public service employees who have contact with blood, as well as staff members in institutions or classrooms for the mentally retarded.

TABLE 162–4. Summary of Reported Cases of Hepatitis B, by Age Group in 1994

Age Group (Years)	Number	Percentage
<1	55	0.44
1–4	73	0.58
5–9	82	0.66
10–14	165	1.32
15–19	807	6.45
20–24	1618	12.93
25–29	1940	15.50
30–39	3615	28.88
40–49	2027	16.19
50–59	840	6.71
≥60	845	6.75
Unknown	450	3.60
Total	12,517	100

Data from Centers for Disease Control and Prevention: Update: Recommendations to prevent hepatitis B virus transmission—United States. M. M. W. R. *44*:574–575, 1995.

Congenital and Neonatal Infections (Vertical Transmission)[40, 73, 106, 107, 189]

Vertical transmission of HBV is common. Transmission may occur transplacentally or during the birth process. Transmission can occur when infection in the pregnant woman is acute or from a chronically infected pregnant women. In studies of chronically infected pregnant women, vertical transmission rates have varied from 73 and 40 per cent in Japan and Taiwan, respectively, to 8.3, 14, and 0 per cent in the United States, United Kingdom, and Denmark, respectively.[189] Transmission from women who had acute infections during pregnancy also is common. The major risk occurs during the third trimester, when transmission rates are greater than 50 per cent.

Transmission is related directly to maternal viral load.[30] Infants born to women positive for HBeAg have a 70 to 90 per cent chance of acquiring perinatal HBV infection, and 85 to 90 per cent of these infected infants become chronic HBV carriers.[163, 164] In 1988, it was estimated that 16,500 births in the United States occurred to HBsAg-positive women each year (about 4300 of these women also were HBeAg-positive), and approximately 3500 of the infants became chronic HBV carriers.[40]

Although transplacental infections do occur, the vast majority of neonatal infections result from exposure during the birth process.

PATHOGENESIS

Evidence to date suggests that HBV does not have a direct cytopathic effect in hepatocytes.[73, 81, 189] Humoral and cell-mediated immune responses appear to contribute to the development of the hepatic and extrahepatic lesions that occur in both acute and chronic phases of HBV disease. HBV has a high degree of specificity in regard to tissue tropism. However, although the liver is the primary site of replication, viral particles and HBV-DNA have been identified in peripheral blood lymphocytes, bile duct epithelial, endothelial and smooth muscle cells, pancreatic acinar cells, corneal tissue, lymph nodes, spleen, gonads, thyroid gland, kidneys, adrenal glands, and bone marrow cells of patients with HBV infection.[22, 54, 72, 115, 142, 148] It appears, however, that extrahepatic cells have a limited ability to replicate infectious virus. The highest concentrations of HBV are in the blood and liver; lower amounts of virus are found in saliva and semen. HBV may be present in a single host in a variety of genotypes (i.e., quasispecies), similar to the case with HIV, although the production of viable mutants is more limited.[78, 81]

The presence of neutralizing antibody to HBsAg is associated strongly with immunity to the virus. Cell-mediated immunity to the surface antigen and the nucleocapsid core also is correlated with immunity.[78] During the initial phase of HBV infection, interferon appears to be the first cytokine produced.[81] Interferon potentially has an antiviral effect by inducing the formation of synthetase enzyme, which inhibits the translation of viral proteins.[11] In a study of chimpanzees acutely infected with HBV, interferon alpha and HBsAg were found concurrently before the appearance of any antibody.[139] An increase in HLA class I antigens on hepatocytes then ensued, with a concomitant increase in transaminases. In humans, a similar increase in HLA class I antigens has been found during acute hepatitis B.[76] Recent studies have shown that disease is related closely to the degree of cytotoxic T-cell response of hepatocytes.[19, 57, 134, 137] HLA class I cytotoxic T lymphocytes (CTLs) directed against nucleocapsid antigens (HBcAg and HBeAg) on the cell surface of hepatocytes along with HLA class I molecules mediate viral clearance and cell injury. HBeAg is a polypeptide encoded by the precore region of the HBV genome. Both HBcAg and HBeAg share an amino acid sequence that confers antigenic relatedness.[78] When antibody to HBeAg develops, it is possible that immunologic selection of mutants that have lost their ability to produce HBeAg and HBcAg occurs, and with this CTL recognition stops. Others have reported that the failure of clearance of infected liver cells by CTLs may be due to induction of anergy in CD4+ cells specific for secreted HBeAg and HBcAg.[26] Other findings in patients with acute HBV infection include increased production of interferon gamma, increased natural killer cell cytotoxicity, and increased levels of interleukin 2.[51, 96, 182]

In studies of patients with acute development of HBV infection, the first immunologic response is directed against pre-S antigens[179] 30 days before liver injury occurs. This is followed by development of IgM antibody to HBcAg 10 days later. Anti-HBsAg antibody develops 10 days before liver disease does. If patients develop chronic HBV infection, no such antibody production is noted.[180] When HBV infection has resolved, HBsAg disappears from the peripheral blood circulation with subsequent development of anti-HBsAg. HBV DNA then is cleared from the blood, and lastly HBV DNA disappears from the liver.[95] Viral mutations have been associated with more fulminant disease courses. Changes in nucleotide sequence of the genome of HBV, which initially occur because of errors in replication, may continue to be propagated because they confer an added advantage to the virions. For example, mutations in the precore region of the C gene inhibit the production of HBeAg without inhibiting viral replication (i.e., patients are HBeAg-negative and HBV DNA–positive).[4, 27, 173] Many other mutations have been identified in the *S*/pre-*S* gene, the *X* gene, and the *P* gene,[21, 31, 33, 184, 186] but their role in the pathogenesis of HBV disease remains to be determined.

Infants who are born to mothers chronically infected with HBV and are HBeAg-positive have a 70 to 90 per cent chance of becoming carriers.[78] HBeAg appears to cross the placenta and induce CD4+ anergy to HBc/HBe antigens.[26] Therefore, CTLs would fail to clear infected hepatocytes, and the carrier state would continue as long as anergy is maintained. Restoration of CTLs could bring about rapid hepatic injury.[78] The rate of HBV carriage decreases as age increases. Among immunocompetent adults, the carrier rate ranges from 1 to 8 per cent.[16, 125, 158] Immunodeficient persons are susceptible to much higher viral carriage rates and chronic HBV infection.[81] Carriers of HBV may have a totally asymptomatic clinical course, may have prolonged asymptomatic periods, or may alternate periods of quiescence and exacerbation of liver disease.

The activity of CTLs directed against viral antigens appears to determine the state of the disease process. Immune responsiveness occurs in chronic active hepatitis with significant hepatocyte destruction. The loss of immune tolerance to HBeAg through viral mutation may account for the pathogenic CTL response. Alteration of the precore gene also is associated with decreased responsiveness to interferon alpha.[155, 188] It is unclear why HBV carriers do not have detectable HBsAg antibody. There have been reports of concurrent antibody and antigen presence, but most often this is not the case.[123, 190] One study demonstrated that HBsAg was captured by B cells and presented on their cell surface only to have these cells destroyed by CTLs, indicating that CTLs potentially could annihilate the cells responsible for antibody production.[10] Other researchers demonstrated that expression of HLA class I antigens was decreased greatly on the cell membranes of liver cells containing HBcAg and HBV DNA in contrast with those expressing HBsAg.[105] This is further evidence of the deleterious effect of CTLs in HBV disease progression.

The major problem associated with chronic carriage of HBV is the development of hepatocarcinoma and cirrhosis of the liver. Studies conducted in Taiwan demonstrated a 100-fold increase in carriers compared with noncarriers.[14, 17] The development of hepatocarcinoma occurs in general many years (at least three decades) after acquisition of HBV infection.[64] Cirrhosis and hepatocarcinoma are two distinct processes. The former results from destruction of the liver parenchyma, and the latter occurs because of oncogenic mutations after integration of the viral DNA into the host cell genome.[81] The vast majority of hepatocarcinomas in persons with HBV infection harbor high levels of integrated viral DNA.[26, 160] The integrated viral DNA is highly mutated,[53, 130] and the host DNA usually is altered as well.[146] The mechanism by which HBV integrates into the host genome is not well understood, particularly because HBV, unlike retroviruses, does not have integrases.[78] It is believed that HBV DNA is incorporated into the nucleus, most probably by host cell mechanisms.[63]

One of the major suspects in HBV cancer induction is the *X* gene, which is a potent transactivator.[34, 41] The X protein is absent in the avian hepadnaviruses, which generally are not associated with hepatocarcinomas.[63] Most oncogenes affect both transcription and signal transduction, which, in the case of HBV, is attributable to the X protein. However, because advanced tumors do express any HBV gene, *X* gene participation in oncogenesis must be an early event with different levels of X expression.[104] Another potential viral product possibly associated with oncogenesis is the truncated M protein, a product of viral integration. However, many tumors do not appear to encode for the M variants, and these proteins have not been shown to induce cell loss of growth control in vitro.[113, 114, 133] Studies of the oncogenic potential of another mammalian hepadnavirus (WHV) have shown that viral sequences contribute *cis*-acting regions rather than coding regions.[90] N-*myc* rearrangements are common in these tumors, and N-*myc* transcription is observed whenever tumors are present.[187] In 40 per cent of cases, the integrated WHV genome is close to the N-*myc* loci.[59, 63] Studies investigating the insertional activation of N-*myc* as a cause of cancer with HBV have failed to reproduce the findings observed with WHV.[130, 171]

Another line of research has investigated the possibility that the HBV-induced liver injury would induce oncogenesis. Because of chronic regeneration, there would be an increased risk of mutagenesis. In this model, HBV participates in the liver injury, but the subsequent development of cancer is due to host factors.[45] Further research is necessary for an adequate understanding of the role of HBV in the development of hepatocarcinomas.

PATHOLOGY

Acute HBV infection is anicteric in approximately 70 per cent of patients. Chronic liver disease follows acute HBV infection in a minority (1 to 8 per cent) of adults.[16, 83] After chronic infection, disease may not manifest itself for years or may progress to cirrhosis and hepatic failure relatively quickly. In the acute phase of disease, the pathologic changes include inflammation and parenchymal abnormalities, generally proximal to the terminal hepatic vein,[1] whereas in the chronic phases, there is a necroinflammatory process that may be accompanied by fibrosis with or without cirrhosis.[20, 81] Other conditions relevant to HBV infection include chronic persistent hepatitis, chronic lobular hepatitis, and chronic active hepatitis.

During the relatively asymptomatic phase of HBV infection, previously designated chronic persistent hepatitis, liver pathology may include a cobblestone pattern across the lobule, which results from disalignment of the normal hepatic arrangement.[81] These findings, however, might be absent, and liver histology in this phase may be normal. Rarely, there are a few selected areas of spotty necrosis with plasma cells, lymphocytes, and eosinophils. The presence of piecemeal necrosis is infrequent, and has a segmental distribution involving less than one-quarter of the limiting plate. Another pathologic variant in HBV disease previously was called chronic lobular hepatitis (or persistent viral hepatitis). Hepatic injury present in this case resembles acute viral hepatitis, with an increased necroinflammatory response in the lobules and portal tracts as well as presence of acidophilic bodies and some ballooning degeneration in the centrolobular region. The presence of many plasma cells characterizes chronic rather than acute hepatitis. Both chronic persistent hepatitis and chronic lobular hepatitis are relatively mild forms of chronic liver disease. Persons with a history of drug use who develop HBV infection may have characteristic hepatic lesions.[94, 129] These include large reticuloendothelial cells surrounded by eosinophils in portal tracts and lobules that may evolve to granulomas. These cells contain foreign material such as talc and other substances used with injectable drugs.

Chronic carriers of HBeAg who are asymptomatic and immunosuppressed patients often display a characteristic finding: "ground-glass hepatocytes."[81] These cells contain increased amounts of HBsAg structures in the smooth endoplasmic reticulum. Such cells are irregular, with an increased size, and have granular, homogeneous, pale eosinophilic cytoplasmic inclusions. Ground-glass hepatocytes are unusual in patients with significant liver disease or in acute viral hepatitis.

Chronic active hepatitis is characterized by a more severe form of liver disease. Piecemeal necrosis resulting from hepatocyte degeneration is significant, with occasional lymphocytic invasion of hepatocytes.[20] There is an increase of plasma cells and lymphocytes in the portal tracts. Hepatocytes initially enlarge, and plasma membranes rupture.[81] Subsequently, there is nuclear lysis with shrinkage and rarefaction followed by formation of apoptotic bodies. Connective tissue surrounds the hepatocytes, with development of fibrous septa, and the limiting plate is eroded greatly. Rosette formation may result from rearrangement of hepatocytes. Progression of hepatic injury leads to development of bridging hepatic necrosis when necrotic involvement extends from portal to portal tracts or from the portal tracts to the terminal hepatic vein. Further involvement leads to panlobular necrosis and eventual progression to macronodular cirrhosis. With the development of cirrhosis, the liver parenchyma is divided by fibrous tissue, creating a nodular appearance. Other findings at this stage include proliferation of the ducts and formation of pseudoducts, erosion of the limiting plate, cholestasis, intense inflammation, and regeneration with formation of thickened hepatic plates. Clinical findings accompany histologic changes. Laboratory abnormalities generally precede the development of hepatic lesions. With onset of severe chronic hepatitis, 40 per cent of persons develop symptoms, and with progression to cirrhosis, 80 per cent of patients have classic findings of hepatic failure.

CLINICAL MANIFESTATIONS

The clinical course of infection with HBV varies extremely; infection may occur without symptoms or be associated with fulminant fatal hepatitis. Manifestations of infection and the development of the carrier state are related to host factors, with age being most important.

Acute Infection[50, 81, 106, 107]

Typical Illness in Children and Adults

There are four clinical phases of acute HBV infection: (1) incubation period, (2) prodromal (preicteric) stage, (3) icteric phase, and (4) convalescent phase.[81] As noted earlier, the incubation period usually is long, lasting an average of 4 months.[39] The prodromal period usually lasts about 7 to 20 days and is characterized by low-grade fever, malaise, anorexia, increased fatigue with exercise, myalgia, nausea, and occasionally vomiting.[81] Weight loss due to anorexia and right upper quadrant pain or discomfort resulting from liver enlargement may occur.

The icteric phase usually begins within 10 days of the prodromal onset. First to appear is the darkening of the urine due to bilirubinemia. Shortly thereafter (1 to several days), jaundice appears as indicated by yellowish discoloration of the skin, mucous membranes, conjunctiva, and sclera. At the same time as jaundice, the stools become pale. Fever that had its onset during the prodromal period usually subsides shortly after the onset of jaundice.

Physical examination reveals an enlarged liver with a firm edge. Five to 15 per cent of patients have splenomegaly in addition to hepatomegaly. Older patients may have palmar erythema and spider angiomata. The convalescent phase begins with the disappearance of jaundice and the return of the liver to normal size.[106] Nausea and vomiting disappear, the appetite returns, and malaise improves. The duration of the convalescent phase varies considerably; in some patients, malaise and easy fatigability persist for months.

Serologic findings (hepatitis B–specific antigens and antibodies) in the course of HBV infection are presented in Figure 55–6 in Chapter 55. In patients with HBV infection, the serum alanine aminotransferase (ALT, SGPT) becomes elevated beginning during the last 2 to 4 weeks of the incubation period; this persists through the icteric phase. The white blood cell count usually is low, with relative lymphocytosis.

Acute Fulminant Hepatitis

Acute fulminant hepatitis is an unusual manifestation of acute HBV infection. Its onset is sudden during the early course of clinical illness. Marked liver necrosis occurs, which results in significant impairment of liver function. Findings include sudden onset of high fever, vomiting, and severe abdominal pain. Jaundice may be marked, and hepatic encephalopathy occurs.

Congenital and Neonatal Infection[189]

The majority of neonates who are infected after vertical transmission have no clinical signs or symptoms of hepatitis. However, as mentioned earlier, 85 to 90 per cent become chronically infected, and laboratory studies often reveal persistently elevated ALT levels; biopsy may reveal signs of chronic hepatitis. Some infected children have clinical signs of hepatitis with jaundice; severe fulminant hepatitis is rare.[18, 150]

Transplacental transmission is rare. Two recently reported infants were small for gestational age and presented with cholestatic hepatitis.[109]

Chronic Infection[81, 106, 189]

Chronic infection with HBV may result from an initial asymptomatic or symptomatic infection. By definition, all chronically infected patients are carriers (a person who is either HBsAg-positive on at least two occasions [at least 6 months apart] or who is HBsAg-positive and IgM anti-HBc–negative when a single serum specimen is tested). Chronic hepatitis can be classified by liver biopsy findings as chronic persistent hepatitis, chronic active hepatitis, or chronic active hepatitis with cirrhosis.

Some patients with chronic persistent hepatitis remain asymptomatic and have no biochemical evidence of liver disease. Others may have mild hepatomegaly and slight or recurring minor elevations of ALT. Patients with chronic active hepatitis also may be asymptomatic but are more likely to complain of easy fatigability, to have malaise, and to be anorexic. Liver ALT is elevated mildly, and jaundice may occur. Illness may involve remissions and relapses.

In a study in adults, the 5-year survival rate of patients with chronic persistent hepatitis was 97 per cent, of patients with chronic active hepatitis 86 per cent, and of patients with chronic active hepatitis with cirrhosis 55 per cent.[185] Some patients with chronic infection develop hepatocellular carcinoma.

In general, chronic infection in infants after vertical transmission has a poor outcome. It has been estimated that more than 25 per cent of these chronically infected children die of primary hepatocellular carcinoma or cirrhosis of the liver.[15]

Extrahepatic Manifestations of Hepatitis B Virus Infection[81, 107]

Extrahepatic manifestations of HBV infections are relatively common and include transient serum sickness–like syndrome, acute necrotizing vasculitis (polyarteritis nodosa), membranous glomerulonephritis, papular acrodermatitis of childhood (Gianotti-Crosti syndrome), and thrombocytopenia and aplastic anemia.

Serum Sickness–Like Syndrome

The serum sickness–like syndrome occurs in the latter part of the incubation period and during the prodromal illness.[107] Findings include fever, exanthem, and polyarthritis.[81] The exanthem is erythematous and macular, maculopapular, or nodular. Urticaria and petechial lesions also occur. The symptoms and signs usually subside with the onset of jaundice but occasionally persist throughout the illness. Virtually all cases have been described in adults; its frequency in children is not known. The illness is due to immune complexes containing HBsAg and antibody to HBsAg as well as cryoprotein and complement components.[6, 135, 183]

Acute Necrotizing Vasculitis (Polyarteritis Nodosa)

This form of vasculitis is a complication of relatively recent HBV infection; HBV can be implicated in one-third to one-half of all patients with polyarteritis nodosa.[81] The illness initially resembles the serum sickness–like syndrome, but the signs and symptoms are more severe and they persist. Findings include high fever, anemia, leukocytosis as well as arthralgia, myalgia, arthritis, renal disease (proteinuria and hematuria), hypertension, pericarditis, acute abdominal pain, and neurologic findings.[81, 107] This illness occurs in both children and adults.[121] It has a high fatality rate.

Membranous Glomerulonephritis

This illness occurs in both adults and children.[81, 107] In contrast with polyarteritis nodosa, which has its onset in association with acute illness, glomerulonephritis occurs in chronic active hepatitis. Illness is found in association with hepatitis B e antigenemia. HBeAg is found in subepithelial immune complexes, and HBsAg immune complexes have a mesangial distribution. The renal lesions resolve with the clearance of HBeAg from the blood.[70, 88, 178]

Papular Acrodermatitis of Childhood (Gianotti-Crosti Syndrome)

This exanthem was reported first in 1955 by Gianotti[69] and further described by Crosti and Gianotti[48] in 1957. Its association with HBV infection was noted in 1973.[68] The exanthem is distributed symmetrically on the face, buttocks, and extremities.[32, 81] Lesions are erythematous, either macular or papular, and about 3 to 5 mm in diameter (lentil-sized). The rash lasts 15 to 25 days and is associated with acute anicteric hepatitis and generalized lymphadenopathy. The illness is thought to be immune complex (HBsAg/anti-HBs)–mediated, and there is a predilection for hepatitis B ayw subtype.[47, 68, 95] The exanthem also has been associated with the following other viral infections: hepatitis A virus, Epstein-Barr virus, cytomegalovirus, and coxsackievirus A16.

Other Extrahepatic Manifestations

Thrombocytopenia and aplastic anemia have been associated with HBV infection.[126, 147] Children who are immunosuppressed are more likely to become persistently infected with HBV and to remain HBeAg-positive.[86]

DIAGNOSIS

Differential Diagnosis

The differential diagnosis of hepatitis is presented in detail in Chapters 55 and 56.

Specific Diagnosis[7, 81, 141] (see also Chapter 244)

Specific diagnosis is made by serologic antigen and antibody tests (see Table 162–1). Assays (radioimmunoassays and enzyme-linked immunoassays) for HBsAg, anti-HBs, anti-HBc, IgM anti-HBc, HBeAg, and anti-HBe are available in most hospital or outside commercial laboratories. The finding of HBsAg in the blood indicates infection, which can be acute or chronic. IgM antibody to HBcAg (IgM anti-HBc) indicates recent infection with HBV; this antibody persists for 4 to 6 months after initial infection. The presence of HBeAg in the blood correlates with HBV replication in high titer and increased infectivity of the serum. Antibody to HBcAg (anti-HBc) indicates prior or present infection with HBV but does not result from immunization. Antibody to HBsAg (anti-HBs) indicates past infection with HBV or an immune response to immunization. A previously infected person who has cleared infection has both anti-HBs and anti-HBc, whereas a previous vaccinee has only anti-HBs.

In acute infection, HBsAg and anti-HBc are noted in the blood. Anti-HBc may be detected alone (without detectable HBsAg or anti-HBs) during early convalescence of acute infection; this is called the window phase.

The demonstration of IgM anti-HBc in the serum is highly specific and sensitive for the diagnosis of acute infection in older children and adults as well as during the window phase of infection. However, this test is less useful (insensitive) in perinatal infections because these infants may not have an IgM antibody response.

TREATMENT (see also Chapter 55)

Acute Uncomplicated Infection

There is no specific treatment for acute HBV infection. Bed rest is not necessary, and routine activities around the home should be encouraged. Careful attention to diet is important. Because of nausea, frequent small meals may be tolerated better than three standard meals. Because nausea usually is less in the morning, it often is wise to provide a bigger meal at this time. Occasionally, hyperalimentation may be necessary early in the illness.

Once improvement begins (e.g., serum bilirubin <2 mg/dL and a reduction in the ALT to less than four times the upper limit of normal), physical activity can be increased gradually. In general, children should have home schooling until they are no longer icteric and their ALT is no more than two times the upper limit of normal.

Patients with acute HBV infection should not be given corticosteroids or hepatitis B immunoglobulin (HBIG). HBIG has no effect, and corticosteroids may increase the risk of relapse or the development of persistent infection.[56, 157]

Acute Fulminant Hepatitis

Children with acute fulminant hepatitis should be admitted to a pediatric intensive care unit. They should be monitored for cerebral edema, cardiopulmonary dysfunction, and secondary microbial infections. Orthotopic liver transplantation may be lifesaving. However, recurrence of HBV infection after transplantation is common and frequently results in graft failure.

Chronic Infection

Although most children with chronic HBV infections are asymptomatic, few clear the infection, and the long-term risk of death due to cirrhosis and hepatocellular carcinoma is substantial.[39, 89] Many drugs and biologic agents have been used in attempts to treat chronic HBV infections, but the only presently approved medication is interferon alpha.[60, 80] In adults, the response rate to interferon alpha is approximately 40 per cent (a response is defined by the loss of HBeAg and HBV DNA in the blood, normalization of the serum ALT, and improvement in the degree of necroinflammatory changes in the liver as noted by biopsy). Although there are fewer data on interferon alpha treatment in children, Torre and Tambini[172] recently carried out a metaanalysis of six randomized pediatric treatment trials.[9, 110, 111, 153, 154, 175] These six trials involved 240 children with chronic HBV infection. In 127 treated patients, HBV DNA was cleared from the blood in 35 per cent. In 7 of 74 patients (8 per cent), HBeAg was cleared from the blood and the interferon alpha treatment normalized serum ALT levels in 39 per cent of 85 treated children.

Improvement persisted after the completion of therapy; HBV DNA and HBeAg clearance from the blood was 29 and 23 per cent, respectively.[172] Prolonged therapy (>6 months) was associated with a better response than was short-duration therapy. High doses of interferon alpha did not improve outcome. According to the data from this metaanalysis as well as other treatment studies, it would seem that an interferon alpha dose of 3 million units/m^2 three times a week for greater than 6 months is appropriate.

Interferon alpha is relatively well tolerated in children. Common side effects include fever, fatigue, myalgia, anorexia, headache, weight loss, and hair loss.[60, 80, 131, 152] Neutropenia and thrombocytopenia also occur, but they usually respond to a reduction in dosage. Premedication with acetaminophen may reduce the common side effects.

PREVENTION (see also Chapters 237 to 240)

General

HBV vaccine use in infants and children is at the forefront of prevention. However, it is important also to stress other general aspects of prevention of HBV transmission. The leading cause of HBV transmission in the United States today is high-risk activities in adolescent and adult populations. Social programs that address high-risk activities should be encouraged.

In the hospital, day care centers, other institutions, and houses with persons who are HBV carriers, universal precautions should be carried out.

For complete information relating to HBV active and passive immunization, the reader is advised to consult the most recent Advisory Committee on Immunization Practices (ACIP) or the Committee on Infectious Diseases of the American Academy of Pediatrics publications. In addition, because vaccines differ by manufacturer, the specific product information also should be consulted. The recommendations listed in the following sections are for the United States and are from the ACIP.[37–40]

Strategy to Eliminate Hepatitis B Virus Transmission[37, 38]

A comprehensive strategy to prevent HBV infection, acute hepatitis B, and the sequelae of HBV infection in the United States must eliminate transmission that occurs during infancy and childhood, as well as during adolescence and adulthood. In the United States, it has become evident that HBV transmission cannot be prevented through vaccinating only the groups at high risk of infection. No current medical treatment reliably eliminates chronic HBV infection and thus eliminates the source of new infections in susceptible persons. Therefore, new infections can be prevented only by immunizing susceptible persons with hepatitis B vaccine. Routine visits for prenatal and well-child care can be used to target hepatitis B prevention. A comprehensive prevention strategy includes (1) prenatal testing of pregnant women for HBsAg to identify newborns who require immunoprophylaxis for the prevention of perinatal infection and to identify household contacts who should be vaccinated, (2) routine vaccination of children born to HBsAg-negative mothers, (3) vaccination of certain older children and adolescents, and (4) vaccination of adults at high risk of infection.

Prophylaxis Against Hepatitis B Virus Infection[38]

Two types of products are available for prophylaxis against HBV infection. Hepatitis B vaccine, which provides long-term protection against HBV infection, is recommended for both pre-exposure and postexposure prophylaxis. HBIG provides temporary protection (i.e., 3 to 6 months) and is indicated only in certain postexposure settings.

Hepatitis B Immunoglobulin

HBIG is prepared from plasma known to contain a high titer of anti-HBs. In the United States, HBIG has an anti-HBs titer of greater than 100,000 by radioimmunoassay. The human plasma from which HBIG is prepared is screened for antibodies to HIV; in addition, the process used to prepare HBIG inactivates and eliminates HIV from the final product. There is no evidence that HIV can be transmitted by HBIG.

Hepatitis B Vaccine

Two types of hepatitis B vaccine have been licensed in the United States. One, which was manufactured from the plasma of chronically infected persons, no longer is produced in the United States. The currently available vaccines are produced by recombinant DNA technology.

The recombinant vaccines are produced by using HBsAg synthesized by *Saccharomyces cerevisiae* (common baker's yeast), into which a plasmid containing the gene for HBsAg has been inserted. Purified HBsAg is obtained by lysing the yeast cells and separating HBsAg from the yeast components by biochemical and biophysical techniques. Hepatitis B vaccines are packaged to contain 10 to 40 μg of HBsAg protein/mL after adsorption to aluminum hydroxide (0.5 mg/mL); thimerosal (1:20,000 concentration) is added as a preservative.

Routes and Sites of Administration

The recommended series of three intramuscular doses of hepatitis B vaccine induces a protective antibody response (anti-HBs ≥10 milli-international units [mIU]/mL in >90 per cent of healthy adults and in >95 per cent of infants, children, and adolescents). Hepatitis B vaccine should be administered only in the deltoid muscle of adults and children or in the anterolateral thigh muscle of neonates and infants; the immunogenicity of the vaccine for adults is substantially lower when injections are administered in the buttock. When hepatitis B vaccine is administered to infants at the same time as other vaccines, separate sites in the anterolateral thigh may be used for the multiple injections. This method is preferable to administering vaccine at sites such as the buttock or deltoid.

Vaccine Use[38]

Pre-exposure Prophylaxis

VACCINATION SCHEDULE AND DOSE. The vaccination schedule most often used for adults and children has been three intramuscular injections, the second and third administered 1 and 6 months, respectively, after the first. An alternative schedule of four doses has been approved for one vaccine that would allow more rapid induction of immunity. However, for preexposure prophylaxis, there is no clear evidence that this regimen provides greater protection than that obtained with the standard three-dose schedule.

Each vaccine has been evaluated to determine the age-specific dose at which an optimal antibody response is achieved. The recommended dose varies by product and the recipient's age and, for infants, by the mother's HBsAg serologic status (Table 162–5). In general, the vaccine dose for children and adolescents is 50 to 75 per cent lower than that required for adults.

In a three-dose schedule, increasing the interval between the first and second doses of hepatitis B vaccine has little effect on immunogenicity or final antibody titer. The third dose confers optimal protection, acting as a booster dose. Longer intervals between the last two doses (4 to 12 months) result in higher final titers of anti-HBs. Several studies have shown that the currently licensed vaccines produce high rates of seroconversion (>95 per cent) and induce adequate levels of anti-HBs when administered to infants at birth, 2 months,

TABLE 162–5. Recommended Doses of Currently Licensed Hepatitis B Vaccines

Group	Recombivax HB*		Engerix-B*	
	Dose (μg)	*(mL)*	*Dose (μg)*	*(mL)*
Infants of HBsAg-negative mothers and children younger than 11 years of age	2.5	(0.25)	10	(0.5)
Infants of HBsAg-positive mothers; prevention of perinatal infection	5	(0.5)	10	(0.5)
Children and adolescents 11 to 19 years of age	5	(0.5)	20	(1.0)
Adults older than 20 years of age	10	(1.0)	20	(1.0)
Dialysis patients and other immunocompromised persons	40	(1.0)†	40	(2.0)§

*Both vaccines routinely are administered in a three-dose series. Engerix-B also has been licensed for a four-dose series administered at 0, 1, 2, and 12 months of age.
†Special formulation.
§Two 1.0-mL doses administered at one site, in a four-dose schedule at 0, 1, 2, and 6 months of age.
HBsAg, hepatitis B surface antigen.

and 6 months of age or at 2, 4, and 6 months of age. When the vaccine is administered in four doses at 0, 1, 2, and 12 months of age, the last dose is necessary to ensure the highest final antibody titer.

Larger vaccine doses or an increased number of doses are required to induce protective antibody in a high proportion of hemodialysis patients and may be necessary for other immunocompromised persons (e.g., those who take immunosuppressive drugs or who are HIV-positive), although few data are available concerning response to higher doses of vaccine by these patients.

POSTVACCINATION TESTING FOR SEROLOGIC RESPONSE. Such testing is not necessary after routine vaccination of infants, children, or adolescents. Testing for immunity is advised only for persons whose subsequent clinical management depends on knowledge of their immune status (e.g., infants born to HBsAg-positive mothers, dialysis patients and staff, persons with HIV infection). Postvaccination testing also should be considered for persons at occupational risk who may have exposures from injuries with sharp instruments, because knowledge of their antibody response helps determine appropriate postexposure prophylaxis. When necessary, postvaccination testing should be performed 1 to 6 months after completion of the vaccine series. Testing after immunoprophylaxis of infants born to HBsAg-positive mothers should be performed from 3 to 9 months after the completion of the vaccination series (see Postexposure Prophylaxis).

REVACCINATION OF NONRESPONDERS. When persons who do not respond to the primary vaccine series are revaccinated, 15 to 25 per cent produce an adequate antibody response after one additional dose, and 30 to 50 per cent do so after three additional doses. Therefore, revaccination with one or more additional doses should be considered for persons who do not respond to vaccination initially.

Postexposure Prophylaxis

After a person has been exposed to HBV, appropriate immunoprophylactic treatment effectively can prevent infection. The mainstay of postexposure immunoprophylaxis is hepatitis B vaccine, but sometimes the addition of HBIG increases protection somewhat. Table 162–6 provides a guide to recommended treatment for various HBV exposures.

Transmission of perinatal HBV infection effectively can be prevented if the HBsAg-positive mother is identified and if her infant receives appropriate immunoprophylaxis. Hepatitis B vaccination and one dose of HBIG, administered within 24 hours after birth, are 85 to 95 per cent effective in preventing both HBV infection and the chronic carrier state. Hepatitis B vaccine administered alone in either a three-dose or four-dose schedule (see Table 162–5) beginning within 24 hours after birth, is 70 to 95 per cent effective in preventing perinatal HBV infections. The infants of women admitted for delivery who have not undergone prenatal HBsAg testing pose problems in clinical management; initiating hepatitis B vaccine at birth in infants born to these women provides adequate postexposure prophylaxis if the mothers indeed are HBsAg-positive. The few infections not prevented by either of these treatment regimens most likely were acquired in utero or may be due to particularly high levels of maternal HBV DNA.

Serologic testing of infants who receive immunoprophylaxis to prevent perinatal infection should be considered as an aid in the long-term medical management of the few infants who become HBV carriers. Testing for anti-HBs and HBsAg at 9 to 15 months of age determines the success of the therapy and, in the case of failure, identifies HBV carriers or infants who may require revaccination.

Vaccine Efficacy and Booster Doses[38]

Clinical trials of the hepatitis B vaccines licensed in the United States have shown that they are 80 to 95 per cent

TABLE 162–6. Guide to Postexposure Immunoprophylaxis for Exposure to Hepatitis B Virus

Type of Exposure	Immunoprophylaxis
Perinatal	Vaccination—HBIG
Sexual—acute infection	HBIG ± vaccination
Sexual—chronic carrier	Vaccination
Household contact—chronic carrier	Vaccination
Household contact—acute case	None unless known exposure
Household contact—acute case, known exposure	HBIG ± vaccination
Infant (younger than 12 months of age)—acute case in primary care	HBIG ± vaccination
Inadvertent—percutaneous/permucosal	Vaccination ± HBIG

Data from Centers for Disease Control: Hepatitis B virus: A comprehensive strategy for eliminating transmission in the United States through Universal Childhood Vaccination. Recommendations of the Immunization Practices Advisory Committee (ACIP). M. M. W. R. *40:*1–25, 1991.
HBIG, hepatitis B immunoglobulin.

effective in preventing HBV infection and clinical hepatitis among susceptible children and adults. If a protective antibody response develops after vaccination, vaccine recipients virtually are 100 per cent protected against clinical illness.

The duration of vaccine-induced immunity has been evaluated in long-term follow-up studies of both adults and children. Only the plasma-derived hepatitis B vaccine has been evaluated because it has had the longest clinical use; however, on the basis of comparable immunogenicity and short-term efficacy, similar results would be expected with recombinant vaccines.

Long-term studies of healthy adults and children indicate that immunologic memory remains intact for at least 9 years and confers protection against chronic HBV infection, even though anti-HBs levels may become low or decline below detectable levels.[118, 181] In these studies, the HBV infections were detected by the presence of anti-HBc. No episodes of clinical hepatitis were reported and HBsAg was not detected, although brief episodes of viremia may not have been detected because of infrequent testing. The mild, inapparent infections among persons who have been previously vaccinated should not produce the sequelae associated with chronic HBV infection and should provide lasting immunity. In general, follow-up studies of children vaccinated at birth to prevent perinatal HBV infection have shown that a continued high level of protection from chronic HBV infections persists at least 5 years.[93]

For children and adults whose immune status is normal, booster doses of vaccine are not recommended, nor is serologic testing to assess antibody levels necessary. The possible need for booster doses will be assessed as additional information becomes available. For hemodialysis patients, vaccine-induced protection may be less complete and may persist only as long as antibody levels are greater than or equal to 10 mIU/mL. For these patients, the need for booster doses should be assessed by annual antibody testing, and a booster dose should be administered when antibody levels decline to less than 10 mIU/mL.

Vaccine Side Effects and Adverse Reactions[38]

Hepatitis B vaccines have been shown to be safe when administered to both adults and children. More than four million adults have been vaccinated in the United States, and at least that many children have received hepatitis B vaccine worldwide.

Vaccine-Associated Side Effects

Pain at the injection site (3 to 29 per cent) and a temperature greater than 37.7° C (1 to 6 per cent) have been among the most frequently reported side effects among adults and children receiving vaccine. In placebo-controlled studies, these side effects were reported no more frequently among vaccinees than among persons receiving a placebo. Among children receiving both hepatitis B vaccine and diphtheria-tetanus-pertussis vaccine, these mild side effects have been observed no more frequently than among children receiving diphtheria-tetanus-pertussis vaccine alone.

Serious Adverse Events

In the United States, surveillance of adverse reactions has shown a possible association between Guillain-Barré syndrome and receipt of the first dose of plasma-derived hepatitis B vaccine (Centers for Disease Control and Prevention, unpublished data). Guillain-Barré syndrome was reported at a low rate (0.5/100,000 vaccinees), no deaths were reported, and all reported cases were among adults. An estimated 2.5 million adults received one or more doses of recombinant hepatitis B vaccine during the period 1986 to 1990. Available data from reporting systems for adverse events do not indicate an association between receipt of recombinant vaccine and Guillain-Barré syndrome (Centers for Disease Control and Prevention, unpublished data).

Recommendations of the Advisory Committee on Immunization Practices

Prevention of Perinatal Hepatitis B Virus Infection[38]

1. All pregnant women should be tested routinely for HBsAg during an early prenatal visit in each pregnancy, preferably at the same time other routine prenatal laboratory testing is performed. HBsAg testing should be repeated late in the pregnancy for women who are HBsAg-negative but who are at high risk of HBV infection (e.g., injecting drug users, those with intercurrent sexually transmitted diseases) or who have had clinically apparent hepatitis. Tests for other HBV markers are not necessary for the purpose of maternal screening. However, HBsAg-positive women identified during screening may have HBV-related liver disease and should be evaluated.
2. Infants born to mothers who are HBsAg-positive should receive the appropriate doses of hepatitis B vaccine (see Table 162–5) and HBIG (0.5 mL) within 12 hours of birth. Both should be administered by intramuscular injection. Hepatitis B vaccine should be administered concurrently with HBIG but at a different site. Subsequent doses of vaccine should be administered according to the recommended schedule (Table 162–7).
3. In women admitted for delivery who have not undergone prenatal HBsAg testing, blood should be drawn for testing. While test results are pending, the infant should receive hepatitis B vaccine within 12 hours of birth, in a dose appropriate for infants born to HBsAg-positive mothers (see Table 162–5).
   a. If the mother is found later to be HBsAg-positive, her infant should receive the additional protection of HBIG as soon as possible and within 7 days of birth, although the efficacy of HBIG administered after 48 hours of age is not known. If HBIG has not been administered, it is important that the infant receive the second dose of hepatitis B vaccine at 1 month and not later than 2 months of age because of the high risk of infection. The last dose should be administered at age 6 months (see Table 162–7).
   b. If the mother is found to be HBsAg-negative, her infant should continue to receive hepatitis B vaccine as part of his or her routine vaccinations (Tables 162–7 and 162–8) in the dose appropriate for infants born to HBsAg-negative mothers (see Table 162–5).
4. In populations in which screening pregnant women for HBsAg is not feasible, all infants should receive their first dose of hepatitis B vaccine within 12 hours of birth, their second dose at 1 to 2 months of age, and their third dose at 6 months of age as a part of their childhood vaccinations and well-child care (see Table 172–7).
5. Household contacts and sex partners of HBsAg-positive women identified through prenatal screening should be vaccinated. Hepatitis B vaccine should be administered at the age-appropriate dose (see Table 162–5) to those determined to be susceptible or judged likely to be susceptible to infection.

TABLE 162–7. Recommended Schedule of Hepatitis B Immunoprophylaxis to Prevent Perinatal Transmission of Hepatitis B Virus Infection

Vaccine Dose†	Age of Infant
Infant Born to Mother Known to Be HBsAg-Positive*	
First	Birth (within 12 hours)
HBIG‡	Birth (within 12 hours)
Second	1 month
Third	6 months§

Vaccine Dose¶	Age of Infant
Infant Born to Mother Not Screened for HBsAg	
First	Birth (within 12 hours)
HBIG‡	If mother is found to be HBsAg-positive, administer dose to infant as soon as possible, not later than 1 week after birth
Second	1 to 2 months**
Third	6 months§

*HBsAg = hepatitis B surface antigen.
†See Table 162–5 for appropriate vaccine dose.
‡Hepatitis B immunoglobulin, 0.5 mL administered intramuscularly at a site different from that used for vaccine.
§If four-dose schedule (Engerix-B) is used, the third dose is administered at 2 months of age and the fourth dose at 12 to 18 months of age.
¶First dose = dose for infant of HBsAg-positive mother (see Table 162–5). If mother is found to be HBsAg-positive, continue that dose; if mother is found to be HBsAg-negative, use approximate dose from Table 162–5.
**Infants of women who are HBsAG-negative can be vaccinated at 2 months of age.

Universal Vaccination of Infants Born to Hepatitis B Surface Antigen–Negative Mothers[38]

1. Hepatitis B vaccination is recommended for all infants, regardless of the HBsAg status of the mother. Hepatitis B vaccine should be incorporated into vaccination schedules for children. The first dose can be administered during the newborn period, preferably before the infant is discharged from the hospital but no later than when the infant is 2 months of age (see Table 162–8). Because the highest titers of anti-HBs are achieved when the last two doses of vaccine are spaced at least 4 months apart, schedules that achieve this spacing may be preferable. However, schedules with 2-month intervals between doses, which conform to schedules for other childhood vaccines, have been shown to produce a good antibody response and may be appropriate in populations in which it is difficult to ensure that infants will be brought back for all their vaccinations. The development of combination vaccines containing HBsAg may lead to other schedules that allow optimal use of combined antigens.
2. Special efforts should be made to ensure that high levels of hepatitis B vaccination are achieved in populations in which HBV infection occurs at high rates among children (Alaskan Natives, Pacific Islanders, and infants of immigrants from countries in which HBV infection is endemic).

TABLE 162–8. Recommended Schedule of Hepatitis B Vaccination for Infants Born to HBsAg-Negative Mothers

Hepatitis B Vaccine	Age of Infant
Option 1	
Dose 1	Birth (before hospital discharge)
Dose 2	1 to 2 months*
Dose 3	6 to 18 months*
Option 2	
Dose 1	1 to 2 months*
Dose 2	4 months*
Dose 3	6 to 18 months*

*Hepatitis B vaccine can be administered simultaneously with diphtheria-tetanus-pertussis, *Haemophilus influenzae* type b conjugate, measles-mumps-rubella, and oral polio vaccines at the same visit.
HBsAg = hepatitis B surface antigen.

Vaccination of Adolescents[38]

All adolescents at high risk of infection because they are injecting drug users or have multiple sex partners (more than one partner every 6 months) should receive hepatitis B vaccine. Widespread use of hepatitis B vaccine is encouraged. Because risk factors are often not identified directly among adolescents, universal hepatitis B vaccination of teenagers should be implemented in communities where injecting drug use, pregnancy among teenagers, or sexually transmitted diseases are common. Adolescents can be vaccinated in school-based clinics, community health centers, family planning clinics, clinics for the treatment of sexually transmitted diseases, and special adolescent clinics.

The 0-, 1-, and 6-month schedule is preferred for vaccinating adolescents with the age-appropriate dose of vaccine (see Table 162–5). However, the choice of vaccination schedule should account for the feasibility of delivering three doses of vaccine over a given period. The use of alternative schedules (e.g., 0, 2, and 4 months) may be advisable to achieve complete vaccination.

Vaccination of All Children 11 to 12 Years of Age[37]

In 1994, the ACIP expanded the vaccination strategy to include the vaccination of all children 11 to 12 years of age who had not received hepatitis B vaccine.

Vaccination of Selected High-Risk Groups[37, 38]

Efforts to vaccinate persons at high risk of HBV infection should follow the vaccine doses shown in Table 162–5. High-risk groups for whom vaccination is recommended include the following.

PERSONS WITH OCCUPATIONAL RISK. HBV infection is an occupational hazard for health care workers and for public-safety workers who are exposed to blood in the workplace. The risk of acquiring HBV infections from occupational exposures depends on the frequency of percutaneous and permucosal exposure to blood or blood-contaminated body fluids. Any health care or public-safety worker may be at risk for HBV exposure, depending on the tasks he or she performs. Workers who perform tasks involving contact with blood or blood-contaminated body fluid should be vaccinated. For public-safety workers whose exposure to blood is infrequent, timely postexposure prophylaxis should be considered rather than routine pre-exposure vaccination. For persons in health care fields, vaccination should be completed during the training in schools of medicine, dentistry, nursing, laboratory technology, and other health professions, before trainees have their first contact with blood.

CLIENTS AND STAFF OF INSTITUTIONS FOR THE DEVELOPMENTALLY DISABLED. Susceptible clients in institutions for the developmentally disabled, as well as staff members who work closely with clients, should be vaccinated. Susceptible clients and staff members who live or work in smaller residential settings with known HBV carriers also should receive hepatitis B vaccine. Clients discharged from residential institutions into community programs should be screened for HBsAg so that appropriate measures can be taken to prevent HBV transmission. These measures should include both environmental controls and appropriate use of vaccine. Staff of nonresidential day care programs for the developmentally disabled (e.g., schools, sheltered workshops) attended by known HBV carriers have a risk of infection comparable with that of health care workers and therefore should be vaccinated. The risk of infection for other clients appears to be lower than the risk for staff members. Vaccination of clients in day care programs may be considered. Vaccination of classroom contacts strongly is encouraged if a classmate who is a HBV carrier behaves aggressively or has special medical problems (e.g., exudative dermatitis, open skin lesions) that increase the risk of exposure to his or her blood or serous secretions.

HEMODIALYSIS PATIENTS. Hepatitis B vaccination is recommended for susceptible hemodialysis patients. Vaccinating patients early in the course of their renal disease is encouraged because patients with uremia who are vaccinated before they require dialysis are more likely to respond to the vaccine. Although their seroconversion rates and anti-HBs titers are lower than those of healthy persons, patients who respond to vaccination are protected from infection, and the need for frequent serologic testing is reduced.

RECIPIENTS OF CERTAIN BLOOD PRODUCTS. Patients who receive clotting-factor concentrates have an increased risk of HBV infection and should be vaccinated as soon as their specific clotting disorder is identified. Prevaccination testing is recommended for patients who already have received multiple infusions of these products.

HOUSEHOLD CONTACTS AND SEX PARTNERS OF HEPATITIS B VIRUS CARRIERS. All household and sexual contacts of persons identified as HBsAg-positive should be vaccinated. Hepatitis B vaccine should be administered at the age-appropriate dose (see Table 162–5) to those determined to be susceptible or judged likely to be susceptible to infection.

ADOPTEES FROM COUNTRIES WHERE HEPATITIS B VIRUS INFECTION IS ENDEMIC. Adopted or fostered orphans or unaccompanied minors from countries where HBV infection is endemic should be screened for HBsAg. If the children are HBsAg-positive, other family members should be vaccinated.

INTERNATIONAL TRAVELERS. Vaccination should be considered for persons who plan to spend more than 6 months in areas with high rates of HBV infection and who will have close contact with the local population. Short-term travelers who are likely to have contact with blood (e.g., in a medical setting) or sexual contact with residents of areas with high or intermediate levels of endemic disease should be vaccinated. Vaccination should begin at least 6 months before travel to allow for completion of the full vaccine series, although a partial series offers some protection. The alternative four-dose schedule (see Table 162–5) should provide protection if the first three doses can be delivered before departure.

INJECTING DRUG USERS. All injecting drug users who are susceptible to HBV infection should be vaccinated as soon as their drug use begins. Because of the high rate of HBV infection in this population, prevaccination screening should be considered. Injecting drug users known to have HIV infection should be tested for anti-HBs response after completion of the vaccine series. Those who do not respond to vaccination should be counseled accordingly.

SEXUALLY ACTIVE HOMOSEXUAL AND BISEXUAL MEN. Susceptible sexually active homosexual and bisexual men should be vaccinated. Because of the high rate of HBV infection in this population, prevaccination screening should be considered. Men known to have HIV infection should be tested for anti-HBs response after completion of the vaccine series. Those who do not respond to vaccination should be counseled accordingly.

SEXUALLY ACTIVE HETEROSEXUAL MEN AND WOMEN. Vaccination is recommended for men and women who are diagnosed as having recently acquired other sexually transmitted diseases, for prostitutes, and for persons who have a history of sexual activity with more than one partner in the previous 6 months. Most patients seen in clinics for sexually transmitted diseases should be considered candidates for vaccination.

INMATES OF LONG-TERM CORRECTIONAL FACILITIES. Prison officials should consider undertaking screening and vaccination programs directed at inmates with histories of high-risk behaviors.

SELECTED CHILDREN YOUNGER THAN 11 YEARS OF AGE. In 1994, the ACIP expanded the vaccination strategy to include the vaccination of all unvaccinated children younger than 11 years of age who are Pacific Islanders or who reside in households of first-generation immigrants from countries where HBV infection is of high or intermediate endemicity.

PROGNOSIS

The outcome of acute HBV infections in the short term generally is good. Acute fulminant hepatitis resulting in death does occur, but it is relatively uncommon. The long-term prognosis in patients who clear their infection is excellent, with no residual problems. However, the long-term prognosis in patients with persistent infection is poor because of the ultimate occurrence of cirrhosis and liver failure or hepatocellular carcinoma.

References

1. Abe, H., Beninger, P. R., Ikejiri, N., et al.: Light microscopic findings of liver biopsy specimens from patients with hepatitis type A and comparison with type B. Gastroenterology *82*:938–947, 1982.
2. Acs, G., Sells, M. A., Purcell, R. H., et al.: Hepatitis B virus produced by transfected Hep G2 cells causes hepatitis in chimpanzees. Proc. Natl. Acad. Sci. U. S. A. *84*:4641–4644, 1987.
3. Aggerback, L. P., and Peterson, D. L.: Electron microscopic and solution X-ray scattering observations on the structure of hepatitis B surface antigen. Virology *141*:155–161, 1985.
4. Akahane, Y., Yamanaka, T., Suzuki, H., et al.: Chronic active hepatitis with hepatitis B virus DNA and antibody against e antigen in the serum. Gastroenterology *99*:1113–1119, 1990.
5. Albin, C., and Robinson, W. S.: Protein kinase activity in hepatitis B virions. J. Virol. *34*:297–302, 1980.
6. Alpert, E., Isselbacher, K. J., and Schur, P. H.: The pathogenesis of arthritis associated with viral hepatitis: Complement-component studies. N. Engl. J. Med. *285*:185–189, 1971.
7. American Academy of Pediatrics: Hepatitis B. *In* Peter, G. (ed.): 1994 Red Book: Report of the Committee on Infectious Diseases. 23rd ed. Elk Grove Village, American Academy of Pediatrics, 1994, pp. 224–238.
8. Argos, P., and Fuller, S. D.: A model for the hepatitis B virus core protein: Prediction of antigenic sites and relationship to RNA virus capsid proteins. EMBO J. *7*:819–824, 1988.
9. Barbera, C., Bortolotti, F., Crivellaro, C., et al.: Recombinant interferon-alpha 2a hastens the rate of HBeAg clearance in children with chronic hepatitis B. Hepatology *20*:287–290, 1994.
10. Barnaba, V., Franco, A., Alberti, A., et al.: Selective killing of hepatitis B

envelope antigen-specific B cells by class I–restricted, exogenous antigen-specific T lymphocytes. Nature *345*:258–260, 1990.
11. Barnaba, V., Franco, A., Alberti, A., et al.: Recognition of hepatitis B virus envelope proteins by liver-infiltrating T lymphocytes in chronic HBV infection. J. Immunol. *143*:2650–2655, 1989.
12. Bartenschlager, R., and Schaller, H.: Hepadnaviral assembly is initiated by polymerase binding to the encapsidation signal in the viral RNA genome. EMBO J. *11*:3413–3420, 1992.
13. Bavand, M., Feitelson, M., and Laub, O.: The hepatitis B virus–associated reverse transcriptase is encoded by the viral pol gene. J. Virol. *63*:1019–1021, 1989.
14. Beasley, R. P.: Hepatitis B virus: The major etiology of hepatocellular carcinoma. Cancer *61*:1941–1956, 1988.
15. Beasley, R. P., and Hwang, L.-Y.: Epidemiology of hepatocellular carcinoma. *In* Vyes, G. N., Dienstag, J. L., and Hoofnagle, J. H. (eds.): Viral Hepatitis and Liver Disease. Orlando, Grune & Stratton, 1984, pp. 209–224.
16. Beasley, R. P., Hwang, L.-Y., Lin, C. C., et al.: Incidence of hepatitis among students at a university in Taiwan. Am. J. Epidemiol. *117*:212–222, 1983.
17. Beasley, R. P., Hwang, L.-Y., Lin, C., et al.: Hepatocellular carcinoma and HBV: A prospective study of 22,707 men in Taiwan. Lancet *2*:1129–1133, 1981.
18. Beath, S. V., Boxall, E. H., Watson, R. M., et al.: Fulminant hepatitis B in infants born to anti-HBe hepatitis B carrier mothers. B. M. J. *304*:1169–1190, 1992.
19. Bertoletti, A., Ferrari, C., Fiaccodori, F., et al.: HLA class I–restricted human cytotoxic T cells recognize endogenously synthesized hepatitis B virus nucleocapsid antigen. Proc. Natl. Acad. Sci. U. S. A. *88*:10445–10449, 1991.
20. Bianchi, L.: Liver biopsy interpretation in hepatitis. Part II. Histopathology and classification of acute and chronic viral hepatitis/differential diagnosis. Pathol. Res. Pract. *178*:180–213, 1983.
21. Blum, H. E.: Hepatitis B virus: Significance of naturally occurring mutants. Intervirology *35*:45–50, 1993.
22. Blum, H. E., Stowring, L., Figus, A., et al.: Detection of hepatitis B virus DNA in hepatocytes, bile duct epithelium, and vascular elements by in situ hybridization. Proc. Natl. Acad. Sci. U. S. A. *80*:6685–6688, 1983.
23. Blumberg, B. S., Gerstley, B. J. S., Hungerford, D. A., et al.: A serum antigen (Australia antigen) in Down's syndrome, leukemia and hepatitis. Ann. Intern. Med. *66*:924–931, 1967.
24. Blumberg, B. S., Alter, H. J., and Visnich, S.: A "new" antigen in leukemia sera. J. A. M. A. *191*:541–546, 1965.
25. Bosch, V., Bartenschlager, R., Radziwell, G., et al.: The duck hepatitis B virus P-gene codes for protein strongly associated with the 5′-end of the viral DNA minus strand. Virology *166*:475–485, 1988.
26. Brechot, C., Pourcel, C., Louise, A., et al.: Presence of integrated hepatitis B virus DNA sequences in cellular DNA in human hepatocellular carcinoma. Nature *286*:533–535, 1980.
27. Brunetto, M. R., Stemler, M., Bonino, F., et al.: A new hepatitis B virus strain in patients with severe anti-HBe positive chronic hepatitis B. Hepatology *10*:258–261, 1990.
28. Brunetto, M. R., Stemley, M., Schodel, F., et al.: Identification of HBV variants which cannot produce precore-derived HBeAg and may be responsible for severe hepatitis. Int. J. Gastroenterol. *21*:151–154, 1989.
29. Bruss, V., and Ganem, D.: The role of envelope proteins in hepatitis B virus assembly. Proc. Natl. Acad. Sci. U. S. A. *88*:1059–1063, 1991.
30. Burk, R. D., Hwang, L.-Y., Ho, G. Y. F., et al.: Outcome of perinatal hepatitis B virus exposure is dependent on maternal virus load. J. Infect. Dis. *170*:1418–1423, 1994.
31. Burrell, C. J., Mackay, P., Greenway, P. J., et al.: Expression in *Escherichia coli* of hepatitis B virus DNA sequences cloned in plasmid pBR322. Nature *279*:43–47, 1979.
32. Caputo, R., Gelmetti, C., Ermacora, E., et al.: Gianotti-Crosti syndrome: A retrospective analysis of 308 cases. J. Am. Acad. Dermatol. *26*:207–210, 1992.
33. Carman, W. F., Zanetti, A. R., Karayiannis, P., et al.: Vaccine-induced escape mutant of hepatitis B virus. Lancet *336*:325–329, 1990.
34. Cattaneo, R., Will, H., Hernandez, N., et al.: Signals regulating hepatitis B surface antigen transcription. Nature *305*:336–338, 1983.
35. Centers for Disease Control and Prevention: Hepatitis Surveillance Report No. 56. Atlanta, 1995, p. 36.
36. Centers for Disease Control and Prevention: Update: Recommendations to prevent hepatitis B virus transmission—United States. M. M. W. R. *44*:574–575, 1995.
37. Centers for Disease Control and Prevention: Summary of notifiable diseases, United States, 1994. M. M. W. R. *43*:1–80, 1994.
38. Centers for Disease Control: Hepatitis B virus: A comprehensive strategy for eliminating transmission in the United States through universal childhood vaccination. Recommendations of the Immunization Practices Advisory Committee (ACIP). M. M. W. R. *40*:1–25, 1991.
39. Centers for Disease Control: Protection against viral hepatitis: Recommendations of the Immunization Practices Advisory Committee (ACIP). M. M. W. R. *39*:1–23, 1990.
40. Centers for Disease Control: Prevention of perinatal transmission of hepatitis B virus: Prenatal screening of all pregnant women for hepatitis B surface antigen. Recommendations of the Immunization Practices Advisory Committee (ACIP). M. M. W. R. *37*:341–346, 1988.
41. Chang, C., Enders, G., Sprengel, R., et al.: Expression of the precore region of an avian hepatitis B virus is not required for viral replication. J. Virol. *61*:3322–3325, 1987.
42. Chang, H.-K., and Ting, L.-P.: The surface gene promoter of the human hepatitis B virus displays a preference for differentiated hepatocytes. Virology *170*:176–183, 1989.
43. Chen, S.-T., LaPorte, P., and Yee, J.-K.: Mutational analysis of hepatitis B virus enhancer 2. Virology *196*:652–659, 1993.
44. Chen, S.-T., Su, H., and Yee, J.-K.: Repression of liver-specific hepatitis B virus enhancer 2 activity by adenovirus EIA proteins. J. Virol. *66*:7452–7460, 1992.
45. Chisari, F. V., and Ferrari, C.: Hepatitis B virus immunopathogenesis. Annu. Rev. Immunol. *13*:29–60, 1995.
46. Chisari, F. V., Filippi, P., Buras, J., et al.: Structural and pathological effects of synthesis of hepatitis B virus large envelope polypeptide in transgenic mice. Proc. Natl. Acad. Sci. U. S. A. *84*:6909–6913, 1987.
47. Columbo, M., Gerber, M. A., Vermace, S. J., et al.: Immune response to hepatitis B virus in children with papular acrodermatitis. Gastroenterology *73*:1103–1106, 1977.
48. Crosti, A., and Gianotti, F.: Dermatose eruptive acro-situee d'origine probablement virosique. Acta Dermatol. Venereol. (Stockh.) *2*:146–149, 1957.
49. Dane, D. S., Cameron, C. H., and Briggs, M.: Virus-like particles in serum of patients with Australia antigen-associated hepatitis. Lancet *1*:695–698, 1970.
50. Deinhardt, F., Gust, I. D., on behalf of the participants in an informal WHO meeting: Viral hepatitis. Bull. W. H. O. *60*:661–691, 1982.
51. Echevarria, S., Casafont, F., Miera, M., et al.: Interleukin-2 and natural killer activity in acute type B hepatitis. Hepato-Gastroenterology *38*:307–310, 1991.
52. Editorial: Jaundice following yellow fever vaccination. J. A. M. A. *119*:1110, 1942.
53. Edman, J., Gray, P., Valenzuela, P., et al.: Integration of hepatitis B virus sequences and their expression in a human hepatoma cell. Nature *286*:535–538, 1980.
54. Elfassi, E., Romet-Lemmone, J. L., Essex, M., et al.: Evidence of extrachromosomal forms of hepatitis B viral DNA in a bone marrow culture obtained from a patient recently infected with hepatitis B virus. Proc. Natl. Acad. Sci. U. S. A. *81*:3526–3528, 1984.
55. Enders, G. H., Ganem, D., and Varmus, H. E.: 5′ terminal sequences influence the segregation of ground squirrel hepatitis virus RNAs into polyribosomes and viral core particles. J. Virol. *61*:35–41, 1987.
56. Evans, A. S., Sprinz, H., and Nelson, R. S.: Adrenal hormone therapy in viral hepatitis. II. The effect of cortisone in the acute disease. Ann. Intern. Med. *38*:1134–1147, 1953.
57. Fiaccadori, F., Bertoletti, A., Penna, A., et al.: The immunopathogenesis of hepatitis B. Ann. Ital. Med. Int. *7*:153–159, 1992.
58. Findlay, G. M., and MacCallum, P. O.: Note on acute hepatitis and yellow fever immunization. Trans. R. Soc. Trop. Med. Hyg. *31*:297–308, 1937.
59. Fourel, G., Trepo, C., Bougueleret, L., et al.: Frequent activation of *N-myc* genes by hepadnavirus insertion in woodchuck liver tumours. Nature *347*:294–298, 1990.
60. Fried, M. W.: Therapy of chronic viral hepatitis. Med. Clin. North Am. *80*:957–972, 1996.
61. Galibert, F., Mandart, E., Fitoussi, F., et al.: Nucleotide sequence of hepatitis B virus genome (subtype ayw) cloned in *E. coli.* Nature *281*:646–650, 1979.
62. Galle, P. R., Schlicht, H., Kuhn, C., et al.: Replication of duck hepatitis B virus in primary duck hepatocytes and its dependence on the state of differentiation of the host cell. Hepatology *10*:459–465, 1989.
63. Ganem, D.: *Hepadnaviridae* and their replication. *In* Fields, B. N., Knipe, D. M., Howley, P. M., et al. (eds.): Fields Virology. 3rd ed. Philadelphia, Lippincott-Raven, 1996, pp. 2703–2737.
64. Ganem, D.: Persistent infection of humans with hepatitis B virus: Mechanisms and consequences. Rev. Infect. Dis. *4*:1026–1047, 1982.
65. Gavilanes, F., Gonzales-Ros, A., and Peterson, D.: Structure of hepatitis B surface antigen: Characterization of the lipid components and their association with the viral proteins. J. Biol. Chem. *257*:7770–7777, 1982.
66. Gerin, J., Purcell, R., Hoggan, M., et al.: Biophysical properties of Australian antigen. J. Virol. *36*:787–795, 1980.
67. Gerlich, W., and Robinson, W. S.: Hepatitis B virus contains protein attached to the 5′ end of its complete strand. Cell *21*:801–811, 1980.
68. Gianotti, F.: Papular acrodermatitis of childhood: An Australia antigen disease. Arch. Dis. Child. *48*:794–799, 1973.
69. Gianotti, F.: Rilievi di'una particolare casisitica tossinfettiva caratterizzata da eurzione eritemto-infiltrativa desquamativa a focolai lenticolari, a sede elettiva acroesposta. G. Ital. Derm. Sif. *96*:678–697, 1955.
70. Gilbert, R. D., and Wiggelinkhuizen, J.: The clinical course of hepatitis B virus-associated nephropathy. Pediatr. Nephrol. *8*:11–14, 1994.
71. Gunther, S., Meisel, H., Reip, A., et al.: Frequent and rapid emergence of mutated pre-C sequences in HBV from e-antigen positive carriers who seroconvert to anti-HBe during interferon treatment. Virology *187*:271–279, 1992.

72. Hadchouel, M., Pasquinelli, C., Fournier, J. G., et al.: Detection of mononuclear cells expressing hepatitis B virus in peripheral blood from HBsAg positive and negative patients by in situ hybridization. J. Med. Virol. *24*:27–32, 1988.
73. Hadler, S. C., and Margolis, H. S.: Viral hepatitis. *In* Evans, A. S. (ed.): Viral Infections of Humans: Epidemiology and Control. 3rd ed. New York, Plenum, 1989, pp. 351–391.
74. Harpaz, R., Von Seidlein, L., Averhoff, F. M., et al.: Transmission of hepatitis B virus to multiple patients from a surgeon without evidence of inadequate infection control. N. Engl. J. Med. *334*:549–554, 1996.
75. Heermann, K. H., Goldmann, U., Schwartz, W., et al.: Large surface proteins of hepatitis B virus containing the pre-S sequence. J. Virol. *52*:396–402, 1984.
76. Heron, I., Hokland, M., and Berg, K.: Enhanced expression of beta2 microglobulin and HLA antigens on human lymphoid cells by interferon. Proc. Natl. Acad. Sci. U. S. A. *75*:6215–6219, 1978.
77. Hertogs, K., Leenders, W. P. J., Depia, E., et al.: Endonexin II present on human liver plasma membranes is a specific binding protein of small hepatitis B virus (HBV) envelope protein. Virology *197*:549–557, 1993.
78. Hilleman, M. R.: Comparative biology and pathogenesis of AIDS and hepatitis B viruses: Related but different. AIDS Res. Hum. Retrovir. *10*:1409–1419, 1994.
79. Hirsch, R., Lavine, J., Chang, L., et al.: Polymerase gene products of hepatitis B viruses are required for genomic RNA packaging as well as for reverse transcription. Nature *344*:552–555, 1990.
80. Hirschman, S. Z.: Current therapeutic approaches to viral hepatitis. Clin. Infect. Dis. *20*:741–746, 1995.
81. Hollinger, F. B.: Hepatitis B virus. *In* Fields, B. N., Knipe, D. M., Howley, P. M., et al. (eds.): Fields Virology. 3rd ed. Philadelphia, Lippincott-Raven, 1996, pp. 2739–2807.
82. Honigwachs, J., Faktor, O., Dikstein, R., et al.: Liver-specific expression of hepatitis B virus is determined by the combined action of the core gene promoter and the enhancer. J. Virol. *63*:919–927, 1989.
83. Hoofnagle, J. H., Seerff, L. B., Bales, Z. B., et al.: Serologic responses in HB. *In* Vyas, G. N., Cohen, S. N., and Schmid, R. (eds.): Viral Hepatitis. Philadelphia, Franklin Institute Press, 1978, pp. 219–244.
84. Hoofnagle, J. H., Gerety, R. J., and Barker, L. F.: Antibody to hepatitis B virus core in man. Lancet *3*:869, 1973.
85. Horwich, A. L., Furtak, K., Pugh, J., et al.: Synthesis of hepadnavirus particles that contain replication-defective duck hepatitis B virus genomes in cultured HuH7 cells. J. Virol. *64*:642–650, 1990.
86. Hovi, L., Saarinen, U. M., Jalanko, H., et al.: Characteristics and outcome of acute infection with hepatitis B virus in children with cancer. Pediatr. Infect. Dis. J. *10*:809–812, 1991.
87. Hruska, J. F., and Robinson, W. S.: The proteins of hepatitis B Dane particle cores. J. Med. Virol. *1*:119–131, 1977.
88. Hsu, H. C., Wu, C. Y., Lin, C. Y., et al.: Membranous nephropathy in 52 hepatitis B surface antigen (HBsAg) carrier children in Taiwan. Kidney Int. *36*:1103–1107, 1989.
89. Hsu, H. Y., Chang, M. H., Lee, C. Y., et al.: Spontaneous loss of HBsAg in children with chronic hepatitis B virus infection. Hepatology *15*:382–386, 1992.
90. Hsu, T., Moroy, T., Etiemble, J., et al.: Activation of *c-myc* by woodchuck hepatitis virus insertion in hepatocellular carcinoma. Cell *55*:627–635, 1988.
91. Hu, K., and Siddiqui, A.: Regulation of the hepatitis B virus gene expression by the enhancer element I. Virology *181*:721–726, 1991.
92. Huovila, A.-P. J., Eder, A. M., and Fuller, S. D.: Hepatitis B surface antigen assembles in a post-ER, pre-Golgi compartment. J. Cell. Biol. *118*:1305–1320, 1992.
93. Hwang, L.-Y., Lee, C.-Y., Beasley, R. P., et al.: Five year follow-up of HBV vaccination with plasma-derived vaccine in neonates: Evaluation of immunogenicity and efficacy against perinatal transmission. *In* Hollinger, F. B., Lemon, S. M., and Margolis, H. S. (eds.): Viral Hepatitis and Liver Disease. Baltimore, Williams & Wilkins, 1991, pp. 759–761.
94. Ishak, K. G.: Light microscopic morphology of viral hepatitis. Am. J. Clin. Pathol. *65*:787–827, 1976.
95. Ishimaru, Y., Ishimaru, H., Toda, G., et al.: An epidemic of infantile papular acrodermatitis (Gianotti's disease) in Japan associated with hepatitis B surface antigen subtype ayw. Lancet *1*:707–709, 1976.
96. Kakumu, S., Ishikawa, T., Wakita, T., et al.: Interferon-gamma production specific for hepatitis B virus antigen by intrahepatic T lymphocytes in patients with acute and chronic hepatitis B. Am. J. Gastroenterol. *89*:92–96, 1994.
97. Kamimura, T., Yoshikawa, A., Ichida, F., et al.: Electron microscopic studies of Dane particles in hepatocytes with special references to intracellular development of Dane particles and their relation with the HBeAg in the serum. Hepatology *1*:392–397, 1981.
98. Kane, M. A., and Lettau, L.: Transmission of HBV from dental personnel to patients. J. Am. Dent. Assoc. *110*:634–636, 1985.
99. Kaplan, P. M., Greenman, R. L., Gerin, J. L., et al.: DNA polymerase associated with human hepatitis B antigen. J. Virol. *12*:995–1005, 1973.
100. Kelly, R.: Pathways of protein secretion in eukaryotes. Science *230*:25–31, 1985.
101. Klingmuller, U., and Schaller, H.: Hepadnavirus infection requires interaction between the viral pre-S domain and a specific hepatocellular receptor. J. Virol. *67*:7414–7422, 1993.
102. Kock, J., and Schlicht, H.-J.: Analysis of the earliest steps of hepadnavirus replication genome repair after infectious entry into hepatocytes does not depend on viral polymerase activity. J. Virol. *67*:4867–4874, 1993.
103. Koff, R. S., and Galambos, J. T.: Viral hepatitis. *In* Schiff, L., and Schiff, E. R. (eds.): Diseases of the Liver. Philadelphia, J. B. Lippincott, 1987, pp. 457–581.
104. Koike, K., Moriya, K., Iino, S., et al.: High-level expression of hepatitis B virus Hbx gene and hepatocarcinogenesis in transgenic mice. Hepatology *19*:810–819, 1994.
105. Koike, K.: Transgenic mouse model for hepatocellular carcinoma in human hepatitis B virus infection. Nippon Rinsho *51*:536–541, 1993.
106. Krugman, S., and Stevens, C. E.: Hepatitis B vaccine. *In* Plotkin, S. A., and Mortimer, E. A. (eds.): Vaccines. 2nd ed. Philadelphia, W. B. Saunders, 1994, pp. 419–437.
107. Krugman, S., and Katz, S. L.: Viral hepatitis: Type A (infectious hepatitis), type B (serum hepatitis), non-A, non-B hepatitis. *In* Krugman, S., and Katz, S. L. (eds.): Infectious Diseases of Children. 7th ed. St. Louis, C. V. Mosby, 1981, pp. 90–129.
108. Krugman, S., Giles, J. P., and Hammond, J.: Infectious hepatitis: Evidence for two distinctive clinical, epidemiological and imunological types of infection. J. A. M. A. *200*:365–373, 1967.
109. Lachaux, A., Lapillonne, A., Bouvier, R., et al.: Transplacental transmission of hepatitis B virus: A familial case. Pediatr. Infect. Dis. J. *14*:60–63, 1995.
110. Lai, C. L., Lin, H.-J., Lau, J. Y.-N., et al.: Effect of recombinant alpha2 interferon with or without prednisone in Chinese HBsAg carrier children. Q. J. Med. *78*:155–163, 1991.
111. Lai, C. L., Lok, A. S.-F., Lin, H. J., et al.: Placebo-controlled trial of recombinant alpha 2-interferon in Chinese HBsAg carrier children. Lancet *2*:877–880, 1987.
112. Laub, O., Rall, L. B., Truett, M., et al.: Synthesis of hepatitis B surface antigen in mammalian cells: Expression of the entire gene and the coding region. J. Virol. *48*:271–280, 1983.
113. Lauer, U., Weiss, L., Lipp, M., et al.: The hepatitis B virus preS2 S-t transactivator utilizes AP-1 and other transcription factors for transactivation. Hepatology *19*:23–31, 1994.
114. Lauer, U., Weiss, L., Hofschneider, P. H., et al.: The hepatitis B virus pre-S/S t transactivator is generated by 3′ truncations within a defined region of the S gene. J. Virol. *66*:5284–5289, 1992.
115. Laure, F., Zagury, D., Saimot, A. G., et al.: Hepatitis B virus DNA sequences in lymphoid cells from patients with AIDS and AIDS-related complex. Science *229*:561–563, 1985.
116. Lein, J. M., Aldrich, C. E., and Mason, W. S.: Evidence that a capped oligoribonucleotide is the primer for duck hepatitis B virus plus-strand DNA synthesis. J. Virol. *57*:229–236, 1986.
117. Lettau, L. A., Smith, J. D., Williams, D., et al.: Transmission of hepatitis B with resultant restriction of surgical practice. J. A. M. A. *255*:934–937, 1986.
118. Lo, K.-J., Lee, S.-D., Tsai, Y.-T., et al.: Long-term immunogenicity and efficacy of hepatitis B vaccine in infants born to HBeAg-positive carrier mothers. Hepatology *8*:1647–1650, 1988.
119. Lopez-Cabrera, M., Letovsky, J., Hu, K. Q., et al.: Transcriptional factor C EBP binds to and transactivates the enhancer element II of the hepatitis B virus. Virology *183*:825–829, 1991.
120. Lurman, A.: Eine icterusepidemic. Berl. Klin. Wochenschr. *22*:20–23, 1885.
121. MacCallum, F. O.: Homologous serum jaundice. Lancet *2*:691–692, 1947.
122. Machida, A., Ohnuma, H., Tsuda, F., et al.: Phosphorylation in the carboxyl-terminal domain of the capsid protein of hepatitis B virus; evaluation with a monoclonal antibody. J. Virol. *65*:6024–6030, 1991.
123. Maruyama, T., McLachlan, A., Iino, S., et al.: The serology of chronic hepatitis B infection revisited. J. Clin. Invest. *91*:2586–2595, 1993.
124. McMahon, B. J., Heyward, W. L., Templin, D. W., et al.: Hepatitis B-associated polyarteritis nodosa in Alaskan Eskimos: Clinical and epidemiologic features and long-term follow-up. Hepatology *9*:97–101, 1989.
125. McMahon, B. J., Alward, W. L., Hall, D. B., et al.: Acute hepatitis B virus infection: Relation of age to the clinical expression of disease and subsequent development of the carrier state. J. Infect. Dis. *151*:599–603, 1985.
126. McSweeney, P. A., Carter, J. M., Green, G. J., et al.: Fatal aplastic anemia associated with hepatitis B viral infection. Am. J. Med. *85*:255–256, 1988.
127. Mehdi, H., Kaplan, M., Anlar, F., et al.: Hepatitis B virus surface antigen binds apolipoprotein H. J. Virol. *68*:2415–2424, 1994.
128. Memorandum prepared by Medical Officers of the Ministry of Health: Homologous serum jaundice. Lancet *1*:83–88, 1943.
129. Min, K.-W., Gyorkey, F., and Cain, D.: Talc granulomata in liver disease in narcotic addicts. Arch. Pathol. *98*:331–335, 1974.
130. Nagaya, T., Nakamura, T., Tokino, T., et al.: The mode of hepatitis B virus DNA integration in chromosomes of human hepatocellular carcinoma. Genes Dev. *1*:773–782, 1987.
131. Narkewicz, M. R., Smith, D., Silverman, A., et al.: Clearance of chronic hepatitis B virus infection in young children after alpha interferon treatment. J. Pediatr. *127*:815–818, 1995.

132. Nassal, M., Galle, P. R., and Schaller, H.: Proteaselike sequence in hepatitis B virus core antigen is not required for e antigen generation and may not be part of an aspartic acid-type protease. J. Virol. *63*:2598–2604, 1989.
133. Natoli, G., Avantaggiani, M. L., Balsano, C., et al.: Characterization of the hepatitis B virus preS/S region encoded transcriptional transactivator. Virology *187*:663–670, 1992.
134. Nayersina, R., Fowler, P., Guilhot, S., et al.: HLA A2 restricted cytotoxic T lymphocyte responses to multiple hepatitis B surface antigen epitopes during hepatitis B virus infection. J. Immunol. *150*:4659–4671, 1993.
135. Onion, D. K., Crumpacker, C. S., and Gilliland, B. C.: Arthritis of hepatitis associated with Australia antigen. Ann. Intern. Med. *75*:29–33, 1971.
136. Pasek, M., Goto, T., Gilbert, W., et al.: Hepatitis B virus genes and their expression in *E. coli*. Nature *282*:575–579, 1978.
137. Penna, A., Chisari, F. V., Bertoletti, A., et al.: Cytotoxic T lymphocytes recognize an HLA-A2 restricted epitope within the hepatitis B virus nucleocapsid antigen. J. Exp. Med. *174*:1565–1570, 1991.
138. Peterson, D.: The structure of hepatitis B surface antigen and its antigenic sites. Bioessays *6*:258–262, 1987.
139. Pignatelli, M., Waters, J., Brown, D., et al.: HLA class I antigens on the hepatocyte membrane during recovery from acute hepatitis B virus infection and during interferon therapy in chronic hepatitis B virus infection. Hepatology *6*:349–353, 1986.
140. Pugh, J. C., and Summers, J. W.: Infection and uptake of duck hepatitis B virus by duck hepatocytes maintained in the presence of dimethyl sulfoxide. Virology *172*:564–572, 1989.
141. Purcell, R., Hoofnagle, J. H., and Gerin, J. L.: Parenterally transmitted hepatitis. *In* Lennette, E. H., Lennette, D. A., and Lennette, E. T. (eds.): Diagnostic Procedures for Viral, Rickettsial, and Chlamydial Infections. Washington, D.C., American Public Health Association, 1995, pp. 331–359.
142. Raber, I. M., and Friedman, H. M.: Hepatitis B surface antigen in corneal donors. Am. J. Ophthalmol. *104*:255–258, 1987.
143. Rigg, R. J., and Schaller, H.: Duck hepatitis B virus infection of hepatocytes is not dependent on low pH. J. Virol. *66*:2829–2836, 1992.
144. Robinson, W. S., and Lutwick, L. I.: The virus of hepatitis type B. N. Engl. J. Med. *295*:1168–1175, 1976.
145. Robinson, W. S., and Greenman, R.: DNA polymerase in the core of the human hepatitis B virus candidate. J. Virol. *13*:1231–1236, 1974.
146. Rogler, C., Sherman, M., Yu, C. J., et al.: Deletion in chromosome 11p associated with a hepatitis B integration site in hepatocellular carcinoma. Science *230*:319–322, 1985.
147. Romero, R., and Kleinman, R. E.: Thrombocytopenia associated with acute hepatitis B infection. Pediatrics *91*:150–152, 1993.
148. Romet-Lemonne, J. L., McLane, M. F., Elfassi, E., et al.: Hepatitis B virus infection in cultured human lymphoblastoid cells. Science *221*:667–669, 1983.
149. Roossinck, M. J., Jameel, S., Loukin, S. H., et al.: Expression of hepatitis B viral core region in mammalian cells. Mol. Cell. Biol. *6*:1393–1400, 1986.
150. Rosh, J. R., Schwersenz, A. H., Grotsman, G., et al.: Fatal fulminant hepatitis B in an infant despite appropriate prophylaxis. Arch. pediatr. Adolesc. Med. *148*:1349–1351, 1994.
151. Rossner, M.: Hepatitis B virus X gene product: A promiscuous transcriptional activator. J. Med. Virol. *36*:101–117, 1992.
152. Ruiz-Moreno, M.: Interferon treatment in children with chronic hepatitis B. J. Hepatol. *22*(Suppl.):49–51, 1995.
153. Ruiz-Moreno, M., Rua, M. J., Molina, J., et al.: Prospective, randomized controlled trial of interferon alpha in children with chronic hepatitis B. Hepatology *13*:1035–1039, 1991.
154. Ruiz-Moreno, M., Jimenez, J., Porres, J. C., et al.: A controlled trial of recombinant interferon alpha in Caucasian children with chronic hepatitis B. Digestion *45*:26–33, 1990.
155. Santantonio, T., Jung, M.-C., Monno, L., et al.: Long-term response to interferon therapy in chronic hepatitis B: Importance of hepatitis B virus heterogeneity. Arch. Virol. *8*(Suppl.):171–178, 1993.
156. Sawyer, W. A., Meyer, K. F., and Eaton, M. D.: Jaundice in army personnel in the western region of the United States and its relation to vaccination against yellow fever. Am. J. Hyg. *39*:337–430, 1944.
157. Schiff, L.: The use of steroids in liver disease. Medicine (Baltimore) *45*:565–573, 1966.
158. Seeff, L. B., Beebe, G. W., Hoofnagle, J. H., et al.: A serologic follow-up of the 1942 epidemic of post-vaccination hepatitis in the United States Army. N. Engl. J. Med. *316*:965–970, 1987.
159. Seeger, C., Ganem, D., and Varmus, H. E.: Genetic and biochemical evidence for the hepatitis B virus replication strategy. Science *232*:477–485, 1986.
160. Shafritz, D., Shouval, D., Sherman, H., et al.: Integration of hepatitis B virus DNA into the genome of liver cell in chronic liver disease and hepatocellular carcinoma. N. Engl. J. Med. *305*:1067–1073, 1981.
161. Siddiqui, A., Jameel, S., and Mapoles, J.: Expression of the hepatitis B virus X gene in mammalian cells. Proc. Natl. Acad. Sci. U. S. A. *84*:2513–2517, 1987.
162. Sprengel, R., Kaleta, E. F., and Will, H.: Isolation and characterization of a hepatitis B virus endemic in herons. J. Virol. *62*:3832–3839, 1988.
163. Stevens, C. E., Toy, P. T., Tong, M. J., et al.: Perinatal hepatitis B virus transmission in the United States: Prevention by passive-active immunization. J. A. M. A. *253*:1740–1746, 1985.
164. Stevens, C. E., Beasley, R. P., Taul, J., et al.: Vertical transmission of hepatitis B antigen in Taiwan. N. Engl. J. Med. *292*:771–774, 1975.
165. Stibbe, W., and Gerlich, W.: Structural relationships between minor and major proteins of hepatitis B surface antigen. J. Virol. *46*:626–628, 1983.
166. Summers, J., and Mason, W. S.: Replication of the genome of a hepatitis B-like virus by reverse transcription of an RNA intermediate. Cell *29*:403–415, 1982.
167. Summers, J., O'Connell, A., Millman, I., et al.: Genome of hepatitis B virus restriction enzyme cleavage and structure of DNA extracted from Dane particles. Proc. Natl. Acad. Sci. U. S. A. *72*:4597–4601, 1975.
168. Takahashi, T., Nakagawa, S., Hashimoto, T., et al.: Large-scale isolation of Dane particles from plasma containing hepatitis B antigen and demonstration of a circular double-stranded DNA molecule extruding directly from their cores. J. Immunol. *227*:1392–1397, 1976.
169. Tavis, J., Perri, S., and Ganem, D.: Hepadnaviral reverse transcription initiates within the RNA stem-loop of the viral encapsidation signal and employs a novel strand transfer. J. Virol. *68*:3536–3543, 1994.
170. Toh, H., Hayashida, H., and Miyasa, T.: Sequence homology between retroviral reverse transcriptase and putative polymerase of hepatitis B virus and cauliflower mosaic virus. Nature *305*:827–829, 1983.
171. Tokino, T., and Matsubara, K.: Chromosomal sites for hepatitis B virus integration in human hepatocellular carcinoma. J. Virol. *65*:6761–6764, 1991.
172. Torre, D., and Tambini, R.: Interferon alpha therapy for chronic hepatitis B in children: A meta-analysis. Clin. Infect. Dis. *23*:131–137, 1996.
173. Tur-Kaspa, R., Klein, A., and Aharanson, S.: Hepatitis B virus precore mutants are identical in carriers from various ethnic origins and are associated with a range of liver disease severity. Hepatology *16*:1338–1342, 1992.
174. Tuttleman, J., Pugh, J. C., and Summers, J. W.: In vitro experimental infection of primary duck hepatocyte cultures with duck hepatitis B virus. J. Virol. *58*:17–25, 1986.
175. Utili, R., Sagnelli, E., Galani, B., et al.: Prolonged treatment of children with chronic hepatitis B with recombinant alpha 2-a interferon: A controlled randomized study. Am. J. Gastroenterol. *86*:327–330, 1991.
176. Valenzuela, P., Quiroga, M., Zaldivar, J., et al.: The nucleotide sequence of the hepatitis B viral genome and the identification of the major viral genes. ICN/UCLA Symposia on Molecular Cellular Biology, 1980, pp. 57–70.
177. Valenzuela, P., Gray, P., Quiroga, M., et al.: Nucleotide sequence of the gene coding for the major protein of hepatitis B virus surface antigen. Nature *280*:815–819, 1979.
178. Venkatasehan, V. S., Lieberman, K., Kim, D. U., et al.: Hepatitis B associated glomerulonephritis: Pathology, pathogenesis, and clinical course. Medicine *69*:200–216, 1990.
179. Vento, S., Rondanelli, E. G., Ranieri, S., et al.: Prospective study of cellular immunity to hepatitis B virus antigens from the early incubation phase of acute hepatitis B. Lancet *2*:119–122, 1987.
180. Vento, S., Hegarty, J. E., Alberti, A., et al.: T lymphocyte sensitization to HBcAg and T-cell mediated unresponsiveness to HBsAg in hepatitis B virus–related chronic liver disease. Hepatology *5*:192–197, 1985.
181. Wainwright, R. B., McMahon, B. J., Bulkow, L. R., et al.: Duration of immunogenicity and efficacy of hepatitis B vaccine in a Yupik Eskimo population. J. A. M. A. *261*:2362–2366, 1989.
182. Wakita, T., Kakumu, S., Yoshioka, K., et al.: Cellular immune responses of peripheral blood mononuclear cells to HBV antigens during chronic and acute HBV infection. Digestion *52*:26–33, 1992.
183. Wands, J. R., Alpert, E., and Isselbacher, K. T.: Arthritis associated with chronic active hepatitis: Complement activation and characterization of circulating immune complexes. Gastroenterology *69*:1286–1291, 1975.
184. Waters, J. A., Kennedy, M., Voet, P., et al.: Loss of the common "a" determinant of hepatitis B surface antigen by a vaccine-induced escape mutant. J. Clin. Invest. *90*:2543–2547, 1992.
185. Weissberg, J. L., Andres, L. L., Smith, C. I., et al.: Survival in chronic hepatitis B: An analysis of 397 patients. Ann. Intern. Med. *101*:613–616, 1984.
186. Yamanaka, T., Akahane, Y., Suzuki, H., et al.: Hepatitis B surface antigen particles with all four subtypic determinants; point mutations of hepatitis B virus DNA inducing phenotype changes or double infection with viruses of different subtypes. Mol. Immunol. *27*:443–449, 1990.
187. Yang, D., Alt, E., and Rogler, C. E.: Coordinate expression of *N-myc* 2 and insulin-like growth factor II in pre-cancerous altered hepatic foci in woodchuck hepatitis virus carriers. Cancer Res. *53*:2020–2027, 1993.
188. Yoffe, B., and Noonan, C. A.: Hepatitis B virus: New and evolving issues. Dig. Dis. Sci. *37*:1–9, 1992.
189. Zeldis, J. B., and Crumpacker, C. S.: Hepatitis. *In* Remington, J. S., and Klein, J. O. (eds.): Infectious Diseases of the Fetus and Newborn Infant. 4th ed. Philadelphia, W. B. Saunders, 1995, pp. 805–834.
190. Zhang, Y. Y., Hansson, B. G., Kuo, L. S., et al.: Hepatitis B virus DNA in serum and liver is commonly found in Chinese patients with chronic liver disease despite the presence of antibodies to HBsAg. Hepatology *17*:538–544, 1993.

Hepatitis D (Delta) Virus

(see also Chapter 55)

Hepatitis D virus (HDV, delta virus) is a defective virus that causes infection only in the presence of active hepatitis B virus (HBV) infection.[13] Infection occurs as either a co-infection with HBV or as a superinfection in a person who is an HBV carrier.[4]

HISTORY

The discovery of HDV was reported in 1977 by Rizzetto and colleagues.[19] They found that fluorescein-labeled immunoglobulin from a patient with HBV infection had antibodies that reacted to liver tissue that did not contain hepatitis B core antigen (HBcAg). Further study revealed that this antibody did not react with any known HBV antigens, but it was noted only in sera of persons who were hepatitis B surface antigen (HBsAg)-positive. Further serologic survey data in Italy, Japan, and the United States confirmed the association of this antibody with HBV infection.[17, 18] Animal studies identified the agent (delta agent) as a separate virus that needed the presence of HBV for infection to occur.[16]

THE VIRUS[13, 21]

HDV is a spherical particle with a 35-nm diameter. It contains a single-stranded RNA genome. The genome is encapsulated with the delta antigen and surface antigen components from the helper HBV. The HBsAg components are pre-S1, pre-S2, and S polypeptides.

EPIDEMIOLOGY[13]

Because HDV infection depends on the presence of HBV, its epidemiology parallels that of HBV. Worldwide, about 5 per cent of the 300 million HBV carriers also are infected with HDV.[15] The prevalence of HDV varies widely even in regions of the world where HBV enjoys a high prevalence. There are two patterns of transmission. In southern Italy, Africa, and South America, which are areas of high endemicity, transmission is thought to occur through person-to-person contact. In contrast, in areas of low endemicity, such as the United States, transmission occurs in groups with frequent percutaneous blood exposures.

In the United States, the prevalence of HDV in the population is low. In blood donors, the prevalence of HBsAg-positive blood is between 0.1 and 0.5 per cent.[10] Of these HBsAg-positive persons, between 1.4 and 12.4 per cent also are infected with HDV.[10, 12] In HBV risk groups, the greatest HDV infection rate is in intravenous drug abusers and hemophiliacs. In general, other high-risk groups have low rates of HDV infection.

Although HDV infection usually is sporadic, outbreaks occur.[5, 8] Outbreaks as co-infections and superinfections both have been observed. Vertical transmission has been reported, but it is rare.[22]

CLINICAL MANIFESTATIONS

HDV infection can occur as a co-infection with HBV or as a superinfection in a person who has an ongoing HBV infection.[13] The acute illnesses in these two types of infections usually are indistinguishable; however, superinfected patients are more likely to develop chronic HDV carriage and more rapid progression to cirrhosis than co-infected patients are.

Co-infection

The symptoms and signs of acute HBV and HDV co-infections are similar to those caused by other viruses. However, a biphasic course is more common, and fulminant hepatitis is significantly more common than its occurrence with HBV alone. After co-infection, the rate of becoming an HBV carrier is low and no greater than that following HBV infection alone.[3, 11] However, in one study, the co-infected patients who became HBV carriers experienced a rapid progression to chronic liver disease and cirrhosis.[3]

Superinfection

Superinfection with HDV in an HBV chronically infected person results in acute hepatitis 50 to 70 per cent of the time.[1, 6, 11] Fulminant hepatitis also occurs as a result of superinfection, and its rate of occurrence is higher than that occurring after infection with HBV alone.[20] The incubation period after a superinfection is relatively short, ranging from 2 to 8 weeks.[16]

DIAGNOSIS

HDV infection can be determined by detecting IgG anti-HD in the serum by radioimmunoassay.[14] This test is commercially available. Other tests available in research settings include hepatitis D antigen in serum, hepatitis D antigen in liver, HDV RNA in serum, HDV RNA in liver, and IgM anti-HD in serum. Co-infection can be differentiated from superinfection by the presence of IgM anti-HBc in the serum during co-infection.

TREATMENT

Interferon alpha has been used to treat both children and adults with chronic HDV infection.[2, 7, 9] In one study involving 23 children, treatment did not alter the clinical, serologic, or histologic course.[2] In another report, one of two children cleared the infection and developed immunity.[9] In a controlled trial in adults, short-term improvement occurred, but relapse was common after treatment.[7]

PREVENTION

The procedures for the prevention of HDV infection are the same as those listed in this chapter for the prevention of HBV infection.

References

1. Bonino, F., Negro, F., Baldi, M., et al.: The natural history of chronic delta hepatitis. Prog. Clin. Biol. Res. *234*:145–152, 1987.
2. Bortolotti, F., DiMarco, V., Vajro, P., et al.: Long-term evolution of chronic delta hepatitis in children. J. Pediatr. *122*:736–738, 1993.
3. Caredda, F., Antinori, S., Re, T., et al.: Course and prognosis of acute HDV hepatitis. Prog. Clin. Biol. Res. *234*:267–276, 1987.
4. Centers for Disease Control: Hepatitis B virus: A comprehensive strategy for eliminating transmission in the United States through universal child-

hood vaccination. Recommendations of the Immunization Practices Advisory Committee (ACIP). M. M. W. R. *40*:1–25, 1991.
5. Centers for Disease Control: Delta hepatitis: Massachusetts. M. M. W. R. *33*:493–494, 1984.
6. Columbo, M., Cambieri, R., Grazia, M., et al.: Long-term delta superinfection in hepatitis B surface antigen carriers and its relationship to the course of chronic hepatitis. Gastroenterology *85*:235–239, 1983.
7. Farci, P., Mandas, A., Colana, A., et al.: Treatment of chronic hepatitis D with interferon alfa-2a. N. Engl. J. Med. *330*:88–94, 1994.
8. Hershow, R. C., Chomel, B. B., Graham, D. R., et al.: Hepatitis D virus infection in Illinois state facilities for the developmentally disabled. Ann. Intern. Med. *110*:779–785, 1989.
9. Kay, M. H., Wyllie, R., Deimler, C., et al.: Alpha interferon therapy in children with chronic active hepatitis B and delta virus infection. J. Pediatr. *123*:1001–1004, 1993.
10. Maynard, J. E., Hadler, S. C., and Fields, H. A.: Delta hepatitis in the Americas: An overview. Prog. Clin. Biol. Res. *234*:493–505, 1987.
11. Moestrup, T., Hansson, B. G., Widell, A., et al.: Clinical aspects of delta infection. B. M. J. *286*:87–90, 1983.
12. Nath, N., Mushahwar, I. K., Fang, C. T., et al.: Antibodies to delta antigen in asymptomatic hepatitis B surface antigen-reactive blood donors in the United States and their association with other markers of hepatitis B virus. Am. J. Epidemiol. *122*:218–225, 1985.
13. Polish, L. B., Gallagher, M., Fields, H. A., et al.: Delta hepatitis: Molecular biology and clinical epidemiological features. Clin. Microbiol. Rev. *6*:211–229, 1993.
14. Purcell, R., Hoofnagle, J. H., and Gerin, J. L.: Parenterally transmitted hepatitis. *In* Lennette, E. H., Lennette, D. A., and Lennette, E. T. (eds.): Diagnostic Procedures for Viral, Rickettsial, and Chlamydial Infections. 7th ed. Washington, D.C., American Public Health Association, 1995, pp. 331–359.
15. Rizzetto, M., Ponzetto, A., and Forzani, L.: Epidemiology of hepatitis delta virus: Overview. Prog. Clin. Biol. Res. *364*:1–20, 1991.
16. Rizzetto, M., Canese, M. G., Gerin, J. L., et al.: Transmission of the hepatitis B virus–associated delta antigen to chimpanzees. J. Infect. Dis. *141*:590–602, 1980.
17. Rizzetto, M., Shih, W.-K., and Gerin, J. L.: The hepatitis B virus-associated delta antigen: Isolation from liver, development of solid phase radioimmunoassays for delta antigen and anti-delta and partial characterization of delta antigen. J. Immunol. *125*:318–324, 1980.
18. Rizzetto, M., Gocke, D. J., Verme, G., et al.: Incidence and significance of antibodies to delta antigen in hepatitis B virus infection. Lancet *2*:986–990, 1979.
19. Rizzetto, M., Canese, M. G., Arico, S., et al.: Immunofluorescence detection of new antigen-antibody system (delta/anti-delta) associated to hepatitis B virus in liver and serum of HBsAg carriers. Gut *18*:997–1003, 1977.
20. Saracco, G., Rosina, F., Brunetto, M. R., et al.: Rapidly progressive HBsAg-positive hepatitis in Italy: The role of hepatitis delta virus infection. J. Hepatitis *5*:274–281, 1988.
21. Taylor, J. M.: Hepatitis delta virus and its replication. *In* Fields, B. N., Knipe, D. M., and Howley, P. M. (eds.): Fields Virology. 3rd ed. Philadelphia, Lippincott-Raven, 1996, pp. 2809–2818.
22. Zanetti, A. R., Ferroni, P., Magliano, E. M., et al.: Perinatal transmission of the hepatitis B virus and of the HBV-associated delta agent from mothers to offspring in northern Italy. J. Med. Virol. *9*:139–148, 1982.

SUBSECTION FIVE

HERPESVIRIDAE

163

HERPES SIMPLEX VIRUS

Steve Kohl

There are eight human herpesviruses. These include herpes simplex virus (HSV types 1 and 2), cytomegalovirus, Epstein-Barr virus, varicella-zoster virus, and human herpesviruses 6, 7, and 8. This chapter deals with infections caused by HSV acquired after the neonatal period.

Herpes means "to creep" in Greek. Initially this term was used as a description of a variety of cutaneous, spreading lesions, including the classic description of fever blisters recorded by Hippocrates and Herodotus. In the 1700s, Astrus described genital herpes lesions, and by the 1800s, the term *herpes* generally was restricted to poxvirus and herpesvirus lesions. With the successful cultivation of HSV from humans on rabbit cornea by Gruter (1912), HSV definitively was differentiated from varicella-zoster virus. Work by Schneweis, Plummer, Nahmias, and Dowdle in Europe and the United States differentiated the antigenic, biologic, and epidemiologic characteristics of HSV-1 and HSV-2.

There are several reasons why HSV has assumed an extraordinary importance to clinicians. It is a ubiquitous virus, infecting the vast majority of humanity. It is the prototype of agents that are able to induce a state of latency in the infected organism, with periodic recurrences, the mechanisms of which remain to be explained. HSV may produce a wide spectrum of illness ranging from the trivial (as fever blisters) to the most severe (as the most common cause of fatal sporadic viral encephalitis). The immune status of the host, to a large extent, determines the severity of the clinical manifestations. As the incidence of genital herpes increases, thereby increasing the incidence of neonatal HSV infection, and as more immunocompromised patients are cared for, the most severe manifestations of HSV are increasing. When misused, some therapies (such as corticosteroids) worsen the manifestations of HSV. On the other hand, a high index of suspicion allows rapid diagnostic testing and increasingly effective and specific antiviral therapy.

THE VIRUS

HSV is a moderately large virus consisting of an icosahedral capsid made of 162 hollow protein subunits or capsomeres enclosing a core of double-stranded DNA and protein, surrounded by a tegument of proteins, enclosed in a lipid-containing envelope.[65, 210, 213] The envelope contains a variety of viral encoded glycoproteins that are important target antigens of the humoral and cellular immune response (gpB, gpC, gpD).[65] Several of these also may function as immunoglobulin Fc receptors (gpE and gpI) or complement receptors (gpC). Most of the glycoproteins are found in both types of HSV with a high degree of homology. gpG is type-specific for HSV-2. There are at least two distinguishable subtypes: type 1 and type 2. Whereas the former is regarded as the "oral" type and the latter as the "genital" type, changing sexual habits and possibly other factors are resulting in a blurring of this distinction. Thus, the virus type is not a reliable indicator of the anatomic site of isolation. Whereas both forms of HSV can infect either oral or genital organs and cells, a definite relationship was demonstrated between HSV-2 and infections below the waist and HSV-1 and infections of the upper torso, head, and neck.[84] It is of interest that HSV-1 is more likely to recur in the oral area and HSV-2 in the genital area in persons initially infected at both sites with the same viral strain.[167] Although a considerable degree of homology (approximately 50 per cent) can be demonstrated between the DNA of types 1 and 2 (they share common sequences), these subtypes can be distinguished biochemically (unique base sequences are present) as well as serologically and biologically. The evolutionary divergence of HSV-1 and HSV-2 required a separation of their biologic niches and may have been the result of the assumption of the upright position that caused changing sexual patterns 8 to 10 million years ago.[107]

HSV attaches to and penetrates cells via glycoproteins B and D, utilizing cell-surface heparin sulfate proteoglycan as a target receptor. Once it is inside the cell, there is an orderly expression of early alpha genes (inhibiting host-cell function), beta genes (encoding regulatory proteins and DNA replication enzymes), and finally gamma genes (encoding the structural proteins). Replication of viral DNA and structural proteins allows viral assembly in the cell nucleus, with envelopment as the naked virus buds through the nuclear membrane. Human HSV can be replicated in tissue cultures derived from a variety of species as well as in embryonated hens' eggs and various laboratory animals. The ready growth of HSV in the laboratory and the lack of species specificity distinguish this virus from the other human herpesviruses. The rapidly progressive and relatively characteristic focal cytopathologic effects induced by HSV in susceptible tissue cultures, coupled with the existence of specific heterologous antisera or monoclonal antibodies and straightforward serologic techniques, permit the simple and inexpensive recovery of this virus and its relatively easy identification. Distinction of HSV-1 and HSV-2 involves performing more specialized procedures using type-specific monoclonal antibody or endonuclease restriction analysis.

The technique of DNA endonuclease restriction analysis, in which the viral DNA is digested enzymatically and then analyzed in gels to produce a pattern of bands of DNA fragments, has demonstrated that essentially all epidemiologically unrelated HSV isolates can be differentiated from one another (unique "viral fingerprint"). This has facilitated epidemiologic analysis and definitively demonstrated transfer from human to human in certain settings (such as nurseries or intensive care settings) and has shown that apparent "outbreaks" of encephalitis were instead random, unrelated case clusters.[42, 125, 179]

The herpesviruses, particularly HSV, have evolved mechanisms to avoid immune surveillance. These mechanisms include elaboration of viral encoded IgG Fc receptors and complement receptors that bind host immune components, down-regulation of major histocompatibility complex class-I antigen (potentially preventing CD8 T-cell recognition of infected cells), and inhibition of lytic activity of natural killer cells.[15]

TRANSMISSION

Although highly infectious, HSV is not transmitted casually from person to person. The enveloped virions are relatively unstable at atmospheric conditions, and close interpersonal contact usually is required for transmission. HSV can be transmitted through body fluids, such as saliva, and certainly can be acquired by direct apposition of infected with uninfected integument or mucous membranes. For example, virus has been transferred directly between wrestlers (herpes gladiatorum)[278] and rugby players (herpes rugbeiorum or "scrum-pox"),[281, 332] probably by the rubbing and abrasion of saliva-contaminated skin. Indeed, one outbreak at a wrestling camp involved 60 of 175 participants.[25, 50] Outbreaks associated with high rates of symptomatic illness have occurred at day care centers.[165] These usually were characterized by gingivostomatitis and occurred in small clusters.[271] Nurses and respiratory therapists may acquire HSV infections of the paronychial region (herpetic whitlow), presumably from working with ungloved hands in contact with oropharyngeal secretions.[110, 250, 297] Health care workers effectively may transfer HSV to their patients and actually cause outbreaks of gingivostomatitis.[185] Children may acquire HSV whitlow while having gingivostomatitis through nail-biting or thumb-sucking. Epidemiologic data have shown that with nonmedical persons with herpetic whitlow, isolation of type 2 virus is most likely, often in association with genital HSV infection.[112] Newborns may acquire HSV infection during passage through a virus-infected birth canal.[209] Genital and anal HSV infections are acquired and transmitted through direct contact with infected genitalia or in connection with oral-genital and oral-anal contacts. In all of these cases, the transmission may occur even when the infected parties are asymptomatic and unaware of the presence of their own HSV infections. The presence of an active lesion is associated with very high titers of virus; this increases the likelihood of transmission. In seronegative or HSV-2 antibody–negative partners of persons who have recurrent genital herpes, the incidence of transmission is 5 to 15 per cent per year.[193, 195] In additional couple studies, transmission occurred in 10 per cent of partners, with higher transmission from males (17 per cent) than from females (4 per cent). In females lacking antibodies to HSV-1 and HSV-2, transmission was 32 per cent; if they had antibodies to type 1, it was 9 per cent.[194] Similar findings of some apparent protection against type 2 genital infection by HSV-1 antibody have been reported more recently.[33, 40] HSV has been isolated from the hands of patients with an oral lesion and has been shown to persist for several hours on inanimate objects or in distilled water. Nevertheless, few data implicate inanimate sources as important reservoirs of virus persistence and spread.[221, 318] HSV has been transmitted through transplanted organs[85] and inseminated donor sperm.[204]

If the uninfected exposed skin or mucous membranes are abraded, damaged, or otherwise altered, the risk of transmission and spread is enhanced. For example, burned skin is much more susceptible to HSV infection than is intact skin, and burn patients are at risk for acquisition of this virus in sites of skin damage.[101] Infants may acquire HSV infections in the area of a diaper rash; babies with eczema are at risk for serious disseminated HSV infections (Kaposi varicelliform eruption),[331] as they are for disseminated vaccinia in those locations and situations in which smallpox immunization still is practiced.

HSV is shed commonly in infected but asymptomatic persons from oral or genital sites. Patients with known recurrent genital disease have been documented to shed HSV as often as 10 per cent of the time during which they appear to be lesion-free.[2] Twelve per cent of women with primary HSV-1 genital infection and 18 per cent with primary genital HSV-2 infection subsequently shed virus asymptomatically, especially in the first 3 months after resolution of primary infection.[150] Two per cent of women attending a sexually transmitted disease clinic shed HSV-2 asymptomatically.[161] In partner studies, transmission of genital herpes appeared to result from sexual contact during periods of asymptomatic viral shedding 70 per cent of the time.[194]

These comments denote the few specific instances of isolation or infection control applied for the containment of HSV. Medical and dental personnel who handle respiratory or oral secretions and administer oropharyngeal and tracheostomy care should wear gloves and wash carefully before and after working with patients and their secretions. Parents and caretakers of infants with eczema or severe diaper rash should be especially careful to avoid making direct or indirect contact of this altered skin with an active HSV lesion. Burn patients should be protected against exposure to or direct contact with personnel or visitors who have active HSV lesions. Immunosuppressed patients who develop evidence of HSV infection usually are manifesting evidence of reactivation of latent virus. Primary HSV infections in immunosuppressed persons, as in neonates, may be especially severe, and it is important to protect these susceptible patients against exposure to HSV lesions. Wrestlers and rugby players who have exposed skin lesions caused by HSV should be excluded from competition.

EPIDEMIOLOGY[211]

Although the susceptible host range of HSV is wide, humans are the primary hosts, and it is the human cell to which HSV has become adapted in the evolutionary sense. The epidemiology of HSV is dominated by symptomatic and asymptomatic infection with resultant transmission and maintenance of a huge pool of latently infected persons. Their symptomatic recurrences and asymptomatic shedding ensure continued spread of HSV because it relies on humanity's need for close contact of both a sexual and an asexual nature. HSV infections are global in distribution. Seroepidemiologic studies have shown that HSV infections are found in all populations, even in the most remote and isolated communities. There is no definite seasonal pattern to HSV infections.

The age distribution of HSV infections is influenced by socioeconomics and race (in both instances, these associations probably are manifestations of related environmental factors), as well as by the subtype of virus. Most neonatal HSV infections are acquired from maternal genital strains and thus usually are caused by HSV-2. After the neonatal period, HSV-1 infections predominate, and depending on social and economic factors, 40 to 60 per cent of young children of lower socioeconomic status are seropositive by 5 years of age. Most of these persons (often more than 90 per cent) exhibit HSV-1 antibodies by adulthood. As noted earlier, such situations as attendance in child care centers, which bring children together in close contact, increase the likelihood of acquisition of HSV-1.[165, 271] Studies of populations of a higher socioeconomic level have revealed seroepidemiologic evidence for HSV-1 infection in 30 to 46 per cent of university students.[109, 344] As a reflection of association with sexual activity, the prevalence of HSV-2 increases at about the time of puberty and early adolescence. Among adults, the percentage of HSV-2 seropositives may range from 20 to 35 per cent, with reports of both lower and higher extremes in certain communities. A study in the United States found a seroprevalence rate for HSV-2 of 16.4 per cent. Prevalence increased with age and was higher in blacks (41 per cent) than in whites (13 per cent).[137] More recent studies have found higher rates of HSV-2 seroprevalence in adults. These include rates of 22 per cent in women attending a family planning clinic in Pittsburgh[33] to as high as 47 per cent in women attending a sexually transmitted disease clinic in Seattle.[161] Most of these women's infections were asymptomatic. The prevalence of HSV-2 infections is higher among promiscuous persons and much lower among sexually inactive persons.[87, 245]

The incidence of HSV genital infection apparently has increased markedly in the last two decades. Although it is not a reportable disease, approximately 3 per cent of visits to clinics specializing in sexually transmitted diseases are related to HSV. Approximately 300,000 new cases a year occur in the United States.[48] The risk of genital HSV infection is increased independently by lower socioeconomic status, early age at first intercourse, increased numbers of sexual partners, female sex, previous marriage, urban living, black race, a history of other sexually transmitted diseases, and renting (not owning) one's residence.[109, 137, 296] In studies of sexually active university students, 4 to 8 per 1000 per year acquire genital HSV infection.[77, 344]

Epidemiology as discussed thus far refers largely to the serologic evidence of infection as evaluated in various populations. The pattern of recurrent HSV infections reflects the influence of different factors. Reactivation of latent HSV is associated with a variety of influences, including exposure to sunlight (ultraviolet), certain febrile illnesses, emotional upsets, menstruation, and immunosuppression. These influences, therefore, define additional epidemiologic factors pertinent to HSV infections.

PATHOGENESIS AND PATHOLOGY

HSV tends to infect cells of ectodermal origin; in most cases, initial viral replication occurs at the portal of entry, usually in skin or mucous membranes. The infected cells swell with intracellular edema and degenerate. The nuclei of affected cells may undergo amitotic division, leading to the formation of multinucleate giant cells. The nuclei of infected cells manifest eosinophilic intranuclear inclusions and marginated nuclear chromatin, often in fixed stained preparations seen as separated from the inclusion by a halo. As the cells manifest injury and local inflammation supervenes, intercellular edema develops and forms vesicles in the affected area. On macroscopic examination, these vesicles are surrounded by erythema. Subsequently, the vesicles pustulate and then dry and crust. These lesions are superficial and do not scar. Vesicles on mucous membranes are transient and usually are seen first as shallow ulcers.

Because HSV has a predilection for cells that originate in embryonic ectoderm, it is not surprising to find that these viruses may involve the central nervous system (CNS). Encephalitis may accompany or follow primary HSV infection but also can be seen in connection with reactivation of latent virus.

The incubation period for primary infection varies from 2 to 20 days in most HSV infections. Although occasionally reported, HSV viremia is difficult to detect in the normal host but may be found more commonly in the immunocompromised person.[123, 295]

After primary HSV infection, the virus remains latent and can be reactivated in the appropriate circumstances. However, it does not appear that HSV remains latent in the same epidermal cells in which the primary infection occurred. HSV resides latent in sensory neural ganglia innervating portions of the skin (mucous membranes) originally involved. The exact state of the virus during latency and the molecular mechanism of reactivation are under active investigation. During latency, no viral particles are produced. There is restricted translation of several latency-associated transcripts. The latency-associated transcripts overlap, in an antisense direction, the viral genes *ICPO* and *ICP* 34.5.[67, 68] It appears that their presence in the virus may be necessary for reactivation from the latency state but is not required to maintain latency.[232] A person with recurrent HSV infection almost always experiences reactivation of the HSV lesions in the identical or virtually identical region. With the appropriate stimulus, the latent HSV is reactivated and moves down the neural elements from the ganglion to the area of skin innervated by this sensory nerve.

The recurrence, in immunologically intact persons, generally is less severe than the primary infection. In persons previously infected with one type of virus (e.g., HSV-1, orally), infection with a second type (e.g., HSV-2, genitally) also is less severe than in a host who has never been infected with either. Similarly, reinfection with the same type occurs occasionally (e.g., a second genital infection with a new strain of HSV-2 in a patient with preexisting genital HSV-2 infection). The reinfection generally is mild and often dismissed as an endogenous recurrence. These can be differentiated only by DNA endonuclease restriction analysis of the viral isolates.[43]

After primary HSV infection, most persons mount a host response. As studied in animals and humans, this consists of an early nonspecific response followed by a specific immunologic response.[146, 152, 210, 252] The nonspecific response consists of mobilization of polymorphonuclear and mononuclear leukocytes to the site of infection, release of interferon and other lymphokines, and activation of macrophages and natural killer cells. This, in several days, is followed by the production of many types of specific antiviral antibody (e.g., neutralizing, complement-fixing, antibody-mediating cellular or complement cytotoxicity, antibody to specific viral glycoproteins). Antibody production may be detected as early as 3 days after HSV inoculation in mice.[156] In the second to third week of infection, one can detect specific cellular immunity as manifested by specific lymphocyte blastogenesis, immune lymphokine production (as interferon-γ, migration inhibitory factor), a positive delayed hypersensitivity skin test, and human leukocyte antigen–restricted T-cell cytotoxicity. In humans or animals with cellular defects (e.g., neonates, severely malnourished infants, patients with the Wiskott-Aldrich syndrome and other primary immunodeficiencies, patients receiving transplants or immunosuppressive chemotherapy), primary HSV infection can be a disseminated, life-threatening syndrome, probably because of a defect in cell-mediated immunity of the nonspecific or specific variety.

The immune response to recurrent infection is less well characterized. It does not appear to be associated with marked alterations in antibody production, although fourfold rises and re-emergence of IgA and IgM antiviral antibody may occur. Natural killer cell activity and lymphokine production increase, and, indeed, relative defects in these and lymphocyte blastogenesis may be associated with frequent or severe recurrent infection. In hosts with cellular defects, such as patients undergoing antitumor chemotherapy or with AIDS, recurrences are common, of long duration, and of increased severity, although often not causing widespread dissemination.

The intrathecal compartmentalized immune response in HSV encephalitis currently is being elucidated.[10, 11] There is an acute-phase elevation of β_2-microglobulin, neopterin, interleukin-6, and interferon-γ. Levels of neopterin correlated with the clinical severity of encephalitis. During convalescence, there was persistence of increased levels of soluble CD8, β_2-microglobulin, neopterin, and specific anti-HSV IgG.

CLINICAL MANIFESTATIONS

HSV is very infectious, and, as already emphasized, most persons have been infected by at least one HSV subtype before reaching adulthood. Most infections do not cause significant or specific symptoms, however, so that the largest percentage of seropositive persons (although still harboring latent HSV) are unaware of ever having encountered these viruses. The spectrum of symptomatic HSV infections ranges from minor localized recurrences, usually at mucocutaneous junctions, to severe and even fatal illnesses.

Gingivostomatitis

This is the most common form of HSV-induced primary illness seen in pediatrics. It has been reported by history in as few as 1 per cent to as many as 31 per cent of seropositive children, the higher percentage being from a study among the Navajo.[21] It usually is seen in young children between 10 months and 3 years of age. In those younger than 10 months of age, the presence of residual maternal antibody probably modifies or prevents the appearance of recognizable symptoms in association with HSV infection. Although acute gingivostomatitis caused by HSV is relatively infrequent, it is common enough that most pediatricians become familiar with the condition and learn to distinguish this infection from herpangina.[227]

The incubation period is brief (a few days), and the illness is ushered in by fretful behavior and fever. During this period of systemic illness, HSV is not cultured from the blood.[123] The infant usually refuses to eat and may even refuse fluids. Thereafter, vesicular lesions appear around and on the lips, along the gingiva, on the anterior tongue, and on the anterior (hard) palate (Figs. 163–1 and 163–2). The vesicles break down rapidly, and when seen, the lesions usually appear as 1- to 3-mm shallow gray ulcers on an erythematous base. The gums generally are mildly swollen, ulcerated, and erythematous. They may appear friable and frequently bleed on contact. It is not uncommon for vesicles to extend about the lips and chin or down the neck in the immunologically normal child. There often is a foul smell to the breath (fetor oris). The child experiences extreme discomfort, cannot or will not eat, and—if fluids are refused as well—may require hospitalization for maintenance of adequate hydration. The risk of dehydration is compounded by the fever that usually accompanies this syndrome. The lesions bleed easily and may become covered with a black crust. Cervical and submental nodes often are swollen and tender. The entire process continues to evolve for 4 to 5 days, and the process of

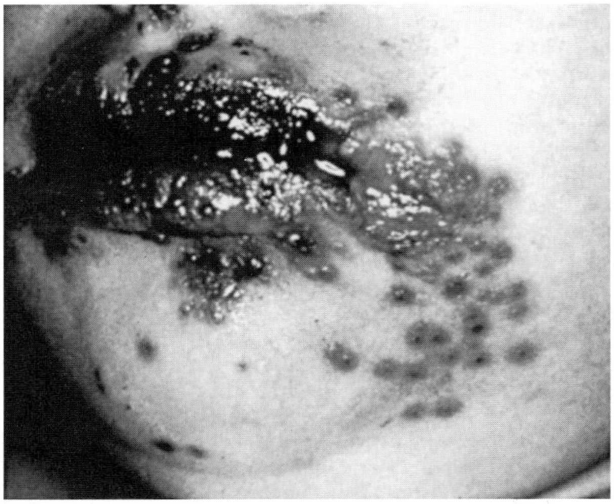

FIGURE 163–1. *Primary HSV gingivostomatitis in a normal toddler; ulcerative-vesicular stage. (Courtesy of Dr. Theodore Rosen, Department of Dermatology, Baylor College of Medicine, Houston, TX.)*

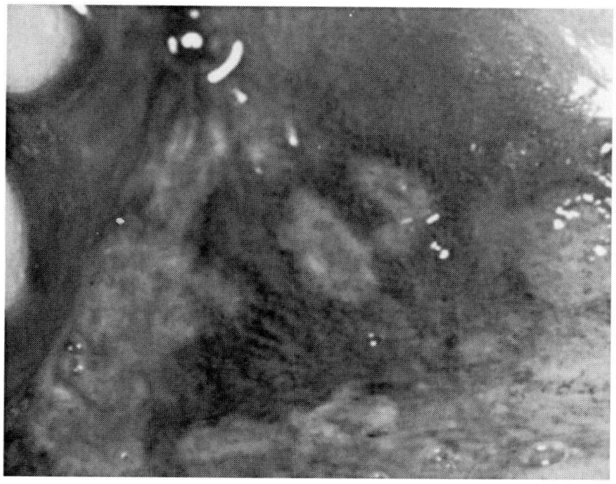

FIGURE 163–2. *Primary HSV gingivostomatitis in a 6-year-old, demonstrating involvement of oral mucosa with ulcers.*

resolution requires at least an additional week. Herpetic epiglottitis[31] and acute otitis media[54] are unusual complications.

HSV gingivostomatitis is differentiated from herpangina, a manifestation of enteroviral infection, by the predominance of ulcers in the anterior and posterior portion of the oropharynx; herpangina usually is a posterior pharyngeal ulcerative condition. In addition, unlike HSV infection, herpangina often has a more acute onset, shorter duration, and seasonal occurrence.[227] Whereas enteroviral-associated hand-foot-mouth disease can present with oral ulcers and a vesicular eruption on the distal portion of extremities, the bilaterally symmetric distribution should differentiate it from HSV gingivostomatitis and concurrent HSV autoinoculation to a digit. Severe Stevens-Johnson syndrome (erythema multiforme) may mimic HSV infection, but the generalized macular rash accompanied by "bull's-eye" lesions is characteristic of erythema multiforme. HSV can be associated with erythema multiforme (see later discussion). Impetigo may be confused with the lesions of HSV.

In adolescents, and especially patients of college age, primary HSV infection not uncommonly presents as a posterior, occasionally exudative pharyngitis. The characteristic findings are shallow tonsillar ulcers with a gray exudate. In this setting, it must be differentiated from streptococcal and Epstein-Barr virus infection and rarely from diphtheria, acute HIV infection, or tularemia-induced pharyngitis. In one study of college students of a higher socioeconomic level, HSV was the etiologic agent of acute pharyngitis (24 per cent) diagnosed most commonly.[111] A more recent study of 613 college students with upper respiratory complaints documented an incidence of 5.7 per cent with positive HSV cultures. Twelve of the 35 students with positive cultures had vesicular lesions on the lips, throat, or gums, and 29 of the 35 had a primary diagnosis of pharyngitis that was indistinguishable from other causes of pharyngitis.[191] This manifestation most often is due to HSV-1, although with increasing frequency of oral-genital sexual practice among both heterosexual and homosexual persons, HSV-2 pharyngitis is more common.

In view of the widespread publicity of HSV infection as a sexually transmitted disease, the physician is advised, when making the diagnosis of HSV oral infection, to anticipate these anxieties, and, unless sexual contact or abuse is suspected, to explain the normal mode of acquisition of oral HSV infection in young children.

Vulvovaginitis

Primary herpetic vulvovaginitis rarely occurs in very young infants and children if HSV is introduced inadvertently when the genital area is handled with contaminated hands. Moreover, genital herpes may reflect sexual abuse of young children. Just as with the occurrence of other potentially sexually transmitted diseases, the occurrence of genital HSV infection in young children warrants a sensitive and careful appraisal of the family dynamics.

The incidence of genital infection has increased markedly in the past two decades.[48, 49, 55] There is a paucity of data concerning the incidence in children. Whereas the mean age of incidence was 30 ± 11 years in males and 26 ± 11 years in females, the incidence was 3 per 100,000 in the 10- to 14-year-old age group and 76 per 100,000 in the 15- to 19-year-old age group in Rochester, Minnesota (a predominantly white, middle-class population of northern European extraction).[55]

Thirty-five to 50 per cent of patients with the first episode of genital herpes are able to give a history of genital HSV infection in their contact. After careful questioning and instruction, 50 to 60 per cent of persons without a history of HSV infection can identify symptoms consistent with previous infection.[170] Even when a careful clinical history is obtained, many HSV-2–seropositive patients are missed unless serologic studies are performed.[38] The transmission rate between sexual partners was approximately 10 to 12 per cent per year.[40, 193–195] HSV-1 accounts for 5 to 25 per cent of primary genital HSV infections in the United States, whereas up to 50 per cent of cases diagnosed in Sheffield, England, were due to type 1. There are indications that, in the United States, HSV-1 is becoming a more common primary genital isolate. The incubation period is 2 to 14 days. Primary illness is accompanied by fever, headache, malaise, and myalgias on 2 or more days in 40 per cent of men and nearly 70 per cent of women.[60, 62] Other systemic symptoms include an aseptic meningitis syndrome (11 to 35 per cent). This is manifested as fever, stiff neck, headache, and photophobia with a cerebrospinal fluid (CSF) lymphocytic cellular response and usually normal glucose.[127] Although HSV-2 may be grown from the CSF occasionally, this syndrome should be differentiated from HSV-1 encephalitis in that it generally is mild, self-limited, and not associated with neurologic residua. Local genital symptoms include severe pain (in 95 per cent of men and 99 per cent of women), itching, dysuria (44 per cent of men and 83 per cent of women), vaginal or urethral discharge, and tender inguinal adenopathy (80 per cent). In primary illness, the lesions begin as vesicles or pustules and progress to wet ulcers and then to healing ulcers with or without crusts (Figs. 163–3, 163–4, and 163–5). Crusts usually occur only on squamous epithelium. Lesions tend to last for 2 to 3 weeks before complete healing (mean, 19 days). They may spread in a wavelike fashion from the initial site to thighs, buttocks, and bladder. Virus shedding occurs for a mean of 11½ days.[60, 62]

Nearly one-third of women with positive cultures for HSV have no or atypical lesions (e.g., fissures, furuncles, excoriations).[161] A standard history and clinical examination only identifies 39 per cent of women with past or current urogenital or anogenital HSV infection.[161] Patients who have primary HSV-1 genital infections may have lesions elsewhere (25 per cent), typically on the hands and face.[26] Those who have HSV-2 primary infections have extragenital lesions (9 per cent), typically on the buttocks.[26]

In addition to an aseptic meningitis syndrome, complications of primary HSV genital infection include sacral autonomic nervous dysfunction (21 per cent of cases, manifested

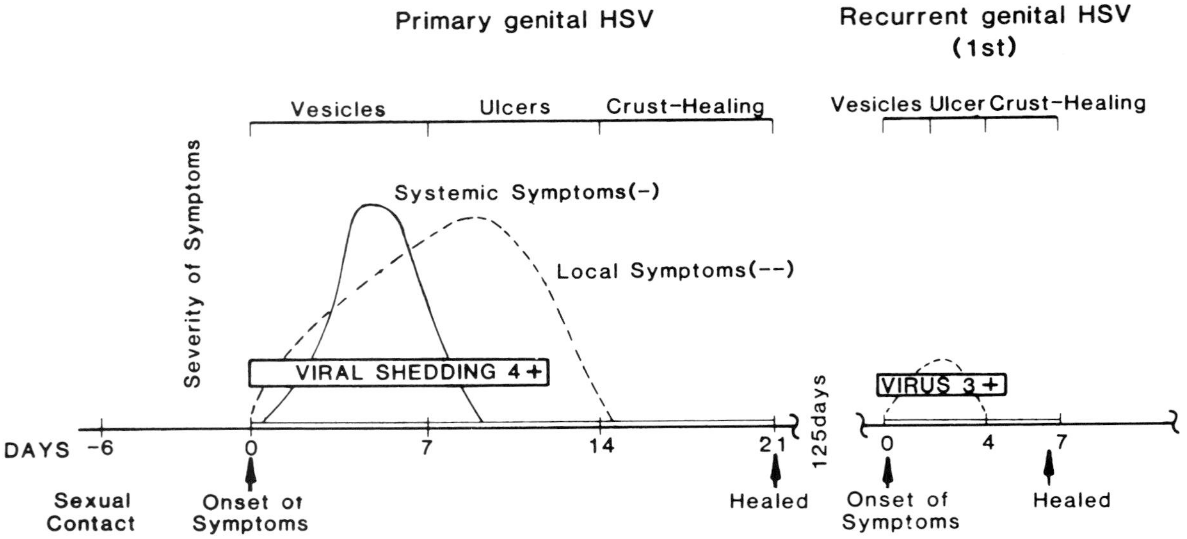

FIGURE 163–3. *Graphic representation of the course of primary and recurrent HSV genital infection. The days illustrated are for the average cases.*

as poor rectal sphincter tone, constipation, sacral anesthesia, urinary retention, or impotence), extragenital lesions (20 per cent, more common in women, often about the buttocks, groin, thighs, or less commonly fingers or conjunctiva, usually occurring in the second week of disease), secondary yeast infections in women (14 per cent), and pharyngitis (19 per cent, usually associated with fever, malaise, myalgia, headache, tender anterior cervical adenopathy, and a mildly erythematous to diffusely ulcerative or exudative posterior pharyngitis; most of these patients have throat cultures positive for HSV).[60, 62] HSV has been associated uncommonly with acute salpingitis[176] or inguinal lymphadenitis.[309] Of critical

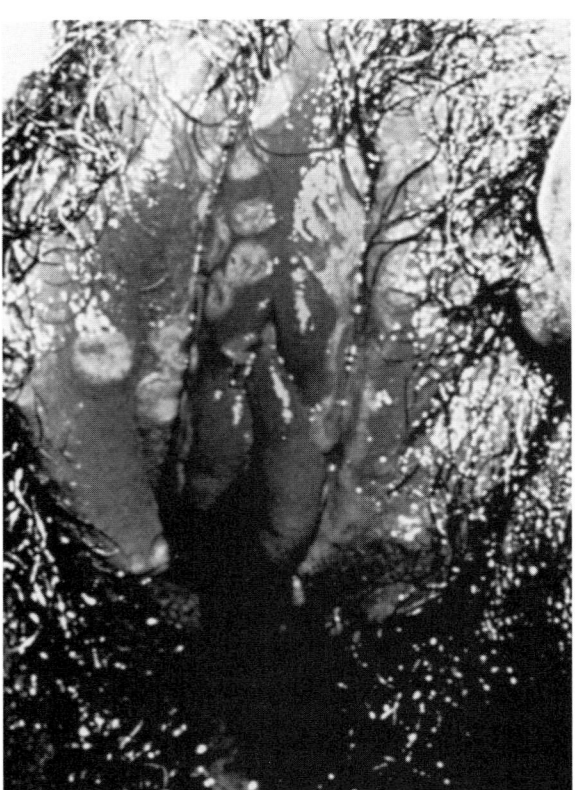

FIGURE 163–4. *Primary genital herpes in a female. (Courtesy of Dr. Theodore Rosen, Department of Dermatology, Baylor College of Medicine, Houston, TX.)*

importance has been the association of prior HSV infection with increased incidence of HIV infection, perhaps due to the genital ulcers of HSV that facilitate HIV transmission.[294]

Beyond the discomfort and embarrassment, the importance of the presence of HSV in the female genital tract relates to (1) the potential impact of the virus on offspring, especially when the child is born in the presence of active genital lesions, particularly in connection with a primary maternal infection (see discussion of prenatal and neonatal herpesvirus infections in Chapter 76), and (2) the possible relevance of these infections to the subsequent appearance of carcinoma of the genital tract.[212]

Perhaps the greatest problem is the effect of genital HSV infection on the self-image of the young, sexually active patient. Whereas some persons have little difficulty coping with the illness and the likelihood of recurrent disease, a sizable group develops a syndrome of profound depression, poor self-esteem, complete abstention from sexual activities, and general withdrawal. This "leper syndrome" must be anticipated, discussed when appropriate, and dealt with in a sensitive and caring manner. Self-help groups of persons who have had genital HSV infection have been found to be useful. They are present in many parts of the United States and can be contacted through the American Social Health Association, Herpes Resource Center, P.O. Box 13827, Research Triangle Park, North Carolina, 27709.

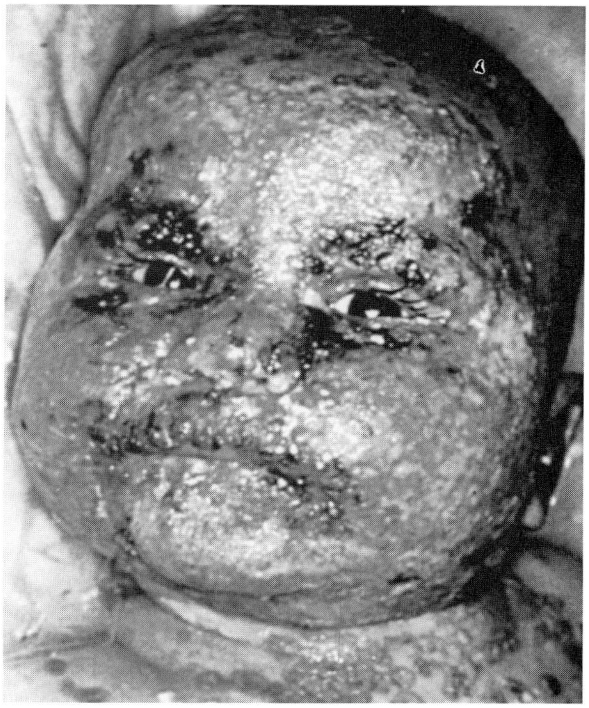

FIGURE 163–6. *Extensive HSV infection in an infant with atopic eczema (Kaposi varicelliform eruption). (Courtesy of Dr. Theodore Rosen, Department of Dermatology, Baylor College of Medicine, Houston, TX.)*

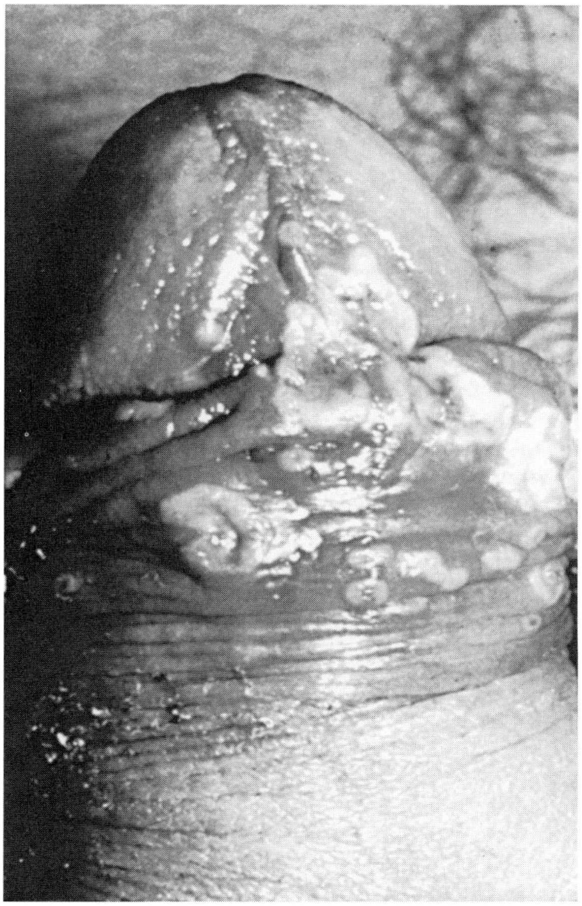

FIGURE 163–5. *Primary genital HSV infection in a male. (Courtesy of Dr. Theodore Rosen, Department of Dermatology, Baylor College of Medicine, Houston, TX.)*

Other Primary Herpes Simplex Virus Skin Infections

Virtually any part of the skin and mucous membranes may be involved in HSV infections. Mucocutaneous junction areas particularly are liable to infection, and, as noted, altered skin often provides a portal of entry for HSV. Vesicular lesions spread throughout the affected skin, usually crusting and resolving in about 1 week. The illness accompanying eczema herpeticum can be severe and even fatal, although in most cases the infection resolves without specific therapy and leaves no sequelae (Fig. 163–6).[32] Similar widespread herpetic lesions may occur in skin altered by thermal or chemical burns. In this situation, usually 1 to several weeks after the initial insult, a secondary fever may occur. Careful inspection of the burn site or adjacent normal tissue may reveal vesicles (Fig. 163–7) or nonspecific ulcerative lesions. Without ther-

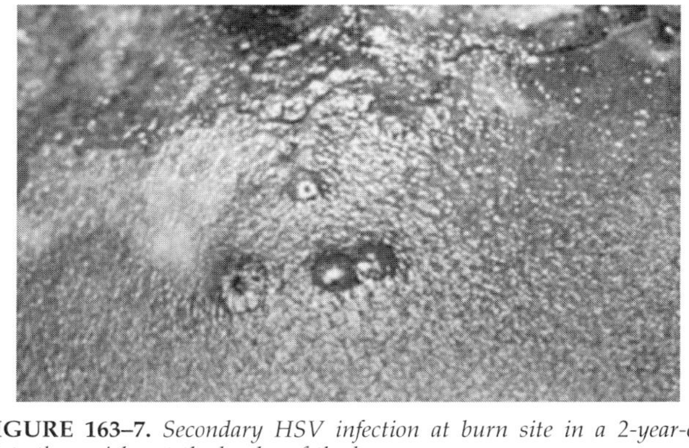

FIGURE 163–7. *Secondary HSV infection at burn site in a 2-year-old. Note the vesicles at the border of the burn.*

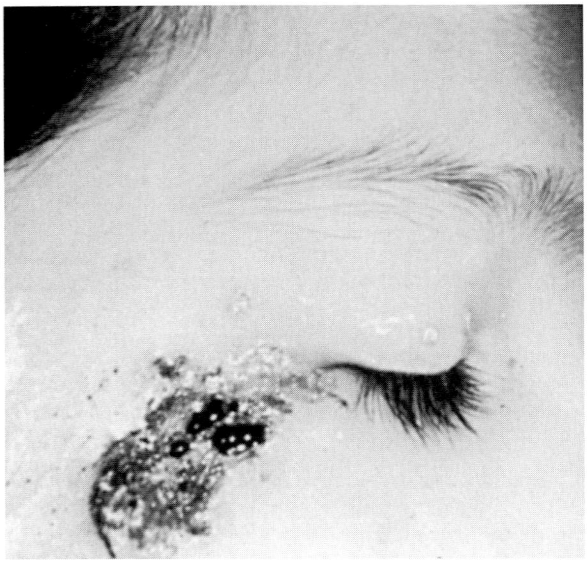

FIGURE 163–8. *Facial HSV infection in a young girl after mild abrasion. (Courtesy of Dr. Johnie Frazier, Department of Pediatrics, University of Texas Medical School, Houston, TX.)*

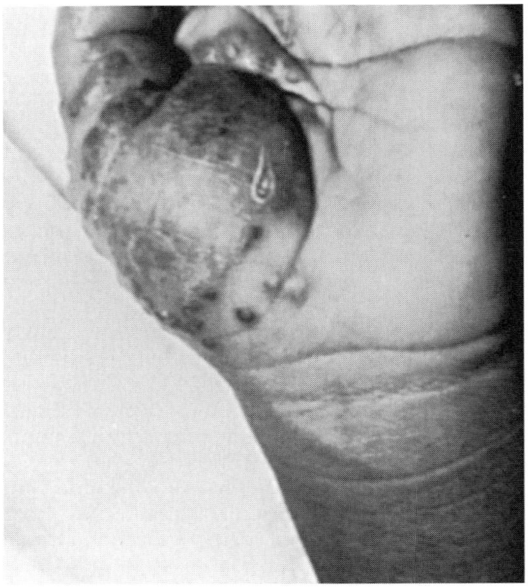

FIGURE 163–9. *Extensive herpetic whitlow in a toddler with oral HSV infection.*

apy, several of these patients have died of disseminated HSV infection.[101] I rarely have seen a similar syndrome in children after simple skin abrasions (Fig. 163–8). Herpetic recurrences may follow in these instances, localized to the particular areas of skin initially invaded. HSV infection has been severe at the site of common diaper rash as a secondary infection.[135]

Herpetic whitlow is a painful, erythematous, swollen lesion occurring at a site of broken skin on the terminal phalanx, usually a damaged cuticle.[23, 110, 250, 297] The fingers (69 per cent) and thumb (21 per cent) are involved most frequently.[110] Less commonly, the palm may be the site of inoculation and major involvement.[265] The painful white swellings appear to be filled with pus but, when opened for drainage, are found to contain little fluid and no purulent material. The white appearance is due to the presence of necrotic epithelial cells. Occasionally, the whitlow, which may persist for 7 to 10 days, is accompanied initially by a few vesicles that may give a clue to the etiologic agent of the primary infection. Less commonly, the whitlow is associated with fever, lymphadenopathy, and lymphangitis.[260]

Whitlows are seen in four typical situations. Most commonly, infants with primary herpetic gingivostomatitis autoinoculate their fingers (Fig. 163–9). At times, whitlows are encountered in infants without obvious oral disease, sometimes due to adults kissing their children's fingers. In these two settings, the viral isolate almost always is HSV-1.[23, 110] In sexually active patients, the whitlow more commonly is a manifestation of concurrent genital disease, which should be sought by appropriate history and physical examination.[112] These most commonly are due to HSV-2. In the fourth setting, persons such as dentists, respiratory therapists, nurses, and pediatricians, who often examine oral cavities or handle secretion-contaminated material without wearing gloves, are at risk for herpetic whitlow (Fig. 163–10). In addition, the same behavior facilitates a well-documented transfer of HSV to other patients, especially in intensive care settings.[3, 96]

It is important that the herpetic condition be diagnosed because it usually is confused with a bacterial felon or paronychia and is incised and drained. This is not indicated in the therapy of HSV whitlow. A needle aspiration and culture are all that are necessary for diagnosis of the whitlow.

In several sports, cutaneous (especially facial) HSV infection is a hazard, particularly in sports with close physical contact, such as wrestling (herpes gladiatorum) and rugby (scrum pox, derived from the line-up of rugby players, the "scrum," or "scrummage").[25, 50, 278, 281, 332] Often, the initial lesions are diagnosed as impetigo, unless HSV is considered. Approximately 3 per cent of wrestlers in high school develop HSV infection, typically on the head and neck but also on the extremities, trunk, and eyes.[50]

Herpes Simplex Virus Infection of the Eye[74, 178, 229, 234, 342]

Primary infection of the eye by HSV may occur as blepharitis or follicular conjunctivitis. This often is accompanied by preauricular lymphadenopathy, corneal injection, watering, discharge, itching, lid swelling, and, in one-third of cases, malaise and fever. If restricted to the conjunctivae, the infection (which can be accompanied by vesicular herpetic lesions elsewhere on the face or in the nose or mouth) usually resolves without sequelae or specific features. Herpetic infection of the eye may, however, progress to involve the cornea with far more serious potential consequences; for this reason,

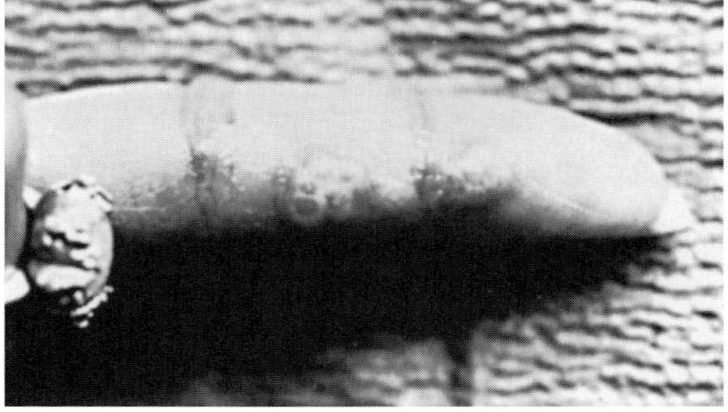

FIGURE 163–10. *Recurrent herpetic whitlow in a pediatrician.*

an ophthalmologic consultant always should examine and evaluate these cases.

Corneal involvement by HSV may be manifested initially by minute vesicles at the corneal margin. The progress of corneal infection (best seen with the use of topical fluorescein dye) is marked by the appearance of branching lesions (a dendritic pattern) or the less diagnostic irregular (ameboid or geographic) ulcer.[24] The child complains of severe photophobia, accompanied in some cases by blurred vision, chemosis, and lacrimation. Primary eye infection may include stromal involvement, uveitis, and rarely retinitis. Retinitis is manifested as multiple, whitish-yellow, punctate retinal lesions. Spontaneous healing, which generally requires 2 to 3 weeks, can be speeded by topical therapy (see later discussion). Corticosteroids are contraindicated. The risk of visual impairment due to direct viral damage, immunopathologic reactions, or both is enhanced greatly if there are recurrences. With each bout of infection, the corneal ulcers become more extensive and are liable to result in scarring and impairment of sight. Herpetic infection of the eye recurs in approximately 32 per cent of patients who have primary symptomatic infection and is more common in younger patients.[341] Recurrences may occur as blepharitis; follicular conjunctivitis with or without lid lesions; or ulcers and keratitis, which more often are accompanied by ulcerations deeper into the corneal stroma (diskiform or necrotizing keratitis) with resultant extensive scarring, irregular astigmatism, and even corneal perforation. Children who have dendritic ulcers have a better prognosis for good vision than do those with geographic or diskiform keratitis.[24] Rarely, in normal and immunocompromised patients (especially those with AIDS), HSV eye infection may result in an acute retinal necrosis.[103] Rarely, an oculoglandular syndrome of conjunctivitis and adenopathy may be due to HSV infection.[45]

Herpes Simplex Virus Infections of the Central Nervous System[153, 155, 206, 215, 216, 264, 284, 337, 339]

HSV is the most common identifiable cause of human acquired sporadic encephalitis and usually is serious as well. It accounts for 2 to 5 per cent of all encephalitis in the United States but for up to 20 per cent of all etiologic diagnoses (60 to 70 per cent of encephalitis remains without an etiologic diagnosis).[47, 242] With the advent of immunization for measles, mumps, rubella, and varicella, the relative incidence of HSV among cases of encephalitis has increased, although absolute numbers remain stable in children.[158, 242] The case-fatality rate associated with untreated HSV encephalitis is approximately 70 per cent,[337, 338] and survivors generally exhibit considerable permanent neurologic disability. Both HSV-1 and HSV-2 have been implicated in the etiology of infection of the CNS caused by HSV.[66] The spread of HSV-1 to the CNS seems to proceed via either neurogenic pathways or hematogenous dissemination or through the cribriform plate from infected nasopharyngeal mucosa in primary infection. Recurrent infection probably results from spread via sensory neurons.[75] HSV-2 meningitis probably follows hematogenous dissemination or neurogenic pathways.

Although HSV encephalitis may involve virtually any area of the brain, there is a striking tendency for this infection to involve the orbital region of the frontal lobes and, with particular frequency, portions of the temporal lobes. Johnson and Mims have suggested that the predilection of HSV to involve regions of the brain governing olfaction suggests that a pathogenetic pathway proceeds from the nasal-respiratory mucosa via the olfactory bulbs and along the subsequent tracts into the brain.[138] Others have suggested that reactivated virus travels from the trigeminal ganglia via the fifth nerve fibers to the meninges of the anterior and middle fossae.[75] More recent studies in children using polymerase chain reaction (PCR) diagnosis and magnetic resonance imaging (MRI) have defined cases with more diffuse cerebral involvement.[266]

It is important to differentiate the HSV-induced aseptic meningitis syndrome, usually caused by HSV-2 and usually a complication of primary genital infection, from HSV encephalitis. In the HSV-induced aseptic meningitis syndrome, signs of meningitis, including headache, photophobia, and stiff neck, appear shortly after genital lesions are noted. This syndrome may occur in young children as well as in adults.[82] HSV-2 meningitis may occur less commonly in the absence of genital lesions[269] or rarely in neonates.[267] Seizures and focal CNS findings usually are absent. The spinal fluid examination reveals lymphocytosis (with 300 to 2600 white blood cells) and may demonstrate low glucose.[60] This syndrome may recur with genital recurrences. Recovery usually is complete without specific therapy. HSV occasionally may be grown from the spinal fluid,[66, 127] although at this time only the PCR test may be diagnostic.[268] Studies using PCR DNA detection analysis have shown that HSV is the major agent responsible for benign recurrent lymphocytic meningitis, also known as Mollaret meningitis.[310] These adult patients had three to nine attacks of recurrent lymphocytic meningitis with 48 to 1600 cells/L, normal glucose, and proteins of 41 to 240 mg/dL in the CSF. PCR analysis detected HSV-2 and, less commonly, HSV-1.[310]

HSV encephalitis, in contrast with meningitis, is a highly lethal disease.[337, 338] In 93 to 96 per cent of cases, it is caused by HSV-1.[13, 216] It may be a result of primary (30 per cent) or recurrent (70 per cent) infection.[216] Although there are no specific data because the prevalence of latent HSV is lower in children than in adults, a larger percentage of HSV encephalitis in younger persons probably is caused by primary infection. One report suggests that primary infection is more likely to be associated with fatal encephalitis.[157] Of 113 cases of biopsy-documented HSV encephalitis, 31 per cent occurred in patients younger than 20 years of age, and 6 to 10 per cent of patients were between 6 months and 10 years of age.[284, 338] As in most manifestations of HSV, but unlike most other common forms of viral encephalitis (enterovirus, arbovirus), HSV encephalitis is not seasonal. It is an acute illness with fever, malaise, irritability, and nonspecific symptoms lasting 1 to 7 days, with progression to signs and symptoms of CNS involvement in 3 to 7 days and finally to coma and death (Table 163–1). A biphasic illness with initial improvement followed by worsening may occur.[251] Any child who has fever and altered behavior should evoke the suspicion of

TABLE 163–1. Historical and Clinical Findings in HSV Encephalitis[18, 284, 338, 339]

Historical Findings		Clinical Findings at Presentations	
Alteration of consciousness	97%	Fever	92%
		Personality changes	85%
Fever	90%	Dysphasia	76%
Headache	81%	Autonomic dysfunction	60%
Persistent seizures	67%	Ataxia	40%
Personality change	71%	Seizures	38%
Vomiting	46%	Focal	28%
Hemiparesis	33%	Generalized	10%
Memory loss	24%	Cranial nerve defects	32%
		Visual field loss	14%
		Papilledema	14%

encephalitis.[215] Meningeal signs are uncommon. There is no correlation between the isolation of HSV from sites extrinsic to the CNS (such as the oropharynx or genital tract) and the diagnosis of HSV encephalitis.[216] Thus, the presence of oral or genital lesions is of no help in diagnosis or exclusion of HSV encephalitis.[216] Identical viruses have been isolated from the brain and oral secretions.[335]

The CSF generally reveals pleocytosis with up to 2000 white blood cells/mm^3, usually (80 per cent of the time) greater than 50 white blood cells/mm^3. In 90 per cent of cases, more than 60 per cent of the cells are lymphocytes. Early in infection, neutrophils may predominate. In 75 to 85 per cent of cases, red blood cells, reflecting the hemorrhagic necrosis, are seen in the CSF. Between 5 and 25 per cent of patients have hypoglycorrhachia, and 80 to 88 per cent have elevated protein levels in the CSF (median, 80 mg/dL), which rise to striking levels as the disease progresses. Two to three per cent of patients who have early HSV encephalitis have normal CSF.[18, 159, 216, 339] A repeated analysis of the CSF usually reveals abnormalities consistent with encephalitis. HSV almost never is grown from lumbar spinal fluid and has been grown rarely from ventricular fluid.[102] Thus, whereas the CSF examination is helpful, it is not at all diagnostic of HSV encephalitis. When CSF from patients with HSV encephalitis is compared with CSF from patients undergoing biopsy for suspected HSV, with other resultant diagnosis, there are no differentiating characteristics of the CSF that could allow one accurately to predict HSV.[338] Some reports describe successful detection of HSV DNA in the CSF of patients who have HSV encephalitis by use of the PCR test.[12, 79, 168, 253, 315]

Neurodiagnostic tests have been of limited assistance. Probably one of the most useful is the electroencephalogram (EEG) (Fig. 163–11).[37, 339] A "typical" pattern of unilateral or bilateral (poor prognosis) periodic focal spikes against a background of slow (flattened) activity (paroxysmal lateral epileptiform discharges, or PLEDS) has been associated with HSV encephalitis. These findings are suggestive but not pathognomonic. Other findings include large-amplitude, irregular, slow activity; sharp waves; and variable spikes. In 80 to 90 per cent of patients, the EEG is not only abnormal but also localizing. In my experience with cases in the pediatric and adult age groups, the EEG was one of the earliest localizing laboratory tests.[80, 117, 155] Less commonly, results of a radionucleotide scan or computed tomography (CT) are abnormal and localizing (50 to 60 per cent of cases). CT results may be characteristic late in illness, with low-density contrast-enhanced lesions in the temporal area, mass effect, edema, and hemorrhage (Fig. 163–12); early in the illness, when diagnosis is critical, CT results more often are unremarkable.[117, 155, 206] Indeed, abnormal CT results are a poor prognostic factor.[206] Reports suggest that the MRI may be abnormal on presentation with HSV encephalitis because of its high sensitivity to changes in brain water content (Fig. 163–13).[273] MRI findings are more sensitive than CT findings for detection of HSV encephalitis.[78] These include hyperintensity on T2 images of temporal areas and Gd enhancement. This also has been my experience. Use of single photon emission CT appears promising.

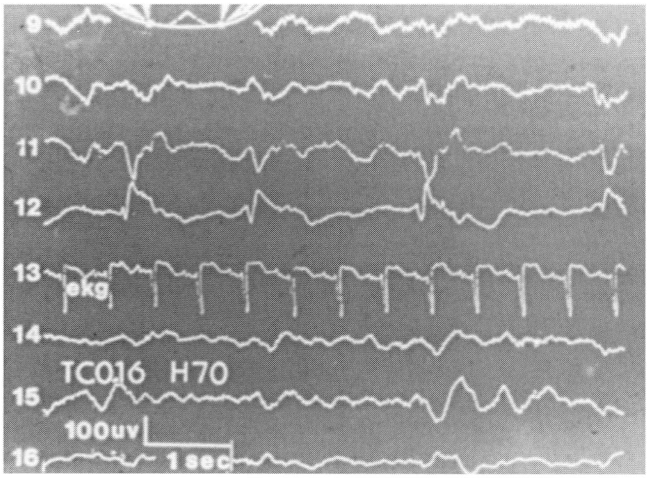

FIGURE 163–11. *Electroencephalogram in a 9-month-old with HSV encephalitis. Note paroxysmal discharges, in lead 12 especially.*

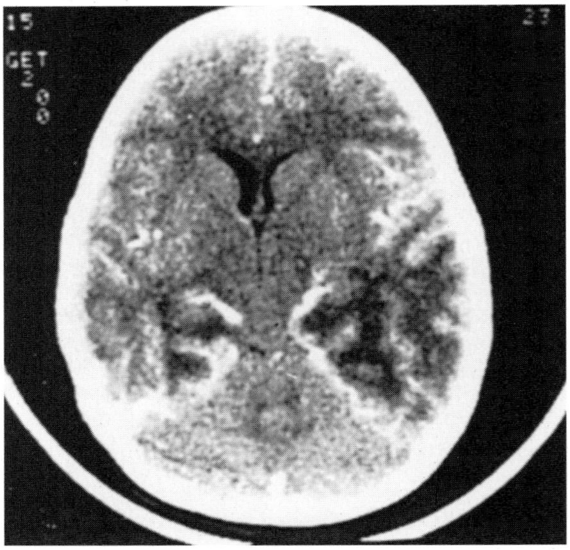

FIGURE 163–12. *Computed tomographic scan 1 week after onset of HSV encephalitis in a 6-year-old. Note bilateral temporal low-density areas with dye enhancement and the greater mass effect on the patient's left side than on the right side.*

The finding of focal abnormality on EEG, CT, MRI, or radionuclide brain scan is significantly more likely in HSV encephalitis than in other illnesses confused with it.[339] All of these findings are biased by our current concept of HSV encephalitis as a focal encephalitis, with very few biopsy data on the etiology of nonfocal encephalitis. It is unknown whether a significant number of cases of HSV encephalitis are milder and nonfocal, because few of these ever come to brain biopsy or even careful retrospective serologic diagnosis. Studies using MRI and PCR technology have identified cases with multifocal brain involvement[267] or mild clinical courses.[79]

Thus, the clinical and laboratory data acquired are valuable only in increasing the index of suspicion for, but not in confirming the diagnosis of, HSV encephalitis. The differential diagnosis of this condition is relatively large, with many treatable conditions (Table 163–2). Especially in the pediatric age range, the ability to discriminate HSV encephalitis from other etiologic agents mimicking it is poor (50 per cent in the national collaborative series in 71 patients younger than 20 years of age[338] and 42 per cent in a smaller series of 12 patients younger than 12 years of age).[155] It remains essential to confirm the specific diagnosis of HSV encephalitis, both to provide optimal aggressive therapy for that condition and, of equal importance, to achieve a diagnosis for the 50 to 60 per cent of patients without HSV infections, roughly 16 per cent of whom would benefit from other specific thera-

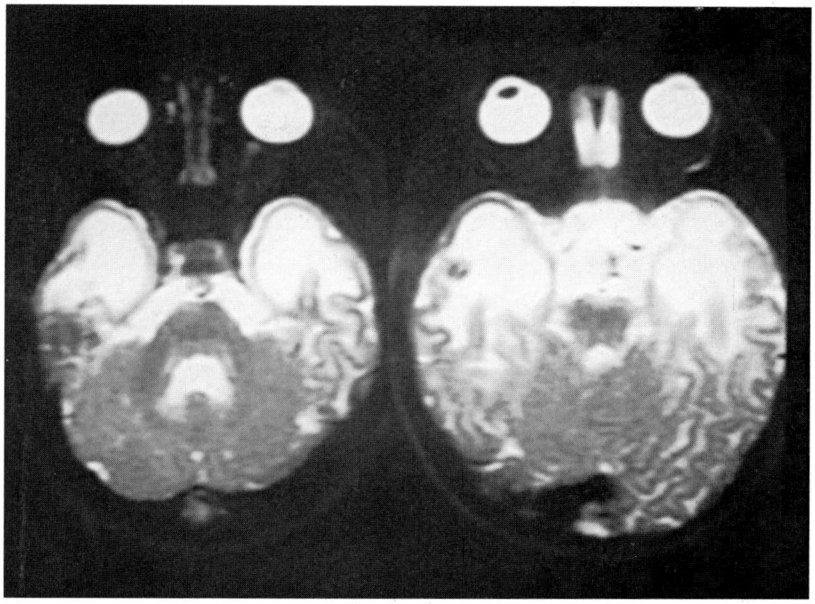

FIGURE 163–13. *Magnetic resonance image in a patient with HSV encephalitis. Note the increased signal intensity bilaterally in the temporal lobes. (From Kohl, S.: Herpes simplex virus encephalitis in children. Pediatr. Clin. North Am. 35:465–483, 1988.)*

pies.[80, 155, 206, 334, 338] In most cases, this can be accomplished by PCR analysis of the CSF.[12, 120, 168, 253, 266, 268, 315, 319] Large studies show PCR analysis to be 98 per cent sensitive and 94 per cent specific when compared with brain biopsy.[168] Some of the 6 per cent "false-positive" results probably were due to poor handling of the biopsy tissue for culture.[168] PCR analysis may yield positive results 1 day after onset of symptoms.[120] PCR primers must be chosen to detect HSV-2, as well as HSV-1, because 4 to 6 per cent of HSV encephalitis cases may be caused by HSV-2.[13] If PCR results are negative in a patient who has symptoms and signs of HSV encephalitis, a brain biopsy may be contemplated.

The risk of brain biopsy is low. In the national collaborative study of 432 biopsies, there were six complications (hemorrhage in three patients and poorly controlled brain edema in three patients; 1.4 per cent complication rate).[334] Roughly 2 to 3 per cent of brain biopsies yielded false-negative results, usually because of biopsy of the wrong site.[334, 338] A decision analysis suggests that biopsy especially is critical in patients with low CSF glucose.[263]

A less acute form of HSV encephalitis in immunocompromised patients has been reported (see later discussion). Also less commonly, HSV has been implicated in brain stem encephalitis.[91] Relapse occurs in approximately 5 per cent of treated patients.[153] Choreoathetosis may be an initial sign of relapse.[327] There are increasingly frequent reports of a postherpectic encephalomyelitis caused by a probable autoimmune or demyelinating etiologic factor[1, 151]; also, there are reports of virus-positive recurrences of HSV encephalitis months after apparently successful therapy.[76, 81] These can be differentiated and documented only by PCR analysis or, if necessary, brain biopsy and appropriate tissue histologic examination and culture.

Herpes Simplex Virus Infection of the Gastrointestinal Tract in Normal Hosts

Whereas infection of visceral organs is well recognized in immunocompromised hosts, less has been written concerning this in apparently normal persons.[225] Several publications have documented HSV esophagitis in normal patients, including several patients from 11 months to 17 years of age.[6, 20, 105, 205] It usually is caused by HSV-1 and associated with primary infection.[105] The presenting symptoms include fever, severe odynophagia, retrosternal and subxiphoid pain, and inability to eat. Skin lesions generally are absent. Esophagoscopy reveals ulcerations and fibrinous, and at times hemorrhagic, exudate. Distal involvement may be more extensive than proximal esophageal findings suggest. Double-contrast esophagography may be diagnostic, although endoscopy and biopsy usually are necessary for definitive diagnosis.[105] Symptoms usually remit in 5 to 7 days, after nonspecific therapy such as antacids, H2-blockers, and hydration.[6, 205]

Of importance is the delineation of involvement of the other end of the gastrointestinal tract with HSV, especially manifesting as an anorectal infection in homosexual males.[116, 238, 329] This syndrome occasionally affects women practicing passive anal intercourse. In most series of HSV proctitis, the younger persons are adolescent males involved in passive anal intercourse. Presenting symptoms include severe anorectal pain, discharge, tenesmus, hematochezia, and, in particular, fever, difficulty in urinating, sacral paresthesias, constipation, and (in 50 to 70 per cent of patients) ulcers or vesicles in the perianal or distal rectal area.[116, 238, 329] The duration of symptoms is 2 to 3 weeks. Primary HSV infection accounts for proctitis in this group in 25 to 30 per cent of cases. Syphilis and infection with *Giardia lamblia, Entamoeba histolytica, Campylobacter fetus, Shigella,* other enteric bacteria, and *Neisseria gonorrhoeae* also must be considered in the differential diagnosis of this entity. Appropriate cultures and histologic analysis are crucial for establishing a specific diagnosis.

Hepatitis caused by HSV in the immunocompetent host is rare. In a review of the literature that found 35 patients who had HSV-associated hepatitis, 14 per cent had no underlying condition. The remainder had various immunocompromising conditions, such as transplantation, steroid administration, pregnancy, burns, primary immunodeficiency, or cancer. These patients tended to have fulminant hepatic necrosis, extremely elevated serum transaminase levels, disseminated intravascular coagulation, and a mortality rate of 86 per cent.[51] In a prospective study of normal young adults who had genital herpes (primary or recurrent), 14 per cent had mild elevations in liver enzyme tests.[197]

TABLE 163–2. Differential Diagnosis of HSV Encephalitis[153, 284, 334, 337, 338]

Infections	Noninfectious Disorders
Fungal	Tumor
Especially *Cyptococcus*	Vascular disease
Bacterial	Arteriovenous malformations
Abscess, cerebritis	Toxins
Listeria monocytogenes meningitis	Alcoholic encephalopathy
Lyme disease	Leukemia
Subdural, epidural empyema	Cerebral infarction
Tuberculosis	Adrenal leukodystrophy
Bacterial endocarditis	
Meningococcal meningitis	
Protozoal	
Toxoplasmosis	
Amebic	
Rickettsial	
Viral	
Mumps virus	
Coxsackievirus, echovirus	
Arbovirus (especially St. Louis, California, and eastern and western equine encephalitis)	
Postinfluenzal encephalitis	
Reye syndrome	
Lymphocytic choriomeningitis virus	
Rabies virus	
Epstein-Barr virus	
Human herpesvirus–6	
Rubella virus	
Cytomegalovirus	
Adenovirus	
Tick-borne encephalitis virus	
Powassan virus	
Subacute sclerosing encephalitis (measles virus)	
Progressive multifocal leukoencephalopathy	

Recurrent Herpes Simplex Virus Infections

All of the sites discussed in connection with primary HSV disease also may be involved in recurrent infections. A striking and important feature of HSV infections is their capacity to establish a state of latency associated with episodes of reactivation in the presence of an apparently adequate immune response. Reactivation of HSV infection with viral shedding may occur in the absence of specific lesions. HSV has been found in the tears of persons with a history of recurrent ophthalmic disease, even in the absence of eye lesions or symptoms, and virus can be recovered from the pharynx and cervix of asymptomatic persons. Indeed, HSV has been recovered from the genital tract of 10 to 26 per cent of women with recurrent genital HSV at a time when there were no clinically apparent lesions.[2, 36] All women who obtained samples on more than 100 days had documented asymptomatic viral shedding.[36] Shedding occurred in 1 per cent of days on which cultures were obtained.[36]

Persons who experience recurrent herpes infections maintain stable levels of serum immunity to HSV and usually do not exhibit significant changes of antibody titer in connection with episodes of reactivation, although a small proportion of patients have significant (fourfold or greater) rises in anti-HSV antibody levels and IgM or IgA responses with recurrences.

Several studies have documented cyclic changes in lymphocyte subset markers and cell-mediated immune functions, including anti-HSV lymphocyte transformation (blastogenesis), interferon production, interleukin-2 production, other lymphokine production, and various cell-mediated cytotoxicity mechanisms.[46, 64, 163, 243] Nevertheless, although immunocompromised persons have more frequent and severe recurrences, there is little evidence to suggest a specific immunodeficiency in otherwise normal persons who have recurrent HSV infection.

The stimulus for reactivation of latent virus may be provided by iatrogenic or naturally occurring episodes of immunosuppression or depression, by endocrine (such as menstruation) or exogenous factors (such as trauma, sun, acupuncture, emotional stress) that influence features of cell-mediated immunity, or by unexplained and as yet unpredictable factors. Ultraviolet light irradiation of persons who have a history of recurrent oral herpes reliably induces recurrences either early (within 48 hours) or 2 to 7 days later.[288]

Skin subject to recurrent HSV infection has been transplanted elsewhere on the body, exchanged with skin taken from the site of graft placement and previously not involved in HSV infections. Subsequent recurrences of HSV infection were found to be localized to the original site, not to the original skin. These studies and others strongly suggest that the virus is not residing latent in the cells of the skin. Currently, most evidence favors the persistence of latent HSV in neural elements innervating the affected areas of skin and mucous membranes.

Evidence related to a possible neural site for latent HSV was presented nearly 80 years ago when Cushing reported the appearance of herpetic vesicles in the trigeminal distribution after rhizotomy of the trigeminal nerve and destruction of the sensory ganglion. Many additional observations have confirmed this evidence, indicating that trigeminal root operation often is followed by the appearance of herpes simplex lesions.[17, 230] Persons who have recurrent HSV infections frequently describe tingling sensations, itching, and burning at the site of recurrence hours before the appearance of clusters of vesicles. Persons who have recurrent genital herpes may experience severe shooting leg pains and even urinary retention before and in connection with recurrent genital herpes infections. Additionally, recurrent HSV skin eruptions may occur in a zosteriform pattern and in a distribution reflecting the sensory innervation of a particular dermatome.

Nevertheless, attempts to recover HSV from suspensions of neural ganglia inoculated into tissue cultures were unsuccessful. Cocultivation techniques have been used to recover HSV from dorsal root ganglia subserving the areas of skin in which persons have experienced recurrent herpes lesions. HSV-1 has been found in trigeminal ganglia, and, appropriately enough, HSV-2 has been recovered from sacral ganglia.[16, 19] Molecular virologic studies have demonstrated limited RNA transcription of latent HSV in neural ganglia.[67, 68] The latency-associated transcripts are antisense relative to viral protein ICPO mRNA.[67, 68, 162] The role of these transcripts in the establishment or maintenance of latency remains to be clarified.[276] The presence of latency-associated transcripts appears to be necessary for efficient reactivation of viral production in vivo.[232]

The clinical manifestations of recurrent HSV infection depend on the area involved. Nearly all types of primary HSV infection cause a state of latency, which then acts as a focus for recurrence. In general, HSV recurrences are milder than the primary illness, although patients may have symptomatic recurrences without having had (or at least having remembered) a clinically apparent primary disease. Also, in general, a person with prior immunity to a heterologous virus (e.g., HSV-1) may have a first attack with HSV-2 that is milder than the typical primary infection, undoubtedly because of cross-reacting immunity.

There are several occasions in the normal host when a recurrent infection may be more severe than the primary. This particularly is true in HSV infection of the eye, in which recurrent illness is associated with deep stromal damage and scarring.[234] This may be related more to the exuberant immune response than to viral damage. HSV encephalitis, which may be a manifestation of recurrent illness (discussed earlier),[216, 335] surely is devastating.

The most common manifestation of recurrent HSV infection is herpes labialis ("cold sores," "fever blisters"). It is estimated to occur in 25 to 50 per cent of persons who have HSV-1 primary oral infection but much less frequently (24 per cent) in those who have HSV-2 primary oral infection.[167] The mean rate of recurrence after primary HSV-1 infection is approximately 0.1 per month.[167] These recurrences often are associated with a variety of febrile illnesses, local trauma, sun, or menstruation. Studies have described carefully the natural history of recurrent HSV labialis in adults.[14, 291] Because there are no similar data in children and no reason to expect differences, these are described.

Most persons experience a prodrome (pain, burning, tingling, or itching) at the site lasting 6 hours to several days. There is then an orderly progression from papules (lasting 12 to 36 hours) to vesicles (usually gone by 48 hours) and finally to ulcers and crust (lasting 2 to 4 days) (Fig. 163–14). The typical lesion size is from 35 to 80 mm^2. Most outbreaks are healed by 5 to 10 days (mean, 200 hours). Most pain occurs during the vesicular stage. Virus is isolated readily from vesicles (80 to 90 per cent of the time) and less commonly from ulcers and crusts (34 per cent of the time). Maximum virus titers (10^7 to 10^8) in lesions are measured in the first day or two, and virus generally is not isolated after 120 hours.[14, 291] Virus also may be detected in the saliva and on the hands of persons with herpes labialis.[318]

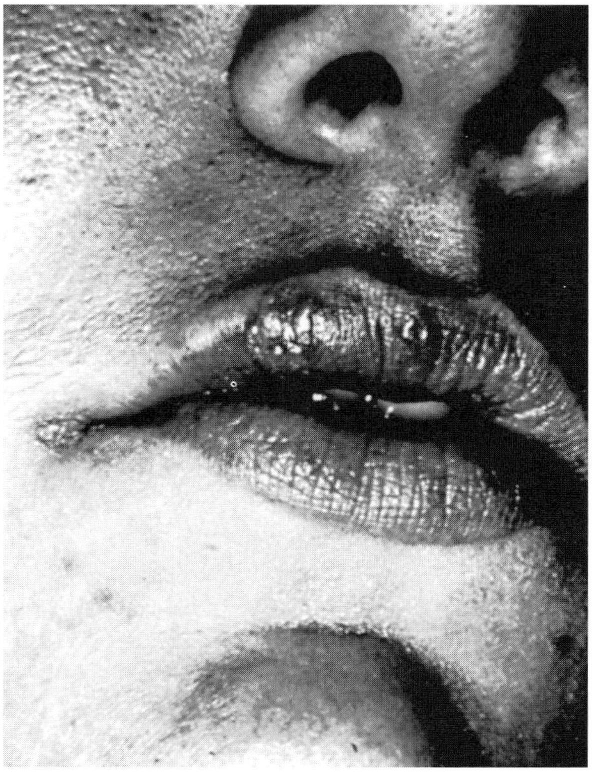

FIGURE 163–14. *Recurrent herpes labialis (cold sore) in an adolescent.*

Recurrences tend to affect the same location or closely related areas. In general, they occur on the lips, mucocutaneous junction, or other parts of the face. Recurrent lesions inside the mouth in normal hosts rarely are caused by HSV and are more likely aphthous lesions. When HSV recurrences are within the mouth, they tend to be on tissue adjacent to bone, such as the gums or palate, and not the lips or buccal mucosa.[288] A differential diagnosis of the condition also includes pemphigus, lichen planus, ulcers caused by cyclic neutropenia and ulcers associated with celiac disease, ulcerative colitis, Crohn disease, pernicious anemia, and Behçet syndrome.

Recurrent genital HSV infection probably is the second most common manifestation of HSV and one of the most bothersome. Studies have elucidated several of the factors increasing the risk of recurrent genital disease after symptomatic primary genital infection. Recurrence rates are much more common after primary HSV-2 (90 per cent) than after primary HSV-1 (25 to 55 per cent) infection.[167, 246] The mean rate of recurrence is 0.02 to 0.1 per month after primary genital HSV-1 and 0.3 per month after primary HSV-2 genital infection.[167, 246] Recurrences are more common in men than in women and after a recurrent lesion than after a first attack.[246] Recurrences are more likely in patients who have high levels of neutralizing antibody. This possibly reflects a high degree of continued antigenic stimulation by more frequently expressed virus.

Only 5 to 12 per cent of persons who have recurrent genital HSV have constitutional symptoms. Local symptoms include pain (average, 4 to 6 days), itching, dysuria (10 to 30 per cent), adenopathy (20 to 30 per cent), lesions (average, 50 to 60 mm^2) lasting 4 to 5 days to crusting, and healing by 9 to 11 days (range, 4 to 29 days) (see Fig. 163–3). Symptoms in females tend to be more severe than those in males. Virus is shed for an average of 3 to 4 days (but in some cases as long as 20 days). Virus generally is shed with titers of 10^2 to 10^4 per lesion. In dry areas, vesicles are seen, but in wet areas, the vesicles rapidly break down into ulcers. Symptoms generally are milder and of shorter duration than in primary genital disease. New lesions not infrequently occur during the course of recurrence. Several authors have remarked on the variation of severity of recurrence among patients and the blending of several discrete recurrences into a single, prolonged recurrence. There are rare cases in which patients have almost continuous recurrences.[39, 60, 62, 121]

With the advent of endonuclease restriction analysis, it has become clear that whereas most recurrences represent endogenous reactivation of the same latent virus, it is possible to be reinfected with a new homologous virus (i.e., HSV-2 and new HSV-2) as well as heterologous virus (i.e., HSV-2 then HSV-1 or vice versa).[43] How common this is remains to be ascertained and surely depends to some degree on the sexual activity and number of partners of the persons studied.[270] This has profound implications regarding the protective value of HSV vaccine.

Other cutaneous recurrences may occur at each anatomic site of primary infection. HSV may recur on the face or trunk in a typical dermatome distribution, such as one associated with varicella-zoster virus. Indeed, frequent repeated attacks of zosteriform-like lesions on any part of the body in a normal host suggest HSV and not varicella-zoster.

Erythema Multiforme and Herpes Simplex Virus Infection[100, 130, 224]

Erythema multiforme is thought to be an allergic response to recurrent HSV infection. It has been associated with the presence of human leukocyte Dqw3 antigen.[141] In several series, approximately 15 to nearly 100 per cent of patients who have erythema multiforme, especially those who have recurrent erythema multiforme, gave a history of recurrent HSV infection before the skin eruption, which may be macular or urticarial.[130] In one series, 5 of 80 patients who had recurrent oral HSV infection experienced a rash (presumably erythema multiforme) 8 to 14 days after the onset of a cold sore.[291] Studies in adults and children have documented HSV antigen-antibody immune complexes and HSV DNA (as detected by PCR analysis and in situ hybridization) in the skin of patients who had erythema multiforme after HSV infection.[34, 35, 224] In a series of 20 children who had erythema multiforme (10 who had antecedent herpes), 16 were documented to have HSV DNA at the site of the rash.[330] The skin manifestations may last 14 to 21 days, and therapy is generally directed toward the allergic and not the viral component of the illness. Suppression of HSV recurrences prevents the associated episodes of erythema multiforme. Indeed, suppressive therapy of erythema multiforme using acyclovir, even in the absence of recurrent HSV infection, completely suppresses clinical manifestations.[272, 308]

Herpes Simplex Virus Infection in the Immunocompromised Host[104]

As the practice of pediatrics continues to include more patients with severe acquired immunodeficiency states brought about by increasingly intensive therapy for malignancies, expanding application of bone marrow and organ transplantation, and HIV infection, the prevalence of severe HSV infection in the immunocompromised host is increasing. Table 163–3 lists the states associated with unusually severe HSV infections. HSV infection in the neonatal period is discussed in Chapter 76. Aside from the several cases of HSV encephalitis in patients with agammaglobulinemia (who also had concomitant infections with enterovirus),[180] the common links in these varied groups are either skin abnormalities

TABLE 163–3. Conditions Contributing to Unusually Severe Herpes Simplex Virus Infections

Newborn period	Pregnancy
Malnutrition	Burns
Malignancy	Trauma
Immunosuppressive therapy	Skin abnormalities
Antineoplastic	Atopic eczema
Transplantation	Bullous impetigo
Corticosteroids or ACTH	Burns
Primary immunodeficiency	Darier disease
Agammaglobulinemia	Ichthyosiform erythroderma
Wiskott-Aldrich syndrome	Pemphigus
Ataxia-telangiectasia	Viral infection
Severe combined immunodeficiency syndrome	Measles
Nucleoside phosphorylase deficiency	Pertussis
Thymoma and hypogammaglobulinemia	Tuberculosis
Common variable agammaglobulinemia	Severe bacterial infection
Chronic mucocutaneous candidiasis	*Haemophilus* meningitis
Natural killer cell defect	Sarcoidosis
AIDS	

(eczema, burns) or immunologic defects, primarily in the cell-mediated aspects of the immune system.[30, 101, 126, 192, 214, 285, 298, 311] This particularly is understandable in light of the ability of HSV to proceed from cell to cell without entering the extracellular environment in which antibody, alone or with complement, can neutralize the virus. Thus, the cell-mediated mechanisms assume special importance. We currently are at too early a stage of research to discern whether the cellular defect is one primarily of the T cell (delayed hypersensitivity, immune lymphokine production, T-cell cytotoxicity), the killer–natural killer cell (antibody-dependent or natural killer cell cytotoxicity or interferon production), the macrophage (antigen processing, primary intrinsic or extrinsic viral resistance, activation, or effector mechanisms), or even other crucial cells or a combination of these cells. As the roles of these cellular mechanisms in resistance of the normal host and their defects in these immunocompromised hosts are defined better, immunomodulation or reconstitution treatments will become a reality.

The incidence of severe HSV infection in these pediatric groups (see Table 163–3) is poorly defined but, in limited series, similar to that seen in adults.[104] Infection usually is a recurrence caused by an endogenous virus. In series of pediatric or adult patients who have renal transplants, marrow transplants, or cardiac transplants, 70 to 90 per cent of seropositive persons excrete HSV, usually from the oropharynx and usually at the time of peak immunosuppression (in the first month after transplantation).[5, 203, 217, 228, 233, 235, 241] Of 68 children undergoing renal transplantation, a herpesvirus was isolated in 43 per cent, with 28 per cent of these being HSV.[314] HSV in cardiac transplant cases causes symptomatic illness in 45 to 85 per cent of seropositive patients, depending on the intensity of immunosuppression.[235, 241] HSV was the most commonly isolated virus in children who underwent bone marrow transplantation (23 per cent).[328] In bone marrow transplantation patients, HSV (often in the absence of cutaneous or mucous membrane lesions) is one of the etiologic agents of interstitial pneumonitis, a disorder that accounts for approximately 5 to 10 per cent of deaths related to this procedure.[220, 240] In children who have leukemia, HSV infection is more common in those with myelocytic than lymphocytic leukemia, and the risk of infection increases with neutropenia and chemotherapy. HSV infection was the most common serious viral infection in children with leukemia. Whereas the greatest number of infections occurred during periods of remission, on a per-day basis, the risk of infection was seven times higher during induction.[343] Of 24 patients who died of infection during remission in the St. Jude's series, 2 (8 per cent) had HSV (one disseminated, one encephalitis).[283] In Africa, many patients suffer from underlying malnutrition and have concomitant measles infection with fatal disseminated HSV infection; such events are rare in industrialized nations.[22, 145, 311]

Chronic mucocutaneous ulcers (persisting for more than 1 month), bronchitis, pneumonitis, and esophagitis caused by HSV are conditions that have been used to categorize the severity of HIV infection.[207] Chronic HSV mucocutaneous diseases or widespread organ involvement was the AIDS-defining condition in 7 of 789 (9 per cent) of HIV-infected children.[317] In series of children with AIDS, 5 to 29 per cent experienced HSV opportunistic infection.[104, 248, 275] In HIV-infected patients, illnesses caused by HSV usually involved chronic mucocutaneous ulcers or extensions to the lungs, bronchi, or esophagus. Dissemination is rare.[239] Multiple recurrences of infection are common as the immunodeficiency worsens. In patients with AIDS, HSV rarely causes a typical[124, 321] or more indolent[7] encephalitis. HSV usually does not cause mortality in HIV-infected patients but causes significant morbidity.[149] HSV genital ulcer disease increases the risks of HIV acquisition[129]; in vitro, HSV can activate HIV.[114]

Several major syndromes are attributable to HSV in immunocompromised patients, with some overlap and occasionally progression from one to the other. The first and most common is a local, chronic, often extensive cutaneous or mucocutaneous infection. The second is infection of one organ, usually contiguous to an orifice (e.g., esophagitis or pneumonitis). The most serious is more widespread dissemination involving distant areas of skin or visceral organs (e.g., lungs, liver, adrenals) and the CNS. There is not enough information to be certain, but except in the most immunocompromised patients, disseminated disease probably most often represents primary infection; the local syndromes may be either a manifestation of primary infection or recurrent illness.

The typical local syndrome begins in the mouth or about the lips, often appearing innocuously as an ordinary herpes labialis recurrence. Over several days, the papules and vesicles progress to bullae, often with hemorrhagic fluid. The bullae or vesicles progress to huge, chronic, bloody, coalescing, ulcerated, oozing lesions, eroding into the subcutaneous tissue and occasionally destroying underlying structures. The tissue is odorous, and the lesions are painful (Fig. 163–15). The lip and palate are the sites most commonly affected. Oral lesions account for approximately 60 per cent of HSV infections in children undergoing transplantation.[314] A similar syndrome may be seen in the perianal or vaginal area, usually caused by HSV-2 infection, and is one of the characteristic syndromes in male homosexuals with AIDS (Fig. 163–16). Untreated, the lesions may lead to death because of local destruction and hemorrhage or may regress as the immune status of the host improves or as antiviral chemotherapy is utilized. A syndrome of herpetic geometric glossitis has been reported in HIV-infected patients.[119] This consists of a tender tongue accompanied by dorsal longitudinal crossed and branching fissures.

In patients with burns, eczema, pemphigus, or abrasions, extensive skin infection may occur, often with conversion of second-degree tissue damage to third-degree damage (see Figs. 163–6 and 163–7). Of 179 children with eczema, 10 developed herpes skin infections, 7 requiring hospitalization.[73] Possibly as a result of the more severe immunodeficiency occurring with several of these conditions, and in the case of primary HSV infection, the local infection may progress to dissemination to visceral organs. The widespread necrotizing lesions commonly are known as Kaposi varicelliform eruption or eczema herpeticum (see Fig. 163–6).

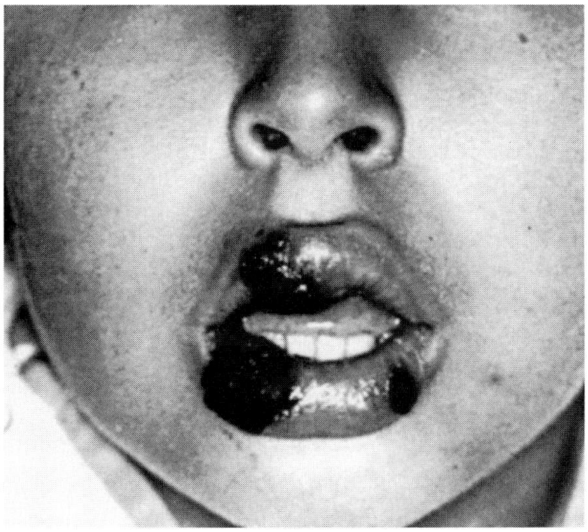

FIGURE 163–15. *Chronic, hemorrhagic HSV infection in a girl with leukemia and a bone marrow transplantation.*

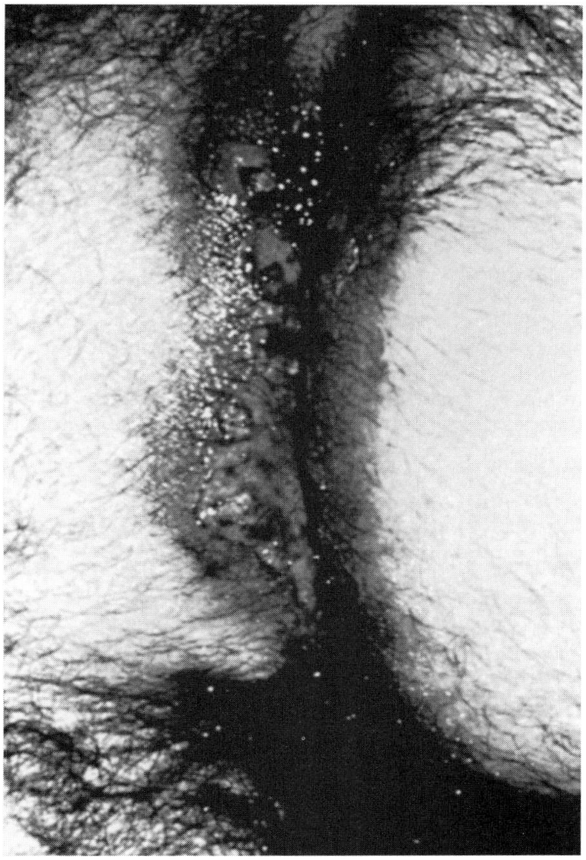

FIGURE 163–16. *HSV proctitis and rectal infection in a male homosexual with AIDS. (Courtesy of Dr. Victor Fainstein, Department of Internal Medicine, M. D. Anderson Cancer Center, Houston, TX.)*

These lesions must be differentiated from bacterial infections caused by gram-positive or gram-negative organisms, chronic fungal infections (as seen with *Mucor,* blastomycosis), other viral infections (vaccinia, varicella), mycobacterial infection, and various noninfectious lesions, such as pyoderma gangrenosum, chemotherapy-induced ulcers, or Sweet syndrome. HSV is the agent most commonly associated with oral lesions in immunocompromised patients.[104]

Esophagitis caused by HSV rarely has been reported in normal children,[20, 225] but it is relatively common in immunocompromised patients. Pathologic studies have suggested that approximately 25 per cent of cases of autopsy-proven esophagitis (1 to 6 per cent of all autopsies) are secondary to HSV infection (14 of 55 cases).[219] Underlying conditions included burns, aplastic anemia, malignancies, transplantation, a variety of other serious medical problems, and postoperative trauma induced by nasogastric tubes.[44, 184, 219] Twenty to 50 per cent of these patients have HSV involvement elsewhere (lungs, trachea, and, less commonly, skin). The esophagitis may be asymptomatic or associated with dysphagia, odynophagia, epigastric discomfort, and retrosternal pain. The characteristic findings in the esophagus are ulcers with raised granular margins. The ulcers often are covered with fibrinous exudate and in advanced cases are confluent, with progression to complete mucosal loss in large segments of the esophagus. Typically, visceral herpes infection is not suspected before death. Uncommonly, involvement of adjacent gastric tissue can be documented. Diagnostic evaluation should include barium swallow, which may demonstrate edema, nodules, and ulceration of the esophagus. Barium studies cannot differentiate HSV from other etiologic agents of esophagitis. Esophagoscopy accompanied by biopsy and viral culture is diagnostic and helps exclude the other common causes of this syndrome, including *Candida,* cytomegalovirus, and possibly other fungi and bacteria or chemotherapy-induced changes.[44, 219]

Probably the second most commonly involved organ in immunocompromised hosts is the lungs. This is a rare premortem diagnosis and almost exclusively occurs in immunocompromised patients. In one series of 1000 consecutive autopsies,[218] HSV pneumonia was identified in 10 cases. HSV pulmonary infection occurred in 3 per cent of children after renal transplantation.[314] In most adult cases, the process is a result of endogenous viral mucocutaneous reactivation and involvement of lung tissue by contiguous spread, causing focal pneumonia (60 per cent of the time), or hematogenous spread from an oral or genital site, resulting in diffuse pneumonitis.[240] Although the largest series primarily was composed of adult patients, three of the patients were 7 years of age or younger (with Down syndrome and congestive heart failure, rhabdomyosarcoma, and pneumococcal pneumonia and a seizure disorder).[131] Patients had cough, dyspnea, fever, and hypoxia, and 50 per cent had rales. Most had other concomitant pulmonary infections with bacteria, *Candida, Aspergillus,* and cytomegalovirus. HSV pneumonia cannot be diagnosed by the association of upper airway cultures with a radiographic picture. It must rest on an aggressive approach utilizing culture and histopathologic examination of involved lung tissue obtained by either biopsy or bronchoscopy.[240]

Meningoencephalitis caused by HSV is not common in immunocompromised patients. It may occur as part of widely disseminated disease or be a localized condition. Several cases have been reported in patients who have agammaglobulinemia in association with concomitant viral infection of the brain.[180] The meningoencephalitis may be fulminant, such as occurs in the normal host.[180] An interesting case, which followed an atypical subacute course accompanied by bilateral brain involvement, has been reported in an anergic patient who had Hodgkin disease.[237] Whereas HSV does not appear to have a predilection for CNS infection in the immunocompromised host, an exception is those patients with AIDS, in whom it may cause ascending myelitis, acute transverse myelitis, and encephalitis.[104, 106, 124, 321]

Hepatitis caused by HSV has been reported most commonly after solid organ or bone marrow transplantation[136, 149, 150] and during pregnancy.[148] Signs include fever, abdominal pain, and elevated liver function test results. Hepatitis usually occurs during the first 3 weeks after transplantation, unless prophylactic acyclovir was given. Mortality is very high (67 to 100 per cent). In at least one case, orthotopic liver transplantation resulted in survival.[279]

The most severe form of HSV in the immunocompromised host is that of widely disseminated disease that can involve liver, adrenals, lungs, spleen, kidney, and often brain. In a large series from South Africa and Kenya,[22, 145, 311] measles and severe malnutrition were frequent cofactors (83 per cent) in children 2 to 25 months of age who had widely disseminated HSV infection. These illnesses represented fatal primary infections. Similar syndromes have been reported; these and other underlying conditions are listed in Table 163–3. Dissemination has been reported coincident with pertussis, *Haemophilus influenzae* meningitis,[134] and other bacterial infections.[22] Disseminated HSV infection occurred in 10 per cent and 25 per cent of children who had HSV infection and who underwent bone marrow and renal transplantation, respectively.[216, 328]

The clinical presentation usually is one of initial fever and skin or mucocutaneous involvement in 80 per cent of cases, which, instead of healing as expected, disseminates. The cutaneous dissemination may involve a widespread vesicular eruption, looking much like varicella, or may involve more local, large, hemorrhagic vesicles and bullae. The major target organs involved, as noted previously, give rise to syndromes of hepatitis, pneumonia, shock, bleeding, disseminated intravascular coagulopathy, seizures, coma, renal failure, hypothermia, and death in days to weeks. The laboratory examination may reveal leukopenia, thrombocytopenia, elevated liver function tests, hyponatremia, azotemia, pneumonitis, hypoglycemia, CSF pleocytosis, abnormal electroencephalogram, and electrocardiographic abnormalities. Death is common in this syndrome (90 per cent), even after the institution of antiviral chemotherapy. Because the liver often is involved and biopsy may be precluded by the tenuous condition of the patient, HSV infection should be considered in all high-risk groups (see Table 163–3) with fulminant hepatitis.

DIAGNOSIS

Before specific diagnostic tests are contemplated, initial attention must be focused on the validity of the specimen regarding the possible syndrome to be diagnosed. Because HSV may be shed in response to fever, other stresses, or immunosuppression, the finding of HSV in certain secretions (e.g., saliva) does not mean the clinical condition (pneumonia, encephalitis, hepatitis) is caused by HSV. In general, the virus must be isolated from the tissue in question for the diagnosis to be confirmed, especially in immunosuppressed hosts. It also is worth emphasizing that in HSV encephalitis, the virus almost never is found in the spinal fluid, and viral DNA detection by PCR analysis or, as a last resort, brain biopsy is crucial to secure the diagnosis as well as exclude other treatable etiologic factors.

Rapid but Nonspecific Methods

There are two rapid and suggestive but not entirely specific modalities of diagnosis. These are electron microscopy, with use of the pseudoreplica or other rapid techniques, and cytologic examination with Giemsa or other tissue stains. Electron microscopy of vesicular fluid or tissue preparations may reveal the characteristic virus of the herpes family (Fig. 163–17). The microscopist cannot differentiate HSV from the other herpesviruses. This is of little importance in some situations, such as in a disseminated vesicular rash in an immunocompromised child, because the antiviral therapy of HSV and varicella-zoster virus infections currently is similar. In contrast, it is important to differentiate HSV from cytomegalovirus in brain, lungs, or liver because therapy differs.

Cytologic examination revealing typical giant cells (Fig. 163–18) and, less commonly, Cowdry type A intranuclear inclusions (Fig. 163–19) is characteristic for HSV but also may be seen with cytomegalovirus and varicella-zoster virus. When performing cytologic examination, it is important that the base of the vesicle (after unroofing) or ulcer be scraped vigorously (with a scalpel or wooden applicator) and the resultant material placed on a slide, air-dried, fixed, and stained, usually with Giemsa or Wright stain (Tzanck smear). In most series, 40 to 80 per cent of culture-positive specimens

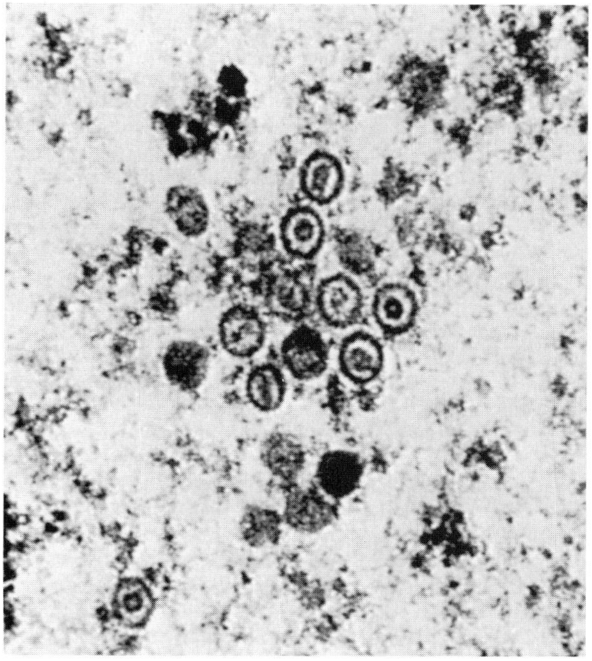

FIGURE 163–17. *Brain biopsy of a 9-month-old with HSV encephalitis, with electron-microscopic demonstration of HSV particles.*

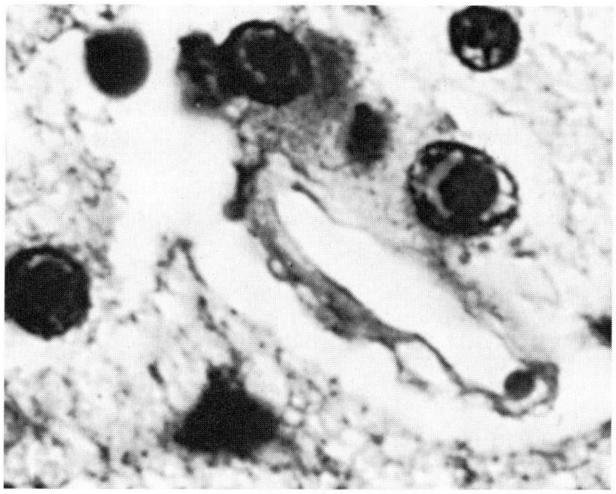

FIGURE 163–19. *Histology of brain biopsy of a 9-month-old with HSV encephalitis. Note the eosinophilic Cowdry type A intranuclear inclusions (H & E stain, × 1000).*

are positive by cytologic study if the examiner is experienced.[223, 287] False-positive results are unusual but do occur.

Rapid and Specific Methods

Several rapid, specific tests depend on immunologic reagents for antigen detection. Fluorescent antibody methods were the original technique, but they have been joined by enzyme-linked immunosorbent assays (ELISA), immunoperoxidase-tagged antibody in ELISA or tissue sections, radiometric tests, and *Staphylococcus* protein A absorption tests.[72, 115, 172, 201, 208, 269, 345] These tests generally employ relatively specific hyperimmune serum to HSV or monoclonal antibodies to specific HSV glycoproteins. Not only are these tests sensitive and generally specific, but with the appropriate reagents, viral typing as well as antigen detection can be made from clinical isolates or young (12- to 24-hour-old) cultures.[115] Studies report a 50 to 90 per cent rate of correlation with cultures. Commercially available kits have been reported to be 90 to 95 per cent sensitive and specific.[72, 173, 345] In general, except for sporadic reports, antigen detection tests for HSV in CSF have been unsuccessful.[153] When the immunologic test results are positive and culture results are negative, the reason may be the presence of nonviable virus.

Polymerase Chain Reaction[12, 53, 90, 253]

The technique of PCR is that of repeated amplification of predetermined (i.e., HSV) DNA by the use of primers and enzymes that denature and then specifically replicate the desired DNA chains in a chemical reaction. This can result in more than a million-fold amplification of the DNA in several hours, possibly allowing the detection of a single copy of DNA in a sample. PCR has been applied successfully to the diagnosis of HSV infection.[12, 53, 253] Currently, it is rather labor-intensive and expensive, although rapid. An additional drawback is that the extreme sensitivity of the assay makes it prone to false-positive results because of poor technique or other avenues of environmental contamination. With appro-

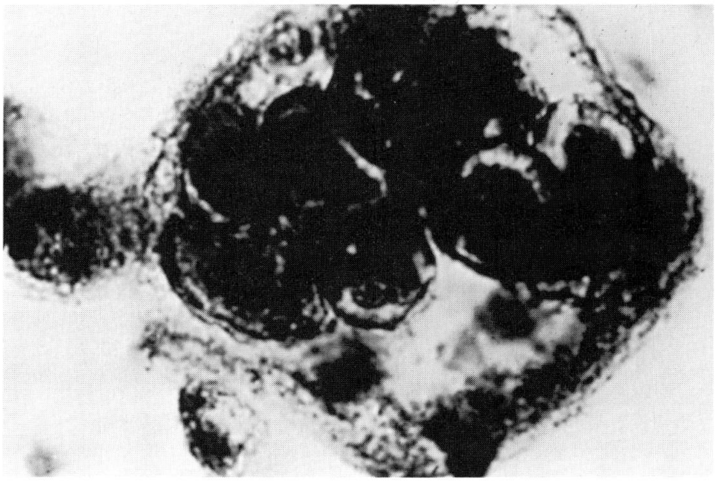

FIGURE 163–18. *Histology of scraping of base of skin vesicle, demonstrating multinucleated giant cell.*

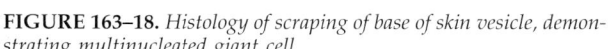

priate controls, this has become the method of choice for detection of low-copy numbers of HSV DNA and of HSV DNA in the CSF for diagnosis of HSV in encephalitis.[12, 253, 315] PCR has made the use of brain biopsy unnecessary in most situations.[168] It also has been used to demonstrate prolonged presence of HSV DNA in genital lesions, although its utility in diagnosing culture-negative mucocutaneous disease still is under study.[59] Reports of HSV myocardial disease diagnosed by PCR await confirmation.[187]

Less Rapid but Specific Methods

The gold standard of HSV diagnosis remains tissue culture.[244] HSV grows rapidly (mean, 2 to 3 days; high-titer samples, 12 to 24 hours; low-titer samples, 5 to 7 days) in human and nonhuman cells, producing a typical cytopathic effect (Fig. 163–20). Human diploid cells (WI-38 or human embryonic lung cells) and primate cells (Vero), as well as a variety of rodent cells, are sensitive to HSV and are used by most diagnostic laboratories. Tentative diagnosis in 95 per cent of isolates can be made by the cell types infected and typical cytopathogenic effect. High-titer specimens of varicella-zoster virus or cytomegalovirus occasionally cause confusion. Sensitivity of culture can be improved by low-speed centrifugation or ultracentrifugation of specimens directly onto monolayers in centrifuge tubes.[312] Speed of diagnosis has been increased by the use of shell vial cultures.[316] Combinations of short-term culture with antigen detection methods applied to the cultures, 14 to 18 hours later, have been promising.[95, 132]

Definitive viral characterization is accomplished by antisera reaction causing neutralization, fluorescent antibody reaction, or several of the antigen detection tests mentioned. HSV-1 and HSV-2 also have biologic differences (replication in chicken embryo cells, effects on baby mice, allantoic membrane pock morphology, and sensitivity to various chemicals).[244] Typing generally is performed by use of specific monoclonal antibodies[115] or endonuclease restriction patterns[108] (see later discussion). Typing may become more important as drugs that are relatively specific for type 1 virus emerge.

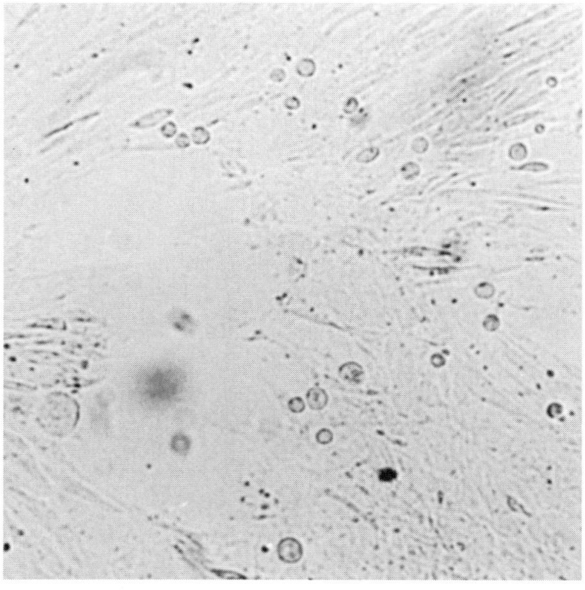

FIGURE 163–20. *Culture of HSV on human fibroblasts demonstrating disruption of cell monolayer and rounding and enlargement of cells to show cytopathogenic effect.*

The patient's immunologic response also can be diagnostic. Whereas cell-mediated responses (lymphocyte blastogenesis, immune lymphokine production) become positive after primary infection, their use is limited to research. A large variety of antibody tests can be used to document primary HSV infection. The classic tests include viral neutralization, complement fixation, indirect hemagglutination, and fluorescent antibody assays. More recent tests involve detection of antibody in ELISA, radioimmunoassays (RIAs), Western blot analysis to detect antibody to specific viral polypeptides, antibody-mediating cellular cytotoxicity (ADCC), and others. Some of these, such as ADCC, may be used to detect early infection (3 to 6 days after the onset of symptoms).[152, 154, 156] Others (such as ELISA or RIA) may be able to separate IgM, IgG, and IgA responses or type-specific viral responses.

Several precautions must be observed when the serologic response is analyzed. Patients who have documented prior HSV infections may have fourfold rises in antibody titer with recurrences and IgM or IgA responses with recurrences. Rarely, severely immunocompromised patients do not produce antibody. Thus, only when a patient's serum converts from negative to positive can a primary infection be diagnosed with confidence. Patients who had HSV infection (symptomatic or asymptomatic) in the past generally maintained positive serologic response for life (probably reflecting existing latency), with minor fluctuations. Finally, although type-specific (e.g., HSV-1 or HSV-2) antibody assays are available in research settings,[137] their commercial availability and reliability at this writing are questionable.[8] In research laboratories, type-specific assays based on purified type-specific glycoproteins (e.g., gpG) or Western blot analysis have been used successfully to determine rates of HSV-2 infection.[33, 137, 161]

Unfortunately, in some of the most important situations, such as in HSV encephalitis or early disseminated HSV infection in the immunosuppressed host, serologic examination is relatively useless because of slow rise or late conversion. In addition, a significant percentage of these conditions represent recurrent and not primary disease. Whereas CSF-serum antibody ratios may be diagnostic in HSV encephalitis, unfortunately they often are not so until several days or weeks into the illness and thus are of limited clinical use.[12, 147, 153, 177, 284, 319]

Endonuclease Restriction Analysis

Each HSV DNA has a specific cleavage pattern or "fingerprint" when digested by endonuclease restriction enzymes and electrophoresed in a gel (Fig. 163–21).[42] These methods can be used to type the virus and to demonstrate relatedness or differences (strains) between isolates for epidemiologic purposes ("outbreaks," nosocomial transmission), between isolates obtained from the same person during one illness from different sites, or over time from the same site.[42, 43, 125, 179, 335] This has added markedly to the understanding of the epidemiology of HSV, the exploration of the possibility of exogenous reinfection versus recurrence, and the recognition of the ability to harbor more than one latent virus at the same site. It has become clear that, in general, the restriction patterns are stable in vivo, although there can be minor changes. In addition, to be sure of identity, several restriction enzymes must be used on each isolate. Thus, this is a powerful tool, but it is time-consuming and requires special expertise beyond that of most viral diagnostic laboratories. Rapid

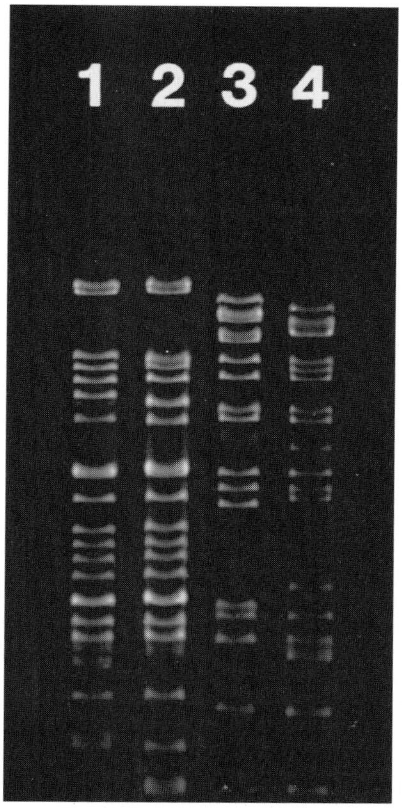

FIGURE 163–21. *Endonuclease restriction analysis. An electrophoretic separation by size of DNA fragments of four HSV isolates, produced by restriction endonuclease enzyme digestion using* BamHI *enzyme. Lanes 1 and 2 are two different HSV-2 clinical isolates, whereas lanes 3 and 4 are two different HSV-1 clinical isolates. The origin of the gel is at the top. (Courtesy of Dr. Saul Kit, Division of Biochemical Virology, Baylor College of Medicine, Houston, TX.)*

restriction analysis of defined PCR products yields viral type identification.[315]

Drug Susceptibility Testing

Although not now in general use, viral culture and sensitivity testing rapidly are becoming available in most centers. With the availability of specific chemotherapy and evolving mechanisms of viral drug resistance, the clinician must rely increasingly on sensitivity tests that resemble in vitro minimal inhibitory concentration tests utilized for bacteria that are performed on cells and not in agar. Evolving clinical data are providing meaningful values for "sensitive and resistant" virus, although the specific numbers vary by assay. In general, ID_{50} levels of more than 3 μg/mL for acyclovir and more than 100 μg/mL for foscarnet denote a resistant isolate.[57, 255, 258] Rapid screening tests that take 3 to 4 days to perform are being developed.[257] In addition, the detection of enzyme characteristics (such as thymidine kinase–negative HSV isolates, which therefore are resistant to acyclovir)[190] will be used, as we routinely analyze *H. influenzae* for the presence of β-lactamase and resultant ampicillin resistance. In the immunocompromised patient, in particular, failure to respond to antiviral therapy should alert the clinician to obtain viral susceptibility testing.

Experimental Methods of Viral Detection

Cocultivation[16, 19]

To date, cocultivation remains a standard technique for detecting latent virus. The tissue to be examined is cultured along with permissive cells for an extended period. In this fashion, latent virus may be identified. This technique has little use in clinical medicine.

Nucleic Acid Hybridization[88, 89, 95, 226]

The development of genetic engineering has permitted production of complementary nucleic acid, which enabled the genetic probing of tissue. This technique may detect virus or incomplete viral DNA or RNA in latent conditions,[276] possibly virus-transformed cells, or sites of low levels of productive infection.

Viral Product Detection[118, 140]

Assays for the detection of virus-specific glycoproteins or enzymes, such as deoxythymidine kinase in clinical specimens, have been developed. Their practical application to the clinical arena remains to be determined.

PROGNOSIS, COMPLICATIONS, AND SEQUELAE

HSV infections occurring beyond the fetal and neonatal periods usually are annoying but not immediately life-threatening. The outcome of eczema herpeticum usually is benign, and there are no sequelae when recovery does occur. There are, however, significant exceptions to these general rules. In particular, the outcome of HSV encephalitis can be serious, ranging from extensive and permanent neurologic disability to death. The case-fatality rate for untreated encephalitis may be as high as 75 per cent.[337, 338] There are increasing case reports of relapses (in approximately 5 per cent of cases) and possibly smoldering CNS damage.[76, 81, 122, 153]

HSV is one of the most common causes of infectious blindness in developed countries. In immunocompromised patients, it is a major cause of morbidity and mortality. Genital HSV infection may not have a life-threatening potential but is a significant cause of physical and psychologic morbidity.

Studies in the early 1970s indicated that cervical infection with HSV-2 might be related directly to the later appearance of cervical carcinoma.[306] The prevalence of HSV-2 antibody was higher among women who had cervical carcinoma than among matched controls. There also has been some success more recently in identifying antibodies in patients with cervical carcinoma to certain nonvirion proteins produced in conjunction with HSV infection.[88, 226] HSV genetic fragments have been detected in cancer tissue. In addition, in vitro studies have shown that the genome of HSV has the capacity to induce morphologic and malignant transformation. However, none of the studies to date clearly has resolved the question of whether HSV is etiologic in any human cancers. It is possible that it may be a cofactor along with the papillomaviruses, but it probably is not an independent cause of cancer.

TREATMENT

Oral Herpes Simplex Virus Infection

Two placebo-controlled trials of primary herpes gingivostomatitis in young children have been described.[4, 86] In one study, the pain and hypersalivation resolved more quickly in acyclovir-treated patients.[86] In a larger study, clinical aspects significantly improved by a 10-day course of oral acyclovir (600 mg/m^2 four times a day) included drooling (4 versus 8 days in placebo), gum swelling (5 versus 7 days), speed of intraoral lesion healing (6 versus 8 days), appearance of new lesions (57 versus 94 per cent), and viral shedding in saliva (4 versus 10 days). Therapy had no effect on the development of subsequent cold sores.[4] I have used intravenous acyclovir in patients who had severe primary gingivostomatitis when the inability to maintain hydration necessitated hospital admission. In these uncommon cases, the illness responded in several days with defervescence and cessation of new lesions.

Symptomatic therapy includes antipyretics and oral hydration with bland liquids and ice slurries. The use of oral anesthetics probably is not indicated and has resulted in cases of self-injury as a result of children's chewing on anesthetized oral mucosa or lips.

There are several conflicting studies regarding the use of topical acyclovir in the treatment of oral herpes recurrences. Whereas there is general agreement that topical acyclovir can decrease the duration of HSV shedding, from 2 to 3 days with placebo treatment to 1 to 2 days,[97, 292, 320] the effect on symptoms is either nil[292] or subtle (1 day fewer of vesicles and a 2- to 3-day speeding of healing).[97, 320] Topical therapy probably is not indicated in recurrent oral HSV infection. Early treatment of recurrent herpes labialis with oral acyclovir (400 mg five times a day) in adults did not affect lesion development but hastened healing and decreased pain significantly.[197] Although there have been no controlled studies, acyclovir therapy has been advocated for the treatment of HSV esophagitis in the normal host.[105]

Herpes Simplex Virus Keratitis[178]

Five topical preparations have been shown to have a beneficial effect on HSV keratitis and probably other superficial ocular HSV infections, such as conjunctivitis and blepharitis.[178] These include idoxuridine (Stoxil, Herplex, Allergan), vidarabine (Vira-A), trifluridine (Viroptic), acyclovir, and interferon. The last two preparations, as of this writing, are not clinically available for use as an ophthalmic medication in the United States, although acyclovir is available in Europe and other parts of the world.

Idoxuridine was the first effective therapy for ocular HSV infections. Its use currently is not suggested because it appears to be less effective and more toxic than the two alternatives.

Trifluridine in a 1 per cent ophthalmic solution is a pyrimidine nucleoside and inhibits HSV DNA synthesis. It probably is the drug of choice for the local therapy of primary and recurrent HSV infection, such as keratitis, keratoconjunctivitis, uveitis, and lid lesions, as well as after operations on eyes previously infected with HSV or when steroid therapy is used in similar eyes. Keratitis appears to respond more rapidly to trifluridine than to either idoxuridine or vidarabine ointment. Ulcers failing to respond to idoxuridine or vidarabine have responded to trifluridine. None of the local therapies affects the rate of recurrence. Trifluridine is used as one drop per eye every 2 hours while awake (maximum nine drops daily per eye) until re-epithelialization of corneal ulcers and then one drop per eye every 5 hours while awake (maximum, five drops daily per eye) for 7 additional days. The maximum duration of therapy is 21 days. Side effects consist of local stinging, burning, and edema (3 to 5 per cent of cases).

Orally administered acyclovir also has been used to treat dendritic keratitis. In a small controlled study, its effects were similar to those of topical acyclovir in the treatment of dendritic corneal ulceration.[58] A small uncontrolled series suggests that oral acyclovir is therapeutic in patients who have stromal keratitis or keratouveitis.[274]

The indications and side effects of vidarabine ophthalmic ointment are similar to those of trifluridine, although the ointment preparation may make this more useful in children. Dosage is ½-inch five times per day (at 3-hour intervals). If there is no improvement in 7 days or lack of complete re-epithelialization in 21 days, trifluridine is indicated.

It is strongly advised that a child with HSV keratitis be cared for in conjunction with an ophthalmologist familiar with this illness. The use of cycloplegic and anti-inflammatory agents in this illness requires practical experience. In severe stromal infection, surgical procedures, including corneal transplant, may be required, often with the concomitant use of corticosteriods and antiviral therapy.

Herpes Simplex Virus Encephalitis

Early studies utilizing vidarabine for the therapy of HSV encephalitis revealed a substantial therapeutic effect (short-term mortality rates of 28 to 33 per cent in drug recipients, compared with 75 per cent in placebo recipients).[337, 338] Younger patients and patients who had less severe neurologic morbidity at the onset of therapy benefited the most from therapy. Two well-controlled clinical studies in Sweden and the United States comparing vidarabine with acyclovir (30 mg/kg/day in three divided doses for 10 to 12 days) have provided evidence that acyclovir is significantly more effective than is vidarabine in treating HSV encephalitis.[284, 333] In the Swedish study, the early mortality rate was 19 per cent in the acyclovir-treated group and 50 per cent in the vidarabine-treated group.[284] The National Institutes of Health collaborative study[333] generated similar data. Intravenous acyclovir (10 mg/kg/dose three times a day for 14 to 21 days) is, therefore, the drug of choice in the treatment of HSV encephalitis after the neonatal period. As seen in the earlier vidarabine studies,[337, 338] the age and mental status at initiation of therapy markedly influence the outcome of HSV encephalitis treated with acyclovir. Lethargic patients have a 15 per cent mortality rate, whereas comatose patients have a 40 per cent mortality rate. The use of long-term therapy remains controversial.[122, 153]

In addition to antiviral therapy, meticulous intensive care is required for optimizing the outcome of these patients. Fluid management for the prevention of overhydration is critical. Often, direct intracranial pressure measurement by ventricular catheter or epidural bolt is necessary for the effective monitoring of increased intracranial pressure and treatment with diuretic agents. The use of steroids is common but remains controversial and unstudied. Anticonvulsant therapy for management of the often severe and prolonged seizures as well as ventilatory support usually is necessary some time during the illness. The use of deep, induced coma (as with a barbiturate) remains unstudied. Isolation of the patient is not necessary.

Genital Herpes Simplex Virus Infection

Acyclovir (Zovirax) is the drug of choice for HSV genital infection. The present problem for the practitioner is how to decide which preparation is best suited for each particular patient.[98, 128, 144]

Acyclovir is one of the more exciting developments in

antiviral chemotherapy. Acyclovir itself is an inactive drug. Inhibition of viral DNA synthesis by inhibition of viral DNA polymerase and DNA chain termination requires its phosphorylation. In this regard, viral thymidine kinase (of HSV in particular) is much more active than is its mammalian counterpart. Thus, acyclovir becomes a specific antiviral agent in the presence of thymidine kinase–positive viruses.[69] Fortunately, thymidine kinase appears to be an important enzyme for viral virulence. Mutant, thymidine kinase–negative virus strains have been recovered in 3 to 10 per cent of patients treated with acyclovir, but the finding of a nearly similar rate of acyclovir-resistant virus in placebo-treated patients has been a surprise.[57, 189] These viral mutants seem less virulent in animal models, and patients who were culture-positive for such mutants often have thymidine kinase–positive HSV isolates in their next recurrence. Thymidine kinase–negative HSV recurrences in immunocompromised patients have been well documented, with demonstration of the ability of these viruses to establish latency and recur.[255] Thus, the clinical significance and epidemiologic importance of these mutants remain to be more fully discerned.[70, 282, 323] (See later discussion regarding resistant viruses.)

Topical acyclovir utilized to treat the first episode of genital herpes decreased the mean duration of viral shedding (4.1 versus 7.0 days with placebo) and time to crusting of lesions (7.1 versus 10.5 days).[63] In the therapy of recurrent genital disease, topical acyclovir generally tended to have a minor effect on duration of viral shedding (from 1 to 2 days in treated patients to 2 to 3 days in placebo recipients), with little or no effect on symptoms.[183, 247] These results were not improved markedly with early use of topical therapy.

Intravenous acyclovir has an impressive effect on primary genital HSV infection. Used in a placebo-controlled, double-blind study at a dose of 5 mg/kg every 8 hours for 5 days, acyclovir decreased duration of viral shedding (2 versus 8 to 13 days in placebo-treated patients), shortened local and systemic symptoms by 2 to 5 days, and shortened time to healing by 7 to 12 days. Complications, such as extragenital lesions or urinary retention, were reduced significantly.[61, 198] The major effect of acyclovir therapy on the first episode of genital HSV infection is seen in those who have true primary disease.[231] Whereas intravenous therapy with acyclovir may shorten viral shedding and duration of symptoms in recurrences, its use is not recommended for therapy of recurrent genital disease.

Oral acyclovir has therapeutic effects on both primary and recurrent HSV infection in adults. In a double-blind, placebo-controlled study of patients who had primary genital infection, using 200 mg five times per day for 5 to 10 days, acyclovir significantly reduced viral shedding (1 to 6 days versus 13 to 15 days with placebo), lesion formation after 48 hours (0 to 4 per cent versus 43 to 44 per cent), the duration of lesions (10 to 12 versus 16 to 21 days), and the duration and severity of symptoms.[41, 222]

In similar studies of adult patients who had recurrent genital HSV infection, acyclovir (200 mg five times per day for 5 days) decreased duration of virus shedding (1 to 2 versus 2 to 4 days), time to healing (5 to 6 versus 6 to 7 days), and new lesion development (2 to 10 per cent versus 19 to 25 per cent), especially when administered early in the recurrence.[222]

In these short-term studies in which patients were cautioned regarding hydration, no significant side effects were noted. Furthermore, no cytogenetic effects were noted.[56] Studies of virus from either placebo or acyclovir recipients showed that 4 to 15 per cent of viruses isolated after therapy were more resistant to acyclovir, regardless of therapy.[57, 189] In several disquieting studies, patients treated with intravenous acyclovir for primary genital herpes failed to make a full range of antibodies (especially to antigen gD and VP66).[9, 27] Those patients who lacked antibody to VP66 had more severe and longer recurrences at the first episode after therapy and then produced a full range of antibodies.[9] Neither oral nor intravenous acyclovir reduces the rate of recurrences when it is used to treat either primary or recurrent genital infection. Oral acyclovir is the drug of choice for patients who have primary genital HSV infection, HSV proctitis,[249] and frequent recurrent disease. Intravenous acyclovir should be reserved for those patients who have severe local or systemic symptoms or complications, such as urinary retention or aseptic meningitis syndrome.[231]

Valacyclovir, which is converted to acyclovir in vivo, and famciclovir, which is converted to penciclovir, are two new antiviral agents that are well absorbed when administered orally (75 to 80 per cent bioavailability). Penciclovir, like acyclovir, is phosphorylated to the active triphosphate with anti-HSV activity similar to that of the acyclovir triphosphate derivative. The major advantage of these agents is less frequent dosing than with acyclovir. Thus, valacyclovir administered two times a day was as efficacious as acyclovir administered five times a day in the treatment of recurrent genital herpes.[133] Similarly, famciclovir administered two times a day was found to be efficacious in the treatment of genital HSV infection but has not been compared with standard acyclovir or valacyclovir treatment.[254]

Studies evaluating interferon, phosphonoformate, 2′-fluoro-5-iodoaracytosine, E-5-(2-iodovinyl)-2′-deoxyuridine, and other nucleoside analogues have appeared promising and, it is hoped, will yield further clinically useful antiherpetic therapy.

Symptomatic therapy of HSV lesions should be directed toward reduction of local discomfort, promotion of healing, and prevention of autoinoculation and superinfection. Nonspecific creams and ointments probably delay healing and increase the risk of maceration and infection. Keeping lesions clean and dry probably is the most important local measure. Urination sometimes is painful and can be made less so by urinating into a bathtub or sitz bath. Some experts advise Burow solution sitz baths or short compress treatments. Prolonged soaking delays healing.

Mucocutaneous Herpes Simplex Virus Infection in the Immunocompromised Host[104]

Therapeutic responses to HSV infection in the immunocompromised host have been difficult to study because of the variable nature of the disease. Nevertheless, several therapies now have proven efficacy in this setting. The most difficult decision for the clinician is how serious the manifestation must be before initiation of therapy, which may require hospitalization. In addition, no comparative studies yet allow cogent decisions regarding the use of vidarabine versus the various forms (topical, intravenous, oral) of acyclovir.

In a randomized, controlled, crossover study of mucocutaneous HSV infection, vidarabine (10 mg/kg/day intravenously in a 12-hour infusion) was shown to decrease pain and induce defervescence in patients older than 40 years of age.[340] None of the 85 patients in this study developed visceral dissemination of HSV. No controlled studies have analyzed the therapeutic effects of vidarabine in a strictly pediatric population, and the relatively low therapeutic index in the cited study would be less than encouraging in that regard. In the only randomized study comparing vidarabine with acyclovir, involving treatment of varicella-zoster infection in the immunocompromised host, acyclovir was superior.[280]

Acyclovir ointment appears to help in decreasing pain, viral shedding, and time to complete lesion healing in immunocompromised persons with mild, non–life-threatening mucocutaneous HSV infection.[336] It has been rendered obsolete by oral acyclovir for mild illness. Patients who have more severe illness should be cared for in a hospital setting with the intravenous preparation. For infection control purposes, the ointment may be applied every 3 hours, six times per day, to cover lesions; a ½-inch ribbon of ointment is sufficient for 4 square inches of lesion area. A rubber glove or finger cot is suggested for avoidance of autoinoculation. Side effects may include pruritus and rash.

Intravenous acyclovir has been analyzed extensively in immunocompromised patients who have mucocutaneous HSV infection.[104] When used early, acyclovir arrests the progression of infection.[277] In several double-blind, placebo-controlled studies, acyclovir has been shown to be highly effective. It decreased time to cessation of new lesions (1 versus 3 days in placebo), time to lesion crusting (3 to 7 versus 9 to 14 days), time to lesion healing (12 to 14 versus 18 to 28 days), cessation of pain (4 to 10 versus 7 to 16 days), and termination of viral shedding (3 versus 14 to 17 days).[200, 325] At this writing, intravenously administered acyclovir is the most effective mode and drug of choice for treating HSV in the immunocompromised host. The dosage is 250 mg/m^2 or 5 mg/kg every 8 hours, infused over 1 hour. In cases of severe disease, the dose may be doubled. The major toxic effect has been renal, with a reversible obstructive nephropathy and transient rises in serum creatinine levels (5 to 10 per cent of patients). Adequate hydration usually prevents this problem. There are guidelines for dosage in patients who have impaired renal function (Table 163–4). One to 5 per cent of patients may experience nausea and vomiting. Less commonly (1 per cent), reversible neurologic symptoms (lethargy, agitation, tremor, disorientation, coma, transient hemiparesthesia) and laboratory abnormalities (abnormal electroencephalogram, increased CSF myelin basic protein) have developed in marrow transplant patients. These patients usually had received interferon and CNS chemoprophylaxis for leukemia.[324] Other less-serious problems include phlebitis (14 per cent) and hives (5 per cent).

Studies have focused on the use of oral acyclovir in this patient population.[303] The 50 per cent virus-inhibiting level of acyclovir for HSV-1 generally is 0.1 to 0.5 μg/mL and for HSV-2 0.5 to 2 μg/mL. Many studies utilize molar concentration; in the case of acyclovir, the dose in micromols divided by 4 equals the dose in micrograms per milliliter. Whereas the peak serum levels with intravenous acyclovir vary from 8 to 15 μg/mL, the levels achieved with oral therapy are considerably lower (1 to 2 μg/mL). In preliminary studies of relatively small populations of immunocompromised adults, oral acyclovir at doses of 200 mg five times per day effectively promoted lesion healing and inhibited viral shedding.[303] Pediatric studies have utilized oral doses of 600 mg/m^2 given four times per day.[305] To date, there are no data comparing the relative efficacy of oral versus intravenous acyclovir in this setting.

To date, all studies about acyclovir in the immunosuppressed patient have documented the marked propensity of recurrence to continue when therapy is withdrawn. Indeed, it has been suggested that because of the blunting effect of acyclovir on both humoral and cellular immune responses to HSV, therapy may predispose patients to HSV recurrences.[322]

TABLE 163–4. Guidelines for Use of Acyclovir in Patients with Renal Impairment*

Creatinine Clearance (mL/min/1.7 m^2)	Dose (mg/kg)	Dose Interval (hours)
50	5	8
25–50	5	12
10–25	5	24
0–10	2.5	24

*A dose (5 mg/kg) should be administered after each dialysis in patients on hemodialysis.

Acyclovir-Resistant Herpes Simplex Virus Infection

After more than a decade of use, acyclovir remains an effective antiviral compound. In the immunocompetent host, acyclovir resistance has been a rare problem, even with prolonged courses of suppressive therapy. Acyclovir-resistant virus occasionally has been shed by immunocompetent patients before, during, or after therapy, yet it usually has not been associated with treatment failure.[174, 175, 189, 304] In pretreatment patients, 3.6 per cent of isolates (31 of 870) were resistant to acyclovir (not inhibited by 3 μg/mL).[57] A similar percentage (3.1 per cent) of resistant isolates were recovered from 663 immunocompetent patients after acyclovir therapy.[57] An immunocompetent patient who had an acyclovir-resistant virus containing an altered thymidine kinase that causes multiple recurrences of genital herpes that are unresponsive to acyclovir therapy was reported.[160] To date, these occurrences are rare in the immunocompetent patient population.

Drug resistance has become more of a problem in the acyclovir-treated immunocompromised population. There are many reports of acyclovir-resistant virus causing local invasive disease, and less commonly dissemination, and even acyclovir-unresponsive meningoencephalitis.[28, 104, 106, 182, 186, 256, 323] Of the three mechanisms of altered sensitivity of HSV to acyclovir (absent thymidine kinase [TK$^-$], altered thymidine kinase [TK^A], and altered viral DNA polymerase), the TK$^-$ type is the problem in the vast majority of cases.[57, 69, 104, 106, 186] These viruses, usually lacking thymidine kinase, cannot phosphorylate acyclovir and convert it to the active triphosphate. Among marrow transplant recipients receiving multiple courses of acyclovir, acyclovir-resistant virus was recovered from 2 per cent of patients during initial therapy and from 9 per cent after treatment for a second recurrence.[323] In a tertiary case center, acyclovir-resistant, clinically significant virus was recovered from 5 per cent of immunocompromised patients (usually after receipt of acyclovir) but from no immunocompetent hosts.[94] Illness caused by the acyclovir-resistant viruses was more severe in pediatric patients and more common in very immunocompromised patients, such as those with AIDS or who had undergone marrow transplantation.[94] Among referred marrow transplant and AIDS patients, after acyclovir therapy, 18 per cent (105 of 582) of their isolates were acyclovir-resistant.[57] In vitro viral susceptibility of HSV has been highly associated with clinical response to acyclovir in HIV-infected patients.[258]

The acyclovir-resistant isolates also are resistant to ganciclovir, which also requires phosphorylation. Although the isolates remain sensitive to vidarabine in vitro, vidarabine has not been a useful drug as therapy for acyclovir-resistant HSV because of both poor response and toxicity.[256] Foscarnet (40 mg/kg every 8 hours) has been used and associated with an excellent clinical response and cessation of viral shedding.[28, 255, 256] The most common side effects of foscarnet are nephrotoxicity (azotemia), alterations in serum calcium and phosphorus, and neutropenia observed in 10 to 25 per cent of patients.[139, 255, 256] In the immunocompromised patient who has HSV infection unresponsive to acyclovir, foscarnet therapy is indicated. Viral susceptibility testing may aid in clinical management.[259]

More recently, in patients receiving chronic or multiple causes of foscarnet, foscarnet-resistant HSV isolates (IC_{50} >100 μg/mL) have been recovered from lesions failing to respond to foscarnet.[28, 258, 259,] Of note, these lesions often responded to acyclovir, alone or in combination with foscarnet.[259] Perhaps the mutation in DNA polymerase responsible for foscarnet resistance was in an area not related to acyclovir activity.[259]

Other experimental strategies used to treat acyclovir-resistant viruses have included high-dose continuous infusion acyclovir (1.5 to 2.0 mg/kg/hour)[92] or the use of intravenous (S)-1-[3-hydroxy-2(phosphonylmethoxy)propyl] cytosine (HPMPC), a nucleotide analogue.[169]

In the case of acyclovir- and foscarnet-resistant viruses, topical HPMPC[287] or a combination of topical trifluorothymidine and interferon-α[29] have been used successfully in a small number of patients who have chronic mucocutaneous lesions.

PREVENTION

Environmental Control or Barrier Prevention

Because HSV is sensitive to heat, light, and lipid solvents, use of antiseptics, soap and hot water, or chlorine decreases the risk of transfer of virus in settings such as the home, spas, pools, wrestling meets, and hospitals. In addition, appropriate use of gloves by respiratory care personnel, dentists, and persons in contact with potentially infected body secretions or skin rashes should decrease acquisition and nosocomial spread of HSV. These are all part of universal body substance precaution policies in place in most health care delivery settings. Wrestlers should be examined, and those who have skin lesions suggestive of herpes should refrain from competition. Although there are no human data, in vitro experiments have shown that condoms retard the passage of viable HSV. The use of cesarean section for preventing neonatal HSV is discussed elsewhere (see Chapter 76).

Immunoprophylaxis

After a dismal history of attempts at vaccination to prevent or ameliorate HSV infection in humans,[193] there finally is a glimmer of hope. When a vaccine containing recombinant glycoprotein D of HSV-2 (gD_2) was used in patients who had established recurrent genital HSV infections, vaccine recipients had one-third fewer genital herpes recurrences than placebo recipients during the study year.[299] It is hoped that recombinant vaccines may be useful in primary HSV infection prevention as well. Recombinant HSV-2 gD_2 and gB_2 have been demonstrated to induce high humoral and cell-mediated immune responses in seronegative and seropositive recipients.[171] Immunomodulation may be the mechanism by which interferon prevented reactivation of HSV in humans undergoing operation of the trigeminal nerve root (see following discussion). Although animal data suggest successful immunomodulation with various agents, such as bacillus Calmette-Guérin, interleukin-2, or immune serum, to date there are no such successes in humans. Agents such as bacillus Calmette-Guérin, smallpox vaccine, lysine, and many other compounds have been shown to be ineffective and at times dangerous. A preliminary report describes the successful use of high-dose intravenous immunoglobulin to suppress frequently recurring genital herpes.[188]

Chemoprophylaxis

Intramuscular human interferon-α administered before and after operation on the trigeminal nerve root significantly decreased the incidence of HSV shedding and clinical reactivation.[230] In similar studies, interferon had no significant effect on HSV shedding or reactivation in renal transplant patients.[52] Intravenous acyclovir has been shown to prevent the reactivation of HSV almost completely in immunosuppressed patients receiving a marrow transplant or antileukemic chemotherapy. Therapy usually is begun at the onset of immunosuppression and continued for 1½ to 3 months. HSV is reactivated in 50 to 70 per cent of these adult patients. Oral acyclovir administered chronically also markedly suppressed recurrence in immunodeficient patients.[236, 261, 262, 301, 307] In children undergoing marrow transplantation, acyclovir dosages of 500 mg/m²/day in three divided doses for 3 weeks, then 250 mg/m²/day for 3 months orally, suppressed HSV infection.[93] The use of prophylactic acyclovir in HSV-seropositive, immunosuppressed pediatric patients is indicated.

Oral acyclovir (200 mg two to five times per day) administered chronically can prevent nearly completely the reactivation of genital HSV in patients suffering frequent recurrences. Recurrences decreased by 50 to 70 per cent, and time to recurrence changed from 14 to 25 days in patients receiving placebo and from 100 to 125 days in those receiving acyclovir.[83, 199, 304] Breakthrough recurrences tended to be mild and to have less viral shedding and rarely were caused by acyclovir-resistant virus. When acyclovir was discontinued (after 12 to 15 weeks of administration), HSV recurrences reverted to the pretreatment frequency. Higher doses of acyclovir suppressed recurrences in those patients experiencing "breakthroughs" on more conventional doses. In patients receiving therapy for 5 years, the number of recurrences declined from the first year (1.7) to the fifth year (0.8).[113] Twenty to 25 per cent of patients are recurrence-free for 4 to 5 years.[113, 143] After prophylactic therapy ended, suppressive therapy was no longer warranted in some patients because of longer time between recurrences.[99, 300] Patients who had resistant virus had reisolation of acyclovir-sensitive virus. Thus, acyclovir suppressed recurrences without eliminating latent virus. A study has reported that acyclovir does not seem to change the rate of asymptomatic viral shedding.[302] A more recent study has demonstrated that acyclovir (400 mg twice a day) resulted in a 95 per cent reduction in subclinical viral shedding when compared with placebo in women with genital herpes.[326] Side effects of chronic acyclovir therapy are limited to an increase in mean corpuscular erythrocyte volume and hemoglobin concentration without anemia or megaloblastic changes, asthenia, and mild gastrointestinal upset.[143, 304] Perhaps the most enjoyable study was that showing a prevention of herpetic recurrences in skiers utilizing a brief course of acyclovir during their ski trip.[290]

There are, as of this writing, few studies concerning the use of prophylactic acyclovir in children. Prophylactic oral acyclovir (30 to 60 mg/kg/day in three to five doses for 1 week) has been shown to decrease seroconversion effectively and to eradicate symptomatic cases of HSV gingivostomatitis in a nursery setting in which outbreaks of HSV primary infection were occurring.[166] Whether the growing child will experience more significant side effects remains to be studied. To date, up to 6 years of therapy in adults has not resulted in new side effects[99, 113, 143, 300] or an increase in the problem of drug-resistant HSV in the normal host.[99] A preliminary report has shown that famciclovir effectively suppressed frequently recurring genital herpes in women using a twice- or once-per-day protocol.[196]

References

1. Abramson, J. S., Roach, E. S., and Levy, H. B.: Postinfectious encephalopathy after treatment of herpes simplex encephalitis with acyclovir. Pediatr. Infect. Dis. *3*:146–147, 1984.
2. Adam, E., Kaufman, R. H., Mirkovic, R. H., et al.: Persistence of virus shedding in asymptomatic women after recovery from herpes genitalis. Obstet. Gynecol. *54*:171–173, 1979.
3. Adams, G., Stover, B. H., Keenlyside, R. A., et al.: Nosocomial herpetic infections in a pediatric intensive care unit. Am. J. Epidemiol. *113*:126–132, 1981.
4. Aoki, F. Y., Law, B. J., Hammond, G. W., et al.: Acyclovir suspension for treatment of acute herpes simplex virus gingivostomatitis in children: A placebo-controlled, double-blind trial. Abstracts of the 33rd Interscience Conference on Antimicrobial Agents and Chemotherapy, 399, 1993.
5. Armstrong, J. A., Evans, A. S., Rao, N., et al.: Viral infections in renal transplant recipients. Infect. Immun. *14*:970–975, 1976.
6. Ashenburg, C., Rothstein, F. C., and Dahms, B. B.: Herpes esophagitis in the immunocompetent child. J. Pediatr. *108*:584–587, 1986.
7. Ashkenazi, S., and Kohl, S. Nervous system abnormalities in pediatric HIV infection and AIDS. Semin. Pediatr. Infect. Dis. *1*:94–106, 1990.
8. Ashley, R., Cent, A., Maggs, V., et al.: Inability of enzyme immunoassays to discriminate between infections with herpes simplex virus types 1 and 2. Ann. Intern. Med. *115*:520–526, 1991.
9. Ashley, R. L., and Corey, L.: Effect of acyclovir treatment of primary genital herpes on the antibody response to herpes simplex virus. J. Clin. Invest. *73*:681–688, 1984.
10. Aurelius, E., Andersson, B., Forsgren, M., et al.: Cytokines and other markers of intrathecal immune response in patients with herpes simplex encephalitis. J. Infect. Dis. *170*:678–680, 1994.
11. Aurelius, E., Fosgren, M., Skoldenberg, B., et al.: Persistent intrathecal immune activation in patients with herpes simplex encephalitis. J. Infect. Dis. *168*:1248–1252, 1993.
12. Aurelius, E., Johansson, B., Skoldenberg, B., et al.: Rapid diagnosis of herpes simplex encephalitis by nested polymerase chain reaction assay of cerebrospinal fluid. Lancet *337*:189–192, 1991.
13. Aurelius, E., Johansson, B., Skoldenberg, B., et al.: Encephalitis in immunocompetent patients due to herpes simplex virus type 1 or 2 as determined by type-specific polymerase chain reaction and antibody assays of cerebrospinal fluid. J. Med. Virol. *39*:179–186, 1993.
14. Bader, C., Crumpacker, C. S., Schnipper, L. E., et al.: The natural history of recurrent facial-oral infection with herpes simplex virus. J. Infect. Dis. *138*:897–905, 1978.
15. Banks, T. A., and Rouse, B. T. Herpes viruses: Immune escape artists? Clin. Infect. Dis. *14*:933–941, 1992.
16. Baringer, J. R.: Recovery of herpes simplex virus from human sacral ganglions. N. Engl. J. Med. *291*:828–830, 1974.
17. Baringer, J. R.: Herpes simplex virus infection of nervous tissue in animals and man. Progr. Med. Virol. *20*:1–26, 1975.
18. Barza, M., and Pauker, S. G.: The decision to biopsy, treat, or wait in suspected herpes encephalitis. Ann. Intern. Med. *92*:641–649, 1980.
19. Bastian, F. O., Rabson, A. S., Yee, C. L., et al.: Herpes-virus hominis: Isolation from human trigeminal ganglion. Science *178*:306–307, 1972.
20. Bastian, J. F., and Kaufman, I. A.: Herpes simplex esophagitis in a healthy 10-year-old boy. J. Pediatr. *100*:426–427, 1982.
21. Becker, T. M., Magder, L., and Harrison, H. R.: The epidemiology of infection with the human herpesviruses in Navajo children. Am. J. Epidemiol. *127*:1071–1078, 1988.
22. Becker, W. B., Kipps, A., and McKenzie, D.: Disseminated herpes simplex virus infection: Its pathogenesis based on virological and pathological studies in 33 cases. Am. J. Dis. Child. *115*:1–8, 1968.
23. Behr, J. T., Daluga, D. J., Light, T. R., et al.: Herpetic infections in the fingers of infants. Report of five cases. J. Bone Joint Surg. [Am.] *69*:137–139, 1987.
24. Beigi, B., Algawi, K., Foley-Nolan, A., et al.: Herpes simplex keratitis in children. Br. J. Ophthalmol. *78*:458–460, 1994.
25. Belongia, E. A., Goodman, J. L., Holland, E. J., et al.: An outbreak of herpes gladiatorum at a high-school wrestling camp. N. Engl. J. Med. *325*:906–910, 1991.
26. Benedetti, J. K., Zeh, J., Selke, S., et al.: Frequency and reactivation of nongenital lesions among patients with genital herpes simplex virus. Am. J. Med. *98*:237–242, 1995.
27. Bernstein, D. I., Lovett, M. A., and Bryson, Y. J.: The effects of acyclovir on antibody response to herpes simplex virus in primary genital herpetic infections. J. Infect. Dis. *150*:7–13, 1984.
28. Birch, C., J., Tachedjian, G., Doherty, R. R., et al.: Altered sensitivity to antiviral drugs of herpes simplex virus isolates from a patient with the acquired immunodeficiency syndrome. J. Infect. Dis. *162*:731–734, 1990.
29. Birch, C. J., Tyssen, D. P., Tachedjian, G., et al.: Clinical effects and in vitro studies of trifluorothymidine combined with interferon-α for treatment of drug-resistant and sensitive herpes simplex virus infections. J. Infect. Dis. *166*:108–112, 1992.
30. Biron, C. A., Byron, K. S., and Sullivan, J. L.: Severe herpes virus infections in an adolescent without natural killer cells. N. Engl. J. Med. *320*:1731–1735, 1989.
31. Bogger-Goren, S.: Acute epiglottitis caused by herpes simplex virus. Pediatr. Infect. Dis. J. *6*:1133–1134, 1987.
32. Brain, R. T.: The clinical vagaries of herpes virus. Br. Med. J. *1*:1061–1068, 1956.
33. Breinig, M. K., Kingsley, L. A., Armstrong, J. A., et al.: Epidemiology of genital herpes in Pittsburgh: Serologic, sexual and racial correlates of apparent and inapparent herpes simplex infections. J. Infect. Dis. *162*:299–305, 1990.
34. Brice, S. L., Krzemien, D., Weston, W. L., et al.: Detection of herpes simplex virus DNA in cutaneous lesions of erythema multiforme. J. Invest. Dermatol. *93*:183–187, 1989.
35. Brice, S. L., Stockert, S. S., Jester, J. D., et al.: Herpes simplex virus–associated erythema multiforme in children. Clin. Res. *38*:182a, 1990.
36. Brock, B. V., Selke, S., Benedetti, J., et al.: Frequency of asymptomatic shedding of herpes simplex virus in women with genital herpes. J. A. M. A. *263*:418–420, 1990.
37. Brodtkorb, E., Lindqvist, M., Johnson, M., et al.: Diagnosis of herpes simplex encephalitis: A comparison between electroencephalography and computed tomography findings. Acta Neurol. Scand. *66*:462–471, 1982.
38. Brown, Z. A., Benedetti, J. D., and Watts, D. H.: A comparison between detailed and simple histories in the diagnosis of genital herpes complicating pregnancy. Am. J. Obstet. Gynecol. *172*:1299–1303, 1995.
39. Brown, Z. A., Kern, E. R., and Spruance, S. L.: Clinical and virologic course of herpes simplex genitalis. West. J. Med. *130*:414–421, 1979.
40. Bryson, Y., Dillon, M., Bernstein, D. I., et al.: Risks of acquisition of genital herpes simplex virus type 2 in sex partners of persons with genital herpes: A prospective couple study. J. Infect. Dis. *167*:942–946, 1993.
41. Bryson, Y. J., Dillon, M., Lovett, M., et al.: Treatment of first episodes of genital herpes simplex virus infection with oral acyclovir. A randomized double-blind controlled trial in normal subjects. N. Engl. J. Med. *308*:916–921, 1983.
42. Buchman, T. G., Roizman, B., Adams, G., et al.: Restriction endonuclease fingerprinting of herpes simplex virus DNA: A novel epidemiological tool applied to a nosocomial outbreak. J. Infect. Dis. *138*:488–498, 1978.
43. Buchman, T. G., Roizman, B., and Nahmias, A. J.: Demonstration of exogenous genital reinfection with herpes simplex virus type 2 by restriction endonuclease fingerprinting of viral DNA. J. Infect. Dis. *140*:295–304, 1979.
44. Buss, D. H., and Scharyj, M.: Herpesvirus infection of the esophagus and other visceral organs in adults: Incidence and clinical significance. Am. J. Med. *66*:457–462, 1979.
45. Caputo, G. M., and Byck, H.: Concomitant oculoglandular and ulceroglandular fever due to herpes simplex type 1. Am. J. Med. *93*:577–580, 1992.
46. Cauda, R., Laghi, V., Tumbarello, M., et al.: Immunological alterations associated with recurrent herpes simplex genitalis. Clin. Immunol. Immunopathol. *51*:294–302, 1989.
47. Centers for Disease Control: Encephalitis surveillance: Annual Summary 1978. U.S. Dept. of Health and Human Services, 1981, pp. 24–25.
48. Centers for Disease Control: Genital herpes infections, United States, 1966–1979. M. M. W. R. *31*:137–139, 1982.
49. Centers for Disease Control: Genital herpes infections, United States, 1966–1984. M. M. W. R. *35*:402–404, 1986.
50. Centers for Disease Control: Herpes gladiatorum at a high school wrestling camp—Minnesota. M. M. W. R. *39*:69–71, 1990.
51. Chase, R. A., Pottage, J. C., Jr., Haber, M. H., et al.: Herpes simplex viral hepatitis in adults: Two case reports and review of the literature. Rev. Infect. Dis. *9*:329–333, 1987.
52. Cheeseman, S. H., Rubin, R. H., Stewart, J. A., et al.: Controlled clinical trial of prophylactic human-leukocyte interferon in renal transplantation. Effect on cytomegalovirus and herpes simplex virus infections. N. Engl. J. Med. *300*:1345–1349, 1979.
53. Cho, M., Xiao, X., Egbert, B., et al.: Rapid detection of cutaneous herpes simplex virus infection with the polymerase chain reaction. J. Invest. Dermatol. *92*:391–392, 1989.
54. Chonmaitree, T., Owen, M., Patel, J., et al.: Presence of cytomegalovirus and herpes simplex virus in middle ear fluids from children with acute otitis media. Clin. Infect. Dis. *15*:650–653, 1992.
55. Chuang, T.-Y., Su, W. P. D., Perry, H. O., et al.: Incidence and trend of herpes progenitalis. A 15-year population study. Mayo Clin. Proc. *58*:436–441, 1983.
56. Clive, D., Corey, L., Reichman, R. C., et al.: A double-blind, placebo-

controlled cytogenetic study of oral acyclovir in patients with recurrent genital herpes. J. Infect. Dis. *164*:753–757, 1991.
57. Collins, P., and Ellis, M. N.: Sensitivity monitoring of clinical isolates of herpes simplex virus to acyclovir. J. Med. Virol. *1*(Suppl.):58–66, 1993.
58. Collum, L. M. T., McGettrick, P., Akhtar, J., et al.: Oral acyclovir (Zovirax) in herpes simplex dendritic corneal ulceration. Br. J. Ophthalmol. *70*:435–438, 1986.
59. Cone, R. W., Hobson, A. C., Palmer, J., et al.: Extended duration of herpes simplex virus DNA in genital lesions detected by the polymerase chain reaction. J. Infect. Dis. *164*:757–760, 1991.
60. Corey, L., Adams, H. G., Brown, Z. A., et al.: Genital herpes simplex virus infections, clinical manifestations, course, and complications. Ann. Intern. Med. *98*:958–972, 1983.
61. Corey, L., Fife, K. H., Benedetti, J. K., et al.: Intravenous acyclovir for the treatment of primary genital herpes. Ann. Intern. Med. *98*:914–921, 1983.
62. Corey, L., and Holmes, K. K.: Genital herpes simplex infections: Current concepts in diagnosis, therapy and prevention. Ann. Intern. Med. *98*:973–983, 1983.
63. Corey, L., Nahmias, A. J., and Guinan, M. E.: A trial of topical acyclovir in genital herpes simplex virus infection. N. Engl. J. Med. *306*:1313–1319, 1982.
64. Corey, L., Reeves, W. C., and Holmes, K. K.: Cellular immune response in genital herpes simplex virus infection. N. Engl. J. Med. *299*:986–991, 1978.
65. Corey, L., and Spear, P. G.: Infections with herpes simplex virus. N. Engl. J. Med. *314*:686–691, 749–757, 1986.
66. Craig, C., and Nahmias, A. J.: Different patterns of neurologic involvement with herpes simplex virus types 1 and 2: Isolation of herpes simplex virus type 2 from the buffy coat of two adults with meningitis. J. Infect. Dis. *127*:365–372, 1973.
67. Croen, K. D., Ostrove, J. M., Dragovic, L. J., et al.: Latent herpes simplex virus in human trigeminal ganglia: Detection of an immediate early gene "anti-sense" transcript by in situ hybridization. N. Engl. J. Med. *317*:1427–1432, 1987.
68. Croen, K. D., Ostrove, S. M., Dragovic, L., et al.: Characterization of herpes simplex virus type 2 latency-associated transcription in human sacral ganglia and in cell culture. J. Infect. Dis. *163*:23–28, 1991.
69. Crumpacker, C. S., II: Molecular targets of antiviral therapy. N. Engl. J. Med. *321*:163–172, 1989.
70. Crumpacker, C. S., Schnipper, L. E., and Marlowe, S. I.: Resistance to antiviral drugs of herpes simplex isolated from a patient treated with acyclovir. N. Engl. J. Med. *306*:343–346, 1982.
71. Darougar, S., Wishart, M. S., and Viswalingam, N. D.: Epidemiological and clinical features of primary herpes simplex virus ocular infection. Br. J. Ophthalmol. *69*:2–6, 1985.
72. Dascal, A., Chan-Thim, J., Morahan, M., et al.: Diagnosis of herpes simplex virus infection in a clinical setting by a direct enzyme immunoassay kit. J. Clin. Microbiol. *27*:700–704, 1989.
73. David, T. J., and Langson, M.: Herpes simplex infection in atopic eczema. Arch. Dis. Child. *60*:338–343, 1985.
74. Davis, L. E., and Johnson, R. T.: An explanation for the localization of herpes simplex encephalitis? Ann. Neurol. *5*:2–5, 1979.
75. Davis, L. E., and McLaren, L. C.: Relapsing herpes simplex encephalitis following antiviral therapy? Ann. Neurol. *13*:192–195, 1983.
76. Dawson, C., Togni, B., and Moore, T. E., Jr.: Structural changes in chronic herpetic keratitis: Studied by light and electron microscopy. Arch. Ophthalmol. *79*:740–747, 1968.
77. Delva, M. D., and McSherry, J. A.: Herpes genitalis in a student population. J. Fam. Pract. *18*:397–400, 1984.
78. Demaeral, P. H., Wilms, G., Robberecht, W., et al.: MRI of herpes simplex encephalitis. Neuroradiology *34*:490–493, 1992.
79. DeVincenzo, J. P., and Thorne, G.: Mild herpes simplex encephalitis diagnosed by polymerase chain reaction: A case report and review. Pediatr. Infect. Dis. J. *13*:662–664, 1994.
80. DiSclafani, A., Kohl, S., and Ostrow, P. T.: The importance of brain biopsy in suspected herpes simplex encephalitis. Surg. Neurol. *17*:101–106, 1982.
81. Dix, R. D., Baringer, J. R., Panitch, H. S., et al.: Recurrent herpes simplex encephalitis: Recovery of virus after Ara-A treatment. Ann. Neurol. *13*:196–200, 1983.
82. Do, A. N., Green, P. A., and Demmler, G. J.: Herpes simplex type 2 meningitis and associated genital lesions in a three-year-old child. Pediatr. Infect. Dis. J. *13*:1014–1016, 1994.
83. Douglas, J. M., Critchlow, C., and Benedetti, J.: A double-blind study of oral acyclovir for suppression of recurrences of genital herpes simplex virus infection. N. Engl. J. Med. *310*:1551–1556, 1984.
84. Dowdle, W. R., Nahmias, A. J., Harwell, R. W., et al.: Association of antigenic type of herpesvirus hominis with site of viral recovery. J. Immunol. *99*:774–780, 1967.
85. Drummer, J. S., Armstrong, J., Somers, J., et al.: Transmission of infection with herpes simplex virus by renal transplantation. J. Infect. Dis. *155*:202–206, 1987.
86. Ducoulombier, H., Cousin, J., Dewilde, A., et al.: A controlled clinical trial versus placebo of acyclovir in the treatment of herpetic gingivostomatitis in children [in French]. Ann. Pediatr. (Paris) *35*:212–216, 1988.
87. Duenas, A., Adam, E., Melnick, J. L., et al.: Herpesvirus type 2 in a prostitute population. Am. J. Epidemiol. *95*:483–489, 1972.
88. Eglin, R. P., Kitchener, H. C., and MacLean, A. B.: The presence of RNA complementary to HSV-2 (herpes simplex virus) DNA in cervical intraepithelial neoplasia after laser therapy. Br. J. Obstet. Gynaecol. *91*:265–269, 1984.
89. Eglin, R. P., Lehner, T., and Subak-Sharpe, J. H.: Detection of RNA complementary to herpes-simplex virus in mononuclear cells from patients with Behcet's syndrome and recurrent oral ulcers. Lancet *2*:1356–1361, 1982.
90. Eisenstein, B. T.: The polymerase chain reaction: A new method of using molecular genetics for medical diagnosis. N. Engl. J. Med. *322*:178–183, 1990.
91. Ellison, P. H., and Hanson, P. A.: Herpes simplex: A possible cause of brain stem encephalitis. Pediatrics *59*:240–243, 1977.
92. Engel, J. P., Englund, J. A., Fletcher, C. V., et al.: Treatment of resistant herpes simplex virus with continuous-infusion acyclovir. J. A. M. A. *263*:1662–1664, 1990.
93. Engelhard, D., Morag, A., Or, R., et al.: Prevention of herpes simplex virus (HSV) infection in recipients of HLA-matched T-lymphocyte–depleted bone marrow allografts. Isr. J. Med. Sci. *24*:145–150, 1988.
94. Englund, J. A., Zimmerman, M. E., Swierhosz, E. M., et al.: Herpes simplex virus resistant to acyclovir: A study in a tertiary care center. Ann. Intern. Med. *112*:416–422, 1990.
95. Espy, M., and Smith, T. F.: Detection of herpes simplex virus in conventional tube cell cultures and in shell vials with a DNA probe kit and monoclonal antibodies. J. Clin. Microbiol. *26*:22–24, 1988.
96. Fedler, H. M., and Long, S. S.: Herpetic whitlow. Epidemiology, clinical characteristics, diagnosis and treatment. Am. J. Dis. Child. *137*:861–863, 1983.
97. Fiddian, A. P., Yeo, J. M., and Clark, A. E.: Treatment of herpes labialis. J. Infect. *6*:41–47, 1983.
98. Field, H. J., and Phillips, I. (eds.): Acyclovir. J. Antimicrob. Chemother. *12*(Suppl. B):1–202, 1983.
99. Fife, K. H., Crumpacker, C. S., and Mertz, G. J.: Recurrence and resistance patterns of herpes simplex virus following cessation of greater than or equal to 6 years of chronic suppression with acyclovir. J. Infect. Dis. *169*:1338–1341, 1994.
100. Fiumara, N. J., and Solomon, J.: Recurrent herpes simplex virus infections and erythema multiforme: A report of three patients. Sex. Transm. Dis. *10*:144–147, 1983.
101. Foley, F. D., Greenwald, K. A., Nash, G., et al.: Herpesvirus infection in burned patients. N. Engl. J. Med. *282*:652–656, 1970.
102. Frank, A. L., and Tucker, G.: Isolation of herpes simplex type 1 from ventricular fluid of an infant with encephalitis. J. Pediatr. *92*:601–602, 1978.
103. Freeman, W. R., Thomas, E. L., Rao, N. A., et al.: Demonstration of herpes group virus in acute retinal necrosis syndrome. Am. J. Ophthalmol. *102*:701–709, 1986.
104. Frenck, R. W., and Kohl, S.: Herpes simplex virus in the immunocompromised child. *In* Patrick, C. C. (ed.): Infections in Immunocompromised Infants and Children. New York, Churchill Livingstone, 1992, pp. 603–624.
105. Galbraith, J. C. T., and Shafran, S.: Herpes simplex esophagitis in the immunocompetent patient: Report of four cases and review. Clin. Infect. Dis. *14*:894–901, 1992.
106. Gateley, A., Gander, R. M., Johnson, P. C., et al.: Herpes simplex virus type 2 meningoencephalitis resistant to acyclovir in a patient with AIDS. J. Infect. Dis. *116*:711–720, 1990.
107. Gentry, G. A., Lowe, M., Alford, G., et al.: Sequence analysis of herpesviral enzymes suggest an ancient origin for human sexual behavior. Proc. Natl. Acad. Sci. U. S. A. *85*:2658–2661, 1988.
108. Gerson, M., Portnoy, J., and Hamelin, C.: Reliable identification of herpes simplex viruses by DNA restriction endonuclease analysis with EcoR-1. Sex. Transm. Dis. *11*:85–90, 1984.
109. Gibson, J. J., Hornung, C. A., Alexander, G. R., et al.: A cross-sectional study of herpes simplex virus types 1 and 2 in college students: Occurrence and determinants of infection. J. Infect. Dis. *162*:306–312, 1990.
110. Gill, M. J., Arlette, J., and Buchan, K.: Herpes simplex virus infection of the hand. A profile of 79 cases. Am. J. Med. *84*:89–93, 1988.
111. Glezen, W. P., Fernald, G. W., and Lohr, J. A.: Acute respiratory disease of university students with special reference to the etiologic role of herpesvirus hominis. Am. J. Epidemiol. *101*:111–121, 1975.
112. Glogau, R., Hanna, L., and Jawetz, E.: Herpetic whitlow as part of genital virus infection. J. Infect. Dis. *136*:689–692, 1977.
113. Goldberg, L. H., Kaufman, R., Kurtz, T. O., et al.: Long-term suppression of recurrent genital herpes with acyclovir: A 5-year benchmark. Arch. Dermatol. *129*:582–587, 1993.
114. Golden, M. P., Kim, S., Hammer, S. M., et al.: Activation of human immunodeficiency virus by herpes simplex virus. J. Infect. Dis. *166*:494–499, 1992.
115. Goldstein, L. C., Corey, L., McDougall, J. K., et al.: Monoclonal antibodies to herpes simplex viruses: Use in antigenic typing and rapid diagnosis. J. Infect. Dis. *147*:829–837, 1983.
116. Goodell, S. E., Quinn, T. C., Mkrtichian, E., et al.: Herpes simplex virus proctitis in homosexual men: Clinical, sigmoidoscopic, and histopathological features. N. Engl. J. Med. *308*:868–871, 1983.
117. Greenberg, S. B., Taber, L., Septimus, E., et al.: Computerized tomography

in brain-biopsy-proven herpes simplex encephalitis: Early normal results. Arch. Neurol. *38*:58–59, 1981.
118. Gronowitz, J. S., and Kallander, C. F.: The use of herpes virus induced dTk as a marker for serological and direct identification of herpes virus infection in man. Dev. Biol. Stand. *52*:193–204, 1982.
119. Grossman, M. E., Stevens, A. W., and Cohen, P. R.: Brief report: Herpetic geometric glossitis. N. Engl. J. Med. *329*:1859–1860, 1993.
120. Guffond, T., Dewilde, A., Lobert, P. E., et al.: Significance and clinical relevance of the detection of herpes simplex virus DNA by polymerase chain reaction in cerebrospinal fluid from patients with presumed encephalitis. Clin. Infect. Dis. *18*:744–749, 1994.
121. Guinan, M. E., MacCalman, J., Kern, E. R., et al.: The course of untreated recurrent genital herpes simplex infection in 27 women. N. Engl. J. Med. *304*:759–763, 1983.
122. Gutman, L. T., Wilfert, C. M., and Eppes, S.: Herpes simplex virus infection in children: Analysis of cerebrospinal fluid and progressive neurodevelopmental deterioration. J. Infect. Dis. *154*:415–421, 1986.
123. Halperin, S. A., Shehab, Z., Thacker, D., et al.: Absence of viremia in primary herpetic gingivostomatitis. Pediatr. Infect. Dis. *2*:452–453, 1983.
124. Hamilton, R. L., Achim, C., Grafe, M. R., et al.: Herpes simplex virus brainstem encephalitis in an AIDS patient. Clin. Neuropathol. *14*:45–50, 1995.
125. Hammer, S. M., Buchman, T. G., D'Angelo, L. J., et al.: Temporal cluster of herpes simplex encephalitis: Investigation by restriction endonuclease cleavage of viral DNA. J. Infect. Dis. *141*:436–440, 1980.
126. Herrod, H. G.: Chronic mucocutaneous candidiasis in childhood and complications of non-Candida infection: A report of the pediatric immunodeficiency study group. J. Pediatr. *116*:377–382, 1990.
127. Hevron, J. E.: Herpes simplex virus type 2 meningitis. Obstet. Gynecol. *49*:622–624, 1977.
128. Hirsch, M. S., and Swartz, M. N.: Antiviral agents. N. Engl. J. Med. *302*:903–907, 949–953, 1980.
129. Hook, E. W. I., Cannon, R. O., Nahmras, A. J., et al.: Herpes simplex virus infection as a risk factor for human immunodeficiency virus infection in heterosexuals. J. Infect. Dis. *165*:251–255, 1992.
130. Huff, J. C., and Weston, W. L.: Recurrent erythema multiforme. Medicine *68*:133–140, 1989.
131. Hull, H. F., Blumhagen, J. D., Benjamin, D., et al.: Herpes simplex viral pneumonitis in childhood. J. Pediatr. *104*:211–215, 1984.
132. Hursh, D. A., Wendt, S. F., Lee, C. F., et al.: Detection of herpes simplex virus by using A549 cells in centrifugation culture with a rapid membrane enzyme immunoassay. J. Clin. Microbiol. *27*:1695–1696, 1989.
133. International Valaciclovir HSV Study Group: Valaciclovir and acyclovir for the treatment of recurrent genital herpes simplex virus infection. Abstracts of the 33rd Interscience Conference on Antimicrobial Agents and Chemotherapy, 341, 1993.
134. Jaworski, M. A., Moffatt, M. E. K., and Ahronheim, G. A.: Disseminated herpes simplex associated with *H. influenzae* infection in a previously healthy child. J. Pediatr. *96*:426–429, 1980.
135. Jenson, H. B., and Shapiro, E. D.: Primary herpes simplex virus infection of a diaper rash. Pediatr. Infect. Dis. J. *6*:1136–1138, 1987.
136. Johnson, J. R., Egaas, S., Gleaves, C. A., et al.: Hepatitis due to herpes simplex virus in marrow-transplant recipients. Clin. Infect. Dis. *14*:38–45, 1992.
137. Johnson, R. E., Nahmias, A. J., Magder, L. S., et al.: A seroepidemiologic survey of the prevalence of herpes simplex virus type 2 infection in the United States. N. Engl. J. Med. *321*:7–12, 1989.
138. Johnson, R. T., and Mims, C. A.: Pathogenesis of viral infections of the nervous system. N. Engl. J. Med. *278*:23–30, 1968.
139. Jones, T. J., and Paul, R.: Disseminated acyclovir-resistant herpes simplex virus type 2 treated successfully with foscarnet. J. Infect. Dis. *171*:508–509, 1995.
140. Kallander, C. F. R., Gronowitz, J. S., and Olding-Stenkvist, E.: Rapid diagnosis of varicella-zoster virus infection by detection of viral deoxythymidine kinase in serum and vesicle fluid. J. Clin. Microbiol. *17*:280–287, 1983.
141. Kampgen, E., Bung, G., and Wank, R.: Association of herpes simplex virus–induced erythema multiforme with the human leukocyte antigen DQW3. Arch. Dermatol. *124*:1372–1375, 1988.
142. Kao, C. H., Wang, S. J., Mak, S. C., et al.: Viral encephalitis in children: Detection with technetium-99mm HMPAO brain single-photon emission CT and its value in prediction of outcome. Am J. Neuroradiol. *15*:1369–1373, 1994.
143. Kaplowitz, L. G., Baker, D., Gelb, L., et al.: Prolonged continuous acyclovir treatment of normal adults with frequently recurring genital herpes simplex virus infection. J. A. M. A. *265*:747–751, 1991.
144. King, D. H., and Galasso, G. (eds.): Proceedings of a symposium on acyclovir. Am. J. Med. *73*:1–392, 1982.
145. Kipps, A., Becker, W., Wainwright, J., et al.: Fatal disseminated primary herpes virus infection in children: Epidemiology based on 93 non-neonatal cases. S. Afr. Med. J. *41*:647–651, 1967.
146. Kirchner, H.: Immunobiology of infection with herpes simplex virus. Monogr. Virol. *13*:1–104, 1982.
147. Klapper, P. E., Laing, I., and Longson, M.: Rapid noninvasive diagnosis of herpes encephalitis. Lancet *2*:607–609, 1981.
148. Klein, N. A., Mabie, W. C., Shaver, D. C., et al.: Herpes simplex virus hepatitis in pregnancy: Two patients successfully treated with acyclovir. Gastroenterology *100*:239–244, 1991.
149. Kline, M. W., Bohannon, B., Kozinetz, C. A., et al.: Characteristics of human immunodeficiency virus–associated mortality in pediatric patients with vertically transmitted infection. Pediatr. Infect. Dis. J. *11*:676–677, 1992.
150. Koelle, D. M., Benedetti, J., Langenberg, A., et al.: Asymptomatic reactivation of herpes simplex virus in women after the first episode of genital herpes. Ann. Intern. Med. *116*:433–437, 1992.
151. Koenig, H., Rabinowitz, S. G., Day, E., et al.: Postinfectious encephalomyelitis after successful treatment of herpes simplex encephalitis with adenine arabinoside: Ultrastructural observations. N. Engl. J. Med. *300*:1089–1093, 1979.
152. Kohl, S.: Human immune response to herpes simplex virus. J. Infect. Dis. *146*:292, 1982.
153. Kohl, S.: Herpes simplex virus encephalitis in children. Pediatr. Clin. North Am. *35*:465–483, 1988.
154. Kohl, S., Adam, E., Matson, D. O., et al.: Kinetics of human antibody responses to primary genital herpes simplex virus infection. Intervirology *18*:164–168, 1982.
155. Kohl, S., and James, A. R.: Herpes simplex virus encephalitis during childhood: The importance of brain biopsy diagnosis. J. Pediatr. *107*:212–215, 1985.
156. Kohl, S., Lawman, M. J. P., Rouse, B. T., et al.: Effect of herpes simplex virus infection on murine antibody-dependent cellular cytotoxicity and natural killer cytotoxicity. Infect. Immun. *31*:704–711, 1981.
157. Koskiniemi, M., Piiparinen, H., Leikola, M., et al.: Poor antibody production in fatal herpes encephalitis. J. Infect. Dis. *171*:1692–1698, 1995.
158. Koskiniemi, M., and Vaheri, A.: Effect of measles, mumps, rubella vaccination on patterns of encephalitis in children. Lancet *1*:31–34, 1989.
159. Koskiniemi, M., Vaheri, A., and Taskinen, E.: Cerebrospinal fluid alterations in herpes simplex virus encephalitis. Rev. Infect. Dis. *6*:608–619, 1984.
160. Kost, R. G., Hill, E. L., Tigges, M., et al.: Brief report: Recurrent acyclovir-resistant genital herpes in an immunocompetent patient. N. Engl. J. Med. *329*:1777–1782, 1993.
161. Koutsky, L. A., Stevens, C. E., Holmes, K. K., et al.: Underdiagnosis of genital herpes by current clinical and viral-isolation procedures. N. Engl. J. Med. *326*:1533–1539, 1992.
162. Krause, P. R., Croen, K. D., Straus, S. E., et al.: Detection and preliminary characterization of herpes simplex virus type 1 transcripts in latently infected human trigeminal ganglia. J. Virol. *62*:4819–4823, 1988.
163. Kuo, Y. C., and Lin, C. U.: Recurrent herpes simplex virus type 1 infection precipitated by the impaired production of interleukin-2, alpha-interferon, and cell-mediated cytotoxicity. J. Med. Virol. *31*:183–189, 1990.
164. Kusne, S., Schwartz, M., Breinig, M. K., et al.: Herpes simplex virus hepatitis after solid organ transplantation in adults. J. Infect. Dis. *163*:1001–1007, 1991.
165. Kuzushima, K., Kimura, H., Kino, Y., et al.: Clinical manifestations of primary herpes simplex virus type 1 infection in a closed community. Pediatrics *87*:152–158, 1991.
166. Kuzushima, K., Kudo, T., Kimura, H., et al.: Prophylactic oral acyclovir in outbreaks of primary herpes simplex virus type 1 infection in a closed community. Pediatrics *89*:379–383, 1992.
167. Lafferty, W. E., Coombs, R. W., Benedetti, J., et al.: Recurrences after oral and genital herpes simplex infection: Influence of site of infection and viral type. N. Engl. J. Med. *316*:1444–1449, 1987.
168. Lakeman, F. D., and Whitley, R. J.: Diagnosis of herpes simplex encephalitis: Application of polymerase chain reaction to cerebrospinal fluid from brain-biopsied patients and correlation with disease. J. Infect. Dis. *171*:857–863, 1995.
169. Lalezari, J. P., Drew, H. L., Glutzer, E., et al.: Treatment with intravenous (S)-1-[3-hydroxy-2-(phosphonylmethoxy) propyl] cytosine of acyclovir-resistant mucocutaneous infection with herpes simplex virus in a patient with AIDS. J. Infect. Dis. *170*:570–572, 1994.
170. Langenberg, A., Benedetti, J., Jenkins, J., et al.: Development of clinically recognizable genital lesions among women previously identified as having "asymptomatic" herpes simplex virus type 2 infection. Ann. Intern. Med. *110*:882–887, 1989.
171. Langenberg, A. G., Burke, R. L., Adair, S. F., et al.: A recombinant glycoprotein vaccine for herpes simplex type 2: Safety and efficacy. Ann. Intern. Med. *122*:889–898, 1995.
172. Lawrence, T. G., Budzko, D. B., Wilcke, B. W., Jr.: Detection of herpes simplex virus in clinical specimens by an enzyme-linked immunosorbent assay. Am. J. Clin. Pathol. *81*:339–341, 1984.
173. Lee, S. F., and Pepose, J. S.: Sandwich enzyme immunoassay and latex agglutination test for herpes simplex virus keratitis. J. Clin. Microbiol. *28*:785–786, 1990.
174. Lehrman, S. N., Douglas, J. M., Corey, L., et al.: Recurrent genital herpes and suppressive oral acyclovir therapy: Relation between clinical outcome and in vitro drug sensitivity. Ann. Intern. Med. *104*:786–790, 1986.
175. Lehrman, S. N., Hill, L., Rooney, J. F., et al.: Extended acyclovir therapy for herpes genitalis: Changes in virus sensitivity and strain variation. J. Antimicrob. Chemother. *18*:85–94, 1986.

176. Lehtinen, M., Runtala, I., Teisala, K., et al.: Detection of herpes simplex virus in women with acute pelvic inflammatory disease. J. Infect. Dis. *152*:78–82, 1985.
177. Levine, D. P., Lauter, C. B., and Lerner, A. M.: Simultaneous serum and CSF antibodies in herpes simplex virus encephalitis. J. A. M. A. *240*:356–360, 1978.
178. Liesegang, T. J.: Ocular herpes simplex infection: Pathogenesis and current therapy. Mayo Clin. Proc. *63*:1092–1105, 1988.
179. Linnemann, C. C., Buchman, T. G., Light, I. J., et al.: Transmission of herpes simplex virus type 1 in a nursery for the newborn: Identification of viral isolates by DNA "fingerprinting." Lancet *1*:964–966, 1978.
180. Linnemann, C. C., May, D. B., Schubert, W. K., et al.: Fatal viral encephalitis in children with X-linked hypogammaglobulinemia. Am. J. Dis. Child. *126*:100–103, 1973.
181. Lipson, S. M., Szabo, K., and Lin, J. H.: Changing patterns of genital herpes simplex virus infections. Zentralbl. Bakteriol. Mikrobiol. Hyg. [A] *268*:57–61, 1988.
182. Ljungman, P., Ellis, M. N., Hackman, R. C., et al.: Acyclovir-resistant herpes simplex virus causing pneumonia after marrow transplantation. J. Infect. Dis. *162*:244–248, 1990.
183. Luby, J. P., Gnann, J. W., Alexander, W. J., et al.: A collaborative study of patient-initiated treatment of recurrent genital herpes with topical acyclovir or placebo. J. Infect. Dis. *150*:1–6, 1984.
184. Lumbreras, C., Fernandez, I., Velosa, J., et al.: Infectious complications following pancreatic transplantation: Incidence, microbiological and clinical characteristics, and outcome. Clin. Infect. Dis. *20*:514–520, 1995.
185. Manzella, J. P., McConville, J. H., Valenti, W., et al.: An outbreak of herpes simplex virus type 1 gingivostomatitis in a dental hygiene practice. J. A. M. A. *256*:2019–2022, 1984.
186. Marks, C. L., Nolan, P. E., Erlich, K. S., et al.: Mucocutaneous dissemination of acyclovir-resistant herpes simplex virus in a patient with AIDS. Rev. Infect. Dis. *11*:474–476, 1989.
187. Martin A. B., Webber, S., Fricker, F. J., et al.: Acute myocarditis: Rapid diagnosis by PCR in children. Circulation *90*:330–339, 1994.
188. Masci, S., DeSimone, C., Famularo, G., et al.: Intravenous immunoglobulins suppress the recurrences of genital herpes simplex virus: A clinical and immunological study. Immunopharmacol. Immunotoxicol. *17*:33–47, 1995.
189. McLaren, C., Corey, L., Dekket, C., et al.: In vitro sensitivity to acyclovir in genital herpes simplex viruses from acyclovir-treated patients. J. Infect. Dis. *148*:868–875, 1983.
190. McLaren, C., Ellis, M. N., and Hunter, G. A.: A colorimetric assay for the measurement of the sensitivity of herpes simplex virus to antiviral agents. Antiviral Res. *3*:223–234, 1983.
191. McMillan, J. A., Weiner, L. B., Higgins, A. M., et al.: Pharyngitis associated with herpes simplex virus in college students. Pediatr. Infect. Dis. J. *12*:280–284, 1993.
192. Merigan, T. C., and Stevens, D. A.: Viral infections in man associated with acquired immunological deficiency states. Fed. Proc. *30*:1858–1864, 1971.
193. Mertz, G. J., Ashley, R., Burke, R. L., et al.: Double-blind, placebo-controlled trial of a herpes simplex virus type 2 glycoprotein vaccine in persons at high risk for genital herpes infection. J. Infect. Dis. *116*:653–660, 1990.
194. Mertz, G. J., Benedetti, J., Ashley, R., et al.: Risk factors for the sexual transmission of genital herpes. Ann. Intern. Med. *116*:197–202, 1992.
195. Mertz, G. J., Coombs, R. W., Ashley, R., et al.: Transmission of genital herpes in couples with one symptomatic and one asymptomatic partner: A prospective study. J. Infect. Dis. *157*:1169–1177, 1988.
196. Mertz, G. J., Loveless, M. O., Krauss, S. J., et al.: Famciclovir for suppression of recurrent genital herpes. Abstracts of the 34th Interscience Conference on Antimicrobial Agents and Chemotherapy, 11, 1994.
197. Minak, G. Y., and Nicolle, L. E.: Genital herpes and hepatitis in healthy young adults. J. Med. Virol. *19*:269–275, 1986.
198. Mindel, A., Adler, M. W., Sutherland, S., et al.: Intravenous acyclovir treatment for primary genital herpes. Lancet *1*:697–700, 1982.
199. Mindel, A., Faherty, A., Hindley, D., et al.: Prophylactic oral acyclovir in recurrent genital herpes. Lancet *2*:57–59, 1984.
200. Mitchell, C. D., Gentry, S. R., Boen, J. R., et al.: Acyclovir therapy for mucocutaneous herpes simplex infections in immunocompromised patients. Lancet *1*:1389–1392, 1981.
201. Mogensen, S. C., and Dishon, T.: Rapid detection of herpes simplex virus and varicella-zoster virus in clinical specimens by the use of *Staphylococcus aureus* rich in protein A. Acta Pathol. Microbiol. Immunol. Scand. *91*:83–88, 1983.
202. Molin, L.: Oral acyclovir prevents herpes simplex virus–associated erythema multiforme. Br. J. Dermatol. *116*:109–111, 1987.
203. Montgomerie, J. Z., Becroft, D. M. O., Croxson, M. C., et al.: Herpes simplex virus infection after renal transplantation. Lancet *2*:867–871, 1969.
204. Moore, D. E., Ashley, R. L., Zarutskie, P. W., et al.: Transmission of genital herpes by donor insemination. J. A. M. A. *261*:3441–3443, 1989.
205. Moore, D. J., Davidson, G. P., and Binns, G. F.: Herpes simplex oesophagitis in young children. Med. J. Aust. *144*:716–717, 1986.
206. Morawetz, R. B., Whitley, R. J., and Murphy, D. M.: Experience with brain biopsy for suspected herpes encephalitis: A review of forty consecutive cases. Neurosurgery *12*:654–657, 1983.
207. Morbidity and Mortality Weekly Report: 1994 Revised classification system for human immunodeficiency virus infection in children less than 13 years of age. M. M. W. R. *43*:1–10, 1994.
208. Moseley, R. D., Corey, L., Benjamin, D., et al.: Comparison of viral isolation, direct immunofluorescence, and indirect immunoperoxidase techniques for detection of genital herpes simplex virus infection. J. Clin. Microbiol. *13*:913–918, 1981.
209. Nahmias, A. J., Alford, C. A., and Korones, S. B.: Infection of the newborn with herpesvirus hominis. Adv. Pediatr. *17*:185–226, 1970.
210. Nahmias, A. J., Dowdle, W. R., Schinazi, R. F. (eds.): The Human Herpes Viruses: An Interdisciplinary Perspective. New York, Elsevier, 1981.
211. Nahmias, A. J., and Josey, W. E.: Epidemiology of herpes simplex viruses 1 and 2. *In* Evans, A. S. (ed.): Viral Infections of Humans: Epidemiology and Control. New York, Plenum, 1982, pp. 351–372.
212. Nahmias, A. J., Naid, Z. N., and Josey, W. E.: Herpesvirus hominis type II infection: Association with cervical cancer and perinatal disease. Perspect. Virol. *7*:73–89, 1971.
213. Nahmias, A. J., and Roizman, B.: Infection with herpes simplex viruses 1 and 2. N. Engl. J. Med. *289*:667–674, 719–725, 781–789, 1973.
214. Nahmias, A. J., Shore, S. L., Kohl, S., et al.: Immunology of herpes simplex virus infection: Relevance to herpes simplex virus vaccines and cervical cancer. Cancer Res. *36*:836–844, 1976.
215. Nahmias, A. J., and Whitley, R. J.: Herpes simplex virus encephalitis in pediatrics. Pediatr. Rev. *2*:259–266, 1981.
216. Nahmias, A. J., Whitley, R. J., Visintine, A. N., et al.: Herpes simplex virus encephalitis: Laboratory evaluations and their diagnostic significance. J. Infect. Dis. *145*:829–836, 1982.
217. Naraqi, S., Jackson, G. G., Jonasson, O., et al.: Prospective study of prevalence, incidence, and source of herpesvirus infections in patients with renal allografts. J. Infect. Dis. *136*:531–540, 1977.
218. Nash, G.: Necrotizing tracheobronchitis and bronchopneumonia consistent with herpetic infection. Hum. Pathol. *3*:283–291, 1972.
219. Nash, G., and Ross, J. S.: Herpetic esophagitis, a common cause of esophageal ulceration. Hum. Pathol. *5*:339–345, 1974.
220. Neiman, P. E., Reeves, W., Ray, G., et al.: A prospective analysis of interstitial pneumonia and opportunistic viral infection among recipients of allogeneic bone marrow grafts. J. Infect. Dis. *136*:754–767, 1977.
221. Nerurkar, L. S., West, F., May, M., et al.: Survival of herpes simplex virus in water specimens collected from hot tubs in spa facilities and on plastic surfaces. J. A. M. A. *250*:3081–3083, 1983.
222. Nilson, A. E., Aasen, T., Halsos, A. M., et al.: Efficacy of oral acyclovir in the treatment of initial and recurrent genital herpes. Lancet *2*:571–573, 1982.
223. Oranje, A. P., Folkers, E., Choufer-Habova, J., et al.: Diagnostic value of Tzanck smear in herpetic and non-herpetic vesicular and bullous skin disorders in pediatric practice. Acta Dermatol. Venereol. *66*:127–133, 1986.
224. Orton, P. W., Huff, J. C., Tonnesen, M. G., et al.: Detection of a herpes simplex viral antigen in skin lesions of erythema multiforme. Ann. Intern. Med. *101*:48–50, 1984.
225. Owensby, L. C., and Stammer, J. L.: Esophagitis associated with herpes simplex infection in an immunocompetent host. Gastroenterology *74*:1305–1306, 1978.
226. Park, M., Lonsdale, D. M., and Timbury, M. C.: Genetic retrieval of viral genome sequences from herpes simplex virus transformed cells. Nature *285*:412–415, 1980.
227. Parrott, R. H., Wolf, S. I., Nudelman, J., et al.: Clinical and laboratory differentiation between herpangina and infectious (herpetic) gingivostomatitis. Pediatrics *14*:122–129, 1954.
228. Pass, R. F., Whitley, R. J., Whelchel, J. D., et al.: Identification of patients with increased risk of infection with herpes simplex virus after renal transplantation. J. Infect. Dis. *140*:487–492, 1979.
229. Pavan-Langston, D., and Brockhurst, R. J.: Herpes simplex panuveitis: A clinical report. Arch. Ophthalmol. *81*:783–787, 1969.
230. Pazin, G. J., Armstrong, J. A., Lam, M. T., et al.: Prevention of reactivated herpes simplex infection by human leukocyte interferon after operation on the trigeminal root. N. Engl. J. Med. *301*:225–230, 1979.
231. Peacock, J. E., Kaplowitz, L. G., Sparling, P. F., et al.: Intravenous acyclovir therapy of first episodes of genital herpes: A multicenter double-blind, placebo controlled trial. Am. J. Med. *85*:301–306, 1988.
232. Perng, G. C., Dunkel, E. C., Geary, P. A., et al.: The latency-associated gene of herpes simplex virus type 1 (HSV-1) is required for efficient in vivo spontaneous reactivation of HSV-1 from latency. J. Virol. *68*:8045–8055, 1994.
233. Pien, F. D., Smith, T. F., Anderson, C. F., et al.: Herpesviruses in renal transplant patients. Transplantation *16*:489–495, 1973.
234. Poirier, R. H.: Herpetic ocular infections of childhood. Arch. Ophthalmol. *98*:704–706, 1980.
235. Pollard, R. B., Arvin, A. M., Gamberg, P., et al.: Specific cell-mediated immunity and infections with herpes viruses in cardiac transplant recipients. Am. J. Med. *73*:679–687, 1982.
236. Prentice, H. G., and Hann, I. M.: Prophylactic studies against herpes infections in severely immunocompromised patients with acyclovir. J. Infect. *6*:17–21, 1983.
237. Price, R., Chernik, N. L., Horta-Barbosa, L., et al.: Herpes simplex encephalitis in an anergic patient. Am. J. Med. *54*:222–228, 1973.

238. Quinn, T. C., Corey, L., Chaffee, R. G., et al.: The etiology of anorectal infections in homosexual men. Am. J. Med. *71*:395–406, 1981.
239. Quinnan, G. V., Masur, H., Rook, A. H., et al.: Herpes virus infections in the acquired immune deficiency syndrome. J. A. M. A. *252*:72–77, 1984.
240. Ramsey, P. G., Fife, K. H., Hackman, R. C., et al.: Herpes simplex virus pneumonia: Clinical, virologic, and pathologic features in 20 patients. Ann. Intern. Med. *97*:813–820, 1982.
241. Rand, K. H., Rasmussen, L. E., Pollard, R. B., et al.: Cellular immunity and herpesvirus infections in cardiac-transplant patients. N. Engl. J. Med. *296*:1372–1377, 1977.
242. Rantala, H., and Uhari, M.: Occurrence of childhood encephalitis: A population based study. Pediatr. Infect. Dis. J. *8*:426–430, 1989.
243. Rasmussen, L. E., Jordan, G. W., Stevens, D. A., et al.: Lymphocyte interferon production and transformation after herpes simplex infections in humans. J. Immunol. *112*:728–736, 1974.
244. Rawls, W. E.: Herpes simplex virus. *In* Lennette, E. H., Belows, A., Hausler, W. I., et al. (eds.): Manual of Clinical Microbiology. Washington, D.C., American Society for Microbiology, 1980, pp. 783–789.
245. Rawls, W. E., Gardner, H. L., Flanders, R. W., et al.: Genital herpes in two social groups. Am. J. Obstet. Gynecol. *110*:682–689, 1971.
246. Reeves, W. C., Corey, L., Adams, H. G., et al.: Risk of recurrence after first episodes of genital herpes: Relation to HSV type antibody response. N. Engl. J. Med. *305*:315–319, 1981.
247. Reichman, R. C., Badger, G. J., Guinan, M. E., et al.: Topically administered acyclovir in the treatment of recurrent herpes simplex genitalis: A controlled trial. J. Infect. Dis. *147*:336–340, 1983.
248. Rogers, M. F., Thomas P. A., Starcher, E. T., et al.: Acquired immunodeficiency syndrome in children: Report of the Centers for Disease Control national surveillance, 1982 to 1985. Pediatrics *79*:1008–1014, 1987.
249. Rompalo, A. M., Mertz, G. J., and Davis, L. G.: Oral acyclovir for treatment of first episode herpes simplex virus proctitis. J. A. M. A. *19*:2879–2881, 1988.
250. Rosato, F. E., Rosato, E. F., and Plotkin, S. A.: Herpetic paronychia: An occupational hazard of medical personnel. N. Engl. J. Med. *283*:804–805, 1970.
251. Rosenfeld, E. A., Radkowski, M. A., Rowley, A. H.: Biphasic course of illness with disparate outcomes in herpes simplex encephalitis in children. Pediatr. Res. *35*:193A, 1994.
252. Rouse, B. T., and Lopez, C. (eds.): Immunobiology of Herpes Simplex Infection. Boca Raton, CRC Press, 1984.
253. Rowley, A. H., Whitley, R. J., Lakeman, F. O., et al.: Rapid detection of herpes-simplex virus DNA in cerebrospinal fluid of patients with herpes simplex encephalitis. Lancet *335*:440–441, 1990.
254. Sacks, S. L., Aok, F. Y., Diaz-Mitoma, F., et al.: Patient-initiated treatment of recurrent genital herpes with oral famciclovir: A Canadian multicenter, placebo-controlled, dose-ranging study. Abstracts of the 34th Interscience Conference on Antimicrobial Agents and Chemotherapy, 11, 1994.
255. Safrin, S., Assaykeen, T., Follansbee, S., et al.: Foscarnet therapy for acyclovir-resistant mucocutaneous herpes simplex virus infection in 26 AIDS patients: Preliminary data. J. Infect. Dis. *161*:1078–1084, 1990.
256. Safrin, S., Crumpaker, C., Chatis, P., et al.: A controlled trial comparing foscarnet with vidarabine for acyclovir-resistant, mucocutaneous herpes simplex in the acquired immunodeficiency syndrome. N. Engl. J. Med. *325*:551–555, 1991.
257. Safrin, S., Elbeik, T., and Mills, J.: A rapid screen test for in vitro susceptibility of clinical herpes simplex virus isolates. J. Infect. Dis. *169*:879–882, 1994.
258. Safrin, S., Elbeik, T., Phan, L., et al.: Correlation between response to acyclovir and foscarnet therapy and in vitro susceptibility results from isolates of herpes simplex virus from human immunodeficiency virus–infected patients. Antimicrob. Agents Chemother. *38*:1246–1250, 1994.
259. Safrin, S., Kemmerly, S., Plotkin, B., et al.: Foscarnet-resistant herpes simplex virus in patients with AIDS. J. Infect. Dis. *169*:193–196, 1994.
260. Sands, M., and Brown, R.: Herpes simplex lymphangitis: Two cases and a review of the literature. Arch. Intern. Med. *148*:2066–2067, 1988.
261. Saral, R., Ambinder, R. F., Burns, W. H., et al.: Acyclovir prophylaxis against herpes simplex virus infection in patients with leukemia: A randomized, double-blind, placebo-controlled study. Ann. Intern. Med. *99*:773–776, 1983.
262. Saral, R., Burns, W. H., Laskin, O. L., et al.: Acyclovir prophylaxis of herpes-simplex-virus infections: A randomized, double-blind, controlled trial in bone-marrow–transplant recipients. N. Engl. J. Med. *305*:63–67, 1981.
263. Sawyer, J., Ellner, J., and Ransohoff, D. F.: To biopsy or not to biopsy in suspected herpes simplex encephalitis: A quantitative analysis. Med. Decis. Making *8*:95–101, 1988.
264. Schauseil-Zipf, U., Harden, A., Hoare, R. D., et al.: Early diagnosis of herpes simplex encephalitis in childhood: Clinical, neurophysiological and neuroradiological studies. Eur. J. Pediatr. *138*:154–161, 1982.
265. Schleiss, M. R., and Fong, W.: Primary palmar herpes simplex virus 1 infection in a ten-year-old girl. Pediatr. Infect. Dis. J. *11*:338–339, 1992.
266. Schlesinger, Y., Buller, R. S., Brunstrom, J. E., et al.: Expanded spectrum of herpes simplex encephalitis in childhood. J. Pediatr. *126*:234–241, 1995.
267. Schlesinger, Y., and Storch, G. A.: Herpes simplex meningitis in infancy. Pediatr. Infect. Dis. J. *13*:141–144, 1994.
268. Schlesinger, Y., Tebas, P., Gaudreault-Keener, M., et al.: Herpes simplex virus type 2 meningitis in the absence of genital lesions: Improved recognition with use of the polymerase chain reaction. Clin. Infect. Dis. *20*:842–848, 1995.
269. Schmidt, N. J., Gallo, D., Devlin, V., et al.: Direct immunofluorescence staining for detection of herpes simplex and varicella-zoster virus antigens in vesicular lesions and certain tissue specimens. J. Clin. Microbiol. *12*:651–655, 1980.
270. Schmidt, O. W., Fife, K. H., and Corey, L.: Reinfection is an uncommon occurrence in patients with symptomatic recurrent genital herpes. J. Infect. Dis. *149*:645–646, 1984.
271. Schmitt, D. L., Johnson, D. W., and Henderson, F. W.: Herpes simplex type 1 infections in group day care. Pediatr. Infect. Dis. J. *10*:729–734, 1991.
272. Schofield, J. K., Tatnall, F. M., and Leigh, I. M.: Recurrent erythema multiforme: Clinical features and treatment in a large series of patients. Br. J. Dermatol. *128*:542–545, 1993.
273. Schroth, G., Gawehn, J., Thorn, A., et al.: Early diagnosis of herpes simplex encephalitis in MRI. Neurology *37*:179–183, 1987.
274. Schwab, I. R.: Oral acyclovir in the management of herpes simplex ocular infection. Ophthalmology *95*:423–430, 1988.
275. Scott, G. B., Buck, B. E., Leterman, J. G., et al.: Acquired immunodeficiency in infants. N. Engl. J. Med. *310*:76–81, 1984.
276. Sedarati, F., Izumi, K. M., Wagner, E. K., et al.: Herpes simplex virus type 1 latency-associated transcription plays no role in establishment of a latent infection in murine sensory neurons. J. Virol. *63*:4455–4458, 1989.
277. Selby, P. J., Jameson, B., Watson, J. G., et al.: Parenteral acyclovir therapy for herpesvirus infections in man. Lancet *2*:1267–1270, 1979.
278. Selling, B., and Kibrick, S.: An outbreak of herpes simplex among wrestlers (herpes gladiatorum). N. Engl. J. Med. *270*:979–982, 1964.
279. Shanley, C. J., Braun, D. K., Brown, K., et al.: Fulminant hepatic failure secondary to herpes simplex virus hepatitis: Successful outcome after orthotopic liver transplantation. Transplantation *59*:145–149, 1995.
280. Shepp, D. H., Dandiker, P. S., and Meyers, J. D.: Treatment of varicella-zoster virus infection in severely immunocompromised patients: A randomized comparison of acyclovir and vidarabine. N. Engl. J. Med. *314*:208–212, 1986.
281. Shute, P., Jeffries, D. J., and Maddocks, A. C.: Scrumpox caused by herpes simplex virus. Br. Med. J. *2*:1629, 1979.
282. Sibrack, C. D., Gutman, L. T., Wilfert, C. M., et al.: Pathogenicity of acyclovir-resistant herpes simplex virus type 1 from an immunodeficient child. J. Infect. Dis. *146*:673–682, 1982.
283. Simone, J. V., Holland, E., and Johnson, W.: Fatalities during remission of childhood leukaemia. Blood *39*:759–770, 1972.
284. Skoldenberg, B., Alestig, K., Burman, L., et al.: Acyclovir versus vidarabine in herpes encephalitis: Randomized, multicentre study in consecutive Swedish patients. Lancet *2*:707–711, 1984.
285. Smego, R. A., Jr., Devoe, P. W., Sampson, H. A., et al.: Candida meningitis in two children with severe combined immunodeficiency. J. Pediatr. *104*:902–904, 1984.
286. Snoeck, R., Andrei, G., Gerard, M., et al.: Successful treatment of progressive mucocutaneous infection due to acyclovir- and foscarnet-resistant herpes simplex virus with (S)-1-(3-hydroxy-2-phosphonylmethyloxypropyl) cytosine (HPMPC). Clin. Infect. Dis. *18*:570–578, 1994.
287. Solomon, A. R., Rasmussen, J. E., Varani, J., et al.: The Tzanck smear in the diagnosis of cutaneous herpes simplex. J. A. M. A. *251*:633–635, 1984.
288. Spruance, S. L.: Pathogenesis of herpes simplex labialis: Excretion of virus in the oral cavity. J. Clin. Microbiol. *19*:675–679, 1984.
289. Spruance, S. L., Freeman, D. J., and Stewart, J. C. B.: The natural history of ultraviolet radiation–induced herpes simplex labialis and response to therapy with peroral and topical formulations of acyclovir. J. Infect. Dis. *163*:728–734, 1991.
290. Spruance, S. L., Hamill, M. L., Hoge, W. S., et al.: Acyclovir prevents reactivation of herpes simplex labialis in skiers. J. A. M. A. *260*:1597–1599, 1988.
291. Spruance, S. L., Overall, J. C., Kern, E. R., et al.: The natural history of recurrent herpes simplex labialis: Implication for antiviral therapy. N. Engl. J. Med. *297*:69–75, 1977.
292. Spruance, S. L., Schnipper, L. E., Overall, J. C., Jr., et al.: Treatment of herpes simplex labialis with topical acyclovir in polyethylene glycol. J. Infect. Dis. *146*:85–90, 1982.
293. Spruance, S. L., Stewart, J. C. B., Rowe, N. H., et al.: Treatment of recurrent herpes simplex labialis with oral acyclovir. J. Infect. Dis. *161*:185–190, 1990.
294. Stamm, W. E., Handsfield, H. H., Rompalo, A. M., et al.: The association between genital ulcer disease and acquisition of HIV infection in homosexual men. J. A. M. A. *260*:1429–1433, 1988.
295. Stanberry, L. R., Floyd-Reising, S. A., Connelly, B. L., et al.: Herpes simplex viremia: Report of eight pediatric cases and review of the literature. Clin. Infect. Dis. *18*:401–407, 1994.
296. Stavraky, K. M., Rawls, W. E., Chiavetta, J., et al.: Sexual and socioeconomic factors affecting the risk of past infections with herpes simplex virus type 2. Am. J. Epidemiol. *118*:109–121, 1983.
297. Stern, H., Elek, S. D., Millar, D. M., et al.: Herpetic whitlow, a form of cross-infection in hospitals. Lancet *2*:871–874, 1959.
298. St. Geme, J. W., Prince, J. T., Burke, B. A., et al.: Impaired cellular

resistance to herpes-simplex virus in Wiskott-Aldrich syndrome. N. Engl. J. Med. *273*:229–234, 1965.
299. Straus, S. E., Corey, L., Burke, R. L., et al.: Placebo-controlled trial of vaccination with recombinant glycoprotein D of herpes simplex virus type 2 for immunotherapy of genital herpes. Lancet *343*:1460–1463, 1994.
300. Straus, S. E., Croen, K. D., Sawyer, M. H., et al.: Acyclovir suppression of frequently recurring genital herpes: Efficacy and diminished need during successive years of treatment. J. A. M. A. *260*:2227–2230, 1988.
301. Straus, S. E., Seidlin, M., Takiff, H., et al.: Oral acyclovir to suppress recurring herpes simplex virus infections in immunodeficient patients. Ann. Intern. Med. *100*:522–524, 1984.
302. Straus, S. E., Seidlin, M., Takiff, H. E., et al.: Effect of oral acyclovir treatment on symptomatic and asymptomatic virus shedding in recurrent genital herpes. Sex. Transm. Dis. *16*:107–113, 1989.
303. Straus, S. E., Smith, H. A., Brickman, C., et al.: Acyclovir for chronic mucocutaneous herpes simplex virus infection in immunosuppressed patients. Ann. Intern. Med. *96*:270–277, 1982.
304. Straus, S. E., Takiff, H. E., Seidlin, M., et al.: Suppression of frequently recurring genital herpes: A placebo-controlled double-blind trial of oral acyclovir. N. Engl. J. Med. *310*:1545–1550, 1984.
305. Sullender, W. M., Arvin, A. M., Diaz, P. S., et al.: Pharmacokinetics of acyclovir suspension in infants and children. Antimicrob. Agents Chemother. *31*:1722–1726, 1987.
306. Symposium: Herpesvirus and cervical cancer. Cancer Res. *33*:1345–1563, 1973.
307. Tang, I. Y. S., Maddax, M. S., Veremis, S. A., et al.: Low-dose oral acyclovir for prevention of herpes simplex virus infection during OKT3 therapy. Transplant. Proc. *21*:1758–1760, 1989.
308. Tatnall, F. M., Schofield, J. K., and Leigh I. M.: A double-blind, placebo-controlled trial of continuous acyclovir therapy in recurrent erythema multiforme. Br. J. Dermatol. *132*:267–270, 1995.
309. Taxy, J. B., Tillaw, I., and Goldman, P. M.: Herpes simplex lymphadenitis. Arch. Pathol. Lab. Med. *109*:1043–1044, 1985.
310. Tedder, D. G., Ashley, R., Tyler, K. L., et al.: Herpes simplex virus infection as a cause of benign recurrent lymphocytic meningitis. Ann. Intern. Med. *121*:334–338, 1994.
311. Templeton, A. C.: Generalized herpes simplex in malnourished children. J. Clin. Pathol. *23*:24–30, 1970.
312. Tenser, R. B., and Dunstan, M. E.: Mechanisms of herpes simplex virus infectivity enhanced by ultracentrifugal inoculation. Infect. Immun. *30*:193–197, 1980.
313. Terni, M., Caccialanza, P., Cassai, E., et al.: Aseptic meningitis in association with herpes progenitalis. N. Engl. J. Med. *285*:503–505, 1971.
314. Trachtman, H., Weiss, R. A., Spigland, I., et al.: Clinical manifestations of herpesvirus infections in pediatric renal transplant recipients. Pediatr. Infect. Dis. J. *4*:480–486, 1985.
315. Troendle-Atkins, J., Demmler, G. J., and Buffone, G. J.: Rapid diagnosis of herpes simplex virus encephalitis by using the polymerase chain reaction. J. Pediatr. *123*:376–380, 1993.
316. Tse, P., Aarnaes, S. L., Dela Meza, L. M., et al.: Detection of herpes simplex virus by 8 H in shell vial cultures with primary rabbit kidney cells. J. Clin. Microbiol. *27*:199–200, 1989.
317. Turner, B. J., Denison, M., Eppes, S. C., et al.: Survival experience of 789 children with the acquired immunodeficiency syndrome. Pediatr. Infect. Dis. J. *12*:310–320, 1993.
318. Turner, R., Shehab, Z., Osborne, K., et al.: Shedding and survival of herpes simplex virus from "fever blisters." Pediatrics *70*:547–549, 1982.
319. Uren, E. C., Johnson, P. D., Montanaro, J., et al.: Herpes simplex virus encephalitis in pediatrics: Diagnosis by detecting antibodies and DNA in cerebrospinal fluid. Pediatr. Infect. Dis. J. *12*:1001–1006, 1993.
320. Van Vloten, W. A., Swart, R. N., and Pot, F.: Topical acyclovir therapy in patients with recurrent orofacial herpes simplex infections. J. Antimicrob. Chemother. *12*:89–93, 1983.
321. Vital, C., Monlun, E., Vital, A., et al.: Concurrent herpes simplex virus type 1 necrotizing encephalitis, cytomegalovirus ventriculoencephalitis and cerebral lymphoma in an AIDS patient. Acta Neuropathol. *89*:105–108, 1995.
322. Wade, J. C., Day, L. M., Crowley, J. J., et al.: Recurrent infection with herpes simplex virus after marrow transplantation: Role of the specific immune response and acyclovir treatment. J. Infect. Dis. *149*:750–756, 1984.
323. Wade, J. C., McLaren, C., and Meyers, J. D.: Frequency and significance of acyclovir-resistant herpes simplex virus isolated from marrow transplant patients receiving multiple courses of treatment with acyclovir. J. Infect. Dis. *148*:1077–1082, 1983.
324. Wade, J. C., and Meyers, J. D.: Neurologic symptoms associated with parenteral acyclovir treatment after marrow transplantation. Ann. Intern. Med. *98*:921–925, 1983.
325. Wade, J. C., Newton, B., McLaren, C., et al.: Intravenous acyclovir to treat mucocutaneous herpes simplex virus infection after marrow transplantation: A double-blind trial. Ann. Intern. Med. *96*:265–269, 1982.
326. Wald, A., Barnum, G., Selke, S., et al.: Acyclovir suppresses asymptomatic shedding of HSV-2 in the genital tract. Abstracts of the 34th Interscience Conference on Antimicrobial Agents and Chemotherapy, 11, 1994.
327. Wang, H. S., Kuo, M. F., Huang, S. C., et al.: Choreoathetosis as an initial sign of relapsing of herpes simplex encephalitis. Pediatr. Neurol. *11*:341–345, 1994.
328. Wasserman, R., August, C. S., and Plotkin, S. A.: Viral infections in pediatric bone marrow transplant patients. Pediatr. Infect. Dis. J. *7*:109–115, 1988.
329. Waugh, M. A.: Anorectal herpesvirus hominis infection in men. J. Am. Vener. Dis. Assoc. *3*:68–70, 1976.
330. Weston, W. L., Brice, S. L., Jester, J. D., et al.: Herpes simplex virus in childhood erythema multiforme. Pediatrics *89*:32–34, 1992.
331. Wheeler, C. E., Jr., and Abele, D. C.: Eczema herpeticum, primary and recurrent. Arch. Dermatol. *93*:162–173, 1966.
332. White, W. B., and Grant-Kels, J. M.: Transmission of herpes simplex virus type 1 infection in rugby players. J. A. M. A. *252*:533–535, 1984.
333. Whitley, R. J., Alford, C. A., Hirsch, M. S., et al.: Vidarabine versus acyclovir therapy in herpes simplex encephalitis. N. Engl. J. Med. *314*:144–149, 1986.
334. Whitley, R. J., Cobbs, C. G., Alford, C. A., Jr., et al.: Diseases that mimic herpes simplex encephalitis: Diagnosis, presentation, and outcome. J. A. M. A. *262*:234–239, 1989.
335. Whitley, R. J., Lakeman, A. D., Nahmias, A., et al.: DNA restriction-enzyme analysis of herpes simplex virus isolates obtained from patients with encephalitis. N. Engl. J. Med. *307*:1060–1062, 1982.
336. Whitley, R. J., Levin, M., Marton, N., et al.: Infections caused by herpes simplex virus in the immunocompromised host: Natural history and topical acyclovir therapy. J. Infect. Dis. *150*:323–329, 1984.
337. Whitley, R. J., Soong, S. J., Dolin, R., et al.: Adenine arabinoside therapy of biopsy-proved herpes simplex encephalitis. N. Engl. J. Med. *297*:289–294, 1977.
338. Whitley, R. J., Soong, S. J., Hirsch, M. S., et al.: Herpes simplex encephalitis: Vidarabine therapy and diagnostic problems. N. Engl. J. Med. *304*:313–318, 1981.
339. Whitley, R. J., Soong, S. J., Linneman, C., Jr., et al.: Herpes simplex encephalitis: Clinical assessment. J. A. M. A. *247*:317–320, 1982.
340. Whitley, R. J., Spruance, S., Hayden, F. G., et al.: Vidarabine therapy for mucocutaneous herpes simplex virus infections in the immunocompromised host. J. Infect. Dis. *149*:1–8, 1984.
341. Wishart, M. S., Darougar, S., and Viswalingam, N. D.: Recurrent herpes simplex virus ocular infection: Epidemiological and clinical features. Br. J. Ophthalmol. *71*:669–672, 1987.
342. Wollensak, J.: Herpes simplex of the eye and possibilities of its therapeutic control. Adv. Ophthalmol. *38*:99–104, 1979.
343. Wood, D. J., and Corbitt, G.: Viral infections in childhood leukemia. J. Infect. Dis. *152*:266–273, 1985.
344. Wu, E., Sayre, J., Wiesmeier, E., et al.: A prospective seroepidemiological survey of herpes simplex (HSV) infections in a college population. Pediatr. Res. *18*:289A, 1984.
345. Wu, T. C., Zaza, S., and Callaway, J.: Evaluation of the DuPont Herpchek herpes simplex virus antigen test with clinical specimens. J. Clin. Microbiol. *27*:1903–1905, 1989.
346. Yamamoto, L. Y., Tedder, D. G., Ashley, R., et al.: Herpes simplex virus type 1 DNA in cerebrospinal fluid of a patient with Mollaret's meningitis. N. Engl. J. Med. *325*:1082–1085, 1991.

164

CYTOMEGALOVIRUS

Gail J. Demmler

Cytomegalovirus (CMV) is a ubiquitous agent that commonly infects persons of all ages from all parts of the world and from all socioeconomic and cultural backgrounds. Although most CMV infections are asymptomatic, certain patient groups are at risk for serious, even life-threatening illness. Discerning which role CMV is playing in a particular patient requires a thorough understanding of the epidemiology, virology, and pathophysiology of the virus and can be difficult, even for the most experienced clinician.

HISTORY

The recorded history of CMV probably began in 1881, when Ribbert described, then later reported in 1904, "protozoan-like cells" in the organs of an infant who died of presumed congenital syphilis.[189] In 1920, Goodpasture and Talbot[97] hypothesized that these swollen cells or "cytomegalia" were host cells that were injured by a virus. During the first half of the twentieth century, CMV was recognizable only by the pathologic changes it produced in infected cells, and because these cells frequently were seen in the salivary glands of animals and humans, CMV originally was called the salivary gland virus.

In 1956, human CMV first was isolated in tissue culture by three independent investigators, Rowe, Smith, and Weller.[194, 208, 245] Because several human and animal viruses subsequently were found to replicate in salivary glands, the descriptive name *cytomegalovirus* was proposed by Weller in 1960. The ability to cultivate CMV in tissue culture led to the development of serologic techniques, which in the 1960s and 1970s led to many important clinical and epidemiologic observations. For example, CMV was found commonly to infect people of all ages throughout the world. By 1962, CMV was established as a significant pathogen of the fetus and newborn, capable of producing a spectrum of clinical manifestations and neurologic sequelae.[246] In 1966, Kaariainen and colleagues[125] reported evidence supporting CMV as a cause of posttransfusion mononucleosis syndrome.

The molecular biology of the virus was explored during the 1970s and 1980s and continues to be explored by many investigators. In addition, during the 1970s and 1980s, CMV emerged as a major cause of morbidity and mortality in immunosuppressed persons, especially patients who underwent organ or marrow transplantation or who had AIDS. In 1976, the first clinical trial of the live attenuated CMV vaccine, Towne 125, was reported; since then, more than 500 renal allograft recipients, as well as healthy young men and women, have received the vaccine under investigational protocols.[86, 172] Also, research on a subunit vaccine based on the glycoproteins of the virus began in the 1980s, and in the 1990s, recombinant vaccines were developed and tested in human volunteers. CMV has become a treatable disease, with two specific antiviral agents, ganciclovir (licensed in 1989) and foscarnet (licensed in 1991), now available to clinicians to treat seriously ill patients.

VIROLOGY

CMV is a member of the *Herpesviridae* family of DNA viruses. This family contains many important human pathogens and is subdivided into three subfamilies: (1) *Alphaherpesvirinae,* the fast-growing, cytolytic viruses that are latent in neurons and include herpes simplex virus types 1 and 2 and varicella-zoster virus; (2) *Betaherpesvirinae,* the slow-growing, cytomegalic viruses that contain the CMVs; and (3) *Gammaherpesvirinae,* the herpesviruses that preferentially grow in lymphocytes and sometimes transform them into malignant states. This subfamily includes Epstein-Barr virus and, tentatively, the newly recognized human herpesviruses 6, 7, and 8.

CMV is the largest member of *Herpesviridae.* The genome is double-stranded DNA, 240 kb in size (150×10^6 daltons; G+C content 58 per cent) and has a unique long sequence and a unique short sequence, both of which are bounded by repetitive sequences that are inverted relative to each other. The genome, therefore, can assume four isomeric forms. The viral particle has a 110-nm icosahedral capsid composed of 162 capsomeres. The entire virion is enclosed by a lipid envelope, giving a final diameter of approximately 200 nm.[224]

The replication of CMV is slow when compared with that of herpes simplex virus. Whereas it takes herpes simplex only 4 to 8 hours to produce infectious progeny virus, CMV requires at least 24 hours. The CMV genome is transcribed slowly in a regulated sequence; on the basis of the appearance of different classes of CMV-specific proteins, the replicative cycle can be divided into three periods: immediate-early, early, and late. The immediate-early period is defined as the first 4 hours after infection. During this period, specific segments of the DNA genome undergo restricted transcription, and certain regulatory proteins that allow the virus to take control of host-cell macromolecular synthesis are produced. The early period of replication begins after the immediate-early phase and persists for almost 20 hours. This period is characterized by replication of viral DNA, production of infected cell proteins, and production of progeny virus. The late period usually is considered to occur 24 hours after infection. During this period, the structural components of the virus are produced, and infectious virus is released from the cell. Monoclonal antibodies against the various immediate-early, early, and late proteins produced by CMV have been used as rapid viral diagnostic tools.

CMV has no distinct serotypes. However, strain relatedness or differences can be determined by molecular analysis of viral DNA. Restriction-enzyme analysis of DNA extracted from CMV isolates that are linked epidemiologically (for example, serial isolates from the same person, mother-infant pairs, or family members experiencing temporally related CMV infections) shows identical or similar DNA fragment-mapping patterns. This technique or modifications of this technique have been applied to the epidemiology of CMV in a variety of patients, such as transplant recipients, congenitally infected infants, and patients whose CMV was transmitted from person to person in hospitals, day care centers, and residences.

EPIDEMIOLOGY

Seroepidemiologic studies have shown that infection with CMV is common and usually is inapparent.[262] The incidence of CMV infection does not appear to be seasonal. However, the prevalence of CMV-IgG antibody is influenced by many factors, including the age, geographic location, cultural and socioeconomic status, and child-rearing practices of the group. For example, in developed countries, such as the United Kingdom and the United States, the prevalence of CMV antibody is 40 to 60 per cent in adult populations of middle-upper socioeconomic status and more than 80 per cent in lower socioeconomic status groups.[102, 220, 260] In contrast, in developing countries, 80 per cent of children acquire CMV by 3 years of age, and almost all persons have been infected by adulthood.[9, 12, 241] Studies on the age-related prevalence of infection with CMV in the United States suggest that there are three periods of increased acquisition: early childhood, adolescence, and the child-bearing years.[9, 247, 261]

Infants and Children

Approximately 1 per cent of all newborns are born congenitally infected with CMV; ranges of 0.2 to 2.5 per cent are reported.[195] Maternal CMV infection that is either primary or recurrent during pregnancy can result in an infant who is infected congenitally with CMV. However, the rate of intrauterine infection with recurrent infection in the mother is less than 1 per cent, whereas transmission to the fetus occurs in 40 to 50 per cent of mothers who primarily are infected with CMV during pregnancy.[220] Although most newborns congenitally infected with CMV are asymptomatic, symptoms and sequelae are much more likely in infants congenitally infected as a result of the mother's primary infection during pregnancy than in those infants congenitally infected from a recurrent maternal infection.

CMV also can be transmitted perinatally from the mother to her infant. The virus can be shed in the mother's cervicovaginal secretions, urine, saliva, and breast milk. The most common and most efficient routes of perinatal transmission are ingestion or aspiration of cervicovaginal secretions at time of delivery or ingestion of breast milk after delivery. CMV-seropositive mothers frequently shed CMV in their breast milk, and up to 53 per cent of children who are breast-fed with milk that contains infectious virus can become infected with CMV.[74] In addition, up to 57 per cent of babies whose mothers shed CMV at or around the time of delivery become infected with CMV.[188]

Children not congenitally or perinatally infected with CMV may be infected during the toddler or preschool years. The acquisition of CMV by children between 1 and 3 years of age is influenced by home exposure to the virus, by the socioeconomic status of the family, and by group day care exposure. Weller[246] suggested that the child-rearing practices in Sweden, where group day care was common practice, accounted for the relatively high prevalence of CMV infection in Swedish children when compared with children in the United States and Great Britain, where day care centers were not common at that time.

Pass and colleagues[165] first reported the prevalence of CMV in day care centers in the United States in 1982.[165] They found that 51 per cent of children who attended a day care center in Alabama excreted CMV in their saliva or urine. In this study, the prevalence of CMV excretion varied with age; 83 per cent of children 13 to 24 months of age shed virus, compared with only 9 per cent of those children younger than 1 year of age. Pass and colleagues concluded that the high prevalence of CMV infection probably was due to horizontal spread between the children in day care. Subsequent studies have confirmed a high prevalence of CMV excretion in children in day care centers across the United States. Overall prevalence rates of 22 to 57 per cent have been observed, the highest prevalence of active CMV infection (29 to 78 per cent) found in children 1 to 3 years of age.[4, 122, 155, 165–167] Children who attend day care centers also shed high titers of virus (up to 10^5 median tissue culture infective dose/mL), with a mean duration of viral shedding of 13 months in urine and 7 months in saliva.[155] This prolonged, generally asymptomatic shedding of large quantities of virus, coupled with mobility and the less than hygienic daily habits notorious in toddler-aged children, no doubt facilitates the transmission of CMV in day care centers.

Several studies support the idea that the high prevalence of CMV infection in young children who attend day care centers is due to horizontal transmission: these studies utilized molecular fingerprinting techniques to show that infected children in contact with each other shed strains of CMV with similar or identical restriction-enzyme banding patterns and that predominant strains of CMV appeared to circulate over a given period in a given day care center.[2, 4, 117] Reinfection with a genetically different stain of CMV also has been observed and may be important in the child-to-child transmission of CMV in the day care center environment.[6] The importance of horizontal spread of CMV has been shown in special care centers for mentally retarded children as well.[204] CMV also has been isolated from plastic toys and from the hands of day care center workers.[79, 117, 165]

Current epidemiologic evidence suggests that CMV-infected children may transmit the virus to the day care center workers who care for them.[1, 2] In addition, children who attend day care centers may transmit CMV to their CMV-seronegative parents. In one study of parents of children who attended one of three day care centers in Alabama, 14 of 67 parents (21 per cent) whose children attended day care seroconverted, compared with none of 31 parents whose children were cared for at home.[168] Excretion of CMV by the child clearly was a key risk factor for parental seroconversion because none of the seroconversions occurred in parents whose children attended the day care center but did not shed CMV. Also, this study revealed a strong trend toward greater risk of CMV infection (seroconversion rate, 45 per cent) in parents of children 18 months of age or younger. Additional evidence implicating young children who attend day care centers as a source of CMV infection for their parents was provided by a study in Virginia day care centers, in which parents of children in day care shed CMV strains identical to those strains shed by their children.[3]

Although early childhood probably is the most rapid period of acquisition of CMV, annual seroconversion rates of only 3 to 6.2 per cent have been observed in older children 3 to 10 years of age in the United States, reflecting an age-related plateau in acquisition of CMV. One identified risk factor for CMV infection in the school age child has been recent or active CMV infection in a family member.[261]

Adolescents

In support of these early findings, a seroepidemiologic study of CMV infection in sexually active adolescent females found a strong association between indicators of sexual activity and serologic evidence of CMV infection and concluded that sexual activity was an important risk factor for CMV infection in adolescent girls.[46, 211] Early cross-sectional epidemiologic studies of CMV implied a gradual increase in CMV antibody prevalence during the teenage years, and this period of rapid acquisition was attributed to the intimate physical contact that is so common during the teenage years.[9] However, these studies were conducted primarily in lower socioeconomic groups. In a seroepidemiologic study of several groups in Houston on the acquisition of CMV infection in late childhood and adolescence, the prevalence of antibody increased with age in subjects of nonwhite races, as it did according to previous studies, but the prevalence of antibody in subjects of white race did not increase with age.[247]

Vertical transmission of CMV acquired during the teenage years may result in congenital infection with CMV in infants born to teenage mothers. In 1984, Kumar and colleagues[134] studied primary CMV infection in more than 3000 pregnant adolescents in Ohio. They found that 57 per cent were CMV-seropositive, that 1 per cent of susceptible pregnant adolescents acquired CMV, and that if primary CMV infection occurred during pregnancy, the risk of intrauterine transmission was 50 per cent. Information provided by the National Registry for CMV Disease and the National Center for Health Statistics suggests that adolescents who are pregnant actually may be at higher risk than older mothers for giving birth to an infant with congenital CMV disease because 34 per cent of mothers who give birth to a baby with congenital CMV disease are younger than 20 years of age; however, this age group makes up only 16 per cent of the mothers giving birth in the United States.[65, 118]

Intrafamilial Transmission

CMV also can be transmitted within the family setting; evidence for intrafamilial transmission of CMV has been provided in the form of case reports, seroepidemiologic studies, and accounts in which molecular analysis of CMV strains was used in tracing transmission of CMV in family members or extended family members with temporally related CMV infections. In most studies, the index case was a child; when a CMV-infected child entered a household, attack rates were 47 to 53 per cent.[229, 257]

Three patterns of intrafamilial transmission have been observed: transmission between siblings, transmission between parents, and transmission between children and parents. Additional support for the intrafamilial transmission of CMV has been provided by published studies in which molecular analysis was performed on CMV isolates from family members or extended family members who experienced temporally related CMV infections. In each of these studies, restriction-enzyme analysis of viral DNA from the CMV isolates from the family members showed that the strain of CMV was the same within each family.[73, 169, 217] New molecular techniques based on the polymerase chain reaction amplification of a hypervariable region of the CMV genome also have corroborated the observation that genetically similar strains of CMV can be transmitted between family members over time.[212]

Sexual Transmission

CMV also appears to be transmitted by heterosexual and homosexual contact. The evidence to support sexual transmission is anecdotal, virologic, serologic, and molecular and, when taken together, suggests that sexual transmission of CMV in certain groups is important. However, because the virus is shed in saliva, cervicovaginal secretions, and semen, it is unclear which form of intimate contact results in transmission between sex partners.[62, 137, 188]

Several observations support the idea that CMV can be transmitted sexually. For example, CMV antibody prevalence increases with age; CMV antibody is more prevalent in sexually active women than celibate women; CMV antibody is associated with indices of sexual activity, such as recent infection with *Chlamydia trachomatis* or *Neisseria gonorrhoeae*; and a strikingly high annual incidence (37 per cent) of primary CMV infection has been observed in young women with a recent first sexual experience.[45, 52, 58, 123, 211, 251] Also, in a longitudinal study of the site-specific shedding of CMV in HIV-seropositive homosexual and bisexual men, CMV was cultured from semen more frequently than from other body sites or fluids.[191] In addition, molecular analysis of viral DNA has shown strains of CMV isolated from sex partners to be identical in most cases analyzed.[62, 108]

Infection of the genital tract can recur by reactivation of an endogenous strain or by reinfection with an exogenous or different strain of CMV.[211] The consequences of such reinfections are unknown but may have important implications, especially if a CMV vaccine is used to control congenital CMV disease in the future.

Nosocomial Transmission

CMV can be transmitted in the hospital setting by blood product transfusion, bone marrow and organ transplantation, and, rarely, by person-to-person transmission. Despite numerous studies that have employed serologic, virologic, and molecular epidemiologic techniques, the transmission of CMV from CMV-infected patient to health care worker has not been documented.[5, 15, 19, 29, 64, 75, 115] Therefore, even though health care workers are exposed to CMV-infected patients, their risk of acquiring CMV appears no greater than that of the general population. And, unlike homes and day care centers, hospitals routinely employ rigorous infection control procedures, including universal precautions, that probably account for the relatively low risk of acquiring CMV, as well as other infections, in the hospital setting. However, infant-to-infant transmission has been shown to occur, albeit infrequently, in crowded hospital units with a high prevalence of CMV excretion in the patients.[64, 214] CMV also can survive on plastic surfaces and has been cultured from inanimate objects in contact with CMV-infected patients in the hospital setting.[64, 179]

Blood products are a well-established source of CMV infection, and the donor-to-recipient transmission of CMV has been documented by restriction-enzyme analysis of viral DNA.[232] Posttransfusion CMV mononucleosis can be seen in adults who receive large volumes of fresh whole blood.[125] In addition, 15 to 17 per cent of CMV-seronegative neonates who receive blood products from CMV-seropositive donors acquire CMV.[258] Posttransfusion CMV infection in newborns, especially premature infants, can cause a syndrome of shock, lymphocytosis, and pneumonitis; CMV infection also appears to hasten the progression to bronchopulmonary dysplasia in these patients.[199, 258]

CMV apparently is transmitted in the residual leukocytes found in whole blood, packed red blood cells, and platelet fractions, as well as by pure leukocyte transfusions. The risk of posttransfusion CMV infection is about 3 per cent per unit transfused, and the risk for symptomatic infection is much higher in CMV-seronegative recipients than in CMV-seropositive recipients.

Immunosuppressed Patients

Primary and reactivation infections, as well as reinfection with CMV, are common in organ and marrow transplant recipients. Active infection with CMV occurs in almost all organ and marrow transplant recipients and usually manifests clinically and virologically 30 to 90 days after transplantation. Rarely, CMV retinitis can occur years after transplantation and usually is associated with chronic CMV viremia.[85] CMV can be transmitted to the recipient by the transplanted organ, by transfused blood products, and, theoretically, also by intimate contact with persons actively infected with CMV.

Infections with CMV are primary when they occur in CMV-seronegative recipients who receive transplants or blood products from CMV-seropositive donors. Recipients who are CMV-seropositive before transplant can experience reactivation of their own endogenous strain of CMV. Also, CMV-seropositive transplant recipients may be superinfected by strains of CMV present in the donor organ.[48] In fact, in one study of renal transplant recipients in the United Kingdom, proven superinfection with the donor strain of CMV was more common than proven reactivation of the recipient strain of virus.[105] Although reactivation, reinfection, and primary CMV infections all can produce symptoms in immunosuppressed transplant recipients, primary CMV infections are much more likely to be severe and even fatal.[177]

The type of transplant also appears to influence the type of CMV disease expressed. For example, the most severe and lethal form of CMV interstitial pneumonitis is seen in bone marrow transplant recipients, especially those experiencing a graft-versus-host reaction. CMV pneumonia also is common after heart, lung, or renal transplantation, but severe CMV hepatitis is a special problem after liver transplantation.

The iatrogenic immunosuppression essential for graft maintenance probably is responsible for the common occurrence of reactivation infections after transplantation, as well as the increased incidence of severe and symptomatic infections seen in primary CMV infections in transplant recipients. Cytotoxic drugs such as cyclophosphamide and azathioprine, in addition to corticosteroids, have been associated with reactivation of latent CMV infection, and the addition of antilymphocyte globulin to an immunosuppressive regimen can increase morbidity of CMV infections.[170] The use of cyclosporine as the primary immunosuppressive agent, even in conjunction with corticosteroids, does not appear to reduce the risk of CMV infection when compared with a regimen of azathioprine and corticosteroids; however, it may decrease the incidence of severe, symptomatic CMV disease in some transplant recipients.[72] The use of OKT3 to treat rejection in certain transplant patients increases the risk for dissemination in patients with primary CMV infection.[206]

The frequency and morbidity of CMV infection in patients with malignancies are not as high as after marrow and organ transplantation; however, the use of chemotherapy, especially in leukemias, is associated with significant CMV disease, especially pneumonitis and persistent fever with viral dissemination. CMV-seropositive patients receiving immunosuppressive therapy for connective tissue disease also can have significant reactivation infection with CMV.[69]

The progressive and profound immunosuppression in adults and children with AIDS also is associated with CMV infection and disease. Although the source of CMV infection in adults with AIDS is most likely heterosexual or homosexual contact, the sources of CMV infection in young children with AIDS have not been determined. It can be hypothesized, however, that many of these infections are acquired from the mother, either congenitally or perinatally. Patients with AIDS also may be infected with multiple strains of CMV.[70, 215]

PATHOLOGY, PATHOGENESIS, AND IMMUNITY

CMV infection causes characteristic type A Cowdry intranuclear inclusions and massive enlargement of the affected cells (Fig. 164–1). It is this property of "cytomegaly" from which CMV acquired its name. The cytomegalic cells (25 to 40 μm in diameter) are two to four times larger than normal cells, and the nucleus usually is more than 10 μm in diameter. The intranuclear inclusion also is large (up to 10 μm in diameter) and is surrounded by an intranuclear halo, then the nuclear membrane, which gives a characteristic "owl's eyes" appearance. Basophilic, granular, intracytoplasmic inclusions (2 to 4 μm in diameter) also may be present in cells that have intranuclear inclusions. These large cells represent productive virus infection, and both the nuclear and cytoplasmic inclusions contain viral nucleocapsids and express virus-specific antigens.[113] These cytomegalic cells frequently are associated with epithelial cells, and their presence generally indicates a productive and symptomatic infection with CMV. Cells also may be infected latently with CMV. These cells may express virus-specific antigen and contain viral nucleic acid without producing typical cytomegaly or cytopathic effect. The significance of these cells must be considered carefully within the clinical context of the patient.

With severe, disseminated CMV disease, involvement can be seen in virtually all organ systems. The salivary glands are infected commonly in both symptomatic and asymptomatic infections, and the ductal epithelium usually is the site of pathologic involvement. The kidneys also commonly are infected in both symptomatic and asymptomatic infections with CMV. In kidneys, cytomegalic cells are pronounced most in the proximal tubules and interstitial cellular infiltrates, and even immune complex deposits can be seen in the glomeruli.

CMV infection often causes prolonged viruria, but it rarely causes significant renal dysfunction. In the lung, the cytomegalic cells are seen in the alveolar and bronchial epithelium and are associated with mononuclear cell inflammation. Pulmonary alveolar macrophages also may express viral antigen and contain CMV DNA. The brain parenchyma can be involved, and a variety of pathologic processes can be observed, including sensorineural hearing loss. Other organs that can be infected or diseased with CMV include the liver, pancreas, adrenals, eye, lymph nodes, heart, skin, bone, male and female genital tracts, esophagus, stomach, intestine, and placenta.

Infections with CMV can be latent and nonproductive, productive yet asymptomatic, or productive and sympto-

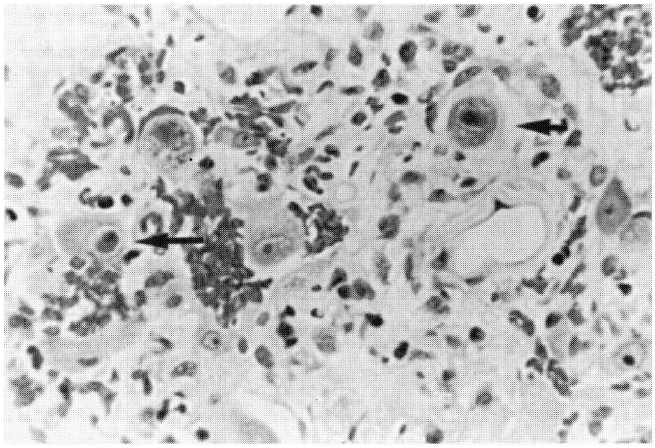

FIGURE 164–1. *Typical cytomegalic inclusion cells seen in lung tissue obtained by open lung biopsy from bone marrow transplant recipient with fatal cytomegalovirus pneumonitis (× 640). (Courtesy of Dr. Milton J. Finegold, Department of Pathology, Texas Children's Hospital, Houston, TX.)*

matic. Therefore, it sometimes is difficult to determine whether a patient is "sick with CMV" or "sick from CMV." Viral strain differences, to date, have not been shown to influence pathogenicity. However, immune responses, including maturity of the immune response, appear to be a major factor exhibiting control over virulence because CMV disease occurs more frequently in fetuses, premature neonates, transplant recipients, and patients with AIDS than in older healthy infants, children, and adults with acquired CMV infection.

The cell-mediated immune response, both specific and nonspecific, is thought to be important in the host defense of CMV. Nonspecific immune mechanisms of natural killer cells and interferon production occur early after CMV infection when early antigens are being produced and before infectious virus is released from the cell. The generation of cytotoxic T cells against CMV early antigens probably is the most important specific host immune response to CMV, and patients who are defective in T-cell response are at high risk for serious CMV disease.[103]

Clinical and laboratory evidence also supports the concept of CMV as an immunosuppressive agent. The proliferative response of T cells to stimulation with mitogens and CMV antigen is suppressed in patients with CMV mononucleosis, and immunosuppressed patients with active CMV disease commonly have other opportunistic infections.[190] In addition, CMV pneumonitis in bone marrow transplant recipients has been hypothesized to result from host cell–mediated events produced in response to chronic viral replication.[263] Homology between certain CMV proteins and class I and II major histocompatibility complex products has been observed. This "molecular mimicry" implies that the severe tissue destruction seen in CMV pneumonitis may be, in part, an autoimmune phenomenon in these patients.

Humoral immunity, on the other hand, does not appear to be a key factor in the host's defense against CMV infection. For example, the fetus can be infected by intrauterine transmission through a reactivated CMV infection in women who are CMV-seropositive prior to pregnancy, and infants commonly are infected perinatally from infected cervicovaginal secretions or breast milk in the presence of passive maternal antibody.[220] In addition, CMV-seropositive transplant recipients can be reinfected with a new strain of CMV from the donor organ, and viruria and viremia occur in transplant recipients, despite high titers of neutralizing antibody against the specific strain of CMV.[48, 49] The presence of CMV antibody, therefore, should be considered a marker of previous or current infection with the virus rather than a measure of immunity per se.

Although humoral immunity does not appear to prevent infection with CMV, it does appear to lessen the severity of symptoms associated with the infection. Infants congenitally infected with CMV as a result of reactivation infection in their mother almost always are asymptomatic, and perinatally infected infants rarely have significant symptoms. Primary infections in transplant recipients are more likely to be symptomatic than reinfection or reactivation. One hypothesis as to how CMV eludes host humoral defenses is that the virus binds to the host protein, β_2-microglobulin, and masks the antigenic determinants that are important for neutralization by antibody.[148]

CLINICAL MANIFESTATIONS

Congenital Infections

Annually, 30,000 to 40,000 babies are born with congenital CMV infection. Of these babies, up to 10 per cent have severe, classic "cytomegalic inclusion disease" characterized by intrauterine growth retardation; jaundice; hepatosplenomegaly; thrombocytopenia with petechiae and purpura; pneumonia; and severe central nervous system damage with microcephaly, intracerebral calcifications, chorioretinitis, and sensorineural hearing loss. Another 5 per cent have atypical involvement, such as ventriculomegaly, periventricular leukomalacia, periventricular cystic malformations with or without calcifications, strabismus, optic atrophy, long-bone osteitis characterized by fine vertical metaphyseal striations, isolated and transient thrombocytopenia and petechiae, cutaneous vasculitis, hemolytic anemia, ascites, and chronic hepatitis. Up to 90 per cent of these infants who are symptomatic at birth later have neurologic sequelae or deafness. However, the range of severity of these sequelae appears broad.

The differential diagnosis of symptomatic congenital CMV disease includes congenital toxoplasmosis, congenital herpes simplex virus infection, congenital syphilis, congenital rubella syndrome, congenital infection with lymphocytic choriomeningitis virus, and congenital HIV infection. In addition, noninfectious causes, such as genetic disorders, metabolic disease, and maternal exposure to drugs and toxins, should be considered.

Most infants who are infected congenitally with CMV are asymptomatic at birth. Yet 10 to 17 per cent of these infants later may have unilateral or bilateral deafness (which often is progressive), differences in higher-level auditory function, and possibly other neurodevelopmental sequelae.[53, 220, 250]

Very low birth weight infants who are infected congenitally with CMV may experience pulmonary and systemic deterioration temporally associated with steroid therapy.[235]

Perinatal Infections

Perinatally acquired infections in healthy infants usually manifest between 4 and 16 weeks of age, and most of these infections are asymptomatic. However, up to one-third of infants exposed to CMV perinatally may have signs and symptoms of disease associated with CMV infection, most often self-limited lymphadenopathy, hepatosplenomegaly, hepatitis, or pneumonitis.[135] Perinatally acquired infection with CMV also can cause severe, protracted pneumonitis and has been associated with the development of bronchopulmonary dysplasia in premature infants.[199] These infections, however, do not appear to cause neurodevelopmental sequelae or deafness.[136] The differential diagnosis includes other perinatally acquired infections, such as *Chlamydia* pneumonitis, hepatitis B virus infection, and infection with HIV, as well as postnatally acquired infections with enteroviruses, adenovirus, and a variety of bacterial pathogens.

Mononucleosis Syndrome

CMV-induced mononucleosis occurs as a primary infection in both immunocompetent and immunosuppressed persons and, occasionally, as a reactivation infection in immunosuppressed patients. It can result from person-to-person transmission of the virus, as well as from transmission by blood products or by organ or marrow transplantation. Although originally described in adults and most often occurring between 20 and 40 years of age, it also can be seen in adolescents, children, and even infants.[145, 164] Typical CMV-induced mononucleosis is characterized by fever and strikingly severe malaise of about 1 to 4 weeks' duration, peripheral lymphocytosis with atypical lymphocytosis, and mild elevation of liver enzymes. In some patients, headache, myalgias, and abdominal pain with diarrhea are prominent symptoms. In premature infants with transfusion-acquired CMV mononucleosis, shock, hepatosplenomegaly, pneumonitis, thrombocytopenia, and renal failure are prominent manifestations.[258] In contrast to Epstein-Barr virus–induced mononucleosis, CMV-induced mononucleosis rarely causes pharyngitis, tonsillitis, or significant splenomegaly, and it does not produce heterophile antibodies.[51, 116] However, like Epstein-Barr virus–induced mononucleosis, it can be associated with a morbilliform rash after ampicillin administration; an elevated erythrocyte sedimentation rate; polyclonal hypergammaglobulinemia; and the production of other antibodies, such as rheumatoid factor, cold agglutinins, and antinuclear antibodies. Complications are rare but include interstitial pneumonitis, myocarditis, pericarditis, hemolytic anemia, thrombocytopenia with or without petechiae or purpura, hemophagocytic syndrome, arthralgias and arthritis, maculopapular rashes, adrenal insufficiency, splenic infarction, ulcerative colitis and proctitis, Guillain-Barré syndrome, and meningoencephalitis.[44, 51, 56, 84, 116, 131, 132, 140] Severe, icteric hepatitis, as well as granulomatous hepatitis, also can occur, but hepatic necrosis and liver failure due to CMV have not been documented convincingly in the normal host.[26, 51, 116, 132, 187]

The differential diagnosis of CMV-induced mononucleosis includes mononucleosis induced by other viruses, such as Epstein-Barr virus, hepatitis A or B virus, and HIV. Also, acquired toxoplasmosis can produce a mononucleosis syndrome in healthy persons.

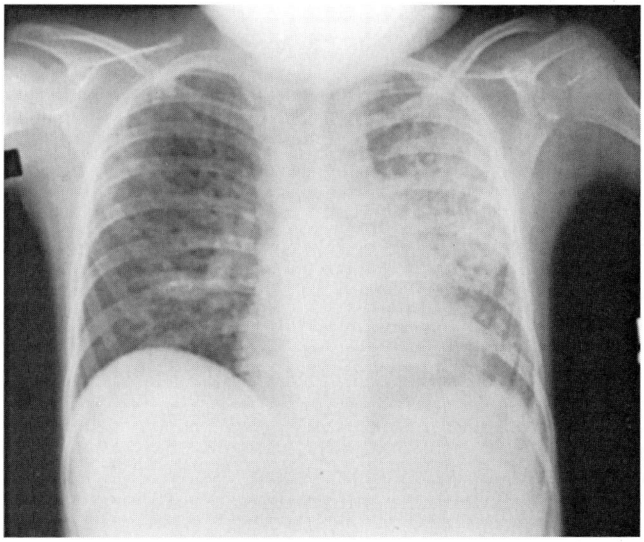

FIGURE 164–2. *Chest radiograph of bone marrow transplant recipient with rapidly fatal cytomegalovirus pneumonitis. Open lung biopsy specimen showed numerous cytomegalic inclusion cells, exhibited cytomegalovirus early antigens by immunoperoxidase staining, and grew cytomegalovirus after inoculation into tissue culture.*

Interstitial Pneumonitis

CMV is a major cause of interstitial pneumonia in both adults and children who are immunosuppressed because of congenital immunodeficiency, AIDS, organ or marrow transplant, or malignancy. In recipients of bone marrow transplantation, CMV accounts for 17 to 70 per cent of interstitial pneumonitis in adult patients but only 10 per cent of pneumonitis in patients younger than 21 years of age.[244] Pneumonia also can occur in apparently immunocompetent young infants with perinatally acquired CMV infection and healthy adults with CMV-induced mononucleosis.[129, 135, 219, 248] Whereas the pneumonia in immunocompetent hosts almost always is benign and self-limited, CMV pneumonia in immunosuppressed patients is a serious, often fatal illness, especially in bone marrow transplant recipients, who have a mortality rate of up to 90 per cent. It also can be particularly troublesome after pediatric heart and lung transplantation.[160] CMV pneumonitis usually occurs 1 to 3 months after transplantation and begins with symptoms of fever and dry, nonproductive cough. It then can progress over 1 to 2 weeks to dyspnea, retractions, wheezing, and hypoxia, which require ventilatory support. It may occur as the only disease manifestation or be part of a disseminated CMV infection. The radiographic appearance of CMV pneumonia most often is diffuse, interstitial infiltrates, but peribronchial infiltrates with hyperinflation and nodular pulmonary infiltrates also have been described (Fig. 164–2).[129, 230] Co-infection with other pathogens, especially gram-negative enteric bacteria and fungal pathogens in transplant recipients and *Pneumocystis carinii* in patients with AIDS, can occur.[240]

Congenitally infected infants also may be born with CMV pneumonitis, which often is severe, requiring ventilatory support, and which usually is part of a multisystem CMV disease process. Very low birth weight infants who are infected congenitally with CMV may experience CMV pneumonitis temporally associated with steroid therapy.[235]

The differential diagnosis of CMV pneumonitis in the immunocompromised patient, including the neonate, is extensive and includes infection with other viruses, such as herpes simplex virus, varicella-zoster virus, measles virus, respiratory syncytial virus, influenza A and B viruses, parainfluenza viruses, and adenoviruses; bacterial pneumonia due to a variety of gram-positive and gram-negative organisms; infection with protozoa, such as *P. carinii* and *Toxoplasma gondii*; *Chlamydia* and *Mycoplasma*; and fungal pneumonia, caused especially by *Candida* and *Aspergillus*. Noninfectious causes of pneumonitis also should be considered, such as pulmonary hemorrhage, aspiration pneumonia, rejection, and pulmonary damage from chemotherapeutic agents.

Retinitis and Other Eye Abnormalities

Chorioretinitis occurs in 17 to 41 per cent of newborns with symptomatic congenital CMV infection and rarely in children born with asymptomatic congenital CMV infection.[27, 195] Although most retinal lesions in congenitally infected infants appear inactive at birth, some observations suggest progression of preexisting lesions and late-onset new lesions, resulting in vision loss, may occur rarely in both symptomatic and asymptomatic congenitally infected infants.[27] Retinitis does not appear to be a prominent part of perinatally acquired infection.[136] CMV retinitis once was a rare manifestation of CMV disease in solid organ transplant recipients with chronic immunosuppression for more than a year and in patients receiving chemotherapy for malignancy.[85] In the 1980s, CMV retinitis emerged as a common manifestation of CMV disease in patients with severe immunosuppression, especially bone marrow transplant recipients and patients with AIDS. It probably is a result of hematogenous spread of the virus to the retina, with continued local viral replication. Despite the common occurrence of CMV retinitis in adults with AIDS, however, it rarely has been reported in children with AIDS.[141]

CMV produces characteristic white, perivascular infiltrates and hemorrhage, with a necrotic, rapidly progressive retinitis. It descriptively has been called cottage cheese and ketchup or brushfire retinitis.[25] Early, peripheral retinitis can be asymptomatic, or the complaints can be minimal and nonspecific; it especially is difficult to ascertain in infants and young children. It does not cause eye pain, photophobia, or conjunctivitis. Once it has progressed, the retinitis can cause blurred vision, decreased visual acuity, visual field defects, and blindness. Young children and infants who have suffered visual loss due to CMV retinitis may exhibit strabismus or failure to fix and follow objects within their visual field. CMV retinitis also can progress rapidly to total blindness if the macula is involved. Immunosuppressed children with CMV disease should receive regular expert ophthalmologic examination to monitor for sight-threatening retinitis. Early diagnosis may allow prompt institution of antiviral therapy that may be sight-saving.[141]

The funduscopic appearance of CMV retinitis usually is characteristic. However, in patients in whom the appearance of the retina is not typical or in whom the retinitis has progressed despite specific antiviral treatment, other causes of retinal lesions should be considered, including cotton-wool spots associated with hypertension, diabetes, connective tissue disease, anemia and leukemia, ocular toxoplasmosis, and candidal infection of the retina, as well as syphilis, herpes simplex virus infections, lymphocytic choriomeningitis virus infection, and varicella-zoster virus infection. Detection of the virus by culture or its DNA by a polymerase chain reaction–based method in vitreous fluid may help diagnose difficult or atypical patients.[82]

Although chorioretinitis is the most common ocular manifestation of CMV disease, CMV also has been associated with other unusual eye abnormalities. In congenitally infected infants, micro-ophthalmia, anophthalmia, optic nerve hypoplasia and coloboma, optic nerve atrophy, Peter anomaly, and irregular retinal pigment have been observed.[89] CMV also has been isolated from tears and has been associated with conjunctivitis in patients with CMV mononucleosis and AIDS, as well as corneal epithelial keratitis and disk neovascularization.[138]

Hepatitis

CMV hepatitis in bone marrow, heart, and lung transplant recipients; patients with cancer or AIDS; and even healthy persons experiencing a primary CMV infection usually is manifested by mild hepatomegaly and mild elevation of serum hepatic enzyme levels and commonly occurs in conjunction with fever, thrombocytopenia, and lymphopenia or lymphocytosis. Jaundice and hyperbilirubinemia usually do not occur, severe hepatitis or cirrhosis is exceedingly rare, and hepatic necrosis and liver failure due to CMV hepatitis have not been documented convincingly in these patients. CMV infection also has been associated with granulomatous hepatitis.[26, 187] In addition, CMV hepatitis is a unique and prominent problem in children who have undergone liver transplantation.[31] Most CMV hepatitis occurs 1 to 2 months after transplantation, but it may occur as early as 2 weeks or as long as 4 months after transplantation.[33] It is more common and more severe after a primary CMV infection and is associated with liver transplantation from a CMV-seropositive donor and the use of OKT3 antibodies for severe rejection.[206] CMV hepatitis in liver transplant recipients is characterized by prolonged fever, leukopenia, thrombocytopenia, elevated liver enzymes, hyperbilirubinemia, and liver failure. It often is difficult, even with a liver biopsy, to distinguish between CMV hepatitis and acute rejection, and the two commonly coexist. CMV infection also has been associated with ascending cholangitis, chronic rejection, and the vanishing bile-duct syndrome in liver transplant recipients.[33, 161]

Infants with congenital CMV disease also may have hepatitis. The liver usually is smooth and nontender and commonly measures 3 to 5 cm below the right costal margin. Ascites may be present prenatally and may persist postnatally for 1 to 2 weeks. The hepatomegaly usually resolves by 3 months of age, and persistence beyond 1 year is highly unusual. Mild hepatitis usually is present, and the transaminase levels in neonatal hepatitis due to CMV rarely exceed 300 IU. Hyperbilirubinemia is present at birth in about one-third of newborns with congenital CMV and may be striking, with conjugated (direct) bilirubin levels up to 30 mg/dL.[118] The abnormal results of liver function tests gradually resolve over the first few weeks of life, and chronic hepatitis due to congenital infection with CMV is unusual but can occur.

The differential diagnosis of CMV hepatitis includes other causes of viral hepatitis, including hepatitis A, B, and C, Epstein-Barr virus, herpes simplex virus, enterovirus, and adenovirus, as well as toxoplasmosis; other infections, such as bacterial ascending cholangitis; and noninfectious causes, such as ischemic injury, vascular thrombosis, hemolysis, rejection, and hepatitis induced by drugs or toxins. In newborns with a significant and persistent direct hyperbilirubinemia, the diagnosis of biliary atresia should be considered as well.

Gastrointestinal Disease

Serious gastrointestinal disease causing esophagitis, gastritis, gastroenteritis, pyloric and small bowel obstruction, duodenitis, colitis, proctitis, pancreatitis, hemorrhage, and acalculous cholecystitis has been associated with CMV infection in immunocompromised patients, especially patients with AIDS and those who have undergone bone marrow, kidney, or liver transplantation.[8, 66–68, 143, 162, 179, 186, 236] Rarely, self-limited CMV gastroenteritis, colitis, and proctitis have been associated with CMV mononucleosis syndrome in apparently normal persons.[51, 116, 180] Characteristic signs and symptoms in infants and children include nausea; vomiting; dysphagia; epigastric pain and tenderness; delayed gastric emptying; watery, guaiac-positive stools or gastrointestinal hemorrhage; and disaccharide and monosaccharide intolerance. Severe disease may cause dehydration and failure to thrive. Endoscopy with biopsy is required for definitive diagnosis and usually shows linear, localized, or punctate ulcers. Hemorrhagic lesions or diffuse erosion can occur in severe disease. Characteristic cytomegalic inclusion cells can be seen in the gastrointestinal endothelium, epithelium, and glandular tissue, and CMV may be cultured from the stool or biopsy specimen, or CMV DNA may be detected by polymerase chain reaction–based methods.[96] In addition, these patients often are viremic and occasionally have evidence of disseminated CMV infection, with involvement of the lungs and retina.

The differential diagnosis of CMV colitis includes infection with other viruses, especially herpes simplex virus and adenovirus, and infection with bacteria, especially *Salmonella, Shigella, Campylobacter,* and *Yersinia,* as well as *Clostridium difficile* and *Mycobacterium avium-intracellulare*. Parasitic infection with *Cryptosporidium, Giardia,* and amebae also should be excluded. The differential diagnosis of CMV esophagitis and gastritis includes herpes simplex virus infection, *Candida* esophagitis, and reflux esophagitis and peptic ulcer disease.

Meningoencephalitis and Other Neurologic Disorders

Central nervous system involvement is well described and is relatively common in infants with symptomatic congenital CMV infection. Although the severity of central nervous system damage during congenital infection varies greatly, postmortem examination of severely affected infants has demonstrated necrotizing encephalitis, especially in the deep periventricular structures, and scattered areas of necrosis and inclusion-bearing cells. Although direct viral infection of neural structures probably plays a major role in central nervous system disease in congenital CMV infection, infectious vasculitis also may occur. Also, because congenital CMV disease can be associated with marked thrombocytopenia, intracranial hemorrhage can contribute to CMV-related central nervous system injury.[17, 39, 109, 239] Clinical manifestations of this disease process include microcephaly, cerebral palsy, intracerebral calcifications, seizures, hemiparesis, developmental delay, ventriculomegaly, paraventricular cysts, intraventricular strands, periventricular leukomalacia, lissencephaly-pachygria, porencephaly, meningoencephalitis, and sensorineural deafness (Fig. 164–3). Remarkably, despite well-documented neuropathology in congenital disease, the isolation of CMV from the cerebrospinal fluid of a congenitally infected child is extremely unusual.[121] CMV DNA has been detected in the cerebrospinal fluid of congenitally infected infants, and its presence at birth appeared to identify infants at risk for a poor neurodevelopmental outcome.[13]

The differential diagnosis of symptomatic congenital CMV infection with neurologic disease includes congenital toxoplasmosis; congenital herpes simplex virus infection; congenital rubella syndrome; congenital infection with lymphocytic choriomeningitis virus; brain tumors, such as craniopharyngioma; and calcified hematoma. Genetic disorders, such as tuberous sclerosis, Sturge-Weber syndrome, and Aicardi syndrome; metabolic conditions, such as hyperthyroidism; alpha$_1$-antitrypsin deficiency; galactosemia; peroxisomal disorders, such as Zellweger syndrome, neonatal adrenoleukodystrophy or infantile Refsum disease; urea cycle deficiencies; organic acidemias; and liposomal storage disorders also may mimic congenital CMV disease involving the central nervous system. Maternal exposure to drugs and toxins, especially isotretinoin, cocaine, and alcohol, also are included in the differential diagnosis. The presence or absence of intracerebral calcification, as well as the pattern of calcifications when present, may be helpful in distinguishing these disorders. In addition, the appropriate microbiologic studies, chromosome analysis, metabolic studies, and drug screens should be performed.

In postnatal life, CMV meningoencephalitis appears to be rare yet well documented.[16] It may present as a complication of CMV mononucleosis, as an isolated manifestation of primary CMV infection in the normal host, or as a primary or recurrent infection in the immunocompromised patient. Symptoms include headache, photophobia, nuchal rigidity, memory deficits, and inability to concentrate. Cerebrospinal fluid findings include mild mononuclear pleocytosis and slightly elevated protein. Although it is exceedingly rare to isolate the virus from the cerebrospinal fluid and brain parenchyma, neuropathologic findings of intranuclear inclusions and microglial nodules are characteristic.

CMV encephalitis may complicate adult immunocompromised transplant recipients, and there is growing recognition of CMV encephalitis in patients with AIDS.[21] Up to 50 per cent of patients with AIDS may demonstrate evidence of CMV infection of the central nervous system at postmortem examination.[157] CMV has been reported to cause a subacute, occasionally progressive encephalitis in patients with AIDS and has been implicated as a cofactor in the pathogenesis of the AIDS dementia complex seen in both adults and children.[55, 112, 154, 209, 249] In this disease, CMV may be isolated from cerebrospinal fluid or CMV DNA may be detected in the fluid or brain by polymerase chain reaction–based methods.[99] In children, this syndrome is characterized by weakness, confusion, and loss of developmental milestones.

The differential diagnosis of CMV encephalitis and meningoencephalitis in the normal host primarily includes other neurotropic viruses, such as herpes simplex virus, Epstein-Barr virus, varicella-zoster virus, enterovirus, and arboviruses. Neurosyphilis and tuberculous meningitis also should be considered. In immunocompromised patients, especially those with AIDS, the following should be added to the differential diagnosis of central nervous system infection: progressive multifocal leukoencephalopathy caused by papovavirus; HIV encephalitis; fungal central nervous system infection caused by *Cryptococcus neoformans, Candida* species, *Aspergillus,* or *Histoplasma*; protozoal infections with *T. gondii* and rarely *P. carinii* and *Strongyloides stercoralis*; bacterial infections with *M. avium-intracellulare* and *Nocardia asteroides*; noninfectious diseases, such as primary cerebral lymphoma and lymphomatoid granulomatosis; and vascular complications, such as hemorrhage and infarction.[10] It is important to remember that in immunosuppressed patients, more than one of these conditions can coexist in the central nervous system.

CMV also can invade the peripheral nervous system and

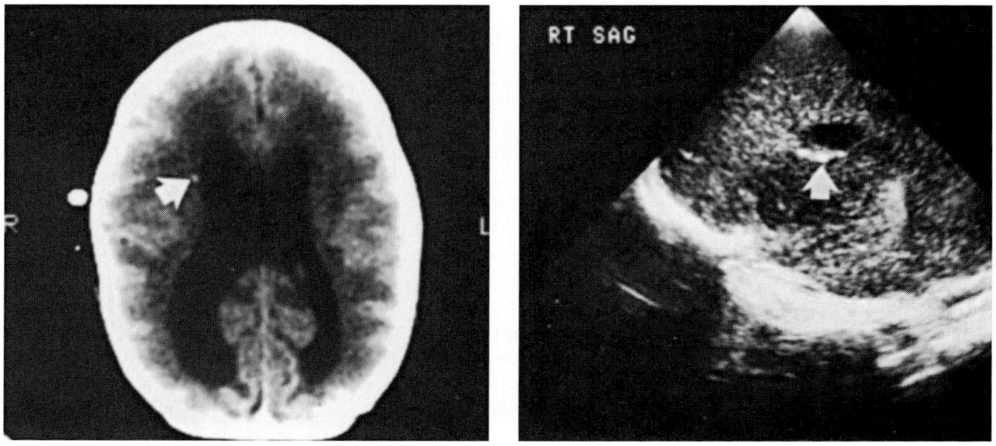

FIGURE 164–3. *Computed tomographic scan* (left) *and ultrasound examination* (right) *of the head of an infant with congenital cytomegalovirus disease. Both tests showed moderate asymmetric enlargement of the lateral ventricles with punctate periventricular calcifications.*

cause a painful peripheral neuropathy in patients with AIDS.[90, 193, 238] Ascending paralysis due to myelitis, with or without vasculitis or necrosis, also can occur and may appear similar to Guillain-Barré syndrome.[238] In addition, CMV polyradiculopathy has been described in adult patients with AIDS and may occur in older children. This disease usually begins with leg pain and sacral paresthesias and may progress to weakness and flaccid paralysis. The cerebrospinal fluid characteristically has a polymorphonuclear pleocytocytosis and moderately elevated protein.[130] The association of CMV infection with infantile spasms, Guillain-Barré syndrome, Charcot-Marie-Tooth disease, Huntington disease, Alzheimer disease, myasthenia gravis, and neuropsychiatric diseases (e.g., schizophrenia) has been reported, but a definite causal relationship between CMV and these diseases remains to be proved.[16]

Deafness and Other Ear Disorders

Hearing loss is present at birth in about 25 to 50 per cent of infants with symptomatic congenital CMV infection and in about 15 per cent of infants with asymptomatic congenital CMV infection.[118] Given that congenital CMV infection affects 30,000 to 40,000 infants annually in the United States, this congenital infection probably is the most common cause of nonhereditary sensorineural deafness. Progression of the hearing loss occurs in at least two-thirds of these children through the preschool years, and it is possible that continued progression may occur through the school age and adolescent years.[250] Although CMV has been detected in the endolabyrinth of infants who died of congenital CMV disease, it still is unclear whether this progressive deafness is due to continued viral replication in the inner ear, reinfection with a new strain of virus, or a complex cascade of immunopathologic events.[59] Mondini dysplasia of the temporal bones has been seen in infants with congenital CMV infection, but the importance of this observation relative to the pathogenesis of the progressive hearing loss so commonly seen in congenitally infected infants is unknown at this time.[22]

CMV has been isolated from middle ear effusions of healthy and immunocompromised children with otitis media.[77] In addition, CMV infection, defined serologically, has been associated with sudden-onset deafness, acute labyrinthitis, and Ménière syndrome.[225, 252] Older children who were born with asymptomatic congenital CMV infection also may exhibit differences in higher auditory function, even though they do not have sensorineural or conductive hearing loss.[53]

Myocarditis and Other Cardiovascular Disorders

Myocarditis has been described as a rare complication of severe congenital CMV disease and CMV mononucleosis in presumably healthy adults and children.[231, 242, 253] CMV myocarditis also has been seen in renal and heart transplant recipients, usually as part of a disseminated CMV infection and associated with graft rejection that was treated with high-dose immunosuppression therapy.[95, 178, 202] Patients can present with heart failure, cardiomegaly, electrocardiographic abnormalities, and poor left ventricular function on echocardiogram; cytomegalic inclusion cells and the presence of CMV DNA can be documented by myocardial biopsy.

The association of CMV infection with other cardiac disorders, such as congenital heart block, structural cardiac anomalies, and pericarditis, is anecdotal, and a cause-and-effect relationship is not well documented.[127] CMV coronary endotheliitis with superimposed thrombosis and myocardial infarct has been described in adult heart transplant recipients and in an infant who died of disseminated CMV disease with an apical ventricular aneurysm.[153, 197] CMV infection also has been postulated to play a role in the pathogenesis of atherosclerosis and coronary artery disease in both normal persons and heart transplant recipients.[100, 147, 149]

Endocrine System

Histopathologic evidence of involvement of the organs of the endocrine system is well described in both congenital and postnatally acquired disseminated CMV infections.[113] Endocrine disorders, such as a Grave disease and diabetes insipidus, have been associated with congenital CMV infection, but these reports may represent coincidental findings.[150, 196] Longitudinal studies are required to determine whether the autoimmune endocrinopathies in children born with congenital rubella parallel findings in children with congenital CMV infection. CMV infection also has been associated with autoimmune type 1 diabetes, although a specific cause-and-effect relationship has not been established.[163] Also, immunosuppressed patients, especially persons with AIDS, may manifest clinical endocrinopathies, such as adrenal insufficiency and adrenal necrosis due to CMV infection.[101] CMV inclusions also have been found in the pituitary gland of patients with AIDS, all of whom showed evidence of CMV encephalitis or disseminated infection elsewhere in the body.[83] In addition, involvement of the thyroid and parathyroid glands with CMV has been reported in adults with AIDS.[88]

Genitourinary System

Disease of the male and female genitourinary system caused by CMV has been reported, and adult patients with AIDS may have symptomatic epididymitis and cystitis due to CMV.[24, 181, 227] CMV also commonly, yet asymptomatically, infects the cervicovaginal secretions and semen of both healthy and immunosuppressed adults.[123, 137]

Skin

Cutaneous manifestations of CMV infection are well described and can occur with both congenital and acquired CMV infection.[140] Infants with symptomatic congenital infection may have nonpalpable petechiae, purpura, or bruises, usually as a result of thrombocytopenia. Violaceous or dark, magenta-colored infiltrative papules or nodules, called "blueberry muffin" lesions, also may occur, but these lesions are more characteristic of congenital rubella syndrome. Skin lesions associated with acquired CMV infection usually are localized cutaneous ulcers or a widespread, exanthematous, maculopapular eruption, although vesiculobullous lesions also have been described.[171] CMV mononucleosis syndrome in adults and children may be accompanied by a maculopapular, rubelliform rash that may be pruritic. In addition, ampicillin-associated rashes may occur with CMV mononucleosis. CMV also may cause a cutaneous, leukoblastic vasculitis.[198] Well-demarcated, ulcerated lesions that show histopathologic evidence of CMV infection may be seen in immunocompromised patients after transplantation or in those who suffer from AIDS. Finally, CMV may play a role in the neoplastic process in Kaposi sarcoma, but definitive proof of a causal relationship remains to be shown.

Unusual Associations

CMV infection, either congenital or acquired, has been detected in association with a wide variety of conditions, including defects in tooth structure and enamel formation, portal vein thrombosis associated with protein S and protein C deficiency, unexplained fevers in burn patients, bacterial sepsis in burn patients, congenital eventration of the diaphragm, inguinal hernia, and fatal *Staphylococcus epidermidis* infection in very low birth weight infants.[11, 23, 126, 133, 144, 222] However, given the common occurrence of CMV infection, it is possible that these associations are coincidental rather than part of a cause-and-effect relationship.

LABORATORY DIAGNOSIS

Detection of the Infectious Agent

CMV can be isolated in tissue culture using fibroblast cell lines, such as human foreskin fibroblasts and human embryonic lung fibroblasts.[200] Specimens that contain a high titer of virus, such as those specimens from congenitally infected infants, may grow in 24 hours. Some specimens, such as those specimens from persons with acquired asymptomatic infections, may require up to 6 weeks to grow, but most cultures grow in 1 to 2 weeks. CMV has been isolated from a variety of specimens, including urine, saliva, nasopharyngeal and sinus washings, conjunctiva, tears, middle ear fluid, breast milk, semen, cervicovaginal secretions, stool, cerebrospinal fluid, white blood cells, amniotic fluid, bronchial lavage samples, and tissue from biopsy or autopsy specimens. All samples (except blood, which should be at room temperature) for virus isolation should be held at 4° C (on wet ice or in a refrigerator) until processed in the virology laboratory. Specimens for virus isolation should be inoculated within hours of collection for an optimal isolation rate. Although isolation of CMV proves that a productive infection is present, it does not confirm an etiologic relationship with the disease process and requires careful interpretation within the patient's clinical context.

An adaptation of tissue culture that now is popular in viral diagnostic laboratories is the low-speed centrifugation enhancement, monoclonal-antibody culture technique, also called shell vial assay. In this test, inoculated tissue-culture cells in small vials are stained with a fluorescein-conjugated monoclonal antibody to either an early or a late CMV antigen (or both). Cells infected with CMV exhibit nuclear and membrane fluorescence 18 to 72 hours after inoculation. This rapid viral diagnostic technique especially is reliable in urine and bronchoalveolar lavage specimens and has been applied with variable results in blood and tissue specimens.[94] However, maximum sensitivity and specificity are obtained when shell vials are used as an adjunct to, and not in place of, routine tissue culture. CMV-infected cells also can be detected by direct immunofluorescence on exfoliated cells in bronchoalveolar lavage specimens or in frozen tissue specimens.[107] This procedure, however, requires a laboratory experienced in direct immunofluorescence technique.

Viral nucleic acid can be detected in clinical specimens by using cloned subgenomic probes that are either radioactively or enzymatically labeled. A variety of DNA hybridization techniques, including dot-blot, Southern blot, and in situ hybridization, have been applied to the clinical diagnosis of CMV infections. For example, detection of CMV DNA in buffy-coat specimens from bone marrow transplant recipients has been shown to be more rapid and more sensitive than viral blood culture and may be predictive of clinically significant CMV viremia and pneumonitis.[216] DNA hybridization also can detect CMV DNA in the urine of patients with a variety of CMV syndromes.[35] In addition, CMV DNA has been detected by in situ hybridization in exfoliated cells in bronchoalveolar lavage samples and peripheral white blood cells of patients with active CMV infection.[57, 93]

Newer technology using primer-mediated DNA amplification techniques (such as polymerase chain reaction) has been applied to the diagnosis of CMV infections in newborns, patients with AIDS, and recipients of transplants.[43, 61, 209] If primer selection and amplification and product detection conditions are chosen carefully, polymerase chain reaction can give results comparable with, and often more sensitive and rapid than, standard tissue culture or cloned probe techniques. However, the exquisite sensitivity of polymerase chain reaction also is its major disadvantage. This extreme sensitivity makes the test vulnerable to false-positive results from contamination and low positive predictive values for CMV disease.

The clinical utility of polymerase chain reaction–based diagnostic tests is evolving, but it does appear that these tests have value in the diagnosis of CMV disease. For example, detection of CMV DNA in the cerebrospinal fluid of patients with AIDS appears to be a reliable diagnostic method for detection of CMV infection of the central nervous system, and detection of CMV DNA in the cerebrospinal fluid of newborns with congenital CMV disease correlates with poor neurodevelopmental outcome.[13, 50, 99, 255] Similarly, detection of CMV DNA by polymerase chain reaction in vitreous fluid provides persuasive evidence that a patient's retinitis is CMV-related.[82] CMV DNA also may be detected in white blood cells of patients with CMV infection, and detection of CMV DNA in plasma or serum of selected groups of patients, such as newborns and immunocompromised patients, appears to correlate with disease severity and viral dissemination.[156, 218]

Another use for polymerase chain reaction–based diagnosis of CMV infection is the very early diagnosis of CMV infection in high-risk patients, such as transplant recipients, before potentially lethal CMV disease such as pneumonitis occurs. This approach may allow pre-emptive antiviral therapy at a time when CMV infection appears active but before overt disease is detected.[36, 256] The role of CMV DNA detection by polymerase chain reaction in monitoring a patient's response to antiviral therapy, however, appears limited because CMV DNA persists for long periods after resolution of CMV-related clinical symptoms in many patients.[91]

CMV antigen also may be detected in the white blood cells of patients with CMV infection and disease, and this CMV antigenemia test is used by some clinical laboratories as a rapid screen for CMV viremia. It is relatively easy to perform, and the degree of antigenemia may be quantitated to monitor response to antiviral therapy.[91]

Exfoliated cells in urine or bronchoalveolar lavage specimens or cells in tissue obtained by biopsy can be examined for histologic evidence of CMV infection. Cells that are infected productively with CMV are enlarged, have type-A Cowdry intranuclear inclusions, and occasionally have perinuclear inclusions. The appearance of these cells is characteristic and has been called owl's eyes. Immunohistochemical staining can be used to augment the detection of these typical cells. The presence of these cells correlates with the presence of active CMV disease and may be useful clinically.

Serology

Standard serologic techniques also can be applied to the diagnosis of CMV infections. CMV-IgG antibody can be determined in serum by several different methods, including complement fixation, hemagglutination inhibition, indirect fluorescent-antibody assay, anticomplement immunofluorescence assay, enzyme-linked immunosorbent assay, latex agglutination, and neutralization tests. The enzyme-linked immunosorbent assay and indirect fluorescent-antibody assay most commonly are employed in clinical virology laboratories. The presence of CMV-IgG antibody in a single serum specimen implies that the patient at some time has been infected with CMV. On the other hand, a negative IgG antibody determination is good evidence against current or past CMV infection because CMV antibody usually is present at the time of infection and persists for life. Severely immunocompromised patients, especially bone marrow transplant patients, however, can lose their ability to make IgG antibody and become CMV-seronegative, even though they are infected actively with CMV. This occurrence has a poor prognosis and usually is a terminal event. A primary infection with CMV is documented best by a clear seroconversion from negative to positive CMV-IgG antibody. A fourfold rise in CMV-IgG antibody titer is not diagnostic of a primary infection because reactivation infection also can cause the titers to fluctuate. In addition, the height of the titer or enzyme-linked immunosorbent assay index in a single serum specimen is not diagnostic.

CMV-IgM antibody can be determined in serum by radioimmunoassay, indirect fluorescent-antibody assay, or enzyme-linked immunosorbent assay. Both the indirect fluorescent-antibody assay and the enzyme-linked immunosorbent assay commonly are employed in clinical laboratories, although some indirect fluorescent-antibody assays have a considerable false-positive rate. Accurate interpretation of CMV-IgM antibody results requires knowledge of the methods employed and careful consideration of the clinical context to exclude diseases that produce cross-reacting antibody or polyclonal responses. Test methods also should remove rheumatoid factor from the test serum, a common cause of false-positive IgM reactions. If the test is performed properly, the presence of CMV-IgM antibody implies a current or recent primary CMV infection. In healthy adults, CMV-IgM antibody usually persists for 6 weeks and may be present up to 3 to 6 months after the primary infection occurs.[63] In immunocompromised adults experiencing clinically significant reactivation infection with CMV, CMV-IgM antibody may be detected for prolonged periods.[158] The sensitivity and specificity of CMV-IgM antibody determination in diagnosing acquired, primary CMV infections or clinically significant reactivation infection in infants and children have not been studied systematically, although clinicians frequently utilize this test for this purpose.

Laboratory Diagnosis of Specific Clinical Syndromes

Congenital

Viral culture is the diagnostic test of choice when considering congenital infection with CMV.[65] The diagnosis is established by isolation of the virus from the urine or saliva in the first 1 to 2 weeks of life. Urine cultures obtained after 3 weeks of life must be interpreted cautiously because perinatally acquired and transfusion-acquired infections with CMV may manifest as early as 3 weeks of age.[199] Detection of nuclear inclusion-bearing renal epithelial cells in the urinary sediment collected in the first 2 weeks of life also implies the presence of congenital infection. This technique is insensitive, however, when compared with tissue culture and is important only historically. Detection of CMV DNA in the urine, serum, or cerebrospinal fluid of newborns by DNA hybridization techniques or DNA amplification techniques also correlates with congenital infection and disease but may be less sensitive than viral isolation.[13, 34, 61, 156]

The diagnosis of fetal intrauterine CMV disease also may be established by isolation of the virus from the amniotic fluid, but a negative culture does not eliminate fetal infection because optimal timing of amniocentesis for these studies is not established. Fetal blood samples that show the presence of CMV-IgM antibody, thrombocytopenia, or leukopenia or elevation of liver function tests also provide supportive evidence of CMV-associated fetal disease. The role of CMV DNA detection by polymerase chain reaction–based methods in amniotic fluid samples is encouraging but requires carefully designed studies before this approach can be recommended over traditional diagnostic tests.

Standard serologic tests also can be applied to diagnose congenital infection with CMV, but this approach is cumbersome and retrospective. The absence of CMV-IgG antibody in the cord blood rules out congenital infection, whereas its presence may imply passive transfer from the mother or indicate a congenital infection. A titer of CMV-IgG antibody in the infant significantly higher than that in the mother may imply a congenital infection, but practically, this difference usually is difficult to ascertain.

Serial serologic specimens also can be obtained at 1, 3, and 6 months of age. If CMV-IgG antibody levels disappear over the first months of life, congenital infection is ruled out. However, if CMV-IgG antibody persists, the infant either was infected congenitally or acquired a CMV infection perinatally or postnatally. The presence of CMV-IgM antibody in cord or infant blood collected in the first 3 weeks of life suggests the diagnosis of a congenital CMV infection.[221] However, care must be taken to determine which technique was used for detecting CMV-IgM antibody. Indirect fluorescent-antibody assay is insensitive when compared with tissue culture (45 to 80 per cent) and has a high frequency (20 to 33 per cent) of false-positive reactions. The detection of CMV-IgM antibody in cord blood by radioimmunoassay is sensitive (89 per cent) and specific (100 per cent) when compared with that by viral culture. In addition, the presence of symptoms and sequelae in congenitally infected infants has been related to the titer of CMV-IgM by radioimmunoassay and enzyme-linked immunosorbent assay.[104, 156] Although radioimmunoassay is sensitive, specific, and useful prognostically, it is not available in most clinical viral diagnostic laboratories. However, a variety of enzyme-linked immunosorbent assays commonly are used by clinical laboratories to detect CMV-IgM antibody. Although apparently specific, enzyme-linked immunosorbent assay may be insensitive (22 per cent) when compared with urine CMV culture for diagnosis of congenital infection, according to one study.[156]

Perinatal and Postnatal

The diagnosis of perinatal infection with CMV is difficult but is documented best by a negative CMV viral culture and CMV-IgM antibody level at birth, a positive viral culture and CMV-IgM antibody at 8 to 16 weeks of age, and persistence of CMV-IgG antibody. Postnatal primary CMV infection is diagnosed by a CMV-IgG seroconversion; presence of CMV-IgM antibody; and viral shedding in saliva, urine, and other bodily fluids.

Cytomegalovirus Syndromes in Immunocompromised Hosts

In immunocompromised patients, the determination of whether serologic or virologic evidence of active CMV infection correlates with disease is difficult because CMV commonly is shed from saliva, urine, and respiratory tract secretions in these patients without clear evidence of a disease process. Therefore, detection of a productive virus infection in the organ system suspected to be involved usually is necessary to establish the diagnosis of CMV disease in the immunocompromised patient. For example, interstitial pneumonitis due to CMV is documented best by an open lung biopsy specimen that shows characteristic CMV histopathology and positive viral culture. Fortunately, studies have shown that detection in bronchoalveolar lavage specimens of viral, infected cells by immunofluorescence, in situ DNA hybridization, cytology, viral culture, or a combination thereof correlates with lung biopsy results.[93] Similarly, the diagnosis of CMV hepatitis or colitis is documented best by the presence of cytomegalic inclusion cells, isolation of CMV from biopsy specimens, or both. In addition, the presence of CMV viremia usually is clinically significant and suggests a disseminated infection. Viremia often precedes or accompanies serious disease, such as CMV pneumonitis in bone marrow transplant patients or CMV retinitis or colitis in patients with AIDS.[216, 237]

Prospective monitoring of high-risk adult patients with serial CMV cultures of urine, blood, or bronchial lavage samples; serial blood samples for evidence of CMV antigenemia or DNAemia; and serum to detect seroconversion by serologic testing usually are indicated because they may allow early pre-emptive therapy with a specific antiviral agent, such as ganciclovir, at a time when CMV infection is active but before overt disease develops.[201] It is likely that high-risk children also would benefit from similar viral surveillance.

TREATMENT

Disease due to CMV now is considered treatable by clinicians. There currently are two antiviral agents, ganciclovir and foscarnet, licensed for treatment of serious CMV disease, and many others are in research and development stages. Ganciclovir, previously called 9-(1,3-dihydroxy-2-propoxymethyl) guanine, or DHPG, was the first antiviral compound licensed specifically for the treatment of life-threatening and sight-threatening infections with CMV. It is a synthetic acyclic nucleotide analog of guanine, structurally similar to acyclovir, and it appears to have in vitro activity against all the human herpesviruses (Fig. 164–4). CMV usually is inhibited by ganciclovir at concentrations of 10 μmol/L or less, making it up to 100 times more active against CMV than acyclovir.[146] The unique in vitro and in vivo activity of ganciclovir against CMV can be explained by both its mechanism of action and its intracellular metabolism and catabolism. When ganciclovir enters a CMV-infected cell, it is converted by cellular enzymes to ganciclovir-5′-triphosphate. This active triphosphate form produces a primary antiviral effect against CMV by competing with deoxyguanosine triphosphate for binding to viral DNA polymerase. This selective inhibition subsequently is enhanced by metabolic factors that allow elevated levels of active ganciclovir-5′-triphosphate to persist in CMV-infected cells.

Ganciclovir is virostatic; therefore, it suppresses active CMV infection but does not produce a cure. It is excreted largely unmetabolized by the kidneys, and total clearance of the drug correlates well with creatinine clearance.[233] Limited data also suggest that hemodialysis reduces levels of ganciclovir by 53 per cent; therefore, the drug probably should be readministered after hemodialysis.[213] Cerebrospinal fluid concentration of the drug usually is 25 to 70 per cent of the plasma concentration. It also penetrates ocular fluids well. Clinical information on this drug in pregnant or lactating women is limited. Ganciclovir is available in both an intravenous and an oral capsular form. However, the oral bioavailability of the capsule form is less than 10 per cent, and a suspension for pediatric use is not licensed yet.

Ganciclovir is indicated for the treatment of CMV retinitis in immunocompromised patients, and it also may be effective in CMV colitis, esophagitis, hepatitis, and meningoencephalitis.[66, 81, 119, 143] Ganciclovir also may improve CMV pneumonia in patients with AIDS and recipients of solid organ transplants, but its effectiveness in treating CMV pneumonitis complicating bone marrow has not been encouraging.[54, 128, 142, 243] Published experience on the use of ganciclovir in children is limited, but the data available imply that the pharmacokinetics, efficacy, and toxicity of ganciclovir in children may be similar to those in adults.[106]

Because of the significant morbidity and mortality associated with symptomatic congenital CMV infection, the pharmacokinetics of intravenous ganciclovir have been studied, and treatment of neonates has been reported. One report of 12 infants evaluated two treatment regimens, 5 mg/kg twice daily for 2 weeks only, and 7.5 mg/kg twice daily for 2 weeks followed by a maintenance regimen of 10 mg/kg three times weekly for 3 months. Unfortunately, the sample size and length of follow-up were inadequate to form a meaningful conclusion from this report about the efficacy of ganciclovir in preventing long-term neurodevelopmental sequelae in congenitally infected infants.[159] A large, multicenter, randomized trial has been in progress for more than 5 years, comparing a dose of 6 mg/kg per dose twice daily for 6 weeks to no antiviral therapy, in congenitally infected infants who have evidence of neurologic involvement at birth. Although the role of ganciclovir treatment of congenitally infected infants, with the intent to improve neurodevelopmental outcome, remains controversial, case reports have suggested that ganciclovir may benefit acutely ill neonates with immediate life-threatening complications of congenital infection, such as pneumonia.[114, 235]

Ganciclovir treatment usually is given in two phases: induction and maintenance. The usual dosage used in adults for induction is 5 mg/kg per dose given intravenously twice daily for 2 to 3 weeks. Because the pharmacokinetics of this drug appear similar in adults and children, this same regimen probably could be used for most children. A variety of other regimens (2.5 to 5 mg/kg per dose given every 8 to 12 hours for 10 to 30 days) also have been shown to be effective in various patient populations. After induction, a maintenance treatment of 5 mg/kg per day given 5 to 7 days is necessary for many patients who remain immunosuppressed, especially patients with AIDS. If disease progresses during maintenance therapy, another course of the induction treatment should be considered. Intravitreal administration of ganciclovir or the use of intraocular devices that deliver a steady amount of drug may help those patients who have severe central retinitis and cannot tolerate systemic ganciclovir treatment.[41, 234] Oral ganciclovir also has been used successfully as maintenance treatment for CMV retinitis in adult patients with AIDS and is considerably more convenient for patients to take than the intravenous form. However, the use of the oral form has not been evaluated yet in infants and children.[71]

The patient's response to ganciclovir should be monitored clinically and virologically. At initiation of therapy, a blood and urine culture for CMV should be obtained and repeated at least weekly during induction and early maintenance therapy to monitor for an antiviral effect. Alternatively, CMV antigenemia tests or detection of CMV DNA in the blood by

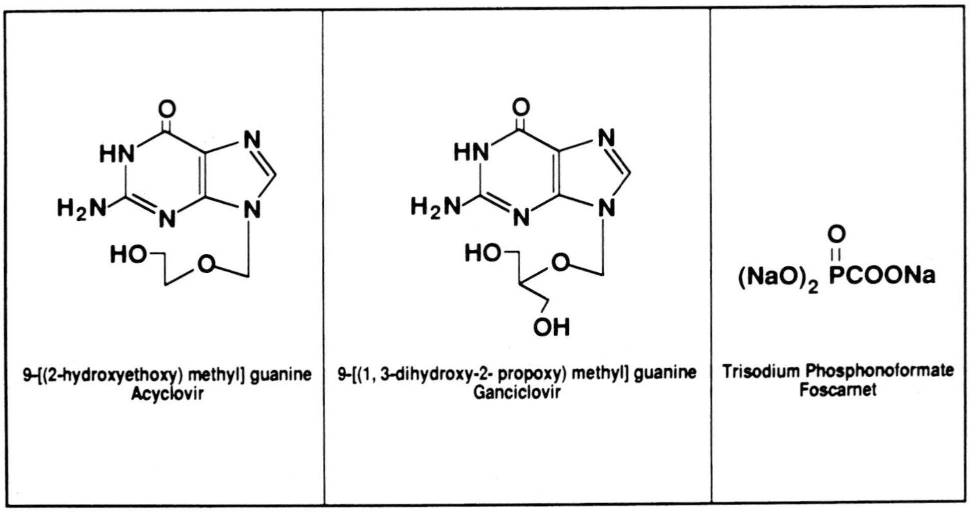

FIGURE 164–4. *Structures of acyclovir, ganciclovir, and foscarnet.*

polymerase chain reaction–based methods may be used to monitor the response in selected patients.[91] However, CMV DNA may be detectable in the blood for weeks or months after apparently successful antiviral treatment. Ganciclovir-resistant strains of CMV also have been reported, and this fact should be considered in patients with proven CMV disease who do not respond to treatment.[78] Weekly ophthalmologic examinations with retinal photographs especially are helpful in documenting regression or progression of CMV retinitis. Because the drug is excreted by the kidneys, the patient's renal function should be monitored while on treatment and the dose adjusted according to creatinine clearance patients with renal insufficiency.

Ganciclovir is myelotoxic and should be used with extreme caution in patients with past or present exposure to myelotoxic drugs, including zidovudine. Daily or every-other-day complete blood counts and platelet counts should be performed, and if they fall to 50 per cent of the baseline count (or an absolute neutrophil count of 500 or a platelet count of less than 25,000), the drug should be suspended. Ganciclovir-induced neutropenia usually is reversible, and recovery commonly occurs within 5 to 7 days after treatment is suspended, at which time a second course of therapy at either the same or a reduced dose may be considered. Ganciclovir also produces testicular atrophy in laboratory animals, and although this toxicity has not yet been observed in humans, it is an important consideration when treatment of children is contemplated.[37]

The combination of ganciclovir with intravenous immunoglobulin or CMV hyper-immunoglobulin in bone marrow transplant recipients with CMV pneumonitis has been shown to increase survival over historical controls who were treated with a variety of other antiviral regimens, including ganciclovir alone, immunoglobulin alone, acyclovir, vidarabine, and interferon. However, differences in methods of diagnosis of CMV pneumonitis, duration of illness, and treatment regimens between study subjects and historical controls obscure interpretation of these studies.[76, 183] Nonetheless, CMV-associated interstitial pneumonitis in bone marrow transplant recipients may be an immunopathologic process, and combination therapy may prevent active virus replication (ganciclovir) while blunting the immune response to viral antigens already expressed on CMV-infected cells (immunoglobulin).[203] In contrast, a small pilot study showed that the addition of CMV hyper-immunoglobulin did not appear to enhance the efficacy of ganciclovir treatment in patients with AIDS-associated CMV retinitis.[120]

Standard immunoglobulin or CMV hyper-immunoglobulin should not be used alone for treatment of established CMV infections in immunocompromised patients.[182] The combination of high-dose corticosteroids with ganciclovir does not appear to improve survival in bone marrow transplant recipients with biopsy-proven CMV pneumonitis.[184] Also, the combination of vidarabine or acyclovir with interferon has not proved efficacious. On the other hand, a regimen combining ganciclovir with hematopoietic growth factor may decrease marrow toxicity.

Foscarnet (trisodium phosphonoformate) now is a licensed antiviral compound that inhibits the DNA polymerase of the human herpesviruses, including CMV. It also is active against HIV-1. Its oral bioavailability is poor, but after intravenous infusion, plasma levels above the mean inhibitory concentration for most strains of CMV are achieved.[7] The drug is excreted in the urine, and up to 30 per cent of each dose may be deposited in bone. It also rapidly distributes into the cerebrospinal fluid. It has been used in adult transplant recipients with life-threatening CMV infections and in patients with AIDS who have CMV retinitis or gastrointestinal disease; clinical and virologic responses were observed in both of these patient groups.[139, 192]

However, information on the pharmacokinetics, safety, and efficacy of the use of foscarnet in children is limited, and published studies are in the form of anecdotal case reports.[38] Foscarnet may be useful as an alternative antiviral agent when CMV disease, such as retinitis, appears to progress while the patient is receiving ganciclovir alone. The drug then may be administered alone or in combination with ganciclovir. Also, intravenous CMV hyper-immunoglobulin may be added to the combination therapy in certain instances. This combination therapy has particular advantage in patients with AIDS who may be infected with multiple strains of CMV with variable susceptibility to antiviral agents.

For patients with AIDS and CMV retinitis, foscarnet may offer a survival advantage over ganciclovir, presumably because of the drug's antiretroviral activity.[226] Foscarnet is nephrotoxic and should be used with caution in patients with impaired renal function.[40] However, unlike ganciclovir, it is not myelosuppressive. The drug also appears to deposit in bone, teeth, and cartilage—an important consideration when treatment of children is contemplated.

Foscarnet usually is administered in two phases, induction and maintenance. The usual dosage used in adults for induction is 60 mg/kg every 8 hours as a 1-hour intravenous infusion for 14 to 21 days. After induction, a maintenance treatment regimen of 90 to 120 mg/kg given once daily is necessary for many patients who remain immunosuppressed, especially patients with AIDS. If disease progresses during maintenance therapy, another course of the foscarnet induction treatment, possibly in combination with ganciclovir, should be considered. Limited experience suggests that similar dosage regimens may be used in children.[38]

The patient's response to foscarnet should be monitored clinically and virologically in a manner similar to that outlined for patients receiving ganciclovir. Foscarnet-resistant strains of CMV have been isolated, and this fact should be considered in patients who do not respond to treatment.[228] Foscarnet generally is less well tolerated than ganciclovir, primarily because it is nephrotoxic. However, although ganciclovir is myelotoxic, foscarnet generally is not. Foscarnet produces a variety of metabolic abnormalities because it binds divalent metal ions, such as calcium.

New, more potent, and longer-acting antiviral compounds, such as (S)-1-(3-hydroxy-2-phosphonylmethoxypropyl) cytosine (HPMPC or cidofovir), show promise and soon may increase the clinician's armamentarium to fight serious CMV disease.[87]

PREVENTION

Because treatment for established CMV disease remains difficult, measures to prevent CMV infection in the fetus, the newborn, and the immunocompromised patient should be employed whenever possible. Approaches to the prevention of CMV disease include the use of CMV-seronegative blood products, CMV-seronegative donor selection for transplant recipients, passive immunoprophylaxis with standard Ig and CMV hyper-Ig prophylactic use of antiviral agents, active immunization with a CMV vaccine, and behavioral strategies.

Blood Product and Transplant Donor Selection

Transplant recipients who are CMV-seronegative and receive solid organ or bone marrow transplants from CMV-seropositive donors are at significant risk for symptomatic primary CMV infection. Therefore, whenever possible, CMV-seronegative recipients should receive transplants from CMV-seronegative donors, and all blood product transfusions should be from CMV-seronegative donors.

Infection with CMV in seriously ill CMV-seronegative neonates can be prevented by using blood products from CMV-seronegative donors or by using frozen deglycerolized red blood cells.[30, 258] Saline-washed red blood cells, however, do not appear to prevent CMV infection in neonates, even though up to 90 per cent of leukocytes can be removed by this method.[60] An alternative method of preparing leukocyte-depleted blood, filtration through a cotton wool filter, appears to prevent posttransfusion-acquired CMV infections in neonates.[92] Many institutions now routinely provide CMV-seronegative or leukocyte-depleted blood products to all neonates or to all low birth weight neonates, regardless of the CMV serostatus of the mother.

Passive Immunoprophylaxis

Although immunoglobulin or CMV hyper-immunoglobulin should not be used alone for the treatment of established CMV disease in immunocompromised patients, these preparations may be used to prevent serious CMV disease in selected immunocompromised patients. Passive immunization remains controversial, however, partially because studies have used different dosages (100 to 200 mg/kg), administered at varying intervals (1 week prior to transplant and every 1 to 3 weeks after transplantation), for varying lengths of time (60 to 120 days). CMV immunoglobulin has been shown to decrease the incidence of symptomatic CMV disease from 60 to 21 per cent in CMV-seronegative renal transplant recipients who received a kidney from a CMV-seropositive donor.[210] CMV immunoprophylaxis also has decreased the incidence of CMV pneumonitis in CMV-seronegative bone marrow transplant recipients who did not receive granulocyte transfusions.[28, 151, 254] The use of immunoglobulin in pregnant women to prevent or ameliorate CMV infection in the fetus has not been studied, and its use cannot be recommended at this time.

Prophylaxis and Early Pre-emptive Therapy with Antiviral Agents

The prophylactic use of antiviral agents in transplant patients has been evaluated and appears in some studies to reduce the incidence of serious CMV disease. However, this approach remains controversial because no regimen has been shown completely to prevent CMV infection or disease. For example, acyclovir is used by some clinicians as prophylaxis for CMV disease in organ transplant recipients, despite evidence that acyclovir is inactive against most strains of CMV and CMV disease occurs despite such prophylaxis.[207] In one study, intravenous acyclovir given 500/mg/m^2 of body surface area per dose every 8 hours for 5 days before and 30 days after transplantation to CMV-seropositive bone marrow transplant recipients appeared to reduce the incidence of CMV disease.[152] High-dose oral acyclovir administered 1 day before and for 12 weeks after transplantation also has been shown to reduce the incidence of CMV disease and infection in renal transplant recipients.[20]

The prophylactic administration of human leukocyte interferon-α has been shown to reduce the incidence of severe CMV disease in renal transplant recipients, but it has no apparent benefit in bone marrow transplant recipients, and it is not used routinely in any patient population.[47, 111, 185] Many clinicians currently favor the prophylactic use of ganciclovir in transplant recipients at high risk for serious CMV disease. Prophylaxis treatment regimens vary, however, and it is difficult to make recommendations about which regimen, if any, is best. Most solid organ recipients appear to benefit from intravenous ganciclovir administered in daily doses between 5 and 10 mg/kg for 2 to 6 weeks after transplant, usually followed by continuing antiviral prophylaxis with acyclovir or a reduced dose of ganciclovir. Prophylactic ganciclovir does not appear, however, to benefit adult lung transplant patients in most published studies. Similarly, administering a short 2-week course of ganciclovir around the time of transplant, without continuing antiviral prophylaxis, does not appear to reduce significantly the incidence of CMV disease in most solid organ transplant recipients studied.[14] The impact of intravenous immunoglobulin or CMV hyperimmunoglobulin, when given with a prophylactic antiviral agent, on the incidence of CMV disease in solid organ recipients is unclear. However, many clinicians administer it concomitantly with an antiviral agent when attempting to prevent CMV disease in certain high-risk transplant recipients. In bone marrow transplant recipients, administration of ganciclovir prophylaxis after marrow engraftment reduced CMV disease but did not appear to reduce significantly overall mortality. In addition, ganciclovir-treated bone marrow transplant recipients experienced prolonged neutropenia.[98]

The strategy of pre-emptive antiviral therapy is relatively new and has certain advantages over strategies that either only treat patients with overt clinical disease or administer prophylactic antiviral agents to many patients at risk, of whom only a few appear to benefit. In addition to preemptive or very early antiviral treatment strategies, clinicians use viral surveillance of blood, urine, and respiratory samples. Viral surveillance of these samples can be by standard viral culture, viral antigen detection, viral nucleic acid detection by polymerase chain reaction, or a combination of these tests. The detection of CMV viremia and culture-positive bronchoalveolar lavage samples has correlated with the development of serious CMV disease in transplant recipients.[36] At least two studies in bone marrow transplant recipients now have documented the efficacy of early intervention with intravenous ganciclovir therapy at the time of positive CMV surveillance cultures but before clinical disease developed.[98, 201] This strategy also appears efficacious in solid organ transplant recipients.[207] Another approach to pre-emptive therapy that does not utilize viral surveillance techniques is to administer an antiviral agent, such as ganciclovir, during times of rejection, when CMV reactivation is likely. This approach has been modestly successful in high-risk renal transplant recipients.[110]

Active Immunization

Another approach to prevention of CMV disease is active immunization with a CMV vaccine. Pregnant women and their fetuses, as well as transplant recipients, would benefit greatly if a safe, effective CMV vaccine became widely available. The ideal CMV vaccine should be safe, effective, immunogenic, and cost-effective. It should prevent primary CMV infection without causing chronic persistent infection. The vaccine also should not be capable of infecting the fetus, and it should not be oncogenic.

In 1975, Plotkin and associates[174] characterized and reported a candidate CMV vaccine strain, Towne 125, that was isolated originally from the urine of a congenitally infected infant named Towne. Since then, more than 500 subjects, including renal transplant recipients and healthy adult male and female volunteers, have received the investigational Towne 125 vaccine.[42, 86, 124, 172–175, 223] Studies of these subjects showed that Towne 125 is attenuated and relatively safe and that it induces humoral and cellular immunity in both healthy and immunosuppressed subjects.

The vaccine also appeared to be protective in a randomized, placebo-controlled study of 91 immunosuppressed renal transplant recipients.[173] In this study, 30 CMV-seronegative vaccine recipients received a kidney from a CMV-seropositive donor, and the incidence of severe CMV disease was significantly lower in the vaccine group than in the placebo group. However, the CMV infection rate did not differ significantly among the groups, and members of both groups experienced mild to moderate CMV disease. Subsequent studies have confirmed that CMV seronegative renal transplant recipients who receive a live attenuated CMV vaccine are more resistant to serious CMV disease.[176] It is not known whether a CMV vaccine given to CMV-seronegative women of child-bearing age before pregnancy protects the fetus from intrauterine infection or disease, but studies that may answer this question are in progress.

While research continues on the live attenuated CMV vaccine, other researchers are exploring vaccine alternatives, such as a genetically engineered subunit vaccine based on the surface glycoproteins of the virus shown to be targets for neutralizing antibody.[32] Clinical trials with human volunteers using recombinant CMV vaccines are in progress. Alternatively, a neutralizing human monoclonal antibody may be developed and used to prepare monoclonal anti-idiotype antibodies that could serve as a CMV vaccine.[80]

Behavioral Strategies to Prevent Primary Cytomegalovirus Infection

Faced with the current complexities associated with the development of a CMV vaccine and the challenges of administering effective antiviral therapy, some investigators believe that an alternative practical option for prevention of CMV infection during pregnancy is education of young women of child-bearing age.[259] Reliable, relatively inexpensive serology is available, so all women contemplating pregnancy should know their CMV serologic status. Also, because epidemiologic studies have shown a major source of CMV infection to be close contact with young children, those women who are CMV-seronegative should be aware that a high percentage of young children are infected actively with CMV and that while pregnant, they should exercise good hygienic practices when in close contact with young children, especially those who attend day care centers or who are known to have an active CMV infection. In fact, some studies have shown that child-to-parent transmission of CMV may be reduced by interventions that identify susceptible pregnant women and educate them about increasing protective behaviors, such as hand washing, and decreasing risky behaviors for acquiring CMV, such as kissing on the mouth and sharing eating utensils.[6a, 85a] In addition, CMV can be transmitted from husband to wife, and if the spouse experiences a CMV mononucleosis syndrome, the CMV-seronegative woman may wish to consider avoiding pregnancy for an individualized period.

References

1. Adler, S. P.: Cytomegalovirus and child day care: Evidence for an increased infection rate among day-care workers. N. Engl. J. Med. *321*:1290–1296, 1989.
2. Adler, S. P.: Cytomegalovirus transmission among children in day care, their mothers and caretakers. Pediatr. Infect. Dis. *7*:279–285, 1988.
3. Adler, S. P.: Molecular epidemiology of cytomegalovirus: Viral transmission among children attending a day care center, their parents, and caretakers. J. Pediatr. *116*:366–372, 1988.
4. Adler, S. P.: The molecular epidemiology of cytomegalovirus transmission among children attending a day care center. J. Infect. Dis. *152*:760–767, 1985.
5. Adler, S. P., Baggett, J., Wilson, M., et al.: Molecular epidemiology of cytomegalovirus in a nursery: Lack of evidence for nosocomial transmission. J. Pediatr. *108*:117–123, 1986.
6. Adler, S. P.: Molecular epidemiology of cytomegalovirus: A study of factors affecting transmission among children at three day-care centers. Pediatr. Infect. Dis. J. *10*:584–590, 1991.

6a. Adler, S. P., Finney, J. W., Manganello, A. M., et al.: Prevention of child-to-mother transmission of cytomegalovirus by changing behaviors: A randomized controlled trial. Pediatr. Infect. Dis. J. *15*:240–246, 1996.

7. Akeeson-Johansson, A., Lernestedt, J. O., Rigden, O., et al.: Sensitivity of cytomegalovirus to intravenous foscarnet treatment. Bone Marrow Transplant. *1*:215–220, 1986.
8. Alexander, J. A., Cuellar, R. E., Fadden, R. J., et al.: Cytomegalovirus infection of the upper gastrointestinal tract before and after liver transplantation. Transplantation *46*:378–382, 1988.
9. Alford, C. A., Stagno, S., Pass, R. F., et al.: Epidemiology of cytomegalovirus infections. *In* Nahmias, A. J., Dowdle, W. R., and Schinazi, R. F. (eds.): The Human Herpesviruses: An Interdisciplinary Perspective. New York, Elsevier North Holland, 1987, pp. 159–171.
10. Anders, K., Steinsapir, K. D., Iverson, D. J., et al.: Neuropathologic findings in the acquired immunodeficiency syndrome (AIDS). Clin. Neuropathol. *5*:1–20, 1986.
11. Arav-Boger, R., Reif, S., Bujanover, Y.: Portal vein thrombosis caused

by protein C and protein S deficiency associated with cytomegalovirus infection. J. Pediatr. *126*:586–588, 1995.

12. Ashraf, S. J., Parande, C. M., and Arya, S. C.: Cytomegalovirus antibodies of patients in the Gizen area of Saudi Arabia. J. Infect. Dis. *152*:1351, 1985.
13. Atkins, J. T., Demmler, G. J., Williamson, W. D., et al.: Polymerase chain reaction to detect cytomegalovirus DNA in the cerebrospinal fluid of neonates with congenital infection. J. Infect. Dis. *169*:1334–1337, 1994.
14. Bailey, T. C., Trulock, E. P., Ettinger, N. A., et al.: Failure of prophylactic ganciclovir to prevent cytomegalovirus disease in recipients of lung transplants. J. Infect. Dis. *165*:548–552, 1992.
15. Balcarek, K. B., Bagley, R., Cloud, G. A., et al.: Cytomegalovirus infection among employees in a children's hospital: No evidence for increased risk associated with patient care. J. A. M. A. *263*:840–844, 1990.
16. Bale, J. F.: Human cytomegalovirus infection and disorders of the nervous system. Arch. Neurol. *41*:310–320, 1984.
17. Bale, J. F., Bray, P. F., and Bell, W. E.: Neuroradiographic abnormalities in congenital cytomegalovirus infection. Pediatr. Neurol. *1*:42–47, 1985.
18. Bale, J.: Conditions mimicking congenital infections. *In* Bale, J. (ed.): Congenital infections of the central nervous system. Semin. Pediatr. Neurol. *1*:63–67, 1994.
19. Balfour, C. L., and Balfour, H. H.: Cytomegalovirus is not an occupational risk for nurses in renal transplant and neonatal units: Results of a prospective surveillance study. J. A. M. A. *256*:1909–1914, 1986.
20. Balfour, H. H., Chace, B. A., Stapleton, J. T., et al.: A randomized, placebo-controlled trial of oral acyclovir for the prevention of cytomegalovirus disease in recipients of renal allografts. N. Engl. J. Med. *320*:1381–1387, 1989.
21. Bamborschke, S., Wullen, T., Huber, M., et al.: Early diagnosis and successful treatment of acute cytomegalovirus encephalitis in a renal transplant recipient. J. Neurol. *239*:205–208, 1992.
22. Bauman, N. M., Kirby-Keyser, L. J., Dolan, K. D., et al.: Mondini dysplasia and congenital cytomegalovirus infection. J. Pediatr. *124*:71–78, 1994.
23. Becraft, D.: Prenatal cytomegalovirus infection and muscular deficiency (eventration) of the diaphragm. J. Pediatr. *94*:74–75, 1979.
24. Benson, M. C., Kaplan, M. S., O'Toole, K., et al.: A report of cytomegalovirus cystitis and a review of other genitourinary manifestations of the acquired immune deficiency syndrome. J. Urol. *140*:153–154, 1988.
25. Bloom, J. N., and Palestine, A. G.: The diagnosis of cytomegalovirus retinitis. Ann. Intern. Med. *109*:963–969, 1988.
26. Bonkowsky, H. L., Lee, R. V., and Klatskin, G.: Acute granulomatous hepatitis: Occurrence in cytomegalovirus mononucleosis. *233*:1284–1288, 1975.
27. Boppana, S., Amos, C., Britt, W., et al.: Late onset and reactivation of chorioretinitis in children with congenital cytomegalovirus infection. Pediatr. Infect. Dis. J. *13*:1139–1142, 1994.
28. Bowden, R. A., Sayers, S., Flournoy, N., et al.: Cytomegalovirus immune globulin and seronegative blood products to prevent primary cytomegalovirus infection after marrow transplantation. N. Engl. J. Med. *16*:1006–1010, 1986.
29. Brady, M. T.: Cytomegalovirus infections: Occupational risk for health professionals. Am. J. Infect. Control *14*:197–203, 1986.
30. Brady, M. T., Milam, J. D., Anderson, D. C., et al.: Use of deglycerolized red blood cells to prevent post transfusion infection with cytomegalovirus in neonates. J. Infect. Dis. *150*:334–339, 1984.
31. Breinig, M. K., Zitelli, B., Starzl, T. E., et al.: Epstein-Barr virus, cytomegalovirus, and other viral infections in children after liver transplantation. J. Infect. Dis. *156*:273–279, 1987.
32. Britt, W. J., Vugler, L., Butfiloski, E. J., et al.: Cell surface expression of human cytomegalovirus (HCMV) gp 55-116(gB): Use of HCMV-recombinant vaccinia virus–infected cells in analysis of the human neutralizing antibody response. J. Virol. *64*:1079–1085, 1990.
33. Bronsther, O., Makowka, L., Jaffe, R., et al.: Occurrence of cytomegalovirus hepatitis in liver transplant patients. J. Med. Virol. *24*:423–434, 1988.
34. Buffone, G. J., Demmler, G. J., Schimbor, C. M., et al.: DNA hybridization assay for congenital cytomegalovirus infection. J. Clin. Microbiol. *26*:2184–2186, 1988.
35. Buffone, G. J., Schimbor, C. M., Demmler, G. J., et al.: Detection of cytomegalovirus in urine by nonisotopic DNA hybridization. J. Infect. Dis. *154*:163–166, 1986.
36. Buffone, G. J., Frost, A., Samo, T., et al.: The diagnosis of CMV pneumonitis in lung and heart/lung transplant patients by PCR compared with traditional laboratory criteria. Transplantation *56*:342–347, 1993.
37. Buhles, W. C., Mastre, J. B., Tinker, A. J., et al.: Ganciclovir treatment of life- or sight-threatening cytomegalovirus infection: Experience in 314 immunocompromised patients. Rev. Infect. Dis. *10*:S495–S506, 1988.
38. Butler, K., DeSmet, M., Husson, R. N., et al.: Treatment of aggressive cytomegalovirus retinitis with ganciclovir in combination with foscarnet in a child infected with human immunodeficiency virus. J. Pediatr. *120*:483–486, 1992.
39. Butt, W., Mackey, R. J., deCrespigny, L. C., et al.: Intracranial lesions of congenital cytomegalovirus infection detected by ultrasound scanning. Pediatrics *73*:611–614, 1984.
40. Cacoub, P., Deray, G., Baumelou, A., et al.: Acute renal failure induced by foscarnet: 4 cases. Clin. Nephrol. *29*:315–318, 1988.
41. Cantrill, H. L., Henry, K., Melroe, N. H., et al.: Treatment of cytomegalovirus retinitis with intravitreal ganciclovir. Ophthalmology *96*:367–374, 1989.
42. Carney, W. P., Hirsch, M. S., Iacoviello, V. R., et al.: T-lymphocyte subsets and proliferative responses following immunization with cytomegalovirus vaccine. J. Infect. Dis. *147*:958–960, 1983.
43. Cassol, S. A., Poon, M. C., Pal, R., et al.: Primer-mediated enzymatic amplification of cytomegalovirus (CMV) DNA: Application to the early diagnosis of CMV infection in marrow transplant recipients. J. Clin. Invest. *83*:1109–1115, 1989.
44. Chanarin, I., and Walford, D. M.: Thrombocytopenic purpura in cytomegalovirus mononucleosis. Lancet *2*:238–239, 1973.
45. Chandler, S. H., Holmes, K. K., Wentworth, B. B., et al.: The epidemiology of cytomegaloviral infection in women attending a sexually transmitted disease clinic. J. Infect. Dis. *152*:597–605, 1985.
46. Chandler, S. H., Handsfield, H. H., and McDougall, J. K.: Isolation of multiple strains of cytomegalovirus from women attending a clinic for sexually transmitted diseases. J. Infect. Dis. *155*:655–660, 1987.
47. Cheeseman, S. H., Rubin, R. H., Stewart, J. A., et al.: Controlled clinical trial of prophylactic human leukocyte interferon in renal transplantation. N. Engl. J. Med. *300*:1345–1349, 1979.
48. Chou, S.: Acquisition of donor strains of cytomegalovirus by renal transplant recipients. N. Engl. J. Med. *314*:1418–1423, 1986.
49. Chou, S.: Neutralizing antibody responses to reinfecting strains of cytomegalovirus in transplant recipients. J. Infect. Dis. *160*:16–21, 1989.
50. Cinque, P., Vago, L., and Brytling, M.: Cytomegalovirus infection of the central nervous system in patients with AIDS: Diagnosis by DNA amplification from cerebrospinal fluid. J. Infect. Dis. *166*:1408–1411, 1992.
51. Cohen, J. I., and Corey, G. R.: Cytomegalovirus infection in the normal host. Medicine *64*:100–114, 1985.
52. Collier, A. C., Handsfield, H. H., Roberts, P. L., et al.: Cytomegalovirus infection in women attending a sexually transmitted disease clinic. J. Infect. Dis. *162*:46–51, 1990.
53. Connolly, P. K., Jerger, S., Williamson, W. D., et al.: Evaluation of higher-level auditory function in children with asymptomatic congenital cytomegalovirus infection. Am. J. Otol. *13*:185–193, 1992.
54. Crumpacker, C., Marlowe, S., Zhang, J. L., et al.: Treatment of cytomegalovirus pneumonia. Rev. Infect. Dis. *10*:S538–S546, 1988.
55. Curless, R. G., Scott, G. B., Post, M. J., et al.: Progressive cytomegalovirus encephalopathy following congenital infection in an infant with acquired immunodeficiency syndrome. Child. Nerv. Syst. *3*:255–257, 1987.
56. Danish, E. H., Dahms, B. B., and Kumar, M. L.: Cytomegalovirus-associated hemophagocytic syndrome. Pediatrics *75*:280–283, 1985.
57. Dankner, W. M., McCutchan, J. A., Richman, D. D., et al.: Localization of human cytomegalovirus in peripheral blood leukocytes by in situ hybridization. J. Infect. Dis. *161*:31–36, 1990.
58. Davis, L. E., Stewart, J. A., and Garvin, S.: Cytomegalovirus infection: A seroepidemiologic comparison of nuns and women from a venereal disease clinic. Am. J. Epidemiol. *102*:327–330, 1975.
59. Davis, G. L., Spector, G. J., Strauss, M., et al.: Cytomegalovirus endolabyrinthitis. Arch. Pathol. Lab. Med. *101*:118–121, 1977.
60. Demmler, G. J., Brady, M. T., Bijou, H., et al.: Post-transfusion cytomegalovirus infection in neonates: Role of saline-washed red blood cells. J. Pediatr. *108*:762–765, 1986.
61. Demmler, G. J., Buffone, G. J., Schimbor, C. M., et al.: Detection of cytomegalovirus in urine from newborns by using polymerase chain reaction DNA amplification. J. Infect. Dis. *158*:1177–1184, 1988.
62. Demmler, G. J., O'Neil, G. W., O'Neil, J. H., et al.: Transmission of cytomegalovirus from husband to wife. J. Infect. Dis. *154*:545–546, 1986.
63. Demmler, G. J., Six, H. R., Hurst, S. M., et al.: Enzyme-linked immunosorbent assay for the detection of IgM-class antibodies to cytomegalovirus. J. Infect. Dis. *153*:1152–1154, 1986.
64. Demmler, G. J., Yow, M. D., Spector, S. A., et al.: Nosocomial cytomegalovirus infections in two hospitals caring for infants and children. J. Infect. Dis. *156*:9–16, 1987.
65. Demmler, G. J.: Summary of a workshop on surveillance for congenital CMV disease. Rev. Infect. Dis *13*:315–329, 1991.
66. Dietrich, D. T., Chachoua, A., Francois, L., et al.: Ganciclovir treatment of gastrointestinal infections caused by cytomegalovirus in patients with AIDS. Rev. Infect. Dis. *10*:S532–S537, 1988.
67. Dimmick, J. E., and Bove K. E.: Cytomegalovirus infection of the bowel in infancy: Pathogenetic and diagnostic significance. Pediatr. Pathol. *2*:95–102, 1984.
68. Dolgin, S. E., Larsen, J. G., Shah, K. D., et al.: CMV enteritis causing hemorrhage and obstruction in an infant with AIDS. J. Pediatr. Surg. *25*:696–698, 1990.
69. Dowling, J. N., Saslow, A. R., Armstrong, J. A., et al.: Cytomegalovirus infection in patients receiving immunosuppressive therapy for rheumatologic disorders. J. Infect. Dis. *133*:399–408, 1976.
70. Drew, W. L., Sweet, E. S., Miner, R. C., et al.: Multiple infections by cytomegalovirus in patients with acquired immunodeficiency syndrome: Documentation by southern blot hybridization. J. Infect. Dis. *150*:952–953, 1984.
71. Drew, W. L., Ives, D., Lalezari, J. P., et al.: Oral ganciclovir as maintenance treatment for cytomegalovirus retinitis in patients with AIDS. N. Engl. J. Med. *333*:615–620, 1995.

72. Dummer, J. S., White, L. T., Ho, M., et al.: Morbidity of cytomegalovirus infection in recipients of heart-lung transplants who received cyclosporine. J. Infect. Dis. *152*:1182–1191, 1985.
73. Dworsky, M., Lakeman, A., and Stagno, S.: Cytomegalovirus transmission within a family. Pediatr. Infect. Dis. *3*:236–238, 1984.
74. Dworsky, M., Yow, M., Stagno, S., et al.: Cytomegalovirus infection of breast milk and transmission in infancy. Pediatrics *72*:295–300, 1983.
75. Dworsky, M. E., Weoch, K., Cassady, G., et al.: Occupational risk for primary cytomegalovirus infection among pediatric health-care workers. N. Engl. J. Med. *309*:950–953, 1983.
76. Emanuel, D., Cunningham, I., Jules-Elysee, K., et al.: Cytomegalovirus pneumonia after bone marrow transplantation successfully treated with the combination of ganciclovir and high-dose intravenous immune globulin. Ann. Intern. Med. *109*:777–782, 1988.
77. Embil, J. A., Goldbloom, A. L., and McFarlane, E. S.: Isolation of cytomegalovirus from middle ear effusion. J. Pediatr. *107*:435–436, 1985.
78. Erice, A., Chou, S., Biron, K. K., et al.: Progressive disease due to ganciclovir-resistant cytomegalovirus in immunocompromised patients. N. Engl. J. Med. *320*:289–293, 1989.
79. Faix, R. G.: Survival of cytomegalovirus on environmental surfaces. J. Pediatr. *106*:649–652, 1985.
80. Farrar, G. H., Bull, J. R., and Greenaway, P. J.: Prospects for the clinical management of human cytomegalovirus infections. Vaccine *4*:217–224, 1986.
81. Felsenstein, E., D'Amico, D. J., Hirsch, M. S., et al.: Treatment of cytomegalovirus retinitis with 9-[2-hydroxy-1-(hydroxymethyl)ethoxymethyl] guanine. Ann. Intern. Med. *103*:377–380, 1985.
82. Fenner, T. E., Garweg, J., Hufert, F. T., et al.: Diagnoses of human cytomegalovirus–induced retinitis in human immunodeficiency virus type-1–infected subjects by using the polymerase chain reaction. J. Clin. Microbiol. *29*:2621–2622, 1991.
83. Ferreiro, J., and Vinters, H. V.: Pathology of the pituitary gland in patients with the acquired immune deficiency syndrome (AIDS). Pathology *20*:211–215, 1988.
84. Fiala, M., and Kattlove, H.: Cytomegalovirus mononucleosis with severe thrombocytopenia. Ann. Intern. Med. *79*:450–451, 1973.
85. Fiala, M., Payne, J. E., Berne, T. V., et al.: Epidemiology of cytomegalovirus infection after transplantation and immunosuppression. J. Infect. Dis. *132*:421–433, 1975.
85a. Finney, J. W., Miller, K. M., and Adler, S. P.: Changing protective and risky behaviors to prevent child-to-parent transmission of cytomegalovirus. J. Appl. Behav. Anal. *26*:471–472, 1993.
86. Fleisher, G. R., Starr, S. E., Friedman, H. M., et al.: Vaccination of pediatric nurses with live attenuated cytomegalovirus. Am. J. Dis. Child. *136*:294–296, 1982.
87. Flores-Aguilar, J., Huang, J. S., Wiley, C. A., et al.: Long-acting therapy of viral retinitis with (S)-1-(3-hydroxy-2-phosphorylmethoxypropyl) cytosine. J. Infect. Dis. *169*:642–647, 1994.
88. Frank, T. S., LiVolsi, V. A., and Connor, A. M.: Cytomegalovirus infection of the thyroid in immunocompromised adults. Yale J. Biol. Med. *60*:1–8, 1987.
89. Frenkel, L. D., Keys, M. P., Hefferen, S. J., et al.: Unusual eye abnormalities associated with congenital cytomegalovirus infection. Pediatrics *5*:763–766, 1980.
90. Fuller, G. N., Jacobs, J. M., and Guiloff, R. J.: Association of painful peripheral neuropathy in AIDS with cytomegalovirus infection. Lancet *2*:937–940, 1989.
91. Gerna, G., Zipeto, D., Parea, M., et al.: Monitoring of human cytomegalovirus infections and ganciclovir treatment in heart transplant recipients by determination of viremia antigenemia and DNAemia. J. Infect. Dis. *164*:488–498, 1991.
92. Gilbert, G. L., Hudson, I. L., Hayes, K., et al.: Prevention of transfusion-acquired cytomegalovirus infection in infants by blood filtration to remove leukocytes. Lancet *1*:1228–1231, 1989.
93. Gleaves, C. A., Myerson, D., Bowden, R. A., et al.: Direct detection of cytomegalovirus from bronchoalveolar lavage samples by using a rapid in situ DNA hybridization assay. J. Clin. Microbiol. *27*:2429–2432, 1989.
94. Gleaves, C. A., Smith, T. F., Shuster, E. A., et al.: Comparison of standard tube and shell vial cell culture techniques for the detection of cytomegalovirus in clinical specimens. J. Clin. Microbiol. *21*:217–221, 1985.
95. Gonwa, T. A., Capehart, J. E., Pilcher, J. W., et al.: Cytomegalovirus myocarditis as a cause of cardiac dysfunction in a heart transplant. Transplantation *47*:197–199, 1989.
96. Goodgame, R. W., Genta, R. M., Estrada, R., et al.: Frequency of positive tests for cytomegalovirus in AIDS patients: Endoscopic lesions compared with normal mucosa. Am. J. Gastroenterol. *88*:338–343, 1993.
97. Goodpasture, E. Q., and Talbot, F. B.: Concerning the nature of "protozoan-like" cells in certain lesions of infancy. Am. J. Dis. Child. *21*:415–425, 1921.
98. Goodrich, J. M., Mori, M., Gleaves, C., et al.: Early treatment with ganciclovir to prevent cytomegalovirus disease after allogeneic bone marrow transplantation. N. Engl. J. Med. *325*:1601–1607, 1991.
99. Gozlan, J., Salord, J. M., Roullet, E., et al.: Rapid detection of cytomegalovirus DNA in cerebrospinal fluid of AIDS patients with neurologic disorders. J. Infect. Dis. *166*:1416–1421, 1992.
100. Grattan, M. T., Moreno-Cabral, C. E., Starnes, V. A., et al.: Cytomegalovirus infection is associated with cardiac allograft rejection and atherosclerosis. J. A. M. A. *261*:3561–3566, 1989.
101. Greene, L. W., Cole, W., Greene, J. B., et al.: Adrenal insufficiency as a complication of the acquired immunodeficiency syndrome. Ann. Intern. Med. *101*:497–498, 1984.
102. Griffiths, P. D., and Baboonian, C.: A prospective study of primary cytomegalovirus infection during pregnancy: Final report. Br. J. Obstet. Gynaecol. *92*:307–315, 1984.
103. Griffiths, P. D., and Grundy, J. E.: Molecular biology and immunology of cytomegalovirus. Biochem. J. *241*:313–324, 1987.
104. Griffiths, P. D., Stagno, S., Pass, R. F., et al.: Congenital cytomegalovirus infection: Diagnostic and prognostic significance of the detection of specific immunoglobulin M antibodies in cord serum. Pediatrics *69*:544–549, 1982.
105. Grundy, J. E., Super, M., Sweny, P., et al.: Symptomatic cytomegalovirus infection in seropositive kidney recipients: Reinfection with donor virus rather than reactivation of recipient virus. Lancet *1*:132–135, 1988.
106. Gudnason, T., Belani, K. K., and Balfour, H. H.: Ganciclovir treatment of cytomegalovirus disease in immunocompromised children. Pediatr. Infect. Dis. *8*:436–440, 1989.
107. Hackman, R. C., Myerson, D., Meyers, J. D., et al.: Rapid diagnosis of cytomegalovirus pneumonia by tissue immunofluorescence with a murine monoclonal antibody. J. Infect. Dis. *151*:325–329, 1985.
108. Handsfield, H. H., Chandler, S. H., Caine, V. A., et al.: Cytomegalovirus infection in sex partners: Evidence for sexual transmission. J. Infect. Dis. *151*:344–348, 1985.
109. Hayward, J. C., Titelbaum, D. S., Clancy, R. R., et al.: Lissencephalypachygyria associated with congenital cytomegalovirus infection. J. Child. Neurol. *6*:109–114, 1991.
110. Hibberd, P. L., Tokoff-Rubin, N. E., Conti, D., et al.: Preemptive ganciclovir therapy to prevent cytomegalovirus disease in cytomegalovirus antibody–positive renal transplant recipients. Ann. Intern. Med. *123*:18–26, 1995.
111. Hirsch, M. S., Schooley, R. T., Cosimi, A. B., et al.: Effects of interferon-alpha on cytomegalovirus reactive syndromes in renal transplant recipients. N. Engl. J. Med. *308*:1489–1493, 1983.
112. Ho, D. D., Bredesen, D. E., Vinters, H. V., et al.: The acquired immunodeficiency sydrome (AIDS) dementia complex. Ann. Intern. Med. *111*:400–410, 1989.
113. Ho, M.: Cytomegalovirus: Biology and infection. *In* Greenough, W. B., and Merigan, T. C. (eds.): New York, Plenum, 1982, pp. 119–129.
114. Hocker, J. R., Cook, L. N., Addams, G., et al.: Ganciclovir therapy of congenital cytomegalovirus pneumonia. Pediatr. Infect. Dis. J. *9*:743–744, 1990.
115. Hokeberg, I., Olding-Stenkvist, E., Grillner, L., et al.: No evidence of hospital-acquired cytomegalovirus infection in a pregnant pediatric nurse using restriction endonuclease analysis. Pediatr. Infect. Dis. J. *7*:812–814, 1988.
116. Horwitz, C. A., Henle, W., Henle, G., et al.: Clinical and laboratory evaluation of cytomegalovirus-induced mononucleosis in previously healthy individuals. Medicine *65*:124–134, 1986.
117. Hutto, C., Little, E. A., Ricks, R., et al.: Isolation of cytomegalovirus from toys and hands in a day care center. J. Infect. Dis. *154*:527–530, 1986.
118. Istas, A. S., Demmler, G. J., Dobbins, J. G., et al.: Surveillance for congenital cytomegalovirus disease: A report from the National Congenital Cytomegalovirus Disease Registry. Clin. Infect. Dis. *20*:665–670, 1995.
119. Jacobson, M. A., and Mills, J.: Serious cytomegalovirus disease in the acquired immunodeficiency syndrome (AIDS). Ann. Intern. Med. *108*:585–594, 1988.
120. Jacobson, M. A., O'Donnel, J. J., Rousell, R., et al.: Failure of adjunctive cytomegalovirus immune globulin to improve efficacy of ganciclovir in patients with acquired immunodeficiency syndrome and cytomegalovirus retinitis: A phase 1 study. Antimicrob. Agents Chemother. *34*:176–178, 1990.
121. Jamison, R. M., and Hathorn, A. W.: Isolation of cytomegalovirus from cerebrospinal fluid of a congenitally infected infant. Am. J. Dis. Child. *132*:63–64, 1978.
122. Jones, L. A., Duke-Duncan, P. M., and Yeager, A. S.: Cytomegaloviral infections in infant-toddler centers: Centers for the developmentally delayed versus regular day care. J. Infect. Dis. *151*:953–955, 1985.
123. Jordan, M. C., Rousseau, W. E., Noble, G. R., et al.: Association of cervical cytomegalovirus with venereal disease. N. Engl. J. Med. *288*:932–934, 1973.
124. Just, M., Buergin-Wolff, A., Emoedi, G., et al.: Immunization trials with live attenuated cytomegalovirus Towne 125. Infection *3*:111–114, 1975.
125. Kaariainen, L., Klemola, E., and Paloheimo, J.: Rise of cytomegalovirus antibodies in an infectious-mononucleosis–like syndrome after transfusion. Br. Med. J. *1*:1270–1272, 1966.
126. Kagan, R. J., Naragi, S., Matsuda, T., et al.: Herpes simplex virus and cytomegalovirus infections in burned patients. J. Trauma *25*:40–45, 1985.
127. Karn, K., Julian, T. M., and Ogburn, P. L.: Fetal heart block associated with congenital cytomegalovirus infection: A case report. J. Reprod. Med. *29*:278–280, 1984.
128. Keay, S., Petersen, E., Icenogle, T., et al.: Ganciclovir treatment of serious

cytomegalovirus infection in heart and heart-lung transplant recipients. Rev. Infect. Dis. *10*:S563–S572, 1988.

129. Kim, Y. J., Gururaj, V. J., and Mirkovic, R. R.: Concomitant diffuse nodular pulmonary infiltration in an infant with cytomegalovirus infection. Pediatr. Infect. Dis. *1*:173–176, 1982.
130. Kim, Y. S., and Hollander, H.: Polyradiculopathy due to cytomegalovirus: Report of two cases in which improvement occurred after prolonged therapy and review of the literature. Clin. Infect. Dis. *17*:32–37, 1993.
131. Klemola, E., Stenstrom, R., and von Essen, R.: Pneumonia as a clinical manifestation of cytomegalovirus infection in previously healthy adults. Scand. J. Infect. Dis. *4*:7–10, 1972.
132. Klemola, E., von Essen, R., Henle, G., et al.: Infectious mononucleosis–like disease with negative heterophil agglutination test: Clinical features in relations to Epstein-Barr virus and cytomegalovirus and antibodies. J. Infect. Dis. *121*:608–614, 1970.
133. Kumar, M. L., Jenson, H. B., Dahms, B. B.: Fatal *Staphylococcal epidermidis* infections in very low–birth-weight infants with cytomegalovirus infection. Pediatrics *76*:110–114, 1985.
134. Kumar, M. L., Gold, E., Jacobs, I. B., et al.: Primary cytomegalovirus infection in adolescent pregnancy. Pediatrics *74*:493–500, 1984.
135. Kumar, M. L., Nankervis, G. A., Cooper, A. R., et al.: Postnatally acquired cytomegalovirus infections in infants of CMV-excreting mothers. J. Pediatr. *104*:669–673, 1984.
136. Kumar, M. L., Nankervis, G. A., Jacobs, I. B., et al.: Congenital and postnatally acquired cytomegalovirus infections: Long-term follow-up. J. Pediatr. *104*:674–679, 1984.
137. Lang, D. J., and Kummer, J. F.: Cytomegalovirus in semen: Observations in selected populations. J. Infect. Dis. *132*:472–473, 1975.
138. Lee, R. W., and Ai, E.: Disc neovascularization in patients with AIDS and cytomegalovirus retinitis. Retina *11*:305–308, 1991.
139. Lehoang, P., Giarard, B., Robinet, M., et al.: Foscarnet in the treatment of cytomegalovirus retinitis in acquired immunodeficiency syndrome. Ophthalmology *96*:865–874, 1989.
140. Lesher, J. L.: Cytomegalovirus infections and the skin. J. Am. Acad. Dermatol. *18*:1333–1338, 1988.
141. Levin, A. V., Zeichner, S., Duker, J. S., et al.: Cytomegalovirus retinitis in an infant with acquired immunodeficiency syndrome. Pediatrics *84*:683–687, 1989.
142. Levin, M.: Current approaches to the prevention and treatment of cytomegalovirus disease after bone marrow transplantation: An overview. Semin. Hematol. *27*:1–4, 1990.
143. Lim, W., Kahn, E., Gupta, A., et al.: Treatment of cytomegalovirus enterocolitis with ganciclovir in an infant with acquired immunodeficiency syndrome. Pediatr. Infect. Dis. *7*:354–357, 1988.
144. Linneman, C. C., and MacMillan, B. G.: Viral infections in pediatric burn patients. Am. J. Dis. Child. *135*:750–753, 1981.
145. Lui, W. Y., and Chang, W. K.: Cytomegalovirus mononucleosis in Chinese infants. Arch. Dis. Child. *47*:643, 1972.
146. Matthews, T., and Boehme, R.: Antiviral activity and mechanism of action of ganciclovir. Rev. Infect. Dis. *10*:S490–S494, 1988.
147. McDonald, K., Rector, T. S., Braunlin, E. A., et al.: Association of coronary artery disease in cardiac transplant recipients with cytomegalovirus infection. Am. J. Cardiol. *64*:359–362, 1989.
148. McKeating, J. A., Griffiths, P. D., and Grundy, J. E.: Cytomegalovirus in urine specimens has host beta 2 microglobulin bound to the viral envelope: A mechanism of evading the host immune response. J. Gen. Virol. *68*:785–792, 1987.
149. Melnick, J. L., Adam, E., and DeBakey, M. E.: Possible role of cytomegalovirus in atherogenesis. J. A. M. A. *263*:2204–2207, 1990.
150. Mena, W., Royal, S., Pass, R. F., et al.: Diabetes insipidus associated with symptomatic congenital cytomegalovirus infection. J. Pediatr. *122*:911–913, 1993.
151. Meyers, J. D., Leszcynski, J., Zaia, J., et al.: Prevention of cytomegalovirus infection by cytomegalovirus immune globulin after marrow transplantation. Ann. Intern. Med. *98*:442–446, 1983.
152. Meyers, J. D., Reed, E. C., Shepp, D. H., et al.: Acyclovir for prevention of cytomegalovirus infection and disease after allogeneic marrow transplantation. N. Engl. J. Med. *318*:70–75, 1988.
153. Millett, R., Tomita, T., Marshall, H. E., et al.: Cytomegalovirus endomyocarditis in a transplanted heart. Arch. Pathol. Lab. Med. *115*:511–515, 1991.
154. Morgello, S., Cho, E. S., Nielsen, S., et al.: Cytomegalovirus encephalitis in patients with acquired immunodeficiency syndrome: An autopsy study of 30 cases and a review of the literature. Hum. Pathol. *18*:289–297, 1987.
155. Murph, J. R., and Bale, J. F.: The natural history of acquired cytomegalovirus infection among children in group day care. Am. J. Dis. Child. *142*:843–846, 1988.
156. Nelson, C. T., Istas, A. S., Wilkerson, M. K., et al.: Polymerase chain reaction detection of cytomegalovirus DNA in serum as a diagnostic test for congenital cytomegalovirus infection. J. Clin. Microbiol. *33*:3317–3318, 1995.
157. Nielsen, S. L., Petito, C. K., Urmacher, C. D., et al.: Subacute encephalitis in acquired immune deficiency syndrome: A postmortem study. Am. J. Clin. Pathol. *82*:678–682, 1984.
158. Nielsen, S. L., Sorensen, I., and Anderson, H. K.: Kinetics of specific immunoglobulins M, E, A and G in congenital, primary and secondary cytomegalovirus infection studied by antibody-capture enzyme-linked immunosorbent assay. J. Clin. Microbiol. *26*:654–661, 1988.
159. Nigro, G., Scholz, H., and Bartman, U.: Ganciclovir therapy for symptomatic congenital cytomegalovirus infection in infants: A two-regimen experience. J. Pediatr. *124*:318–322, 1994.
160. Noyes, B. E., Kurland, G., Orenstein, D. M., et al.: Experience with pediatric lung transplantation. J. Pediatr. *124*:261–268, 1994.
161. O'Grady, J. G., Sutherland, S., Harvey, R. Y., et al.: Cytomegalovirus infection and donor/recipient HLA antigens: Interdependent co-factors in pathogenesis of vanishing bile duct syndrome after liver transplantation. Lancet *2*:302–305, 1988.
162. Ong, E. L., Ellis, M. E., Tweele, D., et al.: Cytomegalovirus cholecystitis and colitis associated with the acquired immunodeficiency syndrome. J. Infect. Dis. *18*:73–75, 1989.
163. Pak, C. Y., McArthur, R., Eun, H. M., et al.: Association of cytomegalovirus infection with autoimmune type 1 diabetes. Lancet *2*:1–4, 1988.
164. Pannuti, C. S., Vilasboas, L. S., Angelo, M., et al.: Cytomegalovirus mononucleosis in children and adults: Differences in clinical presentation. Scand. J. Infect. Dis. *17*:153–156, 1985.
165. Pass, R. F., August, A. M., Dworsky, M., et al.: Cytomegalovirus infection in a day-care center. N. Engl. J. Med. *307*:477–479, 1982.
166. Pass, R. F., and Hutto, C.: Group day care and cytomegaloviral infections of mothers and children. Rev. Infect. Dis. *8*:599–605, 1986.
167. Pass, R. F., Hutto, S. C., Reynolds, D. W., et al.: Increased frequency of cytomegalovirus infection in children in group day care. Pediatrics *74*:121–126, 1984.
168. Pass, R. F., Hutto, S. C., Ricks, R., et al.: Increased rate of cytomegalovirus infection among parents of children attending day-care centers. N. Engl. J. Med. *314*:1414–1418, 1986.
169. Pass, R. F., Little, E. A., Stagno, S., et al.: Young children as a probable source of maternal congenital cytomegalovirus infection. N. Engl. J. Med. *316*:1366–1370, 1987.
170. Pass, R. F., Whitley, R. J., Diethelm, A. G., et al.: Cytomegalovirus infection in patients with renal transplants: Potentiation by antithymocyte globulin and an incompatible graft. J. Infect. Dis. *142*:9–17, 1980.
171. Patterson, J. W., Broecker, A. H., Kornstein, M. J., et al.: Cutaneous cytomegalovirus infection in a liver transplant patient: Diagnosis by in situ DNA hybridization. Am. J. Dermatopathol. *10*:524–530, 1988.
172. Plotkin, S. A., Farquhar, J., and Hornberger, E.: Clinical trials of immunization with the Towne 125 strain of human cytomegalovirus. J. Infect. Dis. *134*:470–475, 1976.
173. Plotkin, S. A., Friedman, H. M., Fleisher, G. R., et al.: Towne-vaccine–induced prevention of cytomegalovirus disease after renal transplants. Lancet *1*:528–530, 1984.
174. Plotkin, S. A., Furukawa, T., Zygraich, N., et al.: Candidate cytomegalovirus strain for human vaccination. Infect. Immun. *12*:521–527, 1975.
175. Plotkin, S. A., Smiley, M. L., Friedman, H. M., et al.: Prevention of cytomegalovirus disease by Towne strain live attenuated vaccine. Birth Defects: Original Article Series *20*:271–287, 1984.
176. Plotkin, S. A., Higgins, R., Kurtz, J. B., et al.: Multicenter trial of Towne strain attenuated virus vaccine in seronegative renal transplant recipients. Transplantation *58*:1176–1178, 1994.
177. Pollard, R. B.: Cytomegalovirus infections in renal, heart, heart-lung and liver transplantation. Pediatr. Infect. Dis. *7*:S97–S102, 1988.
178. Powell, K. F., Bellamy, A. R., Catton, M. G., et al.: Cytomegalovirus myocarditis in a heart transplant recipient: Sensitive monitoring of viral DNA by the polymerase chain reaction. J. Heart Transplant. *8*:465–470, 1989.
179. Proujansky, R., Orenstein, S. R., Kocoshis, S. A., et al.: Cytomegalovirus gastroenteritis after liver transplantation. J. Pediatr. *113*:700–703, 1988.
180. Rabinowitz, M., Bassan, I., and Robinson, M. J.: Sexually transmitted cytomegalovirus proctitis in a woman. Am. J. Gastroenterol. *83*:885–887, 1988.
181. Randazzo, R. F., Hulette, C. M., Gottlieb, M. S., et al.: Cytomegaloviral epididymitis in a patient with the acquired immune deficiency syndrome. J. Urol. *136*:1095–1097, 1986.
182. Reed, E. C., Bowden, R. A., Dandliker, P. S., et al.: Efficacy of cytomegalovirus immunoglobulin in marrow transplant recipients with cytomegalovirus pneumonia. J. Infect. Dis. *156*:641–644, 1987.
183. Reed, E. C., Bowden, R. A., Dandliker, P. S., et al.: Treatment of cytomegalovirus pneumonia with ganciclovir and intravenous cytomegalovirus immune globulin in patients with bone marrow transplants. Ann. Intern. Med. *109*:783–788, 1988.
184. Reed, E. C., Dandliker, P. S., Meyers, J. D., et al.: Treatment of cytomegalovirus pneumonia with 9-[2-hydroxy-1-(hydroxymethyl) ethoxymethyl] guanine and high dose corticosteroids. Ann. Intern. Med. *105*:214–215, 1986.
185. Reed, E. C., and Meyers, J. D.: Treatment of cytomegalovirus infection: Diagnosis and treatment of viral infections. Clin. Lab. Med. *7*:831–852, 1987.
186. Reed, E. C., Wolford, J. L., Kopecky, K. J., et al.: Ganciclovir for the treatment of cytomegalovirus gastroenteritis in bone marrow transplant patients. Ann. Intern. Med. *112*:505–510, 1990.
187. Reller, L. B.: Granulomatous hepatitis associated with acute cytomegalovirus infection. Lancet *1*:20–22, 1973.

188. Reynolds, D. W., Stagno, S., Hosty, T. S., et al.: Maternal CMV excretion and perinatal infection. N. Engl. J. Med. *289*:4–7, 1973.
189. Ribbert, H.: Ueber protozoanartige zellen in der neire eines syphilitischen neugeborenen und in der parotis von kindern. Zentralbl. Allg. Pathol. *15*:945–948, 1904.
190. Rinaldo, C. R., Carney, W. P., Richter, B. S., et al.: Mechanisms of immunosuppression of cytomegalovirus mononucleosis. J. Infect. Dis. *141*:488–495, 1980.
191. Rinaldo, C. R., Kingsley, L. A., Ho, M., et al.: Enhanced shedding of cytomegalovirus in semen of human immunodeficiency virus–seropositive homosexual men. J. Clin. Microbiol. *30*:1148–1155, 1992.
192. Ringden, O., Lonnqvist, B., Paulin, T., et al.: Pharmacokinetics, safety and preliminary clinical experiences using foscarnet in the treatment of cytomegalovirus infections in bone marrow and renal transplant recipients. J. Antimicrob. Chemother. *17*:378–387, 1986.
193. Robert, M. E., Geraghty, J. J., Miles, S. A., et al.: Severe neuropathy in a patient with acquired immune deficiency syndrome (AIDS): Evidence for widespread cytomegalovirus infection of peripheral nerve and human immunodeficiency virus–like immunoreactivity of anterior horn cells. Acta Neuropathol. *79*:255–261, 1989.
194. Rowe, W. P., Hartley, J. W., Waterman, S., et al.: Cytopathogenic agent resembling human salivary gland virus recovered from tissue cultures of human adenoids. Proc. Soc. Exp. Biol. Med. *92*:418–424, 1956.
195. Saigal, S., Luny, K. O., Larke, R., et al.: The outcome in children with congenital cytomegalovirus infection. Am. J. Dis. Child. *136*:896–901, 1982.
196. Salisbury, S., and Embil, J. A.: Graves disease following congenital cytomegalovirus infection. J. Pediatr. *92*:954–955, 1978.
197. Sanchez, G. R., Neches, W. H., and Jaffe, R.: Myocardial aneurysm in association with disseminated cytomegalovirus infection. Pediatr. Cardiol. *2*:63–65, 1982.
198. Sandler, A., and Snedeker, J. D.: Cytomegalovirus infection in an infant presenting with cutaneous vasculitis. Pediatr. Infect. Dis. *6*:422–423, 1987.
199. Sawyer, M. H., Edwards, D. K., and Spector, S. A.: Cytomegalovirus infection and bronchopulmonary dysplasia in premature infants. Am. J. Dis. Child. *141*:303–305, 1987.
200. Schmidt, N. J., and Emmons, R. W.: Diagnostic Procedures for Viral, Rickettsial and Chlamydial Infections. 6th ed. Washington, D.C., American Public Health Association, 1989, pp. 321–378.
201. Schmidt, G. M., Horak, D. A., and Niland, J. C.: A randomized, controlled trial of prophylactic ganciclovir for cytomegalovirus pulmonary infection in recipients of allogeneic bone marrow transplants. N. Engl. J. Med. *324*:1005–1011, 1991.
202. Shabtai, M., Luft, B., Waltzer, W. C., et al.: Massive cytomegalovirus pneumonia and myocarditis in a renal transplant recipient: Successful treatment with DHPG. Transplant. Proc. *20*:562–563, 1988.
203. Shanley, J. D., Via, C. S., Sharrow, S. O., et al.: Interstitial pneumonitis during murine cytomegalovirus infection and graft-versus-host reaction. Transplantation *44*:658–662, 1987.
204. Shen, C., Chang, W., Chang, S., et al.: Cytomegalovirus transmission in special-care centers for mentally retarded children. Pediatrics *91*:79–82, 1993.
205. Shibata, D., Martin, W. J., Appleman, M. D., et al.: Detection of cytomegalovirus DNA in peripheral blood of patients infected with human immunodeficiency virus. J. Infect. Dis. *158*:1185–1192, 1988.
206. Singh, N., Dummer, J. S., Kusne, S., et al.: Infections with cytomegalovirus and other herpesviruses in 121 liver transplant recipients: Transmission by donated organ and the effect of OKT3 antibodies. J. Infect. Dis. *158*:124–131, 1988.
207. Singh, N., Yu, V., Mieles, L., et al.: High-dose acyclovir compared with short-course preemptive ganciclovir therapy to prevent cytomegalovirus disease in liver transplant recipients. Ann. Intern. Med. *120*:375–381, 1994.
208. Smith, M. G.: Propagation in tissue cultures of a cytopathogenic virus from human salivary gland virus (SGV) disease. Proc. Soc. Exp. Biol. Med. *92*:424–430, 1956.
209. Snider, W. D., Simpson, D. M., Nielsen, S., et al.: Neurological complications of acquired immune deficiency syndrome: Analysis of 50 patients. Ann. Neurol. *14*:403–418, 1984.
210. Snydman, D. R., Werner, B. G., Heinze-Lacey, B., et al.: Use of cytomegalovirus immune globulin to prevent cytomegalovirus disease in renal transplant recipients. N. Engl. J. Med. *317*:1049–1054, 1987.
211. Sohn, Y. M., Oh, M. K., Balcarek, K. B., et al.: Cytomegalovirus infection in sexually active adolescents. J. Infect. Dis. *163*:460–463, 1991.
212. Sokol, D. M., Demmler, G. J., and Buffone, G. J.: Rapid epidemiologic analysis of cytomegalovirus by using polymerase chain reaction amplification of the L-S junction region. J. Clin. Microbiol. *30*:839–844, 1992.
213. Sommadossi, J. P., Bevan, R., Ling, T., et al.: Clinical pharmacokinetics of ganciclovir in patients with normal and impaired renal function. Rev. Infect. Dis. *10*:S507–S514, 1988.
214. Spector, S. A.: Transmission of cytomegalovirus among infants in hospital documented by restriction-endonuclease-digestion analyses. Lancet *1*:378–381, 1983.
215. Spector, S. A., Hirata, K. K., and Neuman, T. R.: Identification of multiple cytomegalovirus strains in homosexual men with acquired immunodeficiency syndrome. J. Infect. Dis. *150*:953–956, 1984.
216. Spector, S. A., Rua, J. A., Spector, D. H., et al.: Detection of human cytomegalovirus in clinical specimens by DNA-DNA hybridization. J. Infect. Dis. *150*:121–126, 1984.
217. Spector, S. A., and Spector, D. H.: Molecular epidemiology of cytomegalovirus infections in premature twin infants and their mother. Pediatr. Infect. Dis. *1*:405–409, 1982.
218. Spector, S. A., Merrill, R., Wolf, D., et al.: Detection of human cytomegalovirus in plasma of AIDS patients during acute visceral disease by DNA amplification. J. Clin. Microbiol. *30*:2359–2365, 1992.
219. Stagno, S., Brasfield, D. M., Brown, M. B., et al.: Infant pneumonitis associated with cytomegalovirus, *Chlamydia*, *Pneumocystis*, and *Ureaplasma*: A prospective study. Pediatrics *68*:322–329, 1981.
220. Stagno, S., Pass, R. F., Dworsky, M. E., et al.: Congenital cytomegalovirus infection: The relative importance of primary and recurrent maternal infection. N. Engl. J. Med. *306*:945–949, 1982.
221. Stagno, S., Tinker, M. K., Elrod, C., et al.: Immunoglobulin M antibodies detected by enzyme-linked immunosorbent assay and radioimmunoassay in the diagnosis of cytomegalovirus infections in pregnant women and newborn infants. J. Clin. Microbiol. *21*:930–935, 1985.
222. Stagno, S., Pass, R. F., Thomas, J. P., et al.: Defects of tooth structure in congenital cytomegalovirus infection. Pediatrics *69*:646–648, 1982.
223. Starr, S. E., Glazer, J. P., Friedman, H. M., et al.: Specific cellular and humoral immunity after immunization with live Towne strain cytomegalovirus vaccine. J. Infect. Dis. *143*:585–589, 1981.
224. Stinski, M. F.: Cytomegalovirus and its replication. *In* Fields, B. N. (ed.): Virology. 2nd ed. New York, Raven Press, 1990, pp. 1959–1980.
225. Strauss, M.: Human cytomegalovirus labyrinthitis. Am. J. Otolaryngol. *11*:292–298, 1990.
226. Studies of Ocular Complications of AIDS Research Group, in collaboration with the AIDS Clinical Trials Group: Mortality in patients with the acquired immunodeficiency syndrome treated with either foscarnet or ganciclovir for cytomegalovirus retinitis. N. Engl. J. Med. *326*:213–220, 1992.
227. Subietas, A., Deppisch, L. M., and Astarloa, J.: Cytomegalovirus oophoritis: Ovarian cortical necrosis. Hum. Pathol. *8*:285–292, 1977.
228. Sullivan, V., Coen, D. M.: Isolation of foscarnet-resistant human cytomegalovirus patterns of resistance and sensitivity to other antiviral drugs. J. Infect. Dis. *164*:781–784, 1991.
229. Taber, L. H., Frank, A. L., Yow, M. D., et al.: Acquisition of cytomegaloviral infections in families with young children: A serologic study. J. Infect. Dis. *151*:948–952, 1985.
230. Tanner, D. D., Buckley, P. J., Hong, R., et al.: Fatal cytomegalovirus bronchiolitis in a patient with Nezelof's syndrome. Pediatrics *65*:98–102, 1980.
231. Tiula, E., and Leinikki, P.: Fatal cytomegalovirus infection in a previously healthy boy with myocarditis and consumption coagulopathy as presenting signs. Scand. J. Infect. Dis. *4*:57–60, 1972.
232. Tolpin, M. D., Stewart, J. A., Warren, D., et al.: Transfusion transmission confirmed by restriction endonuclease analysis. J. Pediatr. *107*:953–956, 1985.
233. Trang, J. M., Kidd, L., Gruber, W., et al.: Linear single-dose pharmacokinetics of ganciclovir in newborns with congenital cytomegalovirus infections. Clin. Pharmacol. Ther. *53*:15–21, 1993.
234. Ussery, F. M., Gibson, S. R., Conklin, R. H., et al.: Intravitreal ganciclovir in the treatment of AIDS-associated cytomegalovirus retinitis. Ophthalmology *95*:640–648, 1988.
235. Vallejo, J. G., Englund, J. A., Garcia-Prats, J. A., et al.: Ganciclovir treatment of steroid-associated cytomegalovirus disease in a congenitally infected neonate. Pediatr. Infect. Dis. J. *13*:239–240, 1994.
236. Victoria, M. S., Nangia, B. S., and Jindrak, K.: Cytomegalovirus pyloric obstruction in a child with acquired immunodeficiency syndrome. Pediatr. Infect. Dis. *4*:550–552, 1985.
237. Vilmer, E., Mazeron, M. C., Rabian, C., et al.: Clinical significance of cytomegalovirus viremia in bone marrow transplantation. Transplantation *40*:30–35, 1985.
238. Vinters, H. V., Kwok, M. K., Ho, H. W., et al.: Cytomegalovirus in the nervous system of patients with the acquired immune deficiency syndrome. Brain *112*:245–268, 1989.
239. Virnig, N. L., and Balfour, H. H.: Hemiatrophy and hemiparesis in a patient with congenital cytomegalovirus infection. Am. J. Dis. Child. *129*:1359–1360, 1975.
240. Wang, N. S., Huang, S. N., and Thurkbeck, W. M.: Combined *Pneumocystis carinii* and cytomegalovirus infection. Arch. Pathol. *90*:529–594, 1970.
241. Wang, P. S., and Evans, A. S.: Prevalence of antibodies to Epstein-Barr virus and cytomegalovirus in sera from a group of children in the People's Republic of China. J. Infect. Dis. *153*:150–152, 1986.
242. Waris, E., Rasanen, P., Kreus, K. E., et al.: Fatal cytomegalovirus disease in a previously healthy adult. Scand. J. Infect. Dis. *4*:61–67, 1972.
243. Watson, F. S., O'Connell, J. B., Amber, I. J., et al.: Treatment of cytomegalovirus pneumonia in heart transplant recipients with 9(1, 3-dihydroxy-2-propoxymethyl)-guanine (DHPG). J. Heart Transplant. *7*:102–105, 1988.
244. Weiner, R. S., Bortin, M. M., Gale, R. P., et al.: Interstitial pneumonitis after bone marrow transplantation. Ann. Intern. Med. *104*:168–175, 1986.
245. Weller, T. H., Macauley, J. C., Craig, J. M., et al.: Isolation of intranuclear inclusion-producing agents from infants with illnesses resembling cytomegalic inclusion disease. Proc. Soc. Exp. Biol. Med. *94*:4–12, 1957.

246. Weller, T. H., and Hanshaw, J. B.: Virological and clinical observation of cytomegalic inclusion disease. N. Engl. J. Med. *266*:1233–1344, 1962.
247. White, N. H., Yow, M. D., Demmler, G. J., et al.: Prevalence of cytomegalovirus antibody in subjects between the ages of 6 and 22 years. J. Infect. Dis. *159*:1013–1017, 1989.
248. Whitley, R. J., Brasfield, D., Reynolds, D. W., et al.: Protracted pneumonitis in young infants associated with perinatally acquired cytomegaloviral infection. J. Pediatr. *89*:16–22, 1976.
249. Wiley, C. A., Schrier, R. D., Denaro, F. J., et al.: Localization of cytomegalovirus proteins and genome during fulminant central nervous system infection in an AIDS patient. J. Neuropathol. Exp. Neurol. *45*:127–139, 1986.
250. Williamson, W. D., Demmler, G. J., Percy, A. K., et al.: Progressive hearing loss in infants with asymptomatic congenital cytomegalovirus infection. Pediatrics *90*:862–866, 1992.
251. Wilmott, F. E.: Cytomegalovirus in female patients attending a VD clinic. Br. J. Vener. Dis. *51*:278–280, 1975.
252. Wilson, W. R.: The relationship of the herpesvirus family to sudden hearing loss: A prospective clinical study and literature review. Laryngoscope *96*:870–877, 1986.
253. Wink, K., and Schmitz, H.: Cytomegalovirus myocarditis. Am. Heart J. *100*:667–677, 1980.
254. Winston, D. J., Pollard, R. B., Ho, W. G., et al.: Cytomegalovirus immune plasma in bone marrow transplant recipients. Ann. Intern. Med. *97*:11–18, 1982.
255. Wolf, D. G., and Spector, S. A.: Diagnosis of human cytomegalovirus central nervous system disease in AIDS patients by DNA amplification from cerebrospinal fluid. J. Infect. Dis. *166*:1412–1415, 1992.
256. Wolf, D. G., and Spector, S. A.: Early diagnosis of human cytomegalovirus disease in transplant recipients by DNA amplification in plasma. Transplantation *56*:330–334, 1993.
257. Yeager, A.: Transmission of cytomegalovirus to mothers by infected infants: Another reason to prevent transfusion-acquired infections. Pediatr. Infect. Dis. *2*:295–297, 1983.
258. Yeager, A. S., Grumet, F. C., Hafleigh, E. B., et al.: Prevention of transfusion-acquired cytomegalovirus infections in newborn infants. J. Pediatr. *98*:281–287, 1981.
259. Yow, M. D.: Congenital cytomegalovirus disease: A NOW problem. J. Infect. Dis. *159*:163–167, 1989.
260. Yow, M. D., Williamson, D. W., Leeds, L. J., et al.: Epidemiologic characteristics of cytomegalovirus infection in mothers and their infants. Am. J. Obstet. Gynecol. *158*:1189–1195, 1988.
261. Yow, M. D., White, N. H., Taber, L. H., et al.: Acquisition of cytomegalovirus infection from birth to 10 years: A longitudinal serologic study. J. Pediatr. *110*:37–42, 1987.
262. Zaia, J. A.: Epidemiology and pathogenesis of cytomegalovirus disease. Semin. Hematol. *27*:1–4, 1990.
263. Zaloga, G. P., Chernow, B., and Eil, C.: Hypercalcemia and disseminated cytomegalovirus infection in the acquired immunodeficiency syndrome. Ann. Intern. Med. *102*:331–332, 1985.

165

EPSTEIN-BARR VIRUS

Ciro V. Sumaya

During the 1950s, tumor safaris undertaken by Denis Burkitt[24] led to his description of an endemic childhood cancer of equatorial Africa, subsequently called Burkitt lymphoma (Fig. 165–1*A*). Several years later, Epstein and associates[44] found herpesvirus-like particles in cultured lymphoid cells from Burkitt tumor specimens. These particles were a new human herpesvirus that came to be known as Epstein-Barr virus (EBV). Studies performed mainly by Drs. Werner and Gertrude Henle and Yale University investigators, among others, demonstrated that EBV was the cause of classic infectious mononucleosis.[47, 75, 141] It subsequently was shown that EBV has the capacity to transform ("immortalize") human B lymphocytes in vitro, which allowed the derivation of EBV-transformed B-lymphoblastoid cell lines that can be propagated indefinitely in tissue culture.[77, 152]

The discovery of EBV in Burkitt lymphoma, its ability to growth-transform human B cells in vitro, and its intimate relationship with an increasing array of human cancerous processes[4] have resulted in the designation of EBV as a prime putative human tumor virus and led to intense research efforts on this virus since the 1960s.

This chapter reviews progress in understanding the immunobiology of EBV and EBV's disease associations. Enhanced understanding of EBV is leading to better diagnostic measures, appropriate management of known EBV-induced disorders, and improved evaluation of the role of the virus in other clinical situations as yet etiologically enigmatic.

STRUCTURE AND BIOLOGY

On morphologic examination, EBV is a typical herpesvirus.[43] Electron-microscopic studies reveal an enveloped virus,

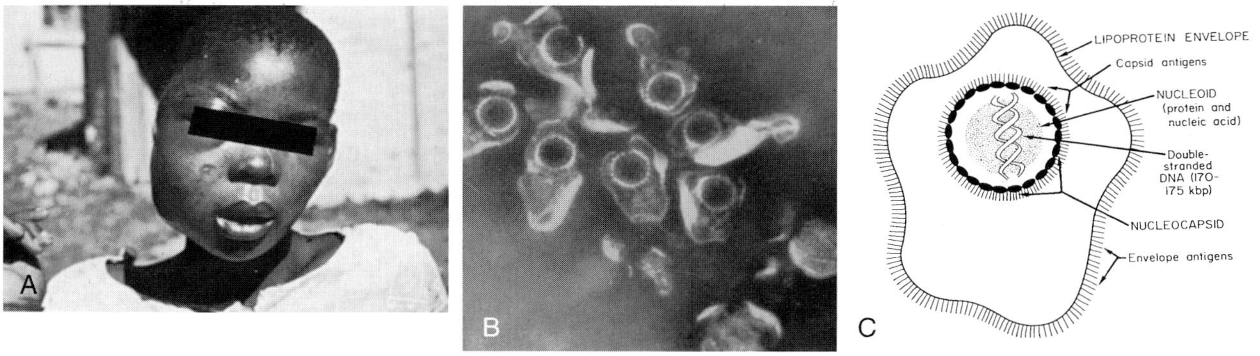

FIGURE 165–1. A, *African boy with Burkitt lymphoma involving the jaw.* B, *Electron micrograph of free, enveloped Epstein-Barr virus particles.* C, *Schematic illustration of components of the free, enveloped Epstein-Barr virus virion. (*A *and* B *courtesy of Dr. George Miller, Yale University.)*

with the nucleocapsid having icosahedral symmetry (162 capsomeres). The nucleocapsid measures 100 to 110 nm in diameter; the whole enveloped virion measures 150 to 220 nm. Inside the nucleocapsid is a nucleoid core containing a double-stranded, linear DNA genome of about 170,000 to 175,000 nucleotide pairs (170 to 175 kilobase pairs, or kb). Figure 165–1*B* and *C* present an electron micrograph and schematic diagram, respectively, depicting enveloped EBV virions.

The initial and predominantly replicative (lytic) infection is likely to occur in epithelial cells of the oropharynx and adjacent structures.[177, 212] Virus then is transmitted to circulating B cells passing through these lymphoepithelial tissues and organs. The EBV virion preferentially infects B lymphocytes, using a cell-surface receptor that probably is the same as the surface moiety functioning as the receptor for the third component of serum complement, that is, the C3d receptor.[49] It appears that EBV enters the B lymphocyte and is transported through the cytoplasm and stripped of its envelope in endocytic vesicles[139]; subsequently, the viral genome circularizes and is maintained in the cell nucleus as a multicopy plasmid.[127]

The EBV-infected human B-lymphocyte populations mainly are latent and have the capacity to induce growth transformation. Some observations indicate that there are various stages of latency with corresponding EBV proteins and genes: (1) immunoblastic cells, seen during the course of infectious mononucleosis, that are highly immunogenic and are eliminated rapidly by virus-specific cytotoxic T-cell responses, (2) infected B cells that progress through the normal pathway of B-cell differentiation and lead to the generation of EBV-carrying memory cells localized in lymphoid follicles, and (3) resting cells that are nonimmunogenic and are likely to form the latent viral reservoir in healthy EBV carriers.[132] Activation of resting cells stimulated by immunosuppression or other triggers could result in greater growth transformation that expands the viral reservoir, homing of infected B cells to germinal centers and protection from cell death, or active viral replication. Thus, the earlier model of EBV persistence in epithelial cells that continually reinfect the host's B-cell pool has been challenged by the more recent findings on the dynamics of EBV infection in B cells. Furthermore, a group of investigators[6] has noted that the latent and productive EBV infection in tonsils occurs in lymphoid cells on the surface of the tonsillar epithelium and within the crypt, but not the epithelial cells. This suggested that the transmission of EBV among persons is due to the transfer of virus from persistently infected EBV lymphoid cells; EBV-infected epithelial cells may not be required for this phenomenon.

EBV can be recovered readily from oropharyngeal secretions of the vast majority of children with mononucleosis[194] and from 6 to 20 per cent of the general population (possibly lower in children compared with adults).[25, 137, 190, 192] EBV DNA, analyzed by polymerase chain reaction, also has been detected in the blood and urine of patients with acute infectious mononucleosis, as well as several months after clinical recovery.[112] An EBV lytic infection of epithelial cells of the uterine cervix also has been reported.[176]

Although EBV productively can infect oropharyngeal and salivary gland epithelial tissue, growth transformation of human epithelial cells by EBV virions has not been well demonstrated yet, a point of some interest in light of the suspected involvement of EBV in undifferentiated nasopharyngeal carcinoma and other carcinomas.[38]

Molecular Biology

The huge size of the EBV genome and the limited ability to propagate free virus from most EBV-infected cell lines hindered the analysis of the viral genome's structure and replicative life cycle for many years. The advent of recombinant DNA methods has led to detailed characterizations of the genomes of several laboratory strains of EBV derived from Burkitt lymphoma cell lines or from marmoset lymphoid cell lines transformed by EBV strains from mononucleosis patients.[35, 50] Nucleotide sequencing of the 172-kb genome of the prototype transforming strain (B95-8) has been performed.[11] These studies have indicated a common general architecture for various strains of EBV, with short and long regions of "unique" nucleotide sequence (regions called U_S and U_L) separated by a major internal repeat region (IR_1) consisting of generally 6 to 12 direct repeats of a 3-kb sequence.[73] The virus also has numerous other regions of repeated nucleotide sequence, including direct repeats of a 0.5-kb sequence at its termini.[11, 107]

Functions are being assigned to various subregions of the viral genome. It is estimated that the EBV genome may encode about 55 to 70 proteins.[11, 30, 90, 104, 206] Viral gene expression in latently infected cells is restricted. At least 11 virally encoded gene products are expressed during latency: two small, nonpolyadenylated RNAs (EBER-1 and EBER-2); six nuclear proteins (EBNA-1, -2, -3A, -3B, and -3C and leader protein [LP]); and three latent membrane proteins (LMP-1, -2a, and -2b).[105]

The regions of the EBV genome responsible for growth transformation of human B lymphocytes have not been discerned fully yet. Certain viral proteins, such as EBNA-2 and perhaps LMP-1, are essential for transformation, although a number of viral gene products appear to be involved in the initiation and maintenance of cell transformation.[62, 74, 83, 103, 134, 197, 204]

Several polypeptides apparently corresponding to traditionally recognized EBV antigens have been mapped to various subregions of the viral genome. The EBV nuclear antigen (EBNA), traditionally defined by anticomplement immunofluorescence,[157] appears to correspond to the presence of at least six virally encoded polypeptides in the cell nucleus.[151] The major antigenic polypeptide of EBNA has been mapped by gene transfer techniques to the *Bam*HI "K" restriction fragment of the EBV strain B95-8 genome.[197] Yates and colleagues[217, 218] have shown that this EBNA-1 (K-EBNA) gene encodes a product that acts via DNA binding at a specific site on the EBV genome (designated *Ori*P) to allow successful replication of the EBV genome as a plasmid in human lymphocytes and other mammalian cells. A separate origin of lytic replication (*Ori*Lyt) is duplicated twice in the genome.

Molecular genetic techniques and hybridoma technology also are being used to expand the identification and characterization of the genes and gene products corresponding to other traditionally recognized EBV antigenic complexes, including viral capsid antigens (VCAs), early antigens (EAs), and membrane antigens (MAs), as well as other virally encoded structural and regulatory proteins.

Virus–Target Cell Interactions

Immunologic analyses of EBV-infected cells and cell cloning studies have indicated that EBV generally transforms relatively mature B lymphocytes, secreting a complete immunoglobulin product (heavy chain plus light chain).[21, 145] It appears that EBV can infect and transform B cells in earlier stages of development, for example, pre-B cells (producing only μ chains) and lymphoid precursors lacking immunoglobulin gene rearrangement.[57, 58, 102] Tumor cells and cell lines from Burkitt lymphomas are B cells, generally expressing small amounts of immunoglobulin, which may be detected as surface immunoglobulin molecules, cytoplasmic/secreted molecules, or both. The major heavy-chain isotype expressed by Burkitt tumors appears to be μ chain (IgM), although IgG-expressing tumors and one IgA-expressing tumor have been reported.[145] Similarly, the EBV-infected cells observed in the blood of persons with mononucleosis and the tumor cells found in immunocompromised persons with EBV-associated lymphoproliferative diseases and lymphomas are B lymphocytes; these EBV-infected cell populations may include cells producing any of the major classes of human immunoglobulin (IgM, IgG, and IgA).[21, 145, 161, 162] Immunoglobulin isotype studies and analyses of immunoglobulin gene rearrangements suggest that the transformed cell populations in immunosuppressed patients with EBV-related malignant lymphoproliferations may be polyclonal, oligoclonal, or monoclonal.[20, 28, 29, 71, 87, 155, 161] It is likely that the lymphoproliferations initially are polyclonal but evolve to oligoclonality or monoclonality. Burkitt lymphomas, on the other hand, always appear to be monoclonal at the time of clinical presentation.[14, 145]

The EBV genome and the expression of EBNAs are found in virtually all Burkitt lymphoma cells derived from African patients and in 10 to 20 per cent of cases of Burkitt lymphoma in Europe or the United States. Burkitt lymphoma cells, but not lymphoid cells found in infectious mononucleosis, exhibit characteristic chromosomal alterations thought to be associated with the enhanced malignant potential of these cells. About 90 per cent of Burkitt tumors exhibit a reciprocal translocation involving the long arms of chromosomes 8 and 14; in almost all of the remaining 10 per cent of Burkitt tumors, translocations involving chromosomes 8 and 2, or 8 and 22, are observed.[108, 166] The region on chromosome 8 that is involved in these translocations contains the c-*myc* proto-oncogene.[34, 198] The chromosomal translocations observed in Burkitt lymphoma cells are believed to result in transcriptional deregulation and overexpression of the c-*myc* oncogene, which possibly accounts for the enhanced malignant potential of Burkitt cells.[33, 116] An EBV immediate early protein was found to activate c-*myc* expression and thus potentially to be relevant to the genesis of Burkitt lymphoma.[67]

Although investigations still are in their infancy, varying patterns of viral gene expressions are being noted in different cancers. Viral strain characterization performed by polymerase chain reaction techniques have detected a type 1 and type 2 virus with differential detection in body fluids and tumors. Future research in this area could yield findings relevant to the development and treatment of oncogenic processes.[4]

PATHOGENESIS OF EPSTEIN-BARR VIRUS–RELATED DISEASES

Partly owing to its tropism for B lymphocytes, EBV elicits protean immunologic responses during human infection. Except in instances of EBV-associated B lymphomas and fatal B-lymphoproliferative diseases, the various components of the immune response may be responsible for or at least contribute to the clinical manifestations of illness associated with EBV infection. After an incubation period of 2 to 7 weeks after exposure, as many as 20 per cent of the circulating B lymphocytes of adolescents or young adults developing infectious mononucleosis are infected with EBV, although more commonly the number is about 1 per cent.[163] The mild EBV-induced B-cell proliferation in the first week or two in mononucleosis patients is aborted quickly by a brisk cellular immune response, which comprises prominent natural killer cell activity, cytotoxic-suppressor (OKT8-positive surface marker) T cells, and antibody-dependent cellular cytotoxicity.[39, 78, 149, 159, 168, 199, 200, 205, 207] The increase in suppressor T lymphocytes during the acute phase of infectious mononucleosis produces a low or "inverted" T4/T8 (helper/suppressor) lymphocytic ratio. The expansion of the T8 lymphocyte population in children with acute infectious mononucleosis may be less marked than that in adult patients.[207] The atypical lymphocytes observed in the blood of mononucleosis patients are thought to be mostly T lymphocytes responding to the B-cell infection. Typically, the immune response reduces the number of circulating EBV-infected B lymphocytes by about 10^4 times, to less than one infected cell per 10^6 B cells, within 4 to 6 weeks.[164]

In patients with various types of immune defects (congenital, acquired, or iatrogenic), the response to primary or chronic EBV infection may be inadequate, with resultant unchecked proliferation of EBV-infected B cells. Such EBV-related B lymphoproliferations may be histologically pleomorphic (B-lymphoproliferative disorders) or relatively uniform (B lymphomas). In organ transplant recipients, no consistent chromosomal translocations are associated with the lymphomas. Many of the lesions regress after withdrawal of immunosuppressive therapy post transplantation.[219] In rare, severe cases, B cells containing EBV DNA and expressing EBNA may become disseminated throughout the body as plasmacytoid cells visible on peripheral blood smears and as B-lymphoid cells potentially invading all organs of the body. Life-threatening EBV infections also may be correlated with an overly strong virus-induced T-cell proliferation that might cause autoaggressive activity, producing hypogammaglobulinemia or other major dysfunctions of body organs.[13]

The pathogenesis of malignant disorders in some settings may be multifactorial, involving a mixture of virologic, genetic, and environmental factors. In nasopharyngeal carcinoma, a genetic predisposed risk is suggested by the human leukocyte antigen linkage of the disease.[124] Furthermore, evidence suggests that an initial viral gene expression from an early EBV infection can result in profound growth stimulating effects, reaching full malignant potential by acquiring cellular genetic changes involving chromosome 3. These secondary genetic alterations could be increased by exposure to environmental carcinogens, such as volatile nitrosamines in dietary salted fish. Increased IgA antibodies to EBV predate the clinical onset of nasopharyngeal carcinoma and define populations at high risk for this cancer.

The evolution of African Burkitt lymphoma appears to be a multistep process involving malaria, EBV, and c-*myc* gene activation resulting from chromosomal translation and perhaps other, as yet unknown steps.[173] EBNA-1, the only viral protein expressed in Burkitt lymphoma, is not recognized by cytotoxic T cells, thus perhaps evading cytotoxic T-cell–mediated viral immune surveillance. Furthermore, EBNA-1 may enhance c-*myc* gene expression in the context of particular chromosomal translocations involving immunoglobulins.[94] There also is evidence that the plant *Euphorbia tirucalli* may be an important environmental risk factor for the genesis of African Burkitt lymphoma.[93] *E. tirucalli* is found in the endemic area for the lymphoma, and it has immunologic properties that enhance EBV infection of B lymphocytes.

Clarification of the possible role played by EBV in the development of virus-associated tumors is hampered by insufficient understanding of the mode of EBV persistence in human B and perhaps T cells. Moreover, the specific stage or stages in the oncogenic process at which EBV activity is essential for malignant formation has not been identified.[144]

EPIDEMIOLOGY

Serologic reactivity to EBV antigens (e.g., the viral capsid antigen) is found in the vast majority of adults in all human populations studied to date, which implies that most adults (80 to 95 per cent) persistently are infected with EBV throughout the world.[80, 195] However, the age of initial (primary) infection varies markedly in different cultural and socioeconomic settings, a fact that has great pertinence to the disease manifestations associated with primary infection. In socioeconomically underprivileged communities or in developing countries, primary infection with EBV occurs early in life, so that 80 to 100 per cent of children are EBV-seropositive by 3 to 6 years of age. In these settings, the vast majority of primary infections are subclinical or only mildly asymptomatic.[54, 97, 189] In privileged communities and in developed countries, primary infection with EBV occurs later in life, for example, often between 10 and 30 years of age. In these settings, primary infections are more likely to induce clinical symptoms, most often a mononucleosis syndrome. An infectious mononucleosis case rate of 50 to 75 per cent with a primary EBV infection was documented in United States college students.[140] An unexpectedly high rate of infectious mononucleosis also has been noted with the eventual primary EBV infection in siblings of a pediatric case of infectious mononucleosis.[192]

It is noteworthy that in populations in which EBV-associated tumors are highly endemic, primary infection with EBV almost universally occurs early in life. African Burkitt lymphoma and undifferentiated nasopharyngeal carcinoma in southern Asia are not manifestations of primary EBV infection. Rather, these tumors occur in patients with a long-standing EBV infection, especially in those persons exhibiting high antibody titers to EBV capsid antigens and persistent antibody titers to the EBV early antigen complex.[37, 38, 80, 135]

Retrospective analysis of sera collected during the 1960s and 1970s suggests that infection with viruses related to those lymphotropic retroviruses that are associated with AIDS has been highly endemic in equatorial regions of Africa for perhaps two decades or more. Thus, these human populations may have been especially susceptible to the endemic, EBV-related form of Burkitt lymphoma. This link also is suggested by the observation that Burkitt lymphomas and other B lymphomas occur with increased frequency in American and European patients with AIDS.[221] It appears that some, and possibly most, of the Burkitt lymphomas and other B lymphomas in AIDS patients may be related to EBV[10, 221]; direct B-cell involvement with other lymphotropic viruses also is possible, however.

TRANSMISSION

The principal route of transmission of EBV appears to be through saliva. Although outbreaks of infectious mononucleosis are uncommon, EBV must spread relatively efficiently because large epidemiologic studies indicate that widespread infections occur in the general population, particularly in lower socioeconomic settings.[57] Higher EBV exposure has been reported in infants residing in nurseries.[26]

However, the transmission of EBV even among close contacts of an acute EBV infection may be slow. In a family study,[192] after the index infectious mononucleosis episode, only 35 per cent of the nonimmune sibling contacts developed EBV antibodies (seroconverted) after an average observation period of 5.6 contact months. Yet, this same study also noted that the eventual seroconversion event in siblings was more likely to be associated with an infectious mononucleosis episode than would be expected in the general population.

The role in viral transmission played by the frequent and prolonged excretion of EBV in oropharyngeal salival secretions from patients with infectious mononucleosis[194] or by the less intense "endemic" prevalence rate (up to the 20 per cent range) of EBV-positive salival secretions in the general population[25, 137, 190, 192] is unclear. There is no requirement for isolation of hospitalized patients with infectious mononucleosis. Treatment of patients with infectious mononucleosis or of EBV-positive persons with such antiviral agents as acyclovir can reduce oropharyngeal virus shedding.[216]

The transmission of EBV through blood products has been described, but its frequency is much lower than that attributed to cytomegalovirus. It customarily is recommended that patients with a recent history of EBV infection or an infectious mononucleosis-like illness should not donate blood.[5] In transplant recipients, the incrimination of the donor organ or blood products as the source of the EBV infection is unclear.[18] However, at least one case involving bone marrow transplantation provides strong evidence that the transplanted material itself may be the source of EBV infection.[170]

The detection of EBV shedding from the uterine cervix raises the possibility of venereal transmission or neonatal infection,[176] but the risk for viral dissemination via this site is unproven.

CLINICAL DISORDERS ASSOCIATED WITH EPSTEIN-BARR VIRUS INFECTION

A number of clinical disorders have been linked to an EBV infection (Table 165–1). Of these, infectious mononucleosis stands out as *the* prototype clinical entity produced by a primary EBV infection. Increasing data indicate that a persis-

TABLE 165–1. Clinical Disorders Associated Etiologically with Epstein-Barr Virus (EBV)

Disorder	Evidence for Etiology*
Acute, Primary Infection	
Infectious mononucleosis	+ + + +
Acute neurologic diseases (Guillain-Barré syndrome, Bell palsy meningoencephalitis)†	+ + +
Acquired agammaglobulinemia, aplastic anemia	+ + +
Tonsillopharyngitis†	+ +
Thrombocytopenia†	+ +
Pneumonia†	+ +
Sudden hearing loss†	+
Reye syndrome	+
Chronic or Putative Reactivated Infection	
Congenital infection with fetal abnormalities‡	+ + +
Lymphoproliferative lesions/lymphomas in immunocompromised states, post organ/bone marrow transplants	+ + +
Burkitt lymphoma, nasopharyngeal carcinoma	+ + +
X-linked lymphoproliferative syndrome	+ + +
Hemophagocytic syndrome	+ +
Chronic mononucleosis or chronic (symptomatic) EBV infection	+ +
Gastric carcinoma	+ +
Chronic fatigue syndrome	+

*Evidence was graded from + + + + (definite) to + (possible).
†Isolated manifestation and not as part of infectious mononucleosis episode.
‡Case reports are extremely rare.

tently active (chronic) EBV infection or reactivation of a previously latent EBV infection can lead to discrete clinical disorders. However, the pathogenesis and validity of these latter associations usually are less definite.

Primary Infections

Asymptomatic, Nonspecific Infections

Primary EBV infection in young children, as noted previously, usually is asymptomatic or accompanied by such mild, nonspecific manifestations as upper respiratory tract infection, tonsillopharyngitis, or prolonged febrile illness with or without lymphadenopathy.[54, 97, 189]

Infectious Mononucleosis

Some young children and many more adolescents and young adults develop the typical signs of infectious mononucleosis during a primary (initial) infection with EBV. The cardinal clinical features of the mononucleosis syndrome (in children as in adults) are fever, sore throat, malaise, and fatigue accompanied by signs of tonsillopharyngitis and lymphadenopathy (Fig. 165–2). There frequently is a prodromal period of 2 to 5 days, consisting of malaise and fatigue (with or without fever), before the onset of the full syndrome. The fever not uncommonly lasts 1 to 2 weeks. The adenopathy in mononucleosis most prominently involves the cervical lymph nodes (anterior and posterior), but diffuse adenopathy often is appreciable, including the occipital, supraclavicular, axillary, epitrochlear, and inguinal chains. The enlarged nodes usually are nontender, or minimally so, and lack overlying skin erythema. Splenomegaly develops in the first 3 weeks of illness in at least 50 per cent of cases, and hepatomegaly develops in about 30 to 50 per cent. The adenopathy and organomegaly most often are prominent in the second to fourth weeks of illness. The tonsillopharyngitis often is severe and exudative but is accompanied by streptococcal infection (group A beta-hemolytic streptococci) in only about 5 per cent of cases. Younger children appear to have higher rates of rashes and abdominal pain than young adults do. An enanthem consisting of petechiae in the soft palate and edema of the eyelids also may occur. The strong correlation noted in young adults between the administration of ampicillin and the subsequent development of a maculopapular rash may not be as apparent among pediatric patients. This may be due, at least in part, to the overall increased rate of cutaneous manifestations in children with infectious mononucleosis. Certain manifestations that seem unique or more closely associated with infectious mononucleosis in the childhood patient, such as failure to thrive, otitis media, and recurrent episodes of tonsillopharyngitis before or after the acute infectious mononucleosis episode, have been noted occasionally.

In one prospective study,[193] significant complications involving mainly the pulmonary, neurologic, and hematologic systems were noted in approximately 20 per cent of the children with infectious mononucleosis (Table 165–2). The childhood patient appeared to develop thrombocytopenia with hemorrhagic manifestations, severe airway obstruction, and neurologic complications more frequently than did adult patients; jaundice occurred less frequently. The thrombocytopenia appears to be due to various mechanisms, including increased destruction by an enlarged spleen, antiplatelet antibodies, and predisposing abnormal platelet function.[27, 41, 175] The intense inflammation and hypertrophy of lymphoid tissue in the Waldeyer ring and surrounding areas probably are responsible for the airway obstruction.[66] Invasion of nervous system tissues is believed to produce the neurologic manifestations.[63, 201] These complications usually develop during or

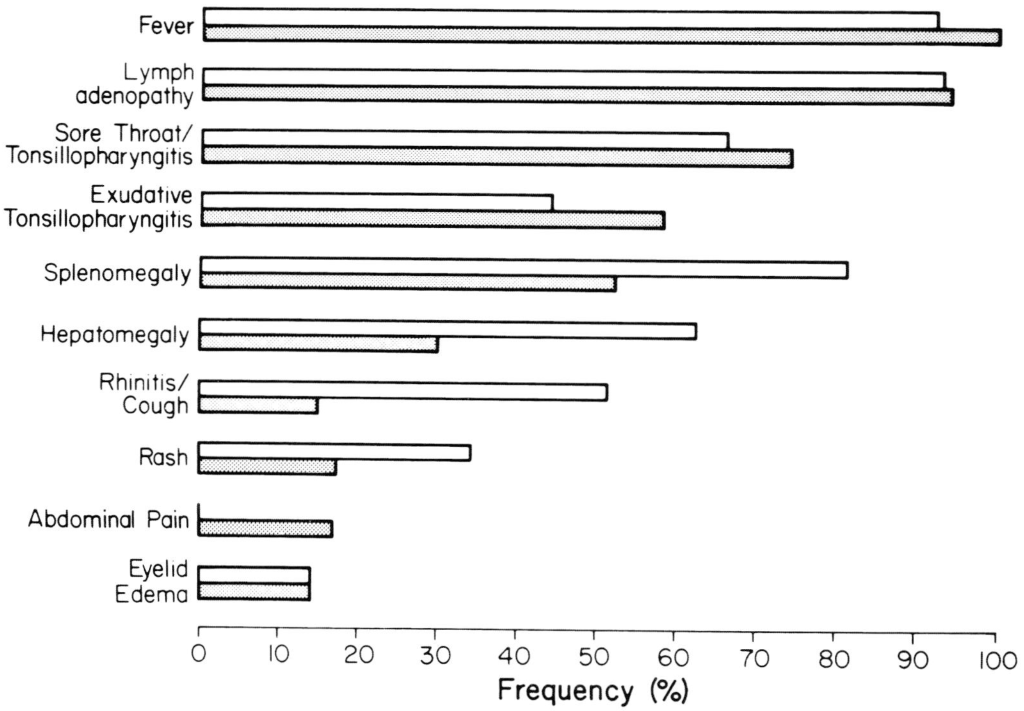

FIGURE 165–2. *Frequency of clinical findings in two age groups of children with documented Epstein-Barr virus infectious mononucleosis: younger than 4 years of age (open bars) and 4 to 16 years of age (dotted bars). (From Sumaya, C. V., and Ench, Y.: Epstein-Barr virus infectious mononucleosis in children. I. Clinical and general laboratory findings. Pediatrics 75:1003–1010, 1985. Reproduced by permission of Pediatrics.)*

TABLE 165–2. Complications Present in Childhood Epstein–Barr Virus Infectious Mononucleosis

Complication	Number of Children (%)
Respiratory tract	
Pneumonia	6 (5.3)
Severe airway obstruction*	4 (3.5)
Neurologic	
Seizures	4 (3.5)
Meningitis/encephalitis	2 (1.8)
Peripheral facial nerve paralysis	1 (0.9)
Guillain-Barré syndrome	1 (0.9)
Hematologic	
Thrombocytopenia with hemorrhages	4 (3.5)
Hemolytic anemia	1 (0.9)
Infectious	
Bacteremia	1 (0.9)
Recurrent tonsillopharyngitis	3 (2.7)
Liver	
Jaundice	2 (1.8)
Renal	
Glomerulonephritis	1 (0.9)
Genital	
Orchitis	1 (0.9)
Total	31†

*Criteria consisted of nasal alar flaring, suprasternal retractions, or stridor.

†Because four children had more than one of these complications, this total is composed of 24 different children, or 21.2 per cent of the study group.

From Sumaya, C. V., and Ench, Y.: Epstein-Barr virus infectious mononucleosis in children. I. Clinical and general laboratory findings. Pediatrics *75*:1003–1010, 1985. Reproduced by permission of Pediatrics.

shortly after the peak of clinical illness, although they may occur in the early or later phases of the infectious mononucleosis episode. Fortunately, complications characteristically are short-lived and produce no permanent sequelae. Splenic rupture is considered a rare event in children, although the actual rate is unknown[3, 193]; a 0.2 per cent rate has been reported in adult patients.[88] Significant bacterial superinfections are rare in spite of the relatively common frequency of significant neutropenia in children with infectious mononucleosis.[193] However, peritonsillar abscess is being recognized as an increasingly frequent bacterial complication.[153] Other uncommon complications in children and young adults include hemolytic or aplastic anemia (the latter being potentially fatal),[113, 193] renal dysfunction,[193, 214] sudden hearing loss,[171, 210] and infantile papular acrodermatitis (Gianotti-Crosti syndrome),[110] among others (for reviews, see references 3, 101, 150, and 193).

Atypical Presentations of Infectious Mononucleosis

Manifestations may be severe in some patients; involvement of organs or systems frequently affected in infectious mononucleosis may be more than usually extensive, or organs or systems that are affected uncommonly may be involved significantly.[188] The diagnosis of infectious mononucleosis may be obscured at times by the intense prominence of some of these manifestations, particularly if they occur early in the course of the disease or even precede the evolution of the more common signs of infectious mononucleosis. For example, the child with infectious mononucleosis may present initially only with hemorrhagic lesions, facial nerve paralysis, seizures, or features indicating severe hepatitis before the more usual signs of infectious mononucleosis develop and are recognized. An Alice-in-Wonderland syndrome manifested by metamorphopsia (i.e., the distortion of apparent sizes, shapes, and spatial relations of objects seen) has been described in a few children.[32, 46]

Other Primary Infections

A number of clinical manifestations that are seen occasionally as part of an infectious mononucleosis episode also may occur as isolated manifestations of a primary EBV infection. These include acute neurologic disorders, such as Bell palsy, Guillain-Barré syndrome, meningoencephalitis, and transverse myelitis.[31, 64] Other clinical disorders, such as Reye syndrome,[55] thrombocytopenia purpura,[41] interstitial pneumonitis,[9] and several recurrent otolaryngologic problems,[1, 171, 203] also have been linked causally to a primary EBV infection, all mainly on the basis of serologic findings.

Chronic, Symptomatic Epstein-Barr Virus Infections

Lymphoproliferative/Malignant Disorders

Persons with various types of immunodeficiency are at increased risk for the development of potentially fatal EBV-related lymphoproliferative diseases, B lymphomas, and severe atypical EBV infections. Most notably, these include male children with the X-linked lymphoproliferative syndrome.[155, 184] Although EBV is found in body fluids and tissues of patients with X-linked lymphoproliferative syndrome, antibody formation to EBV antigens usually is poor or absent. A wide variety of patients with other congenital and acquired immunodeficiency states also are at risk, including patients with severe combined immunodeficiency syndrome, Wiskott-Aldrich syndrome, ataxia telangiectasia, Chédiak-Higashi syndrome, common variable immunodeficiency, AIDS, incompletely characterized congenital immunodeficiencies, and iatrogenic immunosuppression. In patients infected with HIV, EBV often is associated with diffuse large cell/immunoblastic lymphomas and occasionally associated with Burkitt lymphoma. EBV almost always is associated with primary central nervous system lymphomas and usually with Hodgkin disease in the population infected with HIV.[70, 129] Chronic lymphocytic interstitial pneumonitis is a distinctive lesion associated with EBV in children with AIDS, whereas it is uncommon in adults with AIDS.[8] There also are differences in the frequency of other EBV-associated tissue lesions in pediatric compared with adult patients with AIDS. EBV-induced oral "hairy" leukoplakia, a white plaque on the surface of the tongue,[61] and Burkitt lymphoma are uncommon in children with AIDS.[100] It was reported that EBV may be responsible for the unusually high incidence of smooth-muscle tumors (leiomyomas and leiomyosarcomas) found in children with AIDS.[130] Children immunosuppressed for organ transplantation (with steroids, azathioprine, anti–T-cell antibodies, cyclosporine, or a combination thereof) have an increased risk for the development of EBV-related lymphoproliferative syndromes and B lymphomas.[86, 111, 180] Ho and colleagues[86] reported a greater frequency of lymphoproliferative lesions in pediatric transplant recipients (4 per cent) compared with adult transplant recipients (0.8 per cent). Pediatric organ transplant recipients are considered at increased risk for EBV-related disorders because they, more than adult transplant recipients, are seronegative for EBV at transplantation, and primary infection is more likely to progress to lymphoproliferative and other severe EBV-associated disorders in these patients.[86, 87] Children with immunodeficiency disease who have received cultured thymus[17] or bone marrow[170] transplantation also may develop EBV-associated lymphoproliferative disorders. As has been documented recently in some children with AIDS, a few children with liver transplantation and immunosuppression have been found to develop subsequent smooth-muscle tumors.[117] It should be kept in mind, however, that infectious mononucleosis and other forms of EBV infections in immunocompromised children and adults usually run a course similar to that in immunocompetent persons; actually, even in immunosuppressed (and posttransplantation subjects), most EBV infections are silent clinically.[78, 86]

EBV-associated Burkitt lymphoma is a rapidly progressive and fatal tumor that affects predominantly young children in central Africa and Papua New Guinea.[24] About 60 per cent of African patients with Burkitt lymphoma present with jaw masses, with abdominal masses being second most common.[220] It currently is believed that an intense EBV infection during young childhood years is largely responsible for the development of Burkitt lymphoma.[36, 37] The potential role of malaria as a cofactor in this process has been disputed.[15] Non-African patients with Burkitt lymphoma are most likely to present with abdominal masses. Some patients with Burkitt lymphoma and some patients with congenital or acquired immunodeficiencies (including AIDS) present with or develop central nervous system involvement, with intracranial mass lesions of lymphomatous cells or with a pleocytosis malignant cells in the cerebrospinal fluid, or with both.[10, 220, 221] Fatal T-cell lymphomas with evidence of EBV-driven oncogenesis now have been described in several patients.[99, 183] Weiss and colleagues[209] have demonstrated the presence of EBV DNA in Reed-Sternberg cells, which suggests a possible etiologic role for EBV in a subset of patients with Hodgkin disease. The differential incidence distribution of Hodgkin disease in children throughout the world agrees with the age of first EBV infection, increasing in adolescence in developed countries while increasing in earlier childhood in developing countries.[65, 95] Hodgkin disease in children, particularly young children, is at least as strongly linked to EBV as it is in adults.[154]

A growing number of carcinomas, although not being lymphocytic malignancies, have been associated with EBV infections. Nasopharyngeal carcinoma, a tumor seen in adults (although it does affect children) in southern China, has been linked serologically with EBV.[81, 85] The potential etiologic role of EBV became much stronger when Sixbey and colleagues[177] demonstrated that this virus indeed could infect epithelial cells, producing a lytic (productive) state. Polymeric IgA (found predominantly in mucosal secretions) also may promote infection by EBV of otherwise refractory epithelial cells. This important finding suggests the possibility of EBV persistence and "reactivation" in epithelial tissue.[179] Nasopharyngeal carcinoma appears to be a clonal proliferation that develops subsequent to an EBV infection and specific viral genes are expressed consistently within all cells, indicating the probability that EBV gene products are required for tumor growth.[156]

Increasing amounts of data indicate that gastric carcinomas, particularly of the undifferentiated type and in Japanese people, are linked to EBV.[172] EBV also has been implicated in the genesis of other carcinomas, including those of the thymus,[123] parotid gland,[167] and supraglottic larynx.[19]

Severe, Chronic Infections

There are several reports of persistent or reactivated EBV infections, often in persons with no known history of an immunocompromised state, that are believed to be responsible for severe multiorgan or at times unifocal dysfunction. This includes an increasing number of patients who have been described as having prolonged episodes of severe bone marrow aplasias (commonly fatal),[12, 208] pneumonitis, recurrent febrile periods, dysgammaglobulinemias, hepatitis, or neurologic abnormalities.[2, 136, 169] Many of these patients have extremely high antibody titers to antigens of the replicative cycle, that is, EBV viral capsid and early antigen components— a distinctive feature. A malignant lymphoproliferative lesion may develop eventually in some of the patients with the EBV-associated chronic symptoms.

Chronic Fatiguing Disorder

In the early 1980s, a chronic debilitating disorder (now designated chronic fatigue syndrome) began receiving increased publicity and was linked etiologically to EBV.[98, 181] The characteristic manifestations included chronic fatigue (principal finding); neuropsychologic problems; and others, such as recurrent low-grade fever, mild lymphadenopathy, and possibly pharyngitis. The association with EBV was drawn mainly from epidemiologic findings and some abnormal EBV-specific immune responses. Variable general immunologic abnormalities also have been found in the relatively small number of patients studied, but there is no consistency in findings that can explain the pathogenesis of the illness. It is current opinion that EBV probably is involved only peripherally (along with other potential viral agents), if at all, in the triggering of this syndrome; the EBV-related laboratory abnormalities are considered mainly coincidental to other underlying immunologic or metabolic aberrations.[187] Patients with this disorder also may have higher antibody titers against cytomegalovirus, herpes simplex virus, and measles virus.[89] More information on this topic is provided in Chapter 83.

Intrauterine and Newborn Infections

Because the majority of young adults already are EBV-seropositive, primary infection with EBV during pregnancy appears to be a rare occurrence.[51, 91, 92, 114] The low frequency of this event makes it difficult to assess the risk presented to the fetus by primary EBV infection occurring in the mother during gestation. In the few instances in which clinically silent or clinically symptomatic maternal primary infections were detected prospectively, it appeared that the fetuses suffered no adverse effects, and, when studied, EBV infection was not transmitted to the fetus.[53] However, an earlier retrospective study and sporadic case reports suggest the possibility that infants occasionally suffer damage due to maternal EBV infection just before conception[23] or during pregnancy.[59, 96, 138]

At this time, no specific constellation of fetal anomalies has been associated with EBV infection during pregnancy, and the risk for intrauterine transmission of EBV infection appears to be low, even when the mother is symptomatic clinically. Thus, there is no rationale for following routine EBV serologic studies (e.g., anti-VCA) during antenatal care of normal, immunocompetent women. One report suggested the possibility that pregnant women with measurable anti-EA antibody levels had a significant risk for adverse fetal outcomes.[92] A subsequent study found that pregnant women were more likely to have detectable anti-EA antibody titers than were control subjects, but elevated anti-EA titers were not associated with an increased risk for adverse fetal outcomes.[52] Thus, consideration of antiviral drug therapy, in those rare instances in which an expectant woman develops mononucleosis (or other EBV-related disease), should be tempered by the facts that the risk of intrauterine transmission of EBV infection appears to be low and that present antiviral drugs generally are nucleoside analogues with a potential for teratogenic effects. Certainly, however, such a pregnancy should be monitored clinically for continued normal progress, possibly including noninvasive tests, such as abdominal ultrasound examination, for assessment of the possibilities of fetal anomalies or intrauterine growth retardation.

Other Associated Diseases

EBV infections continue to be associated with a variety of usually mild but chronic, recurrent conditions including periodic febrile illnesses,[118] although evidence for EBV causality usually is insufficient.[186] There also have been scattered reports of a relationship between EBV and two chronic neurologic diseases: subacute sclerosing panencephalitis[48] and multiple sclerosis.[196] More recently, a dual infection hypothesis involving a new retrovirus and EBV producing a multiple sclerosis–like disease was proposed.[68] Hemophagocytic syndrome, an entity produced by the proliferation of cytologically nonmalignant hemophagocytic histiocytes in bone marrow, lymph nodes, and other sites, has been associated with EBV in addition to other viral and bacterial agents.[158] A fulminant disease course has been described in patients with an existing EBV-associated peripheral T-cell lymphoma[215] and sometimes in otherwise previously healthy young children.[182]

DIAGNOSIS

General Laboratory Features in Infectious Mononucleosis

Patients with infectious mononucleosis typically demonstrate an absolute lymphocytosis (≥50 per cent lymphocytes, with total leukocytes ≥5000/mm³), prominent atypical lymphocytes (often >10 per cent of total leukocytes), and a positive test result for Paul-Bunnell heterophile antibodies (positive "differential heterophile"). Until specific antiviral therapy is available and shown to be advisable, the specific diagnosis of EBV infection in patients with typical mononucleosis syndromes usually is unnecessary. When the clinical presentation is uncomplicated, a complete blood count (including leukocyte differential) and a test for Paul-Bunnell heterophile antibodies usually suffice. These two tests may need to be repeated periodically during the first 3 to 4 weeks of illness before diagnostic results are achieved. The clinician should be aware that very young (<4 years of age) patients frequently do not develop a detectable heterophile antibody response during EBV-induced illness (Fig. 165–3).

It has been estimated that EBV causes 80 to 95 per cent of mononucleosis syndromes.[191] Other infectious agents, such as cytomegalovirus, *Toxoplasma gondii*, adenoviruses, rubella virus, and hepatitis A virus, occasionally are associated with mononucleosis-like clinical manifestations. These agents are not associated with the presence of Paul-Bunnell heterophile antibodies. However, most non-EBV infectious mononucleosis episodes in children remain of unknown etiology. Reports conflict on the rates of tonsillopharyngitis and cervical adenitis in these non-EBV mononucleosis episodes. In heterophile-negative cases of mononucleosis exhibiting both the clinical and the hematologic characteristics of the syndrome, the most likely known agents are EBV and cytomegalovirus.

Heterophile antibodies classically were measured as sheep erythrocyte agglutinins.[148] Beef, ox, and horse red blood cells also are agglutinated by the heterophile antibodies found in the serum of mononucleosis patients, but these heterophile antibodies do not bind to guinea pig kidney antigen extracts. These properties of mononucleosis heterophile antibodies distinguish them from the naturally occurring Forssman heterophile antibodies and from the heterophile antibodies found in serum sickness and other conditions. Thus, traditional tests for Paul-Bunnell heterophile antibodies employ absorptions of the test serum with beef or ox red blood cells (which remove Paul-Bunnell heterophile antibodies) and guinea pig kidney extract (which does not remove them). Tests in current use (e.g., Mono-Test, Mono-Diff, Mono-Spot) typically use horse red blood cells, which provide a more sensitive assay than sheep erythrocytes do. However, when horse erythrocyte agglutination tests are performed, the specificity of a positive result always should be confirmed by absorption of the serum with at least guinea pig kidney extract or preferably both guinea pig kidney extract and beef (or ox) red blood cells. Materials for the absorption steps are included in many, but not all, of the commercially available kits. Another heterophile antibody test, the beef (or ox) erythrocyte hemolysin assay, does not require absorptions of the test sera but is somewhat less sensitive than is horse erythrocyte agglutination testing. Other tests[56, 69, 121, 133] utilizing purified forms of heterophile antigen do not seem (with the possible exception of the immune adherence test)[119] to offer any significant advantages over the rapid slide test utilizing horse erythrocyte agglutination.

Other laboratory tests in patients with severe mononucleosis syndromes or in patients presenting with atypical clinical manifestations may indicate involvement of major organs of

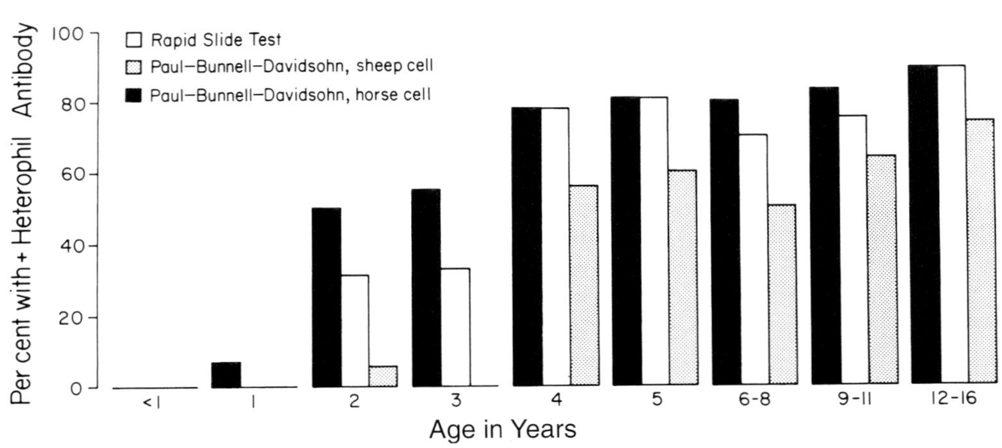

FIGURE 165–3. *Frequency of acute heterophile antibody responses detected in children of varying ages with documented Epstein-Barr virus infectious mononucleosis. Sera were examined by the qualitative method, the rapid slide test, and microtiter modification of a quantitative method (Paul-Bunnell-Davidsohn differential absorption test) utilizing both sheep and horse erythrocytes as agglutination indicator cells. (From Sumaya, C. V., and Ench, Y.: Epstein-Barr virus infectious mononucleosis in children. II. Heterophile antibody and viral-specific responses. Pediatrics 75:1011, 1985. Reproduced by permission of Pediatrics.)*

the body. For example, whereas at least 50 per cent of patients exhibit mild disturbances of liver function (e.g., mildly elevated aspartate and alanine aminotransferases),[193] only a few patients may develop signs of severe liver dysfunction (hyperbilirubinemia and grossly elevated liver enzymes) or even hepatic failure. Similarly, many patients develop antibodies to human erythrocyte antigens (e.g., antibodies to the *i* antigen), but only a few develop significant hemolytic anemia. Also, although neutropenia, at times reaching levels of less than 500/mm^3, is relatively common in the first week of illness, rare patients develop severe and prolonged neutropenias, pancytopenias, or marrow aplasia.

Epstein-Barr Virus Serology

The diagnosis of EBV infection by specific laboratory testing should be reserved for patients with atypical manifestations, lymphoproliferative diseases, or severe illness and for those with negative heterophile tests and prolonged or serious illness. In most cases, serologic (antibody) testing is the preferred mode of obtaining the specific viral diagnosis. Because the biologic activity of EBV is measured classically in lymphocyte transformation assays, virus isolation for EBV is cumbersome and generally impractical. Furthermore, as noted before, healthy children and adults not uncommonly exhibit pharyngeal excretion of EBV at a given time.[25, 137, 190, 192] Thus, positive results in EBV cultivation assays often are of questionable value in diagnosing the patient's disease. In contrast, the demonstration of viral antigens, viral nucleic acid, or virus-bearing cells in larger amounts than those found in normal seropositive persons or their demonstration in pathologic lesions may be of significant etiologic value.

The evolution of serologic response to EBV antigens after an acute EBV infection is depicted in Figure 165–4. By the time of clinical presentation of infectious mononucleosis, and probably other forms of primary EBV infection, most persons have an appreciable antibody response to the EBV VCA.[81, 194] In the case of primary infections (e.g., infectious mononucleosis), the initial serum often contains both IgG and IgM antibodies to VCA. Most children also have, or will shortly develop, antibodies to the EA complex, which sometimes are measured separately as antibodies to the restricted (R) or diffuse (D) components.[54, 194] During the early phase of primary infection, most persons do not have detectable antibodies to EBNA; a few have marginally detectable anti-EBNA titers. Thus, the serologic diagnosis of recent or current primary EBV infection typically comprises positive IgG and IgM anti-VCA response and negative anti-EBNA, with positive results in the anti-EA assay.

When a disease is not a consequence of primary infection but may be related to persistent or reactivated EBV infection (e.g., Burkitt lymphoma, nasopharyngeal carcinoma, some lymphomas of immunocompromised hosts, some chronic or atypical illnesses), the following serologic profile may be observed: positive IgG anti-VCA, often in high titer; usually negative IgM anti-VCA; often elevated anti-EA titer; and a positive anti-EBNA assay (although sometimes in low titer and occasionally undetectable).[71, 79, 80, 155, 184] Additionally, Miller and associates[136] have defined an unusual subgroup of patients with severe, chronic EBV infection whose sera contain a relatively deficient response to selective components of EBNA, EBNA-1 (K-EBNA) in this case.

IgM antibodies to VCA typically disappear within 2 to 3 months, and IgG antibodies to EA usually disappear within 6 to 12 months after infection; IgG anti-VCA and anti-EBNA antibodies persist for life and are indicative of a chronic virus-carrying state.[194] Some studies also have shown the persistence of anti-EA antibodies for several years after an acute EBV infection and the occasional appearance of anti-EA antibodies in healthy seropositive persons; the clinical or virologic import of this finding is not clear. Heterophile antibodies may persist for months, and sometimes a year or more, in persons who have recovered from infectious mononucleosis; they remain detectable longer (usually more than a year) when the more sensitive horse erythrocyte agglutinations and a quantitative method for determining the antibody response are employed.

Some studies[131, 160, 165] suggest that monitoring for decreases in anti-EBNA antibodies, in addition to such increased immunologic mediators as interleukin-4 and soluble CD 23 and increased circulating EBV (see next section, Epstein-Barr Virus Detection), may be useful in providing early serologic signs of EBV-associated tumor development in organ and bone marrow transplant recipients.

Molecular cloning of subregions of the EBV genome into high-expression plasmid vectors presently is being used to generate large amounts of pure proteins containing

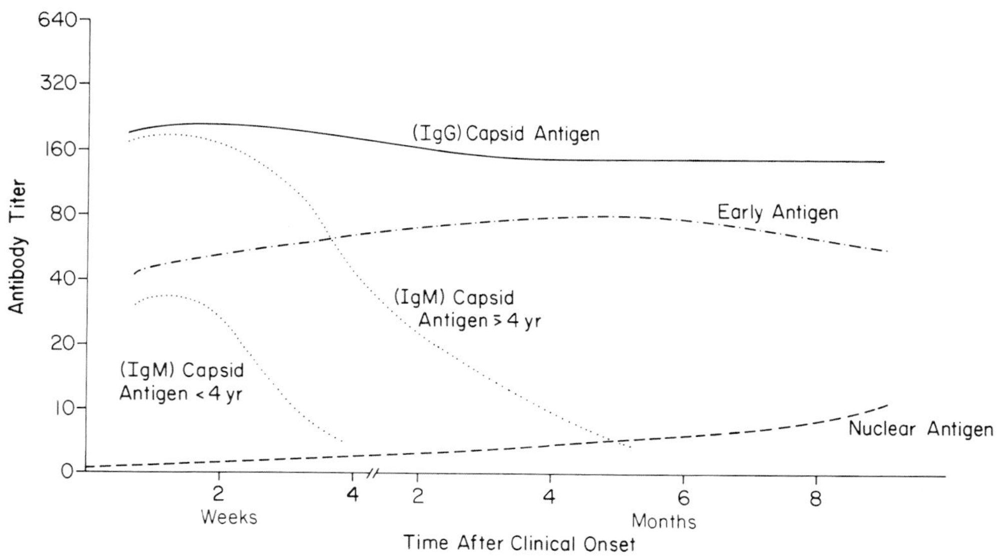

FIGURE 165–4. *Schematic representation of the evolution of various antibodies to various Epstein-Barr virus antigens in children with infectious mononucleosis, the prototype symptomatic primary Epstein-Barr virus infection. The titers are geometric mean values expressed as reciprocals of the serum dilution. The minimal titer tested for antibodies to capsid antigen and early antigen was 10 (1:10) and for nuclear antigen was 2.5 (1:2.5). The IgM response to capsid antigen was divided because of the significant differences noted according to age. (Adapted from Sumaya, C. V., and Ench, Y.: Epstein-Barr virus infectious mononucleosis in children. II. Heterophile antibody and viral-specific responses. Pediatrics 75:1011, 1985. Reproduced by permission of Pediatrics.)*

EBV-encoded polypeptide sequences. These methods are beginning to yield potentially better methods of EBV serodiagnosis. Enzyme-linked immunosorbent assays, for the measurement of antibody responses to a variety of purified EBV-encoded polypeptides, are being constructed. These tests, which have been approved by the Food and Drug Administration, are commercially available but have not been widely tested in children's sera. Because of this circumstance and some published data[122] suggesting problems in interpretation, results from these test kits should be viewed with caution in this age group.

Reliable performance and interpretation of the traditional immunofluorescence assays used in EBV serology require specialized training and experience and the use of appropriate standards and controls in the clinical laboratory. New developments in serologic testing should expand the understanding and definition of interactions between EBV and humans in various states of health and disease. Nevertheless, it will be important to establish the correlations between results obtained by the new tests and those obtained by traditional methods.

Epstein-Barr Virus Detection

In rare patients (e.g., some persons with lymphoproliferative disorders or atypical clinical illness), the serologic response to EBV antigens may be incomplete, lacking, or otherwise not helpful. In such situations, it may be necessary for etiologic purposes to demonstrate the presence of cells carrying EBV antigens (e.g., EBNA) or EBV nucleic acid in tissue sections or in blood.[10, 71, 155]

Immunofluorescence techniques may be used to detect such viral proteins as EBNA and latent membrane proteins in touch imprints of biopsy material or in frozen sections of cryopreserved tissue.[219] Various molecular methods (i.e., dot-blot hybridization, Southern blot hybridization, Western immunoblot, in situ hybridization, and polymerase chain reaction) have been developed to detect EBV genome and encoded proteins.[4] These techniques are useful for diagnostic (disease association and detection), epidemiologic, and pathogenetic (characterizing viral expression in tissues) purposes relevant to EBV infections.

TREATMENT

Supportive therapy usually is all that is required in uncomplicated infectious mononucleosis. This includes rest, fluids, and aspirin or acetaminophen if desired. In some patients who are severely symptomatic, short-term steroids (e.g., prednisone, up to 40 mg/m^2/day) may provide relief, but the long-term consequences of such steroid use are unknown, and most clinicians use steroids cautiously, if at all. A few patients with complicated illnesses (e.g., with stridor due to massively enlarged tonsils or paratracheal adenopathy, or with hematologic or neurologic complications) constitute the group for which steroids more commonly have been used. The small percentage of patients with group A beta-hemolytic streptococcal superinfection of the throat should be treated with appropriate doses of penicillin or erythromycin after documentation of this infection by throat culture or antigen detection. Additionally, it is customary to caution patients against marked physical activity and contact sports during recovery from the acute illness and for the period of significant organomegaly so that the risk of splenic rupture is minimized.

The insertion of an artificial airway may be replacing emergency tonsillectomy as the treatment of choice for complete airway obstruction produced by profound upper respiratory tract inflammation.[213] Nonoperative management of splenic rupture also has been introduced.[40]

Developments in antiviral drug therapy provide hope that effective, specific pharmacologic therapy for EBV infection may be available soon. At present, however, none of the approved antiviral agents has shown impressive activity against EBV. Adenine arabinoside has little significant activity against EBV. Acyclovir has been shown to suppress EBV replication transiently in virus-producing cell lines in vitro, and intravenous acyclovir has been used in large doses (e.g., 1500 mg/m^2/day, divided every 8 hours) in immunosuppressed patients with EBV-related lymphoproliferative disorders, reportedly with beneficial effect in some cases.[71] Acyclovir therapy has been ineffective in a number of other cases of serious illness, however.[146, 185] Trials of acyclovir in patients with mononucleosis resulted in reduced virus shedding in the throat but had little apparent impact on resolution of clinical symptoms.[7, 178, 202] Several other agents, such as congeners of acyclovir, E-5-(2-bromovinyl)-2'-deoxyuridine (BVDU), 9-(1,3-dihydroxy-2-propoxy-methyl) guanine (ganciclovir; DHPG), and several other nucleoside analogues exhibit greater in vitro effect against EBV than does acyclovir,[125, 126] but they have not been evaluated adequately by clinical trials.

Reports of the efficacy in infectious mononucleosis of azoles[72, 128] or cimetidine[60] require greater investigation before their general use is advocated. Preliminary studies with the use of anti–B-cell monoclonal antibodies[16, 115] and irradiated transplant donor leukocytes,[147] along with reduction of the patient's immunosuppressive medication, show that these measures may provide some (albeit variable) benefit in the treatment of severe EBV-induced lymphoproliferation disorders.

CLINICAL COURSE

The clinical course of most patients with infectious mononucleosis is one of gradual, uneventful recovery after an acute phase lasting several days to 3 or 4 weeks. Fever usually resolves within 2 weeks but occasionally lasts longer. Significant organomegaly usually resolves within 1 to 3 months. Recovery from the often severe fatigue can be prompt, but several months often are required for full return of a sense of well-being. Occasionally, the course in patients recovering from mononucleosis may be biphasic, with transient recrudescence of disease manifestations after a period of improvement. The prognosis for patients with unusually complicated courses of severe mononucleosis or for patients with atypical manifestations depends on the nature and severity of their illnesses. An accurate figure for the overall mortality rate from infectious mononucleosis in adults or children is not clear, although mortality is considered rare. In Penman's study[150] of 20 documented deaths, predominantly of young adults, the cause of death included neurologic complications, splenic rupture, secondary infection, hepatic failure, and myocarditis, in that order. EBV-induced aplastic anemia, a rare but dreaded hematologic complication, now is thought to have a better prognosis for eventual recovery if the patient can be supported successfully through the acute stages.[12, 113]

The course of lymphoproliferative disorders in transplant recipients on immunosuppressive therapy is variable, probably related to the heterogeneity among the EBV-driven lymphoid proliferations. Some lymphoproliferative disorders regress after a reduction in immunosuppression, whereas others progress and are lethal, in spite of aggressive therapy.[109, 180]

PREVENTION

Minimal enthusiasm has been generated in developing an EBV vaccine, although such a product could be of use in preventing severe EBV infections and lymphomas in high-risk groups, such as immunodeficient persons, transplant recipients, and those living in areas in which Burkitt lymphoma is endemic. Moreover, it has been considered that, perhaps, a vaccine also could establish causality between EBV and selected human tumors by decreasing tumor incidence among vaccinees. However, some problems are associated with the development of a vaccine, including the inability to produce large quantities of EBV by present techniques, the oncogenic potential of live vaccine strains, and the difficulty of immunizing children in the brief window period between natural viral acquisition and the disappearance of maternally transferable antibodies. With the generation of purified proteins from recombinantly cloned subregions of the EBV genome, potential subunit vaccine products have been identified. Investigations are ongoing with an envelope glycoprotein of EBV, free of viral DNA, that is immunogenic and protective (of lymphoma development) when inoculated in cotton-top tamarins.[42, 142]

References

1. Akaboshi, I., Katuskuki, T., Jamamoto, J., et al.: Unique pattern of Epstein-Barr virus specific antibodies in recurrent parotitis. Lancet *2*:1049, 1983.
2. Alfieri, C., Ghibu, F., and Joncas, J. H.: Lytic, nontransforming Epstein-Barr virus (EBV) from a patient with chronic active EBV infection. Can. Med. Assoc. J. *131*:1249–1252, 1984.
3. Alpert, G., and Fleisher, G. R.: Complications of infection with Epstein-Barr virus during childhood: A study of children admitted to the hospital. Pediatr. Infect. Dis. *3*:304–306, 1984.
4. Ambinder, R. F., and Mann, R. B.: Detection and characterization of Epstein-Barr virus in clinical specimens. Am. J. Pathol. *145*:239–252, 1994.
5. American Academy of Pediatrics: Infectious mononucleosis due to Epstein-Barr virus. *In* Peter, G. (ed.): 1994 Red Book: Report of the Committee on Infectious Diseases. 23rd ed. Elk Grove Village, American Academy of Pediatrics, 1991, pp. 273–275.
6. Anagnostopoulos, I., Hummel, M., Kreschel, C., et al.: Morphology, immunophenotype, and distribution of latently and/or productively Epstein-Barr virus-infected cells in acute infectious mononucleosis: Implications for the interindividual infection route of Epstein-Barr virus. Blood *85*:744–750, 1995.
7. Andersson, J., Britton, S., Ernberg, I., et al.: Effect of acyclovir on infectious mononucleosis: A double-blind, placebo controlled study. J. Infect. Dis. *153*:283–290, 1986.
8. Andiman, W. A., Eastman, R., Martin, K., et al.: Opportunistic lymphoproliferations associated with Epstein-Barr viral DNA in infants and children with AIDS. Lancet 2:1390–1393, 1985.
9. Andiman, W. A., McCarthy, P., Markowitz, R. I., et al.: Clinical, virologic, and serologic evidence of Epstein-Barr virus infections in association with childhood pneumonia. J. Pediatr. *99*:880, 1981.
10. Andiman, W., Gradoville, L., Heston, L., et al.: Use of cloned probes to detect Epstein-Barr viral DNA in tissues of patients with neoplastic and lymphoproliferative diseases. J. Infect. Dis. *148*:967–977, 1983.
11. Baer, R., Bankier, A. T., Biggin, M. D., et al.: DNA sequence and expression of the B95-8 Epstein-Barr virus genome. Nature *310*:207–211, 1984.
12. Barinski, B., Armstrong, G., Truman, J. T., et al.: Epstein-Barr virus in the bone marrow of patients with aplastic anemia. Ann. Intern. Med. *109*:695–704, 1988.
13. Baumgarten, E., Herbst, H., Schmitt, M., et al.: Life-threatening infectious mononucleosis: Is it correlated with virus-induced T cell proliferation? Clin. Infect. Dis. *19*:152–156, 1994.
14. Bechet, J. M., Fialkow, P. J., Nilsson, K., et al.: Immunoglobulin synthesis and glucose-6-phosphate dehydrogenase as cell markers in human lymphoblastoid cell lines. Exp. Cell Res. *89*:275–282, 1974.
15. Biggar, R. J., Gardiner, C., Lennette, E. T., et al.: Malaria, sex, and place of residence as factors in antibody response to Epstein-Barr virus in Ghana, West Africa. Lancet 2:115, 1981.
16. Blanche, S., LeDeist, F., Veber, F., et al.: Treatment of severe Epstein-Barr virus-induced polyclonal B-lymphocyte proliferations by anti-B-cell monoclonal antibodies. Ann. Intern. Med. *108*:199–203, 1988.
17. Borzy, M. S., Hong, R., Horowitz, S. D., et al.: Fatal lymphoma after transplantation of cultured thymus in children with combined immunodeficiency disease. N. Engl. J. Med. *301*:565, 1979.
18. Breinig, M. K., Zitelli, B., Starzl, T., et al.: Epstein-Barr virus, cytomegalovirus and other viral infections in children after liver transplantation. J. Infect. Dis. *156*:273–279, 1987.
19. Brichackek, B., Hirsch, I., Sibl, O., et al.: Association of some supraglottic laryngeal carcinomas with EB virus. Int. J. Cancer *32*:192, 1983.
20. Brown, N. A., Liu, C., Garcia, C. R., et al.: Gene rearrangements in B-lymphocytes cloned from patients with Epstein-Barr virus infections. Clin. Res. *33*:125A, 1985.
21. Brown, N. A., and Miller, G.: Immunoglobulin expression by human B-lymphocytes clonally transformed by Epstein-Barr virus. J. Immunol. *128*:24–29, 1982.
22. Brown, N., Smith, D., Miller, G., et al.: Infectious mononucleosis: A polyclonal transformation *in vivo*. J. Infect. Dis. *150*:517–522, 1984.
23. Brown, Z. A., and Stenchever, M. A.: Infectious mononucleosis and congenital anomalies. Am. J. Obstet. Gynecol. *131*:108–112, 1978.
24. Burkitt, D.: A sarcoma involving the jaws in African children. Br. J. Surg. *46*:218–223, 1958.
25. Chang, R. S., Lewis, J. P., and Abildgaard, C. F.: Prevalence of oropharyngeal excretors of leukocyte-transforming agents among a human population. N. Engl. J. Med. *289*:1325–1329, 1973.
26. Chang, R. S., Rosen, L., and Kapikian, A. Z.: Epstein-Barr virus infections in a nursery. Am. J. Epidemiol. *113*:22–29, 1981.
27. Clancy, R., Jenkins, E., and Firken, B.: Platelet defect of infectious mononucleosis. Br. Med. J. *2*:646, 1971.
28. Cleary, M. L., and Sklar, J.: Lymphoproliferative disorders in cardiac transplant recipients are multiclonal lymphomas. Lancet *2*:489–493, 1984.
29. Cleary, M. L., Warnke, R., and Sklar, J.: Monoclonality of lymphoproliferative lesions in cardiac transplant recipients. N. Engl. J. Med. *310*:477–482, 1984.
30. Cohen, L. K., Speck, S. H., Roberts, B. E., et al.: Identification and mapping of polypeptides encoded by the P3HR-1 strain of Epstein-Barr virus. Proc. Natl. Acad. Sci. U. S. A. *81*:4183–4187, 1984.
31. Connelly, K. P., and DeWitt, L. D.: Neurologic complications of infectious mononucleosis. Pediatr. Neurol. *10*:181–184, 1994.
32. Cooperman, S. M.: "Alice in Wonderland" syndrome as a presenting symptom of infectious mononucleosis in children. Clin. Pediatr. *16*:143–146, 1977.
33. Croce, C. M., Tsujimoto, Y., Erikson, J., et al.: Chromosome translocations and B-cell neoplasia. Lab. Invest. *51*:258–267, 1984.
34. Dalla-Favera, R., Bregni, M., Erikson, J., et al.: Human *c-myc onc* gene is located on the region of chromosome 8 that is translocated in Burkitt lymphoma cells. Proc. Natl. Acad. Sci. U. S. A. *79*:7824–7827, 1982.
35. Dambaugh, T., Raab-Traub, N., Heller, M., et al.: Variation among isolates of Epstein-Barr virus. Ann. N. Y. Acad. Sci. *354*:309–325, 1980.
36. deThe, G.: Is Burkitt's lymphoma related to perinatal infection by Epstein-Barr virus? Lancet *1*:335, 1977.
37. deThe, G., Geser, A., Day, N. E., et al.: Epidemiological evidence for causal relationship between Epstein-Barr virus and Burkitt's lymphoma from Ugandan prospective study. Nature *274*:756–761, 1978.
38. deThe, G., Ho, J. H. L., and Muir, C. S.: Nasopharyngeal carcinoma. *In* Evans, A. S. (ed.): Viral Infections of Humans. 2nd ed. New York, Plenum, 1982, pp. 621–652.
39. DeWaele, M., Thielemans, C., and VanCamp, B. K. G.: Characterization of immunoregulatory T cells in EBV-induced infectious mononucleosis by monoclonal antibodies. N. Engl. J. Med. *304*:460–462, 1981.
40. Ein, S. H., Shandling, B., and Simpson, J. S.: Nonoperative management of traumatic spleen in children: How and why. J. Pediatr. Surg. *113*:117, 1978.
41. Ellman, L., Carvalho, A., Jacobson, B. M., et al.: Platelet autoantibody in a case of infectious mononucleosis presenting as thrombocytopenic purpura. Am. J. Med. *55*:72, 1973.
42. Epstein, M. A.: Vaccination against Epstein-Barr virus: Current progress and future strategies. Lancet *2*:1425–1427, 1986.
43. Epstein, M. A., and Achong, B. G.: Morphology of the virus and of virus-induced cytopathologic changes. *In* Epstein, M. A., and Achong, B. G. (eds.): The Epstein-Barr Virus. New York, Springer-Verlag, 1979, pp. 23–37.
44. Epstein, M. A., Achong, B. G., and Barr, Y. M.: Virus particles in cultured lymphoblasts from Burkitt's lymphoma. Lancet *1*:702–703, 1964.
45. Epstein, M. A., Henle, G., Achong, B. G., et al.: Morphological and biological studies on a virus in cultured lymphoblasts from Burkitt's lymphoma. J. Exp. Med. *121*:761–770, 1965.
46. Eshel, G. M., Eyor, A., Lahat, E., et al.: Alice in Wonderland syndrome, a manifestation of acute Epstein-barr virus infection. Pediatr. Infect. Dis. *6*:68, 1987.
47. Evans, A. S., Niederman, J. C., and McCollum, R. W.: Seroepidemiologic studies of infectious mononucleosis with EB virus. N. Engl. J. Med. *279*:1121–1127, 1968.
48. Feorino, P. M., Humphrey, D., Hochberg, F., et al.: Mononucleosis-associated subacute sclerosing panencephalitis. Lancet *2*:530–532, 1975.
49. Fingeroth, J. D., Weis, J. J., Tedder, T. F., et al.: Epstein-Barr virus receptor

of human B lymphocytes is the C3d receptor CR2. Proc. Natl. Acad. Sci. U. S. A. *81*:4510–4514, 1984.
50. Fischer, D. K., Miller, G., Gradoville, L., et al.: Genome of a mononucleosis Epstein-barr virus contains DNA fragments previously regarded to be unique to Burkitt's lymphoma isolates. Cell *24*:543–553, 1981.
51. Fleisher, G. R., and Bolognese, R.: Epstein-barr virus infection in pregnancy: Report of a prospective study. J. Pediatr. *104*:374–379, 1984.
52. Fleisher, G., and Bolognese, R.: Persistent Epstein-barr virus infection and pregnancy. J. Infect. Dis. *147*:982–986, 1983.
53. Fleisher, G., and Bolognese, R.: Infectious mononucleosis during gestation: Report of three women and their infants studied prospectively. Pediatr. Infect. Dis. *3*:308–311, 1984.
54. Fleisher, G., Henle, W., Henle, G., et al.: Primary infection with Epstein-barr virus in infants in the United States: Clinical and serologic observations. J. Infect. Dis. *139*:553–558, 1979.
55. Fleisher, G., Schwartz, J., and Lennette, E.: Primary Epstein-Barr virus infection in association with Reye's syndrome. J. Pediatr. *97*:935, 1980.
56. Fletcher, M. A., Lo, T. M., Levey, B. A., et al.: Immunochemical studies of infectious mononucleosis. VI. A radioimmunoassay for the detection of infectious mononucleosis heterophil antibody and antigen. J. Immunol. Methods *14*:51, 1977.
57. Fu, S. M., Hurley, J. N., McCune, J. M., et al.: Pre-B cells and other possible precursor lymphoid cell lines derived from patients with X-linked agammaglobulinemia. J. Exp. Med. *152*:1519–1526, 1980.
58. Fu, S. M., and Hurley, J. N.: Human B-cell lines containing Epstein-barr virus but distinct from the common B-cell lymphoblastoid lines. Proc. Natl. Acad. Sci. U. S. A. *76*:6637–6640, 1979.
59. Goldberg, G. N., Fulginiti, V. A., Ray, G., et al.: In utero Epstein-barr virus (infectious mononucleosis) infection. J. A. M. A. *246*:1579–1581, 1981.
60. Goldstein, J. A.: Cimetidine and mononucleosis. Ann. Intern. Med. *99*:410–411, 1983. Letter.
61. Greenspan, J. S., Mastrucci, M. T., Leggott, P. J., et al.: Hairy leukoplakia in a child. AIDS *2*:143, 1988.
62. Grogan, E. A., Summer, W. P., Dowling, S., et al.: Two Epstein-barr viral nuclear neoantigens distinguished by gene transfer, serology and chromosome binding. Proc. Natl. Acad. Sci. U. S. A. *80*:7650–7653, 1983.
63. Grose, C., Gross, S., and Mackey, R.: Neurologic complications. *In* Schlossberg, D. (ed.): Monograph on Infectious Mononucleosis. New York, Springer-Verlag, 1989, pp. 49–68.
64. Grose, C., Henle, W., Henle, G., et al.: Primary Epstein-Barr virus infections in acute neurologic diseases. N. Engl. J. Med. *292*:392, 1975.
65. Gutensohn, N., and Cole, P.: Epidemiology of Hodgkin's disease in the young. Int. J. Cancer *19*:595–604, 1977.
66. Gutgesell, H. P.: Acute airway obstruction in infectious mononucleosis. Pediatrics *47*:141, 1971.
67. Gutsch, D. E., Marcu, K. B., and Kenney, S. C.: The Epstein-barr virus *BRLF1* gene product transactivates the murine and human c-*myc* promoters. Cell. Mol. Biol. *40*:747–760, 1994.
68. Haahr, S., Sommerlund, M., Christensen, T., et al.: A putative new retrovirus associated with multiple sclerosis and the possible involvement of Epstein-barr virus in this disease. Ann. N. Y. Acad. Sci. *724*:148–156, 1994.
69. Halbert, S. P., Anken, M., Henle, W., et al.: Detection of infectious mononucleosis heterophil antibody by a rapid, standardized enzyme-linked immunosorbent assay procedure. J. Clin. Microbiol. *15*:610, 1982.
70. Hamilton-Dutoit, S. J., Pallesen, G., Franzmann, M. B., et al.: AIDS-related lymphoma: Histopathology, immunophenotype, and association with Epstein-barr virus as demonstrated by in situ nucleic acid hybridization. Am. J. Pathol. *138*:149–163, 1991.
71. Hanto, D. W., Gajl-Peczalska, K. J., Frizzera, G., et al.: Epstein-barr virus induced polyclonal and monoclonal B-cell lymphoproliferative diseases occurring after renal transplantation. Ann. Surg. *198*:356–369, 1983.
72. Hedstrom, S. A., Mardh, P. A., and Repa, T.: Treatment of anginose infectious mononucleosis with metronidazole. Scand. J. Infect. Dis. *10*:7, 1978.
73. Heller, M., Dambaugh, T., and Kieff, E.: Epstein-barr virus DNA: Variation among viral DNAs from producer and nonproducer infected cells. J. Virol. *38*:632–648, 1981.
74. Henderson, E., Heston, L., Grogan, E., et al.: Radiobiological inactivation of Epstein-barr virus. J. Virol. *25*:51–59, 1978.
75. Henle, G., Henle, W., and Diehl, V.: Relation of Burkitt tumor associated herpes-type virus to infectious mononucleosis. Proc. Natl. Acad. Sci. U. S. A. *59*:94–101, 1968.
76. Henle, G., and Henle, W.: Immunofluorescence in cells derived from Burkitt's lymphoma. J. Bacteriol. *91*:1248–1256, 1966.
77. Henle, W., Diehl, V., Kohn, G., et al.: Herpes-type virus and chromosome marker in normal leukocytes after growth with irradiated Burkitt cells. Science *157*:1064–1065, 1967.
78. Henle, W., and Henle, G.: Immunology of Epstein-Barr virus. *In* Roizman, B. (ed.): The Herpesviruses. Vol. 1. New York, Plenum, 1982, pp. 209–252.
79. Henle, W., and Henle, G.: Epstein-barr virus–specific serology in immunologically compromised individuals. Cancer Res. *41*:4222–4225, 1981.
80. Henle, W., and Henle, G.: Epidemiologic aspects of Epstein-barr virus (EBV)–associated diseases. Ann. N. Y. Acad. Sci. *354*:326–331, 1980.
81. Henle, W., and Henle, G.: Evidence for an oncogenic potential of the Epstein-Barr virus. Cancer Res. *33*:1419, 1973.
82. Henle, W., Henle, G., and Horwitz, C. A.: Epstein-Barr virus specific diagnostic tests in infectious mononucleosis. Hum. Pathol. *5*:551, 1974.
83. Hennessy, K., and Kieff, E.: A second nuclear protein is encoded by Epstein-Barr virus in latent infection. Science *227*:1238–1240, 1985.
84. Hennessy, K., Fennewald, S., Hummel, M., et al.: A membrane protein encoded by Epstein-Barr virus in latent growth-transforming infection. Proc. Natl. Acad. Sci. U. S. A. *81*:7207–7211, 1984.
85. Ho, H. C., Ng, M. H., Kwan, H. C., et al.: Epstein-Barr virus–specific IgA and IgG serum antibodies in nasopharyngeal carcinoma. Br. J. Cancer *34*:655, 1976.
86. Ho, M., Jaffe, R., Miller, G., et al.: The frequency of Epstein-Barr virus infection and associated lymphoproliferative syndrome after transplantation and its manifestations in children. Transplantation *45*:719–727, 1988.
87. Ho, M., Miller, G., Atchison, R. W., et al.: Epstein-Barr virus infections and DNA hybridization studies in post-transplantation lymphoma and lymphoproliferative lesions: The role of primary infection. J. Infect. Dis. *152*:876, 1985.
88. Hoagland, R. J.: Infectious Mononucleosis. New York, Grune & Stratton, 1967.
89. Holmes, G. P., Kaplan, J. E., Stewart, J. A., et al.: A cluster of patients with a mononucleosis-like syndrome: Is Epstein-Barr virus the cause? J. A. M. A. *25*:2297–2302, 1987.
90. Hummel, M., and Kieff, E.: Mapping of polypeptides encoded by the Epstein-Barr virus genome in productive infection. Proc. Natl. Acad. Sci. U. S. A. *79*:5698–5702, 1982.
91. Hunter, K., Stagno, S., Capps, E., et al.: Prenatal screening of pregnant women for infections caused by cytomegalovirus, Epstein-Barr virus, herpesvirus, rubella, and *Toxoplasma gondii*. Am. J. Obstet. Gynecol. *145*:269–277, 1983.
92. Icart, J., Didier, J., Dalens, M., et al.: Prospective study of Epstein-Barr virus (EBV) infection during pregnancy. Biomedicine *34*:160–165, 1981.
93. Imai, S., Sugiura, M., Mizuno, F., et al.: African Burkitt's lymphoma: A plant, *Euphorbia tirucalli*, reduces Epstein-Barr virus–specific cellular immunity. Anticancer Res. *14*:933–936, 1994.
94. Jain, V. K., Judde, J. G., Max, E. E., et al.: Variable IgH chain enhancer activity in Burkitt's lymphomas suggests an additional, direct mechanism of c-*myc* deregulation. J. Immunol. *150*:5418–5428, 1993.
95. Johansson, B., Klein, G., Henle, W., et al.: Epstein-Barr virus associated antibody pattern in malignant lymphoma and leukemia. 1. Hodgkin's disease. Int. J. Cancer *6*:450–462, 1970.
96. Joncas, J. H., Alfieri, C., Leyritz-Wills, M., et al.: Simultaneous congenital infection with Epstein-Barr virus and cytomegalovirus. N. Engl. J. Med. *304*:1399–1403, 1981.
97. Joncas, J., Boucher, J., Granger-Julien, M., et al.: Epstein-Barr virus infection in the neonatal period and in childhood. Can. Med. Assoc. J. *110*:33, 1974.
98. Jones, J. J., Ray, C. G., Minnich, L. L., et al.: Evidence for active Epstein-Barr virus infection in patients with persistent, unexplained illnesses: Elevated anti-early antigen antibodies. Ann. Intern. Med. *102*:1–7, 1985.
99. Jones, J. F., Shurin, S., Abramowsky, C., et al.: T-cell lymphomas containing Epstein-Barr viral DNA in patients with chronic Epstein-Barr virus infections. N. Engl. J. Med. *318*:733–740, 1988.
100. Kamani, N., Kennedy, J., and Brandsma, J.: Burkitt lymphoma in a child with human immunodeficiency virus infection. J. Pediatr. *112*:241–244, 1988.
101. Karzon, D. T.: Infectious mononucleosis. Adv. Pediatr. *22*:231–265, 1976.
102. Katamine, S., Otsu, M., Tada, K., et al.: Epstein-Barr virus transforms precursor B-cells even before immunoglobulin gene rearrangements. Nature *309*:369–372, 1984.
103. Kaye, K. M., Izumi, K. M., Mosialos, G., et al.: The Epstein-Barr virus LMP1 cytoplasmic carboxy terminus is essential for B-lymphocyte transformation: Fibroblast cocultivation complements a critical function within the terminal 155 residues. J. Virol. *69*:675–683, 1995.
104. Kieff, E., Dambaugh, T., Heller, M., et al.: The biology and chemistry of Epstein-Barr virus. J. Infect. Dis. *146*:506–517, 1982.
105. Kieff, E., and Liebowitz, D.: Epstein-Barr virus and its replication. *In* Fields, B. N., and Knipe, D. M. (eds.): Virology. New York, Raven Press, 1990, pp. 1889–1920.
106. Kikuta, H., Nakanishi, M., Sakiyama, Y., et al.: Chronic active Epstein-Barr virus (EBV) infection is associated with clonotypic intracellular terminal regions of the EBV. J. Infect. Dis. *160*:546–547, 1989.
107. Kintner, C. R., and Sugden, B.: The structure of the termini of the DNA of Epstein-Barr virus. Cell *17*:661–671, 1979.
108. Klein, G.: The role of gene dosage and genetic transpositions in carcinogenesis. Nature *294*:313–318, 1981.
109. Knowles, D. M., Cesarman, E., Chadburn, A., et al.: Correlative morphologic and molecular genetic analysis demonstrates three distinct categories of posttransplantation lymphoproliferative disorders. Blood *85*:552–565, 1995.
110. Konno, M., Kikuta, S., and Shikawa, H.: A possible relationship between hepatitis B antigen negative papular acrodermatitis and Epstein-Barr virus. J. Pediatr. *101*:222–224, 1982.
111. Kurland, G., and Orenstein, D. M. Complications of pediatric lung and heart-lung transplantation. Curr. Opin. Pediatr. *6*:262–271, 1994.
112. Landau, Z., Gross, R., Sanilevich, A., et al.: Presence of infective Epstein-

Barr virus in the urine of patients with infectious mononucleosis. J. Med. Virol. *44*:229–233, 1994.

113. Lazarus, K. H., and Baehner, R. L.: Aplastic anemia complicating infectious mononucleosis: A case report and review of the literature. Pediatrics *67*:907–910, 1981.
114. Le, C. T., Chang, S., and Lysson, M. H.: Epstein-Barr infections in pregnancy: A prospective study and review of the literature. Am. J. Dis. Child. *137*:466–468, 1983.
115. Leblond, V., Sutton, L., Dorent, R., et al.: Lymphoproliferative disorders after organ transplantation: A report of 24 cases observed in a single center. J. Clin. Oncol. *13*:961–968, 1995.
116. Leder, P., Battey, J., Lenoir, G., et al.: Translocations among antibody genes in human cancer. Science *222*:765–771, 1983.
117. Lee, E. S., Locker, J., Nalesnik, M., et al.: The association of Epstein-Barr virus with smooth-muscle tumors occurring after organ transplantation. N. Engl. J. Med. *332*:19–25, 1995.
118. Lekstrom-Himes, J., Dale, J. K., Kingma, D. W., et al.: Periodic illness associated with EBV. Clin. Infect. Dis. *22*:22–27, 1996.
119. Lennette, E. T., Henle, G., Henle, W., et al.: Heterophil antigen in bovine sera detectable by immune adherence hemagglutination with infectious mononucleosis sera. Infect. Immun. *19*:923, 1978.
120. Lerner, M. R., Andrews, N. C., Miller, G., et al.: Two small RNAs encoded by Epstein-Barr virus and complexed with protein are precipitated by antibodies from patients with systemic lupus erythematosus. Proc. Natl. Acad. Sci. U. S. A. *78*:805–809, 1981.
121. Levely, B. A., Lo, T. M., Caldwell, K. W., et al.: Latex test for serodiagnosis of infectious mononucleosis. J. Clin. Microbiol. *11*:256, 1980.
122. Levine, D., Tilton, R. C., Parry, M. F., et al.: False-positive EBNA IgM and IgG antibody tests for infectious mononucleosis in children. Pediatrics *94*:892–894, 1994.
123. Leyvraz, S., Henle, W., Chahinian, A. P., et al.: Association of Epstein-Barr virus with thymic carcinoma. N. Engl. J. Med. *312*:1296, 1985.
124. Liebowitz, D.: Nasopharyngeal carcinoma: The Epstein-Barr virus association. Semin. Oncol. *21*:376–381, 1994.
125. Lin, J. C., Smith, M. C., and Pagano, J. S.: Prolonged inhibitory effect of 9-(1,3-dihydroxy-2-propoxymethyl) guanine against replication of Epstein-Barr virus. J. Virol. *50*:50–55, 1984.
126. Lin, J. C., Smith, M. C., Cheng, Y. C., et al.: Epstein-Barr virus: Inhibition of replication by three new drugs. Science *221*:578–579, 1983.
127. Lindahl, T., Adams, A., Bjursell, G., et al.: Covalently closed circular duplex DNA of Epstein-Barr virus in a human lymphoid cell line. J. Mol. Biol. *102*:511–530, 1976.
128. Lundberg, C., Lonnroth, J., Marklund, G., et al.: Tindazole in the treatment of infections of the upper respiratory tract. Scand. J. Infect. Dis. *26*(Suppl.):130, 1981.
129. MacMahon, E. M. E., Glass, J. D., Hayward, S. D., et al.: Epstein-Barr virus in AIDS-related primary central nervous systems lymphoma. Lancet *338*:969–973, 1991.
130. McClain, K. L., Leach, C. T., Jenson, H. B., et al.: Association of Epstein-Barr virus with leiomyosarcomas in young people with AIDS. N. Engl. J. Med. *332*:12–18, 1995.
131. Martinez, O. M., Villanueva, J., Lawrence-Miyasaki, L., et al.: Viral and immunologic aspects of Epstein-Barr virus infection in pediatric liver transplant recipients. Transplantation *59*:524–529, 1995.
132. Masucci, M. G., and Ernberg, I.: Epstein-Barr virus: Adaptation to a life within the immune system. Trends Microbiol. *2*:12–30, 1994.
133. Milgrom, F., Loza, U., and Kano, K.: Double diffusion in gel tests with Paul–Bunnell antibodies of infectious mononucleosis sera. Int. Arch. Allergy Appl. Immunol. *48*:82, 1975.
134. Miller, G.: Regions of the EBV genome involved in latency and lymphocyte immortalization. Prog. Med. Virol. *30*:107–128, 1984.
135. Miller, G.: Burkitt lymphoma. *In* Evans, A. S. (ed.): Viral Infections of Humans. 2nd ed. New York, Plenum, 1982, pp. 599–619.
136. Miller, G., Grogan, E., Rowe, D., et al.: Selective lack of antibody to a component of EB nuclear antigen in patients with chronic active Epstein-Barr virus infection. J. Infect. Dis. *156*:26–35, 1987.
137. Miller, G., Niederman, J. C., and Andrews, L. L.: Prolonged oropharyngeal excretion of Epstein-Barr virus after infectious mononucleosis. N. Engl. J. Med. *288*:229–232, 1973.
138. Miller, H. C., Clifford, S. H., Smith, C. A., et al.: Study of the relation of congenital malformations to maternal rubella and other infections: Preliminary report. Pediatrics *3*:259–270, 1949.
139. Nemerow, G. R., and Cooper, N. R.: Early events in the infection of human B-lymphocytes by Epstein-Barr virus: The internalization process. Virology *132*:186–198, 1984.
140. Niederman, J. C., Evans, A. S., Subrahmanyan, L., et al.: Prevalence, incidence, and persistence of EB virus antibody in young adults. N. Engl. J. Med. *282*:361, 1970.
141. Niederman, J. C., McCollum, R. W., Henle, G., et al.: Infectious mononucleosis. J. A. M. A. *203*:205–209, 1968.
142. Niedobitek, G., Agathanggelou, A., Finerty, S., et al.: Latent Epstein-Barr virus infection in cottontop tamarins. Am. J. Pathol. *145*:969–978, 1994.
143. Niedobitek, G., Herbst, H., Young, L. S., et al.: Patterns of Epstein-Barr virus infection in non-neoplastic lymphoid tissue. Blood *79*:2520–2526, 1992.
144. Niedobitek, G., and Young, L. S.: Epstein-Barr virus persistence and virus-associated tumours. Lancet *343*:333–335, 1994.
145. Nilsson, K.: The nature of lymphoid cell lines and their relationship to the virus. *In* Epstein, M. A., and Achong, B. G. (eds.): The Epstein-Barr Virus. New York, Springer-Verlag, 1979, pp. 225–281.
146. Pagano, J. S., and Datta, A. K.: Perspectives on interactions of acyclovir with Epstein-Barr and other herpes viruses. *In* King, H., and Galasso, G. (eds.): Acyclovir Symposium. Am. J. Med. *73*(Suppl.):18–26. New York, Technical Publishing, 1982.
147. Papadopoulos, E. B., Ladanyi, M., Emanuel, D., et al.: Infusions of donor leukocytes to treat Epstein-Barr virus–associated lymphoproliferative disorders after allogeneic bone marrow transplantation. N. Engl. J. Med. *330*:1185-1191, 1994.
148. Paul, J. R., and Bunnell, W. W.: The presence of heterophile antibodies in infectious mononucleosis. Am. J. Med. Sci. *183*:90–104, 1932.
149. Pearson, G. R., Neel, B. G., Weiland, L. H., et al.: Antibody-dependent cellular cytotoxicity and disease course in North American patients with nasopharyngeal carcinoma: A prospective study. Int. J. Cancer *33*:777–782, 1984.
150. Penman, H. G.: Fatal infectious mononucleosis: A critical review. J. Clin. Pathol. *23*:765–771, 1970.
151. Petti, L., and Kieff, E.: A sixth Epstein-Barr virus nuclear antigen (EBNA 3B) is expressed in latently infected growth-transformed lymphocytes. J. Virol. *62*:2173–2178, 1988.
152. Pope, J. H., Horne, M. N. K., and Scott, W.: Transformation of foetal human leukocytes *in vitro* by filtrates of a human leukemic cell line containing herpes-like virus. Int. J. Cancer *3*:857–866, 1968.
153. Portman, M., Ingall, D., and Westenfelder, G.: Peritonsillar abscess complicating infectious mononucleosis. J. Pediatr. *104*:742, 1984.
154. Preciado, M. V., De-Matteo, E., Diez, B., et al.: Epstein-Barr virus (EBV) latent membrane protein (LMP) in tumor cells of Hodgkin's disease in pediatric patients. Med. Pediatr. Oncol. *24*:1–5, 1995.
155. Purtilo, D. T., Tatsumi, E., Manolov, G., et al.: Epstein-Barr virus as an etiological agent in the pathogenesis of lymphoproliferative and aproliferative diseases in immune deficient patients. Int. Rev. Exp. Pathol. *27*:112–183, 1985.
156. Raab-Traub, N.: Epstein-Barr virus infection in nasopharyngeal carcinoma. Infect. Agents Dis. *1*:173–184, 1992.
157. Reedman, B. M., and Klein, G.: Cellular localization of an Epstein-Barr virus (EBV)–associated complement-fixing antigen in producer and non-producer lymphoblastoid cell lines. Int. J. Cancer *11*:499–520, 1973.
158. Reisman, M. D., and Greco, M. A.: Virus-associated hemophagocytic syndrome due to Epstein-Barr virus. Hum. Pathol. *15*:290, 1982.
159. Rickinson, A. B., Moss, D. J., Wallace, L. E., et al.: Long-term T-cell–mediated immunity to Epstein-Barr virus. Cancer Res. *41*:4216–4221, 1981.
160. Riddler, S. A., Breinig, M. C., and McKnight, J. L.: Increased levels of circulating Epstein-Barr virus (EBV)–infected lymphocytes and decreased EBV nuclear antigen antibody responses are associated with the development of posttransplant lymphoproliferative disease in solid-organ transplant recipients. Blood *84*:972–984, 1994.
161. Robinson, J. E., Brown, N., Andiman, W., et al.: Diffuse polyclonal lymphoma during primary infection with Epstein-Barr virus. N. Engl. J. Med. *302*:1293–1297, 1980.
162. Robinson, J. E., Smith, D., and Niederman, J.: Plasmacytic differentiation of circulating Epstein-Barr virus–infected B lymphocytes during acute infectious mononucleosis. J. Exp. Med. *153*:235–244, 1981.
163. Robinson, J., Smith, D., and Niederman, J.: Mitotic EBNA-positive lymphocytes in peripheral blood during infectious mononucleosis. Nature *287*:334–335, 1980.
164. Rocchi, G., de Felia, A., Ragona, G., et al.: Quantitative evaluation of Epstein-Barr virus–infected mononuclear peripheral blood leukocytes in infectious mononucleosis. N. Engl. J. Med. *296*:132, 1977.
165. Rooney, C. M., Loftin, S. K., Holladay, M. S., et al.: Early identification of Epstein-Barr virus–associated post-transplantation lymphoproliferative disease. Br. J. Haematol. *89*:98–103, 1995.
166. Rowley, J. D.: Identification of the constant chromosome regions involved in human hematologic malignant disease. Science *216*:749–751, 1982.
167. Saemundsen, A. K., Alback, H., Hansen, J. P. H., et al.: Epstein-Barr virus in nasopharyngeal and salivary gland carcinomas of Greenland Eskimos. Br. J. Cancer *46*:721, 1982.
168. Schooley, R. T., Arbit, D. I., Henle, W., et al.: T-lymphocyte subset interactions in the cell-mediated immune response to Epstein-Barr virus. Cell Immunol. *86*:402–412, 1984.
169. Schooley, R. T., Carey, R. W., Miller, G., et al.: Chronic Epstein-Barr virus infection associated with fever and interstitial pneumonitis. Ann. Intern. Med. *104*:636–643, 1986.
170. Shearer, W. T., Ritz, J., Finegold, M. J., et al.: Epstein-Barr virus–associated B-cell proliferations of diverse clonal origins after bone marrow transplantation in a 12-year-old patient with severe combined immunodeficiency. N. Engl. J. Med. *312*:1151, 1985.
171. Shian, W. J., and Chi, C. S.: Sudden hearing loss caused by Epstein-Barr virus. Pediatr. Infect. Dis. J. *13*:756–758, 1994.
172. Shibata, D., Tokunaga, M., Uemura, Y., et al.: Association of Epstein-Barr virus with undifferentiated gastric carcinomas with intense lymphoid

infiltration: Lymphoepithelioma-like carcinoma. Am. J. Pathol. *139*:467–474, 1991.
173. Shiramizu, B., Barriga, F., Neequaye, J., et al.: Patterns of chromosomal breakpoint locations in Burkitt' lymphoma: Relevance to geography and Epstein-Barr virus association. Blood *77*:1516–1526, 1991.
174. Shope, T., Dechairo, D., and Miller, G.: Malignant lymphoma in cottontop marmosets after inoculation with Epstein-Barr virus. Proc. Natl. Acad. Sci. U. S. A. *70*:2487–2491, 1973.
175. Shurin, S. B.: Infectious mononucleosis. Pediatr. Clin. North Am. *26*:315, 1979.
176. Sixbey, J. W., Lemon, S. M., and Pagano, J. S.: A second site for Epstein-Barr virus shedding: The uterine cervix. Lancet *2*:1122–1124, 1986.
177. Sixbey, J. W., Nedrud, J. G., Raab-Traub, N., et al.: Epstein-Barr virus replication in oropharyngeal epithelial cells. N. Engl. J. Med. *310*:1225–1230, 1984.
178. Sixbey, J. W., Pagano, J. S., and Sullivan, J. L.: Treatment of infectious mononucleosis with intravenous acyclovir. Clin. Res. *31*:542A, 1983.
179. Sixbey, J. W. and Yao, Q. Y.: Immunoglobulin A–induced shift of Epstein-Barr virus tissue tropism. Science *255*:1578–1580, 1992.
180. Sokal, E. M., Caragiozoglou, T., Lamy, M., et al.: Epstein-Barr virus serology and Epstein-Barr virus associated lymphoproliferative disorders in pediatric liver transplant recipients. Transplantation *56*:1394–1398, 1993.
181. Straus, S. E., Tosato, G., Armstrong, G., et al.: Persisting illness and fatigue in adults with evidence of Epstein-Barr virus infection. Ann. Intern. Med. *102*:7–16, 1985.
182. Su, I. J., Chen, R. L., Lin, D. T, et al.: Epstein-Barr virus infects T lymphocytes in childhood EBV-associated hemophagocytic syndrome in Taiwan. Am. J. Pathol. *144*:1219–1225, 1994.
183. Su, I. J., Hsieh, H. C., Lin, K. H., et al.: Aggressive peripheral T-cell lymphomas containing Epstein-Barr viral DNA: A clinicopathologic and molecular analysis. Blood *79*:799–808, 1991.
184. Sullivan, J. L.: Epstein-Barr virus and the X-linked lymphoproliferative syndrome. Adv. Pediatr. *30*:365–399, 1983.
185. Sullivan, J. L., Byron, K. S., Brewster, F. E., et al.: Treatment of life-threatening Epstein-Barr virus infections with acyclovir. *In* King, H., and Galasso, G. (eds.): Acyclovir Symposium. Am. J. Med. *73*(Suppl.):262–266. New York, Technical Publishing, 1982.
186. Sumaya, C. V.: Periodic illness associated with Epstein-Barr virus. Clin. Infect. Dis. *22*:28–29, 1996.
187. Sumaya, C. V.: Serologic and virologic epidemiology of Epstein-Barr virus: Relevance to chronic fatigue syndrome. Rev. Infect. Dis. *13*:S19–S25, 1991.
188. Sumaya, C. V.: Atypical presentations. *In* Schlossberg, D. (ed.): Monograph on Infectious Mononucleosis. New York, Springer-Verlag, 1989, pp. 69–79.
189. Sumaya, C. V.: Primary Epstein-Barr virus infections in children. Pediatrics *59*:15, 1977.
190. Sumaya, C. V.: Epidemiologic study of leukocyte transforming agent in a general population. J. Clin. Microbiol. *2*:520–523, 1975.
191. Sumaya, C. V., and Ench, Y.: Childhood infectious mononucleosis-like illness not associated with Epstein-Barr virus. Pediatr. Res. *21*:336A, 1987.
192. Sumaya, C. V., and Ench, Y.: Epstein-Barr virus in families: The role of children with infectious mononucleosis. J. Infect. Dis. *154*:842, 1986.
193. Sumaya, C. V., and Ench, Y.: Epstein-Barr virus infectious mononucleosis in children. I. Clinical and general laboratory findings. Pediatrics *75*:1003–1010, 1985.
194. Sumaya, C. V., and Ench, Y.: Epstein-Barr virus infectious mononucleosis in children. II. Heterophil antibody and viral-specific responses. Pediatrics *75*:1011, 1985.
195. Sumaya, C. V., Henle, W., Henle, G., et al.: Seroepidemiologic study of Epstein-Barr virus infections in a rural community. J. Infect. Dis. *131*:403, 1975.
196. Sumaya, C. V., Myers, L. W., Ellison, G. W., et al.: Increased prevalence and titer of Epstein-Barr virus antibodies in patients with multiple sclerosis. Ann. Neurol. *17*:371, 1985.
197. Summers, W. I., Grogan, E. A., Shedd, N. D., et al.: Stable expression in mouse cells of a nuclear neoantigen after transfer of a 3.4 megadalton cloned fragment of Epstein-Barr virus DNA. Proc. Natl. Acad. Sci. U. S. A. *79*:5688–5692, 1982.
198. Taub, R., Kirsch, I., Morton, C., et al.: Translocation of the c-*myc* gene into the immunoglobulin heavy chain locus in human Burkitt lymphoma and murine plasmacytoma cells. Proc. Natl. Acad. Sci. U. S. A. *79*:7837–7841, 1982.
199. Thorley-Lawson, D. A., Chess, L., and Strominger, J. L.: Suppression of in vitro Epstein-Barr virus infection: A new role for adult human T-lymphocytes. J. Exp. Med. *146*:495–508, 1977.
200. Tosato, G., Magrath, I., Koski, I., et al.: Activation of suppressor T-cells during Epstein-Barr virus–induced infectious mononucleosis. N. Engl. J. Med. *301*:1133–1137, 1979.
201. Tsutsumi, H., Kamazaki, H., Nakata, S., et al.: Sequential development of acute meningoencephalitis and transverse myelitis caused by Epstein-Barr virus during infectious mononucleosis. Pediatr. Infect. Dis. J. *13*:665–667, 1994.
202. Van Der Horst, C. M., Joncas, J., Ahronheim, G., et al.: Lack of effect of peroral acyclovir for the treatment of acute infectious mononucleosis. J. Infect. Dis. *164*:788–792, 1991.
203. Veltri, R. W., Sprinkle, P. M., and McClung, J. E.: Epstein-Barr virus associated with episodes of recurrent tonsillitis. Arch. Otolaryngol. *101*:552, 1975.
204. Volsky, D. J., Gross, T., Sinangil, F., et al.: Expression of Epstein-Barr virus (EBV) DNA and cloned DNA fragments in human lymphocytes following Sendai virus envelope-mediated gene transfer. Proc. Natl. Acad. Sci. U. S. A. *81*:5926–5930, 1984.
205. Wallace, L. E., Rickinson, A. B., Rowe, M., et al.: Epstein-Barr virus–specific cytotoxic T-cell clones restricted through a single HLA antigen. Nature *297*:413–415, 1982.
206. Weigel, R., and Miller, G.: Major EBV specific cytoplasmic transcripts in a cellular clone of the HR-1 Burkitt lymphoma line during latency and after induction of viral replicative cycle by phorbol esters. Virology *125*:287–298, 1983.
207. Weigle, K. A., Sumaya, C. V., and Montiel, M.: Changes in T lymphocyte subsets in childhood Epstein-Barr virus infectious mononucleosis. J. Clin. Immunol. *3*:151, 1983.
208. Weinblatt, M. E.: Immune thrombocytopenic purpura evolving into aplastic anemia in association with Epstein-Barr virus infection. Am. J. Pediatr. Hematol.-Oncol. *13*:465–469, 1991.
209. Weiss, L. M., Movahed, L. A., Warnke, R. A., et al.: Detection of Epstein-Barr virus genomes in Reed–Sternberg cells of Hodgkin's disease. N. Engl. J. Med. *320*:502–506, 1989.
210. Williams, L. L., Lowery, H. W., and Glaser, R.: Sudden hearing loss following infectious mononucleosis: Possible effect of altered immunoregulation. Pediatrics *75*:102, 1985.
211. Wilson, G., and Miller, G.: Recovery of Epstein-Barr virus from nonproducer neonatal human lymphoid cell transformants. Virology *95*:351–358, 1979.
212. Wolf, H., Haus, M., and Wilmes, E.: Persistence of Epstein-Barr virus in the parotid gland. J. Virol. *51*:795–798, 1984.
213. Wolfe, J. A., and Rowe, L. D.: Upper airway obstruction in infectious mononucleosis. Ann. Otol. Rhinol. Laryngol. *89*:430, 1980.
214. Woodroffe, A. J., Ros, P. G., Meadows, R., et al.: Nephritis in infectious mononucleosis. Q. J. Med. *43*:451, 1974.
215. Yao, M., Cheng, A. L., Su, I. J., et al.: Clinicopathological spectrum of haemophagocytic syndrome in Epstein-Barr virus–associated peripheral T-cell lymphoma. Br. J. Haematol. *87*:535–543, 1994.
216. Yao, Q. Y., Ogan, P., Rowe, M., et al.: The Epstein-Barr virus–host balance in acute infectious mononucleosis patients receiving acyclovir anti-viral therapy. Int. J. Cancer *43*:61–66, 1989.
217. Yates, J. L., Warren, N., and Sugden, B.: Stable replication of plasmids derived from Epstein-Barr virus in various mammalian cells. Nature *313*:812–815, 1985.
218. Yates, J., Warren, N., Reisman, D., et al.: A *cis*-acting element from the Epstein-Barr viral genome that permits stable replication of recombinant plasmids in latently infected cells. Proc. Natl. Acad. Sci. U. S. A. *81*:3806–3810, 1984.
219. Young, L., Alfieri, C., Hennessy, K., et al.: Expression of Epstein-Barr virus transformation-associated genes in tissues of patients with EBV lymphoproliferative disease. N. Engl. J. Med. *21*:1080–1085, 1989.
220. Ziegler, J. L.: Burkitt's lymphoma. N. Engl. J. Med. *305*:735–745, 1981.
221. Ziegler, J. L., Beckstead, J. A., Volberding, P. A., et al.: Non-Hodgkin's lymphoma in 90 homosexual men: Relation to generalized lymphadenopathy and the acquired immunodeficiency syndrome. N. Engl. J. Med. *311*:565–570, 1984.

166

Human Herpesviruses 6, 7, and 8

Charles Grose

Before 1986, there were five known human herpesviruses (HHVs). These included herpes simplex virus (HSV) types 1 (oral) and 2 (genital), cytomegalovirus (CMV), varicella-zoster virus (VZV), and Epstein-Barr virus (EBV). The herpesviruses are important pathogens, causing a variety of childhood diseases that are described in other chapters of this textbook. An inherent characteristic of herpesviruses is their ability to form a latent infection, in which the viral genome continues to reside within the host. When the virus reactivates, it often causes further symptoms and signs. Thus, herpesviruses cause a spectrum of illnesses over the lifetime of the infected human host. Over the last decade, three novel herpesviruses have been discovered. They have been designated as HHV-6 and HHV-7, whereas the newest member of the family tentatively has been called either Kaposi sarcoma–associated herpesvirus (KSHV) or HHV-8. The viruses and the diseases they cause are described in this chapter.

HUMAN HERPESVIRUSES 6 AND 7

One unexpected consequence of the epidemic of AIDS was the discovery of a new human DNA virus. The virus first was isolated from the white blood cells of six patients with lymphoproliferative disorders, two of whom had AIDS.[24] The virus was propagated by subsequent infection of phytohemagglutinin-stimulated human leukocytes. Further electron-microscopic characterization of the cultured virus demonstrated similarities to a herpesvirus, including (1) an icosahedral capsid composed of 162 capsomers covered by a lipid membrane and (2) an enveloped particle with a diameter of 200 nm (Fig. 166–1). Because the virus was isolated originally from B lymphocytes, the agent was designated human B-lymphotropic virus (HBLV). However, this apparent tropism for B lymphocytes was not confirmed by other investigators, who found that the virus preferentially infected T lymphocytes and not B lymphocytes.[16] When they analyzed the virally infected cells with monoclonal antibodies, they discovered that most exhibited the T-cell–associated CD4 molecule. Thus, the initial designation of HBLV seems ill suited. Most virologists have accepted the HHV-6 appellation.

The DNA sequence and the deduced amino acid sequence of a major portion (21 kilobases) of the HHV-6 genome have been published.[13] Calculation of the percentage of amino acid identity shared by HHV-6 proteins with those in other herpesviruses revealed that HHV-6 proteins resembled most closely those of human CMV. Although related, the CMV genome composed of 240-kb pairs is considerably larger than that of HHV-6. The strains of HHV-6 have been divided into group A and group B. The HHV-6 isolates related to prototype strain U1102 have been called group A, whereas those related to strain Z29 have been designated group B. In 1990, while searching for additional strains of HHV-6, Frenkel and coworkers[11] isolated a new T-lymphotropic herpesvirus that was designated HHV-7. HHV-7 is related closely at a genetic level to HHV-6 and to a lesser degree to CMV.[6] All three of these agents are subclassified as beta-herpesviruses.

Most persons contract their primary HHV-6 infection before the age of 5 years; adult populations from the United States, Sweden, and Japan have a seroprevalence rate above 80 per cent. In infants and young children, group B strains of HHV-6 appear to be a major cause of the disease roseola (exanthem subitum). Roseola is discussed at greater length in Chapter 68. Children also may contract a primary HHV-6 infection without manifesting a rash. After acute infection, HHV-6 forms a latent infection, probably in T lymphocytes. Endogenous virus reactivates in adults with immunosuppressive disorders, such as AIDS, although reactivation has not been associated with a specific disease entity. Seronegative recipients of organ transplants may acquire a primary HHV-6 infection from latent virus in the donor organ. In a small number of infants, acute HHV-7 infection appears to cause a roseola illness much like acute HHV-6 infection.

DISEASES CAUSED BY HERPESVIRUSES TYPES 6 AND 7

Soon after the HHV-6 agent was discovered, virologists investigated the seroprevalence of this infection among the United States population. Several hundred sera collected before blood donation by healthy adults from Minneapolis and Kansas City were screened for antibodies to HHV-6; 81 to 88 per cent of the samples had detectable levels of antiviral reactivity. These results clearly showed that the majority of adults in the United States had prior exposure to HHV-6 infection.[25] In a similar serologic survey in Sweden, 97 per cent of adults had detectable HHV-6 antibody.[15] Further stud-

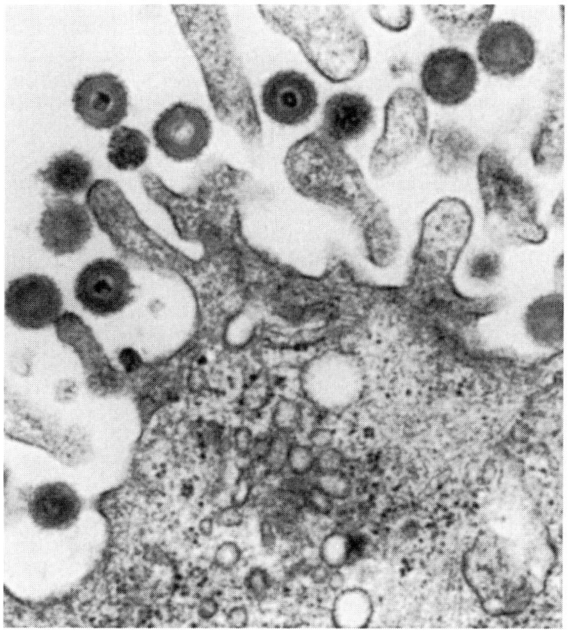

FIGURE 166–1. *Electron micrograph of cultured mononuclear cells infected with HHV-6. Several enveloped viral particles are visible in the extracellular area. (Courtesy of Dr. Y. Asano.)*

ies in a pediatric population in the state of North Carolina demonstrated that most newborn infants had maternally derived anti–HHV-6 antibody, which disappeared by 3 months of age.[25] Thereafter, many young children quickly acquired de novo antibody produced in response to exposure to the infectious agent.[25] The rate of seropositivity reached 100 per cent in some studies in young American children,[3] and in Sweden the percentage was about 60 per cent at 1 year of age and 85 per cent at 5 years of age.[15]

A Japanese study further delineated the nature of the illness associated with acute HHV-6 infection in young children.[31] HHV-6 was cultured from the peripheral blood leukocytes of four infants with presumed roseola (exanthem subitum); each subject was 6 months of age with an acute febrile illness followed by a concurrent fall in temperature and the onset of a rash. The blood samples were collected during the febrile stage of the disease. In a subsequent paper by the same group, two infants (6 and 7 months of age) were described who developed HHV-6 infection *without* a rash.[27] Both infants had been seen by physicians because of a 2- to 3-day history of high fever (38.5° to 39.5° C). The only abnormal clinical finding was congestion of the throat. In both cases, the temperature rapidly returned to normal around day 3 of illness, but no rash was ever observed. Cultures of peripheral blood cells from both infants were positive for HHV-6.[27] Further seroprevalence studies performed in Japan showed that the majority of Japanese (86 per cent) contracted HHV-6 infection by the age of 24 months.[32] Thereafter, there was little increase in seropositivity among the childhood populations. The earlier statistics suggest that HHV-6 infection goes unrecognized in most children.

Primary HHV-6 infection has been implicated in two cases of severe hepatitis. The first case was that of a 21-year-old patient with cystic fibrosis who received a liver transplant.[30] The recipient lacked antibodies to HHV-6, and the organ donor was seropositive. Two weeks after transplantation, the recipient developed fever and grand mal seizures; her hepatic function deteriorated. HHV-6 was cultured from her peripheral blood cells, and herpesviral particles were seen by electron-microscopic examination of a liver biopsy. The patient also developed antibodies to HHV-6 by day 16 after transplantation. The apparent source of infection was the donor liver, from which HHV-6 presumably was reactivated after transplantation. She gradually recovered her hepatic function over several weeks. A fatal case of fulminant HHV-6 hepatitis has been reported in a 3-month-old boy.[5] The infant was admitted to a hospital because of fever, jaundice, convulsions, and loss of consciousness. His serum bilirubin, liver transaminases, and blood ammonia levels were markedly elevated. Within 7 days, he became comatose and died. As part of the diagnostic evaluation, HHV-6 was cultured from his mononuclear cells. Furthermore, HHV-6 DNA was detected in biopsy samples of liver and brain, which were obtained immediately after death. A serum sample drawn before death showed reactivity to HHV-6. On the other hand, the child had no serologic evidence of acute infection with hepatitis A, B, or C or with any other HHV. Thus, these two case reports suggest that HHV-6 can cause severe hepatitis in infants and nonimmune recipients of an organ from an HHV-6–seropositive donor. The virus also may have been the etiologic agent of encephalitis in these two patients.

In one retrospective review of roseola in association with acute HHV-6 infection the signs and symptoms were tabulated.[3] The study population included 94 boys and 82 girls, who ranged in age from 3 weeks to 18 months (Table 166–1). As would be predicted, the two most common clinical findings were fever and rash. The fever often rose to 39° C and persisted for 2 to 4 days. The rash usually appeared when the fever lessened; the rash was papular in 54 per cent, macular in 40 per cent, and maculopapular in the remainder of the children. The exanthem typically persisted for 3 to 4 days and was not followed by desquamation. Diarrhea was surprisingly frequent although not severe. An enanthem called Nagayama spots in Japan consisted of papules on the mucosa of the soft palate and uvula. Of the total study group, 8 per cent developed febrile seizures. More severe central nervous system complications have been documented in children not enrolled in this study. Four children have been diagnosed with HHV-6 encephalitis, all with abnormal electroencephalograms. One of the four children died, and the other three had permanent neurologic sequelae. In the United States in particular, acute HHV-6 infection also appears to be associated with concurrent acute otitis media.[22]

TABLE 166–1. Selected Features in Roseola Associated with Infection in Children

Clinical Findings	%
Prodromal symptoms	14
Fever above 37.5° C	98
Rash	98
Diarrhea	68
Nagayama spots	65
Cough	50
Cervical adenopathy	31
Edematous eyelids	30
Bulging fontanelle	26
Convulsions	8

Data modified from Asano Y., and Grose, C.: Human herpesvirus type 6 infections. *In* Glaser, R., and Jones, J. (eds.): Herpesvirus Infections. New York, Marcel Dekker, 1994, pp. 227–244.

Reactivation of previous HHV-6 infection has been demonstrated in some healthy children and adults who contracted a second herpes-type infection, such as primary EBV infection (infectious mononucleosis) or primary CMV infection.[15] No specific symptoms were attributable to HHV-6 reactivation. A similar serologic survey was performed in 10 renal transplantation patients who initially were HHV-6–seropositive.[19] After transplantation, all 10 showed greater than fourfold rises in antibody to HHV-6. Only 2 of 10 developed a febrile illness, and both of these also had primary CMV infection. However, HHV-6 does not appear to be related causally to Kawasaki disease, because 18 per cent of these patients never showed serologic evidence of HHV-6 infection.[20]

Whether HHV-7 causes a distinct illness has been the subject of many medical investigations since 1990. In general, HHV-7 antibody is acquired by mid-childhood, but there appears to be no corresponding sentinel illness. However, in two infants with roseola, both isolation of HHV-7 and seroconversion to HHV-7 were documented; in addition, another five children with roseola were found to have undergone seroconversion to HHV-7.[29] HHV-7 also has been isolated from one infant with an acute febrile illness.[21] Therefore, in a small number of young children, acute HHV-7 infection may be associated with fever and sometimes a roseola rash.

PATHOGENESIS OF HUMAN HERPESVIRUS 6 INFECTION

The pathogenesis of HHV-6 infection certainly includes a viremia while the child is asymptomatic, although the total duration of the incubation period has not been defined clearly. The prodrome, which signals the end of the incubation period, includes 2 to 4 days of fever, which precedes the onset of the rash.[4] During this period, virtually 100 per cent of peripheral blood cell cultures are positive for HHV-6. By day 3 or 4, when the rash first appears, the viremia is abating. Between 5 and 7 days after the onset of the fever (or 2 to 4 days after appearance of exanthem), viremia persists in less than 20 per cent of the children. Viremia is absent later in convalescence. The serologic response to virus infection is undetectable before the onset of rash but first appears coincidentally with the exanthem.

The mothers of infants with HHV-6 infection have been studied to determine whether they are the source of the infectious agent. Because a majority of mothers are seropositive, the possibility exists that HHV-6 infection could reactivate in the mother, who would then transmit the infection to her child, possibly via exchange of saliva. However, cultures of peripheral blood mononuclear cells and saliva specimens of 14 mothers of infected infants failed to yield any positive results.[33] On the basis of results in this study, mothers do not seem to be the source of contagion. However, in another study, HHV-6 DNA was detected in the vaginal secretions of young adult women, so perinatal HHV-6 transmission remains a possibility.[14] In contrast with HHV-6, HHV-7 is found frequently in the saliva of adults.

RELATIONSHIP OF HUMAN HERPESVIRUS 6 INFECTION TO AIDS

HHV-6 first was isolated from patients with immunosuppressive disorders, including infection with HIV-1. An immediate question, therefore, was the relationship of HHV-6 infection to AIDS. In spite of extensive searches since 1986, no specific syndrome related to HHV-6 infection in AIDS patients has been identified. In HIV-negative homosexual males, no difference in HHV-6 antibody status was noted.[10, 26] Because we now know that most persons first contract roseola as young children, expression of HHV-6 in adults with AIDS probably represents a reactivation of a latent HHV-6 infection. Similar reactivations have been documented with the other herpesviruses (HSV-1, HSV-2, CMV, EBV, and VZV) in the same population of severely immunosuppressed patients.

HHV-6 may play a more subtle role in the pathogenesis of HIV-1 infection than first was imagined. The two viruses appear to infect a similar or overlapping subset of lymphocytes. The phenotypes of the T cells infected by HHV-6 have been determined to be both CD4+, CD8+ and CD4+, CD8−.[28] The virus rarely infected CD4−, CD8+ cells. Both HIV-1 and HHV-6 productively can infect the same CD4+ T lymphocyte under experimental conditions in the laboratory.[17, 18] Moreover, HIV-1 antigen expression was accelerated consistently in cells co-infected with HHV-6, compared with cells lacking HHV-6. The mechanism of this enhancement of HIV-1 replication was related to transactivation of the HIV-1 genome by HHV-6 products.[12, 17] Thus, these in vitro experiments indicate that HHV-6 could be a cofactor in the pathogenesis of AIDS.

DIAGNOSIS

Infection with HHV-6 can be diagnosed by several means; these include (1) measurement of antibody, (2) isolation of virus, (3) detection of viral antigen, and (4) detection of viral DNA. The first method (i.e., the traditional approach for diagnosis of virus infection) usually requires acute and convalescent serum samples for determination of a fourfold or greater rise in titer of virus-specific IgG antibody. Finding IgM specific for HHV-6 in a single serum sample also would indicate an acute infection in a young child. The titer of IgG antibody rises during reactivation of the virus in adults, but it is not known whether IgM antibody to HHV-6 appears regularly at the same time. HHV-6 antibodies usually have been measured by an indirect immunofluorescence method, although neutralization tests also have been performed.[3, 4, 10, 15, 25, 27, 30]

Isolation of HHV-6 was the original technique for identification of this novel herpesvirus.[24] The method is more difficult than those methods commonly used for most herpesviruses (e.g., HSV, CMV, VZV) but similar to that required for isolation of the lymphotropic EBV. The virus usually is isolated in a cell substrate consisting of mononuclear cells obtained from cord blood of a newborn infant. The source of virus in the patient also is the peripheral blood mononuclear cell population. The patient's blood sample is obtained in a heparinized tube, and the mononuclear cells are separated in a density gradient (e.g., Ficoll-Hypaque medium). Cells from the patient are cocultured with cord blood cells in enriched medium supplemented with human interleukin-2.[27] The cultures are observed periodically under light microscopy. If the balloon-like cells are examined by electron microscopy, numerous herpesviral particles are seen, as illustrated in Figure 166–1. Thus, HHV-6 harbored in a patient's mononuclear cells can infect and be propagated in cord blood cells.

Viral genome can be detected in infected tissues by DNA hybridization techniques. Two DNA probes were prepared from the HHV-6 genome hybridized with DNA extracted from the liver of a transplantation patient with a confirmed primary HHV-6 infection.[30] Viral DNA also can be detected in tissue samples by polymerase chain reaction. In one fatal case of HHV-6 infection,[5] DNA was extracted from postmortem liver and brain samples and amplified by polymerase chain reaction with an HHV-6 primer. On direct gel electrophoresis, HHV-6–specific DNA was detected in both the liver and the brain specimens. These studies indicate that HHV-6 infection can be diagnosed by both traditional and newer molecular techniques. Likewise, HHV-7 infection usually is diagnosed by isolation of virus or detection of viral DNA in patient samples. At present, these methods are available mainly in research laboratories.

TREATMENT OF HUMAN HERPESVIRUS 6 INFECTION

In most instances of HHV-6 infection in healthy children, treatment with antiviral medications is indicated. Recovery is complete within a few days after onset of the rash, and sequelae are rare. However, HHV-6 disease in immunocompromised persons may be more persistent or severe. Also, many immunocompromised persons are receiving antiviral medication for other herpesvirus infections and therefore may be modifying their HHV-6 infection unbeknownst to physician or patient. Several groups already have analyzed the in vitro sensitivity of HHV-6 to four antiviral drugs: acyclovir, ganciclovir, phosphonoformic acid, and zidovudine.[1, 23] The first three compounds have been used in treating other herpesvirus infections, and the fourth is the principal therapy for HIV infection. Multiplication of HHV-6 in cell culture is inhibited readily by ganciclovir at a concentration of 2 to 10 μmol/L, easily achievable levels in humans. This effect is of interest because ganciclovir inhibits human CMV to a similar degree; as mentioned earlier, CMV and HHV-6 are related closely at a genomic level. Phosphonoformic acid (foscarnet) at a concentration of 66 μmol/L also is effective against HHV-6 infection. On the other hand, HHV-6 is affected by acyclovir only at concentrations of 50 to 100 μmol/L, considerably higher levels than those required for treatment of HSV-1, HSV-2, and VZV infection and possibly toxic in humans. Likewise, zidovudine has no effect on this herpesvirus. At present, none of the above antiviral drugs has been approved specifically for treatment of HHV-6 infections.

KAPOSI SARCOMA HERPESVIRUS (HUMAN HERPESVIRUS 8)

Yet another consequence of the HIV epidemic in the 1980s was the appearance of Kaposi sarcoma in many people with AIDS. The increase in Kaposi sarcoma especially was puzzling because the tumor occurred more frequently in people who acquired HIV by sexual transmission rather than by infusion of infected blood products, such as factor VIII in hemophiliac patients. The question often arose whether a second infectious agent was involved in the etiology of Kaposi sarcoma. The answer to that question appears to have been provided by a report that was published in late 1994. The authors announced the identification of novel herpesvirus-like DNA sequences collected from AIDS patients in New York.[8] The viral DNA was called Kaposi sarcoma–associated herpesvirus (KSHV). Others have suggested that the agent be called human herpesvirus–8 (HHV-8).

The authors of the original KSHV report discovered the herpesvirus-like DNA sequenced by a combination of genetic techniques, including amplification of DNA by polymerase chain reaction and subsequent representational difference analysis.[8] Thereby, they were able to identify and characterize unique DNA sequences in Kaposi sarcoma that were absent from nonmalignant tissue from the same patient. One such sequence was called KS330*Bam,* and this 330–base pair piece of DNA showed close homology to regions of the genome of herpesvirus saimiri, a simian herpesvirus, and to a lesser degree EBV, the agent that causes infectious mononucleosis. A second DNA fragment called KS631*Bam* was homologous to another region in the herpesvirus saimiri genome. In their study, the authors located one or both of these herpesvirus-like DNA sequences in 20 of 27 different samples of Kaposi sarcoma tissue. The investigators concluded that they had discovered DNA of a previously unknown herpesvirus within Kaposi sarcoma tissues.

Their results were confirmed quickly by other groups. In one study from California, investigators detected the KS330*Bam* DNA sequence in 13 of 13 biopsies of Kaposi sarcoma from AIDS patients.[2] The latter study also found the same sequence in the peripheral blood cells collected from 10 of the 13 patients but not in the blood samples of 20 patients with no history of Kaposi sarcoma. A third study from France found the herpesvirus-like DNA in biopsies from five patients with Mediterranean-type Kaposi sarcoma; all five patients were HIV-seronegative.[9]

Finally, the authors of the original KSHV report found the herpesvirus-like DNA sequences in eight body cavity–based lymphomas from AIDS patients.[7] All eight body cavity lymphomas (pleural, pericardial, and peritoneal) also contained pieces of genome from EBV. Of equal importance, the unusual herpesvirus-like sequences were not found in several other lymphomas or leukemias (e.g., small-lymphocyte lymphoma, monocytoid B-cell lymphoma, follicular lymphoma, diffuse large cell lymphoma, Burkitt lymphoma, lymphoblastic lymphoma, anaplastic large cell lymphoma, multiple myeloma, hairy-cell leukemia, acute lymphoblastic leukemia, cutaneous T-cell lymphoma, Hodgkin disease, posttransplantation lymphoproliferative disorder).

In summary, the herpesvirus-like DNA sequences closely resembling but not identical to portions of the herpesvirus saimiri genome have been detected in Kaposi sarcoma tissues from patients with and without underlying HIV infection and in the rare body cavity lymphoma found in AIDS patients. In contrast with HHV-6 and HHV-7, an intact viral particle containing the KSHV DNA has not been recovered from the tumor tissues. Nevertheless, the finding of this fragment of DNA by newer amplification technology suggests that a previously unknown herpesvirus somewhat related to EBV may be infecting humans worldwide. The epidemiology of this virus is unknown. Studies currently are underway to determine whether children are asymptomatically infected with this virus.

References

1. Agut, H., Collandre, H., Aubin, J. T., et al.: In vitro sensitivity of human herpesvirus-6 to antiviral drugs. Res. Virol. *140*:219–228, 1989.
2. Ambroziak, J. A., Blackbourn, D. J., Herndier, B. G., et al.: Herpes-like sequences in HIV-infected and uninfected Kaposi's sarcoma patients. Science *268*:582–583, 1995.
3. Asano, Y., and Grose, C.: Human herpesvirus type 6 infections. *In* Glaser, R., and Jones, J. (eds.): Herpesvirus Infections. New York, Marcel Dekker, 1994, pp. 227–244.
4. Asano, Y., Yoshikawa, T., Suga, S., et al.: Viremia and neutralizing antibody response in infants with exanthem subitum. J. Pediatr. *114*:535–539, 1989.
5. Asano, Y., Yoshikawa, T., Suga, S., et al.: Fatal fulminant hepatitis in an infant with herpesvirus-6 infection. Lancet *1*:862–863, 1990.
6. Berneman, Z. N., Dharam, V. A., Ge, L., et al.: Human herpesvirus 7 is a T-lymphotropic virus and is related to, but significantly different from, human herpesvirus 6 and human cytomegalovirus. Proc. Natl. Acad. Sci. U. S. A. *89*:10552–10556, 1992.
7. Cesarman, E., Chang, Y., Moore, P. S., et al.: Kaposi's sarcoma–associated herpesvirus-like DNA sequences in AIDS-related body-cavity–based lymphomas. N. Engl. J. Med. *332*:1186–1191, 1995.
8. Chang, Y., Cesarman, E., Pessin, M. S., et al.: Identification of herpesvirus-like DNA sequences in AIDS-associated Kaposi's sarcoma. Science *266*:1865–1869, 1994.
9. Dupin, N., Grandadam, M., Calvez, V., et al.: Herpesvirus-like DNA sequences in patients with Mediterranean Kaposi's sarcoma. Lancet *345*:761–762, 1995.
10. Fox, J., Briggs, M., and Tedder, R. S.: Antibody to human herpesvirus 6 in HIV-1 positive and negative homosexual men. Lancet *2*:396–397, 1988.
11. Frenkel, N., Schirmer, E. C., Wyatt, L. S., et al.: Isolation of a new herpesvirus from CD4+ T cells. Proc. Natl. Acad. Sci. U. S. A. *87*:748–752, 1990.
12. Horvat, R. T., Wood, C., and Balachandran, N.: Transactivation of human immunodeficiency virus promoter by human herpesvirus 6. J. Virol. *63*:970–973, 1989.
13. Lawrence, G. L., Chee, M., Craxton, M. A., et al.: Human herpesvirus 6 is closely related to human cytomegalovirus. J. Virol. *64*:287–299, 1990.
14. Leach, C. T., Newton, E. R., McParlin, S., et al.: Human herpesvirus 6 infection of the female genital tract. J. Infect. Dis. *169*:1281–1283, 1994.
15. Linde, A., Dahl, H., Wahren, B., et al.: IgG antibodies to human herpesvirus-6 in children and adults both in primary Epstein-Barr virus and cytomegalovirus infections. J. Virol. Methods *21*:117–123,1988.
16. Lopez, C., Pellett, P., Stewart, J., et al.: Characteristics of human herpesvirus-6. J. Infect. Dis. *157*:1271–1273, 1988.
17. Lusso, P., Markham, P. D., Tschachler, E., et al.: In vitro cellular tropism of human B-lymphotropic virus (human herpesvirus-6). J. Exp. Med. *167*:1659-1670, 1988.
18. Lusso, P., Ensoli, B., Markham, P. D., et al.: Productive dual infection of human $CD4^+$ T lymphocytes by HIV-1 and HHV-6. Nature *337*:370–373, 1989.
19. Morris, D. J., Littler, E., Arrand, J. R., et al.: Human herpesvirus 6 infection in renal transplant recipients. N. Engl. J. Med. *320*:1560–1561, 1989.
20. Okano, M., Luka, J., Thiele, G. M., et al.: Human herpesvirus 6 infection and Kawasaki disease. J. Clin. Microbiol. *27*:2379–2380, 1989.

21. Portolani, M., Cermelli, C., Mirandola, P., et al.: Isolation of human herpesvirus 7 from an infant with febrile syndrome. J. Med. Virol. *45*:282–283, 1995.
22. Pruksananonda, P., Hall, C. B., Insel R. A., et al.: Primary human herpesvirus 6 infection in young children. N. Engl. J. Med. *326*:1445–1450, 1992.
23. Russler, S. K., Tapper, M. A., and Carrigan, D. R.: Susceptibility of human herpesvirus 6 to acyclovir and ganciclovir. Lancet *2*:382, 1989.
24. Salahuddin, S. Z., Ablashi, D. V., Markham, P. D., et al.: Isolation of a new virus, HBLV, in patients with lymphoproliferative disorders. Science *234*:596–601, 1986.
25. Saxinger, C., Polesky, H., Eby, N., et al.: Antibody reactivity with HBVL (HHV-6) in U.S. populations. J. Virol. Methods *21*:199–208, 1988.
26. Spira, T. J., Bozemann, L. H., Sanderlin, K. C., et al.: Lack of correlation between human herpesvirus-6 infection and the course of human immunodeficiency virus infection. J. Infect. Dis. *161*:567–570, 1990.
27. Suga, S., Yoshikawa, T., Asano, Y., et al.: Human herpesvirus-6 infection (exanthem subitum) without rash. Pediatrics *83*:1003–1006, 1989.
28. Takahashi, K., Sonoda, S., Higashi, K., et al.: Predominant CD4 T-lymphocyte tropism of human herpesvirus 6–related virus. J. Virol. *63*:3161–3163, 1989.
29. Tanaka, K., Kondo, T., Torigoe, S., et al.: Human herpesvirus 7: Another causal agent for roseola (exanthem subitum). J. Pediatr. *125*:1–5, 1994.
30. Ward, K. N., Gray, J. J., and Efstathious, S.: Brief report: Primary human herpesvirus 6 infection in a patient following liver transplantation from a seropositive donor. J. Med. Virol. *28*:69–72, 1989.
31. Yamanishi K., Okuno, T., Shiraki, K., et al.: Identification of human herpesvirus-6 as a causal agent for exanthem subitum. Lancet *1*:1065–1067, 1988.
32. Yoshikawa, T., Suga, S., Asano, Y., et al.: Distribution of antibodies to a causative agent of exanthem subitum (human herpesvirus-6) in healthy individuals. Pediatrics *84*:675–677, 1989.
33. Yoshiyama, H., Suzuki, E., Yoshida, T., et al.: Role of human herpesvirus 6 infection in infants with exanthem subitum. Pediatr. Infect. Dis. J. *9*:71–74, 1990.

167

VARICELLA-ZOSTER VIRUS

Anne A. Gershon

Varicella-zoster virus (VZV) causes two diseases: varicella (chickenpox) and zoster (shingles). Varicella, the primary infection, usually occurs in childhood and is manifested by a pruritic rash accompanied by fever and other systemic signs and symptoms that often are of a mild to moderate nature. Zoster mainly is a disease of adults, although it can occur in children. It develops in a setting of low cell-mediated immunity (CMI) to VZV, which occurs with normal aging or after disease and/or various therapies, such as steroids, cancer chemotherapy, organ transplantation, and irradiation. During varicella, VZV establishes a latent infection in sensory nerve ganglia; zoster results when latent VZV reactivates and returns from the ganglion to infect the skin, resulting in a unilateral dermatomal eruption.

The origin of the name chickenpox is uncertain, but it may may have come from the French *pois chiche*, or chick pea, or from the English *farmyard fowl* (in Old English *cicen* and Middle High German *kuchen*).[21] *Herpes* is the Greek word meaning to creep, and *zoster* comes from the Greek and Latin word meaning girdle or belt.

THE ORGANISM

VZV is an alpha-herpesvirus. It has a DNA core surrounded by a nucleocapsid composed of 162 hexagonal capsomeres that form an icosahedron, with a diameter of about 100 nm.[24] A tegument surrounds this structure, which in turn is surrounded by a lipid-containing envelope. Enveloped virions have a diameter of about 200 nm.

The genome of VZV has been sequenced; it contains 68 unique open-reading frames.[25] The linear double-stranded DNA consists of a long unique segment and a short unique sequence flanked by internal and terminal repeats.[27, 30, 114]

Five open-reading frames (genes 4, 21, 29, 62, and 63) have been detected in human sensory ganglia during latent VZV infection.[25, 65] VZV is synthesized by an orderly cascade of gene expression, consisting of immediate early, early, and finally late lytic structural genes. The genes detectable during latent infection are immediate early and early genes for the most part; it has been postulated that cellular immmunity to VZV normally can control early replication of the virus so that productive or lytic infection does not occur.[65]

During productive infection, VZV synthesizes more than 30 polypeptides; the function of most of these remains unknown, but some are structural and others are nonstructural and presumably have regulatory actions. VZV synthesizes six glycoproteins (gp), gpI through gpVI; they correspond to glycoproteins (g) of herpes simplex virus as follows: gpI (g E), gpII (g B), gpIII (g H), gpIV (g I), gpV (g C), gpVI (g L).[23, 55] The VZV glycoproteins not only provide structure for the virion but also play roles in infectivity, such as mediating adhesion to and promoting entry into uninfected body cells of the virus. The glycoproteins also are antigenic, as is the tegument, and protective aspects of the immune response are directed toward these structures.

There is only one antigenic type of VZV, and there are only minor differences in DNA between various VZV isolates.[87] Wild-type VZV DNA can be distinguished from that of vaccine-type virus by restriction enzyme analysis of DNA from cultured virus or by polymerase chain reaction (PCR).[81, 87]

VZV replicates in the nuclei of infected cells, where the DNA core and capsid are synthesized. The capsid is enveloped by a complex process, after which it traverses the cell in cytoplasmic vesicles.[45] In vitro, VZV grows rather slowly and is highly cell associated; its synthetic pathway entraps it in endosomic vesicles, where it is inactivated before it can be released. In vivo, infectious VZV, however, is released from cells and is highly contagious; VZV avoids the endosomal route in vivo and exits from cells by the secretory pathway.

VZV has an extremely limited host range, infecting mostly primates. Hairless guinea pigs may be infected with VZV; the illness produced is extremely mild, and latent infection occurs only infrequently, but specific immune responses can be demonstrated.[90] A rat model of latent VZV infection has been described.[26]

TRANSMISSION

VZV is spread by the airborne route[83] and requires direct contact with an infected individual for transmission. In varicella, VZV is transmitted from the skin and the respiratory tract; it is isolated readily from skin lesions but is extremely difficult to isolate from the respiratory tract.[92, 116] Spread of VZV from varicella patients before the onset of rash in closed communities has been reported, however, implicating respiratory spread.[53] VZV DNA has been detected by PCR in the nasopharynx of children during pre-eruptive and early varicella.[76, 93, 105] Investigations of leukemic recipients of live attenuated varicella vaccine have implicated spread of VZV from skin. There was no transmission to siblings from vaccinees who had no rash, but there was a 14 per cent transmission rate when siblings were exposed to a child who had a vaccine-associated skin rash.[117] Taken together, these observations suggest that VZV can spread from skin lesions as well as from the respiratory tract. Epidemiologic studies suggest that transmission is most likely to take place in the early stages of varicella.[89]

Zoster is not transmissible per se, but the vesicular lesions of zoster contain infectious VZV and can transmit varicella to others.[19, 78] Zoster is thought to be less contagious than varicella, and whether VZV is spread from the respiratory tract in zoster is unknown.

EPIDEMIOLOGY

VZV infections occur worldwide, and both sexes are affected equally. The virus spreads less efficiently in countries with tropical climates than in those with temperate climates,[77] resulting in a high rate of susceptibility in adults reared in tropical countries. There are about 3.8 million cases of chickenpox annually in the United States, an entire birth cohort. In countries where varicella is a disease of childhood, 8 to 9 per cent of children between 1 and 9 years of age develop the illness annually.[99] These data were collected before the time when many children began to attend day care facilities; it is possible that exposures to VZV in the day care setting might lead to an earlier acquisition of disease.

The link between varicella and zoster first was recognized about a century ago. In the 1870s, von Bokay noticed that cases of varicella often occurred after an exposure to a patient with zoster.[120] In the early part of the 20th century, medical investigators inoculated vesicular fluid from zoster patients into varicella-susceptible children, who then developed chickenpox.[19, 78] Weller first successfully isolated VZV in vitro, gave the virus its name, and demonstrated that viruses isolated from patients with varicella and zoster are identical.[124] Garland proposed that zoster is the result of reactivation of latent VZV.[36] Hope-Simpson presciently recognized the importance of the immune system in preventing reactivation of VZV; he postulated that zoster results when immunity to VZV wanes.[67] The importance of declining CMI to VZV now has been identified in the pathogenesis of zoster.[6, 63] With the use of molecular techniques for DNA analysis, it has been established that the DNA of viruses causing varicella and zoster are the same and that latent VZV is detectable in nuclei of neurons and satellite cells of sensory ganglia of autopsied individuals with a history of varicella.[22, 85, 86, 130] It has been shown that zoster is not acquired from contact with patients with zoster or chickenpox.[40] About 15 per cent of the varicella-immune population develops zoster during their lifetime.[67]

Varicella is highly contagious; 80 to 90 per cent of susceptible people exposed in a household will develop clinical infection.[102] Secondary varicella cases in a family usually are more severe than primary cases.[102] About 75 per cent of adults with no history of varicella have detectable antibodies to VZV,[82] indicating that subclinical varicella can occur. One epidemiologic study suggests that its incidence is about 5 per cent.[102]

Subclinical zoster also may occur, and zoster with dermatomal pain and no rash has been described. Increases in VZV immunity and episodes of viremia shown by PCR in asymptomatic individuals suggest silent reactivation.[42, 56, 132] Asymptomatic shedding of VZV is not known to occur.

Second attacks of varicella are uncommon and may be more frequent in the immunocompromised than in immunologically normal individuals.[47, 73] Immunologic boosting to VZV is common upon re-exposure to the virus.[4, 47] Whether boosting is necessary for long-term maintenance of immunity to VZV is not known.

Adults and children older than 2 years of age who have zoster usually have a history of a previous attack of varicella.[67] Zoster is rare in children, but there is an increased incidence in young children who had varicella either in utero or before reaching their second birthday. [29] Chickenpox in the first year of life increases the risk of childhood zoster by a relative factor between roughly 3 and 21,[58] possibly because of immaturity of the immune response to VZV in young infants.

The incidence of zoster in a population begins to increase sharply at about 50 years of age.[67] The increased incidence of zoster with advancing age is associated with and presumably because of a relative loss of CMI to VZV that occurs naturally with aging.[13, 20]

Zoster occurs with increased frequency in patients with neoplasms and after organ transplantation[84]; severely immunocompromised patients with zoster also may develop disseminated infection with viremia.[32] Spinal trauma, irradiation, and corticosteroid therapy also may be precipitating factors. On occasion, however, healthy young adults who are not immunocompromised may develop zoster, presumably resulting from a transient fall in CMI to VZV caused by a stimulus, such as another viral infection or stress. Because not all immunocompromised persons develop zoster, deficiency of CMI to VZV is a necessary but not sufficient requirement for this illness. The distribution of lesions in chickenpox, which primarily involves the trunk and head, is reflected in a proportionately greater representation of these regions in the dermatomal lesions of zoster.[112] Zoster may recur, either in the same dermatome or in a different dermatome; the chance of developing recurrent zoster is similar to the chance of developing a first attack for a particular age group.[67]

Varicella most commonly occurs in the winter and early spring. In contrast, zoster occurs equally during all seasons of the year.

PATHOGENESIS

The incubation period of varicella ranges from 10 to 23 days (average, 14 days).[53] During the incubation period, VZV is thought to spread to regional lymph nodes, undergo multiplication, and cause a primary low-grade viremic phase after about 5 days that spreads the virus to the viscera, where there is further multiplication of VZV. This results in the second and greater viremic phase that delivers the virus to the skin, where it causes the characteristic skin rash.[57] VZV can be isolated from blood cultures either a few days before onset of rash or within 1 to 2 days after onset in immunocompetent children.[7]

The skin lesions of VZV infection begin as macules and progress rapidly to papules, vesicles, pustules, and scabs. Histologic changes in the skin lesions are similar for chickenpox and zoster. The hallmarks of each are multinucleated giant cells and intranuclear inclusions. In varicella, these are localized primarily in the epidermis, where ballooning degeneration of cells in the deeper layers is accompanied by intercellular edema. As edema progresses, the cornified layers and basal layers separate to form a thin-roofed vesicle. An exudate of mononuclear cells is seen in the dermis.[124]

In zoster, in addition to skin lesions resembling those of varicella, there is a mononuclear inflammatory infiltrate in the dorsal root ganglion of the affected dermatome. There also may be necrosis of ganglion cells and demyelination of the corresponding axon.[31, 85]

Both humoral and CMI responses to VZV develop within a few days after onset of varicella. Peak antibody levels are attained 4 to 8 weeks after onset, remain high for about 6 months, and then decline. Positive IgG VZV antibody titers are detectable in healthy adults decades after varicella occurs.[50, 111, 131] After active immunization against varicella, antibody titers are lower than after natural infection but persist for as long as 20 years in healthy vaccinees immunized as children.[8, 125] Serum IgG, IgA, and IgM develop after both varicella and zoster. Zoster occurs despite high levels of specific antibodies, but significantly higher titers develop during convalescence, reflecting an anamnestic response to VZV in this secondary infection.[17, 119]

CMI is thought to play the major role in host defense against the virus. CMI to VZV can be demonstrated in vitro by stimulation of lymphocytes with VZV antigens,[62, 135] by an intradermal skin test,[82] and by specific lysis of histocompatible target cells by cytotoxic T cells.[5] Natural killer cell and antibody-dependent cellular toxicity to VZV also have been described.[69] CMI responses of normal subjects with remote clinical evidence of varicella are characterized by occasional high activity in the absence of symptoms, suggesting either exposure to VZV with boosting of the immune response or subclinical reactivation of the virus. CMI reactions remain positive for years after varicella occurs, although this response may wane in many individuals older than 50 years of age.[13, 20] The predominant cell in vesicular lesions is the polymorphonuclear leukocyte. Polymorphonuclear leukocytes may play a role in generating interferon in vesicular lesions, which may play a role in recovery.[113]

Exactly how immunity to varicella and zoster is mediated still is unclear. Because patients with isolated agammaglobulinemia do not experience either severe or recurrent varicella, it has been presumed that CMI is more important in host defense than humoral immunity. It generally is thought that T-cell cytotoxicity is crucial in recovery from VZV infection.[3] The response(s) that prevents clinical illness after reinfection with VZV is presumed to be that of cytotoxic T lymphocytes, but antibodies also may play a role. Specific antibodies must have some importance because varicella-zoster immunoglobulin (VZIG) can be used to prevent or modify varicella in people who have been exposed to the virus and are susceptible. However, the issues are not straightforward. Young infants may develop varicella after exposure, despite detectable transplacental antibody titers,[10] and vaccinated leukemic children have developed modified cases of breakthrough varicella, despite measurable humoral and CMI responses measured by lymphocyte stimulation at exposure to VZV.[48, 51] Still, individuals with detectable antibody titers, CMI, or both, at exposure to VZV are far less likely to develop clinical illness than those without antibodies. It seems likely that some forms of CMI and antibodies play roles in host defense against VZV.

NOSOCOMIAL VARICELLA

Nosocomial varicella has become a serious and expensive problem in hospitals, where both patients and employees may be susceptible to chickenpox.[54, 60] Because varicella-susceptible hospital employees may serve as vectors for spread of VZV to susceptible patients, it is appropriate to test serologically employees for immunity to chickenpox if they have no history of clinical varicella and to offer vaccination to those who are susceptible.

The risk of horizontal transmission in maternity wards or the newborn nursery after a hospital exposure to an adult or child is surprisingly low.[37] A few episodes of nursery transmission of varicella have been reported.[35, 41, 59] The low incidence of nursery transmission may be because many infants are in isolettes. Furthermore, most hospital employees and mothers and their newborn infants have antibodies to VZV and are at low risk to develop clinical illness. Even in low birth weight infants, antibodies to VZV usually are detectable.[88, 101]

CLINICAL MANIFESTATIONS OF VARICELLA

Varicella is a highly contagious and usually self-limited systemic infection that is characterized by fever and a generalized pruritic rash, lasting about 5 days. A prodromal phase in children is unusual, but malaise and fever for 1 to 2 days before rash onset in adults are common.[21] The rash is more intense on the trunk and head than on the extremities, and it typically evolves as a series of "crops" over 1 to 2 days in normal hosts. Most children with varicella develop from 250 to 500 superficial skin lesions, many of which are vesicular (Fig. 167–1).[102] Not uncommonly, a few lesions may develop in the mouth, conjunctiva, or other mucosal sites. Residual scarring is exceptional, but depigmented areas of skin may appear in black children. It is not uncommon to observe an increase in hepatic transaminase levels without jaundice during varicella, which is self-limited.[96] Rarely, thrombocytopenia and neutropenia may occur transiently with varicella. Adults are more likely than children to develop more severe infections. Presumably, this is because of lower CMI responses to VZV in adults compared with children.[38, 91] Newborn infants who acquired varicella from their mothers in the few days before delivery also are at risk to develop severe varicella because of immaturity of their CMI response.[38]

COMPLICATIONS OF VARICELLA

The most frequent complication of varicella in normal hosts is bacterial superinfection of the skin, lungs, or bones,

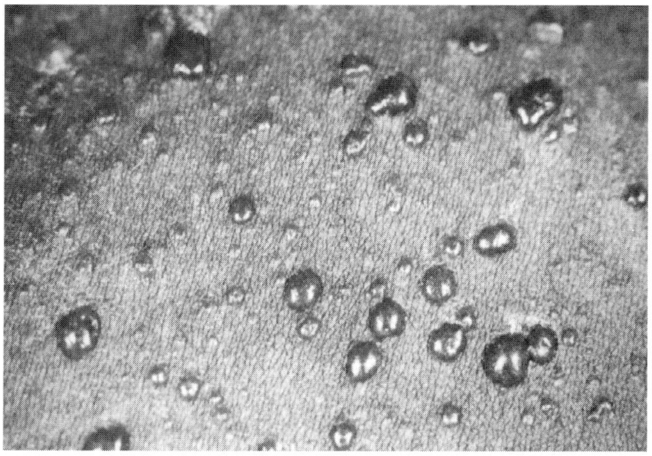

FIGURE 167–1. *Typical skin lesions of varicella.*

most often caused by *Staphylococcus aureus* or group A beta-hemolytic streptococci.[16,133] Central nervous system complications, which may develop before or after varicella, include transient cerebellar ataxia, a severe cerebral encephalitis; aseptic meningitis; and transverse myelitis.[71,72] Encephalopathy due to Reye syndrome has become rare because aspirin no longer is recommended for children with varicella. Other less commonly encountered complications of chickenpox include arthritis, glomerulonephritis, myocarditis, and purpura fulminans.[124]

Varicella may be severe and even fatal in immunocompromised patients, including those with an underlying malignancy or congenital or acquired deficits in CMI, such as in patients who have undergone organ transplantation or have underlying HIV infection, and in children receiving high doses of corticosteroids for any reason (Fig. 167–2).[34] These patients may manifest progressive varicella, with continuing fever and development of new vesicular lesions for 2 weeks or longer. Their skin lesions characteristically are large, umbilicated, and hemorrhagic, and primary varicella pneumonia is a frequent complication. Alternatively, some immunocompromised patients develop an acute form of varicella with disseminated intravascular coagulation that is rapidly fatal, at times before antiviral therapy can be instituted. A 30 per cent rate of dissemination with a 7 per cent fatality rate was reported in leukemic children who developed chickenpox in the pre–antiviral drug era.[33] Severe varicella has been observed in children with underlying HIV infection, especially those classified as having AIDS.[74] Many HIV-infected children, however, develop mild to moderate forms of varicella. Varicella does not seem to be a cofactor for clinical progression of HIV infection to AIDS, although about 5 per cent of these children may develop chronic wart-like hyperkeratotic VZV lesions.[2]

Primary varicella pneumonia accounts for many of the fatalities ascribed to varicella, particularly in immunocompromised patients, in adults, and in neonates.[94] In male military recruits with varicella, radiographic evidence of pneumonia was found in 16 per cent.[123] Symptoms include fever, cough, and dyspnea. Other common symptoms and signs are cyanosis, rales, hemoptysis, and chest pain. The chest x-ray typically reveals a diffuse nodular or miliary pattern, most pronounced in the perihilar region.[115] Blood gas analyses and pulmonary function tests indicate a diffusion defect that may persist in some cases for months after recovery.[15] The availability of antiviral chemotherapy greatly has improved the outcome of this complication.

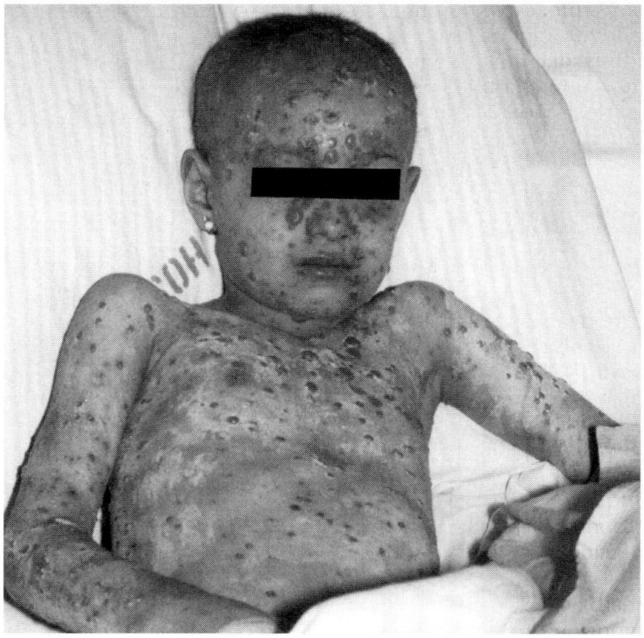

FIGURE 167–2. *Progressive varicella in a 9-year-old child with underlying leukemia.*

CONGENITAL VARICELLA SYNDROME

LaForet and Lynch in 1947 were the first to describe an infant with multiple congenital anomalies after maternal chickenpox.[80] The infant had hypoplasia of the right lower extremity, clubfoot, absent deep tendon reflexes on the right, cerebral cortical atrophy, cerebellar aplasia, chorioretinitis, torticollis, insufficiency of the anal and vesical sphincters, and cicatricial cutaneous lesions of the left lower extremity, which now are recognized to be typical. In 1974, Srabstein and colleagues rediscovered this syndrome.[110] Their report of another case and review of the literature concluded that, although the virus could not be isolated from affected infants, the congenital syndrome consisted of a typical constellation of birth defects as originally described by LaForet and Lynch. This syndrome occurs after maternal VZV infection in the first or second trimester of pregnancy; about 2 per cent of infants of pregnancies so complicated by varicella are affected. About 50 affected infants have been described in the literature; 90 per cent of these cases occurred after maternal varicella and 10 per cent after maternal zoster. It is thought that about 40 affected infants are born yearly in the United States.[37]

Cicatricial scars of the skin are the most prominent stigmata, reported in 70 per cent of cases.[37] Other frequent abnormalities include chorioretinitis, microphthalmia, Horner syndrome, cataract, nystagmus, hypoplastic limbs, cortical atrophy, mental retardation, and early death.

CLINICAL MANIFESTATIONS OF ZOSTER

Zoster usually begins as a localized unilateral vesicular skin eruption involving one to three dermatomal segments (Fig. 167–3). The skin lesions resemble those of varicella but tend more toward confluence and are likely to be painful, especially in adults. Zoster is in general a milder disease in children than in adults.

COMPLICATIONS OF ZOSTER

From 25 to 50 per cent of people older than 50 years of age who develop zoster may develop protracted pain, or postherpetic neuralgia, after healing of rash. Pain may persist for months to years and is described as aching, jabbing, or boring. The cause of postherpetic neuralgia is unknown. Children rarely experience postherpetic neuralgia; both its incidence and duration are related directly to increasing age.[52]

Zoster may be particularly severe and common among bone marrow transplantation recipients, as many as 35 per cent of whom develop zoster in the first year after transplantation.[84]

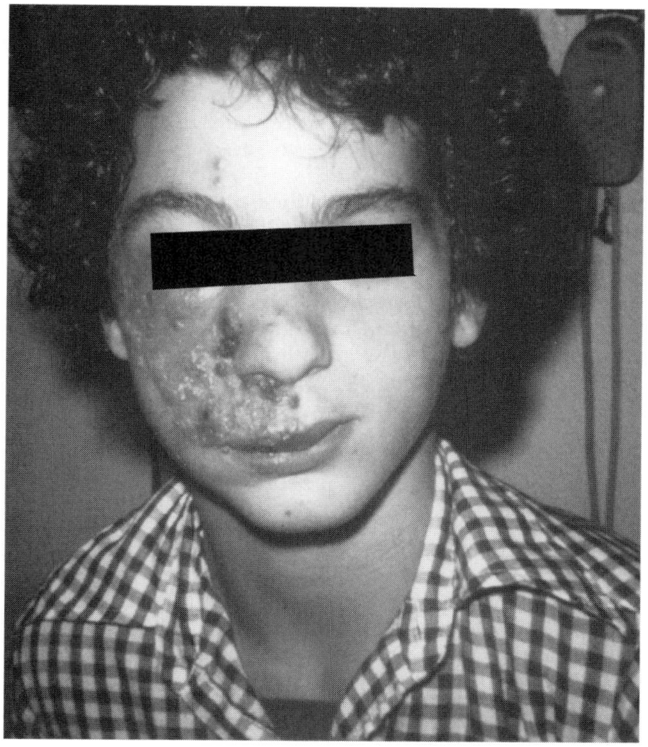

FIGURE 167–3. *Zoster in an otherwise healthy 10-year-old boy.*

CLINICAL DIAGNOSIS OF VARICELLA AND ZOSTER

It usually is not difficult to make a clinical diagnosis of VZV infection because the vesicular rashes are so characteristic. In questionable cases of varicella, epidemiologic information may be useful, such as a history of recent exposure to varicella or zoster and subsequent transmission of varicella to another person. The differential diagnosis of varicella includes generalized herpes simplex virus infection; rickettsialpox; impetigo; allergic reactions, including Stevens-Johnson syndrome and poison ivy; and insect bites. In one study of zoster, 13 per cent of clinically diagnosed cases were proved by culture to be caused by herpes simplex virus.[75] The unilateral rash of zoster most frequently appears on the trunk or face. The trigeminal nerve, most commonly the ophthalmic branch, is an especially significant site because the eye may be involved.

LABORATORY DIAGNOSIS

Laboratory diagnosis of VZV infection is facilitated by the presence of VZV in superficial skin lesions, where it is easily accessible for testing. Diagnosis is best made by demonstration of specific viral antigens in skin scrapings or isolation of VZV from skin vesicles by immunofluorescence, using a commercial monoclonal antibody to VZV that is conjugated to fluorescein.[44] This is a highly sensitive and rapid diagnostic method that can be completed within about an hour.

The diagnosis also may be made by culture of virus from skin lesions. Vesicular fluid for culture should be obtained as early in the course of illness as possible for successful virus isolation. Within several days after onset of varicella, vesicular fluid is no longer likely to be infectious, although viable VZV may be present in zoster lesions for a longer period, especially in immunocompromised patients. It is no longer possible to isolate VZV from skin lesions that have become pustular or dry. Isolation of VZV is a slow method because it takes about 48 hours before the first signs of viral cytopathic effects are seen. Virus isolation is less sensitive than immunofluorescence staining because infectious virus persists for a shorter length of time in vesicles and is more labile than are viral antigens. VZV rarely is isolated from the cerebrospinal fluid and respiratory secretions. Isolation of VZV or demonstration of viral antigen in material obtained from skin or other lesions or from autopsy tissue is diagnostic of a current infection with VZV because, unlike other herpesviruses, there is no known carrier state or shedding of VZV by asymptomatic individuals. For diagnosis of VZV infection, PCR successfully has been employed utilizing skin scrapings, vesicular fluid, respiratory secretions, and cerebrospinal fluid.[81, 100, 105]

A number of serologic tests are useful to measure antibodies to VZV. These include the fluorescent antibody to membrane antigen method,[131, 134] latex agglutination,[111] and enzyme-linked immunosorbent assay.[39, 81, 107] Antibody to VZV develops within a few days after onset of varicella, persists for many years, and is present before the onset of zoster. VZV infections may be documented by a fourfold or greater rise in VZV antibody titer in acute and convalescent serum specimens. Specific IgM in one serum specimen suggests recent VZV infection.[17] Persistence of VZV antibody beyond 8 months of age is highly suggestive of intrauterine varicella.[41] Immunity to varicella is highly likely if a positive antibody titer to VZV is demonstrated on a single serum sample. Serologic methods, however, particularly commercial enzyme-linked immunosorbent assays, may fail to identify individuals who have been immunized.[111]

The value of serologic procedures for diagnosis of zoster is limited. Heterologous increases in antibody titer against VZV in patients with herpes simplex virus infections who previously had varicella may occur, which have been ascribed to antigens common to the two viruses.[106]

TREATMENT OF VARICELLA-ZOSTER VIRUS INFECTIONS

Traditionally, nonspecific measures, such as frequent bathing to discourage bacterial skin infection; antihistamines given orally, calamine lotion applied locally, and oatmeal baths taken to decrease itching; and cutting fingernails short to discourage scratching, have been used to treat varicella. Fever is controlled best with acetaminophen rather than aspirin, which may predispose a child to Reye syndrome.[64]

Useful specific antiviral therapy for VZV became available in the mid-1980s with the introduction of acyclovir (ACV), an inhibitor of DNA polymerase and a DNA chain terminator. The antiviral effect of ACV depends on its being phosphorylated in the body by virus-induced thymidine kinases, accounting for its relative lack of toxicity.[128]

Patients with severe or potentially severe VZV infections should be treated with intravenous ACV (30 mg/kg/day for adults and adolescents and 1500 mg/m^2/day for children, both given in three divided doses). Orally administered ACV is less reliable because only about 20 per cent of this formulation is absorbed from the gastrointestinal tract and there are no published data on its efficacy in high-risk patients. ACV is excreted by the kidneys; patients with creatinine clearances of less than 50 mL/min/1.73 m^2 should receive one-half to one-third of this dosage. Intravenous ACV is infused over at least 1 hour, with maintenance fluids given both before and during the infusion. Adequate hydration is important to prevent renal damage from precipitation of the drug in the renal tubules. Other adverse effects of ACV include phlebitis, rash, nausea, and neurologic manifestations, such as headache and tremor. In general, however, ACV is extremely well tolerated.

Early therapy should be instituted for patients at high risk to develop severe VZV infections, such as leukemic children and children with AIDS, in order to prevent dissemination of VZV.[108, 127] This therapy not only potentially is lifesaving in immunocompromised patients but also prevents considerable morbidity from VZV infections. In zoster patients, use of intravenous ACV is associated with more rapid healing of skin lesions and resolution of acute pain than if no specific treatment is given.[129]

There has been considerable controversy about the role of orally administered ACV for treatment of varicella and zoster in otherwise healthy adults and children because most of these infections are self-limited. Dosages used are 4 g/day (in five divided doses) for adults and 80 mg/kg/day (in four divided doses) for children. Double-blind, placebo-controlled studies in healthy children given 80 mg/kg ACV or placebo a day for 5 days, beginning within 24 hours of onset of the varicella rash, revealed that the number of chickenpox skin lesions was reduced significantly by ACV. There was a modest benefit from ACV; children who received it had about 1 day less of fever, but they did not return to school any more rapidly, nor did they have fewer complications.[12, 28]

There is some indication that early oral ACV therapy may decrease acute pain associated with zoster.[68] However, it is rare to need to administer specific therapy for zoster in otherwise healthy children for whom pain is not a particular problem.

A newer drug, penciclovir, has an action similar to that of ACV.[66] It is administered as famciclovir (FCV), a prodrug that when given orally is converted rapidly to penciclovir in the body. A major advantage of FCV is that it is administered only three times a day (1500 mg/day for adults), whereas ACV is given four to five times daily. Penciclovir has an antiviral action similar to that of ACV. One study suggests that FCV given to elderly patients with zoster early in the course of infection decreases the duration of postherpetic neuralgia, although not its incidence.[118] There are no data about whether varicella may be treated successfully with FCV, nor are there any published data on the use of FCV in immunocompromised patients or in children.

The prodrug of ACV, valacyclovir, also is given orally, reaches blood levels that are about three to four times higher than ACV, and has been shown to be superior to ACV in one study.[14] Valacyclovir is licensed for use in adults (3 g/day divided three times a day) in the United States. Neither valacyclovir nor FCV is licensed for use in children.

Of concern about the potential widespread use of ACV is that drug resistance may develop. At present, resistance is less of a problem with VZV than with herpes simplex virus, but VZV resistance to ACV has been reported in patients with underlying AIDS.[70] Foscarnet was licensed by the Food and Drug Administration for treatment of VZV infections that are resistant to ACV and FCV. Foscarnet inhibits synthesis of VZV DNA polymerase.[103, 104, 109] Intravenous foscarnet has been used at a dosage of 40 mg/kg/day for herpes simplex virus infections and 60 mg/kg/day for retinitis caused by cytomegalovirus in AIDS patients. Its main toxicity is renal.

PROGNOSIS

The prognosis of varicella and zoster is excellent in children without underlying health problems. The outlook for immunocompromised patients receiving antiviral therapy also is good, especially if therapy is begun at an early stage of illness. In general, zoster carries a better prognosis than varicella, possibly because it is a secondary infection. If they are diagnosed promptly, such complications as bacterial superinfections usually can be treated successfully with antimicrobials. Despite the availability of antiviral therapy and passive immunization, however, the Centers for Disease Control and Prevention estimates that there are about 100 VZV-associated deaths annually in the United States, mostly in children with no previous health problems. An epidemiologic study of more than 250,000 health maintenance organization records indicated that the rates of varicella in adolescents and young adults and the complication and hospitalization rates recently have increased by a factor of about 5.[14]

PREVENTION

VZV is such an infectious agent that general measures are not useful for prevention of varicella in people who are susceptible. Some protection, however, can be accomplished by isolation of hospitalized patients, particularly in rooms with negative-pressure ventilation. Hospitalized patients with active VZV infections should be admitted to a private room, and hospital personnel and visitors should wash their hands before and after entering the room and wear masks, gowns, and gloves while in it.

PASSIVE IMMUNIZATION AGAINST VARICELLA WITH VARICELLA-ZOSTER IMMUNOGLOBULIN

Varicella-susceptible children at high risk to develop severe chickenpox should be immunized passively if they are closely exposed to someone with VZV infection. Administration of VZIG may be a lifesaving measure for a high-risk susceptible child; it may modify varicella or prevent it.

VZIG is a licensed product that is distributed in Massachusetts by the Massachusetts Public Health Biological Laboratory and elsewhere by the American Red Cross. Although VZIG has been shown to be effective when given within 3 days and perhaps for as long as 5 days, it should be given as soon as possible.[43] The dose is 1.25 mL (1 vial or 125 units) for each 10 kg of body weight, with a maximum dosage of 6 mL (5 vials or 625 units) intramuscularly. The cost of a vial is about $75. VZIG should be readministered to high-risk, susceptible people who closely are re-exposed 3 weeks after a first exposure.

VZIG is used for prevention of severe varicella in varicella-susceptible children who closely have been exposed to varicella or zoster and are at high risk to develop severe or fatal chickenpox. This includes immunocompromised children with cancer, newborn infants whose mothers have active varicella at the time of delivery, and hospitalized premature infants. High-risk children should be considered to be susceptible to varicella if they have no history of having had chickenpox. False-positive antibody tests may occur in immunocompromised children, and susceptible children thus may be identified serologically as immune; therefore, a history of illness is a preferred indication of immune status for these patients. VZIG should be administered to VZV-exposed adults only if they are proved serologically to be susceptible to chickenpox, because most adults with a negative history for varicella actually are immune.

Patients with HIV infection, and especially those with AIDS, potentially are at high risk to develop severe varicella, and their management should be similar to that of immunocompromised children.[74] Even those children who are receiving intravenous globulin for treatment of HIV infection should receive VZIG if there is no history of varicella and a close exposure has occurred.

Infants whose mothers have the onset of chickenpox 5 days or less before delivery or within 48 hours after delivery should be given one vial of VZIG as soon as possible after birth.[37] The transplacental route of infection and the immaturity of the immune system probably account for the severity of varicella in these infants.[37] Attack rates for varicella as high as 50 per cent in infants exposed to mothers who have varicella have been reported, despite administration of VZIG.[37, 98] Passively immunized infants should be observed closely, but usually they can be managed as outpatients. Intravenous ACV should be reserved for the rare, passively immunized infant with varicella who develops an extensive skin rash (more than 200 vesicles) or possible pneumonia.[11]

It is unnecessary to administer VZIG to full-term infants who are exposed to VZV after they are 48 hours old. VZIG is optional for newborn infants (younger than 1 week of age) if their siblings at home have active varicella. Infants exposed to VZV after birth almost always have mild varicella. Although the reported mortality rate from varicella in children younger than 1 year of age is four times that in older children, both rates are exceedingly low: 8 per 100,000 cases and 2 per 100,000 cases, respectively.[97] The mortality rate for adults and for leukemic children receiving chemotherapy, in contrast, is 20 and 1000 times higher, respectively.[99]

VZIG is not useful to treat or prevent zoster, and it is not known if giving VZIG to pregnant, varicella-susceptible women who have been exposed to VZV will protect their fetus from the congenital varicella syndrome.

ACTIVE IMMUNIZATION AGAINST VARICELLA

Live attenuated varicella vaccine was developed in Japan about 25 years ago. It was licensed for healthy children and adults who are susceptible to varicella in the United States in 1995. It is safe and well tolerated; the most frequent adverse reaction is a mild rash several weeks after vaccination in 5 per cent of healthy children.[49, 50, 125] These rashes are not serious, although there is a potential for transmission of the vaccine virus.[18, 117] Therefore, healthy vaccinees who develop a rash should avoid contact with immunocompromised patients and pregnant women who are susceptible to varicella.[38] The risk of transmission is present while the vaccinee has rash, and it is at least four times less than the chances of transmission of the wild-type virus.[117] The risk from wild-type VZV presumably is greater than the risk from vaccine-type VZV. Weighing potential risks and benefits, it seems prudent to immunize hospital workers and persons whose family members are immunocompromised. If necessary, immunocompromised individuals inadvertently exposed to a vaccinee with rash can be given VZIG if they are susceptible to varicella. Individuals who develop an extensive VZV rash within 2 to 3 weeks after immunization may have wild-type infection. In such situations, PCR and restriction fragment length polymorphism analysis can be used to differentiate between wild-type and vaccine-type VZV.[81, 87]

Live attenuated varicella vaccine is highly protective in healthy and immunocompromised children and in healthy adults, but not all vaccinees are protected completely. From 15 to 30 per cent may manifest a modified breakthrough illness after an intimate exposure. Varicella vaccine has been 100 per cent effective in preventing severe varicella.[51] Varicella vaccine is less effective in adults than in children; even after two doses of vaccine, only 70 per cent of adults are protected completely from varicella.[46, 49] About 85 per cent of healthy children are protected after only one dose of vaccine.[79, 125, 126] Breakthrough varicella almost always is a modified illness, however, with fewer than 50 skin lesions and minimal systemic signs; in one study, children with breakthrough varicella missed on average only 2 days of school.[122]

Leukemic children who are immunized have a 50 per cent chance of developing a vaccine-associated rash about 1 month after vaccination if they still are receiving maintenance chemotherapy; 40 per cent require antiviral therapy for control of this rash.[97] Some leukemic and healthy adult vaccinees lose detectable antibodies after several years, which may indicate some waning immunity to VZV. Antibody loss is rare in healthy vaccinated children, small numbers of whom have been followed for as long as 20 years after immunization.[8, 125] Booster doses of vaccine may be given safely to persons who have lost detectable antibodies, but it is unknown if boosters provide additional protective immunity.[49, 50, 121] Vaccinated leukemic children are at lower risk to develop zoster than are their counterparts who have had natural infection, possibly because they have less opportunity to develop latent infection.[62] Administration of live vaccine after an exposure has been reported[1] but is not recommended by the Food and Drug Administration because it may not be effective.

DRUG PROPHYLAXIS

Prophylaxis of varicella in exposed persons may be achieved by administration of prophylactic ACV. [9] This approach is not recommended, however, because the optimal dosage and timing for administration are unknown; nor is it known whether there is long-term maintenance of immunity. Long-term ACV therapy often is employed to prevent development of zoster in patients who have undergone bone marrow transplantation.[61, 95]

References

1. Arbeter, A. M., Starr, S. E., Preblud, S., et al.: Varicella vaccine trials in healthy children: A summary of comparative follow-up studies. Am. J. Dis. Child. *138*:434–438, 1984.
2. Aronson, J., McSherry, G., Hoyt, L., et al.: Varicella in children with HIV infection. Pediatr. Infect. Dis. J. *11*:1004–1008, 1992.
3. Arvin, A., Koropchak, C., Sharp, M., et al.: The T-lymphocyte response to varicella-zoster viral proteins: Adv. Exp. Med. Biol. 278:71–83, 1990.
4. Arvin, A., Koropchak, C. M., and Wittek, A. E.: Immunologic evidence of reinfection with varicella-zoster virus. J. Infect. Dis. *148*:200–205, 1983.
5. Arvin, A. M.: Cell-mediated immunity to varicella-zoster virus. J. Infect. Dis. *166*:S35–41, 1992.
6. Arvin, A. M., Pollard, R. B., Rasmussen, L., et al.: Selective impairment in lymphocyte reactivity to varicella-zoster antigen among untreated lymphoma patients. J. Infect. Dis. *137*:531–540, 1978.
7. Asano, Y., Itakura, N., Hiroishi, Y., et al.: Viremia is present in incubation period in nonimmunocompromised children with varicella. J Pediatr. *106*:69–71, 1985.
8. Asano, Y., Suga, S., Yoshikawa, T., et al.: Experience and reason: Twenty-year follow up of protective immunity of the Oka strain live varicella vaccine. Pediatrics *94*:524–526, 1994.
9. Asano, Y., Yoshikawa, T., Suga, S., et al.: Postexposure prophylaxis of varicella in family contact by oral acyclovir. Pediatrics *92*:219–222, 1993.
10. Baba, K., Yabuuchi, H., Takahashi, M., et al.: Immunologic and epidemiologic aspects of varicella infection acquired during infancy and early childhood. J. Pediatr. *100*:881–885, 1982.
11. Bakshi, S., Miller, T. C., Kaplan, M., et al.: Failure of VZIG in modification of severe congenital varicella. Pediatr. Infect. Dis. *5*:699–702, 1986.
12. Balfour, H. H., Kelly, J. M., Suarez, C. S., et al.: Acyclovir treatment of varicella in otherwise healthy children. J. Pediatr. *116*:633–639, 1990.
13. Berger, R., Florent, G., and Just, M.: Decrease of the lympho-proliferative response to varicella-zoster virus antigen in the aged. Infect. Immun. *32*:24–27, 1981.

14. Beutner, K. R., Friedman, D. J., Forszpaniak, C., et al.: Valacyclovir compared with acyclovir for improved therapy for herpes zoster in immunocompetent adults. Antimicrob. Agents Chemother. *39*:1546–1553, 1995.
15. Bocles, J. S., Ehrenkranz, N. J., and Marks, A.: Abnormalities of respiratory function in varicella pneumonia. Ann. Intern. Med. *60*:183, 1964.
16. Bradley, J. S., Schlievert, P. M., and Sample, T. G., Jr.: Streptococcal toxic shock–like syndrome as a complication of varicella. Pediatr. Infect. Dis. J. *10*:77–79, 1991.
17. Brunell, P., Gershon, A. A., Uduman, S. A., et al.: Varicella-zoster immunoglobulins during varicella, latency, and zoster. J. Infect. Dis. *132*:49–54, 1975.
18. Brunell, P. A., Shehab, Z., Geiser, C., et al.: Administration of live varicella vaccine to children with leukemia. Lancet *2*:1069–1073, 1982.
19. Bruusgaard, E.: The mutual relation between zoster and varicella. Brit. J. Derm. Syph. *44*:1–24, 1932.
20. Burke, B. L., Steele, R. W., Beard, O. W., et al.: Immune responses to varicella-zoster in the aged. Arch. Intern. Med. *142*:291–293, 1982.
21. Christie, A. B.: Chickenpox. *In* Infectious Diseases: Epidemiology and Clinical Practice. Edinburgh, E. and S. Livingstone, 1969.
22. Croen, K. D., Ostrove, J. M., Dragovic, L. Y., et al.: Patterns of gene expression and sites of latency in human ganglia are different for varicella-zoster and herpes simplex viruses. Proc. Natl. Acad. Sci. U. S. A. *85*:9773–9777, 1988.
23. Davison, A., Edson, C., Ellis, R., et al.: New common nomenclature for glycoprotein genes of varicella-zoster virus and their products. J. Virol. *57*:1195–1197, 1986.
24. Davison, A. J.: Varicella-zoster virus. The Fourteenth Fleming Lecture. J. Gen. Virol. *72*:475–486, 1991.
25. Davison, A. J., and Scott, J. E.: The complete DNA sequence of varicella-zoster virus. J. Gen. Virol. *67*:1759–1816, 1986.
26. Debrus, S., Sadzot-Delvaux, C., Nikkels, A. F., et al.: Varicella-zoster virus gene 63 encodes an immediate-early protein that is abundantly expressed during latency. J. Virol. *69*:3240–3245, 1995.
27. Dumas, A. H., Geelen, J. L. M. C., Weststrate, M. W., et al.: XbaI, PstI, and BglII restriction enzyme maps of the two orientations of the varicella-zoster virus genome. J Virol. *39*:390–400, 1981.
28. Dunkel, L., Arvin, A., Whitley, R., et al.: A controlled trial of oral acyclovir for chickenpox in normal children. N. Engl. J. Med. *325*:1539–1544, 1991.
29. Dworsky, M., Whitely, R., and Alford, C.: Herpes zoster in early infancy. Am. J. Dis. Child. *134*:618–619, 1980.
30. Ecker, J. R., and Hyman, R. W.: Varicella zoster virus DNA exists as two isomers. Proc. Natl. Acad. Sci. U. S. A. *79*:156–160, 1982.
31. Esiri, M., and Tomlinson, A.: Herpes zoster: Demonstration of virus in trigeminal nerve and ganglion by immunofluorescence and electron microscopy. J. Neurol. Sci. *15*:35–48, 1972.
32. Feldman, S., Chaudhary, S., Ossi, M., et al.: A viremic phase for herpes zoster in children with cancer. J. Pediatr. *91*:597–600, 1977.
33. Feldman, S., Hughes, W., and Daniel, C.: Varicella in children with cancer: 77 cases. Pediatrics *80*:388–397, 1975.
34. Feldman, S., and Lott, L.: Varicella in children with cancer: Impact of antiviral therapy and prophylaxis. Pediatrics *80*:465–472, 1987.
35. Friedman, C. A., Temple, D. M., Robbins, K. K., et al.: Outbreak and control of varicella in a neonatal intensive care unit. Pediatr. Infect. Dis. J. *13*:152–154, 1994.
36. Garland, J.: Varicella following exposure to herpes zoster. N. Engl. J. Med. *228*:336–337, 1943.
37. Gershon, A.: Chickenpox, measles, and mumps. *In* Remington, J. S., and Klein, J. O. (eds.): Infectious Diseases of the Fetus and Newborn Infant. 4th ed. Philadelphia, W. B. Saunders, 1994, pp. 565–618.
38. Gershon, A.: Varicella-zoster virus: Prospects for control. Adv. Pediatr. Infect. Dis. *10*:93–124, 1995.
39. Gershon, A., Frey, H., Steinberg, S., et al.: Enzyme-linked immunosorbent assay for measurement of antibody to varicella-zoster virus. Arch. Virol. *70*:169–172, 1981.
40. Gershon, A., LaRussa, P., Steinberg, S., et al.: Varicella vaccine prevents zoster in leukemic recipients of live attenuated varicella vaccine: Effects of more than one immunizing dose. *In* VZV Research Foundation, 2nd International Meeting, Paris, 1994.
41. Gershon, A., Raker, R., Steinberg, S., et al.: Antibody to varicella-zoster virus in parturient women and their offspring during the first year of life. Pediatrics *58*:692–696, 1976.
42. Gershon, A., Steinberg, S., Borkowsky, W., et al.: IgM to varicella-zoster virus: Demonstration in patients with and without clinical zoster. Pediatr. Infect. Dis. *1*:164–167, 1982.
43. Gershon, A., Steinberg, S., and Brunell, P.: Zoster immune globulin: A further assessment. N. Engl. J. Med. *290*:243–245, 1974.
44. Gershon, A., Steinberg, S., and LaRussa, P.: Varicella-zoster virus. *In* Lennette, E. H. (ed.): Laboratory Diagnosis of Viral Infections. 2nd ed. New York, Marcel Dekker, 1992, pp. 749–765.
45. Gershon, A., Zhu, Z., Sherman, D. L., et al.: Intracellular transport of newly synthesized varicella-zoster virus: Final envelopment in the trans-Golgi network. J. Virol. *68*:6372–6390, 1994.
46. Gershon, A. A., LaRussa, P., and Steinberg, S.: Live attenuated varicella vaccine: Current status and future uses. Semin. Pediatr. Infect. Dis. *2*:171–178, 1991.
47. Gershon, A. A., Steinberg, S., Gelb, L., et al.: Clinical reinfection with varicella-zoster virus. J. Infect. Dis. *149*:137–142, 1984.
48. Gershon, A. A., Steinberg, S., Gelb, L., et al.: Live attenuated varicella vaccine: Efficacy for children with leukemia in remission. J. A. M. A. *252*:355–362, 1984.
49. Gershon, A. A., Steinberg, S., LaRussa, P., et al.: Immunization of healthy adults with live attenuated varicella vaccine. J. Infect. Dis. *158*:132–137, 1988.
50. Gershon, A. A., and Steinberg, S. (NIAID Collaborative Varicella Vaccine Study Group): Live attenuated varicella vaccine: Protection in healthy adults in comparison to leukemic children. J. Infect. Dis. *161*:661–666, 1990.
51. Gershon, A. A., and Steinberg, S. (NIAID Collaborative Varicella Vaccine Study Group): Persistence of immunity to varicella in children with leukemia immunized with live attenuated varicella vaccine. N. Engl. J. Med. *320*:892–897, 1989.
52. Gilden, D. H., Dueland, A. N., Cohrs, R., et al.: Postherpetic neuralgia. Neurology *41*:1215–1218, 1991.
53. Gordon, J. E.: Chickenpox: An epidemiologic review. Am. J. Med. Sci. *244*:362–389, 1962.
54. Gray, G. C., Palinkas, L. A., and Kelley, P. W.: Increasing incidence of varicella hospitalizations in United States Army and Navy personnel: Are today's teenagers more susceptible? Should recruits be vaccinated? Pediatrics *86*:867–873, 1990.
55. Grose, C.: Glycoproteins encoded by varicella-zoster virus: Biosynthesis, phosphorylation, and intracellular trafficking. Ann. Rev. Microbiol. *44*:59–80, 1990.
56. Grose, C., and Litwin, V.: Immunology of the varicella-zoster glycoproteins. J. Infect. Dis. *157*:877–881, 1988.
57. Grose, C. H. Variation on a theme by Fenner. Pediatrics 68:735–737, 1981.
58. Guess, H., Broughton, D. D., Melton, L. J., et al.: Epidemiology of herpes zoster in children and adolescents: A population-based study. Pediatrics *76*:512–517, 1985.
59. Gustafson, T. L., Shehab, Z., and Brunell, P.: Outbreak of varicella in a newborn intensive care nursery. Am. J. Dis. Child. *138*:548–550, 1984.
60. Haiduven-Griffeths, D., and Fecko, H.: Varicella in hospital personnel: A challenge for the infection control practitioner. Am. J. Infect. Control *15*:207–211, 1987.
61. Han, C. S., Miller, W., Haake, R., et al.: Varicella zoster infection after bone marrow transplantation: Incidence, risk factors and complications. Bone Marrow Transpl. *13*:277–283, 1994.
62. Hardy, I. B., Gershon, A., and Steinberg, S., et al.: Incidence of zoster after live attenuated varicella vaccine. *In* International Conference on Antimicrobial Agents and Chemotherapy, Chicago, 1991.
63. Hardy, I. B., Gershon, A., Steinberg, S., et al.: The incidence of zoster after immunization with live attenuated varicella vaccine: A study in children with leukemia. N. Engl. J. Med. *325*:1545–1550, 1991.
64. Haverkos, H. W., Amsel, Z., and Drotman, D. P.: Adverse virus-drug interactions. Rev. Infect. Dis. *13*:697–704, 1991.
65. Hay, J., and Ruyechan, W. T.: Varicella-zoster virus: A different kind of herpesvirus latency? Semin. Virol. *5*:241–248, 1994.
66. Hodge, R. A. V.: Famciclovir and penciclovir: The mode of action of famciclovir including its conversion to penciclovir. Antiviral Chem. Chemotherap. *4*:67–84, 1993.
67. Hope-Simpson, R. E.: The nature of herpes zoster: A long-term study and a new hypothesis. Proc. Roy. Soc. Med. *58*:9–20, 1965.
68. Huff, C., Bean, B., Balfour, H., et al.: Therapy of herpes zoster with oral acyclovir. Am. J. Med. *85*(A2A):84–89, 1988.
69. Ihara, T., Starr, S., Ito, M., et al.: Human polymorphonuclear leukocyte–mediated cytotoxicity against varicella-zoster virus–infected fibroblasts. J. Virol. *51*:110–116, 1984.
70. Jacobson, M. A., Berger, T. G., and Fikrig, S.: Acyclovir-resistant varicella-zoster virus infection after chronic oral acyclovir therapy in patients with the acquired immunodeficiency syndrome. Ann. Intern. Med. *112*:187–191, 1990.
71. Jenkins, R. B.: Severe chickenpox encephalopathy. Am. J. Dis. Child. *110*:137, 1965.
72. Johnson, R., and Milbourn, P. E.: Central nervous system manifestations of chickenpox. Can. Med. Assoc. J. *102*:831, 1970.
73. Junker, A. K., Angus, E., and Thomas, E.: Recurrent varicella-zoster virus infections in apparently immunocompetent children. Pediatr. Infect. Dis. J. *10*:569–575, 1991.
74. Jura, E., Chadwick, E., SH, J., et al.: Varicella-zoster virus infections in children infected with human immunodeficiency virus. Pediatr. Infect. Dis. J. *8*:586–590, 1989.
75. Kalman, C. M., and Laskin, O. L. Herpes zoster and zosteriform herpes simplex virus infections in immunocompetent adults. Am. J. Med. *81*:775–778, 1986.
76. Kido, S., Ozaki, T., Asada, H., et al.: Detection of varicella-zoster virus (VZV) DNA in clinical samples from patients with VZV by the polymerase chain reaction. J. Clin. Microbiol. *29*:76–79, 1991.
77. Kjersem, H., and Jepsen, S.: Varicella among immigrants from the tropics: A health problem. Scand. J. Soc. Med. *18*:171–174, 1990.
78. Kundratitz, K.: Experimentelle übertragung von herpes zoster auf den

mensschen und die beziehungen von herpes zoster zu varicellen. Monatsschr. Kinder *29*:516–523, 1925.
79. Kuter, B. J., Weibel, R. E., Guess, H. A., et al.: Oka/Merck varicella vaccine in healthy children: Final report of a 2-year efficacy study and 7-year follow-up studies. Vaccine *9*:643–647, 1991.
80. LaForet, E. G., and Lynch, L. L.: Multiple congenital defects following maternal varicella. N. Engl. J. Med. *236*:534–537, 1947.
81. LaRussa, P., Lungu, O., Hardy, I., et al.: Restriction fragment length polymorphism of polymerase chain reaction products from vaccine and wild-type varicella-zoster virus isolates. J. Virol. *66*:1016–1020, 1992.
82. LaRussa, P., Steinberg, S., Seeman, M. D., et al.: Determination of immunity to varicella by means of an intradermal skin test. J. Infect. Dis. *152*:869–875, 1985.
83. Leclair, J. M., Zaia, J., Levin, M. J., et al.: Airborne transmission of chickenpox in a hospital. N. Engl. J. Med. *302*:450–453, 1980.
84. Locksley, R. M., Flournoy, N., Sullivan, K. M., et al.: Infection with varicella-zoster virus after marrow transplantation. J. Infect. Dis. *152*:1172–1181, 1985.
85. Lungu, O., Annunziato, P., Gershon, A., et al.: Reactivated and latent varicella-zoster virus in human dorsal root ganglia. Proc. Natl. Acad. Sci. U. S. A. *92*:10980–10984, 1995.
86. Mahalingham, R., Wellish, M., Dueland, A. N., et al.: Localization of herpes simplex virus and varicella zoster virus DNA in human ganglia. Ann. Neurol. *31*:444–448, 1992.
87. Martin, J. H., Dohner, D., Wellinghoff, W. J., et al.: Restriction endonuclease analysis of varicella-zoster vaccine virus and wild type DNAs. J. Med. Virol. *9*:69–76, 1982.
88. Mendez, D., Sinclair, M. B., Garcia, S., et al.: Transplacental immunity to varicella-zoster virus in extremely low birthweight infants. Am. J. Perinatol. *9*:236–238, 1992.
89. Moore, D. A., and Hopkins, R. S.: Assessment of a school exclusion policy during a chickenpox outbreak. Am. J. Epidemiol. *133*:1161–1167, 1991.
90. Myers, M., and Connelly, B. L.: Animal models of varicella. J. Infect. Dis. *166*:S48–S50, 1992.
91. Nader, S., Bergen, R., Sharp, M., et al.: Comparison of cell-mediated immunity (CMI) to varicella-zoster virus (VZV) in children and adults immunized with live attenuated varicella vaccine. J. Infect. Dis. *171*:13–17, 1995.
92. Ozaki, T., Matsui, Y., Asano, Y., et al.: Study of virus isolation from pharyngeal swabs in children with varicella. Am. J. Dis. Child. *143*:1448–1450, 1989.
93. Ozaki, T., Miwata, H., Matsui, Y., et al.: Varicella zoster virus DNA in throat swabs. Arch. Dis. Child. *65*:333–334, 1990.
94. Pearson, H. E.: Parturition varicella-zoster. Obstet. Gynecol. *23*:21, 1964.
95. Perren, T., Powles, R., Easton, D., et al.: Prevention of herpes zoster in patients by long-term oral acyclovir after allogeneic bone marrow transplantation. Am. J. Med. *85*(S2A):99–101, 1988.
96. Pitel, P. A., McCormick, K. L., Fitzgerald, E., et al.: Subclinical hepatic changes in varicella infection. Pediatrics *65*:631–633, 1980.
97. Preblud, S., Bregman, D. J., Vernon, L. L.: Deaths from varicella in infants. Pediatr. Infect. Dis. *4*:503–507, 1985.
98. Preblud, S., Nelson, W. L., Levin, M., et al.: Modification of congenital varicella infection with VZIG. *In* Interscience Conference on Antimicrobial Agents and Chemotherapy, New Orleans, 1986.
99. Preblud, S. R. Varicella: Complications and costs. Pediatrics *76*(Suppl.): 728–735, 1986.
100. Puchhammer-Stockl, E., Popow-Kraupp, T., Heinz, F., et al.: Detection of varicella-zoster virus DNA by polymerase chain reaction in the cerebrospinal fluid of patients suffering from neurological complications associated with chicken pox or herpes zoster. J. Clin. Microbiol. *29*:1513–1516, 1991.
101. Raker, R., Steinberg, S., Drusin, L., et al.: Antibody to varicella-zoster virus in low birth weight infants. J. Pediatr. *93*:505–506, 1978.
102. Ross, A. H., Lencher, E., and Reitman, G.: Modification of chickenpox in family contacts by administration of gamma globulin. N. Engl. J. Med. *267*:369–376, 1962.
103. Safrin, S., Berger, T., Gilson, I., et al.: Foscarnet therapy in five patients with AIDS and acyclovir-resistant varicella-zoster infection. Ann. Intern. Med. *115*:19–21, 1991.
104. Safrin, S., Crumpacker, C., Chatis, P. et al.: A controlled trial comparing foscarnet with vidarabine for acyclovir-resistant mucocutaneous herpes simplex in the acquired immunodeficiency syndrome. N. Engl. J. Med. *325*:551–555, 1991.
105. Sawyer, M. H., Wu, Y. N., Chamberlin, C. J., et al.: Detection of varicella-zoster virus DNA in the oropharynx and blood of patients with varicella. J. Infect. Dis. *166*:885–888, 1992.
106. Schmidt, N. J.: Further evidence for common antigens in herpes simplex and varicella-zoster virus. J. Med. Virol. *9*:27–36, 1982.
107. Shehab, Z., Brunell, P.: Enzyme-linked immunosorbent assay for susceptibility to varicella. J. Infect. Dis. *148*:472–476, 1983.
108. Shepp, D. H., Dandliker, P. S., and Meyers, J. D.: Treatment of varicella-zoster virus infection in severely immunocompromised patients: A randomized comparison of acyclovir and vidarabine. N. Engl. J. Med. *314*:208–212, 1986.
109. Smith, K., Kahlter, D. C., Davis, C., et al.: Acyclovir-resistant varicella zoster responsive to foscarnet. Arch. Dermatol. *127*:1069–1071, 1991.
110. Srabstein, J. C., Morris, N., Larke, B., et al.: Is there a congenital varicella syndrome? J. Pediatr. *84*:239–243, 1974.
111. Steinberg, S., and Gershon, A.: Measurement of antibodies to varicella-zoster virus by using a latex agglutination test. J. Clin. Microbiol. 29:1527–1529, 1991.
112. Stern, E. S.: The mechanism of herpes zoster and its relation to chickenpox. Br. J. Dermatol. Syphil. *49*:264–271, 1937.
113. Stevens, D., Ferrington, R., and Jordan, G., et al.: Cellular events in zoster vesicles: Relation to clinical course and immune parameters. J. Infect. Dis. *131*:509–515, 1975.
114. Straus, S. E., Aulakh, H. S., Ruyechan, W. T., et al.: Structure of varicella-zoster virus DNA. J. Virol. *40*:516–526, 1981.
115. Triebwasser, J. H., Harris, R. E., Bryant, R. E., et al.: Varicella pneumonia in adults: Report of seven cases and a review of the literature. Medicine *46*:409–423, 1967.
116. Trlifajova, J., Bryndova, D., and Ryc, M.: Isolation of varicella-zoster virus from pharyngeal and nasal swabs in varicella patients. J. Hyg. Epidemiol. Micro. Immunol. *28*:201–206, 1984.
117. Tsolia, M., Gershon, A., Steinberg, S., et al.: Live attenuated varicella vaccine: Evidence that the virus is attenuated and the importance of skin lesions in transmission of varicella-zoster virus. J. Pediatr. *116*:184–189, 1990.
118. Tyring, S., Barbarash, R. A., Nahlik, J. E., et al.: Famciclovir for the treatment of acute herpes zoster: Effects on acute disease and post herpetic neuralgia. Ann. Intern. Med. *123*:89–96, 1995.
119. Uduman, S. A., Gershon, A. A., and Brunell, P. A.: Should patients with zoster receive zoster immune globulin? J. A. M. A. *234*:1049, 1975.
120. von Bokay, J.: Ueber den aetiologischen zusammenhang der varizellen mit gewissen fallen von herpes zoster. Wien Klin. Wochenschr. *22*:1323–1326, 1909.
121. Watson, B., Boardman, C., Laufer, D., et al.: Humoral and cell-mediated immune responses in healthy children after one or two doses of varicella vaccine. Clin. Infect. Dis. *20*:316–319, 1995.
122. Watson, B. M., Piercy, S. A., Plotkin, S. A., et al.: Modified chickenpox in children immunized with the Oka/Merck varicella vaccine. Pediatrics 91:17–22, 1993.
123. Weber, D. M., and Pellecchia, J. A.: Varicella pneumonia: Study of prevalence in adult men. J. A. M. A. *192*:572, 1965.
124. Weller, T. H.: Varicella and herpes zoster: Changing concepts of the natural history, control, and importance of a not-so-benign virus. N. Engl. J. Med. *309*:1362–1368, 1434–1440, 1983.
125. White, C. J., Kuter, B. J., Hildebrand, C. S., et al.: Varicella vaccine (VARIVAX) in healthy children and adolescents: Results from clinical trials, 1987 to 1989. Pediatrics *87*:604–610, 1991.
126. White, C. J., Kuter, B. J., Ngai, A., et al.: Modified cases of chickenpox after varicella vaccination: Correlation of protection with antibody response. Pediatr. Infect. Dis. J. *11*:19–22, 1992.
127. Whitley, R.: Therapeutic approaches to varicella-zoster virus infections. J. Infect. Dis. *166*:S51–57, 1992.
128. Whitley, R. J., Middlebrooks, M., and Gnann, J. W.: Acyclovir: The past ten years. Adv. Exp. Med. Biol. *278*:243–253, 1990.
129. Whitley, R. J., and Straus, S.: Therapy for varicella-zoster virus infections: Where do we stand? Infect. Dis. Clin. Pract. *2*:100–108, 1993.
130. Williams, D. L., Gershon, A., Gelb, L. D., et al.: Herpes zoster following varicella vaccine in a child with acute lymphocytic leukemia. J. Pediatr. *106*:259–261, 1985.
131. Williams, V., Gershon, A., and Brunell, P.: Serologic response to varicella-zoster membrane antigens measured by indirect immunofluorescence. J. Infect. Dis. *130*:669–672, 1974.
132. Wilson, A., Sharp, M., and Koropchak, C., et al.: Subclinical varicella-zoster virus viremia, herpes zoster, and T lymphocyte immunity to varicella-zoster viral antigens after bone marrow transplantation. J. Infect. Dis. *165*:119–126, 1991.
133. Wilson, G., Talkington, D., Gruber, W., et al.: Group A streptococcal necrotizing fasciitis following varicella in children: Case reports and review. Clin. Infect. Dis. *20*:1333–1338, 1995.
134. Zaia, J., and Oxman, M.: Antibody to varicella-zoster virus–induced membrane antigen: Immunofluorescence assay using monodisperse glutaraldehyde-fixed target cells. J. Infect. Dis. *136*:519–530, 1977.
135. Zaia, J. A., Leary, P. L., and Levin, M. J.: Specificity of the blastogenic response of human mononuclear cells to herpes antigens. Infect. Immun. *20*:646–651, 1978.

❑ ❑ ❑

SUBSECTION SIX

POXVIRIDAE

168

SMALLPOX (VARIOLA VIRUS)

James D. Cherry

Smallpox was a dreaded febrile exanthematous disease caused by the orthopoxvirus variola virus.[2–4, 7] After an extensive decade-long World Health Organization (WHO) program to eradicate smallpox, the world was certified free of smallpox in 1979.[30] This chapter reviews the history and clinical manifestations of smallpox. Virology is presented in Chapter 169.

HISTORY[4, 7, 8, 13, 29]

Evidence suggests that endemic smallpox was occurring before the year A.D. 1000. Three mummies, dating from the eighteenth to the twentieth dynasties in Egypt, had pustular lesions all over their bodies.[8] Reliable written accounts of smallpox first appeared during the fourth century. Smallpox was differentiated from measles in A.D. 340 in China by Ko Hung. At that time in China, smallpox was an established endemic disease that had come from the west 300 years earlier. During the period from A.D. 340 to A.D. 1000, the disease was described in Egypt, India, Korea, Japan, Southern Europe, and North Africa. A major contribution to the spread of smallpox was the great Islamic expansion across North Africa and into Spain in the seventh and eighth centuries.

By the year 1000, smallpox probably was endemic in populated areas of Europe, Asia, and the African Mediterranean countries. Smallpox was established further in Northern Europe by the population movements related to the Crusades. By the sixteenth century, smallpox was a serious disease in Europe, as indicated by death statistics in Geneva, London, and Sweden. In London during the seventeenth century, about 10 per cent of the yearly deaths were attributed to smallpox.

The disease was introduced into the American colonies in 1507 and into Mexico soon thereafter. Epidemics of smallpox posed serious problems for the colonists and for the Native Americans as well. These epidemics may have been important also in certain stages of the American Revolution.[3, 9] Smallpox persisted in the United States and Mexico until the 1940s and 1950s, respectively, despite concerted efforts to eliminate the problem.

Soon after the recognition of this disease, the Chinese are reported to have made efforts to prevent it. The technique used presumably was variolation, which is the intentional intranasal or intracutaneous inoculation of susceptible persons with vesicular fluid or crusts from smallpox patients. This technique apparently originated in China and subsequently was used in many countries, including the United States. As recently as 1968 and 1969, isolated instances of variolation were noted in remote areas of Africa and Asia.[9, 13]

After Jenner's observations in 1796 on the immunity against smallpox that was conferred by prior inoculation with material obtained from cowpox lesions, he extended his observations to include intentional and deliberate exposure of some of those immunized with cowpox. This provided convincing evidence of solid protection against smallpox.[15] Encouraged by the results, he predicted in 1801 the ultimate eradication of smallpox, a remarkable prediction indeed.[9, 11]

The Intensified Smallpox Eradication Program of WHO, set up in 1967, initiated remarkable progress toward the total global eradication of this disease. Several factors were responsible for this rapid progress, including emphasis on surveillance of disease, with containment, rather than on routine vaccination; improved vaccines and vaccination technology; and sound administrative and fiscal support.[9, 10, 12, 18] Of the more than 30 countries in 1967 in which smallpox was endemic, the disease persisted in only 5 in 1975 and in 2 in 1977. The world's last case of endemic smallpox occurred on October 31, 1977, in Merca, Somalia.[6] A year later, in 1978, a photographer working at the University of Birmingham in England was infected and died of infection with a laboratory strain of smallpox virus.[20, 27]

Presently, smallpox virus is retained for research purposes in only two laboratories. One of these is at the Centers for Disease Control and Prevention in Atlanta, and the other is at the Research Institute for Viral Preparations in Moscow.[25]

In recent years, there has been considerable debate as to whether to save or destroy the remaining stocks of smallpox virus.[16, 20] A WHO expert panel had recommended the destruction of the 600 remaining virus samples by December 31, 1993.[21] That date and a subsequent date (June 30, 1995) have come and gone, and no action as yet has been taken.

ETIOLOGY

Smallpox was caused by variola virus, an orthopoxvirus.[7] The virus particles are brick-shaped and measure 250 to 300 × 200 to 250 × 100 nm; the size and shape are similar for all orthopoxviruses. The distinctive appearance is helpful in rapidly identifying members of this virus group by electron microscopy of vesicular fluid or crusts. The virus is stable when dried and may remain viable for long periods in dried crusts and indefinitely under freeze-dry techniques in the laboratory. It is propagated readily on the chorioallantoic membrane of embryonated eggs and in a variety of mammalian cell cultures.

EPIDEMIOLOGY

In infected patients, variola virus was found in respiratory secretions and in vesicular fluid from skin lesions. Transmission most often occurred by close personal contact, but airborne spread also could occur.[28] Patients were contagious during the latter portion of the 7- to 17-day incubation periods, and this contagiousness remained during all stages of illness.

All persons were susceptible to smallpox unless they had had prior infection with variola virus itself or with cowpox or vaccinia virus. Thus, the occurrence of smallpox depended entirely on the presence of a source of infection and the effective exposure of susceptible persons. The age distribution of cases varied in individual countries, depending largely on vaccination practices. Preschool children often were not vaccinated and thus had the greatest prevalence of disease.

The seasonal influence was substantial. This perhaps is shown best by spread of disease after winter and spring introductions of smallpox into Europe; spread of infection was more than 30 times as great after introduction of infection into European nations between December and May, in contrast with substantially less frequent spread after introduction between June and November.[27]

Substantial contrasts in case-fatality rates were recognized between different geographic areas; these differences do not appear to depend on the supportive care available and do not appear to be related to ethnic or specific resistance factors. The only logical explanation for these differences was substantial differences in the virulence of the virus prevalent in the regions. The mildest form of smallpox, described as variola minor or alastrim, was prevalent in Brazil, Ethiopia, and adjacent countries. Case-fatality rates of 1 per cent or less were customary, and permanent residual scarring and blindness were most unusual. In other areas of Africa and Indonesia, the disease appeared to be of intermediate severity, whereas on the Indian subcontinent, case-fatality rates were as high as 30 per cent, with residual permanent scarring, blindness, and other sequelae frequent among those who survived the acute illness.[9]

PATHOLOGY

The characteristic pathologic lesions involved the skin and mucous membranes. They involved the deeper layers of the skin and progressed through macular, papular, vesicular, and pustular stages, resulting in the formation of crusts. Lesions similar to those on the skin also were found in the lower respiratory and gastrointestinal tracts.

Secondary bacterial infection was frequent and often involved the skin and lung. Hemorrhagic complications (hemorrhagic smallpox) were not uncommon.

CLINICAL MANIFESTATIONS

After an incubation period of between 7 and 17 days, the disease began abruptly with fever between 38.9° and 40.5° C (102° and 105° F), headache, and marked malaise. Backache and muscle pains were prominent symptoms. Nausea, vomiting, and abdominal pain also were present.

After these prodromal signs and symptoms were present for 2 to 4 days, the fever usually dropped, and the characteristic cutaneous eruption appeared. The rash was most extensive on the face and extremities, and the individual lesions passed through the stages of macules and papules; by the third or fourth day, they clearly were vesicular. Lesions in a single area of the body characteristically were at the same stage of development.

By the sixth day, the vesicular fluid usually was cloudy and the individual pustules often were umbilicated. Pustules often converged and become confluent. By the tenth day, the individual lesions begin to dry and formed characteristic crusts that remained intact for several days before they were shed. The temperature customarily fell during the early appearance of the rash, although the fever usually returned. Significant fever after the tenth or twelfth day of disease suggested that a bacterial superinfection had occurred.

Although most cases were similar to this description, which was characteristic of the ordinary type of smallpox, other clinical variations were described. The hemorrhagic type was the most severe form, with a case-fatality rate that approached 100 per cent. In this form, hemorrhagic manifestations appeared during the prodromal stage, with extensive cutaneous extravasations of blood and bleeding from the various body orifices. Death usually occurred within the first week of illness, and often few typical diagnostic lesions appeared on the skin surfaces before death. Fortunately, this form of disease only occurred in 2 or 3 per cent of the total cases of variola major in Asia, and it rarely was seen elsewhere.

A flat variety had been reported in approximately 6 per cent of cases observed in India. In this variety, the cutaneous lesions remained flat and soft to the touch, in contrast with the ordinary variety; these lesions characteristically resolved without pustulation. This form was associated with case-fatality rates of 75 to 96 per cent.[9, 26]

A modified form of disease occurred almost exclusively in previously vaccinated persons. Although the prodromal illness often was severe, skin lesions were few, evolved rapidly, and were more superficial; the prognosis was excellent.

The mildest form of the disease, alastrim or variola minor, was caused by a specific variola virus of lesser pathogenicity for humans. Serious forms of the illness, as with variola major, were unusual. The skin lesions tended to be superficial, and the clinical course resembled that of varicella with the exception of the distribution of the cutaneous lesions. These involved the face and extremities, in contrast with the characteristic central body distribution of varicella. Residual scarring, if it occurred at all, usually reflected secondary bacterial infection of individual lesions.

Among recently vaccinated persons, infection with variola virus after exposure had been proved by increases in antibody titer against the virus when acute and convalescent sera were tested. This event was uncommon and was of neither clinical nor epidemiologic significance.

Complications included the hemorrhagic events and various secondary bacterial infections, which included impetigo, pneumonia, empyema, and otitis media. Nephritis and arthritis with permanent joint changes were described.

DIFFERENTIAL DIAGNOSIS

The typical course, the characteristic cutaneous lesions, and the presence of other cases with contact from 7 to 17 days earlier left little doubt of the etiologic agent. Varicella presented the greatest problem in differential diagnosis, particularly from the variola minor or alastrim form of the disease, but the distribution of cutaneous lesions for each was characteristic. Generalized vaccinia or eczema vaccinatum was distinguished by the history of exposure to vaccinia virus, prior skin lesions, and the distribution of the rash. Impetigo (especially the bullous variety due to staphylococcal infection), scabies, secondary syphilis, and yaws were other considerations. Usually, little difficulty was encountered clinically in distinguishing among these infections.

Monkeypox resembled smallpox clinically, but it occurred only in Central and West Africa, primarily in Zaire. Specific laboratory procedures were required for diagnosis.[14]

Noninfectious conditions that were included in the differential diagnosis included erythema multiforme, pityriasis rosea, and the purpuras, which occasionally confused the inexperienced physician.

SPECIFIC DIAGNOSIS

Several laboratory procedures were available to provide specific and accurate diagnosis.

Electron Microscopy

Vesicular fluid, crusts, or scrapings from skin lesions contained the characteristic brick-shaped viral particles of the variola-vaccinia virus group. These orthopoxviruses differed in appearance from those of the herpesviruses, which was the class of infections most frequently confused with smallpox. This technique was precise and rapid and was preferred when facilities for this examination were available.[5]

Precipitation in Gel

In contact with antivaccinial serum in clear agar gel, either vesicular fluid or an emulsified extract of crusts formed a visible line of precipitate. This test could be read within a few hours and was specific for members of the orthopox family.[26]

Complement Fixation

This test could be performed to identify virus antigen in vesicles or crusts and could be used to measure levels of serum antibody.

Fluorescent Antibody Test

This method was used as a rapid diagnostic technique for the identification of orthopoxviruses. It was more subject to error than was electron microscopy, but it was considered a useful adjunctive test.

Isolation and Identification of Virus

Orthopoxviruses may be recovered and propagated on the chorioallantoic membrane of embryonated eggs or in tissue culture. Recovery of the virus required more time (3 to 7 days) than did the direct antigen tests but provided the specific active virus required for differentiation among the various specific orthopoxvirus types.[22, 24, 26]

TREATMENT

Therapy primarily was supportive and symptomatic. The skin was kept clean, the bed linen was changed at regular intervals, and local or systemic therapy was provided for treatment of the frequent bacterial complications. Attention to appropriate fluid and nutritional support was required.

Methisazone, convalescent smallpox serum, and vaccinia immunoglobulin were effective in preventing the disease after exposure, but there was no evidence that these agents altered the course of the disease once symptoms occurred.[17] Idoxuridine was used for corneal lesions.[3]

PREVENTION

Active Immunization

Many strains of vaccinia virus were used in the effective prophylaxis of smallpox. In 1967, at least 15 strains were in use in various countries.[1] In the late 1960s and 1970s, most vaccinations were performed with the New York City Board of Health strain or the Lister (Elstree) strain, which were similar. These were prepared by the freeze-drying process, and inoculation was performed best with use of the bifurcated needle, with 5 (for primary immunization) to 15 (for revaccination) punctures within a small (5 mm in diameter) area of the skin of the upper left deltoid region. The vaccination site was not to be covered tightly, although a loose, dry dressing was applied during the height of the reaction for decreasing the possibility of transfer of vaccinia virus by fingers to the eye or to skin lesions, such as insect bites or impetigo lesions, and so on. A small but definite risk of complications, both local and neurologic, were associated with vaccination.[19, 23]

Passive Immunization and Antiviral Protection

Transient protection after exposure was provided by vaccinia immunoglobulin when available.[17] Because this material often was in short supply, use of methisazone was considered, although this drug was not licensed and was available only on special request. When used prophylactically, this drug provided some measure of protection. Vomiting was a frequent side effect, and dosage presented problems in some persons.

Control of Sources of Infection

All known contacts of cases needed to be vaccinated or revaccinated promptly and kept under surveillance until at least 17 days transpired after the last contact with a known case. When such persons developed fever, prompt isolation was required until the nature of the illness was determined. All personnel in contact with an index case or involved in the surveillance of contacts needed to be vaccinated or revaccinated.

Environmental isolation and disinfection precautions also were required because the virus persisted in crusts for many months. Proper double wrapping and disinfection of all articles leaving the patient's room were necessary. Precautions also were required to prevent transfer of crusts by shoes or clothing of personnel to areas outside the isolation unit. Isolation precautions for the patient were necessary until all crusts had been shed. After recovery or death of the patient, terminal disinfection of the room was required.

References

1. Arita, I.: The control of vaccine quality in the smallpox eradication programme: International Symposium on Smallpox Vaccine, Bilthoven. Symp. Series Immunobiol. Standards *19*:79–87, 1972.
2. Behbehani, A. M.: The smallpox story: Historical perspective. Globally eradicated today, smallpox once killed scores of people over thousands of years. ASM News *57*:571–576, 1991.
3. Benenson, A. S.: Smallpox. *In* Wehrle, P. F., and Top, F. H. (eds.): Communicable and Infectious Diseases. 9th ed. St. Louis, C. V. Mosby, 1982, pp. 577–588.
4. Crosby, A. W.: Smallpox. *In* Kiple, K. F. (ed.): The Cambridge World History of Human Diseases. New York, Cambridge University Press, 1993, pp. 1008–1013.
5. Cruickshank, J. G., Bedson, H. S., and Watson, D. H.: Electron microscopy in the rapid diagnosis of smallpox. Lancet *2*:527, 1966.
6. Deria, A., Jezek, Z., Markvart, K., et al.: The worlds last endemic case of smallpox: Surveillance and containment measures. Bull. W. H. O. *58*:279–283, 1980.
7. Fenner, F.: Poxviruses. *In* Fields, B. N., Knipe, D. M., Howley, P. M., et

al. (eds.): Fields Virology. 3rd ed. Philadelphia, Lippincott-Raven, 1996, pp. 2673–2702.
8. Fenner, F.: Smallpox, "the most dreadful scourge of the human species." Med. J. Aust. Nov. 24, 1984, pp. 728–735.
9. Fenner, F., Henderson, D. A., Arita, I., et al.: Smallpox and Its Eradication. Geneva, World Health Organization, 1988.
10. Foege, W. H., Millar, J. D., and Lane, J. M.: Selective epidemiologic control in smallpox eradication. Am. J. Epidemiol. *94*:311–315, 1971.
11. Henderson, D. A.: Eradication of smallpox: The critical year ahead. Proc. R. Soc. Med. *66*:493–500, 1973.
12. Henderson, D. A., Arita, I., and Shafa, E.: Studies of the bifurcated needle and recommendations for its use. Document SE/72.5. Geneva, Smallpox Eradication Unit of WHO, 1972.
13. Hopkins, D. R.: Princes and Peasants: Smallpox in History. Chicago, University of Chicago Press, 1983.
14. Anonymous: Human monkeypox: The past five years. WHO Chronicle *38*:227–29, 1984.
15. Jenner, E.: The origin of the vaccine inoculation. London, D. N. Shury, 1801. *Cited in* Crookshank, E. M.: History and Pathology of Vaccination. Vol. II. 1889, p. 276.
16. Joklik, W. K., Moss, B., Fields, B. N., et al.: Why the smallpox virus stocks should not be destroyed. Science *262*:1225–1226, 1993.
17. Kempe, C. H., Berge, T. O., and England, B.: Hyperimmune gamma globulin, source, evaluation, and use of prophylaxis and therapy. Pediatrics *18*:177, 1956.
18. Ladnyi, I. D., Ziegler, P., and Kima, F.: A human infection caused by monkeypox virus in Basankusu Territory, Democratic Republic of the Congo. Bull. W. H. O. *46*:593–597, 1972.
19. Lane, J. M., and Millar, J. D.: Risks of smallpox vaccination complications in the United States. Am. J. Epidemiol. *93*:238, 1971.
20. Mahy, B. W. J., Almond, J. W., Berns, K. I., et al.: The remaining stocks of smallpox virus should be destroyed. Science *262*:1223–1224, 1993.
21. Maurice, J.: Virus wins stay of execution. Science *267*:450, 1995.
22. Nakano, J. H., and Bingham, P. G.: Smallpox, vaccinia, and human infections with monkeypox virus. *In* Lennette, E. H., Spaulding, E. H., and Truant, J. P. (eds.): Manual of Clinical Microbiology. 2nd ed. Washington, D.C., American Society for Microbiology, 1974, pp. 782–794.
23. Neff, J., Millar, J. D., Roberto, R. R., et al.: Smallpox vaccination by intradermal jet injection. III. Evaluation in a well vaccinated population. Bull. W. H. O. *41*:771–778, 1969.
24. Nizamuddin, M., and Dumbell, K. R.: A simple laboratory test to distinguish the virus of smallpox from that of alastrim. Lancet *1*:68, 1961.
25. Anonymous: Smallpox: Post-eradication policy—destruction of variola virus stocks. M. M. W. R. *33*:24, 1984.
26. Anonymous: Smallpox in 1974. WHO Chronicle *29*:134–139, 1975.
27. Wehrle, P. F.: Smallpox eradication: A global appraisal. J. A. M. A. *240*:1977–1979, 1978.
28. Wehrle, P. F., Posch, J., Richter, K. H., et al.: Airborne smallpox in a German hospital. Bull. W. H. O. *43*:669–679, 1970.
29. White, P. J., and Shackelford, P. G.: Edward Jenner, MD, and the scourge that was. Am. J. Dis. Child. *137*:864–869, 1983.
30. World Health Organization: The global eradication of smallpox. Final Report of the Global Commission for the Certification of Smallpox Eradication. History of International Public Health No. 4. Geneva, World Health Organization, 1980.

169

OTHER POXVIRUSES

James D. Cherry

Smallpox, which was caused by variola virus (see Chapter 168), was the most important human poxvirus disease. This disease has been eradicated from the world. Today there is only one human poxvirus, molluscum contagiosum virus, that causes specific human illness. In addition, there are nine other poxviruses that can cause human infections. Eight of these viruses are acquired zoonotically, and the other, vaccinia, is a laboratory virus, which is acquired iatrogenically.

PROPERTIES OF THE VIRUSES

Classification[23, 49]

The family *Poxviridae* has two subfamilies: *Chordopoxvirinae* (vertebrate poxviruses) and *Entomopoxviriniae* (insect poxviruses). There are eight genera in the *Chordopoxvirinae* subfamily, and four of these genera contain species that infect humans (Table 169–1).

Structure[5, 49]

Poxviruses are the largest animal viruses and are discernible by light microscopy. In general, by electron microscopy orthopoxviruses appear brick-shaped, with a length of 350 nm and a width of 270 nm. They contain double-stranded DNA genomes that vary from 130 to 300 kbp, depending on the particular species. A 30-nm lipoprotein bilayer (envelope) surrounds the virus core. The envelope contains seven or more distinct glycoproteins. *Parapoxvirus* organisms have a different structure than do *Orthopoxvirus*, *Yatapoxvirus*, and *Molluscipoxvirus* organisms. They are ovoid and vary from 260 × 160 nm for orf virus to 300 × 190 nm for pseudocowpox virus.

SPECIFIC VIRUSES AND THEIR ILLNESSES

Monkeypox Virus[4, 33–35, 39, 50]

Monkeypox virus first was isolated from sick laboratory primates in Copenhagen in 1958.[60] It was found to be a cause of a smallpox-like illness in humans in western and central Africa in 1970. Human disease occurs in a large geographic area from Sierra Leone in the west to Zaire in the east.[33] Illness usually is sporadic, with animals as the source in 72 per cent of cases and human-to-human transmission in the

TABLE 169–1. Poxviruses That Can Cause Human Illness

Genus	Species
Orthopoxvirus	Variola virus
	Monkeypox virus
	Vaccinia virus
	Cowpox virus
Parapoxvirus	Orf virus
	Bovine papular stomatitis virus
	Pseudocowpox virus
Yatapoxvirus	Tanapoxvirus
	Yabapoxvirus
Molluscipoxvirus	Molluscum contagiosum virus

remaining 28 per cent. A number of different monkeys and other primates as well as rodents are thought to be the source of human cases.

Jezek and associates[34] studied 282 patients in Zaire and found that 50 per cent were 4 years of age or younger and 93 per cent were 14 years of age or younger. The clinical features of human monkeypox virus infection are similar to those of smallpox, but overall illness tends to be less severe. Smallpox vaccination markedly lessens the severity of the illness. Illness usually starts with fever for 1 to 3 days before the onset of rash. With fever there is severe headache, backache, general malaise, and prostration.

The skin rash usually appears first on the face. Similar to smallpox lesions, the lesions develop and progress together in the same body region through stages of macules, papules, vesicles, and pustules. The majority of patients have discrete lesions; 23 per cent have semiconfluent and 7 per cent have confluent lesions. Most patients have mucous membrane involvement, and conjunctivitis is common. Lymphadenopathy, particularly involving submaxillary and cervical lymph nodes, is significant; this is not a usual finding in smallpox.

The overall duration of illness is 2 to 4 weeks. Complications include secondary bacterial infections of the skin; pneumonia; vomiting, diarrhea, and dehydration; keratitis and corneal ulceration; septicemia; and encephalitis. The death rate in nonvaccinated patients was 11 per cent in the study reported by Jezek and associates,[34] and all deaths occurred in children 8 years of age or younger. One case of congenital monkeypox infection has been reported.[33] This child's mother had typical illness on August 12, 1983, and the child was born premature on September 23, 1983. At birth, the child had generalized skin lesions; the child died 6 weeks later of malnutrition.

Cowpox Virus[2, 3, 5, 23]

In Europe, a disease with ulcers on the teats of cows (cowpox disease) was recognized for hundreds of years.[23] It was known that milkers who milked cows that were infected often got similar ulcers on their hands. It also was known that milkmaids who had had cowpox were immune to smallpox. This observation led Edward Jenner in May of 1796 to inoculate James Phipps, an 8-year-old boy, with cowpox material obtained from a lesion on a local dairy maid.[3, 31–33] After experimental challenge with material from a smallpox lesion, Phipps did not develop smallpox.

Studies during the last 25 years indicate that bovine cowpox is not a common illness and the cow is not the natural reservoir of the virus in nature.[2, 3, 5] The virus is distributed geographically throughout Western Europe, and the reservoir hosts are wild rodents.

Baxby[2] reported 12 human illnesses due to cowpox virus. Five of the patients were exposed to infected cows, and the other seven patients had no direct contact with cattle. All patients lived in or had visited a rural area prior to illness onset, however. Of 10 patients in whom the lesions were described, 6 had lesions on the hand only, 3 had lesions on the chin or face only, and 1 had involvement of both the face and hand. Most cases had local edema, lymphadenitis, and fever. The lesions were confused with anthrax in two instances.

Vaccinia Virus[5, 23]

Vaccinia virus is the live immunizing antigen successfully used in the global program to eradicate smallpox. This orthopoxvirus is different from cowpox virus, the agent that Jenner and others used for vaccination in the early nineteenth century. Vaccinia virus has been used for vaccination for more than 100 years. Restriction endonuclease studies indicate that strains of vaccinia virus from different parts of the world are similar to each other and distinctly different from cowpox virus.[23] The origin of vaccinia virus is unknown.[5] Four hypotheses as to its origin are (1) it evolved from variola virus through continual passage in the skin of cows or humans, (2) it evolved from cowpox virus through continual passage in the skins of animals, (3) it is a hybrid between cowpox virus and variola virus and, (4) it is a virus from an animal (the natural host) that now is extinct.

Vaccinia virus causes outbreaks of disease in buffaloes in India.[5, 23] However, it is thought that the animal infection originally resulted from contact of buffaloes with vaccinated humans during the smallpox eradication programs and not that the virus is a primary buffalo pathogen.

Because of the original success of the smallpox eradication program, routine vaccinia vaccination in the United States was discontinued in 1971.[7, 16] In 1976, the recommendation for routine vaccination of health care workers also was discontinued.[15] In 1982, the only active licensed producer of vaccinia vaccine in the United States discontinued production for general use, and in 1983, distribution to the civilian populations was discontinued.[10]

For several years, all military personnel continued to be vaccinated routinely. However, only selected groups of military personnel currently are vaccinated against smallpox.

Since January 1982, smallpox vaccination has not been required for international travelers, and International Certificates of Vaccination no longer include smallpox vaccination.[64]

In 1980, the Immunization Practices Advisory Committee (ACIP) recommended the use of vaccinia vaccine to protect laboratory workers from possible infection while working with nonvariola orthopoxviruses (e.g., vaccinia, monkeypox).[14] In 1984, these recommendations were included in guidelines for biosafety in microbiologic and biomedical laboratories.[57] These guidelines expanded the recommendation to include persons working in animal care areas where studies with orthopoxviruses were being conducted and recommended that these workers have documented evidence of satisfactory smallpox vaccination within the preceding 3 years. The Centers for Disease Control and Prevention (CDC) has provided vaccinia vaccine for these laboratory workers since 1983.[11]

Because studies of recombinant vaccinia virus vaccines have been advanced to the stage of clinical trials, health care workers (e.g., physicians, nurses) now may be exposed to vaccinia and recombinant vaccinia viruses and should be considered for vaccinia vaccination.

Vaccinia Vaccine

The vaccinia vaccine currently licensed in the United States is a lyophilized preparation of infectious vaccinia virus (official name: smallpox vaccine, dried; produced as Dryvax by Wyeth Laboratories, Inc., and available only from the CDC). The vaccine was prepared from calf lymph with a seed virus derived from the New York City Board of Health (NYCBOH) strain of vaccinia; it has a concentration of 10^8 pock-forming units per milliliter. Vaccine is administered by using the multiple-puncture technique with a bifurcated needle.

After percutaneous administration of a standard dose of vaccinia vaccine, more than 95 per cent of primary vaccinees (i.e., persons receiving their first dose of vaccine) develop neutralizing or hemagglutination-inhibition antibody at a titer of 1:10 or higher.[17] Neutralizing antibody titers of 1:10 or higher are found among 75 per cent of persons for 10 years after receiving second doses and up to 30 years after receiving three doses of vaccine.[22, 46] The level of antibody required for protection against vaccinia infection is not known. However, when the response to revaccination is used as an indication of immunity, less than 10 per cent of persons with neutralizing titers of 1:10 or higher exhibit a primary-type response at revaccination, compared with greater than 30 per cent of persons with titers of less than 1:10.[48]

Recombinant Vaccinia Virus

Vaccinia virus is the prototype of the genus *Orthopoxvirus*. It is a double-stranded DNA virus that has a broad host range under experimental conditions and rarely is isolated from animals outside the laboratory.[24] There are many strains of vaccinia virus that have different levels of virulence for humans and animals. For example, the Temple of Heaven and Copenhagen vaccinia strains are highly pathogenic in animals, whereas the NYCBOH strain, from which the Wyeth vaccine strain was derived, has relatively low pathogenicity.[25]

Vaccinia virus can be engineered genetically to contain and express foreign DNA without impairing the ability of the virus to replicate. Such foreign DNA can encode protein antigens that induce protection against one or more infectious agents. Recombinant vaccinia viruses have been engineered to express the immunizing antigens of such viruses as herpesvirus, hepatitis B, rabies, influenza, and HIV.[18, 30, 40, 55, 56, 65]

Recombinant vaccinia viruses have been created from several strains of vaccinia virus. In the United States, most recombinants have been made from either the NYCBOH strain or a mouse neuroadapted derivative, the WR strain. Some recombinants have been made from the Copenhagen and Lister vaccinia strains, which are more pathogenic in animals than the NYCBOH strain is. Animal studies generally suggest that recombinants may be no more pathogenic than the parent strain of vaccinia virus. However, no consistently reliable laboratory marker or animal test predicts the attenuation of vaccinia virus or a particular recombinant for humans.[1] Laboratory-acquired infections with vaccinia or recombinant viruses have been reported.[37, 52, 54] However, because no surveillance system has been established to monitor laboratory workers, the risk of infection for persons who handle virus cultures or materials contaminated with these viruses is not known.

With the initiation of human trials of recombinant vaccines, physicians, nurses, and other health care personnel who provide clinical care to recipients of these vaccines could be exposed to both vaccinia and recombinant viruses. This exposure could occur from contact with dressings contaminated with the virus or through exposure to the vaccine. The risk of transmission of recombinant viruses to exposed health care workers is unknown. To date, no reports of transmission to health care personnel from vaccine recipients have been published. If appropriate infection control precautions are observed, health care workers probably are at less risk of infection than laboratory workers because of the smaller volume and lower titer of virus in clinical specimens compared with laboratory material.[27, 63] However, because of the potential for transmission of vaccinia or recombinant vaccinia viruses to such persons, the ACIP suggests that health care personnel who have direct contact with contaminated dressings or other infectious material from volunteers in clinical studies be considered for vaccination.

Laboratory and other health care personnel who work with viral cultures or other infective materials always should observe appropriate biosafety guidelines and adhere to published infection control procedures.[27, 58, 63]

Vaccine Use

Vaccinia vaccine is recommended for laboratory workers who directly handle (1) cultures or (2) animals contaminated or infected with vaccinia, recombinant vaccinia viruses, or other orthopoxviruses that infect humans (e.g., monkeypox, cowpox). Other health care workers (e.g., physicians, nurses) whose contact with these viruses is limited to contaminated materials (e.g., dressings) but who adhere to appropriate infection control measures are at lower risk of inadvertent infection than are laboratory workers. However, because a theoretic risk of infection exists, vaccination may be considered for this group. Because of the low risk of infection, vaccination is not recommended for persons who do not handle virus cultures or materials directly or who do not work with animals contaminated or infected with these viruses.

High seroconversion rates and infrequent adverse events are two benefits of vaccination. Recipients are given controlled percutaneous doses (approximately 2.5×10^5 pock-forming units) of relatively low-pathogenicity vaccinia. The resulting immunity should provide some degree of protection to recipients against infections resulting from uncontrolled, inadvertent inoculation by unusual routes (e.g., eye) with a large dose of virus of higher or unknown pathogenicity. In addition, persons with preexisting immunity to vaccinia may be protected against seroconversion to the foreign antigen expressed by a recombinant virus.[30]

According to available data on the persistence of neutralizing antibody after vaccination, persons working with vaccinia, recombinant vaccinia viruses, or other nonvariola orthopoxviruses should be revaccinated every 10 years.

Side Effects and Adverse Reactions

A papule develops at the site of vaccination 2 to 5 days after percutaneous administration of vaccinia vaccine to a nonimmune person (i.e., primary vaccination). The papule becomes vesicular and then pustular and reaches its maximum size in 8 to 10 days. The pustule dries and forms a scab, which separates within 14 to 21 days after vaccination, leaving a typical scar. Primary vaccination can produce swelling and tenderness of regional lymph nodes, beginning 3 to 10 days after vaccination and persisting for 2 to 4 weeks after the skin lesion has healed. Maximum viral shedding occurs 4 to 14 days after vaccination, but vaccinia can be recovered from the site of vaccination until the scab separates from the skin.[29, 41]

A fever is common after the vaccinia vaccination is administered. Up to 70 per cent of children have 1 or more days of temperature of 37.8° C (100° F) or higher from 4 to 14 days after primary vaccination,[17, 48] and 15 to 20 per cent have temperatures of 38.9° C (102° F) or higher. After revaccination, 35 per cent of children develop temperatures of 37.8° C (100° F) or higher and 5 per cent have temperatures of 38.9° C (102° F) or higher.[29] Fever is less common in adults than in children after vaccination or revaccination.[29]

Erythematous or urticarial rashes may occur approximately 10 days after primary vaccination. The vaccinee usually is afebrile, and the rash resolves spontaneously within 2 to 4 days. Rarely, bullous erythema multiforme (Stevens-Johnson syndrome) occurs.[28]

Inadvertent inoculation at other sites is the most frequent complication of vaccinia vaccination, accounting for about half of all complications of primary vaccination and revaccination. Inadvertent inoculation usually results from autoinoculation of vaccine virus transferred from the site of vaccination. The most common sites involved are the face, eyelid, nose, mouth, genitalia, and rectum. Most lesions heal without specific therapy, but vaccinia immunoglobulin (VIG) may be useful for cases of ocular implantation (see Treatment of Complications of Vaccinia Vaccine).

Generalized vaccinia among persons without underlying illnesses is characterized by a vesicular rash of varying extent. The rash generally is self-limited and requires little or no therapy, except among patients whose conditions appear to be toxic or who have serious underlying illnesses.

More severe complications of vaccinia vaccination include eczema vaccinatum, progressive vaccinia, and postvaccinial encephalitis. These complications occur at least 10 times more often among primary vaccinees than among revaccinees and more frequently among infants than among older children and adults.[42–44]

Eczema vaccinatum is a localized or systemic dissemination of vaccinia virus among persons who have eczema or a history of eczema and other chronic or exfoliative skin conditions (e.g., atopic dermatitis). The illness often is mild and self-limited but may be severe and occasionally fatal. The most serious cases among vaccine recipients occur among primary vaccinees and appear to be independent of the activity of the underlying eczema.[61] Severe cases also have been observed after contact infection.

Progressive vaccinia (vaccinia necrosum) is a severe, potentially fatal illness characterized by progressive necrosis in the area of vaccination, often with metastatic lesions. It occurs almost exclusively among persons with cellular immunodeficiency.

The most serious complication is postvaccinial encephalitis. Most frequently, it affects primary vaccinees younger than 1 year of age. Fifteen to 25 per cent of affected vaccinees with this complication die, and 25 per cent have permanent neurologic sequelae.[28, 43, 44]

Death is rare after vaccinia vaccination, with approximately 1 to 2 deaths per million primary vaccinations and 0.1 deaths per million revaccinations. Death most often is the result of postvaccinial encephalitis or progressive vaccinia.

Vaccinia may be transmitted when a recently vaccinated person has contact with a susceptible person. In the CDC's 10-state survey of complications of smallpox vaccination, the risk of transmission to contacts was 27 infections per million total vaccinations; 44 per cent of these contact cases occurred among children 5 years of age or younger.[43] Since 1980, several occurrences of contact transmission of vaccinia from recently vaccinated military recruits have been reported, including six cases transmitted by a single vaccine recipient.[8, 9, 13]

More than 60 per cent of contact transmission results in uncomplicated inadvertent inoculation. Approximately 30 per cent of contact transmission results in eczema vaccinatum, which may be fatal.[43] Eczema vaccinatum may be more severe among contacts than among vaccinated persons, possibly because of simultaneous multiple inoculations at several sites.[19, 44] Contact transmission rarely results in postvaccinial encephalitis or vaccinia necrosum.

Precautions and Contraindications

Before administering vaccinia vaccine, the physician should take a careful history to document the absence of contraindications to vaccination among both vaccinees and household contacts of vaccinees. Special efforts should be made to identify vaccinees and household contacts who have eczema, a history of eczema, or immunodeficiencies. Vaccinia vaccine should not be administered if these conditions are present among either recipients or household contacts.

Specific precautions and contraindications include history or presence of eczema, pregnancy, altered immunocompetence, infection with HIV, and allergies to vaccine components. The reader is referred to reference 7 for more complete information on contraindications.

Prevention of Contact Transmission of Vaccinia

Vaccinia virus may be cultured from the site of primary vaccination beginning at the time of development of a papule (2 to 5 days after vaccination) until the scab separates from the skin lesion (14 to 21 days after vaccination). During this time, care must be taken to prevent spread of the virus to another area of the body or to another person. The vaccination site should be covered at all times with a porous bandage until the scab has separated and the underlying skin has healed. An occlusive bandage should not be used. The vaccination site should be kept dry. When the vaccinee bathes, the site should be covered with an impermeable bandage.

Vaccinated health care workers may continue to have contact with patients, including those with immunodeficiencies, as long as the vaccination site is covered and a good hand washing technique is maintained.

Semipermeable polyurethane dressings (e.g., Op-Site) are effective barriers to vaccinia and recombinant vaccinia viruses.[18] However, exudate may accumulate beneath the dressing, and care must be taken to prevent viral contamination when the dressing is removed. In addition, accumulation of fluid beneath the dressing may increase the maceration of the vaccination site. Accumulation of exudate may be decreased by first covering the vaccination with dry gauze and then applying the dressing over the gauze. To date, experience with this type of containment dressing has been limited to research protocols, and further investigation is needed before it can be recommended for all vaccinia vaccine recipients.

The most important measure to prevent inadvertent implantation and contact transmission from vaccinia vaccination is thorough hand washing after changing the bandage or after any other contact with the vaccination site.

Treatment of Complications of Vaccinia Vaccine

The only product currently available for the treatment of complications of vaccinia vaccination is VIG. VIG is an isotonic sterile solution of the immunoglobulin fraction of plasma from persons vaccinated with vaccinia vaccine. It is effective for the treatment of eczema vaccinatum and some cases of progressive vaccinia and may be useful in the treatment of ocular vaccinia resulting from inadvertent implantation. VIG also is recommended for severe generalized vaccinia if the patient has a toxic condition or a serious underlying disease. VIG is of no benefit in the treatment of postvaccinial encephalitis.

The recommended dose for treatment of complications is 0.6 mL/kg of body weight. VIG must be administered intramuscularly and should be administered as early as possible after the onset of symptoms. Because therapeutic doses of VIG may be large (e.g., 42 mL for a person weighing 70 kg), the product should be given in divided doses over a 24- to 36-hour period. Doses may be repeated, usually at intervals of 2 to 3 days, until recovery begins (e.g., no new lesions appear).

The CDC is the only source of VIG for civilians.

Misuse of Vaccinia Vaccine

Vaccinia vaccine should never be used therapeutically for any reason. There is no evidence that it has any value in the treatment or prevention of recurrent herpes simplex virus infection, warts, or any disease other than those caused by human orthopoxviruses.[38] Misuse of vaccinia vaccine to treat herpesvirus infections has been associated with severe complications.[12, 59]

Vaccinia Vaccine Availability

The CDC is the only source of vaccinia vaccine and VIG for civilians. The CDC provides vaccinia vaccine to protect laboratory and other health care personnel whose occupations place them at risk of exposure to vaccinia and other closely related orthopoxviruses, including vaccinia recombinants.

Orf Virus[23] (see Table 67–1)

Orf virus is a member of the genus *Parapoxvirus*. Infection with orf virus causes the disease by the same name (orf), which also is called ecthyma contagiosum. The reservoir host of orf virus is sheep, and the virus enjoys worldwide distribution. Orf is an occupationally acquired disease, and most cases occur in adults.[26, 45] Human disease is characterized by single or multiple lesions that most often are located on the hands. The lesions last about 35 to 40 days and progress through six stages[45]: maculopapular, 1 to 7 days; target, 7 to 14 days; acute, 14 to 21 days; regenerative, 21 to 28 days; papillomatous, 28 to 35 days; regressive, 35 to 40 or more days. Patients may have low-grade fever and regional lymphadenitis. Two patients with a widespread papulovesicular eruption, fever, malaise, and lymphadenopathy have been described.[62] A 12-year-old boy, who lived on a farm, developed giant orf granuloma at the site of a rope burn.[51]

Other Parapoxviruses

Human infections with pseudocowpox virus and bovine papular stomatitis virus are, like orf, occupational diseases. Pseudocowpox infections occur on the hands of milkers, and infections with bovine papular stomatitis virus occur on the hands of veterinarians and others with close contact.[6, 23, 47] The lesions of milker's nodule are relatively painless, but they may be pruritic; they initially are red and then become purple. They are firm, do not ulcerate, and last 4 to 6 weeks. The lesions due to bovine papular stomatitis virus are wart-like and last 3 to 4 weeks.

Humans also have been infected with parapoxviruses of camels and seals.[53]

Yatapoxviruses (see Table 67–1)

Tanapox virus and Yabapoxvirus are two monkey viruses that cause human infections.[20, 21, 23, 36] Tanapox in humans first was observed along the Tana River in Kenya in 1957, and outbreaks also were studied in Zaire.[23] The Yabapoxvirus first was isolated from tumors in monkeys in Nigeria. This virus has caused illness in animal handlers in primate centers in the United States, but human infections have not been identified in the field in Africa.

Outbreaks of Tanapox in Africa have involved both children and adults.[36] Illness starts with fever, headache, backache, and mild prostration. Skin lesions occur 2 to 4 days after illness onset. Individual lesions start with itching followed by the development of a pock-like lesion. At 7 days, the lesion is about 10 mm in diameter with surrounding erythema. Local lymphadenitis and regional lymphadenitis occur.

The lesions ulcerate during the second week of illness and they last about 6 weeks. Most patients have a single lesion, but some have from 2 to 10 lesions. Prognosis usually is good, but secondary bacterial infections can occur.

Molluscum Contagiosum Virus
(see Chapter 70 and Table 67–1)

In contrast with the other poxviruses discussed in this chapter, which are zoonotic agents, molluscum contagiosum virus is a human virus that is a common cause of human skin lesions.[23] The virus as yet has not been grown in cell culture, and it does not cause infection in experimental animals.

Although the virus has not been cultivated in the laboratory, large amounts of virus can be extracted from human lesions. Analysis of viral DNA from lesions from patients from different parts of the world indicates that there are two major subtypes and a third, rare subtype.

The clinical aspects of molluscum contagiosum virus infection are presented in Chapter 70.

DIAGNOSIS AND DIFFERENTIAL DIAGNOSIS

Because all but two viruses presented in this chapter are zoonotic agents, careful attention must be given to geographic location and animal exposure. All diseases have local lesions, so that virus for direct identification and culture is readily available. All poxviruses can be identified by the examination of material from lesions by electron microscopy. All viruses except molluscum contagiosum virus grow in one or more tissue culture systems, the chorioallantoic membrane of embryonated eggs, or both. Unusual agents should be referred to specific reference laboratories for species identification.

References

1. Anonymous: Recombinant vaccinia viruses as live virus vectors for vaccine antigens: Memorandum from a W. H. O./USPHS/NIBSC meeting. Bull. W. H. O. *63*:471–477, 1985.
2. Baxby, D.: Is cowpox misnamed? A review of 10 human cases. B. M. J. *1*:1379–1381, 1977.
3. Bennett, M., and Baxby, D.: Cowpox J. Med. Microbiol. *45*:157–158, 1996.
4. Breman, J. G., Ruti, K., Steniowski, M. V., et al.: Human monkeypox, 1970–79. Bull. W. H. O. *58*:165–182, 1980.
5. Buller, R. M. L., and Palumbo, G. J.: Poxvirus pathogenesis. Microbiol. Rev. *55*:80–122, 1991.
6. Carson, C. A., and Kerr, K. M.: Bovine papular stomatitis with apparent transmission to man. J. Am. Vet. Med. Assoc. *151*:183–187, 1987.
7. Centers for Disease Control: Vaccinia (smallpox) vaccine: Recommendations of the Immunization Practices Advisory Committee (ACIP). M. M. W. R. *40*:1–10, 1991.
8. Centers for Disease Control: Contact spread of vaccinia from a National Guard vaccinee: Wisconsin. M. M. W. R. *34*:182–183, 1985.
9. Centers for Disease Control: Contact spread of vaccinia from a recently vaccinated Marine: Louisiana. M. M. W. R. *33*:37–38, 1984.
10. Centers for Disease Control: Smallpox vaccine no longer available for civilians: United States. M. M. W. R. *32*:387, 1983.
11. Centers for Disease Control: Smallpox vaccine available for protection of at-risk laboratory workers. M. M. W. R. *32*:543, 1983.
12. Centers for Disease Control: Vaccinia necrosum after smallpox vaccination: Michigan. M. M. W. R. *31*:501–502, 1982.
13. Centers for Disease Control: Vaccinia outbreak: Newfoundland. M. M. W. R. *30*:453–455, 1981.

14. Centers for Disease Control: Smallpox vaccine: Recommendation of the Immunization Practices Advisory Committee. M. M. W. R. *29*:417–420, 1980.
15. Centers for Disease Control: Recommendation of the Immunization Practices Advisory Committee (ACIP): Smallpox vaccination of hospital and health personnel. M. M. W. R. *25*:9, 1976.
16. Centers for Disease Control: Public Health Service recommendations on smallpox vaccination. M. M. W. R. *20*:339, 1971.
17. Cherry, J. D., McIntosh, K., Connor, J. D., et al.: Primary percutaneous (smallpox) vaccination. J. Infect. Dis. *135*:145–154, 1977.
18. Cooney, E. L., Collier, A. C., Greenberg, P. D., et al.: Safety of and immunological response to a recombinant vaccinia virus vaccine expressing HIV envelope glycoprotein. Lancet *337*:567–572, 1991.
19. Coperman, P. W. M., and Wallace, H. J.: Eczema vaccinatum. B. M. J. *2*:906, 1964.
20. Downie, A. W., and Espaa, C.: A comparative study of tanapox and yaba viruses. J. Gen. Virol. *19*:37–49, 1973.
21. Downie, A. W., Taylor-Robinson, C. H., Caunt, A. E., et al.: Tanapox: A new disease caused by a pox virus. B. M. J. *1*:363–368, 1971.
22. El-Ad, B., Roth, Y., Winder, A., et al.: The persistence of neutralizing antibodies after revaccination against smallpox. J. Infect. Dis. *161*:446–448, 1990.
23. Fenner, F.: Poxviruses. *In* Fields, B. N., Knipe, D. M., Howley, P. M., et al. (eds.): Fields Virology. 3rd ed. Philadelphia, Lippincott-Raven, 1996, pp. 2673–2702.
24. Fenner, F., Wittek, R., and Dumbell, K. R.: The Orthopoxviruses. San Diego, Academic Press, 1989, pp. 10–13.
25. Fenner, F., Henderson, D. A., Arita, I., et al.: Smallpox and Its Eradication. Geneva, World Health Organization, 1988, pp. 581–583.
26. Ganske, J. G., Miller, S. H., and Demuth, R. J.: Ecthyma contagiosum (orf). Plast. Reconstr. Surg. *68*:779–780, 1981.
27. Garner, J. S., and Simmons, B. P.: Guideline for isolation precautions in hospitals. Infect. Cont. *4*(Suppl.):245–325, 1983.
28. Goldstein, J. A., Neff, J. M., Lane, J. M., et al.: Smallpox vaccination reactions, prophylaxis and therapy of complications. Pediatrics *55*:342–347, 1975.
29. Graham, B. S., Belshe, R., Clements, M. L., et al.: HIV-GP-160 recombinant vaccinia vaccination of vaccinia-naive adults followed by RGP160 booster. Abstract. Proceedings of the VI International Conference on AIDS, Florence, June 1991.
30. Graham, B. S., Belshe, R., Clements, M. L., et al.: HIV GP 160 recombinant vaccinia in vaccinia-naive adults. Abstract No. 549. Presented at 30th Interscience Conference for Antimicrobial Agents and Chemotherapy, Atlanta, October 1990.
31. Jenner, E.: Further Observations on the Variolae Vacciniae or Cowpox. London, Sampson Low, 1799.
32. Jenner, E.: An Inquiry into the Causes and Effects of the Variolae Vaccinae, a Disease Discovered in Some of the Western Countries of England, Particularly Gloucestershire, and Known by the Name of the Cowpox. London, Sampson Low, 1798.
33. Jezek, Z., and Fenner, F.: Human monkeypox. *In* Melnick, J. L. (ed.): Monographs in Virology. Vol. 17. Basel, Karger, 1988, pp. 1–140.
34. Jezek, Z., Szczeniowski, M., Paluku, K. M., et al.: Human monkeypox: Clinical features of 282 patients. J. Infect. Dis. *156*:293–298, 1987.
35. Jezek, Z., Marennikova, S. S., Mutumbo, M., et al.: Human monkeypox: A study of 2,510 contacts of 214 patients. J. Infect. Dis. *154*:551–555, 1986.
36. Jezek, Z., Arita, I., Szczeniowski, M., et al.: Human tanapox in Zaire: Clinical and epidemiological observations on cases confirmed by laboratory studies. Bull. W. H. O. *63*:1027–1035, 1985.
37. Jones, L., Ristow, S., Yima, T., et al.: Accidental human vaccination with vaccinia virus expressing nucleoprotein gene. Nature *319*:543, 1986.
38. Kern, A. B., and Schiff, B. L.: Smallpox vaccination in the management of recurrent herpes simplex: A controlled evaluation. J. Invest. Dermatol. *33*:99–102, 1959.
39. Khodakevich, L., Jezek, Z., and Messinger, D.: Monkeypox virus: Ecology and public health significance. Bull. W. H. O. *66*:747–752, 1988.
40. Kieny, M. P., Lathe, R., Drillien, R., et al.: Expression of rabies virus glycoprotein from a recombinant vaccinia virus. Nature *312*:163–166, 1984.
41. Koplan, J. P., and Marton, K. I.: Smallpox vaccination revisited: Some observations on the biology of vaccinia. Am. J. Trop. Med. Hyg. *24*:656–663, 1975.
42. Lane, J. M., Miller, J. D., and Neff, J. M.: Smallpox and smallpox vaccination policy. Annu. Rev. Med. *22*:251–272, 1971.
43. Lane, J. M., Ruben, F. L., Neff, J. M., et al.: Complications of smallpox vaccination, 1968: Results of ten statewide surveys. J. Infect. Dis. *122*:303–309, 1970.
44. Lane, J. M., Huben, F. L., Neff, J. M., et al.: Complications of smallpox vaccination, 1968: National surveillance in the United States. N. Engl. J. Med. *281*:1201–1207, 1969.
45. Leavell, U. W., Jr., McNamara, M. J., Muelling, R., et al.: Orf: Report of 19 human cases with clinical and pathological observations. J. A. M. A. *204*:657–664, 1968.
46. Lublin-Tennenbaum, T., Katzenelson, T., E-Ad, E., et al.: Correlation between cutaneous reaction in vaccinees immunized against smallpox and antibody titer determined by plaque neutralization test and ELISA. Viral Immunol. *3*:19–25, 1990.
47. McEvoy, J. D. S., and Allan, B. C.: Isolation of bovine papular stomatitis virus from humans. Med. J. Austr. *1*:1254–1256, 1972.
48. McIntosh, K., Cherry, J. D., Benenson, A. S., et al.: Standard percutaneous (smallpox) revaccination of children who received primary percutaneous vaccination. J. Infect. Dis. *135*:155–166, 1977.
49. Moss, B.: *Poxviridae:* The viruses and their replication. *In* Fields, B. N., Knipe, D. M., Howley, P. M., et al. (eds.): Fields Virology. 3rd ed. Philadelphia, Lippincott-Raven, 1996, pp. 2637–2671.
50. Mutombo, M. W., Arita, I., and Jezek, Z.: Human monkeypox transmitted by a chimpanzee in a tropical rain-forest area of Zaire. Lancet *1*:735–737, 1983.
51. Pether, J. V. S., Guerrier, C. J. W., Jones, S. M., et al.: Giant orf in a normal individual. Br. J. Dermatol. *115*:497–499, 1986.
52. Pike, R. M.: Laboratory-associated infections: Summary and analysis of 3,921 cases. Health Lab. Sci. *102*:105–114, 1976.
53. Robinson, A. J., and Lyttle, D. J.: Parapoxviruses: Their biology and potential as recombinant vaccines. *In* Binns, M. M., and Smith, G. L. (eds.): Recombinant Poxviruses. Boca Raton, CRC Press, 1992, pp. 285–327.
54. Shimojo, J.: Virus infections in laboratories in Japan. Bibl. Haematol. *40*:771–773, 1975.
55. Smith, G. L., Mackett, M., and Moss, B.: Infectious vaccinia virus recombinants that express hepatitis B virus surface antigen. Nature *302*:490–495, 1983.
56. Smith, G. L., Murphy, B. R., and Moss, B.: Construction and characterization of an infectious vaccinia virus that expresses the influenza hemagglutinin gene and induces resistance to influenza virus infection in hamsters. Proc. Natl. Acad. Sci. U. S. A. *80*:7155–7159, 1983.
57. U. S. Department of Health and Human Services: Biosafety in Microbiological and Biomedical Laboratories. 1st ed. Washington, D.C., U. S. Govt. Printing Office, HHS Publication No. (NIH) 88–8395, 1984, p. 66.
58. U. S. Department of Health and Human Services: Biosafety in Microbiological and Biomedical Laboratories. 2nd ed. Washington, D.C., U. S. Govt. Printing Office, HHS Publication No. (NIH) 88–8396, 1984, pp. 78–79.
59. U. S. Food and Drug Administration: Inappropriate use of smallpox vaccine. FDA Drug Bull. *12*:12, 1982.
60. von Magnus, P., Andersen, E. K., Petersen, K. B., et al.: A pox-like disease in cynomolgus monkeys. Acta Pathol. Microbiol. Scand. *46*:156–176, 1959.
61. Waddington, E., Bray, P. T., Evans, A. D., et al.: Cutaneous complications of mass vaccination in South Wales 1962. Trans. St. Johns Hosp. Dermatol. Soc. *50*:22–42, 1964.
62. Wilkinson, J. D.: Orf: A family with unusual complications. Br. J. Dermatol. *97*:447–450, 1977.
63. Williams, W. W.: Guideline for infection control in hospital personnel. Infect. Cont. *4*(Suppl.):326–349, 1983.
64. World Health Organization: Smallpox vaccination certificates. Wkly. Epidemiol. Rec. *39*:305, 1981.
65. Zagury, D., Leonard, R., Fouchard, M., et al.: Immunization against AIDS in humans. Nature *326*:249–250, 1987.

RNA VIRUSES

❑ ❑ ❑

SUBSECTION ONE

PICORNAVIRIDAE

170

ENTEROVIRUSES: COXSACKIEVIRUSES, ECHOVIRUSES, AND POLIOVIRUSES

James D. Cherry

Enteroviruses—coxsackieviruses, echoviruses, and polioviruses—are responsible for significant and frequent human illnesses with protean clinical manifestations.[117, 118, 170, 285, 460, 496, 501, 653, 736–739, 741] Enteroviruses are a subgroup of picornaviruses.[502] They first were categorized together and named in 1957 by a committee sponsored by the National Foundation for Infantile Paralysis[503]; the human alimentary tract was believed to be the natural habitat of these agents. They are grouped together because of similarities in physical and biochemical properties, as well as shared features in their epidemiology and pathogenesis and the many disease syndromes that they cause.

HISTORY

Poliomyelitis, the first enteroviral disease to be recognized and the most important one, has a long history.[576] The earliest record is an Egyptian stele of the 18th dynasty (1580 to 1350 B.C.), which shows a young priest with a withered, shortened leg, the characteristic deformity of paralytic poliomyelitis.[328, 498] Michael Underwood,[711] a London pediatrician, published the first medical description in 1789 in his *Treatise on Diseases of Children*. During the 19th century, many reports appeared in Europe and the United States describing small clusters of cases of "infantile paralysis." The authors greatly were puzzled as to the nature of the affliction; not until the 1860s and 1870s was the spinal cord firmly established as the seat of the pathologic process. The contagious nature of poliomyelitis was not appreciated until the latter part of the 19th century. Medin, a Swedish pediatrician, was the first to describe the epidemic nature of poliomyelitis (1890), and his pupil Wickman worked out the basic principles of the epidemiology.[743]

The virus first was isolated in monkeys by Landsteiner and Popper in 1908.[432] The availability of a laboratory animal assay system opened up many avenues of research that, in the ensuing 40 years, led to the demonstration that an unrecognized intestinal infection was the usual one and the paralytic disease a relatively uncommon accident.

Coxsackieviruses and echoviruses have had a shorter history. Epidemic pleurodynia was described clinically in 1735 by Hannaeus more than 200 years before the coxsackieviral etiology of this disease was discovered.[298] In 1948, Dalldorf and Sickles[171] first reported the isolation of a coxsackievirus, using suckling mouse inoculation.

In 1949, Enders and associates[202] reported the growth of poliovirus 2 in tissue culture, and their techniques paved the way for the recovery of a large number of other cytopathic viruses. Most of these "new" viruses failed to produce illness in laboratory animals. Because the relationships of many of these newly recovered agents to human disease were unknown, they were called orphan viruses.[501] Later, several agents were grouped together and called *e*nteric *c*ytopathogenic *h*uman *o*rphan viruses, or echoviruses.

THE VIRUSES

Morphology and Classification[215, 499, 500, 502, 626]

The enteroviruses are single-stranded RNA viruses belonging to the family *Picornaviridae* (pico = small). They are grouped together because they share certain physical and biochemical properties. In electron micrographs, the viruses are seen as 24- to 30-nm particles, consisting of naked protein capsids constituting about 70 to 75 per cent of the particles and a dense central core (nucleoid) of RNA. The virion has icosahedral symmetry due to the regular organization of identical protein subunits. The subunits are arranged in axes of fivefold, threefold, and twofold symmetry within the protein shell of the virus. The capsid of enteroviruses is made up of rather indistinct capsomers, the exact number of which has been reported variously as 32, 42, and 60.

All enteroviruses contain polypeptide chains (structural proteins; protomers) VP1, VP2, VP3, and VP4. These coat proteins protect the RNA genome from nucleases and are important determinants of host range and tropism. They determine antigenicity, and they deliver the RNA genome into the cytoplasm of new host cells.

The genome of enteroviruses is a single-stranded, positive-strand RNA molecule.[590] It contains a 5′ noncoding region that is followed by a single long open-reading frame, a short 3′ noncoding region, and a poly (a) tail. The four capsid proteins (VP1 to VP4) and seven nonstructural proteins (2A, 2B, 2C, 3A, 3B, 3C, 3D) result from a cleaved long polyprotein that was translated from genomic RNA.

Viral components and complete virions are formed in the cytoplasm of infected cells. If the rate of virus assembly is rapid and many particles are formed in one area, crystallization may occur.

The classification of human enteroviruses is shown in Table 170–1. The enteroviral subgroups originally were differentiated from each other by their different effects in tissue cultures and in animals. Although these differentiating factors still are useful, many strains now have been isolated that do not conform to such rigid specificities. For example, several coxsackievirus A strains grow and have a cytopathic effect in monkey kidney tissue cultures, and some echovirus strains cause paralysis in mice. Newly characterized enteroviruses now are assigned enterovirus type numbers instead of coxsackievirus or echovirus numbers. Prototype enteroviral

TABLE 170–1. Human Enteroviruses: Animal and Tissue Culture Spectrum*

Virus	Antigenic Types†	Cytopathic Effect: Monkey Kidney Tissue Culture	Cytopathic Effect: Human Tissue Culture	Illness and Pathology: Suckling Mouse	Illness and Pathology: Monkey
Polioviruses	1–3	+	+	−	+
Coxsackieviruses A	1–24‡	−	−	+	−
Coxsackieviruses B	1–6	+	+	+	−
Echoviruses	1–34¶	+	±	−	−

*Many enteroviral stains have been isolated that do not conform to these categories.
†New types, beginning with type 68, now are assigned enterovirus type numbers instead of coxsackievirus or echovirus numbers. Types 68 through 72 have been identified.
‡Type 23 has been found to be the same as echovirus 9.
¶Echovirus 10 is reclassified as a reovirus; echovirus 28 is reclassified as a rhinovirus.
Modified from Cherry, J. D.: Enteroviruses. *In* Remington, J. S., and Klein, J. O. (eds.): Infectious Diseases of the Fetus and Newborn Infant. 3rd ed. Philadelphia, W. B. Saunders, 1990.

strains Fermon, Toluca-1, J670/71, and BrCr have been assigned enteroviral numbers 68 through 71, respectively. Enteroviral types are identified definitively by neutralization with type-specific antiserums.

Complete or partial genetic sequence data are available from several enteroviruses.[181, 399, 590, 591, 595] In general, sequence comparisons partially support the classic subgrouping of enteroviruses as noted in Table 170–1. However, in many instances, genetic relationships do not correlate with these subdivisions.[590] At present, the analysis of different genomic regions of sequenced human enteroviruses reveals two clusters in the 5′ noncoding region and four clusters in the coding region and in the 3′ noncoding region. Therefore, all human enteroviruses with complete or partial sequence data from the coding region fall into four clusters. These clusters are poliovirus-like (C-cluster), enterovirus 70–like (D-cluster), coxsackievirus B–like (B-cluster), and coxsackievirus A–like (A-cluster). The C-cluster includes coxsackieviruses A1, A11, A13, A15, A17, A18, A19, A20, A21, A22, and A24 and polioviruses 1 to 3. The D-cluster contains enteroviruses 68 and 70. The B-cluster contains coxsackieviruses A9, B1, B3, B4, and B5, enterovirus 69, and echoviruses 1, 4, 6, 7, 11, 12, 27, and 30. The A-cluster contains coxsackieviruses A2, A3, A5, A7, A8, A10, A12, A14, and A16 and enterovirus 71.

Characteristics and Host Systems[496, 500]

Enteroviruses are relatively stable viruses in that they retain activity for several days at room temperature and can be stored indefinitely at ordinary freezer temperatures (−20° C). They are inactivated rapidly by heat (>56° C), formaldehyde, chlorination, and ultraviolet light.

Enteroviral strains grow rapidly when adapted to susceptible host systems and cause cytopathology in 3 to 7 days. The typical tissue culture cytopathic effect is shown in Figure 170–1; characteristic pathologic findings in mice are shown in Figures 170–2 and 170–3. Final titers of virus recovered in the laboratory vary markedly among different viral strains and the host system employed; usually, concentrations of 10^3 to 10^7 infectious doses per 0.1 mL of tissue culture fluid or tissue homogenate are obtained. Unadapted viral strains frequently require long periods of incubation. In both tissue cultures and suckling mice, evidence of growth becomes visible. Blind passage occasionally is necessary for cytopathology to become apparent.

Although many different primary and secondary tissue culture systems support the growth of various enteroviruses, generally it is accepted that primary rhesus monkey kidney cultures have the most inclusive spectrum.[83] Other simian kidney tissue cultures also have the same broad spectrum. Tissue cultures of human origin have a more limited spectrum, but several echovirus types have had more consistent primary isolation in human than in monkey kidney cultures.[104, 259, 337] A satisfactory system for the primary recovery of enteroviruses from clinical specimens would include primary rhesus, cynomolgus, or African green monkey kidney; diploid, human embryonic lung fibroblast cell strain; and rhabdomyosarcoma cell line tissue cultures and the intraperitoneal and intracerebral inoculation of suckling mice younger than 24 hours of age.

Antigenic Characteristics[496, 498–500]

Although there are some minor cross-reactions between several coxsackievirus and echovirus types, there are no common group antigens of diagnostic importance. Intratypic strain differences are common, and some strains (prime strains) are neutralized poorly by antiserums to prototype viruses. These prime strains induce antibody in animals that neutralize the specific prototype viruses, however.

The identification of polioviral, coxsackieviral, and echoviral types by neutralization in suckling mice or tissue cultures with antiserum pools is relatively well defined. Neutralization is induced by the epitopes on structural proteins VP1, VP2, and VP3; in particular, several epitopes are clustered on VP1. Prime strains do cause diagnostic difficulties because frequently they are not neutralized by the reference antiserums. This is a particular problem with echoviruses 4, 9, and 11 and enterovirus 71. If these types or other possible prime strains are suspected, this problem can be overcome by employing antiserums in less diluted concentrations or using antiserums prepared against several different strains of problem viruses.

Host Range

It is the general opinion that humans are the only natural hosts of polioviruses, coxsackieviruses, and echoviruses.[252] However, enteroviruses have been recovered in nature from sewage, flies, swine, dogs, a calf, a budgerigar, a fox, mussels, and oysters.[117] In addition, serologic evidence of infection with enteroviruses similar to human strains has been noted in chimpanzees, cattle, rabbits, a fox, a chipmunk, and a marmot.[117] It is probable that infection of these animals results from their direct contact with an infected human or human excreta. The contamination of shellfish also is interest-

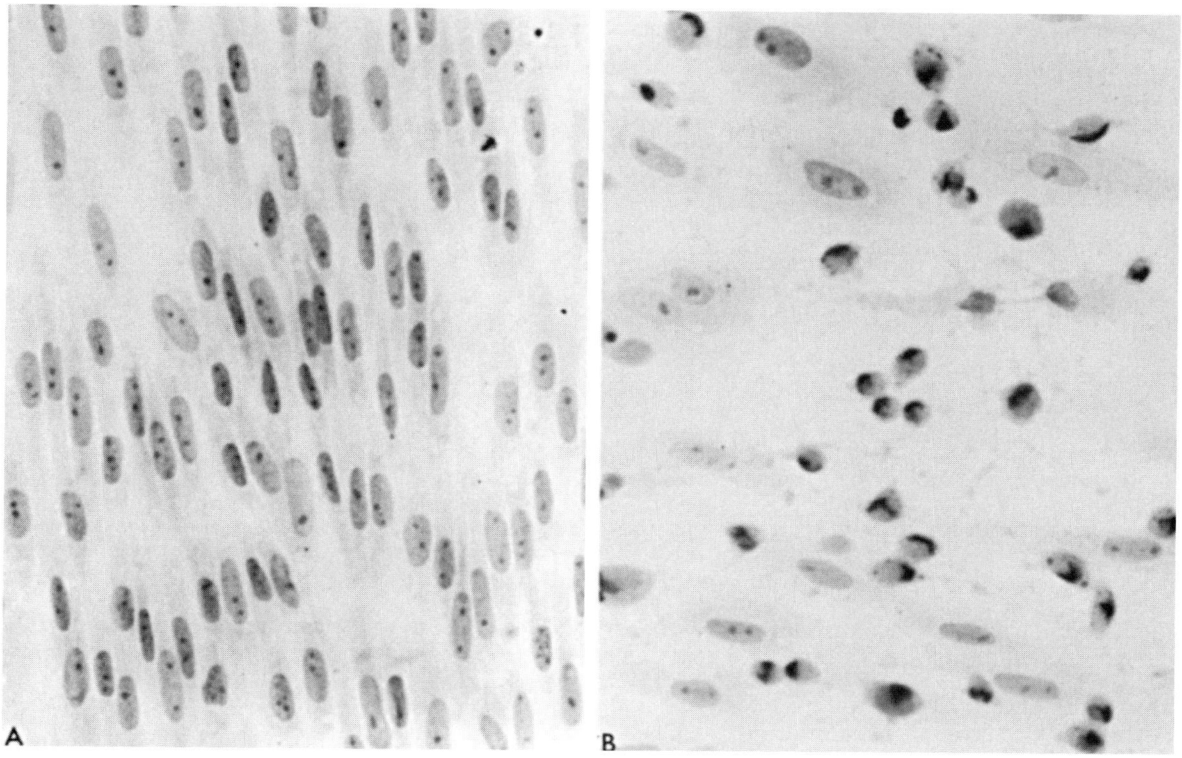

FIGURE 170–1. *Fetal rhesus monkey kidney tissue culture (HL-8).* A, *Uninoculated tissue culture.* B, *Echovirus 11 cytopathic effect. (From Cherry, J. D.: Enteroviruses.* In *Remington, J. S., and Klein, J. O. [eds.]: Infectious Diseases of the Fetus and Newborn Infant. 3rd ed. Philadelphia, W. B. Saunders, 1990.)*

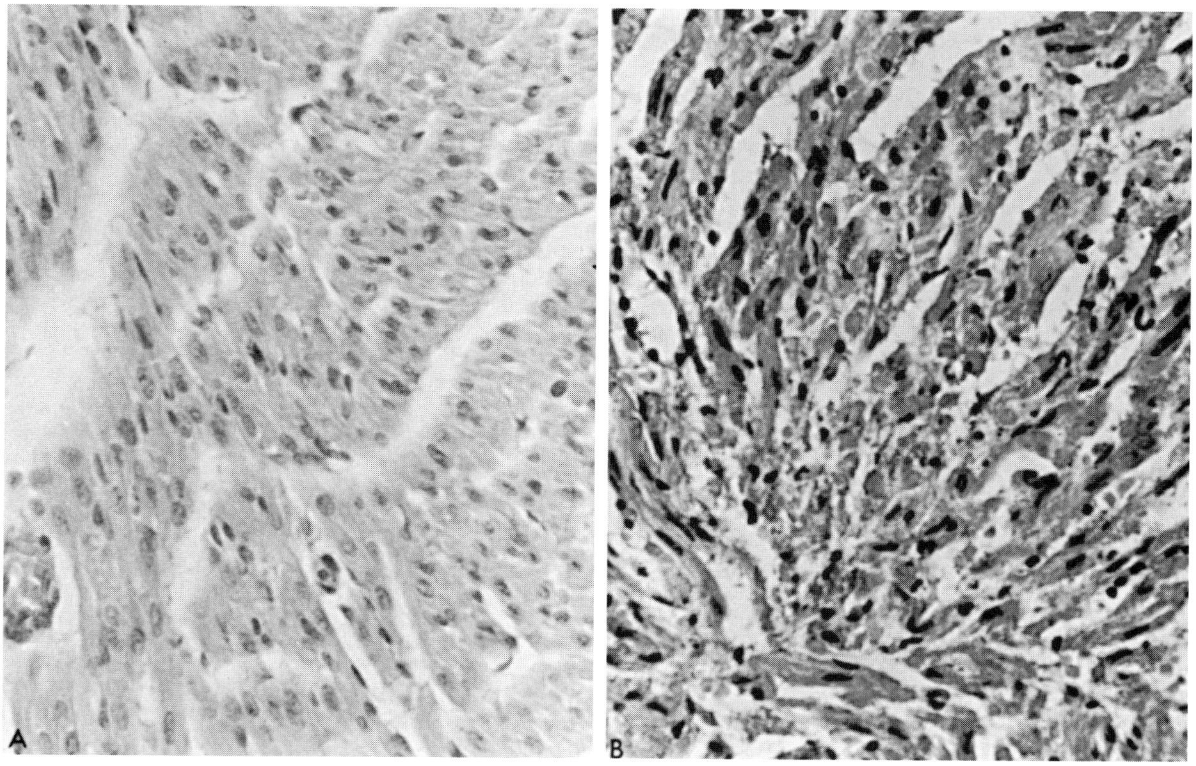

FIGURE 170–2. *Suckling mouse myocardium.* A, *Normal suckling mouse myocardium.* B, *Myocardium of suckling mouse infected with coxsackievirus B1. (From Cherry, J. D.: Enteroviruses.* In *Remington, J. S., and Klein, J. O. [eds.]: Infectious Diseases of the Fetus and Newborn Infant. 3rd ed. Philadelphia, W. B. Saunders, 1990.)*

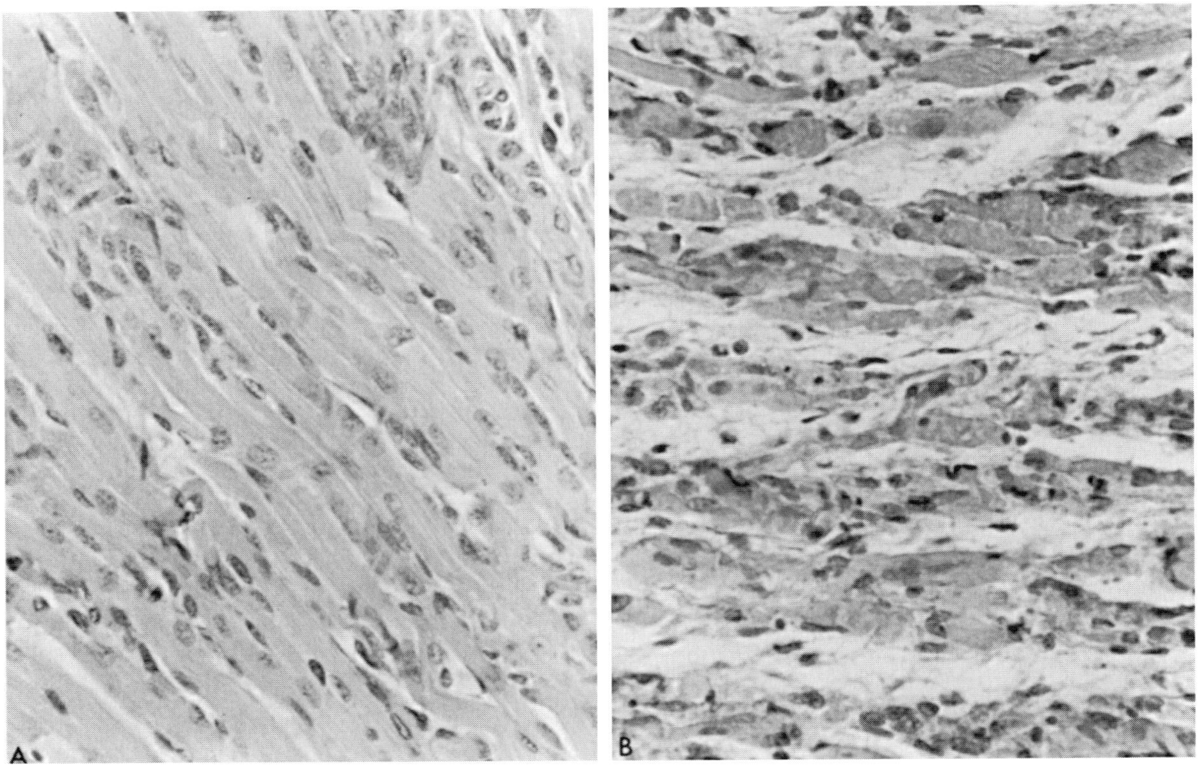

FIGURE 170–3. *Suckling mouse skeletal muscle.* A, *Normal suckling mouse skeletal muscle.* B, *Skeletal muscle of a mouse infected with coxsackievirus A16. (From Cherry, J. D.: Enteroviruses.* In *Remington, J. S., and Klein, J. O. [eds.]: Infectious Diseases of the Fetus and Newborn Infant. 3rd ed. Philadelphia, W. B. Saunders, 1990.)*

ing because, in addition to their possible role in human infection, they offer a source of enteroviral storage during cold-weather periods.[117] Contaminated foods are another possible source of human infection.[115]

EPIDEMIOLOGY

Transmission

Human beings are the only natural hosts of human polioviruses, coxsackieviruses, and echoviruses.[170, 252, 400, 501, 653, 737, 738] Spread is from person to person by fecal-oral and possibly oral-oral (respiratory spread) routes. Swimming and wading pools may serve as a means of spread of enteroviruses during the summertime.[398] Oral-oral transmission by way of the contaminated hands of health care personnel and transmission by fomites have been documented on a chronic care pediatric ward.[370] Enteroviruses have been recovered from trapped flies, and this carriage probably contributes to the spread of human infections, particularly in lower socioeconomic populations that have poor sanitary facilities.[115]

Children are the main susceptible cohort; they are immunologically susceptible, and their unhygienic habits facilitate spread. Spread is from child to child (via feces to skin to mouth) and then within family groups. Recovery of enteroviruses is related inversely to age; prevalence of specific antibodies is related directly to age. The incidence of infections and the prevalence of antibodies do not differ between boys and girls.

Geographic Distribution and Season

Enteroviruses have a worldwide distribution.[115, 228, 252] Neutralizing antibodies for specific viral types have been noted in serologic surveys throughout the world, and most strains have been recovered in worldwide isolation studies. In any one area, there are frequent fluctuations in predominant types. Epidemics probably depend on newly susceptible individuals in the population rather than on reinfections; they may be localized and sporadic and may vary in etiology from place to place in the same year. Pandemic waves of infection also occur.

In temperate climates, enteroviral infections occur primarily in the summer and fall, but in the tropics, they are prevalent all year.[115, 252, 499] A basic concept in understanding their epidemiology concerns the far greater frequency of unrecognized infection compared with clinical disease. This is illustrated by poliomyelitis, which remained an epidemiologic mystery until it was appreciated that unrecognized infections were the main source of contagion. Serologic surveys were instrumental in elucidating the problem: in populations living under conditions of poor sanitation and hygiene, epidemics did not occur, but wide dissemination of polioviruses was confirmed by demonstrating the presence of specific antibodies to all three types in close to 100 per cent of children by 5 years of age.

Epidemics of poliomyelitis first began to appear in Europe and the United States during the latter part of the 19th century; they continued with increasing frequency in the economically advanced countries until the introduction of effective vaccines in the 1950s and 1960s.[71, 140, 328, 576] The evolution from endemic to epidemic follows a characteristic pattern, beginning with collections of a few cases, then higher than usual endemic rates, followed by severe epidemics with high attack rates. The age group attacked in endemic areas and in early epidemics is the youngest one—more than 90 per cent of paralytic cases begin in children younger than 5 years of age. Once this pattern of epidemicity begins, it is irreversible unless preventive vaccination is carried out.

As epidemics recur over a period of years, there is a shift in age incidence, so that relatively fewer cases are in the youngest children; the peak often occurs in the 5- to 14-year-old group, and an increasing proportion is in young adults. These changes are correlated with socioeconomic factors and improved standards of hygiene: when children are protected from immunizing infections in the first few years of life, the pool of susceptible persons builds up and introduction of a virulent strain often is followed by an epidemic. Extensive use of vaccines in the past 30 years has resulted in virtual elimination of paralytic poliomyelitis from large geographic areas, but the disease remains endemic in various parts of the world. Furthermore, first epidemics of true "infantile paralysis" continue to occur, particularly in developing countries where economic and other problems have delayed institution of control measures.[23, 328] Although seasonal periodicity is distinct in temperate climates, some viral activity does take place during the winter months.[115] Infection and acquisition of postinfection immunity occur with greater intensity and at earlier ages among crowded, economically deprived populations with less efficient sanitation.

Recently, molecular techniques have allowed the study of genotypes of specific viral types in populations over time.[185, 352, 458, 533] For example, Mulders and colleagues[533] studied the molecular epidemiology of wild poliovirus 1 in Europe, the Middle East, and the Indian subcontinent. They found that four major genotypes were circulating. Two genotypes were found predominantly in Eastern Europe, a third genotype was circulating mainly in Egypt, and the fourth genotype was dispersed widely. All four genotypes were found in Pakistan.

Prevalence of Different Types

The epidemiologic behavior of coxsackieviruses and echoviruses parallels that of polioviruses, in which unrecognized infections far outnumber those with distinctive symptoms. The agents are disseminated widely throughout the world, and outbreaks due to one or another type occur regularly. These tend to be localized, with different agents being prevalent in different years. In the late 1950s, however, echovirus 9 had a far wider circulation, sweeping through a large part of the world and infecting not only children but also young adults. This behavior has been repeated occasionally with other enteroviruses: after a long absence, a particular agent returns and circulates among the susceptible persons of different ages who have been born since the last epidemic occurred. Other agents remain endemic in a given area, surfacing as sporadic cases and occasionally in small outbreaks. Multiple types frequently are active at the same time, although one agent commonly is predominant in a given locality.

Listed in Table 170–2 are the five most prevalent nonpolio enterovirus isolations per year in the United States from 1961 through 1995.[12, 98, 115, 682] The majority of patients from whom viruses were isolated had neurologic illnesses. It is possible that other enteroviruses also were prevalent but without clinical disease severe enough to cause physicians to submit specimens for study. In addition, probably many coxsackievirus A infections, even in the epidemic situation, went undiagnosed because suckling mouse inoculation frequently is not performed. Although 65 nonpolio enteroviral types are identified, it is of interest that in the 35 years covered in Table 170–2, only 19 different virus types are noted. Echovirus 9 was most common, with echoviruses 6 and 11 and coxsackieviruses B2 and B4 the next most common. Since 1990, echovirus 30 has been the most common circulating viral type.

Although use of live polioviral vaccine has eliminated epidemic poliomyelitis in the United States, it is hard to determine what the effect of polio vaccine viruses has been on enteroviral ecology. In 1970, polioviruses accounted for only 6 per cent of the total enteroviral isolations from patients with neurologic illnesses.[115] Although the figures are not directly comparable, more than one-third of the enteroviral isolations in 1962 from similar patients were polioviruses.[115] However, Horstmann and colleagues[329] studied specimens from sewage and asymptomatic children during the vaccine era and noted that the number of yearly polioviral isolations (presumably vaccine strains) was greater than the number of nonpolioviral enteroviruses. The prevalence of vaccine viruses apparently did not affect the seasonal epidemiology of other enteroviruses.

PATHOGENESIS AND PATHOLOGY

Events During Pathogenesis[71, 117, 496, 630]

Figure 170–4 diagrams the events of pathogenesis. After initial acquisition of virus by the oral or respiratory route, implantation occurs in the pharynx and the lower alimentary tract. Within 1 day, the infection extends to the regional lymph nodes. On about the third day, minor viremia occurs, resulting in involvement of many secondary infection sites. In congenital infections, infection is initiated during the minor viremia phase. Multiplication of virus in secondary infection sites coincides with the onset of clinical symptoms. Illness can vary from minor infections to fatal ones. Major viremia occurs during the period of multiplication of virus in the secondary infection sites; this period usually lasts from the third to the seventh day of infection. In many echovirus and coxsackievirus infections, central nervous system involvement apparently occurs at the same time as other secondary organ involvement does. Occasionally, the central nervous system symptoms of enteroviral infections are delayed, suggesting that seeding occurred later in association with the major viremia.

Cessation of viremia correlates with the appearance of serum antibody. The viral concentration in secondary infection sites begins to diminish on about the seventh day. However, infection continues in the lower intestinal tract for prolonged periods.

In Figure 170–5, clinical and subclinical events in polioviral infections are presented. By 3 to 5 days after exposure, virus can be recovered from blood, throat, and feces. This may be accompanied by symptoms of the "minor illness," or the infection may be unrecognized clinically. The end of the period of viremia coincides with the appearance of antibodies and the onset of clinical signs of central nervous system involvement. Available evidence favors the blood as the main pathway of central nervous system invasion in the natural disease, but experimental infections in monkeys indicate that the virus can travel along axons of peripheral nerves. It is possible that when tonsillectomy is performed on a child with inapparent poliovirus infection, the virus may enter nerve fibers exposed during surgery and spread to the cranial nerve nuclei in the brain, resulting in bulbar paralysis.

Factors That Affect Pathogenesis

The pathogenesis and pathology of enteroviral infections depend on the virulence, tropism, and inoculum concentration of virus, as well as on many specific host factors. It is

TABLE 170–2. Predominant Types of Nonpolio Enteroviral Isolations in the United States: 1961 to 1995*

	Five Most Common Viral Types Per Year				
	First	*Second*	*Third*	*Fourth*	*Fifth*
1961	Coxsackievirus B5	Coxsackievirus B2	Coxsackievirus B4	Echovirus 11	Echovirus 9
1962	Coxsackievirus B3	Echovirus 9	Coxsackievirus B2	Echovirus 4	Coxsackievirus B5
1963	Coxsackievirus B1	Coxsackievirus A9	Echovirus 9	Echovirus 4	Coxsackievirus B4
1964	Coxsackievirus B4	Coxsackievirus B2	Coxsackievirus A9	Echovirus 4	Echovirus 6, Coxsackievirus B1
1965	Echovirus 9	Echovirus 6	Coxsackievirus B2	Coxsackievirus B5	Coxsackievirus B4
1966	Echovirus 9	Coxsackievirus B2	Echovirus 6	Coxsackievirus B5	Coxsackievirus A9, Coxsackievirus A16
1967	Coxsackievirus B5	Echovirus 9	Coxsackievirus A9	Echovirus 6	Coxsackievirus B2
1968	Echovirus 9	Echovirus 30	Coxsackievirus A16	Coxsackievirus B3	Coxsackievirus B4
1969	Echovirus 30	Echovirus 9	Echovirus 18	Echovirus 6	Coxsackievirus B4
1970	Echovirus 3	Echovirus 9	Echovirus 6	Echovirus 4	Coxsackievirus B4
1971	Echovirus 4	Echovirus 9	Echovirus 6	Coxsackievirus B4	Coxsackievirus B2
1972	Coxsackievirus B5	Echovirus 4	Echovirus 6	Echovirus 9	Coxsackievirus B3
1973	Coxsackievirus A9	Echovirus 9	Echovirus 6	Coxsackievirus B2	Coxsackievirus B5, Echovirus 5
1974	Echovirus 11	Echovirus 4	Echovirus 6	Echovirus 9	Echovirus 18
1975	Echovirus 9	Echovirus 4	Echovirus 6	Coxsackievirus A9	Coxsackievirus B4
1976	Coxsackievirus B2	Echovirus 4	Coxsackievirus B4	Coxsackievirus A9	Coxsackievirus B3, Echovirus 6
1977	Echovirus 6	Coxsackievirus B1	Coxsackievirus B3	Echovirus 9	Coxsackievirus A9
1978	Echovirus 9	Echovirus 4	Coxsackievirus A9	Echovirus 30	Coxsackievirus B4
1979	Echovirus 11	Echovirus 7	Echovirus 30	Coxsackievirus B2	Coxsackievirus B4
1980	Echovirus 11	Coxsackievirus B3	Echovirus 30	Coxsackievirus B2	Coxsackievirus A9
1981	Echovirus 30	Echovirus 9	Echovirus 11	Echovirus 3	Coxsackievirus A9, Echovirus 5
1982	Echovirus 11	Echovirus 30	Echovirus 5	Echovirus 9	Coxsackievirus B5
1983	Coxsackievirus B5	Echovirus 30	Echovirus 20	Echovirus 11	Echovirus 24
1984	Echovirus 9	Echovirus 11	Coxsackievirus B5	Echovirus 30	Coxsackievirus B2, A9
1985	Echovirus 11	Echovirus 21	Echovirus 6 & 7†		Coxsackievirus B2
1986	Echovirus 11	Echovirus 4	Echovirus 7	Echovirus 18	Coxsackievirus B5
1987	Echovirus 6	Echovirus 18	Echovirus 11	Coxsackievirus A9	Coxsackievirus B2
1988	Echovirus 11	Echovirus 9	Coxsackievirus B4	Coxsackievirus B2	Echovirus 6
1989	Coxsackievirus B5	Echovirus 9	Echovirus 11	Coxsackievirus B2	Echovirus 6
1990	Echovirus 30	Echovirus 6	Coxsackievirus B2	Coxsackievirus A9	Echovirus 11
1991	Echovirus 30	Echovirus 11	Coxsackievirus B1	Coxsackievirus B2	Echovirus 7
1992	Echovirus 11	Echovirus 30	Echovirus 9	Coxsackievirus B1	Coxsackievirus A9
1993	Echovirus 30	Coxsackievirus B5	Coxsackievirus A9	Coxsackievirus B1	Echovirus 7
1994	Coxsackievirus B2	Coxsackievirus B3	Echovirus E6	Echovirus 30	Coxsackievirus A9
1995	Echovirus 9	Echovirus 11	Coxsackievirus A9	Coxsackievirus B2	Echovirus 30

*The majority of patients from whom viruses were isolated had neurologic illnesses.[12, 98, 115, 244, 682]
†Third and fourth place tie.

obvious that enteroviruses have marked differences in both tropism and virulence. Although some generalizations can be made in regard to tropism, there are marked differences even between strains of specific viral types.

Van Eden and associates[716] studied 17 families during an outbreak of poliomyelitis due to type 1 virus in the Netherlands, and their findings suggested that HLA-encoded genetic factors were important in the occurrence of paralytic disease.

It generally is believed that enterovirus infections of the fetus and neonate are more severe than are similar infections in older persons. This undoubtedly is true in coxsackievirus B infections and probably also true in coxsackievirus A and echovirus infections. Although the reasons for this increased severity are unknown, several aspects of neonatal immune mechanisms have been studied. In addition, the similarity of coxsackievirus B infections in suckling mice to those in human neonates has provided a useful animal model system. Heinberg and associates[310] compared coxsackievirus B1 infections in 24-hour-old suckling mice with similar infections in older mice. They noted that adult mice produced interferon in all infected tissues, whereas suckling mice produced only small amounts of interferon in the liver. They felt that the difference in outcome of coxsackievirus B1 infections in suckling and older mice could be explained by the inability of the cells of the immature animal to elaborate interferon.

Others believe that the increased susceptibility of suckling mice to severe coxsackievirus infections is related to the transplacentally acquired increased concentrations of adrenocortical hormones.[47, 72] Kunin[424] has suggested that the difference in age-specific susceptibility might be explained at the cellular level. He has shown that a variety of tissues of newborn mice bind coxsackievirus B3, whereas tissues of adult mice are virtually inactive in this regard.[424, 425] The progressive loss of receptor-containing cells with increasing age may be the mechanism that accounts for less severe infections in older animals.

In the past, it has been assumed that specific pathology in various organs and tissues in enteroviral infections was due to the direct cytopathic effect and tropism of a particular virus. In more recent years, a large number of studies utilizing murine myocarditis model systems have suggested that

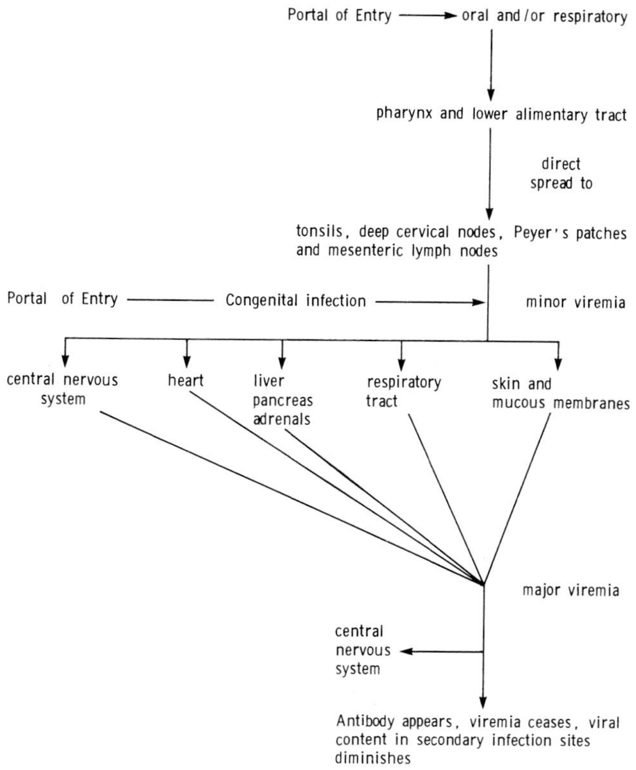

FIGURE 170–4. *The pathogenesis of enteroviral infections. (Modified from Cherry, J. D.: Enteroviruses.* In *Remington, J. S., and Klein, J. O. [eds.]: Infectious Diseases of the Fetus and Newborn Infant. 3rd ed. Philadelphia, W. B. Saunders, 1990.)*

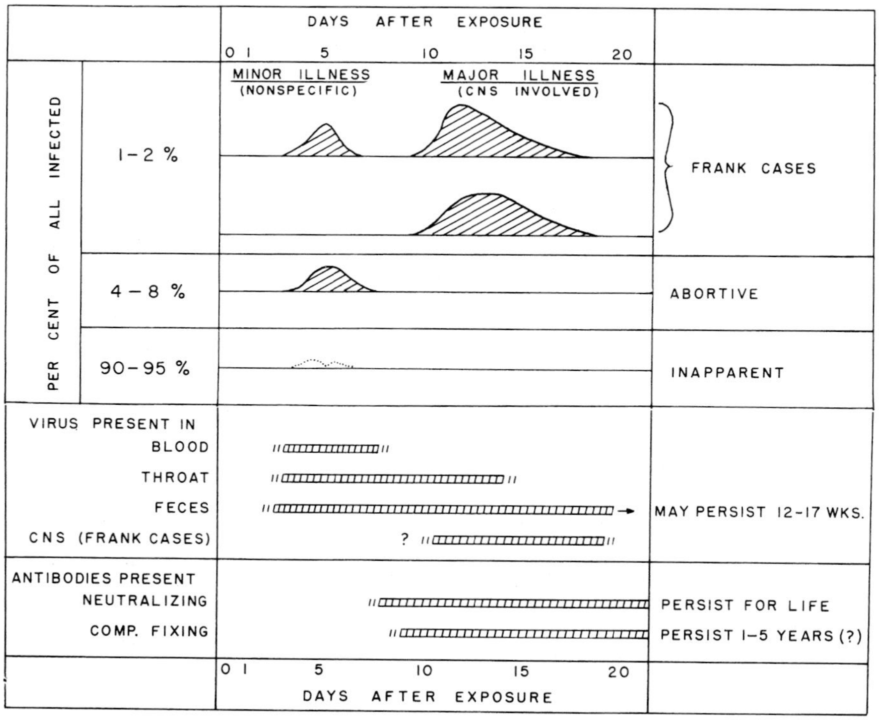

FIGURE 170–5. *The course of clinical and subclinical forms of poliovirus infections in reaction to the presence of virus and the development of antibodies. (From Bodian, D., and Horstmann, D. M.: Poliomyelitis.* In *Horsfall, F. L., and Tamm, I. [eds.]: Viral and Rickettsial Infections of Man. 4th ed. Philadelphia, J. B. Lippincott, 1965, pp. 430–473.)*

host immune responses contribute to the pathology.[19, 246, 247, 314, 317, 333, 433, 546, 571, 597, 655, 754] These studies suggest that T-cell–mediated processes and virus-induced autoimmunity cause both acute and chronic myocardial damage. However, studies by McManus and associates[489] suggest that the primary viral cytopathic effect is responsible for myocardial cell damage and that various T-cell responses are a response to the damage and not the cause of the damage.

Pathology

The clinical signs of enteroviral infections vary widely, so wide variations in pathology also exist. Because pathologic material generally is available only from patients with fatal illnesses, this section discusses only the more severe manifestations. It is worth emphasizing, however, that these fatal infections account for only a small portion of all enteroviral infections. The pathologic findings in children with milder infections, such as nonspecific febrile illness, have not been described.

Coxsackieviruses A

Records of severe illnesses associated with coxsackieviruses A are rare. Gold and colleagues,[267] in a study of sudden unexpected death in infants, recovered coxsackievirus A4 from the brains of three children. In none of these patients were histologic abnormalities noted in the brains or spinal cords. An adult with a fatal coxsackievirus A7 infection had diffuse pancarditis and organized pneumonitis.[32]

Coxsackieviruses B

Of the nonpolio enteroviruses, coxsackieviruses B have been associated most frequently with severe and catastrophic disease. The most common findings in these cases have been myocarditis, meningoencephalitis, or both. Involvement of the adrenals, pancreas, liver, and lungs also has been noted.

HEART.[115, 211, 250, 755] Grossly, the heart usually is enlarged, with dilatation of the chambers and flabby musculature. Microscopically, the pericardium frequently contains some inflammatory cells, and thickening, edema, and the endocardium may have focal infiltrations of inflammatory cells. The myocardium (Fig. 170–6) is congested and contains infiltrations of inflammatory cells (lymphocytes, mononuclear cells, reticulum cells, histiocytes, plasma cells, and polymorphonuclear and eosinophil leukocytes). The involvement of the myocardium often is patchy and focal but occasionally diffuse. The muscle shows loss of striation as well as edema and eosinophilic degeneration. Muscle necrosis without extensive cellular infiltration is common.

BRAIN AND SPINAL CORD.[115, 211, 520, 755] The meninges are congested, edematous, and occasionally mildly infiltrated with inflammatory cells. Lesions in the brain and spinal cord are focal rather than diffuse but frequently involve many different areas. The lesions consist of areas of eosinophilic degeneration of cortical cells, clusters of mononuclear and glial cells (Fig. 170–7), and perivascular cuffing. Two children with fatal coxsackieviral B infections (types 2 and 4, respectively) had, in addition to typical inflammatory encephalitic lesions, widespread multifocal areas of liquefaction necrosis without inflammation.[204]

OTHER ORGANS.[9, 115, 250, 520, 755] The lungs frequently reveal areas of mild focal pneumonitis with peribronchiolar mononuclear cellular infiltrations. The liver frequently is engorged and occasionally contains isolated foci of liver cell necrosis and mononuclear infiltrations. In the pancreas, occasional focal degeneration of the islet cells occurs. Congestion has been observed in the adrenal glands, with mild to severe cortical necrosis; inflammatory cells are present.

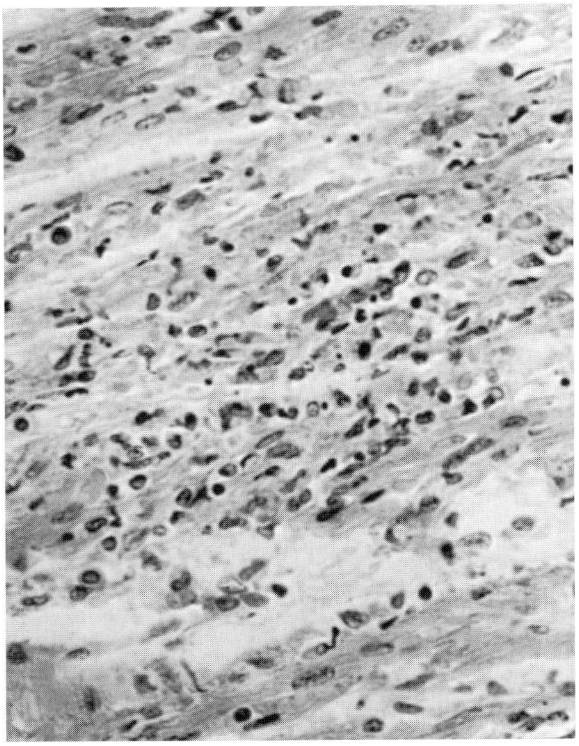

FIGURE 170–6. *Coxsackievirus B4 myocarditis in a 9-day-old infant. Note myocardial necrosis and mononuclear cellular infiltration. (From Cherry, J. D.: Enteroviruses.* In *Remington, J. S., and Klein, J. O. [eds.]: Infectious Diseases of the Fetus and Newborn Infant. 3rd ed. Philadelphia, W. B. Saunders, 1990.)*

Echoviruses

Although frequently responsible for illnesses, echoviruses until relatively recently rarely were associated with fatal infections. Interestingly, in several different reports with eight different echovirus types, hepatic necrosis was a major pathologic finding.[66, 115, 253, 293, 514, 529, 760] Massive hepatic necrosis has been seen with echoviruses 3, 6, 7, 9, 11, 14, 19, and 21. At autopsy, one infant with echovirus 6 infection had cloudy and thickened leptomeninges, liver necrosis, adrenal and renal hemorrhage, and mild interstitial pneumonitis.[115] One infant with echovirus 9 infection had an enlarged and congested liver with marked central necrosis,[115] and another with this virus had interstitial pneumonitis without liver involvement.[115] Three infants with echovirus 11 infections had renal and adrenal hemorrhage and small vessel thrombi in the renal medulla and in both the medulla and inner cortex of the adrenals.[537] These patients' livers were normal. Two infants, one with echovirus 6 and the other with echovirus 31 infection, had only extensive pneumonia.[78, 115]

Polioviruses[71, 140]

The neuropathy of poliomyelitis usually is pathognomonic; only certain cells and areas of the neuraxis are susceptible to the virus. Neuronal damage is due directly to virus multiplication, but not all affected neurons are killed. The injury may be reversible, and function may be restored within 3 to 4

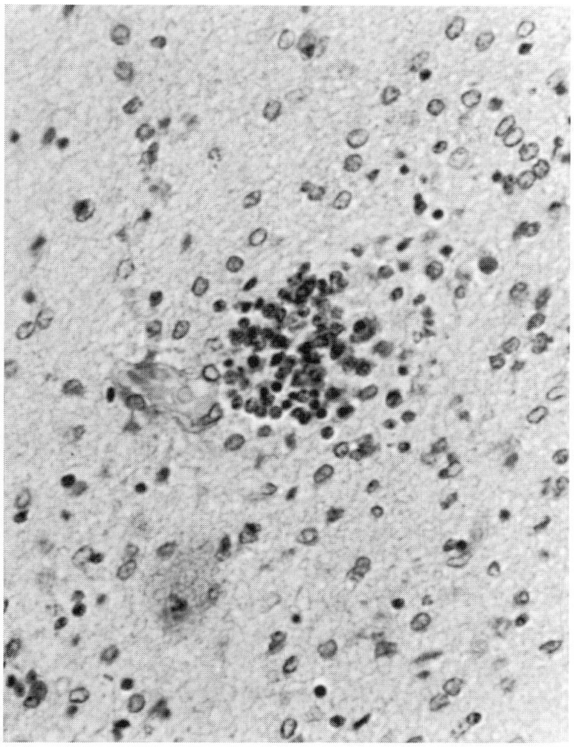

FIGURE 170–7. *Coxsackievirus B4 encephalitis in a 9-day-old infant. Focal infiltrate of mononuclear and glial cells. (From Cherry, J. D.: Enteroviruses.* In *Remington, J. S., and Klein, J. O. [eds.]: Infectious Diseases of the Fetus and Newborn Infant. 3rd ed. Philadelphia, W. B. Saunders, 1990.)*

weeks after onset. There is little histologic evidence of meningeal reaction. Perivascular cuffing and some interstitial glial infiltration are present. Histologic sections generally reveal more widespread lesions than would be estimated from the clinical findings. Scattered neurons may undergo considerable destruction without clinical disability.

The regions in which neuronal lesions occur are the (1) spinal cord (anterior horn cells chiefly and to a lesser degree the intermediate and dorsal horn and dorsal root ganglia), (2) medulla (vestibular nuclei, cranial nerve nuclei, and the reticular formation that contains the vital centers), (3) cerebellum (nuclei in the roof and vermis only), (4) midbrain (chiefly the gray matter but also the substantia nigra and occasionally the red nucleus), (5) thalamus and hypothalamus, (6) pallidum, and (7) cerebral cortex (motor cortex). The viruses spare the following areas: (1) the entire cerebral cortex except the motor area, (2) the cerebellum except the vermis and deep midline nuclei, and (3) the white matter of the spinal cord. This distribution of lesions permits a histologic diagnosis of poliomyelitis.

Extraneural pathology usually is a secondary phenomenon. Bronchopulmonary changes may occur, such as aspiration pneumonia, atelectasis, and purulent bronchitis, because of impairment of cough and decreased thoracic movements. The cardiovascular changes may result in hypertension, cardiac failure, and pulmonary edema. Prolonged immobilization leads to negative nitrogen and calcium balances, with urinary lithiasis, renal failure, hypertension with encephalopathy, and convulsions. Treatment itself may cause untoward complications, such as urinary tract infection (after catheterization), decubitus ulcers, and psychotic disturbances. Ulcerations in the alimentary tract may result in serious bleeding and occasional perforation. Respiratory failure results in respiratory acidosis and anoxic changes.

CLINICAL MANIFESTATIONS—NONPOLIO ENTEROVIRUSES

Nonpolio enteroviral infections are exceedingly common, and the spectrum of disease is protean (Tables 170–3 through 170–16). Many of the clinical-virologic associations listed in Tables 170–3 through 170–16 are based on a limited number of cases. Because coxsackieviruses and echoviruses frequently are carried asymptomatically in the gastrointestinal tract for relatively long periods, some of the observed illnesses and concomitantly recovered viruses may not have a cause-and-effect relationship. However, repeated observations since the 1960s have supported many virus-illness associations, even though their occurrence has been sporadic.

There are few specific enterovirus diseases, but rather a variety of interrelated syndromes and anatomically associated illnesses. Many illnesses and syndromes can be caused by different coxsackieviral and echoviral types, and most types are capable of inducing a variety of clinical syndromes. On the other hand, certain specific coxsackieviral and echoviral types have clinical characteristics that facilitate etiologic diagnosis.

In recent years, there have been few careful studies in which specific clinical findings have been identified with individual enteroviral types. This is unfortunate because specific syndromes likely are related to specific viral types that are being overlooked.

Asymptomatic Infection

Because it is known that 90 to 95 per cent of poliovirus infections are not recognized clinically, it has been assumed that the majority of infections with coxsackieviruses and echoviruses are asymptomatic. This opinion also is strengthened by the fact that coxsackieviruses and echoviruses can be recovered frequently from the stools of normal children. However, relatively few data are available on the rate of asymptomatic infection with nonpolio enteroviruses. All too frequently, the isolation of enteroviruses from the stool is equated with asymptomatic infection. This is an error because illness, if it occurs, happens shortly after virus acquisition and is short-lived; a particular infection may have been associated with nonspecific illness 2 or 3 months prior to collection of a stool specimen obtained in a surveillance program. Unfortunately, in several studies in controlled population groups in which accurate clinical expression rates could have been determined, clinical observations apparently were of secondary importance to the investigators.[115, 251, 252, 254, 416] The data available suggest differences in clinical expression among coxsackieviral and echoviral types.

Table 170–3 lists the approximate frequencies of asymptomatic infections with selected coxsackieviruses and echoviruses. As can be seen, the rates vary among the group as a whole and even within specific types. Overall, it appears that about half and perhaps more of all nonpolio enteroviral infections are associated with clinical manifestations. In general, the more carefully clinical symptoms are examined, the smaller the percentage of truly asymptomatic infections. Clinical expression also is related inversely to age. With coxsackievirus A16, asymptomatic infection occurs in only about 10 per cent of children younger than 5 years of age, whereas rates are higher in older children and adults.[7, 115] Sabin[631] noted no asymptomatic infections in infants with echovirus

TABLE 170–3. Approximate Frequencies of Asymptomatic Infections with Selected Coxsackieviruses and Echoviruses[115]

	Asymptomatic Infection Frequency (Per Cent)
Coxsackieviruses	
A	50
A16	50
B	20
B2	11–50
B3	25–96
B4	30–70
B5	5–40
Echoviruses	50
4	Uncommon—60
6	Rare
9	15–60
18	Rare–20
20	33
25	30
30	50

18, and Nishmi and Yodfat[561] noted less than 20 per cent of infections without illness in children younger than 8 years of age during an echovirus 4 epidemic. At the other extreme, Clemmer and associates[148] reported that 96 per cent of infections with coxsackievirus B3 were asymptomatic. In other studies, the illness rate of coxsackievirus B3 has been 60 to 75 per cent.

Nonspecific Febrile Illness (Table 170–4)

Nonspecific febrile illness is the most common manifestation of coxsackieviral and echoviral infections. All viral types cause this clinical presentation, but the frequency varies considerably among the individual viruses.

The onset of illness usually is abrupt, without prodrome. In young children, the initial finding is fever and associated malaise. In older children, headache usually is noted. The temperature ranges between 38.3° and 40° C (101° and 104° F) and has a mean duration of 3 days. In some instances, the fever is biphasic; it occurs for 1 day, is absent for 2 to 3 days, and then recurs for an additional 2 to 4 days. In many young children, the only manifestation of illness is fever, and its presence is discovered by chance by a parent.

Malaise and anorexia often are related to the degree of temperature elevation, as is headache in older patients. The complaint of sore throat is common, but an inflamed pharynx is not seen on examination. Nausea and vomiting occasionally occur at the onset of illness, as does mild abdominal discomfort. One or two loose stools may be noted. Generalized myalgia also is noted, and children complain of a scratchy feeling in the throat.

Physical examination generally yields benign findings. There may be minimal conjunctivitis, injection on the pharynx, and cervical lymphadenitis. The duration of illness varies from 24 hours to about 6 days, with an average of 3 to 4 days. The white blood cell count is normal.

Respiratory Manifestations (see Table 170–4)

Common Cold

Although numerous coxsackieviruses and echoviruses have been recovered from children with mild upper respiratory infections, only rarely do the illnesses qualify as common colds. (The common cold is an acute illness with nasal stuffiness, rhinitis, no objective evidence of pharyngitis, and no or minimal fever.) In most instances, significant fever (temperature >38.3° C, or >101° F) is associated with enteroviral infections and usually some degree of pharyngitis.

Coxsackievirus A21 is the only enterovirus that clearly qualifies as a common cold virus.[115, 372] This agent has produced epidemics of mild respiratory illness in military populations. In adult volunteers, instillation of this virus in the nose has resulted in the common cold syndrome. Epidemic disease has not been observed in children. Other viruses that have been associated with the common cold syndrome

TABLE 170–4. Coxsackieviruses and Echoviruses Noted in Association with Nonspecific Febrile Illness and Respiratory Disease*

	Virus Types		
Clinical Categories	***Coxsackieviruses A***	***Coxsackieviruses B***	***Echoviruses and Enteroviruses***
Nonspecific febrile illness	All types	All types	All types
Common cold	Mainly 21, 24; rarely other types	Mainly 1–5; rarely 6	Mainly 2, 20; rarely other types
Pharyngitis (pharyngitis, tonsillitis, tonsillopharyngitis, and nasopharyngitis)	Probably all types; mainly 9	Probably all types; mainly 1–5	Probably all types; mainly 2, 4, 6, 9, 11, 16, 19, 25, 30, 71
Herpangina	1–10, 16, 22	1–5	6, 9, 11, 16, 17, 22, 25
Lymphonodular pharyngitis	10		
Stomatitis and other lesions in the anterior mouth	5, 9, 10, 16	2, 5	9, 11, 20, 71
Parotitis	Coxsackievirus A not typed	3, 4	70
Croup	9	4, 5	4, 11, 21
Bronchitis		1, 4	8, 12–14
Bronchiolitis and infectious asthma	Many types	Many types	Many types
Pneumonia	9, 16	1–6	6, 7, 9, 11, 12, 19, 20, 30
Pleurodynia	1, 2, 4, 6, 9, 16	1–6	1–3, 6–9, 11, 12, 14, 16–19, 23–25, 30

include echoviruses 2 and 20 and coxsackieviruses B1, B2, B3, B4, B5, and A24.[115]

Pharyngitis (Pharyngitis, Tonsillitis, Tonsillopharyngitis, and Nasopharyngitis)

Pharyngitis is a common clinical manifestation of coxsackieviral and echoviral infections. Probably all enteroviruses on occasion cause mild pharyngitis. The most common coxsackieviruses and echoviruses associated with pharyngitis are coxsackieviruses A9 and B1, B2, B3, B4, and B5, echoviruses 2, 4, 6, 9, 11, 16, 19, 25, and 30, and enterovirus 71.[115, 125–127, 159, 206, 294, 307, 387, 388, 395, 400, 447, 448, 527, 628, 632, 666] Pharyngitis in coxsackievirus and echovirus infections frequently is associated with other clinical findings, such as meningitis, pleurodynia, or exanthem. These other manifestations become more important than pharyngitis in individual cases in the minds of parents as well as clinicians.

Pharyngitis due to coxsackieviruses and echoviruses usually is abrupt in onset without prodrome. Although pharyngeal involvement is present at the onset of disease, the initial complaint most often is fever. The temperature usually ranges between 38.3° and 40° C (101° and 104° F), but higher temperatures are not unusual. In general, fever tends to be more pronounced in younger patients. Young children have malaise and anorexia. School age children complain of headache and myalgia. Sore throat, coryza and vomiting, diarrhea, or a combination thereof also may be noted.

Examination of the tonsils and pharynx shows varying degrees of erythema. In some cases, only injection is noted, whereas in other cases, severe pharyngitis with patches of exudate is seen. The usual duration of uncomplicated coxsackieviral or echoviral pharyngitis is 3 to 6 days. Routine laboratory study is of minimal value in enteroviral pharyngitis; the total white blood cell count may be normal or slightly elevated with a normal differential determination. A throat culture rules out disease due to group A streptococci.

Other Intraoral Manifestations

HERPANGINA. See Chapter 11.

ACUTE LYMPHONODULAR PHARYNGITIS. In 1962, Steigman and colleagues[674] reported a unique enanthem associated with coxsackievirus A10 infection. The lesions had the typical distribution of herpangina; they were papular, discrete, 3 mm in diameter, and surrounded by a zone of erythema. The lesions were white to yellow and persisted for 6 to 10 days. This entity has not been reported again, although coxsackievirus A10 has been noted in association with hand, foot, and mouth syndrome.[115, 654]

STOMATITIS AND OTHER LESIONS IN THE ANTERIOR MOUTH. The main enteroviral cause of stomatitis and ulcerative lesions in the anterior mouth is coxsackievirus A16, and the clinical entity is the hand, foot, and mouth syndrome. This is presented in detail later in this chapter. It is worth mentioning here, however, that occasionally enanthem occurs without the exanthem and that this enanthem also has been associated with other coxsackieviruses (A5, A9, A10, B2, B5), echovirus 33, and enterovirus 71.[115, 176, 188, 220, 459, 654]

In echovirus 9 infection, Tyrrell and colleagues[710] noted six children with a unique enanthem: painless whitish dots, ulcers, or vesicles were noted on the buccal surfaces near the Stensen duct. They also reported the occasional occurrence of similar lesions under the tongue.

Deseda-Tous and colleagues[180] noted an adolescent with hemorrhagic vesicular lesions on the pharynx, mucosal surfaces, and tongue in association with an echovirus 11 infection. Clarke and Stott[143] reported reddish macules on the buccal mucosa in a patient with echovirus 20 infection, and Cherry and Jahn[123] noted one child with hand, foot, and mouth syndrome in whom buccal lesions suggested Koplik spots, although in this patient the lesions were larger and more yellow.

Parotitis

Parotitis in association with herpangina and coxsackievirus A infection was reported in 1957 by Howlett and associates.[335] In 1960, Kraus[421] reported two additional cases, and Bertaggia and associates[67] and Winsser and Altieri[753] noted parotitis in association with coxsackieviruses B3 and B4, respectively. Three patients with acute hemorrhagic conjunctivitis and parotitis due to enterovirus 70 also have been reported.[643]

Croup

In large studies of respiratory illness in young children, croup sporadically is associated with coxsackieviral and echoviral infections.[111, 115, 230, 259, 740] In general, these illnesses are mild when compared with croup associated with parainfluenza and influenza viruses.

There is one report of an outbreak of croup due to echovirus 11 in a day nursery.[588] In this instance, 17 of 53 ill children were found to be infected with the U strain of echovirus 11. A subsequent study noted the same virus in four children with croup.[581] Croup also is noted in outbreaks of coxsackievirus B5 infection.[30, 157] Other specific agents associated with croup include coxsackieviruses A9 and B4 and echoviruses 4 and 21.[115]

Bronchitis

Acute febrile illness with cough, rhonchi, and referred breath sounds occasionally is a sporadic manifestation of enteroviral infection. A specific association of coxsackieviruses B1 and B4 and echoviruses 8, 12, 13, 14, and 22 has been found.[111, 115, 157, 193, 195]

Bronchiolitis and Infectious Asthma

Coxsackieviruses and echoviruses have been associated sporadically with bronchiolitis, infectious asthma, and the precipitation of asthmatic attacks in atopic children.[111, 115, 193, 230, 259, 278, 326, 740] Epidemic disease has not been observed, and the illnesses usually have been mild.

Pneumonia

In general studies of respiratory infections in children, sporadic coxsackieviruses and echoviruses have been noted in 1 to 7 per cent of the patients with pneumonia with positive viral cultures.[111, 115, 230, 259] Specific virus types include coxsackieviruses A9, A16, B1, B2, B3, B4, B5, and B6, echoviruses 6, 7, 9, 11, 12, 19, 20, and 30, and enterovirus 71.[115, 159, 193, 219, 255, 359, 387, 450, 519, 645, 666, 736]

Only in three instances can it be suggested that an outbreak of pneumonia due to specific viruses occurred. During the summer of 1959, Lerner and colleagues[450] noted that 3 of 15 children infected with coxsackievirus A9 had pneumonia. It is interesting that the three patients with pneumonia had a vesicular rash. The illness in one child was fatal.

Eckert and associates[193] observed six children with coxsackievirus B1 infection and pneumonia during the summer of 1963. These illnesses were not described further, although the mean white blood cell count in 12 children with lower respiratory infections with coxsackieviruses B was reported as 11,383 with a normal differential. All children were hospitalized.

Goldwater[268] reported a coxsackievirus B6 outbreak in South Australia during the summer of 1992 to 1993. Twenty-seven patients had pneumonia associated with high fever and severe cough that lasted several weeks.

In addition to the fatal case with coxsackievirus A9 infection described by Lerner and colleagues,[450] deaths occurred with coxsackieviruses B1, B5, and A16.[219, 359, 761]

Pleurodynia (Bornholm Disease)[31, 115, 170, 273, 281, 400, 518, 690, 727]

Epidemic pleurodynia is an illness that first was noted about 250 years ago by Hannaeus, a Danish physician.[298] Not until the late 19th century, however, did the illness receive further attention in the medical literature. At this time, several epidemics in Scandinavian countries were described.[115, 165, 218] Although Finsen referred to the disease as pleurodynia, others who designated outbreaks used geographic names, such as Skien disease, Bamle disease, Drangedral disease, and Bornholm disease, or descriptive names, such as epidemic myalgia, devil's grippe, epidemic diaphragmatic spasm, or epidemic benign pleurisy.[273] In 1933, Sylvest[690] published the classic monograph on the subject, and from this paper the name Bornholm disease (from Bornholm Island, a Danish island in the Baltic Sea) came to be associated with the illness. The enteroviral etiology of epidemic pleurodynia was established in 1949.[164, 734]

Historically, pleurodynia is an epidemic disease, but sporadic cases do occur. A characteristic incubation period of about 4 days is followed by the sudden onset of fever and pain. The pain typically is located in the chest or upper abdomen and is muscular in origin and of variable intensity. Occasionally, the pain occurs in other areas of the body. Frequently, the pain is excruciatingly severe and sudden and associated with profuse sweating, so that the patient may appear pale and as though in shock. The pain is spasmodic, with durations varying from a few minutes to several hours. Most commonly, the spasmodic periods last about 15 to 30 minutes. During spasms, the respirations usually are rapid, shallow, and grunting, suggesting pneumonia or pleural inflammation. Coughing, sneezing, or deep breathing makes the pain worse. Older children and adults describe the pain as stabbing or knife-like. The older person often fears that a heart attack is occurring.

When pain localizes in the abdomen, it frequently is crampy, suggesting colic in the younger child. The child may double over and refuse to walk or move. Occasionally, the abdominal pain in association with a pale, sweaty, shock-like appearance suggests acute intestinal obstruction. Splinting and guarding of the abdomen also lead to a consideration of appendicitis and peritonitis.

Fever and pain usually last 1 to 2 days. Frequently, however, the illness is biphasic; after the initial febrile period, the patient is asymptomatic for several days, and then pain and fever recur. Rarely, patients have several recurrent episodes over a period of several weeks. In these patients, fever is less prominent.

Tenderness to some degree is present in areas of pain, but frank myositis with muscle swelling is not observed. Pleural friction rubs may be noted on auscultation, and they may appear and disappear with the coming and going of the pain episodes.

In epidemics, both children and adults are afflicted; the majority of cases occur in persons younger than 30 years of age. Most children have other signs of enteroviral infection, such as anorexia, nausea, vomiting, headache, and sore throat. Routine laboratory study is not very helpful. The white blood cell count varies considerably, but an increased percentage of polymorphonuclear neutrophils and band forms is frequent. The erythrocyte sedimentation rate also is inconsistent; normal to extremely high values may be observed. The chest radiograph most often is normal.

Complications in pleurodynia are uncommon. Aseptic meningitis has been noted in some patients, and adult males have experienced orchitis. Cardiac involvement—myocarditis and pericarditis—also may complicate pleurodynia.

The major etiologic agents in epidemic pleurodynia are coxsackieviruses B3 and B5.[31, 115, 338, 628, 650, 666] Other viruses associated with epidemic disease include coxsackieviruses B1 and B2 and echoviruses 1 and 6.[21, 115, 189] Agents associated with sporadic occurrences of pleurodynia include coxsackieviruses A1, A2, A4, A6, A9, A16, B1, B2, B3, B4, B5, and B6 and echoviruses 1, 2, 3, 6, 7, 8, 9, 11, 12, 14, 16, 17, 18, 19, 23, 24, 25, and 30.[49, 115, 157, 190, 294, 382, 405, 486, 518, 556, 688]

In recent years, pleurodynia rarely is reported. Because the enteroviruses that cause pleurodynia still circulate, it is likely that cases are overlooked or misdiagnosed. An outbreak due to coxsackievirus B1 among football players at a public high school was reported.[347] Unfortunately, no clinical data were presented.

Gastrointestinal Manifestations

Gastrointestinal manifestations are common in coxsackieviral and echoviral infections.[24, 25, 115, 136, 170, 281, 326, 400, 477, 480, 484, 486, 501, 518, 521, 522, 556, 602, 653, 737, 738, 741] Clinical manifestations in addition to vomiting and diarrhea are varied; an outline is given in Table 170–5.

Early studies paid particular interest to diarrheal disease of children. However, when specific studies of infantile diarrhea were undertaken, the enteroviral association was far from clear.[46, 115, 272, 573, 772] The association of infection and disease in these studies was compromised by the fact that the main source of culture in study patients and controls was the stool; persistent infection in the bowel made the separation of controls and ill patients impossible.

At present, it seems clear that all coxsackieviruses and echoviruses frequently have one or more symptoms of gastrointestinal involvement as part of their general illnesses. The intensity and spectrum do vary among the specific agents, however, and also among strains of particular viral types. In a review of World Health Organization (WHO) virus reports covering a 4-year period, Assaad and Cockburn[25] noted that the main clinical sign or symptom was gastrointestinal in 12 per cent of coxsackieviral and 6.8 per cent of echoviral infections. In another analysis, Assaad and Borecka[24] noted 16 deaths during the period 1967 to 1975 in those with coxsackievirus and echovirus infections in which the principal clinical association was gastrointestinal.

In a 20-year survey in Wisconsin, Nelson and colleagues[546] noted that gastrointestinal symptoms occurred in about one-third of all patients from whom they recovered nonpolio enteroviruses. Morens and colleagues[521] noted that in 4 per cent of patients from whom nonpolio enteroviruses were recovered during the 1971 to 1975 period, gastrointestinal disease was the major diagnosis. Horn and coworkers,[326] studying respiratory viral infections, noted that 21.2 per cent of those subjects from whom enteroviruses were recovered had gastrointestinal complaints.

Vomiting

Vomiting is a common manifestation of infections with many coxsackieviral and echoviral types, but it rarely is the

TABLE 170–5. Coxsackieviruses and Echoviruses Noted in Association with Gastrointestinal Complaints

Clinical Categories	Virus Types		
	Coxsackieviruses A	*Coxsackieviruses B*	*Echoviruses and Enteroviruses*
Gastrointestinal, not specified	2, 4, 5, 6, 7, 9, 10, 14, 16	1–5	1–9, 11, 12, 14, 16–25, 30, 71
Nausea and vomiting	9, 16	2–5	2, 4, 6, 9, 11, 16, 18–20, 22, 30
Diarrhea	1, 9, 16	2–5	3, 4, 6, 7, 9, 11–14, 16–22, 25, 30
Constipation	9	3–5	4, 6, 9, 11
Abdominal pain	9, 16	2–5	4, 6, 9, 11, 18, 19, 30
Pseudoappendicitis			1, 8, 14
Peritonitis		1	
Mesenteric adenitis		5	7, 9, 11
Appendicitis		2, 5	
Intussusception		3	7, 9
Hepatitis	4, 9, 10, 20, 24	1–5	1, 3, 4, 6, 7, 9, 11, 14, 20, 21, 30
Reye syndrome	2	4	14, 22
Pancreatitis	9	3–5	
Diabetes mellitus		1–5	

major complaint of the patient or the parent.[7, 22, 115, 125, 127, 131, 159, 160, 178, 213, 214, 273, 289, 294, 295, 300, 384, 387, 388, 395, 403, 410, 447, 472, 477, 561, 584, 589, 607, 612, 625, 631, 632, 638, 666, 703, 727, 731, 742, 749, 750] The frequency of vomiting during outbreaks of illness due to coxsackieviruses and echoviruses depends on the specific types of virus and the major manifestation during a particular outbreak. Table 170–6 presents the frequency of vomiting by viral type. In 14 different enteroviral types, vomiting has been noted as a significant aspect of illness during disease outbreaks. Except for coxsackievirus A16 infections—hand, foot, and mouth syndrome—in which it was an uncommon complaint, vomiting occurs in about 50 per cent of all cases in epidemic enteroviral disease. Vomiting is most common in meningitis and least common in pleurodynia and uncomplicated exanthematous disease.

Diarrhea

Diarrhea is common in coxsackieviral and echoviral infections, but it usually is just one of many manifestations of the systemic illness.[7, 21, 22, 63, 82, 84, 115, 123, 157–160, 178, 213, 214, 269, 272, 281, 294, 295, 300, 387, 388, 395, 400, 410, 429, 440, 447, 472, 477, 480, 484, 539, 574, 577, 584, 588, 592, 600–602, 612, 628, 631, 653, 673, 697, 703, 737, 738, 749, 771, 772] Specific studies of diarrheal disease in infants and children have varied results; some studies indicate an enteroviral etiology, whereas in others coxsackieviruses and echoviruses have been recovered from well children with the same prevalence.

Ramos-Alvarez and Olarte[600] carried out an extensive study of diarrheal disease in Mexico City and noted that echoviruses were recovered eight times more frequently from children with diarrhea than from control, nondiarrheal children. They noted that echoviruses 6 and 19 predominated, but types 3, 7, 9, 12, 14, 18, and 21 also were recovered. Pelon and colleagues[577] noted an association between coxsackieviruses B4 and B5 and acute diarrhea; they observed a 42 per cent coxsackievirus B isolation rate in acute diarrhea and a corresponding rate of only 12 per cent in children without diarrhea. Goodwin and associates[272] noted echoviruses in the stools of children with diarrhea at twice the rate observed in normal children. In the study by Yow and colleagues,[771, 772] they could find no association between enteroviruses and infantile diarrhea. Echoviruses were recovered twice as frequently from children ill with diarrhea as from children without gastrointestinal illness.[771] In Canada, McLean and colleagues[484] could find no association between enteroviral infection and gastroenteritis. In a large study of diarrhea in India, coxsackieviruses A9, B3, and B6 and echoviruses 12 and 21 were recovered more commonly from ill patients than from children without diarrhea.[539]

In several studies of specific diarrhea outbreaks, the afflicted persons have been noted to be infected actively with a particular virus type. Goldwater and Laws[269] observed three children younger than 6 months of age infected with echovirus 19 who had gastroenteritis without other signs or symptoms. Klein and colleagues[410] recovered echovirus 11 from the blood of two laboratory workers with acute gastroenteritis. Diarrhea occurred in three of nine volunteers given echovirus 11.[84] Eichenwald and associates[197] and Cramblett and colleagues[157] noted epidemic diarrhea due to echovirus 18 in neonates. An outbreak of diarrhea associated with coxsackievirus A1 was noted in 7 of 14 bone marrow transplantation patients during a 3-week period.[705]

Table 170–7 presents the frequency of diarrhea in outbreaks of specific coxsackieviral and echoviral illnesses. Diarrhea varied among the viruses represented and among different studies with the same agents. Diarrhea in enteroviral disease rarely is severe. In most instances, loose stools occur for a 2- to 4-day period. The stools rarely are watery, never are bloody, and at most number six to eight per day.

Constipation

Some degree of constipation is rather frequent in many acute infectious illnesses, but its evaluation is made difficult by the subjective nature of the complaint. In coxsackievirus and echovirus diseases, a short period of constipation may be associated with fever, vomiting, and anorexia early in the course of the illness. This frequently is followed by mild diarrhea.[84] As noted in Table 170–5, constipation has been reported specifically as a symptom with four coxsackieviral and four echoviral types. Constipation particularly is common in children with enteroviral meningitis; it occurs in 10 to 40 per cent of cases.[115, 213, 214, 387, 388, 427]

Abdominal Pain

Abdominal pain is a common complaint in many coxsackieviral and echoviral infections. Table 170–8 lists the frequency of occurrence of abdominal pain and the main characteristic of the illness by virus type. About 10 per cent of patients with coxsackievirus A16 hand, foot, and mouth syndrome complain of abdominal pain. Meningitis in association with many coxsackieviruses and echoviruses is associated with abdominal pain in about one-fourth of patients.

TABLE 170–6. Frequency of Vomiting in Outbreaks of Illness Due to Coxsackieviruses and Echoviruses

Virus Type	Age Group (Years)	Vomiting (Per Cent)	Main Characteristics of Outbreak	References
Coxsackievirus A9	Mainly children	60–73	Meningitis	115
	Children	14–20	Rash	115, 450
Coxsackievirus A16	Children and adults	3–15	Hand, foot, and mouth syndrome	7, 612
Coxsackievirus B2	Mainly children	50	Meningitis	115
	Mainly children	18–66	Febrile respiratory	115
Coxsackievirus B3	Adults and children	33	Pleurodynia	115
	Children	9	Febrile respiratory	115
	Mainly children	25	Febrile diarrhea	212
Coxsackievirus B4	Mainly children	27	Nonspecific febrile	213
Coxsackievirus B5	Adults and children	31–37	Pleurodynia	273, 666
	Adults and children	50–95	Meningitis	115, 131, 289, 625
	Mainly children	25–33	Nonspecific febrile	131, 625, 749
	Children	45	Febrile respiratory	638
	Mainly children	100	Hepatosplenic syndrome	666
	Children	40	Rash	127
Echovirus 2	Children	12	Respiratory, rash	115
Echovirus 4	Mainly children	70–90	Meningitis	388, 607
	Mainly children	9–50	Epidemic disease including meningitis, minor illness	115, 561
Echovirus 6	Mainly children	55–98	Meningitis	300, 387, 403, 428, 731
	Mainly children	50–75	Epidemic disease including meningitis	115, 749
Echovirus 9	0–4	64–71	Rash, meningitis	115, 632
	5–9	81–83		
	10–19	61–92		
	>20	20–38		
	Mainly children	39–95	Rash, meningitis	115, 589, 731, 742
	Mainly children	26	Pharyngitis	115
	Mainly children	71	Epidemic disease including meningitis	115
Echovirus 11	Not specified	100	Febrile respiratory	115
Echovirus 16	Children	30	Rash	294
Echovirus 19	<0.5	25	Meningitis, upper respiratory, nonspecific febrile	115
	0.5–2	31		
	3–5	37		
	6–12	68		
	13–18	61		
	19–25	53		
	26+	43		
Echovirus 20	Children	67	Febrile respiratory	159
Echovirus 30	Mainly children	15–91	Meningitis	276, 384, 584, 703
	<5	50	Febrile respiratory	115
	>5	70		

The magnitude of abdominal pain as a clinical complaint in coxsackieviral and echoviral infections varies considerably. For example, in aseptic meningitis, headache and other neurologic complaints overshadow the abdominal symptoms. In other situations, fever and abdominal pain are diagnostically troublesome because of the possibility of a surgical abdomen (discussed further in the next paragraph). The pain most often is periumbilical; it may be either constant or colicky. The fever most often is higher than 38.3° C (101° F).

Peritonitis, Pseudoperitonitis, Appendicitis, Pseudoobstruction, Mesenteric Adenitis, and Intussusception

Occasionally, coxsackieviruses and echoviruses are associated with illnesses that suggest severe abdominal involvement. Liebman and St. Geme[455] described two children with abdominal findings suggestive of acute appendicitis (semirigid, tender abdomen, rebound tenderness, rectal tenderness) who had associated infections with echoviruses 1 and 14. McLean and colleagues[487] described a surgical abdomen in one child with coxsackievirus B1 infection. In this case, the virus was recovered from the peritoneal exudate; this boy at operation was found to have peritonitis, but his appendix was normal. Thomas[698] reported a 5-year-old boy with coxsackievirus B5 infection who at operation was found to have excessive clear peritoneal fluid and markedly enlarged mesenteric lymph nodes. A pregnant woman with acute abdominal pain and rebound tenderness associated with echovirus 8 infection has been described.[575]

Tobe[701] has shown in immunofluorescence studies the presence of coxsackievirus B2 and B5 antigens in the mucous membranes and mesenteric lymph nodes of patients with appendicitis more often than in similar studies in control subjects. He has suggested that the virus infection acts as a trigger for the appendicitis. Bell and Steyn[54] recovered echoviruses 7 and 9 from mesenteric lymph nodes in children with intussusception.

Hepatitis[8, 110, 170, 333, 400, 439, 474, 521, 522, 526, 570, 644, 651, 653, 666, 686]

Marked liver involvement is not rare in disseminated coxsackieviral and echoviral infections of neonates.[117] The associ-

TABLE 170–7. Frequency of Diarrhea in Outbreaks of Illness Due to Coxsackieviruses and Echoviruses

Virus Type	Age Group (Years)	Diarrhea (Per Cent)	Main Characteristics of Outbreak	References
Coxsackievirus A9	Adults and children	7–100	Fever, rash	115, 448
Coxsackievirus A16	Mainly children	4–33	Hand, foot, and mouth syndrome	7, 123, 447, 612
Coxsackievirus B2	Mainly children	9–56	Febrile, respiratory	115
	Mainly children	12	Meningitis	472
Coxsackievirus B3	Mainly children	2–5	Pleurodynia	115
	Children	11	Meningitis	157
	Mainly children	54	Nonspecific febrile	212
Coxsackievirus B4	Children	9	Meningitis	158
	Mainly children	8	Febrile, respiratory	214
Coxsackievirus B5	<1	21	Meningitis and febrile, respiratory	588
	1–9	15		
	10–29	3		
	Mainly children	5–9	Meningitis	115, 157, 749
Echovirus 4	Mainly children	5–75	Meningitis	388, 440, 631
	Mainly children	65	Nonspecific febrile	440
Echovirus 6	Mainly children	6–12	Meningitis	115, 300, 387, 631
Echovirus 9	0–4	14	Meningitis, rash	
	5–9	10		
	10–19	8		
	<20	0		
	Mainly children	3–40	Meningitis	115, 160, 631
	Children	15	Rash, fever	187
	Mainly children	5–15	Respiratory	115
Echovirus 11	Adults	33–100	Gastrointestinal	84, 410
	Mainly infants	40	Nonspecific febrile	63
Echovirus 13	Children	11	Respiratory	115
Echovirus 16	Children	20	Rash	294
Echovirus 17	<1–4	100	Fever, diarrhea	115
Echovirus 18	Infants	100	Diarrhea	197
Echovirus 19	<2	30	Meningitis	115
	2–4	7		
	5–11	7		
	12–17	0		
	>18	9		
	Mainly children	3	Meningitis	269
	Mainly children	10	Respiratory	158, 269
	Mainly children	9	Diarrhea	278
Echovirus 20	Children	100	Respiratory, enteric	159
Echovirus 30	<5	12	Meningitis	115
	>5	5		
	Adults and children	7–10	Meningitis	295, 584, 703

ation of hepatitis and enteroviral infections in older children is defined less clearly but probably is more common than generally realized based on the number of individual cases reported. Caution must be exercised in accepting enteroviruses as the exclusive etiologic agent of hepatitis, however, because hepatitis A virus infection has been ruled out in only a few of the available studies.

Morris and associates[527] described an illness suggestive of a coxsackieviral or echoviral infection in an 18-month-old child who had hyperbilirubinemia and abnormal liver function test results. From this child, coxsackievirus A4 was recovered from the blood during the acute illness, and a neutralizing antibody titer rise to the isolated virus was demonstrated. Chang and Weinstein[110] reported a 3-year-old boy with pharyngitis, urinary abnormalities, and neurologic symptoms who had elevated liver enzyme values (SGOT of 1600 and SGPT of 1180). Coxsackievirus A9 was recovered from this child's cerebrospinal fluid, and the child's antibody response to this agent was significant. Coxsackievirus A20 has been associated with clinical hepatitis, and simultaneous infections with coxsackievirus A24 and hepatitis A virus have been demonstrated.[651]

An adult with a coxsackievirus B1 infection had both myocarditis and liver involvement.[4] A similar illness due to coxsackievirus B3 in a 19-year-old girl has been described.[696] An 11-month-old boy had a Reye-like syndrome associated with coxsackievirus B2.[390] Reye syndrome has been associated with echovirus 3 infection.[305] Siegel and colleagues[666] described a hepatosplenic syndrome in which 15 patients had hepatomegaly and coxsackievirus B5 infection. These patients, the majority of whom were children, had otherwise typical enteroviral illnesses. Liver function studies were performed in only three instances, and their results were normal.

Echoviruses 1, 3, 4, 6, 7, 9, 11, 14, 20, 21, and 30 have been associated with hepatitis.[115, 388, 400, 470, 518, 645] Hepatomegaly is common in enteroviral infections.[115, 123, 212, 429, 450] During the period 1971 through 1975, more than 7000 occurrences of nonpolio enteroviruses were reported to the Viral Diseases Division at the Centers for Disease Control and Prevention.[521] In this group, there were 13 instances of hepatitis and 6 of Reye syndrome; coxsackieviruses A2 and B4 and echoviruses 14 and 22 were associated with the latter illness.

Pancreatitis

One of the effects of coxsackievirus B in suckling mice is extensive infection in the pancreas. As with other similarities

TABLE 170–8. Frequency of Abdominal Pain in Outbreaks of Illness Due to Coxsackieviruses and Echoviruses

Virus Type	Age Group (Years)	Abdominal Pain (Per Cent)	Main Characteristics of Outbreak	References
Coxsackievirus A9	Mainly children	7	Meningitis	115
	Children	20	Rash	125
Coxsackievirus A16	Mainly children	12	Hand, foot, and mouth syndrome	450, 612
Coxsackievirus B2	Mainly children	22	Meningitis	472
Coxsackievirus B3	Children and adults	25–90	Pleurodynia	115
Coxsackievirus B4	Children and adults	10	Meningitis	115
	Mainly children	36	Febrile, respiratory	214
Coxsackievirus B5	Mainly children	10	Meningitis	115
	Children	13	Febrile, respiratory	638
	Children and adults	23–67	Pleurodynia	273, 628, 666
Echovirus 4	Mainly children	28–50	Meningitis	115, 388
	Mainly children	13	Febrile, respiratory	561
Echovirus 6	Mainly children	17–43	Meningitis	115, 300, 387, 403
Echovirus 9	0–4	28	Meningitis, rash	115, 131, 447, 632
	5–9	30		
	10–19	25		
	≥20	0		
Echovirus 11	Adults	38	Gastrointestinal	84
Echovirus 16	Children	20	Rash	294
Echovirus 19	<0.5	3	Meningitis	115
	0.5–2	3		
	3–5	27		
	6–12	38		
	13–18	13		
	19–25	9		
	26+	3		
Echovirus 30	Mainly children	17	Meningitis	384, 703

of infection between suckling mice and human neonates, generalized coxsackievirus B infections in neonates also are accompanied frequently by extensive pancreatic damage. Pancreatic involvement in older children and adults is not common.[91, 535, 541, 713] Coxsackieviruses B3, B4, B5, and A9 have been noted.

Diabetes Mellitus

A possible relationship between juvenile diabetes mellitus and the seasonal occurrence of coxsackievirus B4 was suggested in 1969 by Gamble and Taylor.[242] In a second study, Gamble and associates[241] noted higher titers of coxsackievirus B4 antibodies in insulin-dependent diabetic patients within 3 months of onset of disease than in normal subjects or long-term diabetics.

Since the 1960s, many studies in animal models and in children have looked at the relationship between juvenile-onset, type 1 diabetes mellitus (IDDM) and coxsackieviruses B.[34, 35, 107, 146, 163, 182, 311, 320, 407, 508, 649, 715, 748] Between 1973 and 1984, 10 case-control studies examined the prevalence of antibody to various coxsackieviruses B in IDDM patients and in controls. In eight of these studies, the prevalence was greater in the IDDM patients. In three of these studies, IgM antibody to the coxsackieviruses B was examined, and in each the prevalence was greater in the IDDM patients than in the controls. In a Finnish study, it was noted that IDDM patients were more likely to have IgA antibodies to coxsackievirus B4 than were controls.[344]

Recently, Helfand and associates[311] performed a well-done case-control study of IDDM. They found that new-onset cases 13 to 18 years of age were more likely than controls to be IgM-antibody–positive for 9 of the 14 enterovirus serotypes. The serotypes were coxsackieviruses B2, B3, B4, B5, and B6, coxsackievirus A9, and echoviruses 9, 30, and 34.

Cudworth and colleagues[163] noted a correlation between HLA type BW15 and coxsackieviruses B1, B2, B3, and B4 antibodies in insulin-dependent diabetic patients.

In 1979, Yoon and colleagues[769] reported the recovery of coxsackievirus B4 from the pancreas of a previously healthy 10-year-old boy who died after being in a diabetic coma.

Clements and coworkers[146] noted that 9 of 14 serum samples from children with new-onset diabetes were positive for enterovirus RNA tested by polymerase chain reaction. In contrast, only 4 per cent of serum samples from control children had evidence of enterovirus RNA.

Eye Findings

Acute Hemorrhagic Conjunctivitis[65, 97, 115, 263, 277, 281, 319, 417, 641]

Although conjunctivitis has been a frequent occurrence in nonpolio enteroviral illnesses for 42 years, its occurrence as a dominant complaint has been observed only during the last 27 years. In June 1969, Chatterjee and associates[112] noted an epidemic of acute hemorrhagic conjunctivitis in Accra, Ghana. This disease was nicknamed Apollo 11 disease because it coincided with the time of the Apollo 11 moon landing. Since 1969, many epidemics of acute hemorrhagic conjunctivitis have been described. In the majority of epidemics, enterovirus 70 has been the etiologic agent. Similar epidemics have been due to a variant of coxsackievirus A24.[141] In recent years, this virus has been the cause of more epidemics than has enterovirus 70.[97, 263, 607] Most epidemics have occurred in tropical and semitropical countries, but outbreaks have been observed in Minnesota, Moscow, London, and other European cities.[426, 767] In the continental United States, epidemic disease has occurred in Florida and North Carolina.[99] During epidemics, all age groups are affected, but the highest attack rate is in school age children.[728]

Acute hemorrhagic conjunctivitis has a sudden onset, with

severe eye pain and associated photophobia, blurred vision, lacrimation, erythema, and congestion of the eye, as well as edematous and chemotic lids.[319] There are subconjunctival hemorrhages of varying size and frequently a transient punctate epithelial keratitis, conjunctival follicles, and preauricular lymphadenopathy. Eye discharge initially is serous but becomes mucopurulent with secondary bacterial infection. Systemic symptoms, including fever, are rare. Within 2 to 3 days after the onset of illness, patients note some improvement, and recovery usually is complete in 7 to 12 days. In a study in American Samoa, it was found that illness due to coxsackievirus A24 was somewhat different from that caused by enterovirus 70.[641] In cases due to coxsackievirus A24, conjunctival hemorrhage was less severe and upper respiratory and systemic symptoms more common. In a recent study in American Samoa of disease due to enterovirus 70, it was found that children 2 to 10 years of age had the highest attack rate and that antibody from previous infection gave only partial protection against symptomatic reinfection.[65]

Occasionally, findings suggestive of pharyngoconjunctival fever have been noted. A small percentage of patients have had a poliomyelitis-like illness or polyradiculomyeloneuropathy after enterovirus 70 acute hemorrhagic conjunctivitis.[277, 722]

Epidemics are explosive, with spread mainly by the eye-hand-fomite-eye route.

Conjunctivitis Associated with Other Enteroviral Illness

Conjunctivitis is a common minor manifestation of enteroviral illness with several specific agents. Table 170–9 presents the frequency of occurrence of conjunctivitis in selected outbreaks of disease due to coxsackieviruses and echoviruses. Conjunctivitis was most prevalent in coxsackievirus B3 and B5 and echovirus 9 and 30 infections. In addition to the outbreaks reported in Table 157–9, conjunctivitis has been noted in isolated illnesses associated with echoviruses 1, 6, and 20.[400]

Photophobia

As might be expected, photophobia is common in aseptic meningitis due to coxsackieviruses and echoviruses. During epidemic meningitis, it has been noted with the following viruses: coxsackievirus A9 and echoviruses 3, 4, 6, 7, 9, 19, and 30.[53, 115, 273, 278, 383, 384, 387, 388, 403, 447, 470, 584, 703] It is most common with echovirus 9 and 30 infections, but the incidence of this complaint varies greatly among different reports. In one echovirus 30 outbreak, 80 per cent of patients studied had photophobia.[703] On the average, 20 per cent of patients with meningitis have remarkable photophobia. Photophobia also is associated with pleurodynia due to coxsackievirus B infections.[628, 727]

Other Eye Findings

Nodular lesions on the palpebral conjunctiva were observed in some patients with coxsackievirus A10 infection and lymphonodular pharyngitis.[674] A corneal ulcer was observed in one patient with hand, foot, and mouth syndrome,[466] and optic neuritis has been described in a boy with pleurodynia; in this latter case, the enteroviral etiology was not confirmed in the laboratory.[708] Periorbital edema was observed in one patient with echovirus 9 meningitis. An adult woman with panuveitis associated with coxsackievirus B3 infection has been described.[225] Sore eyes and other unspecified eye complaints also have been noted frequently with coxsackievirus and echoviral infections.[115, 210, 223, 289, 440, 464, 549, 640, 644]

Cardiovascular Manifestations

Pericarditis and Myocarditis

Pericarditis, myocarditis, or both have been noted in association with 27 different nonpolio enteroviruses. The relative importance of the different serotypes is presented in Table 170–10. The coxsackieviruses B have been implicated most frequently in heart disease. Coxsackievirus B5 has been the most common causative agent, but types 2, 3, and 4 also have been implicated frequently. Of the echoviruses, type 6 has been associated most frequently with cardiac involvement, but there are few descriptions of the clinical findings with this agent.

With coxsackievirus B cardiac disease, hepatitis, pneumonia, nephritis, meningitis, and orchitis have been occasional associated findings. Occasionally, arrhythmias are the only clinical manifestations of myocarditis.[127, 707] The mortality rate of acute coxsackieviral and echoviral heart disease is unknown, but it is significant. Unfortunately, in recent years, proper virologic study is rare in nonfatal disease.

In the only published follow-up study, it was found that patients who survived acute coxsackievirus myocarditis usually recovered completely without residual disability.[684] However, Bowles and associates[77] found the presence of coxsackievirus B nucleic acid sequences in myocardial biopsy

TABLE 170–9. Frequency of Conjunctivitis in Outbreaks of Illness Due to Coxsackieviruses and Echoviruses

Virus Type	Age Group	Conjunctivitis (Per Cent)	Main Characteristics of Illness	References
Coxsackievirus A9	Children	20	Pharyngitis, rash	450
Coxsackievirus A16	Mainly children	0–18	Hand, foot, and mouth syndrome	112, 466, 612
Coxsackievirus B2	Mainly children	2	Nonspecific febrile, respiratory	115
Coxsackievirus B3	Children	2–42	Upper respiratory	115
Coxsackievirus B4	Children	25	Upper respiratory	115
Coxsackievirus B5	Mainly children	7–50	Rash, meningitis, hepatosplenic, respiratory, pleurodynia	126, 157, 628, 638
Echovirus 2	Children	25	Rhinorrhea	115
Echovirus 4	Children	Rare	Meningitis	470
Echovirus 9	Mainly children	13–30	Rash, meningitis	100, 115, 632
Echovirus 11	Children	15	Rash	126
Echovirus 16	Children	6–10	Rash	294, 550
Echovirus 30	Mainly children	10–60	Meninigitis, nonspecific febrile	115, 295, 703

TABLE 170–10. Nonpolio Enteroviruses Associated with Pericarditis and Myocarditis

Virus Type		Age Group or Age of Individual Patients	Etiologic Importance*	Heart Involvement			Other Aspects of Illness	References
				Pericarditis	*Myocarditis*	*Unspecified*		
Coxsackievirus	A1	Infants and adults	±	+	+			115, 285
	A2	Adults	±			+		25, 115
	A4	Mainly children	+	+	+		Sudden infant death	25, 267, 284, 729
	A5	—	±	+				717
	A7	Adults	±	+	+		Hand, foot, and mouth syndrome	32
	A8	—	±			+		285
	A9	Mainly infants	+		+		High fatality rate	284
	A10	—	±			+		25
	A16	Infants	±		+		High fatality rate	115, 761
Coxsackievirus	B1	Infants, children, and adults	++	+	+		Rare hepatitis	8, 21, 25, 87, 115, 178, 281, 400, 486, 546, 614, 648, 737
	B2	Infants, children, and adults	+++	+	+		Occasional pneumonia	21, 25, 86, 87, 115, 178, 216, 281, 333, 400, 418, 486, 546, 614, 648, 653, 729, 737
	B3	Infants, children, and adults	+++	+	+		Rare hepatitis	25, 29, 52, 86, 87, 115, 178, 281, 333, 400, 418, 453, 546, 614, 653, 686, 726, 729, 737
	B4	Infants, children, and adults	+++	+	+		Occasional pneumonia; myocardial calcifications; rare hepatitis, orchitis, nephritis, hemolytic uremic syndrome	21, 25, 29, 39, 80, 85–87, 115, 178, 216, 281, 333, 400, 418, 546, 605, 614, 688, 707, 729, 737
	B5	Infants, children, and adults	++++	+	+		Occasional pneumonia, pleurodynia, and meningitis; rare orchitis	21, 24, 31, 74, 87, 115, 256, 273, 309, 313, 418, 461, 486, 546, 565, 585, 588, 593, 648, 653, 729, 733, 737, 749
Echovirus	1	Adolescents	±	+	+			25, 644, 737
	4	—	±			+		25, 494
	6	Children and adults	++	+				25, 49, 115, 737
	7	Children and adults	±			+		25, 115, 518
	8	Adolescents	±	+				115, 382
	9	Children and adults	+	+	+			25, 115, 453, 494, 516, 729
	11	Children and adults	+			+		25, 49, 115, 614
	14	—	±			+		518, 717
	17	—	±			+		25
	19	Children and adults	±	+	+			49, 115
	22	Children	±		+			471, 627
	25	Children	±		+			49, 50
	30	—	±			+		25, 453

* ++++ = most common; ± = rare.

samples from several patients with cardiomyopathy. Muir and colleagues[532] found enterovirus-specific IgM antibodies in the sera of nine patients with chronic relapsing pericarditis. Fujioka and colleagues[236] reported positive enteroviral polymerase chain reaction results from endomyocardial biopsies in 6 of 31 patients (19 per cent) with dilated cardiomyopathy. Andreoletti and coworkers[15] noted enterovirus RNA in 18 of 25 samples from heart tissue in patients with dilated cardiomyopathy or ischemic cardiomyopathy. However, in two other well-controlled studies, enteroviral RNA could not be identified in endomyocardial biopsies or in heart tissues from patients undergoing heart transplantation.[149, 456] In 1994, Muir and Archard[530] and Melchers and associates[495] reviewed the evidence for persistent enteroviral infections in chronic medical conditions, including idiopathic dilated cardiomyopathy. Muir and Archard concluded that persistent enterovirus infections are associated causally with chronic medical conditions, whereas Melchers and colleagues concluded that there was no clear evidence for enteroviral persistence and the subsequent development of chronic medical conditions. Constrictive pericarditis occurs occasionally,[478] as do other sequelae.[55, 115, 441, 451]

Other Cardiac Manifestations

Several investigators have studied the possible association of coxsackievirus B infections and myocardial infarctions.[279, 282, 436–438, 515, 554, 559, 587, 756, 758] In many instances, patients with infarctions have been demonstrated to have concomitant coxsackievirus B infections.[279, 282, 437, 438, 515, 554, 559, 567, 756, 758] In controlled studies, the results have varied. Nikoskelainen and associates[559] noted that 9 of 59 patients with acute myocardial infarctions had coxsackievirus B infections, whereas in the control group of 38 patients without infarctions, only 1 patient had evidence of infection. Similarly, Nicholls and Thomas[554] found that 26 per cent of patients had infections, but no infections were found in the control subjects. In contrast, five other studies failed to show an increased rate of infection in patients with myocardial infarction when compared with controls.[279, 282, 567, 587, 756] However, two of these studies were carried out during a nonenteroviral season,[587, 756] and in a third study there apparently was little coxsackievirus B activity in the community during the study period.[279] In analyzing the available studies, it would appear that coxsackievirus B infections have a role in myocardial infarction. In one instance with coxsackievirus B5 infection, there was inferolateral wall myocardial necrosis, but coronary arteriography did not demonstrate obstruction.[179]

Chandy and associates[109] have presented data in which antibody to group B coxsackieviruses was related to rheumatic-like valvular heart disease, and Burch and associates[87] demonstrated coxsackievirus B antigens in rheumatic lesions of the heart. Limson and colleagues[457] could find no association between group B coxsackieviruses and rheumatic fever. Soboleva and associates[670] noted an association between coxsackievirus A13 and rheumatic fever; they reported seven children with concomitant streptococcal and coxsackievirus A13 infections.

Genitourinary Manifestations

Orchitis and Epididymitis

Group B coxsackieviruses are second only to mumps as causative agents of orchitis.[21, 115, 155, 232, 281, 400, 521, 653, 688, 737] Coxsackievirus B5 is the virus most commonly associated with this disease, although coxsackieviruses B2 and B4 also have been implicated on many occasions. In almost all instances, the orchitis is a secondary event in enteroviral infections. The most common association here is with pleurodynia. The illness frequently is biphasic with fever and pleurodynia, and then apparent recovery is followed by orchitis about 2 weeks after the onset. Many patients also have epididymitis. In epidemics of disease due to group B coxsackieviruses, the occurrence of testicular involvement varies considerably. Generally, orchitis is infrequent, but in one coxsackievirus B2 outbreak, 17 per cent of postpubertal males had orchitis, and 7 per cent also had epididymitis.[115] Orchitis also frequently is associated with pericarditis and myocarditis. In one instance, coxsackievirus B5 was recovered from a testicular biopsy.[155]

In virtually all instances, testicular involvement has occurred in postpubertal patients, with most cases appearing in young adults. In addition to coxsackieviruses B2, B4, and B5, other enteroviruses have been implicated: coxsackieviruses B1 and B3[115, 400, 454] and echoviruses 6, 9, and 11.[400, 735] Meningitis and exanthem have been associated with orchitis.

Nephritis

There have been scattered reports of nephritis associated with nonpolio enteroviral infections. Bayatpour and colleagues[44] noted acute glomerulonephritis in a 9-year-old boy with an extensive infection with coxsackievirus B4. This child had a concomitant rise in antistreptolysin O titer. Yuceoglu and colleagues[773] reported twins with echovirus 9 infections and acute glomerulonephritis; Burch and Colcolough[85] observed a patient with progressive, fatal pancarditis and nephritis in whom coxsackievirus B4 antigen was found in the kidneys. Mesangiolytic glomerulonephritis associated with an echovirus 6 infection has been described in an infant with immune deficiency.[336]

Other Genitourinary Findings

Hemolytic uremic syndrome has been associated with virologic or serologic evidence of infection with coxsackieviruses A4, A9, B2, B3, B4, and B5 and echovirus 22.[132, 258, 568, 605, 606] Other abnormal renal or urinary findings in nonpolio enteroviral infections include acute oliguric renal failure with coxsackievirus B5[20]; pyuria, hematuria, or proteinuria with echoviruses 1, 6, and 9 and coxsackievirus B5[115, 387, 447, 632, 644]; and hemorrhagic cystitis.[613]

A 7-year-old girl with coxsackievirus A10 infection had vaginal ulcerative lesions,[509] and Wassermann test results have been falsely positive with echovirus 9 and coxsackievirus B5 infections.[596]

Hematologic Findings

Acute Infectious Lymphocytosis[287, 332]

In 1968, Horwitz and Moore[332] described an outbreak of infectious lymphocytosis during which 27 mentally retarded children were studied. The mean white blood cell count of the study group patients was 57,200; lymphocytes accounted for at least 50 per cent of the total in all cases. About half the patients had low-grade fever, and 15 of 27 had moderate diarrhea. A nontypable enterovirus suggestive of coxsackievirus group A was recovered from ill patients, and 31 per cent of the patients in whom serologic study was performed developed neutralizing antibody to a strain (EVU-16) of the isolated virus.

Muscle and Joint Manifestations

Arthritis

During the period 1971 to 1975, during which enteroviruses were recovered from 7075 persons in the United States, there were nine instances of rheumatic disease[521]; although not clearly specified, apparently three patients had arthritis. Blotzer and Myers[69] noted an adult with an echovirus 9 infection and the concomitant onset of an arthritis that persisted for 3 months. Echovirus 9 has been recovered from the synovial fluid of a man with acute monocytic arthritis,[423] and one adult and one adolescent had serologic evidence of coxsackievirus B4 infections in association with the onset of rheumatoid arthritis–like illnesses.[343]

Myositis

Because group A coxsackieviruses routinely cause myositis in suckling mice, it is reasonable to suspect a similar clinical manifestation in people. Myalgia is a common complaint in illnesses due to many coxsackieviruses and echoviruses as well.[21, 115, 232, 295, 428, 486] However, at present almost no direct evidence (demonstration of virus in muscle) or indirect evidence (muscle enzyme elevations) of muscle involvement in routine enteroviral illnesses exists. Of the nine patients with rheumatic disease noted by Morens and colleagues,[521] six apparently had myositis; in one instance, coxsackievirus A2 was implicated, and in another patient with polymyositis, coxsackievirus A9 was the related agent. Three patients with echovirus 18 infection and polymyositis have been reported.[397] Acute rhabdomyolysis in one adult and myositis, myoglobinemia, and myoglobinuria in another adult have been associated with echovirus 9 infections.[365, 379] Christensen and associates[139] noted that children with dermatomyositis were more likely to have serum antibody to one or more coxsackieviruses B than were control children. Chou and Gutmann[137] noted enterovirus-like particles in the muscles of two patients with fatal dermatomyositis; Tang and colleagues[696] demonstrated coxsackievirus A9 in the muscles of an 11-year-old girl with chronic myopathy. Using both polymerase chain reaction and dot-blot hybridization assays, Fox and colleagues[229] could not find evidence of persistent enteroviral infections in 32 adults with inflammatory muscle disease (1 patient with dermatomyositis and 31 patients with polymyositis).

Skin Manifestations

Nonpolio enteroviruses as a group are a common cause of a variety of skin manifestations.[118, 736, 739] In the summer and fall, they are the leading cause of exanthems. Variation in the clinical expression rate of exanthem is marked among the various viral types and in the age of the host. In general, the expression is related inversely to the age of the infected patient. The frequency of exanthem and common associated illness by viral type are presented in Table 170–11.

Coxsackievirus A2

Rash associated with coxsackievirus A2 has been rare. Febrile illness with exanthem associated with coxsackievirus A2 was observed in Cincinnati in 1957; no details of this outbreak have been presented.[631] Assaad and Cockburn[25] reviewed about 15,000 enteroviral illnesses for the period 1967 to 1970 that were reported to WHO and noted that in 45 instances, skin or mucous membrane lesions associated with coxsackievirus A2 infection were the main clinical manifestations.

Coxsackievirus A3

One case has been reported, but no details are available.[518]

Coxsackievirus A4 (see Fig. 66–15)

Exanthem with coxsackievirus A4 has been noted infrequently.[25, 122, 224, 527, 775] However, many cases may be missed because this virus grows poorly in tissue cultures, and suckling mouse inoculation rarely is employed in present-day diagnostic laboratories. Six children were observed in one outbreak.[224] All patients initially had herpangina, and then with or after defervescence the exanthem appeared. It initially was erythematous, maculopapular, and discrete. In some children the rash resolved within 4 days, but in others it progressed and became vesicular. The vesicular lesions occurred in crops, spread to the extremities but not the palms and soles, and were yellowish, opaque, and 5 to 10 mm in size. They persisted for 1 to 2 weeks and regressed with a brownish discoloration. The lesions easily were confused with resolving bug bites.

Other manifestations of coxsackievirus A4 include an exanthem suggesting combined scarlet fever and rubella,[249] a maculopapular rash that cleared with desquamation,[527] and an anaphylactoid, purpura-like rash (see Fig. 66–15).[122]

Coxsackievirus A5

During the 4-year period studied by Assaad and Cockburn,[25] coxsackievirus A5 was second only to coxsackievirus A16 in the number of instances in which exanthem or mucous membrane involvement was the main clinical manifestation. Even with this apparent frequency, most instances of exanthem have been sporadic rather than part of an outbreak of exanthematous disease. The most common presentation is the hand, foot, and mouth syndrome, which is not clinically discernible from that due to coxsackievirus A16.[162, 220, 224] In one patient, the virus was recovered from vesicular fluid.[220]

Coxsackievirus A7

Coxsackievirus A7 was recovered from one child with a morbilliform rash and aseptic meningitis.[286] An adult with a fatal coxsackievirus 7 infection had pancarditis, pneumonia, and hand, foot, and mouth syndrome.[32]

Coxsackievirus A9 (see Figs. 66–12 and 66–14)

Coxsackievirus A9 is a common cause of exanthem.[25, 115, 122, 125, 331, 340, 374, 377, 405, 450, 521, 564, 747] In contrast with coxsackievirus A16 and echovirus 9, with which clinical expression rates of exanthem are high, the rate of skin manifestations in coxsackievirus A9 infection is low. A review of 259 coxsackievirus A9 infections in 1970 revealed an exanthem rate of 4 per cent.[115] Most cases of coxsackievirus A9 exanthem occur sporadically, although a few outbreaks have been described.[125, 448, 564]

Skin manifestations in coxsackievirus A9 infections have been interesting and varied. The most common rash illness is characterized by fever and an erythematous, maculopapular rash that starts on the face and neck and spreads to the trunk and extremities. Aseptic meningitis is a common associated finding.

In 1960, Lerner and colleagues[450] reported on 11 children with exanthem associated with coxsackievirus A9 infection.

TABLE 170–11. Frequency of Exanthem in Outbreaks of Illness Due to Coxsackievirus and Echoviruses

Virus Type		Age Group	Occurrence of Rash	Characteristics of Rash	Associated Manifestations	References
Coxsackievirus	A2	Children	Rare	Maculopapular	Fever	25, 631
	A4	Children	Rare	Maculopapular, vesicular	Fever, herpangina, hepatitis	25, 122, 224, 527, 775
	A5	Mainly children	Occasional	Hand, foot, and mouth syndrome	Fever	25, 162, 220, 224
	A7	Children and adults	Rare	Morbilliform, hand, foot, and mouth syndrome	Meningitis, pneumonia, pancarditis	32, 286
	A9	Mainly children	4%	Maculopapular, vesicular, urticarial, petechial, hand, foot, and mouth syndrome	Fever, meningitis, pneumonia	25, 115, 122, 125, 331, 340, 374, 377, 405, 450, 521, 564, 746
	A10	Mainly children	Occasional	Hand, foot, and mouth syndrome	Fever	25, 88, 115, 145, 188, 452
	A16	Children and adults	88%, <5 yr 38%, 5–12 yr 11%, adults	Hand, foot, and mouth syndrome	Fever	7, 13, 17, 21, 25, 82, 115, 122, 123, 205, 224, 234, 249, 265, 266, 321–323, 452, 465, 466, 491, 523, 538, 611, 612, 700
	B1	Children	Occasional	Maculopapular, vesicular	Fever, meningitis	25, 115, 122, 124, 176, 463
	B2	Children	Rare	Maculopapular, vesicular, petechial	Fever, herpangina, meningitis	21, 25, 224
	B3	Mainly children	Occasional	Maculopapular, vesicular, petechial	Fever, hepatosplenomegaly	21, 25, 90, 115, 153, 212, 301, 338, 448
	B4	Mainly children	Occasional	Maculopapular, vesicular, urticarial	Fever, respiratory	25, 115, 214, 388, 402
	B5	Mainly children	10%	Maculopapular, petechial, urticarial	Fever, meningitis	25, 74, 115, 127, 153, 178, 289, 308, 546, 562, 585, 588, 638, 666, 679, 683, 689, 749, 763
	B6	Children and adults	20%	Morbilliform	Pneumonia	268
Echovirus	1	Children	Rare	Maculopapular	Conjunctivitis	479
	2	Children	Rare	Macular, maculopapular	Fever, pharyngitis	115, 632, 676
	3	Children	Rare	Petechial	Fever, meningitis	25, 305, 330
	4	Mainly children	10–20%	Macular, maculopapular, petechial	Fever, meningitis	115, 124, 223, 239, 388, 440, 470, 561, 607, 673
	5	Infants and adults	Occasional	Macular	Fever	254, 657
	6	Mainly children	Rare	Maculopapular, macular, papulopustular, vesicular	Fever, meningitis	25, 387, 476, 485, 490, 719, 720, 749
	7	Children	Occasional	Maculopapular	Fever, meningitis	25, 363, 479
	9	Children and adults	57%, <5 yr 41%, 5–9 yr 6%, >10 yr	Maculopapular, petechial, vesicular	Fever, meningitis	25, 59, 115, 144, 151, 160, 174, 210, 221, 240, 243, 306, 331, 361, 374, 381, 400, 402, 412, 427, 446, 464, 488, 521, 546, 558, 589, 594, 603, 624, 632, 671, 680, 693, 742
	11	Mainly children	Occasional	Maculopapular, vesicular, urticarial	Fever, meningitis	25, 84, 115, 126, 180, 653
	13	Children	Rare	Maculopapular		325
	14	Mainly children	Rare	Maculopapular, scarlatiniform	Fever, meningitis	25, 632
	16	Children	Occasional	Roseola-like	Fever, herpangina	118, 154, 294, 548–551
	17	Children	Occasional	Macular, maculopapular, papulovesicular	Fever, diarrhea, herpangina, meningitis	25, 82, 120, 124
	18	Children and adults	Occasional, 1 epidemic	Rubelliform	Fever, meningitis	397, 493, 521, 546
	19	Children and adults	Occasional	Maculopapular	Fever, meningitis, upper respiratory	150, 158, 269
	22	Infants	Rare	Morbilliform	Respiratory	62
	25	Children	Occasional	Maculopapular, hemangioma-like	Fever, pharyngitis	50, 119, 526, 544
	30	Children and adults	Occasional	Macular, maculopapular	Fever, meningitis	25, 115, 384, 703, 764
	32	Children	Rare	Hemangioma-like	Fever	119
	33	—	Rare	—	Meningitis	386, 392
Enterovirus	71	Children	Occasional	Macular, maculopapular, vesicular, hand, foot, and mouth syndrome	Fever, meningitis, encephalitis, paralytic disease	10, 255, 353, 396, 497, 510

Six had vesicular lesions, and two patients had associated viral pneumonia. Since 1960, vesicular exanthem has been noted on several occasions.[115, 125, 340] Most commonly, illnesses have been described as hand, foot, and mouth syndrome, but when the reports were analyzed, the rashes were vesicular but not always in a peripheral pattern.

Papular urticaria and large urticarial lesions have been an occasional manifestation of coxsackievirus A9 infection (see Fig. 66–12).[122, 125] Other manifestations include Stevens-Johnson syndrome and a severe illness simulating meningococcemia (see Fig. 66–14).[122, 521]

Coxsackievirus A10

The most common exanthematous illness associated with coxsackievirus A10 infection is the hand, foot, and mouth syndrome.[88, 115, 145, 188, 354, 452] Stevens-Johnson syndrome has been associated with coxsackievirus A10 infection in one instance,[115] and a child with ulcerative genital lesions also has been reported.[509]

Coxsackievirus A16 (see Figs. 66–9, 66–10, 66–11, and 66–16)

In the WHO review of enteroviral infections for the 4-year period from 1967 through 1970, coxsackievirus A16 was associated with almost half of all skin or mucous membrane diseases. Coxsackievirus A16 is the major cause of the hand, foot, and mouth syndrome (see Figs. 81–9, 81–10, and 81–11). It is of historical interest that the hand, foot, and mouth syndrome apparently was a new clinical entity in 1956.[563] It was noted in sporadic outbreaks until about 1963 and since that time has been a regularly recurring disease throughout the world.[7, 13, 17, 21, 82, 115, 122, 138, 205, 224, 234, 249, 264–266, 321–323, 452, 465, 466, 491, 523, 545, 611, 612, 700] Serologic data suggest that coxsackievirus A16 was not in wide circulation until about 1963.[123]

The symptoms and signs of coxsackievirus A16 hand, foot, and mouth syndrome are recorded in Table 170–12. All illnesses have a typically enteroviral pattern with a short incubation period (4 to 6 days) and a summer and fall seasonal pattern. The clinical expression rate of the enanthem-exanthem complex is high: close to 100 per cent in young children, 38 per cent in school children, and 11 per cent in adults.[523] Exanthem is more common in children, but rash with coxsackievirus A16 in adults is more frequent than with any of the other enteroviral agents.

TABLE 170–12. Symptoms and Signs of Coxsackievirus A16 Illness (Hand, Foot, and Mouth Syndrome)*

Symptoms and Signs	Per Cent of Cases	
Enanthem		90
Buccal	61	
Tongue	44	
Palate, uvula, anterior pillars	36	
Gums	15	
Exanthem		64
Hands	52	
Feet	31	
Buttocks	31	
Legs	13	
Arms	10	
Face	5	
Sore mouth or throat		67
Malaise		61
Anorexia		52
Fever		42
Submandibular and/or cervical adenitis		22
Coryza		11
Cough		11
Diarrhea		10
Nausea and vomiting		3

From Cherry, J. D.: Newer viral exanthems. Adv. Pediatr. *16*:233–286, 1969. Used with permission.
*Data from references 13, 123, 224, 234, 466, 491, 611, 612.

Illness is ushered in with a mild prodromal fever, anorexia, malaise, and frequently a sore mouth. Enanthem occurs 1 to 2 days after the onset of fever, and the exanthem appears shortly thereafter. Of the cutaneous lesions, oral lesions are present more consistently than are those of the skin. Because of this, illness, particularly in adults, mistakenly is identified as aphthous stomatitis (canker sores) or herpes simplex virus infection. The intraoral lesions are ulcerative and average about 4 to 8 mm in size. The tongue and buccal mucosa are involved most frequently.

As noted in Table 157–12, the hands more commonly are involved than are the feet. Buttock lesions also are common, but these usually do not progress to vesiculation. The lesions on the hands and feet usually are vesicular and vary in size from 3 to 7 mm; they generally are more common on the dorsal surfaces but frequently do occur on the palms and soles as well. The vesicles contain virus, but cytologic examination usually does not reveal diagnostic findings. They clear by absorption of the fluid in about 1 week.

Of considerable interest is the frequent association of coxsackievirus A16 with subacute, chronic, and recurring skin lesions.[205, 545] Evans and Waddington[205] noted an 84-year-old woman with chronic recurring skin lesions of more than 2 years' duration. Nankervis and associates[545] noted both subacute and recurring lesions in children. Higgins and Crow[321] described a 31-year-old woman with Darier disease who had a Kaposi varicelliform eruption caused by coxsackievirus A16, and a similar illness was noted in a 1-year-old boy with eczema.[538]

One child with a Gianotti-Crosti–like eruption (papular acrodermatitis of childhood) associated with coxsackievirus A16 infection has been described.[360]

Coxsackievirus B1

Exanthem occasionally occurs in coxsackievirus B1 infections.[25, 115, 122, 124, 176, 463] The most common cutaneous finding is an erythematous maculopapular eruption that is discrete. Two children with illnesses suggestive of hand, foot, and mouth syndrome have been observed.[122]

Coxsackievirus B2

Coxsackievirus B2–associated exanthem is rare. Maculopapular, vesicular, and petechial lesions have been noted.[21, 25, 224]

Coxsackievirus B3

Exanthem occasionally is noted as a sporadic event in coxsackievirus B3 infections, and in one instance a small outbreak occurred.[21, 25, 90, 153, 213, 301, 338, 448, 774] Erythematous maculopapular eruptions are most common, but petechial rash illnesses suggestive of meningococcemia also have been observed. The hand, foot, and mouth syndrome has been observed in one child,[448] and another had a more generalized vesicular eruption. An adult with recurrent hand, foot, and mouth syndrome had a neutralizing antibody titer rise to coxsackievirus B3.[153]

Coxsackievirus B4

Although cutaneous manifestations with coxsackievirus B4 were noted as frequently as those associated with coxsackieviruses B1, B2, and B3,[25, 115] there have been few clinical descriptions.[38, 214, 402] Morbilliform, petechial, and urticarial rashes have been described.

Coxsackievirus B5

Of the group B coxsackieviruses, type B5 is noted most frequently to have skin manifestations.[25, 74, 115, 127, 153, 178, 289, 308, 556, 562, 585, 588, 638, 666, 679, 683, 689, 749] The rash usually is maculopapular; petechial lesions are noted occasionally, and one child with urticaria has been reported.[127] Several children studied by Cherry and colleagues[127] had a roseola-like illness pattern. During outbreaks of coxsackievirus B5 illness, about 10 per cent of young children have exanthem. Many patients have concomitant aseptic meningitis. One adult patient with recurrent hand, foot, and mouth syndrome had serologic evidence of coxsackievirus B5 infection.

Coxsackievirus B6

Goldwater[268] identified 97 children and adults with coxsackievirus B6 infections. The most prominent finding in these cases was cough and pneumonia. Twenty patients had exanthem; the rash was morbilliform and associated with high fever and cough.

Echovirus 1

Exanthem and conjunctivitis have been associated with echovirus 1 infection in several children.[479]

Echovirus 2

Exanthem occasionally occurs with echovirus 2 infection.[632, 676] The rash has been erythematous macular in some instances but usually is maculopapular and discrete. Most children have had associated fever and pharyngitis.

Echovirus 3

Exanthem was noted in 2 of 29 children with echovirus 3 infection.[305] In both instances, the rashes were petechial; most patients in this outbreak had aseptic meningitis. Details of other echovirus 3 infections and exanthems are lacking.[25, 330]

Echovirus 4

Echovirus 4 is a common cause of epidemic aseptic meningitis, and exanthem is an associated finding in 10 to 20 per cent of the pediatric cases.[124, 222, 239, 388, 440, 470, 561, 607, 673] The rash usually is macular or maculopapular, has its onset 1 to 3 days after initial fever, and lasts 1 to 2 days. A child with a petechial rash has been noted.[388]

Echovirus 5

One major outbreak of echovirus 5 infection with exanthem has been described.[254] This outbreak, which involved a maternity unit, resulted in a macular rash in 36 per cent of the infants and 14 per cent of the mothers. The rash was most prominent on the limbs and buttocks, appeared 24 to 36 hours after the onset of fever, and lasted 2 days. Selwyn and Howitt[657] noted a child with a macular rash with a zoster distribution. A neonate with sepsis-like illness and exanthem has been described.[291]

Echovirus 6

Although echovirus 6 has been one of the more prevalent enteroviruses during the last 25 years, it has been associated only sporadically with exanthematous disease. The following manifestations have been observed: morbilliform,[719] maculopapular,[485, 749] macular,[476] and papulopustular exanthems[387]; Stevens-Johnson syndrome[720]; and pityriasis rosea in an adult and in a child.[387] Meade and Chang[490] reported an interesting zoster-like eruption in a 7-year-old boy in whom echovirus 6 was recovered from several bullae.

Echovirus 7

Echovirus 7 has been associated occasionally with exanthem.[25, 363, 518] In one outbreak of aseptic meningitis, 5 of 13 patients had erythematous maculopapular rashes that occurred during fever.[363] One child with a discrete maculopapular rash and thrombocytopenia has been described.[479]

Echovirus 9 (see Fig. 66–13)

For more than 35 years, echovirus 9 has been the most prevalent nonpolio enterovirus, and exanthem is a common clinical manifestation (Table 170–13).[25, 59, 115, 144, 151, 160, 174, 210, 221, 235, 240, 243, 270, 306, 331, 361, 374, 381, 400, 402, 412, 427, 446, 464, 488, 521, 556, 558, 589, 594, 603, 624, 632, 671, 680, 693, 742] Nonspecific febrile illness and aseptic meningitis are the usual major manifestations of echovirus 9 infection. Exanthem occurs in about one-third of cases. Exanthem prevalence is related inversely to age; 57 per cent of children younger than 5 years of age have rash, whereas only 6 per cent of those older than 10 years of age have similar cutaneous findings.[447] The rash usually is rubelliform, but, in addition or as the sole manifestation, petechiae are common. Rash and fever usually appear at about the same time, and frequently the illness closely mimics meningococcemia. The rash usually lasts about 3 to 5 days. In one instance, the rash progressed to a vesicular stage.[446]

Echovirus 11

Exanthem occasionally occurs with echovirus 11 infection, and it varies considerably in appearance.[25, 84, 115, 126, 180, 653] The most notable lesions have been bug bite–like vesicles and urticaria.[126] A child with subacute recurrent vesicular lesions

TABLE 170–13. Signs and Symptoms in Echovirus 9 Disease*

Sign or Symptom	Per Cent of Cases
Fever	92
Headache	85
Nuchal rigidity	83
Nausea and vomiting	71
Pain (neck, back, trunk)	44
Exanthem	35
Nonexudative pharyngitis	28
Cough	24
Sore throat	20
Cervical lymphadenopathy	18
Coryza	18
Abdominal pain	17
Photophobia	16

From Cherry, J. D.: Newer viral exanthems. Adv. Pediatr. *16*:233–286, 1969. Used with permission.
* Modified from references 59, 174, 210, 221, 240, 361, 427, 446, 624, 671, 742.

has been reported.[126] An adult woman with a disseminated vesicular eruption has been reported.[180]

Echovirus 13

One child with a maculopapular eruption has been described.[325]

Echovirus 14

Echovirus 14 is a rare cause of exanthem, and few details are available.[25, 632] One child with a scarlatiniform eruption and aseptic meningitis has been reported.[632]

Echovirus 16

The first of the enteroviral exanthematous diseases to be described was that due to echovirus 16. This initially was studied by Neva and colleagues,[550, 551] and the illness was called Boston exanthem. Two outbreaks of echovirus 16 infection with exanthem were documented by Neva and colleagues in 1951 and 1954[548, 549] and another in Paris in 1960.[154] Since then, Boston exanthem has been reported only once. Seven cases were observed in 1974.[294]

The exanthem associated with echovirus 16 infection is erythematous, maculopapular, and discrete and similar to that of other enteroviral infections. What has been unique with echovirus 16 infection is the relationship of rash to fever. Frequently, the illness is roseola-like in that the rash occurs at the time of or after defervescence.[118, 294] Ulcerative lesions on the soft palate and tonsillar pillars (herpangina) sometimes have been observed.

Echovirus 17

Rash is an occasional occurrence in echovirus 17 infection.[25, 82, 120, 124] In one outbreak, transient erythematous rashes were noted.[82] In cases I have studied, papular, maculopapular, and papulovesicular lesions were noted; two patients had herpangitic enanthems, and one had aseptic meningitis.[120, 122]

Echovirus 18

Kennett and associates[397] described an extensive epidemic of echovirus 18 infection in which aseptic meningitis with or without exanthem was the major finding. In 15 patients, exanthem was the major complaint. The rash was described as rubelliform. The majority of patients were children, but adults also had exanthem.

Echovirus 19

In one extensive epidemic of echovirus 19 infection, exanthem was common.[150] Fifty per cent of children younger than 6 months of age had exanthem, and many of these infants presented a picture of septicemia with peripheral circulatory failure. Rash occurred in adults and older children, but the percentage decreased with age. The rash usually was erythematous, maculopapular, and discrete. It started on the face and upper trunk and spread to the extremities. Fever occurred in all cases, and meningitis and signs of upper respiratory tract involvement were common.

In another outbreak of echovirus 19 infection, 33 per cent of those infected had exanthem,[269] whereas in an outbreak studied by Cramblett and colleagues,[158] exanthem was rare.

Echovirus 21

A 19-day-old infant with aseptic meningitis and rash has been reported.[135]

Echovirus 22

A morbilliform rash was noted in three infants with respiratory disease and echovirus 22 infection.[62]

Echovirus 24

A 4-month-old infant with rash and aseptic meningitis has been presented.[135]

Echovirus 25

Echovirus 25 has been associated with an array of different skin manifestations.[50, 119, 288, 527, 544] In one epidemic of febrile pharyngitis, about one-third of the patients had exanthem.[527] The rash most often was maculopapular and discrete, but occasionally it displayed a morbilliform confluence. The rash most often occurred during the period of defervescence.

Of considerable interest are two children with acute hemangioma-like lesions.[119] The lesions were erythematous and papular and surrounded by a 1- to 4-mm-wide halo of blanched-appearing skin. The center of each lesion had a bright red dot that suggested a dilated capillary or terminal arteriole. The whole lesion would blanch with pinpoint pressure in its middle.

Echovirus 30

Echovirus 30 is a common cause of epidemic aseptic meningitis, and exanthem occasionally is noted concomitantly. The rash is macular or maculopapular.[25, 115, 349, 384, 442, 703, 764]

Echovirus 32

Two children with echovirus 32 infection and hemangioma-like lesions were described by Cherry and colleagues.[119] Some lesions seemed to be composed of many dilated capillaries; they easily blanched with pressure.

Echovirus 33

Four patients with aseptic meningitis and echovirus 33 infection also have had exanthem.[386, 392] Two adults have had vesicular lesions that suggested herpes simplex virus infections.[176]

Enterovirus 71

Kennett and associates[396] studied 49 patients with enterovirus 71 infections and noted exanthem in 11. Six patients had aseptic meningitis, and in five the rash was the predominant complaint. The exanthems varied: some were erythematous maculopapular, some vesicular, and some a combination of lesions. Two children had the hand, foot, and mouth syndrome, and one child had a florid, diffuse, erythematous rash. Outbreaks of hand, foot, and mouth syndrome due to enterovirus 71 have been observed in Japan, Sweden, Australia, and the United States.[255, 353, 497, 570] In many cases, varied neurologic manifestations also occurred.

Clinical Exanthematous Manifestations and Syndromes

The major clinical exanthematous manifestations and syndromes of coxsackieviruses and echoviruses are presented in Table 170–14. Unusual findings include hemangioma-like lesions with echoviruses 25 and 32, anaphylactoid purpura with coxsackievirus A4 and echoviruses 9 and 18, zoster-

TABLE 170–14. Clinical Exanthematous Manifestations of Coxsackieviruses and Echoviruses

	Associated Viral Agents and Prevalence of Manifestations			
Clinical Manifestations	***Virus Subgroup***	***Common***	***Occasional***	***Rare***
Macular rash	Coxsackievirus A			
	B		1, 2, 5	
	Echovirus and enterovirus		2, 4, 5, 13, 14, 17, 19, 30	18, 71
Maculopapular rash	Coxsackievirus A	9	2, 4, 5, 10, 16	6, 7
	B		1–5	
	Echovirus and enterovirus	4, 9	2, 5–7, 11, 16–19, 25, 30, 71	1, 3, 13, 14, 22, 27, 33
Vesicular rash	Coxsackievirus A	5, 16	8–10	4, 7
	B			1–3, 5
	Echovirus and enterovirus		11	6, 9, 17, 71
Petechial or purpuric rash	Coxsackievirus A	9	4	
	B		2–5	
	Echovirus	9	4, 7	3
Urticarial rash	Coxsackievirus A	9	16	
	B		4, 5	
	Echovirus		11	
Erythema multiforme or Stevens-Johnson syndrome	Coxsackievirus A		9	10, 16
	B			4, 5
	Echovirus			6, 11
Exanthem and meningitis	Coxsackievirus A		2, 9	7
	B		1, 2, 4, 5	
	Echovirus and enterovirus	4, 9	6, 11, 17, 18, 25, 30	3, 14, 33, 71
Exanthem and pneumonia	Coxsackievirus A		9	7
	B		6	1
	Echovirus			9, 11
Hand, foot, and mouth syndrome	Coxsackievirus A	16	5, 10	7, 9
	B			1, 3, 5
	Echovirus and enterovirus			71
Hemangioma-like lesions	Coxsackievirus A			
	B			
	Echovirus			25, 32
Herpangina and exanthem	Coxsackievirus A		4	9
	B			2
	Echovirus		16, 17	
Roseola-like illness	Coxsackievirus A			6, 9
	B		5	1, 2, 4
	Echovirus		16, 25	9, 11, 27, 30
Anaphylactoid purpura	Coxsackievirus A			4
	B			
	Echovirus			9, 18
Zoster-like rash	Coxsackievirus A			
	B			
	Echovirus			5, 6
Pityriasis-like rash	Coxsackievirus A			
	B			
	Echovirus			6
Chronic or recurrent rash	Coxsackievirus A	16		
	B			
	Echovirus			11

like rash with echoviruses 5 and 6, pityriasis-like rash with echovirus 6, and chronic or recurrent rash with coxsackievirus A16 and echovirus 11.

Neurologic Manifestations

Neurologic illness is a common manifestation of infections with most coxsackieviruses and echoviruses. The most common illness is aseptic meningitis, but encephalitis and other manifestations also occur. The prevalence of coxsackieviruses and echoviruses in the various clinical syndromes is presented in Table 170–15.

Aseptic Meningitis

Aseptic meningitis due to enteroviruses occurs both in epidemics and as isolated cases. The etiologic agents most often associated with epidemic disease are presented in Table 170–16. Epidemic disease has been most common with coxsackievirus B5 and echoviruses 4, 6, 9, and 30. In general, illness is more common in children, but, if a specific outbreak is large, adults also are involved. Virtually all patients have fever and pharyngitis; other respiratory manifestations are common. Rash is common but varies with the specific viral agents. Between one-third and one-half of all patients with echovirus 9 meningitis have exanthem. Abdominal pain is common in epidemic enteroviral aseptic meningitis.

TABLE 170–15. Neurologic Manifestations of Coxsackieviruses and Echoviruses

	Associated Viral Agents and Prevalence of Manifestations				
Clinical Manifestations	***Virus Subgroup***	***Common***	***Occasional***	***Rare***	***References***
Aseptic meningitis	Coxsackievirus A	9	7	1–6, 8, 10, 11–14, 16–18, 21, 22, 24	10, 11, 59, 64, 102, 115, 174, 192, 201, 210, 221, 239, 240, 270, 281, 290, 297, 312, 361, 363, 367, 374, 393, 394, 400, 427, 441, 442, 447, 482, 485, 497, 499, 518, 524, 610, 615, 617, 624, 631, 653, 658, 661, 671, 714, 742, 746, 764
	B	2, 4, 5	1, 3	6	
	Echovirus	4, 6, 9, 30, 33	3, 11, 12, 14, 16, 18, 19, 25, 31, 71	1, 2, 5, 7, 8, 13, 15, 17, 20–24, 26, 27, 29, 32	
Encephalitis	Coxsackievirus A		9	2, 4–7, 10, 16	115, 281, 308, 353, 400, 420, 430, 511, 518, 647
	B	5	1, 2, 4	3	
	Echovirus	4, 6, 9, 11, 30	3, 25, 71	1, 2, 5, 7, 8, 12, 13, 14, 15, 17–24, 27, 31, 33, 71	10, 617
Paralysis (lower motor neuron involvement)	Coxsackievirus A		4, 7, 9	2, 5, 6, 10, 11, 14, 21	10, 25, 115, 136, 172, 189, 217, 222, 255, 262, 280, 281, 283, 307, 353, 400, 419, 465–467, 497, 586, 604, 637, 653, 675, 721, 722, 767, 774
	B		2, 3	1, 4–6	
	Echovirus	70	9, 11, 30, 71	1–4, 6–8, 12, 14, 16–19, 22, 25, 27, 31, 70, 71	
Guillain-Barré syndrome and transverse myelitis	Coxsackievirus A		9	2, 4, 5, 6, 19	10, 36, 51, 53, 68, 178, 217, 249, 274, 277, 357, 369, 400, 401, 445, 637, 692, 712
	B			1, 4	
	Echovirus		6, 70	5, 7, 19, 22	
Cerebellar ataxia	Coxsackievirus A		9	4, 7	58, 212, 281, 294, 353, 400, 476, 481, 542, 775
	B			3, 4	
	Echovirus		6, 9, 71	16	
Peripheral neuritis	Coxsackievirus A				
	B				653
	Echovirus		9		
Neurologic sequelae and other neurologic illness	Coxsackievirus A		3	9	106, 400, 578, 613, 653, 656, 723, 724, 745, 759
	B		3	2, 4	
	Echovirus		9	19, 25, 30, 33	

Except for rash, herpangina, pleurodynia, or myocarditis, little else occurs clinically to help identify the etiology in a sporadic case of aseptic meningitis. Initial symptoms include fever, headache, malaise, nausea, and vomiting. Headache most often is frontal or generalized; adolescents and adults frequently note retrobulbar pain. Pain in the neck, back, and legs is common. Abdominal pain occurs in about one-fifth of patients, but this symptom varies with the specific etiologic viral type. Photophobia is common.

Physical examination reveals a temperature in the range of 38° to 40° C (100.4° to 104° F). Skin rash is common and most commonly is erythematous, maculopapular, and discrete. Frequently, particularly with echovirus 9 infection, rash is petechial, suggesting meningococcemia. Pharyngitis is common. Generalized muscle stiffness or spasm usually is observed, although the degree varies considerably; Kernig and Brudzinski signs are positive in less than half of cases. Deep tendon reflexes usually are normal. In one study, 9 per cent of children with enteroviral meningitis had the syndrome of inappropriate secretion of antidiuretic hormone.[114] The onset of this syndrome was noted 36 hours after admission to the hospital, and it usually lasted less than 2 days.

Cerebrospinal fluid examination reveals considerable variations among patients and in the same patient on repeated examination. Cerebrospinal fluid leukocyte counts vary from a few cells to a few thousand/mm^3; the median is in the range of 100 to 500 cells/mm^3. The percentage of neutrophils also varies greatly. Initial examinations frequently reveal a predominance of neutrophils but rarely more than 90 per cent, as seen in bacterial disease. Usually, the initial examination reveals between 30 and 60 per cent neutrophils. Repeated cerebrospinal fluid examination demonstrates an

TABLE 170–16. Coxsackieviruses and Echoviruses Associated with Epidemic Aseptic Meningitis

Virus Type		Age Group	Common Nonneurologic Findings	References
Coxsackievirus	A7	Children and adults	Fever	286
	A9	Mainly children	Fever, rash, pharyngitis	115, 450
	B1	Mainly children	Fever, pharyngitis	115
	B2	Children and adults	Fever, pharyngitis, rhinitis, abdominal pain, diarrhea	115, 472
	B3	Children and adults	Fever, pharyngitis, conjunctivitis	115
	B4	Children and adults	Fever, pharyngitis, rash, conjunctivitis	115, 214
	B5	Mainly children	Fever, pharyngitis, rash, pleurodynia, abdominal pain, diarrhea, rhinitis, myocarditis	31, 115, 127, 131, 289, 487, 588, 625, 683, 689, 691
Echovirus	3	Children	Fever, rash	305
	4	Mainly children	Fever, pharyngitis, abdominal pain, rash, conjunctivitis	115, 223, 239, 383, 388, 440, 607, 673
	6	Children and adults	Fever, pharyngitis, abdominal pain, pleurodynia, cardiac involvement	115, 300, 387, 403, 428, 720, 731
		Children	Fever, rash	363
	9	Mainly children	Fever, rash, abdominal pain, pharyngitis	115, 174, 221, 235, 270, 306, 361, 381, 427, 464, 560, 589, 594, 624, 632, 671, 680, 731, 738
	11	Mainly children	Fever, upper respiratory, pneumonia	501
	16	Children	Fever, rash	294
	18	Children and adults	Fever, rash	397
	19	Mainly children	Fever, upper respiratory, rash	150, 269
	25	Children and adults	Fever, rash	50
	30	Children and adults	Fever, pharyngitis, rhinitis, conjunctivitis, rash, abdominal pain	115, 276, 295, 384, 584, 704, 764
	31	Children and adults	Fever	441
	33	Children and adults	Fever, rash	386, 392
Enterovirus	71	Mainly children	Fever, rash	396

increasing percentage of mononuclear cells. Dagan and colleagues[166] observed that the virus isolation rate from the cerebrospinal fluid in enteroviral meningitis was directly proportional to the number of leukocytes in the fluid.

The cerebrospinal fluid protein usually is elevated mildly, and the glucose concentration most often is normal; hypoglycorrhachia is rare.[27, 129, 198, 429, 473, 658, 667, 668, 685] Occasionally, the cerebrospinal fluid findings suggest tuberculosis meningitis with mononuclear pleocytosis, hypoglycorrhachia, and elevated protein.[469] A child with coxsackievirus B4 meningitis had eosinophils in the cerebrospinal fluid.[128] Results of other routine laboratory studies such as the white blood cell count occasionally are abnormal but not helpful diagnostically.

The duration of illness varies significantly. In the majority of patients, the temperature returns to normal within 4 to 6 days, and disability due to neurologic involvement lasts 1 to 2 weeks. Occasionally, the illness pattern is biphasic: an initial period with fever, headache, nausea, vomiting, and muscle aches and pains of a few days' duration followed by general recovery and then return to the same symptoms plus more pronounced neurologic involvement.

Wilfert and associates[744] performed a longitudinal assessment of children who had enteroviral meningitides early in life and found that receptive language functioning was significantly less than that of children in a control group without meningitis. In another study, Sells and colleagues[656] examined the long-term effects of central nervous system enteroviral infections in 19 children. Of this group, 11 were free of detectable abnormalities, 5 had possible defects, and 3 had definite neurologic sequelae. In more recent studies, patients who have had meningitis have performed as well as controls in follow-up developmental evaluations.[60, 615, 617]

Encephalitis

An average of about 2500 cases of encephalitis in the United States per year is reported to the Centers for Disease Control and Prevention.[100] Of this group, only about 2 per cent demonstrate an enteroviral etiology. However, the seasonal pattern of disease and the absence of arboviral activity in many geographic locations suggest that 500 to 1000 cases of enteroviral encephalitis actually occur each year in the United States. The prevalence of coxsackieviruses and echoviruses as etiologic agents in encephalitis is presented in Table 170–15. Echovirus 9 is the most common cause of enteroviral encephalitis. Other commonly associated enteroviral types are echoviruses 4, 6, 11, and 30 and coxsackievirus B5. Of these latter agents, echoviruses 4, 6, and 11 have been noted most frequently over a long period.

In general, the prognosis in encephalitis due to enteroviral infections is good, but fatalities occur. The viral types that have been isolated from the brain or cerebrospinal fluid in fatal cases are coxsackieviruses B3 and B6, echoviruses 2, 9, 17, and 25, and enterovirus 71.[281, 400]

Paralysis

Paralysis based on anterior horn cell disease occasionally results from infection with nonpolio enteroviruses. In contrast with poliovirus prevalence, which in the prevaccine era resulted in epidemic paralytic disease, paralysis due to nonpolio enteroviruses usually is a sporadic event. Coxsackievirus A7 on three occasions has been associated with outbreaks of paralytic disease.[280, 283, 721] Many cases of illness similar to poliomyelitis have occurred during outbreaks and epidemics of illness due to enterovirus 71.[10, 172, 255, 305, 353, 497, 637] Paralytic disease also has been noted during epidemics of acute hemorrhagic conjunctivitis due to enterovirus 70.[722, 767]

Guillain-Barré Syndrome and Transverse Myelitis

From Table 170–15, it is apparent that many coxsackieviruses and echoviruses have been associated with the Guillain-Barré syndrome. In general, there appear to be no specific viral types that cause the disease. Rather, the disease occurs sporadically in association with prevalent enteroviral types.

Other Neurologic Illnesses (see Table 170–15)

Cerebellar ataxia has been associated with coxsackieviruses A4, A7, A9, B3, and B4 and echoviruses 6, 9, and 16. Scott[653] specifically comments on peripheral neuritis with echovirus 9 infection. Coxsackievirus A9 has been associated with focal encephalitis and acute hemiplegia on two occasions,[106, 115] and echovirus 25 infection was noted in a 5-year-old boy with focal encephalitis and subacute hemichorea.[578] Coxsackievirus B4 was isolated from the spinal fluid of a 22-year-old woman with intracranial hypertension,[759] and postencephalitis Parkinson syndrome following coxsackievirus B2 meningoencephalitis has been described.[723] Two children with coxsackievirus B3 infections have had a syndrome of opsoclonus-myoclonis.[422] A 4-year-old boy with Alice in Wonderland syndrome (complex symptoms of perceptual distortion) associated with a coxsackievirus B1 infection has been described.[724]

Phillips and colleagues[583] and Barrett and associates[38] noted the simultaneous occurrence of enteroviral and St. Louis encephalitis viral infections in the same community. In six instances, dual infections occurred, and the afflicted children tended to have more serious illnesses.

Multiple attacks of enteroviral aseptic meningitis in the same individuals have been noted occasionally.[413, 540]

From molecular techniques and antibody prevalence data, it has been suggested that chronic enteroviral infections play a role in the chronic fatigue syndrome and in the postviral fatigue syndrome.[16, 89, 147, 530, 770] However, these findings have not been confirmed by other investigators.[495, 507, 687] Woodall and associates[757] found conserved enteroviral sequences in spinal cords from subjects with sporadic motor neuron disease and from one patient with possible familial motor neuron disease. Behan and associates[45] looked for picornavirus RNA in biopsy specimens from 41 patients with inflammatory myopathy, but all results were negative.[45]

Sudden Infant Death

Balduzzi and Greendyke[33] recovered coxsackievirus A5 from the stool of a 1-month-old child who experienced sudden infant death. In a similar investigation of sudden infant death, Gold and associates[267] recovered coxsackievirus A4 from the brains of three babies. Coxsackievirus A8 also was recovered at the stool of a child in whom anorexia was noted on the day before death. Coxsackievirus B3 was recovered at the autopsy of an infant who died suddenly on the eighth day of life.[33] Morens and colleagues[521] noted sudden infant death eight times in association with enteroviral infection; echovirus 22 was found on two occasions. In a subgroup of infants with sudden unexplained deaths in whom "clinical, biologic, and histologic" findings suggested viral infection, evidence of enterovirus infection was more common than in infants without findings of viral infection.[275] Specifically, enteroviral RNA was found in the respiratory tract in 54 per cent of the viral infection group and in none of the group without findings suggestive of viral infection. These findings were supported by IgM antibodies to coxsackieviruses B in 56 per cent of the first group and in none in the second group.

In five instances of cot death in one study, echovirus 11 was isolated from the lungs in two cases, from the myocardium in one case, and from the nose or feces in the other two cases.[66]

Chronic Enteroviral Infections in Immunocompromised Patients

Patients with cell-mediated and combined immunodeficiencies are susceptible to chronic and often fatal infections with many viruses. Patients with agammaglobulinemias with normal cell-mediated functions generally survive infections with these same viruses. Enteroviruses are the exception, however, in that chronic, unusual infections with a variety of enteroviruses have been reported.[6, 37, 70, 152, 161, 191, 203, 292, 318, 483, 620, 718, 730, 732] The most common illness is meningoencephalitis, but arthritis and polymyositis are other frequent presentations. Echovirus 11 has been the most common cause of chronic infection, but the following other enteroviruses also have been causative: echoviruses 2, 3, 5, 7, 9, 15, 17, 18, 19, 22, 24, 25, 29, 30, and 33 and coxsackieviruses A11, A15, B2, and B3.[483] In addition to the cerebrospinal fluid, enteroviruses have been recovered from many other body sites, such as liver, heart, lung, pancreas, lymph nodes, bone marrow, muscle, throat, and stool.

Several patients with X-linked agammaglobulinemia have had polymyositis or dermatomyositis-like syndromes due to echovirus infections; the following echoviruses have been implicated: types 2, 3, 5, 9, 11, 17, 19, 24, 25, 30, and 33.[37, 161, 492]

A 15-year-old boy with X-linked agammaglobulinemia and chronic arthritis due to echovirus 11 has been described.[6] Enteroviral infections have caused deaths in bone marrow transplant recipients.[238]

Congenital Infections

Abortion

Landsman and associates[431] studied 2631 pregnancies during echovirus 9 epidemic prevalence and could find no difference in antibody to echovirus 9 in women who aborted and in those who delivered term infants. A similar study in Finland revealed no increase in the abortion rate in women infected in early pregnancy with echovirus 9.[603] Although coxsackieviral infections are common, epidemics with specific viral types involving large populations have not been studied.

Two women with coxsackievirus A16 hand, foot, and mouth syndrome had spontaneous abortions.[566] In one instance, coxsackievirus A16 was recovered from the products of conception. Frisk and Diderholm[233] found that 33 per cent of women with abortions had IgM antibody to coxsackieviruses B, whereas only 8 per cent of controls had similar antibody. In a second, larger study, the same research group confirmed their original findings.[28]

Congenital Malformations

In a large prospective study, Brown and Karunas[81] made a serologic search for selected maternal enteroviral infections in association with congenital malformations. Serums from 630 mothers of infants with anomalies and from 1164 mothers of children without defects were studied carefully. Specifically, serologic evidence of infection during the first trimester and during the last 6 months of pregnancy with coxsackieviruses B1, B2, B3, B4, B5, and A9 and with echoviruses 6 and 9 was sought. In this study, infants were examined for 113 specific abnormalities; these anomalies were grouped into 12 categories for analysis. The investigators demonstrated a positive correlation between maternal infection and infant anomaly with coxsackieviruses B2, B3, B4, and A9. The overall anomaly rate associated with first-trimester infections with coxsackievirus B4 was significantly higher than that in controls. Maternal coxsackievirus B2 infection throughout pregnancy, coxsackievirus B4 infections during the first trimester of pregnancy, and infection with at least one of the five coxsackieviruses B during pregnancy all were associated with urogenital anomalies when compared with the controls. Coxsackievirus A9 infection was associated with digestive anomalies, and coxsackieviruses B3 and B4 were associated with cardiovascular defects. When coxsackieviruses B were analyzed as a group (B1 to B5), there was an overall association with congenital heart disease; the likelihood of cardiovascular anomalies was increased when maternal infections with two or more coxsackieviruses B occurred.

Gauntt and colleagues[248] found that the ventricular fluid from 4 of 28 babies with severe anatomic defects contained neutralizing antibody to one or more coxsackievirus B types. In one case, specific IgM antibody to coxsackievirus B6 was demonstrated.

In a serologic study in Scotland, Ross and colleagues[616] found no association between maternal coxsackievirus B infections and fetal developmental anomalies. Elizan and colleagues[199] were unable to find any relationships between maternal infections with coxsackieviruses B and congenital central nervous system malformations. In three studies, no association between maternal echovirus 9 infection and congenital malformation was noted.[411, 431, 603]

Prematurity and Stillbirth

Bates[42] reported an 8-month-old stillborn fetus with calcific pancarditis and hydrops fetalis at autopsy. Fluorescent antibody study revealed coxsackievirus B3 antigen in the myocardium. Burch and colleagues[86] noted three stillborn infants who had fluorescent antibody evidence of coxsackievirus B myocarditis, one each with coxsackieviruses B2, B3, and B4. They also noted a premature boy who had histologic and immunofluorescent evidence of cardiac infection with coxsackieviruses B2, B3, and B4; he lived only 24 hours.

Freedman[231] reported the occurrence of a full-term stillbirth in a woman infected with echovirus 11. Because the baby had no pathologic or virologic evidence of infection, Freedman attributed the event to a secondary consequence of maternal infection due to fever and dehydration rather than primary transplacental infection. In another stillbirth in which echovirus 11 was recovered from the amniotic fluid, the fetus was found to have evidence of focal encephalitis, massive adrenal hemorrhage, and diffuse subarachnoid hemorrhage.[669] Echovirus 27 was recovered from the amniotic fluid in an intrauterine fetal death at 28 weeks' gestation.[554]

Neonatal Infections

Epidemiology and Pathogenesis

Neonatal infection with coxsackieviruses and echoviruses can result from transplacental viral transmission, contact infection during birth, and human-to-human contact after birth. The transplacental passage of coxsackieviruses and echoviruses at term has been noted on many occasions. Benirschke[56] studied the placentas in three cases of congenital coxsackievirus B disease and could find no histologic evidence of infection. In 1956, Kibrick and Benirschke[404] reported the first case of intrauterine infection with coxsackievirus B3. In this instance, the infant was delivered by cesarean section and became symptomatic several hours after birth. Brightman and associates[79] recovered coxsackievirus B5 from the placenta and rectum of a premature infant. No histologic abnormalities of the placenta were noted.

Berkovich and Smithwick[61] noted an asymptomatic neonate who had specific IgM echovirus 22 antibody in the cord blood, suggesting intrauterine infection with this virus. Hughes and colleagues[339] reported a newborn infant with echovirus 14 infection who had markedly elevated IgM (190 mg/dL) on the sixth day of life. It seems likely that this child also was infected in utero. Echovirus 19 also has been noted in a transplacentally acquired infection.[580] Other evidence of intrauterine infection has been presented for coxsackieviruses A4, B1, B2, B3, B4, and B5 and echoviruses 9, 11, and 19.[42, 57, 73, 115, 120, 301, 378, 385, 468, 580]

There is little definitive evidence for either ascending infection or contact infection with coxsackieviruses or echoviruses during birth. However, infection during the birth process seems probable.[120, 385] The fecal carriage rate of enteroviruses in asymptomatic adult patients varies between 0 and 6 per cent or higher in different population groups.[115] Cherry and colleagues[120] noted that in 2 of 55 mothers (4 per cent), enteroviruses were present in the feces shortly after delivery. Coxsackievirus B5 was recovered from the cervices of four women with febrile illnesses during the third trimester of pregnancy.[608] Echovirus 11 was isolated from the cervix of a mother whose baby became ill on the third day of life with a fatal echovirus 11 necrotizing hepatitis.[609]

Several epidemics with coxsackieviruses and echoviruses in newborn nurseries have been studied.[79, 92, 504, 537] Brightman and associates[79] observed an epidemic of coxsackievirus B5 in a premature nursery. Their data suggested that the virus was introduced into this nursery by an asymptomatic infant who had been infected in utero. Secondary infections occurred in 12 babies and 2 nurses. The timing of the secondary cases suggested that three generations had occurred and that the nurses had been infected during the second generation. The investigators suggested that the infection had spread from infant to infant and from infant to nurse.

Javett and associates[364] reported an acute epidemic of myocarditis associated with coxsackievirus B3 infection in a Johannesburg maternity home. Unfortunately, no epidemiologic investigation or search for asymptomatic infected infants was performed. However, in analyzing the dates of the onset of the illnesses, apparently single infections occurred for five generations and then five children became ill within a 3-day period.

Kipps and colleagues[409] carried out epidemiologic investigations in two coxsackievirus B3 nursery epidemics. In the first epidemic, the initial infection probably was transmitted from a mother to her baby; this baby then was the source of five secondary cases in newborn infants and one illness in a nurse. Four of the five secondary cases were located on one side of the nursery, but only one cot was close to the cot of the index baby, and this cot did not adjoin the cots of the three other contact cases. In the second outbreak, a baby who also was infected by his mother probably introduced the virus into the nursery. The three secondary cases geographically were far removed from the primary case.

Cramblett and colleagues[156] reported an outbreak of echovirus 11 disease in four infants in an intensive care nursery. All infants were in enclosed incubators, and three patients became ill within 24 hours; the fourth child became ill 4 days later. Echovirus 11 was recovered from two members of the nursery staff. These data suggest that transmission from personnel to infants occurred because of inadequate washing of hands.

In another outbreak in an intensive care unit, the initial patient was transferred to the nursery because of severe echovirus 11 disease.[527] After transfer, the senior house officer and a psychologist in the unit were infected. It was inferred by the investigators that spread by respiratory droplets to nine other babies occurred from these infected personnel. In another echovirus 11 nursery outbreak, Mertens and colleagues[504] found that the infection spread through close contact between the infected newborns and the nurses in the unit. The spread of infection was interrupted with the installation of vigorous hygienic and isolation measures. In an echovirus 11 outbreak in an intermediate care unit, Kinney and colleagues[408] found that risk of illness was associated with gavage feeding, mouth care, and being a twin.

There have been many other instances of isolated nursery infections and small outbreaks with coxsackieviruses and echoviruses. The most consistent source of original nursery infection seems to be transmission from a mother to her baby,[17, 40, 113, 115, 117, 129, 150, 173, 198, 207, 294, 351, 429, 460, 473, 512, 598, 677, 689] but virus can be introduced into the nursery by personnel.[350, 435, 689]

In a longitudinal study of neonatal enteroviral infections that was carried out during the summer and fall of 1981, Jenista and associates[366] found that the nonpolio enterovirus infection rate was 12.8 per cent. Lower socioeconomic status and the lack of breast feeding were found to be risk factors for infection. Nonpolio enteroviral infections were found to be a significant cause for readmission to the hospital of the cohort neonates. During a community outbreak of echovirus 11 disease, Modlin and colleagues[513] found that the passive transplacental passage of antibody to neonates prevented severe disease, but it did not prevent mucosal infection.

Clinical Manifestations

Coxsackieviral and echoviral infections in neonates result in a wide variety of clinical manifestations, ranging from asymptomatic infection to fatal encephalitis and myocarditis.[117] Unfortunately, enteroviral illnesses have not been examined by specific viral type but in a more generic fashion.[3, 4, 646] An overview by illness category and prevalence is presented in Table 170–17.

INAPPARENT INFECTION. Although it is probable that inapparent infection occasionally occurs with many different enteroviruses, there is little documentation of this assumption. Cherry and colleagues[120] studied 590 normal neonates during a 6-month period and noted only one asymptomatic infection. This was a child infected in utero or immediately thereafter with coxsackievirus B2. The mother had an upper respiratory illness 10 days prior to delivery.

During a survey of perinatal viral infections, 44 babies were found to be infected with echovirus 22 in a study period of May to December 1966.[355] The virus prevalence and the incidence of new infections during this period were fairly uniform. No illness was attributed to echovirus 22 infection, and the virus disappeared from the nursery in mid-December. Asymptomatic infections with echovirus 22 have been noted on two other occasions.[62, 543] Infections without evidence of illness also have been noted with coxsackieviruses A9, B1, B4, and B5 and echoviruses 3, 5, 9, 11, 13, 14, 20, 30, and 31.[115, 117, 196, 208, 254, 356, 366, 528]

MILD, NONSPECIFIC, FEBRILE ILLNESS. In a review of 338 enteroviral infections in early infancy, 9 per cent were classified as nonspecific febrile illnesses.[522] Illness may be sporadic or part of an outbreak with a specific viral type. In the latter case, clinical manifestations vary, depending on the viral type: some infants have aseptic meningitis and other signs and symptoms, and some simply have nonspecific fever. Specific viruses related to nonspecific fever are listed in Table 170–17. Although by definition illness in this category is mild, it is important to be aware that viral infection may be extensive. When sought, virus may be isolated from the blood, urine, and spinal fluid of infants with mild illnesses.[40, 358]

SEPSIS-LIKE ILLNESS. The main diagnostic problem in neonatal enteroviral infections is the differentiation of bacterial from viral disease. Even in the infant with mild nonspecific fever, bacterial disease must be strongly considered. The sepsis-like illness described here is always alarming. Illness is characterized by fever, poor feeding, abdominal distension, irritability, rash, lethargy, and hypotonia.[294, 429] Other findings include diarrhea, vomiting, seizures, and apnea. In severe, frequently fatal illnesses, most often due to echovirus 11 infections, jaundice, hepatitis, disseminated intravascular coagulation, thrombocytopenia, and hypotension occur.[378, 514, 529, 609]

Sepsis-like illness is common. Morens[522] noted its occurrence in one-fifth of 338 enteroviral infections in infants. In an attempt to differentiate bacterial from viral disease, Lake and associates[429] studied 27 infants with enteroviral infections. White blood cell counts were not helpful because the total count, the number of neutrophils, and the number of band form neutrophils were elevated in most. Of most importance were historical data. The majority of mothers had suffered a recent, febrile, viral-like illness. In addition, other factors often associated with bacterial sepsis, such as prolonged rupture of membranes, prematurity, and low Apgar scores, were unusual in the enteroviral infection group.

RESPIRATORY ILLNESS. Respiratory complaints generally are overshadowed by other manifestations of neonatal enteroviral disease. Only 7 per cent of 338 enteroviral infections in early infancy were classified as respiratory illness in one study.[522] Herpangina has been observed and photographed only once; Chawareewong and associates[113] noted several infants with herpangina and coxsackievirus A5 infection.

Hercík and colleagues[315] reported an epidemic of respiratory illness in 22 neonates associated with echovirus 11 infection. All these infants had rhinitis and pharyngitis, 50 per cent had laryngitis, and 32 per cent had interstitial pneumonitis. Berkovich and Pangan[62] studied respiratory illnesses in premature infants and reported 64 babies with illness, 18 of whom had virologic or serologic evidence of echovirus 22 infection. In addition, many had high but constant levels of serum antibody to echovirus 22. Some of these latter infants probably also were infected with echovirus 22. The children with proven echovirus 22 infections could not be differentiated clinically from those without evidence of echovirus 22 infection. Ninety per cent of the infants had coryza, and 39 per cent had radiographic evidence of pneumonia.

Except for echoviruses 11 and 22, respiratory illness associated with enteroviruses has been sporadic. The following other viruses have been noted: coxsackieviruses A5, A9, B1, B4, and B5 and echoviruses 9, 17, 18, 19, 20, 22, and 31. In the review by Morens,[522] only 7 of 338 enteroviral infections of infancy were classified as pneumonia.

Eichenwald and Kostevalov[196] recovered echovirus 20 from four full-term infants younger than 8 days of age. Although these infants were asymptomatic, they were found to be colonized extensively with staphylococci, and they disseminated these organisms into the air around them. Because of this ability to disseminate staphylococci, they were called

TABLE 170–17. Major Manifestations of Neonatal Nonpolio Enteroviral Infections

Specific Involvement	Common	Rare	References
Inapparent infection	Echo 22	Cox A9, B1, B2, B4, B5 Echo 3, 5, 9, 11, 14, 20, 30, 31	61, 115, 120, 196, 208, 254, 356, 528, 543
Mild, nonspecific, febrile illness	Cox B5 Echo 5, 11, 33	Cox B1–B4, A9, A16 Echo 4, 7, 9, 17	17, 40, 63, 75, 115, 120, 173, 198, 254, 303, 358, 386, 460, 517, 537, 664, 709
Sepsis-like illness	Cox B2–B5 Echo 5, 11, 16	Cox B1, A9 Echo 2–4, 6, 9, 14, 19, 21, 22	3, 18, 66, 73, 115, 117, 132, 150, 156, 173, 209, 267, 293, 378, 385, 429, 460, 473, 504, 514, 529, 537, 580, 609, 639, 678, 689, 761
Respiratory illness (general)	Echo 11, 22	Cox B1, B4, B5, A9 Echo 9, 17	120, 315, 339, 356
Herpangina		Cox A5	113
Coryza		Cox A9 Echo 11, 17, 19, 22	61, 158, 315, 543, 647
Pharyngitis		Cox B4 Echo 11, 17, 18	63, 315, 493, 639, 664
Laryngotracheitis or bronchitis		Cox B1, B4 Echo 11	193, 315, 520
Pneumonia		Cox B4, A9 Echo 9, 11, 17, 22, 31	61, 115, 132, 173, 209, 315, 356, 505, 702, 753
Cloud baby		Echo 20	196
Gastrointestinal			
Vomiting or diarrhea	Echo 5, 17, 18	Cox B1, B2, B5 Echo 4, 6, 8, 9, 11, 16, 19, 21, 22	63, 115, 150, 196, 197, 209, 254, 302, 315, 356, 460, 505, 602, 639, 689
Hepatitis	Echo 11, 19	Cox A9, B1, B4 Echo 6, 9, 14, 21	115, 117, 333, 378, 402, 514, 529, 761
Pancreatitis		Cox B3, B4, B5	415, 753
Necrotizing enterocolitis		Cox B2, B3	429
Cardiovascular			
Myocarditis and pericarditis	Cox B1–B4	Cox B5, A9 Echo 11, 19	39, 86, 115, 197, 210, 249, 293, 333, 342, 351, 356, 364, 385, 401, 402, 404, 409, 517, 520, 694, 709, 761
Skin	Cox B5 Echo 5, 17, 22	Cox B1 Echo 4, 9, 11, 16, 18	61, 75, 115, 122, 127, 156, 254, 294, 385, 460, 493, 505, 562, 639
Neurologic			
Aseptic meningitis	Cox B2–B5 Echo 3, 9, 11, 17	Cox A9, A14, B1 Echo 1, 14, 21, 30 Entero 71	63, 75, 115, 117, 127, 156, 184, 196, 209, 293, 301, 305, 306, 374, 385, 473, 504, 505, 562, 646, 647, 652, 678, 689
Encephalitis	Cox B1–B4	Cox B5 Echo 9	129, 207, 208, 306, 652, 761
Paralysis		Cox B2	374
Sudden infant death		Cox B3, A4, A5, A8 Echo 22	33, 267, 521

cloud babies. The investigators felt that these cloud babies contributed to the epidemic spread of staphylococci in the nursery. Because active staphylococcal dissemination occurred only when echovirus 20 could be recovered from the nasopharynx, viral-bacterial synergistic activity was considered to be present.

GASTROINTESTINAL MANIFESTATIONS. Significant gastrointestinal illness occurs in about 7 per cent of enteroviral infections of infancy.[522] Vomiting and diarrhea are common but usually are only part of the overall illness complex and not the major manifestations. In 1958, Eichenwald and associates[197] described epidemic diarrhea associated with echovirus 18 infections. In a nursery unit of premature infants, 12 of 21 babies were mildly ill. Neither temperature elevation nor hypothermia occurred. Six infants were lethargic and listless, and two developed moderate abdominal distension. The diarrhea lasted from 1 to 5 days; there were five or six watery, greenish stools per day, occasionally expelled explosively. In two infants, a small amount of blood was noted in the stools but no mucus or pus cells. Five other babies in another nursery also had similar diarrheal illness. Echovirus 18 was recovered from all ill infants.

In 22 infants with epidemic respiratory disease due to echovirus 11, all had vomiting as a manifestation of the illness.[315] Linnemann and colleagues[460] noted vomiting in 36 per cent and diarrhea in 7 per cent of neonates with echoviral infections. In another study, Lake and associates[429] found diarrhea in 81 per cent and vomiting in 33 per cent of neonates with nonpolio enteroviral infections.

Hepatitis is an important neonatal nonpolio enteroviral illness. Morens[522] noted that 2 per cent of neonates with clinically severe enteroviral disease had hepatitis. Lake and colleagues[429] observed that hepatomegaly was present in 37 per cent of neonates with enteroviral infections, and hepatosplenomegaly was observed by Hercík and associates[315] in 12 of 22 newborns with echovirus 11 respiratory illnesses.

Severe hepatitis, frequently with hepatic necrosis, has been noted with echoviruses 6, 9, 11, 14, 19, and 21.[63, 73, 115, 117, 293, 339, 378, 514, 529, 580] Echovirus 11 most often has been associated with severe and usually fatal hepatitis; findings include disseminated intravascular coagulation and thrombocytopenia, as well as apnea, lethargy, poor feeding, and jaundice.

Philip and Larson[580] reported three catastrophic neonatal echovirus 19 infections that resulted in hepatic necrosis and massive terminal hemorrhage. One infant, infected in utero, was symptomatic at birth. The Apgar score was 3, and multiple petechiae were observed. Generalized ecchymoses and apneic episodes occurred, and the infant died at 3.5 hours of age. Thrombocytopenia was noted, and echovirus 19 was isolated from the brain, liver, spleen, and lymph nodes. The other two infants who died of echovirus 19 infection were twins. They were normal during the first 3 days of life but then became mildly cyanotic and lethargic. Shortly thereafter, apneic episodes occurred and jaundice and petechiae developed. Both twins became oliguric, and they died on the eighth and ninth days of life, respectively, with severe, terminal, gastrointestinal bleeding. Both twins were thrombocytopenic, and virus was recovered from systemic sites in both.

Pancreatitis was noted in three of four newborns with coxsackievirus B5 meningitis[415] and in a coxsackievirus B4 infection at autopsy.[753] In other fatal coxsackievirus B infections, pancreatic involvement has been noted, but clinical manifestations rarely have been observed.

Lake and associates[429] noted three infants with necrotizing enterocolitis. Coxsackievirus B3 was recovered from two of these infants and coxsackievirus B2 from the third.

CARDIOVASCULAR MANIFESTATIONS. In contrast with enteroviral cardiac disease in children and adults, in which pericarditis is common, neonatal disease usually always involves the heart muscle. Most cases of neonatal myocarditis are due to coxsackievirus B infections, and nursery outbreaks have occurred on several occasions. In 1961, Kibrick[401] reviewed the clinical findings in 45 cases of neonatal myocarditis; his findings are summarized in Table 170–18. It is of interest that many of the early experiences, particularly in South Africa, involved catastrophic nursery epidemics. Except for the observation in 1972 of five newborns with echovirus 11 infections and myocarditis, there have been no nursery epidemics.[186]

The illness due to coxsackieviruses B most commonly was abrupt in onset, with symptoms of listlessness, anorexia, and fever. A biphasic pattern was noted in about a third of the patients. Progression was rapid, and signs of circulatory failure appeared in a 2-day period. If death did not occur, recovery occasionally was rapid but usually occurred gradually during an extended period. Most patients had cardiac findings, such as tachycardia, cardiomegaly, electrocardiographic changes, and transitory systolic murmurs. Many patients showed signs of respiratory distress and cyanosis. About one-third of the infants showed signs suggesting neurologic involvement. Of the 45 cases analyzed by Kibrick,[401] only 12 survived.

TABLE 170–18. Signs and Symptoms in Neonatal Coxsackievirus B Myocarditis

Category	Frequency (per cent)
Feeding difficulty	84
Listlessness	81
Cardiac signs	81
Respiratory distress	75
Cyanosis	72
Fever	70
Pharyngitis	64
Hepatosplenomegaly	53
Biphasic course	35
Central nervous system signs	27
Hemorrhage	13
Jaundice	13
Diarrhea	8

Modified from Kibrick, S.: Viral infections of the fetus and newborn. Perspect. Virol. *2*:140, 1961.

In the echovirus 11 nursery outbreak reported by Drew,[186] 5 of 10 babies had tachycardia out of proportion to their fevers. Three of these babies had electrocardiograms; supraventricular tachycardia was noted in all, and ST segment depression was observed in two of the records. Supraventricular tachycardia also has occurred in coxsackievirus B infection.[356] Echovirus 19 also has been associated with myocarditis, and coxsackievirus A9 was noted in a child with pericarditis.[158, 694]

In recent years, neonatal myocarditis due to enteroviruses has been less common than it was in the 1950s and early 1960s. In his review, Morens[522] noted only two instances among 248 severe neonatal enteroviral illnesses.

EXANTHEM. Exanthem as a manifestation of neonatal enteroviral infection has been noted with coxsackieviruses B1 and B5 and echoviruses 4, 5, 9, 11, 16, 17, 18, and 22. In most instances, rash is just a minor manifestation of severe neonatal disease. In 27 infants studied by Lake and colleagues,[429] 41 per cent had exanthem. Cutaneous manifestations usually commence between the third and fifth days of illness. The rash usually is macular or maculopapular. Petechial lesions are noted occasionally. Surprisingly, vesicular lesions have not been described, nor has any rash illness in neonates been associated with coxsackievirus A16. Hall and associates[294] reported two neonates with echovirus 16 infections in which the illnesses were roseola-like. The patients had fevers for 2 and 3 days, defervescence, and then the appearance of maculopapular rashes.

NEUROLOGIC MANIFESTATIONS. As noted in Table 170–17, neurologic illness has been associated with coxsackieviruses B1, B2, B3, B4, and B5 and many echoviruses as well. In neonates, the differentiation of meningitis from meningoencephalitis usually is difficult. Meningoencephalitis is common in infants with sepsis-like illness, and postmortem studies reveal many infants with disseminated viral disease (heart, liver, adrenal glands) in addition to central nervous system involvement. In Moren's review,[522] 50 per cent of the enteroviral infection patients analyzed had encephalitis or meningitis.

The initial clinical findings in neonatal meningitis or meningoencephalitis are similar to those in nonspecific febrile illness or sepsis-like illness. Most often the child is normal and then is noted to be febrile, anorectic, and lethargic. Jaundice frequently is noted in newborns, and vomiting occurs in neonates of all ages. Less common findings include apnea, tremulousness, and general increased tonicity. Seizures occasionally occur.

Cerebrospinal fluid examination reveals considerable variation in protein, glucose, and cellular values. In seven newborns with meningitis due to coxsackievirus B5 studied by Swender and colleagues,[689] the mean cerebrospinal fluid protein value was 244 mg/dL and the highest value was 480 mg/dL. The mean cerebrospinal fluid glucose value was 57 mg/dL, and one of the seven had pronounced hypoglycorrhachia (a value of 12 mg/dL). The mean cerebrospinal fluid leukocyte count in the seven babies was 1069 cells/mm^3 with 67 per cent polymorphonuclear cells. The highest cell count was 4526 cells/mm^3 with 85 per cent polymorphonuclear cells. In another study involving 28 children younger than 2 months of age in which coxsackievirus B5 was the implicated pathogen, 36 per cent of the infants had cerebrospinal fluid leukocyte counts with greater than or equal to 500 cells/mm^3.[473] In this same study, only 13 per cent of the infants had cerebrospinal fluid protein values greater than or equal to 120 mg/dL; 12 per cent of the infants had glucose values less than 40 mg/dL.

In summary, it must be stressed that the cerebrospinal fluid findings in neonatal nonpolio enteroviral infections frequently are similar to those in bacterial disease. In particular, the most consistent finding in bacterial disease, hypoglycorrhachia, is noted in about 10 per cent of newborns with enteroviral meningitis.[129, 198, 429, 473, 689]

Johnson and associates[374] reported a 1-month-old boy with right-sided facial paralysis and loss of abdominal reflexes. The facial paralysis persisted through convalescence; the reflexes returned to normal within 2 weeks. The boy was infected with coxsackievirus B2.

CLINICAL MANIFESTATIONS—POLIOVIRUSES[71, 116, 117, 140, 334]

When a susceptible person has had effective contact with a poliovirus, one of the following responses may occur in this order of frequency: (1) inapparent infection, (2) minor illness (abortive poliomyelitis), (3) nonparalytic poliomyelitis (aseptic meningitis), and (4) paralytic poliomyelitis.

Paralytic poliomyelitis is the most dramatic expression of the infection and the only one clinically recognizable as due to a poliovirus; it accounts for not more than 1 to 2 per cent of infections during epidemics and considerably less under endemic conditions (see Fig. 170–5). The aseptic meningitis syndrome is similarly infrequent; the nonspecific "minor illness" is estimated to occur in 4 to 8 per cent, and 90 to 95 per cent of those infected have inapparent infections. The factors that determine the type of clinical response are poorly understood, but the degree of virulence of the virus and certain host characteristics are important.

Age has a significant effect on patterns of infection; older patients are more likely to have severe paralytic disease and a higher mortality rate. Pregnancy increases the risk, probably owing primarily to hormonal factors but also to the fact that pregnant women may be exposed more to young children, who are the main sources of contagion. Tonsillectomy in the presence of inapparent infection can precipitate bulbar poliomyelitis; there also is evidence that tonsillectomy at any time in the past results in enhanced susceptibility to the bulbar form of the disease. Recent inoculation of diphtheria-tetanus-pertussis vaccine increases the likelihood of paralysis; the site of injection and the site of paralysis appear to be correlated. Physical exertion and trauma around the time of onset also increase the risk of severe paralysis, especially in adults.

Minor Illness (Abortive Poliomyelitis)

The minor illness is mild and nonspecific, with low-grade fever, malaise, anorexia, and sore throat. Physical examination reveals no significant abnormalities, the cerebrospinal fluid is normal, and recovery occurs within 24 to 72 hours. The illness often is so mild that it goes unrecognized, and patients rarely are seen by a physician.

Nonparalytic Poliomyelitis (Aseptic Meningitis)

The onset is with vague malaise followed by fever, headache, aching of the muscles, and sometimes hyperesthesias and paresthesias. Anorexia, nausea, vomiting, constipation, or diarrhea also may be present. The temperature rises to 37.8° to 39.5° C (101° to 103° F); stiffness of the neck, back, and hamstrings soon appears.

Approximately two-thirds of affected children have a short symptom-free interlude between the first phase (minor illness) and the second phase (central nervous system or major illness). This two-phase course is less common in adults, in whom the evolution of symptoms is more insidious. Nuchal and spinal rigidity is necessary for the diagnosis of nonparalytic poliomyelitis during the second phase.

Physical examination reveals nuchal-spinal signs and changes in superficial and deep reflexes. With cooperative patients, the nuchal-spinal signs are sought first by active tests. The child is asked to sit up unassisted. If this causes undue effort, if the knees flex upward, and the patient writhes a bit from side to side in sitting up and uses his or her hands on the bed for the tripod supporting position, there is unmistakable spinal rigidity. Still sitting, the patient is asked to flex chin to chest and is observed for nuchal rigidity. Alternatively, from the supine position, with knees held down gently, the patient is asked to sit up and kiss his or her knees. If the knees draw up sharply or if the maneuver cannot be completed adequately, there is stiffness of the spine due to muscle spasm. If the diagnosis still is uncertain, attempts should be made to elicit Kernig and Brudzinski signs. Gentle forward flexion of the occiput and neck elicits nuchal rigidity, which may precede spinal rigidity. Head drop may be demonstrated by placing the hands under the patient's shoulders and raising the trunk. Normally, the head follows the plane of the trunk, but in poliomyelitis, it often falls backward limply. The frequency of the head-drop sign, even in nonparalytic poliomyelitis, with no subsequent residuals indicates that it is not due to true paresis of the neck flexors. In struggling infants, it may be difficult to distinguish voluntary resistance from clinically important involuntary nuchal rigidity. One may place the infant's shoulders flush with the edge of the table, support the weight of the occiput in the hand, and then flex the head anteriorly. Nuchal rigidity that persists during this maneuver may be interpreted as involuntary. When not closed, the anterior fontanel also may be tense or bulging.

In the early stages, the reflexes normally are active and remain so unless paralysis supervenes. Changes in reflexes, either increased or depressed, may precede weakness by 12 to 24 hours; hence, it is important to detect them, especially in nonparalytic patients managed at home. The superficial reflexes (i.e., cremasteric and abdominal and the reflexes of the spinal and gluteal muscles) usually are the first to be diminished. The spinal and gluteal reflexes are elicited by tapping segmentally downward on each side of the spine and buttocks. These reflexes may disappear before the abdominal and cremasteric ones do. Changes in the deep tendon reflexes, whether exaggerated or depressed, generally occur 8 to 24 hours after depression of superficial reflexes and indicate impending paresis of the extremities.

Laboratory findings consist of a normal or slightly elevated white blood cell count and the characteristic cerebrospinal fluid changes of aseptic meningitis: approximately 20 to 300 cells, predominantly lymphocytes, a normal glucose level, and normal or slightly elevated protein. If a spinal tap is performed in the first few hours after onset, there may be a predominance of polymorphonuclear leukocytes, but this shifts in 6 to 12 hours to more than 90 per cent lymphocytes. If there is no further progression of clinical signs, the disease remains nonparalytic, the temperature falls to normal, and signs of meningeal irritation gradually disappear. Recovery ensues in 3 to 10 days, depending on the severity of the illness.

Paralytic Poliomyelitis

The manifestations of paralytic poliomyelitis are those enumerated earlier for nonparalytic poliomyelitis plus weakness of one or more muscle groups, either skeletal or cranial. Patients destined to develop paralysis often wear an anxious expression; they are extremely alert, restless, and flushed and appear acutely ill. The fever is higher than in abortive disease, and there may be intense muscle pain. Shortly before actual muscle weakness is detected, superficial and deep reflexes often diminish or disappear on the affected side. Frequently, there is a symptom-free interlude of several days between the initial illness phase and the recurrence of symptoms that culminate in paralysis.

The onset of paralysis may be extraordinarily sudden, progressing in a few hours to complete loss of motion of one or more extremities. Asymmetric involvement is typical in the milder cases. More gradual spread of weakness also occurs and may continue over a period of 3 to 5 days. Bladder paralysis of 1 to 3 days' duration occurs in approximately 20 per cent of patients, and bowel atony is common, occasionally to the point of paralytic ileus. In general, when the fever subsides, no further paralysis is likely. Lower limbs are affected more commonly than upper, but in severe cases there may be quadriplegia and loss of function in intercostal, abdominal, and trunk muscles, with resultant respiratory difficulty. Superficial and deep reflexes in the affected limbs are lost; twitchings of the muscles and diffuse fasciculations may be seen transiently. Sensory abnormalities are rare but do occur.

Flaccid paralysis is the most obvious clinical expression of the neuronal changes. The ensuing muscular atrophy is due to denervation plus the atrophy of disuse. The pain, spasticity, nuchal and spinal rigidity, and hypertonia early in the illness probably are due to lesions of the brain stem, spinal ganglia, and posterior columns. Respiratory and cardiac arrhythmias, blood pressure and vasomotor changes, and the like reflect damage to vital centers in the medulla.

On physical examination, the distribution of paralysis is characteristically spotty. To detect mild muscular weakness, it often is necessary to apply gentle resistance in opposition to the muscle group being tested. In the spinal form, there is weakness of some of the muscles of the neck, abdomen, trunk, diaphragm, thorax, or extremities. In the bulbar form, there is weakness in the motor distribution of one or more cranial nerves with or without dysfunction of the vital centers of respiration and circulation. Patients with bulbar disease often are extremely agitated, even delirious, or they may become stuporous. The tenth cranial nerve nuclei most commonly are involved, resulting in paralysis of the pharynx, soft palate, and vocal cords. Facial paralysis is less common; it usually is asymmetric, involving only selected muscle groups. Ocular palsies are unusual.

Components of both bulbar and spinal forms occur together in bulbospinal poliomyelitis. In the encephalitic form of the disease, irritability, disorientation, drowsiness, and coarse tremors not explained by inadequate ventilation are noted. Even during poliomyelitis epidemics, this form can be recognized only if some peripheral or cranial nerve paralysis coexists or ensues. Hypoxia and hypercapnia due to inadequate ventilation from respiratory insufficiency may produce disorientation without true encephalitis.

A number of components acting together may produce insufficiency of ventilation (Table 170–19). The most serious consequences are hypoxia and hypercapnia, which may produce profound effects on many other systems. Respiratory insufficiency should be detected early to diminish its widespread effects, and because the situation may shift rapidly, continued clinical evaluation is essential. Despite weakness of the respiratory muscles, the patient may respond with so much respiratory effort that normal alveolar ventilation is maintained. In fact, the increased effort (associated with anxiety and fear) actually may produce overventilation at the outset, resulting in respiratory alkalosis. Such effort is fatiguing and soon leads to respiratory failure.

For clarity, certain terms characterizing patterns of disease need definition: (1) *Pure spinal poliomyelitis with respiratory insufficiency* refers to tightness, weakness, or paralysis of respiratory muscles (chiefly the diaphragm and intercostals) without discernible clinical involvement of cranial nerves or vital centers. The cervical and thoracic spinal cord segments chiefly are involved. (2) *Pure bulbar poliomyelitis* refers to paralysis of motor cranial nerve nuclei with or without involvement of the vital centers that control respiration, circulation, and body temperature. Involvement of the ninth, tenth, and twelfth cranial nerves is most important because this results in paralysis of the pharynx, tongue, and larynx with consequent airway obstruction. (3) *Bulbospinal poliomyelitis with respiratory insufficiency* refers to involvement of the respiratory muscles with coexisting bulbar paralysis.

The clinical findings resulting from involvement of the respiratory muscles are (1) anxious expression, (2) inability to speak without frequent pauses, resulting in short, jerky, "breathless" sentences, which can be demonstrated by asking the child to count numbers serially, (3) increased respiratory rate, (4) movement of the alae nasi and of the accessory muscles of respiration, (5) inability to cough or sniff with full depth, (6) paradoxic abdominal movements due to diaphragmatic immobility from spasm or weakness of one or both

TABLE 170–19. Common Sources of Hypoxia and Hypercapnia in Poliomyelitis

1. Cranial nerves IX to XII involved, with
   a. Pharyngeal paralysis and pooling of secretions
   b. Laryngeal involvement—either spasm of laryngeal muscles or paralysis of vocal cords
   c. Lingual paralysis
   d. Tracheal accumulation of secretions due to inability to cough
   e. Aspiration of vomitus
2. Vital center involvement with
   a. Inefficient, irregular respiration
   b. Cardiovascular disturbance
   c. Hyperpyrexia causing increased oxygen consumption
3. Cervical and spinal cord involvement causing paresis of the primary and accessory muscles of respiration
4. Pulmonary complications, viz., pneumonia, atelectasis, and edema
5. Contributory factors
   a. Panic
   b. Gastric dilatation
   c. Sedation
   d. Inadequate equipment, viz., small-bore tracheostomy tubes, unsuitable respirator settings, and the like

From Cherry, J. D.: Enteroviruses. *In* Behrman, R. E., and Vaughan, V. C. (eds.): Nelson Textbook of Pediatrics. 12th ed. Philadelphia, W. B. Saunders, 1983, pp. 791–804.

leaves, and (7) relative immobility of the intercostal spaces, which may be segmental, unilateral, or bilateral. When the arms are weak and especially when deltoid paralysis occurs, one should beware of impending respiratory paralysis because the phrenic nerve nuclei are in adjacent areas of the spinal cord. Observing the patient's capacity for thoracic breathing while the abdominal muscles are splinted manually indicates minor degrees of paresis. Light manual splinting of the thoracic cage helps to assess the effectiveness of diaphragmatic movement.

The clinical findings of bulbar poliomyelitis with respiratory difficulty (other than paralysis of extraocular, facial, and masticatory muscles) include (1) nasal twang to the voice or cry due to palatal and pharyngeal weakness (hard-consonant words such as "cookie" or "candy" bring this out best); (2) inability to swallow smoothly, resulting in accumulation of saliva in the pharynx and indicating partial immobility (holding the larynx lightly and asking the patient to swallow confirms immobility); (3) accumulated pharyngeal secretions, which may cause irregular respiration because each inspiration must be "planned" and cannot be "subconscious" in view of the risk of aspirating; the respirations thus may appear interrupted and abnormal even to the point of falsely simulating intercostal or diaphragmatic weakness; (4) the impossibility of effective coughing, with resultant constant fatiguing efforts to clear the throat; (5) nasal regurgitation of saliva and fluids due to palatal paralysis, with inability to separate the oropharynx from the nasopharynx during swallowing; (6) deviation of the palate, uvula, or tongue; (7) involvement of vital centers, manifested by irregularity in rate, depth, and rhythm of respiration; by cardiovascular alterations that include blood pressure changes (especially increased), alternate flushing and mottling of the skin, and cardiac arrhythmias; and by rapid changes in body temperature; (8) paralysis of one or both vocal cords, causing hoarseness, aphonia, and ultimately asphyxia unless recognized by laryngoscopy and managed by immediate tracheostomy; and (9) the "rope sign," an acute angulation between the chin and larynx due to weakness of the hyoid muscles (the hyoid bone is pulled posteriorly, narrowing the hypopharyngeal inlet).

Myocardial failure sometimes develops secondary to pulmonary complications or as a result of acute myocarditis.

The initial presentation of poliovirus infection on occasion can resemble that of Guillain-Barré syndrome.[768]

Congenital Infections

ABORTION. Poliomyelitis is associated with an increased incidence of abortion. Horn[327] noted 43 abortions in 325 pregnancies complicated by maternal poliomyelitis. Abortion was related directly to the severity of the maternal illness, including the degree of fever during the acute phase of illness. However, abortion also occurred in association with mild nonparalytic poliomyelitis. Siegel and Greenberg[665] noted that fetal death occurred in 14 of 30 instances (46.7 per cent) of maternal poliomyelitis during the first trimester. Kaye and associates[391] reviewed the literature in 1953 and noted 19 abortions in 101 cases of poliomyelitis in pregnancy. In a small study in Evanston Hospital, the abortion rate in maternal poliomyelitis was little different from the expected rate.[76]

CONGENITAL MALFORMATIONS. Although isolated instances of congenital malformation and maternal poliomyelitis have been noted, there is little statistical evidence that polioviruses are teratogens. In their review of the literature Kaye and colleagues[391] noted six anomalies in 101 infants born to mothers with poliomyelitis during pregnancy. In the reviews of Horn,[327] Bates,[43] and Siegel and Greenberg,[665] no evidence of maternal polioviral infection–induced anomalies was noted. Similarly, there is no evidence that infection with poliovirus vaccine during pregnancy causes congenital malformations.[302]

PREMATURITY AND STILLBIRTH. In Horn's[327] study of 325 pregnancies, nine infants died in utero. In each instance, the mother was critically ill with poliomyelitis. Horn[327] also noted that 45 infants weighed less than 6 pounds, and 17 of these had a birth weight of less than 5 pounds. These low birth weight infants were born predominantly to mothers who had poliomyelitis early in pregnancy. In New York City, Siegel and Greenberg[665] also noted an increase in prematurity after maternal poliomyelitis infection. This was related specifically to maternal paralytic poliomyelitis.

Neonatal Infections

GENERAL. In the excellent review by Bates[43] in 1955, 58 cases of poliomyelitis in infants younger than 1 month of age were described. Although complete data were not available on many of the cases, 51 had paralysis, died of their disease, or both. Of the total number of infants on whom there were clinical data, only one had nonparalytic disease. More than half of the cases were secondary to maternal disease. Because others have noted congenital infection without symptomatic maternal infection, infection in the mother probably was the source for an even greater percentage of the neonatal illnesses. The incubation period of neonatal poliomyelitis has not been determined, and it therefore is difficult to know how many of the babies were infected in utero. Probably, most illnesses that occurred within the first 5 days of life were congenital.

The majority of the neonates had symptoms of fever, anorexia or dysphagia, and listlessness. Almost half of the infants noted in this review died, and of those surviving, 48 per cent had residual paralysis.

INFECTION ACQUIRED IN UTERO. Elliott and associates[200] described an infant girl in whom "complete flaccidity" was noted at birth. This child's mother had had mild paralytic poliomyelitis, the onset of minor illness occurring 19 days prior to the infant's birth. Fetal movements had ceased 6 days prior to delivery, suggesting that paralysis had occurred at this time. On examination, the baby was severely atonic; when supported under the back, she was passively opisthotonic. Respiratory efforts were abortive and confined to accessory muscles; laryngoscopy revealed complete flaccidity in the larynx.

Johnson and Stimson[371] reported a case in which the mother's probable abortive infection occurred 6 weeks prior to the birth of the baby. The baby initially was thought to be normal but apparently underwent no medical examination until the fourth day of life. At this time, the physician noted right hemiplegia. On the following day, a more complete examination revealed a lateral bulging of the right abdomen accompanied by crying and the maintenance of the lower extremities in a frog-leg position. Adduction and flexion at the hips were weak, and the knee and ankle jerks were absent. Laboratory studies were unremarkable except for the examination of the cerebrospinal fluid. This revealed 20 lymphocytes and a protein count of 169 mg/dL. During a 6-month period, this child's paralysis gradually improved and resulted in only residual weakness of the left lower extremity.

Paresis of the left arm was noted in another child with apparent transplacentally acquired poliomyelitis shortly after birth.[462] At 2 days of age, the baby was quadriplegic, but patellar reflexes were present and there were no respiratory or swallowing difficulties. This child had pneumonia at 3 weeks of age, but aside from this, general neurologic improvement occurred. Examination at 8 weeks of age revealed bilateral atrophy of the shoulder girdle muscles. The cerebrospinal fluid in this case revealed 63 leukocytes/mm^3, 29 per cent of them polymorphonuclear cells, and a protein count of 128 mg/dL.

All three of the infants just discussed apparently were infected in utero several days before birth. Their symptoms were exclusively neurologic; fever, irritability, and vomiting did not occur.

POSTNATALLY ACQUIRED INFECTION. In contrast with infections acquired in utero, those acquired postnatally are more typical of classic poliomyelitis. Shelokov and Weinstein[662] described a child who was asymptomatic at birth. Onset of minor symptoms in the mother occurred 3 weeks, and major symptoms 1 day, prior to delivery. On the sixth day of life, the infant suddenly became ill with watery diarrhea. He looked grayish and pale. On the following day, he was irritable, lethargic, and limp and had a temperature of 38° C. Mild opisthotonus and weakness of both lower extremities developed. He was responsive to sound, light, and touch. The cerebrospinal fluid had an elevated protein level and an increased number of leukocytes. His condition worsened during a total period of 3 days, and then gradual improvement began. At 1 year of age, he had severe residual paralysis of the right leg and moderate weakness in the left leg.

Baskin and associates[41] described two infants with neonatal poliomyelitis. The first child, whose mother had severe poliomyelitis at the time of delivery, was well for 3 days and then developed a temperature of 38.3° C. On the fifth day of life, the boy became listless and cyanotic. Cerebrospinal fluid examination revealed a protein level of 300 mg/dL and 108 leukocyte cells/mm^3. His condition worsened, and extreme flaccidity, irregular respiration, and progressive cyanosis developed; he died on the seventh day of life. The second infant was a boy who was well until he was 8 days old but then became listless and developed a temperature of 38.3° C. During the next 5 days, flaccid quadriplegia developed, as well as irregular, rapid, and shallow respirations and the inability to swallow. The child died on the fourteenth day of life. His mother had developed acute poliomyelitis 6 days before the onset of his symptoms.

Abramson and colleagues[2] reported four children with neonatal poliomyelitis, two of whom died. In three of the children, the illnesses were typical of acute poliomyelitis in older children. The other child died at 13 days of age with generalized paralysis. The onset of his illness was difficult to define, and he was never febrile.

Bates[43] described infants with acute poliomyelitis with clinical illnesses similar to those that occur in older persons.

DIAGNOSIS AND DIFFERENTIAL DIAGNOSIS

Clinical Diagnosis

The clinical differentiation of enteroviral disease frequently is thought to be impossible. Although it is true that treatable bacterial illnesses always should be considered and treated first, it also is true that, when all the circumstances of a particular illness are considered, enteroviral diseases can be suspected on clinical grounds. The most important factors in clinical diagnosis are season of the year, geographic location, exposure, incubation period, and clinical symptoms.

In temperate climates, enteroviral prevalence is distinctly seasonal, so disease usually is seen in the summer and fall. Enteroviral disease is less likely in the winter. In the tropics, enteroviruses are prevalent throughout the year, and the season, therefore, is not diagnostically helpful.

As with all infectious illnesses, the knowledge of exposure and incubation time is important. A careful history of maternal illness is critical in neonatal disease. For example, nonspecific, mild, febrile illness in a mother that occurs in the summer and fall should warn of the possibility of severe neonatal illness. Specific findings (i.e., aseptic meningitis, pleurodynia, herpangina, pericarditis, myocarditis) should alert the clinician to enteroviral illnesses. The short incubation period of enteroviral infections should be considered.

Laboratory Diagnosis

Virus Isolation and Detection Techniques

Most viral diagnostic laboratories have facilities for the recovery of the majority of enteroviruses that cause illness. A three-tissue culture system that includes primary monkey kidney, a diploid, human embryonic lung fibroblast cell strain, and the RD cell line allow the isolation of virtually all coxsackieviruses B and echoviruses and some coxsackieviruses A (e.g., coxsackieviruses A9 and A16). In a study in which Buffalo green monkey kidney cells and subpassages of primary human embryonic kidney cells were used in addition to primary monkey kidney and human diploid fibroblast (MRC-5) cells, the enterovirus recovery rate was increased 11 per cent.[134] For a complete diagnostic isolation spectrum, suckling mouse inoculation also should be performed.

Proper selection and handling of specimens are most important in the isolation of viruses. Enteroviral infections tend to be generalized, so collection of material from multiple sites is important; specimens should be collected from any or all of the following: nose, throat, stool, blood, urine, cerebrospinal fluid, and any other body fluids that are available. Swabs from the nose, throat, and rectum should be placed in a carrying medium containing a small amount of protein. Hanks balanced salt solution with 2 per cent agamma calf serum and antibiotics is satisfactory. Fluid specimens should be collected in sterile vials; specimens of postmortem material are collected best in vials that contain carrying medium. In general, specimens should be refrigerated immediately after collection and during transportation to the laboratory. It is important not to expose specimens to sunlight during transportation. If it is known that an extended period will elapse before a specimen is processed in the laboratory, it is advisable to ship and store it frozen.

Contrary to popular belief, tissue culture evidence of enteroviral growth takes only a few days in many cases and less than a week in most.[316] The use of the spin amplification, shell vial technique, and monoclonal antibodies has been shown to reduce significantly the time of detection in enteroviral cultures.[414, 706] After isolation of an enterovirus, its type identification is performed conventionally by neutralization, and this process, unfortunately, frequently takes a long time.

Nucleic acid techniques with cDNA and RNA probes have been shown to be useful for the direct identification of enteroviruses.[93, 175, 345, 579, 618, 621, 623] Of most importance today, however, has been the development of a number of polymerase chain reaction techniques. Since 1990, innumerable reports have described enteroviral polymerase chain reaction methods and their use in identifying enterovirus RNA in clinical specimens.[1, 5, 15, 130, 146, 147, 149, 194, 229, 236, 296, 456, 475, 495, 530, 555, 617, 619, 640, 646, 659, 660, 663, 687, 695, 699, 757, 765, 766] Polymerase chain reaction has proved most useful for the direct identification of enteroviruses in the cerebrospinal fluid of patients with meningitis.[619, 642, 695, 699, 766] Compared with culture of cerebrospinal fluid specimens, polymerase chain reaction is more rapid and sensitive, and the specificity is equal. The shortcoming of polymerase chain reaction is that enterovirus RNA is identified but the specific enteroviral type is not determined.

Polymerase chain reaction also has proved useful in the identification of enteroviruses in blood, urine, and throat specimens.[5, 555, 660] Enteroviral RNA also has been identified in a number of tissue specimens from patients with chronic medical conditions, such as idiopathic dilated cardiomyopathy. However, as discussed earlier (Cardiovascular Manifestations), the possibility of lack of specificity (false-positive results) is a concern. Polioviruses can be separated from other enteroviruses, and poliovirus vaccine strains can be identified rapidly by polymerase chain reaction.[1, 130, 194, 765]

Serology

Except in special circumstances, the use of serologic techniques in the primary diagnosis of suspected enteroviral infections is impractical. Standard serologic study depends on the demonstration of an antibody titer rise to a specific virus as an indication of infection with that agent. Although hemagglutination inhibition and complement fixation take only a short time to perform, these tests can be performed only after the collection of a second, convalescent-phase blood specimen. These tests also are impractical in searching for the cause of a specific illness in a child because there are so many antigenically different enteroviruses. Because there are no common group antigens, the identification of a particular illness might require the performance of more than 60 individual serologic tests.

In the evaluation of a patient with a suspected enteroviral infection, serum should be collected as soon as possible after the onset of illness and then again 2 to 4 weeks later. This serum should be stored frozen. In most clinical situations, it is not necessary to carry out serologic tests on the collected serum because demonstration of an antibody titer rise in the serum of an infant from whom a specific virus has been isolated from a body fluid obviously is superfluous. However, collected serum can be useful diagnostically if the prevalence of specific enteroviruses in a community is known. In this situation, it is relatively easy to look for antibody titer changes to a selected number of viral types. More rapid diagnosis utilizing a single serum is possible if a search for specific IgM enteroviral antibody is made.[108, 133, 245, 260, 261, 271, 664, 776]

Unfortunately, no enterovirus IgM antibody tests are commercially available. Commercial laboratories do offer enteroviral complement-fixation antibody panels. However, the results of these tests in the clinical setting almost always are meaningless unless acute- and convalescent-phase sera are analyzed.

Histology

There are no specific histologic findings in enteroviral infections such as those seen in cytomegalovirus or herpes simplex virus infections. However, tissues can be examined for specific enteroviral antigens by immunofluorescence.[86]

Differential Diagnosis

The differential diagnosis of enteroviral infections depends on the clinical manifestations. In general, the most important considerations relate to bacterial diseases, such as those commonly associated with pharyngitis, pneumonia, pericarditis, meningitis, and septicemia. Other viruses must be considered in upper respiratory illnesses, gastrointestinal infections, rashes, encephalitis, and neonatal illness.

Paralytic poliomyelitis usually presents no diagnostic problem in the presence of an outbreak, but sporadic cases are another matter, especially in countries such as the United States, where the disease (except for the vaccine-associated form) has disappeared and many pediatricians have never seen a case. Rarely, other enteroviruses have been shown to cause paralytic syndromes that are indistinguishable from poliomyelitis, but the muscle weakness observed usually is brief and not severe.

Several other diseases must be considered in the differential diagnosis of sporadic instances of paralytic illness. Guillain-Barré syndrome is the most common and difficult differential problem. Fever, headache, and meningeal signs usually are less common in Guillain-Barré syndrome; paralysis characteristically is symmetric, and sensory changes are common. Also in Guillain-Barré syndrome, the cerebrospinal fluid contains few cells but a significant elevation of the protein value. Other illnesses confused with paralytic poliomyelitis include peripheral neuritis (postinjection, toxic, herpes zoster), arboviral infections, rabies, tetanus, botulism, and tick paralysis.

TREATMENT

Specific Therapy

No specific therapy for any enteroviral infection commonly is recognized. In severe, catastrophic, and generalized neonatal infection, it is likely that the baby received no specific antibody for the particular virus from the mother. In this situation, it probably is advisable to administer immunoglobulin to the infant because high titers of neutralizing antibodies to many enteroviruses usually are present in immunoglobulin.[167] There is little evidence that this therapy is beneficial; however, it can be expected to stop further organ seeding secondary to continued viremia. Intravenous or intraventricular immunoglobulin and hyperimmune plasma administration have been useful on some occasions and not on others in enteroviral infections in patients with agammaglobulinemia.[6, 70, 161, 191, 203, 292, 318, 483, 492, 718, 732]

Abzug and associates[4] performed a small but controlled study in which nine enterovirus-infected neonates received intravenous immunoglobulin and seven similarly infected infants received supportive care. In this study, there was no significant difference in clinical scores, antibody values, or magnitude of viremia and viruria in those treated compared with the control infants. However, five infants received intravenous immunoglobulin with a high neutralizing antibody titer ($\geq$1:800) to their individual viral isolates, and they experienced a more rapid cessation of viremia and viruria. A neonate with disseminated echovirus 11 infection with hepatitis, pneumonitis, meningitis, disseminated intravascular coagulation, decreased renal function, and anemia who survived after receiving a large dose of intravenous immunoglobulin and supportive care has been described.[376]

Jantausch and associates[362] reported an infant with a disseminated echovirus 11 infection who survived after maternal plasma transfusions. A neonate with fulminant echovirus 11 infection survived after orthotopic liver transplantation.[142]

In severe illnesses such as neonatal myocarditis or encephalitis, it frequently is tempting to administer corticosteroids. Although some workers have felt that this therapy has been beneficial in coxsackieviral myocarditis, I believe that corticosteroids should not be given during acute enteroviral infections. The deleterious effects of these agents in coxsackieviral infections of mice particularly are persuasive factors in this opinion.[406]

Because the possibility of bacterial sepsis cannot be ruled out in many instances of enteroviral infections, antibiotics frequently should be administered for the most likely potential pathogens. Care in antibiotic selection and administration is urged so that drug toxicity is not added to the problems of the patient.

Nonspecific Therapy

Mild, Nonspecific, Febrile Illness

In patients in whom fever is the only symptom, careful observation is important. Many patients who eventually become severely ill initially display 2 to 3 days of fever without other localized findings. Care should be taken to administer adequate fluids to febrile infants, and excessive elevation of temperature should be prevented if possible.

Myocarditis

There is no specific therapy for myocarditis. However, congestive heart failure and arrhythmias occur, and these should be treated by the usual methods. In administering digitalis to patients with enteroviral myocarditis, careful attention to the initial dosage is most important because the heart often is extremely sensitive; frequently, only small amounts of digoxin are necessary.

Meningoencephalitis

In patients with meningoencephalitis, convulsions, cerebral edema, and disturbances of fluid and electrolyte balance all occur frequently and respond to treatment. Seizures are treated best with phenobarbital, phenytoin, or lorazepam. Cerebral edema can be treated with urea, mannitol, or large doses of corticosteroids. As noted, it seems unwise to use corticosteroids in active enteroviral infections because the local benefit might be outweighed by the overall deleterious effects. Fluids should be monitored closely, and serum electrolyte levels should be determined frequently because inappropriate antidiuretic hormone secretion is common.

Poliomyelitis

The broad principles of management are to allay fear, to minimize ensuing skeletal deformities, to anticipate and meet complications in addition to the neuromusculoskeletal ones, and to prepare the child and family for the prolonged treatment that may be required and for permanent disability when this seems likely. Patients with the nonparalytic and mildly paralytic forms may be treated at home.

For the abortive form of poliomyelitis, simple analgesics, sedatives, and attractive diet and bed rest until the child's temperature is normal for several days suffice. Avoidance of exertion for the ensuing 2 weeks is desirable, and there should be careful neuromusculoskeletal examination 2 months later to detect any minor involvement.

Treatment for nonparalytic poliomyelitis is similar to that for the abortive form, relief being indicated in particular for the discomfort of muscle tightness and spasm of the neck, trunk, and extremities. Analgesics alone are not so effective as when combined with the application of hot packs for 15 to 30 minutes every 2 to 4 hours. Hot tub baths sometimes are useful. A firm bed is desirable. A footboard should be used to keep the feet at a right angle to the legs. Muscular discomfort and spasm may continue for some weeks, necessitating hot packs and gentle physical therapy. Such patients also should be examined carefully 2 months after apparent recovery to detect minor residuals that might cause postural problems in later years.

Most patients with paralytic poliomyelitis require hospitalization. A calm atmosphere is desired. Suitable body alignment is necessary to avoid excessive skeletal deformity. A neutral position with the feet at a right angle, knees slightly flexed, and hips and spine straight is achieved by use of boards, sandbags, and, occasionally, light splint shells. Active and passive motions are indicated as soon as the pain has disappeared. Opiates and sedatives are permissible only if no impairment of ventilation is present or impending. Constipation is common, and fecal impaction should be prevented. When bladder paralysis occurs, a parasympathetic stimulant (e.g., bethanechol [Urecholine], 5 to 10 mg orally or 2.5 to 5 mg subcutaneously) may induce voiding in 15 to 30 minutes; some patients do not respond, and others have nausea, vomiting, and palpitation. Bladder paresis rarely lasts more than a few days. If bethanechol fails, manual compression of the bladder and the psychologic effect of running water should be tried. If catheterization must be performed, strict asepsis is essential.

An interesting diet and a relatively high fluid intake should be started at once unless there is vomiting. Additional salt should be provided if the environmental temperature is high or if the application of hot packs induces sweating. Anorexia is common initially. Adequate dietary and fluid intake can be maintained by the placement of a central venous catheter. The orthopedist and the physiatrist should see these patients as early in the illness as possible and assume responsibility before fixed deformities develop.

The management of pure bulbar poliomyelitis consists essentially of maintaining the airway and avoiding all risks of inhalation of saliva, food, or vomitus. Gravity drainage of accumulated secretions is favored by the head-low (foot of the bed elevated 20 to 25 degrees) prone position with the face to one side. Aspirators with rigid or semirigid tips are preferred for direct oral and pharyngeal use, and soft flexible catheters may be used for nasopharyngeal aspiration. Fluid and electrolyte balance is maintained best by intravenous infusion because tube or oral feeding in the first few days may incite vomiting. After the first few days, sips of sterile water may be given from a spoon, with increments as indicated by ability to swallow. In addition to close observation for respiratory insufficiency, the blood pressure should be taken at least twice daily. Hypertension is not uncommon and occasionally leads to hypertensive encephalopathy. Patients with pure bulbar poliomyelitis may require tracheostomy because of vocal cord paralysis or constriction of the hypopharynx. The majority of patients with pure bulbar poliomyelitis who recover have little residual impairment; some patients exhibit mild dysphagia and occasional vocal fatigue with slurring of speech.

Impaired ventilation must be recognized early; mounting anxiety, restlessness, and fatigue are early indications for prompt intervention. Tracheostomy is indicated for some patients with pure bulbar poliomyelitis, spinal respiratory muscle paralysis, and bulbospinal paralysis. Unlike other patients for whom tracheostomy is performed, these patients generally are unable to cough, sometimes for many months. Frequent and swift endotracheal aspiration under aseptic conditions is necessary. Mechanical ventilation often is needed. Patients are fully conscious and aware; terrifying procedures are best carried out in an outward atmosphere of calm. Explaining the procedure and having parents on hand may be helpful. Reduction in thoracic compliance occurs early, and higher-than-expected pressure gradients may be required to achieve adequate ventilation. Weaning a patient from dependency on respiratory assistance is a torturous process, as is total musculoskeletal rehabilitation. Motivation of the patient and of the team of personnel is paramount.

PROGNOSIS

The prognosis in nonpolio enteroviral infections is excellent in the great majority of instances. Virtually all morbidity and mortality are related to cardiac and neurologic disease in older children and to these diseases plus general disseminated infection in neonates.

The prognosis in poliomyelitis varies with the degree of muscle involvement. In patients with mild muscle weakness, complete recovery is the rule. If paralysis is present, recovery of muscle function continues for a period of approximately 18 months to 2 years. By 3 months, about 60 per cent of the ultimate improvement has been achieved, and by 6 months, 80 per cent. The final result depends on the extent and localization of nerve cell damage.

Respiratory failure is responsible for most of the deaths in paralytic poliomyelitis. With the many recent improvements in techniques for handling this complication, the overall mortality rate has been reduced to approximately 4 per cent; in the bulbar form and in adults, it still may be as high as 10 per cent.

Occasionally, patients who have had paralytic poliomyelitis develop new neuromuscular symptoms later in life.[94, 168, 169, 373, 599, 751, 752] Although the cause of this late-onset weakness and muscle atrophy is not completely understood, it is most likely the result of routine attrition of anterior horn cells associated with aging rather than persistent neural infection with polioviruses. However, it is possible that specific immunopathologic mechanisms may play a role in some instances.[257]

Recently, Leparc-Goffant and associates[443] presented data suggesting the presence of poliovirus-specific genomic sequences in the cerebrospinal fluid of patients with postpolio syndrome. However, Muir and colleagues,[531] who performed similar studies, found no association of chronic neurologic disease with the presence of enteroviral RNA in the cerebrospinal fluid.

PREVENTION

Nonpolio Enteroviral Infections

Attenuated viral vaccines for enteroviruses other than polioviruses are not available. However, if a virulent enteroviral type were to emerge, a specific attenuated virus for active immunization probably could be developed.

Passive protection with intravenous immunoglobulin may be useful in preventing disease. In practice, however, this would seem worthwhile only in sudden and virulent nursery outbreaks. For example, if several cases of myocarditis occurred in a nursery, it would seem reasonable to administer intravenous immunoglobulin to all babies in the nursery. Pooled human immunoglobulin in most instances can be expected to contain antibodies against coxsackieviruses B1, B2, B3, B4, and B5, as well as several coxsackieviruses A and echoviruses.[167] Therefore, this procedure would offer protection to those infants without transplacentally acquired specific antibody who had not become infected yet. Immune serum possibly has been useful in the management of two nursery enteroviral outbreaks.[92, 536]

Polioviral Infections

In the United States, the total annual number of paralytic cases fell from an average of 16,000 in the 5 years before the introduction of vaccine to approximately 10 cases per year between 1980 and 1984. The experience in 1979, however, when 26 paralytic cases were reported, served as a reminder that virulent polioviruses still can surface among susceptible persons.[101, 103] Most of the 1979 cases occurred in Pennsylvania and several other states among Amish population groups who had not been immunized. There was a similar epidemic in Connecticut in 1972 involving a pocket of unimmunized students in a Christian Science school.[105] These outbreaks reflect the fact that poliomyelitis still occurs in many parts of the world. The possibility of introduction of virulent strains is ever present, and only through continued and extensive immunization programs can the disease be prevented from reappearing in epidemic form.[23, 328]

The remarkable overall record of decline in paralytic poliomyelitis in the United States is a result of the development and use of two effective vaccines.[328] Inactivated poliovirus vaccine, the first to be licensed, was used extensively beginning in 1955 and considerably reduced the incidence of the disease, although epidemics continued to occur. Live attenuated oral poliovirus vaccine, licensed in 1961 and 1962, subsequently was recommended as the method of choice in the United States, based on its superiority in terms of immunogenic capacity, ability to induce local IgA antibody in the oropharynx and intestinal tract and thus provide greater resistance to reinfection, and ease of administration. Oral poliovirus vaccine gradually supplanted inactivated poliovirus vaccine, and between 1973 and 1978, it was the only vaccine available. Its extraordinary effectiveness at this time, despite reaching only 65 per cent of children younger than 5 years of age with the recommended three doses, suggests that the capacity of the attenuated strains to spread contributes to a much higher immunization rate than is indicated by vaccination statistics. The potential impact of such spread on the immunity of the population is illustrated by the observations of Fox and Hall,[226] who conducted long-term virologic surveillance of middle-income families in Seattle. Polioviruses (vaccine strains) accounted for 50 per cent of the 2937 viral isolates from healthy children, their parents, and others in the community. In an analysis of 611 of the poliovirus isolates, it was found that 75.6 per cent were from vaccinees, 10.5 per cent were from vaccinee contacts, and 14 per cent were in persons without recent contact with vaccine or a vaccinee. These findings provide a vivid picture of the pervasiveness of the attenuated strains and their continuous circulation in the population. This feature also is supported by the almost invariable recovery of polioviruses from weekly samples of sewage collected throughout the year in urban communities.[329]

Despite the striking success of oral vaccine, there have been some problems. One has been the greatly reduced seroconversion rates when the vaccine is given to children living in the tropics: as few as 50 per cent have satisfactory responses in contrast with the more than 95 per cent in the United States and similar countries.[183, 499] Viral interference from other enteroviruses plays some role, and the presence of an inhibitory substance in the oropharynx that prevents significant multiplication of the vaccine strains also may be involved. The seroconversion problem can be lessened by using pulse immunization programs.[368, 629] For example, the strategy of national annual vaccination days twice a year, 2 months apart, has been successful in Cuba, and similar programs that have been well organized at the community level as well as nationally also have been successful.

Another problem with oral poliovirus vaccine and the major problem in the United States has been the occurrence of a small number of vaccine-associated cases of poliomyelitis.[328, 499] The immunogenic effectiveness of the vaccine depends on multiplication of the attenuated strains in the intestinal tract. Because no poliovirus strain is completely stable, progeny of the vaccine strains undergo a certain degree of mutation, which rarely has resulted in increased virulence and in vaccine-associated cases in recipients and in their contacts, most often their parents.

Since 1980, no indigenous cases of wild-poliovirus disease have occurred in the United States.[95, 681] From 1980 to 1989, there were 80 cases of vaccine-associated paralytic poliomyelitis and 5 cases of imported disease. The overall rate of vaccine-associated paralytic poliomyelitis was 1 case per 2.5 million doses of distributed vaccine; the risk for recipients was 1 case per 6.8 million doses, and for household contacts it was 1 case per 6.4 million doses. Of the 80 cases, 30 occurred in vaccinees, 32 occurred in household contacts, 4 were community-acquired, and 14 occurred in immunologically abnormal persons.

Further analysis revealed that the risk associated with the first dose of vaccine was 1 case per 700,000 doses, but it was only 1 case per 6.9 million subsequent doses; for vaccine recipients, the calculated risks were 1 case per 1.4 million initial doses and 1 case per 41.5 million subsequent doses. The calculated risks for contact cases were 1 case per 1.9 million initial doses of vaccine and 1 case per 13.8 million subsequent doses.

Immunodeficient children are at particular risk of acquiring vaccine-associated paralytic poliomyelitis.[104, 681] From 1969 through 1976, 11 per cent of vaccine-associated cases occurred in immunodeficient patients; 10 of 11 of these patients were children and younger than 1 year of age. From 1980 to 1989, 18 per cent of vaccine-associated paralytic poliomyelitis cases occurred in immunodeficient patients.[681]

Although the risks mentioned earlier have been considered acceptable in view of the benefits provided, the question has been raised repeatedly since the 1970s as to whether the United States should return to the use of inactivated poliovirus vaccines, which does not carry a risk of paralytic disease and has been highly successful in several small European countries in which more than 95 per cent of the population has been immunized.[227, 237, 324, 380, 389, 534, 572, 633–636, 681]

The problem was reviewed in detail by a committee of the Institute of Medicine (IOM) of the National Academy of Sciences, which reported its recommendations in April 1977.[557] The conclusion was that given the situation in the United States, in which at that time not more than 65 per cent of susceptible children were vaccinated, oral poliovirus vaccine should continue to be the principal vaccine for routine immunization. Inactivated poliovirus vaccine, on the other hand, should be provided for two groups: immunodeficient persons, because of their greatly enhanced risk of vaccine-associated disease after receiving the oral vaccine, and adults receiving primary immunization, because of their greater susceptibility to paralytic disease. It also was suggested that the inactivated vaccine be available as an alternative for those who prefer it. In addition, a single dose of trivalent oral poliovirus vaccine was suggested for all entrants to the seventh grade of school as a means of added protection for later years when they become parents.

In January 1988, a panel appointed by the IOM again reviewed policy options for vaccination against poliomyelitis in the United States. The IOM panel concluded that no change in policy should be recommended at that time. However, they did recommend that a new enhanced inactivated poliovirus vaccine replace the old vaccine when inactivated vaccine was indicated. They also suggested that when a new enhanced diphtheria-tetanus-pertussis inactivated poliovirus vaccine became available, a regimen of two or more doses of it followed by the oral vaccine be considered.

In 1996, the United States polio vaccine immunization program was evaluated extensively by both the Advisory Committee on Immunization Practices (ACIP) and the Committee on Infectious Diseases of the American Academy of Pediatrics (AAP). The ACIP has recommended that a sequential schedule of inactivated poliovirus vaccine followed by oral poliovirus vaccine be the schedule of choice in the United States.[569] The schedule consists of two doses of the inactivated vaccine at 2 and 4 months of age and two doses of the oral vaccine at 12 to 18 months and 4 to 6 years of age. Both committees indicate that schedules that include all doses of each vaccine also are acceptable.[299, 569] The reader is advised to consult the recommendations of the ACIP and the AAP as well as the manufacturers' literature for a full consideration of contraindications and indications of polio vaccines.

The parents of prospective vaccinees or the vaccinees themselves should be informed of the two available types of polio vaccines and the risks and benefits of the vaccines for both individuals and the community. Inactivated poliovirus vaccine should be given to persons who have contraindications to oral poliovirus vaccine.

Routine primary poliovirus vaccination of adults older than 18 years of age is not carried out in the United States. However, adults at risk of exposure to wild polioviruses (laboratory workers, international travelers, health care workers) should be immunized. For the vaccination of adults, inactivated poliovirus vaccine is recommended.

Patients with immunodeficiency diseases should not be given oral poliovirus vaccine; live virus also should not be used in households in which an immunodeficient person resides.

Global Eradication of Poliomyelitis

WHO established the Expanded Program on Immunization (EPI) in 1974.[341, 725, 762] After this, the use of oral poliovirus vaccine in developing countries vastly increased. In 1980 in Brazil, it had been demonstrated that mass administration of the oral vaccine with National Immunization Days (NIDs) led to a dramatic reduction in poliomyelitis.[177] This led in 1985 to the targeted polio eradication from the Western Hemisphere by 1990. This campaign was successful in that the last confirmed case of paralytic polio caused by wild poliovirus occurred in 1991 in Peru.[95] In September 1994, an international commission convened by the Pan American Health Organization certified that indigenous transmission of wild poliovirus had been interrupted in the Americas.[96]

In 1988, the World Health Assembly established the objective of global polio eradication by 2000.[341] This program is based on four strategies recommended by WHO: (1) maintenance of high vaccination coverage levels among children with at least three doses of oral poliovirus vaccine, (2) development of sensitive systems of epidemiologic and laboratory surveillance, including use of the standard WHO case definition (a confirmed case of polio is defined as acute flaccid paralysis and at least one of the following: laboratory-confirmed wild poliovirus infection, residual paralysis of 60 days, death, or no follow-up investigation at 60 days), (3) administration of supplementary doses of oral poliovirus vaccine to all young children (usually those younger than 5 years of age) during NIDs to interrupt rapidly poliovirus transmission, and (4) "mopping up" vaccination campaigns—localized campaigns targeted at high-risk areas where wild poliovirus transmission is most likely to persist at low levels. NIDs are mass campaigns over a short period (days to weeks) in which two doses of oral poliovirus vaccine are administered to all children in the target age group, regardless of prior vaccination history, with an interval of 4 to 6 weeks between doses.

From 1985 through 1990, worldwide routine vaccination coverage levels increased from 47 to 85 per cent and stabilized at 80 to 81 per cent from 1991 to 1994.[95] From 1985 through 1994, the number of cases reported annually decreased 84 per cent, from 39,361 to 6241. The number of countries reporting polio cases decreased steadily, from 1985 (99 of 196 [51 per cent]) to 1988 (88 of 196 [45 per cent]) and 1994 (51 of 214 [24 per cent]). In addition, the number of countries reporting zero polio cases increased from 1985 (84 [43 per cent]) to 1988 (104 [53 per cent]) and 1994 (145 [68 per cent]). The number of countries with endemic polio that conducted NIDs each year increased from 15 in 1988 to 37 as of April 14, 1995; 24 additional countries scheduled their first NIDs for later in 1995.

A total of 94 countries implemented surveillance for acute flaccid paralysis to detect all cases of polio that meet the standard WHO case definition and to monitor the circulation of wild polioviruses. WHO has certified 12 regional reference laboratories and 60 national laboratories as members of the Global Polio Laboratory Network and has designated six geographic areas as emerging polio-free zones: the Western Hemisphere, Western and Central Europe, North Africa, southern and eastern Africa, the Middle East, and the Western Pacific.

Despite substantial progress toward global eradication of polio, several challenges remain, including (1) increasing vaccination levels in unvaccinated subpopulations, (2) preventing the reintroduction of wild poliovirus into polio-free areas by eliminating reservoirs in polio-endemic countries (particularly in the Indian subcontinent), (3) increasing the awareness of donor agencies and governments in industrialized countries of the substantial financial and humanitarian benefits of global eradication of polio, thus engendering support from unaffected countries beyond that already provided by organizations such as Rotary International, (4) encouraging all countries that remain polio-endemic to make polio eradication a high priority, including the implementation of NIDs and the initiation of acute flaccid paralysis surveillance, and (5) providing support to vaccination program managers for training to develop managerial skills for implementing and maintaining effective vaccination and surveillance programs in all countries.[95] The success of the polio eradication initiative will depend on finding solutions to these financial, managerial, political, and technical challenges.

References

1. Abraham, R., Chonmaitree, T., McCombs, J., et al.: Rapid detection of poliovirus by reverse transcription and polymerase chain amplification: Application for differentiation between poliovirus and nonpoliovirus enteroviruses. J. Clin. Microbiol. *31*:395–399, 1993.
2. Abramson, H., Greenberg, M., and Magee, M. C.: Poliomyelitis in the newborn infant. J. Pediatr. *43*:167–173, 1953.
3. Abzug, M. J., Levin, M. J., and Rotbart, H. A.: Profile of enterovirus disease in the first two weeks of life. Pediatr. Infect. Dis. J. *12*:820–824, 1993.
4. Abzug, M. J., Keyserling, H. L., Lee, M. L., et al.: Neonatal enterovirus infection: Virology, serology and effects of intravenous immune globulin. Clin. Infect. Dis. *20*:1201–1206, 1995.
5. Abzug, M. J., Loeffelholz, M., and Rotbart, H. A.: Diagnosis of neonatal enterovirus infection by polymerase chain reaction. J. Pediatr. *126*:447–450, 1995.
6. Ackerson, B. R., Raghunathan, R., Keller, M. A., et al.: Echovirus 11 arthritis in a patient with X-linked agammaglobulinemia. Pediatr. Infect. Dis. J. *6*:485–488, 1987.
7. Adler, J. L., Mostow, S. R., Mellin, H., et al.: Epidemiologic investigation of hand, foot, and mouth disease. Infection caused by coxsackievirus A16 in Baltimore, June through September 1968, Am. J. Dis. Child. *120*:309–313, 1970.
8. Agranat, A. L.: A near-fatal case of Coxsackie B myocarditis (with pericarditis) in an adult. S. Afr. Med. J. *35*:831–832, 1961.
9. Ahmad, N., and Abraham, A. A.: Pancreatic isleitis with coxasackie virus B5 infection. Hum. Pathol. *13*:661–662, 1982.
10. Alexander, J. P., Jr., Baden, L., Pallansch, M. A., et al.: Enterovirus 71 infections and neurologic disease: United States, 1977–1991. J. Infect. Dis. *169*:905–908, 1994.
11. Alexander, J. P., Jr., Chapman, L. E., Pallansch, M. A., et al.: Coxsackievirus B2 infection and aseptic meningitis: A focal outbreak among members of a high school football team. J. Infect. Dis. *167*:1201–1205, 1993.
12. Alexander, J. P., and Anderson, L. J.: (Respiratory and Enterovirus Branch, Centers for Disease Control). Personal communication, 1990.
13. Alsop, J., Flewett, T. H., and Foster, J. R.: "Hand-foot-and-mouth disease" in Birmingham in 1959. B. M. J. *2*:1708–1711, 1960.
14. American Academy of Pediatrics: Poliovirus infections. *In* Peter, G. (ed.): 1994 Red Book: Report of the Committee on Infectious Diseases. 23rd ed. Elk Grove Village, IL, American Academy of Pediatrics, 1994, pp. 379–386.
15. Andreoletti, L., Wattre, P., Decoene, C., et al.: Detection of enterovirus-specific RNA sequences in explanted myocardium biopsy specimens from patients with dilated or ischemic cardiomyopathy. Clin. Infect. Dis. *21*:1315–1317, 1995.
16. Archard, L. C., Bowles, N. E., Behan, P. O., et al.: Postviral fatigue syndrome: Persistence of enterovirus RNA in muscle and elevated creatinine kinase. J. R. Soc. Med. *81*:326–329, 1988.
17. Archibald, E., and Purdham, D. R.: Coxsackievirus type: A16 infection in a neonate. Arch. Dis. Child. *54*:649, 1979.
18. Arnon, R., Naor, N., Davidson, S., et al.: Fatal outcome of neonatal echovirus 19 infection. Pediatr. Infect. Dis. J. *10*:788–789, 1991.
19. Arola, A., Kalimo, H., Ruuskanen, O., et al.: Experimental myocarditis induced by two different coxsackievirus B3 variants: Aspects of pathogenesis and comparison of diagnostic methods. J. Med. Virol. *47*:251–259, 1995.
20. Aronson, M. D., and Phillips, C. A.: Coxsackievirus B5 infections in acute oliguric renal failure. J. Infect. Dis. *132*:302–306, 1975.
21. Artenstein, M. S., Cadigan, F. C., Jr., and Buescher, E. L.: Clinical and epidemiological features of Coxsackie group B virus infections. Ann. Intern. Med. *63*:597–603, 1965.
22. Ash, I.: Large epidemic outbreak of vomiting associated with meningism and exanthem. B. M. J. *1*:316–318, 1958.
23. Assaad, F., and Ljungars-Esteves, K.: World overview of poliomyelitis: Regional patterns and trends. Rev. Infect. Dis. *6*:S302–S307, 1984.
24. Assaad, F., and Borecka, I.: Nine-year study of WHO virus reports on fatal viral infections. Bull. W. H. O. *55*:445–453, 1977.
25. Assaad, F., and Cockburn, W. C.: Four-year study of WHO virus reports on enteroviruses other than poliovirus. Bull. W. H. O. *46*:329–336, 1972.
26. Austin, T. W., and Ray, C. G.: Coxsackie virus group B infections and the hemolytic-uremic syndrome. J. Infect. Dis. *127*:698–701, 1973.
27. Avner, E. D., Satz, J., and Plotkin, S. A.: Hypoglycorrhachia in young infants with viral meningitis. J. Pediatr. *87*:833–834, 1975.
28. Axelson, C., Bondestam, K., Frisk, G., et al.: coxsackie B virus infection in women with miscarriage. J. Med. Virol. *39*:282–285, 1993.
29. Ayuthya, P. S. N., Jayavasu, J., and Pongpanich, B.: Coxsackie group B virus and primary myocardial disease in infants and children. Am. Heart J. *88*:311–314, 1974.
30. Babb, J. M., Stoneman, M. E. R., and Stern, H.: Myocarditis and croup caused by Coxsackie virus type B5. Arch. Dis. Child. *36*:551–556, 1961.
31. Bain, H. W., McLean, D. M., and Walker, S. J.: Epidemic pleurodynia (Bornholm disease) due to Coxsackie B-5 virus: The interrelationship of pleurodynia, benign pericarditis and aseptic meningitis. Pediatrics *27*:889–903, 1961.
32. Baker, D. A., and Phillips, C. A.: Fatal hand-foot-and-mouth disease in an adult caused by coxsackievirus A7. J. A. M. A. *242*:1065, 1979.
33. Balduzzi, P. C., and Greendyke, R. M.: Sudden unexpected death in infancy and viral infection. Pediatrics *38*:201–206, 1966.
34. Banatvala, J. E.: Insulin-dependent (juvenile onset, type 1) diabetes mellitus: Coxsackie B viruses revisited. Prog. Med. Virol. *34*:33–54, 1987.
35. Banatvala, J. E., Bryant, J., Schernthaner, G., et al.: Coxsackie B, mumps, rubella, and cytomegalovirus specific IgM responses in patients with juvenile-onset insulin-dependent diabetes mellitus in Britain, Austria, and Australia. Lancet *1*:1409–1412, 1985.
36. Barak, Y., and Schwartz, J. F.: Acute transverse myelitis associated with ECHO type 5 infection. Am. J. Dis. Child. *142*:128, 1988.
37. Bardelas, J. A., Winkelstein, J. A., Tsai, S. T., et al.: Fatal ECHO 24 infection in a patient with hypogammaglobulinemia: Relationship to dermatomyositis-like syndrome. J. Pediatr. *90*:396–399, 1977.
38. Barrett, F. F., Yow, M. D., and Phillips, C. A.: St. Louis encephalitis in children during the 1964 Houston epidemic. J. A. M. A. *193*:381–385, 1965.
39. Barson, W. J., Craenen, J., Hosier, D. M., et al.: Survival following myocarditis and myocardial calcification associated with infection by coxsackie virus B4. Pediatrics *68*:79–81, 1981.
40. Barton, L. L.: Febrile neonatal illness associated with echo virus type 5 in the cerebrospinal fluid. Clin. Pediatr. *16*:383–385, 1977.

41. Baskin, J. L., Soule, E. H., and Mills, S. D.: Poliomyelitis of the newborn: Pathologic changes in two cases. Am. J. Dis. Child. *80*:10–21, 1950.
42. Bates, H. R.: Coxsackie virus B3 calcific pancarditis and hydrops fetalis. Am. J. Obstet. Gynecol. *106*:629–630, 1970.
43. Bates, T.: Poliomyelitis in pregnancy, fetus, and newborn. Am. J. Dis. Child. *90*:189–195, 1955.
44. Bayatpour, M., Zbitnew, A., Dempster, G., et al.: Role of coxsackievirus B4 in the pathogenesis of acute glomerulonephritis. Can. Med. Assoc. J. *109*:873–875, 1973.
45. Behan, W. M. H., Gow, J. W., Simpson, K., et al.: Search for picornaviruses at onset of inflammatory myopathy. J. Clin. Pathol. *49*:592–594, 1996.
46. Behbehani, A. M., and Wenner, H. A.: Infantile diarrhea: A study of the etiologic role of viruses. Am. J. Dis. Child. *111*:623–629, 1966.
47. Behbehani, A. A., Sulkin, S. E., and Wallis, C.: Factors influencing susceptibility of mice to Coxsackie virus infection. J. Infect. Dis. *110*:147–154, 1962.
48. Bell, E. J., and Cosgrove, B. P.: Routine enterovirus diagnosis in a human rhabdomyosarcoma cell line. Bull. W. H. O. *58*:423–428, 1980.
49. Bell, E. J., and Grist, N. R.: Echoviruses, carditis and acute pleurodynia. Lancet *1*:326–328, 1970.
50. Bell, E. J., Grist, N. R., and Russell, S. J. M.: Echovirus 25 infections in Scotland, 1961–64. Lancet *2*:464–466, 1965.
51. Bell, E. J., and Russell, S. J. M.: Acute transverse myelopathy and ECHO-2 virus infection. Lancet *2*:1226–1227, 1963.
52. Bell, J. F., and Meis, A.: Pericarditis in infection due to Coxsackie virus group B, type 3. N. Engl. J. Med. *261*:126–128, 1959.
53. Bell, T. M., Clark, N. S., and Chambers, W.: Outbreak of illness associated with E.C.H.O. type 7 virus. B. M. J. *2*:292–294, 1963.
54. Bell, T. M., and Steyn, J. H.: Viruses in lymph nodes of children with mesenteric adenitis and intussusception. B. M. J. *2*:700–702, 1962.
55. Bengtsson, E.: Acute myocarditis and its consequences in Sweden. Postgrad. Med. J. *48*:754–755, 1972.
56. Benirschke, K.: Viral infection of the placenta. *In* Viral Etiology of Congenital Malformations, May 19–20, 1967. Washington, D.C., U.S. Government Printing Office, 1968.
57. Benirschke, K., and Pendleton, M. E.: Coxsackie virus infection: An important complication of pregnancy. Obstet. Gynecol. *12*:305–309, 1958.
58. Berg, R., and Jelke, H.: Acute cerebellar ataxia in children associated with Coxsackie viruses group B. Acta Paediatr. Scand. *54*:497–502, 1965.
59. Berglund, A., Böttiger, M., Johnson, T., et al.: Outbreak of aseptic meningitis with rubella-like rash probably caused by ECHO virus type 9. Arch. Ges. Virusforsch. *8*:294–305, 1958.
60. Bergman, I., Painter, M. J., and Wald, E. R.: Outcome in children with enteroviral meningitis during the first year of life. J. Pediatr. *110*:705–709, 1987.
61. Berkovich, S., and Smithwick, E. M.: Transplacental infection due to ECHO virus type 22. J. Pediatr. *72*:94–96, 1968.
62. Berkovich, S., and Pangan, J.: Recoveries of virus from premature infants during outbreaks of respiratory disease: The relation of ECHO virus type 22 to disease of the upper and lower respiratory tract in the premature infant. Bull. N.Y. Acad. Med. *44*:377–387, 1968.
63. Berkovich, S., and Kibrick, S.: ECHO 11 outbreak in newborn infants and mothers. Pediatrics *33*:534–540, 1964.
64. Berlin, L. E., Rorabaugh, M. L., Heldrich, F., et al.: Aseptic meningitis in infants less than 2 years of age: Diagnosis and etiology. J. Infect. Dis. *168*:888–892, 1993.
65. Bern, C., Pallansch, M. A., Gary, H. E., Jr., et al.: Acute hemorrhagic conjunctivitis due to enterovirus 70 in American Samoa: Serum-neutralizing antibodies and sex-specific protection. Am. J. Epidemiol. *136*:1502–1506, 1992.
66. Berry, P. J., and Nagington, J.: Fatal infection with echovirus 11. Arch. Dis. Child. *57*:22–29, 1982.
67. Bertaggia, A., Meneghetti, F., and Carretta, M.: Observations on a case of parotitis due to Coxsackie virus B3. G. Mal. Infekt. *28*:188–189, 1976.
68. Biren, V. P., and Meitens, C.: Nachweis einer coxsackie B2-infektion bei polyradikulitis (Guillain-Barré syndrom). Ann. Paediatr. *204*:312–322, 1965.
69. Blotzer, J. W., and Myers, A. R.: Echovirus-associated polyarthritis: Report of a case with synovial fluid and synovial histologic characterization. Arthritis Rheum. *21*:978–981, 1978.
70. Bodensteiner, J. B., Morris, H. H., Howell, J. T., et al.: Chronic ECHO type 5 virus meningoencephalitis in X-linked hypogammaglobulinemia: Treatment with immune plasma. Neurology *29*:815–819, 1979.
71. Bodian, D., and Horstmann, D. M.: Poliomyelitis. *In* Horsfall, F. L., and Tamm, I. (eds.): Viral and Rickettsial Infections of Man. 4th ed. Philadelphia, J. B. Lippincott, 1965, pp. 430–473.
72. Boring, W. D., Angevine, D. M., and Walker, D. L.: Factors influencing host-virus interactions. I. A comparison of viral multiplication and histopathology in infant, adult, and cortisone-treated adult mice infected with the Conn-5 strain of Coxsackie virus. J. Exp. Med. *102*:753–766, 1955.
73. Bose, C. L., Gooch, W. M., Sanders, G. O., et al.: Dissimilar manifestations of intrauterine infection with Echovirus II in premature twins. Arch. Pathol. Lab. Med. *107*:361–363, 1983.
74. Bottiger, M., Johnsson, T., and von Zeipel, G.: Family infections with acute pericarditis and myocarditis by Coxsackie virus B5. Arch. Ges. Virusforsch. *13*:153–155, 1963.
75. Bowen, G. S., Fisher, M. C., Deforest, A., et al.: Epidemic of meningitis and febrile illness in neonates caused by ECHO type II virus in Philadelphia. Pediatr. Infect. Dis. *2*:359–363, 1983.
76. Bowers. V. M., Jr., and Danforth, D. N.: The significance of poliomyelitis during pregnancy: An analysis of the literature and presentation of 24 new cases. Am. J. Obstet. Gynecol. *65*:34–39, 1953.
77. Bowles, N. E., Richardson, P. J., Olsen, E. G. J., et al.: Detection of coxsackie B virus-specific RNA sequences in myocardial biopsy samples from patients with myocarditis and dilated cardiomyopathy. Lancet *1*:1120–1122, 1986.
78. Boyd, M. T., Jordan, S. W., and Davis, L. E.: Fatal pneumonitis from congenital echovirus type 6 infection. Pediatr. Infect. Dis. *6*:1138–1139, 1987.
79. Brightman, V. J., Scott, T. F. M., Westphal, M., et al.: An outbreak of Coxsackie B-5 virus infection in a newborn nursery. J. Pediatr. *69*:179–192, 1966.
80. Brodie, H. R., and Marchessault, V.: Acute benign pericarditis caused by Coxsackie virus group B. N. Engl. J. Med. *262*:1278–1280, 1960.
81. Brown, G. C., and Karunas, R. S.: Relationship of congenital anomalies and maternal infection with selected enteroviruses. Am. J. Epidemiol. *95*:207–217, 1972.
82. Brown, J. M., Wright, J. A., and Ogden, W. S.: Hand, foot, and mouth disease. B. M. J. *1*:58, 1964.
83. Bryden, A. S.: Isolation of enteroviruses and adenoviruses in continuous simian cell lines. Med. Lab. Sci. *49*:60–65, 1992.
84. Buckland, F. E., Bynoe, M. L., Philipson, L., et al.: Experimental infection of human volunteers with the U-virus, A strain of ECHO virus type 11. J. Hyg. *57*:274–284, 1959.
85. Burch, G. E., and Colcolough, H. L.: Progressive Coxsackie viral pancarditis and nephritis. Ann. Intern. Med. *71*:963–970, 1969.
86. Burch, G. E., Sun, S. C., Chu, K. C., et al.: Interstitial and coxsackievirus B myocarditis in infants and children. J. A. M. A. *203*:1–8, 1968.
87. Burch, G. E., Sun, S. C., Colcolough, H. L., et al.: Coxsackie B viral myocarditis and valvulitis identified in routine autopsy specimens by immunofluorescent techniques. Am. Heart J. *74*:13–23, 1967.
88. Burry, J. N., Moore, B., and Mattner, C.: Hand, foot and mouth disease in South Australia. Med. J. Aust. *2*:587–589, 1968.
89. Calder, B. D., Warnock, P. J., McCartney, R. A., et al.: Coxsackie B viruses and the post-viral syndrome: A prospective study in general practice. J. R. Coll. Gen. Pract. *37*:11–14, 1987.
90. Canby, J. P.: Petechiae and fever: Infection with Coxsackie virus group B, type 3—Case report. Clin. Pediatr. *2*:187–188, 1963.
91. Capner, P., Lendrum, R., Jeffries, D. J., et al.: Viral antibody studies in pancreatic disease. Gut *16*:866–870, 1975.
92. Carolane, D. J., Long, A. M., McKeever, P. A., et al.: Prevention of spread of echovirus 6 in a special care baby unit. Arch. Dis. Child. *60*:674–676, 1985.
93. Carstens, J. M., Tracy, S., Chapman, N. M., et al.: Detection of enteroviruses in cell cultures by using in situ transcription. J. Clin. Microbiol. *30*:25–35, 1992.
94. Cashman, N. R., Maselli, R., and Wollmann, R. L.: Late denervation in patients with antecedent paralytic poliomyelitis. N. Engl. J. Med. *317*:7–12, 1987.
95. Centers for Disease Control and Prevention: Progress toward global poliomyelitis eradication, 1985–1994. M. M. W. R. *44*:273–281, 1995.
96. Centers for Disease Control and Prevention: Certification of poliomyelitis eradication: The Americas, 1994. M. M. W. R. *43*:720–722, 1994.
97. Centers for Disease Control: Acute hemorrhagic conjunctivitis: Mexico. M. M. W. R. *38*:327–329, 1989.
98. Centers for Disease Control: Enterovirus surveillance: United States, 1985. M. M. W. R. *34*:494–495, 1985.
99. Centers for Disease Control: Acute hemorrhagic conjunctivitis: Florida, North Carolina. M. M. W. R. *30*:501–502, 1982.
100. Centers for Disease Control: Encephalitis surveillance, annual summary 1978. Issued May 1981.
101. Centers for Disease Control: Annual summary 1979: Reported morbidity and mortality in the United States. M. M. W. R. *28*:1–119, 1980.
102. Centers for Disease Control: Aseptic meningitis surveillance: Annual summary 1976. Atlanta, U. S. Dept. H. E. W., issued January 1979.
103. Centers for Disease Control: Follow-up on poliomyelitis: United States, Canada, Netherlands. M. M. W. R. *28*:345–346, 1979.
104. Centers for Disease Control: Poliomyelitis surveillance summary 1974–1976. Issued October 1977.
105. Center for Disease Control: Follow-up on poliomyelitis, Connecticut, New York, Massachusetts, New Hampshire. M. M. W. R. *21*:365–366, 1972.
106. Chalhub, E. G., Devivo, D. C., Seigel, B. A., et al.: Coxsackie A9 focal encephalitis associated with acute infantile hemiplegia and porencephaly. Neurology *27*:574–579, 1977.
107. Champsaur, H. F., Bottazzo, G. F., Bertrams, J., et al.: Virologic, immunologic, and genetic factors in insulin-dependent diabetes mellitus. J. Pediatr. *100*:15–20, 1982.
108. Chan, D., and Hammond, G. W.: Comparison of serodiagnosis of group B coxsackievirus infections by an immunoglobulin M capture enzyme

immunoassay versus microneutralization. J. Clin. Microbiol. *21*:830–834, 1985.
109. Chandy, K. G., John, T. J., Mukundan, P., et al.: Coxsackie B antibodies in "rheumatic" valvular heart-disease. Lancet *1*:381, 1979.
110. Chang, T. W., and Weinstein, L.: Infection of the nervous system by Coxsackie A9 virus. Bull. Tufts N. E. Med. Ctr. *6*:181–193, 1960.
111. Chanock, R. M., and Parrott, R. H.: Acute respiratory disease in infancy and childhood: Present understanding and prospects for prevention. Pediatrics *36*:21–39, 1965.
112. Chatterjee, S., Quarcoopome, C. O., and Apenteng, A.: Unusual type of epidemic conjunctivitis in Ghana. Br. J. Ophthalmol. *54*:628, 1970.
113. Chawareewong, S., Kiangsiri, S., Lokaphadhana, K., et al.: Neonatal herpangina caused by Coxsackie A-5 virus. J. Pediatr. *93*:492–494, 1978.
114. Chemtob, S., Reece, E. R., and Mills, E. L.: Syndrome of inappropriate secretion of antidiuretic hormone in enteroviral meningitis. Am. J. Dis. Child. *139*:292–294, 1985.
115. Cherry, J. D.: Enteroviruses: Polioviruses (poliomyelitis), coxsackieviruses, echoviruses, and enteroviruses. *In* Feigin, R. D., and Cherry, J. D. (eds.): Textbook of Pediatric Infectious Diseases. 2nd ed. Philadelphia, W. B. Saunders, 1987, pp. 1729–1790.
116. Cherry, J. D.: Enteroviruses. *In* Behrman, R. E., and Vaughan, V. C. (eds.): Nelson Textbook of Pediatrics. 12th ed. Philadelphia, W. B. Saunders, 1983, pp. 791–804.
117. Cherry, J. D.: Enteroviruses. *In* Remington, J. S., and Klein, J. O. (eds.): Infectious Diseases of the Fetus and Newborn Infant. 3rd ed. Philadelphia, W. B. Saunders, 1990, pp. 325–366.
118. Cherry, J. D.: Newer viral exanthems. Adv. Pediatr. *116*:233–286, 1969.
119. Cherry, J. D., Bobinski, J. E., Horvath, F. L., et al.: Acute hemangioma-like lesions associated with ECHO viral infections. Pediatrics *44*:498–502, 1969.
120. Cherry, J. D., Soriano, F., and Jahn, C. L.: Search for perinatal viral infection: A prospective, clinical, virologic, and serologic study. Am. J. Dis. Child. *116*:245–250, 1968.
121. Cherry, J. D., Jahn, C. L., and Meyer, T. C.: Paroxysmal atrial tachycardia associated with ECHO 9 virus infection. Am. Heart J. *73*:681–686, 1967.
122. Cherry, J. D., and Jahn, C. L.: Virologic studies of exanthems. J. Pediatr. *68*:204–214, 1966.
123. Cherry, J. D., and Jahn, C. L.: Hand, foot, and mouth syndrome: Report of six cases due to Coxsackie virus, group A, type 16. Pediatrics *37*:637–643, 1966.
124. Cherry, J. D., and Jahn, C. L.: Concomitant enterovirus infection, smallpox vaccination, and exanthem. J. Pediatr. *67*:679–681, 1965.
125. Cherry, J. D., Lerner, A. M., Klein, J. O., et al.: Coxsackie A9 infections with exanthems: With particular reference to urticaria. Pediatrics *31*:819–823, 1963.
126. Cherry, J. D., Lerner, A. M., Klein, J. O., et al.: Echo 11 virus infections associated with exanthems. Pediatrics *32*:509–516, 1963.
127. Cherry, J. D., Lerner, A. M., Klein, J. O., et al.: Coxsackie B5 infections with exanthems. Pediatrics *31*:455–462, 1963.
128. Chesney, J. C., Hoganson, G. E., Wilson, M. H.: CSF eosinophilia during an acute coxsackie B4 viral meningitis. Am. J. Dis. Child. *134*:703, 1980.
129. Chesney, P. J., Quennec, P., and Clark, C.: Hypoglycorrhachia and Coxsackie B3 meningoencephalitis. Am. J. Clin. Pathol. *70*:947–948, 1978.
130. Chezzi, C.: Rapid diagnosis of poliovirus infection by PCR amplification. J. Clin. Microbiol. *34*:1722–1725, 1996.
131. Chin, T. D. Y., Lehan, P. H., Rubin, H., et al.: Epidemiological studies of aseptic meningitis caused by Coxsackie virus B5. Am. J. Public Health *48*:1193–1200, 1958.
132. Cho, C. T., Janelle, J. G., and Behbehani, A.: Severe neonatal illness associated with Echo 9 virus infection. Clin. Pediatr. *12*:304–305, 1973.
133. Chomel, J. J., Thouvenot, D., Fayol, V., et al.: Rapid diagnosis of Echovirus type 33 meningitis by specific IgM detection using an enzyme linked immunosorbent assay (ELISA). J. Virol. Methods *10*:11–19, 1985.
134. Chonmaitree, T., Ford, C., Sanders, C., et al.: Comparison of cell cultures for rapid isolation of enteroviruses. J. Clin. Microbiol. *26*:2576–2580, 1988.
135. Chonmaitree, T., Menegus, M. A., and Powell, K. R.: The clinical relevance of "CSF viral culture": A two-year experience with aseptic meningitis in Rochester, N.Y. J. A. M. A. *247*:1843–1847, 1982.
136. Chonmaitree, T., Menegus, M. A., Schervish-Swierkosz, E. M., et al.: Enterovirus 71 infection: Report of an outbreak with two cases of paralysis and a review of the literature. Pediatrics *67*:489–493, 1981.
137. Chou, S. M., and Gutmann, L.: Picornavirus-like crystals in subacute polymyositis. Neurology *20*:205–213, 1970.
138. Christen, A. G., Crandell, R. A., and Kerstein, M. H.: Hand-foot-and-mouth disease in a father and son. Oral Surg. Oral Med. Oral Pathol. *24*:427–432, 1967.
139. Christensen, M. L., Pachman, L. M., Schneiderman, R., et al.: Prevalence of coxsackie B virus antibodies in patients with juvenile dermatomyositis. Arthritis Rheum. *29*:1365–1370, 1986.
140. Christie, A. B.: Acute poliomyelitis. *In* Infectious Diseases: Epidemiology and Clinical Practice. 2nd ed. Edinburgh, Churchill Livingstone, 1974, pp. 567–614.
141. Christopher, S., Theogaraj, S., Godbole, S., et al.: An epidemic of acute hemorrhagic conjunctivitis due to coxsackievirus A24. J. Infect. Dis. *146*:16–19, 1982.
142. Chuang, E., Maller, E. S., Hoffman, M. A., et al.: Successful treatment of fulminant echovirus 11 infection in a neonate by orthotopic liver transplantation. J. Pediatr. Gastroenterol. Nutr. *17*:211–214, 1993.
143. Clarke, A., and Stott, J.: E.C.H.O. type 20. B. M. J. *1*:900–901, 1961.
144. Clarke, M., Hunter, M., McNaughton, G. A., et al.: Seasonal aseptic meningitis caused by Coxsackie and Echo viruses: Toronto, 1957. Can. Med. Assoc. J. *81*:5–8, 1959.
145. Clarke, S. K. R., Morley, T., and Warin, R. P.: Hand, foot, and mouth disease. B. M. J. *1*:58, 1964.
146. Clements, G. B., Galbraith, D. N., and Taylor, K. W.: Coxsackie B virus infection and onset of childhood diabetes. Lancet *346*:221–223, 1995.
147. Clements, G. B., McGarry, F., Nairn, C., et al.: Detection of enterovirus-specific RNA in serum: The relationship to chronic fatigue. J. Med. Virol. *45*:156–161, 1995.
148. Clemer, D. I., Li, F., LeBlanc, D. R., et al.: An outbreak of subclinical infection with coxsackievirus B3 in southern Louisiana. Am. J. Epidemiol. *83*:123–129, 1966.
149. Cochran, H. R., May, F. E. B., Ashcroft, T., et al.: Enteroviruses and idiopathic dilated cardiomyopathy. J. Pathol. *163*:129–131, 1991.
150. Codd, A. A., Hale, J. H., Bell, T. M., et al.: Epidemic of echovirus 19 in the north-east of England. J. Hyg. (Camb.) *76*:307–317, 1976.
151. Constable, F. L., and Howitt, L. F.: Outbreak of E.C.H.O. type 9 infection in a children's home. B. M. J. *1*:1483–1486, 1961.
152. Cooper, J. B., Pratt, W. R., English, B. K., et al.: Coxsackievirus B3 producing fatal meningoencephalitis in a patient with X-linked agammaglobulinemia. Am. J. Dis. Child. *137*:82–83, 1983.
153. Coucke, C., Kint, A., and Gabriel, P.: Hand, foot and mouth disease in the adult subject. Dermatologica *153*:272–276, 1976.
154. Couvreur, J., Cook, C. M., Chany, C., et al.: Une épidémie d'exanthème à virus ECHO de type 16 en milieu hospitalier avec bilan d'une enquête longitudinale. Arch. Ges. Virusforsch. *13*:215–232, 1963.
155. Craighead, J. E., Mahoney, E. M., Carver, D. H., et al.: Orchitis due to Coxsackie virus group B, type 5: Report of a case with isolation of virus from the testis. N. Engl. J. Med. *267*:498–500, 1962.
156. Cramblett, H. G., Haynes, R. E., Azimi, P. H., et al.: Nosocomial infection with echovirus type 11 in handicapped and premature infants. Pediatrics *51*:603–607, 1973.
157. Cramblett, H. G., Moffet, H. L., Black, J. P., et al.: Coxsackie virus infections: Clinical and laboratory studies. J. Pediatr. *64*:406–414, 1964.
158. Cramblett, H. G., Moffet, H. L., Middleton, G. K., Jr., et al.: Echo 19 virus infections: Clinical and laboratory studies. Arch. Intern. Med. *110*:574–579, 1962.
159. Cramblett, H. G., Rosen, L., Parrott, R. H., et al.: Respiratory illness in six infants infected with a newly recognized echo virus. Pediatrics *21*:168–176, 1958.
160. Crawford, M., Macrae, A. D., and O'Reilly, J. N.: An unusual illness in young children associated with an enteric virus. Arch. Dis. Child. *31*:182–188, 1956.
161. Crennan, J. M., Van Scoy, R. E., McKenna, C. H., et al.: Echovirus poliomyelitis in patients with hypogammaglobulinemia. Am. J. Med. *81*:35–42, 1986.
162. Crow, K. D., Warin, R., and Wilkinson, D. S.: Hand, foot, and mouth disease. B. M. J. *2*:1267–1268, 1963.
163. Cudworth, A. G., White, G. B. B., Woodrow, J. C., et al.: Etiology of juvenile-onset diabetes: A prospective study. Lancet *1*:385–388, 1977.
164. Curnen, E. C., Shaw, E. W., and Melnick, J. L.: Disease resembling nonparalytic poliomyelitis associated with a virus pathogenic for infant mice. J. A. M. A. *141*:894–901, 1949.
165. Daae, A.: Epidemi i drangedal af akut muskelrheumatisme udbredt ved smitte. Norsk Mag. F. Laegevidensk. *2 n. s.*:409–413, 529–542, 1872.
166. Dagan, R., Jenista, J. A., and Menegus, M. A.: Association of clinical presentation, laboratory findings, and virus serotypes with the presence of meningitis in hospitalized infants with enterovirus infection. J. Pediatr. *113*:975–978, 1988.
167. Dagan, R., Prather, S. L., Powell, K. R., et al.: Neutralizing antibodies to non-polio enteroviruses in human immune serum globulin. Pediatr. Infect. Dis. *2*:454–456, 1983.
168. Dalakas, M. C., Elder, G., Hallett, M., et al.: A long-term follow-up study of patients with post-poliomyelitis neuromuscular symptoms. N. Engl. J. Med. *314*:959–963, 1986.
169. Dalakas, M. C., Sever, J. L., Madden, D. L., et al.: Late postpoliomyelitis muscular atrophy: Clinical, virologic, and immunologic studies. Rev. Infect. Dis. *6*:S562–S567, 1984.
170. Dalldorf, F., and Melnick, J. L.: Coxsackie viruses. *In* Horsfall, F. L., and Tamm, I. (eds.): Viral and Rickettsial Infections of Man. Philadelphia, J. B. Lippincott, 1965, pp. 474–512.
171. Dalldorf, G., and Sickles, G. M.: An unidentified, filtrable agent isolated from the feces of children with paralysis. Science *108*:61–62, 1948.
172. DaSilva, E. E., Winkler, M. T., and Pallansch, M. A.: Role of enterovirus 71 in acute flaccid paralysis after the eradication of poliovirus in Brazil. Emerg. Infect. Dis. *2*:231–233, 1996.
173. Davies, D. P., Hughes, C. A., MacVicar, J., et al.: Echovirus-11 infection in a special-care baby unit. Lancet *1*:96–97, 1979.
174. Davies, J. W., McDermott, A., and Severs, D.: Epidemic virus meningitis due to echo 9 virus in Newfoundland. Can. Med. Assoc. J. *79*:162–167, 1958.

175. De, L., Nottay, B., Yang, C. F., et al.: Identification of vaccine-related polioviruses by hybridization with specific RNA probes. J. Clin. Microbiol. *33*:562–571, 1995.
176. Dechamps, C., Peigue-Lafeuille, H. H., Laveran, H., et al.: Four cases of vesicular lesions in adults caused by enterovirus infections. J. Clin. Microbiol. *26*:2182–2183, 1988.
177. DeQuadros, C. A., Andrus, J. K., Olive, J. M., et al.: Eradication of poliomyelitis: Progress in the Americas. Pediatr. Infect. Dis. J. *10*:222–229, 1991.
178. Dery, P., Marks, M. I., and Shapera, R.: Clinical manifestations of coxsackievirus infections in children. Am. J. Dis. Child. *128*:464–468, 1974.
179. Desa'neto, A., Bullington, J. D., Bullington, R. H., et al.: Coxsackie B5 heart disease: Demonstration of inferolateral wall myocardial necrosis. Am. J. Med. *68*:295–298, 1980.
180. Deseda-Tous, J., Bryatt, P. H., and Cherry, J. D.: Vesicular lesions in adults due to echovirus 11 infections. Arch. Dermatol. *113*:1705–1706, 1977.
181. Diedrich, S., Driesel, G., and Schreier, E.: Sequence comparison of echovirus type 30 isolates to other enteroviruses in the 5′ noncoding region. J. Med. Virol. *46*:148–152, 1995.
182. Dippe, S. E., Bennett, P. H., Miller, M., et al.: Lack of causal association between Coxsackie B4 virus infection and diabetes. Lancet *1*:1314–1318, 1975.
183. Domok, I., Balayan, M. S., Fayinka, O. A., et al.: Factors affecting the efficacy of live poliovirus vaccine in warm climates. Bull. W. H. O. *51*:333–347, 1974.
184. Dömök, I., and Molnar, E.: An outbreak of meningoencephalomyocarditis among newborn infants during the epidemic of Bornholm disease in 1958 in Hungary. II. Aetiological findings. Ann. Pediatr. *194*:102–114, 1960.
185. Drebot, M. A., Nguan, C. Y., Campbell, J. J., et al.: Molecular epidemiology of enterovirus outbreaks in Canada during 1991–1992: Identification of echovirus 30 and coxsackievirus B1 strains by amplicon sequencing. J. Med. Virol. *44*:340–347, 1994.
186. Drew, J. H.: ECHO 11 virus outbreak in a nursery associated with myocarditis. Aust. Paediatr. J. *9*:90–95, 1973.
187. Drouhet, V.: Enterovirus infection and associated clinical symptoms in children. Ann. Inst. Pasteur *98*:562–568, 1960.
188. Duff, M. F.: Hand-foot-and-mouth syndrome in humans: Coxsackie A10 infections in New Zealand. B. M. J. *2*:661–664, 1968.
189. Duxbury, A. E., White, J., Lipscomb, B. M., et al.: Illness simulating paralytic poliomyelitis associated with Coxsackie group A type 4 virus infection. Med. J. Aust. *2*:709–711, 1961.
190. Duxbury, A. E., and Warner, P.: Epidemiological and laboratory investigations on Bornholm disease in Adelaide, 1957. Med. J. Aust. *1*:518–523, 1958.
191. Dwyer, J. M., and Erlendsson, K.: Intraventricular gamma-globulin for the management of enterovirus encephalitis. Pediatr. Infect. Dis. J. *7*:S30–S33, 1988.
192. Eckert, G. L., Barron, A. L., and Karzon, D. T.: Aseptic meningitis due to ECHO virus type 18. Am. J. Dis. Child. *99*:1–3, 1960.
193. Eckert, H. L., Portnoy, B., Salvatore, M. A., et al.: Group B, Coxsackie virus infection in infants with acute lower respiratory disease. Pediatrics *39*:526–531, 1967.
194. Egger, D., Pasamontes, L., Ostermayer, M., et al.: Reverse transcription multiplex PCR for differentiation between polio- and enteroviruses from clinical and environmental samples. J. Clin. Microbiol. *33*:1442–1447, 1995.
195. Ehrnst, A., and Eriksson, M.: Epidemiological features of type 22 echovirus infection. Scand. J. Infect. Dis. *25*:275–281, 1993.
196. Eichenwald, H. F., and Kostevalov, O.: Immunologic responses of premature and fullterm infants to infection with certain viruses. Pediatrics *25*:829–839, 1960.
197. Eichenwald, H. F., Ababio, A., Arky, A. M., et al.: Epidemic diarrhea in premature and older infants caused by Echo virus type 18. J. A. M. A. *166*:1563–1566, 1958.
198. Eilard, T., Kyllerman, M., Wennerblom, I., et al.: An outbreak of Coxsackie virus type B2 among neonates in an obstetrical ward. Acta Paediatr. Scand. *63*:103–107, 1974.
199. Elizan, T. S., Ajero-Froechlich, L., Fabiyi, A., et al.: Viral infection in pregnancy and congenital CNS malformations in man. Arch. Neurol. *20*:115–119, 1969.
200. Elliott, G. B., McAllister, J. E., and Alberta, C.: Fetal poliomyelitis. Am. J. Obstet. Gynecol. *72*:896–902, 1956.
201. Elvin-Lewis, M., and Melnick, J. L.: ECHO 11 viruses associated with aseptic meningitis. Proc. Soc. Exp. Biol. Med. *102*:647–649, 1959.
202. Enders, J. R., Weller, T. H., and Robbins, F. C.: Cultivation of the Lansing strain of poliomyelitis virus in cultures of various human embryonic tissues. Science *109*:85–87, 1949.
203. Erlendsson, K., Swartz, T., and Dwyer, J. M.: Successful reversal of echovirus encephalitis in X-linked hypogammaglobulinemia by intraventricular administration of immunoglobulin. N. Engl. J. Med. *312*:351–353, 1985.
204. Estes, M. L., and Rorke, L. B.: Liquefactive necrosis in coxsackie B encephalitis. Arch. Pathol. Lab. Med. *110*:1090–1092, 1986.
205. Evans, A. D., and Waddington, E.: Hand, foot and mouth disease in South Wales, 1964. Br. J. Dermatol. *79*:309–317, 1967.
206. Evans, A. S., and Dick, E. C.: Acute pharyngitis and tonsillitis in University of Wisconsin students. J. A. M. A. *190*:699–708, 1964.
207. Farmer, K., MacArthur, B. A., and Clay, M. M.: A follow-up study of 15 cases of neonatal meningoencephalitis due to Coxsackie virus B5. J. Pediatr. *87*:568–571, 1975.
208. Farmer, K., and Patten, P. T.: An outbreak of Coxsackie B5 infection in a special care unit for newborn infants. N. Z. Med. J. *68*:86–89, 1968.
209. Faulkner, R. S., and Van Rooyen, C. E.: Echovirus type 17 in the neonate. Can. Med. Assoc. J. *108*:878–882, 1973.
210. Faulkner, R. S., MacLeod, A. J., and Van Rooyen, C. E.: Virus meningitis: Seven cases in one family. Can. Med. Assoc. J. *77*:439–444, 1957.
211. Fechner, R. E., Smith, M. G., and Middelkamp, J. N.: Coxsackie B virus infection of the newborn. Am. J. Pathol. *42*:493–505, 1963.
212. Feldman, W., and Larke, R. P. B.: Acute cerebellar ataxia associated with the isolation of coxsackievirus type A9. Can. Med. Assoc. J. *106*:1104–1105, 1972.
213. Felici, A., Archetti, I., Russi, F., et al.: Contribution to the study of diseases caused by the Coxsackie B group of viruses in Italy. III. Arch. Ges. Virusforsch. *11*:592–598, 1961.
214. Felici, A., and Gregorig, B.: Contribution to the study of diseases in Italy caused by the Coxsackie B group of viruses. II. Epidemiological, clinical and virological data obtained in the course of a summer outbreak caused by Coxsackie B4 virus. Arch. Ges. Virusforsch. *9*:317–328, 1959.
215. Fenner, F.: Classification and nomenclature of viruses: Second report of the International Committee on Taxonomy of Viruses. Intervirology *7*:1–115, 1976.
216. Ferreira, A. G., Jr., Ferriera, S. M. A. G., Gomes, M. L. C., et al.: Enteroviruses as a possible cause of myocarditis, pericarditis, and dilated cardiomyopathy in Belém, Brazil. Brazilian J. Med. Biol. Res. *28*:869–874, 1995.
217. Figueroa, J. P., Ashley, D., King, D., et al.: An outbreak of acute flaccid paralysis in Jamaica associated with echovirus type 22. J. Med. Virol. *29*:315–319, 1989.
218. Finsen, J.: Iagttagelser sygdomsforholdeme i Island (Afhandling for den medicinske doktorgrad ved Københavns Universitet). Copenhagen, C. A. Reitzels, 1874, pp. 145–151.
219. Flewett, T. H.: Histological study of two cases of Coxsackie B virus pneumonia in children. J. Clin. Pathol. *18*:743–746, 1965.
220. Flewett, T. H., Warin, R. P., and Clarke, S. K. R.: Hand, foot, and mouth disease associated with Coxsackie A5 virus. J. Clin. Pathol. *16*:53–55, 1963.
221. Flugsrud, L., Abrahamsen, A. M., and Lahelle, O.: An outbreak of aseptic meningitis associated with a virus related to ECHO type 9. Acta Med. Scand. *112*:129–135, 1958.
222. Foley, J. F., Chin, T. D. Y., and Gravelle, C. R.: Paralytic disease due to infection with echo virus type 9. N. Engl. J. Med. *260*:924–926, 1959.
223. Forbes, J. A.: Meningitis in Melbourne due to E.C.H.O. virus. Part I. Clinical aspects. Med. J. Aust. *1*:246–248, 1958.
224. Forman, M. L., and Cherry, J. D.: Enanthems associated with uncommon viral syndromes. Pediatrics *41*:873–882, 1968.
225. Förster, W., Bialasiewicz, A.A., and Busse, H.: Coxsackievirus B3-associated panuveitis. Br. J. Ophthalmol. *77*:182–183, 1993.
226. Fox, J. P., and Hall, C. E.: Viruses in Families. Littleton, PSG Publishing, 1980, pp. 190–195.
227. Fox, J. P.: Eradication of poliomyelitis in the United States: A commentary on the Salk reviews. Rev. Infect. Dis. *2*:277–281, 1980.
228. Fox, J. P.: Epidemiological aspects of coxsackie and ECHO virus infections in tropical areas. Am. J. Public Health *54*:1134–1142, 1964.
229. Fox, S.A., Finklestone, E., Robbins, P.D., et al.: Search for persistent enterovirus infection of muscle in inflammatory myopathies. J. Neurol. Sci. *125*:70–76, 1994.
230. Foy, H. M., Cooney, M. K., Maletzky, A. J., et al.: Incidence and etiology of pneumonia, croup and bronchiolitis in preschool children belonging to a prepaid medical care group over a four-year period. Am. J. Epidemiol. *97*:80–92, 1973.
231. Freedman, P. S.: Echovirus 11 infection and intrauterine death. Lancet *1*:96–97, 1979.
232. Freij, L., Norrby, R., and Olsson, B.: A small outbreak of Coxsackie B5 infection with two cases of cardiac involvement and orchitis followed by testicular atrophy. Acta Med. Scand. *187*:177–181, 1970.
233. Frisk, G., and Diderholm, H.: Increased frequency of coxsackie B virus IgM in women with spontaneous abortion. J. Infect. *24*:141–145, 1992.
234. Froeschle, J. E., Nahmias, A. J., Feorino, P. M., et al.: Hand, foot, and mouth disease (Coxsackie A16) in Atlanta. Am. J. Dis. Child. *114*:278–283, 1967.
235. Frothingham, T. E.: Echo virus type 9 associated with three cases simulating meningococcemia. N. Engl. J. Med. *259*:484–485, 1958.
236. Fujioka, S., Koide, H., Kitaura, Y., et al.: Molecular detection and differentiation of enteroviruses in endomyocardial biopsies and pericardial effusions from dilated cardiomyopathy and myocarditis. Am. Heart J. *131*:760–765, 1996.
237. Fulginiti, V. A.: The problems of poliovirus immunization. Hospital Practice, August 1980, pp. 61–67.
238. Galama, J. M. D., DeLeeuw, N., Wittebol, S., et al.: Prolonged enteroviral infection in a patient who developed pericarditis and heart failure after bone marrow transplantation. Clin. Infect. Dis. *22*:1004–1008, 1996.
239. Gallacher, K., Ghosh, K., Patel, A., et al.: An outbreak of echovirus type 4 infections and its implications for diagnosis and management in general practice. J. Infect. *26*:321–324, 1993.

240. Galpine, J. F., Clayton, T. M., Ardley, J., et al.: Outbreak of aseptic meningitis with exanthem. B. M. J. *1*:319–321, 1958.
241. Gamble, D. R., Kinsley, M. L., FitzGerald, M. G., et al.: Viral antibodies in diabetes mellitus. B. M. J. *3*:627–630, 1969.
242. Gamble, D. R., and Taylor, K. W.: Seasonal incidence of diabetes mellitus. B. M. J. *3*:631–633, 1969.
243. Garnett, D. G., Burlingham, A., and Van Zwanenberg, D.: Outbreak of aseptic meningitis of virus origin in East Suffolk. Lancet *1*:500–502, 1957.
244. Gary, H. (Respiratory and Enteric Viruses Branch, Centers for Disease Control and Prevention): Personal communication. 1996.
245. Gaudin, O.-G., Pozzetto, B., Aouni, M., et al.: Detection of neutralizing IgM antibodies in the diagnosis of enterovirus infections. J. Med. Virol. *28*:200–205, 1989.
246. Gauntt, C. J., Arizpe, H. M., Higdon, A. L., et al.: Molecular mimicry, anti-coxsackievirus B3 neutralizing monoclonal antibodies, and myocarditis. J. Immunol. *154*:2983–2995, 1995.
247. Gauntt, C. J., Higdon, A. L., Arizpe, H. M., et al.: Epitopes shared between coxsackievirus B3 (CVB3) and normal heart tissue contribute to CVB3-induced murine myocarditis. Clin. Immunol. Immunopathol. *68*:129–134, 1993.
248. Gauntt, C. J., Gudvangen, R. J., Brans, Y. W., et al.: Coxsackievirus group B antibodies in the ventricular fluid of infants with severe anatomic defects in the central nervous system. Pediatrics *76*:64–68, 1985.
249. Gear, J.: Coxsackie virus infections in southern Africa. Yale J. Biol. Med. *34*:289–303, 1961/1962.
250. Gear, J. H. S.: Coxsackie virus infections of the newborn. Prog. Med. Virol. *1*:106–121, 1958.
251. Gelfand, H. M., Holguin, A. H., Marchetti, G. E., et al.: A continuing surveillance of enterovirus infections in healthy children in six United States cities. I. Viruses isolated during 1960 and 1961. Am. J. Hyg. *78*:358–375, 1963.
252. Gelfand, H. M.: The occurrence in nature of the Coxsackie and ECHO viruses. Progr. Med. Virol. *3*:193–244, 1961.
253. Georgieff, M. K., Johnson, D. E., Thompson, T. R., et al.: Fulminant hepatic necrosis in an infant with perinatally acquired echovirus 21 infection. Pediatr. Infect. Dis. J. *6*:71–73, 1987.
254. German, L. J., McCracken, A. W., and Wilkie, K. McD.: Outbreak of febrile illness associated with E. C. H. O. virus type 5 in a maternity unit in Singapore. B. M. J. *1*:742–744, 1968.
255. Gilbert, G. L., Dickson, K. E., Waters, M. J., et al.: Outbreak of enterovirus 71 infection in Victoria, Australia, with a high incidence of neurologic involvement. Pediatr. Infect. Dis. J. *7*:484–488, 1988.
256. Gillett, R. L.: Acute benign pericarditis and the Coxsackie viruses. N. Engl. J. Med. *261*:838–845, 1959.
257. Ginsberg, A. H., Gale, M. J., Jr., Rose, L. M., et al.: T-cell alterations in late postpoliomyelitis. Arch. Neurol. *46*:497–501, 1989.
258. Glasgow, L. A., and Balduzzi, P.: Isolation of Coxsackie virus group A, type 4, from a patient with hemolyticuremic syndrome. N. Engl. J. Med. *273*:754–756, 1965.
259. Glezen, W. P., Loda, F. A., Clyde, W. A., Jr., et al.: Epidemiologic patterns of acute lower respiratory disease of children in a pediatric group practice. J. Pediatr. *78*:397–406, 1971.
260. Glimåaker, M., Samuelson, A., Magnius, L., et al.: Early diagnosis of enteroviral meningitis by detection of specific IgM antibodies with a solid-phase reverse immunosorbent test (SPRIST) and μ-capture EIA. J. Med. Virol. *36*:193–201, 1992.
261. Glimåaker, M., Ehrnst, A., Magnius, L., et al.: Early diagnosis of enteroviral meningitis by a solid-phase reverse immunosorbent test and virus isolation. Scand. J. Infect. Dis. *22*:519–526, 1990.
262. Godtfredsen, A., and Hansen, B.: A case of mild paralytic disease due to Echo virus type 11. Acta Pathol. Microbiol. Scand. *53*:111–116, 1961.
263. Goh, K. T., Ooi, P. L., Miyamura, K., et al.: Acute haemorrhagic conjunctivitis: Seroepidemiology of coxsackievirus A24 variant and enterovirus 70 in Singapore. J. Med. Virol. *31*:245–247, 1990.
264. Goh, K. T., Doraisingham, S., Tan, J. L., et al.: An outbreak of hand, foot, and mouth disease in Singapore. Bull. W. H. O. *60*:965–969, 1982.
265. Gohd, R. S., and Gordon, W.: Endemic nature of coxsackievirus A-16. Bacteriol. Proc. *108*:152, 1967.
266. Gohd, R. S., and Faigel, H. C.: Hand-foot-and-mouth disease resembling measles: A life-threatening disease: Case report. Pediatrics *37*:644–648, 1966.
267. Gold, E., Carver, D. H., Heinberg, H., et al.: Viral infection: A possible cause of sudden, unexpected death in infants. N. Engl. J. Med. *264*:53–60, 1961.
268. Goldwater, P. N.: Immunoglobulin M capture immunoassay in investigation of coxsackievirus B5 and B6 outbreaks in South Australia. J. Clin. Microbiol. *33*:1628–1631, 1995.
269. Goldwater, P. N., and Laws, J.: Echovirus 19 outbreak in Auckland, 1975–76. N. Z. Med. J. *597*:319–322, 1977.
270. Gondo, K., Kusuhara, K., Take, H., et al.: Echovirus type 9 epidemic in Kagoshima, southern Japan: Seroepidemiology and clinical observation of aseptic meningitis. Pediatr. Infect. Dis. J. *14*:787–791, 1995.
271. Gong, C. M., Ho, D. W. T., Field, P. R., et al.: Immunoglobulin responses to echovirus type 11 by enzyme linked immunosorbent assay: Single-serum diagnosis of acute infection by specific IgM antibody. J. Virol. Methods *9*:209–221, 1984.
272. Goodwin, M. H., Jr., Love, G. J., Mackel, D. C., et al.: Observations on the association of enteric viruses and bacteria with diarrhea. Am. J. Trop. Med. Hyg. *16*:178–185, 1967.
273. Gordon, R. B., Lennette, E. H., and Sandrock, R. S.: The varied clinical manifestations of Coxsackie virus infections: Observations and comments on an outbreak in California. Arch. Intern. Med. *103*:63–75, 1959.
274. Graber, D., Fossoud, C., Grouteau, E., et al.: Acute transverse myelitis and coxsackie A9 virus infection. Pediatr. Infect. Dis. J. *13*:77, 1994.
275. Grangeot-Keros, L., Broyer, M., Briand, E., et al.: Enterovirus in sudden unexpected deaths in infants. Pediatr. Infect. Dis. J. *15*:123–128, 1996.
276. Gravelle, C. R., Noble, G. R., Feltz, E. T., et al.: An epidemic of echovirus type 30 meningitis in an Arctic community. Am. J. Epidemiol. *99*:368–374, 1974.
277. Green, I. J., Hung, T. P., and Sung, S. M.: Neurologic complications with elevated antibody titer after acute hemorrhagic conjunctivitis. Am. J. Ophthalmol. *80*:832–834, 1975.
278. Gregg, I.: The role of viral infection in asthma and bronchitis. *In* Proudfoot, A. T. (ed.): Symposium on Viral Diseases. Edinburgh Royal College of Physicians, 1975, pp. 82–98.
279. Griffiths, P. D., Hannington, G., and Booth, J. C.: Coxsackie B virus infections and myocardial infarction. Lancet *1*:1387–1389, 1980.
280. Grist, N. R., and Bell, E. J.: Paralytic poliomyelitis and nonpolio enteroviruses: Studies in Scotland. Rev. Infect. Dis. *6*:S385–S386, 1984.
281. Grist, N. R., Bell, E. J., and Assaad, F.: Enteroviruses in human disease. Prog. Med. Virol. *24*:114–157, 1978.
282. Grist, N. R., and Bell, E. J.: A six-year study of coxsackie virus B infections in heart disease. J. Hyg. *73*:165–172, 1974.
283. Grist, N. R., and Bell, E. J.: Enteroviral etiology of the paralytic poliomyelitis syndrome: Studies before and after vaccination. Arch. Environ. Health *21*:382–387, 1970.
284. Grist, N. R., and Bell, E. J.: Coxsackie viruses and the heart. Am. Heart J. *77*:295–300, 1969.
285. Grist, N. R., and Bell, E. J.: Coxsackie virus heart disease. B. M. J. *3*:556, 1968.
286. Grist, N. R.: Further studies of Coxsackie A7 virus infection in the west of Scotland. Lancet *2*:261–263, 1965.
287. Grose, C., and Horwitz, M. S.: Characterization of an enterovirus associated with acute infectious lymphocytosis. J. Gen. Virol. *30*:347–355, 1976.
288. Guidotti, M. B.: An outbreak of skin rash by echovirus 25 in an infant home. J. Infect. *6*:67–70, 1983.
289. Guthrie, N.: Coxsackie B5 meningitis: Report of an outbreak in a high school football squad. J. Tenn. State Med. Assoc. *55*:355–356, 1962.
290. Habel, K., Silverberg, R. J., and Shelokov, A.: Isolation of enteric viruses from cases of aseptic meningitis. Ann. N. Y. Acad. Sci. *67*:223–229, 1957.
291. Haddad, J., Gut, J. P., Wendling, M. J., et al.: Enterovirus infections in neonates: A retrospective study of 21 cases. Eur. J. Med. *2*:209–214, 1993.
292. Hadfield, M. G., Seidlin, M., Houff, S. A., et al.: Echovirus meningomyeloencephalitis with administration of intraventricular immunoglobulin. J. Neuropathol. Exp. Neurol. *44*:520–529, 1985.
293. Halfon, N., and Spector, S. A.: Fatal echovirus type 11 infections. Am. J. Dis. Child. *135*:1017–1020, 1981.
294. Hall, C. B., Cherry, J. D., Hatch, M. H., et al.: The return of Boston exanthem. Am. J. Dis. Child. *131*:323–326, 1977.
295. Hall, C. E., Cooney, M. K., and Fox, J. P.: The Seattle virus watch program. I. Infection and illness experience of virus watch families during a communitywide epidemic of echovirus type 30 aseptic meningitis. Am. J. Public Health *60*:1456–1465, 1970.
296. Halonen, P., Rocha, E., Hierholzer, J., et al.: Detection of enteroviruses and rhinoviruses in clinical specimens by PCR and liquid-phase hybridization. J. Clin. Microbiol. *33*:648–653, 1995.
297. Hammon, W. M., Yohn, D. S., Ludwig, E. H., et al.: A study of certain nonpoliomyelitis and poliomyelitis enterovirus infections: Clinical and serologic associations. J. A. M. A. *167*:727–734, 1958.
298. Hannaeus, G.: Dissertation. Copenhagen, 1735.
299. Hanneman, R. E.: Personal communication, 1996.
300. Hanninen, P., and Pohjonen, R.: Echovirus type 6 meningitis: Clinical and virological observations during an epidemic in Turku in 1968. Scand. J. Infect. Dis. *3*:121–125, 1971.
301. Hanson, L. A., Lundgren, S., Lycke, E., et al.: Clinical and serological observations in cases of Coxsackie B3 infections in early infancy. Acta Paediatr. Scand. *55*:577–583, 1966.
302. Harjulehto, T., Aro, T., Hovi, T., et al.: Congenital malformations and oral poliovirus vaccination during pregnancy. Lancet *1*:771–772, 1989.
303. Hart, E. W., Brunton, G. B., Taylor, C. E. D., et al.: Infection of newborn babies with ECHO virus type 5. Lancet *2*:402, 1962.
304. Hatch, M. H., and Marchetti, G. E.: Isolation of echoviruses with human embryonic lung fibroblast cells. Appl. Microbiol. *22*:736–737, 1971.
305. Haynes, R. E., Cramblett, H. G., Hilty, M. D., et al.: Echo virus type 3 infections in children: Clinical and laboratory studies. J. Pediatr. *80*:589–595, 1972.
306. Haynes, R. E., Cramblett, H. G., and Kronfol, H. J.: Echovirus 9 meningoencephalitis in infants and children. J. A. M. A. *208*:1657–1660, 1969.
307. Hayward, J. C., Gillespie, S. M., Kaplan, K. M., et al.: Outbreak of polio-

myelitis-like paralysis associated with enterovirus 71. Pediatr. Infect. Dis. J. *8*:611–616, 1989.
308. Heathfield, K. W. G., Pilsworth, R., Wall, B. J., et al.: Coxsackie B5 infections in Essex, 1965, with particular reference to the nervous system. Q. J. Med. *144*:579–595, 1967.
309. Hedlung, P., Lycke, E., and Tibblin, G.: The association of acute benign pericarditis in adults with Coxsackie B5 virus infection. Arch. Gesamte. Virusforsch. *13*:156–159, 1963.
310. Heinberg, H., Gold, E., and Robbins, F. C.: Differences in interferon content in tissues of mice of various ages infected with Coxsackie B1 virus. Proc. Soc. Exp. Biol. Med. *115*:947–953, 1964.
311. Helfand, R. F., Gary, H. E., Jr., Freeman, C. V., et al.: Serologic evidence of an association between enteroviruses and the onset of type 1 diabetes mellitus. J. Infect. Dis. *172*:1206–1211, 1995.
312. Helfand, R. F., Khan, A. S., Pallansch, M. A., et al.: Echovirus 30 infection and aseptic meningitis in parents of children attending a child care center. J. Infect. Dis. *169*:1133–1137, 1994.
313. Helin, M., Savola, J., and Lapinleimu, K.: Cardiac manifestations during a Coxsackie B5 epidemic. B. M. J. *3*:97–99, 1968.
314. Henke, A., Huber, S., Stelzner, A., et al.: The role of CD8+ T lymphocytes in coxsackievirus B3–induced myocarditis. J. Virol. *69*:6720–6728, 1995.
315. Hercìk, L., Huml, M., Mimra, J., et al.: Epidemien der respirationstrakterkrankungen bei neugeborenen durch ECHO 11-virus. Zentralbl. Bakteriol. *213*:18–27, 1970.
316. Herrmann, E. C., Jr.: Experience in providing a viral diagnostic laboratory compatible with medical practice. Mayo Clin. Proc. *42*:112–123, 1967.
317. Herskowitz, A., Beisel, K. W., Wolfgram, L. J., et al.: Coxsackievirus B3 murine myocarditis: Wide pathologic spectrum in genetically defined inbred strains. Hum. Pathol. *16*:671–673, 1985.
318. Hertel, N. T., Pedersen, F. K., and Heilmann, C.: Coxsackie B3 virus encephalitis in a patient with agammaglobulinemia. Eur. J. Pediatr. *148*:642–643, 1989.
319. Hierholzer, J. C., Killiard, K. A., and Esposito, J. J.: Serosurvey for "acute hemorrhagic conjunctivitis" virus (enterovirus 70) antibodies in the southeastern United States, with review of the literature and some epidemiologic implications. Am. J. Epidemiol. *102*:533–544, 1975.
320. Hierholzer, J. C., and Farris, W. A.: Follow-up of children infected in a coxsackievirus B-3 and B-4 outbreak: No evidence of diabetes mellitus. J. Infect. Dis. *129*:741–746, 1974.
321. Higgins, P. G., and Crow, K. D.: Recurrent Kaposi's varicelliform eruption in Darier's disease. Br. J. Dermatol. *88*:391–394, 1973.
322. Higgins, P. G., and Warin, R. P.: Hand, foot, and mouth disease: A clinically recognizable virus infection seen mainly in children. Clin. Pediatr. *6*:373–376, 1967.
323. Higgins, P. G., Ellis, E. M., Boston, D. G., et al.: Hand, foot and mouth disease, 1963–64: A study of cases and family contacts. Mo. Bull. Ministry Health (London) *24*:38–45, 1965.
324. Hinman, A. R., Koplan, J. P., Orenstein, W. A., et al.: Live or inactivated poliomyelitis vaccine: An analysis of benefits and risks. Am. J. Public Health *78*:291–295, 1988.
325. Hooft, C., Nihoul, E., Lambert, Y., et al.: Clinical findings during an Echo virus type 13 endemic infection. Helvet. Paediatr. Acta *18*:230–239, 1963.
326. Horn, M. E. C., Brain, E., Gregg, I., et al.: Respiratory viral infection in childhood: A survey in general practice, Roehampton 1967–1972. J. Hyg. (Camb.) *74*:157–168, 1975.
327. Horn, P.: Poliomyelitis in pregnancy: A 20-year report from Los Angeles County, California. Obstet. Gynecol. *6*:121–137, 1955.
328. Horstmann, D. M.: The poliomyelitis story: A scientific hegira. Yale J. Biol. Med. *58*:79–90, 1985.
329. Horstmann, D. M., Emmons, J., Gimpel, L., et al.: Enterovirus surveillance following a community-wide oral poliovirus vaccination program: A seven-year study. Am. J. Epidemiol. *97*:173–186, 1973.
330. Horstmann, D. M.: Viral exanthems and enanthems. Pediatrics *41*:867–870, 1968.
331. Horstmann, D. M.: The new ECHO viruses and their role in human disease. Arch. Intern. Med. *102*:155–162, 1958.
332. Horwitz, M. S., and Moore, G. T.: Acute infectious lymphocytosis: An etiologic and epidemiologic study of an outbreak. N. Engl. J. Med. *279*:399–404, 1968.
333. Hosier, D. M., and Newton, W. A., Jr.: Serious coxsackie infection in infants and children: Myocarditis, meningoencephalitis and hepatitis. Am. J. Dis. Child. *96*:251–267, 1958.
334. Howe, H. A., and Wilson, J. L.: Poliomyelitis. *In* Rivers, T. M., and Horsfall, F. L., Jr. (eds.): Viral and Rickettsial Infections of Man. Philadelphia, J. B. Lippincott, 1959, pp. 432–518.
335. Howlett, J. G., Somlo, F., and Kalz, F.: A new syndrome of parotitis with herpangina caused by the Coxsackie virus. Can. Med. Assoc. *77*:5–7, 1957.
336. Huang, T. W., and Wiegenstein, L. M.: Mesangiolytic glomerulonephritis in an infant with immune deficiency and echovirus infection. Arch. Pathol. Lab. Med. *101*:125–128, 1977.
337. Huber, S. A., Mortensen, A., and Moulton, G.: Modulation of cytokine expression by CD4+ T cells during coxsackievirus B3 infections of BALB/c mice initiated by cells expressing the gamma delta + T-cell receptor. J. Virol. *70*:3039–3044, 1996.
338. Huebner, R. J., Risser, J. A., Bell, J. A., et al.: Epidemic pleurodynia in Texas: A study of 22 cases. N. Engl. J. Med. *248*:267–274, 1953.
339. Hughes, J. R., Wilfert, C. M., Moore, M., et al.: Echovirus 14 infection associated with fatal neonatal hepatic necrosis. Am. J. Dis. Child. *123*:61–67, 1972.
340. Hughes, R. O., and Roberts, C.: Hand, foot, and mouth disease associated with Coxsackie A9 virus. Lancet *2*:751–752, 1972.
341. Hull, H. F., Ward, N. A., Hull, B. P., et al.: Paralytic poliomyelitis: Seasoned strategies, disappearing disease. Lancet *343*:1331–1337, 1994.
342. Hurley, R., Norman, A. P., and Pryse-Davies, J.: Massive pulmonary hemorrhage in the newborn associated with Coxsackie B virus infection. B. M. J. *3*:636–637, 1969.
343. Hurst, N. P., Martynoga, A. G., Nuki, G., et al.: Coxsackie B infection and arthritis. B. M. J. Clin. Res. Ed. *286*:605–607, 1983.
344. Hyoty, H., Huupponen, T., Kotola, L., et al.: Humoral immunity against viral antigens in type 1 diabetes: Altered IgA-class immune response against coxsackie B4 virus. Acta Pathol. Microbiol. Immunol. Scand. *94*:83–88, 1986.
345. Hyypia, T.: Identification of human picornaviruses by nucleic acid probes. Mol. Cell. Probes *3*:329–343, 1989.
346. Hyypia, T., Auvinen, P., and Maaronen, M.: Polymerase chain reaction for human picornaviruses. J. Gen. Virol. *70*:3261–3268, 1989.
347. Ikeda, R. M., Kondrack, S. F., Drabkin, P. D., et al.: Pleurodynia among football players at a high school: An outbreak associated with coxsackievirus B1. J. A. M. A. *270*:2205–2206, 1993.
348. Institute of Medicine: An evaluation of poliomyelitis vaccine policy options. Washington, D.C., National Academy of Sciences, 1988, IOM Publication 88–04.
349. Irvine, D. H., Irvine, A. B. H., and Gardner, P. S.: Outbreak of E. C. H. O. virus type 30 in a general practice. B. M. J. *4*:774–776, 1967.
350. Isaacs, D., Dobson, S. R. M., Wilkinson, A. R., et al.: Conservative management of an echovirus 11 outbreak in a neonatal unit. Lancet *1*:543–545, 1989.
351. Isacsohn, M., Eidelman, A. I., Kaplan, M., et al.: Neonatal coxsackievirus group B infections: Experience of a single department of neonatology. Isr. J. Med. Sci. *30*:371–374, 1994.
352. Ishiko, H., Takeda, N., Miyamura, K., et al.: Phylogenetic analysis of a coxsackievirus A24 variant: The most recent worldwide pandemic was caused by progenies of a virus prevalent around 1981. Virology *187*:748–759, 1992.
353. Ishimaru, Y., Nakano, S., Yamaoka, K., et al.: Outbreaks of hand, foot, and mouth disease by enterovirus 71: High incidence of complication disorders of central nervous system. Arch. Dis. Child. *55*:583–588, 1980.
354. Itagaki, A., Ishihara, J., Mochida, K., et al.: A clustering outbreak of hand, foot, and mouth disease caused by coxsackie virus A10. Microbiol. Immunol. *27*:929–935, 1983.
355. Jack, I., Grutzner, J., Gray, N., et al.: A survey of prenatal virus disease in Melbourne, July 21, 1967. Personal communication.
356. Jack, I., and Townley, R. R. W.: Acute aseptic myocarditis of newborn infants, due to Coxsackie viruses. Med. J. Aust. *2*:265–268, 1961.
357. Jackson, A. L.: A clinical study of the Landry-Guillain-Barré syndrome with reference to aetiology, including the role of Coxsackie virus infections. S. Afr. J. Lab. Clin. Med. *7*:121–137, 1961.
358. Jahn, C. L., and Cherry, J. D.: Mild neonatal illness associated with heavy enterovirus infection. N. Engl. J. Med. *274*:394–395, 1966.
359. Jahn, C. L., Felton, O. L., and Cherry, J. D.: Coxsackie B1 pneumonia in an adult. J. A. M. A. *189*:236–237, 1964.
360. James, W. D., Odom, R. B., and Hatch, M. H.: Gianotti-crosti-like eruption associated with coxsackievirus A16 infection. J. Am. Acad. Dermatol. *6*:862–866, 1982.
361. Jamieson, W. M., Kerr, M., and Sommerville, R. G.: Echo type-9 meningitis in east Scotland. Lancet *1*:581–583, 1958.
362. Jantausch, B. A., Luban, N. L. C., Duffy, L., et al.: Maternal plasma transfusion in the treatment of disseminated neonatal echovirus 11 infection. Pediatr. Infect. Dis. J. *14*:154–155, 1995.
363. Jarvis, W. R., and Tucker, G.: Echovirus type 7 meningitis in young children. Am. J. Dis. Child. *135*:1009–1012, 1981.
364. Javett, S. N., Heymann, S., Mundel, B., et al.: Myocarditis in the newborn infant. J. Pediatr. *48*:1–22, 1956.
365. Jehn, U. W., and Fink, M. K.: Myositis, myoglobinemia, and myoglobinuria associated with enterovirus Echo 9 infection. Arch. Neurol. *37*:457–458, 1980.
366. Jenista, J. A., Powell, K. R., and Menegus, M. A.: Epidemiology of neonatal enterovirus infection. J. Pediatr. *104*:685–690, 1984.
367. Jhala, C. I., Draper, J., and Walcher, D. N.: Aseptic meningitis syndrome due to virus Echo type 23. Am. J. Dis. Child. *102*:868–870, 1961.
368. John, T. J., Pandian, R., Gadomski, A., et al.: Control of poliomyelitis by pulse immunisation in Vellore, India. B. M. J. *286*:31–32, 1983.
369. Johnson, D. A., and Eger, A. W.: Myelitis associated with an echovirus. J. A. M. A. *201*:637–638, 1967.
370. Johnson, I., Hammond, G. W., and Verma, M. R.: Nosocomial coxsackie B4 virus infections in two chronic-care pediatric neurological wards. J. Infect. Dis. *151*:1153–1156, 1985.
371. Johnson, J. F., and Stimson, P. M.: Clinical poliomyelitis in the early neonatal period. J. Pediatr. *40*:733–737, 1956.

372. Johnson, K. M., Bloom, H. H., Forsyth, B., et al.: Relative role of identifiable agents in respiratory disease. II. The role of enteroviruses in respiratory disease. Am. Rev. Respir. Dis. *88*:240–245, 1962.
373. Johnson, R. T.: Late progression of poliomyelitis paralysis: Discussion of pathogenesis. Rev. Infect. Dis. *6*:S568–S570, 1984.
374. Johnson, R. T., Shuey, H. E., and Buescher, E. L.: Epidemic central nervous system disease of mixed enterovirus etiology. I/II. Clinical and epidemiologic description. Am. J. Hyg. *71*:321–330, 331–341, 1960.
375. Johnson, R. T., Portnoy, B., Rogers, N. G., et al.: Acute benign pericarditis: Virologic study of 34 patients. Arch. Intern. Med. *108*:823–832, 1961.
376. Johnston, J. M., and Overall, J. C., Jr.: Intravenous immunoglobulin in disseminated neonatal echovirus 11 infection. Pediatr. Infect. Dis. J. *8*:254–256, 1989.
377. Joncas, J. H., Podoski, M. O., and Pavilanis, V.: Rash associated with Coxsackie A9 infection. Can. Med. Assoc. J. *95*:372–373, 1966.
378. Jones, M. J., Kolb, M., Votava, H. J., et al.: Intrauterine echovirus type 11 infection. Mayo Clin. Proc. *55*:509–512, 1980.
379. Josselson, J., Pula, T., and Sadler, J. H.: Acute rhabdomyolysis associated with an echovirus 9 infection. Arch. Intern. Med. *140*:1671–1672, 1980.
380. Judelsohn, R.: Changing the US polio immunization schedule would be bad public health policy. Pediatrics *98*:115–116, 1996.
381. Kahlmeter, O.: Clinical aspects of Echo viruses. Ciba Found. Symp. *7*:24–36, 1959.
382. Kantor, F. S., and Hsiung, G. D.: Pleurodynia associated with Echo virus type 8. N. Engl. J. Med. *266*:661–663, 1962.
383. Kaplan, G. J., Bender, T. R., Clark, P. S., et al.: Echovirus type 4 meningitis and related febrile illness: Epidemiologic study of an outbreak in two Eskimo communities in 1970. Am. J. Epidemiol. *96*:74–85, 1972.
384. Kaplan, G. J., Clark, P. S., Bender, T. R., et al.: Echovirus type 30 meningitis and related febrile illness: Epidemiologic study of an outbreak in an Eskimo community. Am. J. Epidemiol. *92*:257–265, 1970.
385. Kaplan, M. H., Klein, S. W., McPhee, J., et al.: Group B coxsackievirus infections in infants younger than three months of age: A serious childhood illness. Rev. Infect. Dis. *5*:1019–1032, 1983.
386. Kapsenberg, J. G.: ECHO virus type 33 as a cause of meningitis. Arch. Ges. Virusforsch. *23*:144–147, 1968.
387. Karzon, D. T., and Barron, A. L.: An epidemic of aseptic meningitis syndrome due to Echo virus type 6. I. Correlation of enterovirus isolation with illness. II. Clinical study. III. Sequelae. Pediatrics *29*:409–417, 418–431, 432–437, 1962.
388. Karzon, D. T., Eckert, G. L., Barron, A. L., et al.: Aseptic meningitis epidemic due to Echo 4 virus. Am. J. Dis. Child. *101*:610–622, 1961.
389. Katz, S. L.: Poliovaccine policy: Time for a change. Pediatrics *98*:116–117, 1996.
390. Kaul, A., Cohen, M. E., Broffman, G., et al.: Reye-like syndrome associated with Coxsackie B2 virus infection. J. Pediatr. *94*:67–69, 1979.
391. Kaye, B. M., Rosner, D. C., and Stein, I., Sr.: Viral diseases in pregnancy and their effect upon the embryo and fetus. Am. J. Obstet. Gynecol. *65*:109–118, 1953.
392. Kelen, A. E., Lesiak, J. M., and Labzoffsky, N. A.: Occurrence of Echovirus 33 infections in Ontario. Can. Med. Assoc. J. *98*:985–987, 1968.
393. Kelen, A. E., Lesiak, J. M., and Labzoffsky, N. A.: An outbreak of aseptic meningitis due to Echo 25 virus. Can. Med. Assoc. J. *90*:1349–1351, 1964.
394. Kelen, A. E., Lesiak, J. M., and Labzoffsky, N. A.: Sporadic occurrence of Echo virus types 27 and 31 associated with aseptic meningitis in Ontario. Can. Med. Assoc. J. *91*:1266–1268, 1964.
395. Kendall, E. J. C., Cook, G. T., and Stone, D. M.: Acute respiratory infections in children: Isolation of Coxsackie B virus and adenovirus during a survey in a general practice. B. M. J. *2*:1180–1184, 1960.
396. Kennett, M. L., Birch, C. J., Lewis, F. A., et al.: Enterovirus type 71 infection in Melbourne. Bull. W. H. O. *51*:609–615, 1974.
397. Kennett, M. L., Ellis, A. W., Lewis, F. A., et al.: An epidemic associated with echovirus type 18. J. Hyg. (Camb.) *70*:325–334, 1972.
398. Keswick, B. H., Gerba, C. P., and Goyal, S. M.: Occurrence of enteroviruses in community swimming pools. Am. J. Public Health *71*:1026–1030, 1981.
399. Kew, O. M., Mulders, M. N., Lipskaya, G. Y., et al.: Molecular epidemiology of polioviruses. Virology *6*:401–414, 1995.
400. Kibrick, S.: Current status of Coxsackie and ECHO viruses in human disease. Prog. Med. Virol. *6*:27–70, 1964.
401. Kibrick, S.: Viral infections of the fetus and newborn. Perspect. Virol. *2*:140–159, 1961.
402. Kibrick, S., and Enders, J. F.: Disease due to Echo virus type 9 in Massachusetts. N. Engl. J. Med. *259*:482–484, 1958.
403. Kibrick, S., Melendex, L., and Enders, J. F.: Clinical associations of enteric viruses with particular reference to agents exhibiting properties of the Echo group. Ann. N. Y. Acad. Sci. *67*:311–325, 1957.
404. Kibrick, S., and Benirschke, K.: Acute aseptic myocarditis and meningoencephalitis in the newborn child infected with Coxsackie virus group B, type 3. N. Engl. J. Med. *255*:883–889, 1956.
405. Kilbourne, E. D., and Goldfield, M.: Coxsackie viruses and "virus-like" diseases of the adult: A three-year study in a contagious disease hospital. Am. J. Med. *21*:175–183, 1956.
406. Kilborne, E. D., Wilson, C. B., and Perrier, D.: The induction of gross myocardial lesions by a Coxsackie (pleurodynia) virus and cortisone. J. Clin. Invest. *35*:362–370, 1956.
407. King, M. L., Shaikh, A., Bidwell, D., et al.: Coxsackie B virus specific IgM responses in children with insulin-dependent (juvenile-onset; type 1) diabetes mellitus. Lancet *1*:1397–1399, 1983.
408. Kinney, J. S., McCray, E., Kaplan, J. E., et al.: Risk factors associated with echovirus 11′ infection in a hospital nursery. Pediatr. Infect. Dis. J. *5*:192–197, 1986.
409. Kipps, A., Naude, W. duT., Don, P., et al.: Coxsackie virus myocarditis of the newborn: Epidemiological features. Med. Proc. *4*:401–406, 1958.
410. Klein, J. O., Lerner, A. M., and Finland, M.: Acute gastroenteritis associated with Echo virus, type 11. Am. J. Med. Sci. *240*:749–753, 1960.
411. Kleinman, H., Ramras, D. G., Cooney, M. K., et al.: Aseptic meningitis due to Echo virus type 7. N. Engl. J. Med. *267*:1116–1121, 1962.
412. Kleinman, H., Rogers, D., Ellwood, P. M., Jr., et al.: Epidemic of ECHO 9 aseptic meningitis in Minnesota, 1957, Univ. Minn. Med. Bull. *29*:306, 1958.
413. Klemola, E., and Lapinleimu, K.: Multiple attacks of aseptic meningitis in the same individual. B. M. J. *1*:1087–1090, 1964.
414. Klespies, S. L., Cebula, D. E., Kelley, C. L., et al.: Detection of enteroviruses from clinical specimens by spin amplification shell vial culture and monoclonal antibody assay. J. Clin. Microbiol. *34*:1465–1467, 1996.
415. Koch, V. F., Enders-Ruckle, G., and Wokittel, E.: Coxsackie B-5 infektionen mit signifikanter antikörperentwicklung bei neugeborenen. Arch. Kinderheilk. *165*:245–258, 1962.
416. Kogon, A., Spigland, I., Frothingham, T. E., et al.: The virus watch program: A continuing surveillance of viral infections in metropolitan New York families. VII. Observations on viral excretion, seroimmunity, intrafamilial spread and illness association in Coxsackie and Echovirus infections. Am. J. Epidemiol. *89*:51–61, 1969.
417. Kono, R.: Apollo 11 diseases or acute hemorrhagic conjunctivitis: A pandemic of a new enterovirus infection of the eyes. Am. J. Epidemiol. *101*:383–390, 1975.
418. Koontz, C. H., and Ray, C. G.: The role of Coxsackie group B virus infections in sporadic myopericarditis. Am. Heart J. *82*:750–758, 1971.
419. Kopel, F. B., Shore, B., and Hodes, H. L.: Nonfatal bulbospinal paralysis due to ECHO 4 virus. J. Pediatr. *67*:588–594, 1965.
420. Koskiniemi, M., Paetau, R., and Linnavuori, K.: Severe encephalitis associated with disseminated echovirus 22 infection. Scand. J. Infect. Dis. *21*:463–466, 1989.
421. Kraus, N. S.: La parotite da virus Coxsackie. Estratto Minerva Medica *51*:1379–1381, 1960.
422. Kuban, K. C., Ephros, M. A., Freeman, R. L., et al.: Syndrome of opsoclonus-myoclonus caused by coxsackie B3 infection. Ann. Neurol. *13*:69–71, 1983.
423. Kujala, G., and Newman, J. H.: Isolation of echovirus type 11 from synovial fluid in acute monocytic arthritis. Arthritis Rheum. *28*:98–99, 1985.
424. Kunin, C. M.: Cellular susceptibility to enteroviruses. Bacteriol. Rev. *28*:382–390, 1964.
425. Kunin, C. M.: Virus-tissue union and the pathogenesis of enterovirus infections. J. Immunol. *88*:556–569, 1962.
426. Kuritsky, J. N., Weaver, J. H., Bernard, K. W., et al.: An outbreak of acute hemorrhagic conjunctivitis in central Minnesota. Am. J. Ophthalmol. *96*:449–452, 1983.
427. LaForest, R. A., McNaughton, G. A., Beale, A. J., et al.: Outbreak of aseptic meningitis (meningoencephalitis) with rubelliform rash: Toronto, 1956. Can. Med. Assoc. J. *77*:1–4, 1957.
428. Lahelle, O.: Aseptic meningitis caused by Echo virus. J. Hyg. *55*:475–484, 1957.
429. Lake, A. M., Lauer, B. A., Clark, J. C., et al.: Enterovirus infections in neonates. J. Pediatr. *89*:787–791, 1976.
430. Landry, M. L., Ponseca, S. N. S., Cohen, S., et al.: Fatal enterovirus type 71 infection: Rapid detection and diagnostic pitfalls. Pediatr. Infect. Dis. J. *14*:1095–1100, 1995.
431. Landsman, J. B., Grist, N. R., and Ross, C. A. C.: Echo 9 virus infection and congenital malformations. Br. J. Prev. Soc. Med. *18*:152–156, 1964.
432. Landsteiner, K., and Popper, E.: Übertragung der poliomyelitis acuta auf affen. Z. Immun. Forsch. *2*:377–390, 1909.
433. Lane, J. R., Neumann, D. A., Lafond-Walker, A., et al.: Role of IL-1 and tumor necrosis factor in coxsackie virus-induced autoimmune myocarditis. J. Immunol. *151*:1682–1690, 1993.
434. Lansky, L. L., Krugman, S., and Hug, G.: Anicteric Coxsackie B hepatitis. J. Pediatr. *94*:64–65, 1979.
435. Lapinleimu, K., and Kaski, U.: An outbreak caused by coxsackievirus B5 among newborn infants. Scand. J. Infect. Dis. *4*:27–30, 1972.
436. Lau, R. C. H.: Coxsackie B virus-specific IgM responses in coronary care unit patients. J. Med. Virol. *18*:193–198, 1986.
437. Lau, R. C. H.: Coxsackie B virus infections in New Zealand patients with cardiac and noncardiac diseases. J. Med. Virol. *11*:131–137, 1983.
438. Lau, R. C. H.: Coxsackie B virus infection in acute myocardial infarction and adult heart disease. Med. J. Aust. *2*:520–522, 1982.
439. Leggiadro, R. J., Chwatsky, D. N., and Zucker, S. W.: Echovirus 3 infection associated with anicteric hepatitis Am. J. Dis. Child. *136*:843, 1982.
440. Lehan, P. H., Chick, E. W., Doto, I. L., et al.: An epidemic illness associ-

ated with a recently recognized enteric virus (Echo virus type 4). I. Epidemiologic and clinical features. Am. J. Hyg. *66*:63–75, 1957.

441. Lennette, E. H., Magoffin, R. L., and Knouf, E. G.: Viral central nervous system disease: An etiologic study conducted at the Los Angeles County General Hospital. J. A. M. A. *179*:687–695, 1962.
442. Leonardi, G. P., Greenberg, A. J., Costello, P., et al.: Echovirus type 30 infection associated with aseptic meningitis in Nassau County, New York, USA. Intervirology *36*:53–56, 1993.
443. Leparc-Goffart, I., Julien, J., Fuchs, F., et al.: Evidence of presence of poliovirus genomic sequences in cerebrospinal fluid from patients with postpolio syndrome. J. Clin. Microbiol. *34*:2023–2026, 1996.
444. Lepow, M. L., Coyne, N., Thompson, L. B., et al.: A clinical, epidemiologic and laboratory investigation of aseptic meningitis during the four-year period 1955–1958: II. The clinical disease and its sequelae. N. Engl. J. Med. *266*:1188–1193, 1962.
445. Lepow, M. L. Carver, D. H., Wright, H. T., Jr., et al.: A clinical, epidemiologic and laboratory investigation of aseptic meningitis during the four-year period 1955–1958. I. Observations concerning etiology and epidemiology. N. Engl. J. Med. *266*:1181–1187, 1962.
446. Lepow, M. L., Carver, D. H., and Robbins, F. C.: Clinical and epidemiologic observations on enterovirus infection in a circumscribed community during an epidemic of Echo 9 infection. Pediatrics *26*:12–26, 1960.
447. Lerner, A. M., Klein, J. O., Cherry, J. D., et al.: New viral exanthems. N. Engl. J. Med. *269*:678–686, 736–740, 1963.
448. Lerner, A. M., Klein, J. O., and Finland, M.: Infection with Coxsackie virus group B, type 3, with vesicular eruption: Report of two cases. N. Engl. J. Med. *263*:1305, 1960.
449. Lerner, A. M., Klein, J. O., and Finland, M.: A laboratory outbreak of infections with Coxsackie virus group A, type 9. N. Engl. J. Med. *263*:1302–1304, 1960.
450. Lerner, A. M., Klein, J. O., Levin, H. S., et al.: Infections due to Coxsackie virus group A, type 9, in Boston, 1959, with special reference to exanthems and pneumonia. N. Engl. J. Med. *263*:1265–1272, 1960.
451. Levi, G. F., Proto, C., Quadri, A., et al.: Coxsackie virus heart disease and cardiomyopathy. Am. Heart J. *93*:419–421, 1977.
452. Levin, S., Measroch, V., Pech, W., et al.: Hand-foot-and-mouth disease. S. Afr. Med. J. *55*:502–504, 1962.
453. Lewes, D., Rainford, D. J., and Lane, W. F.: Symptomless myocarditis and myalgia in viral and *Mycoplasma pneumoniae* infections. Br. Heart J. *36*:924–932, 1974.
454. Lewis, H. M., Parry, J. V., Parry, R. P., et al.: Role of viruses in febrile-convulsions. Arch. Dis. Child. *54*:869–876, 1979.
455. Liebman, W. M., and St. Geme, J. W., Jr.: Enteroviral pseudoappendicitis. Am. J. Dis. Child. *120*:77–78, 1970.
456. Liljeqvist, J. A., Bergstrom, T., Holmstrom, S., et al.: Failure to demonstrate enterovirus aetiology in Swedish patients with dilated cardiomyopathy. J. Med. Virol. *39*:6–10, 1993.
457. Limson, B. M., Chan, V. F., Guzman, S. V., et al.: Occurrence of infection with group B coxsackievirus in rheumatic and nonrheumatic Filipino children. J. Infect. Dis. *140*:415–418, 1979.
458. Lin, K.-H., Wang, H.-L., Sheu, M.-M., et al.: Molecular epidemiology of a variant of coxsackievirus A24 in Taiwan: Two epidemics caused by phylogenetically distinct viruses from 1985 to 1989. J. Clin. Microbiol. *31*:1160–1166, 1993.
459. Lindenbaum, J. E., Van Dyck, P. C., and Allen, R. G.: Hand, foot and mouth disease associated with coxsackievirus group B. Scand. J. Infect. Dis. *7*:161–163, 1975.
460. Linnemann, C. C., Jr., Steichen, J., Sherman, W. G., et al.: Febrile illness in early infancy associated with ECHO virus infection. J. Pediatr. *84*:49–54, 1974.
461. Longson, M., Cole, F. M., and Davies, D.: Isolation of a Coxsackie virus group B, type 5, from the heart of a fatal case of myocarditis in an adult. J. Clin. Pathol. *22*:654–658, 1969.
462. Lycke, E., and Nilsson, L. R.: Poliomyelitis in a newborn due to intrauterine infection. Acta Paediatr. *51*:661–664, 1962.
463. Lycke, E., Hiltigardh, A., and Redin, B.: Coxsackie B1 virus and febrile illness with rash. Lancet *1*:1097, 1959.
464. MacLeod, A. J., Faulkner, R. S. and Van Rooyen, C. E.: Echo-9 virus infections in eastern Canada: Clinical and laboratory studies. Can. Med. Assoc. J. *78*:661–665, 1958.
465. Magoffin, R. L., and Lennette, E. H.: Nonpolioviruses and paralytic disease. Calif. Med. *97*:1–7, 1962.
466. Magoffin, R. L., Jackson, E. W., and Lennette, E. H.: Vesicular stomatitis and exanthem: A syndrome associated with Coxsackie virus, type A16. J. A. M. A. *175*:441–445, 1961.
467. Magoffin, R. L., Lennette, E. H., and Schmidt, N. J.: Association of Coxsackie viruses with illnesses resembling mild paralytic poliomyelitis. Pediatrics *28*:602–613, 1961.
468. Makower, H., Skurska, Z., and Halazinska, L.: On transplacental infection with Coxsackie virus. Texas Rep. Biol. Med. *16*:346–353, 1958.
469. Malcolm, B. S., Eiden, J. J., and Hendley, J. O.: ECHO virus type 9 meningitis simulating tuberculous meningitis. Pediatrics *65*:725–726, 1980.
470. Malherbe, H., Harwin, R., and Smith, A. H.: An outbreak of aseptic meningitis associated with Echo virus type 4. S. Afr. Med. J. *31*:1261–1264, 1957.
471. Maller, H. M., Powars, D. F., Horowitz, R. E., et al.: Fatal myocarditis associated with Echo virus, type 22, infection in a child with apparent immunological deficiency. J. Pediatr. *71*:204–210, 1967.
472. Marchessault, V., Pavilanis, V., Podoski, M. O., et al.: An epidemic of aseptic meningitis caused by Coxsackie B type 2 virus. Can. Med. Assoc. J. *85*:123–126, 1961.
473. Marier, R., Rodriguez, W., Chloupek, R. J., et al.: Coxsackievirus B5 infection and aseptic meningitis in neonates and children. Am. J. Dis. Child. *129*:321–325, 1975.
474. Marks, M. I., Joncas, J. H., and Mauer, S. M.: Fatal hepatitis in siblings: Isolation of coxsackievirus B5 and herpes simplex virus. Can. Med. Assoc. J. *102*:1391–1401, 1970.
475. Martino, T. A., Sole, M. J., Penn, L. Z., et al.: Quantitation of enteroviral RNA by competitive polymerase chain reaction. J. Clin. Microbiol. *31*:2634–2640, 1993.
476. Marzetti, G., and Midulla, M.: Acute cerebellar ataxia associated with Echo type 6 infection in two children. Acta Paediatr. Scand. *56*:547–551, 1967.
477. Matsuura, K., Hasegawa, S., Nakayama, T., et al.: Epidemiological studies on echovirus type 18 infection in Toyama Prefecture. Microbiol. Immunol. *27*:359–368, 1983.
478. Matthews, J. D., Cameron, S. J., and George, M.: Constrictive pericarditis following Coxsackie virus infection. Thorax *25*:624–626, 1970.
479. Matumoto, M.: Newer respiratory disease viruses in Japan and some Far Eastern countries. Am. Rev. Respir. Dis. *88*(Part 2):46–55, 1963.
480. McAllister, R. M.: Echo virus infections. Pediatr. Clin. North Am. *7*:927–945, 1960.
481. McAllister, R. M., Hummeler, K., and Coriell, L. L.: Report of a case with isolation of type 9 ECHO virus from the cerebrospinal fluid. N. Engl. J. Med. *261*:1159–1162, 1959.
482. McIntyre, J. P., and Keen, G. A.: Laboratory surveillance of viral meningitis by examination of cerebrospinal fluid in Cape Town, 1981–9. Epidemiol. Infect. *111*:357–371, 1993.
483. McKinney, R. E., Jr., Katz, S. L., and Wilfert, C. M.: Chronic enteroviral meningoencephalitis in agammaglobulinemic patients. Rev. Infect. Dis. *9*:334–356, 1987.
484. McLean, D. M., Catiyanonda, K., Ladyman, S. R., et al.: Gastroenteritis of infants in two Canadian communities. Can. Med. Assoc. J. *102*:1247–1251, 1970.
485. McLean, D. M., Larke, R. P. B., Cobb, C., et al.: Mumps and enteroviral meningitis in Toronto, 1966. Can. Med. Assoc. J. *96*:1355–1361, 1967.
486. McLean, D. M., Larke, R. P. B., McNaughton, G. A., et al.: Enteroviral syndromes in Toronto, 1964. Can. Med. Assoc. J. *92*:658–661, 1965.
487. McLean, D. M.: Patterns of infection with enteroviruses. J. Pediatr. *54*:823–828, 1959.
488. McLean, D. M., and Melnick, J. L.: Association of mouse pathogenic strain of Echo virus type 9 with aseptic meningitis. Proc. Soc. Exp. Biol. Med. *94*:656–660, 1957.
489. McManus, B. M., Chow, L. H., Wilson, J. E., et al.: Direct myocardial injury by enterovirus: A central role in the evolution of murine myocarditis. Clin. Immunol. Immunopathol. *68*:159–169, 1993.
490. Meade, R. H., and Chang, T. W.: Zoster-like eruption due to Echovirus 6. Am. J. Dis. Child. *133*:283–284, 1979.
491. Meadow, S. R.: Hand, foot, and mouth diseases. Arch. Dis. Child. *40*:560–564, 1965.
492. Mease, P. J., Ochs, H. D., and Wedgwood, R. J.: Successful treatment of echovirus meningoencephalitis and myositis-fasciitis with intravenous immune globulin therapy in a patient with X-linked agammaglobulinemia. N. Engl. J. Med. *304*:1278–1281, 1981.
493. Medearis, D. N., Jr., and Kramer, R. A.: Exanthem associated with Echo virus type 18 viremia. J. Pediatr. *55*:367–373, 1959.
494. Meehan, W. F., and Bertrand, C. A.: Ventricular tachycardia associated with echovirus infection. J. A. M. A. *212*:1701–1703, 1970.
495. Melchers, W., Zoll, J., van Kuppeveld, F., et al.: There is no evidence for persistent enterovirus infections in chronic medical conditions in humans. Rev. Med. Virol. *4*:235–243, 1994.
496. Melnick, J. L.: Enteroviruses: Polioviruses, coxsackieviruses, echoviruses and newer enteroviruses. *In* Fields, B. N., and Knipe, D. M. (eds.): Virology. 2nd ed. New York, Raven Press, 1990, pp. 549–605.
497. Melnick, J. L.: Enterovirus type 71 infections: A varied clinical pattern sometimes mimicking paralytic poliomyelitis. Rev. Infect. Dis. *6*:S387–S390, 1984.
498. Melnick, J. L.: Portraits of viruses: The picornaviruses. Intervirology *20*:61–100, 1983.
499. Melnick, J. L.: Enteroviruses. *In* Evans, A. S. (ed.): Viral Infections on Humans: Epidemiology and Control. 3rd ed. New York, Plenum Medical, 1989, pp. 191–263.
500. Melnick, J. L., and Wenner, H. A.: Enteroviruses. *In* Lennette, E. H., and Schmidt, N. J. (eds.): Diagnostic Procedures for Viral and Rickettsial Infections. 4th ed. New York, American Public Health Association, 1969.
501. Melnick, J. L.: Echoviruses. *In* Horsfall, J. R., and Tamm, I. (eds.): Viral and Rickettsial Infections of Man. Philadelphia, J. B. Lippincott, 1965, pp. 513–545.
502. Melnick, J. L., Cockburn, W. C., Dalldorf, G., et al.: Picornavirus group. Virology *19*:114–116, 1963.

503. Melnick, J. L., Dalldorf, G., Enders, J. F., et al.: The enteroviruses. Am. J. Public Health *47*:1556–1566, 1957.
504. Mertens, T., Hager, H., and Eggers, H. J.: Epidemiology of an outbreak in a maternity unit of infections with an antigenic variant of Echovirus 11. J. Med. Virol. *9*:81–91, 1982.
505. Miller, D. G., Gabrielson, M. O., Bart, K. J., et al.: An epidemic of aseptic meningitis, primarily among infants, caused by Echovirus 11-prime. Pediatrics *41*:77–90, 1978.
506. Miller, M. A., Sutter, R. W., Strebel, P. M., et al.: Cost-effectiveness of incorporating inactivated poliovirus vaccine into the routine childhood immunization schedule. J. A. M. A. *276*:967–971, 1996.
507. Miller, N. A., Carmichael, H. A., Calder, B. D., et al.: Antibody to coxsackie B virus in diagnosing postviral fatigue syndrome. B. M. J. *302*:140–141, 1991.
508. Mirkovic, R. R., Varma, S. K., and Yoon, J. W.: Incidence of coxsackievirus B type 4 (CB4) infections concomitant with onset of insulin-dependent diabetes mellitus. J. Med. Virol. *14*:9–16, 1984.
509. Mitchell, S. C., and Dempster, G.: The finding of genital lesions in a case of Coxsackie virus infection. Can. Med. Assoc. J. *72*:117–119, 1955.
510. Miwa, C., Ohtani, M., Watanabe, H., et al.: Epidemic of hand, foot, and mouth disease in Gifu Prefecture in 1978. Jpn. J. Med. Sci. Biol. *33*:167–180, 1980.
511. Modlin, J. F., Dagan, R., Berlin, L. E., et al.: Focal encephalitis with enterovirus infections. Pediatrics *88*:841–845, 1991.
512. Modlin, J. F.: Perinatal echovirus infection: Insights from a literature review of 61 cases of serious infection and 16 outbreaks in nurseries. Rev. Infect. Dis. *8*:918–926, 1986.
513. Modlin, J. F., Polk, B. F., Horton, P., et al.: Perinatal echovirus infection: Risk of transmission during a community outbreak. N. Engl. J. Med. *305*:368–371, 1981.
514. Modlin, J. F.: Fatal echovirus 11 disease in premature neonates. Pediatrics *66*:775–780, 1980.
515. Mokhtar, M. O. E.-H., Banatvala, J. E., and Coltart, D. J.: Coxsackie-B-virus–specific IgM responses in patients with cardiac and other diseases. Lancet *2*:1160–1162, 1980.
516. Monif, G. R. G., Lee, C. W., and Hsiung, G. D.: Isolated myocarditis with recovery of Echo type 9 virus from the myocardium. N. Engl. J. Med. *277*:1353–1355, 1967.
517. Montgomery, J., Gear, J., Prinsloo, F. R., et al.: Myocarditis of the newborn: An outbreak in a maternity home in southern Rhodesia associated with Coxsackie group-B virus infection. S. Afr. Med. J. *29*:608–612, 1955.
518. Moore, M.: Enteroviral disease in the United States, 1970–1979. J. Infect. Dis. *146*:103–108, 1982.
519. Moore, M. L., Hooser, L. E., Davis, E. V., et al.: Sudden unexpected death in infancy: Isolations of ECHO type 7 virus. Proc. Soc. Exp. Biol. Med. *116*:231–234, 1964.
520. Moossy, J., and Geer, J. C.: Encephalomyelitis, myocarditis and adrenal cortical necrosis in Coxsackie B3 virus infection: Distribution of the central nervous system lesions. Arch. Pathol. *70*:614–622, 1960.
521. Morens, D. M., Zweighaft, R. M., and Bryan, J. M.: Nonpolio enterovirus disease in the United States, 1971–1975. Int. J. Epidemiol. *8*:49–54, 1979.
522. Morens, D. M.: Enteroviral disease in early infancy. J. Pediatr. *92*:374–377, 1978.
523. Morgante, O., Wilkinson, D., Burchak, E. C., et al.: Outbreak of hand-foot-and-mouth disease among Indian and Eskimo children in a hospital. J. Infect. Dis. *125*:587–597, 1972.
524. Mori, I., Matsumoto, K., Hatano, M., et al.: An unseasonable winter outbreak of echovirus type 30 meningitis. J. Infect. *31*:219–223, 1995.
525. Morita, H., Kitaura, Y., Deguchi, H., et al.: Coxsackie B5 myopericarditis in a young adult: Clinical course and endomyocardial biopsy findings. Jpn. Circ. J. *47*:1077–1083, 1983.
526. Moritsugu, Y., Sawada, K., Hinohara, M., et al.: An outbreak of type 25 echovirus infection with exanthem in an infant home near Tokyo. Am. J. Epidemiol. *87*:599–608, 1968.
527. Morris, J. A., Elisberg, B. L., Pond, W. L., et al.: Hepatitis associated with Coxsackie virus group A, type 4. N. Engl. J. Med. *267*:1230–1233, 1962.
528. Moscovici, C., and Maisel, J.: Intestinal viruses of newborn and older prematures. Am. J. Dis. Child. *101*:77–777, 1961.
529. Mostoufizadeh, M., Lack, E. E., Gang, D. L., et al.: Postmortem manifestations of echovirus 11 sepsis in five newborn infants. Hum. Pathol. *14*:818–823, 1983.
530. Muir, P., and Archard, L.C.: There is evidence for persistent enterovirus infections in chronic medical conditions in humans. Rev. Med. Virol. *4*:245–250, 1994.
531. Muir, P., Nicholson, F., Spencer, G. T., et al.: Enterovirus infection of the central nervous system of humans: Lack of association with chronic neurological disease. J. Gen. Virol. *77*:1469–1476, 1996.
532. Muir, P., Nicholson, F., Tilzey, A. J., et al.: Chronic relapsing pericarditis and dilated cardiomyopathy: Serological evidence of persistent enterovirus infection. Lancet *1*:804–806, 1989.
533. Mulders, M. N., Lipskaya, G. Y., van der Avoort, H. G. A. M., et al.: Molecular epidemiology of wild poliovirus type 1 in Europe, the Middle East, and the Indian subcontinent. J. Infect. Dis. *171*:1399–1405, 1995.
534. Murdin, A. D., Barreto, L., and Plotkin, S.: Inactivated poliovirus vaccine: Past and present experience. Vaccine *14*:735–746, 1996.
535. Murphy, A. M., and Simmul, R.: Coxsackie B4 virus infections in New South Wales during 1962. Med. J. Aust. *2*:443–445, 1964.
536. Nagington, J., Gandy, G., Walker, J., et al.: Use of normal immunoglobulin in an echovirus 11 outbreak in a special-care baby unit. Lancet *2*:443–446, 1983.
537. Nagington, J., Wreghitt, T. G., Gandy, G., et al.: Fatal Echovirus 11 infections in outbreak in special-care baby unit. Lancet *2*:725–728, 1978.
538. Nahmias, A. J., Froeschle, J. E., Feorino, P. M., et al.: Generalized eruption in a child with eczema due to coxsackievirus A16. Arch. Dermatol. *97*:147–148, 1968.
539. Nair, E., and Kalra, S. L.: Cytopathic enteroviruses in Delhi area. I. From cases of diarrhoea and healthy controls. Indian J. Med. Res. *57*:141–148, 1968.
540. Nakao, T., and Miura, R.: Recurrent virus meningitis. Pediatrics *47*:773–776, 1971.
541. Nakao, T.: Coxsackie viruses and diabetes. Lancet *2*:1423, 1971.
542. Nakao, T., and Horino, K.: Clinical and virological studies of acute cerebellar ataxis in childhood. Tohoku J. Exp. Med. *101*:47–53, 1970.
543. Nakao, T., Miura, R., and Sato, M.: ECHO virus type 22 infection in a premature infant. Tohoku J. Exp. Med. *102*:61–68, 1970.
544. Nakao, T., and Morita, M.: Exanthem associated with ECHO 25 virus. Jika Rinsho *18*:772–773, 1965.
545. Nankervis, G., Starr, J., and Gold, E.: Hand, foot and mouth syndrome in a group of families. Program for the Society for Pediatric Research, May 3–4, 1968, p. 152.
546. Nelson, D., Hiemstra, H., Minor, T., et al.: Non-polio enterovirus activity in Wisconsin based on a 20-year experience in a diagnostic virology laboratory. Am. J. Epidemiol. *109*:352–361, 1979.
547. Neu, N., Beisel, K. W., Traystman, M. D., et al.: Autoantibodies specific for the cardiac myosin isoform are found in mice susceptible to coxsackievirus B3–induced myocarditis. J. Immunol. *138*:2488–2492, 1987.
548. Neva, F. A., and Zuffante, S. M.: Agents isolated from patients with Boston exanthem disease during 1954 in Pittsburgh. J. Lab. Clin. Med. *50*:712–779, 1957.
549. Neva, F. A.: A second outbreak of Boston exanthem disease in Pittsburgh during 1954. N. Engl. J. Med. *254*:838–843, 1956.
550. Neva, F. A., Feemster, R. F., and Gorbach, I. J.: Clinical and epidemiological features of an unusual epidemic exanthem. J. A. M. A. *155*:544–548, 1954.
551. Neva, F. A., and Enders, J. F.: Cytopathogenic agents isolated from patients during an unusual epidemic exanthem. J. Immunol. *72*:307–314, 1954.
552. News and Notes: Epidemiology: Echovirus infections. B. M. J. *3*:594, 1970.
554. Nicholls, A. C., and Thomas, M.: Coxsackie virus infection in acute myocardial infarction. Lancet *1*:883–884, 1977.
555. Nielsen, J. L., Berryman, G. K., and Hankins, G. D. V.: Intrauterine fetal death and the isolation of echovirus 27 from amniotic fluid. J. Infect. Dis. *158*:501–502, 1988.
556. Nielsen, L. P., Modlin, J. F., and Rotbart, H. A.: Detection of enteroviruses by polymerase chain reaction in urine samples of patients with aseptic meningitis. Pediatr. Infect. Dis. J. *15*:625–627, 1996.
557. Nightingale, E. O.: Recommendations for a national policy on poliomyelitis vaccination. N. Engl. J. Med. *297*:249–253, 1977.
558. Nihoul, E., Quersin-Thiry, L., and Weynants, A.: ECHO virus type 9 as the agent responsible for an important outbreak of aseptic meningitis in Belgium. Am. J. Hyg. *66*:102–118, 1957.
559. Nikoskelainen, J., Kalliomaki, J. L., Lapinleimu, K, et al.: Coxsackie B virus antibodies in myocardial infarction. Acta Med. Scand. *214*:29–32, 1983.
560. Nishmi, M., Morr, J., Abrahamov, A., et al.: A winter outbreak of Echo virus type 9 meningitis in Jerusalem, with cases of a simultaneous mixed pneumococcal-viral infection. Israel J. Med. Sci. *7*:1240–1247, 1971.
561. Nishmi, M., and Yodfat, Y.: An outbreak among kibbutz children of a febrile illness associated with Echo virus type 4. Isr. J. Med. Sci. *6*:535–539, 1970.
562. Nogen, A. G., and Lepow, M. L.: Enteroviral meningitis in very young infants. Pediatrics *40*:617–626, 1967.
563. Norton, H.: Report of an outbreak of "hand-foot-and-mouth disease" in Sydney. Med. J. Aust. *2*:570, 1961.
564. Novack, A., Feldman, H. A., Wang, S. S., et al.: A community-wide coxsackievirus A9 outbreak. J. A. M. A. *202*:862–866, 1967.
565. Null, F. C., Jr., and Castle, C. H.: Adult pericarditis and myocarditis due to Coxsackie virus group B, type 5. N. Engl. J. Med. *261*:937–942, 1959.
566. Ogilvie, M. M., and Tearne, C. F.: Spontaneous abortion after hand-foot-and-mouth disease caused by coxsackie virus A16. B. M. J. *281*:1527–1528, 1980.
567. O'Neill, D., McArthur, J. D., Kennedy, J. A., et al.: Coxsackie B virus infection in coronary care unit patients. J. Clin. Pathol. *36*:658–661, 1983.
568. O'Regan, S., Robitaille, P., Mongeau, J. G., et al.: The hemolytic uremic syndrome associated with echo 22 infection. Clin. Pediatr. *19*:125–127, 1980.
569. Orenstein, W. A.: Personal communication, 1996.
570. O'Shaughnessey, W. J., and Buechner, H. A.: Hepatitis associated with a Coxsackie B5 virus infection during late pregnancy. J. A. M. A. *179*:71–72, 1962.

571. Paque, R. E.: Role of anti-idiotypic antibodies in induction, regulation, and expression of coxsackievirus-induced myocarditis. Prog. Med. Virol. *39*:204–227, 1992.
572. Paradiso, P. R.: The future of polio immunization in the United States: Are we ready for change? Pediatr. Infect. Dis. J. *15*:645–649, 1996.
573. Parks, W. P., Queiroga, L. T., and Melnick, J. L.: Studies on infantile diarrhea in Karachi, Pakistan. II. Multiple virus isolations from rectal swabs. Am. J. Epidemiol. *85*:469–478, 1967.
574. Parrott, R. H.: The clinical importance of group A Coxsackie viruses. Ann. N. Y. Acad. Sci. *67*:230–241, 1957.
575. Paterson, W. G., and Smith, I. W.: An unusual acute abdomen in pregnancy: An Echo 8 virus infection. Practitioner *203*:337–339, 1969.
576. Paul, J. R.: A History of Poliomyelitis. New Haven, Yale University Press, 1971.
577. Pelon, W., Villarejos, V. M., Rhim, J. S., et al.: Coxsackie group B virus infection and acute diarrhoea occurring among children in Costa Rica. Arch. Dis. Child. *4*:636–641, 1966.
578. Peters, A. C. B., Vielvoye, G. J., Versteeg, J., et al.: Echo 25 focal encephalitis and subacute hemichorea. Neurology *29*:676–681, 1979.
579. Petitjean, J., Freymuth, F., Kopecka, H., et al.: Detection of enteroviruses in cerebrospinal fluids: Enzymatic amplification and hybridization with a biotinylated riboprobe. Mol. Cell. Probes *8*:15–22, 1994.
580. Philip, A. G. S., and Larson, E. J.: Overwhelming neonatal infection with ECHO 19 virus. J. Pediatr. *82*:391–397, 1973.
581. Philipson, L., and Wesslen, T.: Recovery of a cytopathogenic agent from patients with non-diphtheritic croup and from day-nursery children. Arch. Ges. Virusforsch. *8*:77–94, 1958.
582. Philipson, L.: Association between a recently isolated virus and an epidemic of upper respiratory disease in a day nursery. Arch. Ges. Virusforsch. *8*:204–215, 1958.
583. Phillips, C. A., Melnick, J. L., Barrett, F. F., et al.: Dual virus infections. Simultaneous enteroviral disease and St. Louis encephalitis. J. A. M. A. *197*:169–172, 1966.
584. Plager, H., and Deibel, R.: Echo 30 virus infections: Outbreak in New York State. N. Y. State J. Med. *70*:391–393, 1970.
585. Plager, H., Beebe, R., and Miller, J. K.: Coxsackie B-5 pericarditis in pregnancy. Arch. Intern. Med. *110*:735–738, 1962.
586. Plager, H., and Harrison, F. F.: Paralysis associated with ECHO virus type 9. N. Y. State J. Med. *61*:798–800, 1961.
587. Ponka, A., Jalanki, H., Ponka, T., et al.: Viral and mycoplasmal antibodies in patients with myocardial infarction. Ann. Clin. Res. *13*:429–432, 1981.
588. Pope, J. G., and Pollock, T. M.: Coxsackie B5 virus infections during 1965: A report to the Director of the Public Health Laboratory Service from various laboratories in the United Kingdom. B. M. J. *4*:575–577, 1967.
589. Portnoy, B., Leedom, J. M., Hanes, B., et al.: Aseptic meningitis associated with ECHO virus type 9 infection: With special reference to variability by sex and incidence of paralytic sequelae. Calif. Med. *102*:261–267, 1965.
590. Pöyry, T., Kinnunen, L., Hyypiä, T., et al.: Genetic and phylogenetic clustering of enteroviruses. J. Gen. Virol. *77*:1699–1717, 1996.
591. Pöyry, T., Hyypiä, T., Horsnell, C., et al.: Molecular analysis of coxsackievirus A16 reveals a new genetic group of enteroviruses. Virology *202*:962–967, 1994.
592. Prakash, C. V.: Entero-viruses in infantile diarrhoea in India. I. Investigations carried out in Bombay. Indian J. Med. Res. *250*:343–347, 1962.
593. Price, R. A., Garcia, J. H., and Rightsel, W. A.: Choriomeningitis and myocarditis in an adolescent with isolation of Coxsackie B-5 virus. Am. J. Clin. Pathol. *53*:825–883, 1970.
594. Prince, J. T., St. Geme, J. W., Jr., and Scherer, W. F.: ECHO-9 virus exanthema. J. A. M. A. *167*:691–696, 1958.
595. Pulli, T., Koskimies, P., and Hyypiä, T.: Molecular comparison of coxsackie A virus serotypes. Virology *212*:30–38, 1995.
596. Quaife, R. A., and Gostling, J. V. T.: False positive Wassermann reaction associated with evidence of enterovirus infection. J. Clin. Pathol. *24*:120–121, 197.
597. Rabausch-Starz, I., Schwaiger, A., Grünewald, K., et al.: Persistence of virus and viral genome in myocardium after coxsackievirus B3–induced murine myocarditis. Clin. Exp. Immunol. *96*:69–74, 1994.
598. Rabkin, C. S., Telzak, E. E., Ho, M. S., et al.: Outbreak of echovirus 11 infection in hospitalized neonates. Pediatr. Infect. Dis. J. *7*:186–190, 1988.
599. Ramlow, J., Alexander, M., LaPorte, R., et al.: Epidemiology of the post-polio syndrome. Am. J. Epidemiol. *136*:769–786, 1992.
600. Ramos-Alvarez, M., and Olarte, J.: Diarrheal diseases of children: The occurrence of enteropathogenic viruses and bacteria. Am. J. Dis. Child. *107*:218–231, 1964.
601. Ramos-Alvarez, M., and Sabin, A. B.: Enteropathogenic viruses and bacteria: Role in summer diarrheal diseases of infancy and early childhood. J. A. M. A. *167*:147–156, 1958.
602. Ramos-Alvarez, M.: Cytopathogenic enteric viruses associated with undifferentiated diarrheal syndromes in early childhood. Ann. N. Y. Acad. Sci. *67*:326, 1957.
603. Rantasalo, I., Pentitinen, K., Saxen, L., et al.: Echo 9 virus antibody status after an epidemic period and the possible teratogenic effect of the infection. Ann. Paediatr. Fenn. *6*:175–184, 1960.
604. Ranzenhofer, E. R., Dizon, F. C., Lipton, M. M., et al.: Clinical paralytic poliomyelitis due to Coxsackie virus group A, type 7. N. Engl. J. Med. *259*:182, 1958.
605. Ray, C. G., Portman, J. N., Stamm, S. J., et al.: Hemolytic-uremic syndrome and myocarditis: Association with coxsackievirus B infection. Am. J. Dis. Child. *122*:418–420, 1971.
606. Ray, C. G., Tucker, V. L., Harris, D. J., et al.: Enteroviruses associated with the hemolytic-uremic syndrome. Pediatrics *46*:378–388, 1970.
607. Ray, C. G., McCollough, R. H., Doto, I. L., et al.: Echo 4 illness: Epidemiological, clinical and laboratory studies of an outbreak in a rural community. Am. J. Epidemiol. *84*:253–267, 1966.
608. Reyes, M. P., Zalenski, D., Smith, F., et al.: Coxsackievirus-positive cervices in women with febrile illnesses during the third trimester of pregnancy. Am. J. Obstet. Gynecol. *155*:159–161, 1986.
609. Reyes, M. P., Ostrea, E. M., Jr., Roskamp, J., et al.: Disseminated neonatal echovirus 11 disease following antenatal maternal infection with a virus-positive cervix and virus-negative gastrointestinal tract. J. Med. Virol. *12*:155–159, 1983.
610. Rice, S. K., Heinl, R. E., Thornton, L. L., et al.: Clinical characteristics, management strategies, and cost implications of a statewide outbreak of enterovirus meningitis. Clin. Infect. Dis. *20*:931–937, 1995.
611. Richardson, H. B., Jr., and Leibovitz, A.: Hand, foot, and mouth disease in children. J. Pediatr. *67*:6–12, 1965.
612. Robinson, C. R., Doane, F. W., and Rhodes, A. J.: Report of an outbreak of febrile illness with pharyngeal lesions and exanthem, Toronto, summer 1957: Isolation of group A Coxsackie virus. Can. Med. Assoc. J. *79*:615–621, 1958.
613. Roden, V. J., Cantor, H. E., O'Connor, D. M., et al.: Acute hemiplegia of childhood associated with Coxsackie A9 viral infection. J. Pediatr. *86*:56–58, 1975.
614. Rodriguez-Torres, R., Lin, J. S., and Berkovich, S.: A sensitive electrocardiographic sign in myocarditis associated with viral infection. Pediatrics *43*:846–851, 1969.
615. Rorabaugh, M. L., Berlin, L. E., Heldrich, F., et al.: Aseptic meningitis in infants younger than 2 years of age: Acute illness andneurologic complications. Pediatrics *92*:206–211, 1993.
616. Ross, C. A. C., Bell, E. J., Kerr, M. M., et al.: Infective agents and embryopathy in the west of Scotland 1966–70. Scot. Med. J. *17*:252–258, 1972.
617. Rotbart, H. A.: Enteroviral infections of the central nervous system. Clin. Infect. Dis. *20*:971–981, 1995.
618. Rotbart, H. A.: Nucleic acid detection systems for enteroviruses. Clin. Microbiol. Rev. *4*:156–168, 1991.
619. Rotbart, H. A., Sawyer, M. H., Fast, S., et al.: Diagnosis of enteroviral meningitis by using PCR with a colorimetric microwell detection assay. J. Clin. Microbiol. *32*:2590–2592, 1994.
620. Rotbart, H. A., Kinsella, J. P., and Wasserman, R. L.: Persistent enterovirus infection in culture-negative meningoencephalitis: Demonstration by enzymatic RNA amplification. J. Infect. Dis. *161*:787–791, 1990.
621. Rotbart, H. A.: Enzymatic RNA amplification of the enteroviruses. J. Clin. Microbiol. *28*:438–442, 1990.
622. Rotbart, H. A.: Diagnosis of enteroviral meningitis with the polymerase chain reaction. J. Pediatr. *117*:85–89, 1990.
623. Rotbart, H. A., Abzug, M. J., and Levin, M. J.: Development and application of RNA probes for the study of picornaviruses. Mol. Cell. Probes *2*:65–73, 1988.
624. Rotem, C. E.: Meningitis of virus origin. Lancet *1*:502–504, 1957.
625. Rubin, H., Lehan, P. H., Doto, I. L., et al.: Epidemic infection with Coxsackie virus group B, type 5. I. Clinical and epidemiologic aspects. N. Engl. J. Med. *258*:255–263, 1958.
626. Rueckert, R. R.: *Picornaviridae* and their replication. *In* Fields, B. N., and Knipe, D. M. (eds.): Virology. 2nd ed. New York, Raven Press, 1990, pp. 507–548.
627. Russell, S. J. M., and Bell, E. J.: Echoviruses and carditis. Lancet *1*:784–785, 1970.
628. Ryder, D. E., Doane, F. W., Zbitnew, A., et al.: Report of an outbreak of Bornholm disease, with isolation of Coxsackie B5 virus: Toronto, 1958. Can. J. Public Health *50*:265–269, 1959.
629. Sabin, A. B.: Oral poliovirus vaccine: History of its development and use and current challenge to eliminate poliomyelitis from the world. J. Infect. Dis. *151*:420–436, 1985.
630. Sabin, A. B.: Poliomyelitis. *In* Braude A. I. (ed.): Medical Microbiology and Infectious Diseases. Philadelphia, W. B. Saunders, 1981, pp. 1348–1365.
631. Sabin, A. B.: Role of ECHO viruses in human disease. *In* Rose, H. M. (ed.): Viral Infections of Infancy and Childhood. New York, Hoeber-Harper, 1960, pp. 78–100.
632. Sabin, A. B., Krumbiegel, E. R., and Wigand, R.: ECHO type 9 virus disease: Virologically controlled clinical and epidemiologic observations during a 1957 epidemic in Milwaukee with notes on concurrent similar diseases associated with Coxsackie and other ECHO viruses. Prog. Pediatr. *96*:197–219, 1958.
633. Salk, D.: Polio immunization policy in the United States: A new challenge for a new generation. Am. J. Public Health *78*:296–300, 1988.
634. Salk, D.: Eradication of poliomyelitis in the United States. I. Live virus

vaccine-associated and wild poliovirus disease. Rev. Infect. Dis. *2*:228–242, 1980.
635. Salk, D.: Eradication of poliomyelitis in the United States. II. Experience with killed poliovirus vaccine. Rev. Infect. Dis. *2*:258–257, 1980.
636. Salk, D.: Eradication of poliomyelitis in the United States. III. Poliovaccines. Practical considerations. Rev. Infect. Dis. *2*:258–273, 1980.
637. Samuda, G. M., Chang, W. K., Yeung, C. Y., et al.: Monoplegia caused by enterovirus 71: An outbreak in Hong Kong. Pediatr. Infect. Dis. J. *6*:206–208, 1987.
638. Sanders, D. Y., Powell, R. V., and Smith, A.: Outbreak of Coxsackie B5 virus in a children's home. South. Med. J. *62*:474–476, 1969.
639. Sanders, D. Y., and Cramblett, H. G.: Viral infections in hospitalized neonates. Am. J. Dis. Child. *116*:251–256, 1968.
640. Saslaw, S., Wooley, C. F., and Anderson, G. R.: Aseptic meningitis syndrome: Report of eleven cases with cerebrospinal fluid isolation of enteroviruses. Arch. Intern. Med. *105*:69–75, 1960.
641. Sawyer, L. A., Hershow, R. C., Pallansch, M. A., et al.: An epidemic of acute hemorrhagic conjunctivitis in American Samoa caused by coxsackievirus A24 variant. Am. J. Epidemiol. *130*:1187–1198, 1989.
642. Sawyer, M. H., Holland, D., Aintablian, N., et al.: Diagnosis of enteroviral central nervous system infection by polymerase chain reaction during a large community outbreak. Pediatr. Infect. Dis. J. *13*:177–182, 1994.
643. Saxena, R. C., Bhatia, M., and Chaturvedi, U. C.: Recent epidemic conjunctivitis in Lucknow: A clinical study. Orient. Arch. Ophthal. *10*:253–257, 1982.
644. Schleissner, L. A., and Portnoy, B.: Spectrum of ECHO virus 1 disease in a young diabetic. Chest *63*:457–459, 1973.
645. Schleissner, L. A., and Portnoy, B.: Hepatitis and pneumonia associated with ECHO virus, type 9, infection in two adult siblings. Ann. Intern. Med. *68*:1315–1319, 1968.
646. Schlesinger, Y., Sawyer, M. H., and Storch, G. A.: Enteroviral meningitis in infancy: Potential role for polymerase chain reaction in patient management. Pediatrics *94*:157–162, 1994.
647. Schmidt, N. J., Lennette, E. H., and Ho, H. H.: An apparently new enterovirus isolated from patients with disease of the central nervous system. J. Infect. Dis. *129*:304–309, 1974.
648. Schmidt, N. J., Magoffin, R. L., and Lennette, E. H.: Association of group B coxsackieviruses with cases of pericarditis, myocarditis, or pleurodynia by demonstration of immunoglobulin M antibody. Infect. Immun. *8*:341–348, 1973.
649. Schmidt, W. A. K., Brade, L., Muntefering, H., et al.: Course of Coxsackie B antibodies during juvenile diabetes. Med. Microbiol. Immunol. *164*:291–298, 1978.
650. Schoub, B. D., Johnson, S., McAnerney, J. M., et al.: Epidemic coxsackie B virus infection in Johannesburg, South Africa. J. Hyg. (Camb.) *95*:447–455, 1985.
651. Schultz, W. W., and Weiss, E.: Demonstration of specific antibodies to a Coxsackie-like virus in patients of a hepatitis outbreak. Am. J. Epidemiol. *110*:124–131, 1979.
652. Schürmann, W., Statz, A., Mertens, T., et al.: Two cases of coxsackie B2 infection in neonates: Clinical, virological, and epidemiological aspects. Eur. J. Pediatr. *140*:59–63, 1983.
653. Scott, T. F. M.: Clinical syndromes associated with entero virus and reo virus infections. Adv. Virus Res. *8*:165–197, 1962.
654. Seddon, J. H., and Duff, M. F.: Hand-foot-and-mouth disease: Coxsackie virus types A5, A10 and A16 infections. N. Z. Med. J. *74*:368–373, 1971.
655. Seko, Y., Yoshifumi, E., Yagita, H., et al.: Restricted usage of T-cell receptor Va genes in infiltrating cells in murine hearts with acute myocarditis caused by coxsackie virus B3. J. Pathol. *178*:330–334, 1996.
656. Sells, C. J., Carpenter, R. L., and Ray, C. G.: Sequelae of central nervous system enterovirus infections. N. Engl. J. Med. *293*:1–4, 1975.
657. Selwyn, S., and Howitt, L. F.: A mosaic of enteroviruses: Poliovirus, Coxsackie, and Echo infections in a group of families. Lancet *2*:548–551, 1962.
658. Severien, C., Jacobs, K. H., and Schoenemann, W.: Marked pleocytosis and hypoglycorrhachia in coxsackie meningitis. Pediatr. Infect. Dis. J. *13*:322–323, 1994.
659. Severini, G. M., Mestroni, L., Falaschi, A., et al.: Nested polymerase chain reaction for high-sensitivity detection of enteroviral RNA in biological samples. J. Clin. Microbiol. *31*:1345–1349, 1993.
660. Sharland, M., Hodgson, J., Davies, E. G., et al.: Enteroviral pharyngitis diagnosed by reverse transcriptase-polymerase chain reaction. Arch. Dis. Child. *74*:462–463, 1996.
661. Shelokov, A., and Habel, K.: Viremia in Coxsackie B meningitis. Proc. Soc. Exp. Biol. Med. *94*:782–784, 1957.
662. Shelokov, A., and Weinstein, L.: Poliomyelitis in the early neonatal period: Report of a case of possible intrauterine infection. J. Pediatr. *38*:80–84, 1951.
663. Shimizu, H., Schnurr, D. P., and Burns, J. C.: Comparison of methods to detect enteroviral genome in frozen and fixed myocardium by polymerase chain reaction. Lab. Invest. *71*:612–616, 1994.
664. Sieber, O. F., Jr., Kilgus, A. H., Fulginiti, V. A., et al.: Immunological response of the newborn infant to Coxsackie B-4 infection. Pediatrics *40*:444–446, 1967.
665. Siegel, M., and Greenberg, M.: Poliomyelitis in pregnancy: Effect on fetus and newborn infant. J. Pediatr. *49*:280–288, 1956.
666. Siegel, W., Spencer, F. J., Smith, D. J., et al.: Two new variants of infection with Coxsackie virus group B, type 5, in young children: A syndrome of lymphadenopathy, pharyngitis and hepatomegaly or splenomegaly, or both, and one of pneumonia. N. Engl. J. Med. *268*:1210–1216, 1963.
667. Silver, T. S., and Todd, J. K.: Hypoglycorrhachia in pediatric patients. Pediatrics *58*:67–71, 1976.
668. Singer, J. I., Maur, P. R., Riley, J. P., et al.: Management of central nervous system infections during an epidemic of enteroviral aseptic meningitis. J. Pediatr. *96*:559–563, 1980.
669. Skeels, M. R., Williams, J. J., and Ricker, F. M.: Perinatal echovirus infection. N. Engl. J. Med. *305*:1529–1530, 1981.
670. Soboleva, V. D., Lozovskaya, L. S., Alekseyeva, V. B., et al.: Coxsackie A13 virus in the foci of rheumatism. J. Hyg. Epidemiol. Microbiol. Immunol. (Praha) *22*:195–202, 1978.
671. Solomon, P., Weinstein, L., Chang, T. W., et al.: Epidemiologic, clinical, and laboratory features of an epidemic of type 9 Echo virus meningitis. J. Pediatr. *55*:609–619, 1959.
672. Sommerville, R. G.: Enteroviruses and diarrhea in young persons. Lancet *2*:1347–1349, 1958.
673. Spudis, E. V., and Cramblett, H. G.: ECHO 4 meningoencephalitis. Arch. Neurol. *12*:404–409, 1965.
674. Steigman, A. J., Lipton, M. M., and Braspennickx, H.: Acute lymphonodular pharyngitis: A newly described condition due to Coxsackie A virus. J. Pediatr. *61*:331–336, 1962.
675. Steigman, A. J., and Lipton, M. M.: Fatal bulbospinal paralytic poliomyelitis due to ECHO 11 virus. J. A. M. A. *174*:178–179, 1960.
676. Steigman, A. J.: Poliomyelitis properties of certain non-polio viruses: Enteroviruses and Heine-Medin disease. J. Mt. Sinai Hosp. *25*:391–404, 1958.
677. Steinhoff, M. C.: Viruses and diarrhea: A review. Am. J. Dis. Child. *132*:302–307, 1978.
678. Steinmann, J., and Albrecht, K.: Echovirus 11-epidemie bei fruhgeborenen auf einer neonatal-intensive-station. Zbl. Bakt. Hyg. [A] *259*:284–293, 1985.
679. Stern, H.: Aetiology of central nervous system infections during prevalence of poliovirus and Coxsackie virus: Some clinical manifestations of Coxsackie virus infections. B. M. J. *1*:1061–1066, 1961.
680. Stones, P. B.: Isolation of ECHO virus type 9 during an outbreak of meningo-encephalitis. B. M. J. *2*:1514, 1958.
681. Strebel, P. M., Sutter, R. W., Cochi, S. L., et al.: Epidemiology of poliomyelitis in the United States one decade after the last reported case of indigenous wild virus-associated disease. Clin. Infect. Dis. *14*:568–579, 1992.
682. Strikas, R. A., Anderson, L. J., and Parker, R. A.: Temporal and geographic patterns of isolates of nonpolio enterovirus in the United States, 1970–1983. J. Infect. Dis. *153*:346–351, 1986.
683. Ström, J.: Coxsackie B5 infection causing serous meningitis with exanthema and benign pericarditis with myocarditis in two siblings. Acta Paediatr. *135*(Suppl.):197–202, 1962.
684. Sturup, H.: The long-term prognosis of acute non-specific pericarditis: A follow-up examination including cases of dry pleurisy from an epidemic of Bornholm disease (myalgia epidemica) in 1930–32. Danish Med. Bull. *1*:89–91, 1954.
685. Sumaya, C. V., and Corman, L. I.: Enteroviral meningitis in early infancy: Significance in community outbreaks. Pediatr. Infect. Dis. *1*:151–154, 1982.
686. Sun, N. C., and Smith, V. M.: Hepatitis associated with myocarditis: Unusual manifestation of infection with Coxsackie virus group B, type 3. N. Engl. J. Med. *274*:190–193, 1966.
687. Swanink, C. M. A., Melchers, W. J. G., van der Meer, J. W. M., et al.: Enteroviruses and the chronic fatigue syndrome. Clin. Infect. Dis. *19*:860–864, 1994.
688. Swann, N. H.: Epidemic pleurodynia, orchitis, and myocarditis in an adult due to Coxsackie virus, group B, type 4. Ann. Intern. Med. *54*:1008–1013, 1961.
689. Swender, P. T., Shott, R. J., and Williams, M. L.: A community and intensive care nursery outbreak of coxsackievirus B5 meningitis. Am. J. Dis. Child. *127*:42–45, 1974.
690. Sylvest, E.: Epidemic Myalgia: Bornholm Disease. Translated by H. Andersen. London, Oxford University Press, 1934.
691. Syverton, J. T., McLean, D. M., da Silva, M. M., et al.: Outbreak of aseptic meningitis caused by Coxsackie B5 virus: Laboratory, clinical, and epidemiologic study. J. A. M. A. *164*:2015–2019, 1957.
692. Takahashi, S., Miyamoto, A., Oki, J., et al.: Acute transverse myelitis caused by ECHO virus type 18 infection. Eur. J. Pathol. *154*:378–380, 1995.
693. Takos, M. J., Weil, M., and Sigel, M. M.: Outbreak of ECHO 9 exanthema traced to a children's party. Am. J. Dis. Child. *100*:360–364, 1960.
694. Talsma, M., Vegting, M., and Hess, J.: Generalised coxsackie A9 infection in a neonate presenting with pericarditis. Br. Heart. J. *52*:683–685, 1984.
695. Tanel, R. E., Kao, S.-Y., Niemiec, T. M., et al.: Prospective comparison of culture vs genome detection for diagnosis of enteroviral meningitis in childhood. Arch. Pediatr. Adolesc. Med. *150*:919–924, 1996.
696. Tang, T. T., Sedmak, G. V., Siegesmund, K. A., et al.: Chronic myopathy associated with coxsackievirus type A9: A combined electron microscopical and viral isolation study. N. Engl. J. Med. *292*:608–611, 1975.

697. Tateno, I., Suzuki, S., Kagawa, S., et al.: On an Echo-like agent constantly recoverable from volunteers given Niigata strain of acute epidemic gastroenteritis. Jpn. J. Exp. Med. *26*:125–128, 1956.
698. Thomas, H. M., Jr.: Acute viral peritonitis due to group B Coxsackie viruses. Maryland St. Med. J. *11*:282–285, 1962.
699. Thorén, A., and Widell, A.: PCR for the diagnosis of enteroviral meningitis. Scand. J. Infect. Dis. *26*:249–254, 1994.
700. Tindall, J. P., and Callaway, J. L.: Hand-foot-and-mouth disease: It's more common than you think. Am. J. Dis. Child. *124*:372–375, 1972.
701. Tobe, T.: Inapparent virus infection as a trigger of appendicitis. Lancet *1*:1343–1346, 1965.
702. Toce, S. S., and Keenan, W. K.: Congenital echovirus 11 pneumonia in association with pulmonary hypertension. Pediatr. Infect. Dis. J. *7*:360–361, 1988.
703. Torphy, D. E., Ray, C. G., Thompson, R. S., et al.: An epidemic of aseptic meningitis due to Echo-virus type 30: Epidemiologic features and clinical and laboratory findings. Am. J. Public Health *60*:1447–1455, 1970.
704. Tòth, M., Osvàth, P., Galambos, M., et al.: Kindergarten outbreak of an exanthematous disease caused by echo-virus type 9. Acta Paediatr. Hung. *5*:235–239, 1964.
705. Townsend, T. R., Bolyard, E. A., Yolken, R. H., et al.: Outbreak of coxsackie A1 gastroenteritis: A complication of bone-marrow transplantation. Lancet *1*:820–823, 1982.
706. Trabelsi, A., Grattard, F., Nejmeddine, M., et al.: Evaluation of an enterovirus group-specific anti-VP1 monoclonal antibody, 5-D8/1, in comparison with neutralization and PCR for rapid identification of enteroviruses in cell culture. J. Clin. Microbiol. *33*:2454–1457, 1995.
707. Tubman, T. R. J., Craig, B., and Mulholland, H. C.: Ventricular tachycardia associated with coxsackie B4 virus infection. Acta Paediatr. Scand. *79*:572–575, 1990.
708. Turnbull, D. C.: Optic neuritis: Associated with Bornholm disease. Am. J. Ophthalmol. *46*:81–83, 1958.
709. Tuuteri, L., Lapinleimu, K., and Meurman, L.: Fatal myocarditis associated with Coxsackie B3 infection in the newborn. Ann. Pediatr. Fenn. *9*:56–64, 1963.
710. Tyrrell, D. A. J., Lane, R. R., Snell, B., et al.: Clinical and laboratory studies of a syndrome characterized by meningitis and an exanthem, caused by a virus related to ECHO 9. *In* Rose, H. M. (ed.): Viral Infections of Infancy and Childhood. New York, Hoeber-Harper, 1960, pp. 101–118.
711. Underwood, M.: A Treatise on the Diseases of Children. 2nd ed. London, J. Mathews, 1789.
712. Urano, T., Kawase, T., Kodaira, K., et al.: Gullain-barré syndrome associated with Echo virus type 7 infections. Pediatrics *45*:294–295, 1970.
713. Ursing, B.: Acute pancreatitis in Coxsackie B infection. B. M. J. *3*:524–525, 1973.
714. Utz, J. P., and Shelokov, A. I.: Coxsackie B virus infection: Presence of virus in blood, urine and cerebrospinal fluid. J. A. M. A. *168*:264–267, 1958.
715. Vague, P., Vialettes, B., Prince, M. A., et al.: Coxsackie B viruses and autoimmune diabetes. N. Engl. J. Med. *305*:1157–1158, 1981.
716. Van Eden, W., Persijn, G. G., Bikkerk, H., et al.: Differential resistance to paralytic poliomyelitis controlled by histocompatibility leukocyte antigens. J. Infect. Dis. *147*:422–426, 1983.
717. Van Loon, G. R., and Masson, A. M.: Viral pericarditis: A report of five cases. Can. Med. Assoc. J. *99*:163–168, 1968.
718. Van Maldergem, L., Mascart, F., Ureel, D., et al.: Echovirus meningoencephalitis in X-linked hypogammaglobulinemia. Acta Paediatr. Scand. *78*:325–326, 1989.
719. Verlinde, J. D., Van Tongeren, H. A. E., Wilterdink, J. B., et al.: "Biak fever": An epidemic illness associated with Echo 6 virus. Trop. Geogr. Med. *11*:276–280, 1959.
720. Von Zeipel, G., and Svedmyr, A.: A study of the association of Echo viruses to aseptic meningitis. Arch. Ges. Virusforsch. *7*:355–368, 1957.
721. Voroshilova, M. K., and Chumakov, M. P.: Poliomyelitis-like properties of AB-IV Coxsackie A7 group of viruses. Prog. Med. Virol. *2*:106–170, 1959.
722. Wadia, N. H., Katrak, S. M., Misra, V. P., et al.: Polio-like motor paralysis associated with acute hemorrhagic conjunctivitis in an outbreak in 1981 in Bombay, India: Clinical and serologic studies. J. Infect. Dis. *147*:660–668, 1983.
723. Walters, J. H.: Postencephalitic Parkinson syndrome after meningoencephalitis due to Coxsackie virus group B, type 2. N. Engl. J. Med. *263*:744–747, 1960.
724. Wang, S.-M., Liu, C.-C., Chen, Y.-J., et al.: Alice in Wonderland syndrome caused by coxsackievirus B1. Pediatr. Infect. Dis. J. *15*:470–471, 1996.
725. Ward, C.: Severe arrhythmias in coxsackievirus B3 myopericarditis. Arch. Dis. Child. *53*:174–176, 1978.
726. Ward, N. A., Milstien, J. B., Hull, H. F., et al.: The WHO-EPI initiative for the global eradication of poliomyelitis. Biologicals *21*:327–333, 1993.
727. Warin, J. F., Davies, J. B. M., Sanders, F. K., et al.: Oxford epidemic of Bornholm disease, 1951. B. M. J. *1*:1345–1351, 1953.
728. Waterman, S. H., Casas-Benabe, R., Hatch, M. H., et al.: Acute hemorrhagic conjunctivitis in Puerto Rico, 1981–1982. Am. J. Epidemiol. *120*:395–403, 1984.
729. Waterson, A. P.: Virological investigations in congestive cardiomyopathy. Postgrad. Med. J. *54*:505–507, 1978.
730. Webster, A. D. B., Rotbart, H. A., Warner, T., et al.: Diagnosis of enterovirus brain disease in hypogammaglobulinemic patients by polymerase chain reaction. Clin. Infect. Dis. *17*:657–661, 1993.
731. Wehrle, P. F., Judge, M. E., Parizeau, M. C., et al.: Disability associated with ECHO virus infections. N. Y. State J. Med. *59*:3941–3945, 1959.
732. Weiner, L. S., Howell, J. T., Langford, M. P., et al.: Effect of specific antibodies on chronic echovirus type 5 encephalitis in a patient with hypogammaglobulinemia. J. Infect. Dis. *140*:858–863, 1979.
733. Weinstein, S. B.: Acute benign pericarditis associated with Coxsackie virus group B, type 5. N. Engl. J. Med. *257*:265–267, 1957.
734. Weller, T. H., Enders, J. F., Buckingham, M., et al.: The etiology of epidemic pleurodynia: A study of two viruses isolated from a tropical outbreak. J. Immunol. *65*:337–346, 1950.
735. Welliver, R. C., and Cherry, J. D.: Aseptic meningitis and orchitis associated with echovirus 6 infection. J. Pediatr. *92*:239–240, 1978.
736. Wenner, H. A.: Virus diseases associated with cutaneous eruptions. Prog. Med. Virol. *16*:269–336, 1973.
737. Wenner, H. A.: The enteroviruses. Am. J. Clin. Pathol. *57*:751–761, 1972.
738. Wenner, H. A., and Behbehani, A. M.: ECHO viruses. Monogr. Virol. *1*:1–72, 1968.
739. Wenner, H. A., and Lou, T. Y.: Virus diseases associated with cutaneous eruptions. Progr. Med. Virol. *5*:219–294, 1963.
740. Wenner, H. A., Christodoulopoulou, G., Weston, J., et al.: The etiology of respiratory illnesses occurring in infancy and childhood. Pediatrics *31*:4–17, 1963.
741. Wenner, H. A.: The Echo viruses. Ann. N. Y. Acad. Sci. *10*:398–412, 1962.
742. Wesslén, T., Eriksson, S., Ehinger, A., et al.: Epidemic of aseptic meningitis associated with Echo virus type 9. Arch. Ges. Virusforsch. *8*:183–191, 1958.
743. Wickman, I.: On the epidemiology of Heine-Medin's disease. Rev. Infect. Dis. *2*:319–327, 1980.
744. Wilfert, C. M., Thompson, R. J., Jr., Sunder, T. R., et al.: Longitudinal assessment of children with enteroviral meningitis during the first three months of life. Pediatrics *67*:811–815, 1981.
745. Wilfert, C. M., Buckley, R. H., Mohanakumar, T., et al.: Persistent and fatal central nervous system Echovirus infections in patients with agammaglobulinemia. N. Engl. J. Med. *296*:1485–1489, 1977.
746. Wilkins, A. J. W., Kotze, D. M., Melvin, J., et al.: Meningo-encephalitis due to Coxsackie B virus in Southern Rhodesia. S. Afr. Med. J. *29*:25–28, 1955.
747. Willems, W. R., Hornig, C., Bauer, H., et al.: A case of Coxsackie A9 virus infection with orchitis. J. Med. Virol. *3*:137–140, 1978.
748. Wilson, C., Connolly, J. H., and Thomson, D.: Coxsackie B2 virus infection and acute-onset diabetes in a child. B. M. J. *1*:1008–1009, 1977.
749. Wilt, J. C., Parker, W. L., Owens, A. L., et al.: Enterovirus infections in Manitoba. 1959. Can. Med. Assoc. J. *83*:839–843, 1960.
750. Wilt, J. C., Medovy, H., Besant, D., et al.: Aseptic meningitis in Manitoba, 1957. Can. Med. Assoc. J. *78*:839–842, 1958.
751. Windebank, A. J., Litchy, W. J., Daube, J. R., et al.: Lack of progression of neurologic deficit in survivors of paralytic polio: A 5-year prospective population-based study. Neurology *46*:80–84, 1996.
752. Windebank, A. J., Litchy, W. J., Daube, J. R., et al.: Late effects of paralytic poliomyelitis in Olmsted County, Minnesota. Neurology *41*:501–507, 1991.
753. Winsser, J., and Altieri, R. H.: A three-year study of Coxsackie virus, group B infection in Nassau County. Am. J. Med. Sci. *247*:269–273, 1964.
754. Wolfgram, L. J., and Rose, N. R.: Coxsackievirus infection as a trigger of cardiac autoimmunity. Immunol. Res. *8*:61–80, 1989.
755. Wong, S. N., Tam, A. Y. S., Ng, T. H., et al.: Fatal coxsackie B1 virus infection in neonates. Pediatr. Infect. Dis. J. *8*:638–641, 1989.
756. Wood, S. F., Rogen, A. S., Bell, E. J., et al.: Role of coxsackie B viruses in myocardial infarction. Br. Heart J. *40*:523–525, 1978.
757. Woodall, C. J., Riding, M. H., Graham, D. J., et al.: Sequences specific for enterovirus detected in spinal cord from patients with motor neurone disease. B. M. J. *308*:1541–1543, 1994.
758. Woods, J. D., Nimmo, M. J., and Mackay-Scollay, E. M.: Acute transmural myocardial infarction associated with active Coxsackie virus B infection. Am. Heart J. *89*:283–287, 1975.
759. Wooley, C. F.: Intracranial hypertension associated with recovery of a Coxsackie virus from the cerebrospinal fluid. Neurology *110*:572–574, 1960.
760. Wreghitt, T. G., Sutehall, G. M., King, A., et al.: Fatal echovirus 7 infection during an outbreak in a special care baby unit. J. Infect. *19*:229–236, 1989.
761. Wright, H. T., Jr., Landing, B. H., Lennette, E. H., et al.: Fatal infection in an infant associated with Coxsackie virus group A, type 16. N. Engl. J. Med. *268*:1041–1044, 1963.
762. Wright, P. F., Kim-Farley, R. J., de Quadros, C. A., et al.: Strategies for the global eradication of poliomyelitis by the year 2000. N. Engl. J. Med. *325*:1773–1779, 1991.
763. Yaffee, H. S.: Erythema multiforme caused by Coxsackie B5: A possible association with epidemic pustular stomatitis of children. Arch. Dermatol. *82*:737–739, 1960.
764. Yamashita, K., Miyamura, K., Yamadera, S., et al.: Epidemics of aseptic meningitis due to echovirus 30 in Japan. Jpn. J. Med. Sci. Biol. *47*:221–239, 1994.
765. Yang, C.-F., De, L., Holloway, B. P., et al.: Detection and identification of

vaccine-related polioviruses by the polymerase chain reaction. Viral Res. *20*:159–179, 1991.
766. Yerly, S., Guervaix, A., Simonet, V., et al.: Rapid and sensitive detection of enteroviruses in specimens from patients with aseptic meningitis. J. Clin. Microbiol. *34*:199–201, 1996.
767. Yin-Murphy, M.: Acute hemorrhagic conjunctivitis. Prog. Med. Virol. *29*:23–44, 1984.
768. Yohannan, M. D., Ramia, S., and Al Frayh, A. R. S.: Acute paralytic poliomyelitis presenting as Guillain-Barré syndrome. J. Infect. *22*:129–133, 1991.
769. Yoon, J.-W., Austin, M., Onodera, T., et al.: Virus-induced diabetes mellitus: Isolation of a virus from the pancreas of a child with diabetic ketoacidosis. N. Engl. J. Med. *300*:1173–1179, 1979.
770. Yousef, G. E., Bell, E. J., Mann, G. F., et al.: Chronic enterovirus infection in patients with postviral fatigue syndrome. Lancet *1*:146–150, 1988.
771. Yow, M. D., Melnick, J. L., Phillips, C. A., et al.: An etiologic investigation of infantile diarrhea in Houston during 1962 and 1963. Am. J. Epidemiol. *83*:255–261, 1966.
772. Yow, M. D., Melnick, J. L., Blattner, R. J., et al.: Enteroviruses in infantile diarrhea. Am. J. Hyg. *77*:283–292, 1963.
773. Yuceoglu, A. M., Berkovich, S., and Minkowitz, S.: Acute glomerulonephritis associated with ECHO virus type 9 infection. J. Pediatr. *69*:603–609, 1966.
774. Yui, L. A., and Gledhill, R. F.: Limb paralysis as a manifestation of coxsackie B virus infection. Dev. Med. Child Neurol. *33*:427–438, 1991.
775. Zanetti, A. R.: Enterovirus associated sporadic cases and epidemics. Annali Sclavo *19*:187–192, 1977.
776. Zuniga, M. D. R., Reichardt, J., Braun, W., et al.: Detection of IgM antibodies against coxsackie B viruses by a western blot technique. Acta Virol. *37*:1–10, 1993.

171

RHINOVIRUSES

Elliot C. Dick, Stanley L. Inhorn, and W. Paul Glezen

In 1954, the first recognized rhinovirus (RV) (type 1A) was isolated in monkey kidney cell culture by Mogabgab and associates[188, 203] from a recruit at Great Lakes Naval Training Center (Chicago) during an outbreak of afebrile common colds in his training company. Independently, Price and colleagues[207] reported isolations of an antigenically identical virus from nurses and children with colds. In 1963, the RVs were so named because of their association with illnesses of the nasal passages.[253]

Prior to these actual virus isolations, there was much evidence that viruses cause the common cold. Although there were indications that some cold-like illnesses could be complicated by bacterial infections,[20, 66, 73, 261] bacteria-free nasal filtrates from persons with apparent symptomatic respiratory infections clearly were able to initiate these illnesses. Kruse,[160] in 1914, first demonstrated transmission with apparently sterile filtrates, and, in the late 1920s, his results were confirmed in a series of experiments in humans and chimpanzees by Dochez and associates.[73] In the 1930s, workers from this latter laboratory reported growth of the agent in tissue culture and embryonated eggs, but their results were not confirmed.[8] In the 1940s and 1950s, Andrewes and colleagues[7] at the Common Cold Unit in Salisbury, England, and Dingle and the members of the U.S. Armed Forces Commission on Acute Respiratory Diseases were able to transmit colds from person to person using apparently sterile filtrates.[49] Jackson and colleagues,[142] in Chicago, performed similar experiments and also demonstrated immunity. In 1953, the Salisbury researchers reported isolation of an agent, DC, in serially passaged filtrates of tubed tissue cultures of human embryonic lungs, the virus being detected by its ability to produce colds in humans.[6] (Although these results could not be substantiated at the time, there *was* a virus present; in 1968, the DC filtrates were found to contain RV-9.[51])

The next major advance in growing common cold viruses took place in the late 1950s in Salisbury. Tyrrell and Parsons[254] inoculated human embryonic kidney cells with nasal filtrates and incubated the cultures under conditions simulating those of the nasal passages (e.g., 33° C, neutral pH, and in a roller drum for aeration). Six distinct types of RVs (types 1B to 6)[57] were isolated by observing cytopathic effect.[242] Shortly thereafter, Hamparian and coworkers[57, 117, 155] isolated 18 RVs (types 7 to 12 and 18 to 29) by using a semicontinuous diploid cell strain obtained by Hayflick and Moorhead[122] from human fetal lung cultures. Use of Hayflick's cell lines greatly accelerated isolation and characterization of "new" RVs, and there now officially are 100 serotypes (or 101, if RV-1A and RV-1B are counted as two serologic entities).[116] More remain untyped, although the number of additional serotypes seems limited.[116, 152, 190]

Although the RVs are associated primarily with mild upper respiratory tract disease, they also may be involved in bronchitis, sinusitis, and, on occasion, pneumonia in all age groups. They seem to be precipitants of "infectious asthma" attacks. They cause about 30 to 50 per cent of all acute respiratory illness.[57, 92]

THE ORGANISM

General Description

Rhinovirus is one of three genera of human pathogens in the family *Picornaviridae*.[195] *Enterovirus* includes polioviruses, coxsackieviruses, and echoviruses; hepatitis A virus is the single member of *Hepatovirus*.[131] Like the other picornaviruses, the RVs are small (30 nm), nonenveloped (therefore resistant to lipid solvents, such as ether and chloroform), and icosahedral (20-sided, hexagonal in cross-section), with a genome consisting of single-stranded RNA (molecular weight, -2.5×10^6) 7210 nucleotides long.[220] A picornavirus can be thought of as an RNA genome surrounded by a 20-sided protein coat (the capsid) (Fig. 171–1). The RNA alone is infectious and can serve as messenger.

RVs differ from enteroviruses in being rendered noninfectious at an acidity below pH 5 and by their higher buoyant density in cesium chloride.

Structure of the Virion

Knowledge of the structure of the RVs and of some of the other picornaviruses is approaching near totality. Two serotypes, RV-1A and RV-14, have been described in atomic detail, and many structural observations for these viruses probably can be generalized to all RVs and to all enterovi-

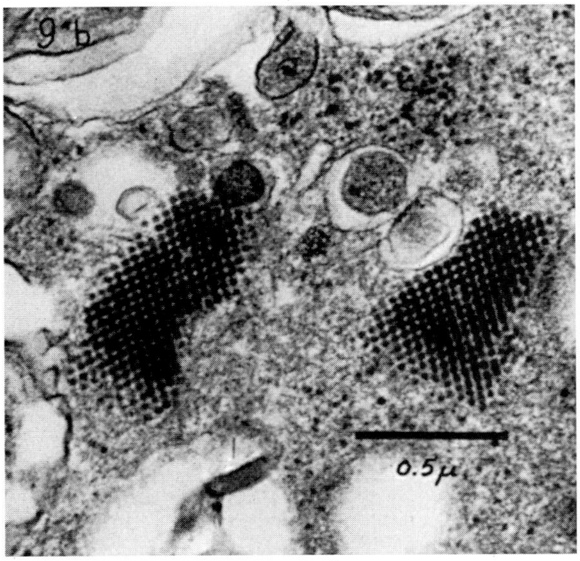

FIGURE 171–1. *Rhinovirus type 2 in human fetal lung cells. Note the hexagonal virus crystals closely packed in a rectangular lattice. (× 40,000.) (From Kawana, R., and Matsumoto, I.: Jpn. J. Microbiol. 15:207–217, 1971.)*

ruses.[11, 18, 130, 156, 217, 218, 220] As viewed in a computer-coded three-dimensional model (Fig. 171–2*A*), the thin (−5-nm) protein capsid has an undulating exterior marked by 12 vertices equally spaced over the surface. Surrounding these vertices is a steep (2.5-nm deep), narrow canyon. At the base of this canyon are loci, called receptor binding sites, by which the virus attaches itself to the receptor on the cell.[217] For all 101 RV serotypes, there are but two different receptor binding sites: 91 serotypes have one (the major receptor group) and 10 the other (the minor receptor group).[1, 255] The canyon is too narrow to accept the Fab arms of immunoglobulins (Fig. 171–2*B*), and that is the reason that there are not just two RV serotypes.[217, 219, 255] Virus-neutralizing antibody prevents virus attachment to cells by adhering to serospecific locations on the upper walls of the canyon, thereby forming a "neutralizing bridge" over the canyon, which blocks the cell receptor from access to its binding site at the canyon base. Thus far, nearly all cell receptor research has been with the major group; presumably, each of the 91 major receptor group RVs has specific amino acid arrangements on the antibody-binding sites on the canyon walls.[10, 48, 220, 227]

The major cell receptor is intercellular adhesion molecule 1 (ICAM-1), which ordinarily functions in immune reactions of various leukocytes.[103, 172, 234, 244] The virus simply has subverted this normal host protein for use as its cell receptor; ICAM-1 fits snugly into the narrow canyon (Fig. 171–2*B*).[217]

A pocket of unknown function whose walls are lined by 17 amino acids that vary with each RV type has been found at the base of the canyon (Fig. 171–2*C*).[9]

These spectacular achievements in molecular virology have stimulated research that may be of use in preventing or controlling picornavirus-caused disease:

1. ICAM-1 itself or portions thereof are being proposed as antiviral agents (e.g., spraying the nasopharynx with ICAM-1 could cause it to adhere to the receptor-binding sites of all "incoming" major group RVs, thereby preventing infection).[21, 173]
2. The pocket at the base of the canyon has been found to bind a variety of organic molecules; when it does, either the virus is prevented from uncoating (necessary to release viral RNA for its translation to viral protein) or the cell receptor is prevented from docking in the canyon.[93, 206] There now are at least 15 drugs, made by several different drug companies in the United States, Europe, and Japan, that are trying to exploit the antipicornavirus potentialities of this pocket.[9] One group of these drugs, the WIN compounds synthesized by Sterling-Winthrop, has had wide scientific exposure[177]; however, clinical trials have been discouraging.[246, 251] One disadvantage to these compounds is that the various RV serotypes vary widely in sensitivity to these organic molecules.[9] Another problem has been the failure to attain effective concentrations of drug at the site of infection.
3. Antibody fragments to cell receptor have blocked RV infection of cells, and application of receptor antibody to the nasopharynx modulated symptoms of RV-39 colds.[52, 121]

Because the structural features of the various picornaviruses seem nearly identical, their genomes demonstrate much cross-homology.[220] At least four RVs have been sequenced completely: RV-1B, RV-2, RV-14, and RV-89.[82, 138, 220, 231, 233] RV-1B and RV-2 are minor receptor group RVs, and their protein homologies are close—74 to 94 per cent. On the other hand, RV-14 proteins are related nearly as closely to those in the poliovirus and enterovirus groups as to those in the RVs.[139, 145, 233] It has been shown in nucleic acid hybridization experiments that cDNA to a segment near the 5′ end of the RV genome reacts with the genomes of many different picornaviruses.[4, 18] How these picornavirus inter-relationships finally develop will become clearer as more are sequenced.

Because the picornaviruses are so homogeneous genetically, it seems possible that an antiviral drug that successfully can treat common colds also may be effective against the many more serious picornavirus illnesses, such as aseptic meningitis, myocardiopathy, and neonatal disease. Many of these common proteins may be virus-coded enzymes used in replication; therefore, common virus-coded replicative enzyme inhibitors could serve as broadly acting picornavirus antiviral agents.

Virus Replication

Replication of the RVs is in the cytoplasm and probably is similar to that of the enteroviruses.[220] Most (90 per cent) RVs attach to the major group receptor, ICAM-1 (see earlier), located in the plasma membrane. The virus then probably is endocytized within a vesicle and the RNA released by an energy-requiring procedure. Although much of the released viral RNA is destroyed by cellular nucleases, sufficient amount remains to attach to ribosomes and provoke translation of the viral genome. The viral RNA is translated directly by host enzymes to a single long polyprotein. This polyprotein is cleaved by virus and (probably) host-coded enzymes to yield viral RNA polymerase, capsid proteins, proteases, and proteins to halt host protein synthesis and other products. Under laboratory conditions, infectious virus first is formed after about 2 hours and reaches a maximum of about 1000 infectious particles per cell at about 7 hours.[220] Infectious virus is, however, a minority of the virus-like particles formed; only about 1 in 200 are complete viruses capable of replicating in cell culture.[220] All viral replication occurs in the cytoplasm, and viruses are released by cell lysis.

Host Range

Animals

RVs have been isolated from natural infections of only cattle, chimpanzees, and humans.[170, 195, 220] Only two bovine

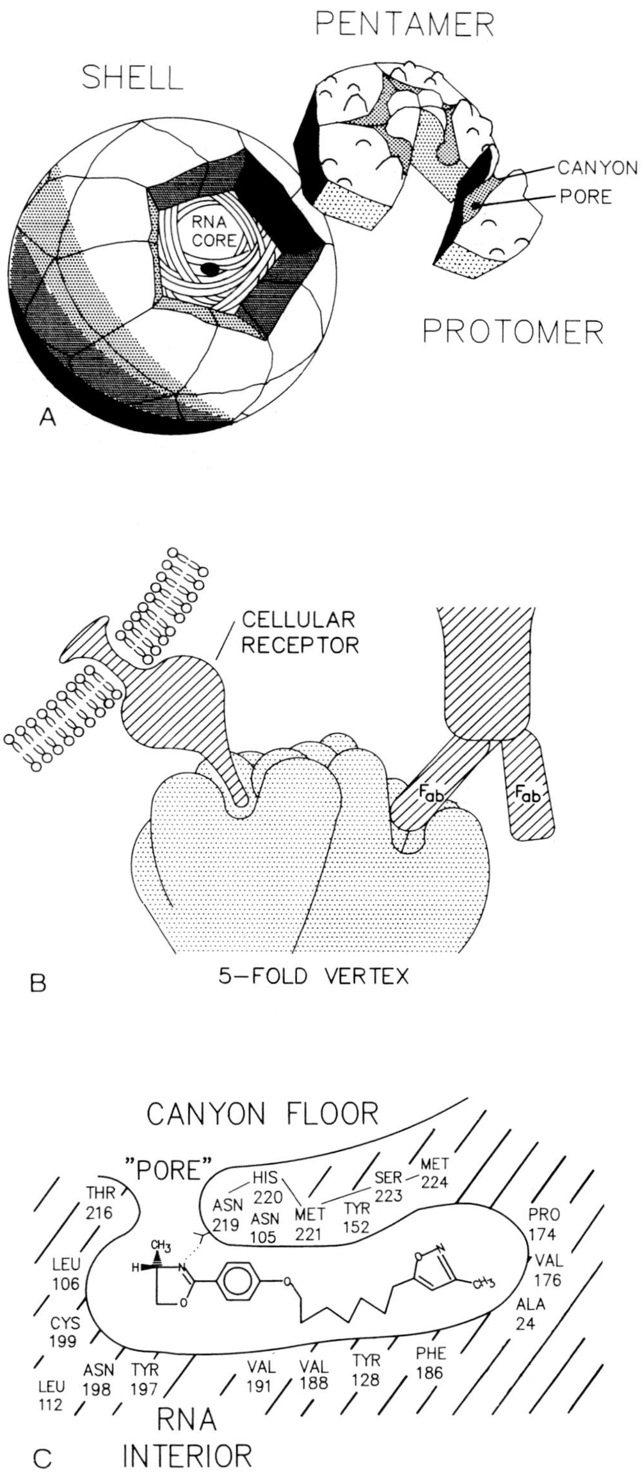

FIGURE 171–2. *Some attributes of a typical rhinovirus. This structure is typical of the entire picornavirus family. A, Exploded diagram of one of the 12 five-sided protein pentamers, which compose the viral coat (capsid). Each pentamer is composed of five interlocking wedge-like pieces, called protomers, one of which is broken away. Surrounding the central vertex of each pentamer is a narrow "canyon," and each protomer, at the bottom of its portion of the canyon, has a cell receptor binding site (not shown) and a pore. B, The cellular receptor for the major rhinovirus receptor group (90 per cent of the 101 rhinoviruses), now known to be intercellular adhesion molecule 1 (ICAM-1), fits snugly into the canyon and attaches to the binding site located at the bottom of the canyon. The Fab arm of an IgG antibody molecule is too large to reach the bottom of the canyon and cannot, therefore, directly neutralize the receptor binding site. To block ICAM-1 from entering the canyon, neutralizing antibody adheres to specific loci high on the canyon wall. C, The pore at the base of the canyon leads to a pocket beneath it. Several experimental antipicornavirus drugs (the one shown is WIN 52084) bind in the pocket, deforming the bottom of the canyon and preventing ICAM-1 attachment. (Adapted from Rueckert, R. R.:* Picornaviridae *and their replication.* In *Fields, B. N., Knipe, D. M., Chanock, R. M., et al. [eds.]: Fields Virology. 2nd ed. New York, Raven Press, 1990, pp. 507–548.)*

RV serotypes have been reported, and they may cause infections ranging from subclinical to overt respiratory disease in epizootics; there is no evidence for human infection.[215] Chimpanzees and humans both are infected with human RVs; chimpanzee infections are subclinical.[68, 228] A natural, subclinical outbreak of RV-31 in chimpanzees has been reported in a primate center.[67, 68]

Many efforts have been made to infect a wide variety of animals with human RVs, but, other than the chimpanzee, only the gibbon has been susceptible, and it is not reliably so.[68] Equine "RVs" have been described, but their taxonomic position in the picornavirus group is uncertain.[198, 220]

Cell and Tissue Cultures

The spectrum of tissue culture cells infected by the human RVs also is narrow.[54, 161] For initial isolation, human embryonic diploid cells usually are used (Fig. 171–3), although, for some RV types, an especially sensitive strain[50] of a continuous cell line, HeLa, serves as well or better.[54, 161] Some RVs only grow in human organ cultures and, perhaps, some only in living human beings.[161]

The first RV (RV-1A) was propagated in primary cell culture from primate kidneys (rhesus monkey cell cultures are used most commonly); surprisingly, chimpanzee kidney cell cultures do not propagate RVs.[64] However, most RVs propagate on original isolation only in cells of human origin, and they are called H strains; others also can be isolated in monkey kidney cell cultures and are called M strains. After laboratory propagation, all RVs seem adaptable to the RV-sensitive HeLa cell strain.[50] When HeLa-grown, RVs attain much higher titers than in the primary human diploid cells used for initial isolation.

Antigenic Properties

An outstanding characteristic of the RV is its great antigenic diversity; there now are at least 101 serotypes.[116] There is evidence that the number of additional serotypes may be limited.[92, 116, 152, 190] Certain serotypes cross-react, but there is little evidence that this could be exploited in vaccination.[53, 90, 187]

RVs often are poor antigens. Up to 50 per cent of patients from whom RVs are isolated may not develop significant (fourfold or greater) increases in serum antibody, and the levels attained often are low.[90–92]

RVs may be undergoing continuous antigenic change.[187] Sufficiently marked antigenic variation has been found for RV-22 and RV-51 to interfere with their typing; however, this drift does not seem to predict a continuing proliferation of RV types.[92, 190, 225, 237]

EPIDEMIOLOGY AND TRANSMISSION

Seasonal Distribution

Over the usual September through May "cold season," RV infections often are predominant at both ends, early fall and mid to late spring (Figs. 171–4 and 171–5). They also are important causes of summer colds. This seasonal pattern seems general because similar findings have been reported from families in Charlottesville, Virginia; Seattle, Washington; and elsewhere.[91, 92, 106, 127] In the southern hemisphere, a similar seasonal pattern occurs, but during opposing months.[148] The general spring-summer-fall seasonal predominance of the RVs does not mean that RVs are absent during the remainder of the year; they are found in varying degrees year-round.[57, 91, 92, 107, 190, 191, 213]

Cycling and Circulation of Individual Rhinovirus Types

Unlike most respiratory viruses (e.g., parainfluenza types 1 and 3 and respiratory syncytial virus), individual RV types seldom repeat within a population from year to year. Several serotypes usually circulate simultaneously,[118] frequently coincident with other respiratory viruses.[65, 133, 191] The various respiratory viruses circulate simultaneously within the neigh-

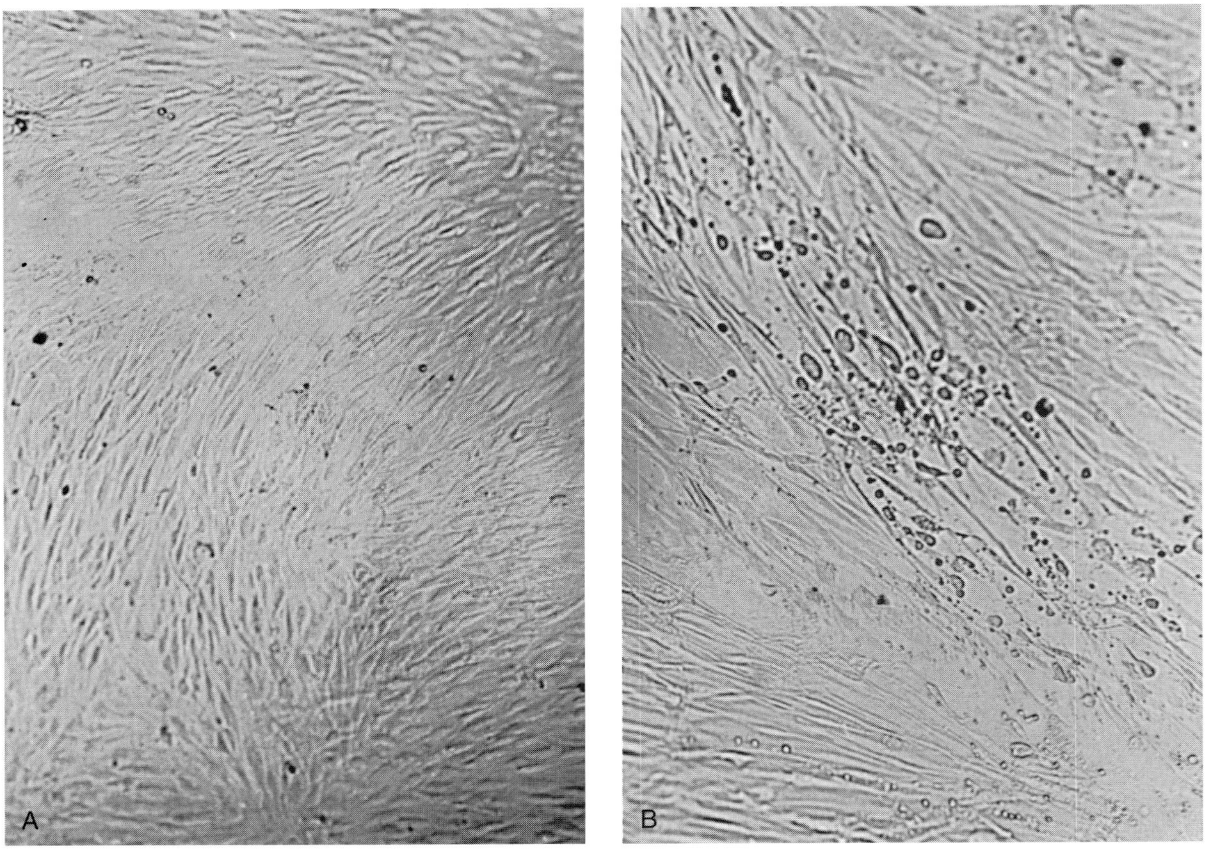

FIGURE 171–3. A, *Normal human diploid (fetal tonsil) cell sheet and* B, *a cell sheet infected for 2 days with rhinovirus type 16. The rounded and misshapen cells are characteristic. (Courtesy of Dr. David M. Warshauer, University of Wisconsin, Madison.)*

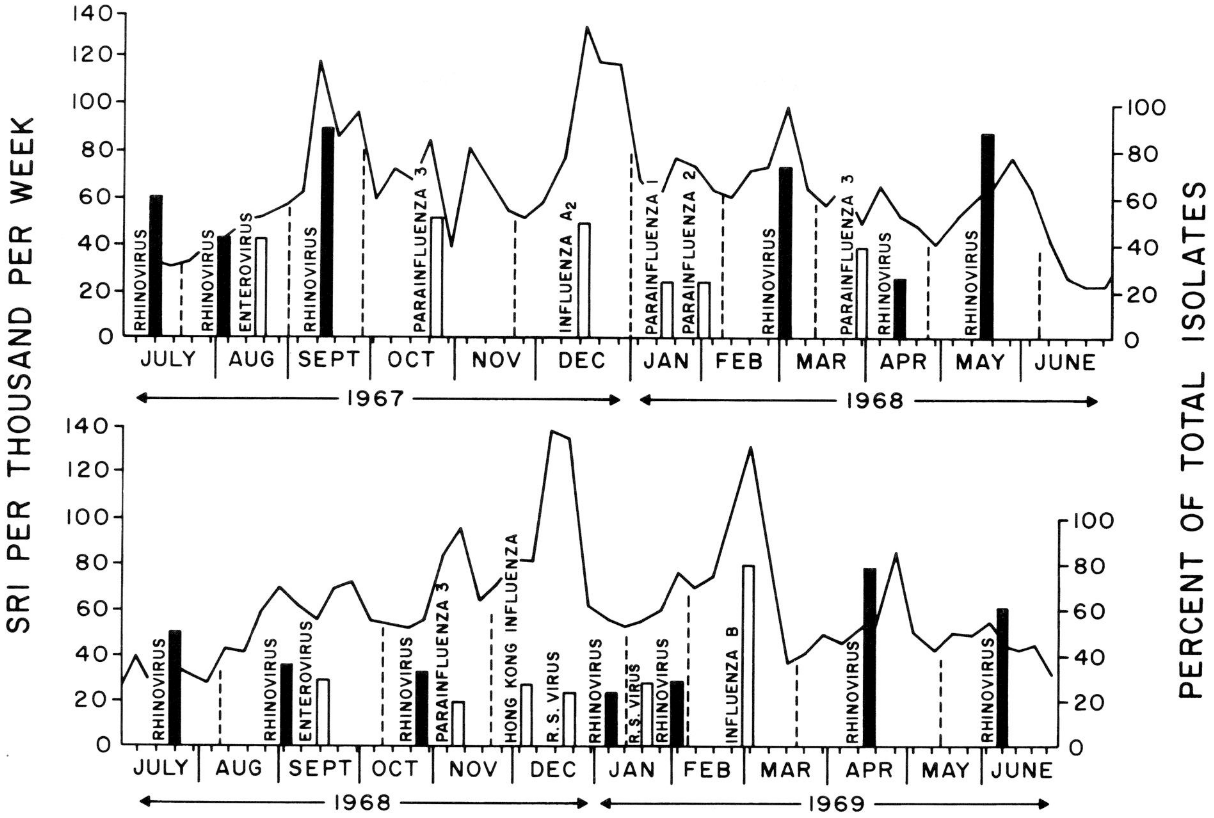

FIGURE 171–4. *Incidence of total symptomatic respiratory infection and predominant isolates in metropolitan Tecumseh, Michigan (population 10,000), 1967–1969. RS, respiratory syncytial. (Adapted from Monto, A. S., and Cavallaro, J. J.: Am. J. Epidemiol. 94:280–289, 1971.)*

borhood, as well as within the larger community. In 24 neighboring Madison, Wisconsin (Eagle Heights), families (Fig. 171–5), 14 different RV types plus several nontypable RVs were found over the 2 academic years 1963 to 1965. Only one type (RV-15) was found both years. The other common respiratory viruses also were present.

Several respiratory viruses may circulate concurrently among close neighbors or even within the family. As an example, from March to May 1963, RV-43 and RV-55, one nontypable RV, parainfluenza types 1 and 3, chickenpox, and poliomyelitis types 2 and 3 (from a community vaccination program) circulated through 10 Eagle Heights families studied in a 12-unit apartment building (Fig. 171–6). In two families, RV-43 and RV-55 were present simultaneously.

The combination of many RV types and nearly annual recycling of other respiratory agents can produce a real welter of different viral infections in individual families (Fig. 171–7).

Circulation Within School Rooms

The mechanism of respiratory virus dissemination throughout the community may be the schoolroom or similar environments. In a Chicago nursery population, Beem[22] observed that some RV types spread extensively, involving up to 77 per cent of the 22 children studied. He observed similar widespread infection with respiratory syncytial virus but not with the parainfluenza and influenza viruses. In an upper middle class Madison second grade schoolroom, results were similar but not identical (Fig. 171–8). The RV types studied infected from 18 to 55 per cent of susceptible children; however, influenza B virus was the agent that circulated most widely.

Although several RV types usually circulate concurrently, all types present are not equal in prevalence. In the aforementioned Chicago nursery school study,[22] 14 different serotypes were isolated over the academic year 1962 to 1963, but 10 of the serotypes did not spread at all. Only three types disseminated widely, infecting greater than 40 per cent of the children. Likewise, in the 1963 to 1965 Madison Eagle Heights village study (see Fig. 171–5), 14 RV types were isolated, but only three types (RV-43, RV-51, and RV-55) were "spreaders." Similar patterns of serologic prevalence have been reported from laboratories in Tecumseh, Michigan[191]; New York City and Seattle[91, 92]; and Charlottesville.[127]

Predominating Rhinovirus Types

Although the pattern of predominating RV types within a circumscribed population and a defined time frame seems well established, predominance of serotypes over large geographic areas or over many years does not seem to occur. This has been studied exhaustively in widely separated locations and over many years: the Gulf South from 1962 to 1970; Tecumseh from 1966 to 1971 and from 1976 to 1981; and Seattle from 1965 to 1969 and from 1975 to 1979.[91, 92, 186, 187, 190, 192] Although there were "common types" (usually the isolation of at least five to eight strains of a serotype over the period studied) during each period and at each place, different types were "common" in different places and times. For

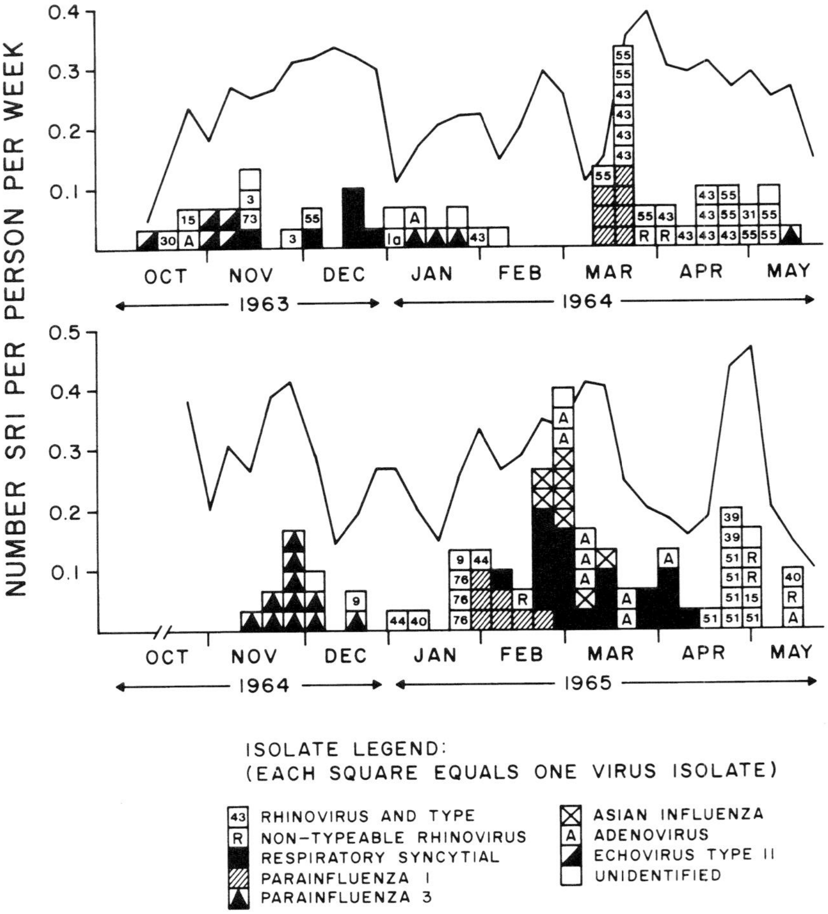

FIGURE 171–5. *Rhinoviruses and other respiratory viruses associated with symptomatic respiratory infection in three neighboring apartment buildings in Eagle Heights, a University of Wisconsin housing village in Madison, Wisconsin (24 to 26 families, about 100 persons), 1963–1965.*

example, at Tecumseh, Monto[187, 192] obtained, during his two 6-year study periods, 475 RV isolates covering 70 serotypes (out of a possible 89 at that time[150]), but only RV-1B, RV-10, RV-28, and RV-58 were common in both periods. They were not that common because only 16, 22, 15, and 18 isolates, respectively, of these four types were found over the 12 years. As shown in Figures 171–5 and 171–9, in the neighboring state of Wisconsin from 1963 to 1965, our common types were RV-43, RV-51, and RV-55—completely different from Michigan. Finally, the late John Fox sifted data from family populations surveyed by him and others in New York City, Seattle, and Tecumseh.[91, 92] He found only four common serotypes (RV-1B, RV-12, RV-15, and RV-38) from among 802 isolates. It would appear, at least in the United States, that dominant RV serotypes often occur locally over relatively short periods but do not extend over decades or over the nation.

PERSON-TO-PERSON TRANSMISSION

Epidemiologic Observations

Individual RV serotypes often disseminate with surprising difficulty, as has been noted previously in Eagle Heights village (see Figs. 171–5 and 171–9), a Madison elementary school (see Fig. 171–8), and a Chicago nursery school.[22] At least within family populations, the most common finding is that a specific RV serotype does not spread from the index case. Hendley and associates,[127] in a study of 19 families in Charlottesville, found that RVs from 10 of 22 index cases did not spread at all, and in only 7 families was there dissemination to at least one other person. In only 4 of the 19 was there further sequential spread. Fox and associates,[91, 92] in a surveillance of more than 200 Seattle families, found intrafamily secondary attack rates in susceptible individuals (no homotypic antibody) to be 44 per cent from 1965 to 1969 and 28 per cent from 1975 to 1979. In both periods, children younger than 5 years of age had the highest secondary attack rate, 60 per cent and 30 per cent, respectively. Monto[189, 193] reported similar findings in 48 Panamanian families: using five RV isolates as antigens, the secondary attack rate varied from 10.5 to 56 per cent.

Our laboratory in Madison examined the inter- and intrafamily dissemination of the three "spreading" RV types—RV-43, RV-51, and RV-55—in the 24 to 26 neighboring families in Eagle Heights village (see Figs. 171–5, 171–6, 171–9, and 171–10). These three serotypes were the only ones of 14 to spread beyond the index family. RV-51 attacked 23 per cent of susceptible individuals, and many family members and close neighbors remained uninfected. RV-43 infected 34 per cent of susceptible individuals; in one building—408—only the families in a single end four-plex became infected. On the other hand, RV-55 caused a miniepidemic in buildings 405 and 408, attaining a 71 per cent attack rate in the latter; several families had all members infected. RV dissemination seemed to focus on the four-plex, probably because, in the winter months, the children played in the hallways and stairs connecting the four-plex apartments (Fig. 171–10). Nevertheless, even the spreading RVs left many susceptible individuals untouched among next-door four-plex neighbors and within many families.

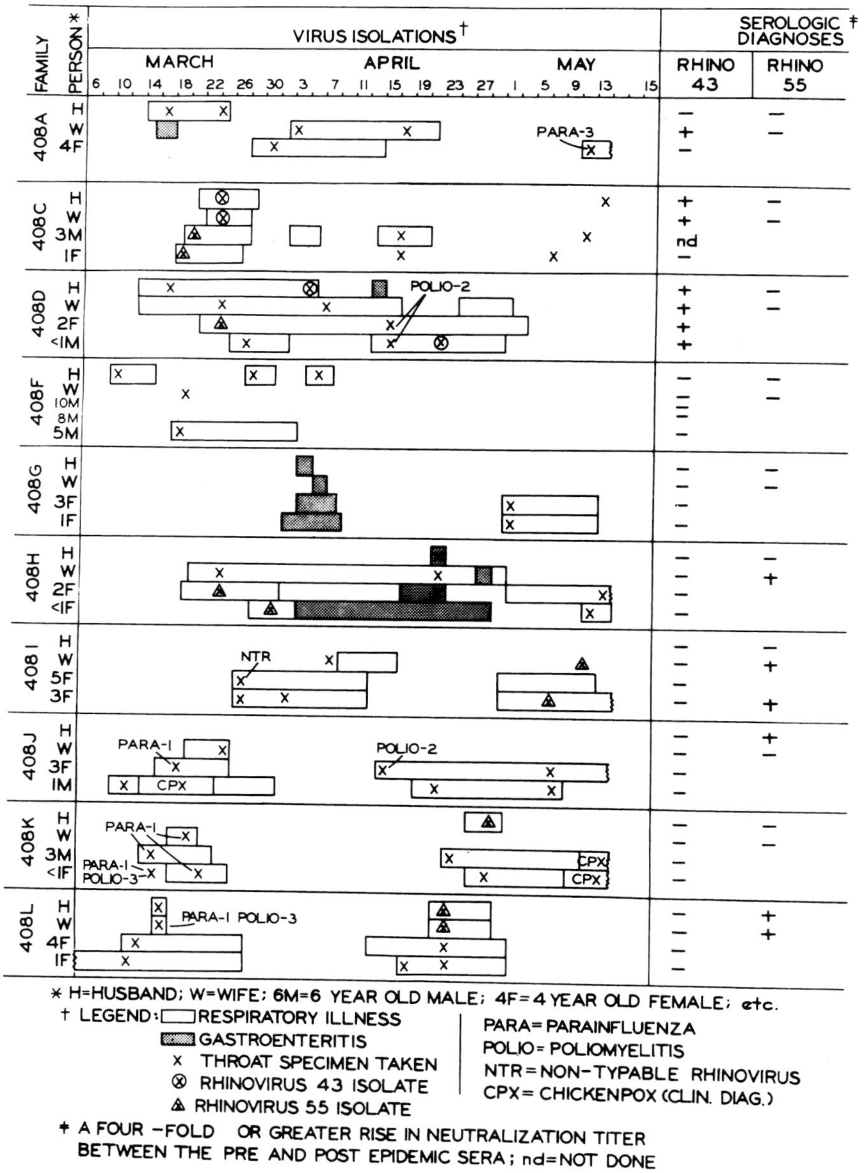

FIGURE 171–6. *Distribution of respiratory viruses in one Eagle Heights apartment building, Madison, Wisconsin, March 6–May 15, 1964. (Adapted from Dick, E. C., Blumer, C. R., Evans, A. S.: Am. J. Epidemiol. 86:386–400, 1967.)*

63-64	64-65	63-64	64-65	63-64	64-65	63-64	64-65	63-64	64-65	63-64	64-65
APT C; 2,1 CHILD		APT D; 2 CHILD		APT G; 2,3 CHILD		APT H; 2 CHILD		APT K; 2 CHILD		APT L; 2,4 CHILD	
E11 R43 R55 Vla	INF A_2 P-1 R44	RS R43 R55 R-NT	INF A_2 RS R15	E11 RS	P-1 P-3 RS R51	RS R55	Ad2 P-3 R40 R44 R51	P-1 R55	NOT DONE	P-1 RS R55	INF A_2 P-1 RS R44
APT A; 1 CHILD		APT B		APT E; 3 CHILD		APT F; 4,2 CHILD		APT I; 2 CHILD		APT J; 2 CHILD	
E11 P-3 R43 R55	NOT DONE	NOT	DONE	NOT DONE	P-3	E11 R15	INF A_2 P-3 RS R9 R44 R51	E11 R55	INF A_2 Ad 8 R40 R44 R-NT	Ad2 P-1 R55 Vla	R51

FIGURE 171–7. *Viral infections in a single Eagle Heights apartment building, Madison, Wisconsin, 1963–1965. Ad, adenovirus; E, echovirus; INF A_2, influenza A (H2N2); NT, nontypable; P, parainfluenza; R, rhinoviruses; RS, respiratory syncytial; Vla, unidentified, virus-like agent. Numbers after letters refer to type (e.g., RV55, rhinovirus type 55). See Figure 171–10 for apartment arrangement.*

	Viral Agent	Number of Susceptible Students *	Number Infected (%)
1968	Non-typeable 'M' Rhinovirus	19	7 (37%)
	Rhinovirus 19	17	3 (18%)
	Rhinovirus 36	11	6 (55%)
	Parainfluenza 3	2	2 (100%)
	Respiratory Syncytial	N.D.	5
1968–69	Rhinovirus 6	24	9 (37%)
	Influenza B	0	13
	Respiratory Syncytial	3	8

*NUMBER WITH NEUTRALIZING ANTIBODY TITERS ≤1:8 AT ONSET OF STUDY

FIGURE 171–8. *Attack rates of several respiratory viruses within a Madison, Wisconsin, second-grade classroom of 26 students. Three semesters, 1968–1969.*

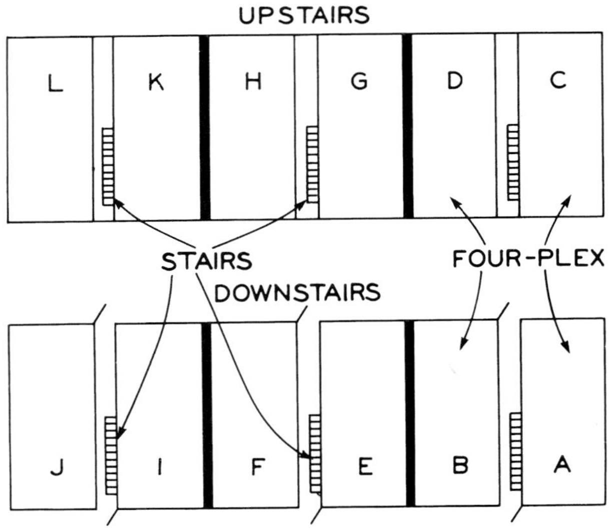

FIGURE 171–10. *Apartment arrangement in an Eagle Heights Village apartment building, Madison, Wisconsin. Each 12-unit building is divided into three four-plexes: two apartments upstairs and two apartments downstairs, accessible inside the unit by stairs. Access to the other four-plexes is only through the doors to the outside.*

As part of the same study, surveillance was carried on for Asian influenza (influenza A [H2N2]), which attacked the population during the 1964 to 1965 winter (see Fig. 171–5), and for parainfluenza type 1. Although the intrafamily attack rates of Asian influenza often were 100 per cent, many persons and families remained uninfected by this usually epidemic virus (Fig. 171–11). The occupants of building 408 had an attack rate of 74 per cent, nearly identical to that associated with RV-55 the previous year. The spread of parainfluenza type 1 was much like that of RV-51 (see Figs. 171–9 and 171–11).

The erratic spreading patterns of these five viruses in Eagle Heights village were perplexing. Although certainly these agents were capable of 100 per cent infection of family members and, occasionally, of near neighbors, it was most provocative that they—even Asian influenza—so often did not transmit at all.

Determination of the reason for such erratic spreading patterns can be sought in well-controlled chain-of-infection experiments with human volunteers. It would not be ethical to carry on such experiments with a virulent influenza virus; however, RVs are one of the few viruses with which healthy, adult humans can be infected safely. RV transmission experiments from several laboratories are described next.

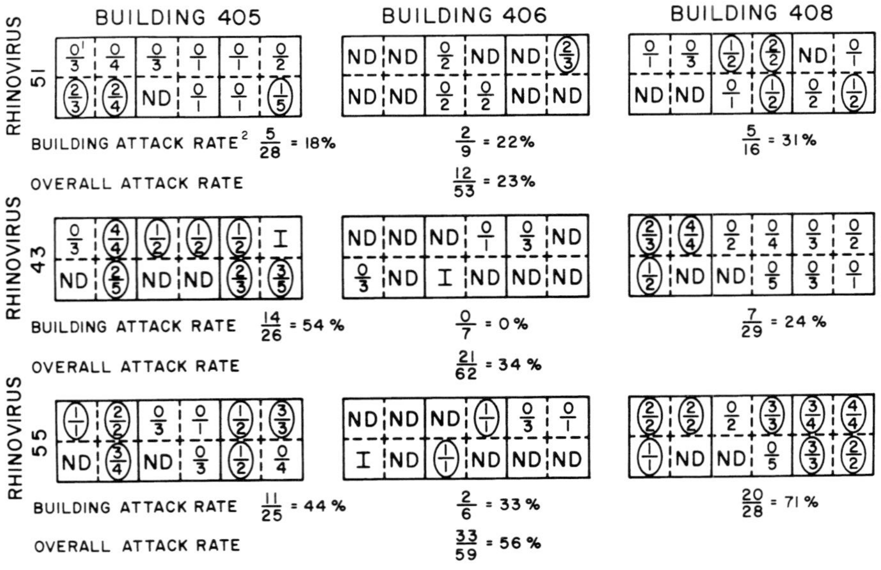

[1] NO. DIAGNOSED CASES / NO. SUSCEPTIBLES (NO DETECTABLE ANTIBODY)

[2] AS DIAGNOSED BY EITHER VIRUS ISOLATION AND/OR A 4-FOLD OR GREATER SEROLOGIC RESPONSE

FIGURE 171–9. *Attack rates of three "spreading" rhinoviruses in three neighboring Eagle Heights apartment buildings, Madison, Wisconsin. I, all members immune; ND, not done; O, family with one or more infected members.*

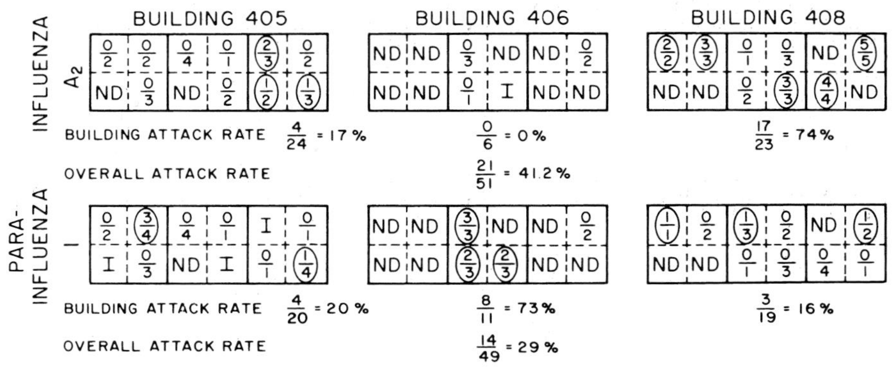

FIGURE 171–11. *Attack rates of two myxoviruses in three neighboring Eagle Heights apartment buildings, Madison, Wisconsin. I, all members immune; ND, not done; O, family with one or more infected members.*

Person-to-Person Transmission Using Human Volunteers

Experiments with Nasal Secretions from Persons with Colds of Unknown Etiology

Experimentation with common colds in human volunteers began at England's Common Cold Unit at Salisbury shortly after World War II.[248, 250] However, the majority of the transmission trials at this unit were performed with nasal secretions prior to the discovery of most of the respiratory viruses, and the results are difficult to interpret. (The adenoviruses first were cultivated about 1953, followed by the parainfluenza viruses, respiratory syncytial virus, RVs [1956], and coronaviruses [1965].) Nonetheless, the general findings of these early experiments were correct; the usual common cold often is surprisingly difficult to transmit.[248]

Early Experiments with Rhinovirus Colds

Even in pure culture, the RVs retained their uncertainty of transmission. Couch and colleagues,[56, 58] trying to repeat with RV-15 a successful cox-A21 aerosol transmission experiment, attained no transmission after housing 15 donors (persons infected intranasally with laboratory-grown virus) with 12 recipients (persons without antibody to the donor's virus) for 26 days. At about the same time, our laboratory carried out transmission trials with RV-55 and RV-16 in a series of experiments ranging in duration from a 1- to 1.5-minute kiss to a 3-day weekend in a dormitory room. In 26 donors and 33 recipients, only two transmissions occurred, one from a 1.5-minute kiss and the other from a weekend in a dormitory.[60] Only when young student married couples were used was a substantial rate attained; among 24 couples, nine donor spouses infected their mates for a transmission rate of 38 per cent.[61]

Human Infectious Dose 50 for Rhinovirus

Judging from RV challenge experiments with laboratory-grown virus administered by nose drops or aerosol, less than one $TCID_{50}$ can initiate infection.[60, 75] Much more (2000 times) is required when placed on the tongue or dried just outside the anterior nares (10,000 times).[60] How accurately these conditions approach the natural state is not known.[125]

Characteristics of a "Good" Rhinovirus Transmitter

In the married couple experiments, a "successful" donor (1) shed enough virus to contaminate his or her environment, (2) exhibited signs and symptoms of a moderate to severe cold, and (3) spent many hours at home with his or her spouse.[61] As illustrative of the effect of high virus shedding, intracouple transmission rates were 71 per cent for donors with nasopharyngeal RV titers of 5000 to more than 80,000 $TCID_{50}$, 33 per cent for those with 1000 to 5000 $TCID_{50}$, and only 18 per cent for those with less ($p = 0.025$). Illustrative of both shedding and production of sufficient nasal secretions was contamination of the hands with RV; those donors whose hands were assayed for virus and who transmitted infections to their spouses all had RV on their hands, whereas none of the nontransmitters did ($p = 0.03$). The amount of time spent together seemed important in transmission ($p = 0.025$) (Table 171–1). Nevertheless, many infectious spouses who spent hours of direct contact with their partners did not infect them.

Some Early Conclusions

The preceding findings both in epidemiologic studies and in human volunteers suggest that, usually, attending a concert or a motion picture with those who have even obvious signs of colds is unlikely to result in infection. (On the other

TABLE 171–1. Relation of the Capacity of Artificially Infected Donors to Transmit Rhinovirus Type 16 to Their Spouses to the Number of Hours Spent Together and to the Number of Hours of Direct Contact

		Number of Hours†	
Donor*	Transmission	*In the Same Air Space*‡	*In Direct Contact*§
A	+	149	10
B	−	142	13
C	+	138	20
D	+	127	39
E	+	122	5
F	−	112	21
G	−	112	12
H	−	105	19
I	−	103	26
J	−	86	6
K	−	63	12

*Listed in order of number of hours in same air space greatest to least. The larger the number of hours spent together, the greater the likelihood of transmission (two-sample Wilcoxon rank test, p is .025).

†During the 7-day period after artificial infection. Total possible number of hours is 168.

‡When the couples were home together.

§Embracing, kissing, and so forth.

Adapted from D'Alessio, D. J., Peterson, J. A., Dick, C. R., et al.: J. Infect. Dis. *133*:28–36, 1976.

hand, students who spend day after day in classrooms may have a higher chance for infection [see Fig. 171–8].) Also, relatively short stays (a few hours) among friends or relatives with RV-caused colds are not liable to cause infection, even if persons embrace briefly. There even is evidence from a group practice in Massachusetts that pediatricians' waiting rooms may *not* be places where respiratory viruses commonly are transferred.[167] These conclusions come with a caveat, however, in that direct experience is only with RVs. Respiratory illnesses in which cough is a large component, such as influenza and measles, can result in substantial dissemination, even in a pediatric clinic.[24, 40, 102] Also, other factors, such as stress, may cause reduced resistance.[47, 239] As a whole, however, the data suggest that healthy persons usually can bank on luck or just plain chance to protect them from the colds that are such a ubiquitous presence wherever humans congregate.

Route of Transmission Experiments

Because RVs and perhaps other respiratory viruses often seem to spread with relative difficulty under many normal circumstances, route of transmission becomes important because controlling transmission of respiratory viruses in various habitats, such as schoolrooms and families, may be feasible by blocking transmission routes.

Since the early 1970s, there has been much human volunteer experimentation on RV transmission routes, chiefly at the University of Virginia, England's Common Cold Unit, and our laboratory at the University of Wisconsin. Gwaltney and Hendley[108] at Charlottesville focused on the possibility that RV colds were disseminated via direct or indirect hand contact. Interest in this approach had been provoked by their inadvertently passing RVs from infected to noninfected persons through the vehicle of a supposedly ethanol-sterilized nasal speculum. Subsequently, they observed that there was a lot of nose picking and eye rubbing among Department of Medicine Grand Rounds participants and Sunday school attendees (infection through conjunctival swabs previously had been reported[31]).[128] They then showed that RV-39 retained infectivity for several hours on various surfaces and could be found on the hands of RV-39–infected persons. They concluded that RV transmission might occur via self-inoculation by environmentally contaminated hands and demonstrated, in human volunteers, RV-39 self-inoculation from an environmental source.[128]

The Charlottesville team then conducted a series of three experiments that, when combined with their prior "self-inoculation" results, greatly influenced the medical community.[35, 55, 110, 128, 146] In two of the experiments, groups of recipients were exposed to RV-infected donors (the RV used was an untypable strain, HH) in circumstances wherein they were exposed naturally in separate closed rooms to large-particle (12 recipients) or small-particle (10 recipients) aerosols produced by donors over periods of 45 minutes (large particles) or 3 days (small particles). One of the large-particle aerosol recipients was infected, and none exposed to small-particle aerosols were. (These essentially negative transmission rates by aerosol exposure were not surprising[108] because, as noted previously, Couch[55] had been unsuccessful via the airborne route over 26 days, and we attained only one RV transmission among 11 recipients after 3 days' exposure in a dormitory.[60]) The third group of Charlottesville recipients was exposed to RV by inoculating themselves with the donor's nasal mucus. The donors blew their noses into their hands. The recipients then stroked the donors' contaminated hands for 10 seconds and then inoculated themselves by deliberately placing their fingers, two or three times, on their nasal and conjunctival mucosa. This inoculation procedure was repeated on 3 successive days. Eleven of the 15 hand-contact recipients (73 per cent) were infected with the donors' RV. The authors concluded that transmission by the hand-contact/self-inoculation route was much more efficient than was the aerosol route and "may be an important natural route of RV transmission."[110] Those conclusions may be correct, but, in our view, there is real doubt whether transmission efficiency can be compared between circumstances in which donors and recipients simply are sharing the same air space over a measured—often brief—period with an experiment in which fresh nasal mucus is transferred purposefully from the donors' to the recipients' mucous membranes on each of 3 days. Nevertheless, Gwaltney did accomplish a high rate of RV transmission using nasal secretions, something that none of the rest of us had been able to accomplish readily in more "natural" experiments.[56, 60] Also in support of hand transmission was our observation in the aforementioned married couple experiments that the ability to transmit was correlated significantly with presence of RV on the donors' hands.[61] As a result of these various pieces of evidence and a lack of compelling evidence to the contrary, hand-to-hand or fomite transmission became the accepted route for RV contagion.[35, 55, 80, 243] However, the hand transmission evidence either was deduced or was contrived (i.e., indirect nose-to-nose mucus transfer); no actual natural transmission of RV by hand contact had been demonstrated.[72, 86]

In later experiments, the Charlottesville group demonstrated approximately 50 per cent transmission via fomites using the same hand-contact/self-inoculation method described earlier, except either a coffee cup handle or a plastic tile was interposed between donors' and recipients' hands.[109]

At England's Common Cold Unit, Reed[211] investigated the likelihood of natural hand-contact transmission among residents (roommates) of several housing units, 38 of whom had been infected with RV-2. Reed[211] found that 16 of the donors had RV on their fingers but none was transmitted to the fingers of their 18 roommates, even though virus could be recovered from some (6 of 40) objects recently handled by RV-2–infected donors. Reed also found that none of 29 virus transfers from virus dried on the fingers could pass through a fomite to a recipient; it was concluded that "spread of colds is unlikely to occur via objects contaminated by the hands of the virus shedder. . . ."

Our laboratory at Wisconsin continued its attempts to devise a natural transmission model to examine routes of transmission and, potentially, methods for interruption of transmission. Although the results of the transmission experiment with married couples were illuminating, the system itself had one great deficiency as an experimental model: the participants could not be observed during their interaction periods.[61] A model was needed in which donors and recipients could be monitored at all times. Ultimately, the scheme for such a system was suggested by two virologic-epidemiologic events in Antarctica, one from a few summer seasons (1975 to 1980) in which Dick studied respiratory virus dissemination in an isolated Antarctic population, and the other from a human volunteer experiment conducted in an Antarctic field party from England's Common Cold Unit.[132, 230, 260] Both experiences suggested that high natural transmission rates after only a few days of exposure could be achieved only in an environment with a high donor-to-recipient ratio and in a population density such as might be found in the classrooms and dormitories of a boarding school. Accordingly, a model was devised whereby donors (with the qualities of a "good" transmitter as described earlier) and recipients interacted during waking hours by card playing, board and video games, and communal studying.[61] During the night, donors and recipients were bunked together in the same or an adjoining room. With such an arrangement, graduate student monitors recorded activities and all clinical signs 24 hours a day. These artifices were successful; with 8 donors and 12 to 16 recipients, a 50 per cent recipient attack rate usually was attained over 12 hours and a 100 per cent rate over a week.[146, 181] Informally, this model, a fully observed monotypic RV mini-epidemic, was named an "Antarctic Hut," from its origins.[126]

Route of Transmission "Blocking" Experiments

Using the Antarctic Hut model, a series of four RV-16 route-of-transmission blocking experiments were conducted to determine whether the virus was spread by hand contact, aerosol, or both.[72, 146] The first three experiments lasted 12 hours, with 8 donors and 12 recipients; the donor-recipient interaction was through variants of stud and draw poker (Fig. 171–12). This interaction mode facilitated both aerosol and fomite–hand-contact transmission. Half of the recipients were blocked completely from any hand contact/self-inoculation by wearing arm restraints (see Fig. 171–12). Evidently, little transmission was by hand or fomite contact because the RV-16 infection rate in the restrained recipients was only slightly lower than in the unrestrained recipients—56 versus 67 per cent, an insignificant reduction ($p = 0.494$). The fourth experiment, using aerosol blocking, commenced immediately after the third. The poker game continued in the original room with eight donors alone, and all the equipment from the third experiment was moved to an identical room across the hall, including the cards (which literally were gummy from the prior 12-hour game), poker chips, pencils, and so forth. (The continuing eight-donor poker game in the room used for the third experiment was refurnished with poker implements.) Then, 12 new recipients entered the second room and began playing poker with the now heavily used cards and other paraphernalia, making exaggerated hand-to-nose self-inoculation movements. Aerosol transmission effectively was blocked by the two brick walls between the rooms. Once each hour the cards, poker chips, and other portables were exchanged between the donor and recipient rooms to maintain a freshly contaminated supply of fomites in the recipient room. The result was extremely surprising; not 1 of the 12 "fomite recipients" caught RV-16. Judging from the results of these four Antarctic Hut experiments, in which fomite–hand-contact and aerosol transmission were blocked alternately, aerosol transmission clearly seems the predominant route, at least for RV-16 among student poker players at the University of Wisconsin. A few months after the 1987 publication of these results, an editorial appeared in *The Lancet* entitled, "Splints Don't Stop Colds—Surprising!"[72, 86] It concluded that ". . . it looks as though coughs and sneezes *do* [italics theirs] spread these diseases more than sticky fingers."

Subsequently, a set of experiments was conducted in our laboratory to determine how RV-16 so surprisingly has disappeared along the five-step fomite transmission chain from nose to hand to fomite to hand to nose.[147] The experiments were a more elaborate version of Reed's prior studies,[211] and we obtained the same results. The virus seems to disappear precipitously at each step in the chain; 10^6 $TCID_{50}$ of RV-16 in the donor's nose is reduced to 0 to 64 $TCID_{50}$ on the card-playing implements, and then the virus nearly disappears upon reaching the recipients' hands.

Putting the results of these various experiments together, we currently lean to the view, at least with the RVs, that natural transmission via the hand-contact/self-inoculation route seems unlikely *unless* the virus actually is suspended in fresh mucus; then little virus is lost in transit.[147, 211] However, judging from the foregoing experiments, wet mucus seems to be passed infrequently from one adult to another, as was predicted by Reed.[211]

We believe, however, that respiratory illnesses may be transmitted by both hand-contact and aerosol routes. Certainly, the evidence presented in favor of the aerosol route as predominant should *not* discourage anyone from careful hand washing, especially around small children in whom transmission by virus in wet mucus indeed could occur. On the other hand, there is a definite likelihood that common respiratory viruses may be carried to patients in aero-

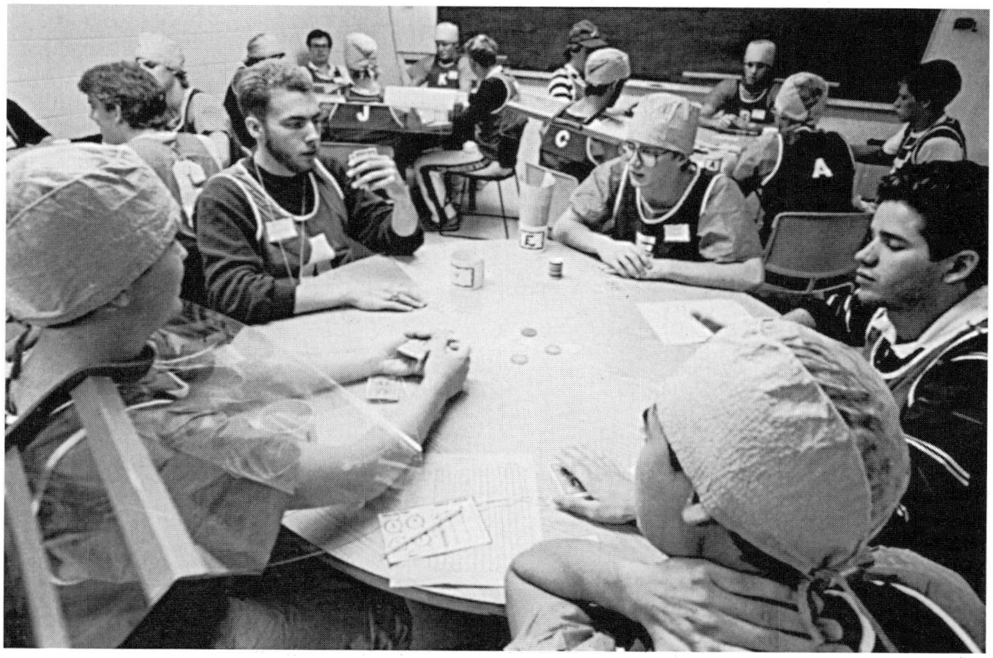

FIGURE 171–12. *A typical "Antarctic Hut" transmission experiment in progress using stud and draw poker as the interaction promoter. At each of four tables are two "donors" (infected with rhinovirus type 16) and three "recipients" (no antibody to rhinovirus type 16) (wearing surgical scrub suits). This particular experiment is one in which hand-contact/self-inoculation transmission is blocked in six of the 12 recipients by their wearing of Thatcher collars. The collars block hand-contact transmission by preventing touching of the face by the hands; therefore, virus can pass from donors to recipients only by aerosol.*

sols.[72, 86, 146, 147, 211] Accordingly, in planning air circulation systems, a medical consultant should consider whether the new air filter technology that claims to be able to remove virus-size particles from large volumes of air might be worthwhile.

Interruption of Transmission

The Virginia team[106, 126] carried out a blocking experiment in the field in which mothers of families attempted to prevent hand contact/self-inoculation by dipping their fingers in iodine. The results of this 1979 to 1982 study were reported twice as segments of two general reviews on RV transmission, and results differed somewhat in the two publications. In the first presentation, the mothers with iodinated fingers had a lower illness rate than did the placebo mothers from 1979 to 1981, but not in 1982.[106] In the second review, the illness rate over the 4 years was reported as 40 per cent lower in the iodine mothers than in the placebo mothers, and the difference was significant ($p = 0.047$).[126] Commendably, the authors speak directly to the difficulty in conducting and interpreting such investigations.[126]

We long have been interested in transmission-interruption methods that could exploit the apparent reluctance of RVs, and perhaps other viruses, to spread from person to person. As part of our general investigation of the epidemiology of respiratory viruses in an isolated (ca. 200 persons) Antarctic population at McMurdo Station, in 1979 we successfully used an iodinated facial tissue for transmission-interruption developed by the S. C. Johnson Company (Johnson's Wax) of Racine, Wisconsin.[69, 230, 260] Three days after all personnel began copious use of these tissues, incidence of respiratory illness dropped rapidly and significantly ($p < 0.01$); in fact, respiratory illness nearly disappeared from the base.[71] Although this effect was striking, the trial only historically could be controlled. However, the apparent success was marked sufficiently to interest the Kimberly-Clark Corporation, makers of Kleenex tissues, in applying virucidal facial tissue technology to interrupt RV-16 transmission in the Antarctic Hut model. Kimberly-Clark Corporation soon made available a nontoxic, highly virucidal facial tissue. The tissues completely stopped RV-16 transmission, compared with transmission rates of 42 and 75 per cent in control recipients using ordinary cotton handkerchiefs ($p < 0.001$) (Table 171–2).[70] Kimberly-Clark Corporation test-marketed these tissues under the brand name "AVERT," but their sales were below expectations. Subsequently, two field trials of AVERT in families were carried out in Charlottesville and Tecumseh with transmission reductions of 5 to 39 per cent.[88, 168] These were disappointing results but not—to us at least—unexpected. We found even in the highly supervised, well-motivated adults in Antarctica that changing established habits of personal nasal sanitation was not easy; it may be impossible in unsupervised children.

TABLE 171–2. Apparent Complete Interruption by Virucidal Tissues of Rhinovirus Type 16 (RV-16) Transmission*

	Cotton Hand'cfs.	Virucidal Tissues		Cotton Hand'cfs.
	Exp. A	*Exp. B*	*Exp. C*	*Exp. D*
Recipients who "caught" RV-16 colds/total (%)†	5/12 (42)	0/12	0/12	9/12 (75)

*In each of four experiments, eight volunteers with RV-16 colds played poker for 12 hours with 12 other volunteers (without RV-16 antibody) using for nasal sanitation either ordinary cotton handkerchiefs (Hand'cfs.) (experiments A and D) or virucidal tissues (B and C). Three-ply KLEENEX tissues were treated, per 100 g, with 9.1 g of citric acid, 4.5 g of malic acid, and 1.8 g of sodium lauryl sulfate. Cotton or paper handkerchiefs were used to clear nasal passages, smother coughs and sneezes, and wipe surfaces. Virucidal tissues were used carefully and copiously.

†Diagnosed by at least one isolation of RV-16 or a fourfold rise in antibody to RV-16 in the convalescent serum sample or both.

Adapted from Dick, E. C., Hossain, S. U., Mink, K. A., et al.: J. Infect. Dis. *153*:352–356, 1986.

PATHOGENESIS AND HOST FACTORS

General Course of Infection

Infection presumably usually is via the respiratory route, although infection by the conjunctival route has been demonstrated.[31, 128] In order to infect via the respiratory tract, a mucus blanket, about 200 times the width of the RV and propelled forward by continuously beating cilia, must be penetrated by as yet unknown means.[125] (It is possible that this is a formidable barrier and may account for the difficulty of RV transmission.) Nonetheless, when given intranasally by pipette, only one $TCID_{50}$ is needed to initiate infection.[60, 75] The incubation period for a cold normally is 2 to 3 days, but up to 7 days has been reported.[76, 127] Ciliary dysfunction can predispose to respiratory infection.[25, 33] RVs replicate well in the upper respiratory tract (see later), but even though lower respiratory symptoms such as cough usually are present even in mild RV colds, there is no incontrovertible evidence of viral replication in the lower respiratory tract.[95, 113, 114]

RVs may be shed in large amounts (1000 to 1,000,000 infectious particles per milliliter of nasal washing) during the first 2 to 3 days of a cold and may be produced for 2 to 3 weeks thereafter.[72, 75, 76, 181] However, the effect on the cells of the nasopharyngeal cavity seems benign, even though there is much local reaction to the virus, which results in the usual signs and symptoms of a cold. Systematic studies of RV-inoculated human volunteers at the University of Virginia demonstrated that damage to the respiratory epithelium was slight, although a few sloughed ciliated epithelial cells did contain RV antigen.[247, 263] Also, using primary monolayer cultures of ciliated and nonciliated epithelial cells, Winther and associates[264] demonstrated that RV, coronavirus, influenza A virus, and adenovirus all grew well in these cell cultures; however, RV and coronavirus produced no discernible cytopathic effect, whereas influenza virus and adenovirus nearly destroyed the cell sheet by 96 hours.

Because the RVs seem to cause only mild pathologic changes in cells of the respiratory tract, attention has turned to various immunologic or inflammatory substances as possible causes of symptomatic illness.[245] It has been known for some years that peripheral blood neutrophils increase in the first 2 to 3 days of illness in RV-infected volunteers.[36, 245] More recently, phagocytes (neutrophils and monocytes) have been demonstrated in large numbers in nasal secretions of RV-infected symptomatic human volunteers.[165] Although the microbe-killing ability of phagocytes is well known, these cells in themselves also could cause cold symptoms through the release of various toxic products, such as superoxide and hydrogen peroxide, during the respiratory burst.[29, 240] In fact, increasing numbers of leukocytes in the peripheral blood correlate with increased symptoms, and in infected non-ill human volunteers, the white blood cell count does not increase.[245] Also, products of cell-mediated immunity, such as the interleukins, can cause varied symptoms of inflammation, such as fever.[137, 208]

A Johns Hopkins–University of Virginia team has been determining the role of individual inflammatory agents as causes of cold symptoms. It found that histamine levels were not increased during experimental or natural colds but that interleukin-1 and kinins (bradykinin and lysyl-bradykinin) were elevated significantly, especially in persons who were symptomatic.[197, 208–210] The kinins are active vasodilators, and their presence correlated with albumin diffusion into the nasal secretions as well as with neutrophil infiltration.[197, 209] Subsequently, it was demonstrated that bradykinin itself could cause cold symptoms in a dose-response progression; however, the first trial with a bradykinin antagonist in RV-infected human volunteers had no effect.[129, 209] This research is continuing.[129] Gwaltney[104] has proposed that a combination of antiviral and antimediator treatment may be effective.

Immunity Due to Serum Antibody

Serum antibody to the various RV types develops with age (presumably from repeated infections), and, by adulthood, antibody may be detected against approximately 50 per cent of RV types tested.[107] The presence of serum antibody correlates positively with immunity, and resistance to infection is related to amount. As examples, in the Eagle Heights families, 21 of 75 persons (28 per cent) without antibody were infected with either RV-43 or RV-55, whereas only 5 of 35 (14 per cent) with homologous antibody to either of these agents were infected.[65] No one was infected who had homologous serum antibody levels above 1:16. Similar results were observed in Charlottesville and Seattle families.[91, 92, 127] However, large doses can overwhelm antibody. At the clinical center at the National Institute of Allergy and Infectious Diseases, where human volunteers were used, 1000 $TCID_{50}$ was found to infect persons with serum antibody titers to 1:256.[37] Judging from the paucity of reports of natural infections in persons with serum antibody titers greater than 1:16, virus inocula in naturally contracted cases must be low.

Immunity Due to Antibody in Nasal Secretions

At the National Institutes of Health, it was found that intranasal administration of RV vaccine produced both serum and nasal antibody, whereas two intramuscular injections of this vaccine produced little, if any, nasal antibody.[38] When the volunteers given the vaccine intranasally were challenged with approximately 100 $TCID_{50}$ of homologous RV, they were protected significantly against both clinical illness and infection, whereas those administered the same vaccine intramuscularly remained susceptible.[204]

On the other hand, other investigators who used the same vaccine preparation but gave it subcutaneously in three injections found nasal antibody responses in 21 of 46 (45 per cent) volunteers.[77] They discovered that, compared with unimmunized, antibody-free controls, challenge of these volunteers with three $TCID_{50}$ of virus produced significantly less virus shedding and reduced duration and severity of illness. (It is possible that this lower infectious dose more closely approximates a natural situation.) This study also showed that protection against infection with the low virus challenge correlated with the magnitude of serum antibody and not with the presence of secretory antibody. The relative roles of serum and secretory antibody in RV infections still are unsettled.

Antibody Appearance over the Course of Infection

A general pattern of the development of humoral (secretory and serum) antibody has emerged from several studies.[30, 79, 216] Approximately 24 hours after infection, there is a sharp increase in nasal IgA secretion. When symptoms begin about 48 hours after infection, rhinorrhea commences, and the transudate is composed of significant amounts of IgG. After approximately 1 week and after the actual episode of illness, virus-specific antibody, predominantly IgA, appears in the nasal passages, the tears, and the parotid saliva. Serum antibody (usually IgG but occasionally IgM) also begins to be formed at 1 week and rises to peak levels at 1 month. Both serum and secretory antibody appear sooner and rise more rapidly in persons with detectable neutralizing antibody in the preinfection serum specimens. Antibody has been detected in nasal secretions and serum approximately 1 year after infection and, judging from the high proportion of the adult population with antibody to many RV serotypes, probably lasts much longer.[28, 107]

Cell-Mediated Immunity

As noted previously, there is substantial evidence that neutrophils increase both in the peripheral blood and in the nasopharynx during the first few days of an RV cold.[36, 262] There also is evidence that peripheral blood lymphocytes actually decrease in the first 2 to 3 days of an RV cold and that there is increased migration of lymphocytes into the nasal secretions at this time.[36, 165] As noted earlier, specific humoral antibody usually is not present in the serum or nasopharynx this early in the illness, which suggests that these in situ nasopharyngeal lymphocytes, through cell-mediated immunity, play an important role in controlling RV proliferation. Hsia and colleagues[137] have examined the ability of peripheral blood lymphocytes to liberate various cytokines (interleukin-2 and interferon-γ) and to participate in other cellular immune processes (cytotoxicity and antigen-stimulated blastogenesis) during the early days of RV colds in experimentally infected human volunteers. They found that, during infection, all of these cell-mediated immunity activities were increased significantly when compared with preinfection levels. Of special interest was their observation that cellular ability to liberate higher levels of interleukin-2 correlated inversely and significantly ($p < 0.02$) with virus shedding and nasal mucus production.

Interference Among Rhinoviruses

Interference between infections with heterotypic RV serotypes, which lasts between 5 and 16 weeks, has been reported in human volunteers.[89] However, subsequent epidemiologic studies in a nursery school population,[22] a military population,[214] and a family population[185] showed sequential heterotypic RV infections occurring frequently, sometimes at intervals as short as 2 days. In the family population, one subject was infected by three different RVs within a 30-day period. On the other hand, we have noted in human volunteer experiments that viral interference clearly can occur; for example, we observed apparent complete resistance to about 2000 $TCID_{50}$ of RV-16 (administered by nasopharyngeal spray) generated by an unsuspected "wild" RV (not typed) infection present at the time of inoculation.[164]

Simultaneous infections with an RV and parainfluenza type 1, respiratory syncytial virus, adenoviruses, various enteroviruses, or other RV serotypes also have been reported.[92, 163]

Influence of a Cold Environment on the Course of Infection

It is widely believed that exposure to cold temperatures either initiates or exacerbates respiratory infections. In fact, chilling of animals has been shown to increase the severity and frequency of viral infection.[259] However, investigations of the effects of chilling on humans infected with "common cold viruses" and with RV-15 have not demonstrated significant effects.[78] In the RV-15 experiments, the conditions were realistic. The subjects (adult males) were cooled sufficiently in air to cause shivering for approximately an hour or were immersed in water long enough to cause a decline in rectal temperatures.

Effect of Age and Sex

There is a much higher prevalence of RV infections in infants and young children than in older persons. In Seattle,[91] the RV infection rate in children 0 to 5 years of age nearly was twice that of older children and adults (0.77 vs. 0.41 infections/person/year); in Tecumseh,[192] the isolation rate in the 1- to 4-year-old group was far higher than in any other age bracket. The high attack rates in these young children were not unexpected because less than 10 per cent of them had antibody to any of the 56 RV types,[107] and children ordinarily are subjected continuously to the family-like environment so conducive to RV transmission. In especially crowded populations, attack rates may be high. In an Alaskan Eskimo village, 70 per cent of 395 children were infected during a spring outbreak of RV-16 infection.[266]

The frequency of RV infection generally declines throughout life. Beginning at the age of school attendance, the number of RV infections declines gradually from 1 to 2 per year to 0.25 per year in the age group older than 60 years.[107, 194] Results from most laboratories have found that persons 20 to 30 years of age account for an exception to the general decline in incidence with age[91, 127, 191, 194]; RV infections as well as infections with other respiratory pathogens increase during this period of life. Because the increase especially is marked in mothers,[91, 127] it probably is due to respiratory illness in small children being transferred to parents.

In Tecumseh, the number of respiratory illnesses per year was consistently higher for females than for males (3 to >60 years of age).[194] If one assumes that RVs account for a similar proportion of disease in each gender, this would indicate that females generally have more RV infections. As noted earlier, women with young children clearly seem to have more RV infections than do others in their age group. In Seattle,[91] mothers had 1.5 times more RV infections than did fathers, and in Charlottesville, females of child-bearing age had approximately 1.2 times more RV illness than did males.[107]

CLINICAL MANIFESTATIONS

Consonant with their benign cytopathology in the respiratory tract, RV infections in any age group usually cause only mild upper respiratory tract illness—that is, common colds.[55] It is estimated that RVs cause 30 to 50 per cent of common colds, at least in adults.[169] In healthy adults, RV infections usually are so innocuous that human volunteers can be infected safely with these agents to study their epidemiology, pathogeneses, and control with experimental drugs.[55, 126, 146, 181, 250] However, even in adults, serious illness is possible: RV-associated, x-ray–positive, atypical pneumonia has been described in military trainees[98] and in adults with underlying illnesses, especially of the respiratory tract.[85, 95, 98, 113, 235, 236]

Nonetheless, it is children—particularly the very young—who most likely are to be subject to serious, sometimes fatal, RV-caused illness. As an example of fatal outcome, a report from Los Angeles described an 11-month-old infant with mild asthma who died, totally unexpectedly during sleep, of apparent acute asthma and interstitial pneumonitis caused by RV-47 (isolated from lung and blood specimens).[162] The authors wrote a special plea to other physicians to be alert for similar exigencies in their own patients. In this respect, two deaths of infants of possible rhinoviremia—one of which occurred during a cold—and six "cot" deaths, diagnosed as bronchiolitis/pneumonia and from which RVs were isolated, may suggest that RV involvement in fatal illnesses in infants is more common than realized.[213, 256]

At least in theory, generalized illness with viremia seems possible with RV infections; the RVs are a division of the larger picornavirus group, which contains many viruses capable of generalized and fatal infection and whose genomes have considerable homology with the RVs (see Structure of the Virion, under Organism).[178]

Spectrum of Respiratory Disease

Early Studies: Severe Disease in Young Children

It has been known since the discovery of the first RV serotypes that these viruses cause considerably more severe illness in children than in adults. In 1959 and 1960, Hamparian, Hilleman, and their associates[118, 212] conducted a clinical and virologic investigation of 15 children (younger than 8 years of age) and 20 adults from the Philadelphia area who had acute respiratory disease and from whom RVs (then called coryzaviruses) had been isolated (Table 171–3). The 20 adults all had typical upper respiratory illness, some with low-grade fever (peak 37.3° C [99.2° F]). In contrast, 60 per cent of the children had fevers higher than 37.7° C (100° F), 20 per cent had otitis, and 53 per cent (eight children) exhibited one or more signs of lower respiratory tract involvement. One had laryngotracheitis (croup); one, bronchitis; two, asthmatic bronchitis; and one, bronchopneumonia. The latter infant was 2 months old, and crepitant rales were heard over the right chest anteriorly and posteriorly; the chest cleared in 2 days.

Shortly thereafter, in 1963, our laboratory began its study of young student families at the Eagle Heights village.[65] Epidemiologic aspects of this investigation have been described previously (see Epidemiology and Transmission). Daily home clinical surveillance was carried out, and although the illnesses generally were mild enough that the participants did not see a physician, the same differential severity between adults and children was present (Table 171–4). With all viruses, including RVs, children were much more likely to be febrile and their symptoms were much more likely to last longer. Overall, however, RV-caused illnesses were milder than those caused by other viruses.

Simultaneous with the aforementioned well-population surveillance, we participated with Dr. J. D. Cherry in a thorough investigation of infants and young children hospitalized with lower respiratory disease at Madison General Hos-

TABLE 171–3. Signs and Symptoms of Respiratory Illness in 20 Adults and 15 Children (2 Months to 8 Years of Age) with Rhinovirus Infections, 1959–1960, Philadelphia, Pennsylvania*

Sign or Symptom	Adults	Children
Fever†	4 (20%)	9 (60%)
Eye, Ear, Nose, and Throat		
Rhinorrhea	18 (90%)	10 (67%)
Purulent nasal discharge	4 (20%)	1 (7%)
Pharyngitis	10 (50%)	5 (33%)
Conjunctival infection	2 (10%)	1 (7%)
Anterior cervical lymphadenopathy	1 (5%)	8 (53%)
Hoarseness	4 (20%)	0
Croup	0	1 (7%)
Infection of the tympanic membrane	0	3 (20%)
Chest		
Cough	8 (40%)	15 (100%)
Dyspnea	0	4 (27%)
Retractions	0	3 (20%)
Rhonchi	0	7 (47%)
Rales	0	2 (13%)
Wheezing	0	4 (27%)

*The children were from the outpatient clinics and the wards of the Children's Hospital of Philadelphia, and the adults were employees of Merck and Company, Inc., Rahway, N.J.

†In adults, 37.2° C (99° F) or above by mouth; peak was 37.3° C (99.2° F). In children, 37.7° C (100° F) or above by rectum; range from 37° C (98.6° F) to 39.1° C (102.4° F); mean 37.9° C (100.4° F).

Adapted from Reilly, C. M., Hoch, S. M., Stokes, J., Jr., et al.: Clinical and laboratory findings in cases of respiratory illness caused by coryzaviruses. Ann. Intern. Med. *57*:515–525, 1962.

pital (Table 171–5).[42] A virus was cultured from 38 per cent of these patients, and RVs predominated (11 of 27 isolates). These children (average age, <1 year) with RV infections were seriously ill: the mean temperature was 39.4° C (103° F), and eight had bronchopneumonia. Six of the virus-infected children yielded a bacterial pathogen in predominance in throat cultures. Five of these—a beta-hemolytic streptococcus, two *Streptococcus pneumoniae,* and two *Haemophilus influenzae*—were present coincidentally with the RV isolates. All the RV-associated cases had antecedent milder respiratory symptoms, especially coryza.

Rhinovirus Pre-eminence in Respiratory Disease of Larger Populations

Two large populations, one a general medical practice in Roehampton, near London, England,[133] and the other a group of families in Tecumseh, a small town in the United States near Detroit,[191] were assayed for the various respiratory viruses in illnesses of differing severity. Each had a pediatric population base of 900 or more. RVs easily were the most common cause of respiratory illness in either population (Table 171–6): 26.3 per cent of isolates in England and 38.1 per cent in Michigan.

In both populations, RVs frequently were associated with lower respiratory tract illness (Table 171–7); the proportion was much higher in the Roehampton clinic. The major RV diagnosis in lower respiratory tract[133] disease was wheezy bronchitis: 42 per cent of all RV isolates in Roehampton and 15 per cent in Tecumseh.[190] Otherwise, severity of disease associated with RV infection often was milder; in Roehampton, none of the RV isolates were from children with bronchiolitis or pneumonia, whereas 8.4 per cent of the respiratory syncytial virus isolates were associated with one of these diagnoses. In Tecumseh, activity restriction was an important differential marker for etiology; only 24.3 per cent of those with RV illness curtailed their normal activities, whereas the percentages often were double that for the other respiratory viruses, varying from 42 per cent for respiratory syncytial virus to 63 per cent for influenza B virus.

Rhinovirus Infections in Hospitalized Children

In Bristol, England, in 1971, 377 infants hospitalized for respiratory disease yielded 199 (53 per cent) viral diagnoses.[143] Respiratory syncytial virus was predominant, accounting for 79 per cent of the diagnoses, but RVs were second at 12 per cent (23 patients). Half of the RV diagnoses were in infants with bronchiolitis or pneumonia. RV illnesses were comparable in severity with those caused by respiratory syncytial virus. One 4-month-old with RV-associated bronchopneumonia died. Except that there were no deaths, similar results were found in 102 hospitalized children in Colorado, where the etiologic diagnosis rate was 85 per cent.[201]

In relatively recent years, serious RV infections in young children have been reported from several locations. Some of

TABLE 171–4. Comparison of the Clinical Illness Attributable to Rhinoviruses with That Attributable to Other Respiratory Viruses Obtained from 24 Families (89 Persons) in the University of Wisconsin's Eagle Heights Village, 1963–1965*

				Per Cent with:				
				Fever (°C)†				
Virus	Age Group	Number of Patients	Average Duration of Illness (Days)	37.7–38.3	<38.3	*Cough*	*Nasal Discharge*	*Sore Throat*
Rhinovirus	Children	26	11	15	4	73	92	15
	Adults	25	9	8	4	68	96	56
Respiratory syncytial	Children	21	10	37	20	90	95	9
	Adults	1	8	0	0	100	100	0
Parainfluenza 1	Children	7	9	0	27	57	100	29
	Adults	6	8	17	0	33	83	67
Parainfluenza 3	Children	10	6	30	60	70	90	40
	Adults	1	6	0	0	0	100	100
Influenza	Children	2	10	100	100	100	100	50
	Adults	3	8	33	66	100	67	67

*The 42 children surveyed varied evenly in age from younger than 1 to 7 years; only three were older than 7.

†37.7° to 38.3° C is 100° to 101° F; less than 38.3° C is less than 101° F.

Adapted from Dick, E. C., Blumer, C. R., and Evans, A. S.: Epidemiology of infections with rhinovirus types 43 and 55 in a group of University of Wisconsin student families. Am J. Epidemiol. *86*:386–400, 1967.

TABLE 171–5. Clinical Findings in 11 Children Hospitalized with Severe Pulmonary Disease in Madison, Wisconsin, from Whom Rhinoviruses Were Isolated, January Through May 15, 1964

	Patients										
Clinical Findings	*A*	*B*	*C*	*D*	*E*	*F*	*G*	*H*	*I*	*J**	*K*
Age (yr)	6/12	6/12	7	4–6/12	1	5	8/12	5/12	5/12	2/12	2
Sex	M	M	M	M	F	F	M	M	F	M	F
History											
Cough	†	†	†				†		†		†
Coryza	†				†	†	†	†	†	†	†
Respiratory distress	†	†		†			†	†		†	
Antibiotics prior to study	†					†	†	†		†	
Physical Findings											
Highest											
Temp (°C)	39.7	40	38.2	39.4	40.5	38.7	40.1	39.3	40.2	38.1	38.3
Temp (°F)	103.6	104	100.8	103	105	101.8	104.2	102.8	104.4	100.6	101
Tonsillitis or pharyngitis				†		†					
Hoarseness or croup											†
Tachypnea	†	†	†					†		†	†
Chest retractions	†							†		†	
Rhonchi							†	†		†	†
Rales			†				†				
Wheezing	†	†	†					†			
Laboratory Studies											
Initial leukocyte count (1000 × mm³)	10	15.5	8.7	11.4	19.8	10	10.7	7.3	30.5	13	11.2
Neutrophils (%)	42	55	93	77	74	79	49	69	72	73	75
Pneumonitis on chest x-ray films	†	†		†		†	†	†	†	†	
Throat culture†	Pn	NF	HI	St	NF	NF	HI	NF	NF	Pn	NF
Diagnosis	BP Br	BP Br	Bron	BP Tons	URI UTI	BP Tons OM	BP	BP	BP	BP Atel	Cr

*Hospitalized since birth with choanal atresia. Right upper lobe pneumonia and atelectasis present for 1 month prior to study.
†Only the predominant organism is recorded. Pn indicates *Streptococcus pneumoniae*; NF, normal flora; HI, *Haemophilus influenzae*; St, beta-hemolytic *Streptococcus*; Br, bronchiolitis; BP, bronchopneumonia; Bron, bronchitis; Tons, tonsillitis; URI, upper respiratory infection; UTI, urinary tract infection; OM, otitis media; Atel, atelectasis; CR, croup.
Adapted from Cherry, J. D., Diddams, J. A., and Dick, E. C.: Rhinovirus infections in hospitalized children. Arch. Environ. Health *14*:390–396, 1967.

these outbreaks have allowed direct comparisons between RV and respiratory syncytial virus infections. In the intensive care nursery of Strong Memorial Hospital in Rochester, New York, eight infants, 2 weeks to 6 months of age, became nosocomially infected, four with RV and four with respiratory syncytial virus, in early February 1980.[257] One of the RV isolates was from an asymptomatic baby. All seven symptomatic babies presented with a dramatic and sudden onset of respiratory illness that included cyanosis, apnea, labored respirations, increased nasal or tracheal secretions, tachypnea, and lethargy. Wheezing, tachycardia, irritability, and cardiac arrest each occurred in a single infant. None of the signs and symptoms differentiated RV and respiratory syncytial virus illnesses.

At St. Anna Children's Hospital in Vienna, Austria, from 1984 to 1986, Kellner and colleagues[154] compared the clinical features of RV and respiratory syncytial virus infections among 519 children, 10 days to 3 years of age (median age, 6.6 months). Viral pathogens were detected in 227 (43 per cent) of the children, and of these, 119 (23 per cent) were respiratory syncytial virus and 60 (12 per cent) were RV. The physical findings (Table 171–8) and the clinical diagnosis (Table 171–9) of those children with RV or respiratory syncytial virus infections were alike, except that RV infections were more likely than respiratory syncytial virus infections to be associated with upper respiratory tract infection.

Two retrospective reviews of clinical and laboratory records also have implicated the RVs as probable causes of lower respiratory illness in infants. In 1982 and 1983, Krilov and associates[159] found 32 RV-infected children who had significant signs of pulmonary disease in Boston hospitals, half with radiologic evidence of new focal infiltrates. From 1984 to 1988, Abzug and associates[2] examined all virus-positive cultures from pneumonias in neonates younger than 30 days of age in Denver hospitals. Definition of pneumonia was strict, including new infiltrates in chest radiographs plus several typical physical signs. Forty patients were found: respiratory syncytial virus was isolated from slightly more than half the cases, and RVs and enteroviruses, at six isolates each, were second most frequent.

Two infants hospitalized at the Children's National Medical Center in Washington, D.C.—a 1-month-old female with bacteriologically negative pertussis syndrome and a 6-month-old male with a prolonged and life-threatening asthma attack—yielded RVs from the lower respiratory tract by bronchoalveolar lavage.[226] No other pathogens were recovered.

Despite the foregoing evidence that RVs can be an important cause of severe lower respiratory tract disease, large studies in Chapel Hill, North Carolina[63]; Huntington, West Virginia[23]; and Tucson, Arizona[265] by experienced investigators yielded the usual respiratory viruses in appropriate numbers, but only 1 to 3 per cent were RVs. These fairly may represent the importance of RV-caused disease in these populations, but negative cultures do not mean absence of

TABLE 171–6. Rhinoviruses and Other Respiratory Viruses Isolated from Some English and American Children Younger than 15 Years of Age with Symptomatic Respiratory Infections

Agent	Roehampton, England*‡	Tecumseh, Michigan U.S.A.†§
Rhinoviruses	162 (26.3)‖	82 (38.1)
Parainfluenza	111 (18.0)	56 (26.0)
Influenza A and B	89 (14.5)	34 (15.8)
Respiratory syncytial virus	56 (9.1)	19 (8.8)
Adenoviruses	45 (7.3)	9 (4.1)
Enteroviruses	66 (10.7)	15 (6.9)
Other agents	58§¶ (9.4)	—
Double isolations	27** (4.4)	—
Total isolates	614	215

*Adapted from Horn, M. E. C., et al.: J. Hyg. (Camb.) *74*:157–168, 1975.
†Adapted from Monto, A. S., and Cavalloro, J. J.: Am. J. Epidemiol. *94*:280–289, 1971.
‡Results from a general practice clinic (919 children) during 1968–1972. Roehampton is a London residential suburb.
§Results from surveillance (472 children) during 1966–1969. Tecumseh is a city of about 10,000, located approximately 50 miles southwest of Detroit.
‖Per cent of total isolates.
¶Mumps, 3; herpes simplex, 17; *Mycoplasma pneumoniae*, 37; psittacosis (serologic diagnosis), 1.
**Includes nine rhinoviruses.

TABLE 171–7. Association of Rhinoviruses with Upper and Lower Respiratory Infection in Some English Children (Roehampton[128]) and American Families (Tecumseh[184])*

	Per Cent of Rhinovirus Isolates	
	Roehampton	*Tecumseh†*
Upper respiratory infection	47	71
Lower respiratory infection	53	21

*See Table 171–6 for virus isolation data and population description.
†Includes rhinovirus isolates from both children and adults (82 isolates from children and 58 isolates from adults).

RVs necessarily. These are difficult viruses to grow, even in supposedly sensitive cell cultures, and often there are few organisms in the specimen (Table 171–10).

In summary, evidence is accumulating that RVs can cause serious lower respiratory illness, especially in young children. In some populations, they may be second to respiratory syncytial virus in importance and cause comparably severe signs and symptoms.

Asthma

A specific lower respiratory illness in which the RVs appear clearly important—perhaps most important—is "wheezy bronchitis" or "infectious asthma." (There really is no widely accepted clinical term to describe the illnesses in which infection and wheezing are present.[124] In this chapter, these two foregoing terms and others are used in an attempt always to reflect the individual investigators' meaning and preference.) The association between RVs and these illnesses first was noted by Horn, Gregg, and their associates[133–135] as part of their previously described 1967 to 1972 Roehampton study of ill children (see Table 171–6). Forty-two per cent of the 162 RV isolates at Roehampton were from children with attacks of wheezy bronchitis, approximately twice the percentage of other viruses causing this syndrome. Many of these children were known to be subject to recurrent episodes.

TABLE 171–8. Physical Findings in Young Children* with Respiratory Illness at the Time of Their Admission to St. Anna Children's Hospital, Vienna, Austria, 1984–1986—Comparison Between Rhinovirus (RV) and Respiratory Syncytial Virus (RSV) Infections

Physical Findings	All Patients† *n* = *519*	RSV *n* = *119*	RV *n* = *60*
Stridor during expiration	67 (13%)	15 (13%)	10 (16%)
Cyanosis	18 (3%)	4 (3%)	2 (3%)
Swollen cervical glands	87 (17%)	17 (14%)	9 (15%)
Red throat	344 (66%)	75 (63%)	41 (68%)
Nasal flaring	75 (14%)	20 (16%)	11 (18%)
Crepitations	20 (4%)	7 (6%)	2 (3%)
Chest x-ray (positive)	260 (50%)	79 (66%)	35 (58%)
Wheezing	113 (22%)	30 (25%)	13 (22%)
Moist rales	174 (34%)	43 (36%)	22 (36%)
Dry rales	49 (9%)	13 (11%)	5 (8%)
Respiratory rate/min			
Median (range)	43 (10–96)	40 (10–84)	36 (10–64)
Body temperature			
Median (range)	38.4° C (36.4°–41.8° C)	39.9° C (36.8°–41.0° C)	38.5° C (36.9°–41.0° C)
Duration of illness			
Median (range)	11.6 days (2–45)	10.5 days (4–42)	12.8 days (3–31)

*10 days to 3 years of age (median age, 6.6 months).
†One hundred twelve (21%) children had upper respiratory tract and 342 (66%) lower respiratory tract illnesses; 471 (91%) were inpatients, and 48 (9%) were outpatients.
Adapted from Kellner, G., Popow-Kraupp, T., Kundi, M., et al.: Clinical manifestations of respiratory tract infections due to respiratory syncytial virus and rhinoviruses in hospitalized children. Acta Paediatr. Scand. *78*:390–394, 1989.

TABLE 171–9. Clinical Diagnosis of Respiratory Illnesses of Young Children* at St. Anna Children's Hospital, Vienna, Austria, 1984–1986—Comparison Between Rhinovirus (RV) and Respiratory Syncytial Virus (RSV) Infections

Clinical Diagnosis	All Patients n = 519	RSV n = 119	RV n = 60
Upper respiratory tract infection			
Rhinitis	65 (12%)	4 (3%)	5 (9%)
Otitis media	10 (2%)	0	
		1 (1%)	2 (3%)
Pharyngitis	23 (4%)	3 (2%)	4 (6%)
Laryngitis	8 (2%)	1 (1%)	2 (3%)
Other diseases	25 (5%)	0	
		9 (7%)	16 (26%)†
Lower respiratory tract infection			
Croup	14 (3%)	4 (3%)	4 (6%)
Tracheobronchitis	100 (19%)	46 (39%)	16 (27%)
Bronchitis	24 (5%)	3 (2%)	0
Obstructive bronchitis‡	78 (15%)	28 (24%)	8 (14%)
Pneumonia	126 (24%)	29 (25%)	15 (25%)
Other diseases	40 (8%)	0	1 (2%)
Total	382 (74%)	110 (93%)	44 (74%)

*See footnotes to Table 171–8.
†RVs were more likely to cause upper respiratory tract infection ($p < .01$).
‡This diagnosis included those children with expiratory wheeze with evidence of air trapping. In a later paper, this same definition was used for wheezy bronchitis.[145]
Adapted from Kellner, G., Popow-Kraupp, T., Kundi, M., et al.: Clinical manifestations of respiratory tract infections due to respiratory syncytial virus and rhinoviruses in hospitalized children. Acta Paediatr. Scand. *78*:390–394, 1989.

During the later years (1971 to 1972) of this period, our Madison laboratory carried out a longitudinal clinical and microbial study (children were sampled at least twice weekly for viral and once monthly for bacterial culture) of 16 nonatopic children with "infectious asthma" and 15 of their normal siblings. A clear temporal relationship was found between (1) the onset of symptomatic respiratory infection, (2) an asthmatic episode, and (3) the presence of viruses—predominantly RVs—in the pharynx (Fig. 171–13).[183, 184] Precipitation of an asthmatic episode was much more frequent during severe symptomatic respiratory infections than during mild ones. RVs caused an asthma attack in 14 of 15 severe symptomatic respiratory infections but in only 1 of 6 mild ones. Subclinical infections never precipitated an attack. Except for one instance, in which *H. influenzae* may have caused asthma, bacterial infections were not associated with asthma attacks, even when they were accompanied by severe symptomatic respiratory infection. (Note that the severe group A streptococcal infections in subjects CC and P did not precipitate asthma, whereas severe RV-49 infections in these two children caused more than three asthma attacks [sufficiently incapacitating for the child to stay home from school].)[184] The asthmatic siblings seemed especially susceptible to symptomatic infection: total infections of probable viral etiology ($p < 0.02$), known viral infections ($p < 0.01$), and RV-caused symptomatic respiratory infections ($p < 0.01$) all significantly were greater in the asthmatic than in the nonasthmatic siblings.[182]

TABLE 171–10. Quantity of Virus Found in 87 Throat Swab Squeezings from Children 3 to 11 Years of Age, Madison, Wisconsin, 1971–1972*

	Per 0.1 mL
1 $TCID_{50}$ or less†	22
>1 to ≥ 50 $TCID_{50}$	46
≥ 50 to <50 $TCID_{50}$	14
>50 to <500 $TCID_{50}$	5

*Fourteen rhinovirus types are represented.
†Median tissue culture infective doses.

A somewhat similar year-long prospective investigation was carried out in England[141] in 30 preschool children with histories of recurrent respiratory infections—often accompanied by wheeze—and in their unaffected siblings. The children with recurring infections had about twice the number of illnesses and of isolated viruses than did the controls. Their illnesses also were much more severe, and they often involved the lower respiratory tract. RVs were heavily preponderant, with 57 per cent of the isolates, and were associated with wheezy bronchitis four times more often than respiratory syncytial viruses were. Atopic children, as measured by positive skin testing and raised serum IgE levels, did not seem especially subject to recurrent infections.

At the University of Colorado, McIntosh and associates[175, 176] demonstrated in 1973 the importance of other respiratory viruses in asthma; later, they suggested that respiratory syncytial virus is the major agent associated with asthma in children younger than 4 years of age and that RVs are preeminent in older children and adults.[175, 176] Subsequent reports have demonstrated the importance of RVs in older children, as well as in many younger children. As examples of RVs in younger children, in recurrent asthmatic patients seen at the pediatric allergy unit in Oslo, Norway, from 1981 to 1983, most of the acute bronchial asthma cases were RV-associated (45 per cent) with respiratory syncytial virus second (19 per cent).[32] Twenty nine per cent of the virus-infected group was between 2 and 3 years of age, with the incidence gradually decreasing to 1 per cent by 15 years of age. Also illustrative of RV in the very young is the prospective study of the 30 English preschool children with recurrent wheezing infections described earlier, in which RVs were most important in those children whose mean age was 2.2 years.[141] Mertsola and colleagues[180] in Turku, Finland, examined children with wheezy bronchitis (mean age, 3.2 years) and found RVs and coronaviruses most important. The comparative importance of respiratory syncytial virus and RV in asthma of infants (median age, 6.6 months) with probable wheezy bronchitis (see "Obstructive bronchitis" in Table 171–9) was examined from 1984 to 1986 by Viennese investigators; 28 isolates yielded respiratory syncytial virus, and only 8 yielded RV.[153] In a later paper from this group covering 1986 to 1990, 179 respiratory syncytial virus isolates and 49 RVs were recovered from these hospitalized infants; the majority of the RVs were recovered from infants with some wheezing.[152] Only three had pneumonia without wheezing.

Virus infection was an important risk factor for wheezing children of all ages presenting for emergent care.[83] Respiratory syncytial virus infection and passive tobacco smoke exposure were associated most frequently with wheezing illness in young children (<2 years of age). Thirty-one per cent of children older than 2 years of age had an accompanying virus infection, usually an RV infection, and were more likely to have IgE antibody to inhalant allergens than were the younger children. This study illustrates the dichotomy of etiologies for wheezing illness in the pediatric age group: respiratory syncytial virus infection is the predominant cause

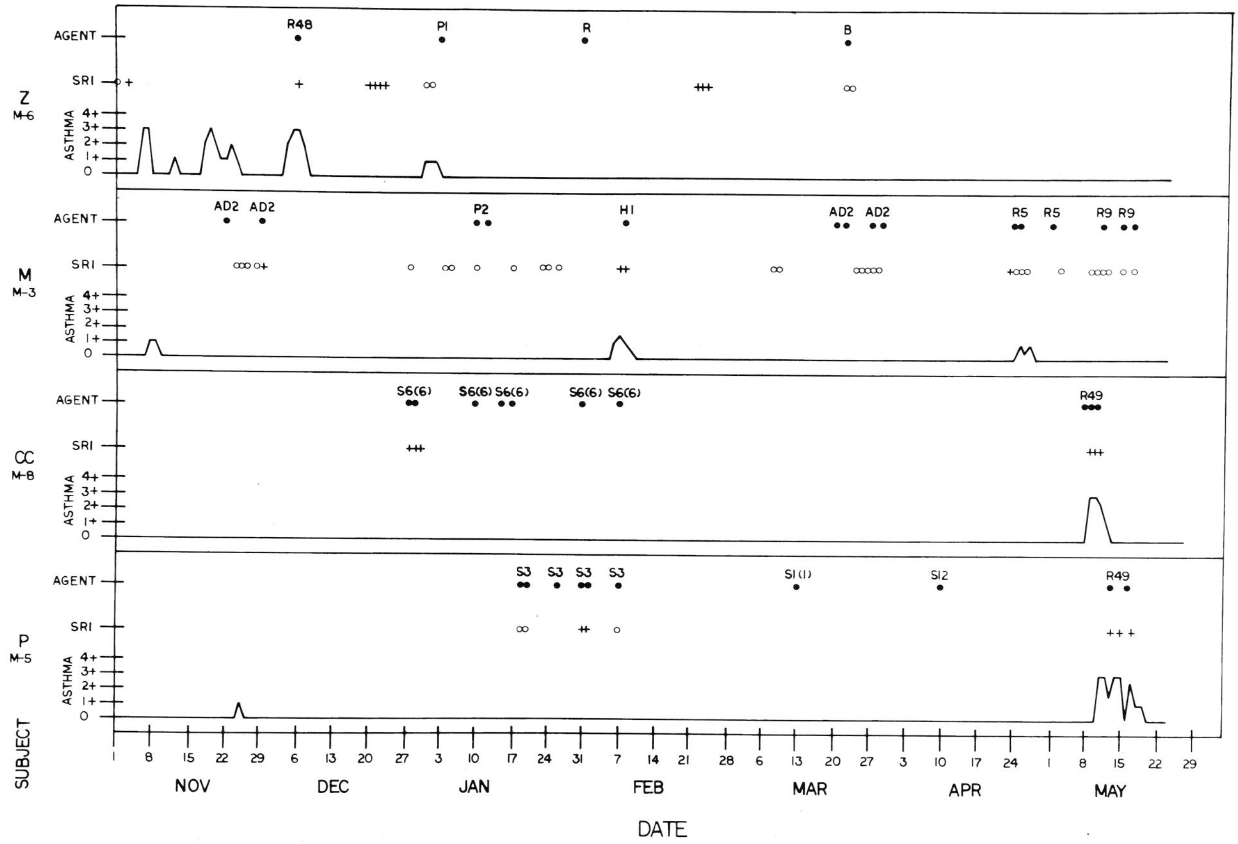

FIGURE 171–13. *Temporal relationship between asthma, symptomatic respiratory infection (SRI), and infectious agent in four children with "infectious" asthma. AD, adenovirus; B, influenza B; HI,* Haemophilus influenzae; *P, parainfluenza; R, rhinovirus; S, group A* Streptococcus; *open circle, mild; +, severe (fever or more than one sign or symptom). Numbers after R and P indicate type; numbers after S indicate T type (M type, if typable, in parentheses). (Adapted from Minor, T. D., Dick, E. C., DeMeo, A. N., et al.: J. A. M. A. 227:292–298, 1974. Copyright 1974, American Medical Association.)*

in infants and atopy combined with virus infection, usually RV infection, in older children.

The Viennese virologists and members of our laboratory serotyped those RVs isolated from children with wheezy bronchitis and found no types to be particularly "asthmagenic"; the Viennese obtained 12 serotypes, and we reported 21.[152, 182–184] Only three—RV-1B, RV-20, and RV-32—overlapped. Therefore, between us, 30 different RV serotypes precipitated asthmatic attacks.

There has been much speculation and research on the mechanism of bronchospasm in virus-infected patients with wheezy bronchitis. Especially provocative is RV-caused wheezing because RVs are thought to be unable to replicate well at the temperature of the lower respiratory tract.[119, 248, 254] Horn and colleagues[136] attempted to address this directly in older Roehampton children (5 to 15 years of age) with acute wheezy bronchitis and whose illnesses chiefly were RV-associated. Sputa and nose and throat swabs were used for virus cultivation, and they found that the virus isolation rate was significantly higher from sputum than from the nasopharyngeal specimens. They found also that the mean day on which cytopathic effect was observed (in HeLa cells) was almost 3 days earlier in sputum samples than from nose and throat swabs. In several patients, virus was isolated only from the sputum. Cytologic examination of sputa demonstrated alveolar macrophages, leukocytes, and eosinophils in a high proportion of samples, which indicated a vigorous local inflammatory response in the lung. These investigators interpreted their virologic and cytologic findings as suggesting that the bronchoconstriction occurring during wheezy bronchitis is a reaction to viral growth in the lower respiratory tract. Although Horn and associates[134] present a strong case for pulmonary RV growth, the issue of RV growth in the lung still is not resolved.[95, 113]

Whether the virus-associated bronchospasm is caused by local viral growth or by replication in the upper respiratory tract, the mechanism for this increased bronchoreactivity has not been resolved, although many reasonable hypotheses have been proposed: diminished beta-adrenergic function, production of virus-specific IgE antibodies, enhanced leukocyte histamine and leukotriene release, and others.[29, 44, 95, 164, 240, 258] Using human volunteers allergic to giant ragweed (who are safer "stand-ins" for asthmatics), we found that experimental RV-16 infection significantly increased bronchial sensitivity to inhaled ragweed antigen and histamine and, perhaps more importantly, induced a late asthmatic response that could be a model for recurrent or chronic asthma.[164]

Chronic Bronchitis

This usually is not a children's disease, but the results are pertinent to the question of RV replication in the lung. Eadie, Stott, and colleagues[85, 236] followed 44 patients with chronic bronchitis for periods of 6 months to 2.5 years between January 1962 and April 1965. RVs by far were the most common virus obtained (isolation of 12 RV strains from 27 exacerbations). Where possible, throat swabs, nasal washings, and sputa were obtained. Interestingly, RVs were isolated from seven specimens of sputum collected during six exacerbations in five patients, and on four of the seven occasions, a throat swab taken at about the same time did not yield an RV. The RV titers in these seven sputum specimens ranged from 130 to 130,000 $TCID_{50}$/mL, which approximated the levels reached in nasopharyngeal washings of RV-infected human volunteers.[61, 72, 75] Stenhouse[235] also found RVs to predominate in chronic bronchitics (18 of 19 virus-positive specimens were RVs), and on occasion RV was recovered from sputum and not from nasal washings or throat swabs. It would appear that RVs can replicate to high titer in the lower respiratory tract, at least in patients with chronic bronchitis.

Otitis Media

Although acute otitis media chiefly is a bacterial disease with about two-thirds of middle ear fluid specimens yielding *S. pneumoniae, H. influenzae,* or both with *Branhamella catarrhalis* and other bacteria playing lesser roles, otitic involvement often is preceded or accompanied by a putative viral upper respiratory tract illness.[13, 15, 105, 157, 166, 221] The majority of the bacterial pathogens found in middle ear fluid are colonizers of the nasopharynx, and bacterial infection of the middle ear is considered to be a direct extension from that area.[157, 166] Clear and comprehensive evidence for viral extension from the nasopharynx to the middle ear has been established. Sarkkinen and coworkers,[224] using antigen detection techniques on middle ear fluid and nasopharyngeal secretions, found respiratory syncytial virus, adenovirus, and parainfluenza viruses in either the middle ear fluid or nasopharyngeal secretions of 58 of 131 children (42 per cent) with acute otitis media. Twenty-four of these children had viruses in the middle ear fluid, and only 1 of the 24 did not have the same viral antigen in both the middle ear fluid and the nasopharyngeal secretions. Most of the sampling was carried out during a local epidemic of respiratory syncytial virus infection, and the curve of the respiratory syncytial virus detections in the middle ear fluid and nasopharyngeal secretions followed the pattern of the respiratory syncytial virus epidemic curve. Others have found similar relationships between the viruses in the middle ear fluid and the nasopharyngeal secretions.[43, 158]

Gwaltney[105] isolated one RV from culture of 16 middle ear fluid specimens in 1971. In 1986, Chonmaitree and colleagues[43] reported three RV isolates in 84 middle ear fluid specimens; then Arola,[12] as part of his 1990 M.D. thesis, carried out a thorough investigation of the role of RVs in this illness.[13–16, 221] In 1987 to 1988, nasopharyngeal secretions were taken from 363 patients (mean age, 2.5 years) with acute otitis media, and viruses were detected in 154 (42 per cent): surprisingly, RV predominated over respiratory syncytial virus, 24 versus 13 per cent.[13] RVs were isolated all through the year, but the usual fall and spring peaks were observed. The patients with respiratory syncytial virus infection generally were sicker with more fever ($p < 0.05$) and cough ($p < 0.01$), but the appearance of the tympanic membrane was similar in both the RV and the respiratory syncytial virus patients. The usual bacterial pathogens were cultured from 82 per cent of the nasopharyngeal secretions, and after 2 days of antimicrobial treatment, fever and earache were reduced sharply in nearly all patients; however, in those with concomitant viral infections, respiratory symptoms remained a week or more with declining intensity. In comparison with RV, cough particularly was long-lasting in the respiratory syncytial virus patients.

Arola and collaborators[15] attempted to detect virus in both nasopharyngeal secretions (116 cases) and middle ear fluid (143 cases) of acute otitis media patients (mean age, 1.5 years) and found it in 33 (28 per cent) and 16 (11 per cent), respectively. RVs were the predominant isolate, with 21 (18 per cent) in the nasopharyngeal secretions and 11 (8 per cent) in the middle ear fluid. Fifty-three per cent of the patients harbored a bacterial pathogen in the middle ear fluid. In the RV-positive group in whom both viral and bacterial cultures were carried out, six of nine middle ear fluid specimens yielded no bacterial pathogens—that is, RV was the only pathogen found. Unfortunately, it was not possible to serotype the RVs to determine whether the same serotype was present in both the nasopharyngeal secretions and the middle ear fluid.

Although, in general, the presence of both bacterial and viral pathogens in the middle ear fluid does not interfere with the effectiveness of antibacterial therapy, in those specific patients whose acute otitis media is refractory to treatment, it may.[16] When measured against a comparison group of 66 "normal" acute otitis media cases (controls), 22 refractory cases harbored significantly ($p < 0.05$) more (68 vs. 41 per cent) viral pathogens than did the controls. Also, when only the middle ear fluid of these groups was examined for the presence of viruses, the refractory cases had virus in 32 per cent of samples compared with 15 per cent in the controls. RVs were the dominant virus in both groups. Bacterial pathogens were grown from the middle ear fluid of 4 of the 22 poor responder group, and all harbored concomitant respiratory viruses, 2 of them RVs; only one of the four bacteria was resistant to the antibacterial used in therapy. These investigators also examined those patients in the 66-patient control group who were refractory to treatment and found significantly more ($p < 0.05$) viruses in the middle ear fluid of this group when compared with those with a good response to therapy. The authors concluded that the presence of viruses in the middle ear fluid of children with acute otitis media can delay response to antibacterial therapy.

Chonmaitree and associates[45] at Galveston, Texas, also investigated the role of viruses in the middle ear fluid as agents that may interfere with antibacterial therapy. In their initial report, viruses were cultured from the middle ear fluid of 11 of 58 children (19 per cent); respiratory syncytial virus and RV were the most frequent isolated at three each. Of those patients in whom therapy failed, significantly more ($p < 0.05$) harbored viruses as well, and of those whose bacteria were susceptible to the treatment antibiotic, significantly more were combined virus-bacterium infections. In two subsequent reports, the highest rate of poor bacteriologic outcome occurred when RV was isolated from middle ear fluid; seven of nine instances of RV infection resulted in bacteriologic treatment failure.[238]

These studies from Finland and Texas suggest that viruses, including RVs, may play a role in acute otitis media, especially in prolonging response to antimicrobial treatment. Perhaps pertinently, McBride and associates[174] at the Universities of Pittsburgh and Virginia, using RV-infected human volunteers, found that the eustachian tube became occluded in 50 per cent of the volunteers and that abnormal middle ear pressure developed for as long as 10 days. These studies were extended by Buchman and colleagues,[27] who inoculated 60 volunteers with RV-39. Middle ear pressures of less than -100 mm H_2O developed in 22 (39 per cent) subjects. Two of three subjects who had pressures of less than -100 mm H_2O developed upper respiratory illnesses with middle ear effusions. This study extends the otologic manifestations of experimental RV infection to include otitis media.

Arola and colleagues[14] examined the role of viruses in 61 children (mean age, 3.2 years) with subacute or chronic asymptomatic otitis media with effusion. Five RVs and one adenovirus were found in the middle ear fluid. The patient with adenovirus infection and two of the RV patients also grew bacterial pathogens. None of these patients with otitis media with effusion was ill with an upper respiratory tract infection at the time the specimen was obtained, and effusion had endured 30 to 60 days prior to myringotomy.

Sinusitis

Like otitis media, sinusitis chiefly is a bacterial disease caused by extension of pathogens that often colonize the upper respiratory tract. Few attempts have been made to recover viruses from the sinuses. In two reports from Virginia, 140 aspirates obtained by direct puncture of the maxillary sinuses yielded 86 positive specimens, only 12 of which contained viruses. Seven of these were RVs, and the remainder were influenza A or parainfluenza viruses.[111, 115] Five of the viruses were isolated in conjunction with bacterial pathogens.

Rhinovirus Infections in Nonindustrialized Populations

There are not many RV surveillance studies in nonindustrialized populations, but those that exist have some unique findings. In the spring of 1967, Wulff and associates[266] observed an outbreak of RV-16 and RV-29 infection in a 93-family (429 children) Eskimo population in Bethel, Alaska. The RV-16 infection outbreak, the larger of the two, was analyzed thoroughly. There were 37 RV-16 isolates, and only 19 of these were from ill children; therefore, nearly half—18 children—had subclinical infections. The ill children often were only mildly so; 12 had common colds, and only 1 had bronchitis and 1 pneumonia. RV-16 spread widely in the population under study, with 70 per cent of antibody-free children demonstrating a fourfold or greater serologic response. Eighty-five of the 93 families were infected with RV-16, and the 8 families that escaped infection had only one to three children each. The amount of RV dissemination was not especially surprising because it was not much higher than RV-55 in the Eagle Heights village (see Fig. 171–9), but it was surprising that half the RV infections were subclinical.

Much subclinical RV infection also was reported in a surveillance of 136 preschool children in two small villages (combined population 1750 in 1982) on an island in the Melanesian nation of Vanuatu, a group of 80 islands located in the South Pacific approximately midway between Australia and Fiji.[241] RVs by far were the predominant viruses (21 isolates), and all were type 16 and all subclinical cases. In addition, pneumococci often were found in conjunction with these symptomless RV-16 cases and rarely otherwise.

These two examples of a high rate of subclinical RV infection are unusual, judging by experience in more industrialized societies. Our own experiences in surveillance of a year-long (1971 to 1972) twice-weekly sampling of 32 children, 3 to 11 years of age, in Madison was much different.[182, 184] As depicted in Figure 171–13 and in Table 171–11, we seldom found asymptomatic shedding, only 11 (0.8 per cent) cases all year. On the other hand, all these children were members of at least middle-class families, and some continental U.S. populations may be analogous to those in underdeveloped nations. Gwaltney[107] notes that overall inapparent RV infection in the continental United States may approach 25 per cent.

However, as emphatically described in reviews by Chretien and associates[46] and Graham,[100] asymptomatic infection with respiratory viruses is not the major problem of families in

TABLE 171–11. Rhinoviruses and Other Viral and Bacterial Pathogens Isolated During Periods of Respiratory Illness and When Illness-Free from 33 Middle-Class Children 3 to 11 Years of Age (Average Age, 6 Years)—Madison, Wisconsin, 1971–1972*

	1971–1972	1972	
	Nov.–Feb.	*Mar.–May*	Total
Illness-Free	753	566	1319
Agents isolated			
Rhinoviruses	4 (0.5)†	7 (1.2)	11 (0.8)
Other viruses‡	10 (1.3)	6 (1.1)	16 (1.2)
Bacterial pathogens§	14 (1.9)	4 (0.7)	18 (1.4)
Total	28 (3.7)	17 (3.0)	45 (3.4)
Respiratory Illness	305	195	500
Agents isolated			
Rhinoviruses	13 (4.3)	57 (29.2)	70 (14)
Other viruses	44 (14.4)	14 (7.2)	58 (11.6)
Bacterial pathogens	35 (11.5)	10 (5.1)	45 (9.0)
Total	92 (30.2)	81 (41.5)	173 (34.6)

*Throat swabs were taken twice weekly and inoculated into three cell lines and a sheep blood agar plate.[175, 177]

†Per cent isolation rate, i.e., 4/753 is 0.5 per cent.

‡Adenoviruses, influenza viruses A and B, parainfluenza virus, herpes simplex virus, and enteroviruses. Coronaviruses would not have been isolated; because they are often midwinter viruses, this may account for the relatively low isolation rate for 1971–1972.

§Chiefly group A streptococci in more than 100 colonies per pour plate.

those communities and nations struggling to raise their children in healthy environments. Graham[100] has estimated that, worldwide, 98 to 99 per cent of deaths from acute respiratory disease occur in the developing nations. A study of children 5 years of age or younger was carried out in such a nation—Kenya.[123] Eight hundred twenty-two children with severe acute respiratory disease were examined etiologically by modern cell culture techniques. Fifty-four per cent of the children yielded viruses (444 isolates), with enterovirus by far the most common (162 isolates), followed by respiratory syncytial virus (98 isolates) and the RVs (54 isolates). Half the RV isolates also were culture-positive for possible bacterial pathogens, and 11 RV isolates were from infants younger than 3 months of age. The authors conclude that RVs may be significant respiratory pathogens in Kenya.

RVs were found to be prevalent in a 29-month household-based study in an impoverished urban population in Fortaleza, Brazil; 175 children younger than 5 weeks of age in 63 families were surveyed for clinical illness and respiratory viruses.[62] There were two major findings: (1) the burden of respiratory illness in these children was so continuous that assigning beginning and ending dates was impossible, and (2) RVs by far were the most common virus isolated, accounting for 46 per cent of all viruses obtained. RV was dominant in all age groups, but overwhelmingly so in those children 0 to 6 months of age. In this age group, only RV and parainfluenza virus were obtained, in a ratio of approximately seven RVs to one parainfluenza virus. The role of RVs in nonindustrialized nations must be assessed carefully; for example, what proportion of RVs in this study in Brazil were just "innocent bystanders," as found in the subclinical infections in Bethel and Vanuatu (see previous discussion)?

DIAGNOSIS OF INFECTION

It is not possible to diagnose RV infections clinically because they cause such a wide spectrum of respiratory illness, particularly in infants and children. However, because of the characteristic spring-summer-fall seasonal pattern of the RVs, it is not unreasonable tentatively to assign RV etiology in cases of mild to moderate respiratory illness during these months.

Culture of the etiologic agent and interpretation of the meaning of a positive specimen can be difficult with the RVs. These viruses often propagate unpredictably, even in the relatively sensitive diploid cell cultures, such as WI-38 and FT cells, or in Ohio strain HeLa cells,[50, 54, 57, 107, 260] and often these cells are highly variable in their susceptibility.[107] RV isolation from children is hampered by the common practice of relying on a throat swab. Inocula from many throat swabs contain one tissue culture infectious virus particle or less and seldom contain infectious particles by the hundreds (see Table 171–10). Hendley and colleagues[127] found nasal specimens to be superior for RV studies, and diagnostic rhinovirologists from many nations successfully use nasal aspirates.[112, 136, 152, 153, 180] Specimens should be placed in cell cultures as soon as possible and without prior freezing and thawing (in our experience, refrigeration [4° C] overnight results in little loss). If freezing is necessary and dry ice is used, great care must be taken to avoid contamination of the specimen with sublimed carbon dioxide because the resultant carbonic acid kills the virus rapidly. Cell cultures should be incubated at 33° C and slowly rolled. Evidence of virus growth usually is seen between 2 days and 2 weeks. Once cytopathic effect is evident, standard techniques for identification are employed.[65, 107, 136, 154, 184, 190] Because of the technical difficulties in isolating RVs, prior to initiating etiologic studies of viral respiratory illness, specimen collection and culture procedures should be developed carefully in collaboration with an experienced respiratory virologist.

It is known that RVs are found in the absence of symptoms, but this is infrequent, at least in industrialized nations. Cherry[41] compiled shedding data from well children who were part of nine independent studies (1798 specimens) and found the total subclinical shedding to be 3 per cent. RV shedding from well children was 5 per cent or less in eight of these studies but was 11 per cent in the remaining survey of a Chicago nursery school population.[22] We cultured 1319 specimens from healthy Madison children, 3 to 11 years of age, and only 11 (0.8 per cent) yielded an RV (see Table 171–11). However, it is known that the rate of subclinical RV shedding can be high—up to 50 per cent—in some third-world populations, so healthy control specimens should be obtained when possible to measure background RV carriage rates.[241, 266]

RVs can be isolated year-round, but highest RV incidence usually is during spring-fall-summer months in both hemispheres.[92, 107, 127, 146, 159, 190, 205, 213]

As described early in this chapter, the RVs have many base sequences in common among the RNA genomes of the various serotypes, especially in the noncoding region at the 5′ end. Several laboratories successfully have used complementary DNA (cDNA) genetic probes to detect RVs in cell culture–grown virus and, experimentally, in clinical specimens. In 1986, Al-Nakib and associates,[4] using a probe from the 5′ end, demonstrated direct cDNA:RNA hybridization with 54 of 56 RVs tested and coxsackievirus A21 but not with influenza A or other taxonomically unrelated viruses. Later, using synthetic cDNA oligonucleotides from the same region, this same group detected with filter hybridization RV-specific RNA in preparations of all 57 serotypes tested and in nasal washings from a human volunteer inoculated with RV-14.[26]

In an effort to increase the sensitivity of this rapid method for use directly with clinical specimens, the genome of the RV suspension being tested was amplified using the polymerase chain reaction (PCR) with specific oligonucleotides from the 5′ noncoding region.[97, 140] In a clinical study of children with acute respiratory illnesses, Johnston and colleagues[149] detected RV by PCR in 146 of 292 samples (50 per cent) that yielded RV in only 47 (16 per cent) by standard culture. The PCR was three times more sensitive than was culture for detecting RV infection. PCR was used for hepatitis A virus, another picornavirus, and the genomic material was detected in a specimen containing virus at less than 1 $TCID_{50}$; this suggests that a similar sensitivity may be possible with RVs.[144] As yet, cDNA probes cannot be used for specific serotyping because, even using cDNA probes from various "specific" locations along RV-2 and RV-14 genomes, the RVs only could be placed in groups of serotypes.[19] PCR, however, can be used to classify picornavirus isolates as enteroviruses or RV; Atmar and Georghiou[17] found 100 per cent concordance between PCR results and acid lability testing.

PREVENTION AND TREATMENT

Prevention and treatment are addressed thoroughly in Chapter 8 and elsewhere, and only measures peculiar to the RVs are added here.[34, 169] Because there are 101 serotypes, a vaccine seems, for the present, to be beyond current technology. However, as more RVs are sequenced, it may be possible to vaccinate with synthetic oligopeptides modeled on the variable proteins high on the canyon walls that may be common to several serotypes; it is known that there are cross-reacting antigenic groupings among the RVs.[53] The section in this text on structure of the virion describes the preventive or therapeutic modalities made possible by taking advantage of current detailed knowledge of RV structure and of specific cell receptors. Some of these preparations have been tested in clinical trials, and one that binds in the pocket at the base of the canyon (see Fig. 171–2C) has been found active in preventing colds caused by RV-9, a virus exquisitely sensitive to the drug.[3, 9] This is the first synthetic drug that effectively has prevented RV-caused common colds.[251] R61837, when incorporated into a cyclodextrin, also exerted a beneficial effect.[199]

The most effective RV cold preventive described to date that has been demonstrated effective in natural RV colds in Australia and the United States is interferon-α, a protein produced as part of the host's natural antiviral defense and now produced for experimentation by genetic recombinant methods.[80, 120] It was administered by nasal spray to other members of the family after symptoms appeared in the index case; 80 per cent of the secondary RV colds were prevented. However, interferon given in this fashion does not seem effective against other respiratory viruses: in a follow-up study in Seattle, interferon-α did not reduce cold incidence using a protocol identical to that used in the prior family studies, chiefly because RV infections were in the minority.[74, 80, 94, 120] Because RVs often have a decided seasonality, a rapid diagnosis of the index case by PCR would be helpful to determine when interferon-α could be used effectively to stop intrafamily spread. A combination of rapid diagnosis and family prophylaxis with interferon-α could be most helpful in such families as those with asthmatic children in whom RV infection may be serious (see Clinical Manifestations). The disadvantage of interferon prophylaxis is that prolonged intranasal administration (>7 days) or repeated treatment produces an inflammatory response with nasal stuffiness, ulceration, and blood-tinged discharge.[223]

Colds usually are treated with mild nonsteroidal anti-inflammatory drugs, sympathomimetics (e.g., phenylpropanolamine), and antihistamines; these are discussed in Chapter 8.[232] Some of these over-the-counter remedies have been tested specifically against RVs in human volunteer studies. Such a trial has been reported from Adelaide, Australia, which examined the anti-inflammatory agents aspirin, acetaminophen, and ibuprofen; none was found to be effective in relieving symptoms.[101] Also, there was a suggestion that aspirin and acetaminophen may suppress the immune response mildly and extend virus shedding. Antihistamines also have been tested against RV colds, and the results are conflicting.[81, 96] Most studies have demonstrated little or no ameliorating effect by antihistamines, which is consistent with evidence that no excess histamine is produced with RV colds; however, chlorpheniramine, an H1 antihistamine with some anticholinergic action, modified symptoms.[81, 196, 197] A combination of antiviral and antimediator preparations may provide effective therapy.[104]

Vitamin C

The scientific literature on vitamin C and the common cold is filled with controversy, especially since the publication in 1970 of *Vitamin C and the Common Cold* by Linus Pauling, winner of Nobel prizes for chemistry in 1954 and for peace in 1962.[202] In prior editions of this book, the evidence, pro and con, was summarized, and it was concluded that there was no clear indication that treatment or prevention of the common cold was affected by this vitamin. We supported this view by citations of reviews written by authorities in the field.[5, 39, 59, 84] Our views have changed somewhat since then as a result of our own research. In 1987, we were asked by a major manufacturer of vitamin C to test the vitamin using our "Antarctic Hut" method,[181] which in reality is just a controlled and monitored small epidemic of monotypic RV colds. Surprisingly, in three repeated trials, vitamin C (500 mg four times daily) markedly, consistently, and significantly ($p = 0.001$ to 0.05) reduced signs and symptoms of RV-16 colds.[229]

Other Restoratives

Because the common cold is such a universal annoyance, a variety of environmental modifications and of drug-like substances have been tested.[232, 243, 249] A warm-air apparatus, the Rhinotherm, which warms the nasal mucous membranes to 43° C, has been tried with positive and negative results on laboratory-given RV colds or on natural colds.[171, 200, 249, 252] Even a sauna has been reported as reducing cold incidence.[87] Perhaps the warm air acts similarly to the legendary effect of chicken soup.[222] For some years, zinc has exhibited a variable therapeutic effect.[232] The variability of results with zinc *may* be due to unintentional use of zinc complexes rather than of ionized zinc; only the ionized element is active in vitro.[179] Godfrey[99] reported significantly reduced symptoms and duration of natural colds in college students in a placebo-controlled trial of 93 per cent ionized zinc tablets used as lozenges; however, the salutary effect of the zinc was delayed for 3 to 4 days.

References

1. Abraham, G., and Colonno, R. J.: Many rhinovirus serotypes share the same cellular receptor. J. Virol. *51*:340–345, 1984.
2. Abzug, M. J., Beam, A. C., Gyorkos, E. A., et al.: Viral pneumonia in the first month of life. Pediatr. Infect. Dis. J. *9*:881–885, 1990.
3. Al-Nakib, W., Higgins, P. G., Barrow, G. I., et al.: Suppression of colds in human volunteers challenged with rhinovirus by a new synthetic drug (R61837). Antimicrob. Agents Chemother. *33*:522–525, 1989.
4. Al-Nakib, W., Stanway, G., Forsyth, M., et al.: Detection of human rhinoviruses and their molecular relationship using cDNA probes. J. Med. Virol. *20*:289–296, 1986.
5. Anderson, T. W.: Vitamin C and the common cold. J. Med. Soc. N. J. *76*:765–766, 1979.
6. Andrewes, C. H., Chaproniere, D. M., Gompels, A. E. H., et al.: Propagation of common-cold virus in tissue cultures. Lancet *2*:546–547, 1953.
7. Andrewes, C. H., Lovelock, J. E., and Sommerville, T.: An experiment on the transmission of colds. Lancet *1*:25–27, 1951.
8. Andrewes, C. H., and Oakley, W. G.: The common cold wins the first round. St. Bartholomew's Hosp. J. *40*:74–75, 1933.
9. Andries, K., Dewindt, B., Snoeks, J., et al.: Two groups of rhinoviruses revealed by a panel of antiviral compounds present sequence divergence and differential pathogenicity. J. Virol. *64*:1117–1123, 1990.
10. Appleyard, G., Russell, S. M., Clarke, B. E., et al.: Neutralization epitopes of human rhinovirus type 2. J. Gen. Virol. *71*:1275–1282, 1990.
11. Arnold, E., and Rossmann, M. G.: Analysis of the structure of a common cold virus, human rhinovirus 14, refined at a resolution of 3 * 0 {dot-A}. J. Mol. Biol. *211*:763–901, 1990.
12. Arola, M.: Respiratory viruses in otitis media. M.D. Thesis. From the Departments of Pediatrics and Virology, University of Turku, Turku, Finland, 1990.
13. Arola, M., Ruuskanen, O., Ziegler, T., et al.: Clinical role of respiratory virus infection in acute otitis media. Pediatrics *86*:848–855, 1990.
14. Arola, M., Ziegler, T., Puhakka, H., et al.: Rhinovirus in otitis media with effusion. Ann. Otol. Rhinol. Laryngol. *99*:451–453, 1990.
15. Arola, M., Ziegler, T., Ruuskanen, O., et al.: Rhinovirus in acute otitis media. J. Pediatr. *113*:693–695, 1988.
16. Arola, M., Ziegler, T., and Ruuskanen, O.: Respiratory virus infection as a cause of prolonged symptoms in acute otitis media. J. Pediatr. *116*:697–701, 1990.
17. Atmar, B. L., and Georghiou, P. R.: Classification of respiratory tract picornavirus isolates as enteroviruses or rhinoviruses by using reverse transcription-polymerase chain reaction. J. Clin. Microbiol. *31*:2544–2546, 1993.
18. Auvinen, P.: Common and specific sequences in picornaviruses. Mol. Cell. Probes *4*:273–284, 1990.
19. Auvinen, P., Ziegler, T., Skern, T., et al.: Identification of rhinoviruses by cDNA probes. J. Virol. Methods *27*:61–68, 1990.
20. Baker, J. W., Hong, R., Dick, E. C., et al.: Asthma, I_gA deficiency, and respiratory infections. J. Allergy Clin. Immunol. *58*:713–721, 1976.
21. Bangham, C. R. M., and McMichael, A. J.: Nosing ahead in the cold war. Nature *344*:16, 1990.
22. Beem, M. O.: Acute respiratory illness in nursery school children: A longitudinal study of the occurrence of illness and respiratory viruses. Am. J. Epidemiol. *90*:30–44, 1969.
23. Belshe, R. B., Van Voris, L. P., and Mufson, M. A.: Impact of viral respiratory diseases on infants and young children in a rural and urban area of southern West Virginia. Am. J. Epidemiol. *117*:467–474, 1983.
24. Bloch, A. B., Orenstein, W. A., Ewing, W. M., et al.: Measles outbreak in a pediatric practice: Airborne transmission in an office setting. Pediatrics *75*:676–683, 1985.
25. Boat, T. F., and Carson, J. L.: Ciliary dysmorphology and dysfunction: Primary or acquired? N. Engl. J. Med. *323*:1700–1702, 1990.
26. Bruce, C. B., Al-Nakib, W., Almond, J. W., et al.: Use of synthetic oligonucleotide probes to detect rhinovirus RNA. Arch. Virol. *105*:179–187, 1989.
27. Buchman, C. A., Doyle, W. J., Skoner, D., et al.: Octologic manifestations of experimental rhinovirus infection. Laryngoscope *104*:1295–1299, 1994.
28. Buscho, R. F., Perkins, J. C., Knopf, H. L. S., et al.: Further characterization of the local respiratory tract antibody response induced by intranasal instillation of inactivated rhinovirus 13 vaccine. J. Immunol. *108*:169–177, 1972.
29. Busse, W. W., Vrtis, R. F., and Dick, E. C.: The role of viral infections in intrinsic asthma: Activation of neutrophil inflammation. Intrinsic Asthma *28*:41–56, 1989.
30. Butler, W. T., Waldmann, T. A., Rossen, R. D., et al.: Changes in I_gA and I_gG concentrations in nasal secretions prior to the appearance of antibody during viral respiratory infection in man. J. Immunol. *105*:584–591, 1970.
31. Bynoe, M. L., Hobson, D., Horner, J., et al.: Inoculation of human volunteers with a strain of virus isolated from a common cold. Lancet *1*:1194–1196, 1961.
32. Carlsen, K. H., Orstavik, I., Leegaard, J., et al.: Respiratory virus infections and aeroallergens in acute bronchial asthma. Arch. Dis. Child. *59*:310–315, 1984.
33. Carson, J. L., Collier, A. M., and Hu, S. S.: Acquired ciliary defects in nasal epithelium of children with acute viral upper respiratory infections. N. Engl. J. Med. *312*:463–468, 1985.
34. Casey, M. J., and Dick, E. C.: Acute respiratory infections. *In* Casey, M. J., Foster, C., and Hixson, E. G. (eds.): Winter Sports Medicine. Philadelphia, F. A. Davis, 1990, pp. 112–128.
35. Cate, T. R.: Self-control of the common cold? Ann. Intern. Med. *88*:569–570, 1978.
36. Cate, T. R., Couch, R. B., and Fleet, W. F., et al.: Production of tracheobron-

chitis in volunteers with rhinovirus in a small-particle aerosol. Am. J. Epidemiol. *81*:95–105, 1965.
37. Cate, T. R., Couch, R. B., and Johnson, K. M.: Studies with rhinoviruses in volunteers: Production of illness, effect of naturally acquired antibody, and demonstration of a protective effect not associated with serum antibody. J. Clin. Invest. *43*:56–67, 1964.
38. Cate, T. R., Rossen, R. D., Douglas, R. G., Jr., et al.: The role of nasal secretion and serum antibody in the rhinovirus common cold. Am. J. Epidemiol. *84*:352–363, 1966.
39. Chalmers, T. C.: Effects of ascorbic acid on the common cold. Am. J. Med. *58*:532–536, 1975.
40. Chen, R. T., Goldbaum, G. M., Wassilak, S. G. F., et al.: An explosive point-source measles outbreak in a highly vaccinated population: Modes of transmission and risk factors for disease. Am. J. Epidemiol. *129*:173–182, 1989.
41. Cherry, J. D.: Newer respiratory viruses: Their role in respiratory illnesses of children. Adv. Pediatr. *20*:225–290, 1973.
42. Cherry, J. D., Diddams, J. A., and Dick, E. C.: Rhinovirus infections in hospitalized children. Arch. Environ. Health *14*:390–396, 1967.
43. Chonmaitree, T., Howie, V. M., and Truant, A. L.: Presence of respiratory viruses in middle ear fluids and nasal wash specimens from children with acute otitis media. Pediatrics *77*:698–702, 1986.
44. Chonmaitree, T., Lett-Brown, M. A., and Grant, J. A.: Respiratory viruses induce production of histamine-releasing factor by mononuclear leukocytes: A possible role in the mechanism of virus-induced asthma. J. Infect. Dis. *164*:592–594, 1991.
45. Chonmaitree, T., Owen, M. J., and Howie, V. M.: Respiratory viruses interfere with bacteriologic response to antibiotic in children with acute otitis media. J. Infect. Dis. *162*:546–549, 1990.
46. Chretien, J., Holland, W., Macklem, P., et al.: Acute respiratory infections in children: A global public-health problem. N. Engl. J. Med. *310*:982–984, 1984.
47. Cohen, S., Tyrrell, D. A. J., and Smith, A. P.: Psychological stress and susceptibility to the common cold. N. Engl. J. Med. *325*:606–612, 1991.
48. Colonno, R. J., Callahan, P. L., and Long, W. J.: Isolation of a monoclonal antibody that blocks attachment of the major group of human rhinovirus. J. Virol. *57*:7–12, 1986.
49. Commission on Acute Respiratory Diseases: Experimental transmission of minor respiratory illness to human volunteers by filter-passing agents. I. Demonstration of two types of illness characterized by long and short incubation periods and different clinical features. J. Clin. Invest. *26*:957–973, 1947.
50. Conant, R. M., and Hamparian, V. V.: Rhinoviruses: Basis for a numbering system. I. HeLa cells for propagation and serologic procedures. J. Immunol. *100*:107–113, 1968.
51. Conant, R. M., Hamparian, V. V., Stott, E. J., et al.: Identification of rhinovirus strain D. C. Nature *217*:1264, 1968.
52. Condra, J. H., Sardana, V. V., Tomassini, J. E., et al.: Bacterial expression of antibody fragments that block human rhinovirus infection of cultured cells. J. Biol. Chem. *265*:2292–2295, 1990.
53. Cooney, M. K., Fox, J. P., and Kenny, G. E.: Antigenic groupings of 90 rhinovirus serotypes. Infect. Immun. *37*:642–647, 1982.
54. Cooney, M. K., and Kenny, G. E.: Demonstration of dual rhinovirus infection in humans by isolation of different serotypes in human heteroploid (HeLa) and human diploid fibroblast cell cultures. J. Clin. Microbiol. *5*:202–207, 1977.
55. Couch, R. B.: The common cold: Control? J. Infect. Dis. *150*:167–173, 1984.
56. Couch, R. B.: Personal communication, 1978.
57. Couch, R. B.: Rhinoviruses. *In* Fields, B. N., Knipe, D. M., Howley, P. M., et al. (eds.): Fields Virology. 3rd ed., Vol. 1. Philadelphia, Lippincott-Raven, 1996, pp. 713–734.
58. Couch, R. B., Douglas, R. G., Jr., Lindgren, K. M., et al.: Airborne transmission of respiratory infection with coxsackievirus A type 21. Am. J. Epidemiol. *91*:78–86, 1970.
59. Coulehan, J. L.: Ascorbic acid and the common cold. Postgrad. Med. *66*:153–160, 1979.
60. D'Alessio, D. J., Meschievitz, C. K., Peterson, J. A., et al.: Short-duration exposure and the transmission of rhinoviral colds. J. Infect. Dis. *150*:189–194, 1984.
61. D'Alessio, D. J., Peterson, J. A., Dick, C. R., et al.: Transmission of experimental rhinovirus colds in volunteer married couples. J. Infect. Dis. *133*:28–36, 1976.
62. de Arruda N. E., Hayden, F. G., McAuliffe, J. F., et al.: Acute respiratory viral infections in ambulatory children of urban northeast Brazil. J. Infect. Dis. *164*:252–258, 1991.
63. Denny, F. W., and Clyde, W. A., Jr.: Acute lower respiratory tract infections in nonhospitalized children. J. Pediatr. *108*:635–646, 1986.
64. Dick, E. C.: Chimpanzee kidney tissue cultures for growth and isolation of viruses. J. Bacteriol. *86*:573–576, 1963.
65. Dick, E. C., Blumer, C. R., and Evans, A. S.: Epidemiology of infections with rhinovirus types 43 and 55 in a group of University of Wisconsin student families. Am. J. Epidemiol. *86*:386–400, 1967.
66. Dick, E. C., and Carr, D. L.: *Haemophilus influenzae*. Arch. Environ. Health *13*:450–453, 1966.
67. Dick, E. C., and Dick, C. R.: A subclinical outbreak of human rhinovirus 31 infection in chimpanzees. Am. J. Epidemiol. *88*:267–272, 1968.
68. Dick, E. C., and Dick, C. R.: Natural and experimental infections of nonhuman primates with respiratory viruses. Lab. Anim. Sci. *24*:177–181, 1974.
69. Dick, E. C., Gavinski, S. S., Mahl, M. C., et al.: A virucidal handkerchief for helping prevent transmission of respiratory infection at McMurdo Station and Scott Base during the winter fly-in period. Antarctic J. U. S. *14*:189–190, 1979.
70. Dick, E. C., Hossain, S. U., Mink, K. A., et al.: Interruption of transmission of rhinovirus colds among human volunteers using virucidal paper handkerchiefs. J. Infect. Dis. *153*:352–356, 1986.
71. Dick, E. C., Jennings, L. C., Meschievitz, C. K., et al.: Possible modification of the normal winter fly-in respiratory disease outbreak at McMurdo Station. Antarctic J. U. S. *15*:173–174, 1980.
72. Dick, E. C., Jennings, L. C., Mink, K. A., et al.: Aerosol transmission of rhinovirus colds. J. Infect. Dis. *156*:442–448, 1987.
73. Dochez, A. R., Shibley, G. S., and Mills, K. C.: Studies in the common cold. IV. Experimental transmission of the common cold to anthropoid apes and human beings by means of a filtrable agent. J. Exp. Med. *52*:701–716, 1930.
74. Douglas, R. G., Jr.: The common cold: Relief at last? N. Engl. J. Med. *314*:114–115, 1986.
75. Douglas, R. G., Jr.: Pathogenesis of rhinovirus common colds in human volunteers. Ann. Otol. Rhinol. Laryngol. *79*:563–571, 1970.
76. Douglas, R. G., Jr., Cate, T. R., Gerone, P. J., et al.: Quantitative rhinovirus shedding patterns in volunteers. Am. Rev. Respir. Dis. *94*:159–167, 1966.
77. Douglas, R. G., Jr., and Couch, R. B.: Parenteral inactivated rhinovirus vaccine: Minimal protective effect. Proc. Soc. Exp. Biol. Med. *139*:899–902, 1972.
78. Douglas, R. G., Jr., Lindgren, K. M., and Couch, R. B.: Exposure to cold environment and rhinovirus common cold: Failure to demonstrate effect. N. Engl. J. Med. *279*:742–747, 1968.
79. Douglas, R. G., Jr., Rossen, R. D., Butler, W. T., et al.: Rhinovirus neutralizing antibody in tears, parotid saliva, nasal secretions and serum. J. Immunol. *99*:297–303, 1967.
80. Douglas, R. M., Moore, B. W., Milles, H. B., et al.: Prophylactic efficacy of intranasal alpha-2 interferon against rhinovirus infections in the family setting. N. Engl. J. Med. *314*:65–70, 1986.
81. Doyle, W. J., McBride, T. P., Skoner, D. P., et al.: A double-blind, placebo-controlled clinical trial of the effect of chlorpheniramine on the response of the nasal airway, middle ear and eustachian tube to provocative rhinovirus challenge. Pediatr. Infect. Dis. J. *7*:215–242, 1988.
82. Duechler, M., Skern, T., Sommergruber, W., et al.: Evolutionary relationships within the human rhinovirus genus: Comparison of serotypes 89, 2, and 14. Proc. Natl. Acad. Sci. U. S. A. *84*:2605–2609, 1987.
83. Duff, A. L., Pomeranz, E. S., Gelber, L. E., et al.: Risk factors for acute wheezing in infants and children: Viruses, passive smoke, and IgE antibodies to inhalant allergens. Pediatrics *92*:535–540, 1993.
84. Dykes, M. H. M., and Meier, P.: Ascorbic acid and the common cold: Evaluation of its efficacy and toxicity. J. A. M. A. *231*:1073–1079, 1975.
85. Eadie, M. B., Stott, E. J., and Grist, N. R.: Virological studies in chronic bronchitis. B. M. J. *2*:671–673, 1966.
86. Editorial: Splints don't stop colds—surprising! Lancet *1*:277–278, 1988.
87. Ernst, E., Pecho, E., Wirz, P., et al.: Regular sauna bathing and the incidence of common colds. Ann. Med. *22*:225–227, 1990.
88. Farr, B. M., Hendley, J. O., Kaiser, D. L., et al.: Two randomized controlled trials of virucidal nasal tissues in the prevention of natural upper respiratory infections. Am. J. Epidemiol. *128*:1162–1172, 1988.
89. Fleet, W. F., Couch, R. B., Cate, T. R., et al.: Homologous and heterologous resistance to rhinovirus common cold. Am. J. Epidemiol. *82*:185–196, 1965.
90. Fox, J. P.: Is a rhinovirus vaccine possible? Am. J. Epidemiol. *103*:345–354, 1976.
91. Fox, J. P., Cooney, M. K., and Hall, C. E.: The Seattle virus watch. V. Epidemiologic observations of rhinovirus infections, 1965–1969, in families with young children. Am. J. Epidemiol. *101*:122–143, 1975.
92. Fox, J. P., Cooney, M. K., Hall, C. E., et al.: Rhinoviruses in Seattle families, 1975–1979. Am. J. Epidemiol. *122*:830–846, 1985.
93. Fox, M. P., Otto, M. J., and McKinlay, M. A.: Prevention of rhinovirus and poliovirus uncoating by WIN 51711, a new antiviral drug. Antimicrob. Agents Chemother. *30*:110–116, 1986.
94. Foy, H. M., Fox, J. P., and Cooney, M. K.: Efficacy of alpha$_2$-interferon against the common cold. N. Engl. J. Med. *315*:513–514, 1986.
95. Frick, W. E., and Busse, W. W.: Respiratory infections: Their role in airway responsiveness and pathogenesis of asthma. Clin. Chest Med. *9*:539–549, 1988.
96. Gaffey, M. J., Gwaltney, J. M., Jr., Sastre, A., et al.: Intranasally and orally administered antihistamine treatment of experimental rhinovirus colds. Am. Rev. Respir. Dis. *136*:556–560, 1987.
97. Gama, R. E., Horsnell, P. R., Hughes, P. J., et al.: Amplification of rhinovirus specific nucleic acids from clinical samples using the polymerase chain reaction. J. Med. Virol. *28*:73–77, 1989.
98. George, R. B., and Mogabgab, W. J.: Atypical pneumonia in young men with rhinovirus infections. Ann. Intern. Med. *71*:1073–1078, 1969.
99. Godfrey, J. C., Conant Sloane, B., Turco, J. H., et al.: Zinc and common

cold: Positive findings in controlled clinical study of a new formulation. Presented at the Thirty-First Interscience Conference on Antimicrobial Agents and Chemotherapy, September 29–October 2, 1991, Chicago. Abstract 1381.

100. Graham, N. M. H.: The epidemiology of acute respiratory infections in children and adults: A global perspective. Epidemiol. Rev. *12*:149–178, 1990.
101. Graham, N. M. H., Burrell, C. J., Douglas, R. M., et al.: Adverse effects of aspirin, acetaminophen, and ibuprofen on immune function, viral shedding, and clinical status in rhinovirus-infected volunteers. J. Infect. Dis. *162*:1277–1282, 1990.
102. Gregg, M. B.: The epidemiology of influenza in humans. Ann. N. Y. Acad. Sci. *353*:45–53, 1980.
103. Greve, J. M., Davis, G., Meyer, A. M., et al.: The major human rhinovirus receptor is ICAM-1. Cell *56*:839–847, 1989.
104. Gwaltney, J. M., Jr.: Combined antiviral and antimediator treatment of rhinovirus colds. J. Infect. Dis. *166*:776–782, 1992.
105. Gwaltney, J. M., Jr.: Virology of middle ear. Ann. Otol. *80*:365–370, 1971.
106. Gwaltney, J. M., Jr.: Understanding and controlling rhinovirus colds. *In* de la Maza, L. M., and Peterson, E. M. (eds.): Medical Virology. Vol. 4. Hillsdale, NJ, Lawrence Erlbaum, 1985, pp. 233–251.
107. Gwaltney, J. M., Jr.: Rhinoviruses. *In* Evans, A. S. (ed.): Viral Infections of Humans: Epidemiology and Control. New York, Plenum Medical, 1989, pp. 593–615.
108. Gwaltney, J. M., Jr., and Hendley, J. O.: Rhinovirus transmission: One if by air, two if by hand. Am. J. Epidemiol. *107*:357–361, 1978.
109. Gwaltney, J. M., Jr., and Hendley, J. O.: Transmission of experimental rhinovirus infection by contaminated surfaces. Am. J. Epidemiol. *116*:828–833, 1982.
110. Gwaltney, J. M., Jr., Moskalski, P. B., and Hendley, J. O.: Hand-to-hand transmission of rhinovirus colds. Ann. Intern. Med. *88*:463–467, 1978.
111. Gwaltney, J. M., Jr., Sydnor, A., Jr., and Sande, M. A.: Etiology and antimicrobial treatment of acute sinusitis. Ann. Otol. Rhinol. Laryngol. *90*(Suppl. 84):68–71, 1981.
112. Hall, C. B., and Douglas, R. G., Jr.: Clinically useful method for the isolation of respiratory syncytial virus. J. Infect. Dis. *131*:1–5, 1975.
113. Halperin, S. A., Eggleston, P. A., Beasley, P., et al.: Exacerbations of asthma in adults during experimental rhinovirus infection. Am. Rev. Respir. Dis. *132*:976–980, 1985.
114. Halperin, S. A., Eggleston, P. A., Hendley, J. O., et al.: Pathogenesis of lower respiratory tract symptoms in experimental rhinovirus infection. Am. Rev. Respir. Dis. *128*:806–810, 1983.
115. Hamory, B. H., Sande, M. A., Sydnor, A., Jr., et al.: Etiology and antimicrobial therapy of acute maxillary sinusitis. J. Infect. Dis. *139*:197–202, 1979.
116. Hamparian, V. V., Colonno, R. J., Cooney, M. K., et al.: A collaborative report: Rhinoviruses—Extension of the numbering system from 89 to 100. Virology *159*:191–192, 1987.
117. Hamparian, V. V., Ketler, A., and Hilleman, M. R.: Recovery of new viruses (coryzaviruses) from cases of common cold in human adults. Proc. Soc. Exp. Biol. Med. *108*:444–453, 1961.
118. Hamparian, V. V., Leagus, M. B., Hilleman, M. R., et al.: Epidemiologic investigations of rhinovirus infections. Proc. Soc. Exp. Biol. Med. *117*:469–476, 1964.
119. Hamre, D.: Rhinoviruses. *In* Melnick, J. L. (ed.): Monographs in Virology. Vol. 1. Basel, Karger, 1968.
120. Hayden, F. G., Albrecht, J. K., Kaiser, D. L., et al.: Prevention of natural colds by contact prophylaxis with intranasal alpha 2-interferon. N. Engl. J. Med. *314*:71–75, 1986.
121. Hayden, F. G., Gwaltney, J. M., Jr., and Colonno, R. J.: Modification of experimental rhinovirus colds by receptor blockade. Antiviral Res. *9*:233–247, 1988.
122. Hayflick, L., and Moorhead, P. S.: The serial cultivation of human diploid cell strains. Exp. Cell Res. *25*:585–621, 1961.
123. Hazlett, D. T. G., Bell, T. M., Tukei, P. M., et al.: Viral etiology and epidemiology of acute respiratory infections in children in Nairobi, Kenya. Am. J. Trop. Med. Hyg. *39*:632–640, 1988.
124. Henderson, F. W., Clyde, W. A., Jr., Collier, A. M., et al.: The etiologic and epidemiologic spectrum of bronchiolitis in pediatric practice. J. Pediatr. *95*:183–190, 1979.
125. Hendley, J. O.: Rhinovirus colds: Immunology and pathogenesis. Eur. J. Respir. Dis. *64*(Suppl. 128):340–343, 1983.
126. Hendley, J. O., and Gwaltney, J. M., Jr.: Mechanisms of transmission of rhinovirus infections. Epidemiol. Rev. *10*:242–258, 1988.
127. Hendley, J. O., Gwaltney, J. M., Jr., and Jordan, W. S., Jr.: Rhinovirus infections in an industrial population. IV. Infections within families of employees during two fall peaks of respiratory illness. Am. J. Epidemiol. *89*:184–196, 1969.
128. Hendley, J. O., Wenzel, R. P., and Gwaltney, J. M., Jr.: Transmission of rhinovirus colds by self-inoculation. N. Engl. J. Med. *288*:1361–1364, 1973.
129. Higgins, P. G., Barrow, G. I., and Tyrrell, D. A. J.: A study of the efficacy of the bradykinin antagonist, NPC 567, in rhinovirus infections in human volunteers. Antiviral Res. *14*:339–344, 1990.
130. Hogle, J. M., Chow, M., and Filman, D. J.: Three-dimensional structure of poliovirus at 2.9 {dot-A} resolution. Science *229*:1358–1365, 1985.
131. Hollinger, F. B., and Ticehurst, J.: Hepatitis A virus. *In* Fields, B. N., Knipe, D. M., et al. (eds.): Virology. New York, Raven Press, 1990, pp. 631–667.
132. Holmes, M. J., Reed, S. E., Stott, R. J., et al.: Studies of experimental rhinovirus type 2 infections in polar isolation and in England. J. Hyg. (Camb.) *76*:379–393, 1976.
133. Horn, M. E. C., Brain, E., Gregg, I., et al.: Respiratory viral infection in childhood: A survey in general practice, Roehampton 1967–1972. J. Hyg. (Camb.) *74*:157–168, 1975.
134. Horn, M. E., Brain, E. A., Gregg, I., et al.: Respiratory viral infection and wheezy bronchitis in childhood. Thorax *34*:23–28, 1979.
135. Horn, M. E. C., and Gregg, I.: Role of viral infection and host factors in acute episodes of asthma and chronic bronchitis. Chest *63*:44s–48s, 1973.
136. Horn, M. E., Reed, S. E., and Taylor, P.: Role of viruses and bacteria in acute wheezy bronchitis in childhood: A study of sputum. Arch. Dis. Child. *54*:587–592, 1979.
137. Hsia, J., Goldstein, A. L., Simon, G. L., et al.: Peripheral blood mononuclear cell interleukin-2 and interferon-γ production, cytotoxicity, and antigen-stimulated blastogenesis during experimental rhinovirus infection. J. Infect. Dis. *162*:591–597, 1990.
138. Hughes, P. J., North, C., Jellis, C. H., et al.: The nucleotide sequence of human rhinovirus 1B: Molecular relationships within the *Rhinovirus* genus. J. Gen. Virol. *69*:49–58, 1988.
139. Hughes, P. J., North, C., Minor, P. D., et al.: The complete nucleotide sequence of coxsackievirus A21. J. Gen. Virol. *70*:2943–2952, 1989.
140. Hyypiä, T., Auvinen, P., and Maaronen, M.: Polymerase chain reaction for human picornaviruses. J. Gen. Virol. *70*:3261–3268, 1989.
141. Isaacs, D., Clarke, J. R., Tyrrell, D. A. J., et al.: Selective infection of lower respiratory tract by respiratory viruses in children with recurrent respiratory tract infections. B. M. J. *284*:1746–1748, 1982.
142. Jackson, G. G., Dowling, H. F., and Anderson, T. O.: Neutralization of common cold agents in volunteers by pooled human globulin. Science *128*:27–28, 1958.
143. Jacobs, J. W., Peacock, D. B., Corner, B. D., et al.: Respiratory syncytial and other viruses associated with respiratory disease in infants. Lancet *1*:871–876, 1971.
144. Jansen, R. W., Siegl, G., and Lemon, S. M.: Molecular epidemiology of human hepatitis A virus defined by an antigen-capture polymerase chain reaction method. Proc. Natl. Acad. Sci. U. S. A. *87*:2867–2871, 1990.
145. Jenkins, O., Booth, J. D., Minor, P. D., et al.: The complete nucleotide sequence of coxsackievirus B4 and its comparison to other members of the picornaviridae. J. Gen. Virol. *68*:1835–1848, 1987.
146. Jennings, L. C., and Dick, E. C.: Transmission and control of rhinovirus colds. Eur. J. Epidemiol. *3*:327–335, 1987.
147. Jennings, L. C., Dick, E. C., Mink, K. A., et al.: Near disappearance of rhinovirus along a fomite transmission chain. J. Infect. Dis. *158*:888–892, 1988.
148. Jennings, L. C., MacDiarmid, R. D., and Miles, J. A. R.: A study of acute respiratory disease in the community of Port Chalmers I. Illnesses within a group of selected families and the relative incidence of respiratory pathogens in the whole community. J. Hyg. (Camb.) *81*:49–66, 1978.
149. Johnston, S. L., Sanderson, G., Pattemore, P. K., et al.: Use of polymerase chain reaction for diagnosis of picornavirus infection in subjects with and without respiratory symptoms. J. Clin. Microbiol. *31*:111–117, 1993.
150. Kapikian, A. Z., Conant, R. M., Hamparian, V. V., et al.: Rhinoviruses: Extension of the numbering system. Virology *43*:524–526, 1971.
151. Kawana, R., and Matsumoto, I.: Electron microscopic study of rhinovirus replication in human fetal lung cells. Jpn. J. Microbiol. *15*:207–217, 1971.
152. Kellner, G., Popow-Kraupp, T., Binder, C., et al.: Respiratory tract infections due to different rhinovirus-serotypes and the influence of maternal antibodies on the clinical expression of the disease in infants. J. Med. Virol. *35*:267–272, 1991.
153. Kellner, G., Popow-Kraupp, T., Kundi, M., et al.: Contribution of rhinoviruses to respiratory viral infections in childhood: A prospective study in a mainly hospitalized infant population. J. Med. Virol. *25*:455–469, 1988.
154. Kellner, G., Popow-Kraupp, T., Kundi, M., et al.: Clinical manifestations of respiratory tract infections due to respiratory syncytial virus and rhinoviruses in hospitalized children. Acta Paediatr. Scand. *78*:390–394, 1989.
155. Ketler, A., Hamparian, V. V., and Hilleman, M. R.: Characterization and classification of ECHO 28-rhinovirus-coryzavirus agents. Proc. Soc. Exp. Biol. Med. *110*:821–831, 1962.
156. Kim, S., Smith, T. J., Chapman, M. S., et al.: Crystal structure of human rhinovirus serotype 1A (HRV1A). J. Mol. Biol. *210*:91–111, 1989.
157. Klein, B. S., Dollette, F. R., and Yolken, R. H.: The role of respiratory syncytial virus and other viral pathogens in acute otitis media. J. Pediatr. *101*:16–20, 1982.
158. Klein, J. O.: Microbiology of otitis media. Ann. Otol. Rhinol. Laryngol. *89*(Suppl. 68):98–101, 1980.
159. Krilov, L., Pierik, L., Keller, E., et al.: Association of rhinoviruses with lower respiratory tract disease in hospitalized patients. J. Med. Virol. *19*:345–352, 1986.
160. Kruse, V. W.: The causative agent of coughs and colds: From the Hygienic Institute of the University of Leipzig. Muenchner Med. Wochenschr. *61*:1547, 1914.
161. Larson, H. E., Reed, S. E., and Tyrrell, D. A. J.: Isolation of rhinoviruses and coronaviruses from 38 colds in adults. J. Med. Virol. *5*:221–229, 1980.

162. Las Heras, J., and Swanson, V. L.: Sudden death of an infant with rhinovirus infection complicating bronchial asthma: Case report. Pediatr. Pathol. *1*:319–323, 1983.
163. Lefkowitz, L. B., Jr., and Jackson, G. G.: Dual respiratory infection with parainfluenza and rhinovirus: The pathogenesis of transmitted infection in volunteers. Am. Rev. Respir. Dis. *93*:519–528, 1966.
164. Lemanske, R. F., Jr., Dick, E. C., Swenson, C. A., et al.: Rhinovirus upper respiratory infection increases airway hyperreactivity and late asthmatic reactions. J. Clin. Invest. *83*:1–10, 1989.
165. Levandowski, R. A., Weaver, C. W., and Jackson, G. G.: Nasal-secretion leukocyte populations determined by flow cytometry during acute rhinovirus infection. J. Med. Virol. *25*:423–432, 1988.
166. Lim, D. J.: Recent advances in otitis media: Report of the Fourth Research Conference. Ann. Otol. Rhinol. Laryngol. *98*(Suppl. 139):1989.
167. Lobovits, A. M., Freeman, J., Goldmann, D. A., et al.: Risk of illness after exposure to a pediatric office. N. Engl. J. Med. *313*:425–428, 1985.
168. Longini, I. M., Jr., and Monto, A. S.: Efficacy of virucidal nasal tissues in interrupting familial transmission of respiratory agents: A field trial in Tecumseh, Michigan. Am. J. Epidemiol. *128*:639–644, 1988.
169. Lowenstein, S. R., and Parrino, T. A.: Management of the common cold. Adv. Intern. Med. *32*:207–234, 1987.
170. Lupton, H. W., Smith, M. H., and Frey, M. L.: Identification and characterization of a bovine rhinovirus isolated from Iowa cattle with acute respiratory tract disease. Am. J. Vet. Res. *41*:1029–1034, 1980.
171. Macknin, M. L., Mathew, S., and Medendorp, S. V. B.: Effect of inhaling heated vapor on symptoms of the common cold. J. A. M. A. *264*:989–991, 1990.
172. Makgoba, M. W., Sanders, M. E., Ginther Luce, G. E., et al.: Functional evidence that intercellular adhesion molecule-1 (ICAM-1) is a ligand for LFA-1–dependent adhesion in T cell–mediated cytotoxicity. Eur. J. Immunol. *18*:637–640, 1988.
173. Marlin, S. D., Staunton, D. E., Springer, T. A., et al.: A soluble form of intercellular adhesion molecule-1 inhibits rhinovirus infection. Nature *344*:70–72, 1990.
174. McBride, T. P., Doyle, W. J., Hayden, F. G., et al.: Alterations of the eustachian tube, middle ear, and nose in rhinovirus infection. Arch. Otolaryngol. Head Neck Surg. *115*:1054–1059, 1989.
175. McIntosh, K.: Bronchiolitis and asthma: Possible common pathogenetic pathways. J. Allergy Clin. Immunol. *57*:595–604, 1976.
176. McIntosh, K., Ellis, E. F., Hoffman, L. S., et al.: The association of viral and bacterial respiratory infections with exacerbations of wheezing in young asthmatic children. J. Pediatr. *82*:578, 1973.
177. McKinlay, M. A., Frank, J. A., Jr., Benziger, D. P., et al.: Use of WIN 51711 to prevent echovirus type 9-induced paralysis in suckling mice. J. Infect. Dis. *154*:676–681, 1986.
178. Melnick, J. L.: Enteroviruses: Polioviruses, coxsackievirus, echoviruses, and newer enteroviruses. *In* Fields, B. N., Knipe, D. M., Chanock, R.M., et al. (eds.): Fields' Virology. 2nd ed. New York, Raven Press, 1990, pp. 549–605.
179. Merluzzi, V. J., Cipriano, D., McNeil, D., et al.: Evaluation of zinc complexes on the replication of rhinovirus 2 in vitro. Res. Commun. Chem. Pathol. Pharmacol. *66*:425–440, 1989.
180. Mertsola, J., Ziegler, T., Ruuskanen, O., et al.: Recurrent wheezy bronchitis and viral respiratory infections. Arch. Dis. Child. *66*:124–129, 1991.
181. Meschievitz, C. K., Schultz, S. B., and Dick, E. C.: A model for obtaining predictable natural transmission of rhinoviruses in human volunteers. J. Infect. Dis. *150*:195–201, 1984.
182. Minor, T. E., Baker, J. W., Dick, E. C., et al.: Greater frequency of viral respiratory infections in asthmatic children as compared with their nonasthmatic siblings. J. Pediatr. *85*:472–477, 1974.
183. Minor, T. E., Dick, E. C., Baker, J. W., et al.: Rhinovirus and influenza type A infections as precipitants of asthma. Am. Rev. Respir. Dis. *113*:149–153, 1976.
184. Minor, T. E., Dick, E. C., DeMeo, A. N., et al.: Viruses as precipitants of asthmatic attacks in children. J. A. M. A. *227*:292–298, 1974.
185. Minor, T. E., Dick, E. C., Peterson, J. A., et al.: Failure of naturally acquired rhinovirus infections to produce temporal immunity to heterologous serotypes. Infect. Immun. *10*:1192–1193, 1974.
186. Mogabgab, W. J.: Prospects for the control of pneumonias. Infect. Dis. Rev. *4*:41–71, 1976.
187. Mogabgab, W. J., Holmes, B. J., and Pollock, B.: Antigenic relationships of common rhinovirus types from disabling upper respiratory illnesses: International Symposium on Immunity to Infections of the Respiratory System in Man and Animals, London, 1974. Dev. Biol. Stand. *28*:400–411, 1975.
188. Mogabgab, W. J., and Pelon, W.: Problems in characterizing and identifying an apparently new virus found in association with mild respiratory disease in recruits. Ann. N. Y. Acad. Sci. *67*:403–412, 1957.
189. Monto, A. S.: A community study of respiratory infections in the tropics. III. Introduction and transmission of infections within families. Am. J. Epidemiol. *88*:69–79, 1968.
190. Monto, A. S., Bryan, E. R., and Ohmit, S.: Rhinovirus infections in Tecumseh, Michigan: Frequency of illness and number of serotypes. J. Infect. Dis. *156*:43–49, 1987.
191. Monto, A. S., and Cavallaro, J. J.: The Tecumseh study of respiratory illness. II. Patterns of occurrence of infection with respiratory pathogens, 1965–1969. Am. J. Epidemiol. *94*:280–289, 1971.
192. Monto, A. S., and Cavallaro, J. J.: The Tecumseh study of respiratory illness. IV. Prevalence of rhinovirus serotypes, 1966–1969. Am. J. Epidemiol. *96*:352–360, 1972.
193. Monto, A. S., and Johnson, K. M.: A community study of respiratory infections in the tropics. II. The spread of six rhinovirus isolates within the community. Am. J. Epidemiol. *88*:55–68, 1968.
194. Monto, A. S., and Ullman, B. M.: Acute respiratory illness in an American community. J. A. M. A. *227*:164–169, 1974.
195. Murphy, F. A., and Kingsbury, D. W.: Virus taxonomy. *In* Fields, B. N., Knipe, D. M., Chanock, R. M., et al. (eds.): Fields' Virology. 2nd ed. New York, Raven Press, 1990, pp. 9–35.
196. Naclerio, R. M., Proud, D., Kagey-Sobotka, A., et al.: Is histamine responsible for the symptoms of rhinovirus colds? A look at the inflammatory mediators following infection. Pediatr. Infect. Dis. *7*:218–242, 1988.
197. Naclerio, R. M., Proud, D., Lichtenstein, L. M., et al.: Kinins are generated during experimental rhinovirus colds. J. Infect. Dis. *157*:133–142, 1988.
198. Newman, J. F. E., Rowlands, D. J., Brown, F., et al.: Physico-chemical characterization of two serologically unrelated equine rhinoviruses. Intervirology *8*:145–154, 1977.
199. Ninomiya, Y., Shimma, N., and Tshitsuka, H.: Comparative studies on the antirhinovirus activity and the mode of action of the rhinovirus capsid binding agents, chalcone amides. Antiviral Res. *13*:61–74, 1990.
200. Ophir, D., and Elad, Y.: Effects of steam inhalation on nasal patency and nasal symptoms in patients with the common cold. Am. J. Otolaryngol. *3*:149–153, 1987.
201. Paisley, J. W., Lauer, B. A., McIntosh, K., et al.: Pathogens associated with acute lower respiratory tract infection in young children. Pediatr. Infect. Dis. *3*:14–19, 1984.
202. Pauling, L. C.: Vitamin C and the Common Cold. San Francisco, W. H. Freeman, 1970.
203. Pelon, W., Mogabgab, W. J., Phillips, I. A., et al.: Cytopathic agents isolated from recruits with mild respiratory illnesses. Bacteriol. Proc. 1956, p. 67. Abstract.
204. Perkins, J. C., Tucker, D. N., Knopf, H. L. S., et al.: Comparison of protective effect of neutralizing antibody in serum and nasal secretions in experimental rhinovirus type 13 illness. Am. J. Epidemiol. *90*:519–526, 1969.
205. Person, D. A., and Herrmann, E. C., Jr.: Experiences in laboratory diagnosis of rhinovirus infections in routine medical practice. Mayo Clin. Proc. *45*:517–526, 1970.
206. Pevear, D. C., Fancher, M. J., Felock, P. J., et al.: Conformational change in the floor of the human rhinovirus canyon blocks absorption to HeLa cell receptors. J. Virol. *63*:2002–2007, 1989.
207. Price, W. H., Emerson, H., Ibler, I., et al.: Studies of the JH and 2060 viruses and their relationship to mild upper respiratory disease in humans. Am. J. Hyg. *69*:224–249, 1959.
208. Proud, D., Gwaltney, J. M., Jr., Hendley, J. O., et al.: Increased levels of interleukin-1 are detected in nasal secretions of volunteers during experimental rhinovirus colds. J. Infect. Dis. *169*:1007–1013, 1994.
209. Proud, D., Hendley, J. O., Gwaltney, J. M., et al.: Recent studies on the rule of kinins in inflammatory diseases of human airways. Adv. Exp. Med. Biol. *247A*:117–123, 1990.
210. Proud, D., Naclerio, R. M., Gwaltney, J. M., et al.: Kinins are generated in nasal secretions during natural rhinovirus colds. J. Infect. Dis. *161*:120–123, 1990.
211. Reed, S. E.: An investigation of the possible transmission of rhinovirus colds through indirect contact. J. Hyg. (Camb.) *75*:249–258, 1975.
212. Reilly, C. M., Hoch, S. M., Stokes, J., Jr., et al.: Clinical and laboratory findings in cases of respiratory illness caused by coryzaviruses. Ann. Intern. Med. *57*:515–525, 1962.
213. Roebuck, M. O.: Rhinoviruses in Britain 1963–1973. J. Hyg. (Camb.) *76*:137–146, 1976.
214. Rosenbaum, M. J., De Berry, P., Sullivan, E. J., et al.: Epidemiology of the common cold in military recruits with emphasis on infections by rhinovirus types 1A, 2, and two unclassified rhinoviruses. Am. J. Epidemiol. *93*:183–193, 1971.
215. Rosenquist, B. D., and Allen, G. K.: Effect of bovine fibroblast interferon on rhinovirus infection in calves. Am. J. Vet. Res. *51*:870–873, 1990.
216. Rossen, R. D., Kasel, J. A., and Couch, R. B.: The secretory immune system: Its relation to respiratory viral infection. Prog. Med. Virol. *13*:194–238, 1971.
217. Rossmann, M. G.: The canyon hypothesis: Hiding the host cell receptor attachment site on a viral surface from immune surveillance. J. Biol. Chem. *264*:14587–14590, 1989.
218. Rossmann, M. G., Arnold, E., Erickson, J. W., et al.: Structure of a human common cold virus and functional relationship to other picornaviruses. Nature *317*:145–153, 1985.
219. Rossmann, M. G., and Palmenberg, A. C.: Conservation of the putative receptor attachment site in picornaviruses. Virology *164*:373–382, 1988.
220. Rueckert, R. R.: *Picornaviridae* and their replication. *In* Fields, B. N., Knipe, D. M., Chanock, R. M., et al. (eds.): Fields Virology. 2nd ed. New York, Raven Press, 1990, pp. 507–548.

221. Ruuskanen, O., Arola, M., Putto-Laurila, A., et al.: Acute otitis media and respiratory virus infections. Pediatr. Infect. Dis. J. *8*:94–99, 1989.
222. Saketkhoo, K., Januszkiewicz, A., and Sackner, M. A.: Effects of drinking hot water, cold water, and chicken soup on nasal mucus velocity and nasal airflow resistance. Chest *74*:408–410, 1978.
223. Samo, T. C., Greenberg, S. B., Couch, R. B., et al.: Efficacy and tolerance of intranasally applied recombinant leukocyte A interferon in normal volunteers. J. Infect. Dis. *148*:535–542, 1983.
224. Sarkkinen, H., Ruuskanen, O., Meurman, O., et al.: Identification of respiratory virus antigens in middle ear fluids of children with acute otitis media. J. Infect. Dis. *151*:444–448, 1985.
225. Schieble, J. H., Lennette, E. H., and Fox, V. L.: Antigenic variation of rhinovirus type 22. Proc. Soc. Exp. Biol. Med. *133*:329–333, 1970.
226. Schmidt, H. J., and Fink, R. J.: Rhinovirus as a lower respiratory tract pathogen in infants. Pediatr. Infect. Dis. J. *10*:700–702, 1991.
227. Sherry, B., Mosser, A. G., Colonno, R. J., et al.: Use of monoclonal antibodies to identify four neutralization immunogens on a common cold picornavirus, human rhinovirus 14. J. Virol. *57*:246–257, 1986.
228. Shipkowitz, N. L., Bower, R. R., Schleicher, J. B., et al.: Antiviral activity of a bis-benzimidazole against experimental rhinovirus infections in chimpanzees. Appl. Microbiol. *23*:117–122, 1972.
229. Shult, P. A., Dick, E. C., Olander, D., et al.: The ameliorating effect of vitamin C supplementation on rhinovirus colds using an experimental epidemiologic model. Presented at the Thirtieth Interscience Conference on Antimicrobial Agents and Chemotherapy, Atlanta, Georgia, 1990. Abstract 1285.
230. Shult, P. A., Polyak, F., Dick, E. C., et al.: Adenovirus 21 infection in an isolated Antarctic station: Transmission of the virus and susceptibility of the population. Am. J. Epidemiol. *133*:599–607, 1991.
231. Skern, T., Sommergruber, W., Blaas, D., et al.: Human rhinovirus 2: Complete nucleotide sequence and proteolytic processing signals in the capsid protein region. Nucleic Acids Res. *13*:2111–2126, 1985.
232. Sperber, S. J., and Hayden, F. G.: Chemotherapy of rhinovirus colds. Antimicrob. Agents Chemother. *32*:409–419, 1988.
233. Stanway, G., Hughes, P. J., Mountford, R. C., et al.: The complete nucleotide sequence of a common cold virus: Human rhinovirus 14. Nucleic Acids Res. *12*:7859–7875, 1984.
234. Staunton, D. E., Dustin, M. L., Erickson, H. P., et al.: The arrangement of the immunoglobulin-like domains of ICAM-1 and the binding sites for LFA-1 and rhinovirus. Cell *61*:243–254, 1990.
235. Stenhouse, A. C.: Rhinovirus infection in acute exacerbations of chronic bronchitis: A controlled prospective study. B. M. J. *3*:461–463, 1967.
236. Stott, E. J., Grist, N. R., and Eadie, M. B.: Rhinovirus infections in chronic bronchitis: Isolation of eight possibly new rhinovirus serotypes. J. Med. Microbiol. *1*:109–117, 1968.
237. Stott, E. J., and Walker, M.: Antigenic variation among strains of rhinovirus type 51. Nature *224*:1311–1312, 1969.
238. Sung, B. S., Chonmaitree, T., Broemeling, L. D., et al.: Association of rhinovirus infection with poor bacteriologic outcome of bacterial-viral otitis media. Clin. Infect. Dis. *17*:38–42, 1993.
239. Swartz, M. N.: Stress and the common cold. N. Engl. J. Med. *325*:654–655, 1991.
240. Taussig, L. M., Busse, W. W., Lemen, R. J., et al.: Models of infectious airway injury in children. Am. Rev. Respir. Dis. *137*:979–984, 1988.
241. Taylor, R., Fauran, C., Berry, P., et al.: The prevalence of viruses and bacteria in the respiratory tract of pre-school children from a Vanuatu village community and the relationship with certain environmental variables. Papua New Guinea Med. J. *31*:19–27, 1988.
242. Taylor-Robinson, D., and Tyrrell, D. A. J.: Serotypes of viruses (rhinoviruses) isolated from common colds. Lancet *1*:452–454, 1962.
243. Thomas, P.: The common cold. Medical World News *32*:24–30, 1991.
244. Tomassini, J. E., Graham, D., DeWitt, C. M., et al.: cDNA cloning reveals that the major group rhinovirus receptor on HeLa cells is intercellular adhesion molecule 1. Proc. Natl. Acad. Sci. U. S. A. *86*:4907–4911, 1989.
245. Turner, R. B.: The role of neutrophils in the pathogenesis of rhinovirus infections. Pediatr. Infect. Dis. J. *9*:832–835, 1990.
246. Turner, R. B., Dutkow, F. J., Goldstein, N. J., et al.: Efficacy of oral WIN 54954 for prophylaxis of experimental rhinovirus infection. Antimicrob. Agents Chemother. *37*:297–300, 1993.
247. Turner, R. B., Hendley, J. O., and Gwaltney, J. M., Jr.: Shedding of infected ciliated epithelial cells in rhinovirus colds. J. Infect. Dis. *145*:849–853, 1982.
248. Tyrrell, D. A. J.: Common Colds and Related Diseases. Baltimore, Williams & Wilkins, 1965.
249. Tyrrell, D. A. J.: Hot news on the common cold. Am. Rev. Microbiol. *42*:35–47, 1988.
250. Tyrrell, D.: The origins of the Common Cold Unit. J. R. Coll. Physicians Lond. *24*:137–140, 1990.
251. Tyrrell, D. A. J., and Al-Nakib, W.: Prophylaxis and treatment of rhinovirus infections. *In* DeClercq, E. (ed.): Clinical Use of Antiviral Drugs. Boston, Martinus Nijhoff, 1988, pp. 241–276.
252. Tyrrell, D., Barrow, I., and Arthur, J.: Local hyperthermia benefits natural and experimental common colds. B. M. J. *298*:1280–1283, 1989.
253. Tyrrell, D. A. J., and Chanock, R. M.: Rhinoviruses: A description. Science *141*:152–153, 1963.
254. Tyrrell, D. A. J., and Parsons, R.: Some virus isolations from common colds: Cytopathic effects in tissue cultures. Lancet *1*:239, 1960.
255. Uncapher, C. R., DeWitt, C. M., and Colonno, R. J.: The major and minor group receptor families contain all but one human rhinovirus serotype. Virology *180*:814–817, 1991.
256. Urquhart, G. E. D., and Stott, E. J.: Rhinoviraemia. B. M. J. *4*:28–30, 1970.
257. Valenti, W. M., Clarke, T. A., Hall, C. B., et al.: Concurrent outbreaks of rhinovirus and respiratory syncytial virus in an intensive care nursery: Epidemiology and associated risk factors. J. Pediatr. *100*:722–726, 1982.
258. Volovitz, B., Faden, H., and Ogra, P. L.: Release of leukotriene C_4 in respiratory tract during acute viral infection. J. Pediatr. *112*:218–222, 1988.
259. Walker, D. L., and Boring, W. D.: Factors influencing host-virus interactions. III. Further studies on alteration of coxsackie virus infection in adult mice by environmental temperature. J. Immunol. *80*:39–44, 1958.
260. Warshauer, D. M., Dick, E. C., Mandel, A. D., et al.: Rhinovirus infections in an isolated Antarctic station: Transmission of the viruses and susceptibility of the population. Am. J. Epidemiol. *129*:319–340, 1989.
261. Webster, L. T., and Clow, A. D.: The association of pneumococci, *H. influenzae* and *Streptococcus hemolyticus* with coryza, pharyngitis, and sinusitis in man. J. Exp. Med. *55*:445–453, 1932.
262. Winther, B., Brofeldt, S., Christensen, B., et al.: Light and scanning electron microscopy of nasal biopsy material from patients with naturally acquired common colds. Acta Otolaryngol. (Stockh.) *97*:309–318, 1984.
263. Winther, B., Farr, B., Turner, R. B., et al.: Histopathologic examination and enumeration of polymorphonuclear leukocytes in the nasal mucosa during experimental rhinovirus colds. Acta Otolaryngol. (Stockh.) *413*(Suppl.):19–24, 1984.
264. Winther, B., Gwaltney, M. J., Jr., and Hendley, J. O.: Respiratory virus infection of monolayer cultures of human nasal epithelial cells. Am. Rev. Respir. Dis. *141*:839–845, 1990.
265. Wright, A. L., Taussig, L. M., Ray, C. G., et al.: The Tucson children's respiratory study. II. Lower respiratory tract illness in the first year of life. Am. J. Epidemiol. *129*:1232–1246, 1989.
266. Wulff, H., Noble, G. R., Maynard, J. E., et al.: An outbreak of respiratory infection in children associated with rhinovirus types 16 and 29. Am. J. Epidemiol. *90*:304–311, 1969.

172

HEPATITIS A VIRUS

Beth P. Bell, Craig N. Shapiro, and Harold S. Margolis

HISTORY

Hepatitis A has been recognized as a clinical entity for centuries, and large epidemics of jaundice occurred during military campaigns in ancient and modern times. During the past several decades, epidemiologic and clinical studies defined the infectious nature of the disease and led to the differentiation of "infectious hepatitis," now designated hepatitis A.[88, 108] Prior to 1970, attempts to isolate a virus associated with hepatitis A uniformly were unsuccessful, and information concerning the clinical course of infection, the fecal-oral route of transmission, and the efficacy of immunoglobulin in preventing disease was obtained from studies conducted in humans.[108, 109, 238] In 1973, hepatitis A virus (HAV) was identified by immune electron microscopy in stool samples of patients with hepatitis A.[62] This discovery led to the development of serologic tests that differentiated acute and resolved infections, characterization of the virus, definition of pathogenetic events during infection, and further definition of the epidemiology of HAV infection. In contrast to the other hepatitis viruses, HAV has been propagated in cell culture,[48, 164, 226] leading to the development and licensure of vaccines shown to be highly efficacious in preventing infection and disease in immunized populations.[32, 93, 225] Ideally, the next chapter in the history of hepatitis A will chronicle the elimination of this vaccine-preventable disease of children and adults.

PROPERTIES

Classification

HAV is a 27-nm, nonenveloped, positive-sense RNA virus belonging to the family *Picornaviradae*. Although HAV initially was classified in the genus *Enterovirus*, nucleotide analysis indicates HAV is distinct from all other picornaviruses.[122, 233] When compared with other enteroviruses, HAV essentially has no nucleotide or amino acid homology, does not have an intestinal replication phase, replicates slowly in cell culture and rarely produces a cytopathic effect, and is relatively resistant to inactivation by heating.[45] For these reasons, HAV has been reclassified in a separate genus designated *Hepatovirus*.[141, 233]

Genomic Organization and Genetic Variation

The HAV genome is composed of a single-stranded, positive-sense RNA of approximately 7500 nucleotides. HAV genomic organization and replication are similar to those of polio and other picornaviruses: (1) the 5′ end is not translated, appears to contain an internal ribosomal entry site, and has a covalently linked protein (VPg); (2) sequences for the structural proteins are located toward the 5′ end followed by sequences encoding nonstructural proteins that include proteases and RNA polymerases; and (3) the viral RNA encodes a single polyprotein from which functional structural and nonstructural proteins are cleaved proteolytically.[122, 227, 233] Each capsid structural motif is composed of three major polypeptides (VP1, VP2, and VP3) of 22,000 to 33,000 daltons, which form an outer shell with icosahedral symmetry. Based on nucleotide sequence, a fourth polypeptide, VP4 (2500 daltons), should be encoded but has not been identified in mature virions.[233]

HAV exists as a single serotype. The neutralization site appears to be conformational and derived from epitopes located on VP1 and VP3 as identified by neutralizing monoclonal antibodies.[146, 161] A high degree of nucleotide conservation exists among geographically diverse human HAV isolates. However, nucleotide variation in VP1 and VP3 has been used to define four human HAV genotypes, and genetic variation has proved useful in tracing unusual patterns of disease transmission.[169, 170] In addition, HAVs have been isolated that appear to be restricted in their primary replication to Old World monkeys.[147, 213] These viruses represent at least three genotypes not identified in humans.[169] Old World monkey HAV is recognized by polyclonal but not monoclonal antibodies to human HAV.

HAV replicates more slowly in cell culture than do other picornaviruses, with wild-type virus requiring many weeks of adaptation before infectious foci or HAV antigen is detected.[11, 120, 189] HAV produces a high ratio of defective to complete (infectious) virus both in cell culture and during infection.[15, 233] Cell culture adaptation is associated with mutations in nonstructural proteins and the 5′-nontranslated region.[58, 59] Cell culture–adapted HAV rarely produces a cytopathic effect, although cytopathic strains have been isolated and serve as a useful model for laboratory studies.[47, 149] Adaptation also results in loss of virulence (attenuation) when evaluated in the chimpanzee model of infectivity.[97]

The HAV virion appears to be extremely stable, although the molecular determinants of this characteristic are not known. HAV is stable in the environment, with only a 100-fold decline in infectivity over 4 weeks at room temperature.[45, 134, 135, 160] The virus retains infectivity when treated with nonionic detergents, organic solvents, and low pH at 38° C for 90 minutes.[45] HAV is more resistant than poliovirus to heat, being only partially inactivated at 60° C for 1 hour,[45] and temperatures of 85° to 95° C for 1 minute are required for complete inactivation of HAV in foods such as shellfish.[45, 140] HAV is inactivated completely by formalin (0.02 per cent at 37° C for 72 hours) but appears to be relatively resistant to free chlorine, especially when the virus is associated with organic matter.[127, 186] Only sodium hypochlorite, 2 per cent glutaraldehyde, and quaternary ammonia compound with 23 per cent hydrogen chloride have been effective in reducing the titer of HAV on contaminated surfaces.[45]

EPIDEMIOLOGY

Routes of Transmission

The routes of HAV transmission are determined by the timing and location of virus replication, circulation, and excretion occurring during infection. HAV replicates in the liver, is excreted in bile, and is found in highest concentrations in stool (up to 10^8 infectious particles/mL). The highest concentrations in stool occur during the 2-week period before jaundice develops or liver enzymes become elevated, followed by a rapid decline after jaundice appears (Fig. 172–1).[62, 194, 207] Children and infants may shed HAV for longer periods than do adults. Through the use of the polymerase chain reaction (PCR) to amplify viral nucleic acid, HAV RNA has been detected in the stools of infected neonates for up to 6 months after infection, and some studies have shown excretion among older children and adults 1 to 3 months after the onset of clinical illness.[93, 172, 236] Chronic shedding of HAV does not occur; however, virus may be present in stool dur-

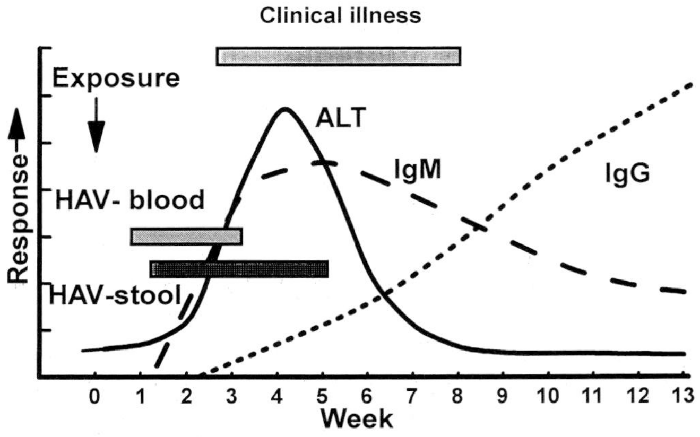

FIGURE 172–1. *Immunologic, virologic, and biochemical events during the course of a typical hepatitis A virus (HAV) infection. ALT, alanine aminotransferase.*

ing relapsing illness (see section on relapsing hepatitis A).[193] Viremia occurs during the prodromal period of the infection and extends into the symptomatic period (Fig. 172–1), with virus concentrations several orders of magnitude less than in stool.[38, 86, 110, 118] In experimentally infected animals, HAV can be detected in saliva during periods of peak excretion in stool,[38] but transmission by saliva has not been demonstrated.

The detection of HAV antigen or HAV RNA in the stool of infected persons by enzyme immunoassays and PCR cannot delineate whether a person is infectious because these assays may detect defective as well as infectious viral particles. Nucleic acid amplification by immunocapture PCR requires the presence of intact virus,[17, 95] and HAV RNA may be detected in stool for months with immunocapture PCR. However, the period of infectivity appears to be shorter than the period when HAV RNA can be detected in stool. Data from epidemiologic studies suggest that peak infectivity occurs during the 2 weeks before the onset of symptoms. For practical purposes, both children and adults with hepatitis A can be assumed to be noninfectious 1 week after jaundice appears.

Because of the high concentrations of virus in the stool of infected persons, HAV transmission primarily is by the fecal-oral route. This occurs most commonly by person-to-person transmission in households and extended family settings and between sexual contacts. Person-to-person transmission results in high rates of infection in young children in developing countries and is the predominant mode of transmission in the United States, particularly during community-wide outbreaks, as well as in outbreaks in child care centers. HAV can remain infectious in the environment,[135] and fecal contamination of food or water can result in common-source outbreaks. HAV has been transmitted by transfusion, but this occurs rarely because the blood donation must occur during the early prodromal stage of the disease or from an asymptomatic person who is viremic.[118] Transmission has not been associated with saliva. Respiratory transmission has not been reported and would be considered an unlikely route of transmission.

The risk of transmission from pregnant women who develop hepatitis A in the third trimester of pregnancy to newborns appears to be low.[211] However, HAV infection in newborns (mother-infant transmission or transfusion-acquired) usually is asymptomatic and is detected by the occurrence of hepatitis A in hospital staff or other persons having contact with the infant.[172, 221] IgG antibodies to HAV (anti-HAV) are transferred passively across the placenta.[66]

Patterns of Disease Worldwide

Worldwide, the endemicity of HAV infection differs markedly among and within countries. Four patterns of HAV infection can be differentiated, each characterized by distinct age-specific profiles of anti-HAV prevalence and hepatitis A incidence and prevailing environmental (hygienic and sanitary) and socioeconomic conditions (Table 172–1).

In areas with a high endemic pattern of infection, represented by the least developed countries (i.e., parts of Africa, Asia, Central and South America), poor socioeconomic conditions allow HAV to spread readily. Most persons are infected as young children, and essentially the entire population becomes infected before reaching adolescence, as demonstrated by the age-specific prevalence of anti-HAV (see Table 172–1).[7, 173, 214] Because virtually all HAV infections occur in age groups in which asymptomatic infection predominates, reported disease rates may be low and outbreaks rare. However, travelers to such areas from countries where HAV infection is of low endemicity are at risk for acquiring disease.

In some geographic areas, sanitary conditions are heterogeneous, HAV is not transmitted as readily, and the predominant age of infection is older than in high-endemic areas. An intermediate endemicity of HAV infection is found in Eastern Europe and parts of the former Soviet Union, Western Europe, the Americas, and Asia.[69, 202] Paradoxically, as the socioeconomic level of a country increases and the endemicity of HAV infection decreases, the overall incidence and average age of reported cases often increase because high levels of HAV transmission may occur in age groups in which symptomatic infection is more common. This has been observed, for example, in Greece, Okinawa, Israel, Iceland, Hong Kong, Thailand, and Italy.[16, 34, 77, 89, 92, 106, 201] Large common-source outbreaks also can occur because of the relatively high rate of virus transmission and large number of susceptible persons, especially among those of higher socioeconomic level. Such an outbreak occurred in Shanghai in 1988, with 250,000 cases associated with consumption of contaminated clams.[83] Nevertheless, person-to-person transmission in community-wide epidemics continues to account for much of the disease in these countries. These outbreaks often show a cyclic pattern; the outbreak subsides when the susceptible population is depleted, only to recur when a new cohort of susceptible children reach an age at which clinical disease occurs more commonly. This pattern can be seen in parts of the United States, such as in Native American communities that experience large outbreaks approximately every 7 years, during which most reported cases occur among children 5 to 15 years of age.[183]

In most areas of North America and Western Europe, sanitary and hygienic conditions are such that the endemicity of HAV infection is low (see Table 172–1). Relatively fewer children are infected, and disease often occurs in the context of community-wide and child care center outbreaks and occa-

TABLE 172–1. Epidemiologic Characteristics of Endemic Patterns of Hepatitis A Virus (HAV) Infection

	Age Group (years) Prevalence of HAV Infection (%)							
Endemicity of Infection	*0–5*	*6–10*	*11–15*	*16–20*	*21–30*	*31–40*	*>40*	**Geographic Areas***
High	40	50–100	80–100	80–100	>85	>85	>85	Africa, Middle East, most of Asia, South America, Central America
Intermediate	20	20–30	30–40	40–50	50–65	75–80	>80	Eastern Europe, former Soviet Union, most Caribbean Islands
Low	0–5	2–5	5–10	5–15	15–20	20–40	>40	Most of Western Europe, Australia, New Zealand, Japan, Canada, United States
Very low	0	0	0–1	1–3	5–10	10–15	15–35	Scandinavian countries

*See Figure 172–4.

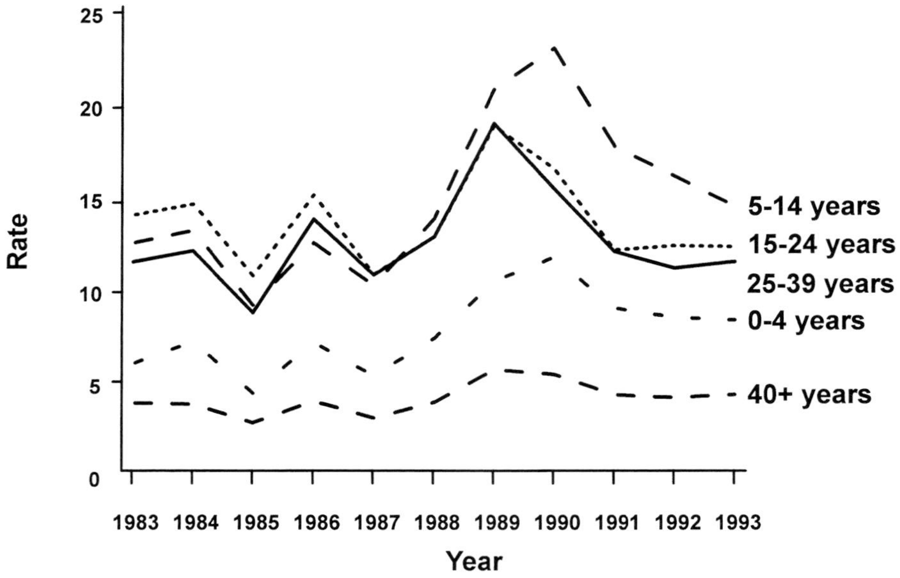

FIGURE 172–2. *Age-specific rates (per 100,000 population) of hepatitis A based on cases reported to the Centers for Disease Control and Prevention (1983–1993).*

sionally as common-source outbreaks.[69, 79, 179, 220] In some countries (e.g., Scandinavia), the endemicity of HAV infection is very low and disease occurs almost exclusively among defined risk groups, such as travelers returning from areas with a high or intermediate endemicity of infection or injecting drug users.[69, 188]

Patterns of Disease in the United States

Large nationwide epidemics have occurred approximately every 10 years, with the most recent peaking in 1989. However, even between these epidemics, disease rates are relatively high and many communities experience periodic epidemics (see section on the epidemiology of hepatitis A in specific settings). In 1994, 26,796 cases were reported to the Centers for Disease Control and Prevention (CDC), which, after correcting for underreporting, represent an estimated 80,000 cases.[27]

Hepatitis A incidence varies by age, race/ethnicity, and geographic region. The highest rates occur among children 5 to 14 years of age (Fig. 172–2), and almost 30 per cent of cases occur among children younger than 15 years of age.[30] Because many children have unrecognized asymptomatic infection, they likely represent a major reservoir for HAV transmission. Among racial/ethnic groups, rates among Native Americans and Alaska Natives are highest, more than 10 times the rate in other racial/ethnic groups. Rates among Hispanics are approximately three times higher than among non-Hispanics (Fig. 172–3). Disease rates are substantially higher in the western United States than in other regions.

Data from disease surveillance systems indicate that the most commonly reported source of infection is household or sexual contact with a person who has hepatitis A (22 to 30 per cent of reported cases).[30, 179] An additional 15 per cent of reported cases occur among children and employees of child care centers and members of their households.[179] International travel (5 to 7 per cent) and suspected food- or waterborne outbreaks (2 to 5 per cent) each account for a small proportion of cases.[30, 179] Nearly 50 per cent of patients with hepatitis A do not have a recognized source of infection[30] but may be contacts of persons, especially children, with asymptomatic infection.

As determined by phase one of the Third National Health

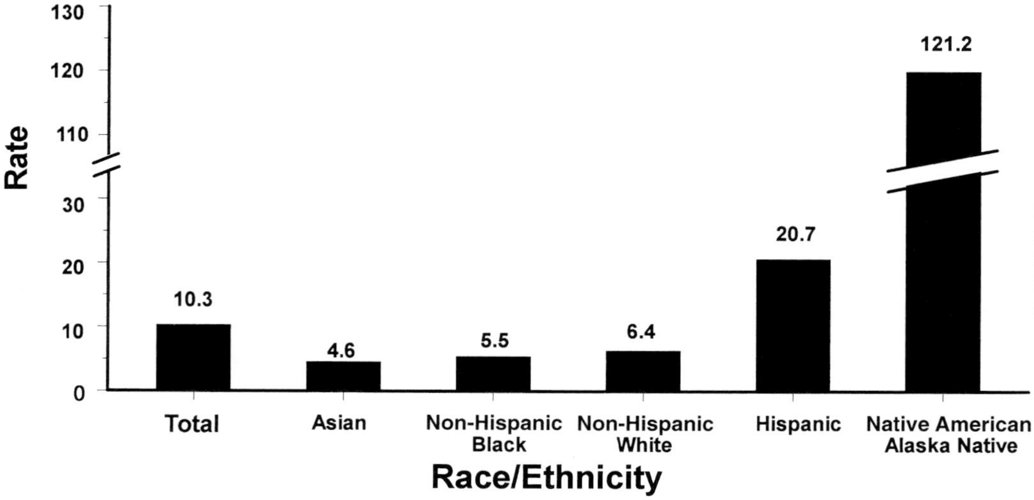

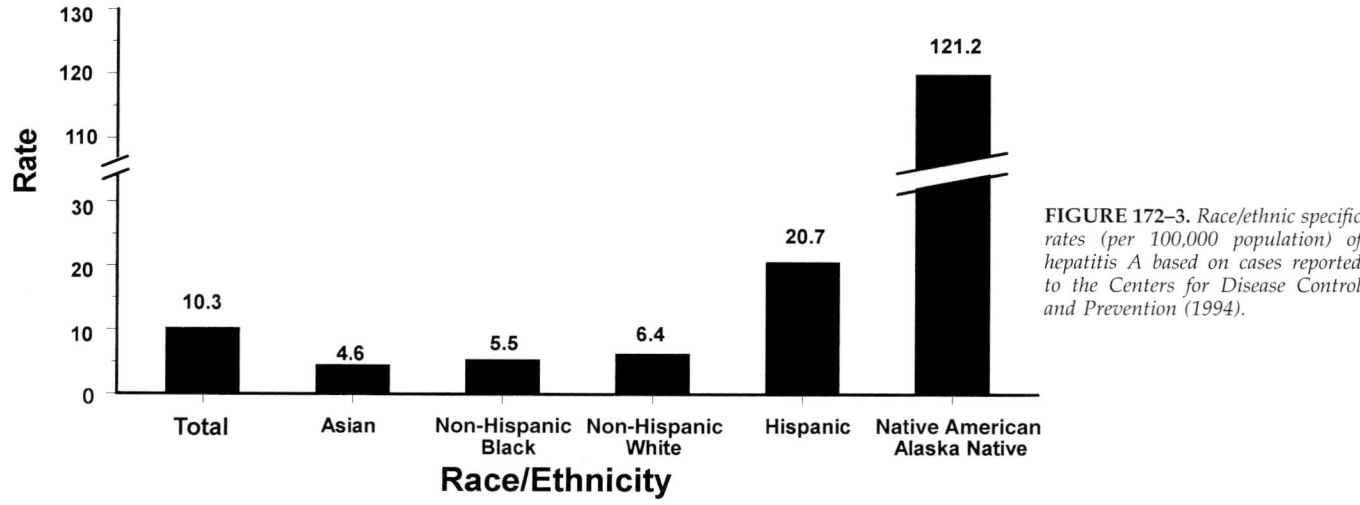

FIGURE 172–3. *Race/ethnic specific rates (per 100,000 population) of hepatitis A based on cases reported to the Centers for Disease Control and Prevention (1994).*

and Nutrition Examination Survey conducted during 1988 to 1991, 33 per cent of the U.S. population has serologic evidence of prior HAV infection (CDC, unpublished data). Anti-HAV prevalence is related directly to age, ranging from 10 per cent among children younger than 10 years of age to 75 per cent among persons older than 70 years of age, and is related inversely to income. Anti-HAV prevalence is highest among Mexican-Americans (67 per cent), compared with non-Hispanic blacks (37 per cent) and whites (29 per cent).

Epidemiology of Hepatitis A in Specific Settings

Community-Wide Outbreaks

Most hepatitis A in the United States appears to occur in the context of community-wide outbreaks during which infection is transmitted person-to-person in households and extended family settings.[23] These outbreaks, often persisting for several years, have been difficult to control by conventional preventive measures such as increasing awareness of the importance of hand washing and postexposure prophylaxis with immunoglobulin.[183, 184] Communities that experience outbreaks can be categorized as high-rate or intermediate-rate based on epidemiologic characteristics such as age-specific rates of infection and temporal patterns of disease incidence (Table 172–2). High-rate communities, as exemplified by Native American or Alaska Native communities, usually are geographically, socially, or ethnically well defined and typically have epidemics every 5 to 10 years.[20, 158, 175, 183, 234] During these outbreaks, disease rates are very high, and most disease occurs among children 5 to 14 years of age[20, 183] because nearly all adults have serologic evidence of prior HAV infection.[183, 231, 234] Outbreaks in intermediate-rate communities generally have less well-defined periodicity and lower overall disease rates.[184] These communities range in size from large metropolitan areas to rural or semirural communities with heterogeneous populations.[5, 67] The highest rates of disease are observed among older children and young adults; however, hepatitis A rates commonly increase among all age and racial/ethnic groups during outbreaks, indicating widespread disease within the community.[8] In addition, disproportionate increases in disease incidence may occur among populations defined by certain demographic characteristics or behaviors that place them at increased risk of infection (e.g., injecting drug users, homosexual men).[8, 24, 26, 84, 176]

Children play an important role in HAV transmission in communities with high or intermediate disease rates. In high-rate communities, the pattern of transmission is similar to that found in countries with an intermediate endemicity of HAV infection (see Table 172–1). Asymptomatic transmission occurs among susceptible young children at low levels during interepidemic periods until a cohort of susceptible children becomes large enough to sustain a community-wide outbreak.[183] Asymptomatic transmission among children also may be important in sustaining outbreaks in some intermediate-rate communities. During such an outbreak, 25 per cent of children younger than 6 years of age who were household contacts of adults with hepatitis A with no identified source of infection were IgM anti-HAV–positive (CDC, unpublished data).

Child Care Centers

The role of children with asymptomatic infection has been recognized in outbreaks in child care centers since the 1970s.[180] Because infection among children usually is mild or asymptomatic, these outbreaks often are not recognized until adult contacts (usually parents) become ill.[82] Outbreaks rarely occur in centers that do not have children in diapers and are more common in larger centers.[82] Both poor hygiene among these children and the need for staff to handle and change diapers contribute to spread. Despite the occurrence of outbreaks when HAV is introduced into a child care center, studies of child care center employees do not show a significantly increased prevalence of HAV infection compared with control populations.[65, 94] Occasionally, outbreaks in child care centers can be the source of more extensive transmission within a community.[51, 81] However, the frequency with which this occurs nationwide has not been determined, and it is likely that most disease within child care centers reflects disease transmission from the community.

Other Groups and Settings

Hepatitis A cases among children in schools usually reflect disease that has been acquired in the community. However, multiple cases among children within a school may indicate a common-source outbreak.[150] Historically, HAV infection was endemic in institutions for the developmentally disabled, but

TABLE 172–2. Features of Communities That Have High and Intermediate Rates of Hepatitis A Virus (HAV) Infection

Community	Anti-HAV Prevalence	Usual Age of Patients	Reported Annual Incidence*	Outbreak Periodicity	Populations	Examples
High rate	30–40% (<5 years old) 70–100% (>15 years old)	5–14 years	700–1000	5–10 years	Well defined geographically or ethnically	Alaska Native villages, Native American reservations, selected Hispanic communities, selected religious communities
Intermediate rate	10–25% (<5 years old) <50% (>15 years old)	5–29 years	50–200	May be periodic	Less defined than in high-rate communities	Zanesville, OH, Oklahoma, St. Louis, MO, selected religious communities

*Typical reported incidence per 100,000 population per year during epidemics, all ages.

From CDC: Prevention of hepatitis A through active or passive immunization: Recommendations of the Advisory Committee on Immunization Practices. M. M. W. R. *45*(RR-15):1–30, 1996.

with smaller facilities and improved conditions, the incidence and prevalence of infection have decreased and outbreaks rarely are reported.[203]

During the two past decades, outbreaks have been reported with increasing frequency among illicit drug users in the United States and Europe.[24, 84, 176] In the United States, these outbreaks often have occurred in the context of a large community-wide outbreak.[8] In the late 1980s, 10 to 19 per cent of persons with hepatitis A reported a history of injecting drug use.[28] The mode of transmission among users of illicit drugs has not been determined. One anecdotal report suggested that a fecally contaminated drug may act as a vehicle for HAV transmission. However, person-to-person transmission because of poor personal hygiene and sanitary conditions is the most likely source of infection. Reuse of needles contaminated with HAV-infected blood may cause some infections.

Hepatitis A outbreaks among men who have sex with men have been reported frequently, most recently in urban areas in the United States, Canada, England, and Australia.[26] These outbreaks may occur in the context of an outbreak in the larger community.[8] In prospective studies, HAV infection rates among men who have sex with men are severalfold higher compared with control populations.[41, 42]

Transfusion-related hepatitis A is rare because the period of viremia during infection is relatively short, HAV does not result in chronic infection, and blood donors are screened for elevated aminotransferase levels. However, outbreaks have been reported in Europe and the United States among patients who received factor VIII and factor IX concentrates prepared using solvent-detergent treatment to inactivate lipid-containing viruses.[31, 128] HAV is resistant to solvent-detergent treatment, and contamination presumably occurred from plasma donors with hepatitis A who donated during the incubation period. The risk of infection in patients with hemophilia is not known, although data from one serologic survey of hemophiliac patients suggest they may be at increased risk for HAV infection.[126] Transmission related to blood transfusions also has resulted in nosocomial outbreaks in neonatal intensive care units. The source of infection was blood donated by persons incubating HAV followed by transmission from transfused, infected infants to other infants and staff.[100, 151, 172] Hepatitis A has been reported in adult cancer patients treated with lymphocytes incubated in serum from a donor with HAV infection.[222]

Nosocomial transmission from adult patients to health care workers usually has been associated with fecal incontinence of the patient.[75, 156] Such transmission is rare, however, because most patients with hepatitis A are hospitalized after the onset of jaundice, when infectivity is low.[194] Health care workers have not been found to have an increased prevalence of anti-HAV compared with control populations in several serologic surveys conducted in the United States.[71, 98]

Persons from developed countries who travel to developing countries with a high or intermediate endemicity of HAV infection are at substantial risk of acquiring hepatitis A.[198] In prospective studies, the risk of infection for travelers who do not receive immunoglobulin was found to be 3 to 5 per 1000 per month of stay,[199] of the same order of magnitude as that for malaria and higher than for cholera or typhoid. The risk may be higher among travelers staying in areas with poor hygienic conditions,[112] varies according to the region and the length of stay, and appears to be increased even among travelers who reported observing protective measures and staying in urban areas or luxury hotels (CDC, unpublished data). In some European countries, returning international travelers with hepatitis A account for a substantial proportion of reported cases (16 to 40 per cent),[35, 228] but only approximately 5 per cent of reported cases in the United States occur in persons with a history of recent international travel.[179]

Food-borne or water-borne hepatitis A outbreaks are relatively uncommon in the United States. Food-borne outbreaks usually are associated with contamination of food during preparation by a food handler with HAV infection. Implicated foods include those not cooked after handling, such as sandwiches and salads, glazed pastries, ice, and cold drinks, as well as partially cooked foods.[21, 25, 80, 113, 125, 142, 145, 157, 195, 223] Control of these outbreaks usually requires intensive public health efforts. However, persons who work as food handlers are not at increased risk for hepatitis A because of their occupation. Food contaminated before retail distribution, such as shellfish harvested from polluted water and lettuce or fruits contaminated at the growing or processing stage, has been responsible for hepatitis A outbreaks.[50, 53, 138, 150, 154, 162, 167, 171] Water-borne hepatitis A outbreaks are rare and related to sewage contamination or inadequate treatment of water.[10, 12, 14, 18, 68]

PATHOGENESIS AND PATHOLOGY

Pathology

Because HAV infection is self-limited and does not result in chronic liver disease, liver biopsy rarely is indicated (see section on the treatment of acute hepatitis A). The light microscopic findings in acute hepatitis A, which include inflammatory cell infiltration, hepatocellular necrosis, and liver cell regeneration, are common to all forms of acute viral hepatitis. These histologic findings vary with the stage and severity of hepatitis. Early biopsy specimens generally show portal infiltration by lymphocytes, plasma cells, and periodic acid–Schiff positive macrophages.[54, 208] Spotty or focal necrosis commonly is seen, as evidenced by balloon degeneration, shrinkage, and fragmentation of hepatocytes.[54] HAV antigen is found primarily in the cytoplasm of hepatocytes but also can be found in liver macrophages.

Differences have been noted in the light microscopic finding of hepatitis A compared with other forms of viral hepatitis, particularly hepatitis B. In addition to degeneration of hepatocytes in the perivenular area, periportal inflammation and destruction of hepatocytes adjacent to the portal area may be more pronounced than in hepatitis B.[1, 155, 208] Findings in some patients may be difficult to distinguish from chronic hepatitis, including extension of the inflammatory infiltration from the periportal area into the hepatic parenchyma and disruption of the limiting plate.[1, 54] Cholestasis may be more prominent than in hepatitis B.[177]

The histologic findings of fulminant hepatitis A are indistinguishable from those in other forms of fulminant viral hepatitis. Examination of pathologic specimens shows massive hepatic necrosis, abnormal architecture of surviving hepatocytes, and a diffuse inflammatory response.[103] Viral antigen can be found in pathologic specimens.

Cellular Immune Response

Unlike other picornaviruses, infection of cultured cells with wild-type HAV has no cytopathic effects. It generally is assumed that HAV infection also is noncytopathic in vivo and therefore that the cytopathic changes in the liver associated with hepatitis A are immune mediated. This is supported by the finding that symptoms and biochemical evidence of liver injury do not occur at the time of maximal virus replication and fecal shedding (during the late incubation period).

Rather, liver injury is associated closely with viral clearance. CD8+, class 1–dependent, cytotoxic, virus-specific T cells that are capable of producing interferon-γ are present in the circulation and the liver.[64, 215, 216] Additional inflammatory cells, recruited to the site of infection by interferon-γ and other cytokines secreted by CD8+ cells, may be responsible for much of the liver injury. Complement has been shown to bind to HAV capsid proteins, and serum complement levels drop during infection, but whether complement-mediated cellular injury occurs is unclear.[131] The mechanism by which infection is resolved remains unclear.

Humoral Immune Response

Antibodies directed against conformational epitopes, displayed on intact virions as well as empty viral capsids, are produced during the later stages of infection (see section on genomic organization and genetic variation). Virus-specific IgM as well as IgG and IgA antibodies are present in serum; IgM anti-HAV first can be detected at the onset of symptoms (see section on serologic events in acute HAV infection). Antibodies that react with nonstructural proteins also have been detected; their presence may differentiate immunity because of prior infection from that gained by immunization (see section on inactivated vaccines).[46, 96]

CLINICAL MANIFESTATIONS

Similar to other forms of viral hepatitis, the clinical manifestations of HAV infection are variable, ranging from asymptomatic anicteric infection to symptoms of acute hepatitis, including fever, malaise, anorexia, nausea, vomiting, and right upper quadrant pain. The likelihood of having symptomatic HAV infection and the severity of the illness are related to the age of the patient. In early childhood, infection usually is asymptomatic, whereas infection in adulthood usually is accompanied by symptoms. The diagnosis of hepatitis A is a serologic diagnosis because no constellation of symptoms is pathognomonic of the disease.

Incubation Period

The average incubation period is 28 to 30 days but can range from 15 to 50 days.[107] The average incubation period has been reported to be shorter among patients who acquired HAV infection by parenteral transmission from contaminated blood products and chimpanzees infected parenterally compared with those infected oral-gastrically.[132, 185]

Spectrum of Illness

HAV infection, evidenced by the detection of IgM anti-HAV in serum, can be inapparent (asymptomatic, with no elevation in serum aminotransferase levels), subclinical (asymptomatic, with elevation of serum aminotransferase levels), or clinically evident (with symptoms). Specific symptoms of liver dysfunction include jaundice and dark urine due to hyperbilirubinemia. However, symptomatic hepatitis A without jaundice (anicteric) occurs. Nonspecific symptoms of acute hepatitis A can include fever, myalgia, anorexia, nausea, right upper quadrant pain or discomfort, diarrhea, and pruritus.

Many acute HAV infections, particularly inapparent and subclinical infection and anicteric hepatitis A, are not recognized as cases of viral hepatitis.[235] The frequency of symptoms with acute infection is influenced strongly by age. Children are less likely to have symptomatic infection compared with adults, and jaundice is rare among children younger than 6 years of age.[73] In one report describing outbreaks in several day care centers, the proportion of infected children without symptoms was 84 per cent among children younger than 3 years of age, 50 per cent among children 3 to 4 years of age, and 20 per cent among children 5 years of age or older.[82] Most adults develop symptoms with acute infection. In a study of two outbreaks among young adult U.S. military personnel, 76 to 97 per cent of infected persons developed symptoms and approximately 55 per cent were icteric.[114]

Clinical Signs and Symptoms

In the individual patient, the clinical symptoms of acute hepatitis A are indistinguishable from those due to other forms of viral hepatitis. Particularly in older children and adults, the onset of illness often is quite abrupt and may consist of fever, myalgia, anorexia, malaise, nausea, intermittent, dull abdominal pain, and vomiting. Fever, rarely higher than 102° F, and headache occur more frequently than in other forms of acute viral hepatitis.[204] Many pediatric patients may have diarrhea or, less commonly, upper respiratory symptoms, such as cough, sore throat, and runny nose, and the diagnosis of hepatitis A might not be considered in children presenting with predominantly respiratory or gastrointestinal symptoms and transient fever without the typical malaise, fatigue, and anorexia.[63, 116] Dark urine followed by jaundice and light-colored stools, if present, will appear within a few days to a week after the onset of the prodromal symptoms.[9, 78, 114, 116] When this icteric phase begins, symptoms often resolve and appetite returns in young children, but older children and adult patients may experience a transient worsening in the prodromal symptoms of anorexia, malaise, and weakness.[103, 144]

In addition to jaundice and scleral icterus, physical findings may include mild hepatomegaly and tenderness, but severe tenderness suggests other diagnoses. The spleen may be palpable in 10 to 20 per cent of patients, and there may be posterior cervical adenopathy.[37, 114, 212] Ascites, peripheral edema, and findings indicative of hepatic encephalopathy suggest the presence of a more severe form of hepatitis (see section on atypical clinical manifestations and complications of hepatitis A). Ultrasonographic findings among children with uncomplicated hepatitis A have included edema of the gallbladder wall, abdominal lymphadenopathy, and, less commonly, transient ascites.[37]

The symptoms of hepatitis A last for several weeks on average and usually not longer than 2 months.[104] Prolonged or relapsing hepatitis A can occur (see section on relapsing hepatitis A).

Laboratory Abnormalities

As in other forms of viral hepatitis, during HAV infection inflammation of the liver is accompanied by abnormalities in serum hepatic enzymes, with increases in serum alanine aminotransferase (ALT), aspartate aminotransferase (AST), alkaline phosphatase, and gamma-glutamyltranspeptidase (GGTP) levels. Elevations of serum ALT and AST occur most consistently and may precede symptoms by a week or more (see Fig. 172–1). Peak levels generally occur 3 to 10 days after the onset of symptoms and are between 200 IU and 5000 IU but can reach as high as 20,000 IU. The level of ALT usually is higher than that of AST because the inflammatory response is destructive particularly to the plasma membrane in acute viral hepatitis. ALT is found in the cytosol of the plasma membrane, whereas AST is located mainly in cell mitochondria.[78]

Serum bilirubin levels, although frequently elevated, usually remain below 10 mg/dL and peak 1 to 2 weeks after illness begins. Higher levels can be seen in some patients, especially when HAV infection is complicated by cholestasis (see section on cholestatic hepatitis A) or hemolysis secondary to an underlying glucose-6-phosphate dehydrogenase (G-6-PD) deficiency state.[33] In patients with G-6-PD deficiency, indirect bilirubin may account for more than 50 per cent of the total bilirubin. Alkaline phosphatase and 5′ nucleotidase activity usually are only mildly elevated, rarely reaching more than two or three times above the normal level. GGTP levels usually are 3 to 10 times the upper limit of normal.

Serum immunoglobulin levels often are elevated, and IgM levels frequently are higher than in acute hepatitis B and non-A, non-B hepatitis.[237] In patients without underlying liver disease, prothrombin time usually is normal. A prolonged prothrombin time, usually associated with severe liver damage, is a prognostic indicator for the development of fulminant hepatitis.[232]

Patients with acute HAV infection usually have a mild lymphocytosis with occasional atypical mononuclear cells.[144] Except in patients who have hemolysis associated with G-6-PD deficiency, the hematocrit is normal.[33, 144]

Except in patients who have relapsing or cholestatic hepatitis A (see section on atypical clinical manifestations and complications of hepatitis A), serum bilirubin and aminotransferase levels usually return to normal by 2 to 3 months after the onset of illness in the majority of patients.[104]

Serologic Events in Acute Hepatitis A Virus Infection

Because the pattern and magnitude of symptoms and hepatic enzyme abnormalities of hepatitis A are not distinctive of hepatitis A, the diagnosis requires serologic detection of specific antibody responses to HAV. Sensitive and specific radioimmunoassays (RIAs) or enzyme immunoassays (EIAs) show that virtually all patients have detectable IgM anti-HAV during the acute or early convalescent phase of HAV infection (see Fig. 172–1).[124] A small proportion (3 per cent) of patients tested within 3 days of the onset of symptoms may be IgM anti-HAV–negative but become IgM anti-HAV–positive within the first 2 weeks of illness.[124] During the first 4 to 8 weeks after the onset of symptoms, the titer of IgM anti-HAV in serum is high.[85] Antibody generally disappears within 6 months, although rarely it can be detected for 2 years or longer.[56, 85, 102, 124] IgM anti-HAV may be detectable for a longer period in patients with symptomatic illness than in those with asymptomatic infection.[85, 195]

IgG anti-HAV is present at a low titer at or shortly after the onset of acute HAV infection, and the titer rises over several weeks as the IgM anti-HAV titer falls (see Fig. 172–1). IgG anti-HAV remains detectable in serum for the lifetime of the individual and confers lasting protection against disease. Secretory IgA antibodies are detected in a minority of humans or primates with acute HAV infection but are unlikely to provide any significant protection against HAV infection.[196]

Commercially available immunoassays (RIAs or EIAs) detect either total (IgG and IgM) antibody against HAV capsid proteins using a competitive inhibition (blocking) format or IgM antibody to capsid proteins using an IgM capture format.[117] These assays do not measure the neutralizing antibodies responsible for biologic activity against HAV, but the detection of total anti-HAV by conventional assays is correlated with the appearance of neutralizing antibodies.[105, 117] Neutralizing antibodies elicited against one strain of HAV have been shown to have biologic activity against other HAV strains.[119]

When tested in parallel with a World Health Organization anti-HAV reference reagent, the lower limit of detection of commercially available assays is approximately 100 mIU/mL of anti-HAV.[70, 117] Administration of small amounts of immunoglobulin provide a high level of protection against hepatitis A, although the antibody concentrations achieved by passive immunization with immunoglobulin or active immunization with vaccine are 10- to 100-fold lower than those produced after natural infection.[117] Antibody concentrations achieved by passive immunization and occasionally by active immunization but known to provide protection against HAV infection both in vivo and in vitro may be below the level of detection of the commercial immunoassays. However, the low levels of neutralizing antibody that provide protection in these situations can be detected by assays that measure the inhibition of HAV in cell culture (i.e., radioimmunofocus inhibition test or plaque assay).[3, 47, 117, 119]

The lower limit of antibody necessary to provide protection against HAV infection is unknown. In vitro studies with cell culture–derived virus suggest that low levels of antibody (e.g., <20 mIU/mL) are neutralizing.[119] Clinical trials that evaluated vaccine efficacy have not provided an estimate of the minimum protective antibody level because vaccine-induced levels of antibody have been very high and few infections have occurred in vaccinees. Experimental studies in chimpanzees indicate that very low levels of passively transferred antibody (<10 mIU/mL) obtained from immunized individuals do not protect against infection but prevent clinical hepatitis and virus shedding.[165]

ATYPICAL CLINICAL MANIFESTATIONS AND COMPLICATIONS OF HEPATITIS A (Table 172–3)

Relapsing Hepatitis A

Relapsing hepatitis is a relatively common manifestation of hepatitis A that occurs in approximately 10 per cent of patients.[178] One to 4 months after the initial episode of acute hepatitis, these patients have a second episode of hepatitis; more than one relapse is rare.[74, 178, 210] Patients with relapsing hepatitis A have no distinctive clinical features of their first disease episode. After the first episode, most patients experi-

TABLE 172–3. Atypical Clinical Manifestations and Complications of Hepatitis A Virus Infection

Relapsing hepatitis A[74, 178, 210]
Fulminant hepatitis A[133, 152, 166, 209]
Extrahepatic manifestations
Transient rash or arthralgias[72, 210]
Papular acrodermatitis of childhood[174]
Cutaneous vasculitis[49, 90, 91]
Cryoglobulinemia[90, 91, 178]
Guillain-Barré syndrome[205]
Other neurologic syndromes (e.g., myeloradiculopathy, mononeuritis, vertigo)[13, 159]
Cholestatic hepatitis A[76, 210]
Hepatitis A triggering autoimmune hepatitis[210, 219]

ence a significant improvement in symptoms and biochemical abnormalities. However, the reported frequency with which serum aminotransferase levels completely normalize during this period has been variable; in one report, this occurred in only one of seven patients with relapsing hepatitis A.[210] The relapse episode of hepatitis rarely is more severe than the initial episode and is accompanied by elevation of serum aminotransferase levels (typically to >1000 mIU/mL) and persistence of IgM anti-HAV. Molecular studies have demonstrated the presence of HAV in stool and HAV RNA in serum during relapse, but whether patients are infectious is unknown.[74] The illness usually lasts a total of 16 to 40 weeks and results in full recovery.[74, 178] Although the pathogenesis of relapsing hepatitis is unknown, it most probably is immunologically mediated.[178] Persistent HAV infection with a relapsing clinical course has been reported in patients after liver transplantation for fulminant hepatitis A; HAV-specific genomic sequences have been identified in the grafts of these patients.[61, 232]

Fulminant Hepatitis A

Only a small proportion of all fulminant hepatitis is due to hepatitis A.[133, 166, 209] Among patients hospitalized with hepatitis A, the case-fatality rate has been estimated to be 0.14 per cent.[78] However, based on all cases of hepatitis A reported in the United States, the case-fatality rate from fulminant hepatitis A is approximately 0.4 per cent (CDC, unpublished data). Host factors reported to be associated with an increased risk of fulminant hepatitis include older age[78, 111] and underlying chronic liver disease.[2, 99, 121, 230] In molecular studies that have examined capsid sequences, fulminant hepatitis A was not associated with viral variants.

There are no distinctive clinical features of fulminant hepatitis A that distinguish it from fulminant hepatic failure from other causes. Within approximately 8 weeks of the onset of illness, patients with no history of prior liver disease develop symptoms of hepatic encephalopathy and a marked prolongation of the prothrombin time.[152] Complications can include cerebral edema, sepsis, gastrointestinal bleeding, and hypoglycemia. The prognosis of fulminant hepatitis A without transplantation is better than that of fulminant disease related to other viral etiologies, and close to 70 per cent of patients without cerebral edema can be expected to recover.[72, 153, 209]

Extrahepatic Manifestations

During acute hepatitis A, transient rash and arthralgias occur in up to 14 per cent and 19 per cent of patients, respectively, particularly during the prodromal period.[72, 210] Urticaria has been reported but occurs less frequently than in acute hepatitis B.[55] Papular acrodermatitis of childhood, the Gianotti-Crosti syndrome, is rare in the United States but has been reported elsewhere in association with HAV infection.[174] The cutaneous lesions, consisting of nonpruritic, symmetric, flat papules on the face, extremities, and buttocks, may persist for several weeks before spontaneously resolving.[57]

Other extrahepatic manifestations that occur chiefly in association with cholestatic or relapsing hepatitis A include cutaneous vasculitis and cryoglobulinemia.[49, 90, 91] The vasculitis, manifested as erythematous maculopapular lesions often affecting the lower extremities and buttocks and typically associated with purpura, appears as leukocytoclastic vasculitis and granular deposits of IgM anti-HAV and complement in blood vessel walls in skin biopsy specimens. Cryoglobulinemia includes cryoglobulins composed of IgG and IgM and IgM anti-HAV antibodies.[49, 90, 91, 178] These manifestations resolve spontaneously with the resolution of hepatitis.

In the absence of fulminant disease, neurologic syndromes have been reported only rarely in association with hepatitis A. Guillain-Barré syndrome has been reported, occurring 3 days to 2 weeks after onset of hepatitis A, as well as myeloradiculopathy, vertigo, mononeuritis (cranial or peripheral nerve), meningoencephalitis, and exacerbation of multiple sclerosis.[13, 159, 205]

Cholestatic Hepatitis A

Cholestatic hepatitis occurs in a small percentage of patients with hepatitis A. These patients are deeply icteric and may have pruritus, fatigue, fever, loose stools, anorexia, dark urine, and weight loss. In two reports of 10 patients with cholestatic hepatitis A, peak serum bilirubin levels generally were higher than 10 mg/dL, reaching as high as 38 mg/dL, and remained elevated for 12 to 16 weeks.[76, 210] Serum aminotransferase levels declined but remained elevated during the period of cholestasis. In one of these reports, five patients had prolonged prothrombin times that normalized with administration of vitamin K.[76]

Cholestatic hepatitis due to hepatitis A can be distinguished from obstructive jaundice by the finding of a normal abdominal ultrasound. Further invasive diagnostic procedures such as liver biopsy or direct forms of cholangiography are not necessary in most cases.[178] Although patients will recover completely without therapy, a course of corticosteroids with a gradual taper over at least 4 weeks has been reported to hasten the relief of symptoms and the resolution of cholestasis.[178]

Hepatitis A Triggering Autoimmune Hepatitis

Several reports have described patients in whom hepatitis A is followed by type 1 autoimmune chronic hepatitis.[210, 219] Laboratory studies demonstrated a T-cell defect in these patients, suggesting a genetic predisposition to the development of autoimmune hepatitis that is "triggered" by HAV infection. These patients have required corticosteroid therapy, sometimes for long periods.

TREATMENT

There is no specific therapy for hepatitis A, and because HAV infection is self-limited and does not result in chronic infection or chronic liver disease, treatment generally is supportive. Hospitalization may be necessary for patients who are dehydrated from nausea and vomiting or who have fulminant hepatic failure. Because there are no conclusive data indicating that bed rest or inactivity influences the course of illness, no restriction of activity is necessary. Similarly, no specific diet is indicated, although many patients may have an intolerance to fatty foods during their illness. Medications should be used with caution, particularly those that have the potential to cause hepatic damage and those that are metabolized by the liver. The half-life of these latter medications may be prolonged.

For fulminant hepatic failure due to hepatitis A, small uncontrolled trials conducted among adults suggest that some patients have benefitted from prostaglandin E and interferon, and amantadine and ribavirin have shown activity in vitro against HAV.[44, 123, 190] There is no evidence that exchange transfusions, plasmapheresis, or corticosteroids are effective.[60, 78] Liver transplantation is successful in some patients.[197, 209, 232] Persistent HAV infection has been demonstrated in some transplant recipients, but whether this affects survival is unknown.[61] Because survival without transplantation among adult and pediatric patients is high[72, 153, 209] and no single factor is predictive of a poor outcome, it has been difficult to establish criteria for choosing candidates for transplantation. Some centers have used the presence of severe coagulopathy and older age, with or without the presence of an elevated bilirubin level and prolonged jaundice,[153, 232] or liver volume on computed tomographic scan and degree of histologic damage on liver biopsy.[218] Survival after transplantation among patients with fulminant hepatitis from all viral causes is 40 to 89 per cent and depends on the severity of liver failure.[115, 209, 232]

PREVENTION

Hepatitis A can be prevented by (1) general measures of good personal hygiene, particularly hand washing, provision of safe drinking water, and proper disposal of sanitary waste; (2) pre- or postexposure immunization with immunoglobulin; and (3) pre-exposure immunization with hepatitis A vaccine.

Immunoglobulin

Immunoglobulin (IG) is a sterile solution of antibodies prepared by a serial cold ethanol precipitation procedure from pooled human plasma that has tested negative for hepatitis B surface antigen, antibody to HIV, and antibody to hepatitis C virus.[39] This precipitation procedure has been shown to inactivate hepatitis B virus and HIV.[22] Since 1995, immunoglobulin prepared in the United States has been required to be negative for hepatitis C virus RNA by PCR amplification or to be produced using a method that ensures additional virus inactivation. When administered before exposure or within 2 weeks after exposure, IG is more than 85 per cent effective in preventing hepatitis A by passive transfer of anti-HAV.[101, 143, 200] Whether IG completely prevents infection or leads to asymptomatic infection and the development of persistent anti-HAV (passive-active immunity) probably is related to the amount of time that has elapsed between exposure and IG administration.[116, 200] Although in recent years IG lots have had slightly lower titers of anti-HAV, probably because of decreasing prevalence of prior HAV infection among plasma donors, no clinical or epidemiologic evidence of decreased efficacy has been reported.[206]

Household and sexual contacts of patients with hepatitis A should receive IG as soon as possible but no later than 2 weeks after exposure.[32] Aggressive use of IG is indicated to control hepatitis A outbreaks in child care centers where a child or employee is diagnosed with hepatitis A (Table 172–4)[32, 181] and in other settings (e.g., hospitals, facilities for developmentally disabled persons) when outbreaks occur.[32] When a food handler is identified with hepatitis A, IG should be administered to other food handlers at the food establishment and under limited circumstances to patrons.[21, 32] Once cases are identified that are associated with a food service establishment, it generally is too late to administer IG to patrons because the 2-week postexposure period during which IG is effective will have passed.

TABLE 172–4. Control of Hepatitis A in Child Care Centers

If a child or employee at a child care center is diagnosed with hepatitis A or hepatitis A cases are identified within a 6-week period in two or more families using the same center, center attendees and employees should receive immunoglobulin.
- If diapered children are at the child care center, immunoglobulin should be given to all children and employees at the center. Immunoglobulin also should be given to newly enrolled children and new employees during the 6 weeks after the last center-associated case is identified.
- If no diapered children are at the child care center, immunoglobulin should be administered only to classroom contacts (children and staff) of the infected child.
- If the child with hepatitis A is an older child with no link to a diapered child, immunoglobulin only for classroom contacts can be considered.

Immunoglobulin administration to household contacts of diapered children in the child care center should be considered if three or more family members are affected or if the outbreak is recognized more than 3 weeks after the first case becomes ill.

Parents should be notified not to transfer their children to another center.

Health care providers should report cases of hepatitis A to local public health authorities and consult with local public health authorities regarding preventive measures.

Adapted from Shapiro, C. N., and Hadler, S. C.: Hepatitis A and hepatitis B virus infections in day care centers. Pediatr. Ann. *20*:435–441, 1991.

IG also may be given to children and adolescents who are traveling to countries with high or intermediate endemicity of HAV infection (Fig. 172–4) instead of or in addition to hepatitis A vaccine.[32] IG should be given to children younger than 2 years of age who are traveling to such countries, because hepatitis A vaccine is not licensed for children in this age group (see section on inactivated vaccines).[32] Although hepatitis A often is asymptomatic in infants and young children, pre-exposure prophylaxis is indicated to prevent the rare severe cases that occur and transmission to others after returning from abroad.

For postexposure prophylaxis, 0.02 mL/kg body weight of IG should be administered intramuscularly. For infants and young children, the injection can be administered in the anterolateral thigh or deltoid muscles; for older children and adolescents, the injection should be administered in the deltoid or gluteus, muscles into which a large volume of IG can be injected.[29] If the IG is administered in the gluteus, the injection should be given in the superior-lateral aspect to avoid sciatic nerve injury.[29]

For pre-exposure prophylaxis of travelers, the dose of IG is 0.02 mL/kg body weight if travel will be for less than 3 months. Because of the decay of passive immunity over time, a dose of 0.06 mL/kg is necessary for persons who will be abroad for 3 to 5 months, and readministration every 5 months is necessary for extended trips. IG does not interfere with the immune response to oral polio virus or yellow fever vaccine or, in general, to inactivated vaccines. However, IG can interfere with the immune response to some live attenuated vaccines (e.g., measles, mumps, rubella, varicella). Administration of these vaccines should be delayed for at least

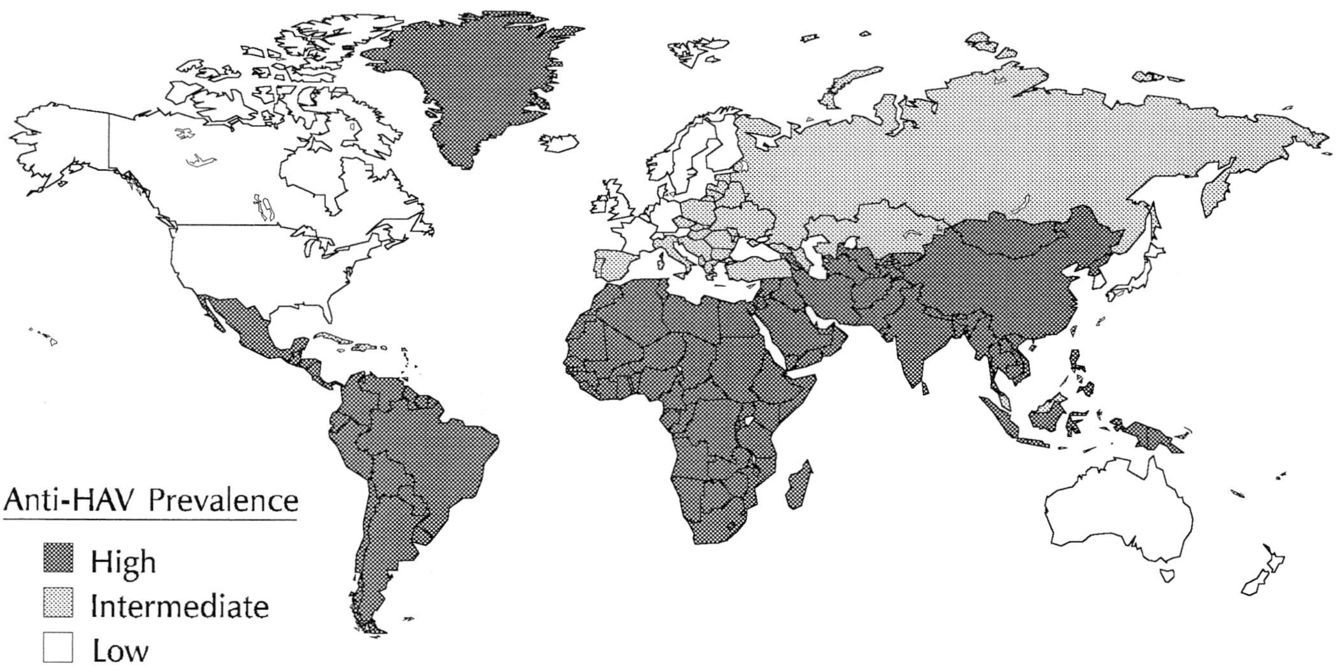

FIGURE 172–4. *Worldwide distribution of patterns of endemicity of hepatitis A virus (HAV) infection. A country's endemicity of infection has been generalized from best available data and may vary within parts of the country.*

5 months after administration of IG, and IG should not be given within 2 weeks after the administration of these vaccines (or within 3 weeks for varicella vaccine).[29] For children younger than 2 years of age traveling to areas of intermediate- or high-HAV endemicity, in whom the use of IG may interfere with the administration of other needed vaccines (e.g., measles, mumps, rubella, varicella), the use of inactivated hepatitis A vaccine could be considered (see section on inactivated vaccines).

Hepatitis A Vaccine

The ability to propagate HAV in cell culture allowed for the development of hepatitis A vaccines. Both inactivated and live attenuated hepatitis A vaccines have been developed, using defined isolates from infected cell lines.[52] However, only inactivated vaccines have been evaluated for efficacy in controlled clinical trials and licensed in the United States and other countries.[93, 225]

Inactivated Vaccines

Inactivated hepatitis A vaccines are prepared by a method similar to that used to prepare inactivated polio vaccine, by propagation of cell culture–adapted virus in human fibroblasts, purification by ultrafiltration or other methods, formalin inactivation, and adsorption to an aluminum hydroxide adjuvant.[4, 36] Inactivated vaccines using the HM175 strain and the CR326F′ strain have been licensed in pediatric and adult formulations for intramuscular administration (Table 172–5).

In extensive studies in children and adults, the inactivated hepatitis A vaccines have been found to be highly immunogenic. In general, after one dose of vaccine, 95 to 100 per cent of children 2 years of age or older and adults respond with levels of antibody considered to be protective; a second dose is necessary 6 to 18 months later to boost antibody levels.[6, 36, 87, 137, 148] Studies in children younger than 2 years of age are limited but suggest that passively transferred maternal antibody may interfere with the immune response. In one study in which vaccine was administered at 2, 4, and 6 months of age, infants whose mothers were anti-HAV–positive had antibody titers at 15 months of age that were one-third the levels among infants who had been administered vaccine on the same schedule but whose mothers were anti-HAV–negative.[182] Further studies are needed to determine the optimum dose and timing of vaccination in children younger than 2 years of age, especially for children living in populations with high rates of HAV infection and whose mothers are likely to be anti-HAV–positive.

Hepatitis A vaccination rarely induces IgM anti-HAV detectable by standard assays. IgM anti-HAV was found in 3 of 15 persons 2 to 3 weeks after receiving VAQTA and in 3 of 311 persons 1 month after completing vaccination with HAVRIX.[187, 191]

Inactivated hepatitis A vaccine has been shown to be highly efficacious in preventing clinically apparent disease. In a study of approximately 40,000 Thai children 1 to 16 years of age, the efficacy of inactivated vaccine (HM175 strain) was 94 per cent after two doses administered 1 month apart.[93] In a study of another inactivated vaccine (CR326F′ strain) conducted among approximately 1000 children 2 to 16 years of age in New York, the efficacy was 100 per cent starting 21 days after administration of one dose.[225]

Several ongoing studies have been evaluating the effectiveness of widespread childhood vaccination in controlling community-wide outbreaks. In communities classified as having a "high rate" of hepatitis A (see Table 172–2) in Alaska, South Dakota, and New York, vaccination of the majority of children, and in some cases adolescents and young adults, resulted in a rapid decline in disease incidence that has lasted for several years of follow-up.[136, 224, 225] There is limited experience using vaccination to control community-wide out-

TABLE 172–5. Recommended Doses of Hepatitis A Vaccines

HAVRIX (Hepatitis A Vaccine, Inactivated, SmithKline Beecham Pharmaceuticals)					
Group	Age	Dose (EL.U.)*	Volume	No. Doses	Schedule (months)†
Children and adolescents§	2–18 years	720	0.5 mL	2	0, 6–12
Adults	>18 years	1440	1.0 mL	2	0, 6–12
VAQTA (Hepatitis A Vaccine, Inactivated, Merck & Co, Inc.)					
Group	Age	Dose (U)£	Volume	No. Doses	Schedule (months)†
Children and adolescents	2–17 years	25 U	0.5 mL	2	0, 6–18
Adults	>17 years	50 U	1.0 mL	2	0, 6

*ELISA units.
†0 months represents timing of the initial dose; subsequent numbers represent months after the initial dose.
§An alternate formulation and schedule (three doses) is available for children and adolescents of 360 EL.U. per 0.5 mL dose at 0, 1, and 6–12 months.
£Units.

breaks in areas classified as having an "intermediate rate" of hepatitis A. It is assumed that vaccination of children, adolescents, and possibly young adults should control these community-wide outbreaks. Specific strategies that target specific populations (e.g., age groups, risk groups) or areas within the community (e.g., census tracts) with the highest rates of disease currently are being evaluated in several communities.[5, 43] It remains to be determined which vaccination strategies will be most effective in these settings. Until hepatitis A vaccine can be incorporated into the routine infant/early childhood immunization schedule, a major challenge in high-rate communities and in intermediate-rate communities that have undertaken vaccination programs will be the ongoing routine vaccination of children at 2 years of age. Combined with catch-up vaccination of older children, routine vaccination of all infants/children has the potential to eliminate HAV transmission in much the same manner that polio was controlled in the United States.

Experience to date indicates that the incidence of adverse events after vaccination is comparable with that after the administration of other widely used vaccines (e.g., hepatitis B vaccine). In clinical studies among children, the most frequently reported side effects included soreness, tenderness, warmth, or induration at the injection site (4 to 19 per cent); feeding problems (8 per cent); and headache (4 per cent).

Antibody has been shown to persist at high levels in vaccine recipients for at least 3 years after vaccination.[217, 229] Estimates based on kinetic models of antibody decline suggest that the duration of protection could be 20 years or longer.[229] Postlicensure surveillance is ongoing to determine whether breakthrough infections occur among vaccinees and to determine the long-term protective efficacy of hepatitis A vaccine. These studies would benefit by the development of diagnostic assays that can distinguish between antibodies resulting from natural infection and vaccination to determine whether ongoing exposure to HAV is occurring in highly vaccinated populations. One assay being evaluated is designed to detect antibody to nonstructural HAV antigens.[46, 96] These proteins are expressed during viral replication but are not present in the purified virus particles (capsid proteins) contained in the inactivated vaccines. Antibody to the nonstructural proteins is produced in response to natural HAV infection, but it is not clear how long after infection these antibodies persist.

In some settings, prevaccination serologic testing may be considered to reduce costs by not vaccinating persons with prior immunity.[19] Testing of children is not indicated because of their expected low prevalence of infection and the lower cost of vaccine for this age group. Testing may be considered for older adolescents in certain population groups with a high prevalence of infection (e.g. Native Americans, Alaska Natives) but should take into account the cost of testing, vaccine cost, and the likelihood that the person will return for vaccination. Postvaccination testing is not indicated because of the high rate of vaccine response. Furthermore, testing methods that can detect the low anti-HAV concentrations generated by immunization have not been licensed for use in the United States.

Recommendations for the use of inactivated hepatitis A vaccines have been developed by the Advisory Committee on Immunization Practices (ACIP) of the U.S. Public Health Service, the American Academy of Pediatrics (AAP), and other groups.[32, 40] These groups recommend vaccination of persons at increased risk of hepatitis A, including travelers to countries where HAV infection is of high or intermediate endemicity (see Fig. 172–4), persons who use illicit drugs and live in communities where local epidemiologic and surveillance data indicate current or past outbreaks among persons with such risk behaviors, sexually active homosexual and bisexual men and adolescents, persons who work with HAV in research settings, and patients with hemophilia and other clotting factor disorders (Table 172–6). In communities with high rates of hepatitis A, routine vaccination of young children beginning at or after 2 years of age and vaccination of previously unvaccinated older children are recommended. Vaccination of persons with chronic liver disease also is recommended because of the increased risk of fulminant hepatitis A. Persons who are awaiting or have received liver transplants also should be vaccinated.

The ACIP and AAP also provide recommendations concerning the use of hepatitis A vaccination to prevent and control outbreaks (see Table 172–6). In high-rate communities experiencing community-wide outbreaks, in addition to continuing ongoing routine vaccination of young children, the recommended vaccination of older children should be accelerated if an outbreak is occurring. In intermediate-rate communities, vaccination should be considered to control hepati-

TABLE 172–6. Recommendations for Use of Hepatitis A Vaccine and Immunoglobulin

Group/Setting	Children*	Adolescents	Adults
Pre-exposure Protection with Hepatitis A Vaccine			
Routine Vaccination			
International travelers†	+§	+	+†
Residents of high-rate communities£	+	+/−	−
Men who have sex with men	na¶	+	+†
Illicit drug users ff	na¶	+	+†
Persons with chronic liver disease	+	+	+†
Persons receiving clotting factors	+	+†	+†
Persons who work with hepatitis A virus in research laboratory settings	na¶	na¶	+
Vaccination to Control Outbreaks			
High-rate communities£	+	+/−	−
Intermediate-rate communities£	+/− f	+/− f	+/− f
Postexposure Protection with Immunoglobulin			
Close personal contact with persons with hepatitis A£	+	+	+
Child care centers‡	+/−	+/−	+/−
Common-source exposure£	+	+	+

*Hepatitis A vaccine is not licensed for children younger than 2 years of age.
+Immunoglobulin may be given in addition to or instead of hepatitis A vaccine.
§Children younger than 2 years of age should receive immunoglobulin.
ff Living in communities where local epidemiologic data indicate current or past outbreaks among such persons.
†Prevaccination serologic testing may be cost-effective.
£See Table 172–2.
¶Not applicable.
f Vaccination program may be targeted to persons in particular age or risk groups.
‡See Table 172–4.
£If immunoglobulin can be given within 2 weeks of exposure.
From CDC: Prevention of hepatitis A through active or passive immunization. Recommendations of the Advisory Committee on Immunization Practices. M. M. W. R. *45*(rr-15):1–30, 1996.

tis A outbreaks, but the precise strategies for use have not been determined.[5, 32, 43]

Although hepatitis A outbreaks occur in child care centers, their frequency is not high enough to warrant routine vaccination of attendees or staff (see section on the epidemiology of hepatitis A in specific settings). When outbreaks are recognized, aggressive use of immunoglobulin is effective in limiting transmission through both postexposure and pre-exposure immunization (see Table 172–4). The use of hepatitis A vaccine to control outbreaks in child care centers or other facilities such as institutions for the developmentally disabled has not been studied. However, in communities where outbreaks in child care centers appear to play a role in sustaining a community-wide hepatitis A outbreak, passive-active immunization with immunoglobulin and hepatitis A vaccine should be considered for children and staff in the involved center or centers.

Hepatitis A vaccine has not been evaluated in clinical trials to determine its efficacy in providing postexposure protection. Limited studies in chimpanzees suggest that active postexposure immunization initiated soon after exposure may provide some protection, including the elimination of virus shedding.[168] In one randomized clinical trial of hepatitis A vaccine efficacy, no cases of hepatitis A occurred in vaccine recipients beginning 21 days after vaccination, indicating that vaccine may have some effectiveness when administered after exposure.[225]

Live Attenuated Hepatitis A Vaccines

Although highly immunogenic and efficacious, inactivated hepatitis A vaccines have several drawbacks, including the necessity of administering multiple doses intramuscularly and that booster doses may be necessary in the future to maintain long-term immunity.

HAV must replicate in the liver to induce an antibody response because extrahepatic replication does not appear to occur and live vaccines have the potential to cause hepatic dysfunction. To reduce this risk, attenuated strains have been developed by serial passages in cell culture. Several such attenuated strains, including two variants of the CR326F′ isolate, the HM175 strain, and the H2 strain of HAV, have been evaluated as vaccine candidates in humans.[129, 163, 192] Seroconversion occurred in most persons who were administered, by the subcutaneous or intramuscular route, one dose of vaccine prepared from the CR326F′ and the HM175 strains.[129, 139, 163, 192] Only the HM175 strains were administered orally and were not effective when given by this route.[129, 192] In some studies, some vaccinees had asymptomatic ALT elevations, were transiently positive for IgM anti-HAV, or had HAV present in the stool.[192] Vaccine prepared from the H2 strain has been studied extensively among children in China. In immunogenicity studies, most vaccinees seroconverted after one dose.[130] During up to 3 years of observation in one city, no hepatitis A cases occurred among 6298 vaccinated children, compared with 495 cases among unvaccinated children. In another city where 90 per cent of children 1 to 15 years of age were vaccinated, the number of reported hepatitis A cases decreased from 12 to 87 cases per year to 0 to 1 case per year.[130]

Although live attenuated vaccines have the potential to overcome the limitations of inactivated vaccines, they do not appear to be immunogenic when administered orally. Unless they are shown to provide long-term protection with a single dose, live attenuated vaccines do not seem to offer a distinct advantage over inactivated vaccines.

References

1. Abe, H., Beninger, P. R., Ikejiri, N., et al.: Light microscopic findings of liver biopsy specimens from patients with hepatitis type A and comparison with type B. Gastroenterology *82*:938–947, 1982.
2. Akriviadis, E. A., and Redeker, A. G.: Fulminant hepatitis A in intravenous drug users with chronic liver disease. Ann. Intern. Med. *110*:838–839, 1989.
3. Anderson, D. A.: Cytopathology, plaque assay, and heat inactivation of hepatitis A strain HM-175. J. Med. Virol. *22*:35–44, 1987.
4. Armstrong, M. E., Giesa, P. A., Davide, J. P., et al.: Development of the formalin-inactivated hepatitis A vaccine VAQTA from the live attenuated virus strain CR326F. J. Hepatol. *18*(Suppl. 2):S20–S26, 1993.
5. Averhoff, F., Shapiro, C., Hyams, I., et al.: The use of inactivated hepatitis A vaccine to interrupt a communitywide hepatitis A outbreak. Interscience Conference on Antimicrobial Agents and Chemotherapy (Abstract H73), 1996.
6. Balcarek, K. B., Bagley, M. R., Pass, R. F., et al.: Safety and immunogenicity of an inactivated hepatitis A vaccine in preschool children. J. Infect. Dis. *171*(Suppl. 1):S70–S72, 1995.
7. Bartoloni, A., Aquilini, D., Roselli, M., et al.: Prevalence of antibody to hepatitis A virus in the Santa Cruz region of Bolivia. J. Trop. Med. Hyg. *92*:279–281, 1989.
8. Bell, B. P., Shapiro, C. N., Mottram, K., et al.: The epidemiology of hepatitis A: Implications for vaccine use. Abstracts of the 1995 Interscience Conference on Antimicrobial Agents and Chemotherapy (Abstract K210):326, 1995.
9. Benenson, M. W., Takafuji, E. T., Bancroft, W. H., et al.: A military community outbreak of hepatitis type A related to transmission in a child care facility. Am. J. Epidemiol. *112*:471–481, 1980.
10. Bergeisen, G. H., Hinds, M. W., and Skaggs, J. W.: A waterborne outbreak of hepatitis A in Meade County, Kentucky. Am. J. Public Health *75*:161–164, 1985.
11. Binn, L. N., Lemon, S. M., Marchwicki, R. H., et al.: Primary isolation and serial passage of hepatitis A virus strains in primate cell cultures. J. Clin. Microbiol. *20*:28–33, 1984.
12. Bloch, A. B., Stramer, S. L., Smith, D., et al.: Recovery of hepatitis A virus from a water supply responsible for a common source outbreak of hepatitis A. Am. J. Public Health *80*:428–430, 1990.
13. Bosch, V. V., Dowling, P. C., and Cook, S. D.: Hepatitis A virus immunoglobulin M antibody in acute neurological disease. Ann. Neurol. *14*:685–7, 1983.
14. Bowen, G. S., and McCarthy, M.: Hepatitis A associated with a hardware store water fountain and a contaminated well in Lancaster County, Pennsylvania, 1980. Am. J. Epidemiol. *117*:695–705, 1983.
15. Bradley, D. W., Fields, H. A., McCaustland, K. A., et al.: Biochemical and biophysical characterization of light and heavy density hepatitis A virus particles: Evidence HAV is an RNA virus. J. Med. Virol. *2*:175–187, 1978.
16. Briem, H.: Declining prevalence of antibodies to hepatitis A virus infection in Iceland. Scand. J. Infect. Dis. *23*:135–138, 1991.
17. Brown, V. K., and Robertson, B. H.: Immunoselection of clinical specimens containing virus followed by polymerase chain reaction amplification and rapid direct sequencing. Biotechniques *8*:10–12, 1990.
18. Bryan, J. A., Lehmann, J. D., Setiady, I. F., et al.: An outbreak of hepatitis A associated with recreational lake water. Am. J. Epidemiol. *99*:145–154, 1974.
19. Bryan, J. P., and Nelson, M.: Testing for antibody to hepatitis A to decrease the cost of hepatitis A prophylaxis with immune globulin or hepatitis A vaccines. Arch. Intern. Med. *154*:663–668, 1994.
20. Bulkow, L. R., Wainwright, R. B., McMahon, B. J., et al.: Secular trends in hepatitis A virus infection among Alaska Natives. J. Infect. Dis. *168*:1017–1020, 1993.
21. Carl, M., Francis, D. P., and Maynard, J. P.: Food-borne hepatitis A: Recommendation for control. J. Infect. Dis. *148*:1133–1135, 1983.
22. CDC: Safety of therapeutic immune globulin preparations with respect to transmission of human T-lymphotropic virus type III/lymphadenopathy-associated virus infection. M. M. W. R. *35*:231–233, 1986.
23. CDC: Communitywide outbreaks of hepatitis A. Hepatitis Surveillance Report *51*:6–8, 1987.
24. CDC: Hepatitis A among drug abusers. M. M. W. R. *37*:297–300,305, 1988.
25. CDC: Foodborne hepatitis A: Alaska, Florida, North Carolina, Washington. M. M. W. R. *39*:228–232, 1990.
26. CDC: Hepatitis A among homosexual men: United States, Canada, and Australia. M. M. W. R. *41*:155, 161–164, 1992.
27. CDC: Summary of Notifiable Diseases, United States, 1996.
28. CDC: Hepatitis Surveillance Report No. 54. Atlanta, (N), 1992.
29. CDC: General recommendations on immunization: Recommendations of the Advisory Committee on Immunization Practices. M. M. W. R. *43*(rr-1):1–38, 1994.
30. CDC: Hepatitis Surveillance Report No. 56. Atlanta, Centers for Disease Control and Prevention, 1996.
31. CDC: Hepatitis A among persons with hemophilia who received clotting factor concentrate: United States, September–December 1995. M. M. W. R. *45*:29–32, 1996.
32. CDC: Prevention of hepatitis A through active or passive immunization: Recommendations of the Advisory Committee on Immunization Practices. M. M. W. R. *45*(rr-15):1–30, 1996.
33. Chan, T. K., and Todd, D.: Hemolysis complicating viral hepatitis in patients with glucose-6-phosphate dehydrogenase deficiency. B. M. J. *1*:131–133, 1975.
34. Chin, K. P., Lok, A. S. F., Wong, L. S. K., et al.: Current seroepidemiology of hepatitis A in Hong Kong. J. Med. Virol. *34*:191–193, 1991.
35. Christenson, B.: Epidemiological aspects of acute viral hepatitis A in Swedish travelers to endemic areas. Scand. J. Infect. Dis. *17*:5–10, 1985.
36. Clemens, R., Safary, A., Hepburn, A., et al.: Clinical experience with an inactivated hepatitis A vaccine. J. Infect. Dis. *17*(Suppl. 1):S44–S49, 1995.
37. Cohen, H. A., Amir, J., Frydman, M., et al.: Infection with the hepatitis A virus associated with ascites in children. Am. J. Dis. Child. *146*:1014–1016, 1992.
38. Cohen, J. I., Feinstone, S., and Purcell, R. H.: Hepatitis A virus infection in a chimpanzee: Duration of viremia and detection of virus in saliva and throat swabs. J. Infect. Dis. *160*:887–890, 1989.
39. Cohn, E. J., Oncley, J. L., Strong, L. E., et al.: Chemical, clinical, and immunological studies on the products of human plasma fractionation. I. The characterization of the protein fractions of human plasma. J. Clin. Invest. *23*:417–432, 1944.
40. Committee on Infectious Disease, American Academy of Pediatrics: Prevention of hepatitis A infections: Guidelines for the use of hepatitis A vaccine and immune globulin. Pediatrics. In press.
41. Corey, L., and Holmes, K. K.: Sexual transmission of hepatitis A in homosexual men. N. Engl. J. Med. *302*:435–438, 1980.
42. Coutinho, R. A., Albrecht-Van Lent, P., Lelie, N., et al.: Prevalence and incidence of hepatitis A among male homosexuals. B. M. J. *287*:1743–1745, 1983.
43. Craig, A. S., Moore, W., Schaffner, W., et al.: Use of hepatitis A vaccine to control a communitywide outbreak. Clin. Infect. Dis. *23*:911, 1996.
44. Crance, J. M., Biziagos, E., Passagot, J., et al.: Inhibition of hepatitis A virus replication in vitro by antiviral compounds. J. Med. Virol. *31*:155–160, 1990.
45. Cromeans, T., Nainan, O. V., Fields, H. A., et al.: Hepatitis A and E viruses. *In* Hui, Y. H., Gorham, J. R., Mucell, K. D., et al. (eds.): Foodborne Disease Handbook. New York, Marcel Dekker, 1994, pp. 1–56.
46. Cromeans, T., Robertson, B. H., Malcolm, B. A., et al.: Detection of antibody to hepatitis A virus (HAV) 3C nonstructural proteins by enzyme immunoassay. IX Triennial International Symposium on Viral Hepatitis and Liver Disease, Rome (Abstract A23), 1996.
47. Cromeans, T., Sobsey, M. D., and Fields, H. A.: Development of a plaque assay for a cytopathic, rapidly replicating isolate of hepatitis A virus. J. Med. Virol. *22*:45–56, 1987.
48. Daemer, R. J., Feinstone, S. M., Gust, I. D., et al.: Propagation of human hepatitis A virus in African green monkey kidney cell culture: Primary isolation and serial passage. Infect. Immun. *32*:388–393, 1981.
49. Dan, M., and Yaniv, R.: Cholestatic hepatitis, cutaneous vasculitis and vascular deposits of immunoglobulin M and complement associated with hepatitis A virus infection. Am. J. Med. *89*:103–104, 1990.
50. Desenclos, J. A., Klontz, K. C., Wilder, M. H., et al.: A multistate outbreak of hepatitis A caused by the consumption of raw oysters. Am. J. Public Health *81*:1268–1272, 1991.
51. Desenclos, J. A., and MacLafferty, L.: Communitywide outbreak of hepatitis A linked to children in day care centers and with increased transmission in young adult men in Florida, 1988–9. J. Epidemiol. Commun. Health *47*:269–273, 1993.
52. D'Hondt, E.: Possible approaches to develop vaccines against hepatitis A. Vaccine *10*(Suppl. 1):S48–S52, 1992.
53. Dienstag, J. L., Lucas, C. R., Gust, I. D., et al.: Mussel-associated viral hepatitis, type A: Serological confirmation. Lancet *1*:561–564, 1976.
54. Dmochowski, L.: Viral type A and type B hepatitis: Morphology, biology, immunology and epidemiology—a review. Am. J. Clin. Pathol. *65*:741–786, 1976.
55. Dollberg, S., Berkun, Y., and Gross-Kisselstein E.: Urticaria in patients with hepatitis A infection. Pediatr. Infect. Dis. J. *10*:702–703, 1991.
56. Dollberg, S., Kerem, E., Klar, A., et al.: Disappearance of IgM antibodies to hepatitis A virus after acute infection in children and adolescents. J. Pediatr. Gastroenterol. Nutr. *10*:307–309, 1990.
57. Draelos, Z. K., Hansen, R. C., and James, W. D.: Gianotti-Crosti syndrome associated with infections other than hepatitis B. J. A. M. A. *256*:2386–2388, 1986.
58. Emerson, S. U., Huang, Y. K., McRill, C., et al.: Mutations in both the 2B and 2C genes of hepatitis A virus are involved in adaptation to growth in cell culture. J. Virol. *66*:650–654, 1992.
59. Emerson, S. U., McRill, C., Rosenblum, B., et al.: Mutations responsible for adaptation of hepatitis A virus to efficient growth in cell culture. J. Virol. *65*:4882–4886, 1991.

60. European Association for the Study of the Liver (EASL): Randomised trial of steroid therapy for acute liver failure. Gut *20*:620–623, 1979.
61. Fagan, E., Yousef, G., Brahm, J., et al.: Persistence of hepatitis A virus in fulminant hepatitis and after liver transplantation. J. Med. Virol. *30*:131–136, 1990.
62. Feinstone, S. M., Kapikian, A. Z., and Purcell, R. H.: Hepatitis A: Detection by immune electron microscopy of a virus-like antigen association with acute illness. Science *182*:1026–1028, 1973.
63. Fishman, L. N., Jonas, M. M., and Lavine, J. E.: Update on viral hepatitis in children. Pediatr. Clin. North Am. *43*:57–74, 1996.
64. Fleischer, B., Fleischer, S., Maier, K., et al.: Clonal analysis of infiltrating T lymphocytes in liver tissue in viral hepatitis A. Immunology *69*:14–19, 1990.
65. Fornasini, M. A., Morrow, A. L., and Pickering, L. K.: Illness and health-related benefits among child daycare providers. American Pediatric Society and Society for Pediatric Research (Abstract 835), 1994.
66. Franzen, C., and Frosner, G.: Placental transfer of hepatitis A antibody. N. Engl. J. Med. *304*:427, 1981.
67. Friedman, C. C.: Communitywide hepatitis A epidemic in St. Louis. Missouri Epidemiol. *XV*:13, 1993.
68. Friedman, L. S., O'Brien, T. F., Morse, L. J., et al.: Revisiting the Holy Cross football team hepatitis outbreak (1969) by serological analysis. J. A. M. A. *254*:774–777, 1985.
69. Frosner, G. G., Papaevangelou, G., Butler, R., et al.: Antibody against hepatitis A in seven European countries. Am. J. Epidemiol. *110*:63–69, 1979.
70. Gerety, R. J., Smallwood, L. A., Finlayson, J. S., et al.: Standardization of the antibody to hepatitis A virus (anti-HAV) content of immunoglobulin. Dev. Biol. Stand. *54*:411–416, 1983.
71. Gibas, A., Biewett, D. R., Schoenfeld, D. A., et al.: Prevalence and incidence of viral hepatitis in health workers in the prehepatitis B vaccination era. Am. J. Epidemiol. *136*:603–610, 1992.
72. Gimson, A. E. S., White, Y. S., Eddleston, A. L. W. F., et al.: Clinical and prognostic differences in fulminant hepatitis type A, B and non-A, non-B. Gut *24*:1194–1198, 1983.
73. Gingrich, G. A., Hadler, S. C., Elder, H. A., et al.: Serologic investigation of an outbreak of hepatitis A in a rural day-care center. Am. J. Public Health *73*:1190–1193, 1983.
74. Glikson, M., Galun, E., Oren, R., et al.: Relapsing hepatitis A: Review of 14 cases and literature survey. Medicine *71*:14–23, 1992.
75. Goodman, R. A.: Nosocomial hepatitis A. Ann. Intern. Med. *103*:452–454, 1985.
76. Gordon, S. C., Reddy, K. R., Schiff, L., et al.: Prolonged intrahepatic cholestasis secondary to acute hepatitis A. Ann. Intern. Med. *101*:635–637, 1984.
77. Green, M. S., Colin, B., and Slater, P. E.: Rise in the incidence of viral hepatitis in Israel despite improved socioeconomic conditions. Rev. Infect. Dis. *2*:464–469, 1989.
78. Gust, I. D., and Feinstone, S. M.: History. *In* Gust, I. D., and Feinstone, S. M. (eds.): Hepatitis. Boca Raton, FL, CRC Press, 1988, pp. 1–19.
79. Gust, I. D., Lewis, F. A., and Lehmann, N. I.: Prevalence of antibody to hepatitis A and polioviruses in an unimmunized urban population. Am. J. Epidemiol. *107*:54–56, 1978.
80. Gustafson, T. L., Hutcheson, R. H., Fricker, R. S., et al.: An outbreak of foodborne hepatitis A: The value of serologic testing and matched case-control analysis. Am. J. Public Health *73*:1191–1201, 1983.
81. Hadler, S. C., Erben, J. J., Matthews, D., et al.: Effect of immunoglobulin on hepatitis A in day-care centers. J. A. M. A. *249*:48–53, 1983.
82. Hadler, S. C., Webster, H., Erben, J. J., et al.: Hepatitis A in day-care centers: A community-wide assessment. N. Engl. J. Med. *302*:1222–1227, 1980.
83. Halliday, M. L., Kang, Lai-Y., Zhou, T., et al.: An epidemic of hepatitis A attributable to the ingestion of raw clams in Shanghai, China. J. Infect. Dis. *164*:852–859, 1991.
84. Harkness, J., Gildon, B., and Istre, G. R.: Outbreaks of hepatitis A among illicit drug users, Oklahoma, 1984–87. Am. J. Public Health *79*:463–466, 1989.
85. Hatzakis, A., and Hadziyannis, S.: Sex-related differences in immunoglobulin M and total antibody response to hepatitis A observed in two epidemics of hepatitis A. Am. J. Epidemiol. *120*:936–942, 1984.
86. Havens, W. P.: Period of infectivity of patients with experimentally induced infectious hepatitis. J. Exp. Med. *83*:251–258, 1946.
87. Horng, Y. C., Chang, M. H., Lee, C. Y., et al.: Safety and immunogenicity of hepatitis A vaccine in healthy children. Pediatr. Infect. Dis. J. *12*:359–362, 1993.
88. Huang, S.-N., Lorenz, D., and Gerety, R. J.: Electron and immunoelectron microscopic study on liver tissues of marmosets infected with hepatitis A virus. Lab. Invest. *41*:63–71, 1979.
89. Ikematsu, H., Seizaburo, K., Hayashi, J., et al.: A seroepidemiologic study of hepatitis A virus infections: Statistical analysis of two independent cross-sectional surveys in Okinawa, Japan. Am. J. Epidemiol. *126*:50–54, 1987.
90. Ilan, Y., Hillman, M., Oren, R., et al.: Vasculitis and cryoglobulinemia associated with persisting cholestatic hepatitis A virus infection. Am. J. Gastroenterol. *85*:586–587, 1990.
91. Inman, R. D., Hodge, M., Johnston, M. E. A., et al.: Arthritis, vasculitis and cryoglobulinemia associated with relapsing hepatitis A virus infection. Ann. Intern. Med. *105*:700–703, 1986.
92. Innis, B. L., Snitbhan, R., Hoke, C. H., et al.: The declining transmission of hepatitis A in Thailand. J. Infect. Dis. *163*:989–995, 1991.
93. Innis, B. L., Snitbhan, R., Kunasol, P., et al.: Protection against hepatitis A by an inactivated vaccine. J. A. M. A. *271*:1328–1334, 1994.
94. Jackson, L. A., Stewart, L. K., Solomon, S., et al.: Seroprevalence of hepatitis A, B, C, measles, varicella and cytomegalovirus among child care providers in King County, Washington. Interscience Conference on Antimicrobial Agents and Chemotherapy (Abstract K178):320, 1995.
95. Jansen, R. W., Newbold, J. E., and Lemon, S. M.: Combined immunoaffinity cDNA-RNA hybridization assay for detection of hepatitis A virus in clinical specimens. J. Clin. Microbiol. *22*:984–989, 1985.
96. Jia, X.-Y., Summers, D. F., and Ehrenfeld, E.: Host antibody response to viral structural and nonstructural proteins after hepatitis A infection. J. Infect. Dis. *165*:273–280, 1992.
97. Karron, R. A., Daemer, R., Ticehurst, J., et al.: Studies of prototype live hepatitis A virus vaccines in primate models. J. Infect. Dis. *157*:338–345, 1988.
98. Kashiwagi, S., Hayashi, J., Ikematsu, H., et al.: Prevalence of immunologic markers of hepatitis A and B infection in hospital personnel in Miyazaki prefecture, Japan. Am. J. Epidemiol. *122*:960–969, 1985.
99. Keefe, E. B.: Is hepatitis A more severe in patients with chronic hepatitis B and other chronic liver diseases? Am. J. Gastroenterol. *90*:201–205, 1995.
100. Klein, B. S., Michaels, J. A., Ryter, M. W., et al.: Nosocomial hepatitis A: A multi-nursery outbreak in Wisconsin. J. A. M. A. *252*:2716–2721, 1984.
101. Kluge, I.: Gamma-globulin in the prevention of viral hepatitis: A study of the effect of medium-size doses. Acta Med. Scand. *174*:469–477, 1963.
102. Koa, H. W., Ashcavai, M., and Redeker, A. G.: Persistence of hepatitis IgM antibody after acute clinical hepatitis A. Hepatology *4*:933–936, 1984.
103. Koff, R. S.: Viral hepatitis. *In* Walker, W. A., et al. (eds.): Pediatric Gastrointestinal Disease: Pathophysiology, Diagnosis, Management. Philadelphia, B. C. Decker, 1991, pp. 857–874.
104. Koff, R. S.: Clinical manifestations and diagnosis of hepatitis A virus infection. Vaccine *10*(Suppl. 1):S15–S17, 1992.
105. Krah, D.: A simplified multiwell plate assay for the measurement of hepatitis A virus infectivity. Biologicals *19*:223–227, 1991.
106. Kremastinou, J., Kalapothaki, V., and Trichopoulos, D.: The changing epidemiologic pattern of hepatitis A infection in urban Greece. Am. J. Epidemiol. *120*:703–706, 1984.
107. Krugman, S., and Giles, J. P.: Viral hepatitis: New light on an old disease. J. A. M. A. *212*:1019–1029, 1970.
108. Krugman, S., Giles, J. P., and Hammond, J.: Infectious hepatitis: Evidence for two distinctive clinical, epidemiological and immunological types of infection. J. A. M. A. *200*:365–373, 1967.
109. Krugman, S., Ward, R., Giles, J. P., et al.: Infectious hepatitis, study on effect of gamma globulin and on the incidence of apparent infection. J. A. M. A. *174*:823–830, 1960.
110. Krugman, S., Ward, R., and Giles, W. P.: The natural history of infectious hepatitis. Am. J. Med. *32*:717–728, 1962.
111. Kumashiro, R., Sata, M., Suzuki, H., et al.: Clinical study of acute hepatitis type A in patients older than 50 years. Acta Hepatol. Jpn. *29*:457–462, 1988.
112. Lange, W. R., and Frame, J. D.: High incidence of viral hepatitis among American missionaries in Africa. Am. J. Trop. Med. Hyg. *43*:527–533, 1990.
113. Latham, R. H., and Schable, C. A.: Foodborne hepatitis A at a family reunion. Am. J. Epidemiol. *115*:640–645, 1982.
114. Lednar, W. M., Lemon, S. M., Kirkpatrick, J. W., et al.: Frequency of illness associated with epidemic hepatitis A virus infection in adults. Am. J. Epidemiol. *122*:226–233, 1985.
115. Lee, H., and Vacanti, J. P.: Liver transplantation and its long-term management in children. Pediatr. Clin. North Am. *43*:99–124, 1996.
116. Lemon, S. M.: Type A viral hepatitis: New developments in an old disease. N. Engl. J. Med. *313*:1059–1067, 1985.
117. Lemon, S. M.: Immunologic approaches to assessing the response to inactivated hepatitis A vaccine. J. Hepatol. *18*(Suppl. 2):S15–S19, 1993.
118. Lemon, S. M.: The natural history of hepatitis A: The potential for transmission by transfusion of blood or blood products. Vox. Sang. *67*(Suppl. 4):19–23, 1994.
119. Lemon, S. M., and Binn, L. N.: Serum neutralizing antibody response to hepatitis A virus. J. Infect. Dis. *148*:1033–1039, 1983.
120. Lemon, S. M., Binn, L. N., and Marchwicki, R. H.: Radioimmunofocus assay for quantitation of hepatitis A virus in cell culture. J. Clin. Micro. *17*:834–839, 1983.
121. Lemon, S. M., and Shapiro, C. N.: The value of immunization against hepatitis A. Infect. Agents Dis. *1*:38–49, 1994.
122. Lemon, S. M., Whetter, L. E., Chang, K. H., et al.: Recent advances in understanding the molecular virology of Hepatoviruses: Contrasts and comparisons with hepatitis C virus. *In* Nishioka, K., Suzuki, H., Mishiro, S., et al. (eds.): Viral Hepatitis and Liver Disease. Tokyo, Springer-Verlag, 1994, pp. 22–27.
123. Levin, S., Leibowitz, E., Torten, J., et al.: Interferon treatment in acute progressive and fulminant hepatitis. Isr. J. Med. Sci. *25*:364–372, 1989.
124. Liaw, Y. F., Yang, C. Y., Chu, C. M., et al.: Appearance and persistence of

hepatitis A IgM antibody in acute clinical hepatitis A observed in an outbreak. Infection *14*:156–158, 1986.
125. Lowry, P. W., Levine, R., Stroup, D. F., et al.: Hepatitis A outbreak on a floating restaurant in Florida, 1986. Am. J. Epidemiol. *129*:155–164, 1989.
126. Mah, M. W., Royce, R. A., Rathouz, P. J., et al.: Prevalence of hepatitis A antibodies in hemophiliacs: Preliminary results from the Southeastern Delta Hepatitis Study. Vox. Sang. *67*(Suppl. 1):21–22, 1994.
127. Mahoney, F. J., Farley, T. A., Kelso, K. Y., et al.: An outbreak of hepatitis A associated with swimming in a public pool. J. Infect. Dis. *165*:613–618, 1992.
128. Mannucci, P. M., Gdovin, S., Gringeri, A., et al.: Transmission of hepatitis A to patients with hemophilia by factor VIII concentrates treated with organic solvent and detergent to inactivate viruses. Ann. Intern. Med. *120*:1–7, 1994.
129. Mao, J. S., Dong, D. X., Zhang, H. Y., et al.: Primary study of attenuated live hepatitis A vaccine (H2 strain) in humans. J. Infect. Dis. *159*:621–624, 1989.
130. Mao, J. S., Dong, D. X., Zhang, S. Y., et al.: Further studies of attenuated live hepatitis A vaccine (strain H2) in humans. *In* Hollinger, F. B., Lemon, S. M., and Margolis, H. S. (eds.): Viral Hepatitis and Liver Disease. Baltimore, Williams & Wilkins, 1991, pp. 110–111.
131. Margolis, H. S., Nainan, O. V., Krawczynski, K., et al.: Appearance of immune complexes during experimental hepatitis A infection in chimpanzees. J. Med. Virol. *26*:315–326, 1988.
132. Margolis, H. S., Nainan, O. V., Krawczynski, K., et al.: Appearance of immune complexes during experimental hepatitis A infection in chimpanzees. J. Med. Virol. *26*:315–326, 1988.
133. Mathiesen, L. R., Skinoj, P., Nielsen, J. O., et al.: Hepatitis type A, B, and non-A non-B in fulminant hepatitis. Gut *21*:72–77, 1980.
134. Mbithi, J. N., Springthorpe, S., Boulet, J. R., et al.: Survival of hepatitis A virus on human hands and its transfer on contact with animate and inanimate surfaces. J. Clin. Microbiol. *30*:757–763, 1992.
135. McCaustland, K. A., Bond, W. W., Bradley, D. W., et al.: Survival of hepatitis A virus in feces after drying and storage for 1 month. J. Clin. Microbiol. *16*:957–958, 1982.
136. McMahon, B. J., Beller, M., Williams, J., et al.: A program to control an outbreak of hepatitis A in Alaska by using an inactivated hepatitis A vaccine. Arch. Pediatr. Adolesc. Med. *150*:733–739, 1996.
137. McMahon, B. J., Williams, J., Bulkow, L., et al.: Immunogenicity of an inactivated hepatitis A vaccine in Alaska Native children and Native and non-Native adults. J. Infect. Dis. *171*:676–679, 1995.
138. Mele, A., Rastelli, M. G., Gill, O. N., et al.: Recurrent epidemic hepatitis A associated with consumption of raw shellfish, probably controlled through public health measures. Am. J. Epidemiol. *130*:540–546, 1989.
139. Midthun, K., Ellerbeck, E., Gershman, K., et al.: Safety and immunogenicity of a live attenuated hepatitis A virus vaccine in seronegative volunteers. J. Infect. Dis. *163*:735–739, 1991.
140. Millard, J., Appleton, H., and Parry, J. V.: Studies on heat inactivation of hepatitis A virus with special reference to shellfish. Part 1. Procedures for infection and recovery of virus from laboratory-maintained cockles. Epidemiol. Infect. *98*:397–414, 1987.
141. Minor, P. D.: *Picornaviridae*. *In* Franki, R. I. B., Fauquet, C. M., Knudson, D. L., et al.: (eds.): Classification and Nomenclature of Viruses: The Fifth Report of the International Committee on Taxonomy of Viruses. Wien, Springer-Verlag, 1991, pp. 320–326.
142. Mishu, B., Hadler, S., Boza, V. A., et al.: Foodborne hepatitis A: Evidence that microwaving reduces risk? J. Infect. Dis. *162*:655–658, 1990.
143. Mosley, J. W., Reisler, D. M., Brachott, D., et al.: Comparison of two lots of immune serum globulin for prophylaxis of infectious hepatitis. Am. J. Epidemiol. *87*:539–550, 1968.
144. Mowat, A. P.: Liver Disorders in Childhood. 3rd ed. Oxford, Butterworth, 1994.
145. Myers, J. D., Romm, F. J., Tihen, W. S., et al.: Foodborne hepatitis A in a general hospital: Epidemiologic study of an outbreak attributed to sandwiches. J. A. M. A. *231*:1049–1053, 1975.
146. Nainan, O. V., Brinton, M. A., and Margolis, H. S.: Identification of amino acids located in the antibody binding sites of human hepatitis A virus. Virology *191*:984–987, 1992.
147. Nainan, O. V., Margolis, H. S., Robertson, B. H., et al.: Sequence analysis of a new hepatitis A virus naturally infecting cynomolgus macaques (Macaca fascicularis). J. Gen. Virol. *72*:1685–1689, 1991.
148. Nalin, D. R.: VAQTA, hepatitis A vaccine, purified, inactivated. Drugs Future *20*:24–29, 1995.
149. Nasser, A. M., and Metcalf, T. G.: Production of cytopathology in FRhK-4 cells by BS-C-1–passaged hepatitis A virus. Appl. Environ. Microbiol. *53*:2967–2971, 1987.
150. Niu, M. T., Polish, L. B., Robertson, B. H., et al.: A multistate outbreak of hepatitis A associated with frozen strawberries. J. Infect. Dis. *166*:518–524, 1992.
151. Noble, R. C., Kane, M. A., Reeves, S. A., et al.: Posttransfusion hepatitis A in a neonatal intensive care unit. J. A. M. A. *252*:2711–2715, 1984.
152. O'Grady, J. G.: Management of acute and fulminant hepatitis A. Vaccine *10*(Suppl. 1):S21–S23, 1992.
153. O'Grady, J. G., Alexander, G. J., Hayllar, K. M., et al.: Early indicators of the prognosis in fulminant hepatic failure. Gastroenterology *97*:439–445, 1989.
154. Ohara, H., Naruto, H., Watanabe, W., et al.: An outbreak of hepatitis A caused by consumption of raw oysters. J. Hyg. (Camb.) *91*:163–165, 1983.
155. Okuno, T., Sano, A., Deguchi, T., et al.: Pathology of acute hepatitis A in humans. Comparison with acute hepatitis B. Am. J. Clin. Pathol. *81*:162–169, 1984.
156. Papaevangelou, G. J., Roumeliotou-Karayannis, A. J., and Contoyannis, P. C.: The risk of hepatitis A and B virus infections from patients under care without isolation precautions. J. Med. Virol. *7*:143–148, 1981.
157. Parkin, W. E., Marzinsky, P., and Griffin, M. R.: Foodborne hepatitis A associated with cheeseburgers. J. Med. Soc. N. J. *80*:612–615, 1983.
158. Pavia, A. T., Nielson, L., Armington, L., et al.: A communitywide outbreak of hepatitis A in a religious community: Impact of mass administration of immune globulin. Am. J. Epidemiol. *131*:1085–1093, 1990.
159. Pelletier, G., Elghozi, D., Trepo, C., et al.: Mononeuritis in acute viral hepatitis. Digestion *32*:5306, 1985.
160. Peterson, D. A., Wolfe, L. G., Larkin, E. P., et al.: Thermal treatment and infectivity of hepatitis A virus in human feces. J. Med. Virol. *2*:201–206, 1978.
161. Ping, L.-H., Jansen, R. W., Stapleton, J. T., et al.: Identification of an immunodominant antigenic site involving the capsid protein VP3 of hepatitis A virus. Proc. Natl. Acad. Sci. U. S. A. *85*:8281–8285, 1988.
162. Portnoy, B. L., Mackowiak, P. A., Caraway, C. T., et al.: Oyster-associated hepatitis failure of shellfish certification programs to prevent outbreaks. J. A. M. A. *233*:1065–1068, 1975.
163. Provost, P. J., Bishop, R. P., Gerety, R. J., et al.: New findings in live, attenuated hepatitis A vaccine development. J. Med. Virol. *20*:165–175, 1986.
164. Provost, P. J., and Hilleman, M. R.: Propagation of human hepatitis A virus in cell culture in vitro. Proc. Soc. Exp. Biol. Med *160*:213–221, 1979.
165. Purcell, R. H., D'Hondt, E., Bradbury, R., et al.: Inactivated hepatitis A vaccine: Active and passive prophylaxis in chimpanzees. Vaccine *10*:S148–S156, 1992.
166. Rakela, J., Redeker, A. G., Edwards, V. M., et al.: Hepatitis A virus infection in fulminant hepatitis and chronic active hepatitis. Gastroenterology *74*:879–882, 1978.
167. Reid, T. M. S., and Robinson, H. G.: Frozen raspberries and hepatitis A. Epidemiol. Infect. *98*:109–112, 1987.
168. Robertson, B. H., D'Hondt, E. H., Spelbring, J., et al.: Effect of postexposure vaccination in a chimpanzee model of hepatitis A virus infection. J. Med. Virol. *43*:249–251, 1994.
169. Robertson, B. H., Jansen, R. W., Khanna, B., et al.: Genetic relatedness of hepatitis A virus strains recovered from different geographical regions. J. Gen. Virol. *73*:1365–1377, 1992.
170. Robertson, B. H., Khanna, B., Nainan, O. V., et al.: Epidemiologic patterns of wild-type hepatitis A virus determined by genetic variation. J. Infect. Dis. *163*:286–292, 1991.
171. Rosenblum, L. S., Mirkin, I. R., Allen, D. T., et al.: A multifocal outbreak of hepatitis A traced to commercially distributed lettuce. Am. J. Public Health *80*:1075, 1990.
172. Rosenblum, L. S., Villarino, M. E., Nainan, O. V., et al.: Hepatitis A outbreak in a neonatal intensive care unit: Risk factors for transmission and evidence of prolonged viral excretion among preterm infants. J. Infect. Dis. *164*:476–482, 1991.
173. Ruiz-Gomez, J., and Bustamante-Calvillo, M. E.: Hepatitis A antibodies: Prevalence and persistence in a group of Mexican children. Am. J. Epidemiol. *121*:116–119, 1985.
174. Sagi, E. F., Linder, N., and Shouval, D.: Papular acrodermatitis of childhood associated with hepatitis A virus infection. Pediatr. Dermatol. *3*:31–33, 1985.
175. Sawyer, J. A., Brown, J. P., Folke, L. E., et al.: Hepatitis A in a border community. Border Health *5*:2–5, 1989.
176. Schade, C. P., and Komorwska, D.: Continuing outbreak of hepatitis A linked with intravenous drug abuse in Multnomah County. Public Health Rep. *103*:452–459, 1988.
177. Scheuer, P. J.: Liver Biopsy Interpretation. 4th ed. London, Bailliere Tindall, 1988.
178. Schiff, E. R.: Atypical clinical manifestations of hepatitis A. Vaccine *10*(Suppl. 1):S18–S20, 1992.
179. Shapiro, C. N., Coleman, P. J., McQuillan, G. M., et al.: Epidemiology of hepatitis A: Seroepidemiology and risk groups in the USA. Vaccine *10*:S59–S62, 1992.
180. Shapiro, C., and Hadler, S.: Significance of hepatitis in children in day care. Semin. Pediatr. Infect. Dis. *1*:270–279, 1990.
181. Shapiro, C. N., and Hadler, S. C.: Hepatitis A and hepatitis B virus infections in day care centers. Pediatr. Ann. *20*:435–441, 1991.
182. Shapiro, C. N., Letson, G. W., Kuehn, D., et al.: Effect of maternal antibody on immunogenicity of hepatitis A vaccine in infants. Interscience Conference on Antimicrobial Agents and Chemotherapy (Abstract H61), 1995.
183. Shaw, F. E. J., Shapiro, C. N., Welty, T. K., et al.: Hepatitis transmission among the Sioux Indians of South Dakota. Am. J. Public Health *80*:1091–1094, 1990.
184. Shaw, F. E., Jr., Sudman, J. H., Smith, S. M., et al.: A community-wide epidemic of hepatitis A in Ohio. Am. J. Epidemiol. *123*:1057–1065, 1986.

185. Sherertz, R. J., Russell, B. A., and Reuman, P. D.: Transmission of hepatitis A by transfusion of blood products. Arch. Intern. Med. *144*:1579–1580, 1984.
186. Shi, G. R., Li, S. Q., and Qian, L.: The epidemiological study on a foodborne outbreak of non-A, non-B hepatitis. J. Chin. Med. Univ. *16*:150, 1987.
187. Shouval, D., Ashur, Y., Adler, R., et al.: Single and booster dose responses to an inactivated hepatitis A virus vaccine: Comparison with immune serum globulin prophylaxis. Vaccine *11*:9–14, 1993.
188. Siebke, J. C., Degre, M., Ritland, S., et al.: Prevalence of hepatitis A antibodies in a normal population and some selected groups of patients in Norway. Am. J. Epidemiol. *115*:185–191, 1982.
189. Simmonds, R. S., Szucs, G., Metcalf, T. G., et al.: Persistently infected cultures as a source of hepatitis A virus. Appl. Environ. Microbiol. *49*:749–755, 1985.
190. Sinclair, S. B., and Levy, G. A.: Treatment of fulminant viral hepatic failure with prostaglandin E: A preliminary report. Dig. Dis. Sci. *36*:791–800, 1991.
191. Sjogren, M. H., Hoke, C. H., Binn, L. N., et al.: Immunogenicity of an inactivated hepatitis A vaccine. Ann. Intern. Med. *114*:470–471, 1991.
192. Sjogren, M. H., Purcell, R. H., McKee, K., et al.: Clinical and laboratory observations following oral or intramuscular administration of a live attenuated hepatitis A vaccine candidate. Vaccine *10*(Suppl. 1):S135–S137, 1992.
193. Sjogren, M. H., Tanno, H., Fay, O., et al.: Hepatitis A virus in stool during clinical relapse. Ann. Intern. Med. *106*:221–226, 1987.
194. Skinhoj, P., Mathiesen, L. R., Kryger, P., et al.: Faecal excretion of hepatitis A virus in patients with symptomatic hepatitis A infection. Scand. J. Gastroenterol. *16*:1057–1059, 1981.
195. Snydman, D. R., Dienstag, J. L., Stedt, B., et al.: Use of IgM-hepatitis A antibody testing: Investigating a common source foodborne outbreak. J. A. M. A. *245*:827–830, 1981.
196. Stapleton, J. T., Lange, D. K., LeDuc, J. W., et al.: The role of secretory immunity in hepatitis A virus infection. J. Infect. Dis. *163*:7–11, 1991.
197. Starzl, T. E., Demetris, A. J., and Van Thiel, D.: Liver transplantation. N. Engl. J. Med. *321*:1014–1022, 1989.
198. Steffen, R., Kane, M. A., Shapiro, C. N., et al.: Epidemiology and prevention of hepatitis A in travelers. J. A. M. A. *272*:885–889, 1994.
199. Steffen, R., Rickenbach, M., Wilhelm, U., et al.: Health problems after travel to developing countries. J. Infect. Dis. *156*:84, 1987.
200. Stokes, J., and Neefe, J. R.: The prevention and attenuation of infectious hepatitis by gamma globulin. J. A. M. A. *127*:144–145, 1945.
201. Stroffolini, T., Franco, E., Mura, I., et al.: Age-specific prevalence of hepatitis A virus infection among teenagers in Sardinia. Microbiologica *14*:21–24, 1991.
202. Szmuness, W., Dienstag, J. L., Purcell, R. H., et al.: The prevalence of antibody to hepatitis A antigen in various parts of the world: A pilot study. Am. J. Epidemiol. *106*:392–398, 1977.
203. Szmuness, W., Purcell, R. H., Dienstag, J. L., et al.: Antibody to hepatitis A antigen in institutionalized mentally retarded patients. J. A. M. A. *237*:1702–1705, 1977.
204. Tabor, E.: Clinical presentation of hepatitis A. *In* Gerety, R. J. (ed.): Hepatitis A. New York, Academic Press, 1984, pp. 47–53.
205. Tabor, E.: Guillain-Barré syndrome and other neurologic syndromes in hepatitis A, B, and non-A, non-B. J. Med. Virol. *21*:207–216, 1987.
206. Tankersley, D. L., and Preston, M. S.: Quality control of immune globulins. *In* Krijnen, H. W., Strengers, P. F. W., and VanAken, X. (eds.): Immunoglobulins: Proceedings of an International Symposium. Amsterdam, Central Laboratory of Netherlands Red Cross Transfusion Service, 1988, pp. 381–399.
207. Tassopoulos, N. C., Papaevangelou, G. J., Ticehurst, J. R., et al.: Fecal excretion of Greek strains of hepatitis A virus in patients with hepatitis A and in experimentally infected chimpanzees. J. Infect. Dis. *154*:231–237, 1986.
208. Teixera, M. R., Jr., Weller, I. V. D., Murray, A., et al.: The pathology of hepatitis A in man. Liver *2*:53–60, 1982.
209. Tibbs, C. J., and Williams, R.: Liver transplantation for acute and chronic hepatitis. J. Viral Hepatol. *2*:65–72, 1995.
210. Tong, M. J., El-Farra, N. S., and Grew, M. I. Clinical manifestations of hepatits A: Recent experience in a community teaching hospital. J. Infect. Dis. *151*(Suppl. 1):S15–S18, 1995.
211. Tong, M. J., Thursby, M., Rakela, J., et al.: Studies on the maternal-infant transmission of the viruses which cause acute hepatitis. Gastroenterology *80*:999–1004, 1981.
212. Toppet, V., Souayah, H., Delplace, O., et al.: Lymph node enlargement as a sign of acute hepatitis A in children. Pediatr. Radiol. *20*:249–252, 1990.
213. Tsarev, S. A., Emerson, S. U., Balayan, M. S., et al.: Simian hepatitis A virus (HAV) strain AGM-27: Comparison of genome structure and growth in cell culture with other HAV strains. J. Gen. Virol. *72*:1677–1683, 1991.
214. Tsega, E., Mengesha, B., Hansson, B. G., et al.: Hepatitis A, B and delta infection in Ethiopia: A serologic survey with demographic data. Am. J. Epidemiol. *123*:344–351, 1986.
215. Vallbracht, A., Fleischer, S., Maier, K., et al.: Clonal analysis of infiltrating T-lymphocytes in liver tissue in viral hepatitis A. Immunology *69*:14–19, 1990.
216. Vallbracht, A., Maier, K., Stierhof, Y. D., et al.: Liver-derived cytotoxic T cells in hepatitis A virus infection. J. Infect. Dis. *160*:209–217, 1989.
217. Van Damme, P., Thoelen, S., Cramm, M., et al.: Inactivated hepatitis A vaccine: Reactogenicity, immunogenicity, and long-term antibody persistence. J. Med. Virol. *44*:446–451, 1994.
218. Van Thiel, D.: When should the decision to proceed with transplantation actually be made in cases of subfulminant liver failure: At admission to hospital or when a donor organ is made available? J. Hepatol. *17*:1–2, 1993.
219. Vento, S., Garofano, T., DiPerri, G., et al.: Identification of hepatitis A virus as a trigger for autoimmune chronic hepatitis type I in susceptible individuals. Lancet *337*:1183–1187, 1991.
220. Vranckx, R., and Muylle, L.: Hepatitis A virus antibodies in Belgium: Relationship between prevalence and age. Infection *18*:48–50, 1990.
221. Watson, J. C., Fleming, D. W., Boretta, A. J., et al.: Vertical transmission of hepatitis A resulting in an outbreak in a neonatal intensive care unit. J. Infect. Dis. *167*:567–571, 1993.
222. Weisfuse, I. B., Graham, D. J., Will, M., et al.: An outbreak of hepatitis A among cancer patients treated with interleukin-2 and lymphokine-activated killer cells. J. Infect. Dis. *161*:647–652, 1990.
223. Weltman, A. C., Bennett, N. M., Ackman, D. A., et al.: An outbreak of hepatitis A associated with a bakery, New York, 1994: The 1968 "West Branch, Michigan" outbreak repeated. Epidemiol. Infect. *117*:333–341, 1996.
224. Welty, T. K., Darling, K., Dye, S., et al.: Guidelines for prevention and control of hepatitis A in American Indian and Alaska Native communities. S. Dak. Med. J. *49*:317–322, 1996.
225. Werzberger, A., Mensch, B., Kuter, B., et al.: A controlled trial of formalin-inactivated hepatitis A vaccine in healthy children. N. Engl. J. Med. *327*:453–457, 1992.
226. Wheeler, C. M., Fields, H. A., Schable, C. A., et al.: Adsorption, purification, and growth characteristics of hepatitis A virus strain HAS-15 propagated in fetal Rhesus monkey kidney cells. J. Clin. Microbiol. *23*:434–440, 1986.
227. Wheeler, C. M., Robertson, B. H., Van Nest, G., et al.: Structure of hepatitis A virion: Peptide mapping of the capsid region. J. Virol. *58*:307–313, 1986.
228. Widell, A., Hansson, B. G., Moestrup, T., et al.: Acute hepatitis A, B and non-A, non-B in a Swedish community studied over a ten-year period. Scand. J. Infect. Dis. *14*:253–259, 1982.
229. Wiens, B. L., Bohidar, N. R., Pigeon, J. G., et al.: Duration of protection from clinical hepatitis A disease after vaccination with VAQTA. J. Med. Virol. *49*:235–241, 1996.
230. Williams, I., Bell, B. P., Kaluba, J., et al.: Association between chronic liver disease and death from hepatitis A, United States, 1989–1992. IX Triennial International Symposium on Viral Hepatitis and Liver Disease, Rome (Abstract A39), 1996.
231. Williams, R.: Prevalence of hepatitis A virus antibody among Navajo school children. Am. J. Public Health *76*:282–283, 1986.
232. Williams, R., and Wendon, J.: Indications for orthotopic liver transplantation in fulminant liver failure. Hepatology *20*:5S–10S, 1994.
233. Wimmer, E., and Murdin, A. D.: Hepatitis A virus and the molecular biology of picornaviruses: A case for a new genus of the family *Picornaviridae*. *In* Hollinger, F. B., Lemon, S. M., and Margolis, H. (eds.): Viral Hepatitis and Liver Disease. Baltimore, Williams & Wilkins, 1991, pp. 31–41.
234. Wong, D. C., Purcell, R. H., and Rosen, L.: Prevalence of antibody to hepatitis A and hepatitis B viruses in selected populations of the South Pacific. Am. J. Epidemiol. *110*:227–236, 1979.
235. Yang, N. Y., Yu, P. H., Mao, Z. Y., et al.: Inapparent infection of hepatitis A virus. Am. J. Epidemiol. *127*:599–604, 1988.
236. Yotsuyanagi, H., Koike, K., Yasuda, K., et al.: Prolonged fecal excretion of hepatitis A virus in adult patients with hepatitis A as determined by polymerase chain reaction. Hepatology *24*:10–13, 1996.
237. Zhuang, H., Kaldor, J., Locarnini, S. A., et al.: Serum immunoglobulin levels in acute A, B, and non-A, non-B hepatitis. Gastroenterology *82*:549–553, 1982.
238. Zuckerman, A. J.: The history of viral hepatitis from antiquity to the present. *In* Deinhardt, F., and Dienhardt, J. (eds.): Viral Hepatitis: Laboratory and Clinical Science. Vol. 3. New York, Marcel Dekker, 1983, pp. 3–32.

❑ ❑ ❑

SUBSECTION TWO

CALICIVIRIDAE

173

CALICIVIRUSES, INCLUDING HEPATITIS E VIRUS

David O. Matson

Caliciviruses currently include several groups of strains that differ in their host of origin, ecologic relationships, and genomic properties. Classification is in flux, and taxonomic decisions in the near future may result in the separation of the family *Caliciviridae* into distinct families of viruses.

Caliciviruses first were recognized to be epidemiologically distinct pathogens in 1932, when outbreaks of a vesicular exanthem restricted to domestic pigs occurred in California (vesicular exanthem of swine virus [VESV] infection).[5] The illness initially was thought to be foot and mouth disease of cattle, which led to extensive programs to eradicate the agent. These programs persisted for decades, with a resulting major impact on the agricultural industry of the West Coast of the United States. VESV strains, when visualized by electron microscopy, had distinctive and unique features (described later), which led to the name calicivirus. A program of sterilization of feed and of restriction of feed types finally stopped the outbreaks. In the 1970s, the source of the outbreaks was suggested to be marine animals fed to pigs, either as offal of marine mammals or as fish meal. The close relationships hypothesized for caliciviruses isolated from marine mammals and VESVs were proved by genome sequencing.[78]

The first recognition of caliciviruses in humans was in 1972, when viral particles were linked to an outbreak of gastroenteritis among schoolchildren, teachers, and their household contacts in Norwalk, Ohio.[54] The Norwalk agent was round and had a rough particle surface when visualized by electron microscopy, but these features did not permit any definitive classification. Many similar small, round-structured viruses (SRSVs) were described subsequently from outbreaks of gastroenteritis around the world. A few experiments with these outbreak agents suggested that at least some of them had physical properties like those of the known animal caliciviruses.[52]

In the 1970s, investigators using electron microscopy to survey diarrhea stool specimens from children visualized particles whose appearance was similar to the previously identified animal caliciviruses.[3, 63, 71] These "typical" caliciviruses occurred in a small percentage of sporadic diarrhea stool specimens and in a few outbreaks of gastroenteritis. Genome sequencing has confirmed that both the SRSVs and human viruses with typical calicivirus morphology are caliciviruses.[49, 61, 70]

Beginning in the 1950s, particularly large outbreaks of hepatitis were described from southern Asia.[42, 56, 72, 102, 106] Because the outbreaks appeared to result from fecal-oral contamination, they initially were attributed to hepatitis A virus. However, the outbreaks frequently were very large, affecting thousands of individuals, had a high mortality rate in pregnant women, and did not show a pattern of person-to-person transmission. In 1987, epidemiologic and laboratory investigation finally succeeded in identifying the cause of these outbreaks to be a new virus—hepatitis E virus—and tentatively classified in *Caliciviridae*.[12, 58, 101]

In 1984, a highly fatal, highly contagious hepatitis was described among European rabbits bred in China.[111] This syndrome spread rapidly across Asia and into Europe, reaching Spain within 4 years. Wild European rabbit populations experienced mortality rates exceeding 90 per cent. Typical calicivirus particles were visualized in infected rabbit livers, and this calicivirus, the rabbit hemorrhagic disease virus, eventually was linked to the syndrome.[80, 83]

These summaries illustrate the diversity of ecologic relationships among caliciviruses, highlight the broad spectrum of illness (from mild gastroenteritis to fatal hepatitis) associated with members of the family, and indicate how recently many of the widespread caliciviruses have been discovered. This chapter presents information on each of the five tentative subfamilies of *Caliciviridae*, with a special focus on the human strains.

PROPERTIES OF CALICIVIRUSES

Structural Features of the Virion

Caliciviruses are nonenveloped RNA viruses classified until 1978 as a genus of *Picornaviridae*.[18] The caliciviral genome is a positive-sense, single-stranded RNA molecule of about 8000 nucleotides. Caliciviruses have a single structural polypeptide with a molecular weight of about 60,000 daltons.[49] Typical calicivirus virion particles are 40.5 nm in diameter and have an icosahedral symmetry with 32 cup-shaped surface depressions ("calici," from chalice; Fig. 173–1).[86] It is not always easy to distinguish the identifying features of a calicivirus in a clinical specimen (Fig. 173–1*b*). Staining of particles, particle integrity, and sample components vary among clinical samples. In one orientation, the surface cups combine to generate a Star of David image under the electron microscope. In another orientation, the depressions are responsible for spike-like projections from the surface.

Cryoelectron microscopy has resolved the three-dimensional structure of typical and SRSV morphologic types to a resolution of 20 Å.[86, 87] Typical virion particles have 90 true arches protruding from the surface of a shell that has a diameter of 27 nm. When such particles are visualized by negative-stain electron microscopy, as in a clinical laboratory, the particles are smaller (30 to 35 nm), presumably from desiccation. The arches form the surface spikes and, when particles are rotated, the walls form the cup-shaped depressions that confer the distinctive Star of David appearance. The SRSVs differ from the typical caliciviruses by having shorter arches; otherwise, the structures of the two forms are quite similar.

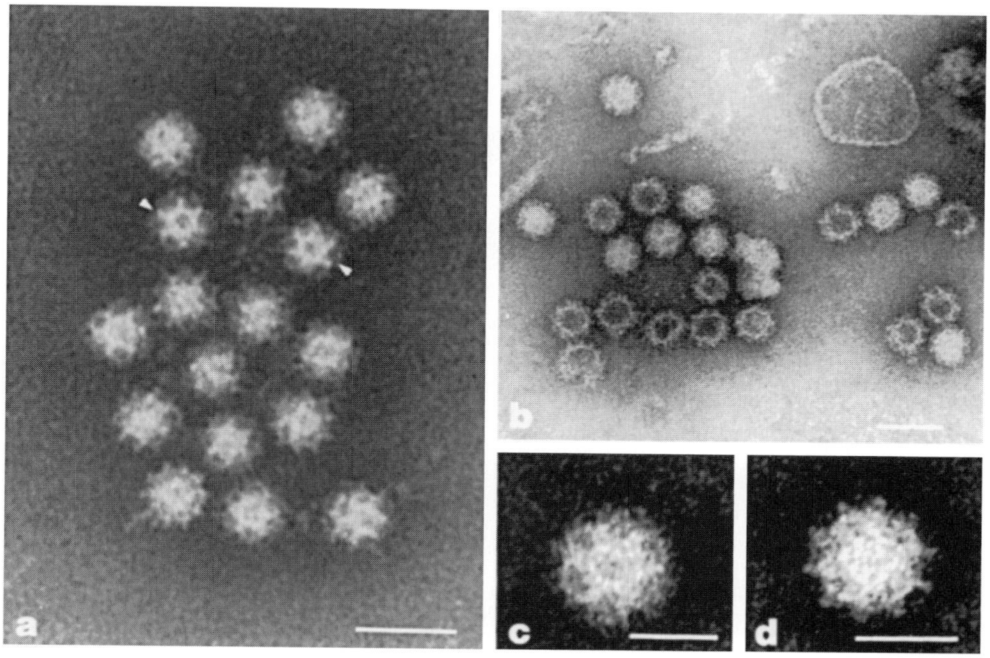

FIGURE 173–1. *Human calicivirus particles visualized by electron microscopy. Particles in a preparation of purified human calicivirus Sapporo strain show distinct surface cups, and the Star of David pattern is visible on some particles* (a, *arrowheads*)*. Particle staining, particle type, and debris in clinical specimens are variable, which makes difficult the recognition of distinct structural features* (b, *specimen from a child from Houston, Texas, infected with an antigenically distinct calicivirus*)*. Two particles at high magnification show the Star of David pattern* (c) *and the 10 surface projections* (d) *characteristic of calicivirus (specimen from a symptomatic child attending a day care center in Phoenix, Arizona). Bar in* a *and* b *= 50 nm; bar in* c *and* d *= 25 nm.*

Taxonomic Relationships Among the Caliciviruses

Prototype Strains and Hosts of Origin

Known caliciviruses can be divided into five genomic groups according to their genomic organization and degree of shared sequence identity (Table 173–1).[6] Strains recovered from natural human infections fall into three genomic groups: SRSVs, which include the Norwalk virus and Snow Mountain virus prototypes; Sapporo-like typical caliciviruses; and hepatitis E viruses. Animal caliciviruses include the rabbit calicivirus–like and VESV-like strains. The VESV-like strains are of marine and terrestrial origin, establishing the hypothesis made in the early 1970s that caliciviruses move between marine and terrestrial reservoirs. Other genomic groups are likely because some clinical specimens containing virus particles have been resistant to genomic characterization.

In addition to the three groups widespread in humans, San Miguel sea lion virus serotype, a member of the VESV-like group, has infected a laboratory worker, producing illness like that observed in the original sea lion host.[5] The VESV-like strains also include a primate calicivirus—Pan-1—isolated from natural infections in several primates.[97] One person exposed to the rabbit hemorrhagic disease virus in a Mexican outbreak developed antibody, suggesting that all five genogroups can infect humans.[41]

Genomic Organization

Caliciviruses have five distinct genomic organizations that match the groups listed in Table 173–1 (Fig. 173–2).[61] Features shared by each of these genomic organizations include a nonstructural polyprotein gene encoded in the 5′ portion of the genome, a capsid gene encoding a single polypeptide and lying 3′ to the nonstructural polyprotein, and consensus amino acid motifs encoded within these two proteins that are markers for significant sequence identity among strains

TABLE 173–1. Genetic Groups Among Human and Animal Caliciviruses

Group	Known Hosts	Examples
Small, round-structured viruses	Human	Norwalk and Snow Mountain viruses
Sapporo-like	Human	Sapporo caliciviruses 82/Japan, 86/Houston, 90/Houston; Manchester and Plymouth viruses
Hepatitis E virus	Human, rodent?	Hepatitis E strains of Burma, Mexico, India, Muslim states of former Soviet Union
Rabbit calicivirus–like	Rabbit, dog?, human?, fox?, mouse?, bird?	Rabbit hemorrhagic disease virus of China, Germany, Spain; European brown hare syndrome virus
Vesicular exanthem of swine virus–like	Pig, cat, chimpanzee, sea lion, dolphin, mussel, sea otter, raccoon, Aruba Island rattlesnake	A48; feline caliciviruses F4, CFI, F9; Pan-1, Tur-1; San Miguel sea lion viruses 1, 4, 5, 9, 13, 15, 16, 17

Data from Berke, T., Golding, B., Smith, A. W., et al.: Phylogenetic relationships among human and animal caliciviruses. 35th Interscience Conference on Antimicrobial Agents and Chemotherapy, San Francisco, October 1995.

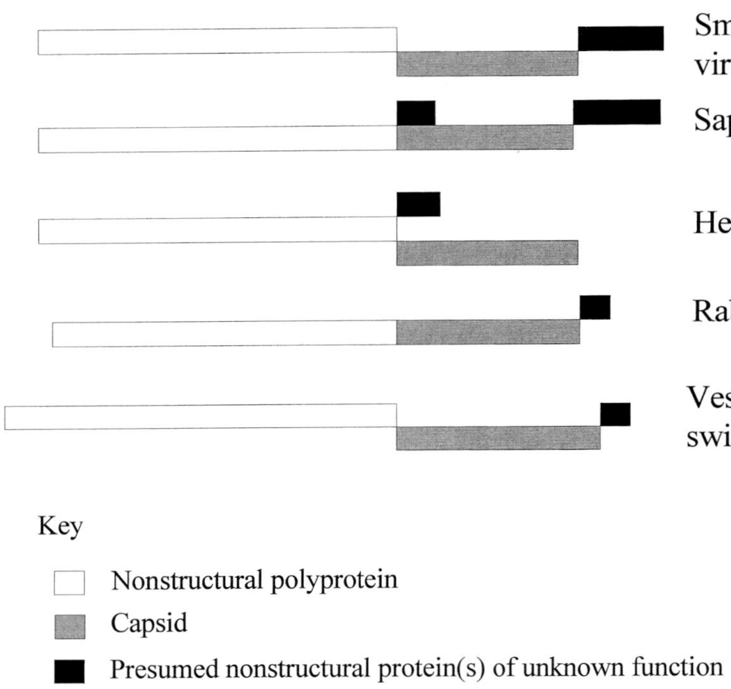

FIGURE 173–2. *Genomic organizations among caliciviruses. Five distinct genomic organizations are known, differing from one another in the size of the capsid gene, the number and location of protein genes, and the location and spacing of consensus amino acid motifs (motifs not shown). (From Matson, D. O.: Caliciviruses. Semin. Pediatr. Infect. Dis. 7:101–106, 1996.)*

in different groups but also with viruses in the picornavirus family (motifs not shown in the figure; see reference 28). The five genomic organizations differ from each other in the length of the capsid gene, in the number and location of third and fourth protein encoding genes, and the presence and spacing of the consensus amino acid motifs. In some strains, a gene lies 3′ to the capsid gene; in other strains, a gene overlies the junction of the nonstructural polyprotein and the capsid gene; and in other strains, both genes are present.

Prior to the description of the genome organization of the Sapporo-like caliciviruses, the genome organization of hepatitis E virus was considered to be sufficiently distinct to warrant separation from *Caliciviridae*. However, the genome organization of Sapporo-like caliciviruses forms a superset for the rabbit calicivirus–like and hepatitis E caliciviruses.[61] This concept of a "superset" derives from the presence in Sapporo-like caliciviruses of the nonstructural polyprotein and capsid gene in the same frame, probably synthesized in one long polyprotein. At the beginning of the capsid gene is another predicted protein product that overlaps the capsid gene in another frame. The function of the protein encoded by this gene is unknown, but we know, at least for hepatitis E virus, that antibody to a protein encoded by a gene at this location is made in natural infections. Another predicted protein is located after the capsid gene in Sapporo-like caliciviruses, meaning that these strains have four genes, rabbit calicivirus–like caliciviruses have three genes in those locations, and hepatitis E virus has a different complement of three genes. The presence of "shared" genes does not imply that the functions of those genes are the same. However, the presence of them and their location require common mechanisms for their expression during replication.

Relationships Established by Comparing Nucleotide and Amino Acid Sequences

Application to calicivirus genome sequences of algorithms that compare nucleotide and amino acid sequences for identity, conservation of substitutions, insertion of gaps, etc., at the primary level sorts strains into the same five groups as does sorting by genome organization.[6] The most informative region of the genome yet analyzed is the hypervariable portion (~1200 nt) of the capsid gene (Fig. 173–3). Based upon these analyses, SRSVs are distinct and distant from other groups and Sapporo-like caliciviruses cluster more closely to rabbit calicivirus–like and VESV-like caliciviruses than to hepatitis E virus or SRSVs. The concordance of assortment of calicivirus strains according to sequence identity or genome organization brings a high level of certainty to the results.

Antigenic Properties of the Virion

The presence of a single structural protein limits the antigenic complexity of the virion. Despite this limitation, circulating caliciviruses are highly diverse. Assays to detect viral antigen and antiviral antibody have been developed for prototype strains within most of the calicivirus genetic groups.[34, 47, 74, 84, 104] Strains from different genetic groups have been distinct antigenically when such testing has been performed, suggesting that different genetic groups represent distinct antigenic groups.

The VESV-like caliciviruses readily are cultivatible in cell culture, whereas cultivation of strains in the other genetic groups has not been successful. The VESV-like caliciviruses include a large number (>30) of distinct serotypes (i.e., neutralization types).[94] It has not been possible to determine whether the other genetic groups include a similar diversity, lacking the ability to test strains for their neutralization characteristics.

Comparisons of paired sera from outbreak-associated cases with outbreak strains and studies of sera from volunteers inoculated with well-characterized prototype strains, using recently developed, sensitive methods, indicate that the Norwalk virus and Snow Mountain virus clusters within the SRSV genogroup are distinct antigenically.[46, 47] Antigenic variants within the Sapporo-like caliciviruses and the other geno-

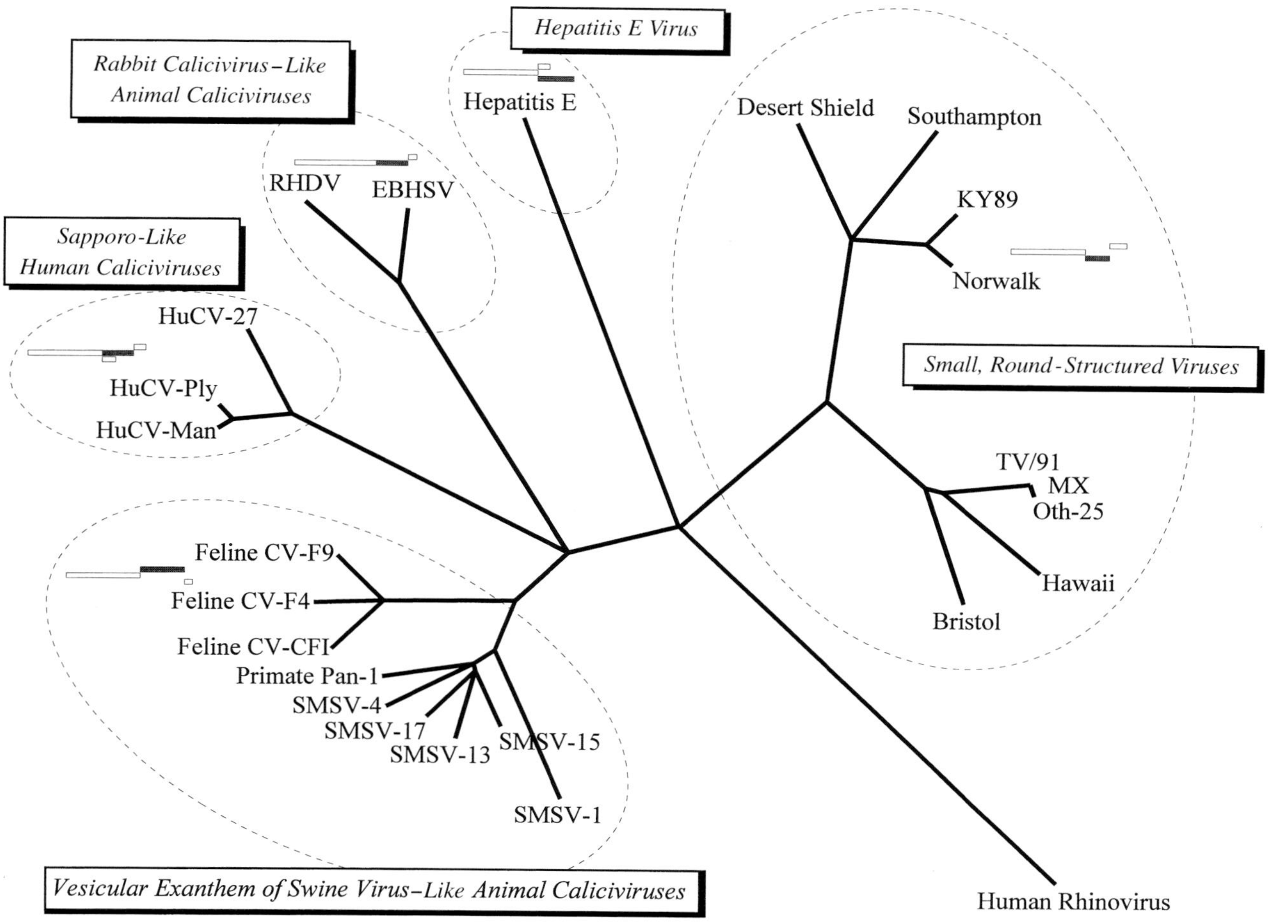

FIGURE 173–3. *Distance tree (Fitch-Margoliash method) constructed from capsid region nucleic acid sequences of selected caliciviruses utilizing 1000 bootstrapped dataset replications and the computer program FITCH of PHYLIP 3.5c. Branch points indicated are those appearing in greater than 95 per cent of the bootstrapped trees. Ovals indicate strains with a common genome organization. Rhinovirus 14 is included as an outgroup. (From Matson, D. O.: Caliciviruses. Semin. Pediatr. Infect. Dis. 7:101–106, 1996.)*

groups that have been studied sufficiently suggest that each genogroup will include a number of serotypes. Type- and group-specific epitopes are present on strains within these clusters, and the degree of genetic distinction associated with distinctiveness of a serotype is not certain.

SMALL, ROUND-STRUCTURED VIRUS–LIKE HUMAN CALICIVIRUSES

Epidemiology

General Prevalence

SRSV-like human caliciviruses have been found wherever sought and probably have a worldwide distribution. Two genetic clusters are known, represented by the Norwalk virus and Snow Mountain virus prototypes (see Fig. 173–3), and studies suggest that large changes in the relative prevalence of these clusters have occurred over the past 30 years. For example, Norwalk virus and closely related strains appear to have been the predominant SRSVs in the 1970s in several regions studied. In the late 1980s and the 1990s, Snow Mountain virus and related strains appear to be predominant and Norwalk virus–like strains are found rarely.[47, 103]

The SRSV-like human caliciviruses are known best for causing outbreaks of gastroenteritis in adults, commonly associated with contaminated water and food, particularly shellfish. The SRSVs may account for about one-third of such outbreaks in North America for which no bacterial or parasitic cause can be found.[40] Multiple antigenic types probably cocirculate in the same region, and regional differences in the prevalence of antibody to specific types exist.

Morbidity and Mortality

The morbidity and mortality of SRSV infections have not been quantified. Death from illness is rare. Attack rates in outbreaks frequently are high: 20 to 90 per cent. These observed attack rates for outbreaks are similar to those from volunteer studies with a single inoculum dose of the Norwalk virus prototype, in which 82 per cent of volunteers were infected and 56 per cent were ill.[37] Although serologic studies indicate that infection is common, with virtually all individuals having antibody by the second decade of life, wherever studied, the portion of sporadic, especially primary, infections resulting in illness and the severity of that illness are uncertain. In general, SRSV infections are considered to be less severe than are rotavirus infections among children. In adults, the severity of SRSV infections appears to be greater, and this trend may be a consequence of the unusual pattern of protective immunity observed for these strains (see later).

Cross-sectional surveys of diarrhea stool specimens from children or adults consistently yield SRSV detections in 0.5 to 2 per cent of samples. The surveys in children are striking for the low rates of detection when compared with the high rates of antibody acquisition in the same age groups. In part, this discrepancy can be attributed to the low concentrations of virus excreted in stool, making virus detection difficult. In addition, assays for antigen detection are highly specific, apparently not detecting group-specific epitopes on the viruses and likely underestimating the prevalence of SRSVs in a survey.

Age Incidence and Prevalence

SRSV infections in developed countries generally have been considered to occur in individuals 4 years of age or older. This tendency was supported by serologic studies that revealed large differences in patterns of age-specific antibody acquisition between developing and developed countries. For example, in Bangladesh, antibody prevalence among 4-year-old children was 100 per cent compared with a prevalence of 19 per cent among children of the same age in the United States.[8, 53] In addition, studies of outbreaks suggested that young children in developed countries were spared.

More recent studies utilizing assays with better sensitivity and specificity are changing these conclusions. For example, among 154 23-month-old infants participating in a vaccine trial in Finland from 1987 to 1989, 73 per cent had anti–Norwalk virus antibody.[60] In England, prevalence of antibody to Norwalk virus in 1991 and 1992 was 48 per cent among 1-year-old toddlers overall, with prevalence in that age group ranging from 12 to 60 per cent among different regions.[38] In South Africa, antibody prevalence in 1992 was 57 per cent among 1-year-old children.[103] These results contrast with those from Hokkaido, Japan, where prevalence of antibody to Norwalk virus among children 1 to 3 years of age was about 6 per cent.[79] In England and Japan, but not in South Africa, a significant increase in antibody prevalence to Norwalk virus was noted among school age children, reaching 80 per cent in England and 70 per cent in Japan by the third decade of life.

Children are likely to be infected with multiple virus types.[22, 69] Testing of a large population-based collection of sera from two cities in Chile for antibody to Norwalk virus and Mx virus (a Snow Mountain–like virus) suggested that these two viruses have different modes of transmission and that exposure to the two types differs in a population.[82] For example, overall prevalence of antibody to Norwalk virus was 83 per cent and to Mx virus was 91 per cent in this age-stratified sample among persons living in Santiago, whereas it was 67 per cent and 90 per cent, respectively, in Punta Arenas ($p < .001$ for Norwalk virus). According to a logistic regression analysis, consumption of uncooked vegetables was an independent risk factor for acquisition of antibody to both viruses in Santiago but only for Mx in Punta Arenas. Consumption of seafood and child care attendance were independent risk factors for acquisition of antibody to both viruses in Punta Arenas but not in Santiago. Results of this kind, to which attributes of the person providing serum, other than just age and location, are matched to the results of antibody testing, are needed for a more complete understanding of modes of transmission and ecologic differences among genetic groups of caliciviruses.

Seasonal Patterns

SRSVs have no recognized seasonality, although infections would be expected to be more common when flooding results in contamination of water supplies and when shellfish are harvested.

Host and Social Factors

SRSV outbreaks tend to be recognized in closed populations where common exposures occur, such as schools, hospitals, summer camps, hotels, and cruise ships. Vehicles of infection in outbreaks include water from regulated and unregulated delivery systems and foods commonly washed, such as salad and fruit. Shellfish are a common source of infection. Person-to-person spread also occurs. Secondary attack rates in common-source outbreaks range from 5 to 30 per cent. New infections can occur over several weeks, with the longest outbreak lasting 3 months. SRSV outbreaks also occur in child care centers.[69]

Pathogenesis and Pathology

Viral Infection

The incubation period after exposure ranges from 10 to 51 hours, with a mean of 24 hours.[9, 29, 30, 90, 110] Illness usually lasts 2 to 3 days.[37] Excretion begins as early as 15 hours after infection, peaks at 25 to 72 hours after infection, and persists at least 7 days after infection.[37] Transmission of infection occurs by fecal-oral spread. Virus also has been detected in vomitus, suggesting the possibility of spread by aerosol or dispersion of vomitus particles.[57]

Pathology

The pathogenic features of SRSV infections have not been determined. The following information is based upon studies of porcine and calf enteric caliciviruses.[36, 43] Enteric animal caliciviruses cause lesions in the proximal small bowel. The first day after inoculation, enterocytes swell along the sides of the microvilli at the base. Damaged enterocytes subsequently slough, resulting in stunted villi. Adjacent villi fuse, which helps to maintain the integrity of the intestinal mucosa. Neutrophils and mononuclear cells infiltrate the epithelium. The peak of pathologic abnormalities is 3 to 7 days after inoculation, after which time gradual healing occurs, restoring normal villus architecture about 10 days after inoculation. Mucosal injury is accompanied by deficiencies of β-galactosidase activity and D-xylose absorption. The capacity for D-xylose absorption recovers by the time normal histologic appearance of the villi is restored, but the β-galactosidase deficiency is delayed for an unknown period thereafter. Individual responses to inoculation vary in both the distribution and severity of lesions.

Norwalk virus causes similar histologic abnormalities, also located in the proximal small bowel.[92] However, the abrupt onset of illness in adults and the consistent finding that individuals with antibody are more likely to be ill than are individuals lacking antibody suggest that an immune mechanism plays a role in illness.

Immunologic Events

Humoral immune responses to SRSV infections are like those for other virus infections. Individuals lacking antibodies show a rapid rise in titers of serum and fecal antibody that persists for months, and individuals with high serum antibody levels are unlikely to show an antibody response when re-exposed to the virus. Children with anti–Norwalk virus antibody appear to be protected against subsequent infection, at least in the short term.[60] A striking and consistent observation is that adult volunteers with higher levels of preexisting serum or fecal antibody are more likely to excrete virus or be ill than are individuals with low or no preexisting antibody.[37] The mechanism is not known for this apparent conflict, with the usual observation that serum or fecal antibody is a marker for protection against infection.

When the symptom profile of 50 Norwalk virus volunteers was assessed, the increased risk of symptoms with higher preexisting antibody titers was statistically significant for those ill subjects who had vomiting as the predominant clinical feature.[37] Because vomiting in the gastroenteritis syndrome may result from a process different from that resulting in diarrhea, this observation suggests an alternative pathogenic mechanism peculiar to the SRSVs. The existence of such an alternative pathogenic mechanism would explain the unusual observation that age-specific morbidity tends to be greatest in adults. One issue unresolved from these studies is whether the antibody assays employed in these volunteer studies measured neutralizing or non-neutralizing anti-Norwalk virus antibody.

Asymptomatic infection is not restricted to those with prior antibody and can occur outside the age range associated with the presence of maternally acquired antibody. Cellular immune responses have not been studied.

Clinical Manifestations

The clinical manifestations of SRSV are those of acute gastroenteritis.[37, 52] In 50 adult volunteers inoculated with Norwalk virus, 59 per cent had diarrhea, 66 per cent nausea, 66 per cent cramps, 66 per cent headache or body ache, 39 per cent vomiting, 24 per cent chills, and 22 per cent fever.[37] As is the case for most other viral pathogens, the majority of SRSV infections in children are likely to be asymptomatic. Extraintestinal infection caused by SRSV is not known.

Diagnosis

Differential Diagnosis

Recognized outbreaks of SRSV infection have tended to be associated with a rapid onset of symptoms and a broad age range of affected persons, especially if associated with common exposure to water or food. Otherwise, the clinical manifestations of SRSV-associated illness are indistinguishable from those caused by other enteric viruses and bacteria. Stool samples should be submitted to a facility skilled in electron microscopy and with individual assays for these pathogens. SRSVs and other caliciviruses are destroyed by repeated freezing and thawing.[21, 44] Therefore, bulk stool samples stored at 4° C and not frozen should be collected early after infection and referred promptly. Consultation with the reference laboratory should precede sample referral.[59] Paired serum samples may be required to detect and confirm the presence of an etiologic agent.

Specific Diagnosis

The diagnosis of SRSVs in stools can be accomplished by electron microscopy, but usually the level of virus excretion is less than the sensitivity of this method ($<10^6$ viral particles per gram of stool). Enzyme-linked immunosorbent assays, reverse transcription–polymerase chain reaction with SRSV-specific primers, and immunosorbent electron microscopy may be used in combination to characterize the infecting SRSV, but only a few laboratories can perform these tests.[46–48]

SAPPORO-LIKE HUMAN CALICIVIRUSES

Epidemiology

General Prevalence

Sapporo-like human caliciviruses have been found wherever sought and probably have a worldwide distribution. Unlike the SRSV-like human caliciviruses, these strains are known primarily from sporadic cases of diarrhea in children described in Japan, England, the United States, Saudi Arabia, and South Africa.[15, 16, 21, 45, 76, 109] Typical caliciviruses in stool specimens not yet characterized to type may fall into this genetic group.[19–21, 24–26, 39, 44, 71, 81, 98] Antigenically distinct strains appear to cocirculate in some regions.[45, 69, 109]

Morbidity and Mortality

The morbidity and mortality of Sapporo-like human calicivirus infections are defined poorly. In one longitudinal study of diarrhea in children attending child care centers, Sapporo-like caliciviruses were detected in 2.9 per cent of diarrhea episodes, a rate half that of rotavirus detection in the same study.[67] Cross-sectional surveys of diarrhea stool specimens from children, most of whom were hospitalized, have found caliciviruses with typical morphology in 0.2 to 6.6 per cent of samples.[31, 36, 73, 85, 89] The rate of hospitalization for children with Sapporo-like calicivirus infection is unknown, but serious illness does occur.[35, 66] No case of Sapporo-like calicivirus infection resulting in hospitalization or death has been confirmed serologically or histologically.

Age Incidence and Prevalence

Most Sapporo-like calicivirus infections have been detected in children younger than 4 years of age. Serologic studies confirm that children acquire infection soon after birth and that virtually all are infected by 4 years of age.[23, 77, 90] Children are likely to be infected with multiple typical calicivirus types during this period.[23, 68] Outbreaks have been described among infants and young children. The prevalence of antibody to Sapporo-like caliciviruses exceeds 70 per cent in adults studied in Asia, Australia, Africa, Europe, and North America.[23, 75, 77]

Seasonal Patterns

A distinct seasonal prevalence of Sapporo-like calicivirus–associated illness is not apparent from two studies that have reported such information. Among 39 samples referred from Northwest London to a calicivirus research laboratory, 22 were collected in the winter.[22] In a longitudinal population-based study in Phoenix, Arizona, more positive samples were observed in the late summer and fall.[67]

Host and Social Factors

Like other enteric viruses, Sapporo-like caliciviruses are likely to cause outbreaks of illness in settings in which the potential for fecal-oral contamination and person-to-person transmission is high. Outbreaks tend to occur in closed populations and have a high attack rate. Most of the exposed in these reported outbreaks are infected and ill. Sapporo-like calicivirus infections appear to be common in child care centers.[67, 68] New infections with typical caliciviruses in an outbreak may occur over a period of several weeks, which indicates that person-to-person transmission has a role in the virus spread.[15, 68] This pattern also suggests that asymptomatic individuals can transmit the virus. Asymptomatic Sapporo-like calicivirus infections have been noted in association with four human calicivirus outbreaks.[15, 24, 68, 76] In one study, 11 of 14 children infected in an outbreak were asymptomatic. Two outbreaks have been associated with the consumption of seafood.[2, 20]

Pathogenesis and Pathology

Viral Infection

The incubation period after exposure to Sapporo-like caliciviruses is 1 to 4 days.[16, 68, 91, 98] Excretion lasts 5 to 7 days after the onset of symptoms in half of the children and can extend up to 13 days.[16, 98] It is possible that virus excretion may be longer because the detection methods used in these studies are relatively insensitive. Transmission of infection is likely to occur by fecal-oral spread.

Pathology

The pathogenic features of Sapporo-like calicivirus infections have not been determined and are presumed to be the same as for SRSV caliciviruses.

Immunologic Events

Humoral immune responses to Sapporo-like calicivirus infection follow patterns common to many human viral illnesses.[76] Children with high levels of serum antibody are protected against subsequent infection.[24, 76] Asymptomatic infection is not restricted to those with prior antibody and can occur outside the age range associated with the presence of maternally acquired antibody. Cellular immune responses and immunologic events in the intestine have not been studied.

Clinical Manifestations

Intestinal Infection

The clinical manifestations of Sapporo-like calicivirus infection generally are mild and are those usually associated with gastroenteritis.[22, 67] Diarrhea, vomiting, anorexia, and fever are common. Respiratory symptoms may occur in about a third of patients. The constellation of symptoms associated with Sapporo-like calicivirus gastroenteritis has been indistinguishable from that associated with rotavirus gastroenteritis in both hospitalized and nonhospitalized children. As is the case for most other viral pathogens, the majority of Sapporo-like calicivirus infections are likely to be asymptomatic.

A few children hospitalized with Sapporo-like calicivirus infections have been recognized. Findings in these children include prolonged malabsorption, frank rectal bleeding, severe dehydration and acidosis, and transient leukopenia. Three children with combined immunodeficiency infected with typical calicivirus early in life have been reported.[10, 19] Typical caliciviruses have been the only identified pathogen in the stool specimens of a few children who died of gastroenteritis, but little information describing the illness or pathologic findings in these children has been reported.[19, 35]

Extraintestinal Infection

Extraintestinal infection caused by Sapporo-like caliciviruses is not known. Sapporo-like caliciviruses share genomic features with the rabbit hemorrhagic disease virus and hepatitis E virus, as reviewed earlier. The Sapporo-like caliciviruses also are closer to animal caliciviruses than to other human caliciviruses when phylogenetic trees are constructed, as described earlier. These findings suggest that Sapporo-like caliciviruses may cause a broader spectrum of illness, as has been recognized for animal calicivirus infections.

Diagnosis

Differential Diagnosis

The known clinical manifestations of Sapporo-like calicivirus–associated illness are indistinguishable from those caused by rotaviruses and other enteric viruses. As for SRSVs, fresh, unfrozen samples should be submitted to a diagnostic facility with expertise in this area.

Specific Diagnosis

The diagnosis of Sapporo-like calicivirus in stools can be accomplished by electron microscopy, enzyme-linked immunosorbent assays, reverse transcription–polymerase chain reaction, and immunosorbent electron microscopy, but only a few laboratories can perform these tests.[67]

HEPATITIS E VIRUS

Epidemiology

General Prevalence

Hepatitis E is known from outbreak and sporadic cases of hepatitis in Asia, Africa, Australia, and Latin America. These outbreaks are intermittent and can involve thousands of cases. Known transmission is by contaminated drinking water, but the intermittent nature of the outbreaks suggests that additional factors, such as an animal reservoir, may be important. Imported cases to Europe and North America are known; however, hepatitis E is not endemic in these regions. Ten hepatitis E cases were reported to the Centers for Disease Control and Prevention in 1995.

Morbidity and Mortality

Hepatitis E causes acute hepatitis, like hepatitis A, with a mortality rate of 0.5 to 3.0 per cent in the general population.[107] Mortality particularly is high in pregnant women, approaching 20 to 25 per cent in them. Hepatitis E is the principal cause of enterically transmitted acute hepatitis in some cross-sectional surveys, occurring 10 to 20 times more frequently than hepatitis A.[17] Whether this is a general trend or reflects the waxing and waning occurrence of hepatitis A and E from year to year in some regions will need to be determined from longitudinal studies.

Hepatitis E outbreaks can be intense. During one epidemic period in Kanpur, India, 111 hepatitis cases occurred among 2018 members of 343 families, for a hepatitis attack rate of 5.5 per cent in the individuals.[1] Eighty-two (24 per cent) of the 343 monitored households were affected. The pattern of secondary cases suggested that person-to-person spread did not occur. In an epidemic period in Somalia, 11,413 cases and 346 deaths occurred among 245,312 persons in 142 villages during a 20-month period, for an attack rate of 4.6 per cent and case fatality rate of 3 per cent.[7]

Age Incidence and Prevalence

Seroepidemiologic studies in endemic regions suggest that hepatitis E virus infection occurs primarily after the first decade of life. In Pune, India, antibody prevalence was less than 5 per cent in the first decade of life and reached a peak prevalence of 30 to 40 per cent in the third and fourth decades of life.[4] This contrasted with seroprevalence rates for hepatitis A, for which virtually all children were infected by the second decade of life. These patterns were the same in 1982 and 1992, indicating that there were no significant changes in virus circulation that might be expected from acquisition of herd immunity or other factors. In the study from Somalia cited earlier, the infection rate was 5 per cent among children 1 to 4 years of age, 13 per cent in children 5 to 15 years of age, and 20 per cent among older individuals. The female:male ratio among cases was 1.5:1.[4]

Seasonal Patterns

A distinct seasonal prevalence of hepatitis E virus infections is not apparent. Cases are more likely to be more common in seasons when flooding results in contamination of drinking water supplies by sewage disposal systems.

Host and Social Factors

Risk factors for sporadic cases of hepatitis E have not been described. Person-to-person spread is not a common mode of transmission. Nosocomial transmission has occurred.[88] Disease occurrence is greatest in regions with the poorest water treatment procedures, and the virus has been detected in treated water and sewage.[51] The intermittent occurrence of hepatitis E outbreaks and the failure to discover person-to-person transmission have suggested the possibility that hepatitis E is a zoonosis. In one attempt to discover such reservoirs during a hepatitis E outbreak, rodents of 23 species caught within 1 km of an affected village were studied.[55] Five of the 23 species had hepatitis E virus viremia, and white mice have been infected enterically in the laboratory.

Pathogenesis and Pathology

Viral Infection

The incubation period after exposure is 15 to 60 days, with an average of 40 days.[56, 72] Excretion lasts up to 14 days at levels detectable by enzyme immunoassay but probably is longer at lower and infectious levels because viral antigen persists in the liver for about 6 weeks after infection and virus is excreted in the bile.[11]

Pathology

The pathogenic features of hepatitis E virus infection are of an acute viral hepatitis, with focal hepatocellular necrosis, cholestatic inflammation, and acidophilic hepatocellular degeneration.[42, 56, 72]

Immunologic Events

Humoral immune responses to hepatitis E virus infection follow patterns common to many viral illnesses.[11] Individuals lacking antibodies are at increased risk of illness and show a rapid rise in titers of serum antibody that persists for months. Individuals with high serum antibody levels are unlikely to show an antibody response or to become ill when re-exposed to the virus. Asymptomatic and subclinical infection is common. Cellular immune responses have not been studied.

Immunoglobulin prepared from donors living in endemic regions may protect naive patients from infection, but such preparations have not been standardized for this purpose.[13]

Clinical Manifestations

Hepatitis E virus probably causes a mild gastroenteritis, but the symptoms of that infection would occur weeks before jaundice. Longitudinal studies to determine the features of primary infection have not been conducted. Hepatitis E virus–infected patients with hepatitis frequently have malaise (95 to 100 per cent), anorexia (66 to 100 per cent), abdominal pain (37 to 82 per cent), hepatomegaly (10 to 85 per cent), nausea and vomiting (29 to 100 per cent), fever (23 to 97 per cent), and pruritus (14 to 47 per cent).[56, 72] Resolution of illness occurs 1 to 6 weeks after onset. Chronic disease has not been observed.

Diagnosis

Differential Diagnosis

Hepatitis E is indistinguishable clinically from hepatitis caused by other viruses and a variety of noninfectious causes. Clinicians should obtain serial blood samples for serologic assays and submit fresh, unfrozen sequential stool specimens to a reference laboratory skilled in the detection of hepatitis E virus.

Specific Diagnosis

The pattern of onset of illness, epidemiologic features such as recent travel history or other exposures, and the presence of serologic markers will help determine that hepatitis E is the cause of an acute hepatitis. As for other calicivirus genetic groups, virus is excreted at low levels, and electron microscopy is a poor technique for hepatitis E virus detection. Enzyme-linked immunosorbent assays and molecular techniques have been developed for detection of viral antigen and antiviral antibody, as well as for detection of viral nucleic acid in clinical specimens. Specimens for such testing should be submitted to a reference laboratory after consultation.[11, 33]

VESICULAR EXANTHEM OF SWINE VIRUS–LIKE ANIMAL CALICIVIRUSES

Epidemiology

General Prevalence

VESV-like caliciviruses include a large number of animal caliciviruses isolated from many different hosts, including pig, cow, cat, dog, sea lion, sea otter, walrus, whale, several snakes, pygmy chimpanzee, and gorilla. These viruses probably have a worldwide distribution in terrestrial and marine environments.[94] VESV-like caliciviruses include at least 30 neutralization types (serotypes). The prevalence of these serotypes in different regions has not been studied very much.

Morbidity and Mortality

VESV-like caliciviruses cause a variety of severe illnesses in animals. The morbidity and mortality of individual strains differ from species to species in experimental infections. Several laboratory workers had subclinical infection with marine calicivirus serotypes.[5, 96] One laboratory worker was infected with San Miguel sea lion virus serotype 5 and experienced a flu-like illness, followed by viremia and vesicular exanthem over the next several days like that observed in the original host.[5]

Host and Social Factors

Although animal caliciviruses cause a variety of diseases, only a few cause gastroenteritis, a feature common to human caliciviruses.[32] Among the animal caliciviruses are a number that exhibit a broad host range. For example, the San Miguel sea lion virus serotype 5 has been found to infect sea lions, seals, opaleye fish, pigs, cattle, and laboratory workers.[100]

Pathogenesis and Pathology

Viral Infection

Animal caliciviruses cause infection on mucosal surfaces (pneumonia, aphthous ulcers) and disease after viremia (generalized vesicular eruption, encephalitis, hepatitis, spontaneous abortion). The incubation period after exposure is short: 1 to 4 days.[100] Excretion is variable between species. For three cultivatable animal caliciviruses, asymptomatic and persistent virus excretion has been detected for months after primary infection.[50, 95, 97]

Pathology

The pathogenic features of VESV-like calicivirus infection are variable, according to the syndrome of the affected animal.

Diagnosis

Differential Diagnosis

The known clinical manifestations in humans from VESV-like calicivirus infection are limited to those of the single laboratory worker. Because VESV-like caliciviruses cause a variety of illnesses in animals and these viruses occur naturally in primates, the potential spectrum of illness in humans is broad. Groups at greatest risk of infection likely would be zoo workers, indigenous populations handling marine mammals, veterinarians, and laboratory workers, but studies of these groups have been limited.[96] VESV-like caliciviruses are heat-labile, and clinical samples should be submitted promptly and unfrozen.

Specific Diagnosis

Many VESV-like caliciviruses can be cultivated in cell culture, and many are at high concentrations in clinical samples. This permits the use of electron microscopy and classic virologic methods for detection of infecting viruses. Other strains have resisted cultivation, and molecular techniques are being developed for them.[65, 93]

RABBIT HEMORRHAGIC DISEASE VIRUS

Epidemiology

General Prevalence

Rabbit hemorrhagic disease virus (RHDV) has been epidemic in Asia and Europe since its first recognition in China in 1984. Rabbits in more than 40 countries have been affected. Disease spreads rapidly and appears to "leap" large distances in a short period. Ability of the virus to spread rapidly across large bodies of water (e.g., English Channel) suggests that arthropods or other flying vectors have a role in transmission.[14] One outbreak in Mexico was traced to a shipment of rabbit meat from Asia, resulting in an extensive slaughter of rabbits in Mexico to eradicate the agent. In that outbreak, one human developed antibody. Studies of zoo workers, rabbit breeders, foresters, and others with an occupation risk of rabbit calicivirus–like calicivirus exposure have not been reported to assess the potential for human infection during this epidemic.

RHDV was released in field studies in Australia in 1995. The virus escaped from the study site the same year and spread widely throughout that continent. The rabbit calicivirus–like caliciviruses include the genetically distinct European brown hare syndrome virus. Antigenic diversity in this genetic group has been described, and the number of serotypes in the group is unknown.[108]

Morbidity and Mortality

RHDV infections are highly fatal (>80 per cent) in wild and domesticated European rabbits. Subclinical infections occur in young rabbits, and this infection appears to attenuate later exposures. The human infection in the Mexican outbreak apparently was subclinical.

Host and Social Factors

The host range of rabbit calicivirus–like caliciviruses and the source of the RHDV prior to its recognition in China are unknown. In Australian studies, a number of Australian animal species challenged with a subimmunogenic dose of RHDV had no antibody response. On the other hand, kiwis, mice, dogs, and foxes did develop antibodies; in the case of the fox, serum antibody response was to oral feeding.[17a] Natural spread in rabbits is enhanced by their colony breeding behavior.

Pathogenesis and Pathology

The incubation period after exposure is 1 to 3 days.[105] Rabbit calcivirus–like caliciviruses cause a fatal hepatitis, resulting in disseminated intravascular coagulation and diffuse hemorrhage. Death is rapid: 6 to 12 hours after illness onset. RHDV and European brown hare syndrome virus appear to be sufficiently distinct that animals infected with the latter are not protected against subsequent exposure to RHDV.

Diagnosis

Because the infection in the Mexican worker exposed during the RHDV outbreak apparently was subclinical, the spectrum of potential infection in humans is unknown. Samples from suspected infections should be submitted to reference laboratories after consultation. Diagnosis is possible through immunologic and molecular techniques.

TREATMENT AND PREVENTION

No specific treatment for calicivirus infections has been reported. The existence of an effective vaccine for the feline calicivirus indicates that this prevention method would work for human caliciviruses, and vaccine development for hepatitis E virus is in progress. Children with diarrhea are more likely to be excreting enteric viruses than are children without diarrhea, which reflects an association between the incidence of diarrhea and cleanliness of the environment. This principle is likely to hold for caliciviruses as well. For children in care settings with other children, a few infection control measures are likely to reduce the spread of infection. These measures include trained personnel, cleanliness of the surfaces and food preparation areas, exclusion of ill or carrier care providers, adequate hand washing, and exclusion or cohorting of ill children.[27] Laboratory workers exposed to caliciviruses should be aware of the risk of infection.

PROGNOSIS

Understanding of the features of calicivirus infections has increased rapidly since 1990, when molecular tools for studying the viruses became available. Knowledge in this area will increase rapidly. The availability of abundant diagnostic reagents will permit an accurate assessment of the extent and variety of calicivirus-associated illness.

Acknowledgment

Supported by U.S. Public Health Service grants A128544, HD13021, and A137093.

References

1. Aggarwal, R., and Naik, S. R.: Hepatitis E: Intrafamilial transmission versus waterborne spread. J. Hepatol. *21*:718–723, 1994.
2. Appleton, H.: Small round viruses: Classification and role in food-borne infections. *In* Bock, G., and Whelan, J. (eds.): Novel Diarrhoea Viruses. Chichester, Wiley, 1987, pp. 238–249.
3. Appleton, H., and Higgins, P. G.: Viruses and gastroenteritis in infants. Lancet *1*:1297, 1975.
4. Arankalle, V. A., Tsarev, S. A., Chadha, M. S., et al.: Age-specific prevalence of antibodies to hepatitis A and E viruses in Pune, India, 1982 and 1992. J. Infect. Dis. *171*:447–50, 1995.
5. Barlough, J. E., Berry, E. S., Skilling, D. E., et al.: The marine calicivirus story. Compendium on Continuing Education for the Practicing Veterinarian *8*:F5–F14, F75–F82, 1986.
6. Berke, T., Golding, B., Smith, A. W., et al.: Phylogenetic relationships among human and animal caliciviruses. 35th Interscience Conference on Antimicrobial Agents and Chemotherapy, San Francisco, October 1995.
7. Bile, K., Isse, A., Mohamud, O., et al.: Contrasting roles of rivers and wells as sources of drinking water on attack and fatality rates in a hepatitis E epidemic in Somalia. Am. J. Trop. Med. Hyg. *51*:466–74, 1994.
8. Black, R. E., Greenberg, H. B., Kapikian, A. Z., et al.: Acquisition of serum antibody to Norwalk virus and rotavirus and relation to diarrhea in a longitudinal study of young children in rural Bangladesh. J. Infect. Dis. *145*:483–489, 1982.
9. Blacklow, N. R., Dolin, R., Fedson, D. S., et al.: Acute infectious nonbacterial gastroenteritis: Etiology and pathogenesis. A combined clinical staff conference at the Clinical Center of the National Institutes of Health. Ann. Intern. Med. *76*:993–1008, 1972.
10. Booth, I. W., Chrystie, I. L., Levinsky, R. J., et al.: Protracted diarrhoea, immunodeficiency and viruses. Eur. J. Pediatr. *138*:271–272, 1982.
11. Bradley, D. W.: Hepatitis E virus: A brief review of the biology, molecular virology, and immunology of a novel virus. J. Hepatol. *22*:140–145, 1995.
12. Bradley, D. W., Krawczynski, K., Cook, E. H., et al.: Enterically transmitted non-A, non-B hepatitis: Serial passage of disease in cynomolgous macaques and tamarins and recovery of disease-associated viruslike particles. Proc. Natl. Acad. Sci. U. S. A. *84*:6277–6281, 1987.
13. Bryan, J. P., Tsarev, S. A., Iqbal, M., et al.: Epidemic hepatitis E in Pakistan: Patterns of serologic response and evidence that antibody to hepatitis E virus protects against disease. J. Infect. Dis. *170*:517–521, 1994.
14. Chasey, D.: Possible origin of rabbit haemorrhagic disease in the United Kingdom. Vet. Rec. *135*:496–499, 1994.
15. Chiba, S., Sakuma, Y., Kogasaka, R., et al.: An outbreak of gastroenteritis associated with calicivirus in an infant home. J. Med. Virol. *4*:249–254, 1979.
16. Chiba, S., Sakuma, Y., Kogasaka, R., et al.: Fecal shedding of virus in relation to the days of illness in infantile gastroenteritis due to calicivirus. J. Infect. Dis. *142*:247–249, 1980.
17. Clayson, E. T., Innis, B. L., Myint, K. S., et al.: Short report: Relative risk of hepatitis A and E among foreigners in Nepal. Am. J. Trop. Med. Hyg. *52*:506–507, 1995.
17a. Coman, B. J.: Environmental impact associated with the proposed use of rabbit calicivirus disease for integrated rabbit control in Australia. Australia and New Zealand Rabbit Calicivirus Program, Sydney, February 1996.
18. Cooper, P. D., Agol, V. I., Bachrach, H. L., et al.: *Picornaviridae*: Second report. Intervirology *10*:165, 1978.
19. Cubitt, W. D.: Human caliciviruses: Characterization and epidemiology. Dissertation, Middlesex Hospital Medical School, London, 1985.
20. Cubitt, W. D.: The candidate caliciviruses. *In* Bock, G., and Whelan, J. (eds.): Novel Diarrhoea Viruses. Chichester, Wiley, 1987, pp. 126–143.
21. Cubitt, W. D., Blacklow, N. R., Herrmann, J. E., et al.: Antigenic relationships between human caliciviruses and Norwalk virus. J. Infect. Dis. *156*:806–814, 1987.
22. Cubitt, W. D., and McSwiggan, D. A.: Calicivirus gastroenteritis in north west London. Lancet *2*:975–977, 1981.
23. Cubitt, W. D., and McSwiggan, D. A.: Seroepidemiological survey of the prevalence of antibodies to a strain of human calicivirus. J. Med. Virol. *21*:361–368, 1987.
24. Cubitt, W. D., McSwiggan, D. A., and Arstall, S.: An outbreak of calicivirus infection in a mother and baby unit. J. Clin. Pathol. *33*:1095–1098, 1980.
25. Cubitt, W. D., McSwiggan, D. A., and Moore, W.: Winter vomiting disease caused by calicivirus. J. Clin. Pathol. *32*:786–793, 1979.
26. Cubitt, W. D., Pead, P. J., and Saeed, A. A.: A new serotype of calicivirus associated with an outbreak of gastroenteritis in a residential home for the elderly. J. Clin. Pathol. *34*:924–926, 1981.
27. Cummings, G. D.: Epidemic diarrhea of the newborn from the point of view of the epidemiologist and bacteriologist. J. Pediatr. *30*:706–710, 1947.
28. Dinulos, M. B., and Matson, D. O.: Recent developments with human caliciviruses. Pediatr. Infect. Dis. J. *13*:998–1003, 1994.
29. Dolin, R., Blacklow, N. R., Dupont, H., et al.: Biological properties of Norwalk agent of acute infectious nonbacterial gastroenteritis. Proc. Soc. Exp. Biol. Med. *140*:578–583, 1972.
30. Dolin, R., Blacklow, N. R., Dupont, H., et al.: Transmission of acute infectious nonbacterial gastroenteritis to volunteers by oral administration of stool filtrates. J. Infect. Dis. *123*:307–312, 1971.
31. Ellis, M. E., Watson, B., Mandal, B. K., et al.: Micro-organisms in gastroenteritis. Arch. Dis. Child. *59*:848–855, 1984.
32. Evermann, J. F., McKeirnan, A. J., Smith, A. W., et al.: Isolation and identification of caliciviruses from dogs with enteric infections. Am. J. Vet. Res. *46*:218–220, 1985.
33. Favorov, M. O., Fields, H. A., Purdy, M. A., et al.: Serologic identification of hepatitis E virus infections in epidemic and endemic settings. J. Med. Virol. *36*:246–250, 1992.
34. Favorov, M. O., Khudyakov, Y. E., Fields, H. A., et al.: Enzyme immunoassay for the detection of antibody to hepatitis E virus based on synthetic peptides. J. Virol. Methods *46*:237–250, 1994.
35. Flewett, T. H., and Davies, H.: Caliciviruses in man. Lancet *1*:311, 1976.
36. Flynn, W. T., Saif, L. J., and Moorhead, P. D.: Pathogenesis of porcine enteric calicivirus-like virus in four-day-old gnotobiotic piglets. Am. J. Vet. Res. *49*:819–825, 1988.
37. Graham, D. Y., Jiang, X., Tanaka, T., et al.: Norwalk virus infection of volunteers: New insights based on improved assays. J. Infect. Dis. *170*:34–43, 1994.
38. Gray, J. J., Jiang, X., Morgan-Capner, P., et al.: Prevalence of antibodies to Norwalk virus in England: Detection by enzyme-linked immunosorbent assay using baculovirus-expressed Norwalk virus capsid antigen. J. Clin. Microbiol. *31*:1022–1025, 1993.
39. Gray, J. J., Wreghitt, T. G., Cubitt, W. D., et al.: An outbreak of gastroenteritis in a home for the elderly associated with astrovirus type 1 and human calicivirus. J. Med. Virol. *23*:377–381, 1987.
40. Greenberg, H. B., Valdesuso, J., Yolken, R. H., et al.: Role of Norwalk virus in outbreaks of nonbacterial gastroenteritis. J. Infect. Dis. *139*:564–568, 1979.
41. Gregg, D. A., House, C., Meyer, R., et al.: Viral haemorrhagic disease of rabbits in Mexico: Epidemiology and viral characterization. Rev. Sci. Tech. *10*:435–451, 1991.
42. Gupta, D. N., and Smetana, H. F.: The histopathology of viral hepatitis as seen in the Delhi epidemics (1955–56). Indian J. Med. Res. *45*(Suppl.):101–113, 1957.
43. Hall, G. A., Bridger, J. C., Brooker, B. E., et al.: Lesions of gnotobiotic calves experimentally infected with a calicivirus-like (Newbury) agent. Vet. Pathol. *21*:208–215, 1984.
44. Humphrey, T. J., Cruickshank, J. G., and Cubitt, W. D.: An outbreak of calicivirus associated gastroenteritis in an elderly persons home: A possible zoonosis? J. Hyg. Camb. *92*:293–299, 1984.
45. Jiang, X., Berke, T., Zhong, W., et al.: Molecular characterization of two genetic and antigenically distinct strains of the Sapporo genogroup of human caliciviruses. Submitted.
46. Jiang, X., Cubitt, D., Hu, J., et al.: Development of a type-specific EIA for detection of Snow Mountain agent–like human caliciviruses in stool specimens. J. Gen. Virol. *76*:2739–2747, 1995.
47. Jiang, X., Turf, E., Hu, J., et al.: Outbreaks of gastroenteritis in elderly nursing homes and retirement facilities associated with human caliciviruses. J. Med. Virol. *50*:335–341, 1996.
48. Jiang, X., Wang, J., Graham, D. Y., et al.: Detection of Norwalk virus in stool by polymerase chain reaction. J. Clin. Microbiol. *30*:2529–2534, 1992.
49. Jiang, X., Wang, M., Wang, K., et al.: Sequence and genomic organization of Norwalk virus. Virology *195*:51–61, 1993.
50. Johnson, R. P., and Povey, R. C.: Feline calicivirus infection in kittens borne by cats persistently infected with the virus. Res. Vet. Sci. *37*:114–119, 1984.

51. Jothikumar, N., Aparna, K., Kamatchiammal, S., et al.: Detection of hepatitis E virus in raw and treated wastewater with the polymerase chain reaction. Appl. Environ. Microbiol. *59*:2558–2562, 1993.
52. Kapikian, A. Z., and Chanock, R. M.: Norwalk group of viruses. *In* Fields, B. N., and Knipe, D. M. (eds.): Virology. New York, Raven Press, 1990, pp. 671–693.
53. Kapikian, A. Z., Greenberg, H. B., Cline, W. L., et al.: Prevalence of antibody to the Norwalk agent by a newly developed immune adherence assay. J. Med. Virol. *2*:281–294, 1978.
54. Kapikian, A. Z., Wyatt, R. G., Dolin, R., et al.: Visualization by immune electron microscopy of a 27-nm particle associated with acute infectious non-bacterial gastroenteritis. J. Virol. *10*:1075–1081, 1972.
55. Karetnyi, I. V., Dzhumalieva, D. I., Usmanov, R. K., et al.: The possible involvement of rodents in the spread of viral hepatitis E. Zh. Mikrobiol. Epidemiol. Immunobiol. *4*:52–56, 1993.
56. Khuroo, M. S.: Study of an epidemic of non-A, non-B hepatitis: Possibility of another human hepatitis virus distinct from post-transfusion non-A, non-B type. Am. J. Med. *68*:818–824, 1980.
57. Kilgore, P. E., Belay, E. D., Hamlin, D. M., et al.: A university outbreak of gastroenteritis due to a small round-structured virus: Application of molecular diagnostics to identify the etiologic agent and patterns of transmission. J. Infect. Dis. *173*:787–793, 1996.
58. Krawcrynski, K., and Bradley, D. W.: Enterically transmitted non-A, non-B hepatitis: Identification of virus-associated antigen in experimentally infected cynomolgus macaques. J. Infect. Dis. *159*:1042–1049, 1989.
59. LeBaron, C. W., Furutan, N. P., Lew, J. F., et al.: Viral agents of gastroenteritis: Public health importance and outbreak management. M. M. W. R. *39*(RR-5):1–24, 1990.
60. Lew, J. F., Valdesuso, J., Vesikari, T., et al.: Detection of Norwalk virus or Norwalk-like virus infections in Finnish infants and young children. J. Infect. Dis. *169*:1364–1367, 1994.
61. Liu, B. L., Clarke, I. N., Caul, E. O., et al.: Human enteric caliciviruses have a unique genome structure and are distinct from the Norwalk-like viruses. Arch. Virol. *140*:1–12, 1995.
62. Longer, C. F., Denny, S. L., Caudill, J. D., et al.: Experimental hepatitis E: Pathogenesis in cynomolgus macaques (*Macaca fascicularis*). J. Infect. Dis. *168*:602–609, 1993.
63. Madeley, C. R., and Cosgrove, B. P.: Caliciviruses in man. Lancet *2*:199, 1976.
64. Matson, D. O.: Caliciviruses. Semin. Pediatr. Infect. Dis. *7*:101–106, 1996.
65. Matson, D. O., Berke, T., Dinulos, M. B., et al.: Partial characterization of the genome of nine animal caliciviruses. Arch Virol. *141*:2443–2456, 1996.
66. Matson, D. O., and Estes, M. K.: Unpublished data.
67. Matson, D. O., Estes, M. K., Glass, R. I., et al.: Human calicivirus–associated diarrhea in children attending day care centers. J. Infect. Dis. *159*:71–78, 1989.
68. Matson, D. O., Estes, M. K., Tanaka, T., et al.: Asymptomatic human calicivirus infection in a day care center. Pediatr. Infect. Dis. J. *9*:190–196, 1990.
69. Matson, D. O., Mitchell, D. K., Van, R., et al.: Enteric viral pathogens as causes of outbreaks of diarrhea among children attending day care centers during one year of observation. Pediatr. Res. *37*:826, 1995.
70. Matson, D. O., Zhong, W. M., Nakata, S. et al.: Molecular characterization of a human calicivirus with sequence relationships closer to animal caliciviruses than other known human caliciviruses. J. Med. Virol. *45*:215–222, 1995.
71. McSwiggan, D. A., Cubitt, W. D., and Moore, W.: Calicivirus associated with winter vomiting disease. Lancet *1*:1215, 1978.
72. Morrow, R. H., Smetana, H. F., Sai, F. T., et al.: Unusual features of viral hepatitis in Accra, Ghana. Ann. Intern. Med. *68*:250–264, 1968.
73. Murphy, A.: An etiology of viral gastroenteritis: A review. Med. J. Aust. *2*:177–182, 1981.
74. Nagesha, H. S., Wang, L. F., Hyatt, A. D., et al.: Self-assembly, antigenicity, and immunogenicity of the rabbit haemorrhagic disease virus (Czechoslovakian strain V-351) capsid protein expressed in baculovirus. Arch. Virol. *140*:1095–1108, 1995.
75. Nakata, S., Chiba, S., Terashima, H., et al.: Prevalence of antibody to human calicivirus in Japan and Southeast Asia determined by radioimmunoassay. J. Clin. Microbiol. *22*:519–521, 1985.
76. Nakata, S., Chiba, S., Terashima, H., et al.: Humoral immunity in infants with gastroenteritis caused by human calicivirus. J. Infect. Dis. *152*:274–279, 1985.
77. Nakata, S., Estes, M. K., and Chiba, S.: Detection of human calicivirus antigen and antibody by enzyme-linked immunosorbent assays. J. Clin. Microbiol. *26*:2001–2005, 1988.
78. Neill, J. D., Meyer, R. F., and Seal, B. S.: Genetic relatedness of the caliciviruses: San Miguel sea lion and vesicular exanthema of swine viruses constitute a single genotype within the *Caliciviridae*. J. Virol. *69*:4484–4488, 1995.
79. Numata, K., Nakata, S., Jiang, X., et al.: Epidemiological study of Norwalk virus infections in Japan and Southeast Asia by enzyme-linked immunosorbent assays with Norwalk virus capsid protein produced by the baculovirus expression system. J. Clin. Microbiol. *32*:121–126, 1994.
80. Ohlinger, V. F., and Thiel, H. J.: Identification of the viral haemorrhagic disease virus of rabbits as a calicivirus. Rev. Sci. Tech. *10*:311–323, 1991.
81. Oishi, I., Maeda, A., Yamazaki, K., et al.: Calicivirus detected in outbreaks of acute gastroenteritis in school children. Biken J. *23*:163–168, 1980.
82. O'Ryan, M. L., Mamani, N., Vial, P., et al.: Epidemiological differences of two human caliciviruses in two widely separated cities of the same country. 36th Interscience Conference on Antimicrobial Agents and Chemotherapy, New Orleans, October 1996.
83. Parra, F., and Prieto, M.: Purification and characterization of a calicivirus as the causative agent of a lethal hemorrhagic disease in rabbits. J. Virol. *64*:4013–4015, 1990.
84. Paul, D. A., Knigge, M. F., Ritter, A., et al.: Determination of hepatitis E virus seroprevalence by using recombinant fusion proteins and synthetic peptides. J. Infect. Dis. *169*:801–806, 1994.
85. Payne, C. M., Ray, C. G., Borduin, V., et al.: An eight-year study of the viral agents of acute gastroenteritis in humans: Ultrastructural observations and seasonal distribution with major emphasis on coronavirus-like particles. Diagn. Microbiol. Infect. Dis. *5*:39–54, 1986.
86. Prasad, B. V. V., Matson, D. O., and Smith, A. W.: Three-dimensional structure of the primate calicivirus. J. Mol. Biol. *240*:256–264, 1994.
87. Prasad, B. V. V., Rothnagel, R., Jiang, X., et al.: Three-dimensional structure of baculovirus-expressed Norwalk virus capsids. J. Virol. *68*:5117–5125, 1994.
88. Robson, S. C., Adams, S., Brink, N., et al.: Hospital outbreak of hepatitis E. Lancet *339*:1424–1425, 1992.
89. Riepenhoff-Talty, M., Saif, L. J., Barrett, H. J., et al.: Potential spectrum of etiological agents of viral enteritis in hospitalized infants. J. Clin. Microbiol. *17*:352–356, 1983.
90. Sakuma, Y., Chiba, S., Kogasaka, R., et al.: Prevalence of antibody to human calicivirus in general population of northern Japan. J. Med. Virol. *7*:221–225, 1981.
91. Sawyer, L. A., Murphy, J. J., Kaplan, J. E., et al.: 25–30-nm virus particle associated with a hospital outbreak of acute gastroenteritis with evidence for airborne transmission. Am. J. Epidemiol. *127*:1261–1271, 1988.
92. Schreiber, D. S., Blacklow, N. R., and Trier, J. S.: The mucosal lesion of the proximal small intestine in acute infectious nonbacterial gastroenteritis. N. Engl. J. Med. *288*:1318–1323, 1973.
93. Seal, B. S., Lutze-Wallace, C., Kreutz, L. C., et al.: Isolation of caliciviruses from skunks that are antigenically and genotypically related to San Miguel sea lion virus. Virus Res. *37*:1–12, 1995.
94. Smith, A. W., and Boyt, P. M.: Caliciviruses of ocean origin: A review. J. Zoo. Wildl. Med. *21*:3–23, 1990.
95. Smith, A. W., Mattson, D. E., Skilling, D. E., et al.: Isolation and partial characterization of a calicivirus from calves. Am. J. Vet. Res. *44*:851–855, 1983.
96. Smith, A. W., Prato, C., and Skilling, D. E.: Caliciviruses infecting monkeys and possibly man. Am. J. Vet. Res. *39*:287–289, 1978.
97. Smith, A. W., Skilling, D. E., Ensley, P. K., et al.: Calicivirus isolation and persistence in a pygmy chimpanzee (*Pan paniscus*). Science *221*:79–81, 1983.
98. Spratt, H. C., Marks, M. I., Gomersall, M., et al.: Nosocomial infantile gastroenteritis associated with minirotavirus and calicivirus. J. Pediatr. *93*:922–926, 1978.
99. Steinhoff, M. C., Douglas, R. G., Jr., Greenberg, H. B., et al.: Bismuth subsalicylate therapy of viral gastroenteritis. Gastroenterology *78*:1495–1499, 1980.
100. Studdert, M. J.: Caliciviruses. Arch. Virol. *58*:157–191, 1978.
101. Tam, A. W., Smith, M. W., Guerra, M. E., et al.: Hepatitis E virus (HEV): Molecular cloning and sequencing of the full-length viral genome. Virology *185*:120–131, 1991.
102. Tandon, B. N., Joshi, Y. K., Jain, S. K., et al.: An epidemic of non-A, non-B hepatitis in north India. Indian J. Med. Res. *75*:739–744, 1982.
103. Taylor, M. B., Parker, S., Grabow, W. O. K., et al.: An epidemiological investigation of Norwalk virus infection in South Africa. Epidemiol. Infect. *116*:203–206, 1996.
104. Tsarev, S. A., Tsareva, T. S., Emerson, S. U., et al.: ELISA for antibody to hepatitis E virus (HEV) based on complete open-reading frame–2 protein expressed in insect cells: Identification of HEV in primates. J. Infect. Dis. *168*:369–378, 1993.
105. Ueda, K., Park, J. H., Ochiai, K., et al.: Disseminated intravascular coagulation (DIC) in rabbit haemorrhagic disease. Jpn. J. Vet. Res. *40*:133–141, 1992.
106. Viswanathan, R.: Infectious hepatitis in Delhi (1955–56): Epidemiology. Indian J. Med. Res. *45*:71–76, 1957.
107. Wattre, P.: Hepatitis E virus. Ann. Biol. Clin. *52*:507–513, 1994.
108. Wirblich, C., Meyers, G., Ohlinger, V. F., et al.: European brown hare syndrome virus: Relationship to rabbit hemorrhagic disease virus and other caliciviruses. J. Virol. *68*:5164–5173, 1994.
109. Wolfaardt, M., Taylor, M. B., Berke, T., et al.: Detection of human caliciviruses with sequence relationships closer to animal caliciviruses in South Africa. Submitted.
110. Wyatt, R. G., Dolin, R., Blacklow, N. R., et al.: Comparison of three agents of acute infectious nonbacterial gastroenteritis by cross-challenge in volunteers. J. Infect. Dis. *129*:709–714, 1974.
111. Xu, Z. J., and Chen, W. X.: Viral hemorrhagic disease in rabbits: A review. Vet. Res. Commun. *13*:205–212, 1989.

❑ ❑ ❑

SUBSECTION THREE

REOVIRIDAE

174

REOVIRUSES

James D. Cherry

Reoviruses are ubiquitous in nature, but their role in human disease is vague. After their classification in 1959, a number of reports noted their association with human disease.[54, 66] Since that time, these viruses have been evaluated extensively in laboratory animal studies, but there have been few reports of human disease during the last two decades.

HISTORY

On the basis of its cytopathic effect in monkey kidney tissue culture and its recovery from stool specimens at a time of enterovirus surveillance, the first recovered reovirus was designated ECHO virus type 10.[9, 10] This virus and four similar strains were recovered in 1954 from the stools of healthy children in Cincinnati and Mexico.[50, 51] By 1959, it was apparent that ECHO 10 viral strains had many characteristics that were different from enteroviruses, such as large size and unique cytopathic effect, so they were withdrawn from this grouping. The term *reovirus* was chosen to stress the association of these agents with both the respiratory *(r)* and enteric *(e)* tracts. The *o* for orphan was retained in the designation. In the early 1960s, reoviral infections were noted in association with human illness.[15, 26, 33, 58, 59, 72, 81]

PROPERTIES[8, 53, 54, 64, 77, 78]

Reoviruses are members of the family *Reoviridae*.[17] All mammalian reoviruses are related by a common, group-specific, complement-fixing antigen.[62, 78] Three distinct human serotypes can be identified by neutralization or hemagglutination inhibition.[60]

Reovirus particles are composed of an inner protein shell (core) with a diameter of 60 nm that is surrounded by an outer protein shell (outer capsid) measuring 81 nm in diameter.[64] The outer capsid has icosahedral symmetry and is composed of between 92 and 180 hexagonal and pentagonal subunits (capsomeres). The outer capsid is composed of three proteins: sigma-1, sigma-3, and M1C. The following functions have been ascribed to sigma-1: cell attachment, hemagglutinin, antigen for neutralizing antibody production, T-cell–dependent delayed-type hypersensitivity, suppressor T-cell generation, cytotoxic T-cell generation, tropism and specific cell uptake and injury, pathways of spread, growth in intestine, interaction with host-cell microtubules, and inhibition of host-cell DNA replication.

Functions or properties of sigma-3 protein are affinity for double-stranded RNA, zinc metalloprotein, inhibition of cellular RNA and protein synthesis, establishment of persistent infection, and regulation of viral transcription and translation.[64] The properties and functions of M1C protein include in vivo resistance of outer capsid to protease, modulation of virulence within a serotype, and induction of tolerance after oral inoculation.

The reovirus core is 60 nm in diameter, and in its center are contained 10 double-stranded RNA genome segments.[64] The core is composed of three major (lambda-1, lambda-2, and sigma-2) and several minor proteins. Lambda-2 protein is a core spike with projections that extend to the outer surface of the virion. The core proteins are responsible for transcriptase and replicase activities.

The virion also contains three nonstructural proteins. The molecular weight of the virion is 129.5×10^6 daltons; about 11.5 to 16.5 per cent of the weight is RNA.

Reoviruses are moderately heat-stable. The half-life at 56° C of a type 3 strain is 1.6 minutes; at 37° C, it is about 2.5 hours. Reoviruses are inactivated by visible light in the presence of heterocyclic dyes. They are inactivated by ultraviolet light but are more resistant to this treatment than are RNA viruses with single-stranded nucleic acid. Reoviruses are stable through a wide pH range and also are stable as aerosols, particularly when the relative humidity is high. They are relatively resistant to 3 per cent formaldehyde solution, 1 per cent hydrogen peroxide, and 1 per cent phenol but are inactivated completely by 70 per cent ethyl alcohol at room temperature for 1 hour. Brief exposure to 70 per cent ethanol is ineffective in disinfecting reoviruses, but brief exposure to 95 per cent ethanol or sodium hypochlorite is effective.

Reoviruses replicate with a cytopathic effect in a large number of tissue culture systems of both primate and other animal origin. For recovery from clinical material, monkey kidney tissue culture is satisfactory. Cytopathic effect is enhanced in rolled compared with stationary cultures.[33] Infected cells develop characteristic cytoplasmic inclusions that contain double-stranded RNA, virus-specific proteins, and complete and incomplete viral particles. All three serotypes agglutinate human erythrocytes, and this virus-cell interaction is stable in a wide temperature and pH range.

Of all viruses that naturally infect humans, reoviruses have the broadest host range. They have been recovered from natural infections in cattle, chimpanzees, monkeys, mice, dogs, turkeys, sheep, pigs, chickens, and cats.[11, 20, 22, 37–40, 55, 63, 79, 80] In addition, hemagglutination-inhibiting and neutralizing antibodies to one or more of the three reoviral serotypes have been found in the serums of rabbits, horses, trout, guinea pigs, antelopes, zebras, warthogs, bats, wallabies, quokkas, kangaroos, and several genera of New World monkeys.[44, 57, 60, 62, 70, 71]

Because of their widespread prevalence in nature and the ease of infection in laboratory animals, reoviruses have been used widely in pathogenicity studies. The following unique illnesses have been observed: diabetes mellitus in mice; hydrocephalus in hamsters, ferrets, rats, and mice; encephalitis in mice; chronic infection with runting in mice; myocarditis in mice; chronic obstructive jaundice associated with choledochal obliteration in mice; and lymphomas in mice with chronic infection.[24, 28, 36, 46, 48, 67, 69, 73]

EPIDEMIOLOGY

From the serologic data presented in the preceding section of this chapter, it is obvious that reoviruses are prevalent infectious agents in the animal world. Similarly, surveys of sera collected from humans indicate worldwide human infection.[4–6, 18, 27, 31, 32, 34, 47, 61, 65, 74, 76] The occurrence in nature of identical viruses in many different animals and humans leads to consideration of possible transmission from species to species. At present, this transmission has not been demonstrated.

Reoviruses are recovered frequently from sewage.[16, 25, 29, 35, 38, 45] In San Diego, reoviruses more consistently than any other virus have been recovered throughout the year from sewage.[16] This finding suggests that reoviral infection is endemic in humans in the San Diego area.

The type 2 hemagglutination-inhibiting antibody prevalence pattern by age in sera collected in Boston from 1959 to 1962 is presented in Table 174–1. It is seen that antibody is transmitted transplacentally to the newborn. During the first year of life, this acquired antibody wanes. After this, antibody prevalence increases with increasing age. About 50 per cent of school age children have hemagglutination-inhibiting antibody titers greater than or equal to 1:20 to type 2 reovirus; about 80 per cent of adults have similar titers.

The method of transmission of reoviruses is unknown. However, because they are recovered most frequently from the feces, it seems most likely that primary spread is similar to that of enteroviruses by the fecal-oral route. Because the reoviruses are stable in aerosols and because respiratory illness has been associated with reovirus infections, this route is an additional possibility.

CLINICAL MANIFESTATIONS

The role of reoviral infections in human disease is far from clear. In most instances, virologic or serologic evidence of reoviral infection has been a sporadic finding in human illness, so that cause and effect are impossible to establish; there always is the possibility that the observed illness is due to an unrecognized infectious agent and the reoviral infection is concomitant but not pathogenic.

The prevalence of antibody to all three reoviral types in humans and the frequency of reovirus isolation from human sewage indicate that human infection is common, but the relative paucity of virus recovery during studies of community disease suggests that most infections are inapparent or associated with trivial illness.

TABLE 174–1. Hemagglutination-Inhibition (HI) Antibodies to Reovirus Type 2 in 253 Serum Specimens Collected in Boston from 1959 to 1962

Age Group	Percentage with HI Titer ≥1 : 20
Premature newborn	68
0–6 months	25
7–12 months	9
13–24 months	27
2–5 years	37
6–10 years	52
11–20 years	54
21–40 years	34
41–60 years	83
>60 years	73

From Lerner, A. M., Cherry, J. D., Klein, J. O., et al.: Infections with reoviruses. N. Engl. J. Med. *267*:947–952, 1962. Reprinted, with permission, from the New England Journal of Medicine.

Upper Respiratory Illness

In the winter of 1957, Rosen and colleagues[58] noted an outbreak of infection with reovirus type 1 in nursery children in a welfare institution. Illness was noted in 16 of 22 infected children and was characterized by low-grade fever (rectal temperatures from 38.1° to 38.6° C; 100.6° to 101.5° F), rhinorrhea, and pharyngitis. The average duration of fever was 2.2 days; in nine children, the duration was only 1 day. Three children had diarrhea, and three had mild otitis media. In another study at the same institution during the winter of 1955 to 1956, four children with reovirus type 3 infection and illness were noted.[59] One child had a temperature of 38.9° C (102° F), coryza, and tonsillitis; another child had fever (temperature 38.2° C; 100.8° F), cough, and diarrhea; and two children had only coryza. During another reovirus type 3 outbreak in the fall of 1957, all six infected infants had symptoms. Five children had mild fever, five had coryza, and four had diarrhea. Pharyngitis was not observed in any of the infected children.

Other sporadic instances of similar mild upper respiratory illnesses have been described.[12, 21, 23, 68, 72] In volunteer trials in young adults, reovirus type 1 infection was associated with malaise, rhinorrhea, cough, sneezing, pharyngitis, and headache in some subjects in one study,[56] and cold-like illness was observed in 37 per cent of subjects in another trial.[23] In both volunteer studies and natural infection, mild diarrhea occurred with the upper respiratory illness.

Pneumonia

Tillotson and Lerner[75] reported a 5-year-old girl who had extensive pneumonia and died after 15 days of illness. This child initially had fever, cough, rhinorrhea, and a generalized maculopapular rash. When admitted to the hospital on the tenth day of illness, the child was cyanotic and in marked respiratory distress; rash was present no longer, but mild pharyngitis and conjunctivitis were. A chest radiograph revealed a diffuse confluent pneumonia, and reovirus type 3 was recovered from the lungs, adrenals, liver, spleen, kidney, a lymph node, heart, brain, and blood.

Joske and associates[26] noted a 10-month-old girl who died after a respiratory illness of 4 days' duration. A reovirus type 1 was recovered from the stool and brain of this child, and postmortem study revealed interstitial pneumonia, myocarditis, hepatitis, and encephalitis. El-Rai and Evans[15] reported the case of an 18-year-old boy who had fever (temperature of 39.4° C; 103° F), nausea, vomiting, cough, and patchy pneumonia. He had serologic evidence of infection with reovirus type 1. Pneumonia has been noted in another child with reovirus type 3 infection.[72]

Gastrointestinal Manifestations

Mild diarrhea has been noted both in association with upper respiratory illness and as an isolated event.[49, 56, 58, 59, 63] Because reovirus type 3 consistently produces steatorrhea in mice, this clinical manifestation has been sought in illnesses of children and noted in six.[62, 72] Three patients with hepatitis and encephalitis have been reported.[26] Zalan and associates[81] have noted two patients in whom abdominal pain and cramps were prominent.

In 1980, Bangaru and associates[1] reported the similarity of induced hepatobiliary injury in mice due to reovirus type 3 infection and biliary atresia in human infants. Subsequent to this observation, Morecki and colleagues[19, 42, 43] looked for an association between reovirus type 3 infection and biliary atresia in humans. In their first report, they found that 17 of 25 patients (68 per cent) with biliary atresia had antibodies (indirect immunofluorescent antibody technique) to reovirus type 3, whereas similar antibodies were recovered in only 3 of 37 control sera.[42] In a second study, they found that 62 per cent of babies with extrahepatic biliary atresia and 52 per cent of infants with idiopathic neonatal hepatitis had antibodies to reovirus type 3; only 12 per cent of control children had similar antibodies.[19] In an ultrastructural and immunocytochemical study, they found evidence of reovirus type 3 in the porta hepatis of an infant with extrahepatic biliary atresia.[43]

Using similar serologic techniques, Dussaix and associates[13] were unable to find any relationship between reovirus type 3 antibody and either biliary atresia or neonatal hepatitis. They found reovirus type 3 antibody in sera from 45 per cent of infants with biliary atresia, 50 per cent of infants with neonatal hepatitis, and 50 per cent of control infants. Minuk and colleagues[41] found no association between reovirus type 3 infection and idiopathic cholestatic liver disease in adults. Brown and colleagues[7] reported a relatively large study of reovirus type 3 infection and extrahepatic biliary atresia and neonatal hepatitis. They interpreted their data as demonstrating no correlation between the virus and the illnesses studied. However, the geometric mean antibody value in the combined biliary atresia and neonatal hepatitis groups was significantly higher than that of the control group. Recently, Richardson and associates[52] reported a study in which they examined the percentage of IgG, IgA, and IgM serum antibodies to reovirus type 3 in 40 infants with extrahepatic biliary atresia, 59 infants with neonatal hepatitis, 61 infants with cholestatic liver disease due to causes other than extrahepatic biliary atresia or neonatal hepatitis, and 138 control infants with no liver disease. They found no difference in the prevalence of IgG and IgA antibodies between the liver disease groups and the controls. They did, however, note a greater prevalence of IgM antibody in each of the liver disease groups compared with the rate in the control group. However, it seems unlikely that this virus could play a role in such a wide variety of illnesses. It seems most likely that, by some unknown mechanism related to liver disease, the increased prevalence is due to false-positive findings. The results would be more plausible if recurring infections in some of the subjects had been documented by virus isolation.

Exanthem

Exanthem has been a common manifestation of clinically apparent reoviral infections.[15, 26, 32, 75] Lerner and associates[32] noted exanthem in six of seven children infected with reovirus type 2. Predominant symptoms in these patients included fever, malaise, anorexia, and pharyngitis. Two children had adenopathy, and one child had diarrhea. The rash was maculopapular in five patients and vesicular in one child. One child had a measles-like illness with photophobia, conjunctivitis, cervical lymphadenopathy, and a confluent maculopapular rash that lasted about 1 week.

Exanthem has been noted in a 5-year-old girl with pneumonia and type 3 reovirus infection, a 28-month-old girl with encephalitis and type 2 infection, and an 18-year-old boy with pharyngitis and cervical and posterior occipital lymph node enlargement and type 2 infection.[15, 26, 75]

Neuromuscular Disease

Joske and colleagues[26] noted three cases of hepatitis encephalitis syndrome with reoviral infections. All had abnormal liver function test results and clinical and laboratory evidence of meningeal and cerebral involvement. One child died, one had mild neurologic residua at 6-week follow-up, and one recovered without difficulty. Two patients were infected with reovirus type 2 and one with reovirus type 3.

El-Rai and Evans[15] found serologic evidence of reovirus type 2 infection in two children with aseptic meningitis, and Zalan and colleagues[81] noted two children with reovirus type 2 infections associated with leg weakness and pain. Krainer and Aronso[30] reported a 29-year-old woman who died of disseminated demyelinating encephalomyelitis in which a reovirus was recovered from the cerebrospinal fluid and brain.

Other Manifestations

A 25-year-old man with Hodgkin disease had persistent reovirus type 1 viruria for a 5-week period, but no associated clinical illness was demonstrated.[13] Reoviruses have been recovered from biopsy material from patients with Burkitt lymphoma.[2, 3] One child with hemorrhagic bullous myringitis was infected with reovirus type 2.[81]

DIAGNOSIS

No specific clinical features suggest reoviral infection, so virologic and serologic study is necessary for diagnosis. Reoviruses can be recovered from clinical material, in primary monkey kidney tissue culture.[53] Care must be taken in interpreting results, however, because reoviruses can be contaminants of monkey tissue cultures. Cytopathic effect in tissue culture is enhanced by rolling during incubation.[33] Virus identification is made by neutralization; the distinctive cytopathic effect should be helpful in selecting strains for study with reovirus antisera. Paired serum specimens can be examined for antibody titer rise to reoviruses by neutralization, indirect immunofluorescent antibody technique, enzyme-linked immunosorbent assay, or hemagglutination inhibition.

References

1. Bangaru, B., Morecki, R., Glaser, J. H., et al.: Comparative studies of biliary atresia in the human newborn and reovirus-induced cholangitis in weaning mice. Lab. Invest. *43*:456–462, 1980.
2. Bell, T. M., Massie, A., Ross, M. G. R., et al.: Further isolations of reovirus type 3 from cases of Burkitt's lymphoma. B. M. J. *1*:1514–1517, 1966.
3. Bell, T. M., Massie, A., Ross, M. G. R., et al.: Isolation of a reovirus from a case of Burkitt's lymphoma. B. M. J. *1*:1212–1213, 1964.
4. Berger, R. H., and Brody, J. A.: Reovirus antibody patterns in Alaska. Am. J. Epidemiol. *86*:724–735, 1967.
5. Bricout, F. J. R., and Duval, J.: Pouvoir pathogéne et diffusion des reovirus. Ann. Pediatr. *41*:43–48, 1965.
6. Brown, P. K., and Taylor-Robinson, D.: Respiratory virus antibodies in sera of persons living in isolated communities. Bull. W. H. O. *34*:895–900, 1966.
7. Brown, W. R., Sokol, R. J., Levin, M. J., et al.: Lack of correlation between infection with reovirus 3 and extrahepatic biliary atresia or neonatal hepatitis. J. Pediatr. *113*:670–676, 1988.
8. Cohen, J. A., Williams, W. V., Weiner, D. B., et al.: Reoviruses. *In* von Regenmortel, M. H. V., and Neurath, A. R. (eds.): Immunochemistry of Viruses, II: The Basis for Serodiagnosis and Vaccines. New York, Elsevier Science Publishers, 1990, pp. 381–401.

9. Committee on the ECHO Viruses. Science *122*:1187, 1955.
10. Committee on the Enteroviruses. Am. J. Public Health *47*:1556, 1957.
11. Csiza, C. K.: Characterization and serotyping of three feline reovirus isolates. Infect. Immun. *9*:159–166, 1974.
12. deLavergne, E., Olive, D., and LeMoyne, M. T.: Les reovirus: Les difficultés de la mise en évidence de leur pouvoir pathogéne chez l'homme. Presse Méd. *73*:951–956, 1965.
13. Dussaix, E., Hadchouel, M., Tardieu, M., et al.: Biliary atresia and reovirus type 3 infection. N. Engl. J. Med. *310*:658, 1984.
14. Edmonson, J. H., Millian, S. J., Goodenow, M., et al.: Persistent viruria due to reovirus in a patient treated for Hodgkin's disease in a protected environment. J. Infect. Dis. *121*:438–441, 1970.
15. El-Rai, F. M., and Evans, A. S.: Reovirus infections in children and young adults. Arch. Environ. Health *7*:700–704, 1963.
16. England, B.: Concentration of reovirus and adenovirus from sewage and effluents by protamine sulfate (Salmine) treatment. Appl. Microbiol. *24*:510–512, 1972.
17. Fenner, F.: Classification and nomenclature of viruses: Second report of the International Committee on Taxonomy of Viruses. Intervirology *7*:34, 1976.
18. George, S., and John, T. J.: Reovirus antibodies in human sera in South India. Indian J. Med. Res. *58*:1680–1685, 1970.
19. Glaser, J. H., Balistreri, W. F., and Morecki, R.: Role of reovirus type 2 in persistent infantile cholestasis. J. Pediatr. *105*:912–915, 1984.
20. Hartley, J. W., Rowe, W. P., and Huebner, R. J.: Recovery of reoviruses from wild and laboratory mice. Proc. Soc. Exp. Biol. Med. *108*:390–395, 1961.
21. Hilleman, M. R., Hamparian, V. V., Ketler, A., et al.: Acute respiratory illnesses among children and adults. J. A. M. A. *180*:445–453, 1962.
22. Hull, R. N., Minner, J. R., and Smith, J. W.: New viral agents recovered from tissue cultures of monkey kidney cells. I. Origin and properties of cytopathogenic agents S.V.1, S.V.2, S.V.4, S.V.5, S.V.6, S.V.11, S.V.12, and S.V.15. Am. J. Hyg. *63*:204–215, 1956.
23. Jackson, G. G., Muldoon, R. L., and Cooper, G. S.: Reovirus type 1 as an etiologic agent of the common cold. J. Clin. Invest. *40*:1051, 1961.
24. Jenson, A. B., Rabin, E. R., Phillips, C. A., et al.: Reovirus encephalitis in newborn mice: An electron microscopic and virus assay study. Am. J. Pathol. *47*:223–239, 1965.
25. Jopkiewics, T. K., Krzeminska, K., and Stachowska, Z.: Virologic survey of sewage in the city of Bydgoszcz (English summary). Przegl. Epidemiol. *22*:521–527, 1968.
26. Joske, R. A., Keall, D. D., Leak, P. J., et al.: Hepatitis-encephalitis in humans with reovirus infection. Arch. Intern. Med. *113*:811–816, 1964.
27. Kalra, S. L., Nair, E., and Nair, C. M. G.: Reovirus antibodies in Delhi. Indian J. Med. Res. *57*:1–4, 1969.
28. Kilham, L., and Margolis, G.: Hydrocephalus in hamsters, ferrets, rats, and mice following inoculations with reovirus type 1. I. Virologic studies. Lab. Invest. *21*:183–188, 1969.
29. Knocke, K. W., Pittler, H., and Hoepken, W.: Nachweis von reovirus in abwassern (English summary). Zentralbl. Bakteriol. Parasitol. Infektionskr. Hyg. *203*:417–421, 1967.
30. Krainer, L., and Aronson, B. E.: Disseminated encephalomyelitis in humans with recovery of hepato-encephalitis virus (HEV). J. Neuropathol. Exp. Neurol. *18*:339–342, 1969.
31. Leers, W. D., and Rozee, K. R.: A survey of reovirus antibodies in sera of urban children. Can. Med. Assoc. J. *94*:1040–1042, 1966.
32. Lerner, A. M., Cherry, J. D., Klein, J. O., et al.: Infections with reoviruses. N. Engl. J. Med. *267*:947–952, 1962.
33. Lerner, A. M., Cherry, J. D., and Finland, M.: Enhancement of cytopathic effects of reoviruses in rolled cultures of rhesus kidney. Proc. Soc. Exp. Biol. Med. *110*:727–729, 1962.
34. Levy, J. A., Tanabe, E., and Curnen, E. C.: Occurrence of reovirus antibodies in healthy African children and in children with Burkitt's lymphoma. Cancer *21*:53–57, 1968.
35. Malherbe, H. H., and Strickland-Cholmley, M.: Quantitative studies on viral survival in sewage purification processes. *In* Berg, G. (ed.): Transmission of Viruses by the Water Route. New York, John Wiley & Sons, 1967, pp. 379–387.
36. Margolis, G., and Kilham, L.: Hydrocephalus in hamsters, ferrets, rats, and mice following inoculations with reovirus type I. II. Pathologic studies. Lab. Invest. *21*:189–192, 1969.
37. Massie, E. L., and Shaw, E. D.: Reovirus type 1 in laboratory dogs. Am. J. Vet. Res. *27*:783–787, 1966.
38. Matsuura, K., Ishikura, M., Nakayama, T., et al.: Ecological studies on reovirus pollution of rivers in Toyama Prefecture. II. Molecular epidemiological study of reoviruses isolated from river water. Microbiol. Immunol. *37*:305–310, 1993.
39. McFerran, J. B., Nelson, R., and Clarke, J. K.: Isolation and characterization of reoviruses isolated from sheep. Arch. Ges. Virusforsch. *40*:72–81, 1973.
40. McFerran, J. B., and Connor, T.: A reovirus isolated from a pig. Res. Vet. Sci. *11*:388–390, 1970.
41. Minuk, G. Y., Paul, R. W., and Lee, P. W. K.: The prevalence of antibodies to reovirus type 3 in adults with idiopathic cholestatic liver disease. J. Med. Virol. *16*:55–60, 1985.
42. Morecki, R., Glaser, J. H., Cho, S., et al.: Biliary atresia and reovirus type 3 infection. N. Engl. J. Med. *307*:481–484, 1982.
43. Morecki, R., Glaser, J. H., Johnson, A. B., et al.: Detection of reovirus type 3 in the porta hepatis of an infant with extrahepatic biliary atresia: Ultrastructural and immunocytochemical study. Hepatology *4*:1137–1142, 1984.
44. Munz, E., Reimann, M., and Ackerman, E.: Serologische untersuchungen zur epidemiologie von reovirus-infektionen bei menschen, nutz- und wildtieren in Tanzania. Acta Trop. *36*:277–288, 1979.
45. Nupen, E. M.: Virus studies on the Windhoek waste-water reclamation plant (southwest Africa). Water Res. *4*:661–672, 1970.
46. Onodera, T., Jenson, A. B., Yoon, J. W., et al.: Virus-induced diabetes mellitus: Reovirus infection of pancreatic B cells in mice. Science *201*:529–530, 1978.
47. Pal, S. R., and Agarwal, S. C.: Sero-epidemiological study of reovirus infection amongst the normal population of the Chandigarh area: Northern India. J. Hyg. (Camb.) *66*:519–529, 1968.
48. Phillips, P. A., Keast, D., Walters, M. N.-I., et al.: Murine lymphoma induced by reovirus 3. Pathology *3*:133–138, 1971.
49. Ramos-Alvarez, M., and Sabin, A. B.: Enteropathogenic viruses and bacteria: Role in summer diarrheal diseases of infancy and early childhood. J. A. M. A. *167*:147–156, 1958.
50. Ramos-Alvarez, M., and Sabin, A. B.: Intestinal viral flora of healthy children demonstrable by monkey kidney tissue culture. Am. J. Public Health *46*:295–299, 1956.
51. Ramos-Alvarez, M., and Sabin, A. B.: Characteristics of poliomyelitis and other enteric viruses recovered in tissue culture from healthy American children. Proc. Soc. Exp. Biol. Med. *87*:655–661, 1954.
52. Richardson, S. C., Bishop, R. F., and Smith, A. L.: Reovirus serotype 3 infection in infants with extrahepatic biliary atresia or neonatal hepatitis. J. Gastroenterol. Hepatol. *9*:264–268, 1994.
53. Rosen, L.: Reoviruses. *In* Lennette, E. H., and Schmidt, N. J. (eds.): Diagnostic Procedures for Viral and Rickettsial Infections. 4th ed. New York, American Public Health Association, 1969, pp. 354–363.
54. Rosen, L.: Reoviruses. *In* Wenner, H. A., Behbehani, A. M., and Rosen, L. (eds.): Virology Monographs. New York, Springer-Verlag, 1968, pp. 74–107.
55. Rosen, L., Abinati, F. R., and Hovis, J. F.: Further observations on the natural infection of cattle with reoviruses. Am. J. Hyg. *77*:38–48, 1963.
56. Rosen, L., Evans, H. E., and Spickard, A.: Reovirus infections in human volunteers. Am. J. Hyg. *77*:29–37, 1963.
57. Rosen, L.: Reoviruses in animals other than man. Ann. N. Y. Acad. Sci. *101*:461–465, 1962.
58. Rosen, L., Hovis, J. F., Mastrota, F. M., et al.: An outbreak of infection with a type 1 reovirus among children in an institution. Am. J. Hyg. *71*:266–274, 1960.
59. Rosen, L., Hovis, J. F., Mastrota, F. M., et al.: Observations on a newly recognized virus (Abney) of the reovirus family. Am. J. Hyg. *71*:258–265, 1960.
60. Rosen, L.: Serologic grouping of reoviruses by hemagglutination-inhibition. Am. J. Hyg. *71*:242–249, 1960.
61. Ruiz-Gomez, J., Faingezicht-Gutman, I., and Sosa-Martinez, J.: Virus reo: Investigación de anticuerpos en individuos de diferentes edades. Bol. Méd. Hosp. Infant (Méx.) *22*:359–363, 1965.
62. Sabin, A. B.: Reoviruses: A new group of respiratory and enteric viruses formerly classified as ECHO type 10 is described. Science *130*:1387–1389, 1959.
63. Sabin, A. B.: The significance of viruses recovered from the intestinal tracts of healthy infants and children. Ann. N. Y. Acad. Sci. *66*:226–230, 1956.
64. Schiff, L. A., and Fields, B. N.: Reoviruses and their replication. *In* Fields, B. N., Knipe, D. M., Chanock, R. M., et al. (eds.): Fields' Virology. 2nd ed. New York, Raven Press, 1990, pp. 1275–1306.
65. Schmidt, J., Tauchnitz, C., and Kühn, O.: Untersuchungen über das vorkommen hämagglutinationschemmender antikörper gegen die reovirustypen 1 und 2 in der bevölkerung. Z. Hyg. Infektionskr. *150*:269–279, 1965.
66. Scott, T. F. M.: Clinical syndromes associated with entero virus and reo virus infections. Adv. Virus Res. *8*:165–197, 1962.
67. Sherry, B., and Blum, M. A.: Multiple viral core proteins are determinants of reovirus-induced acute myocarditis. J. Virol. *68*:8461–8465, 1994.
68. Stanley, N. F.: Reoviruses. Br. Med. Bull. *23*:150–155, 1967.
69. Stanley, N. F., Leak, P. J., Walter, M. N. I., et al.: Murine infection with reovirus. II. The chronic disease following reovirus type 3 infection. Br. J. Exp. Pathol. *95*:142–149, 1964.
70. Stanley, N. F., Leak, P. J., Grieve, G. M., et al.: The ecology and epidemiology of reovirus. Aust. J. Exp. Biol. Med. Sci. *42*:373–384, 1964.
71. Stanley, N. F., and Leak, P. J.: The serologic epidemiology of reovirus infection with special reference to the Rottnest Island quokka *(Setonix brachyurus)*. Am. J. Hyg. *78*:82–88, 1963.
72. Stanley, N. F.: Reovirus: A ubiquitous orphan. Med. J. Aust. *2*:815–818, 1961.
73. Stanley, N. F., Dorman, D. C., and Ponsford, J.: Studies on the pathogenesis of a hitherto undescribed virus (hepato-encephalomyelitis) producing unusual symptoms in suckling mice. Aust. J. Exp. Biol. Med. Sci. *31*:147–160, 1953.
74. Taylor-Robinson, D.: Respiratory virus antibodies in human sera from different regions of the world. Bull. W. H. O. *32*:833–847, 1965.
75. Tillotson, J. R., and Lerner, A. M.: Reovirus type 3 associated with fatal pneumonia. N. Engl. J. Med. *276*:1060–1063, 1967.

76. Toth, M., and Honty, A.: Age-incidence of haemagglutination-inhibiting antibodies to reovirus types 1, 2 and 3. Acta Microbiol. Acad. Sci. Hung. *13*:119–126, 1966.
77. Tyler, K. L., and Fields, B. N.: Reoviruses. *In* Fields, B. N., Knipe, D. M., Chanock, R. M., et al. (eds.): Fields' Virology. 2nd ed. New York, Raven Press, 1990, pp. 1307–1328.
78. Tyler, K. L., and Fields, B. N.: *Reoviridae:* A brief introduction. *In* Fields, B. N., Knipe, D. M., et al. (eds.): Virology. 2nd ed. New York, Raven Press, 1990, pp. 1271–1273.
79. Walker, E. R., Friedman, M. H., and Olson, N. O.: Electron microscopic study of an avian reovirus that causes arthritis. J. Ultrastruct. Res. *41*:67–79, 1972.
80. Wooley, R. E., Dees, T. A., Cromack, A. S., et al.: Infectious enteritis of turkeys: Characterization of two reoviruses isolated by sucrose density gradient centrifugation from turkeys with infectious enteritis. Am. J. Vet. Res. *33*:157–164, 1972.
81. Zalan, E., Leers, W. D., and Labzoffsky, N. A.: Occurrence of reovirus infection in Ontario. Can. Med. Assoc. J. *87*:714–715, 1962.

175

ORBIVIRUSES AND COLTIVIRUSES

Theodore F. Tsai

Viruses in the genera *Orbivirus* and *Coltivirus* differ from those in the family *Reoviridae* structurally, in physicochemical properties, and by their arthropod mode of transmission.[34–36] More than 100 orbiviruses are classified within 14 serogroups defined by relationships in complement fixation, agar gel precipitation, and immunofluorescent assays. Additional serocomplex relationships are recognized; individual viruses are differentiated by neutralization tests. These principally are animal pathogens (e.g., the bluetongue viruses); only viruses in the Kemorovo, Orungo, Lebombo, and Changuinola serogroups have been recognized to cause human illness. Four coltiviruses are recognized to be human pathogens: Colorado tick fever (CTF) virus, Salmon River virus, Banna virus, and WX3 virus.

The orbiviruses are spherical nonenveloped viruses with two protein shells: an outer shell (capsid) approximately 86 nm in diameter and an inner shell (core) 69 nm in diameter. The inner core VP7 protein, arranged in trimers, contains group-reactive antigens, and outer capsid VP2 or VP5 proteins bear serotype-specific antigens. The viruses are acid-labile, and some exhibit sensitivity to lipid solvents. The double-stranded RNA viral genome is composed of 10 segments associated with viral structural and nonstructural proteins. Their complete nucleotide sequences and coding assignments have been determined for a bluetongue virus, and partial information is available for others. Generally, reassortments of genomic segments among viruses within serogroups are viable but not between groups, validating the broad serogroup classification. Genetic relationships (e.g., RNA hybridization) among viruses within serogroups diverge from antigenic relationships in some instances, providing an additional basis for taxonomic classification.

The coltiviruses resemble the orbiviruses in size and in having two capsids. Virions have a smoother surface morphology, and the genome is organized into 12 RNA segments.[28] The taxon was established from the genus *Orbivirus* in 1991.

COLORADO TICK FEVER VIRUS

CTF is an acute tick-borne febrile illness caused by a coltivirus.[4, 13, 18, 19, 34, 43]

Eyach virus, isolated from *Ixodes* ticks in France and Germany, S6-1403, isolated in California from a gray squirrel, and mosquito strains from Indonesia are related to but distinct from CTF virus and have not been associated with human disease.[3, 27] The closely related Salmon River virus was isolated from a viremic person with a CTF-like illness who most likely acquired her infection while camping on the middle fork of Idaho's Salmon River. The majority of CTF-like illnesses in Idaho and Montana are likely to be infections with Salmon River virus (unpublished observations, T. F. Tsai). RNA hybridization studies of CTF viral strains from a 33-year interval found a minor heterogeneity, suggesting that a single gene pool has been maintained by mixing of viral strains and by constraints of viral replication within tick vectors and vertebrate hosts.[2] A wide variety of small and large mammals are infected naturally with the virus, but only humans develop clinical illness. Experimental infections of rhesus monkeys, hamsters, and mice produce hematologic changes similar to those occurring in human infections.[21]

Epidemiology

Cases occur principally in association with the habitats and activity patterns of the wood tick. Most cases occur in May and June, when adult ticks are most active, but infections from March to November have been reported. Infections are acquired principally in the western United States and Canada in the known geographic distribution of the vector, *Dermacentor andersoni* (Fig. 175–1).[8, 11–13, 34] CTF viral antibodies have been found in serosurveys in South Korea, but no viral isolates have been recovered (unpublished observations, C. H. Calisher).

In rare cases, CTF has occurred in persons who had not traveled to areas of known risk, for example, in persons exposed to ticks brought home on clothing of family members and, in one case, by transfusion.[7, 38, 43]

CTF virus is maintained in a 2- to 3-year cycle among small mammals, principally rodents, and *D. andersoni* ticks (Fig. 175–2).[4, 13] Once infected in the larval stage, ticks remain infected through the nymphal and adult stages (transstadial transmission). Larvae are infected from viremic rodents. After molting, they carry the virus through the winter, and as nymphs, they infect other rodents and renew the cycle of transmission the following spring. Humans become infected incidentally by the bite of infected adult ticks.

The least chipmunk (*Eutamias minimus*), the golden-mantled ground squirrel (*Spermophilus lateralis*), and the porcupine (*Erethizon dorsatum*) appeared to be the primary hosts for larval, nymphal, and adult *D. andersoni*; secondary hosts include rock mice (*Peromyscus maniculatus*), meadow voles

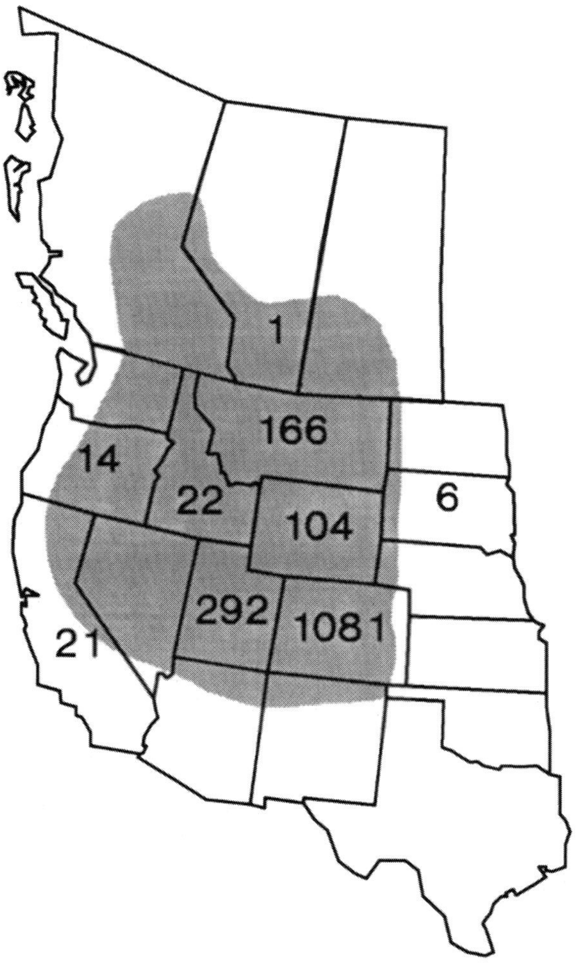

FIGURE 175–1. *Geographic distribution of* Dermacentor andersoni *ticks and reported cases of Colorado tick fever, 1980–1991.*

(*Microtus pennsylvanicus*), and pine squirrels (*Tamiasciurus hudsonicus*).[6]

D. andersoni is found exclusively in the geographic distribution previously mentioned in high plains and mountainous terrain between 4000 and 10,000 feet in altitude. The specific microhabitats where infected ticks are most prevalent are south-facing slopes with open stands of ponderosa pine, moderate shrubs, and rocky surfaces that provide favorable habitats for the intermediate rodent hosts.[6, 32] Both male and female adult ticks can transmit infection to humans, and the period of attachment required for transmission of the virus may be very brief.

Clinical Manifestations

A history of tick bite or tick exposure is given by more than 90 per cent of patients.[23] The incubation period usually is 3 to 4 days, with a range of 0 to 14 days after known exposure to a tick.[32] The onset typically is abrupt, with fever, chills, malaise, headache, retro-orbital pain, myalgias, lumbar pain, and hyperesthesia. Nausea, vomiting, and abdominal pain occur less frequently. Upper respiratory symptoms usually are absent. Conjunctival injection may be present; lymphadenopathy and hepatosplenomegaly are found in some patients. Maculopapular and petechial eruptions have been observed in 5 to 12 per cent of cases.[42]

The disease classically is diphasic: an initial attack lasting 2 to 3 days is followed by an equal interval of defervescence, followed by a second, and rarely a third, recurrence. However, this saddleback pattern is absent in more than 50 per cent of cases. Symptoms resolve several days after the second bout of fever, but prolonged asthenia for several weeks is typical, especially in adults.[22]

Leukopenia is a hallmark of the illness. The mean initial leukocyte count is 3900/mm^3. Leukopenia reaches its nadir 5 to 6 days after the onset of illness, often during the period of remission. A left shift with an absolute neutropenia and relative lymphocytosis is usual. Examination of bone marrow aspirates shows a maturational arrest in the granulocytic series with absent mature forms and numerous metamyelocytes and myelocytes. Megakaryocytes are depleted. A reduced platelet count ($<$150,000/mm^3) is found in the majority of patients; however, thrombocytopenia rarely reaches a level of clinical significance.[33]

An uncomplicated recovery is the rule. Epididymoorchitis, pneumonitis, hepatitis, and pericarditis have been reported as complications, but the most serious complications are encephalitis and hemorrhage,[16, 20, 22, 24, 31] which have been reported nearly exclusively in children younger than 10 years of age.[11, 22, 40, 42] Three deaths have been reported, all in children who exhibited signs of generalized bleeding accompanied by a reduced platelet count.[10, 22] Examination of the bone marrow in one child disclosed a generalized depression of myeloid and erythroid elements and a marked reduction in megakaryocytes. Central nervous system signs consistent with meningitis and encephalitis have been reported in both children and adults. Examination of the cerebrospinal fluid disclosed elevated protein and mononuclear cell pleocytosis in the few cases that have been described.

D. andersoni is a vector for both CTF and Rocky Mountain spotted fever.[4] Although dual isolations of CTF virus and *Rickettsia rickettsii* from the same tick have not been reported, a concurrent rickettsial infection could not be discounted in all of the previously mentioned fatal cases attributed to CTF. Furthermore, an individual exposed to more than one tick could develop a dual infection.

CTF virus is teratogenic in experimentally infected mice.[23] One pregnant woman aborted 2 weeks after illness. An infant delivered 6 days after its mother had onset of CTF and developed a febrile illness with leukopenia at 3 days of age, indicating a possible vertically acquired infection. In a single

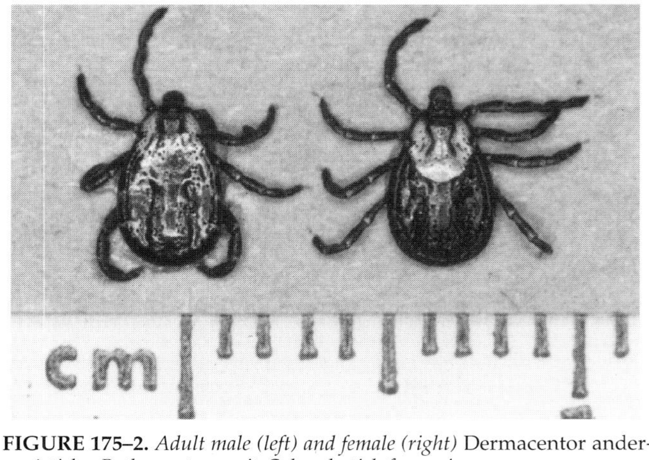

FIGURE 175–2. *Adult male (left) and female (right)* Dermacentor andersoni *ticks. Both can transmit Colorado tick fever virus.*

instance, a second attack of CTF was documented, which indicates that immunity may not be permanent.[22]

The combined historical elements of tick exposure and outdoor activity in an enzootic area should suggest the diagnosis in patients with a spring-summer grippe-like illness. Abdominal pain, pharyngitis, and rash are less common in patients with CTF, compared with patients with other illnesses. Rocky Mountain spotted fever is rare in the states in which CTF is prevalent. Moreover, a petechial rash occurs infrequently in CTF; its biphasic course also differs. Tick-borne relapsing fever also follows a remitting course. However, it has a more acute and toxic onset, splenomegaly is common, and remission is by crisis. The geographic distribution of the diseases overlaps; however, human encounters with the argasid (soft) tick vectors of relapsing fever (*Ornithodoros* ticks) are likely to be in cabins and other protected areas.

Pathophysiology

Infection with the virus of CTF is unusual because of the hematopoietic tropism of the virus.[14, 15, 26] Experimental infections of rhesus monkeys, rodents,[14, 15, 26] and human marrow cells in vitro have shown that virus infects erythropoietic elements (erythroblasts to reticulocytes) at an early stage of infection.[9, 36, 39] After the infected cells mature and are released into the peripheral circulation, virus persists intracellularly, where it is stabilized or protected from circulating antibody.[36] Virus can be cultured from circulating erythrocytes up to 120 days after onset of illness.[25] After natural infection, virus has been visualized within erythrocytes and reticulocytes by electron microscopy, and intraerythrocytic viral antigen has been demonstrated by immunofluorescence.[15, 36] Red cell survival evidently is not shortened, and infected cells circulate in the presence of neutralizing antibody. The virus titer of the red cell fraction is equal to or greater than that of whole blood. Prolonged viremia has not been associated with either a prolonged or a more severe course of illness. Viral replication also is seen in CD34+ progenitor cells. Patients exhibit impaired mononuclear cell production of colony-stimulating factors.[39] High levels of serum interferon-γ correlate with fever during the acute phase of illness.[1]

Laboratory Diagnosis

Direct immunofluorescent examination of blood smears for intraerythrocytic viral antigen is the most rapid approach to laboratory diagnosis.[14] This procedure should be accompanied by attempts to isolate virus from blood. Ninety-six per cent of all cases diagnosed by seroconversion are identified by viral isolation. Freezing and thawing the clot should be avoided. Virus has been isolated from a blood clot that had been refrigerated for 14 months. Blood from acute- or convalescent-phase samples can be inoculated into suckling mice or susceptible cell cultures (BHK or Vero cells). Virus isolates are identified by immunofluorescent examination.[9, 14] Serologic diagnosis by demonstration of fourfold rises in neutralizing, complement-fixation, immunofluorescent, or enzyme-linked immunosorbent assay antibody is confirmatory.[5] Neutralizing antibody rises slowly; only one-third of patients had detectable neutralizing antibody 10 days after onset. Fourfold rises in neutralizing antibody appear within 30 days of onset in 92 per cent of patients with the disease.

Treatment

No specific therapy is available. Because thrombocytopenia may occur and hemorrhage is a reported complication in children, antipyretics that interfere with coagulation should not be used.

Prevention

Repellents containing permethrin should be sprayed on clothing, and DEET-containing repellents should be applied to exposed skin (Table 175–1). Long pants should be tucked into socks, and shirts should be worn tucked in. Clothing, gear, and skin should be inspected frequently for attached ticks. It is easier to identify ticks on light-colored clothing. One case of human-to-human transmission by transfusion of infected blood has been reported.[7] Persons with documented CTF should be prohibited from blood donation until the often prolonged viremia has cleared.[38]

BANNA AND WX-3 VIRUSES

Banna and WX-3 viruses have been associated with febrile illness and encephalitis in China. Both have 12 RNA segments; WX-3 and several related strains are cross-reactive antigenically but distinct from CTF, S6-1403, and Eyach viruses (coltiviruses from the Rocky Mountain region, California, and Germany). The antigenic relationship of Banna and M-14 strains has not been reported. Banna virus was isolated from encephalitis patients in Yunnan province in southern China and later from 98 patients with fever, headache, and arthralgias from Xinjiang province in western China.[29] WX-3 and nine related strains, segregating into four distinct RNA electropherotypes, were isolated from *Culex tritaeniorhynchus* mosquitoes in Gansu province and the suburbs of Beijing in 1991.[41] Serologic evidence of recent infection with the strains was found in 50 per cent of encephalitis patients in Henan province and in 17 per cent of patients in Jiangsu province, suggesting that these coltiviruses may be a leading cause of summer viral encephalitis after Japanese encephalitis. Details of the clinical illness and epidemiology of infection have not been reported.

TABLE 175–1. Precautions for Minimizing Potential for Adverse Reactions from Repellents

Apply repellent sparingly only to exposed skin or clothing.
Avoid applying high-concentration (>30% DEET) products to the skin, particularly of children.
Do not inhale or ingest repellents or get them into the eyes.
Wear long sleeves and long pants, when possible, and apply repellents (e.g., permethrin) to clothing for reducing exposure to DEET.
Avoid applying repellents to portions of children's hands that are likely to have contact with eyes or mouth.
Pregnant and nursing women should minimize use of repellents.
Never use repellents on wounds or irritated skin.
Use repellent sparingly; one application will last 4 to 8 hours. Saturation does not increase efficacy.
Wash repellent-treated skin after coming indoors.
If a suspected reaction to insect repellents occurs, wash treated skin and call a physician. Take the repellent can to the physician.

Adapted from Centers for Disease Control: Seizures temporarily associated with use of DEET insect repellent: New York and Connecticut. M. M. W. R. *38*:678–680, 1989.

KEMEROVO AND RELATED VIRUSES

The Kemerovo serogroup contains more than 50 viruses divided into four serocomplexes. The viruses are unique among the orbiviruses in being tick-borne. Many are associated with bird ticks. Only Kemerovo, Tribec, and Lipovnik viruses have been associated with human illness. Kemerovo virus was isolated from the cerebrospinal fluid of two encephalitis patients and ticks in the Kemerovo region of Russia; seroconversions were demonstrated in 10 other meningoencephalitis patients with tick bites in whom Russian spring-summer encephalitis was excluded.[8] Subsequent reports have not been published. The virus is transmitted in an *Ixodes persulcatus*–rodent cycle. In studies from the former Czechoslovakia, where flaviviral tick-borne encephalitis is endemic, half of the encephalitis patients in one study showed seroconversions to Lipovnik virus, two-thirds seroconverted to Lipovnik virus alone, and in the others, dual infection with tick-borne encephalitis and Lipovnik viruses was suspected.[30] This seems plausible because both viruses are transmitted by *Ixodes ricinus* ticks, and multiple exposures with singly infected ticks or infection with a dually infected tick may be possible. In addition, serologic evidence of Lipovnik or Tribec infection was reported in patients with chronic polyradiculoneuritis; however, spirochetal infection was not ruled out in these cases.

On the basis of serologic rises in patients with acute febrile illness diagnosed clinically as Rocky Mountain spotted fever, a Kemerovo-related virus is suspected to occur in the southwestern United States. Patients with a history of tick bite or tick exposure, whose sera were negative for *R. rickettsii*, demonstrated fourfold or greater changes in immunofluorescent titers to Lipovnik and Six Gun City viruses (Kemerovo group). Rises in immunofluorescent antibody titers to 128–512 suggested recent infection with a Kemerovo-related virus, possibly a novel agent or related to rabbit syncytium virus, which is enzootic in the United States. The patients had acute febrile illnesses with myalgias, vomiting, and severe abdominal pain, with leukopenia, thrombocytopenia, and anemia resembling Rocky Mountain spotted fever. No agent has been isolated. Serologic evidence of infection was found in a cotton rat in the vicinity of one case. The syndrome tentatively is called Oklahoma tick fever.

ORUNGO VIRUS

Orungo virus is unrelated antigenically to other orbiviruses. Infection is prevalent in West, Central, and East Africa, apparently transmitted in a sylvatic monkey–*Aedes* mosquito cycle similar to that of yellow fever. Human-to-human transmission by *Anopheles* mosquitoes is speculated to occur. The virus has been isolated from patients with fever and headache, and serologic evidence of infection has been reported in outbreaks of illness characterized by fever, headache, myalgia, nausea, and vomiting. Seroconversions have been observed in patients studied during yellow fever outbreaks, presumably because of concurrent transmission of the viruses. The virus also was isolated from the blood of a child with convulsions and flaccid paralysis.[17, 35]

LEBOMBO VIRUS

Lebombo virus is not grouped antigenically. The virus first was isolated from *Aedes circumluteolus* mosquitoes in South Africa. Subsequently, the virus was recovered from a Nigerian child with nonspecific febrile illness. The virus also has been isolated from rodents and mosquitoes in Nigeria.[35]

CHANGUINOLA VIRUS

Changuinola virus belongs to an antigenic complex of 12 principally phlebotomine-borne orbiviruses. The virus is transmitted in Panama among forest mammals and phlebotomine flies. Only one human case has been reported—a nonspecific febrile illness in a mosquito catcher.[34]

References

1. Ater, J. L., Overall, J. C., Yeh, T. J., et al.: Circulating interferon and clinical symptoms in Colorado tick fever. J. Infect. Dis. *151*:966, 1985.
2. Brown, S. E., Miller, B. R., McLean, R. G., et al.: Cocirculation of multiple Colorado tick fever genotypes in nature. Am. J. Trop. Med. Hyg. *40*:94–101, 1989.
3. Brown, S. E., Gorman, B. M., Tesh, R. B., et al.: Coltiviruses isolated from mosquitoes collected in Indonesia. Virology *196*:363–367, 1993.
4. Burgdorfer, W.: Tick-borne diseases in the United States: Rocky Mountain spotted fever and Coloardo tick fever: A review. Acta Trop. *34*:103, 1977.
5. Calisher, C. H., Poland, J. D., Calisher, S. B., et al.: Diagnosis of Colorado tick fever virus infection by enzyme immunoassays for immunoglobulin M and G antibodies. J. Clin. Microbiol. *22*:84, 1985.
6. Carey, A. B., McLean, R. B., and Maupin, G. O.: The structure of a Coloardo tick fever ecosystem. Ecol. Monogr. *50*:131–151, 1980.
7. Centers for Disease Control: U. S. P. H.: Transmission of Colorado tick fever virus by blood transfusion: Montana. M. M. W. R. *24*:422–427, 1975.
8. Chumakov, M. P., Karpovich, L. G., Sarmanova, E. S., et al.: Report on the isolation from *Ixodes persulcatus* ticks and from patients in western Siberia of a virus differing from the agent of tick-borne encephalitis. Arch. Virol. *7*:82–83, 1993.
9. Earnest, M. P., Breckinridge, J. C., Barr, R. J., et al.: Colorado tick fever: Clinical and epidemiologic features and evaluation of diagnostic methods. Rocky Mtn. Med. J. *68*:60–62, 1971.
10. Eklund, C. M., and Kennedy, R. C.: Preliminary studies of pathogenesis of Colorado tick fever virus infection in mice. *In* Libikova, H. (ed.): Biology of Viruses of the Tick-Borne Encephalitis Complex. London, Academic Press, 1962, pp. 286–293.
11. Eklund, C. M., Kennedy, R. C., and Casey, M.: Colorado tick fever. Rocky Mtn. Med. J. *58*:21–25, 1961.
12. Eklund, C. M., Kohls, G. M., and Brennan, J. M.: Distribution of Colorado tick fever and virus-carrying ticks. J. A. M. A. *157*:335–337, 1955.
13. Emmons, R. W.: Ecology of Colorado tick fever. Annu. Rev. Microbiol. *42*:49, 1988.
14. Emmons, R. W., and Lennette, E. H.: Immunofluorescent staining in the laboratory diagnosis of Colorado tick fever. J. Lab. Clin. Med. *68*:923–929, 1966.
15. Emmons, R. W., Oshiro, L. S., Johnson, H. N., et al.: Intra-erythrocytic location of Colorado tick fever virus. J. Gen. Virol. *17*:185–195, 1972.
16. Emmons, R. W., and Schade, H. I.: Colorado tick fever simulating acute myocardial infarction. J. A. M. A. *222*:87–88, 1972.
17. Familusi, J. B., Moore, D. L., Fomufod, A. K., et al.: Virus isolates from children with febrile convulsions in Nigeria: A correlation study of clinical and laboratory observations. Clin. Pediatr. *11*:272–276, 1972.
18. Florio, L., Mugrage, E. R., and Stewart, M. O.: Colorado tick fever. Ann. Intern. Med. *25*:466–471, 1946.
19. Florio, L., Stewart, M.O., and Mugrage, E. R.: The etiology of Colorado tick fever. J. Exp. Med. *83*:1–10, 1946.
20. Fraser, C. H., and Schiff, D. W.: Colorado tick fever encephalitis. Pediatrics *29*:187–190, 1962.
21. Gerloff, R. K., and Larson, C. L.: Experimental infection of rhesus monkeys with Colorado tick fever virus. Am. J. Pathol. *35*:1043–1054, 1959.
22. Goodpasture, H. C., Poland, J. D., Francy, D. B., et al.: Colorado tick fever: Clinical, epidemiologic and laboratory aspects of 228 cases in Colorado in 1973–1974. Ann. Intern. Med. *88*:303–310, 1978.
23. Harris R. E., Morahan, P., and Coleman, P.: Teratogenic effects of Colorado tick fever virus in mice. J. Infect. Dis. *131*:397–402, 1975.
24. Hierholzer, W. J., Jr., and Barry, D. W.: Colorado tick fever pericarditis. J. A. M. A. *217*:825, 1971.
25. Hughes, L. E., Casper, E. A., and Clifford, C. M.: Persistence of Colorado tick fever virus in red blood cells. Am. J. Trop. Med. Hyg. *23*:530–532, 1974.
26. Johnson, E. S., Napoli, V. M., and White, W. C.: Colorado tick fever as a hematologic problem. Am. J. Clin. Pathol. *34*:118–124, 1960.
27. Karabatos, N., Poland, J. D., Emmons, R. W., et al.: Antigenic variants of Colorado tick fever virus. J. Virol. *68*:1463, 1987.
28. Knudson, D. L.: Genome of Colorado tick fever virus. Virology *112*:361–364, 1981.
29. Li, Q. P., Shei, S. T., Hua, C., et al.: First isolation of 8 strains of new orbivirus (Banna) from patients with innominate fever in Xinjiang. Endemic Dis. Bull. *7*:77–82, 1993.
30. Libikova, H., Heinz, F., Ujhazyova, D., et al.: Orbivirses of the Kemerovo complex and neurological diseases. Med. Microbiol. Immunol. *116*:255–263, 1978.

31. Loge, R. V.: Acute hepatitis associated with Colorado tick fever. West. J. Med. *142*:91, 1985.
32. McLean, R. G., Shriner, R. B., Pokorny, K. S., et al.: The ecology of Colorado tick fever in Rocky Mountain National Park in 1974. III. Habitats supporting the virus. Am. J. Trop. Med. Hyg. *40*:86, 1989.
33. Markovitz, A.: Thrombocytopenia in Colorado tick fever. Arch. Intern. Med. *111*:307–308, 1963.
34. Monath, T. P., and Guirakhoo, F.: Orbiviruses and coltiviruses. *In* Fields, B. N., Knipe, D. M., and Horsley, P. M. (eds.): Virology. 3rd ed. Philadelphia, Lippincott-Raven, 1996, pp. 1709–1734.
35. Moore, D. E., Causey, O. R., and Carey, D. E.: Arthropod-borne viral infections of man in Nigeria, 1964–1970. Ann. Trop. Med. Parasitol. *69*:49–64, 1975.
36. Murphy, F. A., Faugvet, C. M., Bishop, D. K., et al.: Virus taxonomy: Classification and nomenclature of viruses: Sixth report of the International committee on taxonomy of viruses. Arch. Virol. *10*(Suppl.):208–225, 1995.
37. Oshiro, L. S., Dondero, D. V., Emmons, R. W., et al.: The development of Colorado tick fever virus within cells of the haemopoietic system. J. Gen. Virol. *39*:73–79, 1978.
38. Philip, C. S., Callaway, C., Chu, M. C., et al.: Replication of Colorado tick fever virus within human hematopoietic progenitor cells. J. Virol. *67*:2389–2395, 1993.
39. Philip, R. N., Casper, E. A., Cory, J., et al.: The potential for transmission of arboviruses by blood transfusion with particular references to Colorado tick fever. *In* Greenwalt, T. J., and Jamieson, G. A. (eds.): Transmissible Disease and Blood Transfusion. New York, Grune & Stratton, 1975, pp. 175–195.
40. Silver, H. K., Meiklejohn, G., and Kempe, C. H.: Colorado tick fever. Am. J. Dis. Child. *101*:30–36, 1961.
41. Song, L. T., Chen, B. Q., and Zhao, Z. J.: Isolation and identification of new members of coltivirus from mosquitoes collected in China. J. Clin. Exp. Virol. China *9*:7–10, 1995.
42. Spruance, S. L., and Bailey, A.: Colorado tick fever. Arch. Intern. Med. *131*:288–293, 1973.
43. Tsai, T. F.: Arboviral infections in the United States. Infect. Dis. Clin. North Am. *5*:73–102, 1991.

176

ROTAVIRUSES

David I. Bernstein and Richard L. Ward

Rotaviruses are recognized as the single most important cause of severe infantile gastroenteritis worldwide.[104, 185, 224] In the United States alone, these viruses are estimated to cause between 24,000 and 110,000 hospitalizations in young children annually[114, 159, 198, 199, 280, 392] and between 75 and 125 deaths.[159, 198, 199] Costs associated with rotavirus disease in the United States have been estimated to be between $100 and $400 million annually.[6, 280] On a world scale, rotaviruses are estimated to be responsible for nearly 1 million deaths each year.[213, 224] For these reasons, rotaviruses have received a high priority as a target for vaccine development.[213, 382]

Rotavirus transmission occurs by the fecal-oral route, providing a highly efficient mechanism for universal exposure that has circumvented differences in regional and national cultural practices and public health standards. The symptoms associated with rotavirus disease typically are diarrhea and vomiting accompanied by fever, nausea, anorexia, cramping, and malaise that can be mild and of short duration or produce severe dehydration.[113, 223, 229, 248, 359, 362, 390, 402, 440, 452, 473] Severe disease occurs primarily in young children, most commonly between 6 and 24 months of age. Approximately 90 per cent of children in both developed and developing countries experience a rotavirus infection by 3 years of age.[223, 224] Rotavirus infection normally provides short-term protection and immunity against subsequent severe illnesses but does not provide lifelong immunity; furthermore, there are numerous reports of sequential illnesses.[26, 31, 62, 76, 101, 139, 141, 149, 179, 261, 279, 341, 383, 427, 518, 525] Neonates also can experience rotavirus infections, and these occur endemically in some settings but typically are asymptomatic.[23, 26, 27, 30, 65, 176, 184, 187, 311, 356, 434, 467] These neonatal infections have been reported to reduce the morbidity associated with a subsequent rotavirus infection.[23, 26] Rotavirus illnesses also occur in adults[111, 206, 239, 391, 508] and the elderly,[92, 189, 276, 438] but, as with other sequential rotavirus infections, the symptoms usually are mild.

Because of the frequency of rotavirus infections and the reduced severity of illness typically associated with sequential infections, a realistic goal for a rotavirus vaccine may be to protect against severe disease. Several vaccine candidates have been developed and evaluated in infants with promising results.[18, 68, 71, 137, 252, 304, 483, 486] Incorporation of an effective rotavirus vaccine into the infant immunization schedule in developed countries could reduce hospitalizations due to dehydrating diarrhea in young children by 40 to 60 per cent.[382] More importantly, worldwide use of such a vaccine could decrease total diarrheal deaths by approximately 10 to 20 per cent.[104, 213, 492] Until an effective vaccine is available, control of rotavirus disease is limited to nonspecific methods, particularly rehydration therapy for replacement of body fluids and electrolytes.

HISTORY

Viruses with morphologic features later associated with rotaviruses first were observed in 1963 in intestinal tissues and rectal swab specimens from mice and monkeys by electron microscopy.[1, 274] These agents, called epizootic diarrhea of infant mice virus and simian agent 11, respectively, were described as 70-nm particles that had a wheel-like appearance. Hence, they later were designated as "rota" viruses from the Latin for wheel.[127, 517] In 1969, Mebus and colleagues[297] demonstrated the presence of these particles in stools of calves with diarrhea, thus associating these viruses with a diarrheal disease in cattle. The correlation between these viruses and human diarrheal disease first was reported in 1973 by Bishop and colleagues.[28] They used electron microscopy to examine biopsy specimens of duodenal mucosa from children with acute gastroenteritis. Within a short time, these and other investigators confirmed the association between the presence of rotavirus in feces and acute gastroenteritis.[29, 50, 96, 112, 126, 228, 302] In addition to their distinctive morphologies, these human viruses along with their animal rotavirus counterparts later were shown to share a group antigen[226, 301, 511] and have been classified as members of the *Rotavirus* genus within the *Reoviridae* family.[285] In 1980, particles that were indistinguishable morphologically from established rotavirus strains but lacked the common group antigen were discovered in pigs.[36, 406] This subsequently led to the identification of rotaviruses belonging to six additional groups (B to G) based on a common group antigen, with the original rotavirus strains classified as group A.[407] Only groups A to C have been associated with human diseases, and most known cases of rotavirus gastroenteritis have been caused by group A strains. However, non–group A rotaviruses have been associated with large outbreaks in China[210, 211] and Japan,[283] which suggests that they could become major pathogens in the future.

PROPERTIES

Visualization of the rotavirus particle by conventional electron microscopy revealed a double-shelled structure with icosahedral symmetry.[117, 200, 242, 269, 277, 396, 436] The outer shell is composed of two structural proteins, VP4 and VP7, which form capsomers that radiate from the inner capsid composed of the major structural protein VP6.[120, 224] This inner shell surrounds a core containing the viral genome and three additional structural proteins: VP1, VP2, and VP3.

Much greater structural definition was obtained using cryoelectron microscopy (Fig. 176–1). With this technique, it was shown that the rotavirus core is surrounded by a third protein shell composed of VP2,[369, 423] which can self-assemble into core-like particles when expressed in insect cells by a baculovirus recombinant.[90, 526] Thus, the mature rotavirus particle contains three protein shells with radii of 21 to 26.5 nm (inner shell), 26.5 to 35 nm (intermediate shell), and 35 to 38 nm (outer shell). Detailed analysis of the outer shell suggests that it is composed primarily of the VP7 glycoprotein (780 molecules/virus), which contains 132 aqueous channels that are positioned over 132 channels within the perforated VP6 intermediate shell, also composed of 780 molecules/virus.[371, 520] Sixty dimers of the VP4 protein, 20 nm in length, are anchored to the VP6 shell and form spike-like projections as they extend through and 11 to 12 nm beyond the VP7 shell.[368, 369, 423, 519] Thus, the full diameter of the mature rotavirus particle, including the VP4 spikes, is approximately 100 nm.

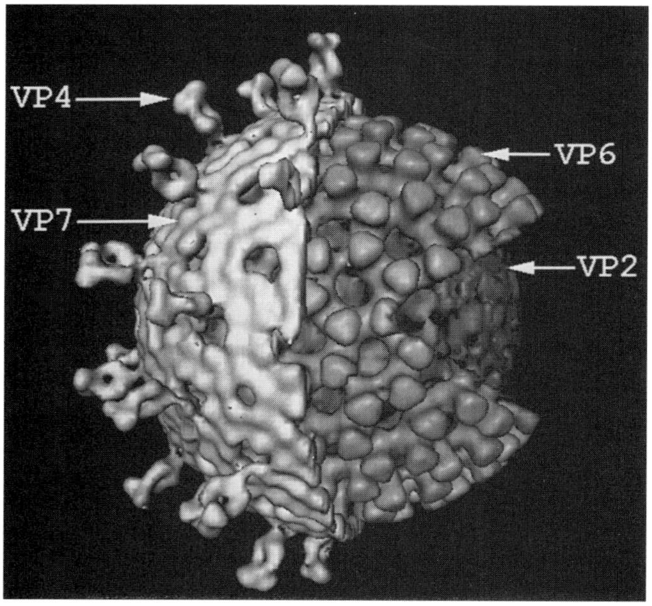

FIGURE 176–1. *Computer-generated image of the triple-shelled rotavirus particle obtained by cryoelectron microscopy. The cut-away diagram shows the outer capsid composed of VP4 spikes and VP7 shell, intermediate VP6 shell, and inner VP2 shell surrounding the core containing the 11 double-stranded RNA segments and VP1 and VP3 proteins. (Courtesy of Dr. B. V. V. Prasad, Baylor College of Medicine, Houston, TX.)*

Further examination of the rotavirus structure by cryoelectron microscopy has indicated that the inner shell composed of VP2 molecules not only encloses the viral genome but interacts with it as well.[370] This interaction has been found to cause significant conformational changes in the VP2 structure. Furthermore, it has been proposed that VP1 and VP3 form a complex below the VP2 layer that interacts with ordered portions of the genome.[370]

The genome of rotavirus is composed of 11 segments of double-stranded RNA that encode the six structural proteins—VP1 to 4, VP6, and VP7—and five nonstructural proteins designated NSP1 to 5.[120] Each segment encodes one known rotavirus protein whose functions have been investigated but, in some cases, remain poorly defined.[5, 33, 60, 120, 207, 233, 251, 264, 275, 346, 347, 363, 364, 481, 482] The genome segments range in size from approximately 660 to 3300 base pairs, and their encoded proteins, whose known functions briefly are described in Table 176–1, have molecular weights of approximately 22,000 to 125,000 daltons.

The RNA genome segments of rotavirus can be extracted from viral particles and separated by polyacrylamide gel electrophoresis into 11 distinct bands visualized by ethidium bromide or silver staining (Fig. 176–2). Each rotavirus strain has a characteristic RNA profile or electropherotype, a property that has been used extensively in epidemiologic studies of these viruses.[72, 107, 218, 232, 361, 376, 388, 389, 399, 417, 439, 451, 453, 497] The characteristic RNA electrophoretic pattern of group A rotaviruses consists of four size classes containing segments 1 to 4, 5 and 6, 7 to 9, and 10 and 11. RNA segments of strains belonging to less well-characterized rotavirus groups (i.e., groups B to G) also can be separated into four size classes, but the distribution of segments within these classes differs from group to group.[37, 287, 294, 352, 353, 405, 407, 463]

REPLICATION

Rotaviruses are activated by cleavage of the outer capsid VP4 protein by trypsin-like proteases into proteins VP5* and VP8*, which remain virus-associated.[74, 119, 121, 265] After attachment to receptors on the cytoplasmic membrane,[12, 13, 142, 235, 299, 321, 395, 400, 446, 450, 524] probably via association with protein VP8*,[398] the activated virion passes directly through this membrane into the cytoplasm.[11, 143, 221, 447, 448] Either during membrane penetration[448] or soon thereafter, the outer capsid proteins are removed, thus stimulating the RNA-dependent RNA polymerase (transcriptase) associated with the inner shell to synthesize the 11 viral mRNAs that are translated into viral proteins.[78, 79, 116, 133, 194, 278, 288, 346, 348, 433, 435] Once viral proteins accumulate within the cytoplasm, large inclusions or viroplasms are formed in which the assembly of virion precursors is initiated.[4, 58, 118] The earliest particles detected contain the complete complement of single-stranded plus-sense RNAs (i.e., one molecule of each mRNA) together with VP1, VP3, NSP1, NSP2, NSP3, and NSP5.[144, 346] This initial replication intermediate then loses its NSP1 proteins and becomes a core replication intermediate with the addition of VP2. Still later, core replication intermediates become double-shelled particles with the addition of VP6 and loss of most of the remaining nonstructural proteins. During these assembly steps, an RNA polymerase (replicase) associated with the replication intermediates uses the single-stranded mRNAs within the particles as a template for minus-strand synthesis and formation of the double-stranded RNA genome segments.[60, 275, 345, 347] The double-shelled particles then associate with VP4 and bud into the rough endoplasmic reticulum

TABLE 176–1. Sizes of Rotavirus Gene Segments and Properties of Encoded Proteins

RNA Segment	No. of Base Pairs	Encoded Protein	Molecular Weight of Protein (× 10⁻⁴)	Properties of Protein
1	3300	VP1	12.5	Inner core protein, RNA polymerase?
2	2700	VP2	10.2	Inner capsid protein, RNA binding, leucine zipper
3	2600	VP3	9.8	Inner core protein, guanylyltransferase
4	2360	VP4	8.7	Outer capsid protein, hemagglutinin, neutralization protein, receptor binding, fusogenic protein
5	1600	NSP1	5.9	Nonstructural protein, contains zinc fingers
6	1360	VP6	4.5	Intermediate capsid protein, group and subgroup antigen
7	1100	NSP3	3.5	Nonstructural protein, RNA binding
8	1060	NSP2	3.7	Nonstructural protein, RNA binding
9	1060	VP7	3.7	Outer capsid glycoprotein, neutralization protein
10	750	NSP4	2.0	Nonstructural glycoprotein, transmembrane protein
11	660	NSP5	2.2	Nonstructural protein, phosphorylated

after their transient association with the NSP4 transmembrane glycoprotein.[16, 34, 57, 270, 300, 365, 458] The other rotavirus glycoprotein VP7, which becomes sequestered within the rough endoplasmic reticulum, then is added to complete the formation of mature viral particles.[75, 270, 271, 366, 444, 445, 509] These mature viruses accumulate within the lumen of the rough endoplasmic reticulum until cell lysis occurs. In cell culture, maximum production of infectious rotaviruses is found at approximately 12 hours after infection is initiated.[73, 288, 372]

EPIDEMIOLOGY

Reassortant Formation and Genogrouping

A variety of classification schemes have been used to characterize rotaviruses for epidemiologic purposes. Each scheme, however, is intertwined with a unique property of viruses with segmented genomes—that is, the ability to form reassortants. During the rotavirus replication cycle, newly formed plus-sense viral mRNAs are free within the viroplasm prior to incorporation into replication intermediates in the first stages of virion assembly.[375] From these genomic precursors are selected the appropriate number and combination of segments for assembly of progeny virions. Co-infection of cells with more than one virion permits reassortment of the mRNAs from both parents. If co-infection is between different strains of virus, reassortment of mRNAs results in progeny that are genetic mosaics of the co-infecting strains (Fig. 176–3). These new strains, or reassortants, are identified by their specific array of genome segments, usually through their electrophoretic mobilities during polyacrylamide gel electrophoresis (i.e., electropherotypes). The properties of the new virus strains depend on which segments are inherited from which parent and the functional behavior of each particular combination of segments and their protein products.

Rotavirus reassortants form readily in cell culture[59, 145, 167, 374, 478, 498, 499, 501] and in co-infected experimental animals,[44, 160] which at least partially is responsible for the variety of rotavirus strains found in nature.[164] Reassortant formation between rotavirus strains is, however, not a universal phenomenon. For example, there is no evidence that reassortants form between strains belonging to different rotavirus groups.[521] Even within group A rotaviruses, there are severe limitations within strain combinations that are capable of forming stable reassortants, limitations that appear to be related directly to the degree of genetic variation between strains.[375]

One outcome of restricted reassortant formation between rotavirus strains is the concept of genetic families[138] or genogroups.[318] A genogroup is composed of rotavirus strains

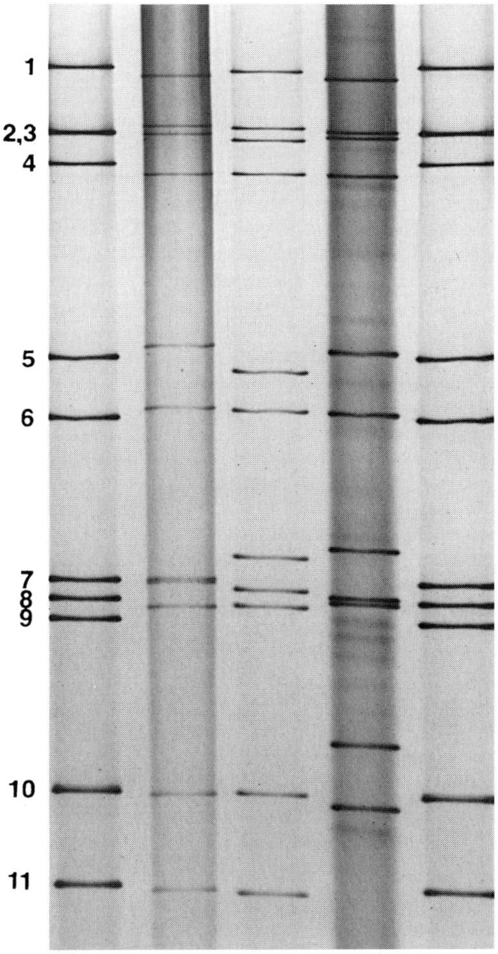

FIGURE 176–2. *Polyacrylamide gel electrophoretic patterns of genomic RNAs obtained from group A human rotaviruses and visualized by silver staining. The patterns demonstrate the characteristic four size classes of RNA separated into groups of 4, 2, 3, and 2 segments each. Human rotavirus strains included (from left to right) lane 1, Wa; lane 2, 248 strain; lane 3, 456 strain; lane 4, DS-1; lane 5, Wa.*

whose gene segments form interstrain RNA-RNA hybrids of sufficient stability to migrate as defined bands during polyacrylamide gel electrophoresis.[318] Thus, members of a genogroup share a high degree of genetic relatedness and have significantly less genetic homology with members of

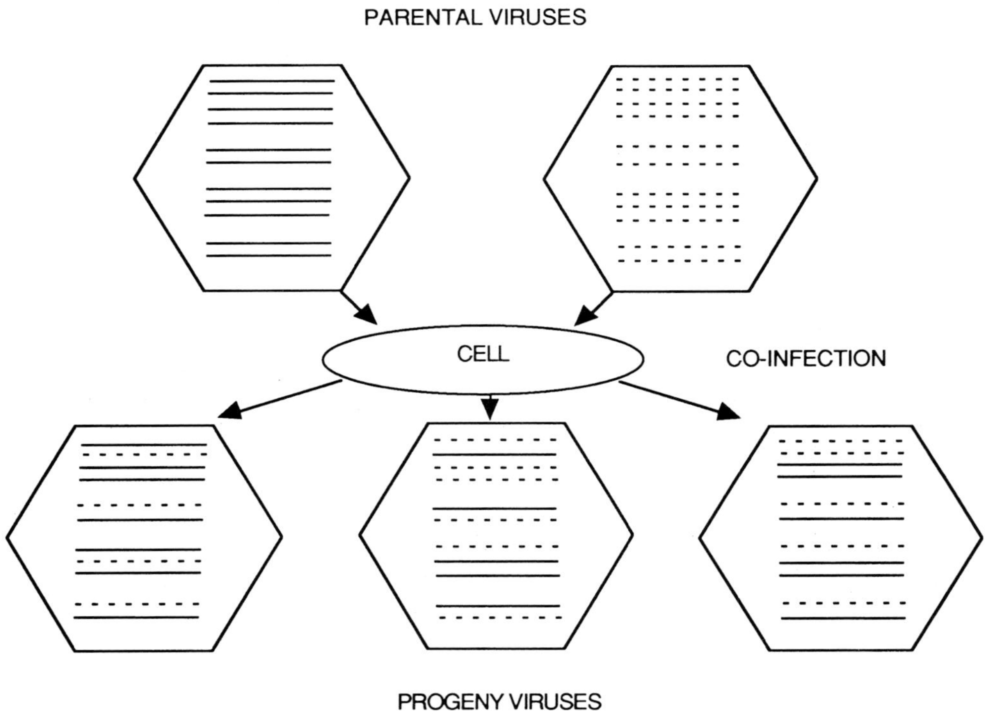

FIGURE 176–3. *Diagram of the formation of reassortant progeny rotaviruses after co-infection of a cell with two different (parental) strains of rotavirus.*

other genogroups. Because rotavirus genogroups appear to be species-specific,[48, 130, 317, 318] interspecies transmission of rotaviruses should be detectable readily by genogroup analyses. Almost all human rotaviruses belong to the Wa or DS-1 genogroup,[136, 138, 316, 507] a designation developed from these prototype strains. The concept of genogroup has been used extensively to determine the origin of rotaviruses causing human infections and disease, particularly to detect viruses or reassortants with gene segments of animal origin.[47, 95, 108, 151, 152, 312–315, 319, 339, 425, 476]

Serotypes and Genetic Linkage

Both outer capsid proteins of rotavirus, VP4 and VP7, contain neutralization epitopes, and, thereby, both are involved in serotype determination.[172, 174, 204, 220, 327] Originally, serotyping was based solely on differences in the VP7 protein because animals hyperimmunized with rotaviruses develop most neutralizing antibody to this protein. Cross-neutralization studies conducted with these hyperimmune sera readily separated the strains into VP7 serotypes.[205, 515] When it was found later that VP4 could, in some cases, be the dominant neutralization protein,[69, 355, 503, 504] a dual serotyping scheme was required. Although VP7 serotypes could be determined readily by cross-neutralization studies, this was more difficult for VP4.[87, 154, 162, 272, 344, 429, 454] Therefore, two numeric systems were devised to classify the VP4 protein in rotavirus strains. One is based on comparative nucleic hybridization and sequence analyses (genotypes),[120, 146, 154, 166, 260, 514] and the second is based on neutralization (serotypes) using antisera against baculovirus-expressed VP4 proteins[162] or reassortants with specific VP4 genes.[201, 214, 429]

Rotavirus classification based on VP4 and VP7 is designated P and G types to describe the protease sensitivity and glycosylated structure of these two proteins, respectively.[120] Although the numbers continue to grow, 14 G types[45, 46, 120, 455] and 20 P types[147, 191, 208, 214, 419, 424, 457, 477] have been identified. Human rotaviruses belonging to 11 G serotypes have been isolated,[155] but the vast majority have been identified as G1, G2, G3, or G4, and strains belonging to these G types commonly have been designated as serotype 1, 2, 3, or 4, respectively.[224] The severity of illness among viruses belonging to these four serotypes has varied little if at all.[10, 17, 378] Likewise, 7 P genotypes have been found in humans, but almost all illnesses have been associated with P genotypes 4 and 8.[224] However, other G and P types have been the most frequently isolated in some settings.[147, 309, 442, 462]

If the G and P types of rotaviruses found in humans could associate freely because of reassortant formation, it is anticipated that the combinations of types for these proteins would be generated randomly. However, this is clearly not the case. For example, G1P8 and G2P4 rotaviruses similar to the prototype Wa and DS-1 strains, respectively, frequently are isolated but belong to two distinct genogroups of human rotaviruses.[318] Therefore, they rarely should form reassortants, an assumption that has been substantiated through analyses of numerous rotavirus strains.

Other associations between gene segments also have been found. The VP6 protein or group antigen can be divided into two subgroups (I and II), based on antigenic differences within this protein.[173, 456] Almost all G2 and G8 human rotaviruses belong to subgroup I, whereas G1, G3, G4, and G9 human rotaviruses belong almost solely to subgroup II.[3, 70, 148, 205, 225, 388, 451] G3 also is a common serotype in animal strains, but in contrast with results found with G3 human strains, almost all G3 animal rotaviruses belong to subgroup I. In addition, subgroup I human, but not animal, strains have been found to have a characteristic "short" electropherotype associated with an inversion in the migration order of segments 10 and 11.[219, 250] Thus, distinct genetic linkages have been found by serotype, genotype, subtype, and electropherotype analysis as well as by genogroup determination.

Cross-Species Rotavirus Infections

Rotaviruses have an extremely wide host range, but natural cross-species infections may be rare, particularly those between animals and humans. However, a number of human isolates appear to be animal strains or animal-human rotavirus reassortants, as determined by genogroup and sequence analyses.[47, 95, 108, 151, 152, 312–315, 319, 339, 425, 476] The importance of these strains in human disease may be limited. It has been suggested, however, that once adapted to replication in humans, such strains may become important human pathogens.[318]

The property of host restriction has been utilized extensively to develop rotavirus vaccines for humans from naturally attenuated bovine and simian rotaviruses. Oral immunization of infants with these experimental live virus vaccines has resulted in low levels of intestinal replication and partial protection against human rotavirus illnesses.[18, 68, 71, 137, 252, 304, 483, 486] Thus, the barrier of host restriction can be bypassed sufficiently under these controlled conditions to permit the development of protective immune responses in a heterologous host. Experimental studies in animals have shown that intestinal replication of rotaviruses in heterologous species generally is limited, and, if shedding of progeny viruses is detectable, it often occurs only when animals are inoculated with very high doses of the heterologous viruses.[44, 52, 83, 124, 291, 332, 373, 505, 506]

The basis for host range restriction is unknown and probably involves the collective properties of at least several genes. When reassortants between a murine and a simian rotavirus were used in a mouse model, however, a significant linkage to host range restriction was associated with gene 5 encoding NSP1.[44] Other studies also report nonrandom selection of gene 5 in progeny after co-infection of cells in culture[167] and in mice,[160] thus suggesting a possible growth advantage associated with this gene. This gene also shows a high amount of sequence divergence between rotaviruses of different species,[120] which supports its possible role in host restriction.

Age-Dependent Susceptibility to Rotavirus Disease

In addition to restrictions in interspecies transmission of rotaviruses, age restrictions are associated with rotavirus disease. In animals, rotavirus illness appears to be limited to the first days or weeks of life. Mice are susceptible to rotavirus disease for only their first 15 days of life but can experience a rotavirus infection for their entire lifetime.[293] Similarly, piglets and calves are most susceptible to rotavirus diarrhea during their first days of life.[38, 240] In contrast, severe human rotavirus disease is most common between 6 and 24 months of age (Fig. 176–4),[393] but milder rotavirus illnesses occur throughout our lifetimes.

Causes for the reduced severity of rotavirus disease before 6 months and after the first years of life are subjects of intense investigation. Possibly, nonimmunologic, age-dependent changes occur within the intestine that could account for this reduced severity, including an observed decrease in virus-specific receptors on enterocytes between suckling and adult mice.[386] This also may explain why human infants are more susceptible to rotavirus illnesses than older children or adults. Decreased concentrations of proteases needed to cleave the VP4 protein in intestinal secretions of newborns relative to older infants also could help explain the resistance of neonates to rotavirus disease.[255]

Neonatal rotavirus infections are common and in some newborn nurseries appear to be endemic.[26, 65, 356, 388] Based on sequence analyses, it was proposed that neonatal strains possess unique VP4 genes, which have been classified as genotype P6.[120, 132, 161] Because neonatal rotavirus infections also typically are asymptomatic, rotaviruses containing P6 VP4 genes were designated as neonatal or asymptomatic strains. Further epidemiologic studies have shown that these descriptions, however, are not totally accurate; asymptomatic neonatal infections sometimes are caused by non-P6 strains,[94] and many symptomatic infections of older infants in some settings are due to P6 strains.[147, 309, 442, 462] It is, therefore, unclear why most neonatal rotavirus infections are due to P6 strains and whether the P6 genotype is in any way responsible for the asymptomatic phenotype of these infections.

It has been reported that the onset of rotavirus disease in infants coincided with the decline of maternal antibody titers to low concentrations.[528] Therefore, the commonly asymptomatic nature of neonatal rotavirus infections at least partially may be due to protection from transplacental antibody that may persist for the first months of life.[22] Mechanisms by which transplacental maternal antibody might protect against intestinal infection are unclear. Passive transfer of neutralizing antibody to the intestine of both humans and animals is associated with protection,[39, 54, 99, 109, 110, 196, 258, 408, 416, 428, 430] but circulating antirotavirus IgG appears to confer little, if any, protection in animals.[330, 430, 431] Possibly, maternal IgG in humans is taken into the intestine where it neutralizes rotaviruses prior to infection. Regardless of why rotavirus infection of neonates typically is asymptomatic, these infections have been found to reduce the severity of rotavirus illnesses in older infants.[23, 26] For these reasons, at least two rotavirus strains obtained from neonates have been developed as vaccine candidates.[9, 304]

The reduced severity of rotavirus disease in older children and adults probably is due primarily to immune responses stimulated by previous rotavirus infections. Almost all humans experience at least one rotavirus infection by 3 years of age in developed as well as developing countries, and circulating rotavirus antibody remains detectable indefinitely.[223, 224] Protection against rotavirus infection and disease in adults has been correlated with titers of both circulating and intestinal rotavirus antibody.[169, 230, 231, 494, 495] Although these antibodies have not been established as the effectors of protection, their presence indicates a natural infection that has elicited a protective immune response.

Rotavirus Seasonality and Sources of Epidemic Strains

As with other respiratory and enteric viruses, distinct seasonality is associated with rotavirus disease.[86, 182, 185, 228] This particularly is evident in temperate climates, where rotaviruses probably are responsible for the large increase in diarrheal deaths found during the winter season.[159, 198, 199, 254] The seasonality of rotavirus disease is less apparent in tropical climates but still is more prevalent in the drier, cooler months.[185] The cause for the seasonality of rotavirus disease is a topic of considerable interest but remains unknown.

The transmission of rotavirus infections is believed to be fecal-oral, with little evidence of airborne transmission. Yet a unique pattern of rotavirus infections is observed annually in North America that follows the general direction of the prevailing winds.[254] These infections begin in Mexico and the southwestern United States in mid to late fall and travel systematically across the continent, ending in the northeastern United States and maritime provinces of Canada in the spring (Fig. 176–5). This is the only description of a repetitive geographic sequence for the seasonal epidemic activity of a viral agent. There are no satisfactory explanations for this annual event, including wind movements. The phenomenon appears to be independent of latitude, which argues against

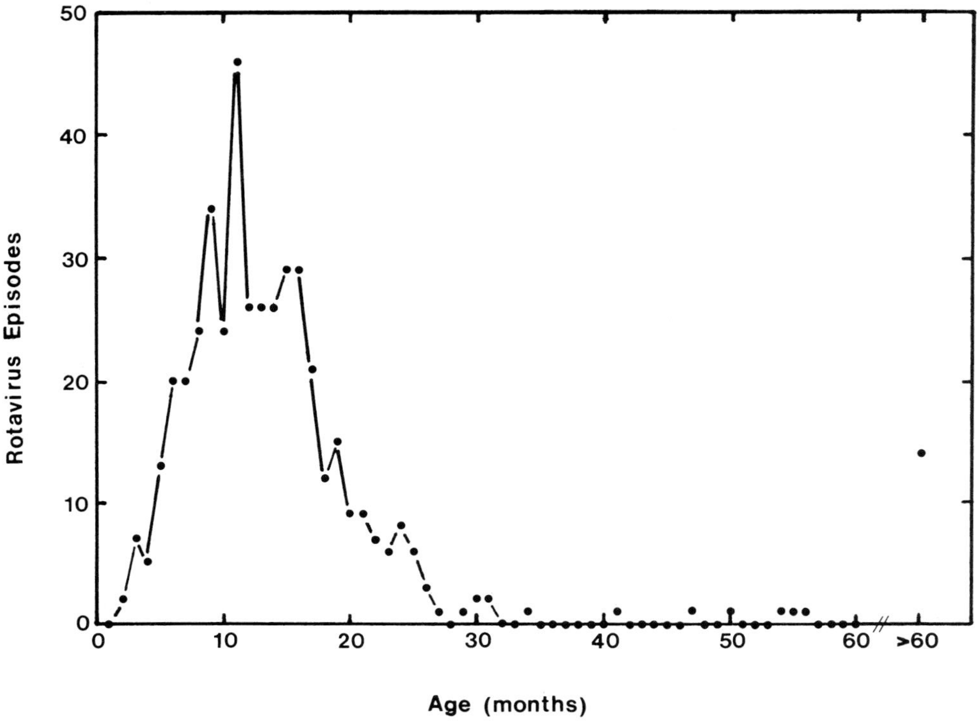

FIGURE 176–4. *Age-related incidence of clinically significant rotavirus episodes in the Matlab region of Bangladesh for residents under surveillance in 1985 and 1986. (From Ward, R. L., et al.: J. Clin. Microbiol. 29:1915–1923, 1991.)*

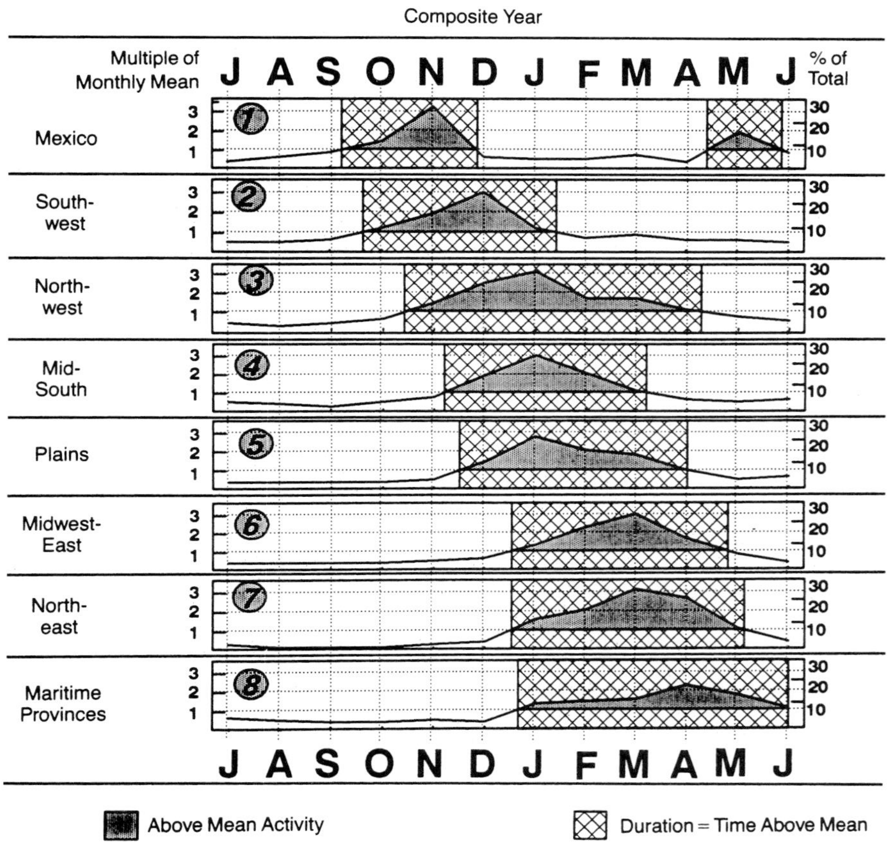

FIGURE 176–5. *West-to-east movement of annual rotavirus epidemics in North America based on a monthly average of rotavirus illnesses between 1984 and 1988. Results are from 88 centers in Canada, Mexico, and the United States. (From LeBaron, C. W., et al.: J. A. M. A. 264:983–988, 1990.)*

temperature-dependent associations and humidity. Furthermore, the electropherotypes and serotypes of isolates found in different geographic locations can vary,[493] a counterindication for a gradual, physical transmission of rotavirus infections as a wave to the north and east.

Because rotavirus illnesses occur with seasonal regularity and decrease to almost undetectable levels during the off-season, the virus must be retained in a less active state during the majority of each year. It is unlikely that human rotavirus is retained in animal reservoirs between seasons because of the low interspecies transmissibility associated with this virus, as already discussed. Therefore, the virus may continue to replicate at low levels in humans until conditions are favorable for the annual epidemic. The occasional rotavirus illnesses that occur in the off-season support the suggestion that humans are a reservoir. It also is possible that the virus survives in the environment that provides continuous exposure throughout the year but results in sustained rotavirus illnesses only during seasonal epidemics. Rotaviruses are shed in extremely high concentrations (i.e., approximately 10^{11} particles/g of human feces),[502] retain their infectivities for many months at ambient temperatures,[122, 237, 307] and readily are detectable on environmental surfaces.[53] Therefore, the environment could be a reservoir for human rotavirus and a possible source for the initiation of seasonal epidemics.

To provide clues regarding the origin of rotavirus strains responsible for epidemics, many extensive studies have been performed to characterize the circulating viruses, primarily using electropherotypes and serotypes. From these, it has been determined that rotavirus strains in a specific locale can vary little over sequential seasons or change dramatically, even within a single season.[72, 232, 361, 376, 388, 399, 417, 439, 451, 453, 497] Furthermore, multiple strains often are present within a region at any period during an epidemic. Because gene reassortment can be extensive after rotavirus co-infection,[164] it is difficult to identify the source of new strains within a defined geographic area. They could be derived from outside sources, they could be obtained from local reservoirs, or they could arise by gene reassortment of circulating strains. Clearly, if the source of virus responsible for initiating annual rotavirus epidemics could be identified, much would be learned about the epidemiology of rotavirus.

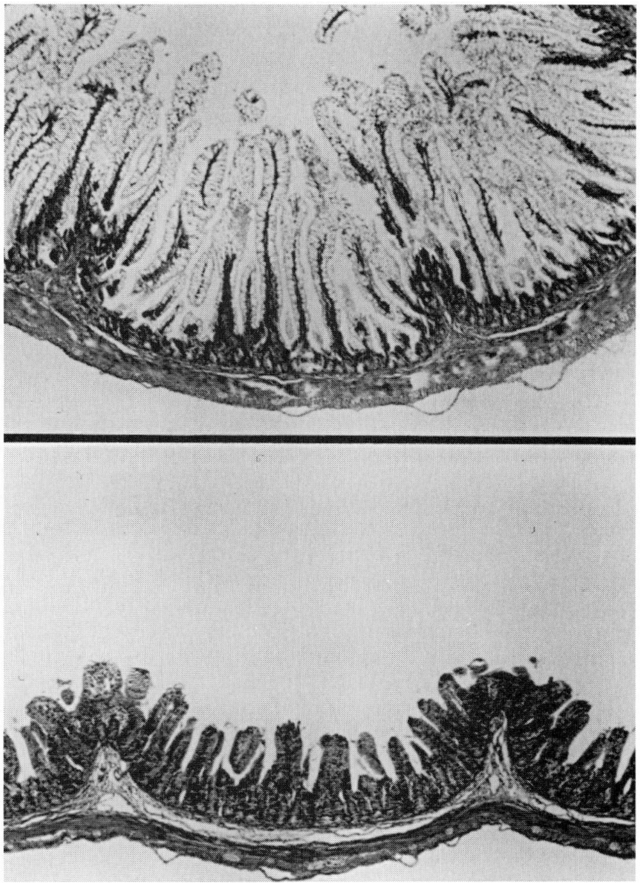

FIGURE 176–6. Top, *Normal histologic appearance of ileum from an 8-day-old gnotobiotic pig. Normal mature vacuolate absorptive cells cover the villi. Hematoxylin and eosin (H & E) stain.* Bottom, *Ileum from an 8-day-old gnotobiotic pig after oral inoculation with virulent human rotavirus (Wa strain). Severe villous atrophy and early crypt hyperplasia are evident. H & E stain. (Courtesy of Dr. L. A. Ward, Ohio Agricultural Research and Development Center, The Ohio State University, Wooster, OH.)*

PATHOLOGY AND PATHOGENESIS

Histologic and Structural Changes in Intestinal Villi

After fecal-oral transmission of rotavirus, infection is initiated in the upper intestine and typically leads to a series of histologic and physiologic changes. These changes have been examined extensively, particularly through experimental infections of animals (Fig. 176–6). Studies in calves revealed that rotavirus infection caused the villus epithelium to change from columnar to cuboidal, which resulted in shortening and stunting of the villi.[295, 296, 298, 351] The cells at the villus tips became denuded, while in the underlying lamina propria, the numbers of reticulum-like cells increased and mononuclear cell infiltration was observed. The infection started at the proximal end of the small intestine and advanced distally. The most pronounced changes usually, but not always,[464] were associated with the proximal small intestine. When bovine rotaviruses of different virulence were compared, it was reported that a low-virulence strain infected the proximal small intestine poorly but infected more villus enterocytes in the mid and distal intestine than the high-virulence strain.[41, 188] Although the low-virulence strain replicated in these cells and caused cytopathic effects, it did not damage intestinal structure or affect function. Similar observations were made after rotavirus infection of piglets.[80, 91, 171, 256, 257, 322, 349, 350, 367, 459, 465]

The pathology of murine rotavirus infection also has been examined in several studies, and the results are similar to those found in larger animals.[2, 8, 15, 77, 163, 249, 262, 263, 343, 394, 437] Many of these studies have been conducted with heterologous rotavirus strains that require orders of magnitude more virus because of their restricted replication in mice.[15, 44, 124, 163, 175, 332, 373, 506] The histologic changes induced by these heterologous strains are similar to those found after murine rotavirus infection, even though viral replication is limited after oral inoculation with these viruses. Studies with the mouse model also have revealed a potential hazard associated with the possible use of heterologous viruses as vaccine candidates. Although replication of the homologous strains appeared to be restricted to the intestine, oral inoculation of either severe combined immune deficiency (SCID) or normal mice with a simian rotavirus resulted in its spread to the liver and induction of hepatitis.[474, 475] Because of evidence for abnormal liver function during natural rotavirus infection in humans,[177, 180, 247] this observation has caused concern over the use of animal strains as vaccine candidates. However, no significant alteration of liver function has been associated with any rotavirus vaccine candidate after extensive investigations, even though most candidates have been derived from animal rotavirus strains.

A few studies have examined the pathologic changes in the intestines of humans, but the results appeared to be similar to those found in animals.[200, 449] Tissue tropism for rotavirus infection in humans also appeared to be restricted normally to villi of the small intestine. Sporadic instances of nongastrointestinal rotavirus-associated disease have been reported, including the association with abnormal liver function mentioned earlier, as well as respiratory and nervous system involvement.[183, 193, 217, 234, 245, 259, 284, 310, 323, 409, 452, 474, 475, 480, 510, 523, 527] However, because no consistent evidence of extraintestinal replication of rotavirus has been forthcoming, it generally is assumed that rotavirus pathology strictly is intestinal.

As with host-range restriction, the molecular basis for pathogenicity has not been established. Offit and coworkers[328] reported that the virulence of reassortants generated between heterologous rotaviruses and tested in a mouse model correlated with the presence of the VP4 protein from the more virulent virus. Neither rotavirus strain used in his study (a simian and a bovine strain) replicated efficiently in mice, however, which suggested that the observation may have limited applicability. A later study with murine-simian rotavirus reassortants revealed no association between the VP4 protein and virulence.[44] In that study, the strongest association between virulence and a gene product was with NSP1, a nonstructural protein.

Associations between virulence and specific gene segments also were examined in piglets. Virulence variants that appeared to differ only in their VP4 genes were isolated from the feces of an infected pig.[40, 51] However, differences in other gene products could not be eliminated as determinants of virulence. In a more extensive study with reassortants between a virulent porcine virus and a human strain attenuated for piglets, it was found that the porcine rotavirus genes encoding VP3, VP4, VP7, and NSP4 all were required for virulence in piglets.[202] Whether this observation has general applicability or pertains only to a limited combination of rotavirus strains because of specific interactions between their proteins remains to be determined. It was observed that passage of a porcine rotavirus in piglets dramatically increased its virulence,[40] whereas passage of a virulent porcine rotavirus in cell culture attenuated this virus.[472] Thus, the associations between specific rotavirus genes and virulence can be altered readily by natural selection through mutation.

Mechanisms of Diarrhea

Although rotaviruses cause severe diarrhea in numerous species, including humans, the mechanisms responsible have not been determined and may be due to multiple factors. An early study in piglets indicated that net Na^+ and Cl^- fluxes were not different between control and infected animals, but glucose-mediated sodium adsorption was diminished by rotavirus infection.[97] Based on this and other physiologic changes, the authors concluded that retarded differentiation of uninfected enterocytes that migrated at an accelerated rate from the crypts after the virus had invaded villus cells was responsible for adsorptive abnormalities. Another study with piglets led to the conclusion that destruction of the villus tip cells causes carbohydrate maladsorption and osmotic diarrhea.[168] In mice it has been reported that carbohydrate maladsorption did not occur as in piglets, and, therefore, crypt cell secretions may be the cause of fluid loss.[81] Additional studies in animals and humans concerning changes in the adsorption of macromolecules across the intestinal surface after rotavirus infection have revealed no general pattern.[171, 195, 212, 286, 325] Uptake of some molecules, such as horseradish peroxidase and 2-rhamnose, is increased; uptake of other molecules, such as lactulose and D-xylose, is decreased. Therefore, the relationship between the absorptive properties of intestinal mucosa induced by rotavirus infection and development of diarrhea remains unclear.

The importance of virus replication for induction of rotavirus diarrhea also has been challenged. It had been observed that inoculation of mice with heterologous rotaviruses produced diarrhea only when mice were inoculated with large quantities of these viruses, and in these cases diarrhea occurred despite a lack of efficient viral replication.[44, 332, 373, 506] It subsequently was reported that inoculation with a large number of inactivated particles from a heterologous rotavirus also resulted in diarrhea.[421] The authors suggested that rotavirus attachment or entry into cells was sufficient to induce diarrhea in this model and that the mechanism of rotavirus-induced diarrhea was consistent with a viral toxin-like effect exerted during virus-cell contact.

Diarrhea also has been induced in infant mice and rats by intraperitoneal inoculation with the rotavirus NSP4 protein as well as with a 22–amino acid peptide derived from this protein.[7] It was observed that this protein and its peptide caused an increase in Ca^{2+} concentration in insect cells when added exogenously.[461] Thus, binding of these molecules to intestinal epithelium after their release from infected cells may contribute to altered ion transport and diarrhea. Whether this is a major mechanism of diarrhea occurring after rotavirus infection remains to be determined.

IMMUNITY

Much has been learned about the immune response to rotavirus, but the key question of what provides protection from infection or disease remains unanswered. It is clear that rotavirus infections induce a humoral immune response beginning with production of IgM antibodies and later including IgA and IgG antibody.[98, 178, 289, 384] Infection also induces local, intestinal antibodies that predominantly are IgA but also include IgG and IgM initially.[20, 89, 98, 178, 281, 289, 384] After infection in mice, up to 50 per cent of all IgA cells in the lamina propria of the intestine can be rotavirus-specific.[422] Cell-mediated immunity including lymphoproliferative responses also is detected easily after infection in animals and humans,[336, 337, 387, 466] and a brisk cytolytic T-cell response (CD8+) has been found in the intestine and spleen of infected mice.[333, 334]

The most immunogenic protein appears to be VP6. Thus, antibodies measured by enzyme-linked immunosorbent assay (ELISA) are directed mainly at this protein and may not be neutralizing.[420] Some evidence suggests, however, that IgA antibodies directed at VP6 can be protective by as yet incompletely understood mechanisms.[426] Antibodies directed at either the VP4 or the VP7 proteins can neutralize virus and provide protection when given passively to animals.[282, 338] Although a number of problems are associated with measuring the VP4- and VP7-specific responses in humans,[326] the preponderance of information suggests that after infection, the predominant response appears to be to the VP4 protein,[49, 153, 503, 504] and VP7 antibodies were more common after vaccination with a poorly replicating vaccine: WC3.[500] Both VP4 and VP7 proteins can induce both type-specific and cross-reactive serotype responses, although most of the

VP7 responses are type-specific, whereas those directed at VP4, especially the VP5* region, are more likely to be cross-reactive.[162, 170, 272, 308, 454] These findings have important implications for vaccine development, as will be discussed.

Rotavirus-specific cytotoxic T lymphocytes recognize VP7 better than VP4 and are not serotype-specific.[329, 333] Adoptive transfer of splenic lymphocytes from mice infected with homologous or heterologous rotavirus strains can protect suckling mice.[335] Protection is major histocompatibility complex–restricted and depends on the presence of CD8+ lymphocytes. Similarly, CD8+ splenic or intraepithelial lymphocytes obtained from the intestine of rotavirus-infected mice can eliminate the chronic rotavirus shedding seen in SCID mice.[106] Adoptive transfer of CD8+ cells from mice immunized with baculovirus recombinants expressing VP1, VP4, VP6, or VP7 also can terminate the chronic shedding in SCID mice.[105] Any possible role of cytolytic T cells in human rotavirus infections remains to be determined.

An obvious place to begin to understand rotavirus immunity is to determine the effectiveness of previous rotavirus infections in prevention of subsequent infections and disease. The important questions relate not only to the degree of protection but whether protection is serotype-specific. As discussed earlier in this chapter, multiple serotypes of human rotavirus are based on neutralization epitopes on the VP4 (P serotypes) and VP7 (G serotypes) outer capsid proteins. Thus, protection may be limited to those strains that share neutralization epitopes, or it may be associated with the development of other B- or T-cell immune responses to shared epitopes.

A number of investigators have reported that natural rotavirus infections produce incomplete protection, but there is little doubt that previous infections protect against severe reinfections.[21, 26, 31, 61, 62, 76, 101, 139, 141, 149, 179, 279, 341, 383, 401, 427, 493, 518] Sequential infections even with the same serotype have, however, been reported. In the initial study reporting rotavirus disease with reinfection by the same serotype, the investigators noted that protection of young children in a Japanese orphanage lasted 6 months then declined after 1 year.[62] This study noted a close correlation between titers of serotype-specific antibody and protection. Animal studies also support a role for serotype-specific infection. Thus, in a study with piglets, immunization with reassortant viruses containing either the VP4 or the VP7 protein of the same serotype was protective, whereas immunization with reassortants containing heterotypic genes for these proteins was not protective.[203] In other studies using mice, this association was not as clear,[506] and protection was correlated better to serum and intestinal levels of IgA.[124, 291, 293]

Although, as discussed earlier, reinfections with rotavirus appear to be common, other studies have shown protection that lasts at least 1 year.[21, 26, 493] Neonates infected within the first 2 weeks of life were protected against severe disease but not against reinfection in one study.[26] In another, infants who developed a symptomatic or an asymptomatic rotavirus infection during the first year of study were protected against a subsequent rotavirus illness or even an asymptomatic reinfection during the following year.[21] Similarly, when the placebo recipients of a large vaccine trial were followed, a natural rotavirus infection in the first year was found to be 93 per cent protective against a symptomatic reinfection in the second year.[493] This occurred even though the G1 strains that circulated during the first year were responsible for only 66 per cent of rotavirus disease in the second year. Other studies conducted in less-developed countries and in day care centers have not shown the same degree of protection.[31, 76, 179, 279, 383, 427] Differences in these studies may be due to the variation in circulating strains, the dose of exposure, or the duration of protection.

Protection has been correlated to both serum and stool antibody titers produced after natural rotavirus infection.[31, 62, 76, 88, 281, 342, 403, 494] Studies reporting a correlation with serotype-specific neutralizing antibody and protection[61, 342] have not been supported in other larger studies.[197, 496, 528] In the largest study, which was conducted in Bangladesh over a 2-year period when all four G serotypes circulated, the titers of both homologous and heterologous neutralizing antibody were significantly lower in patients with acute rotavirus disease compared with those of matched controls.[496] However, further analysis could not find a correlation with serotype-specific neutralizing antibody. Thus, protection seemed to be correlated better with the magnitude of the response rather than with specific neutralizing responses. Similarly, animal studies in both calves and mice have shown that protection can occur in the absence of virus-specific neutralizing antibodies in the serum, feces, or intestinal washes.[42, 291, 292, 506, 513]

Some results from rotavirus vaccine trials also fail to support a role for serum neutralizing antibody and protection. Thus, immunization with heterologous animal rotavirus vaccines has provided protection in some studies without inducing serum neutralizing antibody to human serotypes.[67, 484] In other studies that failed to demonstrate overall efficacy, protection was seen in those who developed the highest antibody titers to the heterologous vaccine,[22] again implicating the magnitude of the response rather than specific neutralizing antibody titers. It is possible that these measures of serum antibody are a marker for the true protective responses in the intestine.

Studies evaluating the protective role of previous infections and the mechanism of protection have used adults in challenge studies. Although essentially all adults have been infected previously with rotavirus, they are susceptible to reinfection and mild disease upon natural exposure.[206, 508] Initial challenge studies revealed an association between the preinoculation titer of serotype-specific neutralizing serum antibody and protection.[230, 231] These studies later were extended to show a correlation between VP7 antibody and protection but failed to establish a relationship between intestinal antibodies and protection.[169] When similar studies were conducted with a larger group of adults, the correlation between both serum and intestinal antibody became clearer.[494, 495] The most significant correlations were found to be between serum rotavirus IgG and shedding and between intestinal neutralizing antibody and illness. However, some subjects with high titers of antibody became infected and ill, whereas some subjects with low titers appeared to be protected.

Animal models also have proven useful for examining protective immune responses. Initially, large animals, such as piglets and calves, were used, whereas mouse models were limited to the study of passive protection because mice are susceptible to rotavirus diarrhea for only the first 15 days of life. These studies have been extended to the study of protection from infection using adult mice, which allows evaluation of both passive and active immunization.[505]

Initial studies of passive immunization including cross-fostering studies in mice found that gastrointestinal but not circulating antibodies were protective and that secretory IgA was more effective than IgG at providing protection.[39, 258, 268, 330, 408, 416, 428] Animals can be protected with antibodies directed at either VP4 or VP7.[331, 338] Similarly, active immunization against both homotypic and heterotypic challenge has been demonstrated in mice, calves, pigs, and rabbits.[42, 82, 84, 203, 292, 506, 512, 513] Protection has been seen after both oral and parenteral immunization, although it is not clear what provides protection. In studies of mice, although no correlation could be found between protection and either serum or intestinal neutralizing antibody, levels of serum or fecal rotavirus IgA did correlate to protection.[124, 291] The use of these models has been extended to gene knockout mice in order to distinguish the role of CD8+ cells and antibody in protection. These studies have particular relevance to vaccines. From these studies it appears that CD8+ cytolytic cells are important for resolution of an infection, but only antibody could provide protection from a subsequent challenge.[140, 290] The levels, location, and targets of this protective antibody, as well as the proteins against which it is directed, are of immediate importance, provided the results found in mice are relevant to larger animals and humans.

Information on protective immune responses continues to become available and should prove useful in the development of rotavirus vaccines. The absence, to date, of a reliable immunologic marker of protection, however, continues to make vaccine trials more difficult.

VACCINES

The development of rotavirus vaccines is a high priority for public health institutions. Based on the belief that protection from rotavirus is achieved best by inducing local intestinal immune responses, vaccine efforts have been directed mostly at the development of live attenuated rotavirus vaccines.[25, 85, 131, 158] Most of these efforts have concentrated on the use of animal rotavirus strains, called the Jennerian approach[342] because it relies on the natural attenuation of animal viruses in humans for safety and largely heterotypic immune responses for protection. More recently, human rotavirus genes have been introduced into these animal strains by creating reassortant viruses as described earlier to increase the relatedness of the vaccine to human rotaviruses. This is called the modified Jennerian approach.[131] Table 176–2 lists some of the major efficacy trials conducted to date.

Just 10 years after the identification of rotavirus as an agent of severe diarrhea, the first vaccine trials were performed.[484] The initial study utilized RIT4237, a bovine rotavirus. Since then, other vaccine candidates, including a rhesus monkey rotavirus (RRV or MMU 18006), another bovine rotavirus, WC3, and animal/human reassortants using RRV and WC3, have been evaluated. Less extensive studies also have been performed using neonatal human viruses M37 and RV3[9, 25, 85, 131, 135, 326, 490] that are believed to be naturally attenuated, human rotavirus strain 89-12 attenuated by multiple passages in tissue culture (Bernstein, unreported), and cold-adapted rotavirus strains.[131]

The initial studies of RIT vaccine produced variable results. The vaccine was safe and effective in Finland, providing a protective efficacy of about 50 per cent against all disease and a greater than 80 per cent protection against severe disease.[483, 485, 486] Later studies in developing countries, however, were disappointing,[102, 190, 252] showing little or no efficacy. Similarly, the vaccines failed to provide protection in a study performed on a Navajo reservation in Arizona.[413]

The WC3 rotavirus vaccine similarly is of bovine origin and also appears to be free of side effects. It replicates poorly in humans, but infants develop a neutralizing antibody response to WC3 and both rotavirus IgA and IgG antibody.[22] The initial studies conducted in Philadelphia appeared prom-

TABLE 176–2. Selected Vaccine Studies

Vaccine	Country	No. of Subjects	No. of Doses	Protection* (Overall/ Severe Disease)	Reference
RTT 4237	Finland	178	1	50/88	486
	Finland	328	2	58/82	485
	Rwanda	245	3	0/0	102
	Gambia	185	3	0/37	190
	Peru	391	3	40/75	252
WC3	USA (Philadelphia, PA)	104	1	43/89	67
	USA (Cincinnati, OH)	206	1	17/41	22
	Central African Republic	472	2	0/36	150
RRV	USA (Rochester, NY)	176	1	0/0	63
	Venezuela	247	1	68/100	128
	Finland	200	1	38/67	488
	Venezuela	320	1	64/90	357
	USA (Rochester, NY)	223	1	66/ND	273
RRV	USA (Indian reservation)	321	1	0/ND	413
RRV/human reassortants					
RRV G1	Finland	359	1	67/ND	489
RRV G2	Finland			66/ND	
RRV G1	USA (Rochester, NY)	223	1	77/ND	273
RRV G1	USA	898	3	69/73	18
RRV TV				64/82	
RRV G1	USA	1,187	3	54/69	379
RRV TV				49/80	
WC3 reassortants					
WC3 G1	USA (Rochester, NY)	325	3	64/87	468
WC3 TV	USA	417	3	73/73	71

*Measured in the first year after vaccination.
ND, not done.

ising,[67] but later trials in Cincinnati[22] and less-developed countries[150] did not show significant protection. This vaccine virus is being used to make reassortants containing rotavirus genes encoding the VP7 and VP4 proteins of human serotypes discussed later.

There have been more trials of RRV than any of the other vaccine candidates. RRV replicates better in humans than do the bovine vaccine strains, perhaps because it is a G3 serotype, but it also produces mild side effects, including low-grade fever and mild diarrhea, especially when given to older children who have lost maternal antibodies.[267, 358, 487] RRV induces serum rotavirus IgG and IgA, intestinal rotavirus IgA, and RRV neutralizing antibody but not G1-specific neutralizing antibody.[63, 268, 358] Protection with this vaccine has been inconsistent, ranging from greater than 50 per cent, even in developing countries,[128, 273, 357, 380] to moderate (20 to 50 per cent),[381, 488] to nonexistent.[63, 413] Although some evidence suggests that protection predominantly was against G3 but not G1 outbreaks,[85, 131] the evidence is not conclusive.

Because of the belief that homotypic immunity might increase the protection seen with rotavirus vaccines and because of a lack of consistent protection with the animal strains, most recent efforts have been directed toward creating vaccines that contain the VP7 or the VP7 and VP4 proteins of human rotavirus strains. As discussed earlier, these proteins were chosen because they induce neutralizing antibody. One goal of this strategy is to create a multivalent vaccine containing viruses with human rotavirus genes representing the main human serotypes. Reassortant vaccines have been developed with both RRV[303, 305] and WC3[68, 468] as the animal strain. The RRV/human VP7 rotavirus reassortants contain 10 genes from RRV and a single human rotavirus gene that specifies the neutralization protein VP7 (Fig. 176–7). A monovalent RRV vaccine containing the G1 VP7 reassortant or a bivalent preparation containing the G1 and G2 reassortants has been evaluated.[273, 489] The tetravalent preparation, however, is the one being advanced for licensure. This vaccine contains RRV and reassortants with the VP7 genes of G1, G2, or G4 serotypes. The G3 serotype virus of this vaccine is RRV. Vaccination produces a rotavirus IgG and IgA serum antibody response, but neutralizing antibodies are produced predominantly to RRV rather than the human serotypes.[18, 134, 306, 355, 379] This appears to be consistent with the experiments showing that VP4 rather than VP7 is more immunogenic after natural infection.[503, 504]

Extensive evaluations of RRV reassortants have been completed.[18, 273, 379, 489] In two large trials conducted at centers across the United States,[18, 379] the tetravalent vaccine was safe, with a slight increase in fever after the first dose. The efficacy of the vaccine against rotavirus disease for the first year was 49 to 64 per cent and 57 per cent over 2 years. Protection was increased against more severe disease to a level of about 80 per cent for severe disease. Vaccination also significantly decreased the number of medical office visits for rotavirus gastroenteritis or dehydration. Vaccination appeared to provide protection against both G1 and G3 serotypes. Large safety studies presently are being conducted with the tetravalent vaccine in final preparation for licensure applications.

WC3-based reassortants also have been evaluated. A monovalent vaccine containing the VP7 protein of a human G1 rotavirus provided 64 per cent efficacy against all symptomatic rotavirus disease and 87 per cent efficacy against more severe disease during a predominantly serotype G1 outbreak in Rochester.[468] The WC3-based reassortant quadrivalent vaccine includes both VP7 and VP4 human rotavirus gene substitutions[71] with G1, G2, G3, or P8 substitutions and most other segments from WC3. In studies conducted at multiple centers in the United States, it was shown to be safe, with

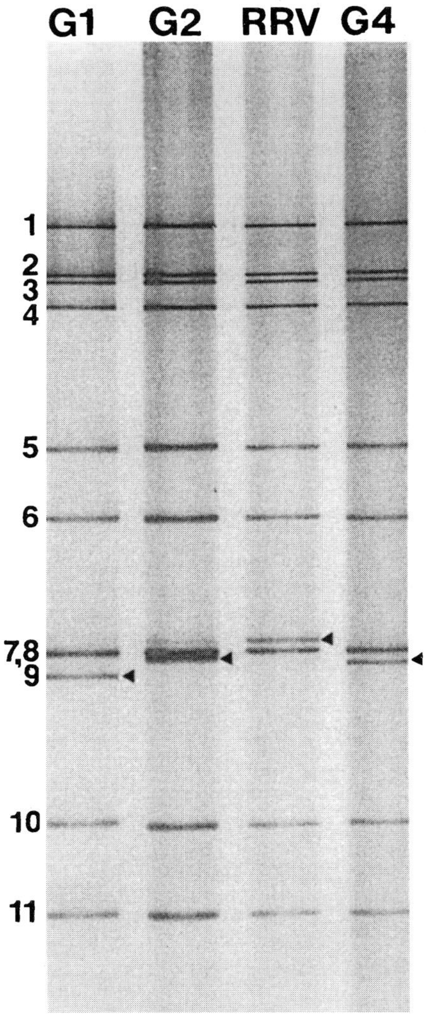

FIGURE 176–7. *Polyacrylamide gel electrophoretic patterns of the genome segments from RRV and the G1, G2, and G4 reassortant strains that compose the tetravalent RRV-based vaccine. The strains all contain 10 RRV genes and differ only in the gene segment encoding the VP7 protein, which migrates in the seventh (RRV) or ninth (reassortants) position, as designated by arrowheads.*

only a slight increase in diarrhea after the first dose.[71] The vaccine was 73 per cent effective against all cases of rotavirus gastroenteritis and 73 per cent effective against more severe cases.

Other approaches to rotavirus vaccines including the use of attenuated human viruses also are being evaluated. The initial evaluation of M37, a strain isolated from an asymptomatic newborn, showed reduced immunogenicity and a lack of efficacy,[135, 490] and evaluations of another neonatal strain (RV3) are just beginning.[9] A phase I trial of human strain 89-12, which was protective after natural infection and attenuated by multiple tissue culture passages, is underway (Bernstein, unreported), as are trials of a temperature-sensitive mutant.[131] Subunit vaccines, various expression vectors, synthetic peptides, and baculovirus-expressed capsids also are being considered as alternative strategies.[25, 85, 131]

CLINICAL MANIFESTATIONS

Rotavirus is the most common cause of dehydrating diarrhea in children in the United States and worldwide and infects nearly every child in the first few years of life.[104, 185, 223, 224] About 20 per cent of summer diarrhea is associated with rotavirus infection, compared with about 70 to 80 per cent of winter cases.[443] In a surveillance study of diarrhea across the United States, the percentage of specimens positive for rotavirus increased from 6 per cent in October to 36 per cent in February.[55] In the United States, more than 1 million cases of severe diarrhea are caused annually by rotavirus, resulting in 75 to 125 deaths.[159, 198, 199] In one study,[280] it was estimated that 8.5 per 1000 children per year are hospitalized in the United States for rotavirus illness in the first 2 years of life. An estimated 870,000 deaths are associated with rotavirus infection worldwide.[104, 213, 224] The incidence of rotavirus infections is highest in children between 6 and 24 months of age,[393] but the age may be lower in less-developed countries.[186, 378] Adults, including elderly patients, also are susceptible to reinfection, which can cause mild disease.[92, 111, 189, 206, 239, 276, 391, 508]

After an incubation period of about 2 to 4 days, there is an abrupt onset of vomiting and diarrhea. Vomiting may precede the diarrhea in about half the cases.[183] The disease usually is self-limited, lasting 4 to 8 days, although in a Guatemalan study the range of symptoms was between 2 and 22 days.[518] When hospitalization is required, usually the stay also is brief, with an average of 4 days and a range of 2 to 14 days.[390] Recovery usually is complete, but persistent diarrhea associated with lactose intolerance has been described.[14, 238]

In general, rotavirus infections are more severe than those due to other viral agents.[32, 390] In developing countries, 20 to 40 per cent of hospitalizations for diarrhea are due to rotavirus infections,[104] whereas in the United States, it is estimated that rotavirus accounts for between one-third and two-thirds of admissions for diarrhea in children.[35, 392] Vomiting, dehydration, and hospitalization all occur significantly more often in rotavirus-infected patients, compared with those with other causes of diarrhea.[390, 452, 473] In one study,[390] vomiting and diarrhea also lasted longer in rotavirus-infected patients (2.6 versus 0.9 days and 5.0 versus 2.6 days, respectively). In another study, the severity score for rotavirus diarrhea was almost twice that of disease due to other causes.[401] Rotavirus infections, however, also frequently can be asymptomatic,[378, 528] and a carrier state has been defined.[56] Reports of neonatal infections that are asymptomatic in selected settings also are common.[23, 26, 27, 30, 65, 176, 184, 187, 311, 356, 434, 467]

Other clinical findings include fever, abdominal distress, and mild dehydration. Fever occurs commonly during rotavirus illness, with estimates of between 45 and 84 per cent of patients.[248, 390, 443, 473] Dehydration due to rotavirus reportedly was more likely to be isotonic than dehydration caused by other agents,[390] although in another study one-fourth of the rotavirus-infected patients presented with hypernatremic dehydration.[248] Other findings include irritability and pharyngeal or tympanic membrane erythema. Numerous reports associate respiratory symptoms, such as cough, pharyngitis, otitis media, and pneumonia, with rotavirus infections, but the relationship of these symptoms to rotavirus is unclear, and the ability to isolate rotavirus from respiratory secretions has varied among studies.[183, 246, 259, 390, 414, 452, 527] Laboratory findings are related mostly to the extent of dehydration and can include elevated blood urea nitrogen and evidence of mild metabolic acidosis.

The diarrheal stools usually are loose and watery, with up to 10 stools per day. Mucus is found in about 20 per cent of stools, but blood is rare.[183] Fecal leukocytes also are uncommon.[209, 360] The peak viral shedding in stools occurs about day 3 of illness and then declines rapidly.[96, 244, 491] Persistent viral shedding has been reported for up to 5 weeks in Guatemala and also is associated with immunodeficiency.[64, 279, 415]

Other clinical manifestations associated either etiologically or incidentally with rotavirus infection include encephalitis and meningitis[217, 234, 409, 480, 510]; various upper and lower respiratory infections, including otitis media, laryngitis, pharyngitis, and pneumonia[246, 259, 324, 390, 414, 452, 527]; intussusception[245, 310, 452]; Kawasaki syndrome[284]; sudden infant death syndrome[523]; hepatic abscess[180, 452]; and pancreatitis.[323] Elevated liver function test results also have been reported during rotavirus infection.[177, 180, 247] Perhaps the strongest link is to neonatal necrotizing enterocolitis.[100, 236, 397] However, the difficulty of false-positive reactions with some ELISA tests in neonates must be considered.[66, 377, 469] Rotavirus infections can be more severe in immunosuppressed persons, including bone marrow transplant recipients, patients infected with HIV, and those who are malnourished,[93, 115, 157, 215, 222, 522] and they may spread to the liver and kidney.[157]

LABORATORY DIAGNOSIS

It is not possible to diagnose rotavirus infection on clinical presentation, even when combined with stool examination and nonspecific laboratory tests. Therefore, specific tests have been developed. Findings suggestive of rotavirus infection include a mildly febrile illness with vomiting and watery diarrhea that is occurring in the winter months in temperate climates, especially in patients 6 to 24 months of age. The presence of more severe dehydration also is suggestive. In the initial epidemiologic studies, electron microscopy was used for identification because of the large number of particles present in stools ($>10^{10}$) and the characteristic appearance of rotavirus. This technique largely has been replaced by enzyme immunoassay–based and latex agglutination tests, for which kits are available commercially. Both have good sensitivity when compared with electron microscopy.[103, 115, 156, 243, 460] One problem that has been noted in the past was false-positive results in neonatal stools with certain ELISA kits.[66, 377, 469] Inclusion of a rotavirus-negative capture antibody as a control in these kits should eliminate these false-positive reactions.

Rotavirus also can be grown in tissue culture,[24, 192, 502, 516] although the methods used for routine viral cultures do not detect rotavirus. The serotype (G type) of cultured strains then can be identified using monoclonal antibodies.[229] Genotypes can be identified as a surrogate for serotypes using DNA probes[129, 253, 441] and by reverse transcription polymerase chain reaction.[146, 165] Electrophoresis of extracted RNA also can be used to identify rotavirus by its characteristic 11 segments and is used to define electropherotypes.[218, 389, 410, 417] All these methods have proved useful as epidemiologic tools and in vaccine studies. Identification of electropherotypes especially is useful for epidemiologic studies because it allows identification of specific strains.

Rotavirus infection, both symptomatic and asymptomatic, also can be identified by changes in rotavirus antibody. ELISA assays are used most commonly to measure serum IgM, IgA, and IgG levels, as well as stool and intestinal antibodies. Specific neutralizing titers also can be measured for each serotype of rotavirus by plaque reduction[205, 515] or focus reduction assays.[19, 43] One ELISA-based antigen reduction neutralization assay has been found to be better-suited for the analyses of large numbers of specimens.[241] Serologic detection of infection is more difficult in the first months of life because of the presence of maternal antibodies. Detection of IgA, which does not cross the placenta, has been used as a marker for previous infection in the first months of life.

TREATMENT

Treatment of rotavirus gastroenteritis is aimed largely at restoring the proper fluid balance in dehydrated patients. Emphasis has shifted from intravenous rehydration to oral rehydration using glucose electrolyte solutions. The glucose in the solution enhances sodium and, therefore, water absorption in the intestine.[320] Several studies have shown the utility of this approach for rotavirus gastroenteritis.[404, 411, 412] The solution accepted by the World Health Organization contains 30 mEq/L of sodium, 30 mEq/L of potassium, and 30 mEq/L of bicarbonate, which is similar to other oral rehydrating solutions available commercially. Should oral rehydration efforts fail, or in cases of severe dehydration and shock, intravenous fluid administration should be used.

Other experimental approaches to treatment are based on the success of passive oral therapy in animals. Chronic rotavirus shedding has been treated successfully with human milk that contained rotavirus antibody.[415] Treatment and prophylaxis of normal children with immune colostrum, immunoglobulin, or milk from rotavirus-immunized cows also have been evaluated with some success.[99, 110, 196, 266, 471] The treatment of normal children with one dose of human serum immunoglobulin given orally was reported to be effective in reducing the mean duration of diarrhea, viral excretion, and hospital stay,[181] and prophylaxis with bovine antibody–supplemented formula decreased the number of days with rotavirus diarrhea.[471] Trials of bismuth subsalicylate also have been conducted with some reported success.[125, 432]

NON–GROUP A ROTAVIRUSES

As described earlier, rotaviruses can be classified into seven groups (A to G). All seven groups are associated with diarrhea in animals, although only groups A, B, and C have been associated with disease in humans.[407] Of these, group A causes the majority of illness. Major epidemics of group B rotavirus have, however, been reported in China[123, 210] and appear to occur as yearly epidemics. Group C infections largely have been reported from Japan[283, 340, 479] but also have been detected in the United States.[216] Seroprevalence studies have identified group B rotavirus infections in Hong Kong, Burma, Thailand, Australia, Canada, England, Kenya, and the United States, although the prevalence is lower than in the epidemic regions of China.[407] Group C rotavirus infections may be distributed more widely, although the evidence is uncertain because of the poor assays that are available. Evidence of infection has been reported in Asia, Australia, Europe, Central and South America,[354, 407, 470] and the United States.[216]

Outbreaks due to water-borne or food-borne spread of group B rotavirus in China[211] and group C rotavirus in Japan have been reported, although person-to-person spread also has been implicated.[123] Outbreaks usually involve older children and adults,[123, 210, 340] but infants apparently can be infected.[216] Group C rotaviruses have been associated with extrahepatic biliary atresia.[385, 418] If infection is suspected, the diagnosis is suggested by electron microscopic detection of the typical rotavirus particles with a negative test result for rotavirus by the routine assays that only detect group A rotaviruses. The detection of typical RNA migration patterns by polyacrylamide gel electrophoresis of RNA also is suggestive. Both tests require confirmation by ELISA or immune electron microscopy using specific reagents.

References

1. Adams, W. R., and Kraft, L. M.: Epizootic diarrhea of infant mice: Identification of the etiologic agent. Science *141*:359–360, 1963.
2. Adams, W. R., and Kraft, L. M.: Electron microscopic study of the intestinal epithelium of mice infected with the agent of epizootic diarrhea of infant mice (EDIM virus). Am. J. Pathol. *51*:39–60, 1967.
3. Albert, M. J., Unicomb, L. E., and Bishop, R. F.: Cultivation and characterization of human rotaviruses with "super short" RNA patterns. J. Clin. Microbiol. *25*:183–185, 1987.
4. Altenburg, B. C., Graham, D. Y., and Estes, M. K.: Ultrastructural study of rotavirus replication in cultured cells. J. Gen. Virol. *46*:75–85, 1980.
5. Au, K.-S., Mattion, N. M., and Estes, M. K.: A subviral particle binding domain on the rotavirus nonstructural glycoprotein NS28. Virology *194*:665–673, 1993.
6. Avendano, P., Matson, D. O., Long, J., et al.: Costs associated with office visits for diarrhea in infants and toddlers. Pediatr. Infect. Dis. J. *12*:897–902, 1993.
7. Ball, J. M., Peng, T., and Estes, M. K.: Rotavirus nonstructural protein, NSP4, induces diarrhea. Abstract. American Society for Virology, Austin, TX, July 8–12, 1995, p. 146.
8. Banfield, W. G., Kasnic, G., and Blackwell, J. H.: Further observations on the virus of epizootic diarrhea of infant mice: An electron microscopic study. Virology *36*:411–417, 1968.
9. Barnes, G., Bishop, R., Lund, J., et al.: Phase I trial of a neonatal strain (RV3) rotavirus vaccine candidate. Abstract. Fifth Rotavirus Vaccine Workshop, Atlanta, October 16–17, 1995.
10. Barnes, G. L., Unicomb, L., and Bishop, R. F.: Severity of rotavirus infection in relation to serotype, monotype and electropherotype. J. Paediatr. Child. Health *28*:54–57, 1992.
11. Bass, D. M., Baylor, M. R., Chen, C., et al.: Liposome-mediated transfection of intact viral particles reveals that plasma membrane penetration determines permissivity of tissue culture cells to rotavirus. J. Clin. Invest. *90*:2313–2320, 1992.
12. Bass, D. M., and Greenberg, H. B.: Strategies for the identification of icosahedral virus receptors. J. Clin. Invest. *89*:3–9, 1992.
13. Bass, D. M., Mackow, E. R., and Greenberg, H. B.: Identification and partial characterization of a rhesus rotavirus binding glycoprotein on murine enterocytes. Virology *183*:602–610, 1991.
14. Beattie, R. M., Vieira, M. C., Phillips, A. D., et al.: Carbohydrate intolerance after rotavirus gastroenteritis: A rare problem in the 1990's. Arch. Dis. Child. *72*:446, 1995.
15. Bell, L. M., Clark, H. F., O'Brien, E. A., et al.: Gastroenteritis caused by human rotaviruses (serotype three) in a suckling mouse model. Proc. Soc. Exp. Biol. Med. *184*:127–132, 1987.
16. Bergmann, C. C., Maass, D., Poruchynsky, M. S., et al.: Topology of the non-structural rotavirus receptor glycoprotein NS28 in the rough endoplasmic reticulum. EMBO J. *8*:1695–1703, 1989.
17. Bern, C., Unicomb, L., Gentsch, J. R., et al.: Rotavirus diarrhea in Bangladeshi children: Correlation of disease severity with serotypes. J. Clin. Microbiol. *30*:3234–3238, 1992.
18. Bernstein, D. I., Glass R., Rodgers, G., et al.: Evaluation of rhesus rotavirus monovalent and tetravalent reassortant vaccines in U.S. children. J. A. M. A. *273*:1191–1196, 1995.
19. Bernstein, D. I., Kacica, M. A., McNeal, M. M., et al.: Local and systemic antibody response to rotavirus WC3 vaccine in adult volunteers. Antiviral Res. *12*:293–300, 1989.
20. Bernstein, D. I., McNeal, M. M., Schiff, G. M., et al.: Induction and persistence of local anti-rotavirus antibody in relation to serum antibodies. J. Med. Virol. *28*:90–95, 1989.
21. Bernstein, D. I., Sander, D. S., Smith, V., et al.: Protection from rotavirus reinfection: Two-year prospective study. J. Infect. Dis. *164*:277–283, 1991.
22. Bernstein, D. I., Smith, V., Sander, D., et al.: Evaluation of WC3 rotavirus vaccine and correlates of protection in healthy infants. J. Infect. Dis. *162*:1055–1062, 1990.
23. Bhan, M. K., Lew, J. F., Sazawal, S., et al.: Protection conferred by neonatal rotavirus infection against subsequent rotavirus diarrhea. J. Infect. Dis. *168*:282–287, 1993.
24. Birch, C. J., Rodgers, S. M., Marshall, J. A., et al.: Replication of human rotavirus in cell culture. J. Med. Virol. *11*:241–250, 1983.
25. Bishop, R. F.: Development of candidate rotavirus vaccines. Vaccine *11*:247–254, 1993.
26. Bishop, R., Barnes, G., Cipriani, E., et al.: Clinical immunity after neonatal rotavirus infection: A prospective longitudinal study in young children. N. Engl. J. Med. *309*:72–76, 1983.
27. Bishop, R. F., Cameron, D. J. S., Veenstra, A. A., et al.: Diarrhea and rotavirus infection associated with differing regimens of postnatal care of newborn babies. J. Clin. Microbiol. *9*:525–529, 1979.
28. Bishop, R. F., Davidson, G. P., Holmes, I. H., et al.: Virus particles in epithelial cells of duodenal mucosa from children with acute gastroenteritis. Lancet *2*:1281–1283, 1973.
29. Bishop, R. F., Davidson, G. P., Holmes, I. H., et al.: Detection of a new virus by electron microsocpy of faecal extracts from children with acute gastroenteritis. Lancet *1*:149–151, 1974.
30. Bishop, R. F., Hewstone, A. S., Davidson, G. P., et al.: An epidemic

of diarrheoa in human neonates involving a reovirus-like agent and "enteropathogenic" serotypes of *Escherichia coli*. J. Clin. Pathol. *29*:46–49, 1976.
31. Black, R., Greenberg, H., Kapikian, A., et al.: Acquisition of serum antibody to Norwalk virus and rotavirus in relation to diarrhea in a longitudinal study of young children in rural Bangladesh. J. Infect. Dis. *145*:483–489, 1982.
32. Black, R. E., Merson, M. H., Huq, I., et al.: Incidence and severity of rotavirus and *Escherichia coli* diarrhoea in rural Bangladesh: Implications for vaccine development. Lancet *1*:141–143, 1981.
33. Both, G. W., Bellamy, A. R., and Mitchell, D. B.: Rotavirus protein structure and function. Curr. Top. Microbiol. Immunol. *185*:67–105, 1994.
34. Both, G. W., Siegman, L. J., Bellamy, A. R., et al.: Coding assignment and nucleotide sequence of simian rotavirus SA11 gene segment 10: Location of glycosylation sites suggests that the signal peptide is not cleaved. J. Virol. *48*:335–339, 1983.
35. Brandt, C. D., Kim, H. W., Rodriguez, W. J., et al.: Gastroenteritis—a human reovirus-like agent infection during the 1975–76 outbreak: An electron microscopic study. Clin. Proc. Child. Hosp. *33*:21–26, 1977.
36. Bridger, J. C.: Detection by electron microscopy of caliciviruses, astroviruses and rotavirus-like particles in the faeces of piglets with diarrhoea. Vet. Rec. *107*:532, 1980.
37. Bridger, J. C.: Novel rotaviruses in animals and man. Ciba Found. Symp. *128*:5–23, 1987.
38. Bridger, J. C.: A definition of bovine rotavirus virulence. J. Gen. Virol. *75*:2807–2812, 1994.
39. Bridger, J. C., and Brown, J.F.: Development of immunity to porcine rotavirus in piglets protected from disease by bovine colostrum. Infect. Immun. *31*:906–910, 1981.
40. Bridger, J. C., Burke, B., Beards, G. M., et al.: The pathogenicity of two porcine rotaviruses differing in their in vitro growth characteristics and gene 4. J. Gen. Virol. *73*:3011–3015, 1992.
41. Bridger, J. C., Hall, G. A., and Parsons, K. R.: A study of the basis of virulence variation of bovine rotaviruses. Vet. Microbiol. *33*:169–174, 1992.
42. Bridger, J., Oldham, G., Howard, C., et al.: In vivo depletion of CD8+ but not CD4+ or BOWC1+ lymphocytes increases primary rotavirus excretion in calves. Abstract. Fourth International Symposium of Double-Stranded RNA Viruses, Scottsdale, AZ, 1987, pp. S6–S7.
43. Bridger, J. C., and Woode, G. N.: Neonatal calf diarrhea: Identification of a reovirus-like (rotavirus)* agent in faeces by immunofluorescence and immune electron microscopy. Br. Vet. J. *131*:528–535, 1975.
44. Broome, R. L., Vo, P. T., Ward, R. L., et al.: Murine rotavirus genes encoding outer capsid proteins VP4 and VP7 are not major determinants of host range restriction and virulence. J. Virol. *67*:2448–2455, 1993.
45. Browning, G. F., Chalmers, R. M., Fitzgerald, T. A., et al.: Serological and genomic characterization of L338, a novel equine group A rotavirus G serotype. J. Gen. Virol. *72*:1059–1064, 1991.
46. Browning, G. F., Fitzgerald, T. A., Chalmers, R. M., et al.: A novel group A rotavirus G serotype: Serological and genomic characterization of equine isolate F123. J. Clin. Microbiol. *29*:2043–2046, 1991.
47. Browning, G. F., Snodgrass, D. R., Nakagomi, O., et al.: Human and bovine serotype G8 rotaviruses may be derived by reassortment. Arch. Virol. *125*:121–128, 1992.
48. Brüssow, H., Nakagomi, O., Minamoto, N., et al.: Rotavirus 993/83, isolated from calf feces, closely resembles an avian rotavirus. J. Gen. Virol. *73*:1873–1875, 1992.
49. Brussow, H., Offit, P., Gerna, G., et al.: Polypeptide specificity of antiviral serum antibodies in children naturally infected with human rotavirus. J. Virol. *64*:4130–4136, 1990.
50. Bryden, A. S., Davies, H. A., Hadley, R. E., et al.: Rotavirus enteritis in the west midlands during 1974. Lancet 2:241–243, 1975.
51. Burke, B., McCrae, M. A., Desselberger, U.: Sequence analysis of two porcine rotaviruses differing in growth in vitro and in pathogenicity: Distinct VP4 sequences and conservation of NS53, VP6 and VP7 genes. J. Gen. Virol. *75*:2205–2212, 1994.
52. Burns, J. W., Krishnaney, A. A., Vo, P. T., et al.: Analyses of homologous rotavirus infection in the mouse model. Virology *207*:143–153, 1995.
53. Butz, A. M., Fosarelli, P., Dick, J., et al.: Prevalence of rotavirus on high-risk fomites in daycare facilities. Pediatrics *92*:202–205, 1993.
54. Castrucci, G., Frigeri, F., Ferrari, M., et al.: The protection of newborn calves against experimental rotavirus infection by feeding mammary secretions from vaccinated cows. Microbiologica *11*:379–385, 1988.
55. Centers for Disease Control: Rotavirus surveillance: United States, 1989–1990. M. M. W. R. *40*:80–87, 1991.
56. Champosaur, H., Questiaux, E., Prevot, J., et al.: Rotavirus carriage asymptomatic infection and disease in the first two years of life. I. Virus shedding. J. Infect. Dis. *149*:667–674 1984.
57. Chan, W.-K., Au, K.-S., and Estes, M. K.: Topography of the simian rotavirus nonstructural glycoprotein (NS28) in the endoplasmic reticulum membrane. Virology *164*:435–442, 1988.
58. Chasey, D.: Different particle types in tissue culture and intestinal epithelium infected with rotavirus. J. Gen. Virol. *37*:443–451, 1977.
59. Chen, D., Burns, J. W., Estes, M. K., et al.: Phenotypes of rotavirus reassortants depend upon the recipient genetic background. Proc. Natl. Acad. Sci. U. S. A. *86*:3743–3747, 1989.
60. Chen, D., Zeng, C. Q.-Y., Wentz, M. J., et al.: Template-dependent, in vitro replication of rotavirus RNA. J. Virol. *68*:7030–7039, 1994.
61. Chiba, S., Nakata, S., Ukae, S., et al.: Virological and serological aspects of immune resistance to rotavirus gastroenteritis. Clin. Infect. Dis. *16*(Suppl. 2):S117–S121, 1993.
62. Chiba, S., Nakata, S., Urasawa, T., et al.: Protective effect of naturally acquired homotypic and heterotypic rotavirus antibodies. Lancet *1*:417–421, 1986.
63. Christy, C., Madore, P., Pichichero, M., et al.: Field trials of rhesus rotavirus vaccine in infants. Pediatr. Infect. Dis. J. *7*:645–650, 1988.
64. Chrystie, I. L., Booth, I. W., Kidd, A. H., et al.: Multiple faecal virus excretion in immunodeficiency. Lancet *1*:282, 1982.
65. Chrystie, I. L., Totterdel, B., Baker, M. J., et al.: Rotavirus infections in a maternity unit. Lancet *2*:79, 1975.
66. Chrystie, I. L., Totterdell, B. M., and Banatvala, J. E.: False positive rotazyme tests on faecal samples from babies. Lancet *2*:1028, 1983.
67. Clark, H., Borian, F., Bell, L., et al.: Protective effect of WC3 vaccine against rotavirus diarrhea in infants during a predominantly serotype 1 rotavirus season. J. Infect. Dis. *158*:570–587, 1988.
68. Clark, H. F., Borian, F. E., Modesto, K., et al.: Serotype 1 reassortant of bovine rotavirus WC3 strain, strain W179-9, induces a polytypic antibody response in infants. Vaccine *8*:327–332, 1990.
69. Clark, H. F., Borian, F. E., and Plotkin, S. A.: Immune protection of infants against rotavirus gastroenteritis by a serotype 1 reassortant of bovine rotavirus WC3. J. Infect. Dis. *161*:1099–1104, 1990.
70. Clark, H. F., Hoshino, Y., Bell, L. M., et al.: Rotavirus isolate WI61 representing a presumptive new human serotype. J. Clin. Microbiol. *25*:1757–1762, 1987.
71. Clark, H., White, C. J., Offit, P. A., et al.: Preliminary evaluation of safety and efficacy of quadrivalent human-bovine reassortant rotavirus vaccine (QHBRV). Pediatr. Res. *37*:172A, 1995.
72. Clark, J. D., Hill, S. M., and Phillips, A. D.: Investigation of hospital-acquired rotavirus gastroenteritis using RNA electrophoresis. J. Med. Virol. *26*:289–299, 1988.
73. Clark, S. M., Barnett, B. B., and Spendlove, R. S.: Production of high-titer bovine rotavirus with trypsin. J. Clin. Microbiol. *9*:413–417, 1979.
74. Clark, S. M., Roth, J. R., Clark, M. L., et al.: Trypsin enhancement of rotavirus infectivity: Mechanism of enhancement. J. Virol. *39*:816–822, 1981.
75. Clarke, M. L., Lockett, L. J., and Both, G. W.: Membrane binding and endoplasmic reticulum retention sequences of rotavirus VP7 are distinct: Role of carboxy-terminal and other residues in membrane binding. J. Virol. *69*:6473–6478, 1995.
76. Clemens, J. D., Ward, R. L., Rao, M. R., et al.: Seroepidemiologic evaluation of antibodies to rotavirus as correlates of the risk of clinically significant rotavirus diarrhea in rural Bangladesh. J. Infect. Dis. *165*:161–165, 1992.
77. Coelho, K. I. R., Bryden, A. S., Hall, C., et al.: Pathology of rotavirus infection in suckling mice: A study by conventional histology, immunofluorescence, ultrathin sections, and scanning electron microscopy. Ultrastruct. Pathol. *2*:59–69, 1981.
78. Cohen, J.: Ribonucleic acid polymerase activity associated with purified calf rotavirus. J. Gen. Virol. *36*:395–402, 1977.
79. Cohen, J., Laporte, J., Charpilienne, A., et al.: Activation of rotavirus RNA polymerase by calcium chelation. Arch. Virol. *60*:177–186, 1979.
80. Collins, J. E., Benfield, D. A., and Duimstra, J. R.: Comparative virulence of two porcine group-A rotavirus isolates in gnotobiotic pigs. Am. J. Vet. Res. *50*:827–835, 1989.
81. Collins, J., Starkey, W. G., Wallis, T. S., et al.: Intestinal enzyme profiles in normal and rotavirus-infected mice. J. Pediatr. Gastroenterol. Nutr. *7*:264–272, 1988.
82. Conner, M. E., Crawford, S. E., Barone, C., et al.: Rotavirus vaccine administered parenterally induces protective immunity. J. Virol. *67*:6633–6641, 1993.
83. Conner, M. E., Estes, M. K., and Graham, D. Y.: Rabbit model of rotavirus infection. J. Virol. *62*:1625–1633, 1988.
84. Conner, M., Gilger, M., Estes, M., et al.: Serologic and mucosal immune response to rotavirus infection in the rabbit model. J. Virol. *65*:2562–2571, 1991.
85. Conner, M. E., Matson, D. O., and Estes, M. K.: Rotavirus vaccines and vaccination potential. *In* Ramig, R. F. (ed.): Rotaviruses. Berlin/Heidelberg, Springer-Verlag, 1994, pp. 285–337.
86. Cook, S. M., Glass, R. I., LeBaron, C. W., et al.: Global seasonality of rotavirus infections. Bull. W. H. O. *68*:171–177, 1990.
87. Coulson, B. S.: Typing of human rotavirus VP4 by an enzyme immunoassay using monoclonal antibodies. J. Clin. Microbiol. *31*:1–8, 1993.
88. Coulson, B. S., Grimwood, K., Hudson, I. L., et al.: Role of coproantibody in clinical protection of children during reinfection with rotavirus. J. Clin. Microbiol. *30*:1678–1684, 1992.
89. Coulson, B. S., Grimwood, K., Masendycz, P. J., et al.: Comparison of rotavirus immunoglobulin A coproconversion with other indices of rotavirus infection in a longitudinal study in childhood. J. Clin. Microbiol. *28*:1367–1374, 1990.
90. Crawford, S. E., Labbé, M., Cohen, J., et al.: Characterization of virus-like

particles produced by the expression of rotavirus capsid proteins in insect cells. J. Virol. *68*:5945–5952, 1994.
91. Crouch, C. F., and Woode, G. N.: Serial studies of virus multiplication and intestinal damage in gnotobiotic piglets infected with rotavirus. J. Med. Microbiol. *11*:325–334, 1978.
92. Cubitt, W. D., and Holzel, H.: An outbreak of rotavirus infection in a long-stay ward of a geriatric hospital. J. Clin. Pathol. *33*:306–308, 1980.
93. Dagan, R., Bar-David, Y., Sarov, B., et al.: Rotavirus diarrhea in Jewish and Bedouin children in the Negev region of Israel: Epidemiology, clinical aspects and possible role of malnutrition in severity of illness. Pediatr. Infect. Dis. J. *9*:314–321, 1990.
94. Das, B. K., Gentsch, J. R., Cicirello, H. G., et al.: Characterization of rotavirus strains from newborns in New Delhi, India. J. Clin. Microbiol. *32*:1820–1822, 1994.
95. Das, B. K., Gentsch, J. R., Hoshino, Y., et al.: Characterization of the G serotype and genogroup of New Delhi newborn rotavirus strain 116E. Virology *197*:99–107, 1993.
96. Davidson, G. P., Bishop, R. F., Townley, R. R. W., et al.: Importance of a new virus in acute sporadic enteritis in children. Lancet *1*:242–245, 1975.
97. Davidson, G. P., Gall, D. G., Petric, M., et al.: Human rotavirus enteritis induced in conventional piglets: Intestinal structure and transport. J. Clin. Invest. *60*:1402–1409, 1977.
98. Davidson, G. P., Hogg, R., and Kirabakaran, C: Serum and intestinal immune response to rotavirus enteritis in children. Infect. Immun. *40*:447–452, 1983.
99. Davidson, G. P., Whyte, P. B. D., Daniels, E., et al.: Passive immunization of children with bovine colostrum containing antibodies to human rotavirus. Lancet *2*:709–712, 1989.
100. Dearlove, J., Latham, P., Dearlove, B., et al.: Clinical range of neonatal rotavirus gastroenteritis. Br. Med. J. *286*:1473–1475, 1983.
101. DeChamps, C., Laveran, H., Peigue-Lafeville, H., et al.: Sequential rotavirus infections: Characterization of serotypes and electropherotypes. Res. Virol. *142*:39–45, 1991.
102. DeMol, P., Zissis, G., Tubzler, J. P., et al.: Failure of live attenuated oral rotavirus vaccine. Lancet *2*:108, 1986.
103. Dennehy, P. H., Schutzbank, T. E., and Thorne, G. M.: Evaluation of an automated immunodiagnostic assay, VIDAS Rotavirus, for detection of rotavirus in fecal specimens. J. Clin. Microbiol. *32*:825–827, 1994.
104. De Zoysa, I., and Feachem, R. G.: Interventions for the control of diarrhoeal diseases among young children: Rotavirus and cholera immunization. Bull. W. H. O. *63*:569–583, 1985.
105. Dharakul, T., Labbe, M., Cohen, J., et al.: Immunization with baculovirus-expressed recombinant rotavirus proteins VP1, VP4, VP6 and VP7 induces $CD8^+$ T lymphocytes that mediate clearance of chronic rotavirus infection in SCID mice. J. Virol. *65*:5928–5932, 1991.
106. Dharakul, T., Rott, L., and Greenberg, H.: Recovery from chronic rotavirus infection in mice with severe combined immunodeficiency: Virus clearance mediated by adoptive transfer of immune $CD8^+$ T lymphocytes. J. Virol. *64*:4375–4382, 1990.
107. Dolan, K. T., Twist, E. M., Horton-Slight, P., et al.: Epidemiology of rotavirus electropherotypes determined by a simplified diagnostic technique with RNA analysis. J. Clin. Microbiol. *21*:753–758, 1985.
108. Dunn, S. J., Greenberg, H. B., Ward, R. L., et al.: Serotypic and genotypic characterization of human serotype 10 rotaviruses from asymptomatic neonates. J. Clin. Microbiol. *31*:165–169, 1993.
109. Ebina, T., Ohta, M., Kanamaru, Y., et al.: Passive immunizations of suckling mice and infants with bovine colostrum containing antibodies to human rotavirus. J. Med. Virol *38*:117–123, 1992.
110. Ebina, T., Sato, A., Umezu, K., et al.: Prevention of rotavirus infection by oral administration of cow colostrum containing antihuman rotavirus antibody. Med. Microbiol. Immunol. *174*:177–185, 1985.
111. Echeverria, P., Blacklow, N. R., Cukor, G. G., et al.: Rotavirus as a cause of severe gastroenteritis in adults. J. Clin. Microbiol. *18*:663–667, 1983.
112. Echeverria, P., Blacklow, N. R., and Smith, D. H.: Role of heat-labile toxigenic *Escherichia coli* and reovirus-like agent in diarrhoea in Boston children. Lancet *2*:1113–1116, 1975.
113. Echeverria, P., Ho, M. T., Blacklow, N. R., et al.: Relative importance of viruses and bacteria in the etiology of pediatric diarrhea in Taiwan. J. Infect. Dis. *136*:383–390, 1977.
114. Edelman, R., Klish, W. J., Middleton, P. J., et al.: Prospects for immunizing against rotavirus. *In* Committee on Issues and Priorities for New Vaccine Development (eds.): New Vaccine Development: Establishing Priorities. Vol. 1. Washington, D.C., National Academy Press, 1985, pp. 410–423.
115. Eiden, J., Losonsky, G. A., Johnson, J., et al.: Rotavirus RNA variation during chronic infection of immunocompromised children. Pediatr. Infect. Dis. *4*:632–637, 1985.
116. Ericson, B. L., Graham, D. Y., Mason, B. B., et al.: Identification, synthesis and modifications of simian rotavirus SA11 polypeptides in infected cells. J. Virol. *42*:825–839, 1982.
117. Esparza, J., and Gil, F.: A study on the ultrastructure of human rotavirus. Virology *91*:141–150, 1978.
118. Esparza, J., Gorziglia, M., Gil, F., et al.: Multiplication of human rotaviruses in cultured cells: An electron microscopic study. J. Gen. Virol. *47*:461–472, 1980.
119. Espejo, R. T., López, S., and Arias, C. F.: Structural polypeptides of simian rotavirus SA11 and the effect of trypsin. J. Virol. *37*:156–160, 1981.
120. Estes, M. K., and Cohen, J.: Rotavirus gene structure and function. Microbiol. Rev. *53*:410–449, 1989.
121. Estes, M. K., Graham, D. Y., and Mason, B. B.: Proteolytic enhancement of rotavirus infectivity: Molecular mechanisms. J. Virol. *39*:879–888, 1981.
122. Estes, M. K., Graham, D. Y., Smith, E. M., et al.: Rotavirus stability and inactivation. J. Gen. Virol. *43*:403–409, 1979.
123. Fang Z.-Y., Ye, Q., Ho, M.-S., et al.: Investigation of an outbreak of adult diarrhea rotavirus in China. J. Infect. Dis. *160*:948–953, 1989.
124. Feng, N., Burns, J. W., Bracy, L., et al.: Comparison of mucosal and systemic humoral immune responses and subsequent protection in mice orally inoculated with a homologous or a heterologous rotavirus. J. Virol. *68*:7766–7773, 1994.
125. Figueroa-Qunitanilla, D., Salazar-Lindo, E., Sack, R. B., et al.: A controlled trial of bismuth subsalicylate in infants with acute watery diarrheal disease. N. Engl. J. Med. *328*:1653–1658, 1993.
126. Flewett, T. H., Bryden, A. S., and Davies, H.: Virus particles in gastroenteritis. Lancet *2*:1497, 1973.
127. Flewett, T. H., Bryden, A. S., Davies, H., et al.: Relation between viruses from acute gastroenteritis of children and newborn calves. Lancet *2*:61–63, 1974.
128. Flores, J., Gonzalez, M., Perez, M., et al.: Protection against severe rotavirus diarrhoea by rhesus rotavirus vaccine in Venezuelan infants. Lancet *1*:882–884, 1987.
129. Flores, J., Green, K., Garcia, D., et al.: Dot hybridization assay for distinction of rotavirus serotypes. J. Clin. Microbiol. *27*:29–34, 1989.
130. Flores, J., Hoshino, Y., Boeggeman, E., et al.: Genetic relatedness among animal rotaviruses. Arch. Virol. *87*:273–285, 1986.
131. Flores, J., and Kapikian, A. Z.: Vaccines against rotavirus. *In* Woodrow, G. C., and Levine M. M. (eds.): New Generation Vaccines. New York/Basel, Marcel Dekker, 1990, pp. 765–788.
132. Flores, J., Midthun, K., Hoshino, Y., et al.: Conservation of the fourth gene among rotaviruses recovered from asymptomatic newborn infants and its possible role in attenuation. J. Virol. *60*:972–979, 1986.
133. Flores, J., Myslinski, J., Kalica, A. R., et al.: *In vitro* transcription of two human rotaviruses. J. Virol. *43*:1032–1037, 1982.
134. Flores, J., Perez-Schael, I., Blanco, M., et al.: Reactions to and antigenicity of two human-rhesus rotavirus reassortant vaccine candidates of serotypes 1 and 2 in Venezuelan infants. J. Clin. Microbiol. *27*:512–518, 1989.
135. Flores, J., Perez-Schael, I., Blanco, M., et al.: Comparison of reactogenicity and antigenicity of M37 rotavirus vaccine and rhesus-rotavirus-based quadrivalent vaccine. Lancet *2*:330–334, 1990.
136. Flores, J., Perez-Schael, I., Boeggeman, E., et al.: Genetic relatedness among human rotaviruses. J. Med. Virol. *17*:135–143, 1985.
137. Flores, J., Perez-Schael, I., Gonzalez, M., et al.: Protection against severe rotavirus diarrhoea by rhesus rotavirus vaccine in Venezuelan infants. Lancet *1*:882–884, 1987.
138. Flores, J., Perez, I., White, L., et al.: Genetic relatedness among human rotaviruses as determined by RNA hybridization. Infect. Immun. *37*:648–655, 1982.
139. Fonteyne, J., Zissis, G., and Lambert, J. P.: Recurrent rotavirus gastroenteritis. Lancet *1*:1983, 1978.
140. Franco, M. A., and Greenberg, H. B.: Role of B cells and cytotoxic T lymphocytes in clearance of and immunity to rotavirus infection in mice. J. Virol. *69*:7800–7806, 1995.
141. Friedman, M., Gaul, A., Sarov, B., et al.: Two sequential outbreaks of rotavirus gastroenteritis: Evidence of symptomatic and asymptomatic reinfection. J. Infect. Dis. *158*:814–822, 1988.
142. Fukudome, K., Yoshie, O., and Konno, T.: Comparison of human, simian, and bovine rotaviruses for requirement of sialic acid in hemagglutination and cell adsorption. Virology *172*:196–205, 1989.
143. Fukuhara, N., Yoshie, O., Kitaoka, S., et al.: Role of VP3 in human rotavirus internalization after target cell attachment via VP7. Virology *62*:2209–2218, 1988.
144. Gallegos, C. O., and Patton, J. T.: Characterization of rotavirus replication intermediates: A model for the assembly of single-shelled particles. Virology *172*:616–627, 1989.
145. Garbarg-Chenon, A., Bricout, F., and Nicolas, J. C.: Study of genetic reassortments between two human rotaviruses. Virology *139*:358–365, 1984.
146. Gentsch, J. R., Glass, R. I., Woods, P., et al.: Identification of group A rotavirus gene 4 types by polymerase chain reaction. J. Clin. Microbiol. *30*:1365–1373, 1992.
147. Gentsch, J. R., Ramachandran, M., Das, B. K., et al.: Review of G and P typing results from a global collection of strains: Implications for vaccine development. Abstract. Fifth Rotavirus Vaccine Workshop, Atlanta, October 16–17, 1995.
148. Georges-Courbot, M. C., Beraud, A. M., Beards, G. M., et al.: Subgroups, serotypes, and electropherotypes of rotavirus isolated from children in Bangui, Central African Republic. J. Clin. Microbiol. *26*:668–671, 1988.
149. Georges-Courbot, M., Monges, J., Beraud-Cassel, A., et al.: Prospective longitudinal study of rotavirus infections in children from birth to two years of age in Central Africa. Ann. Inst. Pasteur/Virol. *139*:421–428, 1988.
150. Georges-Courbot, M., Monges, J., Siopathis, M., et al.: Evaluation of the

efficacy of a low-passage bovine rotavirus (strain WC3) vaccine in children in Central Africa. Res. Virol. *142*:405–411, 1991.
151. Gerna, G., Sarasini, A., Di Matteo, A., et al.: Serotype 3 human rotavirus strains with subgroup I specificity. J. Clin. Microbiol. *28*:1342–1347, 1990.
152. Gerna, G., Saransini, A., Parea, M., et al.: Isolation and characterization of two distinct human rotavirus strains with G6 specificity. J. Clin. Microbiol. *30*:9–16, 1992.
153. Gerna, G., Sarasini, Z., Torsellini, M., et al.: Group- and type-specific serologic response in infants and children with primary rotavirus infections and gastroenteritis caused by a strain of known serotype. J. Infect. Dis. *161*:1105–1111, 1990.
154. Gerna, G., Sears, J., Hoshino, Y., et al.: Identification of a new VP4 serotype of human rotaviruses. Virology *200*:66–71, 1994.
155. Gerna, G., Steele, A. D., Hoshino, Y., et al.: A comparison of the VP7 gene sequences of human and bovine rotaviruses. J. Gen. Virol. *75*:1781–1784, 1994.
156. Gilchrist, M. J. R., Bretl, T. S., Moultney, et al.: Comparison of seven kits for detection of rotavirus in fecal specimens with a sensitive, specific enzyme immunoassay. Diagn. Microbiol. Infect. Dis. *8*:221–228, 1987.
157. Gilger, M. A., Matson, D. O., Conner, M. E., et al.: Extraintestinal rotavirus infections in children with immunodeficiency. J. Pediatr. *120*:912–917, 1992.
158. Glass, R. I., Gentsch, J. R., Smith, J. C.: Rotavirus vaccines: Success by reassortment? Science *265*:1389–1391, 1994.
159. Glass, R. I., Lew, J. F., Gangarosa, R. E., et al.: Estimates of morbidity and mortality rates for diarrheal diseases in American children. J. Pediatr. S27–S33, 1991.
160. Gombold, J. L., and Ramig, R. F.: Analysis of reassortment of genome segments in mice mixedly infected with rotaviruses SA11 and RRV. J. Virol. *57*:110–116, 1986.
161. Gorziglia, M., Hoshino, Y., Buckler-White, A., et al.: Conservation of amino acid sequence of VP8 and cleavage region of 84-kDa outer capsid protein among rotaviruses recovered from asymptomatic neonatal infection. Proc. Natl. Acad. Sci. U. S. A. *83*:7039–7043, 1986.
162. Gorziglia, M., Larralde, G., Kapikian, A. Z., et al.: Antigenic relationships among human rotaviruses as determined by outer capsid protein VP4. Proc. Natl. Acad. Sci. U. S. A. *87*:7155–7159, 1990.
163. Gouvea, V. S., Alencar, A. A., Barth, O. M., et al.: Diarrhoea in mice infected with a human rotavirus. J. Gen. Virol. *67*:577–581, 1986.
164. Gouvea, V., and Brantley, M.: Is rotavirus a population of reassortants? Trends Microbiol. *3*:159–162, 1995.
165. Gouvea, V., Ramirez, C., Li, B., et al.: Restriction endonuclease analysis of the VP7 genes of human and animal rotaviruses. J. Clin. Microbiol. *31*:917–923, 1993.
166. Gouvea, V., Santos, N., and Timenetsky, M. C.: VP4 typing of bovine and porcine group A rotaviruses by PCR. J. Clin. Microbiol. *32*:1333–1337, 1994.
167. Graham, A., Kudesia, G., Allen, A. M., et al.: Reassortment of human rotavirus possessing genome rearrangements with bovine rotavirus: Evidence of host cell selection. J. Gen. Virol. *68*:115–122, 1987.
168. Graham, D. Y., Sackman, J. W., and Estes, M. K.: Pathogenesis of rotavirus-induced diarrhea: Preliminary studies in miniature swine piglet. Dig. Dis. Sci. *29*:1028–1035, 1984.
169. Green, K. Y., and Kapikian, A. Z.: Identification of VP7 epitopes associated with protection against human rotavirus illness or shedding in volunteers. J. Virol. *66*:548–553, 1992.
170. Green, K. Y., Sarasini, A., Qian, Y., et al.: Genetic variation in rotavirus serotype 4 subtypes. Virology *188*:362–368, 1992.
171. Greenberg, H. B., Clark, H. F., and Offit, P. A.: Rotavirus pathology and pathophysiology. Curr. Top. Microbiol. Immunol. *185*:255–283, 1994.
172. Greenberg, H. B., Flores, J., Kalica, A. R., et al.: Gene coding assignments for growth restriction, neutralization and subgroup specificities of the W and DS-1 strains of human rotavirus. J. Gen. Virol. *64*:313–320, 1983.
173. Greenberg, H. B., McAuliffe, V., Valdesuso, J., et al.: Serological analysis of the subgroup protein of rotaviruses, using monoclonal antibodies. Infect. Immun. *39*:91–99, 1983.
174. Greenberg, H. B., Valdesuso, J., Van Wyke, K., et al.: Production and preliminary characterization of monoclonal antibodies directed at two surface proteins of rhesus rotavirus. J. Virol. *47*:267–275, 1983.
175. Greenberg, H. B., Vo, P. T., and Jones, R.: Cultivation and characterization of three strains of murine rotavirus. J. Virol. *57*:585–590, 1986.
176. Grillner, L., Broberger, U., Chrystie, I., et al.: Rotavirus infections in newborns: An epidemiological and clinical study. Scand. J. Infect. Dis. *17*:349–355, 1985.
177. Grimwood, K., Coakley, J. C., Hudson, I. L., et al.: Serum aspartate aminotransferase levels after rotavirus gastroenteritis. J. Pediatr. *112*:597–600, 1988.
178. Grimwood, K., Lund, J., Coulson, B., et al.: Comparison of serum and mucosal antibody responses following severe acute rotavirus gastroenteritis in young children. J. Clin. Microbiol. *26*:732–738, 1988.
179. Grinstein, S., Gomez, J., Bercovich, J., et al.: Epidemiology of rotavirus infection and gastroenteritis in prospectively monitored Argentine families with young children. Am. J. Epidemiol. *130*:300–308, 1989.
180. Grunow, J. E., Dunton, S. F., and Wanter, J. L.: Human rotavirus-like particle in a hepatic abscess. J. Pediatr. *106*:73–76, 1985.
181. Guarino, A., Canani, R. B., Russo, S., et al.: Oral immunoglobulins for treatment of acute rotaviral gastroenteritis. Pediatrics *93*:12–61, 1994.
182. Gurwith, M. J., and Williams, T. W.: Gastroenteritis in children: A two-year review in Manitoba. 1. Etiology. J. Infect. Dis. *136*:239–247, 1977.
183. Haffejee, I. E.: The pathophysiology, clinical features and management of rotavirus diarrhoea. Q. J. Med. *288*:289–299, 1991.
184. Haffejee, I. E.: Neonatal rotavirus infections. Rev. Infect. Dis. *13*:957–962, 1991.
185. Haffejee, I. E.: The epidemiology of rotavirus infections: A global perspective. J. Pediatr. Gastroent. Nutr. *20*:275–286, 1995.
186. Haffejee, I. E., and Moosa, A.: Rotavirus studies in Indian (Asian) South African infants with acute gastroenteritis. I. Microbiological and epidemiological aspects. Ann. Trop. Paediatr. *10*:165–172, 1990.
187. Haffejee, I. E., Moosa, A., and Windsor, I.: Circulating and breastmilk anti-rotaviral antibodies and neonatal rotavirus infections: A maternal-neonatal study. Ann. Trop. Paediatr. *10*:3–14, 1990.
188. Hall, G. A., Bridger, J. C., Parsons, K. R., et al.: Variation in rotavirus virulence: A comparison of pathogenesis in calves between two rotaviruses of different virulence. Vet. Pathol. *30*:223–233, 1993.
189. Halvorsrud, J., and Orstavik, I.: An epidemic of rotavirus-associated gastroenteritis in a nursing home for the elderly. Scand. J. Infect. Dis. *12*:161–164, 1980.
190. Hanlon, P., Marsh, V., Shenton, F., et al.: Trial of an attenuated bovine rotavirus vaccine (RIT 4237) in Gambian infants. Lancet *1*:1342–1345, 1987.
191. Hardy, M. E., Gorziglia, M., and Woode, G. N.: The outer capsid protein VP4 of equine rotavirus strain H-2 represents a unique VP4 type by amino acid analysis. Virology *193*:492–497, 1993.
192. Hasegawa, A., Matsuno, S., Inouye, S., et al.: Isolation of human rotaviruses in primary cultures of monkey kidney cells. J. Clin. Microbiol. *16*:387–390, 1982.
193. Hattori, H., Torii, S., Nagafuji, H., et al.: Benign acute myositis associated with rotavirus gastroenteritis. J. Pediatr. *121*:748–749, 1992.
194. Helmberger-Jones, M., and Patton, J. T.: Characterization of subviral particles in cells infected with simian rotavirus SA11. Virology *155*:655–665, 1986.
195. Heyman, M., Corthier, G., Petit, A., et al.: Intestinal absorption of macromolecules during viral enteritis: An experimental study on rotavirus-infected conventional and germ-free mice. Pediatr. Res. *22*:72–78, 1987.
196. Hilpert, H., Brussow, H., Mietens, C., et al.: Use of bovine milk concentrate containing antibody to rotavirus to treat rotavirus gastroenteritis in infants. J. Infect. Dis. *156*:158–166, 1987.
197. Hjelt, K., Graubelle, P. C., Paerregaard, A., et al.: Protective effect of preexisting rotavirus-specific immunoglobulin against naturally acquired rotavirus infection in children. J. Med. Virol. *21*:39–47, 1987.
198. Ho, M.-S., Glass, R. I., Pinsky, P. F., et al.: Rotavirus as a cause of diarrheal morbidity and mortality in the United States. J. Infect. Dis. *158*:1112–1116, 1988.
199. Ho, M.-S., Glass, R. I., Pinsky, P. F., et al.: Diarrheal deaths in American children. Are they preventable? J. A. M. A. *260*:3281–3285, 1988.
200. Holmes, I. H., Ruck, B. J., Bishop, R. F., et al.: Infantile enteritis viruses: Morphogenesis and morphology. J. Virol. *16*:937–943, 1975.
201. Hoshino, Y., and Kapikian, A. Z.: Rotavirus vaccine development for prevention of severe diarrhea in infants and young children. Trends Microbiol. *2*:242–249, 1994.
202. Hoshino, Y., Saif, L. J., Kang, S.-Y., et al.: Identification of group A rotavirus genes associated with virulence of a porcine rotavirus and host range restriction of a human rotavirus in the gnotobiotic piglet model. Virology *209*:274–280, 1995.
203. Hoshino, Y., Saif, L., Sereno, M., et al.: Infection immunity of piglets to either VP3 or VP7 outer capsid protein confers resistance to challenge with a virulent rotavirus bearing the corresponding antigen. J. Virol. *62*:744–748, 1988.
204. Hoshino, Y., Sereno, M. M., Midthun, K., et al.: Independent segregation of two antigenic specificities (VP3 and VP7) involved in neutralization of rotavirus infectivity. Proc. Natl. Acad. Sci. U. S. A. *82*:8701–8704, 1985.
205. Hoshino, Y., Wyatt, R. G., Greenberg, H. B., et al.: Serotypic similarity and diversity of rotaviruses of mammalian and avian origin as studied by plaque-reduction neutralization. J. Infect. Dis. *149*:694–702, 1984.
206. Hrdy, D. B.: Epidemiology of rotaviral infection in adults. Rev. Infect. Dis. *9*:461–469, 1987.
207. Hua, J., Chen, X., and Patton, J. T.: Deletion mapping of the rotavirus metalloprotein NS53 (NSP1): The conserved cysteine-rich region is essential for virus–specific RNA binding. J. Virol. *68*:3990–4000, 1994.
208. Huang, J., Nagesha, H. S., and Holmes, I. H.: Comparative sequence analysis of VP4s from five Australian porcine rotaviruses: Implication of an apparent new P type. Virology *196*:319–327, 1993.
209. Huicho, L., Sanchez, D., Contreras, M., et al.: Occult blood and fecal leukocytes as screening tests in childhood infectious diarrhea: An old problem revisited. Pediatr. Infect. Dis. J. *12*:474–477, 1993.
210. Hung, T.: Rotavirus and adullt diarrhea. Adv. Virus Res. *35*:193–218, 1988.
211. Hung, T., Chen, G., Wang, C., et al.: Waterborne outbreak of rotavirus diarrhoea in adults in China caused by a novel rotavirus. Lancet *2*:1139–1142, 1984.
212. Ijaz, M. K., Sabara, M. I., Frenchick, P. J., et al.: Assessment of intestinal

damage in rotavirus infected neonatal mice by a D-xylose absorption test. J. Virol. Methods *18*:153–157, 1987.
213. Institute of Medicine: Prospects for immunizing against rotavirus. *In* New Vaccine Development: Establishing Priorities: Diseases of Importance in Developing Countries. Vol. 2. Washington, D.C., National Academy Press, 1986, pp. 308–318.
214. Isa, P., and Snodgrass, D. R.: Serological and genomic characterization of equine rotavirus VP4 proteins identifies three different P serotypes. Virology *201*:364–372, 1994.
215. Jarvis, W. R., Middleton, P. J., and Gelfand, E. W.: Significance of viral infections in severe combined immunodeficiency disease. Pediatr. Infect. Dis. 2:187–192, 1983.
216. Jiang, B., Dennehy, P. H., Spangenberger, S., et al.: First detection of group C rotavirus in fecal specimens of children with diarrhea in the United States. J. Infect. Dis. *172*:45–50, 1995.
217. Jones, P. D., Roddick, L. G., and Wilkinson, I. A.: Rotavirus and seizures. Med. J. Austr. *162*:223, 1995.
218. Kalica, A. R., Garon, C. F., Wyatt, R. G., et al.: Differentiation of human and calf reovirus-like agents associated with diarrhea using polyacrylamide gel electrophoresis of RNA. Virology *74*:86–92, 1976.
219. Kalica, A. R., Greenberg, H. B., Espejo, R. T., et al.: Distinctive ribonucleic acid patterns of human rotavirus subgroups 1 and 2. Infect. Immun. *33*:958–961, 1981.
220. Kalica, A. R., Greenberg, H. B., Wyatt, R. G., et al.: Genes of human (strain Wa) and bovine (strain UK) rotavirus that code for neutralization and subgroup antigens. Virology *112*:385–390, 1981.
221. Kaljot, T. K., Shaw, R. D., Rubin, D. H., et al.: Infectious rotavirus enters cells by direct cell membrane penetration, not by endocytosis. J. Virol. *62*:1136–1144, 1988.
222. Kanfer, E. J., Abrahamson, G., Taylor, J., et al.: Severe rotavirus-associated diarrhoea following bone marrow transplantation: Treatment with oral immunoglobulin. Bone Marrow Transpl. *14*:651–652, 1994.
223. Kapikian, A. Z.: Viral gastroenteritis. J. A. M. A. *269*:627–630, 1993.
224. Kapikian, A.Z., and Chanock, R. M.: Rotaviruses. *In* Fields, B. N., Knipe, D. M., Chanock, R. M., et al. (eds.): Virology. Vol. 2. 2nd ed. New York, Raven Press, 1990, pp. 1353–1404.
225. Kapikian, A. Z., Cline, W. L., Greenberg, H. B., et al.: Antigenic characterization of human and animal rotaviruses by immune adherence hemagglutination assay (IAHA): Evidence for distinctness of IAHA and neutralization antigens. Infect. Immun. *33*:415–425, 1981.
226. Kapikian, A. Z., Cline, W. L., Kim, H. W., et al.: Antigenic relationships among five reovirus-like (RVL) agents by complement fixation (CF) and development of new substitute CF antigens for the human RVL agent of infantile gastroenteritis. Proc. Soc. Exp. Biol. Med. *152*:535–539, 1976.
227. Kapikian, A. Z., Flores, J., Hoshino, Y., et al.: Rotavirus: The major etiologic agent of severe infantile diarrhea may be controllable by a "Jennerian" approach to vaccination. J. Infect. Dis. *153*:815–822, 1986.
228. Kapikian, A. Z., Kim, H. W., Wyatt, R. G., et al.: Reovirus-like agent in stools: Association with infantile diarrhea and development of serologic tests. Science *185*:1049–1053, 1974.
229. Kapikian, A. Z., Kim, H. W., Wyatt, R. G., et al.: Human reovirus-like agent as the major pathogen associated with "winter" gastroenteritis in hospitalized infants and young children. N. Engl. J. Med. *294*:965–972, 1976.
230. Kapikian, A. Z., Wyatt, R. G., Levine, M. M., et al.: Oral administration of human rotavirus to volunteers: Induction of illness and correlates of resistance. J. Infect. Dis. *147*:95–106, 1983.
231. Kapikian, A. Z., Wyatt, R. G., Levine, M. M., et al.: Studies in volunteers with human rotaviruses. International Symposium Enteric Infections in Man and Animals: Standardization of Immunological Procedures, Dublin, Ireland, 1982, Dev. Biol. Standard. Basel, S. Karger, 1983, pp. 209–218.
232. Kasempimolporn, S., Louisirirotchanakul, S., Sinarachatanant, P., et al.: Polyacrylamide gel electrophoresis and silver staining for detection of rotavirus in stools from diarrheic patients in Thailand. J. Clin. Microbiol. *26*:158–160, 1988.
233. Kattoura, M. D., Chen, Z., and Patton, J. T.: The rotavirus RNA-binding protein NS35 (NSP2) forms 10S multimers and interacts with the viral RNA polymerase. Virology *202*:803–813, 1994.
234. Keidan, I., Shif, I., Keren, G., et al.: Rotavirus encephalopathy: Evidence of central nervous system involvement during rotavirus infection. Pediatr. Infect. Dis. J. *11*:773–775, 1992.
235. Keljo, D. J., and Smith, A. K.: Characterization of binding of simian rotavirus SA-11 to cultured epithelial cells. J. Pediatr. Gastroent. Nutr. *7*:257–263, 1988.
236. Keller, K. M., Schmidt, H., Wirth, S., et al.: Differences in the clinical and radiologic patterns of rotavirus and non-rotavirus necrotizing enterocolitis. Pediatr. Infect. Dis. J. *10*:734–738, 1991.
237. Keswick, B. H., Pickering, L. K., Dupont, H. L., et al.: Survival and detection of rotaviruses on environmental surfaces in day care centers. Appl. Environ. Microbiol. *46*:813–816, 1983.
238. Khoshoo, V., Bhan, M. K., Jayashree, S., et al.: Rotavirus infection and persistent diarrhea in young children. Lancet 2:1314–1315, 1990.
239. Kim, H. W., Brandt, C. D., Kapikian, A. Z., et al.: Human reovirus-like agent infection: Occurrence in adult contacts of pediatric patients with gastroenteritis. J. A. M. A. *238*:404–407, 1977.
240. Kirstein, C. G., Clare, D. A., and Lecce, J. G.: Development of resistance of enterocytes to rotavirus in neonatal agammaglobulinemic piglets. J. Virol. *55*:567–573, 1985.
241. Knowlton, D. R., Spector, D. M., and Ward, R. L.: Development of an improved method for measuring neutralizing antibody to rotavirus. J. Virol. Methods *33*:127–134, 1991.
242. Kogasaka, R., Akihara, M., Horino, K., et al.: A morphological study of human rotavirus. Arch. Virol. *61*:41–48, 1979.
243. Kohli, E., Pothier, P., Denis, F., et al.: Multicentre evaluation of a new commercial latex agglutination test using a monoclonal antibody for rotavirus detection. Eur. J. Clin. Microbiol. Infect. Dis. *8*:251–253, 1989.
244. Konno, T., Suzuki, H., Imai, A., et al.: Reovirus-like agent in acute epidemic gastroenteritis in Japanese infants: Fecal shedding and serologic response. J. Infect. Dis. *135*:259–266, 1977.
245. Konno, T., Suzuki, H., Kutsuzawa, T., et al.: Human rotavirus and intussusception. N. Engl. J. Med. *297*:945, 1977.
246. Koopman, J. S., and Monto, A. S.: The Tecumseh Study. XV. Rotavirus infection and pathogenicity. Am. J. Epidemiol. *130*:750–759, 1989.
247. Kovacs, A., Chan, L., Hotrakitya, C., et al.: Serum transaminase elevations in infants with rotavirus gastroenteritis. J. Pediatr. Gastroenterol. Nutr. *5*:873–877, 1986.
248. Kovacs, A., Chan, L., Hotrakitya, C., et al.: Rotavirus gastroenteritis. Am. J. Dis. Child. *141*:161–166, 1987.
249. Kubelka, C. F., Marchevsky, R. S., Stephens, P. R. S., et al.: Murine experimental infection with rotavirus SA-11: Clinical and immunohistological characteristics. Exp. Toxic Pathol. *45*:433–438, 1993.
250. Kutsuzawa, T., Konno, T., Suzuki, H., et al.: Two distinct electrophoretic migration patterns of RNA segments of human rotaviruses prevalent in Japan in relation to their serotypes. Microbiol. Immunol. *26*:271–273, 1982.
251. Labbé, M., Baudoux, P., Charpilienne, A., et al.: Identification of the nucleic acid binding domain of the rotavirus VP2 protein. J. Gen. Virol. *75*:3423–3430, 1994.
252. Lanata, C., Black, R., Del Aguila, R., et al.: Protection of Peruvian children against rotavirus diarrhea of specific serotypes by one, two or three doses of the RIT 4237 attenuated bovine rotavirus vaccine. J. Infect. Dis. *159*:452–459, 1989.
253. Larralde, G., and Flores, J.: Identification of gene alleles among human rotaviruses by polymerase chain reaction derived probes. Virology *179*:469–473, 1990.
254. LeBaron, C. W., Lew, J., Glass, R. I., et al.: Annual rotavirus epidemic patterns in North America. J. A. M. A. *264*:983–988, 1990.
255. Lebenthal, E., and Lee, P. C.: Development of functional response in human exocrine pancreas. Pediatrics *66*:556–560, 1980.
256. Leece, J. G., and King, M. W.: Role of rotavirus (reo-like) in weanling diarrhea of pigs. J. Clin. Microbiol. *8*:454–458, 1978.
257. Leece, J. G., King, M. W., and Mock, R.: Reovirus-like agent associated with fatal diarrhea in neonatal pigs. Infect. Immun. *14*:816–825, 1976.
258. Leece, J. G., Leary, H. L., Jr., Clare, D. A., et al.: Protection of agammaglobulinemic piglets from porcine rotavirus infection by antibody against simian rotavirus SA-11. J. Clin. Microbiol. *29*:1382–1386, 1991.
259. Lewis, H. M., Parry, J. V., Davies, H. A., et al.: A year's experience of the rotavirus syndrome and its association with respiratory illness. Arch. Dis. Child. *54*:339–346, 1979.
260. Li, B., Larralde, G., and Gorziglia, M.: Human rotavirus K8 strain represents a new VP4 serotype. J. Virol. *67*:617–620, 1993.
261. Linares, A., Gabbay, Y., Mascarenhas, J., et al.: Epidemiology of rotavirus subgroups and serotypes in Belem, Brazil: A three-year study. Ann. Inst. Pasteur/Virol. *139*:89–99, 1988.
262. Little, L. M., and Shadduck, J. A.: Pathogenesis of rotavirus infection in mice. Infect. Immun. *38*:755–763, 1982.
263. Little, L. M., and Shadduck, J. A.: Pathogenesis of rotavirus infections. Prog. Food Nutr. Sci. *7*:179–187, 1983.
264. Liu, M., Mattion, N. M., and Estes, M. K.: Rotavirus VP3 expressed in insect cells possesses guanylyltransferase activity. Virology *188*:77–84, 1992.
265. López, S., Arias, C. F., Bell, J. R., et al.: Primary structure of the cleavage site associated with trypsin enhancement of rotavirus SA11 infectivity. Virology *144*:11–19, 1985.
266. Losonsky, G. A., Johnson, G. P., Winkelstein, J. A., et al.: The oral administration of human serum immunoglobulin in immunodeficiency patients with viral gastroenteritis: A pharmacokinetic and functional analysis. J. Clin. Invest. *76*:2362–2367, 1985.
267. Losonsky, G. A., Rennels, M. B., Kapikian, A. Z., et al.: Safety, infectivity transmissibility, and immunogenicity of rhesus rotavirus vaccine (MMU 18006) in infants. Pediatr. Infect. Dis. *5*:25, 1986.
268. Losonsky, G., Vonderfecht, S., Eiden, J., et al.: Homotypic and heterotypic antibodies for prevention of experimental rotavirus gastroenteritis. J. Clin. Microbiol. *24*:1041–1044, 1986.
269. Ludert, J. E., Michalangeli, F., Gil, F., et al.: Penetration and uncoating of rotaviruses in cultured cells. Intervirology *27*:95–101, 1987.
270. Maass, D. R., and Atkinson, P. H.: Rotavirus proteins VP7, NS28, and VP4 form oligomeric structures. J. Virol. *64*:2632–2641, 1990.
271. Maass, D. R., and Atkinson, P. H.: Retention by the endoplasmic reticulum of rotavirus VP7 is controlled by three adjacent amino-terminal residues. J. Virol. *68*:366–378, 1994.

272. Mackow, E. R., Shaw, R. D, Matsui, S. M., et al.: The rhesus rotavirus gene encoding VP3: Location of amino acids involved in homologous and heterologous rotavirus neutralization and identification of a putative fusion region. Proc. Natl. Acad. Sci. U. S. A. *85*:645–649, 1988.
273. Madore, H., Christy, C., Pichichero, M., et al.: Field trial of rhesus rotavirus or human-rhesus rotavirus reassortant vaccine of VP7 serotype 3 or 1 specificity in infants. J. Infect. Dis. *166*:235–243, 1992.
274. Malherbe, H. H., Harwin, R., and Ulrich, M.: The cytopathic effect of vervet monkey viruses. S. Afr. Med. J. *37*:407–411, 1963.
275. Mansell, E. A., and Patton, J. T.: Rotavirus RNA replication: VP2, but not VP6, is necessary for viral replicase activity. J. Virol. *64*:4988–4996, 1990.
276. Marrie, T. J., Lee, S. H. S., Faulkner, R. S., et al.: Rotavirus infection in a geriatric population. Arch. Intern. Med. *142*:313–316, 1982.
277. Martin, M. L., Palmer, E. L., and Middleton, P. J.: Ultrastructure of infantile gastroenteritis virus. Virology *68*:146–153, 1975.
278. Mason, B. B., Graham, D. Y., and Estes, M. K.: In vitro transcription and translation of simian rotavirus SA11 gene products. J. Virol. *33*:1111–1121, 1980.
279. Mata, L., Simhon, A., Urrutia, J. J., et al.: Epidemiology of rotavirus in a cohort of 45 Guatemalan Mayan Indian children observed from birth to the age of three years. J. Infect. Dis. *148*:452–461, 1980.
280. Matson, D. O., and Estes, M. K.: Impact of rotavirus infection at a large pediatric hospital. J. Infect. Dis. *162*:598–604, 1990.
281. Matson, D. O., O'Ryan, M. L., Herrera, I., et al.: Fecal antibody responses to symptomatic and asymptomatic rotavirus infections. J. Infect. Dis. *167*:577–583, 1993.
282. Matsui, S., Offit, P., Vo, P., et al.: Passive protection against rotavirus-induced diarrhea by monoclonal antibodies to the heterotypic neutralization domain of VP7 and the VP8 fragment of VP4. J. Clin. Microbiol. *27*:780–782, 1989.
283. Matsumoto, K., Hatano, M., Kobayashi, K., et al.: An outbreak of gastroenteritis associated with acute rotaviral infection in school children. J. Infect. Dis. *160*:611–615, 1989.
284. Matsuno, S., Utagawa, E., and Sugiura, A.: Association of rotavirus infection with Kawasaki syndrome. J. Infect. Dis. *148*:177, 1983.
285. Matthews, R. E. F.: The classification and nomenclature of viruses: Summary of results of meetings of The International Committee on Taxonomy of Viruses in The Hague, September, 1978. Intervirology *11*:133, 135.
286. Mavrovichalis, J., Evans, N., McNeish, A. S., et al.: Intestinal damage in rotavirus and adenovirus gastroenteritis assessed by D-xylose malabsorption. Arch. Dis. Child. *52*:589–591, 1977.
287. McCrae, M. A.: Nucleic acid-based analysis of non-group A rotaviruses. Ciba Found. Symp. *128*:24–48, 1987.
288. McCrae, M. A., and Faulkner-Valle, G. P.: Molecular biology of rotaviruses. J. Virol. *39*:490–496, 1981.
289. McLean, B., Sonza, S., and Holmes, I. H.: Measurement of immunoglobulin A, G and M class rotavirus antibodies in serum and mucosal secretions. J. Clin. Microbiol. *12*:314–319, 1980.
290. McNeal, M. M., Barone, K. S., Rae, M. N., et al.: Effector functions of antibody and $CD8^+$ cells in resolution of rotavirus infection and protection against reinfection in mice. Virology *214*:387–397, 1995.
291. McNeal, M. M., Broome, R. L., and Ward, R. L.: Active immunity against rotavirus infection in mice is correlated with viral replication and titers of serum rotavirus IgA following vaccination. Virology *204*:642–650, 1994.
292. McNeal, M., Sheridan, J., and Ward, R.: Active protection against rotavirus infection of mice following intraperitoneal immunization. Virology *191*:150–157, 1992.
293. McNeal, M. M., and Ward, R. L.: Long-term production of rotavirus antibody and protection against reinfection following a single infection of neonatal mice with murine rotavirus. Virology *211*:474–480, 1995.
294. McNulty, M. S., Todd, D., Allan, G. M., et al.: Epidemiology of rotavirus infection in broiler chickens: Recognition of four serogroups. Arch. Virol. *81*:113–121, 1984.
295. Mebus, C. A.: Reovirus-like calf enteritis. Dig. Dis. *21*:592–598, 1976.
296. Mebus, C. A., Stair, E. L., Underdahl, N. R., et al.: Pathology of neonatal calf diarrhea induced by a reo-like virus. Vet. Pathol. *8*:490–505, 1974.
297. Mebus, C. A., Underdahl, N. R., Rhodes, M. B., et al.: Calf diarrhea (scours): Reproduced with a virus from a field outbreak. Univ. Nebraska Res. Bull. *233*:1–16, 1969.
298. Mebus, C. A., Wyatt, R. G., and Kapikian, A. Z.: Intestinal lesions induced in gnotobiotic calves by the virus of human infantile gastroenteritis. Vet. Pathol. *14*:273–282, 1977.
299. Méndez, E., Arias, C. F., and López, S.: Binding to sialic acids is not an essential step for the entry of animal rotaviruses to epithelial cells in culture. J. Virol. *67*:5253–5259, 1993.
300. Meyer, J. C., Bergmann, C. C., and Bellamy, A. R.: Interaction of rotavirus cores with the nonstructural glycoprotein NS28. Virology *171*:98–107, 1989.
301. Middleton, P. J., Holdaway, M. D., Petric, M., et al.: Solid-phase radioimmunoassay for the detection of rotavirus. Infect. Immun. *16*:439–444, 1977.
302. Middleton, P. J., Szymanski, M. T., Abbott, G. D., et al.: Orbivirus acute gastroenteritis of infancy. Lancet *1*:1241–1244, 1974.
303. Midthun, K., Greenberg, H., Hoshino, Y., et al.: Reassortant rotaviruses as potential live rotavirus vaccine candidates. J. Virol. *53*:949–954, 1985.
304. Midthun, K., Halsey, N. A., Jett-Goheen, M., et al.: Safety and immunogenicity of human rotavirus vaccine strain M37 in adults, children, and infants. J. Infect. Dis. *164*:792–796, 1991.
305. Midthun, K., Hoshino, Y., Kapikian, A., et al.: Single gene substitution rotavirus reassortants containing the major neutralization protein (VP7) of human rotavirus serotype 4. J. Clin. Microbiol. *24*:822–826, 1986.
306. Midthun, K., Pang, L., Flores, J., et al.: Comparison of immunoglobulin A (IgA), IgG, and IgM enzyme-linked immunosorbent assays, plaque-reduction neutralization assay, and complement fixation in detecting seroresponses to rotavirus vaccine candidates. J. Clin. Microbiol. *27*:2799–2804, 1989.
307. Moe, K., and Shirley, J. A.: The effect of relative humidity and temperature on the survival of human rotavirus in faeces. Arch. Virol. *72*:179–186, 1982.
308. Morita, Y., Taniguchi, K., Urasawa, T., et al.: Analysis of serotype-specific neutralization epitopes on VP7 of human rotavirus by the use of neutralizing monoclonal antibodies and antigenic variants. J. Gen. Virol. *69*:451–458, 1988.
309. Mphahlele, M. J., and Steele, A. D.: Relative frequency of human rotavirus VP4 (P) genotypes recovered over a ten-year period from South African children with diarrhea. J. Med. Virol. *47*:1–5, 1995.
310. Mulcahy, D. L., Kamath, K. R., de Silva, L. M., et al.: A two-part study of the aetiological role of rotavirus in intussusception. J. Med. Virol. *9*:51–55, 1982.
311. Murphy, A. M., Albrey, M. B., and Hay, P. J.: Rotavirus infections in neonates. Lancet *2*:452–453, 1975.
312. Nakagomi, O., Isegawa, Y., Ward, R. L., et al.: Naturally occurring dual infection with human and bovine rotaviruses as suggested by the recovery of G1P8 and G1P5 rotaviruses from a single patient. Arch. Virol. *137*:381–388, 1994.
313. Nakagomi, O., Kaga, E., Gerna, G., et al.: Subgroup I serotype 3 human rotavirus strains with long RNA pattern as a result of naturally occurring reassortment between members of the bovine and AU-1 genogroups. Arch. Virol. *126*:337–342, 1992.
314. Nakagomi, O., Mochizuki, M., Aboudy, Y., et al.: Hemagglutination by a human rotavirus isolate as evidence for transmission of animal rotaviruses to humans. J. Clin. Microbiol. *30*:1011–1013, 1992.
315. Nakagomi, O., Oyamada, H., Kuroki, S., et al.: Molecular identification of a novel human rotavirus in relation to subgroup and electropherotype of genomic RNA. J. Med. Virol. *28*:163–168, 1989.
316. Nakagomi, O., and Nakagomi, T.: Molecular evidence for naturally occurring single VP7 gene substitution reassortant between human rotaviruses belonging to two different genogroups. Arch. Virol. *119*:67–81, 1991.
317. Nakagomi, O., and Nakagomi, T.: Genetic diversity and similarity among mammalian rotaviruses in relation to interspecies transmission of rotavirus. Arch. Virol. *120*:43–55, 1991.
318. Nakagomi, O., and Nakagomi, T.: Interspecies transmission of rotaviruses studied from the perspective of genogroup. Microbiol. Immunol. *37*:337–348, 1993.
319. Nakagomi, T., and Nakagomi, O.: RNA-RNA hybridization identifies a human rotavirus that is genetically related to feline rotavirus. J. Virol. *63*:1431–1434, 1989.
320. Nalin, D. R., Levine, M. M., Mata, L., et al.: Comparison of sucrose with glucose in oral therapy of infant diarrhea. Lancet *2*:277–279, 1978.
321. Nandi, P., Charpilienne, A., and Cohen, J.: Interaction of rotavirus particles with liposomes. J. Virol. *66*:3363–3367, 1992.
322. Narita, M., Fukusho, A., and Shimizu, Y.: Electron microscopy of the intestine of gnotobiotic piglets infected with porcine rotavirus. J. Comp. Pathol. *92*:589–597, 1982.
323. Nigro, G.: Pancreatitis with hypoglycemia-associate convulsions following rotavirus gastroenteritis. J. Pediatr. Gastroent. Nutr. *12*:280–282, 1991.
324. Nigro, G., and Midulla, M.: Acute laryngitis associated with rotavirus gastroenteritis. J. Infect. Dis. *7*:81–82, 1983.
325. Noone, C., Menzies, I. S., Banatvala, J. E., et al.: Intestinal permeability and lactose hydrolysis in human rotaviral gastroenteritis assessed simultaneously by non-invasive differential sugar permeation. Eur. J. Clin. Invest. *16*:217–225, 1986.
326. Offit, P. A.: Rotaviruses: Immunological determinants of protection against infection and disease. Adv. Virus Res. *44*:161–202, 1994.
327. Offit, P. A., and Blavat, G.: Identification of the two rotavirus genes determining neutralization specificities. J. Virol. *57*:376–378, 1986.
328. Offit, P. A., Blavat, G., Greenberg, H. B., et al.: Molecular basis of rotavirus virulence role of gene segment 4. J. Virol. *57*:46–49, 1986.
329. Offit, P., Boyle, D., Both, G., et al.: Outer capsid glycoprotein VP7 is recognized by cross-reactive rotavirus-specific cytotoxic T lymphocytes. Virology *184*:563–568, 1991.
330. Offit, P., and Clark, H.: Protection against rotavirus-induced gastroenteritis in a murine model by passively acquired gastrointestinal but not circulating antibodies. J. Virol. *54*:58–64, 1985.
331. Offit, P., Clark, H., Blavat, G., et al.: Reassortant rotaviruses containing structural proteins VP3 and VP7 from different parents induce antibodies protective against each parental serotype. J. Virol. *60*:491–496, 1986.
332. Offit, P., Clark, H., Kornstein, M., et al.: A murine model for oral infection with a primate rotavirus (simian SA11). J. Virol. *51*:233–236, 1984.
333. Offit, P. A., and Dudzik, K.: Rotavirus-specific cytotoxic T lymphocytes

cross-react with target cells infected with different rotavirus serotypes. J. Virol. *62*:127–131, 1988.
334. Offit, P. A., and Dudzik, K.: Rotavirus-specific cytotoxic T lymphocytes appear at the intestinal mucosal surface after rotavirus infection. J. Virol. *63*:3507–3512, 1989.
335. Offit, P., and Dudzik, K.: Rotavirus-specific cytotoxic T lymphocytes passively protect against gastroenteritis in suckling mice. J. Virol. *64*:6325–6328, 1990.
336. Offit, P. A., Hoffenberg, E. J., Pia, E. S., et al.: Rotavirus-specific helper T cell responses in newborns, infants, children and adults. J. Infect. Dis. *165*:1107–1111, 1992.
337. Offit, P. A., Hoffenberg, E. J., Santos, N., et al.: Rotavirus-specific humoral and cellular immune response after primary symptomatic infection. J. Infect. Dis. *167*:1436–1440, 1993.
338. Offit, P., Shaw, R., and Greenberg, H.: Passive protection against rotavirus-induced diarrhea by monoclonal antibodies to surface proteins VP3 and VP7. J. Virol. *58*:700–703, 1986.
339. Ohshima, A., Takagi, T., Nakagomi, T., et al.: Molecular characterization by RNA-RNA hybridization of serotype 8 human rotavirus with "super-short" RNA electropherotype. J. Med. Virol. *30*:107–112, 1990.
340. Oishi, I., Yamazaki, K., and Minekawa, Y.: An occurrence of diarrheal cases associated with group C rotavirus in adults. Microbiol. Immunol. *37*:505–509, 1993.
341. O'Ryan, M., Matson, D., Estes, M., et al.: Molecular epidemiology of rotavirus in young children attending day care centers in Houston. J. Infect. Dis. *162*:810–816, 1990.
342. O'Ryan, M. L., Matson, D. O., Estes, M. K., et al.: Anti-rotavirus G type-specific and isotype-specific antibodies in children with natural rotavirus infections. J. Infect. Dis. *169*:504–511, 1994.
343. Osborne, M. P., Haddon, S. J., Spencer, A. J., et al.: An electron microscopic investigation of time-related changes in the intestine of neonatal mice infected with murine rotavirus. J. Pediatr. Gastroenterol. Nutr. *7*:236–248, 1988.
344. Padilla-Noriega, L., Fiore, L., Rennels, M. B., et al.: Humoral immune responses to VP4 and its cleavage products VP5* and VP8* in infants vaccinated with rhesus rotavirus. J. Clin. Microbiol. *30*:1392–1397, 1992.
345. Patton, J. T.: Synthesis of simian rotavirus SA11 double-stranded RNA in a cell-free system. Virus Res. *6*:217–233, 1986.
346. Patton, J. T.: Rotavirus replication. Curr. Top. Microbiol. Immunol. *185*:107–127, 1994.
347. Patton, J. T., and Gallegos, C. O.: Structure and protein composition of the rotavirus replicase particle. Virology *166*:358–365, 1988.
348. Patton, J. T., and Gallegos, C. O.: Rotavirus RNA replication: Single-stranded RNA extends from the replicase particle. J. Gen. Virol. *71*:1087–1094, 1990.
349. Pearson, G. R., and McNulty, M. S.: Pathological changes in the small intestine of neonatal pigs infected with a pig reovirus-like agent (rotavirus). J. Comp. Pathol. *87*:363–375, 1977.
350. Pearson, G. R., and McNulty, M. S.: Ultrastructural changes in small intestinal epithelium of neonatal pigs infected with pig rotavirus. Arch. Virol. *59*:127–136, 1979.
351. Pearson, G. R., McNulty, M. S., and Logan, E. F.: Pathological changes in the small intestine of neonatal calves naturally infected with reo-like virus (rotavirus). Vet. Rec. *102*:454–458, 1978.
352. Pedley, S., Bridger, J. C., Brown, J. F., et al.: Molecular characterization of rotaviruses with distinct group antigens. J. Gen. Virol. *64*:2093–2101, 1983.
353. Pedley, S., Bridger, J. C., Chasey, D., et al.: Definition of two new groups of atypical rotaviruses. J. Gen. Virol. *67*:131–137, 1986.
354. Penaranda, M. E., Cubitt, W. D., Sinarachatanant, P., et al.: Group C rotavirus infections in patients with diarrhea in Thailand, Nepal, and England. J. Infect. Dis. *160*:392–297, 1989.
355. Perez-Schael, I., Blanco, M., Vilar, M., et al.: Clinical studies of a quadrivalent rotavirus vaccine in Venezuelan infants. J. Clin. Microbiol. *28*:553–558, 1990.
356. Perez-Schael, I., Daoud, G., White, L., et al.: Rotavirus shedding by newborn children. J. Med. Virol. *14*:127–136, 1984.
357. Perez-Schael, I., Garcia, D., Gonzalez, M., et al.: Prospective study of diarrheal diseases in Venezuelan children to evaluate the efficacy of rhesus rotavirus vaccine. J. Med. Virol. *30*:219–229, 1990.
358. Perez-Schael, I., Gonzalez, M., Daoud, N., et al.: Reactogenicity and antigenicity of the rhesus rotavirus vaccine MMU 18006 in Venezuelan children. J. Infect. Dis. *155*:34, 1987.
359. Persson, B. L., Thoren, A., Tufvesson, B., et al.: Diarrhoea in Swedish infants: Aetiology and clinical appearance. Acta Paediatr. Scand. *71*:909–913, 1982.
360. Pickering, L. K., DuPont, H. L., Olarte, J., et al.: Fecal leukocytes in enteric infections. Am. J. Clin. Pathol. *68*:562–565, 1977.
361. Pipittajan, P., Kasempimolporn, S., Ikegami, N., et al.: Molecular epidemiology of rotaviruses associated with pediatric diarrhea in Bangkok, Thailand. J. Clin. Microbiol. *29*:617–624, 1991.
362. Pitson, G. A., Grimwood, K., Coulson, B. S., et al.: Comparison between children treated at home and those requiring hospital admission for rotavirus and other enteric pathogens associated with acute diarrhea in Melbourne, Australia. J. Clin. Microbiol. *24*:395–399, 1986.
363. Pizarro, J. L., Sandino, A. M., Pizarro, J. M., et al.: Characterization of rotavirus guanylyltransferase activity associated with polypeptide VP3. J. Gen. Virol. *72*:325–332, 1991.
364. Poncet, D., Laurent, S., and Cohen, J.: Four nucleotides are the minimal requirement for RNA recognition by rotavirus non-structural protein NSP3. EMBO J. *13*:4165–4173, 1994.
365. Poruchynsky, M. A., and Atkinson, P. H.: Rotavirus protein rearrangements in purified membrane-enveloped intermediate particles. J. Virol. *65*:4720–4727, 1991.
366. Poruchynsky, M. A., Tyndall, C., Both, G. W., et al.: Deletions into an NH_2-terminal hydrophobic domain result in secretion of rotavirus VP7, a resident endoplasmic reticulum membrane glycoprotein. J. Cell Biol. *101*:2199–2209, 1985.
367. Pospiscil, A., Hess, R. G., and Bachmann, P. A.: Morphology of intestinal changes in pigs experimentally infected with porcine rotavirus and two porcine corona viruses. Scand. J. Gastroenterol. *74*(Suppl.):167–169, 1982.
368. Prasad, B. V. V., Burns, J. W., Marietta, E., et al.: Localization of VP4 neutralization sites in rotavirus by three-dimensional cryo-electron microscopy. Nature *343*:476–479, 1990.
369. Prasad, B. V. V., and Chiu, W.: Structure of rotavirus. Curr. Top. Microbiol. Immunol. *185*:9–29, 1994.
370. Prasad, B. V. V, Rothnagel, R., Zeng, C. Q.-Y., et al.: Rotavirus structure by electron cryomicroscopy. Abstract. 5th Rotavirus Vaccine Workshop, Atlanta, October 16–17, 1995.
371. Prasad, B. V. V., Wang, G. J., Clerx, J. P. M., et al.: Three-dimensional structure of rotavirus. J. Mol. Biol. *199*:269–275, 1988.
372. Ramig, R. F.: Isolation and genetic characterization of temperature-sensitive mutants of simian rotavirus SA11. Virology *120*:93–105, 1982.
373. Ramig, R. F.: The effects of host age, virus dose, and virus strain on heterologous rotavirus infection of suckling mice. Microbiol. Pathol. *4*:189–202, 1984.
374. Ramig, R. F.: Superinfecting rotaviruses are not excluded from genetic interactions during asynchronous mixed infections *in vitro*. Virology *176*:308–310, 1990.
375. Ramig, R. F., and Ward, R. L.: Genomic segment reassortment in rotaviruses and other Reoviridae. Adv. Virus Res. *39*:163–207, 1991.
376. Rasool, N., Othman, R. Y., Adenan, M. I., et al.: Temporal variation of Malaysian rotavirus electropherotypes. J. Clin. Microbiol. *27*:785–787, 1989.
377. Ratnam, S., Tobin, A. M., Flemming, J. B., et al.: False positive rotazyme results. Lancet *1*:345–346, 1984.
378. Raul-Velazquez, F., Calva, J. J., Lourdes-Guerrero, M., et al.: Cohort study of rotavirus serotype patterns in symptomatic and asymptomatic infections in Mexican children. Pediatr. Infect. Dis. J. *12*:54–61, 1993.
379. Rennels, M. B., Glass, R. I., Dennehy, et al.: Safety and efficacy of high dose rhesus-human reassortant rotavirus vaccines: Report of the national multicenter trial. Pediatrics *97*:7–13, 1996.
380. Rennels, M., Losonsky, G., Levine, M., et al.: Preliminary evaluation of the efficacy of rhesus rotavirus vaccine strain MMU 18006 in young children. Pediatr. Infect. Dis. J. *5*:587–588, 1986.
381. Rennels, M., Losonsky, G., Young, A., et al.: An efficacy trial of the rhesus rotavirus vaccine in Maryland. Am. J. Dis. Child. *144*:601–604, 1990.
382. Research priorities for diarrhoeal diseases vaccines: Memorandum from a WHO meeting. Bull. W. H. O. *69*:667–676, 1991.
383. Reves, R., Hossain, M., Midthun, K., et al.: An observational study of naturally acquired immunity to rotavirus diarrhea in a cohort of 363 Egyptian children. Am. J. Epidemiol. *130*:981–988, 1989.
384. Riepenhoff-Talty, M., Bogger-Goren, S., Li, P., et al.: Development of serum and intestinal antibody response to rotavirus after naturally acquired rotavirus infection in man. J. Med. Virol. *8*:215–222, 1981.
385. Riepenhoff-Talty, M., Gouvea, V., Evans, M. J., et al.: Group C rotavirus (ROTA C) detected by liquid hybridization on PCR products of liver samples from four infants with extrahepatic biliary atresia (EHBA). *In* Program and Abstracts of the IXth International Congress of Virology, Glasgow, 1993.
386. Riepenhoff-Talty, M., Lee, P. C., Carmody, P. J., et al.: Age-dependent rotavirus-enterocyte interactions. Proc. Soc. Exp. Biol. Med. *170*:146–154, 1982.
387. Riepenhoff-Talty, M., Suzuki, H., and Ogra, P. L.: Characteristics of the cell-mediated immune response to rotavirus in suckling mice. Abstract. International Symposium on Enteric Infections in Man and Animals: Standardization of Immunological Procedures, Dublin, Ireland, 1982, Dev. Biol. Standard, Vol. 53. Basel, S. Karger, 1983, pp. 263–268.
388. Rodger, S. M., Bishop, R. F., Birch, C., et al.: Molecular epidemiology of human rotaviruses in Melbourne, Australia, from 1973 to 1979, as determined by electrophoresis of genome ribonucleic acid. J. Clin. Microbiol. *13*:272–278, 1981.
389. Rodger, S. M., and Holmes, I. H.: Comparison of the genomes of simian, bovine, and human rotaviruses by gel electrophoresis and detection of genomic variation among bovine isolates. J. Virol. *30*:839–846, 1979.
390. Rodriguez, W. J., Kim, H. W., Arrobio, J. O., et al.: Clinical features of acute gastroenteritis associated with human reovirus-like agent in infants and young children. J. Pediatr. *91*:188–193, 1977.
391. Rodriguez, W. J., Kim, H. W., Brandt, C. D., et al.: Common exposure outbreak of gastroenteritis due to type 2 rotavirus with high secondary attack rate within families. J. Infect. Dis. *140*:353–357, 1979.

392. Rodriquez, W. J., Kim, H. W., Brandt, C., et al.: Rotavirus gastroenteritis in the Washington, D.C., area. Am. J. Dis. Child. *134*:777–779, 1980.
393. Rodriguez, W. J., Kim, H. W., Brandt, C. D., et al.: Longitudinal study of rotavirus infection and gastroenteritis in families served by a pediatric medical practice: Clinical and epidemiologic observations. Pediatr. Infect. Dis. J. *6*:170–176, 1987.
394. Rodriquez-Toro, G.: Natural epizootic diarrhea of infant mice (EDIM): A light and electron microscope study. Exp. Mol. Pathol. *32*:241–252, 1980.
395. Rolsma, M. D., Gelberg, H. B., and Kuhlenschmidt, M. S.: Assay for evaluation of rotavirus-cell interactions: Identification of an enterocyte ganglioside fraction that mediates group A porcine rotavirus recognition. J. Virol. *68*:258–268, 1994.
396. Roseto, A., Escaig, J., Delain, E., et al.: Structure of rotaviruses as studied by the freeze-drying technique. Virology *98*:471–475, 1979.
397. Rotbart, H. A., Nelson, W. L., Glode, M. P., et al.: Neonatal rotavirus associated necrotizing enterocolitis: Case control study and prospective surveillance during an outbreak. J. Pediatr. *112*:87–93, 1988.
398. Ruggeri, F. M., and Greenberg, H. B.: Antibodies to the trypsin cleavage peptide VP8 neutralize rotavirus by inhibiting binding of virions to target cells in culture. J. Virol. *65*:2211–2219, 1991.
399. Ruggeri, F. M., Marziano, M. L., Tinari, A., et al.: Four-year study of rotavirus electropherotypes from cases of infantile diarrhea in Rome. J. Clin. Microbiol. *27*:1522–1526, 1989.
400. Ruiz, M.-C., Alonso-Torre, S. R., Charpilienne, A., et al.: Rotavirus interaction with isolated membrane vesicles. J. Virol. *68*:4009–4016, 1994.
401. Ruuska, T., and Vesikari, T.: A prospective study of acute diarrhoea in Finnish children from birth to 2½ years of age. Acta Paediatr. Scand. *80*:500–507, 1991.
402. Ryder, R. W., Sack, D. A., Kapikian, A. Z., et al.: Enterotoxigenic *Escherichia coli* and reovirus-like agent in rural Bangladesh. Lancet *1*:659–662, 1976.
403. Ryder, R. W., Singh, N., Reeves, W. C., et al.: Evidence of immunity induced by naturally acquired rotavirus and Norwalk virus infection on two remote Panamanian islands. J. Infect. Dis. *151*:99–105, 1985.
404. Sack, D. A., Chowdhury, A. M. A. K., Eusof, A., et al.: Oral hydration in rotavirus diarrhoea: A double blind comparison of sucrose with glucose electrolyte solution. Lancet *2*:280–283, 1978.
405. Saif, L. J.: Nongroup A rotaviruses. *In* Saif, L. J., and Theil, K. W. (eds.): Viral Diarrheas of Man and Animals. Boca Raton, CRC Press, 1990, pp. 73–95.
406. Saif, L. J., Bohl, E. H., Theil, K. W., et al.: Rotavirus-like, calcivirus-like, and 23-nm virus-like particles associated with diarrhea in young pigs. J. Clin. Microbiol. *12*:105–111, 1980.
407. Saif, L. J., and Jiang, B.: Nongroup A rotaviruses of humans and animals. Curr. Top. Microbiol. Immunol. *185*:339–371, 1994.
408. Saif, L. J., Redman, D. R., Smith, K. L., et al.: Passive immunity to bovine rotavirus in newborn calves fed colostrum supplements from immunized or non-immunized cows. Infect. Immun. *41*:1118–1131, 1983.
409. Salmi, T. T., Arstila, P., and Koivkko, A.: Central nervous system involvement in patients with rotavirus gastroenteritis. Scand. J. Infect. Dis. *10*:29–31, 1978.
410. Santos, N., and Gouvea, N.: Improved method for purification of viral RNA from fecal specimens for rotavirus detection. J. Virol. Meth. *46*:11–21, 1994.
411. Santosham, M., Burns, B., Nadkarni, V., et al.: Oral rehydration therapy for acute diarrhea in ambulatory children in the United States: A double-blind comparison of four different solutions. Pediatrics *76*:159–166, 1985.
412. Santosham, M., Daum, R. S., Dillman, L., et al: Oral rehydration therapy of infantile diarrhea: A controlled study of well-nourished children hospitalized in the United States and Panama. N. Engl. J. Med. *306*:1070–1076, 1982.
413. Santosham, M., Letson, G. W., Wolff, M., et al.: A field study of the safety and efficacy of two candidate vaccines in a Native American population. J. Infect. Dis. *163*:483–487, 1991.
414. Santosham, M., Yolken R. H., Quiroz, E., et al.: Detection of rotavirus in respiratory secretions of children with pneumonia. J. Pediatr. *103*:58, 1983.
415. Saulsbury, F. T., Winkelstein, J. A., and Yolken, R. H.: Chronic rotavirus infection in immunodeficiency. J. Pediatr. *97*:661–665, 1980.
416. Schaller, J. P., Saif, L. J., Cordle, C. T., et al.: Prevention of human rotavirus-induced diarrhea in gnotobiotic piglets using bovine antibody. J. Infect. Dis. 165:623–630, 1992.
417. Schnagl, R. D., Rodger, S. M., and Holmes, I. H.: Variation in human rotavirus electropherotypes occurring between rotavirus gastroenteritis epidemics in central Australia. Infect. Immun. *33*:17–21, 1981.
418. Schreiber, R. A., and Kleinman, R. E.: Genetics, immunology, and biliary atresia: An opening or a division? J. Pediatr. Gastroenterol. Nutr. *16*:111–113, 1993.
419. Sereno, M. M., and Gorziglia, M. I.: The outer capsid protein VP4 of murine rotavirus strain Eb represents a tentative new P type. Virology *199*:500–504, 1994.
420. Shaw, R., Groene, W., Mackow, E., et al.: VP4-specific intestinal antibody response to rotavirus in a murine model of heterotypic protection. J. Virol. *65*:3052–3059, 1991.
421. Shaw, R. D., Hempson, S. J., and Mackow, E. R.: Rotavirus diarrhea is caused by nonreplicating viral particles. J. Virol. *69*:5946–5950, 1995.
422. Shaw, R., Merchant, A., Groene, W., et al.: Persistence of intestinal antibody response to heterologous rotavirus infection in a murine model beyond 1 year. J. Clin. Microbiol. *31*:188–191, 1993.
423. Shaw, A. L., Rothnagel, R., Chen, D., et al.: Three-dimensional visualization of the rotavirus hemagglutinin structure. Cell *74*:693–701, 1993.
424. Shen, S., Burke, B., and Desselberger, U.: Nucleotide sequences of the VP4 and VP7 genes of a Chinese lamb rotavirus: Evidence for a new P type in a G10 type virus. Virology *197*:497–500, 1993.
425. Shif, I., Iizuka, M., Silberstein, I., et al.: Rotaviruses belonging to the AU-1 genogroup recovered from Israeli infants with diarrhea. Arch. Virol. *138*:357–364, 1994.
426. Siadatpajouh, M., Burns, J. W., Ruggeri, F., et al.: Novel protection of rotavirus murine model by an anti-VP6 IgA monoclonal antibody. *In* Abstracts of the American Society of Virology 14th Annual Meeting, No. P25–P27, 1995, p. 174.
427. Simhon, A., Mata, L., Vives, M., et al.: Low endemicity and low pathogenicity of rotaviruses among rural children in Costa Rica. J. Infect. Dis. *152*:1134–1142, 1985.
428. Snodgrass, D., Fahey, K., Wells, P., et al.: Passive immunity in calf rotavirus infections: Maternal vaccination increases and prolongs immunoglobulin G1 antibody secretion in milk. Infect. Immun. *28*:344–349, 1980.
429. Snodgrass, D. R., Hoshino, Y., Fitzgerald, T. A., et al.: Identification of four VP4 serological types (P serotypes) of bovine rotavirus using viral reassortants. J. Gen. Virol. *73*:2319–2325, 1992.
430. Snodgrass, D. R., amd Wells, P. W.: Rotavirus infection in lambs: Studies on passive protection. Arch. Virol. *52*:201–205, 1976.
431. Snodgrass, D., and Wells, P.: Passive immmunity in rotaviral infections. J. Am. Vet. Med. Assoc. *173*:565–568, 1978.
432. Soriano Brücher, H. E., Avendāno, P., O'Ryan, M., et al.: Use of bismuth subsalicylate in acute diarrhea in children. Rev. Infect. Dis. *12*:S51–S56, 1990.
433. Spencer, E., and Arias, M. I.: In vitro transcription catalyzed by heat-treated human rotavirus. J. Virol. *40*:1–10, 1981.
434. Srinivasan, G., Azarcon, E., Muldoon, M. R. L., et al.: Rotavirus infection in normal nursery: Epidemic and surveillance. Infect. Control. *5*:478–481, 1984.
435. Stacy-Phipps, S., and Patton, J. T.: Synthesis of plus- and minus-strand RNA in rotavirus-infected cells. J. Virol. *61*:3479–3484, 1987.
436. Stannard, L. M., and Schoub, B. D.: Observations on the morphology of two rotaviruses. J. Gen. Virol. *37*:435–439, 1977.
437. Starkey, W. G., Collins, J., Wallis, T. S., et al.: Kinetics, tissue specificity and pathological changes in murine rotavirus infection of mice. J. Gen. Virol. *67*:2625–2634, 1986.
438. Steel, H. M., Garnham, S., Beards, G. M., et al.: Investigation of an outbreak of rotavirus infection in geriatric patients by serotyping and polyacrylamide gel electrophoresis (PAGE). J. Med. Virol. *37*:132–136, 1992.
439. Steele, A. D., and Alexander, J. J.: Molecular epidemiology of rotavirus in black infants in South Africa. J. Clin. Microbiol. *25*:2384–2387, 1987.
440. Steele, A. D., Bos, P., and Alexander, J. J.: Clinical features of acute infantile gastroenteritis associated with human rotavirus subgroups I and II. J. Clin. Microbiol. *26*:2647–2649, 1988.
441. Steele, A. D., Garcia D., Sears J., et al.: Distribution of VP4 gene alleles in human rotaviruses by using probes to the hyperdivergent region of the VP4 gene. J. Clin. Microbiol. *31*:1735–1740, 1993.
442. Steele, A. D., van Niekerk, M. C., and Mphahlele, M. J.: Geographic distribution of human rotavirus VP4 genotypes and VP7 serotypes in five South African regions. J. Clin. Microbiol. 33:1516–1519, 1995.
443. Steinhoff, M. C.: Rotavirus: The first five years. J. Pediatr. 96:611–622, 1980.
444. Stirazaker, S. C., and Both, G. W.: The signal peptide of the rotavirus glycoprotein VP7 is essential for its retention in the ER as an integral membrane protein. Cell *56*:741–747, 1989.
445. Stirazaker, S. C., Whitfield, P. L., Christie, D. L., et al.: Processing of rotavirus glycoprotein VP7: Implications for the retention of the protein in the endoplasmic reticulum. J. Cell Biol. *105*:2897–2903, 1987.
446. Superti, F., and Donelli, G.: Gangliosides as binding sites in SA-11 rotavirus infection of LLC-MK2 cells. J. Gen. Virol. *72*:2467–2474, 1991.
447. Suzuki, H., Kitaoka, S., Konno, T., et al.: Two modes of human rotavirus entry into MA104 cells. Arch. Virol. *85*:25–34, 1985.
448. Suzuki, H., Kitaoka, S., Sato, T., et al.: Further investigation on the mode of entry of human rotavirus into cells. Arch. Virol. 91:135–144, 1986.
449. Suzuki, H., and Konno, T.: Reovirus-like particles in jejunal mucosa of a Japanese infant with acute infectious non-bacterial gastroenteritis. Tohoku J. Exp. Med. *115*:199–221, 1975.
450. Svensson, L.: Group C rotavirus requires sialic acid for erythrocyte and cell receptor binding. J. Virol. *66*:5582–5585, 1992.
451. Svensson, L., Uhnoo, I., Grandien, M., et al.: Molecular epidemiology of rotavirus infections in Uppsala, Sweden, 1981: Disappearance of a predominant electropherotype. J. Med. Virol. *18*:101–111, 1986.
452. Tallet, S., MacKenzie, C., Middleton, P., et al.: Clinical laboratory and epidemiological features of a viral gastroenteritis in infants and children. Pediatrics *60*:217–222, 1977.
453. Tam, J. S., Kum, W. W. S., Lam, B., et al.: Molecular epidemiology of human rotavirus infection in children in Hong Kong. J. Clin. Microbiol. *23*:660–664, 1986.

454. Taniguchi, K., Maloy, W., Nishikawa, K., et al.: Identification of cross-reactive and serotype 2–specific neutralization epitopes on VP3 of human rotavirus. J. Virol. *62*:2421–2426, 1988.
455. Taniguchi, K., Urasawa, T., Kobayashi, N., et al.: Nucleotide sequence of VP4 and VP7 genes of human rotaviruses with subgroup 1 specificity and long RNA pattern: Implication for new serotype G specificity. J. Virol. *64*:5640–5644, 1990.
456. Taniguchi, K., Urasawa, T., Urasawa, S., et al.: Production of subgroup-specific monoclonal antibodies to an enzyme-linked immunosorbent assay for subgroup determination. J. Med. Virol. *14*:115–125, 1984.
457. Taniguchi, K., Urasawa, T., and Urasawa, S.: Species specificity and interspecies relatedness in VP4 genotypes demonstrated by VP4 sequence analysis of equine, feline, and canine rotavirus strains. Virology *200*:390–400, 1994.
458. Taylor, J. A., Meyer, J. C., Legge, M. A., et al.: Transient expression and mutational analysis of the rotavirus intracellular receptor: The C-terminal methionine residue is essential for ligand binding. J. Virol. *66*:3566–3572, 1992.
459. Theil, K. W., Bohl, E. H., Cross, R. F., et al.: Pathogenesis of porcine rotaviral infection in experimentally inoculated gnotobiotic pigs. Am. J. Vet. Res. *39*:213–220, 1978.
460. Thomas, E. E., Puterman, M. L., Kawano, E., et al.: Evaluation of seven immunoassays for detection of rotavirus in pediatric stool samples. J. Clin. Microbiol. *26*:1189–1193, 1988.
461. Tian, P., Estes, M. K., Hu, Y., et al.: The rotavirus nonstructural glycoprotein NSP4 mobilizes Ca^{2+} from the endoplasmic reticulum. J. Virol. *69*:5763–5772, 1995.
462. Timenetsky, M. C. S. T., Santos, N., and Gouvea, V.: Survey of rotavirus G and P types associated with human gastroenteritis in São Paulo, Brazil, from 1986 to 1992. J. Clin. Microbiol. *32*:2622–2624, 1994.
463. Todd, D., and McNulty, M. S.: Electrophoretic variation of avian rotavirus RNA in polyacrylamide gel. Avian Pathol. *15*:149, 1986.
464. Torres-Medina, A.: Effect of combined rotavirus and *Escherichia coli* in neonatal gnotobiotic calves. Am. J. Vet. Res. *45*:643–651, 1984.
465. Torres-Medina, A., and Underdahl, N. R.: Scanning electron microscopy of intestine of gnotobiotic piglets infected with porcine rotavirus. Can. J. Comp. Med. *44*:403–411, 1980.
466. Totterdell, B. M., Banatvala, J. E., Chrystie, I. L., et al.: Systemic lymphoproliferative responses to rotavirus. J. Med. Virol. *25*:37–44, 1988.
467. Totterdell, B. M., Chrystie, I. L., and Banatvala, J. E.: Rotavirus infections in a maternity unit. Arch. Dis. Child. *51*:924–928, 1976.
468. Treanor, J. J., Clark, H. F., Pichichero, M., et al.: Evaluation of the protective efficacy of a serotype 1 bovine-human rotavirus reassortant vaccine in infants. Pediatr. Infect. Dis. J. *14*:301–307, 1995.
469. Troonen, H.: False positive rotazyme results. Lancet *1*:345, 1984.
470. Tsunemitsu, H., Jiang, B., and Saif, L. J.: Detection of group C rotavirus antigens and antibodies in animals and humans by ELISA. J. Clin Microbiol. *30*:2129–2134, 1992.
471. Turner, R. B., and Kelsey, D. K.: Passive immunization for prevention of rotavirus illness in healthy infants. Pediatr. Infect. Dis. J. *12*:718–722, 1993.
472. Tzipori, S., Unicomb, L., Bishop, R., et al.: Studies on attenuation of rotavirus: A comparison in piglets between virulent virus and its attenuated derivative. Arch. Virol. *109*:197–205, 1989.
473. Uhnoo, I., Olding-Stenkvist, E., and Kreuger, A.: Clinical features of acute gastroenteritis associated with rotavirus, enteric adenoviruses, and bacteria. Arch. Dis. Child. *61*:732–738, 1986.
474. Uhnoo, I., Riepenhoff-Talty, M., Chegas, P., et al.: Effect of malnutrition on extraintestinal spread of rotavirus and development of hepatitis in mice. Nutr. Res. *10*:1419–1429, 1990.
475. Uhnoo, I., Riepenhoff-Talty, M., Dharakul, T., et al.: Extramucosal spread and development of hepatitis with rhesus rotavirus in immunodeficient and normal mice. J. Virol. *64*:361–368, 1990.
476. Urasawa, S., Hasegawa, A., Urasawa, T., et al.: Antigenic and genetic analyses of human rotaviruses in Chiang Mai, Thailand: Evidence for a close relationship between human and animal rotaviruses. J. Infect. Dis. *166*:227–234, 1992.
477. Urasawa, T., Taniguchi, K., Kobayashi, N., et al.: Nucleotide sequence of VP4 and VP7 genes of a unique human rotavirus strain Mc35 with subgroup 1 and serotype 10 specificity. Virology *195*:766–771, 1993.
478. Urasawa, S., Urasawa, T., and Taniguchi, K.: Genetic reassortment between two human rotaviruses having different serotype and subgroup specificities. J. Gen. Virol. *67*:1551–1559, 1986.
479. Ushijima, H., Honma, H., Mukoyama, A., et al.: Detection of group C rotaviruses in Tokyo. J. Med. Virol. *27*:299–303, 1989.
480. Ushiyima, H., Tajima, T., Tagaya, M., et al.: Rotavirus and central nervous system. Brain. Dev. *6*:215, 1984.
481. Valenzuela, S., Pizarro, J., Sandino, A. M., et al.: Photoaffinity labeling of rotavirus VP1 with 8-Azido-ATP: Identification of the viral RNA polymerase. J. Virol. *65*:3964–3967, 1991.
482. Vásquez, M., Sandino, A. M., Pizarro, J. M., et al.: Function of rotavirus VP3 polypeptide in viral morphogenesis. J. Gen. Virol. *74*:937–941, 1993.
483. Vesikari, T.: Clinical trials of live oral rotavirus vaccines: The Finnish experience. Vaccine *11*:255–261, 1993.
484. Vesikari, T., Isolauri, E., Delem, A., et al.: Immunogenicity and safety of live oral attenuated bovine rotavirus vaccine strain RIT 4237 in adults and young children. Lancet *2*:807–811, 1983.
485. Vesikari, T., Isolauri, E., Delem, A., et al.: Clinical efficacy of the RIT 4237 live attenuated bovine rotavirus vaccine in infants vaccinated before a rotavirus epidemic. J. Pediatr. *107*:189–194, 1985.
486. Vesikari, T., Isolauri, E., D'Hondt, E., et al.: Protection of infants against rotavirus diarrhoea by RIT 4237 attenuated bovine rotavirus strain vaccine. Lancet *1*:977–981, 1984.
487. Vesikari, T., Kapikian, A. Z., Delem, A., et al.: A comparative trail of rhesus monkey (RRV-1) and bovine (RIT 4237) oral rotavirus vaccines in young children. J. Infect. Dis. *153*:832, 1986.
488. Vesikari, T., Rautanen, T., Varis, T., et al.: Rhesus rotavirus candidate vaccine: Clinical trial in children vaccinated between 2 and 5 months of age. Am. J. Dis. Child. *144*:285–289, 1990.
489. Vesikari, T., Ruuska, T., Green, K., et al.: Protective efficacy against serotype 1 rotavirus diarrhea by live oral rhesus-human reassortant rotavirus vaccines with human rotavirus VP7 serotype 1 or 2 specificity. Pediatr. Infect. Dis. J. *11*:535–542, 1992.
490. Vesikari, T., Ruuska, T., Koivu, H., et al.: Evaluation of the M37 human rotavirus vaccine in 2- to 6-month-old infants. Pediatr. Infect. Dis. J. *10*:912–917, 1991.
491. Vesikari, T., Sarkkinen, H. K., and Maki, M.: Quantitative aspects of rotavirus excretion in childhood. Acta Pediatr. Scand. *70*:717–721, 1981.
492. Walsh, J. A., and Warren, K. S.: An interim strategy for disease control in developing countries. N. Engl. J.Med. *301*:967–974, 1979.
493. Ward, R. L., Bernstein, D. I., and U.S. Rotavirus Vaccine Efficacy Group: Protection against rotavirus disease following natural rotavirus infection. J. Infect. Dis. *169*:900–904, 1994.
494. Ward, R. L., Bernstein, D. I., Shukla, R., et al.: Effects of antibody to rotavirus on protection of adults challenged with a human rotavirus. J. Infect. Dis. *159*:79–88, 1989.
495. Ward, R. L., Bernstein, D. I., Shukla, R., et al.: Protection of adults rechallenged with a human rotavirus. J. Infect. Dis. *161*:440–445, 1990.
496. Ward, R. L., Clemens, J. D., Knowlton, D. R., et al.: Evidence that protection against rotavirus diarrhea after natural infection is not dependent on serotype-specific neutralizing antibody. J. Infect. Dis. *166*:1251–1257, 1992.
497. Ward, R. L., Clemens, J. D., Sack, D. A., et al.: Culture adaptation and characterization of group A rotaviruses causing diarrheal illnesses in Bangladesh from 1985 to 1986. J. Clin. Microbiol. *29*:1915–1923, 1991.
498. Ward, R. L., and Knowlton, D. R.: Genotypic selection following coinfection of cultured cells with subgroup 1 and subgroup 2 human rotaviruses. J. Gen. Virol. *70*:1691–1699, 1989.
499. Ward, R. L., Knowlton, D. R., and Greenberg, H. B.: Phenotypic mixing during coinfection of cells with two strains of human rotavirus. J. Virol. *62*:4358–4361, 1988.
500. Ward, R. L., Knowlton, D. R., Greenberg, H. B., et al.: Serum neutralizing antibody to VP4 and VP7 proteins in infants following vaccination with WC3 bovine rotavirus. J. Virol. *64*:2687–2691, 1990.
501. Ward, R. L., Knowlton, D. R., Hurst, P.-F. L.: Reassortant formation and selection following coinfection of cultured cells with subgroup 2 human rotaviruses. J. Gen. Virol. *69*:149–162, 1988.
502. Ward, R. L., Knowlton, D. R., and Pierce, M. J.: Efficiency of human rotavirus propagation in cell culture. J. Clin. Microbiol. *19*:748–753, 1984.
503. Ward, R., Knowlton, D., Schiff, G., et al.: Relative concentrations of serum neutralizing antibody to VP3 and VP7 proteins in adults infected with a human rotavirus. J. Virol. *62*:1543–1549, 1988.
504. Ward, R. L., McNeal, M. M., Sander, D. S., et al.: Immunodominance of the VP4 neutralization protein of rotavirus in protective natural infections of young children. J. Virol. *67*:464–468, 1993.
505. Ward, R. L., McNeal, M. M., and Sheridan, J. F.: Development of an adult mouse model for studies on protection against rotavirus. J. Virol. *64*:5070–5075, 1990.
506. Ward, R. L., McNeal, M. M., and Sheridan, J.: Evidence that active protection following oral immunization of mice with live rotavirus is not dependent on neutralizing antibody. Virology *188*:57–66, 1992.
507. Ward, R. L., Nakagomi, O., Knowlton, D. R., et al.: Evidence for natural reassortants of human rotaviruses belonging to different genogroups. J. Virol. *64*:3219–3225, 1990.
508. Wenman, W. M., Hinde, D., Feltham, S., et al.: Rotavirus infection in adults. N. Engl. J. Med. *301*:303–306, 1979.
509. Whitfield, P. L., Tyndall, C., Stirazaker, S. C., et al.: Location of signal sequences within the rotavirus SA11 glycoprotein VP7 which direct it to the endoplasmic reticulum. Mol. Cell. Biol. *7*:2491–2497, 1987.
510. Wong, C. J., Price, Z., and Bruckner, D. A.: Aseptic meningitis in an infant with rotavirus gastroenteritis. Pediatr. Infect. Dis. *3*:244–246, 1984.
511. Woode, G. N., Bridger, J. C., Jones, J. M., et al.: Morphological and antigenic relationships between viruses (rotaviruses) from acute gastroenteritis of children, calves, piglets, mice, and foals. Infect. Immun. *14*:804–810, 1976.
512. Woode, G., Kelso, N., Simpson, T., et al.: Antigenic relationships among some bovine rotaviruses: Serum neutralization and cross-protection in gnotobiotic calves. J. Clin. Microbiol. *18*:358–364, 1983.
513. Woode, G., Zheng, S., Rosen, B., et al.: Protection between different

serotypes of bovine rotavirus in gnotobiotic calves: Specificity of serum antibody and coproantibody responses. J. Clin. Microbiol. *25*:1052–1058, 1987.
514. Wu, H., Taniguchi, K., Wakasugi, F., et al.: Survey on the distribution of the gene 4 alleles of human rotaviruses by polymerase chain reaction. Epidemiol. Infect. *112*:615–622, 1994.
515. Wyatt, R. G., Greenberg, H. B., James, W. D., et al.: Definition of human rotavirus serotypes by plaque reduction assay. Infect. Immun. *37*:110–115, 1982.
516. Wyatt, R. G., James, H. D., Jr., Pittman, A. L., et al.: Direct isolation in cell culture of human rotaviruses and their characterization into four serotypes. J. Clin. Microbiol. *18*:310–317, 1983.
517. Wyatt, R. G., Kalica, A. R., Mebus, C. A., et al.: Reovirus-like agents (rotaviruses) associated with diarrheal illness in animals and man. *In* Pollard, M. (ed.): Perspectives in Virology. New York, Raven Press, 1978, pp. 121–145.
518. Wyatt, R. G., Yolken, R. H., Urrutia, J. J., et al.: Diarrhea associated with rotavirus in rural Guatemala: A longitudinal study of 24 infants and young children. Am. J. Trop. Med. Hyg. *28*:325–328, 1979.
519. Yeager, M., Berriman, J. A., Baker, T. S., et al.: Three-dimensional structure of the rotavirus haemagglutinin VP4 by cryo-electron microscopy and difference map analysis. EMBO J. *13*:1011–1018, 1994.
520. Yeager, M., Dryden, K. A., Olson, N. H., et al.: Three-dimensional structure of rhesus rotavirus by cryo-electron microscopy and image reconstruction. J. Cell Biol. *110*:2133–2144, 1990.
521. Yolken, R., Arango-Jaramillo, S., Eiden, J., et al.: Lack of genomic reassortment following infection of infant rats with group A and group B rotaviruses. J. Infect. Dis. *158*:1120–1123, 1988.
522. Yolken, R. H., Bishop, C. A., Townsend, T. R., et al.: Infectious gastroenteritis in bone-marrow transplant recipients. N. Engl. J. Med. *306*:1009–1012, 1982.
523. Yolken, R. H., and Murphy, M.: Sudden infant death syndrome associated with rotavirus infection. J. Med. Virol. *10*:291–296, 1982.
524. Yolken, R. H., Willoughby, R., Wee, S.-B., et al.: Sialic acid glycoproteins inhibit in vitro and in vivo replication of rotaviruses. J. Clin. Invest. *79*:148–154, 1987.
525. Yolken, R., Wyatt, R., and Zissis, G.: Epidemiology of human rotavirus types 1 and 2 as studied by enzyme-linked immunosorbent assay. N. Engl. J. Med. *299*:1156–1161, 1978.
526. Zeng, C. Q.-Y., Labbé, M., Cohen, J., et al.: Characterization of rotavirus VP2 particles. Virology *201*:55–65, 1994.
527. Zheng, B. J., Chang, R. X., Ma, G. Z., et al.: Rotavirus infection of the oropharynx and respiratory tract in young children. J. Med. Virol. *34*:29–37, 1991.
528. Zheng, B. J., Lo, S. K. F., Tam, J. S. L., et al.: Prospective study of community-acquired rotavirus infection. J. Clin. Microbiol. *27*:2083–2090, 1989.

❑ ❑ ❑

SUBSECTION FOUR

TOGAVIRIDAE

177

RUBELLA VIRUS

James D. Cherry

Rubella (German measles) is a generally mild, exanthematous, infectious illness in which morbidity and mortality usually are minimal. However, infection in pregnancy may result in fetal infection as well, and this usually is associated with considerable adversities for the developing infant. The rubella virus has only one known type.

HISTORY

In ancient history, rubella as a disease is lost among the other prominent exanthematous diseases (i.e., scarlet fever, measles, and smallpox). In an extensive review, Griffith[180] suggested that rubella was known to the early Arabian physicians under the name *al-hamikah;* they considered rubella a form of measles, however. Two German physicians, de Bergen in 1752 and Orlow in 1758, generally are credited with the first clinical descriptions of rubella as a specific entity.[180, 503] In early writings, rubella generally was called *Rötheln.*[140, 503] However, because of the great interest of German physicians in the disease during the period from the mid-18th to the mid-19th centuries, the name *German measles* frequently was employed in other countries.

In 1866, a Scottish physician named Veale described 30 cases of German measles. In his paper, he gave the illness its present name, rubella. It was his opinion that the German name, Rötheln, was too harsh and foreign and that other possible names—rubeola notha and rosalia idiopathica—were too long for general use and could be confused with measles.[140, 480] Other historical synonyms of rubella include rubeola, rubeola sine catarrho, rubeola epidemica, rubeola morbillosa, rubeola scarlatinosa, rosania, roseola, roseola epidemica, rosalia, scarlatina morbillosa, scarlatina hybrida, morbilli scarlatinosi, feuer masern, roséole, roséole idiopathique, rubéole, rougéole fausse, French measles, false measles, bastard measles, hybrid measles, and bastard scarlatina.[180]

In 1881 at the International Congress of Medicine in London, a consensus was reached that rubella was a distinct disease. Rubella was felt to be similar in some respects but not identical to measles or scarlatina. By the beginning of the 20th century, the clinical description of rubella was complete, except that joint manifestations had received curiously little notation.[13, 99, 140, 180, 299, 390, 465]

Rubella gained its present-day importance in 1941 when Gregg,[179] an Australian ophthalmologist, reported congenital defects in babies of mothers who had rubella during early pregnancy. In spite of considerable skepticism, Gregg's observations were confirmed quickly by Swan and colleagues[449, 450] in Australia and other investigators in the United States[126, 368, 373] and the United Kingdom. By 1947, 28 communications describing 500 children with severe congenital defects associated with maternal rubella had appeared in the literature.[503]

In 1938, Hiro and Tasaka[214] demonstrated that rubella was a disease of viral etiology by transmission of disease in humans by the subcutaneous injection of filtered nasal washings. In 1942, Habel[187] was able to infect monkeys with nasal washings and blood from human cases. In 1962, rubella virus first was propagated in the laboratory; two investigative teams, Weller and Neva[502] and Parkman and colleagues,[340] using different techniques, reported the growth of rubella virus in tissue culture.

The isolation of rubella virus in 1962 paved the way for definitive study of the 1964 rubella pandemic. The results of extensive virologic, serologic, and epidemiologic investigation were presented at a Rubella Symposium in May 1965.[251] After the isolation of rubella virus in tissue culture, an intensive worldwide effort to develop vaccines was mounted. The accumulation of these experiences resulted in an extensive body of knowledge related to rubella and rubella immunization, which was presented at the International Conference on Rubella Immunization in February 1969.[250] Live attenuated rubella virus vaccines were licensed for use in mid-1969 in the United States.[298] In the 28-year period since licensure, an estimated 182 million doses of rubella vaccine were distributed in the United States, and rubella activity decreased by about 99 per cent.[58, 59, 61, 62, 360]

PROPERTIES

Classification

Rubella virus is placed in the *Rubivirus* genus of the family *Togaviridae*.[134, 512] At present, it is the only species in this genus. The virus is similar physiochemically to the other members of its family (alphavirus, flavivirus, and pestivirus) but is unrelated serologically. Rubella virus has no invertebrate host (a characteristic of all alphavirus and most flavivirus types), and humans are the only known vertebrate host.

Physical Properties

The rubella virion is spherical, with a diameter of 60 to 70 nm, and it contains three major polypeptides—E1, E2, and C.[281, 347, 512] E1 (relative molecular weight 58,000) and E2 (relative molecular weight 42,000 to 47,000) are glycosylated and are located on the viral surface membrane. E1 is the viral hemagglutinin that is found on 5- to 6-nm surface projections.[216, 347] The nucleocapsid has a diameter of 30 to 40 nm and is composed of polypeptide (C protein) and the genomic RNA. The nucleic acid of rubella virus is single-stranded RNA with a molecular weight of 3.2 to 3.8 × 10^6.[407] The outer coat of the virus (envelope) is lipoprotein in nature with host-cell lipid and virus-specified polypeptides.

Rubella virus is relatively sensitive to heat; it generally has been found to lose infectivity within 30 minutes at 56° C.[132, 339, 355] However, Kistler and Sapatino[242] have observed that some infectivity persists even after heating for 60 minutes at 70° C. At 37° C in the presence of 2 per cent serum, 90 per cent is inactivated in 3 hours.[339] At 4° C, with protein stabilization, viral titers are maintained for 7 or more days. The virus is stable indefinitely at −60° C and below but labile at normal (−10° to −20° C) refrigeration temperatures. When stabilized with protein, the virus can survive several rapid freeze-thaw cycles without significant loss of titer.[393]

Rubella virus is sensitive to ultraviolet light. In 1 hour, a high-titered cell-free virus suspension was inactivated by an intensity of 1350 $\mu W/cm^2$; on the other hand, a tissue culture suspension of virus was not inactivated completely when it was exposed to a similar intensity of radiation.[242] Rubella virus also is sensitive to visible light, and this photosensitivity can be potentiated by the basic dye proflavine.[40]

The virus also is sensitive to pH extremes of less than 6.8 and greater than 8.1.[68] The following chemicals rapidly inactivate rubella virus: ether, acetone, chloroform, deoxycholate, formalin, β-propiolactone, ethylene oxide, free chlorine, and 70 per cent alcohol.[355] It is resistant to thimerosal.

Antigenic Composition

Rubella virus infection of tissue culture cells results in the production of infectious virus that can be neutralized by specific antiserum. Specific viral antibodies can be identified by hemagglutination inhibition (HI), complement fixation (CF), precipitation in gel, platelet aggregation, passive hemagglutination (PH), single radial hemolysis, latex agglutination (LA), enzyme-linked immunosorbent assay (ELISA), and immunofluorescence.[27, 33, 70, 72, 73, 124, 125, 135, 147, 210, 262, 263, 282, 344, 355, 386, 387, 478, 512, 520] Neutralization and HI identify antibodies that inhibit specific biologic functions of the virus, whereas the other assays only identify the formation of antigen-antibody complexes. The E1 glycoprotein is the predominant erythrocyte-binding and neutralization site of the virus.[467, 496] Weak neuraminidase activity also has been associated with purified rubella virus.[20]

In 1967, Stewart and associates[441] reported that tissue culture–grown rubella virus produced hemagglutination of erythrocytes from chickens that were younger than 1 day of age and from one goose and one lamb, but no hemagglutination was observed with adult chicken, guinea pig, and other commonly employed red cell preparations. Subsequently, techniques employing careful control of test system diluents have revealed that red cells from many different animals are agglutinated by rubella virus.[270, 400] Viral hemagglutinin is stable at −20° C for months and at 4° C for several weeks but is destroyed rapidly by heat.[156, 189]

Sever and colleagues[418] first demonstrated that supernatant fluid from primary African green monkey kidney (AGMK) and RK-13 rabbit kidney tissue cultures contained useful complement-fixing antigens. There are two distinct rubella complement-fixing antigens.[403] One of the antigens is similar in size and weight to both the hemagglutinin and infectious virus; the other "soluble" antigen is smaller, with a buoyant density of 1.08 g/mL. The soluble antigen is noninfectious and does not contain nucleic acid.[355] Rubella complement-fixing antigens retain their antigenicity after ether treatment.

Two major small-particle antigens have been identified in the medium of tissue culture–infected cells by immunodiffusion.[263, 402] These two soluble antigens are structural components of the virion, and natural infection with rubella virus results in the formation of serum precipitating antibodies. These antigens have been designated theta and iota. Their importance lies in the fact that antibody to the iota antigen rarely is noted in the serum of recipients of some rubella vaccines; therefore, they may be of value in studying vaccine-induced immunity.[52, 262]

Tissue Culture Growth

Rubella virus grows in many different tissue cultures, including cell strains, cell lines, and primary cells.[106, 285, 339, 355, 511, 512] Cell sources include mature and embryonic tissue from humans and other primates, rabbits, swine, dogs, birds, hamsters, and cattle. In tissue culture, rubella virus growth can be identified by either cytopathic effect or the ability to produce interference of the growth of another tissue culture–susceptible virus.

For primary isolation of rubella virus from clinical material, the most commonly used method is the interference technique employing primary AGMK cells.[339] In this system, nonadapted rubella virus grows readily but does not produce cytopathic effect. Infection is demonstrated in the AGMK tissue culture by the failure of typical enterovirus cytopathic effect to occur after challenge of the culture with echovirus 11 or another suitable enterovirus. A common alternative to the AGMK–echovirus 11 interference system for primary rubella virus isolation is the use of the RK-13 rabbit kidney cell line, in which infection can be identified by cytopathic effect. For laboratory study and neutralizing antibody determinations, many different cell lines (such as RK-13, BHK-21, and LLC-MK_2) can be employed. The highest titers of rubella virus are produced in the BHK-21 and Vero cell lines.

Kinetic studies in tissue culture indicate that virus adsorption is complete within 90 minutes, and the eclipse period lasts about 12 hours. The first new virus noted is cell-associated, and this is followed in 2 to 4 hours by extracellular virus. In primary cell culture, titers of both cell-associated and free virus reach 10^3 $TCID_{50}$/mL by the fourth day; maximum titers (10^5 $TCID_{50}$/mL) are not attained until about the seventeenth day. In all cell systems, chronic infection occurs but is limited in some cultures by the cytopathic effect. Rubella virus plaques in several cell lines.

Animal Susceptibility

Although natural infection is known to occur only in humans, several other primates have been infected experimentally.[285, 339, 355] In addition to primates, rabbits, hamsters, ferrets, guinea pigs, and suckling mice all have been infected with rubella virus.

EPIDEMIOLOGY

In contrast with measles and other diseases with clearly apparent dramatic cycles, knowledge of rubella epidemiology has been acquired primarily over the last 65 years. Major events during this period that stimulated epidemiologic interest were the observation of teratogenicity in 1941,[179] the isolation of the virus in the early 1960s,[340, 502] and the pandemic of 1964. Unfortunately, rubella was not a reportable disease in the United States until 1966, so there are considerable gaps in available information. At present, we are in a new epidemiologic era because of the widespread use of rubella vaccine. Predicting rubella today must take into account the extent and method of vaccine use in the population under surveillance.

Incidence and Prevalence

Epidemic Behavior

The epidemic pattern of rubella incidence in selected areas of the United States in the prevaccine era is presented in Figure 177–1.[66] It generally is stated that the rubella epidemic cycle is one of 6- to 9-year intervals, with each cycle consisting of a build-up and fall in incidence over a 3- to 4-year period.[222, 224] However, a close look at Figure 177–1 suggests that the basic pattern in the prevaccine era was a 3.6-year cycle. Of the 11 peaks from 1928 to 1968, all but two occurred in a 2- to 4-year span with a median of 3 years. Over and above the 3-year cycle is the better known 6- to 9-year cycle of major disease. Pandemics occurred in the periods 1941 to 1944 and 1963 to 1965.

Since the introduction and widespread use of rubella vaccine in the United States, epidemic rubella on a national scale has not occurred. However, in countries in which universal childhood immunization has not been carried out, periodic epidemics continue to occur. Epidemic rubella was documented in the former Czechoslovakia in 1972; in Australia in 1969 to 1970 and 1975 to 1976; in Israel in 1972, 1979, and 1983; in Japan in 1975 to 1977; in Brazil in 1981; and in the United Kingdom in 1971 to 1973, 1978, and 1983.[139, 170, 196, 221, 240, 290, 391, 430, 451, 452]

The incidence of rubella varies with the epidemic cycle, the number of susceptibles within a population group, and the intrapersonal contact within the group. In closed populations such as military training centers and institutions for the mentally handicapped, the attack rate after disease introduction approaches 100 per cent of susceptibles.[225, 226, 265] Disease introduction in the family also affects virtually all susceptibles.[157, 158] In community epidemics, attack rates in susceptibles are estimated to range from 50 to 90 per cent.

Age Groups

The age distribution of reported rubella cases and estimated incidence rates in Illinois, Massachusetts, and New York City for 1966 through 1968 and the entire United States for 1985 through 1987[62] are presented in Table 177–1. In the period immediately before vaccine introduction (1966 to 1968), the attack rate was highest in the 5- to 9-year-old age group, and the incidence was high in preschool age children. The overall reduction in the rate of rubella from the prevaccine era to 1987 was 99.2 per cent. However, 50.2 per cent of the cases reported in the 1985 through 1988 period were in persons older than 19 years of age; in the prevaccine period (1966 through 1968), the percentage in this age group was 10.2. During the last 15 years, rubella outbreaks have occurred in prisons,[65] in colleges and universities,[64] in hospi-

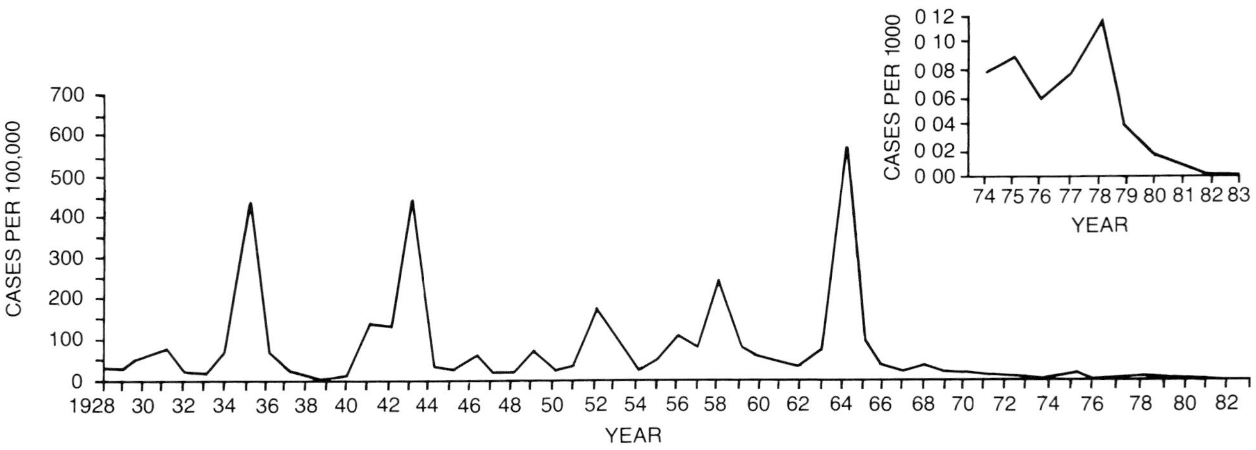

FIGURE 177–1. *Rubella incidence in ten selected areas (Maine, Rhode Island, Connecticut, New York City, Ohio, Illinois, Wisconsin, Maryland, Washington, and Massachusetts) of the United States, 1928 to 1983. (From the Centers for Disease Control: CDC Surveillance Summaries, 1984: Rubellan and congenital rubella surveillance, 1983. M. M. W. R. 33:1SS–10SS, 1984.)*

TABLE 177–1. Age Distribution of Reported Rubella Cases and Estimated Incidence Rates*—Illinois, Massachusetts, and New York City, 1966–1968,† and Total United States, 1985–1987†

Age Group (years)	1966–1968 Average‡		1985–1987 Average§		Rate Change‖ (%) 1966–1987
	%	Rate	%	Rate	
<5	21.6	63.3	24.8	0.6	−99.1
5–9	38.5	101.3	11.8	0.3	−99.7
10–14	17.0	44.0	5.2	0.1	−99.7
15–19	12.7	35.7	8.0	0.2	−99.5
≥20	10.2	3.7	50.2	0.1	−96.5
Total	100.0	24.3	100.0	0.2	−99.2

*Reported cases per 100,000 population. Patients with unknown age are excluded.

†Average annual figures over 3-year period.

‡Represents prevaccine years. National age data were not available before 1975 and were not reported consistently (i.e., >75 per cent of cases) until 1980.

§Total United States data (1986 population projections) are used for 1985–1987; because the overall number of reported rubella cases currently is small, fluctuations (such as the epidemic in New York City in 1985) in only these three reporting areas skewed the data for this period.

‖Based on actual rates.

From Centers for Disease Control: Rubella and congenital rubella syndrome—United States 1985–1988. M. M. W. R. *38*:173–178, 1989.

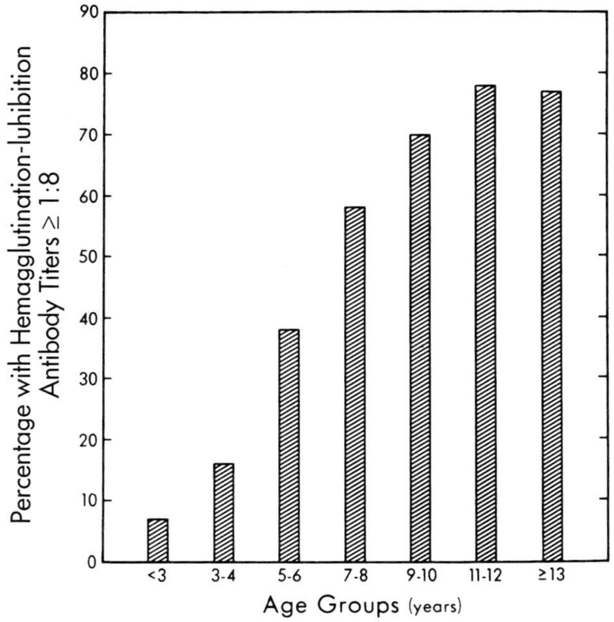

FIGURE 177–2. *The percentage of children with rubella hemagglutination-inhibition antibody titers ≥1:8 in a St. Louis study in 1969. (From Cherry, J. D.: Rubella: Past, present and future. Volta Rev. 76:461–465, 1974. Reprinted with permission from* The Volta Review. *Copyright © 1974 by the Alexander Graham Bell Association for the Deaf, 3417 Volta Place, NW, Washington, DC 20007.)*

tals,[359, 443] among office workers,[63, 67, 171] and among the Amish in six areas of the United States.[60]

Because rubella was not a reportable disease in the United States until 1966, few age-specific incidence or prevalence data relating to epidemic disease are available. In Table 177–2, age-specific attack rates in two communities during epidemic rubella in 1964 are presented.[90] The attack rate curves during epidemic rubella in 1964 are similar to the curve for the prevaccine nonepidemic period from 1966 to 1968 seen in Table 177–1. The overall attack rate during the 1964 epidemic in the two communities was 23 per cent. Eighty-six per cent of the cases occurred in children younger than 15 years of age. In 1993, there were 190 cases of rubella reported in the United States, and of the 187 with known ages, 62.5 per cent occurred in persons 20 years of age or older.[58]

Antibody prevalence by age group in the prevaccine era in the St. Louis area is presented in Figure 177–2.[75] As can be seen, rubella HI antibody prevalence went from less than 10 per cent in children younger than 3 years of age to almost 80 per cent in preadolescents. Surveys of adolescents and young women of child-bearing age conducted before 1969 generally have indicated an immunity rate (HI antibody titer ≥1:8) of about 75 to 85 per cent.[89]

Immunity to rubella as indicated by the curve in Figure 177–2 obviously is affected by epidemic periods. With epidemic disease, the curve itself most probably maintains the same slope, but it moves to the left; antibody prevalence in each age group of children increases significantly (perhaps 10 to 30 per cent). However, studies in the prevaccine era on sera from young adults indicate that the percentage of susceptibles in this age group is affected only slightly by epidemic disease.[89, 139, 412, 419, 511] In a survey of sera from 600 pregnant women in 1962, Sever and associates[419] noted that 17.5 per cent had no detectable antibody. In a similar study in 1966 in which the mean age was slightly less (23.6 vs. 25.6 years), the percentage without detectable antibody was 7.8. Other surveys of rubella antibody in sera of young adults acquired after the 1964 pandemic indicate susceptibility per-

TABLE 177–2. Age-Specific Attack Rates in Two Communities During Epidemic Rubella in 1964

Age Group (years)	Doraville, Georgia			Kingston, Tennessee		
	Total Population	Cases	Attack Rate (%)	Total Population	Cases	Attack Rate (%)
0–4	87	32	36.8	69	30	43.5
5–9	206	104	50.5	127	90	70.9
10–14	208	59	28.4	127	68	53.5
15–19	78	9	11.5	90	25	27.8
20+	427	11	2.6	487	19	3.9
Unknown	8	—	—			
Total	1014	215	21.2	900	232	25.8

From Communicable Disease Center: Morbidity and Mortality Weekly Report *13*:349–360, 1964.

centages in the 15 to 20 per cent range, similar to pre-1964 data.[89, 414, 419]

Effect of Vaccination

Rubella vaccine was licensed for use in the United States and many other countries in 1969, and it has been used extensively for more than 20 years; more than 182 million doses have been administered in the United States.[58, 61, 360] The immunization effort in the United States initially focused on children.[89] A secondary goal was to immunize seronegative postpubertal girls and women of child-bearing age, but little effort was extended in this area until 1978. The overall effect of the immunization effort in the United States on the young adult population is difficult to interpret. As noted in Table 177–1 and subsequent data, the reported number of cases and incidence of rubella decreased significantly from the prevaccine period until the present.[58] There also has been a marked reduction in the number of reported cases of congenital rubella since 1969 (Table 177–3). However, the actual number of cases and incidence of rubella in adolescents and young adults did not decrease until 1981, and 58.2 per cent of all cases in the 1985 through 1987 period were 15 years of age or older (see Table 177–1). Also alarming was the marked upswing in the number of congenital rubella cases in 1990 and 1991.[58] Antibody survey data during the last 17 years indicate that 5 to 25 per cent of the adolescent and young adult population in the United States is susceptible to rubella.[107, 118, 147, 238, 258, 333, 334, 372, 405, 439, 444, 488] In four studies in which rubella antibody prevalence was analyzed by the vaccination status of the participants, differences were significant.[258, 333, 372] Between 87 and 96 per cent of vaccinated persons had rubella antibody, whereas only 70 to 80 per cent of nonvaccinated persons had antibody.

In contrast with the immunization program in the United States, which focused on children and the elimination of epidemic rubella, the immunization efforts in the United Kingdom and many other countries were aimed at girls 11 to 14 years of age and the selective immunization of women of child-bearing age. This approach would not be expected to disrupt the epidemic pattern of rubella but only to decrease disease in young adult women. Serologic surveys in the United Kingdom indicate a significant reduction in the number of seronegative persons in the target population.[85, 190, 304–306, 377, 462] In one study, in which 10,000 serum samples were analyzed, 93 to 96 per cent of females born after 1956 (who would have been offered rubella vaccine in school) were found to have antibody, whereas only 80 to 89 per cent of those born before 1954 were found to have antibody.[85] In spite of the high level of antibody prevalence in women of child-bearing age, rubella infection in pregnancy and congenital rubella continued to be a major problem in the United Kingdom.[306, 462] From 1971 to 1982, there were 625 cases of congenital rubella, and from 1974 to 1981, 3273 women had their pregnancies terminated because of rubella infections or contact with a person with rubella in England and Wales.[462]

In Finland, where initial immunization in 1975 involved 11- to 13-year-old girls, and since 1982, when a two-dose program involving all children was started, the susceptibility in 1992 for 16- to 19-year-old females was 3 to 5 per cent, whereas for males it was 30 per cent.[474]

Congenital Rubella

Congenital rubella was not a reportable disease until 1966, so good data on incidence and prevalence during epidemics of rubella are not available. In the 1964 to 1965 rubella epidemic in the United States, there were 20,000 cases of congenital rubella, 5000 therapeutic abortions performed, an excess in fetal wastage of 6250, and an excess in neonatal deaths of 2100.[89] The National Register for Congenital Rubella was established in 1966, and data for a 25-year period are presented in Table 177–3.

Estimates of the risk of congenital rubella after maternal infection vary considerably among different studies. In general, studies done before 1964, which included nonepidemic periods, tended to underestimate the risk, whereas early retrospective studies after epidemics resulted in high incidence values.[140] Clearly, however, individual risk of congenital rubella depends on the month of pregnancy in which maternal infection occurs. Sallomi[385] analyzed eight published studies that met his rigid criteria and noted the following rates of anomalies by gestational age when maternal infection occurred: weeks 1 to 4, 61 per cent; weeks 5 to 8, 26 per cent; and weeks 9 to 12, 8 per cent. In pregnancies complicated by rubella in weeks 1 to 8, only 36 per cent ended in normal

TABLE 177–3. Number of Cases and Incidence Rates* of Congenital Rubella Syndrome (CRS)† Reported to the National CRS Registry—United States, 1969–1993§

Year	No. Cases	Incidence Rate	Year	No. Cases	Incidence Rate
1969	62	1.7	1982	13	0.4
1970	67	1.8	1983	7	0.2
1971	44	1.2	1984	2	<0.1
1972	32	1.0	1985	2	<0.1
1973	30	1.0	1986	13	0.4
1974	22	0.7	1987	3	<0.1
1975	32	1.0	1988	2	<0.1
1976	22	0.7	1989	1	<0.1
1977	29	0.9	1990	25	0.6
1978	30	0.9	1991	31	0.8
1979	57	1.6	1992	5	0.1
1980	14	0.4	1993	0	0
1981	10	0.3			

*Per 100,000 live births.
†Confirmed and compatible cases reported by year of birth.
§Excluded are the following imported cases: 1984 (one), 1985 (one), 1986 (two), 1987 (three), 1988 (two), 1990 (six), 1991 (two), 1992 (five), and 1993 (one).
From Centers for Disease Control and Prevention: Rubella and congenital rubella syndrome—United States, January 1, 1991–May 7, 1994. M. M. W. R. *43*:391–401, 1994.

live births; 39 per cent ended in abortion or stillbirth, and 25 per cent produced gross fetal anomalies. Peckham[343] noted that 85 per cent of infants born to mothers infected during the first 8 weeks of pregnancy had detectable defects during the first 4 years of life. Infection at other times during pregnancy revealed the following rates of detectable defects: 9 to 12 weeks, 52 per cent; 13 to 20 weeks, 16 per cent; and after 20 weeks, no defect. Other studies indicate a risk of malformations of 3 per cent and a risk of abortion and stillbirth of 4 per cent in situations of conception-rubella intervals greater than 12 weeks.[87]

Infection with rubella virus confers lifelong immunity against clinical illness, but asymptomatic and symptomatic reinfection occurs. Asymptomatic reinfection is common in pregnant women, but this generally has not been considered a risk to the fetus. However, in rare instances, reinfection has resulted in severely damaged babies.[108, 371, 498]

Transmission

It generally is assumed that rubella infection is spread by the respiratory route. Although definitive evidence supporting this assumption is not available, data from volunteer projects and the study of natural disease strongly support this view.[178, 209, 398] Infected persons regularly shed large concentrations of virus in the nose and throat, and droplets of secretions are released into the environment, which allows respiratory-to-respiratory transmission. It also is possible that the initial host may contaminate his or her own hands and then transmit the infectious agent to environmental surfaces or directly to contacts. Under this circumstance, the new host can acquire infection via the fomite-hand-respiratory or hand-hand-respiratory route.

In experimental transmission studies, Green and colleagues[178] noted that efficient transmission of infection to susceptible persons required prolonged, repeated contact; after a brief, single contact, only 1 of 5 children acquired disease, whereas of 17 subjects with prolonged, repeated contact, all but 1 were infected. Although the period of communicability has never been determined accurately, it was noted almost 100 years ago that the period of infectivity preceded the eruptive phase of illness.[180] Volunteer studies indicate the presence of rubella virus in nasopharyngeal secretions from 7 days before to 14 days after the onset of rash.[178, 209] Maximum shedding and presumably maximal transmissibility occur for an 11-day period of 5 days before to 6 days after the appearance of rash. Infants with congenital rubella shed virus from the nose and throat for many months and have been responsible for spread of virus to susceptible contacts.[227, 396]

Seasonal Patterns

Rubella is a winter and spring disease, with the largest number of cases in March, April, and May in the United States.[89, 90] This seasonal pattern occurs in years of both high and low rubella incidence. Presumably, some transmission and sporadic illness occur throughout the year in large urban areas.

Geographic Distribution

Although clinical rubella has gone unrecognized in many countries in Africa, Asia, and South and Central America, serologic surveillance indicates its presence throughout the world.[87] In remote islands, rubella may not be endemic, so that large segments of the population may be susceptible.[43, 212] In these locales, the introduction of rubella results in epidemic infection that involves about 90 per cent of the susceptible population. In populated areas of the world, rubella is both endemic and epidemic, and between 80 and 90 per cent of the adult population have serum rubella antibody.[87] It is interesting to note that in several well-populated large islands (Jamaica, Taiwan, Barbados, Trinidad, Hawaii, and Japan) that are not remote, a smaller percentage of the total population has antibody, and rubella is not endemic.[87, 131, 158, 175]

Other Factors

Sex

The incidence of clinical rubella is similar in boys and girls.[89, 90] In adults, more cases of rubella are reported in women.[89] This finding possibly is the result of interest and concern relating to congenital rubella rather than a true difference on the basis of sex. It is of interest that in rubella vaccine trials, girls have been noted to have higher geometric mean convalescent-phase antibody titers than do boys.[301, 431]

Mitchell and associates[310] studied the IgG, IgM, and IgA antibody responses in men and women to rubella virus structural proteins (E1, E2, and C). Men did not develop IgA E2 antibodies, but women did. Men had lower IgG antibody to E2, an earlier onset of E1-specific IgG and IgM antibodies, and a greater proportion of total antibody against E1 than did women.

Genetics

Hattis and associates[205] showed that individuals differ in their ability to transmit rubella. During a rubella epidemic, they noted a small number of persons who had a high potential for transmitting virus to susceptible persons ("spreaders"). The majority of persons demonstrated only minimal virus transmission ("nonspreaders"). Honeyman and colleagues[217, 218] have suggested that the ability to spread rubella virus is favored by cell-surface antigen HL-A1 or the combination HL-A1 and HL-A8. In a rubella vaccine trial, Spencer and associates[431] noted that 44 per cent of persons with high rubella HI antibody titer (≥1:512) responses had HL-A28. In this study, it also was noted that high convalescent-phase geometric mean antibody titer occurred in subjects with AB blood type.

PATHOLOGY AND PATHOGENESIS

Viral Infection

The sequence of events in uncomplicated, postnatally acquired rubella is presented in Table 177–4. Although much is known about rubella infection in humans, considerable gaps regarding specific events exist.[178, 207–209, 398] Estimates for the timing of events in rubella infection (see Table 177–4) have come from volunteer inoculation studies. In many instances, artificial inoculation has resulted in a reduction in the length of the incubation period of clinical disease. This finding suggests that the size of inoculum is important in the initial generation of human infection. It also helps explain the rather wide boundaries of incubation period noted in many clinical studies.[180, 299, 390]

The primary site of infection is the respiratory epithelium of the nasopharynx. Initial infection of the respiratory epithe-

TABLE 177–4. The Sequence of Rubella Viral Infection in Uncomplicated Primary Disease

Day	Event
0	Rubella virus from the respiratory secretions of an infected person comes in contact with the epithelial surface of the nasopharynx of a susceptible person. Localized infection in the respiratory epithelium is established, and virus spreads via lymphatics and possibly by transient viremia to regional lymph nodes
1–22	Viral replication in localized areas of nasopharynx and regional lymph nodes
3–8	First evidence of nasopharyngeal viral shedding
6–20	Viremia (virus free in serum and associated with leukocytes)
8–14	Establishment of infection in the skin and other viremic sites, including generalized nasopharyngeal involvement
10–17	Maximum viremia and viruria
10–24	Maximum nasopharyngeal viral shedding
17–19	Viremia decreases and then ceases. Viral content at viremic sites rapidly diminishes

From references 178, 207–209, 398.

lium apparently is minor; a more important event is the early spread of virus to the regional lymphatics. In volunteers given 100 $TCID_{50}$ of rubella virus intranasally, viral multiplication at the respiratory site was noted on the third day.[398] After viremia, extensive nasopharyngeal infection occurs. In persons who have received either attenuated or unattenuated virus via the subcutaneous route, nasopharyngeal shedding in varying concentration always occurs.[77, 78, 178, 398] Concentrations of virus generally are greater in specimens collected from the nose than from the throat.

Viremia peaks just before the onset of exanthem and disappears shortly thereafter. In contrast, virus continues to be present consistently in the nasopharynx for a 6-day period after the onset of rash and occasionally for an additional week thereafter.[178] In addition to the blood and nasopharynx, rubella virus has been recovered from the following sites: lymph node,[155] urine,[398] cerebrospinal fluid,[435] conjunctival sac,[207] breast milk,[49] synovial fluid,[211] and lung.[420] Rubella virus was recovered from the skin of rubella patients at sites with rash and without rash.[207, 208]

Immunologic Events

Antibody

After natural or vaccine rubella viral infection, an antibody response regularly occurs. Serum antibodies to different rubella viral antigens can be measured by HI, CF, neutralization, immunofluorescence, precipitation, radioimmunoassay, ELISA, single radial hemolysis, PH, LA, and platelet aggregation.[12, 33, 72, 135, 173, 210, 262, 267, 282, 296, 298, 308, 322, 344, 354, 413, 418, 481, 485, 520] In natural postnatal rubella infection, HI and neutralizing antibodies appear 14 to 18 days after exposure, at the time of the rash. HI antibody titers usually peak about 2 weeks after the onset of clinical illness, stay at a high level for several weeks, decrease about fourfold over a year's time, and then generally persist for life. Immunofluorescence, ELISA, radioimmunoassay, and LA reveal antibody patterns similar to those determined by HI.[210] Antibody detected by PH does not appear until 3 to 4 weeks after illness onset, and that detected by single radial hemolysis is delayed until 1 to 2 weeks after illness onset. In an Amazon Indian tribe, the geometric mean rubella HI antibody titer 12 years after infection, with no intercurrent rubella exposure, was 1:33.[35] The pattern of the neutralizing antibody response is similar to the HI antibody response, except that the peak is delayed slightly. Brody and colleagues[43] noted that all but 10 per cent of an island population had rubella neutralizing antibody 22 years after the time of epidemic illness.

CF antibody first appears about a week after HI and neutralizing antibody, peaks about 1 month after illness, and in general does not persist as long as either HI or neutralizing antibody. Occasionally, the CF antibody response is delayed, appearing 1 month after exanthem, with peak titers 2 to 5 months later. Sever and colleagues[415] noted CF antibodies in only 44 per cent of persons with neutralizing antibody who were studied 10 to 20 years after illness. The employment of an antigen prepared by alkaline extraction has increased the sensitivity of CF, but low levels of antibody still are best identified by HI or neutralization.[354, 401]

After natural infection, precipitating antibodies to both the theta and iota antigens occur.[263] Antibody to the theta antigen appears early, parallels HI antibody, and is persistent. In contrast, the response to the iota antigen is delayed, with a slow rise in concentration over a 2- to 3-month period. Five years after infection, anti-iota antibody cannot be detected.

After immunization, the antibody response pattern varies according to the type of vaccine employed.[34, 262, 330, 353, 354, 394, 492] With RA 27/3 vaccine, the serum antibody response is similar to that after natural disease, except that the peak HI and neutralizing antibody titers attained usually are lower. The serum antibody responses after HPV-77 and Cendehill vaccine viral infections are different from natural infection in that CF and anti-iota antibodies are noted only irregularly and then in minimal concentrations.

Primary rubella virus infection, either naturally acquired or vaccine-induced, is characterized by the initial appearance of antibody in the IgM and IgG serum components.[24, 32, 102, 114, 186, 341, 342, 436] In general, the IgM-specific response is short-lived and not detectable more than 8 weeks after the onset of infection. Occasionally, it has been detected in the serum for extended periods.

IgA nasal HI and neutralizing antibody also regularly occurs after natural viral infection. After immunization, the nasal antibody response varies with the type of vaccine and the route of administration.[7, 103, 104, 330, 354] After subcutaneous immunization with HPV-77 vaccine, rubella-specific nasal IgA antibody is rare; it occurs in most subjects who receive RA 27/3 vaccine administered intranasally and in about half of those vaccinated with this vaccine by the subcutaneous route.

Specific Cell-Mediated Responses

Rubella-specific cell-mediated lymphocyte responses regularly occur after infection with rubella virus.[71, 218, 236, 274, 277, 287, 309, 318, 336, 379, 429, 438, 483, 484] Steele and associates,[438] using an in vitro lymphocyte-mediated cytotoxicity assay, first noted that lymphocytes from persons who previously had rubella caused cell destruction in a tissue culture chronically infected with rubella virus. Rubella antigen-specific cell-mediated immunity also has been demonstrated in lymphocyte cultures by blast transformation, migration-inhibition factor production, and interferon production.[50, 219, 318, 429, 457, 483, 484] With vaccination, rubella-specific cell-mediated immunity first was noted to occur 7 days after immunization, with peak responses at 3 weeks.[483, 484] Honeyman and associates[219] noted that the rubella antigen-specific cell-mediated response commenced 1 week before the humoral immune response in both natural and vaccine-induced rubella viral infections. They also noted that the cell-mediated response was of greater magnitude and duration after natural disease than after immunization. Rossier and associates[378] studied cloistered nuns and noted that specific cell-mediated immunity to rubella virus persisted until 79 years of age in the probable absence of reinfection.

Morag and colleagues[318] demonstrated the specific appearance of cell-mediated immunity in tonsillar lymphoid tissue after natural infection or intranasal immunization with rubella vaccine. This responsiveness was conspicuously low after vaccination by the subcutaneous route. In most instances, the presence of cell-mediated responsiveness correlates with the presence of antibody; specific rubella lymphocyte transformation has been noted in the absence of antibody, however.[429] The magnitude of the rubella-specific cell-mediated response is suppressed during pregnancy.[457]

McCarthy and colleagues[287] identified potential determinants of human cellular immunity to rubella virus using synthetic peptides representing well-defined sequences of rubella virus structural proteins. They employed the following peptide subsequences: two capsid domains (C_1 to C_{29} and C_{64} to C_{97}), a glycoprotein E1 domain ($E1_{202}$ to $E1_{283}$), and a glycoprotein E2 domain ($E2_{31}$ to $E2_{105}$). All but C_{64} to C_{97} subsequences stimulated specific lymphoproliferative responses in peripheral blood mononuclear cells in 25 to 50 per cent of immune subjects. The immunodominant T-proliferative epitope (C_{14} to C_{29}) was recognized by only 50 per cent of the peripheral blood mononuclear cells of the study population. Relatively immunodominant T-cell epitopes vary among different persons.

Nonspecific Responses

A large number of nonspecific, immunologically related responses can be demonstrated during rubella virus infections. Niwa and Kanoh[325] carried out a comprehensive study of these responses in 85 children and adults during a rubella epidemic. They noted a decreased number of total leukocytes, neutrophils, and T cells initially, which returned to normal values within 1 week. Some patients had slightly elevated levels of serum IgM, and total hemolytic complement was elevated in 12 of 30 patients. Marked increases of C_4 and C_9 also were noted. They also noted a marked insensitivity to dinitrochlorobenzene and purified-protein derivative in many patients. Atypical lymphocytes, autoantibodies, and reduced blastogenesis as measured by PHA stimulation were noted in some patients. Other studies consistently have demonstrated a reduction in lymphocyte response to PH.[47, 53, 159, 231, 255, 277, 289] In general, this reduction lasts less than 1 month, and infections with attenuated strains of rubella vaccine virus are less immunosuppressive than are infections with unattenuated rubella virus.

Hyypiä and colleagues[231] noted that during rubella virus infection, the proportion of suppressor-cytotoxic T cells was increased and the proportion of helper-inducer T cells was decreased. Polyclonal activation of B cells was associated with these findings.[230]

Zaknun and coworkers[518] noted a marked increase in urine neopterin levels in two children with acute rubella. Their levels increased dramatically 4 days before the onset of exanthem.

Fetal Events

Viral Infection

A considerable amount of information about fetal infection became available from extensive studies during the 1964 rubella epidemic,[6, 55, 80, 93, 97, 121, 195, 198, 199, 227, 312–315, 350, 366, 396, 397, 442] and further information has been obtained more recently from both natural and vaccine viral infections.[37, 115, 123, 257, 349, 409, 478, 507, 516] In spite of the number and extent of investigations performed to date, we know little about virus transmission to the fetus in maternal infections in the latter half of pregnancy.

With maternal infection during the first trimester, placental infection regularly occurs and often persists throughout the remainder of the pregnancy. In the therapeutic abortion studies of Alford and associates,[6] fetal infection occurred in about 50 per cent of placental infections. However, other studies have revealed almost identical isolation rates from both placental and fetal tissues.[365, 456] Persistent infection is the usual occurrence of first trimester fetal infection. This fetal infection usually involves multiple organs, and at birth, virus regularly can be isolated from the throat, rectum, and urine.[227, 350]

Little is known about events in second and third trimester maternal rubella infections. It is most probable that placental infection is a regular occurrence, and transmission of virus to the infant in utero also may occur regularly. Because few infants born after maternal rubella in the second and third trimesters have defects, careful search for rubella infection in these infants by virologic or serologic methods has been rare. Random studies seem to indicate that virus often does get to the fetus after the first trimester, and occasionally the infection becomes persistent.[100, 115, 199, 227, 316, 486, 505] Other studies have failed to show virologic or serologic evidence of infection in infants in whom maternal rubella occurred in the second and third trimesters.[80, 314, 442]

With maternal rubella infection, the cervix also is involved, so that fetal infection could occur by the ascending route as well as by primary placental infection.[409, 477] Fetal infection also has resulted from maternal disease that occurred before conception.[138, 507, 516]

Rubella virus can be recovered regularly from infants with congenital rubella after their birth. The percentage of infants with persistent infection decreases over the first year of life; by the first birthday, between 10 and 20 per cent of children still shed virus in nasopharyngeal secretions.[97, 366] Rawls and colleagues[366] were unable to isolate virus from the throats of 15 congenitally infected infants after they reached 18 months of age, and Sever and Monif[416] and Cooper and Krugman[97] were unable to demonstrate nasopharyngeal virus persistence in older children. A 4.5-year-old boy with congenital rubella was found on one occasion to be shedding rubella virus in the throat.[421]

Immunologic Findings

SPECIFIC ANTIBODY. Humoral antibody in the congenitally infected fetus is acquired transplacentally from the mother and actively is produced by the fetus. In the normal maternal-fetus relationship, the transport of antibody to the fetus is minimal until the midpoint of the second trimester (16 to 20 weeks).[5, 6] With first trimester maternal infections (transplacentally acquired), rubella antibody titers in serum amount to only about 5 per cent of maternal values. The fetal immune system becomes functional during the second trimester,[259] and small amounts of specific rubella fetal IgM antibody can be detected. From the midpoint of pregnancy, antibody levels in the developing fetus rise so that at birth the maternal and infant values are similar. Although the values of total antibody are similar, the composition is different. Maternal antibody at the time of delivery usually is composed entirely of IgG. In contrast, the infant titer is composed of fetal IgM, presumably fetal IgG, and occasionally fetal IgA and transplacentally derived maternal IgG.

Long-term rubella antibody patterns in congenitally infected infants after birth are different from those of their mothers or from those of a group of children with acquired disease.[94, 198, 240, 471] Cooper and colleagues[94] followed a group of 223 mothers of children with congenital rubella and noted that at the end of 5 years, all still had detectable HI antibody, and the geometric mean titer for the group had undergone a fourfold reduction. In contrast, 5-year follow-up of the congenitally infected infants revealed a 16-fold decline in geometric mean titer; 8 of 29 infants had serum HI antibody titers of less than 1:8 when they were examined at 5 years of age. Others have observed similar declines in rubella antibody titers of congenitally infected infants.[198, 240, 471]

Another unique aspect of rubella antibody in congenitally infected infants is the persistence of specific IgM. Cradock-Watson and colleagues[101] studied 40 infants with congenital rubella and noted that IgM antibody persisted for about 6 months in the majority of cases and up to 2 years in a few children. de Mazancourt and colleagues[283] studied the antibody response to the rubella virus structural proteins in infants with congenital rubella syndrome and found that the immunoprecipitation patterns were different from those in sera from postnatally infected adults. The sera from the congenitally infected infants had little or no C-specific antibody, occasionally only antibody to E1 was precipitated, the E1 protein was precipitated in relative excess of the E2 protein, and the relative amount of E2 antibody was greater than the antibody to E1.

SPECIFIC CELL-MEDIATED IMMUNITY. Rubella-specific cell-mediated immune responses have been studied in children with congenital rubella by the following assays: lymphocyte-mediated cytotoxicity, lymphocyte transformation, lymphocyte interferon production, and leukocyte migration-inhibition factor production.[48, 154] By all methods of study, infants with congenital rubella have decreased rubella-specific cell-mediated responses, compared with persons with previous postnatally acquired rubella. Buimovici-Klein and associates[48] noted that the degree of suppression correlated with the time of in utero infection: the earlier in pregnancy the maternal infection, the greater the depression of specific cell-mediated responses. In the study of an infant with late-onset congenital rubella syndrome, Verder and associates[482] noted decreased activity of killer and natural-killer cells and alloreactive direct cytotoxic cells. Their data indicated that defective cytotoxic effector cell function was the primary cause for the failure to eliminate virus in the illness.

NONSPECIFIC RESPONSES. Desmyter and colleagues[113] noted that infants with congenital rubella produced normal amounts of interferon after measles immunization. They also noted that the clinical response and antibody development in these measles-vaccinated children were similar to those that occurred in normal children. Lebon and associates[260] have noted that sera collected from rubella-infected fetuses and infants with congenital rubella contain an acid-labile interferon. Michaels[300] observed that infants with congenital rubella who still were shedding virus in their throat or urine had depressed antibody responses to diphtheria and tetanus toxoids. White and colleagues[506] noted decreased in vitro lymphocyte blast transformation responses to vaccinia and diphtheria toxoid antigens in children with congenital rubella, compared with normal children. They also noted depressed skin reactivity to intradermal *Candida* antigen in the congenital rubella group. Buimovici-Klein and associates[48] observed a marked reduction in lymphocyte transformation after PH stimulation in their congenital rubella group. The most marked defect was noted in children in whom maternal rubella occurred during the first 8 weeks of pregnancy.

Pathology

Postnatally Acquired Disease

Almost no data relating to the histologic findings in uncomplicated rubella are available, but occasionally postmortem tissue has been studied from patients with encephalitis. Giuliani and associates[168] studied lymph nodes from rubella patients and noted edema, reticulum cell hyperplasia, and loss of the usual follicular morphologic features. Sherman and associates[420] reported six cases of rubella encephalitis and noted the autopsy findings in three cases. They specifically searched all organs for inclusion bodies, syncytial giant cells, focal cellular necrosis, and unusual proliferative changes, but none was found. Only mild, nonspecific, follicular hyperplasia in the spleen and lymph nodes was seen. Histologic examination of the brain of a 7-year-old girl who died of encephalitis revealed diffuse swelling; nonspecific degeneration; and a sparse, mononuclear, perivascular, and meningeal exudate.

The synovial biopsy specimen in a woman with rubella arthritis revealed scattered areas of fibrinopurulent exudate and synovial cell hyperplasia; there was inflammatory cell infiltration composed mainly of lymphocytic cells, and vascularity was increased.[517]

Congenital Infection

In contrast with postnatal rubella, the pathologic process of congenital infection has been studied extensively.[3, 4, 25, 39, 45, 54, 84, 93, 119, 127–130, 145, 150, 151, 183, 192, 194, 195, 237, 243–245, 271, 313, 323, 335, 348, 356, 357, 363, 367, 369, 374, 375, 381, 408, 425, 426, 432, 440, 445, 458, 464, 494, 497, 504, 515] Table 177–5 summarizes the main pathologic findings by anatomic location or system in congenital rubella. As noted, defects in congenital rubella result from both specific cell damage and cellular deficiency. Although specific cellular necrosis is important in certain early lesions, such as the inner ear, of greater overall importance are the secondary effects of generalized vascular damage. Also of presumed major importance is the noncytolytic cellular infection characteristic of rubella virus. This results in mitotic arrest and a reduction in total cells in many organs.

CLINICAL MANIFESTATIONS

Postnatal Illness[74, 79, 137, 140, 178, 182, 248, 256, 299, 390, 398, 469, 503]

Although clinical rubella is a distinctive exanthematous disease, its features are not as clearly discernible as are those of measles or chickenpox. Exanthematous illnesses due to enteroviruses, adenoviruses, and other common respiratory viruses often are clinically similar or identical to rubella (see Chapter 67). Because of these other viral illnesses that simulate rubella, descriptions of clinical rubella made before the availability of modern virologic diagnostic techniques are not always accurate; this particularly is true when rubella in infants and young children is described because exanthems due to other viruses are most common in these age groups. Unfortunately, in spite of the availability of a vast amount of clinical material during the rubella epidemic of 1964, the majority of clinical knowledge relating to postnatally acquired rubella was formulated before the present virologic era.

Incubation Period

Although prodromal complaints and lymphadenopathy frequently precede the exanthem in rubella, the incubation period in most studies has been calculated from the time of exposure to the onset of rash. More than 70 years ago, Michael[299] reviewed the incubation periods in 59 different reports and noted a variation of 5 days to 4 weeks. However, in the majority of reports, the minimum incubation time was

TABLE 177–5. Pathologic Findings in Congenital Rubella

Anatomic Location or System	Gross and Microscopic Findings	References
Placenta	Perivascular mononuclear cellular infiltration in the decidua	335
	Edema, fibrosis, and necrosis of villi; cytoplasmic inclusion bodies noted in swollen Hofbauer cells in villous stroma	
	Perivasculitis, endovasculitis, and perivascular fibrosis also noted	
Generalized growth retardation	Subnormal number of cells in many organs	323
Nervous system	Chronic meningitis with infiltrates of large mononuclear cells, lymphocytes, and plasma cells in the leptomeninges	374, 375, 426, 458
	Vascular degeneration, ischemic lesions, and retardation of myelinization throughout brain	
Eye	Lens: cataract, cortical liquefaction, and spherophakia	39
	Iris and ciliary body: necrosis of ciliary body, iridocyclitis, iris atrophy, and pigmentation defects	
	Retina: posterior pigmentary disturbances	
	Cornea: usually normal; occasional endothelial degeneration	
	Optic nerve: posterior bowing	
Ear	Hemorrhage in the fetal cochlea resulting in epithelial necrosis	150, 151, 494
	Inflammatory cells in the stria vascularis	
	Adhesions between Reissner membrane and the tectorial membrane	
	Sacculocochlear degeneration of Scheibe (strial atrophy, collapse of Reissner membrane, atrophy of the organ of Corti, rolled-up tectorial membranes, and collapse and degeneration of the sacculus) noted after birth	
Cardiovascular	Common heart defects in order of frequency: patent ductus arteriosus, pulmonary artery stenosis, ventricular septal defect, and atrial septal defect (These rubella-induced lesions do not differ from similar nonrubella-induced lesions.)	3, 130, 145, 244, 245, 497
	Myocarditis with swelling of muscle fibers and loss of striations; necrosis	
	Intimal proliferation of major arteries	
Pulmonary	Chronic interstitial pneumonia with large mononuclear cells, lymphocytes, and plasma cells within the interstitial spaces and within the alveoli	245, 348, 426
Liver	Hyalinization and swelling of hepatocytes, hematopoiesis, and multinucleated giant cells	127, 129, 440, 445
	Bile stasis	
Skin	Purpuric lesion: focal areas of erythropoiesis in the dermis and upper subcutaneous adipose tissue	54, 243
	Chronic reticulated rash: acute and chronic inflammatory cells and histiocytes in the dermis	
	Edema in the dermal papillae	
Bone	Thinning of the metaphyseal trabeculae and decrease in the number of osteoblasts and osteoclasts	367, 381, 408, 504
	Many plasma cells in the metaphyses and cartilaginous epiphyses and around vessels	
	Occasional giant cells with cytoplasmic inclusions	
	Thinning of cartilage	
Muscle	Focal abnormalities: very small fibers with darkly staining nuclei and muscle bundles containing empty connective tissue tubes	432
Teeth	Necrosis of the enamel-forming epithelial cells	183, 464
Hematologic	Transient thrombocytopenia with decreased megakaryocytes in bone marrow; increased platelet adhesiveness and platelet agglutinins	25, 84, 357, 363
	Lymph node consistent with histiocytosis; unorganized cell mass made up of mononuclear cells with dense round nuclei and irregularly shaped cytoplasm	
	Spleen: fibrosis	
Immunologic	Loss of normal architecture and absence of germinal centers in spleen and lymph nodes; dysgammaglobulinemia usually with decreased IgG and IgA and elevated IgM	84, 192, 356, 369

14 days or more, and the maximum was 17 to 21 days. The mean incubation period from modern reviews is considered to be 18 ± 3 days.

In carefully controlled studies, Green and colleagues[178] noted an incubation time of 13 to 15 days to the onset of rash after the intramuscular inoculation of serum from rubella-infected patients and a longer incubation time (16 to 21 days) in cases acquired by contact with ill patients. In similar volunteer studies in young adults, Schiff and colleagues[398] noted that the onset of rash occurred 11 to 12 days after the administration of 100 $TCID_{50}$ of tissue culture–grown rubella virus. The investigators attributed this shorter incubation period to a larger inoculum than that occurring in natural transmission.

Prodromal Period

Complaints before the onset of rash in rubella vary with age. In young children, the first evidence of disease usually is the appearance of rash. Occasionally, mild coryza and diarrhea precede exanthem in the younger patient. In contrast with the lack of prodrome in the child, the adolescent and adult usually have symptoms before the onset of rash.[74, 137, 182] In one study, 94 per cent of college students with rubella had prodromal complaints. In decreasing order of frequency, the reported symptoms were eye pain, sore throat, headache, swollen glands, fever, aches, chills, anorexia, and nausea.[137] Gross and associates[182] reported prodromal upper respiratory complaints in 65 per cent of an infected adolescent study group, with malaise, cough, sore throat, red eyes, and runny nose noted.

Prodromal symptoms usually precede rash by 1 to 5 days. In the studies with volunteers of Green and associates,[178] onset of lymphadenopathy commonly was noted 5 to 7 days before the onset of rash. In contrast, Schiff and colleagues[398] observed the appearance of lymphadenopathy only 1 day before rash; fever was noted 1 to 4 days before rash, and most of the volunteers also had malaise and sore throat. Pain on lateral and upward eye movement is common and occasionally distressing.[74, 137]

Exanthem Period

The rubella exanthem appears first on the face. The spread of the rash is centrifugal from the head toward the hands and feet. The progression, extent, and duration of the exanthem vary considerably. In a typical case, the rash involves the entire body during the first 24 hours, begins to fade on the face during the second day, and has disappeared throughout the body by the end of the third day. The characteristic rash is erythematous, maculopapular, and discrete (see Fig. 67–3). Its appearance on the adolescent's face occasionally initially is confused with an exacerbation of acne. Frequently, the rash is only macular with a scarlatiniform appearance. In some, the rash is present for less than a day, although sometimes it persists for 5 days or more. Particularly in the adult, the exanthem frequently is pruritic. This complaint is troublesome because it often leads the patient as well as the physician to attribute the rash to an allergic cause rather than to rubella virus infection.

Occasionally, the exanthem progresses to confluence with a morbilliform appearance. Here the rash usually is less coppery and pinker than measles and heals without desquamation or brownish discoloration. The typical picture of erythema infectiosum (slapped-cheek appearance and reticular rash) has been observed in rubella-infected patients. Balfour and associates[18] reported eight children with erythema infectiosum from whom rubella virus was recovered concurrently and two additional children with serologic evidence of rubella infection. The preliminary results of volunteer studies with a virus recovered from one of the patients in this study produced a slapped-cheek appearance but nonreticulated rash in four of five men. One 3-year-old child from whom the author recovered rubella virus had typical erythema infectiosum.[74] A 14-month-old girl had a roseola-like illness and arthritis.[211]

In the volunteer studies of Schiff and associates,[398] the rash was noted to be pink-red and maculopapular. It appeared initially on the face, chest, upper arms, and shoulders and then spread rapidly over the abdomen, back, and thighs. It developed into an erythematous blush on the face and abdomen. The median duration was 3 days, with extremes of 2 and 5 days. No pruritus was noted.

Rubella infection without rash is rather common. In some, the infection is without symptoms; in other persons, careful questioning reveals prodromal symptoms, and lymphadenopathy is found on examination. Green and associates[178] noted that about 25 per cent of exposed children who became infected had subclinical infection. In an intensive study of 46 susceptible children and adults, all but one subject had clinical symptoms with infection[417]; 60 per cent of the group had both rash and characteristic posterior auricular or suboccipital lymphadenopathy, and 40 per cent had lymphadenopathy without rash. In another study of rubella in an institution for retarded children, Horstmann and associates[226] noted that only about half the children who became infected had rash. Of nine children without rash, five developed significant posterior auricular lymph node enlargement. Buescher[46] reported a subclinical-to-clinical infection ratio in a military recruit population of 6.5:1.

Lymphadenopathy is a major clinical manifestation of rubella. The most characteristic enlargement occurs in the suboccipital and posterior auricular nodes, but there is generalized involvement as well. In the volunteer studies of Schiff and colleagues,[398] the lymph node enlargement usually lasted between 5 and 8 days. In two outbreak studies involving adolescents and young adults, posterior auricular and suboccipital lymphadenopathy was noted in all patients with rash.[137, 182] In contrast with these findings, Landrigan and associates[256] noted that only 47 per cent of children and 58 per cent of adolescents had similar lymph node enlargement during epidemic rubella illness. Although it frequently is suggested that the finding of exanthem and suboccipital lymphadenopathy is pathognomonic for rubella, this is incorrect. In the young child, similar involvement is common with enteroviral and adenoviral infections. In the adolescent and young adult, the association more strongly indicates rubella, but infectious mononucleosis, *Mycoplasma pneumoniae* infection, acquired toxoplasmosis, and other possibilities also must be considered.

The occurrence of fever in rubella varies; when it occurs, the temperature usually is elevated only minimally. In children with experimentally induced rubella, Krugman and Ward[252] noted that 5 of 13 had temperatures of greater than or equal to 38° C (100.4° F). Two children had maximum temperatures of 38.5° C (101.6° F). Schiff and colleagues[398] noted that all nine infected volunteers had fever, with a median duration of 5 days. Landrigan and colleagues[256] found fever in 74 per cent of children and only 47 per cent of adolescents; Gross and associates[182] observed fever in only 6 of 17 adolescents. Occasionally, children with apparent rubella have been noted to have markedly elevated temperatures. Few such cases have undergone virologic study, so some doubt must be raised as to whether the illnesses were induced by rubella virus or were due to other viral agents more commonly associated with marked febrile responses, such as enteroviruses or adenoviruses. The author has seen an 8-year-old boy with virologically and serologically confirmed rubella with a temperature of 40° C (104° F) on the day before the appearance of his rash. The 14-month-old girl with arthritis described by Hildebrandt and Maassab[211] had a temperature as high as 40.5° C (105° F).

In 1898, Forchheimer[141] described what he thought was the enanthem of German measles. He described pinhead-sized macular lesions of a rose-red color on the soft palate and uvula, which appeared at about the time of the exanthem and lasted less than 24 hours. This exanthem has not been identified in children examined by the author; however, petechial lesions on the soft palate and uvula have been seen occasionally. Mild pharyngitis is not uncommon. Other symptoms and signs in rubella include mild conjunctivitis, sore throat, coryza, cough, and headache.

The duration of illness in uncomplicated rubella varies considerably. The majority of patients would continue normal activity if the rash were not present. In general, full return to normal activity occurs within 3 days. A small number of adults are bothered by persistent headache, eye pain, and pruritus for 7 to 10 days.

The white blood cell count in rubella tends to be low. Schiff and colleagues[398] found leukopenia in all nine volunteers. In these subjects, leukopenia paralleled the fever pattern with its onset 24 hours before rash and persistence for 4 to 5 days. Before rubella could be confirmed by both specific serologic and virologic methods, many experts thought that rubella could be confirmed accurately by characteristics of the white blood cell count.[213, 229] Leukopenia was found at the onset of disease; the total count rose to a high-normal value over a 10-day period. Relative neutropenia was noted by Hynes[229] in many patients; one patient had a neutrophil count of 868 cells/mm^3 on the first day of illness. Plasma cells, Türk cells, or both were noted in acute rubella in all cases studied by Hynes[229] and Hillenbrand.[213] A Türk cell is a developing plasma cell that is 25 to 40 μm in diameter and contains a 15- to 30-μm nucleus. The nucleus has two to five prominent nucleoli and a well-defined, light reticulum. The cytoplasm often is vacuolated. Twenty-five per cent of the patients studied by Hynes[229] had elevated erythrocyte sedimentation rates during the first week of illness.

Complications

JOINT INVOLVEMENT. The incidence of reported arthritis and arthralgia varies considerably among different studies.[29, 69, 160, 182, 235, 256, 424, 473, 503] In general, both arthralgia and arthritis are more common in adults than in prepubertal children. Women are afflicted more often than men. In a large outbreak in Bermuda in 1971, 42 per cent of 125 patients studied complained of joint pain or discomfort.[235] Three patients had joint swelling. The prevalence of joint symptoms increased from 18 per cent in the 0- to 9-year-old age group by about 20 per cent increments per decade; 73 per cent of those older than 30 years of age had symptoms. Joint complaints generally were more common in females than in males older than 10 years of age. This difference was most marked in the 10- to 20-year-old age group. Landrigan and associates[256] studied the location of joint symptoms in adolescents and found that the fingers were involved most often; knees and wrists also were implicated commonly.

Yanez and associates[517] studied 11 patients with rubella arthritis. In all instances, multiple joints were involved. The onset of arthritis occurred 1 to 6 days after the beginning of exanthem and lasted 3 to 28 days (mean, 9 days). The erythrocyte sedimentation rate was elevated in three of seven cases, and one patient had markedly positive latex test results. The white blood cell count was below 5000 cells/mm^3 in five of seven patients. One woman had bilateral carpal tunnel syndrome. Four children with transient carpal tunnel syndrome accompanying rubella virus infection have been reported.[36] Panush[338] noted serum hypocomplementemia with rubella arthritis in a 25-year-old woman.

The possibility that rubella viral infection is related to rheumatoid arthritis has been studied on several occasions.[110, 280, 329] Martenis and colleagues[280] reported a 21-year-old woman in whom rheumatoid arthritis evolved after typical rubella with arthritis. Deinard and associates[110] found that all serum specimens from 80 patients with rheumatoid arthritis contained rubella HI antibody. In contrast, only 86 per cent of an equal number of nonarthritic controls and a group of persons with other forms of arthritis had measurable rubella antibody titers. Ogra and associates[329] noted that patients with juvenile rheumatoid arthritis had IgM and IgG serum rubella antibody levels that were four to six times higher than those observed in controls during rubella infection. They also noted specific staining for rubella virus antigen in the synovial fluid of 33 per cent of these patients with juvenile rheumatoid arthritis. Grahame and associates[172] repeatedly recovered rubella virus from the synovial fluid from six cases of inflammatory oligoarthritis or polyarthritis over a 2-year period.

NEUROLOGIC MANIFESTATIONS. Encephalitis is a rare complication of rubella.[2, 23, 42, 83, 91, 109, 122, 279, 295, 324, 376, 420, 435, 490, 509] Sherman and colleagues[420] noted six cases of encephalitis in an epidemic during the spring of 1964, which involved approximately 30,000 children. This rate of encephalitis (1 per 5000 cases) is similar to the rate of 1 per 6000 noted in Detroit in 1942.[279] Rubella encephalitis is similar clinically to encephalitis resulting from measles virus infection but is thought to be less severe. Mortality and morbidity have varied considerably. Sherman and colleagues[420] noted that three of six children studied in Pittsburgh died with this complication during the spring of 1964, whereas in Atlanta during the same epidemic period, six patients recovered uneventfully.

The onset of encephalitis most often occurs 2 to 4 days after the appearance of rash, but occasionally rash and neurologic symptoms occur at the same time; in other instances, the appearance of encephalitis is delayed as much as 1 week after the onset of illness. Examination of the cerebrospinal fluid usually reveals mild pleocytosis (20 to 100 cells/mm^3), with the majority of cells being lymphocytes. The protein is normal or slightly elevated, and the sugar concentration is normal.

Kenny and associates[239] studied seven survivors of rubella encephalitis 1 year after illness and could find no significant loss of intellectual function. Five of the seven had abnormalities on electroencephalography, and two patients had minor neurologic abnormalities. Gibbs and colleagues[164] found abnormal electroencephalographic tracings in 6 of 45 children with uncomplicated rubella.

Other neurologic complications associated with rubella include progressive panencephalitis, carotid artery thrombosis, myelitis, optic neuritis, Guillain-Barré syndrome, and peripheral neuritis.[2, 16, 69, 91, 153, 202, 206, 215, 384, 463, 510, 513, 514]

Of particular interest is the common occurrence of numbness, tingling, and other symptoms consistent with neuritis during rubella infection. Cuetter and John[105] studied 20 patients with complaints of neuritis during rubella and could find no objective sensory deficits or nerve conduction abnormalities.

Wolinsky and colleagues[514] and Lebon and Lyon[261] have described a slowly progressive and fatal nervous system disorder with rubella similar to subacute sclerosing panencephalitis.

THROMBOCYTOPENIA. Thrombocytopenic purpura occurs in rubella with an incidence of 1 per 3000 cases.[25] Children are afflicted more frequently than adults, and girls are affected more often than boys.[18, 185, 273, 319, 337, 437, 438, 495] The median interval between the onset of exanthem and the occurrence of purpura is about 4 days. Occasionally, rash and purpura occur simultaneously; often, the hemorrhagic manifestations do not become apparent until 2 weeks after the exanthem. The illness usually is self-limited, but duration varies from a few days to several months; although deaths due to hemorrhagic complications have occurred, recovery is the general rule.

OTHER COMPLICATIONS. Myocarditis and pericarditis are rare complications of rubella.[155] A 30-year-old woman was noted to have erythema multiforme exudativum and arthritis with apparent clinical rubella.[152] In an outbreak that involved 46 military recruits, testicular pain was a complaint in 25 per cent.[399]

During a rubella epidemic in Japan in 1976 in which 79 patients were studied, 71 per cent were noted to have mild catarrhal or follicular conjunctivitis.[196] Six patients had epithelial keratitis that persisted for 2 to 7 days. Seventeen patients had preauricular lymph node swelling in association with their eye findings. During the same epidemic, 13 cases of hemolytic anemia (including two cases of hemolytic uremic syndrome) were noted after rubella virus infection.[468] During a rubella epidemic in Japan, Sugaya and colleagues[447] found that 7.5 per cent of 241 patients had liver involvement.

Congenital Rubella

From Gregg's original observation in 1941 of congenital defects in babies born to mothers who had rubella during early pregnancy until the pandemic of 1964, the congenital rubella syndrome was considered only to include some combination of abnormalities involving the eyes, ears, brain, and heart. However, observations in 1964, supported by new virologic and serologic techniques, revealed a far more complex congenital rubella syndrome picture: the rubella syndrome was expanded to include many new anatomic findings and to acknowledge the reality of chronic persistent infection.

Congenital rubella is the result of in utero fetal infection, which usually occurs during the first 12 weeks of pregnancy. The fetal infection usually is subacute or chronic and may result in abortion; stillbirth; congenital malformations; active processes at birth, such as thrombocytopenia, encephalitis, or hepatitis; and, rarely, infected infants without defects. Table 177–6 summarizes clinical findings in congenital rubella, an estimation of their frequency, and main characteristics.

General: Infant Death and Growth Retardation[15, 82, 96, 146, 176, 197, 227, 244, 266, 275, 292, 302, 341, 351, 381, 382, 385, 397, 411, 426, 458]

The most common manifestation of congenital rubella, readily apparent at birth, is generalized growth retardation. Between 50 and 85 per cent of all babies weigh less than 2500 g, although gestational age is normal. Virtually all babies with intrauterine growth retardation have one or more other stigmata of congenital rubella. After birth, babies with intrauterine growth retardation often demonstrate continued growth retardation. In some, this is a severe failure to thrive. Others show a normal growth pattern, but the child is proportionally small. The mortality rate of children with congenital rubella during the first year of life is high. Death is related specifically to congenital pneumonia, heart defects and myocarditis, hepatitis, thrombocytopenia, encephalitis, immune deficiency, and failure to thrive.

Eye Findings[15, 26, 39, 88, 92, 96, 128, 146, 162, 169, 176, 197, 199, 201, 227, 244–247, 292, 321, 332, 380–382, 393, 397, 406, 411, 426, 458, 466, 470, 472]

About one-third of all babies with congenital rubella have cataracts. Cataracts may be bilateral or unilateral and are either central in location with a surrounding clear zone or diffuse. In most instances, cataracts are present at birth, but occasionally they are not observed until later in infancy. Retinopathy consisting of pigmentary defects is common in congenital rubella and is useful diagnostically but rarely adversely affects visual acuity. Microphthalmia is relatively common and most often unilateral. Cataracts frequently are associated with microphthalmia.

Congenital glaucoma occurs in about 5 per cent of congenitally infected infants. This defect usually is present at birth, but often it is overlooked. Early diagnosis is important if sight is to be preserved.

Auditory Defects[15, 41, 111, 128, 146, 176, 184, 195, 197, 201, 254, 292, 307, 346, 351, 370, 397, 411, 470, 472, 475]

Sensorineural deafness is the most common manifestation of congenital rubella; almost all patients have some degree of hearing impairment. Hearing loss most often is bilateral but may be unilateral. Frequently, the only manifestation of congenital infection is deafness. It is important to note that deafness is overlooked frequently in infancy, and children incorrectly are considered to be mentally retarded. All children born to mothers who had rubella during the first half of pregnancy should undergo hearing evaluation several times during the first 5 years of life, whether or not they have other manifestations of congenital infection.

Neurologic Findings[15, 92, 98, 111, 112, 133, 176, 195, 197, 201, 227, 244, 245, 292, 346, 348, 351, 375, 376, 381, 382, 387, 388, 397, 411, 426, 446, 458, 466, 493, 500, 501, 508, 509]

Between 10 and 20 per cent of all infants with congenital rubella have active meningoencephalitis at birth. Manifestations of this infection include one or more of the following: a full anterior fontanelle, irritability, hypotonia, seizures, lethargy, and head retraction and arching of the back. Cerebrospinal fluid examination reveals elevated protein and mild pleocytosis. Later neurologic disease, such as mental and motor retardation, can be related to the severity and persistence of the initial meningoencephalitis. Active central nervous system infection has been demonstrated for a year or more.

Behavior disorders are common in children with deafness and often cannot be associated with apparent meningoencephalitis. Congenital rubella children, with generalized growth retardation but a proportionally small head size, often have normal intelligence. In contrast, the prognosis for mental development in a child with true microcephaly is poor.

A small number of adolescents with congenital rubella have developed chronic progressive panencephalitis similar to measles-related subacute sclerosing panencephalitis.

Cardiovascular Findings[3, 15, 16, 128, 130, 145, 146, 197, 201, 204, 225, 233, 244, 245, 316, 411, 422, 423, 426, 458, 470, 487, 497]

In severe congenital rubella with multisystem involvement, myocarditis occurs and often is a cause of death. Of the structural defects of the heart, patent ductus arteriosus is most common. It may be the only lesion noted, but two-thirds of patients have other lesions as well. Pulmonary artery stenosis is the next most common defect. This may involve the main pulmonary artery or its branches. Pulmonary valvular stenosis is the third most frequent defect. Pulmonic valvular or artery stenosis and patent ductus arteriosus commonly occur together.

Other Manifestations[1, 8, 11, 15, 25, 26, 30, 38, 39, 51, 54, 74, 86, 87, 92, 96, 98, 117, 128–130, 144, 146, 166, 176, 191, 192, 194, 195, 200, 201, 227, 234, 243–245, 253, 272, 291, 292, 294, 311, 312, 315, 316, 328, 346, 348, 351, 356, 357, 361–364, 367, 369, 375, 381–383, 397, 408, 410, 411, 425, 426, 432, 440, 445, 458, 489, 493, 504, 508]

The other manifestations of congenital rubella can be separated into three categories: manifestations that are related to

TABLE 177–6. Frequency and Main Characteristics of Clinical Findings in Congenital Rubella Virus Infection

Clinical Findings	Frequency (%)	Main Characteristics	Selected References
General			
In utero death	10–30	Spontaneous abortion; stillbirth	176, 197, 385
Intrauterine growth retardation	50–85	Generalized effect	15, 82, 146, 197, 201, 227, 244, 266, 275, 292, 351, 381, 382, 397, 426, 458
Extrauterine growth retardation	10	Failure to thrive	201, 266, 292, 302, 341, 458
Neonatal and infant deaths	10	Due to pneumonia, heart disease, hepatitis, thrombocytopenia, failure to thrive, immune deficiency, encephalitis	96, 176, 197, 244, 381, 397, 458
Eye			
Cataracts	35	Present at birth	15, 26, 39, 96, 128, 146, 162, 176, 197, 201, 227, 244, 245, 292, 321, 382, 392, 397, 426, 458, 470, 472
Retinopathy	35	Present at birth; usually does not cause problems with vision	39, 88, 96, 162, 176, 197, 227, 246, 247, 292, 470, 472
Microphthalmia	5	Usually associated with cataract	39, 128, 162, 227, 292, 382, 458
Glaucoma	5	Usually present at birth	39, 96, 197, 201, 227, 244, 381, 406, 411
Cloudy cornea	Rare	Usually present at birth; resolves spontaneously	39, 201
Severe myopia	Rare	Usually present at birth; defect may progress	92
Hypoplasia of the iris	Rare	Present at birth	39, 380
Strabismus	5	Associated with other eye defects	199, 292, 332
Iridocyclitis	Rare	Transient; associated with other eye defects	426
Auditory			
Nerve deafness	80–90	May be bilateral or unilateral; moderate or severe; often not recognized early	15, 41, 111, 128, 146, 176, 184, 197, 201, 254, 292, 307, 346, 351, 397, 411, 470, 472, 475
Central deafness	5	Often associated with other central nervous system defects	195
Middle ear damage	5	Usually associated with nerve deafness	370
Intraoral, nasal, and facial			
Cleft palate or lip	Rare		128, 176, 397
Dental abnormalities	Rare		54, 183, 292
Micrognathia	Rare		224, 397
Chronic rhinitis	Rare	Transitory finding	351
High-arched palate	Rare		197
Neurologic			
Motor defects	10	Associated with mental and other neurologic defects	292, 411, 519
Hyperirritability (tremors)	Rare	Transitory finding	376
Microcephaly	Rare		15, 201, 227, 292, 411, 458, 493, 508
Mental retardation	10–20	Associated with other stigmata	92, 176, 195, 197, 290, 411, 446
Full anterior fontanelle	10	Transitory finding related to meningoencephalitis	98, 382
Meningoencephalitis	10–20	Transitory finding but may last for 1 year	112, 201, 244, 245, 351, 381, 426, 458
Spastic diplegia and quadriparesis	Rare	Associated with other stigmata	98, 112
Seizures	Rare	Frequently transitory and related to meningoencephalitis	112, 201, 292, 351
Hypotania	Rare	Transitory defect	111, 112
Brain calcification	Rare		346, 348, 426, 458
Cerebral arterial stenosis	Rare		195
Anencephaly	Rare		397
Encephalocele	Rare		397
Meningomyelocele	Rare		446
Behavior disorders	10–20	Frequently related to deafness	92, 111
Central language disorders	5		133, 176, 501
Autism	5		92, 133, 195
Aqueductal occlusion and/or hydrocephalus	Rare		176, 388
Poor balance	Rare		111, 519
Progressive panencephalitis	Very rare	Has onset during adolescence	466, 500
Cardiovascular			
Patent ductus arteriosus	30	Frequently associated with other defects	15, 26, 128, 146, 197, 201, 204, 233, 245, 316, 411, 426, 458, 470, 497
Pulmonary arterial hypoplasia, supravalvular stenosis, valvular stenosis, and peripheral branch stenosis	25	Frequently associated with other defects	146, 197, 201, 204, 233, 411, 423, 470, 497
Aortic stenosis	2–5		145, 204, 422, 487, 497
Ventricular and atrial septal defects	2–5		26, 128, 411, 470, 497
Tetralogy of Fallot	2–5		128, 201
Myocarditis and myocardial necrosis	10		3, 128, 244, 245, 316, 458, 497
Intimal fibromuscular proliferation of many arteries	5		130
Ventricular aneurysm	Rare		225, 479

Table continued on following page

TABLE 177–6. Frequency and Main Characteristics of Clinical Findings in Congenital Rubella Virus Infection *Continued*

Clinical Findings	Frequency (%)	Main Characteristics	Selected References
Pulmonary			
Interstitial pneumonitis	5–10	May be acute, subacute, or chronic	38, 128, 201, 244, 245, 316, 346, 348, 351, 397, 426, 458, 508
Tracheoesophageal fistula	Rare		397
Respiratory distress	Rare	Secondary to acute pneumonia	292
Gastrointestinal			
Esophageal atresia	Rare		227
Hepatitis	5–10	Associated with other evidence of disseminated disease	15, 128, 129, 201, 312, 315, 440, 458, 501
Obstructive jaundice	5		244, 245, 316, 375, 426
Chronic diarrhea	Rare	Related to failure to thrive and immune deficiency	351, 458
Pancreatitis	Rare	May lead to diabetes in later life	51, 117
Jejunal or rectal atresia	Rare		128
Genitourinary			
Undescended testicle	Rare	Cause-and-effect relationship with rubella infection in doubt	292, 426
Polycystic kidney, ectopic kidney, renal agenesis, or bilobed kidney	Rare	Cause-and-effect relationship with rubella infection in doubt	128, 130, 291
Hypospadias	Rare	Cause-and-effect relationship with rubella infection in doubt	39, 146, 426
Duplication of ureter	Rare	Cause-and-effect relationship with rubella infection in doubt	26
Renal artery stenosis	Rare		294
Hydroureter and hydronephrosis	Rare	Cause-and-effect relationship with rubella in doubt	375
Inguinal hernia	Rare	Cause-and-effect relationship with rubella in doubt	200, 346, 411, 426
Nephritis and nephrocalcinosis	Rare		426, 458
Testicular agenesis	Rare	Cause-and-effect relationship with rubella in doubt	128
Orthopedic			
Bone radiolucencies	10–20	Radiolucencies in metaphyses of long bones	201, 292, 346, 357, 364, 367, 381, 382, 408, 493, 504, 508
Pathologic fractures	Rare		383
Bone deformities	Rare		74, 176, 272
Club foot	Rare		397
Myositis	Rare	Transitory defect	432
Skin			
Dermal erythropoiesis (blueberry muffin syndrome)	5	Transitory defect; usually associated with severe disease	243
Chronic rash	Rare		54, 194
Dermatoglyphic abnormalities	5		361, 362
Dimples	Rare		191
Endocrine			
Diabetes mellitus	Rare		144, 234, 291
Thyroid disorder	Rare		92
Precocious puberty	Rare		92
Growth hormone deficiency	Rare		361
Hematologic			
Thrombocytopenic purpura	5–10	Usually associated with severe disease with high death rate; transitory	15, 25, 26, 30, 96, 146, 201, 227, 244, 253, 292, 346, 351, 357, 363, 364, 381, 382, 397, 411, 489
Hemolytic anemia	Rare	Transitory	311, 346, 363
Hypoplastic anemia	Rare	Transitory	98, 253
Extramedullary hematopoiesis	5–10	Usually associated with severe disease	458
Immunologic			
Thymic hypoplasia	Rare		195
Dysgammaglobulinemia	Rare		87, 192, 356, 369, 425
Asplenia	Rare		222
Reticuloendothelial			
Generalized lymphadenopathy	10		98, 146, 194, 458
Hepatosplenomegaly	10–20	Usually associated with severe disease; transitory	26, 244, 357, 382, 397, 411
Genetic			
Chromosomal abnormalities	Rare	Cause-and-effect relationship with rubella not established	11, 328

active persistent infection, structural defects, and delayed manifestations of congenital rubella.

MANIFESTATIONS RELATED TO PERSISTENT INFECTION. In this category is a broad constellation of clinical events that largely were unknown before the pandemic of 1964. Collectively they frequently are called the expanded congenital rubella syndrome and include interstitial pneumonitis, hepatitis, nephritis, bone radiolucencies, myositis, dermal erythropoiesis, chronic rash, thrombocytopenic purpura, hemolytic and hypoplastic anemia, immunologic deficiency, generalized lymphadenopathy, hepatosplenomegaly, meningoencephalitis, and myocarditis. Most infants with the expanded rubella syndrome clinically have low birth weight; exanthem due to thrombocytopenia, dermal erythropoiesis, or both; hepatosplenomegaly; and jaundice. Radiographs usually reveal long bone radiolucencies. Respiratory distress, due to both diffuse pulmonary disease and myocarditis, is common, and meningoencephalitis usually is evident. The duration of chronic infection in these babies varies. About 20 per cent of the survivors still are shedding virus at 1 year of age. Between 10 and 20 per cent of babies with hepatosplenomegaly and thrombocytopenia die during the first year of life.

CONGENITAL ANOMALIES. Other than deafness, eye defects, and cardiac anomalies, which have been discussed previously, the association of other malformations with congenital rubella infection is less well established. Malformations such as tracheoesophageal fistula, jejunal atresia, inguinal hernia, and others recorded in Table 177–6 occur frequently without evidence of in utero infection. Because they are noted only sporadically in babies after maternal rubella, it is possible that they are chance associations rather than cause-and-effect relationships.

DELAYED MANIFESTATIONS. The following delayed manifestations of congenital rubella that were not present in early life have been noted: endocrinopathies, deafness, ocular damage, vascular effects, and progressive rubella panencephalitis.[410] Of particular importance is the association between endocrine abnormalities and autoimmunity.[86] In one study of 201 deaf adolescents with congenital rubella, 23.3 per cent had positive thyroid microsomal or thyroglobulin antibodies, and of these patients, 19.6 per cent had thyroid gland dysfunction. Patients with congenital rubella have an increased incidence of insulin-dependent diabetes mellitus.[166]

DIAGNOSIS

Differential Diagnosis

Postnatally Acquired Disease (See also Chapter 67.)

Because there is no pathognomonic finding in rubella, the clinical diagnosis in the individual case often is difficult. However, as with other exanthematous diseases, the key to diagnosis is the careful elicitation of historical data. Rubella is an epidemic disease with a high clinical expression rate of exanthem. Therefore, it is unusual, when proper investigation is carried out, not to find the contact case or other cases in the community. Season also is an important consideration. Rubella generally occurs in the winter and spring, whereas enteroviral exanthems, which are the greatest masqueraders in young children, mainly occur in the summer and fall.

The incubation period also is important in separating German measles from exanthems due to common enteroviruses or respiratory viruses. In rubella, the incubation period is long (18 ± 3 days), whereas in the other illnesses, the period usually is short (from 3 to 7 days). Age is important. Today, rubella mainly is an illness of adolescents and young adults, and enteroviral exanthems are uncommon in these ages.

The nature of fever is useful in the diagnosis of rubella. Fever greater than 38.5° C (101.5° F) is unusual in rubella but common with enteroviral exanthems, measles, and *M. pneumoniae* infection. Generally, a past history of rubella infection is not particularly reliable. However, if a past illness can be documented by year, season, and symptoms, accurate information may be obtained. Useful characteristics of the rubella exanthem are its mild, erythematous, maculopapular, and discrete nature; marked pruritus in adolescents and adults; and an acneiform appearance on the face in adolescents.

Although suboccipital and posterior auricular lymphadenopathy often is thought by some to be pathognomonic, its presence in nonrubella exanthems often leads to undue concern. In general, in the young child, suboccipital and posterior auricular lymphadenopathy is as common with enteroviral illnesses as with rubella. In young adults, however, this lymphadenopathy is much more useful because the enteroviral differential consideration is less of a problem. Similar lymphadenopathy does occur with acquired toxoplasmosis, infectious mononucleosis, and *M. pneumoniae* infection. A major problem in differential diagnosis in the adult is allergy. However, fever (even low-grade), lymphadenopathy, headache, and eye pain, which are common in rubella, rarely should occur in contact or other simple allergies.

Congenital Rubella

The diagnosis of congenital rubella in known maternal exposure generally is not difficult. However, it is important to examine an apparently normal child at periodic intervals during the first few years of life so that deafness and subtle neurologic defects are not missed. The diagnosis of congenital rubella after an uneventful pregnancy is more difficult. All babies with evidence of intrauterine growth retardation or stigmata suggestive of congenital infection should undergo virologic and serologic study for rubella as well as for other infectious agents. Determination of the amount of serum IgM also can be useful in the study of babies with intrauterine growth retardation or babies born to mothers in whom suspected rubella or other infection occurred during pregnancy.[442] Values greater than 21 mg/dL during the first week of life strongly indicate congenital infection; normal values do not rule out congenital infection, however.

Specific Diagnosis

Postnatally Acquired Disease

Rubella viral infection can be diagnosed specifically by viral isolation from nasal or throat specimens in AGMK tissue culture or other sensitive tissue culture systems; by the observation of a significant change in value of HI, ELISA, immunofluorescence, CF, or neutralizing antibody in two sequential serum samples; or by the demonstration of specific rubella IgM antibody in a single serum sample. Most often today, the diagnosis of rubella is attempted by the use of a single serum test for identifying rubella IgM antibody.[10, 19, 27, 28, 56, 70, 73, 104, 125, 136, 143, 167, 220, 278, 297, 320, 342, 404, 427, 481] Although this is practical, it should be realized that the specificity and sensitivity of all routinely used tests is not 100 per cent. False-positive results are all too frequent and commonly lead to unnecessary interventions. When the diagnosis is critical, such as with suspected rubella in pregnancy, it is wise to study IgG antibody in paired sera collected 1 to 2 weeks apart in addition to IgM antibody determination.

HI has been the standard serologic diagnostic test, and the demonstration of a fourfold or greater titer rise is reliable evidence of rubella infection. Today, however, HI rarely is available to the clinician. The usual test available is ELISA, and in most commercial laboratories, the ability to determine a significant change in value from acute phase to convalescent phase should be questioned.

Congenital Rubella

The best method for the definitive diagnosis of congenital rubella is viral isolation. Specimens for viral culture should be obtained from the nose, throat, urine, buffy coat of the blood, and cerebrospinal fluid. Because of the transplacental passage of maternal IgG, the establishment of the diagnosis of congenital rubella in the neonatal period by serologic methods is fraught with difficulty. Usually, specific rubella IgM antibody can be demonstrated with presently available techniques. In questionable cases, follow-up studies comparing infant and maternal antibody values often establish the diagnosis. If the infant's value solely is the result of transplacentally acquired antibody, it should drop fourfold to eightfold by 3 months of age and continue to fall to nondetectable values by 6 to 8 months of age. However, the antibody value in some congenital infections also may fall, so that the disappearance of antibody in the serum does not rule out in utero infection completely.

Qualitative Demonstration of Rubella Antibody

The original screening method for rubella antibody was HI. Today, HI has been replaced by more rapid and easier tests. These tests employ enzyme immunoassays, erythrocyte agglutination, and LA. In general, all are both highly sensitive and specific.[72, 135]

TREATMENT

Postnatally Acquired Disease

Uncomplicated Rubella

No specific therapy is necessary or indicated in uncomplicated rubella. Starch baths may be useful for the adult with troublesome pruritus. It is important that the affected patient understand that he or she is contagious and that transmission of infection to a pregnant woman could have serious consequences.

Complications of Rubella

Occasionally, in adults, arthritis can be severe. When weight-bearing joints are affected, rest is encouraged. Symptoms readily respond to aspirin therapy; corticosteroids are not indicated. In rubella encephalitis, care is supportive, with adequate maintenance of fluids and electrolytes.

Thrombocytopenia usually is self-limited; however, severe bleeding has occurred on occasion. Splenectomy is not indicated. Corticosteroid therapy often is employed, but there is little evidence of specific benefit in the rubella-infected patient. In patients who do not recover rapidly and in those with severe bleeding, treatment with intravenous immunoglobulin should be considered.

Management of the Exposed Pregnant Woman

Ideally, all pregnant women previously should have received rubella vaccine or been shown to have rubella antibody by an appropriate serologic test. If a pregnant woman is exposed to a person with rubella and the history of previous immunization or antibody presence is unknown, an immediate blood specimen should be obtained and a rubella antibody test performed. If antibody to rubella is demonstrated, no action is necessary. Susceptible rubella-exposed women should undergo careful clinical observation for fever, lymphadenopathy, or exanthem for a 4-week period. If illness occurs, a nasal specimen should be cultured for rubella virus and serum should be examined for rubella IgM antibody. A second serum specimen should be submitted for rubella antibody examination. If illness occurred, this should be collected 1 to 2 weeks later; if the women had no illness, the second serum should be collected 6 to 8 weeks after the exposure. If rubella antibody seroconversion is noted or specific IgM antibody demonstrated, there is considerable risk for fetal infection and malformation. Because false-positive rubella IgM antibody test results are not rare, it is wise to repeat all tests that yield positive results (by another assay and in another laboratory if possible) for confirmation. The patient should be so advised and therapeutic abortion contemplated.

In situations of known exposure of a susceptible pregnant woman in which therapeutic abortion is not possible and exposure can be documented to have taken place within 72 hours, it is the author's opinion that 20 mL of immunoglobulin should be administered immediately. The use of immunoglobulin is controversial, but in certain controlled situations, it has been effective in preventing disease.[43, 303, 395, 476]

Management of the Pregnant Woman with an Exanthem Thought to Be Rubella

In this circumstance, if previous rubella serologic study results are available, they are extremely useful. If previous serum antibody has been noted, the mother should be reassured that the present illness is not likely to be rubella. However, because false-positive rubella screening results do occur, it is wise to carry out rubella serologic study and, when possible, also viral culture. An acute-phase serum should be examined for rubella-specific IgM antibody. A second serum specimen should be collected 1 to 2 weeks after the disappearance of the rash. If rubella antibody rose significantly or IgM antibody was demonstrated, it is highly likely that congenital infection has occurred and that anomalies may result. Again, it is wise to confirm IgM-positive test results. In this circumstance, the woman should be counseled about therapeutic abortion.

If a previous serum rubella antibody value is not available, a serum should be collected immediately and another 2 to 3 weeks later. These sera should be examined as paired specimens for rubella antibody and examined for specific rubella IgM antibody. If a rubella antibody rise is demonstrated or the presence of rubella IgM is noted, it must be assumed that an acute rubella viral infection has occurred, and the patient should be advised about the risk of congenital infection and the possibility of therapeutic abortion.

Management of Children with Congenital Rubella

Isolation Procedures

Most babies with congenital rubella still are infected actively at the time of birth, are contagious, and, therefore, should be placed in isolation. Room isolation and urine precautions are the major necessities. The isolated baby should be cared for only by persons known to be seropositive for rubella. Because rubella viral shedding has been known to occur for a year or more in some babies, isolation of infants with congenital rubella should be continued for this duration unless repeated viral cultures have proved negative.

After discharge from the hospital, no special precautions are necessary in the household setting. However, the parents should be advised of the potential risk to pregnant visitors.

Neonatal Period

As noted, the clinical manifestations of congenital rubella are varied, and in many infants, no symptoms are manifested during the first few months of life. In these apparently asymptomatic infants, no particular management problems are encountered. In other neonates, the symptoms of the continued viral infection readily are apparent and frequently are severe. In these infants, the following findings are important: pneumonia, thrombocytopenia, eye findings, heart defects, hyperbilirubinemia, and hepatosplenomegaly.

Although purpura and petechiae secondary to thrombocytopenia may be impressively severe in these infants, true hemorrhagic difficulties have not been a major problem. Corticosteroid therapy does not seem indicated, but it might be worthwhile to consider treating with intravenous immunoglobulin. Careful evaluation of the eyes is important. Of immediate concern is the search for corneal clouding because this probably indicates infantile glaucoma. Cataracts and retinopathy also should be sought carefully. Infants with glaucoma should be referred immediately for ophthalmologic evaluation and therapy. Children with cataracts or retinopathy also should be referred, but therapy for cataracts best is delayed until a later age.

Respiratory distress secondary to extensive viral involvement should be managed similarly to other neonatal respiratory disease: assisted ventilation and careful attention to arterial blood gas pressures and pH. Although jaundice secondary to congenital rubella infection rarely is severe, standard criteria for the treatment of hyperbilirubinemia should be followed. Hepatosplenomegaly may be marked in some instances but is of no therapeutic concern.

Cardiac evaluation should be the same as in affected infants without rubella. Specifically, congestive cardiac failure should be treated vigorously; in malignant conditions (patent ductus arteriosus, coarctation of the aorta), lifesaving surgery should be contemplated.

Long-Term Problems

DEAFNESS. Hearing disability is the most frequent abnormality after congenital rubella infection; more than 80 per cent of infected infants have some degree of hearing disability. In many instances, deafness is the only clinical manifestation of congenital rubella, and because of the difficulty in making this diagnosis in early infancy, diagnosis frequently is delayed. However, early diagnosis of deafness and the institution of proper educational programs are the most productive aspects in long-term management of children with congenital rubella. All too frequently, poor medical advice has delayed appropriate diagnosis and therapy. Any time that a mother suspects that her child is deaf, specific audiometric testing should be performed. Many general practitioners, pediatricians, and even otolaryngologists believe that hearing cannot be tested in infants. This concept must be discouraged vigorously; at proper centers, the severely deaf child can be recognized in virtually all instances.

If deafness is diagnosed, the child should be referred immediately to a training program. Information about training programs can be obtained from the Alexander Graham Bell Association for the Deaf, Inc., 1537 35th Street, N.W., Washington, DC 20007; and The John Tracy Clinic, Inc., 806 West Adams Boulevard, Los Angeles, CA 90007. In virtually all instances, severely deaf children should be enrolled in an education program before or during the second year of life, and the child should be fitted with a proper auditory amplification device. Although deafness in congenital rubella is sensorineural, it is surprising that conduction defects also are noted in many older children. For these, other aspects of otolaryngologic care may be indicated.

EYE PROBLEMS. All children with eye problems (cloudy cornea, glaucoma, cataracts, retinitis, strabismus) should be referred at an early age for ophthalmologic evaluation. Glaucoma needs immediate attention. Cataract surgery should be left to the discretion of the ophthalmologist but in general is well deferred until after the end of the first year. Retinopathy, although frequently impressive on ophthalmoscopic examination, rarely causes much visual defect. Strabismus is managed as it is in children without rubella. Advice on eye problems in congenital rubella can be obtained from the American Foundation for the Blind, Inc., 15 West 16th Street, New York, NY 10011.

HEART PROBLEMS. Congenital heart disease secondary to in utero rubella infection should be managed as heart disease is in children without rubella. It is important that the children be referred to cardiac centers where sophisticated diagnostic techniques and cardiac surgery facilities for correctable lesions are available.

MUSCULOSKELETAL PROBLEMS. Isolated musculoskeletal defects are relatively uncommon in congenital rubella. However, when the symptoms indicate, referral to a cerebral palsy clinic is useful, both for specific therapeutic modalities and for the camaraderie of group therapy for the children as well as the parents.

CENTRAL NERVOUS SYSTEM PROBLEMS. A careful analysis of available data suggests that many infants who have been labeled retarded really are children with auditory or visual defects who have not had proper diagnosis and training for their handicaps. No child with congenital rubella should be labeled mentally subnormal until extensive audiologic and ophthalmologic investigations and perhaps specific therapy have been performed. Probably only about 10 per cent of all congenitally infected rubella children have a central nervous system defect that precludes normal development.

IMMUNOLOGIC DEFECTS. A small number of children with congenital rubella have been noted with specifically low levels of serum IgG. These infants have systemic continued viral infection and in general do poorly. Although outcome studies are not available, it seems prudent to administer immune serum globulin (intramuscular or intravenous immunoglobulin) to these infants periodically.

MULTIPLE HANDICAPS. All too frequently, children infected in utero with rubella virus suffer from one or more of the handicaps mentioned. The care of these infants and children requires many different resources and modalities of therapy. Frequently, it is the physician who is called upon to coordinate both the diagnostic and long-term educational efforts that are necessary for the optimal progress of an affected child. In addition to the Alexander Graham Bell Association for the Deaf, The John Tracy Clinic, and the American Foundation for the Blind, already mentioned, the following agencies may be helpful to the physicians or parents of congenital rubella children: United Cerebral Palsy Research and Educational Foundation, Inc., 66 East 34th Street, New York, NY 10016; Easter Seal Research Foundation, 2023 West Ogden Avenue, Chicago, IL 60612; National Association for Retarded Citizens, Research and Demonstration Institute, 2709 Avenue E East, Arlington, TX 76011; Bureau of Education for the Handicapped, Office of Education, 400 Maryland Avenue, S.W., Washington, DC 20202; and Maternal and Child Health Division, Department of Health and Human Services, Parklawn Building, 5600 Fishers Lane, Rockville, MD 20852.

PREVENTION

Active Immunization: Live Attenuated Rubella Virus Vaccine

At present, one attenuated rubella virus vaccine is available for use in the United States (RA 27/3 strain grown in

WI38 human embryonic lung tissue culture). Vaccination can be expected to produce antibodies in more than 95 per cent of those immunized.[17, 269, 394, 431, 492] Antibody titers after RA 27/3 vaccine are slightly lower than those after natural infection, but they have been demonstrated to persist for an 11- to 15-year period with a pattern similar to that following natural infection, even in the absence of re-exposure to rubella virus.[34, 223, 352]

Because of universal immunization, rubella in the United States currently is at an all-time low, but indigenous cases still occur.[58] Finland's vigorous two-dose immunization program has resulted in the elimination of indigenous rubella.[345]

Recommendations for Use

For complete information regarding rubella immunization, the reader is referred to the most recent recommendations of the Immunization Practices Advisory Committee of the U.S. Public Health Service,[57, 61] the recommendations of the Committee on Infectious Diseases of the American Academy of Pediatrics,[9] and the vaccine manufacturer's product information.

Rubella vaccine is recommended for all children 12 months of age or older, adolescents, and adults, particularly women, unless it otherwise is contraindicated. The vaccination of children protects them from rubella and thus prevents their subsequently spreading it. Vaccinating susceptible postpubertal women confers individual protection from rubella-induced fetal injury. Vaccinating adolescents or adults in population groups such as those in colleges, places of employment, or military bases protects them from rubella and reduces the chance of epidemics in partially immune groups.

Rubella vaccine should not be administered to infants younger than 1 year of age because persisting maternal antibodies may interfere with seroconversion. When the rubella vaccine is part of a combination vaccine that includes the measles antigen, it should be administered to children about 12 to 15 months of age. A second dose of measles-mumps-rubella vaccine is recommended at school entry. Children who have not received rubella vaccine at the optimal age should be vaccinated promptly. Because a history of rubella is not a reliable indicator of immunity, all children for whom vaccine is not contraindicated should be vaccinated.

Vaccinating all unimmunized prepubertal children and adolescents as well as adult females in the child-bearing age group must be emphasized. Because of the theoretic risk to the fetus, females of child-bearing age should receive vaccine only if they are not pregnant and understand that they should not become pregnant for 3 months after vaccination.

Educational and training institutions, such as colleges, universities, and military bases, should seek proof of rubella immunity (a positive serologic test or documentation of previous rubella vaccination) from all students and employees in the child-bearing age. Nonpregnant women who lack proof of immunity should be vaccinated unless contraindications exist.

For the protection of susceptible female patients and female employees, persons working in hospitals and clinics who might contract rubella from infected patients or who, if infected, might transmit rubella to pregnant patients either should have serologically demonstrated immunity to rubella or should receive the vaccine.

Routine premarital serologic testing for rubella immunity would enhance efforts to identify susceptible women before pregnancy. Prenatal or antepartum screening for rubella susceptibility should be undertaken and vaccine administered in the immediate postpartum period—before hospital discharge. Previous administration of anti-Rho (D) immunoglobulin (human) or blood products is not a contraindication to vaccination; however, 6- to 8-week postvaccination serologic testing should be performed on those few who have received the globulin or blood products for confirming seroconversion. Obtaining laboratory evidence of seroconversion in other vaccinees is not necessary.

There is no evidence that live rubella virus vaccine given after exposure prevents illness or that vaccinating a person incubating rubella is harmful. However, because a single exposure may not result in infection and postexposure vaccination would protect a person in the event of future exposure, vaccination is recommended unless it otherwise is contraindicated.

Adverse Reactions

Vaccination in young children rarely is associated with any symptoms. Occasionally, rash, lymphadenopathy, mild fever, and upper respiratory symptoms have been observed.

More severe reactions have been noted rarely in children but have been an occasional problem in adults. Most of these complications were reported in association with the previously available vaccines, but complications with RA 27/3 vaccine have been noted.[17, 120] Particularly troublesome are arthralgia and arthritis.[14, 22, 95, 174, 268, 317, 331, 358, 434, 453–455, 462, 491] These complaints are most common in adults. Approximately 25 per cent of susceptible postpubertal females develop arthralgia after RA 27/3 vaccination, and approximately 10 per cent have been reported to have arthritis-like signs and symptoms.[31, 181, 358] Infrequently, susceptible vaccinees, primarily adult women, reportedly have developed chronic or recurrent arthralgias, sometimes with arthritis or neurologic symptoms, including paresthesias, carpal tunnel syndrome, and blurred vision.[61, 228] One group of investigators has reported the frequency of chronic joint symptoms and signs in adult women to be as high as 5 to 11 per cent[459–461]; however, other data from the United States and other countries suggest that such occurrences due to RA 27/3 vaccine are rare or perhaps nonexistent.[95, 142, 148, 203, 327, 428, 433]

Other complications mainly with vaccines other than RA 27/3 include polyneuropathies (catcher's crouch, carpal tunnel syndrome, neuritis, and myeloradiculoneuritis),[76, 81, 165, 188, 241, 326, 389] marked lymphadenopathy,[74] and vasculitis and myositis.[193]

Geiger and associates[161] noted a persistent rubella virus infection in 16-year-old boy with acute lymphoblastic leukemia in remission who was vaccinated. The virus was identified in the patient's peripheral blood mononuclear cells 8 months after immunization. In contrast, persistent infection could not be demonstrated in 10 children with symptomatic HIV-1 infection.[149]

Contraindications

Live rubella virus vaccine is contraindicated in pregnancy; in altered immune states, such as immunodeficiency, leukemia, lymphoma, and generalized malignancy; or in therapy with steroids, alkylating drugs, antimetabolites, and radiation. Also, rubella vaccination should not be performed during febrile illnesses or when viral interference from another agent might preclude a "take" from the rubella immunization. Rubella immunization also, in most instances, should be deferred for 3 months after the administration of blood products, including immune serum globulin.

Inadvertent Rubella Immunization in Pregnancy

From January 1971 to April 1989, the Centers for Disease Control and Prevention followed to term 321 known rubella-susceptible pregnant women who had been vaccinated with rubella vaccine within 3 months before or 3 months after conception.[61] Ninety-four women received HPV-77 or Cendehill vaccines; 1 received vaccine of unknown strain; and 226 received RA 27/3 vaccine. None of the 324 infants born to these pregnancies had malformations compatible with congenital rubella, but 5 of the infants had serologic evidence of subclinical infection.

Passive Immunization

The use of immunoglobulin for the prevention of rubella has been controversial for many years.[21, 44, 116, 177, 276, 284, 288, 303, 395, 476] However, it is the author's opinion that its use is indicated under certain circumstances. The specific indication for immune serum globulin is for the prevention of rubella in a woman thought to be susceptible to rubella who is in the first 20 weeks of pregnancy. If an exposure can be documented clearly as one to a specific, single person with rubella and the immunoglobulin is given within 72 hours of that exposure, prevention of both maternal disease and congenital infection is likely. On the other hand, if the exposure were more general in nature (a school teacher exposed to a child or children in the school setting), it is likely that the woman actually was exposed a considerable period of time before her realization of that exposure. Therefore, administration of immunoglobulin probably will be too late (well into the incubation period of her disease and after viremia), so congenital infection is unlikely to be prevented. The dose of immunoglobulin for the prevention of rubella during pregnancy is 20 mL intramuscularly.

Quarantine and Disease Containment

Patients with rubella should not have contact with susceptible persons until the rash has disappeared. Rubella containment is a vital part of the prevention policy in the United States today. Rubella is a reportable disease, and compliance is the obligation of all physicians and other health professionals. Rubella reporting enables public health workers to organize vaccination programs so that small outbreaks of disease can be prevented from developing into major epidemics.

References

1. Achs, R., Harper, R. T., and Siegel, M.: Unusual dermatoglyphic findings associated with rubella embryopathy. N. Engl. J. Med. *274*:148–150, 1966.
2. Aguado, J. M., Posada, I., Gonzalez, M., et al: Meningoencephalitis and polyradiculoneuritis in adults: Don't forget rubella. Clin. Infect. Dis. *17*:785–786, 1993.
3. Ainger, L. E., Lawyer, N. G., and Fitch, C. W.: Neonatal rubella myocarditis. Br. Heart J. *28*:691–697, 1966.
4. Alford, B. R.: Rubella: La bête noire de la médecine. Laryngoscope *78*:1623–1659, 1968.
5. Alford, C. A., Jr.: Studies on antibody in congenital rubella infections. I. Physicochemical and immunologic investigations of rubella-neutralizing antibody. Am. J. Dis. Child. *110*:455–463, 1964.
6. Alford, C. A., Jr., Neva, F. A., and Weller, T. H.: Virologic and serologic studies on human products of conception after maternal rubella. N. Engl. J. Med. *271*:1275–1281, 1964.
7. Al-Nakib, W., Best, J. M., and Banatvala, J. E.: Rubella-specific serum and nasopharyngeal immunoglobulin responses following naturally acquired and vaccine-induced infection: Prolonged persistence of virus-specific IgM. Lancet *1*:182–185, 1975.
8. Alter, M., and Schulenberg, R.: Dermatoglyphics in the rubella syndrome. J. A. M. A. *197*:685–688, 1966.
9. American Academy of Pediatrics: Section 1 and rubella. *In* Peter, G. (ed.): 1994 Red Book: Report of the Committee on Infectious Diseases. 23rd ed. Elk Grove Village, American Academy of Pediatrics, 1994, pp. 7–72; 406–412.
10. Ankerst, J., Christensen, P., Kjellen, L., et al.: A routine diagnostic test for IgA and IgM antibodies to rubella virus: Absorption of IgG with *Staphylococcus aureus*. J. Infect. Dis. *130*:268–273, 1974.
11. Ansari, B. M., and Mason, M. K.: Chromosomal abnormality in congenital rubella. Pediatrics *59*:13–15, 1977.
12. Appleton, P. N., and Macrae, A. D.: Comparison of radial haemolysis with haemagglutination inhibition in estimating rubella antibody. J. Clin. Pathol. *31*:479–482, 1978.
13. Atkinson, I. E.: Rubella (Rotheln). Am. J. Med. Sci. *93*:17–34, 1887.
14. Austin, S. M., Altman, R., Barnes, E. K., et al.: Joint reactions in children vaccinated against rubella. Study I: Comparison of two vaccines. Am. J. Epidemiol. *95*:53–66, 1972.
15. Avery, G. B., Monif, G. G. R., Sever, J. L., et al.: Rubella syndrome after inapparent maternal illness. Am. J. Dis. Child. *110*:444–446, 1965.
16. Bailey, G.: Carpal-tunnel syndrome. B. M. J. *1*:1207, 1962.
17. Balfour, H. H., Jr., Balfour, C. L., Edelman, C. K., et al.: Evaluation of Wistar RA27/3 rubella virus vaccine in children. Am. J. Dis. Child. *130*:1089–1091, 1976.
18. Balfour, H. H., Jr., May, D. B., Rotte, T. C., et al.: A study of erythema infectiosum: Recovery of rubella virus and echovirus-12. Pediatrics *50*:285–290, 1972.
19. Banatvala, J. E., Best, J. M., Bertrand, J., et al.: Serological assessment of rubella during pregnancy. B. M. J. *3*:247–250, 1970.
20. Bardeletti, G., Kessler, N., and Aymard-Henry, M.: Morphology, biochemical analysis and neuraminidase activity of rubella virus. Arch. Virol. *49*:175–186, 1975.
21. Barenberg, L. H., Levy, W., Greenstein, N. M., et al.: Prophylactic use of human serum against contagion in a pediatric ward: Further observations, with special reference to measles and rubella. Am. J. Dis. Child. *63*:1101–1109, 1942.
22. Barnes, E. K., Altman, R., Austin, S. M., et al.: Joint reactions in children vaccinated against rubella. Study II: Comparison of three vaccines. Am. J. Epidemiol. *95*:59–66, 1972.
23. Barraclough, W. W.: German measles encephalomyelitis. Can. Med. Assoc. J. *36*:511–513, 1937.
24. Baublis, J. V., and Brown, G. C.: Specific response of the immunoglobulins to rubella infection. Proc. Soc. Exp. Biol. Med. *128*:206–210, 1968.
25. Bayer, W. L., Sherman, F. E., Michaels, R. H., et al.: Purpura in congenital and acquired rubella. N. Engl. J. Med. *273*:1362–1366, 1390–1391, 1965.
26. Bellanti, J. A., Artenstein, M. S., Olson, L. C., et al.: Congenital rubella: Clinicopathologic, virologic, and immunologic studies. Am. J. Dis. Child. *110*:464–471, 1965.
27. Bellany, K., Rousseau, S. A., and Gardner, P. S.: The development of an M antibody capture ELISA for rubella IgM. J. Virol. Methods *14*:243–251, 1986.
28. Bellin, E., Safyer, S., and Braslow, C.: False-positive IgM-rubella enzyme linked immunoassay in three first trimester pregnant patients. Pediatr. Infect. Dis. J. *9*:671–672, 1990.
29. Bennett, R. A., and Copeman, W. S. C.: Notes on rubella: With special reference to certain rheumatic sequelae. B. M. J. *1*:924–926, 1940.
30. Berge, T., Brunnhage, F., and Nilsson, L. R.: Congenital hypoplastic thrombocytopenia in rubella embryopathy. Acta Paediatr. (Stockh.) *52*:349–352, 1963.
31. Best, J. M., Banatvala, J. E., and Bowen, J. M.: New Japanese rubella vaccine: Comparative trials. B. M. J. *3*:221–224, 1974.
32. Best, J. M., Banatvala, J. E., and Watson, D.: Serum IgM and IgG response in postnatally acquired rubella. Lancet *2*:65–68, 1969.
33. Birch, C. J., Glaun, B. P., Hunt, V., et al.: Comparison of passive haemagglutination and haemagglutination-inhibition techniques for detection of antibodies to rubella virus. J. Clin. Pathol. *32*:128–131, 1979.
34. Black, F. L., Lamm, S. H., Emmons, J. E., et al.: Durability of antibody titers induced by RA27/3 rubella virus vaccine. J. Infect. Dis. *137*:322–323, 1978.
35. Black, F. L., Lamm, S. H., Emmons, J. E., et al.: Reactions to rubella vaccine and persistence of antibody in virgin-soil populations after vaccination and wild virus-induced immunization. J. Infect. Dis. *133*:393–398, 1976.
36. Blennow, G., Bekassy, A. N., Eriksson, M., et al.: Transient carpal tunnel syndrome accompanying rubella infection. Acta Paediatr. Scand. *71*:1025–1028, 1982.
37. Bolognese, R. J., Corson, S. L., Fuccillo, D. A., et al.: Evaluation of possible transplacental infection with rubella vaccination during pregnancy. Am. J. Obstet. Gynecol. *117*:939–941, 1973.
38. Boner, A., Wilmott, R. W., Dinwiddie, R., et al.: Desquamative interstitial pneumonia and antigen-antibody complexes in two infants with congenital rubella. Pediatrics *72*:835–839, 1983.
39. Boniuk, M., and Zimmerman, L. E.: Ocular pathology in the rubella syndrome. Arch. Ophthalmol. *77*:455–473, 1967.

40. Booth, J. C., and Stern, H.: Photodynamic inactivation of rubella virus. J. Med. Microbiol. *5*:515–528, 1972.
41. Borton, T. E., and Stark, E. W.: Audiological findings in hearing loss secondary to maternal rubella. Pediatrics *45*:225–229, 1970.
42. Bradford, R. I. C.: Two cases of rubella meningoencephalitis. B. M. J. *1*:312–313, 1943.
43. Brody, J. A., Sever, J. L., and Schiff, G. M.: Prevention of rubella by gamma globulin during an epidemic in Barrow, Alaska in 1964. N. Engl. J. Med. *272*:127–129, 1965.
44. Brody, J. A., Sever, J. L., McAllister, R., et al.: Rubella epidemic on St. Paul Island in the Pribilofs, 1963. J. A. M. A. *191*:619–623, 1965.
45. Brookhouser, P. E., and Bordley, J. E.: Congenital rubella deafness: Pathology and pathogenesis. Arch. Otolaryngol. *98*:252–257, 1973.
46. Buescher, E. L.: Behavior of rubella virus in adult populations. Arch. Ges. Virusforsch. *16*:470–476, 1965.
47. Buimovici-Klein, E., and Cooper, L. Z.: Immunosuppression and isolation of rubella virus from human lymphocytes after vaccination with two rubella vaccines. Infect. Immun. *25*:352–356, 1979.
48. Buimovici-Klein, E., Lang, P. B., Ziring, P. R., et al.: Impaired cell-mediated immune response in patients with congenital rubella: Correlation with gestational age at time of infection. Pediatrics *64*:620–626, 1979.
49. Buimovici-Klein, E., Hite, R. L., Byrne, T., et al.: Isolation of rubella virus in milk after postpartum immunization. J. Pediatr. *91*:939–941, 1977.
50. Buimovici-Klein, E., Weiss, K. E., and Cooper, L. Z.: Interferon production in lymphocyte cultures after rubella infection in humans. J. Infect. Dis. *135*:380–385, 1977.
51. Bunnell, C. E., and Monif, G. R. G.: Interstitial pancreatitis in the congenital rubella syndrome. J. Pediatr. *80*:465–466, 1972.
52. Cappel, R., Schluederberg, A., and Horstmann, D. M.: Large-scale production of rubella precipitinogens and their use in the diagnostic laboratory. J. Clin. Microbiol. *1*:201–205, 1975.
53. Cappel, R.: Cell-mediated immunity in experimental rubella infections. Arch. Virol. *47*:375–379, 1975.
54. Castrow, F. F., II, and Beukelaer, M. D.: Congenital rubella syndrome: Unusual cutaneous manifestations. Arch. Dermatol. *98*:260–262, 1968.
55. Catalano, L. W., Jr., Fuccillo, D. A., Traub, R. E., et al.: Isolation of rubella virus from placentas and throat cultures of infants: A prospective study after the 1964–65 epidemic. Obstet. Gynecol. *38*:6–14, 1971.
56. Caul, E. O., Smyth, G. W., and Clarke, S. K. R.: A simplified method for the detection of rubella-specific IgM employing sucrose density fractionation and 2-mercaptoethanol. J. Hyg. (Camb.) *73*:329–340, 1974.
57. Centers for Disease Control and Prevention: Recommended childhood immunization schedule—United States, January–June, 1996. M. M. W. R. *44*:940–944, 1996.
58. Centers for Disease Control and Prevention: Rubella and congenital rubella syndrome—United States, January 1, 1991–May 7, 1994. M. M. W. R. *43*:391–401, 1994.
59. Centers for Disease Control: Increase in rubella and congenital rubella syndrome—United States, 1988–1990. M. M. W. R. *40*:93–99, 1991.
60. Centers for Disease Control: Outbreaks of rubella among the Amish—United States, 1991. M. M. W. R. *40*:264–265, 1991.
61. Centers for Disease Control: Rubella prevention: Recommendations of the Immunization Practices Advisory Committee (ACIP). M. M. W. R. *39*:RR–15, 1990.
62. Centers for Disease Control: Rubella and congenital rubella syndrome—United States, 1985–1988. M. M. W. R. *38*:173–178, 1989.
63. Centers for Disease Control: Rubella outbreak among office workers—New York City. M. M. W. R. *34*:455–459, 1985.
64. Centers for Disease Control: Rubella in colleges—United States, 1983–1984. M. M. W. R. *34*:228–230, 1985.
65. Centers for Disease Control: Rubella outbreaks in prisons—New York City, West Virginia, California. M. M. W. R. *34*:615–618, 1985.
66. Centers for Disease Control: CDC Surveillance Summaries, 1984: Rubella and congenital rubella surveillance, 1983. M. M. W. R. *33*:1SS–10SS, 1984.
67. Centers for Disease Control: Rubella in hospitals—California. M. M. W. R. *32*:37–39, 1983.
68. Chagnon, A., and Laflamme, P.: Effect of acidity on rubella virus. Can. J. Microbiol. *10*:501–503, 1964.
69. Chambers, R. J., and Bywaters, E. G.: Rubella synovitis. Ann. Rheum. Dis. *22*:263–268, 1963.
70. Champsaur, H., Fattal-German, M., and Arranhado, R.: Sensitivity and specificity of viral immunoglobulin M determination by indirect enzyme-linked immunosorbent assay. J. Clin. Microbiol. *26*:328–331, 1988.
71. Chaye, H., Ou, D., Chong, P., et al.: Human T- and B-cell epitopes of E1 glycoprotein of rubella virus. J. Clin. Immunol. *13*:93–100, 1993.
72. Chernesky, M. A., DeLong, D. J., Mahony, J. B., et al.: Differences in antibody responses with rapid agglutination tests for the detection of rubella antibodies. J. Clin. Microbiol. *23*:772–776, 1986.
73. Chernesky, M. A., Wyman, L., Mahony, J. B., et al.: Clinical evaluation of the sensitivity and specificity of a commercially available enzyme immunoassay for detection of rubella virus–specific immunoglobulin M. J. Clin. Microbiol. *20*:400–404, 1984.
74. Cherry, J. D.: Unpublished data.
75. Cherry, J. D.: Rubella: Past, present, and future. Volta Rev. *76*:461–465, 1974.
76. Cherry, J. D.: Peripheral pain syndromes following rubella immunization. J. Pediatr. *80*:541–542, 1972.
77. Cherry, J. D., Horvath, F. L., Comerci, G. D., et al.: Clinical trials with Cendehill strain attenuated rubella virus vaccine. Antimicrob. Agents Chemother. *9*:357–363, 1970.
78. Cherry, J. D., Bobinski, J. E., and Comerci, G. D.: A clinical trial with live attenuated rubella virus vaccine (Cendehill 51 strain). J. Pediatr. *75*:79–86, 1969.
79. Cherry, J. D.: Newer viral exanthems. Adv. Pediatr. *16*:233–286, 1969.
80. Cherry, J. D., Soriano, F., and Jahn, C. L.: Search for perinatal viral infection: A prospective, clinical, virologic and serologic study. Am. J. Dis. Child. *116*:245–250, 1968.
81. Chin, J., and Werner, S. B.: Neuritis and arthritis following rubella immunization. J. A. M. A. *215*:485–486, 1971.
82. Chiriboga-Klein, S., Oberfield, S. E., Casullo, A. M., et al.: Growth in congenital rubella syndrome and correlation with clinical manifestations. J. Pediatr. *115*:251–255, 1989.
83. Cifarelli, P. S., and Freireich, A. W.: Rubella encephalitis. N. Y. State J. Med. *66*:1117–1122, 1966.
84. Claman, H. N., Suvatte, V., Githens, J. H., et al.: Histiocytic reaction in dysgammaglobulinemia and congenital rubella. Pediatrics *46*:89–96, 1970.
85. Clarke, M., Boustred, J., Schild, G. C., et al.: Effect of rubella vaccination programme on serological status of young adults in United Kingdom. Lancet *1*:1224–1226, 1979.
86. Clarke, W. L., Shaver, K. A., Bright, G. M., et al.: Autoimmunity in congenital rubella syndrome. J. Pediatr. *104*:370–373, 1984.
87. Cockburn, W. C.: World aspects of the epidemiology of rubella. Am. J. Dis. Child. *118*:112–122, 1969.
88. Collis, W. J., and Cohen, D. N.: Rubella retinopathy: A progressive disorder. Arch. Ophthalmol. *84*:33–35, 1970.
89. Communicable Disease Center: Rubella surveillance. June, 1969.
90. Communicable Disease Center: Morbidity and Mortality Weekly Report *13*:349–360, 1964.
91. Connolly, J. H., Hitchinson, W. M., Allen, I. V., et al.: Carotid artery thrombosis, encephalitis, myelitis and optic neuritis associated with rubella virus infections. Brain *98*:583–594, 1975.
92. Cooper, L. Z.: Congenital rubella in the United States. *In* Krugman, S., and Gershon, A. A. (eds.): Progress in Clinical Biological Research. Vol. 3. Infections of the Fetus and the Newborn Infant. New York, A. R. Liss, 1975, pp. 1–22.
93. Cooper, L. Z., Preblud, S. R., and Alford, C. A., Jr.: Rubella. *In* Remington, J. S., and Klein, J. O. (eds.): Infectious Diseases of the Fetus and Newborn Infants. Philadelphia, W. B. Saunders, 1995, pp. 268–311.
94. Cooper, L. Z., Florman, A. L., Ziring, P. R., et al.: Loss of rubella hemagglutination inhibition antibody in congenital rubella: Failure of seronegative children with congenital rubella to respond to HPV-77 rubella vaccine. Am. J. Dis. Child. *122*:397–403, 1971.
95. Cooper, L. Z., Ziring, P. R., Weiss, H. J., et al.: Transient arthritis after rubella vaccination. Am. J. Dis. Child. *118*:218–225, 1969.
96. Cooper, L. Z., Ziring, P. R., Ockerse, A. B., et al.: Rubella: Clinical manifestations and management. Am. J. Dis. Child. *118*:18–29, 1969.
97. Cooper, L. Z., and Krugman, S.: Clinical manifestations of postnatal and congenital rubella. Arch. Ophthalmol. *77*:434–439, 1967.
98. Cooper, L. Z., and Krugman, S.: Diagnosis and management: Congenital rubella. Pediatrics *37*:335–338, 1966.
99. Corlett, W. T.: A Treatise on the Acute Infectious Exanthemata, Including Rubeola, Rubella, Scarlatina, Varicella and Vaccinia, with Especial Reference to Diagnosis and Treatment. Philadelphia, F. A. Davis, 1902, pp. 348–371.
100. Cradock-Watson, J. E., Ridehalgh, M. K. S., Anderson, M. J., et al.: Fetal infection resulting from maternal rubella after the first trimester of pregnancy. J. Hyg. (Camb.) *85*:381–391, 1980.
101. Cradock-Watson, J. E., Ridehalgh, M. K. S., and Chantler, S.: Specific immunoglobulins in infants with the congenital rubella syndrome. J. Hyg. (Camb.) *76*:109–123, 1976.
102. Cradock-Watson, J. E., Macdonald, H., Ridehalgh, M. K. S., et al.: Specific immunoglobulin response in serum and nasal secretions after the administration of attenuated rubella vaccine. J. Hyg. (Camb.) *73*:127–141, 1974.
103. Cradock-Watson, J. E., Ridehalgh, M. K. S., Bourne, M. S., et al.: Nasal immunoglobulin responses in acute rubella determined by the immunofluorescent technique. J. Hyg. (Camb.) *71*:603–617, 1973.
104. Cradock-Watson, J. E., Bourne, N. S., and Vandervelde, E. M.: IgG, IgA and IgM responses in acute rubella determined by the immunofluorescent technique. J. Hyg. (Camb.) *70*:473–485, 1972.
105. Cuetter, A. C., and John, J. F.: Nerve conduction studies in natural rubella. Ann. Neurol. *1*:199–200, 1977.
106. Cunningham, A. L., and Fraser, J. R. E.: Persistent rubella virus infection of human synovial cells cultured in vitro. J. Infect. Dis. *151*:638–645, 1985.
107. Dales, L. G., and Chin, J.: Public health implications of rubella antibody levels in California. Am. J. Public Health *72*:167–172, 1982.
108. Das, B. D., Lakhani, P., Kurtz, J. B., et al.: Congenital rubella after previous maternal immunity. Arch. Dis. Child. *65*:545–546, 1990.
109. Davison, C., and Friedfeld, L.: Acute encephalomyelitis following German measles. Am. J. Dis. Child. *55*:496–510, 1938.

110. Deinard, A. S., Bilka, P. J., Venters, H. D., et al.: Rubella-antibody titres in rheumatoid arthritis. Lancet *1*:526–528, 1974.
111. Desmond, M. M., Fisher, E. S., Vorderman, A. L., et al.: The longitudinal course of congenital rubella encephalitis in nonretarded children. J. Pediatr. *93*:584–591, 1978.
112. Desmond, M. M., Wilson, G. S., Melnick, J. L., et al.: Congenital rubella encephalitis. J. Pediatr. *71*:311–331, 1967.
113. Desmyter, J., Rawls, W. E., Melnick, J. L., et al.: Interferon in congenital rubella: Response to live attenuated measles vaccine. J. Immunol. *99*:771–777, 1967.
114. Dibbert, H.-J.: Diagnosis of rubella by demonstrating rubella-specific 19 S and 7 S antibodies. Zentralbl. Bakteriol. Hyg. *A234*:145–158, 1976.
115. Division of Maternal and Perinatal Studies, Department of Health, Sydney: Report on pregnancy complicated by wild rubella—Spring, 1971. Med. J. Aust. 2:545–547, 1973.
116. Doege, T. C., and Kim, K. S. W.: Studies of rubella and its prevention with immune globulin. J. A. M. A. *200*:584–590, 1967.
117. Donowitz, M., and Gryboski, J. D.: Pancreatic insufficiency and the congenital rubella syndrome. J. Pediatr. *87*:241–243, 1975.
118. Dorfman, S. F., and Bowers, C. H., Jr.: Rubella susceptibility among prenatal and family planning clinic populations. Mt. Sinai J. Med. *52*:248–252, 1985.
119. Driscoll, S. G.: Histopathology of gestational rubella. Am. J. Dis. Child. *118*:49–53, 1969.
120. Dudgeon, J. A., Marshall, W. C., and Peckham, C. S.: Rubella vaccine trials in adults and children: Comparison of three attenuated vaccines. Am. J. Dis. Child. *118*:237–246, 1969.
121. Dudgeon, J. A.: Congenital rubella: Pathogenesis and immunology. Am. J. Dis. Child. *118*:35–44, 1969.
122. Dwyer, D. E., Hueston, L., Field, P. R., et al.: Acute encephalitis complicating rubella virus infection. Pediatr. Infect. Dis. J. *11*:238–239, 1992.
123. Ebbin, A. J., Wilson, M. G., Chandor, S. B., et al.: Inadvertent rubella immunization in pregnancy. Am. J. Obstet. Gynecol. *117*:505–512, 1973.
124. Enders, G., and Knotek, F.: Detection of IgM antibodies against rubella virus: Comparison of two indirect ELISAs and an anti-IgM capture immunoassay. J. Med. Virol. *19*:377–386, 1986.
125. Enders, G., Knotek, F., and Pacher, U.: Comparison of various serological methods and diagnostic kits for the detection of acute, recent, and previous rubella infection, vaccination, and congenital infections. J. Med. Virol. *16*:219–232, 1985.
126. Erickson, C. A.: Rubella early in pregnancy causing congenital malformations of eyes and heart. J. Pediatr. *25*:281–283, 1944.
127. Esterly, J. R., and Oppenheimer, E. H.: The pathologic manifestations of intrauterine rubella infection. Arch. Otolaryngol. *98*:246–248, 1973.
128. Esterly, J. R., and Oppenheimer, E. H.: Pathological lesions due to congenital rubella. Arch. Pathol. *87*:380–388, 1969.
129. Esterly, J. R., Slusser, R. J., Slusser, R. J., et al.: Hepatic lesions in the congenital rubella syndrome. J. Pediatr. *71*:676–685, 1967.
130. Esterly, J. R., and Oppenheimer, E. H.: Vascular lesions in infants with congenital rubella. Circulation *36*:544–554, 1967.
131. Evans, A. S., Cox, F., Nankervis, G., et al.: A health and seroepidemiological survey of a community in Barbados. Int. J. Epidemiol. *3*:167–175, 1974.
132. Fabiyi, A., Sever, J. L., Ratner, N., et al.: Rubella virus: Growth characteristics and stability of infectious virus and complement-fixing antigen. Proc. Soc. Exp. Biol. Med. *122*:392–396, 1966.
133. Feldman, R. B., Pinsky, L., Mendelson, J., et al.: Can language disorder not due to peripheral deafness be an isolated expression of prenatal rubella? Pediatrics *52*:296–299, 1973.
134. Fenner, F.: Classification and nomenclature of viruses: Second report of the International Committee on Taxonomy of Viruses. Intervirology *7*:1–115, 1976.
135. Ferraro, M. J., Kallas, W. M., Welch, K. P., et al.: Comparison of a new, rapid enzyme immunoassay with a latex agglutination test for qualitative detection of rubella antibodies. J. Clin. Microbiol. *25*:1722–1724, 1987.
136. Field, P. R., and Gong, C. M.: Diagnosis of postnatally acquired rubella by use of three enzyme-linked immunosorbent assays for specific immunoglobulins G and M and single radial hemolysis for specific immunoglobulin G. J. Clin. Microbiol. *20*:951–958, 1984.
137. Finklea, J. F., Sandifer, S. H., and Moore, G. T., Jr.: Epidemic rubella at the Citadel. Am. J. Epidemiol. *87*:367–372, 1968.
138. Fleet, W. F., Jr., Benz, E. W., Jr., Karzon, D. T., et al.: Fetal consequences of maternal rubella immunization. J. A. M. A. *227*:621–627, 1974.
139. Fogel, A., Gerichter, C. B., Rannon, L., et al.: Serologic studies in 11,460 pregnant women during the 1972 rubella epidemic in Israel. Am. J. Epidemiol. *103*:51–59, 1976.
140. Forbes, J. A.: Rubella: Historical aspects. Am. J. Dis. Child. *118*:5–11, 1969.
141. Forcheimer, F.: The enanthem of German measles. Trans. Am. Pediatr. Soc. *10*:118–128, 1898.
142. Ford, D. K., Reid, G. D., Tingle, A. J., et al.: Sequential follow up observations of a patient with rubella associated persistent arthritis. Ann. Rheum. Dis. *51*:407–410, 1992.
143. Forghani, B., Schmidt, N. J., and Lennette, E. H.: Demonstration of rubella IgM antibody by indirect fluorescent antibody staining, sucrose density gradient centrifugation and mercaptoethanol reduction. Intervirology *1*:48–59, 1973.
144. Forrest, J. M., Menser, M. A., and Harley, J. D.: Diabetes mellitus and congenital rubella. Pediatrics *44*:445–447, 1969.
145. Fortuin, N. J., Morrow, A. G., and Roberts, W. C.: Late vascular manifestations of the rubella syndrome. Am. J. Med. *51*:134–140, 1971.
146. Franco, S. A., Riley, H. D., Jr., and Chitwood, L. A.: The congenital rubella syndrome. South. Med. J. *63*:825–830, 1970.
147. Fraser, V., Spitznagel, E., Medoff, G., et al.: Results of a rubella screening program for hospital employees: A five-year review (1986–1990). Am. J. Epidemiol. *138*:756–764, 1993.
148. Frenkel, L. M., Nielsen, K., Garakian, A., et al.: A search for persistent rubella virus infection in persons with chronic symptoms after rubella and rubella immunization and in patients with juvenile rheumatoid arthritis. Clin. Infect. Dis. *22*:287–294, 1996.
149. Frenkel, L. M., Nielsen, K., Garakian, A., et al.: A search for persistent measles, mumps, and rubella vaccine virus in children with human immunodeficiency virus type 1 infection. Arch. Pediatr. Adolesc. Med. *148*:57–60, 1994.
150. Friedmann, I.: Cochlear pathology in viral disease. Adv. Otorhinolaryngol. *20*:155–177, 1973.
151. Friedmann, I., and Wright, M. I.: Histopathological changes in the foetal and infantile inner ear caused by maternal rubella. B. M. J. 2:20–23, 1966.
152. Fruehan, A. E.: Erythema multiforme exudativum and arthritis following infection with rubella. N. Y. State J. Med. *63*:859–863, 1963.
153. Fry, J., Dillane, J. B., and Fry, L.: Rubella, 1962. B. M. J. 2:833–834, 1962.
154. Fucillo, D. A., Steele, R. W., Hensen, S. A., et al.: Impaired cellular immunity to rubella virus in congenital rubella. Infect. Immun. *9*:81–84, 1974.
155. Fujimoto, T., Katoh, C., Hayakawa, H., et al.: Two cases of rubella infection with cardiac involvement. Jpn. Heart J. *20*:227–235, 1979.
156. Furukawa, T., Plotkin, S. A., Sedwick, W. D., et al.: Studies on hemagglutination by rubella virus. Proc. Soc. Exp. Biol. Med. *126*:745–750, 1967.
157. Gale, J. L., Detels, R., Kim, K. S. W., et al.: The epidemiology of rubella on Taiwan. III. Family studies in cities of high and low attack rates. Int. J. Epidemiol. *1*:261–265, 1973.
158. Gale, J. L., Grayston, J. T., Beasley, R. P., et al.: The epidemiology of rubella on Taiwan. II. 1968–1969 epidemic. Int. J. Epidemiol. *1*:253–260, 1973.
159. Ganguly, R., Cusumano, C. L., and Waldman, R. H.: Suppression of cell-mediated immunity after infection with attenuated rubella virus. Infect. Immun. *13*:464–469, 1976.
160. Geiger, J. C.: Epidemic of German measles in a city adjacent to an army cantonment, and its probable relation thereto. J. A. M. A. *70*:1818–1820, 1918.
161. Geiger, R., Fink, F. M., Sölder, B., et al.: Persistent rubella infection after erroneous vaccination in an immunocompromised patient with acute lymphoblastic leukemia in remission. J. Med. Virol. *47*:442–444, 1995.
162. Geltzer, A. I., Guber, D., and Sears, M. L.: Ocular manifestations of the 1964–65 rubella epidemic. Am. J. Ophthalmol. *63*:221–229, 1967.
163. Gerna, G., Zannino, M., Revello, M. G., et al.: Development and evaluation of a capture enzyme-linked immunosorbent assay for determination of rubella immunoglobulin M using monoclonal antibodies. J. Clin. Microbiol. *25*:1033–1038, 1987.
164. Gibbs, F. A., Gibbs, E. L., Carpenter, P. R., et al.: Electroencephalographic abnormality in "uncomplicated" childhood diseases. J. A. M. A. *171*:1050–1055, 1959.
165. Gilmartin, R. C., Jr., Jabbour, J. T., and Duenas, D. A.: Rubella vaccine myeloradiculoneuritis. J. Pediatr. *80*:406–412, 1972.
166. Ginsberg-Fellner, F., Witt, M. E., Fedun, B., et al.: Diabetes mellitus and autoimmunity in patients with the congenital rubella syndrome. Rev. Infect. Dis. *7*:S170–S176, 1985.
167. Gispen, R., Nagel, J., Brand-Saathof, B., et al.: Immunofluorescence test for IgM rubella antibodies in whole serum after absorption with anti-yFc. Clin. Exp. Immunol. *22*:431–437, 1975.
168. Giuliani, G., Angela, G. C., Baglione, L., et al.: German measles: Acute benign viral lymphoreticulosis. The haemato-humoral and histological aspects of rubella. Panminerva Med. 2:585–602, 1960.
169. Givens, K. T., Lee, D. A., Jones, T., et al.: Congenital rubella syndrome: Ophthalmic manifestations and associated systemic disorders. Br. J. Ophthalmol. *77*:358–363, 1993.
170. Goldwater, P. N., Quiney, J. R., and Banatvala, J. E.: Maternal rubella at St. Thomas' hospital: Is there a need to change British vaccination policy? Lancet 2:1298–1230, 1978.
171. Goodman, A. K., Friedman, S. M., Beatrice, S. T., et al.: Rubella in the workplace: The need for employee immunization. Am. J. Public Health *77*:725–726, 1987.
172. Grahame, R., Armstrong, R., Simmons, N., et al.: Chronic arthritis associated with the presence of intrasynovial rubella virus. Ann. Rheum. Dis. *42*:2–13, 1983.
173. Granberg, C., and Meurman, O.: Performance of two new enzyme immunoassays for the detection of IgM and IgG antibodies to rubella. Eur. J. Clin. Microbiol. Infect. Dis. *13*:512–516, 1994.
174. Grand, M. G., Wyll, S. A., Gehlbach, S. H., et al.: Clinical reactions following rubella vaccination: A prospective analysis of joint, muscular and neuritis symptoms. J. A. M. A. *220*:1569–1572, 1972.
175. Grayston, J. T., Gale, J. L., and Watten, R. H.: The epidemiology of rubella

on Taiwan. I. Introduction and description of the 1957–1958 epidemic. Int. J. Epidemiol. *1*:245–252, 1972.
176. Grayston, J. T., Peng, J. Y., and Lee, G. C. Y.: Congenital abnormalities following gestational rubella in Chinese: Report of a prospective study including five-year follow-up examinations after the 1957–1958 rubella epidemic on Taiwan (Formosa). J. A. M. A. *202*:1–6, 1967.
177. Green, R. H., Balsamo, M. R., Giles, J. P., et al.: Experimental studies with rubella: Evaluation of gamma globulin for prophylaxis. Arch. Ges. Virusforsch. *16*:513–516, 1965.
178. Green, R. H., Balsamo, M. R., Giles, J. P., et al.: Studies of the natural history and prevention of rubella. Am. J. Dis. Child. *110*:348–365, 1965.
179. Gregg, N. M.: Congenital cataract following German measles in the mother. Trans. Ophthalmol. Soc. Aust. *3*:35–46, 1941.
180. Griffith, J. P. C.: Rubella (rotheln: German measles): With a report of one hundred and fifty cases. Med. Rec. *32*:11–41, 1887.
181. Grillner, L., Hedstrom, E.-E., Bergstrom, H., et al.: Vaccination against rubella of newly delivered women. Scand. J. Infect. Dis. *5*:237–241, 1973.
182. Gross, P. A., Portnoy, B., Mathies, A. W., Jr., et al.: A rubella outbreak among adolescent boys. Am. J. Dis. Child. *119*:326–331, 1970.
183. Guggenheimer, J., Nowak, A. J., and Michaels, R. H.: Dental manifestations of the rubella syndrome. Oral Surg. Oral Med. Oral Pathol. *32*:30–37, 1971.
184. Gumpel, S. M., Hayes, K., and Dudgeon, J. A.: Congenital perceptive deafness: Role of intrauterine rubella. B. M. J. *2*:300–304, 1971.
185. Gunn, W.: A case of rubella complicated by purpura haemorrhagica. Br. J. Child. Dis. *30*:111–117, 1933.
186. Gupta, J. D., Peterson, V. J., and Murphy, A. M.: Differential immune response to attenuated rubella virus vaccine. Infect. Immun. *5*:151–154, 1972.
187. Habel, K.: Transmission of rubella to *Macacus mulatta* monkeys. Public Health Rep. *57*:1126–1139, 1942.
188. Hale, M. S., and Ruderman, J. E.: Carpal tunnel syndrome associated with rubella immunization. Am. J. Phys. Med. *52*:189–193, 1973.
189. Halonen, P. E., Ryan, J. M., and Stewart, J. A.: Rubella hemagglutinin prepared with alkaline extraction of virus grown in suspension culture of BHK-21 cells. Proc. Soc. Exp. Biol. Med. *125*:162–167, 1967.
190. Hambling, M. H.: Effect of a vaccination programme on the distribution of rubella antibodies in women of childbearing age. Lancet *1*:1130–1138, 1975.
191. Hammond, K.: Skin dimples and rubella. Pediatrics *39*:291–292, 1967.
192. Hancock, M. P., Huntley, C. C., and Sever, J. L.: Congenital rubella syndrome with immunoglobulin disorder. J. Pediatr. *72*:636–645, 1968.
193. Hannissian, A. S., Martinez, A. J., Jabbour, J. T., et al.: Vasculitis and myositis secondary to rubella vaccination. Arch. Neurol. *28*:202–204, 1973.
194. Hannissian, A. S., and Hashimoto, K.: Paramyxovirus-like inclusions in rubella syndrome. J. Pediatr. *81*:231–237, 1972.
195. Hanshaw, J. B., and Dudgeon, J. A.: Rubella. *In* Viral Diseases of the Fetus and Newborn. Philadelphia, W. B. Saunders, 1978, pp. 17–96.
196. Hara, J., Fujimoto, F., Ishibashi, T., et al.: Ocular manifestations of the 1976 rubella epidemic in Japan. Am. J. Ophthalmol. *87*:642–645, 1979.
197. Hardy, J. B.: Clinical and developmental aspects of congenital rubella. Arch. Otolaryngol. *98*:230–236, 1973.
198. Hardy, J. B., Sever, J. L., and Gilkeson, M. R.: Declining antibody titers in children with congenital rubella. J. Pediatr. *75*:213–220, 1969.
199. Hardy, J. B., McCracken, G. H., Jr., Gilkeson, M. R., et al.: Adverse fetal outcome following maternal rubella after the first trimester of pregnancy. J. A. M. A. *207*:2414–2420, 1969.
200. Hardy, J. B., and Sever, J. L.: Indirect inguinal hernia in congenital rubella. J. Pediatr. *73*:416–418, 1968.
201. Hardy, J. B., Monif, G. R. G., and Sever, J. L.: Studies in congenital rubella, Baltimore, 1964–65. Bull. Johns Hopkins Hosp. *118*:97–108, 1966.
202. Harrison, B. L.: Neuritis following rubella. B. M. J. *1*:637, 1940.
203. Hart, H., and Marmion, B. P.: Rubella virus and rheumatoid arthritis. Ann. Rheum. Dis. *36*: 3–12, 1977.
204. Hastreiter, A. R., Joorabchi, B., Pujatti, G., et al.: Cardiovascular lesions associated with congenital rubella. J. Pediatr. *71*:59–65, 1967.
205. Hattis, R. P., Halstead, S. B., Hermann, K. L., et al.: Rubella in an immunized island population. J. A. M. A. *223*:1019–1021, 1973.
206. Heathfield, K. W. G.: Carpal-tunnel syndrome. B. M. J. *2*:58, 1962.
207. Heggie, A. D.: Pathogenesis of the rubella exanthem: Distribution of rubella virus in the skin during rubella with and without rash. J. Infect. Dis. *137*:74–77, 1978.
208. Heggie, A. D.: Pathogenesis of the rubella exanthem: Isolation of rubella virus from the skin. N. Engl. J. Med. *285*:664–666, 1971.
209. Heggie, A. D., and Robbins, F. C.: Natural rubella acquired after birth: Clinical features and complications. Am. J. Dis. Child. *118*:12–17, 1969.
210. Herrmann, K. L.: Available rubella serologic tests. Rev. Infect. Dis. *7*:S108–S112, 1985.
211. Hildebrandt, H. M., and Maassab, H. F.: Rubella synovitis in a one-year-old patient. N. Engl. J. Med. *274*:1428–1430, 1966.
212. Hillenbrand, F. K. M.: Rubella in a remote community. Lancet *2*:64–66, 1956.
213. Hillenbrand, F. K. M.: The blood picture in rubella: Its place in diagnosis. Lancet *2*:66–68, 1956.
214. Hiro, V. Y., and Tasaka, S.: Die rotheln sind eine viruskrankheit. Monatsschr. Kinderheilk. *76*:328–332, 1938.
215. Hodges, G. M.: Neuritis following rubella. B. M. J. *1*:830–831, 1940.
216. Holmes, I. H., Wark, M. C., and Warburton, M. F.: Is rubella an arbovirus? II. Ultrastructural morphology and development. Virology *37*:15–25, 1969.
217. Honeyman, M. C., Dorman, D. C., Menser, M. A., et al.: HL-A antigens in congenital rubella and the role of antigens 1 and 8 in the epidemiology of natural rubella. Tissue Antigens *5*:12–18, 1975.
218. Honeyman, M. C., and Menser, M. A.: Ethnicity is a significant factor in the epidemiology of rubella and Hodgkin's disease. Nature *251*:441–442, 1974.
219. Honeyman, M. C., Forrest, J. M., Dorman, D. C.: Cell-mediated immune response following natural rubella and rubella vaccination. Clin. Exp. Immunol. *17*:665–671, 1974.
220. Hornsleth, A., Leerhoy, J., Grauballe, P., et al.: Rubella-virus–specific IgM- and IgA-antibodies: The indirect immunofluorescence (IF) technique applied to sera with reduced IgG concentration. Acta Pathol. Microbiol. Scand. [B] *82*:742–744, 1974.
221. Hornstein, L., and Ben-Porath, E.: Rubella antibodies in women of childbearing age during an epidemic and the two years thereafter. Isr. J. Med. Sci. *12*:1189–1193, 1976.
222. Horstmann, D. M.: Rubella. *In* Evans, A. S. (ed.): Viral Infections of Humans: Epidemiology and Control. 3rd ed. New York, Plenum Medical, 1990, pp. 617–631.
223. Horstmann, D. M., Schluederberg, A., Emmons, J. E., et al.: Persistence of vaccine-induced immune responses to rubella: Comparison with natural infection. Rev. Infect. Dis. *7*:S80–S85, 1985.
224. Horstmann, D. M.: Problems in measles and rubella. Disease-a-Month *24*:3–52, 1978.
225. Horstmann, D. M., Liebhaber, H., LeBouvier, G. L., et al.: Rubella: Reinfection of vaccinated and naturally immune persons exposed in an epidemic. N. Engl. J. Med. *283*:771–778, 1970.
226. Horstmann, D. M., Riordan, J. T., Ohtawara, M., et al.: A natural epidemic of rubella in a closed population: Virological and epidemiological observations. Arch. Ges. Virusforsch. *16*:483–487, 1965.
227. Horstmann, D. M., Banatvala, J. E., Riordan, J. T., et al.: Maternal rubella and the rubella syndrome in infants: Epidemiologic, clinical, and virologic observations. Am. J. Dis. Child. *110*:408–415, 1965.
228. Howson, C. P., Katz, M., Johnston, R. B., Jr., et al.: Chronic arthritis after rubella vaccination. Clin. Infect. Dis. *15*:307–312, 1992.
229. Hynes, M.: Leucocyte count in rubella. Lancet *2*:679–680, 1940.
230. Hyypiä T., Eskola, J., Laine, M., et al.: Polyclonal activation of B cells during rubella infection. Scand. J. Immunol. *21*:615–617, 1985.
231. Hyypiä, T., Eskola, J., Laine, M., et al.: B-cell function in vitro during rubella infection. Infect. Immun. *43*:589–592, 1984.
232. Jeffries, D. J., Johnson, A. H., and Mowbray, J. F.: Abnormal responses to rubella infection. J. Clin. Pathol. *29*:1003–1006, 1976.
233. Jeresaty, R. M., and Russell, W.: Hepatosplenomegaly and heart disease in the congenital rubella syndrome: Report of eight cases. Pediatrics *39*:36–42, 1967.
234. Johnson, G. M., and Tudor, R. B.: Diabetes mellitus and congenital rubella infection. Am. J. Dis. Child. *120*:453–455, 1970.
235. Judelsohn, R. G., and Wyll, S. A.: Rubella in Bermuda: Termination of an epidemic by mass vaccination. J. A. M. A. *223*:401–406, 1973.
236. Kanra, G. Y., and Vesikari, T.: Cytotoxic activity against rubella-infected cells in the supernatants of human lymphocyte cultures stimulated by rubella virus. Clin. Exp. Immunol. *19*:17–32, 1975.
237. Kelemen, G.: Rubella and deafness. Arch. Otolaryngol. *83*:520–532, 1966.
238. Kelley, P. W., Petrucelli, B. P., Stehr-Green, P., et al.: The susceptibility of young adult Americans to vaccine-preventable infections: A national serosurvey of US army recruits. J. A. M. A. *266*:2724–2729, 1991.
239. Kenny, F. M., Michaels, R. H., and Davis, K. S.: Rubella encephalopathy: Later psychometric, neurologic, and encephalographic evaluation of seven survivors. Am. J. Dis. Child. *110*:374–380, 1965.
240. Kenrick, K. G., Slinn, R. F., Dorman, D. C., et al.: Immunoglobulins and rubella-virus antibodies in adults with congenital rubella. Lancet *1*:548–551, 1968.
241. Kilroy, A. W., Schaffner, W., Fleet, W. F., Jr., et al.: Two syndromes following rubella immunization: Clinical observations and epidemiological studies. J. A. M. A. *214*:2287–2292, 1970.
242. Kistler, G. S., and Sapatino, V.: Temperature- and UV-light resistance of rubella virus infectivity. Arch. Ges. Virusforsch. *38*:11–16, 1972.
243. Klein, H. Z., and Markarian, M.: Dermal erythropoiesis in congenital rubella: Description of an infected newborn who had purpura associated with marked extramedullary erythropoiesis in the skin and elsewhere. Clin. Pediatr. *8*:604–607, 1969.
244. Korones, S. B., Ainger, L. E., Monif, G. R. G., et al.: Congenital rubella syndrome: Study of 22 infants. Am. J. Dis. Child. *110*:434–440, 1965.
245. Korones, S. B., Ainger, L. E., Monif, G. R. G., et al.: Congenital rubella syndrome: New clinical aspects with recovery of virus from affected infants. J. Pediatr. *67*:166–181, 1965.
246. Kresky, B., and Nauheim, J. S.: Rubella retinitis. Am. J. Dis. Child. *114*:305–310, 1967.
247. Krill, A. E.: The retinal disease of rubella. Arch. Ophthalmol. *77*:445–449, 1967.

248. Krugman, S., Ward, R., and Katz, S. L.: Rubella (German measles). *In* Infectious Diseases of Children. 6th ed. St. Louis, C. V. Mosby, 1977, pp. 274–292.
249. Krugman, S.: Present status of measles and rubella immunization in the United States: A medical progress report. J. Pediatr. *90*:1–12, 1977.
250. Krugman, S. (ed.): International Conference on Rubella Immunization. Am. J. Dis. Child. *118*:2–410, 1969.
251. Krugman, S. (ed.): Rubella Symposium. Am. J. Dis. Child. *110*:345–476, 1965.
252. Krugman, S., and Ward, R.: The rubella problem: Clinical aspects, risk of fetal abnormality and methods of prevention. J. Pediatr. *44*:489–498, 1954.
253. Lafer, C. Z., and Morrison, A. N.: Thrombocytopenic purpura progressing to transient hypoplastic anemia in a newborn with rubella syndrome. Pediatrics *38*:499–501, 1966.
254. Laguaite, J. K., and Joseph, M.: A study of children with communication problems associated with maternal rubella. South. Med. J. *58*:231–235, 1965.
255. Lalla, M., Vesikari, T., and Virolainen, M.: Lymphoblast proliferation and humoral antibody response after rubella vaccination. Clin. Exp. Immunol. *15*:193–202, 1973.
256. Landrigan, P. J., Stoffels, M. A., Anderson, E., et al.: Epidemic rubella in adolescent boys: Clinical features and results of vaccination. J. A. M. A. *227*:1283–1287, 1974.
257. Larson, H. E., Parkman, P. D., Davis, W. J., et al.: Inadvertent rubella virus vaccination during pregnancy. N. Engl. J. Med. *284*:870–873, 1971.
258. Lawless, M. R., Abramson, J. S., Harlan, J. E., et al.: Rubella susceptibility in sixth graders: Effectiveness of current immunization practice. Pediatrics *65*:1086–1089, 1980.
259. Lawton, A. R., Self, K. S., Royal, S. A., et al.: Ontogeny of B-lymphocytes in the human fetus. Clin. Immunol. Immunopathol. *1*:84–93, 1972.
260. Lebon, P., Daffos, F., Checoury, A., et al.: Presence of an acid-labile alpha-interferon in sera from fetuses and children with congenital rubella. J. Clin. Microbiol. *21*:775–778, 1985.
261. Lebon, P., and Lyon, G.: Non-congenital rubella encephalitis. Lancet *2*:468, 1974.
262. LeBouvier, G. L., and Plotkin, S. A.: Precipitin responses to rubella vaccine RA 27/3. J. Infect. Dis. *123*:220–223, 1971.
263. LeBouvier, G. L.: Rubella precipitins. International Symposium on Rubella Vaccines, London, 1968. Symposium Series in Immunobiological Standardization. Vol. 11. Basel/New York, Karger, 1969, pp. 113–138.
264. LeBouvier, G. L.: Precipitinogens of rubella virus–infected cells. Proc. Soc. Exp. Biol. Med. *130*:51–54, 1969.
265. Lehane, D. E., Newberg, N. R., and Beam, W. E., Jr.: Evaluation of rubella herd immunity during epidemic. J. A. M. A. *213*:2236–2239, 1970.
266. Lejarraga, H., and Peckham, C. S.: Birthweight and subsequent growth of children exposed to rubella infection in utero. Arch. Dis. Child. *49*:50–54, 1974.
267. Lennette, E. H., Schmidt, N. J., and Magoffin, R. L.: The hemagglutination inhibition test for rubella: A comparison of its sensitivity to that of neutralization, complement-fixation and fluorescent antibody tests for diagnosis of infection and determination of immunity status. J. Immunol. *99*:785–793, 1967.
268. Lerman, S. J., Nankervis, G. A., Heggie, A. D., et al.: Immunologic response, virus excretion, and joint reactions with rubella vaccine: A study of adolescent girls and young women given live attenuated virus vaccine (HPV-77:DE-5). Ann. Intern. Med. *74*:67–73, 1971.
269. Liebhaber, H., Ingalls, T. H., LeBouvier, G. L., et al.: Vaccination with RA 27/3 rubella vaccine: Persistence of immunity and resistance to challenge after two years. Am. J. Dis. Child. *123*:133–136, 1972.
270. Liebhaber, H.: Measurement of rubella antibody by hemagglutination inhibition. I. Variables affecting rubella hemagglutination. J. Immunol. *104*:818–825, 1970.
271. Lindquist, J. M., Plotkin, S. A., Shaw, L., et al.: Congenital rubella syndrome as a systemic infection: Studies of affected infants born in Philadelphia. U. S. A. Med. J. *2*:1401–1406, 1965.
272. Lock, F. R., Gatling, H. B., and Wells, H. B.: Difficulties in the diagnosis of congenital abnormalities: Experience in a study of the effect of rubella on pregnancy. J. A. M. A. *178*:711–714, 1961.
273. Lokietz, H., and Reynolds, F. A.: Postrubella thrombocytopenic purpura: Report of nine new cases and review of published cases. Lancet *85*:226–230, 1965.
274. Lovett, A. E., Hahn, C. S., Rice, C. M., et al.: Rubella virus–specific cytotoxic T-lymphocyte responses: Identification of the capsid as a target of major histocompatibility complex class I–restricted lysis and definition of two epitopes. J. Virol. *67*:5849–5858, 1993.
275. Macfarlane, D. W., Boyd, R. D., Dodrill, C. B., et al.: Intrauterine rubella, head size, and intellect. Pediatrics *55*:797–801, 1975.
276. Macrae, A. D., Mogford, H., Reid, D., et al.: Studies of the effect of immunoglobulin on rubella in pregnancy: Report of the Public Health Laboratory Service Working Party on Rubella. B. M. J. *2*:497–500, 1970.
277. Maller, R., Fryden, A., and Soren, L.: Mitogen stimulation and distribution of T- and B-lymphocytes during natural rubella infection. Acta Pathol. Microbiol. Scand. [C] *86*:93–98, 1978.
278. Mallinson, H., Roberts, C., and White, G. B. B.: Staphylococcal protein A: Its preparation and an application to rubella serology. J. Clin. Pathol. *29*:99–102, 1976.
279. Margolis, F. J., Wilson, J. L., and Top, F. H.: Postrubella encephalomyelitis: Report of cases in Detroit and review of literature. J. Pediatr. *23*:158–165, 1943.
280. Martenis, T. W., Bland, J. H., and Phillips, C. A.: Rheumatoid arthritis after rubella. Arthritis Rheum. *11*:683–687, 1968.
281. Matsumoto, A., and Higashi, N.: Electron microscopic studies on the morphology and the morphogenesis of togaviruses. Ann. Rep. Inst. Virus Res. Kyoto Univ. *17*:11–22, 1974.
282. Matter, L., Gorgievski-Hrisoho, M., and Germann, D.: Comparison of four enzyme immunoassays for detection of immunoglobulin M antibodies against rubella virus. J. Clin. Microbiol. *32*:2134–2139, 1994.
283. de Mazancourt, A., Waxham, M. N., Nicolas, J. C., et al.: Antibody response to the rubella virus structural proteins in infants with the congenital rubella syndrome. J. Med. Virol. *19*:111–122, 1986.
284. McCallin, P. F., Fuccillo, D. A., Ley, A. C., et al.: Gammaglobulin as prophylaxis against rubella-induced congenital anomalies. Obstet. Gynecol. *39*:185–189, 1972.
285. McCarthy, K., and Taylor-Robinson, C. H.: Rubella. Br. Med. Bull. *23*:185–191, 1967.
286. McCarthy, K., Taylor-Robinson, C. H., and Pillinger, S. E.: Isolation of rubella virus from cases in Britain. Lancet *2*:593–598, 1963.
287. McCarthy, M., Lovett, A., Kerman, R. H., et al.: Immunodominant T-cell epitopes of rubella virus structural proteins defined by synthetic peptides. J. Virol. *67*:673–681, 1993.
288. McDonald, J. C., and Peckham, C. S.: Gammaglobulin in prevention of rubella and congenital defect: A study of 30,000 pregnancies. B. M. J. *3*:633–637, 1967.
289. McMorrow, L. E., Vesikari, T., Wolman, S. R., et al.: Suppression of the response of lymphocytes to phytohemagglutinin in rubella. J. Infect. Dis. *130*:464–469, 1974.
290. Menser, M. A., Hudson, J. R., Murphy, A. M., et al.: Epidemiology of congenital rubella and results of rubella vaccination in Australia. Rev. Infect. Dis. *7*:S37–S41, 1985.
291. Menser, M. A., Forrest, J. M., and Bransby, R. D.: Rubella infection and diabetes mellitus. Lancet *1*:57–60, 1978.
292. Menser, M. A., and Forrest, J. M.: Rubella: High incidence of defects in children considered normal at birth. Med. J. Aust. *1*:123–126, 1974.
293. Menser, M. A., Robertson, S. E. J., Dorman, D. C., et al.: Renal lesions in congenital rubella. Pediatrics *40*:901–904, 1967.
294. Menser, M. A., Dorman, D. C., Reye, R. D. K., et al.: Renal-artery stenosis in the rubella syndrome. Lancet *1*:790–792, 1966.
295. Merritt, H. H., and Koskoff, Y. D.: Encephalomyelitis following German measles. Am. J. Med. Sci. *191*:690–696, 1936.
296. Meurman, O. H.: Antibody responses in patients with rubella infection determined by passive hemagglutination, hemagglutination inhibition, complement fixation, and solid-phase radioimmunoassay tests. Infect. Immun. *19*:369–372, 1978.
297. Meurman, O. H., Viljanen, M. K., and Granfors, K.: Solid-phase radioimmunoassay of rubella virus immunoglobulin M antibodies: Comparison with sucrose density gradient centrifugation test. J. Clin. Microbiol. *5*:257–262, 1977.
298. Meyer, H. M., Hopps, H. E., Parkman, P. D., et al.: Control of measles and rubella through use of attenuated vaccines. Am. J. Clin. Pathol. *70*:128–135, 1978.
299. Michael, M.: Rubella: A report of an epidemic of eighty cases. Arch. Pediatr. *25*:598–606, 1908.
300. Michaels, R. H.: Suppression of antibody response in congenital rubella. J. Pediatr. *80*:583–588, 1972.
301. Michaels, R. H., and Rogers, K. D.: A sex difference in immunologic responsiveness. Pediatrics *47*:120–123, 1971.
302. Michaels, R. H., and Kenny, R. M.: Postnatal growth retardation in congenital rubella. Pediatrics *43*:251–259, 1969.
303. Miller, C. H., Dowd, J. M., Rytel, M. W., et al.: Prevention of rubella with γ-globulin. J. A. M. A. *201*:560–561, 1967.
304. Miller, C. L., Miller, E., and Waight, P. A.: Rubella susceptibility and the continuing risk of infection in pregnancy. B. M. J. *294*:1277–1278, 1987.
305. Miller, C. L., Miller, E., Sequeira, P. J. L., et al.: Effect of selective vaccination on rubella susceptibility and infection in pregnancy. B. M. J. *291*:1398–1401, 1985.
306. Miller, K. A., and Zager, T. D.: Rubella susceptibility in an adolescent female population. Mayo Clin. Proc. *59*:31–34, 1984.
307. Miller, M. H., Rabinowitz, M., and Cohen, M.: Pure-tone audiometry in prenatal rubella. Arch. Otolaryngol. *94*:25–29, 1971.
308. Millian, S. J., and Wegman, D.: Rubella serology: Applications, limitations and interpretations. Am. J. Public Health *62*:171–176, 1972.
309. Mitchell, L. A., Zhang, T., and Tingle, A. J.: Differential antibody responses to rubella virus infection in males and females. J. Infect. Dis. *166*:1258–1265, 1992.
310. Mitchell, L. A., De'carie, D., Tingle, A. J., et al.: Use of synthetic peptides to map regions of rubella virus capsid protein recognized by human T lymphcoytes. Vaccine *12*:639–646, 1994.
311. Miyazaki, S., Ohtsuka, M., Ueda, K., et al.: Coombs-positive hemolytic anemia in congenital rubella. J. Pediatr. *94*:759–760, 1979.

312. Monif, G. R. G.: Congenital rubella. *In* Monif, G. R. G. (ed.): Viral Infections of the Human Fetus. London, Macmillan, 1969, pp. 104–132.
313. Monif, G. R. G., Asofsky, R., and Sever, J. L.: Hepatic dysfunction in the congenital rubella syndrome. B. M. J. *1*:1086–1088, 1966.
314. Monif, G. R. G., Hardy, J. B., and Sever, J. L.: Studies in congenital rubella, Baltimore 1964–65. I. Epidemiologic and virologic. Bull. Johns Hopkins Hosp. *118*:85–96, 1966.
315. Monif, G. R. G., Sever, J. L., Schiff, G. M., et al.: Isolation of rubella virus from products of conception. Am. J. Obstet. Gynecol. *91*:1143–1146, 1965.
316. Monif, G. R. G., Avery, G. B., Korones, S. B., et al.: Postmortem isolation of rubella virus from three children with rubella-syndrome defects. Lancet *1*:723–724, 1965.
317. Monto, A. S., Cavallaro, J. J., and Whale, E. H.: Frequency of arthralgia in women receiving one of three rubella vaccines. Arch. Intern. Med. *126*:635–639, 1970.
318. Morag, A., Morag, B., Bernstein, J. M., et al.: In vitro correlates of cell-mediated immunity in human tonsils after natural or induced rubella virus infection. J. Infect. Dis. *131*:409–416, 1975.
319. Morse, E. E., Zinkham, W. H., and Jackson, D. P.: Thrombocytopenic purpura following rubella infection in children and adults. Arch. Intern. Med. *117*:573–579, 1966.
320. Murphy, A. M., Field, P. R., and Collins, E.: The value of specific IgM tests in the early diagnosis of congenital rubella. Med. J. Aust. *2*:290–293, 1978.
321. Murphy, A. M., Reid, R. R., Pollard, I., et al.: Rubella cataracts: Further clinical and virologic observations. Am. J. Ophthalmol. *64*:1109–1119, 1967.
322. Myllyla, G., Vaheri, A., Vesikari, T., et al.: Interaction between human blood platelets, viruses and antibodies. IV. Post-rubella thrombocytopenic purpura and platelet aggregation by rubella antigen-antibody interaction. Clin. Exp. Immunol. *4*:323–332, 1969.
323. Naeye, R. L., and Blanc, W.: Pathogenesis of congenital rubella. J. A. M. A. *194*:1277–1283, 1965.
324. Naveh, Y., and Friedman, A.: Rubella encephalitis successfully treated with corticosteroids. Clin. Pediatr. *14*:286–287, 1975.
325. Niwa, Y., and Kanoh, T.: Immunological behaviour following rubella infection. Clin. Exp. Immunol. *37*:470–476, 1979.
326. Noble, J. S., and Wand, M.: Catcher's crouch and rubella immunization. J. A. M. A. *217*:212, 1971.
327. Norval, M., and Smith, C.: Search for viral nucleic sequences in rheumatoid cells. Ann. Rheum. Dis. *38*:456–462, 1979.
328. Nusbacher, J., Hirschhorn, K., and Cooper, L. Z.: Chromosomal abnormalities in congenital rubella. N. Engl. J. Med. *276*:1409–1413, 1967.
329. Ogra, P. L., Ogra, S. S., Chiba, Y., et al.: Rubella-virus infection in juvenile rheumatoid arthritis. Lancet *1*:1157–1168, 1975.
330. Ogra, P. L., Kerr-Grant, D., Umana, G., et al.: Antibody response in serum and nasopharynx after naturally acquired and vaccine-induced infection with rubella virus. N. Engl. J. Med. *285*:1333–1339, 1971.
331. Ogra, P. L., and Herd, J. K.: Arthritis associated with induced rubella infection. J. Immunol. *107*:810–813, 1971.
332. O'Neill, J. F.: Strabismus in congenital rubella: Management in the presence of brain damage. Arch. Ophthalmol. *77*:450–454, 1967.
333. Orenstein, W. A., Herrmann, K. L., Holmgreen, P., et al.: Prevalence of rubella antibodies in Massachusetts school children. Am. J. Epidemiol. *124*:290–298, 1986.
334. Orenstein, W. A., Heseltine, P. N. R., LeGagnoux, S. J., et al.: Rubella vaccine and susceptible hospital employees: Poor physician participation. J. A. M. A. *245*:711–713, 1981.
335. Ornoy, A., Segal, S., Nishmi, M., et al.: Fetal and placental pathology in gestational rubella. Am. J. Obstet. Gynecol. *116*:949–956, 1973.
336. Ou, D., Chong, P., Tripet, B., et al.: Analysis of T- and B-cell epitopes of capsid protein of rubella virus by using synthetic peptides. J. Virol. *66*:1674–1681, 1992.
337. Ozsoylu, S., Kanra, G., and Savas, G.: Thrombocytopenic purpura related to rubella infection. Pediatrics *62*:567–569, 1978.
338. Panush, R. S.: Serum hypocomplementemia with rubella arthritis: Case report. Mil. Med. *140*:117–118, 1975.
339. Parkman, P. D., Buescher, E. L., Artenstein, M. S., et al.: Studies of rubella. I. Properties of the virus. J. Immunol. *93*:595–617, 1964.
340. Parkman, P. D., Buescher, E. L., and Artenstein, M. S.: Recovery of rubella virus from Army recruits. Proc. Soc. Exp. Biol. Med. *111*:225–230, 1962.
341. Pattison, J. R., Dane, D. S., and Mace, J. E.: Persistence of specific IgM after natural infection with rubella virus. Lancet *1*:185–190, 1975.
342. Pattison, J. R., and Mace, J. E.: The detection of specific IgM antibodies following infection with rubella virus. J. Clin. Pathol. *28*:377–382, 1975.
343. Peckham, C. S.: Clinical and laboratory study of children exposed in utero to maternal rubella. Arch. Dis. Child. *47*:571–577, 1972.
344. Pedneault, L., Zrein, M., Robillard, L., et al.: Comparison of novel synthetic peptide-based DETECT-RUBELLA enzyme immunoassays with enzygnost and IMx for detection of rubella-specific immunoglobulin G. J. Clin. Microbiol. *32*:1085–1087, 1994.
345. Peltola, H., Heinonen, O. P., Valle, M., et al.: The elimination of indigenous measles, mumps, and rubella from Finland by a 12-year, two-dose vaccination program. N. Engl. J. Med. *331*:1397–1402, 1994.
346. Peters, E. R., and Davis, R. L.: Congenital rubella syndrome: Cerebral mineralizations and subperiosteal new bone formation as expressions of this disorder. Clin. Pediatr. *5*:743–746, 1966.
347. Pettersson, R. F., Oker-Blom, C., Kalkkinen, N., et al.: Molecular and antigenic characteristics and synthesis of rubella virus structural proteins. Rev. Infect. Dis. *7*:S140–S149, 1985.
348. Phelan, P., and Campbell, P.: Pulmonary complications of rubella embryopathy. J. Pediatr. *75*:202–212, 1969.
349. Phillips, C. A., Maeck, J. V. S., Rogers, W. A., et al.: Intrauterine rubella infection following immunization with rubella vaccine. J. A. M. A. *213*:624–625, 1970.
350. Phillips, C. A., Melnick, J. L., Yow, M. D., et al.: Persistence of virus in infants with congenital rubella and in normal infants with a history of maternal rubella. J. A. M. A. *193*:1027–1029, 1965.
351. Pineda, R. G., Desmond, M. M., Rudolph, A. J., et al.: Impact of the 1964 rubella epidemic on a clinic population. Am. J. Obstet. Gynecol. *100*:1139–1146, 1968.
352. Plotkin, S. A., and Buser, F.: History of RA27/3 rubella vaccine. Rev. Infect. Dis. *7*:S77–S78, 1985.
353. Plotkin, S. A., Farquhar, J. D., and Ogra, P. L.: Immunologic properties of RA 27/3 rubella virus vaccine: A comparison with strains presently licensed in the United States. J. A. M. A. *225*:585–590, 1973.
354. Plotkin, S. A., and Farquhar, J. D.: Immunity to rubella: Comparison between naturally and artificially induced resistance. Postgrad. Med. J. *48*(Suppl. 3):47–59, 1972.
355. Plotkin, S. A.: Rubella virus. *In* Lennette, E. H., and Schmidt, N. J. (eds.): Diagnostic Procedures for Viral and Rickettsial Infections. New York, American Public Health Association, 1969, pp. 364–413.
356. Plotkin, S. A., Klaus, R. M., and Whitley, J. P.: Hypogammaglobulinemia in an infant with congenital rubella syndrome: Failure of 1-adamantanamine to stop virus excretion. J. Pediatr. *69*:1085–1091, 1966.
357. Plotkin, S. A., Oski, F. A., Hartnett, E. M., et al.: Some recently recognized manifestations of the rubella syndrome. J. Pediatr. *67*:182–191, 1965.
358. Polk, B. F., Modlin, J. F., White, J. A., et al.: A controlled comparison of joint reactions among women receiving one of two rubella vaccines. Am. J. Epidemiol. *115*:19–25, 1982.
359. Polk, B. F., White, J. A., DeGirolami, P. C., et al.: An outbreak of rubella among hospital personnel. N. Engl. J. Med. *303*:541–545, 1980.
360. Preblud, S. R., and Alford, C. A., Jr.: Rubella. *In* Remington, J. S., and Klein, J. O. (eds.): Infectious Diseases of the Fetus and Newborn Infant. 3rd ed. Philadelphia, W. B. Saunders, 1990, pp. 196–240.
361. Preece, M. A., Kearney, P. J., and Marshall, W. C.: Growth-hormone deficiency in congenital rubella. Lancet *2*:842–844, 1977.
362. Purvis-Smith, S. G., Howard, P. R., and Menser, M. A.: Dermatoglyphic defects and rubella teratogenesis. J. A. M. A. *209*:1865–1868, 1969.
363. Rausen, A. R., Richter, P., Tallal, L., et al.: Hematologic effects of intrauterine rubella. J. A. M. A. *199*:75–78, 1967.
364. Rausen, A. R., London, R. D., Mizrahi, A., et al.: Generalized bone changes and thrombocytopenic purpura in association with intrauterine rubella. Pediatrics *36*:264–267, 1965.
365. Rawls, W. E., Desmyter, J., and Melnick, J. L.: Serological diagnosis and fetal involvement in maternal rubella. J. A. M. A. *203*:627–631, 1968.
366. Rawls, W. E., Phillips, C. A., Melnick, J. L., et al.: Persistent virus infection in congenital rubella. Arch. Ophthalmol. *77*:430–433, 1967.
367. Reed, G. B., Jr.: Rubella bone lesions. J. Pediatr. *74*:208–213, 1969.
368. Reese, A. B.: Congenital cataract and other anomalies following German measles in the mother. Am. J. Ophthalmol. *27*:483–487, 1944.
369. Ribon, A., and Wasserman, E.: Immunodeficiency with congenital rubella. Ann. Allergy *32*:35–40, 1974.
370. Richards, C. S.: Middle ear changes in rubella deafness. Arch. Otolaryngol. *80*:48–59, 1964.
371. Robinson, J., Lemay, M., and Vaudry, W. L.: Congenital rubella after anticipated maternal immunity: Two cases and a review of the literature. Pediatr. Infect. Dis. J. *13*:812–815, 1994.
372. Robinson, R. G., Dudenhoeffer, F. E., Holroyd, H. J., et al.: Rubella immunity in older children, teenagers, and young adults: A comparison of immunity in those previously immunized with those unimmunized. J. Pediatr. *101*:188–191, 1982.
373. Rones, B.: The relationship of German measles during pregnancy to congenital ocular defects. Med. Ann. D. C. *13*:285–287, 1944.
374. Rorke, L. B.: Nervous system lesions in the congenital rubella syndrome. Arch. Otolaryngol. *98*:249–252, 1973.
375. Rorke, L. B., and Spiro, A. J.: Cerebral lesions in congenital rubella syndrome. J. Pediatr. *70*:243–255, 1967.
376. Rose, H. D.: Fatal rubella encephalitis. Am. J. Med. Sci. *268*:287–290, 1974.
377. Ross, A. C., and McCartney, A.: Progress of rubella immunity in pregnant women. B. M. J. *1*:1636, 1979.
378. Rossier, E., Phipps, P. H., Weber, J. M., et al.: Persistence of humoral and cell-mediated immunity to rubella virus in cloistered nuns and in schoolteachers. J. Infect. Dis. *144*:137–141, 1981.
379. Rossier, E., Phipps, P. H., Polley, J. R., et al.: Absence of cell-mediated immunity to rubella virus 5 years after rubella vaccination. Can. Med. Assoc. J. *116*:481–484, 1977.
380. Roy, F. H., Hiatt, R. L., Korones, S. B., et al.: Ocular manifestations of

congenital rubella syndrome: Recovery of virus from affected infants. Arch. Ophthalmol. *75*:601–607, 1966.
381. Rudolph, A. J., Singleton, E. B., Rosenberg, H. S., et al.: Osseous manifestations of the congenital rubella syndrome. Am. J. Dis. Child. *110*:428–433, 1965.
382. Rudolph, A. J., Yow, M. D., Phillips, C. A., et al.: Transplacental rubella infection in newly born infants. J. A. M. A. *191*:843–845, 1965.
383. Sacks, R., and Habermann, E. T.: Pathological fracture in congenital rubella: A case report. J. Bone Joint Surg. [Am.] *59*:557–559, 1977.
384. Saeed, A. A., and Lange, L. S.: Guillain-Barré syndrome after rubella. Postgrad. Med. J. *54*:333–334, 1978.
385. Sallomi, S. J.: Rubella in pregnancy: A review of prospective studies from the literature. Obstet. Gynecol. *27*:252–256, 1966.
386. Salmi, A. A.: Characterization of a structural antigen of rubella virus reacting by gel precipitation. Acta Pathol. Microbiol. Scand. *80*:534–544, 1972.
387. Salmi, A. A.: Gel precipitation reactions between alkaline-extracted rubella antigens and human sera. Acta Pathol. Microbiol. Scand. *76*:271–278, 1969.
388. Sarwar, M., Azar-Kia, B., Schechter, M. M., et al.: Aqueductal occlusion in the congenital rubella syndrome. Neurology *24*:198–201, 1974.
389. Schaffner, W., Fleet, W. F., Kilroy, A. W., et al.: Poly-neuropathy following rubella immunization: A follow-up study and review of the problem. Am. J. Dis. Child. *127*:684–687, 1974.
390. Schamberg, J. F., and Kolmer, J. A.: The treatment of measles. *In* Acute Infectious Diseases. 2nd ed. Philadelphia, Lea & Febiger, 1928, pp. 545–573.
391. Schatzmayr, H. G.: Aspects of rubella infection in Brazil. Rev. Infect. Dis. *7*:S53–S55, 1985.
392. Scheie, H. G., Schaffer, D. B., Plotkin, S. A., et al.: Congenital rubella cataracts: Surgical results and virus recovery from intraocular tissue. Arch. Ophthalmol. *77*:440–444, 1967.
393. Schell, K., and Wong, K. T.: Stability and storage of rubella complement-fixing antigen. Nature *212*:621–622, 1966.
394. Schiff, G. M., Linnemann, C. C., Shea, L., et al.: Evaluation of RA 27/3 rubella vaccine. J. Pediatr. *85*:379–381, 1974.
395. Schiff, G. M.: Titered lots of immune globulin (Ig): Efficacy in the prevention of rubella. Am. J. Dis. Child. *118*:322–327, 1969.
396. Schiff, G. M., and Dine, M. S.: Transmission of rubella from newborns: A controlled study among young adult women and report of an unusual case. Am. J. Dis. Child. *110*:447–451, 1965.
397. Schiff, G. M., Sutherland, J. M., Light, I. J., et al.: Studies on congenital rubella: Preliminary results on the frequency and significance of presence of rubella virus in the newborn and the effect of γ-globulin in preventing congenital rubella. Am. J. Dis. Child. *110*:441–443, 1965.
398. Schiff, G. M., Sever, J. L., and Huebner, R. J.: Experimental rubella: Clinical and laboratory findings. Arch. Intern. Med. *116*:537–543, 1965.
399. Schlossberg, D., and Topolosky, M. K.: Military rubella. J. A. M. A. *238*:1273–1274, 1977.
400. Schmidt, N. J., Dennis, J., and Lennette, E. H.: Rubella virus hemagglutination with a wide variety of erythrocyte species. Appl. Microbiol. *22*:469–470, 1971.
401. Schmidt, N. J., and Lennette, E. H.: Complement-fixing and fluorescent antibody responses to an attenuated rubella virus vaccine. Am. J. Epidemiol. *91*:351–354, 1970.
402. Schmidt, N. J., and Styk, B.: Immunodiffusion reactions with rubella antigens. J. Immunol. *101*:210–216, 1968.
403. Schmidt, N. J., Lennette, E. H., and Gee, P. S.: Demonstration of rubella complement-fixing antigens of two distinct particle sizes by gel filtration of Sephadex G-200. Proc. Soc. Exp. Biol. Med. *123*:758–762, 1966.
404. Schmitz, H., Shinizu, H., Kampa, D., et al.: Rapid method to detect rubella immunoglobulin M and immunoglobulin A antibodies. J. Clin. Microbiol. *1*:132–135, 1975.
405. Schum, T. R., Nelson, D. B., Duma, M. A., et al.: Increasing rubella seronegativity despite a compulsory school law. Am. J. Public Health *80*:66–69, 1990.
406. Sears, M. L.: Congenital glaucoma in neonatal rubella. J. Ophthalmol. *51*:744–748, 1967.
407. Sedwick, W. D., and Sokol, F.: Nucleic acid of rubella virus and its replication in hamster kidney cells. J. Virol. *5*:478–481, 1970.
408. Sekeles, E., and Ornoy, A.: Osseous manifestations of gestational rubella in young human fetuses. Am. J. Obstet. Gynecol. *122*:307–312, 1975.
409. Seppala, M., and Vaheri, A.: Natural rubella infection of the female genital tract. Lancet *1*:46–47, 1974.
410. Sever, J. L., South, M. A., and Shaver, K. A.: Delayed manifestations of congenital rubella. Rev. Infect. Dis. *7*:S164–S169, 1985.
411. Sever, J. L., Hardy, J. B., Nelson, K. B., et al.: Rubella in the collaborative perinatal research study. II. Clinical and laboratory findings in children through 3 years of age. Am. J. Dis. Child. *118*:123–132, 1969.
412. Sever, J. L., Fuccillo, D. A., Gilkeson, M. R., et al.: Changing susceptibility to rubella. Obstet. Gynecol. *32*:365–369, 1968.
413. Sever, J. L., Fuccillo, D. A., Gitnick, G. L., et al.: Rubella antibody determinations. Pediatrics *40*:789–797, 1967.
414. Sever, J. L.: The epidemiology of rubella. Arch. Ophthalmol. *77*:427–429, 1967.
415. Sever, J. L., Huebner, R. J., Fabiyi, A., et al.: Antibody responses in acute and chronic rubella. Proc. Soc. Exp. Biol. Med. *122*:513–516, 1966.
416. Sever, J. L., and Monif, G.: Limited persistence of virus in congenital rubella. Am. J. Dis. Child. *110*:452–454, 1965.
417. Sever, J. L., Brody, J. A., Schiff, G. M., et al.: Rubella epidemic on St. Paul Island in the Pribilofs, 1963. J. A. M. A. *191*:624–626, 1965.
418. Sever, J. L., Huebner, R. J., Castellano, G. A., et al.: Rubella complement fixation test. Science *148*:385–387, 1965.
419. Sever, J. L., Schiff, G. M., and Huebner, R. J.: Frequency of rubella antibody among pregnant women and other human and animal populations. Obstet. Gynecol. *23*:153–159, 1964.
420. Sherman, F. E., Michaels, R. H., and Kenny, F. M.: Acute encephalopathy (encephalitis) complicating rubella. J. A. M. A. *192*:675–681, 1965.
421. Shewmon, D. A., Cherry, J. D., and Kirby, S. E.: Shedding of rubella virus in a 4½-year-old boy with congenital rubella. Pediatr. Infect. Dis. *1*:342–343, 1982.
422. Siassi, B., Klyman, G., and Emmanouilides, G. C.: Hypoplasia of the abdominal aorta associated with the rubella syndrome. Am. J. Dis. Child. *120*:476–479, 1970.
423. Simpson, J. W., Nora, J. J., Singer, D. B., et al.: Multiple valvular sclerosis in Turner phenotypes and rubella syndrome. Am. J. Cardiol. *23*:94–97, 1969.
424. Simpson, R. E. H.: Rubella and polyarthritis. B. M. J. *1*:830–831, 1940.
425. Singer, D. B., Rudolph, A. J., Rosenberg, H. S., et al.: Pathology of the congenital rubella syndrome: J. Pediatr. *71*:665–675, 1967.
426. Singer, D. B., South, M. A., Montgomery, J. R., et al.: Congenital rubella syndrome: Lymphoid tissue and immunologic status. Am. J. Dis. Child. *118*:54–61, 1969.
427. Skaug, K., and Gaarer, P. I.: An indirect immunofluorescent antibody test for determination of rubella virus–specific IgM antibodies. Acta Pathol. Microbiol. Scand. [C] *86*:33–35, 1978.
428. Slater, P. E., Ben-Zvi, T., Fogel, A., et al.: Absence of an association between rubella vaccination and arthritis in underimmune postpartum women. Vaccine *13*:1529–1532, 1995.
429. Smith, K. A., Chess, L., and Mardiney, M. R., Jr.: The relationship between rubella hemagglutination inhibition antibody (HIA) and rubella-induced in vitro lymphocyte tritiated thymidine incorporation. Cell. Immunol. *8*:321–327, 1973.
430. Smithells, R. W., Sheppard, S., Holzel, H., et al.: National congenital rubella surveillance programme, 1 July 1971–30 June 1984. B. M. J. *291*:40–41, 1985.
431. Spencer, M. J., Cherry, J. D., Powell, K. R., et al.: Antibody responses following rubella immunization analyzed by HLA and ABO types. Immunogenetics *4*:365–372, 1977.
432. Spiro, A. J., and Rorke, L. B.: Skeletal muscle lesions in congenital rubella syndrome. Am. J. Dis. Child. *112*:427–428, 1966.
433. Spruance, S. L., Metcalf, R., Smith, C. B., et al.: Chronic arthropathy associated with rubella vaccination. Arthritis Rheum. *20*:741–747, 1977.
434. Spruance, S. L., and Smith, C. B.: Joint complications associated with derivatives of HPV-77 rubella virus vaccine. Am. J. Dis. Child. *122*:105–112, 1971.
435. Squadrini, F., Taparelli, F., DeRienzo, B., et al.: Rubella virus isolation from cerebrospinal fluid in postnatal rubella encephalitis. B. M. J. *2*:1329–1330, 1977.
436. Stallman, N. D., Allan, B. C., and Sutherland, C. J.: Prolonged rubella IgM antibody response. Med. J. Aust. *2*:629–631, 1974.
437. Staub, H. P.: Postrubella thrombocytopenic purpura: A report of eight cases with discussion of hemorrhagic manifestations of rubella. Clin. Pediatr. *7*:350–356, 1968.
438. Steele, R. W., Hensen, S. A., Vincent, M. M., et al.: A ^{51}Cr microassay technique for cell-mediated immunity to viruses. J. Immunol. *110*:1502–1510, 1973.
439. Stehr-Green, P. A., Cochi, S. L., Preblud, S. R., et al.: Evidence against increasing rubella seronegativity among adolescent girls. Am. J. Public Health *80*:88, 1990.
440. Stern, H., and Williams, B. M.: Isolation of rubella virus in a case of neonatal giant-cell hepatitis. Lancet *1*:293–295, 1966.
441. Stewart, G. L., Parkman, P. D., Hopps, H. E., et al.: Rubella-virus hemagglutination-inhibition test. N. Engl. J. Med. *276*:554–557, 1967.
442. Stiehm, E. R., Ammann, A. J., and Cherry, J. D.: Elevated cord macroglobulins in the diagnosis of intrauterine infections. N. Engl. J. Med. *275*:971–977, 1966.
443. Storch, G. A., Gruber, C., Benz, B., et al.: A rubella outbreak among dental students: Description of the outbreak and analysis of control measures. Infect. Control *6*:150–156, 1985.
444. Strassburg, M. A., Imagawa, D. T., Fannin, S. L., et al.: A rubella outbreak among hospital employees with exposure to women in early pregnancy. Obstet. Gynecol. *57*:283–288, 1981.
445. Strauss, L., and Bernstein, J.: Neonatal hepatitis in congenital rubella. Arch. Pathol. *86*:317–327, 1968.
446. Streissguth, A. P., Vanderveer, B. B., and Shepard, T. H.: Mental development of children with congenital rubella syndrome. Am. J. Obstet. Gynecol. *108*:391–399, 1970.
447. Sugaya, N., Nirasawa, M., Mitamura, K., et al.: Hepatitis in acquired rubella infection in children. Am. J. Dis. Child. *142*:817–818, 1988.

448. Svenningsen, N. W.: Thrombocytopenia after rubella (report of two cases). Acta Paediatr. Scand. *54*:97–100, 1965.
449. Swan, C., Tostevin, A. L., Mayo, H., et al.: Further observations on congenital defects in infants following infectious diseases during pregnancy, with special reference to rubella. Med. J. Aust. *1*:409–413, 1944.
450. Swan, C., Tostevin, A. L., Moore, B., et al.: Congenital defects in infants following infectious diseases during pregnancy: With special reference to the relationship between German measles and cataract, deaf-mutism, heart disease and microcephaly, and to the period of pregnancy in which the occurrence of rubella is followed by congenital abnormalities. Med. J. Aust. *11*:201–210, 1943.
451. Swartz, T. A., Hornstein, L., and Epstein, I.: Epidemiology of rubella and congenital rubella infection in Israel, a country with a selective immunization program. Rev. Infect. Dis. *7*:S42–S46, 1985.
452. Swartz, T. A.: An extensive rubella epidemic in Israel, 1972: Selected epidemiologic characteristics. Am. J. Epidemiol. *103*:60–66, 1976.
453. Swartz, T. A., Klingberg, W., Goldwasser, R. A., et al.: Clinical manifestations according to age, among females given HPV-77 duck rubella vaccine. Am. J. Epidemiol. *94*:246–251, 1971.
454. Thompson, G. R., Weiss, J. J., Shillis, J. L., et al.: Intermittent arthritis following rubella vaccination: A three-year follow-up. Am. J. Dis. Child. *125*:526–530, 1973.
455. Thompson, G. R., Ferreyra, A., Brackett, R. G.: Acute arthritis complicating rubella vaccination: Arthritis Rheum. *14*:19–26, 1971.
456. Thompson, K. M., and Tobin, J. O.: Isolation of rubella virus from abortion material. B. M. J. *1*:264–266, 1970.
457. Thong, Y. H., Steele, R. W., Vincent, M. M., et al.: Impaired in vitro cell-mediated immunity to rubella virus during pregnancy. N. Engl. J. Med. *289*:604–606, 1973.
458. Thorburn, M. J., and Miller, C. G.: Pathology of congenital rubella in Jamaica. Arch. Dis. Child. *42*:389–396, 1967.
459. Tingle, A. J., Allen, M., Petty, R. E., et al.: Rubella associated arthritis. I. Comparative study of joint manifestations associated with natural rubella infection and RA 27/3 rubella immunization. Ann. Rheum. Dis. *45*:110–114, 1986.
460. Tingle, A. J., Chantler, J. K., Pot, K. H., et al.: Postpartum rubella immunization: Association with development of prolonged arthritis, neurological sequelae, and chronic rubella viremia. J. Infect. Dis. *152*:606–612, 1985.
461. Tingle, A. J., Yang, T., Allen, M., et al.: Prospective immunological assessment of arthritis induced by rubella vaccine. Infect. Immun. *40*:22–28, 1983.
462. Tobin, J. O., Sheppard, S., Smithells, R. W., et al.: Rubella in the United Kingdom, 1970–1983. Rev. Infect. Dis. *7*:S47–S52, 1985.
463. Tomlinson, I. W.: Rubella polyneuropathy. Postgrad. Med. J. *51*:30–32, 1975.
464. Tondury, G., and Smith, D.: Fetal rubella pathology. J. Pediatr. *68*:867–879, 1966.
465. Townsend, C. W.: Concerning German measles. Boston Med. Surg. J. *150*:403–404, 1904.
466. Townsend, J. J., Baringer, J. R., Wolinsky, J. S., et al.: Progressive rubella panencephalitis: Late onset after congenital rubella. N. Engl. J. Med. *292*:990–993, 1975.
467. Trudel, M., Nadon, F., Sequin, C., et al.: E1 glycoprotein of rubella virus carries an epitope that binds a neutralizing antibody. J. Virol. Methods *12*:243–250, 1985.
468. Ueda, K., Shingaki, Y., Sato, T., et al.: Hemolytic anemia following postnatally acquired rubella during the 1975–1977 rubella epidemic in Japan. Clin. Pediatr. *24*:155–157, 1985.
469. Ueda, K., Sasaki, F., Tokugawa, K., et al.: The 1976–1977 rubella epidemic in Fukuoka City in Southern Japan: Epidemiology and incidences of complications among 80,000 persons who were school children at 28 primary schools and their family members. Biken J. *27*:161–168, 1984.
470. Ueda, K., Nishida, Y., Oshima, K., et al.: Congenital rubella syndrome: Correlation of gestational age at time of maternal rubella with type of defect. J. Pediatr. *94*:763–765, 1979.
471. Ueda, K., Nishida, Y., Oshima, K., et al.: Seven-year follow-up study of rubella syndrome in Ryukyu with special reference to persistence of rubella hemagglutination inhibition antibodies. Jpn. J. Microbiol. *19*:181–185, 1975.
472. Ueda, K., Nishida, Y., Kano, M., et al.: Clinical studies of patients with rubella syndrome occurring in a high incidence in the Ryukyu Islands in 1965: On the diagnostic significance of clinical manifestations. Acta Paediatr. Jpn. *14*:9–16, 1972.
473. Ueno, Y.: Rubella arthritis: An outbreak in Tokyo J. Rheumatol. *21*:874–876, 1994.
474. Ukkonen, P.: Rubella immunity and morbidity: Impact of different vaccination programs in Finland 1979–1992. Scand. J. Infect. Dis. *28*:31–35, 1996.
475. Upfold, L. J.: Deafness following rubella in pregnancy. Med. J. Aust. *1*:420–424, 1970.
476. Urquhart, G. E. D., Crawford, R. J., and Wallace, J.: Trial of high-titre human rubella immunoglobulin. B. M. J. *2*:1331–1332, 1978.
477. Vaheri, A., Vesikari, T., Oker-Blom, N., et al.: Isolation of attenuated rubella-vaccine virus from human products of conception and uterine cervix. N. Engl. J. Med. *286*:1071–1074, 1972.
478. Vaheri, A., and Vesikari, T.: Small size rubella virus antigens and soluble immune complexes: Analysis by the platelet aggregation technique. Arch. Ges. Virusforsch. *35*:10–24, 1971.
479. Van der Horst, R. L., and Gotsman, M. S.: Left ventricular aneurysm in rubella heart disease. Am. J. Dis. Child. *120*:248–251, 1970.
480. Veale, H.: History of an epidemic of Rotheln, with observations on its pathology. Edinburgh Med. J. *12*:404–414, 1866.
481. Vejtorp, M., Fanoe, E., and Leerhoy, J.: Diagnosis of postnatal rubella by the enzyme-linked immunosorbent assay for rubella IgM and IgG antibodies. Acta Pathol. Microbiol. Scand. [B] *87*:155–160, 1979.
482. Verder, H., Dickmeiss, E., Haahr, S., et al.: Late-onset rubella syndrome: Coexistence of immune complex disease and defective cytotoxic effector cell function. Clin. Exp. Immunol. *63*:367–375, 1986.
483. Vesikari, T., Kanra, G. Y., Buimovici-Klein, E., et al.: Cell-mediated immunity in rubella assayed by cytotoxicity of supernatants from rubella virus-stimulated human lymphocyte cultures. Clin. Exp. Immunol. *19*:33–43, 1975.
484. Vesikari, T., and Buimovici-Klein, E.: Lymphocyte responses to rubella antigen and phytohemagglutinin after administration of the RA 27/3 strain of live attenuated rubella vaccine. Infect. Immun. *11*:748–753, 1975.
485. Vesikari, T., Vaheri, A., and Leinikki, P.: Antibody response to rubella virion (V) and soluble (S) antigens in rubella infection and following vaccination with live attenuated rubella virus. Arch. Ges. Virusforsch. *35*:25–37, 1971.
486. Vesikari, T., Vaheri, A., Pettay, O., et al.: Congenital rubella: Immune response of the neonate and diagnosis by demonstration of specific IgM antibodies. J. Pediatr. *75*:658–664, 1969.
487. Vince, D. J.: The role of rubella in the etiology of supravalvular aortic stenosis. Can. Med. Assoc. J. *103*:1157–1160, 1970.
488. Vogt, R. L., and Clark, S. W.: Premarital rubella vaccination program. Am. J. Public Health *75*:1088–1089, 1985.
489. Vossaugh, P., Leikin, S., Avery, G., et al.: Neonatal thrombocytopenia in association with rubella. Acta Haematol. *35*:158–162, 1966.
490. Walker, J. M., and Nahmias, A. J.: Neurologic sequelae of rubella infection. Clin. Pediatr. *5*:699–702, 1966.
491. Wallace, R. B., Libert, P., Ibrahim, M., et al.: Joint symptoms following an area-wide rubella immunization campaign: Report of a survey. Am. J. Public Health *62*:658–661, 1972.
492. Wallace, R. B., and Isacson, P.: Comparative trial of HPV-77, DE-5 and RA 27/3 live-attenuated rubella vaccines. Am. J. Dis. Child. *124*:536–538, 1972.
493. Walls, W. L., Altman, D. H., Gair, D. R., et al.: Roentgenological findings in congenital rubella. Clin. Pediatr. *4*:704–708, 1965.
494. Ward, P. H., Honrubia, V., and Moore, B. S.: Inner ear pathology in deafness due to maternal rubella. Arch. Otolaryngol. *87*:40–46, 1968.
495. Warren, H. D., Rogliand, F. T., and Potsubay, S. F.: Thrombocytopenic purpura following rubella. Med. Clin. North Am. *30*:401–404, 1946.
496. Waxham, M. N., and Wolinsky, J. S.: Immunochemical identification of rubella virus hemagglutinin. Virology *126*:194–203, 1983.
497. Way, R. C.: Cardiovascular defects and the rubella syndrome. Can. Med. Assoc. J. *97*:1329–1334, 1967.
498. Weber, B., Enders, G., Schlößer, R., et al.: Congenital rubella syndrome after maternal reinfection. Infection *21*:118–121, 1993.
499. Weibel, R. E., Stokes, J., Jr., Buynak, E. B., et al.: Live rubella vaccines in adults and children: HPV-77 and Merck-Benoit strains. Am. J. Dis. Child. *118*:226–229, 1969.
500. Weil, M. L., Itabashi, H. H., Cremer, N. E., et al.: Chronic progressive panencephalitis due to rubella virus simulating subacute sclerosing panencephalitis. N. Engl. J. Med. *292*:994–998, 1975.
501. Weinberger, M. M., Masland, M. W., Asbed, R. A., et al.: Congenital rubella presenting as retarded language development. Am. J. Dis. Child. *120*:125–128, 1970.
502. Weller, T. H., and Neva, F. A.: Propagation in tissue culture of cytopathic agents from patients with rubella-like illness. Proc. Soc. Exp. Biol. Med. *111*:215–225, 1962.
503. Wesselhoeft, C.: Rubella (German measles). N. Engl. J. Med. *236*:943–950, 978–988, 1947.
504. Whalen, J. P., Winchester, P., Krook, L., et al.: Neonatal transplacental rubella syndrome: Its effect on normal maturation of the diaphysis. Am. J. Roentgenol. Rad. Ther. Nucl. Med. *121*:166–172, 1974.
505. White, L. R., Sever, J. L., and Alepa, F. P.: Maternal and congenital rubella before 1964: Frequency, clinical features, and search for isoimmune phenomena. J. Pediatr. *74*:198–207, 1969.
506. White, L. R., Leikin, S., Villavicencio, O., et al.: Immune competence in congenital rubella: Lymphocyte transformation, delayed hypersensitivity, and response to vaccination. J. Pediatr. *73*:229–234, 1968.
507. Whitehouse, W. L.: Rubella before conception as a cause of foetal abnormality. Lancet *1*:139, 1963.
508. Williams, H. J., and Carey, L. S.: Rubella embryopathy: Roentgenologic features. Am. J. Roentgenol. Rad. Ther. Nucl. Med. *97*:92–99, 1966.
509. Wingo, S. M.: Encephalomyelitis complicating rubella: Report of a case. U. S. Naval Med. Bull. *45*:546–547, 1945.
510. Witney, E. W.: Neuritis following rubella. B. M. J. *1*:831, 1940.

511. Witte, J. J., Karchmer, A. W., Case, G., et al.: Epidemiology of rubella. Am. J. Dis. Child. *118*:107–111, 1969.
512. Wolinsky, J. S.: Rubella. *In* Fields, B. N., Knipe, D. M., Howley, P. M., et al. (eds.): Fields Virology. 2nd ed. New York, Raven Press, 1990, pp. 815–838.
513. Wolinsky, J. S., Dau, P. C., Buimovici-Klein, E., et al.: Progressive rubella panencephalitis: Immunovirological studies and results of isoprinosine therapy. Clin. Exp. Immunol. *35*:397–404, 1979.
514. Wolinsky, J. S., Berg, B. O., and Maitland, C. J.: Progressive rubella panencephalitis. Arch. Neurol. *33*:722–723, 1976.
515. Wolman, S. R., McMorrow, L. E., Ziring, P. R., et al.: Lack of chromosomal breakage in congenital rubella. Pediatrics *52*:213–220, 1973.
516. Wyll, S. A., and Herrmann, K. L.: Inadvertent rubella vaccination of pregnant women: Fetal risk in 215 cases. J. A. M. A. *225*:1472–1476, 1973.
517. Yanez, J. E., Thompson, G. R., Mikkelsen, W. M., et al.: Rubella arthritis. Ann. Intern. Med. *64*:772–777, 1966.
518. Zaknun, D., Weiss, G., Glatzl, J., et al.: Neopterin levels during acute rubella in children. Clin. Infect. Dis. *17*:521–522, 1993.
519. Zausmer, E.: Congenital rubella: Pathogenesis of motor deficits. Pediatrics *47*:16–26, 1971.
520. Zrein, M., Joncas, J. H., Pedneault, L., et al.: Comparison of a whole-virus enzyme immunoassay (EIA) with a peptide-based EIA for detecting rubella virus immunoglobulin G antibodies following rubella vaccination. J. Clin. Microbiol. *31*:1521–1524, 1993.

178

ALPHAVIRUSES

❑ ❑ ❑

CHAPTER 178 (A)

Eastern Equine Encephalitis

Theodore F. Tsai

Eastern equine encephalitis (EEE) is an arthropod-borne viral infection of humans, horses, and other vertebrates occurring in North and South America. In North America, infections recur in highly focal, primarily coastal locations in association with the habitat of *Culiseta melanura,* the enzootic vector. Birds are the amplifying hosts, and humans and horses are infected incidentally.

ETIOLOGIC AGENT

EEE virus is an antigenically distinct member of the *Alphavirus* genus in the *Togaviridae* family. On the basis of nucleotide differences, EEE and Venezuelan equine encephalitis may have diverged 1000 to 2000 years ago, with a subsequent division of EEE virus into North and South American varieties.[48, 50, 51] South American strains can be differentiated by monoclonal antibodies and by short-incubation hemagglutination-inhibition tests.

North American strains collected over a broad geographic and temporal span indicate remarkable genetic stability in one or two major lineages, with minor local divergences within isolated geographic loci. South American strains genetically are heterogeneous. South American strains have been isolated in northward-migrating birds captured in the United States, but they have never been shown to become established.[8]

ECOLOGY

Equine cases have been reported as far north as Quebec, Ontario, and Alberta provinces and New Hampshire; in South America, EEE viral activity has been reported from the Caribbean, Mexico, Guatemala, Honduras, Panama, Colombia, Venezuela, Peru, Guyana, Brazil, and as far south as Argentina.[9, 39, 48] The viral transmission cycles in the Caribbean and South America are not well characterized but apparently involve small mammals, birds, and *Culex (Melanolonion)* species mosquitoes.[45]

In North America, the distribution of virus activity closely follows the distribution of freshwater swamps on the Eastern Seaboard, Gulf Coast, and other inland areas, corresponding to the distribution of the principal enzootic vector *C. melanura.*[21, 39, 45] *C. melanura* feeds nearly exclusively on birds.[42] Various epizootic (bridging) vectors are responsible for infecting humans and horses, including *Coquillettidia perturbans, Aedes sollicitans, Aedes vexans,* and *Aedes canadensis.*[18, 21, 39, 45, 46, 48]

Infection and viremia are subclinical in most native birds; whooping cranes and exotic birds, such as sparrows, ring-necked pheasants, Pekin ducks, and Chukar partridges, may become ill and die of infection.[3, 13] Large outbreaks resulting in thousands of deaths have occurred in commercial pheasant flocks. In some instances, transmission was perpetuated by cannibalistic pecking or preening of persistently infected quills.[3] Humans and horses are the most conspicuous incidental hosts, but illness and deaths in emus, whooping cranes, pigs, goats, calves, rodents, and other mammals also have been reported.[13, 22, 39, 45]

C. melanura is found in and near fresh-water swamps, where larval stages breed in acidic waters associated with mucky peat soils. These foci are associated with upland red maple, coastal white cedar, and southern loblolly bay biotypes.[21, 39, 45, 48] *C. melanura* is distributed in scattered areas of the eastern United States and Canada, except in elevated mountainous locations.

The overwintering mechanism has not been elucidated. Although EEE virus has been isolated from northward-migrating birds, the identification of these strains as South American varieties argues against this hypothesis. Furthermore, virus activity in local birds has been documented to precede annual migratory movements. Neither survival of the virus in overwintering larvae nor transovarial transmission has been demonstrated conclusively. The winter maintenance of virus in persistently infected permanent resident birds has been proposed.[11] The remarkable permanence of endemic foci is a strong argument for overwintering in local reservoirs.[38, 50, 51]

EPIDEMIOLOGY

EEE is a disease of low incidence, with a median of three cases occurring annually in the United States (Fig. 178–1).[35]

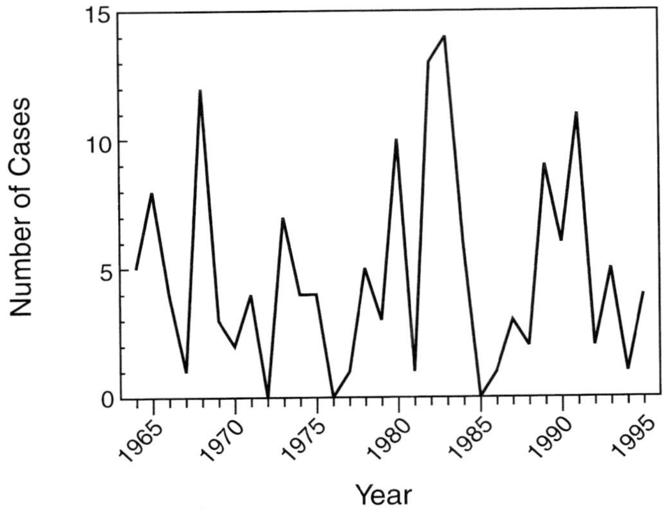

FIGURE 178–1. *Reported cases of eastern equine encephalitis by year, 1964 to 1995.*

The states with the highest rates of infection show an average annual incidence of 0.012 (New Jersey and Massachusetts) to 0.020 to 0.026 per 100,000 (Florida and Delaware) (Fig. 178–2). However, these estimates of incidence obscure the remarkably consistent and focal distribution of cases on the Atlantic and Gulf Coasts, from New Hampshire to Texas, and in isolated pockets of activity inland. For example, until 1995, all human cases in Massachusetts had occurred east of Highway 495 in Essex, Norfolk, Plymouth, Bristol, and Middlesex Counties; the six southernmost counties account for most of the epizootic activity in New Jersey; and foci of EEE viral activity recur in upstate New York counties near Syracuse, southwestern Michigan, northeastern Indiana, and northeastern Florida.[31, 48] Outbreaks of human cases, due to North American viral strains, have been reported from Jamaica, Trinidad, and the Dominican Republic. Isolated epizootics with sporadic human cases have been reported from South America.[6, 15, 47]

Viral transmission, reflected in equine cases, occurs all year in Florida, although the peak occurrence is from May to September.[7] Human cases have appeared as early as February and as late as December in Florida, but most cases occur from June to August in that state.[7] In the Northeast, cases usually appear in late summer, from August to September and as late as the third week in October.[29, 33]

Cases occur chiefly at the extremes of age. However, serologic studies during the New Jersey outbreak disclosed that infection occurred with equal frequency in all age groups, indicating that biologic responses to infection, rather than factors associated with exposure, were responsible for lower attack rates in young and middle-aged adults.[27] The ratio of inapparent infections to cases was highest in the middle years of life (29:1) and lowest in children younger than 4 years of age (8:1) and in adults older than 55 years of age (16:1).[27]

Family clusters were observed in this epidemic and in the 1947 Louisiana outbreak.[29] Family members of cases had twice the rate of inapparent infections as did the general population in the New Jersey study.[26] Two fatal cases and two seropositive members were observed in the same family in the southern Louisiana outbreak. Clusters of equine cases on a single premise are reported frequently.

Asymptomatic infections are uncommon. Long-term residence in an enzootic area leads to a slight increase in population immunity. Only 7 per cent of persons who had resided in southern coastal New Jersey 45 years or more had neutralizing antibody.[24] However, the New Jersey studies may reflect an unusually active focus. In serosurveys of endemic foci in Massachusetts, evidence of past infections was found in 0.5 to 0.7 per cent of residents.[19, 44] A serosurvey of Connecticut pheasant farmers, working in areas that had experienced repeated outbreaks, showed no evidence of infections.[37]

Specific behavioral risk factors have not been described; however, residence or outdoor activity near swampy habitats has been reported anecdotally.

CLINICAL MANIFESTATIONS

EEE is a fulminant encephalitis with a rapid progression to coma and death in one-third of cases.[1,2, 7, 12, 15–17, 20, 35, 36, 40, 42, 44, 49, 52, 53] In infants and children, an abrupt onset of fever, irritability, and headache is followed closely by lethargy, confusion, seizures, and coma. A bulging fontanelle, meningismus, high temperature, and generalized flaccid or spastic paralysis are found on examination.[1, 16, 17, 20, 52, 53] Some patients present in status epilepticus. The prodrome in adults and older children may be brief, with nonspecific symptoms of fever, headache, and dizziness followed by clouding of the

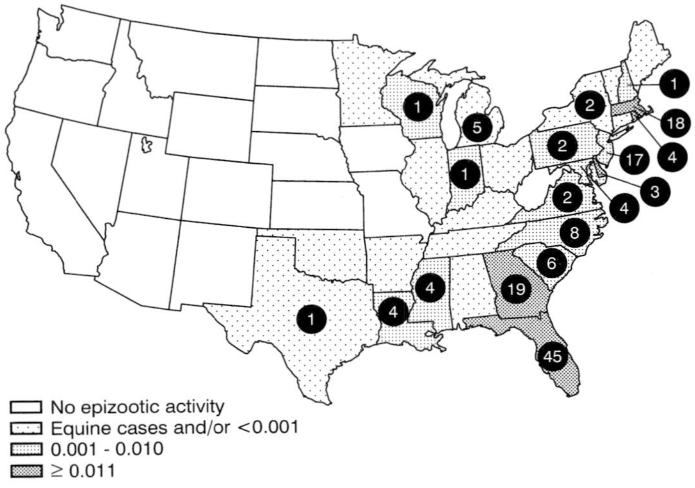

FIGURE 178–2. *Reported cases and average annual incidence (per 100,000) of eastern equine encephalitis by state, 1964 to 1995.*

sensorium and rapid deterioration to coma. However, some patients have a prolonged prodrome lasting more than a week, with a waxing and waning course of nonspecific symptoms in some cases.[44] Various neurologic defects have been described; in some cases, unilateral seizures, hemiparesis, hemiplegia, and aphasia have indicated focal areas of involvement.[40, 42]

The peripheral leukocyte count usually is elevated, with a shift to the left. White blood cell counts of 20,000/mm^3 are typical and range as high as 60,000, with 55 to 89 per cent neutrophils.[44] The cerebrospinal fluid usually shows a polymorphonuclear pleocytosis with a total leukocyte count ranging from 500 to 2000/mm^3. The initial neutrophilic pleocytosis of 60 to 100 per cent may persist into the second week before shifting toward a predominance of mononuclear cells.[44] The cerebrospinal fluid protein is elevated and the glucose reduced in the majority of cases. Erythrocyte counts higher than 500/mm^3 are found in some cases.

Imaging studies disclose only cerebral edema in three-quarters of cases. However, focal rim enhancing lesions and areas of low alteration with mass effect have been observed on computed tomographic scans in the frontal cortex, thalami, midbrain, and lentiform nuclei.[40, 42] Electroencephalographic tracings with focal or background slowing were associated with a favorable outcome; disorganized background activity, a burst-suppression pattern, or high-voltage delta slowing was associated with a poor prognosis.[44]

Mild nonencephalitic illnesses usually are not diagnosed. However, in the 1959 outbreak in New Jersey, fever, headache, nausea, vomiting, and sore throat were common symptoms in 19 patients who had serologic evidence of infection. One-third of the patients had illnesses severe enough to motivate a visit to a physician.[26] Other cases with bladder dysfunction, dysethesias, weakness, and signs of myelitis have been reported.[10, 34] One case of infection during pregnancy has been reported. The third trimester infection produced encephalitis and coma, but the woman recovered and delivered an apparently normal baby. Serologic studies of the neonate's blood were not performed.

PATHOLOGY

Pathologic changes in the brain are characterized by lesions in the cortical and deep gray matter. Viral antigen is found predominantly in neurons and only occasionally in astrocytes.[45] The degree of neuronal loss varies from mild involvement to extensive necrotic lesions. Neutrophils predominate in cellular infiltrates in the meninges, vascular cuffs, and foci of tissue damage in the cortex and brain nuclei.[2, 14, 16, 41, 53] The predominance of neutrophils probably reflects the rapid course of infection. In patients who die at later stages, neutrophilic infiltrates are replaced by mononuclear cells. Immunohistochemical examination of one case disclosed a predominance of helper T cells in perivascular infiltrates with some B lymphocytes. The most intense inflammatory reaction occurred in areas where antigen-positive neurons were absent, presumably where cell lysis already had occurred. Perivascular macrophages contained cleared viral antigen, but antigen could not be demonstrated in vascular endothelial cells.[43] Severe leptomeningeal reactions simulating acute pyogenic meningitis are observed in some cases. Rare viral particles have been identified by electron microscopy in principally extracellular locations.[2, 32]

PATHOGENESIS

After peripheral inoculation of experimental animals, local viral replication occurs at a low level or may be undetectable. After a brief period, viremia develops, followed by appearance of virus in viscera: spleen, liver, and kidney in monkeys and guinea pigs and spleen, heart, and lung in mice. Infectivity can be demonstrated in brain only after viremia and infection in viscera are established. These observations suggest that central nervous system invasion occurs by hematogenous spread.

The immune response in the human case presumably is similar to that observed in experimental alphaviral infections of mice, in which host resistance depends on the rapid elaboration of a humoral immune response. The rapidity of lytic EEE viral infection may underlie its marked virulence.

TREATMENT

Specific treatment is unavailable. Therapy aimed at supporting cardiorespiratory function, homeostasis of fluid, and electrolyte balance and control of cerebral edema and convulsions may be lifesaving.

PROGNOSIS AND SEQUELAE

The case-fatality ratio is 33 per cent among reported cases.[35] In previous reports, fatality rates have been even higher, approaching 75 per cent in some outbreaks. The age-specific case-fatality rate is highest in the elderly; outcome is best in young adults 20 to 59 years of age, in whom the case-fatality rate is 24 per cent. Outcome is better in patients with a long prodromal illness (>4 days), which is consistent with the protective effect of a peripheral antibody response in the preneuroinvasive phase.[44]

Residual neurologic damage is observed more often in young children. Serious sequelae were seen in 4 of 7 survivors younger than 5 years of age and in 1 of 10 survivors in other age groups in a Florida series.[7] Similar findings were reported in a follow-up of epidemic cases in Massachusetts: 7 of 8 survivors younger than 3 years of age had neurologic sequelae, and only 1 of 4 surviving adults had residua.[1, 17] Neurologic impairment ranged from mild unilateral spasticity to profound mental retardation, seizure disorders, and quadriplegia.

DIAGNOSIS

The specific laboratory diagnosis usually is made from serologic determinations. Isolations of virus from cerebrospinal fluid are unusual. The virus should be sought from brain biopsy tissue or autopsy material. EEE virus grows rapidly on Vero cells, causing widespread cytopathic effect in several days. Specific identification of viral isolates can be accomplished rapidly by immunofluorescent or immunoperoxidase techniques. EEE virus has been identified by immunofluorescence and by electron microscopy in brain tissue.[2, 32] Viral antigen can be detected directly by antigen capture enzyme-linked immunosorbent assay. This technique has been used to identify viremic bird blood, infected mosquito pools, and infected equine brains.

Serologic testing is available in many state laboratories. Virus-specific IgM usually can be detected in acute serum and cerebrospinal fluid samples. Indirect immunofluorescence, neutralization, and hemagglutination inhibition (HI) also are sensitive procedures. Antibodies often are present in the first week of illness. Neutralizing antibody appears 3 to 4 days after onset of illness, and HI antibody appears with almost equal rapidity.[23] Both HI and neutralizing antibodies appear to be long lived.[25] Complement-fixing (CF) antibody is slower to rise, appearing 11 days after onset, with diagnostic fourfold rises often appearing only in the third week after onset.[23] The peaks of both HI and CF titers are observed 3 to 4 weeks after onset.[26] CF antibody declines more rapidly. Measurable CF antibodies were found in approximately 50 per cent of persons infected 8 years earlier in one study, although the effects of re-exposures could not be ruled out in this endemic area.[25]

The low prevalence of EEE antibody in the general population suggests that EEE viral antibody found in the acute serum of a patient with encephalitis indicates a high probability of that diagnosis. Applying Bayes theorem, if the "rate" of EEE is 1 in every 2000 cases of encephalitis, if HI antibody to EEE is present in 100 per cent of cases in the first week of illness, and if the prevalence of HI antibody in the general population is 0.05 per cent, then the probability of EEE in an encephalitis patient who has demonstrable EEE antibody in a single serum specimen is a certainty. Thus, there is a high probability of the diagnosis when specific antibody is found in any (i.e., acute) serum specimen.

DIFFERENTIAL DIAGNOSIS

The fulminant clinical course of EEE and the laboratory findings of neutrophilic leukocytosis and a polymorphonuclear pleocytosis in the cerebrospinal fluid may suggest bacterial cerebritis or meningitis. Detection of bacterial antigens by latex agglutination or other means and the identification of bacteria in cerebrospinal fluid by acridine orange staining may facilitate a rapid diagnosis of bacterial meningitis.

PREVENTION

An effective killed vaccine is available for horses. A killed vaccine, available under investigatory permit, is used to protect laboratory personnel. Vaccination of the general public is not feasible as a public health measure because of the low incidence of disease.

Climatologic studies have shown a correlation between outbreaks and heavy rainfall in the summer of an epidemic year and in the preceding fall.[28, 30, 35] Although such predictors would have considerable utility in guiding control measures, outbreaks of EEE have been too few for their validity to be tested. Isolations of Highlands J virus, which shares a common enzootic cycle with EEE virus, often peak 2 to 3 weeks before the appearance of EEE virus in *C. melanura*.

Surveillance and public health interventions to prevent EEE cases have been shown to be economic when balanced against the direct and indirect costs of even one human case.[49] Larviciding swampland to control *C. melanura* is difficult because of the large areas involved, the potential toxic effects for fish and other wildlife, and the relative inaccessibility of the larvae. Emergency applications of adulticides to control epizootic vectors are indicated where viral, mosquito, and animal surveillance suggest a risk for epizootic transmission. Public health advisories to avoid outdoor activity near enzootic foci and the closure of campgrounds and parks in these locations may be necessary when viral transmission indices suggest a high level of risk. The use of repellents and avoidance of outdoor activity 1 to 2 hours after sunset when many mosquitoes are most active may reduce exposure; however, some vector *Aedes* species are daytime biters.

References

1. Ayres, J. C., and Feemster, R. F.: The sequelae of eastern equine encephalomyelitis. N. Engl. J. Med. *240*:960–962, 1949.
2. Bastian, F. O., Wende, R. D., Singer, D. B., et al.: Eastern equine encephalomyelitis: Histopathologic and ultrastructural changes with isolation of the virus in a human case. Am. J. Clin. Pathol. *64*:10–13, 1975.
3. Beaudette, F. R., Black, J. J., Hudson, C. B., et al.: Equine encephalomyelitis in pheasants from 1947 to 1951. J. Am. Vet. Med. Assoc. *121*:478–483, 1952.
4. Bellavance, R., Rossier, E., and Le Maitre, M. P.: Eastern equine encephalitis in eastern Canada: 1972. Can. J. Public Health *64*:189–190, 1973.
5. Belle, E. A., Grant, L. S., and Thorburn, M. J.: An outbreak of eastern equine encephalomyelitis in Jamaica. II. Laboratory diagnosis and pathology of eastern equine encephalomyelitis in Jamaica. Am. J. Trop. Med. Hyg. *13*:335–341, 1964.
6. Bigler, W. J., Lassing, E. B., Buff, E. E., et al.: Endemic eastern equine encephalomyelitis in Florida: A twenty-year analysis, 1955–1974. Am. J. Trop. Med. Hyg. *25*:884–890, 1976.
7. Calisher, C. H., Maness, K. S. C., Lord, R. D., et al.: Identification of two South American strains of eastern equine encephalomyelitis virus from migrant birds captured on the Mississippi delta. Am. J. Epidemiol. *94*:172–178, 1971.
8. Carman, P. S., Artsob, H., Emery S., et al.: Eastern equine encephalitis in a horse from southwestern Ontario. Can. Vet. J. *36*:170–172, 1995.
9. Clarke, D. H.: Two nonfatal human infections with the virus of eastern encephalitis. Am. J. Trop. Med. Hyg. *10*:67–70, 1961.
10. Crans, W. J., Caccamise, D. F., and McNelly, J. R.: Eastern equine encephalomyelitis virus in relation to the avian community of a coastal cedar swamp. J. Med. Entomol. *31*:711–728, 1994.
11. Davenport, D. S., Batts, D. H., and Carter, J. W.: Eastern equine encephalitis in Michigan. Arch. Neurol. *39*:322–323, 1982.
12. Dein, F. J., Carpenter, J. W., Clark, G. G., et al.: Mortality of captive whooping cranes caused by eastern equine encephalitis virus. J. Am. Vet. Med. Assoc. *9*:1006–1010, 1986.
13. de la Monte, S. M.: Selective vulnerability of particular central nervous system regions to eastern equine encephalitis virus in humans. J. Neuropathol. Exp. Neurol. *44*:358, 1985.
14. Eklund, C. M., Bell, J. F., and Brennan, J. M.: Antibody survey following an outbreak of human and equine disease in the Dominican Republic, caused by the eastern strain of equine encephalomyelitis virus. Am. J. Trop. Med. Hyg. *31*:312–328, 1951.
15. Farber, S., Hill, A., Connerly, M. L., et al.: Encephalitis in infants and children. J. A. M. A. *114*:1725–1731, 1940.
16. Feemster, R. F.: Equine encephalitis in Massachusetts. N. Engl. J. Med. *257*:701–704, 1957.
17. Feemster, R. F., and Getting, V. A.: Distribution of the vectors of equine encephalomyelitis in Massachusetts. Am. J. Public Health *31*:791–802, 1941.
18. Feemster, R. F., Wheeler, R. E., Daniels, J. B., et al.: Field and laboratory studies on equine encephalitis. N. Engl. J. Med. *259*:107–113, 1958.
19. Getting, V. A.: Equine encephalomyelitis in Massachusetts. N. Engl. J. Med. *24*:999–1006, 1941.
20. Gibbs, P. J., and Tsai, T.: Eastern encephalitis. *In* Beran, G. (ed.): Handbook of Zoonoses: Section B, Viral. Boca Raton, FL, CRC Press, 1994.
21. Goldfield, M., Sussman, O., Black, H. C., et al.: Arbovirus infection of animals in New Jersey. J. Am. Vet. Med. Assoc. *153*:1780–1787, 1968.
22. Goldfield, M., Taylor, B. F., and Welsh, J. N.: The 1959 outbreak of eastern encephalitis in New Jersey. 3. Serologic studies on clinical cases. Am. J. Epidemiol. *87*:18–22, 1968.
23. Goldfield, M., Taylor, B. F., and Welsh, J. N.: The 1959 outbreak of eastern encephalitis in New Jersey. 6. The frequency of prior infection. Am. J. Epidemiol. *87*:39–49, 1968.
24. Goldfield, M., Taylor, B. F., Welsh, J. N., et al.: The persistence of eastern encephalitis serologic reactivity following overt and inapparent human infection: An eight-year followup. Am. J. Epidemiol. *87*:50–57, 1968.
25. Goldfield, M., Welsh, J. N., and Taylor, B. F.: The 1959 outbreak of eastern encephalitis in New Jersey. 4. CF reactivity following overt and inapparent infection. Am. J. Epidemiol. *87*:23–31, 1968.
26. Goldfield, M., Welsh, J. N., and Taylor, B. F.: The 1959 outbreak of eastern encephalitis in New Jersey. 5. The inapparent infection: Disease ratio. Am. J. Epidemiol. *87*:32–38, 1968.
27. Grady, G. F., Maxfield, H. K., Hildreth, S. W., et al.: Eastern equine encephalitis in Massachusetts, 1957–1976: A prospective study centered upon analyses of mosquitoes. Am. J. Epidemiol. *107*:170–178, 1978.
28. Hauser, G. H.: Human equine encephalomyelitis, eastern type, in Louisiana. New Orleans Med. Surg. J. *100*:551–558, 1948.
29. Hayes, R. O., and Hess, A. D.: Climatological conditions associated with outbreaks of eastern encephalitis. Am. J. Trop. Med. Hyg. *13*:851–858, 1964.
30. Howard, J. J., Morris, C. D., Emord, D. E., et al.: Epizootiology of eastern equine encephalitis virus in upstate New York, USA: Virus surveillance 1978–1985, description of 1983 outbreak, and series conclusions. J. Med. Entomol. *25*:501–514, 1988.
31. Kim, J. H., Booss, J., Manvelidis, E. E., et al.: Human eastern equine encephalitis: Electron microscopic study of a brain biopsy. Am. J. Clin. Pathol. *84*:223–227, 1985.
32. Komar, N., and Spielman, A.: Emergence of eastern encephalitis in Massachusetts. Ann. N. Y. Acad. Sci. *740*:157–168, 1995.
33. Lavoie, S. R., Markowitz, S. and Kapadia, S. J.: Eastern equine encephalomyelitis with hematuria and bladder dysfunction. South. Med. J. *86*:812–814, 1993.

34. Letson, G. W., Bailey, R. E., and Pearson, J., et al.: Eastern equine encephalitis (EEE): A description of the 1989 outbreak, recent epidemiologic trends, and the association of rainfall with EEE occurrence. Am. J. Trop. Med. Hyg. *49*:677–685, 1993.
35. Levitt, L. P., Lovejoy, F. H., and Daniels, J. B.: Eastern equine encephalitis in Massachusetts: First human case in 14 years. N. Engl. J. Med. *284*:540, 1971.
36. Liao, S. J.: Eastern equine encephalitis in Connecticut: A serological survey of pheasant farmers. Yale J. Biol. Med. *27*:287–296, 1955.
37. McLean, R. G., Frier, G., Parham, G. L., et al.: Investigations of the vertebrate hosts of eastern equine encephalitis during an epizootic in Michigan. Am. J. Trop. Med. Hyg. *34*:1190–1202, 1985.
38. Morris, C. D.: Eastern equine encephalomyelitis. *In* Monath, T. P. (ed.): The Arboviruses: Epidemiology and Ecology. Vol. 3. Boca Raton, CRC Press, 1988, pp. 1–20.
39. Morse, R. P., Bennish, M.L., and Darras, B. T.: Eastern equine encephalitis presenting with a focal brain lesion. Pediatr. Neurol. *8*:473–475, 1992.
40. Nathanson, N., Stolley, P. D., and Boolukos, P. J.: Eastern equine encephalitis: Distribution of central nervous system lesions in man and rhesus monkeys. J. Comp. Pathol. *79*:109–115, 1969.
41. Piliero, P. J., Brody, J., Zamani, A., et al.: Eastern equine encephalitis presenting as focal neuroradiographic abnormalities: Case report and review. Clin. Infect. Dis. *18*:985–988, 1994.
42. Powers, J. M., Tsai, T. F., Garen, P. D., et al.: Eastern equine encephalitis: Immunohistochemical and ultrastructural distribution of virus. J. Neuropathol. Exp. Neurol. *47*:304, 1988.
43. Przelomski, M. M., O'Rourke, E., Grady, G. F., et al.: Eastern equine encephalitis in Massachusetts: A report of 16 cases 1970–1984. Neurology *38*:736–739, 1988.
44. Scott, T. W., and Weaver, S. C.: Eastern equine encephalomyelitis virus: Epidemiology and evolution of mosquito transmission. Adv. Virus Res. *37*:277–328, 1989.
45. Sudia, W. D., Stamm, D. D., Chamberlain, R. W., et al.: Transmission of eastern equine encephalitis to horses by *Aedes sollicitans* mosquitoes. Am. J. Trop. Med. Hyg. *5*:802–808, 1956.
46. Tikasingh, E. S., Ardoin, P., Everard, C. O. R., et al.: Eastern equine encephalitis in Trinidad, epidemiological investigations following two human cases of South American strain in Santa Cruz. Trop. Georgr. Med. *25*:355–361, 1973.
47. Tsai, T. F.: Arboviral infections in the United States. Infect. Dis. Clin. North Am. *5*:73–102, 1991.
48. Villari, P., Spielman, A., Komar, N., et al.: The economic burden imposed by a residual case of eastern encephalitis. Am. J. Trop. Med. Hyg. 52:8–13, 1995.
49. Weaver, S. C., Scott, T. W., and Rico-Hesse, R.: Molecular evolution of eastern equine encephalomyelitis virus in North America. Virology *182*:774–784, 1991.
50. Weaver, S. C., Bellew, L. A., Govsett, L., et al.: Diversity within natural populations of eastern encephalomyelitis virus. Virology *195*:700–709, 1993.
51. Wesselhoeff, C., Smith, E. C., and Branch, C. F.: Human encephalitis: Eight fatal cases with four due to virus of equine encephalomyelitis. J. A. M. A. *111*:1735–1741, 1938.
52. Winter, W. D., Jr.: Eastern equine encephalomyelitis in Massachusetts in 1955. N. Engl. J. Med. *255*:262–270, 1956.

❑ ❑ ❑

CHAPTER 178 (B)

Western Equine Encephalitis

Theodore F. Tsai

Western equine encephalitis (WEE) is an endemic and enzootic acute central nervous system infection of humans and horses in the western United States, Canada, Mexico, and parts of South America. In North America, *Culex tarsalis*, the principal mosquito vector, also maintains the virus in an avian enzootic cycle.

ETIOLOGIC AGENT

WEE and other alphaviruses (group A arboviruses) form a genus of principally mosquito-borne viruses in the family *Togaviridae*.[63] Three of the eight viruses constituting the WEE antigenic complex are found in North America: Highlands J, Fort Morgan, and WEE viruses; among them, only WEE virus is a human pathogen. Much of what is known about the molecular biology of alphaviruses is inferred from studies of Sindbis (the type species and a member of the WEE complex) and Semliki Forest viruses.

Alphaviruses are small, enveloped, positive-stranded RNA viruses. Virions are spherical and 69 nm in diameter (including the length of glycoprotein spikes), with a lipid bilayer enveloping a nucleocapsid core containing the 11.7-kb RNA viral genome. Glycoprotein spikes, embedded in the viral envelope, bind to cell membrane receptors, initiating infection by endocytotic fusion. The viral and lysosomal membranes fuse in a pH-dependent step, releasing the viral nucleocapsid into the cell cytoplasm, where RNA and protein synthesis occurs. The 5′ terminal two-thirds of the RNA genome encodes four nonstructural proteins, and the 3′ terminal one-third of the RNA genome encodes the three structural proteins. The 30-kd nucleocapsid and two 50-kDa glycoproteins—E1 and E2—are translated as a polyprotein from subgenomic 26S RNA. The envelope proteins—E1 and E2—are assembled in trimers of a single E2 protein and an E1 dimer. Eighty such trimer spikes are arranged in an icosahedral lattice on the virion surface.[11] Capsid proteins assemble with the viral genome in the cytoplasm and bud through the virally modified cell membrane, acquiring an envelope.

The E1 glycoprotein possesses a group-reactive hemagglutinin and group-reactive epitopes linked to cross-protection and cell-mediated cytotoxic effects. E1 also mediates viral cellular membrane fusion. Epitopes on E2 are linked to cell receptor recognition, viral neutralization and clearance, and neurovirulence.[21, 66, 69]

Molecular genetic studies indicate that WEE virus arose more than 1000 years ago as a recombinant of eastern equine virus and an ancestral, now extinct, Sindbis-like virus acquiring the neurotropic potential of eastern equine virus while retaining antigenic characteristics of the non-neurotropic Sindbis virus.[22] Alphaviruses are believed to have originated in the New World with separate introductions, presumably by birds, to the Old World, resulting in establishments of present day Sindbis-like viruses and Semliki Forest–related viruses.[55, 67] Oligonucleotide fingerprints of individual WEE strains generally are similar, and lineages of other alphaviruses show remarkable stability. A slow rate of evolution, circa 10^{-4} nucleotide changes/year (compared with 10^{-2}/year for other RNA viruses), probably reflects natural pressures on viruses constrained to replicate in both insect and vertebrate cells.[68]

ECOLOGY

WEE virus is transmitted in an enzootic cycle among mosquitoes and birds and other vertebrate hosts.[46, 47, 49] Horses and humans are dead-end hosts, but they may develop severe central nervous system infections. Although WEE is a public health and veterinary problem, primarily in the western United States and Canada, the geographic range of the virus includes Mexico, Guyana, Brazil, Uruguay, and Argentina. Epizootics in horses, accompanied by small numbers of human cases, were reported in Argentina in 1972 and 1983. The virus apparently is transmitted by *Aedes albifasciatus* among introduced European hares and possibly birds. In addition, a distinct sylvatic subtype of WEE virus is transmitted in the subtropical Chaco province.[2, 4]

In the United States, *C. tarsalis* is the principal vector. Its geographic distribution includes the western and central United States, southern Canada, and Mexico. A related virus—Highlands J virus, isolated from *Culiseta melanura* in the eastern United States—now is known to be distinct from but related to WEE virus.[63] An overlap in the range of WEE and Highlands J viruses appears in the east central United States. Highlands J virus causes encephalitis in horses but is not known to cause human illness.

In the western United States, *C. tarsalis* breeds in ground pools found on pasture lands, in irrigation wastewater, and at the margins of lakes, ponds, marshes, and flooded riversides. Some of these aquatic habitats are shared by birds that participate in the amplification of virus in nature.[46, 47, 49]

The female mosquito becomes infected after feeding on a viremic bird (or mammal). After an extrinsic incubation period of 7 to 9 days, when the virus propagates in the mosquito and the salivary glands become infected, the mosquito can transmit virus to other birds or mammals (amplifying hosts) or to humans and horses (dead-end hosts). The peak period of feeding activity is during twilight hours, especially in the first hour after sunset.

Passerine (perching) birds, especially sparrows and finches, have proved to be particularly important in virus amplification. In midsummer, the mosquito shifts its host seeking to mammals. The shift may be influenced by an increase in the defensive behavior of nestling birds, which are its preferred host.[7] The shift corresponds temporally to the appearance of cases in horses and people and appears to be a critical element enabling *C. tarsalis* to function as both an enzootic and an epizootic vector. In California, an auxiliary *Aedes melanimon–jackrabbit (Lepus californicus)* cycle has been demonstrated.[24]

The overwintering mechanism for WEE virus has not been elucidated. However, virus has been recovered from adult *Aedes dorsalis* mosquitoes collected as larvae from a coastal area of California, indicating a possible role for vertical transmission of the virus in mosquitoes.[18] Arguments also have been advanced for viral overwintering in adult mosquitoes and in persistently infected mammals, birds, and poikilotherms (snakes, frogs, and turtles). In Canada, *Aedes* species and *Culiseta inornata,* which are potential vectors of WEE, emerge at an earlier stage in the spring than does *C. tarsalis* and have been proposed as early amplifying vectors.[35, 36]

Numerous climatologic and biologic indices have been shown to correlate with the occurrence of WEE outbreaks. Vector population size, mosquito infection rates, and virus transmission rates to sentinel chickens or wild-caught sparrows have shown various degrees of predictive value. These transmission indices are monitored in surveillance activities by public health agencies; however, their sensitivity, specificity, and predictive value for forecasting epidemics have not been evaluated rigorously. A retrospective analysis of a 21-year experience in California showed correlation between average daily numbers of *C. tarsalis* females and the occurrence of human encephalitis.[43] In a Texas study, house sparrow infection and antibody rates were the best predictors of human disease, and *C. tarsalis* light trap indices were of borderline significance.[28]

Physical measures associated with disease incidence in humans or virus transmission to sentinels include ambient air temperature, snow pack in mountains providing runoff water, river flow rate, soil temperature inversion date (the date the surface soil temperature exceeds the subsurface soil temperature), and the date when 50 or more days of 70° F (21° C) temperature have accumulated. Snow pack and river flow rate are associated with abundance of irrigation water and flooding, which in turn are associated with the availability of breeding habitats and mosquito population size.[5, 7, 27, 46, 47]

Longitudinal and intraseasonal observations show that high temperatures are associated with reduced risk of human disease. High ambient air temperature (>89.6° F [32° C]) decreases mosquito survival, adversely affects the competence of *C. tarsalis* to become infected with and transmit WEE virus, and limits host-seeking activity.[51] In a model of global warming, higher temperatures are predicted to move the range of WEE viral transmission northward.[48]

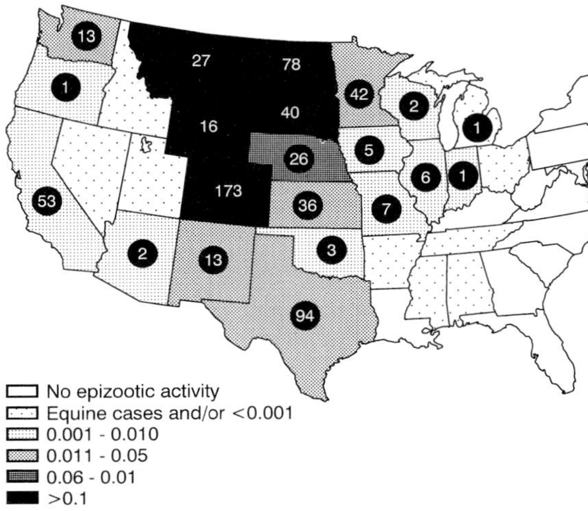

FIGURE 178–3. *Reported cases of average annual incidence (per 100,000) of western equine encephalitis by state, 1964 to 1995.*

EPIDEMIOLOGY

WEE occurs sporadically and in epidemic form, principally in Canadian provinces and states west of the Mississippi River (Figs. 178–3 and 178–4).[64] Cases occur mainly in rural areas, where water impoundments, irrigated farmland, and naturally flooded sites provide *C. tarsalis* breeding habitats. The annual median number of cases between 1964 and 1995 was only four; however, periodic outbreaks can lead to scores or hundreds of cases (see Fig. 178–4).

Recurrent endemic and epidemic transmission has been recorded in the Yakima Valley, Washington (1939 to 1942); California's Central Valley (1939 to 1952); North Central States and Canadian provinces, including Minnesota, North and South Dakota, Alberta, Manitoba, and Saskatchewan

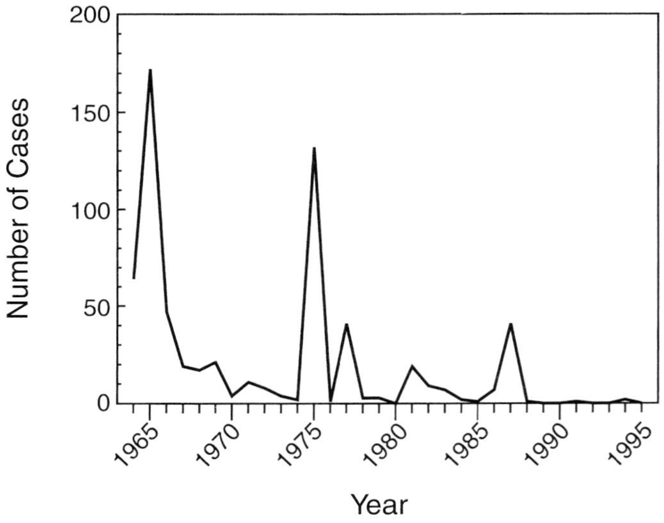

FIGURE 178–4. *Reported cases of western equine encephalitis by year, 1964 to 1995.*

(1941 and 1975); and the high plains panhandle of Texas (1963 to 1966).[15, 23, 29, 45] The largest outbreak on record, in 1941, resulted in more than 3400 human cases in Minnesota, North and South Dakota, Nebraska, Montana, Alberta, Manitoba, and Saskatchewan; equine cases were estimated in the hundreds of thousands. The outbreak centered in North Dakota, where the attack rate for the state was 167 cases per 100,000.[15, 32] In 1952, an outbreak in California's Central Valley led to 348 reported cases, an incidence of 36 cases per 100,000 residents.[29] More recent outbreaks led to 277 cases in the central United States and Manitoba in 1975 and to 40 cases in the Central and Mountain States in 1987.[13, 33, 36]

The majority of cases occur between June and September (Fig. 178–5). Cases in horses often precede human cases by several weeks. Surveillance of equine cases is a widely used approach to assess the risk for epidemic transmission. However, the low frequency of laboratory-confirmed diagnoses, vaccination, and underreporting limit the precision of equine surveillance as a predictive marker.[44]

Several risk factors for acquiring WEE have been identified:[64]

1. Attack rates usually are highest at the extremes of age (Fig. 178–6).[10] The experience from the 1952 California outbreak showed that one-third of cases occurred in infants younger than 1 year of age.[29, 46] Other reports confirm the bimodal pattern of an elevated risk in infants, a declining risk in children and in young adults, and a gradual increase in risk in the elderly.
2. Attack rates in males are twofold higher than in females in every age group (see Fig. 178–5).[10] Biologic differences in susceptibility to infection may account for the observed disparity in infancy and greater occupational and recreational exposures outdoors for the differences in adults. In the 1981 outbreak in Manitoba, 21 of 25 cases were in males; the 4 affected females were widows who maintained their premises alone.[13]
3. Rural residence is associated with attack rates 1.5 to 5 times higher than for urban residence (Table 178–1). Counties lying in major river drainages and with more irrigated acreage have had the highest incidence of equine and human disease (Fig. 178–7).[10]

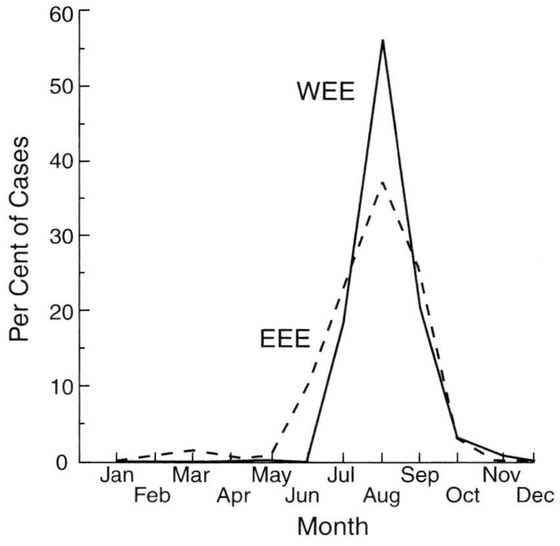

FIGURE 178–5. *Reported cases of western and eastern equine encephalitis by month, 1972 to 1989.*

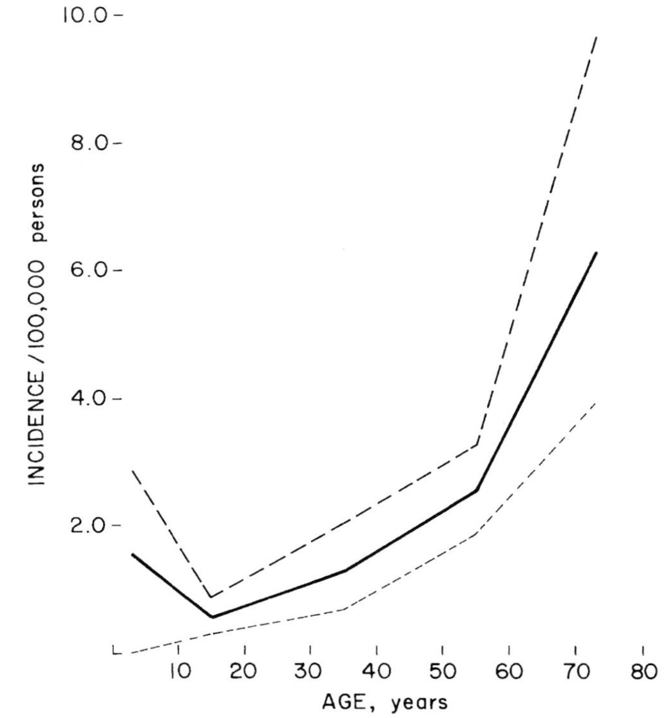

FIGURE 178–6. *Age- and sex-specific incidence of western equine encephalitis, Colorado, 1987. – –, male; ___, total; --- , female.*

4. Agricultural occupation has been suggested as a risk factor in several studies.
5. Length of residence in areas where WEE is endemic is associated inversely with risk of illness. Acquired immunity, through asymptomatic or mild infections, accumulates with length of residence; in endemic areas, the point prevalence of specific antibody approaches 20 per cent by adulthood.[46, 47]

CLINICAL MANIFESTATIONS

The clinical expression of illness ranges from a viral syndrome of headache and fever to aseptic meningitis, meningoencephalitis, and frank encephalitis. The estimated case-infection ratio is 1:58 in children 1 to 4 years of age, which declines to 1:1150 in adults.[17, 46, 49]

The onset of illness typically is abrupt, with a sudden onset of fever, headache, malaise, chills, and nausea and vomiting.[3, 15, 26, 45] Occasionally, the prodrome may include signs of an upper respiratory infection. Signs of central ner-

TABLE 178–1. Western Equine Encephalitis Epidemic Attack Rates by Population Density*

	Minnesota, 1941	Kern County, CA, 1952	Hale County, TX, 1963–1966	Manitoba, 1975
Rural	15.8–22.0	149.2	2.62	10.8
Small town	2.3–5.6			2.4
Urban		28.5	1.0	0.9

*Per 100,000.

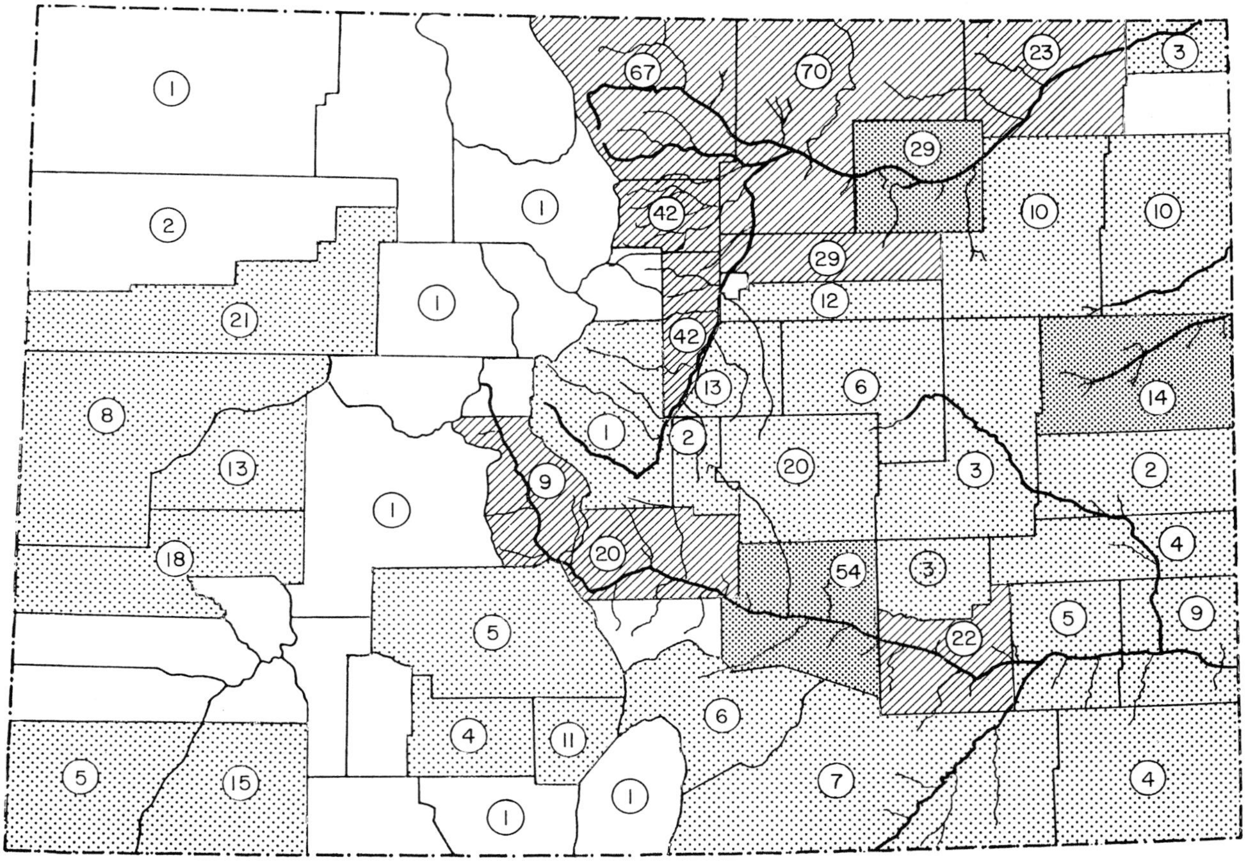

FIGURE 178–7. *Reported equine cases and incidence of western equine encephalitis by county, Colorado, 1975 to 1988.*

vous system infection gradually become evident, as dizziness, drowsiness, increasing headache, stiff neck, and disorientation develop over the course of hours or days. Infants typically present with a sudden cessation in feeding, fussiness, fever, and protracted vomiting. The prodromal interval is abbreviated, and convulsions and a lethargic unresponsive state develop rapidly.

On examination, patients appear somnolent and may have signs of meningeal irritation. The sensorium is depressed, and patients may alternate between agitation and somnolence. Generalized muscular weakness is present, and deep tendon reflexes are diminished. Focal neurologic signs in WEE patients, leading to confusion with herpes encephalitis, have been reported in few cases.[1, 6] Only 3 of 226 cases reported from the 1941 Minnesota outbreak had unilateral weakness.[15]

In infants, the fontanelle may be tense or bulging. Contrary to the course of illness in adults and children, spastic paresis and generalized convulsions typify the course of illness in infants. The frequency of seizures is related inversely to age. Convulsions occur with greatest frequency in infants younger than 3 months of age (75 to 80 per cent of cases). In 2- to 4-year-old children, seizures occur in 15 per cent of cases.[37]

The peripheral leukocyte count is unremarkable. Cerebrospinal fluid obtained at an early stage in the illness generally exhibits a normal glucose, elevated protein concentration, and a leukocyte count between 10 and 300/mm^3.[33] Mononuclear cells usually predominate.

Five instances of late third-trimester infection in pregnant women resulted in perinatal illness or encephalitis.[12, 37] The mothers' illnesses had onset 0 to 10 days before delivery, and the infants became ill on the fifth and sixth postpartum days. Teratogenic effects of infections earlier in gestation have not been reported for WEE virus but are suspected for other group A arboviruses.[38]

PATHOLOGY

Specific pathologic changes are confined to the central nervous system.[3, 33, 41] Grossly, the brain appears normal or may be congested and swollen. Minimal changes are observed in the meninges. Microscopic lesions affecting gray and white matter appear throughout the brain but predominate in the basal ganglia. Disseminated small focal abscesses infiltrated with neutrophils are a distinctive feature. The vessels appear congested, and small focal hemorrhages or diffuse extravasations of erythrocytes are present with neutrophilic infiltration of the vascular wall and endarteritis. Vascular lumina may be occluded by endothelial proliferation and swelling.

Extensive patchy areas of demyelination are found throughout the brain. Older lesions appear as sharply circumscribed punched-out plaques. Secondary microglial reaction in demyelinated areas is minimal.

The spinal cord is affected in the same fashion, with focal, perivascular, and diffuse lesions involving both polymorphonuclear and mononuclear cells. Lesions predominate in the central gray matter.

PATHOGENESIS

Peripheral inoculation of experimental animals with WEE virus is followed by viral replication in various extraneural sites before invasion of the central nervous system.[21, 30, 34, 42, 60, 71] The peripheral site of inoculation, viscera, muscle, and perhaps vascular endothelial cells support viral replication, leading to viremia, before the appearance of central nervous system infection and symptoms.

Host resistance and recovery from infection depend chiefly on an effective antibody response.[21] Antibody contributes to recovery by a variety of means, including viral neutralization and antibody-mediated restriction of viral gene expression.[21, 69] Interferon may contribute to the containment of local viral spread in the central nervous system. Antibodies are protective and may be cross-protective to other alphaviruses. Antibodies to the E2 glycoprotein typically are virus-specific and associated with neutralization and protection. Antibodies to E1 exhibit greater cross-reactivity with other alphaviruses.[63]Immune serum given to monkeys prophylactically protects them from challenge with WEE virus, and passive protection has been demonstrated in monkeys inoculated with WEE virus and treated with immune serum within 24 hours.[71] However, immunotherapy of monkeys uniformly is unsuccessful in preventing death once signs of central nervous system infection have appeared. In guinea pigs peripherally inoculated with WEE virus, immunotherapy given within 24 to 48 hours of inoculation leads to survival of some animals and delayed deaths in others.[42] However, in one human case, passive immunization led to a delayed antibody response and was followed by the development of parkinsonism.[19]

Age-dependent virulence of specific Sindbis virus strains has been linked to the immaturity of the suckling mouse T- and B-cell repertoire.[60] Fibroblasts from newborn mice but not weanling mice are susceptible to Sindbis virus infection, which suggests a cellular basis for increased susceptibility to these viruses in immature mice as well. Sindbis viral infection of immature mouse neurons leads to apoptotic cell death. Mature neurons are protected against apoptosis by induction of the *bcl-2* oncogene, whose products convert the infection to a persistent nonlytic infection. Viral persistence in brain of recovered mice is modulated by antibody.[21, 66, 69]

TREATMENT

Specific antiviral therapy is not available. Supportive treatment of acutely ill patients includes monitoring of cardiorespiratory function, fluid and electrolyte balance, and intracranial pressure. A case of laboratory infection treated with immune equine serum resulted in recovery; however, the patient developed acute Parkinson syndrome, which coincided temporally with serum sickness resulting from immunotherapy.[19]

PROGNOSIS

Major neurologic sequelae of WEE have been reported in approximately 13 per cent of cases, including quadriplegia, hemiplegia, spasticity, intracerebral calcifications, developmental delay and retardation in children, and epilepsy.[14, 16, 26, 72] The risk of serious neurologic sequelae in infants is triple that of other age groups, and 30 per cent of recovered infants younger than 1 year of age remain seriously impaired.[14, 16, 59] In infants younger than 1 year of age, convulsions during the acute phase of illness were associated with a greater risk of poor long-term outcome, including continued seizures. Multiple intracranial calcifications were observed in one recovered infant with persistent seizures.[59] Central apnea has been reported as a complication of encephalitis in two adult cases. In one instance, chronic sleep-associated apnea was a long-term sequela.[70] Minor psychiatric or neurologic deficits remained in about one-fourth of children and adults followed 18 months after infection.[16]

Parkinson syndrome has been a residual of adults surviving WEE in at least 15 cases.[19, 40, 57, 58] Onset may be immediate or delayed for several years after recovery from the illness. Investigations of patients with idiopathic Parkinson disease found no difference between cases and controls in seroprevalences to several arboviruses, including WEE virus.

The case-fatality rate among reported cases in the United States from 1955 to 1978 was 3 to 4 per cent. In outbreaks in the central United States and Canada in 1941, 1975, and 1981, approximately 7 to 9 per cent of patients died; age-specific fatality rates were highest in the elderly.

DIAGNOSIS

Virus rarely can be recovered from blood or cerebrospinal fluid, but it can be isolated readily from the brain of fatal cases. In a few attempts, WEE virus has been isolated from brain biopsy material; in principle, a rapid diagnosis can be made by the identification of WEE viral antigen in brain biopsy tissue by immunofluorescence. The virus can be isolated readily in Vero cell culture or in suckling mice.[58]

IgM capture enzyme-linked immunosorbent assay (ELISA) is the preferred serologic procedure.[8] IgM antibody usually is present in acute serum within a week after the onset of illness, and its presence is presumptive evidence of recent infection. IgM often can be detected in cerebrospinal fluid before it can be identified in serum.[8] The presence of specific IgM in cerebrospinal fluid, which indicates intrathecal production of antibody, confirms a recent central nervous system infection. Identification of virus-specific IgM in serum and cerebrospinal fluid by immunofluorescence also is possible; however, this approach is somewhat less sensitive than is IgM capture ELISA and may be confounded by effects of rheumatoid factor.

Hemagglutination-inhibition (HI) and neutralizing antibody are elevated in the first week of illness in most cases, and a diagnostic fourfold rise in titer usually is observed in the second week. Complement-fixing (CF) antibody is slower to rise, with fourfold changes delayed until the third to fifth weeks after onset. The CF response may be blunted in older patients.[62]

Neutralizing and HI antibody titers have considerable longevity, with minimal decay noted 30 months after onset. In contrast, CF antibody is relatively short lived, and its presence is a useful indicator of recent infection, particularly in endemic areas where long-term residents may have neutralizing and HI antibody from previous exposures. Only two-thirds of patients are estimated to show CF antibody 2 years after onset, and less than 15 per cent have residual CF antibody after 5 years.[62]

DIFFERENTIAL DIAGNOSIS

The clinical presentation of patients with encephalitis seldom sufficiently is characteristic that a specific diagnosis can be made on clinical grounds alone. Fever, vomiting, signs of meningeal irritation, and confusion are nonspecific features of encephalitis and cerebral edema. In infants, early symptoms, such as fever, lethargy, and vomiting, may be even less specific.[31]

The peak occurrence of arboviral infections in midsummer to late summer temporally is juxtaposed with the seasonal occurrence of other central nervous system infections from enteroviruses, leptospires, and free-living ameba. Central nervous system signs may be prominent in other summertime diseases, such as Rocky Mountain spotted fever, heat stroke, shigellosis, and lead encephalopathy.

The clinical differentiation of enteroviral central nervous system infections from arboviral infections may be difficult. Furthermore, numerous instances of dual infections of enteroviruses with St. Louis encephalitis, Powassan, La Crosse, or WEE viruses have been reported.

Other causes of central nervous system infection without an established summertime seasonality that should be considered in the differential diagnosis include fungal, mycobacterial, and partially treated bacterial meningitis; brain abscess and infected subdural collections; bacterial endocarditis; toxoplasmosis; cat-scratch disease; and infections with rabies, mumps, herpes simplex, Epstein-Barr, human herpesvirus 6, adenovirus, lymphocytic choriomeningitis, and HIV viruses.[61] Parainfectious disorders, such as postinfectious viral encephalitis, acute cerebellar ataxia of childhood, mycoplasmal infection, neuroblastoma presenting with opsoclonus, and Reye syndrome, also may enter into the differential diagnosis. Vascular disorders formed the largest single group of disorders mimicking herpes encephalitis in several studies. Drugs such as trimethoprim-sulfamethoxazole, penicillin, isoniazid, phenazopyridine, ibuprofen, tolmetin, sulindac, carbamazepine, high doses of bismuth, OKT3 antibody, and vidarabine also may cause aseptic meningitis or encephalopathy.[20]

Diethylmethylbenzamide (DEET)–containing insect repellents have been implicated as a cause of seizures and encephalopathy after brief cutaneous exposure (see later).

Valuable clues to the diagnosis of an arbovirus infection are gleaned from a history of travel, residence, or occupational and recreational activities within the appropriate incubation period. Suspected cases should be reported to public health officials.

PREVENTION

Killed vaccine prepared in chick embryo fibroblast culture is available in the United States under an investigatory permit for laboratory and field personnel who are at risk for occupational exposures. Effective killed vaccines are available for horses and usually are administered in bivalent or multivalent formulations (with eastern equine encephalitis, Venezuelan equine encephalitis, and influenza viruses). Vaccination of the general public, even in endemic areas, is not a practical consideration because of the low risk of disease. Personal protective measures include avoiding outdoor activity during the hours of peak mosquito activity at dusk and using repellents.

The most effective repellents contain DEET as the active ingredient, but they should be used with caution, especially in children.[9, 65] DEET is absorbed readily through the skin; in seven cases, encephalopathy was reported in children after cutaneous exposure.[52, 53, 65] Three cases were fatal. In one recovered case, encephalopathy and seizures developed after only two applications.[65] In an additional case, seizures and encephalopathy occurred after cutaneous and respiratory exposure to DEET in an automobile with closed windows. Additional cases of seizures in patients using small quantities of DEET have been reported, but it is unclear whether these were coincidental events in populations in which the prevalence of DEET usage is high.[9] DEET may have an effect on ammonia metabolism; in one case, encephalopathy occurred in a patient with partial ornithine carbamyltransferase deficiency.[25] DEET is a proven neurotoxin when it is ingested. The incidence of neurologic side effects after cutaneous exposure is unknown. Nevertheless, it is prudent to avoid formulations containing DEET in high concentrations. Precautions listed in Table 178–2 should be followed to minimize exposure.[9, 65]

Permethrin, a synthetic pyrethroid available as a 0.5 per cent aerosol (Permanone), is both insecticidal and a repellent.[56, 65] Permethrin is extremely effective in reducing bites of mosquitoes and ticks when it is sprayed on clothing and shoes, and it also can be applied to tents, mosquito nets, and other gear.[56] Its use on the skin is not approved, except as treatment for scabies and head lice.

Prevention is focused primarily on interrupting the transmission of virus from mosquitoes to humans. In many localities where WEE is endemic, mosquito abatement districts monitor mosquito populations, virus infection rates in the vector population, and/or evidence of transmission of virus

TABLE 178–2. Precautions to Minimize Potential Adverse Reactions from Repellents

- Apply repellent sparingly only to exposed skin or clothing.
- Avoid applying high-concentration products (>35% DEET) to the skin, particularly of children.
- Do not inhale or ingest repellents or get them into the eyes.
- Wear long-sleeved shirts and long pants when possible; apply repellents (e.g., permethrin) to clothing to reduce skin exposure to DEET.
- Avoid applying repellents to children's hands to reduce mucosal and oral contact.
- Pregnant and nursing women should minimize use of repellents.
- Never use repellents on wounds or irritated skin.
- Use repellent sparingly; one application will last several hours. Saturation does not increase efficacy.
- Wash repellent-treated skin after coming indoors.
- If a suspected reaction to insect repellents occurs, wash treated skin and call a physician. Bring the repellent container to a physician.

Adapted from Centers for Disease Control: Seizures temporally associated with use of DEET insect repellent: New York and Connecticut. M. M. W. R. *38*:678–680, 1989; Tsai, T. F.: Arboviral infections: General considerations for prevention, diagnosis and treatment in travelers. Semin. Pediatr. Infect. Dis. *3*:62–69, 1992.

to wild or sentinel birds and chickens. These surveillance efforts provide a basis for predicting epidemic transmission and for emergency mosquito control.[39, 50]

As a general rule, *C. tarsalis* densities exceeding 10 to 15 females per trap night and mosquito infection rates greater than 5 to 10 per 1000 signal a risk for epizootic transmission. Evidence of seroconversions in sentinel chickens and observations of equine cases are further indications that human cases may occur.

References

1. Anderson, B. A.: Focal neurologic signs in western equine encephalitis. Can. Med. Assoc. J. *130*:1019–1021, 1984.
2. Aviles, G., Sabattini, M. S., and Mitchell, C. J.: Transmission of western equine encephalomyelitis virus by Argentine *Aedes albifasciatus.* J. Med. Entomol. *29*:850–853, 1992.
3. Baker, A. B., and Noran, H. H.: Western variety of equine encephalitis in man: A clinicopathologic study. Arch. Neurol. Psychiatr. *47*:565–587, 1942.
4. Bianchi, T. I., Aviles, G., Monath, T.P., et al.: Western equine encephalomyelitis: Virulence markers and their epidemiologic significance. Am. J. Trop. Med. Hyg. *49*:322–328, 1993.
5. Bennington, E. E., and Sherman, I. L.: A note on reported cases of encephalitis and soil temperatures in Colorado. Mosq. News *20*:191–195, 1960.
6. Bia, F. J., Thornton, G. F., Main, A. J., et al.: Western equine encephalitis mimicking herpes simplex encephalitis. J. A. M. A. *244*:367–369, 1980.
7. Blackmore, J. S., and Dow, R. P.: Differential feeding of *Culex tarsalis* on nestling and adult birds. Mosq. News *18*:15–17, 1958.
8. Calisher, C. H., Meurman, O., Brummer-Korvenkontio, M., et al.: Sensitive enzyme immunoassay for detecting immunoglobulin M antibodies to Sindbis virus and further evidence that Pogosta disease is caused by a western equine encephalitis complex virus. J. Clin. Microbiol. *22*:566–571, 1985.
9. Centers for Disease Control: Seizures temporally associated with use of DEET insect repellent: New York and Connecticut. M. M. W. R. *38*:678–680, 1989.
10. Centers for Disease Control: Arboviral infections of the central nervous system: United States, 1987. M. M. W. R. *37*:506, 1988.
11. Cheng, R. H., Kuhn, R. J., Olson, N. H., et al.: Nucleocapsid and glycoprotein organization in an enveloped virus. Cell *80*:621–630, 1995.
12. Copps, S. C., and Giddings, L. E.: Transplacental transmission of western equine encephalitis. Pediatrics *24*:31–33, 1959.
13. Eadie, J. A., and Friesen, B.: Epidemiological study of western equine encephalitis. *In* Sekla, L. (ed.): Western Equine Encephalitis in Manitoba. Winnipeg, Province of Manitoba, 1982, pp. 142–155.
14. Earnest, M. P., Goolishian, H. A., Calverley, J. R., et al.: Neurologic, intellectual, and psychologic sequelae following western encephalitis: A follow-up study of 35 cases. Neurology *21*:969–974, 1971.
15. Eklund, C. M.: Human encephalitis of the western equine type in Minnesota in 1941: Clinical and epidemiological study of serologically positive cases. Am. J. Hyg. *43*:171–193, 1946.
16. Finley, K. H., Longshore, W. A., Jr., Palmer, R. J., et al.: Western equine and St. Louis encephalitis: Preliminary report of a clinical follow-up study in California. Neurology *5*:223–235, 1955.
17. Froeschle, J. E., and Reeves, W. C.: Serologic epidemiology of western equine and St. Louis encephalitis virus infection in California. II. Analysis of inapparent infections in residents of an endemic area. Am. J. Epidemiol. *81*:44–51, 1965.
18. Fulhorst, C. F., Hardy, J. L., Eldridge, B. F., et al.: Natural vertical transmission of western equine encephalomyelitis virus in mosquitoes. Science *263*:676–678, 1994.
19. Gold, H., and Hampil, B.: Equine encephalomyelitis in a laboratory technician with recovery. Ann. Intern. Med. *16*:556–569, 1942.
20. Gordon, M. F., Allon, M., and Coyle, P. K.: Drug-induced meningitis. Neurology *40*:163–164, 1990.
21. Griffin, D. E., Levine, B., Ubul, S., et al.: The effects of alphavirus infection on neurons. Ann. Neurol. *35*:523, 1994.
22. Hahn, C. S., Lustig, S., Strauss, E. G., et al.: Western equine encephalitis virus is a recombinant virus. Proc. Natl. Acad. Sci. U. S. A. *85*:5997–6001, 1988.
23. Hammon, W., McD., Reeves, W. C., Benner, S. R., et al.: Human encephalitis in the Yakima Valley, Washington, 1942. J. A. M. A. *128*:1133–1139, 1945.
24. Hardy, J. L., Milby, M. M., Wright, M. E., et al.: Natural and experimental arboviral infections in a population of blacktail jackrabbits along the Sacramento River in Butte County, California (1971–1974). J. Wildl. Dis. *13*:383–392, 1977.
25. Heick, H. M. C., Peterson, R. G., Dalpe-Scott, M., et al.: Insect repellent, N,N-diethyl-m-toluamide, effect on ammonia metabolism. Pediatrics *82*:373–376, 1988.
26. Herzon, H., Shelton, J. T., and Bruyn, H. B.: Sequelae of western equine and other arthropod-borne encephalitides. Neurology *7*:535–548, 1957.
27. Hess, A. D., Cherubin, C. E., and LaMotte, L. C.: Relation of temperature to activity of western and St. Louis encephalitis viruses. Am. J. Trop. Med. Hyg. *12*:657–667, 1963.
28. Holden, P., Hayes, R. O., Mitchell, C. J., et al.: House sparrows, *Passer domesticus* (L.), as hosts of arboviruses in Hale County, Texas. I. Field studies, 1965–1969. Am. J. Trop. Med. Hyg. *22*:244–253, 1973.
29. Hollister, A. C., Longshore, W. A., Jr., Dean, B. H., et al.: The 1952 outbreak of encephalitis in California. Epidemiologic aspects. Calif. Med. *79*:84–90, 1953.
30. Hurst, W.: Infection of the Rhesus monkey *(Macaca mulatta)* and the guinea pig with the virus of equine encephalomyelitis. J. Pathol. Bacteriol. *42*:271–302, 1936.
31. Kokernot, R. H., Shinefield, H. R., and Longshore, W. A.: The 1952 outbreak of encephalitis in California: Differential diagnosis. Calif. Med. *79*:73, 1953.
32. Leake, J. P.: Epidemic of infectious encephalitis. Public Health Rep. *56*:1902–1905, 1941.
33. Leech, R. W., Harris, J. C., and Johnson, R. M.: 1975 encephalitis epidemic in North Dakota and western Minnesota: An epidemiologic, clinical, and neuropathologic study. Minn. Med. *64*:545–548, 1981.
34. Liu, C., Voth, D. W., Rodina, P., et al.: A comparative study of the pathogenesis of western equine encephalitis and eastern equine encephalomyelitis viral infections in mice by intracerebral and subcutaneous inoculations. J. Infect. Dis. *122*:53–63, 1970.
35. McLintock, J., Burton, A. N., McKiel, J. A., et al.: Known mosquito hosts of western encephalitis virus in Saskatchewan. J. Med. Entomol. *7*:446–454, 1970.
36. Medovy, H.: II. The history of western encephalomyelitis in Manitoba. Can. J. Public Health *67*(Suppl. 1):13–14, 1976.
37. Medovy, H.: Western equine encephalomyelitis in infants. J. Pediatr. *22*:308, 1943.
38. Milner, A. R., and Marshall, I. D.: Pathogenesis of in utero infections with abortogenic and nonabortogenic alphaviruses in mice. J. Virol. *50*:66–72, 1984.
39. Mitchell, C. J., Hayes, R. O., Holden, P., et al.: Effects of ultra-low volume applications of malathion in Hale County, Texas. I. Western encephalitis virus activity in treated and untreated towns. J. Med. Entomol. *6*:155–162, 1969.
40. Mulder, D. W., Parrott, M., and Thaler, M.: Sequelae of western equine encephalitis. Neurology *1*:318–327, 1951.
41. Noran, H. H., and Baker, A. B.: Sequels of equine encephalomyelitis. Arch. Neurol. Psychiatr. *49*:398–413, 1943.
42. Olitsky, P. K., Schlesinger, R. W., and Morgan, I. M.: Induced resistance of the central nervous system to experimental infection with equine encephalomyelitis virus. J. Exp. Med. *77*:359–375, 1943.
43. Olson, J. G., Reeves, W. C., Emmons, R. W., et al.: Correlation of *Culex tarsalis* population indices with the incidence of St. Louis encephalitis and western equine encephalomyelitis in California. Am. J. Trop. Med. Hyg. *28*:335–343, 1979.
44. Potter, M. E., Currier, R. W., II, Pearson, J. E., et al.: Western equine encephalomyelitis in horses in the northern Red River Valley, 1975. J. Am. Vet. Med. Assoc. *170*:1396–1399, 1977.
45. Ray, C. G., Sciple, G. W., Holden, P., et al.: Acute, febrile CNS illnesses in an endemic area of Texas: Epidemiologic and serologic findings, 1965. Public Health Rep. *82*:785–793, 1967.
46. Reeves, W. C., and Hammon, W., McD.: Epidemiology of the Arthropod-Borne Viral Encephalitides in Kern County, California, 1943–1952. Berkeley, University of California Press, 1962, pp. 1–257.
47. Reeves, W. C.: Epidemiology and control of mosquito borne arboviruses in California, 1943–1987. Sacramento, California Mosquito Vector Control Association, 1990.
48. Reeves, W. C., Hardy, J. L., Reisen, W. K., et al.: Potential effect of global warming on mosquito-borne arboviruses. J. Med. Entomol. *31*:323–332, 1994.
49. Reisen, W. K., and Monath, T. P.: Western equine encephalitis. *In* Monath, T. P. (ed.): The Arboviruses: Epidemiology and Ecology. Vol. 5. Boca Raton, FL, CRC Press, 1990, pp. 89–137.
50. Reisen, W. K., Yoshimura, G., Reeves, W. C., et al.: The impact of aerial applications of ultra-low volume adulticides on *Culex tarsalis* populations (Diptera:Culicidae) in Kern County, California, USA, 1982. J. Med. Entomol. *21*:573–585, 1984.
51. Reisen, W. K., Meyer, R. P., Presser, S. B., et al.: Effect of temperature on the transmission of western equine encephalomyelitis and St. Louis encephalitis viruses by *C. tarsalis*. J. Med. Entomol. *30*:151–160, 1993.
52. Robbins, P. J., and Cherniack, M. G.: Review of the biodistribution and toxicity of the insect repellent N,N-diethyl-m-toluamide (DEET). J. Toxicol. Environ. Health *18*:503–525, 1986.
53. Roland, E. H., Jan, J. E., and Rigg, J. M.: Toxic encephalopathy in a child after brief exposure to insect repellents. Can. Med. Assoc. J. *132*:155–156, 1985.
54. Rowley, A. H., Whitley, R. J., Lakeman, F. D., et al.: Rapid detection of herpes-simplex-virus DNA in cerebrospinal fluid of patients with herpes simplex encephalitis. Lancet *335*:440–441, 1990.
55. Rumenapf, T., Strauss, E. G., and Strauss, J. H.: Aura virus is a new world representative of sindbis-like viruses. Virology *208*:621, 1995.
56. Schreck, C. E., and Kline, D. L.: Personal protection afforded by controlled-

release topical repellents and permethrin-treated clothing against natural populations of *Aedes taeniorhynchus*. J. Am. Mosq. Contr. Assoc. *5*:77–80, 1989.
57. Schultz, D. R., Barthal, J. S., and Garrett, C.: Western equine encephalitis with rapid onset of Parkinsonism. Neurology *27*:1095–1096, 1977.
58. Sciple, G. W., Ray, G., LaMotte, L. C., et al.: Western encephalitis with recovery of virus from cerebrospinal fluid. Neurology *17*:169–171, 1967.
59. Somekh, E., Glode, M. P., Reilly, T. T., et al.: Multiple intracranial calcifications after western equine encephalitis. Pediatr. Infect. Dis. *10*:408, 1991.
60. Sherman, L. A., and Griffin, D. E.: Pathogenesis of encephalitis induced in newborn mice by virulent and avirulent strains of Sindbis virus. J. Virol. *64*:2041–2046, 1990.
61. Spanos, A., Harrell, F. E., and Durack, D. T.: Differential diagnosis of acute meningitis. J. A. M. A. *262*:2700–2707, 1989.
62. Stallones, R. A., Reeves, W. C., and Lennette, E. H.: Serologic epidemiology of western equine and St. Louis encephalitis virus infection in California. I. Persistence of complement-fixing antibody following clinical illness. Am. J. Hyg. *79*:16–28, 1964.
63. Strauss, J. H., and Strauss, E. G.: The alphaviruses: Gene expression, replication and evolution. Microbiol. Rev. *58*:491, 1994.
64. Tsai, T. F.: Arboviral infections in the United States. Infect. Dis. Clin. North Am. *5*:73–102, 1991.
65. Tsai, T. F.: Arboviral infections: General considerations for prevention, diagnosis and treatment in travelers. Semin. Pediatr. Infect. Dis. *3*:62–69, 1992.
66. Ubol, S., Tucker, P. Griffin, D. E., et al.: Neurovirulent strains of *Alphavirus* induce apoptosis in *bcl-2* expressing cells: Role of a single amino acid change in the E2 glycoprotein. Proc. Natl. Acad. Sci. U. S. A. *91*:5202, 1994.
67. Weaver, S. C., Hagenbaugh, A., Bellow, L.A., et al.: A comparison of the nucleotide sequences of eastern and western equine encephalomyelitis viruses with those of other alphaviruses and related RNA viruses. Virology *197*:375–90, 1993.
68. Weaver, S. C., Rico-Hesse, R., and Scott T. W.: Genetic diversity and slow rates of evolution in New World alphaviruses. Curr. Top. Microbiol. Immunol. *176*:99–117, 1992.
69. Wesseling, S. L., and Griffin, D. E.: Local cytokine responses during acute and chronic viral infections to the central nervous system. Semin. Virol. *5*:457, 1994.
70. White, D. P., Miller, F., and Erickson, R. W.: Sleep apnea and nocturnal hypoventilation after western equine encephalitis. Am. Rev. Respir. Dis. *127*:132–133, 1983.
71. Wyckoff, R. W. G., and Tesar, W. C.: Equine encephalomyelitis in monkeys. J. Immunol. *37*:329–343, 1939.
72. Zeifert, M., Pennell, W. H., Finley, K. H., et al.: The electroencephalogram following western and St. Louis encephalitis. Neurology *12*:311–319, 1962.

❑ ❑ ❑

CHAPTER 178 (C)

Venezuelan Equine Encephalitis

Theodore F. Tsai

Mosquito-borne Venezuelan equine encephalitis (VEE) arguably is the most important viral zoonosis of Latin America. Periodic outbreaks of equine encephalitis have been reported from northern South America since the last century. The disease, known locally as "peste loca," has occurred in combined epizootics and epidemics at regular intervals since the 1920s, sometimes leading to hundreds of thousands of human and equine cases. Between 1935 and 1961, 11 outbreaks were reported, and from 1962 to 1973, epizootics recurred in every year except 1965.[15] The virus was isolated in 1938 during an outbreak in Venezuela from horse brain. Although outbreaks have arisen principally in northern South America, especially from Colombia and Venezuela, in a remarkable period between 1969 and 1971, epizootics and epidemics were reported from Colombia, Venezuela, Ecuador, Peru, all the countries of Central America (except Panama), Mexico, and the state of Texas.[22, 35, 36] No major epizootics/epidemics had been recognized since 1973, leading to speculation that epizootic VEE virus strains (IAB, IC) had become extinct. But a major outbreak in 1995 due to IC virus and recent molecular phylogenetic analyses suggest that epizootic strains might arise spontaneously from sylvatic viral strains circulating silently in nature.[6, 18, 25, 37, 38, 40]

ETIOLOGIC AGENT

VEE virus is distinct antigenically from other alphaviruses but is itself a complex of antigenically and ecologically distinct viral subtypes (Table 178–3).[40] Epizootic subtypes IAB and IC are so named because they have been associated with major outbreaks in horses. Sylvatic viral subtypes circulate in silent cycles of rodent/bird-mosquito transmission and in general do not cause encephalitis in equines. Both epizootic and sylvatic viral strains cause human illness.[22, 35]

VEE virus is believed to have evolved approximately 1400 years ago from a now extinct ancestral alphavirus, in one of two extant lineages of New World alphaviruses represented by eastern equine encephalomyelitis and VEE viruses.[27, 29, 38] Because epizootic VEE viral strains had never been isolated from nature except during epizootics, their reservoirs and the mechanisms by which they emerged to cause outbreaks had remained a puzzle. However, recent molecular phylogenetic analyses have found a close genetic relationship between epizootic IC and sylvatic ID strains, suggesting that these epizootic strains might arise spontaneously by mutation from naturally circulating ID virus.

Comparisons of the attenuated TC-83 vaccine strain of VEE virus and the epizootic IAB parent virus and mutations of virulent infectious clones have shown that changes associated with attenuation occur principally in genes encoding the E2 and E1 glycoproteins but also in the 5′ nontranslated region.[14, 17] Attenuation is associated with reduced neuroinvasiveness (faster clearance from blood and lower viremia levels), as well as reduced neurovirulence (minimal histopathologic changes after intracerebral inoculation of horses).

VEE virus rapidly produces cytopathic effects in a variety of cell cultures, including Vero, LLCMK-2, BHK-21, and primary chicken and duck embryo cells. Epizootic strains cause lethal infections in horses, donkeys, mules, rabbits, and dogs. In certain guinea pig strains, pathogenicity is correlated with equine virulence.

EPIDEMIOLOGY AND ECOLOGY

Epizootics and concurrent epidemics of VEE due to the IAB and IC strains typically have led to thousands and, on at least one occasion, hundreds of thousands of cases in humans and equines. The majority of such outbreaks have occurred in Venezuela and Colombia and have been caused by IC viruses (Fig. 178–8).[26, 29] The virus' interepidemic reservoir had not been elucidated, despite intensive field investigations, but recent molecular phylogenetic studies suggest that these viruses may arise from closely related enzootic ID viruses circulating in nature. The circumstances leading to the emergence of outbreaks are poorly understood, but outbreaks often have occurred in arid areas during years of heavy rainfall and flooding, especially during the dry season.[35] The importance of a nonimmune horse population to amplify the virus has been underscored in the most recent outbreak in 1995, occurring in areas of Colombia and Venezuela where equine immunizations had lapsed.[6, 7] Equines are the most important vertebrate amplifying host because they develop and sustain high levels of viremia and because they provide a large surface area for biting mosquitoes. Numerous species of mosquitoes and other blood-feeding insects can transmit the virus from horse to horse and from horses to humans, among them *Aedes taeniorhychus*, a salt marsh mosquito, and *Psorophora confinnis*, found in ground pools.[32]

TABLE 178–3. Viruses in the Venezuelan Equine Encephalomyelitis Complex

Subtype	Variety	Pattern of Transmission	Location	Transmission Cycle
I	AB	Epizootic	South, Central, and North America	Various mosquitoes and biting insects/equines
	C	Epizootic	Northern South America	Various mosquitoes and biting insects/equines
	D	Enzootic	Ecuador, Panama, Colombia, and Venezuela	*Culex* (*Melanoconion*) *ocossa* and *panocossa*/ rodents, aquatic birds
	E	Enzootic	Central America	*Culex* (*Melanoconion*) *taeniopus*/rodents
	F	Enzootic	Brazil	Unknown
II (Everglades)		Enzootic	Southern Florida	*Culex* (*Melanoconion*) *cedecei*/rodents
III	A			
	Mucambo	Enzootic	South America	*Culex* (*Melanoconion*) *portesi*/rodents
	B			
	Tonate	Enzootic	South America	Unknown
	Bijou Bridge	Unknown	Western North America	*Oeciacus vicarius*/birds
	C	Enzootic	Peru	Unknown
IV (Pixuna)		Enzootic	Brazil	Unknown
V (Cabassou)		Enzootic	French Guiana	Unknown
VI		Enzootic	Argentina	Unknown

Infections are transmitted rapidly among animals and to people, and the movement of outbreaks has been measured at rates of several miles per day. The epidemic curve of human cases usually follows the equine epizootic by several weeks, and epidemic transmission ceases when the number of susceptible horses has been exhausted by immunization or natural infection.[13, 35]

The role of other animals, including humans, in sustaining epidemic viral transmission has been investigated in urban outbreaks, during which household clustering of cases has been observed, and in recent outbreaks, during which few horses were kept in the community. VEE virus levels in human blood are high enough to infect mosquitoes, and virus also has been isolated from the pharynx of ill persons, indicating the possibilities of person-to-person transmission by mosquitoes, such as *Aedes aegypti*, or by direct close contact.[4, 31] Although such transmission mechanisms may account for some cases, a recent household survey found rates of apparent secondary transmission no higher than the underlying community attack rate.[7] Community attack rates of 20 to 50 per cent have been recorded, with the course of epidemics completed in intervals as short as 1 month, underscoring the considerable force of epidemic transmission.

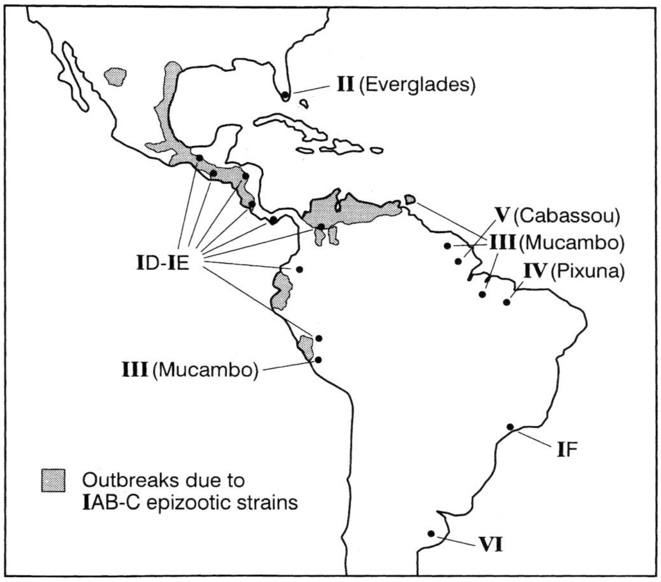

FIGURE 178–8. *Locations of Venezuelan equine encephalitis (VEE) outbreaks due to IAB-IC epizootic strains and locations where VEE sylvatic subtypes have been recognized.*

The series of epizootics, beginning in Guatemala in 1969 and that reached Texas in 1971, was caused by an IAB virus that nearly is identical genetically to the 1943 Trinidad donkey (epizootic IAB) virus used in inactivated vaccines, leading to speculation that these were iatrogenic outbreaks due to use of inadequately inactivated equine vaccines.[16] A similar outbreak in Argentina was traced to a similar etiology.

In contrast to the epizootic strains, sylvatic VEE viruses are avirulent in horses, causing a low level of viremia after infection, subclinical or mild illness, and minimal inflammatory change after direct intracerebral inoculation.[34] However, outbreaks of enzootic IE-like viruses rarely have caused outbreaks and deaths in horses (e.g., in Chiapas, Mexico, in 1993). The viruses are maintained in mosquitoes, rodents, and aquatic birds principally by *Culex melaconion* species mosquitoes in marshy coastal lowlands. In coastal lagoons in Panama, ibises (*Endocinus albus*) and spoon-billed ducks (*Cochlearius cochlearius*) appear to serve as intermediate hosts.[1] VEE subtype II virus, Everglades virus, is enzootic among cotton rats and other small mammals on hammocks in the Everglades swamp and rarely has caused human illnesses in Florida.[10] The other VEE virus found in the United States, Bijou Bridge virus, is unique in its enzootic transmission among birds by swallow bugs. The virus is believed to have evolved from South American subtype III virus transferred as recently as 40 years ago, probably by a migrating bird. No human illness has been associated with Bijou Bridge virus.

VEE infections due to sylvatic strains can be considered "diseases of place," occurring sporadically in persons who enter sylvatic habitats where the viruses are maintained.[9]

Sporadic cases and rare outbreaks among soldiers in field bivouacs have been reported.[28] Many infections undoubtedly are undiagnosed. Bridge vectors, mosquitoes that feed on mammals in the enzootic transmission cycle and subsequently on humans, usually are responsible for these infections.

Numerous cases and outbreaks of VEE have occurred in laboratories when infective aerosols have been generated in laboratory procedures.[19] Laboratory manipulations should be undertaken only in BL-3 laboratories and by immunized personnel.

CLINICAL MANIFESTATIONS

The incubation period is brief—2 to 5 days—and in many accounts, the onset of illness is so sudden that it can be timed to an exact hour.[19] Fever, chills, headache, myalgias, and malaise are the earliest symptoms, and illness quickly leads to prostration. Photophobia, neck stiffness, backache, conjunctivitis, and sore throat also are common symptoms, occurring in about one-quarter or more of cases. Gastrointestinal complaints, especially nausea and vomiting, and, to a lesser degree, loose stools or diarrhea, are reported frequently.[2]

Physical examination discloses severe prostration and few specific findings. The face may appear hyperemic, inflammation of the pharynx is common, and sometimes tonsillitis, palatal ulcers, or petechiae are observed. The cervical lymph nodes may be enlarged and tender. Conjunctivitis and conjunctival suffusion are observed frequently. Nuchal rigidity can be elicited in 10 per cent of cases, more often in children. Confusion, agitation, and mild disturbances of consciousness suggesting encephalitis are present in 5 to 10 per cent of cases, but patients with significant neurologic findings, such as cranial nerve palsy, motor weakness and paralysis, seizures, and coma, usually constitute less than 5 per cent of all cases.[2, 26] In epidemics, neurologic findings and encephalitis have been more common in children; however, sporadic cases, including encephalitis cases due to VEE subtype II (Everglades) virus, have occurred in middle-aged or elderly adults.[10] The fatality rate among patients with encephalitis is 10 to 25 per cent, or about 0.5 per cent of all cases.[26]

In many cases, the illness has an apparent biphasic course with seizures, projectile vomiting, and ataxia occurring several days after the onset of fever, with complete and rapid resolution thereafter. Sequelae, such as nervousness, forgetfulness, recurrent headache, and easy fatigability, are common and may persist for months or even up to 1 year. Motor abnormalities usually resolve without residual deficit; however, rarely, sensory and motor abnormalities may persist. Long-term effects on psychometric examination have been reported.[20]

Experimental observations in animals suggest that congenital infection may lead to central nervous system anomalies, such as porencephaly, micrencephaly, and hydrocephalus. A similar pattern of central nervous system structural abnormalities has been observed in fetuses aborted during outbreaks, and VEE virus has been isolated from fetal brain.[39] Pancreatic beta-cell infection occurs in experimentally infected animals, leading to speculation that VEE may be followed by diabetes, but epidemiologic studies have failed to find an association.[3, 22, 24]

The principal clinical laboratory finding is leukopenia ($<4500/mm^3$), occurring at its nadir on the fourth day of illness.[2, 9] After the onset of illness, the absolute neutrophil count declines from normal values to 500 to 2000; total lymphocytes are depressed at the onset of illness and gradually recover after 1 week. The platelet count may be diminished below 100,000 mm^3, and lactic dehydrogenase and hepatic transaminases may be elevated moderately. The cerebrospinal fluid shows a lymphocytic pleocytosis with up to several hundred cells, a moderately elevated protein, and normal or slightly depressed glucose.

PATHOLOGY AND PATHOGENESIS

VEE virus is both lymphotropic and neurotropic.[22, 33] Pathologic changes are observed consistently in lymph nodes, spleen, lungs, liver, gastrointestinal lymphoid tissue, and brain. Inflammatory infiltrates are a mixture of mononuclear and polymorphonuclear cells. Lymph nodes and spleen show pronounced lymphoid depletion and necrosis of germinal centers, with neutrophilic infiltration and lymphophagocytosis. The selective depletion of lymphoid follicles, sparing paracortical areas and the thymus, suggests that VEE virus principally destroys B cells. These histopathologic changes are reflected in the early lymphopenia seen in the peripheral blood. The liver shows patchy hepatocellular degeneration typical of viral hepatitis. A diffuse interstitial pneumonia with a mixed intraseptal inflammatory cell infiltrate is a consistent finding, and some cases also exhibit intra-alveolar hemorrhages and/or secondary bronchopnemonia. The brain shows only congestion and edema in the majority of cases. Mild, often focal meningitis and changes associated with encephalitis, perivascular inflammatory infiltrates, and neuronal degeneration are found in a large number of cases.[8] The consistent findings of congestion and edema in various organs and necrotizing vasculitis seen in some cases suggest that vascular endothelial cells may be a target of infection. VEE viral antigen can be found in vascular endothelial cells of experimentally infected animals. Secondary immune-mediated destruction of infected vascular endothelia and lymphoid cells may account for later-appearing clinical manifestations.

LABORATORY DIAGNOSIS

VEE virus can be recovered from blood during the first 3 days of illness in at least 75 per cent of cases, although isolates have been made after 6 days.[4] Virus also has been recovered from throat swabs in about 25 per cent of cases.[23] Specimens should be inoculated onto Vero or other susceptible cell cultures but only in a laboratory with BL-3 level containment because of the possibility of laboratory aerosol-associated infection. As an alternative to viral isolation, genomic sequences in acute viremic blood can be detected rapidly and with high sensitivity by polymerase chain reaction. It is vital to establish the subtype of VEE viral isolates because subtypes IAB and IC have the potential for epidemic spread. Isolates can be identified rapidly with monoclonal antibodies having subtype specificity.

IgM capture enzyme-linked immunosorbent assay is the recommended serologic procedure. Both serum or cerebrospinal fluid specimens can be tested by this means. Elevated viral-specific IgM in a single serum or cerebrospinal fluid specimen is diagnostic, often obviating the need for a second paired serum. Alternative available serologic procedures in increasing order of specificity include IgG enzyme-linked immunosorbent assay, hemagglutination inhibition, complement fixation, and neutralization.

DIFFERENTIAL DIAGNOSIS

The self-limited acute febrile illness that characterizes most VEE cases resembles infection due to dengue, Oropouche, Mayaro, group C bunyaviruses, and various other arboviruses. The epidemic occurrence of cases may suggest dengue or Oropouche; however, the absence of rash and hemorrhagic manifestations and an association with equine deaths strongly indicate VEE until disproved. Eastern and western equine encephalitis overlap with VEE in some areas of Latin America, but only sporadic human cases have been recognized. Clinical recognition of sporadic VEE due to sylvatic viruses is difficult; the diagnosis should be entertained in patients with central nervous system infection and appropriate exposure history.

TREATMENT AND PREVENTION

No specific treatment is available. Symptomatic treatment with antipyretics and fluids alone is sufficient in most cases. In patients with encephalitis, anticonvulsants may be needed, and intensive supportive care, especially recognition and treatment of secondary pneumonia, may improve outcome.

Immunization with experimental live attenuated TC-83 vaccine is indicated for laboratory and field personnel with a high risk of exposure to VEE virus.[5] However, the vaccine is immunogenic in only 85 per cent of vaccinees, and about 20 per cent of vaccinees develop significant side effects of fever, stiff neck, malaise, and myalgias.[11] Approximately 75 per cent of persons who fail to respond will develop antibody after immunization with experimental inactivated TC-84 vaccine.[11]

Immunization of equines with TC-83 vaccine is the best approach to preventing the emergence of outbreaks. Inadequately inactivated vaccine prepared from epizootic IAB strains poses a danger of producing iatrogenic outbreaks and should only be used if appropriate safety and quality assurance standards of vaccine production have been met. Because the live vaccine provides rapid immunity after a single dose, it is the most effective approach in combating outbreaks. Attenuated vaccine is commercially available in certain Latin American countries, but in the United States, only inactivated vaccine, formulated with western and eastern equine encephalitis and equine influenza and tetanus antigens, is available.

Mosquito control, with a combination of larvicides and adulticides, may be indicated to mitigate large outbreaks. Taking precautions against mosquito bites, such as using repellents, staying in well-screened or air-conditioned areas when possible, and wearing long-sleeved shirts and long pants, are advised for persons who cannot avoid traveling to areas experiencing epidemics.

References

1. Adames, A. J., Dutary, B., Tejera, H., et al.: Relacion entre mosquitos vectores y aves acuaticas en la transmision potencial de dos arbovirus. Rev. Med. Panama *18*:106–119, 1993.
2. Bowen, G. S., Fashinell, T. R., Dean, P. B., et al.: Clinical aspects of human Venezuelan equine encephalitis in Texas. Bull. Pan. Am. Health Org. *10*:46–57, 1976.
3. Bowen, G. S., Rayfield, E. J., Monath, T. P., et al.: Studies of glucose metabolism in Rhesus monkeys after Venezuelan equine encephalitis virus infection. J. Med. Virol. *6*:227–234, 1980.
4. Bowen, G. S., and Calisher, C. H.: Virological and serological studies in Venezuelan equine encephalomyelitis in humans. J. Clin. Microbiol. *4*:22–27, 1976.
5. Burke, D. S., Ramsburg, H. H., and Edelman, R.: Persistence in humans of antibody to subtypes of Venezuelan equine encephalomyelitis (VEE) virus after immunization with attenuated (TC-83) VEE virus vaccine. J. Infect. Dis. *136*:354–359, 1977.
6. Centers for Disease Control and Prevention: Venezuelan equine encephalitis: Colombia, 1995. M. M .W. R. *44*:721–724, 1995.
7. Centers for Disease Control and Prevention: Update: Venezuelan equine encephalitis: Colombia, 1995. M. M. W. R. *44*:775–777, 1995.
8. Charles, P. C., Walters, E., Margolis, F., et al.: Mechanism of neuroinvasion of Venezuelan equine encephalitis virus in the mouse. Virology *208*:662–671, 1995.
9. Dietz, W. H., Peralta, P. H., and Johnson, K. M.: Ten clinical cases of human infection with Venezuelan equine encephalomyelitis virus, subtype I-D. Am. J. Trop. Med. Hyg. *28*:329–334, 1979.
10. Ehrenkranz, N. J., and Ventura, A. K.: Venezuelan equine encephalitis virus infection in man. Ann. Rev. Med. *25*:9–14, 1974.
11. Engler, R. J. M., Mangiafico, J. A., Jahrling, P., et al.: Venezuelan equine encephalitis–specific immunoglobulin responses: Live attenuated TC-83 versus inactivated C-84 vaccine. J. Med. Virol. *38*:305–310, 1992.
12. Franck, P. T., and Johnson, K. M.: An outbreak of Venezuelan equine encephalomyelitis in Central America. Am. J. Epidemiol. *94*:487–495, 1971.
13. Gutierrez, V. E., Monath, T. P., Alava, A. A., et al.: Epidemiologic investigations of the 1969 epidemic of Venezuelan encephalitis in Ecuador. Am. J. Epidemiol. *102*:400–413, 1975.
14. Johnson, B. J. B., Brubaker, J. R., Roehrig, J. T., et al.: Variants of Venezuelan equine encephalitis virus that resist neutralization define a domain of the E2 glycoprotein. Virology *177*:676–683, 1990.
15. Johnson, K. M., and Martin, D. H.: Venezuelan equine encephalitis. Adv. Vet. Sci. Comp. Med. *18*:79–116, 1974.
16. Kinney, R. M., Tsuchiya, K. R., Sneider, J. M., et al.: Molecular evidence for the origin of the widespread Venezuelan equine encephalitis epizootic of 1969 to 1972. J. Gen. Virol. *73*:3301–3305, 1992.
17. Kinney, R. M., Chang, G.-J., Tsuchiya, K. R., et al.: Attenuation of Venezuelan equine encephalitis virus strain TC-83 is encoded by the 5′-noncoding region and the E2 envelope glycoprotein. J. Virol. *67*:1269–1277, 1993.
18. Kinney, R. M., Tsuchiya, K. R., Sneider, J. M., et al.: Genetic evidence that epizootic Venezuelan equine encephalitis (VEE) viruses may have evolved from enzootic VEE subtype I-D virus. Virology *191*:569–580, 1992.
19. Koprowski, H., and Cox, H. R.: Human laboratory infection with Venezuelan equine encephalomyelitis virus. N. Engl. J. Med. *236*:647–654, 1947.
20. Leon, C. A., Jaramillo, R., Martinez, A., et al.: Sequelae of Venezuelan equine encephalitis in humans: A four-year follow-up. Int. J. Epidemiol. *4*:131–140, 1975.
21. London, W. T., Levitt, N. H., Kent, S. G., et al.: Congenital cerebral and ocular malformations induced in Rhesus monkeys by Venezuelan equine encephalitis virus. Teratology *16*:285–296, 1977.
22. Monte de la, S. M., Castro, F., Bonilla, N. J., et al.: The systemic pathology of Venezuelan equine encephalitis virus infection in humans. Am. J. Trop. Med. Hyg. *34*:194–202, 1985.
23. Pan American Health Organization: Venezuelan encephalitis. Proceedings of the Workshop Symposium on Venezuelan Encephalitis Virus, Washington, D.C., Scientific Publication 243, 1972, pp. 1–416.
24. Rayfield, E. J., Seto, Y., Goldberg, S. L., et al.: Venezuelan encephalitis virus-induced alterations in carbohydrate metabolism in genetically diabetic mice. Diabetes *28*:799–803, 1979.
25. Rico-Hesse, R., Weaver, S. C., Siger de, J., et al.: Emergence of a new epidemic/epizootic Venezuelan equine encephalitis virus in South America. Proc. Natl. Acad. Sci. U. S. A. *92*:5278–5281, 1995.
26. Rossi, A. L. B.: Rural epidemic encephalitis in Venezuelan caused by a group A arbovirus (VEE). Progr. Med. Virol. *9*:176–203, 1967.
27. Rumenapf, T., Strauss, E. G., and Strauss, J. H.: Aura virus is a New World representative of Sindbis-like viruses. Virology *208*:621–633, 1995.
28. Sanchez, J. L., Lednar, W. M., Macasaet, F. F., et al.: Venezuelan equine encephalomyelitis: Report of an outbreak associated with jungle exposure. Mil. Med. *149*:618–621, 1984.
29. Sanmartin-Barberi, C., Groot, H., and Osorno-Mesa, E.: Human epidemic in Colombia caused by the Venezuelan equine encephalomyelitis virus. Am. J. Trop. Med. Hyg. *3*:283–293, 1954.
30. Strauss, J. H., and Strauss, E. G.: The alphaviruses: Gene expression, replication and evolution. Microbiol. Rev. *58*:491–562, 1994.
31. Suarez, O. M., and Bergold, G. H.: Investigations of an outbreak of Venezuelan equine encephalitis in towns of eastern Venezuela. Am. J. Trop. Med. Hyg. *17*:875–880, 1968.
32. Sudia, W. D., and Newhouse, V. F.: Epidemic Venezuelan equine encephalitis in North America: A summary of virus-vector-host relationships. Am. J. Epidemiol. *101*:1–58, 1975.
33. Walker, D. H., Harrison, A., Murphy, K., et al.: Lymphoreticular and myeloid pathogenesis of Venezuelan equine encephalitis in hamsters. Am. J. Pathol. *84*:351–370, 1976.
34. Walton, T. E., Alvarez, O., Buckwalter, R. M., et al.: Experimental infection of horses with enzootic and epizootic strains of Venezuelan equine encephalomyelitis virus. J. Infect. Dis. *128*:271–282, 1973.
35. Walton, T. E., and Grayson, M. A.: Venezuelan equine encephalitis. *In* Monath, T. P. (ed.): The Arboviruses: Epidemiology and Ecology. Vol. 4. Boca Raton, FL, CRC Press, 1989, pp. 203–231.
36. Walton, T. E.: Venezuelan, eastern and western encephalomyelitis. *In* Gibbs,

E. P. J. (ed.): Virus Disease Mamographs. Vol. 2. New York, Academic Press, 1981, pp. 587–625.
37. Weaver, S. C., Bellew, L. A., and Rico-Hesse, R.: Phylogenetic analysis of alphaviruses in the Venezuelan equine encephalitis complex and identification of the source of epizootic viruses. Virology *191*:282–290, 1992.
38. Weaver, S. C., Rico-Hesse, R., and Scott, T. W.: Genetic diversity and slow rates of evolution in New World alphaviruses. Curr. Top. Microbiol. Immunol. *176*:99–117, 1992.
39. Wenger, F.: Venezuelan equine encephalitis. Teratology *16*:359–362, 1977.
40. Young, N. A., and Johnson, K. M.: Antigenic variants of Venezuelan equine encephalitis virus: Their geographic distribution and epidemiologic significance. Am. J. Epidemiol. *89*:286–307, 1969.

❑ ❑ ❑

CHAPTER 178 (D)

Chikungunya

Scott B. Halstead

Chikungunya is a benign, dengue-like syndrome characterized by abrupt onset of fever, arthralgia, maculopapular rash, and leukopenia. The term in Swahili means "that which bends up," referring to the characteristic symptom of arthralgia.[38] In historical times, the terms knokkel koorts, abu rokab, mal de genoux, dengue, dyenga, and 3-day fever have been given to epidemics probably caused by chikungunya virus.[8]

The classic account, widely cited as being the initial description of epidemic dengue fever, is that of David Bylon, who was "staads chirurgyn" to the City of Batavia (Jakarta) in the year 1779.[4] Dr. Bylon, who himself contracted the illness, wrote:

> It was last May 25, in the afternoon at 5:00 when I noted while talking with two good friends of mine, a growing pain in my right hand, and the joints of the lower arm, which step by step proceeded upward to the shoulder and then continued onto all my limbs; so much so that at 9:00 that same evening I was already in my bed with a high fever. . . .
>
> It's now been three weeks since I . . . was stricken by the illness, and because of that had to stay home for 5 days; but even until today I have continuously pain and stiffness in the joints of both feet, with swelling of both ankles; so much so, that when I get up in the morning, or have sat up for a while and start to move again, I can not do so very well and going up and down stairs is very painful.

This account of a febrile illness of acute onset with involvement of the joints clearly suggests that the disease was chikungunya (see the section on clinical manifestations).

In the same year in Cairo and Alexandria, Egypt, another outbreak of disease occurred that bears a close resemblance to chikungunya.[8]

An important pandemic of "dengue" occurred in the years 1870 to 1873, when it appeared first on the East African coast, then on the Arabian coast and in Port Said, Egypt. From there, it was carried to Bombay and Calcutta, India, and Java. The 1870 outbreak led to the discovery that the Swahili word for this disease was ki-dinga pepo.[12] The term denga or dyenga had been used to designate the disease in Africa in an earlier outbreak in 1823. In this pandemic, dengue had spread with the slave trade to the Caribbean, where in 1827 and 1828 an extensive outbreak occurred in the West Indies. It was in Cuba that the Spanish homonym dengue was used first. There is written or serologic evidence of chikungunya pandemics in India in 1824 and 1825, 1871 and 1872, 1923, and 1964 and 1965.[8]

Chikungunya virus was isolated first by inoculation of suckling mice from an explosive dengue-like epidemic in Tanganyika in 1952.[39]

ETIOLOGIC AGENT

Classification

According to epidemiologic criteria, chikungunya virus is arthropod-borne because it is transmitted by several species of mosquito. With the use of antigenic relationships demonstrated by hemagglutination inhibition and complement fixation, chikungunya is placed in the *Alphavirus* genus of the family *Togaviridae*.[24] Antisera prepared to chikungunya virus show strong cross-reactions by complement fixation and virus-dilution neutralization with o'nyong nyong. Mayaro and Semliki Forest viruses, however, demonstrate only weak cross-reactions by hemagglutination inhibition and no reactions by complement fixation with chikungunya antigen. Cross-comparisons by plaque-reduction neutralization tests have shown little relatedness among alphaviruses.[43] Similar results have been obtained by fluorescent antibody technique.

African and Asian strains of chikungunya virus are not separable antigenically by use of mouse immune sera.[33] Although differences in plaque size and heat stability have been described between these strains, there is a possibility that these might be due to the high number of mouse passages received by the prototype African strain. Wild-type strains from both geographic regions share the property of autointerference and production of hemorrhagic enteritis (Halstead, S. B., unpublished data, 1978).

Morphology

Chikungunya virions are spherical particles approximately 42 nm in diameter.[21] They possess a lipid-containing envelope with fine projections. The central core, approximately 25 to 30 nm in diameter, is roughly hexagonal in cross-section and contains a nucleocapsid of uncertain symmetry. Together with other alphaviruses, the genome is a positive-sense, single-stranded RNA of 12 kb that is messenger-active and specifies the viral structural and nonstructural protein, including the polymerase. After an initial round of RNA replication, a subgenomic RNA of approximately 4 kb (26 sRNA) is produced. This RNA encodes the viral structural proteins, which include two envelope and capsid proteins.[22] The gene is translated from the 5′ end, where genes for nonstructural proteins are located. Assembly of virus particles at the cell surface occurs by a budding process involving incorporation of the "core" virus precursor into virus particles.[21] Host cell membranes are modified during infection and contain viral antigen when incorporated into viral envelopes. The protein hemagglutinin spikes are mounted on a phospholipid envelope.

Growth

Chikungunya virus produces death in infant mice, rats, and hamsters after intracerebral inoculation. Serial passage of the virus in mice has resulted in the selection of a strain with a short incubation period that is lethal to weanling mice.[39] Virus grows to titers of 10^8 to 10^9 infectious doses per mL. Low-passage material is highly infectious for humans during routine laboratory handling. Appropriate precautions should be taken by laboratory workers.

If a mouse brain seed suspension is prepared of low-passage virus and inoculated into other mice at a 1:5 or 1:10 final concentration, deaths may be delayed significantly, may be sporadic, or may not occur at all. This is due to autointerference. Low-passage strains recovered in suckling mice characteristically demonstrate autointerference when inoculated at dilutions below 1:100.

Chikungunya virus produces a cytopathic effect in primary hamster kidney cells and in BHK-21, BSC-1, Vero, FL, HeLa, and rhesus kidney cells.[24] Virus multiplies in *Aedes aegypti, Aedes vittatus, Aedes albopictus, Anopheles stephensi*, and *Culex fatigans* continuous cell lines and in a cell line derived from *Drosophila*. Plaque assays have been described in LLC-MK2, Vero, and BHK-21 cells and in duck and chick embryos.[24]

TRANSMISSION

Chikungunya virus has been recovered from wild *A. aegypti* in Tanzania, Nigeria, India, and Thailand; from *Aedes africanus* in Uganda and Bangui; and from *Aedes luteocephalus* in Senegal.[1, 13, 27] Occasional isolates have been made from *Mansonia fuscopennata* in Uganda and from *C. fatigans* in Thailand and Tanzania.

Transmission to humans has been demonstrated with the *Aedes furcifer-taylori* group; transmission to monkeys or mice has been demonstrated with *A. aegypti, A. albopictus, Aedes calceatus, Aedes triseriatus, Aedes togoi, Aedes pseudoscutellaris, Aedes polynesiensis, Anopheles albinanus, Mansonia africana, Eretmapodites chrysogaster*, and *Aedes apicoargenteus*.[24, 29, 36, 41]

Tesh and colleagues[44] examined *A. albopictus* strains from 13 geographic locations from Hawaii to Africa, finding considerable variation in susceptibility to infection by oral feeding. The 50 per cent oral ID_{50} of a Hawaiian *A. albopictus* for a wild-type virus from India was $10^{5.4}$ plaque-forming units per mL. The amount of virus replicated by different mosquito strains varied between $10^{4.6}$ and $10^{7.4}$ plaque-forming units per mosquito. These observations, plus a mathematical model of chikungunya virus transmission developed by deMoor and Steffens,[14] suggest that major factors in determining endemicity of chikungunya may be arthropod related. Tesh and associates[44] suggest that susceptibility to oral infection and amount of virus replicated may be under genetic control, whereas deMoor and Steffens[14] found mosquito longevity to be the most important determinant in epidemic transmission of chikungunya.

Almost all recorded chikungunya infections in people occur in areas infested with *A. aegypti*. The epidemiology, therefore, is similar to that of other *A. aegypti*–borne diseases and parallels the distribution of the vector. When the mosquitoes are abundant in occupied dwellings, infection rates can be expected to be highest in women and children who are at home during daylight hours. When *A. aegypti* is found in public buildings, schools, and hospitals, outbreaks may involve persons in occupational patterns. Characteristically, chikungunya pandemics are explosive. Studying *A. aegypti* in laboratory mice, Rao and colleagues[37] have documented mechanical transmission. Viremia in humans may be as high as 10^8 infectious doses per mL.[37] Because the extrinsic incubation period in *A. aegypti* is relatively long, the explosive nature of chikungunya outbreaks is explained best by mechanical transmission.

EPIDEMIOLOGY

Host Range

Chikungunya virus has the ability to replicate in a broad spectrum of vertebrate species. Newborn mice, hamsters, rats, rabbits, guinea pigs, and kittens all can be infected by subcutaneous inoculation of field strains of chikungunya virus.[9] This produces viremia, sickness, and, in most instances, death. Adult rabbits, mice, rats, and chickens inoculated peripherally have an asymptomatic viremia followed by antibody response. Neutralizing or hemagglutination-inhibition antibodies to chikungunya have been recovered occasionally from sera obtained from ungulates. Attempts to infect cattle, goats, sheep, or horses experimentally failed to produce either viremia or antibody response.[26] Vervet monkeys and baboons are infected readily. Rhesus monkeys were infected by intravenous and intramuscular inoculation of animals, with viremia titers in excess of 10^7 mouse LD_{50}. *A. aegypti* transmitted virus to rhesus monkeys and could be infected by biting viremic animals.

Chikungunya antibodies have been found in vervet monkeys, baboons, chimpanzees, and red-tailed monkeys in Zimbabwe, South Africa, and Uganda.[28] The zoonotic status of chikungunya virus in Asia has not been studied carefully.

In Africa, zoonotic transmission to subhuman primates is surmised to take place in a wide variety of habitats, with transmission occurring in the forest canopy, at ground level, or both.[30] Chikungunya appears to be enzootic throughout much of eastern, central, southern, and western Africa.[24] Subhuman primate populations are involved in epizootics, which involve critical numbers of the susceptible population, followed by disappearance of virus. Thus, chikungunya may maintain itself in wildlife populations by constantly moving epizootic activity, in much the same fashion as respiratory and enteric virus infections are maintained in humans. It seems reasonable to expect that intercurrent and epidemic human infections in Africa are related to epizootic activity. Many putative or identified chikungunya vectors feed on people as well as on subhuman primates.

Geographic Distribution

When susceptible human and *A. aegypti* populations are above the threshold level required for transmission, a person-mosquito-person cycle is established. This cycle probably is responsible for most of the large urban outbreaks of chikungunya studied during the past 40 years. In Africa, chikungunya outbreaks have been reported from Uganda, Tanzania, Zimbabwe, South Africa, Angola, Zaire, Nigeria, and Senegal.[24] This distribution best fits the present location of virus research laboratories. A reasonable assumption is that chikungunya is endemic throughout sub-Saharan Africa.

There is historical evidence that chikungunya has spread from the African enzootic focus, causing large pandemics throughout both the American and Asian tropics.[8, 12, 42] In North America during summer months, outbreaks have extended up the Atlantic Coast as far as Philadelphia, Pennsylvania, and up the Asian Coast to Hong Kong.[12] Pandemics have swept India in 1824, 1871, 1902, 1923, and 1963 and 1964, reaching Sri Lanka (formerly Ceylon) in 1965.[8] During the late 1950s and early 1960s, chikungunya appears to have established itself endemically in Southeast Asia and was transmitted continuously in urban populations in Thailand, Cambodia, and South Vietnam, possibly into the 1970s.[10, 17, 46] Involvement of urban populations in Burma appears to have been intermittent, with outbreaks recorded in 1963 and from 1970 to 1973.[31] There is serologic evidence of chikungunya virus infection throughout the Philippines, possibly during World War II; since then, localized outbreaks have occurred in Manila, Philippines, in 1967 and Negros, Philippines, in 1968[3, 6, 25] and as recently as 1986.[2] In the nineteenth century, chikungunya epidemics were reported in the Indonesian archipelago. An extensive serologic survey using the plaque-reduction neutralization test has suggested chikungunya activity possibly during World War II in Kalimantan and Sulawesi, Indonesia. A large chikungunya epidemic involved much of Indonesia in 1983 and 1984 and Burma in 1984 and

TABLE 178–4. Chikungunya and Dengue in Children: Comparison of Onset of Illness

	Hospitalized				Outpatient			
	Chikungunya (32 cases)		*Dengue (523 cases)**		*Chikungunya (17 cases)*		*Primary Dengue (29 cases)*	
Day of Illness	Number	Per Cent	Number	Per Cent	Number	Per Cent	Number	Per Cent
0	8	25	2	0.4	0	0	0	0
1	15	47	44	8	11	65	8	27
2	5	16	67	13	1	6	5	17
3	2	6	145	28	2	12	3	10
4	1	3	148	28	0	0	7	24
5			84	16	3	17	4	14
6			20	4			2	
7	1	3	11	2			7	
8 or more			3	0.6				

*Includes primary and secondary infections.
Data modified from Nimmannitya et al.[35] and Halstead et al.[16] Patients with simultaneous dengue and chikungunya are excluded from analysis.

1985 (Slemons, R. D., personal communication). Chikungunya virus was isolated in Australia in 1989.[18] From 1990 to 1995, chikungunya remained endemic at low levels in Thailand, Myanmar (formerly Burma), and Indonesia. Little or no chikungunya virus infection has been reported in the twentieth century in New Guinea, the Solomon Islands, Vanuatu (formerly New Hebrides), the Caroline Islands, the Pacific Islands, or any of the American tropics.[43]

It is pertinent to ask why it is that chikungunya and dengue viruses, both transmitted by *A. aegypti*, do not have an identical geographic distribution. The question may be answered partially by differences in the transmission of chikungunya and dengue. The threshold for infection of chikungunya virus in *A. aegypti* is relatively high: approximately $10^{5.6}$ mouse infectious doses are required to infect 50 per cent of adult females.[44] The infection threshold of female *A. aegypti* for dengue virus is rather similar. However, *A. aegypti* infected with chikungunya virus transmits virus to vertebrates poorly, whereas dengue-infected mosquitoes transmit with great regularity.[15] Thus, the transmission of chikungunya virus would be expected to occur only in areas with high human susceptibility rates and consistently high densities of *A. aegypti* and possibly by mechanical transmission.

CLINICAL MANIFESTATIONS

The incubation period of chikungunya fever usually is 2 to 4 days. In infants, the disease typically begins with the abrupt onset of fever, followed by flushing of the skin. Febrile convulsions may occur in as many as one-third of patients. After 3 to 5 days of fever, a generalized maculopapular rash and lymphadenopathy are noted. Conjunctival injection, swelling of the eyelids, pharyngitis, and symptoms and signs of upper respiratory tract disease are common. There is no enanthem. Some infants have a biphasic fever curve. Arthralgia may be quite severe, although it is not seen frequently.[7, 16, 23, 35]

In older children, fever develops acutely and is accompanied by headache, myalgia, and arthralgia involving various joints. Residual arthralgia is uncommon. An early macular blush and a maculopapular rash accompany or immediately precede defervescence. At this same time, there is marked lymphadenopathy. Febrile convulsions are common. Hemorrhagic findings, including a positive tourniquet test, are rare.[7, 16, 23, 35]

Arthralgia or arthritis is the most conspicuous feature of chikungunya in adults. Usually, they can identify the precise time and the joint first affected in a chikungunya illness. Swelling and redness of joints and even the pinnae of the ear may occur.[7]

Although dengue and chikungunya illnesses are similar, important distinguishing features are summarized in Tables 178–4 through 178–8 from clinical data obtained from children in Thailand.[16, 35]

Table 178–4 shows the abrupt onset and early severity of chikungunya compared with dengue illnesses, many of

TABLE 178–5. Chikungunya and Dengue in Children: Comparison of Duration of Illness

Duration of Fever (Days)	Chikungunya (32 cases)		Dengue (241 cases)*	
	Number	*Per Cent*	*Number*	*Per Cent*
2	11	34.4	8	3.3
3	4	12.5	16	6.6
4	5	15.6	33	13.7
5	5	15.6	52	21.6
6	2	6.3	52	21.6
7	3	9.4	38	15.8
8 or more	2	6.3	42	17.4
	Mean 4 days		Mean 5.85 days	

*Includes primary and secondary dengue infections.
After Nimmannitya, S., Halstead, S. B., Cohen, S. N., et al.: Dengue and chikungunya virus infection in man in Thailand, 1962–1964. I. Observations on hospitalized patients with hemorrhagic fever. Am. J. Trop. Med. Hyg. *18*:954–971, 1969.

TABLE 178–6. Chikungunya and Dengue in Children: Comparison of Frequency of Clinical Findings

	Hospitalized Cases				Outpatient Cases			
	Chikungunya (32 cases)		*Dengue* (142 cases)*		*Chikungunya (17 cases)*		*Primary Dengue* (27 cases)*	
Findings	Number†	Per Cent	Number†	Per Cent	Number	Per Cent	Number	Per Cent
Headache	13/19	68	37/83	45	2	12	4	15
Injected pharynx	28/31	90	121/125	97	12	71	27	100
Enanthem	3/27	11	7/84	8	0		0	
Rhinitis	3/31	6	6/47	13	4	24	6	22
Cough	7/30	22	17/79	22	1	6	11	41
Vomiting	19/32	59	73/126	58	6	35	15	56
Constipation	12/30	40	16/30	53	0		4	15
Diarrhea	5/32	16	5/78	6	1	6	1	4
Abdominal pain	6/19	32	38/76	50	3	18	2	7
Lymphadenopathy	8/26	31	32/79	41				
Restlessness	10/30	33	17/79	22				

*Includes primary and secondary dengue infections.
†Number with finding/number with observations recorded.
Adapted from Nimmannitya, S., Halstead, S. B., Cohen, S. N., et al.: Dengue and chikungunya virus infection in man in Thailand, 1962–1964. I. Observations on hospitalized patients with hemorrhagic fever. Am. J. Trop. Med. Hyg. *18*:954–971, 1969; and Halstead, S. B., Nimmannitya, S., and Margiotta, M. R.: Dengue and chikungunya virus infection in man in Thailand, 1962–1964. II. Observations on disease in outpatients. Am. J. Trop. Med. Hyg. *18*:972–983, 1969.

which came to medical attention only several days after onset of fever.

Chikungunya virus infections are shorter in duration than dengue virus infections (Table 178–5). Almost one-half of children with chikungunya had a fever that ended within 72 hours after onset, whereas the median duration of dengue fever was 2 days longer.

Many constitutional signs and symptoms occur with similar frequency in chikungunya and dengue viral infections and cannot be used to differentiate illnesses clinically (Table 178–6). However, a terminal maculopapular rash, arthralgia or arthritis, and conjunctival injection were more common in chikungunya than in dengue (Table 178–7). Shock has been reported infrequently in chikungunya.[7, 40, 45] It was not observed in Thai cases.[35] Changes in taste perception, post-illness bradycardia, and post-illness depression or asthenia are found rarely in chikungunya; these manifestations are distinctive findings in patients with dengue.

Hemorrhagic phenomena rarely occur with chikungunya virus infection. The frequency of hemorrhagic findings among chikungunya and primary and secondary dengue viral infections in Thai children is compared in Table 178–8. The frequency of minor hemorrhagic manifestations in outpatient and inpatient dengue did not differ significantly from that in chikungunya cases. However, only hospitalized dengue cases developed a petechial rash and spontaneous hematemesis or melena.

PATHOGENESIS AND PATHOLOGY

The pathologic process of fatal human chikungunya illnesses has not been studied extensively.[45]

DIAGNOSIS

The differential diagnosis includes the viral causes of the dengue fever syndrome. In Australia and the western Pacific area, Ross River fever is a frequent cause of epidemic, arthropod-borne, viral arthralgia.

With use of the classic test methods, diagnosis depends on demonstrating the development of a significant increase in antibody after an illness. Ordinarily, a serum sample collected within 5 days of the onset of fever will not contain hemagglutination-inhibition, complement-fixation, and neutralizing antibodies.[7, 16] Neutralizing and hemagglutination-inhibition antibodies generally are present in samples collected 2 weeks or more after onset of fever. From a single serum sample collected 7 or more days after onset, it is possible to detect antibodies of the IgM class using an IgM–capture enzyme-linked immunosorbent assay. Neutralizing antibody can be measured by the virus dilution method in suckling mice (or weanling mice, with use of the Ross high mouse passage strain) or by the serum dilution method with use of any one of a variety of tissue cultures or plaque assay methods.

TABLE 178–7. Chikungunya and Dengue in Children: Clinical Findings Occurring with Different Frequency

	Chikungunya (32 cases)		Dengue* (32 cases)		
Manifestation	*Number†*	*Per Cent*	*Number†*	*Per Cent*	**Significance**
Maculopapular rash	19/32	59.4	16/132	12.1	$p < .001$
Conjunctival injection	15/27	55.6	20/61	32.8	$.05 > p < .01$
Myalgia/arthralgia	8/20	40.0	9/75	12.0	$.05 > p < .01$

*Includes primary and secondary dengue infections.
†Number positive/number of observations.
From Nimmannitya, S., Halstead, S. B., Cohen, S. N., et al.: Dengue and chikungunya virus infection in man in Thailand, 1962–1964. I. Observations on hospitalized patients with hemorrhagic fever. Am. J. Trop. Med. Hyg. *18*:954–971, 1969.

TABLE 178–8. Chikungunya and Dengue in Children: Comparison of Hemorrhagic Manifestations

	Chikungunya				Primary Dengue		Secondary Dengue	
	Outpatients (17 cases)		*Inpatients (32 cases)*		*Outpatients (27 cases)*		*Inpatients (135 cases)*	
Finding	Number*	Per Cent	Number*	Per Cent	Number*	Per Cent	Number*	Per Cent
Positive tourniquet test	3/17	18.0	24/31	77.4	4/27	14.8	94/112	83.9
Petechiae, scattered	0/17	0	10/32	31.2	4/27	7.4	60/129	46.5
Petechial rash	—		0/32	0			13/129	10.1
Maculopapular rash	0/17	0	19/32	59.4	2/27	7.4	16/132	12.1
Epistaxis	0/17	0	4/32	12.5	1/27	3.7	20/106	18.9
Gum bleeding			0/32	0			2/135	1.5
Melena/hematemesis	0/17	0	0/32	0	0/27	0	14/119	11.8

*Number positive/number of observations.
After Nimmannitya, S., Halstead, S. B., Cohen, S. N., et al.: Dengue and chikungunya virus infection in man in Thailand, 1962–1964. I. Observations on hospitalized patients with hemorrhagic fever. Am. J. Trop. Med. Hyg. *18*:954–971, 1969; and Halstead, S. B., Nimmannitya, S., and Margiotta, M. R.: Dengue and chikungunya virus infection in man in Thailand, 1962–1964. II. Observations on disease in outpatients. Am. J. Trop. Med. Hyg. *18*:972–983, 1969.

Virus isolation may be made by inoculating acute-phase serum or other suspect materials intracerebrally in 1- to 2-day-old mice or in tissue cultures. On initial passage, death may occur within 2 to 5 days after inoculation. An autointerference phenomenon is noted if low-dilution passages of infected mouse brain are made. Passage at 10^{-3} dilution or higher avoids this effect.

Vero cells and suckling mice equally are effective for primary isolation.

TREATMENT

1. Treatment is supportive.
2. Bed rest is advised during the febrile period. Antipyretics or cold sponging should be used to keep the body temperature below 40° C (104° F).
3. Analgesics or mild sedation may be required to control pain. Post-illness arthritis may require continued treatment with anti-inflammatory agents and graduated physiotherapy.
4. Salicylates, because of their hemorrhagic potential, are contraindicated.
5. Febrile convulsions are treated with phenobarbital given intravenously or orally and continued until the temperature is normal. Severe or intractable convulsions may respond to intravenous diazepam.
6. Children who have lost excessive fluid because of vomiting, fasting, or thirsting and who cannot take oral fluids may require oral rehydration. Individuals with severe hemorrhagic phenomena should be studied for underlying hemostatic disorder.

PROGNOSIS

In a few instances, isolation or serologic evidence of recent infection has been obtained for persons with severe hemorrhagic findings or for individuals dying during an acute febrile illness.[7, 23, 32, 40, 45] In addition to hemorrhage, neurologic and myocardial involvement has been reported during chikungunya infections in adults.[7, 11] In adults, arthralgia may persist for weeks. Exercise may prolong this symptom. Typically, pains shift from joint to joint and are worse in the morning and upon first use of the joint. Swelling of ankles, wrists, and fingers is frequent. In older patients, the sequelae may resemble rheumatoid arthritis. Chikungunya virus infection might coincide with other pathologic processes, resulting in the death of the individual.[32] Carefully studied, virologically documented cases have shown neither thrombocytopenia nor severe neutropenia.[23] Until more is known of the pathogenesis of chikungunya virus infection, it will be difficult to estimate the frequency with which death can be attributed directly to chikungunya fever.

Infants with chikungunya may experience residual neurologic deficits after febrile convulsions.

PREVENTION

Formalin-treated chikungunya virus (Ross strain) grown in African green monkey kidney cells produces satisfactory immune response and resistance to challenge when administered in three divided doses in monkeys.[19] A vaccine prepared under similar conditions produced hemagglutination-inhibition, complement-fixation, and neutralizing antibody responses in susceptible human volunteers.[20] A comparative study from the same laboratory was made of formalin-inactivated chikungunya vaccines prepared from the virus propagated in African green monkey kidney monolayers and concentrated chick embryo suspension cultures.[47] The latter vaccine was significantly more protective to mice against live homologous virus challenge and stimulated the production of four to five times more circulating antibodies than was and did the vaccine prepared with virus grown in African green monkey kidney cultures. Nakao and Hotta,[34] studying chikungunya grown in BHK-21 cells, found that ultraviolet-inactivated preparations were significantly more immunogenic than were formalin-treated virus. Tween-ether–extracted virus preparations also have been found to be immunogenic. Commercial production of chikungunya vaccine, however, has not been attempted. In view of the low mortality associated with chikungunya virus infections, the production of a chikungunya vaccine probably will have a low public health priority.

At present, prevention consists of avoiding mosquito bites. For urban outbreaks in most of the Asian and African tropics, the regimen for individual protection and for chronic and emergency control is the same as has been described for dengue. When other vectors are involved, measures designed to combat *A. aegypti* may fail. In such outbreaks, expert entomologic advice will be needed to design appropriate preventive measures.

For control of mosquitoes, epidemic measures, and health education, see Chapter 179.

References

1. Anderson, C. R., Singh, K. R. P., and Sarkar, J. K.: Isolation of chikungunya virus from *Aedes aegypti* fed on naturally infected humans in Calcutta. Curr. Sci. *34*:579–580, 1965.
2. Anonymous: Chikungunya fever among U.S. Peace Corps volunteers: Republic of the Philippines. M. M. W. R. *35*:573–574, 1986.
3. Basaca-Sevilla, V., and Halstead, S. B.: Recent virological studies of haemorrhagic fever and other arthropod-borne virus infections in the Philippines. J. Trop. Med. Hyg. *69*:203–208, 1966.
4. Bylon, D.: Korte aatekening, wegens eene algemeene ziekte, doorgans genaamd de knokkel-koorts. Verhandelungen van het Bataviaasch Genootschop der Konsten in Wetenschappen *2*:17–30, 1780.
5. Calisher, C. H., el-Kafrawi, A. O., Al-Deen Mahmud, M. I., et al.: Complex-specific immunoglobulin M antibody patterns in humans infected with alphaviruses. J. Clin. Microbiol. *23*:155–159, 1986.
6. Campos, L. E., San Juan, A., Cenabre, L. C., et al.: Isolation of chikungunya virus in the Philippines. Acta Med. Philippina *5*:152–155, 1969.
7. Carey, D. E., Myers, R. M., Deranitz, C. M., et al.: The 1964 chikungunya epidemic at Vellore, South India, including observations on concurrent dengue. Trans. R. Soc. Trop. Med. Hyg. *63*:434–445, 1969.
8. Carey, D. E.: Chikungunya and dengue: A case of mistaken identity? J. Hist. Med. Allied Sci. *26*:243–262, 1971.
9. Chakravarty, S. K., and Sarkar, J. K.: Susceptibility of newborn and adult laboratory animals to chikungunya virus. Indian J. Med. Res. *57*:1157–1164, 1969.
10. Chastel, C.: Human infections in Cambodia with chikungunya or a closely allied virus. III. Epidemiology. Bull. Soc. Pathol. Exot. *57*:65–82, 1964.
11. Chatterjee, S. N., Chakravarti, S. K., Mitra, A. C., et al.: Virological investigation of cases with neurological complications during the outbreak of haemorrhagic fever in Calcutta. J. Indian Med. Assoc. *45*:314–316, 1965.
12. Christie, J.: Remarks on "kidinga Pepo": A peculiar form of exanthematous disease. Br. Med. J. *1*:577–579, 1872.
13. Cornet, M., and Chateau, R.: Quelques données biologiques sur *Aedes* (Stegomyia) *luteocephalus* (Newstead) en zone de savane soudanienne dans l'ouest du Senegal. Cah. Off. Recherche Sci. Tech. Outre-Mer. Entomol. Méd. Parasitol. *12*:97–109, 1974.
14. deMoor, P. P., and Steffens, F. E.: A computer-simulated model of an arthropod-borne virus transmission cycle, with special reference to chikungunya virus. Trans. R. Soc. Trop. Med. Hyg. *64*:927–934, 1970.
15. Gubler, D. J., Nalim, S., Tan, R., et al.: Variation in susceptibility to oral infection with dengue viruses among geographic strains of *Aedes aegypti*. Am. J. Trop. Med. Hyg. *28*:1045–1052, 1979.
16. Halstead, S. B., Nimmannitya, S., and Margiotta, M. R.: Dengue and chikungunya virus infection in man in Thailand, 1962–1964. II. Observations on disease in outpatients. Am. J. Trop. Med. Hyg. *18*:972–983, 1969.
17. Halstead, S. B., Scanlon, J. E., Umpaivit, P., et al.: Dengue and chikungunya virus infection in man in Thailand, 1962–1964. IV. Epidemiologic studies in the Bangkok metropolitan area. Am. J. Trop. Med. Hyg. *18*:987–1021, 1969.
18. Harnett, G. B., and Bucens, M. R.: Isolation of chikungunya virus in Australia. Med. J. Aust. *152*:328–329, 1990.
19. Harrison, V. R., Binn, L. N., and Randall, R.: Comparative immunogenicities of chikungunya vaccines prepared in avian and mammalian tissues. Am. J. Trop. Med. Hyg. *16*:786–791, 1967.
20. Harrison, V. R., Eckels, K. H., Bartelloni, P. J., et al.: Production and evaluation of a formalin-killed chikungunya vaccine. J. Immunol. *107*:643–647, 1971.
21. Higashi, N., Matsumoto, A., Tabata, K., et al.: Electron microscope study of development of chikungunya virus in green monkey kidney stable (VERO) cells. Virology *35*:55–59, 1967.
22. Igarashi, A., Fukuoka, T., Nithiuthai, P., et al.: Structural components of chikungunya virus. Biken J. *13*:93–110, 1970.
23. Jadhav, M., Namboodripad, M., Carman, R. H., et al.: Chikungunya disease in infants and children in Vellore: A report on clinical and haematological features of virologically proved cases. Indian J. Med. Res. *53*:764–776, 1965.
24. Karabatsos, N. (ed.): International Catalog of Arbovirus 1985. Ft. Collins, CO, American Society of Tropical Medicine and Hygiene, 1985.
25. Macasaet, F. F., Villamil, P. T., Wexler, S., et al.: Epidemiology of arbovirus infections in Negros Oriental. II. Serologic findings of the epidemic in Amlan. J. Philippine Med. Assoc. *45*:311–317, 1969.
26. McIntosh, B. M., Paterson, H. E., Donaldson, J. M., et al.: Chikungunya virus: Viral susceptibility and transmission studies with some vertebrates and mosquitoes. S. Afr. J. Med. Sci. *28*:45–52, 1963.
27. McIntosh, B. M., Paterson, H. E., McGillivray, G., et al.: Further studies on the chikungunya outbreak in Southern Rhodesia in 1962. I. Mosquitoes, wild primates and birds in relation to the epidemic. Ann. Trop. Med. Parasitol. *58*:45–51, 1964.
28. McIntosh, B. M.: Antibody against chikungunya virus in wild primates in southern Africa. S. Afr. J. Med. Sci. *35*:65–74, 1970.
29. McIntosh, B. M., and Jupp, P. G.: Attempts to transmit chikungunya virus with six species of mosquito. J. Med. Entomol. *7*:615–618, 1970.
30. McIntosh, B. M., Jupp, P. G., and DeSouza, J.: Mosquitoes feeding at two horizontal levels in gallery forest in Natal, South Africa, with reference to possible vectors of chikungunya virus. J. Entomol. Soc. S. Afr. *35*:81–90, 1972.
31. Ming, C. K., Thein, S., Thaung, U. T., et al.: Clinical laboratory studies on haemorrhagic fever in Burma, 1970–1972. Bull. W. H. O. *51*:227–236, 1974.
32. Munasinghe, D. R., and Rajasuriya, K.: Haemorrhage in Christmas disease following dengue-like fever. Ceylon Med. J. *11*:39–40, 1966.
33. Nakao, E.: Biological and immunological studies on chikungunya virus: A comparative observation of two strains of African and Asian origins. Kobe J. Med. Sci. *18*:133–141, 1972.
34. Nakao, E., and Hotta, S.: Immunogenicity of purified, inactivated chikungunya virus in monkeys. Bull. W. H. O. *48*:559–562, 1973.
35. Nimmannitya, S., Halstead, S. B., Cohen, S. N., et al.: Dengue and chikungunya virus infection in man in Thailand, 1962–1964. I. Observations on hospitalized patients with hemorrhagic fever. Am. J. Trop. Med. Hyg. *18*:954–971, 1969.
36. Paterson, H. E., and McIntosh, B. M.: Further studies on the chikungunya outbreak in southern Rhodesia in 1962. II. Transmission experiments with the *Aedes furcifertaylori* group of mosquitoes and with a member of the *Anopheles gambiae* complex. Ann. Trop. Med. Parasitol. *58*:52–55, 1964.
37. Rao, T. R., Devi, P. S., and Singh, K. R. P.: Experimental studies on the mechanical transmission of chikungunya virus by *Aedes aegypti*. Mosq. News *28*:406–408, 1968.
38. Robinson, M. C.: An epidemic of virus disease in Southern Province, Tanganyika Territory, in 1952–1953. I. Clinical features. Trans. R. Soc. Trop. Med. Hyg. *49*:28–32, 1955.
39. Ross, R. W.: The Newala epidemic. III. The virus: Isolation, pathogenic properties and relationship to the epidemic. J. Hyg. *54*:177–191, 1956.
40. Sarkar, J. K., Chatterjee, S. N., Chakrevarti, S. K., et al.: Chikungunya virus infection with haemorrhagic manifestations. Indian J. Med. Res. *53*:921–925, 1965.
41. Shah, K. V., Gilotra, S. K., Gibbs, C. J., Jr., et al.: Laboratory studies of transmission of chikungunya virus by mosquitoes. Indian J. Med. Res. *52*:703–709, 1964.
42. Siler, J. F., Hall, M. W., and Hitchens, A. P.: Dengue: Its history, epidemiology, mechanisms of transmission, etiology, clinical manifestations, immunity and prevention. Philippine J. Sci. *29*:1–305, 1926.
43. Tesh, R. B., Gadjusek, D. C., Garruto, R. M., et al.: The distribution and prevalence of group A arbovirus neutralizing antibodies among human populations in Southeast Asia and the Pacific Islands. Am. J. Trop. Med. Hyg. *24*:664–675, 1975.
44. Tesh, R. B., Gubler, D. J., and Rosen, L.: Variation among geographic strains of *Aedes albopictus* in susceptibility to infection with chikungunya virus. Am. J. Trop. Med. Hyg. *25*:326–335, 1976.
45. Thiruvengadam, K. V., Kalyanasundaram, V., and Rajgopal, J.: Clinical and pathological studies on chikungunya fever in Madras City. Indian J. Med. Res. *53*:720–728, 1965.
46. Vu-Qui, D., Nguyen-Thi, K. T., and Ly, Q. B.: Antibodies to chikungunya virus in Vietnamese children in Saigon. Bull. Soc. Pathol. Exot. *60*:353–359, 1967.
47. White, A., Berman, S., and Lowenthal, J. P.: Comparative immunogenicities of chikungunya vaccines propagated in monkey kidney monolayers and chick embryo suspension cultures. Appl. Microbiol. *23*:951–952, 1972.

❑ ❑ ❑

CHAPTER 178 (E)

Ross River Virus Arthritis

John G. Aaskov

Epidemics of a benign disease with polyarthralgia and rash have been described in Australia since 1927.[47] Between 4000 and 5000 cases of epidemic polyarthritis are diagnosed now in Australia each year. Investigations of an epidemic of polyarthritis in southern Australia in 1956[10, 52] suggested that an alphavirus was the causative agent. This was confirmed when Ross River virus was isolated from *Aedes vigilax* mosquitoes in Townsville in northern Australia, and shown, on serologic grounds, to be the causative agent of epidemic polyarthritis.[20, 23] Although the first isolation of virus from a human was from a febrile child without arthritis,[19] subsequent use of mosquito cell lines enabled numerous isolations of Ross River virus from epidemic polyarthritis patients in Australia and the Pacific Islands.[9, 50, 53]

Some confusion has been generated recently by the use of the term Ross River fever to describe clinical Ross River virus infections (more than half of those with clinical disease do not develop a fever).[45] Additional confusion has been generated by efforts to call any polyarthritis caused by Australian arboviruses epidemic polyarthritis. It is proposed that the term epidemic polyarthritis be used to describe clinical disease caused by Ross River virus and only Ross River virus.

ETIOLOGIC AGENT

Ross River virus is related serologically to Getah and Bebaru viruses in the Semliki Forest virus subgroup.[17] Nucleotide sequencing has confirmed this close relationship between Ross River, Getah, and Semliki Forest viruses.[24] Cryoelectron microscopic studies[13] suggest that the nucleocapsid is approximately 400 Å in diameter and has a T=4 quaternary structure. It is surrounded by a membrane bilayer that is penetrated by 80 spikes also arranged in a T=4 lattice. Each spike is a trimer of heterodimers of envelope glycoproteins E1 and E2.

Oligonucleotide mapping and limited nucleotide sequencing suggest that there may be four topotypes of Ross River virus.[43] This mirrors the extensive biologic variation (e.g., plaque size, mouse neurovirulence) observed with different isolates.[9, 25, 35] The virus grows to high titer in the muscle and brain of day-old mice, causing paralysis and death,[44, 46] and it also grows to high titer in vertebrate and mosquito cell lines.[9]

TRANSMISSION AND EPIDEMIOLOGY

Ross River virus is endemic in all mainland states of Australia and in Papua New Guinea and possibly New Caledonia. There has been no disease reported from those island states involved in the 1979 to 1980 epidemic (Fiji, Samoa, Tonga, Cook Islands)[6, 41, 50, 53] since that time.

The isolation of Ross River virus from mosquitoes, especially *A. vigillax*[23, 35] and *Culex annulirostris*,[22, 35] and the widespread occurrence of antibody to the virus in mammals[21] suggested a mammal-mosquito cycle with humans as an incidental host.

However, with improved laboratory diagnostic services, it now is apparent that clinical infection in humans occurs year-round, although most occur in the late summer and in autumn, and that the majority of patients are city dwellers.[8, 45] Taken together with the explosive spread of disease during the 1979 to 1980 epidemic of Ross River virus infection in the Pacific,[6, 50, 53] it appears that this virus may be maintained in either of two cycles, mammal-mosquito-mammal or human-mosquito-human, with occasional movement of virus between the two.

Evidence also has been presented of transovarial transmission of Ross River virus in *Aedes* mosquitoes.[40, 42]

Patients may be viremic for up to 7 days after onset of symptoms,[9, 50] and the incubation time from infection to onset of symptoms may vary from 1 to 27 days, 7 to 9 days being the usual interval in endemic areas.[28]

In endemic areas, the ratio of subclinical to clinical infections is high (approximately 50:1),[8] but during epidemics the ratio may be reduced to 4:1 or less.[6, 37] The subclinical infection rate for most of northern Australia is approximately 1.5 per cent per annum,[8] but there are areas where this is even higher.[15, 16]

Although infection rates are the same in both sexes, clinical disease is more common in women, particularly among those 18 to 45 years of age.[18, 45] An association between HLA-DR7 and clinical disease also has been observed.[34]

Epidemic polyarthritis has been reported in residents of the United States and Europe after visits to Australia and the Pacific Islands, indicating a role for air transport in the spread of this virus.

Ross River also has been shown to cross the placenta in mice[4] and humans.[7] In mice, this may result in extensive postpartum mortality,[4] but in humans there is no evidence of morbidity or mortality in children infected in utero.

CLINICAL MANIFESTATIONS[10, 18, 20, 36, 45]

Epidemic polyarthritis occurs as a mild to severe illness characterized by joint pain, particularly in the knees and the small joints of the hands and feet. Joint pain often is accompanied by a maculopapular or vesicular rash on the trunk and limbs and sometimes by fever and/or chills. Sore throat, lymphadenopathy, paraesthesia and tenderness of palms and soles, exanthema, and, more rarely, petechiae have been observed. Most patients experience several weeks of painful arthritis, followed by a slow decrease in the severity of symptoms over the 30 to 40 weeks required by most for recovery.[3] Infrequently, symptoms may persist for a year or more,[26] and some patients may experience episodes of severe arthritis during convalescence. A small proportion of patients (<0.1 per cent) may develop clinical disease without arthritis.[19] There also are rare reports of glomerulonephritis,[31] hematuria,[11] and central nervous system symptoms[1, 49] accompanying Ross River virus infection in humans.

PATHOLOGY

The only synovial biopsy to date to yield pathologic tissue showed a marked mononuclear leucocyte infiltrate with small amounts of fibrin deposition and synovial-cell hyperplasia.[38] No virus or viral antigen could be detected. Fluid from affected joints consists almost entirely of mononuclear leukocytes at all stages of disease.[14, 27, 30] There is no evidence of immune complexes or complement activation in arthritic joints, and viral antigen can be detected (in macrophages) for only 5 to 7 days after onset of symptoms, despite the persistence of arthritis for 30 to 40 weeks.[29] No significant levels of anticollagen antibodies could be detected in serum from epidemic polyarthritis patients.[33] The primary, virus-specific, cell-mediated immune response to Ross River virus infection in mice is weak,[2] and it does not correlate with the presence or absence of arthritis in human infections.[5] In humans, a nonspecific (natural killer cell) immunologic response correlated well with the presence or absence of arthritic symptoms.[3, 5] Functional natural killer cells have been recovered from the knee of a patient with epidemic polyarthritis,[38] and natural killer cells have been found to kill autologous synovial tissue in vitro.[3]

Prolonged infection of human synovial cells, incubated in vitro at 32° C,[39] suggests that Ross River virus also may be able to persist in the synovium of peripheral joints, perhaps at levels below the sensitivity of the detection systems used to date.

Approximately 30 per cent of epidemic polyarthritis patients develop a rash.[45] The dermis underlying these lesions contains a perivascular infiltrate of suppressor-cytotoxic T cells and some monocytes and macrophages.[32] No immunoglobulin or complement deposition has been observed in these lesions, although Ross River virus antigen was detected in the basal epidermal and eccrine duct epithelial cells.

DIAGNOSIS

Most epidemic polyarthritis patients are diagnosed using an indirect enzyme-linked immunosorbent assay (ELISA)[48] to detect Ross River virus–specific IgM antibodies in serum collected 7 to 10 days after the onset of symptoms. The IgM can be detected for approximately 3 months after the onset of disease.[8]

In rare cases, IgM production may persist for years. It has been suggested that assays for serum anti–Ross River virus IgA might be an alternative to IgM assays.[12] More recently, indirect ELISA assays that measure the avidity of anti–Ross River virus antibody have been shown to be able to discriminate between recent and old infections with this virus.

Although virus sometimes can be isolated from seronegative, acute-phase sera,[6, 9, 50, 53] this is not a procedure performed in most routine diagnostic laboratories.

Because epidemic polyarthritis is an arthritic disease, care must be taken to avoid false-positive results in indirect ELISA because of the presence of rheumatoid factor either by absorbing out any rheumatoid factor before testing sera or by performing latex agglutination or Rose-Waaler tests in parallel with the ELISA.

Other sources of false-positive diagnoses include the following:

1. Production of anti–Ross River virus IgM due to polyclonal B-cell activation after infection with Epstein-Barr virus, cytomegalovirus, or *Coxiella burnetti.*
2. Detection of IgM produced during a subclinical Ross River virus infection.

Other viral infections to be considered when a patient presents with suspected epidemic polyarthritis include those with Barmah Forest, Sindbis, Kunjin, or rubella viruses.

TREATMENT AND PROGNOSIS

No specific antiviral therapy is available, although there is experimental evidence that interferon-α may ameliorate acute disease.[51] Patients with more severe or more prolonged symptoms have been given either steroids or nonsteroidal anti-inflammatory medication, but the value of this treatment is not clear. Rest, while maintaining mobility and muscle tone, appears to provide greatest relief.

Epidemic polyarthritis has not been shown to progress to chronic joint disease.

PREVENTION

A killed vaccine is under development.[54] In urban areas, public health mosquito control programs reduce mosquito numbers, but it is impossible to eliminate mosquito exposure for those with outdoor occupations and pastimes. Personal protection (insect screening of houses, wearing protective clothing, and using of insect repellents) is the only reliable way to avoid infection.

References

1. Aaskov, J. G.: Ross River virus disease. *In* St. George, T. D., and French, E. L. (eds.): Arbovirus Research in Australia. Proceedings, Second Symposium, July 17–19, 1979. Commonwealth Scientific and Industrial Organisation and Queensland Institute of Medical Research, p. 166.
2. Aaskov, J. G., Dalglish, D. A., Davies, C. E. A., et al.: Cell-mediated immune response to Ross River virus in mice: Evidence for a defective effector-cell response. Aust. J. Exp. Biol. Med. Sci. *61*:529–540, 1983.
3. Aaskov, J. G., Dalglish, D. A., Harper, J. J., et al.: Natural killer (NK) cells in viral arthritis. Clin. Exp. Immunol. *68*:23–32, 1987.
4. Aaskov, J. G., Davies, C. E. A., Tucker, M., et al.: Effect on mice of infection during pregnancy with three Australian arboviruses. Am. J. Trop. Med. Hyg. *30*:198–203, 1981.
5. Aaskov, J. G., Fraser, J. R. E., and Dalglish, D. A.: Specific and non-specific immunological changes in epidemic polyarthritis in patients. Aust. J. Exp. Biol. Med. Sci. *55*:599–608, 1981.
6. Aaskov, J. G., Mataika, J. U., Lawrence, G. W., et al: An epidemic of Ross River virus infection in Fiji, 1979. Am. J. Trop. Med. Hyg. *30*:1053–1059, 1981.
7. Aaskov, J. G., Nair, K., Lawrence, G. W., et al.: Evidence for transplacental transmission of Ross River virus in humans. Med. J. Aust. *2*:20–21, 1981.
8. Aaskov, J. G., Ross, P., Davies, C. E. A., et al.: Epidemic polyarthritis in northeastern Australia, 1978–1979. Med. J. Aust. *2*:17–19, 1981.
9. Aaskov, J. G., Ross, P. V., Harper, J. J., et al: Isolation of Ross River virus from epidemic polyarthritis patients in Australia. Aust. J. Exp. Biol. Med. Sci. *63*:587–597, 1985.
10. Anderson, S. G., and French, E. L.: An epidemic exanthem associated with polyarthritis in the Murray Valley, 1956. Med. J. Aust. *2*:113–117, 1957.
11. Anstey, N., Currie, B., and Tai, K. S.: Ross River virus disease presenting with hematuria. Southeast Asian J. Trop. Med. Public Health *22*:281–283, 1991.
12. Carter, I. W. J., Fraser, J. R. E., and Cloonan, M. J.: Specific IgA antibody response in Ross River virus infection. Immunol. Cell. Biol. *65*:511–513, 1987.
13. Cheng, R. H., Kuhn, R. J., Olson, N. H., et al.: Nucleocapsid and glycoprotein organisation in an enveloped virus. Cell *80*:621–630. 1995.
14. Clarris, B. J., Doherty, R. L., Fraser, J. R. E., et al.: Epidemic polyarthritis: A cytological, virological and immunochemical study. Aust. N. Z. J. Med. *5*:450–457, 1975.
15. Doherty, R. L.: Arboviruses of Australia. Aust. Vet. J. *48*:172–180, 1972.
16. Doherty, R. L.: Surveys of haemagglutination-inhibiting antibody to arboviruses in Aborigines and other population groups in northern Australia. Trans. R. Soc. Trop. Med. Hyg. *67*:197–205, 1973.
17. Doherty, R. L.: Ross River virus. *In* Karabatsos, N. (ed.): International Catalogue of Arboviruses Including Certain Other Viruses of Vertebrates. 3rd ed. San Antonio, American Society for Tropical Medicine and Hygiene, 1985.
18. Doherty, R. L., Barrett, E. J., Gorman, B. M., et al.: Epidemic polyarthritis in eastern Australia 1959–1970. Med. J. Aust. *1*:5–8, 1971.
19. Doherty, R. L., Carley, J. G., and Best, J. C.: Isolation of Ross River virus from man. Med. J. Aust. *1*:1083–1084, 1972.
20. Doherty, R. L., Gorman, B. M., Whitehead, R. H., et al.: Studies of epidemic polyarthritis: The significance of three group A arboviruses isolated from mosquitoes in Queensland. Australasian. Ann. Med. *13*:322–327, 1964.
21. Doherty, R. L., Gorman, B. M., Whitehead, R. H., et al.: Studies of arthropod-borne virus infections in Queensland. V. Survey of the antibodies to group A arboviruses in man and animals. Aust. J. Exp. Biol. Med. Sci. *44*:365–377, 1966.
22. Doherty, R. L., Standfast, H. A., Domrow, R., et al.: Studies of the epidemiology of arthropod-borne virus infections at Mitchell River Mission, Cape York Peninsula, north Queensland. IV. Arbovirus infections of mosquitoes and mammals, 1967-1969. Trans. R. Soc. Trop. Med. Hyg. *65*:504–513, 1971.
23. Doherty, R. L., Whitehead, R. H., Gorman, B. M., et al.: The isolation of a third group A arbovirus in Australia, with preliminary observations on its relationship to epidemic polyarthritis. Aust. J. Sci. *26*:183–184, 1963.
24. Farragher, S. G., Meek, A. D. J., Rice, C. M., et al.: Genome sequence of a mouse avirulent and a mouse virulent strain of Ross River virus. Virology *163*:509–526, 1988.
25. Fauran, P., Donaldson, M., Harper, J., et al.: Characterisation of Ross River viruses isolated from patients with polyarthritis in New Caledonia and Wallis and Futuna islands. Am. J. Trop. Med. Hyg. *33*:1228–1231, 1984.
26. Fraser, J. R. E: Epidemic polyarthritis and Ross River virus disease. Clin. Rheum. Dis. 12:369–388, 1986.
27. Fraser, J. R. E., and Becker, G. J.: Mononuclear cell types in chronic synovial effusions of Ross River virus disease. Aust. N. Z. J. Med. *14*:505, 1984.
28. Fraser, J. R. E., and Cunningham, A. L.: Incubation time of epidemic polyarthritis. Med. J. Aust. *1*:550–551, 1980.
29. Fraser, J. R. E., Cunningham, A. L., Mathews, J. D., et al.: Immune complexes and Ross River virus disease (epidemic polyarthritis). Rheumatol. Int. *8*:113–117, 1988.
30. Fraser, J. R. E., Cunningham, A. L., Clarris, B. J., et al.: Cytology of synovial effusions in epidemic polyarthritis. Aust. N. Z. J. Med. *11*:168–173, 1981.
31. Fraser, J. R. E., Cunningham, A. L., Muller, H. K., et al.: Glomerulonephritis in the acute phase of Ross River virus disease (epidemic polyarthritis). Clin. Nephrol. *29*:149–152, 1988.
32. Fraser, J. R. E., Ratnamohan, A. M., Dowling, J. P. G., et al.: The exanthem of Ross River virus infection: Histology, location of virus antigen and the nature of inflammatory infiltrate. J. Clin. Pathol. *36*:1256–1263, 1983.
33. Fraser, J. R. E., Rowley, M. J., and Tait, B.: Collagen antibodies in Ross River virus disease (epidemic polyarthritis). Rheumatol. Int. *7*:267–269, 1987.
34. Fraser, J. R. E., Tait, T., Aaskov, J. G., et al.: Possible genetic determinants in epidemic polyarthritis caused by Ross River virus infection. Aust. N. Z. J. Med. *10*:597–603, 1980.
35. Gard, G., Marshall, I. D., and Woodroofe, G. M.: Annually recurrent epidemic polyarthritis and Ross River virus activity in a coastal area of New South Wales. II. Mosquitoes, viruses and wildlife. Am. J. Trop. Med. Hyg. *22*:551–560, 1973.

36. Halliday, J. H., and Horan, J. P.: An epidemic of polyarthritis in the Northern Territory. Med. J. Aust. 2:293–295, 1943.
37. Hawkes, R. A., Boughton, C. R., Naim, H. M., et al.: A major outbreak of epidemic polyarthritis in New South Wales during the summer of 1983–1984. Med. J. Aust. *143*:330–333, 1985.
38. Hazelton, R. A., Hughes, C., and Aaskov, J. G: The inflammatory response in the synovium of a patient with Ross River arbovirus infection. Aust. N. Z. J. Med. *15*:336–339, 1985.
39. Journeaux, S. F., Brown, W. B., and Aaskov, J. G.: Prolonged infection of human synovial cells with Ross River virus. J. Gen. Virol. *68*:3165–3169, 1987.
40. Kay, B. H.: Three modes of transmission of Ross River virus by *Aedes vigilax* (Skuse). Aust. J. Exp. Biol. Med. Sci. *60*:339–344, 1982.
41. Kay, B. H.: Assignment Report, WHO Regional Office for the South Pacific, 1983.
42. Lindsay, M. D. A., Broom, A. K., Wright, A. E., et al.: Ross River virus isolations from mosquitoes in arid regions of Western Australia: Implication of vertical transmission as a means of persistence of the virus. Am. J. Trop. Med. Hyg. *49*:686–696, 1993.
43. Lindsay, M. D., Coelen, R. J., and Mackenzie, J. S.: Genetic heterogeneity among isolates of Ross River virus from different geographical regions. J. Virol. *67*:3576–3585, 1995.
44. Mims, C. A., Murphy, F. A., Taylor, W. P., et al.: Pathogenesis of Ross River virus infection in mice. I. Ependymal infection, cortical thinning, and hydrocephalus. J. Infect. Dis. *127*:121–128, 1973.
45. Mudge, P. R., and Aaskov, J. G.: Epidemic polyarthritis in Australia, 1980–1981. Med. J. Aust. 2:269–273, 1983.
46. Murphy, F. A., Taylor, W. P., Mims, C. A., et al.: Pathogenesis of Ross River virus infection in mice. II. Muscle, heart and brown fat lesions. J. Infect. Dis. *127*:129–138, 1973.
47. Nimmo, J. R.: An unusual epidemic. Med. J. Aust. *1*:549–550, 1928.
48. Oseni, R. A., Donaldson, M. D., Dalglish, D. A., et al.: Detection by ELISA of IgM antibodies to Ross River virus in serum from patients with suspected epidemic polyarthritis. Bull. W. H. O. *61*:703–708, 1983.
49. Penna, J. E., and Irving, L. G.: Evidence for meningitis in Ross River virus infection. Med. J. Aust. *159*:492–493, 1993.
50. Rosen, L., Gubler, D. J., and Bennett, P. H.: Epidemic polyarthritis (Ross River) virus infection in the Cook Islands. Am. J. Trop. Med. Hyg. *30*:1294–1302, 1981.
51. Seay, A. R., Kern, E. R., and Murray, R. S.: Interferon treatment of experimental Ross River virus polymyositis. Neurology *37*:1189–1193, 1987.
52. Shope, R. E., and Anderson, S. G.: The virus aetiology of epidemic exanthem and polyarthritis. Med. J. Aust. *1*:156–158, 1960.
53. Tesh, R. B., McLean, R. G., Shrover, D. A., et al.: Ross River virus (Togaviridae: *Alphavirus*) infection (epidemic polyarthritis) in American Samoa. Trans. R. Soc. Trop. Med. Hyg. *75*:426–431, 1981.
54. Yu, S., and Aaskov, J. G.: Development of a candidate vaccine against Ross River virus infection. Vaccine *12*:1118–1124, 1994.

❑ ❑ ❑

CHAPTER 178 (F)

Other Alphaviral Infections

Theodore F. Tsai

O'NYONG NYONG

The virus name derives from the Acholi term meaning "very painful and weak," which describes the acute constitutional symptoms and polyarthritis associated with the disease of the same name.[12] The virus is unique in several respects: it is related closely to chikungunya virus but unlike most alphaviruses does not kill suckling mice inoculated intracerebrally. On initial passages, infected mice develop alopecia and runting, and fatal infections occur only after adaptation. The virus is transmitted by anopheline mosquitoes (unusual for any arbovirus) in an interhuman cycle, analogous to that of malaria in rural Africa. Apart from the human-to-human epidemic cycle, the natural transmission cycle and involvement of other vertebrate hosts are unknown. The disease first came to attention in, arguably, the largest arboviral epidemic ever recorded. After emerging in Uganda in 1959, the epidemic spread to South and West Africa, producing an estimated 2 million cases before the outbreak died out spontaneously 3 years later. The disease apparently had disappeared from East Africa, although sporadic viral isolations have been made from mosquitoes until 1996, when only the second outbreak appeared in Uganda. Factors underlying the virus' emergence, its natural reservoir, and the reasons for its disappearance only can be surmised. The exhaustion of susceptible human hosts may explain the disappearance of the initial epidemic. Clinically, the disease is similar to chikungunya, although lymphadenopathy is more pronounced. In some cases, the enlargement of cervical lymph nodes mimicked the lymphadenopathy of sleeping sickness. Virus can be isolated from acute-phase blood samples, or the diagnosis can be confirmed serologically by detecting specific IgM. Personal protective measures against malaria (e.g., using bednets) should be effective against acquiring infection.

IGBO-ORA FEVER

Igbo-Ora virus is related closely to chikungunya and o'nyong nyong viruses and, like the latter, is transmitted by anopheline mosquitoes and (without adaptation) is nonpathogenic for suckling mice.[16] The viral transmission cycle has not been defined. Sporadic cases and small outbreaks have been reported from Igbo-Ora and Ibadan, Nigeria, Ivory Coast, and Central African Republic. Based on a single case description, the illness consists of fever, polyarthritis, and pharyngitis.

BARMAH FOREST FEVER

Barmah Forest fever occurs only in Australia, where it has been a sporadic and occasionally hyperendemic infection in the southeastern, eastern, and northern parts.[2, 10] Evidently, the virus was introduced recently to western Australia, where hyperendemic transmission has followed. The viral transmission cycle seems to share features with that of Ross River virus; however, independent outbreaks have occurred in locations where both viruses are enzootic, indicating differences in their transmission cycles or human susceptibility. Seroprevalence to Barmah Forest virus generally is lower. Clinically, the illnesses are indistinguishable. Serologic diagnosis is straightforward in most cases, with little cross-reaction between the viruses.

SINDBIS FEVER

Sindbis virus was named after a district north of Cairo, Egypt, where it first was isolated. It is the prototype of an antigenic complex that also includes western equine encephalitis virus. Several Sindbis viral subtypes have been described, including the Ockelbo and related strains isolated from Scandinavia and the Babanki strain from West Africa. Two genotypes have been defined, comprising South African/Scandinavian strains and Australian/Asian strains.[19] The close genetic relationship of South African and Scandinavian strains indicates a recent introduction to Europe, possibly by a migrating bird.

The virus is distributed widely over four continents, although only sporadic cases have been reported from Asia and Australia. Transmission is endemic and occasionally hyperendemic in Africa and Fennoscandinavia. The virus is transmitted to birds by various species of *Culex* mosquitoes. Humans are infected when virus transmission "spills out" of the enzootic cycle, e.g., with the intervention of bridging vectors that feed on viremic birds and later on humans.

Endemic infections occur with varying intensity in areas

of Africa.[9, 14] Seroprevalence rates range from a few per cent to 20 per cent in some areas. Outbreaks producing hundreds to thousands of cases have been described. Concurrent transmission with West Nile virus, transmitted in the same avian cycle, is common. In South Africa, transmission occurs during the austral summer from December to April.

An endemic focus in Scandinavia (between 60° and 63° latitude in Sweden) was recognized after a series of outbreaks in 1981 led to several hundred cases in Sweden, Norway, Finland, and adjacent areas of western Russia.[4, 11] Seroprevalence is low, circa 5 per cent. Estimating from seroprevalence rates, 600 to 1200 clinical cases may occur annually in Sweden alone. Most cases occur in the summer (July to September) among middle-aged adults exposed to forested areas while picking berries or mushrooms or during other recreational activities.

Acute arthralgias and rash are the principal features of the illness. They may be preceded by mild fever, headache, and myalgias, but patients may present with arthralgias alone. The joints are involved symmetrically, especially the ankles, wrists, knees, fingers, and toes and less often the hips, shoulders, elbows, neck, and back. The joints appear swollen, and movement is limited. Achilles and wrist tendons may be inflamed as well, sometimes causing nerve entrapment and paresthesias. Some patients are confined to bed and unable to walk, but, typically, joint pain and stiffness lead to a lesser degree of discomfort and compromised function. A fine papular rash appears on the trunk and extremities (including the palms and soles), usually sparing the face and head, and after a few days develops a stained appearance and disappears. Lesions on the hands and feet may vesiculate. Joint symptoms resolve within 3 to 4 months in about 60 per cent of cases; however, in one-third of patients, symptoms may persist for 3 to 4 years. Serologic evidence of infection has been reported in patients with central nervous system infections in China.[5]

The illness is not differentiated easily from West Nile fever, which is transmitted in similar epidemiologic circumstances. Other infections presenting with acute arthralgias were mentioned earlier. The diagnosis is confirmed serologically by detecting specific IgM in acute-phase serum samples. IgM is detectable for months in some patients.[15] The virus can be isolated, but not reliably, from acute-phase capillary blood and from skin lesions. Viral genomic products can be detected in skin biopsy samples.[7]

Treatment is symptomatic. Persons who choose to enter sylvatic transmission foci in the summer should apply mosquito repellents and dress appropriately.

MAYARO FEVER

Infections are highly prevalent in forested areas of South and Central America, where Mayaro virus is transmitted among *Hemagogus* mosquitoes, marsupials, and small mammals, somewhat analogous to the jungle cycle of yellow fever. Seroprevalence rates increase with age to higher than 50 per cent in native peoples in some locations. The virus was isolated from sporadic fever cases on Trinidad and named after the island's Mayaro district.[1] Outbreaks have occurred in Bolivia, Pará (a state in Brazil), and Surinam, principally among men exposed occupationally to forested sites and among residents of adjoining villages.[3, 8, 17, 18] The virus is placed in the Semliki Forest antigenic complex; its Una subtype causes arthritis in horses.

The illness consists of acute polyarthritis and rash. Joint swelling, pain, and stiffness involve principally the hands, wrists, ankles, toes, elbows, and knees. The hands may be so swollen that they cannot be closed and joints of the lower extremities so painful that patients limp or are unable to walk. Milder cases may occur. The morbilliform rash is difficult to distinguish from rubella; individual or coalescent papular lesions occur on the trunk and extremities, usually sparing the face. Rash occurs more often in children than in adults. Mild fever, pharyngitis, conjunctivitis, headache, and lymphadenitis occur in some patients. Constitutional symptoms resolve rapidly, but joint symptoms may wax and wane over several weeks or months. Pneumonitis and renal dysfunction have been described in some cases, but they may have been caused by concurrent infections. Transient leukopenia is usual; some patients have had mild elevations of liver enzymes and bilirubin. A fatal case of yellow fever was reported in a patient recovering from Mayaro fever.

The illness is differentiated from other tropical febrile illnesses with rash and musculoskeletal pains by the specific involvement of the joints and the sylvatic setting of exposure. The illness closely resembles rubella. Virus can be isolated from acute-phase blood specimens, but laboratory confirmation by IgM serology is sensitive, specific, and more practical. Symptoms are treated with nonsteroidal anti-inflammatory drugs and rest. Repellents should be used when sylvatic-enzootic foci cannot be avoided.

SEMLIKI FOREST VIRAL INFECTION

Febrile illnesses with severe persistent headache have been reported from Central and West Africa, where Semliki Forest virus is transmitted principally by forest *Aedes* mosquitoes.[13] The virus appears to be a common cause of infection among horses as well. The MeTri subtype has been implicated serologically in encephalitis cases in Vietnam; its transmission cycle has not been described. A fatal case of encephalitis was reported in a laboratory worker.[6]

References

1. Anderson, C. R., Downs, W. G., Wattley, G. H., et al.: Mayaro virus: A new human disease agent. II. Isolation from blood of patients in Trinidad, B. W. I. Am. J. Trop. Med. Hyg. *6*:1012, 1957.
2. Anonymous: Barmah Forest virus. Lancet *337*:948, 1991.
3. Causey, O. R., and Maroja, O. M.: Mayaro virus: A new human disease agent. III. Investigation of an epidemic of acute febrile illness on the River Guama in Para, Brazil, and isloation of Mayaro virus as causative agent. Am. J. Trop. Med. Hyg. *6*:1017, 1957.
4. Espmark, A., and Niklasson, B.: Ockelbo disease in Sweden: Epidemiological, clinical and virological data from the 1982 outbreak. Am. J. Trop. Med. Hyg. *33*:1203, 1984.
5. Gu, H. X., Artsob, H., Lin, Y. Z., et al.: Arboviruses as aetiological agents of encephalitis in the People's Republic of China. Trans. R. Soc. Trop. Med. Hyg. *86*:198, 1992.
6. Ha, D. Q., Calisher, C. H., Tien, P. H., et al.: Isolation of a newly recognized alphavirus from mosquitoes in Vietnam and evidence for human infection and disease. Am. J. Trop. Med. Hyg. *53*:100, 1995.
7. Horling, J., Vene, S., Franzen, C., et al.: Detection of Ockelbo virus RNA in skin biopsies by polymerase chain reaction. J. Clin. Microbiol. *31*:2004, 1993.
8. Jonkers, A. H., Spence, L., and Karbaat, J.: Arbovirus infections in Dutch military personnel stationed in Surinam: Further studies. Trop. Geogr. Med. *20*:251, 1968.
9. Jupp, P. G., Blackburn, N. K., Thompson, D. L., et al.: Sindbis and West Nile virus infection in the Witwatersrand-Pretoria region. S. Afr. Med. J. *70*:218, 1986.
10. Lindsay, M. D. A., Johansen, C. A., Smith, D. W., et al.: An outbreak of Barmah Forest virus disease in the south-west of Western Australia. Med. J. Aust. *162*:291, 1995.
11. Lundstrom, J. O., Vene, S., Espmark, A. et al.: Geographical and temporal distribution of Ockelbo disease in Sweden. Epidemiol. Infect. *106*:567, 1991.
12. Mangi, R. J.: Viral arthritis: The great masquerader. Bull. Rheum. Dis. *43*:5, 1994.

13. Mathiot, C. C., Grimaud, G., Bouquety, G. P., et al.: An outbreak of human Semliki Forest virus infections in Central African Republic. Am. J. Trop. Med. Hyg. *42*:386, 1990.
14. McIntosh, B. M., McGuilivray, G. M., and Dickinson, D. B.: Illness caused by Sindbis and West Nile viruses in South Africa. S. Afr. Med. J. *38*:219, 1964.
15. Niklasson, B., Espmark, A., and Lundstrom, J.: Occurrence of arthralgia and specific IgM antibodies three to four years after Ockelbo disease. J. Infect. Dis. *157*:832, 1988.
16. Olaleye, O. D., Omilabu, S. A., and Fagbami, A. H.: Igbo-Ora virus (an alphavirus isolated in Nigeria): A serological survey for haemagglutination inhibiting antibody in humans and domestic animals. Trans. R. Soc. Trop. Med. Hyg. *82*:905, 1988.
17. Pinheiro, F. P., Freitas, R. B., Travassos da Rosa, J. F. S., et al.: An outbreak of Mayaro virus disease in Belterra, Brazil. I. Clinical and virological findings. Am. J. Trop. Med. Hyg. *30*:674, 1981.
18. Schaeffer, M., Gajdusek, D. C., Lema, A. B., et al.: Epidemic jungle fevers among Okinawan colonists in Bolivian rain forest. I. Epidemiology. Am. J. Trop. Med. Hyg. *8*:372, 1959.
19. Yukio, S., Niklasson, B., Dalrymple, J. M., et al.: Structure of the Ockelbo virus genome and its relationship to other Sindbis viruses. Virology *182*:753, 1991.

❑ ❑ ❑

SUBSECTION FIVE

FLAVIVIRIDAE

179

FLAVIVIRUSES

❑ ❑ ❑

CHAPTER 179 (A)

St. Louis Encephalitis

Theodore F. Tsai

St. Louis encephalitis (SLE) is the most important arboviral infection in the United States because of its potential to occur in massive epidemics. Encephalitis is the principal clinical manifestation, although milder central nervous system syndromes occur, especially in children. The virus is transmitted between birds and *Culex* mosquitoes; humans are incidental hosts.

ETIOLOGIC AGENT

The SLE virus is a member of the family *Flaviviridae* (group B arboviruses).[15, 36] Characteristics of the virus and its replicative strategy are described in the yellow fever subchapter. SLE virus is placed in an antigenic complex with Japanese encephalitis, Murray Valley encephalitis, and West Nile viruses.

Analyses of the E glycoprotein sequences of strains from the United States and Central and South America have designated three genotypes corresponding to origins in the eastern and western United States and South America. Strains from a more than 60-year interval diverge by less than 10 per cent in the total *E* gene nucleotide sequence, indicating a highly constrained viral adaptation to vector and vertebrate hosts. Strains from the three genotypes differ in biologic characteristics, such as capacity to produce significant viremia in sparrows and virulence in 3-week-old mice.[37, 59] Epidemic-associated strains from the Ohio and Mississippi river basins and Florida are more virulent for mice and produce higher viremias in sparrows, a principal amplifying host, than do strains from the western United States associated with an endemic pattern of transmission.

ECOLOGY

SLE virus is transmitted in an enzootic cycle among birds and *Culex* mosquitoes. Three distinct enzootic cycles exist in the United States in association with the four principal vector species: *C. tarsalis* in the western and central United States, *C. pipiens* and *C. quinquefasciatus* in the east-central and Atlantic states, and *C. nigripalpus* in Florida. *C. salinarius* and *C. restuans* may have accessory roles in viral amplification and transmission (Fig. 179–1).[32, 35, 60, 64]

In the western United States, *C. tarsalis,* which also is the vector of western equine encephalitis (WEE), serves as both an enzootic and epizootic vector. This species feeds chiefly on birds early in the summer and switches to mammalian hosts, including humans, in midsummer. Although SLE and WEE viruses coexist in endemic areas of the West, the peak of SLE virus activity appears about 2 months after the peak period of WEE virus activity. The relative delay in SLE virus transmission may be related to higher temperatures required for the virus' extrinsic incubation in vector mosquitoes. Sparrows, finches, and other small birds, and especially their nestlings, are the principal amplifying hosts.[33] Human infections result from encounters with the vector near collections of water along natural and artificial waterways, irrigated farmland, and other breeding sites found chiefly in rural agricultural areas (see the yellow fever subchapter).

In the Ohio and Mississippi valleys and on the Gulf Coast, *C. pipiens* and *C. quinquefasciatus* are, respectively, the enzootic vectors in northern and southern states, overlapping around the latitude of Memphis. *C. pipiens* does not bite humans readily, and other species, such as *C. restuans* and *C. salinarius,* may be important bridging vectors, infecting humans from viremic birds.[64] *C. pipiens* complex mosquitoes breed preferentially in polluted water rich in organic material, commonly found in sewage ditches and peridomestic collections of water. Viral amplification occurs in passerine (perching) or columbiforme (pigeon-like) birds (e.g., sparrows, blue jays, doves, other species prolific in residential areas), so both vectors and amplifying hosts are found in close proximity to human dwellings and other sites of human activity.[33] *C. restuans,* which is most active in cool weather, plays a role in viral amplification in early spring and after cool spells in the summer. The mechanism by which the virus overwinters is not known; however, several observations suggest that the virus persists locally in winter and is not reintroduced annually. Persistent infection in a resident vertebrate host (e.g., birds, bats) is a possibility. Virus has

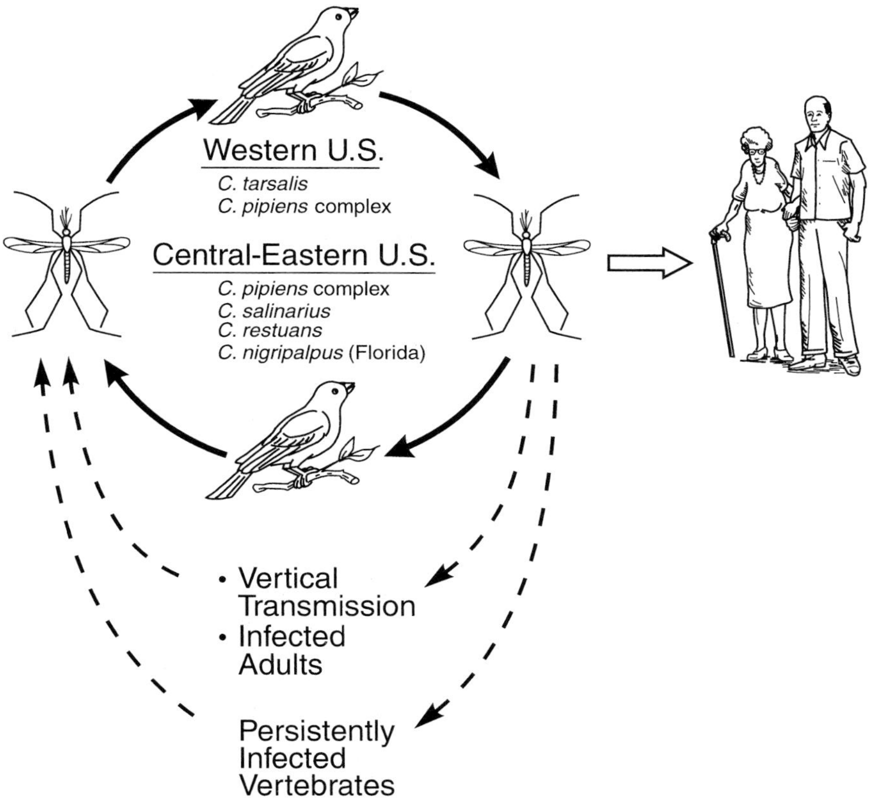

FIGURE 179–1. *Transmission cycles of St. Louis encephalitis virus in North America.* Culex *mosquito vectors differ geographically:* C. tarsalis *in the West;* C. pipiens *and* C. quinquefasciatus *in the Ohio and Mississippi valleys;* C. nigripalpus *in Florida. Epidemics occur when intense viral transmission in the enzootic cycle "spills over," resulting in human infections. The viral overwintering mechanism, possibly in mosquitoes or persistently infected vertebrates, has not been proved (broken lines).*

been recovered from hibernating bats through the winter, with recrudescent viremia after awakening.[2] Other data suggest that the virus could overwinter by transovarial (vertical) transmission in *C. pipiens* complex mosquitoes or in overwintering adult mosquitoes.[5, 40]

C. nigripalpus is both an enzootic and an epizootic vector in Florida.[18, 19, 47] It breeds in a variety of water sources, including ditches, grassy swales, and other temporary collections from April to December. In the summer, adult mosquitoes are active after sunset and rest during the day in humid vegetated locations. Viral amplification occurs in birds, but the mosquito feeds on dogs, cattle, and other mammalian hosts as well. SLE virus also has been isolated from *C. nigripalpus* in the Caribbean and South America.[57]

SLE virus has been recovered from various birds, mammals, and mosquitoes in widely scattered areas of Central and South America. In some areas, the virus is transmitted in a sylvan cycle involving aquatic birds.[1, 57]

Studies to elucidate the intermittent occurrence of urban SLE outbreaks have shown that climatic factors, such as antecedent mild winter, wet spring, and dry hot summer, have prevailed in epidemic years; however, the predictive value of this combination of conditions in foretelling outbreaks has not been evaluated.[35] In a model of global warming, SLE transmission is predicted to move to northern latitudes and, in existing endemic areas, to develop a spring-fall seasonality.[49, 50]

EPIDEMIOLOGY

Although cases of SLE occur sporadically in the United States each year and SLE has the potential to cause major epidemics leading to thousands of cases for many states, cumulative reported cases represent activity confined to a single series of epidemic years (Fig. 179–2).

The epidemiologic patterns of SLE virus transmission reflect human interactions with the virus' reservoirs and its principal mosquito vectors.[28, 32, 35, 60, 64] In western states, perennial WEE and SLE virus transmission leads to an endemic pattern of transmission; epidemics may occur, but their scale is limited by a high level of immunity in the population. Infections occur chiefly in rural areas in association with the habitat of the vector. Combined WEE-SLE outbreaks have occurred typically in rural agricultural areas and their small towns. Large recurrent outbreaks were reported from the

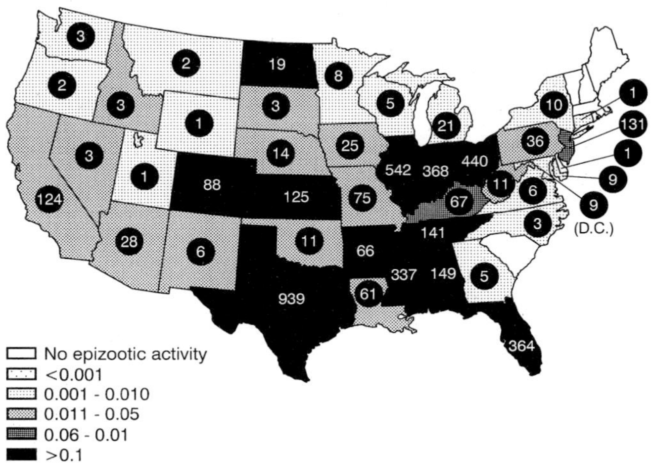

FIGURE 179–2. *St. Louis encephalitis. Reported cases and crude incidence/10,000 by state, 1964–1994.*

Yakima Valley from 1939 to 1942, the Central Valley of California from 1950 to 1959, and the Red River Valley in 1941 and 1975.[27, 35] In 1984, the first urban SLE outbreak in the West led to 27 cases from urban and suburban areas of Los Angeles and Orange counties; in successive years, sporadic human cases and viral transmission in birds and mosquitoes have recurred.[13, 51] Studies in Texas indicate that the urban and rural cycles can overlap. An urban outbreak in Dallas was attributed to introduction of virus to the urban *C. quinquefasciatus* cycle from rural *C. tarsalis*.[25, 28, 32]

In the east-central United States, discrete and occasionally widespread outbreaks occur intermittently, followed by variable, often lengthy periods with no evidence of viral transmission (Fig. 179–3). In some instances, a small premonitory outbreak has been followed by a larger outbreak the next year in the same location, viral amplification presumably beginning at a higher level in the second of the 2 years. Because virus activity occurs intermittently, the human population is immunologically susceptible, and when epidemics erupt, they may be explosive. The physical, ecologic, and epidemiologic conditions leading to the intermittent appearance of outbreaks are not understood.

Epidemics frequently have occurred in urban locations or their peripheries. In 1975, a nationwide epidemic led to outbreaks in Houston, Chicago, Memphis, and Detroit as well as smaller outbreaks in rural towns throughout the South and Midwest. Outbreaks in large urban centers generally have been associated with attack rates of less than 40 cases per 100,000 residents.

Epidemic cases often have clustered in delimited areas where environmental factors are associated with increased mosquito breeding or exposure to mosquitoes. Often, these are low socioeconomic status areas, where dwellings are built on open foundations or where open sewage ditches are present.[46] In recent urban outbreaks, homelessness and HIV infection have been the principal risk factors for acquiring SLE.[43] In the St. Louis outbreak in 1933, the highest attack rates were associated with wealthy areas of low housing density, where open sewers, streams, ponds, and weeds were prevalent. In other outbreaks, lush vegetation around houses, which provides shelter for *C. nigripalpus*, and closed sewer systems clogged with grass clippings were factors associated with high attack rates in upper socioeconomic areas.

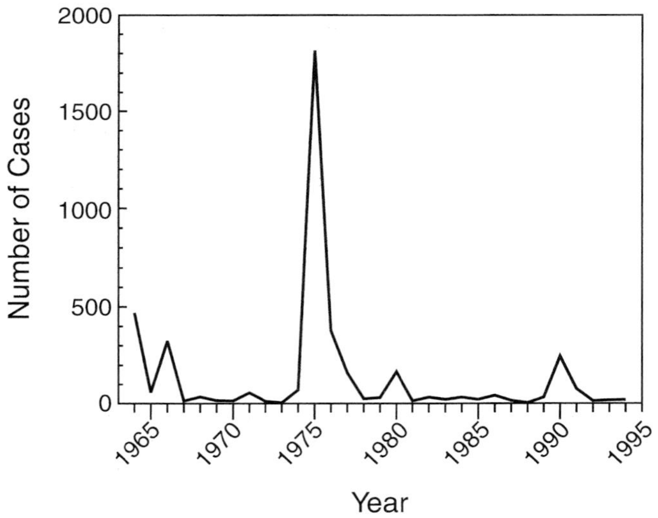

FIGURE 179–3. *Reported St. Louis encephalitis cases by year, United States, 1964–1994. A nationwide epidemic in 1975 produced more than 2000 cases.*

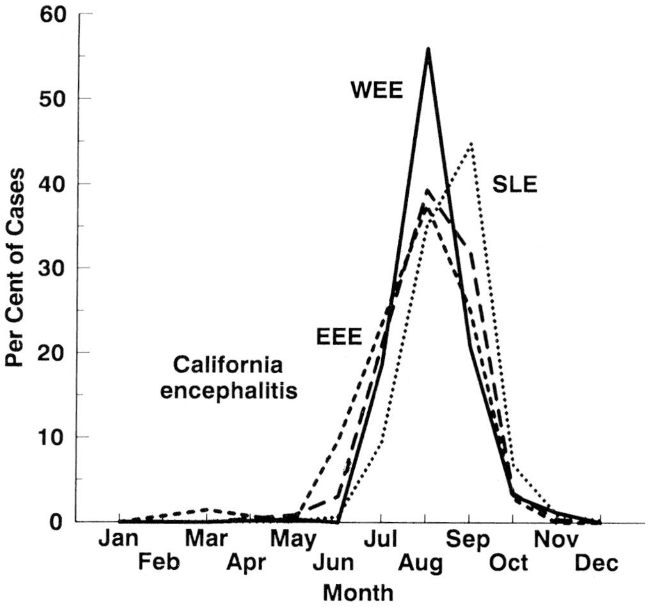

FIGURE 179–4. *Reported arboviral encephalitis by etiology and month of onset, United States, 1972–1989.*

C. pipiens and *C. quinquefasciatus* are highly domesticated species and bite inside and around houses. Risk factors associated with increased exposure to the vectors include the absence or disrepair of screens and the absence of air conditioning. Epidemic attack rates are 1.2 to 3 times higher in females than in males, possibly reflecting increased exposure of females to the peridomestic vector.

In the West, where *C. tarsalis* is the vector, risk is associated with rural outdoor exposure. Attack rates in males usually are higher than in females. A similar observation has been made in Florida, where SLE attack rates are highest in working-age males.[41] *C. quinquefasciatus, C. nigripalpus,* and *C. tarsalis* all are most active in twilight hours, and outdoor activity during these periods is associated with a greater risk for exposure.[14]

Most cases of SLE occur in late summer or early fall (Fig. 179–4). However, where *C. nigripalpus* is active until the beginning of winter, epidemics have continued through mid-December. In the 1975 nationwide epidemic, outbreaks appeared first in southeastern states in June, followed by the appearance of outbreaks in northern foci later in the summer and fall.[35, 64]

The most important risk factor for neuroinvasive SLE is advanced age.[29, 34] Age-specific attack rates are lowest in children and rise steadily in adulthood, with attack rates 5 to 40 times higher in persons older than 60 years of age than in those younger than 10 years of age. During outbreaks, infections occur uniformly in all age groups, with as many as 300 asymptomatic infections for each clinically apparent case. Therefore, higher clinical attack rates in the elderly are a function of susceptibility and not of exposure.[29, 34] The clinical expression of illness is more severe and the case-fatality rate also is highest in the elderly. The biologic basis for increased risk in the elderly has not been elucidated. Immunologic factors may play a role; however, hypertension and factors associated with cerebrovascular integrity also may be important.[11] A second peak of increased risk also is seen in infants.[62]

In the West, where SLE infections are endemic, an increasing level of immunity, associated with length of residence in these areas, leads to an adult population with low susceptibility.[35, 60] Consequently, cases often are seen in children and young adults. Immunity to other flaviviruses (mainly dengue) also was shown to protect against acquiring SLE in a Florida outbreak.[8]

SLE cases acquired in tropical America (Jamaica, Surinam, French Guiana, and northern Argentina) principally have resulted in mild febrile illnesses. A single encephalitis outbreak was reported from northern Mexico.[17, 57]

CLINICAL MANIFESTATIONS

Clinical manifestations range from a mild "flu-like" illness to fatal encephalitis.[9, 48, 66] An epidemiologic case definition that stratifies cases into clinical syndromes of encephalitis, aseptic meningitis, and febrile headache (Table 179–1)[9] has proved useful (Fig. 179–5). Although children as a group exhibit milder symptoms, more than half of confirmed and presumptive cases develop encephalitis, and 95 per cent have objective clinical signs of central nervous system infection.[66, 67]

SLE cannot be differentiated easily clinically from other viral central nervous system infections. Photophobia, headache, fever, nausea and vomiting, malaise, and neck stiffness are typical early symptoms. In about half of reported cases, there may be an abrupt onset of weakness, incoordination, disturbed sensorium, or other neurologic signs. Equally often, patients show nonspecific symptoms and subtle changes in coordination or mentation during a prodromal phase lasting several days to more than a week.

In addition to fever and signs of meningeal irritation, patients nearly uniformly exhibit alterations in state of consciousness, such as restlessness, confusion, lethargy, delirium, or coma. The neurologic examination usually reveals general weakness, hyperreflexia, and tremulousness, but focal weakness and other deficits are unusual. Cranial nerve palsies, especially of cranial nerves VII, IX, and X, occur in 10 to 25 per cent of cases.[9] Clinical signs of increased intracranial pressure have been reported in few patients. However, unusual localizing neurologic signs have been reported in patients with involvement of the midbrain, thalamus, or brain stem. In a 4-year-old girl, paralysis of upward gaze was associated with a brain stem infection.[26] Ataxia has been observed in one-fourth of the cases in children, and opsoclonus has been reported in several cases in young adults.[21, 22] Convulsions occur infrequently in adult patients; in children, however, seizures may be more common. In a series of 26 SLE cases in children, convulsions occurred in 8, 6 of whom had focal seizures. However, concurrent isolations of enteroviruses were made in 5 of the 8 patients.[6, 45] In most cases, fever defervesces 4 to 7 days after onset, and clinical improvement is evident early in the second week of illness.

The peripheral leukocyte count is elevated modestly, with a shift to the left in most patients. The cerebrospinal fluid cell count usually is less than 100 leukocytes/mm^3, with a median value between 100 and 200. However, in some cases, less than 10 cells and occasionally no cells are discovered in the cerebrospinal fluid. Varying ratios of polymorphonuclear and mononuclear cells are present, depending on the interval from the onset of illness. An increasing ratio of mononuclear to polymorphonuclear cells is observed on successive examinations. Cerebrospinal fluid protein rarely exceeds 200 mg/dL, and hypoglycorrhachia is unusual.[9]

In one series, elevated serum aldolase levels suggested a myopathic process, and muscle biopsies and electromyograms disclosed lower motor neuron dysfunction, possibly from spinal root involvement. Moderate elevations of transaminase have been reported in 19 to 48 per cent of adult patients. Decreased serum osmolality attributed to inappropriate secretion of antidiuretic hormone was observed in one-fourth to one-third of cases in two series.[9, 10]

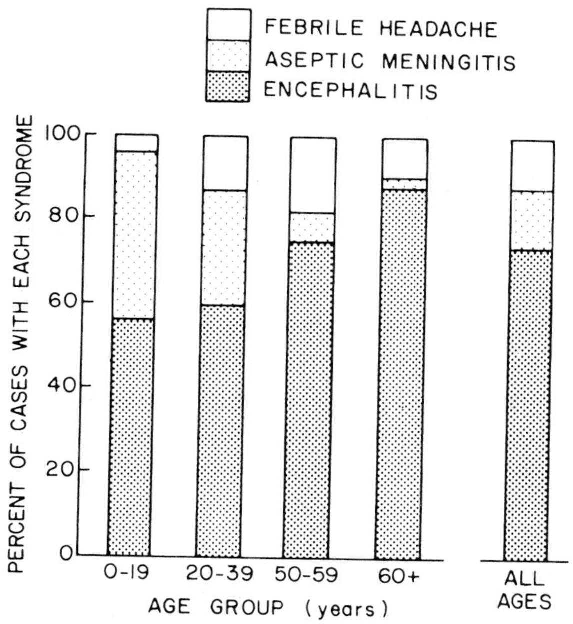

FIGURE 179–5. *Distribution of St. Louis encephalitis cases by clinical syndrome and age. Although mortality rates and disease severity increase with age, the majority of cases in children are clinical encephalitis. (Data from Zweighaft, R. M., et al.: St. Louis encephalitis: The Chicago experience. Am. J. Trop. Med. Hyg. 28:114–118, 1979.)*

TABLE 179–1. Definitions of Clinical Syndromes in St. Louis Encephalitis

I. Encephalitis* (including meningoencephalitis and encephalomyelitis)
   A. Acute febrile illness (oral temperature ≥37.8° C [≥100° F])
   B. One or more signs in either of the following categories:
      1. Altered level of consciousness (confusion, disorientation, delirium, lethargy, stupor, coma)
      2. Objective signs of neurologic dysfunction (convulsion, cranial nerve palsy, dysarthria, rigidity, paresis, paralysis, abnormal reflexes, tremor)

II. Aseptic meningitis*
   A. Acute febrile illness
   B. Sign(s) of meningeal irritation (stiff neck with or without positive Kernig or Brudzinski sign)
   C. No objective signs of neurologic dysfunction

III. Febrile headache*
   A. Acute febrile illness
   B. Headache (also may have other systemic symptoms, such as nausea or vomiting)
   C. No signs of meningeal irritation or neurologic dysfunction

*Cerebrospinal fluid pleocytosis is present in patients with encephalitis and aseptic meningitis; it also may be found in patients with the syndrome of febrile headache.

From Brinker, K. R., and Monath, T. P.: The acute disease. *In* Monath, T. P. (ed.): St. Louis Encephalitis. Washington, D.C., American Public Health Association, 1980, pp. 503–534.

Urinary incontinence, frequency, or retention and pyuria or proteinuria have been reported in some patients, and viral antigen was detected on cells in the urinary sediment by immunofluorescence in one report.[30] Lower motor neuron lesions may have been the mechanism for bladder symptoms in some patients.

Electroencephalographic tracings were abnormal in five of six children who were studied in the 1964 Houston outbreak. One patient had a focal abnormality in the temporal lobe. Five patients exhibited diffuse changes: two with associated focal discharges, and one with a spike abnormality.[6] Electroencephalograms in most adult patients show diffuse generalized slowing.[10] Computed tomographic and magnetic resonance imaging scans of a few patients found no abnormalities other than premorbid findings, in contrast to thalamic lesions typifying Japanese encephalitis.[24, 56] In related Japanese encephalitis cases, areas of low density and abnormal signal intensity are found most frequently in the thalamus and basal ganglia.

PATHOLOGY

Pathologic changes are found predominantly in the midbrain, thalamus, and brain stem but also in the cerebral cortex and cerebellum. Lesions are observed in the spinal cord in some cases.[52, 55, 58, 65] The leptomeninges are affected to a variable degree with edema, small hemorrhages, and round-cell infiltration.

Perivascular and parenchymal inflammation is prevalent in the brain nuclei but also is scattered in the white matter of the brain stem and spinal cord and subcortical and deep cerebral areas. Nodular collections of inflammatory cells composed of lymphocytes, microglial cells, and monocytes are found in proximity to or surrounding degenerating neurons. Eccentric nuclear displacement, nuclear pyknosis, and cellular contraction are evidence of neuronal loss. Vascular infiltrations and thrombosis have not been described, as they have in WEE and EEE. Focal demyelination, which is observed in WEE, is not characteristic of SLE.

Immunofluorescent examination of frozen sections of brain, obtained at autopsy, disclosed widely scattered infected cells in a few samples.[52] Antigen-positive sections corresponded to histopathologically involved areas from which virus was isolated successfully.

PATHOGENESIS

After infection, viral replication occurs locally and in regional lymph nodes. After this eclipse phase, blood-borne (viremic) dissemination occurs to secondary sites of replication in muscle, endocrine, lymphoreticular, and other tissues. Less than 1 per cent of infections lead to neuroinvasive disease. Vascular endothelial cells may have a role in actively transporting virus from the capillary lumen to the brain and in supporting secondary viral replication.[20] Conditions that compromise cerebrovascular integrity and disrupt the blood-brain barrier may predispose to neuroinvasion; for example, concurrent central nervous system cysticercosis may be a risk factor for Japanese encephalitis, a related flaviviral infection. Although some experimental studies suggest that central nervous system invasion occurs through the olfactory epithelium, pathologic studies of Japanese encephalitis cases indicate widespread involvement of the brain stem, deep nuclei, and cortex, most consistent with hematogenous infection.[38]

Recovery from flaviviral encephalitis depends on the early intrathecal synthesis of antibodies and viral clearance by macrophages. The inflammatory response in related central nervous system infections consists of helper-inducer T cells and, to a lesser degree, B lymphocytes, infiltrating the perivascular space and parenchyma from the blood. Macrophages and activated microglial cells in the perivascular space and parenchyma, respectively, are responsible for viral clearance. Outcome is determined by the comparative rates of viral spread and neuronal infection and the migration of inflammatory cells into the central nervous system. Presumably, outcome in SLE also is correlated with the dynamics of the antibody response. Production of interferon is elicited in the brain of human SLE patients, but its role in limiting the spread of virus in the central nervous system is unknown.[31] The clinical course of SLE in HIV-infected persons has not been significantly different from other cases; however, few patients have been studied.

Resistance and susceptibility to some flaviviral infections in mice have been linked to autosomal dominant genes associated with permissiveness to infection and immune response. Environmental factors that influence susceptibility to flaviviral infections in experimental models include stress from cold or isolation, reticuloendothelial cell blockade, and heavy metal intoxication.

DIAGNOSIS

The laboratory diagnosis of SLE usually is made serologically, although virus has been recovered from acute blood in six reported instances.[28] Virus should be sought from brain and other organs obtained by biopsy or at autopsy by inoculating Vero cell cultures and suckling mice intracerebrally.[12, 16] SLE viral antigen was detected in cells from urinary sediment in one report.[30] Viral antigen has been demonstrated in brain sections examined at autopsy by immunofluorescence.[52] Viral antigen can be detected directly by capture enzyme immunoassay in infected mosquitoes, but the technique has not been evaluated in clinical specimens.[61]

IgM-capture enzyme-linked immunosorbent assay (ELISA) is the preferred serologic procedure.[39] Intrathecal production of virus-specific IgM reflects recent infection, and a positive result confirms the diagnosis. Virus-specific IgM can be detected in acute serum or cerebrospinal fluid in 75 per cent or more of specimens obtained within 4 days of onset. In most patients, IgM levels decline in the convalescent sample and disappear about 4 months after onset, although IgM persisted at high titer in a few patients for 6 months.[63] In areas where SLE is endemic, virus-specific IgM carried over from the previous transmission season potentially could lead to an erroneous diagnosis. The indirect immunofluorescent antibody procedure offers a similar capacity for rapid diagnosis; however, it is less sensitive than is ELISA, and IgM rheumatoid factor can lead to a false-positive result.

Hemagglutination-inhibition and neutralizing antibodies rise rapidly after infection (often within 2 to 5 days after onset), reach a peak in the second week, and persist for years after recovery.[12] An elevated titer (≥80) is presumptive evidence of recent infection. Complement-fixation antibody may not appear until the second week after onset and rises more slowly and to lower levels. Complement-fixation antibody declines more rapidly (only one-half of patients followed 3 years after infection have measurable complement-fixation antibody) and is useful as a measure of recent infection.[10] However, no complement-fixation antibody was detected in 20 per cent of confirmed, principally elderly SLE patients from Memphis.[17] Although complement fixation has utility in the diagnosis of recent infection, the test is insensitive and is inadequate as the sole test for serologic diagnosis.

The serologic response in a primary flavivirus infection usually is type-specific; however, repeated infections lead to broad heterologous responses, which often are difficult to interpret. Fortunately, in the United States, human infections with indigenous flaviviruses (e.g., Rio Bravo, Powassan) other than SLE are rare. However, in patients with antecedent yellow fever immunization or infections with dengue virus acquired in areas of the United States where dengue previously was endemic (e.g., Texas, Florida) or acquired in travel or residence abroad, a broadly reactive flavivirus antibody response may appear. Incremental increases in specificity are associated with hemagglutination inhibition, complement fixation, and neutralization, but often a specific diagnosis may not be possible, even after the completion of cross-neutralization tests.

DIFFERENTIAL DIAGNOSIS

In an endemic setting, clinicians should consider SLE principally in the differential diagnosis of patients with aseptic meningitis or acute encephalitis. However, in the context of an outbreak, the diagnostic threshold should be lowered to include patients with less specific presentations, especially acute febrile illnesses with headache, and patients who exhibit confusion or are encephalopathic without fever. Increased suspicion of SLE in mildly ill patients should be directed particularly at children and young adults, in whom the infection often presents without meningoencephalitis.

The clinical presentation of SLE cannot be distinguished easily from other central nervous system infections. Fever, headache, and confusion are nonspecific signs of cerebral inflammation. However, focal neurologic deficits are not characteristic of SLE and should suggest other diagnoses. The combination of global confusion and tremulousness in SLE may suggest a metabolic encephalopathy; however, fever, meningismus, and cerebrospinal fluid pleocytosis should point to infection as an underlying process. In elderly patients, the initial presentation of SLE can overlap signs and symptoms of a cerebrovascular accident.

The progression of symptoms and localizing signs associated with herpes encephalitis contrasts sharply with the clinical presentation in SLE, in which localizing signs are rare. Enteroviral infections have an overlapping summer seasonality but often are associated with clustering of illness in families and other epidemiologic clues of person-to-person spread. Skin eruptions, respiratory symptoms, pericarditis, myocarditis, and conjunctivitis are helpful distinguishing characteristics. Concurrent enterovirus infection and SLE may be associated with an increased risk of convulsions during the acute phase of illness.[6, 45] Enteroviral infections can be confirmed by detecting viral genomic sequences in cerebrospinal fluid by polymerase chain reaction, by IgM-capture ELISA, or by recovering virus from stool or cerebrospinal fluid. Primary HIV, human herpesvirus 6, and mumps virus infections are other common infections that should be entertained in the differential diagnosis. One-third of patients with mumps encephalitis do not have associated parotid gland swelling.

Adenovirus encephalitis is a rare infection in children, more severe than is SLE, and associated sometimes with hepatic and other extraneural sites of infection. The presence of lymphoreticular involvement and typical hematologic features should suggest the clinical diagnosis of Epstein-Barr virus infection.

Partially treated bacterial meningitis and parameningeal pyogenic infections are the principal bacterial causes to exclude. Cat-scratch fever can present with fever and encephalopathy mimicking arboviral encephalitis.[42] Convulsions associated with *Shigella* enteritis and ataxia associated with typhoid fever potentially could be interpreted as a primary central nervous system infection. Tuberculous meningitis typically is a subacute illness; evidence of active extraneural sites of infection should be sought. A low cerebrospinal fluid glucose level is a clue to the diagnosis.

In urban areas, or where there may be parental occupational exposure, lead intoxication remains an important potential cause of encephalopathy in summer. Hyperthermia, associated with sustained exposure to elevated environmental temperature, may lead to encephalopathy with convulsions and signs of raised intracranial pressure. A history of hyperpyrexia and evidence of hepatic dysfunction are clues to the diagnosis. This constellation of symptoms also may suggest Reye syndrome. However, Reye syndrome typically occurs in winter and spring after a respiratory viral infection, and laboratory features such as hypoglycemia and elevated blood ammonia are characteristic. Patients with salicylism exhibit similar clinical findings. A history of salicylate ingestion, an elevated anion gap early in the course of illness, and an elevated blood salicylate level suggest the diagnosis.

TREATMENT

Supportive therapy, as outlined in the earlier sections, should be aimed at maintaining cardiorespiratory function and fluid and electrolyte balance, controlling convulsions, and monitoring and maintaining normal intracranial pressure. No specific antiviral therapy is available.

PROGNOSIS

The principal risk factor for a fatal outcome is advanced age (see Fig. 179–5).[28, 35, 63, 64] Among all cases reported to the Centers for Disease Control and Prevention from 1955 to 1971, 8 per cent died, but the age-specific mortality rate in persons 60 years of age or older was 19.5 per cent. Fatality rates as high as 38 to 80 per cent were recorded in the 1933 St. Louis outbreak in patients who were 60 to 89 years of age. Mortality in children has ranged from 2 to 5 per cent, with the highest risk in children younger than 5 years of age. The overall case-fatality rate in an outbreak in Hermosillo, Sonora (involving principally children), was 20 per cent.[17] The high fatality rate in this instance is anomalous because fatality rates usually are lower in *C. tarsalis*–borne SLE outbreaks in the West. The role of neurocysticercosis as a risk factor for SLE should be examined in view of its potential involvement as a risk factor in Japanese encephalitis (see Japanese encephalitis subchapter).

Among adults, presentation in coma, a low cerebrospinal fluid leukocyte count ($<$100 cells/mm^3), and underlying hypertensive vascular disease have been factors associated with a fatal outcome.[11] However, the factors that lead to higher mortality and more severe disease with age remain obscure. Risk factors for mortality in children have not been described.

Recovery from SLE usually is complete or associated with soft sequelae, such as emotional disturbances, dizziness, headache, memory impairment, and tremor.[4, 23] In one study[4, 23] of 193 cases, 25 per cent of children who were 1 to 4 years of age at the time of infection had serious neurologic sequelae, the highest rate of any age group.[44] The incidence of sequelae was 10 per cent in children from 5 to 9 years of age. Children who were younger than 1 year of age at the time of infection appeared to be spared of any serious sequelae. Deficits in motor and intellectual function were reported in some cases.

Convulsions were not a significant residual abnormality. However, the same cohort followed for intervals from 6 months to 14 years later had no perceptible differences in intelligence quotient, compared with the normal population. In a case report, persistent ataxia of the extremities and trunk and dysarthria were reported as residual effects in a 4-year-old patient.[26]

No deleterious effects of SLE on the outcome of pregnancy have been reported. However, infection with Japanese encephalitis virus in the second trimester results in transplacental viral transmission and abortion. Infection in the third trimester is not associated with fetal damage. In experimentally infected mice, vertical transmission led to learning deficits in congenitally infected pups.[3]

PREVENTION

Preventive public health efforts have focused on surveillance of viral activity in the enzootic cycle to predict epidemic activity. In many east-central states, serologic surveys are conducted weekly on captured wild birds and sentinel chickens. Rising seroprevalence rates, associated with viral amplification,[40] may precede the appearance of human infections by several weeks. The abundance of female vector mosquitoes and viral infection rates in vectors also have been correlated with risk of human infection.

When viral activity is elevated, ground and aerial applications of insecticides are aimed at reducing the infected adult vector population. If they are applied early enough, viral amplification potentially could be attenuated and epidemic transmission could be aborted.

Avoidance of outdoor activity during twilight and evening hours, the appropriate use of repellents (Table 179–2), and repairing screens or installing air conditioners in residences are simple but effective measures that reduce exposure to adult mosquitoes. Improving drainage and removing containers that could serve as mosquito breeding sites are important steps in preventing the disease.

A vaccine is not available. Vaccination of the general public is not a realistic preventive measure because of low attack rates and the intermittent and focal nature of outbreaks. However, if a vaccine or chemoprophylactic were available, selective administration to a targeted population, particularly the elderly, might be appropriate in an outbreak.

TABLE 179–2. Precautions to Minimize Potential Adverse Reactions from Repellents

Apply repellent sparingly only to exposed skin or clothing.
Avoid applying high-concentration (>30% DEET) products to the skin, particularly of children.
Do not inhale or ingest repellents or get them into the eyes.
Wear long sleeves and long pants, when possible, and apply repellents (e.g., permethrin) to clothing for reducing exposure to DEET.
Avoid applying repellents to portions of children's hands that are likely to have contact with eyes or mouth.
Pregnant and nursing women should minimize the use of repellents.
Never use repellents on wounds or irritated skin.
Use repellent sparingly; one application will last 4 to 8 hours. Saturation does not increase efficacy.
Wash repellent-treated skin after coming indoors.
If a suspected reaction to insect repellents occurs, wash treated skin and call a physician. Take the repellent can to the physician.

Adapted from Centers for Disease Control: Seizures temporarily associated with use of DEET insect repellent: New York and Connecticut. M. M. W. R. *38*:678–680, 1989.

References

1. Adames, A. J., Dutary, B., Tejera, H., et al.: Relocion entre mosquitos vectores y aves acuaticas en la transmission potencial de dos arbovirus. Revista Medica de Panama *18*:106–119, 1993.
2. Allen, R., Taylor, S. K., and Sulkin, S. E.: Studies of arthropod-borne virus infections in Chiroptera. VIII. Evidence of natural St. Louis encephalitis virus infection in bats. Am. J. Trop. Med. Hyg. *19*:851–859, 1970.
3. Andersen, A. A., and Hanson, R. P.: Intrauterine infection of mice with St. Louis encephalitis virus: Immunological, physiological, neurological, and behavioral effects on progeny. Infect. Immun. *12*:1173–1183, 1975.
4. Azar, G. J., Bond, J. O., Chappell, G. L., et al.: Follow up studies of St. Louis encephalitis in Florida: Sensorimotor findings. Am. J. Public Health *56*:1074–1081, 1966.
5. Bailey, C. L., Eldridge, B. F., Hayes, D. E., et al.: Isolation of St. Louis encephalitis virus from overwintering *Culex pipiens* mosquitoes. Science *199*:1346–1349, 1978.
6. Barrett, F. F., Yow, M. D., and Phillips, C. A.: St. Louis encephalitis in children during the 1964 epidemic. J. A. M. A. *193*:381–385, 1965.
7. Blattner, R. J., and Heys, F. M.: St. Louis encephalitis: Occurrence in children in the St. Louis area during nonepidemic years 1939–1944. J. A. M. A. *129*:854–857, 1945.
8. Bond, J. O., and Hammon, W. McD.: Epidemiologic studies of possible cross protection between dengue and St. Louis encephalitis arboviruses in Florida. Am. J. Epidemiol. *92*:321–329, 1970.
9. Brinker, K. R., and Monath, T. P.: The acute disease. *In* Monath, T. P. (ed.): St. Louis Encephalitis. Washington, D.C., American Public Health Association, 1980, pp. 503–534.
10. Brinker, K. R., Paulson, G., Monath, T. P., et al.: St. Louis encephalitis in Ohio, September 1975: Clinical and EEG studies in 16 cases. Arch. Intern. Med. *139*:561–566, 1979.
11. Broun, G. O.: Relationship of hypertensive vascular disease to mortality in cases of St. Louis encephalitis. Med. Bull. St. Louis Univ. *4*:32–37, 1952.
12. Calisher, C. H., and Poland, J. D.: Laboratory diagnosis. *In* Monath, T. P. (ed.): St. Louis Encephalitis. Washington, D.C., American Public Health Association, 1980, pp. 571–601.
13. Centers for Disease Control: Arboviral infections of the central nervous system: United States, 1987. M. M. W. R. *37*:506–515, 1988.
14. Centers for Disease Control: St. Louis encephalitis: Florida and Texas, 1990. M. M. W. R. *39*:756–759, 1990.
15. Chambers, T. J., Hahn, C. S., Galler, R., et al.: Flavivirus genome organization, expression and replication. Annu. Rev. Microbiol. *44*:649–688, 1990.
16. Coleman, P. H., Lewis, A. L., Schneider, N. J., et al.: Isolations of St. Louis encephalitis virus from postmortem tissues of human cases in the 1962 Florida epidemic. Am. J. Epidemiol. *87*:530–538, 1968.
17. Cortes, A. G., Aquino, M. L. Z., Bahena, J. G., et al.: St. Louis encephalomyelitis in Hermosillo, Sonora, Mexico. Pan American Health Organization Bull. *9*:306–316, 1975.
18. Day, J. F., and Curtis, G. A.: Annual emergence patterns of *Culex nigripalpus* females before, during or after a widespread St. Louis encephalitis epidemic in south Florida. J. Am. Mosq. Control Assoc. *9*:249–255, 1993.
19. Day, J. F.: A review of the 1990 St. Louis encephalitis virus epidemic in Indian river country, Florida. New Jersey Mosquito Control Assoc. Inc. 32–39, 1990.
20. Dropulic, B., and Masters, C. L.: Entry of neurotropic arboviruses into the central nervous system: An in vitro study using mouse brain endothelium. J. Infect. Dis. *161*:685–691, 1990.
21. Estrin, W. J.: The serological diagnosis of St. Louis encephalitis in a patient with the syndrome of opsoclonia, body tremulousness, and benign encephalitis. Ann. Neurol. *1*:596–598, 1977.
22. Evans, R. W., and Welch, K.: Opsoclonus in a confirmed case of St. Louis encephalitis. J. Neurol. Neurosurg. Psychiatry *45*:660–661, 1982.
23. Finley, K. H., and Riggs, N.: Convalescence and sequelae. *In* Monath, T. P. (ed.): St. Louis Encephalitis. Washington, D.C., American Public Health Association, 1980, pp. 535–550.
24. Fleckenstein, J. L., Cerna, F., Mehrad, B., et al.: St. Louis encephalitis: MRI/CT evaluation (in press).
25. Hopkins, C. C., Hollinger, F. B., Johnson, R. F., et al.: The epidemiology of St. Louis encephalitis in Dallas, Texas, 1966. Am. J. Epidemiol. *102*:1–15, 1975.
26. Kaplan, A. M., and Koveleski, J. T.: St. Louis encephalitis with particular involvement of the brain stem. Arch. Neurol. *35*:45–46, 1978.
27. Longshore, W. A., Stevens, I. M., Hollister, A. C., et al.: Epidemiologic observations on acute infectious encephalitis in California, with special reference to the 1952 outbreak. Am. J. Hyg. *63*:69–86, 1956.
28. Luby, J. P.: St. Louis encephalitis. Epidemiol. Rev. *1*:55–73, 1979.
29. Luby, J. P., Miller, G., Gardner, P., et al.: The epidemiology of St. Louis encephalitis in Houston, Texas, 1964. Am. J. Epidemiol. *86*:584–597, 1967.
30. Luby, J. P., Murphy, F. K., Gilliam, J. N., et al.: Antigenuria in St. Louis encephalitis. Am. J. Trop. Med. Hyg. *29*:265–268, 1980.

31. Luby, J. P., Stewart, W. E., Sulkin, S. E., et al.: Interferon in human infections with St. Louis encephalitis virus. Ann. Intern. Med. *71*:703–709, 1969.
32. Luby, J. P.: St. Louis encephalitis. *In* Beran, G. W. (ed.): Handbook of Zoonoses. 2nd ed. Section B: Viral. Boca Raton, CRC Press, 1994, p. 47.
33. McLean, R. G.: Arboviruses of wild birds and mammals. Bull. Soc. Vector Ecol. *16*:3–16, 1991.
34. Marfin, A. A., Bleed, D. M., Lofgren, J. P., et al.: Epidemiological aspects of a St. Louis encephalitis epidemic in Jefferson County, Arkansas. Am. J. Trop. Med. Hyg. *49*:30–37, 1993.
35. Monath, T. P.: Epidemiology. *In* Monath, T. P. (ed.): St. Louis Encephalitis. Washington, D.C., American Public Health Association, 1980, pp. 239–312.
36. Monath, T. P.: Flaviviruses. *In* Fields, B. N., Knipe, D. M., and Howley, P. M. (eds.): Virology. 3rd ed. New York, Lippincott-Raven Press, 1996, pp. 961–1034.
37. Monath, T. P., Cropp, C. B., Bowen, G. S., et al.: Variation in virulence for mice and rhesus monkeys among St. Louis encephalitis virus strains of different origin. Am. J. Trop. Med. Hyg. *29*:948–962, 1980.
38. Monath, T. P., Cropp, C. B., and Harrison, A. K.: Mode of entry of a neurotropic arbovirus into the central nervous system. Lab. Invest. *48*:399–410, 1983.
39. Monath, T. P., Nystrom, R. R., Bailey, R. E., et al.: Immunoglobulin M antibody capture enzyme-linked immunosorbent assay for diagnosis of St. Louis encephalitis. J. Clin. Microbiol. *20*:784–790, 1984.
40. Monath, T. P., and Tsai, T. F.: St. Louis encephalitis: Lessons from the last decade. Am. J. Trop. Med. Hyg. *37*:40S–59S, 1987.
41. Nelson, D. B., Kappus, K. D., Janowski, J. T., et al.: St. Louis encephalitis, Florida 1977: Patterns of a widespread outbreak. Am. J. Trop. Med. Hyg. *32*:412–418, 1983.
42. Noah, D. L., Bresee, J. S., Gorensek, M. J., et al.: Cluster of five children with acute encephalopathy associated with cat-scratch disease in South Florida. Pediatr. Infect. Dis. J. *14*:866–869, 1995.
43. Okhuysen, P. C., Crane, J. K., and Pappas, J.: St. Louis encephalitis in patients with human immunodeficiency virus infection. Clin. Infect. Dis. *17*:140–141, 1993.
44. Palmer, R. J., and Finley, K. H.: Sequelae of encephalitis: Report of a study after the California epidemic. Calif. Med. *84*:98–100, 1956.
45. Phillips, C. A., Melnick, J. L., Barrett, F. F., et al.: Dual virus infections: Simultaneous enteroviral disease and St. Louis encephalitis. J. A. M. A. *197*:169–172, 1966.
46. Powell, K. E., and Blakey, D. L.: St. Louis encephalitis: The 1975 epidemic in Mississippi. J. A. M. A. *237*:2294–2298, 1977.
47. Provost, M. W.: The natural history of *Culex nigripalpus*. *In* St. Louis Encephalitis in Florida, Ten Years of Research, Surveillance, and Control Programs. Florida State Board of Health, Monograph 12. Jacksonville, Fla., 1969, pp. 46–62.
48. Quick, D. T., Thompson, J. M., Bond, J. O., et al.: The 1962 epidemic of St. Louis encephalitis in Florida. II. Clinical features of cases in the Tampa Bay area. Am. J. Epidemiol. *81*:415–424, 1965.
49. Reeves, W. C., Hardy, J. L., Reisin, W. K., et al.: Potential effect of global warming on mosquito-borne arboviruses. J. Med. Entomol. *31*:323–332, 1994.
50. Reisin, W. K., Meyer, R. P., Presser, S. B., et al.: Effect of temperature on the transmission of western equine encephalomyelitis and St. Louis encephalitis viruses by *Culex tarsalis* (Diptera: Culicidae) J. Med. Entomol. *30*:151–160, 1994.
51. Reisin, W. K., Milby, M. M., Presser, S. B., et al.: Ecology of mosquitoes and St. Louis encephalitis virus in the Los Angeles basin of California. J. Med. Entomol. *29*:582–587, 1992.
52. Reyes, M. G., Gardner, J. J., Poland, J. D., et al.: St. Louis encephalitis: Quantitative histologic and immunofluorescent studies. Arch. Neurol. *38*:329–334, 1981.
53. Riggs, S., Smith, D. L., and Phillips, C. A.: St. Louis encephalitis in adults during the 1964 Houston epidemic. J. Am. Med. Assoc. *193*:284, 1965.
54. Sanders, M., Blumberg, A., and Haymaker, W.: Polyradiculopathy in man produced by St. Louis encephalitis (SLE). South. Med. J. *69*:1121–1125, 1976.
55. Shinner, J. J.: St. Louis virus encephalomyelitis. Arch. Pathol. *75*:311–322, 1963.
56. Shoji, H., Hiraki, Y., Kuwasaki, N., et al.: Japanese encephalitis in the Kurume region of Japan: CT and MRI findings. J. Neurol. *236*:255–259, 1989.
57. Spence, L. P.: St. Louis encephalitis in tropical America. *In* Monath, T. P. (ed.): St. Louis Encephalitis. Washington, D.C., American Public Health Association, 1980, pp. 451–471.
58. Suzuki, M., and Phillips, C. A.: St. Louis encephalitis: A histopathologic study of the fatal cases from the Houston epidemic in 1964. Arch. Pathol. *81*:47–54, 1966.
59. Trent, D. W., Monath, T. P., Bowen G. S., et al.: Variation among strains of St. Louis encephalitis virus: Basis for a genetic, pathogenic and epidermologic classification. Ann. N. Y. Acad. Sci. *354*:219, 1980.
60. Tsai, T. F.: Arboviral infections in the United States. Infect. Dis. Clin. North Am. *5*:73–102, 1991.
61. Tsai, T. F., Bolin, R. A., Montoya, M., et al.: Detection of St. Louis encephalitis virus antigen in mosquitoes by capture enzyme immunoassay. J. Clin. Microbiol. *25*:370–376, 1987.
62. Tsai, T. F., Canfield, M. A., Reed, C. M., et al.: Epidemiologic aspects of a St. Louis encephalitis outbreak in Harris County, Texas, 1986. J. Infect. Dis. *157*:351–356, 1988.
63. Tsai, T. F., Cobb, W. B., Bolin, R. A., et al.: Epidemiologic aspects of a St. Louis encephalitis outbreak in Mesa County. Am. J. Epidemiol. *126*:460–473, 1987.
64. Tsai, T. F., and Mitchell, C. J.: St. Louis encephalitis. *In* Monath, T. P. (ed.): The Arbovirus: Epidemiology and Ecology. Vol 4. Boca Raton, CRC Press, 1989, pp. 113–144.
65. Weil, A.: Histopathology of the central nervous system in epidemic encephalitis (St. Louis epidemic). Arch. Neurol. Psychiatry *31*:1139–1152, 1934.
66. Zweighaft, R. M., Rasmussen, C., Brolnitsky, O., et al.: St. Louis encephalitis: The Chicago experience. Am. J. Trop. Med. Hyg. *28*:114–118, 1979.

❑ ❑ ❑

CHAPTER 179 (B)

Yellow Fever

Duane J. Gubler

Yellow fever is a mosquito-borne viral disease of humans and lower primates. It occurs naturally in tropical Africa and the Americas (Fig. 179–6). Epidemics, which can occur in both urban and rural areas, often are associated with severe hemorrhagic disease and high fatality rates.

HISTORY

Yellow fever first was described as a disease entity in 1648 in the Yucatan, Mexico. This apparently was part of a larger regional epidemic that affected the Caribbean Islands and Central America from Barbados to Mexico from 1647 to 1649.[7] Although first described in the Americas, yellow fever virus most likely originated in Africa and was introduced to the New World via the slave trade, along with its principal epidemic mosquito vector, *Aedes aegypti*. During the seventeenth, eighteenth, nineteenth, and early twentieth centuries, yellow fever was a major public health problem. Large epidemics occurred in tropical America as well as in the United States (as far north as Boston) and Europe (as far north as England).[11] Epidemics occurred primarily in port cities, reflecting the primary mode of spread: sailing vessels and commerce.

After mosquito transmission had been documented by Reed and the Yellow Fever Commission in Cuba,[10] major efforts were made to control the disease by mosquito control. The first yellow fever virus was isolated in 1927. By 1938, an effective vaccine had been developed. Yellow fever was controlled in the Americas by eradication of the mosquito vector of urban disease, *A. aegypti*, from most Central and South American countries. In West Africa, yellow fever was controlled by mass vaccination programs. The result was the disappearance of major urban epidemics of yellow fever in both Africa and the Americas during the 1950s, 1960s, and 1970s. In recent years, however, the urban form of disease has re-emerged in West Africa, with major epidemics in Nigeria and increased transmission in other countries.[5] Kenya experienced its first epidemic in history in 1993. In the Americas, *A. aegypti* has reinfested most Central and South American countries from which it had been eradicated, placing urban centers of the American tropics at the highest risk for epidemic urban yellow fever in more than 50 years.[1] Thus, the disease continues to be an important public health problem in both Africa and the Americas. Yellow fever has never been recognized in Asia or the Pacific.

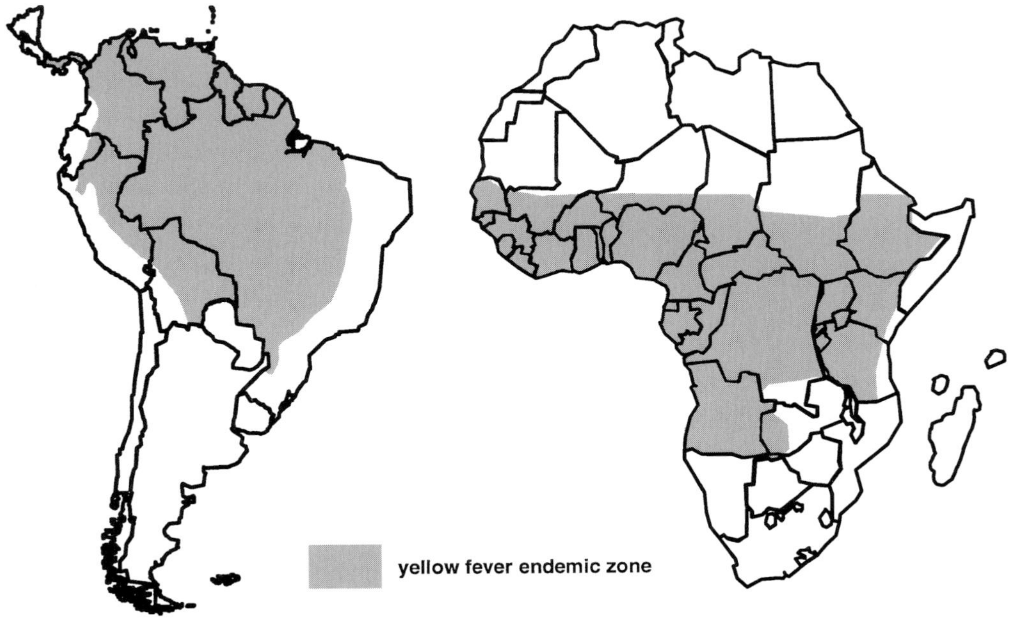

FIGURE 179–6. *Geographic distribution of yellow fever in Africa and the Americas.*

ETIOLOGIC AGENT

Yellow fever is caused by yellow fever virus, the prototype of the genus *Flavivirus*, family *Flaviviridae*. The genus *Flavivirus* contains 69 viruses, which are small (40 to 50 nm in diameter), spherical, and enveloped, with a single-stranded RNA about 11 kb in length.[3] Many of the flaviviruses are very closely related antigenically, resulting in extensive cross-reactivity in most serologic tests. This makes laboratory diagnosis difficult.

EPIDEMIOLOGY

Yellow fever viruses are maintained in natural zoonotic cycles involving lower primates and canopy-dwelling mosquitoes that breed in tree holes in the rain forests of both Africa and the Americas.[5, 7, 11] This is called the jungle or sylvatic cycle of yellow fever. Humans become involved accidentally only when they encroach on this cycle in the forest. Humans so infected may take the virus back to a village or city during incubation. If the infected persons are fed upon by urban *A. aegypti*, the virus can then be transmitted from human to human. Major urban epidemics are transmitted by this highly domesticated mosquito, which lives in close association with humans in most tropical cities of the world.

Yellow fever occurs throughout much of sub-Saharan Africa and tropical America in the sylvatic cycle (see Fig. 179–6). In Africa, cercopithecid and celobid monkeys are the main vertebrate hosts; infection rarely causes illness and death in these species. Year-round enzootic transmission by *A. africanus* occurs in the rain forests. In wet savannah areas bordering the rain forests of West and Central Africa, transmission increases during the rainy season and decreases during the dry season. *A. furcifer*, *A. africanus*, and *A. leuteocephalus* are the main mosquito vectors in this "zone of emergence," transmitting the virus from monkey to monkey, monkey to human, and human to human. In the dry savannah zones, yellow fever activity is intermittent, occurring mainly during the rainy season, but it also occurs in major epidemics in urban areas, where stored water provides the ideal larval habitat for *A. aegypti*. In East Africa, *A. simpsoni* (*A. bromeliae*) provides the link between the *A. africanus* sylvatic cycle and humans in areas bordering gallery forests.

In tropical America, howler, spider, squirrel, owl, capuchin, and wooly monkeys all act as vertebrate hosts for yellow fever virus. Mosquitoes of the genus *Haemagogus* are the principal vectors in tropical American rain forests, feeding in the canopy as well as at ground level. Other mosquito species, such as *Sabethes chloropterus*, *A. leucocelaenus*, and *A. fulvus*, may play secondary roles. The enzootic zone includes the rain forests of at least six countries (Colombia, Ecuador, Peru, Bolivia, Brazil, and Venezuela) and involves "wandering" enzootic transmission among the monkey populations. The humans involved mainly are adult males who work in the forest.

Vertical transmission of yellow fever virus from an infected female mosquito through the eggs to her offspring plays an important role in the survival and maintenance of yellow fever virus in the enzootic cycles and has been demonstrated in nature in West Africa by isolation of the virus from male *A. furcifer* mosquitoes. Experimentally, *Haemagogus* and *A. aegypti* mosquitoes have been shown to be capable of vertical transmission. This mechanism is thought to be of major importance in survival of the virus during prolonged dry periods in both enzootic regions.

Urban epidemics of yellow fever have reappeared in West Africa in the past 10 years.[9] Unfortunately, surveillance is very poor, and the actual number of cases reported is thought to be grossly underestimated. For example, in Nigeria in 1986 and 1987, the numbers of reported cases and deaths during epidemics were 2612 and 973, respectively. Seroepidemiologic studies, however, estimated that the actual numbers of cases and deaths were 130,000 and 29,000, respectively.

In the Americas, urban yellow fever has not occurred in more than 50 years. The reinvasion of American tropical urban centers by *A. aegypti*, however, has placed more than 300 million susceptible individuals at risk. It is expected that urban yellow fever epidemics will occur in the near future unless vaccination or effective mosquito control programs are implemented.

Yellow fever has never been reported in Asia. The reason for this is not known, but both variation in mosquito vector competence and partial protection by heterotypic flavivirus antibody have been suggested as reasons why this virus has never become established in that part of the world.

CLINICAL MANIFESTATIONS

Infection with yellow fever virus causes a spectrum of illness, ranging from inapparent infection to severe yellow fever with the classic triad of symptoms, jaundice, hemorrhage, and albuminuria, associated with a high case-fatality rate. The majority of yellow fever infections present clinically as mild to severe viral syndrome without the symptoms of intoxication; 10 to 20 per cent of infections may present as classic yellow fever.

The incubation period may be as long as 13 days but generally is 3 to 6 days.[7] Onset of illness is abrupt, with fever, headache, backache, myalgias, nausea, and other nonspecific signs and symptoms. In mild cases, the illness will last for several days, after which recovery is uneventful and complete. In severe cases, prostration is common, and examination reveals congestion of the skin, conjunctivae, and mucous membranes. The pulse rate usually increases early in the illness, and blood pressure is normal. Leukopenia is common, and there may be a mild albuminuria. The temperature usually is between 38.5° and 40° C. Nausea and vomiting are common. There may be minor hemorrhagic manifestations, such as epistaxis and bleeding gums. This period of infection may last for about 3 days, when the congestion declines, and there may be a relative bradycardia, despite the elevated temperature (Faget sign). The temperature falls to or below normal, and the patient feels better.

In the majority of patients, this period of remission signals the beginning of convalescence, but in severe cases, it may last only a few hours, at which point the patient enters a period of intoxication characterized by venous congestion and extreme bradycardia, despite a secondary rise in temperature. Nausea and vomiting are severe and associated with epigastric pain. There is prostration, jaundice, marked albuminuria, and anuria. Hemorrhage includes hematemesis and melena.

Jaundice in some patients is not striking; it is difficult to detect in early disease and often not detected until after death. The severity of hemorrhagic manifestations also varies greatly, but some hemorrhage can be found in most cases. As indicated earlier, minor hemorrhagic manifestations may be observed in the early stage of illness; the severe hemorrhage usually develops late in the illness, although in fulminant cases, it may occur as early as the second or third day. Hemorrhage may be so severe as to cause shock and death from blood loss. Albuminuria is one of the most common findings in yellow fever and occurs in all but the very mild cases. It occurs early in the illness and may increase rapidly. It probably is related to renal involvement during the period of infection. Anuria, on the other hand, appears to be related to hepatic involvement and is never seen in the absence of other signs of liver infection.

Death may occur as early as 2 to 4 days after onset but usually occurs after 7 to 10 days of illness in 20 to 50 per cent of severe cases. In cases in which death occurs later than this, autopsy usually reveals a cause other than yellow fever. Severe cases often have lowered resistance to secondary infection, which may develop at the time of convalescence. Other complications include kidney abscesses, pneumonia, subgenerative parotitis, and skin infections. Convalescence usually is rapid and complete except for a general weakness that may last for several weeks. Permanent damage to the liver or kidneys is not apparent.

PATHOLOGY

The gross pathology in fatal cases of yellow fever is not striking.[8] The skin, sclerae, serosa, some internal organs, and subcutaneous fat usually have moderate icterus. There often are serous effusions, edema, and hemorrhages, including petechiae and purpuric lesions on the skin, conjunctivae, mucous membranes, stomach, duodenum, and bladder. Gastrointestinal hemorrhage may be prominent.

The most characteristic lesions caused by yellow fever virus are seen in the liver, although liver failure usually is not the cause of death. The liver may have a yellowish color and be enlarged and fatty in consistency. In typical cases, there is a marked necrosis of the midzone of the lobule. The necrosis extends both centrally and peripherally, involving, on average, 80 per cent of the lobule in fatal cases.[4, 8] The cells bordering the central vein and portal areas usually are spared. Councilman and Torres bodies can be observed in hepatocytes. There is little or no inflammatory response, and the reticulin framework is preserved.

The kidneys usually are tense and swollen. Glomerular changes are minor, but acute tubular necrosis and fatty metamorphosis may be significant. There may be cloudy swelling, degeneration, and fatty infiltration in the myocardial fibers. The spleen and lymph nodes are depleted of lymphocytes, and mononucleocytes or histiocytes accumulate in the follicles of the spleen. Edema and petechiae may be observed in the brain.

LABORATORY FINDINGS

Leukopenia and albuminuria are common in early disease. In severe cases, prolonged prothrombin and partial thromboplastin times, thrombocytopenia, fibrin split products, and elevated liver enzymes will be observed. Total and conjugated serum bilirubin levels are elevated. Albumin levels in the urine usually are less than 5 g/L, but in rare cases may reach 40 g/L. The urine contains bile. The cerebrospinal fluid usually is normal but may be under increased pressure.

DIFFERENTIAL DIAGNOSIS

Clinically, yellow fever is difficult to differentiate from many other viral, bacterial, and parasitic infections, including other viral hemorrhagic fevers, such as Lassa, Ebola, Marburg, Rift Valley, and dengue hemorrhagic fevers, and other diseases that cause fever and jaundice, such as viral hepatitis, leptospirosis, falciparum malaria, tick-borne relapsing fever, typhus, typhoid, and Q fever. A definitive diagnosis of yellow fever can be made only by using the appropriate laboratory test.

LABORATORY DIAGNOSIS

Specific laboratory diagnosis requires isolation of the virus, serology, or immunohistochemical tests. Virus can be isolated most easily from the acute-phase serum taken during the first 4 days of illness, but it has been isolated as long as 14 days after onset of illness as well as from the liver after death.[8] The most sensitive method of virus isolation is inoculation of mosquitoes followed by the use of AP-61 cell cultures from *A. pseudoscutellaris* mosquitoes. Vero cells and inoculation of suckling mice also can be used but are less sensitive. Viral antigen can be demonstrated in the liver by immunohistochemical methods.[2] Either fresh or formalin-fixed tissue can be used with these techniques, which can be used to establish a virologic diagnosis after virus has been cleared from the blood.

Serologic diagnosis depends on the collection of properly timed acute- and convalescent-phase serum samples in order to demonstrate a rise in specific antibody. Serologic tests commonly used to diagnose yellow fever include hemagglutination inhibition (HI), complement fixation (CF), and plaque-reduction neutralization (PRN), as well as newer tests, such as the enzyme-linked immunosorbent assay (ELISA) for both IgG and IgM antibodies. The immunofluorescent assay (IFA) is used in some laboratories.

Antibodies detected by HI, PRN, IFA, and IgM-capture ELISA appear within 5 to 7 days after onset of illness, whereas the CF antibodies appear later, usually after 10 to 14 days. The HI and PRN antibodies persist at detectable levels for many years (>50) in most patients, whereas the duration of CF and IgM antibodies is uncertain but probably wanes to undetectable levels after 12 to 18 months.

PRN is the most sensitive and specific of the serologic tests. In patients who have had no prior flavivirus infection, this test can be used to make a specific yellow fever diagnosis, as can IgM-capture ELISA. Cross-reaction between yellow fever antigen and antibodies to other related flaviviruses complicates the serodiagnosis of this and other flavivirus diseases. HI, IFA, and IgG ELISA all are nonspecific tests in which there is considerable cross-reactivity with heterologous flavivirus antibodies.

The use of yellow fever 17D vaccine in disease-endemic areas also may complicate serologic diagnosis. Vaccination induces HI and neutralizing antibodies detectable at low titers (1:10 to 1:40) but no detectable IF or CF antibodies. Vaccination also induces IgM antibody, which may remain at detectable levels for up to 18 months. Vaccination of individuals who have had a previous flavivirus infection induces an anamnestic response of heterotypic flavivirus antibodies at high titers (≥1:1280).

TREATMENT

Treatment of yellow fever is supportive because no specific therapy exists.[4, 6] Antiviral drugs are not effective. Patients with severe disease requiring hospitalization should have complete bed rest with good nursing care and close monitoring of vital organ functions. Salicylates should be avoided, but mild sedatives may be helpful. Maintaining fluid and electrolyte balance is critical. Guidelines for intensive care of severe yellow fever cases have not been established. Secondary bacterial infections may occur and should be treated with appropriate antibiotics.

PROGNOSIS

Mortality in all yellow fever infections is low (<5%), but in severe cases requiring hospitalization, mortality may be 20 to 50 per cent.[4, 8] The prognosis is poor for patients who enter a period of intoxication with rapidly increasing albuminuria, jaundice, and fever and with severe hemorrhage. Patients in the terminal stage of illness usually are somnolent, have below-normal temperature, and may have intractable hiccups.

PREVENTION AND CONTROL

The most practical and cost-effective method of yellow fever prevention is vaccination. A single dose of 17D vaccine provides effective, long-term (10 years) protection and should be used in the World Health Organization Expanded Program of Immunization in endemic countries of Africa and the Americas.

The 17D vaccine is prepared from infected chicken embryos and produces effective immunity in more than 95 per cent of recipients.[8] Adverse reactions are rare, although infants younger than 4 months of age have a high risk of encephalitis. Infants should not be vaccinated with 17D vaccine until 9 months of age. Pregnant women also should avoid vaccination because vaccine virus may infect the developing fetus, although the risk of adverse events associated with congenital infection is unknown. Finally, 17D vaccine should not be given to persons who are allergic to eggs or to persons who are immunodeficient or are receiving immunosuppressive drugs.

The other method of yellow fever prevention is mosquito control, especially during epidemic activity. The principal mosquito vector of urban yellow fever, *A. aegypti*, is a highly domesticated species that lives in and around the houses of humans. It breeds primarily in artificial containers that collect rain water or in domestic water storage containers. The most effective control, therefore, is source reduction, that is, to control or discard the larval habitats in the domestic environment.[1] This is a labor-intensive process but can be done with the help of the citizens in the community.

Some authorities recommend adult mosquito control using insecticide space sprays, primarily ultra low volume. Recent field trials, however, have shown this approach to be ineffective unless portable sprayers are used to treat the inside of each dwelling. Because of the excessive cost and lack of efficacy of ultra-low–volume application of insecticides, this method is not recommended.

Patients suspected of having yellow fever should be protected from mosquitoes. The most effective protection is to use a mosquito net on the bed. Alternatively, patients can be kept in screened rooms.

References

1. Gubler, D. J.: *Aedes aegypti* and *Aedes aegypti*-borne disease control in the 1990's: Top down or bottom up. Am J. Trop. Med. Hyg. *40*:571–578, 1989.
2. Hall, W. C., Crowell, T. P., Watts, D. M., et al.: Demonstration of yellow fever and dengue antigens in formalin-fixed paraffin-embedded human liver by immunohistochemical analysis. Am. J. Trop. Med. Hyg. *145*:408–417, 1991.
3. Karabatos, N.: International catalogue of arboviruses, including certain other viruses of vertebrates. American Society of Tropical Medicine and Hygiene, San Antonio, TX, 1985.
4. McKee, K. T., and Monath, T. P.: Arboviruses of Africa. *In* Feigin, R. D., and Cherry, J. D. (eds.): Textbook of Pediatric Infectious Diseases. Vol. II. 3rd ed. Philadelphia, W. B. Saunders, 1990, pp. 1435–1456.
5. Meegan, J. M.: Yellow fever. *In* Beran, G. W., and Steele, J. H. (eds.): Handbook of Zoonoses. 2nd ed. Boca Raton, CRC Press, 1994, pp. 111–124.
6. Monath, T. P.: Yellow fever: A medically neglected disease. Report on a seminar. Rev. Infect. Dis. *9*:165–175, 1987.
7. Monath, T. P.: Yellow fever. *In* Monath, T. P. (ed.): The Arboviruses: Epidemiology and Ecology. Vol. V. Boca Raton, CRC Press, 1988, pp. 139–231.
8. Monath, T. P.: Yellow fever. *In* Strickland, G. T. (ed.): Hunter's Tropical Medicine. Philadelphia, W. B. Saunders, 1991, pp. 233–238.
9. Nasidi, A., Monath, T. P., DeCock, K., et al.: Urban yellow fever epidemic in western Nigeria, 1987. Trans. R. Soc. Trop. Med. Hyg. *83*:401, 1989.
10. Reed, W.: Recent researches concerning etiology, propagation and prevention of yellow fever, by the United States Army Commission. J. Hyg. 2:101–119, 1902.
11. Strode, G. K.: Yellow Fever. New York, McGraw Hill, 1951.

❑ ❑ ❑

CHAPTER 179 (C)

Dengue and Dengue Hemorrhagic Fever

Scott B. Halstead

Dengue fever is an acute febrile illness syndrome caused by several arthropod-borne viruses and characterized by biphasic fever, myalgia or arthralgia, rash, leukopenia, and lymphadenopathy. Synonyms are dengue and breakbone fever. Dengue hemorrhagic fever (DHF), a febrile disease caused by dengue viruses, is characterized by hemoconcentration, by abnormalities of hemostasis, and, in the most severe cases, by a fluid- and protein-losing shock syndrome (dengue shock syndrome, DSS). It is thought to have an immunopathologic basis. Synonyms are hemorrhagic dengue; acute infectious thrombocytopenic purpura; and Philippine, Thai, and Singapore hemorrhagic fever.

There are four antigenically distinct members of the dengue subgroup.[13, 14, 36, 64] From 1956, according to reports received by the World Health Organization, dengue viruses were thought to be responsible for more than 4,000,000 hospital admissions and 50,000 deaths in Southeast Asia, South China, India, Sri Lanka, Pakistan, Cuba, Venezuela, Colombia, Guyana, Brazil, Puerto Rico, and Nicaragua, mostly among vital, healthy children. In Southeast Asian countries, dengue is among the 10 leading causes of death in children 1 to 14 years of age.

The first outbreak that resembles a disease now recognized as dengue fever was that described by Benjamin Rush in Philadelphia, Pennsylvania, in 1780.[9, 72] Epidemics probably due to dengue were common from the eighteenth to the twentieth centuries among the inhabitants of the Atlantic coast of the United States, the Caribbean Islands, and the Mississippi basin.[72] Dengue viruses almost certainly were the cause of the 5- and 7-day fevers that occurred among European colonists in tropical Asia.[9] Similar epidemics were common among settlers in tropical Australia, where, in 1905, *Aedes aegypti* was identified as a dengue vector by Bancroft.[46] Ashburn and Craig[72] found the etiologic agent in human blood and showed that it could pass through a diatomaceous earth filter. An intrinsic incubation period in humans of 3 to 8 days, an extrinsic incubation period in mosquitoes of 8 to 11 days, immunity in people and monkeys, and the nonsusceptibility of most domestic animals were demonstrated in the classic studies of Siler and Simmons and their coworkers[72, 73] between 1924 and 1930. When dengue viruses were isolated in laboratory mice in 1943 and 1944, the modern era of dengue research began.[37, 66] Two strains from Hawaii and New Guinea failed to cross-protect humans. From this experiment, it was recognized that there were at least two different dengue viruses; these were named dengue virus type 1 and type 2.[67]

During most of the previrologic era, dengue viruses were thought to be the cause of a generally benign, self-limited, febrile exanthem. However, deaths, shock, and severe hemorrhagic manifestations had accompanied classic dengue fever outbreaks in Australia in 1897 and for 15 years thereafter. Similar phenomena were recorded in Greece in 1928 and in Formosa in 1931.[35] This "new" syndrome was recognized again in Manila in 1954. It was called *Philippine hemorrhagic fever* because of a resemblance to the epidemic hemorrhagic fever then occurring among United Nations troops in the Korean Peninsula.[32] In 1956, Philippine hemorrhagic fever was associated with dengue when types 3 and 4 were recovered.[32] It now has become endemic throughout tropical Asia.[21, 25] Since 1967, the terms *dengue hemorrhagic fever* and *dengue shock syndrome* have come into general use.[22]

In 1981, Cuba reported a severe outbreak with more than 116,000 patients hospitalized within 3 months, of whom 10,000 had DHF/DSS.[39] In 1986, an epidemic of DHF/DSS occurred on Hainan Island, China[54]; in 1988, the Maldive Islands, Sri Lanka, and India were involved.[74, 81] From about 1987, DHF/DSS outbreaks have occurred in Venezuela, Brazil, Colombia, and on a lesser scale in Puerto Rico and Nicaragua.[55]

By epidemiologic criteria, dengue viruses are arthropod-borne (arboviruses) because they are transmitted biologically by various members of the genus *Stegomyia*.[72, 73] Gene structure, replicative strategy, and antigenic relatedness place the dengue viruses in the family *Flaviviridae*.[36, 83] At present, there are 68 members of the flavivirus family, 29 of which are established as human pathogens.[36] Cross-comparisons by plaque-reduction neutralization tests have shown dengue viruses to be an antigenic subgroup with little relationship to other flaviviruses.[14] In addition to their antigenic relatedness and their ability to be transmitted by *Stegomyia*, each type of dengue virus produces a closely similar clinical syndrome in susceptible human beings.[23 68, 72, 73]

Dengue virions are spherical particles approximately 50 nm in diameter. The central core, approximately 25 nm in diameter, has icosahedral symmetry and contains a single plus strand of RNA. Dengue RNA consists of about 11,000 nucleotides coding from the 5′ end for core, premembrane, envelope, and five nonstructural proteins.[20] The envelope, studded with poorly resolved projections, is composed of many replicates of the envelope protein (54 kDa) embedded in a lipid bilayer. When assembled on the virion, the envelope protein bears epitopes unique to serotypes. Antibodies to these epitopes neutralize by hindering viral entry into cells. Other epitopes are shared between dengue viruses (dengue subgroup antigens) and other flaviviruses (group antigens).

Four clearly defined types exist, based on plaque-reduction neutralization tests using antibodies raised by infection of monkeys and by genetic relatedness.[14, 64, 83] Different strains of each dengue serotype show a degree of genetic heterogeneity.[12, 42, 58, 79] However, sequences of the envelope region gene of viruses from the same geographic area exhibited genetic homogeneity.[11, 79] The most sharply divergent strains are dengue viruses type 2 recovered from African monkeys.[58, 59] Of particular interest, Jamaica 1981, 1982, and 1983 dengue viruses type 2 are related closely to Southeast Asian topotypes.[58] It has been speculated that these dengue viruses type 2 are identical to those that caused the 1981 Cuban outbreak.[58]

Dengue virus can be grown in 1- to 2-day-old mice or hamsters by intracerebral inoculation or in various mosquitoes by oral or parenteral inoculation. High mouse-passaged virus grows and produces deaths in weanling mice. Various tissue cultures of vertebrate and invertebrate origin support dengue virus growth in vitro, as reviewed in the following section.

TRANSMISSION

A. aegypti, a daytime-biting mosquito, is the principal vector. All four virus types have been recovered from naturally infected *A. aegypti*.[21, 30] In most tropical areas, *A. aegypti* is highly domesticated, breeding in water stored for drinking, washing, or bathing or in any container collecting fresh water. Dengue viruses also have been recovered from naturally infected *A. albopictus*, which breeds outdoors in vegetation.[21, 30] Outbreaks in the Pacific area have been attributed to *A. scutellaris* and *A. polynesiensis*.

In urban areas, dengue transmission may be explosive, involving as much as 70 to 80 per cent of the population.[72] Because *A. aegypti* has a limited flight range, spread of virus mainly is via mobile viremic human beings.

Dengue viruses replicate in the gut, brain, and salivary glands of infected mosquitoes without apparent harm to adult mosquitoes.[60] Mosquitoes are infectious for a lifetime and as long as 70 days in experimental circumstances.[73] Because female mosquitoes take repeated blood meals, long-lived female mosquitoes have great potency as vectors. Several species of *Stegomyia* and *Toxorhynchites* are infected readily by intrathoracic inoculation, although the threshold of infection by oral feeding is higher.[60, 61] *A. aegypti* and *Culex quinquefasciatus* can transmit dengue mechanically by interrupted feeding.[73] The contribution of mechanical feeding to the spread of dengue virus during epidemics has never been measured, but because of the "skittishness" of *A. aegypti* and its habit of feeding during the day when its intended victim is awake and often moving, interrupted feeding and thus mechanical transmission must be common.

A. aegypti feeds preferentially on people and hence is most abundant in and around human habitations. The mosquito breeds preferentially in clean water. Biting activity is reduced at temperatures below a wet bulb temperature of 14° C.[15] Dengue transmission in temperate countries is interrupted during winter weather, and dengue has not established itself endemically at latitudes above 25° north or south. Breeding sites may be provided by humans through living habits, as in Thailand, where water is stored in and around homes in large earthenware jars.[21, 30] In contrast, *A. aegypti* is not abundant in some parts of India because only small amounts of water are brought to homes from village wells for immediate use. Water in flower vases, household offerings, ant traps, coconut husks, tin cans, and rubber tires may supply breeding sites for *A. aegypti*.[30, 46]

In the tropics, dengue outbreaks generally coincide with the monsoon season. Eggs, which resist desiccation, are deposited inside water containers above the water line.[30] With the beginning of monsoon rains, a large number of eggs laid outdoors are hatched. Indoor populations do not show seasonal change. There is evidence that biting rates increase with increased temperature and relative humidity.[71]

Isolations in sylvan settings have been made from three subgenera of *Aedes*, namely, *Stegomyia, Diceromyia,* and *Finlaya*, some in circumstances suggesting the existence of transovarial transmission.[62] This phenomenon has been demonstrated experimentally.[62]

EPIDEMIOLOGY

Host Range

Inoculation of dengue strains of known human pathogenicity does not produce demonstrable infection in adult chickens, lizards, guinea pigs, rabbits, hamsters, or cotton rats.[70, 72]

Subhuman primates generally are susceptible to infection by dengue viruses. A number of species belonging to *Macacus, Pongidae, Cercopithecus, Cercocebus, Papio, Hylobates,* and *Pan* can be infected by bites of virus-infected mosquitoes or by injection of infectious virus preparations.[70, 73] Infection essentially is asymptomatic. Viremia occurs at levels sufficient to infect mosquitoes. Simmons and colleagues[73] were the first to note that wild-caught *Macaca philippinensis* resisted dengue infection, whereas *Macaca fuscatus* (Japanese macaque) was susceptible. Work by Rudnick[63] in Malaysia has revealed a jungle cycle of dengue transmission involving canopy-feeding monkeys and *A. niveus*, a species that feeds on both monkeys and humans. Although the existence of a jungle dengue cycle in the Malaysian rain forest has been documented, the full geographic range of the subhuman primate zoonotic reservoir is not known. In the early 1980s, there appeared to have been an extensive epizootic of dengue virus type 2 involving subhuman primates over wide areas of West Africa.[59] From genetic and epidemiologic studies, it has been concluded that urban human dengue and jungle monkey dengue are relatively compartmentalized.[58] Urban dengue is vectored by anthropophilic mosquitoes, and virus travels along routes of transportation. *A. aegypti* and susceptible humans are so abundant and so widespread that the impact of the exchange of dengue viruses between humans and monkeys is hardly discernible. If urban dengue ever were eliminated, the reintroduction of virus from a jungle cycle could become important.

Geographic Distribution

Dengue fever outbreaks have been documented on every continent except Antarctica.[25] Evidence suggests that human dengue may have originated from enzootic or endemic foci in tropical Asia.[48] The probable spread during historical times of *A. aegypti* from Africa throughout the world provided an ecologic niche quickly occupied by several human viral pathogens: yellow fever, chikungunya, and the dengue viruses. During the eighteenth and nineteenth centuries, epidemics occurred in newly settled lands, largely because of the necessity for domestic water storage in frontier areas. Isolated shipboard or garrison outbreaks often confined to nonindigenous settlers or visitors were reported in Africa, the Indian subcontinent, and Southeast Asia.[9, 46, 72] During World War II, dengue virus infections were common in combatants of the Pacific War, spreading to staging areas not infected normally: Japan, Hawaii, and Polynesia.[70] During the past 20 years, major epidemics of all four dengue serotypes have occurred on Caribbean and Pacific islands.[1, 25, 26, 30] After its introduction in 1977, dengue virus type 1 appears to have remained in the region. Endemic dengue transmission occurs on the larger Caribbean islands, coastal central America, and tropical areas of Colombia.[25, 30] A sharp dengue virus type 2 epidemic in Cuba in 1981 led to island-wide *A. aegypti* control and apparent eradication of the virus.[40] In 1986 and 1987, dengue virus type 1 spread through most of coastal Brazil and from there to Paraguay and to Peru and Ecuador.[18] In 1990, more than 9000 dengue cases were reported from Venezuela; 2600 of them were classified as dengue hemorrhagic fever, and 74 deaths were associated with the epidemic.[55] Dengue virus types 1, 2, and 4 were isolated.[3] In 1995, dengue virus type 3 was introduced into the region.[3]

Dengue virus types 1 and 2 have been recovered from humans with mild clinical illness in Nigeria in the absence of epidemic disease.[25] In 1983, dengue virus type 3 was recovered from Mozambique.[31]

DHF-like disease was described clinically in Thailand beginning in 1950 and in the Philippines from 1953 and subsequently confirmed as DHF/DSS in 1958 and 1956, respectively. DHF first was described in Singapore and Malaysia in 1962, Vietnam in 1963, India in 1963, Ceylon (Sri Lanka) in 1965, Indonesia in 1969, Burma in 1970, China in 1985, and Kampuchea and Laos from about 1985 and has sustained major outbreaks in Sri Lanka and India from 1988 and from French Polynesia since 1990.[17, 25, 26, 54, 74, 81, 84] DHF has occurred at consistently high endemicity in Thailand, Burma, and Vietnam and at a lower level in Indonesia.[25] In Thailand, it is the third ranking cause of hospitalization and deaths in children. Intermittent epidemics have involved Malaysia and the Philippines. The sharpest outbreak in history, involving 116,000 hospitalizations in a 3-month period, occurred in Cuba in 1981.[36] A small outbreak of DHF/DSS occurred in Venezuela in 1989 and 1990.[55] Since then, DHF/DSS has spread to Colombia, French Guiana, Guyana, and Brazil and to a smaller extent to Puerto Rico and Nicaragua.[53, 55, 56]

CLINICAL MANIFESTATIONS

Dengue Fever

Biphasic fever and rash are the most characteristic features of the dengue fever syndrome.[13, 68, 72, 73] Manifestations vary with age and from patient to patient. In infants and young children, the disease may be undifferentiated or characterized by a 1- to 5-day fever, pharyngeal inflammation, rhinitis, and mild cough. A distinctive mean incubation period, duration of illness, and spectrum of clinical findings may characterize disease with different dengue types, although as yet there are not enough confirmatory studies to document this.[23] Differences in mild dengue syndromes, hospitalized dengue cases (predominantly during secondary dengue virus infections), and chikungunya illnesses are illustrated in the section on chikungunya (see Tables 178–4 through 178–8).

Chikungunya virus infections result in the dengue fever syndrome. Chikungunya illnesses begin more abruptly and are of shorter duration than dengue. Maculopapular rash, conjunctival injection, and myalgia or arthralgia occur more frequently in chikungunya than in dengue illnesses, but other features associated with both viruses are remarkably similar. DHF syndrome is differentiated from dengue fever by its association with thrombocytopenia and capillary leakage.

In classic dengue fever, after an incubation period of 2 to 7 days, there is a sudden onset of fever, which rapidly rises to 39.5° to 41.4° C (103° to 106° F), usually accompanied by frontal or retro-orbital headache. Occasionally, back pain precedes the fever. A transient, macular, generalized rash that blanches under pressure may be seen during the first 24 to 48 hours of fever. The pulse rate may be slow in proportion to the degree of fever. Myalgia or bone pain occurs soon after onset and increases in severity. During the second to the sixth day of fever, nausea and vomiting are apt to occur; during this phase, generalized lymphadenopathy, cutaneous hyperesthesia or hyperalgesia, taste aberrations, and pronounced anorexia may develop.

Coincident with or 1 or 2 days after defervescence, a generalized, morbilliform, maculopapular rash appears, sparing the palms and soles. It disappears in 1 to 5 days. In some cases, there is edema of the palms and soles. Desquamation may occur. About the time of appearance of this second rash, the body temperature, which has fallen to normal, may become elevated slightly and establish the biphasic temperature curve.

Epistaxis, petechiae, and purpuric lesions, although uncommon, may occur at any stage of the disease. Swallowed blood from epistaxis may be passed by the rectum or vomited and could be interpreted as bleeding of gastrointestinal origin. Gastrointestinal bleeding, menorrhagia, and bleeding from other organs have been observed in some dengue fever outbreaks.[57, 80, 82] There is very clear evidence that peptic ulcer predisposes to gastrointestinal hemorrhage; in some cases, patients may exanguinate during an otherwise normal dengue fever.[80] This false DHF contributes greatly to confusion over pathogenic mechanisms of DHF/DSS. The pathogenesis of hemorrhagic diathesis during dengue virus infections is not known, but speculation centers on platelet abnormalities.

After the febrile stage, prolonged asthenia, mental depression, bradycardia, and ventricular extrasystoles are common in adults.

Dengue Hemorrhagic Fever/Dengue Shock Syndrome

This is an acute vascular permeability syndrome accompanied by abnormal hemostasis. The incubation period of DHF/DSS is unknown but is presumed to be that of dengue fever. In children, the progression of the illness is characteristic.[10, 50, 51, 85] A relatively mild first phase with abrupt onset of fever, malaise, vomiting, headache, anorexia, and cough may be followed after 2 to 5 days by rapid deterioration and physical collapse. In Thailand, the median day of admission to hospital after onset of fever is day 4. In this second phase, the patient usually manifests cold, clammy extremities, a warm trunk, flushed face, and diaphoresis. Patients are restless and irritable and complain of midepigastric pain. There frequently are scattered petechiae on the forehead and extremities, spontaneous ecchymoses may appear, and easy bruisability and bleeding at sites of venipuncture are common. There may be circumoral and peripheral cyanosis. Respirations are rapid and often labored. The pulse is weak, rapid, and thready, and the heart sounds are faint. The pulse pressure frequently is narrow ($\leq$20 mm Hg); the systolic and diastolic pressures may be low or unobtainable. The liver may become palpable two or three fingerbreadths below the costal margin and usually is firm and nontender. A chest radiograph shows unilateral (right) or bilateral pleural effusions. Approximately 10 per cent of patients manifest gross ecchymosis or gastrointestinal bleeding. After a 24- or 36-hour period of crisis, convalescence is fairly rapid in children who recover. The temperature may return to normal before or during the stage of shock.

PATHOGENESIS AND PATHOLOGY

In experimental studies of dengue virus infection in rhesus monkeys, after subcutaneous inoculation, virus was disseminated rapidly to regional lymph nodes and then to lymphatic tissue throughout the body.[47] Early in the viremic period, virus could be recovered only from lymph nodes, whereas 2 to 3 days later there was evidence of dissemination to skin and other tissues. Virus was recovered from skin, lymph nodes, and several leukocyte-rich tissues for up to 3 days after termination of viremia. Virus can be recovered from circulating leukocytes and from the skin only at the end of the viremic period. The number of sites of virus recovery increases as the infection progresses. Intracellular infection is terminated abruptly 2 to 3 days after viremia ceases.

Animals infected with dengue virus type 1, 3, or 4 and then infected with dengue virus type 2 circulated virus at higher titer than when the same strain was inoculated into susceptible animals.[29] This phenomenon, in vivo immunologic enhancement of dengue virus infection, forms the basis for a hypothesis of the immunopathogenesis of dengue in humans. Epidemiologic, clinical, and virologic studies of DHF/DSS in humans have shown a significant association between severe illness and infection in the presence of circulating dengue antibody, whether passively acquired of maternal origin or actively acquired from previous infection.[7, 19, 22, 38, 39, 65, 69] This circulating antibody has two biologic activities: viral neutralization and infection enhancement.[38, 39] Infants in Thailand developed DHF/DSS during dengue virus type 2 infections only when maternal neutralizing antibody had catabolized to low titer, leaving only infection-enhancing antibodies in circulation.[39] Similarly, in a prospective study of dengue virus infections in Thai children, DHF/DSS occurred in children who were circulating enhancing antibodies from a previous single dengue virus infection but did not occur in children whose first infection left them with low levels of cross-reactive dengue virus type 2 neutralizing antibodies at the time of second dengue virus infections.[38] In vitro studies of dengue virus type 2 demonstrated enhanced growth in cultures of human mononuclear phagocytes that were supplemented with very small quantities of dengue antibodies.[24] Both immunofluorescent study and virus isolation from human autopsy tissues suggest that dengue virus replicates in mononuclear phagocytes and lymphatic tissues.[4, 26–29, 31, 52] It has been proposed that the number of infected mononuclear phagocytes in individuals with naturally or passively acquired antibody may exceed that in nonimmune individuals. In this concept, increased production of infected cells may contribute to shock, possibly through the release of cytokines, themselves the products of the immune elimination of virus-infected mononuclear phagocytes through cell-mediated mechanisms.[26, 27, 29, 41] It is thought that the reduced risk to DHF/DSS of protein-calorie malnourished children and increased risk of girls compared with boys are consistent with the hypothesis that a competent immune-elimination system generates the cytokines that produce DHF/DSS.[27, 72]

Epidemiologic studies of the 1981 Cuban outbreak demonstrated a higher risk of developing DHF/DSS for whites than for blacks.[19, 40] Early in the acute stage of secondary dengue virus infection, there is rapid activation of the complement system.[6, 49] During shock, blood levels of C1q, C3, C4, C5, C6, C7, C8, and C3 proactivator are depressed and C3 catabolic rates elevated. The blood clotting and fibrinolytic systems are activated. As yet, neither the mediator of vascular permeability nor the complete mechanism of bleeding has been identified. The kinin system apparently is not involved. Recent studies suggest a role for tumor necrosis factor and interferon-gamma.[41, 81] Capillary damage allows fluid, electrolytes, protein, and, in some instances, red blood cells to leak into intravascular spaces. This internal redistribution of fluid, together with deficits due to fasting, thirsting, and vomiting, results in hemoconcentration, hypovolemia, increased cardiac work, tissue hypoxia, metabolic acidosis, and hyponatremia. A mild degree of disseminated intravascular coagulation, plus liver damage and thrombocytopenia, could contribute additively to produce hemorrhage.

If tissue culture or suckling mice are used for virus recovery, dengue virus almost invariably is absent in tissues at the time of death.[52] Tissue suspensions contain large quantities of dengue-neutralizing substances. With mosquito inoculation techniques, in some instances, virus isolation rates from tissues are improved.[76]

On pathologic examination, there usually are no gross or microscopic lesions found that might account for death.[4] In rare instances, death may be due to gastrointestinal or intracranial hemorrhages. Minimal to moderate hemorrhages are seen in the upper gastrointestinal tract, and petechial hemorrhages are frequent in the intraventricular septum of the heart, on the pericardium, and on the subserosal surfaces of major viscera. Focal hemorrhages occasionally are seen in the lungs, liver, adrenals, and subarachnoid space. The liver usually is enlarged, often with fatty changes. Yellow, watery, at times blood-tinged effusions are present in serous cavities in about three-fourths of patients. Retroperitoneal tissues are markedly edematous.

On microscopic examination, there is perivascular edema in the soft tissues and widespread diapedesis of red blood cells. There may be maturational arrest of megakaryocytes in the bone marrow, and increased numbers of them are seen in capillaries of the lungs, in renal glomeruli, and in sinusoids of the liver and spleen. Proliferation of lymphocytoid and plasmacytoid cells, lymphocytolysis, and lymphophagocytosis occur in the spleen and lymph nodes. In the spleen, malpighian corpuscle germinal centers are necrotic. There is depletion of lymphocytes in the thymus. In the liver, there are varying degrees of fatty metamorphosis, focal midzonal necrosis, and hyperplasia of the Kupffer cells. Nonnucleated cells, with vacuolated acidophilic cytoplasm resembling Councilman bodies, are seen in the sinusoids. There is a mild, proliferative glomerulonephritis. Biopsies of the skin rash reveal swelling and minimal necrosis of endothelial cells, subcutaneous deposits of fibrinogen, and, in a few cases, dengue antigen in extravascular mononuclear cells and on blood vessel walls.[28]

DIAGNOSIS

Dengue Fever

Clinical diagnosis derives from a high index of suspicion and a knowledge of the geographic distribution and ecology of dengue viruses. Activities of the patient during the period preceding the onset of illness may give important clues to the possibility of infection.

Differential diagnosis includes many viral, respiratory, and influenza-like diseases and the early stages of malaria, typhoid fever, scrub typhus, hepatitis, and leptospirosis. Abortive forms of these latter diseases may never evolve beyond a dengue-like stage. Four arbovirus diseases are dengue-like: chikungunya and o'nyong nyong fevers (togaviruses), West Nile fever (flavivirus), and Oropouche (bunyavirus). Four others are dengue-like but without rash: Colorado tick fever, sandfly fever, Ross River fever, and the mild form of Rift Valley fever. Because of the variation in clinical findings and the multiplicity of possible causative agents, the descriptive term *dengue-like disease* should be used until a specific etiologic diagnosis is provided by the laboratory.

Dengue Hemorrhagic Fever/Dengue Shock Syndrome

According to World Health Organization criteria, DHF is a dengue illness accompanied by thrombocytopenia (≤100,000 mm^3) and hemoconcentration (hematocrit ≥ 20% of recovery value). Pleural or peritoneal effusions virtually are pathognomonic. DSS is diagnosed when these manifestations are accompanied by hypotension or narrow pulse pressure (≤20 mm Hg). In areas endemic for dengue, hemorrhagic fever should be suspected in children with a febrile illness who exhibit shock and hemoconcentration with thrombocytopenia. Hypoproteinemia, hemorrhagic manifestations, and hepatic enlargement are frequent accompanying findings. Because many rickettsial diseases, meningococcemia, and other severe illnesses caused by a variety of agents may produce a similar clinical picture, the diagnosis should be made only when epidemiologic or serologic evidence suggests the possibility of dengue. Hemorrhagic manifestations have been described in other diseases of viral origin; these include the arenavirus hemorrhagic fevers of Argentina, Bolivia, and West Africa (Lassa fever); the tick-borne hemorrhagic fevers of India and the former Soviet Union; hemorrhagic fever with renal syndrome, which occurs across northern Eurasia, that is, from Scandinavia to Korea; and Marburg and Ebola virus infections in central Africa.

LABORATORY STUDIES

Etiologic diagnosis can be made by serologic study of a properly collected serum sample or by isolation of the virus.[34, 85] Blood should be obtained during or after the febrile period but before 1 month elapses after onset of illness. The acute-phase serum or plasma collected for virus isolation should be stored optimally at −65° C or colder. Serologic diagnosis depends on a fourfold or greater increase in antibody titer by hemagglutination inhibition, complement fixation, radioimmunoassay, enzyme-linked immunosorbent assay, or neutralization. IgM-capture enzyme-linked immunosorbent assay has revolutionized dengue serology. Primary and sequential (secondary) dengue virus infections result in the production of dengue-reactive IgM antibodies, which appear during the acute phase and disappear within 60 days of infection.[34] Secondary or primary dengue virus infections can be confirmed in a single serum specimen by quantitating IgM-IgG antibody ratios. IgG antibody concentrations are abundant in secondary but minimal in primary dengue virus infections. Sequential infections with dengue virus followed by Japanese encephalitis, or vice versa, produce relatively specific IgM antibodies to the recent infecting virus.[34]

A large number of techniques are available for the recovery and identification of dengue viruses.[70] Recommendations for general use have been made by a World Health Organization expert committee.[85] Acute-phase serum, mosquito suspensions, or other materials thought to contain dengue virus may be inoculated into suckling mice, which may be examined for sickness or subtle neurologic signs or challenged at 14 days with a neurovirulent dengue virus. Repeated subpassage markedly increases neurovirulence of dengue virus. Alternatively, materials may be inoculated into any of several tissue cultures of mammalian or mosquito origin and examined for plaques under agar or methyl cellulose overlay, for cytopathic effect or resistance to a challenge cytopathic virus by use of a fluid overlay, or for fluorescence or other markers with use of an appropriate detection system. Intrathoracic inoculation of *A. albopictus, A. aegypti*, or *Toxorhynchites* species is a highly sensitive dengue virus recovery system.[60, 61] The presence of virus in mosquitoes may be detected by a fluorescent antibody test, complement fixation, or inoculation of mosquito suspension in tissue culture.

TREATMENT

Dengue Fever

Treatment is supportive. Bed rest is advised during the febrile period. Antipyretics or cold sponging should be used to keep the body temperature below 40° C (104° F). Analgesics or mild sedation may be required to control pain. Fluid and electrolyte replacement therapy is required when there are deficits due to sweating, fasting, thirsting, vomiting, or diarrhea. Because of the dengue hemorrhagic diathesis, aspirin should not be given to reduce fever or control pain.

Dengue Hemorrhagic Fever/Dengue Shock Syndrome

Explicit recommendations for management of DSS have been made by a World Health Organization expert committee.[85] These, plus earlier recommendations by Cohen and Halstead,[10] are the basis of this section.

There is no specific antiviral treatment, but in DHF/DSS, symptomatic and supportive measures are effective.

The major pathophysiologic abnormality seen in DHF/DSS is an acute increase in vascular permeability that leads to leakage of plasma. Plasma volume studies revealed a reduction of more than 20 per cent in severe cases. Supporting evidence of plasma leakage includes pleural effusion on chest radiograph, hemoconcentration, and hypoproteinemia.

In the absence of increased vascular permeability, clinically significant hemoconcentration may result from thirst, dehydration, fever, anorexia, and vomiting. Fluid intake by mouth should be as ample as tolerated. Electrolyte and dextrose solution (as used in diarrheal disease) or fruit juice or both are preferable to plain water. With high fever there is a risk of convulsion, and antipyretic drugs may be indicated in patients. *Salicylates should be avoided* because they are known to cause bleeding and acidosis. Acetaminophen is preferable at the following doses: younger than 1 year of age, 60 mg/dose; 1 to 3 years of age, 60 to 120 mg/dose; 3 to 6 years of age, 120 mg/dose; 6 to 12 years of age, 240 mg/dose.

Children should be observed closely for early signs of shock. The critical period is the transition from the febrile to the afebrile phase. Frequent hematocrit determinations are essential because they reflect the degree of plasma leakage and the need for intravenous fluid. Hemoconcentration usually precedes blood pressure and pulse changes. Hematocrit should be determined daily from the third day until the temperature becomes normal for 1 or 2 days.

Oral or parenteral fluid therapy can be administered in an outpatient rehydration unit for correction of dehydration or acidosis or when there are signs of hemoconcentration. The volume of fluid and its composition are similar to the fluids used in the treatment of diarrhea with moderate dehydration. The schedule in Table 179–3 is recommended as a guideline. The fluids should consist of the following:

- One-third to one-half of the total fluid as physiologic saline solution.
- One-half to two-thirds of the remainder as 5 per cent glucose in water.
- For acidosis: one-fourth of the total fluids should be one-sixth molar sodium bicarbonate.
- Solution for fluid therapy in DHF: lactated Ringer, 5 per cent glucose in one-half physiologic saline solution, 5 per cent glucose in one-half lactated Ringer, 5 per cent glucose in one-third physiologic saline solution.
- Fluids as listed are calculated to be given over a 24-hour period. If the child seems severely dehydrated, half of the calculated fluid is given in the first 8 hours and the second half in the next 16 hours. During rapid administration of fluids, it especially is important to watch for signs of cardiac failure.

Written orders should be explicit about the type of solution and the rate of administration. A rough estimate of flow may be derived from the formula

$$\text{mL/hour} = \text{drops/minute} \times 3$$

Management of Shock

Patients should be hospitalized and immediately treated when there are any of the following signs and symptoms of shock: restlessness/lethargy, cold extremities and circumoral cyanosis, rapid and feeble pulse, narrowing of pulse pressure (≤20 mm Hg) or hypotension, and sudden rise of hematocrit

TABLE 179–3. Fluid Therapy*

	mL/kg Body Weight/24 Hours		
Weight on Admission	*First Day*	*Second Day*	*Third Day*
<7 kg	220	165	132
7–11 kg	165	132	88
12–18 kg	132	88	88
>18 kg	88	88	88

*See text for composition of fluids.

or continuously elevated hematocrit, despite administration of intravenous fluid.

Shock is a medical emergency. *An immediate administration of intravenous fluid for expanding plasma volume is essential.* Children may develop or recover from shock over a 48-hour period. Close observation 24 hours a day is imperative. Patients with similar degrees of severity should be grouped together. Those with shock require intensive 24-hour care by nurses and physicians. Paramedical workers or parents can assist in oral fluid therapy or in surveillance of the rate of intravenous fluid administration and general status of the patient.

Initial fluid therapy with lactated Ringer or isotonic saline solution (20 mL/kg intravenously) infused as rapidly as possible may be required. Positive pressure may be necessary. In continued or profound shock, plasma or plasma expanders (dextran, medium-sized molecular weight in normal saline) may be given to replace initial fluid and administered at a rate of 10 to 20 mL/kg/hour or more until improvement of vital signs is apparent. In most cases, not more than 20 to 30 mL/kg of plasma is needed.

Intravenous fluids (5% dextrose, one-half lactated Ringer or one-half normal saline) are continued, even after improvement of vital signs and a declining hematocrit. The rate of fluid replacement should be adjusted as judged by the rate of plasma loss. Plasma loss may continue for 24 or 48 hours. Microhematocrit determination is a simple and reliable index for estimating plasma leakage. Monitoring of central venous pressure may be necessary in the management of severe cases of shock that are not easily reversible.

Intravenous fluids *should be discontinued* when the hematocrit level drops to around 40 per cent and the patient's appetite improves. A good urine flow indicates sufficient circulating volume. In general, there is no need for fluid therapy beyond 48 hours after shock terminates. Resorption of extravasated plasma takes place, manifested by a further drop in hematocrit after intravenous fluid is stopped, and may cause hypervolemia, pulmonary edema, or heart failure if more fluid is given. It is important that a drop of hematocrit at this stage not be viewed as a sign of internal hemorrhage. Strong pulse and blood pressure, with wide pulse pressure, and diuresis are good vital signs found at this resorption phase. They rule out the likelihood of gastrointestinal hemorrhage, which occurs mostly during the shock stage.

Hyponatremia and commonly metabolic acidosis occur. Electrolyte and blood gas determinations should be made periodically in severely ill patients as well as in patients who do not seem to respond as promptly as expected. This will provide an estimate of the sodium deficit and help determine the presence and degree of acidosis. Acidosis, in particular, if uncorrected may lead to disseminated intravascular coagulation. The use of heparin may be indicated in some of these cases, but *extreme caution* should be exercised in its use. In general, early volume replacement and early correction of acidosis with sodium bicarbonate result in a favorable outcome, and heparin is not required. Heparin should be reserved for cases with laboratory evidence of consumptive coagulopathy (disseminated intravascular coagulation) or intractable bleeding.

Sedatives are needed in some cases because of marked agitation. Hepatotoxic drugs should be avoided. Chloral hydrate orally or rectally is recommended in a dose of 30 to 50 mg/kg as a *single hypnotic dose* (maximum dose, 1 g). In cases without pulmonary complications, paraldehyde, 0.1 mL/kg intramuscularly (maximum dose, 10 mL), also may be used.

Oxygen therapy should be given to all patients in shock. The oxygen mask or tent may increase apprehension.

Blood transfusion is indicated *only in cases with severe bleeding (e.g., gastrointestinal bleeding, hematemesis, melena).* Fresh whole blood is preferable. Blood grouping and matching for prompt treatment should be carried out as a *routine precaution* for every patient in shock.

Generally, steroids do not shorten the duration of disease or improve the prognosis in children receiving careful supportive therapy.[77]

Frequent recording of vital signs and determination of hematocrit are important in evaluating results of treatment. If patients show any signs of shock, vigorous antishock therapy should be instituted promptly. Patients should be monitored constantly until there is a reasonable certainty that the danger has passed. In practice:

1. Pulse, blood pressure, respiratory rate, and temperature should be taken every 15 to 30 minutes or more often, until shock resolves.
2. Hematocrit or hemoglobin studies should be performed every 2 hours for the first 6 hours, then every 4 hours thereafter until the patient is stable.
3. An accurate record of intake and output including the type of fluid given should be made. The frequency and volume of urine output should be recorded.

A pro forma sheet for recording symptoms, signs, and treatment of DHF and DSS cases is useful.

Management of Epidemic Dengue Hemorrhagic Fever

During epidemics, outpatient and inpatient facilities may be overwhelmed. Under these conditions, it is essential that only children requiring hospital care be admitted. A recently elevated body temperature and positive tourniquet test are sufficient to suggest DHF; when possible, a microhematocrit and platelet count should be done in the outpatient department. Patients with thrombocytopenia and elevated hematocrit counts should be sent to a rehydration ward or, if hematocrit does not fall or rises in the face of fluid therapy, admitted to hospital. If a patient lives a long distance from the hospital and nearby accommodations are not available, admission for observation may be necessary.

Triage can be done by properly instructed paramedical workers. Competent laboratory assistance is essential.

Cool extremities, skin congestion, circumoral cyanosis, and a rapid pulse are signs that suggest the need for hospitalization. Patients should be hospitalized until 2 days after fever terminates.

Regulatory Measures

Dengue diseases are not subject to international quarantine or surveillance regulations. An intensive and effective voluntary reporting system has been devised by the regional offices of the World Health Organization.

PROGNOSIS

It is not necessary to hospitalize all suspect cases of DHF because circulatory failure and shock may develop in only about a third of patients. Mild and moderate cases may be treated on an outpatient basis. For the purpose of early recognition of shock, parents should be advised to bring the patient back if there is evidence of clinical deterioration or such warning signs as restlessness with or without lethargy, severe abdominal pain, cold extremities, and skin congestion that occur on or after the third day after onset of fever.

In most cases, early and effective replacement of lost plasma with plasma, plasma expanders, and/or fluid and electrolyte solutions results in a favorable outcome. The acute onset of shock and the rapid, often dramatic clinical recovery, together with the fact that no destructive or inflammatory vascular lesions are observed, suggest that the disease is produced by transient functional vascular changes due to short-acting pharmacologic mediators.

Sequelae in dengue or in DHF have not been studied systematically. Common sequelae of mild and uncomplicated dengue virus infections include bradycardia and ventricular extrasystoles during the convalescent stage, often persisting for several weeks. A profound asthenia with or without mental depression has been described. In DHF/DSS, great care must be taken to reduce invasive procedures for managing shock. Nosocomial infections, such as gram-negative sepsis, can masquerade as DHF/DSS. Overhydration during the shock resuscitation phase may lead to heart failure and a complicated, stormy postshock stage. Infrequently, there is residual brain damage, apparently due either to prolonged shock or, occasionally, to intracranial hemorrhage. Children who develop profound shock rapidly with no detectable diastolic pressure or with unobtainable blood pressure, children in shock with delayed admission to hospital, or children in shock with gastrointestinal hemorrhage have a poor prognosis. Mortality rates may exceed 50 per cent in these groups.

PREVENTION

Tissue culture–based vaccines for dengue virus types 1, 2, 3, and 4 are immunogenic but not available for general use.[5] Prophylaxis depends on use of insecticides, repellents, body protective clothing, and screening of houses to avoid the bite of the mosquito. Destruction of *A. aegypti* breeding sites also is effective.[18] If water storage is mandatory, a tight-fitting lid or a thin layer of oil may prevent egg deposits or hatching. A larvicide, such as Abate, available as a 1 per cent sand granule formulation and effective at a concentration of 1 part per million, may be added safely to drinking water.

Epidemic Measures

World Health Organization recommendations are as follows. On the basis of epidemiologic and entomologic information, the size of the area that requires adult mosquito abatement should be determined. With technical malathion or fenitrothion at 438 mL/ha, two adulticidal treatments at a 10-day interval should be made by use of a vehicle-mounted or portable ultra-low–volume aerosol generator or mist blower.[45, 85] Cities of moderate size should stockpile at least one vehicle-mounted aerosol generator, five mist blowers, 10 swing fog machines, and 1000 liters of ultra-low–volume insecticides to be prepared to carry out adulticidal operations over a 20-km^2 area rapidly. With limited funds, such equipment and insecticides can be stockpiled centrally for rapid transportation where required. Priority areas for launching ground applications are those having a concentration of cases. Special attention should be focused on areas where people congregate during daylight hours, for example, hospitals and schools. If necessary, ultra-low–volume insecticides may be applied from aircraft. C47 or similar aircraft, smaller agricultural spray planes, and helicopters have been used to make aerial applications.

During the early stages of epidemics, ultra-low–volume spray of 4 per cent malathion in diesel oil or kerosene may be used to spray all houses within a 100-m radius of the residence of DHF patients.

Eradication and Control

A. aegypti was eradicated successfully from countries and whole continents with use of the techniques pioneered by the Rockefeller Foundation in its worldwide program to control urban yellow fever.[75] With time, the species successfully reestablished itself in much of its former range. An eradication campaign in the United States was abandoned and was replaced by a program of disease surveillance and containment of introduced virus.

Mosquito control or eradication programs require the simultaneous use of two approaches: reduction in breeding sites and application of larvicides. Alternatively, a significant reduction in population may be effected by closely spaced application of adulticides.[2]

Source reduction requires the support of the population either by legal sanctions or with voluntary actions (see the following section). Source reduction campaigns should be well organized, supervised, and evaluated. This includes proper disposal of discarded cans, bottles, tires, and other potential breeding sites not used for storage of drinking or bathing water. Sides of water storage containers should be scrubbed to remove eggs when water level is low. Drinking and bathing water storage containers and flower vases should be emptied completely once weekly. Water containers that can not be emptied should be treated with Abate 1 per cent sand granules at a dosage of 1 ppm (e.g., 10 g of sand to 100 L of water). Treatments should be repeated at intervals of 2 to 3 months.

Vehicle-mounted or portable ultra-low–volume aerosol generators or mist blowers can be used to apply technical grade malathion or fenitrothion at 438 mL/ha. Three applications made at 1-week intervals can suppress *A. aegypti* populations for about 2 months.

Health Education

A. aegypti control has been maintained effectively in some tropical areas through the simple expedient of emptying water containers once a week. During the yellow fever campaigns, strong sanitary laws made the breeding of mosquitoes on premises a crime punishable by fine or jail.[75] In the modern era, Singapore and Cuba have adopted these measures successfully. Health education through mass media or through the schools has been attempted in Burma, Thailand, Malaysia, and Indonesia without spectacular success. The goals of health education and community participation approaches are to make the population aware of the identity of the vector of DHF, to describe its biting habits (daytime feeding) and its breeding habits (containers holding clean water), and to motivate people to reduce breeding sources by emptying water from containers on a regular basis.[18] The use of piped water rather than of water storage should be encouraged. Studies in Malaysia after the 1973 epidemic of DHF indicated a very low level of functional knowledge among the inhabitants of Kuala Lumpur, Malaysia, about the vector of DHF.[16] Discouragingly, those persons who were informed correctly, in most instances, took no action to protect themselves against mosquito breeding in their homes. This may be contrasted with the present situation in Singapore, where stiff fines and frequent inspections have reduced infestation by *A. aegypti* drastically. Extensive efforts are being made to apply social science methods to gain the voluntary participation of the population in sustained mosquito control programs.[44]

References

1. Anonymous: Dengue in the Caribbean, 1977. Proceedings of a Workshop held in Montego Bay, Jamaica, May 8–11, 1978. Scientific Publication No. 375. Pan American Health Organization. Washington, D.C., 1979, 186 pp.
2. Anonymous: Programma de eliminacion del dengue y erradicacion del Aedes aegypti en Cuba. Boletin Epidemiologico PAHO 3:7–10, 1982.
3. Anonymous: Isolation of dengue type 3 virus prompts concern and action. Bull. Pan Am. Health Org. *29*:184–185, 1995.
4. Bhamarapravati, N., Toochinda, P., and Boonyapaknavik, V.: Pathology of Thailand hemorrhagic fever: A study of 100 autopsy cases. Ann. Trop. Med. Parasitol. *61*:500–510, 1967.
5. Bhamarapravati, N., Yoksan, S., Chayaniyayothin, T., et al.: Immunization with a live attenuated dengue-2-virus candidate vaccine (16681-PDK 53): Clinical, immunological and biological responses in adult volunteers. Bull. W. H. O. *65*:189–195, 1987.
6. Bokisch, V. A., Top, F. H., Jr., Russell, P. K., et al.: The potential pathogenic role of complement in dengue hemorrhagic shock syndrome. N. Engl. J. Med. *289*:996–1000, 1973.
7. Burke, D. S., Nisalak, A., Johnson, D. E., et al.: A prospective study of dengue infections in Bangkok. Am. J. Trop. Med. Hyg. *38*:172–180, 1988.
8. Carey, D. E., Myers, R. M., and Reuben, R.: Studies on dengue in Vellore, South India. Am J. Trop. Med. Hyg. *15*:580–587, 1966.
9. Carey, S. E.: Chikungunya and dengue: A case of mistaken identity? J. Hist. Med. Allied Sci. *26*:243–262, 1971.
10. Cohen, S. N., and Halstead, S. B.: Shock associated with dengue infection. I. The clinical and physiologic manifestations of dengue hemorrhagic fever in Thailand, 1964. J. Pediatr. *68*:448–456, 1966.
11. Chungue, E., Deubel, V., Cassar, O., et al.: Molecular epidemiology of dengue 3 viruses and genetic relatedness among dengue 3 strains isolated from patients with mild or severe form of dengue fever in French Polynesia. J. Gen. Virol. *74*:1765–1770, 1993.
12. Chungue, E., Cassar, O., Drouet, M. T. et al.: Molecular epidemiology of dengue-1 and dengue-4 viruses. J. Gen. Virol. *76*:1877–1884, 1995.
13. Deller, J. J., Jr., and Russell, P. K.: Fevers of unknown origin in American soldiers in Vietnam. Ann. Intern. Med. *66*:1129–1143, 1967.
14. DeMadrid, A. T., and Porterfield, J. S.: The flaviviruses (group B arboviruses): A cross neutralization study. J. Gen. Virol. *23*:91–96, 1974.
15. Derrick, E. H., and Bicks, V. A.: The limiting temperature for the transmission of dengue. Australian Ann. Med. *7*:102, 1958.
16. Dobbins, J. G., and Else, J. G.: Knowledge, attitudes and practices related to control of dengue hemorrhagic fever in an urban Malay kampung. Southeast Asian J. Trop. Med. Public Health *6*:120–126, 1975.
17. Glaziou, P., Chungue, E., Gestas P., et al.: Dengue fever and dengue shock syndrome in French Polynesia. Southeast Asian J. Trop. Med. Public Health *23*:531–532, 1992.
18. Gubler, D. J.: *Aedes aegypti* and *Aedes aegypti*–borne disease control in the 1990's: Top down or bottom up. Am. J. Trop. Med. Hyg. *40*:571–578, 1989.
19. Guzman, M. G., Kouri, G. P., Bravo, J., et al.: Dengue hemorrhagic fever in Cuba, 1981: A retrospective seroepidemiologic study. Am. J. Trop. Med. Hyg. *42*:179–184, 1990.
20. Hahn, Y. S., Galler, R., Hunkapiller, T., et al.: Nucleotide sequence of dengue 2 RNA and comparison of the encoded proteins with those of other flaviviruses. Virology *162*:167–180, 1988.
21. Halstead, S. B.: Mosquito-borne haemorrhagic fevers of South and Southeast Asia. Bull. W. H. O. *35*:3–15, 1966.
22. Halstead, S. B., Nimmannitya, S., Yamarat, C., et al.: Hemorrhagic fever in Thailand: Newer knowledge regarding etiology. Jpn. J. Med. Sci. Biol. *20*(Suppl.):96–102, 1967.
23. Halstead, S. B.: Etiologies of the experimental dengue of Siler and Simmons. Am. J. Trop. Med. Hyg. *23*:974–982, 1974.
24. Halstead, S. B., and O'Rourke, E. J.: Dengue viruses and mononuclear phagocytes. I. Infection enhancement by non-neutralizing antibody. J. Exp. Med. *146*:201–217, 1977.
25. Halstead, S. B.: Dengue haemorrhagic fever: A public health problem and a field for research. Bull. W. H. O. *58*:1–21, 1980.
26. Halstead, S. B.: Immunological parameters of togavirus disease syndromes. *In* Schlesinger, R. W. (ed.): The Togaviruses, Biology, Structure, Replication. New York, Academic Press, 1980, pp. 107–173.
27. Halstead, S. B.: The pathogenesis of dengue: Molecular epidemiology in infectious disease. The Alexander D. Langmuir Lecture. Am. J. Epidemiol. *114*:632–648, 1981.
28. Halstead, S. B.: Dengue: Hematologic aspects. Semin. Hematol. *19*:116–131, 1982.
29. Halstead, S. B.: Immune enhancement of viral infection. Prog. Allergy *31*:301–364, 1982.
30. Halstead, S. B.: Selective primary health care: Strategies for control of disease in the developing world. XI. Dengue. Rev. Infect. Dis. *6*:251–264, 1984.
31. Halstead, S. B.: Pathogenesis of dengue: Challenges of molecular biology. Science *239*:476–481, 1988.
32. Hammon, W. McD., Rudnick, A., and Sather, G. E.: Viruses associated with hemorrhagic fevers of the Philippines and Thailand. Science *131*:1102–1103, 1960.
33. He, R. T., Innis, B. L., Nisalak, A., et al.: Antibodies that block virus attachment to Vero cells are a major component of the human neutralizing antibody response against dengue virus type 2. J. Med. Virol. *45*:452–461, 1995.
34. Innis, B. L., Nisalak, A., Nimmannitya, S., et al.: An enzyme-linked immunosorbent assay to characterize dengue infections where dengue and Japanese encephalitis co-circulate. Am. J. Trop. Med. Hyg. *40*:418–427, 1989.
35. Johnson, K. M., Halstead, S. B., and Cohen, S. N.: Hemorrhagic fevers of Southeast Asia and South America: A comparative appraisal. Prog. Med. Virol. *9*:105–158, 1967.
36. Karabatsos, N. (ed.): International Catalog of Arbovirus 1985. Ft. Collins, CO, American Society of Tropical Medicine and Hygiene, 1985.
37. Kimura, R., and Hotta, S.: On the inoculation of dengue virus into mice. Nippon Igaku *3379*:629–633, 1944.
38. Kliks, S., Nisalak, A., Brandt, W. E., et al.: Evidence that maternal dengue antibodies are important in the development of dengue hemorrhagic fever in infants. Am. J. Trop. Med. Hyg. *38*:411–419, 1988.
39. Kliks, S. C., Nisalak, A., Brandt, W. E., et al.: Antibody dependent enhancement of dengue virus growth in human monocytes as a risk factor for dengue hemorrhagic fever. Am. J. Trop. Med. Hyg. *40*:444–451, 1989.
40. Kouri, G. P., Guzman, M. G., Bravo, J. R., et al.: Dengue haemorrhagic fever/dengue shock syndrome: Lessons from the Cuban epidemic. Bull. W. H. O. *67*:375–380, 1989.
41. Kurane, I., and Ennis, F. A.: Cytokines in dengue virus infections: Role of cytokines in the pathogenesis of dengue hemorrhagic fever. Semin. Virol. *5*:443–448, 1994.
42. Lewis, J. G., Chang, G. J., Lanciotti, R. S., et al.: Phylogenic relationships of dengue-2 viruses. Virology *197*:216–224, 1993.
43. La Russa, V. F., and Innis, B. L.: Mechanisms of dengue virus-induced bone marrow suppression. Baillieres Clin. Haematol. *8*:249–270, 1995.
44. Lloyd, L. S., Winch, P., Ortega-Canto, J., et al.: The design of a community-based health education intervention for the control of *Aedes aegypti*. Am. J. Trop. Med. Hyg. *50*:401–411, 1994.
45. Lofgren, C. S., Ford, H. R., Tonn, R. J., et al.: The effectiveness of ultra-low volume applications of malathion at a rate of 6 fluid ounces per acre in controlling *Aedes aegypti* in a large-scale test at Nakohn Sawan, Thailand. Bull. W. H. O. *42*:15–25, 1970.
46. Lumley, G. F., and Taylor, F. H.: Dengue. School of Public Health and Tropical Medicine Service Publication Number 3. Glebe, N. S. W., Australasian Medical Publishing Company, 1943, p. 74.
47. Marchette, N. J., Halstead, S. B., Falkler, W. A., Jr., et al.: Studies on the pathogenesis of dengue infection in monkeys. III. Sequential distribution of virus in primary and heterologous infections. J. Infect. Dis. *128*:23–30, 1973.
48. Mattingly, P. F.: Symposium on the evolution of arbovirus diseases. II. Ecological aspects of the evolution of mosquito-borne virus diseases. Trans. Soc. Trop. Med. Hyg. *54*:97–112, 1960.
49. Memoranda: Pathogenetic mechanisms in dengue haemorrhagic fever: Report of an international collaborative study. Bull. W. H. O. *48*:117–133, 1973.
50. Nimmannitya, S., Halstead, S. B., Cohen, S. N., et al.: Dengue and chikungunya virus infections in man in Thailand, 1962–1964. I. Observations on hospitalized patients with hemorrhagic fever. Am. J. Trop. Med. Hyg. *18*:954–971, 1969.
51. Nimmannitya S: Clinical spectrum and management of dengue hemorrhagic fever. Southeast Asia J. Trop. Med. Public Health 3:392–97, 1987.
52. Nisalak, A., Halstead, S. B., Singharaj, P., et al.: Observations related to pathogenesis of dengue hemorrhagic fever. III. Virologic studies of fatal disease. Yale J. Biol. Med. *42*:293–310, 1970.
53. Nogueira, R. M., Zagner, S. M., Martins, I. S., et al.: Dengue haemorrhagic fever/dengue shock syndrome (DHF/DSS) caused by serotype 2 in Brazil. Mem. Inst. Oswaldo Cruz *86*:269, 1991.
54. Qui, F. X., Gubler, D. J., Liu, D. J. et al.: Dengue in China: A clinical review. Bull. W. H. O. *71*:349–359, 1993.
55. Ramirez-Ronda, C. H., and Garcia, C. D.: Dengue in the western hemisphere. Infect. Dis. Clin. North Am. *8*:107–128, 1994.
56. Reynes, J. M., Laurent, A., Deubel, V., et al.,: The first epidemic of dengue hemorrhagic fever in French Guiana. Am. J. Trop. Med. Hyg. *51*:545–553, 1994.
57. Rice, L.: Dengue fever: A clinical report of the Galveston epidemic of 1922. Am. J. Trop. Med. *3*:73–90, 1923.
58. Rico-Hesse, R.: Molecular evolution and distribution of dengue viruses type 1 and 2 in nature. Virology *174*:479–493, 1990.
59. Roche, J. C., Cordellier, R., Hervey, J. P., et al.: Isolement de 96 souches de virus dengue 2: A partier de moustique captures en Cote-D'Ivoire et Haute-Volta. Ann. Virol. (Inst. Pasteur) *134E*:233–244, 1983.
60. Rosen, L., and Gubler, D.: The use of mosquitoes to detect and propagate dengue viruses. Am. J. Trop. Med. Hyg. *23*:1153–1160, 1974.
61. Rosen, L.: The use of *Toxorhynchites* mosquitoes to detect and propagate dengue and other arboviruses. Am. J. Trop. Med. Hyg. *30*:177–183, 1981.

62. Rosen, L., Shroyer, D. A., Tesh, R. B., et al.: Transovarial transmission of dengue viruses by mosquitoes *Aedes albopictus* and *Aedes aegypti*. Am. J. Trop. Med. Hyg. *32*:1108–1119, 1983.
63. Rudnick, A.: Ecology of Dengue Virus. Conference on DHF. Oct. 24–28, 1977, Singapore. Asian J. Infect. Dis. *2*:156–160, 1978.
64. Russell, P. K., and Nisalak, A.: Dengue virus identification by the plaque reduction neutralization test. J. Immunol. *99*:291, 1967.
65. Russell, P. K., Yuill, T. M., Nisalak, A., et al.: An insular outbreak of dengue hemorrhagic fever. II. Virologic and serologic studies. Am. J. Trop. Med. Hyg. *17*:600–608, 1968.
66. Sabin, A. B., and Schlesinger, R. W.: Production of immunity to dengue with virus modified by propagation in mice. Science *101*:640–642, 1945.
67. Sabin, A. B.: The dengue group of viruses and its family relationships. Bacteriol. Rev. *14*:225–232, 1950.
68. Sabin, A. B.: Research on dengue during World War II. Am. J. Trop. Med. Hyg. *1*:30–50, 1952.
69. Sangkawibha, N., Rojansuphot, S., Ahandrik, S., et al.: Risk factors in dengue shock syndrome: A prospective epidemiologic study in Rayong, Thailand. Am. J. Epidemiol. *120*:653–669, 1984.
70. Schlesinger, R. W.: Dengue Viruses. Virology Monograph 16. Vienna, Springer, 1977.
71. Sheppard, P. M., MacDonald, W. W., Tonn, R. J., et al.: The dynamics of an adult population of *Aedes aegypti* in relation to dengue haemorrhagic fever in Bangkok. J. Anim. Ecol. *38*:661–702, 1969.
72. Siler, J. F., Hall, M. W., and Hitchens, A. P.: Dengue: Its history, epidemiology, mechanisms of transmission, etiology, clinical manifestations, immunity and prevention. Philippine J. Sci. *29*:1–304, 1926.
73. Simmons, J. S., St. John, J. H., and Reynolds, F. H. K.: Experimental studies of dengue. Philippine J. Sci. *44*:1–247, 1931.
74. Srivastava, V. K., Suri, S., Bhasin, A., et al.: An epidemic of dengue haemorrhagic fever and dengue shock syndrome in Delhi: A clinical study. Ann. Trop. Paediatr. *10*:329–334, 1990.
75. Strode, G. K. (ed.): Yellow Fever. New York, McGraw-Hill, 1951.
76. Sumarmo, Wulur, H., Jahja, E., et al.: Clinical observations on virologically confirmed fatal dengue infections in Jakarta, Indonesia. Bull. W. H. O. *61*:693–701, 1983.
77. Tassniyom, S., Vasanawathana, V., Chirawatkul, A., et al.: Failure of high-dose methylprednisolone in established dengue shock synrome: A placebo-controlled, double-blind study. Pediatrics *92*:111–115, 1993.
78. Thisyakorn, U., and Nimmannitya, S.: Nutritional status of children with dengue hemorrhagic fever. Clin. Infect. Dis. *16*:295–297, 1993.
79. Trent, D. W., Grant, J. A., Monath, T. P., et al.: Genetic variation and microevolution of dengue 2 virus in Southeast Asia. Virology *172*:523–535, 1989.
80. Tsai, J. C., Kuo, C. H., and Chen, P. C.: Upper gastrointestinal bleeding in dengue fever. Am. J. Gastroenterol. *86*:33–35, 1991.
81. Vitarana, T., and Jayasekara, N.: Dengue haemorrhagic fever outbreak in Sri Lanka. Southeast Asian J. Trop. Med. Public Health *21*:682, 1990.
82. Wen, K. H., Sheu, M. M., Chung, C. B., et al.: The ocular fundus findings in dengue fever. Kaohsiung. J. Med. Sci. *5*:24–30, 1989.
83. Westaway, E. G., Brinton, M. A., Gaidamovich, S. Y. A., et al.: *Flaviviridae*. Intervirology *24*:183–192, 1985.
84. Western Pacific regional Officer, WHO: Personal communication, 1995.
85. World Health Organization: Dengue Haemorrhagic Fever: Diagnosis, Treatment Prevention and Control. Geneva, World Health Organization, 1994.

❑ ❑ ❑

CHAPTER 179 (D)

Japanese Encephalitis

Theodore F. Tsai

Japanese encephalitis (JE), a mosquito-borne flaviviral infection, is the leading cause of childhood viral encephalitis in Asia.

HISTORY

JE first was recognized after an outbreak in Japan in 1924 led to 6125 cases. The disease was differentiated from von Economo's encephalitis, which had a different seasonality and clinical features, by being designated Japanese B encephalitis. In retrospect, similar summer-autumn outbreaks were recognized as early as 1871 to 1873. In 1933, Hayashi recovered the virus in monkeys and from the brain of a patient and, in 1938, Mitamura confirmed its mosquito-borne mode of transmission by isolating the virus from *Culex tritaeniorhynchus*.[31] Inactivated vaccine prepared from infected mouse brain was licensed in Japan in 1956, and its use has led to control of the disease in developed Asian countries.[61] Because poliomyelitis has been brought under control in Asia, JE has become the leading viral central nervous system infection on that continent.

ETIOLOGIC AGENT

JE virus is a member of an antigenic complex that includes St. Louis, Murray Valley, Kunjin encephalitis, and West Nile viruses.[9, 54] Molecular taxonomic studies based on nucleotide sequences of the E protein gene or the preM region have segregated JE strains into four genotypes that can be mapped roughly to regions of epidemic and endemic transmission in temperate Asia and India or Southeast Asia (three types, including one limited to Indonesia).[11] A correspondence of genotype to human virulence has not been demonstrated epidemiologically. Sequence analysis has been helpful in tracing the potential origins of epidemic strains.

Strains isolated from nature exhibit a range of virulence for mice; with repeated cell culture passage, neuroattenuated strains have been produced for use as vaccines. Combinations of mutations in genes of the E glycoprotein, nonstructural proteins, and noncoding regions have been associated with attenuation of the live vaccine strain SA 14-14-2.[21, 57] Comparisons of neurovirulent and attenuated viruses have found that single codon changes (resulting in amino acid changes in the E protein) are sufficient to make fully replicative viruses avirulent.[78] The development of candidate vaccines, engineered by the introduction of attenuating mutations, has been aided greatly by the development of infectious clones derived from ligated cDNA templates.

As with other flaviviruses, important biologic functions, such as viral neutralization, are associated with the E glycoprotein. Its proper processing in conjunction with other viral proteins is necessary for authentic presentation. Canarypox and vaccinia recombinant viruses containing the sequences of JE prM, E, and NS1 genes protect mice from challenge and have been immunogenic in swine. These recombinant viruses also may have utility as synthetic antigens in diagnostic assays.[40]

ECOLOGY

In its basic transmission cycle, JE virus is transmitted between birds, especially certain egrets and herons, and *Culex* mosquitoes.[4, 8, 69] However, pigs, where they are present, are the most important source of viral amplification (Fig. 179–7). Pigs develop high sustained viremias and may be hosts to thousands of mosquitoes in a single night, providing an abundant source of infected mosquitoes that can transmit the infection further. In the typical setting in rural Asia, the onset of human cases each summer follows shortly after infections in pigs.[1, 63, 85] The importance of pigs to epidemic transmission can be seen in countries such as Bangladesh, Malaysia, and Indonesia, where JE occurs principally among the non-Moslem population who do not eschew pigs. Ducklings, pigeons, sparrows, and possibly other small birds found near human residences may play a role in viral amplification. JE outbreaks have occurred in areas devoid of pigs, where avians have been the principal amplifying hosts.[3, 18, 68]

C. tritaeniorhynchus is the principal mosquito vector in most areas of Asia, although in various regions, related species

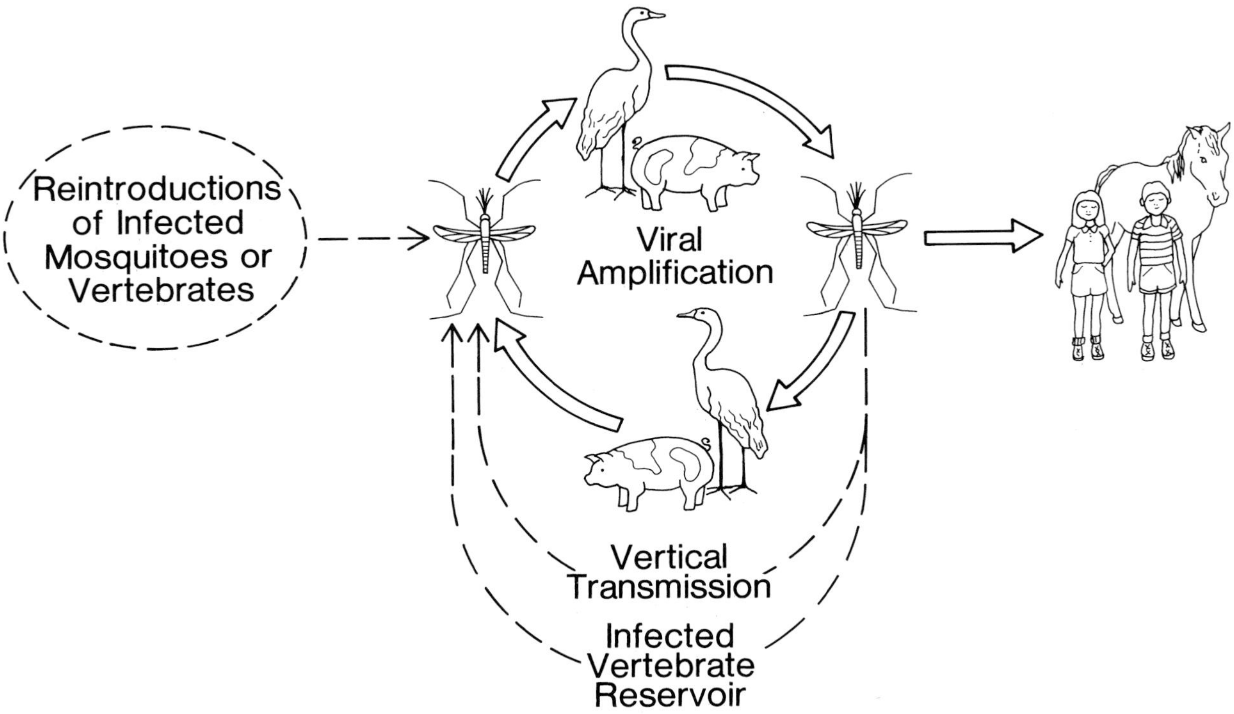

FIGURE 179–7. *Transmission cycle of Japanese encephalitis virus. Speculative portions of the cycle are shown in broken lines.*

(*C. pseudovishnui, C. vishnui, C. gelidus, C. fuscocephalus,* and *C. bitaeniorhynchus*) are important locally.[69, 77] Certain anophelines may contribute to JE transmission in northeastern India. The principal *Culex* vectors use ground pools and especially rice paddies in their preadult stages. Immense numbers of vector mosquitoes are produced from flooded rice paddies that frequently surround individual residences and villages. With the custom of keeping pigs near or inside houses, all elements of the viral transmission cycle are found in close proximity to human activity. *C. tritaeniorhynchus* is zoophilic and prefers to feed on large animals over humans. The mosquito is most active in the evening and night and feeds outdoors.

Domestic animals, such as dogs and cattle, can be infected but do not develop sufficient viremias to support further transmission. Because they are attractive to JE vectors, their presence may divert mosquitoes from humans (zooprophylaxis). Horses develop clinical illness after infection; equine vaccines are administered in China, Mongolia, and Japan to prevent cases and periodic outbreaks. Adult pigs remain asymptomatic after infection; however, sows infected during pregnancy abort or deliver piglets with lethal congenital malformations.

The overwintering mechanism for JE virus has not been defined clearly, although there is considerable evidence to suggest a carryover of virus in mosquito eggs with reestablishment of the transmission cycle by vertically infected mosquitoes.[15, 69] Viral persistence in local mammalian reservoirs such as bats and reintroductions from external sources by migrating birds or windblown mosquitoes also have been proposed.

EPIDEMIOLOGY

The disease occurs mainly in rural areas, where high levels of virus transmission lead to infection at an early age. Nearly all cases occur in children younger than 10 years of age, with a slight predominance in boys.[83] More than 99 per cent of infections are subclinical, and cumulative exposures with age lead to seroprevalence rates of 80 per cent or more by adulthood.[19] In Japan and other developed Asian countries, where children are protected by mass vaccination, adult cases occur principally in the elderly. Waning immunity or other biologic factors associated with aging have been speculated to be risk factors.[38]

Transmission is seasonal, spanning the late summer and early fall in temperate regions (July to September), with a longer interval in southern China and Southeast Asia (April to November). The seasonality is more complex in tropical areas, where mosquito abundance follows monsoonal rains with a possibility of two epidemic seasons or year-round transmission in some tropical locations. Although mosquito abundance usually corresponds to the rainy season, in many locations, vector populations now follow irrigation-controlled schedules of rice field flooding.[59, 60]

JE occurs in nearly every country of Asia (Fig. 179–8).[29] Currently, 30,000 to 50,000 cases are reported annually from the region. Transmission is endemic, with annual incidence rates of 1 to 10 per 100,000 population in China and most areas of Southeast Asia. Epidemic attack rates as high as 100 per 100,000 population have been reported. Only sporadic cases are reported from Indonesia, Malaysia, and the Philippines, and periodic, often sizable, outbreaks typify transmission in India. Rare outbreaks have occurred in Oceania, on Guam and Saipan in 1949 and 1989, respectively, and in the Torres Strait, between Australia and New Guinea, in 1995.[22, 62] These outbreaks appeared to have followed introductions of the virus by migrating birds or other means, coupled with unusual conditions of human activity or weather patterns. Few cases currently are reported from countries where vaccination rates are high (e.g., Japan, Korea, Taiwan) and where development through urbanization, decreased land under cultivation, and an improved standard of living have reduced human exposure. The use of agricultural pesticides and centralized pig rearing also may have contributed to a decline of infected vectors in these countries.[72] Despite the significant reduction in human cases, JE persists in focal sites of enzootic viral transmission.

Although economic development has paralleled a decline of JE in some countries, in other areas, development, in the form of deforestation, construction of dams, and irrigation schemes, has led to increases in JE virus transmission or its emergence in areas where the disease had not occurred previously. Examples include development projects in the Terai of southern Nepal and the Mahaweli Valley in Sri Lanka, where JE and malaria have become hyperendemic after large-scale programs of deforestation and agricultural development.

Travelers to areas where JE is endemic may be at risk for acquiring the illness.[84] However, risk among the general traveling public is low: fewer than 30 cases have been reported among travelers from North America, Europe, and Australia in the last 20 years, many of them in military personnel and their family members. Risk has been estimated in the range of 1 per 15,000 to 1 per 150,000 person-months of exposure. This low rate can be understood by factoring the probability of developing an illness after a single mosquito bite: only certain vector species transmit the virus, less than 3 per cent of vector mosquitoes usually are infected, and only one in several hundred infections leads to clinical illness. Because the principal vector species are found in rural areas and they mainly feed outdoors and in the evening and night, risk is low among the vast majority of travelers who can avoid these circumstances of exposure.

CLINICAL MANIFESTATIONS

Only one of several hundred infections leads to clinical illness, and the overwhelming majority of infections are inapparent or manifest as mild self-limited illnesses. Patients who come to medical attention may have aseptic meningitis or encephalitis, of whom 5 to 25 per cent die. After an incubation period of 4 to 14 days, the earliest symptoms are lethargy, nausea or abdominal pain, headache, and feverishness (Fig. 179–9). Over a period of 2 to 3 days, lethargy increases and the child may exhibit uncharacteristic patterns of behavior.[2, 35, 42, 46, 48, 64, 65, 79] In other cases, there may be a long prodrome of a week or more. Vomiting is common, and there may be periods of confusion or agitation and unsteadiness. The child may develop a sudden convulsion. Unusual presentations, such as acute psychosis and Guillain-Barré syndrome, have been reported.[67, 76]

The principal physical findings are high fever and obvious alterations of consciousness, ranging from mild mental clouding to frank disorientation and delirium to coma. Some children exhibit bizarre behaviors, including shouting, spitting, and other personality changes. Mutism is a presenting feature in some cases. Signs of meningeal irritation can be elicited in one-third to two-thirds of cases. Cranial nerve palsies, mainly disconjugate gaze and central facial paralysis, are observed in one-third of cases. Muscular weakness, either flaccid or spastic, is usual. Weakness may be generalized or in many cases is asymmetric, with hemiparesis or unusual distributions of flaccid and spastic paralysis. Muscular tone usually is increased with hyperreflexia and ankle clonus; Babinski sign and other abnormal reflexes are variable. Some patients exhibit erratic flailing movements. Tremor, rigidity,

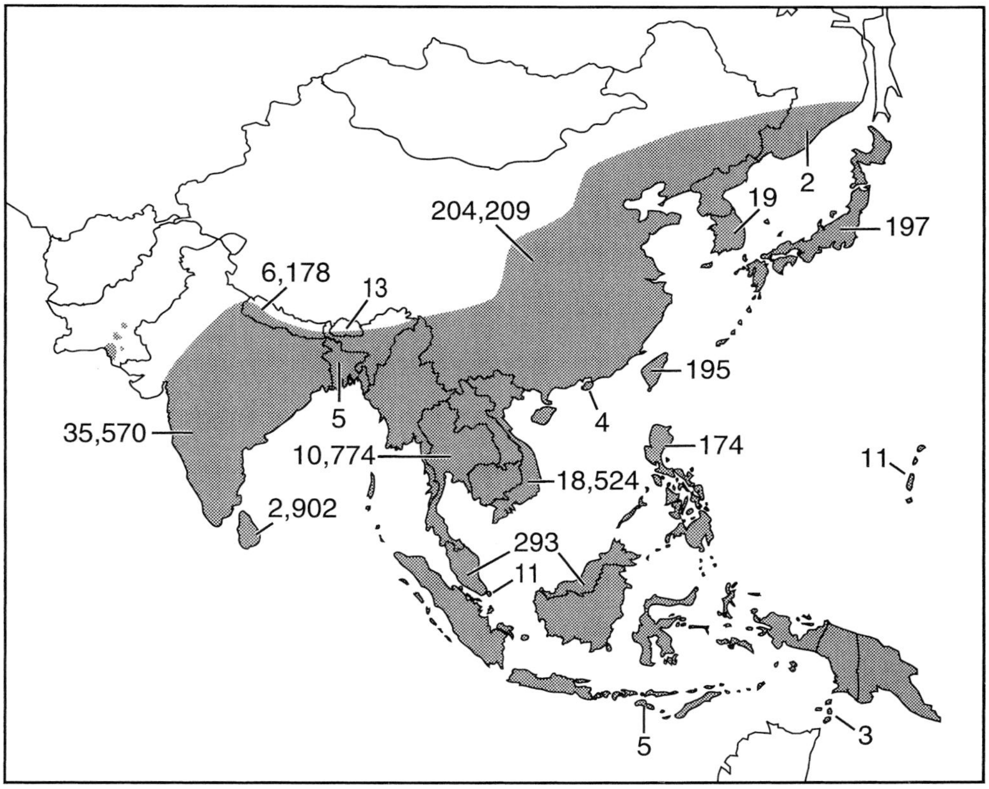

FIGURE 179–8. *Geographic distribution of Japanese encephalitis and reported cases 1985 to 1994. Torres Strait cases are from 1995.*

Clinical Stages of Japanese Encephalitis

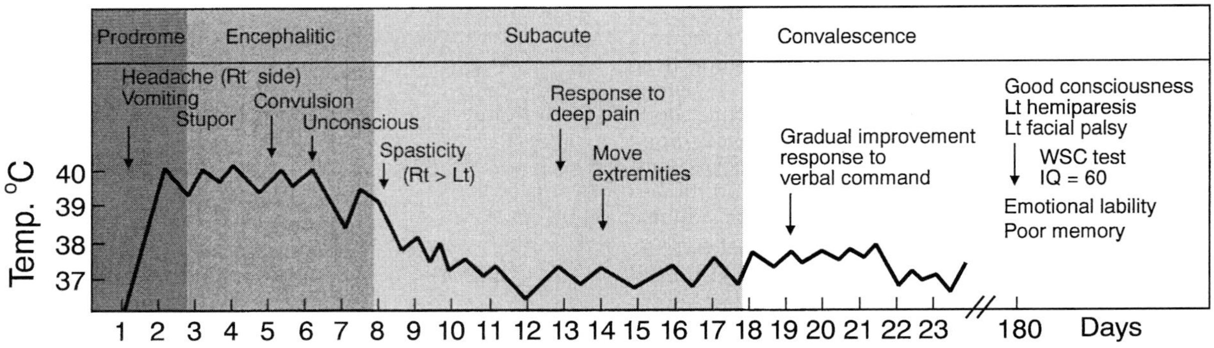

WBC	13800	12800	4050		2650
PMN %	97	86	36		69
L%	1	14	55		20
M%	2		6		
Plt.	172,000	adequate			adequate
CSF Cells		304		4	
Mononuclear		93%			
Protein		68 mg %			
Sugar		64 mg %			
CSF MAC JE		72		490	
GAC JE		100		>889	

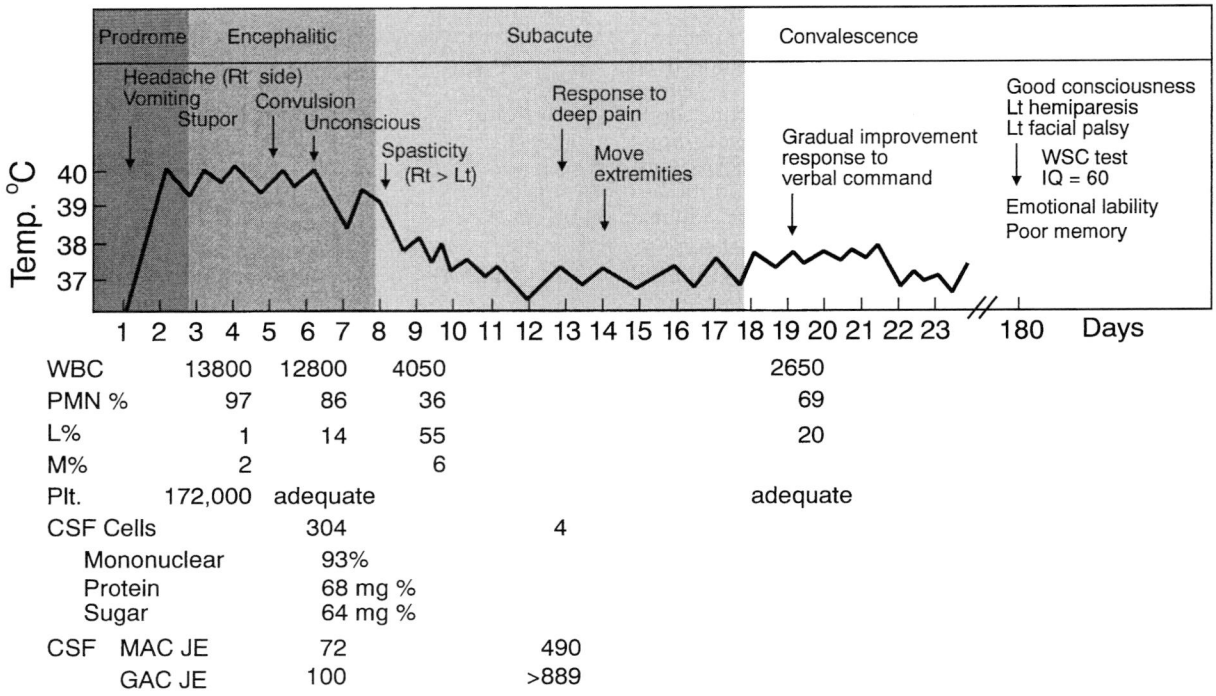

FIGURE 179–9. *Clinical stages of a typical Japanese encephalitis case.*

expressionless facies, or thick slurred speech may be presenting features, but it is more usual for choreoathetosis and other extrapyramidal signs to become evident in the second week of illness. Fifty to 75 per cent of cases develop focal or generalized convulsions. Papilledema is seen in 10 per cent of cases, and patients occasionally may be hypertensive. Patients with fulminant infections usually die during the 5 days of illness.

In the majority of other cases, fever defervesces during the next week and neurologic function gradually improves over several weeks. Further recovery of motor function occurs over the next several months to years. In more than one-third of patients, coma and respiratory failure necessitate ventilatory support. During this prolonged period of recovery from coma and paralysis, stasis ulcers, urinary tract infections, pneumonia, and bacteremia are frequent complications and may be secondary causes of death.

Routine laboratory studies initially show a peripheral leukocytosis, often with a left shift; the total leukocyte count may be as high as 30,000/mm^3. Opening pressures on lumbar puncture usually are normal or slightly elevated. Cerebrospinal fluid pleocytosis ranges from less than 10 cells to several thousand, with a median of several hundred/mm^3. A lymphocytic pleocytosis is typical, but in some cases there is an initial predominance of polymorphonuclear cells. The cerebrospinal fluid sugar and protein typically are normal (80 per cent of cases); when elevated, protein levels rarely exceed 100 mg per cent.

Electroencephalograms typically show diffuse delta wave activity; spike and seizure discharges are uncommon. Computed tomograms show diffuse white matter edema and nonenhancing low-density areas, mainly in the thalamus, basal ganglia, and pons.[44, 53, 75] Thalamic lesions frequently are associated with unilateral or bilateral hemorrhages. A thalamic location of involvement is consistent with the electroencephalogram's pattern of slowing. Magnetic resonance imaging studies show a similar distribution of abnormalities, with high signal intensity lesions in the thalamus, basal ganglia, cerebellum, pons, midbrain, and spinal cord.[36, 53] Electromyograms show a neurogenic pattern consistent with anterior horn cell involvement. Central motor conduction times are prolonged, indicating diffuse subcortical damage.[53]

PATHOLOGY

Pathologic changes are found in lungs and viscera in addition to the brain.[14, 26, 33, 34, 47, 73, 87] Grossly, the brain appears swollen, and the meninges may be congested. Punctate hemorrhages may be visible macroscopically. Microscopic examination discloses a moderate inflammatory response in the meninges. Foci of neuronal degeneration with parenchymal and perivascular inflammatory response are found principally in the thalamus and brain stem and also in the hippocampus, the temporal cortex, cerebellum, and spinal cord. Microglial nodules surround areas of neuronophagia. Sharply defined round areas of softening or necrolysis without an inflammatory response often are seen. Loss of Purkinje cells and glial shrubs may be seen in the cerebellum.

PATHOPHYSIOLOGY

After virus is introduced by a mosquito bite, replication locally and within regional lymphatic tissues leads to a secondary amplified viremia and infection of various organs and the brain. Neuroinvasion is believed to occur through cerebral capillaries, with infection crossing from the vascular side of the endothelial cell to the perivascular space with subsequent neuronal infection.[16] Neurons show evidence of viral antigen in the cell body, axons, and dendrites, and virus spreads within the brain from cell to cell.[14, 34] Infiltrating T cells elicit a broad inflammatory response, with B and T cells and macrophages in perivascular cuffs and macrophages and T cells in the parenchyma. Neuronophagia proceeds with the formation of microglial nodules and the eventual disappearance of neurons, leaving ghost-like remnants and antigen accumulated within macrophages.[34]

The rapidity of the neutralizing antibody response is believed to be a principal determinant of outcome.[34, 56] Most fatal cases occur in the first 5 days after onset of illness, and no antibody can be detected in the cerebrospinal fluid. In experimentally infected animals, passive immunization reduces mortality, even when given 4 to 5 days after inoculation.[56, 58] However, other studies have found that antigen persists in neurons for extensive periods in the presence of intrathecal antibody and immune complexes, suggesting a failure of antibody-mediated viral clearance.[14] A role for immunopathologic mechanisms, including development of antineurofilament antibodies, has been proposed as an alternate correlate of outcome.[13]

Why the majority of JE virus infections are subclinical or lead to no signs of central nervous system infection is unclear. Epidemiologic observations indicate an elevated risk for acquiring the disease among the elderly and increased severity in young children, but the biologic basis for these increased susceptibilities has not been defined. Previous dengue virus infections, providing cross-reactive flaviviral immunity, may modulate the severity of JE in some cases.[17] Pathologic observations have shown a higher prevalence of neurocysticercosis in fatal JE cases than in deaths from other causes, suggesting that physical and/or physiologic disruptions of the brain architecture by infection or other mechanisms could facilitate neuroinvasion.[12, 49] Experimental dual infections of animals with JE virus and other agents support this hypothesis.[50] Other host factors associated with risk of illness and poor outcome in experimental animals include a specific gene defining resistance, age, sex hormones, and cold and stress response.[37, 39]

COMPLICATIONS

The principal complications are secondary bacterial infections and stress-induced gastrointestinal hemorrhage occurring in the acute and subacute phases of illness. Hyponatremia due to inappropriate antidiuretic hormone secretion is common. Concurrent malaria and other parasitic or bacterial infections may complicate management.

Cases of clinical relapse, with seizures, coma, and weakness, several occurring 6 to 9 months after recovery from acute illness, have been reported. These patients and other asymptomatic recovered patients had evidence of persistent JE virus infection of peripheral blood mononuclear cells.[74] A study of 253 patients found laboratory evidence of subacute central nervous system infection in 5 per cent of cases, with persistent intrathecal production of JE virus–specific IgM beyond 50 to 180 days or cerebrospinal fluid containing JE virus antigen or virus more than 3 weeks after recovery.[66] Further studies are needed to confirm and characterize JE virus persistence and its clinical significance.

JE acquired during the first two trimesters of pregnancy may lead to fetal infection and miscarriage. JE virus has been isolated from products of conception in a few cases. Infections acquired during the third trimester have not been associated with adverse outcomes to the pregnancy.[10, 52] It is unknown whether congenital JE virus infections are associated with sublethal malformations in humans or whether congenital infections follow subclinical JE virus infection.

LABORATORY DIAGNOSIS

A specific diagnosis can be confirmed serologically by identifying JE virus–specific IgM antibody in serum or cerebrospinal fluid by enzyme-linked immunosorbent assay (ELISA) or by demonstrating fourfold titer changes in neutralization, hemagglutination inhibition, complement fixation, or immunofluorescent antibodies between acute- and convalescent-phase serum samples.[6, 82] Serologic cross-reactions with dengue virus and other flaviviruses are a common problem that sometimes can be resolved with cross-neutralization. Some laboratories have established empiric ELISA absorbance cutoffs that differentiate dengue and JE virus infections.[32] IgM can be detected in serum and/or cerebrospinal fluid of nearly all cases by 1 week after onset of illness.[6] Patients who are moribund or are severely ill on admission may be seronegative. It is principally from these patients, who have not mounted an immunologic response, in whom viral isolation from cerebrospinal fluid is most likely to be successful.[7] Limited experience with polymerase chain reaction suggests a sensitivity of less than 10 per cent with cerebrospinal fluid samples.[55] Immunofluorescent staining of cerebrospinal fluid mononuclear cells can provide a specific diagnosis within several hours after a lumbar puncture, but this procedure has a reported sensitivity of only 60 per cent.[51]

JE virus occasionally can be isolated from the blood of patients in the preneuroinvasive phase of illness, usually no later than 6 to 7 days after onset. Virus can be recovered from brain biopsy and autopsy material by intracerebral inoculation of baby mice and in various cell cultures, such as primary chick or duck embryo cells, and lines of Vero, LLCMK-2, C6-36, and AP61 cells.[82]

DIFFERENTIAL DIAGNOSIS

In rural Asia, the principal considerations include tuberculous and pyogenic meningitis; typhoid fever manifesting with tremors and ataxia[80]; cerebral malaria; dengue virus infection with encephalopathy[25]; and herpes simplex and measles viruses, enterovirus, HIV, and other causes of viral encephalitis. In a series from Lucknow, India, in which 394 children 6 months to 12 years of age with acute encephalopathic illness underwent virologic studies, 23 per cent had JE.[43] Some scrub typhus patients develop meningitis or encephalitis; rash, adenopathy, and an eschar, if present, are helpful diagnostic signs. Acute encephalitis with convulsions is encountered in two-thirds of patients with neurocysticercosis, which may be detected by brain imaging. Neurocysticercosis itself may increase risk for JE (see Pathophysiology).

Noninfectious causes of acute encephalopathy to consider include heat stroke, vascular occlusions and intracranial hemorrhage, acute electrolyte disturbances, lead encephalopathy and other poisonings, especially due to insect repellents, and inherited metabolic disorders.

TABLE 179–4. Risk of Japanese Encephalitis (JE) by Country, Region, and Season

Country	Affected Areas/Jurisdictions	Transmission Season	Comments
Bangladesh	Few data, probably widespread	Possibly July–December as in northern India	Outbreak reported from Tangail district, Dacca division; sporadic cases in Rajshahi division
Bhutan	No data	No data	Not applicable
Brunei	Presumed to be sporadic—endemic as in Malaysia	Presumed year-round transmission	
Burma	Presumed to be endemic—hyperendemic countrywide	Presumed to be May–October	Repeated outbreaks in Shan State in Chiang Mai Valley
Cambodia	Presumed to be endemic—hyperendemic countrywide	Presumed to be May–October	Cases reported from Phnom Penh
Hong Kong	Rare cases in new territories	April–October	Vaccine not routinely recommended
India	Reported cases from all states except Arunachal, Dadra, Daman, Diu, Gujarat, Himachal, Jammu, Kashmir, Lakshadweep, Meghalaya, Nagar Haveli, Orissa, Punjab, Rajasthan, and Sikkim	*South India:* May–October in Goa; July–January in Tamil Nadu August–December in Karnataka; second peak April–June in Mandya district *Andrha Pradesh:* September–December *North India:* July–December	Outbreaks in West Bengal, Bihar, Karnataka, Tamil Nadu, Andrha Pradesh, Kerala, Assam, Uttar Pradesh, Manipure, and Goa Urban cases reported, e.g., Lucknow
Indonesia	Kalimantan, Bali, Nusa Tenggara, Sulawesi, Mollucas, West Irian Java, and Lombok	Probably year-round risk; varies by island; peak risks associated with rainfall, rice cultivation, and presence of pigs Peak periods of risk November–March; June–July in some years	Human cases recognized on Bali and Java only
Japan*	Rare—sporadic cases on all islands except Hokkaido	June–September except Ryukyu Islands (Okinawa): April–October	Vaccine not routinely recommended for travel to Tokyo and other major cities; enzootic transmission without human cases observed on Hokkaido
Korea	No data from North Korea; South Korea sporadic—endemic with occasional outbreaks	July–October	Last major outbreaks in 1982–1983
Laos	Presumed to be endemic—hyperendemic countrywide	Presumed to be May–October	No data available
Malaysia	Sporadic—endemic in all states of Peninsula, Sarawak, and probably Sabah	No seasonal pattern; year-round transmission	Most cases from Penang, Perak, Salangor, Johore, and Sarawak
Nepal	Hyperendemic in southern lowlands (Terai); first outbreak in Katmandu valley in 1995	July–December	Vaccine recommended for travelers to lowland areas and persons with outdoor exposure in Katmandu valley
People's Republic of China	Cases in all provinces except Xizang (Tibet), Xinjiang, and Qinghai Hyperendemic in southern China; endemic—periodically epidemic in temperate areas	*Northern China:* May–September *Southern China:* April–October (Guangshi, Yunnan, Gwangdong, and southern Fujian, Szechuan, Guizhou, Hunan, and Jiangsi provinces)	Vaccine not routinely recommended for travelers to urban areas only
Pakistan	May be transmitted in central deltas	Presumed to be June–January	Cases reported near Karachi; endemic areas overlap those for West Nile virus
Philippines	Presumed to be endemic on all islands	Uncertain, speculations based on locations and agroecosystems: *West Luzon, Mindoro, Negro Palowan:* April–November; *Elsewhere:* year-round; greatest risk April–January	Outbreaks described in Nueva Ecija, Luzon, and Manila
Russia	Far eastern maritime areas south of Khabarousk	Peak period July–September	First human cases in 30 years recently reported
Singapore	Rare cases	Year-round transmission; April peak	Vaccine not routinely recommended

TABLE 179–4. Risk of Japanese Encephalitis (JE) by Country, Region, and Season *Continued*

Country	Affected Areas/Jurisdictions	Transmission Season	Comments
Sri Lanka	Endemic in all but mountainous areas; periodically epidemic in northern and central provinces	October–January; secondary peak of enzootic transmission May–June	Recent outbreaks in central (Anuradhapura) and northwestern provinces
Taiwan*	Endemic, sporadic cases; island-wide	April–October; June peak	Cases reported in and around Taipei
Thailand	Hyperendemic in north; sporadic—endemic in south	May–October	Annual outbreaks in Chiang Mai Valley; sporadic cases in Bangkok suburbs
Vietnam	Endemic, hyperendemic in all provinces	May–October	Highest rates in and near Hanoi
Western Pacific and Australia	Epidemics reported in Guam, Saipan (northern Mariana Islands) and Torres Strait Islands (Australia)	September–January in the Pacific; February–April in the Torres Strait	Enzootic cycle may not be sustainable; epidemics only follow introductions of virus

*Local JE incidence rates may not reflect risks to nonimmune visitors accurately because of high immunization rates in local populations. Humans are incidental to the transmission cycle. High levels of viral transmission may occur in the absence of human disease.

Note: Assessments are based on publications, surveillance reports, and personal correspondence. Extrapolations have been made from available data. Transmission patterns may change.

From Tsai, T. F., and Yu, Y. X.: Japanese encephalitis vaccines. *In* Plotkin, S., and Mortimer, E. A. (eds.): Vaccines. 2nd ed. Philadelphia, W. B. Saunders, 1995, pp. 671–713.

TREATMENT

No specific antiviral therapy is available. A few patients have been treated with alpha interferon, but efficacy has not been evaluated in wider trials.[23, 24] Supportive care is critical to outcome, and control of intracranial pressure is believed to be an important risk factor. Mannitol is used routinely in many areas of Asia, but early high-dose dexamethasone therapy was shown to have no clinical efficacy in a prospective controlled clinical trial.[28] Corticosteroids also have been given, without apparent benefit, in late stages of illness as empiric therapy of late neurologic changes that were presumed to have an immunopathologic basis.[13] Other supportive measures, including control of fever and convulsions, attention to fluid balance, respiratory support, and prevention and treatment of secondary infections, have contributed to increased survival and improved outcomes.

PROGNOSIS

The case fatality ratio varies from 10 to 35 per cent, depending on the accessibility and quality of supportive care. Younger children (<10 years of age) are more likely to die of the infection and to have more serious neurologic complications acutely and as sequelae. Gross neurologic impairment, such as paralysis, weakness, abnormal muscular tone, seizures, ataxia, and extrapyramidal movement disorders, are found in about one-third to one-half of recovered patients several months to a year after onset.[45, 71] Electroencephalogram abnormalities have been detected in more than 50 per cent of surviving children 1 year after recovery. Behavioral disorders and subnormal performance on psychologic testing may be found in up to 75 per cent of surviving patients 5 years after onset. Thus, in areas where the disease is prevalent, JE may account for substantial disability among the resident population.

PREVENTION

In areas of Asia where JE is endemic, the disease is prevented by childhood immunization.[84] Three JE vaccines are used, of which the most widely distributed is an inactivated vaccine produced from infected mouse brain.[61] The others, a killed primary hamster kidney cell–derived vaccine and a live vaccine, made from the attenuated SA14-14-2 strain, are available exclusively in the People's Republic of China.[86] Inactivated mouse brain–derived JE vaccine is distributed in the United States and internationally for use in travelers. Two doses, the schedule recommended in Asia, have a protective efficacy of 91 per cent.[27] However, three subcutaneous doses of 1.0 mL (days 0, 7, and 30 or 0, 7, and 14) are needed to produce adequate neutralizing antibody levels in persons from developed countries. The additional dose appears to be necessary because previous flaviviral immunity, generally lacking in residents of developed countries, primes the immune response to vaccination.[84] High antibody titers are sustained for at least 3 years, after which a booster dose may be given.[20] The dose for children 1 to 3 years of age is 0.5 mL; the vaccine is not approved for use in children younger than 1 year of age. JE vaccine has been given concurrently with hepatitis A and diptheria-tetanus-pertussis vaccines without interference.[41]

Local reactions and mild systemic reactions, such as fever, headache, and myalgias, occur in 10 to 25 per cent of vaccines.[30] Allergic reactions, consisting of generalized urticaria and facial and peripheral angioedema, have been a cause of concern because of the potential for respiratory obstruction and anaphylaxis and because the onset of reactions typically has been delayed for 12 to 72 hours after vaccine administration.[1, 70, 84] In addition to antihistamines, parenteral corticosteroid therapy often has been needed. Allergic side effects are estimated to occur in 0.6 per cent of vaccinees, a sufficiently high rate that the vaccine should not be considered a routine immunization for travel to Asia.[84] Current recommendations specify that the vaccine be reserved for expatriates, for persons spending 30 days or more in an endemic area during the transmission season, and for persons with briefer itineraries if they have a high risk of exposure (Table 179–4). The course of immunization should be completed 7 to 10 days before the onset of travel.[30]

Avoidance of outdoor activities during evening hours, staying in screened or air-conditioned quarters, and sleeping under a bednet will reduce the risk of exposure to vector mosquitoes. Long-sleeved shirts, long pants, and mosquito repellents applied to clothing and exposed skin are recommended for outdoor activities.[81]

The production of vector mosquitoes in rice fields has been controlled by scheduled changes in water levels, applications of larvicides and larval predators, and nontargeted effects of agricultural pesticides.

References

1. Andersen, M. M., and Ronne, T.: Side effects with Japanese encephalitis vaccine. Lancet *337*:1044, 1991.
2. Benakappa, D. G., Anvekar, G. A., Viswanath, D., et al.: Japanese encephalitis. Indian J. Pediatr. *21*:811–815, 1994.
3. Bhattacharya, S., Chakraborty, S. K., Chakraborty, S., et al.: Density of *Culex vishnui* and appearance of JE antibody in sentinel chicks and wild birds in relation to Japanese encephalitis cases. Trop. Geogr. Med. *38*:46–50, 1986.
4. Buescher, E. L., and Scherer, W. F.: Ecologic studies of Japanese encephalitis virus in Japan. Am. J. Trop. Med. Hyg. *8*:719–722, 1959.
5. Burke, D. S., Lorsomrudee, W., Leake, C. J., et al.: Fatal outcome in Japanese encephalitis. Am. J. Trop. Med. Hyg. *34*:1203–1210, 1985.
6. Burke, D. S., Nisalak, A., Ussery, M. A., et al.: Kinetics of IgM and IgG responses to Japanese encephalitis virus in human serum and cerebrospinal fluid. J. Infect. Dis. *151*:1093–1099, 1985.
7. Burke, D. S., and Morrill, J. C.: Levels of interferon in the plasma and cerebrospinal fluid of patients with acute Japanese encephalitis. J. Infect. Dis. *155*:797–799, 1987.
8. Burke, D. S., and Leake, C. J.: Japanese encephalitis. *In* Monath, T. P. (ed.): The Arboviruses: Epidemiology and Ecology. Vol 3. Boca Raton, CRC Press, 1988, pp. 63–92.
9. Calisher, C. H., Karabatsos, N., Dalrymple, J. M., et al.: Antigenic relationships among flaviviruses as determined by cross-neutralizing tests with polyclonal antisera. J. Gen. Virol. *70*:37–43, 1989.
10. Chaturvedi, U. C., Mathur, A., Chandra, A., et al.: Transplacental infection with Japanese encephalitis virus. J. Infect. Dis. *141*:712–715, 1980.
11. Chen, W. R., Rico-Hesse, R., and Tesh, R. B.: A new genotype of Japanese encephalitis virus from Indonesia. Am. J. Trop. Med. Hyg. *47*:61–69, 1992.
12. Das, S. K., Nityanand, S., Sood, K., et al.: Japanese B encephalitis with neurocysticercosis. J. Assoc. Physicians India *39*:643–644, 1991.
13. Desai, A., Ravi, V., Guru, S. C., et al.: Detection of autoantibodies to neural antigens in the CSF of Japanese encephalitis patients and correlation of findings with the outcome. J. Neurol. Sci. *122*:109–116, 1994.
14. Desai, A., Shankar, S. K., Ravi, V., et al.: Japanese encephalitis virus antigen in the human brain and its topographic distribution. Acta Neuropathol. *89*:368–373, 1995.
15. Dhanda, V., Mourya, D. T., Mishra, A. C., et al.: Japanese encephalitis virus infection in mosquito reared from field-collected immatures and in wild-caught males. Am. J. Trop. Med. Hyg. *41*:732–736, 1989.
16. Dropulic, B., and Masters, C. L.: Entry of neurotropic arboviruses into the central nervous system: An in vitro study using brain endothelium. J. Infect. Dis. *161*:685–691, 1990.
17. Edelman, R., Schneider, R. J., Chieowanich, P., et al.: The effect of dengue virus infection on the clinical sequelae of Japanese encephalitis: A one-year follow-up study in Thailand. Southeast Asian J. Trop. Med. Public Health *6*:308–315, 1975.
18. Fang, R., Hus, D. R., and Lim, T. W.: Investigation of a suspected outbreak of Japanese encephalitis in Pulau Langkawi. Malaysia J. Pathol. *3*:23–30, 1980.
19. Gajanana, A., Thenmozhi, V., Samuel, P. P., et al.: A community-based study of subclinical flavivirus infections in children in an area of Tamil Nadu, India, where Japanese encephalitis is endemic. Bull. W. H. O. *73*:237–244, 1995.
20. Gambel, J. M., DeFraites, R., Hoke, C., Jr., et al.: Japanese encephalitis vaccine: Persistence of antibody up to 3 years after a three-dose primary series. J. Infect. Dis. *171*:1074, 1995.
21. Gritsun, T. S., Holmes, E. C., and Gould, E. A.: Analysis of flavivirus envelope proteins reveals variable domains that reflect their antigenicity and may determine their pathogenesis. Virus Res. *35*:307–321, 1995.
22. Hanna, J., Ritchie, S., Loewenthal, M., et al.: Probable Japanese encephalitis acquired in the Torres Strait. Commun. Dis. Intell. *19*:206–208, 1995.
23. Harinasuta, C., Nimmanitya, S., and Titsyakorn, U.: The effect of interferon-alpha A on two cases of Japanese encephalitis in Thailand. Southeast Asian J. Trop. Med. Public Health *16*:332–336, 1985.
24. Harrington, D. G., Hilmas, D. E., Elwell, M. L., et al.: Intranasal infection of monkeys with Japanese encephalitis virus: Clinical response and treatment with a nuclease-resistant derivative of poly (I)-poly (C). Am. J. Trop. Med. Hyg. *25*:1191–1198, 1977.
25. Hendarto, S. K., and Hadinegoro, S. R.: Dengue encephalopathy. Acta Paediatr. Jpn. *34*:350–357, 1992.
26. Hiyake, M.: The pathology of Japanese encephalitis. Bull. W. H. O. *30*:153–160, 1964.
27. Hoke, C. H., Nisalak, A., Sangawhipa, N, et al.: Protection against Japanese encephalitis by inactivated vaccines. N. Engl. J. Med. *319*:609–614, 1989.
28. Hoke, C. H., Vaughn, D. W., Nisalak, A., et al.: Effect of high-dose dexamethasone on the outcome of acute encephalitis due to Japanese encephalitis virus. J. Infect. Dis. *165*:631–637, 1992.
29. Igarashi, A.: Epidemiology and conrol of Japanese encephalitis. World Health Stat. Q. *45*:299–305, 1992.
30. Immunization Practices Advisory Committee (ACIP): Inactivated Japanese encephalitis virus vaccine: Recommendations of the ACIP. M. M. W. R. *42*(RR-1):1–15, 1993.
31. Inada, R.: Compte rendu des recherches sur l'encephalite epidemique au Japon. Offic Internat d'hyg Pub. Bull. Mens. *29*:1389–1401, 1937.
32. Innis, B. L., Nisalak, A., Nimmannitya, S., et al.: An enzyme-linked immunosorbent assay to characterize dengue infections where dengue and Japanese encephalitis cocirculate. Am. J. Trop. Med. Hyg. *40*:418–427, 1989.
33. Ishii, T., Matsushita, M., and Hamada, S.: Characteristic residual neuropatholoigcal features of Japanese B encephalitis. Acta Neuropathol. *38*:181–186, 1977.
34. Johnson, R. T., Burke, D. S., Elwell, M., et al.: Japanese encephalitis: Immunocytochemical studies of viral antigen and inflammatory cells in fatal cases. Ann. Neurol. *18*:567–573, 1985.
35. Kamala, C. S., Venkatwshwara, R. M., George, S., et al.: Japanese encephalitis in children in Bellary Karnataka. Indian Pediatr. *26*:445–452, 1989.
36. Kao, C.-H., Wang, S.-J., Mak, S.-C., et al.: Viral encephalitis in children: Detection with technetium-99m HMPAO brain single-photon emission CT and its value in prediction of outcome. Am. J. Neuroradiol. *15*:1369–1373, 1994.
37. Kimura-Kuroda, J., Ichikawa, M., Ogata, A., et al.: Specific tropism of Japanese encephalitis virus for developing neurons in primary rat brain culture. Arch. Virol. *130*:477–484, 1993.
38. Kitaoka, M.: Shift of age distribution of cases of Japanese encephalitis in Japan during the period 1950 to 1967. *In* Hammon, McD. W., Kitaoka, M., and Downs, W. G. (eds.): Immunization for Japanese Encephalitis. Amsterdam, Excerpta Medica, 1972, pp. 285–291.
39. Kiura, K., Onodera, T., Nishida, A., et al.: A single gene controls resistance to Japanese encephalitis virus in mice. Arch. Virol. *112*:261–270, 1990.
40. Konishi, E., Pincus, S., Paoletti, E., et al.: Avipox virus–vectored Japanese encephalitis virus vaccines: Use as vaccine candidates in combination with purified subunit immunogens. Vaccine *12*:633–638, 1994.
41. Kruppenbacker, J., Bienzle, U., Bock, H. L., et al.: Co-administration of an inactivated hepatitis A vaccine with other travelers' vaccines: Interference with the immune response. *In* American Society of Microbiologists: Proceedings of the 34th Interscience Conference on Antimicrobial Agents and Chemotherapy. Washington, D.C., 1994, p. 256.
42. Kumar, R., Mathur, A., Kumar, A., et al.: Clinical features and prognostic indicators of Japanese encephalitis in children in Lucknow (India). Indian J. Med. Res. *91*:321–327, 1990.
43. Kumar, R., Mathur, A., Kumar, A., et al.: Virological investigations of acute encephalopathy in India. Indian Council Med. Res. 1228–1230, 1990.
44. Kumar, R., Kohli, N., Mathur, A., et al.: Use of the computed tomographic scan in Japanese encephalitis. Ann. Trop. Med. Parasitol. *86*:777–781, 1992.
45. Kumar, R., Mathur, A., Singh, K. B., et al.: Clinical sequelae of Japanese encephalitis in children. Indian J. Med. Res. *97*:9–13, 1993.
46. Kumar, R., Selvan, A. S., Sharma, S., et al.: Clinical predictors of Japanese encephalitis. Neuroepidemiology *13*:97–102, 1994.
47. Li, Z. S., Hong, S. F., and Gong, N. L.: Immunohistochemical study of Japanese B encephalitis. Chinese Med. J. *101*:768–771, 1988.
48. Lincoln, A. F., and Sivertson, S. E.: Acute phase of Japanese B encephalitis: Two hundred and one cases in American soldiers, Korea, 1960. J. Med. Assoc. *150*:268–273, 1952.
49. Liu, Y. F., Teng, C. L., and Liu, K.: Cerebral cysticercosis as a factor aggravating Japanese B encephalitis. Chinese Med. J. *75*:1010, 1957.
50. Lubinieski, A. S., Cypress, C. H., and Lucas, J. P.: Synergistic interaction of two agents in mice: Japanese B encephalitis virus and *Trichinella spiralis*. Am. J. Trop. Med. Hyg. *23*:235–241, 1974.
51. Mathur, A., Kumar, R., Sharma, S., et al.: Rapid diagnosis of Japanese encephalitis by immunofluorescent examination of cerebrospinal fluid. Indian J. Med. Res. *91*:1–4, 1990.
52. Mathur, A., Tandon, H. O., Mathur, K. R., et al.: Japanese encephalitis infection during pregnancy. Indian J. Med. Res. *81*:9–12, 1985.
53. Misra, U. K., Kalita, J., Jain, S. K., et al.: Radiological and neurophysiological changes in Japanese encephalitis. J. Neurol. Neurosurg. Psychiatry *57*:1484–1487, 1994.
54. Monath, T. P., and Heinz, F. X.: Flaviviruses. *In* Fields, B. N., Knipe D. M., and Howley, P. M. (eds.). Virology. 3rd ed. New York, Raven Press, 1995.
55. Morita, K.: Principle of PCR and its application for the diagnosis of dengue and Japanese encephalitis. Trop. Med. *36*:228–234, 1994.
56. Nathanson, N., and Cole, G. A.: Fatal Japanese encephalitis virus infection in immunosuppressed spider monkeys. Clin. Exp. Immunol. *6*:161–166, 1970.
57. Ni, H., Chang, G.-J., Xie, H., et al.: Molecular basis of attenuation of neurovirulence of wild-type Japanese encephalitis virus strain SA14. J. Gen. Virol. *76*:409–413, 1995.

58. Ohyama, A., Ishiga, A., Fujita, N., et al.: Effect of human gamma globulin upon encephalitis viruses. Jpn. J. Microbiol. *3*:159–169, 1959.
59. Olson, J. G., Atmosoedjono, S., Lee, V. H., et al.: Correlation between population indices of *Culex tritaeniohynchus* and *Cx. Gelidus* (Culicidae: Diptera) and rainfall in Kapuk, Indonesia. J. Med. Entomol. *20*:108–109, 1983.
60. Olson, J. G., Ksiazek, T. G., Tan, R., et al.: Correlation of population indices of female *Culex tritaeniorhynchus* with Japanese encephalitis viral activity in Kapuk, Indonesia. Southeast Asian J. Trop. Med. Public Health *16*:337–340, 1985.
61. Oya, A.: Japanese encephalitis vaccine. Acta Pediatr. Jpn. *30*:175–184, 1988.
62. Paul, W. S., Moore, P. S., Karabatsos, N., et al.: Outbreak of Japanese encephalitis on the island of Saipan, 1990. J. Infect. Dis. *167*:1053–1058, 1993.
63. Peiris, J. S. M., Amerasinghe, F. P., Amerasinghe, P. H., et al.: Japanese encephalitis in Sri Lanka. I. The study of an epidemic-vector incrimination, porcine infection and human disease. Trans. R. Soc. Trop. Med. Hyg. *86*:307–323, 1992.
64. Poneprasert B.: Japanese encephalitis in children in northern Thailand. Southeast J. Trop. Med. Public Health 20:599–603, 1989.
65. Rathi, A. K., Kushwaha, K. P., Singh, Y. D., et al.: JE virus enephalitis: 1988 epidemic at Gorakhpur. Indian Pediatr. *30*:325–333, 1993.
66. Ravi, V., Desai, A. S., Shenoy, P. K., et al.: Persistence of Japanese encephalitis virus in the human nervous system. J. Med. Virol. *40*:326–329, 1993.
67. Ravi, V., Taly, A. B., Shankar, S. K., et al.: Association of Japanese encephalitis virus infection with Guillain-Barré syndrome in endemic areas of South India. Acta Neurol. Scand. *90*:67–72, 1994.
68. Rodgriues, F. M., Guttikar, S. N., and Pinto, B. D.: Prevalence of antibodies to Japanese encephalitis and West Nile viruses among wild birds in the Krishna-Godavari Delta, Andhra Pradesh, India. Trans. R. Soc. Trop. Med. Hyg. *75*:258–262, 1981.
69. Rosen, L.: The natural history of Japanese encephalitis virus. Annu. Rev. Microbiol. *40*:395–414, 1986.
70. Ruff, T. A., Eisen, D., Fuller, A., et al.: Adverse reactions to Japanese encephalitis vaccine. Lancet *338*:881–882, 1991.
71. Schneider, R. J., Fireston, M. H., Edelman, R., et al.: Japanese encephaliltis: A one-year follow-up study in Thailand. Southeast Asian J. Trop. Med. Public Health *5*:560–568, 1974.
72. Service, M. W.: Agricultural development and arthropod-borne disease: A review. Rev. Saude Publica *25*:165–178, 1991.
73. Shankar, S. K., Rao, T. V., Mruthyunjayanna, B. P., et al.: Autopsy study of brains during an epidemic of Japanese encephalitis in Karnataka. Indian J. Med. Res. *78*:431–440, 1983.
74. Sharma, S., Mathur, A., Prakash, R., et al.: Japanese encephalitis virus latency in peripheral blood lymphocytes and recurrence of infection in children. Clin. Exp. Immunol. *85*:85–89, 1991.
75. Shoji, H., Hiraki, Y., Kuwasaki, Y., et al.: Japanese encephalitis in the Kurume region of Japan: CT and MRI findings. J. Neurol. *236*:255–259, 1989.
76. Srikanth, S., Ravi, V., Poornima, S., et al.: Viral antibodies in recent onset, nonorganic psychoses: Correspondence with symptomatic severity. Soc. Biol. Psychiatry *36*:517–521, 1994.
77. Sucharit, S., Surathin, K., and Shrestha, S. R.: Vectors of Japanese encephalitis virus (JEV): Species complexes of the vectors. Southeast Asian J. Trop. Med. Public Health *20*:611–621, 1989.
78. Sumiyoshi, H., Tignor, G. H., and Shope, R. E.: Characterization of a highly attenuated Japanese encephalitis virus generated from molecularly cloned cDNA. J. Infect. Dis. *171*:1144–1151, 1995.
79. Thisyakorn, U. S. A., and Nimmannitya, S.: Japanese encephalitis in Thai children, Bangkok, Thailand. Southeast Asian J. Trop. Med. Public Health *16*:93–97, 1985.
80. Trevett, A. J., Nwokolo, N., Lightfoot, D., et al.: Ataxia in patients infected with *Salmonella typhi* phage type D2: Clinical, biochemical and immunohistochemical studies. Trans. R. Soc. Trop. Med. Hyg. *88*:565–568, 1994.
81. Tsai, T. F.: Arboviral infections: General considerations for prevention, diagnosis and treatment in travelers. Semin. Pediatr. Infect. Dis. *3*:62–69, 1992.
82. Tsai, T. F.: Arboviruses. *In* Murray, P. R. (ed.): Manual of Clinical Microbiology. Washington, D.C., American Society for Microbiology, 1995, pp. 980–996.
83. Tsai, T. F., Nadhirat, S., and Rojanasuphot, S.: Regional workshop on control strategies for Japanese encephalitis. Southeast Asian J. Trop. Med. Public Health *26*(Suppl. 3):1–59, 1995.
84. Tsai, T. F., and Yu, Y. X.: Japanese encephalitis vaccines. *In* Plotkin, S., and Mortimer, E. (eds.): Vaccines. 2nd ed. Philadelphia, W. B. Saunders, 1995, p. 713.
85. Vaughn, D. W., and Hoke, C. H.: The epidemiology of Japanese encephalitis: Prospects for prevention. Epidemiol. Rev. *14*:197–221, 1992.
86. Yu, Y. X., Ming, A. G., Pen, G. Y., et al.: Safety of a live-attenuated Japanese encephalitis virus vaccine (SA14-14-2) for children. Am. J. Trop. Med. Hyg. *39*:214–217, 1988.
87. Zimmerman, H. M.: The pathology of Japanese B encephalitis. Am. J. Pathol. *22*:965–991, 1946.

❑ ❑ ❑

CHAPTER 179 (E)

Murray Valley Encephalitis

John Aaskov

Epidemics of an acute, severe, encephalitic illness clinically similar to Japanese and St. Louis encephalitis occurred in rural areas of southeastern Australia in 1917, 1918, 1922, 1925, 1951, 1956, 1971, and 1974[1, 13, 14] and in the north of western Australia in 1978 and 1981.[7] They are believed to represent a single entity for which various names (Australian X disease, Murray Valley encephalitis, Australian encephalitis) have been used. About 350 cases were reported in the 10 epidemics.

Case fatality rates, as high as 60 per cent in early years, declined to 20 per cent in the 1974 outbreak and have remained at this level since then. The presence of this disease in New Guinea was confirmed in 1956.[18] The causative virus was transmitted to experimental animals as early as 1918,[5, 9] although those strains could not be maintained. The definitive isolation and characterization of Murray Valley encephalitis virus in 1951[17] led to epidemiologic studies that suggested its survival in bird-mosquito cycles in northern Australia but not in the area of epidemic occurrence in southern Australia.[1]

In an effort to dissociate a regional disease from a specific locality, the term Australian encephalitis was proposed by residents of the Murray Valley for the disease caused by Murray Valley encephalitis virus. Some subsequently have attempted to expand the term Australian encephalitis to include encephalitis caused by any Australian arbovirus. Because the term Australian encephalitis has no scientific validity, it should not be used.

ETIOLOGIC AGENT

Murray Valley encephalitis virus was isolated from the brains of patients with fatal cases in 1951[17] and 1974[20] and shown to be related antigenically to Japanese encephalitis virus.[17, 20]

A partial nucleotide sequence of Murray Valley encephalitis virus[25] has confirmed the previous classification of this virus, on serologic grounds, as a member of the Japanese encephalitis, St. Louis encephalitis, West Nile fever subgroup of flaviviruses. It has been possible to distinguish Australian strains of Murray Valley encephalitis virus from those isolated in Papua New Guinea on the basis of limited nucleotide sequencing.[10, 21]

TRANSMISSION AND EPIDEMIOLOGY

The mosquito *Culex annulirostris* is believed to be the major vector of Murray Valley encephalitis virus, [14, 15, 23] although other mosquitoes, such as *Anopheles normanensis* and *C. quinquefasciatus*, also may be involved.

Murray Valley encephalitis virus is believed to survive in cycles of infection between birds and mosquitoes in northern Australia and Papua New Guinea,[1] where regular infection of humans and other animals is indicated by seroconversion in the summer-autumn "wet" season.[12] Cases of overt disease have been rare in that area, presumably because of the sparse population and the low ratio of clinical to subclinical infection (perhaps 1:1000). Epidemics that occurred in more populous areas of southeastern Australia were believed to follow the introduction of virus when abnormal spring rainfall allowed chains of bird-mosquito transmission through northern Australia.[2]

However, several studies have suggested interepidemic survival of virus in southern Australia.[19] Isolation of Murray Valley encephalitis virus from wild-caught male *A. tremulus* mosquitoes[6] suggests vertical transmission may be one mechanism by which this is achieved.

In early epidemics, disease occurred most commonly in children, but since the 1974 outbreak, clinical infection has occurred in individuals of all ages.[1, 3, 7, 14, 22]

CLINICAL MANIFESTATIONS[4, 8, 27]

An initial period of nonspecific prodromal symptoms and signs—fever, headache, nausea, vomiting, muscle pain, and photophobia—is followed within 2 to 5 days by drowsiness, mental obtundation, confusion, disorientation, incongruous behavior, ataxia, disturbance of speech, or convulsions, sometimes of grand mal character. Neurologic signs were present in most cases on admission to hospital, and additional signs appeared as the disease progressed. In some cases, signs fluctuated from hour to hour. Bennett[4] recognized three groups of patients according to eventual clinical outcome:

1. Mild cases commonly showed disturbed mentation short of coma, incoherent or slurred speech, aphasia, speech perseveration, incontinence, neck stiffness, intention tremor, and limb hypertonicity but rarely required assistance for respiration. The neurologic changes stabilized in 5 to 10 days, and the patients improved.
2. Severe cases showed more profound central nervous system involvement, with impairment of consciousness to coma, more marked signs of upper motor neuron involvement, and pharyngeal or respiratory paralysis requiring artificial respiration.
3. Fatal cases showed either spastic quadriplegia progressing to almost complete loss of nervous function or severe disease with superimposed infection.

PATHOLOGY

It is likely that a period of viremia precedes infection of the central nervous system, but this has not been demonstrated. Pathologic changes in fatal cases were restricted to the central nervous system. These included extensive perivascular cuffing, especially in the cortex, lymphocytic infiltration of the meninges, and neuron degeneration and neuronophagia in the cerebellum and spinal cord. Evidence of repair, including calcification, was described in patients who died late in the disease.[5, 9, 24, 26] These pathologic changes do not distinguish Murray Valley encephalitis from other arthropod-borne encephalitides.

DIAGNOSIS

Clinical and epidemologic features may suggest the diagnosis of Murray Valley encephalitis, especially during recognized epidemics, but individual cases may be difficult to distinguish from cases of encephalitis or encephalopathy due to other causes (e.g., herpesvirus).[4] Specific diagnosis depends on serologic evidence of infection concurrent with disease. The detection of IgM antibody that reacts with Murray Valley encephalitis virus in hemagglutination inhibition[16, 28] or in enzyme-linked immunosorbent assay[71] is the most useful indication of recent infection. Other flaviviruses, especially Kunjin virus, may cause encephalitis, subclinical infection, or minor illness during epidemics of Murray Valley encephalitis, and interpretation of serologic cross-reactions may require specific tests (e.g., neutralization) with several viruses.[14]

Virus isolation has not been successful for antemortem diagnosis.

TREATMENT AND PROGNOSIS

No specific antiviral therapy is available. Administration of corticosteroids is recommended during the acute phase of the illness to reduce brain edema. Antibiotics are used to prevent or treat secondary bacterial infections. Artificial respiration has been lifesaving, and all patients should be transported to base hospitals with facilities for management of patients with respiratory paralysis.[4]

Early epidemics left some neurologic and psychiatric sequelae, but the lower case-fatality rate in a recent epidemic, presumably due to modern intensive care techniques, was associated with a high rate of residual disability. Bennett[4] reviewed 18 patients up to 16 months after infection. Four of 11 mild cases had emotional problems and mild degrees of impaired motor coordination and mental acuity. All seven severe cases had serious defects, including paraplegia or quadriplegia and mental disturbance.

This pattern of high residual disability has continued to the present.

PREVENTION

The irregularity of epidemics and the large areas in which they occur make preventive measures difficult. However, both government and personal programs for restriction of exposure of humans to the common mosquito vector, *C. annulirostris*, are likely to minimize disease.

There is no vaccine available, and, although the killed Japanese encephalitis vaccine elicits antibodies that neutralize Murray Valley encephalitis virus in vitro, it is not known whether a Japanese encephalitis vaccine would offer any cross-protection in humans infected with Murray Valley encephalitis virus.

References

1. Anderson, S. G.: Murray Valley encephalitis and Australian X disease. J. Hyg. (Camb.). *52*:447–468, 1954.
2. Anderson, S. G., and Eagle, M.: Murray Valley encephalitis: The contrasting epidemiological picture in 1951 and 1952. Med. J. Aust. *1*:478–481, 1953.
3. Anonymous: Annual report of the National Notifiable Diseases Surveillance System, 1993. Comm. Dis. Int. Bull. *18*:518–547, 1994.
4. Bennett, N. M.: Murray Valley encephalitis, 1974: Clinical features. Med. J. Aust. *2*:446–450, 1976.
5. Breinl, A.: Clinical pathological and experimental observations on the "mysterious disease," a clinically aberrant form of acute poliomyelitis. Med. J. Aust. *1*:209–213, 1918.
6. Broom, A. K., Lindsay, M. D. A., Johansen, C. A. et al.: Two possible mechanisms for survival and initiation of Murray Valley encephalitis virus activity in the Kimberley region of Western Australia. Am. J. Trop. Med. Hyg. *53*:95–99, 1995.
7. Bucens, M.: Arbovirus infections diagnosed in Perth, 1981. *In* St. George, T. D., and Kay, B. H. (eds.): Arbovirus Research in Australia. Proceedings, 3rd Symposium, February 15–17, 1982. Commonwealth Scientific and Industrial Research Organisation and Queensland Institute of Medical Research, p. 171.
8. Burnell, G. H.: The Broken Hill epidemic. Med. J. Aust. *2*:157–161, 1917.
9. Cleland, J. B., Campbell, A. W., and Bradley, B.: Rep. Dir. Gen. Public Health N. S. W., 1917. 1918, pp. 150–280.
10. Coelen, R. J., and MacKenzie, J. S.: The 5′-terminal non-coding region of Murray Valley encephalitis virus RNA is highly conserved. J. Gen. Virol. *71*:241–245, 1990.

11. Dalgarno, L., Trent, D. W., Strauss, J. H., et al.: Partial nucleotide sequence of the Murray Valley encephalitis virus genome: Comparison of the encoded polypeptides with yellow fever virus structural and non-structural proteins. J. Mol. Biol. *187*:309–329, 1986.
12. Doherty, R. L.: Arthropod-borne viruses in Australia and their relation to infection and disease. Prog. Med. Virol. *17*:136-192, 1974.
13. Doherty, R. L., Carley, J. G., Cremer, M. R., et al.: Murray Valley encephalitis in eastern Australia, 1971. Med. J. Aust. 2:1170–1173, 1972.
14. Doherty, R. L., Carley, J. G., Filippich, C., et al.: Murray Valley encephalitis in Australia, 1974: Antibody response in cases and community. Aust. N. Z. J. Med. *6*:446–453, 1976.
15. Doherty, R. L., Carley, J. G., Kay, B. H., et al.: Murray Valley encephalitis virus infection in mosquitoes and domestic fowls in Queensland, 1974. Aust. J. Exp. Biol. Med. Sci. *54*:237–243, 1976.
16. Field, P. R., and Murphy, A. M.: The role of specific IgM globulin estimations in the diagnosis of acquired rubella. Med. J. Aust. 2:1244–1248, 1972.
17. French, E. L.: Murray Valley encephalitis: Isolation and characterisation of aetiological agent. Med. J. Aust. *1*:100–103, 1992.
18. French, E. L., Anderson, S. G., Price, A. V. G., et al.: Murray Valley encephalitis in New Guinea. 1. Isolation of Murray Valley encephalitis virus from the brain of a fatal case of encephalitis occurring in a Papuan native. Am. J. Trop. Med. Hyg. *6*:827–834, 1957.
19. Gard, G. P., Giles, J. R., Dwyer-Gray, R. J., et al.: Serological evidence of interepidemic infection of feral pigs in New South Wales with Murray Valley encephalitis virus. Aust. J. Exp. Biol. Med. Sci. *54*:297–302, 1976.
20. Lehmann, N. I., Gust, I. D., and Doherty, R.: Isolation of Murray Valley encephalitis virus from the brains of three patients with encephalitis. Med. J. Aust. 2:450–454, 1976.
21. Lobigs, M., Marshall, I. D., Weir, R. C., et al.: Murray Valley encephalitis virus field strains from Australia and Papua New Guinea: Studies on the sequence of the major envelope protein gene and virulence for mice. Virology *165*:245–255, 1988.
22. Mackenzie, J. S., Smith, D. W., Broom, A. K. et al: Australian encephalitis in Western Australia, 1979-1991. Med. J. Aust. *158*:591–595, 1993.
23. Marshall, I. D., Woodroofe, G. M., and Hirsch, S.: Viruses recovered from mosquitoes and wildlife serum collected in the Murray Valley of southeastern Australia, February, 1974, during an epidemic of encephalitis. Aust. J. Exp. Biol. Med. Sci. *60*:457–470, 1982.
24. Pedrau, J. R.: The Australian epidemics of encephalomyelitis (X-disease). J. Pathol. Bacteriol. *42*:59–65, 1936.
25. Pond, W. L., Russ, S. B., Rogers, N. G., et al.: Murray Valley encephalitis virus: Its serological relationship to the Japanese-West Nile-St. Louis encephalitis group of viruses. J. Immunol. *75*:78–84, 1955.
26. Robertson, E. G.: Murray Valley encephalitis: Pathological aspects. Med. J. Aust. *1*:107–110, 1952.
27. Robertson, E. G., and McLorinan, H.: Murray Valley encephalitis: Clinical aspects. Med. J. Aust. *1*:103–107, 1952.
28. Wiemers, M. A., and Stallman, N. D.: Immunoglobulin M in Murray Valley encephalitis. Pathology *7*:187–191, 1975.

❑ ❑ ❑

CHAPTER 179 (F)

Tick-borne Encephalitis

Christoph Aebi and Theodore F. Tsai

Tick-borne encephalitis refers here to the neurotropic tick-transmitted flaviviral infections that occur across the Eurasian land mass from the Far East to Western Europe. The Far Eastern form of the disease frequently is called Russian spring-summer encephalitis (RSSE) and in Europe, where the disease distinctly is milder and often biphasic, simply tick-borne encephalitis (TBE), spring-summer meningoencephalitis (Frühsommer Meningoenzephalitis), biphasic meningoencephalitis, central European encephalitis, or, because it sometimes is transmitted by raw infected milk, biphasic milk fever.[8, 28, 43, 49]

HISTORY

After an outbreak of encephalitis in the Far Eastern region of Russia in 1932, Zilber isolated the virus from viremic humans and from *Ixodes persulcatus* ticks. A milder form of the disease with a similar seasonality previously had been described in Sweden and in Austria, but its etiology was not defined until 1948, when the virus was isolated in the Czech Republic and Slovakia. Milk-borne transmission of TBE from infected livestock animals first was recognized in an outbreak in 1951 and 1952.

ETIOLOGIC AGENT

TBE virus and the closely related viruses of RSSE and Powassan encephalitis are flaviviruses placed antigenically within a complex of tick-borne flaviviruses that also includes the agents of Kyasanur Forest disease, Omsk hemorrhagic fever, and an encephalomyelitis syndrome in sheep, called variously louping ill in the British Isles and Spanish, Greek, or Turkish sheep encephalomyelitis in their respective countries.[15, 32] Molecular taxonomic studies based on nucleotide sequence differences in the virus' E protein gene show a correlation between geographic and genetic distances, with a continuous east to west cline consistent with an evolutionary origin of TBE viruses in the Far East with dispersion westward to Europe and the British Isles (Fig. 179–10).[50]

ECOLOGY

The viruses of RSSE and TBE are transmitted principally by hard ticks in the *I. ricinus* complex: *I. ricinus* in Europe and *I. persulcatus* in the Far East.[8, 28, 43, 45, 49] Other tick vectors include *I. arbicola*, *I. hexagonus*, *Haemaphysalis punctata*, *H. concinna*, *Dermacentor marginatus*, and *D. reticulatus*. Viral circulation is maintained by continuous horizontal infections between ticks and animals and through the winter by vertical transmission in vector ticks and by latent infections in hibernating animals. The viruses are transmitted transtadially from larval to nymphal to adult tick stages and transovarially. All stages of the tick and both male and female ticks transmit infections to animals and humans. Ixodid ticks feed on three hosts, one for each of the stages, during the typical 3-year life cycle. Larval and nymphal ticks feed preferentially on birds and small mammals, such as wild mice, voles, and dormice, and adult ticks on larger mammals, such as roe deer, hedgehogs, foxes, hares, badgers, deer, domestic livestock (pigs, goats, sheep, and cows), dogs, cats, and humans. Infections in animals, except occasionally in dogs, are asymptomatic, and viremias are brief. Therefore, a large population of susceptible vertebrate hosts is needed to maintain viral transmission. Human infections are incidental to the natural cycle of transmission. Birds and large mammals contribute to the spread of vector ticks and viral foci.

Ticks in the *I. ricinus* complex require high soil and ambient humidity (>80–90 per cent relative humidity) and moderate temperatures, within the 8° C isotherm. They typically are found in the transitional vegetation zone from forest edge to fields or meadows or in areas where dense brush or ground vegetation provides a sheltered microenvironment. Vector ticks are absent from mountainous areas with an elevation greater than 1000 m. Foci of TBE transmission are restricted geographically and ecologically to these biotopes and tend to be highly stable from year to year.

Tick activity varies with seasonal temperature and humidity. In central Europe, activity begins in March and April, reaches a peak in May, and declines during the summer in July and August. With the return of cooler temperatures, a second peak of activity occurs in September.[6, 7, 11] In temperate regions, tick activity begins later and is greatest in the summer months. In Mediterranean climates, ticks are most active from November to January.

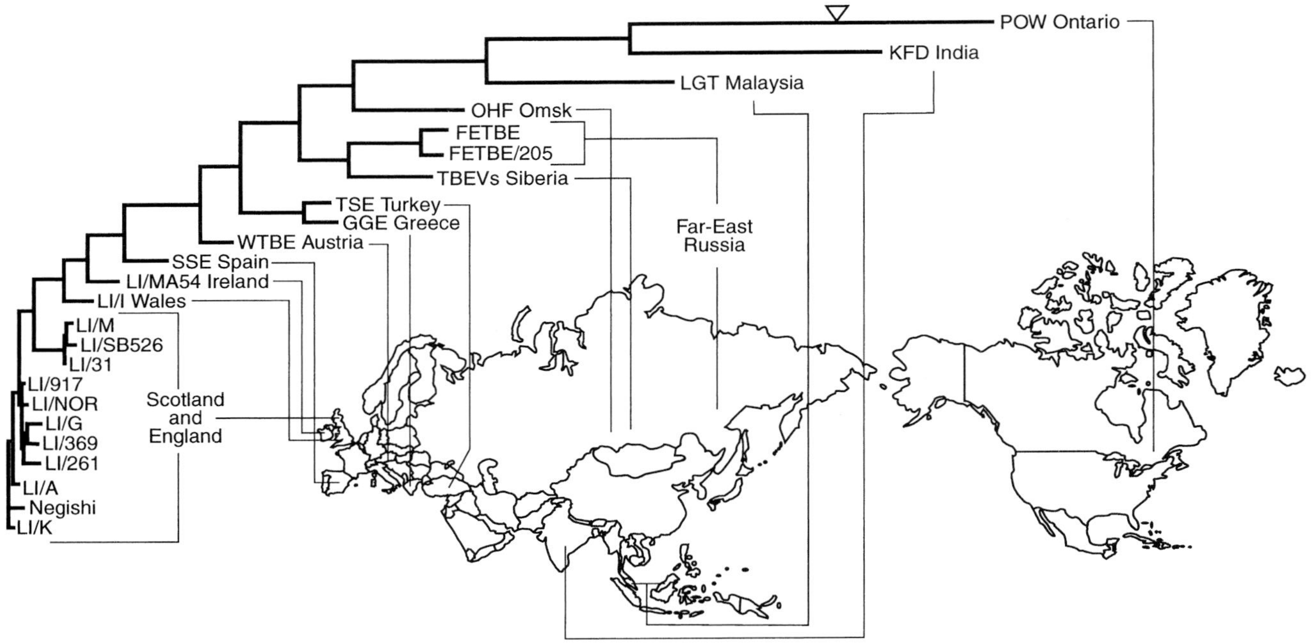

FIGURE 179–10. *Cladogram of tick-borne encephalitis complex viruses based upon* E *gene sequences, from west to east with respect to louping ill (LI) virus. SSE, Spain sheep encephalitis; WTBE, western tick-borne encephalitis; GGE, Greek goat encephalitis; TSE, Turkey sheep encephalitis; FETBE, Far Eastern tick-borne encephalitis; OHF, Omsk hemorrhagic fever; LGT, Langat; KFD, Kyasanur Forest disease; POW, Powassan encephalitis. Phylogenetics of these and other mosquito-borne flaviviruses are rooted in the Powassan branch indicated by the triangle. (From Zanotto, P. M., Gao, G. F., Gritsun, T., et al.: An arbovirus cline across the Northern Hemisphere. Virology 210:152–159, 1995.)*

In foci with hyperendemic transmission, tick density may exceed one per square meter. Viral infection rates in ticks generally are in the range of 0.1 to 5 per cent. These rates typically are 10-fold lower than *Borrelia burgdorferi* (sensu lato) infection rates in *I. ricinus* in the same areas.[20] The reason for this difference is unclear, but it may be that brief TBE viremias in animals, lasting only a few days, result in a reduced chance of viral transmission to feeding ticks while *B. burgdorferi* infections of rodents are persistent, so that tick feedings are more likely to result in infection. Another possibility is that the principal reservoir hosts for the respective infectious agents differ, with a more limited and focal distribution of important hosts for TBE virus, such as goats.

The geographic distributions of RSSE and European TBE correspond to the ranges of their principal tick vectors; however, transmission is highly focal within this range, reflecting the locations of biotopes that support viral circulation (Fig. 179–11). New foci are reported periodically, reflecting better recognition of the disease, its natural spread, and human modifications of the landscape.

EPIDEMIOLOGY

TBE has been recognized in all the countries of Europe except Portugal and the Benelux countries, but endemic transmission is most intense in central Europe.[8, 20, 28, 43, 49] TBE incidence previously ranged as high as 50 per 100,000 population in Austria, Poland, Hungary, Russia, the Czech Republic, Slovakia, and the former Yugoslavia, and, in certain areas, similar levels of transmission still may prevail. Vaccination has reduced disease incidence locally, especially in Austria, where a national program of immunization in effect for 15 years had brought incidence to less than 1 per 100,000 population. Currently, isolated cases are reported from France, Greece, and Lichtenstein, and fewer than 100 sporadic cases are reported annually in Sweden, Germany, Switzerland, Italy, and Austria. Reporting from other countries of Eastern and central Europe is less certain, but several hundred cases a year have been reported recently in Slovenia. In the Far East, RSSE cases occur principally among forest workers. The disease is recognized in Russia and China, and recently the first cases acquired in Japan were reported.

Within each country, the distribution of cases is highly focal in certain cantons or districts; local seroprevalence may exceed 20 per cent, but general seroprevalence usually is less than 1 per 100,000 population. Frequent exposures during long-term residence lead to a general trend of increasing seroprevalence with age. Seroprevalence rates as high as 50 per cent have been observed among groups at high risk of exposure, such as farmers and forestry workers. Adults 20 to 50 years of age characteristically have made up the majority of cases. In some studies, cases in males (adults and children) predominate by a ratio of 2:1.[1, 6, 11] Cases have occurred in children as young as 3 months of age, but, generally, risk in children increases with age, reflecting their increased mobility and activity in the sylvatic environment. These epidemiologic patterns are changing in areas with high immunization coverage. Vaccination efforts have been focused principally on hyperendemic areas and at high-risk occupational groups, such as forestry workers. The low numbers of cases currently reported from areas where vaccination coverage is high belie the continued transmission of virus in these locations.

Cases may be acquired during outdoor activities, such as berry picking and mushroom gathering, and infections occasionally have been acquired from ticks brought from endemic areas on Christmas trees and other objects. One study found that seroprevalence in Swedish orienteers (1 per cent) was not substantially different from general seroprevalence in residents of Stockholm County (5 per cent), an area where TBE is endemic.[4] The absence of a higher TBE risk among persons with occasional sylvatic exposure reflects the low infection rate of ticks and generally low risk to persons with sporadic or short-term exposure. A study of American soldiers stationed in central Europe found no cases and one seroconversion in 3297 person-months of exposure, an infection rate of 0.9 per 1000 person-months.[34] With the dissolution of the former Soviet Union and increasing commerce with Eastern Europe, there has been increased interest in the risk of TBE among travelers to Europe and Russia. The available data suggest that risk is low for most travelers and that vaccination is not indicated except under unusual circumstances of prolonged stay in an endemic area.

The seasonal distribution of cases lags roughly 1 month behind that of tick activity, extending from April until November. Peak incidence in Sweden is in August and in Austria, in June and July, with a secondary rise in October.

Milk-borne TBE previously accounted for 10 to 20 per cent of all cases in central Europe. Infections frequently were acquired from consuming unpasteurized milk or cheese from infected goats, sheep, and cows, and outbreaks resulting in thousands of cases have been reported. Transmission from infected milk now is rare, but as recently as 1994, an outbreak in Slovakia led to seven cases among a group that regularly

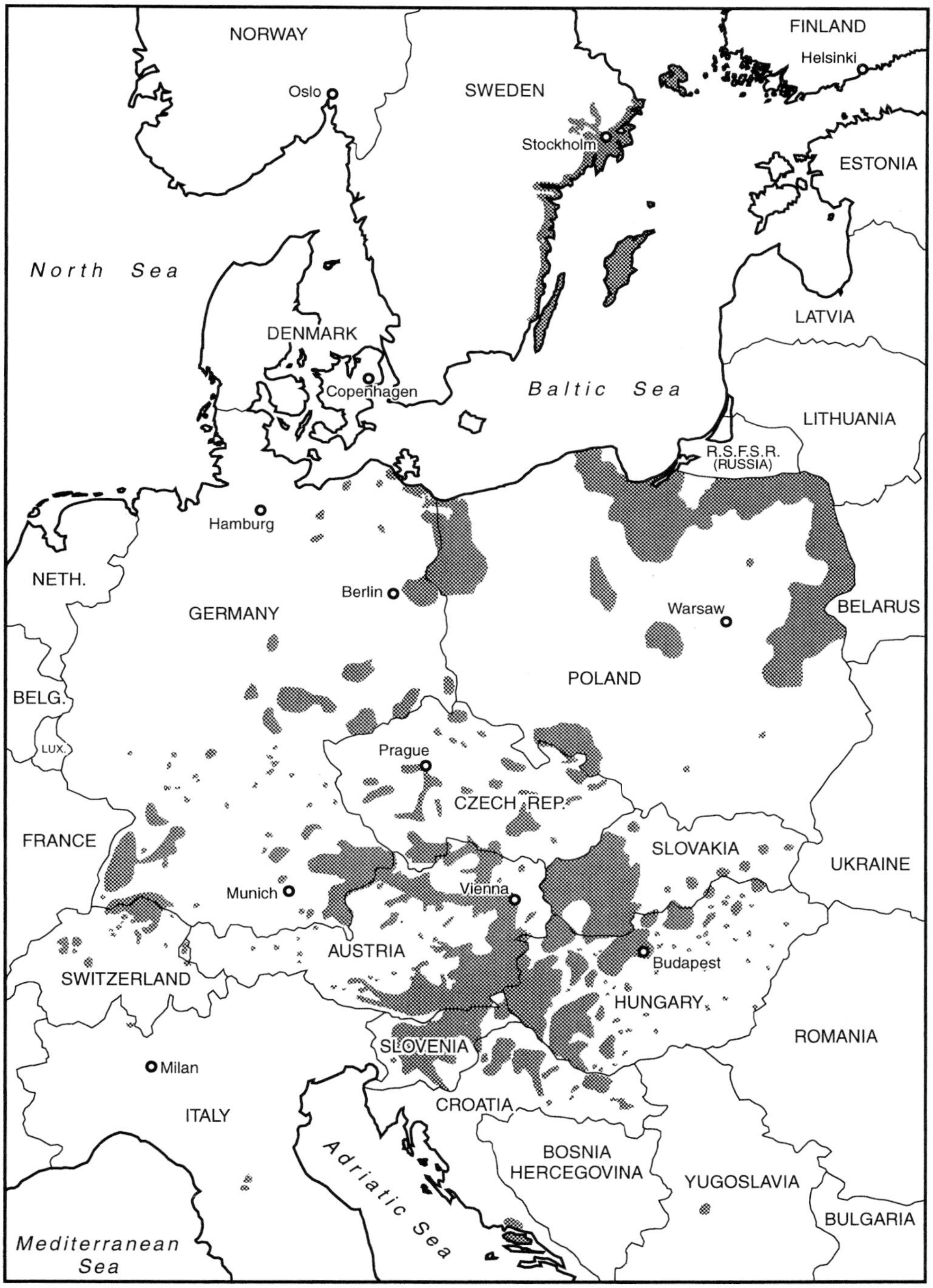

FIGURE 179–11. *Recognized foci of tick-borne encephalitis in Western and Central Europe. Foci tend to be delimited and relatively stable.*

drank raw milk from a family goat.[48] Contact infection, acquired during slaughter of an infected goat, also has been reported.

CLINICAL MANIFESTATIONS

The European form of TBE is an acute febrile illness characterized by a biphasic course consisting of a nonspecific prodromal syndrome that is followed by central nervous system disease in 5 to 30 per cent of infected patients.[7, 47] Infection with Far Eastern viral strains results in a more severe illness, progressing directly to neurologic involvement and a poorer prognosis for survival and full recovery. TBE has been observed in all age groups, with the exception of neonates. Congenital infection has not been reported. The youngest patient with serologically documented TBE described in the literature was a 3-month-old infant.[10] Severe acute disease and persistent neurologic sequelae are rare in children and occur most commonly in elderly patients.

The diagnosis of TBE should be suspected if the patient reports a recent tick exposure in an endemic area or presents with a biphasic course of fever. The clinical presentation itself is nonspecific. After an incubation period of 2 to 28 days, in most cases 7 to 14 days,[6, 11, 47] the patient may present with a prodromal illness consisting of fever, malaise, nausea and vomiting, headache, myalgia, and occasionally upper respiratory tract symptoms.[6, 11, 22, 47] Defervescence occurs after 2 to 7 days, and the patient subsequently remains asymptomatic for 1 to 20 days, usually 2 to 8 days.[6, 11, 22] This prodromal illness may be absent in the majority of children. Harasek[11] observed a biphasic course in 11 of 38 (29 per cent) pediatric cases. Abrupt onset of fever higher than 39° C, headache, and emesis herald the onset of the second phase of disease. The majority of children (66 to 85 per cent) present with aseptic meningitis without clinical evidence of parenchymal central nervous system involvement.[11, 21, 25, 35, 41] In adult patients, by contrast, aseptic meningitis without encephalitis occurs in 17 to 56 per cent of cases.[2, 22, 39] On physical examination, irritability, signs of meningeal irritation, and photophobia are the most common features in patients with meningitis. In these uncomplicated cases, patients usually defervesce within 3 to 4 days.[11] Encephalitis and/or myelitis manifested by altered state of consciousness, seizures, and focal neurologic signs is less common in children. Among 13 pediatric patients with encephalitis (34 per cent of the case series), Harasek[11] observed ataxia in 10, somnolence in 4, paresthesias and seizures in 2 each, and central facial palsy and nystagmus in 1 each. In two of these patients, transient unilateral shoulder girdle weakness occurring during the second week of central nervous system disease suggested cervical anterior horn involvement or radiculitis. Children with encephalitis may remain febrile for a longer period, although rarely for more than 1 week.[11]

In large case series with predominantly adult patients, a paralytic course secondary to myelitic and/or radiculoneuritic involvement was observed in 5 to 25 per cent of cases.[33, 47, 51] Transient unilateral paralysis of an upper extremity is the most common manifestation of lower motor neuron disease complicating TBE.[33, 37, 47, 51] Involvement of the cranial nerves is less common and usually manifested by external ocular muscle paralysis (usually cranial nerve III), peripheral facial palsy (VII), or involvement of the pharyngeal muscles (IX, X, XI).[6, 33, 44] Lower extremity weakness and, occasionally, autonomic nervous system involvement manifested by bladder dysfunction also may occur.[6, 44] No data regarding the incidence of a paralytic course are available for pediatric cases of TBE.

Seizures during the acute stage of illness are uncommon in adults and have been observed in 0.3 per cent of 679 cases reported by Duniewicz[6]; Harasek[11] reported convulsions in 2 of 38 (5 per cent) children with TBE.

The peripheral leukocyte count is not altered characteristically. Although it usually is in the normal range, both leukopenia and moderate leukocytosis may occur.[11, 44] In adult populations, several investigators observed leukopenia during the viremic prodrome and normal or moderately elevated white blood cell counts during the second phase of illness.[22, 30] In a recent report evaluating peripheral blood values during the prodromal phase of TBE, 23 of 28 (82 per cent) adult patients were shown to have mild to moderate thrombocytopenia (60 to 130 $\times$ 10^9/L), with values returning to normal during the second phase of illness.[30] Cerebrospinal fluid analysis in children with serologically documented TBE reveals pleocytosis with mononuclear predominance in almost all patients. Typically, a cerebrospinal fluid white blood cell count of 100 to 1000 cells/mm^3 is found.[11, 24, 44] Occasionally, lower blood cell counts occur, as reported by Krausler and colleagues,[21] who found blood cell counts of less than 100/mm^3 in 24 of 75 (32 per cent) pediatric cases. Wahlberg and colleagues[47] found no pleocytosis in 17 of 94 (18 per cent) adult patients examined. Harasek[11] reported the lack of correlation between the cerebrospinal fluid leukocyte count and the severity of clinical disease. Pleocytosis disappears within 4 to 5 weeks of the onset of acute central nervous system disease. The cerebrospinal fluid glucose concentration is normal, and the protein concentration rarely exceeds 100 mg/dL.[11, 22, 44] Electroencephalographic examination during acute TBE usually is abnormal and characterized by nonspecific reduction of rhythmic background activity, bilateral periodic slowing, and, rarely, focal abnormalities.[11, 16, 46] Attenuation of background activity with periodic delta groups has been shown to correlate with parenchymal central nervous system involvement in adult TBE patients.[46] Reorganization of electroencephalographic activity commonly lags behind clinical improvement, and abnormalities may persist for months to years.[11, 16] The diagnostic and prognostic value of neuroimaging studies in children with TBE is unknown to date.

PATHOLOGY

Central nervous system findings mainly are those of acute meningeal inflammation and focal gray matter encephalomyelitis. The white matter rarely is involved. Macroscopic findings include congestion of the leptomeninges and swelling and hyperemia of the cerebral parenchyma, particularly in the brain stem and cervical region of the spinal cord.[23] Petechial hemorrhages are seen in the brain stem, the anterior horns of the spinal cord, and, less consistently, in the cerebellum and the anterior central region of the cortex. Histologic changes are dominated by infiltration and ganglion cell damage in the gray matter of these same areas. Changes particularly are pronounced in the anterior horns of the cervical spine, the medulla oblongata, the cranial nerve nuclei of the pons, and the Purkinje cell layer of the cerebellum.[23] Inflammatory foci are characterized by lymphocytic perivascular infiltration and various stages of degenerative changes of neuronal cells. Areas of neuronal necrosis are characterized by perifocal edema, lymphocytic and neutrophilic infiltration, and, at a later stage, nodular microglial proliferation at sites of complete neuronophagia. Rarely, spinal nerve roots, spinal ganglia, and peripheral nerves are involved. Spongiform changes, particularly after protracted illness, appear as sharply defined areas of softening with minimal inflammatory reaction. In the Far Eastern form of the disease, extensive poliomyelitis of the spinal cord is noted with destruction of anterior horn cells, particularly in the upper cervical and lower lumbar areas, and of the brain stem.

PATHOGENESIS

Infection of local dermal cells is followed by seeding of regional lymph nodes and further replication. Viremia leads to generalized infection, especially of reticuloendothelial cells, followed by a secondary viremia that leads to neuroinvasion. Viral entry to the central nervous system occurs through capillary endothelia and by infected infiltrating mononuclear cells. Presumably, patients who develop only the primary nonspecific febrile illness in the European form of TBE are able to clear the systemic infection before neuroinvasion occurs.

The inflammatory response initially is composed of granulocytes and macrophages and is followed by lymphocytic and mononuclear infiltration and microglial reaction.

LABORATORY DIAGNOSIS

Because clinical presentation and cerebrospinal fluid findings do not differentiate TBE from other causes of aseptic meningitis or meningoencephalitis, the diagnosis of TBE rests on the demonstration of specific antibody by serologic testing. Virus can be recovered from blood by culture, but because viremia occurs during the prodromal stage (when the diagnosis of TBE seldom is considered), viral culture is not useful clinically in diagnosis. Virus also can be recovered from the brain tissue of patients who died at an early stage of disease.[5] The demonstration of a significant titer rise in specific antibody or the presence of specific IgM is the diagnostic mainstay for TBE. Enzyme-linked immunosorbent assay (ELISA) largely has replaced complement fixation, hemagglutination inhibition, and neutralization.[13] ELISA has been shown to offer increased sensitivity, reliably differentiates between IgM and IgG antibodies, and, as opposed to neutralization, uses nonviable viral antigens.[12, 41] For the detection of specific anti-TBE IgM, an IgM-capture ELISA system has proved to be more sensitive and specific than has the conventional three-layer ELISA system because high titers of specific IgG and rheumatoid factor do not interfere with IgM binding.[12, 41] Specific IgM and IgG also can be measured by ELISA in the cerebrospinal fluid.[12, 41] Through use of the highly sensitive capture ELISA format, the presence of anti-TBE IgM can be determined, even in serum samples obtained late during the acute illness, when high titers of specific IgG already are present. With this method, specific IgM virtually always can be demonstrated during the acute illness and may persist for up to 9 months thereafter.[14, 41]

DIFFERENTIAL DIAGNOSIS

The clinical course of TBE is nonspecific in the majority of cases, and a history of tick exposure in an endemic area can be elicited in 33 to 47 per cent of pediatric patients only.[11, 35, 42] Because serologic confirmation of the diagnosis is not available immediately in most cases, the differential diagnosis includes a wide spectrum of diseases presenting with fever and central nervous system manifestations.

Although uncommon in childhood, herpes simplex encephalitis is the most important differential diagnosis, and therapy with intravenous acyclovir needs to be initiated without delay. Early in the course of disease, localizing signs observed by neurologic examination, electroencephalography, and magnetic resonance imaging suggest herpes encephalitis and are uncharacteristic of TBE. The diagnosis of herpes simplex virus infection is confirmed by viral culture, brain biopsy, and, more recently, polymerase chain reaction (PCR) testing of the spinal fluid.[29] Infections caused by enteroviruses are an important alternative because seasonal incidence and clinical presentation overlap with that of TBE. Enteroviral infections may present with a biphasic fever course reminiscent of that of TBE. Lack of skin manifestations, mucosal changes, and involvement of organs other than the central nervous system in TBE may be helpful in differentiating the two entities. Enteroviral infections are diagnosed most readily by viral cultures from cerebrospinal fluid and mucosal surfaces or by PCR.

Other possible viral etiologies include the common respiratory tract viruses, such as influenza, parainfluenza, and respiratory syncytial viruses, Epstein-Barr virus, adenovirus, and mumps virus. Partially treated bacterial meningitis, *Mycoplasma pneumoniae* infection, and encephalitis in association with cat-scratch disease may present similarly. Tuberculous meningitis runs a subacute course. Although near-normal cerebrospinal fluid glucose and protein concentration may be measured very early in the disease, glucose characteristically is very low, and protein continuously rises to very high levels.

At least three cases of concomitant infection with the TBE virus and *B. burgdorferi* have been reported in the literature.[1, 20, 23, 38] It has been suggested[23] that in some cases of TBE, persistent or late-appearing limb paralysis may be attributed to concomitant but undiagnosed borrelial radiculoneuritis rather than to TBE-related myelitis with anterior horn-cell involvement. In this situation, diagnostic evidence for Lyme borreliosis should be sought because this condition requires specific antimicrobial therapy.

TREATMENT

No specific antiviral therapy currently is available to treat TBE. TBE hyperimmunoglobulin is indicated exclusively for passive immunization within 96 hours after tick exposure and should not be administered during acute disease. Clinical evidence suggests that administration of TBE hyperimmunoglobulin thereafter may have a detrimental effect on the course of disease.[3, 17, 26, 28] In severe cases, supportive therapy is aimed at preventing sequelae related to increased intracranial pressure, seizures, and bulbar dysfunction. After the acute stage, neurorehabilitation may be necessary for patients with motor, cognitive, or emotional disturbances. Because TBE rarely causes a chronic seizure disorder, prolonged anticonvulsive therapy seldom is indicated in patients who had convulsions during acute disease.

PROGNOSIS

The main risk factor for neurologic residua and fatal outcome of TBE appears to be advanced age.[2] Persistent sequelae appear to be exceedingly rare in children,[11, 25] although no long-term follow-up studies of TBE patients have been performed to date. In adult patient populations, residua are observed in 2 to 10 per cent of patients with clinical evidence of parenchymal involvement during the acute illness.[2, 7, 18, 47] Patients presenting with meningitis alone rarely have long-lasting residua.[2] Ill-defined manifestations, such as chronic fatigue, headache, sleep disorders, and emotional disturbances, are reported most commonly by continuously symptomatic adults.[6] Muscular weakness and atrophy are the most common persistent findings on neurologic examination.[2, 6, 31] Chronic unilateral upper limb palsy has been observed in a 10-month-old infant with serologically documented TBE.[47] In some patients, the electroencephalogram may remain abnormal for prolonged periods, occasionally demonstrating seizure activity.[11] Most of these patients are asymptomatic, although epilepsy secondary to TBE has been reported infrequently.[11, 36] The reported case-fatality rate in adult TBE patients is approximately 1 per cent in large series,[2, 6, 7, 18, 31] the majority of deaths being attributed to severe bulbar encephalitis or related to underlying cardiovascular disease in elderly patients.[6]

PREVENTION

Inactivated vaccines for TBE are produced in Austria (Immuno), Germany (Bering), and Russia. The vaccines are made from different central European viral strains and are produced by concentrating and purifying cell culture fluid from infected chick embryo cells. Adjuvant and thimerosal are added to the formalin-inactivated cell culture fluid. The Russian vaccine is an inactivated unconcentrated cell culture fluid from infected African green monkey kidney cells. Vaccine is available in the United States under investigational drug exemption to military personnel. A commercial immunoglobulin for pre-exposure and postexposure immunoprophylaxis is available in Europe.[3]

References

1. Abshagen, R., and Bahr, J.: Doppelinfektion *Borrelia burgdorferi*: FSME-virus. Kinderaerztliche Praxis *60*:103–104, 1992.
2. Ackermann, R., Krueger, K., Roggendorf, M., et al.: Die verbreitung der fruehsommer-meningoenzephalitis in der Bundesrepublik Deutschland. Dtsch. Med. Wochenschr. *111*:927–933, 1986.
3. Aebi, C., and Schaad, U. B.: FSME immunoglobulin: Eine kritische beurteilung der wirksamkeit. Schweiz. Med. Wochenschr. *124*:1837–1840, 1994.
4. Berglund, J., and Eitrem R.: Tick-borne borreliosis in the archipelago of southern Sweden. Scand. J. Infect. Dis. *25*:67–72, 1993.
5. Clarke, D. H., and Casals, J.: Arboviruses: Group B. *In* Horsfall, F. L., and Tamer, I. (eds.): Viral and Rickettsial Infections in Man. Philadelphia, Lippincott, 1965, pp. 606–658.
6. Duniewicz, M.: Klinisches bild der zentraleuropaeischen zeckenenzephalitis. Muench. Med. Wochenschr. *118*:1609–1613, 1976.
7. Gold, R., Wiethoelter, H., Rihs, I., et al.: Fruehsommer-meningoenzephalitis-impfung. Dtsch. Med. Wochenschr. *117*:112–116, 1992.
8. Gresikova, M., and Calisher, C. H.: Tick-borne encephalitis. *In* Monath, T. P. (ed.): The Arboviruses: Epidemiology and Ecology. Boca Raton, CRC, 1989, pp. 177–201.
9. Grinschgl, G.: Virus-meningo-encephalitis in Austria. Bull. W. H. O. *12*:535–564, 1955.
10. Grubbauer, H. M., Dornbusch, H. J., Spork, D., et al.: Tick-borne encephalitis in a 3-month-old child. Eur. J. Pediatr. *151*:743–744, 1992.
11. Harasek, G.: Zeckenenzephalitis im kindesalter. Dtsch. Med. Wochenschr. *99*:1965–1970, 1974.
12. Heinz, F. X., Roggendorf, M., Hofmann, H., et al.: Comparison of two different enzyme immunoassays for detection of immunoglobulin M antibodies against tick-borne encephalitis virus in serum and cerebrospinal fluid. J. Clin. Microbiol. *14*:141–146, 1981.
13. Hofmann, H., Frisch-Niggemeyer, W., and Heinz, F.: Rapid diagnosis of tick-borne encephalitis by means of enzyme linked immunosorbent assay. J. Gen. Virol. *42*:505–511, 1979.
14. Hofmann, H., Kunz, C., Heinz, F. X., et al.: Detectability of IgM antibodies against TBE virus after natural infection and after vaccination. Infection *11*:164–166, 1983.
15. Holzmann, H., Vorobyova, M. S., Ladyzhenskaya, I. P., et al.: Molecular epidemiology of tick-borne encephalitis virus: Cross-protection between European and Far Eastern subtypes. Vaccine *10*:345–349, 1992.
16. Juhasz, C., and Szirmai, I.: Spectral EEG parameters in patients with tick-borne encephalitis: A follow-up study. Clin. Electroencephalogr. *24*:53–58, 1993.
17. Kluger, G., Schottler, A., Waldvogel, K., et al.: Tickborne encephalitis despite specific immunoglobulin prophylaxis. Lancet *346*:1502, 1995.
18. Koeck, T., Stuenzner, D., Freidl, W., et al.: Zur klinik der fruehsommermeningoenzephalitis (FSME) in der steiermark. Nervenarzt *63*:205–208, 1992.
19. Koernyey S.: Contribution to the histology of tick-borne encephalitis. Acta Neuropathol. *43*:179–183, 1978.
20. Korenberg, E. I.: Comparative ecology and epidemiology of Lyme disease and tick-borne encephalitis in the former Soviet Union. Parasitol. Today *10*:157–160, 1994.
21. Krausler, J., Kraus, P., and Moritsch, H.: Klinische und virologisch-serologische untersuchungsergebnisse bei FSME und anderen virusinfektionen des zentralnervensystems im bezirk neunkirchen. Wien. Klin. Wochenschr. *70*:634–40, 1958.
22. Krech, U., Jung, F., and Jung, M.: Zentraleuropaeische zeckenzephalitis in der Schweiz. Schweiz. Med. Wochenschr. *99*:282–285, 1969.
23. Kristoferitsch, W., Stanek, G., and Kunz, C.: Doppelinfektion mit fruehsommermeningoenzephalitis- (FSME-) virus und *Borrelia burgdorferi*. Dtsch. Med. Wochenschr. *111*:861–864, 1986.
24. Kunz, C.: Arbovirus B–infektionen. *In* Grumbach, A., and Bonin, O. (eds.): Die Infektionskrankheiten des Menschen und Ihre Erreger. Stuttgart, Thieme, 1969.
25. Kunz, C.: Die fruehsommer-meningoenzephalitis. Paediatr. Praxis *14*:189–192, 1974.
26. Kunz, C., Hofmann, H., Kundi, M., et al.: Zur wirksamkeit von FSME-immunglobulin. Wien. Klin. Wochenschr. *93*:665–667, 1981.
27. Kunz, C., Bosch, R., and Richter, H.: Zur wirksamkeit von FSME-immunglobulin. Die Ellipse *10*:109–111, 1987.
28. Kunz, C.: Tick-borne encephalitis in Europe. Acta Leidensia *60*:1–14, 1992.
29. Lakeman, F. D., and Whitley, R. J.: Diagnosis of herpes simplex encephalitis: Application of polymerase chain reaction to cerebrospinal fluid from brain-biopsied patients and correlation with disease. J. Infect. Dis. *171*:857–863, 1995.
30. Lotric-Furlan, S., and Strle, F.: Thrombocytopenia: A common finding in the initial phase of tick-borne encephalitis. Infection *23*:203–206, 1995.
31. Mamoli, B., and Pelzl, G.: Residualschaeden nach FSME. Oesterr. Aerzteztg. *45*:45–51, 1990.
32. Marin, M. S., McKenzie, J., Gao, G. F., et al.: The virus causing encephalomyelitis in sheep in Spain: A new member of the tick-borne encephalitis group. Res. Vet. Sci. *58*:11–13, 1995.
33. McNair, A. N. B., and Brown J. L.: Tick-borne encephalitis complicated by monoplegia and sensorineural deafness. J. Infect. *22*:81–86, 1991.
34. McNeil, J. G., Lednar, W. M., Stansfield, S. K., et al.: Central European tick-borne encephalitis: Assessment of risk for persons in the Armed Forces and vacationers. J. Infect. Dis. *152*:650–651, 1985.
35. Moritsch, H.: Durch arthropoden uebertragene virusinfektionen des zentralnervensystems in Europa. Ergebn. Inn. Med. Kinderheilk. *17*:1, 1962.
36. Moritsch, H.: Die arboviren. *In* Haas, R., and Vivell, O. (eds.): Die Virus- und Rickettsieninfektionen des Menschen. Muenschen, Lehmann, 1965.
37. Ogawa, M., Okubo, H., Tsuji, Y., et al.: Chronic progressive encephalitis occurring 13 years after Russian spring-summer encephalitis. J. Neurol. Sci. *19*:363–373, 1973.
38. Oksi, J., Viljanen, M. K., Kalimo, H., et al.: Fatal encephalitis caused by concomitant infection with tick-borne encephalitis virus and *Borrelia burgdorferi*. Clin. Infect. Dis. *16*:392–396, 1993.
39. Rehse-Kuepper, B., Danielova, V., Klenk, W., et al.: Epidemiologie der zentraleuropaeischen enzephalitis. Muench. Med. Wochenschr. *118*:1615–1616, 1976.
40. Richling, E.: Virus-meningo-encephalitis in Austria. Bull. W. H. O. *12*:521, 1955.
41. Roggendorf, M., Heinz, F., Deinhardt, F., et al.: Serological diagnosis of acute tick-borne encephalitis by demonstration of antibodies of the IgM class. J. Med. Virol. *7*:41–50, 1981.
42. Scholz, H., and Summer, K.: Tick-borne encephalitis 1970 in Styria. *In* XIII. Symposium de l'Association Européenne contre la Poliomyelite, Helsinki, 1971. Brussels, Imprimerie des Sciences, 1972.
43. Silber, L. A., and Soloviev, V. D.: Far Eastern tick-borne spring-summer (spring) encephalitis. *In* Davis, B. D., and Fisher, S. H. (eds.): American Review of Soviet Medicine. New York, America-Soviet Medical Society, 1946, pp. 1–75.
44. Spiess, H., Mumenthaler, M., Burkhardt, S., et al.: Zentraleuropaeische enzephalitis (zeckenenzephalitis) in der Schweiz. Schweiz. Med. Wochenschr. *99*:277–282, 1969.
45. Suss, J., Sinnecker, H., Sinnecker, R., et al.: Epidemiology and ecology of tick-borne encephalitis in the eastern part of Germany between 1960 and 1990 and studies on the dynamics of a natural focus of tick-borne encephalitis. Zentralbl. Bakteriol. *277*:224–235, 1992.
46. Szirmai, I.: Elektroenzephalographische befunde bei der zeckenenzephalitis. Z. EEG-EMG *15*:138–141, 1984.
47. Wahlberg, P., Saikku, G., and Grummer-Korvenkontio, M.: Tick-borne viral encephalitis in Finland: The clinical features of Kumlinge disease during 1959–1987. J. Intern. Med. *225*:173–177, 1989.
48. World Health Organization: Outbreak of tick-borne encephalitis, presumably milk-borne. Wkly. Epidemiol. Record *19*:140, 1994.
49. World Health Organization: Tick-borne encephalitis and haemorrhagic fever with renal syndrome in Europe. *In* World Health Organization, Regional Office for Europe, Copenhagen, 1983, pp. 1–50.

50. Zanotto, P. M., Gao, G. F., Gritsun, T., et al.: An arbovirus cline across the Northern Hemisphere. Virology *210*:152–159, 1995.
51. Zeipel, G. V., Svedmyr, A., Holmgren, B., et al.: Tick-borne meningoencephalomyelitis in Sweden. Lancet *ii*:104, 1959.

❑ ❑ ❑

CHAPTER 179 (G)

Other Flaviviral Infections

Theodore F. Tsai

POWASSAN ENCEPHALITIS

Powassan virus is placed within the antigenic complex of tick-borne flaviviruses. The complete viral genomic sequence shows Powassan virus to be the most divergent of viruses in the antigenic complex.[21] Clinical and pathologic signs of encephalitis have been produced in experimentally infected horses.

Epidemiology and Ecology

Twenty-one cases of naturally acquired Powassan encephalitis have been reported from North America and 11 from Russia. Two cases of laboratory-acquired Powassan infections have been reported as well. Cases from North America have occurred primarily in children: 15 in children younger than 15 years of age, 2 in teenagers 15 to 19 years of age, and 4 in adults. Thirteen of the cases were in males. With one exception, infections have occurred in the summer or early fall; one case had onset in December.[25]

The probable sites of exposure of cases have been confined to eastern states and provinces: Ontario (six cases), Quebec (four cases), New York (nine cases), Pennsylvania (one case), and Massachusetts (one case).[3, 8, 16, 25, 31, 32, 36, 37] However, the known and suspected geographic distribution of the virus is wider, with viral isolations recorded from Connecticut, Massachusetts, West Virginia, Colorado, South Dakota, and California, and serologic evidence of infection in humans or animals from Maine, Wyoming, North Dakota, British Columbia, Alberta, and Sonora, Mexico. Viral isolates have been recovered from ticks, mosquitoes, and birds from southeastern Russia, and there is evidence of viral transmission in China and Southeast Asia.[20]

In North America, the virus is transmitted by *Ixodes cookei, I. marxi, I. spinipalpis*, and *Dermacentor andersoni* to small mammals (ground hogs, *Marmota monax*; red squirrels, *Tamiasciurus hudsonicus*; weasels, *Mustela*; skunks, *Mephitis* species; foxes, *Vulpes* species; chipmunks, *Tamias straiatus*; mice, *Peromyscus* species; snowshoe hares, *Lepus americanus*; voles, *Microtus* species; and gray squirrels, *Scurius carolensis*).[3] In Russia, the virus is transmitted by *I. persulcatus* and various *Haemaphysalis* species ticks; *Apodemus* mice and *Microtus* species voles are the principal vertebrate hosts.[20] Powassan virus is transmitted transstadially in *D. andersoni* and *I. pacificus*, and transovarial transmission has been shown in other species. Powassan virus infections in humans probably are rare because the implicated ixodid ticks infrequently bite people. Human infections are associated with outdoor activities and subsequent exposure to infected ticks. In one case involving a 13-month-old infant, however, the infecting tick was brought into the home by a domestic cat.[36] Animal serosurveys indicate that infections occur among dogs, and exposure to ticks on domestic animals may be an alternative source of infection. In a human serosurvey from Ontario, 3 per cent had Powassan antibody; however, in other areas, the prevalence of antibody has been less than 1 per cent.[3] Experimental studies have shown that *I. scapularis*, the vector of Lyme disease, can transmit Powassan virus, and a field isolate has been reported. The absence of a Powassan epidemic paralleling that of Lyme disease suggests differences in the agents' transmission cycles.

Although no Powassan cases have been attributed to milk-borne transmission, experimental studies have shown that domestic goats can be infected with Powassan virus and can shed virus into milk. In a survey of New York goats, 2 per cent had serologic evidence of past Powassan virus infection, which indicates the possibility of milk-borne Powassan virus infections in the United States.[37]

Clinical Manifestations

The incubation period may be several weeks after known exposure to a tick. Fever, headache, lethargy, retro-orbital pain, and photophobia are early symptoms that may be followed abruptly by changes in sensorium, generalized or focal seizures, paresis, and paralysis. A presentation with focal neurologic signs has been observed in 6 of the 11 patients in whom clinical descriptions have been reported. In one patient, olfactory hallucinations, focal seizures, and localizing electroencephalographic irregularities were concordant, which suggested a temporal lobe focus.[9]

Of 16 patients in whom outcome and follow-up were reported, 2 deaths occurred, and significant neurologic sequelae (hemiplegia, quadriplegia, aphasia) were reported in 7 individuals. Residual shoulder girdle atrophy and weakness analogous to sequelae after European and Far Eastern tick-borne encephalitis were reported in one recovered patient with Powassan encephalitis; in another, wasting and weakness of a leg consistent with a lumbosacral poliomyelitis were reported.[6, 16]

Clinical and experimental observations of tick-borne encephalitis suggest that chronic central nervous system infection, characterized by a convulsive disorder (epilepsia partialis continua), weakness, and dementia, may follow recovery from the acute phase of illness. A retrospective study of 22 Canadian patients with a similar clinical syndrome, and in whom histologic changes in brain resembled those of chronic tick-borne encephalitis, showed no evidence of Powassan virus infection. However, none of these patients had a history of acute encephalitis.

Laboratory Diagnosis

Virus has been recovered from the brain of patients with fatal cases of the disease. A serologic diagnosis can be achieved more rapidly by detecting specific IgM antibody in acute-phase serum or spinal fluid.[3] Serologic diagnosis by hemagglutination inhibition and complement fixation is specific in most instances, but heterologous antibodies from other flavivirus infections (e.g., dengue, St. Louis encephalitis) or vaccinations (yellow fever) may obscure the results.

Differential Diagnosis

The clinical presentation of encephalitis in a patient with a history of tick bite acquired in an endemic area should suggest the possibility of Powassan encephalitis. However, ixodid tick bites may be inconspicuous, so that a negative history does not exclude the diagnosis. Other viral agents of encephalitis, especially eastern equine encephalitis virus and

California group viruses, which are prevalent in New York state and eastern Canada, should be considered in the differential diagnosis. Lyme disease, because of its known geographic distribution and association with a tick vector, also may present with neurologic complications; however, a history of typical rash and arthritis should differentiate the conditions. An imported case of tick-borne encephalitis, encountered in Ohio but acquired in Austria, underscores the value of obtaining a travel history.

Treatment and Prevention

No specific therapy for Powassan encephalitis is available. Personal protective measures to avoid tick bites are advised (see Colorado tick fever section in Chapter 175). The consumption of unpasteurized goat milk should be avoided because of the theoretical risk of Powassan virus infection and the well-documented risks of other infections.[24, 32] Commercial inactivated tick-borne encephalitis vaccine does not cross-protect against Powassan virus infection.

WEST NILE FEVER

West Nile fever virus was isolated from an ill viremic person in the West Nile district of Uganda in 1937. Antigenic characterization disclosed its relationship to viruses in the Japanese encephalitis antigenic complex of flaviviruses. Its geographic distribution is among the most extensive of all arboviruses, encompassing southern, central, eastern, and western Africa, areas of Europe and Russia, the Middle East, Pakistan, India, Southeast Asia, and Australia.[11, 26] Strains from various geographic regions have been differentiated antigenically and genetically.[29] However, associated differences in human virulence have not been described. Natural infections have been described in a wide variety of birds and mammals; encephalitis outbreaks have been reported in horses, mild febrile illness with myopathy in dogs, and disseminated viscera and neurotropic infection in a wild pigeon.

In most areas, the virus is transmitted in an avian–*Culex* mosquito cycle: *C. univittatus* in Africa, *C. modestus* and *C. pipiens* in the Middle East and Europe, and *C. tritaenirhynchus* and *C. vishnui* complex mosquitoes in Asia.[23] Transmission between birds and their mites or ticks also has been demonstrated, providing a potential viral overwintering mechanism. Migrating birds may be responsible for transferring the virus over long distances. Sindbis virus, an alphavirus, is transmitted in identical avian-mosquito cycles in overlapping geographic areas; combined epidemics have occurred frequently in South Africa.

Seroprevalence rates vary widely according to location and ecologic conditions. For example, seroprevalence rates higher than 80 per cent, indicating a high level of endemic infection, were found in residents near Lake Chad (with an extensive avian population), but 300 km south, seroprevalence rates declined to less than 30 per cent. Epidemics have been reported from South Africa, Israel, Algeria, Bulgaria, France, and Romania. The latter outbreak, in 1996, led to nearly 400 neurologic cases, principally in elderly residents of Bucharest. Conditions that led to epidemic transmission in South Africa included heavy early season rainfall and warm temperatures, which led to expanded mosquito breeding habitat and accelerated viral extrinsic incubation in infected vectors, which led to high vector infection rates.

Subclinical infections are common.[22] The incubation period is 1 to 6 days, after which there is an abrupt onset of fever, headache, muscle aches, conjunctivitis, pharyngitis, and gastrointestinal symptoms. Headache often is severe and may be accompanied by ocular pain. Grippe symptoms are followed by a morbilliform rash affecting the trunk and extremities in about 50 per cent of cases. Lymphadenopathy may be prominent. Arthralgias have been an important component of the illness in some outbreaks. Defervescence usually occurs within 5 days, but like dengue, may be followed by a recrudescence of fever and symptoms in some cases. Treatment is symptomatic.

Meningoencephalitis is the most common complication.[11, 12, 34] Neurologic signs may be the initial manifestation of illness or can follow the initial grippe prodrome. Neurologic infection has resulted in aseptic meningitis; an encephalitis syndrome with mental status changes, cranial nerve and bulbar palsies, motor weakness, and abnormal reflexes; and myelitis.[15] Optic neuritis and polyradiculitis also have been reported. During outbreaks in Israel and Romania, central nervous system infection occurred most frequently in the elderly; however, encephalitis cases have been reported in children in Asia. The case fatality ratio in neurologic cases is approximately 10 per cent, with higher rates in the elderly. Myocarditis, pancreatitis, and fatal hepatitis also have been reported as complications.[2, 13, 27] Peripheral leukopenia and lymphocytosis are usual. In patients with central nervous system infection, pleocytosis and elevated protein are found in the cerebrospinal fluid.

The uncomplicated illness cannot be differentiated clinically from dengue and other febrile illnesses with nonspecific symptoms. The diagnosis also should be suspected in patients with illnesses featuring hepatitis or encephalitis. The virus can be isolated from blood taken early in the illness. Virus can be recovered from three-quarters of samples taken on the first day of onset, whereas only 25 per cent of samples from the second or third postillness day are positive. Virus also has been isolated from cerebrospinal fluid, from liver biopsies, and from brain and other organs at autopsy. Vero cells and continuous mosquito cell lines usually are employed. Intracerebral inoculation of suckling mice is a sensitive system for viral isolation used in reference laboratories.

Serologic procedures can provide a diagnosis in most cases. Detection of viral-specific IgM in serum is presumptive evidence of recent infection; presence of IgM in cerebrospinal fluid indicates intrathecal production and confirms a recent infection. Cases also can be confirmed by demonstrating fourfold or greater changes in antibody titer by hemagglutination, complement fixation, immunofluorescence, or neutralization. Cross-reactions with dengue and other flaviviruses (Banzi, yellow fever, Wesselsbron, and others in Africa; Japanese encephalitis, Zika, and others in Asia) can complicate interpretation of serologic results. Neutralizing antibody titers are most specific.

An experimental inactivated vaccine is under development. Personal protection consists of avoiding outdoor activity during the crepuscular periods (when vector mosquitoes are most active) and applying mosquito repellents.

ROCIO ENCEPHALITIS

Rocio encephalitis virus was isolated from human brain of a fatal encephalitis case occurring during an outbreak in 1975.[19, 24, 28] The virus is related peripherally to viruses in the Japanese encephalitis viral antigenic complex. The disease has occurred exclusively in the coastal São Paulo State and adjacent Parana State, Brazil, principally in the Ribiera Valley and Santista lowlands. More than 1000 cases were documented in outbreaks between 1975 and 1977; only 1 symptomatic case (in an infant) has been recognized subsequently, although recent infections (IgM in asymptomatic individuals) were documented in serosurveys between 1983 and 1987. Thus, the virus may be transmitted undetected in the Ribiera Valley. The viral transmission cycle has not been elucidated; however, field and laboratory observations suggest transmission between birds and *Psorophora* or *Aedes* mosquitoes. Humans are dead-end hosts. Human cases have occurred principally in men with outdoor occupations, especially fishermen.

The incubation period is estimated to be 7 to 14 days. Prodromal symptoms of fever, headache, malaise, vomiting, and conjunctivitis are followed by mental status changes, meningismus, and motor impairment. Cerebellar signs are common. Signs of bulbar involvement also are seen. Coma and fatal outcome are most common in children (30 per cent) and in the elderly; overall, 10 per cent of cases are fatal and 20 per cent have neuropsychiatric sequelae. Pathologic findings of encephalitis involve principally the thalamus, cerebellar dentate nucleus, brain nuclei, brain stem, and spinal cord.

The diagnosis should be suspected in acute encephalitis patients with a consistent history of exposure. Virus has been isolated from autopsy brain specimens. Presence of viral-specific IgM in cerebrospinal fluid or fourfold changes in serum antibody titer confirm a case. IgM in serum is presumptive evidence of recent infection. Treatment is supportive. Emergency applications of adulticides and larvicides have been used in epidemic control.

LOUPING ILL

Louping ill virus derives its name from an old Scots term describing the leaping motions of encephalitic sheep. Historical accounts of the disease in sheep date from 1795, and the virus was isolated from ill sheep in 1931. The virus, a member of the antigenic complex of tick-borne flaviviruses, is transmitted by *I. ricinus* to sheep, deer, small mammals, and grouse. The disease is enzootic in pasturelands of Scotland, England, Wales, and Ireland. Naturally acquired human infections have occurred mainly in sheep farmers, veterinarians, and abattoir workers or butchers with direct animal contact. Antibody prevalence is 10 per cent among abattoir workers in enzootic areas. Laboratory-acquired infections are common, accounting for half of all reported human cases. These observations suggest that infections are transmitted easily by direct mucous membrane or respiratory infection. Tick-transmitted cases also have been reported. Hospital surveillance in an enzootic area found louping ill to be rare, accounting for less than 0.5 per cent of encephalitis cases. Related tick-borne viruses in Spain, Greece, Norway, and Turkey have not been associated with human disease. The virus is shed in sheep and goat milk, but, unlike tick-borne encephalitis, milk-transmitted cases have not been reported.

The incubation period can be as short as 3 days. Three clinical syndromes have been described.[7] About one-third of patients have a self-limited flu-like illness with fever, headache, dizziness, and myalgias. The febrile illness is followed by clinical improvement and a second encephalitic phase in more than one-half of cases. Neurologic symptoms include meningismus, severe headache, vomiting, drowsiness, and tremor; one fatal case was reported. A poliomyelitis syndrome with muscular weakness or paralysis has been described in a few cases. A case of hemorrhagic fever also was reported in one atypical laboratory-acquired case.

The diagnosis should be suspected in febrile patients with occupational or other exposure, especially if central nervous system symptoms are present. The diagnosis is confirmed serologically by demonstrating viral-specific IgM in cerebrospinal fluid or serum or with fourfold antibody rises by other techniques. Treatment is symptomatic. Unpasteurized milk products should be avoided. Persons with outdoor exposure in enzootic areas are advised to use repellents and other protective measures against tick bites.

KYASANUR FOREST DISEASE

Kyasanur Forest virus was isolated in 1957 after an outbreak of hemorrhagic fever, initially suspected to be the first outbreak of yellow fever in Asia, appeared in India in the Kyasanur Forest of Mysore (now Karnataka).[4] The virus is a member of the tick-borne flaviviral antigenic complex. The virus is transmitted by *Haemaphysalis spinigera* (among numerous other ixodid ticks) to forest rodents, insectivors, and possibly bats; cattle and other large animals are important tick hosts but do not appear to amplify the virus. Langur monkeys sicken in epizootics and die of the infection. Human cases occur in dry season epidemics, chiefly among persons with forest contact. The disease has spread contiguously as villagers clear forests for pastureland. Between 1982 and 1988, 1847 cases were reported, 254 fatal.

After an incubation period of 3 to 8 days, illness begins abruptly with fever, headache, myalgias, chills, and gastrointestinal symptoms.[30, 33] Facial hyperemia, conjunctival suffusion, lymphadenopathy, hepatomegaly, papulovesicular enanthem, and petechiae are the principal physical findings. Bradycardia and hypotension are present and may progress to become life-threatening. Epistaxis, hemoptysis, and gastrointestinal bleeding may be prominent. Bronchopneumonia and hemorrhagic pulmonary edema complicate the illness in 40 per cent of cases. Renal failure may develop. After the resolution of symptoms and an afebrile interval of 1 to 3 weeks, fever, a recurrence of symptoms, and meningoencephalitis develop in 15 to 50 per cent of cases, as occurs in tick-borne encephalitis. Leukopenia with a left shift, thrombocytopenia, and elevated hematocrit, reflecting hemoconcentration, are seen. Elevations in liver enzymes are common. The case-fatality ratio is 3 to 15 per cent; keratitis and iritis occur as sequelae. Virus frequently can be isolated from acute-phase blood specimens (<12 days after onset), or the diagnosis can be confirmed serologically. A formalin-inactivated chick embryo cell culture vaccine is distributed in epidemic areas.

OMSK HEMORRHAGIC FEVER

Omsk hemorrhagic fever virus was isolated from a viremic human during a series of outbreaks in the Omsk region of western Siberia from 1945 to 1949.[20] Between 1945 and 1958, approximately 1500 cases were reported in the forest-steppe zones within the Omsk, Novosibirsk, Kurgan, and Tjumen regions. The virus is related antigenically and genetically to other tick-borne flaviviruses. The virus circulates among microtine rodents and *Dermacentor* ticks, leading to a spring–early summer peak of infected ticks with a smaller peak in early autumn. The disease epidemiology changed after muskrats were introduced to the region; extensive muskrat epizootics occurred, leading to an increase in human cases and geographic spread of the disease. Muskrat trappers, who may be infected by direct contact with infected tissues or blood, continue to account for the majority of cases, but tick-borne infections also occur among other local residents, including children. Seroprevalence rates range to higher than 30 per cent in some locations. Laboratory-associated cases

TABLE 179–5. Less Commonly Recognized Flaviviral Infections

Virus and Reference	Clinical Syndrome	Geographic Distribution	Transmission Cycle	Mode of Transmission
Alma-Arasan[21]	Febrile illness, meningitis	Kazakhstan	*Ixodes persulcatus*—?	V
Apoi[19]	Encephalitis	Japan	Rodent—?	L
Banzi[18]	Nonspecific febrile illness	South, East Africa	*Culex rubinotus*—rodent	V
Bussuquara[31]	Fever, arthralgias	Brazil, Colombia, Panama	*Culex melaconion* species—rodent	V
Edge Hill[1]	Fever, polyarthritis	Australia	*Aedes vigilax*—marsupial	V
Ilheus[31]	Fever, myalgia, encephalitis	Argentina, Brazil, Colombia, Guatemala, Panama, Trinidad	*Psorophora ferox*—bird	V,E
Karshi[21]	Nonspecific febrile illness	Uzbekistan	Various ticks—rodent	V
Kokobera[23]	Fever, polyarthralgia	Australia, Papua New Guinea	*Culex annulirostris*—? marsupial	V
Koutango[27]	Fever, rash, arthralgia	West and Central Africa	Tick—rodent	L
Kunjin[23]	Fever, polyarthralgia, encephalitis	Australia, Malaysia, Thailand	*Culex annulirostris*—bird	V
Langat[27]	Fever, encephalitis	Malaysia, Thailand, Russia	*Ixodes* tick—rodent	L
Modoc[27]	Aseptic meningitis	Western United States, Canada	Rodent—rodent	Z
Negishi[27]	Encephalitis	Japan, China, Russia	Tick—unknown	L,V
Rio Bravo[39]	Nonspecific febrile illness, meningitis	Western United States, Canada	Bat—bat	Z,L
Sepik[23]	Nonspecific febrile illness	Papua New Guinea	*Mansonia* species—?	V
Spondweni[18]	Fever, arthralgia, rash	South and West Africa	*Aedes* species—?	L,V
Usutu[27]	Fever, rash	South and central Africa	*Culex* species—bird	V
Wesselsbron[18]	Fever, arthralgia, rash, encephalitis	Sub-Saharan Africa, Thailand	*Aedes* species—?	V,L,DC?
Zika[18]	Fever, rash, arthralgia	West, East, and central Africa; Indonesia, Malaysia	*Aedes* species—monkey	V

L, laboratory-acquired infection; V, vector-borne infection; E, experimental infection; Z, zoonotic infection; DC, direct contact with infected sheep.

frequently have occurred in workers not immunized with tick-borne encephalitis vaccine.

The incubation period may be as brief as 2 to 4 days. The illness is similar to Kyasanur Forest disease, with an earlier onset of hemorrhagic phenomena (e.g., epistaxis).[33] Hemorrhages tend to be less severe, neurologic complications are less frequent, and overall mortality is lower (less than 3 per cent). Neuropsychiatric sequelae, however, are common. Uncomplicated cases usually resolve within 7 to 10 days. The diagnosis is made serologically. Vaccine produced against tick-borne encephalitis virus is reported to provide some degree of cross-protection.

OTHER FLAVIVIRAL INFECTIONS

Flaviviral infections of lesser public health importance or that are recognized less frequently are listed in Table 179–5. Several of the viruses are known to cause human illness only because of laboratory exposures. The clinical manifestations of these infections may differ from naturally acquired infections because of their mode of transmission by respiratory, mucosal, or other routes of infection. Others that cause nonspecific syndromes of febrile illness were discovered through fever surveys; although few cases may have been reported, their prevalence may be underestimated because few cases are recognized. Of the zoonotic flaviviruses (transmitted from animal to animal without the agency of an arthropod vector), only Rio Bravo and Modoc viruses are known to cause human illness.

References

1. Aaskov, J. G., Phillips, D. A., and Wiemers, M. A.: Possible clinical infection with Edge Hill virus. Trans. R. Soc. Trop. Med. Hyg. *87*:452–453, 1993.
2. Albagali, C., and Chaimoff, R.: A case of West Nile myocarditis. Hare Fuah *57*:274–275, 1959.
3. Artsob, H.: Powassan encephalitis. *In* Monath, T. P. (ed.): The Arboviruses: Epidemiology and Ecology. Boca Raton, CRC Press, 1989, pp. 29–49.
4. Bannerjee, K.: Kyasanur forest disease. *In* Monath, T. P. (ed.): The Arboviruses: Epidemiology and Ecology. Boca Raton, CRC Press, 1989, p. 198.
5. Boughton, C. R., Hawkes, R. A., and Naim, H. M.: Illness caused by a kokobera-like virus in southeastern Australia. Med. J. Aust. *145*:90–97, 1986.
6. Conway, D., Rossier, E., Spence, L., et al.: A case report: Powassan virus encephalitis with shoulder girdle involvement. Can. Dis. Weekly Rep. *2-22*:85–87, 1976.
7. Davidson, M. M., Williams, H., and MacLeod, A. J.: Louping ill in man: A forgotten disease. J. Infect. *23*:241–249, 1991.
8. Deibel, R., Srihongse, S., and Woodall, J.P.: Arboviruses in New York State. Am. J. Trop. Med. Hyg. *28*:577–582, 1979.
9. Embil, J., Camfield, P., Artsob, H., et al.: Powassan virus encephalitis resembling herpes simplex encephalitis. Arch. Intern. Med. *143*:341–343, 1983.
10. Essed, W. C. A. H., Van, T., and Ongeran, H. A. E.: Arthropod-borne virus infections in New Guinea. 1. Report of a case of Murray Valley encephalitis in a Papvan woman. Trop. Geogr. Med. *1*:52–55, 1965.
11. Flatau, E., Kohr, D., Daker, O., et al.: West Nile fever encephalitis. Isr. J. Med. Sci. *17*:1057–1059, 1981.
12. George S., Prasad, S. R., Rao, J. A., et al.: Isolation of Japanese encephalitis and West Nile viruses from fatal cases of encephalitis. Indian J. Med. Res. *86*:131, 1987.
13. Georges, A. J., Lesbordes, J. L., Georges-Courbot, M. C., et al.: Fatal hepatitis from West Nile virus. Ann. Inst. Pasteur. Virol. *138*:234–237, 1988.
14. Goldfield, M., Austin, S. M., Black, H. C., et al.: A nonfatal human case of Powassan virus encephalitis. Am. J. Trop. Med. Hyg. *22*:78–81, 1973.
15. Gradoth, N., Weitzman, S. and Lehmann, E. E.: Acute anterior myelitis complicating West Nile fever. Arch. Neurol. *36*:172–173, 1979.
16. Jackson, A. C.: Leg weakness associated with Powassan virus infection-Ontario. Can. Dis. Weekly Rep. *15*:123, 1989.
17. Juff, P. G.: Arboviral zoonoses of Africa. *In* Beran, G. W. (ed.): Handbook of Zoonoses. 2nd ed. Section B: Viral. Boca Raton, CRC Press, 1994, pp. 261–273.
18. Karabatsos, N.: International catalogue of arboviruses and certain other viruses of vertebrates. Am. Soc. Trop. Med. Hyg. San Antonio, 1987.
19. Lopes, O., Sacchetta, L. de A., Coimbra, T. L. M., et al.: Emergence of a

new arbovirus disease in Brazil. II. Epidemiologic studies on 1975 epidemic. Am. J. Epidemiol. *108*:394–401, 1978.
20. Lvov, D. K.: Arboviral zoonoses of northern Eurasia (Eastern Europe and The Commonwealth of Independent States). *In* Beran, G. W. (ed.): Handbook of Zoonoses. 2nd ed. Boca Raton, CRC Press, 1994, pp. 237–260.
21. Mandl, C. W., Holzman, N., Kunz, C., et al.: Complete genomic sequence of Powassan virus: Evaluation of genetic elements in tick-borne versus mosquito-borne flaviviruses. Virology *194*:173–184, 1993.
22. Marberg, K., Golblum, N., Sterk, V. V., et al.: The natural history of West Nile fever. I. Clinical observations during an epidemic in Israel. Am. J. Hyg. *64*:259–265, 1956.
23. McIntosh, B. M., Jupp, P. G., Dos Santos I., et al.: Epidemics of West Nile and Sindbis viruses in South Africa with *Culex univittatus* Theobald as a vector. S. Afr. J. Sci. *72*:295, 1976
24. Monath, T. P., and Heinz, F.: Flaviviruses. *In* Fields, B. N., Knipe, D. M., and Howley, P. (eds.): Fields Virology. 3rd ed. Philadelphia, Lippincott-Raven, 1996, pp. 961–1034.
25. Partington, M. W., Thomson, V., and O'Shaughnessy, M. V.: Powassan virus encephalitis in southeastern Ontario. Can. Med. Assoc. J. *123*:603–604, 1980.
26. Peiris, J. S. M., and Amerasinghe, F. P.: West Nile fever. *In* Beran, G. W. (ed.): Handbook of Zoonoses. 2nd ed. Boca Raton, CRC Press, 1994, pp. 139–148.
27. Perelman, A., and Stern, J.: Acute pancreatitis in West Nile fever. Am. J. Trop. Med. Hyg. *23*:1150–1152, 1974.
28. Pinheiro, F. P.: Arboviral zoonoses of Central and South America. *In* Beran, G. W. (ed.): Handbook of Zoonoses. 2nd ed. Boca Raton, CRC Press, 1994, pp. 201–225.
29. Porter, K. R., Summers, P. L., DuBois, D., et al.: Detection of West Nile virus by the polymerase chain reaction and analysis of nucleotide sequence variation. Am. J. Trop. Med. Hyg. *48*:440–446, 1993.
30. Prabha, A., Prabhu, M. G., Raghuvcer, C. V., et al.: Clinical study of 100 cases of Kyasanur Forest disease with clinicopathological correlation. Indian J. Med. Sci. *47*:124–130, 1993.
31. Rossier, E., Harrison, R. J., and Lemieux, B.: A case of Powassan virus encephalitis. Can. Med. Assoc. J. *110*:1173–1180, 1974.
32. Smith, R., Woodall, J. P., Whitney, E., et al.: Powassan virus infection: A report of three human cases of encephalitis. Am. J. Dis. Child. *127*:691–693, 1974.
33. Smorodintsev, A. A., Kazbintsev, and Chudakov, V. G.: Virus Hemorrhagic Fevers: Israel Program for Scientific Translations. Jerusalem, 1964, pp. 175–192.
34. Southam, C. M., and Moore, A. E.: Induced virus infections in man by the Egypt isolates of West Nile virus. Am. J. Trop. Med. Hyg. *3*:19–50, 1954.
35. Sulkin, S. E., Burns, K. F., Shelton, D. F., et al.: Bal salivary gland virus: Infections of man. Tx. Rep. Biol. Med. *20*:113–127, 1962.
36. Wilson, M. S., Wherrett, B. A., and Mahdy, M. S.: Powassan virus meningoencephalitis: A case report. Can. Med. Assoc. J. *121*:320–323, 1979.
37. Woodall, J. P., and Roz, A.: Experimental milk-borne transmission of Powassan virus in the goat. Am. J. Trop. Med. Hyg. *26*:190–192, 1977.
38. Wolff, M. S., Calishan, C. H., and McGuire, K.: Spondweni virus infection in a foreign resident of Upper Volta. Lancet *2*:1306–1307, 1982.

180

HEPATITIS C VIRUS

Miriam J. Alter, Eric E. Mast, and Harold S. Margolis

HISTORY

Hepatitis C virus (HCV) was discovered in 1988 and was shown to be the primary etiologic agent of parenterally transmitted non-A, non-B hepatitis worldwide.[12, 36, 87] The term non-A, non-B hepatitis was applied to those cases of acute hepatitis for which other specific etiologies (hepatitis A virus, hepatitis B virus, Epstein-Barr virus, cytomegalovirus, and a variety of other infectious and noninfectious agents that can cause liver inflammation) reliably could be excluded.[7] Because currently licensed tests for HCV infection cannot distinguish between recent and past or resolved and active infection, exclusion of other etiologies for liver inflammation continues to be necessary. Although HCV infection first was recognized to be associated commonly with blood transfusion, it now is known to be an important cause of acute and chronic community-acquired viral hepatitis.[16, 18]

PROPERTIES OF THE VIRUS

Classification

HCV has been classified as a separate genus—*Hepacivirus*—in the family *Flaviviridae* because of similarities to the flavivirus and pestivirus genomes.[43] The HCV genome is a single-stranded, positive-sense RNA molecule, composed of approximately 9400 nucleotides encoding a single open-reading frame.[28, 77] The 5′ end encodes the core and envelope proteins, followed by the nonstructural proteins that extend to the 3′ end of the genome (see Fig. 55–7).

Genomic Organization

The 5′ end of the large open-reading frame begins with an untranslated region (UTR), which has a high degree of sequence conservation, indicating that it may play a major role in virus replication. The 5′ UTR is followed by codes for the putative structural proteins of the virus. In vitro translation of this region indicates that it is processed into a minimum of four proteins.[28, 77] The amino-terminal end is cleaved to produce an unglycosylated core protein (p22), followed by two envelope glycoproteins, designated E1 and E2. The amino-terminal end of E2 exhibits up to 58 per cent variation among geographically distinct virus isolates and has been termed the hypervariable region. Following E2 is the extremely hydrophobic NS2 region, for which no function has been ascertained.

The NS3 region encodes a protein that contains consensus sequences for two distinct enzymatic functions, which may be involved in polyprotein processing (protease) and in unwinding the RNA genome for replication (helicase). Like NS2, NS4 is very hydrophobic and of unknown function. The NS5 region encodes a protein that contains RNA-dependent RNA polymerase that replicates the RNA genome. Like its pestivirus and flavivirus relatives, HCV does not appear to produce DNA replication intermediates, and integrated forms of the viral genome in the host genome have not been detected.[28, 77]

The HCV genome exhibits substantial heterogeneity as a result of mutations occurring during viral replication.[33, 125, 153] Comparative nucleotide sequence analysis of different HCV isolates indicates the existence of at least six genetically distinct major groups (genotypes) and more than 30 subgroups. In a single infected individual, rapid mutation results in a population of heterogeneous but closely related HCV sequences (quasispecies).[32] The quasispecies nature of certain RNA viruses is known to represent a mechanism by which such viruses escape immune surveillance by undergoing sequential mutations leading to antigenetically distinct epitopes. Furthermore, the genetic heterogeneity of the envelope proteins of the different genotypes of HCV is so great that it is likely that the proteins are distinct immunologically as well.[32] In an HCV-infected individual, the quasispecies population of heterogeneous RNA sequences centers around one dominant sequence. The dominant sequence, as well as the consensus sequence, changes sequentially during the course of infection. A hypervariable region (HVR1) within one of the envelope proteins of HCV (E2) evolves very rapidly. Patients infected with HCV mount a humoral immune response to epitopes of HVR1. However, sequential changes in the consensus sequence of HVR1 during infection result in the generation of variants that are not recognized by preexisting antibodies. This might represent a mechanism by which HCV evades host immune surveillance and establishes and maintains persistent infection.

LABORATORY METHODS FOR DETECTING INFECTION

Serologic Assays

The first version of the enzyme immunoassays (EIA-1) for antibody to HCV (anti-HCV) detected antibody to the c100-3 antigen, a nonstructural recombinant protein located in the NS4 region of the HCV genome. The second version of the EIAs (EIA-2) for anti-HCV use three recombinant proteins: two from nonstructural regions (NS3 and NS4) of the genome (c100–3 and c33c) and one from the core region of the genome (c22–3).[5] On the basis of these assays, anti-HCV has been detected in an average of 70 to 90 per cent of patients with non-A, non-B hepatitis.[8, 18, 57] The greater sensitivity of the EIA-2 compared with the EIA-1 resulted in a 6 to 32 per cent increase in the antibody detection rate among patients with non-A, non-B hepatitis[1, 6, 16, 18, 92] and in a 59 per cent increase among volunteer blood donors.[87] In this latter group, the EIA-2 detected an additional 1.4 HCV-positive donors per 1000 tested.

The EIA-2 detects anti-HCV in approximately 90 to 95 per cent of patients with HCV infection.[18] In addition to its greater sensitivity, the EIA-2 detects antibody earlier in the course of HCV infection:[162] 5 to 6 weeks after onset of hepatitis in 80 per cent of patients versus 40 to 60 per cent with EIA-1.[18, 19] Anti-HCV remains detectable by EIA-2 long after the primary infection; in contrast, in many patients anti-HCV became undetectable by EIA-1 within a few years after disease onset.[18, 23, 59] In addition to assays that detect antibodies to recombinant HCV proteins, assays have been developed that detect antibodies to synthetic peptides alone or in combination with recombinant proteins.[5]

Interpretation of the results of EIAs that screen for anti-HCV is limited by several factors: (1) these assays will not detect anti-HCV in approximately 5 to 10 per cent of persons infected with HCV; (2) these assays do not distinguish between acute and chronic or past infection; (3) in the acute phase of hepatitis C, there may be a prolonged interval between onset of illness and seroconversion; and (4) in populations with a low prevalence of infection, the rate of false positivity for anti-HCV is high.

As with any screening test, the proportion of repeatedly reactive EIA results that are falsely positive varies depending on the prevalence of infection in the population screened. Although no true confirmatory test has been developed, supplemental tests for specificity are available. The Recombinant Immunoblot Assay (RIBA, Chiron Corp., Emeryville, CA), which is a commercially available licensed assay, and the MATRIX HCV Assay (Abbott Laboratories, North Chicago, IL), which is available on a research-use basis, use different formats and expression systems to evaluate repeatedly reactive results obtained from the screening assays.[87, 112] On the basis of these supplemental assays, 70 to 100 per cent of repeatedly reactive anti-HCV results in persons at high risk for HCV infection, such as patients with clinically diagnosed hepatitis C, injecting drug users, and persons with a history of blood transfusion, are judged true-positives.[18, 36] In contrast, less than 50 per cent of repeatedly reactive anti-HCV results in persons at low risk of HCV infection, such as volunteer blood donors, are judged true-positives.[36, 87]

Nucleic Acid Detection

The diagnosis of HCV infection also is possible by detecting HCV RNA using polymerase chain reaction (PCR) techniques to amplify reverse-transcribed cDNA.[77] Primers specific for the 5′ UTR are the most sensitive because this region is highly conserved among all HCV isolates studied to date. Although PCR assays for HCV RNA are available from several commercial laboratories on a research-use basis, they are not standardized and the cost is high. In one study in which a reference panel containing known HCV RNA–positive and HCV RNA–negative sera was provided to 86 laboratories worldwide,[98] only 50 per cent were considered to have performed adequately (missing one weak positive sample), and only 16 per cent reported faultless results. Both false-positive and false-negative results can occur from improper collection, handling, and storage of the test samples.[46, 171] To prevent false-positive results from cross-contamination, a separate designated area in the laboratory should be used when separating and aliquoting serum; the aliquoting area should be decontaminated with a 1 per cent bleach solution between specimen batches and if any spills occur; one specimen should be open at a time; a positive-displacement pipette with a separate sterile disposable pipette tip for each specimen should be used to aliquot all serum specimens; and gloves should be changed if they become contaminated with serum. False-positive results also may occur because the extraction and handling of the viral RNA easily is subject to contamination. To prevent false-negative results, serum should be separated and frozen at −20° C (short-term storage) or −70° C (long-term storage) within 2 to 4 hours of collection in a non–frost-free freezer; if shipping is required, samples should be packed in dry ice. In addition, the detection of HCV RNA may be intermittent, and the meaning of a single negative PCR test result is not conclusive.[18]

Tests also have been developed to quantitate HCV RNA in serum, including a branched-chain DNA assay (Quantiplex HCV RNA Assay [bDNA], Chiron Corp., Emeryville, CA)[49] and quantitative PCR (Roche Amplicor HCV Monitor, Roche Molecular Systems, Branchburg, NJ)[134]; however, the applicability of these tests in the clinical setting has not been determined. These quantitative tests are less sensitive than standard PCR assays[72, 120]; thus, they should not be used as a primary test to confirm or exclude the diagnosis of HCV infection or to monitor the end-point of treatment.

Several different nucleic acid detection methods have been developed to group isolates of HCV based on genotypes, including genomic amplification of certain genomic regions and nucleotide sequencing, PCR with genotype-specific primers, restriction fragment length polymorphism analysis of the PCR amplicons, differential hybridization, and serologic genotyping.[97] In general, a high level of concordance has been found between these different genotyping methods.

EPIDEMIOLOGY

Prevalence

The prevalence of HCV infection as measured by anti-HCV is highly variable in the population.[11, 102] Worldwide, the highest rates are found among those with large or repeated direct percutaneous exposures, such as injecting drug users and hemophilia patients (60 to 90 per cent); moderate rates are found among those with smaller but repeated direct or inapparent percutaneous exposures, such as hemodialysis patients (20 per cent); and lower rates are found among those with inapparent parenteral or mucosal exposures, such as persons with high-risk sexual behaviors and sexual and household contacts of persons with chronic HCV infection (1 to 10 per cent), as well as among those with sporadic percutaneous exposures, such as health care workers (1 to 2 per cent). The lowest rates of anti-HCV are found among those with no high-risk characteristics, such as volunteer blood donors (0.01 to 1 per cent). Infection rates in blood donor populations are not representative of the infection rates in the general population because donors generally are highly selected groups that have been screened for risk factors and serologic markers associated with a variety of infectious diseases. There are few studies on the prevalence of HCV infection in representative samples of the general population. In the United States, a serologic survey of a population-based sample of more than 20,000 civilian noninstitutionalized persons conducted from 1988 to 1994 found an anti-HCV prevalence of 1.8 per cent,[109] sixfold higher than that observed in volunteer blood donors. Among children younger than 12 years of age, the prevalence is 0.2 per cent (Centers for Disease Control and Prevention [CDC]; unpublished data).

Incidence

Most studies on the incidence of HCV infection have been limited to transfusion recipients. Prior to 1986, worldwide incidence rates of posttransfusion hepatitis C ranged from 5 to 13 per cent.[1, 24, 54, 55, 83, 117, 118, 146] From 1986 to 1990, these rates declined to between 1.5 and 9 per cent,[54, 57, 83, 108, 117] and subsequent to anti-HCV screening of donors in 1990 in the United States, posttransfusion hepatitis C rates have been reported to be less than 0.1 per cent per recipient or 0.01 to 0.001 per cent per unit transfused.[12, 54, 117, 141]

Although most studies of hepatitis C have focused on transfusion recipients, most HCV infections are acquired outside the transfusion setting.[16, 18] In the United States, an average of 15 per cent of the acute viral hepatitis reported during 1982 to 1995 was due to HCV. The estimated incidence of acute hepatitis C remained relatively stable through much of the 1980s, with an average annual rate of 15 per 100,000 (corrected for underreporting),[17] but declined by more than 80 per cent between 1989 and 1995 (Fig. 180–1).[11, 16] After correcting for underreporting and asymptomatic infections, the CDC estimated that an average of 120,000 (range, 30,000 to 180,000) HCV infections occurred annually in the United States during the past decade. The number of cases of transfusion-associated hepatitis C declined significantly after 1985, but this change had little impact on overall disease incidence. The dramatic decline observed since 1989 correlates with a decrease in cases associated with injecting drug use, which

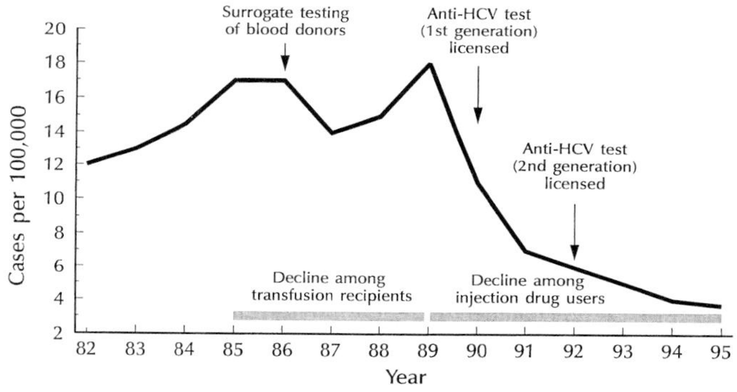

FIGURE 180–1. *Estimated incidence of acute hepatitis C, 1982–1995, United States. (Source: Centers for Disease Control and Prevention.)*

may be due to HCV infection saturation of the susceptible population and possibly to safer needle-using practices.

Geographic Distribution

Worldwide, estimates of HCV infection prevalence are available mainly from studies of blood donors (Fig. 180–2).[11, 102] The lowest anti-HCV prevalence rates have been reported from the United Kingdom (0.075 to 0.1 per cent) and Scandinavia (0.01 to 0.1 per cent), and the highest rates have been reported from Egypt (>5 per cent). Geographic clustering of high prevalence rates of anti-HCV has been reported from Japan and Egypt in populations lacking commonly recognized risk factors for acquiring hepatitis C.[74, 79, 154] The reasons for such clustering have not been ascertained, but hypotheses include traditional and nontraditional medical treatment with contaminated equipment and familial aggregation as a result of perinatal and horizontal transmission.

The distribution of the different genotypes of HCV also varies geographically.[32, 33, 47, 97] Genotypes 1 and 2 are distributed widely throughout the world. Genotype 1 is predominant in North and South America, Europe, and Asia, although the relative frequencies of the different subtypes vary; 1a and 1b both are common in the first three continents, but only 1b is predominant in Asia. Type 3 also is distributed widely, and subtype 3a has been seen with increasing frequency among persons who acquired their infection recently.[121] However, subtype 3b has been identified only in Japan, Nepal, Thailand, and Indonesia. Type 4 is predominant in northern and central African countries and type 5 in southern Africa. Type 6 has been found in 20 to 30 per cent of isolates studied in Hong Kong and Vietnam.

Seasonal Patterns

Studies of community-acquired hepatitis C show no evidence of seasonality or of epidemic cycles.

Host and Social Factors

Acute and chronic hepatitis C may occur in all age groups. Most cases of acute hepatitis C occur among young adults.[16, 18, 39] Clinical illness is uncommon among children, but among adults older than 40 years of age, HCV infection often is the most common cause of acute and chronic hepatitis.[39] This age distribution of disease likely is related to patterns of exposure (injecting drug use in young adults and in prior

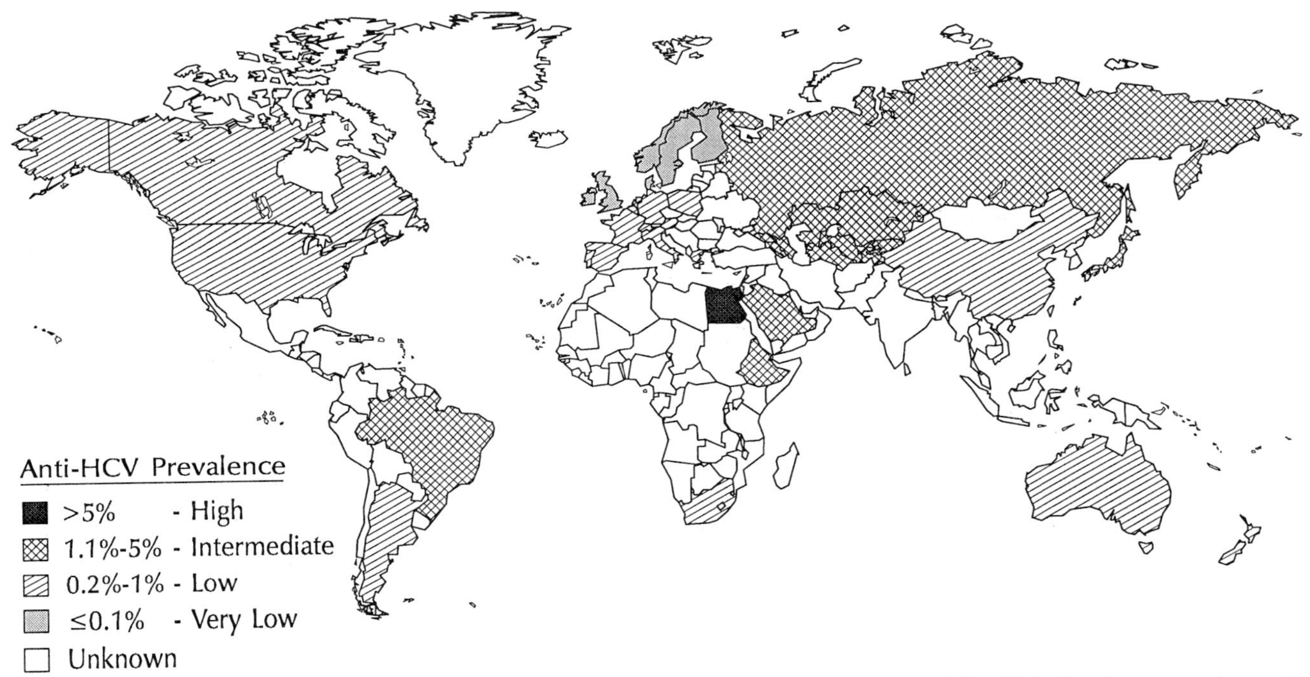

FIGURE 180–2. *Prevalence of antibody to hepatitis C virus (anti-HCV) in volunteer blood donors. Anti-HCV positivity based on enzyme immunoassays and supplemental testing. (Source: Centers for Disease Control and Prevention.)*

years transfusions in older adults) and possibly to age-specific variations in clinical expression of disease. The male to female ratio for hepatitis C generally is 2:1,[16, 18, 39] with a higher frequency of cases among men related to injecting drug use. Hepatitis C occurs worldwide in all racial/ethnic groups studied. In the United States, the highest proportion of cases is among whites, but the incidence of disease is highest in nonwhite racial/ethnic groups, particularly Hispanics.[16]

Spread of Infection

Direct percutaneous exposures, such as transfusion of blood or blood products or transplantation of organs or tissues from infectious donors and sharing of contaminated needles among injection drug users, are associated with the most efficient transmission of HCV.[11, 25, 96, 128, 133, 136, 158] Exposure to blood and blood products historically has been the most common identifiable source of infection among children and adolescents. HCV now is transmitted infrequently by transfusion because of screening tests that exclude infectious donors.

In 1994, the first outbreak of hepatitis C associated with contaminated intravenous immunoglobulin was reported in the United States.[38] This outbreak involved recipients of a single product, Gammagard (Baxter Healthcare Corporation, Deerfield, IL), received between April 1, 1993, and February 23, 1994, when the product was withdrawn from the market. Infection was associated with lots of Gammagard produced from plasma screened by second-version anti-HCV assays that were positive for HCV RNA, and the risk increased with increasing quantities of HCV RNA in the lots infused.[29] Intramuscular immunoglobulin has never been associated with the transmission of any infectious disease in the United States. Currently, all immunoglobulin products (intravenous and intramuscular) commercially available in the United States must undergo an inactivation procedure or be HCV RNA–negative before release.

Other persons at risk as a result of exposure to infectious blood are hemodialysis patients and health care workers.[11, 115, 129] The average risk of acquiring HCV infection after a needle-stick contaminated with anti-HCV–positive blood is 3.5 per cent.[20, 39] Epidemiologic and seroprevalence studies have suggested that sexual and household exposure to an infected contact, exposure to multiple partners, and perinatal exposure also may be associated with the transmission of HCV, although the efficiency of transmission in these settings appears to be low.[11] Among cases of acute non-A, non-B hepatitis (most of which presumably are due to HCV infection) in persons younger than 15 years of age reported to the CDC in the years prior to donor screening, about 5 per cent reported a history of blood transfusion in the 6 months preceding onset of their illness, 4 per cent a history of exposure to a contact with hepatitis, 1 per cent hemodialysis, and the vast majority (90 per cent) no known source for their infection.[37] In 1995, however, no transfusion-associated cases were reported in this age group; 14 per cent reported exposure to a household contact who had hepatitis, and 86 per cent were unable to identify a specific source.[40]

The strongest evidence in support of the transmission of HCV between sexual partners and household contacts is derived from epidemiologic studies of non-A, non-B hepatitis conducted prior to the development of an assay to detect anti-HCV. Two case-control studies found that non-A, non-B hepatitis patients with no history of parenteral exposures were significantly more likely than control patients without liver disease to have a history of exposure to a sexual partner or household contact who had hepatitis in the past; one of these studies also found a significant association between acquiring disease and a history of exposure to multiple heterosexual partners.[14, 15] Among eight seroprevalence studies of long-term spouses of patients with chronic hepatitis C who had no other risk factors, the average anti-HCV prevalence was 5 per cent[13]; however, five of these studies found none of the spouses to be anti-HCV–positive, and three studies found that the prevalence of anti-HCV ranged from 2 to

15 per cent. Among nine seroprevalence studies of nonsexual household contacts of patients with chronic hepatitis C, the average anti-HCV prevalence also was 4 per cent[13]; two of these studies found none of the household contacts to be anti-HCV–positive, and seven studies found that the prevalence of anti-HCV ranged from 1 to 11 per cent. The presumed mechanism of transmission was inapparent percutaneous or permucosal exposure to infectious blood or body fluids containing blood. Although the infected contacts reported no other commonly recognized risk factors for hepatitis C, most of these studies were conducted in countries where it has been suggested that transmission of HCV infection may be associated with common exposures in the community resulting from contaminated equipment used in traditional and nontraditional medical procedures in the past.

Perinatal transmission of HCV infection from anti-HCV–positive, anti-HIV–negative women has been documented in an average of 5 per cent of their infants based on detection of anti-HCV and in a similar proportion (6 per cent) based on detection of HCV RNA (Table 180–1).[106] Substantial and/or persistent elevations in alanine aminotransferase (ALT) levels as evidence of hepatitis developed in an average of 4 per cent of all the infants followed and 67 per cent of the HCV-infected infants. Among the studies of infants born to women co-infected with HCV and HIV, the average transmission rate was higher: 14 per cent based on detection of anti-HCV and 17 per cent based on detection of HCV RNA (Table 180–1).[106] Hepatitis developed in 21 per cent of all the infants followed and in 100 per cent of the HCV-infected infants.

In all of the studies that determined the HCV RNA status of the mother at the time of delivery, only mothers who were HCV RNA–positive transmitted HCV to their infants (Table 180–1).[106] The apparent higher HCV transmission rate to infants from women co-infected with HIV may be the result of higher titers of HCV RNA compared with those in women infected only with HCV. In two studies of HCV-positive, HIV-negative women, the transmission of HCV to their infants was related to the titer of HCV RNA in the women at the time of delivery.[100, 123] In one of these studies, transmission occurred only from women with titers $\geq 10^6$ copies per mL[123]; in the other, transmission occurred only from one woman with a titer of 10^{10}.[100]

The data on the risk of HCV transmission from breast feeding are limited but suggest that breast feeding does not play a role in the transmission of this virus. In the five studies that have evaluated breast feeding among infants born to HCV-infected women, the average rate of infection was 4 per cent in both breast-fed and bottle-fed infants (Table 180–1).[106] Although in one study the duration of breast feeding was longer for infants who became infected compared with those who did not (mean, 6.6 vs. 3.3 months), evidence of HCV infection (HCV RNA positivity) first was detected in all of the infected infants within 1 to 2 months of age, an incubation period shorter than the duration of breast feeding in the uninfected infants.[122]

PATHOGENESIS AND IMMUNITY

Infection and Pathology

The primary site of infection is the liver. In experimentally infected chimpanzees, HCV RNA can be detected in serum and HCV RNA and HCV antigen in liver within 48 to 72 hours after inoculation.[76, 93, 116] In human recipients of blood from infectious donors, viremia is detectable within 2 weeks after exposure. All of the hepatotropic viruses produce liver cell injury and necrosis during the acute infection, including ballooning degeneration, focal necrosis, and acidophilic bodies.[71]

Histopathologic features commonly observed in biopsy specimens from patients with chronic HCV infection include bile duct damage, bile duct loss, steatosis, and lymphoid cell aggregation (follicles).[21, 69, 140] Severe lobular necrosis and inflammation and piecemeal necrosis are seen less often. Chronic hepatocellular inflammation and cirrhosis may be the key factor in the development of primary hepatocellular carcinoma.[110]

Immunologic Events

The extraordinarily high rates of chronic disease and persistent viremia observed in humans suggest that HCV fails to induce an effective neutralizing antibody response. Experimental studies in animals have shown that after a primary HCV infection, rechallenge of convalescent (i.e., HCV RNA–negative) chimpanzees with the same or different strains of HCV resulted in the reappearance of viremia, which was due to infection with the subsequent challenge virus.[59] This reappearance of viremia was associated with mild ALT elevations and histopathologic signs of acute hepatitis. Reinfection or superinfection with HCV may be a possible explanation for the apparent episodes of posttransfusion or posttransplant hepatitis observed among recipients who were anti-HCV–positive before they received blood or organs from an HCV-infected donor.[24, 128]

Although antibodies to the E2 region of the HCV genome have been identified as potential neutralizing antibodies,

TABLE 180–1. Summary of Studies of Perinatal Transmission of Hepatitis C Virus (HCV)

	Number/Total Infants Infected by HIV Status of Mother	
Infants of HCV-Infected Mothers	***HIV-Negative (%) (Range)***	***HIV-Positive (%) (Range)***
Total infected		
Anti-HCV-positive	16/295 (5) (0–25)	18/128 (14) (5–36)
HCV RNA–positive	19/312 (6) (0–25)	29/169 (17) (5–36)
HCV RNA status of mother		
Positive	17/194 (9) (0–42)	14/44 (32) (13–44)
Negative	0/95 (0)	0/14 (0)
Type of feeding		
Breast	5/124 (4) (0–25)	Not done
Bottle	2/44 (4) (0–20)	

*Infection in infants defined as loss of passively acquired anti-HCV with subsequent seroconversion to anti-HCV based on second-generation enzyme immunoassay and supplemental testing and/or detection of HCV RNA in a venous sample at 1 month of age or older. All but two studies followed infants for 12 or more months.

their effectiveness is extremely limited and their role in protection has not been demonstrated.[61, 151] Historically, several studies attempted to assess the value of prophylaxis with immunoglobulins against posttransfusion non-A, non-B hepatitis. In some of these studies, immunoglobulins seemed to reduce the rate of clinical disease but not overall infection rates[88, 138, 147]; in one, patients receiving immunoglobulin were less likely to develop chronic hepatitis.[138]

None of these data have been reanalyzed since anti-HCV testing became available, and in only one study was the first dose of immunoglobulin given after, rather than before, the exposure (i.e., transfusion), making it difficult to assess its value for postexposure prophylaxis. In 1992, the Food and Drug Administration recommended that all plasma be screened for anti-HCV. If protective antibody does exist, such screening may affect its presence in immunoglobulin manufactured from screened plasma pools. In an experimental study in chimpanzees,[94] neither infection nor disease was prevented by treatment with commercially prepared immunoglobulin manufactured from screened plasma or a preparation of hepatitis C immunoglobulin manufactured from plasma containing high titers of anti-HCV given 1 hour after inoculation.

DIAGNOSIS

Diagnosis of HCV infection generally is made on the basis of detection of anti-HCV in serum by EIAs, with supplemental testing of repeatedly reactive sera by an immunoblot assay (e.g., RIBA, MATRIX).[19] In adults with acute infection, 70 to 80 per cent have anti-HCV detectable at the time of clinical presentation and 90 per cent have anti-HCV detectable by 12 weeks after onset of hepatitis.[18] In patients with posttransfusion HCV infection, anti-HCV is detectable in 40 per cent within 10 weeks of exposure, in 80 per cent within 15 weeks, and in virtually all patients within 6 months.[162] Because the appearance of anti-HCV may be delayed in patients with acute infection, testing should be repeated if hepatitis C is suspected in a patient and initial testing is negative for anti-HCV. Criteria for diagnosing perinatal HCV infection using anti-HCV tests have not been established. A variety of patterns of anti-HCV detection have been observed in both infected and uninfected infants of anti-HCV–positive mothers. However, it is unlikely that passively acquired maternal antibody would persist for more than 12 months.

HCV infection also can be diagnosed by detecting HCV RNA in serum by PCR. HCV RNA can be detected within 1 to 2 weeks after exposure to the virus, weeks before the onset of ALT elevations or the appearance of anti-HCV. In some persons, HCV RNA may be the only evidence of HCV infection. As mentioned previously, both false-positive and false-negative PCR results can occur if appropriate specimen collection, handling, and storage procedures are not used. In addition, there is substantial laboratory-to-laboratory variation in the performance of PCR, and HCV RNA may be detected intermittently in a patient over time.[18, 46, 98, 171]

No tests are available to differentiate acute from chronic infection or active from resolved infection, and the diagnosis of chronic hepatitis C in an HCV-infected individual generally is based on the presence of elevated ALT activity for 6 or more months. However, HCV causes persistent infection even in the absence of chronic ALT elevations.[18]

CLINICAL MANIFESTATIONS

The incubation period for acute hepatitis C after transfusion or accidental needle-stick has been reported to average 6 to 7 weeks but may range from 2 to 26 weeks.[92, 105, 143, 170] Children and adults with acute hepatitis C typically either are asymptomatic or have a mild clinical illness. The most commonly reported symptoms among children include anorexia, asthenia, and abdominal pain. In one case series of children (mean age, 4 years) with hepatitis C, only 17 per cent had symptomatic illness and 4 per cent had jaundice.[25] However, symptomatic infection was reported in 70 per cent of children with immunodeficiency disorders.[29; CDC, unpublished data] In adults with hepatitis C, up to 40 per cent had symptomatic illness and 15 to 30 per cent had jaundice.[1, 8, 91] Clinical illness in patients who seek medical care with acute hepatitis C is similar to that of other types of viral hepatitis, and serologic testing is necessary to determine the etiology of hepatitis in an individual patient.

Fulminant hepatic failure after acute HCV infection is rare.[165] Several cases of fulminant hepatitis C among adults have been reported in the medical literature,[60, 137, 168] and one case has been reported in an infant born to an HCV-infected mother.[90] However, evidence of HCV infection rarely has been found in several case series of patients with fulminant non-A, non-B hepatitis.[63, 99, 166]

Persistent HCV infection develops in most (85 per cent or more) adults after acute hepatitis C,[18, 45] and evidence of chronic hepatitis with persistently elevated ALT levels more than 6 months after illness onset develops in an average of 67 per cent (range, 58 to 81 per cent).[1, 8, 55, 92, 108, 119, 132, 155, 157] In studies among children, similar rates of chronic infection and persistently elevated liver enzymes have been found.[25, 41, 107, 118] No clinical or epidemiologic features among patients with acute infection have been found to be predictive of either persistent infection or chronic liver disease. Moreover, a variety of ALT patterns have been observed in these patients during follow-up, and some patients may have prolonged periods (12 or more months) of normal ALT activity even though they have histologically confirmed chronic hepatitis.[18] Thus, long-term follow-up of patients with acute HCV infection is needed to determine the consequences of infection in these patients.

HCV may result in persistent infection even in the absence of biochemical evidence of chronic liver disease. Among patients with community-acquired hepatitis C who apparently had resolved their disease, all persistently were HCV RNA–positive up to 4 years after onset of their acute illness, although in four patients detection of HCV RNA was intermittent.[18] HCV RNA also has been detected in anti-HCV–positive blood donors with normal ALT levels.[4, 30, 45, 58, 68, 87, 149, 172] Among those who also were HCV RNA–positive, liver biopsies showed chronic hepatitis.[4, 58, 149]

In prospective studies of adults presenting with signs and symptoms of acute hepatitis C who were followed up with liver biopsies, 26 to 50 per cent had chronic active hepatitis and 3 to 26 per cent had cirrhosis within several years after acute infection.[18, 155, 157] Similar histologic findings have been reported among children.[25, 78] In addition, anti-HCV–positive persons have been found to have a 5- to 50-fold higher risk of primary hepatocellular carcinoma than anti-HCV–negative patients in case-control studies.[52, 84, 170] However, in most persons with chronic HCV infection, disease progresses indolently over decades with little clinical evidence of liver disease, even among patients with histologic evidence of chronic active hepatitis or cirrhosis.

The long-term consequences of chronic HCV infection have not been determined fully. In cohort studies of patients with posttransfusion hepatitis C, 3 to 5 per cent died of hepatitis C–related liver disease after 16 to 23 years of follow-up.[10, 53, 91, 144, 145] In one of these studies, 20 per cent of patients had clinical evidence of cirrhosis after a mean interval of 16 years.[91] However, long-term outcome data from patients with transfusion-associated hepatitis may not be generalizable to all patients with HCV infection because it is possible that patients with transfusion-associated hepatitis C may have more severe disease in the form of chronic active hepatitis compared with patients with a history of other exposures.[18, 155] In addition, longer-term follow-up studies will be needed to assess the lifetime consequences of chronic hepatitis C because disease related to hepatitis C progresses slowly over decades. In one study, the mean interval between blood transfusion and the clinical recognition of hepatocellular carcinoma was 30 years (range, 15 to 60 years).[86]

A variety of factors may influence the progression of liver disease in patients with chronic HCV infection. In several studies, an association between disease severity and genotype has been found; patients infected with genotype 1b were more likely to have elevated ALT levels and liver biopsy evidence of chronic liver disease than were patients infected with other genotypes.[121] However, this finding may reflect differences in viral titer and duration of infection associated with different genotypes rather than differences in strain virulence. One factor strongly correlated with severe disease is alcohol-induced liver injury.[89] Other factors that may influence the progression of chronic hepatitis C include immunodeficiency disorders, route of transmission, age at infection, and co-infection with other viruses.

EXTRAHEPATIC MANIFESTATIONS

Type II Cryoglobulinemia

Type II cryoglobulinemia (essential mixed cryoglobulinemia) is a vasculitis characterized by cryoglobulins consisting of polyclonal IgG and monoclonal IgM rheumatoid factors. Typical clinical manifestations include arthralgias, Raynaud syndrome, and purpura; peripheral neuropathy and glomerulonephritis occur occasionally. In several studies, 80 to 95 per cent of patients with type II cryoglobulinemia have been found to have evidence of HCV infection, whereas patients with type I cryoglobulinemia (monoclonal only) had no evidence of infection.[2, 64, 104, 113] Although immune-mediated disorders develop in only a minority of HCV-infected patients, immunologic abnormalities including cryoglobulinemia (36 per cent), serum rheumatoid factor (71 per cent), and serum antitissue antibody (41 per cent) frequently have been found among these patients.[127] Further evidence of a causal association of type II cryoglobulinemia with HCV infection includes the presence of anti-HCV and HCV RNA concentrated 10-fold and 1000-fold, respectively, in cryoprecipitate[2] and immunohistochemical evidence of HCV antigens in skin biopsy specimens from patients with this disorder.[139] In addition, substantial improvement in cutaneous vasculitis has been observed in HCV-infected patients who responded to interferon treatment, and clinical relapse occurred in patients whose HCV infection recurred after interferon treatment was discontinued.[65, 114]

Membranoproliferative Glomerulonephritis

The findings of several studies suggest that membranoproliferative glomerulonephritis may be mediated by HCV infection.[80, 167] Characteristic histopathologic findings of membranoproliferative glomerulonephritis, including deposition of IgG, IgM, and C3 in glomeruli, have been observed in renal biopsy specimens of patients with HCV infection and proteinuria. In addition, cryoglobulin-like structures have been found by electron microscopy in renal biopsy specimens from these patients, and cryoprecipitates have been found to contain HCV RNA and anti-HCV. Improvement in renal function has been noted in HCV-infected patients who initially responded to interferon, but viremia and renal disease relapsed after cessation of therapy.[80]

Porphyria Cutanea Tarda

A strong association has been found between HCV infection and sporadic (nonfamilial) porphyria cutanea tarda (PCT), a disease caused by a deficiency of hepatic uroporphyrinogen decarboxylase. In studies of patients with sporadic PCT, 60 to 80 per cent have been found to be infected with HCV, whereas patients with familial PCT had no evidence of infection.[50, 62, 73] Typical clinical manifestations in patients with PCT include hepatic dysfunction and lesions on light-exposed areas of the skin, consisting of enhanced facial pigmentation, increased fragility to trauma, erythema, and ulcerative lesions. Extrinsic factors, such as alcohol consumption, estrogens, and iron overload, appear to be required to trigger clinical illness in predisposed persons. HCV infection also may act as one of these triggering factors, which could account for the long-standing association of PCT with chronic liver disease. No data are available to assess the efficacy of interferon treatment in patients with PCT and chronic hepatitis C.

Other Conditions

Other extrahepatic conditions have been reported in patients with HCV infection, including Sjögren syndrome,[127] autoimmune thyroiditis,[156] lichen planus,[82] Mooren corneal ulcers,[164] and idiopathic pulmonary fibrosis.[161] However, definitive associations of these conditions with HCV infection have not been established. Diseases with possible infectious etiologies that have not been found to be associated with HCV infection include aplastic anemia and biliary atresia.[3, 75]

TREATMENT

For acute hepatitis, there is no specific therapy that currently is of proven benefit. In studies that administered interferon during the acute phase of HCV infection, rapid improvement in serum aminotransferase levels and a decrease in the proportion of patients developing chronic hepatitis were demonstrated.[66] However, in general, the majority of patients treated still developed chronic hepatitis C, and it is unclear whether therapy during the acute phase offered additional benefit over delayed therapy during the chronic phase.[66]

Interferon-α has been licensed in the United States for the treatment of adults with chronic hepatitis C and generally is recommended for patients with well-compensated disease, persistently elevated liver enzymes, and chronic hepatitis on liver biopsy.[48, 66] There is little evidence supporting any long-term benefit of interferon treatment for patients with persistently normal liver enzymes[148] or for patients with advanced cirrhosis who may be at risk for decompensation with therapy. Initially, the standard recommended regimen of interferon-α based on the results of randomized, controlled treatment trials in the United States and Europe was 3 million units administered subcutaneously three times per week for 24 weeks.[51, 66, 103] With this regimen, approximately 50 per cent of treated patients have a complete response, with normalization of serum aminotransferases and a loss or decrease of HCV RNA in serum at the end of therapy; most of these patients respond within the first 12 weeks of treatment, and most are associated with histologic improvement in liver pathology.[66] However, more than half of the patients who respond to treatment will experience relapse with recurrence of elevated serum aminotransferases and reappearance of HCV RNA in serum after interferon is discontinued. Thus, only 10 to 25 per cent of treated patients will have a sustained, beneficial response with persistent normalization of serum aminotransferases; usually these patients have no detectable HCV RNA in serum by PCR. The absence of HCV RNA by PCR at the end of therapy has been found to be predictive of long-term response.[42] Higher rates of sustained response have been observed after longer duration of therapy, and a 12-month treatment regimen of interferon-α (same dosage and interval) recently was licensed in the United States.

Improved interferon response rates have been found to be associated with virologic factors including lower serum and hepatic HCV RNA titers, HCV genotypes other than genotype 1, and the presence of mutations in the NS5 region of the viral genome.[56, 101, 121, 124, 152, 169] However, it is unclear whether the effect of genotype is related independently to interferon response or whether this finding reflects higher HCV RNA titers and longer duration of disease that generally are found in patients with genotype 1. Response rates also have been found to be better in patients with shorter duration of disease, and the results of trials to evaluate interferon treatment in patients with acute hepatitis C are encouraging.[34] Additional factors that have been found to predict a favorable response to interferon include host factors such as younger age, mild to moderate liver inflammation, absence of cirrhosis, and lower hepatic iron content.[35, 81, 126, 159]

The optimum dose and duration of treatment have not been determined; however, data suggest that higher initial interferon doses, longer duration of treatment, and gradual reduction in dose may improve sustained response rates.[85, 130, 131, 150] Limitations of alternative dosing strategies may include cost with marginal additional response rates, side effects of higher interferon doses, the possible selection of resistant mutants, and the development of neutralizing antibodies to interferon.[111, 151] Additional strategies that have been used in an attempt to increase response rates to interferon include selecting patients with pretreatment variables that predict a good response,[66] use of interferon in combination with other drugs, such as ribavirin,[27, 31, 142] and reduction of hepatic iron content with phlebotomy.[22] Further data are needed before recommendations can be made regarding use of these alternative treatment approaches.

Experience is limited using interferon to treat children with chronic hepatitis C, and interferon is not approved by the Food and Drug Administration for persons younger than 18 years of age. Data from preliminary interferon trials among children with chronic hepatitis C are promising, with sustained responses in 45 to 55 per cent of treated children.[26, 67, 135] In one of these studies, children with pretreatment HCV RNA titers of $\leq 10^7$ copies/mL were more likely to respond to treatment than were those with higher HCV RNA titers.[67] However, definitive recommendations for the use of interferon in children with hepatitis C cannot be made until the long-term effects of treatment on symptoms and progression have been documented and more data are available regarding side effects of treatment in children.[44, 106] Treatment under a research protocol may be considered for patients with disabling symptoms of disease or histologically advanced pathology (e.g., bridging necrosis, active cirrhosis).

PREVENTION

Development of a vaccine against hepatitis C is proving to be difficult because of the genetic diversity of HCV, the rapid development of mutations in a critical region of the envelope protein, and the failure of antibody elicited by infection to prevent reinfection with either heterologous or homologous virus strains. Postexposure prophylaxis with immunoglobulin does not appear to be effective in preventing HCV infection and is not recommended by the Advisory Committee on Immunization Practices.[39] There is no information regarding the use of antiviral agents (e.g., interferon-α) for postexposure prophylaxis, and such treatment is not recommended.[39]

In the absence of immunoprophylaxis, the primary measures available to prevent hepatitis C are screening of blood, organ, and tissue donors; modification of high-risk behaviors; and use of blood and body fluid precautions. Blood donor screening will prevent only a small proportion of disease in the United States because less than 10 per cent of hepatitis C cases were associated with transfusion before anti-HCV tests became available.

At the present, no measures are available to prevent perinatal transmission of HCV and there is no licensed therapy or guidelines for the treatment of HCV-infected infants or children. Thus, screening of pregnant women for evidence of HCV infection is not recommended. If an infant is born to a woman who is known to be infected with HCV, testing of the infant for evidence of HCV infection should be considered.[44, 106] However, there are no data to support discouraging either pregnancy or breast feeding for women based on their HCV infection status alone.[36, 44]

All persons with HCV infection should be considered potentially infectious and should be counseled regarding available measures to prevent transmission to others.[36] They should not donate blood, body organs, or other tissue, or semen. Cuts or skin lesions should be kept covered, and personal articles such as toothbrushes and razors that could be contaminated with blood should not be shared. Although there are no recommendations for changes in sexual practices for persons with a steady sex partner, infected persons should be informed of the potential risk of sexual transmission so that they can decide if they wish to take precautions. Persons with multiple sex partners should follow safer sex practices, including reducing the number of sex partners and using barriers (e.g., latex condoms) to prevent contact with body fluids. Epidemiologic studies to define the risk of and the factors facilitating HCV transmission in these settings need to be conducted to develop more specific recommendations to prevent most disease acquisition.

References

1. Aach, R. D., Stevens, C. E., Hollinger, F. B., et al.: Hepatitis C virus infection in post-transfusion hepatitis: An analysis with first- and second-generation assays. N. Engl. J. Med. *325*:1325–1329, 1991.
2. Agnello, V., Chung, R. T., and Kaplan, L. M.: A role for hepatitis C virus infection in type II cryoglobulinemia. N. Engl. J. Med. *327*:1490–1495, 1992.
3. A-Kader, H. H., Nowicki, M. J., Kuramoto, K. I., et al.: Evaluation of the role of hepatitis C virus in biliary atresia. Pediatr. Infect. Dis. J. *13*:657–659, 1994.
4. Alberti, A., Chemello, L., Cavalletto, D., et al.: Antibody to hepatitis C virus and liver disease in volunteer blood donors. Ann. Intern. Med. *114*:1010–1012, 1991.
5. Alter, H. J.: New kit on the block: Evaluation of second-generation assays for detection of antibody to the hepatitis C virus. Hepatology *15*:350–353, 1992.
6. Alter, H. J.: Post-transfusion hepatitis (PTH) in the United States. *In* Nishioka, K., Suzuki, H., Mishiro, S., Oda, T. (eds.): Viral Hepatitis and Liver Disease. Tokyo, Springer-Verlag, 1994, pp. 551–553.

7. Alter, H.J., Holland, P. V., Morrow, A. G., et al.: Clinical and serological analysis of transfusion-associated hepatitis. Lancet *2*:838–841, 1975.
8. Alter, H. J., Jett, B. W., Polito, A. J., et al.: Analysis of the role of hepatitis C virus in transfusion-associated hepatitis. *In* Hollinger, F. B., Lemon, S. M., and Margolis, H. S. (eds.): Viral Hepatitis and Liver Disease. Baltimore, Williams & Wilkins, 1991, pp. 396–402.
9. Alter, H. J., Purcell, R. H., Shih, J. W., et al.: Detection of antibody to hepatitis C virus in prospectively followed transfusion recipients with acute and chronic non-A, non-B hepatitis. N. Engl. J. Med. *321*:1494–1500, 1989.
10. Alter, H. J.: To C or not to C: These are the questions. Blood *85*:1681–1695, 1995.
11. Alter, M. J.: Epidemiology of hepatitis C in the West. Semin. Liver Dis. *15*:5–14, 1995.
12. Alter, M. J.: Residual risk of transfusion-associated hepatitis. NIH Consensus Development Conference on Infectious Disease Testing for Blood Transfusions. Bethesda, MD, National Institutes of Health, 1995, pp. 23–27.
13. Alter, M. J.: Epidemiology of hepatitis C. Eur. J. Gastroenterol. Hepatol. *8*:1–5, 1996.
14. Alter, M. J., Coleman, P. J., Alexander, W. J., et al.: Importance of heterosexual activity in the transmission of hepatitis B and non-A, non-B hepatitis. J. A. M. A. *262*:1201–1205, 1989.
15. Alter, M. J., Gerety, R. J., Smallwood, L., et al.: Sporadic non-A, non-B hepatitis: Frequency and epidemiology in an urban United States population. J. Infect. Dis. *145*:886–893, 1982.
16. Alter, M. J., Hadler, S. C., Judson, F. N., et al.: Risk factors for acute non-A, non-B hepatitis in the United States and association with hepatitis C virus infection. J. A. M. A. *264*:2231–2235, 1990.
17. Alter, M. J., Mares, A., Hadler, S. C., et al.: The effect of underreporting on the apparent incidence and epidemiology of acute viral hepatitis. Am. J. Epidemiol. *125*:133–139, 1987.
18. Alter, M. J., Margolis, H. S., Krawczynski, K., et al.: The natural history of community-acquired hepatitis C in the United States. N. Engl. J. Med. *327*:1899–1905, 1992.
19. Alter, M. J.: Review of serologic testing for hepatitis C virus infection and risk of posttransfusion hepatitis C. Arch. Pathol. Lab. Med. *118*:342–345, 1994.
20. Alter, M. J.: Occupational exposure to hepatitis C virus: A dilemma. Infect. Control Hosp. Epidemiol. *15*:742–744, 1994.
21. Bach, N., Thung, S. N., and Schaffner, F.: The histological features of chronic hepatitis C and autoimmune chronic hepatitis: A comparative analysis. Hepatology *15*:572–577, 1992.
22. Bacon, B. R., Rebholz, A. E., Fried, M. W., et al.: Beneficial effect of iron reduction therapy in patients with chronic hepatitis C who failed to respond to interferon therapy. Hepatology *18*:371, 1993.
23. Beach, M. J., Meeks, E. L., Mimms, L. T., et al.: Temporal relationships of hepatitis C virus RNA and antibody responses following experimental infection of chimpanzees. J. Med. Virol. *36*:226–237, 1992.
24. Berrera, J. M., Brugera, M., Guadalupe, E., et al.: Incidence of non-A, non-B hepatitis after screening blood donors for antibodies for hepatitis C virus and surrogate markers. Ann. Intern. Med. *115*:596–600, 1991.
25. Bortolotti, F., Jara, P., Diaz, C., et al.: Posttransfusion and community-acquired hepatitis C in childhood. J. Pediatr. Gastroenterol. Nutr. *18*:279–283, 1994.
26. Bortolotti, F., Giacchino, R., Vajro, P., et al.: Recombinant interferon-alpha therapy in children with chronic hepatitis C. Hepatology *22*:1623–1627, 1995.
27. Braconier, J. H., Paulsen, O., Engman, K., et al.: Combined alpha-interferon and ribavirin treatment in chronic hepatitis C: A pilot study. Scand. J. Infect. Dis. *27*:325–329, 1995.
28. Bradley, D. W., Beach, M. J., and Purdy, M. A.: Recent developments in the molecular cloning and characterization of hepatitis C and E viruses. Microb. Pathog. *12*:391–398, 1992.
29. Bresee, J. S., Mast, E. E., Coleman, P. J., et al.: Hepatitis C virus infection associated with administration of intravenous immune globulin. J. A. M. A. *276*:1563–1567, 1996.
30. Brillanti, S., Gaiani, S., Miglioli, M., et al.: Persistent hepatitis C viraemia without liver disease. Lancet *341*:464–465, 1993.
31. Brillanti, S., Garson, J., Foli, M., et al.: A pilot study of combination therapy with ribavirin plus interferon alpha for interferon alpha–resistant chronic hepatitis C. Gastroenterology *107*:812–817, 1994.
32. Bukh, J., Miller, R. H., and Purcell R. H.: Genetic heterogeneity of hepatitis C virus: Quasispecies and genotypes. Semin. Liver Dis. *15*:41–63, 1995.
33. Bukh, J., Purcell, R. H., and Miller R. H.: At least 12 genotypes of hepatitis C virus predicted by sequence analysis of the putative E1 gene of isolates collected worldwide. Proc. Natl. Acad. Sci. U. S. A. *90*:8234–8238, 1993.
34. Camma, C., Almasio P., and Craxi, A.: Interferon as treatment for acute hepatitis C: A meta-analysis. Dig. Dis. Sci. *41*:1248–1255, 1996.
35. Camps J., Crisostomo S., Garcia-Granero M., et al.: Prediction of the response of chronic hepatitis C to interferon alpha: A statistical analysis of pretreatment variables. Gut *34*:1714–1717, 1993.
36. Centers for Disease Control: Public Health Service inter-agency guidelines for screening donors of blood, plasma, organs, tissues, and semen for evidence of hepatitis B and hepatitis C. M. M. W. R. *40*(RR-4):1–17, 1991.
37. Centers for Disease Control: Hepatitis Surveillance Report No. 54. Atlanta, 1992.
38. Centers for Disease Control and Prevention: Outbreak of hepatitis C associated with intravenous immunoglobulin administration: United States, October 1993–June 1994. M. M. W. R. *43*:505–509, 1994.
39. Centers for Disease Control and Prevention: Hepatitis Surveillance Report No. 56. Atlanta, 1996.
40. Centers for Disease Control and Prevention: Hepatitis Surveillance Report No. 57. Atlanta (in press).
41. Chang, M. H., Ni, Y. H., Hwang, L. H., et al.: Long-term clinical and virologic outcome of primary hepatitis C virus infection in children: A prospective study. Pediatr. Infect. Dis. J. *13*:769–773, 1994.
42. Chemello, L., Cavalletto, L., Casarin, C., et al.: Persistent hepatitis C viremia predicts late relapse after sustained response to interferon-alpha in chronic hepatitis C. Ann. Intern. Med. *124*:1058–1060, 1996.
43. Choo, Q. L., Kuo, G., Weiner, A. J., et al.: Isolation of a cDNA clone derived from a bloodborne non-A, non-B viral hepatitis genome. Science *244*:359–362, 1989.
44. Committee on Infectious Diseases: 1997 Redbook: Report of the Committee on Infectious Diseases. Elk Grove Village, IL, American Academy of Pediatrics. In press.
45. Conry-Cantilena, C., VanRaden, M., Gibble, J., et al.: Routes of infection, viremia, and liver disease in blood donors found to have hepatitis C virus infection. N. Engl. J. Med. *334*:1691–1696, 1996.
46. Cuypers, H. T. M., Bresters, D., Winkel, I. N., et al.: Storage conditions of blood samples and primer selection affect yield of cDNA polymerase chain reaction products of hepatitis C virus. J. Clin. Microbiol. *30*:3320–3324, 1992.
47. Davidson, F., Simmonds, P., Ferguson, J. C., et al.: Survey of major genotypes and subtypes of hepatitis C virus using RFLP of sequences amplified from the 5′ non-coding region. J. Gen. Virol. *76*:1197–1204, 1995.
48. Davis, G. L., Lau, J. Y., and Lim, H. L.: Therapy for chronic hepatitis C. Gastroenterol. Clin. North Am. *23*:603–613, 1994.
49. Davis, G. L., Lau, J. Y., Urdea, M. S., et al.: Quantitative detection of hepatitis C virus RNA with a solid-phase signal amplification method: Definition of optimal conditions for specimen collection and clinical application in interferon-treated patients. Hepatology *19*:1337–1341, 1994.
50. DeCastro, M., Sanchez, J., Herrera, J. F., et al.: Hepatitis C virus antibodies and liver disease in patients with porphyria cutanea tarda. Hepatology *17*:551–557, 1993.
51. Di Bisceglie, A. M., Martin, P., Kassianides, C., et al.: Recombinant interferon alpha therapy for chronic hepatitis C: A randomized, double-blind, placebo-controlled trial. N. Engl. J. Med. *321*:1506–1510, 1989.
52. Di Bisceglie, A. M., Order, S. E., Klein, J. L., et al.: The role of chronic viral hepatitis in hepatocellular carcinoma in the United States. Am. J. Gastroenterol. *86*:335–338, 1991.
53. Di Bisceglie, A. M., Goodman, Z. D., Ishak, K. G., et al.: Long-term clinical and histopathological follow-up of chronic posttransfusion hepatitis. Hepatology *14*:969–974, 1991.
54. Donahue, J. G., Munoz, A., Ness, P. M., et al.: The declining risk of post-transfusion hepatitis C virus infection. N. Engl. J. Med. *327*:369–373, 1992.
55. Elia, G. F., Magnani, G., Belli, L., et al.: Incidence of anti–hepatitis C virus antibodies in non-A, non-B post-transfusion hepatitis in an area of northern Italy. Infection *19*:336–339, 1991.
56. Enomoto, M., Sakuma, I., Asahina, Y., et al.: Mutations in the nonstructural protein 5A and response to interferon in patients with chronic hepatitis C virus 1b infection. N. Engl. J. Med. *334*:77–81, 1996.
57. Esteban, J. I., Gonzalez, A., Hernandez, J. M., et al.: Evaluation of antibodies to hepatitis C virus in a study of transfusion-associated hepatitis. N. Engl. J. Med. *323*:1107–1112, 1990.
58. Esteban, J. I., Lopez-Talavera, J. C., Genesca, J., et al.: High rate of infectivity and liver disease in blood donors with antibodies to hepatitis C virus. Ann. Intern. Med. *115*:443–449, 1991.
59. Farci, P., Alter, H. J., Govindarajan, S., et al.: Lack of protective immunity against reinfection with hepatitis C virus. Science *258*:135–140, 1992.
60. Farci, P., Munoz S., Alter, H. J., et al.: Hepatitis C virus–associated fulminant hepatitis failure. N. Engl. J. Med. *335*:631–634, 1996.
61. Farci, P., Alter, H. J., Wong, D. C., et al.: Prevention of hepatitis C virus infection in chimpanzees after antibody-mediated in vitro neutralization. Proc. Natl. Acad. Sci. U. S. A. *91*:7792–7796, 1994.
62. Fargion, S., Piperno, A., Cappellini, M. D., et al.: Hepatitis C virus and porphyria cutanea tarda: Evidence of a strong association. Hepatology *16*:1322–1326, 1992.
63. Feray, C., Gigou, M., Samuel, D., et al.: Hepatitis C virus RNA and hepatitis B virus DNA in serum and liver of patients with fulminant hepatitis. Gastroenterology *103*:549–555, 1992.
64. Ferri, C., Greco, F., Longombardo, G., et al.: Antibodies to hepatitis C virus in patients with mixed cryoglobulinemia. Arthritis Rheum. *34*:1606–1610, 1991.
65. Ferri, C., Marzo, E., Longombardo, G., et al.: Interferon-alpha in mixed cryoglobulinemia patients: A randomized, crossover-controlled trial. Blood *81*:1132–1136, 1993.
66. Fried, M. W., and Hoofnagle, J. H.: Therapy of hepatitis C. Semin. Liver Dis. *15*:82–91, 1995.

67. Fujisawa, T., Inui, A., Ohkawa, T., et al.: Response to interferon therapy in children with chronic hepatitis C. J. Pediatr. *127*:660–662, 1995.
68. Garson, J. A., Tedder, R. S., Briggs, M., et al.: Detection of hepatitis C viral sequences in blood donations by "nested" polymerase chain reaction and prediction infectivity. Lancet *335*:1419–1422, 1990.
69. Gerber, M. A., Krawczynski, K., Alter, M. J., et al.: Histopathology of community acquired chronic hepatitis C. Mod. Pathol. *5*:483–486, 1992.
70. Giovannini, M., Tagger, A., Ribero, M. L., et al.: Maternal-infant transmission of hepatitis C virus and HIV infections: A possible interaction. Lancet *335*:1166, 1990.
71. Goodman, Z. D., and Ishak, K. G.: Histopathology of hepatitis C virus infection. Semin. Liver Dis. *15*:70–81, 1995.
72. Gretch, D. R., dela Rosa, C., Carithers, R. L., et al.: Assessment of hepatitis C viremia using molecular amplification technologies: Correlations and clinical implications. Ann. Intern. Med. *123*:321–329, 1995.
73. Herrero, C., Vicente, A., Bruguera, M., et al.: Is hepatitis C virus infection a trigger of porphyria cutanea tarda? Lancet *341*:788–789, 1993.
74. Hibbs, R. G., Corwin, A. L., Hassan, N. F., et al.: The epidemiology of antibody to hepatitis C in Egypt. J. Infect. Dis. *168*:789–790, 1993.
75. Hibbs, J. R., Frickhofen, N., Rosenfeld, S. J., et al.: Aplastic anemia and viral hepatitis: Non-A, non-B, non-C? J. A. M. A. *267*:2051–2054, 1992.
76. Hosoda, K., Omata, M., Yokosuka, O., et al.: Non-A, non-B chronic hepatitis is chronic hepatitis C: A sensitive assay for detection of hepatitis C virus RNA in the liver. Hepatology *15*:777–781, 1992.
77. Houghton, M., Weiner, A., Han, J., et al.: Molecular biology of the hepatitis C viruses: Implications for diagnosis, development and control of viral disease. Hepatology *14*:381–388, 1991.
78. Inui, A., Fujisawa, T., Miyagawa, Y., et al.: Histologic activity of the liver in children with transfusion-associated chronic hepatitis C. J. Hepatol. *21*:748–753, 1994.
79. Ito, S.-I., Ito, M., Cho, M.-J., et al.: Massive sero-epidemiological survey of hepatitis C virus: Clustering of carriers on the southwest coast of Tsushima, Japan. Jpn. J. Cancer Res. *82*:1–3, 1991.
80. Johnson, R. J., Gretch, D. R., Yamabe, H., et al.: Membranoproliferative glomerulonephritis associated with hepatitis C virus infection. N. Engl. J. Med. *328*:465–70, 1993.
81. Jouet, P., Roudot-Thoraval, F., Dhumeaux, D., et al.: Comparative efficacy of interferon alpha in cirrhotic and noncirrhotic patients with non-A, non-B, C hepatitis. Gastroenterology *106*:686–690, 1994.
82. Jubert, C., Pawlotsky, J. M., Pouget, F., et al.: Lichen planus and hepatitis C virus–related chronic active hepatitis. Arch. Dermatol. *130*:73–76, 1994.
83. Jullien, A. M., Courouce, A. M., Massari, V., et al.: Impact of screening donor blood for alanine aminotransferase and antibody to hepatitis B core antigen on the risk of hepatitis C virus transmission. Eur. J. Clin. Microbiol. Infect. Dis. *12*:668–672, 1993.
84. Kaklamani, E., Trichopoulos, D., Tzonou, A., et al.: Hepatitis B and C viruses and their interaction in the origin of hepatocellular carcinoma. J. A. M. A. *265*:1974–1976, 1991.
85. Kasahara, A., Hayashi, N., Hiramatsu, N., et al.: Ability of prolonged interferon treatment to suppress relapse after cessation of therapy in patients with chronic hepatitis C: A multicenter randomized controlled trial. Hepatology *21*:291–297, 1995.
86. Kiyosawa, K., Sodeyama, T., Tanaka, E., et al.: Interrelationship of blood transfusion, non-A, non-B hepatitis and hepatocellular carcinoma: Analysis by detection of antibody to hepatitis C virus. Hepatology *12*:671–675, 1990.
87. Kleinman, S., Alter, H., Busch, M., et al.: Increased detection of hepatitis C virus (HCV)–infected blood donors by a multiple-antigen HCV enzyme immunoassay. Transfusion *32*:805–813, 1992.
88. Knodell, R. G., Conrad, M. E., Ginsburg, A. L., et al.: Efficacy of prophylactic gammaglobulin in preventing non-A, non-B post-transfusion hepatitis. Lancet *1*:557–561, 1976.
89. Koff, R. S., and Dienstag, J. L.: Extrahepatic manifestations of hepatitis C and the association with alcoholic liver disease. Semin. Liver Dis. *15*:101–109, 1995.
90. Kong, M.-S., and Chung, J.-L.: Fatal hepatitis C in and infant born to a hepatitis C positive mother. J. Pediatr. Gastroenterol. Nutr. *19*:460–463, 1994.
91. Koretz, R. L., Abbey, H., Coleman, E., et al.: Non-A, non-B post-transfusion hepatitis: Looking back in the second decade. Ann. Intern. Med. *119*:110–115, 1993.
92. Koretz, R. L., Brezina, M., Polito, A. J., et al.: Non-A, non-B posttransfusion hepatitis: Comparing C and non-C hepatitis. Hepatology *17*:361–365, 1993.
93. Krawczynski, K., Beach, M. J., Bradley, D. W., et al.: Hepatitis C virus antigen in hepatocytes: Immunomorphologic detection and identification. Gastroenterology *103*:622–629, 1992.
94. Krawczynski, K., Alter, M. J., Tankersly, D. L., et al.: Effect of immune globulin on the prevention of experimental hepatiis C virus infection. J. Infect. Dis. *173*:822–828, 1996.
95. Kuo, G., Choo, Q. L., Alter, H. J., et al.: An assay for circulating antibodies to a major etiologic virus of human non-A, non-B hepatitis. Science *244*:362–364, 1989.
96. Lai, M. E., Mazzoleni, A. P., Argiolu, F., et al.: Hepatitis C virus in multiple episodes of acute hepatitis in polytransfused thalassaemic children. Lancet *343*:388–390, 1994.
97. Lau, J. Y., Mizokami, M., Kolberg, J. A., et al.: Application of six hepatitis C virus genotyping systems to sera from chronic hepatitis C patients in the United States. J. Infect. Dis. *171*:281–289, 1995.
98. Lelie, M., Damen, H. T. M., Cuypers, H. L., et al.: International collaborative study on the second Eurohep HCV-RNA reference panel. Proceedings of the IX International Symposium on Viral Hepatitis and Liver Disease, Rome, 1996, p. 25.
99. Liang, T. J., Jeffers, L., Reddy, R. K., et al.: Fulminant or subfulminant non-A, non-B hepatitis: Hepatitis C and E viruses. Gastroenterology *103*:556–562, 1992.
100. Lin, H. H., Kao, J. H., Hsu, H. Y., et al.: Possible role of high-titer maternal viremia in perinatal transmission of hepatitis C virus. J. Infect. Dis. *169*:638–641, 1994.
101. Mahaney, K., Tedeschi, V., Maertens, G., et al.: Genotypic analysis of hepatitis C virus in American patients. Hepatology *20*:1405–1411, 1994.
102. Mansell, C. J., and Locarnini, S. A.: Epidemiology of hepatitis C in the East. Semin. Liver Dis. *15*:15–32, 1995.
103. Marcellin, P., Boyer, N., Giostra, E., et al.: Recombinant human alpha-interferon in patients with chronic non-A, non-B hepatitis: A multicenter randomized controlled trial from France. Hepatology *13*:393–397, 1991.
104. Marcellin, P., Descamps, V., Martinot-Peignoux, M., et al.: Cryoglobulinemia with vasculitis associated with hepatitis C infection. Gastroenterology *104*:272–277, 1993.
105. Marranconi, F., Mecenero, V., Pellizzer, G. P., et al.: HCV infection after accidental needlestick injury in health-care workers. Infection *20*:111, 1992.
106. Mast, E. E., and Alter, M. J.: Hepatitis C. Semin. Pediatr. Infect. Dis. *8*:1–7, 1997.
107. Matsuoka, S., Tatara, K., Hayabuchi, Y., et al.: Serologic, virologic and histologic characteristics of chronic phase hepatitis C virus disease in children infected by transfusion. Pediatrics *94*:919–922, 1994.
108. Mattsson, L., Grillner, L., von Sydow, M., et al.: Seroconversion to hepatitis C virus antibodies in patients with acute posttransfusion non-A, non-B hepatitis in Sweden. Infection *19*:309–312, 1991.
109. McQuillan, G., Alter, M., Moyer, L., et al.: A population based serologic study of hepatitis C virus infection in the United States. Proceedings of the IX International Symposium on Viral Hepatitis and Liver Disease, Rome, 1996, p. 8.
110. Mendenhall, D. L., Seeff, L., Diehl, A. M., et al.: Antibodies to hepatitis B virus and hepatitis C virus in alcoholic hepatitis and cirrhosis: Their prevalence and clinical relevance. Hepatology *14*:581–589, 1991.
111. Milella, M., Antonelli, G., Santantonio, T., et al.: Neutralizing antibodies to recombinant alpha-interferon and response to therapy in chronic hepatitis C virus infection. Liver *13*:146–150, 1993.
112. Mimms, L., Vallari, D., Ducharme, L., et al.: Specificity of anti-HCV ELISA assessed by reactivity to three immunodominant HCV regions. Lancet *336*:1590–1591, 1990.
113. Misiani, R., Bellavita, P., Fenili, D., et al.: Hepatitis C virus infection in patients with essential mixed cryoglobulinemia. Ann. Intern. Med. *117*:573–577, 1992.
114. Misiani, R., Bellavita, P., Fenili, D., et al.: Interferon alpha-2a therapy in cryoglobulinemia associated with hepatitis C virus. N. Engl. J. Med. *330*:751–756, 1994.
115. Moyer, L. A., and Alter, M. J.: Hepatitis C virus in the hemodialysis setting: A review with recommendations for control. Semin. Dialysis *7*:124–127, 1994.
116. Negro, F., Pacchioni, D., Shimizu, Y., et al.: Detection of intrahepatic replication of hepatitis C virus RNA by in situ hybridization and comparison with histopathology. Proc. Natl. Acad. Sci. U. S. A. *89*:2247–2251, 1992.
117. Nelson, K. E., Ahmed, F., Ness, P., et al.: Comparison of first and second generation ELISA screening tests in detecting HCV infections in transfused cardiac surgery patients. Program and Abstracts of the International Symposium on Viral Hepatitis and Liver Disease, Tokyo, 1993, p. 50.
118. Ni, Y. H., Chang, M. H., Lue, H. C., et al.: Posttransfusion hepatitis C virus infection in children. J. Pediatr. *124*:709–713, 1994
119. Nishioka, K., Watanabe, J., Furuta, S., et al.: Antibody to the hepatitis C virus in acute hepatitis and chronic liver diseases in Japan. Liver *11*:65–70, 1991.
120. Nolte, F. S., Thurmond, C., and Fried, M. W.: Preclinical evaluation of AMPLICOR hepatitis C virus test for detection of hepatitis C virus RNA. J. Clin. Microbiol. *33*:1775–1778, 1995.
121. Nousbaum, J. B., Pol, S., Nalpas, B., et al.: Hepatitis C virus type 1b (II) infection in France and Italy. Ann. Intern. Med. *122*:161–168, 1995.
122. Ohto, H., Okamoto, H., and Mishiro, S.: Vertical transmission of hepatitis C virus. N. Engl. J. Med. *331*:400, 1994.
123. Ohto, H., Terazawa, S., Sasaki, N., et al.: Transmission of hepatitis C virus from mothers to infants. N. Engl. J. Med. *330*:744–750, 1994.
124. Okada, S., Akahane, Y., Suzuki, H., et al.: The degree of variability in the amino terminal region of the E2/NS1 protein of hepatitis C virus correlates with responsiveness to interferon therapy in viremic patients. Hepatology *16*:619–624, 1992.
125. Okamoto, H., Kurai, K., Okada, S., et al.: Full-length sequence of a hepatitis C virus genome having poor homology to reported isolates: Comparative study of four distinct genotypes. Virology *188*:331–341, 1992.

126. Olynyk, J. K., Reddy, K. R., Di Bisceglie, A. M., et al.: Hepatic iron concentration as a predictor of response to interferon alpha therapy in chronic hepatitis C. Gastroenterology *108*:1104–1109, 1995.
127. Pawlotsky, J. M., Roudot-Thoraval, F., Simmonds, P., et al.: Extrahepatic immunologic manifestations in chronic hepatitis C and hepatitis C virus serotypes. Ann. Intern. Med. *122*:169–173, 1995.
128. Pereira, B. J. G, Milford, E. L., Kirkman, R. L., et al.: Prevalence of hepatitis C virus RNA in organ donors positive for hepatitis C antibody and in the recipients of their organs. N. Engl. J. Med. *327*:910–915, 1992.
129. Polish, L. B., Tong, M. J., Co, R. L., et al.: Risk factors for hepatitis C virus infection among health care personnel in a community hospital. Am. J. Infect. Control *21*:196–200, 1993.
130. Poynard, T., Bedossa, P., Chevallier, M., et al.: A comparison of three interferon alfa-2b regimens for the long-term treatment of chronic non-A, non-B hepatitis: Multicenter Study Group. N. Engl. J. Med. *332*:1457–1462, 1995.
131. Reichard, O., Foberg, U., Fryden, A., et al.: High sustained response rate and clearance of viremia in chronic hepatitis C after treatment with interferon-alpha 2b for 60 weeks. Hepatology *19*:280–285, 1994.
132. Rodriguez, M., Riestra, S., San Roman, F., et al.: Prevalence of antibody to hepatitis C virus in prospectively followed acute non-A, non-B hepatitis, from different epidemiological categories. Liver *11*:129–133, 1991.
133. Roth, D., Fernandez, J. A., Babischkin, S., et al.: Detection of hepatitis C virus infection among cadaver organ donors: Evidence for low transmission of disease. Ann. Intern. Med. *117*:470–475, 1992.
134. Roth, W. K., Lee, J.-H., Rüster, B., et al.: Comparison of two quantitative hepatitis C virus reverse transcriptase PCR assays. J. Clin. Microbiol. *34*:261–264, 1996.
135. Ruiz-Moreno, M., Rua, M. J., Castillo, I., et al.: Treatment of children with chronic hepatitis C with recombinant interferon-α: A pilot study. Hepatology *16*:882–885, 1992.
136. Rumi, M. G., Colombo, M., Gringeri, A., et al.: High prevalence of antibody to hepatitis C virus in multitransfused haemophilacs with normal transaminase levels. Ann. Intern. Med. *112*:379–380, 1990.
137. Sacher, R. A., Melpolder, J. J., and Alter, H. J.: Hepatitis C virus and fulminant hepatitis. Ann. Intern. Med. *115*:984–985, 1991.
138. Sanchez-Quijano, A., Pineda, J. A., Lissen, E., et al.: Prevention of post-transfusion non-A, non-B hepatitis by non-specific immunoglobulin in heart surgery patients. Lancet *1*:1245–1249, 1988.
139. Sansonno, D., Cornacchiulo, V., Iacobelli, A. R., et al.: Localization of hepatitis C virus antigens in liver and skin tissues of chronic hepatitis C virus–infected patients with mixed cryoglobulinemia. Hepatology *21*:305–12, 1995.
140. Scheuer, P. J., Ashrafzadeh, P., Sherlock, S., et al.: The pathology of hepatitis C. Hepatology *15*:567–571, 1992.
141. Schreiber, G. B., Busch, M. P., Kleinman, S. H., et al.: The risk of transfusion-transmitted viral infections. N. Engl. J. Med. *334*:1685–1690, 1996.
142. Schvarcz, R., Yun, Z. B., Sonnerborg, A., et. al.: Combined treatment with interferon alpha-2b and ribavirin for chronic hepatitis C in patients with a previous non-response or non-sustained response to interferon alone. J. Med. Virol. *46*:43–47, 1995.
143. Seeff, L. B.: Hepatitis C from a needlestick injury. Ann. Intern. Med. *115*:411, 1991.
144. Seeff, L. B., Buskell-Bales, Z., Wright, E. C., et al.: Long-term mortality after transfusion-associated non-A, non-B hepatitis. N. Engl. J. Med. *327*:1906–1911, 1992.
145. Seeff, L. B., and the National Heart, Lung, and Blood Institute Study Group: Sequelae of transfusion-associated non-A, non-B (TA-NANB) hepatitis. Program and Abstracts of the Fourth International Symposium on HCV, Tokyo, May 7–9, 1993, p. 29.
146. Seeff, L. B., Wright, E. C., Zimmerman, H. J., et al.: VA cooperative study of posttransfusion hepatitis, 1969–1974: Incidence and characteristics of hepatitis and responsible risk factors. Am. J. Med. Sci. *270*:355–362, 1975.
147. Seeff, L. B., Zimmerman, J. H., Wright, E. L., et al.: A randomized double-blind controlled trial of the efficacy of immune serum globulin for the prevention of post-transfusion hepatitis: A Veterans Administration cooperative study. Gastroenterology *72*:111–121, 1977.
148. Serfaty, L., Chazouilleres, O., Pawlotsky, J. M., et al.: Interferon alfa therapy in patients with chronic hepatitis C and persistently normal aminotransferase activity. Gastroenterology *110*:291–295, 1996.
149. Shakil, A. O., Conry-Cantilena, C., Alter, H. J., et al.: Volunteer blood donors with antibody to hepatitis C virus: Clinical, biochemical, virologic, and histologic features. Ann. Intern. Med. *123*:330–337, 1995.
150. Shiffman, M. L., Hofmann, C. M., Luketic, V. A., et al.: Improved sustained response following treatment of chronic hepatitis C by gradual reduction in the interferon dose. Hepatology *24*:21–26, 1996.
151. Shimizu, Y. K., Hijikata, M., Iwamoto, A., et al.: Neutralizing antibodies against hepatitis C virus and the emergence of neutralization escape mutant viruses. J. Virol. *68*:1494–1500, 1994.
152. Shindo, M., Arai, K., Sokawa, Y., et al.: Hepatic hepatitis C virus RNA as a predictor of a long-term response to interferon-alpha therapy. Ann. Intern. Med. *122*:586–591, 1995.
153. Simmonds, P., Smith, D. B., McOmish, F., et al.: Identification of genotypes of hepatitis C virus by sequence comparisons in the core, E1 and NS-5 regions. J. Gen. Virol. *75*:1053–1061, 1994.
154. Tajima, K., Shimotohno, K., and Oki, S.: Natural horizontal transmission of HCV in microepidemic town in Japan. Lancet *337*:1410–1411, 1991.
155. Tassopoulos, N. C., Hatzakis, A., Delladetsima, I., et al.: Role of hepatitis C virus in acute non-A, non-B hepatitis in Greece: A 5-year prospective study. Gastroenterology *102*:969–972, 1992.
156. Tran, A., Quaranta, J. F., Benzaken, S., et al.: High prevalence of thyroid autoantibodies in a prospective series of patients with chronic hepatitis C before interferon therapy. Hepatology *18*:253–257, 1993.
157. Tremolada, F., Casarin, C., Tagger, A., et al.: Antibody to hepatitis C virus in post-transfusion hepatitis. Ann. Intern. Med. *114*:277–281, 1991.
158. Troisi, C. L., Hollinger, F. B., Hoots, W. K., et al.: A multicenter study of viral hepatitis in a United States hemophilic population. Blood *81*:412–418, 1993.
159. Tsubota, A., Chayama, K., Ikeda, K., et al.: Factors predictive of response to interferon-alpha therapy in hepatitis C virus infection. Hepatology *19*:1088–1094, 1994.
160. Tsude, K., Fujiyama S., Sato, S., et al.: Two cases of accidental transmission of hepatitis C to medical staff. Hepato-Gastroenterology *39*:73–75, 1992.
161. Ueda, T., Ohta, K., Suzuki, N., et al.: Idiopathic pulmonary fibrosis and high prevalence of serum antibodies to hepatitis C virus. Am. Rev. Resp. Dis. *146*:266–268, 1992.
162. Vallari, D. S., Jett, B. W., Alter, H. J., et al.: Serological markers of post-transfusion hepatitis C viral infection. J. Clin. Microbiol. *30*:552–556, 1992.
163. Van den Hoek, J. A. R., Van Haastrecht, H. J. A., Goudsmit, J., et al.: Prevalence, incidence, and risk factors of hepatitis C virus infection among drug users in Amsterdam. J. Infect. Dis. *160*:823–826, 1990.
164. Wilson, S. E., Lee, W. M., Murakami, C., et al.: Mooren-type hepatitis C virus–associated corneal ulceration. Ophthamology *101*:736–745, 1994.
165. Wright, T. L.: Etiology of fulminant hepatic failure: Is another virus involved. Gastroenterology *104*:640–653, 1993.
166. Wright, T. L, Hsu, H., Donegan, E., et al.: Hepatitis C virus not found in fulminant non-A, non-B hepatitis. Ann. Intern. Med. *115*:111–112, 1991.
167. Yamabe, H., Johnson, R. J., Gretch, D. R., et al.: Hepatitis C virus and membranoproliferative glomerulonephritis in Japan. J. Am. Soc. Nephrol. *6*:220–223, 1995.
168. Yanagi, M., Kaneko, S., Unoura, M., et al.: Hepatitis C virus in fulminant liver failure. N. Engl. J. Med. *324*:1895–1896, 1991.
169. Yoshioka, K., Kakumu, S., Wakita, T., et al.: Detection of hepatitis C virus by polymerase chain reaction and response to interferon-alpha therapy: Relationship to genotypes of hepatitis C virus. Hepatology *16*:293–299, 1992.
170. Yu, M. C., Tong, M. J., Coursaget, P., et al.: Prevalence of hepatitis B and C viral markers in black and white patients with hepatocellular carcinoma in the United States. J. Natl. Cancer Inst. *82*:1038–1041, 1990.
171. Zaaijer, H. L., Cuypers, H. T., Reesink, H. W., et al.: Reliability of polymerase chain reaction for detection of hepatitis C virus. Lancet *341*:722–724, 1993.
172. Zanetti, A. R., Tanzi, E., Zehender, G., et al.: Hepatitis C virus RNA in symptomless donors implicated in post-transfusion non-A, non-B hepatitis. Lancet *336*:448, 1990.

❑ ❑ ❑

SUBSECTION SIX

ORTHOMYXOVIRIDAE

181

INFLUENZA VIRUSES

W. Paul Glezen

Influenza is an acute respiratory infection caused by strains of the orthomyxoviruses. The first of the human respiratory viruses to be isolated and characterized,[261] influenza viruses also have been studied the most extensively and are the best understood of these agents from a biologic, epidemiologic, and clinical standpoint.[106, 154, 268] Yet, despite great sophistication in our understanding of it as a disease, influenza remains "the last great plague of man."[154]

With improvements in living standards and the introduction of antibiotics, the overall impact of influenza on mortality rates has not diminished. The possibility of a recurrence of the catastrophic 1918–1919 epidemic, in which an estimated 550,000 deaths occurred in the United States alone,[51] therefore seems remote. Nevertheless, an estimated 47,500 excess deaths and $3.8 billion in economic losses[150] were ascribed to the U.S. pandemic of 1968–1969. Annual epidemics have continued unabated. Each year, the peak of influenza virus activity coincides with the peak of health care visits and hospitalizations for acute respiratory tract disease.[49] Despite the decline in overall pneumonia mortality, an average of 20,000 excess deaths are attributed to influenza each year.[175]

As other agents capable of causing respiratory tract infection in children have been identified, influenza has received relatively less attention. Yet the morbidity and mortality of influenza in children can be considerable, and the spectrum of clinical manifestations resulting from influenza viral infections is broad.

HISTORY

Although the authenticity of influenza in medical antiquity is difficult to establish, apparently the disease has existed for 2000 years. The epidemic in 412 B.C. described by Hippocrates and Livy was probably influenza.[235, 274] This outbreak started in December, occurred after a change in the weather, and was complicated by pneumonia. Epidemic influenza-like disease occurred in Europe in the 6th and 10th centuries, but the first generally accepted influenza epidemic occurred in December 1173.[53, 133, 274] Hirsch[133] noted 299 epidemics of influenza between 1173 and 1875. Major epidemics occurred in 1411, 1414, 1427, 1510, and 1557.[274] The first pandemic involving Europe, Asia, and North Africa occurred in 1580, and the first epidemic in the Western Hemisphere occurred in 1647. From 1580 until 1918, there were at least eight influenza pandemics.[235]

In recent times, pandemics of influenza due to different influenza A subtypes occurred in 1874, 1889, 1900, 1918, 1957, 1968, and 1977. The most noteworthy of all influenza pandemics occurred in 1918. This event has the dubious distinction of the greatest morbidity and mortality of all time; there were more than 20 million deaths in the world.[163]

The term *influenza* may have come from the Latin word *influo*, "to flow in," perhaps indicating its airborne transmission. It may be Italian, relating to an "influence," such as the weather, or mystical astrologic causes.[163, 235]

PROPERTIES OF THE VIRUS

Classification

Classified taxonomically as orthomyxoviruses, the influenza viruses are negative-stranded RNA viruses of three major antigenic types—A, B, and C—and multiple antigenic subtypes.[74, 154, 268] Influenza A and B viruses are most important in human disease and have been studied far more extensively than influenza C viruses. All have the property of hemagglutination and, with the possible exception of influenza C, possess the enzyme neuraminidase. The current World Health Organization (WHO) system of nomenclature for influenza virus strains specifies type, host (for strains of animal origin), geographic source, strain number, and year of isolation, to which code designations of hemagglutinin and neuraminidase subtypes are appended.[293] Thus, the "Russian" influenza A strain is designated A/USSR/90/77 (H1N1); the "Philippines" influenza A strain is designated A/Philippines/2/82 (H3N2). Strains are characterized and named at the WHO influenza reference centers in Atlanta, Georgia (Centers for Disease Control and Prevention), London, England, and Melbourne, Australia.

Physical Properties

In electron-microscopic preparations, influenza viruses are irregular spherical particles 80 to 120 nm in diameter that also may exhibit filamentous or icosahedral structures[256, 300] (Fig. 181–1). Numerous hemagglutinin and neuraminidase "spikes" bristle from their surfaces. Inside fragmented viral particles, helical nucleocapsids are discernible.

Influenza A and B viruses are composed of approximately 1 per cent RNA, 7 per cent carbohydrate, 22 per cent lipid, and 70 per cent protein.[37] The virion proteins are all specified by the viral genome, but the lipid bilayer and the carbohydrate constituents of glycoproteins and glycolipids in the viral envelope are derived from the host cell (Fig. 181–2). Besides the "surface" hemagglutinin and neuraminidase, eight other virus-coded proteins have been characterized (Table 181–1). Matrix, or membrane protein (M1), is the most abundant protein and is the major structural component of the viral envelope. The M2 protein is a smaller tetrameric protein that acts as an ion channel extending through the viral envelope. M2 has an important role in the penetration and release of viral RNA into the host cell.[269] Nucleoprotein (NP) is associated with the RNA genome of the virus in ribonucleoprotein complexes in which multiple NP molecules are associated with single-stranded RNA. Proteins PB2, PB1, and PA, the largest proteins of the virus, are so designated because two are basic proteins and one is an acidic protein. They are involved with the synthesis of three differ-

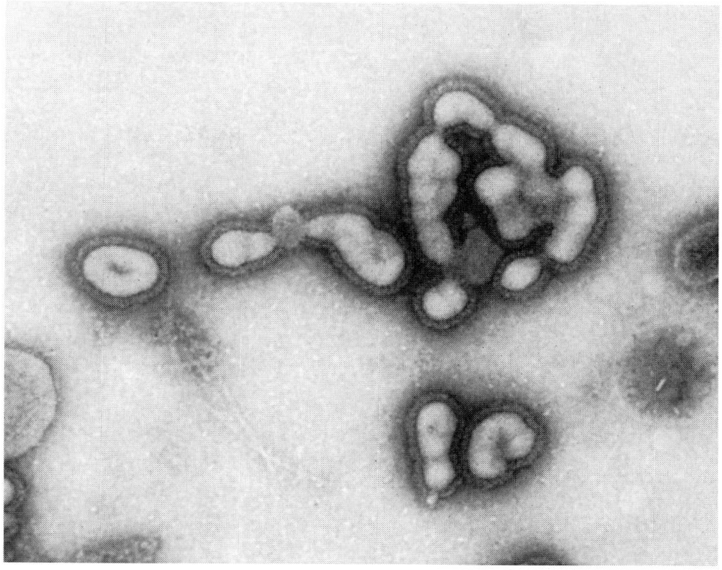

FIGURE 181–1. *Influenza A/USSR/90/77 (H1N1). Note hemagglutinin and neuraminidase "spikes" and occasional filamentous forms. (×189,000.) (Courtesy of G. R. Noble, M.D., Centers for Disease Control and Prevention.)*

ent kinds of virus-specific RNAs. Evidence suggests that the PB2 protein is the cap-recognizing protein and that PB1 and PA are involved in chain initiation or in chain elongation.[14, 15, 165, 227, 276] Nonstructural proteins, although not incorporated into viral progeny, are virus-coded proteins of unknown function found in infected host cells.

The biologic and antigenic diversity of influenza viruses is attributable in part to their unique, segmented RNA genome. This peculiarity of influenza viruses was suggested by the early genetic experiments of Burnet and Lind,[22] in which, for example, the frequency of recombinants recovered after simultaneous infection with two distinctive influenza A strains, A/Melbourne/35 (H1N1) and a neurotropic variant of A/WS/33 (H1N1), was 37 per cent. Interchange of corresponding segments of a linear genome, in the traditional sense of genetic recombination, did not account for this extraordinarily high frequency. Hirst,[134] in 1962, proposed the hypothesis that the influenza genome consists of subgenomic pieces capable of semiautonomous replication and random "reassortment" during the process of assembly. This theory accounted for observed recombination frequencies and subsequently was supported by the finding that the RNA of influenza virions was indeed segmented when analyzed by polyacrylamide gel electrophoresis.[233] More refined electrophoretic studies in urea-polyacrylamide gels have established that the influenza A genome consists of eight pieces. By the association of single discrepant antigenic or biochemical attributes of otherwise similar recombinant viruses with discrepant RNA lines in electrophoretic tracks, the genomes of influenza A/HK/1/68 and A/PR/8/34 were mapped by Ritchey, Palese, and Schulman (Fig. 181–3).[240] By means of RNA-protein hybridization techniques, Inglis and associates[144, 145] independently arrived at virtually identical findings.

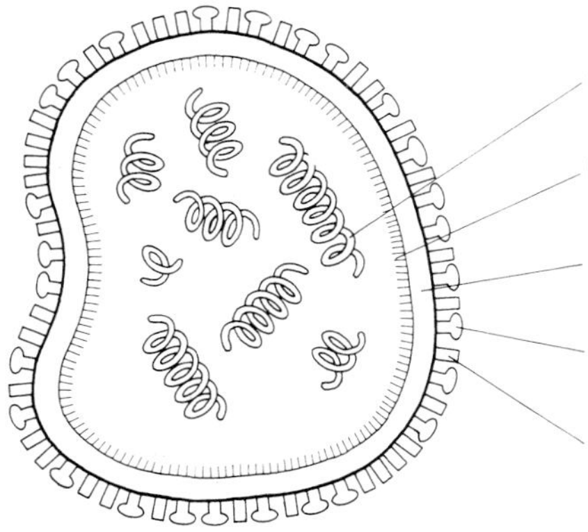

FIGURE 181–2. *An influenza virion. Nucleocapsid structures consist of segmented RNA complexed with nucleoprotein and P proteins.*

Antigenic Composition

Of the protein constituents of influenza viruses, four are known antigens. The "internal" nucleoprotein and matrix protein are antigenically type-specific and stable. Nucleoprotein is the antigenic basis for typing of strains as A, B, or C and is the predominant constituent of the "soluble" antigen employed for complement-fixation serologic testing. Although antibody against nucleoprotein is formed regularly after natural infection and antibody against matrix protein has been detected after severe illness, these antibodies are short lived and appear to have no protective value.[205]

In contrast, hemagglutinin and neuraminidase antigens are subtype-specific and variable. Hemagglutinin is required for attachment of infecting virus to host-cell membranes. Hemagglutination-inhibiting antibodies neutralize viral infectivity

TABLE 181–1. Virus-Coded Proteins of Influenza Virus

Gene Segment	Protein Designation	Function	Antigenicity
1	PB2	RNA synthesis	?
2	PB1	RNA synthesis	?
3	PA	RNA synthesis	?
4	HA	Hemagglutinin	Subtype-specific
5	NA	Neuraminidase	Subtype-specific
6	NP	RNA synthesis	Type-specific
7	M1,M2	Matrix	Type-Specific
8	NS1,NS2	Nonstructural	?

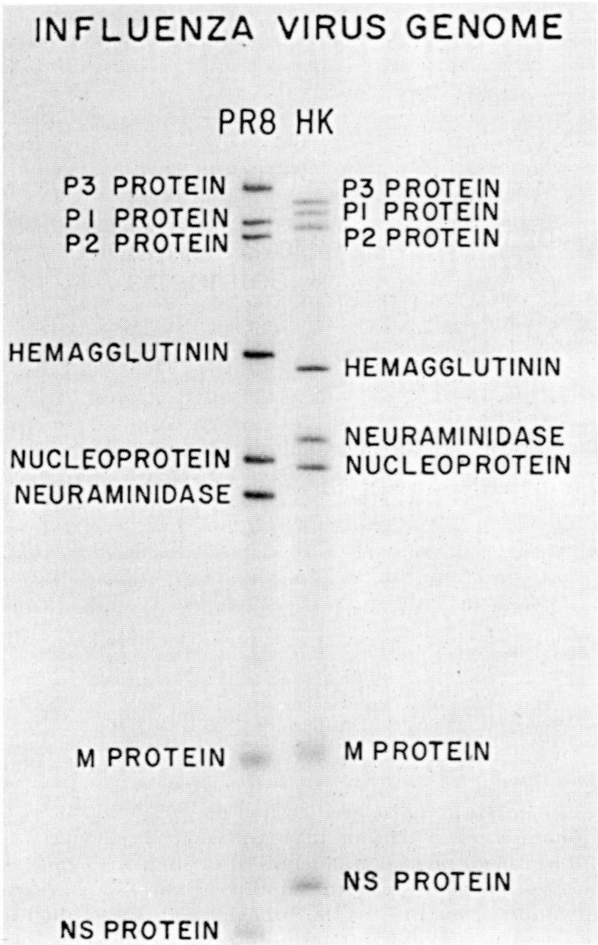

FIGURE 181–3. *Polyacrylamide urea gel electrophoretic maps of the RNA genome of influenza A/PR/8/34 (H0N1) and A/HK/68 (H3N2). (From Ritchey, M. B., Palese, P., and Schulman, J. L.: Mapping of the influenza virus genome. III. Identification of genes coding for nucleoprotein, membrane protein, and nonstructural protein. J. Virol.* 20:307–313, 1976.)

and are the most important index of immunity against influenza in humans.[135] Neuraminidase appears to be required for release of virus from infected cells. Specific antineuraminidase antibodies reduce plaque size, mitigate the pathogenic effects of influenza in experimentally infected mice, and correlate inversely with viral shedding and illness severity.[211] Thus far, three separate hemagglutinins, H1, H2, and H3, and two separate neuraminidases, N1 and N2, have been recognized in influenza A viruses affecting humans.

Variation in hemagglutinin and neuraminidase specificity is the basis for antigenic "drift" and "shift" in prevalent viruses. Drift implies a minor change in either antigen, without a change in subtype; shift implies a major change in either or both antigens, with a change in subtype. Antigenic drift occurs in influenza A and B viruses; antigenic shift occurs only in influenza A.

Antigenic drift is the result of point mutation. Selective pressure in an immune population results in selection of mutant viruses with altered antigenic determinants that allow a growth advantage in the presence of prevalent antibody. Supporting this concept are the in vitro studies of Laver and Webster,[168] in which antigenic mutants isolated by serial egg passage in the presence of low-avidity antiserum develop changes in the peptide make-up of their hemagglutinin subunits.

Antigenic shift occurs when an influenza A virus acquires hemagglutinin or neuraminidase components that differ from antecedent strains by a quantum jump. The phenomenon has been well studied in influenza A (H3N2) viruses. Their H3 hemagglutinins, by chromatographic analysis of peptide composition, are sufficiently distinctive to make highly improbable their emergence by point mutation from the H2 hemagglutinin of preceding Asian strains.[169]

Considerable evidence suggests that antigenic shift strains could arise by reassortment of gene segments between human and animal influenza viruses during chance simultaneous infection. It is known that the H3 hemagglutinin of influenza A/Hong Kong/1/68 is antigenically and biochemically similar to the hemagglutinins of two influenza A viruses of animal origin: A/equine/Miami/1/63 (H3N2) and A/duck/Ukraine/1/63 (H3N2).[170] Moreover, reassortment of gene segments between human and animal strains has been demonstrated under experimental conditions. In one study, sty mates of pigs experimentally infected with either A/HK/1/68 (H3N2) or A/swine/Iowa/15/30 (H1N1) developed infections from which recombinant as well as wild-type virus could be recovered.[284] An analogous event initially was suspected as the origin of the swine-like A/New Jersey/8/76 (H1N1) virus recovered from infections in Fort Dix military recruits in 1976. However, the RNA genome of A/NJ now has been shown to be virtually identical by polyacrylamide gel chromatography to other strains of influenza virus isolated from swine.[222] It shows no RNA homology to human strains. Thus, the emergence from animal reservoirs of influenza strains with sufficient virulence to cause widespread human epidemics remains an attractive theory.

Tissue Culture and Chicken Embryo Growth

Influenza viruses grow well in a variety of culture systems, although embryonated chicken eggs and the Madin-Darby canine kidney cell line are used most widely. Primary rhesus monkey kidney tissue culture and other monkey cell lines are alternative choices for influenza virus isolation. Intra-amniotic and intra-allantoic inoculation of 10- to 11-day-old eggs is followed by incubation for 3 to 4 days at 33° C. Fluid samples are harvested and tested for the presence of hemagglutinating virus by addition of guinea pig or chicken red blood cells. Monkey kidney cells have maximum sensitivity to influenza viruses when they are maintained after inoculation in a serum-free medium. Subtle cytopathic effects may appear but are variable. Detection of virus is carried out best after 3 to 5 days of incubation at 34° C in the Madin-Darby canine kidney cells or after 7 to 10 days of incubation at 33° C with use of the rhesus kidney cell line, then hemadsorbing with guinea pig red blood cells. Influenza C viruses grow best in eggs; Madin-Darby canine kidney and monkey kidney cells generally give higher yields of influenza A and B viruses. "Blind" repassages may result in an isolation in either system when the initial passage is negative, but the yield drops off sharply. Although parainfluenza viruses also may be isolated in these tissue culture lines, they can be distinguished from influenza viruses by their characteristic syncytial cytopathogenicity and their poor growth in embryonated eggs.[89, 90] Definitive identification of virus isolates is carried out by indirect immunofluorescence or hemagglutination inhibition with use of specific antisera. Antigen detection and identification of influenza viruses by use of enzyme-linked immunosorbent assays have been valuable additions to the diagnostic laboratory.[11, 62, 128, 248, 283]

Animal Susceptibility

Influenza virus types readily grow and produce disease in ferrets.[241] This animal commonly is used for experimental studies. Influenza viruses also can be adapted to grow in mice for research purposes. Other animals, including hamsters, guinea pigs, monkeys, squirrels, chipmunks, and mink, have varying degrees of susceptibility to influenza viruses.

Horses, swine, and birds are infected naturally by type A influenza viruses. In most instances, these animal strains are different from those of human origin.

EPIDEMIOLOGY

Incidence and Prevalence

The epidemiology of influenza is truly "the study of epidemics."[173] Outbreaks may be localized, nationwide, or global; sporadic cases are unusual. On the whole, influenza joins other, more recently characterized agents (respiratory syncytial virus, parainfluenza viruses, and *Mycoplasma pneumoniae*) to account for the majority of respiratory tract illness in children.[101, 153, 186] During periods of epidemic or pandemic spread, however, respiratory tract infections by influenza viruses exceed those caused by all other etiologic agents. In the peak month of a composite of 11 consecutive influenza A virus outbreaks observed in Washington, D.C., influenza A virus was isolated from 68 per cent of croup patients and 36 per cent of all hospitalized children with respiratory tract disease.[157] Influenza viruses are the most important causes of acute respiratory tract illnesses leading to hospitalization of schoolchildren.[108, 228]

Although local outbreaks and individual cases of influenza are optionally reportable in all states, information about disease activity as it varies from year to year derives mainly from ongoing surveillance in public health departments and university medical centers.[178] Longitudinal studies of viral respiratory tract illnesses in families,[122, 147] in hospitalized children,[111, 156] in private pediatric practices,[109, 110, 120] and in public clinics[105] have provided useful data regarding the community impact of influenza infections. Detection of new influenza variants and their spread is facilitated by reporting of virus isolations and serologic responses in specimens submitted to an international network of WHO laboratories.[27]

Weekly tabulations of deaths from "pneumonia" and "influenza" from larger cities in the United States provide a valuable index of mortality from influenza. Several methods have been used to estimate the expected number of deaths in the absence of influenza so that excess mortality can be derived from the observed number during epidemics. Reported deaths in excess of an epidemic threshold usually correlate well with the occurrence of widespread influenza activity (Fig. 181–4).[112, 166, 175]

The highest attack rates of influenza occur in children and tend to proceed to secondary peaks of illness in adult populations.[103–105] Although case-fatality has been considered to occur most frequently at both extremes of age, increases in pneumonia-influenza deaths in recent years have been most clear-cut in the elderly.[85, 140] Regardless of age, influenza is fatal more frequently in persons with preexisting heart disease, chronic pulmonary disorders, diabetes mellitus, chronic renal disease, neuromuscular disorders, and neoplasms.[70]

A remarkable ecologic feature of influenza viruses is the tendency of one particular virus subtype to achieve worldwide distribution at the same time its predecessor disappears from human circulation. Since their first isolation in the 1930s, three major subtypes of influenza A viruses are known to have circulated widely. At the transition years of these "influenza eras," a major antigenic drift or shift has occurred. The prototypic strains for these time intervals are 1933 to 1957, influenza A/Puerto Rico/8/34 (H1N1); 1957 to 1967,

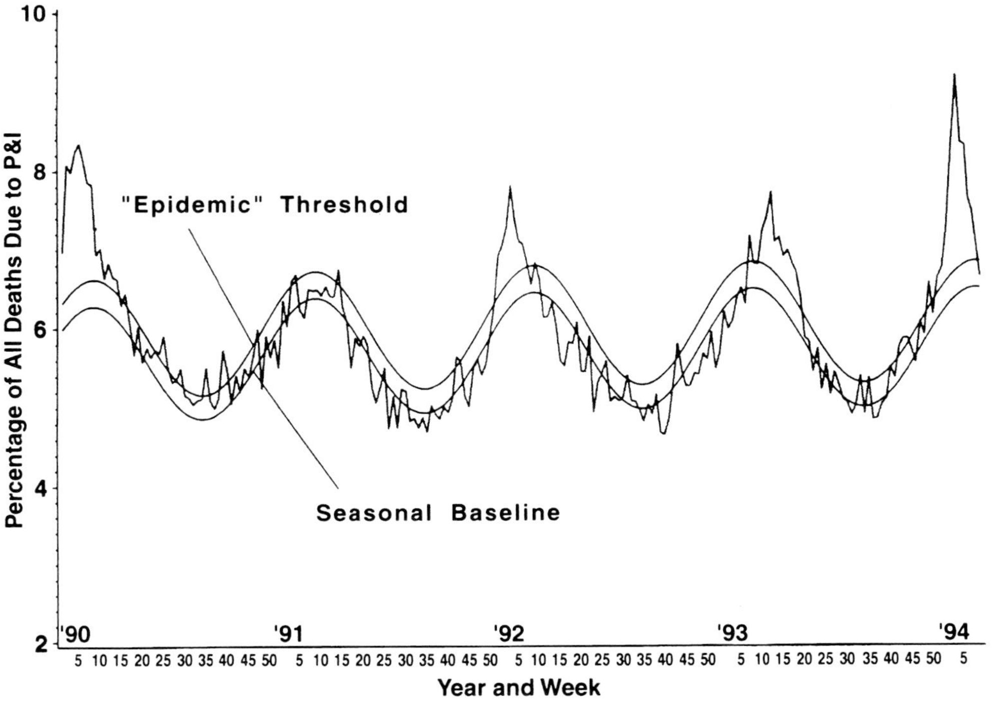

FIGURE 181–4. *Percentage of deaths attributed to pneumonia and influenza in 121 cities, United States, 1990–1994. (From Centers for Disease Control and Prevention: United States Influenza Surveillance, March 4, 1994.)*

influenza A/Japan/305/57 (H2N2); and 1968 to 1977, influenza A/Hong Kong/8/68 (H3N2). In 1977, influenza A/USSR/90/77 (H1N1) made its appearance; since then, both H1N1 and H3N2 strains have been prevalent.

The antigenic make-up of viruses prevalent before the 1930s has been inferred by seroepidemiologic studies. By this means, it has been determined that persons born before 1924 have a high prevalence of antibodies against the swine-like H1 hemagglutinin.[258] Similarly, in serum specimens collected before the emergence of H2N2 and H3N2 strains, high prevalences of antibody against the H3 hemagglutinin were found in persons born before 1889.[188] Thus, it appears that the number of major variants of influenza A viruses may be finite and that the major subtypes may recycle periodically. This concept is supported by the re-emergence of A/USSR/90/77 (H1N1). Antigenically and genetically, this strain of influenza A was identical to influenza A/Fort Warren/1/50 (H1N1), the virus subtype prevalent between 1950 and 1953.[215, 307]

Seasonal and Geographic Patterns

Influenza infections have marked seasonality. In temperate climates, epidemics occur almost exclusively in winter months. Off-season infections are documented infrequently. Winter circulation in the Southern Hemisphere probably maintains influenza viruses during northern summer months. Geographic variations in the incidence of influenza also may reflect global patterns of spread of new virus strains. Isolated populations may escape the dispersion of new viruses. When outbreaks do occur in such highly susceptible populations, explosive spread and high attack rates in all age groups have been observed.[21, 94]

Transmission

Droplet spread, with inhalation of airborne particles produced by coughing and sneezing, generally is accepted as the most common mode of natural influenza transmission. Spread also may occur by direct contact, indirect contact, and fine-particle aerosols. Small-particle aerosol, by which virus particles are deposited directly into the lower respiratory tract, is the most efficient means of inducing influenza in volunteer studies. In one such study, a human infectious dose (HID_{50}) of influenza A/Bethesda/10/63 (H2N2) by aerosol was equivalent to 0.6 to 3.0 tissue culture infectious doses ($TCID_{50}$).[1] In contrast, studies in which influenza A/Aichi/2/68 (H3N2) was given by direct instillation or coarse spray into the nose revealed a range of HID_{50} of 127 to 320 $TCID_{50}$.[46, 54] The contribution of small-particle aerosol to transmission of influenza under natural conditions remains uncertain but could be important in the pathogenesis of primary influenza pneumonia.[106]

Once infection is established, peak virus shedding coincides with clinical symptoms. Virus may be recovered for a day before the onset of symptoms with influenza B and up to 6 days in the case of influenza A. Virus shedding is detected for a variable period of time in children but usually exists for a week or less for influenza A and up to 2 weeks after influenza B infection.[93] At the height of illness, respiratory tract secretions commonly contain 10^6 or more infectious viral particles per milliliter.[210]

The incubation period of influenza ranges from 1 to 7 days but commonly is 2 to 3 days. This brief incubation period, coupled with the large amounts of infectious virus in secretions and the relatively small dose necessary for infection of susceptibles, accounts for the sharpness of influenza outbreaks. Spread is most rapid in institutions, such as schools, colleges, military barracks, and nursing homes. In community outbreaks, school age children usually have the highest attack rates, with secondary spread to their parents and younger siblings (Fig. 181–5).[33, 56, 103, 104]

Nosocomial infection may occur during community epidemics of influenza and has been documented in hospitalized adults,[16] infants,[119] and premature infants.[192] In hospital settings, it is reasonable to separate physically highly susceptible patients from other patients and personnel with acute respiratory tract illness. Room isolation generally is sufficient for patients with influenzal illness. Personnel with respiratory tract illness compatible with influenza should be excused from work.

PATHOGENESIS AND IMMUNITY

Viral Infection and Pathogenesis

To establish infection, influenza viruses must penetrate the mucous blanket lining the respiratory tract and escape inactivation by nonspecific inhibitors as well as specific local antibodies. The major site of infection is the ciliated columnar epithelial cell.[131, 282, 308] Necrosis of ciliated epithelial cells occurs as early as the first day after the onset of symptoms. Local edema and cellular infiltration by lymphocytes, histiocytes, plasma cells, and polymorphonuclear cells follow. Repair of the epithelium begins between the third and fifth days, as indicated by mitoses in the surviving basal cells. A pseudometaplastic response of undifferentiated epithelium occurs, which reaches its maximum 9 to 15 days after the onset of the infection. After 15 days, cilia and mucus production reappear.[282] With secondary bacterial infection, more extensive inflammatory cell infiltration and destruction of the basal cell layer and basement membrane are seen, with consequent delay in regeneration of the ciliated epithelium.

Pneumonia associated with influenza virus infection may occur as a result of primary viral infection, bacterial superinfection, or combined bacterial-viral infection.[180] Fatal primary influenza pneumonia, fortunately rare in children, is characterized at autopsy by diffuse hemorrhagic alveolar exudates, necrosis of bronchiolar epithelium, peribronchial lymphocytic infiltration, and marked lymphocytic infiltration of the alveolar walls and interstitial lung tissue.[208]

Although the major pathologic process in influenza is in the respiratory tract, focal and diffuse myocarditis, mediastinal lymph node disorganization and necrosis, and diffuse cerebral edema also have been noted in fatal cases. In recent years, the pathologic entity of diffuse encephalopathy and fatty degeneration of the liver (Reye syndrome) has been established as a potential complication of influenza, particularly type B, in children.[172]

Immunologic Events

Immunity against influenza results from a complex interplay of humoral, secretory, and cell-mediated mechanisms. Because of the brief incubation period of the disease, anamnestic stimulation of antibody affords little protection. Thus, some degree of preexisting antibody appears to be essential to prevent infection. The sequential antigenic changes that occur in the virus in the course of antigenic drift afford each new variant a selective advantage in establishing infection; the major antigenic changes that accompany antigenic shifts render larger populations susceptible and account for pandemic spread.

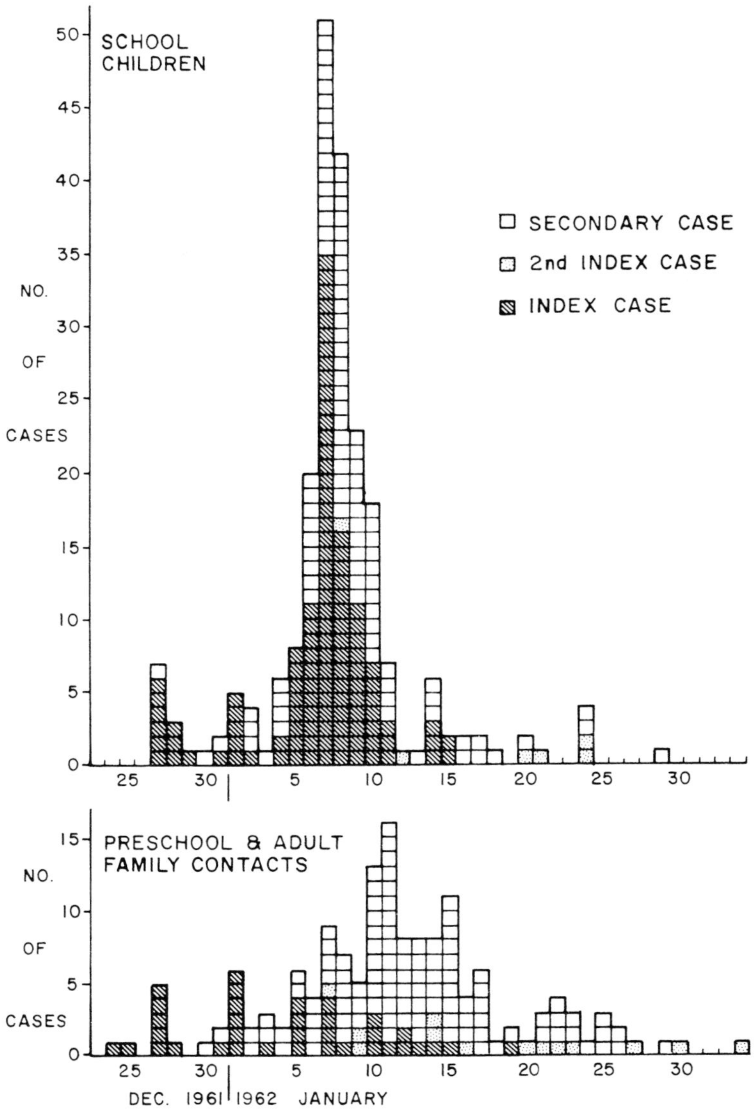

FIGURE 181–5. *Epidemic curve of infections by influenza B, in Hazleton, Iowa, 1961–1962. Note that the epidemic wave in school age children precedes the epidemic wave in household contacts. (From Chin, T. D. Y., Mosley, W. H., Poland, J. D., et al.: Epidemiologic studies of type B influenza in 1961–1962. Am. J. Public Health 53:1068–1074, 1963.)*

After natural influenza infection, both local and humoral antibodies are elicited against hemagglutinin, neuraminidase, nucleocapsid, and matrix protein antigens. Hemagglutination-inhibiting antibodies are critical for virus neutralization. Antibodies against neuraminidase are associated with diminished illness severity and reduced rates of person-to-person transmission. Antibodies against nucleocapsid and matrix protein do not appear to provide protection or modify transmission.

Because influenza is a respiratory epithelial surface infection rather than a systemic infection, some uncertainty exists regarding the relative degree of protection afforded by local and humoral antibodies. Neutralizing antibodies in respiratory tract secretions were demonstrated first in 1941 by Francis and Brightman.[87] Protection against experimental infection of hyperimmunized mice subsequently was demonstrated, by Fazekas de St. Groth and Donnelley,[73] to correlate better with the antibody titer of respiratory tract secretions than with that of serum. Studies in human volunteers, however, have yielded conflicting results. Couch and colleagues[47] demonstrated good protection against experimental challenge by influenza A/HK/1/68 in subjects possessing serum antibodies but who lacked nasal antibodies. In subjects challenged by influenza B/Eng/65, Downie and Stuart-Harris[66] also demonstrated a better correlation of protection with serum antibody levels than with nasal antibodies. Moreover, in a large experience with volunteers summarized by Hobson and associates,[135] an impressive linear correlation between serum hemagglutination-inhibiting antibody titers and protection was evident. Thus, although an important role for local antibodies as a "first line of defense" against influenza is accepted, serum antibodies clearly contribute to resistance.

Waldman and colleagues[280] have demonstrated that the predominant influenza-neutralizing antibody in nasal secretions is secretory IgA, whereas the predominant neutralizing antibody present in tracheobronchial secretions is IgG. A synthesis of the available data suggests that local secretory IgA in nasal secretions may be important in the prevention of infection transmitted by droplet spread and originating in the upper respiratory tract. Serum and local IgG antibodies appear to be of greater importance in neutralizing infection transmitted directly to the lower respiratory tract by aerosol or in preventing extension of upper respiratory tract infection to the lungs.

Cell-mediated immune mechanisms of several varieties have been demonstrated in influenza infection and vaccination. A T-cell "helper" function has been demonstrated in strain-specific humoral antibody response against hemagglutinin.[279] Both nonspecific and specific mechanisms of lymphocyte cytotoxicity have been found in model systems,[72, 309] but only type-specific cytotoxic T cells have been found in humans.[12, 17, 69] Cytotoxic T lymphocytes are important for recovery from infection in susceptible hosts. Antibody-dependent cell-mediated cytotoxicity has been shown to correlate with the titer of serum anti-HA antibody.[114] This mechanism also may play a role in recovery.[60, 254]

The immunologic imprint made by the first influenza infection of childhood has lasting effects. According to the "doctrine of original antigenic sin," developed by Francis and colleagues[88] from seroepidemiologic data, hemagglutination-inhibiting antibody against the strain of first infection is recapitulated with each subsequent infection by an antigenically distinctive strain of influenza A. It has been found since 1957, however, that infections or immunizations with H2N2 or H3N2 strains do not recall antibody against earlier strains in persons primed by H1N1 viruses.[185] Therefore, the doctrine only holds within broad groups of influenza A strains possessing some degree of homology of antigens. Virelizier and associates[278] analyzed the basis for the phenomenon using irradiated mice immunologically reconstituted with bone marrow from immune donors. Their studies indicate that antigenic "original sin" derives from cross-stimulation of a population of committed memory B lymphocytes that persist after primary infection.

After natural infection, the duration of immunity and the degree of protection against challenge by heterologous variants appear to be variable. On the basis of clinical experience in a Yorkshire general practice, Pickles and associates[229] concluded that natural immunity against influenza A strains lasted at least 4 years. On the other hand, serologic reinfection rates of 2 per cent and 12 per cent against influenza A and influenza B, respectively, were noted by Hall and colleagues[122] during a 3-year observation period in Seattle children. Frank and colleagues[91, 95] reported that variations in reinfection among young children may be multifactorial but, most important, may be related to the age at first infection and the antigenic differences of virus variants in subsequent challenges. Thus, protection against clinical disease appears to persist for a number of years after influenza infection in older children but may be of much shorter duration in infants and very young children; subclinical reinfection probably occurs after much shorter intervals. A gradual increase in duration and breadth of immunity against related virus strains probably occurs over a period of years. Unlike the findings for influenza A (H3N2) infections, Frank and associates[92] found that infection with influenza B virus provided consistent protection for most persons against infection with the next influenza B variant. The protection decreased somewhat for subsequent variants and longer intervals. This may account for the relative infrequency of influenza B infections in adults because only antigenic drift has been documented for this virus. The major antigenic changes occurring in antigenic shifts, however, have the potential to circumvent cumulative immunity in all age groups.

CLINICAL MANIFESTATIONS

Disease due to epidemic influenza A virus is unique in that persons of all ages in a population become ill with febrile respiratory tract complaints. In contrast, whereas other respiratory tract viral agents (respiratory syncytial virus, rhinoviruses, parainfluenza viruses) also may cause community epidemics that involve both children and adults, the illness is different in the two age groups; young children with primary viral infections with noninfluenzal agents have febrile illnesses, whereas older children and adults with similar infections most commonly have common colds and other upper respiratory tract involvement with little or no fever.

The symptoms and signs of type A influenza in children and adults due to the Asian subtype (H2N2) are compared in Table 181–2.[147] The following findings have been significantly more common in children: sudden onset, anorexia, abdominal pain, vomiting, nausea, cervical adenopathy, and temperature higher than 38.9° C. Influenza C viruses cause illnesses similar to influenza A infection, but the severity of disease usually is less and the duration shorter. In addition, because antigenic changes in influenza B viruses are less pronounced, there frequently is a greater difference in illness between children and adults. Influenza B may cause an epidemic in which children will have typical influenza with fever, but many adults in the population will have only respiratory

TABLE 181–2. Frequency of Symptoms and Signs of Proven Influenza A (H2N2) in Children (0–14 Years of Age) and Adults*

Symptoms	Percentage with Symptom or Sign: *Children (N = 95)*	*Adults (N = 30)*
Sudden onset	66*	46
Systemic symptoms		
Feverishness	93	71
Headache	81	72
Anorexia	69*	37
Malaise	68	67
Chilliness	37	64†
Myalgia	33	62†
Respiratory symptoms		
Cough	86	90
Nasal discharge	67	82
Sore throat	62	62
Nasal obstruction	54	52
Sneezing	38	67†
Hoarseness	22	37
Sputum production	19	41†
Other symptoms		
Abdominal pain	31*	0
Vomiting	26*	7
Nausea	23*	4
Diarrhea	2	0
Maximum Temperature		
≤37.7° C	11	13
37.8 to 38.8° C	29	58†
≥38.9° C	60*	29
Conjunctival abnormalities	61	56
Pharyngeal injection	60	68
Nasal injection/edema	50	64
Nasal discharge	38	20
Cervical adenopathy	38*	8
Rhonchi and/or rales	2	0
Pharyngeal exudate	1	0

*Significantly more frequent in children ($p < .05$, Fisher's Exact test).

†Significantly more frequent in adults ($p < .05$, Fisher's Exact test).

Data from Jordan, W. S., Denny, F. W., Badger, G. F., et al.: A study of illness in a group of Cleveland families. XVII. The occurrence of Asian influenza. Am. J. Hyg. *68*:190–212, 1958.

TABLE 181–3. Relative Frequency of Symptoms and Signs During Classic Influenza in Older Children and Adolescents

	Occurrence*
Symptoms	
Chilly sensation	+ + + +
Cough	+ + +
Headache	+ + +
Sore throat	+ + +
Prostration	+ +
Nasal stuffiness	+ +
Dizziness	+
Eye irritation or pain	+
Vomiting	+
Myalgia	+
Signs	
Fever	+ + + +
Pharyngitis	+ + +
Conjunctivitis (mild)	+ +
Rhinitis	+ +
Cervical adenitis	+
Pulmonary rales; wheezes or rhonchi	+

*+ + + +, 76 to 100 per cent; + + +, 51 to 75 per cent; + +, 26 to 50 per cent; and +, 1 to 25 per cent.

From Cherry, J. D.: Influenza viral infections. *In* Vaughan, V., McKay, R., and Behrman, R (eds.): Nelson Textbook of Pediatrics. 14th ed. Philadelphia, W. B. Saunders Company, 1987, pp. 675–678.

tract[107] illnesses without significant fever. In other outbreaks due to antigenically variant influenza B virus, significant illness has been identified in adults.[28, 124]

Older Children and Adolescents (Classic Influenza)

The symptoms and signs of classic influenza in older children and adolescents are presented in Table 181–3. The onset of illness is abrupt, with fever and associated flushed face, chills, headache, myalgia, and malaise.[4, 23, 33, 34, 231, 238, 247, 255] The temperature range is between 39° and 41° C (102° to 106° F), with a general inverse correlation with age. The systemic symptoms are reported to be more severe in older patients, probably because of their ability to describe them. Although a dry cough and coryza also are early manifestations of influenza, these symptoms go unobserved by the patients because of the severity of the systemic manifestations. Sore throat occurs in more than half the cases and usually is associated with a not otherwise remarkable nonexudative pharyngitis. Ocular symptoms include tearing, photophobia, burning, and pain with eye movement.

In uncomplicated illness, the fever usually persists for 2 to 3 days but may last up to 5 days. A biphasic temperature pattern may occur, even without apparent secondary bacterial complications. By the second to the fourth day, respiratory tract symptoms become more prominent and the systemic complaints begin to subside. The cough is dry and hacking and usually persists for 4 to 7 days; cough, in association with some degree of general malaise, occasionally will persist for 1 or 2 weeks after the rest of the illness has subsided. Illness due to influenza B virus generally is associated with more prominent nasal and eye complaints and fewer systemic findings, such as dizziness and prostration, than is influenza A illness. In a study in which both influenza A (H1N1) and influenza C were noted in a population of young adults, the illnesses could not be differentiated by clinical findings.[67]

In uncomplicated classic influenza, the leukocyte count most often is normal, but leukopenia (<4500 cells/mm^3) has been noted in about 25 per cent of cases. The differential cell count is of no diagnostic value, for about one-third of patients will have normal values; one-third, relative lymphopenia; and one-third, relative neutropenia. The relative proportion of each white cell type may depend on the time during the course of infection that the differential count is determined.[162] Approximately 10 per cent of older children and adolescents will have clinical signs and roentgenographic evidence of pulmonary involvement.

Younger Children

GENERAL. Clinical expression of influenza in younger children and infants has been studied intensively, a reflection of increasingly sensitive and specific respiratory tract viral diagnosis. With some exceptions,[83, 84, 86, 91, 95, 108, 136, 139, 159, 177, 199, 200, 250] most studies have contained disproportionate numbers of hospitalized patients[20, 25, 30, 31, 82, 137, 176, 181, 182, 207, 216, 223, 224, 232, 277, 301] and thus may tend to exaggerate the more severe end of the influenza spectrum.

In younger children, the manifestations of influenza viral infections frequently are similar to those resulting from other respiratory tract viruses (parainfluenza, respiratory syncytial, rhinovirus, and adenovirus) (Table 181–4). Laryngotracheitis, bronchitis, bronchiolitis, pneumonia, and the common cold all occur. Clinical descriptions of these illnesses are presented in Chapters 8, 9, and 10. The overall rate of hospitalization of children with lower respiratory tract involvement is the same for influenza virus infections as for other viruses, but influenza tends to affect older children.

Primary infection with influenza A in these age categories typically is seen as an undifferentiated febrile upper respiratory tract illness.[294] Hospitalization of infants younger than

TABLE 181–4. Relative Frequency of Clinical Manifestations of Influenza Viral Infections in Children Younger Than 5 Years of Age

	Occurrence*
Major Clinical Category	
Upper respiratory tract illness	+ + + +
Laryngotracheitis	+
Bronchitis	+
Bronchiolitis	+
Pneumonia	+
Symptoms	
Cough	+ + + +
Anorexia	+ +
Coryza	+ +
Vomiting	+ +
Diarrhea	+
Sore throat	+
Signs	
Fever	+ + + +
Pharyngitis	+ + +
Cervical adenitis	+ +
Otitis media	+ +
Convulsions	+
Exanthem	+
Generalized adenitis	+

*+ + + +, 76 to 100 per cent; + + +, 51 to 75 per cent; + +, 26 to 50 per cent; and +, 1 to 25 per cent.

From Cherry, J. D.: Influenza viral infections. *In* Vaughan, V., McKay, R., and Behrman, R (eds.): Nelson Textbook of Pediatrics. 14th ed. Philadelphia, W. B. Saunders Company, 1987, pp. 675–678.

2 months of age for ruling out bacterial sepsis is common, particularly when influenza A (H3N2) viruses are epidemic.[111] Fever tends to be quite high and, in the majority of patients, will exceed 39.5° C. Affected children appear moderately toxic, with clear nasal discharge, cough, and irritability as almost constant findings. Pharyngitis usually is present, with diffuse erythema and boggy, enlarged tonsillar tissue. Between 5 and 10 per cent of those infected will have some degree of pulmonary involvement; in hospitalized children, this percentage may be as high as 50 per cent. Vomiting, diarrhea, otitis media, pneumonitis, and croup frequently are associated findings, and fleeting erythematous, macular or maculopapular discrete rashes occasionally are observed.

GASTROINTESTINAL SYMPTOMS. In contrast to illness symptoms in older children and adults, gastrointestinal symptoms have been noted in several studies of influenza infection in young children. Among 68 children admitted to hospital during a community epidemic of influenza B/Hong Kong/72 in 1974, Kerr and colleagues[152] encountered acute abdominal pain, with minimal associated respiratory tract symptoms, as the presenting complaint in 37 patients. This symptom was most frequent in children 4 to 10 years of age and led to unnecessary laparotomy in two patients. In infants, infection by influenza A virus may elicit diarrhea and vomiting. Of 18 infants 6 months of age or younger with proven influenza A/HK/68 infections, Price and associates[234] noted prominent anorexia, diarrhea, or vomiting in 13 (72 per cent), and only 5 (23 per cent) had respiratory tract symptoms alone. Five of the infants with gastrointestinal disturbance had moderate to severe dehydration. Similarly, among 53 hospitalized infants younger than 1 year of age with infections by influenza A, Paisley and associates[220] found diarrhea to be a prominent symptom in 18 patients (34 per cent). Thus, unlike adults with influenza, infants and young children indeed may display "gastric flu."

FEBRILE CONVULSIONS. Febrile convulsions precipitated by fever of abrupt onset have been cited as common presenting complaints in several studies of hospitalized children with influenza. Among 75 children with infections by influenza A/Hong Kong/68 (H3N2), 26 (35 per cent) of the patients reported by Price and associates[234] presented with a febrile convulsion. Of the 77 hospitalized children reported by Brocklebank and colleagues,[20] 31 (40 per cent) had convulsions at onset; 27 of the children in this series were 3 years of age or younger, a distribution consistent with the usual age-specific susceptibility pattern of febrile seizures.

CROUP. Acute laryngotracheobronchitis (croup) has been noted as a prominent feature of influenza A in young children during the H3N2 era. Illness tends to be more severe than is the rule for the croup syndrome induced by parainfluenza viruses, and tenacious tracheal secretions may necessitate tracheostomy or endotracheal intubation in a higher proportion of hospitalized patients. During the peak month of a composite of 13 consecutive influenza A outbreaks, influenza A virus was demonstrated in 68 per cent of croup patients hospitalized in Washington, D.C.[157] Of 10 infants requiring tracheostomy for severe laryngotracheobronchitis during a Dallas outbreak in 1972, Howard and associates[141] found serologic evidence of infection by influenza A/Hong Kong/68 (H3N2) in 8 patients. Among 79 croup patients studied by Eller and colleagues[71] in 1968 and 1969, 8 of 11 children (73 per cent) infected with influenza A/Hong Kong/68 (H3N2) had "severe" respiratory tract distress, whereas only 8 of 48 children (17 per cent) infected with other viral respiratory tract pathogens (predominantly parainfluenza type 1) had a similarly severe course.

Neonates

In neonates, influenza infection may suggest bacterial sepsis: lethargy, poor feeding, petechiae, poor peripheral circulation with mottling of the skin, and apneic spells. Bauer and colleagues[7] and Meibalane and associates[192] have reported nosocomial influenza A outbreaks in neonatal nurseries in association with symptomatic illnesses among nursery staff and parents. Six of the eight infants in the latter study had apneic spells. Two infants required mechanical ventilation for frequent apneic spells for a period of 6 to 8 days.

High-Risk Children

Other host characteristics generally considered to influence the clinical expression of influenza include preexisting chronic pulmonary, cardiac, and neuromuscular disease. Most deaths occur in these vulnerable patients.[275] The basis for this doctrine, however, derives almost exclusively from pathologic and epidemiologic analysis of influenza in adult patients.[70, 132] In children with chronic illness, the available data are surprisingly meager. Among the 77 hospitalized children with influenza A reported by Brocklebank and colleagues,[20] 13 of 23 (56 per cent) with chronic diseases or congenital malformations developed lower respiratory tract infection, compared with 10 of 54 (19 per cent) without preexisting chronic conditions. The few comprehensive virologic studies carried out in asthmatic children have yielded conflicting results. In a longitudinal study of young children (younger than 3 years of age) hospitalized for prolonged periods because of severe extrinsic asthma, McIntosh and associates[190] serologically documented 11 episodes of infection by influenza A/Hong Kong/68, all of which were mild and none of which were associated with exacerbations of wheezing. Studies of pediatric outpatients older than 3 years of age with intrinsic asthma have found an important role for influenza virus infections in triggering asthma attacks. In these studies, Minor and associates[196, 197] documented influenza A/Hong Kong/68 infections by virus isolation as well as by seroconversion in 11 children. Ten of the 11 virus isolations were associated with febrile illness and exacerbations of asthmatic symptoms. Roldaan and Masurel[242] followed a group of older (9 to 16 years of age) asthmatic children housed in Davos, Switzerland, and demonstrated significant respiratory tract compromise associated with influenza virus infections. The preponderance of clinical studies incriminates influenza virus infection as an important instigator of asthma attacks in children.[102] Kempe and colleagues[151] studied influenza virus infection in children with malignancies and found that affected children had both more frequent and more severe influenza-related illness than did their healthy contacts or age-matched controls.

DIAGNOSIS

Infection with influenza virus can be deduced more accurately from epidemiologic features than from clinical presentation. Epidemics occur each winter and usually begin with a sudden increase in presentation to primary care facilities of school age children with febrile respiratory tract illnesses.[100] Routine laboratory studies provide little help in the differentiation of influenza from other viral respiratory tract diseases. Serial monitoring of induced infections in adults has revealed a characteristic moderate increase in total white blood cell count, with relative lymphopenia, during the height of symptoms and low serum iron values.[61, 63, 75] In children, however, hematologic manifestations are variable, with marked leukocytosis frequently observed in infants.[119] Chest radiographs are useful primarily for determining the presence of complicating interstitial or lobar pneumonia. Transient alterations in tests of pulmonary function have been documented in a high percentage of normal adults with uncomplicated influenza.[123] Thus, arterial blood gas determinations may be useful in hospitalized children with influenza and clinical evidence of lower respiratory tract involvement, even if chest radiographs do not show infiltrates.

Definite diagnosis of influenza depends on either virus isolation from respiratory tract secretions or a significant rise in serum antibody during convalescence. In contrast to shedding of adenoviruses or herpes simplex virus from the respiratory tract, asymptomatic carriage of influenza viruses is rare. Thus, virus isolation alone is considered conclusive evidence for an etiologic role in an illness. Hemagglutinating agents often can be detected in embryonated eggs, Madin-Darby canine kidney, or monkey kidney tissue culture within 72 hours of inoculation. However, longer incubation and serial passage are required before cultures can be regarded as negative.[64] Rapid detection of influenza antigens in nasopharyngeal epithelial cells with specific fluorescent antibody conjugates has been successful in a number of studies.[174, 218] Enzyme immunoassay can be used for early detection of influenza A antigen.[62, 283] A composite approach employs short-term incubation of clinical specimens in tissue culture, followed by rapid identification of hemagglutinating viruses with fluorescent antibody.[8]

Serologic diagnosis may be accomplished by use of either complement-fixation or hemagglutination-inhibition techniques.[64] The complement-fixation test detects antibody against the "soluble" nucleoprotein antigens that are common to all strains of influenza A or influenza B. Reagents are commercially available, and the test is provided by most clinical laboratories. Complement-fixing antibodies are of relatively brief duration; titers wane within 6 months of infection. Hemagglutination-inhibiting antibodies, which are subtype-specific, provide more definitive evidence of infection. However, subtype-specific reagents are required and are less widely available in clinical laboratories. Titers persist for years and are boosted by infection with related strains. The hemagglutination-inhibition test has the added advantage of greater sensitivity. Neutralizing antibodies correlate best with protection against reinfection and are more sensitive indicators. Rises in neuraminidase-inhibiting antibody also may be detected after infection, but such studies are technically cumbersome and restricted to specialized applications. A versatile method for measuring antibodies against influenza hemagglutinins employs the enzyme-linked immunosorbent assay.[13, 213] This system is technically simple and has the advantage of permitting specific identification of IgA and IgM antibodies as well as IgG subclasses.

The differential diagnosis of influenza includes an extensive list of febrile conditions, most commonly caused by other respiratory tract viruses and *Streptococcus pyogenes*. In common pediatric practice, influenza and other common respiratory tract viral illnesses too often are lumped casually as "viral upper respiratory tract infection." Definitive diagnosis of influenza in even a few children greatly increases the likelihood that other pediatric respiratory tract illness is caused by the same agent and may be useful in forecasting the development of epidemic influenza in adult populations.

COMPLICATIONS

Bacterial Infections

The most frequent complications of influenza are bacterial infections of the respiratory tract (particularly pneumonia), otitis media, and sinusitis.[77, 78, 98, 130, 147, 148, 160, 179, 180, 184, 201, 220, 257, 259, 266, 267, 280, 303] Characteristically, these complications arise in early convalescence, with bacterial invasion of portions of the respiratory tract with denuded ciliated epithelium and defective mucociliary transport. Of 37 young infants experiencing their first infections by influenza A viruses, Wright and colleagues[294] noted otitis media in 10 and pneumonia in 7. Of 12 patients who developed nosocomial infection by influenza A on an infant ward, most with underlying chronic cardiorespiratory disease, Hall and Douglas[119] documented complicating bacterial pneumonia in 5. The incidence of complicating bacterial infections in community studies, including children of all ages, is approximately 10 per cent, with otitis media the most frequent finding.[147, 303] A 14-year longitudinal study of young children demonstrated a 28 per cent incidence of otitis media after influenza A and B virus infections and an increased risk of recurrent disease.[130]

Although most cases of bacterial pneumonia complicating influenza are pneumococcal,[257] the two most feared pulmonary complications are progressive primary viral pneumonia and staphylococcal pneumonia.[180] Progressive primary viral pneumonia has been observed most frequently in adult patients with preexisting rheumatic heart disease but may occur in previously healthy children as well.[148, 220] It is characterized radiographically by diffuse bronchopneumonic infiltrates and clinically by intense dyspnea and a relentless downhill course, despite antimicrobial and supportive therapy. Staphylococcal pneumonia may occur as a postinfluenzal lobar pneumonia progressing to pneumatoceles and empyema. More characteristically, staphylococcal pneumonia in association with influenza occurs as a fulminant, synergistic, viral-bacterial process with diffuse involvement on radiographs, leukopenia, intense dyspnea, blood-tinged sputum, and rapid death. Necrotizing pneumonitis with microabscesses and positive lung cultures for both influenza A virus and *Staphylococcus aureus* are characteristic.[180]

Three children have been described in whom orbital cellulitis developed as a complication of influenza.[127] An adult patient with septicemic infection has been described. This case is of interest because it appears to have been the activation of a latent *Pseudomonas pseudomallei* infection that had been acquired 6 years previously.[184] Two adults have had fatal fungal infections after influenza A viral infections.[79]

Acute Myositis

Acute myositis occurs in the setting of early convalescence from a typical influenzal illness.[6, 59, 195] Severe pain and tenderness in the calves of both legs come on suddenly, often with refusal to walk. Other muscle groups may be involved as well, but the gastrocnemius and soleus muscles are affected in virtually all cases. Elevation of serum creatine kinase and aspartate aminotransferase is characteristic. Influenza B virus has been isolated in 20 of 26 such cases by Middleton and associates[195] and in 11 of 17 cases by Dietzman and colleagues.[59] Infection by influenza A has been documented in one case of the former series. The condition generally is self-limited, but rhabdomyolysis with myoglobinuria and acute renal failure has been described in severe adult cases occurring in association with influenza A.[58, 198, 204, 306]

Reye Syndrome and Encephalopathy

Reye syndrome is a condition of obscure pathogenesis characterized by fatty degeneration of the liver and diffuse cerebral edema.[44, 239] Although the condition has been recognized under varying nomenclatures since its partial description by Brain and colleagues[18] in 1929, only somewhat recently has influenza infection been implicated as an inciting factor. Of 85 patients treated at Cincinnati Children's Hospital, 74 (87 per cent) had a respiratory tract prodrome clinically indistinguishable from influenza and 11 patients (13 per cent) had varicella.[225] During the 1974 outbreak in Cincinnati, influenza B/HK/8/73 was isolated from the nasopharyngeal secretions of 9 of 23 affected children, with serologic evidence of influenza B in an additional 3 children.[172] Numerous other reports have demonstrated similar associations of influenza A (H1N1 and H3N2) as well as influenza B with subsequent outbreaks of Reye syndrome.[126, 143, 270, 292] Surveillance data indicate a significant decline in both the incidence and mortality ratio.[3, 5] In a survivor of Reye syndrome, who was studied intensively by Partin and colleagues,[225] influenza A/Vic/3/75 (H3N2) virus was recovered from nasotracheal secretions, cerebrospinal fluid, liver, and skeletal (gastrocnemius) muscle, which led the investigators to postulate visceral dissemination of virus as an element in the pathogenesis of this condition. Clinically, Reye syndrome, most common in white male school age children, is marked by nausea, vomiting, and stupor during convalescence from a viral illness, most commonly characterized by respiratory tract symptoms.[3, 5] In this setting, the finding of elevated serum transaminase and blood ammonia levels, with unremarkable cerebrospinal fluid, is sufficient for diagnosis.[44] During the 1974 outbreak, Reye syndrome was estimated to have occurred at a rate of 31 to 58 cases per 100,000 infections with influenza B in children,[43, 45] although a lower incidence was reported among Colorado children in association with the 1978–1979 H1N1 outbreak.[126] The most recent case:fatality ratio is 26 per cent.

An ever-increasing body of data have revealed a strong association between the use of salicylates or salicylate-containing medications and Reye syndrome, with resultant strict warnings against the use of salicylates in children with influenza.[35, 125, 142, 265, 281, 290, 304] The decreased use of aspirin for children with influenza and varicella has paralleled the decline in reporting of cases of Reye syndrome.[3]

Encephalopathy may occur without fatty degeneration of the liver. An encephalitis-like picture is not uncommon among children hospitalized with influenza virus infection.[57]

Other Complications

NEUROLOGIC DISEASE. Apart from encephalopathy or Reye syndrome, other severe neurologic illnesses have been noted rarely in association with influenza viral infections.[57, 68, 81, 193, 219, 249] As noted, the most common manifestation is an encephalitis in association with a respiratory tract illness. In most instances, there is no evidence of a concomitant meningitis. Guillain-Barré syndrome and a transverse myelitis are also rare complications of influenza.[68, 81] Epidemiologic and laboratory evidence indicates that some cases of Parkinson disease are the result of influenza viral infections.[96, 203]

CARDIAC DISEASE. Pericarditis and myocarditis have been noted rarely in association with influenza viral infections.[42, 201, 219, 266, 267] This cardiac involvement has occurred in normal children and adults as well as in those with preexisting heart disease.

SUDDEN DEATHS. During influenza epidemics, sudden unexpected deaths are observed occasionally.[219] These occur in persons of all ages, and postmortem examination most frequently indicates respiratory tract involvement. Cases of sudden infant death syndrome have been associated with influenza viral infection.[65, 271]

OTHER OBSERVATIONS. Glomerulonephritis and renal failure have been associated with influenza viral infections.[286, 288] In two instances, acute parotitis has occurred with influenza A infection.[19] Although there is evidence of the transplacental passage of influenza virus to a 30-week-old male fetus, there is no epidemiologic evidence of influenza virus teratogenicity.[183, 289, 302]

TREATMENT

Because most influenza infections are unpleasant but uncomplicated illnesses, symptomatic treatment is the cornerstone of management. Bed rest, adequate hydration with oral fluids, control of fever and myalgia with acetaminophen, and maintenance of comfortable breathing by means of nasal decongestants and humidified air suffice in most cases. Prophylactic administration of antibiotics should be discouraged. Persistent irritative cough during convalescence often can be relieved with dextromethorphan or codeine.

Complicated illnesses demand the physician's clinical judgment in the use of other therapeutic modalities. Bacterial infections, suggested by a prolonged febrile course or recrudescence of fever during early convalescence, should be identified as to site, and appropriate cultures should be obtained. Antibiotic therapy then is indicated and should be guided and modified by Gram stain findings and the results of cultures. Because most infections are caused by *S. pneumoniae*, *Haemophilus influenzae*, and *S. pyogenes*, therapy with ampicillin or amoxicillin is adequate for most cases of otitis media or lobar pneumonia. The possibility of penicillin-resistant pneumococci and of other agents, particularly *S. aureus* and opportunistic gram-negative pathogens, should be entertained in fulminant or protracted pneumonias.

Inhalation therapy is an integral part of the management of patients with illnesses complicated by airway compromise (croup), apneic spells, or diffuse pneumonia. Such patients should be monitored carefully. Humidified air is the most important element in management of croup, but nasotracheal intubation or tracheostomy has been required in a high percentage of patients with croup due to influenza.[141] Provision of supplemental oxygen and, as indicated by arterial blood gas analysis, continuous positive airway pressure or mechanical ventilation may be required in infants and children with apnea or significant alveolar-capillary block due to pneumonia.

The antiviral agent amantadine hydrochloride is active in vitro against influenza A viruses and has been shown to provide prophylactic and therapeutic benefit in adults.[146, 263] Amantadine lacks activity against influenza B viruses. A number of studies also have documented the prophylactic effect of amantadine or its analogue, rimantadine, in community-acquired influenza A in children.[40, 50, 76, 226, 237, 243, 244, 287, 296] There are, however, few pediatric data regarding therapeutic efficacy.[80, 158] Treatment with rimantadine of young children who probably lacked prior experience with the infecting subtype has resulted in emergence of resistant viruses.[10, 118] In some instances, the resistant viruses have been noted to infect susceptible contacts.[129]

A newer, broad-spectrum antiviral agent, ribavirin, has been used successfully in the treatment of both influenza A and B in adult patients when it is administered as an aerosol.[161, 164, 189, 291] Experience with this treatment modality in children is limited to other viruses but has resulted in no significant adverse reactions.[97, 121, 191, 273]

PROGNOSIS

The prognosis for clinical recovery from uncomplicated influenza generally is considered to be excellent. Of the complications of influenza, primary influenza pneumonia, staphylococcal pneumonia, and Reye syndrome have a guarded prognosis. However, a bewildering array of chronic pulmonary conditions has been noted to begin with undifferentiated childhood respiratory tract infections, among which "influenza" often is cited but infrequently proved.[167, 251] These conditions include lobar atelectasis; localized and generalized bronchiectasis; and such clinicopathologic entities as Swyer-James syndrome (unilateral hyperlucent lung), bronchiolitis obliterans, Hamman-Rich syndrome (diffuse interstitial pneumonia), and desquamative interstitial pneumonitis. Only precise virologic diagnosis of acute respiratory tract disease, especially viral pneumonia, will delineate the long-term complications that may occur in a small proportion of cases.

PREVENTION

Immunization offers the best hope for prevention of influenza. Yet epidemiologic, technologic, pharmacologic, logistic, and political difficulties have hampered widespread implementation of such programs, as witnessed by the storm of controversy that greeted the A/New Jersey/76 "swine flu" vaccine campaign of 1976.[245] Prediction of the epidemic potential of new influenza virus variants and their potential for epidemic spread is a major difficulty. In order to be effective, vaccines must contain antigens similar to those of the potential infecting agent. In years when a new variant arises and causes widespread outbreaks, the available vaccine may contain a previous variant with only modest heterologous immunizing potential. Conversely, in years in which new variants do not arise, vaccines may be formulated ideally but the epidemic potential of virus strains that have already circulated may be minimal. Thus, by virtue of changes in either virus antigens or prevalences of natural immunity, prevention of epidemics through the widespread use of vaccine has been difficult.

Only inactivated (formalin-treated) influenza vaccines currently are licensed for use in the United States. A number of improvements have been made in these vaccines since their introduction in the late 1930s.[194, 246] These innovations have included enhanced vaccine production by use of reassortment virus strains that grow rapidly in eggs,[221] exclusion of host antigens and other toxic impurities by zonal ultracentrifugation (current "whole-virus" vaccines),[206] disruption of viral particles with ether or detergents (current "split-product" vaccines),[54] and, most recently, physical purification of hemagglutinin and neuraminidase (HANA or "subunit" vaccines).[48, 171]

In supposedly equivalent dosages, the antigenicity and reactogenicity of whole-virus and split-product vaccines were studied extensively in children during the trials of A/New Jersey/76 (H1N1) monovalent and A/New Jersey/76 (H1N1)–A/Victoria/75 (H3N2) bivalent vaccines in 1976.[4, 297, 272] Whole-virus vaccines were more antigenic and, at the same time, more reactogenic than were split-product vaccines because they contained a greater concentration of antigens. In two-dose regimens, the split-product vaccines produced adequate antibody levels without acute reactions. The A/Victoria/75 component of the bivalent vaccines had significantly greater antigenicity than did the A/New Jersey/76 component in children, which reflects previous priming by H3N2 viral strains but a lack of previous exposure to H1N1-like viruses. The consensus of these studies was that split-product vaccines, by virtue of their minimal reactogenicity, should be preferred for vaccination of children. Similar large-scale trials evaluating monovalent A/USSR/77 (H1N1) and trivalent A/USSR/77 (H1N1), A/Texas/77 (H3N2), and B/Hong Kong/72 inactivated influenza virus vaccines were in agreement with previous results.[299] However, proof of protective efficacy, which with whole-virus vaccines has ranged from 50 to 95 per cent after homologous challenge,[52, 155] is limited for split-product vaccines,[115, 236] particularly against antigenic shift virus strains. Gruber and associates[117] have reported a protective rate of 60 per cent with B/USSR/83 vaccine against the next variant, B/Ann Arbor/86.

The side effects of vaccination with inactivated vaccines in children deserve further comment. Such reactions, when they occur, include fever, "flu-like" symptoms of malaise and myalgia, and local tenderness at the site of inoculation.[297] Febrile convulsions have been cited as a particular risk of vaccination in the very young.[187, 295] In the extensive trials cited, however, 813 children aged 6 months to 5 years received varying doses of whole-virus and split-product vaccines.[115, 297] None of these children had febrile convulsions. During the 1978 trials with subunit vaccines standardized for hemagglutinin content, local and systemic reactions were minimal in high-risk children.

Guillain-Barré syndrome occurred in roughly 1 in 100,000 adult recipients of the A/New Jersey/76 vaccine in the National Influenza Immunization Program.[26, 194, 252] Its risk after natural influenza infection is unknown, but, although sporadic cases after influenza have been reported, it is not felt to be an important agent triggering this syndrome.[68, 81, 253, 285] The incidence of this complication among pediatric vaccine recipients as well as those members of the military younger than 25 years of age was not increased. Surveillance of subsequent vaccine years has revealed no association of an increased frequency of Guillain-Barré syndrome and influenza vaccine.[29, 149]

Other influenza vaccines remain experimental in the United States. Neuraminidase-specific inactivated vaccines offer some degree of protection against severe illness, diminish virus shedding and subsequent transmission, and would be expected to be outdated less frequently by antigenic drift.[217] Addition of adjuvants to inactivated vaccines enhances the height, duration, and breadth of the antibody response they elicit.[246, 292] Candidate live virus vaccines have employed strains spontaneously attenuated after serial passage ("spontaneous" mutants),[262] strains resistant to nonspecific inhibitors present in normal horse serum ("inhibitor-resistant" mutants),[264] strains incapable of replication at 37° C ("temperature-sensitive" mutants),[209] and strains adapted to incubation temperatures of 25° C ("cold-adapted" mutants).[55] Live vaccines, administered intranasally, correspond most closely to natural infection in their capacity to produce both secretory and humoral immunity. The most promising are the cold-adapted reassortment influenza virus vaccines. These vaccines have been administered to adults and children; both local and systemic antibody responses resulted with no significant side effects.[24, 38, 212, 299, 305] They also have been shown to be safe and nontransmissible in both of these populations and result in protection against challenge with wild influenza virus.[24, 32, 39, 214, 298] Live attenuated vaccines appear to be the most promising new approaches.

The strategy of vaccination against influenza remains perhaps the most controversial aspect of prevention. Vaccination of normal children, who have the highest attack rates during epidemics, has not been advocated routinely in the United States, except for household contacts of high-risk patients.[99] The risk of hospitalization of children younger than 5 years of age is almost as high as for elderly persons and, unlike the elderly, less than 20 per cent of young hospitalized children have a chronic underlying condition.[228] Because children are the most important population group in the propagation of epidemics, a vaccine strategy aimed at epidemic prevention would necessarily be focused on this age group. Supporting this concept, mass vaccination of schoolchildren had a measurable effect on the overall incidence of A/HK/68 in Tecumseh, Michigan, during the 1968 epidemic.[202] The protective effect was most evident in adults 20 to 30 years of age, which suggests that immunization of children lowered the incidence of influenza in their parents. Universal immunization of children in school or day care not only would reduce serious morbidity significantly in this age group but also would have the potential for dampening epidemics and reducing risk of exposure to virus for vulnerable high-risk patients. The cold-adapted attenuated vaccine developed by Maassab has broader and longer lasting immunity for children younger than 10 years of age. The administration by nosedrops is accepted better by children and easier to administer than the inactivated vaccine given by injection. The cold-adapted vaccine warrants testing in children as an approach to epidemic control.

The emphasis of current vaccination strategy is focused on the prevention of complicated illness not only in population groups at highest risk of death from pneumonia or influenza during epidemics but also in physicians, nurses, and household contacts of these high-risk patients. Mortality rates are highest in persons with cardiovascular disorders, such as rheumatic, congenital, or ischemic heart disease; chronic bronchopulmonary disease, such as emphysema, asthma, bronchitis, and bronchiectasis; chronic metabolic diseases, such as diabetes mellitus; chronic glomerulonephritis and nephrosis; and chronic neurologic disorders, especially those associated with weak or paralyzed respiratory tract muscles.[29] In addition, it seems judicious to consider vaccination of children with various illnesses requiring long-term salicylate therapy (i.e., Kawasaki disease, juvenile rheumatoid arthritis, acute rheumatic fever, and others). It is clear from experience that judicious dosage of inactivated vaccines in children of all ages can produce acceptable levels of antibody with minimal side effects.

References

1. Alford, R. M., Kasel, J. A., Gerone, P. J., et al.: Human influenza resulting from aerosol inhalation. Proc. Soc. Exp. Biol. Med. *122*:800–804, 1966.
2. Alling, D. W., Blackwelder, W. C., and Stuart-Harris, C. H.: A study of excess mortality during influenza epidemics in the United States, 1968–1976. Am. J. Epidemiol. *113*:30–43, 1981.
3. Arrowsmith, J. B., Kennedy, D. L., Kuritsky, J. N., et al.: National patterns of aspirin use and Reye syndrome reporting, United States, 1980 to 1985. Pediatrics *79*:858–863, 1987.
4. Banatvala, J. E., Reiss, B. B., Anderson, T. B., et al.: Asian influenza in 1963 in two general practices in Cambridge, England. Can. Med. Assoc. J. *93*:593–597, 1965.
5. Barrett, M. J., Hurwitz, E. S., Schonberger, L. B., et al.: Changing epidemiology of Reye syndrome in the United States. Pediatrics *77*:598–602, 1986.
6. Barton, L. L., and Chalhub, E. G.: Myositis associated with influenza A infection. J. Pediatr. *87*:1003–1004, 1975.
7. Bauer, C. K., Elie, K., Spence, L., et al.: Hong Kong influenza in a neonatal unit. J. A. M. A. *223*:1233–1235, 1973.
8. Baxter, B. D., Couch, R. B., Greenberg, S. B., et al.: Maintenance of viability and comparison of identification methods for influenza and other respiratory viruses of humans. J. Clin. Microbiol. *6*:19–22, 1977.
9. Bell, W. E., McKee, A. P., and Utterback, R. A.: Asian influenza virus as the cause of acute encephalitis. Neurology *8*:500–502, 1958.
10. Belshe, R. B., Smith, M. H., Hall, C. B., et al.: Genetic basis of resistance to rimantadine emerging during treatment of influenza virus infection. J. Virol. *62*:1508–1512, 1988.
11. Berg, R. A., Yolken, R. H., Rennard, S. I., et al.: New enzyme immunoassays for measurement of influenza A/Victoria/3/75 virus in nasal washes. Lancet *2*:851–853, 1980.
12. Biddison, W. E., Shaw, S., and Nelson, D. L.: Virus specificity of human influenza virus immune cytotoxic T cells. J. Immunol. *122*:660–664, 1979.
13. Bishai, F. R., and Galli, R.: Enzyme-linked immunosorbent assay for detection of antibodies to influenza A and B and parainfluenza type 1 in sera of patients. J. Clin. Microbiol. *8*:648–656, 1978.
14. Blass, D., Patzelt, E., and Kuechler, E.: Identification of the cap binding protein of influenza virus. Nucleic Acids Res. *10*:4803–4812, 1982.
15. Blass, D., Patzelt, E., and Kuechler, E.: Cap recognizing protein of influenza virus. Virology *116*:339–348, 1982.
16. Blumenfeld, L., II, Kilbourne, E. D., Louria, D. B., et al.: Studies on influenza in the pandemic of 1957–1958. I. An investigation of an intrahospital epidemic, with a note on vaccine efficacy. J. Clin. Invest. *38*:199–212, 1959.
17. Braciale, T. J.: Immunologic recognition of influenza-infected cells. 1. Generation of virus strain specific and cross-reactive subpopulations of cytotoxic T cells in response to type A influenza virus infection of different subtypes. Cell. Immunol. *33*:423–426, 1977.
18. Brain, W. R., Hunter, D., and Turnball, H. M.: Acute meningoencephalitis of childhood. Lancet *1*:221–227, 1929.
19. Brill, S. J., and Gilfillan, R. F.: Acute parotitis associated with influenza type A. N. Engl. J. Med. *296*:1391–1392, 1977.
20. Brocklebank, J. T., Coust, S. D. M., McQuillan, J., et al.: Influenza A infections in children. Lancet *2*:497–500, 1972.
21. Brown, P., Gajdusek, D. C., and Morris, J. A.: Epidemic A_2 influenza in isolated Pacific Island populations without pre-epidemic antibody to influenza types A and B, and the discovery of other still unexposed populations. Am. J. Epidemiol. *83*:176–188, 1966.
22. Burnet, F. M., and Lind, P. E.: Studies on recombination with influenza viruses in the chick embryo. III. Reciprocal genetic interaction between two influenza virus strains. Aust. J. Exp. Biol. Med. Sci. *30*:469–477, 1952.
23. Carey, D. E., Dunn, F. L., Robinson, R. Q., et al.: Community-wide epidemic of Asian strain influenza: Clinical and subclinical illnesses among school children. J. A. M. A. *167*:1459–1463, 1958.
24. Cate, T. R., and Couch, R. B.: Live influenza A/Victoria/75 (H3N2) virus vaccines: Reactogenicity, immunogenicity, and protection against wild-type virus challenge. Infect. Immun. *38*:141–146, 1982.
25. Caul, E. O., Waller, D. K., Clarke, S. K. R., et al.: A comparison of influenza and respiratory syncytial virus infections among infants admitted to hospital with acute respiratory infections. J. Hyg. (Camb.) *77*:383–392, 1976.
26. Centers for Disease Control: Followup on Guillain-Barré syndrome—United States. M. M. W. R. *25*:430, 1977.
27. Centers for Disease Control: Influenza surveillance report No. 91, 1977.
28. Centers for Disease Control: Influenza—United States. M. M. W. R. *29*:71–72, 1980.
29. Centers for Disease Control: Recommendation of the Public Health Service Advisory Committee on Immunization Practices. Influenza vaccine. M. M. W. R. *33*:253–266, 1984.
30. Chanock, R. M., and Parrott, R. H.: Acute respiratory disease in infancy and childhood: Present understanding and prospects for prevention. Pediatrics *36*:21–39, 1965.
31. Chanock, R. M., Chambon, L., Chang, W., et al.: WHO respiratory disease survey in children: A serological study. Bull. World Health Org. *37*:363–369, 1967.
32. Chanock, R. M., and Murphy, B. R.: Use of temperature-sensitive and cold-adapted mutant viruses in immunoprophylaxis of acute respiratory tract disease. Rev. Infect. Dis. *2*:421–432, 1980.
33. Cherry, J. D.: Newer respiratory viruses: Their role in respiratory illnesses of children. *In* Schulman I. (ed.): Advances in Pediatrics. Vol. 20. Chicago, Year Book Medical Publishers, 1973, pp. 225–289.
34. Cherry, J. D.: Influenza viral infections. *In* Vaughan, V., McKay, R., and Behrman, R. (eds.): Nelson Textbook of Pediatrics. 14th ed. Philadelphia, W. B. Saunders, 1987, pp. 675–678.
35. Chin, T. D. Y., Mosley, W. H., Poland, J. D., et al.: Epidemiologic studies of type B influenza in 1961–1962. Am. J. Public Health *53*:1068–1074, 1963.
36. Choi, K., and Thacker, S. B.: Mortality during influenza epidemics in the United States, 1967–1978. Am. J. Public Health *72*:1280–1283, 1982.
37. Choppin, P. W., and Compans, R. W.: The structure of influenza virus. *In* Kilbourne, E. D. (ed.): The Influenza Viruses and Influenza. New York, Academic Press, 1975, pp. 15–52.
38. Clements, M. L., O'Donnell, S., Levine, M. M., et al.: Dose response of A/Alaska/6/77 (H3N2) cold-adapted reassortant vaccine virus in adult volunteers: Role of local antibody in resistance to infection with vaccine. Infect. Immun. *40*:1044–1051, 1983.
39. Clements, M. L., Betts, R. F., and Murphy, B. R.: Advantage of live attenuated cold-adapted influenza A virus over inactivated vaccine for A/Washington/80 (H3N2) wild-type virus infection. Lancet *1*:705–708, 1984.
40. Clover, R. D., Crawford, S. A., Abell, T. D., et al.: Effectiveness of rimantadine prophylaxis of children in families. Am. J. Dis. Child. *140*:706–709, 1986.
41. Clover, R. D., Crawford, S., Glezen, W. P., et al.: Comparison of heterotypic protection against influenza A/Taiwan/86 (H1N1) by attenuated and inactivated vaccines to A/Chile/83-like viruses. J. Infect. Dis. *163*:300–304, 1991.
42. Coltman, Jr., C. A.: Influenza myocarditis. Report of a case with observations on serum glutamic oxaloacetic transaminase. J. A. M. A. *180*:204–208, 1962.
43. Corey, L., Rubin, R. J., and Hattwick, M.: A nationwide outbreak of Reye's

syndrome: Its epidemiologic relationship to influenza B. Am. J. Med. *61*:615–626, 1976.
44. Corey, L., Rubin, R. J., Bregman, D., et al.: Diagnostic criteria for influenza B–associated Reye's syndrome: Clinical vs. pathologic criteria. Pediatrics *60*:702–714, 1977.
45. Corey, L., Rubin, R. J., Thompson, T. R., et al.: Influenza B–associated Reye's syndrome: Incidence in Michigan and potential for prevention. J. Infect. Dis. *135*:398–407, 1977.
46. Couch, R. B., Douglas, R. G., Fedson, D. S., et al.: Correlated studies of a recombinant influenza-virus vaccine. III. Protection against experimental influenza in man. J. Infect. Dis. *124*:473–480, 1971.
47. Couch, R. B., Douglas, R. G., Rossen, R., et al.: Role of secretory antibody in influenza. *In* The Secretory Immunologic System. Washington, D.C., U.S. Department of Health, Education and Welfare, 1969, pp. 93–112.
48. Couch, R. B., Kasel, J. A., Gerin, J. L., et al.: Induction of partial immunity to influenza by a neuraminidase-specific vaccine. J. Infect. Dis. *129*:411–420, 1974.
49. Couch, R. B., Kasel, J. A., Glezen, W. P., et al.: Influenza: Its control in persons and populations. J. Infect. Dis. *153*:431–440, 1986.
50. Crawford, S. A., Clover, R. D., Abell, T. D., et al.: Rimantadine prophylaxis in children: A follow-up study. Pediatr. Infect. Dis. J. *7*:379–383, 1988.
51. Crosby, A. W.: Epidemic and Peace, 1918. Westport, CT, Greenwood Press, 1976.
52. Davenport, F. M.: Inactivated influenza virus vaccine. Past, present and future. Am. Rev. Respir. Dis. *83*(Suppl.):146–156, 1961.
53. Davenport, F. M.: Influenza viruses. *In* Evans, A. S. (ed.): Viral Infections of Humans: Epidemiology and Control. New York, Plenum Press, 1976, pp. 273–296.
54. Davenport, F. M., Hennessy, A. V., Brandon, F. M., et al.: Comparisons of serologic and febrile responses in humans to vaccination with influenza A viruses or their hemagglutinins. J. Lab. Clin. Med. *63*:5–13, 1964.
55. Davenport, F. M., Hennessy, A. V., Maassab, H. F., et al.: Pilot studies on recombinant cold-adapted live type A and B influenza virus vaccines. J. Infect. Dis. *136*:17–25, 1977.
56. Davis, L. E., Caldwell, G. G., Lynch, R. E., et al.: Hong Kong influenza: The epidemiologic features of a high school family study analyzed and compared with a similar study during the 1957 Asian influenza epidemic. Am. J. Epidemiol. *92*:240–247, 1970.
57. Delorme, L., and Middleton, P. J.: Influenza A virus associated with acute encephalopathy. Am. J. Dis. Child. *133*:822–824, 1979.
58. DiBona, F. J., and Morens, D. M.: Rhabdomyolysis associated with influenza A: Report of a case with unusual fluid and electrolyte abnormalities. J. Pediatr. *91*:943–945, 1977.
59. Dietzman, D. E., Schaller, J. G., Ray, C. G., et al.: Acute myositis associated with influenza B infection. Pediatrics *57*:255–258, 1976.
60. Dolin, R., Murphy, B. R., and Caplan, E. A.: Lymphocyte blastogenic responses to influenza virus antigens after influenza infection and vaccination in humans. Infect. Immun. *19*:867–874, 1978.
61. Dolin, R., Richman, D. D., Murphy, B. R., et al.: Cell-mediated immune responses following induced influenza in humans. J. Infect. Dis. *177*:714–719, 1977.
62. Dominguez, E. A., Taber, L. H., and Couch, R. B.: Comparison of rapid diagnostic techniques for respiratory syncytial and influenza A virus respiratory infections in young children. J. Clin. Microbiol. *31*:2286–2290, 1993.
63. Douglas, R. G., Jr., Alford, R. H., Cate, T. K., et al.: The leukocyte response during viral respiratory illness in man. Ann. Intern. Med. *64*:521–530, 1966.
64. Dowdle, W. A., Kendal, A. P., and Noble, G. R.: Influenza viruses. *In* Lennette, E. H., and Schmidt, N. J. (eds.): Diagnostic Procedures for Viral, Rickettsial and Chlamydial Infections. Washington, D.C., American Public Health Association, 1979, p. 593.
65. Downham, M. A. P. S., Gardner, P. S., McQuillin, J., et al.: Role of respiratory viruses in childhood mortality. Br. Med. J. *1*:235–239, 1975.
66. Downie, J. C., and Stuart-Harris, C. H.: The production of neutralizing activity in serum and nasal secretion following immunization with influenza B virus. J. Hyg. *68*:233–244, 1970.
67. Dykes, A. C., Cherry, J. D., and Nolan, C. E.: A clinical, epidemiologic, serologic, and virologic study of influenza C virus infection. Arch. Intern. Med. *140*:1295–1298, 1980.
68. Editorial: Influenza and the nervous system. Br. Med. J. *5745*:357–358, 1971.
69. Effros, R. B., Doherty, P. C., Gerhard, W. E., et al.: Generation of both cross-reactive and virus specific cytotoxic T cell population after immunization with serologically distinct influenza A viruses. J. Exp. Med. *145*:557–558, 1977.
70. Eickhoff, T. C., Sherman, I. L., and Serfling, R. E.: Observations on excess mortality associated with epidemic influenza. J. A. M. A. *176*:776–782, 1961.
71. Eller, J. J., Fulginiti, V. A., Plunket, D. C., et al.: Attack rates for hospitalized croup in children in a military population: Importance of A_2 influenza infection. Pediatr. Res. *6*:386, 1972.
72. Ennis, F. A., Martin, W. J., Verbonitz, M. W., et al.: Specificity studies on cytotoxic thymus-derived lymphocytes reactive with influenza virus–infected cells: Evidence for dual recognition of H-2 and viral hemagglutinin antigens. Proc. Natl. Acad. Sci. U. S. A. *74*:3006–3010, 1977.
73. Fazekas de St. Groth, S., and Donnelley, M.: Studies in experimental immunology of influenza. IV. The protective effect of active immunization. Aust. J. Exp. Biol. Med. Sci. *28*:62–75, 1950.
74. Fenner, F.: Classification and nomenclature of viruses. Intervirology *7*:1–115, 1976.
75. Fernandez, H.: Low serum iron in influenza. N. Engl. J. Med. *302*:865, 1980.
76. Finklea, J. F., Hennessey, A. B., and Davenport, F. M.: A field trial of amantadine chemoprophylaxis in respiratory disease. Am. J. Epidemiol. *85*:403–412, 1967.
77. Finland, M., Strauss, E., and Peterson, O. L.: Staphylococcal pneumonia occurring during an epidemic of clinical influenza. Trans. Assoc. Am. Physicians *56*:139–146, 1941.
78. Finland, M., Ory, E. M., Meads, M., et al.: Influenza and pneumonia. Serologic studies during and after an outbreak of influenza B. J. Lab. Clin. Med. *33*:32–46, 1948.
79. Fischer, J. J., and Walker, D. H.: Invasive pulmonary aspergillosis associated with influenza. J. A. M. A. *241*:1493–1494, 1979.
80. Fishaut, M., and Mostow, S. R.: Amantadine for severe influenza A pneumonia in infancy. Am. J. Dis. Child. *134*:321–322, 1980.
81. Flewett, T. H., and Hoult, J. G.: Influenzal encephalopathy and postinfluenzal encephalitis. Lancet *1*:11–15, 1958.
82. Forbes, J. A.: Severe effects of influenza virus infection. Med. J. Aust. July:75–79, 1958.
83. Foy, H. M., Cooney, M. K., Maletzky, A. J., et al.: Incidence and etiology of pneumonia, croup and bronchiolitis in preschool children belonging to a prepaid medical care group over a four-year period. Am. J. Epidemiol. *97*:80–92, 1973.
84. Foy, H. M., Cooney, M. K., McMahan, R., et al.: Viral and mycoplasmal pneumonia in a prepaid medical care group during an eight-year period. Am. J. Epidemiol. *97*:93–102, 1973.
85. Foy, H. M., Cooney, M. K., Allan, I., et al.: Rates of pneumonia during influenza epidemics in Seattle, 1964–1975. J. A. M. A. *241*:253–258, 1979.
86. Fox, J. P., Hall, C. E., Cooney, M. K., et al.: Influenza virus infections in Seattle families, 1975–1979. Am. J. Epidemiol. *116*:212–227, 1982.
87. Francis, T., and Brightman, I. J.: Virus-inactivating capacity of nasal secretions in the acute and convalescent stages of influenza. Proc. Soc. Exp. Biol. Med. *48*:116–117, 1941.
88. Francis, T., Davenport, F. M., and Hennessy, A. V.: A serological recapitulation of human infection with different strains of influenza virus. Trans. Assoc. Am. Physicians *66*:231–239, 1953.
89. Frank, A. L., Couch, R. B., Griffis, C. A., et al.: Comparison of different tissue cultures for isolation and quantitation of influenza and parainfluenza viruses. J. Clin. Microbiol. *10*:32–36, 1979.
90. Frank, A. L., Puck, J., Hughes, B. J., et al.: Microneutralization test for influenza A and B and parainfluenza 1 and 2 viruses that uses continuous cell lines and fresh serum enhancement. J. Clin. Microbiol. *12*:426–432, 1980.
91. Frank, A. L., Taber, L. H., Glezen, W. P., et al.: Reinfection with influenza A (H3N2) virus in young children and their families. J. Infect. Dis. *140*:829–836, 1979.
92. Frank, A. L., Taber, L. H., and Porter, C. M.: Influenza B virus reinfection. Am J. Epidemiol. *125*:576–586, 1987.
93. Frank, A. L, Taber, L. H., Wells, C. R., et al.: Patterns of shedding of myxoviruses and paramyxoviruses in children. J. Infect. Dis. *144*:433–441, 1981.
94. Frank, A. L.: Selected laboratory aspects of influenza surveillance. Yale J. Biol. Med. *55*:201–205, 1982.
95. Frank, A. L., and Taber, L. H.: Variation in frequency of natural reinfection with influenza A viruses. J. Med. Virol. *12*:17–23, 1983.
96. Gamboa, E. T., Wolf, A., and Yahr, M. D.: Influenza virus antigen in postencephalitic parkinsonism brain. Arch. Neurol. *31*:228–232, 1974.
97. Gelfand, E. W., McCurdy, D., Rao, C. R., et al.: Treatment of viral pneumonitis with ribavirin in severe-combined immunodeficiency disease. Lancet *2*:732–733, 1983.
98. Gerber, G. J., Farmer, W. C., and Fulkerson, L. L.: β-Hemolytic streptococcal pneumonia following influenza. J. A. M. A. *240*:242–243, 1978.
99. Glezen, W. P.: Consideration of the risk of influenza in children and indications for prophylaxis. Rev. Infect. Dis. *2*:408–420, 1980.
100. Glezen, W. P.: Serious morbidity and mortality associated with influenza epidemics. Epidemiol. Rev. *4*:25–44, 1982.
101. Glezen, W. P.: Viral pneumonia as a cause and result of hospitalization. J. Infect. Dis. *147*:765–770, 1983.
102. Glezen, W. P.: Reactive airway disorders in children: Role of respiratory viruses. Clin. Chest Med. *5*:635–643, 1984.
103. Glezen, W. P.: The pediatrician's role in influenza control. Pediatr. Infect. Dis. J. *5*:615–618, 1986.
104. Glezen, W. P.: Influenza surveillance in an urban area. Can. J. Infect. Dis. *4*:272–274, 1993.
105. Glezen, W. P., and Couch, R. B.: Interpandemic influenza in the Houston area, 1974–76. N. Engl. J. Med. *298*:587–592, 1978.
106. Glezen, W. P., and Couch, R. B.: Influenza viruses. *In* Evans, A. S. (ed.):

Viral Infections of Humans: Epidemiology and Control. 3rd ed. New York, Plenum Press, 1989, pp. 419–449.
107. Glezen, W. P., Couch, R. B., Taber, L. H., et al.: Epidemiologic observations of influenza B virus infections in Houston, Texas, 1976–1977. Am. J. Epidemiol. *111*:13–22, 1980.
108. Glezen, W. P., Decker, M., Joseph, S. W., et al.: Acute respiratory disease associated with influenza epidemics in Houston, 1982–1983. J. Infect. Dis. *155*:1119–1126, 1987.
109. Glezen, W. P., and Denny, F. W.: Epidemiology of acute lower respiratory disease in children. N. Engl. J. Med. *288*:498–505, 1973.
110. Glezen, W. P., Loda, F. A., Clyde, W. A., Jr., et al.: Epidemiologic patterns of acute lower respiratory disease of children in a pediatric group practice. J. Pediatr. *78*:397–406, 1971.
111. Glezen, W. P., Paredes, A., and Taber, L. H.: Influenza in children related to other respiratory agents. J. A. M. A. *243*:1345–1349, 1980.
112. Glezen, W. P., Payne, A. A., Synder, D. N., et al.: Mortality and influenza. J. Infect. Dis. *146*:313–321, 1982.
113. Glezen, W. P., Six, H. R., Perrotta, D. M., et al.: Epidemics and their causative viruses: Community experience. *In* Stuart-Harris, C. H., and Potter, C. W. (eds.): The Molecular Virology and Epidemiology of Influenza. London, Academic Press, 1984, pp. 17–38.
114. Greenberg, S. B., Criswell, B. S., and Couch, R. B.: Lymphocyte cytotoxicity to influenza virus–infected cells: Response to vaccination and virus infection. Infect. Immun. *20*:640–645, 1978.
115. Gross, P. A.: Reactogenicity and immunogenicity of bivalent influenza vaccine in one- and two-dose trials in children: A summary. J. Infect. Dis. *136*:S616–S625, 1977.
116. Gross, P. A., Quinnan, G. V., Gaerlaw, P. F., et al.: Influenza vaccines in children: Comparison of a new cetrimonium bromide and standard ether-treated vaccines. Am. J. Dis. Child. *137*:26–28, 1983.
117. Gruber, W. C., Taber, L. H., Glezen, W. P., et al.: Live attenuated and inactivated influenza vaccine in school-age children. Am. J. Dis. Child. *144*:595–600, 1990.
118. Hall, C. G., Dolin, R., Gala, C. L., et al.: Children with influenza A infection: Treatment with rimantadine. Pediatrics *80*:275–282, 1987.
119. Hall, C. B., and Douglas, R. G., Jr.: Nosocomial influenza infection as a cause of intercurrent fevers in infants. Pediatrics *55*:673–677, 1975.
120. Hall, C. B., and Douglas, R. S.: Respiratory syncytial virus and influenza: Practical community surveillance. Am. J. Dis. Child. *130*:615–620, 1976.
121. Hall, C. B., McBride, J. T., Walsh, E. E., et al.: Aerosolized ribavirin treatment of infants with respiratory syncytial viral infections. N. Engl. J. Med. *308*:1443–1447, 1983.
122. Hall, C. E., Cooney, M. K., and Fox, J. P.: The Seattle virus watch. IV. Comparative epidemiologic observations of infections with influenza A and B viruses, 1965–69, in families with young children. Am. J. Epidemiol. *98*:365–380, 1973.
123. Hall, W. J., Douglas, R. G., Jr., Hyde, R. W., et al.: Pulmonary mechanics during uncomplicated influenza A infection. Am. Rev. Respir. Dis. *113*:141–153, 1976.
124. Hall, W. N., Goodman, R. A., Noble, G. R., et al.: An outbreak of influenza B in an elderly population. J. Infect. Dis. *144*:297–302, 1981.
125. Halpin, T. J., Holtzhauer, F. J., Campbell, R. J., et al.: Reye's syndrome and medication use. J. A. M. A. *248*:687–691, 1982.
126. Halsey, N. A., Hurwitz, E. S., Meiklejohn, G., et al.: An epidemic of Reye syndrome associated with influenza A (H1N1) in Colorado. J. Pediatr. *97*:535–539, 1980.
127. Harley, M. J., and Guerier, T. H.: Orbital cellulitis related to an influenza A virus epidemic. Br. Med. J. *2*:13–14, 1978.
128. Harmon, M. W., and Pawlik, K. M.: Enzyme immunoassay for direct detection of influenza type A and adenovirus antigens in clinical specimens. J. Clin. Microbiol. *15*:5–11, 1982.
129. Hayden, F. G., Belshe, R. B., Clover, R. D., et al.: Emergence and apparent transmission of rimantadine-resistant influenza A virus in families. N. Engl. J. Med. *321*:1696–1702, 1989.
130. Henderson, F. W., Collier, A. M., Sanyal, M. A., et al.: A longitudinal study of respiratory viruses and bacteria in the etiology of acute otitis media with effusion. N. Engl. J. Med. *306*:1377–1383, 1982.
131. Hers, J. F. P.: Disturbances of the ciliated epithelium due to influenza virus. Am. Rev. Respir. Dis. *93*:162–171, 1966.
132. Hers, J. F. P., Masurel, N., and Mulder, J.: Bacteriology and histopathology of the respiratory tract and lungs in fatal Asian influenza. Lancet *2*:1141–1143, 1958.
133. Hirsch, A.: *In* Creighton, C. (ed.): Handbook of Geographical and Historical Pathology. Vol. 1. London, New Sydenham Society, 1883, pp. 7–17.
134. Hirst, G. K.: Genetic recombination with Newcastle disease virus, polioviruses, and influenza. Cold Spring Harbor Symp. Quant. Biol. *27*:303–308, 1962.
135. Hobson, D., Curry, R. L., Beare, A. S., et al.: The role of serum hemagglutination-inhibiting antibody in protection against challenge infection with influenza A2 and B viruses. J. Hyg. *70*:767–777, 1972.
136. Hoekstra, R. E., Herrmann, Jr., E. C., and O'Connell, E. J.: Virus infections in children. Clinical comparison of overlapping outbreaks of influenza A2/HongKong/68 and respiratory syncytial virus infections. Am. J. Dis. Child. *120*:14–16, 1970.
137. Holzel, A., Parker, L., Patterson, W. H., et al.: Virus isolations from throats of children admitted to hospital with respiratory and other diseases, Manchester 1962–4. Br. Med. J. *1*:614–619, 1965.
138. Horisberger, M. A.: The large P proteins of influenza A viruses are composed of one acidic and two basic polypeptides. Virology *107*:302–305, 1980.
139. Horn, M. E. C., Brain, E., Gregg, I., et al.: Respiratory viral infection in childhood: A survey in general practice, Roehampton 1967–1972. J. Hyg. (Camb.) *74*:157–168, 1975.
140. Housworth, W. J., and Langmuir, A. D.: Excess mortality from epidemic influenza, 1957–1966. Am. J. Epidemiol. *100*:40–48, 1974.
141. Howard, J. B., McCracken, G. H., and Luby, J. P.: Influenza A_2 virus as a cause of croup requiring tracheostomy. J. Pediatr. *81*:1148–1149, 1972.
142. Hurwitz, E. S., Barrett, M. J., and Bregnan, D.: Public Health Service study of Reye's syndrome and medication: Report of the main study. J. A. M. A. *257*:1905–1911, 1987.
143. Hurwitz, E. S., Nelson, D. B., Davis, C., et al.: National surveillance for Reye syndrome: A five year review. Pediatrics *70*:895–900, 1982.
144. Inglis, S. C., Carroll, A. R., Lamb, R. A., et al.: Polypeptides specified by the influenza virus genome. 1. Evidence for eight distinct gene products specified by fowl plague virus. Virology *74*:489–503, 1976.
145. Inglis, S. C., McGeoch, D. J., and Mahy, B. W. J.: Polypeptides specified by the influenza virus genome. 2. Assignment of protein coding functions to individual genome segments by in vitro translation. Virology *78*:522–536, 1977.
146. Jackson, G. G., Muldoon, R. L., and Ahern, L. W.: Serological evidence for prevention of influenzal infection in volunteers by an anti-influenzal drug: Amantadine hydrochloride. Antimicrob. Agents Chemother. *120*:703–707, 1963.
147. Jordan, W. S., Denny, F. W., Badger, G. F., et al.: A study of illness in a group of Cleveland families. XVII. The occurrence of Asian influenza. Am. J. Hyg. *68*:190–212, 1958.
148. Joshi, V. V., Escobar, M. R., Stewart, L., et al.: Fatal influenza A_2 viral pneumonia in a newborn infant. Am. J. Dis. Child. *126*:839–840, 1973.
149. Kaplan, J. E., Katona, P., Hurwitz, E. S., et al.: Guillain-Barré syndrome in the United States, 1979–80 and 1980–81: Lack of an association with influenza vaccination. J. A. M. A. *248*:698–700, 1982.
150. Kavet, J.: Influenza and public policy. Doctoral thesis, Harvard School of Public Health, Boston, 1973, p. 369.
151. Kempe, A., Hall, C. B., MacDonald, N. E., et al.: Influenza in children with cancer. J. Pediatr. *115*:33–39, 1989.
152. Kerr, A. A., Downham, M. A. P. S., McQuillin, J., et al.: Gastric flu: Influenza B causing abdominal symptoms in children. Lancet *1*:291–295, 1975.
153. Khamapirad, T., and Glezen, W. P.: Clinical and radiographic assessment of acute lower respiratory tract disease in infants and children. Semin. Respir. Infect. 2:130–144, 1987.
154. Kilbourne, E. D.: Influenza. New York, Plenum, 1987.
155. Kilbourne, E. D., Chanock, R. M., Choppin, P. W., et al.: Influenza vaccine: Summary of influenza workshop V. J. Infect. Dis. *129*:750–771, 1974.
156. Kim, H. W., Brandt, C. D., Arrobio, J. O., et al.: Virus infections in respiratory disease patients during 1974. Clin. Proc. Child. Hosp. Natl. Med. Cent. *32*:56–58, 1976.
157. Kim, H. W., Brandt, C. D., Arrobio, J. O., et al.: Influenza A and B virus infection in infants and young children during the years 1957–1976. Am. J. Epidemiol. *109*:464–479, 1979.
158. Kitamoto, O.: Therapeutic effectiveness of amantadine hydrochloride in influenza A2: Double blind studies. Jpn. J. Tuberc. Chest Dis. *15*:1–7, 1968.
159. Klein, J. D., Collier, A. M., and Glezen, W. P.: An influenza B epidemic among children in day care. Pediatrics *58*:340–345, 1976.
160. Klimek, J. J., Lindenberg, L. B., Cole, S., et al.: Fatal case of influenza pneumonia with suprainfection by multiple bacteria and herpes simplex virus. Am. Rev. Respir. Dis. *113*:683–688, 1976.
161. Knight, V.: Ribavirin aerosol treatment of influenza. *In* Leive, L., and Schlessinger, D. (eds.): Microbiology. Washington, D.C., American Society for Microbiology, 1984, pp. 416–417.
162. Knight, V., and Gilbert, B. E.: Ribavirin aerosol treatment of influenza. Infect. Dis. Clin. North Am. *1*:441–457, 1987.
163. Knight, V., and Kasel, J. A.: Influenza viruses. *In* Knight, V. (ed.): Viral and Mycoplasmal Infections of the Respiratory Tract. Philadelphia, Lea & Febiger, 1973, pp. 87–123.
164. Knight, V., McClung, H. W., Wilson, S. Z., et al.: Ribavirin small-particle aerosol treatment of influenza. Lancet *2*:945–949, 1981.
165. Krug, R. M.: Priming of influenza viral RNA transcription by capped heterologous RNAs. Curr. Top. Microbiol. Immunol. *93*:125–150, 1981.
166. Langmuir, A. D., and Housworth, J.: A critical evaluation of influenza surveillance. Bull. W. H. O. *41*:393–398, 1969.
167. Laraya-Cuasay, L. R., DeForest, A., Huff, D., et al.: Chronic pulmonary complications of early influenza virus infection in children. Am. Rev. Respir. Dis. *116*:617–625, 1977.
168. Laver, W. G., and Webster, R. G.: Selection of antigenic mutants of influenza viruses: Isolation and peptide mapping of their hemagglutinating proteins. Virology *34*:193–202, 1968.
169. Laver, W. G., and Webster, R. G.: Studies on the origin of pandemic influenza. II. Peptide maps of the light and heavy polypeptide chains from the hemagglutinin subunits of A2 influenza viruses isolated before

and after the appearance of Hong Kong influenza. Virology *48*:445–455, 1972.

170. Laver, W. G., and Webster, R. G.: Studies on the origin of pandemic influenza. III. Evidence implicating duck and equine influenza viruses as possible progenitors of the Hong Kong strain of human influenza. Virology *51*:383–391, 1973.
171. Laver, W. G., and Webster, R. G.: Preparation and immunogenicity of an influenza virus hemagglutinin and neuraminidase subunit vaccine. Virology *69*:511–522, 1976.
172. Linnemann, C. C., Shea, L., Kauffman, C. A., et al.: Association of Reye's syndrome with viral infection. Lancet *2*:179–182, 1974.
173. Little, J. W., Hall, W. J., Douglas, R. G., Jr., et al.: Airway hyperreactivity and peripheral airway dysfunction in influenza A infection. Am. Rev. Respir. Dis. *118*:295–303, 1978.
174. Liu, C.: Diagnosis of influenzal infection by means of fluorescent antibody staining. International Conference on Asian Influenza. Am. Rev. Respir. Dis. *83*(Suppl.):130–138, 1960.
175. Liu, K. J., and Kendal, A. P.: Impact of influenza epidemics on mortality in the United States from October 1972 to May 1985. Am. J. Public Health *77*:712–716, 1987.
176. Loda, F. A., Clyde, W. A., Jr., Glezen, W. P., et al.: Studies on the role of viruses, bacteria, and *M. pneumoniae* as causes of lower respiratory tract infections in children. J. Pediatr. *72*:161–176, 1968.
177. Loda, F. A., Glezen, W. P., and Clyde, W. A., Jr.: Respiratory disease in group day care. Pediatrics *49*:428–437, 1972.
178. Longini, I. M., Koopman, J. S., Monto, A. S., et al.: Estimating household and community transmission parameters for influenza. Am. J. Epidemiol. *115*:736–751, 1982.
179. Loosli, C. G.: Influenza and the interaction of viruses and bacteria in respiratory infections. Medicine *52*:369–384, 1973.
180. Louria, D. B., Blumenfeld, H. L., Ellis, J. T., et al.: Studies on influenza in the pandemic of 1957–58. II. Pulmonary complications of influenza. J. Clin. Invest. *38*:213–265, 1959.
181. Lubkiewicz, K., Elie, K., Spence, L., et al.: Laboratory and clinical features of influenza A2 1971–72 in Montreal. Chest *66*:671–674, 1974.
182. Macasaet, F. F., Kidd, P. A., Bolano, C. R., et al.: The etiology of acute respiratory infections. III. The role of viruses and bacteria. J. Pediatr. *72*:829–839, 1968.
183. MacKenzie, J. S., and Houghton, M.: Influenza infections during pregnancy: Association with congenital malformations and with subsequent neoplasms in children, and potential hazards of live virus vaccines. Bacteriol. Rev. *38*:356–370, 1974.
184. Mackowiak, P. A., and Smith, J. W.: Septicemic melioidosis: Occurrence following acute influenza A six years after exposure in Vietnam. J. A. M. A. *240*:764–766, 1978.
185. Maito, M., Soto, T., and Ischida, N.: Antigenic memory in man in response to sequential infections with influenza A viruses. J. Infect. Dis. *126*:61–68, 1972.
186. Maletzky, A. J., Cooney, M. K., Luce, R., et al.: Epidemiology of viral and mycoplasmal agents associated with childhood lower respiratory illness in a civilian population. J. Pediatr. *78*:407–414, 1971.
187. Marine, W. M., and Stuart-Harris, C.: Reactions and serologic responses in young children and infants after administration of inactivated monovalent influenza A vaccine. J. Pediatr. *88*:26–30, 1976.
188. Masurel, N., and Marine, W. M.: Recycling of Asian and Hong Kong influenza A virus hemagglutinins in man. Am. J. Epidemiol. *97*:44–49, 1973.
189. McClung, H. W., Knight, V., Gilbert, B. E., et al.: Ribavirin aerosol treatment of influenza virus B infection. J. A. M. A. *249*:2671–2674, 1983.
190. McIntosh, K., Ellis, E. F., Hoffman, L. S., et al.: The association of viral and bacterial respiratory infections with exacerbations of wheezing in young asthmatic children. J. Pediatr. *82*:578–590, 1974.
191. McIntosh, K., Kurachek, S. C., Cairns, L. M., et al.: Treatment of respiratory syncytial viral infection in an immunodeficient infant with ribavirin aerosol. Am. J. Dis. Child. *138*:305–308, 1984.
192. Meibalane, R., Sedinak, G. V., Sasidharan, P., et al.: Outbreak of influenza in a neonatal intensive care unit. J. Pediatr. *91*:974–976, 1977.
193. Mellman, W. J.: Influenza encephalitis. J. Pediatr. *53*:292, 1958.
194. Meyer, H. M., Hopps, H. E., Parkman, P. D., et al.: Review of existing vaccines for influenza. Am. J. Clin. Pathol. *70*:146–151, 1978.
195. Middleton, P. J., Alexander, R. M., and Szymonski, M. T.: Severe myositis during recovery from influenza. Lancet *2*:533–535, 1970.
196. Minor, T. E., Dick, E. C., Baker, J. W., et al.: Rhinovirus and influenza type A infections as precipitants of asthma. Am. Rev. Respir. Dis. *113*:149–153, 1976.
197. Minor, T. E., Dick, E. C., DeMeo, A. N., et al.: Virus as precipitants of asthmatic attacks in children. J. A. M. A. *227*:292–298, 1974.
198. Minow, R. A., Gorbach, S., Johnson, B. L., et al.: Myoglobinuria associated with influenza A infection. Ann. Intern. Med. *80*:359–361, 1974.
199. Moffet, H. L., Cramblett, H. G., and Dobbins, J.: Outbreak of influenza A2 among immunized children. J. A. M. A. *190*:806–810, 1964.
200. Moffet, H. L., Cramblett, H. G., Middleton, Jr., G. K., et al.: Outbreak of influenza B in a children's home. J. A. M. A. *182*:834–838, 1962.
201. Mogabgab, W. J.: The complications of influenza. Med. Clin. North Am. *47*:1191–1199, 1963.
202. Monto, A. S., Davenport, F. M., Napier, S. A., et al.: Effect of vaccination of a school age population upon the course of an A2/Hong Kong influenza epidemic. Bull. W. H. O. *41*:537–542, 1969.
203. Moore, G.: Influenza and Parkinson's disease. Public Health Rep. *92*:79–80, 1977.
204. Morgensen, J. L.: Myoglobinuria and renal failure associated with influenza. Ann. Intern. Med. *80*:362–363, 1974.
205. Mostow, S. R., Schild, G. C., Dowdle, W. R., et al.: Applications of the single-radial-diffusion test for the assay of influenza type A viruses. J. Clin. Microbiol. *2*:531–540, 1975.
206. Mostow, S. R., Schoenbaum, S. C., Dowdle, W. R., et al.: Studies with inactivated influenza vaccine purified by zonal ultracentrifugation. I. Adverse reactions and serological responses. Bull. W. H. O. *41*:525–530, 1969.
207. Mufson, M. A., Krause, H. E., Mocega, H. E., et al.: Viruses, *Mycoplasma pneumoniae* and bacteria associated with lower respiratory tract disease among infants. Am. J. Epidemiol. *91*:192–202, 1970.
208. Mulder, J., and Hers, J. F. P.: Influenza. Leiden, The Netherlands, Walters-Noordhoff, International School Book Service, 1972.
209. Murphy, B. R., Chalhub, E. G., Nusinoff, S. R., et al.: Temperature-sensitive mutants of influenza virus. II. Attenuation of its recombinants for man. J. Infect. Dis. *126*:170–178, 1972.
210. Murphy, B. R., Chalhub, E. G., Nusinoff, S. R., et al.: Temperature-sensitive mutants of influenza virus. III. Further characterization of the ts-1 (E) influenza A recombinant (H3N2) virus in man. J. Infect. Dis. *128*:479–487, 1973.
211. Murphy, B. R., Kasel, J. A., and Chanock, R. M.: Association of serum antineuraminidase antibody with resistance to influenza in man. N. Engl. J. Med. *286*:1329–1332, 1972.
212. Murphy, B. R., Rennels, M. B., Douglas, R. G., Jr., et al.: Evaluation of influenza A/Hong Kong/123/77 (H1N1) ts-1A2 and cold-adapted recombinant viruses in sero-negative adult volunteers. Infect. Immun. *29*:348–355, 1980.
213. Murphy, B. R., Phelan, M. A., Nelson, D. L., et al.: Hemagglutinin-specific enzyme-linked immunosorbent assay for antibodies to influenza A and B viruses. J. Clin. Microbiol. *13*:554–560, 1981.
214. Murphy, B. R., Clements, M. L., Madore, H. P., et al.: Dose response of cold-adapted, reassortant influenza A/California/10/78 virus. J. Infect. Dis. *149*:816, 1984.
215. Nakajima, K., Desselberger, U., and Palese, P.: Recent human influenza A (H1N1) viruses are closely related genetically to strains isolated in 1950. Nature *274*:334–339, 1978.
216. Nichol, K. P., and Cherry, J. D.: Bacterial-viral interrelations in respiratory infections of children. N. Engl. J. Med. *277*:667–672, 1967.
217. Ogra, P. L., Chow, T., Beutner, K. R., et al.: Clinical and immunologic evaluation of neuraminidase-specific influenza A virus vaccine in humans. J. Infect. Dis. *135*:499–506, 1977.
218. Olding-Stenkvist, E., and Grandhen, M.: Rapid diagnosis of influenza A infection by immunofluorescence. Acta Pathol. Microbiol. Scand. [B] *85*:296–302, 1977.
219. Oseasohn, R., Adelson, L., and Kaji, M.: Clinicopathologic study of thirty-three fatal cases of Asian influenza. N. Engl. J. Med. *260*:509–518, 1959.
220. Paisley, J. W., Bruker, F. W., Laner, B. A., et al.: Type A2 influenza viral infections in children. Am. J. Dis. Child. *132*:34–36, 1978.
221. Palese, P., Ritchey, M. B., Schulman, J. L., et al.: Genetic composition of a high-yielding influenza virus recombinant: A vaccine strain against "swine" influenza. Science *194*:334–335, 1976.
222. Palese, P., and Schulman, J. L.: RNA pattern of "swine" influenza virus isolated from man is similar to those of other swine influenza viruses. Nature *263*:528–530, 1976.
223. Parrott, R. H., Kim, H. W., Vargosko, A. J., et al.: Serious respiratory tract illness as a result of Asian influenza and influenza B infections in children. J. Pediatr. *61*:205–213, 1962.
224. Parrott, R. H.: Viral respiratory tract illnesses in children. Bull. W. H. O. *39*:629–648, 1963.
225. Partin, J. C., Schubert, J. C., Partin, J. S., et al.: Isolation of influenza virus from liver and muscle biopsy specimens from a surviving case of Reye's syndrome. Lancet *2*:599–602, 1976.
226. Payler, D. K., and Purdham, P. A.: Influenza A prophylaxis with amantadine in a boarding school. Lancet *1*:502–504, 1984.
227. Penn, C. R., Blaas, D., Kuechler, E., et al.: Identification of the cap-binding protein of two strains of influenza A/FPV. J. Gen. Virol. *62*:177–180, 1982.
228. Perrotta, D. M., Decker, M., and Glezen, W. P.: Acute respiratory disease hospitalizations as a measure of impact of epidemic influenza. Am. J. Epidemiol. *122*:468–476, 1985.
229. Pickles, W. N., Burnet, F. M., and McArthur, M.: Epidemic respiratory infection in a rural population with special reference to the influenza A epidemics of 1933, 1936–37, and 1943–44. J. Hyg. *45*:469–473, 1947.
230. Piedra, P. A., and Glezen, W. P.: Influenza in children: Epidemiology, immunity, and vaccines. Semin. Pediatr. Infect. Dis. *2*:140–146, 1991.
231. Podosin, R. L., and Felton, W. L.: The clinical picture of Far East influenza occurring at the fourth National Boy Scout Jamboree. N. Engl. J. Med. *258*:778–782, 1958.
232. Poland, J. D., Welton, E. R., and Chin, T. D. Y.: Influenza virus B as cause of acute croup syndrome. Am. J. Dis. Child. *107*:54–57, 1964.

233. Pons, U. W., and Hirst, G. K.: Polyacrylamide gel electrophoresis of influenza virus RNA. Virology *34*:385–388, 1968.
234. Price, D. A., Postlethwaite, R. J., and Longson, M.: Influenza virus A2 infections presenting with febrile convulsions and gastrointestinal symptoms in young children. Clin. Pediatr. *15*:361–367, 1976.
235. Pryor, H. B.: Influenza: That extraordinary malady: Notes on its history and epidemiology. Clin. Pediatr. *3*:19–24, 1964.
236. Pyrhönen, S., Suni, J., and Romo, M.: Clinical trial of a subunit influenza vaccine. Scand. J. Infect. Dis. *13*:95–99, 1981.
237. Quilligan, J. J., Hirayama, M., and Bernstein, H. D.: The suppression of A2 influenza in children by the chemoprophylactic use of amantadine. J. Pediatr. *69*:572–575, 1966.
238. Rebhan, A. W.: An outbreak of Asian influenza in a girl's camp. Can. Med. Assoc. J. *77*:797–799, 1957.
239. Reye, R. D. K., Morgan, G., and Baral, J.: Encephalopathy and fatty degeneration of the viscera. A disease entity in childhood. Lancet *1*:749–752, 1963.
240. Ritchey, M. B., Palese, P., and Schulman, J. L.: Mapping of the influenza virus genome. III. Identification of genes coding for nucleoprotein, membrane protein, and nonstructural protein. J. Virol. *20*:307–313, 1976.
241. Robinson, R. Q., and Dowdle, W. R.: Influenza viruses. *In* Lennette, E. H., and Schmidt, N. J. (eds.): Diagnostic Procedures for Viral and Rickettsial Infections. New York, American Public Health Association, 1969, pp. 414–433.
242. Roldaan, A. C., and Masurel, N.: Viral respiratory infections in asthmatic children staying in a mountain resort. Eur. J. Respir. Dis. *63*:140–150, 1982.
243. Rose, H. J.: The use of amantadine and influenza vaccine in a type A influenza epidemic in a boarding school. J. R. Coll. Gen. Pract. *30*:619–621, 1980.
244. Rose, H. J.: Use of amantadine in influenza: A second report. J. R. Coll. Gen. Pract. *33*:651–653, 1983.
245. Rubin, D. M., and Hendy, V.: Swine influenza and the news media. Ann. Intern. Med. *87*:769–774, 1977.
246. Salk, J. E., and Salk, D.: Control of influenza and poliomyelitis with killed virus vaccines. Science *195*:834–847, 1977.
247. Sanders, D. Y., Carroll, N. B., Jeffreys, L. U., et al.: Outbreak of influenza A2 (Hong Kong strain) in a children's home. South. Med. J. *63*:414–416, 1970.
248. Sarkkinen, H. K., Halonen, P. E., and Salmi, A. A.: Detection of influenza A virus by radioimmunoassay and enzyme-immunoassay from nasopharyngeal specimens. J. Med. Virol. *7*:213–220, 1981.
249. Schambelan, M., and Sussman, S.: Encephalitis and purpura with influenza infection. Am. J. Dis. Child. *111*:302–303, 1966.
250. Schmidt, J. P., Metcalf, T. G., and Miltenberger, F. W.: An epidemic of Asian influenza in children at Ladd Air Force Base, Alaska, 1960. J. Pediatr. *61*:214–220, 1962.
251. Schneider, R. M., Nevins, D. B., and Brown, H. Z.: Desquamative interstitial pneumonia in a four year old child. N. Engl. J. Med. *277*:1056–1058, 1967.
252. Schonberger, L. B., Bregman, D. J., Sullivan-Bolyai, J. Z., et al.: Guillain-Barré syndrome following vaccination in the national influenza immunization program, United States, 1976–1977. Am. J. Epidemiol. *110*:105–123, 1979.
253. Schonberger, L. B., Hurwitz, E. S., Katona, P., et al.: Guillain-Barré syndrome: Its epidemiology and associations with influenza vaccination. Ann. Neurol. *9*(Suppl.):31–38, 1981.
254. Schulman, J. L., Petigrow, C., and Woodruff, J.: Effects of cell-mediated immunity in influenza virus infection in mice. Dev. Biol. Stand. *39*:385–395, 1977.
255. Schultz, I., Gundelfinger, B., Rosenbaum, M., et al.: Comparison of clinical manifestations of respiratory illness due to Asian strain influenza, adenovirus, and unknown cause. J. Lab. Clin. Med. *55*:497–509, 1960.
256. Schulze, I. T.: The structure of influenza virus. II. A model based on the morphology and composition of subviral particles. Virology *47*:181–196, 1972.
257. Schwarzmann, S. W., Adler, J. L., Sullivan, R. L., Jr., et al.: Bacterial pneumonia during the Hong Kong influenza epidemic of 1968–69. Arch. Intern. Med. *127*:1037–1041, 1971.
258. Shope, R. E.: The incidence of neutralizing antibodies for swine influenza virus in the sera of human beings of different ages. J. Exp. Med. *63*:669–684, 1936.
259. Sinclair, D. J., Stuart, F. G., and Ritchie, G. W.: Pulmonary complications of influenza: A radiological review of 30 cases. Can. Med. Assoc. J. *101*:780–784, 1969.
260. Six, H. R., Glezen, W. P., Kasel, J. A., et al.: Heterogeneity of influenza viruses isolated from the Houston community during defined epidemic periods. *In* Nayack, D., and Cox, C. F. (eds.): Genetic Variation among Influenza Viruses. New York, Academic Press, 1981, pp. 505–513.
261. Smith, W., Andrewes, C. H., and Laidlaw, P. P.: A virus obtained from influenza patients. Lancet *2*:66–68, 1933.
262. Smorodintsev, A. A.: The efficacy of live influenza vaccines. Bull. W. H. O. *41*:585–588, 1969.
263. Smorodintsev, A. A., Zlydnikov, D. M., Kiseleva, A. M., et al.: Evaluation of amantadine in artificially induced A2 and B influenza. J. A. M. A. *213*:1448–1454, 1970.
264. Spencer, M. J., Cherry, J. D., Powell, K. R., et al.: Clinical trials with "Alice" strain, live attenuated serum inhibitor-resistant intranasal influenza A vaccine. J. Infect. Dis. *132*:415–420, 1975.
265. Starko, K. M., Ray, C.G., Dominguez, L. B., et al.: Reye's syndrome and salicylate use. Pediatrics *66*:859–864, 1980.
266. Stuart-Harris, C. H.: The complications of influenza. Postgrad. Med. J. *39*:578–581, 1963.
267. Stuart-Harris, C. H.: Influenza and its complications. Br. Med. J. *1*:149–150, 1966.
268. Stuart-Harris, C. H., and Schild, G. L.: Influenza: The Viruses and the Disease. London, Arnold, 1976.
269. Sugrue, R. J., and Hay, A. J.: Structural characteristics of the M2 protein of influenza A viruses: Evidence that it forms a tetrameric channel. Virology *180*:617–624, 1991.
270. Sullivan-Bolyai, J. Z., Mark, J., Johnson, D., et al.: Reye syndrome in Ohio 1973–77. Am. J. Epidemiol. *112*:629, 1980.
271. Sutton, R. N. P., and Emery, J. L.: Sudden death in infancy: A microbiological and epidemiological study. Arch. Dis. Child. *41*:674–677, 1966.
272. Taber, L. H., Paredes, A., Glezen, W. P., et al.: Infection with influenza A/Victoria virus in Houston families, 1976. J. Hyg. (Lond.) *86*:303–313, 1981.
273. Taber, L. H., Knight, V., Gilbert, B. E., et al.: Ribavirin aerosol treatment of bronchiolitis associated with respiratory syncytial virus infection in infants. Pediatrics *72*:613–618, 1983.
274. Thomson, D.: Influenza (Part I): With special reference to the part played by Pfeiffer's bacillus, streptococci, pneumococci, etc. and the virus theory. Ann. Picket-Thomson Res. Lab. *9*:1–42, 1933.
275. Troendle, J. F., Demmler, G. J., Glezen, W. P., et al.: Fatal influenza B virus pneumonia in pediatric patients. Pediatr. Infect. Dis. J. *11*:117–121, 1992.
276. Ulmanen, I., Broni, B. A., and Krug, R. M.: Role of two of the influenza virus core P proteins in recognizing cap 1 structure (m^7GpppNm) on RNAs and in initiating viral RNA transcription. Proc. Natl. Acad. Sci. U. S. A. *78*:7355–7359, 1981.
277. Vargosko, A. J., Chanock, R. M., Huebner, R. J., et al.: Association of type 2 hemadsorption (parainfluenza 1) virus and Asian influenza A virus with infectious croup. N. Engl. J. Med. *261*:1–10, 1959.
278. Virelizier, J. L., Allison, A. C., and Schild, G. C.: Antibody responses to antigenic determinants of influenza virus hemagglutinin. II. Original antigenic sin is a bone marrow–derived lymphocyte memory phenomenon modulated by thymus-derived lymphocytes. J. Exp. Med. *140*:1571–1578, 1974.
279. Virelizier, J. L., Postlethwaite, R., Schild, G. C., et al.: Antibody responses to antigenic determinants of influenza virus hemagglutinin. I. Thymus dependence of antibody formation and thymus independence of immunologic memory. J. Exp. Med. *140*:1559–1570, 1974.
280. Waldman, R. H., Gadal, N., Olsen, G. N., et al.: Respiratory tract cell-mediated immunity to influenza. Symp. Ser. Immunobiol. Stand. *20*:222–231, 1973.
281. Waldman, R. J., Hall, W. N., McGee, H., et al.: Aspirin as a risk factor in Reye's syndrome. J. A. M. A. *247*:3089–3094, 1982.
282. Walsh, J. J., Dietlein, L. F., Low, F. N., et al.: Bronchotracheal response in human influenza. Arch. Intern. Med. *108*:376–388, 1961.
283. Waner, J. L., Todd, S. J., Shalaby, H., et al.: Comparison of Directogen FLU-A with viral isolation and direct immunofluorescence for the rapid detection and identification of influenza A virus. J. Clin. Microbiol. *29*:479–482, 1991.
284. Webster, R. G., Campbell, C. H., and Granoff, A.: The "in vivo" production of "new" influenza viruses. III. Isolation of recombinant influenza viruses under simulated conditions of natural transmission. Virology *51*:149–162, 1973.
285. Wells, C. E. C., James, W. K. L., and Evans, A. D.: Guillain-Barré syndrome and virus of influenza A (Asian strain). Arch. Neurol. Psychiatr. *81*:699–705, 1959.
286. Whitaker, A. N., and Bunce, I.: Disseminated intravascular coagulation and acute renal failure in influenza A2 infection. Med. J. Aust. *2*:196–201, 1974.
287. Williams, S. W.: Prevention and treatment of respiratory viral infections in children. Del. Med. J. *1*:315, 1971.
288. Wilson, C. B., and Smith, R. C.: Goodpasture's syndrome associated with influenza A2 virus infection. Ann. Intern. Med. *76*:91–94, 1972.
289. Wilson, M. G., and Stein, A. M.: Teratogenic effects of Asian influenza. An extended study. J. A. M. A. *210*:336–337, 1969.
290. Wilson, R., Miller, J., Greene, H., et al.: Reye's syndrome in three siblings. Am. J. Dis. Child. *134*:1032–1034, 1980.
291. Wilson, S. Z., Gilbert, B. E., Quarles, J. M., et al.: Treatment of influenza A (H1N1) virus infection with ribavirin aerosol. Antimicrob. Agents Chemother. *26*:200–203, 1984.
292. Woodhour, A. F., Friedman, A., Weibel, R. E., et al.: Clinical and laboratory studies of improved adjuvant 65 influenza vaccines. Symp. Ser. Immunobiol. Stand. *20*:125–132, 1972.
293. World Health Organization: Influenza nomenclature. W. H. O. Weekly Epidemiol. Rec. *54*:294–295, 1980.
294. Wright, P. F., Rose, K. B., Thompson, J., et al.: Influenza A infections in young children: Primary natural infection and protective efficacy of live-vaccine-induced or naturally acquired immunity. N. Engl. J. Med. *296*:829–834, 1977.

295. Wright, P. F., Sell, S. H. W., Thompson, J., et al.: Clinical reactions and serologic response following inactivated monovalent influenza type B vaccine in young children and infants. J. Pediatr. *88*:31–35, 1976.
296. Wright, P. F., Khaw, K. T., Oxman, M. N., et al.: Evaluation of the safety of amantadine-HCI and the rate of respiratory viral infections in children with cystic fibrosis. J. Infect. Dis. *134*:144–149, 1976.
297. Wright, P. F., Thompson, J., Vaughn, W. K., et al.: Trials of influenza A/New Jersey/76 virus vaccine in normal children: An overview of age-related antigenicity and reactogenicity. J. Infect. Dis. *136*:S731–S741, 1977.
298. Wright, P. F., Okabe, N., Mckee, K. T., Jr., et al.: Cold-adapted recombinant influenza A virus vaccines in seronegative young children. J. Infect. Dis. *146*:71–79, 1982.
299. Wright, P. F., Cherry, J. D., Foy, H. M., et al.: Antigenicity and reactogenicity of influenza A/USSR/77 virus vaccine in children: A multicentered evaluation of dosage and safety. Rev. Infect. Dis. *5*:758–764, 1983.
300. Wrigley, N. G.: Electron microscopy of influenza virus. Br. Med. Bull. *35*:35–38, 1979.
301. Wulff, H., Kidd, P., and Wenner, H. A.: Etiology of respiratory infections: Further studies during infancy and childhood. Pediatrics *33*:30–44, 1964.
302. Yawn, D. H., Pyeatte, J. C., Joseph, M., et al.: Transplacental transfer of influenza virus. J. A. M. A. *216*:1022–1023, 1971.
303. Yodfat, Y., and Nishmi, M.: Epidemiologic and clinical observations in six outbreaks of viral disease in a kibbutz, 1968–1971. Am. J. Epidemiol. *97*:415–423, 1973.
304. Young, R. S., Torretti, D., Williams, R. H., et al.: Reye's syndrome associated with long-term aspirin therapy. J. A. M. A. *251*:754–756, 1984.
305. Zahradnik, J. M., Kasel, J. A., Martin, R. R., et al.: Immune responses in serum and respiratory secretions following vaccination with a live cold-recombinant (CR35) and inactivated A/USSR/77 (H1N1) influenza virus vaccine. J. Med. Virol. *11*:277–285, 1983.
306. Zamkoff, K., and Rosen, N.: Influenza and myoglobinuria in brothers. Neurology *29*:340–345, 1979.
307. Zhdanov, V. M., Lvov, D. K., Zakstelskaya, L. Y., et al.: Return of epidemic A1 (H1N1) influenza virus. Lancet *1*:294–295, 1978.
308. Zinserling, A.: Peculiarities of lesions in viral and mycoplasma infections of the respiratory tract. Virchows Arch. (Pathol. Anat.) *356*:259–273, 1972.
309. Zwernick, H. S., Courtneidge, S. A., Skekel, J. J., et al.: Cytotoxic T cells kill influenza virus infected cells but do not distinguish between serologically distinct type A viruses. Nature *267*:354–356, 1977.

❑ ❑ ❑

SUBSECTION SEVEN

PARAMYXOVIRIDAE

182

PARAINFLUENZA VIRUSES

Caroline Breese Hall

Physical ills are the taxes laid upon this wretched life; some are taxed higher, and some lower, but all pay something.

Philip Stanhope, Lord Chesterfield
Letter to the Bishop of Waterford, 1757

The parainfluenza viruses (PIVs) are ubiquitous agents with well-earned recognition as being among the most important viral respiratory pathogens of humans. They are capable of causing upper respiratory tract infections at all ages and are major contributors, subordinate only to respiratory syncytial virus, to the sizable morbidity caused by acute lower respiratory tract disease in infants and young children. Among the agents of acute laryngotracheobronchitis, the PIVs are second to none. The frequently epidemic nature of PIVs types 1 and 2, the prolonged seasonal occurrence of type 3, and the ability of all types to cause repeated infections indicate why their import has not been diminished despite the technologic advances available toward control of viral diseases.

HISTORY

The historical delineation of the parainfluenza viral family is intertwined with the discovery of the related animal viruses and marked by the colorful names descriptive of their origin (Table 182–1). The first strain of PIV was discovered in Japan and named Sendai, or the hemagglutinating virus of Japan (HVJ).[115] This agent was recovered from mice that had been inoculated with postmortem lung tissue of infants with pneumonia. The first PIV from human sources was recovered several years later by Chanock from infants with croup and thus became known as the "croup-associated (CA) virus."[21] Subsequently, three additional PIVs that were distinct antigenically were isolated from children with acute respiratory illness.[25, 102] In contrast to the CA virus, which was recognized by its ability to produce syncytia in tissue culture, the strains of the next two types of PIVs produced little or no cytopathic effect but were recognized by their ability to cause hemadsorption of guinea pig erythrocytes to infected tissue culture. These viruses thus were called "hemadsorption type 1 (HA-1)" and "hemadsorption type 2 (HA-2) viruses."

Once the familial characteristics of the CA virus with the other three viruses were recognized, they were renamed as the PIVs: type 1 (HA-2), type 2 (CA), and type 3 (HA-1).[5] The fourth human PIV, discovered subsequent to this reclassification, is without a sobriquet and simply is termed "PIV-4," with two subtypes, A and B. The first type 4 strain was recovered in monkey kidney cell culture from a college student afflicted with a common cold.[102]

Several animal species appear to be natural hosts to the PIVs (see Table 182–1), with the exception of PIV-4, which has been found only in humans. In animals, PIVs may be important pathogens. Bovine PIV, similar to human PIV-3, often in combination with infection by *Pasteurella* organisms, causes the illness of considerable morbidity and cost in cattle called "shipping fever."[1] Naturally acquired antibodies to the PIVs are found not only in cows but also in rodents, monkeys, rabbits, and other mammals. A variety of rodents, along with ferrets, dogs, and lambs, have been used for experimental infection.

CHARACTERIZATION OF THE VIRUSES

Classification

Human PIVs belong to the genus *Paramyxovirus* and to the *Paramyxoviridae* family. They are distinct from the orthomyxo-

TABLE 182–1. Parainfluenza Viruses

Parainfluenza Virus Type/ Related Animal Virus	Natural Host	Experimental Infection	Preferred Tissue Culture for Initial Isolation	Cytopathic Effect: *Initial Isolation*	Cytopathic Effect: *Passage*
Parainfluenza type 1, hemadsorption type 2 (HA-2)	Human, guinea pig, rabbit, monkey, marmoset	Hamster, ferret	Primary monkey kidney, LLC human diploid, human embryonic kidney	+ –	Rounding, cell destruction
Sendai, hemagglutinating virus of Japan (HVJ)	Mouse, pig				
Parainfluenza type 2	Human, monkey, rabbit, guinea pig	Hamster, dog	Primary monkey kidney, human embryonic kidney	+ (Syncytial on monkey and human cells)	Syncytial, "Swiss cheese"
Simian virus 5 (SV 5)	Monkey				
Simian virus 41 (SV 41)	Monkey				
Parainfluenza type 3, hemadsorption type 1 (HA-1)	Human, guinea pig, monkey	Hamster, ferret, cotton rat, mouse, lamb	Primary monkey kidney, human embryonic kidney, LLC	±	In monkey cells—elongated, detachment of cell sheet In human cells—syncytial
Shipping fever (SF-4)	Cow				
Parainfluenza type 4	Human	Hamster, guinea pig	Primary monkey kidney	±	Rounding, granular, vacuolated

viruses in size, nucleocapsid structure (nonsegmented), antigenic composition, and laboratory growth characteristics.

Composition and Properties

Human PIVs are single, negative-stranded RNA viruses appearing as pleomorphic enveloped particles with an average diameter of 150 to 300 nm.[23, 111] The genome of all the human PIVs, which consists of an average of 15,000 nucleotides, codes for at least six structural proteins (Fig. 182–1). Enclosed within the spherical virion is the helical nucleocapsid with its herringbone core tightly wrapped by the nucleocapsid protein (NP). This is surrounded by the host-cell–derived lipid envelope, which is studded with spikes of surface glycoproteins, the hemagglutinin-neuraminidase

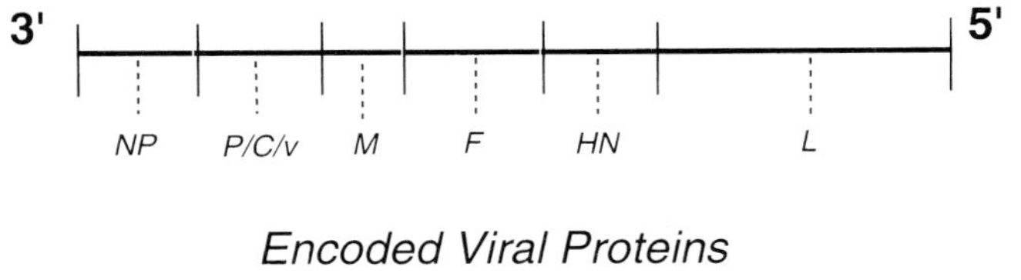

FIGURE 182–1. *Schematic representation of the genomic RNA structure of PIV-3.*[80] *NP, nucleocapsid protein; P, phosphoprotein; C, nonstructural protein (not contained in virion but found in infected cells); v, nonstructural protein encoded by human PIV-2; M, matrix protein; F, fusion protein; HN, hemagglutinin-neuraminidase protein; L, large protein.*

(HN) and fusion (F) proteins. The large (L) protein and phosphoprotein (P) also form clusters within the nucleocapsid structure. The sixth structural protein is the matrix (M) protein, which facilitates the interaction between the nucleocapsid and the surface glycoprotein by the attachment and insertion of the surface glycoproteins to the host cell and recruitment of the completed nucleocapsid to the budding sites of new virions. The NP appears to function along with P and L protein in the replication of the human PIV genome. The NP forms the template for the transcription of the messenger RNA by the L protein (RNA polymerase) and P. The HN protein mediates the attachment of the virus to the host cell and also is necessary for complete fusion with the host cell.[44] The HN protein is a dimer of two polypeptide portions held together by a disulfide link in the hydrophilic region and at the bases by hydrophobic bonds. Neuraminidase activity also is located on the HN protein but at a different site than the hemagglutination activity.[139, 196]

The F protein effects the entry of virus by fusing the host and viral cellular membranes. Once adsorption of the virus occurs, the F protein precursor, FO, is cleaved by host proteases into the active F1 and F2 protein fragments, which mediate penetration of the virus into the cell, with subsequent fusion of the viral and cell membranes and hemolysis. Sequences of oligopeptides that mimic the N-terminus of the F1 protein have been shown to inhibit the penetration of the virus and membrane fusion.[29, 156] The amino terminus of the F1 protein subunit appears to be conserved highly for the first 25 amino acids among the PIVs.[166] A nonstructural protein (C protein), found in infected cells, is encoded by the human PIVs-1, -2, and -3 genomes, and a "v" protein is encoded by the human PIV-2 genome.

The PIVs replicate in the cytoplasm of the host cells. The crop of completed virions is released from the cell surface by evagination of the plasma membrane. The buds contain the surface glycoproteins, allowing the characteristic hemadsorption of red blood cells observed in infected tissue.

Human PIVs share common antigens but also may be differentiated into two antigenic groups, with human PIV-1 and human PIV-3 in one group and human PIV-2, human PIV-4, and mumps virus in the other.[83, 172] Their common antigenicity is illustrated by the heterotypic antibody responses to infection with human PIV-1, -2, and -3 and mumps virus.[140] Although the human PIVs do not undergo the major antigenic alterations in their surface antigens similar to influenza virus, genetic and antigenic variations within all four types have been detected, and their evolution can be determined by analysis of strains obtained over time.[32, 83, 85, 113, 150, 172, 197]

The PIVs are inactivated rapidly by acid at a pH of 3.0 and by exposure to lipid solvents, such as ether or chloroform, which destroy the envelope of the virus. They also are relatively labile to temperatures higher than 37° C.[40, 42] Media containing protein, however, tend to protect against loss of infectivity when the virus is exposed to heat and when frozen at −70° C.[40, 93]

Isolation and Identification

The preferred cell cultures for the growth of PIV are primary or continuous monkey kidney cells, such as LLC-MK, a continuous line of mucoepidermoid human lung carcinoma cells, NCI-H292, and human embryonic kidney cells.[80, 133] PIV-1 also will grow well in human embryonic lung and less well in diploid fibroblastic lines. In other types of kidney tissue, the growth of the PIVs is more variable. PIV-3 replicates in bovine and canine kidney cells and PIV-4 in bovine and hamster kidney cells. After passage, PIV can be propagated in a variety of other cell lines. Persistent infection of some cell lines has been observed with PIV-1, -2, and -3. HeLa cells have been infected continually with PIV-1, BHK-21 with PIV-2, and KB cells with PIV-3.[52, 62, 96] Cells persistently infected with PIV-3 have little or no cytopathic effect that is related to the lack of cell fusion, despite the production of large amounts of the cleaved active form of the F1 protein.[183] The growth of the PIVs in embryonated eggs is poor or variable, according to the type and strain. PIV-1, -2, and -3, but not PIV-4, have been adapted to grow in the amniotic cavity of embryonated chicken eggs, although some strains appear resistant to such adaptation.[100, 133]

The production and type of cytopathic effect in tissue culture are variable with PIV (see Table 182–1). PIV-1 and -3 on initial isolation are unlikely to demonstrate distinctive cytopathic effect. On passage, cytopathic effect may be observed, depending upon the cell line. With PIV-1, cells become rounded and no longer adherent to the glass surface. PIV-3 in primary cell lines tends to produce a "stringy" and fragmented cell sheet, whereas in continuous cell lines, syncytial formation is more common. Initial isolation of PIV-2 may demonstrate cytopathic effect, which characteristically is syncytial. PIV-4 is the most difficult PIV to grow in tissue culture. It produces no cytopathic effect and may require 2 to 4 weeks before identification by hemadsorption is possible.

The ability of the PIVs to hemadsorb erythrocytes has been the major mode of recognizing these viruses in tissue culture. Hemadsorption involves the interaction of the viral hemagglutinin with specific receptors on the erythrocytes. Guinea pig, human group O, or chicken erythrocytes at 4° or 25° C are used most commonly.[92, 133] PIV-4 hemagglutinates guinea pig and human erythrocytes but not chicken erythrocytes.

Staining of infected tissue demonstrates eosinophilic intracytoplasmic inclusions that are the excess nucleocapsids. Specific identification of PIV in tissue culture may be accomplished by testing the hemadsorbing isolates by hemadsorption inhibition, hemagglutination inhibition, or complement-fixation assays.[133] Of these, hemadsorption inhibition, which is specific and sensitive, generally is preferred but often requires days for passage of the isolate in cell culture in order to obtain sufficient antigen. More rapid identification, often within a couple of days of inoculation, may be made by antigen detection with assays using immunologic reagents. In tissue culture, these rapid assays, generally using polyclonal or monoclonal antibodies, are both sensitive and specific.[15, 87, 151, 167]

EPIDEMIOLOGY

Geographic Distribution

The ubiquitous nature of the PIVs has been illustrated by many serologic and viral isolation studies in varied populations, in many parts of the world, and in differing climates.[2, 4, 65, 69, 74, 89, 91, 116, 118, 122, 123, 125, 131, 175, 193] Despite the wide variation in climate and geography, experience with the PIVs is similar in most countries.

Prevalence and Age of Infection

The frequency and impact of PIV infections are greatest in preschool age children and are estimated to account for about one-third of the lower respiratory tract infections in this age group.[41, 65, 84, 112] Acquisition of PIV-3 usually occurs first, followed by PIV-1 and PIV-2 (Fig. 182–2). The epidemiology of PIV-4 is understood less well. Infection with PIV-4A and -4B appears to be relatively common in the preschool years, with 50 per cent or more of 5-year-old children possessing antibodies.[60, 109] Infections with PIV-4B, however, may be less common, with one-third or more of adults being seronegative.[60, 109]

Infection with PIV-3 occurs early in life. One-half to two-thirds of infants by 12 months of age have acquired infection.[64, 65, 89] Experience with PIV-1 and -2 is more gradual. In Washington, D.C., neutralizing antibody was present in less than 10 per cent of infants 6 to 12 months of age, in one-third of children 4 years of age, and in about three-fourths of school age children.[144] By adulthood, virtually all have hemagglutination-inhibition antibody to PIV-1 and -3, but acquisition of antibody to PIV-2 is more variable, ranging from 50 to 90 per cent.[21, 145]

The frequency of PIV infection in the young has been illustrated clearly by the Houston Family Studies, in which infections were detected by both viral isolation and serology in children followed since birth.[64, 65, 68] By 2 years of age, 92 per cent of the children had experienced at least one infection with PIV-3 and 32 per cent had been infected more than once. Serious illness occurs most frequently with primary infection. Infection with lower respiratory tract illness occurring in hospitalized infants most frequently is from PIV-3, and in hospitalized children 2 to 6 years of age, most likely from PIV-1 and -2. The age distribution of children with PIV-1 and -3 viral infections seen in private pediatric practice, however, may overlap substantially (see Fig. 182–2). Approximately one-half of the PIV-3 viral infections occurred in children younger than 24 months of age, compared with about one-third of the PIV-1 infections. In children 2 to 5 years of age, the reverse was true, with one-half of the PIV-1 infec-

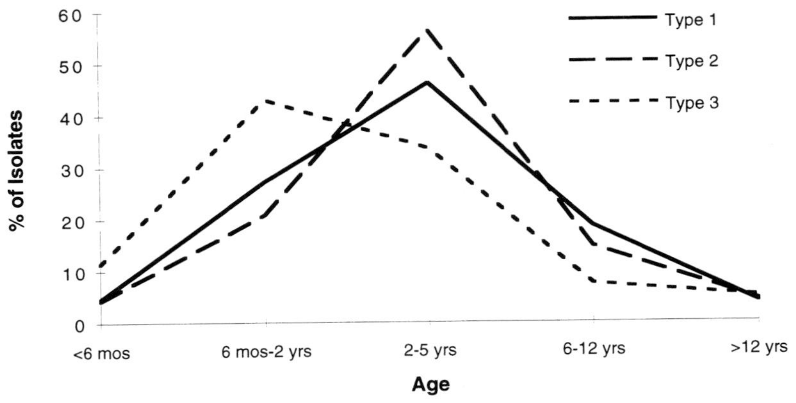

FIGURE 182–2. *Age distribution of PIV-1, -2, and -3 infections in outpatient children in Rochester, New York, from 1976 to 1992. (From Knott, A., et al.: Parainfluenza viral infections in pediatric outpatients: Seasonal patterns and clinical characteristics. Pediatr. Infect. Dis. J. 13:269–273, 1994.)*

tions and about one-third of the PIV-3 infections occurring in this older age group (see Fig. 182–2).

Seasonal Occurrence

The seasonal patterns of the PIVs vary somewhat with the location and the year but in general are distinctive in their predictable and repetitive behavior. Prior to the early 1960s, the PIVs appeared mostly endemic.[24] Since the mid-1960s, however, PIV-1 changed its preference by confining most of its activities to the fall. Subsequently, sizable outbreaks of PIV-1 infection were observed to occur every other year, in the even-numbered years, until the 1970s. Then, for unknown reasons, PIV-1 developed temporarily a sporadic nature for a couple of years before settling into its current pattern of causing outbreaks in fall of the odd-numbered years.[4, 65, 66, 68, 69]

PIV-2 has been more erratic in its behavior than PIV-1.[65, 112] Over 16 years of surveillance in Rochester, New York, PIV-2 sporadically appeared in low numbers at the end of PIV-1 outbreaks in the odd-numbered years (Fig. 182–3).[112] Only twice during the 16 years did PIV-2 appear in outbreak form and both were recent years, suggesting that PIV-2 again may be altering its pattern of activity. PIV-3 predominantly has been endemic but has become more epidemic in nature, with swells of activity in the spring to fall.[65, 112] Although 75 per cent of PIV-3 isolates obtained over the 16 years of surveillance were recovered in the spring and summer, in the autumn of even-numbered years, when PIV-1 was absent, PIV-3 moved into the fall.[112]

PATHOGENESIS

Transmission

Clinical and experimental observations suggest that the PIVs spread readily and effectively.[6, 13, 64, 73, 107, 127, 129, 134, 163] Person-to-person contact appears necessary, allowing direct exposure to infected secretions through large droplets or through self-inoculation. The contagiousness, therefore, will depend upon (1) the quantities of virus contained in the nasal secretions[13, 73]; (2) how effectively the infected secretions are propelled into the environment, such as through sneezing and coughing[127, 163]; and (3) how well the infectious virus can survive in the environment.[6, 13, 127, 129] The PIVs appear to be able to survive in the environment for hours.[6, 13, 142, 143] On

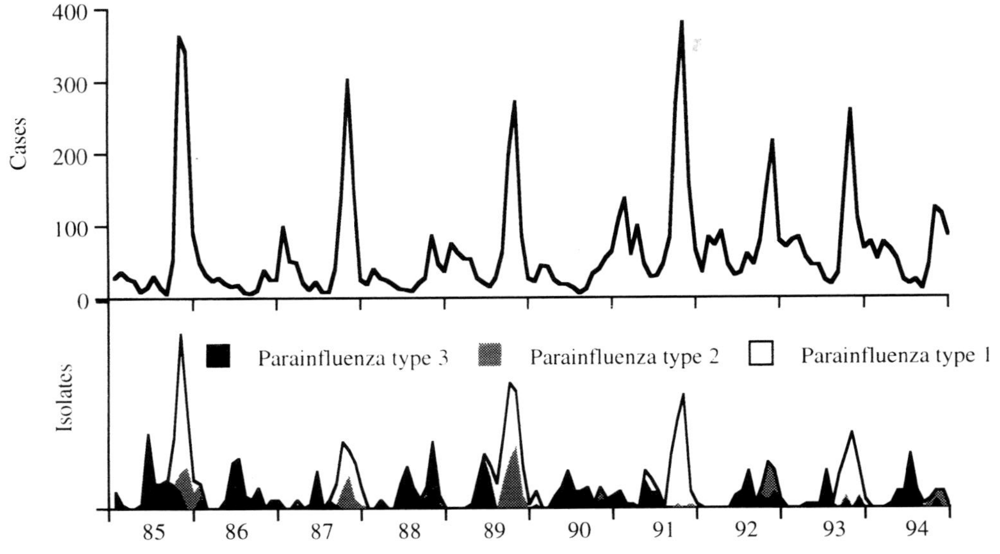

FIGURE 182–3. *Number of cases of croup reported by the primary care physicians in Rochester and Monroe County, New York, from 1985 through 1994 to the Community Infectious Disease Surveillance Program of the University of Rochester School of Medicine, Rochester, NY, shown in relation to the periods of isolation of the parainfluenza viruses.*

nonporous surfaces, the PIVs remain infectious for up to 10 hours and on porous surfaces for up to 4 hours, but survival may be diminished by drying.[13] PIVs may be transferred to hands from environmental surfaces, suggesting that fomites may play a role in dissemination.[6, 13] Infectivity of PIVs on skin, however, declines more rapidly than on nonporous surfaces.[6]

Children with primary infection due to PIV-1 have considerable quantities of infectious virus in their nasal secretions, an average of approximately 1000 median tissue culture–infective doses ($TCID_{50}$) per mL.[73] Because the PIVs tend to cause acute respiratory syndromes often associated with frequent sneezing, coughing, and profuse nasal discharge, contamination of the environment of infected young children likely occurs readily and effectively. Although PIV-3 has been shown to remain viable for 1 hour in a small-particle aerosol experimentally produced,[127] the secretions disseminated through coughs and sneezes probably mostly are in the form of large-particle aerosols, which tend to be greater than 15 μm in diameter. In order for particles of this size to be inhaled, close person-to-person contact is required. The routes of inoculation that occur naturally have not been studied completely. Adults have been infected experimentally by intranasal and oropharyngeal inoculation, but the eye and anterior oral cavity as sites of inoculation have not been examined similarly, which may be important portals in self-inoculation from contaminated hands.[104, 174]

Pathology

Inoculation of the PIVs in the upper respiratory tract is followed by infection of the nasal epithelium and nasopharynx and the appearance of clinical signs after an incubation period of 2 to 4 days. Specific receptors on the cell membrane of the respiratory epithelium allow attachment of the virus to the cell, with subsequent penetration by fusion and phagocytosis.[78, 191] After production of the nucleocapsid in the cytoplasm and final assembly of the virus near the cell membrane, the virus is extruded by budding. This process may occur without destruction of the cell and thus allow continued release of the virus.

The observed pathologic changes generally have been confined to the respiratory tract. Several reports, however, have suggested that spread of the virus may occur not only by cell-to-cell transfer but also occasionally by viremia after both primary and secondary infection.[70, 158] In rodents, viremia and penetration of PIV-1 in migratory mononuclear cells have been observed.[101, 191]

Pathologic studies of children with PIV infections are limited. The few cases of confirmed PIV infection studied pathologically have shown that in the young child with primary infection, inflammation (marked by necrosis of the epithelium) is evident throughout the respiratory tract. The subglottic tissues may appear particularly involved, but the conducting airways at all levels and the alveoli may be affected.[22, 200]

Viral shedding tends to be most abundant and prolonged in young children with primary and severe disease.[73] Children with PIV-1 infections shed the virus for an average of 4 to 7 days but up to 12 days.[51] In PIV-3 infections, shedding tends to be longer, occasionally 2 to 3 weeks.[51] In adults with chronic lung disease, viral shedding may be both prolonged and intermittent.[70] In healthy, young adults stationed at the South Pole, PIVs were shed throughout an 8.5-month winter period of isolation, suggesting that persistent infection may occur with continued shedding under extreme environmental conditions.[132]

Experimental infection of animals with the PIVs has provided a model for the study of the pathophysiology of these infections. Inoculation of rodents with PIV-3 has produced histologically evident, but usually asymptomatic, interstitial pneumonitis or bronchiolitis.[19, 58, 63, 80, 136, 148, 152, 161] In newborn ferrets, PIV infection is progressive and often fatal.[128] Pathologic changes involve the bronchi and peribronchial areas with hyperplasia of the epithelium and surrounding infiltration with pneumocytes and macrophages, causing obliteration of the alveolar spaces. A canine model of PIV-2 into the respiratory tract has produced clinical signs of cough and rhinitis.[182] Histologic changes observed were of denudation of the ciliated epithelium and peribronchial and peribronchiolar lymphocytic infiltrates affecting airways of all sizes.

Immune Response: Role in Pathogenesis and Protection

Whether illness in PIV infections is related mostly to the direct effects of viral replication or compounded by an immunologic reaction is not clear. Clinical severity appears to be related to the degree of viral replication,[73] but cellular destruction and pathology also may be engendered by antigen-antibody complexes, IgE antibody, augmented delayed-type hypersensitivity, cytotoxic cellular responses, and release of cytokines and a cascade of other inflammatory mediators.

In contrast to infection from PIV-1 and -2, the most serious form of illness with PIV-3 infection occurs in the first year of life, when infants may possess maternally derived specific antibody, suggesting that the interactions of maternal antibody and virus may be detrimental.[59, 123] In experimental animals, however, passively administered antibody appears to be protective during PIV-3 infection. Monoclonal antibodies against F and HN proteins offered significant protection in hamsters against challenge, whereas protection from antibody directed against a single surface glycoprotein produced diminished protection.[154, 161] Hamsters administered specific antibody have been observed to develop less severe pulmonary infiltrates when infected with PIV-3 than did the animals without passive antibody. When reinfected, however, they developed more severe pulmonary involvement than did animals who had not received antibody during primary infection.[67]

The clinical observation that lower respiratory tract disease from PIV-1 and -2 rarely occurs in the first few months of life suggests a protective role for passively derived antibodies.[67] For all the PIVs, serum antibody appears to afford some, but not complete, resistance to infection.[54, 68, 144, 165, 186] In the Houston Family Studies,[64, 68] the level of passively acquired maternal antibody to PIV-3 in the cord blood correlated inversely with the risk of infection. In addition, preexisting serum antibody has been shown to result in diminished quantities of virus shed from the oropharynx in adults with PIV infections.[12]

Antibody to the F protein, more than to the HN protein, has been suggested as important in immunity to infection.[29] In cord sera, antibody to the HN protein is present consistently, whereas antibody to the F protein and neutralizing antibody are more variable.[80] After primary infection with PIV-3, infants produce antibody to the HN protein more frequently and at higher levels than to F protein, and antifusion activity tends to be found only in sera having relatively high levels of neutralizing antibody.[108] In most young children with primary PIV-3 infection, the antibody response to HN protein has been shown to be directed to four of six antigenic sites examined on the HN protein, three of which were neutralizing sites.[178] The response to the F protein, whether with primary or recurrent infection, generally was more variable in magnitude and restricted in terms of antigenic sites. The presence of maternal antibody, however, appeared inhibitory to the infant's ability to produce specific humoral antibody.[178]

The more severe illness occurring during reinfection in experimental animals generally has not been shown for children. In a group of young children prospectively followed, a second PIV infection with a heterotypic or homotypic strain occurred in approximately one-half by 30 months of age.[186] Although previous infection with a heterotypic strain did not produce significant protection against the development of lower respiratory tract disease, previous homotypic infection did provide a brief period of such immunity. In Glezen and colleagues' studies,[64, 68] the risk of reinfection was related inversely to the serum-neutralizing antibody titer persisting from a previous infection, and the rate of lower respiratory tract disease decreased with reinfection.

The role of secretory antibody in the protection or pathogenesis of PIV infections in children is not clear. In experimentally infected adults, neutralizing activity in the nasopharyngeal secretions has been demonstrated to correlate better than the level of serum antibody with protection against PIV reinfection.[171] In children, however, no relation appears to exist between neutralizing activity in the nasopharyngeal secretions and specific secretory IgA antibody.[195] Most young children infected with PIV produce IgA antibody to the homologous strain.[186, 195] Primary and secondary infections with a heterotypic strain result in low and transient levels of IgA antibody, whereas homotypic reinfection produces an enhanced response.[186]

Specific IgE antibody in the nasopharyngeal secretions in children with PIV illness has been correlated with more severe disease.[184, 185, 187, 188] Greater levels of virus-specific IgE antibody and release of histamine in the nasopharyngeal secretions were found in children who developed croup or wheezing, suggesting a pathogenic mechanism for the development of hyperreactive airways during PIV infection in some children with a genetic or atopic predisposition.

Genetic and immunologic factors have been suggested as being particularly integral in children who manifest their PIV infections as croup. An abnormal cell-mediated response to PIV in children developing croup has been suggested by their increased lymphoproliferative responses and decreased histamine-induced suppression of lymphocyte transformation responses to PIV when compared with children with PIV infection that is manifest as an upper respiratory tract infection.[185] Furthermore, an atopic state, as well as diminished serum IgA levels, has been correlated with a propensity to develop recurrent croup.[198, 199]

Interferon's importance in recovery from PIV infections has not been delineated well. Children with acute PIV-1 infections, however, produce interferon in their nasal secretions.[73] The role of local cell-mediated immunity has not been examined in humans, but evidence from animal studies suggests that it may be important. In rodents with PIV-3 pneumonia, the development of a cellular cytotoxic response in the lung was associated temporally with the cessation of viral shedding[81] and recovery from the interstitial pneumonitis was correlated with the development of systemic cell-mediated immunity.[152]

CLINICAL MANIFESTATIONS

The types of illnesses caused by PIV infections have characteristic associations with the age of the child, season, and PIV serotype (Table 182–2; see also Figs. 182–2 and 182–5).[64–66, 68, 69, 112] In general, most primary infections are symptomatic, and a high proportion affect the lower respiratory tract, particularly when the initial infection occurs in the second year of life.[68, 112] Of the primary infections that involve only the upper respiratory tract, fever and laryngeal or tracheal involvement are common. Reinfections frequently occur at all ages and primarily are mild, involving the upper respiratory tract, or sometimes they even are asymptomatic.[68] In a general practice in Britain, the attack rate of PIV infections in the first 4 years of life was 43.2 per thousand people, at 5 to 14 years of age the rate was 12 per thousand, and in patients 40 years of age or older the rate fell to 3.7 per thousand.[9] In the Tecumseh study, PIVs ranked second only to the rhinoviruses as the most frequently identified agents of upper respiratory tract infections.[131] In persons 20 to 50

TABLE 182–2. Proportion of Respiratory Syndromes Caused by the Parainfluenza Viruses in Various Studies

		Per Cent of Cases Caused by Parainfluenza Viruses		
Syndrome	**Patient Source**	***Type 1***	***Type 2***	***Type 3***
Croup[18, 26, 30, 39, 69, 112]	Inpatient	10–31	0.5–8	3–8
	Outpatient	7–31	2–4	2–9
Bronchiolitis[26, 30, 69]	Inpatient	1–3	0.4–4	1–13
	Outpatient	2–11	0–2	3–11
Pneumonia[26, 30, 69]	Inpatient	1–3	0.4–4	1–13
	Outpatient	2–11	0–2	3–11
Tracheobronchitis[26, 30, 69]	Inpatient	1–4	0.2–2	2–12
	Outpatient	1–5	0.2–3	4–5
Upper respiratory tract infections[26, 30, 157, 162]	Inpatient	4–12	1–2	5–12
	Outpatient	2–10	0–2	0.4–4
Total upper and lower respiratory tract illnesses[26, 30]	Inpatient	2–5	0.7–2	2–13
	Outpatient	5	2	13

years of age, 16 to 28 per cent were shown to be infected each year.

The PIVs cause a greater proportion of respiratory illnesses in outpatients than of the respiratory illnesses in hospitalized children.[112] Of all the viral respiratory illnesses examined in a pediatric practice, the PIVs caused approximately two-thirds of the croup cases, one-fourth of the tracheobronchitis cases, and about one-half of the upper respiratory tract illnesses, including colds, laryngitis, pharyngitis, and otitis media.

The proportion of hospitalized cases of lower respiratory tract illnesses caused by the PIVs varies according to the year and the age of the children. The risk of hospitalization for PIV lower respiratory tract disease is greatest during the fall outbreaks from PIV-1 and -2 in the odd-numbered years and from PIV-3 during the spring.[65] Infants hospitalized with PIV infection, especially those with bronchiolitis or pneumonia, most likely are to be infected by PIV-3. Hospitalization of children beyond 1 year of age through 5 years of age mainly results from PIV-1 and to a much lesser extent from PIV-2 infections.[64–66, 68, 69]

The various respiratory syndromes associated with PIV-1, -2, and -3 are shown in Table 182–2 and Figures 182–4 and 182–5. Although variation occurs according to the population and diagnostic method (viral isolation, serology, or both) used for identification of infection, all studies indicate that PIVs are the major cause of croup and an important, but less frequent, cause of the other lower respiratory tract syndromes in children (see Figs. 182–3 and 182–4). PIV-1 and -2 primarily are associated with croup, especially in hospitalized patients (see Table 182–2).[65, 112] PIV-3 is manifested most frequently in hospitalized patients as pneumonia or bronchiolitis and in outpatients as upper respiratory tract illness.[65, 112] In outpatients, upper respiratory tract infections are produced by all three types of PIV in approximately 40 to 66 per cent of cases (Figs. 182–4 and 182–5).[112] PIVs have been isolated from middle ear aspirates and may play a primary or secondary role of predisposing to bacterial middle ear infection. Otitis media has been shown to complicate upper respiratory tract infections in about 10 per cent of patients, most frequently in infants younger than 6 months of age. Otitis media from PIV-1 accounted for 17 per cent of cases and PIV-3 for 9 per cent of cases.[28, 77, 82, 112, 160] Of the children 6 years of age or older seen in pediatric practice with a PIV infection, 60 per cent had an upper respiratory tract infection (one-half of these infections primarily were pharyngitis), 14 per cent had croup, 9 per cent had laryngitis, and 4 per cent had tracheobronchitis. Infection with PIV-1, -2, and -3 also may result in an undifferentiated febrile illness without noticeable respiratory signs in 5 to 7 per cent of cases.

In the 11-year study of croup in a pediatric practice in Chapel Hill, North Carolina, the PIVs constituted three-fourths of the agents isolated. The majority (65 per cent) were type 1.[39] Fifty-eight per cent of the lower respiratory tract infections from PIV-1 and 60 per cent of those from PIV-2 were manifest as croup, compared with 29 per cent of the PIV-3 lower respiratory tract infections.[39] The type and proportion of illnesses associated with PIV-2 are similar to those seen with PIV-1. PIV-2 infections, however, occur five times less frequently; thus, their impact on health care is less noticeable.[39, 69, 112]

The clinical manifestations associated with PIV-4 are much less well described. This in part may be due to the technical difficulty of isolating PIV-4. According to one study, however, PIV-4 may account for 3 per cent of respiratory disease.[20] Most PIV-4 isolates have been associated with a mild, usually afebrile, upper respiratory tract infection.[20, 86] The diseases associated with 17 PIV-4 strains submitted from various laboratories in England, however, were more serious.[60] In this selected group, more than one-half of the isolates came from children hospitalized with respiratory tract disease or febrile convulsions. In larger, unselected groups of patients, only mild upper respiratory tract signs have been associated with PIV-4 infections.[20, 86]

The onset of the typical primary PIV infection generally is acute and associated with upper respiratory signs, such as rhinitis and sore throat. Cough and hoarseness frequently are prominent.[9, 73, 86] Most children with PIV-1 infection during a community outbreak seen in a practice setting had fever, upper respiratory tract signs, and tracheobronchial or tracheolaryngeal signs of croup.[73] Fever occurred in 75 per cent and frequently was high. Only 12 per cent had an afebrile upper respiratory tract illness.[73]

The onset of croup usually is preceded by upper respiratory tract signs. Subsequently, a harsh cough develops, followed by stridor, retractions of the chest wall, and dyspnea. The course of croup characteristically is variable, with an unpredictable waxing and waning in the intensity of the stridor and dyspnea. The acute symptoms usually last for 3 to 4 days. In the more severely ill, hypoxemia may occur from viral involvement of the lung parenchyma.[137] This, although important in management, may not be recognized because of the focus on the apparent major site of inflammation, the subglottic area. Rarely, PIV infection in children has resulted in the manifestations of adult respiratory distress syndrome and as acute parotitis.[36, 90, 201]

Reinfections are common with PIV infections and usually are milder, often a common cold. In adults, PIV-1, -2, and -3 constitute about 2 to 5 per cent of the upper respiratory tract infections, but one-fifth or more may be asymptomatic.[12, 43, 86, 117] Of those with clinical illness, approximately 30 to 92 per cent develop fever commonly with malaise, sore throat, and cough.[12, 43, 86] Rhinorrhea is less common in adults than in children, occurring in less than 25 per cent of the adult infections.

PIV infection may cause an exacerbation of symptoms in both children and adults with chronic lung disease, including chronic bronchitis and asthma.[48, 49, 79, 124, 130] Occasionally, as in military recruits, pneumonia has been described with adult PIV infections but is most unusual in a normal population.[46, 190] Exacerbations of nephrotic syndrome also have been engendered by PIV infections.[121]

PIV infections may result in serious morbidity in immunocompromised hosts. Children with combined immunodeficiency disorders can develop severe, often fatal, disease, with prolonged viral shedding and dissemination of the virus.[33, 38, 51, 99, 105, 119] At autopsy, multinucleated giant cells have been found in the lung. PIV infection often is acquired nosocomially and particularly can be hazardous in transplant units.[37, 189] Of bone marrow transplant patients studied from 1974 to 1990, PIV infections were documented in 2.2 per cent (15 children and 12 adults).[189] Lower respiratory tract disease occurred in 70 per cent of these 27 patients and respiratory failure and death in 22 per cent. Diagnosis often was difficult because only in about one-third of those with lower respiratory tract involvement was PIV isolated from the upper respiratory tract. Bronchoalveolar lavage was required to obtain a culture positive for PIV in 20 per cent.

The association of acute PIV infections with nonrespiratory illness is rare, as is the isolation of PIV from sites other than the respiratory tract. A number of case reports have associated PIV infections with disease of the central nervous system.[7, 8, 97, 98, 159, 180, 192] Among these case reports, involving both children and adults, are cases of meningitis, Guillain-Barré syndrome, demyelinating disease, and nonspecific neurologic signs associated with acute infections. Rarely, PIV has been

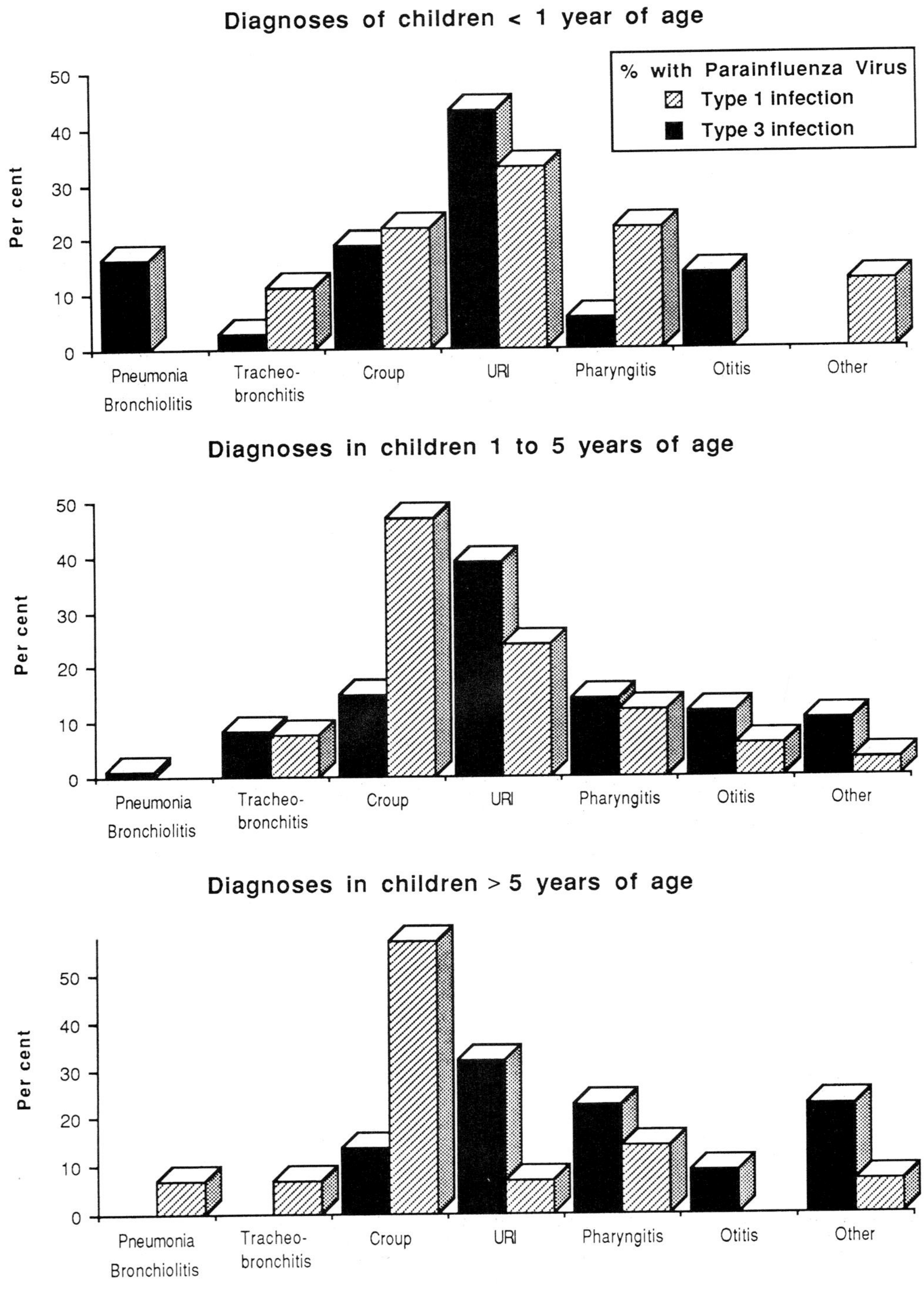

FIGURE 182–4. *Type of illness with PIV-1 compared with PIV-3 according to age in outpatients from private pediatric practices presenting with acute respiratory and/or febrile illnesses. URI, upper respiratory tract infection. (Data obtained 1984 through 1988 from the Community Infectious Disease Surveillance Program of the University of Rochester School of Medicine, Rochester, NY.)*

isolated from the cerebrospinal fluid.[98, 159, 180] Anecdotal reports also have associated PIV infection with collagen vascular diseases and a sporadic severe hepatitis, characterized histologically by syncytial giant hepatocytes.[146, 147]

DIAGNOSIS

The diagnosis of PIV infections often may be surmised on clinical and epidemiologic grounds, such as the patient's age, type of illness, and the seasonal patterns of PIV in the community. Specific diagnosis may be made during the acute phase of the illness by viral isolation, by identification of the viral antigen in patient specimens or in culture, and during convalescence by serologic assays. PIVs, as noted previously, usually are detected in tissue culture by their ability to hemadsorb erythrocytes. Most PIV-1 and -3 strains obtained from acutely ill children may be recognized by hemadsorption within the first 3 to 7 days. PIV-2 and -4 may require longer periods. Specific identification requires subsequent confirmation using type-specific serologic assays or one of the rapid techniques for identifying specific viral antigen in tissue culture (see the subsection on isolation and identification).

Serologic diagnosis requiring acute and convalescent sera may be accomplished by a number of assays, including complement fixation, hemagglutination inhibition, hemadsorption inhibition, neutralizing and enzyme immunoassay, and immunofluorescence.[50, 133] Most of these are relatively sensitive, but heterotypic antibody rises commonly are produced by PIV and related viruses.[50, 133] How often heterologous antibody rises are detected depends in part on the assay.[50] During reinfection, homotypic and/or heterotypic antibody rises may occur, or even no antibody response may be measured, despite virus being shed from the nasopharynx.[12, 117, 142] Less is known about the antibody response to PIV-4 infection, but in primary infection, a homotypic response is usual.[109] Detection of specific IgM antibodies, which usually persist for 2 to 11 weeks after infection, has been of limited success as a diagnostic technique.[176, 181]

DIFFERENTIAL DIAGNOSIS

Most of the other major respiratory viral pathogens at times can mimic the illnesses from PIV infections. Differentiation clinically rarely is possible; more helpful are epidemiologic clues, such as the differing seasonal patterns of the respiratory viruses.[72]

Croup from PIVs or any other virus must be differentiated from bacterial tracheitis and epiglottitis, with their rapidly progressive course and potentially fatal outcome. Fortunately, with the widespread use of the *Haemophilus influenzae* type b vaccine, epiglottitis now is rare. In contrast, PIV croup usually has a more gradual onset with a preceding upper respiratory tract infection. Its fluctuating course and prominent "seal's bark" cough without drooling help differentiate it from epiglottitis and bacterial tracheitis. In PIV croup, the peripheral white blood cell count may be normal or initially show a slight elevation and left shift, whereas in these bacterial causes of stridor, the left shift usually is marked. In view of the recent outbreaks of diphtheria in some countries, laryngeal diphtheria may be a consideration in an unimmunized child. In contrast to bacterial tracheitis and epiglottitis, however, laryngeal diphtheria usually is gradual in onset and presents with the characteristic membranous pharyngitis. Stridor and other signs of croup also may be present in children with aspiration of a foreign body, tracheomalacia, and acute angioneurotic edema.

TREATMENT

Specific therapy is not available yet for PIV infections. The antiviral drug ribavirin inhibits PIV replication in tissue culture and has appeared beneficial in controlling overwhelming PIV infection occurring in infants with severe immunodeficiency.[17, 61, 126, 149]

In experimental animals, therapeutic approaches utilizing immunomodulators against Sendai virus have been explored.[57, 94, 95] Nonspecific stimulation of the host cytokines, as well as administration of such mediators as interferon-α, human interleukin-1β, and human granulocyte colony-stimulating factor, has appeared to be beneficial in the rodent model. Passive topical administration of IgG, which contains neutralizing antibody to PIV, also has appeared beneficial against PIV-3 infection in the cotton rat.[141]

Most PIV infections are self-limited and require no treatment. In the more severely affected children with lower respiratory tract disease, supportive therapy can play an important role in the outcome.[34]

The treatment of croup has been varied and often anecdotal, ranging from cold night air to steam to antiemetics. Yet no such home therapies have proved to be beneficial. After several days of a fluctuating course, most children with croup will improve spontaneously. The more severely affected requiring hospitalization may require monitoring for oxygenation and hypercapnia.[34] The hypoxemia usually is responsive to relatively low concentrations of oxygen.

Rapid improvement in the airway obstruction and respiratory distress for the child who is hospitalized or being monitored in the emergency department may be achieved with aerosolized bronchodilators, such as racemic epinephrine.[34] The relief, however, is transient, and the hypoxemia, if present, is not affected.[164] Children who continue to have respiratory distress are candidates for corticosteroids. The dose of steroids is important and likely explains the conflicting results of previous studies using varied doses of corticosteroids.[103, 173] High doses of dexamethasone (>0.3 mg/kg) or its equivalent or oral prednisone appear necessary to produce the beneficial effect.[34, 103, 168] A single dose of 0.6 mg/kg intramuscularly or intravenously has been recommended to be given in the emergency department to patients requiring hospital admission for croup.[10] One study also has found 0.6 mg/kg of dexamethasone to be beneficial in the therapy of outpatient croup.[35] The treatment of croup is discussed more thoroughly in Chapter 22.

Antibiotic therapy should be reserved for documented episodes of secondary bacterial infection, which is an infrequent occurrence in PIV infections.

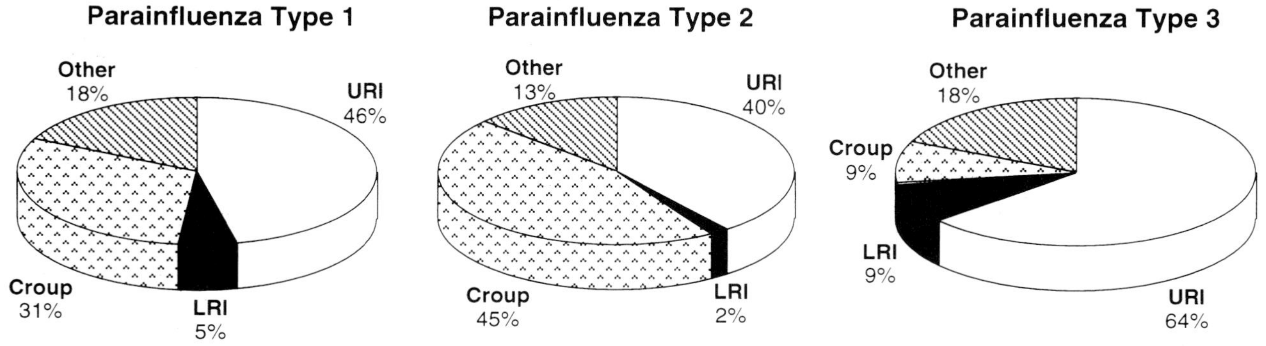

FIGURE 182–5. *Clinical manifestations of parainfluenza virus infections according to serotype in pediatric outpatients in Rochester, New York (1976–1992). URI, upper respiratory tract infection (including otitis, colds, pharyngitis); LRI, lower respiratory tract infection other than croup. (From Knott, A., et al.: Parainfluenza viral infections in pediatric outpatients: Seasonal patterns and clinical characteristics. Pediatr. Infect. Dis. J. 13:269–273, 1994.)*

PROGNOSIS

The majority of children who previously were healthy recover completely and without complication from PIV infections. The acute complications, morbidity, and mortality relate to the presence of an underlying condition, especially a cardiopulmonary or immunodeficiency disease. Of children hospitalized with PIV infection studied over a 4-year period, 35 per cent had preexisting pulmonary or cardiac abnormalities, prematurity, or asthma.[79] When compared with the children who previously were normal, the children with underlying conditions had significantly more severe disease and more complicated courses requiring longer hospitalization. Immunodeficient patients, as described previously, have particular difficulty in controlling and clearing PIV infections, resulting in complicated, prolonged, and recurrent respiratory infections.

Prolonged or persistent infection with PIVs also has been noted in some patients with chronic bronchitis, possibly related to the lack of sufficient response of specific antibody in the sputum.[70] The possibility that PIV-like viruses also may be latent in the human central nervous system has been suggested by the occasional detection of such viruses in the central nervous system of patients with chronic neurologic conditions, such as multiple sclerosis.[16, 114, 138, 170] PIV-1 isolated from the brain tissue of a multiple sclerosis patient has been inoculated intracerebrally into newborn hamsters and shown to produce hydrocephalus with aqueductal stenosis.[53] Viral antigen could be identified in the ependyma and the meninges. Persistent PIV infection also has been established in vitro, and abnormalities in the function of the F protein have been observed, and in human cells, but not in bovine cells, the virus became cell associated with no viral antigen detectable by serologic or immunofluorescent methods.[183, 194] Although long-term follow-up studies of children with proven PIV infection early in life are lacking, subsequent studies of children who have had croup suggest that pulmonary function abnormalities may persist in some of these children.[71, 120] Studies evaluating children with a history of acute laryngotracheobronchitis, for which the viral etiology was unknown, have suggested that an appreciable proportion later have increased bronchial reactivity, which appears to be independent of an atopic predisposition.[71, 120]

PREVENTION

For decades, attempts to prevent PIV infections have focused on the development of effective vaccines. A variety of formalin-inactivated, parenteral PIV vaccines have been developed and evaluated in clinical trials.[27, 55, 56, 110, 169, 179] Most of these vaccines have been grown in embryonated hens' eggs and prepared as an aqueous suspension. One vaccine was grown in monkey kidney cell cultures and prepared in alum formulation.[179] The vaccines, whether monovalent, trivalent, or combined with other respiratory vaccines, were able to induce an excellent humoral antibody response but were not protective.[27, 56] Subsequent natural PIV infection in the vaccinees, however, did not result in more severe disease, as occurred with the alum-precipitated respiratory syncytial viral vaccine.[27, 56]

Alternative means of immunization have been sought.[80, 135] Live attenuated vaccines compared with inactivated or subunit vaccines have the potential advantages of inducing immunity more closely mimicking natural infection with the production of both humoral and mucosal immunity and a longer duration of protection. The potential disadvantages of a live vaccine are the adverse or symptomatic reactions, the possible transmission of the vaccine virus, and its stability, i.e., whether reversion from its attenuated to a more virulent state is possible. Cold-adapted mutant PIV-3 strains have been produced that appear stable and grow well at the lower temperatures of the nasal passages but not at the higher temperatures of the lower respiratory tract.[80, 135] Two cold-adapted candidate vaccines of low passages, however, were ineffective in adult volunteers, and one of these was not attenuated sufficiently in children.[11, 31] A more highly passaged, cold-adapted PIV-3 mutant used to immunize chimpanzees, however, has proved to be protective and is being explored as a possible candidate vaccine for children.[76]

A second approach has been the use of a strain of virus from another species that is related to the human PIV. Focus has been on the bovine PIV-3 because of its close antigenic relationship to human PIV. The F and HN proteins of the two viruses show more than 75 per cent amino acid homology and, more importantly, have high levels of antigenic relatedness.[80, 135, 177] Immunization with the bovine PIV-3 in rodents and primates has resulted in protection of the upper and lower respiratory tract against challenge with human PIV-3, but in adult volunteers, it was avirulent and poorly infectious.[31, 135, 177] Evaluation of an attenuated bovine PIV-3 vaccine in seronegative children, nevertheless, appeared safe and immunogenic with hemagglutination-inhibition antibody induced to bovine PIV-3 in 92 per cent of the children and to human PIV-3 in 61 per cent of the vaccines.[106]

Subunit vaccines containing HN and F proteins are being explored concurrently. These glycoproteins have been produced through viral purification procedures and by expression of recombinant viruses using vaccinia and baculovirus vectors.[3, 14, 44, 45, 47, 75, 80, 88, 135] Neutralizing antibodies are produced by vaccination with either the HN or the F proteins, but protection against infection may require immunization with both glycoproteins.[75, 135, 153, 154] Studies evaluating these subunit vaccines in rodents and in primates have been encouraging. Several creative approaches are being investigated to enhance the immune response from immunization with PIV proteins, including incorporation of PIV-3 into liposomes and microspheres of a biodegradable DL-lactide and glycolide copolymer, and addition of various adjuvants.[47, 155]

References

1. Abinanti, F. R., Chanock, R. M., Cook, M. K., et al.: Relationship of human and bovine strains of myxovirus para-influenza 3. (26371). Proc. Soc. Exp. Biol. Med. *106*:466–469, 1961.
2. Agarwal, S. C., and Schgal, S.: Para-influenza virus infection in respiratory illnesses of infants and children. Indian J. Med. Res. *59*:206–212, 1971.
3. Ambrose, M. W., Wyde, P. R., Ewasyshyn, M., et al.: Evaluation of the immunogenicity and protective efficacy of a candidate parainfluenza virus type 3 subunit vaccine in cotton rats. Vaccine *9*:505–511, 1991.
4. Anderson, L. J., Parker, R. A., and Strikas, R. L.: Association between respiratory syncytial virus outbreaks and lower respiratory tract deaths of infants and young children. J. Infect. Dis. *161*:640–646, 1990.
5. Andrewes, C. H., Bang, F. B., Chanock, R. M., et al.: Parainfluenza viruses 1, 2, and 3: Suggested names for recently described myxoviruses. Biology *8*:129–130, 1959.
6. Ansari, S. A., Springthorpe, V. S., Sattar, S. A., et al.: Potential role of hands in the spread of respiratory viral infections: Studies with human parainfluenza virus 3 and rhinovirus 14. J. Clin. Microbiol. *29*:2115–2119, 1991.
7. Arguedas, A., Stutman, H. R., and Blanding, J. G.: Parainfluenza type 3 meningitis: Report of two cases and review of the literature. Clin. Pediatr. *29*:175–178, 1990.
8. Arisoy, E. S., Demmler, G. J., Thakar, S., et al.: Meningitis due to parainfluenza virus type 3: Report of two cases and review. Clin. Infect. Dis. *17*:995–997, 1993.
9. Banatavala, J. E.: Parainfluenza infections in the community. Br. Med. J. *1*:537–540, 1964.
10. Barkin, R. M.: Pediatric Emergency Medicine: Concepts and Clinical Practice. St. Louis, C. V. Mosby, 1992, p. 1002.
11. Belshe, R. B., Karron, R. A., Newman, F. K., et al.: Evaluation of a live

attenuated, cold-adapted parainfluenza virus type 3 vaccine in children. J. Clin. Microbiol. *30*:2064–2070, 1992.

12. Bloom, H. H., Johnson, K. M., Jacobsen, R., et al.: Recovery of parainfluenza viruses from adults with upper respiratory illness. Am. J. Hyg. *74*:50–59, 1961.
13. Brady, M. T., Evans, J., and Cuartas, J.: Survival and disinfection of parainfluenza viruses on environmental surfaces. Am. J. Infect. Control *18*:18–23, 1990.
14. Brideau, R. J., Oien, N. L., Lehman, D. J., et al.: Protection of cotton rats against human parainfluenza virus type 3 by vaccination with a chimeric FHN subunit glycoprotein. J. Gen. Virol. *74*:471–477, 1993.
15. Brinker, J. P., and Doern, G. V.: A comparison of commercially available monoclonal antibodies for direct and indirect immunofluorescence culture confirmation and direct detection of parainfluenza viruses. Diagn. Microbiol. Infect. Dis. *15*:669–672, 1992.
16. Brody, J. A.: Epidemiology of multiple sclerosis and a possible virus aetiology. Lancet *2*:173–176, 1972.
17. Browne, M. J.: Comparative inhibition of influenza and parainfluenza virus replication by ribavirin in MDCK cells. Antibmicrob. Agents Chemother. *19*:712–715, 1981.
18. Buchan, K. A., Marten, K. W., and Kennedy, D. H.: Aetiology and epidemiology of viral croup in Glasgow, 1966–1972. J. Hyg. *73*:143–150, 1974.
19. Buthala, D. A., and Soret, M. G.: Parainfluenza type 3 virus infection in hamsters: Virologic, serologic, and pathologic studies. J. Infect. Dis. *114*:226–234, 1964.
20. Canchola, J., Vargosko, A. J., Kim, H. W., et al.: Antigenic variation among newly isolated strains of parainfluenza type 4 virus. Am. J. Hyg. *79*:357–364, 1964.
21. Chanock, R. M.: Association of a new type of cytopathogenic myxovirus with infantile croup. J. Exp. Med. *104*:555–576, 1965.
22. Chanock, R. M., Bell, J. A., and Parrott, R. H.: Natural history of parainfluenza infection. Perspect. Virol. *2*:126–139, 1961.
23. Chanock, R. M., and McIntosh, K.: Parainfluenza viruses. *In* Fields, B. N., Knipe, D. M., Chanock, R. M., et al. (eds.): Virology. New York, Raven Press, 1990, pp. 963–988.
24. Chanock, R. M., and Parrott, R. H.: Acute respiratory disease in infancy and childhood: Present understanding and prospects for prevention. Pediatrics *36*:21–39, 1965.
25. Chanock, R. M., Parrott, R. H., Cook, K., et al.: Newly recognized myxoviruses from children with respiratory disease. N. Engl. J. Med. *258*:207–213, 1958.
26. Chanock, R. M., Parrott, R. H., Johnson, K. M., et al.: Myxoviruses: Parainfluenza. Am. Rev. Resp. Dis. *88*:152–166, 1963.
27. Chin, J., Magoffin, R. L., Shearer, L. A., et al.: Field evaluation of a respiratory syncytial virus vaccine and a trivalent parainfluenza virus vaccine in a pediatric population. Am. J. Epidemiol. *89*:449–463, 1969.
28. Chonmaitree, T.: Viral otitis media. Pediatr. Ann. *19*:522–523, 1990.
29. Choppin, P. W., Richardson, C. D., Merz, D. C., et al.: The functions and inhibitions of the membrane glycoproteins of the paramyxoviruses and myxoviruses and the role of the measles virus M protein in subacute sclerosing panencephalitis. J. Infect. Dis. *143*:501–503, 1981.
30. Clarke, S. K. R.: Parainfluenza virus infections. Postgrad. Med. J. *49*:792–797, 1973.
31. Clements, M. L., Belshe, R. B., King, J., et al.: Evaluation of bovine, cold-adapted human, and wild-type human parainfluenza type 3 virus in adult volunteer and in chimpanzees. J. Clin. Microbiol. *29*:1175–1182, 1991.
32. Coelingh K. V., Winter, C. C., and Murphy, B. R.: Antigenic variation in the hemagglutinin-neuraminidase protein of human parainfluenza type 3 virus. Virology *143*:569–582, 1985.
33. Craft, A. W., Reid, M. M., Gardner, P. S., et al.: Virus infections in children with acute lymphoblastic leukemia. Arch. Dis. Child. *54*:755–759, 1979.
34. Cressman, W. R., and Myer, C. C., III: Diagnosis and management of croup and epiglottitis. Pediatr. Clin. North Am. *41*:265–276, 1994.
35. Cruz, M. N., Stewart, G., and Rosenberg, N.: Use of dexamethasone in the outpatient management of acute laryngotracheitis. Pediatrics *96*:220–223, 1995.
36. Cullen, S. J., and Baublis, J. V.: Parinfluenza parotitis in two immunodeficient children. J. Pediatr. *96*:437-438, 1980.
37. Defabritus, A. M., Riggio, R. R., David, D. S., et al.: Parainfluenza type 3 in a transplant unit. J. A. M. A. *241*:384–386, 1979.
38. Delage, G., Brochu, P., Pelletier, M., et al.: Giant-cell pneumonia caused by parainfluenza virus. J. Pediatr. *94*:426–429, 1979.
39. Denny, F. W.: Croup: An 11-year study in a pediatric practice. Pediatrics *71*:871–876, 1983.
40. Denny, Jr., F. W.: Certain biologic characteristics of myxovirus parainfluenza 3. Fed. Proc. *19*:409, 1960.
41. Denny, F.W., and Clyde, W. A., Jr.: Acute lower respiratory infections in nonhospitalized children. J. Pediatr. *108*:635–646, 1986.
42. Dick, E. C., and Mogabgab, W. J.: Characteristics of parainfluenza 1 (HA-2) virus. III. Antigenic relationships, growth, interaction with erythrocytes and physical properties. J. Bacteriol. *85*:561–571, 1962.
43. Dick, E. C., Mogabgab, W. J., and Holmes, B.: Characteristics of parainfluenza 1 (HA-2) virus 1. Incidence of infection and clinical features in adults. Am. J. Hyg. *73*:263–272, 1961.
44. Ebata, S. N., Cote, M. J., Kang, C. Y., et al.: The fusion and hemagglutinin-neuraminidase glycoproteins of human parainfluenza virus 3 are both required for fusion. Virology *183*:437–441, 1991.
45. Ebata, S. N., Prevec, L., Graham, F. L., et al.: Function and immunogenicity of human parainfluenza virus 3 glycoproteins expressed by recombinant adenoviruses. Virus Res. *24*:21–33, 1992.
46. Evans, A. S., and Brobst, M.: Bronchitis, pneumonitis and pneumonia in University of Wisconsin students. N. Engl. J. Med. *265*:401–409, 1961.
47. Ewasyshyn, M., Caplan, B., Bonneau, A. M., et al.: Comparative analysis of the immunostimulatory properties of different adjuvants on the immunogenicity of prototype parainfluenza virus type 3 subunit vaccine. Vaccine *10*:412–420, 1992.
48. Falsey, A. R.: Noninfluenza respiratory virus infection in long-term care facilities. Infect. Control Hosp. Epidemiol. *12*:602–608, 1991.
49. Falsey, A. R., Cunningham, C. K., Barker, W. H., et al.: Respiratory syncytial virus and influenza A infections in the hospitalized elderly. J. Infect. Dis. *172*:389–394, 1995.
50. Fedova, D., Novotny, J., and Kubinova, I.: Serological diagnosis of parainfluenza virus infections: Verification of the sensitivity and specificity of the haemagglutination-inhibition (HI), complement-fixation (CF), immunofluorescence (IFA) tests and enzyme immunoassay (ELISA). Acta Virol. *36*:304–312, 1992.
51. Fishaut, M., Tubergen, D., and McIntosh, K.: Cellular response to respiratory viruses with particular reference to children with disorders of cell-mediated immunity. J. Pediatr. *96*:179–180, 1980.
52. Fraser, K. B., and Anderson, J.: Persistent non-cytocidal infection in BHK 21 cells by human parainfluenza type 2 virus. J. Gen. Microbiol. *44*:47–58, 1966.
53. Friedman, H. M., Gilden, D. H., Lief, F. S., et al.: Hydrocephalus produced by the 6/94 virus: A parainfluenza type 1 isolate from multiple sclerosis brain tissue. Arch. Neurol. *32*:408–413, 1975.
54. Fukumi, H.: Meaning of circulating antibody titers in the infections of parainfluenza 3 virus and RS virus. Dev. Biol. Stand. *28*:159–166, 1975.
55. Fulginiti, V. A., Amer, J., Eller, J. J., et al.: Parainfluenza virus immunization. IV. Simultaneous immunization with parainfluenza types 1, 2, and 3 aqueous vaccines. Am. J. Dis. Child. *114*:26–28, 1967.
56. Fulginiti, V. A., Eller, J. J., Sieber, O. F., et al.: Respiratory virus immunization. I. A field trial of two inactivated respiratory vaccines; an aqueous trivalent parainfluenza virus vaccine and an alum-precipitated respiratory syncytial virus vaccine. Am. J. Epidemiol. *89*:435–448, 1969.
57. Fulton, R. W., Burge L. J., and McCraken, J. S.: Effect of recombinant DNA-derived bovine and human interferons on replication of bovine herpesvirus-1, parainfluenza-3, and respiratory syncytial virus. Am. J. Vet. Res. *47*:751–753, 1986.
58. Galinski, M. S., Mink, M. A., Lambert, D. M., et al.: Molecular cloning and sequence analysis of the human parainfluenza 3 virus gene encoding the matrix protein. Virology *157*:24–30, 1987.
59. Gardner, P. S., McQuillin, J., McGuckin, R., et al.: Observations on clinical and immunofluorescent diagnosis of parainfluenza virus infections. Br. Med. J. *2*:7–12, 1971.
60. Gardner, S. D.: The isolation of parainfluenza 4 subtypes A and B in England and serological studies of their prevalence. J. Hyg. *67*:545–550, 1969.
61. Gelfand, E. W., McCurdy, D., Rao, C. P., et al.: Ribavirin treatment of viral pneumonitis in severe combined immunodeficiency disease. Lancet *2*:732–733, 1983.
62. Genest, P., and Daniel, P.: Genomic modifications in cell line cultures chronically infected with a myxovirus. Proc. Soc. Exp. Biol. Med. *123*:722-725, 1966.
63. Giddens, Jr., W. E., Van Hoosier, Jr., G. L., and Garlinghouse, L. E.: Experimental Sendai virus infection in laboratory rats. II. Pathology and immunohistochemistry. Lab. Anim. Sci. *37*:442–448, 1987.
64. Glezen, W. P.: Incidence of respiratory syncytial and parainfluenza type 3 viruses in an urban setting. Pediatr. Virol. *2*:1–4, 1987.
65. Glezen, W. P.: Serious morbidity associated with the major respiratory viruses. Pediatr. Ann. *19*:535–542, 1990.
66. Glezen, W. P., and Denny, F. W.: Epidemiology of acute lower respiratory disease in children. N. Engl. J. Med. *288*:498–505, 1973.
67. Glezen, W. P., and Fernald, G. W.: Effect of passive antibody on parainfluenza virus type 3 pneumonia in hamsters. Infect. Immun. *14*:212–216, 1976.
68. Glezen, W. P., Frank, A. L., Taber, L. H., et al.: Parainfluenza virus type 3: Seasonality and risk of infection in young children. J. Infect. Dis. *150*:851–857, 1984.
69. Glezen, W. P., Loda, F. A., Clyde, W. A., Jr., et al.: Epidemiologic patterns of acute lower respiratory disease of children in pediatric group practice. J. Pediatr. *78*:397–406, 1971.
70. Gross, P. A., Green, R. H., and Curnen, M. G. M.: Persistent infection with parainfluenza type 3 virus in man. Am. Rev. Resp. Dis. *108*:894–898, 1973.
71. Gurwitz, D., Corey, M., and Levison, H.: Pulmonary function and bronchial reactivity in children after croup. Am. Rev. Resp. Dis. *122*:95–99, 1980.
72. Hall, C. B., and Douglas, R. G., Jr.: Respiratory syncytial virus and influenza: Practical community surveillance. Am. J. Dis. Child. *130*:615–620, 1976.
73. Hall, C. B., Geiman, J. M., Breese, B. B., et al.: Parainfluenza viral infec-

tions in children: Correlation of shedding with clinical manifestations. J. Pediatr. *91*:194–198, 1977.
74. Hall, C. E., Brandt, C. D., Frothingham, T. E., et al.: The virus watch program: A continuing surveillance of viral infections in metropolitan New York families. IX. A comparison of infections with several respiratory pathogens in New York and New Orleans families. Am. J. Epidemiol. *94*:367–385, 1971.
75. Hall, S. L., Murphy, B. R., and van Wyke Coelingh, K. L.: Protection of cotton rats by immunization with the human parainfluenza virus type 3 fusion (F) glycoprotein expressed on the surface of insect cells infected with a recombinant baculovirus. Vaccine *9*:659–667, 1991.
76. Hall, S. L., Sarris, C. M., Tierney, E. L., et al.: A cold-adapted mutant of parainfluenza virus type 3 is attenuated and protective in chimpanzees. J. Infect. Dis. *167*:958–962, 1993.
77. Halsted, C., Lepow, M. L., Balassanian, N, et al.: Otitis media: Clinical observations, microbiology and evaluation of therapy. Am. J. Dis. Child, *115*:524–551, 1968.
78. Haywood, A. M.: Phagocytosis of Sendai virus by model membranes. J. Gen. Virol. *29*:63–68, 1975.
79. Heidemann, S. M.: Clinical characteristics of parainfluenza virus infection in hospital children. Pediatr. Pulmonol. *13*:86–89, 1992.
80. Heilman, C. A.: Respiratory syncytial and parainfluenza viruses. J. Infect. Dis. *161*:402–406, 1990.
81. Henderson, F. W.: Pulmonary cell-mediated cytotoxicity in hamsters with parainfluenza virus type 3 pneumonia. Am. Rev. Resp. Dis. *120*:41–47, 1979.
82. Henderson, F. W., Collier, A. M., Sanyal, M. A., et al.: A longitudinal study of respiratory viruses and bacteria in the etiology of acute otitis media. N. Engl. J. Med. *306*:1377–1383, 1982.
83. Henrickson, K. J.: Monoclonal antibodies to human parainfluenza virus type 1 detect major antigenic changes in clinical isolates. J. Infect. Dis. *164*:1128–1134, 1991.
84. Henrickson, K. J., Kuhn, S. M., and Savatski, L. L.: Epidemiology and cost of human parainfluenza virus type one and two infections in young children. Clin. Infect. Dis. *18*:770–779, 1994.
85. Henrickson, K. J., and Savatski, L. L.: Genetic variation and evolution of human parainfluenza virus type 1 hemagglutinin neuraminidase: Analysis of 12 clinical isolates. J. Infect. Dis. *166*:995–1005, 1992.
86. Herrmann, E. C., and Hable, K. A.: Experiences in laboratory diagnosis of parainfluenza viruses in routine medical practice. Mayo Clin. Proc. *45*:177–188, 1970.
87. Hierholzer, J. C., Bingham, P. G., Coombs, R. A., et al.: Comparison of monoclonal antibody time-resolved fluoroimmunoassay with monoclonal antibody capture–biotinylated detector enzyme immunoassay for respiratory syncytial virus and parainfluenza virus antigen detection. J. Clin. Microbiol. *27*:1243–1249, 1989.
88. Homa, F. L., Brideau, R. J., Lehman, D. J., et al.: Development of a novel subunit vaccine that protects cotton rats against both human respiratory syncytial virus and human parainfluenza virus type 3. J. Gen. Virol. *74*:1995–1999, 1993.
89. Hope-Simpson, R. E.: Parainfluenza virus infections in the Cirencester survey: Seasonal and other characteristics. J. Hyg. *87*:393–406, 1981.
90. Hotez, P. J., Goldstein, B., Ziegler, J., et al.: Adult respiratory distress syndrome associated with parainfluenza virus type 1 in children. Pediatr. Infect. Dis. J. *9*:750–752, 1990.
91. Hruskova, J., Fedpva, D., Syrucek, L., et al.: Antibody to parainfluenza virus types 1, 2 and 3 in sera and nasal secretions of persons of different age. J. Hyg. Epidemiol. Microbiol. Immunol. *25*:65–70, 1981.
92. Hsiung, G. D.: Myxoviruses. *In* Hsiung, G. D., Fong, C. K. Y., and Landry, M. L. (eds.): Hsiung's Diagnostic Virology. New Haven, CT, Yale University Press, 1973, pp. 84–92.
93. Hurrell, J. M.: Methods of storing viruses at low temperatures with particular reference to the myxovirus group. J. Med. Lab. Technol. *24*:30–41, 1967.
94. Iida, J., Ishihara, C., Mizukoshi, M., et al.: Prophylactic activity of dihydrohepatrenol, a synthetic polyprenol derivative, against Sendai virus infection in mice. Vaccine *8*:376–380, 1990.
95. Iida, J., Saiki, I., Ishihara, C., et al.: Prophylactic activity against Sendai virus infection and macrophage activation with lipophilic derivatives of N-acetylglucosaminylmuramyl tri- or tetrapeptides. Vaccine *7*:225–228, 1989.
96. Ishida, N., Homma, M., Osato, T., et al.: Persistent infection in the HeLa cells with hemadsorption virus type 2. Virology *24*:670–672, 1964.
97. Jackson, M. A., Olson, L. C., Burry, V. F., et al.: Parainfluenza virus and neurologic signs. Pediatr. Infect. Dis. J. *13*:759–760, 1994.
98. Jantausch, B. A., Wiedermann, B. L., and Jeffries, B.: Parainfluenza virus type 2 meningitis and parotitis in an 11-year-old child. South. Med. J. *88*:230–231, 1995.
99. Jarvis, W. R., Middleton, P. J., and Gelfand, E. W.: Parainfluenza pneumonia in severe combined immunodeficiency disease. J. Pediatr. *94*:423–425, 1979.
100. Jensen, K. E.: Adaptation of parainfluenza virus types 1 and 3 to eggs and rodents. Bacteriol. Proc. *60*:90, 1960.
101. Johnson, D. P., and Green, R. H.: Viremia during parainfluenza type 3 virus infection of hamsters. Proc. Soc. Exp. Biol. Med. *144*:745–748, 1973.
102. Johnson, K. M., Chanock, R. M., Cook, M. K., et al.: Studies of a new human hemadsorption virus. I. Isolation, properties, and characterization. Am. J. Hyg. *71*:81–92, 1960.
103. Kairys, S. W., Olmstead, E. M., and O'Connor, G. T.: Steroid treatment of laryngotracheitis: A meta-analysis of the evidence from randomized trials. Pediatrics *83*:683–693, 1989.
104. Kapikian, A. Z., Chanock, R. M., Reichelderfer, T. E., et al.: Inoculation of human volunteers with parainfluenza virus type 3. J. A. M. A. *178*:537–541, 1961.
105. Karp, D., Willis, J., and Wilfert, C.: Parainfluenza virus II and the immunocompromised host. Am. J. Dis. Child. *127*:592–593, 1974.
106. Karron, R. A., Wright, P. F., Hall, S. L., et al.: A live attenuated bovine parainfluenza virus type 3 vaccine is safe, infectious, immunogenic, and phenotypically stable in infants and children. J. Infect. Dis. *171*:1107–1114, 1995.
107. Karron R. A., O'Brien, K. L., Froehlich, J. L., et al.: Molecular epidemiology of a parainfluenza type 3 virus outbreak on a pediatric ward. J. Infect. Dis. *167*:1441–1445, 1993.
108. Kasel, J. A., Frank, A. L., Keitel, W. A., et al.: Acquisition of serum antibodies to specific viral glycoproteins of parainfluenza virus 3 in children. J. Virol. *52*:828–832, 1984.
109. Killgore, G. E., and Dowdle, W. R.: Antigenic characterization of parainfluenza 4A and 4B by the hemagglutination-inhibition test and distribution of HI antibody in human sera. Am. J. Epidemiol. *91*:306–316, 1970.
110. Kim, H. W., Canchola, J. G., Vargosko, A. J., et al.: Immunogenicity of inactivated parainfluenza type 1, type 2, and type 3 vaccines in infants. J. A. M. A. *196*:819–824, 1966.
111. Kingsbury, D. W.: Paramyxoviridae and their replication. *In* Fields, B. N., Knipe, D. M., Chanock, R. M., et al. (eds.): Virology. New York, Raven Press, 1990, pp. 945–962.
112. Knott, A., Long, C. E., and Hall, C. B.: Parainfluenza viral infections in pediatric outpatients: Seasonal patterns and clinical characteristics. Pediatr. Infect. Dis. J. *13*:269–273, 1994.
113. Komada, H., Kusagawa, S., Orvell, C., et al.: Antigenic diversity of human parainfluenza virus type 1 isolates and their immunological relationship with Sendai virus revealed by monoclonal antibodies. J. Gen. Virol. *73*:875–884, 1992.
114. Koprowski, H., and ter Meulen, V.: Multiple sclerosis and parainfluenza 1 virus: History of the isolation of the virus and expression of phenotypic differences between the isolated virus and Sendai virus. J. Neurol. *208*:175–190, 1975.
115. Kuroya, M., Ishida, N., and Shirator, T.: New born virus pneumonitis (type Sendai). II. The isolation of a new virus possessing hemagglutination activity. Yokohama M. Bull. *4*:217–233, 1953.
116. LaPlaca, M., and Moscovici, C.: Distribution of parainfluenza antibodies in different groups of population. J. Immunol. *88*:72–77, 1962.
117. Lefkowitz, L. J., Jr., and Jackson, G. G.: Dual respiratory infection with parainfluenza and rhinovirus: The pathogenesis of transmitted infection in volunteers. Am. Rev. Respir. Dis. *93*:519–528, 1966.
118. Leogrande, G.: Studies on the epidemiology of child infections 3 parainfluenza viruses (types 1-4) and respiratory syncytial virus infections. Microbiol. 72:55–63, 1992.
119. Little, B. W., Tihen, W. S., Dickerman, J. D., et al.: Giant-cell pneumonia associated with parainfluenza virus type 3 infection. Hum. Pathol. *12*:478–481, 1981.
120. Loughlin, G., and Taussig, L. M.: Pulmonary function in children with a history of laryngotracheobronchitis. J. Pediatr. *94*:365–369, 1979.
121. MacDonald, N. E., Wolfish, N., McLaine, P., et al.: Role of respiratory viruses in exacerbations of primary nephrotic syndrome. J. Pediatr. *108*:378–382, 1986.
122. Maynard, J. E., Feltz, E. T., Wulff, H., et al.: Surveillance of respiratory virus infections among Alaskan Eskimo children. J. A. M. A. *200*:927–931, 1967.
123. McIntosh, K.: Pathogenesis of severe acute respiratory infections in the developing world: Respiratory syncytial virus and parainfluenza virus. Rev. Infect. Dis. *13*(Suppl.):S492–S500, 1991.
124. McIntosh, K., Ellis, E. F., Hoffman, L. S., et al.: The association of viral and bacterial respiratory infections with exacerbations of wheezing in young asthmatic children. J. Pediatr. *82*:578–590, 1973.
125. McIntosh, K., Halonen, P., and Ruuskanen, O.: Report of a workshop on respiratory viral infections: Epidemiology, diagnosis, treatment, and prevention. Clin. Infect. Dis. *16*:151–164, 1993.
126. McIntosh, K., Kurachek, S. C., Cairns, L. M., et al.: Treatment of respiratory viral infection in an immunodeficient infant with ribavirin aerosol. Am. J. Dis. Child. *138*:305–308, 1984.
127. McLean, D. M., Bannatyne, R. M., and Givan, K. F.: Myxovirus dissemination by air. Can. Med. Assoc. J. *96*:1449–1453, 1967.
128. Metzgar, D. P., Gower, T. A., Larson, E. J., et al.: The effect of parainfluenza virus type 3 on newborn ferrets. J. Biol. Stand. *2*:273–282, 1974.
129. Miller, W. S., and Artenstein, M. S.: Aerosol stability of three acute respiratory disease viruses. Proc. Soc. Exp. Biol. Med. *125*:222–227, 1967.
130. Minor, T. E., Baker, J. W., Dick, E. C., et al.: Greater frequency of viral respiratory infections in asthmatic children as compared with their non-asthmatic siblings. J. Pediatr. *85*:472–477, 1974.
131. Monto, A. S.: The Tecumseh study of respiratory illness. V. Patterns of

infection with the parainfluenza viruses. Am. J. Epidemiol. *97*:338–348, 1973.
132. Muchmore, H. C., Parkinson, A. J., Humphries, J. E., et al.: Persistent parainfluenza viruses shedding during isolation at the South Pole. Nature *289*:187–189, 1981.
133. Mufson, M. A.: Parainfluenza viruses, mumps virus, and Newcastle disease virus. *In* Schmidt, N. J., and Emmons, R. W, (eds.): Diagnostic Procedure for Viral and Rikettsial Infections. New York, American Public Health Association, 1989, pp. 669–712.
134. Mufson, M. A., Mocega, H. E., and Krause, H. E.: Acquisition of parainfluenza 3 virus infection by hospitalized children. I. Frequencies, rates, and temporal data. J. Infect. Dis. *128*:141–147, 1973.
135. Murphy, B. R.: Current approaches to the development of vaccines effective against parainfluenza viruses. Bull. World Health Org. *66*:391–397, 1988.
136. Murphy, T. F., Dubovi, E. J., and Clyde, W. A., Jr.: The cotton rat as an experimental model of human parainfluenza virus type 3 disease. Exp. Lung. Res. *2*:97–109, 1981.
137. Newth, C. J., Levinson, H., and Byron, A. C.: The respiratory status of children with croup. J. Pediatr. *81*:1068–1073, 1972.
138. Norrby, E., Link, H., Olsson, J. E., et al.: Comparison of antibodies against different viruses in cerebrospinal fluid and serum samples from patients with multiple sclerosis. Infect. Immun. *10*:688–694, 1974.
139. Orvell, C., and Grandien, M.: The effects of monoclonal antibodies on biologic activities of structural proteins on Sendai virus. J. Immunol. *129*:2779–2787, 1982.
140. Orvell, C., and Norrby, E.: Antigenic structure of paramyxoviruses. *In* Van Regenmortel, E. M. H. V., and Neurath, A. R. (eds.): Immunochemistry of Viruses: The Basis for Serodiagnosis and Vaccines. Amsterdam, Elsevier Science, 1985, pp. 241–264.
141. Ottolini, M. G., Hemming, V. G., Piazza, F. M., et al.: Topical immunoglobulin is an effective therapy for parainfluenza type 3 in a cotton rat model. J. Infect. Dis. *243*–245, 1995.
142. Parkinson, A. J., Muchmore, H. G., Scott, L. V., et al.: Parainfluenza virus upper respiratory tract illness in partially immune adult human subjects: A study at an Antarctic station. Am. J. Epidemiol. *110*:753–763, 1979.
143. Parkinson, A. J., Muchmore, H. G., Scott, E. N., et al.: Survival of human parainfluenza viruses in the South Polar environment. Appl. Environ. Microbiol. *46*:901–905, 1983.
144. Parrott, R. H., Vargosko, A. J., Kim, H. W., et al.: Acute respiratory diseases of viral etiology. III. Myxoviruses: Parainfluenza. Am. J. Public Health *52*:907–917, 1962.
145. Pereira, M. S., and Fisher, O. D.: An outbreak of acute laryngotracheobronchitis associated with parainfluenza 2 virus. Lancet *2*:790–791, 1960.
146. Phillips, M. J., Blendis, L. M., Poucell, S., et al.: Sporadic hepatitis with distinctive pathological features, a severe clinical course, and paramyxoviral features. N. Engl. J. Med. *324*:455–460, 1991.
147. Phillips, P. E., and Christian, C. L.: Myxovirus antibody increases in human connective tissue disease. Science *168*:982–984, 1970.
148. Porter, D. D., Prince, G. A., Hemming, V. G., et al.: Pathogenesis of human parainfluenza virus 3 infection in two species of cotton rats: *Sigmodon hispidus* develops bronchiolitis, while *Sigmodon fulviventer* develops interstitial pneumonia. J. Virol. *65*:103–111, 1991.
149. Povey, C.: *In vitro* antiviral efficacy of ribavirin against feline calcivirus, feline viral rhinotracheitis virus and canine parainfluenza virus. Am. J. Vet. Res. *39*:175–178, 1978.
150. Prinoski, K., Cote, M. J., Kang, C. Y., et al.: Evolution of the fusion protein gene of human parainfluenza virus 3. Virus Res. *22*:55–69, 1992.
151. Rabalais, G. P., Stout, G. G., Ladd, K. L., et al.: Rapid diagnosis of respiratory viral infections by using a shell vial assay and monoclonal antibody pool. J. Clin. Microbiol. *30*:505–508, 1992.
152. Ramakrishnan, I., and Agarwal, S. C.: Cell-mediated immunity in experimental parainfluenza type 3 virus infection. Med. Microbiol. *13*:527–534, 1980.
153. Ray, R., Galinski, M., and Compans, R. W.: Expression of the fusion glycoprotein of human parainfluenza type 3 virus in insect cells by a recombinant baculovirus and analysis of its immunogenic property. Virus Res. *12*:169–180, 1989.
154. Ray, R., Glaze, B. J., and Compans, R. W.: Role of individual glycoproteins of human parainfluenza virus type 3 in the induction of a protective immune response. J. Virol. *62*:783–787, 1988.
155. Ray, R., Novak, M., Duncan, J. D., et al.: Microencapsulated human parainfluenza virus induces a protective immune response. J. Infect. Dis. *167*:752–755, 1993.
156. Richardson, C. D., and Choppin, P. W.: Oligopeptides that specifically inhibit membrane fusion by paramyxoviruses: Studies on the site of action. Virology *131*:518–532, 1983.
157. Robinson, R. Q., Hoshiwara, I., Schaeffer, M., et al.: A survey of respiratory illnesses in a population. I. Viral studies. Am. J. Hyg. *75*:18–27, 1962.
158. Rocchi, G., Arangio-Ruiz, G., Giannini, V., et al.: Detection of viraemia in acute respiratory disease of man. Acta Virol. *14*:405–407, 1970.
159. Roman, G., Phillips, C. A., and Poser, C. M.: Parainfluenza viruses type 3: Isolation from CSF of a patient with Guillain-Barré syndrome. J. A. M. A. *240*:1613–1615, 1978.
160. Ruuskanen, O., Arola, M., Heikkinen, T., et al.: Viruses in acute otitis media: Increasing evidence for clinical significance. Pediatr. Infect Dis. J. *10*:425–427, 1991.
161. Rydbeck, R., Love, A., and Norrby, E.: Protective effects of monoclonal antibodies against parainfluenza virus type 3 induced brain infection in hamsters. J. Gen. Virol. *69*:1019–1024, 1988.
162. Sarkkihen, H. C., Haloren, P. E., Arstita, P. P., et al.: Detection of respiratory syncytial, parainfluenza type 3, and adenovirus antigens by radioimmunoassay and enzyme immunoassay in nasopharyngeal specimens from children with acute respiratory disease. J. Clin. Microbiol. *13*:258–265, 1981.
163. Singh-naz, N., Willy, M., and Riggs, N.: Outbreak of parainfluenza virus type 3 in a neonatal nursery. Pediatr. Infect. Dis. J. *9*:31–33, 1990.
164. Skolnik, N. S.: Treatment of croup: A critical review. Am. J. Dis. Child. *143*:1045–1049, 1989.
165. Smith, C. B., Purcell, R. H., Bellanti, J. A., et al.: Protective effect of antibody to parainfluenza type 1 virus. N. Engl. J. Med. *275*:1145–1152, 1966.
166. Spriggs, M. K., Olmsted, R. A., Venkatesan, S., et al.: Fusion glycoprotein of human parainfluenza virus type 3: Nucleotide sequence of the gene, direct identification of the cleavage-activation site, and comparison with other paramyxoviruses (published erratum appears in Virology *158*:263, 1987). Virology *152*:241–251, 1986.
167. Stout, C., Murphy, M. D., Lawrence, S., et al.: Evaluation of a monoclonal antibody pool for rapid diagnosis of respiratory viral infections. J. Clin. Microbiol. *27*:448–452, 1989.
168. Super, D. M., and Cartelli, N. A.: A prospective randomized double-blind study to evaluate the effect of dexamethasone in acute laryngotracheitis. J. Pediatr. *115*:323–329, 1989.
169. Sweet, B. H., Tyrell, A. A., Potash, L., et al.: Respiratory virus vaccine. III. Pentavalent respiratory syncytial–parainfluenza–*Mycoplasma pneumoniae* vaccine. Am. Rev. Resp. Dis. *94*:340–349, 1966.
170. ter Meulen, V., Koprowski, H., Iwasaki, Y., et al: Fusion of cultured multiple sclerosis brain cells with indicator cells: Presence of nucleocapsids and virions and isolation of parainfluenza-type virus. Lancet *2*:1–5, 1972.
171. Tremonti, L. P., Lin, J. S., and Jackson, G. G.: Neutralizing activity in nasal secretions and serum in resistance of volunteers to parainfluenza virus type 2. J. Immunol. *101*:572–577, 1968.
172. Tsurudome, M., Nishio, M., Komada, H., et al.: Extensive antigenic diversity among human parainfluenza 2 virus isolates and immunological relationships among paramyxoviruses revealed by monoclonal antibodies. Virology *171*:38–48, 1989.
173. Tunnessen, W. W., and Feinstein, A. R.: The steroid-croup controversy: An analytic review of methodologic problems. J. Pediatr. *96*:751–756, 1980.
174. Tyrrell, D. A. J., Bynoe, M. L., Birkum, K., et al.: Inoculation of human volunteers with parainfluenza viruses 1 and 3 (HA2 and HA1). Br. Med. J. *2*:909–911, 1959.
175. Ukkonen, P., Hovl, T., Von Bonsdorff, C. H., et al.: Age-specific prevalence of complement fixing antibodies to sixteen viral antigens: A computer analysis of 58,500 patients covering a period of 8 years. J. Med. Virol. *13*:131–148, 1984.
176. van der Logt, J. T., van Loon, A. M., Heessen, F. W., et al.: Diagnosis of parainfluenza virus infection in children and older patients by detection of specific IgM antibody. J. Med. Virol. *16*:191–199, 1985.
177. van Wyke Coelingh, K. L., Winter, C. C., Tierney, E. L., et al.: Attenuation of bovine parainfluenza virus type 3 in nonhuman primates and its ability to confer immunity to human parainfluenza virus type 3 challenge. J. Infect. Dis. *157*:655–662, 1988.
178. van Wyke Coelingh, K. L., Winter, C. C., Tierney, E. L., et al.: Antibody responses of humans and nonhuman primates to individual antigenic sites of the hemagglutinin-neuraminidase and fusion glycoproteins after primary infection or reinfection with parainfluenza type 3 virus. J. Virol. *64*:3833–3843, 1990.
179. Vella, P. P., Weibel, R. E., Woodhour, A. F., et al.: Respiratory virus vaccines. VIII. Field evaluation of trivalent parainfluenza virus vaccine among preschool children in families, 1967–1968. Am. Rev. Resp. Dis. *99*:526–541, 1969.
180. Vreede, R. W., Schellekens, H., and Zuijderwijk, M.: Isolation of parainfluenza virus type 3 from cerebrospinal fluid. J. Infect. Dis. *165*:1166, 1992.
181. Vuorinen, T., and Meurman, O.: Enzyme immunoassays for detection of IgG and IgM antibodies to parainfluenza types 1, 2, and 3. J. Virol. Methods *23*:63–70, 1989.
182. Wagener, J. S., Minnich, L., Sobonya, R., et al.: Parainfluenza type II infection in dogs: A model of viral respiratory tract infection in humans. Am. Rev. Resp. Dis. *127*:771–775, 1983.
183. Wechsler, S. L., Lambert, D. M., Galinski, M. S., et al.: Immediate persistent infection by human parainfluenza virus 3: Unique fusion properties of the persistently infected cells. J. Gen. Virol. *68*:1737–1748, 1987.
184. Welliver, R. C.: Advances in the understanding of croup. Pediatr. Virol. *2*:1–4, 1988.
185. Welliver, R. C., Sun, M., and Rinaldo, D.: Defective regulation of immune response in croup due to parainfluenza virus. Pediatr. Res. *19*:716–720, 1985.
186. Welliver, R., Wong, D. T., Choi, T. S., et al.: Natural history of parainfluenza virus infection in childhood. J. Pediatr. *101*:180–187, 1982.

187. Welliver, R. C., Wong D. T., Middleton, E., Jr., et al.: Role of parainfluenza virus–specific IgE in pathogenesis of croup and wheezing subsequent to infection. J. Pediatr. *101*:889–896, 1982.
188. Welliver, R. C., Wong, D. T., Sun, M., et al.: Parainfluenza virus bronchiolitis: Epidemiology and pathogenesis. Am. J. Dis. Child. *140*:34–40, 1986.
189. Wendt, C. H., Weisdorf, D. J., Jordan, M. C., et al.: Parainfluenza virus respiratory infection after bone marrow transplantation. N. Engl. J. Med. *326*:921–926, 1992.
190. Wenzel, R. P., McCormick, D. P., and Beam, W. E., Jr.: Parainfluenza pneumonia in adults. J. A. M. A. 221:294-295, 1972.
191. Wolinsky, J. S., and Gilden, D. H.: *In vivo* studies of parainfluenza I (6/94) virus: Mononuclear cell interactions. Arch. Virol. *49*:25–31, 1975.
192. Wong, V. K., Steinberg, E., and Warford, A.: Parainfluenza virus type 3 meningitis in an 11-month-old infant. Pediatr. Infect. Dis. J. *7*:300–301, 1988.
193. Wright, A. L., Taussig, L. M., Ray, C. G., et al.: The Tucson children's respiratory study. II. Lower respiratory tract illness in the first year of life. Am. J. Epidemiol. *129*:1232–1246, 1989.
194. Wroblewska, Z., Santoli, D., Gilden, D., et al: Persistent parainfluenza type 1 (6/94) infection of brain cells in tissue culture. Arch. Virol. *50*:287–303, 1976.
195. Yanagihara, R., and McIntosh, K.: Secretory immunological response in infants and children to parainfluenza types 1 and 2. Infect. Immun. *30*:23–28, 1980.
196. Yewdell, J., and Gerhard, W.: Delineation of four antigenic sites on a paramyxovirus glycoprotein via which monoclonal antibodies mediate distinct antiviral activities. J. Immunol. *128*:2570–2575, 1982.
197. Yurlova, T. I., Sverkunova, M. V., Furaeva, V. A., et al.: Studies of natural population variability of parainfluenza viruses during their epidemic circulation. Acta Virol. *25*:64–70, 1991.
198. Zach, M., Erban, A., and Olinsky, A.: Croup, recurrent croup, allergy, and airways hyperreactivity. Arch. Dis. Child. *56*:336–341, 1981.
199. Zach, M., and Messner, H.: Serum IgA in recurrent croup. Am. J. Dis. Child. *137*:184–185, 1983.
200. Zinserling, A.: Peculiarities of lesions in viral and mycoplasma infections of the respiratory tract. Virchows Arch. Pathol. Anat. *356*:259–273, 1972.
201. Zollar, L. M., and Mufson, M. A.: Acute parotitis associated with parainfluenza 3 virus infection. Am. J. Dis. Child. *119*:147–148, 1970.

183

MEASLES VIRUS

James D. Cherry

Measles virus is a singular agent that causes a relatively distinct, exanthematous disease characterized by fever, cough, coryza, conjunctivitis, an erythematous maculopapular confluent rash, and a pathognomonic enanthem. Clinical measles is an epidemic disease, the incidence of which in the United States has been reduced from 315 cases per 100,000 population in the prevaccine era to less than 2 per 100,000 since 1981 by the use of attenuated vaccines. However, measles still is a major problem because of its worldwide prevalence and its changing epidemiologic pattern in the United States and in those countries where vaccine use has been widespread.

HISTORY

In antiquity, measles and smallpox frequently were confused with each other as well as with other exanthematous diseases.[20, 265] Major epidemics of both measles and smallpox occurred 1800 years ago in the Roman Empire and in China.[30, 231] The first written record of measles generally is credited to Rhazes, a tenth century Persian physician[20, 30, 180, 365]; however, Rhazes quoted writers, including El Yahudi, a famous Hebrew physician, who lived 300 years earlier.[30] Rhazes identified measles as an entity distinct from smallpox.

During the Middle Ages in Europe, smallpox and measles continued to be confused. By the beginning of the seventeenth century, however, the differentiation between the two diseases was relatively clear; death reports of the parish clerks of London in 1629 listed measles and smallpox separately.[365] Repeated epidemics of measles were described in the English medical literature during the seventeenth and eighteenth centuries.[180]

The first account of measles in America was by John Hall, who described epidemic disease in Boston in the fall of 1657.[47] The next epidemic in Colonial America was reported in 1687. Over the next 150 years, the epidemic interval in Boston gradually decreased from 30 years to about 3 years. Epidemics during the seventeenth and eighteenth centuries involved persons of all ages, including neonates; coincident with the reduction in epidemic interval was a reduction in measles age incidence. The reduction in epidemic interval can be attributed to the increased importation of measles owing to more and faster ships crossing the Atlantic and the gradual increase in population density in North America. By the turn of the nineteenth century, both Boston and Philadelphia had sufficient populations for measles to propagate itself.

The first recognition of the contagiousness of measles is unclear. Shakespeare in *Coriolanus* was aware of its human-to-human transmission.[365] Home[161] in 1758 attempted to immunize against measles by a technique similar to variolation in smallpox.[293] In 1911, Goldberger and Anderson[128] produced clinical measles in monkeys by injecting filtered material from acute cases of human disease.

The classic epidemiologic study of measles was the account of the 1846 Faroe Islands epidemic by Panum.[284] In this study, Panum confirmed that spread solely was through human-to-human contagion via the respiratory route, the incubation period was 14 days, and infection conveyed lifelong immunity.

The enanthem of measles, which is pathognomonic, was described carefully and presented by Koplik in 1896, 1898, and 1899.[29, 193–195] However, it is clear that Koplik spots were recognized specifically about a century earlier by John Quier, a physician in Jamaica,[29, 126] and by Richard Hazeltine, a general practitioner in rural Maine.[47]

Although Plotz[294] reported cultivation of measles virus in 1938 and Rake and Shaffer[297] noted similar findings in 1940, reliable tissue culture methods were not available until about 10 years later. In 1954, Enders and Peebles[98] isolated eight agents (from cases of measles) in human or simian renal cell cultures. They also demonstrated the ability of convalescent-phase serum from a measles patient to neutralize the viral cytopathogenic effect. The stage for vaccine development was set by the tissue culture recovery of the virus,[98] the adaptation of viral growth in chicken embryos,[238] and, finally, the cultivation of the virus in chicken embryo tissue culture cells.[182]

After extensive trial from 1958 through 1962, tissue culture–grown inactivated ("killed") and attenuated ("live") measles viral vaccines became available for general use in 1963.[66, 181, 201] In the United States, a nationwide immunization effort was instituted in 1965 and 1966. This led to a dramatic reduction in epidemic measles for several years. Epidemic measles recurred in 1971, 1977, and 1989 but at lesser overall levels than in the prevaccine era.[56, 57, 66, 200] After the Childhood Immunization Initiative, which began in 1977, and the Measles Elimination Program, which began in 1978, the incidence of measles in the United States fell in 1981 to less than 1.5 cases per 100,000 population and remained at this low level until 1986.[49–51] In 1990, the rate was 11.2 cases per 100,000 population, which was the highest it had been since 1977. Since 1990, there has been a substantial decline in measles to an all-time low of 301 confirmed cases in 1995.[48] However, about 1 million children worldwide die of measles each year.[123, 279]

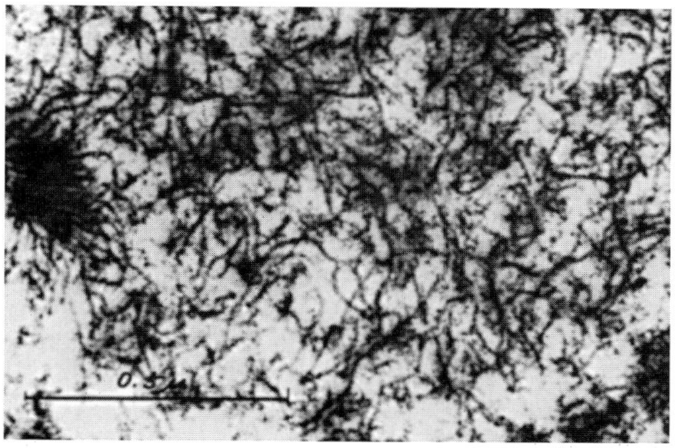

FIGURE 183–1. *Nucleocapsid fragments. Electron micrograph. (Courtesy of Dr. John M. Adams.)*

PROPERTIES

Classification

Measles virus is a relatively large virus with helical capsid symmetry and an RNA genome.[26, 100, 234] It is a singular virus, but antigenically it is related closely to canine distemper. These agents, as well as peste des petits ruminants virus and rinderpest virus, presently are included in the genus *Morbillivirus*; they are members of the family *Paramyxoviridae*. During the last decade, several candidate new members of the genus were recovered from aquatic mammals and horses.[26, 87, 253, 282, 320] Measles virus differs from the other paramyxoviruses in that it does not possess specific neuraminidase activity and it does not adsorb to neuraminic acid–containing cellular receptors.[247, 274, 291, 356] Measles virus hemagglutinates, whereas the other members of its genus do not.

Physical Properties

Measles virus is a roughly spherical but pleomorphic virus that ranges from 100 to 250 nm in diameter.[26, 100, 234, 258, 265, 356, 357] The virion is composed of an outer lipoprotein envelope and an internal helical nucleocapsid. The virion contains six structural proteins; three of these proteins are complexed with viral RNA, and three are related to the virus envelope. The outer viral envelope is 10 to 22 nm thick, has short surface projections (peplomers), and contains three virus-coded proteins (F, H, and M).[70, 247, 265] The F protein is a dumbbell-shaped peplomer that causes membrane fusion of virus and host cell and enables penetration of the virus into the host cell. The H protein is the hemagglutinin and is a conical peplomer. The M (matrix) protein is nonglycosylated and is associated with the inner lipid bilayer of the envelope. It plays an important role in virus maturation.

The nucleocapsid (N) protein (Fig. 183–1) is a coiled rod, with a diameter of 18 nm and a length of 1 μm, that contains the viral genomic RNA.[265, 268, 272, 354, 356] The N protein has a molecular weight of about 60 kDa. About 5 per cent of the nucleocapsid is RNA.[151, 348, 355] The other internal proteins of the virus are the L (large) and P (phospho) proteins, which are parts of the transcription complex.[265]

The virus genome has a molecular weight of 4.5×10^6 daltons; it is a linear, single strand of RNA that contains about 15,900 nucleotides.

Measles virus is labile.[179, 180, 254] It is inactivated rapidly by heat, ultraviolet light, lipid solvents such as ether and chloroform, and extreme degrees of acidity and alkalinity (i.e., pH <5 and >10). Longevity is prolonged when protein is in the viral suspending medium and when the virus is lyophilized with a protein stabilizer. Protein specifically protects against the adverse effects of heat and light. Protein-stabilized measles virus can be stored at −70° C for 5 or more years without significant loss of infectivity. At room temperature, there is a 60 per cent loss in titer in 3 to 5 days; inactivation occurs within 30 minutes at 56° C.[35, 254]

Antigenic Composition

Clinical and epidemiologic data and early laboratory study suggested antigenic homogeneity of all measles strains.[179] Recent nucleotide sequence analyses have identified distinct lineages among wild-type measles virus isolates.[26, 342] The following properties have been associated with measles virus: a hemagglutinin (for simian cells), complement-fixing antigens, hemolytic activity, and a giant cell–inducing factor.[41, 150, 179, 180, 266, 269, 273, 291, 319] Human measles virus infection results in serum antibodies that are capable of neutralizing viral infectivity, fixing complement with viral antigen, and inhibiting viral hemagglutination and hemolysis.

There is cross-seroreactivity among three members of the genus *Morbillivirus* but not with other members of the family *Paramyxoviridae*.[36, 44, 168] Measles virus serum antibody in humans reacts with distemper virus, but canine serum after distemper does not react with measles virus. A two-way cross between measles and rinderpest viruses has been demonstrated.

Tissue Culture Growth

Measles virus can be propagated in many different primary and cell line tissue cultures.[36, 179, 227] However, for isolation of virus from specimens from patients, primary human and monkey kidney cultures have been most successful over the years. In one study, an Epstein-Barr virus–transformed marmoset lymphocytic line (B95-8) was found to be superior to primary monkey kidney cell cultures for the isolation of virus from nasopharyngeal specimens.[190] In tissue culture, measles virus has two distinct cytopathogenic effects. With initial isolation, syncytial formation occurs; this is the result of cell fusion in which the resulting giant cells may contain 10 to 50 or more nuclei (Fig. 183–2). On stained preparation, both the nuclei and cytoplasm contain eosinophilic inclusions. The second form of cytopathogenic effect is characterized by the

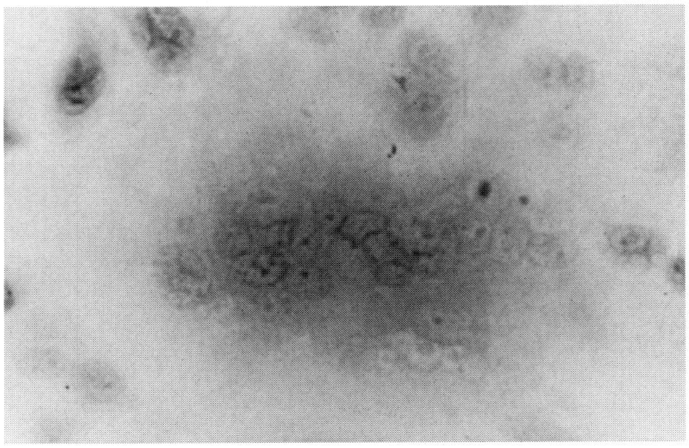

FIGURE 183–2. *Measles virus cytopathogenic effect in monkey kidney tissue culture. Giant cell with approximately 20 nuclei.*

alteration of single cells into spindle shapes or stellate forms. In general, tissue culture–adapted measles viral strains are more likely to cause this cytopathogenic effect than is giant cell formation. In most cultures, both forms of cytopathogenic effect are evident, and changes in medium composition make one or the other type predominate.

Infection in tissue culture is associated with an attachment-adsorption phase of about 1 hour and an eclipse period of 6 to 12 hours.[227, 247] Antigen first is noted in the cytoplasm perinuclearly at 12 hours; by 24 hours, it is noted throughout the cytoplasm. By 30 hours, most antigen is detected at the cell surface. In mature cultures, there is more cell-associated virus than is found free within the medium.

Animal Susceptibility

Humans are the natural hosts of measles virus, but with human contact, monkeys also are infected easily.[236] Laboratory strains of measles virus have been adapted to suckling mice and hamsters.[40, 45, 169, 352]

EPIDEMIOLOGY

Prevalence

The prevalence of measles throughout history has been affected markedly by population density and, during the last 33 years, by the use of measles vaccine. The reported cases of measles in the United States from 1960 to 1994, analyzed by year, are presented in Figure 183–3. After the widespread use of measles vaccine, which began in 1965, the number of cases in the United States fell to 22,231 in 1968.[48] In 1971 and 1977, modest epidemics occurred; then, after a national commitment to measles immunization, the number of cases of measles fell to an all-time low of 1497 cases reported in 1983. Beginning in 1986, the number of measles cases again increased, reaching 27,786 reported cases in 1990. Since 1990, measles in the United States has declined, reaching an all-time low of 301 cases in 1995.[48] In this century, before the widespread use of measles vaccine, between 200,000 and 600,000 cases of measles were reported annually in the United States.[75, 207] Careful survey suggests that reported cases account for only about 15 per cent of the actual number of cases of measles.[66]

In the prevaccine era in the United States and in other concentrated populations of the world, measles epidemics regularly occurred. In the United States, urban-centered measles epidemics occurred every 2 to 5 years, with each epidemic lasting 3 to 4 months.[20, 30, 148, 156, 214, 360, 373] In general, the larger the community size, the shorter the interval between epidemics. In the vaccine era, the epidemic pattern has been changed. As noted in Figure 183–3, the total number of cases has been reduced, and the cycle between peaks has lengthened.

Age Incidence and Prevalence

In modern times in populous areas, measles has been a disease of children. The age-specific incidence in the United States for selected years is presented in Table 183–1. In the prevaccine era during the twentieth century, the highest measles attack rate occurred in children 5 to 9 years of age.[20, 30, 156, 364] In the period 1960 and 1964, the data from five re-

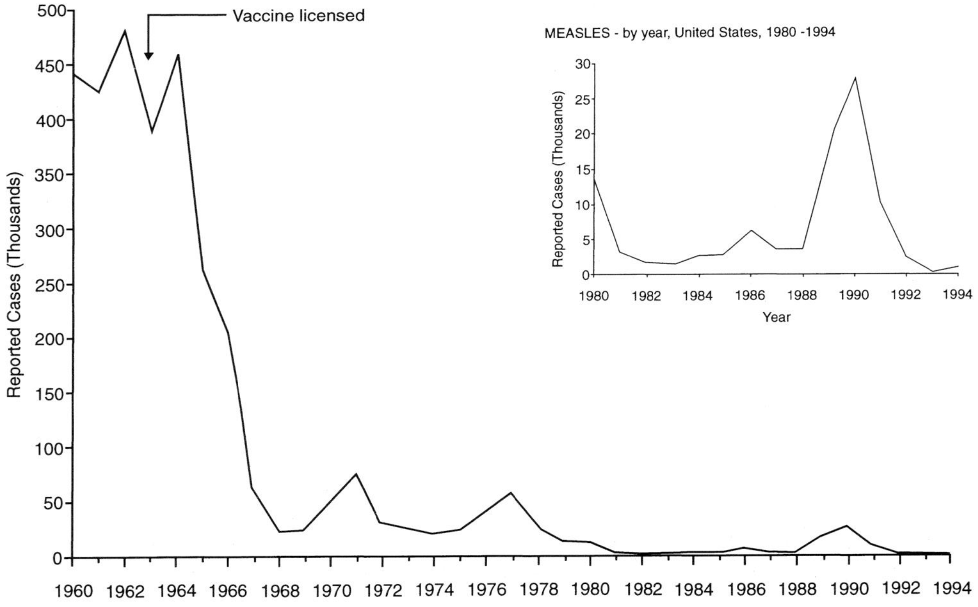

FIGURE 183–3. *Reported measles cases, by year—United States, 1960–1994. (From Centers for Disease Control and Prevention: Summary of notifiable diseases, United States 1994. M. M. W. R. 43:40, 1995.)*

TABLE 183–1. Incidence and Per Cent Distribution of Reported Measles Cases by Age Group in Selected Years, United States[50, 53, 57, 152]

Age Group	1960–64* Cases	1960–64* %	1960–64* Incidence†	1974 Cases	1974 %	1974 Incidence†	1979 Cases	1979 %	1979 Incidence†	1991 Cases	1991 %	1991 Incidence†
<1–4	93,653	37.2	766	5,899	26.7	36	2,331	20.7	18.0	4,756	49.3	24.7
5–9	132,956	52.8	1,237	5,391	24.4	30	2,473	21.9	18.1	991	10.2	5.5
10–14	16,403	6.5	169	7,799	35.3	38	3,054	27.1	20.4	905	9.4	5.3
15–19	8,635	3.4	10	2,475	11.2	12	2,633	23.3	15.2	1,102	11.4	6.2
20+				552	2.5	>1	786	7.0	0.6	1,890	19.6	1.8
Totals	251,647			22,094			11,277			9,643		

*Data from four reporting areas: Washington, D.C., New York City, Illinois (including Chicago), and Massachusetts.
†Incidence, cases per 100,000 population, extrapolated from age distribution of known cases.

porting areas showed that more than one-half of all measles cases occurred in this age group.[152] Before the present vaccine era, infections and epidemic loci centered in elementary schools. Younger children acquired measles as secondary cases from their school-attending older siblings. In rural areas, the interval between measles epidemics tended to be greater; therefore, there was a greater age spread in the percentage of measles cases. In a nationwide serum survey of U.S. military recruits in 1962, Black[32] found that 99 per cent had measles antibody.

As noted in Table 183–1, the age incidence and percentage of measles cases by age group have changed markedly since 1964. In 1991, more than 40 per cent of measles cases occurred in persons older than 10 years of age; in the period from 1960 to 1964, less than 10 per cent of the cases were older than 10 years of age. About one-third of the cases in 1991 were in adolescents and young adults. Evidence also indicates high primary measles attack rates in 0- to 4-year-old children in areas of suboptimal vaccine utilization.[48, 50, 66, 113, 154] In 1995, the number of reported measles cases was a historic low (301 cases); 39 per cent of the cases occurred in adults (20 years of age or older), and 11 per cent of the cases were international importations.[48] However, the study of measles virus genotypes suggests that the majority of cases of measles in the United States in 1994 and 1995 resulted from international importation of virus.[310]

In 1989 in the United States, the setting of measles transmission was the following: 46.8 per cent acquired measles in primary or secondary schools; 19.6 per cent in colleges or universities; 15.5 per cent at home; 6.1 per cent in medical settings; 2.2 per cent in day care; and 9.8 per cent in a variety of other settings, including work, church, and the military.[52] Of the 6880 patients with measles during the first 26 weeks of 1989, 51.2 per cent had been vaccinated on or after their first birthday. The age distribution of measles patients in 1989 by vaccine status is presented in Figure 183–4. Most vaccine failures occurred in 12- to 19-year-olds. Of the measles patients who were unvaccinated, the vaccine was indicated in 55.5 per cent; most of these cases occurred in children 16 months to 4 years of age and in persons 20 years of age or older.

Measles in heavily populated but underdeveloped countries has its greatest incidence in children younger than 2 years of age.[72, 107, 155, 250, 276]

Geographic Distribution

In the twentieth century, measles has occurred regularly throughout the world in all but the most remote areas.[20, 30] In island and other isolated populations, interepidemic periods can be 10 years or more, and disease occurrence depends on the introduction of disease from the outside.

Seasonal Patterns

Epidemic measles is a winter-spring disease in temperate climates, with peak activity in the Northern Hemisphere occurring in March or April. In equatorial regions, epidemics of measles are less marked but tend to occur in the hot, dry seasons.[20, 249, 305, 341]

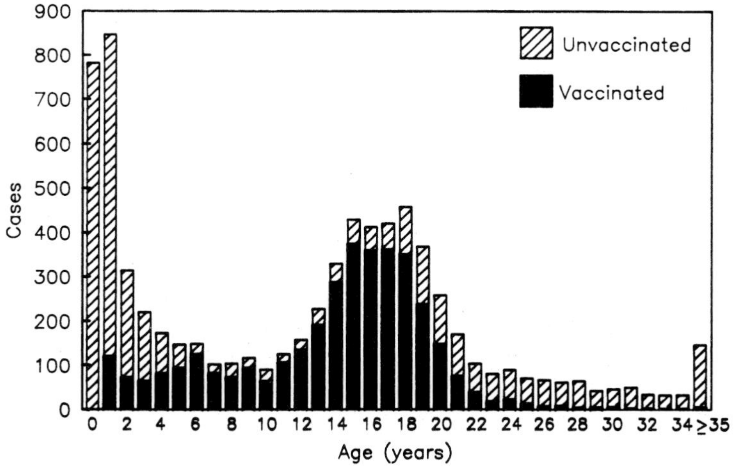

FIGURE 183–4. *Age distribution of measles patients, by vaccine status—United States, 1989. (From Centers for Disease Control: Measles: United States, first 26 weeks, 1989. M. M. W. R. 38:863–871, 1989.)*

Host and Social Factors

There is no difference between males and females in measles incidence. There is a suggestion, however, that complication rates are higher in males than in females. Tidstrom[344] found that acute laryngitis was more than twice as common in males as in females. In other studies, otitis media, pneumonia, and deaths were slightly more common in males.[20, 275] Miller,[237] in a large survey in England in 1963, found no difference in the incidence of complications between males and females. Christensen and associates,[71] in studies of an epidemic in Greenland, noted a greater number of complications in females among patients older than 15 years of age; this mainly was due to an increased incidence of pneumonia. In a review of 375 confirmed cases of subacute sclerosing panencephalitis, the male-to-female ratio was 2.4:1.[243] According to Black,[30] antibody titers are slightly higher in women than in men. Our studies involving young adults failed to reveal a similar sex difference in antibody levels, however.[329]

Recently, Green and associates[135] noted that a group of adult women had a higher postimmunization geometric mean antibody titer than did vaccinated men.

Measles susceptibility does not vary by race. Although severity of disease in certain populations appears to suggest differences based on race, this probably is the result of nutritional and other environmental factors. Deseda-Tous and associates[86] were unable to demonstrate any differences in measles antibody by HLA or ABO blood types.

In the prevaccine era, the age of patients at measles infection was related inversely to the number of siblings in the family.[20, 30, 369] In general, measles occurred at an earlier age in city dwellers and in lower socioeconomic classes, compared with rural families and well-educated upper income groups.

In the present era of antibiotics and other medical modalities, the greatest factors in measles morbidity and mortality are age and nutritional status. Measles mortality is highest in children younger than 2 years of age and in adults.[20, 30] Severity of measles and mortality correlate in general with the severity of malnutrition.[30, 276] However, extensive investigations by Aaby and others[2, 3, 122] during the last 15 years suggest that overcrowding and intensive exposure are more important determinants of measles mortality than is nutritional status.

Studies of measles early in the twentieth century and in developing countries have indicated that secondary cases in households are likely to be more severe than are primary cases.[1–3, 122] However, recent studies in the United States have found no difference in severity between primary and secondary cases in families.[42, 359]

Spread of Infection

Measles is a highly contagious disease in nonimmune persons. It is spread from the infected ill person to the new host by the respiratory route.[20, 30, 303, 304, 306] Although monkeys can acquire measles from humans, practically speaking there is no animal reservoir.[236] Available evidence suggests that infection is spread by persons ill with measles. Asymptomatic contagious carriers are unknown, and persons with acute asymptomatic infections probably are not contagious or are only minimally so. The period of greatest contagion occurs during the prodromal period.[128]

Transmission of measles is thought to occur mainly by aerosolized droplets of respiratory secretions. The acquisition of infection by the new host is by the nose and possibly the conjunctivae.[285] Infection can occur by small-droplet nuclei, which stay suspended in air for considerable periods, or by direct hits of large droplets at close range.[37, 301] It also seems possible that spread involves close person-to-person contact in young children, with large virus-containing droplets of nasal secretions being picked up on the hands of the future host and then applied to the nose.

PATHOGENESIS AND PATHOLOGY

Viral Infection

The sequence of viral events in uncomplicated measles is presented in Table 183–2.[138–140, 146, 177, 183, 188, 210, 264, 278, 290, 306, 312, 321, 371] Although much is known about measles virus infection in humans, considerable gaps exist regarding specific events. Experimental studies in other primates have been utilized in an attempt to fill in the gaps and therefore give a more complete picture.[177, 264, 278, 321, 371] The primary site of infection appears to be the respiratory epithelium of the nasopharynx. Measles vaccine virus instilled in the nose or by aerosol results in infection.[34, 197] Papp[285] reported studies suggesting that infection resulted from conjunctival contact and suggested that this was the primary portal of entry. However, experiments with vaccine virus generally have been unsuccessful when conjunctival inoculation has been carried out.[34] It appears that initial infection of the respiratory epithelium is minimal; a more important event is the early spread of virus to regional lymphatics. After this, it is presumed from data derived from Fenner's ectromelia-mouse experimental model[101] that primary viremia occurs. After initial viremia, extensive multiplication of virus occurs in the reticuloendothelial system at both regional and distant sites. Virus multiplication also continues at the site of initial infection.

During the fifth to seventh days of infection, extensive secondary viremia occurs, which results in the establishment of generalized measles viral infection. The skin, conjunctivae, and respiratory tract are obvious sites of infection, but other organs may be involved as well. From the eleventh to the fourteenth days, the viral content of the blood, respiratory tract, and other organs peaks and then rapidly diminishes over the ensuing 2- to 3-day period.

In immunologically compromised patients with defects of

TABLE 183–2. Sequence of Measles Virus Infection in Uncomplicated Primary Disease

Day	Event
0	Measles virus in droplet nuclei or large droplet comes in contact with the epithelial surface of the nasopharynx or possibly the conjunctiva
	Infection of epithelial cells and virus multiplication
1–2	Extension of infection to regional lymphoid tissue
2–3	Primary viremia
3–5	Multiplication of measles virus in respiratory epithelium at site of initial infection and in the reticuloendothelial system regionally and at distant sites
5–7	Secondary viremia
7–11	Establishment of infection in the skin and other viremic sites, including the respiratory tract
11–14	Virus in blood, respiratory tract, skin, and other organs
15–17	Viremia decreases and then ceases
	Viral content in organs rapidly diminishes

From references 138, 139, 146, 177, 183, 188, 210, 264, 278, 290, 306, 312, 321, 371.

cell-mediated factors, measles virus is not cleared from the secondary infection sites, and progressive, frequently fatal illnesses occur.[7, 97, 241, 242, 252]

During infection, measles virus replicates in endothelial cells, epithelial cells, and monocytes and macrophages.[140, 244] The cell receptor for measles virus infection is CD46 (membrane cofactor protein).[88, 218, 219, 259]

Pathology

The characteristic pathologic feature of measles is the widespread distribution of multinucleated giant cells, which are the result of cell fusion.[36, 177, 180, 210, 227, 264, 278, 307, 321, 371] Two main types of giant cells occur in measles: (1) the Warthin-Finkeldey cells, which are found in the reticuloendothelium, and (2) the epithelial giant cells (Fig. 183–5), which occur principally in the respiratory epithelium but also on other epithelial surfaces.[210]

Warthin-Finkeldey giant cells are found throughout the reticuloendothelial system in adenoids, tonsils, Peyer patches, appendix, lymph nodes, spleen, and thymus. They vary in size and contain up to 100 or more nuclei. The cells contain both cytoplasmic and intranuclear eosinophilic inclusions, with the cytoplasmic inclusions being more common than the intranuclear lesions.

During prodromal measles, epithelial giant cells regularly are present on respiratory surfaces and frequently are sloughed free (see Fig. 183–5).

Measles Exanthem

Hematoxylin and eosin–stained sections of skin biopsies have revealed typical epithelial syncytial giant cells with nuclear and cytoplasmic inclusions.[188, 338] The giant cells contain 3 to 26 nuclei. Other findings include the following: focal parakeratosis, dyskeratosis, spongiosis, and intracellular edema. The superficial blood vessels are dilated with a sparse, surrounding lymphohistiocytic infiltrate.

Koplik Spots

Suringa and colleagues[338] noted that the histopathologic features of Koplik spots were similar to those of the skin rash. They noted more giant cells with more nuclei, a greater degree of edema, and a lessened inflammatory response in the enanthem biopsy, however.

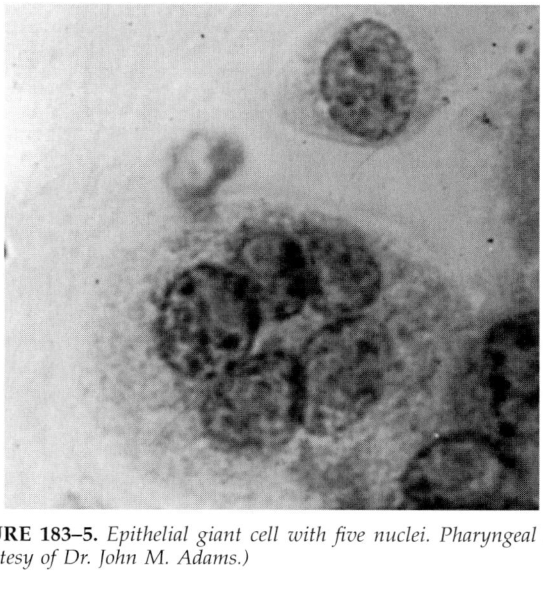

FIGURE 183–5. *Epithelial giant cell with five nuclei. Pharyngeal smear. (Courtesy of Dr. John M. Adams.)*

Respiratory Tract

The extent of respiratory involvement in uncomplicated measles is not known. However, clinical symptoms and the extensive radiographic studies of Kohn and Koiransky[192] suggest that pharyngitis, tracheitis, bronchitis, and pulmonary infiltration are the rule rather than the exception. Unfortunately, the human pathologic data available have been obtained mainly from complicated cases, so that the findings cannot be considered representative.[84, 307] In a study in monkeys, Nii and colleagues[264] noted giant cells in the mucosal epithelium of the trachea, bronchi, and bronchioli. The lumina of these airways contained sloughed syncytial cells. Warthin-Finkeldey cells were found in the adjacent lymphatics.

In the lungs of experimentally infected monkeys, interstitial pneumonitis was observed with giant-cell formation.[264] Infiltration of neutrophils, eosinophils, and mononuclear cells also was noted.

Immunologic Events

After natural or attenuated measles virus infection, a large number of specific and nonspecific immunologic responses occur. There still are many unanswered questions relating to immunity in measles, but on the other hand, a considerable body of knowledge has been gathered over the last 45 years.

Antibody

After measles viral infection, an antibody response regularly occurs. Serum antibodies to N, F, H, and M proteins of measles virus can be demonstrated after infection.[119, 133, 202, 267, 269] The presence of serum antibody can be demonstrated by hemagglutination inhibition (HI), complement fixation (CF), neutralization, immune precipitation, hemolysin inhibition (HLI), enzyme-linked immunosorbent assay (ELISA), and fluorescent antibody (FA) methods.[119, 133, 189, 202, 260] Antibody-dependent cellular cytotoxicity (ADCC) and antibody-dependent complement-mediated lysis (ADCML) also can be demonstrated by chromium-release assays.[111, 112, 186] In natural infection, HI and neutralizing antibodies appear at about the fourteenth day, peak at about 4 to 6 weeks, and decrease about fourfold from the peak over a year's time. The vast majority of naturally infected persons have demonstrable HI and neutralizing antibodies for life. Krugman[200] noted an average 16-fold reduction in HI antibody titer 15 years after natural infection in a group of children who had no measles exposure during the observation period.

After immunization, both HI and neutralizing antibodies are present by the fourteenth day.[119, 202] CF antibody appears slightly later than HI antibody and in general does not persist as long as either HI or neutralizing antibody. Primary infection is characterized by the initial appearance of antibody in the IgM and IgG serum components.[109, 157, 317, 318, 346] The IgM-specific response is short-lived, and rarely can measles antibody in this fraction be demonstrated more than 9 weeks after infection.

IgA secretory antibody also regularly occurs after vaccine viral infection and after natural infection.[25, 116]

IgG antibody appearing after infection primarily is subclasses IgG-1 and IgG-4.[225] Antibody detected by neutralization and by HI mainly is to the H protein and correlates with clinical protection against illness.[140, 269] Antibody to the N protein is the main antibody detected by CF.[269] Antibody to fusion protein is demonstrated by inhibition of the hemolysis of monkey erythrocytes by measles virus or by immunoprecipitation.[266, 267] Antibody to F protein may contribute to neutralization by disrupting the fusion of virus membrane with host-cell membranes. Only small amounts of antibody to M protein are elicited after infection with wild virus or vaccine virus.[133]

Specific Cell-Mediated Responses

It was recognized 30 years ago that patients with defective cellular resistance factors frequently died of progressive measles virus infections.[257] Twenty years ago, techniques became available that demonstrated measles-specific lymphocyte sensitization.[121, 134, 136, 196, 205, 311] Graziano and colleagues[134] found that lymphocytes in vitro from persons who previously had measles had a blastogenic response when they were incubated with measles antigen. Labowskie and associates,[205] utilizing an in vitro lymphocyte-mediated cytotoxicity assay, noted that lymphocytes from persons who previously had measles caused cell destruction in a tissue culture chronically infected with measles virus. Ruckdeschel and colleagues[311] observed that two physicians without detectable measles antibody, who had had repeated recent exposure to measles without illness, had strong in vitro cellular responsiveness to measles virus. Krause and associates[196] demonstrated excessive measles-specific lymphocyte blastogenic responses in some persons previously immunized with killed measles vaccine.

Today it is appreciated that T cells are important in both the B-cell antiviral antibody responses and as effector cells for the clearance of virus-infected cells from tissues.[140] Both helper (CD4+) and suppressor (CD8+) cells participate in the cellular response.[353] During infection, CD8+ T cells eliminate virus-infected cells by major histocompatibility complex class I–restricted cytotoxic mechanisms.[140] CD4+ T cells respond to measles virus infection by the secretion of cytokines. Upon initial virus exposure, CD4+ T cells respond with a Th-1 response. Before rash occurs, there is an increase in plasma interferon-gamma (INF-γ), and with rash, interleukin-2 (IL-2) appears. With clinical recovery, plasma levels of IL-4 increase (a Th-2 response) and stay elevated for several weeks, whereas the initial Th-1 responses subside.

Upon re-exposure, Th-1 and Th-2 responses occur as indicated by the production of INF-γ, IL-2 and tumor necrosis factor–beta (TNF-β), IL-4, IL-5, and IL-10. The Th-1 cytokine response is important for macrophage activation (due to INF-γ), lymphocyte proliferation (due to IL-2), and major histocompatibility complex class II–restricted cytotoxicity (due to TNF-β). The Th-2 cytokine response is important for macrophage deactivation (due to IL-4 and IL-10) and B-cell help (due to IL-4, IL-5, and IL-10).

Other Responses

Listed in Table 183–3 are nonspecific, immunologically related responses that can be demonstrated during natural or vaccine measles virus infections. Anderson and colleagues[14] demonstrated a temporary defect in neutrophil motility during acute measles that resolved by the eleventh day after the onset of rash. Leukopenia has been observed in natural measles[27] and after immunization.[31] With immunization, both neutrophil and lymphocyte numbers are reduced; this reduction lasts about 1 week, with its onset about 7 days after vaccination. Coovadia and colleagues[76, 77] have shown that the numbers of T, B, and null cells of the lymphocyte population are reduced. With the reduction of the number of T lymphocytes, there is no change in the ratio between helper-cell and suppressor cytotoxic-cell phenotypes.[9, 16, 175]

Thrombocytopenia occasionally has been associated with natural measles[166] and vaccination.[10, 362] Oski and Naiman[281] noted a mild reduction in the peripheral platelet count during routine measles immunization. Transitory complement defects vary in measles; Charlesworth and associates[59] noted evidence of pathologic complement activation in 20 of 50 patients studied. Coovadia and colleagues[76] noted slight but significant reductions in serum IgA levels and elevations of IgM values in acute measles virus infections. They found the IgG concentrations to be normal. Increased levels of serum or plasma IgE have been noted in two studies.[144, 322] Delayed hypersensitivity responses in skin are suppressed in both natural and vaccine measles virus infections[104, 331]; similarly, in vitro lymphocyte blastogenic responses to common antigens are suppressed.[363]

TABLE 183–3. Nonspecific, Immunologically Related Responses During Measles Virus Infection

Category	Finding	Reference
Leukocytes	Defective neutrophil motility	14
	Leukopenia (both lymphocytes and neutrophils)	27, 30
	Decreased T, B, and null lymphocytes	9, 16, 76, 77, 175
	Decreased natural killer–cell activity	141
	Decreased helper T cells	82, 187
	Prolonged depression of virus-specific interferon-alpha production	258a
Interferon-alpha	Elevated plasma levels	143
Neopterin	Elevated plasma levels	143
Interleukin-2 receptor (soluble)	Elevated plasma levels	142
Platelets	Reduction in peripheral count	281
Complement	Frequent pathologic activation of the complement system; reduction of C1q, C4, C3, and C5	59
Serum immunoglobulins	IgA reduced and IgE and IgM elevated	76, 144, 322
In vitro lymphocyte response to phytohemagglutinin	Suppressed in presence of autologous serum; normal in presence of calf serum	361
In vitro lymphocyte response to *Candida*	Suppressed	361
Cutaneous delayed hypersensitivity	Depressed	104
C-reactive protein	Elevated at onset of rash	145
Circulating immune complexes	Noted in 25% of patients 7 to 13 days after rash onset	377

Mechanisms in Recovery from Measles Viral Infection

Acute clinical measles is characterized by viral multiplication in many organs of the body, then rapid subsidence of the infection by the seventeenth day. As noted earlier, measles virus infection is associated with both serum and secretory antibody responses and specific cell-mediated responses that coincide with clinical recovery. It would appear that all three factors should be important in recovery in acute measles virus infection, but confusing bits of information cloud the issue. For example, it has been noted that children with simple agammaglobulinemia who do not develop measurable measles antibodies with measles virus infection recover from the disease normally.[130] This finding suggests that measles antibody development is not important for recovery from acute infection. However, utilizing a sensitive plaque-reduction measles neutralizing antibody technique, Black[33] found small amounts of antibody in the sera of three agammaglobulinemic patients.

In contrast with antibody data, it is clear that patients with defects in the cell-mediated immune system do poorly with measles virus infections and frequently succumb to progressive infection, despite administration of large doses of measles antibody–containing immunoglobulin. T cells (both CD4+ and CD8+) clear virus-infected cells from tissues by cytotoxicity. INF-α, which is released by a variety of cells, including T cells, inhibits spread of virus infection.

Mechanisms in Prevention of Repeat Illness in Persons Previously Infected with Measles Virus

In contrast with mechanisms of recovery in acute measles, the role of serum antibody in the protection against recurrent disease is solid. Before the present vaccine era, it was demonstrated repeatedly that the administration of measles antibody containing immunoglobulin could prevent clinical measles.[171, 336] Similarly, infants with transplacentally acquired measles antibody are immune.[202] Whether other factors also are important in the protection against reinfection is not clear. It often is cited that patients with agammaglobulinemia do not have repeated measles virus infections, so other factors must be involved.[130] Ruckdeschel and colleagues[311] reported two physicians who frequently were exposed to measles but in whom no serum antibody could be demonstrated. Both of these subjects had measles-specific cell-mediated responses.

It is of interest that patients have been described in whom antibody after immunization with killed measles vaccine did not prevent atypical measles.[212] The data of Krause and associates[196] suggest that persons in whom the capacity for exaggerated measles-specific lymphocyte activity persists (some previous killed-vaccine recipients) may be subject to illness in spite of the presence of antibody. However, the antibody after killed measles vaccine was incomplete; it lacked specific antibody to the F protein.[70] Black[33] noted one child with a low measles neutralizing antibody titer, presumably from natural measles virus infection, who later developed measles. Chen and coinvestigators[61] found that some students with measurable but low neutralizing antibody titers were not protected from clinical measles upon exposure.

CLINICAL MANIFESTATIONS

Before the present vaccine era, measles was an inevitable disease of childhood that was recognized readily by parents and other lay persons as well as by physicians. Although occasional confusion with other exanthematous diseases occurred,[68] the epidemic character of measles usually resulted in accurate diagnosis. Currently in North America, the epidemiologic pattern of measles has changed, as has the general knowledge of the disease by a new generation of parents, physicians, and other medical personnel.

Typical Illness[20, 63, 66, 180, 199, 306, 335]

Incubation Period

The incubation period of measles is about 10 (8 to 12) days. Although extensive virologic and immunologic events are occurring during this period, there virtually is no outward sign of illness. Goodall[131] suggested (and Partington and Quinton[286] have presented supporting data) that some patients have mild transient respiratory symptoms and fever shortly after initial acquisition of the virus.

Prodromal Period

The prodrome of measles lasts about 3 (2 to 4) days. Initial symptoms are respiratory and suggest the possibility of a cold except for the fact that fever is an early sign. In fact, in situations of close observation, slight temperature elevation has occurred and then subsided for a day or two before the appearance of typical respiratory symptoms.[335]

The onset of clinical measles is characterized by general malaise, fever, coryza, conjunctivitis, and cough. These symptoms worsen over a 2- to 4-day period. Early in the prodromal period, a transitory rash occasionally has been observed. This has been urticarial or macular, has occurred with the initial onset of fever, and has disappeared before the onset of the typical exanthem.

During the prodromal period, the temperature increases gradually to a value of 39.5° ± 1.1° C (103° ± 2° F) over a 4-day period. The nasal symptoms are similar to those of other respiratory viral infections and similar to those of the common cold or acute nasopharyngitis. Sneezing, rhinitis, and congestion are common. The degree of prodromal conjunctivitis varies considerably. Initially, the conjunctival injection is divided by a transverse marginal line across the lower lids.[334] The conjunctivitis is associated with considerable lacrimation, and older patients in particular are bothered by photophobia, which frequently is severe. Slit-lamp examination reveals both corneal and conjunctival lesions.[19, 106]

The cough in prodromal measles frequently is troublesome. It worsens throughout the period and often has a brassy quality, suggesting laryngeal and tracheal involvement. On about day 10 ± 1, Koplik spots, the pathognomonic enanthem of measles, first appear (see Fig. 67–1). Koplik[193–195] originally described the lesions as bluish-white specks on a bright-red mucosal surface. In my experience, the lesions always have appeared white, and a blue component has not been observed. Koplik spots first appear on the buccal mucosa opposite the lower molars but usually quickly spread to involve most of the buccal and lower labial mucosa. The lesions initially are about 1 mm in size but occasionally seem to coalesce into larger lesions. Initially there are only a few lesions, but within 12 hours the number usually is uncountable. Of equal importance in diagnosis is the appearance of the background mucosal surface. This always is bright red and granular. Frequently, 1-mm lesions (Fordyce aphthae), which commonly occur normally in adolescents and adults, are confused with Koplik spots.[69] These lesions, however, can be differentiated easily because they appear on a normal pale mucosal surface rather than the bright red background of measles.

During the prodromal period, erythematous maculopapular lesions also are observed occasionally on the palate. At the end of the prodromal period, the posterior pharyngeal wall usually is erythematous and injected, and the patient may complain of a sore throat.

Exanthem Period

In typical measles, the exanthem appears on about the fourteenth day after exposure. The exanthem occurs at about the peak of the respiratory symptoms and when the temperature usually is about 39.5° C (103° F). At this time the Koplik spots have peaked, and over the next 3 days they disappear. However, after the specific white spots have disappeared, the red, sandpapery mucosal background still is present for a day or two.

The measles exanthem first appears behind the ears and on the forehead at the hair line. The spread of the rash is centrifugal from the head to the feet. By the third day, the rash sequentially has involved the face, neck, trunk, upper extremities, buttocks, and lower extremities. The rash initially is erythematous and maculopapular but progresses to confluence in the same centrifugal manner as it is spread. Confluence always is more prominent on the face; frequently, the lesions on the lower extremities remain discrete. At the height of the rash, the appearance suggests microvesicles on top of a generalized erythematous confluent base (see Fig. 67–2).

The exanthem begins to clear on the third to fourth day, again following the centrifugal course of progression. During the initial stages of the rash, its color is red and it readily blanches on pressure. As the rash fades, it takes on a coppery appearance. After this, brownish discoloration occurs that does not clear with pressure. With healing, a fine desquamation frequently occurs in confluent areas with brownish discoloration. The duration of the exanthem usually is 6 to 7 days.

During the exanthem period, the fever usually peaks on about the second or third day of the rash and then falls by lysis over a 24-hour period. Fever that persists after the third or fourth day of exanthem usually is an indication of a complication. Conjunctivitis and nasal symptoms usually subside at about the time of defervescence. Continued nasal discharge, whether purulent or not, suggests bacterial secondary infection. With the appearance of the rash, the cough loosens up, and in older persons it frequently becomes productive. It is not uncommon for the cough to persist for 10 days or more.

Pharyngitis is common during the exanthem period, as is cervical lymph node enlargement. Generalized lymphadenopathy with suboccipital and postauricular involvement is not an uncommon finding, nor is splenomegaly. Young children occasionally have diarrhea, vomiting, laryngitis, and croup. Abdominal pain also can be troublesome.

Laboratory Findings

Laboratory studies rarely are indicated in acute uncomplicated typical measles because the diagnosis can be established on a clinical and epidemiologic basis and the results of studies rarely affect patient management. During the periods of prodrome and rash, the total leukocyte count is low. The numbers of neutrophils and lymphocytes are reduced, but the most marked reduction, when absolute counts are considered, is in the number of lymphocytes.[27] In difficult cases, such as the first apparent case in a particular locality, specific diagnosis can be made by serologic study. This is done most easily by measles CF or HI antibody studies. If an acute serum sample is obtained during the prodrome and a second serum sample is obtained 7 to 10 days later, a fourfold antibody titer rise usually is demonstrated. At the time of the rash, the identification of measles antibody in the IgM fraction also is a useful test.

Modified Illness[20, 23, 61, 64, 66, 93, 120, 171, 199, 302, 316]

Modified measles is an infection that occurs in the partially immune person. It is characterized by a generally mild illness that usually follows the regular sequence of events in measles. The prodromal period is shorter; cough, coryza, and fever are minimal. Koplik spots are few and transient; they frequently do not occur. The exanthem follows the progression pattern of regular measles, but confluence of the lesions does not occur. Because serologic studies reveal some children with measles antibody who had never had clinical disease suggestive of measles, it is probable that some modified infections occur without exanthem and perhaps without overt symptoms at all.[33, 203]

Modified measles occurs under a variety of circumstances, the most important of which historically was the result of intentional disease alteration by the administration of immune serum globulin to the exposed susceptible child. Naturally occurring modified measles occasionally is seen in infants younger than 9 months of age because of the presence of transplacentally acquired maternal measles antibody.

Although the magnitude of the problem is unknown, modified measles also occurs as an occasional manifestation of live vaccine failure. In these instances, patients have had modified illness but demonstrated a secondary measles serum antibody response (only IgG antibody).[64, 66, 327] With increasing time from immunization, it is possible that this will occur more frequently.[85] However, there currently are few data to support this possibility.

Recurrent measles also rarely results in modified illness. The frequency of recurrent measles is unknown. In general, most authorities have discounted recurrent measles and suggested that the recorded experiences were the result of confusion due to infections with other exanthem-producing agents.[68, 132] However, Cherry and colleagues,[66] Schaffner and colleagues,[315] and Schluederberg[317] have described children with modified illnesses, secondary immunologic responses, and well-documented instances of previous measles.

Atypical Measles

Atypical measles is a clearly defined clinical syndrome that occurs in some previously immunized persons after exposure to natural measles. The overwhelming majority of cases have occurred in persons who initially received inactivated (killed) measles viral vaccines, but some cases also have been noted in children who received only live measles vaccines.[65, 212, 261]

Historical Aspects

Initial studies with inactivated measles vaccines in the early 1960s demonstrated that multiple doses were necessary for the stimulation of an antibody response and that measurable serum antibody levels were short-lived.[120, 147, 178, 202, 366] In the initial trials, it soon became apparent that some killed-vaccine study participants still were susceptible to measles. On exposure to natural measles, some children developed typical measles and others, a mild modified illness.[120] Because of this, regimens were developed in which children were immunized with two or three doses of killed vaccine at monthly intervals, followed in a month or more by a single dose of Edmonston B live measles vaccine (KKL or KKKL). Studies at the time demonstrated good antibody levels after both regimens. After measles vaccine licensure in 1963, killed-live measles vaccine regimens enjoyed modest popularity in the United States (as well as in other countries) because live Edmonston B strain vaccine frequently was associated with alarming febrile responses and occasional febrile convulsions.

In 1965, Rauh and Schmidt[299] reported the occurrence of an unusual illness after exposure to natural measles in some children who had received killed vaccine 2 years previously. The significance of their findings became more apparent during the following 2 years when Fulginiti and colleagues[118] and Nader and colleagues[256] noted many instances of "atypical measles" in previous recipients of KKK and KKL vaccination regimens. In these two instances, original immunization had taken place 4 to 6 years before the occurrence of atypical illness.

In 1968, killed measles vaccine was taken off the market in the United States after the distribution of approximately 1.8 million doses of the vaccine in the period from 1963 to 1968.[280] During the 23-year period from 1968 to 1991, atypical measles was observed frequently.[15, 39, 60, 117, 127, 149, 159, 165, 208, 228, 239, 261, 263, 270, 358, 359, 374, 375] Presently, it is a disease of adults and it likely is misdiagnosed because the history of killed measles vaccine is not uncovered and specific antibody studies are not performed. I have observed one 26-year-old physician and a 28-year-old nurse with the syndrome.

In 1971, during study of an extensive measles epidemic, Cherry and colleagues[65] observed six children who had relatively mild atypical measles-like illnesses but who had received only live measles vaccines. Linnemann and colleagues[212] also noted two children with atypical measles-like illnesses who had received only live measles vaccines. Nichols[261] and St. Geme and associates[333] also have reported bizarre measles illnesses in former live vaccine recipients.

Clinical Characteristics[39, 61, 63, 65, 117, 118, 127, 149, 159, 165, 208, 228, 239, 256, 261, 263, 270, 271, 299, 358, 359, 374, 375]

Atypical measles was a common illness from 1967 to 1978. Because killed measles vaccines have not been available in the United States for the last 19 years, two obvious facts need to be mentioned: with each passing year, potential patients and actual patients with atypical measles will be 1 year older and also 1 year farther from the time of primary killed measles vaccine immunization series. Both of these aspects raise concern about whether the clinical manifestations of the syndrome will remain the same today as when the illness first was described. It was my opinion in 1981 that the syndrome had changed slightly but still was recognizable from the original illness descriptions.[63]

The incubation period of atypical measles is similar to that of typical measles—between 7 and 14 days in duration. The prodromal period is characterized by the sudden onset of high fever (39.5° to 40.6° C; 103° to 105° F) and usually headache. Abdominal pain and myalgia also are common complaints. Dry, nonproductive cough is noted in most and vomiting in about a third of those afflicted. Pleuritic chest pain and weakness also are common complaints. Although there are a few reports to the contrary, Koplik spots appear to be rare in atypical measles.

Two to 3 days after the onset of the illness, the rash appears. It is unique in that it first appears on the distal extremities and progresses in a cephalad direction. The rash usually initially is erythematous and maculopapular. I have been impressed by a slight yellowish hue to the exanthem, compared with that of typical measles. The rash particularly is prominent on the wrists and ankles; it involves the palms and soles. The spread of the rash varies considerably. In some patients, only the wrists and ankles are involved, whereas in others, the entire extremities as well as the lower trunk are affected. In a peculiar fashion, the rash frequently seems to end its cephalad progression in a line at the level of the nipples. Occasionally, a few erythematous, maculopapular but discrete lesions are on the face. In some cases, the rash becomes vesicular, with the lesions being about 2 to 3 mm in diameter; they do not go on to scab formation as in varicella, but occasionally pruritus is a problem so that excoriation occurs from scratching. The exanthem frequently has a petechial or purpuric component, and urticaria also is frequent. Edema of the extremities has been a frequent finding.

Although coryza has been noted in a few reports, it is not a prominent finding, nor is conjunctivitis. Respiratory distress with dyspnea and rales is common, and radiographic examination reveals pulmonary involvement in virtually all cases. Most patients have hilar adenopathy and pneumonia. Pleural effusion also is common. The pneumonia in atypical measles usually is lobular or segmental, with the lesions frequently appearing nodular (Fig. 183–6). Although the initial descriptions of the syndrome suggested an illness of about a week's duration, more recent observations indicate illnesses of 2 weeks or more. In one case, fatigue and other symptoms persisted for more than 1½ years.

In the original description by Rauh and Schmidt,[299] one patient had an exanthem that was biphasic; initially, a transitory rash suggested modified measles. Two weeks later, the more typical atypical exanthem developed. The same observers also noted a second case with a biphasic exanthem in which the first lesions were vesicular and occurred when the child had little fever. The second exanthem was maculopapular and associated with a febrile response. Zahradnik and colleagues[375] also noted a similar sequence in two young adults. Two patients who had received killed measles vaccine in the past have had radiographic evidence of characteristic pulmonary findings but have not developed the typical exanthem.[270, 374]

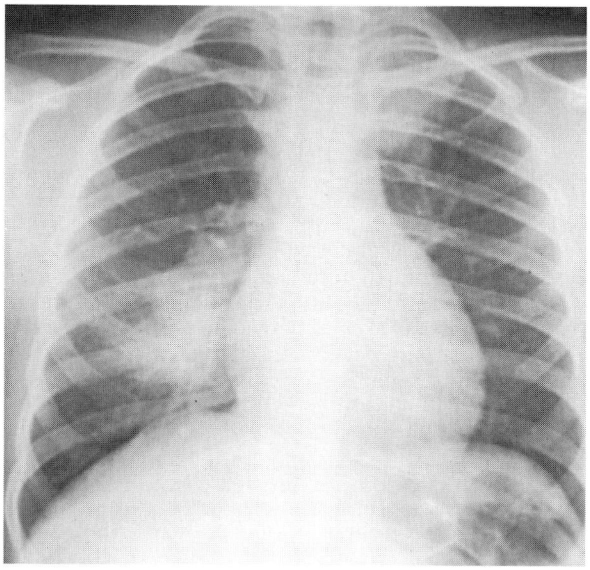

FIGURE 183–6. *Nodular pulmonary infiltrates in a child with atypical measles.*

Other findings in atypical measles include marked hepatosplenomegaly,[299] marked hyperesthesia,[256] weakness,[208] and numbness and paresthesia.[228] Personal observations of cases in adolescents and young adults suggest that the exanthem is less prominent than in past cases and the fever and overall morbidity are of greater duration.[63] Follow-up radiographic studies have demonstrated the persistence of nodular pulmonary lesions for more than 1 year in several patients and up to 6 years in one patient.[208, 239, 374]

Measles antibody studies in atypical measles are remarkably diagnostic. If an initial serum is obtained before or at the onset of the exanthem, the CF and HI titers usually are less than 1:5. By the tenth day of illness, both titers are elevated markedly, with most being greater than or equal to 1:1280. In contrast, in typical natural measles at the tenth day of illness, the titer rarely is greater than 1:160.

To date, measles virus has not been recovered from a patient with atypical measles, but only a few adequately performed studies have been carried out. Epidemiologic data presently available suggest that patients with atypical measles are not contagious. Other laboratory studies are not particularly useful in atypical measles. The erythrocyte sedimentation rate is elevated. When serial blood counts have been performed, slight early leukopenia and late eosinophilia have been noted.[118]

Unusual Manifestations and Complications of Measles

In addition to typical measles, modified measles, and atypical measles, there are many other clinical manifestations and complications that have a broad range of frequency. By definition, unusual manifestations are the direct result of the primary viral infection, whereas complications are the result of damage by a secondary infection with another microorganism. In many instances, it is difficult to determine whether a particular manifestation is just viral or involved with a second agent. Combinations of infections are common.

In general, complications due to secondary infections are not as common today as they were before the antibiotic era; there is no evidence to suggest that unusual manifestations of illness are less frequent today than formerly. To demonstrate the magnitude of the problem today, the findings in a 1970–1971 hospital survey in St. Louis are revealing.[66, 67] In this period, an extensive epidemic with 10,000 cases of measles occurred. In eight area hospitals, 130 children (1.3 per cent) were admitted; 66 cases of pneumonia with 6 fatalities occurred, and 6 children had encephalitis.

The records of measles patients in three hospitals were reviewed carefully. Of this group of 71 patients, 53 had pneumonia; 37 of the pneumonia patients had either previous cardiorespiratory or other chronic systemic disorders. Two children had mediastinal and subcutaneous emphysema. All six deaths were due to fulminant pneumonia. Of the six children with encephalitis, three developed severe residual neurologic damage. One child had acute measles appendicitis with perforation and peritonitis, and another patient had mesenteric lymphadenitis.

Pneumonia

Pulmonary involvement in measles, due to the viral infection, probably is the rule rather than the exception. Kohn and Koiransky[192] performed careful radiographic studies in 130 children with measles and noted that 55 per cent had pneumonic infiltration and 74 per cent had hilar adenopathy. In the majority of instances, the pneumonia was observed early in the course of the illness, which suggested primary viral involvement rather than secondary bacterial infection. In the 1970–1971 St. Louis measles epidemic, about 1 in every 150 patients with measles was hospitalized because of pneumonia.

Pneumonia in measles has varied radiographic manifestations.[5, 67, 137, 192, 213, 217, 224, 275, 340] Clearly, viral pneumonia is characterized by bilateral hyperinflation with diffuse fluffy infiltrates that are more confluent at the hilum. Unilateral, segmental, and lobar pneumonias also are observed. Gremillion and Crawford[137] reviewed 106 instances of pneumonia that occurred in 3220 cases of measles in Air Force recruits between 1976 and 1979. Illnesses were severe, but no deaths occurred. Bacterial superinfection was documented in 30.3 per cent of the cases; bronchospasm occurred in 17 per cent of the recruits with pneumonia. In one study, seven children with massive and bilateral lung consolidations had clinical findings consistent with adult respiratory distress syndrome.[5]

Clinically, young infants have a picture of bronchiolitis with expiratory distress. In severe cases at all ages, there is a marked ventilation-perfusion deficit.[213, 287] Patients with defects in the cell-mediated immune system particularly are prone to progressive fatal bilateral infections.[97, 191, 241, 242, 326, 328]

Secondary bacterial pneumonias are the result of common respiratory pathogens, particularly *Streptococcus pneumoniae, Haemophilus influenzae, Streptococcus pyogenes,* and *Staphylococcus aureus.*

Other Respiratory Manifestations

Otitis media is the most common complication and is age-related. In the immediate prevaccine era in the United States, about 5 to 15 per cent of patients with measles developed otitis media. Now it is a lesser problem because of the change in age incidence of measles. The bacterial pathogens in otitis media associated with measles are similar to those in otitis media in children without measles. Mastoiditis was a common complication of measles in the era before antibiotics, but fortunately today it is rare.

Laryngitis and mild laryngotracheitis are common. Occasionally, frank, severe laryngotracheobronchitis occurs and requires tracheotomy.[308] Measles-associated bacterial tracheitis is not uncommon.[73] Secondary bacterial infection of cervical lymph nodes and secondary bacterial pharyngitis also are rather frequent complications of measles. Field[102] attributed 3.2 per cent of the cases of childhood bronchiectasis to former measles virus infections.[102] Measles also has a deleterious effect on the course of tuberculosis.

Cardiac Manifestations

Myocarditis and pericarditis occasionally occur in measles.[84, 103] Nonspecific, transient electrocardiographic abnormalities were noted in more than half of 71 children with measles in one study.[309] In another study, 19 per cent of patients had transient but clear-cut abnormalities, including T-wave changes, atrioventricular conduction defects, and premature auricular contractions.[129] Although cardiac involvement appears to be common in measles, clinical consequences of this involvement are rare.

Neurologic Manifestations

Neurologic involvement is not uncommon in measles.[4, 20, 28, 94, 99, 125, 132, 204, 215, 229, 283, 295, 347, 376] Gibbs and associates[125] noted that 51 per cent of 680 measles patients without clinical evidence of encephalitis had abnormal electroencephalographic results during acute or immediate postacute illness.

Although the incidence varies, clinically evident encephalitis occurs in about 0.5 to 1 of every 1000 measles cases.[20, 55, 63, 94, 181] From 1962 to 1979, the average measles encephalitis-to-case ratio was 0.73:1000.[55] Both mortality and incidence of sequelae have varied among the available reports. LaBoccetta and Tornay[204] noted a mortality rate of 32 per cent in 50 patients in a group seen before 1947 and a rate of 11.5 per cent in a group seen between 1947 and 1957. Ziegra[376] noted only two deaths in a group of 38 cases. Long-term morbidity data also vary considerably. In general, between 20 and 40 per cent of the patients who recover from measles encephalitis have manifestations of brain damage. Douglas[89] could find no evidence of later subnormal school performance in a group of children who had uncomplicated measles.

Symptoms of encephalitis usually occur during the period of the measles exanthem and within 8 days of the onset of illness.[4, 204, 307] Occasionally, the onset of central nervous system signs and symptoms occurs during the prodromal period. LaBoccetta and Tornay[204] noted the following frequencies of signs and symptoms at the onset of measles encephalitis: convulsions, 56 per cent; lethargy, 46 per cent; coma, 28 per cent; and irritability, 26 per cent. Patients with encephalitis frequently have multiple findings: headache, abnormalities of respiratory rate and rhythm, twitching and other involuntary movements, and disorientation. Cerebellar ataxia, myelitis, retrobulbar neuritis, transient mental disorders, and hemiplegia are findings noted during subacute stages of illness. Long-term sequelae include various degrees of retardation and selective brain damages, recurrent seizures, deafness, and hemiplegia and paraplegia.

Cerebrospinal fluid findings in measles encephalitis usually reveal mild pleocytosis with a predominance of mononuclear cells, mildly elevated protein values, and a normal glucose level.[204, 229, 277, 347] In one study, 15 per cent of the cases did not have cerebrospinal fluid pleocytosis.[204]

Considerable controversy relates to the mechanisms in measles encephalitis.[6, 105, 108, 124, 140, 142, 143, 176, 184, 229, 235, 244, 289, 292] Some investigators have failed to isolate measles virus or to demonstrate measles virus RNA or other viral antigens in the brains of affected patients.[124, 176, 184, 244] These findings have led to the widespread belief that the illness is autoimmune and that viral invasion of the central nervous system is unnecessary. However, other investigators have recovered measles virus from the cerebrospinal fluid and brain of affected patients, which indicates that the virus may be involved directly in the process.[99, 108, 229, 235]

Other Manifestations

Measles has been associated with many other manifestations and complications. Of historical interest was the occurrence of a severe, often fatal, form of measles called black measles, which was characterized by a confluent hemorrhagic skin eruption.[199] Patients with this illness had signs of both encephalitis or encephalopathy and pneumonia. Extensive bleeding from the mouth, nose, and bowel were common. Severe hemorrhagic measles rarely is seen today, and little is known about the pathogenesis. Disseminated intravascular coagulation would appear to play a role.

Another measles complication involving bleeding is thrombocytopenic purpura.[5, 166] This is a postinfectious illness and different from hemorrhagic measles. Although bleeding is extensive on occasion, the ultimate prognosis usually is good. Stevens-Johnson syndrome has been noted occasionally in measles[220]; other manifestations include pneumomediastinum, subcutaneous emphysema, hepatitis, appendicitis, ileocolitis, mesenteric lymphadenitis, cervicitis, acute glomerulonephritis, corneal ulceration, and gangrene of the extremities.[114, 158, 181, 185, 199, 211, 230, 245, 262, 325, 345, 370]

Measles in pregnancy results in significant maternal and fetal morbidity and mortality.[18, 92, 174, 251, 332] Jespersen and associates[174] retrospectively reviewed 10 epidemics of measles in Greenland; they obtained adequate data on 327 women infected during pregnancy, and they also were able to examine 252 of the offspring. Thirty-two per cent of women infected during the first trimester had spontaneous abortions, and 9 per cent of these pregnancies that continued to term resulted in stillbirths. Congenital malformations occurred in 8 of 300 liveborn infants.[174] Pneumonia is a common maternal complication of measles during pregnancy.[18, 92]

Subacute Sclerosing Panencephalitis

Subacute sclerosing panencephalitis (SSPE) is a rare degenerative central nervous system disease of children and adolescents due to a persistent measles virus infection. It was described first by Dawson[83] in 1933; he proposed a viral etiologic agent because of the occurrence of inclusion bodies in the neurons of patients dying of the disease. In 1967, Connolly and colleagues[74] reported the observation of measles viral antigen in the brain of a patient with SSPE. They also noted high measles HI and CF titers in the sera and spinal fluids of three afflicted patients. Shortly thereafter, cultures of brain cells from patients with SSPE resulted in syncytial formation and the presence of measles antigen.[24] By cocultivation, measles virus was recovered from the brains of patients with SSPE.[163, 164, 288]

The risk of SSPE in children who previously had natural measles is between 0.6 and 2.2 per 100,000 infections.[53, 243] However, the risk is greater in patients who acquire measles at an early age. The mean incubation period from measles illness to onset of SSPE is 7 years. In contrast with natural measles, the risk of SSPE after measles immunization is about one per million. In vaccinees who developed SSPE, the mean incubation period was 3.3 years.

SSPE has an insidious onset.[58, 343] There is progressive behavioral and intellectual deterioration. Symptoms frequently are bizarre and complex and include psychic difficulties, motor incoordination, seizures of various types but most often myoclonic jerks, visual impairment, and difficulties with speech. Progression of the disease leads to stupor, dementia, mutism, central blindness, and, finally, decorticate rigidity.

Electroencephalography shows a periodic suppression burst pattern with synchronous myoclonic jerks. Laboratory studies reveal a markedly elevated cerebrospinal fluid globulin that is predominantly IgG. The serum measles HI and CF antibody titers are exceptionally high (>1:1280), although serial determinations occasionally are necessary to demonstrate this.[162] Measles antibody (HI and CF) can be determined in the cerebrospinal fluid.

There is at present no effective treatment for SSPE. The average duration of illness from onset to death is about 6 to 9 months. A variety of antiviral and immunomodulatory agents have been tried in the treatment of individual patients. Inosiplex and intrathecal INF-α seem to elicit transient improvement in some patients.[90, 91, 216] The incidence of SSPE in the United States decreased dramatically because of the extensive use of measles vaccine.[243]

Measles in Developing Countries

Measles has been and continues to be a staggering problem in developing countries. The mortality rate in much of Africa is about 10 per cent,[276] and it is reasonable to assume that the rate is similar in much of Central and South America and Asia.[246, 305, 341] In developing countries, measles is a disease of young children. For example, in Kenya, 25 to 30 per cent of children contract measles before their first birthday, 55 to 60 per cent before they are 2 years of age; virtually all children have had measles by 4 years of age.[155] In Kenyan children, mortality peaked in the 17- to 20-month age group, and the median age for hospital admission was 14 months.

Although many factors, such as age of infection, suboptimal medical facilities, and failure to seek medical care, contribute to the excessive morbidity and mortality in children of developing countries, the single overriding factor generally has been thought to be the nutritional status of the infected children.[248, 249, 276] The data of O'Donovan[276] clearly indicate a direct relationship between malnutrition and hospital admissions for measles and deaths. Studies by Coovadia and colleagues[78] and Carney and associates[46] indicate both humoral and cell-mediated defects in protein-calorie malnutrition. The clinical picture of measles in children with malnutrition frequently is similar to that in patients with known defects of cell-mediated functions.

It has been found that low serum retinol concentrations nearly always are present in children with measles in developing countries.[22, 80, 167, 170, 222, 300, 349] Low retinol levels correlate directly with measles mortality, and treatment with vitamin A reduces this mortality.[22, 167, 222]

Studies during the last decade indicate that intensive exposure that occurs in children in developing countries is a major factor in measles mortality.[2, 3, 124]

Clinical Manifestations

Measles in children in developing countries is characterized by two different types of severe disease. One type of illness is a fulminant, toxic illness without apparent localizing complications. The other is a more prolonged illness with obvious complications; the complications may be due to infection with secondary bacterial or other infectious agents, persistent measles viral infection, or a combination of both.

In a group of 507 hospitalized children, O'Donovan[276] noted that 301 had pneumonia; 96, gastroenteritis; 36, croup; 11, convulsions; 67, two or more complications; and 140, nonlocalized systemic toxic effects. The measles rash in malnourished children tends to go to greater confluence and progresses to a dark red and then violet color.[249] Desquamation is marked and occurs in large scales.[316] After desquamation, patchy depigmentation lasts for some weeks. Another common problem is stomatitis and a resultant sore mouth, which leads to further loss of nutritional intake. Acute corneal ulceration, which occurs after measles in malnourished children, is a common cause of blindness.[313] Multiple skin abscesses and noma (cancrum oris) are rare secondary infectious problems.[181]

Measles in the Immunocompromised Host

Today, because of the extensive use of immunosuppressive therapeutic modalities and greater duration of survival in a number of rapidly fatal diseases, a sizable population of children and adults is immunologically compromised. Measles virus infection in the patient with disease-induced or iatrogenically caused immune deficiency usually is severe and protracted and frequently is fatal.

The most common severe measles virus infection in the immunocompromised host is giant-cell pneumonia.[97, 191, 232, 240, 242, 298, 326] The mode of presentation of this illness varies. Some patients initially have severe but otherwise typical measles after a normal incubation period. Clinical findings at the time of the exanthem indicate pulmonary involvement and respiratory distress, and radiographic findings become rapidly worse over a period of about a week or less. Other patients initially have rather vague illness, frequently without rash. In these cases, the pulmonary process may progress over a month or longer. Siegel and associates[326] reported a child with leukemia who recovered from typical measles and then the following year died of diffuse interstitial pneumonia in which characteristic measles giant cells were seen.

A unique form of measles encephalitis also is manifested in immunosuppressed patients.[7, 153, 233, 252, 255, 296, 367] Although the symptoms in different described cases varied, the illness appears to be intermediate between acute encephalitis that occurs in patients without known immunodefect and the chronic picture of SSPE. The incubation period has varied between 5 weeks and 6 months.[7] Convulsions frequently are the initial symptom, and they are a prominent aspect of the illness. The seizures have been focal, unilateral, or permanent localized twitching. Other findings include hemiplegia, stupor, coma, hypertonia, and slurred speech. Most cases have been fatal, and the duration of illness has been from 1 week to 2 months.

DIAGNOSIS

Differential Diagnosis

(See also Chapter 67.) The differential diagnosis of typical measles must include all illnesses in which an erythematous maculopapular rash occurs. Of most importance in establishing the diagnosis of measles is a consideration of possible exposure; the duration of the incubation period; the presence of Koplik spots; the presence of the typical febrile prodrome with cough, coryza, and conjunctivitis; and the progression of the rash in a caudal direction. The brown discoloration and the intensity of the measles rash are such that the illness usually should not be confused with rubella, erythema infectiosum, roseola infantum, or enteroviral infection. Of greatest differential difficulty are the exanthems of infectious mononucleosis, *Mycoplasma pneumoniae* infection, and drug eruptions.

Atypical measles has caused great difficulty in diagnosis. Today, this is a disease of adults. The key to diagnosis in this illness is the careful elicitation of an accurate vaccination history. Even if it is not known whether the vaccination that the patient received as a child was live or killed vaccine, this usually can be determined by the number of doses given; if a child received more than one dose, it almost is certain that killed vaccine was administered. The differential considerations in atypical measles include Rocky Mountain spotted fever, anaphylactoid purpura, *M. pneumoniae* infection, and drug eruptions.

Specific Diagnosis

Measles virus infection can be diagnosed specifically by viral isolation in an appropriate tissue culture system; by demonstration of measles antigen in exfoliated cells and tissues by FA techniques or the polymerase chain reaction[226]; or by the demonstration of HI, CF, ELISA, FA, or neutralizing antibody titer rise in two sequential serum samples or specific measles IgM antibody in a single serum sample (see Chapter 245). For practical purposes, most measles cases can be diagnosed by the demonstration of specific IgM antibody in an acute-phase serum specimen. It should be noted that false-positive IgM ELISA results may occur.[173]

TREATMENT

Uncomplicated Measles

There is no specific treatment for uncomplicated measles. During the febrile period of illness, activity should be discouraged, and fluids should be maintained by the liberal provision of soft drinks and ice. Fever may be controlled with acetaminophen. Cough frequently is distressing and can be managed by judicious use of common antitussives. Room humidification also is useful in controlling the cough and generally can be expected to make the patient more comfortable. As the fever disappears, a gradual return to normal activity is indicated. However, measles virus infection is associated with considerable damage to the ciliated epithelium of the respiratory tract; therefore, too-early resumption of normal activities and exposure to other children and their bacterial pathogens can be associated with severe secondary infection.

Children in developing countries frequently have vitamin A deficiency. Measles morbidity correlates with this deficiency, and treatment with vitamin A is beneficial.[22, 80, 167, 170, 222, 300, 349] Recent studies in the United States indicate that vitamin A levels are low in a substantial number of measles cases and that morbidity is increased in these deficient children.[12, 17, 43, 115] It also has been shown that vitamin A supplementation enhances IgG antibody levels and total lymphocyte numbers.[79] In 1993, the Committee on Infectious Diseases of the American Academy of Pediatrics recommended vitamin A supplementation in children with measles in selected circumstances.[12] Vitamin A was recommended for children 6 months to 2 years of age who require hospitalization and all patients 6 months of age or older with immune deficiencies or possible vitamin A deficiency. The dose of vitamin A is 100,000 IU for children 6 months to 1 year of age and 200,000 IU for children 1 year of age or older. The dose should be repeated 24 hours and 4 weeks after the first dose in children with ophthalmologic evidence of vitamin A deficiency.

Atypical Measles

The most important aspect of therapy of atypical measles is proper diagnosis. Patients with atypical measles frequently are diagnosed erroneously as having Rocky Mountain spotted fever, other septic conditions, lymphoma, or collagen vascular disease, and their work-up is associated with extensive blood cultures, other diagnostic procedures, and vigorous antibiotic therapy. Careful attention to a history of prior administration of killed measles vaccine should clarify the diagnosis and prevent the unnecessary trauma associated with extensive diagnostic and therapeutic procedures.

In atypical measles, chest radiographs always should be obtained because the pneumonia that these patients usually develop frequently is much more extensive than the clinical findings would indicate. Activity should be discouraged in the acutely ill patient, and follow-up chest radiographs should be used as a guide to the resumption of normal activity. In some patients, pulmonary abnormalities have persisted for a considerable period.

Complications of Measles

Otitis Media

Otitis media is the most frequent complication of measles. The infectious agent of otitis media in measles is no different from that in other children without measles of comparable ages, so conventional antibiotic therapy is all that is necessary (see Chapter 19).

Laryngotracheitis

The management of laryngotracheitis due to measles virus infection is similar to that in other patients with croup due to other viral etiologic agents. The mainstay of therapy is the administration of humidified air and a concerted effort to relieve the apprehension of the patient. The administration of corticosteroids is contraindicated in measles, and the administration of antibiotics is indicated only if there is laboratory or clinical evidence of secondary bacterial infection (see Chapter 22).

Pneumonia

Pneumonia is a common complication of measles, and it is the leading cause of death. Pneumonia may be a manifestation of primary viral infection, or it may result from a superimposed bacterial infection. The differential diagnosis between primary viral and superimposed bacterial disease cannot be made with certainty. Because the diagnosis of viral pneumonia often is uncertain, most cases should be treated with antibiotics (see Chapters 26 and 27). In a primary viral pneumonia, treatment with aerosolized ribavirin should be considered.

In one uncontrolled study in adult patients, it was found that intravenous ribavirin was well tolerated, and its use was associated with clinical improvement.[110] In a study in pregnant women, Atmar and associates[18] were unable to demonstrate clear clinical benefit with aerosolized ribavirin.

Encephalitis

The course of measles encephalitis is unpredictable, and the treatment is symptomatic and supportive. Trained nursing care is essential. Careful attention to fluid and electrolyte balance is necessary. In prolonged states of coma, parenteral hyperalimentation is indicated. Status epilepticus should be treated vigorously with the use of a structured protocol for ensuring optimal control (see Chapter 43). Controlled studies have shown that corticosteroids in relatively low dosage offer no benefit. In severe intractable seizures or other evidence of cerebral edema, the use of intravenous mannitol therapy (0.25 to 1 g/kg of a 20 per cent solution in 30 to 60 minutes) is indicated. In occasional circumstances, respiratory arrest is a problem, and artificial ventilators should be used to tide patients over until respirations become normal. Mustafa and coworkers[255] noted improvement in an immunocompromised child with subacute measles encephalitis who was treated with intravenously administered ribavirin.

Appendicitis

Acute abdominal pain is an occasional occurrence in primary measles, and this can be caused by a generalized mesenteric adenitis due to measles virus or to appendicitis. In appendicitis, there is evidence of measles virus involvement of the appendix. However, therapy should be similar to that in other cases of appendicitis; removal of the appendix is indicated because measles appendicitis perforates with a frequency equal to that in nonmeasles virus infection cases.

Crohn Disease

Wakefield and associates[95, 96, 350, 351] have presented data suggesting that congenital measles virus infection may be a cause of Crohn disease.

PREVENTION

Active Immunization: Live Attenuated Measles Virus Vaccine

Attenuated measles vaccines are prepared in chicken embryo tissue cultures. Vaccination produces a mild or inapparent noncommunicable infection that induces active immunity in more than 95 per cent of recipients. Vaccine-induced antibodies persist for many years, and although reinfection with illness has been noted on occasion in apparently successfully immunized children, it does not appear that waning immunity is of significant epidemiologic importance.[13, 64, 66, 85, 200] Symptoms associated with measles immunization are minimal and are limited to fever, mild malaise, and occasionally a faint rash occurring approximately 1 week after immunization. For complete information and recommendations relating to measles immunization, the reader is referred to the most recent recommendations of the Advisory Committee on Immunization Practices,[51] the Committee on Infectious Diseases of the American Academy of Pediatrics,[11] and the manufacturer's package insert. Only a summary of recommendations is presented here.

Recommendations for Use

The widespread epidemics of measles in the United States in 1989 to 1991 were the result of the failure to immunize children at the appropriate age and the increased number of susceptible older children and adults due to vaccine failure.[49–52, 209, 221, 223] Therefore, the future eradication of measles in the United States depends on programs that (1) enroll all children of initial vaccination age and (2) allow the revaccination of all persons whose primary vaccine failed. Because routine immunity testing is not a viable public health option, the revaccination of primary vaccine failures can be accomplished only by universal reimmunization.

Presently, live measles vaccine is recommended in a two-dose schedule.[11, 51, 221] The Advisory Committee on Immunization Practices (ACIP) and the Committee on Infectious Diseases of the American Academy of Pediatrics recommend different ages for the second dose. However, these differences are not important. What is important is that all vaccinees receive two doses of vaccine. A shortcoming of both recommendations is that some persons older than the designated second-dose age still are susceptible and are not being vaccinated. Until provisions are made to immunize all potentially susceptible children and adults, sporadic measles will continue to occur. In general, live measles vaccine should be administered at 12 to 15 months of age.[8, 11, 54, 198, 323, 363, 372] Children who have not received vaccine during infancy may be immunized at any age, and adults who have not had natural measles also should be immunized. When measles is endemic or epidemic in a community, all children 6 months of age or older should be immunized. In children who initially were vaccinated before 12 months of age, a second vaccination should be administered at 15 months of age or before the next measles season because the likelihood of protection in children vaccinated during the first year of life is far from optimal.

Precautions

Measles vaccination should be deferred at times of febrile illnesses or when interference from another viral infection might cause measles vaccine failure. Measles immunization also should be postponed for 3 to 11 months in persons who have received whole blood, blood plasma, or immunoglobulin because these products may contain sufficient measles antibody to neutralize the vaccine virus. The duration of postponement depends on the product administered and the dose.[11] Children treated with intravenous immunoglobulin for Kawasaki disease should not receive measles vaccine until 11 months after the immunoglobulin, whereas 3 months' time is adequate for children given immunoglobulin for hepatitis A prophylaxis.

Contraindications

Live measles vaccine should not be administered to pregnant women or to some persons with diseases or therapeutic programs associated with impaired cell-mediated immunity. These conditions in general include leukemia; lymphoma or other generalized malignancies; primary and secondary immunologic disorders; and therapy with steroids, radiation, antimetabolites, or alkylating agents. In all instances, the risk of measles in the patient should be compared with the risk of immunization. For example, measles in children with HIV infection frequently is progressive and fatal, whereas to date immunization has not been associated with severe or unusual adverse events.[11, 51] Therefore, children with HIV infection should be immunized.

Complications

Serious complications associated with measles vaccine administration are exceedingly rare. Serious neurologic disease (encephalitis, Reye syndrome, cranial nerve palsy, cerebellar ataxia, and Guillain-Barré syndrome) occurring within 30 days of immunization happens at a rate of about one case per million doses of vaccine administered.[57, 206] This rate actually is below the rate of occurrence of encephalitis of unknown cause in children for any 30-day period. However, the recovery of measles virus from the cerebrospinal fluid of a vaccinated child with encephalitis indicates that rare vaccine-induced neurologic disease may occur.[108]

Thrombocytopenic purpura, anaphylaxis, hearing loss, and toxic epidermal necrolysis also have been associated with measles immunization.[10, 21, 172, 314, 324, 337, 362]

In developing countries, high-titered measles vaccines were employed to induce seroconversion at a young age.[368] However, follow-up studies noted that mortality was increased in female recipients of these high-titer vaccines over a 3-year period compared with children who received conventional doses of vaccine.[160]

Quarantine and Disease Containment

Before the widespread use of measles vaccines, quarantine measures were practiced widely but largely were ineffective in preventing the spread of measles. However, disease containment is practical today because the widespread use of measles vaccine has reduced the general number of susceptible young children, which in turn has decreased the rapidity of epidemic development. Epidemic measles now generally involves a greater age range of the population (cases in adolescents and young adults are frequent), and progression of disease from one age group to another is slower than in epidemics that involve one uniform, largely susceptible population.

Containment is a vital part of the measles prevention policy in the United States. Measles is a reportable disease throughout the United States, and compliance is the obligation of all physicians. After early reports of sporadic measles, health department workers can organize local immunization clinics so that disease often can be contained in a small geographic area rather than developing into a widespread epidemic.

Passive Immunization: Immunoglobulin

In the present vaccine era, there should be little need for passive immunization. However, when a known susceptible child has had definite exposure to measles, immunoglobulin should be administered in a dose of 0.25 mg/kg (maximum dose, 15 mL). If this is performed within 5 days of exposure, prevention of infection and disease can be expected. The administration of immunoglobulin later in the incubation period may modify illness but does not prevent it. The use of immunoglobulin particularly is important in those children who have not been immunized because of the contraindications to vaccination mentioned. In these children, immunoglobulin (0.5 mL/kg; maximum dose, 15 mL) should be administered when measles is epidemic in the community in which they reside. Dosage should be repeated every 4 weeks until the epidemic subsides. Intravenous immunoglobulin may be used.

References

1. Aaby, P.: Patterns of exposure and severity of measles infection: Copenhagen 1915–1925. Ann. Epidemiol. *2*:257–262, 1992.
2. Aaby, P.: Malnutrition and overcrowding/intensive exposure in severe measles infection: Review of community studies. Rev. Infect. Dis. *10*:478–491, 1988.
3. Aaby, P., Bukh, J., Lisse, I. M., et al.: Overcrowding and intensive exposure as determinants of measles mortality. Am. J. Epidemiol. *120*:49–63, 1984.
4. Aarli, J. A.: Nervous complications of measles: Clinical manifestations and prognosis. Eur. Neurol. *12*:79–93, 1974.
5. Abramson, O., Dagan, R., Tal, A., et al.: Severe complications of measles requiring intensive care in infants and young children. Arch. Pediatr. Adolesc. Med. *149*:1237–1240, 1995.
6. Adams, J. M., Baird, C., and Filloy, L.: Inclusion bodies in measles encephalitis. J. A. M. A. *195*:290–298, 1966.
7. Aicardi, J., Goutieres, F., Arsenio-Nunes, M. L., et al.: Acute measles encephalitis in children with immunosuppression. Pediatrics *59*:232–239, 1977.
8. Albrecht, P., Ennis, F. A., Saltzman, E. J., et al.: Persistence of maternal antibody in infants beyond 12 months: Mechanism of measles vaccine failure. J. Pediatr. *91*:715–718, 1977.
9. Alpert, G., Liebovitz, L., and Danon, Y. L.: Analysis of T-lymphocyte subsets in measles. J. Infect. Dis. *149*:1018, 1984.
10. Alter, H. J., Scanlon, R. T., and Schechter, G. P.: Thrombocytopenic purpura following vaccination with attenuated measles virus. Am. J. Dis. Child. *115*:111–113, 1968.
11. American Academy of Pediatrics: Active immunization: Measles. *In* Peter, G. (ed.): 1994 Red Book: Report of the Committee on Infectious Diseases. 23rd ed. Elk Grove Village, American Academy of Pediatrics, 1994, pp. 7–72, 308–322.
12. American Academy of Pediatrics, Committee on Infectious Diseases, 1992–1993: Vitamin A treatment of measles. Pediatrics *91*:1014–1015, 1993.
13. Anders, J. F., Jacobson, R. M., Poland, G. A., et al.: Secondary failure rates of measles vaccines: A metaanalysis of published studies. Pediatr. Infect. Dis. J. *15*:62–66, 1996.
14. Anderson, R., Rabson, A. R., Sher, R., et al.: Defective neutrophil motility in children with measles. J. Pediatr. *89*:27–32, 1976.
15. Annunziato, D., Kaplan, M. H., Hall, W. W., et al.: Atypical measles syndrome: Pathologic and serologic findings. Pediatrics *70*:203–209, 1982.
16. Arneborn, P., and Biberfeld, G.: T-lymphocyte subpopulations in relation to immunosuppression in measles and varicella. Infect. Immun. *39*:29–37, 1983.
17. Arrieta, A. C., Zaleska, M., Stutman, H. R., et al.: Vitamin A levels in children with measles in Long Beach, California. J. Pediatr. *121*:75–78, 1992.
18. Atmar, R. L., Englund J. A., and Hammill, H.: Complications of measles during pregnancy. Clin. Infect. Dis. *14*:217–226, 1992.
19. Azizi, A., and Krakovsky, D.: Keratoconjunctivitis as a constant sign of measles. Ann. Pediatr. *204*:397–405, 1965.
20. Babbott, F. L., Jr., and Gordon, J. E.: Modern measles. Am. J. Med. Sci. *228*:334–361, 1954.
21. Bachard, A. J., Rubenstein, J., and Morrison, A. N.: Thrombocytopenic purpura following live measles vaccine. Am. J. Dis. Child. *118*:283–285, 1967.
22. Barclay, A. J. G., Foster, A., and Sommer, A.: Retinol supplements and mortality related to measles: A randomised clinical trial. B. M. J. *294*:294–296, 1987.
23. Barsegar, B., Hofmann, H., and Zweymuller, E.: The diagnosis of measles in the newborn and infant age groups. Z. Kinderheilk. *113*:175–184, 1972.
24. Baublis, J. V., and Payne, F. E.: Measles antigen and syncytium formation in brain cell cultures from subacute sclerosing panencephalitis (SSPE). Proc. Soc. Exp. Biol. Med. *129*:593–597, 1968.
25. Bellanti, J. A., Sanga, R. L., Klutinis, B., et al.: Antibody responses in serum and nasal secretions of children immunized with inactivated and attenuated measles-virus vaccines. N. Engl. J. Med. *280*:628–633, 666–667, 1969.
26. Bellini, W. J., Rota, J. S., and Rota, P. A.: Virology of measles virus. J. Infect. Dis. *170*(Suppl. 1):S15–S23, 1994.
27. Benjamin, B., and Ward, S. M.: Leukocytic response to measles. Am. J. Dis. Child. *44*:921–963, 1932.
28. Berkovich, S., and Schneck, L.: Ascending paralysis associated with measles. J. Pediatr. *64*:88–93, 1964.
29. Berm, J.: Koplik spots for the record: An illustrated historical note. Clin. Pediatr. *11*:161–163, 1972.
30. Black, F. L.: *In* Evans, A. S. (ed.): Viral Infections of Humans: Epidemiology and Control. 3rd ed. New York, Plenum Medical, 1989, pp. 451–469.
31. Black, F. L., and Sheridan, S. R.: Blood leukocyte response to live measles vaccine. Am. J. Dis. Child. *113*:301–304, 1967.
32. Black, F. L.: A nationwide serum survey of United States military recruits, 1962, III. Measles and mumps antibodies. Am. J. Hyg. *80*:304–307, 1964.
33. Black, F. L.: Discussion of paper by Karelitz, S.: Measles vaccine and immunity. N. Y. J. Med. *63*:519–528, 1963.
34. Black, F. L., and Sheridan, S. R.: Studies on an attenuated measles-virus vaccine. IV. Administration of vaccine by several routes. N. Engl. J. Med. *263*:165–169, 1960.
35. Black, F. L.: Growth and stability of measles virus. Virology *7*:184–192, 1959.
36. Black, F. L., Reissig, M., and Melnick, J. L.: Measles virus. Adv. Virus Res. *6*:205–277, 1959.
37. Bloch, A. B., Orenstein, W. A., Ewing, W. M., et al.: Measles outbreak in a pediatric practice: Airborne transmission in an office setting. Pediatrics *75*:676–683, 1985.
38. Boteler, W. L., Luipersbeck, P. M., Fuccillo, D. A., et al.: Enzyme-linked immunosorbent assay for detection of measles antibody. J. Clin. Microbiol. *17*:814–818, 1983.
39. Brodsky, A. L.: Atypical measles: Severe illness in recipients of killed measles virus vaccine upon exposure to natural infection. J. A. M. A. *222*:1415–1416, 1972.
40. Burnstein, T., Frankel, J. W., and Jensen, J. H.: Adaptation of measles virus to suckling hamsters. Fed. Proc. *17*:507, 1958.
41. Bussell, R. H., and Karzon, D. T.: Measles-canine distemper-rinderpest group. *In* Prier, J. E. (ed.): Basic Medical Virology. Baltimore, Williams & Wilkins, 1966, pp. 313–336.
42. Butler, J. C., Proctor, M. E., Fessler, K., et al.: Household-acquisition of measles and illness severity in an urban community in the United States. Epidemiol. Infect. *112*:569–577, 1994.
43. Butler, J. C., Havens, P. L., Sowell, A. L., et al.: Measles severity and serum retinol (vitamin A) concentration among children in the United States. Pediatrics *91*:1176–1181, 1993.
44. Carlstrom, G.: Relation of measles to other viruses. Am. J. Dis. Child. *103*:287–291, 1962.
45. Carlstrom, G.: Comparative studies on measles and distemper viruses in suckling mice. Arch. Virusforsch. *8*:527–538, 1958.
46. Carney, J., Stiehm, E. R., Cherry, J. D., et al.: Unpublished data, 1978.
47. Caulfield, E.: Early measles epidemics in America. Yale J. Biol. Med. *15*:531–536, 1943.
48. Centers for Disease Control and Prevention: Measles: United States, 1995. M. M. W. R. *45*:305–307, 1996.
49. Centers for Disease Control and Prevention: Summary of notifiable diseases, United States, 1994. M. M. W. R. *43*:1–80, 1995.
50. Centers for Disease Control and Prevention: Measles surveillance: United States, 1991. M. M. W. R. *41*(No. SS-6):1–12, 1992.
51. Centers for Disease Control: Measles prevention: Recommendations of the Immunization Practices Advisory Committee (ACIP). M. M. W. R. *38*:1–18, 1989.
52. Centers for Disease Control: Measles: United States, first 26 weeks, 1989. M. M. W. R. *38*:863–871, 1989.

53. Centers for Disease Control: Measles prevention. M. M. W. R. *31*:217–231, 1982.
54. Centers for Disease Control: Measles surveillance, 1977–1981. Issued September 1982.
55. Centers for Disease Control: Measles encephalitis: United States, 1962–1979, M. M. W. R. *30*:362–364, 1981.
56. Centers for Disease Control: Measles prevention. M. M. W. R. *27*:427–437, 1978.
57. Centers for Disease Control: Measles Surveillance Report No. 10, 1973–1976. July 1977.
58. Chao, D.: Subacute inclusion body encephalitis. J. Pediatr. *61*:501–510, 1962.
59. Charlesworth, J. A., Pussell, B. A., Roy, L. P., et al.: Measles infection: Involvement of the complement system. Clin. Exp. Immunol. *24*:401–406, 1976.
60. Chatterji, M., and Mankad, V.: Failure of attenuated viral vaccine in prevention of atypical measles. J. A. M. A. *238*:2635, 1977.
61. Chen, R. T., Markowitz, L. E., Albrecht, P., et al.: Measles antibody: Reevaluation of protective titers. J. Infect. Dis. *162*:1036–1041, 1990.
62. Cherry, J. D.: The "new" epidemiology of measles and rubella. Hosp. Prac. *115*:49–57, 1980.
63. Cherry, J. D.: Personal observations, 1978.
64. Cherry, J. D., Feigin, R. D., Shackelford, P. G., et al.: A clinical and serologic study of 103 children with measles vaccine failure. J. Pediatr. *82*:802–808, 1973.
65. Cherry, J. D., Feigin, R. D., Lobes, L. A., Jr., et al.: Atypical measles in children previously immunized with attenuated measles virus vaccines. Pediatrics *50*:712–717, 1972.
66. Cherry, J. D., Feigin, R. D., Lobes, L. A., Jr., et al.: Urban measles in the vaccine era: A clinical, epidemiologic, and serologic study. J. Pediatr. *81*:217–230, 1972.
67. Cherry, J. D., Feigin, R. D., Lobes, L. A., Jr., et al.: Unpublished data, 1971.
68. Cherry, J. D.: Newer viral exanthems. Adv. Pediatr. *16*:233–286, 1969.
69. Cherry, J. D.: Lesions of the lips and mouth. *In* Gellis, S. S., and Kagan, B. M. (eds.): Current Pediatric Therapy: 3. Philadelphia, W. B. Saunders, 1968, pp. 257–260.
70. Choppin, P. W., Richardson, C. D., Merz, D. C., et al.: The functions and inhibition of the membrane glycoproteins of paramyxoviruses and myxoviruses and the role of the measles virus M protein in subacute sclerosing panencephalitis. J. Infect. Dis. *143*:352–363, 1981.
71. Christensen, P. E., Schmidt, H., Bang, H. O., et al.: An epidemic of measles in southern Greenland, 1951: Measles in virgin soil. II. The epidemic proper. Acta Med. Scand. *144*:430–449, 1953.
72. Cobban, K.: Measles in Nigerian children. West Afr. Med. J. *12*:18–23, 1963.
73. Conley, S. F., Beste, D. J., and Hoffmann, R. G.: Measles-associated bacterial tracheitis. Pediatr. Infect. Dis. J. *12*:414–415, 1993.
74. Connolly, J. H., Allen, I. V., Hurwitz, L. J., et al.: Measles-virus antibody and antigen in subacute sclerosing panencephalitis. Lancet *1*:542–544, 1967.
75. Conrad, J. L., Wallace, R., and Witte, J. J.: The epidemiologic rationale for the failure to eradicate measles in the United States. Am. J. Public Health *61*:2304–2310, 1971.
76. Coovadia, H. M., Wesley, A., Henderson, L. G., et al.: Alterations in immune responsiveness in acute measles and chronic post-measles chest disease. Int. Arch. Allergy Appl. Immunol. *56*:14–23, 1978.
77. Coovadia, H. M., Brain, P., Hallett, A. F., et al.: Immunoparesis and outcome in measles. Lancet *1*:619–621, 1977.
78. Coovadia, H. M., Parent, M. A., Loening, W. E. K., et al.: An evaluation of factors associated with the depression of immunity in malnutrition and in measles. Am. J. Clin. Nutr. *27*:665–669, 1974.
79. Coutsoudis, A., Kiepiela, P., Coovadia, H. M., et al.: Vitamin A supplementation enhances specific IgG antibody levels and total lymphocyte numbers while improving morbidity in measles. Pediatr. Infect. Dis. J. *11*:203–209, 1992.
80. Coutsoudis, A., Broughton, M., and Coovadia, H. M.: Retinol supplementation reduces morbidity in young African children: A randomised placebo-controlled, double-blind trial. Am. J. Clin. Nutr. *54*:890–895, 1991.
81. Cremer, N. E., Cossen, C. K., Shell, G., et al.: Enzyme immunoassay versus plaque neutralization and other methods for determination of immune status to measles and varicella-zoster viruses versus complement fixation for serodiagnosis of infections with those viruses. J. Clin. Microbiol. *21*:869–874, 1985.
82. Dagan, R., Phillip, M., Sarov, I., et al.: Cellular immunity and T-lymphocyte subsets in young children with acute measles. J. Med. Virol. *22*:175–182, 1987.
83. Dawson, J. R., Jr.: Cellular inclusions in cerebral lesions of lethargic encephalitis. Am. J. Pathol. *9*:7–16, 1933.
84. Degen, J. A., Jr.: Visceral pathology in measles: A clinicopathologic study of 100 fatal cases. Am. J. Med. Sci. *194*:104–111, 1937.
85. Deseda-Tous, J., Cherry, J. D., Spencer, M. J., et al.: Measles revaccination: Persistence and degree of antibody titer by type of immune response. Am. J. Dis. Child. *132*:287–290, 1978.
86. Deseda-Tous, J. E., Spencer, M. J., Cherry, J. D., et al.: Measles antibody in healthy adults analyzed by HLA and ABO blood types. 16th Interscience Conference on Antimicrobial Agents and Chemotherapy, Chicago, October 1976. Abstract.
87. DeSwart, R. L., Harder, T. C., Ross, P. S., et al.: Morbilliviruses and morbillivirus disease of marine mammals. Infect. Agents Dis. *4*:125–130, 1995.
88. Döring, R. E. A., Marcil, A., Chopra, A., et al.: The human CD46 molecule is a receptor for measles virus (Edmonson strain). Cell *75*:295–305, 1993.
89. Douglas, J. W. B.: Ability and adjustment of children who have had measles. B. M. J. *2*:1301–1303, 1964.
90. Dunn, R. A.: Subacute sclerosing panencephalitis. Pediatr. Infect. Dis. J. *10*:68–72, 1991.
91. Durant, R. H., Dyken, P. R., and Swift, A. V.: The influence of Inosiplex treatment on the neurological disability of patients with subacute sclerosing panencephalitis. J. Pediatr. *101*:288–293, 1982.
92. Eberhart-Phillips, J. E., Frederick, P. D., Baron, R. C., et al.: Measles in pregnancy: A descriptive study of 58 cases. Obstet. Gynecol. *82*:797–801, 1993.
93. Edmonson, M. B., Addiss, D. G., McPherson, T., et al.: Mild measles and secondary vaccine failure during a sustained outbreak in a highly vaccinated population. J. A. M. A. *263*:2467–2471, 1990.
94. Ehrengut, W.: Measles encephalitis: Age disposition and vaccination. Arch. Virusforsch. *16*:1–5, 1965.
95. Ekbom, A., Daszak, P., Kraaz, W., et al.: Crohn's disease after in-utero measles virus exposure. Lancet *348*:515–517, 1996.
96. Ekbom, A., Wakefield, A. J., Zack, M., et al.: Perinatal measles infection and subsequent Crohn's disease. Lancet *344*:508–510, 1994.
97. Enders, J. F., McCarthy, K., Mitus, A., et al.: Isolation of measles virus at autopsy in cases of giant-cell pneumonia without rash. N. Engl. J. Med. *261*:875–896, 1959.
98. Enders, J. F., and Peebles, T. C.: Propagation in tissue cultures of cytopathogenic agents from patients with measles. Proc. Soc. Exp. Biol. Med. *86*:277–286, 1954.
99. Esolen, L. M., Takahashi, K., Johnson, R. T., et al.: Brain endothelial cell infection in children with acute fatal measles. J. Clin. Invest. *96*:2478–2481, 1995.
100. Fenner, F.: Classification and nomenclature of viruses: Second report of the International Committee on Taxonomy of Viruses. Intervirology *7*:1–115, 1976.
101. Fenner, F.: The pathogenesis of the acute exanthems. Lancet *2*:915–920, 1948.
102. Field, C. E.: Bronchiectasis in childhood. I. Clinical survey of 160 cases. Pediatrics *4*:21–46, 1949.
103. Finkel, H. E.: Measles myocarditis. Am. Heart J. *67*:679–683, 1964.
104. Fireman, P., Friday, G., and Kumate, J.: Effect of measles vaccine on immunologic responsiveness. Pediatrics *43*:264–272, 1969.
105. Fleischer, B., and Kreth, H. W.: Clonal expansion and functional analysis of virus-specific T lymphocytes from cerebrospinal fluid in measles encephalitis. Hum. Immunol. *7*:239–248, 1983.
106. Florman, A. L., and Agatston, H. J.: Keratoconjunctivitis as a diagnostic aid in measles. J. A. M. A. *179*:192–194, 1962.
107. Foege, W. H.: Measles control in West and Central Africa. Eighth Annual Immunology Conference, Kansas City, Missouri, March 1971.
108. Foreman, M. L., and Cherry, J. D.: Isolation of measles virus from the cerebrospinal fluid of a child with encephalitis following measles vaccination. Program for the American Pediatric Society, 1967. Abstract.
109. Forghani, B., Myoraku, C. K., and Schmidt, N. J.: Use of monoclonal antibodies to human immunoglobulin M in "capture" assays for measles and rubella immunoglobulin M. J. Clin. Microbiol. *18*:652–657, 1983.
110. Forni, A. L., Schluger, N. W., and Roberts, R. B.: Severe measles pneumonitis in adults: Evaluation of clinical characteristics and therapy with intravenous ribavirin. Clin. Infect. Dis. *19*:454–462, 1994.
111. Forthal, D. N., Landucci, G., Habis, A., et al.: Measles virus-specific functional antibody responses and viremia during acute measles. J. Infect. Dis. *169*:1377–1380, 1994.
112. Forthal, D. N., Landucci, G., Katz, J., et al.: Comparison of measles virus-specific antibodies with antibody-dependent cellular cytotoxicity and neutralizing functions. J. Infect. Dis. *168*:1020–1023, 1993.
113. Frank, J. A., Jr., Orenstein, W. A., Bart, K. J., et al.: Major impediments to measles elimination: The modern epidemiology of an ancient disease. Am. J. Dis. Child. *139*:881–888, 1985.
114. Frederique, G., Howard, R. O., and Boniuk, V.: Corneal ulcers in rubeola. Am. J. Ophthalmol. *68*:996–1003, 1969.
115. Frieden, T. R., Sowell, A. L., Henning, K. J., et al.: Vitamin A levels and severity of measles: New York City. Am. J. Dis. Child. *146*:182–186, 1992.
116. Friedman, M. G., Phillip, M., and Dagan, R.: Virus-specific IgA in serum, saliva, and tears of children with measles. Clin. Exp. Immunol. *75*:58–63, 1989.
117. Fulginiti, V. A., and Helfer, R. E.: Atypical measles in adolescent siblings 16 years after killed measles virus vaccine. J. A. M. A. *244*:804–806, 1980.
118. Fulginiti, V. A., Eller, J. J., Downie, A. W., et al.: Altered reactivity to measles virus: Atypical measles in children previously immunized with inactivated measles virus vaccines. J. A. M. A. *202*:1075–1080, 1967.
119. Fulginiti, V. A., and Kempe, C. H.: A comparison of measles neutralizing and hemagglutination-inhibition antibody titers in individual sera. Am. J. Epidemiol. *82*:135–142, 1965.

120. Fulginiti, V. A., and Kempe, C. H.: Measles exposure among vaccine recipients: Response to measles exposure and antibody persistence among recipients of measles vaccines. Am. J. Dis. Child. *106*:450–461, 1963.
121. Gallagher, M. R., Welliver, R., Yamanaka, T., et al.: Cell-mediated immune responsiveness to measles: Its occurrence as a result of naturally acquired or vaccine-induced infection and in infants of immune mothers. Am. J. Dis. Child. *135*:48–51, 1981.
122. Garenne, M., and Aaby, P.: Pattern of exposure and measles mortality in Senegal. J. Infect. Dis. *161*:1088–1094, 1990.
123. Gellin, B. G., and Katz, S. L.: Putting a stop to a serial killer: Measles. J. Infect. Dis. *170*(Suppl. 1):S1–S2, 1994.
124. Gendelman, H. E., Wolinsky, J. S., Johnson, R. T., et al.: Measles encephalomyelitis: Lack of evidence of viral invasion of the central nervous system and quantitative study of the nature of demyelination. Ann. Neurol. *15*:353–360, 1984.
125. Gibbs, F. A., Gibbs, E. L., Carpenter, P. R., et al.: Electroencephalographic abnormality in "uncomplicated" childhood diseases. J. A. M. A. *72*:1050–1055, 1959.
126. Goerka, H.: The life and scientific works of Mr. John Quier. West Indian Med. J. *V*:23, 1956.
127. Gokiert, J. G., and Beamish, W. E.: Altered reactivity to measles virus in previously vaccinated children. Can. Med. Assoc. J. *103*:724–727, 1970.
128. Goldberger, J., and Anderson, J. F.: An experimental demonstration of the presence of the virus of measles in the mixed buccal and nasal secretions. J. A. M. A. *57*:476–478, 1911.
129. Goldfield, M., Boyer, N. H., and Weinstein, L.: Electrocardiographic changes during the course of measles. J. Pediatr. *46*:30–35, 1955.
130. Good, R. A., and Zak, S. J.: Disturbances in gamma globulin synthesis as "experiments of nature." Pediatrics *18*:109–149, 1956.
131. Goodall, E. W.: Measles with an "illness of infection." Clin. J. *54*:69, 1925.
132. Grattan-Smith, P. J., Procopis, P. G., Wise, G. A., et al.: Serious neurological complications of measles: A continuing preventable problem. Med. J. Aust. *143*:385–387, 1985.
133. Graves, M., Griffin, D. E., Johnson, R. T., et al.: Development of antibody to measles virus polypeptides during complicated and uncomplicated measles virus infections. J. Virol. *49*:409–412, 1984.
134. Graziano, K. D., Ruckdeschel, J. C., and Mardiney, M. R., Jr.: Cell-associated immunity to measles (rubeola): The demonstration of in vitro lymphocyte tritiated thymidine incorporation in response to measles complement fixation antigen. Cell. Immunol. *15*:347–359, 1975.
135. Green, M. S., Shohat, T., and Lerman, Y.: Sex differences in the humoral antibody response to live measles vaccine in young adults. Int. J. Epidemiol. *23*:1078–1081, 1994.
136. Greenstein, J. I., and McFarland, H. F.: Response of human lymphocytes to measles virus after natural infection. Infect. Immun. *40*:198–204, 1983.
137. Gremillion, D. H., and Crawford, G. E.: Measles pneumonia in young adults: An analysis of 106 cases. Am. J. Med. *71*:539–542, 1981.
138. Gresser, I., and Chany, C.: Isolation of measles virus from the washed leucocytic fraction of blood. Proc. Soc. Exp. Biol. Med. *113*:695–698, 1963.
139. Gresser, I., and Katz, S. L.: Isolation of measles virus from urine. N. Engl. J. Med. *263*:452–454, 1960.
140. Griffin, D. E., Ward, B. J., and Esolen, L. M.: Pathogenesis of measles virus infection: An hypothesis for altered immune responses. J. Infect. Dis. *170*(Suppl. 1):S24–S31, 1994.
141. Griffin, D. E., Ward, B. J., Jauregui, E., et al.: Natural killer cell activity during measles. Clin. Exp. Immunol. *81*:218–224, 1990.
142. Griffin, D. E., Ward, B. J., Jauregui, E., et al.: Immune activation in measles. N. Engl. J. Med. *320*:1667–1672, 1989.
143. Griffin, D. E., Ward, B. J., Jauregui, E., et al.: Immune activation during measles: Interferon-α and neopterin in plasma and cerebrospinal fluid in complicated and uncomplicated disease. J. Infect. Dis. *161*:449–453, 1990.
144. Griffin, D. E., Cooper, S. J., Hirsch, R. L., et al.: Changes in plasma IgE levels during complicated and uncomplicated measles virus infections. J. Allergy Clin. Immunol. *76*:206–213, 1985.
145. Griffin, D. E., Hirsch, R. L., Johnson, R. T., et al.: Changes in serum C-reactive protein during complicated and uncomplicated measles virus infections. Infect. Immun. *41*:861–864, 1983.
146. Grist, N. R.: The pathogenesis of measles: Review of the literature and discussion of the problem. Glasgow Med. J. *31*:431–441, 1950.
147. Guinee, V. F., Henderson, D. A., Casey, H. L., et al.: Cooperative measles vaccine field trial. I. Clinical efficacy. II. Serologic studies. Pediatrics *37*:649–657, 657–665, 1966.
148. Gunn, W.: Control of common fevers: Measles. Lancet *1*:795–799, 1938.
149. Haas, E. J., and Wendt, V. E.: Atypical measles 14 years after immunization. J. A. M. A. *236*:1050, 1976.
150. Hall, W. W., and Martin, S. J.: Structure and function relationships of the envelope of measles virus. Med. Microbiol. Immunol. *160*:143–154, 1974.
151. Hall, W. W., and Martin, S. J.: Purification and characterization of measles virus. J. Gen. Virol. *19*:175–188, 1973.
152. Halsey, N. A., Nieburg, P. I., Preblud, S. R., et al.: Recent trends in reported measles cases and deaths. Effectiveness of measles vaccine administered at 12 months of age. Simultaneous administration of measles vaccine and DPT antigens. Prepared for the American Academy of Pediatrics Committee on Infectious Diseases, Red Book Committee and Advisory Committee on Immunization Practices. Atlanta, U.S. DHEW, Public Health Service, Centers for Disease Control, 1978.
153. Haltia, M., Tarkkanen, A., Vaheri, A., et al.: Measles retinopathy during immunosuppression. Br. J. Ophthalmol. *62*:356–360, 1978.
154. Hardy, G. E., Jr., Kassanoff, I., Orbach, H. G., et al.: The failure of a school immunization campaign to terminate an urban epidemic of measles. Am. J. Epidemiol. *91*:286–293, 1970.
155. Hayden, R. J.: The epidemiology and nature of measles in Nairobi before the impact of measles immunization. East Afr. Med. J. *51*:199–205, 1974.
156. Hedrich, A. W.: The corrected average attack rate from measles among city children. Am. J. Hyg. *11*:576–600, 1930.
157. Heffner, R. R., Jr., and Schluederberg, A.: Specificity of the primary and secondary antibody responses to myxoviruses. J. Immunol. *98*:668–672, 1967.
158. Heimann, A., Scanlon, R., Gentile, J., et al.: Measles cervicitis: Report of a case with cytologic and molecular biologic analysis. Acta Cytol. *36*:727–730, 1992.
159. Henderson, J. A. M., and Hammond, D. I.: Delayed diagnosis in atypical measles syndrome. Can. Med. Assoc. J. *133*:211–213, 1985.
160. Holt, E. A., Moulton, L. H., Siberry, G. K., et al.: Differential mortality by measles vaccine titer and sex. J. Infect. Dis. *168*:1087–1096, 1993.
161. Home, F.: Medical Facts and Experiments. London, A. Millar, 1759.
162. Horta-Barbosa, L., Krebs, H., Ley, A., et al.: Progressive increase in cerebrospinal fluid measles antibody levels in subacute sclerosing panencephalitis. Pediatrics *47*:782–783, 1971.
163. Horta-Barbosa, L., Fuccillo, D. A., and Sever, J. L.: Subacute sclerosing panencephalitis: Isolation of measles virus from a brain biopsy. Nature *221*:974, 1969.
164. Horta-Barbosa, L., Fuccillo, D. A., London, W. T., et al.: Isolation of measles virus from brain cell cultures of two patients with subacute sclerosing panencephalitis. Proc. Soc. Exp. Biol. Med. *132*:272–277, 1969.
165. Horwitz, M. S., Grose, C., and Fisher, M.: Atypical measles rash mimicking Rocky Mountain spotted fever. N. Engl. J. Med. *289*:1203–1204, 1973.
166. Hudson, J. B., Weinstein, L., and Chang, T. W.: Thrombocytopenic purpura in measles. J. Pediatr. *48*:48–56, 1956.
167. Hussey, G. D., and Klein, M.: A randomized, controlled trial of vitamin A in children with severe measles. N. Engl. J. Med. *323*:160–164, 1990.
168. Imagawa, D. T.: Relationships among measles, canine distemper and rinderpest viruses. Prog. Med. Virol. *10*:160–193, 1968.
169. Imagawa, D. T., and Adams, J. M.: Propagation of measles virus in suckling mice. Proc. Soc. Exp. Biol. *98*:567–569, 1958.
170. Inua, M., Duggan, M. B., West, C. E., et al.: Postmeasles corneal ulceration in children in northern Nigeria: The role of retinol, malnutrition, and measles. Ann. Trop. Pediatr. *3*:181–191, 1983.
171. Janeway, C. A.: Use of concentrated human serum γ-globulin in the prevention and attenuation of measles. Bull. N. Y. Acad. Med. *21*:202–222, 1945.
172. Jayarajan, V., and Sedler, P. A.: Hearing loss following measles vaccination. J. Infect. *30*:184–185, 1995.
173. Jenkerson, S. A., Beller, M., Middaugh, J. P., et al.: False-positive rubeola IgM tests. N. Engl. J. Med. *332*:1103–1104, 1995.
174. Jespersen, C. S., Littauer, J., and Sagild, U.: Measles as a cause of fetal defects: A retrospective study of ten measles epidemics in Greenland. Acta Pediatr. Scand. *66*:367–372, 1977.
175. Joffe, M. I., Sukha, N. R., and Rabson, A. R.: Lymphocyte subsets in measles: Depressed helper/inducer subpopulation reversed by in vitro treatment with levamisole and ascorbic acid. J. Clin. Invest. *72*:971–980, 1983.
176. Johnson, R. T., Griffin, D. E., Hirsch, R. L., et al.: Measles encephalomyelitis: Clinical and immunologic studies. N. Engl. J. Med. *310*:137–141, 1984.
177. Kamahora, J., and Nii, S.: Pathological and immunological studies of monkeys infected with measles virus. Arch. Virusforsch. *16*:161–167, 1965.
178. Karzon, D. T., Rush, D., and Winkelstein, W., Jr.: Immunization with inactivated measles virus vaccine: Effect of booster dose and response to natural challenge. Pediatrics *36*:40–50, 1965.
179. Katz, S. L., and Enders, J. F.: Measles virus. *In* Lennette, E. H., and Schmidt, N. J. (eds.): Diagnostic Procedures for Viral and Rickettsial Infections. Washington, D.C., American Public Health Association, 1969, pp. 504–528.
180. Katz, S. L., and Enders, J. F.: Measles virus. *In* Horsfall, F. L., Jr., and Tamm, T. (eds.): Viral and Rickettsial Infections of Man. Philadelphia, J. B. Lippincott, 1965, pp. 784–801.
181. Katz, S. L.: Measles: Its complications, treatment and prophylaxis. Med. Clin. North Am. *46*:1163–1175, 1962.
182. Katz, S. L., Milovanovic, M. V., and Enders, J. F.: Propagation of measles virus in cultures of chick embryo cells. Proc. Soc. Exp. Biol. Med. *97*:23–29, 1958.
183. Kempe, C. H., and Fulginiti, V. A.: The pathogenesis of measles virus infection. Arch. Virusforsch. *16*:103–128, 1965.
184. Kennedy, C. R., and Webster, A. D. B.: Measles encephalitis. N. Engl. J. Med. *311*:330–331, 1984.
185. Khatib, R., Siddique, M., and Abbas, M.: Measles-associated hepatobiliary disease: An overview. Infection *21*:112–114, 1993.
186. Kibler, R., and TerMeulen, V.: Antibody-mediated cytotoxicity after measles virus infection. J. Immunol. *114*:93–98, 1975.

187. Kiepiela, P., Coovadia, H. M., and Coward, P.: T helper cell defect related to severity in measles. Scand. J. Infect. Dis. *19*:185–192, 1987.
188. Kimura, A., Tosaka, K., and Nakao, T.: Measles rash. I. Light and electron microscopic study of skin eruptions. Arch. Virol. *47*:295–307, 1975.
189. Kleiman, M. B., Blackburn, C. K. L., Zimmerman, S. E., et al.: Comparison of enzyme-linked immunosorbent assay for acute measles with hemagglutination inhibition, complement fixation, and fluorescent antibody methods. J. Clin. Microbiol. *14*:147–152, 1981.
190. Kobune, F., Sakata, H., and Sugiura, A.: Marmoset lymphoblastoid cells as a sensitive host for isolation of measles virus. J. Virol. *64*:700–705, 1990.
191. Koffler, D.: Giant cell pneumonia: Fluorescent antibody and histochemical studies on alveolar giant cells. Arch. Pathol. *78*:267–273, 1964.
192. Kohn, J. L., and Koiransky, H.: Successive roentgenograms of the chest of children during measles. Am. J. Dis. Child. *38*:258–270, 1929.
193. Koplik, H.: The new diagnostic spots of measles on the buccal and labial mucous membrane. Med. News *74*:673, 1899.
194. Koplik, H.: A new diagnostic sign of measles. Med. Rec. *53*:505, 1898.
195. Koplik, H.: The diagnosis of the invasion of measles from a study of the exanthema as it appears on the buccal mucous membrane. Arch. Pediatr. *13*:918, 1896.
196. Krause, P. J., Cherry, J. D., Naiditch, M. J., et al.: Revaccination of previous recipients of killed measles vaccine: Clinical and immunologic studies. J. Pediatr. *93*:565–571, 1978.
197. Kress, S., Schluederberg, A. E., Hornick, R. B., et al.: Studies with live attenuated measles-virus vaccine. II. Clinical and immunologic response of children in an open community. Am. J. Dis. Child. *101*:701–707, 1961.
198. Krugman, R. D., Rosenberg, R., McIntosh, K., et al.: Further attenuated live measles vaccines: The need for revised recommendations. J. Pediatr. *91*:766–767, 1977.
199. Krugman, S., Ward, R., and Katz, S. L.: Measles (rubeola). *In* Krugman, S., Ward, R., and Katz, S. L. (eds.): Infectious Diseases of Children. 6th ed. St. Louis, C. V. Mosby, 1977, pp. 132–148.
200. Krugman, S.: Present status of measles and rubella immunization in the United States: A medical progress report. J. Pediatr. *90*:1–12, 1977.
201. Krugman, S.: Present status of measles and rubella immunization in the United States: A medical progress report. J. Pediatr. *78*:1–16, 1971.
202. Krugman, S., Giles, J. P., Friedman, H., et al.: Studies on immunity to measles. J. Pediatr. *66*:471–488, 1965.
203. Krugman, S., Giles, J. P., Jacobs, A. M., et al.: Studies with live attenuated measles-virus vaccine. Am. J. Dis. Child. *103*:353–363, 1962.
204. LaBoccetta, A. C., and Tornay, A. S.: Measles encephalitis: Report of 61 cases. Am. J. Dis. Child. *107*:247–255, 1964.
205. Labowskie, R. J., Edelman, R., Rustigian, R., et al.: Studies of cell-mediated immunity to measles virus by in vitro lymphocyte-mediated cytotoxicity. J. Infect. Dis. *129*:233–239, 1974.
206. Landrigan, P. J., and Witte, J. J.: Neurologic disorders following live measles-virus vaccination. J. A. M. A. *223*:1459–1462, 1973.
207. Langmuir, A. D.: Medical importance of measles. Am. J. Dis. Child. *103*:224–226, 1962.
208. Laptook, A., Wind, E., Nussbaum, M., et al.: Pulmonary lesions in atypical measles. Pediatrics *62*:42–46, 1978.
209. Levy, D. L.: The future of measles in highly immunized populations. Am. J. Epidemiol. *120*:39–48, 1984.
210. Lightwood, R., Nolan, R., Franco, M., et al.: Epithelial giant cells in measles as an aid in diagnosis. J. Pediatr. *77*:59–64, 1970.
211. Lin, C.-Y., and Hsu, H.-C.: Measles and acute glomerulonephritis. Pediatrics *71*:398–401, 1983.
212. Linnemann, C. C., Jr., Rotte, T. C., Schiff, G. M., et al.: A seroepidemiologic study of a measles epidemic in a highly immunized population. Am. J. Epidemiol. *95*:238–246, 1972.
213. Lobes, L. A., Jr., and Cherry, J. D.: Fatal measles pneumonia in a child with chickenpox pneumonia. J. A. M. A. *223*:1143–1144, 1973.
214. London, W. P., and Yorke, J. A.: Recurrent outbreaks of measles, chickenpox and mumps. I. Seasonal variation in contact rates. Am. J. Epidemiol. *98*:453–468, 1973.
215. Lyon, G., Ponsot, G., and Lebon, P.: Acute measles encephalitis of the delayed type. Ann. Neurol. 2:322–327, 1977.
216. Maimone, D., Grimaldi, L. M. E., Incorpora, G., et al.: Intrathecal interferon in subacute sclerosing panencephalitis. Acta Neurol. Scand. *78*:161–166, 1988.
217. Makhene, M. K., and Diaz, P. S.: Clinical presentations and complications of suspected measles in hospitalized children. Pediatr. Infect. Dis. J. *12*:836–840, 1993.
218. Manchester, M., Valsamakis, A., Kaufman, R., et al.: Measles virus and C3 binding sites are distinct on membrane cofactor protein (CD46). Proc. Natl. Acad. Sci. U. S. A. *92*:2303–2307, 1995.
219. Manchester, M., Lisszewski, M. K., Atkinson, J. P., et al.: Multiple isoforms of CD46 (membrane cofactor protein) serve as receptors for measles virus. Proc. Natl. Acad. Sci. U. S. A. *91*:2161–2165, 1994.
220. Maretic, Z., Stihovic, L. J., Ogrizek, M., et al.: Stevens-Johnson syndrome in the course of measles. J. Trop. Med. Hyg. *68*:50–52, 1965.
221. Markowitz, L. E., and Orenstein, W. A.: Measles vaccines. Pediatr. Clin. North Am. *37*:603–625, 1990.
222. Markowitz, L. E., Nzilambi, N., Driskell, W. H., et al.: Retinol concentration and mortality among hospitalized measles patients, Kinshasa, Zaire. J. Trop. Pediatr. *35*:109–112, 1989.
223. Markowitz, L. E., Preblud, S. R., Orenstein, W. A., et al.: Patterns of transmission in measles outbreaks in the United States, 1985–1986. N. Engl. J. Med. *320*:75–81, 1989.
224. Mason, W. H., Ross, L. A., Lanson, J., et al.: Epidemic measles in the postvaccine era: Evaluation of epidemiology, clinical presentation and complications during an urban outbreak. Pediatr. Infect. Dis. J. *12*:42–48, 1993.
225. Mathiesen, T., Hammarstrom, L., Fridell, E., et al. Aberrant IgG subclass distribution to measles in healthy seropositive individuals, in patients with SSPE and in immunoglobulin-deficient patients. Clin. Exp. Immunol. *80*:202–205, 1990.
226. Matszuzono, Y., Narita, M., Ishiguro, N., et al.: Detection of measles virus from clinical samples using the polymerase chain reaction. Arch. Pediatr. Adolesc. Med. *148*:289–293, 1994.
227. Matumoto, M.: Multiplication of measles virus in cell cultures. Bacteriol. Rev. *30*:152–176, 1966.
228. McLean, D. M., Kettyls, G. D. M., Hingston, J., et al.: Atypical measles following immunization with killed measles vaccine. Can. Med. Assoc. J. *103*:743–744, 1970.
229. McLean, D. M., Best, J. M., Smith, P. A., et al.: Viral infections of Toronto children during 1965. II. Measles encephalitis and other complications. Can. Med. Assoc. J. *94*:905–910, 1966.
230. McLellan, R. K., and Gleiner, J. A.: Acute hepatitis in an adult with rubeola. J. A. M. A. *247*:2000–2001, 1982.
231. McNeill, W. H.: Plagues and Peoples. Garden City, New York, Anchor Press–Doubleday, 1976, pp. 105, 119.
232. Meadow, S. R., Weller, R. O., and Archibald, R. W. R.: Fatal systemic measles in a child receiving cyclophosphamide for nephrotic syndrome. Lancet *2*:876–878, 1969.
233. Mellor, D. H., and Purcell, M.: Unusual encephalitic illnesses in a child with acute leukaemia in remission: Possible role of measles virus and *Toxoplasma gondii.* Neuropaediatrie *7*:423–430, 1976.
234. Melnick, J. L.: Taxonomy of viruses, 1976. Prog. Med. Virol. *22*:211–221, 1976.
235. Meulen, V. T., Kackell, Y., Muller, D., et al.: Isolation of infectious measles virus in measles encephalitis. Lancet *2*:1172–1175, 1972.
236. Meyer, H. M., Jr., Brooks, B. E., Douglas, R. D., et al.: Ecology of measles in monkeys. Am. J. Dis. Child. *103*:307–313, 1962.
237. Miller, D. L.: Frequency of complications of measles, 1963. B. M. J. *2*:75–78, 1964.
238. Milovanovic, M. V., Enders, J. F., and Mitus, A.: Cultivation of measles virus in human amnion cells and in developing chick embryo. Proc. Soc. Exp. Biol. Med. *95*:120–127, 1957.
239. Mitnick, J., Becker, M. H., Rothberg, M., et al.: Nodular residua of atypical measles pneumonia. AJR Am. J. Roentgenol. *134*:257–260, 1980.
240. Mitus, A., Enders, J. F., Edsall, G., et al.: Measles in children with malignancy problems and prevention. Arch. Virusforsch. *16*:331–337, 1965.
241. Mitus, A., Holloway, A., Evans, A. E., et al.: Attenuated measles vaccine in children with acute leukemia. Am. J. Dis. Child. *103*:413–418, 1962.
242. Mitus, A., Enders, J. F., Craig, J. M., et al.: Persistence of measles virus and depression of antibody formation in patients with giant-cell pneumonia after measles. N. Engl. J. Med. *261*:882–889, 1959.
243. Modlin, J. F., Jabbour, J. T., Witte, J. J., et al.: Epidemiologic studies of measles, measles vaccine, and subacute sclerosing panencephalitis. Pediatrics *59*:505–512, 1977.
244. Moench, T. R., Griffin, D. E., Obriecht, C. R., et al.: Acute measles in patients with and without neurological involvement: Distribution of measles virus antigen and RNA. J. Infect. Dis. *158*:433–442, 1988.
245. Monif, G. R. G., and Hood, G. I.: Ileocolitis associated with measles (rubeola). Am. J. Dis. Child. *120*:245–247, 1970.
246. Moraes, N. D. A.: Medical importance of measles in Brazil. Am. J. Dis. Child. *103*:233–236, 1962.
247. Morgan, E. M., and Rapp, F.: Measles virus and its associated diseases. Bacteriol. Rev. *41*:636–666, 1977.
248. Morley, D. C., Martin, W. J., and Allen, I.: Measles in East and Central Africa. East Afr. Med. J. *44*:497–508, 1967.
249. Morley, D., Woodland, M., and Martin, W. J.: Measles in Nigerian children: A study of the disease in West Africa, and its manifestations in England and other countries during different epochs. J. Hyg. (Camb.) *61*:115–134, 1963.
250. Morley, D. C.: Measles in Nigeria. Am. J. Dis. Child. *103*:230–233, 1962.
251. Moroi, K., Saito, S., Kurata, T., et al.: Fetal death associated with measles virus infection of the placenta. Am. J. Obstet. Gynecol. *164*:1107–1108, 1991.
252. Murphy, J. V., and Yunis, E. J.: Encephalopathy following measles infection in children with chronic illness. J. Pediatr. *88*:937–942, 1976.
253. Murray, K., Selleck, P., Hooper, P., et al.: A morbillivirus that caused fatal disease in horses and humans. Science *268*:94–97, 1995.
254. Musser, S. J., and Underwood, G. E.: Studies on measles virus. II. Physical properties and inactivation studies of measles virus. J. Immunol. *85*:292–297, 1960.
255. Mustafa, M. M., Weitman, S. D., Winick, N. J., et al.: Subacute measles encephalitis in the young immunocompromised host: Report of two cases

diagnosed by polymerase chain reaction and treated with ribavirin and review of the literature. Clin. Infect. Dis. *16*:654–660, 1993.

256. Nader, P. R., Horwitz, M. S., and Rousseau, J.: Atypical exanthem following exposure to natural measles: Eleven cases in children previously inoculated with killed vaccine. J. Pediatr. *72*:22–28, 1968.
257. Nahmias, A. J., Griffith, D., Salsbury, C., et al.: Thymic aplasia with lymphopenia, plasma cells, and normal immunoglobulins. J. A. M. A. *201*:729–734, 1967.
258. Nakai, M., and Imagawa, D. T.: Electron microscopy of measles virus replication. J. Virol. *3*:187–197, 1969.
258a. Nakayama, T., Urano, T., Osano, M., et al.: Long-term regulation of interferon production by lymphocytes from children inoculated with live measles virus vaccine. J. Infect. Dis. *158*:1386–1390, 1988.
259. Naniche, D., Varior-Krisnan, G., Cervoni, F., et al.: Human membrane cofactor protein (CD46) acts as a cellular receptor for measles virus. J. Virol. *67*:6025–6032, 1993.
260. Neumann, P. W., Weber, J. M., Jessamine, A. G., et al.: Comparison of measles antihemolysin test, enzyme-linked immunosorbent assay, and hemagglutination inhibition test with neutralization test for determination of immune status. J. Clin. Microbiol. *22*:296–298, 1985.
261. Nichols, E. M.: Atypical measles syndrome: A continuing problem. Am. J. Public Health *69*:160–164, 1979.
262. Nickell, M. D., Cannady, P. B., Jr., and Schwitzer, G. A.: Subclinical hepatitis in rubeola infections in young adults. Ann. Intern. Med. *90*:354–355, 1979.
263. Nieburg, P. I., D'Angelo, L. J., and Herrmann, K. L.: Measles in patients suspected of having Rocky Mountain spotted fever. J. A. M. A. *244*:808–809, 1980.
264. Nii, S., Kamahora, J., Mori, Y., et al.: Experimental pathology of measles in monkeys. Biken J. *6*:271–297, 1964.
265. Norrby, L., and Oxman, M. N.: Measles virus. *In* Fields, B. N., Knipe, D. M., Chanock, R., M., et al. (eds.): Virology. 2nd ed. New York, Raven Press, 1990, pp. 1013–1044.
266. Norrby, E., and Gollmar, Y.: Identification of measles virus-specific hemolysis-inhibiting antibodies separate from hemagglutination-inhibiting antibodies. Infect. Immun. *11*:231–239, 1975.
267. Norrby, E., Enders-Ruckle, G., and ter Meulen, V.: The significance of hemolysing-inhibiting antibodies in protection against measles. Med. Microbiol. Immunol. *160*:232, 1974.
268. Norrby, E., and Hammarskjold, B.: Structural components of measles virus. Microbios *5*:17–29, 1972.
269. Norrby, E., and Gollmar, Y.: Appearance and persistence of antibodies against different virus components after regular measles infections. Infect. Immun. *6*:240–247, 1972.
270. Norrby, E., Lagercrantz, R., and Gard, S.: Measles vaccination. VII. Followup studies in children immunized with four doses of inactivated vaccine. Acta Pediatr. Scand. *58*:261–267, 1969.
271. Norrby, E., Lagercrantz, R., and Gard, S.: Measles vaccination. IV. Responses to two different types of preparations given as a fourth dose of vaccine. B. M. J. *1*:813–817, 1965.
272. Norrby, E. C. J., and Magnusson, P.: Some morphological characteristics of the internal component of measles virus. Arch. Virusforsch. *17*:443–447, 1965.
273. Norrby, E. C. J., Magnusson, P., Falksveden, L. G., et al.: Separation of measles virus components by equilibrium centrifugation in CsCI gradiants. II. Studies on the large and the small hemagglutinin. Arch. Virusforsch. *14*:462–473, 1964.
274. Norrby, E.: Hemagglutination by measles virus. II. Properties of the hemagglutinin and of the receptors on the erythrocytes. Arch. Virusforsch. *12*:164–172, 1962.
275. O'Donovan, C., and Barua, K. N.: Measles pneumonia. Am. J. Trop. Med. Hyg. *22*:73–77, 1973.
276. O'Donovan, C.: Measles in Kenyan children. East Afr. Med. J. *48*:526–532, 1971.
277. Ojala, A.: On changes in the cerebrospinal fluid during measles. Ann. Med. Fenn. *36*:321–331, 1947.
278. Ono, K., Iwa, N., Kato, S., et al.: Demonstration of viral antigen in giant cells formed in monkeys experimentally infected with measles virus. Biken J. *13*:329–337, 1970.
279. Orenstein, W. A., Markowitz, L. E., Atkinson, W. L., et al.: Worldwide measles prevention. Israel J. Med. Sci. *30*:469–481, 1994.
280. Orenstein, W. A., Halsey, N. A., Hayden, G. F., et al.: Current status of measles in the United States, 1973–1977. J. Infect. Dis. *137*:847–853, 1978.
281. Oski, F. A., and Naiman, J. L.: Effect of live measles vaccine on the platelet count. N. Engl. J. Med. *275*:352–356, 1966.
282. Osterhaus, A. D. M. E., deVries, P., and van Binnendjik, R. S.: Measles vaccines: Novel generations and new strategies. J. Infect. Dis. *70*:(Suppl. 1):S42–S45, 1994.
283. Pampiglione, G.: Prodromal phase of measles: Some neurophysiological studies. B. M. J. *2*:1296–1300, 1964.
284. Panum, P. L.: Observations made during the epidemic of measles on the Faroe Islands in the year 1846. Med. Classics *3*:829–886, 1939.
285. Papp, K.: Experiences prouvant que la voie d'infection de la rougeole est la contamination de la muqueuse conjonctivale. Rev. Immunol. Ther. Anti-Microb. *20*:27–36, 1956.
286. Partington, M. W., and Quinton, J. F. P.: The preeruptive illness of measles. Arch. Dis. Child. *34*:149–153, 1959.
287. Pather, M., Wesley, A. G., Schonland, M., et al.: Severe measles-associated pneumonia treated with assisted ventilation. S. Afr. Med. J. *50*:1600–1603, 1976.
288. Payne, F. E., Baublis, J. V., and Itabashi, H. H.: Isolation of measles virus from cell cultures of brain from a patient with subacute sclerosing panencephalitis. N. Engl. J. Med. *281*:585–589, 1969.
289. Pearl, P. L., Abu-Farshak, H., Starke, J. R., et al.: Neuropathology of two fatal cases of measles in the 1988–1989 Houston epidemic. Pediatr. Neurol. *6*:126–130, 1990.
290. Peebles, T. C.: Distribution of virus in blood components during the viremia of measles. Arch. Virusforsch. *22*:43–47, 1967.
291. Peries, J. R., and Chany, C.: Studies on measles viral hemagglutination. Proc. Soc. Exp. Biol. Med. *110*:477–482, 1962.
292. Phillips, C. A.: Inclusion bodies in measles encephalitis. J. A. M. A. *195*:167–168, 1966.
293. Plotkin, S. A.: Vaccination against measles in the 18th century. Clin. Pediatr. *6*:312–315, 1967.
294. Plotz, H.: Culture "in vitro" du virus de la rougeole. Bull. Acad. Méd. Paris, *119*:598, 1938.
295. Pollack, M. A., Grose, C., and Friend, H.: Measles associated with Bell palsy. Am. J. Dis. Child. *129*:747, 1975.
296. Pullan, C., Noble, T. C., Scott, D. J., et al.: Atypical measles infections in leukaemic children on immunosuppressive treatment. B. M. J. *1*:1562–1565, 1976.
297. Rake, G., and Shaffer, M. F.: Studies on measles. I. The use of the chorio-allantois of the developing chicken embryo. J. Immunol. *38*:177–200, 1940.
298. Rand, K. H., Emmons, R. W., and Merigan, T. C.: Measles in adults: An unforeseen consequence of immunization? J. A. M. A. *236*:1028–1031, 1976.
299. Rauh, L. W., and Schmidt, R.: Measles immunization with killed virus vaccine: Serum antibody titers and experience with exposure to measles epidemic. Am. J. Dis. Child. *109*:232–237, 1965.
300. Reddy, V., Bhaskaram, P., Raghuramulu, N., et al.: Relationship between measles, malnutrition, and blindness: A prospective study in Indian children. Am. J. Clin. Nutr. *44*:924–930, 1986.
301. Remington, P. L., Hall, W. N., Davis, I. H., et al.: Airborne transmission of measles in a physician's office. J. A. M. A. *253*:1574–1577, 1985.
302. Reyes, M. A., DeBorrero, M. F., Roa, J., et al.: Measles vaccine failure after documented seroconversion. Pediatr. Infect. Dis. J. *6*:848–851, 1987.
303. Riley, E. C., Murphy, G., and Riley, R. L.: Airborne spread of measles in a suburban elementary school. Am. J. Epidemiol. *107*:421–432, 1978.
304. Riley, R. L.: Airborne infection. Am. J. Med. *57*:466–475, 1974.
305. Ristori, C., Boccardo, H., Borgono, J. M., et al.: Medical importance of measles in Chile. Am. J. Dis. Child. *103*:236–241, 1962.
306. Robbins, F. C.: Measles: Clinical features. Pathogenesis, pathology and complications. Am. J. Dis. Child. *103*:266–273, 1962.
307. Roberts, G. B. S., and Bain, A. D.: The pathology of measles. J. Pathol. Immunol. *76*:111–118, 1958.
308. Ross, L. A., Mason, W. H., Lanson, J., et al.: Laryngotracheobronchitis as a complication of measles during an urban epidemic. J. Pediatr. *121*:511–515, 1992.
309. Ross, L. J.: Electrocardiographic findings in measles. Am. J. Dis. Child. *83*:282–291, 1952.
310. Rota, P. A., Rota, J. S., and Bellini, W. J.: Molecular epidemiology of measles virus. Virology *6*:379–386, 1995.
311. Ruckdeschel, J. C., Graziano, K. D., and Mardiney, M. R., Jr.: Additional evidence that the cell-associated immune system is the primary host defense against measles (rubeola). Cell. Immunol. *17*:11–18, 1975.
312. Ruckle, G., and Rogers, K. D.: Studies with measles virus. II. Isolation of virus and immunologic studies in persons who have had the natural disease. J. Immunol. *78*:341–355, 1957.
313. Sandford-Smith, J. H., and Whittle, H. C.: Corneal ulceration following measles in Nigerian children. Br. J. Ophthalmol. *63*:720–724, 1979.
314. Saxton, N. L.: Thrombocytopenic purpura following the administration of attenuated live measles vaccine. J. Iowa Med. Soc. *57*:1017–1018, 1967.
315. Schaffner, W., Schluederberg, A. E. S., and Byrne, E. B.: Clinical epidemiology of sporadic measles in a highly immunized population. N. Engl. J. Med. *279*:783–789, 1968.
316. Scheifele, D. W., and Forbes, C. E.: Prolonged giant cell excretion in severe African measles. Pediatrics *50*:867–873, 1972.
317. Schluederberg, A.: Modification of immune response by previous experience with measles. Arch. Ges. Virusforsch. *16*:347–350, 1965.
318. Schluederberg, A.: Immune globulins in human viral infections. Nature *205*:1232, 1965.
319. Schluederberg, A.: Separation of measles virus particles in density gradients. Am. J. Dis. Child. *103*:291–296, 1962.
320. Selvey, L. A., Wells, R. M., McCormack, J. G., et al.: Infection of humans and horses by a newly described morbillivirus. Med. J. Aust. *162*:642–645, 1995.
321. Sergiev, P. G., Ryazantseva, N. E., and Shroit, I. G.: The dynamics of pathological processes in experimental measles in monkeys. Acta Virol. *4*:265–273, 1960.

322. Shalit, M., Ackerman, Z., Wollner, S., et al.: Immunoglobulin E response during measles. Int. Arch. Allergy Appl. Immun. *75*:84–86, 1984.
323. Shasby, D. M., Shope, T. C., Downs, H., et al.: Epidemic measles in a highly vaccinated population. N. Engl. J. Med. *296*:585–589, 1977.
324. Shoss, R. G., and Rayhanzadeh, S.: Toxic epidermal necrolysis following measles vaccination. Arch. Dermatol. *110*:766–770, 1974.
325. Siegel, D., and Hirschman, S. Z.: Hepatic dysfunction in acute measles infection of adults. Arch. Intern. Med. *137*:1178–1179, 1977.
326. Siegel, M. M., Walter, T. K., and Ablin, A. R.: Measles pneumonia in childhood leukemia. Pediatrics *60*:38–40, 1977.
327. Smith, F. R., Curran, A. S., Raciti, K. A., et al.: Reported measles in persons immunologically primed by prior vaccination. J. Pediatr. *101*:391–393, 1982.
328. Sobonya, R. E., Hiller, F. C., Pingleton, W., et al.: Fatal measles (rubeola) pneumonia in adults. Arch. Pathol. Lab. Med. *102*:366–371, 1978.
329. Spencer, M. J., and Cherry, J. D.: Unpublished data, 1976.
330. Starr, S., and Berkovich, S.: The effect of measles, gamma globulin modified measles, and attenuated measles vaccine on the course of treated tuberculosis in children. Pediatrics *35*:97–102, 1965.
331. Starr, S., and Berkovich, S.: Effects of measles, gamma-globulin–modified measles and vaccine measles on the tuberculin test. N. Engl. J. Med. *270*:386–391, 1964.
332. Stein, S. J., and Greenspoon, J. S.: Rubeola during pregnancy. Obstet. Gynecol. *78*:925–929, 1991.
333. St. Geme, J. W., Jr., George, B. L., and Bush, B. M.: Exaggerated natural measles following attenuated virus immunization. Pediatrics *57*:148–150, 1976.
334. Stimson, P. M.: The earlier diagnosis of measles. J. A. M. A. *90*:660–663, 1928.
335. Stokes, J., Jr.: Viral infections, including those presumed to be caused by viruses: Measles (rubeola). *In* Nelson, W. E. (ed.): Textbook of Pediatrics. 6th ed. Philadelphia, W. B. Saunders, 1954, pp. 466–471.
336. Stokes, J., Jr., Maris, E. P., and Gellis, S. S.: Chemical, clinical, and immunological studies on the products of human plasma fractionation. XI. The use of concentrated normal human serum gamma globulin (human immune serum globulin) in the prophylaxis and treatment of measles. J. Clin. Invest. *23*:531–540, 1944.
337. Stratton, K. R., Howe, C. J., and Johnston, R. B., Jr.: Adverse events associated with childhood vaccines other than pertussis and rubella: Summary of a report from the Institute of Medicine. J. A. M. A. *271*:1602–1605, 1994.
338. Suringa, D. W. R., Bank, L. J., and Ackerman, A. B.: Role of measles virus in skin lesions and Koplik's spots. N. Engl. J. Med. *283*:1139–1142, 1970.
339. Sutter, R. W., Markowitz, L. E., Bennetch, J. M., et al.: Measles among the Amish: A comparative study of measles severity in primary and secondary cases in households. J. Infect. Dis. *163*:12–16, 1991.
340. Swift, J. D., Barruga, M. C., Perkin, R. M., et al.: Respiratory failure complicating rubeola. Chest *104*:1786–1787, 1993.
341. Taneja, P. N., Ghal, O. P., and Bhakoo, O. N.: Importance of measles in India. Am. J. Dis. Child. *103*:226–229, 1962.
342. Taylor, M. J., Godfrey, E., Baczko, K., et al.: Identification of several different lineages of measles virus. J. Gen. Virol. *72*:83–88, 1991.
343. Tellez-Nagel, I., and Harter, D. H.: Subacute sclerosing leukoencephalitis. I. Clinico-pathological, electron microscopic and virological observations. J. Neuropathol. Exp. Neurol. *25*:560–581, 1966.
344. Tidstrom, B.: Complications in measles with special reference to encephalitis. Acta Med. Scand. *184*:411–415, 1968.
345. Tishler, M., and Abramov, A. L.: Liver involvement in measles infection of young adults. Is. J. Med. Sci. *19*:791–793, 1983.
346. Tuokko, H., and Salmi, A.: Detection of IgM antibodies to measles virus by enzyme-immunoassay. Med. Microbiol. Immunol. *171*:187–198, 1983.
347. Tyler, H. R.: Neurological complications of rubeola (measles). Medicine *36*:147–167, 1957.
348. Udem, S. A., and Cook, K. A.: Isolation and characterization of measles virus intracellular nucleocapsid RNA. J. Virol. *49*:57–65, 1984.
349. Varavithya, W., Stoecker, B., Chaiyaratana, W., et al.: Retinol status of Thai children with measles. Trop. Geogr. Med. *38*:359–361, 1986.
350. Wakefield, A. J., Ekbom, A., Dhillon, A. P., et al.: Crohn's disease: Pathogenesis and persistent measles virus infection. Gastroenterology *108*:911–916, 1995.
351. Wakefield, A. J., Pittilo, R. M., Sim, R., et al.: Evidence of persistent measles virus infection in Crohn's disease. J. Med. Virol. *39*:345–353, 1993.
352. Waksman, B. H., Burnstein, T., and Adams, R. D.: Histologic study of the encephalomyelitis produced in hamsters by a neurotropic strain of measles. J. Neuropathol. Exp. Neurol. *21*:25, 1962.
353. Ward, B. J., Johnson, R. T., Vaisberg, A., et al.: Spontaneous proliferation of peripheral mononuclear cells in natural measles virus infection: Identification of dividing cells and correlation with mitogen responsiveness. Clin. Immunol. Immunopathol. *55*:315–326, 1990.
354. Waters, D. J., and Bussell, R. H.: Isolation and comparative study of the nucleocapsids of measles and canine distemper viruses from infected cells. Virology *61*:64–79, 1974.
355. Waters, D. J., Hersh, R. T., and Bussell, R. H.: Isolation and characterization of measles nucleocapsid from infected cells. Virology *48*:278–281, 1972.
356. Waterson, A. P.: Measles virus. Arch. Ges. Virusforsch. *16*:57–80, 1965.
357. Waterson, A. P., Cruickshank, J. G., Lawrence, G. D., et al.: The nature of measles virus. Virology *15*:379–382, 1961.
358. Weiner, L. B., Corwin, R. M., Nieburg, P. I., et al.: A measles outbreak among adolescents. J. Pediatr. *90*:17–20, 1977.
359. Welliver, R. C., Cherry, J. D., and Holtzman, A. E.: Typical, modified, and atypical measles. Arch. Intern. Med. *137*:39–41, 1977.
360. Wells, M. W.: The seasonal patterns of measles and chicken pox. Am. J. Hyg. *40*:279–317, 1944.
361. Whittle, H. C., Dossetor, J., Oduloju, A., et al.: Cell-mediated immunity during natural measles infection. J. Clin. Invest. *62*:678–685, 1978.
362. Wilhelm, D. J., and Paegle, R. D.: Thrombocytopenic purpura and pneumonia following measles vaccination. Am. J. Dis. Child. *113*:534–537, 1967.
363. Wilkins, J., and Wehrle, P. F.: Evidence for reinstatement of infants 12 to 14 months of age into routine measles immunization programs. Am. J. Dis. Child. *132*:164–166, 1978.
364. Wilson, E. B., and Worcester, J.: Contact with measles. Proc. Natl. Acad. Sci. U. S. A. *27*:7–13, 1941.
365. Wilson, G. S.: Measles as a universal disease. Am. J. Dis. Child. *103*:219–223, 1962.
366. Winkelstein, W., Jr., Karzon, D. T., Rush, D., et al.: A field trial of inactivated measles virus vaccine in young school children. J. A. M. A. *194*:106–110, 1965.
367. Wolinsky, J. S., Swoveland, P., Johnson, K. P., et al.: Subacute measles encephalitis complicating Hodgkin's disease in an adult. Ann. Neurol. *1*:452–457, 1977.
368. World Health Organization Expanded Programme of Immunizations: Global Advisory Group. Wkly. Epidemiol. Rec. *65*:5–12, 1990.
369. Wright, G. P., and Wright, H. P.: The influence of social conditions upon diphtheria, measles, tuberculosis and whooping cough in early childhood in London. J. Hyg. *42*:451–473, 1942.
370. Wynne, J. M., Williams, G. L., and Ellman, B. A. H.: Gangrene of the extremities in measles. S. Afr. Med. J. *52*:117–121, 1977.
371. Yamanouchi, K., Egashira, Y., Uchida, N., et al.: Giant cell formation in lymphoid tissues of monkeys inoculated with various strains of measles virus. Jpn. J. Med. Sci. Biol. *23*:131–145, 1970.
372. Yeager, A. S., Davis, J. H., Ross, L. A., et al.: Measles immunization: Successes and failures. J. A. M. A. *237*:347–351, 1977.
373. Yorke, J. A., and London, W. P.: Recurrent outbreaks of measles, chickenpox, and mumps. II. Systematic differences in contact rates and stochastic effects. Am. J. Epidemiol. *98*:469–482, 1973.
374. Young, L. W., Smith, D. I., and Glasgow, L. A.: Pneumonia of atypical measles: Residual nodular lesions. Am. J. Roentgenol. Radium Ther. Nucl. Med. *110*:439–448, 1970.
375. Zahradnik, J. M., Cherry, J. D., and Rachelefsky, G.: Atypical measles acquired abroad: Foreign travel and pseudoexotic disease. J. A. M. A. *241*:1711–1712, 1979.
376. Ziegra, S. R.: Corticosteroid treatment for measles encephalitis. J. Pediatr. *59*:322–323, 1961.
377. Ziola, B., Lund, G., Muerman, O., et al.: Circulating immune complexes in patients with acute measles and rubella virus infections. Infect. Immun. *41*:578–583, 1983.

184

Mumps Virus

James D. Cherry

Mumps (epidemic parotitis) is an acute communicable disease caused by the mumps virus, a member of the genus *Paramyxovirus*. As a result of universal childhood immunization, mumps is an uncommon disease in the United States today.

HISTORY[58, 102]

In the 5th century B.C., Hippocrates described an outbreak on the island of Thasus.[58] He noted that most patients had bilateral swelling near the ears and that the others had unilateral swelling. He also noted that some patients had bilateral or unilateral pain and swelling of the testicles. The origin of the name mumps is not known. It may be from the English noun *mump* which means "a lump" or the English verb *mump*, one of whose definitions is "mumble." This latter possible origin is based on the mumbling speech that patients with significant parotitis may have.

In 1790, Robert Hamilton presented an extensive study of mumps in which he noted orchitis, associated the illness with neurologic involvement, and described the neuropathology of a fatal case.[43, 44] In 1886, Hirsch[51] noted that mumps occurred throughout the world and that it was a major cause of morbidity among Confederate troops during the American Civil War. In the first half of the present century, it was recognized that mumps virus infection involved multiple organs, and the causative agent was shown to be a filterable virus by Johnson and Goodpasture in 1934.[28, 53]

The growth of mumps virus in embryonated eggs was reported in 1945, and 10 years later its propagation in tissue culture was noted.[42, 46] This latter development led to the development and licensure of live attenuated mumps vaccine in 1967.[12]

PROPERTIES

Classification

Mumps virus is a member of the genus *Paramyxovirus* in the family *Paramyxoviridae*.[102] It contains a single-stranded, nonsegmented, negative-sense RNA genome that is surrounded by a helical nucleocapsid and a surface envelope.

Physical Properties[61, 102]

The virus generally is spherical, but marked pleomorphism occurs. Its size varies from 100 to 600 nm. There are six major structural proteins. These are nucleocapsid-associated protein (NP), a phosphoprotein (P), a high-molecular-weight protein (L), a matrix or membrane protein (M), a hemagglutinin-neuraminidase glycoprotein (HN), and a fusion glycoprotein (F). The viral envelope is studded with 12- to 15-nm projections that contain either of the two structural glycoproteins (HN or F).

The P structural protein is associated with the nucleocapsid, and an RNA-dependent RNA polymerase is located within the nucleocapsid structure. The envelope has a high lipid content, and it contains the M protein.

Mumps virus infectivity is destroyed by heat (56° C for 20 minutes), and its infectivity is reduced by ultraviolet light, Tween 80, ether, and formalin. The virus is stable at 4° C for several days, and when placed in a buffered salt solution (such as Hank) with 1 to 2 per cent inactivated fetal calf serum, it can be stored indefinitely at −70° C.

Antigenic Composition[61]

The three major antigenic components of mumps virus are the two glycoproteins (HN or V antigen and F) and the nucleocapsid protein (NP or S antigen). The glycoproteins that project from the viral surface are the antigenic target for specific antibodies. Host antibodies to HN and F proteins confer protective immunity against the virus. Mumps viral particles agglutinate erythrocytes of several mammalian and avian species (human, avian, rodent, and simian); at 37° C, the virus causes partial hemolysis of susceptible erythrocytes when the virus is attached to cellular surface receptors. Specific antibody blocks hemagglutination, hemadsorption, and hemolysis.

Mumps virus is considered to have a single immunotype. However, polyclonal antibodies to parainfluenza and Newcastle disease viral antigens cross-react with antibodies to mumps virus in complement fixation and hemagglutination inhibition. With monoclonal antibodies, an antigenic relationship between NH and NP proteins of Sendai virus (a murine parainfluenza type 1 virus) and mumps virus has been demonstrated.[75]

Tissue Culture Growth and Animal Susceptibility[61]

Mumps virus can be propagated in many different primary and cell line tissue cultures. For virus isolation, primary monkey kidney cells usually are employed. Cytopathic effect is similar to that of other paramyxoviruses. When stained, multinucleated giant cells and cytoplasmic eosinophilic inclusions may be observed. In culture, the addition of erythrocytes results in hemadsorption to surface virus.

Mumps virus infects monkeys, rabbits, dogs, cats, and rodents. The virus readily is isolated after the inoculation of the amniotic sac of 7- to 8-day-old chicken embryos.

EPIDEMIOLOGY

Incidence

In the United States, mumps was a reportable disease from 1922 to 1950 and has been again since 1967.[18] Between 1950 and 1967, incidence data were gathered from voluntary reporting by cooperating states. Incidence data from 1922 to 1982 are presented in Figure 184–1, and vaccine era data are presented in Figure 184–2.[11, 18] In the prevaccine era, mumps

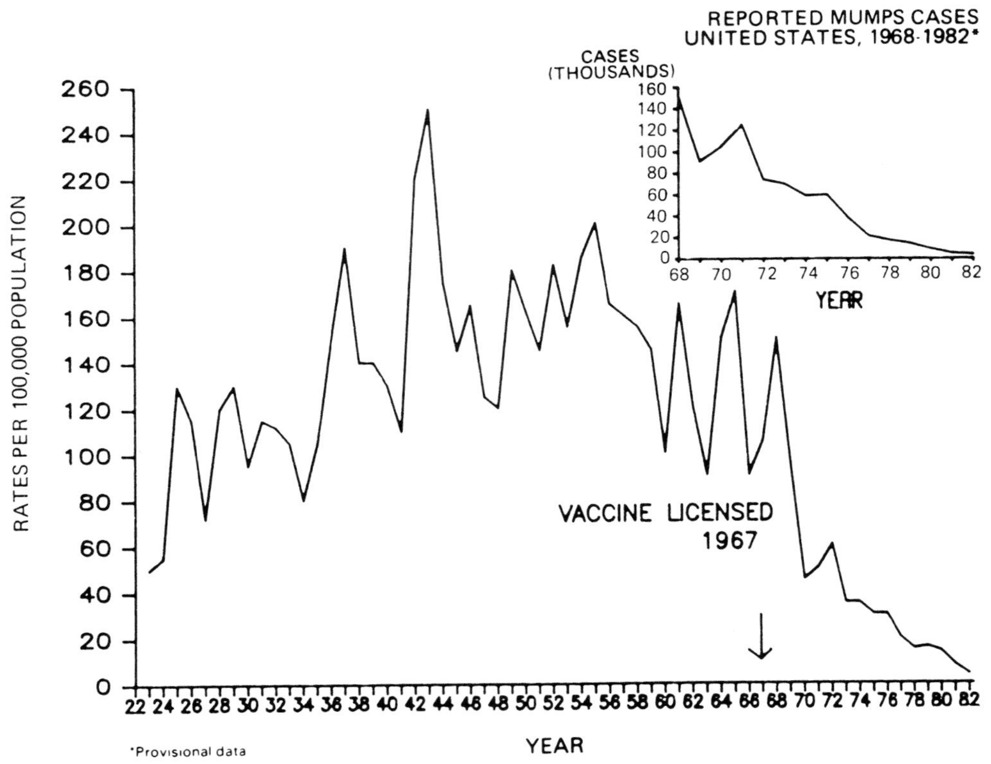

FIGURE 184–1. *Incidence of reported mumps in the United States from 1922 to 1982 and the number of reported cases from 1968 to 1982. (From Centers for Disease Control: Mumps surveillance, January 1977–December 1982. Issued September 1984.)*

was a yearly disease, with epidemic peaks occurring about every 4 years. The peak epidemic year was 1944, when the rate was 250 per 100,000 population.

In the prevaccine era, mumps predominantly was a disease of young children.[18] However, mumps outbreaks were a significant problem in young adults in the military.[38, 69] The age distribution of mumps in the United States during selected years is presented in Table 184–1. After the licensure of mumps vaccine in 1967, mumps remained predominantly a disease of young children from 1967 to 1971. However, by 1981, the majority of reported cases were 10 years of age or older. In 1987, 76 per cent of the cases occurred in persons 10 years of age or older (see Table 184–1). In 1994, 1537 cases were reported—the lowest number ever reported in the United States—and of those with age noted, 21.8 per cent were 20 years of age or older. The increase in reported cases that occurred in 1987 (see Fig. 184–2) was due to a marked increase in cases in unimmunized persons 10 to 19 years of

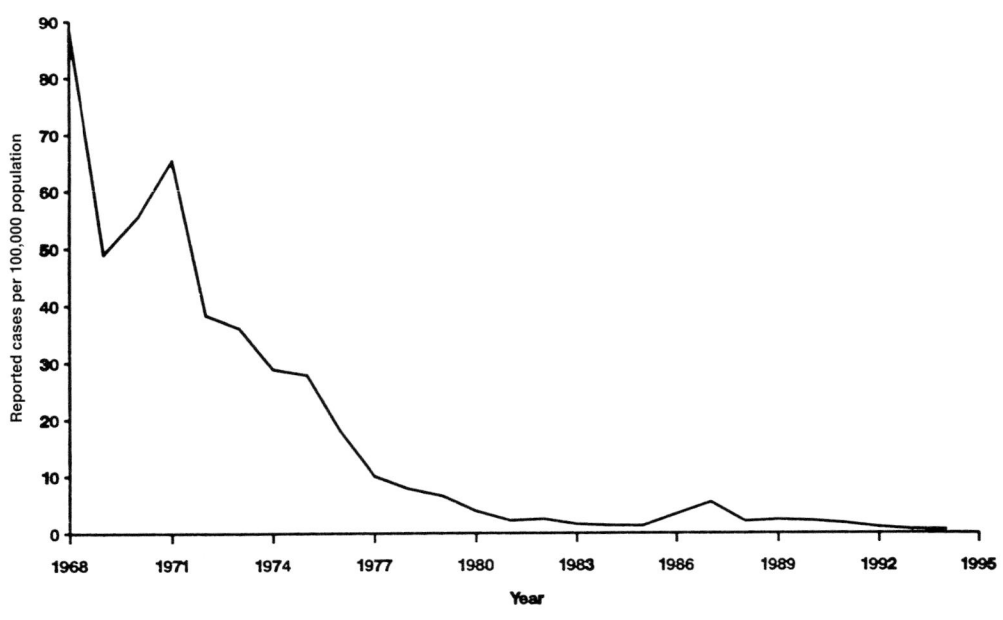

FIGURE 184–2. *Incidence of reported mumps in the United States from 1968 to 1994. (From Centers for Disease Control and Prevention: CDC Surveillance Summaries; Mumps surveillance, United States, 1988–1993. M. M. W. R. 44:1–14, 1995.)*

TABLE 184–1. Age Distribution of Mumps Cases in the United States During Selected Years[11, 14, 18]

Age Group (years)	1967–1971*		1987		1994	
	Cases	%	Cases	%	Cases	%
<5	2932	17.1	804	6.5	250	17.4
5–9	10413	60.8	2196	17.9	473	33.0
10–14	2372	13.8	4567	37.3	271	18.9
15–19	1418†	8.3	3455	28.2	128	8.9
≥20			1235	10.1	312	20.8

*Average annual reported cases for California, Massachusetts, and New York City.
†Includes all reported cases 15 years of age or older.
Data from references 11, 14, and 18.

age. This group had been protected for a time by herd immunity because of the rapidly declining incidence of mumps due to routine vaccine use beginning in 1977.[23]

In the prevaccine era, the peak occurrence of mumps occurred in the winter and spring months, and this continued well into the vaccine era.[18] Since 1989, there has been little seasonal variation in cases.[11, 13]

Morbidity and Mortality

The most common clinical manifestations of mumps virus infection are fever and parotitis. However, about 30 per cent of infections do not involve parotitis and are not recognized.[64] Epididymo-orchitis occurs in 20 to 30 per cent of clinical cases in postpubertal males. About 60 per cent of clinical mumps cases involve cerebrospinal fluid pleocytosis, but only one-sixth of these have meningeal symptoms.[3] In 1966, there were 628 cases of encephalitis (0.5 per cent), and of these, 10 (1.6 per cent) had a fatal outcome.[18] Encephalitis is more common in males (61 per cent), and the rate of occurrence is greatest in adults. Deafness post mumps has been estimated to occur in 0.5 to 5.0 per 100,000 cases.[29, 96]

From 1966 to 1975, 200 mumps-associated deaths were reported.[18] Of these, 44 (22 per cent) were in patients with encephalitis; in the others, the causes of death were not identified. Forty-one per cent of the deaths occurred in adults 40 years of age or older.

Spread of Infection

Mumps virus is contagious in nonimmune persons. It is spread from the infected person to the new host by the respiratory route. The virus can be isolated from the saliva of infected patients from 7 days before the onset of parotitis to 9 days after its onset.[61] Transmission is greatest during a 7-day period beginning 2 days before the onset of parotitis. Asymptomatically infected persons also can transmit the viruses. The fact that outbreaks of mumps occurred in young adult populations in the prevaccine era suggests that mumps virus is less contagious than measles; a significant number of persons passed through childhood without being infected with mumps virus. A serologic study by Black[6] noted that 24 per cent of army recruits lacked hemagglutination-inhibition antibody to mumps, whereas only 1 per cent lacked measles antibody.

The incubation period most often is 16 to 18 days, although it can vary from 12 to 25 days.[61]

PATHOGENESIS AND PATHOLOGY

Viral Infection[30, 61, 102]

After respiratory or perhaps oral acquisition of the virus, primary viral replication occurs in the upper respiratory mucosal epithelium.[102] Virus multiplies and is spread via drainage to local lymph nodes.[30] Subsequently, viremia occurs.[57, 76] As a result of viremia, infection occurs in multiple secondary infection sites. Most prominent is infection of the salivary glands, resulting in inflammation and swelling. This infection results in virus shedding for 1 to 2 weeks. Other secondary infection sites include the inner ear (cochlea), pancreas, heart, nervous system (meninges and brain), joints, kidneys, liver, gonads, and thyroid.

Pathology[102]

In the salivary glands, virus infects the ductal epithelium, causing periductal interstitial edema and a local inflammatory reaction involving lymphocytes and macrophages.[100] Tissue damage occurs, and the involved cells desquamate. Virus enters the central nervous system by the choroid plexus via infected mononuclear cells. Virus multiplies in choroid and ependymal cells on the ventricular surfaces, and these cells desquamate into the cerebrospinal fluid, resulting in meningitis. In encephalitis, perivascular infiltration with mononuclear cells, scattered foci of neuronophagia, and microglial rod-cell proliferation occurs.[9] Periventricular demyelination also occurs.

In the male gonad, the primary site of viral replication occurs in the seminiferous tubules; this infection results in lymphocytic infiltration and edema of interstitial tissues.

Immunologic Events

Infection gives rise to serum antibodies to the HN glycoprotein (V antigen), the F antigen, and the NP protein (S antigen).[61] Antibody to the NP protein develops first, occurring 3 to 7 days after onset of symptoms. The antibodies to the NP protein are short-lived and usually are absent after 6 months; they cross-react with parainfluenza viruses. Antibodies to the HN glycoprotein develop 2 to 4 weeks after illness onset and persist for long periods after infection.

IgG and IgM antibody responses (determined by enzyme-linked immunosorbent assay [ELISA]) regularly occur after infection.[94] The IgG antibody levels measured by ELISA correlate best with those derived by complement fixation and hemolysis-in-gel assays. IgM antibodies develop early (second day of illness) in infection, peak within the first week of illness, and usually are undetectable 3 months after illness onset; occasionally mumps-specific IgM antibody persists for 5 to 6 months.[61, 94] Mumps-specific IgG antibody appears at the end of the first week of illness, peaks 3 weeks later, and persists throughout life. The IgG response mainly is IgG1 subclass.[81] Salivary IgA antibodies to mumps virus regularly appear after infection.[34]

During infection with vaccine virus, the cell-mediated response to tuberculin is diminished for up to 4 weeks.[65] During the same period, a mumps-specific, cell-mediated immune response develops.[61, 102] This has been demonstrated by skin-test hypersensitivity, in vitro lymphocyte-proliferative responses, and cytotoxic T-lymphocyte studies.[8, 10, 63]

CLINICAL MANIFESTATIONS

In epidemics of mumps, cases can be separated into five groups: (1) those with a short course whose signs and symptoms are nonspecific, (2) those in which the disease is full-blown with salivary swelling but with no complications, (3) those with severe mumps with complications (epididymo-orchitis or meningoencephalitis or both or other complications), (4) those with no apparent symptoms but with typical antibody responses, and (5) those with meningoencephalitis or orchitis without involvement of the salivary glands.[89] Approximately 75 per cent of all cases of apparent mumps in children belong to the full-blown type without complications. Involvement of the gonads is rare before puberty.

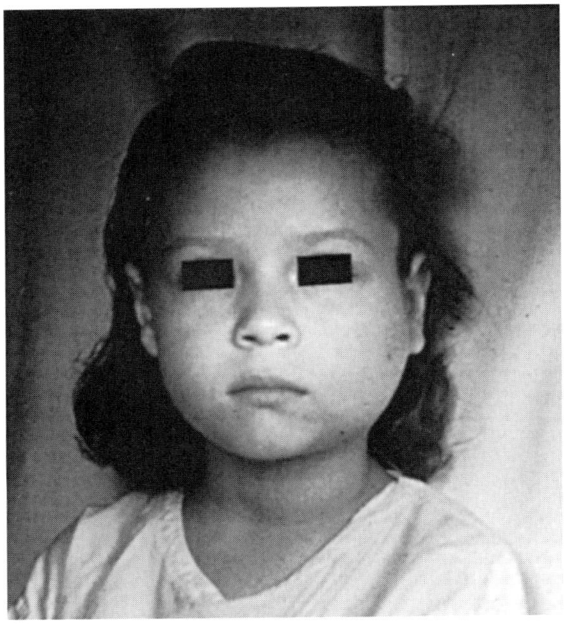

FIGURE 184–3. *Note swelling of the left side of the face related to parotitis secondary to mumps virus infection. The left ear protrudes from the side of the head.*

Typical Mumps Without Complications[89]

The average case in children has a prodromal period of 1 to 2 days, with fever, anorexia, headache, vomiting, and generalized aches and pains. The headache often particularly is marked and probably is due to mild meningoencephalitis.[32] The temperature usually rises slowly to 102° F or 103° F (38.9° C or 39.4° C) as the disease becomes full-blown, but at times fever is only slight or absent.

After the prodromal period, one or both parotid glands begin to enlarge (Fig. 184–3). Mumps is bilateral in approximately 70 to 80 per cent of cases. A few days to a week or more may intervene between the swellings of the two sides. A distinctive "puckering" sensation is experienced at the angle of the jaw in the early stage, and this may be increased by application to the tongue of sour liquids, such as lemon juice or vinegar. This sign, when present, may be useful in the early diagnosis. The swelling of the gland also is distinctive in that a brawny type of edema occurs about the parotid gland, the borders of which are not discrete, in contrast with the discrete swelling typical of lymphadenitis, in which the node usually easily is outlined. The lobe of the ear is in the center of the swelling, which usually cannot be separated by palpation from the angle of the mandible. Pressure is painful, and it often is difficult to open the jaw.

The swelling of an individual gland reaches its maximum in about 3 days, remains at its peak for approximately 2 days, and then slowly recedes. The extent of the swelling varies considerably but at times is sufficient to distort completely the outline of the face and head. The submaxillary and sublingual glands may be involved separately or with the parotids in any combination.

During the prodromal phase, slight redness of the orifices of Stensen or Wharton ducts, when present, has diagnostic significance. The amount of saliva usually is unchanged, although the mouth may be dry or salivation may be extreme. Gellis and Peters[37] described a few cases with edema over the upper part of the sternum, apparently due to pressure on the lymphatics in the neck.

In uncomplicated mumps, the white blood cell count usually is low with slight relative lymphocytosis. The serum amylase usually is elevated.

Meningitis, Meningoencephalitis, and Encephalitis

Meningitis and mild meningoencephalitis are the most frequent complications of mumps in children. Azimi and Cramblett[2] reviewed 51 children with mumps meningoencephalitis admitted to Columbus Children's Hospital between July 1964 and December 1967. Of this group of patients, the frequency of signs and symptoms was fever, 94 per cent; vomiting, 84 per cent; nuchal rigidity, 71 per cent; lethargy, 69 per cent; parotid swelling, 47 per cent; headache, 47 per cent; convulsions, 18 per cent; abdominal pain, 14 per cent; sore throat, 8 per cent; diarrhea, 8 per cent; and delirium, 6 per cent.

Clinical findings in neurologic illness due to mumps virus infection differ by patient age. Meningeal signs are recognized more readily in older children, adolescents, and adults, whereas nonspecific findings such as drowsiness and lethargy are more common in young children.[102] Although seizures occur in 20 to 30 per cent of hospitalized patients, electroencephalogram results usually are normal. Even in patients with severe obturation, the electroencephalogram only reveals diffuse slowing with increased voltage. Focal findings are rare. The outlook in mumps meningoencephalitis generally is good and usually is better than in encephalitis due to other viral causes (see Chapter 43). Even patients with profound obturation generally recover without residual damage. Rare deaths do occur, however.[18]

In the typical case, the cerebrospinal fluid has normal glucose and elevated protein levels and pleocytosis. The glucose is slightly low in about 20 per cent of cases. At the onset of symptoms, there is modest mononuclear pleocytosis. The cerebrospinal fluid cell count peaks on the third day of illness; counts average 250/mm^3, but counts greater than 1000/mm^3 are not uncommon.

Mumps meningitis usually develops in patients with parotitis about 5 days after illness onset, but central nervous system findings can precede parotid findings and can occur without any salivary gland involvement.

Herndon and colleagues[48] noted that ependymitis regularly occurs in mumps meningitis. A rare complication of mumps appears to be acquired aqueductal stenosis, and it has been suggested that this may be due to the preceding ependymitis.[48, 74, 88, 93]

Gonadal Infection (Epididymo-orchitis and Oophoritis)

Epididymo-orchitis and oophoritis almost never occur before puberty.[89] However, in adolescent and adult males, epididymo-orchitis is second only to parotitis as a manifestation of mumps virus infection.[64] Cases of orchitis have been reported in children as young as 3 years of age.[79] In postpubertal males, 30 to 38 per cent with mumps develop orchitis.[4, 77] The rate of orchitis is highest in those 15 to 29 years of age. The greatest number of cases occur during the second, third, and fourth decades of life. Approximately 80 per cent of cases of epididymo-orchitis appear during the first 8 days of salivary gland involvement, but a few cases occur a considerable time after the parotitis has subsided.[89]

The onset of testicular involvement usually is with a chill, recurrence of fever, and swelling of the testes. Pain over the renal area or in the lower abdomen, bilateral or unilateral, may precede or accompany orchitis. Occasionally, this pain, if on the right side, may suggest appendicitis.

The involvement most often is unilateral, but bilateral involvement has been reported to occur in 17 to 38 per cent of cases.[4, 77] Although atrophy may occur after orchitis, in unilateral involvement sterility is not a concern. Sterility has resulted after some cases of bilateral orchitis. Development of malignancies in affected testes has been reported.[4, 55]

Oophoritis occurs in about 7 per cent of postpubertal females. Pelvic pain and tenderness are noted.[82]

Pancreatitis

In a retrospective survey of 2482 hospitalized mumps patients, pancreatitis was noted in 75 (3 per cent).[1] Cases occurred in children and adults, and occurrence was 1.6 times more common in males than females. Severe involvement of the pancreas is rare, but mild or subclinical infection may be more common than is recognized.[82] It may be unassociated with salivary gland manifestations and misdiagnosed as gastroenteritis. Epigastric pain and tenderness are suggestive; these may be accompanied by fever, chills, vomiting, and prostration. A child with acute hemorrhagic pancreatitis and pseudocyst due to mumps virus infection has been reported.[31]

Diabetes Mellitus[18]

Diabetes mellitus long has been suspected to be associated with antecedent mumps.[45] In experimental animals, mumps virus infection has been associated with hyperglycemia and histologic lesions of the pancreatic islets. Mumps virus can invade the human pancreas and can infect and destroy human and rhesus beta cells in vitro,[78] but pancreatic damage has never been documented in reported cases of diabetes after mumps or mumps vaccination.[87]

In humans, many cases of temporal association have been described both in individuals and in siblings,[25, 26, 60, 71, 73] and outbreaks of diabetes mellitus a few months or years after outbreaks of mumps have been reported.[41, 70, 92] Although evidence has not established a causal association in these cases, a study in Surrey, England, suggested that a small proportion, if any, of diabetes cases that start in childhood (only 15 of the 1663 patients in the study, or <1 per cent) may have resulted from a recent mumps virus infection.[35] Antibody studies have shown fewer positive titers for mumps in diabetics than in normal subjects, even in children.[80] Infection might contribute to the development of diabetes either by specifically damaging the islet cells or by precipitating diabetes in patients whose disease is latent.

Nephritis

Viruria is common in uncomplicated mumps, and mild abnormalities of renal function occur.[95] Severe and fatal nephritis has been reported as a rare complication of mumps occurring 10 to 14 days after parotitis.[82]

Deafness

Deafness is an important but rare complication of mumps virus infection.[18] Its incidence has been estimated to be from 0.5 to 5.0 per 100,000 cases of mumps.[29, 96] However, the incidence rate of minor degrees of hearing impairment, such as high-tone hearing loss, probably is much higher.[21]

Mumps-associated deafness occurs with or without meningoencephalitis and may occur after asymptomatic infection.[18, 29, 72] Deafness usually is unilateral and often is permanent. Twenty-two of 103 cases (21 per cent) reviewed by Everberg[29] were bilateral. Mumps virus has been isolated from perilymph fluid in a case of sudden-onset, unilateral, complete deafness that began 2 days after the onset of mumps.[101] Vertigo also is noted occasionally in patients with mumps; this is most common in patients who develop deafness.[53]

Mumps and Pregnancy[18]

The incidence of mumps during pregnancy was estimated at 0.8 to 10 cases per 10,000 pregnancies[83] prior to vaccine licensure. No vaccine-era data are available for comparison. Maternal complications such as mastitis,[77] aseptic meningitis,[7] and fatal glomerulonephritis[27] have been reported. Mumps virus has been isolated from human breast milk.[56]

Increased fetal mortality was reported in women who contracted mumps during the first trimester. In a large prospective case-control study, there was a 27.3 per cent rate of fetal wastage in women with mumps during the first trimester versus a 13.0 per cent rate in matched, nonill controls during the first trimester.[85] No significant differences in birth weight were noted among the live births.[86] Because fetal loss usually occurs in such cases within 2 weeks of maternal infection, it was postulated that factors related to maternal gonadal infection with resulting hormonal changes might be responsible. A histopathologic study of the products of conception in mothers with gestational mumps revealed severe proliferative necrotic villitis and vasculitis in the placentas and viral inclusions, as seen in mumps infection, in the fetal tissues.[36] Mumps virus has been isolated from a spontaneously aborted 10-week-old human fetus.[66]

There is no evidence that gestational mumps in humans increases the risk of fetal malformations,[84] although there are a few case reports of various congenital malformations showing no consistent pattern.[53]

Other Manifestations

Other rare clinical manifestations include exanthem and enanthem,[20] arthritis,[39] myocarditis,[5] thrombocytopenia,[67] lower respiratory tract infection,[33] and other glandular involvement (thyroiditis, mastitis, dacryoadenitis, and bartholinitis).[64]

DIAGNOSIS

Differential Diagnosis

Not all patients with mumps have parotid swelling, and mumps virus is not the only cause of parotitis. Mumps virus infection must be considered in all children with aseptic meningitis, meningoencephalitis, and encephalitis (see Chapters 42 and 43). In addition to mumps virus infection, a number of other infectious agents and noninfectious conditions are associated with parotitis or parotid swelling (see Chapter 16). Purulent parotitis can be differentiated from mumps by the exquisite tenderness of the region, an elevated white blood cell count, and the observation of pus coming from the Stensen duct. Other viral causes of parotitis can be differentiated by the respective epidemiologic and clinical characteristics of specific agents and appropriate culture, serologic study, or both.

Enlargement of lymph nodes in proximity to the parotid gland must be differentiated from parotid enlargement (see Chapter 15). Cervical lymph nodes are below the ramus of the mandible. Preparotid nodes usually are anterior to the parotid, and their enlargement usually is associated with conjunctivitis. Occasionally, an enlarged lymph node within the parotid gland may cause some confusion.

Lesions of the ramus of the mandible, such as osteomyelitis, occasionally have been mistaken for parotid enlargement. In this case, the enlargement usually is persistent.

Specific Diagnosis

In the epidemic situation, the diagnosis of mumps is straightforward clinically and laboratory tests are unnecessary. The critical points are an exposure history, an incubation period of 2 to 3 weeks, and a typical clinical picture with fever and parotitis. In the sporadic case or in a previously vaccinated child, it is important to confirm the etiology by laboratory study. Mumps virus as well as most other viruses that cause parotitis can be isolated readily from saliva, throat swabs, or mouth washings during acute illness. In patients with meningoencephalitis, virus also can be recovered from the cerebrospinal fluid. Virus is isolated in primary monkey kidney tissue culture (see Chapter 244).

Mumps virus infection also can be confirmed by demonstrating a significant antibody titer rise in paired serum specimens by complement fixation, hemagglutination inhibition, or ELISA. However, because mumps cross-reacts with parainfluenza viruses, this method is not ideal. Mumps-specific IgM antibody also can be determined by ELISA; its presence indicates a recent infection.

In unusual cases in which the source of facial swelling is obscure, the determination of a serum amylase level may be helpful; a high value would indicate parotid involvement.

TREATMENT

Conservative therapy is indicated in the treatment of mumps. Adequate attention to hydration and alimentation of patients is important. Patients may have difficulty with acid foods, such as orange juice. In addition, orange juice may cause vomiting in an already nauseated patient. The diet should be light with a generous offering of fluids.

Occasionally, analgesics are necessary for severe headache or discomfort due to parotitis. Stronger analgesics, such as codeine or Demerol, rarely are required for headache but may be useful in orchitis. It is unusual for vomiting to be severe enough to require intravenous fluids. In these instances, however, electrolytes lost by vomiting should be replaced.

Although lumbar punctures frequently are not necessary for diagnosis in patients with meningoencephalitis accompanying mumps, patients often indicate that they have experienced relief of headache after this procedure.

There is no antiviral agent appropriate or indicated for the treatment of mumps, which is a self-limited illness.

PROGNOSIS

The overall prognosis in uncomplicated mumps is excellent. The outlook in meningoencephalitis also generally is favorable, but death and neurologic damage can occur. Deafness and sterility are rare complications.

PREVENTION

Immunization

A summary of the Advisory Committee on Immunization Practices (ACIP) recommendations for mumps vaccine use follows.[15] For more complete information, the reader should consult the most recent ACIP statement or the Report of the Committee on Infectious Diseases of the American Academy of Pediatrics.

Mumps virus vaccine (official name: mumps virus vaccine, live) Jeryl-Lynn strain is prepared in chick embryo cell culture. More than 84 million doses were distributed in the United States from its introduction in December 1967 through 1988. The vaccine produces a subclinical, noncommunicable infection with few side effects. Mumps vaccine is available both in monovalent (mumps only) form and in combinations: mumps-rubella and measles-mumps-rubella (MMR) vaccines.

The vaccine is approximately 95 per cent efficacious in preventing mumps disease[50, 90]; more than 97 per cent of persons known to be susceptible to mumps develop measurable antibody after vaccination.[99] Vaccine-induced antibody is protective and long-lasting,[97, 98] although of considerably lower titer than antibody resulting from natural infection.[99] The duration of vaccine-induced immunity is unknown, but serologic and epidemiologic data collected during 20 years of live vaccine use indicate both the persistence of antibody and continuing protection against infection. Estimates of clinical vaccine efficacy ranging from 75 to 95 per cent have been calculated from data collected in outbreak settings using different epidemiologic study designs.[19]

General Recommendations

Susceptible children, adolescents, and adults should be vaccinated against mumps unless vaccination is contraindicated. Mumps vaccine is of particular value for children approaching puberty and for adolescents and adults who have not had mumps. MMR vaccine is the vaccine of choice for routine administration and should be used in all situations in which recipients also are likely to be susceptible to measles, rubella, or both. The favorable benefit/cost ratio for routine mumps immunization is more marked when vaccine is administered as MMR.[62] Persons should be considered susceptible to mumps unless they have documentation of (1) physician-diagnosed mumps, (2) adequate immunization with live mumps virus vaccine on or after their first birthday, or (3) laboratory evidence of immunity.

Persons who are unsure of their mumps disease history or mumps vaccination history should be vaccinated. There is no evidence that persons who previously either received mumps vaccine or had mumps are at any increased risk of local or systemic reactions from receiving live mumps vaccine. Testing for susceptibility before vaccination, especially among adolescents and young adults, is not necessary. In addition to the expense, some tests (e.g., mumps skin test, complement-fixation antibody test) may be unreliable, and tests with established reliability (e.g., neutralization, enzyme immunoassay, radial hemolysis antibody test) are not readily available.

Dosage

A single dose of vaccine in the volume specified by the manufacturer should be administered subcutaneously.

Age

Live mumps virus vaccine is recommended at any age on or after the first birthday for all susceptible persons, unless a contraindication exists. Under routine circumstances, mumps vaccine should be given in combination with measles and rubella vaccines as MMR, following the currently recommended schedule for administration of measles vaccine. It should not be administered to infants younger than 12 months of age because persisting maternal antibody might interfere with seroconversion. To ensure immunity, all persons vaccinated before their first birthday should be revaccinated on or after their first birthday.

Persons Exposed to Mumps

Use of Vaccine

When given after exposure to mumps, live mumps virus vaccine may not provide protection. However, if the exposure did not result in infection, vaccine should induce protection against infection from subsequent exposures. There is no evidence that the risk of vaccine-associated adverse events increases if vaccine is administered to persons incubating disease.

Use of Immunoglobulin

Immunoglobulin has not been demonstrated to be of established value in postexposure prophylaxis and is not recommended.

Adverse Effects of Vaccine Use

In field trials before licensure, illnesses did not occur more often in vaccinees than in unvaccinated controls.[49] Reports of illnesses following mumps vaccination mainly have been episodes of parotitis and low-grade fever. Allergic reactions, including rash, pruritus, and purpura, have been associated temporally with mumps vaccination but are uncommon and usually mild and of brief duration. The reported occurrence of encephalitis within 30 days of receipt of a mumps-containing vaccine in the United States (0.4 per million doses) is not greater than the observed background incidence rate of central nervous system dysfunction in the normal population. Other manifestations of central nervous system involvement in the United States, such as febrile seizures and deafness, also have been reported infrequently. Complete recovery is usual. Reports of nervous system illness following mumps vaccination do not denote necessarily an etiologic relationship between the illness and the vaccine.

In parts of Europe, Canada, and Japan, where different mumps vaccines (Leningrad 3 strain and Urabe Am 9 strain) have been used, the rates of vaccine-induced aseptic meningitis have been high.[22, 24, 68, 91]

Contraindications to Vaccine Use

Pregnancy

Although mumps vaccine virus has been shown to infect placenta and fetus,[103] there is no evidence that it causes congenital malformations in humans. However, because of the theoretic risk of fetal damage, it is prudent to avoid giving live virus vaccine to pregnant women. Vaccinated women should avoid pregnancy for 3 months after vaccination. Routine precautions for vaccinating postpubertal women include asking if they are or may be pregnant, excluding those who say they are, and explaining the theoretic risk to those who plan to receive the vaccine. Vaccination during pregnancy should not be considered an indication for termination of pregnancy. However, the final decision about interruption of pregnancy must rest with the individual patient and her physician.

Severe Febrile Illness

Vaccine administration should not be postponed because of minor or intercurrent febrile illnesses, such as mild upper respiratory infections. However, vaccination of persons with severe febrile illnesses generally should be deferred until they have recovered.

Allergies

Because live mumps vaccine is produced in chick embryo cell culture, persons with a history of anaphylactic reactions (e.g., hives, swelling of the mouth and throat, difficulty breathing, hypotension, shock) after egg ingestion should be vaccinated only with caution using published protocols.[40, 47] Known allergic children should not leave the vaccination site for 20 minutes. Evidence indicates that persons are not at increased risk if they have egg allergies that are not anaphylactic. Such persons may be vaccinated in the usual manner. There is no evidence to indicate that persons with allergies to chickens or feathers are at increased risk of reaction to the vaccine.

Because mumps vaccine contains trace amounts of neomycin (25 μg), persons who have experienced anaphylactic reactions to topically or systemically administered neomycin should not receive mumps vaccine. Most often, neomycin allergy is manifested as contact dermatitis, which is a delayed-type (cell-mediated) immune response, rather than anaphylaxis. In such persons, the adverse reaction, if any, to 25 μg of neomycin in the vaccine would be an erythematous, pruritic nodule or papule at 48 to 96 hours. A history of contact dermatitis to neomycin is not a contraindication to receiving mumps vaccine. Live mumps virus vaccine does not contain penicillin.

Recent Immunoglobulin Injection

Passively acquired antibody can interfere with the response to live attenuated virus vaccines. Therefore, mumps vaccine should be given at least 2 weeks before the administration of immunoglobulin or deferred until approximately 3 months after the administration of immunoglobulin.

Altered Immunity

In theory, replication of the mumps vaccine virus may be potentiated in patients with immune deficiency disease and by the suppressed immune responses that occur with leukemia, lymphoma, or generalized malignancy or with therapy with corticosteroids, alkylating drugs, antimetabolites, or radiation. In general, patients with such conditions should not be given live mumps virus vaccine. Because vaccinated persons do not transmit mumps vaccine virus, the risk of mumps exposure for those patients may be reduced by vaccinating their close susceptible contacts.

An exception to these general recommendations is in children infected with HIV: all asymptomatic HIV-infected children should receive MMR at 15 months of age.[17] If measles vaccine is administered to symptomatic HIV-infected children, the combination MMR vaccine generally is preferred.[16]

Patients with leukemia in remission whose chemotherapy has been terminated for at least 3 months also may receive live mumps virus vaccine. Short-term (less than 2 weeks' duration) corticosteroid therapy, topical steroid therapy (e.g., nasal, skin), and intraarticular, bursal, or tendon injection with corticosteroids do not contraindicate mumps vaccine administration. However, mumps vaccine should be avoided if systemic immunosuppressive levels are reached by prolonged, extensive, topical application.

Disease Containment

Containment is important in mumps prevention in the United States. Mumps is a reportable disease, and compliance is the obligation of all physicians. After early reports of sporadic mumps cases, health department workers can organize local immunization clinics and exclusion of susceptible students from schools so that disease can be contained in a small geographic area.

References

1. Association for the Study of Infectious Diseases: A retrospective survey of the complications of mumps. J. R. Coll. Gen. Pract. *24*:552–556, 1974.
2. Azimi, P. H., and Cramblett, H. G.: Mumps meningoencephalitis in children. J. A. M. A. *207*:509–512, 1969.
3. Bang, H. O., and Bang, J.: Involvement of the central nervous system in mumps. Bull. Hyg. *19*:503–504, 1944.
4. Beard, C. M., Benson, R. C., Jr., Kelalis, P. P., et al.: The incidence and outcome of mumps orchitis in Rochester, Minnesota, 1935 to 1974. Mayo Clin. Proc. *52*:3–7, 1977.
5. Bengtsson, E., and Orndahl, G.: Complications of mumps with special reference to the incidence of myocarditis. Acta Med. Scand. *149*:381–389, 1954.
6. Black, F. L.: A nationwide serum survey of United States military recruits, 1962. III. Measles and mumps antibodies. Am. J. Hyg. *80*:304–307, 1964.
7. Bowers, D.: Mumps during pregnancy. West. J. Surg. Obstet. Gynecol. *61*:72, 1953.
8. Bruserud, O., and Thorsby, E.: HLA control of the proliferative T lymphocyte response to antigenic determinants on mumps virus: Studies of healthy individuals and patients with type 1 diabetes. Scand. J. Immunol. *22*:509–518, 1985.
9. Bruyn, H. B., Sexton, H. M., and Brainerd, H. D.: Mumps meningoencephalitis: A clinical review of 119 cases with one death. Calif. Med. *86*:155–160, 1957.
10. Callaghan, J. T., Petersen, B. H., Smith, W. C., et al.: Delayed hypersensitivity to mumps antigen in humans. Clin. Immunol. Immunopathol. *26*:102–110, 1983.
11. Centers for Disease Control and Prevention: CDC Surveillance Summaries; Mumps surveillance, United States, 1988–1993. M. M. W. R. *44*:1–14, 1995.
12. Centers for Disease Control and Prevention: Summary of notifiable diseases, United States, 1994. M. M. W. R. *43*:1–80, 1995.
13. Centers for Disease Control: Summary of notifiable diseases, United States, 1989. M. M. W. R. *38*:1–59, 1990.
14. Centers for Disease Control: Mumps—United States, 1985–1988. M. M. W. R. *38*:101–105, 1989.
15. Centers for Disease Control: ACIP: Mumps prevention. M. M. W. R. *38*:388–400, 1989.
16. Centers for Disease Control: ACIP, Immunization of children infected with human immunodeficiency virus: Supplementary ACIP statement. M. M. W. R. *37*:181–183, 1988.
17. Centers for Disease Control: ACIP, Immunization of children infected with human T-lymphotrophic virus type III/lymphadenopathy-associated virus. M. M. W. R. *35*:595–596, 603–606, 1986.
18. Centers for Disease Control: Mumps surveillance, January 1977–December 1982. Issued September 1984.
19. Chalken, B. P., Williams, N. M., Preblud, S. R., et al.: The effect of a school entry law on mumps activity in a school district. J. A. M. A. *257*:2455–2456, 1987.
20. Cherry, J. D., and Jahn, C. L.: Exanthem and enanthem associated with mumps virus infection. Arch. Environ. Health *12*:518–521, 1966.
21. Chuden, H. G., Michtl, W., and Stehr, K.: Hearing loss due to mumps. Laryngol. Rhinol. Otol. *57*:745–750, 1978.
22. Cizman, M., Mozetic, M., Radescek-Rakar, R., et al.: Aseptic meningitis after vaccination against measles and mumps. Pediatr. Infect. Dis. J. *8*:302–308, 1989.
23. Cochi, S. L., Preblud, S. R., and Orenstein, W. A.: Perspectives on the relative resurgence of mumps in the United States. Am. J. Dis. Child. *142*:499–507, 1988.
24. Colville, A., and Pugh, S.: Mumps meningitis and measles, mumps and rubella vaccine. Lancet *340*:876, 1992.
25. Craighead, J. E.: The role of viruses in the pathogenesis of pancreatic disease and diabetes mellitus. *In* Melnick, J. L. (ed.): Progress in Medical Virology. Vol. 19. Basel, S. Kargen, 1975, pp. 162–214.
26. Dacau-Voutetakis, C., Constantinidis, M., Moschos, A., et al.: Diabetes mellitus following mumps. Am. J. Dis. Child. *127*:890–891, 1974.
27. Dutta, P. C.: A fatal case of pregnancy complicated with mumps. J. Obst. Gyn. Br. Emp. *42*:869, 1935.
28. Enders, J. F.: Mumps. *In* Rivers, T. M., and Horsfall, F. L., Jr. (eds.): Viral and Rickettsial Infections of Man. 3rd ed. Philadelphia, J. B. Lippincott, 1959, pp. 780–789.
29. Everberg, G.: Deafness following mumps. Acta Otolaryngol. *48*:397–403, 1957.
30. Feldman, H. A.: Mumps. *In* Evans, A. S. (ed.): Viral Infections of Humans: Epidemiology and Control. 3rd ed. New York, Plenum, 1989, pp. 471–491.
31. Feldstein, J. D., Johnson, F. R., Kallick, C. A., and Doolas, A.: Acute hemorrhagic pancreatitis and pseudocyst due to mumps. Ann. Surg. *180*:85–88, 1974.
32. Finkelstein, H.: Meningo-encephalitis in mumps. J. A. M. A. *3*:17–19, 1938.
33. Foy, H. M., Cooney, M. K., Hall, C. E., et al.: Isolation of mumps virus from children with acute lower respiratory tract disease. Am. J. Epidemiol. *94*:467–471, 1971.
34. Friedman, M. G.: Salivary IgA antibodies to mumps virus during and after mumps. J. Infect. Dis. *143*:617, 1981.
35. Gamble, D. R.: Relationship of antecedent illness to development of diabetes in children. B. M. J. *12*:99–101, 1980.
36. Garcia, A. G., Pereira, J. M., Vidigal, N., et al.: Intrauterine infection with mumps virus. Obstet. Gynecol. *56*:756–759, 1980.
37. Gellis, S. S., and Peters, M.: Mumps with presternal edema. Bull. Johns Hopkins Hosp. *75*:241, 1944.
38. Gordon, J. E.: The epidemiology of mumps. Am. J. Med. Sci. *200*:412–428, 1940.
39. Gordon, S. C., and Lauter, C. B.: Mumps arthritis: A review of the literature. Rev. Infect. Dis. *6*:338–344, 1984.
40. Greenberg, M. A., and Birx, D. L.: Safe administration of mumps-measles-rubella vaccine in egg-allergic children. J. Pediatr. *113*:504–506, 1988.
41. Gundersen, E.: Is diabetes of infectious origin? J. Infect. Dis. *41*:198–202, 1927.
42. Habel, K.: Cultivation of mumps virus in the developing chick embryo and its application to studies of immunity to mumps in man. Public Health Rep. *60*:201–212, 1945.
43. Hamilton, R.: An account of distemper by the common people of England vulgarly called the mumps. London Med. J. *11*:190–211, 1790.
44. Hamilton, R.: An account of a distemper, by the common people in England vulgarly called the mumps. Trans. Royal Soc. Edinburgh *2*:59–72, 1790.
45. Hams, H. F.: A case of diabetes quickly following mumps. Boston Med. Surg. J. *140*:465–469, 1899.
46. Henle, G., and Deinhardt, F.: Propagation and primary isolation of mumps virus in tissue culture. Proc. Soc. Exp. Biol. Med. *89*:556–560, 1955.

47. Herman, J. J., Radin, R., and Schneiderman, R.: Allergic reactions to measles (rubeola) vaccine in patients hypersensitive to egg protein. J. Pediatr. *102*:196–199, 1983.
48. Herndon, R. M., Johnson, R. T., Davis, L. E., and Descalzi, L. R.: Ependymitis in mumps virus meningitis. Arch. Neurol. *30*:475–479, 1974.
49. Hilleman, M. R., Buynak, E. B., Weibel, R. E., and Stokes, J., Jr.: Live, attenuated mumps-virus vaccine. N. Engl. J. Med. *278*:227–232, 1968.
50. Hilleman, M. R., Weibel, R. E., Buynak, E. B., et al.: Live, attenuated mumps-virus vaccine. 4. Protective efficacy as measured in a field evaluation. N. Engl. J. Med. *276*:252–258, 1967.
51. Hirsch, A.: Handbook of Historical and Geographical Pathology. Translated by Charles Creighton. London, 1886.
52. Holowach, J., Thurston, D. L., and Becker, B.: Congenital defects in infants following mumps during pregnancy: A review of the literature and a report of chorioretinitis due to fetal infection. J. Pediatr. *50*:689–694, 1957.
53. Hyden, D., Odkvist, L. M., and Kylen, P.: Vestibular symptoms in mumps deafness. Acta Otolaryngol. *360*(Suppl.):182–183, 1979.
54. Johnson, C. D., and Goodpasture, E. W.: The etiology of mumps. Am. J. Hyg. *21*:46–57, 1935.
55. Kaufman, J. J., and Bruce, P. T.: Testicular atrophy following mumps: A cause of testis tumor? Br. J. Urol. *35*:67–69, 1963.
56. Kilham, L.: Mumps virus in human milk and in milk of infected monkey. J. A. M. A. *146*:1231, 1951.
57. Kilham, L.: Isolation of mumps virus from the blood of a patient. Proc. Soc. Exp. Biol. Med. *69*:99–100, 1948.
58. Kim-Farley, R. J.: Mumps. *In* Kiple, K. F. (ed.): The Cambridge World History of Human Disease. Cambridge, England, Cambridge University Press, 1993, pp. 887–889.
59. Kim-Farley, R., Bart, S., Stetler, H., et al.: Clinical mumps vaccine efficacy. Am. J. Epidemiol. *121*:593–597, 1985.
60. King, R. C.: Mumps followed by diabetes. Lancet *2*:1055, 1962.
61. Kleiman, M. B., and Leland, D. S.: Mumps virus and Newcastle disease virus. *In* Lennette, E. H., Lennette, D. A., and Lennette, E. T. (eds.): Diagnostic Procedures for Viral, Rickettsial, and Chlamydial Infections. 7th ed. Washington, D. C., American Public Health Association, 1995, pp. 455–463.
62. Koplan, J. P., and Preblud, S. R.: A benefit-cost analysis of mumps vaccine. Am. J. Dis. Child. *136*:362–364, 1982.
63. Kress, H. G., and Kreth, H. W.: HLA restriction of secondary mumps-specific cytotoxic T lymphocytes. J. Immunol. *129*:844–849, 1982.
64. Krugman, S.: Mumps (epidemic parotitis). *In* Krugman, S. (ed.): Infectious Diseases of Children. 7th ed. St. Louis, Mosby, 1981, pp. 195–207.
65. Kupers, T. A., Petrich, J. M., Holloway, A. W., and St. Geme, J. W., Jr.: Depression of tuberculin delayed hypersensitivity by live attenuated mumps virus. J. Pediatr. *76*:716–721, 1970.
66. Kurtz, J. B., Tomlinson, A. H., and Pearson, J.: Mumps virus isolated from a fetus. B. M. J. *394*:471, 1982.
67. Lacour, M., Mahyerzi, M., Vienny, H., and Suter, S.: Thrombocytopenia in a case of neonatal mumps infection: Evidence for further clinical presentations. Eur. J. Pediatr. *152*:739–741, 1993.
68. McDonald, J. C., Moore, D. L., and Quennec, P.: Clinical and epidemiologic features of mumps meningoencephalitis and possible vaccine-related disease. Pediatr. Infect. Dis. J. *8*:751–755, 1989.
69. McGuinness, A. C., and Gall, E. A.: Mumps at army camps in 1943. War Med. *5*:95–104, 1944.
70. Melin, K., and Ursung, B.: Diabetes mellitus som komplikation till parotitis: Epidemia. Nord. Med. *60*:1715–1717, 1958.
71. Messaritikas, J., Karabula, C., Kattamis, C., and Matsaniotis, N.: Diabetes following mumps in sibs. Arch. Dis. Child. *46*:561–562, 1971.
72. Nomura, Y., Harada, T., Sakata, H., and Sugiura, A.: Sudden deafness and asymptomatic mumps. Acta Otolaryngol. (Stockh.) *456*(Suppl.):9–11, 1988.
73. Notkins, A. L.: Virus-induced diabetes mellitus: Brief review. Arch. Virol. *54*:1–17, 1977.
74. Ogata, H., Oka, K., and Mitsudome, A.: Hydrocephalus due to acute aqueductal stenosis following mumps infection: Report of a case and review of the literature. Brain Dev. *14*:417–419, 1992.
75. Örvell, C., Rydbeck, R., and Löve, A.: Immunological relationships between mumps virus and parainfluenza viruses studied with monoclonal antibodies. J. Gen. Virol. *67*:1929–1939, 1986.
76. Overman, J. R.: Viremia in human mumps virus infections. Arch. Intern. Med. *102*:354–356, 1958.
77. Philip, R. N., Reinhard, K. R., and Lackman, D. B.: Observations on a mumps epidemic in a "virgin" population. Am. J. Hyg. *69*:91–111, 1959.
78. Prince, G. A., Henson, A. B., Billiups, L. C., and Notkins, A. L.: Infection of human pancreatic beta cell cultures with mumps virus. Nature *271*:158–161, 1978.
79. Reed, D., Brown, G., Merrick, R., et al.: A mumps epidemic on St. George Island, Alaska. J. A. M. A. *199*:967–971, 1967.
80. Samantray, S. K., Christopher, S., Mukundan, P., and Jonson, S. C.: Lack of relationship between viruses and human diabetes mellitus. Aust. N. Z. Med. *7*:139, 1977.
81. Sarnesto, A., Julkunen, I., and Makela, O.: Proportion of Ig classes and subclasses in mumps antibodies. Scand. J. Immunol. *22*:345–350, 1985.
82. Scott, T. F. M.: Mumps (epidemic parotitis). *In* Nelson, W. E., Vaughan, V. C., and McKay, R. J. (eds.): Textbook of Pediatrics. 9th ed. Philadelphia, W. B. Saunders, 1969, pp. 647–651.
83. Sever, J., and White, L. R.: Intrauterine viral infections. Ann. Rev. Med. *19*:471, 1968.
84. Siegel, M.: Congenital malformations following chickenpox, measles, mumps, and hepatitis: Results of a cohort study. J. A. M. A. *226*:1521–1524, 1973.
85. Siegel, M., Fuerst, H. T., and Peress, N. S.: Comparative fetal mortality in maternal virus diseases: A prospective study on rubella, measles, mumps and chickenpox and hepatitis. N. Engl. J. Med. *274*:768–771, 1966.
86. Siegel, M., and Fuerst, H. T.: Low birth weight and maternal virus diseases: A prospective study of rubella, measles, mumps, chickenpox, and hepatitis. J. A. M. A. *197*:88, 1966.
87. Sinaniotos, C. A., Daskalopoulou, E., Lapatsanis, P., and Doxiadis, S.: Diabetes mellitus after mumps vaccination. Arch. Dis. Child. *50*:749, 1975.
88. Spartaro, R. F., Lin, S-R., Horner, F. A., et al.: Aqueductal stenosis and hydrocephalus: Rare sequelae of mumps virus infection. Neuroradiology *12*:11–13, 1976.
89. Stokes, J., Jr.: Mumps (epidemic parotitis). *In* Nelson, W. E. (ed.): Textbook of Pediatrics. 7th ed. Philadelphia, W. B. Saunders, 1959, pp. 505–508.
90. Sugg, W. C., Finger, J. A., Levine, R. H., and Pagano, J. S.: Field evaluation of live virus mumps vaccine. J. Pediatr. *72*:461–466, 1968.
91. Sugiura, A., and Yamada, A.: Aseptic meningitis as a complication of mumps vaccination. Pediatr. Infect. Dis. J. *10*:209–213, 1991.
92. Sultz, H. A., Hart, B. A., Zielezny, M., and Schlesinger, E. R.: Is mumps virus an etiological factor in juvenile diabetes mellitus? Preliminary report. J. Pediatr. *86*:654–656, 1975.
93. Thompson, J. A.: Mumps: A cause of acquired aqueductal stenosis. J. Pediatr. *94*:923–924, 1979.
94. Ukkonen, P., Granström, M. L., and Penttinen, K.: Mumps-specific immunoglobulin M and G antibodies in natural mumps infection as measured by enzyme-linked immunosorbent assay. J. Med. Virol. *8*:131–142, 1981.
95. Utz, J. P., and Alling, D.: Clinical and laboratory studies of mumps. IV. Viruria and abnormal renal function. N. Engl. J. Med. *270*:1283–1286, 1964.
96. Vuori, M., Lahikainen, E. A., and Peltonen, T.: Perceptive deafness in connection with mumps: A study of 298 servicemen suffering from mumps. Acta Otolaryngol. *55*:231–236, 1962.
97. Weibel, R. E., Buynak, E. B., McLean, A. A., et al.: Persistence of antibody in human subjects for 7 to 10 years following administration of combined live attenuated measles, mumps and rubella virus vaccines. Proc. Soc. Exp. Biol. Med. *165*:260–263, 1980.
98. Weibel, R. E., Buynak, E. B., McLean, A. A., et al.: Follow-up surveillance for antibody in human subjects following live attenuated measles, mumps and rubella virus vaccines. Proc. Soc. Exp. Biol. Med. *162*:328–332, 1979.
99. Weibel, R. E., Stokes, J., Jr., Buynak, E. B., et al.: Live, attenuated mumps-virus vaccine. 3. Clinical and serologic aspects in a field evaluation. N. Engl. J. Med. *276*:245–251, 1967.
100. Weller, T. H., and Craig, J. R.: Isolation of mumps virus at autopsy. Am. J. Pathol. *25*:1105–1125, 1949.
101. Westmore, G. A., Pickard, B. H., and Stern, H.: Isolation of mumps virus from the inner ear after sudden deafness. B. M. J. *1*:14–15, 1979.
102. Wolinsky, J. S.: Mumps virus. *In* Fields, B. N., and Howley, P. M. (eds.): Fields Virology. 3rd ed. Philadelphia, Lippincott-Raven, 1996, pp. 1243–1265.
103. Yamauchi, T., Wilson, C., and St. Geme, J. W., Jr.: Transmission of live, attenuated mumps virus to the human placenta. N. Engl. J. Med. *290*:710–712, 1974.

185

Respiratory Syncytial Virus

Caroline Breese Hall

As by one bow on varied strings, the tune is played,
By both the microbe and the host, disease is made.

C. B. H.

Respiratory syncytial virus (RSV), a singular virus, is the most important respiratory pathogen of infancy and early childhood.[55, 81, 172, 276, 382] Each year approximately 91,000 infants are hospitalized with RSV infection in the United States at a cost of 300 million dollars, according to the estimates of the Institute of Medicine.[224] This virus is the only viral agent that produces its most severe disease in the first few weeks to months of life, when specific maternal antibody is present uniformly in the infant's serum. It circulates with an incompletely understood efficiency, causing sizable outbreaks each year, such that it infects virtually all children in their first years of life. Most all of these first infections are symptomatic, and an appreciable proportion involve the lower respiratory tract. RSV does not respect age, continuing to cause symptomatic infections throughout life, nor does it heed geographic boundaries.

HISTORY

In 1956, Morris and associates[348] noted a cropping of colds with coryza in a colony of chimpanzees that had been under observation for the previous 3 to 24 weeks. From 1 of the 14 afflicted chimpanzees a new virus was recovered and appropriately named "chimpanzee coryza agent" (CCA). The remaining 13 animals developed specific antibody to the CCA agent during convalescence; thus, the attack rate was 100 per cent. A person working with these chimpanzees also developed an upper respiratory tract infection and convalescent antibody to CCA. Viral isolation, however, was unsuccessful. Subsequently, susceptible chimpanzees, inoculated with the new agent grown in tissue culture, developed a coryzal illness after 3 days.

The human origin of the chimpanzees' agent was suspected; this was confirmed when Chanock and Finberg[78] recovered two agents indistinguishable from the CCA virus from the throat swabs of an infant with bronchopneumonia (Long strain) and a child with laryngotracheobronchitis (Snyder strain). They[78] studied the rise of antibody to these viruses among patients with respiratory disease and noted that 80 per cent of children by 4 years of age possessed neutralizing antibody for the Long virus. Nevertheless, they could not determine a definite etiologic association between the virus and the lower respiratory tract disease in their young patients. They proposed to call this group of viruses (Long, Snyder, and CCA) "respiratory syncytial virus" because of its manifestations clinically and in tissue culture. Confirmation of RSV as a major agent in respiratory disease soon accumulated from studies throughout the United States.[67, 80, 218, 267, 358, 413] Subsequently, investigators from many countries have confirmed and further delineated RSV's importance and have been enticed by its enigmatic ways.[40, 46, 55, 79, 81, 160, 161, 172, 276, 382, 472]

PROPERTIES

A tiny thistle—
Of coiled spine
and outer quill . . .

C. B. H.

Classification

The original classification of RSV with the Newcastle disease and parainfluenza group of viruses was due to their similar internal particle structure, eosinophilic inclusions, and syncytial appearance in tissue cultures. However, RSV is distinct antigenically and does not hemagglutinate erythrocytes.[512] Subsequently, the diameter of the nucleocapsid of RSV was determined to be between that of the larger paramyxoviruses and that of the smaller influenza viruses. Further studies of RSV's structure have resulted in its current classification within the order *Mononegavirales*, which contains the nonsegmented negative strand RNA viruses, and within the family of *Paramyxoviridae* and genus of *Pneumovirus*.[403, 405] Classified with RSV in *Pneumovirus* are the closely related bovine RSV, ovine RSV, caprine RSV, turkey rhinotracheitis virus, and pneumonia virus of mice.

Structural and Antigenic Properties

The virion of RSV consists of a nucleocapsid enclosed within a bilayer lipid envelope. Under electron microscope, the virions are heterogeneous, spherical, and filamentous, with the diameter ranging from 80 to 350 nm.[29, 266, 367] RSV has been demonstrated to bud from the cytoplasm, but an appreciable portion of the viral particles may remain attached. This, plus the heterogeneous shape of the virions, has impeded the purification and characterization of the structure of RSV.

The last few years, nevertheless, have witnessed major advances in deciphering and divulging the molecular soul and secrets of RSV. The transcriptional map of the RSV's genome has been delineated, and most of the genome has been sequenced (Fig. 185–1).[92, 94, 96, 100–102, 124, 248, 433, 434, 535] The surface glycoproteins have been purified; monoclonal antibodies have been produced; and the products of the RSV gene have been expressed individually in vaccinia, baculoviral, and adenoviral vectors.[31, 376, 465, 466, 479, 511, 515–517, 521, 535]

These studies have revealed that the genome of RSV is composed of a single strand of RNA of negative polarity that is transcribed into 10 major mRNAs, each encoding for the 10 viral proteins (Table 185–1).[92, 95, 98, 168, 248, 377, 515, 517] Eight of these are structural proteins, including the seven largest, (L, G, F, N, P, M, and SH), and two are nonstructural proteins (NS1 and NS2).[248] Three of the structural proteins are transmembrane surface proteins, the glycosylated F (fusion) and G (attachment) proteins and the small, nonglycosylated hy-

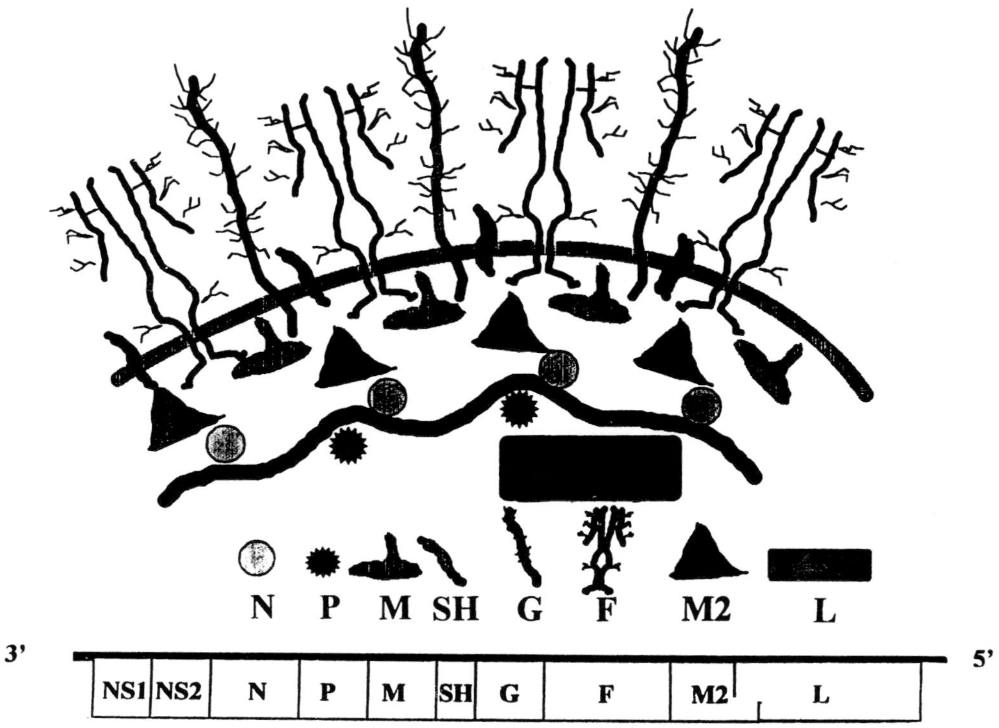

FIGURE 185–1. *Schematic representation of the genomic structure of respiratory syncytial virus (RSV). The 10 proteins of RSV are F, G, and SH (surface glycoproteins); M and M2 (matrix proteins); N, P, and L (nucleocapsid-associated proteins); and NS1 and NS2 (nonstructural proteins). (Adapted from Walsh, E. E., and Hall, C. B.: Approaches to the respiratory syncytial virus vaccine.* In *Meyers, R. A., Beaubien, M. P., and Kraus, H.-J. (eds.): Encyclopedia of Molecular Biology and Molecular Medicine. New York, VCH Publishers [in press]. With permission of VCH Publishers, Inc.)*

drophobic SH (or 1A) protein.[377] Three proteins, associated with the genomic mRNA, form the viral capsid proteins, N (nucleoprotein), P (phosphoprotein), and L (polymerase). Two matrix proteins, in contrast with the other paramyxoviruses, also are present in RSV, the nonglycosylated M and M2 (membrane-associated proteins). The complete sequence of the genes of the A2 strain now has been determined (Fig. 185–1).

Significant strain variation among RSV isolates has resulted in strains being divided into two major groups.[20, 22, 168, 354] These two major groups, A and B, have inter- and intragroup variations in several proteins, including F, G, P, and N

TABLE 185–1. Respiratory Syncytial Virus: Characteristics and Differences According to Strain Group

Viral Protein	Gene Length (Nucleotides)	Percentage Difference of Strain Groups A vs. B*		Protein Induces
		Nucleotides	*Amino Acids*	
Structural				
Surface				
F	1903	79	89	Viral penetration, major protection, NA, FIA, CTL
G	923	67	53	Viral attachment, strain group protection, NA, no CTL
SH (1A)	410	78	76	Unknown function, CTL, no NA
Matrix				
M	958	—	—†	?Nucleocapsid to envelope, CTL, no NA
M2 (22k)	961	78	92	Unique to pneumoviruses, unknown function, CTL, no NA
Nucleocapsid-Associated				
N	1203	86	96	Major RNA-binding, nucleocapsid protein, CTL, no NA
P	914	80	90	Major phosphoprotein, CTL, no NA
L	6578	—	—†	Major polymerase subunit, immune response unknown
Nonstructural				
NS1 (1C)	532	78	92	Unique to pneumoviruses, unknown function, CTL
NS2 (1B)	503	78	87	Unique to pneumoviruses, unknown function, no CTL

NA, neutralizing antibody; FIA, fusion-inhibiting antibody; CTL, cytotoxic lymphocyte response (in humans).
*Percentage difference between strain A2 (group A) and strain 18537 (group B).
†Dash (—) = difference between strain groups not yet determined.

(Table 185–1). The primary difference is in the largest surface glycoprotein, the G protein. The F protein, along with the N, P, M2, NS1, and NS2 proteins, are conserved relatively well, and antibody to the F protein is cross-reactive between the two groups.[222, 262, 263, 510] The F proteins of prototype strains from groups A and B have a greater than 90 per cent amino acid homology and a high degree of antigenic relatedness. In comparison, the amino acid homology between the G proteins of the two groups is 55 per cent, and the antigenic relatedness is only about 3 to 7 per cent.[262, 263, 510] Amino acid diversity for G protein within a group has varied from about 12 per cent for group B to about 20 per cent for group A.[66]

Laboratory Growth

RSV is relatively labile, which has hampered its purification. At 55° C, it is destroyed rapidly; at 37° C for 24 hours, only 10 per cent of infectivity remains; and at 4° C for 1 week, 1 per cent remains.[217]

The viability of RSV depends in part on the salt and protein content of the media. At 4° C, the addition of 1 molar of magnesium sulfate maintains viral stability for 5 weeks.[135] The virus withstands freezing and thawing poorly.[217, 512] Preservation is enhanced by rapid freezing in a dry ice and alcohol bath and by the addition of sucrose or glycerin to the storage media.[512] Infectivity also is influenced by the pH of the medium, rapidly diminishing at less than 5. The optimal pH for preservation is 7.5.[217] RSV is inactivated rapidly by detergents, such as 0.1 per cent sodium deoxycholate, sodium dodecyl sulfate, and Triton-X 100, as well as by chloroform and ether. On sucrose gradients, a method often used for purification, RSV has a density of 1.18 g/cm^3.[135]

RSV generally grows best in cultures of human heteroploid cells, such as HEp-2 and HeLa cells. However, the sensitivity of these cell lines is variable, especially with passage, and must be monitored constantly. Other suitable but generally less sensitive cell lines include monkey kidney, human kidney, and amnion and human diploid fibroblastic cell lines. The characteristic cytopathic effect of RSV in continuous cell lines is syncytial formation containing eosinophilic cytoplasmic inclusions. The syncytia usually are evident 2 to 7 days after inoculation and progress to complete degeneration within about 4 days.[194] The cytopathic effect, however, depends on the strain of virus, the medium, the sensitivity and thickness of the cell cultures, and the number of passages.[264, 512] In HEp-2 cultures, syncytia formation and the amount of fusion protein produced appear to depend on the presence of calcium and glutamine in the medium.[440] Syncytia tend to be less evident in fibroblast cell lines, and in some primary cell cultures, RSV may produce rounded, refractile cells. In human and animal infections, syncytia may be evident in epithelial cells of the respiratory tract, although syncytia appear to be unnecessary for the pathologic process because most infected cells are not syncytial but contain only one nucleus.

The growth cycle of RSV has been shown to consist of a period of adsorption with 50 per cent of the inoculum adsorbing in 2 hours, followed by an eclipse period of 12 hours. New virus appears shortly thereafter and enters a log phase of replication lasting for approximately 10 hours.[309] Viral antigen can be documented 7 to 10 hours after inoculation in the cytoplasm by fluorescent antibody staining. Shortly thereafter, cell-free virus may be demonstrated in the culture medium, but 50 to 90 per cent of the virus remains cell-associated on the cell surface at the time when maximal titers of the virus are obtained.[264, 309] Most of the cell-associated virus consists of incomplete virions that failed to bud entirely and may be released by agitation and sonication. An appreciable portion of the cell-free virus consists of noninfectious, empty virions and of aggregated virus, as demonstrated by the 99 per cent diminished infectivity after processing through a 0.45-μm filter.[29] With the laboratory Long strain (group A), peak titers are reached generally in 48 hours. For each infected cell, about 10 plaque-forming units usually result. Titers of virus are enhanced by inoculation of cell monolayers that are not confluent yet.[391] With continued high passage or propagation of temperature-sensitive mutants of RSV at nonpermissive temperatures, persistent infection may occur, associated with a loss of cytopathic effect and the amount of cell-free virus.[134, 406]

Animal Susceptibility

The natural hosts for symptomatic RSV infection primarily are humans, chimpanzees, and cows. RSV also has been recovered from asymptomatic goats and sheep. Closely related bovine strains have been isolated from cattle with respiratory disease and, when reinoculated into cattle, sometimes have produced fever and rhinitis.[64, 250, 341, 467, 498, 501] Susceptible animals that could serve as a model for the lower respiratory tract disease of infants have been sought for some time. Although RSV grows in animals, such as baboons, guinea pigs, mice, ferrets, mink, chinchillas, marmosets, and hamsters, direct inoculation into their respiratory tract generally produces infection that is silent clinically and pathologically. Other domestic animals, such as dogs, cats, sheep, and goats, have been found to possess antibody to RSV, the significance of which is unclear.[51, 312, 418] Several animals have been used as models for studying different aspects of RSV disease, but all have limitations, most frequently diminished replication of RSV and lack of symptomatic infection. Chimpanzees resemble most closely humans in their clinical response to RSV.[42] The cebus and owl monkeys are other nonhuman primates that may be made to develop some degree of clinical disease.[403, 417, 418] Other monkeys, such as the squirrel and newborn rhesus, shed only small quantities of virus from the nasopharynx.[42] Infection in ferrets is age-dependent, with adults developing a limited histopathology of the nasal turbinates and trachea. In infant ferrets, however, the virus replicates in the lung.[401, 470]

The cotton rat has been the most widely used animal model.[396, 398, 400, 402] With intranasal inoculation, viral titers peak in the lung and nasal turbinates after 4 to 5 days. Histologic changes in the lung generally are minimal and inconsistent, and only a small portion of cells appear to have productive infection. Inoculation of inbred mice similarly results in replication of virus in the lung, although the quantity and consistency of the infection may vary with the type and age of the mouse.[180, 397, 481] Marked pulmonary pathology may occur in BALB/c mice after high-titered, large-volume inocula, and in older mice this is accompanied by evidence of clinical illness.[180] A lamb model also has been developed, which after challenge with ovine, bovine, or human RSV results in pathologic changes in the lung.[302, 506] Intrathecal or intranasal inoculation of human RSV in one study using the lamb model produced fever and tachypnea more frequently in lambs receiving RSV than in control lambs.[302] The lack of a suitable animal model for human RSV infection has resulted in an increased interest in the natural model of bovine RSV in cattle. Despite the appreciable morbidity that occurs naturally with bovine RSV, experimental infection in cattle has been difficult, variable, and unreliable.[282]

EPIDEMIOLOGY

What occult power pries loose the lid
to give you winter flight,
But with the lengthening light of spring
gives cloak and leaden wing?

C. B. H.

Geographic Distribution

RSV shows no prejudice toward country or climate but does have a particular preference for the very young in each area of the world in which the patterns of RSV infection have been examined. Experience with RSV is ecumenical and the manifestations similar.[50, 142, 143, 155, 172, 175, 183, 223, 340, 343, 347, 382, 458, 471, 472]

Seasonal Patterns

RSV has the distinction of being the only viral respiratory pathogen that regularly produces each year an important outbreak of infection in urban areas.[155, 276, 353, 382] The outbreaks usually are sharp in onset and limited in length, lasting 2 to 5 months.[55, 155, 170, 172, 276, 343, 353, 382] In general, the epidemics tend to recur annually at regular, predictable intervals. In temperate climates, RSV activity usually peaks in the winter and extends into the spring. In the United Kingdom, the peaks of illness have been observed in January through March.[155] In Chicago and Seattle, the peak varied from December to April, with 13-month intervals for 3 years followed by a 9-month interval.[145, 170, 353] In the more tropical climes of Trinidad and Hong Kong, the epidemics have occurred during the rainy season.[458, 471] In American Samoa, however, RSV infections have not correlated with the rainfall.[223]

Over 11 consecutive years, the annual arrival of RSV in Washington, D.C., has been associated with a regular increase in the number of children admitted to the hospital with acute lower respiratory tract disease. The yearly number of admissions did not vary by more than 2.7 times.[276] The consistent ramifications of this pathogen in a community have been used to detect its presence. The peak period of admissions for children with lower respiratory tract disease each year is associated mainly with RSV activity.[170, 171, 183, 197, 276, 353] A rise in the number of cases of bronchiolitis or pediatric pneumonia reported from the outpatient offices in a community also is predictive of RSV's arrival (Fig. 185–2).[197] Similar to RSV, influenza A virus and sometimes parainfluenza virus

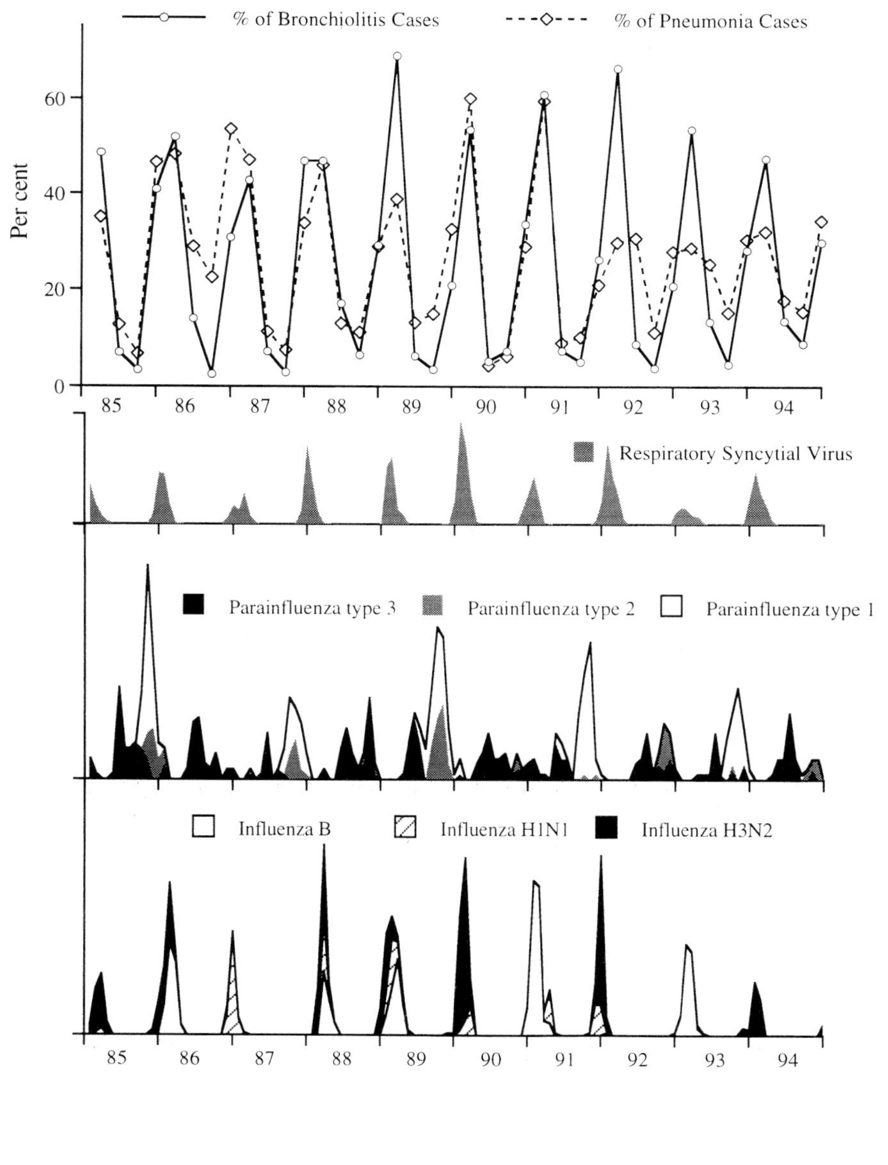

FIGURE 185–2. *The proportion of cases of pediatric bronchiolitis and pneumonia in children younger than 2 years of age reported in Rochester, New York, from 1985 through 1994 is shown in relation to the periods of the three major respiratory viral pathogens, respiratory syncytial virus, the parainfluenza viruses, and the influenza viruses. The cases are reported weekly by private offices and clinics to the Community Infectious Diseases Surveillance system. The major peaks of bronchiolitis and pneumonia occurred simultaneously and in association with the periods of respiratory syncytial virus isolation.*

may cause an increase in the number of respiratory tract infections in children in the community, but they do not cause consistently a rise in the number of hospital admissions for respiratory disease.

Usually, RSV captures the center stage during its peak activity in a community, with the other major respiratory pathogens absent or unnoticed.[25, 172] Although outbreaks of RSV and influenza A infections may overlap, the peaks of the epidemics uncommonly coincide.[25, 145, 197, 242]

Strain Variation

Although RSV is consistent in its ability to cause an annual outbreak of respiratory illness, the severity of the outbreaks may vary from year to year.[215] Variation in circulating strains has been suggested as partly accounting for the fluctuating clinical impact of RSV epidemics. The two major strain groups, A and B, circulate simultaneously during an outbreak, but the proportion of strains from each group may vary by season and geography, as do the predominance of the subgroups of A and B strains.[8, 22, 168, 215, 235, 351, 354, 368, 464, 478, 492] In Rochester, over a 20-year period, group A strains predominated in 11 years, and group A and B strains were relatively equal in another 5 years (Fig. 185–3).[215] In only four seasons did group B strains make up more than 75 per cent of the year's isolates (Fig. 185–3). In Cain, France, however, B strains predominated in 4 of 8 years and accounted overall for 64 per cent of isolates.[148] The strains from 14 cities across the United States over two consecutive seasons were shown to vary greatly, suggesting the influence of local, rather than national, factors.[20] Homotypic immunity, as suggested by several small studies, may play a role.[19, 352, 520]

The relationship between the circulating strain group and the size of an RSV outbreak does not appear to be strong or consistent.[215] The correlation of strain group with clinical severity requires further study, but in several, although not all, of the reports examining this, evidence suggested that group A strains may be associated with greater clinical severity.[215, 324, 331, 378, 478]

Incidence and Prevalence

RSV is the major cause of inpatient and outpatient pneumonia and bronchiolitis in infancy and early childhood. Infection with RSV in the young infant produces the greatest morbidity. RSV accounts for approximately 50 per cent of all pneumonia in infancy and 50 to 90 per cent of the cases of bronchiolitis.[55, 81, 155, 169, 173, 229, 255, 311, 313, 317, 323, 363, 383, 497] It also has been associated with 10 to 30 per cent of the cases of pediatric bronchitis.[255, 276] In contrast, only a relatively small proportion, less than 10 per cent, of croup cases have been associated with RSV infection.[155, 173, 255, 276, 311] RSV is isolated rarely from patients (from <1 per cent) without respiratory disease.[80, 276]

Specific neutralizing antibody passively received from the mother is present in the sera of all newborns.[38, 382] The level of antibody in the term newborn is similar to the maternal level, with gradual decline of the passive antibody over the first 6 months of life. After 7 months of age, detectable specific serum antibody usually is the result of natural infection. During the first year of life, about 50 to 70 per cent or more of infants acquire RSV infection, most all during the subsequent season.[38, 119, 169, 174, 175, 245, 385, 472, 495] Essentially all children by 3 years of age and all adults possess specific serum antibody.

Three generalizations may be made about the relation of age to the incidence and type of RSV disease: (1) lower respiratory tract disease (pneumonia and bronchiolitis) almost entirely is confined to the child younger than 3 years, (2) the occurrence of RSV lower respiratory tract disease during the first 3 to 4 weeks of life is relatively uncommon, and (3) reinfections are frequent in both older children and adults.[91, 157, 169, 170, 174, 175, 214, 230, 249, 276, 345, 382]

The proportion of RSV infections in infants that involve the lower respiratory tract is strikingly high but greatest during the first few months of life. The peak incidence of hospitalized cases of RSV bronchiolitis and pneumonia occurs in children 2 to 5 months of age.[157, 171, 228, 382] In Washington, D.C., approximately 40 per cent of primary infections involved the lower respiratory tract, and of every 100 primary RSV infections, one resulted in a hospital admission for bronchiolitis. In the Houston family studies, lower respiratory tract disease was the manifestation of 33 per cent of the infections in the first year of life and of 16 to 23 per cent of the RSV infections in the subsequent 3 years (Table 185–2).[169, 175] The risk of hospitalization for an infant infected with RSV during the first 12 months of life was 1.6 per cent.

Infants from better socioeconomic environments tend to be older when they first acquire lower respiratory tract disease from RSV and less frequently have severe disease.[323] In a private practice in Chapel Hill, only 13 per cent of the bron-

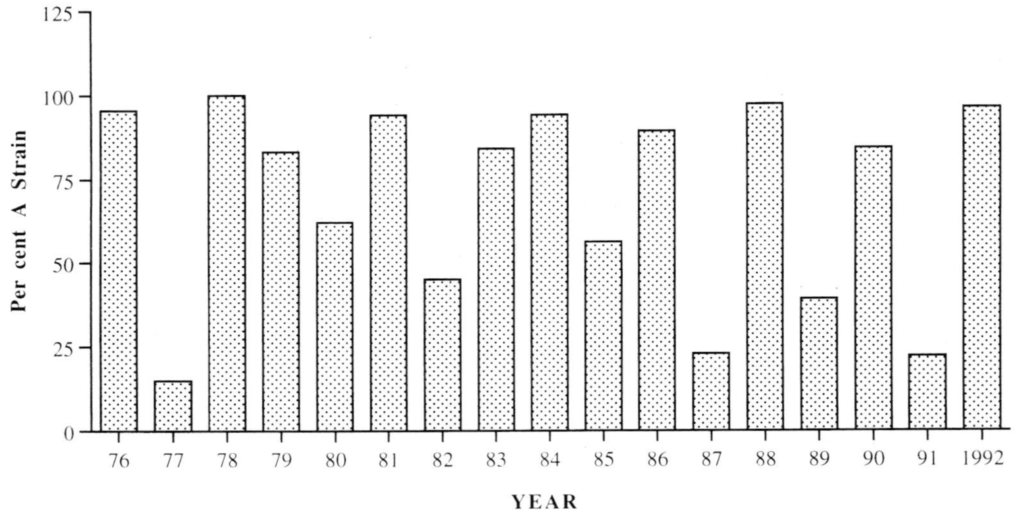

FIGURE 185–3. *The proportion of yearly (1976–1992) isolates of respiratory syncytial virus from Rochester, New York, area that were group A strains. Data were obtained from 1619 respiratory syncytial virus isolates from hospitalized children and from outpatient children included in the Community Surveillance Program of the University of Rochester School of Medicine.*

TABLE 185–2. Frequency of Respiratory Syncytial Virus Infection Among Children Studied from Birth*

Age, Months	No. of Child Years	No. with Respiratory Syncytial Virus: Primary	Reinfection	Total (Rate/100 Child Years)	LRD† (Rate/100 Child Years)	LRD† (Rate/100 Infections
0–12	125	85	1	86 (68.8)	28 (22.4)	32.6
13–24	92	33	43	76 (82.6)	12 (13.0)	15.8
25–36	65	1	29	30 (46.2)	7 (10.8)	23.3
37–48	39	0	13	13 (33.3)	3 (7.7)	23.1
49–60	24	0	12	12 (50.0)	0 (0)	—
Total	**345**	**119**	**98**	**217 (62.9)**	**50 (14.5)**	**23.0**

*Houston Family Study, 1975 through 1980.
†LRD indicates lower respiratory tract disease.
Reprinted with permission from Glezen, W. P., Taber, L. H., Frank, A. L., et al.: Risk of primary infection and reinfection with respiratory syncytial virus. Am. J. Dis. Child. *140*:543–546, 1986. Copyright 1986, American Medical Association.

chiolitis patients were younger than 6 months of age, compared with 40 per cent in the day care center and 56 per cent of hospitalized cases.[119] The risk of hospitalization with RSV disease for infants from middle-income families in Chapel Hill was less than 1 per 1000, compared with a 5- to 10-fold greater risk for infants of low-income families in Houston and Washington, D.C.[169, 170, 174, 175] Similarly, rates of hospitalization for RSV disease have been lower in children from middle-income families in Seattle and from a less urban area in Michigan.[145, 345] However, in Huntington, the risk of hospitalization with RSV during the first year of life was 1 per 88 live births.[44] In England, crowding and unemployment also seem to augment the risk of hospital admission.[414, 446] In the urban environs of Tyneside, 1 of every 50 infants during the first year of life required hospital admission for RSV infection.

In most studies of children hospitalized with RSV disease, males predominate in a ratio of about 2:1.[194, 382] However, in children with milder RSV illness, boys and girls are affected about equally, suggesting that gender influences the expression rather than the rate of illness, with boys developing more severe disease.[31, 119, 170]

RSV infection in older age groups is common. In Tecumseh, RSV infection, detected by the relatively insensitive complement-fixation antibody test, was most frequent in school age children.[345] Twenty per cent of the children 5 to 9 years of age were shown to be infected within 1 year. The rate fell to 10 per cent in family members 15 to 19 years of age, and to 3 to 6 per cent in those 20 to 50 years of age. When infection is assessed by viral isolation, the attack rate in family members exposed to young children with RSV infection is appreciable at all ages (Table 185–3).[175, 202] In school age children and adult family members, the attack rate during an RSV epidemic varied between 38 and 43 per cent.

Spread of Infections

Each breath's toll is virus spread and shed . . .*

RSV spreads effectively through exposed families, and introduction of the virus into the family appears to occur most commonly through a school age child.[45, 202, 343, 345] The serious disease of infancy, therefore, is likely to follow a mild "cold" of an older sibling.[202] In a prospective study of families with an infant and one or more older siblings, 44 per cent of the families became infected with RSV during a 3-month epidemic. In most all these families, older siblings (2 to 16 years of age) introduced the virus into the family, and the infants became infected secondarily. Furthermore, intrafamilial spread of the virus, according to the Tecumseh study, was related to the number of family members.[345] Families with six members had approximately three times the rate of infection observed in families with three members.

The conundrum of how this labile virus can spread so effectively has not been solved. Transmission by small-particle aerosols seems unlikely according to epidemiologic observations.[198] Small-particle aerosols of RSV are unstable at the low relative humidity of 20 to 30 per cent usually encountered indoors during winter months.[411] At relative humidities of 30 and 80 per cent, RSV in aerosols was inactivated maximally. Maximal stability occurred at 60 per cent relative humidity.

Spread may occur, however, through large droplets of secretions or through contact with contaminated secretions, as has been shown for rhinoviruses.[192, 233] RSV in the nasal secretions of infants with acute infection remains infectious on countertops for more than 6 hours and on cloth and paper tissue for 30 minutes.[204] Furthermore, these nasal secretions remain infectious after transfer from objects or hands to the hands of another person. This suggests that contact with clothing, furniture, or tissues contaminated by secretions of infected children may be one means of spread. This mode of spread has been supported by studies demonstrating that infection may occur in volunteers who touch surfaces contaminated by secretions and then their eyes or nasal mucosa.[195] In contrast, no infections developed in volunteers exposed to infected infants at a distance of greater than 6 feet, suggesting that small-particle aerosol spread of RSV was not a major mode of transmission. The spread of RSV, therefore, most frequently results from close contact with infected people or their infectious secretions, which tend to be profuse and prolonged in young and old, and less dependent on the long-distance travel of small-particle aerosols.

PATHOLOGY AND PATHOGENESIS

The newly born
from mother shorn
With seeds unsown
and shield unknown . . .

C. B. H.

The incubation period of illness from RSV has been reported variably as being between 2 and 8 days, with 4 to 6

*From Hall, C. B.: The shedding and spreading of respiratory syncytial virus. Pediatr. Res. *11*:235–239, 1977.

Table 185–3. Attack Rate of Respiratory Syncytial Virus (RSV) in Families According to Age

Age (Years)	Attack Rate* Crude Rate No.†	%	In RSV-Positive Families No.†	%	Secondary Rate No.†	%
<1	10/34	29.4	10/16	62.5	5/11	45.4
1–<2	2/7	28.6	2/5	40.0	0/3	0.0
2–<5	9/34	26.4	9/19	47.0	2/12	16.6
5–<17	9/48	18.7	9/24	38.0	4/19	21.0
17–45	9/55	16.8	9/21	43.0	6/18	33.3
Total	39/178	21.9	39/85	45.9	17/63	27.0

*Crude attack rate according to age is shown for all family members studied and for members of RSV-positive families. The secondary attack rate is also shown for members of RSV-positive families, excluding all primary and coprimary cases.
†No. of persons infected with RSV/total no. of persons exposed.
From Hall, C. B., Geiman, J. M., Biggar, R., et al.: Respiratory syncytial virus infection within families. N. Engl. J. Med. *294*:414–419, 1976.

days being the most common.[158, 267, 305, 463] Experimental infection in adult volunteers produced an average incubation period of 5 days.[261, 292] Inoculation is through the upper respiratory tract, and infection occurs in the respiratory epithelium. Both the eye and the nose appear to be equally sensitive routes of inoculation.[201] In contrast, inoculation by mouth results much less frequently in infection. Spread along the respiratory tract occurs mainly by cell-to-cell transfer of the virus along intracytoplasmic bridges. Spread from the upper to lower respiratory tract may involve the conducting airways at all levels.

The major pathologic findings as shown in infants dying with RSV bronchiolitis are (1) peribronchiolar mononuclear infiltration, (2) necrosis of the epithelium of the small airways, (3) plugging of the lumens, and (4) hyperinflation and atelectasis (Fig. 185–4).[4, 7, 122, 136, 155, 160, 161, 496] The initial lesions in bronchiolitis occur in the small airways (75 to 300 μm).[7] Lymphocytic peribronchiolar infiltration develops, along with edema of the walls, the submucosa, and the adventitial tissue. Subsequently, the epithelium of the bronchioles undergoes striking necrosis, sometimes with proliferation of the epithelium into the lumen. The necrotic material is sloughed into the lumen of these small airways, impeding the flow of air. In addition, the virus stimulates increased mucus secretion, which compounds the obstruction. The small lumens of the infant's airways especially are vulnerable to the obstruction caused by the edema and exudate.

Peripheral to the sites of partial occlusion, air trapping occurs, similar to a ball and valve mechanism. During the negative intrapleural pressure of inspiration, air can flow past the site of partial obstruction. On expiration, however, the positive pressure narrows the lumen, resulting in more complete obstruction and hyperinflation. In areas where the bronchiolar lumens become obstructed completely, the trapped air may be absorbed, resulting in multiple areas of focal atelectasis. These pathologic changes adversely affect the mechanics of the infant's respiration by causing a markedly increased lung volume and higher expiratory resistance.[540, 541]

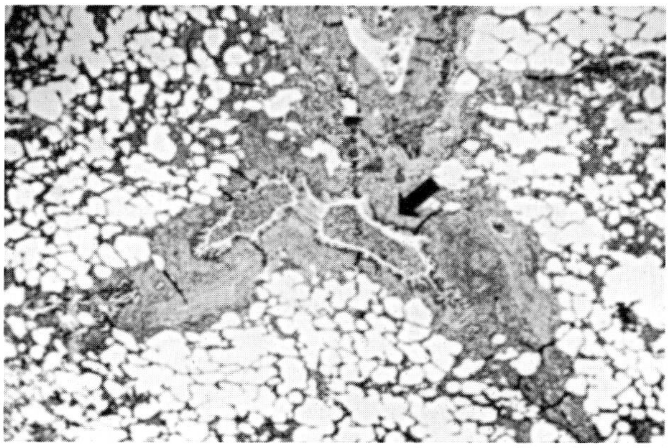

FIGURE 185–4. *Histologic examination of an infant dying with respiratory syncytial virus bronchiolitis. The arrow denotes a bronchiole filled with inflammatory exudate with comparatively normal alveoli.*

Recovery from acute bronchiolitis may be noted histologically within a few days, but complete restoration may take weeks, and some morphologic changes remain.[7, 412] Regeneration of the bronchiolar epithelium may begin in 3 to 4 days, but ciliated cells rarely are present before 2 weeks.[7] The enlarged submucosal glands, augmented numbers of goblet cells, and muscular hypertrophy that often accompany acute bronchiolitis may persist.[412, 540, 541] Although complete clinical recovery is the rule, bronchiolitis may have a rowen of subtle pathologic changes.

In RSV pneumonia, the characteristic finding is an interstitial infiltration of mononuclear cells.[7, 161] In some cases, lymphocytic infiltration of the bronchiolar walls also is present. The lung parenchyma appears edematous with areas of necrosis, leading to alveolar filling, consolidation, and collapse.[7]

Role of the Immune Response in Pathogenesis

The cabal of the immune response of the infant with RSV disease has evoked several theories of pathogenesis. Several observations have suggested that immunologic mechanisms may be the key to the severity of RSV lower respiratory tract disease in infancy. First, the most severe disease occurs during the period when the infant possesses specific maternal antibody. Second, this also is the period when the infant is immature immunologically. Third, children with high levels of circulating antibody induced by the inactivated RSV vaccine had more severe disease than their unvaccinated counterparts when naturally infected with RSV.[7, 152, 268, 279] In addition, the clinical expression of their disease, although exaggerated, was typical of the natural lower respiratory tract disease of infancy. Fourth, shedding of the virus frequently is abundant and prolonged in the youngest and most severely affected infants.[199, 200] Immunologic reaction and injury are most likely in infections in which the antigen persists for prolonged periods.[40]

From such observations, several hypotheses have evolved to explain the severity of RSV lower respiratory tract disease in the first few months of life: (1) an immune complex (type III) reaction occurs in the lung, involving the viral antigen and the maternally acquired IgG antibody in an infant who lacks IgA secretory antibody[77, 79]; (2) a cell-mediated (type IV) immune reaction occurs in the lung of these infants[280]; (3) an IgE-mediated (type I) response is evoked in the lungs of infants with bronchiolitis or wheezing[160, 527, 533, 548]; (4) the immature development of the immune system of the young infant is related to the disease's severity; and (5) the clinical expression of the disease is related mostly to the virulence of the virus and the age of development of the airway at the time of the first RSV infection.

The first theory emphasizes the detrimental role of maternally acquired antibody in an infant who has an imbalance of serum antibody compared with the other components of immunity that would be derived though natural infection, such as secretory antibody.[79] In favor of such a theory are the observations that disease tends to be most severe when maternal antibody is present and that disease was exaggerated in vaccinated children. The inactivated vaccine tended to produce high levels of serum antibody, not all of which was functional antibody, and a poor secretory antibody response.[79, 359, 360] Countering this theory are the observations that the level of maternal antibody cannot be related directly to the severity or expression of illness and that disease may be severe in infants with no detectable antibody.[63, 79, 257, 268, 296, 382] More recent studies have suggested a protective role for specific maternal antibody.[174, 369, 519] Furthermore, complement cannot be detected in the lungs of infants dying with RSV disease, nor do the levels of complement fall during the acute phase of illness, as may be expected in an immune-complex disease.[15] The detrimental role of antibody, however, may not be enacted via this immune-complex mechanism but rather by enhancement of viral replication.[293] Monoclonal antibodies to the F and G proteins have been found to augment the in vitro infection of macrophages by RSV.

The second hypothesis invoking a cell-mediated immune reaction is difficult to prove directly. No technique currently available can evaluate a cell-mediated reaction in the human lung. Natural RSV infection stimulates systemic cell-mediated immunity, and in children with more severe disease after receiving the formalin-inactivated vaccine, this cell-mediated immune response was augmented.[52, 79, 133, 253, 280, 339, 438, 528] In experimental animals, the inactivated RSV vaccine elicited dermal delayed hypersensitivity, which appeared to be a prerequisite to the development of lower respiratory tract disease.[125] Because a cell-mediated response to RSV may be demonstrated in the cord blood lymphocytes of some infants, specific sensitization of the lymphocytes of the infant derived from the mother has been suggested.[40, 111, 438, 441, 528]

An IgE-mediated (type I) reaction initially was suggested by Gardner and his colleagues,[160] based on their studies of the pathology of RSV bronchiolitis and pneumonia. Scarce RSV antigen was detected by immunofluorescence in the lungs of infants dying with bronchiolitis, compared with abundant antigen present in infants dying with RSV pneumonia. From this they hypothesized that in bronchiolitis, the major pathology was from an allergic response in a host previously sensitized to the virus rather than from viral replication.[122, 136, 160] Epidemiologic observations, however, do not support this theory. The peak occurrence of bronchiolitis during an RSV epidemic is not later than that of pneumonia, as would be expected if bronchiolitis developed only after repeated exposure to the virus.[55] Infants with bronchiolitis also do not have an accelerated serologic response characteristic of primed subjects.[529] Nevertheless, specific IgE antibody in the serum and secretions identified on exfoliated nasopharyngeal epithelial cells frequently is formed in RSV disease.[65, 527, 533] A pathogenic role for the IgE antibody is suggested by the correlation of the IgE antibody titer and the histamine content in the secretions to RSV infection associated with wheezing. A similar correlation to wheezing has been shown for specific IgE and IgG4 humoral antibody.[65]

Immunologic immaturity partly related to the presence of maternal antibody also has been proposed as the pivotal deficit in infants with RSV disease. The infant's ability to respond serologically is related inversely to the amount of passively transferred antibody, and the inhibition may be not only quantitative but also qualitative.[63, 356, 357, 426, 487] The immune response of cotton rats to the glycoproteins of RSV has been suppressed by the passive transfer of specific antibody, resulting in their increased susceptibility to infection and in the production of antibodies with abnormally low neutralizing activity.[358] The presence of maternal antibody also may inhibit an early, local antibody response in the lung, which could be integral to the initial control of viral replication.[54] The absence of the secretory component in some infants with fatal RSV disease suggests that the secretory component, with or without IgA antibody, may offer nonspecific protection.[370, 371] The correlation of abundant and prolonged shedding of RSV with younger age and in immunocompromised patients with more severe disease also suggests immunologic immaturity or deficiency.[140, 199, 200, 211, 441]

The last of the proposed theories necessitates no immunologic mechanism to explain the severity of RSV disease in infancy. Maternal antibody may offer some protection to the infant, but when matched against a large inoculating dose of RSV, this may be of limited efficacy.[170] The level of maternal antibody, nevertheless, may be important, as suggested by the diminished occurrence of serious lower respiratory tract disease in the first 4 weeks of life and by the correlation of maternal antibody with protection against the rate and severity of infection.[133, 174, 208, 296, 369, 382, 519]

The anatomy of the small infant's airway engenders more severe physiologic consequences from the inflammation and obstruction of infection because the proportion of the total pulmonary flow resistance derived from the small peripheral airways is much greater than that in older children.[243] Anatomic differences in the developing lung also may render it more susceptible to the pathologic sequelae of a viral infection.[412, 540] The submucosal glands of the infant are relatively larger and the collateral ventilation poorer. Hypoxemia, characteristic of RSV infection, tends to produce pulmonary vasoconstriction, which may interfere with the normal development of the arterial wall during the first several months of life. The infantile lung may be not only more vulnerable but also less able to compensate for the insult of RSV inflammation.

Components from each of these theories may contribute in varying degrees to the pathogenicity of RSV in individual infants. The incontrovertible factors associated with potentially severe RSV disease, however, may be summarized as (1) young age, (2) immunologic immaturity or deficiency, (3) preexisting maternal antibody, which may be just a marker of young age, (4) certain underlying diseases, especially prematurity and functionally significant cardiopulmonary diseases, (5) abundant and prolonged viral shedding, and (6) administration of the formalin-inactivated vaccine. The conundrum, nevertheless, remains whether these are intertwining correlates or causes.

IMMUNE RESPONSE

The focus of much recent investigation to delineate the cabal of the immune response to RSV has revealed integral new pieces of the mosaic of immunity. These are likely to aid the development of an effective vaccine and control of RSV infection.

Immunity to RSV infection is variable, incomplete, and not durable. Repetitive infections occur throughout life and sometimes even within the same season. Infants may have repetitive lower respiratory tract infections, but the subsequent infections rarely are as severe as primary infection. This, plus the observation that RSV infection after the first several years of life involves primarily the upper respiratory tract, indicates that immunity, although not perfect, does develop.

Serum Antibody

After several days, infants undergoing primary infection produce specific serum IgM antibody, which is detectable only for a few weeks.[246, 529] Immunoglobulin antibody subsequently appears in the second week, peaks in the fourth week, and declines after 1 to 2 months. The IgA serum antibody response in infants tends to be limited and may not be detectable, depending on the assay.[110, 246, 356, 529] After reinfection, the serum antibody response in all three immunoglobulin classes is enhanced, and antibody titers reach levels similar to those of adults after approximately three infections. Although high levels of IgG antibody to RSV tend to be associated with protection against infection, the correlation of the level of specific humoral antibody to susceptibility and clinical severity is poor and not consistently predictive.[215]

The benefits afforded by specific antibody depend on a number of factors other than titer level, which include the type, function, and protein specificity. The two surface glycoproteins, F and G, clearly are integral in the immune response. Neutralizing epitopes are present on both F and G, and a fusion epitope also is present on F.[510, 514, 515] Monoclonal antibodies to the F and G proteins but not to the internal proteins N, P, and M, when passively transferred to rodents, afford protection against subsequent RSV challenge.[399, 479, 514, 516] The protection primarily is observed in the lung rather than in the nose and upper respiratory tract.[399, 479, 516] In animal models, the degree of protection for the lower respiratory tract tends to correlate with the levels of neutralizing antibody to the F and G proteins.[398, 399]

Immunization with the F, G, and N proteins in experimental animals also produces lower respiratory tract resistance, but the degree of protection varies according to the animal model.[93, 99, 240] Although immunization of baboons with the F protein afforded lower respiratory tract protection, in the chimpanzee, vaccination with F and G was less immunogenic and not protective. The rodent model has verified the broader, heterologous immunity induced by the F protein, whereas antibody induced by the G protein has provided little protection against challenge with a heterologous strain.[262, 376, 514, 536] Immunization with the G but not the F protein also can result in an eosinophilic pathology in the mouse lung.[379]

In humans, the roles of F and G proteins also appear integral in the development of immunity to RSV. The response to these proteins in infants, however, is affected by several factors. The quantitative and qualitative humoral response of the infant is influenced by the presence of preexisting maternal antibody, by age, and by the particular viral antigens. Young children are able to produce after infection antibodies against both of the major surface glycoproteins, F and G, but the responses are inconsistent, especially to the G protein, in the youngest infants.[234, 357, 487, 519, 531] The heavily glycosylated G protein is a poorer immunogen in the young, and preexisting serum antibody appears to have a greater dampening effect on the response to the G than to the F protein.[234, 356, 357] The effect of young age, however, is greater on the F and IgG antibody responses than on the development of IgM antibody.[356, 487]

The subclass of antibody formed to the F and G proteins mainly is IgG1 and IgG3, the subclasses primarily associated with antibodies to proteins, rather than IgG2, the subclass associated with antibody to carbohydrates. Because the F and G proteins are glycosylated heavily, the lack of the IgG2 response is notable.[350, 505] Much less is known in humans, especially in infants with primary infection, about the role of antibodies to the F and G proteins in protection against infection, reinfection, or illness. The humoral response of infants to the formalin-inactivated vaccine characterized by a deficiency in neutralizing antibody to the F protein and in fusion antibody supports the importance of functional F antibody in a normal, protective response.[359, 360] In adults who were challenged with RSV after natural infection, levels of antibody to the F and homologous G proteins and of neutralizing antibodies to the homologous strain correlated with resistance to reinfection.[214] Protection against symptomatic infection correlated more with antibody to the homologous G protein. The infecting strain also is likely to be a factor in determining the immune, and possibly the clinical, response. During primary infection, the homologous and heterologous antibody responses to the F proteins of both major subgroups appear to be similar, but there is little heterologous response to the G proteins.[234] Limited data suggest that prior infection with group A strains provides more resistance to reinfection with the homologous or heterologous strain.[234, 350, 352]

Local Humoral Response

Because RSV spreads from cell to cell, it may escape mostly the net of serum neutralizing antibody, emphasizing the possible importance of the local humoral and cell-mediated immune responses. In animal models, circulating specific antibody generally has not ablated viral replication in the upper respiratory tract, although the administration of high titers of IgG antibodies has diminished nasal titers and afforded lower respiratory tract protection.[399, 431, 516] Viral replication has been diminished more effectively in the rodent respiratory tract by local IgA antibody than by serum IgG antibody, but the IgA response and any associated protection is relatively short-lived, less than 8 months, whereas IgG antibody in the lower respiratory tract is more durable.[181, 399] Although the neutralizing activity in the nasal secretions of children with RSV infection has been examined, a correlation with protection from infection or severe disease has not been consistent.[77, 279, 329, 338, 437] In many infants, neutralizing activity was present in the nasal secretions at the time of the infant's admission. Second, the neutralizing activity appeared nonspecific, not relating to susceptibility to infection but to diminished viral shedding.[77, 329, 338] Specific IgA antibody, however, can be detected in the nasal secretions of infants of all ages in response to RSV infection, but it may not be neutralizing and does not appear to have a clear role in recovery or in protection against reinfection.[214, 271, 327, 329]

Specific IgA, IgG, IgM, and transiently IgE antibodies are present in the secretions of most infected infants.[159, 329, 330, 525] With primary infection, specific IgA, IgG, and IgM antibodies are present in the nasal secretions by 3 days in half or more of infants.[246, 271] Immunoglobulin antibody appears early, with IgM and IgG antibodies peaking in the second week. All three usually disappear within 1 to 3 months. These secretory antibodies are directed to the F, G, and N proteins in both the IgG and IgA isotypes in the nasal washes of infants undergoing primary infection, but IgA tends to dominate.[357] In younger infants, nasal antibody is present less often and in lower quantities. After secondary infection, levels are boosted and more persistent.[246, 271] Small amounts of specific IgE antibody also are produced frequently in the secretions of infants in the early days of acute primary infection.[65, 527, 533] Higher and more persistent titers of IgE and histamine, however, appear to be pathogenic and associated with wheezing and more severe disease acutely and with subsequent airway hyperreactivity.[527, 532, 533] Specific IgE antibody may stimulate a cascade of inflammatory mediators, producing the clinical manifestations of wheezing and hyperreactivity.[162, 503, 504, 530, 531] In vitro and clinical evidence suggests that the production of specific antibody results in the release of bronchoactive leukotrienes, including LTC4 and eosinophil cationic protein, and these may be in elevated quantities in bronchiolitis.[16, 162, 442, 503, 504, 530, 531]

Cellular Immunity

Some studies have helped delineate the components and contributions of the cellular response to immunity. Although these studies almost entirely have been in experimental animals, the findings may provide understanding and guidelines for the development of vaccines for infants. The type of cellular response to RSV has been clarified further and may be critical to the outcome from infection. Active viral infections, such as with natural RSV infection, usually stimulate T-helper cells with a Th1 cytokine profile (interleukin-2, interferon-γ). In contrast, inactivated or nonreplicating antigens characteristically evoke a Th2 cytokine pattern (interleukins 4 to 6). Th1-type response usually requires the antigen to be processed in context with class I histocompatibility proteins, resulting in the production of IgG2a neutralizing antibody and CD8+ cytotoxic T lymphocytes (CTLs). Th2 responses, on the other hand, process antigens in association with class II histocompatibility proteins with the subsequent synthesis of IgG1 but without CTLs. Rodent models have demonstrated that Th1 responses are evoked by live RSV infection. Specific CTLs have been identified in the liver and spleen of mice after RSV challenge.[33, 480] The Th1 response has been demonstrated in vitro to occur in both adults and children.[24] Specific CTLs have been demonstrated in the peripheral blood of adults infected previously.[34] Experimental inoculation of volunteers with live RSV produced specific CTL responses that were associated with diminished clinical symptoms.[252] Limited data in infants with primary infection suggest that a cell-mediated response with specific CTLs is evoked variably within 10 days of infection.[86, 253]

The N, F, and M2 proteins are targets for CTLs in both rodents and humans.[34, 67, 85, 366, 380, 388] SH, M, and NS2 proteins additionally have been shown to be recognized by human CTLs. CTL responses to G, F, N, and M2 have been associated with resistance to infection in mice, but the protective effect to the N and M2 proteins tends to be transient.[104, 106]

The contributions of the various T-cell subsets to the clearance and convalescence from RSV infection remain confusing, complicated, and contrasting. In mice, the response to RSV infection has been characterized as a Th1 pattern with the production of CD4+ cells, the characteristic Th1 cytokines, IgG2a, and CTLs. Both group A and B strains evoke CD8+ CTLs and are correlated with clearance of RSV.[32, 34, 67, 69, 355] Furthermore, RSV-specific CTL lines or clones when infused into normal or nude mice result in clearance of the virus.[68, 69, 178, 355]

Graham and colleagues[178, 179, 181] have characterized carefully in mice the evoked T-cell subsets and their functional contributions. Mice depleted of CD4+ or CD8+ cells demonstrated somewhat prolonged viral shedding but were able to clear the virus. If both subsets were depleted, viral shedding remained high and prolonged. In immune mice depleted of CD4+ cells, CD8+ cells, or both, rechallenge with RSV resulted in little effect on the ability to clear the infection. Experiments that passively transferred RSV-specific CD4+ or CD8+ cells diminish viral replication in the lung but in some studies have been associated with an increase in both morbidity and pathology.[13, 68, 355] The variable degree of pathologic findings in these studies in the murine model may relate to the quantity, timing, specificity, and types of T cells infused or evoked.

Of note for vaccine development is that the type of antigen used for primary immunization can produce different T-helper cytokine mRNA expression in the lungs of mice subsequently challenged with RSV. Immunization with a live virus, whether intramuscular or intranasal, stimulates a Th1-type response, in contrast with the Th2 pattern resulting from challenge with the inactivated virus.[182] These specific Th responses, however, are affected by the specific RSV proteins. Immunization with F protein stimulates a Th1 cytokine response and CD4+ and CD8+ cells. On the other hand, immunization with G produces a Th2 cytokine pattern with only CD4+ cells.[11, 12] After M2 inoculation, only CD8+ cells are produced.

These studies in experimental animals offer a possible and piquant explanation for the exaggerated disease observed in infants who had received the formalin-inactivated vaccine. The vaccine, altered from live virus by formalin inactivation, produced an abnormal and unbalanced primary immunization in infants that possibly entailed multiple components of the immune response. First, the inactivated antigen stimulated little or no antibody. Second, although the vaccine was immunogenic, the humoral antibody quantitatively was awry, with diminished neutralizing and fusion functions. In vivo studies, however, do not suggest that humoral antibody is the sole factor in producing the pathogenic response because passive transfer of antibody induced by the formalin-inactivated vaccine in mice did not result in a similar pathologic pulmonary picture. The altered antigens of the killed vaccine shifted the cellular immune response to a Th2 rather than a Th1 CTL response. In mice immunized with formalin-inactivated vaccine, specific viral memory T cells were produced abundantly but consisted of CD4 cells, which could be visualized in the pulmonary pathology. The plethora of CD4 cells was not accompanied by the specific CTL response of CD8+ cells. On reinfection with wild RSV, therefore, the memory cells present and able to respond were CD4+ cells. Their rapid proliferation and characteristic inflammatory effects would be unchecked by CD8+ cells, important in the clearance of infection, and also would be unmodified by the presence of local secretory antibody or adequate function of serum antibodies.

The pattern of T-cell and cytokine responses evoked in humans is delineated less well. In vitro infection of human peripheral blood mononuclear cells with RSV produces not only interleukin-1, but also inhibitors to interleukin-1.[421] The impaired lymphoproliferative response is evoked only by live, replicating RSV and consisted of a cell-cycle arrest and no proliferative response to mitogens or nonviral antigens. Inactivated virus or live influenza does not result in a similar inhibition.[393, 421, 429, 430] These findings may be hypothesized as partly explaining the susceptibility to repetitive RSV infections. Such a cellular inhibitory response not only may be detrimental to recovery from acute RSV but also may dampen the secondary immune response upon reinfection.

CLINICAL MANIFESTATIONS

We view their chests ballooning, with the fears
that they're "pink puffers" of more tender years.*

Primary Infection

An infant's first encounter with RSV almost always is apparent, but the symptoms may range from those of a mild cold to severe bronchiolitis or pneumonia.[80, 276, 382] RSV is isolated rarely from children with no signs of respiratory illness.[80, 276] The risk of lower respiratory tract disease occurring during this initial experience is high but varies with the setting. Parrott and his associates[382] have estimated that 40 per cent of primary infections result in febrile pneumonitis. Only a small portion of these require hospital admission. According to their estimates, 1 per cent of all primary RSV infections led to a hospital admission for bronchiolitis.[276] Considering the universal nature of RSV infection, even a small percentage magnifies into the appreciable health and economic problem of an estimated 91,000 infants hospitalized for RSV infection each year in the United States alone.[224]

In closed populations of young children, the entrance of RSV often has been followed by even higher rates of lower respiratory tract disease. In a welfare nursery of 90 infants with and without previous infection, an outbreak of RSV resulted in pneumonia in 40 per cent and a febrile upper respiratory tract illness in 53 per cent.[267] When RSV recirculated in this nursery 6 years later, only 10 per cent of the young children developed pneumonia. In similar facilities in other countries, outbreaks of RSV infection have resulted in lower respiratory tract involvement in up to 89 per cent of the children.[305, 325, 458, 463] Primary infections were associated with lower respiratory tract infection in more than half of normal children followed longitudinally in a day care center.[230] Even second infections in these children produced lower respiratory tract disease in 25 and 17 per cent of those with third and fourth infections, respectively.

In the longitudinal Houston family studies, 69 per cent of children in their first year acquired RSV infection, and one-third of these infections were lower respiratory tract illnesses (Table 185–2).[175] By 24 months of age, essentially all children had been infected at least once, and half had had two infections, such that the rate of infections during the second year of life was 83 per cent. The proportion of RSV infections involving the lower respiratory tract remains appreciable during the second, third, and fourth years of life, but the severity decreases (Tables 185–2 and 185–3). Pneumonia and bronchiolitis occur with diminishing frequency and are replaced by tracheobronchitis or reactive airway disease.[175]

Pneumonia appears to be the most common manifestation of lower respiratory tract disease with RSV. Croup is least common, usually accounting for less than 5 per cent of cases.[382] In studies from several different locations, the ratio of pneumonia to bronchiolitis cases has ranged from 1:1 to 7:1.[170] This variability may stem partly from a lack of standard criteria to differentiate clinical bronchiolitis from pneumonia. Wheezing may occur in both syndromes, as may infiltrates on chest radiographs.[155, 170, 275] In bronchiolitis, these shadows mostly are the result of atelectasis rather than from the interstitial inflammation and alveolar filling of pneumonia. Radiographic differentiation of the pathogenesis of the observed infiltrates often is impossible. Bronchiolitis usually is defined clinically by the presence of the two cardinal signs: wheezing and hyperinflation of the lung. In pneumonia, the infiltrates on chest radiograph may be accompanied by rales and rhonchi, with or without wheezing. Often, the two syndromes are combined, and pneumonia appears to be a continuum of bronchiolitis.

The signs associated with lower respiratory tract illness due to RSV are shown in Table 185–4. Upper respiratory tract symptoms commonly precede by several days the lower respiratory tract involvement. Fever is common in the initial phase of the illness, but by the time of hospitalization, it may be low-grade or have disappeared. In a study of 565 hospitalized children with RSV infection, less than half had fever higher than 38° C at the time of admission.[212] The duration of fever usually is 2 to 7 days and tends to be lower in infants younger than 6 months of age, compared with those 6 to 12 months of age. Although fever is more common in primary infections, approximately 20 to 40 per cent of children with their second, third, or fourth infections are febrile.[230]

Cough also becomes a consistent and prominent finding. An increased cough may herald the lower respiratory tract involvement. The retractions of the chest wall and dyspnea are common, especially in bronchiolitis. Rales and rhonchi commonly accompany the wheezing and hyperinflation of bronchiolitis.[206, 229, 413] In pneumonia, rales and sometimes wheezes are present bilaterally. The duration of illness usually is 7 to 12 days.[46, 200] Most infants hospitalized with bronchiolitis or pneumonia show clinical improvement after 3 to 4 days, and most are discharged after an average of 4 to 7 days.[199, 206, 333] The typical course of an infant with pneumonia from RSV is illustrated in Figure 185–5.

The clinical appearance of improvement, however, often belies the continued inflammation and prolonged physiologic abnormalities in the young infant.[199, 200, 333] In infants hospitalized with lower respiratory tract disease, viral shedding commonly continues, despite clinical improvement, and usually is accompanied by continued abnormalities in the infant's

TABLE 185–4. Signs in Children with Respiratory Syncytial Viral Infections

	Percentage of Hospitalized Infants*	Percentage of Ambulatory Infants and Young Children†
Fever	45–65	74–100
Cough	97–100	83–100
Rhinitis	56–82	45–73
Pharyngitis	45–54	20–30
Hoarseness	—	6–20
Dyspnea	50–78	70–90
Retractions	36–68	40–100
Cyanosis	11–25	—
Wheezing	45–76	17–34
Rales	27–72	60–75
Rhonchi	59–78	15–90
Otitis	31	10–34
Conjunctivitis	9	15–30
Vomiting	45–52	20–27

*Data from ref. 46 (93% of infants had lower respiratory tract disease), ref. 157 (87% of infants had lower respiratory tract disease), and Hall, C. B. (unpublished data on 637 hospitalized infants with lower respiratory tract disease).

†Data from ref. 413 (outpatients with bronchiolitis and pneumonia), ref. 493 (patients from a British practice survey, two-thirds with lower respiratory tract disease), and Hall, C. B. (unpublished data on 434 outpatient children, one-third with lower respiratory tract disease).

*From Hall, C. B.: The shedding and spreading of respiratory syncytial virus. Pediatr. Res. *11*:235–239, 1977.

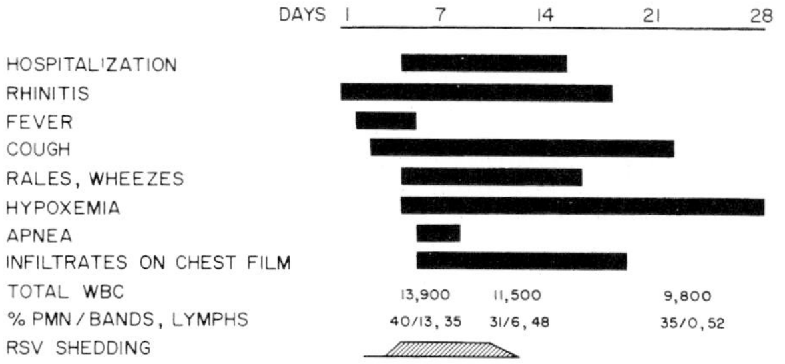

FIGURE 185–5. *The course of this 8-week-old infant with pneumonia due to respiratory syncytial virus (RSV) is characteristic of the course of young infants hospitalized with RSV lower respiratory tract disease. WBC, total white blood cell count per mm³; % PMN/Bands, Lymphs, percentage of polymorphonuclear cells, bands, and lymphocytes in the peripheral white blood cell count.*

gas exchange.[199, 200, 206, 212] The degree of hypoxemia may fluctuate within hours as well as day to day. At discharge, infants may continue to have some degree of hypoxemia and do not recover completely until weeks later, as would be expected from the histologic studies of the regeneration of the bronchiolar epithelium (see Pathology and Pathogenesis).

Clinical evaluation of the severity of RSV lower respiratory tract disease in young infants is difficult.[206, 333, 415] Less than one-third of these infants have cyanosis.[206, 415] Moderate to severe degrees of hypoxemia, nevertheless, may exist without evidence of cyanosis.[206] An increased respiratory rate has been correlated with the degree of hypoxemia but only if obtained in a standard manner when the infant is asleep or peaceful and if the effect of fever is recognized.[415] The severity of retractions, wheezing, irritability, and lethargy generally correlates poorly with the degree of hypoxemia. The hypoxemia most likely arises from an abnormally low ratio of ventilation to perfusion rather than from shunting.[206, 415, 540] Despite the often prolonged and severe hypoxemia in these young infants, alveolar hypoventilation with progressive hypercarbia is uncommon in those given good supportive care.[206, 540]

The radiographic findings in infants hospitalized with RSV lower respiratory tract disease yield a variety of patterns.[151, 155, 275, 416, 445] The most typical finding is a diffuse interstitial pneumonitis, commonly accompanied by hyperinflation of the lung.[416] In nearly 66 per cent of cases, the interstitial infiltrates are present in all lobes, and in about 20 per cent of the cases, they are present in only one lobe.[416] Hyperaeration was observed in more than 50 per cent and peribronchial thickening in 39 per cent of those children hospitalized in Newcastle-upon-Tyne with RSV bronchiolitis, pneumonia, or both.[155, 445] Air trapping particularly is indicative of RSV infection and may be the only abnormality. Peribronchial thickening also may be the only finding, but its presence in the Newcastle studies did not correlate more with RSV than with other infections. Alveolar pneumonia, appearing as lobar or segmental consolidations, is evident in about one-fourth of children with RSV lower respiratory tract disease, especially in infants younger than 6 months of age.[151, 155, 445] Lobar or segmental consolidation was noted in about one-fifth of the children hospitalized in Chapel Hill, and the right upper lobe was involved in all cases.[416] Collapse of the lung or demonstrable pleural fluid development is rare. The radiographic abnormalities tend to last longer than the clinical symptoms and signs, with consolidated areas being the slowest to clear.[416]

The other common forms of primary infection are tracheobronchitis and upper respiratory tract infections. The accompanying signs and symptoms tend to be moderately severe, with predominant cough and sometimes fever. Otitis media frequently is associated with RSV infections in young children, particularly in children younger than 1 year of age.[26, 27, 46, 47, 89, 202, 231, 232, 286, 482, 494] RSV has been detected in middle ear aspirates, alone, or simultaneously with a bacterial pathogen, suggesting that RSV may play both a primary and a secondary role in the pathogenesis of otitis media.[26, 27, 47, 89, 231, 374, 375, 386] RSV-induced otitis media also has been associated with prolonged symptoms and apparent failure of therapy.[26, 27]

Repeated Infection

In Children

Repeated experiences with RSV are common.[37, 119, 175, 202, 230, 249, 270, 345] Between 6 and 83 per cent of children followed longitudinally have been reinfected each year.[119, 175, 230, 270] The interval between infections may be no longer than the period between successive outbreaks of RSV infection or even less.[37, 175, 230] The repeated experience with RSV usually is milder, consisting of tracheobronchitis or an upper respiratory tract infection.[119, 169, 175] Children, nevertheless, may experience repeated bouts of RSV lower respiratory tract disease. In preschool children, 20 to more than 50 per cent of the repeated infections involve the lower respiratory tract.[37, 230]

In the longitudinal study of children in a Chapel Hill day care center, the attack rate for the first infection was 98 per cent and for the second and third infections, 75 and 65 per cent, respectively.[230] Of note was the finding that immunity resulting from a single infection appeared to have no ameliorating effect on illness associated with reinfection 1 year later. Not until the third infection was severity reduced appreciably, suggesting that both age and immune factors are important. It should be recognized, however, that because the illnesses in this study were in children in day care centers, the illnesses were relatively mild. Infants with first infections severe enough to require hospitalization rarely appear to have second or repeated infections of equal severity, unless they have an underlying disease that places them at high risk for complications.

In the Houston longitudinal studies, infants in families had similarly high rates of reinfection.[169, 175] Of babies experiencing primary infection during the first year of life, 76 per cent were reinfected by 24 months of age. One-fourth of these second infections involved the lower respiratory tract, but they tended to be mild. Most children had lower respiratory tract illness only once. Those with repetitive lower respiratory tract infections tended to have reactive airway disease.

In Adults

RSV most commonly evokes a "common cold" in adults. In the 1960s, Beem[37] isolated RSV from adults, and Hamre and Procknow[218] recovered the virus from 15 medical students with naturally acquired upper respiratory infections. RSV accounted for more than one-fourth of the viruses recovered from these students with colds. In about two-thirds of military recruits, RSV infection was manifested as a mild upper respiratory tract infection, whereas the rest were asymptomatic.[260] These older studies and those of experimental infection in adult volunteers, therefore, suggested that in the healthy adult, RSV infection is either asymptomatic or limited to upper respiratory tract manifestations.[261, 292]

Subsequently, however, RSV has been shown to produce more severe illness, such as bronchitis or an influenza-like illness, in some healthy adults, especially parents and hospital staff caring for young infants with RSV infection.[198, 202, 207, 214] In these groups, most infections appear to be symptomatic, consisting of upper respiratory tract infections with or without fever and tracheobronchitis. About 70 per cent have had an illness more severe and prolonged than the usual "cold" from other causes.[198] Malaise, nasal congestion, and cough may persist for an average of 10 to 14 days.[202, 207] Studies by Smith and colleagues[452] from the Cambridge Health Psychology Research Unit have indicated by visual perception tests in experimentally infected volunteers that susceptibility to more symptomatic illness from RSV, but not from other viruses, may be related to behavioral measures. Lower respiratory tract abnormalities also have been detected in young, previously healthy adults by pulmonary function studies, predominantly hyper-reactivity of the airway to cholinergic stimulus.[207] The more severe disease sometimes seen in these groups of adults may relate partly to a high challenge dose from the intimate exposure to infants with primary infection who shed the virus abundantly.[170] More severe illness, however, also has been described in institutionalized young adults.[138]

Interest in RSV's role in illness in the elderly recently has expanded. Early in RSV's clinical career, a few reports noted that RSV could cause acute exacerbations of illness in patients with chronic bronchitis.[72, 344, 455] RSV subsequently was recognized in the elderly as a cause of acute and often severe lower respiratory tract disease requiring hospitalization.[147, 281, 502] It also may cause illness in the elderly living at home, but most of the knowledge about RSV's pathogenic potential in the geriatric population has come from the increasing recognition of outbreaks in nursing homes or in other groups of the institutionalized elderly. Various manifestations of RSV may occur in this population, ranging from mostly asymptomatic and mild upper respiratory infections to severe, even fatal, respiratory tract infection.[6, 28, 53, 75, 130–132, 141, 222, 322, 346, 381] In one outbreak on geriatric wards housing 68 patients, 52 acquired RSV illness.[6] The most frequent clinical manifestations, occurring in 96 per cent of patients, were fever and intensive coughing, which was productive in about two-thirds. Most patients gradually improved over a period of 5 to 7 days, but complications occurred in 15 per cent. Pneumonia in this elderly population may result from RSV infection either alone or combined with bacterial infection.[346, 502] Severe or fatal disease in previously healthy adults living at home has been reported but is rare.[307]

With the increasing numbers of immunocompromised patients, RSV's pathogenicity in high-risk adult patients has been a growing concern and the hazard of its nosocomial transmission emphasized.[18, 127, 128, 144, 190, 237, 361, 449, 475, 538] Outbreaks in bone marrow transplant units may be devastating and expensive in terms of the diagnostic work-up and infection control. The clinical findings, often diffuse pulmonary interstitial infiltrates and hypoxemia that even can be consistent with the adult respiratory distress syndrome, usually are not attributed initially to RSV in this setting.

Infection in Neonates

Infection with RSV in the first 4 weeks of life appears to be relatively infrequent.[280, 338] In Washington, D.C., the incidence of RSV infection during the first month of life was noted to be only one-third of that during the second month of life.[338] The protected environment of newborns and their diminished exposure to others, as well as the high levels of maternal antibody or other early immune factors, may explain partly the lower incidence of illness. The clinical expression of RSV infection during this period, nevertheless, may be variable, with few or no respiratory signs.[208]

In early studies, the infants in nurseries were older than 1 month of age, and their illnesses generally were characteristic of RSV infection in this age group.[48, 56, 267, 305, 463] Studies of premature and term neonates with RSV infection have described atypical clinical features, resulting in delayed diagnosis.[177, 208, 337, 349] In a Newcastle nursery, eight babies were infected, and all became symptomatic, usually in the second week of life. The illness generally was mild in these infants, consisting of upper respiratory tract symptoms and cough. Only one infant had radiographic evidence of pneumonia, although three had mild wheezing. In Rochester, 25 per cent of infants in a neonatal special care unit for more than 6 days acquired RSV infection during the 3 months that RSV was prevalent in the community.[208] Premature infants particularly were susceptible, illness often was atypical, and the manifestations appeared to be related to age. Infants older than 3 weeks of age tended to have the classic lower respiratory tract disease and apnea, whereas babies in the first 3 weeks of life uncommonly had clinical evidence of lower respiratory tract involvement. Less than half of these younger neonates had upper respiratory tract signs. Most had nonspecific signs, such as poor feeding, lethargy, and irritability. Nevertheless, four (17 per cent) died, and death was sudden and unexpected in two.

Nosocomial Infection

More than half a century ago in 1941, Adams[2] described an epidemic of pneumonitis that occurred in January through February in the nurseries of two Minneapolis hospitals. Thirty-two infants, mostly in the second and third months of life, were affected, and 29 per cent died. Cytoplasmic inclusions in the bronchial epithelium were observed in all fatal cases. The distinctive epidemiology, clinical syndrome, and pathology of these cases led Adams to propose a viral etiology. Twenty years later, he and his colleagues described a markedly similar epidemic of respiratory illness in infants during which they identified RSV as the cause.[3, 4] RSV thus was indicted as the agent of the earlier, first described nosocomial outbreak, although proof was not possible.

Nosocomial infection from RSV now has become recognized as a problem of increasing magnitude, especially in immunocompromised patients.[120, 121, 154, 158, 176, 190, 193, 198, 237, 298, 301, 304, 337, 447, 454, 475, 538] During RSV epidemics, infants hospitalized with RSV lower respiratory tract disease pose a particular hazard to the other young infants admitted with compromising illnesses. If RSV is not recognized as a potential nosocomial hazard and specific infection control procedures employed, morbidity and mortality may be appreciable. One-third or more of infants nosocomially infected have developed pneumonia or bronchiolitis, significantly prolonging their hospital stay.[155, 198] The risk of acquiring nosocomial infection is related to the child's age, the underlying disease, the length of hospitalization, and clearly the adherence to proper infection control procedures. Forty-five per cent of the infants hospitalized for 1 week or more have become infected, and open wards with infants younger than 1 year of age particularly are fertile grounds for frequent cross-infections.[120, 158, 198]

Nosocomial infections in immunocompromised children and adults particularly may be serious and difficult to control.[127, 138, 190, 221, 237, 449, 475, 538] Outbreaks on transplant units have been associated with a high mortality rate and prolonged transmission. The diagnosis of RSV infection often is not suspected until spread already has occurred. Furthermore, the shedding of RSV from such patients often is abundant and prolonged but may be intermittent.

Hospital staff acquire infection readily and may be important in its spread to patients. Staff may transmit the virus not only by becoming infected and shedding the virus but also by carrying contaminated secretions on hands, clothing, and objects between patients.[5, 154, 176, 192, 193, 195, 198, 203, 298, 304, 538] About half of the personnel on an infants' ward have become infected during periods of RSV prevalence. Most are symptomatic and require restricted activity and absenteeism, resulting in both medical and economic burdens.

Prevention of Nosocomial Infection

Nosocomial acquisition of RSV requires close contact with an infected person or with surfaces contaminated by secretions.[195] Spread occurs by direct inoculation of large particles (droplets) or by self-inoculation after touching contaminated secretions.[154, 192, 195, 198, 204] The risk of nosocomial infection in an infants' ward has been diminished by a variety of infection control procedures.[9, 121, 195, 196, 203, 254, 316] The most important, however, is careful hand washing by all persons entering and leaving an infant's room. The success of additional barrier precautions, such as gowns, gloves, and masks, has been variable in different settings.[5, 154, 196, 304, 362, 454] When hand washing cannot be enforced strictly, gloves may be effective. In two controlled studies, the routine use of gowns and masks did not add further benefit to conscientious hand washing and other infection control procedures.[196, 362] Others have reduced the nosocomial infection rate with procedures that include the use of gowns, gloves, and masks while emphasizing the importance of staff compliance.[304, 454] Because RSV seems to infect mostly via the eyes and nose, regular nose-mouth masks are of limited benefit, especially because touching or rubbing the eyes appears to be a major mode of self-inoculation.[154, 195, 201] Eye-nose goggles or goggles plus a mask have been evaluated and shown to be effective in diminishing nosocomial infection in both staff and infants.[5, 154]

Care in the handling of objects and materials contaminated by the infant's secretions also is advisable. As facilities allow, infants with respiratory signs should be isolated. With the use of techniques allowing rapid viral diagnosis, infants with RSV infection may be isolated in the same room.[291] Cohorting of staff to infants with RSV infection also may be helpful. Staff with any respiratory signs preferably should not care for infants at risk for nosocomial infection, at least those at highest risk, and isolation of the most vulnerable infants may be beneficial. Visitors, especially young children, should be limited and possibly screened for illness during community outbreaks of RSV infection.

Unusual Manifestations of Disease

RSV rarely has been associated with central nervous system disorders.[274] Acute RSV infection has been demonstrated in case reports of children with meningitis, myelitis, ataxia, hemiplegia, and facial palsy.[70, 274, 508] In several of these children with central nervous system disorders, antibody to RSV has been demonstrated in the cerebrospinal fluid, suggesting local production. In general, however, the role of RSV in central nervous system disease has been difficult to assess.[70, 274] Neurotropism of the virus has been suggested experimentally by the production of a neuropathic strain of RSV in mice.[74] By intracerebral inoculation of suckling mice, a strain of RSV was adapted to produce encephalitis. The pathology depended on the age of the mouse and only could be produced by an intracerebral route of inoculation.

Isolated case reports describe RSV infection in association with cardiac disease, including myocarditis and complete heart block occurring in previously normal children.[30, 167] An exanthem also has been reported occasionally in association with RSV infection.[49] In these cases, the rash has been described variably but as predominantly involving the trunk and appearing as a mild erythema, confluent macules and papules, or mixed macules and petechiae. A causal relationship to RSV, however, is lacking.

DIAGNOSIS

Though minuscule
of micron measure,
It leaves its scent
and prints precise;
A fleeing hare
for hunt and snare . . .

C. B. H.

Clinical and Epidemiologic Diagnosis

Because RSV has a repetitive and distinctive behavior, diagnosis often may be determined with reasonable accuracy by knowing three factors: (1) the age of the infected child, (2) the clinical syndrome, and (3) the local seasonal patterns of RSV. An infant acquiring lower respiratory tract disease, especially bronchiolitis, in the winter certainly would be suspected of having RSV infection. Recognition of the historical habits and arrival of RSV in a community may help, such as by surveillance programs monitoring RSV's activity and the number of bronchiolitis cases or hospital admissions for respiratory illness in young children.[170, 183, 197, 276, 305]

Specific Diagnosis

Specific diagnosis of RSV infection preferably is made by isolation of virus or detection of antigen from respiratory secretions.[272, 273, 512] The relative lability of the virus necessitates that specimens be transported quickly in proper media[259] and not subject to freezing, thawing, temperature, and pH changes. By quantitative assays, a nasal wash is more sensitive than a nasopharyngeal swab specimen in the recovery of RSV.[194] Nasal wash specimens may be obtained by suction apparatus or simply by the use of a tapered rubber bulb (Fig. 185–6).[194] Specimens thus obtained and inoculated onto sensitive HEp-2 cells have allowed identification of the characteristic cytopathic effect of RSV in an average of 3 to 4 days. Identification may be expedited by the use of shell vials and the detection of antigen in cell culture by rapid techniques, such as enzyme-linked immunoassay (EIA) and immunofluorescence assay (IFA). The sensitivity of viral isolation as a means of diagnosis varies markedly among laboratories[543] and relates in part to improper specimen collection, transport, or the use of cell cultures that are relatively insensitive or too dense, which mask the characteristic syncytial appearance.

Many assays and commercial kits are available for rapid diagnosis by antigen detection, including IFA, EIA, radioimmunoassays, DNA-RNA hybridization, and RNA–polymerase chain reaction.[117, 216, 499] Most involve IFA or EIA on either nasopharyngeal swab or wash specimens and employ polyclonal or monoclonal antibodies. The sensitivities of IFA

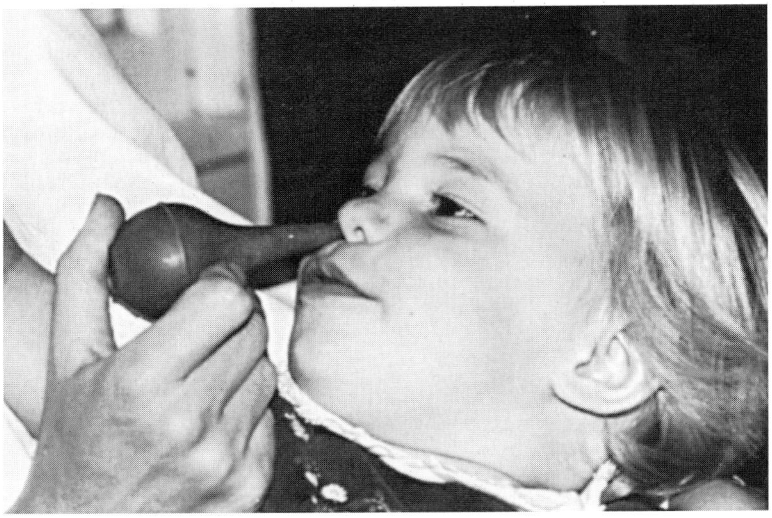

FIGURE 185–6. *Simple method for obtaining nasal wash specimens from young children. A 1-ounce, tapered rubber bulb is used to inject and collect 5 to 10 mL of saline with one squeeze. (From Hall, C. B., and Douglas, R. G., Jr.: Clinically useful method for the isolation of respiratory syncytial virus. J. Infect. Dis. 131:1–5, 1975. University of Chicago, Publisher.)*

and EIA generally are equivalent but have ranged from 32 to 98 per cent (most in the range of 70 to 90 per cent), with IFA tending to be the more sensitive and specific rapid diagnostic technique. IFA has the advantage of allowing morphologic distinctions.[60, 272, 273, 473, 512, 525] Monoclonal antibodies to the nucleocapsid or phosphoprotein produce a picture of discrete, large and small cytoplasmic inclusions, whereas monoclonal antibodies to the F protein result in a diffuse and dust-like staining of the cytoplasm.[39, 84, 512, 525] The reported sensitivity of these antigen tests may be falsely high if compared with that of less than optimal tissue culture techniques.[543]

Serologic diagnosis rarely aids clinical management of the patient. Not only does the requirement of a convalescent serum make the diagnosis retrospective, but a serologic response may not be detectable in young infants, despite severe infection.[356] In addition, repeated infections in older groups may not be associated with detectable seroconversion.[45, 214, 218, 261] In older children, a serologic response may be measured by the complement-fixation, EIA, neutralization, indirect IFA, fusion inhibition, immunoprecipitation, and Western blot assays.[512] Several of these tests, most frequently EIA and IFA, may be used to detect class-specific antibodies directed to the purified viral proteins.[129, 334, 356, 531] The complement-fixation test generally is less sensitive than EIA or neutralization tests, especially in infants.[525] Solid-phase EIA is preferable for young infants.[420] A neutralization test combined with an EIA in microtiter plates has simplified the assay for neutralizing antibodies and appears to be as sensitive as the standard neutralization and plaque-reduction assays.[21]

TREATMENT

The treatment of RSV lower respiratory tract disease mainly is supportive, and the outcome of the severely affected infant has been related directly to the quality of this supportive care.[364, 518] The diminished mortality in high-risk infants over the past decade mainly has resulted from such technical and physiologic advancements in supportive care for these infants.[364] Because most of these infants are hypoxemic, supplemental oxygen is integral to their therapy.[206] Most respond to relatively low concentrations of oxygen because the physiologic abnormality mostly is one of an unequal ratio of ventilation to perfusion.[540] In the more severely ill, arterial blood gas monitoring may be necessary to detect hypercarbia. Progressive hypercarbia, hypoxemia unresponsive to oxygen administration, and recurrent apnea are potential indications for airway intervention.

Therapy with bronchodilating agents, corticosteroids, and antibiotics has been evaluated in infants with RSV infection. Each agent has been shown to be of limited or no benefit. Despite this, a study of Canadian hospitals showed that therapy used for RSV infection included bronchodilators in 68 to 93 per cent of cases, corticosteroids in 3 to 69 per cent of low-risk infants, and antibiotics in 69 per cent of high-risk infants and in 58 per cent of low-risk infants.[303]

The use of bronchodilating agents in infants with bronchiolitis is controversial. The results of the many studies using bronchodilators parenterally, orally, or by nebulization have been conflicting.[153, 285, 318, 392, 432, 435, 439, 451, 540, 541] Some studies have indicated that younger infants are least likely to respond to bronchodilators, and some have documented no change in pulmonary resistance with their use or even have noted a detrimental paradoxical response.[58, 389, 392, 427, 541] Others have suggested a better response if both alpha- and beta-receptor agonists are combined in the therapy.[432, 541] Because a subgroup of infants may respond to these agents, many experts advise a carefully monitored trial of bronchodilators, usually aerosolized, in the more severely affected infant older than 6 months of age.[540]

The use of corticosteroids in the treatment of bronchiolitis has been shown to be of no benefit in controlled studies.[306, 460, 462] Although no adverse effect of such therapy has been demonstrated for RSV infection, evidence in primate infections and in children receiving immunosuppressive therapy suggests that as a possibility.[211, 441, 484]

The only specific treatment currently approved for children hospitalized with RSV infections is ribavirin (1-β-D-ribofuranosyl-1,2,4-triazole-3-carboxamide). This synthetic nucleoside has been administered as a small-particle aerosol for 12 to 22 hours per day for 3 or more days, usually about 3 days. Therapy, however, may be for only 1 day or for more than 3 days because the end-point is clinical improvement. Much shorter, intermittent courses of higher doses also appear to be an acceptable mode of administration.[126] Use of this nucleotide has diminished clinical severity and improved arterial oxygen saturation in all placebo-controlled studies in which they were measured.[36, 71, 108, 164, 188, 209, 210, 213, 287, 288, 310, 328, 422, 423, 425, 453, 459, 474] One placebo-controlled study in ventilated infants who were an average age of 1 month showed significant improvements in length of ventilation, oxygenation, and hospitalization.[453] The total number of patients in these controlled studies, however, is small, and the expense of this drug indicates that it should be reserved primarily for those infants at high risk for severe disease, as suggested by the American Academy of Pediatrics.[14]

Ribavirin therapy has been correlated with decreased levels of RSV-specific IgE and IgA antibodies and leukotrienes in the secretions of treated infants.[425, 503] RSV-specific IgE antibody and leukotrienes in the secretions of infected infants have been associated with worse disease, hypoxia, and the development of wheezing.

Viral resistance to ribavirin has not been demonstrated. Clinical trials testing additional antiviral therapy for RSV are lacking currently. Vitamin A supplementation has been suggested as adjunctive therapy in severely ill infants.[365] Interferon-α-2a has been administered in controlled studies intramuscularly to infants with RSV bronchiolitis[88] and intranasally to volunteers without measurable benefit.[238]

Interest has grown in the potential prophylactic and therapeutic benefit to young infants of passively administered immunoglobulin containing high levels of specific RSV antibody (RSVIG).[82, 184, 186, 187, 225, 308] In experimental animals, commercial gamma-globulin containing RSV neutralizing antibody has been administered parenterally and intranasally, resulting in a protective effect against pulmonary infection after challenge with RSV.[189, 226, 394–396, 399] Subsequently, infants hospitalized with RSV lower respiratory tract disease were treated with placebo or intravenous gamma-globulin (2 g/kg of body weight). No adverse reactions occurred, and in the treated infants, viral shedding in the nasal secretions was diminished significantly, and arterial oxygenation improved.[227] Possessing high titers of neutralizing antibody, RSVIG, given as prophylaxis against RSV disease in high-risk infants, also has been shown to ameliorate or prevent clinical disease.[184, 186, 187] Monoclonal antibodies, particularly human monoclonal Fab fragments, are being explored as a means of potentially more feasible and effective therapy and prophylaxis for infants.[35, 116]

PROGNOSIS AND COMPLICATIONS

Thus, if infected at this tender stage
will they become "blue bloaters" as they age?*

Information on the mortality caused by RSV infection is limited. In patients hospitalized with RSV infection or with bronchiolitis, the recent mortality rate has been reported as 1 to 3 per cent but varies greatly with the population, increasing in those with certain underlying diseases, especially cardiac, pulmonary, and immunodeficient conditions.[303, 342, 364, 469] Of infants dying with acute respiratory infection, RSV remains the major cause in developed countries. In less developed areas, RSV remains a major cause of mortality, in part from complicating bacterial infection, which is rare in the United States.[122, 156, 161, 251, 257, 325, 446]

In 1978 and 1979, newspaper headlines described an outbreak of a "mystery disease" ("il male oscuro") in Naples, Italy, which killed more than 60 young children in the fall and winter months.[297, 436] Investigations by Italian researchers and the World Health Organization revealed that the deaths occurring in the winter were associated with an outbreak of respiratory infection in young children. Virologic studies were not extensive, but several viruses were isolated, the major one being RSV, and bacteria did not appear to play a role. Although RSV thus was implicated, a mystery remains as to why the mortality rate was so high and why the average age of the fatal cases (about 1 year) was older than that expected for fatal RSV cases. Although crowding, impoverished living conditions, and the use of nonprescription drugs, such as steroids, have been offered as explanations, none has been proved as such, and knowledge of the previous epidemiologic characteristics of RSV in this population of Naples and the surrounding area was limited.

The risk of severe or fatal RSV infection has varied appreciably among countries and to some extent from year to year within a community, but the major risk factors for the individual infant are the presence of underlying disease, including prematurity and young age.[118, 303, 333, 335, 336, 364, 378, 444] Approximately 30 to 70 per cent of infants hospitalized with RSV infection in large medical centers have an underlying disease.[211, 303, 364] In more than 1200 infants hospitalized in Rochester with RSV infection, 63 per cent had one or more underlying conditions, of which 21 per cent were prematurity and 11 per cent were cardiac abnormalities. Environmental factors, including lower socioeconomic status, passive smoking, crowding, lack of breast feeding, and attendance in day care, and possibly also variations in the virus itself, have been associated with poorer prognosis.[215, 244, 245, 319, 324, 364, 476, 478, 518] The proportion of children hospitalized in Rochester with RSV infection who have required intensive care each season has varied between 5 and 25 per cent over a 15-year period.[215] Although the reasons for this wide annual variation are not entirely clear, the strain of virus circulating in the community may play a role. Children hospitalized with strain group A infections had a significantly increased risk of being admitted to the intensive care unit, and during years in which group A strains strongly predominated in the community, the rate of intensive care admission for RSV was significantly greater than during the years when B strains were highly dominant.[215]

Infants in the first few months of life with functionally important cardiac disease, lung disease, or both are at the greatest risk, and an appreciable proportion acquire the RSV infection nosocomially.[1, 118, 185, 211, 303, 314, 315, 333, 335, 336, 364, 446] In a prospective study in the early 1980s of hospitalized infants with cardiac lesions, the mortality rate was 37 per cent.[314] If the infant's cardiac lesion was complicated by pulmonary hypertension, the mortality rate doubled. Since then, the mortality rate has diminished in infants with cardiac disease, partly because of early surgical correction, advanced techniques, and recognition of the risk associated with RSV infection and of acquiring it nosocomially. The risk of severe infection, nevertheless, remains appreciable in these infants.[342, 364] One Canadian study estimates the mortality rate in infants with cardiac disease to be 3 to 4 per cent.[364]

Premature infants with lung disease and complicated neonatal courses have a propensity not only for complicated primary infection but also for severe reinfections extending into subsequent seasons, as long as their pulmonary function remains compromised.[118, 185, 335, 336, 444, 476] In one prospective study of 30 children younger than 2 years of age with bronchopulmonary dysplasia, RSV infection was documented in 59 per cent during a single season, and two-thirds of these children required hospitalization.[185] The chance of more severe disease requiring hospitalization was increased in children who were on home oxygen therapy or had required oxygen therapy within the last 3 months. The chance that a premature infant will be rehospitalized with RSV infection is considerable. In Syracuse, 36 per cent of preterm infants (<32 weeks' gestation) were rehospitalized, compared with 2.5 per cent of term babies; rehospitalization occurred within 4 months of discharge in 80 per cent.[118]

The risk of severe or complicated infection from RSV for

*From Hall, C. B.: The shedding and spreading of respiratory syncytial virus. Pediatr. Res. *11*:236–239, 1977.

children with immunocompromising conditions varies with the degree of immunosuppression. Patients with severe forms of congenital immunodeficiency and with transplants are at particular risk.[59, 61, 109, 128, 140, 211, 258, 372, 390, 469, 542] Such patients at any age may develop severe lower respiratory tract disease. The normal immune mechanisms to control spread of the virus appear to be diminished, resulting in prolonged and often repeated periods of shedding. Information on the effect of human immunodeficiency virus infection on RSV infection is limited thus far, but an increased mortality rate has not been demonstrated. Shedding of RSV, however, can be prolonged markedly and is likely to be an unrecognized source of nosocomial infection.[76, 284, 361, 387, 461]

Infection with RSV also may be detrimental to the course of the underlying chronic disease in young children. Exacerbations of nephrotic syndrome have been documented with upper respiratory tract infections, the most frequent cause of which was RSV.[315] Similarly, RSV infection occurring in young infants with cystic fibrosis has been shown to aggravate their pulmonary status and to be an important cause of early acute morbidity.[1]

Infection with RSV has been implicated in "cot deaths" and the sudden infant death syndrome in a number of studies, especially in the United Kingdom.[122, 136, 155, 371, 446, 457, 539] About one-third of the cases of cot deaths in these studies were associated with viral infections, mostly RSV, and had a bronchiolar lymphocytic reaction histologically, as in bronchiolitis. In one 9-year study, viruses were found in the respiratory tract in 200 of 763 cases of sudden infant death syndrome, with the incidence highest in those older than 3 months of age (39 per cent), compared with those infants who were younger (14 per cent).[539] RSV was the common virus in these older infants and present more often than in a control group of live infants.

Ogra and colleagues[371] identified RSV by IFA in the pulmonary tissues of five of eight cases of sudden infant death syndrome and in none of the controls. Furthermore, in all sudden infant death syndrome infants, the secretory component in the bronchopulmonary epithelium was absent or markedly reduced, suggesting a defect in the defense of the respiratory mucosa. In addition, pathologic studies using IFA by Raven and colleagues[410] demonstrated bound IgG in lung sections of 22 sudden infant death syndrome victims, and 4 of these also contained RSV antigen. The current definition and more recent studies of sudden infant death syndrome, however, indicate that RSV and other viral infections do not have a primary role.

Some of these unexpected infant deaths or cot deaths associated with RSV actually may have resulted from apnea, which may be the initial sign of RSV infection before respiratory signs are recognized.[17, 62, 90, 206] Twenty per cent of the infants younger than 6 months of age hospitalized with RSV infection in Denver demonstrated apnea.[62] Apnea is most likely in the youngest infants, those born prematurely, those with a young postnatal age, and those with a history of apnea of prematurity.[90] The apnea tends to develop at the beginning of the RSV infection, to be short-lived, and to be nonobstructive.[17] The prognosis of infants who develop apnea in conjunction with their RSV infection is not well defined, but in most infants apnea does not recur, even with subsequent respiratory infections.[90] Infants with apnea or periodic breathing associated with RSV infection require monitoring during the acute phase of their illness, but the subsequent prognosis for the normal infant is good.

Secondary bacterial infection appears to be an unusual complication of RSV infection in the United States. A number of clinical and pathologic studies suggest that RSV infection rarely predisposes to bacterial superinfection.[46, 48, 212, 413] In a 9-year prospective study of 565 children hospitalized with RSV lower respiratory tract disease, the rate of subsequent bacterial infection was 1.2 per cent in the total group of children infected with RSV and 0.6 per cent in the 352 children who received no antibiotics.[212] The highest rate (11 per cent) of subsequent bacterial infections occurred in infants who received broad-spectrum parenteral antibiotics for 5 or more days. Controlled studies with randomized antibiotic treatment of bronchiolitis and pneumonia mostly caused by RSV have shown no difference in severity or duration of the illness or in outcome.[137, 150]

Development of Chronic Lung Disease

Infection with RSV in early infancy has been implicated as predisposing to the development of chronic lung disease in later life. Infants with bronchiolitis and particularly those hospitalized with lower respiratory tract disease documented to be from RSV have been shown to be at high risk for subsequent recurrent wheezing or other respiratory disease. The reasons for this appear multifactorial. Although RSV infection clearly is associated, it is not necessarily causal.[73, 205, 236, 289, 290, 299, 300, 407, 424, 443, 448, 450, 456, 483, 524, 534, 548] Recurrent clinical respiratory problems have been noted on follow-up to occur in half or more of such infants and tend to be most frequent in the first couple of years after discharge. Although the frequency of clinical disease may diminish subsequently, a number of studies have documented the persistence of pulmonary function abnormalities in asymptomatic children.[205, 269, 289, 290, 407, 448, 483] How great a role atopy plays in producing these sequelae is unclear. Some studies have noted an increased incidence of atopic manifestations in these children or in their first-degree relatives, but others have not been able to indict allergic diathesis as a major risk factor.[191, 236, 290, 295, 450, 456, 524, 526] Atopy does, however, appear to play a significant role in a subgroup of these children, who tend to have more severe clinical manifestations and pulmonary function abnormalities.[236, 290, 428, 526]

A genetic, not necessarily atopic predisposition toward hyperreactivity of the lung has been suggested as a selective factor by the demonstration of an increased incidence of airway hyperreactivity in these children and their close relatives.[191, 289, 526] Whether a genetic airway responsiveness is the cause of chronic airway abnormalities or the viral infection is synergistic or primary in causing these lung abnormalities in a previously normal host remains abstruse.[299, 300, 412] Some studies suggest that normal young infants have nonspecific airway reactivity, which may predate any injury to the lung and which normally diminishes with age. Viral infections as well as other factors, such as environmental pollutants, may interfere with this normal physiologic decline and thus act to maintain a hyperreactive state of the airways.[165, 320, 321, 477]

PREVENTION

With perseverance
And the dreamer's scanning scope,
Reality is made of distant hope . . .

C. B. H.

Prevention of RSV infection currently is not possible. Control must await a successful means of immunization. In the interim, alternative methods of prevention are being sought that may at least offer temporary protection during the most vulnerable periods of an infant's life. If high levels of maternal antibody prove to be protective, the antibodies in pregnant women could be boosted by immunization, as suggested by Glezen.[170] Similarly, high-titered intravenous immunoglobulin and specifically targeted monoclonal antibodies, as mentioned previously, may be useful prophylactically.

Breast feeding may offer some protection against RSV infection, but the degree and type of such protection remain unclear.[23, 123, 146, 170, 245, 408, 446] Both in England and in the United States, the proportion of breast-fed infants has been noted to be lower in those hospitalized with RSV infection than in controls.[23, 123, 170, 408] Specific IgA antibodies and to a lesser extent IgG and IgM antibodies to RSV have been identified in human colostrum and milk.[123, 139, 294, 486] The IgA-specific antibody may persist for prolonged periods in the products of lactation and may be boosted by maternal reinfection.[139, 485] Neutralization of RSV by breast milk appears to be mediated by both immunoglobulin and non-immunoglobulin components.[294] Direct evidence for the protective effect of breast feeding for RSV disease, nevertheless, is lacking. Studies in experimental animals, however, have demonstrated that breast feeding by infant ferrets from an immune natural or foster mother confers protection, whereas passive serum antibody offers no such protection against RSV infection.[470]

Vaccines

The control of RSV long has lured but eluded investigators. Although the outcome of infants with RSV infection has improved greatly in recent years with a marked decrease in the mortality rate, the burden on health care that RSV imposes yearly remains notable. This burden may be alleviated only through immunization. The singular characteristics of RSV, however, have posed barriers to the successful development of a vaccine, despite more than three decades of effort.

Among these problems is the past experience with the formalin-inactivated vaccine, the shroud of which slows current development with concern and caution. That devastating experience, nevertheless, has stimulated research that has divulged information useful to the development of future vaccines. Although most of the information is derived from rodent models, the exaggerated disease and lung pathologies have been related to several factors that are likely to be applied to the information required for progress toward a vaccine. The type of immunizing agent clearly influences the immune response.[105, 107, 114, 500] The formalin-inactivated vaccine induced a Th2-type response, characteristic of nonreplicating immunogens, suggesting that a successful vaccine should produce a Th1 response with both CD4+ and CTL cells. Furthermore, the specific antigens to be included in a vaccine potentially will alter the immune response. In mice, immunization with the G protein has been associated with more lung pathology than has immunization with the F protein.[10, 12] Broad and effective immunity may require inclusion of both of these surface glycoproteins, however. The lack of an adequate model to test candidate vaccines remains a significant barrier.

An RSV vaccine also would have to both reflect and improve the immunity afforded by natural infection. The variable and nondurable protection engendered by natural disease, especially in infants, should be prevented or at least the clinical severity reduced. The vaccine also would have to be administered in the first few weeks of life because the most severe disease occurs in these youngest infants. Immunization with live viruses within the neonatal period is a step yet to be explored and likely to be influenced greatly by the immature and variably developed immune system of the neonate. In addition, maternal antibody would be most abundant at this period. Passive antibody clearly has been shown to diminish the infant's antibody response. Furthermore, the effect of the multiple antigens of other immunizing agents administered to infants is unknown.

Although an inactivated vaccine has been immunogenic and safe in cattle, the experience with the formalin-inactivated vaccine in children turned the path of subsequent research toward the development of an attenuated live vaccine.[43, 83, 149, 166, 241, 256, 277, 278, 326, 332, 384, 417, 465, 468, 544–546] Candidate vaccines were derived using cold-adapted strains from temperature-sensitive mutants. Trials with these candidate vaccines generally produced promising results in adult volunteers and seropositive children but proved to be unsuitable for infants and young, seronegative children. These vaccines produced unacceptable degrees of illness, were overattenuated and not protective, or were not stable genetically, resulting in the shedding of wild-type virus.[82, 83, 241, 277, 278, 326, 384, 544, 546] Research has continued toward the development of live attenuated vaccines with the identification of other mutants. Interest has been stimulated in this approach by the potential advantages of immunization with a live virus, which include the production of local, humoral, and cell-mediated responses to all of the important viral proteins, and the putative diminished risk of enhanced disease upon reinfection.[112, 113, 115, 404, 409]

Concurrent effort has been directed toward the development of a nonreplicating subunit vaccine. Most candidate vaccines have contained the two major surface glycoproteins, F and G, as purified proteins alone or in combination.[57, 99, 114, 247, 283, 376, 466, 485, 489, 491, 514, 521, 536, 537] Potential vaccines of these RSV proteins also have been constructed from incorporating the genes coding for specific RSV proteins into viral vectors, including vaccinia, baculovirus, and adenovirus.[82, 103, 115, 225, 247, 376, 466, 521, 537] Although these recombinant vaccines generally have appeared to be promising in most experimental animals, they have not been so in chimpanzees. The response has appeared to vary according to the animal model, as well as to the proteins and type of vector.[99, 114, 247, 537] One of the subunit vaccines, containing the F protein, has been evaluated in adults and young children.[41, 488, 489] Although efficacy could not be determined because of the limited number of vaccines, the vaccine appeared to be immunogenic and has not resulted in exaggerated disease during the subsequent 2 years.

The components of a subunit vaccine chosen will be important in their efficacy and safety. The concern that any inactivated or subunit vaccine may hinder responses on reinfection in infants derives not only from the experience with the formalin-inactivated vaccine but also from some, but not all, studies in experimental animals. Lung pathology on rechallenge after subunit immunization has been increased in some rodent studies.[103, 219, 239, 265, 500, 522] The F glycoprotein appears to be essential to a subunit vaccine. The F glycoprotein is conserved well between the major strain groups, and among the subgroups it induces both neutralizing and fusion-inhibiting antibody and is a target for CTLs. Whether and which other proteins should be included requires further investigation.

Successful control of RSV morbidity through immunization likely will require creative and combined approaches. In recognition of the beneficial effect of passive specific antibody, maternal immunization has been suggested as one approach. Novel adjuvants are being investigated; some can shift the immune response evoked by subunit vaccines from a Th2- to Th1-type response in experimental animals. Some induce mucosal as well as systemic immunity and potentially allow routes of administration that are preferable to the parenteral route.[373, 509] Both enterically active adjuvants and carriers, such as liposomes and biodegradable microspheres, are being evaluated. New adjuvants, such as quil A in the form of vesicles of immunostimulating complexes may enhance immunogenicity, which may be necessary for the fainéant T cells of neonates.[220, 490, 507] Immune response possibly could be enhanced through specific cytokine stimulators or inhibitors.[163] Peptide fragments of F and G may provide potential vaccines that allow the inclusion of desirable epitopes and precise targeting of specific B- and T-cell responses.[112, 491] The rapidly advancing technology suggests that construction of infectious DNA clones of viral RNA could improve the precision of immunization, attenuation, and evaluation.[92, 547]

A single oral vaccine that incorporates all the desired immunizing agents and that could be administered to newborns is the goal of soothsayer and scientist. In the interim, the novel development of individual vaccines and approaches is being explored, reducing the hurdles and detours on the road toward successful control of RSV. Limited and stepwise protection from disease in the infant, as well as in the elderly, may be necessary to diminish morbidity and RSV's human and financial costs.

References

1. Abman, S. H., Ogle, J. N., Butler-Simon, N., et al.: Role of respiratory syncytial virus in early hospitalization for respiratory distress of young infants with cystic fibrosis. J. Pediatr. *113*:826–830, 1988.
2. Adams, J. M.: Primary virus pneumonitis with cytoplasmic inclusion bodies: A study of an epidemic involving thirty-two infants with nine deaths. J. A. M. A. *116*:925–933, 1941.
3. Adams, J. M., Imagawa, D. T., and Zike, K.: Epidemic bronchiolitis and pneumonitis related to respiratory syncytial virus. J. A. M. A. *176*:1037–1039, 1961.
4. Adams, J. M., Imagawa, D. T., and Zike, K.: Relationship of pneumonitis in infants to respiratory syncytial virus. Lancet *81*:502–506, 1961.
5. Agah, R., Cherry, J. D., Garakian, A. J., et al.: Respiratory syncytial virus (RSV) infection rate in personnel caring for children with RSV infections. Am. J. Dis. Child. *141*:695–697, 1987.
6. Agius, G., Dindinaud, G., Biggar, R. J., et al.: An epidemic of respiratory syncytial virus in elderly people: Clinical and serological findings. J. Med. Virol. *30*:117–127, 1990.
7. Aherne, W., Bird, T., Court, S. D. M., et al.: Pathological changes in virus infections of the lower respiratory tract in children. J. Clin. Pathol. *23*:7–18, 1970.
8. Akerlind, B., and Norrby, E.: Occurrence of respiratory syncytial virus subtypes A and B strains in Sweden. J. Med. Virol. *19*:241–247, 1986.
9. Allen, U., and Ford-Jones, E. L.: Nosocomial infections in the pediatric patient: An update. Am. J. Infect. Control *18*:176–193, 1990.
10. Alwan, W. H., Kozlowska, W. J., and Openshaw, P. J.: Distinct types of lung disease caused by functional subsets of antiviral T cells. J. Exp. Med. *179*:81–89, 1994.
11. Alwan, W. H., and Openshaw, P. J.: Distinct patterns of T- and B-cell immunity to respiratory syncytial virus induced by individual viral proteins. Vaccine *11*:431–437, 1993.
12. Alwan, W. H., Record, F. M., and Openshaw, P. J.: Phenotypic and functional characterization of T cell lines specific for individual respiratory syncytial virus proteins. J. Immunol. *150*:5211–5218, 1993.
13. Alwan, W. H., Record, F. M., and Openshaw, P. J.: $CD4^+$ T cells clear virus but augment disease in mice infected with respiratory syncytial virus: Comparison with the effects of $CD8^+$ T cells. Clin. Exp. Immunol. *88*:527–536, 1992.
14. American Academy of Pediatrics: Use of ribavirin in the treatment of respiratory syncytial virus infection. *In* 1994 Red Book: Report of the Committee on Infectious Diseases. 23rd ed. Elk Grove Village, IL, American Academy of Pediatrics, 1994, pp. 570–573.
15. Ana, P. P. S., Arrobio, J. O., and Kim, H. W.: Serum complement in acute bronchiolitis. Proc. Soc. Exp. Biol. Med. *134*:499–503, 1970.
16. Ananaba, G. A., and Anderson, L. J.: Antibody enhancement of respiratory syncytial virus stimulation of leukotriene production by a macrophagelike cell line. J. Virol. *65*:5052–5060, 1991.
17. Anas, N., Boettrich, C., Hall C. B., et al.: The association of apnea and respiratory syncytial virus in infants. J. Pediatr. *101*:65–68, 1982.
18. Anderson, J. J., Norden, J., Saunders, D., et al.: Analysis of the local and systemic immune responses induced in BALB/c mice by experimental respiratory syncytial virus infection. J. Gen. Virol. *71*:1561–1570, 1990.
19. Anderson, L. J., and Heilman, C. A.: Protective and disease-enhancing immune responses to respiratory syncytial virus. J. Infect. Dis. *171*:1–7, 1995.
20. Anderson, L. J., Hendry, R. M., Pierik, L. T., et al.: Multicenter study of strains of respiratory syncytial virus. J. Infect. Dis. *163*:687–692, 1991.
21. Anderson, L. J., Hierholzer, J. C., Bingham, P. G., et al.: Microneutralization test for respiratory syncytial virus based on an enzyme immunoassay. J. Clin. Microbiol. *22*:1050–1052, 1985.
22. Anderson, L. J., Hierholzer, J. C., Tsou, C., et al.: Antigenic characterization of respiratory syncytial virus strains with monoclonal antibodies. J. Infect. Dis. *151*:626–632, 1985.
23. Anderson, L. J., Parker, R. A., Strikas, R. A., et al.: Day-care center attendance and hospitalization for lower respiratory tract illness. Pediatrics *82*:300–308, 1988.
24. Anderson, L. J., Tsou, C., Potter, C., et. al.: Cytokine response to respiratory syncytial virus stimulation of human peripheral blood mononuclear cells. J. Infect. Dis. *170*:1201–1208, 1994.
25. Anestad, G.: Interference between outbreaks of respiratory syncytial virus and influenza virus infection. Lancet 2:502, 1982.
26. Arola, M., Ruuskanen, O., Ziegler, T., et al.: Clinical role of respiratory virus infection in acute otitis media. Pediatrics *86*:848–855, 1990.
27. Arola, M., Ziegler, T., and Ruuskanen, O.: Respiratory virus infection as a cause of prolonged symptoms in acute otitis media. J. Pediatr. *116*:697–701, 1990.
28. Arroyo, J. C., Jordan, W., and Milligan, L.: Upper respiratory tract infection and serum antibody responses in nursing home patients. Am. J. Infect. Control *16*:152–158, 1988.
29. Bachi, T.: Direct observation of the budding and fusion of an enveloped virus by video microscopy. J. Cell. Biol. *197*:1689–1695, 1973.
30. Bairan, A. C., Cherry, J. D., Fagan, L. F., et al.: Complete heart block and respiratory syncytial virus. Am. J. Dis. Child. *127*:264–265, 1974.
31. Ball, L. A., Young, K. K. Y., Anderson, K., et al.: Expression of the major glycoprotein G of human respiratory syncytial virus from recombinant vaccinia virus vectors. Proc. Natl. Acad. Sci. U. S. A. *83*:246–250, 1986.
32. Bangham, C. R. M., and Askonas, B. A.: Murine cytotoxic T cells specific to respiratory syncytial virus recognize different antigenic subtypes of the virus. J. Gen. Virol. *67*:623–629, 1986.
33. Bangham, C. R. M., Cannon, M. J., Karzon, D. T., et. al.: Cytotoxic T-cell response to respiratory syncytial virus in mice. J. Virol. *56*:55–59, 1985.
34. Bangham, C. R. M., Openshaw, P. J. M., Ball, L. A., et al.: Human and murine cytotoxic T cells specific to respiratory syncytial virus recognize the viral nucleoprotein (N), but not the major glycoprotein (G), expressed by vaccinia virus recombinants. J. Immunol. *137*:3973–3977, 1986.
35. Barbas, C. F., III, Crowe, J. E., Jr., Cababa, D., et. al.: Human monoclonal Fab fragments derived from a combinatorial library bind to respiratory syncytial virus F glycoprotein and neutralize infectivity. Proc. Natl. Acad. Sci. U. S. A. *89*:10164–10168, 1992.
36. Barry, W., Cockburn, F., Cornall, R., et al.: Ribavirin aerosol for acute bronchiolitis. Arch. Dis. Child. *61*:593–594, 1986.
37. Beem, M.: Repeated infections with respiratory syncytial virus. J. Immunol. *98*:1115–1122, 1967.
38. Beem, M., Egerer, R., and Anderson, J.: Respiratory syncytial virus neutralizing antibodies in persons residing in Chicago, Illinois. Pediatrics *34*:761–770, 1964.
39. Bell, D. M., Walsh, E. E., Hruska, J. F., et al.: Rapid detection of respiratory syncytial virus with a monoclonal antibody. J. Clin. Microbiol. *17*:1099–1101, 1983.
40. Bellanti, J. A.: Development of nonimmunologic, nonspecific mechanisms and specific immunologic mechanisms in resistance to airways and pulmonary infections in infants and children. Pediatr. Res. *11*:224–227, 1977.
41. Belshe, R. B., Anderson, E. L., and Walsh, E. E.: Immunogenicity of purified F glycoprotein of respiratory syncytial virus: Clinical and immune responses to subsequent natural infection in children. J. Infect. Dis. *168*:1024–1029, 1993.
42. Belshe, R. B., Richardson, L. S., London, W. T., et al.: Experimental respiratory syncytial virus infection of four species of primates. J. Med. Virol. *1*:157–162, 1977.
43. Belshe, R. B., Richardson, L. S., London, W. T., et al.: Evaluation of five temperature sensitive mutants of respiratory syncytial virus in primates. II. Genetic analysis of virus recovered during infection. J. Med. Virol. *3*:101–110, 1978.
44. Belshe, R. B., VanVoris, L. P., Mufson, M. A., et al.: Epidemiology of severe respiratory syncytial virus infections in Huntington, West Virginia. West Virginia Med. J. *77*:49–52, 1981.
45. Berglund, B.: Respiratory syncytial virus infection in families: A study of family members of children hospitalized for acute respiratory disease. Acta Pediatr. Scand. *56*:395–404, 1967.
46. Berglund, B.: Studies on respiratory syncytial virus infection. Acta Paediatr. Scand. *176*(Suppl.):1–40, 1967.
47. Berglund, B., Salmivalli, A., Toivanen, P., et al.: Isolation of respiratory syncytial virus from middle ear exudates of infants. Arch. Dis. Child. *41*:554–555, 1966.
48. Berkovich, S.: Acute respiratory illness in the premature nursery associated with respiratory syncytial virus infections. Pediatrics *34*:753–760, 1964.
49. Berkovich, S., and Kibrick, S.: Exanthem associated with respiratory syncytial virus infection. J. Pediatr. *65*:368–370, 1964.

50. Berman, S.: Epidemiology of acute respiratory infections in children of developing countries. Rev. Infect. Dis. *13*(Suppl. 6):S454–S462, 1991.
51. Berthiaume, L., Joncas, L., Boulay, G. et al.: Serologic evidence of respiratory syncytial virus infection in sheep. Vet. Rec. *93*:337–338, 1973.
52. Bertotto, A., Stagni, G., Caprino, D., et al.: Cell-mediated immunity in RSV bronchiolitis. J. Pediatr. *97*:334–335, 1980.
53. Black-Payne, C.: Respiratory syncytial virus infection among families and within hospitals: Infancy to the aged. Schumpert. Med. Q. *9*:203–219, 1992.
54. Blandford, G., and Heath, R. B.: Studies on the immune response and pathogenesis of Sendai virus infection of mice. Immunology *22*:637–650, 1972.
55. Brandt, C. D., Kim, H. W., Arrobio, J. O., et al.: Epidemiology of respiratory syncytial virus infection in Washington, D.C. III. Composite analysis of eleven consecutive yearly epidemics. Am. J. Epidemiol. *98*:355–364, 1973.
56. Breton, A., Samaille, J., Gaudier, B., et al.: Isolement du virus syncytial (virus C.C.A. de Morris) au cours de manifestations respiratoires benignes épidémiques chez des prématures. Arch. Franc. Pediatr. *18*:459–467, 1961.
57. Brideau, R. J., and Wathen, M. W.: A chimeric glycoprotein of human respiratory syncytial virus termed FG induces T-cell mediated immunity in mice. Vaccine *9*:863–864, 1991.
58. Brooks, J., and Cropp, G. J. A.: Theophylline therapy in bronchiolitis. Am. J. Dis. Child. *135*:934–936, 1981.
59. Bruce, E., Reid, M. M., Craft, A. W., et al.: Multiple virus isolations in children with acute lymphoblastic leukemia. J. Infect. *1*:243–248, 1979.
60. Bruckova, M., Grandien, M., Pettersson, C. A., et al.: Use of nasal and pharyngeal swabs for rapid detection of respiratory syncytial virus and adenovirus antigens by enzyme-linked immunosorbent assay. J. Clin. Microbiol. *27*:1867–1869, 1989.
61. Brugman, S., and Hutter, J. L.: Respiratory syncytial virus (RSV) pneumonitis in acute leukemia. Am. J. Hematol. Oncol. *2*:371–374, 1980.
62. Bruhn, F. W., Mokrohisky, S. T., and McIntosh, K.: Apnea associated with respiratory syncytial virus infection in young infants. J. Pediatr. *90*:382–386, 1977.
63. Bruhn, F. W., and Yeager, A. S.: Respiratory syncytial virus in early infancy. Am. J. Dis. Child. *131*:145–148, 1977.
64. Bryson, D. G., McNulty, M. S., Logan, E. F., et al.: Respiratory syncytial virus pneumonia in young calves: Clinical pathologic findings. Am. J. Vet. Res. *44*:1648–1655, 1983.
65. Bui, R. H. D., Molinaro, G. A., Kettering, J. D., et al.: Virus-specific IgE and IgG4 antibodies in serum of children infected with respiratory syncytial virus. J. Pediatr. *110*:87–90, 1987.
66. Cane, P. A., and Pringle, C. R.: Evolution of subgroup A respiratory syncytial virus: Evidence for progressive accumulation of amino acid changes in the attachment protein. J. Virol. *69*:2918–2925, 1995.
67. Cannon, M. J., and Bangham, C. R. M.: Recognition of respiratory syncytial virus fusion protein by mouse cytotoxic T cell clones and a human cytotoxic T cell line. J. Gen. Virol. *70*:79–87, 1989.
68. Cannon, M. J., Openshaw, P. J. M., and Askonas, B. A.: Cytotoxic T cells clear virus but augment lung pathology in mice infected with respiratory syncytial virus. J. Exp. Med. *163*:1163–1168, 1988.
69. Cannon, M. J., Stott, E. J., Taylor, G., et al.: Clearance of persistent respiratory syncytial virus infections in immunodeficient mice following transfer of primed T cells. Immunology *62*:133–138, 1987.
70. Cappel, R., Thiry, L., and Clinet, G.: Viral antibodies in the CSF after acute CNS infections. Arch. Neurol. *32*:629–631, 1975.
71. Caramia, G., and Palazzini, E.: Efficacy of ribavirin aerosol treatment for respiratory syncytial virus bronchiolitis in infants. J. Int. Med. Res. *15*:227–233, 1987.
72. Carilli, A. D., Gohd, R. S., and Gordon, W.: A virologic study of chronic bronchitis. N. Engl. J. Med. *270*:123–127, 1964.
73. Carlsen, K. H., Larsen, S., Bjerve, O., et al.: Acute bronchiolitis: Predisposing factors and characterization of infants at risk. Pediatr. Pulmonol. *3*:153–160, 1987.
74. Cavallaro, J. J., Maassab, H. F., and Abrams, G. D.: An immunofluorescent and histopathological study of respiratory syncytial (RS) virus encephalitis in suckling mice. Proc. Soc. Exp. Biol. Med. *124*:1059–1064, 1967.
75. Cesario, T. C., and Yousefi, S.: Viral infections. Clin. Geriatr. Med. *8*:735–743, 1992.
76. Chandwani, S., Borkowsky, W., Krasinski, K., et. al.: Respiratory syncytial virus infection in human immunodeficiency virus–infected children. J. Pediatr. *117*:251–254, 1990.
77. Chanock, R. M.: Control of acute mycoplasmal and viral respiratory tract disease. Science *169*:248–256, 1970.
78. Chanock, R. M. and Finberg, L.: Recovery from infants with respiratory illness of a virus related to chimpanzee coryza agent (CCA). II. Epidemiologic aspects of infection in infants and young children. Am. J. Hyg. *66*:291–300, 1957.
79. Chanock, R. M., Kapikian, A. Z, Mills, J., et al.: Influence of immunological factors in respiratory syncytial virus disease of the lower respiratory tract. Arch. Environ. Health *21*:347–355, 1970.
80. Chanock, R. M., Kim, H. W., Vargosko, A. J., et al.: Respiratory syncytial virus. I. Virus recovery and other observations during 1960 outbreak of bronchiolitis, pneumonia, and minor respiratory diseases in children. J. A. M. A. *176*:647–653, 1961.
81. Chanock, R. M., and Parrott, R. H.: Acute respiratory disease in infancy and childhood: Present understanding and prospects for prevention. Pediatrics *36*:21–39, 1965.
82. Chanock, R. M., Parrott, R. H., Connors, M., et. al.: Serious respiratory tract disease caused by respiratory syncytial virus: Prospects for improved therapy and effective immunization. Pediatrics *90*:137–143, 1992.
83. Chanock, R. M., Richardson, L. S., Belshe, R. B., et al.: Prospects for prevention of bronchiolitis caused by respiratory syncytial virus. Pediatr. Res. *11*:264–267, 1977.
84. Cheeseman, S. H., Pierik, L. T., Leombruno, D., et al.: Evaluation of a commercially available direct immunofluorescent staining reagent for the detection of respiratory syncytial virus in respiratory secretions. J. Clin. Microbiol. *24*:155–156, 1986.
85. Cherrie, A. H., Anderson, K., and Wertz, G. W.: Human cytotoxic T cells stimulated by antigen on dendritic cells recognize the N, SH, F, M, 22K, and 1b proteins of respiratory syncytial virus. J. Virol. *66*:2102–2110, 1992.
86. Chiba, Y., Higashidato, Y., Suga, K., et al.: Development of cell-mediated cytotoxic immunity to respiratory syncytial virus in human infants following naturally acquired infection. J. Med. Virol. *28*:133–139, 1989.
87. Chin, J., Magoffin, R. L., Shearer, L. A., et al.: Field evaluation of a respiratory syncytial virus vaccine and a trivalent parainfluenza virus vaccine in a pediatric population. Am. J. Epidemiol. *89*:449–463, 1969.
88. Chipps, B. E., Sullivan, W. F., and Portnoy, J. M.: Alpha-2a-interferon for treatment of bronchiolitis caused by respiratory syncytial virus. Pediatr. Infect. Dis. J. *12*:653–658, 1993.
89. Chonmaitree, T., Owen, M. J., Patel, J. A., et al.: Effect of viral respiratory tract infection on outcome of acute otitis media. J. Pediatr. *120*:856–862, 1992.
90. Church, N. R., Anas, N. G., Hall, C. B., et al.: Respiratory syncytial virus–related apnea in infants: Demographics and outcome. Am. J. Dis. Child. *138*:247–250, 1984.
91. Coates, H. V., and Chanock, R. M.: Clinical significance of respiratory syncytial virus. Postgrad. Med. *35*:460–465, 1964.
92. Collins, P. L., Anderson, K., Langer, S. J., et al.: Correct sequence for the major nucleocapsid protein mRNA of respiratory syncytial virus. Virology *146*:69–77, 1985.
93. Collins, P. L., Davis, A., Lubeck, M., et al.: Evaluation of the protective efficacy of recombinant vaccinia viruses and adenoviruses that express respiratory syncytial virus glycoproteins. Modern Approaches to New Vaccines Including Prevention of AIDS. Abstracts of 1989 meeting, September 20–24, 1989. Cold Spring Harbor Laboratory, Cold Spring Harbor, New York, p. 26.
94. Collins, P. L., Dickens, L. E., Buckler-White, A., et al.: Nucleotide sequences for the gene functions of human respiratory syncytial virus reveal distinctive features of intergenic structure and gene order. Proc. Natl. Acad. Sci. U. S. A. *83*:4594–4598, 1986.
95. Collins, P. L., Huang, Y. T., and Wertz, G. W.: Identification of a tenth mRNA of respiratory syncytial virus and assignment of polypeptides to viral genes. J. Virol. *49*:572–578, 1984.
96. Collins, P. L., Huang, Y. T., and Wertz, G. W.: Nucleotide sequence of the gene encoding the fusion (F) glycoprotein of human respiratory syncytial virus. Proc. Natl. Acad. Sci. U. S. A. *81*:7683–7687, 1984.
97. Collins, P. L., Mink, M. A., Hill, M. G., et al.: Rescue of a 7502-nucleotide (49.3% of full-length) synthetic analog of respiratory syncytial virus genomic RNA. Virology *195*:252–256, 1993.
98. Collins, P. L., and Mottet, G.: Membrane orientation and oligomerization of the small hydrophobic protein of human respiratory syncytial virus. J. Gen. Virol. *74*:1445–1450, 1993.
99. Collins, P. L., Purcell, R. H., London, W. T., et al.: Evaluation in chimpanzees of vaccinia virus recombinants that express the surface glycoproteins of human respiratory syncytial virus. Vaccine *8*:164–168, 1990.
100. Collins, P. L. and Wertz, G. W.: The envelope-associated 22K protein of human respiratory syncytial virus: Nucleotide sequence of the mRNA and a related polytranscript. J. Virol. *54*:65–71, 1985.
101. Collins, P. L., and Wertz, G. W.: Nucleotide sequences of the 1B and 1C nonstructural protein mRNAs of human respiratory syncytial virus. Virology *143*:442–451, 1985.
102. Collins, P. L., and Wertz, G. W.: The 1A protein gene of human respiratory syncytial virus: Nucleotide sequence of the mRNA and a related polycistronic transcript. Virology *141*:283–291, 1985.
103. Connors, M., Collins, P. L., Firestone, C. Y., et al.: Cotton rats previously immunized with a chimeric RSV FG glycoprotein develop enhanced pulmonary pathology when infected with RSV, a phenomenon not encountered following immunization with vaccinia–RSV recombinants or RSV. Vaccine *10*:475–484, 1992.
104. Connors, M., Collins, P. L., Firestone, C. Y., et al.: Respiratory syncytial virus (RSV) F, G, M2 (22K), and N proteins each induce resistance to RSV challenge, but resistance induced by M2 and N proteins is relatively short-lived. J. Virol. *65*:1634–1637, 1991.
105. Connors, M., Giese, N. A., Kulkarni, A. B., et al.: Enhanced pulmonary histopathology induced by respiratory syncytial virus (RSV) challenge of formalin-inactivated RSV-immunized BALB/c mice is abrogated by depletion of interleukin-4 (IL-4) and IL-10. J. Virol. *68*:5321–5325, 1994.
106. Connors, M., Kulkarni, A. B., Collins, P. L., et al.: Resistance to respiratory syncytial virus (RSV) challenge induced by infection with a vaccinia virus

recombinant expressing the RSV M2 protein (Vac-M2) is mediated by CD8+ T cells, while that induced by Vac-F or Vac-G recombinants is mediated by antibodies. J. Virol. 66:1277–1281, 1992.
107. Connors, M., Kulkarni, A. B., Firestone, C. Y., et al.: Pulmonary histopathology induced by respiratory syncytial virus (RSV) challenge of formalin-inactivated RSV-immunized BALB/c mice is abrogated by depletion of CD4+ T cells. J. Virol. 66:7444–7451, 1992.
108. Conrad, D. A., Christenson, J. C., Waner, J. L. et al.: Aerosolized ribavirin treatment of respiratory syncytial virus infection in infants hospitalized during an epidemic. Pediatr. Infect. Dis. J. 6:152–158, 1987.
109. Craft, A. W., Reid, M. M., Gardner, P. S., et al.: Virus infections in children with acute lymphoblastic leukemia. Arch. Dis. Child. 54:755–759, 1979.
110. Cranage, M. P., and Gardner, P. S.: Systemic cell-mediated and antibody responses in infants with respiratory syncytial virus infections. J. Med. Virol. 5:161–170, 1980.
111. Cranage, M. P., Gardner, P. S., and McIntosh, K.: ADCC in secretions from infants recovering from RSV bronchiolitis. Pediatr. Res. 14:556, 1980.
112. Crowe, J. E., Jr.: Current approaches to the development of vaccines against disease caused by respiratory syncytial virus (RSV) and parainfluenza virus (PIV). Vaccine 13:415–421, 1995.
113. Crowe, J. E., Jr., Bui, P. T., Davis, A. L., et al.: A further attenuated derivative of cold-passaged temperature-sensitive mutant of human respiratory syncytial virus retains immunogenicity and protective efficacy against wild-type challenge in seronegative chimpanzees. Vaccine 12:783–790, 1994.
114. Crowe, J. E., Jr., Bui, P. T., Karron, P. A., et al.: Live attenuated mutants of respiratory syncytial virus (RSV): In vitro markers and replication in mice or chimpanzees correlate with level of attenuation for seronegative human infants. Pediatr. Res. 37:172A, 1995.
115. Crowe, J. E., Jr., Bui, P. T., London, W. T., et al.: Satisfactorily attenuated and protective mutants derived from a partially attenuated cold-passaged respiratory syncytial virus mutant by introduction of additional attenuating mutations during chemical mutagenesis. Vaccine 12:691–699, 1994.
116. Crowe, J. E., Jr., Murphy, B. R., Chanock, R. M., et al.: Recombinant human respiratory syncytial virus (RSV) monoclonal antibody Fab is effective therapeutically when introduced directly into the lungs of RSV-infected mice. Proc. Natl. Acad. Sci. U. S. A. 91:1386–1390, 1994.
117. Cubie, H. A., Inglis, J. M., and McGowan, A. M.: Detection of respiratory syncytial virus antigen and nucleic acid in clinical specimens using synthetic oligonucleotides. J. Virol. Methods 34:27–35, 1991.
118. Cunningham, C. K., McMillan, J. A., and Gross, S. J.: Rehospitalization for respiratory illness in infants of less than 32 weeks' gestation. Pediatrics 88:527–532, 1991.
119. Denny, F. W., Collier, A. M., Henderson, F. W., et al.: The epidemiology of bronchiolitis. Pediatr. Res. 11:234–236, 1977.
120. Ditchburn, R. K., McQuillin, J., Gardner, P. S., et al.: Respiratory syncytial virus in hospital cross-infection. Br. Med. J. 3:671–673, 1971.
121. Donowitz, L. G.: Hospital-acquired infections in children. N. Engl. J. Med. 323:1836–1837, 1990.
122. Downham, M. A., Gardner, P. S., McQuillin, J., et al.: Role of respiratory viruses in childhood mortality. Br. Med. J. 1:235–239, 1975.
123. Downham, M. A., Scott, R., Sims, D. G., et al.: Breast-feeding protects against respiratory syncytial virus infections. Br. Med. J. 2:274–276, 1976.
124. Elango, N., Satake, M., and Venkatesan, S.: mRNA sequence of three respiratory syncytial virus genes encoding two nonstructural proteins and a 22K structural protein. J. Virol. 55:101–110, 1985.
125. Eller, J. J.: Infectious agents of importance in airways and parenchymal diseases in infants and children with particular emphasis on bronchiolitis. Pediatr. Res. 11:247–249, 1977.
126. Englund, J. A.: Passive protection against respiratory syncytial virus disease in infants: The role of maternal antibody. Pediatr. Infect. Dis. J. 13:449–453, 1994.
127. Englund, J. A., Anderson, L. J., and Rhame, F. S.: Nosocomial transmission of respiratory syncytial virus in immunocompromised adults. J. Clin. Microbiol. 29:115–119, 1991.
128. Englund, J. A., Sullivan, C. J., Jordan, C., et al.: Respiratory syncytial virus infection in immunocompromised adults. Ann. Intern. Med. 109:203–208, 1988.
129. Erdman, D. D., and Anderson, L. J.: Monoclonal antibody–based capture enzyme immunoassays for specific serum immunoglobulin G (IgG), IgA, and IgM antibodies to respiratory syncytial virus. J. Clin. Microbiol. 28:2744–2749, 1990.
130. Falsey, A. R.: Noninfluenza respiratory virus infection in long-term care facilities. Infect. Control Hosp. Epidemiol. 12:602–608, 1991.
131. Falsey, A. R., Cunningham, C. K., Barker, W. H., et al.: Respiratory syncytial virus and influenza A infections in the hospitalized elderly. J. Infect. Dis. 172:389–394, 1995.
132. Falsey, A. R., Treanor, J. J., Betts, R. F., et al.: Viral respiratory infections in the institutionalized elderly: Clinical and epidemiologic findings. J. Am. Geriatr. Soc. 40:115–119, 1992.
133. Fernald, G. W., Almond, J. R., and Henderson, F. W.: Cellular and humoral immunity in recurrent respiratory syncytial virus infections. Pediatr. Res. 17:753–758, 1983.
134. Fernie, B. F., Ford E. C., and Gerin, J. L.: The development of Balb/c cells persistently infected with respiratory syncytial virus: Presence of ribonucleoprotein on the cell surface. Proc. Soc. Exp. Biol. Med. 167:83–86, 1981.
135. Fernie, B. F., and Gerin, J. L.: The stabilization and purification of respiratory syncytial virus using $MgSO_4$. Virology 106:141–144, 1980.
136. Ferris, J. A. J., Aherne, W. A., Locke, W. S., et al.: Sudden and unexpected deaths in infants: Histology and virology. Br. Med. J. 2:439–442, 1973.
137. Field, C. M. B., Connolly, J. H., Murtagh, G., et al.: Antibiotic treatment of epidemic bronchiolitis: A double-blind trial. Br. Med. J. 1:83–85, 1966.
138. Finger, R., Anderson, L. J., Dicker, R. C., et al.: Epidemic infections caused by respiratory syncytial virus in institutionalized young adults. J. Infect. Dis. 155:1335–1339, 1987.
139. Fishaut, M., Murphy, D., Neifert, M., et al.: Bronchomammary axis in the immune response to respiratory syncytial virus. J. Pediatr. 99:186–191, 1981.
140. Fishaut, M., Tubergen, D., and McIntosh, K.: Cellular response to respiratory viruses with particular reference to children with disorders of cell-mediated immunity. J. Pediatr. 96:179–186, 1980.
141. Fleming, D. M., and Cross, K. W.: Respiratory syncytial virus or influenza? Lancet 342:1507–1510, 1993.
142. Forbes, J. A., Bennett, N., McK., and Gray, N. J.: Epidemic bronchiolitis caused by respiratory syncytial virus: Clinical aspects. Med. J. Aust. 2:933–935, 1961.
143. Forgie, I. M., Campbell, H., Lloyd-Evans, N., et al.: Etiology of acute lower respiratory tract infections in children in a rural community in the Gambia. Pediatr. Infect. Dis. J. 11:466–473, 1992.
144. Fouillard, L., Mouthon, L., Laporte, J. P., et al.: Severe respiratory syncytial virus pneumonia after autologous bone marrow transplantation: A report of three cases and review. Bone Marrow Transplant. 9:97–100, 1992.
145. Foy, H. M., Cooney, M. K., Maletzky, A. J., et al.: Incidence and etiology of pneumonia, croup, and bronchiolitis in preschool children belonging to a prepaid medical care group over a four-year period. Am. J. Epidemiol. 97:80–92, 1973.
146. Frank, A. L., Taber, L. H., Glezen, W. P., et al.: Breast feeding and respiratory virus infections. Pediatrics 70:239–245, 1982.
147. Fransen, H., Sterner, G., Forsgren, M., et al.: Acute lower respiratory illness in elderly patients with respiratory syncytial virus infection. Acta Med. Scand. 182:323–330, 1967.
148. Freymuth, F., Petitjean, J., Pothier, P., et al.: Prevalence of respiratory syncytial virus subgroups A and B in France from 1982 to 1990. J. Clin. Microbiol. 29:653–655, 1991.
149. Friedewald, W. J., Forsyth, B. R., Smith, C. B., et al.: Low-temperature–grown RS virus in adult volunteers. J. A. M. A. 204:690–694, 1968.
150. Friis, B., Anderson, P., Brenoe, E., et al.: Antibiotic treatment of pneumonia and bronchiolitis: A prospective randomized study. Arch. Dis. Child. 59:1038–1045, 1984.
151. Friis, B., Eiken, M., Hornsleth, A., et al.: Chest x-ray appearances in pneumonia and bronchiolitis. Acta Paediatr. Scand. 79:219–225, 1990.
152. Fulginiti, V. A., Eller, J. J., Sieber, O. F., et al.: Respiratory virus immunization. I. A field trial of two inactivated respiratory virus vaccines: An aqueous trivalent parainfluenza virus vaccine, and an alum-precipitated respiratory syncytial virus vaccine. Am. J. Epidemiol. 89:435–448, 1969.
153. Gadomski, A. M., Lichenstein, R., Horton, L., et al.: Efficacy of albuterol in the management of bronchiolitis. Pediatrics 93:907–912, 1994.
154. Gala, C. L., Hall, C. B., Schnabel, K. C., et al.: The use of eye-nose goggles to control nosocomial respiratory syncytial virus infection. J. A. M. A. 256:2706–2708, 1986.
155. Gardner, P. S.: How etiologic, pathologic, and clinical diagnoses can be made in a correlated fashion. Pediatr. Res. 11:254–261, 1977.
156. Gardner, P. S.: Rapid diagnostic techniques in clinical virology. *In* Heath, R. B., and Waterson, A. P. (eds.): Modern Trends in Medical Virology. Vol. 2. New York, Appleton-Century-Crofts, 1970, pp. 15–50.
157. Gardner, P. S.: Respiratory syncytial virus infections. Postgrad. Med. J. 49:788–791, 1973.
158. Gardner, P. S., Court, S. D. M., Brocklebank, J. T., et al.: Virus cross-infection in paediatric wards. Br. Med. J. 2:571–575, 1973.
159. Gardner, P. S., and McQuillin, J.: The coating of respiratory syncytial (RS) virus–infected cells in the respiratory tract by immunoglobulins. J. Med. Virol. 2:165–173, 1978.
160. Gardner, P., McQuillin, J., and Court, S. D. M.: Speculation on pathogenesis in death from respiratory syncytial virus infection. Br. Med. J. 1:327–330, 1970.
161. Gardner, P. S., Turk, D. C., Aherne, W. A., et al.: Deaths associated with respiratory tract infection in childhood. Br. Med. J. 4:316–320, 1967.
162. Garofalo, R., Kimpen, J. L. L., Welliver, R. C., et al.: Eosinophil degranulation in the respiratory tract during naturally acquired respiratory syncytial virus infection. J. Pediatr. 120:28–32, 1992.
163. Garside, P., and Mowat, A. M.: Polarization of Th-cell responses: A phylogenetic consequence of nonspecific immune defence? Immunol. Today 16:220–223, 1995.
164. Gelfand, E. W., McCurdy, D., Rao, P., et al.: Ribavirin treatment of viral pneumonitis in severe combined immunodeficiency disease. Lancet 2:732–733, 1983.
165. Geller, D. E., Morgan, W. J., Cota, K. A., et al.: Airway responsiveness to cold, dry air in normal infants. Pediatr. Pulmonol. 4:90–97, 1988.

166. Gharpure, M. A., Wright, P. F., and Chanock, R. M.: Temperature-sensitive mutant of respiratory syncytial virus. J. Virol. *3*:414–421, 1969.
167. Giles, T. D., and Gohd, R. S.: Respiratory syncytial virus and heart disease. J. A. M. A. *236*:1128–1130, 1976.
168. Gimenez, H. B., Cash, P., and Melvin, T.: Monoclonal antibodies to human respiratory syncytial virus and their use in comparison of different virus isolates. J. Gen. Virol. *65*:963–971, 1984.
169. Glezen, W. P.: Incidence of respiratory syncytial and parainfluenza type 3 viruses in an urban setting. Pediatr. Virol. *2*:1–4, 1987.
170. Glezen, W. P.: Pathogenesis of bronchiolitis: Epidemiologic considerations. Pediatr. Res. *11*:239–243, 1977.
171. Glezen, W. P.: Viral pneumonia as a cause and result of hospitalization. J. Infect. Dis. *4*:765–770, 1983.
172. Glezen, W. P., and Denny, F. W.: Epidemiology of acute lower respiratory disease in children. N. Engl. J. Med. *288*:498–505, 1973.
173. Glezen, W. P., Loda, F. A., Clyde, W. A., et al.: Epidemiologic patterns of acute lower respiratory disease of children in the pediatric group practice. J. Pediatr. *78*:397–406, 1971.
174. Glezen, W. P., Paredes, A., Allison, J. E., et al.: Risk of respiratory syncytial virus infection from low-income families in relationship to age, sex, ethnic group and maternal antibody group. J. Pediatr. *98*:708–715, 1981.
175. Glezen, W. P., Taber, L. H., Frank, A. L., et al.: Risk of primary infection and reinfection with respiratory syncytial virus. Am. J. Dis. Child. *140*:543–546, 1986.
176. Goldmann, D. A.: Transmission of infectious diseases in children. Pediatr. Rev. *13*:283–294, 1992.
177. Goldson, E. J., McCarthy, J. T., Welling, M. A., et al.: A respiratory syncytial virus outbreak in a transitional care nursery. Am. J. Dis. Child. *133*:1280–1282, 1979.
178. Graham, B. S., Bunton, L. A., Rowland, J., et al.: Respiratory syncytial virus infection in anti-μ treated mice. J. Virol. *65*:4936–4942, 1991.
179. Graham, B. S., Bunton, L. A., Wright, P. F., et al.: The role of T lymphocyte subsets in the pathogenesis of primary RSV infection and rechallenge in mice. J. Clin. Invest. *88*:1026–1033, 1991.
180. Graham, B. S., Perkins, M. D., Wright, P. F., et al.: Primary respiratory syncytial virus infection in mice. J. Med. Virol. *26*:153–162, 1988.
181. Graham, B. S., Bunton, L. A., Wright, P. F., et al.: Reinfection of mice with respiratory syncytial virus. J. Med. Virol. *34*:7–13, 1991.
182. Graham, B. S., Henderson, G. S., Tang, Y.-W., et al.: Priming immunization determines T helper cytokine mRNA expression patterns in lungs of mice challenged with respiratory syncytial virus. J. Immunol. *151*:2032–2040, 1993.
183. Grist, N. R., Ross, C. A. C., and Stott, E. J.: Influenza, respiratory syncytial virus, and pneumonia in Glasgow, 1962–1965. Br. Med. J. *1*:456–457, 1967.
184. Groothuis, J. R.: Role of antibody and use of respiratory syncytial virus (RSV) immune globulin to prevent severe RSV disease in high-risk children. J. Pediatr. *124*:S28–S32, 1994.
185. Groothuis, J. R., Gutierrez, K. M., and Lauer, B. A.: Respiratory syncytial virus infection in children with bronchopulmonary dysplasia. Pediatrics *82*:199–203, 1988.
186. Groothuis, J. R., Simoes, E. A. F., and Hemming, V. G.: Respiratory syncytial virus (RSV) infection in preterm infants and the protective effects of RSV immune globulin (RSVIG). Pediatrics *95*:463–467, 1995.
187. Groothuis, J. R., Simoes, E. A. F., Levin, M. J., et al.: Prophylactic administration of respiratory syncytial virus immune globulin to high-risk infants and young children. N. Engl. J. Med. *329*:1524–1530, 1993.
188. Groothuis, J. R., Woodin, K. A., Katz, R., et al.: Early ribavirin treatment of respiratory syncytial viral infection in high-risk children. J. Pediatr. *117*:792–798, 1990.
189. Gruber, W. C., Wilson, S. Z., Throop, B. J., et al.: Immunoglobulin administration and ribavirin therapy: Efficacy in respiratory syncytial virus infection in the cotton rat. Pediatr. Res. *21*:270–274, 1987.
190. Guidry, G. G., Black-Payne, C. A., Payne, D. K., et al.: Respiratory syncytial virus infection among intubated adults in a university medical intensive care unit. Chest *100*:1377–1384, 1991.
191. Gurwitz, D., Mindorff, C., and Levison, H.: Increased incidence of bronchial reactivity in children with a history of bronchiolitis. J. Pediatr. *98*:551–555, 1981.
192. Hall, C. B.: The nosocomial spread of respiratory syncytial virus infections. Ann. Rev. Med. *34*:311–319, 1983.
193. Hall, C. B.: The shedding and spreading of respiratory syncytial virus. Pediatr. Res. *11*:236–239, 1977.
194. Hall, C. B., and Douglas, R. G., Jr.: Clinically useful method for the isolation of respiratory syncytial virus. J. Infect. Dis. *131*:1–5, 1975.
195. Hall, C. B., and Douglas, R. G., Jr.: Modes of transmission of respiratory syncytial virus. J. Pediatr. *99*:100–103, 1981.
196. Hall, C. B., and Douglas, R. G., Jr.: Nosocomial respiratory syncytial viral infections: Should gowns and masks be used? Am. J. Dis. Child. *135*:512–515, 1981.
197. Hall, C. B., and Douglas, R. G., Jr.: Respiratory syncytial virus and influenza: Practical community surveillance. Am. J. Dis. Child. *130*:615–620, 1976.
198. Hall, C. B., Douglas, R. G., Jr., Geiman, J. M., et al.: Nosocomial respiratory syncytial virus infections. N. Engl. J. Med. *293*:1343–1346, 1975.
199. Hall, C. B., Douglas, R. G., Jr., and Geiman, J. M.: Quantitative shedding patterns of respiratory syncytial virus in infants. J. Infect. Dis. *132*:151–156, 1975.
200. Hall, C. B., Douglas, R. G., Jr., and Geiman, J. M.: Respiratory syncytial virus infection in infants: Quantitation and duration of shedding. J. Pediatr. *89*:11–15, 1976.
201. Hall, C. B., Douglas, R. G., Jr., Schnabel, K. C., et al.: Infectivity of respiratory syncytial virus by various routes of inoculation. Infect. Immun. *33*:779–783, 1981.
202. Hall, C. B., Geiman, J. M., Biggar, R., et al.: Respiratory syncytial virus infection within families. N. Engl. J. Med. *294*:414–419, 1976.
203. Hall, C. B., Geiman, J. M., Douglas, R. G., Jr., et al.: Control of nosocomial respiratory syncytial viral infection. Pediatrics *62*:728–731, 1978.
204. Hall, C. B., Geiman, J. M., and Douglas, R. G., Jr.: Possible transmission by fomites of respiratory syncytial virus. J. Infect. Dis. *141*:98–102, 1980.
205. Hall, C. B., Hall, W. J., Gala, C. L., et al.: A long term prospective study of children following respiratory syncytial virus infection. J. Pediatr. 105:358–364, 1984.
206. Hall, C. B., Hall, W. J., and Speers, D. M.: Clinical and physiological manifestations of bronchiolitis and pneumonia: Outcome of respiratory syncytial virus. Am. J. Dis. Child. *133*:798–802, 1979.
207. Hall, W. J., Hall, C. B., and Speers, D. M.: Respiratory syncytial virus infections in adults: Clinical, virologic, and serial pulmonary function studies. Ann. Intern. Med. *88*:203–205, 1978.
208. Hall, C. B., Kopelman, A. E., Douglas, R. G., Jr., et al.: Neonatal respiratory syncytial virus infection. N. Engl. J. Med. 300:393–396, 1979.
209. Hall, C. B., McBride, J. T., Gala, C. L., et al.: Ribavirin aerosol treatment of respiratory syncytial viral infection in infants with underlying cardiac and pulmonary disease. J. A. M. A. *254*:3047–3051, 1985.
210. Hall, C. B., McBride, J. T., Walsh, E. E., et al.: Aerosolized ribavirin treatment of infants with respiratory syncytial viral infection. N. Engl. J. Med. *308*:1443–1447, 1983.
211. Hall, C. B., Powell, K. R., MacDonald, N. E., et al.: Respiratory syncytial viral infection in children with compromised immune function. N. Engl. J. Med. *315*:77–80, 1986.
212. Hall, C. B., Powell, K. R., Schnabel, K. C., et al.: Risk of secondary bacterial infection in infants hospitalized with respiratory syncytial viral infection. J. Pediatr. *113*:266–271, 1988.
213. Hall, C. B., Walsh, E. E., Hruska, J. F., et al.: Ribavirin aerosol treatment of experimental respiratory syncytial viral infection in young adults: A controlled double blind study. J. A. M. A. *249*:2666–2670, 1983.
214. Hall, C. B., Walsh, E. E., Long, C. G., et al.: Immunity and frequency of reinfection with respiratory syncytial virus. J. Infect. Dis. *163*:693–698, 1991.
215. Hall, C. B., Walsh, E. E., Schnabel, K. C., et al.: The occurrence of groups A and B of respiratory syncytial virus over 15 years: The associated epidemiologic and clinical characteristics in hospitalized and ambulatory children. J. Infect. Dis. *162*:1283–1290, 1990.
216. Halstead, D. C., Todd, S., and Fritch, G.: Evaluation of five methods for respiratory syncytial virus detection. J. Clin. Microbiol. *28*:1021–1025, 1990.
217. Hambling, M. H.: Survival of the respiratory syncytial virus during storage under various conditions. Br. J. Exp. Pathol. *45*:647–655, 1964.
218. Hamre, D., and Procknow, J. J.: Viruses isolated from natural common colds in the U.S.A. Br. Med. J. *2*:1382–1385, 1961.
219. Hancock, G. E., Hahn, D. J., Speelman, D. J., et al.: The pulmonary immune response of Balb/c mice vaccinated with the fusion protein of respiratory syncytial virus. Vaccine *12*:267–274, 1994.
220. Hancock, G. E., Speelman, D. J., Frenchick, P. J., et al.: Formulation of the purified fusion protein of respiratory syncytial virus with the saponin QS-21 induces protective immune responses in Balb/c mice that are similar to those generated by experimental infection. Vaccine *13*:391–400, 1995.
221. Harrington, R. D., Hooton, T. M., Hackman, R. C., et al.: An outbreak of respiratory syncytial virus in a bone marrow transplant center. J. Infect. Dis. *165*:987–993, 1992.
222. Hart, R. J. C.: An outbreak of respiratory syncytial virus infection in an old people's home. J. Infect. *8*:259–261, 1984.
223. Hayes, E. B., Hurwitz, E. S., Schonberger, L. B., et al.: Respiratory syncytial virus outbreak on American Samoa. Am. J. Dis. Child. 143:316–321, 1989.
224. Heilman, C. A.: Respiratory syncytial and parainfluenza viruses. J. Infect. Dis. *161*:402–406, 1990.
225. Hemming, V. G., and Prince, G. A.: Respiratory syncytial virus: Babies and antibodies. Infect. Agents Dis. *1*:24–32, 1992.
226. Hemming, V. G., Prince, G. A., London, W. T., et al.: Topically administered immunoglobulin reduces pulmonary respiratory syncytial virus shedding in owl monkeys. Antimicrob. Agents Chemother. *32*:1269–1270, 1988.
227. Hemming, V. G., Rodriguez, W., Kim, H. W., et al.: Intravenous immunoglobulin treatment of respiratory syncytial virus infections in infants and young children. Antimicrob. Agents Chemother. *31*:1882–1886, 1987.
228. Henderson, F. W.: Pulmonary infections with respiratory syncytial virus and the parainfluenza viruses. Semin. Respir. Infect. *2*:112–121, 1987.
229. Henderson, F. W., Clyde, W. A., Jr., Collier, A. M., et al.: The etiologic and

epidemiologic spectrum of bronchiolitis in pediatric practice. J. Pediatr. *95*:183–190, 1979.

230. Henderson, F. W., Collier, A. M., Clyde, W. A., Jr., et al.: Respiratory syncytial virus infections, reinfections and immunity: A prospective longitudinal study in young children. N. Engl. J. Med. *300*:530–534, 1979.
231. Henderson, F. W., Collier, A. M., Sanyal, M. A., et al.: A longitudinal study of respiratory viruses and bacteria in the etiology of acute otitis media with effusion. N. Engl. J. Med. *306*:1377–1383, 1982.
232. Henderson, F. W., and Giebink, G. S.: Otitis media among children in day care: Epidemiology and pathogenesis. Rev. Infect. Dis. *8*:533–538, 1986.
233. Hendley, J. O., Wenzel, R. P., and Gwaltney, J. M., Jr.: Transmission of rhinovirus colds by self-inoculation. N. Engl. J. Med. *288*:1361–1364, 1973.
234. Hendry, R. M., Burns, J. C., Walsh, E. E., et al.: Strain-specific serum antibody responses in infants undergoing primary infection with respiratory syncytial virus. J. Infect. Dis. *157*:640–647, 1988.
235. Hendry, R. M., Pierik, L. T., and McIntosh, K.: Prevalence of respiratory syncytial virus subgroups over six consecutive outbreaks: 1981–1987. J. Infect. Dis. *160*:185–190, 1989.
236. Henry, R. L., Hodges, I. G. C., Milner, A. D., et al.: Respiratory problems 2 years after acute bronchiolitis. Arch. Dis. Child. *58*:713–716, 1983.
237. Hertz, M. I., Englund, J. A., Snover, D., et al.: Respiratory syncytial virus–induced acute lung injury in adult patients with bone marrow transplants: A clinical approach and review of the literature. Medicine *68*:269–281, 1989.
238. Higgins, P. G., Barrow, G. I., Tyrrell, D. A., et al.: The efficacy of intranasal interferon alpha–2a in respiratory syncytial virus infection in volunteers. Antiviral Res. *14*:3–10, 1990.
239. Hildreth, S. W., Baggs, R. R., Brownstein, D. G., et al:. Lack of detectable enhanced pulmonary histopathology in cotton rats immunized with purified F glycoprotein of respiratory syncytial virus (RSV) when challenged at 3–6 months after immunization. Vaccine *11*:615–618, 1993.
240. Hildreth, S. W., Baggs, R. B., Eichberg, J. W., et al.: A parenterally administered subunit RSV vaccine: Safety studies in animals and adult humans. Pediatr. Res. *25*:180A, 1989.
241. Hodes, D. S., Kim, H. W., Parrott, R. H., et al.: Genetic alteration in a temperature-sensitive mutant of respiratory syncytial virus after replication *in vivo*. Proc. Soc. Exp. Biol. Med. *145*:1158–1164, 1974.
242. Hoekstra, R. E., Herrmann, E. C., and O'Connell, E. J.: Virus infections in children. Am. J. Dis. Child. *120*:14–16, 1970.
243. Hogg, J. C., Williams, J., Richardson, J. B., et al.: Age as a factor in the distribution of lower-airway conductance and in the pathologic anatomy of obstructive lung disease. N. Engl. J. Med. *282*:1283–1287, 1970.
244. Holberg, C. J., Wright, A. L., Martinez, F. D., et al.: Child day care, smoking by caregivers, and lower respiratory tract illness in the first 3 years of life. Pediatrics *91*:885–892, 1993.
245. Holberg, C. J., Wright, A. L., Martinez, F. D., et al.: Risk factors for respiratory syncytial virus–associated lower respiratory illnesses in the first year of life. Am. J. Epidemiol. *133*:1135–1151, 1991.
246. Hornsleth, A., Friis, B., Grauballe, P. C., et al.: Detection by ELISA of IgA and IgM antibodies in secretion and IgM antibodies in serum in primary lower respiratory syncytial virus infection. J. Med. Virol. *13*:149–161, 1984.
247. Hsu, K. H., Lubeck, M. D., Davis, A. R., et al.: Immunogenicity of recombinant adenovirus–respiratory syncytial virus vaccines with adenovirus types 4, 5, and 7 vectors in dogs and a chimpanzee. J. Infect. Dis. *166*:769–775, 1992.
248. Huang, Y. T., Collins, P. L., and Wertz, G. W.: Characterization of the 10 proteins of human respiratory syncytial virus: Identification of a fourth envelope-associated protein. Virus Res. *2*:157–173, 1985.
249. Hurrell, G. D., Sturdy, P. M., Frood, J. D. L., et al.: Viruses in families. Lancet *1*:769–774, 1971.
250. Inabu, Y., Tanaka, Y., Sato, K., et al.: Bovine respiratory syncytial virus: Studies on an outbreak in Japan, 1968–1969. Jpn. J. Microbiol. *16*:373–383, 1972.
251. Institute of Medicine: ARI and meningococcal meningitis in the developing world. *In* Pearson, G. W. (ed.): The Children's Vaccine Initiative: Continuing Activities. A Summary of Two Workshops held September 12–13, 1994, and October 25–26, 1994. Washington, D.C., Institute of Medicine, National Academy Press, 1995, pp. 2–5.
252. Isaacs, D.: Viral subunit vaccines. Lancet *337*:1223–1224, 1991.
253. Isaacs, D., Bangham, C. R. M., and McMichael, A. J.: Cell-mediated cytotoxic response to respiratory syncytial virus in infants with bronchiolitis. Lancet *2*:769–771, 1987.
254. Isaacs, D., Dickson, H., O'Callaghan, C., et al.: Handwashing and cohorting in prevention of hospital acquired infections with respiratory syncytial virus. Arch. Dis. Child. *66*:227–231, 1991.
255. Jackson, G. G., and Muldoon, R. L.: Viruses causing common respiratory infections in man. III. Respiratory syncytial viruses and coronaviruses. J. Infect. Dis. *128*:674–692, 1973.
256. Jacobs, J. W.: Immunity to infections of the respiratory system in man and animals. Dev. Biol. Stand. *28*:609–616, 1975.
257. Jacobs, J. W., Peacock, D. B., Corner, B. D., et al.: Respiratory syncytial and other viruses associated with respiratory disease in infants. Lancet *1*:871–876, 1971.
258. Jarvis, W. R., Middleton, P. J., and Gelfand, E. W.: Significance of viral infections in severe combined immunodeficiency disease. Pediatr. Infect. Dis. *2*:187–192, 1983.
259. Jensen, C., and Johnson, F. B.: Comparison of various transport media for viability maintenance of herpes simplex virus, respiratory syncytial virus, and adenovirus. Diagn. Microbiol. Infect. Dis. *19*:137–142, 1994.
260. Johnson, K. M., Bloom, H. H., Mufson, M. A., et al.: Natural reinfection of adults by respiratory syncytial virus: Possible relation to mild upper respiratory disease. N. Engl. J. Med. *267*:68–72, 1962.
261. Johnson, K. M., Chanock, R. M., Rifkind, D., et al.: Respiratory syncytial virus. IV. Correlation of virus shedding, serologic response, and illness in adult volunteers. J. A. M. A. *176*:663–667, 1961.
262. Johnson, P. R., Olmsted, R. A., Prince, G. A., et al.: Antigenic relatedness between glycoproteins of human respiratory syncytial virus subgroups A and B: Evaluation of the contributions of F and G glycoproteins to immunity. J. Virol. *10*:3163–3166, 1987.
263. Johnson, P. R., Spriggs, M. K., Olmsted, R. A., et al.: The G glycoprotein of human respiratory syncytial viruses of subgroups A and B: Extensive sequence divergence between antigenically related proteins. Proc. Natl. Acad. Sci. U. S. A. *84*:5625–5629, 1987.
264. Jordan, W. S., Jr.: Growth characteristics of respiratory syncytial virus. J. Immunol. *88*:581–590, 1962.
265. Kakuk, T. J., Soike, K., Brideau, R. J., et al.: A human respiratory syncytial virus (RSV) primate model of enhanced pulmonary pathology induced with a formalin-inactivated RSV vaccine but not a recombinant FG subunit vaccine. J. Infect. Dis. *167*:533–561, 1993.
266. Kalica, A. R., Wright, P. F., Hetrick, F. M., et al.: Electron microscopic studies of respiratory syncytial temperature sensitive mutants. Arch. Ges. Virusforsch. *41*:248–258, 1973.
267. Kapikian, A. Z., Bell, J. A., Mastrota, F. M., et al.: An outbreak of febrile illness and pneumonia associated with respiratory syncytial virus infection. Am. J. Hyg. *74*:234–248, 1961.
268. Kapikian, A. Z., Mitchell, R. H., Chanock, R. M., et al.: An epidemiologic study of altered clinical reactivity to respiratory syncytial (RS) virus infection in children previously vaccinated with an inactivated RSV virus vaccine. Am. J. Epidemiol. *89*:405–421, 1969.
269. Kattan, M., Keens, L. G., Lapierre, J. G., et al.: Pulmonary function abnormalities in symptom-free children after bronchiolitis. Pediatrics *59*:683–688, 1977.
270. Kaul, T. N., Welliver, R. C., and Ogra, P. L.: Development of antibody-dependent cell-mediated cytotoxicity in the respiratory tract after natural infection with respiratory syncytial virus. Infect. Immun. *37*:492–497, 1982.
271. Kaul, T. N., Welliver, R. C., Wong, D. T., et al.: Secretory and antibody response to respiratory syncytial virus infection. Am. J. Dis. Child. *135*:1013–1016, 1981.
272. Kellogg, J. A.: Culture vs direct antigen assays for detection of microbial pathogens from lower respiratory tract specimens suspected of containing the respiratory syncytial virus. Arch. Pathol. Lab. Med. *115*:451–458, 1991.
273. Kellogg, J. A.: Culture vs direct antigen assay for the detection of respiratory syncytial virus (RSV). Pan Am. Group Rapid Viral Diagn. *17*:1–4, 1991.
274. Kennedy, C. R., Chrzanowska, K., Robinson, R. O., et al.: A major role for viruses in acute childhood encephalopathy. Lancet *1*:989–991, 1986.
275. Khamapirad, T., and Glezen, W. P.: Clinical and radiographic assessment of acute lower respiratory tract disease in infants and children. Semin. Resp. Infect. *2*:130–144, 1987.
276. Kim, H. W., Arrobio, J. O., Brandt, C. D., et al.: Epidemiology of respiratory syncytial virus infection in Washington, D.C. I. Importance of the virus in different respiratory disease syndromes and temporal distribution of infection. Am J. Epidemiol. *98*:216–225, 1973.
277. Kim, H. W., Arrobio, J. O., Brandt, C. D., et al.: Safety and antigenicity of temperature sensitive (TS) mutant respiratory syncytial virus (RSV) in infants and children. Pediatrics *52*:56–79, 1973.
278. Kim, H. W., Arrobio, J. O., Pyles, G., et al.: Clinical and immunological response of infants and children to administration of low-temperature adapted respiratory syncytial virus. Pediatrics *48*:745–755, 1971.
279. Kim, H. W., Canchola, J. G., Brandt, C. D., et al.: Respiratory syncytial virus disease in infants despite prior administration of antigenic inactivated vaccine. Am. J. Epidemiol. *89*:422–434, 1969.
280. Kim, H. W., Leikin, S. L., Arrobio, J., et al.: Cell-mediated immunity to respiratory syncytial virus induced by inactivated vaccine or by infection. Pediatr. Res. *10*:75–78, 1976.
281. Kimball, A. M., Foy, H. M., Cooney, M. K., et al.: Isolation of respiratory syncytial and influenza viruses from the sputum of patients hospitalized with pneumonia. J. Infect. Dis. *147*:181–184, 1983.
282. Kimman, T. G., Westenbrink, F., Schreuder, B. E. C., et al.: Local and systemic antibody response to bovine respiratory syncytial virus infection and reinfection in calves with and without maternal antibodies. J. Clin. Microbiol. *25*:1097–1106, 1987.
283. King, A. M. Q., Stott, E. J., Langer, S. J., et al.: Recombinant vaccinia viruses carrying the N gene of human respiratory syncytial virus: Studies of gene expression in cell culture and immune response in mice. J. Virol. *61*:2885–2889, 1987.
284. King, J. C., Burke, A. R., Clemens, J. D., et al.: Respiratory syncytial virus illnesses in human immunodeficiency virus and noninfected children. Pediatr. Infect. Dis. J. *12*:733–739, 1993.

285. Klassen, T. P., Rowe, P. C., Sutcliffe, T., et al.: Randomized trial of salbutamol in acute bronchiolitis. J. Pediatr. *118*:807–811, 1991.
286. Klein, B. S., Dollete, F. R., and Yolken, R. H.: The role of respiratory syncytial virus and other viral pathogens in acute otitis media. J. Pediatr. *101*:16–20, 1982.
287. Knight, V., and Gilbert, B. E.: Chemotherapy of respiratory viruses. Adv. Intern. Med. *31*:95–118, 1986.
288. Knight, V., Yu, C. P., Gilbert, B. E., et al.: Ribavirin aerosol treatment: Emerging technical and clinical summary. Royal Society of Medicine Services Limited. International Congress and Symposium Series, No. 145, 1988, pp. 69–84.
289. Korppi, M., Kuikka, L., Reijonen, T., et al.: Bronchial asthma and hyperreactivity after early childhood bronchiolitis or pneumonia: An 8-year follow-up study. Arch. Pediatr. Adolesc. Med. *148*:1079–1084, 1994.
290. Korppi, M., Reijonen, T., Pöysä, L., et al.: A 2- to 3-year outcome after bronchiolitis. Am. J. Dis. Child. *147*:628–631, 1993.
291. Krasinski, K., LaCouture, R., Holzman, R. S., et al.: Screening for respiratory syncytial virus and assignment to a cohort at admission to reduce nosocomial transmission. J. Pediatr. *116*:894–898, 1990.
292. Kravetz, H. M., Knight, V., Chanock, R. M., et al.: Respiratory syncytial virus. III. Production of illness and clinical observations in adult volunteers. J. A. M. A. *176*:657–667, 1961.
293. Krilov, L. R., Anderson, L. J., Marcoux, L., et al.: Antibody-mediated enhancement of respiratory syncytial virus infection in two monocyte/macrophage cell lines. J. Infect. Dis *160*:777–782, 1989.
294. Laegreid, A., Kolsto Otnaess, A. B., Orstavik, I., et al.: Neutralizing activity in human milk fractions against respiratory syncytial virus. Acta Paediatr. Scand. *75*:696–701, 1986.
295. Laing, I., Riedel, F., Yap, P. L., et al.: Atopy predisposing to acute bronchiolitis during an epidemic of respiratory syncytial virus. Br. Med. J. *284*:1070–1072, 1982.
296. Lamprecht, C. L., Krause, H. E., and Mufson, M. A.: Role of maternal antibody in pneumonia and bronchiolitis due to respiratory syncytial virus. J. Infect. Dis. *134*:211–217, 1976.
297. Lancet Editorial: Male Oscuro|R.S.V.? The Lancet *1*:651–652, 1979.
298. Lancet Editorial: Nosocomial infection with respiratory syncytial virus. Lancet *340*:1071–1072, 1992.
299. Landau, L. I.: Bronchiolitis and asthma: Are they related? Thorax *49*:293–296, 1994.
300. Landau, L. I., Morgan, W., McCoy, K. S., et al.: Gender related differences in airway tone in children. Pediatr. Pulmonol. *16*:31–35, 1993.
301. Landry, M. L.: Multiple viral infections in the immunocompromised host: Recognition and interpretation. Clin. Diagn. Virol. *2*:313–321, 1994.
302. Lapin, C. D., Hiatt, P. W., Langston, C., et al.: A lamb model for human respiratory syncytial virus infection. Pediatr. Pulmonol. *15*:151–156, 1993.
303. Law, B., and Carvalho, V. D.: Respiratory syncytial virus infections in hospitalized Canadian children: Regional differences in patient populations and management practices. Pediatr. Infect. Dis. J. *12*:659–663, 1993.
304. LeClair, J. M., Freeman, J., Sullivan, B. F., et al.: Prevention of nosocomial respiratory syncytial virus infections through compliance with glove and gown isolation precautions. N. Engl. J. Med. *317*:329–334, 1987.
305. Lee, G. C.-Y., Funk, G. A., Chen, S. T., et al.: An outbreak of respiratory syncytial virus infection in an infant nursery. J. Formosan Med. Assoc. *72*:39–46, 1973.
306. Leer, J. A., Jr., Green, J. L., Heimlich, E. M., et al.: Corticosteroid treatment in bronchiolitis. Am. J. Dis. Child. *117*:495–503, 1969.
307. Levenson, R. M., and Kantor, O. S.: Fatal pneumonia in an adult due to respiratory syncytial virus. Arch. Intern. Med. *147*:791–792, 1987.
308. Levin, M. J.: Treatment and prevention options for respiratory syncytial virus infections. J. Pediatr. *124*:S22–S27, 1994.
309. Levine, S., and Hamilton, R.: Kinetics of the respiratory syncytial virus growth cycle in HeLa cells. Arch. Ges. Virusforsch. *28*:122–132, 1969.
310. Liss, H. P., and Bernstein, J.: Ribavirin aerosol in the elderly. Chest *93*:1239–1241, 1988.
311. Loda, F. A., Clyde, W. A., Glezen, W. P., et al.: Studies of the role of viruses, bacteria, and *M. pneumoniae* as causes of lower respiratory tract infections in children. J. Pediatr. *72*:161–176, 1968.
312. Lundgren, D. L., Magnuson, M. G., and Clapper, W. E.: A serologic survey in dogs for antibody to human respiratory viruses. Lab. Anim. Care *19*:352–359, 1969.
313. Macasaet, F. F., Kidd, P. A., Balano, C. R., et al.: The etiology of acute respiratory infections. III. The role of viruses and bacteria. J. Pediatr. *72*:829–839, 1968.
314. MacDonald, N. E., Hall, C. B., Suffin, S. C., et al.: Respiratory syncytial viral infection in infants with congenital heart disease. N. Engl. J. Med. *307*:397–400, 1982.
315. MacDonald, N. E., Wolfish, N., McLaine, P., et al.: Role of respiratory viruses in exacerbations of primary nephrotic syndrome. J. Pediatr. *108*:378–382, 1986.
316. Madge, P.: Controlling RSV requires a three-pronged approach. Infect. Dis. Alert *12*:58–59, 1993.
317. Maletzky, A. J., Cooney, M. K., Luce, R., et al.: Epidemiology of viral and mycoplasmal agents associated with childhood lower respiratory illness in a civilian population. J. Pediatr. *78*:407–414, 1971.
318. Mallory, G. B., Motoyama, E. K., Koumbourlis, A. C., et al.: Bronchial reactivity in infants in acute respiratory failure with viral bronchiolitis. Pediatr. Pulmonol. *6*:253–259, 1989.
319. Margolis, P. A., Greenberg, R. A., Keyes, L. L., et al.: Lower respiratory illness in infants and low socioeconomic status. Am. J. Public Health *82*:1119–1126, 1992.
320. Martinez, F. D., Morgan, W. J., Wright, A. L., et al.: Diminished lung function as a predisposing factor for wheezing respiratory illness in infants. N. Engl. J. Med. *319*:1112–1117, 1988.
321. Martinez, F. D., Morgan, W. J., Wright, A. L., et al.: Initial airway function is a risk factor for recurrent wheezing respiratory illnesses during the first three years of life. Am. Rev. Respir. Dis. *143*:312–316, 1991.
322. Mathur, U., Bentley, D. W., and Hall, C. B.: Concurrent outbreaks of respiratory syncytial virus and influenza A/Texas/77 infection in the institutionalized, elderly, and chronically ill. Ann. Intern. Med. *93*:49–52, 1980.
323. McConnochie, K. M., Hall, C. B., and Barker, W. H.: Lower respiratory tract illness in the first 2 years of life: Epidemiologic patterns and costs in a suburban pediatric practice. Am. J. Public Health *78*:34–39, 1988.
324. McConnochie, K. M., Hall, C. B., Walsh, E. E., et al: Variation in severity of respiratory syncytial virus infection with subtype. J. Pediatr. *117*:52–62, 1990.
325. McIntosh, K.: Pathogenesis of severe acute respiratory infections in the developing world: Respiratory syncytial virus and parainfluenza virus. Rev. Infect. Dis. *13*:S492–S500, 1991.
326. McIntosh, K., Arbeter, A. M., Stahl, M. K., et al.: Attenuated respiratory syncytial virus vaccines in asthmatic children. Pediatr. Res. *8*:689–690, 1974.
327. McIntosh, K., Hendry, R. M., Fahnestock, M. L. et al.: Enzyme-linked immunosorbent assay for detection of respiratory syncytial virus infection: Application to clinical samples. J. Clin. Microbiol. *16*:329–333, 1982.
328. McIntosh, K., Kurachek, S. C., Cairns, L. M., et al.: Treatment of respiratory viral infection in an immunodeficient infant with ribavirin aerosol. Am. J. Dis. Child. *138*:305–308, 1984.
329. McIntosh, K., Masters, H. B., Orr, I., et al.: The immunologic response to infection with respiratory syncytial virus in infants. J. Infect. Dis. *138*:24–32, 1978.
330. McIntosh, K., McQuillin, J., and Gardner, P. S.: Secretory immunologic response to respiratory syncytial virus infection in infants: Antibody on and off epithelial cells. Pediatr. Res. *12*:495, 1978.
331. McIntosh, K., Pierik, L. T., and Hendry, R. M.: Virulence of the two major antigenic subgroups of respiratory syncytial virus in hospitalized infants. Pediatr. Res. *23*:292A, 1988.
332. McKay, E., Higgins, P., Tyrrell, D., et al.: Immunogenicity and pathogenicity of temperature-sensitive modified respiratory syncytial virus in adult volunteers. J. Med. Virol. *25*:411–421, 1988.
333. McMillan, J. A., Tristram, D. A., Weiner, L. B., et al.: Prediction of the duration of hospitalization in patients with respiratory syncytial virus: Use of clinical parameters. Pediatrics *81*:22–26, 1988.
334. Meddens, M. J. M., Herbrink, P., Lindeman, J., et al.: Serodiagnosis of respiratory syncytial virus (RSV) infection in children as measured by detection of RSV-specific immunoglobulins G, M, and A, with enzyme-linked immunosorbent assay. J. Clin. Microbiol. *28*:152–155, 1990.
335. Meert, K., Heidemann, S., Abella, B., et al.: Does prematurity alter the course of respiratory syncytial virus infection? Crit. Care Med. *18*:1357–1359, 1990.
336. Meert, K., Heidemann, S., Lieh-Lai, M., et al.: Clinical characteristics of respiratory syncytial virus infections in healthy versus previously compromised host. Pediatr. Pulmonol. *7*:167–170, 1989.
337. Meissner, H. C., Murray, S. A., Kiernan, M. A., et al.: A simultaneous outbreak of respiratory syncytial virus and parainfluenza virus type 3 in a newborn nursery. J. Pediatr. *104*:680–684, 1984.
338. Mills, J. V., VanKirk, J. E., Wright, P. F., et al.: Experimental respiratory syncytial virus infection of adults: Possible mechanisms of resistance to infection and illness. J. Immunol. *107*:123–130, 1971.
339. Mito, K., Chiba, Y., Suga, K., et al.: Cellular immune response to infection with respiratory syncytial virus and influence of breast-feeding on the response. J. Med. Virol. *14*:323–332, 1984.
340. Mlinaric-Galinovic, G., Ugrcic, I., and Bozikov, J.: Respiratory syncytial virus infections in SR Croatia, Yugoslavia. Pediatr. Pulmonol. *3*:304–308, 1987.
341. Mohanty, S. B., Lillie, M. G., and Ingling, A. L.: Effect of serum and nasal neutralizing antibodies on bovine respiratory syncytial virus infection in calves. J. Infect. Dis. *134*:409–413, 1976.
342. Moler, F. W., Khan, A. S., Meliones, J. N., et al.: Respiratory syncytial virus morbidity and mortality estimates in congenital heart disease patients: A recent experience. Crit. Care Med. *20*:1406–1413, 1992.
343. Monto, A. S., and Cavallaro, J. J.: The Tecumseh study of respiratory illness. II. Patterns of occurrence of infection with respiratory pathogens, 1965–1969. Am. J. Epidemiol. *94*:280–289, 1971.
344. Monto, A. S., Higgins, M. W., and Ross, H. W.: The Tecumseh study of respiratory illness. VIII. Acute infection in chronic respiratory disease and comparison groups. Am. Rev. Respir. Dis. *111*:27–36, 1975.
345. Monto, A. S., and Lim, S. K.: The Tecumseh study of respiratory illness. III. Incidence and periodicity of respiratory syncytial virus and *Mycoplasma pneumoniae* infections. Am. J. Epidemiol. *94*:290–301, 1971.

346. Morales, F., Calder, M. A., Inglis, J. M., et al.: A study of respiratory infections in the elderly to assess the role of respiratory syncytial virus. J. Infect. *7*:236–247, 1983.
347. Morrell, R. E., Marks, M. I., Champlin, R., et al.: An outbreak of severe pneumonia due to respiratory syncytial virus in isolated arctic population. Am. J. Epidemiol. *101*:231–237, 1975.
348. Morris, J. A., Blount, R. E., and Savage, R. E.: An outbreak of severe pneumonia due to respiratory syncytial virus in isolated arctic population. Am. J. Epidemiol. *101*:231–237, 1975.
349. Morton, R. E., Dinwiddie, R., Marshall, W. C., et al.: Respiratory syncytial virus infection causing neurological disorder in neonates. Lancet *1*:1426–1427, 1981.
350. Muelenaer, P. M., Henderson, F. W., Hemming, V. G., et al.: Group-specific serum antibody responses in children with primary and recurrent respiratory syncytial virus infections. J. Infect. Dis. *164*:15–21, 1991.
351. Mufson, M. A., Belshe, R. B., Örvell C., et al.: Respiratory syncytial virus epidemics: Variable dominance of subgroups A and B strains among children, 1981–1986. J. Infect. Dis. *157*:143–148, 1988.
352. Mufson, M. A., Belshe, R. B., Örvell, C., et al.: Subgroup characteristics of respiratory syncytial virus strains recovered from children with two consecutive infections. J. Clin. Microbiol. *25*:1535–1539, 1987.
353. Mufson, M. A., Levine, H. D., Wasil, R. E., et al.: Epidemiology of respiratory syncytial virus infection among infants and children in Chicago. Am. J. Epidemiol. *98*:88–95, 1973.
354. Mufson, M. A., Orvell, C., Rafner, B., et al.: Two distinct subtypes of human respiratory syncytial virus. J. Gen. Virol. *66*:2111–2124, 1985.
355. Munoz, J. L., McCarthy, C. A., Clark, M. E., et al.: Respiratory syncytial virus infection in C57BL/6 mice: Clearance of virus from the lungs with virus-specific cytotoxic T cells. J. Virol. *65*:4494–4497, 1991.
356. Murphy, B. R., Alling, D. W., Snyder, M. H., et al.: Effect of age and preexisting antibody on serum antibody response of infants and children to the F and G glycoproteins during respiratory syncytial virus infection. J. Clin. Microbiol. *24*:894–898, 1986.
357. Murphy, B. R., Graham, B. S., Prince, G. A., et al.: Serum and nasal-wash immunoglobulin G and A antibody response of infants and children to respiratory syncytial virus F and G glycoproteins following primary infection. J. Clin. Microbiol. *23*:1009–1014, 1986.
358. Murphy, B. R., Olmsted, R. A., Collins, P. L., et al.: Passive transfer of respiratory syncytial virus (RSV) antiserum suppresses the immune response to the RSV fusion (F) and large (G) glycoproteins expressed by recombinant vaccinia viruses. J. Virol. *62*:3907–3910, 1988.
359. Murphy, B. R., Prince, G. A., Walsh, E. E., et al.: Dissociation between serum neutralizing and glycoprotein antibody responses of infants and children who received inactivated respiratory syncytial virus vaccine. J. Clin. Microbiol. *24*:197–202, 1986.
360. Murphy, B. R., and Walsh, E. E.: Formalin-inactivated respiratory syncytial virus vaccine induces antibodies to the fusion glycoproteins that are deficient in fusion-inhibiting activity. J. Clin. Microbiol. *26*:1595–1597, 1988.
361. Murphy, D., and Rose, R. C.: Respiratory syncytial virus pneumonia in a human immunodeficiency virus-infected man. J. A. M. A. *261*:1147, 1989.
362. Murphy, D., Todd, J. R., Chao, R. R., et al.: The use of gowns and masks to control respiratory illness in pediatric hospital personnel. J. Pediatr. *99*:746–750, 1981.
363. Murphy, T. F., Henderson, F. W., Clyde, W. C., Jr., et al.: Pneumonia: An eleven-year study in a pediatric practice. Am. J. Epidemiol. *113*:12–21, 1981.
364. Navas, L., Wang, E., de Carvalho, V., et al.: Improved outcome of respiratory syncytial virus infection in a high-risk hospitalized population of Canadian children. J. Pediatr. *121*:348–354, 1992.
365. Neuzil, K. M., Gruber, W. C., Chytil, F., et al.: Serum vitamin A levels in respiratory syncytial virus infection. J. Pediatr. *124*:433–436, 1994.
366. Nicholas, J. A., Rubino, K. L., Levely, M. E., et al.: Cytolytic T-lymphocyte responses to respiratory syncytial virus: Effector cell phenotype and target proteins. J. Virol. *64*:4232–4241, 1990.
367. Norrby, E., Marisyk, H., and Orvel, C.: Moylogenesis of respiratory syncytial virus in a green monkey kidney cell line (vero). J. Virol. *6*:237–242, 1970.
368. Norrby, E., Mufson, M. A., and Hooshmand, S.: Structural differences between subtype A and B strains of respiratory syncytial virus. J. Gen. Virol. *67*:2721–2729, 1986.
369. Ogilivie, M. M., Vatheneo, S., Radford, M., et al.: Maternal antibody and respiratory syncytial virus infection in infancy. J. Med. Virol. *7*:263–271, 1981.
370. Ogra, P. L., Morag, A., Ogra, S. S., et al.: Host defense mechanisms in viral respiratory infections. Pediatr. Res. *11*:231–233, 1977.
371. Ogra, P. L., Ogra, S. S., and Coppola, P. R.: Secretory component and sudden-infant-death syndrome. Lancet *2*:387–390, 1975.
372. Ogra, P. L., and Patel, J.: Respiratory syncytial virus infection and the immunocompromised host. Pediatr. Infect. Dis. J. *7*:246–249, 1988.
373. Oien, N. L., Brideau, R. J., Walsh, E., et al.: Induction of local and systemic immunity against human respiratory syncytial virus using a chimeric FG glycoprotein and cholera toxin B subunit. Vaccine *12*:731–735, 1994.
374. Okamoto, Y., Kudo, K., Ishikawa, K., et al.: Presence of respiratory syncytial virus genomic sequences in middle ear fluid and its relationship to expression of cytokines and cell adhesion molecules. J. Infect. Dis. *168*:1277–1281, 1993.
375. Okamoto, Y., Kudo, K., Shirotori, K., et al.: Detection of genomic sequences of respiratory syncytial virus in otitis media with effusion in children. Ann. Otol. Rhinol. Laryngol. *157*:(Suppl.)7–10, 1992.
376. Olmsted, R. A., Elango, N., Prince, G. A., et al.: Expression of the F glycoprotein of respiratory syncytial virus by a recombinant vaccinia virus: Comparison of the individual contributions of the F and G glycoproteins to host immunity. Proc. Natl. Acad. Sci. U. S. A. *83*:7462–7466, 1986.
377. Olmsted, R. A., and Collins, P. L.: The 1A protein of respiratory syncytial virus is an integral membrane protein present as multiple, structurally distinct species. J. Virol. *63*:2019–2029, 1989.
378. Opavsky, M. A., Stephens, D., Wang, E. E.-L., et al.: Testing models predicting severity of respiratory syncytial virus infection on the PICNIC RSV database. Arch. Pediatr. Adolesc. Med. *149*:1217–1220, 1995.
379. Openshaw, P. J., Clarke, S. L., and Record, F. M.: Pulmonary eosinophilic response to respiratory syncytial virus infection in mice sensitized to the major surface glycoprotein G. Int. Immunol. *4*:493–500, 1992.
380. Openshaw, P. J. M., Anderson, K., Wertz, G. W., et al.: The 22,000-kilodalton protein of respiratory syncytial virus is a major target for Kd-restricted cytotoxic T lymphocytes from mice primed by infection. J. Virol. *64*:1683–1689, 1990.
381. Osterweil, D., and Norman, D.: An outbreak of an influenza-like illness in a nursing home. J. Am. Geriatr. Soc. *38*:659–662, 1990.
382. Parrott, R. H., Kim, H. W., Arrobio, J. O., et al.: Epidemiology of respiratory syncytial virus infection in Washington, D.C. II. Infection and disease with respect to age, immunologic status, race, and sex. Am. J. Epidemiol. *98*:289–300, 1973.
383. Parrott, R. H., Kim, H. W., Brandt, C. D., et al.: Respiratory syncytial virus in infants and children. Prev. Med. *3*:473–480, 1974.
384. Parrott, R. H., Kim, H. W., Brandt, C. D., et al.: Potential of attenuated respiratory syncytial virus vaccine for infants and children. Dev. Biol. Stand. *28*:389–399, 1975.
385. Parrott, R. H., Vargosko, A. J., Kim, H. W., et al.: Respiratory syncytial virus. II. Serologic studies over a 34-month period of children with bronchiolitis, pneumonia, and minor respiratory diseases. J. A. M. A. *176*:653–657, 1961.
386. Patel, J., Faden, H., Sharma, S., et al.: Effect of respiratory syncytial virus on adherence, colonization and immunity of non-typable *Haemophilus influenzae*: Implications for otitis media. Int. J. Pediatr. Otorhinolaryngol. *23*:15–23, 1992.
387. Peigue-Lafeuille, H., Gazuy, N., Mignot, P., et al.: Severe respiratory syncytial virus pneumonia in an adult renal transplant recipient: Successful treatment with ribavirin. Scand. J. Infect. Dis. *22*:87–89, 1990.
388. Pemberton, R. M., Cannon, M. J., Openshaw, P. J., et al.: Cytotoxic T cell specificity for respiratory syncytial virus proteins: Fusion protein is an important target antigen. J. Gen. Virol. *68*:2177–2182, 1987.
389. Phelan, P. D., Williams, H. E., and Freeman, M.: The disturbances of ventilation in acute viral bronchiolitis. Aust. Paediatr. J. *4*:96–104, 1968.
390. Pohl, C., Green, M., Wald, E. R., et al.: Respiratory syncytial virus infections in pediatric liver transplant recipients. J. Infect. Dis. *165*:166–169, 1992.
391. Pons, M. W., Lambert, A. L., Lambert, D. M., et al.: Improvement of respiratory syncytial virus replication in actively growing HEp-2 cells. J. Virol. Methods *7*:217–221, 1983.
392. Prendiville, A., Green, S., and Silverman, M.: Paradoxical response to nebulized salbutamol in wheezy infants, assessed by partial expiratory flow-volume curves. Thorax *42*:86–91, 1987.
393. Preston, F. M., Beier, P. L., and Pope, J. H.: Infectious respiratory syncytial virus (RSV) effectively inhibits the proliferative T cell response to inactivated RSV *in vitro*. J. Infect. Dis. *165*:819–825, 1992.
394. Prince, G. A., Hemming, V. G., and Chanock, R. M.: The use of purified immunoglobulin in the therapy of respiratory syncytial virus infection. Pediatr. Infect. Dis. *5*:5201–5206, 1986.
395. Prince, G. A., Hemming, V. G., Horswood, R. L., et al.: Effectiveness of topically administered neutralizing antibodies in experimental immunotherapy of respiratory syncytial virus infection in cotton rats. J. Virol. *61*:1851–1854, 1987.
396. Prince, G. A., Hemming, V. G., Horswood, R. L., et al.: Immunoprophylaxis and immunotherapy of respiratory syncytial virus infection in the cotton rat. Virus Res. *3*:193–206, 1985.
397. Prince, G. A., Horswood, R. L., Berndt, J., et al.: Respiratory syncytial virus infection in inbred mice. Infect. Immun. *26*:764, 1979.
398. Prince, G. A., Horswood, R. L., Camargo, E., et al.: Mechanisms of immunology to respiratory syncytial virus in cotton rats. Infect. Immun. *42*:81–87, 1983.
399. Prince, G. A., Horswood, R. L., and Chanock, R. M.: Quantitative aspects of passive immunity to respiratory syncytial virus infection in infant cotton rats. J. Virol. *55*:517, 1985.
400. Prince, G. A., Jenson, A. B., Horswood, R. L., et al.: The pathogenesis of respiratory syncytial virus infection in cotton rats. Am. J. Pathol. *93*:771–792, 1978.
401. Prince, G. A., and Porter, D. D.: The pathogenesis of respiratory syncytial virus infection in infant ferrets. Am. J. Pathol. *82*:339–352, 1976.

402. Prince, G. A., Potash, L., Horswood, R. L., et al.: Intramuscular inoculation of live respiratory syncytial virus induces immunity in cotton rats. Infect. Immun. *23*:723–728, 1979.
403. Prince, G. A., Suffin, S. C., Prevar, D. A., et al.: Respiratory syncytial viral infection in owl monkeys: Viral shedding, immunological response, and associated illness caused by wild-type virus and two temperature-sensitive mutants. Infect. Immun. *26*:1009–1013, 1979.
404. Pringle, C. R., Filipiuk, A. H., Robinson, B. S., et al.: Immunogenicity and pathogenicity of a triple temperature-sensitive modified respiratory syncytial virus in adult volunteers. Vaccine *11*:473–478, 1993.
405. Pringle, C. R.: The order *Mononegavirales*. Arch. Virol. *117*:137–140, 1991.
406. Pringle, C. R., Shirodaria, P. V., Cash, P., et al.: Initiation and maintenance of persistent infection by respiratory syncytial virus. J. Virol. *28*:199–211, 1978.
407. Pullan, C. R., and Hey, E. N.: Wheezing, asthma, and pulmonary dysfunction 10 years after infection with respiratory syncytial virus in infancy. Br. Med. J. *284*:1665–1669, 1982.
408. Pullan, C. R., Toms, G. L., Martin, A. J., et al.: Breast feeding and respiratory syncytial virus infection. Br. Med. J. *281*:1034–1036, 1980.
409. Randolph, V. B., Kandis, M., Stemler-Higgins, P., et al.: Attenuated temperature-sensitive respiratory syncytial virus mutants generated by cold adaptation. Virus Res. *33*:241–591, 1994.
410. Raven, C., Maverokis, N. H., Eveland, W. C., et al.: The sudden infant death syndrome: A possible hypersensitivity reaction determined by distribution of IgG in lungs. J. Forensic Sci. *23*:116–138, 1978.
411. Rechsteiner, J., and Winkler, K. C.: Inactivation of respiratory syncytial virus in aerosol. J. Gen. Virol. *5*:405–410, 1969.
412. Reid, L.: Influence of the pattern of structural growth of lung on susceptibility to specific infectious diseases in infants and children. Pediatr. Res. *11*:210–215, 1977.
413. Reilly, C. M., Stokes, J., Jr., McClelland, L., et al.: Studies of acute respiratory illness caused by respiratory syncytial virus. 3. Clinical and laboratory findings. N. Engl. J. Med. *264*:1176–1182, 1961.
414. Report to the Medical Research Council Subcommittee on Respiratory Syncytial virus Infection: Admissions to hospitals in industrial, urban and rural areas. Br. Med. J. *2*:796–798, 1978.
415. Reynolds, E. O. R.: Arterial blood gas tensions in acute disease of lower respiratory tract in infancy. Br. Med. J. *1*:1192–1195, 1963.
416. Rice, R. P., and Loda, F.: A roentgenographic analysis of respiratory syncytial virus pneumonia in infants. Radiology *87*:1021–1027, 1966.
417. Richardson, L. S., Belshe, R. B., London, W. T., et al.: Evaluation of five temperature sensitive mutants of respiratory syncytial virus in primates. I. Viral shedding, immunologic response and associated illness. Med. Virol. *3*:91–100, 1978.
418. Richardson, L. S., Belshe, R. B., London, W. T., et al.: Respiratory syncytial virus antibodies in nonhuman primates and domestic animals. Lab. Animal Sci. *31*:413–415, 1981.
419. Richardson, L. S., Belshe, R. B., Sly, D. L., et al.: Experimental respiratory syncytial virus pneumonia in cubus monkeys. J. Med. Virol. *2*:45–59, 1978.
420. Richardson, L. S., Yolken, R. H., Belshe, R. B., et al.: Enzyme linked immunosorbent assay for measurement of serological response to respiratory syncytial virus infection. Infect. Immunol. *20*:660–664, 1978.
421. Roberts, N. J., Jr., Prill, A. H., and Mann, T. N.: Interleukin 1 and interleukin 1 inhibitor production by human macrophages exposed to influenza virus or respiratory syncytial virus: Respiratory syncytial virus is a potent inducer of inhibitor activity. J. Exp. Med. *163*:511–519, 1986.
422. Rodriguez, W. J., Kim, H. W., Brandt, C. D., et al.: Aerosolized ribavirin in the treatment of patients with respiratory syncytial virus disease. Pediatr. Infect. Dis. J. *6*:159–163, 1987.
423. Rodriguez, W. J., and Parrott, R. H.: Ribavirin aerosol treatment of serious respiratory syncytial virus infection in infants. Infect. Dis. Clin. North Am. *1*:425–439, 1987.
424. Rooney, J. C., and Williams, H. E.: The relationship between proved viral bronchiolitis and subsequent wheezing. J. Pediatr. *79*:744–747, 1971.
425. Rosner, I. K., Welliver, R. C., Edelson, P. J., et al.: Effect of ribavirin therapy on respiratory syncytial virus-specific IgE and IgA responses after infection. J. Infect. Dis. *155*:1043–1047, 1987.
426. Ross, C. A., Pinkerton, I. W., and Assaad, F. A.: Pathogenesis of respiratory syncytial virus diseases in infancy. Arch. Dis. Child. *46*:702–704, 1971.
427. Rutter, N., Milner, A. D., and Hiller, E. J.: Effect of bronchodilators of respiratory resistance in infants and young children with bronchiolitis and wheezy bronchiolitis. Arch. Dis. Child. *50*:719–722, 1975.
428. Rylander, E., Eriksson, M., and Freyschuss, U.: Risk factors for occasional and recurrent wheezing after RSV infection in infancy. Acta Paediatr. Scand. *77*:711–715, 1988.
429. Salkind, A. R., McCarthy, D. O., Nichols, J. E., et al.: Interleukin-1–inhibitor activity induced by respiratory syncytial virus: Abrogation of virus-specific and alternate human lymphocyte proliferative responses. J. Infect. Dis. *163*:71–77, 1991.
430. Salkind, A. R., Nichols, J. E., and Roberts, N. J., Jr.: Suppressed expression of ICAM-1 and LFA-1 and abrogation of leukocyte collaboration after exposure of human mononuclear leukocytes to respiratory syncytial virus in vitro. Comparison with exposure to influenza virus. J. Clin. Invest. *88*:505–511, 1991.
431. Sami, I. R., Piazza, F. M., Johnson, S. A., et al.: Systemic immunoprophylaxis of nasal respiratory syncytial virus infection in cotton rats. J. Infect. Dis. *171*:440–443, 1995.
432. Sanchez, I., DeKoster, J., Powell, R. E., et al.: Effect of racemic epinephrine and salbutamol on clinical score and pulmonary mechanics in infants with bronchiolitis. J. Pediatr. *122*:145–151, 1993.
433. Satake, M., Elango, N., and Venkatesan, S.: Sequence analysis of the respiratory syncytial virus phosphoprotein gene. J. Virol. *52*:991–994, 1984.
434. Satake, M., and Venkatesan, S.: Nucleotide sequence of the gene encoding respiratory syncytial virus matrix protein. J. Virol. *50*:92–99, 1984.
435. Schuh, S., Canny, G., Reisman, J. J., et al.: Nebulized albuterol in acute bronchiolitis. J. Pediatr. *117*:633–637, 1990.
436. Marshall, E.: Visiting experts find the "mystery disease" of Naples is a common virus. Science *203*:908–981, 1979.
437. Scott, R., and Gardner, P. S.: Respiratory syncytial virus neutralizing activity in nasopharyngeal secretions. J. Hyg. *68*:581–588, 1970.
438. Scott, R., Pullan, C. R., Scott, M., et al.: Cell-mediated immunity in respiratory syncytial virus disease. J. Med. Virol. *13*:105–114, 1984.
439. Serwint, J.: Efficacy of albuterol in the management of bronchiolitis. Pediatrics *95*:320, 1995.
440. Shahrabadi, M. S., and Lee, P. W. K.: Calcium requirement for syncytium formation in HEp-2 cells by respiratory syncytial virus. J. Clin. Microbiol. *26*:139–141, 1988.
441. Sieber, O. F.: Immunologic factors in infectious diseases of the airways and lung in infants and children with particular emphasis on bronchiolitis. Comments Pediatr. Res. *11*:230, 1977.
442. Sigurs, N., Bjarnason, R., and Sigurbergsson, F.: Eosinophil cationic protein in nasal secretion and in serum and myeloperoxidase in serum in respiratory syncytial virus bronchiolitis: Relation to asthma and atopy. Acta Pediatr. *83*:1151–1155, 1994.
443. Sigurs, N., Bjarnason, R., Sigurbergsson, F., et al.: Asthma and immunoglobulin E antibodies after respiratory syncytial virus bronchiolitis: A prospective cohort study with matched controls. Pediatrics *95*:500–505, 1995.
444. Simoes, E. A. F., King, S. J., Lehr, M. V., et al.: Preterm twins and triplets: A high-risk group for severe respiratory syncytial virus infection. Am. J. Dis. Child. *147*:303–306, 1993.
445. Simpson, W., Hacking, P. M., Court, S. D. M., et al.: The radiological findings in respiratory syncytial virus infection in children. Part II. The correlation of radiological categories with clinical and virological findings. Pediatr. Radiol. *2*:155–160, 1974.
446. Sims, D. G., Downham, M. A. P. S., McQuillin, J., et al.: Respiratory syncytial virus infection in north-east England. Br. Med. J. *2*:1095–1098, 1976.
447. Sims, D. G., Downham, M. A. P. S., Webb, J. K. G., et al.: Hospital cross-infection on children's wards with respiratory syncytial virus and the role of adult carriage. Acta Paediatr. Scand. *64*:541–545, 1975.
448. Sims, D. G., Gardner, P. S., Weightman, D., et al.: Atopy does not predispose to RSV bronchiolitis or postbronchiolitic wheezing. Br. Med. J. *282*:2086–2088, 1981.
449. Sinnott, J. T., IV, Cullison, J. P., Sweeney, M. S., et al.: Respiratory syncytial virus pneumonia in a cardiac transplant recipient. J. Infect. Dis. *158*:650–651, 1988.
450. Sly, P. D., and Hibbert, M. D.: Childhood asthma following hospitalization with acute viral bronchiolitis in infancy. Pediatr. Pulmonol. *7*:153–158, 1989.
451. Sly, P. D., Lanteri, C. J., and Raven, J. M.: Do wheezy infants recovering from bronchiolitis respond to inhaled salbutamol? Pediatr. Pulmonol. *10*:36–39, 1991.
452. Smith, A. P., Tyrrell, D. A. J., Barrow, G. I., et al.: The common cold, pattern sensitivity and contrast sensitivity. Psychol. Med. *22*:487–494, 1992.
453. Smith, D. W., Frankel, L. R., Mathers, L. H., et al.: A controlled trial of aerosolized ribavirin in infants receiving mechanical ventilation for severe respiratory syncytial virus infection. N. Engl. J. Med. *325*:24–29, 1991.
454. Snyderman, D. R., Greer, C., Meissner, H. C., et al.: Prevention of nosocomial transmission of respiratory syncytial virus in a newborn nursery. Infect. Control Hosp. Epidemiol. *9*:105–108, 1988.
455. Sommerville, R. G.: Respiratory syncytial virus in acute exacerbations of chronic bronchitis. Lancet *2*:1247–1248, 1963.
456. Soto, M. E., Sly, P. E., Uren, E., et al.: Bronchodilator response during acute viral bronchiolitis in infancy. Pediatr. Pulmonol. *1*:85–90, 1985.
457. Southall, D. P.: Role of apnea in the sudden infant death syndrome: A personal view. Pediatr. *81*:73–84, 1988.
458. Spence, L., and Barratt, N.: Respiratory syncytial virus associated with acute respiratory infections in Trinidadian patients. Am. J. Epidemiol. *88*:257–266, 1968.
459. Spinelli, M., Geraci-Ciardullo, K., Palumbo, P. E., et al.: Efficacy of ribavirin for treating respiratory syncytial virus (RSV) pneumonia in high risk infants. Pediatr. Res. *19*:304A, 1985.
460. Springer, C., Bar-Yishay, E., Uwayyed, K., et al.: Corticosteroids do not affect the clinical or physiological status of infants with bronchiolitis. Pediatr. Pulmonol. *9*:181–185, 1990.
461. Sriskandan, S., and Shaunak, S.: Respiratory syncytial virus infection in an adult with AIDS. Clin. Infect. Dis. *17*:1065, 1993.

462. Stecenko, A. A.: Treatment of viral bronchiolitis: Do steroids make sense? Contemp. Pediatr. *4*:121–130, 1987.
463. Sterner, G., Wolontis, S., Bloth, B., et al.: Respiratory syncytial virus: An outbreak of acute respiratory illness in a home for infants. Acta Paediatr. Scand. *55*:273–279, 1966.
464. Storch, G. A., and Park, C. S.: Monoclonal antibodies demonstrate heterogeneity in the G glycoprotein of prototype strains and clinical isolates or respiratory syncytial virus. J. Med. Virol. *22*:345–356, 1987.
465. Stott, E. J., Ball, L. A., Young, K. K., et al.: Human respiratory syncytial virus glycoprotein G expressed from a recombinant vaccinia virus vector protects mice against live-virus challenge. J. Virol. *60*:607–613, 1986.
466. Stott, E. J., Taylor, G., Ball, L. A., et al.: Immune and histopathological responses in animals vaccinated with recombinant vaccinia viruses that express individual genes of human respiratory syncytial virus. J. Virol. *61*:3855–3861, 1987.
467. Stott, E. J., Thomas, L. H., Collins, A. P., et al.: A survey of virus infections of the respiratory tract of cattle and their association with disease. J. Hyg. *85*:257–270, 1980.
468. Stott, E. J., Thomas, L. H., Howard, C. J., et al.: Field trial of a quadrivalent vaccine against calf respiratory disease. Vet. Rec. *121*:342–347, 1987.
469. Stretton, M., Ajizian, S. J., Mitchell, I., et al.: Intensive care course and outcome of patients infected with respiratory syncytial virus. Pediatr. Pulmonol. *13*:143–150, 1992.
470. Suffin, S. C., Prince, G. A., Muck, K. B., et al.: Immunoprophylaxis of respiratory syncytial virus infection in the infant ferret. J. Immunol. *23*:10–14, 1979.
471. Sung, R. Y. T., Murray, H. G. S., Chan, R. C. K., et al.: Seasonal patterns of respiratory syncytial virus infection in Hong Kong: A preliminary report. J. Infect. Dis. *156*:527–528, 1987.
472. Suto, T., Yano, N., Ikeda, M., et al.: Respiratory syncytial virus infection and its serologic epidemiology. Am. J. Epidemiol. *82*:211–224, 1965.
473. Swenson, P. D., and Kaplan, M.: Rapid detection of respiratory syncytial virus in nasopharyngeal aspirates by a commercial enzyme immunoassay. J. Clin. Microbiol. *23*:485–488, 1986.
474. Taber, L. H., Knight, V., Gilbert, B. E., et al.: Ribavirin aerosol treatment of bronchiolitis due to respiratory syncytial virus infection in infants. Pediatrics *72*:613–618, 1983.
475. Takimoto, C. H., Cram, D. L., and Root, R. K.: Respiratory syncytial virus infections on an adult medical ward. Arch. Intern. Med. *151*:706–708, 1991.
476. Tammela, O. K.: First-year infections after initial hospitalization in low birth weight infants with and without bronchopulmonary dysplasia. Scand. J. Infect. Dis. *24*:515–524, 1992.
477. Taussig, L. M., Busse, W. W., Lemen, R. J., et al.: NHLB Workshop Summary: Models of infectious airway injury in children. Am. Rev. Respir. Dis. *137*:979–984, 1988.
478. Taylor, C. E., Morrow, S., Scott, M., et al.: Comparative virulence of respiratory syncytial virus subgroups A and B. Lancet *1*:777–778, 1989.
479. Taylor, G., Stott, E. J., Bew, M., et al.: Monoclonal antibodies protect mice against respiratory syncytial virus infection in mice. Immunology *52*:137–142, 1984.
480. Taylor, G., Stott, E. J., and Hayle, A. J.: Cytotoxic lymphocytes in the lungs of mice infected with respiratory syncytial virus. J. Gen. Virol. *66*:2533–2538, 1985.
481. Taylor, G., Stott, E. J., Hughes, M., et al.: Respiratory syncytial virus infection in mice. Infect. Immun. *43*:649–655, 1984.
482. Teele, D. W.: Respiratory syncytial virus and otitis media with effusion. J. Pediatr. *101*:61–62, 1982.
483. Tepper, R. S., Rosenberg, D., and Eigen, H.: Airway responsiveness in infants following bronchiolitis. Pediatr. Pulmonol. *13*:6–10, 1992.
484. Thomas, L. H., Stott, E. J., Collins, A. P., et al.: Infection with gnotobiotic calves with a bovine and human isolate of respiratory syncytial virus: Modification of the response by dexamethasone. Arch. Virol. *79*:67–77, 1984.
485. Toms, G. L.: Respiratory syncytial virus: Virology, diagnosis, and vaccination. Lung *168*(Suppl.):388–395, 1990.
486. Toms, G. L., Gardner, P. S., Pullan, C. R., et al.: Secretion of RSV inhibitors and antibody in human milk throughout lactation. J. Med. Virol. *5*:351–360, 1980.
487. Toms, G. L., Webb, M. S. C., Milner, P. D., et al.: IgG and IgM antibodies of viral glycoproteins in respiratory syncytial virus infections of graded severity. Arch. Dis. Child. *64*:1661–1665, 1989.
488. Tristram, D. A., Welliver, R. C., Hogerman, D. A., et al.: Second-year surveillance of recipients of a respiratory syncytial virus (RSV) F protein subunit vaccine, PFP-1: Evaluation of antibody persistence and possible disease enhancement. Vaccine *12*:551–556, 1994.
489. Tristram, D. A., Welliver, R. C., Mohar, C. K., et al.: Immunogenicity and safety of respiratory syncytial virus subunit vaccine in seropositive children 18–36 months old. J. Infect. Dis. *167*:191–195, 1993.
490. Trudel, M., Nadon, F., Seguin, C., et al.: Initiation of cytotoxic T-cell response and protection of Balb/c mice by vaccination with an experimental ISCOMs respiratory syncytial virus subunit vaccine. Vaccine *10*:107–112, 1992.
491. Trudel, M., Nadon, F., Seguin, C., et al.: Protection of BALB/c mice from respiratory syncytial virus infection by immunization with a synthetic peptide derived from the G glycoprotein. Virology *185*:749–757, 1991.
492. Tsutsumi, H., Onuma, M., Suga, K., et al.: Occurrence of respiratory syncytial virus subgroup A and B strains in Japan, 1980 to 1987. J. Clin. Microbiol. *26*:1171–1174, 1988.
493. Tyrrell, D. A. J.: Discovering and defining the etiology of acute respiratory disease. Am. Rev. Respir. Dis. *88*:77–84, 1963.
494. Uhari, M., Hietala, J., and Tuokko, H.: Risk of acute otitis media in relation to the viral etiology of infections in children. Clin. Infect. Dis. *20*:521–524, 1995.
495. Ukkonen, P., Hovl, T., VonBonsdorff, C. H., et al.: Age-specific prevalence of complement fixing antibodies to sixteen viral antigens: A computer analysis of 58,500 patients covering a period of 8 years. J. Med. Virol. *13*:131–148, 1984.
496. Urquhart, G. E. D., and Gibson, A. A. M.: RSV infections and infant deaths. Br. Med. J. *3*:110, 1970.
497. Urquhart, G. E. D., and Walker, G. H.: Immunofluorescence for routine diagnosis of respiratory syncytial virus infection. J. Clin. Pathol. *25*:843–845, 1972.
498. VanDenIngh, T. S. G. A. M., Averhoeff, J., and VanNieuwstadt, A. P. K. M. I.: Clinical and pathological observations on spontaneous bovine respiratory syncytial virus infections in calves. Res. Vet. Sci. *33*:152–158, 1982.
499. van Milaan, A. J., Sprenger, M. J. W., Rothbarth, P. H., et al.: Detection of respiratory syncytial virus by RNA-polymerase chain reaction and differentiation of subgroups with oligonucleotide probes. J. Med. Virol. *44*:80–87, 1994.
500. Vaux-Peretz, F., Chapsal, J. M., and Meignier, B.: Comparison of the ability of formalin-inactivated respiratory syncytial virus, immunopurified F, G and N proteins and cell lysate to enhance pulmonary changes in Balb/c mice. Vaccine *10*:113–118, 1992.
501. Verhoeff, J., Wierda, A., and Boon, J. H.: Clinical signs following experimental lungworm infection and natural bovine respiratory syncytial virus infection in calves. Vet. Rec. *123*:346–350, 1988.
502. Vikerfors, T., Grandien, M., and Olcen, P.: Respiratory syncytial viral infection in adults. Am. Rev. Respir. Dis. *136*:561–564, 1987.
503. Volovitz, B., Faden, H., and Ogra, P. L.: Releases of leukotriene C4 in respiratory tract during acute viral infection. J. Pediatr. *112*:218–222, 1988.
504. Volovitz, B., Welliver, R. C., de Castro, G., et al.: The release of leukotrienes in the respiratory tract during infection with respiratory syncytial virus: Role in obstructive airway disease. Pediatr. Res. *24*:504–507, 1988.
505. Wagner, D. K., Graham, B. S., Wright, P. F., et al.: Serum immunoglobulin G antibody subclass responses to respiratory syncytial virus F and G glycoproteins after primary infection. J. Clin. Microbiol. *24*:304–306, 1986.
506. Wagner, M. H., Evermann, J. F., Gaskin, J., et al.: Subacute effects of respiratory syncytial virus infection on lung function in lambs. Pediatr. Pulmonol. *11*:56–64, 1991.
507. Walker, R.I.: New strategies for using mucosal vaccination to achieve more effective immunization. Vaccine *12*:387–400, 1994.
508. Wallace, S. J., and Zealley, H.: Neurological, electroencephalographic, and virological findings in febrile children. Arch. Dis. Child. *45*:611–623, 1970.
509. Walsh, E. E.: Mucosal immunization with a subunit respiratory syncytial virus vaccine in mice. Vaccine *11*:1135–1138, 1993.
510. Walsh, E. E., Brandriss, M. W., and Schlesinger, J. J.: Immunological differences between the envelope glycoproteins of two strains of human respiratory syncytial virus. J. Gen. Virol. *68*:2169–2176, 1987.
511. Walsh, E. E., Brandriss, M. W., and Schlesinger, J. J.: Purification and characterization of the respiratory syncytial virus fusion protein. J. Gen. Virol. *66*:409–415, 1985.
512. Walsh, E. E., and Hall, C. B.: Respiratory syncytial virus. *In* Schmidt, N.J., and Emmons, R.W. (eds.): Diagnostic Procedures for Viral and Rickettsial Infections. New York, American Public Health Association, 1989, pp. 693–712.
513. Walsh, E. E., and Hall, C. B.: Approaches to the respiratory syncytial virus vaccine. *In* Meyers, R. A., Beaubien, M. P., and Kraus, H.-J. (eds.): Encyclopedia of Molecular Biology and Molecular Medicine. New York, VCH Publishers, in press.
514. Walsh, E. E., Hall, C. B., Briselli, M., et al.: Protection from respiratory syncytial viral infection in cotton rats by viral glycoprotein subunit immunization. J. Infect. Dis. *55*:1198–1204, 1987.
515. Walsh, E. E., and Hruska, J. F.: Monoclonal antibodies to respiratory syncytial virus proteins: Identification of the fusion protein. J. Virol. *47*:171–177, 1983.
516. Walsh, E. E., Schlesinger, J. J., and Brandriss, M. W.: Protection from respiratory syncytial virus infection in cotton rats by passive transfer of monoclonal antibodies. Infect. Immun. *43*:756–758, 1984.
517. Walsh, E. E., Schlesinger, J. J., and Brandriss, M. W.: Purification and characterization of GP90, one of the envelope glycoproteins of respiratory syncytial virus. J. Gen. Virol. *65*:1–7, 1984.
518. Wang, F., Brytting, M., Bratt, G., et al.: Continuous detection of CMV DNA in plasma of patients with advanced HIV infection implies the poorest prognosis. Clin. Diagn. Virol. *3*:371–375, 1995.
519. Ward, K. A., Lambden, P. R., Ogilivie, M. M., et al.: Antibodies to RSV polypeptides and their significance in human infection. J. Gen. Virol. *64*:1867–1876, 1983.

520. Waris, M.: Pattern of respiratory syncytial virus epidemics in Finland: Two-year cycles with alternating prevalence of groups A and B. J. Infect. Dis. *163*:464–469, 1991.
521. Wathen, M. W., Brideau, R. J., and Thomsen, D. R.: Immunization of cotton rats with the human respiratory syncytial virus F glycoprotein produced using a baculovirus vector. J. Infect. Dis. *159*:255–264, 1989.
522. Wathen, M. W., Kakuk, T. J., Brideau, R. J., et al.: Vaccination of cotton rats with a chimeric FG glycoprotein of human respiratory syncytial virus induces minimal pulmonary pathology on challenge. J. Infect. Dis. *163*:477–482, 1991.
523. Watt, P. J., Robinson, B. S., Pringle, C. R., et al.: Determinants of susceptibility to challenge and the antibody response of adult volunteers given experimental respiratory syncytial virus vaccines. Vaccine *8*:231–236, 1990.
524. Webb, M. S. C., Henry, R. L., Milner, A. D., et al.: Continuing respiratory problems three and a half years after acute viral bronchiolitis. Arch. Dis. Child. *60*:1064–1067, 1985.
525. Welliver, R. C.: Detection, pathogenesis, and therapy of respiratory syncytial virus infections. Clin. Microbiol. Rev. *1*:27–39, 1988.
526. Welliver, R. C., and Duffy, L.: The relationship of RSV-specific immunoglobulin E antibody responses in infancy, recurrent wheezing, and pulmonary function at age 7–8 years. Pediatr. Pulmonol. *15*:19–27, 1993.
527. Welliver, R. C., Kaul, T. N., and Ogra, P. L.: The appearance of cell-bound IgE in respiratory-tract epithelium after respiratory syncytial virus infection. N. Engl. J. Med. *303*:1198–1202, 1980.
528. Welliver, R. C., Kaul, A., and Ogra, P. L.: Cell-mediated immune response to respiratory syncytial virus infection: Relationship to the development of reactive airway disease. J. Pediatr. *94*:370–375, 1979.
529. Welliver, R. C., Kaul, T. N., Putnam, T. I., et al.: The antibody response to primary and secondary infection with respiratory syncytial virus: Kinetics of class specific response. J. Pediatr. *96*:808–813, 1980.
530. Welliver, R. C., Kaul, T. N., Sun, M., et al.: Defective regulation of immune response in respiratory syncytial virus infection. J. Immunol. *133*:1925–1930, 1984.
531. Welliver, R. C., Sun, M., Hildreth, S. W., et al.: Respiratory syncytial virus–specific antibody responses in immunoglobulin A and E isotypes to the F and G proteins and to intact virus after natural infection. J. Clin. Microbiol. *27*:295–299, 1989.
532. Welliver, R. C., Sun, M., Rinaldo, D., et al.: Predictive value of respiratory syncytial virus specific IgE responses for recurrent wheezing following bronchiolitis. J. Pediatr. *109*:776–790, 1986.
533. Welliver, R. C., Wong, D. T., Sun, M., et al.: The development of respiratory syncytial virus-specific IgE and the release of histamine in nasopharyngeal secretions after infection. N. Engl. J. Med. *305*:841–846, 1981.
534. Wennergren, G., Hansson, S., Engstrom, I., et al.: Characteristics and prognosis of hospital-treated obstructive bronchitis in children aged less than two years. Acta Paediatr. *81*:40–45, 1992.
535. Wertz, G. W., Collins, P. L., Huang, Y. T., et al.: Nucleotide sequence of the G protein gene of human respiratory syncytial virus reveals an unusual type of viral membrane protein. Proc. Natl. Acad. Sci. U. S. A. *82*:4075–4079, 1985.
536. Wertz, G. W., Stott, E. J., Young, K. K. Y., et al.: Expression of the fusion protein of human respiratory syncytial virus from recombinant vaccinia virus vectors and protection of vaccinated mice. J. Virol. *61*:293–301, 1987.
537. Wertz, G. W., and Sullender, W. M.: Approaches to immunization against respiratory syncytial virus. Biotechnology *20*:151–176, 1992.
538. Whimbey, E., and Bodey, G. P.: Viral pneumonia in the immunocompromised adult with neoplastic disease: The role of common community respiratory viruses. Semin. Respir. Infect. *7*:122–131, 1992.
539. Williams, A. L., Uren, E. C., and Bretherton, L.: Respiratory viruses and sudden infant death. Br. Med. J. *288*:1491–1493, 1984.
540. Wohl, M. E. B.: Bronchiolitis. Pediatr. Ann. *15*:307–313, 1986.
541. Wohl, M. E. B., and Chernick, V.: Bronchiolitis. Am. Rev. Respir. Dis. *118*:759–781, 1978.
542. Wong, D. T., Rosenband, M., Hovey, K., et al.: Respiratory syncytial virus infection in immunosuppressed animals: Implications in human infection. J. Med. Virol. *17*:359–370, 1985.
543. Woodin, K. A., Hall, C. B., Leibenguth, K. C., et al.: Variables affecting the rapid diagnosis of respiratory syncytial virus (RSV). 28th Interscience Conference on Antimicrobial Agents and Chemotherapy, 1988, p. 145, Abstract No. 204.
544. Wright, P. F., Belshe, R. B., Kim, H. W., et al.: Administration of a highly attenuated live respiratory syncytial virus vaccine to adults and children. Infect. Immun. *37*:397–400, 1982.
545. Wright, P. F., Mills, J., and Chanock, R. M.: Evaluation of a temperature-sensitive mutant of respiratory syncytial virus in adults. J. Infect. Dis. *124*:505–511, 1971.
546. Wright, P. F., Shinozaki, T., Fleet, W., et al.: Evaluation of a live, attenuated respiratory syncytial virus vaccine in infants. J. Pediatr. *88*:931–936, 1976.
547. Yu, Q., Hardy, R. W, and Wertz, G. W.: Functional cDNA clones of the human respiratory syncytial (RS) virus N, P, and L proteins support replication of RS virus genomic RNA analogs and define minimal trans-acting requirements for RNA replication. J. Virol. *69*:2412–2419, 1995.
548. Zweiman, B., Schoenwetter, W. F, and Hildreth, E. A.: The relationship between bronchiolitis and allergic asthma. J. Allergy *37*:48, 1966.

❑ ❑ ❑

SUBSECTION EIGHT

RHABDOVIRIDAE

186

RABIES VIRUS

Stanley A. Plotkin and H. Fred Clark

Rabies is a viral infection of the central nervous system transmitted from animals to people. Introduction of the agent by bite, scratch, or aerosol enables it to attach to and travel up the nerves to the brain. The encephalitis so caused is characterized by hydrophobia and almost always is fatal.

HISTORY[72, 123]

Rabies has a long and colorful history. The Greeks called it *lyssa*, and Democritus is thought to have made the first description of rabies in the dog in 500 B.C. The ultimate derivation of the English word *rabies* is from the Sanskrit word *rabhas*, which means "to do violence." Early writers believed that rabies followed the rising of the star Sirius, and the disease became associated with the dog days of summer.

Celsus, the Roman physician, writing in A.D. 100, displayed an accurate understanding of the disease by attributing infection to a "virus" (i.e., a poison) in the saliva. He advocated cauterization of the wounds produced by rabid animals. Galen, writing a century later, advised surgical resection as the method for preventing rabies.

Rabies was well known in Europe during medieval times, and the great Mohammedan physicians also mention it in their writings. Epizootics, however, were not recorded until 1271, when rabid wolves attacked people in Franconia. Epizootics associated with wolves then occurred frequently in various areas of Europe until early in the 18th century, when epizootics of rabies in domestic dogs began in cities. Rabies probably was transmitted from Europe to the New World, where it became common in North America and the West Indies by the 18th century and spread to South America early in the 19th century. The history of the disease in Asia is not as well known, but rabies clearly has been present since ancient times in China and India.

The scientific study of rabies began with the demonstration by Zinke in 1803 that saliva transmitted the disease. As is well known, it was the work of Louis Pasteur in the 1880s that made possible modern prevention of rabies. He showed that rabies could be transmitted by intracerebral inoculation of a preparation made from the brain of a rabid dog into uninfected rabbits or dogs and then serially transmitted by intracerebral inoculation. He thus demonstrated that rabies is a disease of the central nervous system. Among Pasteur's other discoveries were the differentiation of furious and dumb rabies, the production of rabies by the intravenous route, and the attenuation of rabies virus in the dried spinal cords of infected rabbits. The famous episode of Joseph Meister, the French boy who received rabies vaccine in 1885, demonstrated that serial inoculations of dried infected rabbit spinal cord, proceeding from most attenuated to least attenuated, in principle could protect against rabies.

Vaccination with nerve-tissue vaccines quickly became standard, with important modifications being introduced by Roux, Fermi, and Semple. Semple vaccines, composed of infected sheep or goat brain tissue suspensions in which virus completely was inactivated by phenol, became the standard vaccine in the 1920s.

THE VIRUS

The rabies virus apparently can infect all species of mammals, although wide variations in the sensitivity of different species have been observed. Laboratory propagation may be accomplished readily in mice or other standard laboratory animals; in vitro in neuroblastoma or certain hamster cell cultures; or, after adaptation, in certain other cell lines of human or other mammalian origin.[148]

Electron-microscopic studies reveal that rabies is a bullet-shaped virus typically maturing at cytoplasmic plasma membranes and intracellular membranes of the endoplasmic reticulum in infected cultured cells (Fig. 186–1).[91] Standard virions are approximately 75 nm in diameter and 160 to 180 nm in length. Regular arrays of standard-sized virions maturing from plasma membranes are observed in infected salivary glands. Budding of virus from plasma membrane is much less pronounced in neurons of the central nervous system than in cell culture or salivary gland cells. However, meticulous electron-microscopic examination of experimentally and naturally infected brains has revealed that budding from membranes of perikarya and dendrites as well as presence of virus in intracellular spaces of brain (especially at synaptic junctions) occurs regularly.[70] In addition, central nervous system neurons often exhibit both typical and bizarre morphologic forms of virus maturing in cytoplasm. Cytoplasmic forms often develop in proximity to nucleocapsid matrix inclusions (Negri bodies).[84]

The gross morphologic characteristics and biochemical composition of rabies virus place it within the rhabdovirus group. Until recently, no other rhabdoviruses bearing related antigens were known. However, several recently isolated rhabdoviruses of Old World origin exhibit an antigenic relationship to rabies primarily on the basis of similarities of nucleoprotein components detected by complement fixation and fluorescent antibody tests and by reaction with monoclonal antibodies directed against nucleocapsid epitopes. Therefore, distinct antigenic types, of which six now are recognized (and more are anticipated), have been designated by the World Health Organization. Rabies virus is a *Lyssavirus* type 1 and continues to account for the vast preponderance of isolates. Type 3 (Mokola virus), type 4 (Duvenhage virus subtypes), and type 5 are represented by very rare isolates from humans or animals in Africa or Europe. *Lyssavirus* type 2 and type 6 have not been associated with human disease.[108] However, *Lyssavirus* type 2 (Lagos bat virus) and *Lyssavirus* type 3 (Mokola virus) were isolated from a rabid dog and from a rabid cat, respectively, in Ethiopia.[85]

The rabies virion now is recognized to be of a molecular composition similar to that of the rhabdovirus prototype virus, vesicular stomatitis virus. It is composed of a helical nucleocapsid core, which contains the RNA genome coupled to nucleoprotein, the transcriptase-associated protein, and a large protein presumably representing the RNA transcriptase replicase.[35] The core is surrounded by a lipoprotein envelope, which contains two matrix proteins, a single glycoprotein, and lipids (primarily phospholipids and cholesterol).[19, 122] The genome is a single-stranded RNA molecule containing 11,932 nucleotides with a molecular weight of approximately 4.0×10^6 daltons.[18] It is a negative-stranded genome, that is, it

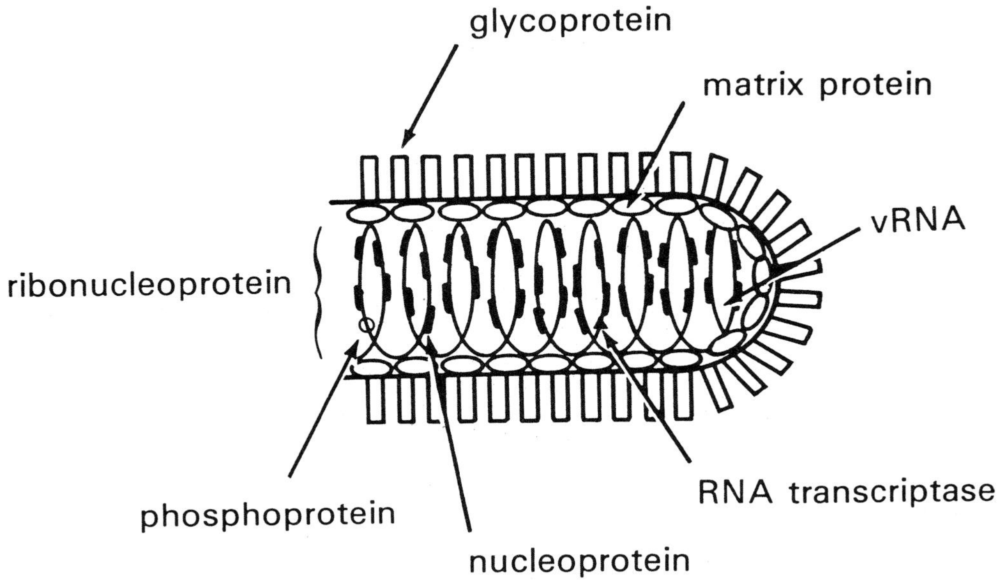

FIGURE 186–1. *Cartoon of the rabies virus. (Courtesy of Dr. William Wunner, Wistar Institute, Philadelphia, PA.)*

rabies); the more common encephalitic depression symptom is associated with early, very widespread infection in the brain. In either case, infection rapidly spreads to infect nearly all brain neurons within a few days of the onset of brain infection and central nervous system symptoms. Brain infection leads rapidly to death by mechanisms that are poorly understood. Fatal cases of encephalitis reveal little damage of neuronal cells, despite the ubiquitous neuronal infection. On the other hand, persons kept alive by vigorous supportive therapy for lengthy periods after onset of disease may develop severe histopathologic encephalitic lesions.

The entire manner of progression of the infecting virus, particularly those points in its transit vulnerable to immune intervention, remains to be determined fully. It is clear that preexisting humoral antibody protects, apparently by inactivating virus before it gains entry to the nervous system. After an immunized person is exposed to rabies, disease can be delayed or prevented in some cases by passive antibody, interferon treatment, or both,[71] but protection becomes efficient only when active immunization with potent vaccine accompanies such treatment. More sophisticated understanding of rabies pathogenesis is required before ideal combinations of immunotherapeutic procedures, possibly including interferon, finally can be formulated.

That neutralizing antibodies are key to protection against rabies has been obvious for many years. However, recent studies have demonstrated the complexity of the immune response.[94] Although the importance of cellular immunity is unclear, the induction of cytotoxic activity against virus-infected cells by vaccination was shown to correlate with protection. Interestingly, rabies-specific cytotoxic T lymphocytes do not develop during the disease, and wild rabies virus may act as an immunosuppressor. Moreover, chemical immunosuppression enhances the development of experimental rabies. Interferon[11] and interleukin-2,[96] both important immunomodulators produced by cells, enhance protection against rabies.

The reverse side of the coin is shown by the "early death" phenomenon, in which exposed animals or humans developed earlier onset of rabies if they partly had been immunized previously. Sugamata and associates[124] have shown that early death depends on the presence of T cells, indicating that it is mediated by an immunopathologic cellular response.

CLINICAL MANIFESTATIONS

In Animals

Rabies encephalitis in animals is expressed in either a paralytic ("dumb") or "furious" syndrome. Typical infections are characterized by behavioral changes and a rapid clinical course leading to coma and death, but occasionally encephalitis can be nonfatal.[8] Because literally millions of animal bites of humans occur annually in the United States, the identification of aberrant behavior is a critical factor in many decisions to treat or not to treat immunoprophylactically for rabies.

The prodromal stage of disease is marked by nonspecific signs, such as restlessness and malaise. Subsequently, placid dogs, cats, cattle, or horses may become vicious. Fear of humans and of areas frequented by them may be lost by wild animals. Thus, rabid foxes, normally nocturnal, may be seen wandering abroad in daylight, even in populous areas. Similarly, rabid bats often have been encountered flying in daytime hours. Early behavioral changes are not accompanied by paralysis.

The clinical course rapidly progresses to either dumb or furious disease. Dumb rabies typically is a depressed encephalitic disease. In addition to lethargy, selectively severe paralysis of throat muscles may be observed, which causes drooling of saliva because of difficulty in swallowing. Hydrophobia is not noted in animals.

Furious rabies is characterized by an unusual state of alertness in which any visual or sound stimulation may incite an attack. Animals may roam indiscriminately, frequently feeding on stones, twigs, and other inanimate objects. Pets alternatively may exhibit unusually affectionate and playful behavior and then viciously bite those playing with them. Biting behavior may be noted by herbivores such as horses, mules, and cattle, as well as by normally carnivorous pets and wild animals.

Both dumb and furious rabies have a rapid clinical course in domestic and wild animals. The period between onset of prodromal signs and death caused by respiratory paralysis rarely exceeds 7 to 10 days. Although 10 days usually is given as the limit of virus excretion in the saliva of dogs before death supervenes, rare exceptions involving prolonged or chronic excretion have been reported experimentally and in animals observed in both Africa and Asia.[47, 139]

In Humans[141, 143, 149, 160]

The incubation period of rabies in some cases may be so long as to qualify it as a slow virus disease. Well-documented cases have occurred as long as 6 years after the bite.[141] However, most cases occur within 20 to 90 days after exposure. The shortest incubation period appears to be 10 days.

It is well known that incubation periods are longer after bites on the legs than after bites on the face. The reason for this appears to be related not to the length of the nerve that the virus must traverse, because it travels rapidly even from the farthest site, but to the extent of innervation of different parts of the body. Bites on the tips of the fingers or on the genitalia have relatively short incubation periods for this reason. Children in general tend to have shorter incubation periods. Curiously, cases of vaccination failure tend to have shorter incubation periods, a fact that also is observed in experimental trials in animals. This "early death" effect is discussed under Pathogenesis.

The first symptoms of rabies usually are vague and insidious. The patient simply may feel unwell or have anxiety or depression. There may be some fever or nausea. The most striking prodromal symptom is itching, pain, or tingling at the site of the bite. This paresthesia is not present always and may take various forms, but its localization is a definite harbinger of rabies. The prodrome lasts 2 to 10 days, when the acute neurologic phase begins. The symptoms of this second phase must be divided into furious versus paralytic rabies, the majority of cases being in the furious category.

In furious rabies, the emphasis is on agitation, hyperactivity, fluctuating consciousness, bizarre behavior, and perhaps nuchal rigidity. Sore throat and hypersalivation are prominent complaints, and laryngospasm may cause hoarseness.

The legendary, but all too real, pathognomonic sign of furious rabies is hydrophobia. Initial attempts to swallow liquid result in painful spasms of the pharyngeal and laryngeal muscles, with aspiration of the liquid into the trachea. A conditioned response appears to be created, in which fear exacerbates the actual spasms. Warrell and associates[142] have hypothesized that brain stem encephalitis leads to destruction of inhibitors of inspiratory motor neurons. Respiratory tract instant reflexes are exaggerated, leading to inspiratory spasms. There is an important psychologic element to the hydrophobia. In an extreme case, spasms occur if the patient merely is approached with water. Also frequently present is aerophobia, in which spasms occur when a current of air is fanned across the face.

The neurologic examination in rabies is not uniform. Meningismus is a common abnormality. Even more common are cranial nerve signs, particularly paralysis of the palate and vocal cords. The voice may develop a hoarse, barking quality. The reflexes may vary from hyperactive to absent, and involuntary movements are prominent.

A distinct pattern of neurologic involvement is shown by approximately 20 to 30 per cent of rabies patients, particularly those bitten by vampire bats. Flaccid paralysis may start in the limb that was bitten originally and spread to other limbs. The cranial nerves become involved, and the face, rather than showing agitation, becomes expressionless. Hydrophobia is not a feature. Paralytic rabies is confused easily with Guillain-Barré syndrome. Hemachuda and colleagues[66] emphasize the importance of fever, intact sensation, urinary incontinence, and percussion myoedema in the former.

The cerebrospinal fluid is abnormal in a minority of patients, particularly those in whom meningismus is present clinically. When abnormal, the cerebrospinal fluid shows a mild pleocytosis, mainly mononuclear. The peripheral white blood cell count shows increased polymorphonuclear cells.

Death due to rabies in the acute stage occurs because of cardiac or respiratory problems. Cardiac arrhythmias with circulatory collapse are common, and virus may be recovered at autopsy from the heart, which shows pathologic evidence of myocarditis. Respiration becomes increasingly labored, and death may occur during a laryngeal spasm or aspiration.

The acute neurologic phase lasts 2 to 10 days, with eventual deterioration of the patient's mental status into coma. The patient may survive in this state for 2 weeks, particularly in dumb rabies. Before the final deterioration, the patient may have alternating periods of wild agitation and alert cooperation. During the alert state, patients may be able to discuss their own illnesses and express fear of impending death. However, most often, death rapidly follows onset of coma, unless intubation and ventilatory assistance are offered, in which case survival may be prolonged for months. During the comatose state, there may be a variety of problems, including cerebral edema; inappropriate antidiuretic hormone secretion; diabetes insipidus; and other manifestations of hypothalamic dysfunction, hypotension or arrhythmia, and pneumonia.

DIAGNOSIS

The diagnosis of rabies in humans begins with its diagnosis in the animal. The technique now most commonly used is to stain the brain of the previously apprehended animal with a fluorescein-labeled antibody to rabies. More recently, enzyme-coupled antibodies have been introduced, allowing the colored product to be seen under the light microscope. Rabies RNA also can be detected by dot hybridization or by polymerase chain reaction amplification.[73] Virus isolation is used for confirmation, either by the classic procedure of intracerebral inoculation in mice or by inoculation of neuroblastoma cells followed by fluorescent antibody staining for rabies antigen.

Unfortunately, there are no known methods for the identification of rabies virus infection before the onset of clinical signs. Although the clinical expression of the disease often is characteristic and diagnosis is simplified by history of known exposure to an animal bite, encephalitic illness may occur, in which rabies virus involvement cannot be diagnosed with certainty without laboratory assistance.

When a patient has a history of being bitten by an animal, paresthesia at the wound site, and hydrophobia, a clinical diagnosis of rabies is not difficult. Other diseases in which there is encephalitis, such as those caused by arboviruses, enteroviruses, and herpes simplex virus, occasionally may cause confusion. However, if one finds signs of brain stem involvement in a patient whose sensorium basically is clear and who has no signs of a space-occupying lesion, the other diagnoses usually can be set aside.

Paralytic rabies may be misdiagnosed as Guillain-Barré syndrome, poliomyelitis, or post–rabies vaccine encephalomyelitis. Careful neurologic examination and analysis of the cerebrospinal fluid often help to rule out these diagnoses.

The spasms of tetanus can cause momentary confusion, but trismus is not part of rabies, and hydrophobia is not part of tetanus. Botulism (wound or ingestion) will cause paralysis, but the absence of sensory changes should exclude rabies.

Postvaccination encephalitis after nerve tissue vaccine poses a diagnostic problem in countries in which it still is used and may require the performance of laboratory tests described later.[42]

Perhaps the most confusing differential problem is hysteria in a person who thinks he or she has rabies. Normal blood gas analyses and the absence of variation in bizarre behavior suggest pseudorabies. Psychiatric and drug-induced reactions also may cause transient diagnostic problems.

Laboratory diagnosis now is possible before death. The virus may be demonstrated by fluorescent antibody stain of smears of corneal epithelial cells[78, 113] or sections of skin from the neck at the hairline.[21, 121] These test results are positive because virus migrates down the nerves from the brain, and both the cornea and hair follicles are richly innervated.

Serologic diagnosis also is possible if the patient survives beyond the acute period. In persons not given postexposure immunoprophylactic treatment, only low levels of antibodies appear.[65] In contrast, patients who have received vaccine show a rapid rise in titer of virus-neutralizing antibodies between 6 and 10 days after the onset of symptoms.[59] Such antibodies are detected most rapidly by an in vitro fluorescent antibody rapid fluorescent focus-inhibition test or by mouse or plaque-reduction neutralization tests. Rabies may be diagnosed in immunized persons by a rise in titer after the onset of clinical symptoms and is suggested by any antibody titer greater than or equal to 1:5000, a level not usually achieved by vaccines. High antibody levels in cerebrospinal fluid are characteristic late in the course of rabies encephalitis; cerebrospinal fluid antibody is not induced efficiently by vaccination.[59, 144]

Rabies virus has been isolated from human saliva between days 4 and 24 after onset of disease.[59] Virus also may be isolated in some cases from cerebrospinal fluid, brain tissue, or urine sediment during the first 2 weeks of illness. In persons surviving longer than this, isolation of virus from body tissues or fluids (or from postmortem brain) may be impossible, presumably because of virus neutralization by humoral antibody.

Postmortem diagnosis can be confirmed by the presence of pathognomonic cytoplasmic inclusions (Negri bodies) in brain tissue, but these are present in less than 80 per cent of cases. Rabies antigen may be detected by fluorescent antibody examination, with higher frequency in brain tissues of persons dying after a brief, acute course of disease. In postmortem tissues, histochemical staining with monoclonal antibody to rabies virus ribonucleoprotein especially may be useful because ribonucleoprotein possesses epitopes resistant to the formalin fixation and the paraffin-embedding process.[88] However, as in the case of virus isolation attempts, identification of virus antigen in brains of persons kept alive for prolonged periods after onset of disease may be extremely difficult.

Rabies now has been recognized post mortem in patients whose history included transplantation of corneas from donors dying of encephalitis. All cases of undiagnosed fatal encephalitis therefore should be studied for rabies, and tissue from such patients should not be used for transplantation.[99]

PROGNOSIS

The recovery of a 6-year-old boy from Ohio who developed rabies after a bat bite fueled optimism that survival in rabies might be possible with intensive care.[103] Other rare survivals have been reported,[1, 25, 61, 105] but the optimism seems to be unjustified. Many other patients now have been treated intensively and nevertheless have died after a prolonged clinical course.[17, 56] Antirabies antibodies, interferon and its inducers, and various antivirals all have been used without evident success. However, the fact that all survivors have had vaccine administered before or after the bite suggests that some immune mechanism may operate to reduce rabies virus replication or inhibit virus-induced pathophysiologic changes.

POSTEXPOSURE PREVENTION[98]

Local Treatment

Removal of saliva containing rabies virus is a crucial part of treatment and should be undertaken urgently. The wound should be flushed copiously with soap and water. Some authors, including ourselves, would follow flushing with a local application of ethyl alcohol in whatever form is immediately available. The concentration of ethanol is important; 43 per cent (86 proof) or higher gives the best results.[150]

Experimental data suggest that, regardless of the solution used, adequate flushing is important, particularly in puncture wounds. Catheters should be inserted into puncture wounds and fluid instilled by means of an attached syringe.[39, 116] If this proves too painful, the area can be anesthetized safely with local procaine-type anesthetics.[74, 150] Suturing should be done in line with good surgical practice but avoided when unnecessary.

Equine Rabies Immunoglobulin

An experimental basis for the desirability of combining antiserum with vaccine was established in 1954.[79] A field test of combined vaccine-serum protection was made possible by a natural disaster, the attack of a rabid wolf on 29 Iranian villagers, 18 of whom were bitten on the head and neck.[13] Rabies developed in three of five persons who were treated with nerve-tissue vaccine only but in only 1 of 13 persons who were given antiserum with nerve-tissue vaccine.

Animal rabies serum is no longer available in the United States. However, an immunoglobulin has been prepared from the serum of rabies-immunized horses (equine rabies immunoglobulin) and now is used extensively outside of the United States because of its lower price and greater availability (compared with human rabies immunoglobulin).[159] The product is dispensed at a concentration of 200 IU/mL, and the dose that should be administered is 40 IU/kg, half of which, if possible, should be infiltrated into the wound. Administration of higher doses dampens the active immune response. To reduce allergic reactions, pepsin digestion is used to convert the equine globulin to a Fab'2 preparation. The manufacturers recommend an intradermal skin test with the equine rabies immunoglobulin, but the sensitivity and specificity of the test for prediction of subsequent allergic reactions are poor, and abandonment of the skin test has been proposed.[158] At least one preparation of equine rabies immunoglobulin was purified sufficiently so that the allergic reaction rate was less than 1 per cent,[156] whereas another yielded a 6 per cent reaction rate.[157]

Human Rabies Immunoglobulin

To avoid possible reactions to animal proteins, gamma-globulin was prepared from the plasma of volunteers hyperimmunized with rabies vaccine. Although expensive, human rabies immunoglobulin is preferable in the United States to equine rabies immunoglobulin for use in postexposure treatment. Because the gamma-globulin is homologous in humans, human rabies immunoglobulin persists longer in the circulation of inoculated persons but for this reason may have an even greater dampening effect on active immunization. Thus, Hattwick and associates[60] found that 23 doses of duck embryo vaccine were needed to overcome the suppressive effect on antibody production of 15 to 40 units of human rabies immunoglobulin per kilogram.

Pharmacokinetic measurements[64, 83, 86, 107] resulted in a recommendation to give 20 IU of human rabies immunoglobulin per kilogram immediately, with approximately half being injected locally if feasible. No further dose is necessary or desirable because excessive antibody diminishes the active response to vaccine. Moreover, if human rabies immunoglobulin is not available immediately, vaccination should be started immediately, followed by administration of human rabies immunoglobulin if it arrives within a week.[75a] Because of the expense and occasional difficulty in obtaining adequate supplies of human rabies immunoglobulin, the World Health Organization now is exploring the possibility of using instead "cocktail" mixtures of neutralizing monoclonal antibodies to rabies virus prepared in either murine[115] or human[42] hybridoma cell cultures.

Nerve-Tissue Vaccine

Most of the rabies vaccine produced in the world today is of nervous tissue origin. Vaccines made in sheep brain or goat brain are used throughout Asia and Africa but are associated with a definite incidence of postvaccinal encephalitis.[7] Suckling mouse brain vaccines are used in South America and Russia to decrease sensitization to myelinated adult nerve tissue, which is the cause of autoimmune allergic encephalitis.[54]

The efficacy of nerve-tissue vaccine in humans has not been evaluated by controlled studies. The Pasteur Institute of Southern India analyzed the incidence of disease in vaccinated and unvaccinated people bitten by animals that were proved rabid by the transmission of rabies to other animals or humans. Fifty-six per cent of untreated persons developed rabies, compared with only 7 per cent of vaccinated persons, for an efficacy of about 88 per cent.[138]

On the other hand, vaccination with nerve-tissue vaccine of persons bitten on the head or neck by rabid wolves in Iran still was followed by a 40 per cent overall mortality rate. In comparison, 15 of 32 villagers (47 per cent) who failed to seek treatment after being attacked by a rabid wolf developed rabies.[68]

Nerve-tissue vaccines are not used in the United States.

Duck Embryo Vaccine

Duck embryo vaccine was developed to overcome the problem of encephalitic reactions to nerve-tissue vaccine. In this respect, it was successful; the incidence of neuroparalytic reactions fell from 1 in 1000 with nerve-tissue vaccine to 1 in 25,000 with duck embryo vaccine.[98, 106, 112] Unfortunately, a high price was paid in immunogenicity. In postexposure treatment of Americans, Corey and associates[37] found that 8 per cent of those given courses of duck embryo vaccine failed to respond with the production of measurable antibody. Even more disturbing was the fact that 23 per cent of recipients of duck embryo vaccine plus rabies antiserum did not develop antibody. Duck embryo vaccine contained enough duck protein to produce a significant number of allergic reactions.[106]

Human Diploid-Cell Vaccine[100]

The ideal solution to the problems of antigenicity and safety of rabies vaccine clearly lay in the development of vaccines prepared from rabies virus grown in cell culture free of neural tissue. For avoiding inclusion of foreign host proteins in the vaccine, the optimal tissue culture would be of human cells.

The basic ingredients for the production of human diploid-cell vaccine were the development of the WI-38 normal human fibroblast cell line by Hayflick and Moorhead[62] and the adaptation of the Pitman-Moore strain of rabies virus to growth in WI-38 by Wiktor and associates.[153] Virus grown in WI-38 or other human fibroblasts is concentrated by ultrafiltration to increase antigen content and then inactivated by β-propiolactone.

After various schedules of human diploid-cell vaccine were tried, it was found that three properly spaced intramuscular doses invariably produced an immune response. A similar schedule of duck embryo vaccine resulted in titers 10 to 20 times lower. The excellent immunogenicity of human diploid-cell virus has been confirmed amply,[6, 22, 38, 55, 102, 104, 137, 155] and it has become the gold standard against which other vaccines are measured.

Table 186–2 shows the serologic data of three persons who received postexposure immunization from one of the authors.[101]

Even with human diploid-cell vaccine, antibodies fall off rapidly after initial immunization, although most who receive human diploid-cell vaccines have some detectable antibody at 2 years after initial vaccination. One booster of human diploid-cell vaccine given to previously vaccinated persons results in a dramatic anamnestic response, with titers rising from 2.8 units to 94 units at 14 days and more than 100 units in 35 days.

The crucial test of a rabies vaccine is protection of those actually exposed to the virus. In Europe, the human diploid-cell vaccine has been used to treat thousands of people exposed to possible rabies. However, it particularly is important to consider those situations in which rabies was confirmed in the biting animal. Kuwert and associates,[81, 82] in Essen, vaccinated 68 persons after exposure to dogs, cats, cows, or wild animals with laboratory-confirmed rabies virus infection or exposed as a result of laboratory accident. The schedule used was 1 mL intramuscularly on days 0, 3, 7, 14, 30, and 90. There were no failures of protection, no significant reactions, and excellent neutralizing and complement-fixing antibody responses.

Bahmanyar and associates in Iran[12] conducted another test of human diploid-cell vaccine. Forty-five persons who were bitten by rabid wolves or dogs were given rabies antiserum, followed by the same schedule of vaccine as that used in Germany. Once again, no rabies was seen in vaccinees, despite a 40 per cent risk (estimated from previous experience) if they had remained unvaccinated. Antibody measurements showed mean titers as follows: 7 days, 1.1 IU; 14 days, 10.7 IU; 30 days, 49 IU; and 100 days, 312 IU.

The Centers for Disease Control and Prevention distributed human diploid-cell vaccine of American manufacture after exposure to persons whose exposure to rabies was established.[2] No vaccine failure occurred, and all who received the full schedule of five 1-mL doses intramuscularly responded with antibodies.

Although a small number of vaccine failures have been reported in other countries after administration of the human diploid-cell vaccine, ancillary treatment recommendations were not followed scrupulously in each case.[4] The failure rate is estimated to be at most 1 in 12,000 courses of vaccination given in high rabies risk countries such as Thailand.[95] General anesthetics given during wound repair may increase the risk of vaccine failure.[49]

Three types of rabies vaccine are available in the United States: human diploid-cell vaccine for intramuscular use; hu-

TABLE 186–2. Antibody Response in Three Children to Postexposure Rabies Vaccination with Human Diploid-Cell Vaccine

Time After Vaccination	Antibody Titers (IU) by Rapid Fluorescent Focus-Inhibition Test					
	Inoculation Schedule	*Case 1*	*Inoculation Schedule*	*Case 2*	*Inoculation Schedule*	*Case 3*
0 day*	V (+ 1 day)†	<0.5	V (+ 3 days)†	<0.4	V (+ 5 days)†	<0.3
3 days	V				V	
7 days	V	<0.1	V	0.6	V	<0.3
14 days	V	13.5	V	1.1	V	0.4
21 days			V			
28 days				17	V	27
30 days	V	20				
38 days		30				
42 days				90		30
3 months		35				
4 months				22		7
7 months						
18 months				2.4		

*Day of first vaccination is day 0.
†Number of days after bite on which human diploid-cell vaccine first was administered.

TABLE 186–3. Schedule of Human Diploid-Cell Vaccine for Immunization Against Rabies

Situation	Vaccine Dosage		
	Route	*Volume*	*Schedule (days)*
Postexposure			
United States	IM	1.0 mL	0, 3, 7, 14, 28
WHO	IM	1.0 mL	0, 3, 7, 14, 30, 90
Rapid*	ID	0.1 mL	0 (8 doses), 7 (4 doses), 28, 91
PVRV	ID	0.1 mL	0 (2 doses), 3 (2 doses), 7 (2 doses), 30, 90
Rapid*	IM	1.0 mL	0 (2 doses), 7, 21
Previously vaccinated	IM	1.0 mL	0, 3
Pre-exposure			
Primary	IM	1.0 mL	0, 7, 21, or 28
	ID	0.1 mL	0, 7, 21, or 28
Booster	IM	1.0 mL	0
	ID	0.1 mL	0

*Not for United States.

man diploid-cell vaccine for intradermal use; and a tissue culture vaccine made in fetal rhesus diploid cells by the Michigan State Department of Health, called rabies vaccine adsorbed.[15] Human diploid-cell vaccine or rabies vaccine adsorbed is recommended for postexposure immunization when given by the intramuscular route according to the regimens listed in Table 186–3. Note that only five doses are recommended in the United States, although the World Health Organization recommends six.[57] The dose should not be reduced for children.[5] Decreased immune responses have been noted in vaccinees given injections in the gluteal area,[52] and therefore all intramuscular injections of rabies vaccine should be given in the deltoids. Although rabies has never been reported in persons with any prior history of vaccination, in the event of re-exposure they should be given two intramuscular booster doses, as also stated in Table 186–3.

The effectiveness of current rabies vaccines to protect against rabies-related lyssaviruses is doubtful.[67]

Alternative Vaccines to Human Diploid-Cell Vaccine

An effort has been made to produce vaccines with the desirable properties of human diploid-cell vaccine at a lower cost that would make them broadly available in the developing nations, where the risk of human rabies is most severe. Their products have been produced in Europe and used primarily in Europe or Asia.

Purified Vero rabies vaccine is the Pasteur strain of rabies (as used in human diploid-cell vaccine) grown in the Vero cell line in industrial fermenters. The virus is concentrated, inactivated, and purified. Purified Vero rabies vaccine has an immunogenic potency similar to that of human diploid-cell vaccine. Successful postexposure experience has been reported in Tunisia[30] and in Thailand, even after severe exposure.[126, 129]

Purified chick embryo-cell rabies vaccine is produced in primary chick embryo-cell culture with use of the Flury LEP strain of rabies virus. It is inactivated, concentrated, and purified, yielding a vaccine preparation of antigenic potency similar to that of purified Vero rabies and human diploid-cell vaccines.[14] Purified chick embyro-cell rabies vaccine was uniformly successful in preventing rabies in postexposure trials in the former Yugoslavia, including subjects who were exposed by wolf bite.[36]

Purified duck embryo-cell rabies vaccine is produced in embryonated duck eggs. The Pitman-Moore virus harvested from the eggs is purified, concentrated, and inactivated.[75]

It is regrettable that although the new vaccines are considerably less expensive than human diploid-cell vaccines, their cost still places them out of reach of many poorer countries. Therefore, because of expensive purification procedures whose need is open to doubt, these less affluent nations often continue to use predominantly nerve-tissue vaccines of high reactogenic potential and variable antigenic potency.

An argument has been made that a potent rabies virus might be made at low cost in BHK-21 cells and, if it were inactivated with β-propiolactone, the β-propiolactone would so damage the cell DNA that the theoretic danger posed by cell DNA in vaccine would be eliminated totally.[90]

A number of regimens have been developed for rapid immunization of exposed patients in poor countries who may seek medical help late or who may not return for subsequent doses.[125, 140] These regimens also are listed in Table 186–3 and have the advantage of being less expensive.

Decisions To Vaccinate

The physician must take into account a number of human and zoologic factors in deciding when to vaccinate, although reluctance to use vaccine now is based more on cost than on the pain of injections. Among the factors to be considered are the following.

Geography

Bites in most large urban areas in the developed world are unlikely to be from rabid animals, although Philadelphia, Baltimore, and Washington, D.C., have become part of the raccoon epizootic, with transfer of disease to urban cats.

Type of Animal

Cats always are suspect if they go out of their way to bite. Dogs near the Mexican border are more suspect than are those farther north. Skunks, foxes, and raccoons involved in biting incidents must be considered rabid until proven otherwise. With the exception of woodchucks, rodents such as squirrels are unlikely to be rabid. Contact with a bat, if there was opportunity for a bite, must be considered an indication for vaccination.

Circumstances of Bite

The attempt to feed an undomesticated animal always must be considered provocative behavior. Invasion of an animal's territory may result in an attack, which is less suspicious of rabies than is an attack by an animal that invades human environments. However, judgment as to whether or not a bite was provoked is poorly predictive of rabies in enzootic areas.[117]

Animal Vaccination

Rabies is extremely rare in properly vaccinated animals.

Table 186–4 summarizes recommendations by the Advisory Committee on Immunization Practices (ACIP) on vaccination against rabies.[28] Advice can be sought from state and local health departments (particularly with regard to the occurrence of rabies in animals) and from the Centers directly.

TABLE 186–4. Pre-Exposure Immunization Against Rabies

	Criteria for Pre-Exposure Immunization		
Risk Category	***Nature of Risk***	***Typical Populations***	***Pre-Exposure Regimen***
Continuous	Virus present continuously, often in high concentrations Aerosol, mucous membrane, bite, or nonbite exposure Specific exposures may go unrecognized	Rabies research lab workers Rabies biologics production workers	Primary pre-exposure immunization course Serologic study every 6 months Booster immunization when antibody titer falls below acceptable level†
Frequent	Exposure usually episodic, with source recognized, but exposure also may be unrecognized Aerosol, mucous membrane, bite, or nonbite exposure	Rabies diagnostic lab workers, spelunkers, veterinarians and staff, and animal control and wildlife workers in rabies epizootic areas Travelers to foreign rabies enzootic areas for more than 30 days	Primary pre-exposure immunization course Booster immunization or serologic study every 2 years†
Infrequent (greater than population at large)	Exposure nearly always episodic with source recognized Mucous membrane, bite, or nonbite exposure	Veterinarians and animal control and wildlife workers in areas of low rabies enzooticity Veterinary students	Primary pre-exposure immunization No routine booster immunization or serologic study
Rare (population at large)	Exposure always episodic Mucous membrane, or bite with source recognized	United States population at large, including individuals in rabies epizootic areas	No pre-exposure immunization‡

Pre-exposure immunization consists of three doses of HDCV or RVA, 1.0 mL, IM (deltoid area); or three doses of HDCV, 0.1 mL, ID, one each on days 0, 7, and 21 or 28.

†Minimum acceptable antibody level is complete virus neutralization of a 1:5 serum dilution by RFFIT. Booster dose should be administered if the titer falls below this level.

‡Consideration now is being given to pre-exposure vaccination of children in countries where exposure to rabies is common.

Modified from the Public Health Service Advisory Committee on Immunization Practices, Atlanta, Georgia: Rabies: Prevention—United States, 1991. M. M. W. R. *40*:RR-3, 1–19, 1991.

PRE-EXPOSURE IMMUNIZATION

The development of human diploid-cell vaccine has made immunization of persons at risk of coming into contact with rabies virus possible before the actual exposure. Veterinarians, animal handlers, laboratory workers, and spelunkers need pre-exposure immunization. Large numbers of veterinary students have been vaccinated with human diploid-cell vaccine under a three-dose schedule at 0, 7, and 21 or 28 days. Rabies antibody titers were determined on the serum of each veterinary student. Nearly 100 per cent developed antibodies, with geometric mean titers of 10 IU or greater, which is equivalent to a neutralizing antibody titer of at least 1:400.[80, 105] The three-dose regimen listed in Table 186–3 induces antibodies in 100 per cent of recipients if the precautions are taken into account. Pre-exposure immunization may be given with use of human diploid-cell vaccine or rabies vaccine absorbed by intramuscular administration (see Table 186–4). Alternatively, and more cheaply, immunization may be performed intradermally with the human diploid-cell vaccine intradermal formulation, according to the same schedule. Intradermal vaccine should not be used for postexposure immunization in the United States; in poor countries, however, considerations of cost may force its use, and alternative schedules have been developed (discussed later). The success of intradermal vaccination depends on technique that ensures intradermal rather than subcutaneous injection, but there is a margin of error.[16, 51]

Although antibody responses are sufficiently regular that postimmunization testing usually is unnecessary, if a test is obtained, neutralizing antibody titers of 1/25 or 0.5 IU are considered protective.

Intradermal Vaccination

The place of intradermal vaccination in rabies prophylaxis is somewhat controversial. For pre-exposure use, the intradermal route is considered an acceptable alternative, with the important proviso that persons receiving antimalarial or other immunosuppressive agents and perhaps older persons should have their titers checked after vaccination or receive the injections by the intramuscular route. Trimarchi and Safford[133] reported that about 7 per cent of persons failed to develop rabies neutralizing antibodies after intradermal vaccination.

Intradermal vaccination for postexposure use to reduce the costs of vaccination has become popular in developing countries. Although single-dose preparations are not available for the intradermal route, extensive experience in Thailand and elsewhere has validated the successful prevention of rabies using this route.[45, 135, 145, 146] However, attention must be paid to the correct administration of the dose into the skin, the sterility of unused portions of the vial, and the antigenic content of the vaccine used. For example, purified duck embryo–cell vaccine must be used in a 0.2-mL dose because of its lower antigenic content.[117]

Poor responses to intradermal vaccine have been noted in those concurrently receiving chloroquine or immunosuppressives, such as corticosteroids.[28, 97] Therefore, persons who must be vaccinated while they are taking chloroquine or related antimalarials should be given injections into the deltoid muscle, and postvaccination rabies serologic studies should be obtained on those patients and others who are immunosuppressed.

Alternative Schedules

Although the American and World Health Organization (sometimes called Essen) schedules firmly are established for the induction of optimal immune responses, other schedules have been tested extensively to reduce the number of vaccination visits, particularly in the developing world. The most popular of these are the 2-1-1 schedule, in which a double dose is given intramuscularly at day 0, followed by single doses on days 7 and 21,[34, 89] and the regimen developed by Warrell and associates,[145] consisting of eight intradermal doses on day 0, four intradermal doses on day 7, and single doses on days 28 and 91.[45]

Booster Doses

Once an immune response to rabies vaccine has developed, a person probably is sensitized forever. Nevertheless, even with human diploid-cell vaccine, antibodies fall off rapidly after initial immunization, although most human diploid-cell vaccines have some detectable antibody at 2 years after initial vaccination. One booster of human diploid-cell vaccine given to previously vaccinated persons results in a dramatic anamnestic response, with titers in one study rising from 2.8 IU to 94 IU at 14 days and more than 100 IU in 35 days.[100] As mentioned, with exposure to rabies in a previously vaccinated person, two intramuscular booster doses are recommended to provide a margin of safety. Single intramuscular or intradermal boosters are given to maintain immunity in those chronically exposed to rabies according to the recommendations made by the Centers for Disease Control and Prevention in Table 186–5.

In persons who have received pre-exposure immunization to rabies, the necessity of boosters is an important issue. Those who definitely are exposed to a rabid animal should receive two booster doses of vaccine by the intramuscular route. Those who are likely to be exposed, such as rabies laboratory workers, are boosted to maintain their antibody titers above 0.5 IU. Booster vaccination is not recommended for others who are less exposed, but a follow-up study by Briggs and Schwenke[20] is interesting. They found maintenance of an adequate titer (>0.5 IU) at 1.5 to 2 years after vaccination in 99 per cent of subjects who received vaccine by the intramuscular route and in 93 per cent who received vaccine by the intradermal route. Peace Corps volunteers, who are exposed to immunosuppressive drugs, showed adequate antibody levels in 88 per cent after intramuscular vaccination but only 64 per cent after intradermal vaccination. On the other hand, Thraenhart and associates[130] observed 100 per cent positive antibodies in 18 subjects studied between 2 and 14 years after vaccination.

Adverse Reactions

The available tissue culture vaccines are well tolerated. In more than 1770 human volunteers receiving pre-exposure immunization with human diploid-cell vaccine intramuscularly, sore arm was noted in about 20 per cent, headache in about 8 per cent, malaise in 5 per cent, and allergic edema in 0.1 per cent.[100] Pregnancy is not a contraindication to modern rabies vaccines.[33] Guillain-Barré syndrome and other neurologic problems have been rare, and their relationship to human diploid-cell vaccine is uncertain.[77] Guillain-Barré syndrome after nerve-tissue vaccine is associated with antibodies to myelin basic protein.[66]

In contrast, booster vaccinations with human diploid-cell vaccine have been associated with allergic reactions in about 6 per cent of subjects.[29] These reactions are due to the presence in the vaccine of human albumin that has been altered by the β-propiolactone used to inactivate the virus.[3, 128, 147]

TABLE 186–5. Rabies Postexposure Prophylaxis Guide

Animal Species	Condition of Animal at Time of Attack	Treatment of Exposed Person*
Dog and cat	Healthy and available for 10 days' observation	None, unless animal develops symptoms of rabies
	Rabid or suspected rabid	HRIG and HDCV†
	Unknown (escaped)	Consult public health officials; if treatment is indicated, give HRIG and HDCV†
Skunk, raccoon, fox, bat, and other carnivores; woodchucks	Regard as rabid unless proven negative by laboratory tests‡	HRIG and HDCV†
Livestock, rodents, and lagomorphs (rabbits and hares)	Consider individually. Local and state public health officials should be consulted on questions about the need for rabies prophylaxis. Bites of squirrels, hamsters, guinea pigs, gerbils, chipmunks, rats, mice, other rodents, rabbits, and hares almost never call for antirabies prophylaxis.	

These recommendations are only a guide. In applying them, take into account the animal species involved, the circumstances of the exposure, the vaccination status of the animal, and the presence of rabies in the region. Local or state public health officials should be consulted if questions arise about the need for rabies prophylaxis.

*All bites and wounds should be cleansed thoroughly immediately with soap and water. If antirabies treatment is indicated, HRIG and rabies vaccine should be given as soon as possible, regardless of the interval from exposure. Local reactions to vaccines are common and do not contraindicate continuing treatment. Discontinue vaccine if immunofluoresence tests of the animal are negative.

During the usual holding period of 10 days, begin treatment with HRIG and HDCV or RVA at first sign of rabies in a dog or cat that has bitten someone. The symptomatic animal should be killed immediately and tested.

†RVA or PVRV are alternatives to HDCV (see text).

‡The animal should be killed and tested as soon as possible. Holding for observation is not recommended. Rabies postexposure prophylaxis (PEP) is recommended for all persons with bite, scratch, or mucous membrane exposure to a bat, unless the bat is available for testing and is negative for evidence of rabies. The inability of care providers to elicit information surrounding potential exposures may be influenced by the limited injury inflicted by a bat bite (compared with lesions inflicted by terrestrial carnivores) or by circumstances that hinder accurate recall of events. Therefore, PEP also is appropriate even in the absence of a demonstrable bite or scratch and in situations in which there is reasonable probability that such contact occurred (e.g., a sleeping individual awakes to find a bat in the room, an adult witnesses a bat in the room with a previously unattended child, mentally challenged person, intoxicated individual, etc.).

Modified from the Public Health Service Advisory Committee on Immunization Practices, Atlanta, Georgia: Rabies: Prevention—United States, 1984 (and 1991). M. M. W. R. *33*:393–402, 1984 and M. M. W. R. *40*:RR-3, 1–19, 1991.

The reactions are of the immune complex type (type III), with urticaria, edema, joint manifestations, fever, and malaise. Centers for Disease Control and Prevention data suggest that when primary vaccination is given intramuscularly and booster intradermally or vice-versa, reactions are more common than if all vaccination is by the same route.[53] Because the reaction is associated with the particular formulation of human diploid-cell vaccine rather than with the rabies antigen itself, additional boosters may be given if necessary with rabies vaccine absorbed or human diploid-cell vaccine manufactured in Canada (Connaught).[50]

FUTURE DEVELOPMENTS

The world of rabies is far from static. Table 186–6 shows the progress of rabies vaccine development for humans. Perhaps the most dramatic future prospect is the development of vaccines in which the gene for rabies glycoprotein has been inserted into a viral vector, such as vaccinia.[111] Amazingly, these vaccines are safe and highly immunogenic when fed to a large variety of animal species.[109] In field studies, raccoons and other wild animals already have been immunized successfully with baits containing rabies recombinant vaccine. Other avenues being pursued include the use of potent adjuvants to enhance the immunogenicity of subunit vaccine,[48] the addition of the internal ribonucleoprotein to enhance protection through induction of cellular immune responses and higher antibody responses,[131] animal poxvirus vectors in which the rabies glycoprotein gene has been inserted,[23] synthetic peptides constructed from epitopes of the single glycoprotein and nucleoprotein,[41] and plasmid vectors containing cDNA of the single glycoprotein genes.[162] Rabies continues to stimulate scientists, particularly in vaccinology.

TABLE 186–6. Some Rabies Vaccines Developed for Humans

Vaccine Types	Remarks
Pasteur: dried rabbit spinal cord	Residual live virus
Fermi: phenolized sheep or goat brain	Residual live virus
Semple: phenol-inactivated sheep or goat brain	Contains nerve tissue
Fuenzalida: phenol-inactivated suckling mouse brain	Contains less myelin
Duck embryo: β-propiolactone (BPL)–inactivated	Allergy to duck proteins
Human diploid (HDCV): BPL-inactivated fetal human cell culture vaccine	Current standard Booster allergic reactions
Rhesus diploid (RVA): fetal rhesus cell culture BPL-inactivated	Fewer allergic reactions
Vero cell (PVRV): BPL-inactivated virus grown in Vero monkey kidney cell line	Purified by density gradient centrifugation
PCEC rabies vaccine: inactivated virus grown in chick embryo cells	Purified as with PVRV
Vaccinia recombinant (VRG): genetic construct expressing rabies glycoprotein	Probably will be used only in animals (see text)

References

1. Alvarez, L., Fajardo, R., Lopez, E., et al.: Partial recovery from rabies in a nine-year-old boy. Pediatr. Infect. Dis. J. *13*:1154–1155, 1994.
2. Anderson, L. J., Sikes, R. K., Langkop, C. W., et al.: Postexposure trial of a human diploid cell strain rabies vaccine. J. Infect. Dis. *142*:133–137, 1980.
3. Anderson, M. C., Baer, H., Frazier, D. J., et al.: The role of specific IgE and beta-propiolactone in reactions resulting from booster doses of human diploid cell rabies vaccine. J. Allergy Clin. Immunol. *80*:861–868, 1987.
4. Anonymous: Rabies vaccine failures. Lancet *1*:912, 1988.
5. Aoki, F. Y., Rubin, M. E., and Fast, M. V.: Rabies neutralizing antibody in serum of children compared to adults following post-exposure prophylaxis. Biologicals *20*:283–287, 1992.
6. Aoki, F. Y., Tyrrell, D. A. J., Hill, L. E., et al.: Immunogenicity and acceptability of a human diploid-cell culture rabies vaccine in volunteers. Lancet *1*:660–662, 1975.
7. Applebaum, E., Greenberg, M., and Nelson, J.: Neurological complications following antirabies vaccine. J. A. M. A. *151*:188–191, 1953.
8. Arko, R. J., Schneider, L. G., and Baer, G. M.: Nonfatal canine rabies. Am. J. Vet Res. *34*:937–938, 1973.
9. Arrellano-Sota, C.: Biology, ecology, and control of the vampire bat. Rev. Infect. Dis. *10*(Suppl. 4):S615–S619, 1988.
10. Baer, G. M., and Cleary, V. F.: A model in mice for the pathogenesis and treatment of rabies. J. Infect. Dis. *125*:520–527, 1972.
11. Baer, G. M., Moore, S. A., Shaddock, J. H., et al.: An effective rabies treatment in exposed rabies monkeys. Bull. W. H. O. *57*:807–813, 1979.
12. Bahmanyar, M., Fayaz, A., Nour-Salehi, S., et al.: Successful protection of humans exposed to rabies infection: Postexposure treatment with the new human diploid cell rabies vaccine and antirabies serum. J. A. M. A. *236*:2751–2754, 1976.
13. Baltazard, M., Bahmanyar, M., Ghodssi, M., et al.: Essai pratique du serum antirabique les mordus par loups enrage. Bull. W. H. O. *13*:747–772, 1955.
14. Barth, R., Gruschkau, H., Bijok, U., et al.: A new inactivated tissue culture rabies vaccine for use in man: Evaluation of PCEC-vaccine by laboratory test. J. Biol. Stand. *12*:29–46, 1984.
15. Berlin, B. S., Mitchell, J. R., Burgoyne, G. H., et al.: Rhesus diploid rabies vaccine (adsorbed): A new rabies vaccine. J. A. M. A. *249*:2663–2665, 1983.
16. Bernard, K. W., Mallonee, J., Wright, J. C., et al.: Preexposure immunization with intradermal human diploid cell rabies vaccine. J. A. M. A. *257*:1059–1063, 1987.
17. Bhatt, D. R., Hattwick, M. A. W., Gerdsen, R., et al.: Human rabies: Diagnosis, complications, and management. Am. J. Dis. Child. *127*:862–869, 1974.
18. Bishop, D. H. L., Aaslestad, H. G., Clark, H. F., et al.: Evidence for the sequence homology and genome size of rhabdovirus RNA's. *In* Mahy, B. W. J., and Barry, R. D. (eds.): Negative Strand Viruses. Vol. 1. New York, Academic Press, 1975, pp. 259–292.
19. Blough, H. A., Tiffany, J. M., and Aaslestad, H. G.: Lipids of rabies virus and BHK-21 cell membranes. J. Virol. *21*:950–955, 1977.
20. Briggs, D. J., and Schwenke, J. R.: Longevity of rabies antibody titre in recipients of human diploid cell rabies vaccine. Vaccine *10*:125–129, 1992.
21. Bryceson, A. D. M., Breenwood, B. M., Warrell, D. A., et al.: Demonstration during life of rabies antigen in humans. J. Infect. Dis. *131*:71–74, 1975.
22. Cabasso, V. J., Dobkin, M. B., Roby, R. E., et al.: Antibody response to a human diploid cell rabies vaccine. Appl. Microbiol. *27*:553–561, 1974.
23. Cadoz, M., Strady, A., Meignier, B., et al.: Immunisation with canarypox virus expressing rables glycoprotein. Lancet *339*:1429–1432, 1992.
24. Celis, E., Ou, D., Dietzschold, B., et al.: Recognition of rabies and rabies-related viruses by T cells derived from human vaccine recipients. J. Virol. *62*:3128–3134, 1988.
25. Centers for Disease Control: Rabies in a laboratory worker: New York. M. M. W. R. *26*:183, 1977.
26. Centers for Disease Control: Rabies Surveillance: Annual Summary, 1975. Issued August 1976.
27. Centers for Disease Control: Rabies Surveillance: Annual Summary, 1976. Issued October 1977.
28. Centers for Disease Control: Recommendation of the Immunization Practices Advisory Committee, Rabies Prevention—United States, 1990.
29. Centers for Disease Control: Systemic allergic reactions following immunization with human diploid cell rabies vaccine. M. M. W. R. *33*:185–187, 1984.
30. Chadli, A., Merieux, C., Arrouji, A., et al.: Study on the efficacy of a vaccine produced from rabies virus cultivated on Vero cells. *In* Vodopija, I., Nicholson, K. G., Smerdel, S., et al. (eds.): Improvements in Rabies Post-Exposure Treatment. Zagreb, Zagreb Institute of Public Health, 1985, pp. 129–136.

31. Charlton, K. M.: The pathogenesis of rabies and other lyssaviral infections: Recent studies. Curr. Top. Microbiol. Immunol. *187*:95–119, 1994.
32. Charlton, K. M., and Casey, G. A.: Experimental rabies in skunks: Immunofluorescence light and electron microscopic studies. Lab. Invest. *41*:36–44, 1979.
33. Chutivongse, S., Wilde, H., Benjavongkulchai, M., et al.: Postexposure rabies vaccination during pregnancy: Effect on 202 women and their infants. Clin. Infect. Dis. *20*:818–820, 1995.
34. Chutivongse, S., Wilde, H., Fishbein, D. B., et al.: One-year study of the 2-1-1 intramuscular postexposure rabies vaccine regimen in 100 severely exposed Thai patients using rabies immune globulin and Vero cell rabies vaccine. Vaccine *9*:573–576, 1991.
35. Clark, H. F., and Prabhakar, B. S.: Rabies. *In* Olsen, R. G., Krakowka, G. S., and Blakesle, J. R. (eds.): Comparative Pathobiology of Viral Disease. Vol. 2. Boca Raton, CRC Press, 1985, pp. 165–214.
36. Clark, H. F., and Vodapija, I.: Human vaccination against rabies. *In* Baer, G. (ed.): Natural History of Rabies. 2nd ed., Vol. 2. Boca Raton, CRC Press, 1990.
37. Corey, L., Hattwick, M. A. W., Baer, G. W., et al.: Serum neutralizing antibody after rabies postexposure prophylaxis. Ann. Intern. Med. *85*:170–176, 1976.
38. Cox, J. H., and Schneider, L. G.: Prophylactic immunization of humans against rabies by intradermal inoculation of human diploid cell culture vaccine. J. Clin. Microbiol. *3*:96–101, 1976.
39. Dean, D. J., Baer, G. M., and Thompson, W. R.: Studies on the local treatment of rabies-infected wounds. Bull. W. H. O. *28*:477–486, 1963.
40. Dietzschold, B.: Oligosaccharides of the glycoprotein of rabies virus. J. Virol. *23*:293–296, 1977.
41. Dietzschold, B., and Ertl, H. C. J.: New developments in the pre-exposure and post-exposure treatment of rabies. Crit. Rev. Immunol. *10*:427–440, 1991.
42. Dietzschold, B., Gore, M., Casali, P., et al.: Biological characterization of human monoclonal antibodies to rabies virus. J. Virol. *64*:3087–3090, 1990.
43. Dietzschold, B., Rupprecht, C. E., Tollis, M., et al.: Antigenic diversity of the glycoprotein and nucleocapsid proteins of rabies and rabies-related viruses: Implications for epidemiology and control of rabies. Rev. Infect. Dis. *10*:S785–S798, 1988.
44. Dietzschold, B., Wang, H., Rupprecht, C. E., et al.: Induction of protective immunity against rabies by immunization with rabies virus ribonucleoprotein. Proc. Natl. Acad. Sci. U. S. A. *84*:9165–9169, 1987.
45. Dutta, J. K., Warrell, M. J., and Dutta, T. K.: Intradermal rabies immunization for pre- and post-exposure prophylaxis. Natl. Med. J. India *7*:119–122, 1994.
46. Eng, T. R., Fishbein, D. B., Talamante, H. E., et al.: Urban epizootic of rabies in Mexico: Epidemiology and impact of animal bite injuries. Bull. W. H. O. *71*:615–624, 1993.
47. Fekadu, M.: Pathogenesis of rabies virus infection in dogs. Rev. Infect. Dis. *10*:S678–S683, 1988.
48. Fekadu, M., Shaddock, J. H., Ekstrom, J., et al.: An immune stimulating complex (ISCOM) subunit rabies vaccine protects dogs and mice against street rabies challenge. Vaccine *10*:192–197, 1992.
49. Fescharek, R., Franke, V., and Samuel, M. R.: Do anaesthetics and surgical stress increase the risk of post-exposure rabies treatment failure? Vaccine *12*:12–13, 1994.
50. Fishbein, D. B., Dreesen, D. W., Holmes, D. F., et al.: Human diploid cell rabies vaccine purified by zonal centrifugation: A controlled study of antibody response and side effects following primary and booster pre-exposure immunizations. Vaccine *7*:437–442, 1988.
51. Fishbein, D. B., Pacer, R. E., Holmes, D. F., et al.: Rabies preexposure prophylaxis with human diploid cell rabies vaccine: A dose-response study. J. Infect. Dis. *156*:50–55, 1987.
52. Fishbein, D. B., Sawyer, L. A., Reid-Sanden, F. L., et al.: Administration of human diploid-cell rabies vaccine in the gluteal area. N. Engl. J. Med. *318*:124–125, 1988.
53. Fishbein, D. B., Yenne, K. M., Dreesen, D. W., et al.: Risk factors for systemic hypersensitivity reactions after booster vaccinations with human diploid cell rabies vaccine: A nationwide prospective study. Vaccine *11*:1390–1394, 1993.
54. Fuenzalida, E., Palacios, R., and Borgono, J. M.: Antirabies antibody response in man to vaccine made from infected suckling-mouse brains. Bull. W. H. O. *30*:431–436, 1964.
55. Garner, W. O., Jones, D. O., and Pratt, E.: Problems associated with rabies pre-exposure prophylaxis. J. A. M. A. *235*:1131–1132, 1976.
56. Gode, G. R., Jayalakshami, T. S., Raju, A. V., et al.: Intensive care in rabies therapy: Clinical observations. Lancet *2*:6–8, 1976.
57. Gross, E. M., Belmaker, I., and Torok, V.: Diploid cell rabies vaccine, six doses or five? Lancet *2*:1339, 1987.
58. Halonen, P. E., Murphy, F. A., Fields, B. N., et al.: Hemagglutinin of rabies and some other bullet-shaped viruses. Proc. Soc. Exp. Biol. Med. *127*:1037–1042, 1968.
59. Hattwick, M. A. W., and Gregg, M. B.: The disease in man. *In* Baer, G. M. (ed.): The Natural History of Rabies. New York, Academic Press, 1975, pp. 281–304.
60. Hattwick, M. A. W., Rubin, R. H., Music, S., et al.: Postexposure rabies prophylaxis with human rabies immune globulin. J. A. M. A. *227*:407–410, 1974.
61. Hattwick, M. A. W., Weis, T. T., Stechaschulte, C. J., et al.: Recovery from rabies in man. Ann. Intern. Med. *76*:931–942, 1972.
62. Hayflick, L., and Moorhead, P. S.: The serial cultivation of human diploid cell strains. Exp. Cell. Res. *25*:585–621, 1961.
63. Heick, A.: Prince Dracula, rabies, and the vampire legend. Ann. Intern. Med. *117*:172–173, 1920.
64. Helmick, C., Johnstone, C., Sumner, J., et al.: A clinical study of Merieux human rabies immune globulin. J. Biol. Stand. *10*:357–367, 1982.
65. Hemachuda, T.: Human rabies: Clinical aspects, pathogenesis, and potential therapy. Curr. Top. Microbiol. Immunol. *187*:121–143, 1994.
66. Hemachuda, T., Griffin, D. E., Chen, W. W., et al.: Immunologic studies of rabies vaccination–induced Guillain-Barré syndrome. Neurology *38*:375–378, 1988.
67. Hertzog, M., Fritzell, C., Lafage, M., et al.: T and B cell human responses to European bat lyssaviruses after postexposure rabies vaccination. Clin. Exp. Immunol. *85*:224–230, 1991.
68. Hildreth, E. A.: Prevention of rabies, or the decline of Sirius. Ann. Intern. Med. *58*:833–896, 1963.
69. Houff, S. A., Burton, R. C., Wilson, R. W., et al.: Human-to-human transmission of rabies virus by corneal transplant. N. Engl. J. Med. *300*:603–604, 1979.
70. Iwasaki, Y., Liu, D. S., Yamamoto, T., et al.: The replication and spread of rabies virus in the human central nervous system. J. Neuropathol. Exp. Neurol. *44*:185–195, 1985.
71. Janis, B., and Habel, K.: Rabies in rabbits and mice: Protective effect of polyribosinic-polyribocytidylic acid. J. Infect. Dis. *125*:345–352, 1972.
72. Johnson, H. N.: Rabies virus. *In* Horsfall, F., and Tamm, I. (eds.): Viral and Rickettsial Diseases of Man. Philadelphia, J. B. Lippincott, 1965.
73. Kamolvarin, N., Tirawatnpong, T., Rattanasiwamoke, R., et al.: Diagnosis of rabies by polymerase chain reaction with nested primers. J. Infect. Dis. *167*:207–210, 1993.
74. Kaplan, M. M., Cohen, D., Koprowski, H., et al.: Studies on the local treatment of wounds for the prevention of rabies. Bull. W. H. O. *26*:765–775, 1962.
75. Khawplod, P., Glueck, R., Wilde, H., et al.: Immunogenicity of purified duck embryo rabies vaccine (Lyssavac-N) with use of the WHO-approved intradermal postexposure regimen. Clin. Infect. Dis. *20*:646–651, 1995.
75a. Khawplod, P., Wilde, H., Chomchey, P., et al.: What is an acceptable delay in rabies immune globulin administration when vaccine alone had been given previously? Vaccine *14*:389–391, 1996.
76. King, A. A., and Turner, G. S.: Rabies: A review. J. Comp. Pathol. *108*:1–39, 1993.
77. Knittel, T., Ramadori, G., Mayet, W. J., et al.: Guillain-Barré syndrome and human diploid cell rabies vaccine. Lancet *1*:1334–1335, 1989.
78. Koch, F. J., Sagartz, J. W., Davidson, D. E., et al.: Diagnosis of human rabies by the cornea test. Am. J. Clin. Pathol. *63*:509–515, 1975.
79. Koprowski, H., and Black, J.: Studies on chick-embryo–adapted rabies virus. V. Protection of animals with antiserum and living attenuated virus after exposure to street strain of rabies virus. J. Immunol. *72*:84–93, 1954.
80. Kramer, T. T.: Personal communication, 1978.
81. Kuwert, E. K., Marcus, I., and Hoher, P. G.: Neutralizing and complement-fixing antibody responses on pre- and postexposure vaccines to a rabies vaccine produced in human diploid cells. J. Biol. Stand. *4*:249–262, 1976.
82. Kuwert, E. K., Werner, J., Marcus, I., et al.: Immunization against rabies with rabies immune globulin, human (RIGH) and a human diploid cell strain (HDCS) rabies vaccine. J. Biol. Stand. *6*:211–219, 1978.
83. Loofbourow, J., Cabasso, V., Roby, R., et al.: Human rabies immune globulin: Clinical trials and dose determination. J. A. M. A. *217*:1825–1831, 1971.
84. Matsumoto, S.: Electron microscopy of central nervous system infection. *In* Baer, G. M. (ed.): The Natural History of Rabies. New York, Academic Press, 1975, pp. 33–61.
85. Mebatsion, T., Cox, J. H., and Frost, J. W.: Isolation and characterization of 115 street rabies virus isolates from Ethiopia by using monoclonal antibodies: Identification of two isolates as Mokola and Lagos bat virus. J. Infect. Dis. *166*:972–797, 1992.
86. Mertz, G. J., Nelson, K. E., Vithayasai, V., et al.: Antibody responses to human diploid cell vaccine for rabies with and without human rabies immune globulin. J. Infect. Dis. *145*:720–727, 1982.
87. Meslin, F. X., Fishbein, D. B., and Matter, H. C.: Rationale and prospects for rabies elimination in developing countries. Curr. Top. Cell Regul. *187*:1–26, 1994.
88. Metze, K., and Feiden, W.: Demonstration of rabies virus antigen at autopsy. Hum. Pathol. *24*:930, 1993.
89. Meyer, J. P., Tissot, J., Estavoyer, J. M., et al.: Efficacy and immunogenicity of reduced anti-rabies vaccination schedule in subjects in contact with rabies-infected animals. Presse Med. *21*:319, 1992.
90. Morgeaux, S., Tordo, N., Gonteur, C., et al.: Propiolactone treatment impairs the biological activity of residual DNA from BHK-21 cells infected with rabies virus. Vaccine *11*:82–90, 1993.
91. Murphy, F. A.: Morphology and morphogenesis. *In* Baer, G. M. (ed.): The Natural History of Rabies. New York, Academic Press, 1975, pp. 33–61.

92. Murphy, F. A.: Rabies pathogenesis: A brief review. Arch. Virol. *54*:279–297, 1977.
93. Murphy, F. A., and Bauer, S. P.: Early street rabies virus infection in striated muscle and later progression to the central nervous system. Intervirology *3*:256–268, 1974.
94. Nathanson, N., and Ganzalez, S. F.: Immune response to rabies virus. 145–161, 1991.
95. Nicholson, K. G.: Modern vaccines. Lancet *335*:1201–1205, 1990.
96. Numberg, J., II, Doyle, M. U., York, S. M., et al.: Interleukin-2 acts as an adjuvant to increase the potency of inactivated rabies virus vaccines. Proc. Natl. Acad. Sci. U. S. A. *86*:4240–4243, 1989.
97. Pappaioanou, M., Fishbein, D. B., Dreesen, D. W., et al.: Antibody response to preexposure human diploid-cell rabies vaccine given concurrently with chloroquine. N. Engl. J. Med. *314*:280–284, 1986.
98. Plotkin, S. A., and Clark, H. F.: Committee on immunization: Prevention of rabies in man. J. Infect. Dis. *123*:227–240, 1971.
99. Plotkin, S. A., and Koprowski, H.: Phobia of hydrophobia justified. N. Engl. J. Med. *300*:620–622, 1979.
100. Plotkin, S. A., and Wiktor, T. J.: Rabies vaccination. Annu. Rev. Med. *29*:583–591, 1978.
101. Plotkin, S. A., and Wiktor, T. J.: Vaccination of children with human cell culture rabies vaccine. Pediatrics *63*:219–221, 1979.
102. Plotkin, S. A., Wiktor, T. J., Koprowski, H., et al.: Immunization schedules for the new human diploid cell vaccine against rabies. Am. J. Epidemiol. *103*:75–80, 1976.
103. Porras, C., Barboza, J. J., Fuenzalida, E., et al.: Recovery from rabies: A case report. Ann. Intern. Med. *85*:44–48, 1976.
104. Public Health Service Advisory Committee on Immunization Practices, Atlanta, Georgia: Rabies: Prevention—United States. M. M. W. R. *33*:393–402, 1984.
105. Rosanoff, E., and Tint, H.: Responses to human diploid cell rabies vaccine: Neutralizing antibody responses of vaccinees receiving booster doses of human diploid cell rabies vaccine. Am. J. Epidemiol. *110*:322–327, 1978.
106. Rubin, R. H., Hattwick, M. A. W., Jones, S., et al.: Adverse reactions to duck embryo rabies vaccine. Ann. Intern. Med. *78*:643–649, 1973.
107. Rubin, R., Kikes, K., Gregg, M.: Human rabies immune globulin: Clinical trials and effects on serum anti-globulins. J. A. M. A. *224*:871–874, 1973.
108. Rupprecht, C. E., Dietzschold, B., Wunner, W. H., et al.: Antigenic relationship of lyssaviruses. *In* Baer, G. (ed.): Natural History of Rabies. 2nd ed., Vol. 1. Boca Raton, CRC Press, 1990.
109. Rupprecht, C. E., Hamir, A. N., Johnston, D. H., et al.: Efficacy of a vaccinia-rabies glycoprotein recombinant virus vaccine in raccoons (Procyon lotor). Rev. Infect. Dis. *10*:S803–S809, 1988.
110. Rupprecht, C. E., and Wiktor, T. J.: Personal communication.
111. Rupprecht, C. E., Wiktor, T. J., Johnston, D. H., et al.: Oral immunization and protection of raccoons (Procyon lotor) with a vaccinia-rabies glycoprotein recombinant virus vaccine. Proc. Natl. Acad. Sci. U. S. A. *83*:7947–7950, 1986.
112. Schlenska, G. K.: Neurological complications following rabies duck embryo vaccination. J. Neurol. *214*:71–74, 1976.
113. Schneider, L. G.: Spread of virus from the central nervous system. *In* Baer, G. M. (ed.): The Natural History of Rabies. New York, Academic Press, 1975, pp. 273–301.
114. Schneider, L. G.: Spread of virus within the central nervous system. *In* Baer, G. M. (ed.): The Natural History of Rabies. New York, Academic Press, 1975, pp. 199–216.
115. Schumacher, C. L., Dietzschold, B., Ertl, H. C. J., et al.: Use of mouse anti-rabies monoclonal antibodies in postexposure treatment of rabies. J. Clin. Invest. *84*:971–975, 1989.
116. Shaughnessy, J. K., and Zichis, J.: Treatment of wounds inflicted by rabid animals. Bull. W. H. O. *10*:805–813, 1954.
117. Siwasontiwat, D., Lumlertdacha, B., Polsuwan, C., et al.: Rabies: Is provocation of the biting dog relevant for risk assessment? Trans. Roy. Med. Soc. Trop. Med. Hyg. *86*:443, 1992.
118. Smith, J. S., Fishbein, D. B., Rupprecht, C. E., et al.: Unexplained rabies in three immigrants in the United States. N. Engl. J. Med. *324*:205–211, 1991.
119. Smith, J. S., Orciari, L. A., Yager, P. A., et al.: Epidemiologic and historical relationships among 87 rabies virus isolates a determined by limited sequence analysis. J. Infect. Dis. *166*:296–307, 1992.
120. Smith, J. S., Seidel, H. D.: Rabies: A new look at an old disease. Prog. Med. Virol. *40*:82–106, 1993.
121. Smith, W. B., Blenden, D. C., Fuh, T., et al.: Diagnosis of rabies by immunofluorescent staining of frozen sections of skin. J. Am. Vet. Med. Assoc. *161*:1495–1501, 1972.
122. Sokol, F.: Recent advances in microbiology. *In* Perez-Miravete, A., and Pelez, D. (eds.): Xth International Congress of Microbiology. Association Mexicana de Microbiologia, Mexico City, Mexico, 1971, pp. 551–562.
123. Steele, J. H.: History of rabies. *In* Baer, G. M. (ed.): The Natural History of Rabies. New York, Academic Press, 1975, pp. 1–29.
124. Sugamata, M., Miyazawa, M., Mori, S., et al.: Paralysis of street rabies virus-infected mice is dependent on T lymphocytes. J. Virol. *66*:1252–1260, 1992.
125. Suntharasamai, P., Warrell, M. J., Warrell, D. A., et al.: Early antibody responses to rabies post-exposure vaccine regimens. Am. J. Trop. Med. *36*:160–165, 1987.
126. Suntharasamai, P., Warrell, M. J., Warrell, D. A., et al.: New purified Vero-cell vaccine prevents rabies in patients bitten by rabid animals. Lancet *2*:129–131, 1986.
127. Sureau, P., Rollin, P., and Wiktor, T. J.: Epidemiologic analysis of antigenic variations of street rabies virus: Detection by monoclonal antibodies. Am. J. Epidemiol. *117*:605–609, 1983.
128. Swanson, M. C., Rosanoff, E., Gurwith, M., et al.: IgE and IgG antibodies to β-propiolactone and human serum albumin associated with urticarial reactions to rabies vaccine. J. Infect. Dis. *155*:909–913, 1987.
129. Thongcharoen, P., Wasi, C., Chaitprasithikul, P., et al.: Immunogenicity of a purified Vero cell rabies vaccine. Virus Info Exchange Newsletter for SE Asia *3*:80, 1986.
130. Thraenhart, O., Kreuzfelder, E., Hillebrandt, M., et al.: Long-term humoral and cellular immunity after vaccination with cell culture rabies vaccines in man. Clin. Immunol. Immunopathol. *71*:287–292, 1994.
131. Tollis, M., Dietzschold, B., Volia, C. B., et al.: Immunization of monkeys with rabies ribonucleoprotein (RNP) confers protective immunity against rabies. Vaccine *9*:134–136, 1991.
132. Tordo, N, Poch, O., Ermine, A., et al.: Completion of the rabies virus genome sequence determination: Highly conserved domains among the l. (polymerase) proteins of unsegmented negative-strand RNA viruses. Virology *165*:565–576, 1988.
133. Trimarchi, C. V., and Safford, M., Jr.: Poor response to rabies vaccination by the intradermal route. J. A. M. A. *268*:874, 1992.
134. Tsiang, H.: Pathophysiology of rabies virus infection of the nervous system. Adv. Virus Res. *42*:375–412, 1993.
135. Turner, G. S., Aoki, F. Y., Nicholson, K. G., et al.: Human diploid cell strain rabies vaccines: Rapid prophylactic immunization of volunteers with small doses. Lancet *1*:1379–1381, 1976.
136. Turner, G. S.: A review of the world epidemiology of rabies. Trans. R. Soc. Trop. Med. Hyg. *70*:175–178, 1976.
137. Turner, G. S., Aoki, F. Y., Nicholson, K. G., et al.: Human diploid cell strain rabies vaccine: Rapid prophylactic immunisation of volunteers with small doses. Lancet *1*:1379–1381, 1976.
138. Veeraghavan, N.: Scientific Report for 1968 of the Pasteur Institute of Southern India. Madras, India, 1969.
139. Veeraraghavan, N., Ganajana, A., Rangasami, R., et al.: Studies on the salivary excretion of rabies virus by the dog from Surandai. *In* Anonymous (ed.): Pasteur Institute Annual Report of the Director 1968, and Science Report 1969. Coonoor, Pasteur Institute, 1970, pp. 68–70.
140. Vodopija, I., Sureau, P., Lafon, M., et al.: An evaluation of second generation tissue culture rabies vaccines for use in man: A four-vaccine comparative immunogenicity study using a pre-exposure vaccination schedule and an abbreviated 2-1-1 postexposure schedule. Vaccine *4*:245–248, 1986.
141. Warrell, D. A.: The clinical picture of rabies in man. Trans. R. Soc. Trop. Med. Hyg. *70*:175–178, 1976.
142. Warrell, D. A., Davidson, N. McD., Pope, H. M., et al.: Pathophysiologic studies in human rabies. Am. J. Med. *60*:180–190, 1976.
143. Warrell, D. A., and Warrell, M. J.: Human rabies and its prevention: An overview. Rev. Infect. Dis. *10*:S726–S731, 1988.
144. Warrell, M. J., Looareesuwan, S., Manatsathit, S., et al.: Rapid diagnosis of rabies and post-vaccinal encephalitides. Clin. Exp. Immunol. *71*:229–234, 1988.
145. Warrell, M. J., Nicholson, K. G., Warrell, D. A., et al.: Economical multiple-site intradermal immunisation with human diploid-cell strain vaccine is effective for post-exposure rabies prophylaxis. Lancet *1*:1059–1062, 1985.
146. Warrell, M. J., Warrell, D. A., Svatbarasamai, P., et al.: An economical regimen of human diploid cell strain anti-rabies vaccine for post-exposure prophylaxis. Lancet *2*:301–304,1983.
147. Warrington, R. J., Martens, C. J., Rubin, M., et al.: Immunologic studies in subjects with a serum sickness-like illness after immunization with human diploid cell rabies vaccine. J. Allergy Clin. Immunol. *79*:605–610, 1987.
148. Wiktor, T. J., and Clark, H. F.: Growth of rabies virus in cell culture. *In* Baer, G. M. (ed.): The Natural History of Rabies. New York, Academic Press, 1975, pp. 155–179.
149. Wiktor, T. J., and Hattwick, M. A. W.: Rhabdoviruses: Rabies and rabies-related viruses. *In* Kurstak, E., and Kurstak, C. (eds.): Comparative Diagnosis of Viral Diseases. New York, Academic Press, 1977.
150. Wiktor, T. J., and Koprowski, H.: Action locale de certains medicaments sur l'infection rabique de la souris. Bull. W. H. O. *28*:487–494, 1963.
151. Wiktor, T. J., and Koprowski, H.: Antigenic variants of rabies virus. J. Exp. Med. *152*:99–112, 1980.
152. Wiktor, T. J., and Koprowski, H.: Monoclonal antibodies against rabies virus produced by somatic cell hybridization: Detection of antigenic variants. Proc. Natl. Acad. Sci. U. S. A. *75*:3938–3942, 1978.
153. Wiktor, T. J., Fernandes, M. V., and Koprowski, H.: Cultivation of rabies virus in human diploid cell strain WI-38. J. Immunol. *93*:353–366, 1964.
154. Wiktor, T. J., Gyorgy, E., Schlumberger, H. D., et al.: Antigenic properties of rabies virus components. J. Immunol. *110*:269–276, 1973.
155. Wiktor, T. J., Plotkin, S. A., and Grella, D. W.: Human cell culture rabies vaccine. J. A. M. A. *224*:1170–1171, 1973.

156. Wilde, H., Chomchey, P., Prakongsri, S., et al.: Adverse effects of equine rabies immune globulin. Vaccine 7:10–11, 1989.
157. Wilde, H., Chomkasien, P,. Prakongsri, S., et al.: Safety of equine rabies immune globulin. Lancet 2:1275, 1987.
158. Wilde, H., and Chutivongse, P.: Equine rabies immune globulin: A product with an underserved poor reputation. Am. J. Trop. Med. Hyg. *42*:175–178, 1990.
159. Wilde, H., Chomchey, P., Punyaratabandhu, P., et al.: Purified equine rabies immune globulin: A safe and affordable alternative to human rabies immune globulin (experience with 3156 patients). Bull. W. H. O. *67*:731–736, 1989.
160. Wilson, J. M., Hettiarachchi, J., and Wijesuriya, L. M.: Presenting features and diagnosis of rabies. Lancet 2:1139–1140, 1975.
161. World Health Organization: Guidelines for Dog Rabies Control. Geneva, March 1984.
162. Xiang, Z. Q., Spitalnik, S., Tran, M., et al.: Vaccination with a plasmid vector carrying the rabies virus glycoprotein gene induces protective immunity against rabies virus. Virology *199*:132–140, 1994.

SUBSECTION NINE

FILOVIRIDAE

187

ARENAVIRAL AND FILOVIRAL HEMORRHAGIC FEVERS

Karl M. Johnson

HISTORY

Argentine hemorrhagic fever (AHF) clinically was described in 1955, and the causative Junin virus was isolated in 1958.[40] Initially recognized in the western Buenos Aires province of Argentina, this disease slowly expanded into north-central Argentina over several decades, until it finally was controlled by use of a live vaccine developed in the 1980s. In 1959, a similar disease was recognized in the Beni Department of eastern Bolivia, but in 1963 an isolate recovered from the spleen of a 2-year-old child was found to be related to, but distinct from, Junin virus. This was named Machupo virus.[23] Lassa fever (LF) first was described definitively in Nigeria in 1969, and the etiologic virus was identified during that same year.[2] This disease occurs also in Sierra Leone, Liberia, and possibly other countries of West Africa. Hemorrhagic disease was reported from central Venezuela in 1991, and another arenavirus, called Guanarito, was recovered a year later.[48] Yet another agent, given the name Sabia virus, was recovered from a fatal human infection near Sao Paulo, Brazil, in 1994. This virus has since caused serious, but nonfatal, illness in two laboratory workers. The epidemiology and the natural reservoirs of this virus remain unknown.

In their classic form, these arenaviral infections are potentially fatal diseases with insidious onsets, high fever, severe myalgia, focal hemorrhagic manifestations, and hypovolemic shock. The Argentine and Bolivian fevers also may be marked by encephalopathic changes, such as intention tremor, cerebellar signs, convulsions, and coma. A few patients with LF manifest classic signs of meningitis, and virus has been recovered from spinal fluid in these patients but not in those infected with the South American agents.

ETIOLOGIC AGENTS

The arenaviruses have been divided on the basis of immunologic and geographic characteristics into New and Old World sets. At least 16 individual viruses are recognized. Lassa virus is the only Old World taxon that causes human hemorrhagic fever, but four members of the family, Junin, Machupo, Guanarito, and Sabia, have been associated with the syndrome in South America. Arenaviruses have two genome segments, the smaller of which (S) codes for three virion structural proteins (G1, G2, and N) and the larger (L) of which codes for a viral polymerase and nonstructural proteins. Nucleocapsid antigens are shared by most of these viruses, and quantitative relationships show the basic split between the viruses of Africa and the Western Hemisphere. Individual viruses immunologically are distinct by neutralization test, which depends on the specificity of epitopes contained in the sugar-containing (G) envelope proteins.

Patterns of experimental infection in natural rodent hosts generally are similar for several arenaviruses that have been studied. Unlike the prototype virus of the family, lymphocytic choriomeningitis, which causes acute lethal disease when inoculated into the brain of albino laboratory mice, Lassa, Junin, and Machupo viruses do not cause death of their main natural rodent reservoir species when administered by any route or any dose to animals of any age. All very young hosts experience chronic infection with continuous viremia and viruria. As adults, such mice chronically infected with Machupo or Junin viruses virtually are infertile because embryos die during the last week of gestation.[24] In contrast, the chronically infected rodent host of Lassa virus gives birth to viable offspring, which immediately are infected via maternal milk. This chronic infection has an apparent element of immune tolerance because antiviral antibodies rarely are detectable in such animals. Rodents infected as adults (venereal transmission has been documented experimentally and is suspected in nature) may respond either with a tolerant type of infection in which much virus continuously is excreted in urine or with a more immunocompetent pattern in which viremia is controlled, antibodies to the virus are formed, and shedding of virus in urine drastically is curtailed.

Other animals have provided reasonable models for the clinical disease seen in humans. Junin virus causes fatal hemorrhagic disease in guinea pigs, rhesus monkeys are good models for Lassa[17] and Machupo virus infections, and marmosets *(Callithrix jacchus)* reproduce the pathogenesis of Junin virus. Indeed, rhesus monkeys were used to predict the effectiveness of the antiviral drug, ribavirin, to treat LF, and guinea pigs were instrumental in the development of an attenuated vaccine for AHF.

Arenaviruses are isolated most readily by use of Vero cells. Although cytopathic effects often are minimal or absent, immunofluorescence or viral plaques can be used to detect and eventually identify these agents. The recent development of enzyme-linked immunosorbent assay (ELISA) has provided a powerful and portable tool to detect viral antigens in blood and tissues of animals and patients.[44] Polymerase chain reaction methods are under development and promise to be the most sensitive means for arenavirus diagnosis yet achieved. Arenaviruses can be inactivated by gamma irradiation, betapropriolactone treatment, or heating for 60 minutes at 60° C.[29]

Because humans can be infected by the respiratory route (although this rarely occurs under natural conditions), the pathogenic arenaviruses are classed as level 4 agents, requiring maximum containment laboratories for their safe manipulation. Materials for viral diagnosis should be sent to one of the few such facilities in the world (the Centers for Disease Control and Prevention in Atlanta, Georgia, and the U.S. Army Medical Research Institute for Infectious Disease in Frederick, Maryland).

EPIDEMIOLOGY

The epidemiology of the arenaviral hemorrhagic fevers has few common features and many important differences among individual syndromes. Some comparative elements of the epidemiology of these diseases are given in Table 187–1.

All of these fevers are transmitted to humans primarily by excreta of chronically infected rodents, either as aerosols or by ingestion of contaminated food stuffs. Usually, only one or two rodent species are important as vectors of infection. Mortality in these diseases also is similar, ranging from about 10 to 20 per cent in the absence of specific therapy. Beyond this basic biology, there is much divergence in the particulars of epidemiologic patterns. Most of these diseases occur in tropical ecosystems, but AHF occurs on the rich temperate pampa of Argentina. Bolivian hemorrhagic fever (BHF) and LF usually are acquired in or very close to homes, but AHF is a disease acquired during harvest of maize, and Venezuelan hemorrhagic fever (VHF) usually is contracted in gardens and fields close to, but not inside, houses. These patterns reflect the behavior of the respective main virus reservoir rodents: *Mastomys natalensis* for LF,[42] *Calomys musculinus* for AHF, *Calomys callosus* for BHF, and *Sigmodon alstoni* for VHF.[54]

Both sexes and all ages contract LF and BHF, which are important pediatric diseases, but AHF largely is restricted to adult male agricultural workers.[32, 40] Similarly, VHF so far has been mainly a disease of adults, but both sexes are affected equally. In Argentina, there is a strong seasonal pattern of infection linked to the austral fall harvest of maize (March to June). The late rainy season from February to July defines peak transmission of BHF, and LF is a true endemic disease with cases occurring without major peaks or valleys throughout the year.[12, 37] These features are determined by the patterns of reproduction and invasion of habitat by the different rodent reservoirs or humans.

Inapparent or mild infections as a ratio to clinically severe disease also differ. Such infections are not common in American hemorrhagic fever patients but are notable findings in LF patients. Antibody prevalence in Sierra Leone ranges to 50 per cent, and prospective studies showed that seroconversion occurred in village populations at rates of 5 to 22 per cent per year.[37] It is estimated that about 20 mild Lassa virus infections occur for each hospitalized case of LF. Nevertheless, at one hospital in Sierra Leone, about 40 per cent of all febrile medical admissions (10 to 16 per cent of *all* medical illness) were for LF, and more than 20 per cent of pediatric admissions were diagnosed as having LF, with 12 to 14 per cent fatality.[56] LF also is an important cause of fetal death and abortion, especially in the third trimester. Mortality is increased in such pregnant women as well, unless uterine evacuation is carried out without delay.[47]

PERSON-TO-PERSON TRANSMISSION

LF is thought to be transmitted on occasion from person to person as result of intimate contact—sexual, by caring for the sick, or from mother to nursing infant. The virus has been recovered from maternal milk. Virus also has been recovered from throat secretions, but its presence or absence in semen and vaginal fluid remains unknown. Recognition of this disease originally was highlighted by serial transmission among three missionary nurses in Nigeria.[11] Explosive nosocomial outbreaks totaling 26 secondary and 3 tertiary cases occurred in Jos, Nigeria, and Zorzor, Liberia, in 1970 and 1972, respectively.[4, 39] Close, often unprotected contact with an index case of unknown etiology was important in the spread of illness in all of these episodes, and in the Jos outbreak there was evidence suggestive of airborne transmission. Surgical, obstetric, and autopsy procedures, needlesticks, cuts, contamination of ungloved hands by blood and

TABLE 187–1. Some Epidemiologic Features of Arenaviral Hemorrhagic Fevers

Fever	Virus	Case, Season, or Place, Pattern	Annual Incidence	Geographic Distribution	Ecology	Reservoir	Comment
Argentine hemorrhagic fever	Junin	Males; corn harvest; March–June	20–200	North-central Argentina	Temperate pampa	Mouse, *Calomys musculinus*	3- to 4-year rodent-disease cycle
Bolivian hemorrhagic fever	Machupo	All ages, both sexes; villages; February–July	<10	Northeast Bolivia	Tropical savanna	Mouse, *Calomys callosus*	Rodent control successful
Venezuelan hemorrhagic fever	Guanarito	All ages, both sexes equally affected; house, gardens; no seasonality	0–100	Central Venezuela	Tropical mixed savanna	Mouse, *Sigmodon alstoni*	Recently described
Lassa fever	Lassa	All ages, both sexes; villages; no seasonality	10,000	West Africa	Tropical forest savanna	Mouse, *Mastomys natalensis*	No long-term cycle; nosocomial infections

TABLE 187–2. Some Laboratory Findings in Arenaviral Hemorrhagic Fevers

Disease	Viremia	RBC Increase	WBC	Urine Protein	AST/ALT
Argentine hemorrhagic fever	+	+ +	↓ ↓	+	N-200
Bolivian hemorrhagic fever	±	+ +	↓ ↓	+	N-200
Venezuelan hemorrhagic fever	+ +	+ +	↓ ↓	+	??
Lassa fever	+ + + +	+ +	N- ↑	+ +	100–1500

ALT, alanine aminotransferase; AST, aspartate aminotransferase; RBC, red blood cell; WBC, white blood cell.

body fluids, and droplet exposure during tracheostomy management are the most common apparent modes for nosocomial acquisition of infection. Good barrier nursing and protection of personnel by use of gloves, gowns, and eye shields have reduced the incidence of such infection in recent years. Although LF has been imported into several countries outside West Africa, to date there has not been a single instance of secondary infection.

The South American hemorrhagic fevers rarely are transmitted from person to person. Isolated instances of such infection between spouses have been recorded for BHF, and in one unusual outbreak in Cochabamba, Bolivia, an index case from the Beni Department led to five secondary cases among the hospital staff.[46]

CLINICAL MANIFESTATIONS

After an incubation period of about 8 to 14 days, patients suffer the usually insidious onset of progressive fever and generalized myalgia.[11, 25, 32, 53] Hyperesthesia of the skin is common in AHF and BHF patients, and retrosternal pain often is a major complaint in LF patients. Abdominal pain has led to ill-advised surgical exploration in some instances. Vomiting and diarrhea may occur, and enanthem of the hard palate is common. LF patients complain of sore throat, and pharyngeal inflammation, sometimes with frank purulent discharge, may occur. In white patients, general suffusion of the skin of the face and upper trunk is notable, and this readily blanches on pressure. Patients commonly present with injected conjunctival membranes, but respiratory symptoms are not prominent.

Petechiae of the skin and hemorrhages from the gums, vagina, and gastrointestinal tract beginning about the fourth day of illness herald the advent of hypovolemic clinical shock. Blood loss usually is minor, so hematocrits generally increase as the capillary leak syndrome, which is the hallmark of these diseases, becomes more severe. Bleeding and prothrombin time now may be prolonged, and reductions of factors II and VII of the coagulation cascade have been noted in AHF patients. Renal function generally is preserved until shock occurs, but urinary protein may be high, especially in American hemorrhagic fever patients. In LF patients, fever may be high and unremitting for more than 2 weeks prior to the advent of hypovolemic shock. In this disease, up to 5 per cent of patients also suffer permanent eighth nerve damage, either unilateral or bilateral, with deafness. Some male patients also experience signs of epicarditis.

Neurologic manifestations are prominent in AHF and BHF patients. Intention tremor of the hands and inability to swallow or to speak clearly may develop, and these can progress to grand mal convulsions, coma, and death in the absence of significant capillary leak or hemorrhagic signs. Death usually occurs 7 to 12 days after onset. Those who survive generally recover completely without permanent sequelae, although transient loss of scalp hair and Beau lines in digital nails are a common consequence of the high and sustained fever.

Lassa virus, unlike the agents of the American hemorrhagic fevers, also attacks the liver. There is widespread hepatic necrosis, but little inflammatory reaction; thus, jaundice is unusual. Blood aminotransferases strongly are elevated, but liver failure is never apparent clinically. The virus also replicates to enormous levels in the placenta of pregnant women, a fact that has been offered as partial explanation for the excessive mortality associated with LF in these patients.

Leukopenia and thrombocytopenia characterize some, but not all, of these viral hemorrhagic fevers. Some clinical laboratory findings in the various syndromes are compared in Table 187–2.

Clinical disease among children generally is similar to that in adults. Systematic data are available only for LF patients. Fever, vomiting, diarrhea, and cough are common presenting complaints, but bleeding manifestations are less conspicuous among children than among adults, making the clinical differential diagnosis much more difficult. Pulmonary signs, including rales and pleural effusion, are more common in children than in adults. Among very young children, especially those infected ante partum, an unusual syndrome called swollen baby has been described. This is marked by abdominal distention, widespread edema, and spontaneous bleeding.[43]

PATHOGENESIS AND PATHOLOGY

With the exception of the hepatitis peculiar to LF, the pathology of arenaviral hemorrhagic fever is notable for the general lack of parenchymal histologic damage. Edema of tissues and focal hemorrhages in mucosal surfaces and fascia of many organs are common. It is rare to find blood clots large enough to be of clinical significance per se. Minor foci of necrosis with acidophilic inclusions (Councilman bodies) have been reported in BHF patients,[8] and erythroid hypoplasia of bone marrow, as well as lymphoid depletion of nodes and spleen, may be present in patients with these fevers. Histologic evidence for disseminated intravascular coagulation generally is absent. Inflammatory lesions of the central nervous system are lacking, except for the rare LF patient with clinical evidence for meningeal involvement. Mild inflammation of the myocardium has been noted in BHF patients.

Thus, it appears that the crucial and life-threatening lesion in these diseases is the capillary leak. How this lesion is produced, in which plasma protein and fluid escape the circulation at a much higher rate than erythrocytes, still is not clear. Macrophages and lymphocytes or their precursors are infected in AHF and BHF patients, and it seems likely that such infections activate the complex cytokine cascade, which can cause endothelial cells of small capillaries to lose the tight continuity that keeps protein and red cells inside the circulation. As part of this cascade, levels of interferon-α have been elevated in patients with AHF, and this molecule also may play a role in the fever, myalgia, and chills seen. Both Junin and Machupo viruses appear to be immunosuppressive; specific antibodies may not appear until almost 30 days after the onset of clinical symptoms. Cell-mediated immune function has not been assessed, but it is clear that viral antigen-antibody complexes play no role in the pathogenesis of infection.[31] Preliminary studies of VHF suggest that this disease resembles its other South American relatives.[48]

Direct damage to circulating leukocytes in LF patients is problematic, and thrombocytopenia does not occur. The longer duration of fever prior to clinical evidence for capillary leak and the increase in segmented white blood cells often seen as disease worsens further cloud the mechanism involved in the induction of shock in these patients. Immune responses to infection in LF patients also are unique. More than one-third of patients have antibodies to the nucleocapsid of the virus on admission to hospital. These antibodies do not neutralize the virus, which is found in blood in concentrations much higher in severe infection than in any of the other arenaviral diseases. During convalescence, viral neutralizing antibodies evolve slowly (for months) and rarely reach levels even one-tenth of those that develop after infection with the other viruses in this group. Thus, in the LF patient, it seems reasonable to speculate that compromise of cell-mediated immunity is responsible for uncontrolled virus replication and functional capillary collapse. Studies in rhesus monkeys, which reproduce the clinical and virologic spectrum of human disease, have not been performed to elucidate the humoral and molecular events leading to shock and death.

DIAGNOSIS AND DIFFERENTIAL DIAGNOSIS

Because arenaviral hemorrhagic fevers usually are undifferentiated early in disease, laboratory diagnosis is essential. When disease is encountered in endemic areas, many other infectious causes for fever must be considered. Chief among these are malaria, enteric bacteria, leptospirosis, and rickettsiosis. Lymphocytic choriomeningitis has been confused with AHF, and patients finally shown to have LF have been diagnosed on clinical grounds as having dengue, meningococcemia, typhoid fever, diphtheria, and streptococcal pharyngitis. In one prospective study in which 40 per cent of febrile admissions were shown to have LF on laboratory grounds, triads of symptoms and signs composed of either pharyngitis, retrosternal pain, and proteinuria or of pharyngitis, retrosternal pain, and vomiting had positive predictive values of about 85 per cent, but only about half of confirmed infections had these findings.[35] Thus, it is clear that specific diagnostic procedures are necessary. In nonendemic settings, the key to diagnosis of these diseases is a history of travel and activity in the 3 weeks prior to onset of fever.

Nearly half of LF patients have specific IgM antibodies when admitted to the hospital. These can be assayed by immunofluorescence or by ELISA.[44, 59] Viral antigens also have been detected by ELISA in LF and in BHF patients. Virus can be detected in blood and at times in secretions of most LF, AHF, and VHF patients but only sporadically in BHF patients. Because antibody production is delayed in this disease, final diagnosis of BHF may be delayed well into convalescence, although lymphoid tissues are uniformly positive from specimens obtained at necropsy.

TREATMENT AND PROGNOSIS

Treatment of arenaviral hemorrhagic fever begins with supportive measures directed at reversal of dehydration, management of electrolyte and acid-base balance, and recognition and control of hemoconcentration and hypotension (human albumin and fluid replacement) before the advent of clinical shock. In AHF and BHF patients, the only variable predictive of ultimate outcome of infection is duration of symptoms prior to admission to hospital. Patients arriving for treatment more than 5 days after onset of disease have higher mortality than do those seen earlier. Dehydration and hypovolemia seem to be the likely factors involved.

Specific treatment of AHF patients with human convalescent plasma has been shown to be lifesaving if initiated within 7 days of the onset of illness.[30] In a prospective, placebo-controlled trial, the mortality rate was reduced from 16 to 1 per cent. Such therapy, if available, likely would benefit patients suffering from the other American hemorrhagic fevers. Plasma therapy also has been tried in LF patients, but with equivocal results, probably because virus-neutralizing antibodies in convalescent patients are quantitatively much inferior to those in AHF patients.[17]

During trials of ribavirin in LF patients in Sierra Leone, it was discovered that viremia and aspartate aminotransferase levels on admission were powerful objective predictors of outcome of infection.[21, 35] Patients having at least 150 IU/L of aspartate aminotransferase experienced a 50 per cent mortality rate; 73 per cent of those with greater than $10^{3.6}$ $TCID_{50}$/mL of virus in the blood died, and if both conditions were present the risk of death was 80 per cent. With the aspartate aminotransferase value of 150 IU/L, the mortality rate in patients treated with intravenous ribavirin beginning 6 days or less after onset was reduced from 61 to 5 per cent, the most dramatic antiviral efficacy on record. In adults, treatment was initiated with a loading dose of 30 mg/kg, followed by 15 mg/kg each 6 hours for 4 days, and finally 15 mg/kg every 8 hours for an additional 6 days.[36] Treatment begun after 6 days of illness was less effective but still of clear value.

No data are available yet for ribavirin treatment of LF in children, but a regimen based on surface area relative to weight in adults appears to be cautiously reasonable. The principal side effect of ribavirin therapy is anemia. Although hematocrits in adult patients often decreased to concentrations of 25 per cent or lower, blood transfusion was never required, and normal red blood cell mass was achieved within 6 weeks after therapy was complete.

PREVENTION AND CONTROL

Person-to-person spread of infection is limited largely to LF patients, and few clinical features are of use in assessing this risk. Pregnant patients and those with spontaneous bleeding, significant diarrhea, or pulmonary symptoms appear to be the greatest hazard to others, primarily caregivers. Experience in endemic areas suggests that barrier-nursing techniques effectively prevent such transmission. In nonendemic areas, strict isolation should be observed, with attention directed especially to risks imposed by diagnostic samples and invasive procedures.[5] A recommended, but unproven, prophylactic regimen for persons intimately exposed to LF patients or who suffer invasive accidents is oral ribavirin, 500 mg four times daily for 7 days. A corresponding pediatric dose is 6 to 8 mg/kg. If employed, this regimen should be followed closely during and after treatment.[16, 19]

Control of disease in endemic areas ranges from none in the case of LF to nearly complete for AHF and BHF. In Bolivia, it was discovered that the *Calomys* reservoir could be trapped successfully in homes. This led to termination of a major epidemic in the town of San Joaquin, where nearly one-third of the population had been infected during an interval of 18 months. Chronically infected rodents were found to have hemolytic anemia and enlarged spleens. This marker has been used with such effect during recent decades that fewer than 10 cases of BHF occur per year.[38] Rodent control is not feasible for AHF, in which the *Calomys* reservoir is sylvatic, and it was found that the *Mastomys* reservoir of LF, although resident in human dwellings, was not sufficiently trappable to make disease control by this means effective.[26]

An attenuated vaccine for AHF has been developed in recent years and shown to be effective, and it now is used in persons exposed to the agricultural occupational hazards that characterize high risk for this disease. Work on a genetically engineered vaccine for LF still is in early stages and has languished for want of funding.[10]

FILOVIRAL HEMORRHAGIC FEVERS: MARBURG AND EBOLA FEVERS

Marburg and Ebola viruses are African viruses maintained in nature through unknown mechanisms and capable of inducing a severe and highly lethal hemorrhagic fever syndrome in humans. The mortality rate of Ebola fever may be as high as 90 per cent. Recent outbreaks of Ebola disease in nonhuman primates from the Philippine Islands have provided clues to the eventual solution of the mystery of filovirus maintenance in nature.

History

In 1967, simultaneous outbreaks of a previously unknown hemorrhagic fever occurred in Marburg and Frankfurt, Germany, and Belgrade, Serbia. Infection was traced to contact with African green monkeys *(Cercopithecus aethiops)* from a primate export facility in Entebbe, Uganda. There were 31 cases, including 6 of secondary transmission. Seven deaths occurred in primary cases.[34, 52] An infectious agent unlike any previously seen was recovered in England from the blood and organs of these persons, and the name Marburg virus was ascribed to it.[50] Since that time, sporadic cases of this disease have occurred in southern Africa and in Kenya.[13, 20, 51]

In 1976, two nearly simultaneous and explosive outbreaks of a similar illness occurred in northwestern Zaire and in southern Sudan. Viruses morphologically similar to, but antigenically distinct from, Marburg virus were recovered from patient blood specimens. This agent was named Ebola virus after a small river near the epicenter of the epidemic in Zaire.[1, 22] More than 500 persons were affected, and the mortality rate was high: 88 per cent in Zaire and 53 per cent in Sudan.[57, 58] A single case of fatal infection was documented in Tandala, Zaire, in 1977,[15] and another outbreak occurred in the same area of Sudan in 1979,[55] in which 22 of 34 illnesses were fatal. In 1995, a major epidemic with a mortality rate of more than 75 per cent among 310 patients was recorded in the Kikwit region of Zaire, about 600 miles southwest of the original site in the Bumba province of Zaire.[7]

An isolated and nonfatal Ebola virus infection occurred in 1994 in an anthropologist who was observing chimpanzees in a national park in the Ivory Coast.[28] This researcher noted that some of these animals were suffering from a hemorrhagic illness; her infection most likely was acquired in the course of performing an autopsy of one of the chimpanzees.

In 1989, it suddenly became apparent that Ebola virus was not restricted to the African continent. A group of cynomolgus monkeys *(Macaca fascicularis)* from the Philippines quarantined in a Reston, Virginia, laboratory experienced lethal hemorrhagic disease. Virions antigenically similar to those of Ebola virus were observed in tissues and confirmed by culture in Vero cells.[18] Over the next several weeks, further introductions of new monkeys and spread of infection to several rooms in the facility made it necessary to kill the entire cohort of more than 400 animals. The building was fumigated and abandoned. The virus was recovered from another macaque in Philadelphia and later in a laboratory in Italy. Although no human disease was associated with these episodes, several monkey handlers in the United States were infected, as confirmed by serologic conversion from negative to positive for Ebola antibodies.[14]

Etiologic Agents

The *Filoviridae* family now comprises Marburg virus and four antigenically and genetically related subtypes of Ebola virus: Zaire, Sudan, Ivory Coast, and Reston. The viruses have a similar morphology. Long filamentous particles often have bizarre configurations (Fig. 187–1) and may be as long as 14,000 nm. They always are 80 nm in width and contain a single negative-sense genome that codes for seven polypeptides. An excellent review of the molecular organization and replication strategy of this virus group and comparison with other closely related families has been published recently.[45]

The filoviruses replicate readily in Vero, MA-104, or SW-13 cell cultures, although given subtypes seem to prefer individual lines, all of which were derived from primates. The viruses also are highly pathogenic for macaques, producing a hemorrhagic disease that usually is more than 75 per cent fatal and that offers the only useful pathophysiological model for human infection.

There virtually is no antigenic relationship between Marburg and any of the Ebola viruses. The latter, however, exhibit extensive immunologic cross-reactivity, as detected by immunofluorescence or ELISA. Virus neutralization, in contrast, virtually has been impossible to measure for any of the filoviruses, and this difficulty has proved to be an important obstacle to understanding the epidemiology and ecology of these agents.

With the possible exception of the Reston Ebola virus, the filoviruses are highly pathogenic organisms that must be handled only in special laboratories under maximum biologic containment. Advice regarding management of patients and specimens suspected of having these viruses has been published.[6] Further detail is available constantly from the Centers for Disease Control and Prevention in Atlanta.

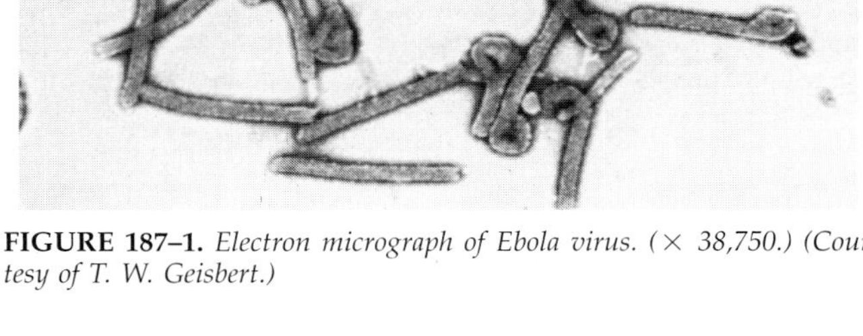

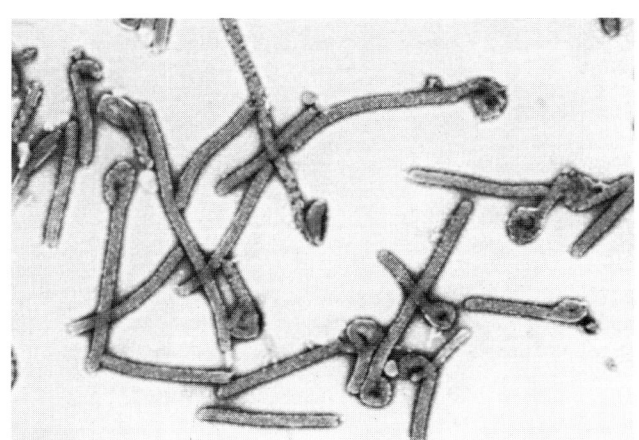

FIGURE 187–1. *Electron micrograph of Ebola virus.* ($\times$ *38,750.) (Courtesy of T. W. Geisbert.)*

Epidemiology

Partly because of the infrequent occurrence of filoviruses in humans, the natural reservoirs and vectors (if any) of filoviruses remain a mystery 30 years after first recognition. Limited surveys of vertebrates and certain arthropods at or near sites of human outbreaks have failed to yield even a first clue. The inability to develop a method for serologic search for infection having uniform sensitivity in diverse species is a continuing problem. Such surveys in human populations using immunofluorescent techniques appear to add to the confusion. Much has been published to indicate that humans may be infected without serious disease to prevalence levels of up to 40 per cent. Work with ELISA employing purified recombinant antigen suggests that such infection actually is rare.[27]

The origin of every index case of human filovirus disease is unknown. Thus, all outbreaks so far identified are based on person-to-person transmission. Such transmission is fueled by the high and persistent viremia that marks the syndrome and by the presence of virus in other body fluids, especially when contaminated by blood. Tissues of monkeys used to prepare cell culture for manufacture of poliovirus vaccine were the source of the original Marburg outbreak, and secondary infection largely was limited to medical workers who initially failed to take precautions designed to prevent direct skin contact with body fluids. The 1976 Ebola outbreaks were spread primarily by use of contaminated needles, and the recent Kikwit, Bandundu, epidemic was fomented by ill-advised surgical procedures carried out without any protection whatsoever.

Intimate family contact also is an important factor in spread of infection, and this occurs primarily among persons providing direct care to patients in the home and those preparing corpses for burial. Up to 17 per cent of infections in Zaire were so documented, and this fraction was even higher in the 1995 outbreak. Although these factors mitigate against pediatric disease, it is of interest that 20 per cent of patients in the 1976 Zaire epidemic were younger than 15 years of age.[58]

Aerosol has not been implicated frequently in human infections. However, aerosols have been shown to be infectious for primates, and there is one anecdotal report from the original Marburg epidemic.[33] In addition, there is strong evidence that dissemination of the Reston Ebola virus among monkeys and to monkey handlers at least partially was attributable to respiratory infection.

Clinical Manifestations

The African filoviruses induce a similar syndrome in humans after an incubation period roughly estimated to range from 2 to 21 days, with a modal range of 6 to 9 days.[33, 52] Onset is abrupt and marked by fever, myalgia, chills, and headache. Pharyngitis, nausea, vomiting, diarrhea, and abdominal pain appear within about 3 days. Dry cough is common but apparently not highly infectious. Relative bradycardia and pharyngeal and conjunctival injection are common, and there may be exudates or ulcers on the posterior pharynx. By the fifth day of illness, patients are apathetic; a maculopapular rash appears on the trunk and spreads to the extremities. At this time, bleeding into the skin and from venipuncture sites begins, and mucosal hemorrhages, especially in the gastrointestinal tract, become prominent. Severe hemorrhage and neurologic signs (disorientation and coma) are poor prognostic findings, and death usually occurs between days 6 and 12. Capillary leak with hypovolemia is prominent, but patients appear simply to fade away without abrupt onset of a shock syndrome reminiscent of arenaviral or bacterial septic disease. In those who survive, fever generally abates by the end of the first week of disease. The rash desquamates. Pancreatitis and orchitis may occur as acute complications, and orchitis and uveitis have been recorded as late events. Virus has been isolated from semen and anterior eye chamber fluid several weeks after recovery, and semen was implicated as a mode of transmission in one instance of Marburg virus infection.[33]

Mild leukopenia with a left shift is common early in disease, but leukocytosis may appear later, reflecting secondary bacterial infection that most often is pulmonary. Thrombocytopenia below 100,000 platelets/nm^3 is uniform, and as bleeding begins, coagulation studies are abnormal. Fibrin split products indicative of disseminated intravascular coagulation have been observed in a few cases. Serum transaminases markedly are elevated, but increased bilirubin and clinical jaundice rarely are noted. Serum protein levels are depressed, hematocrits are increased, and proteinuria is a common finding.

Pathogenesis and Pathology

Although many tissues at autopsy contain large amounts of virus, direct evidence of such replication in capillary endothelium remains elusive. Thus, the final trigger for the capillary leak syndrome is not known. In vitro studies, however, show that Marburg virus replicates to high titers in cultured human vascular endothelium.[49] Pathologic examination reveals diffuse hemorrhage involving most organ systems, and there are histologic findings compatible with those of disseminated intravascular coagulation. Lymph nodes and spleen show mild enlargement, edema, and areas of lymphoid necrosis. Diffuse hepatitis with focal necrosis, virtually no inflammatory response, and many Councilman-like bodies invariably is present. Electron microscopy shows that hepatocytic inclusions consist of massive arrays of virus particles.

Diagnosis and Differential Diagnosis

Marburg and Ebola fevers must be differentiated from other viral hemorrhagic diseases in Africa as well as from the many bacterial, rickettsial, and protozoal diseases that may present in a similar manner early in clinical disease. The absence of jaundice helps to eliminate yellow fever and Rift Valley fever. For patients seen outside Africa, a travel history is the single most important diagnostic tool available to physicians.

Specific diagnosis is established by virus isolation because antibodies to these agents usually are not present prior to death or defervescence. An ELISA method has been developed that correlates well with viral presence in blood.[27] Methods based on polymerase chain reaction have proved to be successful in the recent Kikwit epidemic of Ebola fever. Infection can be confirmed in survivors by the use of ELISA or Western blot technology.

Treatment and Prevention

There exists no more deadly viral disease for which there is no specific treatment. Ribavirin and interferon have no effect on filoviruses, and the search for other antiviral compounds has had low priority until recently. Convalescent plasma has been used on occasion without proven effect. One person infected with Ebola-Sudan virus after a laboratory accident survived after receiving such plasma from Ebola-Zaire survivors.[9] Several patients are thought to have had milder Marburg disease after early treatment with plasma.[33] There also are recent reports that hyperimmunoglobulin prepared in horses protected baboons in experimental studies.[41] Still, most attempts to protect monkeys with serum antibodies have failed, and it is unclear which, if any, specific viral epitopes confer immunity against infection or disease. Thus, there is no firm basis for the development of a vaccine for any filovirus.

References

1. Bowen, E. T. W., Lloyd, G., Harris, W. J., et al.: Viral haemorrhagic fever in southern Sudan and northern Zaire. Lancet *1*:571–573, 1977.
2. Buckley, S. M., and Casals, J.: Lassa fever, a new virus of man from West Africa. III. Isolation and characterization of the virus. Am. J. Trop. Med. Hyg. *19*:680–691, 1970.
3. Buckley, S. M., and Casals, J.: Pathobiology of Lassa fever. Int. Rev. Exp. Pathol. *18*:97–136, 1978.
4. Carey, D. C., Kemp, G. E., White, H. A., et al.: Lassa fever: Epidemiological aspects of the 1970 epidemic, Jos, Nigeria. Trans. R. Soc. Trop. Med. Hyg. *66*:402–408, 1972.
5. Centers for Disease Control: Management of patients with suspected viral hemorrhagic fever. M. M. W. R. *37*:1–16, 1988.
6. Centers for Disease Control and Prevention: Update: Management of patients with suspected viral hemorrhagic fever. M. M. W. R. *44*:475–479, 1995.
7. Centers for Disease Control and Prevention: Update: Outbreak of Ebola virus hemorrhagic fever—Zaire, 1995. M. M. W. R. *44*:399, 1995.
8. Child, P. L., Mackenzie, R. B., Valverde, L. R., et al.: Bolivian haemorrhagic fever: A pathologic description. Arch. Pathol. *83*:434–445, 1967.
9. Edmond, R. T. D., Evans, B., Bowen, E. T., et al.: A case of Ebola virus infection. B. M. J. *2*:541–544, 1977.
10. Fisher-Hoch, S. P., McCormick, J. B., Auperin, D., et al.: Protection of rhesus monkeys from fatal Lassa fever by vaccination with a recombinant vaccinia virus containing the Lassa virus glycoprotein gene. Proc. Natl. Acad. Sci. U. S. A. *85*:1–6, 1988.
11. Frame, J. D., Baldwin, J. M., Jr., Gocke, D. J., et al.: Lassa fever, a new virus disease of man from West Africa: Clinical description and pathological findings. Am. J. Trop. Med. Hyg. *19*:670–676, 1970.
12. Fraser, D. W., Campbell, C. C., Monath, T. P., et al.: Lassa fever in the eastern province of Sierra Leone, 1970–1972. I. Epidemiologic studies. Am. J. Trop. Med. Hyg. *23*:1131–1139, 1974.
13. Gear, J. S. S., Cassell, G. A., Gear, A. J., et al.: Outbreak of Marburg virus disease in Johannesburg. B. M. J. *4*:489–493, 1975.
14. Hayes, C. G., Burans, J. P., Ksiazek, T. G., et al.: Outbreak of fatal illness among captive macaques in the Philippines caused by an Ebola-related filovirus. Am. J. Trop. Med. Hyg. *46*:664–671, 1992.
15. Heymann, D. C., Weisfeld, J. S., Webb, P. A., et al.: Ebola hemorrhagic fever, Tandala, Zaire, 1977–1978. J. Infect. Dis. *142*:372–376, 1980.
16. Holmes, G. P., McCormick, J. B., Trock, S. C., et al.: Lassa fever in the United States: Investigation of a case and new guidelines for management. N. Engl. J. Med. *323*:1120–1123, 1990.
17. Jahrling, P. B., and Peters, C. J.: Passive antibody therapy of Lassa fever in cynomolgus monkeys: Importance of neutralizing antibody and Lassa virus strain. Infect. Immun. *44*:528–533, 1984.
18. Jahrling, P. B., Geisbert, T. W., Dalgard, D. W., et al.: Preliminary report: Isolation of Ebola virus from monkeys imported to USA. Lancet *335*:502–505, 1990.
19. Johnson, K. M., and Monath, T. P.: Imported Lassa fever: Reexamining the algorithms. N. Engl. J. Med. *323*:1139–1141, 1990.
20. Johnson, E. D., Roimet, E., Gitau, L. G., et al.: Marburg virus disease: An environmental health threat in Kenya. *In* Kinoti, S. H., Waiyoki, P. G., and Were, B. D. (eds.): Proceedings of the 11th Annual Medical Scientific Conference. Nairobi, Kenya, African Medical Research Foundation, 1990.
21. Johnson, K. M., McCormick, J. B., Webb, P. A., et al.: Clinical virology of Lassa fever in hospitalized patients. J. Infect. Dis. *155*:456–464, 1987.
22. Johnson, K. M., Webb, P. A., Lange, J., et al.: Isolation and partial characterization of a new virus causing acute haemorrhagic fever in Zaire. Lancet *1*:569–571, 1977.
23. Johnson, K. M., Wiebenga, N. H., Mackenzie, R. B., et al.: Virus isolations from human cases of hemorrhagic fever in Bolivia. Proc. Soc. Exp. Biol. Med. *118*:113–118, 1965.
24. Johnson, K. M.: Hemorrhagic fevers of Southeast Asia and South America: A comparative appraisal. Prog. Med. Virol. *9*:105–158, 1967.
25. Keane, E., and Gilles, H. M.: Lassa fever in Panguma Hospital, Sierra Leone, 1973–1976. B. M. J. *1*:1399–1402, 1977.
26. Keenlyside, R. A., McCormick, J. B., Webb, P. A., et al.: Case-control study of *Mastomys natalensis* and humans in Lassa virus–infected households in Sierra Leone. Am. J. Trop. Med. Hyg. *32*:829–837, 1983.
27. Ksiazek, T. G., Rollin, P. E., Jahrling, P. B., et al.: Enzyme immunosorbent assay for Ebola virus antigens in tissues of infected primates. J. Clin. Microbiol. *30*:947–950, 1992.
28. Le Guenno, B., Formentry, P., Wyers, M., et al.: Isolation and partial characterization of a new strain of Ebola virus. Lancet *345*:1271–1274.
29. Lloyd, G., Bowen, E. T. W., and Slade, J. H. R.: Physical and chemical methods of inactivating Lassa virus. Lancet *1*:1046–1048, 1982.
30. Maiztegui, J. I., Fernandez, N. J., and de Damilano, A. J.: Efficacy of immune plasma in treatment of Argentine hemorrhagic fever and association between treatment and a late neurological syndrome. Lancet *2*:1216–1217, 1979.
31. Maiztegui, J. I., Laguens, R. P., Cossio, P. M., et al.: Ultrastructural and immunohistochemical studies in five cases of Argentine hemorrhagic fever. J. Infect. Dis. *132*:35–43, 1975.
32. Maiztegui, J. I.: Clinical and epidemiological patterns of Argentine haemorrhagic fever. Bull. W. H. O. *52*:567–576, 1975.
33. Martini, G. A., and Siegert, R. (eds.): Marburg Virus Disease. New York, Springer-Verlag, 1971.
34. Martini, G. A., Knauff, H. G., Schmidt, H. A., et al.: A previously unknown infectious disease contracted from monkeys: Marburg virus disease. Dtsch. Med. Wochenschr. *93*:559–571, 1968.
35. McCormick, J. B., King, I. J., Webb, P. A., et al.: A case-control study of the clinical diagnosis and course of Lassa fever. J. Infect. Dis. *155*:445–455, 1987.
36. McCormick, J. B., King, I. J., Webb, P. A., et al.: Lassa fever: Effective therapy with ribavirin. N. Engl. J. Med. *314*:20–26, 1986.
37. McCormick, J. B., Webb, P. A., Krebs, J. W., et al.: A prospective study of the epidemiology and ecology of Lassa fever. J. Infect. Dis. *155*:437–444, 1987.
38. Mercado, R.: Rodent control programmes in areas affected by Bolivian haemorrhagic fever. Bull. W. H. O. *52*:691–695, 1975.
39. Mertens, P. E., Patton, R., Baum, J. J., et al.: Clinical presentation of Lassa fever during the hospital epidemic of Zorzor, Liberia, March–April 1972. Am. J. Trop. Med. Hyg. *22*:780–784, 1973.
40. Mettler, N. E.: Argentine hemorrhagic fever: Current knowledge. Sci. Publ. No. 183. Washington, D.C., Pan American Health Organization, 1969.
41. Mikhailov, V. V., Borisevich, I. V., Chernikov, N. K., et al.: The evaluation in hamadryas baboons of the possibility for the specific prevention of Ebola fever. Vopr. Virusol. *39*:82–84, 1994.
42. Monath, T. P., Newhouse, V. F., Kemp, G. E., et al.: Lassa virus isolation from *Mastomys natalensis* rodents during an epidemic in Sierra Leone. Science *185*:263–265, 1974.
43. Monson, M. H., Cole, A. K., Frame, J. D., et al.: Pediatric Lassa fever: A review of 33 Liberian cases. Am. J. Trop. Med. Hyg. *36*:408–415, 1987.
44. Niklasson, B. S., Jahrling, P. B., and Peters, C. J.: Detection of Lassa fever antigens and Lassa-specific immunoglobulin G and M by enzyme-linked immunosorbent assay. J. Clin. Microbiol. *20*:239–244, 1984.
45. Peters, C. J., Sanchez, A., Rollin, P. E., et al.: *Filoviridae:* Marburg and Ebola viruses. *In* Belshe, B. (ed.): Textbook of Human Virology. 4th ed. St. Louis, Mosby–Year Book, 1996, p. 699.
46. Peters, C. J., Kuehne, R. W., Mercado, R. R., et al.: Hemorrhagic fever in Cochabamba, Bolivia, 1971. Am. J. Epidemiol. *99*:425–433, 1974.
47. Price, M. E., Fisher-Hoch, S. P., Craven, R. B., et al.: A prospective study of maternal and fetal outcome in acute Lassa fever infection during pregnancy. B. M. J. *297*:584–587, 1988.
48. Salas, R., de Manzione, N., Tesh, R. B., et al.: Venezuelan haemorrhagic fever. Lancet *338*:1033–1036, 1991.
49. Schnittler, H. J., Mahner, F., Drenckhaln, D., et al.: Replication of Marburg virus in human endothelial cells: A possible mechanism for the development of viral hemorrhagic disease. J. Clin. Invest. *91*:1301–1309, 1993.
50. Smith, C. E. G., Simpson, D. I. H., Bowen, E. T. W., et al.: Fatal human disease from vervet monkeys. Lancet *2*:1119–1121, 1967.
51. Smith, D. H., Johnson, B. K., Isaacson, M., et al.: Marburg virus disease in Kenya. Lancet *1*:816–820, 1982.
52. Stille, W., Boehle, E., Heim, E., et al.: An infectious disease transmitted by *Cercopthecus aethiops*. Dtsch. Med. Wochenschr. *93*:572–582, 1968.
53. Stinebaugh, B. J., Schloeder, F. X., Johnson, K. M., et al.: Bolivian hemorrhagic fever. Am. J. Med. *40*:217–230, 1966.
54. Tesh, R. B., Wilson, M. L., Salas, R., et al.: Field studies on the epidemiology of Venezuelan hemorrhagic fever: Implication of the cotton rat *Sigmodon alstoni* as the probable rodent reservoir. Am. J. Trop. Med. Hyg. *49*:227–235, 1993.
55. Viral haemorrhagic fever surveillance. Wkly. Epidemiol. Rec. No. 44, November 1979, p. 2.
56. Webb, P. A., McCormick, J. B., King, I. J., et al.: Lassa fever in children in Sierra Leone, West Africa. Trans. R. Soc. Trop. Med. Hyg. *80*:577–582, 1986.
57. WHO/International Commission Report: Ebola haemorrhagic fever in Sudan, 1976. Bull. W. H. O. *56*:247–270, 1978.
58. WHO/International Commission Report: Ebola haemorrhagic fever in Zaire, 1976. Bull. W. H. O. *56*:271–293, 1978.
59. Wulff, H., and Johnson, K. M.: Immunoglobulin M and G responses measured by immuno-fluorescence in patients with Lassa or Marburg virus infections. Bull. W. H. O. *57*:631–635, 1979.

❑ ❑ ❑

SUBSECTION TEN

CORONAVIRIDAE

188

CORONAVIRUSES

Elliot C. Dick, Stanley L. Inhorn, and Robert L. Atmar

Since the first report of human coronavirus (HCV) isolation in 1965,[130] the HCV group of RNA viruses has been confirmed as a frequent cause of the common cold in children and adults. Determining the role of coronaviruses in other diseases has been hindered by the great difficulty in isolating these fastidious organisms from clinical material. Therefore, much of our current information about the significance of HCV in infectious disease comes from electron-microscopic and seroepidemiologic studies. For the latter, antigens from only two different HCVs, HCV-229E and HCV-OC43, are available. Although it is possible that these two contain antigens representative of many HCV serotypes,[71, 101] several isolates do not seem to fit into these antigenic groups.[75–77, 86] With these limited tools, HCVs have been implicated as possible contributors in lower respiratory disease of children and adults, gastroenteritis, and central nervous system disorders in addition to the common cold.

A clue to the potential range of pathogenicity of HCV rests in the large number of serious and widespread coronavirus infections found in animals. These include infectious bronchitis and nephrosis of chickens, gastroenteritis and encephalitis in young piglets, infectious diarrhea of turkeys, diarrhea in newborn calves, hepatitis and encephalitis in mice, enteritis in dogs, pneumonitis and sialodacryoadenitis in rats, and infectious peritonitis in domestic and exotic cats.[75–77, 124, 134]

The first HCV was cultivated by Tyrrell and Bynoe[130] at the Common Cold Unit in Salisbury, England, through the introduction of human embryonic tracheal and nasal epithelial mucosal organ culture. They were able to produce colds regularly in volunteers inoculated with organ culture fluids from the first and later passages of an agent, B814, obtained from a boy with a cold. All attempts to isolate this agent in cell culture had been unsuccessful.[49]

Working independently, Hamre and Procknow[44] at the University of Chicago described in 1966 the isolation of five viruses, including prototype strain HCV-229E, from primary human embryonic kidney cell cultures. Four of these agents were obtained from secretions of medical students with upper respiratory illnesses and one from a healthy student. These viruses produced a cytopathic effect in human embryonic kidney cells after an initial blind passage and could be adapted to grow and produce a cytopathic effect in human diploid cell strain WI-38.

Growth of six additional HCVs, including the second human prototype, HCV-OC43, was reported in 1967 by McIntosh and his associates[78, 80] at the National Institutes of Health, using human embryonic tracheal organ culture to culture adult upper respiratory infections.

It soon became evident that the HCVs were related to similar agents known to infect animals. By electron microscopy, the tissue culture isolate, 229E, and the organ culture isolate, B814, were demonstrated by Almeida and Tyrrell[2] to be morphologically identical with each other and with avian infectious bronchitis virus. Subsequently, mouse hepatitis virus was demonstrated to be very similar morphologically and related antigenically to HCV-OC43.[75, 78, 82] Shortly thereafter, it was suggested[1] and accepted[129] that these and similar agents be placed in the genus *Coronavirus* of the family *Coronaviridae*. Infectious bronchitis virus was named the type species for reasons of priority, being described in 1936[5] and grown in eggs and further characterized in 1937.[7] Recently, a second genus, *Torovirus*, has been added to the *Coronaviridae* family.[25] Toroviruses have been associated with gastroenteritis in animals.[6]

Poor growth and a lack of cytopathic effect in cell culture have been major deterrents to HCV research. Although animal coronaviruses are quite host-specific in their requirements for cell culture, they will grow, often well and with a cytopathic effect, in primary cell cultures from their host species or, with adaptation, in continuous cell lines.[134] In contrast, HCVs must be isolated—if they can be grown at all—in either human organ culture or human embryonic tissue cultures; because of this handicap, probably fewer than 60 HCVs have been isolated to date.[57, 58, 65, 82, 93, 101, 107] Where sufficient virus can be recovered for characterization, most isolates have proved to be similar, either HCV-229E–like or HCV-OC43–like,[71] although several HCVs remain antigenically uncharacterized, including the very first isolate, HCV-B814.[12, 14, 75, 82, 86, 107]

Both HCV-OC43 and HCV-229E have been adapted to host systems capable of supporting good growth and allowing relative ease of virus detection. HCV-OC43 has been propagated in suckling mouse brain[78] and shown to agglutinate[59] and hemadsorb erythrocytes,[58] and both viruses have been adapted to cell lines producing sufficient virus for biochemical studies.[108, 109, 112] With the use of these two different HCVs for serologic epidemiology and animal coronaviruses for basic immunologic, genetic, and biochemical investigations, much has been learned.

ETIOLOGIC AGENT

The biologic properties of coronaviruses now are quite well defined.[49, 77, 86, 134] They are medium to large (80 to 220 nm),[49, 77, 113, 134] pleomorphic, spherical, or elliptical enveloped RNA viruses. Their most distinctive characteristic is the widely spaced, petal-shaped, 20-nm-long projections that stud the envelope surface and give the virus particle the appearance of a solar corona. As is typical of enveloped viruses, coronaviruses are labile to heat, lipid solvents, and acid pH. The genome is 27 to 32 kb (large for an RNA virus), single-stranded, and positive-sense RNA and is, in itself, infective (in common with other positive-sense RNA viruses). The infectious bronchitis virus and 229E genomes have been sequenced completely, and the genomes of several other coronaviruses have been sequenced partially.[11, 47, 49] The genome and its surrounding capsid are arranged in helical symmetry and enclosed within a lipoprotein envelope.

The internal structure of coronaviruses and their antigenic and genetic interrelationships also have yielded to study.[49, 112, 113] A nucleoprotein (N) surrounds the RNA genome, and together they appear as a coiled tubular helix within the bilayer lipid-containing envelope. The envelope contains two or three glycoproteins: (1) a matrix protein M (or E1), which is embedded in the envelope; (2) a surface component S (or E2), which is the structural protein of the petal-shaped spikes; and (3) a hemagglutinin HE (or E3), which is found in several of the group II viruses (see later), including HCV-OC43, and seems closely related to the influenza C hemagglutinin.[133] The antigenic interrelationships of these four proteins have permitted arrangement of both the animal coronaviruses and HCVs into three groups. The two known HCV serotypes, each along with several other mammalian coronaviruses, have been placed in group I (HCV-229E) or II (HCV-OC43), and an avian (chicken) strain is the single member of group III.[49, 86, 113] Evidence from RNA base sequencing strengthens the intercoronavirus relationship.[112]

In coronavirus replication, as with other single-stranded, positive-sense viruses, all processes take place in the cytoplasm.[49, 77, 113] In the first step, the virus attaches to the cell membrane, using its HE or S protein in the petal-shaped spike. HCV 229E uses aminopeptidase N as a receptor,[138] whereas HCV-OC43 interacts with MHC class I molecules to establish infection.[28, 29] Penetration occurs as a result of S protein–mediated fusion of the viral envelope with the plasma membrane. The genome then is translated into (probably) one large polyprotein, which contains an RNA-dependent RNA polymerase. Using the genome RNA as a template, this virus-coded polymerase synthesizes a negative-stranded RNA. In turn, through use of the negative-stranded RNA as a template, the polymerase synthesizes new positive-stranded genomic RNA and several subgenomic RNAs. Through use of one of the latter, N is synthesized on free ribosomes, forming a helical nucleocapsid surrounding the newly formed genomic RNA. Other small RNAs migrate to membrane-bound ribosomes, where they translate the structural proteins M, S, and HE. Virions then are assembled by budding into cytoplasmic vesicles in the rough endoplasmic reticulum and Golgi region. Virus particles are released by cell lysis or fusion of post-Golgi, virion-containing vesicles with the plasma membrane.

EPIDEMIOLOGY

Because of the difficulty in isolating HCV, the majority of epidemiologic data are derived from serologic surveillance (chiefly complement fixation, hemagglutination inhibition, neutralization, and/or enzyme-linked immunosorbent assay [ELISA]),[18, 64, 68, 70, 76, 86, 107] with HCV-229E or HCV-OC43 viruses as antigens. Because enteric HCVs rarely have been propagated in culture, epidemiologic study of these latter agents is hindered further by lack of antigens for seroepidemiology; those epidemiologic data that exist for enteric HCVs—mostly electron-microscopic studies—will be described in the section on clinical manifestations.

Geographic Prevalence

Coronavirus infections seem to be present worldwide. Seroprevalence studies for HCV-229E and HCV-OC43 infection have been conducted in the United States,[24, 46, 60, 61, 83] England,[14] Germany,[106] Brazil,[20] Finland,[131] and Iraq.[45] In any population, prevalence estimates will vary with the sensitivity of the serologic tests used. Complement fixation is the least sensitive, and the titers often are transient, reflecting only fairly recent infection, whereas hemagglutination inhibition, neutralization, and ELISA often reflect infection months or years in the past. Whatever test is employed, 50 to 60 per cent of adults older than 30 years of age usually have antibody to both serotypes; with ELISA, antibody prevalence may approach 90 to 100 per cent.[45]

Seasonal Incidence and Annual Recycling Pattern

The majority of HCV infections occur in midwinter to early spring.[16, 24, 43, 46, 57, 60, 61, 65, 76, 78, 83, 86, 88] Also, individual serotypes typically may predominate in one year and then be followed by one or more years of low activity.[76, 86] However, there have been some significant exceptions to these generalizations.[60, 61, 68, 79, 80] For example, in healthy children in Atlanta, Georgia, prospectively examined for HCV-229E and HCV-OC43 infection from 1960 through 1968 (Fig. 188–1), the incidence of autumn infections approached that of spring infections, and there usually were a few infections in the summer. Also, although there was a very considerable HCV-229E outbreak in 1961 to 1962, followed by 2 years with low incidence, in the remaining 4 years incidence was quite similar from year to year.[60, 61]

Whatever the season, a single HCV serotype can cause, at least locally, a high incidence of infection, e.g., HCV-229E in Atlanta children in 1961 to 1962 (see Fig. 188–1). HCV-229E also was associated with a very significant outbreak in University of Chicago, Chicago, Illinois, medical students in 1966 and 1967.[43] Very substantial portions of the population can be infected during these exacerbations. Among the Chicago medical students, 66 (35 per cent) of 191 were infected. In Tecumseh, Michigan,[24] a 10,000-person community just southwest of Detroit, Michigan, a large HCV-229E outbreak between January and April 1967 affected 68 per cent of 38 families and 34 per cent of 159 individuals tested. Sharp outbreaks also can occur in certain hospitalized infants: At National Jewish Hospital in Denver, Colorado, 16 of 20 hospitalized asthmatic infants were infected with HCV-OC43 in December 1968.[81]

Ratio of Clinical to Subclinical Illness

In healthy children and adults, HCVs often are shed asymptomatically. In the 8.5-year surveillance of healthy older children in Atlanta (see Fig. 188–1), only 63 (38 per cent) of 168 with HCV-229E seroconversion reported respiratory illness, and the ratio for HCV-OC43 was 44:93, or 47 per cent. Among a group of infants and young children in metropolitan Washington, D.C., tested for HCV-OC43 seroconversion, at least 50 per cent of the infections were subclinical[83]; in the 133 HCV-229E infections in the Chicago medical students just described, 43 per cent were in asymptomatic individuals. In a study of premature infants in a neonatal intensive care unit in Brest, France, nosocomial acquisition of coronavirus infection was demonstrated in 10 infants; however, the incidence of clinical symptomatology, such as apnea or bradycardia, was the same as in uninfected infants.[117]

Susceptibility to HCV-induced diseases may be much greater in certain populations. In the Denver children hospitalized with atopic asthma, 19 were infected with either HCV-229E or HCV-OC43 and 17 were symptomatic.[81]

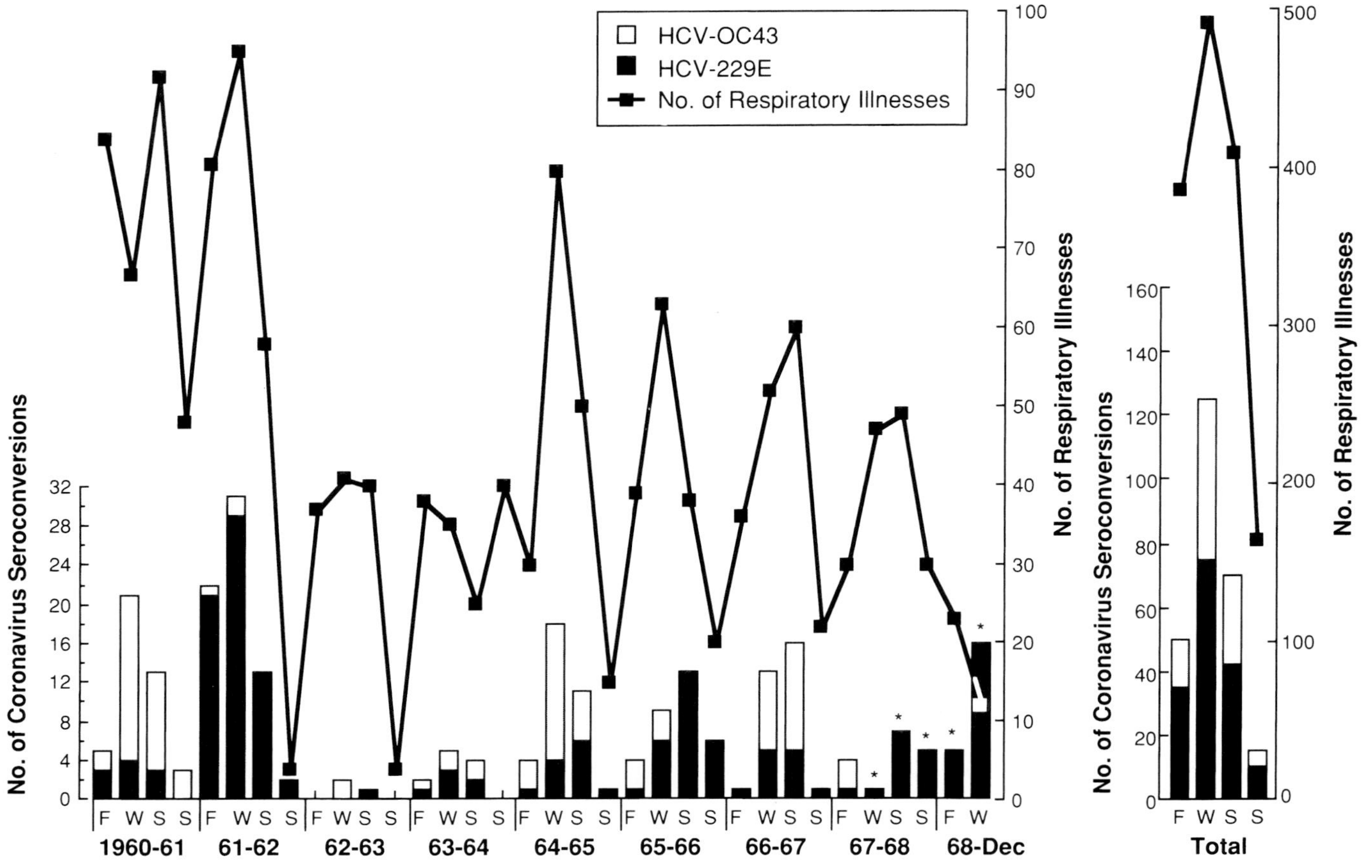

* HCV-OC43 diagnoses were not continued past fall of 1967

FIGURE 188–1. *Seasonal distribution of seroconversions to human coronaviruses OC43 and 229E, 1960 through 1968, in a group of children's cottages in Atlanta, Georgia (120 to 175 children, 5 to 19 years of age). Forty-one per cent of the seroconversions were associated with respiratory illness. (Adapted from Kaye, H. S., Marsh, H. B., and Dowdle, W. R.: Seroepidemiologic survey of coronavirus [strain OC43] related infections in a children's population. Am. J. Epidemiol. 94:43–49, 1971; and Kaye, H. S., and Dowdle, W. R.: Seroepidemiologic survey of coronavirus [strain 229E] infections in a population of children. Am. J. Epidemiol. 101:238–244, 1975.)*

Age Specificity of Infection

Unlike the other respiratory viruses, which are most likely to infect the very young, HCVs do not demonstrate much age specificity. In the Tecumseh families studied during a community-wide HCV-229E epidemic in 1967,[24] only 3 of 54 infections were in children younger than 4 years of age. The attack rate then rose to a peak of 14 per cent between 15 and 29 years of age and then slowly fell off to 8 per cent in those 40 years of age or older. Peculiarly, the results were different in a 1968 to 1969 Tecumseh community-wide outbreak of HCV-OC43 infection. With this virus, the highest rate, 29 per cent, was in children 4 years of age or younger, and the rates decreased very little even into the adult years, when the incidence was 22 per cent.[88]

Transmission

Human volunteers can be infected readily via nose drops and develop a typical cold 2 to 3 days later, and it is assumed, therefore, that natural infections can occur through the respiratory route.[86] A natural transmission experiment in human volunteers, with a model system similar to that previously used for such studies with rhinoviruses,[31] demonstrated that HCV-229E spread (1) apparently was unimpeded when direct contact by self-inoculation was blocked by arm restraints and (2) readily was accomplished by small-particle aerosol.[126] Monto[86] favors aerosol transmission of HCV because, like influenza viruses, HCVs often cause sharp and widespread outbreaks, and influenza epidemics may spread chiefly by the aerosol route.[10, 41] Whatever the means of transmission, HCVs do not spread easily, at least within families.[24]

INFECTION AND IMMUNITY

Pathogenesis, Incubation Period, and Serologic Response

In a healthy adult, HCVs seem to replicate only in the upper respiratory tract and to produce little damage to the host. In human embryonic tracheal organ culture, a decline in ciliary activity after serial passage was the only cytopathic effect observed.[78, 130] This was confirmed in a modified organ culture system, in which, in contrast to influenza virus and adenovirus infections that produced destruction of the cells, HCV-229E and rhinoviruses had no effect, even though these viruses were replicating.[137] HCVs have been detected in nasopharyngeal cells,[84, 94, 95] and HCV-229E virus titers from 10 to more than 1000 $TCID_{50}$ were found for a week or more in nasopharyngeal washings.[92] Bende and associates[9] studied the course of HCV-229E colds in 24 volunteers and delineated typical signs, symptoms, and virus shedding patterns; 8 volunteers were asymptomatic. HCV colds usually last about 1 week but can endure for nearly 3 weeks.[13, 77] In human volunteers, the incubation period is 2 to 3 days, with a range of 1 to 5 days.[13, 77, 101]

In as many as 50 per cent of HCV infections, diagnostic rises in antibody titer do not occur; when they do, those with absent or low titers are more likely to seroconvert.[13]

Reinfection

Repeated infection with HCVs is very common. Among Atlanta children who seroconverted to HCV-229E, 35 per cent had preinfection antibody titers of 1:10 or higher, and 8 per cent had 1:20 or higher.[60] Antibody against HCV-OC43 was equally ineffective.[61] There also was no evidence that antibody ameliorated clinical illness. In the Tecumseh family study described earlier, 81.5 per cent of the infections occurred despite the presence of neutralizing antibody.[88]

There is, however, evidence from human volunteer experiments that strain-specific antibody can be protective. Reed[101] infected volunteers with one of several HCV-229E–like HCVs. She found immunity to homotypic challenge to endure at least 1 year, but the immunity to heterotypic HCV-229E strains in these same volunteers was much lower.

Quantity of specific antibody may be important. Callow,[17] also working with previously HCV-229E–infected volunteers, found that when rechallenged, those individuals who did not become infected or who had asymptomatic infections possessed six times or more the serum neutralizing antibody of those who became ill. High specific secretory IgA levels also were associated with milder symptoms.

Little is known about the role of cell-mediated immunity in resistance to HCV infection. In mice, cytotoxic T cells are generated to the mouse hepatitis virus N protein, and both CD4+ and CD8+ T cells are involved in virus clearance.[122] HCV-229E will replicate in human macrophages,[98] but the role of these cells and of cell-mediated immunity in limiting infection is not understood at present.

CLINICAL MANIFESTATIONS OF RESPIRATORY TRACT INFECTIONS

The Common Cold and Other Chiefly Upper Respiratory Tract Illnesses

A significant association of HCVs with respiratory illnesses—most of them cold-like—has been demonstrated in prospective studies of adults and of families with children. In the Chicago medical students described earlier, HCV-229E attack rates were 31 per cent during "illness periods" and only 9 per cent in "wellness periods" ($p < .001$); the illnesses did not differ significantly from undifferentiated acute respiratory infections caused by respiratory syncytial virus, parainfluenza viruses, or rhinoviruses.[43] In the Tecumseh families described earlier, the illness in the family index HCV-229E cases was compared with that of matched controls; the illness rate in the index cases was nearly twice (1.8 times) that in the controls. Whereas most (58 per cent) of the families had illnesses that were cold-like, the remainder had lower respiratory tract symptoms, including productive cough, wheezing, or pain on respiration.[24]

The symptoms in the adults in the two investigations cited earlier were much like those in human volunteers who were "given" HCV colds by means of many different HCV isolates.[9, 13, 14, 17, 18, 101] These were very typical common colds, with perhaps more rhinorrhea than in rhinovirus colds; sore throat, cough, malaise, and headache were present in approximately 50 per cent of volunteers. Twenty per cent of volunteers had definite pyrexia.[13, 77]

In a surveillance at England's Common Cold Unit, 18 per cent of adult colds were caused by HCV,[65] a figure that agrees generally with other estimates.[75, 127]

Clinical findings in children also are typical of colds, although the manifestations can be more severe. In a group of Atlanta children (Table 188–1), pharyngeal injection (72 to 82 per cent) and sore throat (30 to 66 per cent) were prominent; 34 to 40 per cent had fevers higher than 37.6° C (99.6° F), and 8 to 21 per cent of the fevers exceeded 39° C (102.2° F). One-third of the cases reported cervical adenitis, and a few had pulmonary signs.

The proportion of total respiratory disease or of colds attributable to HCV varies markedly by season and from

TABLE 188–1. Clinical Findings in 61 and 43 Atlanta, Georgia, Children* Who Seroconverted† to HCV-229E and HCV-OC43, Respectively, 1960 to 1968

Presenting Complaints	Virus (%)		Physical Findings	Virus (%)	
	229E	*OC43*		*229E*	*OC43*
Sore throat	66	30	Pharyngeal injection	82	72
Coryza	52	19	Coryza	64	49
Cough	43	30	Fever, 37.6° C (99.6° F) and higher	34	40
Fever	21	9			
Headache	15	NR‡	Fever, 39° C (102.2° F) and higher	8	21
			Cervical adenitis	30	35
			Pulmonary rales (or dullness)	NR	5
			Rash	NR	2

*A changing population of 120 to 175 white children, 5 to 19 years of age (median, 9 to 11 years of age) in a church-sponsored home, 1960 to 1968. The children were housed in cottages of 8 to 12 persons, assigned on the basis of age and gender.

†Paired acute and convalescent sera (2 to 3 weeks) showing fourfold or greater antibody rises by indirect hemagglutination (HCV-229E) or hemagglutination-inhibition (HCV-OC43).

‡Not reported.

Adapted from Kaye, H. S., Marsh, H. B., and Dowdle, W. R.: Seroepidemiologic survey of coronavirus (strain OC43) related infections in a children's population. Am. J. Epidemiol. *94*:43–49, 1971; and Kaye, H. S., and Dowdle, W. R.: Seroepidemiologic survey of coronavirus (strain 229E) infections in a population of children. Am. J. Epidemiol. *101*:238–244, 1975.

year to year. In the 8.5-year long Atlanta study (see Fig. 188–1), 7 per cent of all respiratory disease was associated with HCV seroconversion, but in the winter of the epidemic year 1961 to 1962, approximately 16 per cent of respiratory illness was associated with HCV.

Lower Respiratory Tract Disease

Asthma and Recurrent Wheezing

There is substantial evidence that HCVs can precipitate asthma attacks.[52, 55, 81, 85, 93, 96, 97] In a 2-year surveillance (1967 to 1969)[81] of 32 mostly atopic children 1 to 5 years of age hospitalized in Denver for severe, recurrent bouts of wheezing, 19 HCV infections were diagnosed, 16 of them in a typical sharp HCV epidemic (December 1968). Six simultaneously were infected with either parainfluenza virus 2 or respiratory syncytial virus. Of the remaining 13 HCV "pure culture cases," all were symptomatic, 3 had mild wheezing, and 7 had acute asthma attacks, 2 of which required intravenous therapy. Three had pneumonia accompanied by radiographic changes, and four were febrile (>38° C [>100° F]). HCVs were not as likely to cause wheezing as was respiratory syncytial virus and were more likely to cause only coldlike illnesses and fewer fevers.

The capacity of HCVs to cause wheezing in asthmatics was confirmed in a study in 1979 to 1981 of young (younger than 6 years of age) English children especially subject to rather severe recurrent respiratory disease.[52] Compared with a normal control population, these "susceptible" children were much more likely to have attacks of wheezing, as well as fever, cervical adenitis, rales, and other signs and symptoms of more serious respiratory disease. Thirty per cent of infections were diagnosed as HCV-caused. Those children who suffered from recurrent respiratory infections seemed less able to localize HCVs or other respiratory viruses to the nasal area.[51, 52] In Turku, Finland, HCVs were found to be the most common viruses in children, 1 to 6 years of age, who were prone to episodes of wheezing.[85]

Pertinently, among HCV-229E–infected human volunteers, persons who were atopic had much more severe colds than did those who were not ($p < .001$).[19]

Pneumonia and Other Severe Lower Respiratory Tract Infections

As noted earlier, children who are prone to recurrent respiratory infections, including those caused by HCV, seem also likely to have more severe disease, including that of the lower airways.[51, 52] However, evidence for HCV involvement in children actually hospitalized for respiratory disease is not as clear. The reasons for this uncertainty are threefold: (1) there are very few studies of HCV in this setting[77, 86]; (2) HCVs can be nearly absent from the population in some years (see Fig. 188–1)[84]; and (3) about 50 per cent of HCV infections are asymptomatic.[60, 61, 83] The last reason has been a particular problem in those few attempts that have been made to establish the etiologic role of HCV in lower respiratory tract disease. For example, among pediatric patients with lower respiratory tract disease at Children's Hospital, Washington, D.C., the HCV incidence in ill children, 3.5 per cent, actually was lower than in control patients with nonrespiratory disease, 8.2 per cent.[83]

Better evidence for causation was found in 417 Cook County infants hospitalized for lower respiratory tract disease during 1967 to 1970.[79] Both HCV-229E and HCV-OC43 were found, and HCV was the third most important virus (behind respiratory syncytial virus and parainfluenza virus 3), both in incidence and in specific association with pneumonia and bronchiolitis (Table 188–2). Many of these HCV-infected infants were in sufficient respiratory distress to require oxygen or to exhibit intercostal retractions. In two "periods of increased incidence," HCVs were diagnosed in 16 to 19 per cent of cases and were the dominant type of virus. Finally, HCV-229E was cultivated from oropharyngeal swabs from two infants with pneumonia in August 1967.

HCV-associated lower respiratory tract disease has been found in adults. The clearest association is with chronic obstructive pulmonary disease. Three controlled studies, in Burlington, Vermont[42]; Chicago[16]; and Salt Lake City, Utah,[118] found significant association between acute exacerbations ($.001 < p < .05$) and/or attacks of acute respiratory disease ($p < .01$) and HCV infection. A sharp outbreak of acute respiratory disease sufficient to cause hospitalization of United States Marine recruits has been attributed at least partially to HCV-OC43.[136]

OTHER HUMAN DISEASES ASSOCIATED WITH HUMAN CORONAVIRUSES

As described early in this chapter, coronaviruses cause a wide spectrum of disease in animals. Whereas, as in humans, coronavirus-caused respiratory disease is important in animals, enteric disease is at least as important, especially in the young. Diseases of the liver and the nervous system also are prevalent in some species.[89, 124]

Enteric Human Coronavirus Infections

The first reports of HCV as a possible cause of human gastroenteritis appeared in 1975; coronavirus-like particles (CVLPs) were found by electron microscopy in stools of young English adults in three sharp outbreaks of nonbacterial gastroenteritis.[21, 23] In the same year, CVLPs were reported in

TABLE 188–2. Relative Incidence of Various Respiratory Virus Infections in Infants with Pneumonia or Bronchiolitis, Cook County Hospital, Chicago, Illinois, 1967 to 1970

	Number of Infants with Indicated Condition Who Were Positive for Virus (%)		
Virus	***Pneumonia***	***Bronchiolitis***	***Total***
Respiratory syncytial	58 (25.1)	48 (32.2)	106 (27.9)
Parainfluenza 3	54 (23.4)	28 (18.8)	82 (21.6)
Coronavirus*	20 (8.7)	10 (6.7)	30 (7.9)
Adenovirus	11 (4.8)	15 (10.1)	26 (6.8)
Parainfluenza 1	11 (4.8)	9 (6.0)	20 (5.3)
Influenza A	10 (4.3)	5 (3.4)	15 (4.0)
Rhinovirus	6 (2.6)	2 (1.3)	8 (2.1)
Parainfluenza 2	3 (1.3)	3 (2.0)	6 (1.6)
Total	126 (55.0)	83 (55.7)	209

*Both HCV-229E and HCV-OC43.

Note: Infants were considered positive if virus was recovered or if there was serologic evidence of infection; 231 infants with pneumonia and 149 infants with bronchiolitis were tested. Some infants were positive for more than one virus.

From McIntosh, K., Chao, R. K., Krause, H. E., et al.: Coronavirus infection in acute lower respiratory tract disease of infants. J. Infect. Dis. *130*:502–507, 1974. University of Chicago, publisher.

the stools of *healthy* adults in India.[73] These rather contrasting publications from England and from India heralded the beginning of a continuing controversy on the etiologic importance of these agents as enteric pathogens.[27, 69, 72]

The firmest link of CVLPs to human enteric disease is with gastroenteritis in the very young, especially neonatal necrotizing enterocolitis (NEC). In Paris, France, a controlled epidemiologic investigation of NEC was conducted in two hospitals—one with and one without an NEC outbreak.[26] Within each hospital, newborns with "no pathologic occurrence" were used as controls. In the NEC-free hospital, no CVLPs were found in the stools of 21 controls, but two patients with mild diarrhea had CVLPs. In the NEC hospital, 23 of the 32 (72 per cent) NEC patients had fecal CVLPs, whereas only 3 of 26 (11.5 per cent) controls were positive ($p < .02$). In Dallas, Texas, CVLPs were observed in infants who were part of an NEC outbreak in a hospital special care nursery.[102] CVLP-caused gastroenteritis, even if not typical NEC, also may be important, at least in the southwestern United States. In September 1979, an episode of acute, severe (bloody stools, bilious gastric aspirates, abdominal distention) gastroenteritis occurred in the neonatal intensive care unit of the University of Arizona Medical Center, Tucson, Arizona, and several clinical signs were associated significantly ($p = .002$ to $.05$) with CVLPs in patients' stools.[132] Subsequently, CVLPs were found in older Arizona children (1 month to 12 years of age) hospitalized for gastroenteritis.[89] Finally, in an 8-year (1976 to 1984) electron-microscopic surveillance of primarily hospitalized gastroenteritis patients from southern Arizona,[99] 41 per cent of stools from 862 patients were positive for some virus-like particle, and the majority, 70 per cent, were CVLPs. Rotaviruses were second with 17 per cent, and the remaining four putative enteritis-causing viruses (adenoviruses, picorna/parvoviruses, astroviruses, caliciviruses) were present in less than 5 per cent of positive specimens. Only 2.8 per cent of samples contained more than one agent.

In Pavia, Italy, a case-control study of infants and young children with enteritis found a significant difference in fecal CVLP presence between the ill and control groups: 16.3 per cent in ill children and 1.6 per cent in controls ($p < .01$).[39]

At least three possible CVLP-related deaths have been reported, two of sepsis in Arizona[132] and one of severe enteritis in an Oklahoma City, Oklahoma, infant.[103] In the latter case, a careful electron-microscopic examination was made of the epithelial cells of the distal small bowel; the location, size, shape, and arrangement of the virus-like particles were identical to those described for coronavirus infections in puppies, calves, and mice.

Despite the foregoing evidence for a causal relationship between CVLPs and gastrointestinal disease, there still is reservation about the role of CVLPs in children's enteric disease,[27, 56, 69, 76, 86] chiefly because CVLPs so often are found in the feces of healthy children.[63, 69, 111, 115, 116] For example, in India, electron-microscopic surveillance of 426 hospitalized children—half with diarrhea and half control—found that only 8.9 per cent of the ill patients had positive test results, whereas 23 per cent of the controls had positive results. In contrast, the distribution of fecal rotaviruses, a proven enteric pathogen,[56] among these children was nearly exactly the converse: 28.6 per cent in children with diarrhea and 1.4 per cent in the controls.[115] However, prolonged CVLP shedding after acute illness clouds the meaning of "healthy controls." Although CVLPs usually disappear from stools within a month of the cessation of illness, shedding for several months to nearly 2 years has been reported.[39, 69, 99] It also is possible, because the immune response to CVLPs is not well-understood, that chronic shedding is due to asymptomatic reinfection.[27, 99]

Evidence for CVLP-caused enteritis in adults and older children, even those with AIDS, is inconclusive.[35, 62, 69, 72, 111] In a recent 69-month survey of CVLPs in various social groups in Australia, a strong association was shown only between CVLP shedding and unhygienic living or working conditions ($p < .0005$). There is some provocative evidence that CVLPs could be, at least partially, responsible for the enteropathy typical of tropical sprue.[3, 74]

CVLP shedding seems to show little seasonality, even in the endemic southwestern United States area.[99] In this environment, they seem to be present year-round, with a slight preference for the autumn months.[89, 99] However, in nonendemic areas, there seems to be no seasonal pattern; for example, no CVLPs were detected in the 4 years prior to the September 1979 to March 1980 CVLP-associated NEC epidemic in the Paris hospital cited previously.[26]

Attempts have been made to cultivate CVLP in cell and organ culture and to compare the resultant virus suspensions antigenically with other HCVs or animal coronaviruses. A partial motivation for both efforts rests in demonstrating the very nature of CVLP; they are so bizarre and pleomorphic in electron-microscopic preparations that questions of their viral authenticity have been raised.[27, 33, 69, 89, 99] Although there have been convincing reports of human CVLP growth in human fetal organ cultures from patients with gastroenteritis[21, 22] and NEC,[102] the investigators have not reported further. These organ culture–grown viruses were more regular in form than were the viruses directly visualized in feces, and typical coronavirus replication with budding into cisternae of endoplasmic reticulum was illustrated.[22] The cultivated NEC virus was not related antigenically to HCV-229E or HCV-OC43 or to two animal toroviruses, Breda virus of calves and Berne virus of horses.[102] More recently, a hemagglutinating coronavirus antigenically and genetically related to a bovine coronavirus, BCV-LY138, was isolated from a 6-year-old child with severe diarrhea.[139] A continuous cell line, HRT, derived from a human rectal adenocarcinoma was used for virus isolation.

Because of the great difficulty in culturing CVLPs, investigators[4, 39] at the University of Pavia purified CVLPs from NEC infants' fecal suspensions for use as antigen to raise antisera and to react with acute and convalescent sera of NEC patients. These viruses were related antigenically to HCV-OC43, and specific antibody was present in the convalescent sera.

Neurologic Diseases

As described earlier, coronaviruses are the cause of some animal neurologic disorders,[124] including murine demyelination.[36] In humans, a serosurvey of HCV infection in southern Finland discovered HCV-OC43 association with six cases of acute neurologic episodes, including one with polyradiculitis.[104] Because of some immunologic responses[105] and temporal associations with symptoms of infectious diseases,[54] multiple sclerosis long has been thought to have a viral cause.[37, 53] Several observations have suggested a possible role of coronavirus infection in this disease: (1) the isolation of coronaviruses (SK + SD) from central nervous system tissue of two patients wih multiple sclerosis[15]; (2) the demonstration that coronavirus SD can cause demyelination in a primate model[91]; (3) the direct visualization of CVLPs in the brain of a patient with multiple sclerosis[123]; (4) the identification of coronavirus RNA in the brains of multiple sclerosis patients by in situ hybridization or polymerase chain reaction[90, 121];

and (5) correlations of multiple sclerosis with colds and HCV-229E infections.[54] However, coronaviruses SK and SD are antigenically[37, 38] and genetically[135] very similar to mouse hepatitis virus and were isolated using mouse tissues[15]; the possibility that these isolates were of mouse origin has not been excluded. In addition, other studies have failed to demonstrate coronavirus RNA in central nervous system tissues of multiple sclerosis patients[120] or differences in serologic responses to HCVs in multiple sclerosis patients.[37, 50] Further investigation will be needed to establish whether HCVs causally are related to any neurologic disease in humans.

LABORATORY DIAGNOSIS

Virus Isolation

Respiratory Coronaviruses

Because it is so difficult, isolation of HCVs from clinical material has been limited to a few research laboratories.[44, 57, 65, 78, 101] On primary isolation, some HCV-229E–type strains will replicate and produce a cytopathic effect in certain diploid cell lines: WI-38,[43] MRC-5,[54] and MA-177.[57] The cells become "stringy" after several days' incubation in a roller drum at 33° C or upon subsequent passage. However, some HCV-229E–like strains require organ culture.[65, 71, 101] HCV-OC43–like strains all seem to require organ culture, usually human embryonic trachea or nasal mucosa.[65] The cytopathic effect often is indistinct, and the presence of virus often must be detected by electron microscopy.

Enteric Coronavirus-like Particles

Growth of these agents in cell or organ culture has been reported,[22, 102, 139] but the results need confirmation.

Virus Detection Techniques

Most of the direct methods determine whether HCV-229E or HCV-OC43 antigens are present in nasal or nasopharyngeal washings, aspirates, and/or swabs from individuals who describe symptoms of viral respiratory illness. There is evidence that antigens in these two viruses may be representative of the respiratory HCV group as a whole.[71, 101] The usual procedure is to fix the specimen to a glass slide or the flat-bottomed well of a plastic microtiter plate and then cover the specimen with specific HCV antiserum. The antibody reacts with the antigen in the specimen and continues to adhere during subsequent rinsing. Then labeled (with an immunofluorescent or otherwise pigmented dye), species-specific (e.g., antirabbit) antiserum is added. Depending on the label, the test is read by a microscope equipped to read fluorescence or by a photometer that will measure absorbance of specific wave lengths of transmitted light, such as ELISA. Both immunofluorescence[84] and ELISA have been used successfully for HCV diagnosis.[52, 69, 70, 85] These methods of virus detection can be rapid and very sensitive, but great care must be taken to rule out false-positive results.

Because at present HCV diagnosis seldom is carried out other than in research laboratories, antigens and antisera specifically for HCV must be prepared by the laboratory seeking to make HCV diagnoses. However, preparation of these reagents is well within the capability of experienced, large virus laboratories serving states, provinces, cities, and similar population units. Both HCV-229E and HCV-OC43 can be grown to high titer in certain continuous cell lines, MRCc,[70] human rhabdomyosarcoma cells,[108, 109] and others.[86] HCV-OC43 grows well in mouse brain.[61, 80] Specific antisera to HCV-229E and HCV-OC43 have been raised in rabbits.[70, 108]

Detection of the HCV genome has been reported. A cDNA probe composed of the base sequence coding for the HCV-229E nucleocapsid protein may detect as few as 10 $TCID_{50}$; this probe did not cross-hybridize with HCV-OC43.[92, 94] Polymerase chain reaction amplification of both HCV-229E and HCV-OC43 from respiratory secretions also has been described.[93]

An antigen-detection ELISA for enteric coronavirus has been described[66] and applied to fecal specimens from healthy and diarrheal subjects in Thailand.[67] Findings were similar to the electron-microscopic stool studies from India: coronavirus excretion was higher in healthy subjects, and excretion of viral antigen was observed occasionally to persist for months. Other studies of this assay have not been reported.

Serodiagnosis

By using antigen prepared as just described, the usual serologic tests can be performed by standard procedures: complement fixation,[24, 79, 88, 104] hemagglutination inhibition (for HCV-OC43 only[61]), neutralization,[17, 24] ELISA,[18, 40, 64, 71] indirect hemagglutination,[60] and Western blot.[100]

We are not aware of any serodiagnostic techniques for CVLPs, but, if some are related to HCV-OC43,[39] serodiagnosis may be possible in the future.

PREVENTION AND TREATMENT

Even if it were possible to prepare sufficient antigen for vaccine preparation, the high reinfection rate for these viruses suggests that a vaccine may be ineffective in preventing HCV-caused respiratory illness. At present, not enough is known about the putative enteric HCV to consider vaccine development. There is evidence from the other common cold viruses, the rhinoviruses, that environmental control of respiratory illness may be possible, either by use of virucidal facial tissues[30] or by air filtration.[31] Prevention of symptoms of respiratory HCV infection by alpha-interferon may be possible, although side effects of nasal bleeding often are present and protection from natural colds has not been demonstrated.[32, 48, 125] A broad-spectrum antiviral drug, ribavirin, has some in vitro activity against coronavirus[119] and has been shown to reduce markedly hepatitis in mice infected with mouse hepatitis virus, a coronavirus related antigenically to HCV-OC43.[82]

References

1. Almeida, J. D., Berry, D. M., Cunningham, C. H., et al.: Coronaviruses. Nature *220*:650, 1968.
2. Almeida, J. D., and Tyrrell, D. A. J.: The morphology of three previously uncharacterized human respiratory viruses that grow in organ culture. J. Gen. Virol. *1*:175–178, 1967.
3. Baker, S. J., Mathan, M., Mathan, V. I., et al.: Chronic enterocyte infection with coronavirus. Dig. Dis. Sci. *27*:1039–1043, 1982.
4. Battaglia, M., Passarani, N., Di Matteo, A., et al.: Human enteric coronaviruses: Further characterization and immunoblotting of viral proteins. J. Infect. Dis. *155*:140–143, 1987.
5. Beach, J. R., and Schalm, O. W.: A filterable virus, distinct from that of laryngotracheitis, the cause of a respiratory disease of chicks. Poultry Sci. *15*:199–206, 1936.
6. Beards, G. M., Hall, C., Green, J., et al.: An enveloped virus in stools of

children and adults with gastroenteritis that resembles the Breda virus of calves. Lancet *1*:1050–1052, 1984.
7. Beaudette, F. R., and Hudson, C. B.: Cultivation of the virus of infectious bronchitis. J. Am. Vet. Med. Assoc. *90*:51–60, 1937.
8. Becker, W. B., McIntosh, K., Dees, J. H., et al.: Morphogenesis of avian infectious bronchitis virus and a related human virus (strain 229E). J. Virol. *1*:1019–1027, 1967.
9. Bende, M., Barrow, I., Heptonstall, J., et al.: Changes in human nasal mucosa during experimental coronavirus common colds. Acta Otolaryngol. (Stockholm) *107*:262–269, 1989.
10. Betts, R. F.: Influenza virus. *In* Mandell, G. L., Bennett, J. E., and Dolin R. (eds.): Principles and Practice of Infectious Diseases. 4th ed. New York, Churchill Livingstone, 1995, pp. 1546–1567.
11. Boursnell, M. E. G., Brown, T. D. K., Foulds, I. J., et al.: Completion of the sequence of the genome of the coronavirus avian infectious bronchitis virus. J. Gen. Virol. *68*:57–77, 1987.
12. Bradburne, A. F.: Antigenic relationships amongst coronaviruses. Arch. Virol. *31*:352–364, 1970.
13. Bradburne, A. F., Bynoe, M. L., and Tyrrell, D. A. J.: Effects of a "new" human respiratory virus in volunteers. Br. Med. J. *3*:767–769, 1967.
14. Bradburne, A. F., and Somerset, B. A.: Coronavirus antibody titres in sera of healthy adults and experimentally infected volunteers. J. Hyg. (Camb.) *70*:235–244, 1972.
15. Burks, J. S., DeVale, B. L., Jankovsk, L. D., et al: Two coronaviruses isolated from central nervous system tissue of two multiple sclerosis patients. Science *209*:933–934, 1980.
16. Buscho, R. O., Saxtan, D., Schultz, P. S., et al.: Infections with viruses and *Mycoplasma pneumoniae* during exacerbations of chronic bronchitis. J. Infect. Dis. *137*:377–383, 1978.
17. Callow, K. A.: Effect of specific humoral immunity and some non-specific factors on resistance of volunteers to respiratory coronavirus infection. J. Hyg. (Camb.) *95*:173–189, 1985.
18. Callow, K. A., Parry, H. F., Sergeant, M., et al.: The time course of the immune response to experimental coronavirus infection of man. Epidemiol. Infect. *105*:435–446, 1990.
19. Callow, K. A., Tyrrell, D. A. J., Shaw, R. J., et al.: Influence of atopy on the clinical manifestations of coronavirus infection in adult volunteers. Clin. Allergy *18*:119–129, 1988.
20. Candeias, J. A. N., Carvalho, R. P. de S., and Antonacio, F.: Seroepidemiologic study of coronavirus infection in Brazilian children and civilian adults. Rev. Inst. Med. Trop. *14*:121–125, 1972.
21. Caul, E. O., and Clarke, S. K. R.: Coronavirus propagated from patient with non-bacterial gastroenteritis. Lancet 2:953–954, 1975.
22. Caul, E. O., and Egglestone, S. I.: Further studies on human enteric coronaviruses. Arch. Virol. *54*:107–117, 1977.
23. Caul, E. O., Paver, W. K., and Clarke, S. K. R.: Coronavirus particles in faeces from patients with gastroenteritis. Lancet *1*:1192, 1975.
24. Cavallaro, J. J., and Monto, A. S.: Community-wide outbreak of infection with a 229E-like coronavirus in Tecumseh, Michigan. J. Infect. Dis. *122*:272–279, 1970.
25. Cavanagh D., Brian, D. A., Brinton, M. A., et al.: The *Coronaviridae* now comprises two genera, *Coronavirus* and *Torovirus:* Report of the *Coronaviridae* Study Group. Adv. Exp. Med. Biol. *342*:255–257, 1993.
26. Chany, C., Moscovici, O., Lebon, P., et al.: Association of coronavirus infection with neonatal necrotizing enterocolitis. Pediatrics *69*:209–214, 1982.
27. Christensen, M. L.: Human viral gastroenteritis. Clin. Microbiol. Rev. 2:51–89, 1989.
28. Collins, A.: Human coronavirus OC43 interacts with major histocompatibility complex class I molecules at the cell surface to establish infection. Immunol. Invest. *23*:313–321, 1994.
29. Collins, A. R.: Interferon gamma potentiates human coronavirus OC43 infection of neuronal cells by modulation of HLA class I expression. Immunol. Invest. *24*:977–986, 1995.
30. Dick, E. C., Hossain, S. U., and Mink, K. A., et al.: Interruption of transmission of rhinovirus colds among human volunteers using virucidal paper handkerchiefs. J. Infect. Dis. *153*:352–356, 1986.
31. Dick, E. C., Jennings, L. C., and Mink, K. A., et al.: Aerosol transmission of rhinovirus colds. J. Infect. Dis. *156*:442–448, 1987.
32. Douglas, R. M., Moore, B. W., Miles, H. B., et al.: Prophylactic efficacy of intranasal alpha$_2$-interferon against rhinovirus infections in the family setting. N. Engl. J. Med. *314*:65–70, 1986.
33. Dourmashkin, R. R., Davies, H. A., Smith, H., et al.: Are coronavirus-like particles seen in diarrhoea stools really viruses? Lancet *2*:971–972, 1980.
34. Editorial: Splints don't stop colds—surprising! Lancet *1*:277–278, 1988.
35. Eis-Hübinger, A. M., Stifter, G., and Schneweis, K. E.: Opportunistic infections with coronavirus-like particles in patients infected with the human immunodeficiency virus? Int. J. Med. Microbiol. *271*:351–355, 1989.
36. Erlich, S. S., Fleming, J. O., Stohlman, S. A., et al.: Experimental neuropathology of chronic demyelination induced by a JHM virus variant (DS). Arch. Neurol. *44*:839–842, 1987.
37. Fleming, J. O., El Zaatari, F. A. K., Gilmore, W., et al.: Antigenic assessment of coronaviruses isolated from patients with multiple sclerosis. Arch. Neurol. *45*:629–633, 1988.
38. Gerdes, J. C., Klein, I., DeVald, B. L., et al.: Coronavirus isolates SK and SD from multiple sclerosis patients are serologically related to murine coronaviuses A59 and JHM and human coronavirus OC43, but not to human coronavirus 229E. J. Virol. *38*:231–238, 1981.
39. Gerna, G., Passarani, N., Battaglia, M., et al.: Human enteric coronaviruses: Antigenic relatedness to human coronavirus OC43 and possible etiologic role in viral gastroenteritis. J. Infect. Dis. *151*:796–803, 1985.
40. Gill, E. P., Dominguez, E. A., Greenberg, S. B., et al.: Development and application of an enzyme immunoassay for coronavirus OC43 antibody in acute respiratory illness. J. Clin. Microbiol. *32*:2372–2376, 1994.
41. Gregg, M. B.: The epidemiology of influenza in humans. Ann. N. Y. Acad. Sci. *353*:45–53, 1980.
42. Gump, D. W., Phillips, C. A., Forsyth, B. R., et al.: Role of infection in chronic bronchitis. Am. Rev. Respir. Dis. *113*:465–474, 1976.
43. Hamre, D., and Beem, M.: Virologic studies of acute respiratory disease in young adults. Am. J. Epidemiol. *96*:94–106, 1972.
44. Hamre, D., and Procknow, J. J.: A new virus isolated from the human respiratory tract. Proc. Soc. Exp. Biol. Med. *121*:190–193, 1966.
45. Hasony, H. J., and Macnaughton, M. R.: Prevalence of human coronavirus antibody in the population of southern Iraq. J. Med. Virol. *9*:209–216, 1982.
46. Hendley, J. O., Fishburne, H. B., and Gwaltney, J. M.: Coronavirus infections in working adults. Am. Rev. Respir. Dis. *105*:805–811, 1972.
47. Herold J., Raabe, T., and Siddell, S.: Molecular analysis of the human coronavirus (strain 229E) genome. Arch. Virol. *7*(Suppl.):63–74, 1993.
48. Higgins, P. G., Phillpotts, R. J., Scott, G. M., et al.: Intranasal interferon as protection against experimental respiratory coronavirus infection in volunteers. Antimicrob. Agents Chemother. *24*:713–715, 1983.
49. Holmes, K. V., and Lai, M. M. C.: *Coronaviridae*: The viruses and their replication. *In* Fields, B. N., Knipe, D. M., Howley, P. M., et al. (eds.): Fields Virology. 3rd ed. New York, Raven Press, 1996, pp. 1075–1093.
50. Hovanec, D. L., and Flanagan, T. D.: Detection of antibodies to human coronaviruses 229E and OC43 in the sera of multiple sclerosis patients and normal subjects. Infect. Immun. *41*:426–429, 1983.
51. Isaacs, D., Clarke, J. R., Tyrrell, D. A. J., et al.: Selective infection of lower respiratory tract by respiratory viruses in children with recurrent respiratory tract infections. Br. Med. J. *284*:1746–1748, 1982.
52. Isaacs, D., Flowers, D., Clarke, J. R., et al.: Epidemiology of coronavirus respiratory infections. Arch. Dis. Child. *58*:500–503, 1983.
53. Johnson, R. T.: The possible viral etiology of multiple sclerosis. Adv. Neurol. *13*:1–46, 1975.
54. Johnson-Lussenburg, C. M., and Zheng, Q.: Coronavirus and multiple sclerosis: Results of a case/control longitudinal serological study. *In* Lai, M., and Stohlman, S. (eds.): Coronaviruses. New York, Plenum, 1987, pp. 421–429.
55. Johnston, S. L., Pattemore, P. K., Sanderson, G., et al.: Community study of the role of viral infections in exacerbations of asthma in 9–11 year old chilren. Br. Med. J. *310*:1225–1229, 1995.
56. Kapikian, A. Z., and Chanock, R. M.: Viral gastroenteritis. *In* Evans, A. S. (ed.): Viral Infections of Humans. 3rd ed. New York, Plenum, 1989, pp. 293–340.
57. Kapikian, A. Z., James, H. D., Kelly, S. J., et al.: Isolation from man of "avian infectious bronchitis virus-like" viruses (coronaviruses) similar to 229E virus, with some epidemiological observations. J. Infect. Dis. *119*:282–290, 1969.
58. Kapikian, A. Z., James, H. D., Kelly, S. J., et al.: Hemadsorption by coronavirus strain OC43 (36105). Proc. Soc. Exp. Biol. Med. *139*:179–186, 1972.
59. Kaye, H. S., and Dowdle, W. R.: Some characteristics of hemagglutination of certain strains of "IBV-like" virus. J. Infect. Dis. *120*:576–581, 1969.
60. Kaye, H. S., and Dowdle, W. R.: Seroepidemiologic survey of coronavirus (strain 229E) infections in a population of children. Am. J. Epidemiol. *101*:238–244, 1975.
61. Kaye, H. S., Marsh, H. B., and Dowdle, W. R.: Seroepidemiologic survey of coronavirus (strain OC43) related infections in a children's population. Am. J. Epidemiol. *94*:43–49, 1971.
62. Kern, P., Müller, G., Schmitz, H., et al.: Detection of coronavirus-like particles in homosexual men with acquired immunodeficiency and related lymphadenopathy syndrome. Klin. Wochenschr. *63*:68–72, 1985.
63. Kidd, A. H., Esrey, S. A., and Ujfalusi, M. J.: Shedding of coronavirus-like particles by children in Lesotho. J. Med. Virol. *27*:164–169, 1989.
64. Kraaijeveld, C. A., Reed, S. E., and Macnaughton, M. R.: Enzyme-linked immunosorbent assay for detection of antibody in volunteers experimentally infected with human coronavirus strain 229E. J. Clin. Microbiol. *12*:493–497, 1980.
65. Larson, H. E., Reed, S. E., and Tyrrell, D. A. J.: Isolation of rhinoviruses and coronaviruses from 38 colds in adults. J. Med. Virol. *5*:221–229, 1980.
66. Leechanachai, P., Yoosook, C., and Matangkasombut, P.: Epidemiological study of enteric coronavirus excretion by an enzyme-linked immunosorbent assay. J. Med. Assoc Thai. 72:452–457, 1989.
67. Leechanachai, P., Yoosook, C., Saguanwongse, S., et al.: Comparison of a modified enzyme-linked immunosorbent assay with immunosorbent electron microscopy to detect coronavirus in human faecal specimens. J. Diarrhoeal Dis. Res. *5*:24–29, 1987.
68. Macnaughton, M. R.: Occurrence and frequency of coronavirus infections in humans as determined by enzyme-linked immunosorbent assay. Infect. Immun. *38*:419–423, 1982.

69. Macnaughton, M. R., and Davies, H. A.: Human enteric coronaviruses. Arch. Virol. *70*:301–313, 1981.
70. Macnaughton, M. R., Flowers, D., and Isaacs, D.: Diagnosis of human coronavirus infections in children using enzyme-linked immunosorbent assay. J. Med. Virol. *11*:319–325, 1983.
71. Macnaughton, M. R., Madge, M. H., and Reed, S. E.: Two antigenic groups of human coronaviruses detected by using enzyme-linked immunosorbent assay. Infect. Immun. *33*:734–737, 1981.
72. Marshall, J. A., Thompson, W. L., and Gust, I. D.: Coronavirus-like particles in adults in Melbourne, Australia. J. Med. Virol. *29*:238–243, 1989.
73. Mathan, M., Mathan, V. I., Swaminathan, S. P., et al.: Pleomorphic virus-like particles in human faeces. Lancet *1*:1068–1069, 1975.
74. Mathan, V. I.: Tropical sprue in southern India. Trans. R. Soc. Trop. Med. Hyg. *82*:10–14, 1988.
75. McIntosh, K.: Coronaviruses: A comparative review. Curr. Top. Microbiol. Immunol. *63*:86–129, 1974.
76. McIntosh, K.: Coronaviruses. *In* Fields, B. N., Knipe, D. M., Howley, P. M., et al. (eds.): Fields Virology. 3rd ed. New York, Raven Press, 1996, pp. 1095–1103.
77. McIntosh, K.: Coronavirus. *In* Mandell, G. L., Bennett, J. E., and Dolin, R. (eds.): Principles and Practice of Infectious Diseases. 4th ed. New York, Churchill Livingstone, 1995, pp. 1486–1489.
78. McIntosh, K., Becker, W. B., and Chanock, R. M.: Growth in suckling-mouse brain of "IBV-like" viruses from patients with upper respiratory tract disease. Proc. Natl. Acad. Sci. U. S. A. *58*:2268–2273, 1967.
79. McIntosh, K., Chao, R. K., Krause, H. E., et al.: Coronavirus infection in acute lower respiratory tract disease of infants. J. Infect. Dis. *130*:502–507, 1974.
80. McIntosh, K., Dees, J. H., Becker, W. B., et al.: Recovery in tracheal organ cultures of novel viruses from patients with respiratory disease. Proc. Natl. Acad. Sci. U. S. A. *57*:933–940, 1967.
81. McIntosh, K., Ellis, E. F., Hoffman, L. S., et al.: The association of viral and bacterial respiratory infections with exacerbations of wheezing in young asthmatic children. J. Pediatr. *82*:578–590, 1973.
82. McIntosh, K., Kapikian, A. Z., Hardison, K. A., et al.: Antigenic relationships among the coronaviruses of man and between human and animal coronaviruses. J. Immunol. *102*:1109–1118, 1969.
83. McIntosh, K., Kapikian, A. Z., Turner, H. C., et al.: Seroepidemiologic studies of coronavirus infection in adults and children. Am. J. Epidemiol. *91*:585–592, 1970.
84. McIntosh, K., McQuillin, J., Reed, S. E., et al.: Diagnosis of human coronavirus infection by immunofluorescence: Method and application to respiratory disease in hospitalized children. J. Med. Virol. *2*:341–346, 1978.
85. Mertsola, J., Ziegler, T., and Ruuskanen, O., et al: Recurrent wheezy bronchitis and viral respiratory infections. Arch. Dis. Child. *66*:124–129, 1991.
86. Monto, A. S.: Coronaviruses. *In* Evans, A. S. (ed.): Viral Infections of Humans. 3rd ed. New York, Plenum, 1989, pp. 153–167.
87. Monto, A. S., Higgins, M. W., and Ross, H. W.: The Tecumseh study of respiratory illness. VIII. Acute infection in chronic respiratory disease and comparison groups. Am. Rev. Respir. Dis. *111*:27–36, 1975.
88. Monto, A. S., and Lim, S. K.: The Tecumseh study of respiratory illness. VI. Frequency of and relationship between outbreaks of coronavirus infection. J. Infect. Dis. *129*:271–276, 1974.
89. Mortensen, M. L., Ray, C. G., Payne, C. M., et al.: Coronaviruslike particles in human gastrointestinal disease. Am. J. Dis. Child. *139*:928–934, 1985.
90. Murray, R. S., Brown, B., Brian, D., et al.: Detection of coronavirus RNA and antigen in multiple sclerosis brain. Ann. Neurol. *31*:525–533, 1992.
91. Murray, R. S., Cai, G.-Y., Hoel, K., et al.: Coronavirus infects and causes demyelination in primate central nervous system. Virology *188*:274–284, 1992.
92. Myint, S., Harmsen, D., Raabe, T., et al.: Characterization of a nucleic acid probe for the diagnosis of human coronavirus 229E infections. J. Med. Virol. *31*:165–172, 1990.
93. Myint, S., Johnston, S., Sanderson, G., et al.: Evaluation of nested polymerase chain methods for the detection of human coronaviruses 229E and OC43. Mol. Cell. Probes *8*:357–364, 1994.
94. Myint, S., Siddell, S., and Tyrrell, D.: Detection of human coronavirus 229E in nasal washings using RNA:RNA hybridisation. J. Med. Virol. *29*:70–73, 1989.
95. Myint, S., Siddell, S., and Tyrrell, D.: The use of nucleic acid hybridization to detect human coronaviruses. Arch. Virol. *104*:335–337, 1989.
96. Nicholson, K. G., Kent, J., and Ireland, D. C.: Respiratory viruses and exacerbations of asthma in adults. Br. Med. J. *307*:982–986, 1993.
97. Pattemore, P. K., Johnston, S. L., and Bardin, P. G.: Virses as precipitants of asthma symptoms. I. Epidemiology. Clin. Exp. Allergy *22*:325–336, 1992.
98. Patterson, S., and Macnaughton, M. R.: Replication of human respiratory coronavirus strain 229E in human macrophages. J. Gen. Virol. *60*:307–314, 1982.
99. Payne, C. M., Ray, G. C., Borduin, V., et al.: An eight-year study of the viral agents of acute gastroenteritis in humans: Ultrastructural observations and seasonal distribution with a major emphasis on coronavirus-like particles. Diagn. Microbiol. Infect. Dis. *5*:39–54, 1986.
100. Pohl-Koppe, A., Raabe, T., Siddell, S. G., et al.: Detection of human coronavirus 229E-specific antibodies using recombinant fusion proteins. J. Virol. Methods *55*:175–183, 1995.
101. Reed, S. E.: The behaviour of recent isolates of human respiratory coronavirus in vitro and in volunteers: Evidence of heterogeneity among 229E-related strains. J. Med. Virol. *13*:179–192, 1984.
102. Resta, S., Luby, J. P., Rosenfeld, C. R., et al.: Isolation and propagation of a human enteric coronavirus. Science *229*:978–981, 1985.
103. Rettig, P. J., and Altshuler, G. P.: Fatal gastroenteritis associated with coronaviruslike particles. Am. J. Dis. Child. *139*:245–248, 1985.
104. Riski, H., and Hovi, T.: Coronavirus infections of man associated with diseases other than the common cold. J. Med. Virol. *6*:259–265, 1980.
105. Salmi, A., Reunanen, M., Ilonen, J., et al.: Intrathecal antibody synthesis to virus antigens in multiple sclerosis. Clin. Exp. Immunol. *52*:241–249, 1983.
106. Sarateanu, D. E., and Ehrengut, W.: A two-year serological surveillance of coronavirus infections in Hamburg. Infection *8*:70–72, 1980.
107. Schieble, J. H.: Coronaviruses. *In* Schmidt, N. J., and Emmons, R. W. (eds.): Diagnostic Procedures for Viral, Rickettsial and Chlamydial Infections. 6th ed. Washington, D.C., American Public Health Association, 1989, pp. 615–630.
108. Schmidt, O. W.: Antigenic characterization of human coronaviruses 229E and OC43 by enzyme-linked immunosorbent assay. J. Clin. Microbiol. *20*:175–180, 1984.
109. Schmidt, O. W., Cooney, M. K., and Kenny, G. E.: Plaque assay and improved yield of human coronaviruses in a human rhabdomyosarcoma cell line. J. Clin. Microbiol. *9*:722–728, 1979.
110. Schmidt, O. W., and Kenny, G. E.: Immunogenicity and antigenicity of human coronaviruses 229E and OC43. Infect. Immun. *32*:1000–1006, 1981.
111. Schnagl, R. D., Holmes, I. H., and Mackay-Scollay, E. M.: Coronavirus-like particles in aboriginals and non-aboriginals in western Australia. Med. J. Aust. *1*:307–309, 1978.
112. Schreiber, S. S., Kamahora, T., and Lai, M. M.: Sequence analysis of the nucleocapsid protein gene of human coronavirus 229E. Virology *169*:142–151, 1989.
113. Siddell, S., Wege, H., and Ter Meulen, V.: The biology of coronaviruses. J. Gen. Virol. *64*:761–776, 1983.
114. Sidwell, R. W., Huffman, J. H., Campbell, N., et al.: Effect of ribavirin on viral hepatitis in laboratory animals. Ann. N. Y. Acad. Sci. *284*:239–246, 1977.
115. Singh, P. B., Sreenivasan, M. A., and Pavri, K. M.: Viruses in acute gastroenteritis in children in Pune, India. Epidemiol. Infect. *102*:345–353, 1989.
116. Sitbon, M.: Human-enteric-coronaviruslike particles (CVLP) with different epidemiological characteristics. J. Med. Virol. *16*:67–76, 1985.
117. Sizun, J., Soupre, D., Legrand, M. C., et al.: Neonatal nosocomial respiratory infection with coronavirus: A prospective study in a neonatal intensive care unit. Acta Paediatr. *84*:617–620, 1995.
118. Smith, C. B., Golden, C. A., Kanner, R. E., et al.: Association of viral and *Mycoplasma pneumoniae* infections with acute respiratory illness in patients with chronic obstructive pulmonary diseases. Am. Rev. Respir. Dis. *121*:225–232, 1980.
119. Smith, R. A., and Kirkpatrick, W. (eds.): Ribavirin, Broad Spectrum Antiviral Agent. New York, Academic Press, 1980.
120. Sorensen, O., Collins, A., Flintoff, W., et al.: Probing for the human coronavirus OC43 in multiple sclerosis. Neurology 36:1604–1606, 1986.
121. Stewart, J. N., Mounir, S., and Talbot, P. J.: Human coronavirus gene expression in the brains of multiple sclerosis patients. Virology *191*:502–505, 1992.
122. Stohlman, S. A., Kyuwa, S., Polo, J. M., et al.: Characterization of mouse hepatitis virus-specific cytotoxic T cells derived from the central nervous system of mice infected with the JHM strain. J. Virol. *67*:7050–7059, 1993.
123. Tanaka, R., Iwasaki, Y., and Koprowski, H.: Intracisternal virus-like particles in brain of a multiple sclerosis patient. J. Neurol. Sci. *28*:121–126, 1976.
124. Timoney, J. F., Gillespie, J. H., Scott, F. W., et al.: The *Coronaviridae*. *In* Timoney J. F., Gillespie, J., Scott, F. W., et al. (eds.): Hagan and Bruner's Microbiology and Infectious Diseases of Domestic Animals. 8th ed. Ithaca, Comstock Publishing Associates, 1988, pp. 886–911.
125. Turner, R. B., Felton, A., Kosak, K., et al.: Prevention of experimental coronavirus colds with intranasal alpha-2b interferon. J. Infect. Dis. *154*:443–447, 1986.
126. Turner, R. B., Meschievitz, C. K., Streisand, A. C., et al.: Mechanism of transmission of coronavirus 229E in human volunteers. Clin. Res. *35*:145A, 1987.
127. Tyrrell, D. A. J.: Rhinoviruses and coronaviruses: Virological aspects of their role in causing colds in man. Eur. J. Respir. Dis. *64*(Suppl. 128):332–335, 1983.
128. Tyrrell, D. A. J.: Common colds. Intervirology *25*:177–189, 1986.
129. Tyrrell, D. A. J., Almeida, J. D., Cunningham, C. H., et al.: *Coronaviridae*. Intervirology *5*:76–82, 1975.
130. Tyrrell, D. A. J., and Bynoe, M. L.: Cultivation of a novel type of common-cold virus in organ cultures. Br. Med. J. *1*:1467–1470, 1965.
131. Ukkonen, P., Hovi, T., von Bonsdorff, C.-H., et al.: Age-specific prevalence of complement-fixing antibodies to sixteen viral antigens: A computer analysis of 58,500 patients covering a period of eight years. J. Med. Virol. *13*:131–148, 1984.
132. Vaucher, Y. E., Ray, C. G., Minnich, L. L., et al.: Pleomorphic, enveloped,

virus-like particles associated with gastrointestinal illness in neonates. J. Infect. Dis. *145*:27–36, 1982.
133. Vlasak, R., Luytjes, W., Spaan, W., et al.: Human and bovine coronaviruses recognize sialic acid-containing receptors similar to those of influenza C viruses. Proc. Natl. Acad. Sci. U. S. A. *85*:4526–4529, 1988.
134. Wege, H., Siddell, S., and Ter Meulen, V.: The biology and pathogenesis of coronaviruses. Curr. Top. Microbiol. Immunol. *99*:165–200, 1982.
135. Weiss, S. R.: Coronaviruses SD and SK share extensive nucleotide homology with murine coronavirus MHV-A59, more than that shared between human and murine coronaviruses. Virology *126*:669–677, 1983.
136. Wenzel, R. P., Hendley, J. O., Davies, J. A., et al.: Coronavirus infections in military recruits: Three-year study with coronavirus strains OC43 and 229E. Am. Rev. Respir. Dis. *109*:621–624, 1974.
137. Winther, B., Gwaltney, J. M., and Hendley, J. O.: Respiratory virus infection of monolayer cultures of human nasal epithelial cells. Am. Rev. Respir. Dis. *141*:839–845, 1990.
138. Yeager, C. L., Ashmun, R. A., Williams, R. K., et al.: Human aminopeptidase N is a receptor for human coronavirus 229E. Nature *357*:420–422, 1992.
139. Zhang, X. M., Herbst, W., Kousoulas, K. G., et al.: Biological and genetic characterization of a hemagglutinating coronavirus isolated from a diarrhoeic child. J. Med. Virol. *44*:152–161, 1994.

❑ ❑ ❑

SUBSECTION ELEVEN

BUNYAVIRIDAE

189

HANTAVIRUSES

Louisa E. Chapman, Kelly T. McKee, Jr., and C. J. Peters

HISTORICAL PERSPECTIVE

Hantaviruses are the etiologic agents of a diverse group of rodent-borne hemorrhagic fevers that are responsible for considerable morbidity and mortality worldwide. Although recognized by so-called modern medicine only relatively recently, clinical syndromes now known to be associated with these viruses have been described by traditional practitioners across the globe from antiquity.[14, 60, 74] In the twentieth century, Soviet scientists described sporadic outbreaks of febrile renal failure with hemorrhage in the eastern Soviet Union between 1913 and 1930,[8] and Japanese and Soviet scientists recognized annual outbreaks of a similar syndrome in Manchuria and Siberia between 1932 and 1935.[30, 73, 101, 107] In 1934, Swedish scientists described a novel disorder characterized by fever, abdominal and back pain, and renal abnormalities[78, 121]; epidemic disease with these features occurred among German and Finnish troops stationed in Lapland during World War II.[43, 104]

North American medical practitioners initially became acquainted with a similar syndrome in the early 1950s, when thousands of soldiers serving with United Nation forces during the Korean War developed a previously unrecognized febrile illness characterized by shock, hemorrhage, and renal failure. Physicians called this syndrome, which had a mortality rate of 5 to 15 per cent, epidemic hemorrhagic fever.[25, 75]

In 1953, Gajdusek[29] noted similarities among epidemic hemorrhagic fever, the severe and frequently fatal Far Eastern diseases described by Soviet and Japanese scientists, and the Scandinavian disorder and proposed a common etiology. Subsequent validation of this hypothesis (see The Organism) ultimately prompted adoption of the collective term hemorrhagic fever with renal syndrome (HFRS) to describe this clinical entity characterized by varying degrees of renal dysfunction and hemorrhage with fever.

In June 1993, the investigation of a cluster of unexplained respiratory deaths in previously healthy young adult residents of rural areas in the southwestern United States led to recognition of a "new" hemorrhagic fever in North America. Application of sophisticated serologic and virologic tools to diagnostic specimens from patients with this mysterious disease quickly pointed to a hantavirus related to, but distinct from, those causing HFRS.[56, 80] This disorder, now called hantavirus pulmonary syndrome (HPS), proved to be different clinically from classic HFRS, but as virologic and epidemiologic studies of the etiologic agent and its reservoirs were completed, similarities to other hantaviruses became apparent.

THE ORGANISM

Classification and Antigenic Composition

The genus *Hantavirus* of the family *Bunyaviridae* was defined in 1985.[95, 96] The members of the *Hantavirus* genus are classified among the bunyaviruses because of their shared morphologic, physicochemical, and molecular properties. Like other members of the family *Bunyaviridae*, hantaviruses are negative-stranded, lipid-enveloped RNA viruses with tripartite genomes; genomic segments are designated as large (L), medium (M), and small (S). Also like other bunyaviruses, they display a Golgi-associated morphogenesis and usually acquire their envelopes by budding into intracytoplasmic vacuoles.[94] However, they are distinct serologically from other family members and possess unique terminal genome sequences.[95] The *Hantavirus* genus contains the only members of *Bunyaviridae* that lack arthropod vectors. Each hantavirus is adapted highly to a specific rodent species and depends on persistent asymptomatic infections in wild rodents for its maintenance in nature.

Physical Properties

Morphologically, hantaviruses are spherical, are 80 to 120 nm in diameter, and have surface glycoprotein projections that are embedded in a lipid bilayer envelope. Elongated particles (110 to 120 nm long) often are observed, and they display a characteristic grid-like pattern on their surfaces.[35, 94]

Susceptibility

Hantaviruses are inactivated readily by lipid solvents and most disinfectants, including dilute hypochlorite solutions, detergents, ethyl alcohol (70 per cent), most general-purpose household disinfectants, and beta-propiolactone (0.1 per cent at 4° C for 3 days).[36, 55, 91] Limited studies with Hantaan virus have shown sensitivity to a pH of 5 or less and to temperatures of 56° C or higher.[36, 62] The survival time in the environment in the absence of disinfection is not known, but limited studies have shown persistent infectivity in dried cell culture medium for up to 2 days and in neutral solutions for several hours at 37° C or several days at lower temperatures.[10]

Laboratory Propagation and Tissue Culture Growth

Hantaviruses are fastidious but can be grown in culture through serial blind passage. They routinely establish persistent, noncytolytic infections and generally do not replicate to high titer.[36, 94] The prototype member of the group, Hantaan virus, was isolated in 1978[67] and was propagated successfully in cell culture in the A-549 cell line in 1981.[28] However, Vero E-6 cells subsequently were found to be a better cell culture system for this and other hantaviruses.[36] Hantaviruses have been isolated and propagated successfully through direct inoculation of homogenates of infected tissue from wild-caught rodent hosts onto cell lines or after amplification through serially infected, colonized rodent hosts.[26, 28, 34, 36, 67, 82, 93, 117] Recovery of hantaviruses from human specimens has been difficult and infrequent. More than 20 hantaviruses currently are recognized, 9 of which have been linked definitively to human disease. The major viruses are listed in Table 189–1. All have been isolated in cell culture except Andes virus (known only from genetic sequences amplified from human tissue) and New York 1 (passed in *Peromyscus leucopus* in the laboratory). This list will be expanded and modified as our knowledge of classification and new viruses expands. Laboratory infections of persons working with cell culture–adapted Hantaan virus as well as laboratory transmission of hantaviruses from infected rodents to humans are well documented.[22, 23, 48, 63, 64, 71, 109, 110] Consequently, attempts to propagate the virus should be carried out only when using biosafety level 3 or 4 facilities and practices.[10, 13]

Transmission

Hantaviruses are zoonotic; each hantavirus is associated with a distinct rodent species in which it establishes a chronic, inapparent infection. Hantavirus infection of rodents produces a short viremia, resulting in dissemination of virus to lungs, salivary glands, and kidneys. Once infected, the rodent sheds virus in urine, saliva, and (to a lesser extent) feces throughout its life, despite the development of neutralizing antibodies.[65] Infection does not diminish the longevity or the reproductive potential of the infected rodent; vertical transmission has not been demonstrated. Enzootic infection appears to be maintained by exposure to nesting materials contaminated with infectious secretions, grooming behaviors, and intraspecies biting.[63, 65]

It generally is accepted that humans become infected with hantaviruses after contact with contaminated secreta or excreta of infected rodents via inhalation of small-particle aerosols or, rarely, percutaneous inoculation of infected materials. The primacy of respiratory droplets or airborne particles as the mode of transmission to humans is supported by evidence from outbreaks of disease among laboratory workers as well as sporadic cases resulting from brief exposures to rodent-infected habitats.[13, 22, 23, 48, 63–65, 71, 109, 110, 115, 120]

The risk of human hantavirus infection is a function of the density of the local rodent reservoir population, the prevalence of infection among rodents, and the frequency of activities that result in contact between humans and rodent excreta. Individual hantavirus infections usually occur when humans disturb rodent habitats or rodents enter human housing. Epidemics generally are associated with either changes in the behavior of human populations that result in large-scale exposure of persons to rodent-infected areas (e.g., military maneuvers, agricultural or forestry activities) or environmental changes that result in rapid increases in the density of the rodent population (e.g., proliferation of food sources). Person-to-person transmission of hantaviruses associated with HFRS has not been demonstrated. Experience to date with HPS has been similar,[112] although interpersonal spread may have occurred during a single outbreak in South America.[26a, 113a] If subsequent investigations support this observation, a reappraisal of transmission risks associated with South American hantaviruses may be necessary.

EPIDEMIOLOGY

Geographic Distribution

Hantaviruses have been found on every continent except Antarctica. With the exception of HFRS caused by Seoul

TABLE 189–1. Some Currently Recognized Hantaviruses

Virus Strain	Principal Reservoir	Distribution	Disease Association
Hantaan	*Apodemus agrarius*	Far East Northern Asia Balkans	HFRS (severe)
Seoul	*Rattus norvegicus*	Worldwide	HFRS (mild/moderate)
Dobrava	*Apodemus flavicollis*	Balkans	HFRS (severe)
Puumala	*Clethrionomys glareolus*	Scandinavia Northern Europe Balkans	HFRS (mild) (Nephropathia epidemica)
Thailand	*Bandicota indica*	Thailand	None recognized
Prospect Hill	*Microtus pennsylvanicus*	United States	None recognized
Sin Nombre	*Peromyscus maniculatus*	United States	HPS
New York 1	*Peromyscus leucopus*	United States	HPS
Black Creek Canal	*Sigmodon hispidus*	United States	HPS
Bayou	*Oryzomys palustris*	United States	HPS
Andes	Unknown	South America	HPS
Thottapalayam	*Suncus marinus*	India	None recognized

HFRS, hemorrhagic fever with renal syndrome; HPS, hantavirus pulmonary syndrome.

virus, hantavirus diseases occur almost exclusively in rural areas. Hantaan virus, the cause of "classic" HFRS found in northern Asia and the Orient, is carried by the striped field mouse, *Apodemus agrarius.* This rodent is distributed across eastern Russia, China, and the Korean Peninsula.[115] The principal reservoir for Puumala virus, etiologic agent of a milder HFRS variant found in Scandinavia, northern Europe, and Russia west of the Ural Mountains, is the bank vole *Clethrionomys glareolus.*[66, 98]

In the Balkans, at least three viruses have been linked etiologically with HFRS: Puumala, Hantaan, and Dobrava; the latter two agents are associated with *Apodemus flavicollis,* the yellow-necked field mouse.[2, 4, 5, 34] *Rattus* species (primarily *R. norvegicus)* serve as reservoirs for Seoul-like viruses identified worldwide; human infections have been seen most frequently in eastern Asia. Outbreaks of severe and occasionally fatal HFRS among animal handlers and laboratory scientists have been caused by inapparent infections of laboratory rats with Seoul-like viruses.[61]

At least six, and probably more, hantaviruses are known to exist in the United States. Seoul-like agents have been associated with human infections in several large cities, but acute (HFRS-like) disease has not been confirmed.[32, 33, 59] Prospect Hill virus has been recovered from meadow voles *(Microtus pennsylvanicus)* in Maryland, and related but distinct hantaviruses are inferred to be present in other voles by detection of genetic sequences, using reverse transcriptase polymerase chain reaction. Another hantavirus, El Moro Canyon virus, has been identified in the harvest mouse *(Reithrodontomys megalotis),* also using reverse transcriptase polymerase chain reaction. No human infections have been documented with these viruses, and their disease potential, if any, is unknown.[38, 115, 116] The deer mouse *Peromyscus maniculatus* is the reservoir rodent for Sin Nombre virus, the agent most frequently associated with human disease in the Western Hemisphere.[17] This rodent is distributed widely over the United States, Canada, and parts of Mexico. Additionally, HPS cases in the Northeast have been associated with a virus called New York 1, which is either a variant of Sin Nombre virus or another distinct virus. This virus has been found in *P. leucopus* (white-footed mouse) as well as *P. maniculatus.*[40, 102] Clinical HPS has been recognized in areas outside the known ranges of *P. maniculatus* and *P. leucopus,* however, and a search for other virus-rodent pairings has yielded at least two additional United States hantaviruses, Black Creek Canal virus from *Sigmodon hispidus* (cotton rat) and Bayou virus from *Oryzomys palustris* (rice rat).[39, 50, 53, 79, 92, 106]

The recognition of clinical HPS in Canada and Central and South America clearly has established HPS as a panhemispheric, rather than a geographically circumscribed, disease.[38, 42, 72, 79, 84, 103, 113, 114] However, all HPS agents identified or suspected to date belong to a single genetic group of hantaviruses and are associated with rodents of the family *Muridae,* subfamily *Sigmodontinae.* These rodent species are restricted to the Americas, suggesting that HPS ultimately may prove to be an exclusively Western Hemisphere disease.[88]

Seasonal Patterns

The natural population cycles of rodents and the seasonal nature of certain human behaviors result in a pattern of human hantavirus disease that varies both seasonally and annually.[8, 13, 14, 30, 60, 74, 107] Although the incidence of disease varies by season, cases of hantavirus-associated human diseases are recognized year-round in all disease-endemic areas.[12, 51, 61, 98]

In the Far East and Russia east of the Ural Mountains, HFRS occurs primarily during the late fall and early winter, with smaller peaks during the spring and summer. Most Scandinavian HFRS occurs between the late summer and early spring, whereas European HFRS in warmer regions (e.g., France, Belgium) tends to peak in the spring.[111] In the Balkans, the presence of multiple viral strains results in a more diffuse seasonal distribution of human disease. Persons whose occupations or avocations bring them to rural settings, such as agricultural workers, foresters, biologists, hunters, campers, and soldiers stationed in the field, are at greatest risk for contracting HFRS.

HFRS due to Seoul virus tends to occur throughout the year. Descriptions of a seasonal occurrence of Seoul virus infection have conflicted.[16, 68] Cases of Seoul virus disease also are distributed more evenly among the ages and genders than are rural hantavirus infections, presumably because of the peridomestic nature of the agent's reservoir.

The temporal distribution of HPS cases identified as of July 1, 1996, through national surveillance conducted at the Centers for Disease Control and Prevention (CDC) suggests a mild spring-summer seasonality of human disease, with about 45 per cent of all United States cases since 1993 recognized during May through July. However, these surveillance data are influenced strongly by the epidemic of human disease associated with an ecologically circumscribed rapid increase in the population density of infected deer mice in the southwestern United States in the spring of 1993.[85] Spring-summer seasonality is less evident in subsequent years.[12] Additional surveillance is necessary to confirm a consistently seasonal nature to hantavirus infections in the United States.

Prevalence

Worldwide, human hantavirus infections number in the hundreds of thousands of cases annually.[115] Because of the predominantly rural nature of the diseases and their prevalence in developing regions of the Eurasian land mass (e.g., rural China), accurate case reporting (and statistical data) for HFRS is limited. It is estimated that more than 100,000 cases of HFRS occur each year in China[115]; one report suggested an incidence of 1.6 to 29.6 per 100,000 population during 1980.[47] In the former Soviet Union, more than 4000 cases per year were recorded between 1978 and 1989, 96 per cent of which occurred in "European" republics. The rates in western regions near the Ural Mountains were higher (20 to 40 per 100,000 population) than those in eastern districts (2 to 5 per 100,000 population).[105] In Korea, about 500 persons with HFRS are hospitalized annually,[105] about half of whom are soldiers. In central and northern Sweden, a mean annual incidence of 4.3 per 100,000 population has been reported, although northern locales have rates of more than 20 per 100,000 population.[98] CDC surveillance identified 141 cases of HPS with clinical onset between July 1959 and June 1996. These cases were infected in 25 states dispersed throughout the continental United States.

Demographic Features

Hantavirus infections are recognized infrequently in the pediatric age group.[3, 31, 51, 52, 98, 105, 118] The peak incidence of HFRS in Europe, the Balkans, and the Far East occurs in those 20 to 50 years of age.[57, 61, 86, 107] Few cases have been reported in children younger than 10 years of age. Both HFRS and HPS cases in young children often are recognized in association with cases among other family members.[3, 31, 57, 77, 86] A male preponderance of cases has been observed for both severe (Korean) and milder (European) forms of HFRS in children.[1, 54, 77, 118] Although this pattern, also seen in adults with HFRS, suggests a differential susceptibility or risk of exposure by gender, the absolute number of recorded cases, particularly in the youngest age groups, is too small to draw firm conclusions.

The age distribution of HPS cases identified by CDC surveillance through June 1996 is 11 to 69 years (mean age, 36 years). Twelve (8.5 per cent) cases have been diagnosed in persons younger than 20 years of age, of whom 6 (4.2 per cent) were younger than 15 years of age. Although the disease initially was distributed evenly by gender, a slight male preponderance may be emerging with ongoing surveillance (58.9 per cent male preponderance overall as of July 1, 1996).

The underrepresentation of children recognized to have HFRS and HPS may not be explained entirely by age-related avoidance of activities resulting in exposure. The limited data available (see Clinical Manifestations) suggest that hantavirus infections in children may induce milder disease than that seen in adults. Comprehensive population-based serosurveys are few and have been inadequate to define age-associated infection rates. It is possible that the apparently immune-mediated pathology of this disease (see Pathogenesis and Pathology) is more evident in persons experiencing infection in adulthood.

CLINICAL MANIFESTATIONS

Hemorrhagic Fever with Renal Syndrome

Two major clinical variants of HFRS have been recognized traditionally. Severe disease associated with high morbidity and mortality occurs primarily in areas of the world where Hantaan and Dobrava viruses are endemic: across the northern half of Asia, China, the Korean Peninsula, and the Balkan nations. Milder illness with little mortality occurs in areas where Puumala virus has been recovered; this latter disease, known also as nephropathia epidemica, is found throughout northern Europe, Scandinavia, and western areas of the former Soviet Union. In the Balkans, Puumala virus–like strains coexist with viruses causing more serious disease, resulting in a mixture of clinical presentations in former Yugoslavia and neighboring countries. Benign presentations of HFRS are well recognized in many regions where Hantaan virus is found, however, and clinically severe disease occasionally results from Puumala virus infection.[89] It thus is important to appreciate the protean nature of this disorder and to recognize the potential for disease of any severity whenever and wherever human infection with hantavirus occurs.

HFRS associated with Hantaan virus (and Dobrava virus) is a complex, multiphase disorder presenting substantial challenges in patient management. The clinical course of HFRS caused by Hantaan virus in adults spans a wide spectrum from mildly symptomatic disease to severe hemorrhagic fever and death. Subclinical infections probably are infrequent.[90, 118] In the majority of cases, the clinical course is relatively benign; approximately 20 to 30 per cent develop severe disease. Modern day case-fatality rates range from 2 to 7 per cent. In Korea, about a third of recognized Hantaan virus infections follow a clinical course consisting of progression through five clinically and pathophysiologically defined stages: febrile, hypotensive, oliguric, diuretic, and convalescent.[68, 99] Phases often blur, however, and in milder cases one or more phases may not be seen. After an incubation period of 2 to 3 weeks (range, 4 to 42 days), most patients report the abrupt onset of high fever, headache, chills, dizziness, myalgias, anorexia, and backache. About a third of patients experience prodromal mild respiratory or gastrointestinal symptoms. Nausea, vomiting, abdominal pain, and intense thirst may be evident at presentation but increase in severity over succeeding days. Photophobia, blurred vision, and eyeball pain commonly are reported. Physical examination reveals a restless, acutely ill patient with flushing of the face, neck, and upper thorax. Relative bradycardia is present. Conjunctival and pharyngeal injection, together with facial puffiness, is characteristic. More than 90 per cent of patients develop petechiae on the soft palate, axillae, lateral thorax, conjunctivae, or face, generally between the third and sixth days of illness. Tenderness over the costovertebral angles and diffusely throughout the abdomen is common. Hematologic studies in the first 3 to 4 days of illness reveal leukocytosis with a left shift in more than 90 per cent and thrombocytopenia almost universally; the hematocrit at this stage generally is normal or slightly increased. Proteinuria develops by the third to fourth day, and microscopic hematuria, hyposthenuria, and mild pyuria are reported in most patients; fibrin clots in the urine are a characteristic finding.

This febrile phase generally lasts about a week, followed by abrupt defervescence. About 40 per cent of patients then become hypotensive; in most cases, the drop in blood pressure is mild and brief, but in severely ill persons (30 to 50 per cent of hypotensive patients), clinical shock develops. Tachycardia replaces bradycardia, the pulse pressure narrows, and cyanosis and mental confusion may be seen. The hypotensive phase may last from a few hours to 3 days, and 30 to 40 per cent of deaths occur during this period.

As patients recover from hypotension, they enter a period of oliguria. This phase occurs in about 60 per cent of patients and generally lasts for several days. Anuria develops in about 10 per cent of patients. Blood pressure normalizes, and hypertension often develops. Clinical manifestations of uremia, including protracted vomiting and hiccups, may be seen. More extensive hemorrhagic manifestations become evident during the oliguric phase, with ecchymoses, hemoptysis, hematemesis, melena, gross hematuria, and, rarely, bleeding of the central nervous system. Striking elevations of blood urea nitrogen and creatinine levels are common. Biochemical disturbances (electrolyte derangements, metabolic acidosis, uremia) may be severe, and dialysis may be lifesaving. About half of fatalities occur during the oliguric phase.

Between 10 and 14 days into the illness, renal function is restored spontaneously in most patients, and a period of diuresis follows. Polyuria may be substantial, and the urine output frequently exceeds 3 to 6 liters a day. With the onset of diuresis, clinical recovery is initiated; however, the rapid change in fluid status may precipitate further electrolyte disturbances, so close monitoring remains necessary.

Convalescence typically lasts from 3 to 6 weeks, but in many cases a longer period passes before health is restored completely. Weight gain and strength are recovered slowly. Proteinuria resolves, but hyposthenuria persists for months. Most patients recover completely, although permanent sequelae may result from such complications as anterior pituitary or other central nervous system hemorrhage.

The disease has been reported infrequently in children.[31, 54, 118] However, available data indicate that clinical manifestations are similar to, and perhaps somewhat less severe than, those observed in adults. In a series of 63 children identified retrospectively over a 15-year period in Korea, fever was universal, whereas abdominal pain, headache, and vomiting were present in 73 per cent or more patients[118] (Table 189–2). Proteinuria (100 per cent), leukocytosis (71 per cent), thrombocytopenia (80 per cent), hypocholesterolemia (87 per cent), and elevations of creatinine (94 per cent), blood urea nitrogen (94 per cent), and alanine amino transaminase (80 per cent) were the most commonly found laboratory abnormalities.

TABLE 189–2. Prominent Clinical and Laboratory Features of Hemorrhagic Fever with Renal Syndrome in Children

Features	Korea[118] (%)	Sweden[1] (%)	Finland[77] (%)
Fever	100	100	100
Headache	76	100	59
Anorexia	33	100	NR
Nausea	62	86	81
Vomiting	73	91	72
Abdominal pain	91	93	59
Back/costovertebral angle pain	35	76	63
Dizziness	21	73	9
Thirst	NR	75	NR
Polyuria	NR	57	NR
Diarrhea	NR	57	9
Petechiae	38	NR	NR
Conjunctival hemorrhage	35	NR	3
Proteinuria	100	100	97
Hematuria	67	80	73
Pyuria	8	43	44
Glucosuria	NR	26	12
Casts	NR	33	NR
Leukocytosis	71	22	41
Thrombocytopenia	80	68	87
Elevated hemoglobin	39	NR	28
Elevated C-reactive protein	NR	28	89
Elevated erythrocyte sedimentation rate	NR	58	74
Elevated alanine amino transaminase	80	NR	53
Elevated creatinine	94	76	84

NR, not recorded.

Petechiae and hypotension occurred infrequently (38 per cent and 11 per cent, respectively), and frank hemorrhage was rare. Eleven patients (18 per cent) required dialysis. The mortality rate was 5 per cent, and the remaining patients recovered without sequelae.

HFRS occurring after infection with Seoul virus resembles that described for Hantaan virus infection, but clinical manifestations generally are much milder.[68] Fever and constitutional symptoms are similar between the two types of infections, but hypotension is infrequent in persons infected with Seoul virus (10 per cent of cases) and clinical shock is rare. The frequency and severity of thrombocytopenia are less in Seoul virus infection, whereas elevations of transaminases are common (more than 60 per cent of cases). The mortality rate for HFRS due to Seoul virus is 1 per cent or less.

The Scandinavian or European form of HFRS (nephropathia epidemica) generally is a much more benign disease than that attributed to Hantaan virus, and mortality virtually is nonexistent (although recent reports of severe Puumala virus–associated disease in Germany[89] and elsewhere challenge this assertion). In contrast with the findings with Hantaan virus, subclinical infection apparently is common with Puumala virus; one report suggests a case-to-infection ratio of 1:10.[83]

Nephropathia epidemica typically is a biphasic disease of 1 to 3 weeks' duration.[20, 86, 111] Onset usually is abrupt, with no apparent prodrome. High fever is the initial presenting symptom in 95 per cent of patients. On examination, a facial flush is usual. This febrile phase lasts from 3 to 6 days. The development of nausea, vomiting, abdominal pain, back pain, somnolence, and occasionally joint pain heralds the onset of the second, or renal, phase. Abdominal pain may be of such severity and character that an acute abdomen is suspected, and many patients have undergone surgery for suspected appendicitis prior to receiving a diagnosis of nephropathia epidemica. Visual disturbances are common, and hypotension, if it develops, usually is mild. Petechiae are relatively infrequent. The renal stage generally lasts 1 to 2 weeks and is characterized by development of oliguria, proteinuria, hematuria, and hyposthenuria. Modest elevations in blood urea nitrogen and creatinine (in most cases to but a fraction of the levels seen in severe forms of HFRS) accompany the oliguria, which typically lasts for no more than a few days before diuresis begins. Mild leukocytosis and thrombocytopenia occur during the renal phase, whereas electrolyte disturbances sufficient to require dialysis are infrequent. As with other forms of HFRS, convalescence may be prolonged, and hyposthenuria may persist for many months. Recovery typically is complete.[58, 81]

As with Hantaan virus–associated HFRS, nephropathia epidemica in children is recognized infrequently. Clinically, the disease also appears to be similar to, and in most cases milder than, that seen in adults. Among 32 Swedish cases reported (18 identified retrospectively and 14 prospectively), fever (100 per cent), headache (100 per cent), anorexia (100 per cent), abdominal pain (93 per cent), vomiting (91 per cent), nausea (86 per cent), and back pain (76 per cent) were the most prevalent symptoms[1] (see Table 189–2). Proteinuria (100 per cent), microscopic hematuria (80 per cent), elevated serum creatinine (76 per cent), and thrombocytopenia (68 per cent) were the most frequently found laboratory abnormalities. Leukocytosis was relatively infrequent in this series (22 per cent). Six children (19 per cent) had hemorrhagic manifestations, and one complained of blurred vision. In a separate 32-patient series from Finland, fever (100 per cent), nausea (81 per cent), vomiting (72 per cent), and back pain (63 per cent) again were prevalent, but headache and abdominal pain (59 per cent each) were reported less frequently[77] (see Table 189–2). Proteinuria (97 per cent), hematuria (73 per cent), and elevated serum creatinine (84 per cent) were common. Thrombocytopenia (87 per cent) was reported more prominently among Finnish than Swedish children. About a quarter of Finnish children displayed hemorrhagic manifestations. The proportion of transient visual blurring was identical to that seen in adults (25 per cent). No children in this series required dialysis.

Hantavirus Pulmonary Syndrome

Classic HPS in adults is a biphasic illness that challenges the diagnostic acumen and clinical management skills of the physician. The clinical features of the prodrome phase are not pathognomonic, and the diagnosis rarely is suspected prior to the abrupt clinical deterioration that heralds onset of the cardiopulmonary phase. HPS characteristically begins with a prodrome that lasts on average 3 to 4 days but may extend up to a week or more.[24, 70] This phase is characterized by fever and myalgias, particularly of the back or lower extremities. Although a cough may develop as the prodrome progresses, illnesses initially characterized predominantly by upper respiratory symptoms, such as cough and coryza, are unlikely to be HPS.[24, 70, 76] More than half of HPS patients manifest gastrointestinal symptoms (e.g., nausea, vomiting, diarrhea) as well, which usually are mild.[24] Occasionally, HPS-associated gastrointestinal symptoms have been mistaken for an acute surgical abdomen or another intra-abdominal process. The presence of thrombocytopenia in the context of a compatible prodrome is highly discriminatory for HPS.[100]

The onset of the cardiopulmonary phase is abrupt and often life-threatening. Patients usually are hospitalized within

12 to 24 hours of first presenting for medical evaluation, and most deaths occur during the first 24 to 48 hours in the hospital.[11, 24, 70] Clear chest radiographs have progressed to diffuse bilateral pulmonary involvement over the course of several hours. Interstitial edema, present in only 5 per cent of adult respiratory distress syndrome patients, is present in the majority of HPS patients on initial radiograph, and alveolar flooding that usually is indistinguishable from the peripheral pattern seen in the acute phase of adult respiratory distress syndrome develops in most patients.[49] This noncardiogenic pulmonary edema, resulting from a diffuse pulmonary capillary leak, can be differentiated from cardiac (hydrostatic) pulmonary edema by the presence of low pulmonary artery occlusion pressures and an increased protein content in edema fluid.[37] Secretions recovered when HPS patients are intubated generally are acellular, resemble plasma or pulmonary edema fluid, and have been observed to clot in severe cases.[24, 37] The presence of significant numbers of polymorphonuclear leukocytes in pulmonary secretions suggests an alternative etiology.

The pulmonary decline usually is accompanied by onset of shock due to myocardial dysfunction and hypovolemia.[37, 70] In severe cases, hemodynamic measurements show a high systemic vascular resistance combined with low cardiac and stroke volume indices. Progression to death is associated with worsening cardiac dysfunction unresponsive to treatment, sometimes despite adequate oxygenation.[37]

Thrombocytopenia may be present in the late prodrome and almost always is present in the cardiopulmonary phase. Additional laboratory abnormalities in hospitalized patients include hemoconcentration, prolonged prothrombin and partial thromboplastin times, elevated serum lactate dehydrogenase concentration, decreased serum protein concentration, mild leukocytosis with a marked left shift, and the frequent presence of myeloid precursors on the peripheral smear.[24, 70] Proteinuria is common. Serum creatinine often is elevated modestly in severe cases, although renal failure is not characteristic of infection with Sin Nombre virus, despite episodes of hypotension and other predisposing conditions in many patients. Among patients who survive, recovery may be as dramatic as decline; survivors frequently are extubated within 72 hours after admission to the intensive care unit and may be discharged from the hospital within 1 week after admission.

Renal failure has been more prominent in two reported cases of HPS due to Black Creek Canal virus and Bayou virus infections.[24, 53] Hantavirus disease associated with Andes virus[72] in Argentina and Chile and that from as-yet-unidentified viral species in Brazil[79] and Paraguay[114] closely resembles Sin Nombre virus disease. Renal failure has accompanied some cases in a focus in northern Argentina.[84]

Subclinical or mild disease rarely is associated with Sin Nombre virus infection.[100] However, although initial case-fatality rates of 70 to 80 per cent were reported in 1993, a wider clinical spectrum has been recognized as clinicians have developed a heightened suspicion and diagnostic assays have become available more readily. Although the overall case-fatality rate among HPS cases identified through CDC surveillance was 50.4 per cent, the fatality rate among 62 cases identified after January 1, 1994, was only 40.3 per cent. This apparent decline in mortality may reflect improvement in survival due to improved clinical management. However, it undoubtedly also reflects a decrease in a bias toward suspecting this diagnosis only with fatal and near-fatal disease that existed early in the clinical understanding of this syndrome.

HPS has been recognized infrequently among children younger than 17 years of age. In one review of nine pediatric HPS patients identified through CDC surveillance, the geographic distribution, clinical course, and mortality rates were similar to those described for adult patients.[7] Pediatric patients in this small series were significantly less likely than adults to describe chills or myalgias during the prodrome phase. Hospital stays of pediatric patients were shorter than those of adults, though this difference was not statistically significant. Although all of three identified prepubertal patients survived without intubation and it has been suggested that the mortality rate might be lower among prepubertal cases, more observations are needed to conclude that infections produce milder disease in children than in adults.[3, 7]

Only two case reports of HPS in pediatric patients have been published. The first described a fatal illness in a 14-year-old adolescent that largely was indistinguishable from adult disease.[52] However, in addition to the dizziness frequently described in adults, this patient exhibited a vestibular component not described elsewhere.[3, 24, 70, 76] The second case report described seroconversion to IgM temporally associated with fever, cough, and earache in a 4-year-old child. Ten days after this child was diagnosed with "bronchitis and nasal congestion," his mother was hospitalized and died of HPS after 1 week of prodrome. The child underwent serologic assessment as part of an investigation of household contacts and not because of clinical suspicion of hantavirus disease.[3]

COMPLICATIONS

In general, human infection with HFRS-associated hantaviruses results in an acute illness with prolonged incapacitation followed by complete recovery. Unless complicated by organ hemorrhage (e.g., central nervous system bleeding), residua have not been observed. However, epidemiologic associations between hypertensive renal disease and evidence of prior United States hantavirus infection have been reported.[32, 33] These data suggest that sequelae in fact may be a feature of hantavirus infection in humans. Further study clearly is needed to determine the significance of these observations.

Although prolonged prothrombin and partial thromboplastin times are common among hospitalized HPS patients, overt disseminated intravascular coagulation is not, and overt hemorrhage is rare.[119] Patients in whom disseminated intravascular coagulation is established rarely survive more than 48 hours. One patient who did survive a cardiopulmonary phase accompanied by overt disseminated intravascular coagulation died 3 weeks later from gangrenous complications.

PATHOGENESIS AND PATHOLOGY

Serum antibodies develop within 3 to 7 days of onset of illness in patients infected with hantaviruses. Early clinical events are presumed to be accompanied by a viremia; however, significant signs and symptoms develop in temporal association with the onset of a measurable antibody response. Pathologic studies of fatal HFRS cases indicate that multiple organ systems are involved, but a triad of lesions consisting of hemorrhagic necrosis of the renal medulla, anterior pituitary, and cardiac right atrium is described as characteristic.[45] In HPS, multiple organ involvement with variable degrees of vascular congestion is noted in all fatal cases. However, the predominant findings at autopsy have involved the lungs, with pulmonary edema and serous effusions seen grossly and interstitial pneumonitis with a mononuclear cell infiltrate, intra-alveolar edema, and focal hyaline membrane formation described microscopically. Immunohistochemical studies demonstrate widespread presence of hantavirus antigens in endothelial cells of the microvasculature, particularly in the lung but also in the kidney, heart, spleen, pancreas, lymph nodes, skeletal muscle intestine, adrenal gland, adipose tissue, urinary bladder, and brain. However, few histologic changes have been noted in the kidney, brain, and heart of autopsied HPS patients.[119]

The underlying pathologic lesion leading to hemodynamic alterations in hantavirus infections is damage to the vascular endothelium. The cause of injury is unknown, but both cellular and humoral immune-mediated mechanisms have been implicated.[21, 25, 45, 108, 119] Soluble factors acting on hematologic and immunologic systems also are released. The abrupt onset of noncardiogenic pulmonary edema in HPS follows the development of an immune response directed against viral antigen present throughout the endothelial cells lining the pulmonary capillaries, leading to a pulmonary capillary leak syndrome.[87]

DIAGNOSIS AND DIFFERENTIAL DIAGNOSIS

A high index of suspicion is essential to the recognition of hantavirus infections among persons living or traveling in disease-endemic areas. The protean nature of the disease in children is such that almost any ill-defined febrile disease associated with abdominal or back pain in an appropriate geographic setting should stimulate consideration of the diagnosis. This particularly is true if the clinical syndrome is accompanied by myalgias, if thrombocytopenia or proteinuria is present, or if a history of exposure to rodents or rural environments is obtained in disease-endemic areas.[100]

The differential diagnosis of HFRS includes rickettsial disease, leptospirosis, meningococcemia, other viral diseases, poststreptococcal syndromes, pyelonephritis, leukemia, and hemolytic uremic syndrome. Differentiation from an acute intra-abdominal or pelvic process, such as appendicitis, may be extremely difficult on clinical grounds.

The differential diagnosis of HPS includes legionellosis, *Yersinia pestis* infection (plague), meningococcemia, brucellosis, rickettsial diseases, mycoplasma and fungal pneumonias (including *Coccidioides immitis* and *Histoplasma* pneumonias), tularemia, psittacosis, pancreatitis accompanied by adult respiratory distress syndrome, and autoimmune disorders (including thrombotic thrombocytopenia purpura). A prominent cough or sore throat or a localized infiltrate on chest radiograph that does not generalize within hours argues for a nonhantaviral etiology.[76] A constellation of the absence of a cough in the presence of dizziness, nausea or vomiting, a low platelet count, a low serum bicarbonate level, and an elevated hematocrit discriminated HPS from similar patients with unexplained adult respiratory distress syndrome in one study.[76]

Laboratory diagnosis of HFRS or HPS is made by demonstration of specific antihantavirus IgM antibodies in acute-phase serum by enzyme immunoassay in the IgM capture format. A fourfold or greater rise in specific IgG antibodies by enzyme immunoassay or immunofluorescence[56, 69] in sequential sera (ideally obtained 2 or more weeks apart) also is useful. The availability of purified recombinant hantavirus antigens has enhanced the diagnostic specificity in both enzyme immunoassay and Western blot assay systems.[27, 46, 122] Enzyme-linked immunosorbent assay and indirect fluorescent antibody tests are broadly cross-reactive, particularly among viruses from rodents of the same subfamily.[18, 19] For example, a recombinant Sin Nombre virus antigen detects antibodies against Bayou, Black Creek Canal, Andes, and several other viruses from Sigmodontine rodents, and it maintains reactivity with antibodies directed against Arvicolid rodent–associated viruses (e.g., Puumala and Prospect Hill). Neutralizing antibody assays are more specific, but technical requirements preclude their routine use. Immunohistochemical techniques have been applied to tissue samples from patients infected with hantaviruses.[119] Nucleic acid primers from several hantavirus strains have been generated, enabling nucleotide sequences from fresh or frozen tissues to be amplified using reverse transcriptase polymerase chain reaction. Reverse transcriptase polymerase chain reaction usually is successful on whole blood or blood clots obtained within the first 7 to 10 days of illness. However, the expense and effort of the method are not justified unless the resulting genetic sequence information is needed for viral strain definition or epidemiologic studies.[2, 80] Attempts to isolate hantaviruses from human specimens generally are unrewarding.

TREATMENT

Cautious fluid management and hemodynamic and intensive care unit support are the most important aspects of the clinical management of any hantavirus disease.[37, 70] Early hospitalization and avoidance of even minor trauma are essential to maintaining the integrity of damaged vascular beds in these patients. Transport of patients should be minimized; barotrauma associated with transport in underpressurized aircraft particularly may be hazardous.[6] Attention to fluid management and metabolic status especially is critical. In HFRS, fluid restriction may be necessary early in the disease course as renal function diminishes, but large inputs may be required later during diuresis to cover massive losses. Electrolyte abnormalities and metabolic acidosis are common. Peritoneal or hemodialysis may be lifesaving in severe cases.[6] In HPS, the nature of the pulmonary pathology predisposes to iatrogenic pulmonary edema; careful attention must be given to maintaining appropriate central venous and pulmonary arterial pressures to avoid such complications. Tissue perfusion and adequate oxygenation are the goals of supportive therapy with this syndrome. Oxygen supplementation and mechanical ventilation almost always are required. Inotropic agents may be necessary to maintain tissue perfusion.[37, 70]

Hantaan and Sin Nombre viruses exhibit similar in vitro sensitivity to ribavirin. One prospective, placebo-controlled trial suggested that intravenous ribavirin was effective in reducing the mortality and morbidity associated with HFRS in China.[44] In contrast, although 30 HPS patients who received investigational, open-label intravenous ribavirin generally tolerated it well, treatment was accompanied by a low frequency of clearly drug-associated adverse events, most significantly anemia and resulting transfusion, and no clear evidence of benefit was obtained.[15] This contrast in clinical experience is not explained by differences in dosing schedules; patients in both protocols were dosed identically.[15, 44] The lack of any dramatic effects by intravenous ribavirin in HPS may be due in part to the rapidity of disease progression; HPS-associated deaths usually occur within the first 48 hours after admission and therapeutic intervention.[11, 15, 24, 37, 44, 70]

Ribavirin is not licensed for intravenous use in the United States. Teratogenic concerns mandate careful informed consent if use of this drug is considered in children, pregnant women, or nursing mothers. A placebo-controlled trial, necessary to ascertain whether intravenous ribavirin has efficacy for HPS and whether other adverse events noted during open-label use were associated etiologically or merely temporally,[15] is ongoing.

PREVENTION

Primary Prevention

The most effective preventive measure available for hantavirus infection is the avoidance of rodents and their habitats. However, eradication of the rodent reservoir hosts in disease-endemic areas is not feasible. Prevention efforts are directed more appropriately toward reducing the frequency of rodent-human interactions through environmental hygiene practices that minimize rodent density in home and work environments and avoidance of known rodent-infested areas and activities that increase the risk of human exposure to aerosolized infectious rodent excreta.

Detailed guidelines on measures appropriate to eliminate rodents from homes in disease-endemic areas, to clean up rodent-contaminated areas safely, and to minimize the risks for workers occupationally exposed to rodents and participants in outdoor recreational activities have been published.[9] Although rodent ectoparasites do not transmit hantaviruses, in the southwestern United States several rodent species also are hosts to fleas that transmit *Y. pestis*. In such areas, insecticides should be used in conjunction with rodent extermination measures because eradication of rodents without concurrent control of the associated fleas may increase the risk of human plague.[9]

Vaccine Prospects

Inactivated vaccines to Hantaan and Seoul viruses have been developed in South Korea and China. Some of these vaccines induce neutralizing antibody responses in humans and are being tested in field studies. A recombinant vaccinia strain expressing Hantaan antigens has been tested in human volunteers in the United States and also induces a serum neutralizing antibody response.[97] There is an immediate need for a vaccine effective against Hantaan virus, but there are several obstacles to accepting the aforementioned candidates as yet. There is no realistic animal model of human disease that permits full preclinical evaluation, the disease process is immunopathologic, and some monoclonal antibodies can enhance macrophage infection. Thus, even more than with other viral vaccines, double-blind, placebo-controlled trials urgently are needed to provide definitive evidence of protection and to exclude adverse effects.

Hospital Infection Control

The use of universal precautions in handling blood and body fluids of all patients constitutes prudent practice. In addition, a certified biologic safety cabinet should be used for all handling of human body fluids where splatter or aerosolization is possible.[10] Viral antigens can be detected in necropsy specimens, and reverse polymerase chain reaction readily detects viral genetic material in necropsy tissue and in blood and plasma obtained from hantavirus-infected persons early in the course of the disease.[41, 119] However, secondary transmission of hantaviruses associated with HFRS has never been documented after contact with acutely ill persons or exposure to their clinical laboratory specimens. The experience with American hantaviruses linked to HPS has been similar,[10, 112] although a single report has suggested person-to-person spread during an outbreak in South America.[26a, 113a] This latter incident notwithstanding, the many years of experience with HFRS and HPS indicate that once the diagnosis has been confirmed, isolation of hospitalized patients to prevent nosocomial transmission generally is not required. Sera and other specimens from hantavirus-infected persons can be handled safely by using biosafety level 2 facilities and practices. Higher biosafety levels are recommended for attempts to propagate hantaviruses.[10, 13]

References

1. Ahlm, C., Settergren, B., Gothefors L., et al.: Nephropathia epidemica (hemorrhagic fever with renal syndrome) in children: Clinical characteristics. Pediatr. Infect. Dis. J. *13*:45, 1994.
2. Antoniadis, A., Stylianakis, A., Papa, A., et al.: Direct genetic detection of Dobrava virus in Greek and Albanian haemorrhagic fever with renal syndrome (HFRS) patients. J. Infect. Dis. *174*:407, 1996.
3. Armstrong, L. R., Bryan, R. T., Sarisky, J., et al.: Mild hantaviral disease caused by Sin Nombre virus in a four-year-old child. Pediatr. Infect. Dis. J. *14*:1108, 1995.
4. Avsic-Zupnac, T., Likar, M., Novakovic, S., et al.: Evidence of the presence of two hantaviruses in Slovenia. Arch. Virol. *115*(Suppl. 1):87, 1990.
5. Avsic-Zupanc, T., Xiao, S.-Y., Stojanovic, R., et al.: Characterization of Dobrava virus: A hantavirus from Slovenia. J. Med. Virol. *38*:132, 1992.
6. Bruno, P., Hassell, L. H., Brown, J., et al.: The protean manifestations of hemorrhagic fever with renal syndrome: A retrospective review of 26 cases from Korea. Ann. Intern. Med. *113*:385, 1990.
7. Bryan, R. T., Doyle, T. J., Moolenaar, R. L., et al.: Hantavirus pulmonary syndrome in children. Semin. Pediatr. Infect. Dis. *8*:1–7, 1997.
8. Casals, J., Henderson, B. E., Hoogstraal, H., et al.: A review of Soviet viral hemorrhagic fever 1969. J. Infect. Dis. *122*:437, 1970.
9. Centers for Disease Control and Prevention: Hantavirus infection—Southwestern United States: Interim recommendations for risk reduction. M. M. W. R. *42*(RR-11):1–13, 1993.
10. Centers for Disease Control and Prevention: Laboratory management of agents associated with hantavirus pulmonary syndrome: Interim biosafety guidelines. M. M. W. R. *43*(RR-7):1, 1994.
11. Centers for Disease Control and Prevention: Intravenous ribavirin in the treatment of hantavirus pulmonary syndrome in the United States: Annual report to FDA on IND No. 17,186. Amendment No. 6. June 4, 1995.
12. Centers for Disease Control and Prevention: Hantavirus pulmonary syndrome: United States, 1995 and 1996. M. M. W. R. *45*:291, 1996.
13. Centers for Disease Control and Prevention/National Institutes of Health: Biosafety in Microbiological and Biomedical Laboratories. 3rd ed. Washington, D.C.: U.S. Department of Health and Human Services, Public Health Service, 1993. HHS Publication No. (CDC) 93-8395.
14. Chapman, L. E., and Khabbaz, R. F.: Review: Etiology and epidemiology of the Four Corners hantavirus outbreak. Infect. Agents Dis. *3*:234, 1994.
15. Chapman, L. E., Mertz, G., Khan, A. S., et al.: Open label intravenous ribavirin for hantavirus pulmonary syndrome. Abstract No. H111. Program and Abstracts of the 34th Interscience Conference on Antimicrobial Agents and Chemotherapy. Orlando, American Society of Microbiologists, 1994.
16. Chen, H.-X., Qiu, F.-X., Dong, B.-J., et al.: Epidemiological studies on hemorrhagic fever with renal syndrome in China. J. Infect. Dis. *154*:394, 1986.
17. Childs, J. E., Ksiazek, T. G., Spiropoulou, C. F., et al.: Serologic and genetic identification of *Peromyscus maniculatus* as the primary rodent reservoir for a new hantavirus in the southwestern United States. J. Infect. Dis. *169*:1271, 1994.
18. Chu, Y. K., Jennings, G., Schmaljohn, A., et al.: Cross-neutralization of hantaviruses with immune sera from experimentally infected animals and from hemorrhagic fever with renal syndrome and hantavirus pulmonary syndrome patients. J. Infect. Dis. *172*:1581, 1995.
19. Chu, Y. K., Rossi, C., LeDuc, J. W., et al.: Serological relationships among viruses in the *Hantavirus* genus, family *Bunyaviridae*. Virology *198*:196, 1994.
20. Collan, Y., Mihatsch, M. J., Lahdevirta, J., et al.: Nephropathia epidemica: Mild variant of hemorrhagic fever with renal syndrome. Kidney Int. *40*(Suppl. 35):S62, 1991.
21. Cosgriff, T. M.: Mechanisms of disease in hantavirus infection: Pathophysiology of hemorrhagic fever with renal syndrome. Rev. Infect. Dis. *13*:97, 1991.
22. Desmyter, J., LeDuc, J. W., Johnson, K. M., et al.: Laboratory rat associated outbreak of haemorrhagic fever with renal syndrome due to Hantaan-like virus in Belgium. Lancet *2*:445, 1983.
23. Dournon, E., Moriniere, B., Matheron, S., et al.: HFRS after a wild rodent bite in the Haute-Savoie and risk of exposure to Hantaan-like virus in a Paris laboratory. Lancet *1*:676, 1984.
24. Duchin, J. S., Koster, F. T., Peters, C. J., et al.: Hantavirus pulmonary

syndrome: A clinical description of 17 patients with a newly recognized disease. N. Engl. J. Med. *330*:949, 1994.

25. Earle, D. P.: Symposium on epidemic hemorrhagic fever. Am. J. Med. *16*:619, 1954.
26. Elliott, L., Ksiazek T. G., Rollin P. E., et al.: Isolation of the causative agent of hantavirus pulmonary syndrome. Am. J. Trop. Med. Hyg. *51*:102, 1994.

26a. Enria, D., Padula, P., Segura, E. L., et al.: Hantavirus pulmonary syndrome in Argentina: Possibility of person-to-person transmission. Medicina *56*:709–711, 1996.

27. Feldmann, H., Sanchez, A., Morzunov, S., et al.: Utilization of autopsy RNA for the synthesis of the nucleocapsid antigen of a newly recognized virus associated with hantavirus pulmonary syndrome. Virus Res. *30*:351, 1993.
28. French, G. R., Foulke, R. S., Brand, O. A., et al.: Korean hemorrhagic fever: Propagation of the etiologic agent in a cell line of human origin. Science *211*:1046, 1981.
29. Gajdusek, D. C.: Acute infectious hemorrhagic fevers and mycotoxicoses in the Union of Soviet Socialist Republics. Medical Science Publication No. 2. Washington, D.C., Army Medical Service Graduate School, Walter Reed Army Medical Center, 1953.
30. Gajdusek, D. C.: Hemorrhagic fevers in Asia: A problem in medical ecology. Geogr. Rev. *41*:20, 1956.
31. Gajdusek, D. C.: Virus hemorrhagic fevers: Special reference to hemorrhagic fever with renal syndrome (epidemic hemorrhagic fever). J. Pediatr. *60*:841, 1962.
32. Glass, G. E., Watson, A. J., LeDuc, J. W., et al.: Infection with rat borne hantavirus in U.S. residents is consistently associated with hypertensive renal disease. J. Infect. Dis. *167*:614, 1993.
33. Glass, G. E., Watson, A. J., LeDuc, J. W., et al.: Domestic cases of hemorrhagic fever with renal syndrome in the United States. Nephron *68*:48, 1994.
34. Gligic, A., Dimkovic, N., Xiao, S.-Y., et al.: Belgrade virus: A new hantavirus causing severe hemorrhagic fever with renal syndrome in Yugoslavia. J. Infect. Dis. *166*:113, 1992.
35. Goldsmith, C. S., Elliot, L. H., Peters, C. J., et al.: Ultrastructural characteristics of Sin Nombre virus, causative agent of hantavirus pulmonary syndrome. Arch. Virol. *140*:2107, 1995.
36. Gonzalez-Scarano, F., and Nathanson, N.: *Bunyaviridae*. *In* Fields, B. N., Knipe, D. M., Howley, P. M., et al. (eds.): Fields' Virology. 3rd ed. Philadelphia, Lippincott-Raven, 1996, pp. 1473–1504.
37. Hallin, G. W., Simpson, S. Q., Crowell, R. E., et al.: Cardiopulmonary manifestations of hantavirus pulmonary syndrome. Crit. Care Med. *24*:252, 1996.
38. Hjelle, B., Chavez-Giles, F., Torrez-Martinez, N., et al.: Genetic identification of a novel hantavirus of the harvest mouse *Reithrodontomys megalotis*. J. Virol. *68*:6751, 1994.
39. Hjelle, B., Goade, D., Torrez-Martinez, N., et al.: Hantavirus pulmonary syndrome, renal insufficiency and myositis associated with infection by Bayou hantavirus. Clin. Infect. Dis. *23*:495–500, 1996.
40. Hjelle, B., Krolikowski, J., Torrez-Martinez, N., et al.: Phylogenetically distinct hantavirus implicated in a case of hantavirus pulmonary syndrome in the northeastern United States. J. Med. Virol. *46*:21, 1995.
41. Hjelle, B., Spiropoulou, C. F., Torrez-Martinez, N., et al.: Detection of Muerto Canyon virus RNA in peripheral blood mononuclear cells from patients with hantavirus pulmonary syndrome. J. Infect. Dis. *170*:1013, 1994.
42. Hjelle, B., Torrez-Martinez, N., and Koster, F. T.: Hantavirus pulmonary syndrome–related virus from Bolivia. Lancet *347*:57, 1996.
43. Hortling, H.: En epidemi av falteben in finska Lappland. Nord. Med. *30*:1001, 1946.
44. Huggins, J. W., Hsiang, C. M., Cosgriff, T. M., et al.: Prospective, double-blind, concurrent, placebo-controlled clinical trial of intravenous ribavirin therapy of hemorrhagic fever with renal syndrome. J. Infect. Dis. *164*:1119, 1991.
45. Hullinghorst, R. L., and Steer, A.: Pathology of epidemic hemorrhagic fever. Ann. Intern. Med. *38*:77, 1953.
46. Jenison, S., Yamada, T., Morris, C., et al.: Characterization of human antibody responses to Four Corners hantavirus infections among patients with hantavirus pulmonary syndrome. J. Virol. *68*:3000, 1994.
47. Jiang, Y.-T.: A preliminary report on hemorrhagic fever with renal syndrome in China. Chin. Med. J. *96*:265, 1983.
48. Kawamata, J., Yamanouchi, T., Dohmae, K., et al.: Control of laboratory acquired hemorrhagic fever with renal syndrome (HFRS) in Japan. Lab. Anim. Sci. *37*:431, 1987.
49. Ketai, L. H., Williamson, M. R., Telepak, R. J., et al.: Hantavirus pulmonary syndrome: Radiographic findings in 16 patients. Radiology *191*:665, 1994.
50. Khan, A. S., Gaviria, M., Rollin, P. E., et al.: Hantavirus pulmonary syndrome in Florida: Association with the newly identified Black Creek Canal virus. Am. J. Med. *100*:46, 1996.
51. Khan, A. S., Khabbaz, R. F., Armstrong, L. R., et al.: Hantavirus pulmonary syndrome: The first 100 U.S. cases. J. Infect. Dis. *173*:1297, 1996.
52. Khan, A. S., Ksiazek, T. G., Zaki, S. R., et al.: Fatal hantavirus pulmonary syndrome in an adolescent. Pediatrics *95*:276, 1995.
53. Khan, A. S., Spiropoulou, C. F., Morzunov, S., et al.: Fatal illness associated with a new hantavirus in Louisiana. J. Med. Virol. *46*:281, 1995.
54. Ko, K. W.: Korean hemorrhagic fever in Korean children. *In* Murakami K., and Sakai Y. (eds.): Recent Advances in Pediatric Nephrology. Amsterdam, Elsevier Science Publishers, 1987, pp. 643–646.
55. Kolman, J.: Some physical and chemical properties of Uukuniemi virus, strain Potepli-63. Acta Virol. *14*:159, 1970.
56. Ksiazek, T. G., Peters, C. J., Rollin, P. E., et al.: Identification of a new North American hantavirus that causes acute pulmonary insufficiency. Am. J. Trop. Med. Hyg. *52*:117, 1995.
57. Lahdevirta, J.: Nephropathia epidemica in Finland: A clinical, histological and epidemiological study. Ann. Clin. Res. *3*(Suppl. 8):1, 1971.
58. Lahdevirta, J., Collan, Y. K., Jokinen, E. J., et al.: Renal sequelae to nephropathia epidemica. Acta Patholol. Microbiol. Scand. *86*:265, 1978.
59. LeDuc, J. W., Childs, J. E., and Glass, G. E.: The hantaviruses, etiologic agents of hemorrhagic fever with renal syndrome: A possible cause of hypertension and chronic renal disease in the United States. Annu. Rev. Public Health *13*:79, 1992.
60. Lee, H. W.: Epidemiologic features of Korean hemorrhagic fever and research activities on this disease in the Republic of Korea. Tokyo, WHO Working Group on Hemorrhagic Fever with Renal Syndrome, February 1982.
61. Lee, H. W.: Epidemiology. *In* Lee, H. W., and Dalrymple, J. M. (eds.): Manual of Hemorrhagic Fever with Renal Syndrome. Seoul, Korea University, World Health Organization Collaborating Center for Virus Reference and Research Institute for Viral Diseases, 1989, pp. 39–48.
62. Lee, H. W., Baek, L. J., Seong, I. W., et al.: Physico-chemical properties of Hantaan virus. II. The effect of temperature and pH on infectivity of Hantaan virus. J. Korean Soc. Virol. *13*:23, 1983.
63. Lee, H. W., French, G. R., Lee, P. W., et al.: Observations on natural and laboratory infection of rodents with the etiologic agent of Korean hemorrhagic fever. Am. J. Trop. Med. Hyg. *30*:477, 1981.
64. Lee, H. W., and Johnson, K. M.: Laboratory-acquired infections with Hantaan virus, the etiologic agent of Korean hemorrhagic fever. J. Infect. Dis. *146*:645, 1982.
65. Lee, H. W., Lee, P. W., Baek, L. J., et al.: Intraspecific transmission of Hantaan virus, etiologic agent of Korean hemorrhagic fever, in the rodent *Apodemus agrarius*. Am. J. Trop. Med. Hyg. *30*:1106, 1981.
66. Lee, H. W., Lee, P. W., Baek, L. J., et al.: Geographical distribution of hemorrhagic fever with renal syndrome and hantaviruses. Arch. Virol. *115*(Suppl. 1):5, 1990.
67. Lee, H. W., Lee, P. W., and Johnson, K. M.: Isolation of the etiologic agent of Korean hemorrhagic fever. J. Infect. Dis. *137*:298, 1978.
68. Lee, J. S.: Clinical features of hemorrhagic fever with renal syndrome in Korea. Kidney Int. *40*(Suppl. 35):S88, 1991.
69. Lee, P. W., Meegan, J. M., LeDuc, J. W., et al.: Serologic techniques for detection of Hantaan virus infection, related antigens and antibodies. *In* Lee, H. W., and Dalrymple, J. M. (eds.): Manual of Hemorrhagic Fever with Renal Syndrome. Seoul, Korea University, World Health Organization Collaborating Center for Virus Reference and Research Institute for Viral Diseases, 1989, pp. 36–38.
70. Levy, H., and Simpson, S. Q.: Hantavirus pulmonary syndrome. Am. J. Respir. Crit. Care Med. *149*:1710, 1994.
71. Lloyd, G., Bowen, E. T. W., Jones N., et al.: HFRS outbreak associated with laboratory rats in UK. Lancet *1*:175, 1984.
72. Lopez, N., Padula, P., Rossi, C., et al.: Genetic identification of a new hantavirus causing severe pulmonary syndrome in Argentina. Virology *220*:223, 1996.
73. Mayer, C. F.: Epidemic hemorrhagic fever of the Far East, or endemic hemorrhagic nephroso-nephritis, a short outline of the disease, with supplemental data on the results of experimental inoculation of human volunteers. Milit. Surg. *110*:276, 1952.
74. McKee, K. T., Jr., LeDuc, J. W., and Peters, C. J.: Hantaviruses. *In* Belshe, R. B. (ed.): Textbook of Human Virology. 2nd ed. Littleton, MA, PSG Publishing, 1991, pp. 615–632.
75. McNinch, J. H.: Far East command conference on epidemic hemorrhagic fever. Ann. Intern. Med. *38*:53, 1953.
76. Moolenaar, R. L., Dalton, C., Lipman, H. B., et al.: Clinical features that differentiate hantavirus pulmonary syndrome from three other acute respiratory illnesses. Clin. Infect. Dis. *21*:643, 1995.
77. Mustonen, J., Huttunen, N.-P., Brummer-Korvenkontio, M., et al.: Clinical picture of nephropathia epidemica in children. Acta Pediatr. *83*:526, 1994.
78. Myhrman, G.: En njursjukdorn med egenartad symptombild. Nord. Med. Tidskr. *7*:793, 1934.
79. Nichol, S. T., Rollin, P. E., Ksiazek, T. G., et al.: Hantavirus pulmonary syndrome and newly described hantaviruses in the United States. *In* Elliott, R. H. (ed.): *Bunyaviridae*. New York, Plenum, 1996, pp. 269–280.
80. Nichol, S. T., Spiropoulou, C. F., Morzunov, S., et al.: Genetic identification of a hantavirus associated with an outbreak of acute respiratory illness. Science *262*:914, 1993.
81. Niklasson, B., Hellsten, G., and LeDuc, J.: Hemorrhagic fever with renal syndrome: A study of sequelae following nephropathia epidemica. Arch. Virol. *137*:241, 1994.
82. Niklasson, B., and LeDuc, J. W.: Isolation of the nephropathia epidemica agent in Sweden. Lancet *1*:1012, 1984.

83. Niklasson, B., LeDuc, J., Nystrom, K., et al.: Nephropathia epidemica: Incidence of clinical cases and antibody prevalence in an endemic area of Sweden. Epidemiol. Infect. *99*:559, 1987.
84. Parisi, M. D. N., Enria, D. A., Piri, N. C., et al.: Retrospective detection of clinical infection caused by hantavirus in Argentina. Medicina *56*:1, 1996.
85. Parmenter, R. R., Brunt, J. W., Moore, D. I., et al.: The hantavirus epidemic in the Southwest: Rodent population dynamics and the implications for transmission of hantavirus-associated adult respiratory distress syndrome (HARDS) in the Four Corners region. Sevilleta LTER Publications Nos. 41 and 45. Albuquerque, University of New Mexico, 1993.
86. Peco-Antic, A., Popovic-Rolovic, M., Gligic, A., et al.: Clinical characteristics of haemorrhagic fever with renal syndrome in children. Pediatr. Nephrol. *6*:335, 1992.
87. Peters, C. J.: Pathogenesis of viral hemorrhagic fevers. *In* Nathanson, N., Ahmed, R., Gonzalez-Scarano, F., et al. (eds.): Viral Pathogenesis. Philadelphia, Lippincott-Raven, 1996, pp. 779–800.
88. Peters, C. J., Khan, A. S., and Zaki, S. R.: Hantaviruses in the United States. Arch. Intern. Med. *156*:705, 1996.
89. Pilaski, J., Feldman, H., Morzunov, S., et al.: Genetic identification of a new Puumala virus strain causing severe hemorrhagic fever with renal syndrome in Germany. J. Infect. Dis. *170*:1456, 1994.
90. Pon, E., McKee, K. T., Jr., Diniega, B. M., et al.: Outbreak of hemorrhagic fever with renal syndrome among U.S. Marines in Korea. Am. J. Trop. Med. Hyg. *42*:612, 1990.
91. Prince, H. N., Prince, D. L., and Prince, R. N.: Principles of viral control and transmission. *In* Block, S. S. (ed.): Disinfection, Sterilization, and Preservation. 4th ed. Philadelphia, Lea & Febiger, 1991, pp. 411–444.
92. Rollin, P. E., Ksiazek, T. G., Elliot, L. H., et al.: Isolation of Black Creek Canal virus, a new hantavirus from *Sigmodon hispidus* in Florida. J. Med. Virol. *46*:35, 1995.
93. Schmaljohn, A., Li, D., Negley, D. L., et al.: Isolation and initial characterization of a new found hantavirus from California. Virology *206*:963, 1995.
94. Schmaljohn, C. S.: *Bunyaviridae:* The viruses and their replication. *In* Fields, B. N., Knipe, D. M., Howley, P. M., et al. (eds.): Fields' Virology. 3rd ed. Philadelphia, Lippincott-Raven, 1996, pp. 1447–1471.
95. Schmaljohn, C. S., and Dalrymple, J. M.: Analysis of Hantaan virus RNA: Evidence for a new genus of *Bunyaviridae.* Virology *131*:482, 1983.
96. Schmaljohn, C. S., Hasty, S. E., Dalrymple, J. M., et al.: Antigenic and genetic properties of viruses linked to hemorrhagic fever with renal syndrome. Science *227*:1041, 1985.
97. Schmaljohn, C. S., Hasty, S. E., and Dalrymple, J. M.: Preparation of candidate vaccinia-vectored vaccines for haemorrhagic fever with renal syndrome. Vaccine *10*:10, 1992.
98. Settergren, B.: Nephropathia epidemica (hemorrhagic fever with renal syndrome) in Scandinavia. Rev. Infect. Dis. *13*:736, 1991.
99. Sheedy, J. A., Froed, B. F., Batson, H. A., et al.: The clinical course of epidemic hemorrhagic fever. Am. J. Med. *16*:619, 1954.
100. Simonsen, L., Dalton, M. J., Breiman, R. F., et al.: Evaluation of the magnitude of the 1993 hantavirus outbreak in the southwestern United States. J. Infect. Dis. *172*:729, 1995.
101. Smorodintsev, A. A., Kazbintsev, L. I., and Chudakov, V. G.: Viral hemorrhagic fevers. Washington, D.C., Office of Technical Services, U.S. Department of Commerce, 1964, p. 1.
102. Song, J. W., Back, L. J., Gajdusek, D. C., et al.: Isolation of pathogenic hantavirus from white-footed mouse *(Peromyscus leucopus).* Lancet *344*:1637, 1994.
103. Stevens, C., Johnson, M., and Bell, A.: First reported cases of hantavirus pulmonary syndrome in Canada. Can. Commun. Dis. Rep. *20*:121, 1994.
104. Stuhlfauth, K.: Bericht über ein neues schlammtieberahnliches krankheitsbild bei deutschen truppen in Lappland. Dtsch. Med. Wochenschr. *69*:439, 1973.
105. Tkachenko, E. A., and Lee, H. W.: Etiology and epidemiology of hemorrhagic fever with renal syndrome. Kidney Int. *40*(Suppl. 35):S54, 1991.
106. Torrez-Martinez, N., and Hjelle, B.: Enzootic of Bayou hantavirus in rice rats *(Oryzomys palustris)* in 1983. Lancet *346*:780, 1995.
107. Trencseni, T., and Keleti, B.: Clinical Aspects and Epidemiology of Haemorrhagic Fever with Renal Syndrome. Budapest, Akademiai Kiado, 1971.
108. Tsai, T. F.: Hemorrhagic fever with renal syndrome: Clinical aspects. Lab. Anim. Sci. *37*:419, 1987.
109. Tsai, T. F.: Hemorrhagic fever with renal syndrome: Mode of transmission to humans. Lab. Anim. Sci. *37*:428, 1987.
110. Umenai, T., Lee, H. W., Lee, P. W., et al.: Korean haemorrhagic fever in staff in an animal laboratory. Lancet *1*:314, 1979.
111. van Ypersele de Strihou, C.: Clinical features of hemorrhagic fever with renal syndrome in Europe. Kidney Int. *40*(Suppl. 35):S80, 1991.
112. Vitek, C. R., Breiman, R. F., Ksiazek, T. G., et al.: Evidence against person-to-person transmission of hantavirus to health-care workers. Clin. Infect. Dis. *22*:824, 1996.
113. Weissenbacher, M. C., Cura, E., Segura, E. L., et al.: Serological evidence of human hantavirus infection in Argentina, Bolivia, and Uruguay. Medicina *56*:17, 1996.
113a. Wells, R. M., Sosa Estani, S., Yadon, Z. E., et al.: Epidemiologic features of an unusual hantavirus outbreak in southern Argentina. Emerg. Infect. Dis. (in press).
114. Williams, R. J., Bryan, R. T., Mills, J. N., et al.: An outbreak of hantavirus pulmonary syndrome among Mennonite colonies in western Paraguay. Am. J. Trop. Med: Hyg. (in press).
115. Yanagihara, R.: Hantavirus infection in the United States: Epizootiology and epidemiology. Rev. Infect. Dis. *12*:449, 1990.
116. Yanagihara, R., Gajdusek, D. C., Gibbs, C. J., Jr., et al.: Prospect Hill virus: Serological evidence for infection in mammologists. N. Engl. J. Med. *310*:1325, 1984.
117. Yanagihara, R., Goldgaber, D., Lee, P. W., et al.: Propagation of nephropathia epidemica in cell culture. Lancet *1*:1013, 1984.
118. Yoo, K. H., Choi, Y., and the Korean Society of Pediatric Nephrology: Haemorrhagic fever with renal syndrome in Korean children. Pediatr. Nephrol. *8*:540, 1994.
119. Zaki, S. R., Greer, P. W., Coffield, L. M. et al.: Hantavirus pulmonary syndrome: Pathogenesis of an emerging infectious disease. Am. J. Pathol. *146*:552, 1995.
120. Zeizt, P. S., Butler, J. C., Cheek, J. E., et al.: A case-control study of hantavirus pulmonary syndrome during an outbreak in the southwestern United States. J. Infect. Dis. *171*:864, 1995.
121. Zetterholm, S. G.: Akuta mefriter simulerande akuta bukfall. Svenska Lakartidningen *31*:425, 1934.
122. Zoller, L., Yang, S., Gott, P., et al.: Use of recombinant nucleocapsid proteins of the Hantaan and nephropathia epidemica serotypes of hantaviruses as immunodiagnostic antigens. J. Med. Virol. *39*:200, 1993.

190

CALIFORNIA/LA CROSSE ENCEPHALITIS

James E. McJunkin, Linda L. Minnich, and Theodore F. Tsai

TERMINOLOGY

The name of the California serogroup does not reflect the widespread geographic distribution of viruses in the serogroup but simply the name of the initially discovered prototype virus in California in 1943. In fact, California encephalitis (CE) virus has been shown to be questionable as a central nervous system pathogen, with reports of encephalitis limited to three original cases.[13, 39, 45, 84] Furthermore, La Crosse (LAC) virus, the most prevalent and pathogenic member of the California serogroup, produces disease in the midwest and eastern United States but not in the west coast region. Because of its prevalence and virulence, LAC virus has been the most studied member of the group and is the major focus of this chapter. Other members of the serogroup will be covered briefly as well.

ETIOLOGIC AGENT

In 1960, a 4-year-old girl died of "rural encephalitis" in a hospital in La Crosse County, Wisconsin. Four years later,

Dr. Wayne Thompson isolated a novel virus from frozen hemogenates of the child's brain by intracerebral inoculation of suckling mice.[16, 20] In the past three decades, we have come to appreciate that LAC encephalitis is the most prevalent arboviral infection of children in the United States and can occur at a rate rivaling that of bacterial meningitis in endemic foci found in midwestern and mid-Atlantic states.[1, 2] Soon after its discovery, LAC virus was identified as a member of the California serogroup and is one of five (prototype CE, LAC, snowshoe hare, Jamestown Canyon [JC], and trivittatus) viruses causing human disease in North America. Inkoo and Tahyna viruses are members of the California serogroup distributed in Europe.

The California serogroup is 1 of 16 in the *Bunyavirus* genus. Bunyaviruses are spherical particles 75 to 115 nm in diameter, with nucleocapsid cores 60 to 70 nm in diameter enveloped by a membrane bilayer 4 nm thick.[79] Virions bud directly by vesicular fusion from cisternae of Golgi or endoplasmic reticulum. The genome is composed of three pieces of negative-sense, single-stranded circularized RNA. Each of the three RNA segments—L, M, and S—is associated with a nucleoprotein, encoded by the S segment, and small quantities of the L protein, a viral polymerase, which form the three nucleocapsids.[39, 41, 47] The circular, helical nucleocapsids are enclosed in a lipid envelope in which the G1 and G2 glycoproteins are located on 5- to 10-nm long spikes.

The M RNA segment that encodes the G1 and G2 glycoproteins is a major determinant of viral neuroinvasiveness in mice and susceptibility of *Aedes triseriatus* mosquitoes to oral and intrathoracic infection.[7, 38, 39, 75] Neuroinvasiveness may be linked to cell receptor and fusion functions associated with glycoproteins.[37, 38] The G1 protein of LAC virus is involved in viral attachment to mammalian cell receptors, hemagglutination, and viral neutralization.[38, 39, 60, 61, 75] Truncated G1 protein may prove to be important in vaccine development (see Prevention). Group and LAC virus–specific epitopes are present on G1. The G2 glycoprotein mediates viral attachment to insect cells,[64] but recent work emphasizes that G1 also is required for infection of mosquito cells (in vitro and in vivo).[48] Antibodies to the nucleocapsid protein neither hemagglutinate nor neutralize.

Although the M segment genome via its glycoprotein products (especially G1) largely determines *neuroinvasiveness* (i.e., the ability to invade the central nervous system from an extraneural site), recent evidence using viral reassortants of different virulence implicates the L segment as a major factor in determining *neurovirulence* (i.e., the ability to infect central nervous system tissue after direct cerebral injection).[33] Nevertheless, the concept of neuroinvasiveness, particularly as it relates to G1 glycoprotein, has significant clinical implications. Recent work shows that a truncated G1 protein preparation induces a protective immune response in the suckling mouse model via neutralizing antibody (see Prevention).[71] Apparently, neuroinvasion is prevented by interruption of the transient viremia, which occurs just after virus inoculation.

Oligonucleotide maps of LAC viral isolates from various areas of the United States have grouped the viruses into three types. Upper Midwest viral strains are of two types, A and B, and type C varieties are found in scattered areas of the eastern United States.[32, 62] Strain variation indicates that changes in the viral genome occur by genetic drift. Genetic reassortment, through exchanges of RNA segments, also has been demonstrated in nature.

ECOLOGY

A. triseriatus, the treehole mosquito, is the reservoir of LAC virus in nature and the vector for transmission of infection to humans.[45, 86, 87] Humans do not maintain prolonged viremias and therefore are dead-end hosts. The mosquito is distributed principally in eastern hardwood deciduous forests, where it breeds in treeholes; however, it also is adapted to breeding in small artificial containers that hold rainwater, such as discarded cans, bottles, and tires. The mosquito is diurnal and feeds actively during the day. Although they disperse over a wide area, fairly permanent foci of infected mosquitoes are observed in sharply delimited areas, and virus isolations and human cases recur each summer in established foci.[45]

LAC virus is maintained in nature vertically by transovarial transmission in *A. triseriatus* and horizontally by venereal transmission among the vector mosquitoes and through amplification of virus in vertebrate hosts. The virus overwinters in infected eggs, providing the mechanism of recurrent disease each summer in endemic areas. The fact that not all progeny are infected after vertical transmission may relate to differences in the mesenteric barrier to infection in the developing mosquito, which result from differences in larval rearing conditions, especially nutrition.[45, 70] Supplemental horizontal transmission appears to contribute to viral maintenance in nature as well.[67, 86, 87] The principal amplifying hosts are chipmunks (*Tamias striatus*) and squirrels (*Sciurus carolensis* and *Sciurus niger*).[91] Other wild vertebrates (foxes, *Vulpes fulva* and *Urocyon cinereoargenteus*; and woodchucks, *Marmota monax*) also may contribute to amplification, but domestic dogs, cats, and livestock do not. [35] Although domestic livestock and pets do not contribute to horizontal amplification of the virus, certain species do show seroconversion to California serogroup viruses, and such species may prove to be useful markers of viral presence in a given area.[35] Outbreaks of fatal encephalitis have occurred in puppies; dogs have been used in an animal model of central nervous system infection.[11]

Aedes canadensis is an important secondary vector in Ohio.[9] LAC virus varieties with a type C oligonucleotide pattern are found in this species in Ohio and New York. *Aedes albopictus*, the Asian Tiger mosquito that has been shown experimentally to transmit LAC virus efficiently, presents a major concern as a potential vector.[24] The mosquito, which is dispersed widely in the southeastern United States, potentially could enter the transmission cycle for LAC or one of the other California serogroup viruses, expanding the geographic range and circumstances in which the viruses might be transmitted.[23, 43]

Although JC virus first was isolated in Colorado and it is distributed widely in the West and Midwest, most cases of human illness have been reported in New York, New England, Ontario, and the upper Midwest. Various *Aedes* mosquitoes (e.g., *Aedes communis* in the West, *Aedes stimulans* in the upper Midwest, *Aedes abserratus* in Connecticut) function as vectors.[27, 42, 44, 45] As opposed to LAC virus, in which large mammals do not play a role in viral propagation in nature, deer are the primary amplifying host of JC virus, with up to 80 per cent seroconversion found in adult deer populations in endemic areas.[69] The overwintering mechanism has not been elucidated, although transovarial transmission in *Aedes provocans* has been demonstrated.[10]

Snowshoe hare virus is distributed throughout Canada, including the Yukon and Northwest Territories, in adjacent northern states, and in Russia and China. *Culiseta inornata* and various *Aedes* species transmit the virus to snowshoe hares (*Lepus americanus*), ground squirrels (*Citellus undulatus*), and other mammals. Transovarial transmission in *Aedes* mosquitoes has been demonstrated.[50]

Trivittatus virus is transmitted and maintained by vertical transmission by *Aedes* trivittatus in the Midwest and is vectored in the South by *Aedes infirmatus*. CE virus is distributed in the western United States, where *Aedes melanimon* and *Aedes dorsalis* are the principal vectors.[45, 49, 73, 83] Inkoo and Tahyna viruses cause febrile illness with central nervous system and respiratory tract infection, respectively, in Scandinavia, Central Europe, and western Russia. Viral recombinants have been demonstrated.[29]

EPIDEMIOLOGY

The annual incidence of LAC virus central nervous system infection, estimated in population studies of endemic counties, is approximately 10 per 100,000. This rate is similar to the incidence of bacterial meningitis of all causes. From 1971 to 1983, reported cases of LAC encephalitis nearly equaled reports of herpes encephalitis (Fig. 190–1). LAC virus infections are endemic in the United States, with sporadic infections occurring annually from July to September or October (depending on the first frost), chiefly in rural areas of the east-central states (Fig. 190–2).[58, 84] The geographic distribution of LAC virus infections corresponds to natural divisions where beech, oak, and maple woodlots are prevalent.[45] Although LAC encephalitis has been considered a disease of midwestern and mid-Atlantic states (with highly endemic zones in Minnesota, Wisconsin, Illinois, Iowa, Ohio, and West Virginia), sporadic cases have been found in more than 20 states, as far south as Louisiana and as far east as Connecticut (see Fig. 190–1). Active surveillance efforts can increase case finding markedly, as seen recently in West Virginia,[10, 59] where after the death of a child from LAC encephalitis in 1987, more than 150 cases were diagnosed over the next 8 years (compared with only 15 cases ever previously reported in West Virginia) (unpublished data from the West Virginia State Health Department). Therefore, the public health importance of LAC encephalitis nationally is not known fully because the virus is distributed discontinuously in the eastern United States, where the disease could be endemic.[8, 54, 89] However, these observations suggest that its importance as a cause of childhood morbidity has been underestimated.

LAC encephalitis principally is a disease of children. Among reported cases in the United States from 1972 to 1981, 75 per cent were in children younger than 10 years of age, and only 3 per cent occurred in persons 20 years of age or older.[58] The majority of cases are in males, with a ratio of 1.8:1. The proportion of seropositive males in rural areas (32 per cent) is about 10 per cent higher than in females in persons between 5 and 39 years of age. In those younger than 5 years of age or older than 40 years of age, no differences were found, and seropositivity rates are similar in males and females from urban areas. These findings indicate that males are at a higher risk of infection because of factors associated with exposure to sylvan vectors. This conclusion is supported by observations of wildlife workers with heavy

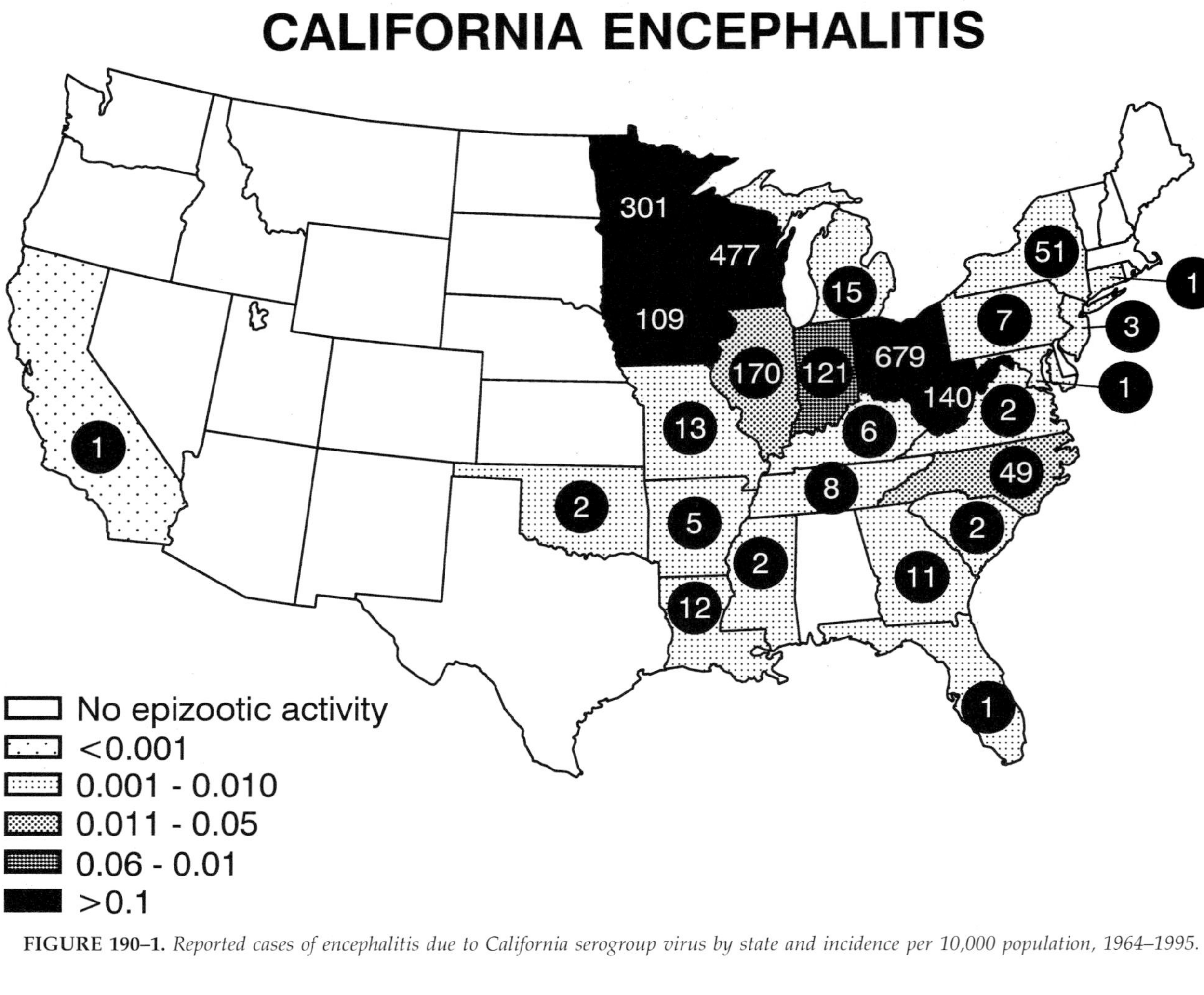

FIGURE 190–1. *Reported cases of encephalitis due to California serogroup virus by state and incidence per 10,000 population, 1964–1995.*

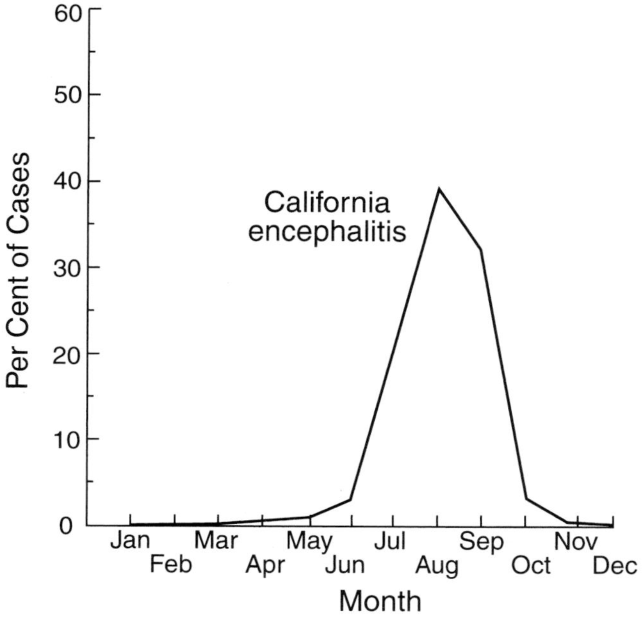

FIGURE 190–2. *Reported cases of encephalitis due to California serogroup virus by month of onset, 1972–1989.*

exposure to forested areas who had threefold higher antibody prevalence rates than did controls.[68, 81]

A case-control study done in a highly endemic county found several characteristics of the peridomestic environment associated with risk of acquiring LAC encephalitis: treeholes on the residential premise, proximity of the house to the forest edge, and the presence of artificial containers and large numbers of discarded tires. Various behaviors (e.g., time spent outdoors, air-conditioner use) were not risk factors. These observations point to the proximity and abundance of natural and artificial mosquito breeding sites as the principal risk factors for sporadic infection.[89]

Inapparent infections are frequent, which result in rising seroprevalence with age. Point prevalence rates vary in endemic locations from 30 per cent in rural areas to 15 per cent in urban locations.[68] Although the risk appears highest in rural areas, many cases occur in suburban residential locations, and travel to forested recreational areas in endemic regions is given in the history of other patients.[28, 82] However, a study of LAC encephalitis in endemic areas of Minnesota and Wisconsin failed to find a significant difference in attack rates in urban and rural locations.[54]

Serosurveys indicate JC virus seroprevalence rates of 5 to 40 per cent in the upper Midwest. The preponderance of reported cases (21 of 29 in one series) is in males.[77] Unlike LAC encephalitis, cases occur in all age groups. Human infections with snowshoe hare virus have been documented by serosurveys in Alaska and throughout Canada.[45] Antibody prevalence rates were more than 30 per cent in some areas; seroprevalence in males was double the rate in females. Sporadic infections with CE viruses probably are frequent in the western United States.[73] The prevalence of seroreactors was approximately one-third in a study of Kern County, California, residents. However, symptomatic cases are rare.

PATHOGENESIS

LAC virus, which infects the salivary glands of the mosquito vector, is introduced into the host's skin and subcutaneous tissue during feeding. Probing alone is infectious. The completion of a blood meal is not necessary for transmission. Local viral replication in adjacent muscle tissue leads to a systemic viremia that seeds the reticuloendothelial system, muscle, and chondrocytes, leading to further amplication of viremia, which allows central nervous system invasion.[37, 55, 56] Entrance to the central nervous system probably is gained via infection of vascular endothelial cells initially, followed by infection of neurons and glial cells.[55, 56] Recent case reports suggest that vascular involvement in human LAC encephalitis may be important in the pathogenesis of focal deficits (from stroke) and of more generalized cerebral edema (from vasogenic edema).[63, 66]

Studies indicate that the extraneural phase of viral replication and neuroinvasiveness largely are mediated by the M RNA segment primarily via G1 glycoprotein, which has cell receptor and fusion functions.[38, 39, 37, 75] A more recent study in adult mice indicates that once the virus has gained access to the central nervous system, replication in central nervous system tissue, that is, neurovirulence, is mediated largely by the L RNA segment, probably via viral polymerase.[33, 36] Previous work had implicated the M segment in neurovirulence as well, but in that study neurovirulence was defined as time to death after intracutaneous inoculation.[75] The host immune response involves neutralizing antibody, which mediates viral aggregation, inhibition of viral attachment to cells, and inhibition of viral penetration and uncoating.[61]

CLINICAL MANIFESTATIONS

The clinical spectrum of illness in LAC virus infections ranges from inapparent infection or a mild febrile illness to aseptic meningitis and fatal encephalitis.[4, 18, 19, 22, 46, 51, 80, 90] The ratio of inapparent to clinical infections has ranged from 26:1 to 322:1.[58] Most infections are associated with signs and symptoms of meningoencephalitis. The case-fatality rate is less than 1 per cent overall[84] but approaches 1 per cent of hospitalized cases.

Children typically present with a 2- to 3-day prodrome of fever, malaise, headache, and vomiting. Despite the presence of vomiting during the prodrome, diarrhea usually is absent, providing a clue that the symptoms are not due to merely a gastroenteritis. The illness further evolves with clouding of the sensorium, increasing temperature, and lethargy. In more fulminant cases, an abrupt onset of fever and headache may be associated with the sudden onset of focal or generalized seizures.

On examination, a temperature of 39° to 40° C (102.2° to 104° F) is not uncommon. Most children, even those presenting with transient seizures initially, are lethargic but not frankly disoriented at admission. The development of disorientation represents an important sign in the patient's course because the child who develops this sign (which in preverbal patients usually is seen as lack of recognition of parents) is at greater risk for neurologic deterioration to further seizures and/or coma. Although obvious signs of increased intracranial pressure (ICP) are rare, children with LAC encephalitis who develop disorientation and/or coma should be considered at risk for development of increased ICP. The Glasgow Coma Score provides the best systematic measure of changes in level of consciousness and is the most important clinical tool in evaluating these children serially in the hospital. Signs of meningeal irritation are found in only about 50 per cent of cases.[4] Most patients have an uncomplicated course, in which fever, headache, and lethargy gradually resolve over 7 to 8 days. In others, the course of illness is complicated by seizures and coma. As opposed to herpes simplex encephalitis, the presence of deep coma does not portend poor outcome necessarily. Focal neurologic signs, principally focal seizures, paresis, aphasia, and abnormal reflexes, are found in 16 to 25 per cent of cases of LAC encephalitis. Focal and generalized seizures occur in 42 to 62 per cent of cases, and 10 to 15 per cent of cases develop status epilepticus. Focal neurologic signs, whether found on physical or on electroencephalographic or imaging studies, generally should be taken as evidence of presumptive herpes simplex encephalitis until a diagnosis of LAC encephalitis can be confirmed.[88]

JC virus infections often present with prodromal respiratory symptoms in conjunction with aseptic meningitis or clinical encephalitis. Among 39 patients with proven or suspected central nervous system infection with JC virus, 10 had encephalitis and 7 reported upper respiratory symptoms or pneumonia.[45, 77]

The few reported cases of snowshoe hare virus infection have had presentations ranging from an influenza-like illness to aseptic meningitis and fatal encephalitis. One fatality was reported in a 14-year-old girl who presented with symptoms and signs that suggested Reye syndrome.[30] In a 59-year-old man, radiologic and electroencephalographic findings showed a temporal lobe focus, which led to brain biopsy and a clinical and pathologic diagnosis of herpes encephalitis, although herpes virus was not isolated.[2] Serologic examination later confirmed the diagnosis of snowshoe hare virus infection. Mild febrile illnesses attributed to infection with trivittatus virus have been described in some patients, and central nervous system infections have been identified in others.[68] Three cases of infection attributed to prototype CE virus have been reported. All three patients had signs and symptoms of encephalitis.[49]

Laboratory examinations in LAC virus infections are not diagnostic. The peripheral leukocyte count may be slightly elevated, and a neutrophilia may be present. Examination of the cerebrospinal fluid shows changes typical of viral meningoencephalitis, with a pleocytosis and a wide range of differential counts of polymorphonuclear and mononuclear cells.[4, 18, 22, 51] The total cerebrospinal fluid leukocyte count generally is not high (in one series, the median white blood cell count was 47), and 10 per cent of cases had red blood cells in the cerebrospinal fluid. An elevated protein is observed in less than one-third of cases.[4, 18, 22, 51] An occasional child will have negative or equivocal findings on initial cerebrospinal fluid analysis, only to have numerous white blood cells within 24 to 48 hours on repeat lumbar puncture.

Results of imaging techniques are not diagnostic in most cases. Computed tomography (CT) generally is normal or nonspecific, showing decreased ventricular size from cerebral edema. In 95 confirmed and presumptive LAC encephalitis cases reported from 1981 to 1983 in Ohio, 51 had CT; 4 had definite focal changes of mass effect or localized inflammation, and 8 others showed generalized inflammation or edema. Focal abnormalities were localized to the frontal or temporal lobes. Two patients, one with a focal abnormality and one with generalized inflammation, underwent brain biopsy, and four patients were treated with vidarabine. Focal abnormalities were demonstrated by technetium-99m pertechnetate scans in four patients (in the temporal and parietal areas) in another series of 66 patients,[4] and a mass was found by CT in a fatal case of a patient with a hematoma. Recent case reports suggest superiority of magnetic resonance imaging (MRI) over CT in defining lesions in LAC encephalitis, with new insights into the pathology of the disease. In a case of a 20-month-old with right hemiparesis, CT on admission was negative, but MRI on day 1 showed evidence of acute infarction of the left basal ganglia.[63] In another case of a 12-month-old child with clinical evidence of a neurodegenerative clinical picture, MRI showed areas of increased signal intensity in the periventricular white matter, even though the initial CT had been negative.[34] In a third recent case, the CT was normal initially but when repeated in 48 hours (due to clinical deterioration), multiple hypodense lesions were present in both hemispheres (Fig. 190–3). In this case, MRI showed multiple areas of increased signal intensity in the same areas defined as hypodense lesions on CT.[66] *It must be emphasized, however, that the technical difficulties in obtaining MRI in children (including the need for sedation/anesthesia in most cases) still favor CT as the initial imaging study.*

Descriptions of electroencephalographic abnormalities have been emphasized because of the frequency of convulsions during the illness: more than 90 per cent of patients exhibit electroencephalographic abnormalities consisting of generalized or symmetric slow waves. Focal electroencephalographic findings, usually slowing, may appear in as many as 40 per cent of patients. Recent evidence indicates that periodic lateralizing epileptiform discharges previously thought virtually pathognomonic of herpes simplex encephalitis also are seen in cases of LAC encephalitis. These instances usually have been severe cases that also resembled herpes simplex encephalitis clinically.[25]

DIAGNOSIS

It especially is important for clinicians to communicate with virology laboratory colleagues in choosing diagnostic tests for encephalitis and in understanding the limitations of these tests. Information about the clinical presentation and

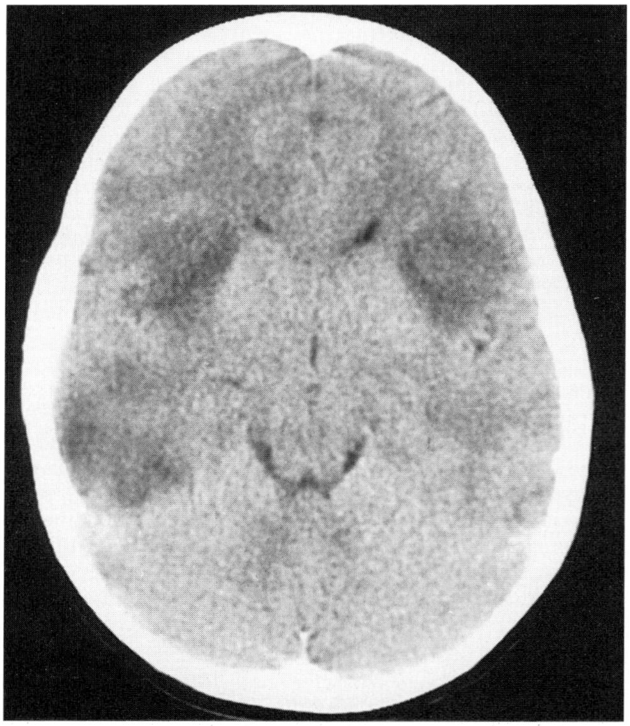

FIGURE 190–3. *Computed tomographic scan of unusually severe case of La Crosse encephalitis shows small ventricles and multifocal hypodense lesions with loss of gray-white differentiation in right frontotemporoparietal and left temporal regions. Computed tomographic scans usually are negative in La Crosse encephalitis (see text).*

travel history must be combined with knowledge of the local epidemiology and natural history of viral infections to select appropriate laboratory tests.

Although the preferred approach to diagnosis of viral encephalitis is to identify the viral agent by isolation or detection of antigen or nucleic acid in cerebrospinal fluid, limitations of these procedures for LAC virus require the diagnosis to be made by serologic methods. To our knowledge, LAC virus has never been cultured from human cerebrospinal fluid, even though it has been isolated from brain on three occasions (two post mortem and one via brain biopsy in a surviving patient).[66, 83] No isolations from cerebrospinal fluid were reported in a series of 34 LAC encephalitis patients.[85] Identification of viral antigen in infected mosquitoes or brain autopsy or biopsy specimens can be accomplished by immunohistochemical techniques such as immunofluorescence and immunoperoxidase.[17] Viral genome components can be identified by hybridization. Polymerase chain reaction assays have been developed but have not been evaluated clinically.[14]

Given the limitations for identification of virus in cerebrospinal fluid, serologic methods remain the diagnostic method of choice. IgM-specific antibody to LAC virus can be detected by an IgM-capture enzyme-linked immunosorbent assay (ELISA) or by indirect immunofluorescence in cerebrospinal fluid and serum specimens. IgM-capture ELISA is a sensitive serologic test that detects virus-specific IgM in 83 to 100 per cent of cases.[5, 6, 12, 31] Absorbance usually is higher in cerebrospinal fluid than serum, but serum may be positive for IgM-specific antibody earlier in the course of infection than may cerebrospinal fluid. Cerebrospinal fluid should be tested to confirm that a positive serum result is associated with acute infection because serum IgM can persist for 9 months after primary infection in about one-third of patients and for 1 to 7 years after acute infection in patients with postencephalitic seizures. It is not clear whether this is due to persistence of viral infection in patients with central nervous system sequelae.

The only diagnostic serologic kit approved by the Food and Drug Administration is an indirect immunofluorescence test for LAC, eastern equine, western equine, and St. Louis encephalitis viruses (Hillcrest Laboratories). Despite the cost of reagents, this technique is suited better for rapid (same-day) results and processing of single specimens. Although the procedure is not difficult technically for individuals familiar with immunofluorescence procedures, experience and observation of strict criteria for positive readings especially are critical for the IgM-specific tests. Pretreatment of the serum to remove or inactivate IgG, comparison of reactivity among the four viral antigens, and requirement of intracytoplasmic inclusions are essential to maintaining specificity of the test. Sensitivity is lower than that of IgM-capture ELISA, with about 60 to 80 per cent of cases positive for IgM at the time of hospital admission. Sensitivity can be enhanced further (to more than 90 per cent) by repeat serologic testing 3 to 7 days later in cases in which initial testing is negative but clinical suspicion remains because IgM serology frequently will become positive in such cases. (Note that a similar relationship between timing of testing and sensitivity applies to IgM-capture ELISA as well.) Specificity is related directly to observation of reading criteria but approaches 100 per cent in a laboratory with experienced technologists.

For all diagnostic tests for LAC encephalitis, false-positive results (compromised specificity) remain the key clinical issue. A false-positive test could result in serious consequences if, for example, antiviral therapy for herpes simplex virus infection erroneously was discontinued or if antibiotic therapy for a partially treated bacterial meningitis were discontinued similarly. Therefore, clinicians should be in direct communication with laboratory colleagues concerning specificity data for their laboratory, particularly in cases in which treatable alternative diagnoses, such as herpes simplex encephalitis or partially treated meningitis, remain in the differential diagnosis on clinical grounds.

Fourfold or greater changes in hemagglutination-inhibition and neutralization antibody titers confirm a repeat infection. A stable or single elevated serum IgG titer of 128/160 or higher by immunofluorescence or 64/80 or higher by hemagglutination or neutralization is presumptive evidence of recent infection. Complement fixation, although less expensive to perform and frequently offered by commercial laboratories, never should be used alone due to lack of sensitivity.

DIFFERENTIAL DIAGNOSIS

The principal consideration in differential diagnosis is herpes simplex encephalitis. Early clinical descriptions disclosed a high rate of focal findings in LAC encephalitis (approximately 20 per cent). The frontal and temporal lobe locations of abnormalities detected by electroencephalography, radionuclide scan, and CT indicated that many patients had a clinical appearance typical of herpes simplex encephalitis.[4] Recently, five patients with LAC encephalitis were described with electroencephalographic findings of periodic lateralizing epileptiform discharges, thought previously to be highly indicative of herpes simplex encephalitis.[26] Because late institution of therapy in herpes simplex encephalitis is associated with poor outcome, it is reasonable to make an early diagnosis of presumptive herpes simplex encephalitis in cases of encephalitis with focal findings, pending definitive diagnosis.[88]

In patients with less fulminant signs of central nervous system infection, enteroviral aseptic meningitis is a common consideration, especially because it occurs in summer and early fall as well. The presence of rash, pharyngitis, myocarditis, or conjunctivitis is a clue to enterovirus and is not characteristic of LAC virus infection. In areas of the Midwest where immunizations are eschewed for religious reasons, poliomyelitis remains an important diagnostic consideration. Mumps encephalitis is another consideration, even in the absence of parotid swelling, and low cerebrospinal glucose level may be a clue to this diagnosis.[1]

Zoonotic infections that cause meningitis or encephalitis should be considered carefully in the differential diagnosis because of the rural distribution of LAC virus infections. Patients with Rocky Mountain spotted fever exhibit signs of central nervous system disturbance, but the disorder usually is characterized by rash and/or evidence of viscerotrophic infection. Leptospirosis can be differentiated by the presence of rash, conjunctivitis, and pulmonary and cardiac involvement. Listeria encephalitis, in nonimmunocompromised patients, occurs principally at the extremes of age. Encephalomyocarditis virus infections of the central nervous system have been reported in Europe; in the United States, antibody to the virus has been found in human serosurveys, but clinical evidence of disease has not been documented. Cat-scratch encephalopathy should be brought into the differential, especially in southeastern states, where the disease is most prevalent. Rabies should be considered in the differential diagnosis because patients may present with signs of encephalitis in the absence of hydrophobia and without a history of animal bite. Drug-induced aseptic meningitis and neurotoxic reactions to DEET insect repellent also should be considered in the differential diagnosis (see earlier and Table 178–2). *Mycoplasma pneumoniae* rarely causes encephalitis.

TREATMENT

General pediatric and pediatric critical care measures remain the mainstay for the treatment of these patients. It is a reasonable general strategy to assess these patients as one would assess the child with closed head injury because in both instances (1) changes in level of consciousness can not be assumed to be due to a normal need to sleep and therefore need to be monitored serially and (2) changes in the level of consciousness generally are the best and earliest indicators of evolving intracranial pathology as opposed to brain stem signs (e.g., pupillary abnormalities, bradycardia with hypertension), which usually indicate impending cerebral herniation. Therefore, serial monitoring of the level of consciousness is the most important aspect of neurologic monitoring (using the Glasgow Coma Score), even if the child has minimal change in level of consciousness at the time of admission. Note that the development of mental status changes or focal findings may represent ictal (or postictal) events, emphasizing the need for electroencephalography and neurologic consultation in such cases.

Seizure control especially is important because continued seizures in a child with brain inflammation and edema could increase cerebral metabolic rate and also might compromise the airway and ventilation. Fever control also is important to prevent unnecessary increases in cerebral metabolic rate. It is important to maintain normal serum osmolality by avoiding hypotonic intravenous fluids and by monitoring for hyponatremia, which may signal developing inappropriate antidiuretic hormone syndrome.

With the above basic supportive measures in place, there are three particularly important decision points in management that depend on the presence or absence of (1) disorientation, (2) focal findings, and (3) deterioration in the Glasgow Coma Score. Children who remain lethargic but do not progress to disorientation may be observed carefully on the general pediatric floor. Once the child becomes disoriented, as shown by mental status changes in the older child or shown by a lack of recognition of parents in the infant, the child should be transferred to the pediatric intensive care unit. Those cases that suggest herpes simplex encephalitis due to focal findings and/or deep coma warrant presumptive treatment with acyclovir until the diagnosis of LAC virus infection is confirmed (see Diagnosis).

Children whose Glasgow Coma Score falls to 8 or lower warrant strong consideration for endotracheal intubation, using appropriate premedication to prevent possible increases in ICP. Once intubated, the patient requires frequent ongoing sedation to prevent increased ICP, which might be exacerbated with pain or coughing. The patient generally is ventilated to a partial carbon dioxide pressure in the low-normal range to prevent cerebral vasodilatation with exacerbation of possible increased ICP. Hemodynamic stability is essential, often including central venous pressure monitoring (and in some patients infusions of vasoactive drugs) to maintain adequate mean arterial pressure in the face of sedation and/or neurologic deterioration and possible increased ICP. Although there are little current data on the use of ICP monitoring in LAC encephalitis, in one recent case report ICP monitoring was a useful adjunct in directing therapy. In this case, there was radiographic evidence of cerebral edema along with clinical symptoms of increased ICP.[66]

Ribavirin can inhibit the replication of LAC in vitro (primarily by direct effect on viral polymerase activity) at levels potentially achievable in cerebrospinal fluid. It also is relevant to the potential use of ribavirin in LAC encephalitis that other bunyaviruses are sensitive to ribavirin in vitro and/or in animal studies.[21, 52, 53, 63, 72, 76, 78] Hantaan virus, for example, which causes lethal encephalitis in the suckling mouse model (as does LAC virus), produces less viremia and mortality in mice treated with ribavirin.[52] Intravenous ribavirin has been used on a compassionate-use basis in at least one case of severe LAC encephalitis without adverse effects.[66] Recently, a randomized, double-blind, placebo-controlled clinical trial of intravenous ribavirin was started in the highly endemic region of southern West Virginia, where its use has been limited to severe cases.

It is important to keep in perspective the generally benign outcome of LAC encephalitis without antiviral therapy. It especially is important to recognize that the supportive measures outlined previously remain the mainstay of therapy for these patients.

OUTCOME

LAC and JC virus infections are associated with a case-fatality ratio of less than 1 per cent.

Six to 15 per cent of recovered LAC encephalitis patients exhibit recurrent seizures.[19, 26] The risk of a recurrent convulsive disorder was about 25 per cent in patients who experienced a seizure during the acute phase of illness.[26, 40] The interval between the onset of recurrent seizures and recovery from acute infection ranged from a few days to years (mean, 4 years).[26] Persistent hemiparesis was a residual abnormality in 2 of 151 patients followed up to 6 years after recovery, but 1 patient had a brain biopsy of the opposite hemisphere.[19]

Unilateral infarction of basal ganglia and hemiparesis was described recently in an infant case.[63] Another infant presented with an apparent neurodegenerative disease secondary to acute disseminated encephalomyelitis associated with a presumed case.[34] Psychometric evaluations of recovered patients have failed to show significant differences in standard tests of cognitive ability, compared with controls. However, changes in performance in tests administered before and after illness suggest some effects in children who were most seriously ill. Abnormalities in visual-motor function and intellectual impairment were observed more often in patients who had focal abnormalities in the acute illness; however, the number studied was small.[65, 74] Recent work suggests that susceptibility and complications of LAC encephalitis have an immunogenic component based on the association of illness and seizures with certain human leukocyte antigens.[15]

PATHOLOGY

Pathologic descriptions of two fatal cases have been reported.[57] In gross appearance, the brain is swollen and meninges are congested. The principal brain lesions are neuronal degeneration, patchy inflammatory lesions, and vasculitis. The cerebrum and basal ganglia are the principal sites of involvement, but petechial hemorrhages and edema were noted in the spinal cord of one case. In both cases, lesions in the cerebrum were confined to the frontal, parietal, and temporal lobes and the cerebellum was uninvolved.

Focal inflammatory lesions and perivascular reactions are composed primarily of mononuclear cells. Neuronolysis and neuronophagia are observed in foci of inflammation and necrosis, with reactive polymorphonuclear, mononuclear, and microglial responses. Small extravasations of erythrocytes may appear as well. Lymphocytic perivascular cuffs are seen. Inclusion bodies are not seen. In one case, a focal area of necrosis and hemorrhage and hematoma formation were present in the temporal lobe, which corresponded to a mass lesion seen with CT.

In a recent case, brain biopsy material examined by indirect immunofluorescence demonstrated LAC viral antigen in neurons and perhaps in endothelial cells. The same biopsy material from this case showed minimal necrosis and perivascular cuffing on light microscopy.[66] The finding of minimal necrosis despite abnormal CT findings and deep coma is interesting in view of the generally benign outcome of LAC encephalitis, even in patients who experience deep coma or who exhibit CT abnormalities. This is in marked contradistinction to herpes simplex encephalitis, in which the presence of either deep coma or CT lesions would be very poor prognostic factors consistent with the extensive necrosis seen pathologically.[88]

PREVENTION

Public health prevention has focused on elimination of breeding sites of *A. triseriatus*. Sealing tree holes with cement and removal of used tires and other containers that provide breeding sites for the vector have been elements of an active public health program in many endemic areas.[89] The sheer number of such potential breeding sites necessitates intervention on a community-wide basis.[82] Public health education has been directed at communities at risk and at children through magazines such as *Ranger Rick*.[3] In La Crosse, Wisconsin, these measures were coordinated in an intensive mosquito program, supplemented with ovitraps and adulticiding when populations of the adult mosquito reached critical levels. Since the program's inception in 1978, a gradual reduction in the number of cases has been observed and no cases have been reported in the county in 3 years. However, surrounding, untreated counties have experienced a similar decline in incidence (W. Thompson, personal communication).

The proper use of repellents (see Table 178–2), playing in open, sunny fields, and avoidance of tree-shaded areas may confer a reduction in risk by minimizing exposure to the vector. Insect repellents for use in children should contain less than 10 per cent DEET and can be applied to the child's clothing and then in lesser amounts to areas of exposed skin.

Potential for vaccine development comes from recent work with a truncated G1 protein preparation that induces a protective immune response in suckling mice via neutralizing antibody.[71] Protection against neuroinvasion was afforded by interruption of the transient viremia, which occurs just after virus inoculation. Should ecologic preventive measures fail to lower disease rates in endemic areas, vaccine development for use in persons living in these areas may prove worthwhile.

References

1. Anonymous: Mumps meningitis and MMR vaccination. Lancet *2*:1015–1016, 1989.
2. Artsob, H., and Spence, L.: California encephalitis: Quebec. Can. Dis. Wkly. Rep. *7*:194–195, 1981.
3. Athey, E., and Thomas, N.: Fight that bite! Ranger Rick *18*:13–15, 1984.
4. Balfour, H. H., Fr., Siem, R. A., Bauer, H., et al.: California arbovirus (La Crosse) infections. I. Clinical and laboratory findings in 66 children with meningoencephalitis. Pediatrics *52*:680–691, 1973.
5. Beaty, B. J., Casals, J., Brown, K. L., et al.: Indirect fluorescent-antibody technique for serological diagnosis of La Crosse (California) virus infections. J. Clin. Microbiol. *15*:429–434, 1982.
6. Beaty, B. J., Jamnback T. L., Hildreth, S. W., et al.: Rapid diagnosis of La Crosse virus infections: Evaluation of serologic and antigen detection techniques for the clinically relevant diagnosis of La Crosse encephalitis. *In* Thompson, W. H., and Calisher, C. H. (eds.): California Serogroup Viruses. New York, Alan R. Liss, 1983, pp. 293–302.
7. Beaty, B., and Bishop, D. H. L.: Bunyavirus-vector interactions. Virus Res. *10*:289–302, 1988.
8. Beghi, E., Nicolosi, A., Kurland, L. T., et al.: Encephalitis and aseptic meningitis, Olmsted County, Minnesota, 1950–1981. I. Epidemiology. Ann. Neurol. *16*:283–294, 1984.
9. Berry, R. L., Parsons, M. A., LaLonde-Weigert, B. J., et al.: *Aedes canadensis*, a vector of La Crosse virus (California serogroup) in Ohio. J. Am. Mosq. Contr. Assoc. *2*:73, 1986.
10. Berry, R. L., Weigert, J. L., Calisher, C. H., et al.: Evidence for transovarial transmission of Jamestown Canyon virus in Ohio. Mosq. News *37*:494–496, 1977.
11. Black, S. S., Harrison, L. R., Purcell, A. R., et al.: Necrotizing panencephalitis in puppies infected with LaCrosse virus. J. Vet. Diagn. Invest. *6*:250–254, 1994.
12. Calisher, C. H., Pretzman, C. I., Muth, D. J., et al.: Serodiagnosis of La Crosse virus infections in humans by detection of immunoglobulin M class antibodies. J. Clin. Microbiol. *23*:667–671, 1976.
13. Campbell, G. L., Reeves, W. D, Hardy, J. L., et al.: Seroepidemiology of California and bunyamwera serogroup bunyavirus infections in humans in California. Am. J. Epidemiol. *136*:308–319, 1992.
14. Campbell, W. P., and Huang, C.: Detection of California serogroup viruses using universal primers and reverse transcription-polymerase chain reaction. J. Virol. Methods *53*:55–61, 1995.
15. Case, K. L, West, R. M., and Smith, M. J.: Histocompatibility antigens and La Crosse encephalitis. J. Infect. Dis. *168*:358–360, 1993.
16. Cassidy, L. F., and Patterson, J. L.: Mechanism of La Crosse virus inhibition by ribavirin. Antimicrob. Agents Chemother. *33*:2009–2011, 1989.
17. Chandler, L. J., Beaty, B. J., Bishop, D. H. L., et al.: Detection of La Crosse and Snowshoe hare viral nucleic acids by in situ hybridization. Am. J. Trop. Med. Hyg. *40*:561–568, 1989.
18. Chun, R. W. M., Thompson, W. H., Grabow, J. D., et al.: California arbovirus encephalitis in children. Neurology *18*:369–375, 1968.
19. Chun, R. W. M.: Clinical aspects of La Crosse encephalitis: Neurological and psychological sequelae. *In* Thompson, W. H., and Calisher, C. H. (eds.): California Serogroup Viruses. New York, Alan R. Liss, 1983, pp. 193–201.
20. Calisher, C. H., Pretzman, C. I., Muth, D. J., et al.: Serodiagnosis of La Crosse virus infections in humans by detection of immunoglobulin M class antibodies. J. Clin. Microbiol. *23*:667–671, 1986.
21. Connor, E., Morrison, S., Lane, J., et al.: Safety tolerance and pharmacokinetics of systemic ribavirin in children with human immunodeficiency virus infection. Antimicrob. Agents Chemother. *37*:532–539, 1993.
22. Cramblett, H. G., Stegmiller, H., and Spencer, C.: California encephalitis virus infections in children: Clinical and laboratory studies. J. A. M. A. *198*:128–132, 1966.
23. Craven, R. B., Eliason, D. A., Francy, D. B., et al.: Importation of *Aedes albopictus* and other exotic mosquito species into the United States in used tires from Asia. J. Am. Mosq. Contr. Assoc. *4*:138–142, 1988.
24. Cully, J. F., and Streit, T. G.: Transmission of La Crosse virus by four strains of *Aedes albopictus* to and from the eastern chipmunk (tamias striatus). J. Am. Mosq. Control. Assoc. *8*:237–240, 1992.
25. de los Reyes, E., Glauser, T. A., McJunkin, J. E., et al.: Periodic lateralizing epileptiform discharges and La Crosse encephalitis: Diagnostic and public health implications. Neurology *46*:150–151, 1996.
26. Deering, W. M.: Neurologic aspects and treatment of La Crosse encephalitis. *In* Thompson, W. H., and Calisher, C. H. (eds.): California Serogroup Viruses. New York, Alan R. Liss, 1983, pp. 187–191.
27. Deibel, R., Srihongse, S., and Grayson, M. A.: Jamestown Canyon virus: The etiologic agent of an emerging human disease? *In* Thompson, W. H., and Calisher, C. H. (eds.): California Serogroup Viruses. New York, Alan R. Liss, 1983, pp. 313–325.
28. Deibel, R., Srihongse, S., and Woodall, J. P.: Arboviruses in New York State: An attempt to determine the role of arboviruses in patients with viral encephalitis and meningitis. Am. J. Trop. Med. Hyg. *28*:577–582, 1979.
29. Demikhov, V. G., Chaitsev, V. G., Dutenko, A. M., et al.: California serogroup virus infections in the Ryazan region of the USSR. Am. J. Trop. Med. Hyg. *45*:371–376, 1991.
30. Disease Control and Epidemiology Service, Ontario Ministry of Health: Surveillance of arboviruses in Ontario in 1983: The increased detection of seropositive cases to the California group viruses (CGV). Ontario Dis. Surveill. Rep. *5*:394–400, 1984.
31. Dykers, T. I., Brown, K. L., Gundersen, C. B., et al.: Rapid diagnosis of La Crosse encephalitis: Detection of specific immunoglobulin M in cerebrospinal fluid. J. Clin. Microbiol. *22*:740–744, 1985.
32. El Said, L. H., Vorndam, V., Gentsch, J. R., et al.: A comparison of La Crosse virus isolates obtained from different ecological niches and an analysis of the structural components of California encephalitis serogroup viruses and other bunyaviruses. Am. J. Trop. Med. Hyg. *28*:364–386, 1979.
33. Endres, M. J., Griot, C., Gonzalez-Scarano, F., et al.: Neuroattenuation of an avirulent bunyavirus variant maps to the L RNA segment. J. Virol. *65*:5465–5470, 1991.
34. Garg, B. P., and Kleiman, M. B.: Acute disseminated encephalomyelitis presenting as a neurodegenerative disease in infancy. Pediatr. Neurol. *11*:57–58, 1994.
35. Godsey, M. S., Amoo, F., Yuill, T. M., et al.: California serogroup virus infections in Wisconsin domestic animals. Am. J. Trop. Med. Hyg. *39*:409–416, 1988.
36. Gonzalez-Scarano, F., Endres, M. J., and Nathanson, N.: *Bunyaviridae*: Pathogenesis. Curr. Top. Microbiol. Immunol. *169*:217–249, 1991.

37. Gonzalez-Scarano, F., Pobjecky, N., and Nathanson, N.: La Crosse bunyavirus can mediate pH-dependent fusion from without. Virology *132*:222–225, 1984.
38. Gonzalez-Scarano, F., Beaty, B. J., Sudin D., et al.: Genetic determinants of the virulence and infectivity of La Crosse virus. Microb. Pathog. *4*:1–7, 1988.
39. Gonzalez-Scarano, F., Pobjecky, N., and Nathanson, N.: Bunyaviruses. *In* Fields, B. N., and Knipe, D. M. (eds.): Virology. New York, Raven Press, 1990, pp. 1195–1228.
40. Grabow, J. D., Matthews, C. G., Chun, R. W. M., et al.: The electroencephalogram and clinical sequelae of California arbovirus encephalitis. Neurology *19*:394–404, 1969.
41. Grady, L. J., Sanders, M. L., and Campbell, W. P.: The sequence of the M RNA of an isolate La Crosse virus. J. Gen. Virol. *68*:3057–3071, 1987.
42. Grimstad, P. R., Haroff, R. N., Wentworth, B. B., et al.: Jamestown Canyon virus (California serogroup) is the etiologic agent of widespread infection in Michigan humans. Am. J. Trop. Med. Hyg. *35*:376–386, 1986.
43. Grimstad, P. R., Kobayashi, J. F., Zhand, M., et al.: Recently introduced *Aedes albopictus* in the United States: Potential vector of La Crosse virus (*Bunyaviridae*: California serogroup). J. Am. Mosq. Contr. Assoc. *5*:422–426, 1989.
44. Grimstad, P. R., Shabino, C. L., Calisher, C. H., et al.: A case of encephalitis in a human associated with a serologic rise of Jamestown Canyon virus. Am. J. Trop. Med. Hyg. *31*:1238–1244, 1982.
45. Grimstad, P. R.: California group virus disease. *In* Monath, T. P. (ed.): The Arbovirus: Epidemiology and Ecology. Vol. 2. Boca Raton, CRC Press, 1988, pp. 99–136.
46. Gundersen, C. B., and Brow, K. L.: Clinical aspects of La Crosse encephalitis: Preliminary report. *In* Thompson, W. H., and Calisher, C. H. (eds.): California Serogroup Viruses. New York, Alan R. Liss, 1983, pp. 169–177.
47. Hacker, D., Rochat, S., and Kolakofsky, D.: Anti-mRNAs in La Crosse bunyaviruses-infected cells. J. Virol. *64*:5051–5057, 1990.
48. Hacker, J. K., Volkman, L. E., and Hardy, J. L.: Requirement for the G1 protein of California encephalitis virus in infection in vitro and in vivo. Virology *206*:945–953, 1995.
49. Hammon, W. McD., and Reeves, W. C.: California encephalitis virus: A newly described agent. California Med. *77*:303–309, 1952.
50. Heard, P. B., Zhang, M. B., and Grimstad, P. R.: Laboratory transmission of Jamestown Canyon and snowshoe hare viruses (*Bunyaviridae*: California serogroup) by several species of mosquitoes. J. Am. Mosq. Control. Assoc. *7*:94–102, 1991.
51. Hilty, M. D., Haynes, R. E., Azimi, P. H., et al.: California encephalitis in children. Am. J. Dis. Child. *124*:530–533, 1972.
52. Huggins, J. W., Jahrling, P., Kende, M., et al.: Efficacy of ribavirin against virulent RNA virus infections. *In* Smith, R. A., Knight, V., and Smith, J. A. D. (eds.): Clinical Applications of Ribavirin. Orlando, Academic Press, 1984, pp. 49–63.
53. Huggins, J. W., Kim, G. R., Brand, O. M., et al.: Ribavirin therapy for Hantaan virus infection in suckling mice. J. Infect. Dis. *153*:489–497, 1986.
54. Hurwitz, E. S., Schell, W., Nelson, D., et al.: Surveillance of California encephalitis group virus illness in Wisconsin and Minnesota, 1978. Am. J. Trop. Med. Hyg. *32*:595–601, 1983.
55. Janssen, R., Gonzalez-Scarano, F., and Nathanson, N.: Mechanisms of bunyavirus virulence: Comparative pathogenesis of a virulent strain of La Crosse and an avirulent strain of Tahyna virus. Lab. Invest. *50*:447–455, 1984.
56. Johnson, K. P., and Johnson, R. T.: California encephalitis. II. Studies of experimental infection in the mouse. J. Neuropathol. Exp. Neurol. *27*:390–400, 1968.
57. Kalfayan, B.: Pathology of La Crosse virus infection in humans. *In* Thompson, W. H., and Calisher, C. H. (eds.): California Serogroup Viruses. New York, Alan R. Liss, 1983, pp. 179–186.
58. Kappus, K. D., Monath, T. P., Kaminski, R. M., et al.: Reported encephalitis associated with California serogroup virus infections in the United States, 1963–1981. *In* Thompson, W. H., and Calisher, C. H. (eds.): California Serogroup Viruses. New York, Alan R. Liss, 1983, pp. 31–41.
59. Kindle, A. A., McJunkin, J. E., Meek, J. R., et al.: La Crosse encephalitis in West Virginia. M. M. W. R. *37*:1449–1453, 1988.
60. Kingsford, L., and Boucquey, K. H.: Monoclonal antibodies specific for the G1 glycoprotein of La Crosse virus that react with other California serogroup viruses. J. Gen. Virol. *71*:523–530, 1990.
61. Kingsford, L., Boucquey, K. H., and Cardoso, T. P.: Effects of specific monoclonal antibodies on La Crosse virus neutralization: Aggregation, inactivation by Fab fragments, and inhibition of attachment to baby hamster kidney cells. Virology *181*:591–601, 1991.
62. Klimas, R. A., Thompson, W. H., Calisher, C. H., et al.: Genotypic varieties of La Crosse isolated from different geographic regions of the continental United States and evidence for naturally occurring intertypic recombinant La Crosse virus. Am. J. Epidemiol. *114*:112–131, 1981.
63. Leber, S. M., Brunberg, J. A., and Pavkovic, I. M.: Infarction of basal ganglia associated with California encephalitis virus. Pediatr. Neurol. *12*:346–349, 1995.
64. Ludwig, G., Israel, B. A., Christensen, B. M., et al.: Role of La Crosse virus glycoproteins in attachment of virus to host cells. Virology *181*:564–571, 1991.
65. Matthews, C. G., Chun, R. W. M., Grabow, J. D., et al.: Psychological sequelae in children following California arbovirus encephalitis. Neurology *18*:1023–1030, 1968.
66. McJunkin, J. E., Minnich, L. L., Khan, R., et al.: Treatment of severe case of La Crosse encephalitis with IV ribavirin following diagnosis by brain biopsy. Pediatrics (in press)
67. Miller, B. R., DeFoliart, G. R., and Yuill, T. M.: Vertical transmission of La Crosse virus (California encephalitis group): Transovarial and filial infection rates in *Aedes triseriatus (Diptera: Culicidae)*. J. Med. Entomol. *14*:437–440, 1977.
68. Monath, T. P., Nuckolls, J. G., Berall, J., et al.: Studies on California encephalitis in Minnesota. Am. J. Epidemiol. *92*:40–50, 1970.
69. Neitzel, D. F., and Grimstad, P. R.: Serological evidence of California group and Cache Valley virus infection in Minnesota white-tailed deer. J. Wildl. Dis. *27*:230–237, 1991.
70. Paulson, S. L., and Hawley, W. A.: Effect of body size on the vector competence of field and laboratory populations of *Aedes triseriatus* for La Crosse virus. J. Am. Mosq. Control. Assoc. *7*:170–175, 1991.
71. Perkosz, A., Griot, C., Stillmock, K., et al.: Protection from La Crosse virus encephalitis with recombinant glycoproteins: Role of neutralizing anti-G1 antibodies. J. Virol. *69*:3475–3481, 1995.
72. Peters, C. J., Reynolds, J. A., Slone, T. W., et al.: Prophylaxis of Rift Valley fever with antiviral drugs, immune serum, interferon inducer, and a macrophage activator. Antiviral Res. *6*:285–297, 1986.
73. Reeves, W. C., Emmons, R. W., and Hardy, J. L.: Historical perspectives on California encephalitis virus in California. *In* Thompson, W. H., and Calisher, C. H. (eds.): California Serogroup Viruses. New York, Alan R. Liss, 1983, pp. 19–29.
74. Rie, H. E., Hilty, M. D., and Cramblett, H. G.: Intelligence and coordination following California encephalitis. Am. J. Dis. Child. *125*:824–827, 1973.
75. Shope, R. E., Rozhon, E. J., and Bishop, D. H. L.: Role of the middle-sized bunyavirus RNA segment in mouse virulence. Virology *114*:273–276, 1981.
76. Sidwell, R. W., Huffman, J. H., Barnett, B. B., et al.: In vitro and in vivo phlebovirus inhibition by ribavirin. Antimicrob. Agents Chemother. *32*:331–336, 1988.
77. Srihongse, S., Grayson, M. A., and Deibel, R.: California serogroup viruses in New York State: The role of subtypes in human infections. Am. J. Trop. Med. Hyg. *33*:1218–1227, 1984.
78. Stephen, E. L., Jones, D. E., Peters, C. J., et al.: Ribavirin treatment of toga- arena- and bunyavirus infection in subhuman primates and other laboratory animal species. *In* Smith, R. A., and Kirkpatrick, W. (eds.): Ribavirin: A Broad-Spectrum Antiviral Agent. New York, Academic Press, 1980, pp. 169–183.
79. Talmon, Y., Pradad, B. V. V., Clerx, J. P. M., et al.: Electron microscopy of vitrified-hydrated La Crosse virus. J. Virol. *61*:2319–2321, 1987.
80. Taylor, M. R., Carpenter, D. E., Currier, R. D., et al.: California encephalitis virus causes subacute encephalomyelitis in an adult. Arch. Neurol. *42*:88–89, 1985.
81. Thompson, W. H., and Evans, A. S.: California encephalitis virus studies in Wisconsin. Am. J. Epidemiol. *81*:230–244, 1965.
82. Thompson, W. H., and Gundersen, C. B.: La Crosse encephalitis: Occurrence of disease and control in a suburban area. *In* Thompson, W. H., and Calisher, C. H. (eds.): California Serogroup Viruses. New York, Alan R. Liss, 1983, pp. 225–236.
83. Thompson, W. H., Kalfayan, B., and Anslow, R. O.: Isolation of California encephalitis group virus from a fatal human illness. Am. J. Epidemiol. *81*:245–263, 1965.
84. Tsai, T. F.: Arboviral infection in the United States. Infect. Dis. Clin. North Am. *5*:73–102, 1991.
85. Tsai, T. F.: Arboviruses. *In* Murray, P. R. (ed.): Manual of Clinical Microbiology. 6th ed. Washington, D. C., ASM Press, 1995, pp. 980–993.
86. Watts, D. M., Pantuwatana, S., Yuill, T. M., et al.: Transovarial transmission of La Crosse virus in *Aedes triseriatus*. Ann. N. Y. Acad. Sci. *266*:135–143, 1975.
87. Watts, D. M., Thompson, W. H., Yuill, T. M., et al.: Overwintering of La Crosse virus in *Aedes triseriatus*. Am. J. Trop. Med. Hyg. *23*:694–700, 1974.
88. Whitley, R. J.: Viral encephalitis. N. Engl. J. Med. *323*:242–250, 1990.
89. Woodruff, B. A., Baron, R. C., and Tsai, T. F.: Symptomatic La Crosse viral infections in the central nervous system: A study of risk factors in an endemic area. Am. J. Epidemiol. *136*:320–327, 1992.
90. Young, D. J.: California encephalitis virus: Report of three cases and review of the literature. Ann. Intern. Med. *65*:419–428, 1966.
91. Yuill, T. M.: The role of mammals in the maintenance and dissemination of La Crosse virus. *In* Thompson, W. H., and Calisher, C. H. (eds.): California Serogroup Viruses. New York, Alan R. Liss, 1983, pp. 77–87.

191

OTHER BUNYAVIRUSES

❑ ❑ ❑

CHAPTER 191 (A)

Rift Valley Fever

Robert E. Shope

Rift Valley fever (RVF) primarily is a disease of sheep and cattle. It is transmitted by mosquitoes and caused by a virus with a selective affinity for the parenchymal cells of the liver, which undergo characteristic eosinophilic degeneration. Infection with RVF virus causes a short but severe disease in sheep and cattle. Most pregnant ewes and cows abort, and more than 90 per cent of newborn lambs die. The mortality rates in older sheep and cattle are lower, but nonetheless significant. People usually acquire the infection from aerosols generated from body fluids and tissues of animals dying of the disease and less commonly from bites of infected mosquitoes, especially during epidemics.

HISTORY

RVF probably has occurred for many years in Africa and first was recognized at the beginning of the twentieth century with the introduction of intensive livestock husbandry. In 1912, large numbers of newborn lambs died of an unknown disease in the Rift Valley of Kenya, and the following year the clinical features first were described. Daubney and associates[2] proved that the causal agent was a filterable virus, which they suspected was transmitted by mosquitoes because animals protected by screens did not contract the disease. In 1944, the virus was isolated from mosquitoes caught in the Semliki Forest in western Uganda, and it was proved later that *Eretmapodites chrysogaster* was able to transmit the infection under experimental conditions. Between 1950 and 1974, there were at least 15 major epizootics of RVF in livestock in various areas of sub-Saharan Africa. During 1975, an extensive epizootic of RVF occurred in South Africa, with many human cases and several deaths documented.[3]

An extensive epizootic of RVF also occurred in lower Egypt in 1977. Hundreds of thousands of domestic animals, including cattle, buffaloes, goats, and sheep, were lost. Associated with this epizootic was the largest human epidemic of the disease ever known, in which 200,000 humans were infected and 600 died.[4] This outbreak emphasized the increasing threat of RVF to humans and domestic animals and showed that RVF virus infection was an important cause of hemorrhagic fever in Africa. In 1987, an epidemic of RVF occurred in Mauritania after flooding of the Senegal River basin that followed completion of a dam; at least 1200 human cases and 200 deaths occurred in one affected area alone. The most recent epizootics were reported in Madagascar in 1990[6] and Egypt in 1993.[1]

Based on virus isolations, RVF probably occurs sporadically throughout most of sub-Saharan Africa. Zinga virus, previously described as a cause of sporadic human disease in central Africa, has been shown to be a strain of RVF virus.

ETIOLOGIC AGENT

RVF virus is destroyed by solvents such as ether and is inactivated readily by formalin; it is destroyed by 56° C heat for 40 minutes. When stored at 4° C or −10° C, the virus loses its infectivity in about 3 months. The virus can be preserved indefinitely on dry ice at −70° C or in lyophilized form.

The fully formed virions are spherical and about 94 nm in diameter. They mature in the cytoplasm, although intranuclear inclusions occur in vivo and in cell cultures. The virus multiplies readily in a variety of cell lines of animal and human origin. RVF virus has been assigned to the *Phlebovirus* genus of the family *Bunyaviridae.*

The virus is highly pathogenic for mice, young rats, and hamsters, and death occurs in 95 to 100 per cent of these animals 36 to 96 hours after inoculation.

VECTORS

In studies in South Africa, the virus has been transmitted experimentally by *Culex theileri, C. zombaensis, C. neavei, Aedes juppi,* and *Eretmapodites quinquevittatus.* Epizootics of RVF have occurred in years of unusually heavy rains, which fill natural depressions in the land (pans or dambos), favoring the proliferation of flood-water mosquitoes. Studies in Kenya have shown that transovarial transmission of the virus in pan-breeding *Aedes* of the subgenus *Neomelanoconion* is the probable mechanism for virus maintenance and periodic recrudescence. *C. pipiens* was implicated as a vector in Egypt during the epidemic of 1977 and 1978. During epizootics, domestic livestock serve as viremic, amplifying hosts in the transmission cycle.

CLINICAL MANIFESTATIONS

Humans are very susceptible to RVF virus. During the epizootics in South Africa, most veterinarians and many farmers engaged in work with sick sheep and cattle became infected. In most cases, the infection was associated with direct contact with carcasses, tissues, and organs of animals that died of RVF. Transmission probably was by aerosolized body fluids of the animals. Some patients gave no history of such contact; in these cases, it is presumed that infection was transmitted by mosquitoes or possibly acquired by drinking infected milk. The virus can be transmitted readily to laboratory personnel by direct contact with infected animals or by the respiratory route from aerosol droplet infection.

The incubation period of RVF is 3 to 7 days; onset is sudden, with chills, myalgia, joint pains, headache, and a biphasic fever that lasts about 1 week. The patient often feels nauseated and may vomit or complain of abdominal fullness and pain. The face is flushed, conjunctivae are injected, and the tongue is furred. There is bradycardia, and there may be slight tenderness over the liver, which may be enlarged. Many patients become delirious, and some have hallucinations. In a small proportion (<1 per cent) of patients, the infection is complicated by retinitis. Late in the course of the illness or early in convalescence, unclear vision may be noted and the patient may have a central blind spot. This visual defect is associated with a cotton-wool exudate on the macula. Both eyes are involved occasionally, and the loss of vision is a severe handicap. These lesions gradually resolve, and the patient's vision returns to normal in most cases. Meningoencephalitis may occur as a complication in less than 1 per cent of patients during or after the second wave of fever, manifesting as intense headache, confusion, and stupor. Lumbar puncture relieves the headache. The cerebrospinal fluid shows a slight pleocytosis, mostly of lymphocytes, a normal glucose, and a slightly increased protein content. Antibody to RVF virus may be demonstrated in the fluid. Few patients with encephalitis die. Recovery usually is complete but may be prolonged. Occasionally, the patient is left with permanent sequelae.

Approximately 1 per cent of patients with RVF develop hemorrhagic fever, a complication with a case-fatality rate of 15 per cent. Mortality was disproportionately less in children than adults during the 1977 Egyptian epidemic. In cases of severe illness, the patient may develop a hemorrhagic diathesis that includes epistaxis, hematemesis, and melena. Sometimes cerebral hemorrhage occurs. Profuse gastrointestinal hemorrhage may be fatal. Jaundice may be evident.

LABORATORY FINDINGS

There is an initial leukocytosis that is followed by leukopenia. A profound thrombocytopenia and other defects in coagulation may be observed. Disturbance of liver and kidney function also may be documented.

The diagnosis of RVF is suggested when human beings suffer from an acute, severe, but short febrile illness at the same time that an epizootic with a high mortality occurs among sheep.

The diagnosis usually can be confirmed by the isolation of virus from blood and, in fatal cases, from the liver. The development of antibodies can be demonstrated by immunofluorescence, IgM enzyme-linked immunosorbent assay, hemagglutination inhibition, complement fixation, and neutralization. In patients with encephalitis, IgM antibodies are detectable in cerebrospinal fluid.

TREATMENT

Treatment is symptomatic. When a hemorrhagic diathesis develops, treatment should be directed toward controlling bleeding. Transfusions of fresh frozen plasma and platelets may be beneficial. Disseminated intravascular coagulation has been documented in a monkey model, but its role in human disease is uncertain.

PREVENTION

RVF mainly is a disease of adults and usually is acquired occupationally. It is a serious hazard faced by veterinarians, ranchers, and laboratory personnel in the course of their work. Because RVF usually is acquired by direct contact with the tissues of infected sheep and cattle, risk of infection can be reduced by wearing gloves, protective masks, and goggles when postmortem examinations are carried out on animals that have died of unknown causes. Because of the value of domestic animals in many economically depressed areas of Africa, sheep and cattle often are housed within family compounds. Sick or dying animals usually are killed to salvage their meat. In this peridomestic environment, children also can be exposed to virus aerosols and infected readily. Infection from a mosquito bite also is possible but less common.

The primary strategy for RVF for both humans and animals relies on vaccination of sheep and cattle, which are the amplifying hosts. Attenuated strains of the virus have been developed and have been used successfully on a mass scale to immunize livestock. Their use is associated with some abortions in pregnant ewes and cows. An inactivated vaccine is safe and is in widespread use in Africa.

A new, live attenuated vaccine designated MP-12 has been developed by passage of RVF virus in the presence of the mutagen 5-fluorouracil.[5] The vaccine has proved safe for use in domestic livestock and does not produce abortions. It offers considerable promise as a veterinary and human vaccine. Formalin-inactivated vaccines produced in cell cultures[7] have been used on an investigational basis in more than 3000 persons, with greater than 95 per cent seroconversion. A single case of Guillain-Barré syndrome has been reported, but the relationship to vaccination is uncertain. Human vaccination is recommended for high-risk occupational groups. Various genetically engineered vaccine candidates are under development.

References

1. Arthur, R. R., el-Sharkawy, M. S., Cope, S. E., et al.: Recurrence of Rift Valley fever in Egypt. Lancet *342*:1149–1150, 1993.
2. Daubney, R., Hudson, J. R., and Garnham, P. C.: Enzootic hepatitis or Rift Valley fever: An undescribed virus disease of sheep, cattle and man from East Africa. J. Pathol. Bacteriol. *34*:545–579, 1931.
3. Gear, J.: Hemorrhagic fevers in South Africa: An account of two recent outbreaks. J. S. Afr. Vet. Assoc. *48*:5–8, 1977.
4. Meegan, J. M.: Rift Valley fever in Egypt: An overview of the epizootics in 1977 and 1978. Contrib. Epidemiol. Biostat. *3*:100–113, 1981.
5. Morrill, J. C., Jennings, G. B., Caplen, H., et al.: Pathogenicity and immunogenicity of a mutagen-attenuated Rift Valley fever virus immunogen in pregnant ewes. Am. J. Vet. Res. *48*:1042–1047, 1987.
6. Morvan, J., Rollin, P. E., Laventure, S., et al.: Rift Valley fever epizootic in the central highlands of Madagascar. Res. Virol. *143*:407–415, 1992.
7. Randall, R., Gibbs, C. J., Anlisio, C. G., et al.: The development of a formalin-killed Rift Valley fever vaccine for use in man. J. Immunol. *89*:660–671, 1962.

❑ ❑ ❑

CHAPTER 191 (B)

Crimean-Congo Hemorrhagic Fever

Robert B. Tesh

Crimean-Congo hemorrhagic fever (CCHF) is an acute febrile viral illness, often with severe hemorrhagic manifestations. The clinical entity and its viral etiology first were described by Chumakov in 1945,[5] but the agent was not propagated or available for study until 1967. Since then, CCHF has been reported from many countries in eastern Europe, central Asia, and Africa. Ticks or contact with the blood of infected livestock is the usual source of infection, but a number of nosocomial outbreaks of CCHF also have been reported.

ETIOLOGIC AGENT

CCHF virus, the etiologic agent, is a member of the genus *Nairovirus*, family *Bunyaviridae*. It is lethal to newborn mice and rats after intracerebral inoculation. CCHF virus replicates in a number of vertebrate cell lines, but it usually does not cause discernible cytopathogenic effect under fluid overlay. Thus, indirect methods, such as immunofluorescence, must be used to detect viral infection/antigen in the cells.

Persons with CCHF develop a relatively high level of viremia (up to 6.2 $\log_{10}$ LD_{50}/mL) that persists for 8 to 12 days after the onset of illness. Blood from CCHF patients is quite infectious, and a number of nosocomial infections have occurred among hospital personnel caring for acutely ill patients with hemorrhagic symptoms.[5] CCHF virus is relatively stable in blood or serum and has been recovered from specimens stored for as long as 2 or 3 weeks at 4° C.

EPIDEMIOLOGY

CCHF virus is known to occur over a wide geographic area including Eastern Europe, central Asia, and much of Africa. The endemic zone of CCHF has been well delineated in Russia and other states of the former Soviet Union and in South Africa, but in other regions of central Asia and Africa, most cases of the disease probably are unrecognized as a result of their sporadic occurrence and largely rural distribution.

The epidemiology of CCHF is complex and not well understood because of the variety of tick and mammalian species that have been found naturally infected with the virus. The basic transmission cycle of the virus varies from region to region, depending upon the developmental stage and species of ticks involved and their preferred mammalian hosts. In addition, transovarial and transstadial transmission of CCHF virus also has been demonstrated in some tick vectors. In general, human cases of CCHF usually are associated with periods of tick abundance and feeding activity. For example, in Eastern Europe, cases of CCHF typically occur between May and August, when the tick population is active. The disease usually is rural in distribution and occurs mainly among farm workers, many of whom report a history of tick bite or of crushing ticks with their fingers. Although cases of CCHF occur among children, the disease mainly affects adults, probably because of their greater occupational exposure.

A number of nosocomial outbreaks of CCHF have occurred among hospital workers and laboratory technicians.[1, 2, 5] All of these persons had direct contact with the blood of CCHF patients. Cases of the disease also have been reported in persons slaughtering or performing autopsies on infected and presumedly viremic domestic animals.[5]

CLINICAL MANIFESTATIONS

The incubation period for CCHF is 3 to 6 days.[4, 5] The disease begins suddenly with fever, nausea, severe headache, dizziness, myalgia, and general toxemia. Vomiting, abdominal pain, diarrhea, and depression also are common. Patients often are flushed and conjunctivae are injected. Hepatomegaly is present in about 50 per cent of cases. In general, hemorrhagic manifestations do not appear before the third or fourth day of the illness, at which point the patient's condition markedly deteriorates. Patients typically become asthenic, apathetic, and sometimes delirious during this stage. Central nervous system changes characterized clinically by loss of consciousness, agitated or myotonic movements, decreased tendon reflexes, and meningeal symptoms are quite common. The appearance of purpura on the skin and mucous membranes indicates the onset of the hemorrhagic phase of this disease, which generally lasts 3 to 6 days. Hemorrhages, varying in size from petechiae to large hematomas, develop on mucous membranes and the skin of the trunk and extremities, especially at the site of injections, trauma, or tight clothing. Bleeding from the nose, gums, and buccal cavity also is common. In severe cases of CCHF, gastric, uterine, intestinal, genitourinary, and pulmonary hemorrhages occur in decreasing frequency. In patients with profuse hemorrhage, tachycardia, shock, and death may occur. If the patient survives the hemorrhagic phase of the disease, by the ninth or tenth day recovery begins and a 2- to 6-week period of slow convalescence follows. Viremia is intense and prolonged in CCHF, especially in fatal cases, so blood from these patients should be treated with extreme care.

Leukopenia and thrombocytopenia are a consistent feature of CCHF and occur early in the disease.[4] Other abnormal laboratory findings usually include elevated levels of serum aspartate and alanine aminotransaminases, lactic dehydrogenase, bilirubin, creatinine, and urea. Clinical studies of CCHF patients in South Africa[4] found markedly elevated values for prothrombin ratio, activated partial thromboplastin time, thrombin time, and fibrin degradation products, indicative of disseminated intravascular coagulopathy. Many of these abnormal clinical laboratory values were evident early in the disease and had a high predictive value for the outcome.

PATHOGENESIS

Fluorescent antibody studies on organs of fatal cases of CCHF show a concentration of viral antigen in reticuloendothelial cells of the liver and spleen, suggesting that these cells are a major site of virus replication.[4] Other pathologic changes observed at autopsy include generalized vascular lesions with endothelial damage, giving rise to scattered focal hemorrhages and edema in most organs. In severe cases, marked renal involvement and kidney failure may occur.

DIAGNOSIS

The clinical diagnosis of CCHF is difficult to make before the onset of hemorrhagic manifestations because the initial symptoms are nonspecific and cases usually are sporadic in occurrence. Because of the frequency and severity of abdominal pain associated with the prodromal phase of CCHF, it sometimes is misdiagnosed as appendicitis or gastric ulcer, and patients are subjected to unnecessary surgery, which can be fatal to both the patient and the attending medical personnel.[1, 2, 5] Once hemorrhagic manifestations appear, the differential diagnosis would include erythema multiforme (Stevens-Johnson syndrome), leptospirosis, hemorrhagic fever with renal syndrome, Ebola virus infection, Lassa fever, and yellow fever, depending upon the region of the world where the patient was exposed.

A definitive diagnosis of CCHF can be made by isolation of the virus from the patient's blood during the first weeks of illness. IgG and IgM antibodies become demonstrable 7 to 10 days after onset of symptoms in nonfatal cases.[3]

TREATMENT

The treatment of CCHF is symptomatic but should include immediate hospitalization and strict bed rest.[5] Because death usually results from acute blood loss and shock, transfusions of fresh blood, platelets, and/or plasma may be necessary. Administration of immune plasma obtained from convalescent donors also is recommended early in the illness or to persons such as hospital personnel, who inadvertently are exposed to the virus. In severe cases of the disease, steroids sometimes are used.

PROGNOSIS

The mortality rate of CCHF varies from about 10 to 50 per cent.[4, 5] If the patient survives the hemorrhagic phase of the disease, recovery is complete and permanent immunity results.

PREVENTION

A killed CCHF virus vaccine, prepared in mouse brain, has been used experimentally in Russia and Bulgaria.[5] It is recommended for use in laboratory and hospital personnel and in other high-risk populations; however, few data are available on its efficacy.

Strict isolation should be maintained in caring for all CCHF patients in order to protect hospital personnel.

Other measures designed to prevent CCHF include insecticide spraying of fields and animals for tick control, use of personal insect repellents and protective clothing to prevent tick bites, and public education about the epidemiology of CCHF.

References

1. Burney, M. I., Ghafoor, A., Saleen, M., et al.: Nosocomial outbreak of viral hemorrhagic fever caused by Crimean hemorrhagic fever–Congo virus in Pakistan, January 1976. Am. J. Trop. Med. Hyg. *29*:941–947, 1980.
2. Joubert, J. R., King, J. B., Rossouw, D. J., et al.: A nosocomial outbreak of Crimean-Congo hemorrhagic fever at Tygerberg Hospital. Part 3. Clinical pathology and pathogenesis. S. Afr. Med. J. *68*:772–778, 1985.
3. Shepherd, A. J., Swanepoel, R., and Leman, P. A.: Antibody response in Crimean-Congo hemorrhagic fever. Rev. Infect. Dis. *11*(Suppl. 4):S801–S806, 1989.
4. Swanepoel, R., Gill, D. E., Shepherd, A. J., et al.: The clinical pathology of Crimean-Congo hemorrhagic fever. Rev. Infect. Dis. *11*(Suppl. 4):S794–S800, 1989.
5. Watts, D. M., Ksiazek, T. G., Linthicum, K. J., et al.: Crimean-Congo hemorrhagic fever. *In* Monath, T. P. (ed.): The Arboviruses: Epidemiology and Ecology. Vol. 2. Boca Raton, CRC Press, 1989, pp. 177–222.

❑ ❑ ❑

CHAPTER 191 (C)

Phlebotomus Fever (Sandfly Fever)

Robert B. Tesh

Phlebotomus fever, an acute, self-limited, febrile illness of 2 to 4 days' duration, is acquired from the bite of infected phlebotomine sandflies. Phlebotomus fever also is known as sandfly fever, pappataci fever, and 3-day fever. The disease is endemic in many areas of central Asia, northern Africa, and southern Europe. Historically, phlebotomus fever has been largely of military interest because the introduction of large numbers of susceptible troops into endemic areas often has resulted in epidemics of the disease[7]; more recently, the disease has been reported with increasing frequency among tourists visiting endemic areas.[2, 6]

In 1909, Doerr and associates first demonstrated that the causative agent of the illness was a virus transmitted by *Phlebotomus papatasii*, but it was not until 1954 that Sabin successfully adapted the agent to mice and described two distinct serologic types, designated as the Naples and Sicilian strains.[7] Subsequently, 44 additional phlebotomus fever virus serotypes that show varying degrees of antigenic relatedness have been isolated from various regions of the world. Although most of the viruses in the phlebotomus fever serogroup probably are capable of producing human illness, the discussion here is limited to the three (Naples, Sicilian, and Toscana) that most commonly are associated with the disease. Rift Valley fever virus also is a member of this serogroup and frequently causes a phlebotomus fever–like illness in infected persons.[4] However, humans generally acquire Rift Valley fever from the bite of infected mosquitoes or from aerosol, and the sequelae of the latter disease are more severe and occasionally fatal.

ETIOLOGIC AGENT

The phlebotomus fever serogroup viruses are members of the genus *Phlebovirus*, family *Bunyaviridae*. They are RNA-containing viruses, spherical in shape, and 90 to 100 nm in diameter.[7] The Naples, Sicilian, and Toscana viruses produce a cytopathic effect as well as plaques in Vero cells. Most laboratory animals are not susceptible to infection with these viruses, although they can be adapted to newborn mice by serial passage intracerebrally. For this reason, tissue culture is recommended for primary isolation of these agents.

EPIDEMIOLOGY

The geographic distribution of the Naples and Sicilian virus types in the Old World closely parallels that of their presumed vector, *P. papatasii* (Fig. 191–1).[7] Toscana virus has been isolated in Portugal, Spain, Italy, and Cyprus[6] and has been associated with two other peridomestic sandfly species, *P. perniciosus* and *P. perfiliewi.*

These phlebotomine species are tiny, sand-colored biting flies about 2 to 3 mm long. Because of their small size, they have little difficulty in squeezing through ordinary screens and mosquito netting. They usually are nocturnal in their activity, and only the female bites. Sandflies move in short hops and rarely travel more than a few hundred meters from their resting and breeding sites. During the day, peridomestic species such as *P. papatasii* and *P. perniciosus* rest in dark corners and crevices, often within houses. The larvae develop in loose soil and organic debris in stone walls, animal sheds, privies, open wells, and gardens. Because of their indoor habits, these peridomestic species are quite vulnerable to residual insecticides.

In central Asia and the Mediterranean region, sandflies are active during the late spring and summer. The incidence of phlebotomus fever follows the same seasonal pattern.

Many phlebotomus fever viruses appear to be maintained in the sandfly population by transovarial (vertical) transmission.[7] Thus, sandflies appear to serve as both vectors and reservoirs of these viruses. Unlike most other arboviruses, whose activity depends on the presence of susceptible and viremic vertebrate hosts, phlebotomus fever viruses probably are active continuously during each sandfly season. Serologic studies among persons living in endemic areas of the disease indicate that most of the residents are infected early in life.[7] In these communities, sporadic cases of phlebotomus fever occur among children because most of the adult population already is immune. However, because of the benign nature of the disease, its sporadic occurrence, and its similarity

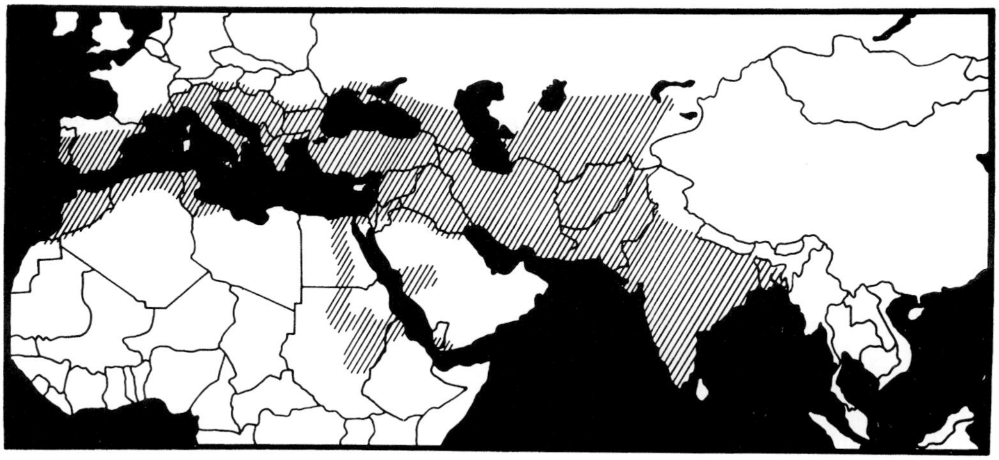

FIGURE 191–1. *The known geographic distribution of* Phlebotomus papatasii, *principal vector of the Naples and Sicilian types of phlebotomus fever virus. (Modified from Tesh, R. B., Saidi, S., Gajdamovic, S. J., et al.: Serological studies on the epidemiology of sandfly fever in the Old World. Bull. W. H. O. 54:663–674, 1976.)*

to many other viral diseases of childhood, most cases are unrecognized. Still, when a large number of susceptible persons (soldiers, tourists, refugees, and so on) enter an endemic area of phlebotomus fever, bite transmission occurs and an epidemic of the disease quickly appears.[6, 7]

CLINICAL MANIFESTATIONS

The incubation period for phlebotomus fever averages 3 to 5 days.[1, 7] The illness begins suddenly with fever, severe frontal headache, retro-orbital pain, conjunctival injection, photophobia, malaise, anorexia, nausea, vomiting, myalgia, and lower back pain. The face may be flushed, but a true rash is absent. The disease is self-limited, and symptoms usually disappear within 1 to 3 days; however, a general feeling of weakness and depression is not uncommon for a week or more after the illness.

A number of cases of meningitis and meningoencephalitis have been described in persons with Toscana virus infection.[5, 6] In addition to the classic symptoms of phlebotomus fever, these patients exhibit nuchal ridigity, positive Kernig sign, clouded sensorium, and occasionally nystagmus and tremor. To date, no deaths have been recorded. Childhood cases of the meningoencephalitic form of Toscana virus infection have not been reported yet, but this simply may be a reflection of the populations studied.[5, 6]

One attack of phlebotomus fever usually confers lifelong immunity against the infecting virus type but not against heterologous serotypes.[7] For this reason, second cases of the disease have been reported in the same individual in areas where more than one virus serotype are active.

A marked leukopenia usually is observed with phlebotomus fever.[1] It is characterized by an initial lymphopenia, followed by a protracted neutropenia (Fig. 191–2). In patients with central nervous system involvement, pleocytosis and elevated protein content are observed in the cerebrospinal fluid.

PATHOLOGY

Fatalities due to phlebotomus fever have not been reported, and little is known of the pathologic changes produced by these viruses.

DIAGNOSIS

The diagnosis of phlebotomus fever usually is made on the basis of clinical and epidemiologic evidence. A sudden outbreak during the summer months of a short febrile illness with severe headache among visitors or other newcomers to an endemic area where sandflies are abundant should suggest the disease. Depending on the region, the differential diagnosis might include dengue, West Nile fever, malaria, influenza, and a number of other respiratory and enterovirus infections.

A transient viremia (24 to 36 hours) occurs during this illness, which means isolation of the virus from blood is unusual. In a few instances, Toscana virus has been isolated directly from cerebrospinal fluid of persons with central nervous system symptoms.[5] Serologic tests offer the simplest method for specific diagnosis of phlebotomus fever. Antibodies are present in the serum 7 to 14 days after infection

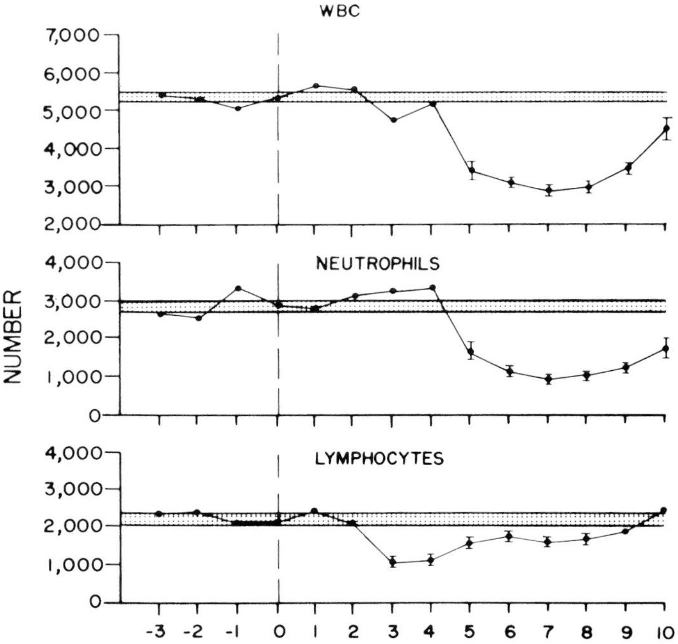

FIGURE 191–2. *Mean total leukocyte count as well as absolute neutrophil and lymphocyte counts on 11 adult volunteers inoculated (day 0) with Sicilian serotype of phlebotomus fever virus. The average incubation period in the subjects was about 70 hours. (Modified from Bartelloni, P. J., and Tesh, R. B.: Clinical and serologic responses of volunteers infected with phlebotomus fever virus [Sicilian type]. Am. J. Trop. Med. Hyg. 25:456–462, 1976.)*

and can be demonstrated by immunofluorescence,[2] enzyme immunoassay,[3] or neutralization.[1] A fourfold rise in antibody titers from acute to convalescent sera or the presence of specific IgM antibodies would provide presumptive evidence of a recent phlebotomus fever virus infection. At present, these serologic tests generally are not available and usually are performed in only a few arbovirus laboratories.

TREATMENT

Treatment is symptomatic, and hospitalization usually is not necessary. Occasionally, narcotics are required to relieve the severe headache associated with the disease.

PROGNOSIS

Phlebotomus fever is a self-limited, nonfatal disease. Recovery is complete.

PREVENTION

Control measures are directed primarily against the vector. Household spraying with residual insecticides is quite effective in reducing peridomestic vector populations and controlling the disease. The use of personal insect repellents (e.g., diethyltoluamide) and fine mesh bed nets also is effective in avoiding sandfly bites.

References

1. Bartelloni, P. J., and Tesh, R. B.: Clinical and serologic responses of volunteers infected with phlebotomus fever virus (Sicilian type). Am. J. Trop. Med. Hyg. *25*:456–462, 1976.
2. Eitrem, R., Niklasson, B., and Weiland, O.: Sandfly fever among Swedish tourists. Scand. J. Infect. Dis. *23*:451–457, 1991.
3. Eitrem, R., Vene, S., and Niklasson, B.: ELISA for detection of IgM and IgG antibodies to sandfly fever Sicilian virus. Res. Virol. *142*:387–394, 1991.
4. Meagan, J. M., and Bailey, C. L: Rift Valley fever. *In* Monath, T. P. (ed.): The Arboviruses: Epidemiology and Ecology. Vol. 4. Boca Raton, CRC Press, 1989, pp. 51–76.
5. Nicoletti, L., Verani, P., and Caciolli, S., et al.: Central nervous system involvement during infection by *Phlebovirus* Toscana of residents in natural foci in central Italy (1977–1988). Am. J. Trop. Med. Hyg. *45*:429–434, 1991.
6. Schwarz, T. F., Gilch, S., and Jager, G.: Aseptic meningitis caused by sandfly fever virus, serotype Toscana. Clin. Infect. Dis. *21*:669, 1995.
7. Tesh, R. B.: Phlebotomus fever. *In* Monath, T. P. (ed.): The Arboviruses: Epidemiology and Ecology. Vol. 4. Boca Raton, CRC Press, 1989, pp. 15–27.
8. Tesh, R. B., Saidi, S., Gajdamovic, S. J., et al.: Serological studies on the epidemiology of sandfly fever in the Old World. Bull. W. H. O. *54*:663–674, 1976.

❑ ❑ ❑

CHAPTER 191 (D)

Oropouche Fever

Francisco P. Pinheiro,
Amelia P. A. Travassos da Rosa,
and Pedro F. C. Vasconcelos

Oropouche fever is an arbovirus infection manifesting itself in the form of an acute febrile episode, accompanied by headache, myalgia, arthralgia, and other systemic symptoms. The symptoms usually recur a few days after the end of the first febrile episode, at which time they generally are less severe. Some patients may develop aseptic meningitis. Patients make a full recovery, without any apparent aftereffects, even in the most serious cases. There are no records of any confirmed fatalities attributable to Oropouche fever. One of the most striking characteristics of Oropouche virus is its ability to produce epidemics in urban population centers, most of which reportedly have occurred in the Brazilian Amazon region. A number of these outbreaks have had a major impact on the stricken cities.

The first case of the disease was described in a resident of Vega de Oropouche, Trinidad, in 1955, from whose blood the agent was isolated.[1] The disease was detected again in 1961, this time in the city of Belém, Pará State, northern Brazil, where it caused an epidemic that affected at least 11,000 people.[13] This was followed by the occurrence of many epidemics, several of an explosive nature, in urban population centers throughout the Brazilian states of Pará, Amapá, Amazonas, Tocantins, Maranhão, and Rondônia.[6, 10, 13–15, 23, 24] Outside of Brazil, epidemics of Oropouche fever were reported in Panama in 1989 (Quiroz, E., and associates, Panama, unpublished data, 1989) and in the Amazon region of Peru in 1992[4] and in 1994 (Ministry of Health, Peru, and U.S. Naval Medical Research Institute Detachment, NAMRID, Lima, 1994).

ETIOLOGIC AGENT

Oropouche fever is caused by the Oropouche arbovirus belonging to the genus *Bunyavirus* of the family *Bunyaviridae*.[21] The virus has enveloped spherical particles 90 to 100 nm in diameter, the capsid has helical symmetry, and the RNA contains three segments.[11, 21] Antigenically, it belongs to the Simbu group, which, in turn, is part of the Bunyamwera supergroup of arboviruses. The virus has a hemagglutinin that is active against geese erythrocytes, which can be recovered from infected hamster serum treated with acetone (Travassos da Rosa, Belém, unpublished data, 1969). Intracerebral and intraperitoneal inoculations of the Oropouche virus into baby mice and intracerebral, intraperitoneal, and subcutaneous inoculations of the virus into adult hamsters produce lethal infections. The virus replicates in a number of cell cultures, such as Vero, BHK-21, and primary chicken embryo fibroblast, causing a cytopathic effect.[21] The agent is sensitive to the action of sodium deoxycholate.[9]

EPIDEMIOLOGY

Geographic Distribution

So far, the only reported cases of Oropouche fever have been in Brazil, Panama, Peru, and Trinidad (Fig. 191–3). However, most occurrences of the disease have been limited to the Brazilian Amazon region, with no cases of the disease reported in other areas of Brazil.

With a few exceptions, all occurrences of Oropouche fever have been in the form of urban epidemics, including those in Belém and Manaus, the largest cities of the Brazilian Amazon region. The city of Belém, capital of Pará State, was struck by three major epidemics over a 20-year period. The city of Santarém and surrounding villages also were affected by a major epidemic in 1974 and 1975.[14] The first epidemics occurring outside the State of Pará were reported early in the 1980s, striking the cities of Manaus and Barcelos in the State of Amazonas[3] and the city of Mazagão in what was then the Amapá Territory.[19] After a period of silence lasting until 1988, new outbreaks of the disease struck the cities of Porto Franco and Tocantinópolis in the states of Maranhão and Tocantins, respectively.[24] The next reported epidemics occurred in 1991,

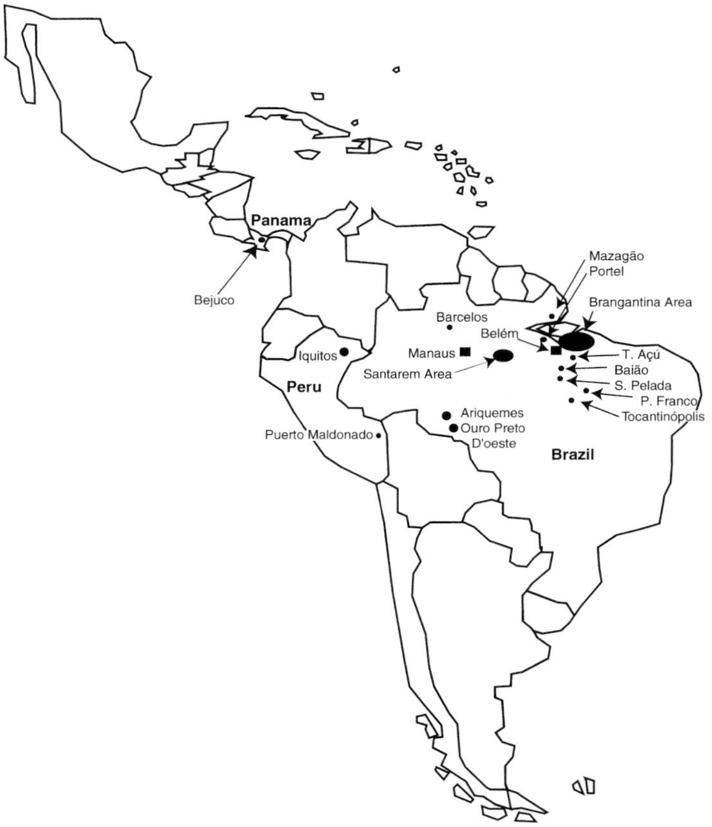

FIGURE 191–3. *Outbreaks of Oropouche fever reported in the Americas from 1961 to 1994.*

this time in more distant locations, namely in the cities of Ariquemes and Ouro Preto D'Oeste in the State of Rondônia; the epidemic's impact on these cities was so great that it was reported in the national press. The last reported outbreak in Brazil occurred in Serra Pelada, Pará State, in 1994, during which 83 per cent of its 6000 inhabitants were infected with the agent.[23]

In addition to the above-mentioned epidemic areas, there are countless small villages scattered throughout virtually the entire Amazon region whose residents show hemagglutination-inhibition antibodies against the Oropouche virus. In general, the prevalence of these antibodies is less than 3 per cent, with the exception of Ilha de Gurupá, where the prevalence is 10.7 per cent.[15]

Outside of Brazil, outbreaks were reported in Panama and in Peru. The outbreak in Panama occurred in 1989, striking the village of Bejuco approximately 50 kilometers west of the capital (Quiroz, E., and associates, Panama, unpublished data, 1989). The first epidemic in Peru was reported in 1992 in the city of Iquitos in the Peruvian Amazon region[4]; subsequently, an outbreak occurred in Puerto Maldonado, Madre de Dios, also in the Peruvian Amazon region (Ministry of Health, Peru, and U.S. Naval Medical Research Institute Detachment, NAMRID, Lima, 1994). Evidence of immunity to the Oropouche virus was detected in nonhuman primates in Colombia, suggesting its presence in that country as well.[9]

Incidence

Because Oropouche fever is not a reportable disease, it is difficult to estimate its incidence. Therefore, serologic surveys have been useful to determine the incidence of Oropouche fever during outbreaks. In most surveys, sera were tested for the presence of hemagglutination-inhibiting antibodies against Oropouche virus.[6, 15, 19, 20] According to these surveys, at least 357,000 individuals are estimated to have been infected with the Oropouche virus between 1961 and 1994. However, this estimate actually is quite conservative, considering that the incidence of the viral disease had not been computed in a number of major outbreaks (Belém, 1968; Porto Franco and Tocantinópolis, 1988). Accordingly, it is possible that more than half a million people in the Brazilian Amazon region may have been infected with the Oropouche virus since the beginning of the 1960s.

Gender-specific attack rates vary, with female rates slightly higher than attack rates for males in villages in the Bragantina area, Eastern Pará State, struck by the virus in 1979,[6] with the opposite true in the outbreak in Belém that same year. However, in the reported epidemics in Santarém, the infection struck females twice as often as males.[5] Oropouche fever strikes all age groups, although, in certain outbreaks, its incidence was higher among children and young adults.

Diffusion of Epidemics

As indicated earlier, Oropouche fever epidemics have struck different locations at varying intervals. However, a number of outbreaks were marked by bona fide epidemic sweeps, with countless numbers of villages within a particular geographic area affected by the virus. This diffusion phenomenon was observed in Braganca in 1967, in Santarém in 1974 and 1975, and, even more so, in Belém and in the Bragantina area from 1978 to 1980 (where at least 10 towns were stricken), as well as in Rondônia in 1991. Virus spread most likely is due to the movement of viremic individuals throughout areas in which the virus vector is present.

Seasonal Fluctuation

Most epidemics of Oropouche fever typically occur during the rainy season, which, in the case of the State of Pará, corresponds to the period between the months of January and June. However, a number of epidemics also have extended into the dry season, although with less intensity. The seasonal nature of Oropouche fever is linked most likely to the higher density of populations of *Culicoides paraensis*, commonly known as biting midge, the urban virus vector, in months with higher levels of rainfall, combined with a higher concentration of exposed individuals. Downward trends in epidemics of Oropouche fever generally are associated with the arrival of the dry season and the resulting lower density of biting midge populations and smaller numbers of exposed individuals.

Transmission Mechanism

Laboratory studies and broad-based surveys conducted by the Evandro Chagas Institute during the course of epidemics point to the importance of the insect *C. paraensis* belonging to the *Ceratopogonidae* family as the urban vector for the Oropouche virus.[16, 17] These tiny insects, commonly known as maruins (biting midges) in the Amazon region, are active during the day, particularly in the late afternoon hours. They crave human blood, biting people inside as well as outside their homes.[8, 14, 22] The disease is transmitted by the bites of infected midges inoculating the virus into exposed individuals.

Transmission Cycles

Studies conducted by the Evandro Chagas Institute[15] suggest that the Oropouche virus is perpetuated in nature through two different cycles, namely an urban cycle and a wild cycle.

In the urban or epidemic cycle, the virus is transmitted from person to person by the bite of *C. paraensis*. One of the most conclusive pieces of evidence attesting to the truth of this assertion lies in the demonstration of the ability of *C. paraensis*, after feeding on the blood of viremic patients, to transmit the virus to hamsters bitten by the midges 5 or more days later.[17] Moreover, these midges typically are found in high densities during periods of epidemics. They breed mostly in decomposing trunks of felled banana trees, in rotting husks of cocoa beans[7] and in piles of detritus formed in tree hollows.[12] They are scattered throughout tropical and subtropical areas of the Americas.[12]

Attempts to transmit the virus from one hamster to another through the bite of the *Culex p. quinquefasciatus* mosquito (a species commonly found in urban areas throughout the Amazon region) showed that it was transmitted only in the presence of extremely high levels of viremia, which is rare in infected humans.[16] Thus, this finding virtually rules out all likelihood of the epidemic vector being *C. p. quinquefasciatus*. Curiously enough, the virus isolation rate from *C. paraensis* during periods of epidemics is only 1:12,500,[11] which suggests that we are dealing with a low-efficiency vector. Apparently, humans are the only vertebrate involved in the urban cycle of Oropouche virus because studies of domestic animals conducted during the course of a number of outbreaks ruled out the possibility of these animals playing an amplifying role.

As far as its wild, silent cycle is concerned, there is evidence that, among the vertebrates, the Edentata (sloths), nonhuman primates, and possibly certain species of wild birds serve as hosts. Although the vector still is unknown, the possible involvement of biting midges in the virus' wild cycle nevertheless should be investigated.

The link between the two cycles is most likely humans themselves, who, after contracting the infection in enzootic forested areas and then returning to an urban setting during the viremic phase, become a source of infection for biting midges. The virus replicates in the tissues of biting midges, which, after the extrinsic incubation period, bite and infect exposed individuals, who, in turn, serve as a source of infection for other midges, thereby forming a chain of transmission, resulting in the unleashing of an epidemic.

Incubation Period

Observations conducted during a number of epidemics suggest that the incubation period ranges from 4 to 8 days. A laboratory worker who accidentally was infected orally exhibited symptoms of the viral disease 3 days later, while another technician fell ill 4 days after probably being infected through the respiratory route.[15]

Transmissibility Period

The blood of infected patients is infectious to *C. paraensis* during the first 3 or 4 days after the onset of symptoms, when the level of viremia is high enough to infect the midges. Experimental studies show the length of the extrinsic incubation period as 5 or more days.[17] The virus is not transmitted directly from one person to another.

Ratio of Symptomatic Cases

A prospective study conducted in the city of Santa Izabel in the State of Pará during the course of the epidemic of 1979 showed the ratio of symptomatic to asymptomatic cases to be roughly 2:1.[6] The study was carried out over the period from March through June of that year, covering a group of 274 individuals exposed to the virus who were monitored on a weekly basis throughout the study period through clinical examinations and laboratory testing. By the end of the study period, 78 (28.5 per cent) of these individuals had serologic evidence of Oropouche virus infection, with 49 (63 per cent) of the 78 developing clinical manifestations of the disease.

CLINICAL MANIFESTATIONS

In most cases of Oropouche fever, the infection manifests itself in the form of an acute febrile episode, which runs its course. However, certain patients may show typical signs and symptoms of aseptic meningitis, which also runs its course without complications.

"Classic" Febrile Form

This form of the disease is characterized by the sudden onset of symptoms after an incubation period ranging from 4 to 8 days. The first symptoms to appear are fever, headache, chills, dizziness, muscular pain, arthralgia, and photophobia. There also may be retro-ocular pain and congestion of the conjunctiva. Some patients also suffer from nausea, which may be accompanied by episodes of vomiting. It is not uncommon for patients to suffer from severe anorexia and insomnia. Sometimes, patients also will have cough and coryza, although these manifestations may be due to intercurrent infections. Certain patients complain of fleeting burning or stinging sensations in different parts of their body. The presence of exanthema is rare. Two accidentally infected laboratory workers reported a longer and heavier than usual menstrual flow.[14, 15, 24] The fever can be quite high, that is, 39° or 40° C, and, in some cases, may be higher than 40° C. The headache usually is localized in the front or back part of the head, although it also may be diffuse. It generally is severe and, in some cases, may not respond readily to common analgesics. There is generalized myalgia, sharpest in the neck, along the vertebral column and in the area of the sacrum. The pain may be extremely strong, causing the patient a great deal of discomfort. Patients generally describe feeling as if their body had been crushed or as if they had been beaten. Usually, there also is generalized arthralgia. Certain patients suffer from dizzy spells so severe that, in some cases, it causes them to collapse. Any epigastralgia generally is mild. There is no sign of jaundice, hepatomegaly, or splenomegaly. Occasionally, there may be swollen lymph nodes in the submaxillary and occipital regions, which totally could be unrelated to the virus infection.

The intensity of the clinical symptoms varies. In some cases, symptoms are quite severe and even may cause prostration, whereas, in others, they can be rather mild. Many patients are bedridden and, in the case of certain epidemics, flood area hospitals, causing serious overcrowding.

The acute phase of the disease generally lasts from 2 to 5 days but could run as long as a week. The myalgia, on the other hand, may persist for a period of 3 to 5 days after the fever has disappeared. Some patients report prolonged asthenia for as long as a month. Certain patients complain of a persistent headache lasting as long as several weeks.

Nearly 60 per cent of all patients suffer one or more recurrences during the course of the first or second week after the disappearance of the manifestations of the acute phase of the disease.[6, 16, 19] Relapses may take the form of reappearance of all the acute-phase symptoms of the disease or may be limited strictly to fever, asthenia, and dizziness. In some patients, relapses were accompanied by a urinary tract infection of bacterial origin. One particular patient developed an abscess in the oropharynx, most likely of bacterial origin, approximately 10 days after recovering from the original febrile condition. In some cases, patients may suffer a series of relapses over a period of 2 to 3 weeks.[15]

Observations made during the course of the 1980 outbreak in Belém revealed that about 5 per cent of all laboratory-confirmed cases developed an exanthema.[19] The exanthema appeared between the third and sixth day after the onset of the fever, disappearing 2 or 3 days later, and mainly involved the thorax, back, arms, and legs.[19, 20] During the outbreak in Manaus, a number of patients exhibited a maculopapular exanthema, beginning on the torso and subsequently spreading to the upper and lower extremities.[3] In another rare case, a 4-year-old child whose infection with the virus was confirmed by serodiagnosis experienced nystagmus, generalized tremors, and somnolence.[6] These symptoms lasted approximately 8 days, with the child apparently making a full recovery.

The effects of Oropouche fever on pregnancy essentially are unknown. The only available data in this regard come from studies conducted in Manaus of nine pregnant patients, two of whom, both in the second month of their pregnancy at the time, suffered miscarriages.[3]

Aseptic Meningitis[18]

At first, patients exhibit manifestations typical of the initial acute phase of the infection. As the illness progresses, a few days later, the headache and dizziness become increasingly severe and certain patients begin to experience other neurologic symptoms, at which point they seek medical care. This generally occurs during the second week of the illness. The main complaints cited by patients are fever, extremely severe headache in the back of the head, and dizziness. Roughly one-third of all patients complain of nausea and vomiting. Some patients suffer from moderate lethargy. They also may have trouble holding themselves in an upright position. Certain patients complain of double vision or diplopia. They generally try to keep from moving their head to avoid aggravation of their pain. In most cases, a physical examination of these patients reveals varying degrees of stiffness of the neck but no signs of paresis or paralysis. Some patients experience nystagmus. Despite the seriousness of these neurologic symptoms, patients make a full recovery. Encephalograms taken of four patients showed no abnormalities. The incidence of meningitis among patients who seek medical care is less than 5 per cent.[18]

PATHOGENESIS

Little is known about the pathogenesis of Oropouche fever. Apparently, the agent produces a systemic infection in humans, which induces a viremic phase. However, it is not known in which organ or organs the virus replicates itself. Virtually all infected patients exhibit viremia during the first 2 days of their illness. By the third day, the viremia level drops to 72 per cent, falling to 44 and 23 per cent by the fourth and fifth days, respectively. Viremia titers generally are above 3.0 $\log_{10}$ DL_{50}/0.02 mL in mice, with approximately 10 per cent of patients exhibiting virus titers as high as 5.0 to 5.3 $\log_{10}$ DL_{50}/0.02 mL during the course of the first 2 days of their illness. By the third day, virus titers are 1 log lower than in the first 2 days, with virus titers plummeting by the fourth day.[15]

Likewise, little is known about the pathogenesis of relapses, which are common in cases of Oropouche fever. The fact that no sign of viremia could be detected in any of the countless patients examined while suffering from relapses is noteworthy.

The fact that the Oropouche virus is capable of causing aseptic meningitis, combined with the fact that it was isolated from the cerebrospinal fluid in one case of meningitis,[18] suggests that the virus has the ability to penetrate the blood-brain barrier.

With no known confirmed fatalities attributable to the Oropouche virus, there are no available data on possible organic lesions caused by this agent in humans.

Laboratory tests using young hamsters inoculated with Oropouche virus show it as having essentially hepatoviscerotropic properties, with isolated necrosis of hepatocytes or focal necrosis, and the involvement of Kupffer cells exhibiting reactive hyperplasia; the animals invariably succumb to the infection. In newborn mice, the virus exhibits marked neurotropism, with the animals showing signs of focal encephalitis within 24 to 48 hours after inoculation.[2]

LABORATORY FINDINGS

Leukopenia associated with neutropenia is found commonly, although in certain cases there may be moderate leukocytosis. The leukopenia can be severe, with reports of counts showing a mere 2000 leukocytes per mm^3. There are no signs of cell abnormalities. Glutamic-oxalacetic and glutamic-pyruvic transaminase levels are normal or may show a moderate increase, but in no case do they exceed 135 units per mL of serum. Platelet counts usually are normal but occasionally may be slightly low. Sedimentation rates and levels of urea, creatinine, and glucose in the blood are normal, as are urine tests.[15]

The cerebrospinal fluid of patients with aseptic meningitis shows pleocytosis and an increased concentration of proteins.[18] The cell count varies from 7 to 310 cells per cubic millimeter of cerebrospinal fluid; both segmented and mononuclear cells are present, with a predominance of segmented cells. In one case, the cell count in the cerebrospinal fluid fell from 130 to 30 in a 1-week period, and another patient's cell count fell from 70 to 10 cells over a 3-week interval. In general, there is a moderate increase in protein levels in the cerebrospinal fluid, although one patient's protein level was more than 100 mg/mL of cerebrospinal fluid. Sugar levels remain normal.

LABORATORY DIAGNOSIS

A specific confirmation of the infection is made by isolating the virus from patients' blood or by performing Oropouche virus–specific serologic assays.[21] In order to isolate the virus, the blood samples need to be taken during the first 5 days of the illness, preferably in the first 2 days, when viremia is present in virtually all cases. The virus can be isolated by means of intracerebral or intraperitoneal inoculations of serum from infected patients into baby mice or young hamsters (in this case subcutaneous inoculations also can be used). Viral isolates also can be recovered in different cell cultures, such as Vero and BHK-21. The virus is identified by complement fixation or neutralization using Oropouche virus–specific ascitic fluid or antisera. The serodiagnosis is made by the demonstration of an antibody rise in paired serum samples taken during the acute and convalescent phases of the disease using hemagglutination inhibition, complement fixation, or neutralization. A positive IgM antibody–capture enzyme-linked immunosorbent assay on a single serum sample provides a presumptive diagnosis of recent infection, particularly in the presence of a clinical picture consistent with the disease; the test usually is positive after the fifth day of illness.

DIFFERENTIAL DIAGNOSIS

Among the main pathologies to be taken into consideration for purposes of a differential diagnosis of classic febrile forms of Oropouche fever are malaria and dengue. In fact, malaria or dengue initially were suspected as the cause of a number of epidemics of Oropouche fever. Detailed clinical records, combined with epidemiologic data, can help establish a differential diagnosis, whose certitude hinges on the absence of plasmodia in blood samples and the lack of laboratory evidence of dengue infection. Other viral and bacterial febrile diseases need to be considered in making a differential diagnosis. Accordingly, clinical and epidemiologic data and nonspecific tests will need to be taken into account, although an accurate diagnosis will require specific tests.

Febrile forms of the disease accompanied by exanthema need to be distinguished from other exanthematous febrile symptoms caused by dengue, measles, enteroviruses, and allergies to medication.

Lastly, differentiating cases of aseptic meningitis associated with the Oropouche virus infection from cases of aseptic meningitis associated with other causative agents will require a specific etiologic diagnosis.

TREATMENT

Because there is no specific treatment for Oropouche fever, the only type of treatment for the virus infection is symptomatic. Rest is important and should be continued several days after the disappearance of its initial acute manifestations because relapses are suspected of occurring more often in patients prematurely resuming their regular activities, particularly strenuous activities. Aspirin or another antipyretic should be used to lower the fever, with the use of ordinary analgesics recommended against headache, myalgia, and arthralgia. However, certain patients whose headaches failed to respond to this treatment have been treated with morphine derivatives. It also is recommended that patients be given fruit juices or glucose solutions. Cases of severe dehydration may be treated by administering intravenous fluids.

PREVENTION AND CONTROL

The most effective way to prevent, avert, or curb the impact of epidemics of Oropouche fever is to combat its vector *C. paraensis*. In order to be effective, vector control efforts will need to focus on the midge's adult and larval forms. Considering how *C. paraensis* habitually is active during the day, applications of insecticides to its habitats through thermonebulization or ultra-low–volume aerosolization may help reduce adult biting midge populations. Because this *Culicoides* species is most active during the late afternoon hours,[22] ultra-low–volume spraying may be more effective during this period of the day. However, carefully planned-out studies are needed to assess how to maximize the effectiveness of spraying in order to determine the type and concentration of insecticide to be used, the necessary volume of insecticide per treatment area, the size of the droplets, the frequency and timing of applications, etc. At the same time, it is essential that an effort be made to control its larvae by larviciding corresponding habitats or, better yet, by conducting drives to eliminate or burn breeding sites, such as rotting cocoa bean husks and decomposing trunks of felled banana trees.[7] Obviously, the success of these measures will be dependent largely on community involvement. Proper community education, thus, is important. Individuals can protect themselves by applying insecticides directly to the skin. However, these types of products provide only temporary action, and they may be unaffordable to the poor.

There is no vaccine against Oropouche fever at this time. In light of the relatively benign nature of this viral disease, it is hard to justify developing a general-purpose vaccine for at-risk populations living in areas where they are exposed to the disease.

References

1. Anderson, C. R., Spence, L., Downs, W. G., et al.: Oropouche virus: A new human disease agent from Trinidad, West Indies. Am. J. Trop. Med. Hyg. *10*:574–578, 1961.
2. Araújo, R., Pinheiro, F. P., Araújo, M. T., et al.: Patogenia das lesões hepáticas na infeccão experimental com o vírus Oropouche (BeAn 19991): Análise comparativa das curvas virêmica e de infectividade com as alterações ultra-estruturais. Hiléia Médica Belém *1*:7–12, 1979.
3. Borborema, C. A. T., Pinheiro, F. P., Albuquerque, B. C., et al.: Primeiro registro de epidemias causadas pelo vírus Oropouche no Estado do Amazonas. Rev. Inst. Med. Trop. São Paulo *24*:132–139, 1982.
4. Chavez, R., Colan, E., and Phillips I.: Fiebre de Oropouche en Iquitos: Reporte preliminar de 5 casos. Rev. Farmacol. Terap. 2:12–14, 1992.
5. Dixon, K. E., Travassos da Rosa, A. P. A., Travassos da Rosa, J. F. S., et al.: Oropouche virus. II. Epidemiological observations during an epidemic in Santarém, Pará, Brazil, in 1975. Am. J. Trop. Med. Hyg. *30*:161–164, 1981.
6. Freitas, R. B., Pinheiro, F. P., Santos, M. A. V., et al.: Epidemia de vírus Oropouche no leste do Estado do Pará, 1979. *In* Pinheiro, F. P. (ed.):

International Symposium on Tropical Arboviruses and Haemorrhagic Fevers, Rio de Janeiro. Academia Brasileira de Ciencias, 1982, pp. 419–439.
7. Hoch, A. L., Roberts, D. R., and Pinheiro, F. D. P.: Breeding sites of *Culicoides paraensis*, and other options for control by environmental management. Bull. Pan Am. Health Org. *20*:284–293, 1986.
8. Hoch, A. L., Roberts, D. R., and Pinheiro, F. P.: Host-seeking behavior and seasonal abundance of *Culicoides paraensis* (Diptera: Ceratopogonidae) in Brazil. J. Am. Mosq. Control Assoc. *6*:110–114, 1990.
9. Karabatsos, N. (ed.): International Catalogue of Arboviruses, 1985. 3rd ed. San Antonio, American Society of Tropical Medicine and Hygiene, 1985.
10. LeDuc, J. W., Hoch, A. L., Pinheiro, F. P., et al.: Epidemic Oropouche virus disease in northern Brazil. Bull. Pan Am. Health Org. *15*:97–103, 1981.
11. LeDuc, J. W., and Pinheiro, F. P.: Oropouche fever. *In* Monath, T. P. (ed.): The Arboviruses: Epidemiology and Ecology. Vol. IV. Boca Raton, CRC Press, 1986, pp. 1–14.
12. Linley, J. R., Hoch, A. L., and Pinheiro, F. P.: Biting midges (Diptera: Ceratopogonidae) and human health. J. Med. Entomol. *20*:347–364, 1983.
13. Pinheiro, F. P., Pinheiro, M., Bensabath, G., et al.: Epidemia de vírus Oropouche em Belém. Rev. Serv. Esp. Saúde Publ. *12*:15–23, 1962.
14. Pinheiro, F. P., Travassos da Rosa, A. P. A., Travassos da Rosa, J. F., et al.: An outbreak of Oropouche virus disease in the vicinity of Santarém, Pará, Brazil. Tropenmed. Parasitol. *27*:213–223, 1976.
15. Pinheiro, F. P., Travassos da Rosa, A. P. A., Travassos da Rosa, J. F., et al.: Oropouche virus. I. A review of clinical, epidemiological and ecological findings. Am. J. Trop. Med. Hyg. *30*:149–160, 1981.
16. Pinheiro, F. P., Hoch, A. L., Gomes, M. L. C., et al.: Oropouche virus. IV. Laboratory transmission by *Culicoides paraensis*. Am. J. Trop. Med. Hyg. *30*:172–176, 1981.
17. Pinheiro, F. P., Travassos da Rosa, A. P. A., Gomes, M. L. C., et al.: Transmission of Oropouche virus from man to hamster by the midge *Culicoides paraensis*. Science *215*:1251–1253, 1982.
18. Pinheiro, F. P., Rocha, A. G., Freitas, R. B., et al.: Meningite associada às infecções por vírus Oropouche. Rev. Inst. Med. Trop. São Paulo *24*:246–251, 1982.
19. Pinheiro, F. P.: Febre do Oropouche. J. Brasil. Med. *44*:46–62, 1983.
20. Pinheiro, F. P., Travassos da Rosa, A. P. A., Freitas, R. B., et al.: *In* Instituto Evandro Chagas, 50 Anos de Contribuição às Ciências Biológicas e à Medicina Tropical. Fundação Serviços de Saúde Pública, 1986, pp. 349–357.
21. Pinheiro, F. P., Travassos da Rosa, A. P. A. and Vasconcelos, P. F. C.: Arboviral zoonoses of Central and South America. Part G. Oropouche fever. *In* Beran, G. W. (ed.): Handbook of Zoonoses. 2nd ed. Boca Raton, CRC Press, 1994, pp. 214–217.
22. Roberts, D. R., Hoch, A. L., Dixon, K. E., et al.: Oropouche virus. III. Entomological observations from three epidemics in Pará, Brazil, 1975. Am. J. Trop. Med. Hyg. *30*:165–171, 1981.
23. Travassos da Rosa, A. P. A., Rodrigues, S. G., Nunes, M. R., et al.: Epidemia de febre do Oropouche em Serra Pelada, Município de Curionópolis, Pará, 1994. Rev. Soc. Bras. Medic. Trop. *29*:537–541, 1996.
24. Vasconcelos, P. F. C., Travassos da Rosa, J. F. S., Guerreiro, S. C., et al.: Primeiro registro de epidemias causadas pelo vírus Oropouche nos estados do Maranhão e Goiás, Brasil. Rev. Inst. Med. Trop. São Paulo *31*:271–278, 1989.

❑ ❑ ❑

SUBSECTION TWELVE

RETROVIRIDAE

192

HUMAN RETROVIRUSES

Lynne M. Mofenson

In the decade and a half since the first recognition of AIDS in 1981, remarkable progress has been made. In 1983, the causative agent was identified as a human retrovirus, HIV-1, and by 1985, diagnostic assays were developed to detect HIV-1 antibodies. The first antiretroviral therapeutic agent, zidovudine (ZDV), was approved in the United States in 1987 for adult use and in 1990 for pediatric use. In 1994, the hypothesis that prophylaxis against HIV transmission might be feasible became a reality when a regimen of ZDV given to infected pregnant women and their newborns was shown to prevent perinatal HIV transmission.[137] As of 1996, at least seven therapeutic agents have been approved, and the intricacies of viral pathogenesis and elements of an effective host immune response are being unraveled. However, important gaps in knowledge remain, frustrating the development of a curative therapy, preventive vaccine, and effective behavioral intervention efforts. HIV-1 infection has continued its global spread and has emerged as a primary cause of mortality among adults and children in both the developed and developing world; HIV-1 has been the most common cause of death among persons 25 to 44 years of age in the United States since 1993.[106]

AIDS has redirected scientific attention to human retroviruses and their possible pathologic effects. Retroviruses first were recognized in the early 1900s as pathogens causing malignancies in animals. The first human retrovirus, human T-cell lymphotropic virus (HTLV) type I, was identified by Gallo and coworkers in 1979 and subsequently defined as the etiologic agent of adult T-cell leukemia/lymphoma.[243] HTLV-I also has been associated with a chronic degenerative neurologic disease, HTLV-I–associated myelopathy/tropical spastic paraparesis (HAM/TSP), and infective dermatitis, a chronic eczema associated with *Staphylococcus aureus* and beta-hemolytic *Streptococcus* seen in infected children.[108] In 1982, a second antigenically related retrovirus, HTLV-II, was identified from a patient with a T-cell variant of hairy-cell leukemia. After the identification of HIV-1 as the cause of AIDS in 1983, a second antigenic variant, HIV-2, was identified in 1986 in patients with AIDS from West Africa.[408]

With the explosion of information concerning the molecular, biologic, clinical, and epidemiologic aspects of these viruses, an important model for exploring the pathobiology of a number of human diseases, ranging from neoplastic disorders to autoimmune and immunodeficiency syndromes, has been provided. It is likely, given the rapid pace of breakthroughs in retrovirology, that continued new isolations will result in the discovery of additional examples of these types of viruses, perhaps unlocking secrets of some human diseases whose etiology currently is unknown.

THE VIRUSES

Classification

Retroviruses form a family of single-stranded RNA viruses that are unusual because they contain a diploid RNA genome that replicates through a DNA intermediate; the name retrovirus is derived from this characteristic. This unique capability is due to the presence of a virally coded RNA-dependent

DNA polymerase, reverse transcriptase, that catalyzes the reverse transcription of viral RNA into a double-stranded DNA copy. This viral DNA intermediary becomes integrated into host-cell DNA by a specialized recombination mechanism requiring another viral protein, integrase. This capacity for genomic integration correlates with the capability of retroviruses to cause lifelong infection, evade the usual mechanisms of immune clearance, and produce chronic diseases in the host that become manifest only after a long asymptomatic period that may last years to decades.

Retroviruses can be grouped into two broad categories, classical/simple and complex, based on complexity of the viral genome and replication mechanisms[228, 663] (Table 192–1). Simple retroviruses contain only three genes (*env*, *gag*, and *pol*), which encode for two classes of transcripts, genomic RNA (coding for *env*, *gag*, and *pol*) and spliced RNAs that code for viral enzymes or structural components. These viruses cause disease in animals and will not be discussed further in this chapter. Complex retroviruses have a more complicated genome that encodes for a number of regulatory genes that are involved in modulating viral replication. These retroviruses are divided into three subfamilies on the basis of nucleotide sequences and genetic organization. The subfamilies are the *Oncovirinae* (oncogenic or transforming viruses, which include HTLV-I and HTLV-II); the *Lentivirinae* (slow viruses with cytopathic effects, which include HIV-1 and HIV-2); and the *Spumavirinae* (foamy viruses). Although sharing some similarities in genomic structure and life cycle, the different subfamilies of retroviruses have distinct in vitro and in vivo effects and different strategies for evading host immunity. Oncoviruses generally transform cells in culture, stimulate target-cell proliferation, and cause tumors in their hosts. Lentiviruses cause cell fusion, multinucleated giant-cell formation, and cytopathic effect in culture and cause slow infections characterized by immunodeficiency in their hosts. The spumaviruses also are cytopathic for susceptible cells, inducing syncytial giant cells and vacuolation in cells in vitro.[228] Transgenic mice carrying the spumavirus *bel* gene were found to express the transgene in the central nervous system and smooth muscle and to develop a progressive degenerative encephalopathy and myopathy.[51] However, the relevance of spumaviruses as human pathogens is not known, and they will not be discussed further in this chapter.

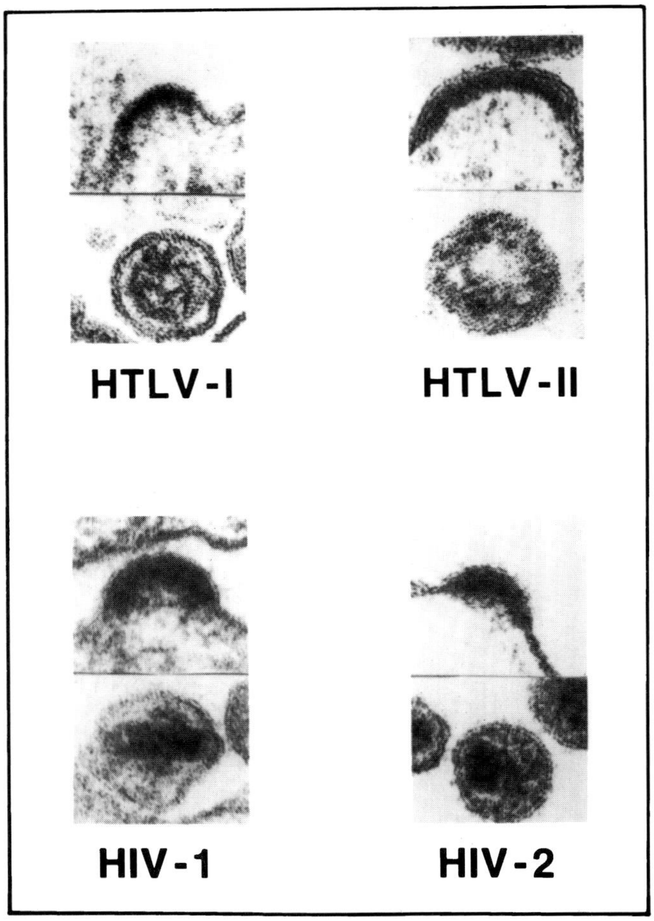

FIGURE 192–1. *Electron micrographs of HTLV-I, HTLV-II, HIV-1, and HIV-2. In the upper panel for each virus is shown the budding particle; in the lower panel, the mature virion. (From Blattner, W. A.: Retroviruses. In Evans, A. S. (ed.): Viral Infections of Human Epidemiology and Control. 3rd ed. New York, Plenum, 1989, pp. 545–592.)*

Morphology/Genomic Structure

Retroviruses have a distinct morphology. They are enveloped RNA viruses with diameters of 80 to 120 nm and have a thin electron-dense outer envelope and an electron-dense core that is either spherical (HTLV-I and HTLV-II) or cylindrical (HIV-1 and HIV-2) (Fig. 192–1). The surface of the virus is made up of projections of viral envelope glycoproteins containing lipids partially derived from the cell surface during budding of mature virions. The core protein encloses a ribonucleoprotein complex of genomic RNA complexed with viral reverse transcriptase and integrase.[121]

TABLE 192–1. *Retroviridae* Family

Type of Retrovirus	Prototype Viruses
Classical (or Simple) Retroviruses	
D-type retroviruses	Mason-Pfizer monkey virus
B-type retroviruses	Mouse mammary tumor virus
C-type retroviruses a	Rous sarcoma virus
C-type retroviruses b	Murine leukemia virus
Complex Retroviruses	
Oncoviruses	Human T-cell lymphotropic virus types I and II
Lentiviruses	HIV-1 and HIV-2
Spumaviruses	Human spuma retrovirus

The RNA genome is a messenger-sense, linear, single-stranded RNA composed of two identical subunits held together by hydrogen bonds at their 5′ ends. The 5′ and 3′ ends of the RNA contain repeated sequences, called long terminal repeats (LTRs), which are required for integration of viral DNA into the host genome and for efficient replication. The LTR can be divided functionally into modulatory, core, and transactivation-response (TAR) domains.[551, 704] These domains contain binding sites for cellular transcription factors that initially are required for viral mRNA transcription. For example, sites in the modulatory domain bind the potent transcription up-regulator nuclear factor kappa B (NF-κB) proteins. The core promoter domain also contains binding sites for other cellular proteins (such as SP-1), the transcription initiator site, and a TATA motif that mediates interactions between transcription factors and host-cell RNA polymerase. The TAR domain contains binding sites for other cellular and viral DNA- and RNA-binding proteins that regulate transcription, such as the viral tat protein. Thus, clus-

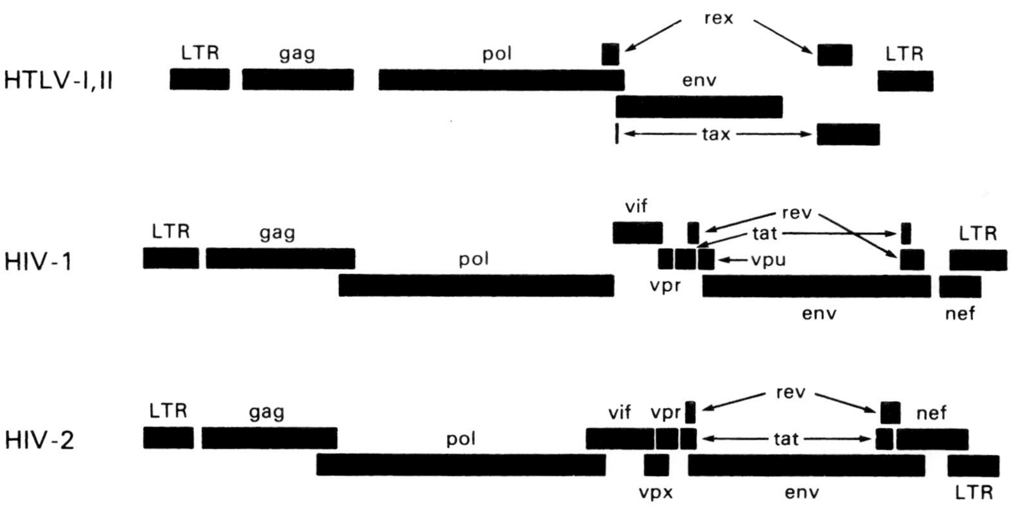

FIGURE 192–2. *Retroviral genome. The schematic depiction of the HTLV and HIV genomes shows that HTLV has a more complex genome than do most animal retroviruses and that HIV in turn has additional regulatory genes. The details of the function of each of these genes are summarized in the text. (From Gallo, R. C., Wong-Staal, F., Montagnier, L., et al.: HIV/HTLV gene nomenclature. Nature 333:504, 1988. Copyright 1988 Macmillan Magazines, Ltd.)*

tered near the ends of the RNA are the sequences that regulate the structural transformation of the viral genome—signals for initiation and progression of DNA synthesis and proviral integration, for transcription and processing of viral RNA, and for packaging of RNA and protein products into new viral particles. Between these regions are the genes that encode the major structural proteins of the virus, the enzymes found in the viral particles, and additional proteins with specialized intracellular functions.

All retroviruses contain three genes, *gag* (group-specific antigen), *pol* (polymerase), and *env* (envelope), arranged in 5′ to 3′ order, with LTRs at each end (Fig. 192–2). The *gag* gene encodes the protein products that form the core particle of the virus, including nucleocapsid, capsid, and matrix proteins. The *pol* gene products include the viral reverse transcriptase, as well as the protease, endonuclease (ribonuclease), and integrase enzymes. The *env* gene encodes the major components of the viral coat, the surface, and the transmembrane glycoproteins. Retroviral genes generally are expressed first as large overlapping polyproteins that undergo processing into functional peptide products by the virally encoded protease. A complex array of additional genes with various regulatory functions also is present (Table 192–2).

The oncoviruses HTLV-I and HTLV-II have a unique region at the 3′ end of the genome called the pX region; genes in this region encode proteins that are important for viral replication and activation of host genes.[289] One gene, known as *tax* (transactivator), encodes a protein that regulates transcription of both viral and host genes downstream of the LTR region of the viral genome. This gene may be involved in malignant transformation of infected T cells, possibly through activation of host oncogenes and increased expression of host-cell interleukin-2 (IL-2) genes or receptors.[12, 663] The second gene, called *rex* (regulator of expression of virion proteins), acts to down-regulate *tax*-mediated transactivation,

TABLE 192–2. Retroviral Genome Terminology

Name	Function
Major Structural Genes (all retroviruses)	
gag	Nucleocapsid, capsid, and matrix proteins
pol	Reverse transcriptase, polymerase, endonuclease, and integrase enzymes
env	Envelope surface and transmembrane glycoproteins
Accessory Regulatory Genes (onco- and lenti-retroviruses only)	
HTLV-I and HTLV-II	
tax	Binds to promoter region of long terminal repeat to enhance transcription
rex	Directs selective transport of unspliced genomic and partially spliced RNA from nucleus to cytoplasm
HIV-1 and HIV-2	
tat	Binds to promoter region of long terminal repeat to enhance transcription
rev	Directs selective transport of unspliced genomic and partially spliced RNA from nucleus to cytoplasm
nef	Suppresses CD4+ expression on cell surface; facilitates expression of envelope proteins on cell surface?
vif	Affects processing/transport of viral nucleoprotein core; facilitates viral infectivity and spread
vpr	Affects cellular events after uncoating, localization of preintegrated viral DNA to nucleus; present in virion
vpu (HIV-1 only)	Induces intracellular degradation of the cytoplasmic domain of CD4+; important in virion assembly and release
vpx (HIV-2 only)	Affects efficiency of early replication events; present in virion

possibly promoting viral latency. The rex protein also effects mRNA splicing and export from nucleus to cytoplasm and promotes viral mRNA translation into viral proteins.

The lentiviruses HIV-1 and HIV-2 have even more complex genomes containing at least eight regulatory genes in addition to *env, gag,* and *pol*. Some of the regulatory genes function through interacting with cellular proteins that bind to the LTR region and thereby influence viral replication (see Table 192–2). Lentiviral genes corresponding to the oncoviral *tax* and *rex* are called *tat* and *rev,* which are expressed early and appear essential for replication. The *tat* gene product binds to the promoter region of the integrated proviral DNA LTR and enhances transcription of viral mRNA, and the rev protein appears to direct the selective transport of spliced and genomic mRNA to the cytoplasm for translation into viral proteins and mature particles.[121, 704] The remaining accessory regulatory genes, which include *nef, vif, vpr, vpu* (HIV-1 only), and *vpx* (HIV-2 and simian immunodeficiency virus [SIV]), provide fine-tuning by diminishing or, more commonly, enhancing viral replication. The *nef* gene is expressed early, like *tat* and *rev,* and may play a role in suppression of CD4+ on the surface of the host cell, which could facilitate expression of env proteins on the cell surface.[13] The *vif* and *vpu* accessory genes are expressed late, along with the structural and enzymatic proteins. The *vif* gene product facilitates viral infectivity and spread and appears to affect processing and/or transport of the viral nucleoprotein core; the vpu protein induces intracellular degradation of the cytoplasmic domain of CD4 and may be important in virion assembly and particle release.[115, 247, 683] The vpr protein is present in the virion itself, may act to regulate cellular events after virus penetration and uncoating to facilitate permissiveness for viral replication, and may be involved in efficient localization of the preintegrated viral DNA into the nucleus; similarly, HIV-2 *vpx* is found in the virus particle and appears to affect the efficiency of early replication events, but the precise mechanism is unknown.[121, 274, 375]

Viral Replication

There are two phases of the retroviral life cycle: an infection phase (including viral attachment, entry, reverse transcription, and proviral integration) and an expression phase (including transcription, translation, assembly, and budding of the virion)[121] (Fig. 192–3).

Retroviruses attach to cells through recognition and binding of viral outer envelope proteins to specific proteins present on the surface of the host cell; the cell-surface receptor specificity may account for the species and cellular tropism of the viruses.[310] The major receptor for HIV-1 is the CD4 molecule on the surface of T lymphocytes and monocytes/macrophages; another potential receptor for HIV-1 is galactosyl ceramide found on cells derived from the central nervous system.[270] For HTLV-I, a yet-to-be-defined T-cell marker, perhaps of activated T cells, is suspected.

Interaction of the virus with cellular receptors causes a conformational change in the viral transmembrane glycoprotein, exposing a fusogenic domain of gp41.[483] Viral entry appears to be mediated by fusion of the viral envelope to the host-cell membrane with release of the viral RNA-protein complex into the cytoplasm.[260, 663] RNA to DNA transcriptional events are initiated through the action of viral enzymes reverse transcriptase (RNA-directed DNA polymerase) and ribonuclease. Viral single-stranded (ss) RNA is transcribed into a viral RNA/DNA hybrid complex by the DNA polymerase; the ribonuclease then destroys the original RNA and permits the DNA polymerase to complete transcription of a second DNA strand to form a linear double-stranded (ds) DNA copy of the original viral RNA.[260] Activation of T lymphocytes is required for completion of viral DNA synthesis, suggesting that inducible host-cell factors may play an important role in early replication steps.[121, 663] The dsDNA is translocated to the nucleus, where the viral integrase enzyme inserts the viral DNA duplex into the host genome. This may occur via recognition by integrase of the LTR segments at the

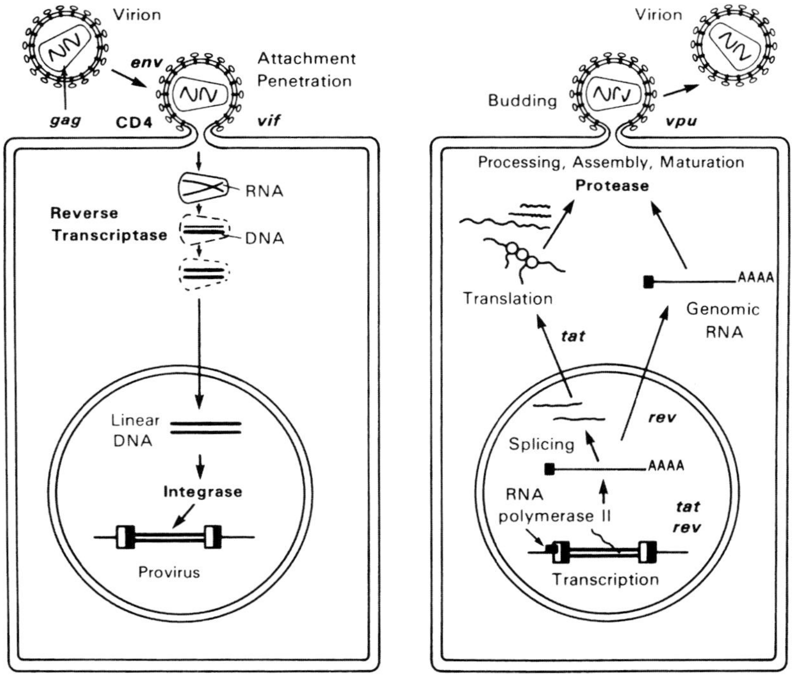

FIGURE 192–3. *Life cycle of HIV-1. The left panel shows the process of viral attachment and integration. The right panel shows the process whereby new infectious virions are produced. Details of these processes are discussed in the text. (From Gallo, R. C.: Mechanisms of disease induction by HIV. J. AIDS 3:380–389, 1990. Copyright 1988 Macmillan Magazines, Ltd.)*

ends of the viral DNA molecules; integration appears to be random but may be influenced by host chromatic factors.[266]

Once viral DNA is integrated into the host cell, the virus becomes highly dependent on the host cell for further replication. The virus can remain in a latent state for prolonged periods with very little viral RNA or protein production, thus remaining invisible to the host immune system. The signals that induce productive replication in a latently infected cell are incompletely understood but probably involve control at the level of cellular activation. Cell activation induces expression of a variety of host-cell transcriptional factors, such as the NF-κB family of enhancer binding proteins. These factors normally regulate expression of a variety of cellular genes involved in cell growth. Host-cell endogenous or inducible factors also can interact with promoter-enhancer gene sequences in the viral LTR, which regulate HIV replication or gene expression, and stimulate early HIV-1 regulatory gene expression.[121, 260] Disparities in the types of endogenous or inducible transcriptional factors present in different host cells may be associated with viral cellular tropism.[310] The early phase of gene expression is characterized by the presence of spliced and unspliced viral RNAs in the nucleus but only fully spliced mRNAs in the cytoplasm; the mRNAs serve to direct production of the tat, rev, and nef proteins. These protein products then modulate the production and splicing of mRNA and viral proteins.

The transition from early regulatory gene to late structural protein gene expression is characterized by the selective transport of unspliced and partially spliced viral mRNA in the cytoplasm and is dependent on the presence of sufficient amounts of the rev protein.[121, 663] The polyproteins translated from these viral mRNAs then are split into their final structural viral protein components by the action of viral and host-cell proteolytic enzymes. The viral envelope proteins are synthesized as a gp160 precursor that is cleaved by a cellular protease to gp120 and gp41. The gag protein is derived similarly from a larger precursor protein, divided by the viral protease to form p24, p17, p9, and p7 proteins. The pol protein is translated via a unique ribosomal frame-shifting mechanism from the same mRNA transcript as the *gag* precursor and is cleaved to the viral enzymes reverse transcriptase, integrase, ribonuclease, and protease.[260]

Virion assembly involves aggregation of the ribonucleoprotein core in the cytoplasm. In HIV-1 (but not other retroviruses), a host-cell protein, cyclophilin A, interacts with the viral gag protein and is incorporated into the virion.[233, 649] This host factor appears to be required for the formation of infectious virions, possibly by playing an essential role in virion morphogenesis or facilitating conformation changes in capsid proteins necessary for uncoating.[147] The assembled core moves to the cell surface and buds through the plasma membrane, incorporating viral envelope and transmembrane proteins. During the process of budding, substantial amounts of cellular surface antigens, such as β-2 microglobulin and human leukocyte antigen (HLA)–DR, are incorporated into the viral envelope. Myristylation of the p17 gag protein occurs during the budding process, as does final cleavage of viral proteins by the HIV protease. Viral accessory gene products, vif and vpu, appear to promote release of the budding virion.

Genetic Variation

Retroviruses, particularly the lentiviruses, may undergo significant antigenic drift with strain variation within an individual viral type. Because replication of retroviruses involves several conversions of genetic material and the virally encoded reverse transcriptase is error-prone, potential for mutation is great.

HIV-1 infection is a dynamic process, with rapid turnover of virus. Kinetic studies of viral replication have shown that the estimated half-life of free virus in plasma is only 6 hours and that the half-life of infected cells with actively replicating virus is less than 2 days.[285, 484, 692] These data indicate that at least 30 per cent of free plasma virus is replaced daily; at least 10^9 virions are estimated to be produced daily. The combination of extremely rapid viral turnover with an error-prone replication process yields a virus with great capacity for genetic mutation. Accumulation of genetic mutations over time secondary to immunologic or drug pressure causes the virus to evolve into a complex mix of divergent but related populations of viral genomes (called viral swarms or quasispecies) within a single individual.[294] This allows HIV-1 to evade the host immune response effectively and to develop drug resistance rapidly.

In contrast, the genome of HTLV is fairly stable, perhaps reflecting the low proliferation rate of this virus. For HTLV-I, the strategies by which this relatively stable virus evades immune surveillance are not characterized fully but may involve a lower level of virus proliferation, altered immune response due to viral effects on immune recognition, and/or more frequent cell-to-cell transmission in order to avoid immune surveillance.

A phylogenetic tree of HIV-1 subtypes has been developed based on nucleotide sequencing of the *env* gene. At least nine subtypes, designated A through I, have been identified and form a major HIV-1 group of genetically related viruses called group M.[294] HIV-1 strains that are significantly dissimilar to group M have been categorized as group O, which contains a separate diverse group of genetically related isolates. The global distribution of subtypes varies. In some areas of the world, one subtype predominates, such as subtype B in the United States and Europe. Other areas have cocirculation of multiple subtypes, such as subtypes A, C, and D in Africa and B and E in Thailand. In one study, differences in viral genotype were correlated with distinct neutralization serotypes, and cross-reactivity, although seen, appeared to be uncommon.[413] Additionally, dual infection with distinct subtypes (B and E) has been described in a few individuals.[20] These data suggest that infection with one subtype of virus may not protect fully against infection with the other and that a multivalent vaccine will be necessary for HIV-1. The genetic variation of HIV also has important implications for the sensitivity and specificity of diagnostic tests, suggesting that subtype-specific serologic tests may be required in some areas of the world.[294] Possible differences in cell tropism and transmissibility between subtypes have been suggested by in vitro findings that HIV-1 subtype E may grow more efficiently in Langerhans cells from genital tract mucosa than may subtype B and by epidemiologic findings that suggest more efficient sexual transmission of subtype E than B.[127, 351, 414]

GENERAL METHODS OF DIAGNOSIS OF RETROVIRAL INFECTIONS

Detection of retroviral antibody has been the most widely used test to diagnose infection in older children and adults. However, due to transplacental passage of maternal antibody, antibody testing during infancy is not diagnostic of infection in the infant, and direct viral detection methods are necessary for diagnosis.

Antibody testing for retroviruses most frequently involves use of an initial screening test followed by a more specific confirmatory test. Initial screening generally is performed using viral antigens from disrupted whole virus or synthetic or recombinant viral antigens in an enzyme-linked immunosorbent assay (ELISA). A positive ELISA is confirmed by the more specific immunoblot (or Western blot), which measures the presence of antibodies to a number of virus-associated proteins, both structural and nonstructural. Viral antigens (from disrupted whole virus or synthetic or recombinant antigens) undergo electrophoresis through a polyacrylamide gel, separating the antigens by size. The separated antigens then are transferred to nitrocellulose paper, incubated with the patients' serum, and then incubated with enzyme-linked antihuman antibody and chromogenic substrate, which results in visible bands where patient antibodies are bound by antigens. Analysis of band pattern permits more specific identification of the virus. Other techniques used to measure antibodies to retroviruses include indirect immunofluorescence (IFA), radioimmunoprecipitation assay (RIPA), and biologic assays for antibody to envelope glycoproteins (neutralization or syncytium inhibition assays).

Because of antigenic differences between HIV-1 and HIV-2, HIV-1 screening tests are not reliable for detection of HIV-2. A commercial HIV-1/HIV-2 combination assay is available that has high sensitivity for detection of both viruses; a supplemental immunoblot assay is used to confirm viral subtype.[92, 408] Serologic diagnosis of HTLV infection is similar to that of HIV, involving a screening enzyme immunoassay (EIA) and confirmatory immunoblot or RIPA. However, these tests do not distinguish between antibodies directed to HTLV-I or HTLV-II.[108] In those patients with positive serology, virologic detection tests, such as proviral amplification by polymerase chain reaction (PCR) or viral isolation, have been used. Assays containing several synthetic peptides and recombinant proteins have been developed that appear to be capable of differentiating between HTLV-I and HTLV-II.[48, 562]

Direct detection of virus by culture is intensive, expensive, and time-consuming, often requiring several weeks for results. The ability to isolate HTLV and HIV is dependent on disease state, immune status, and viral load. The ability to culture retroviruses has been improved by cocultivation of patient cells with human peripheral blood mononuclear cells that have been stimulated in vitro with mitogens (e.g., phytohemagglutinin) and growth factors (e.g., IL-2), as well as by removal of patient CD8+ (suppressor) cells from the coculture. In infants and children, the small volume of blood available for culture and low virus load in some cases make virus isolation especially challenging.

Other methods used for detection of virus include (1) antigen-capture assays to detect free circulating viral antigens (e.g., p24 HIV-1 core antigen); (2) IFA and immunohistochemistry to detect viral antigens in tissue; (3) detection of viral nucleic acids by Southern blot analysis; (4) in situ hybridization or dot blots; and (5) PCR to detect proviral DNA in leukocytes or tissue or RNA in plasma. PCR can be used to quantitate virus and is the most sensitive virologic test to detect virus because it is capable of amplifying tiny quantities of viral nucleic acids enzymatically to detectable levels using a system of specific nucleotide primers and probes. This technique can be modified to detect viral RNA by using reverse transcription to convert viral RNA to DNA and performing PCR on the DNA product or other techniques, such as branched chain amplification or nucleic acid sequence-based amplification.[79, 501, 614]

VIRAL PATHOGENESIS

The pathogenesis of HIV-1 infection has been studied in more detail than that of other retroviruses. Variation in the biologic properties of HIV-1 isolates, such as cytotropism (lymphocyte vs. monocyte/macrophage), syncytium-inducing capacity, and replication rate (rapid/high vs. slow/low), may influence pathogenicity.[167, 343] Viral biologic phenotype combined with the route of exposure also may be an important determinant of transmissibility. Nonsyncytia-inducing, macrophage-tropic virus appears to be the predominant form of HIV-1 that is transmitted sexually and perinatally.[492, 554, 671]

Once transmission has occurred, there is an initial 2- to 6-week stage of systemic viral dissemination that is characterized by high levels of viremia, drop in CD4+ lymphocyte count, and, in some patients, a "mononucleosis-like" clinical syndrome.[510] As HIV-1–specific humoral and cellular immune responses develop, the amount of circulating virus decreases to low levels, CD4+ lymphocytes increase, and a long period of clinical latency ensues. However, despite clinical latency and a seemingly effective immune response, active replication of HIV-1, particularly in lymphoid tissues, is occurring during all stages of infection.[509]

Initial establishment of HIV-1 infection in lymphoid organs occurs very early in infection.[200] Immune complexes of virus, antibody, and complement become trapped on follicular dendritic cells in the germinal centers of lymph nodes.[509] The microenvironment of the germinal center is highly conducive to HIV infection; CD4+ lymphocytes migrate through lymphoid tissue in close contact with follicular dendritic cells, and the elevated cytokines found in activated lymph nodes act to increase CD4+ cell susceptibility to infection as well as induce HIV replication within latently infected cells.[273] Free virus and latently infected cells may remain sequestered within the lymphoid tissue, providing a stimulus for continued activation and immune responses and a reservoir for persistent viral production.

During this period of ongoing infection in lymphoid tissue, high levels of viral production are maintained (approximately 10^9 virions daily), and an equilibrium between viral production and elimination is felt to exist.[285, 692] Turnover of CD4+ lymphocytes is occurring at a similar rapid rate. The half-life of a productively infected CD4+ cell has been estimated to be only 2 days, and an estimated mean of 1.8×10^9 cells are destroyed daily.[285] Therefore, to maintain the CD4+ lymphocyte number, CD4+ cell replenishment must be maintained at chronically high levels; these levels may become difficult to sustain if viral replication increases. Although the primary factor in CD4+ cell loss appears to be a direct cell lysis from viral infection, a number of other mechanisms also are postulated to cause CD4+ cell destruction in HIV-1 infection, including HIV-induced programmed cell death (apoptosis), host HIV-specific immune responses (HIV-1–specific cytotoxic T lymphocytes, antibody-dependent cellular cytotoxicity mediated by natural killer cells), HIV-mediated fusion and syncytium formation, autoimmune phenomenon, and disruption of normal immunoregulatory pathways.[11, 510]

The high level of HIV-1 production and turnover facilitates the generation of immune escape mutants, requiring the host immune response to "catch up" with a pathogen that continually is changing antigenically.[639, 708] The constant lag between the host immune response and viral genotype allows viral persistence even in a seemingly immunologically competent host. Mutations leading to drug resistance or more virulent phenotypes also may occur.[257] In addition, even nonproductive infection with HIV-1 results in disruption of normal immune function and impairs normal cytokine production.[603] Some cytokines are necessary for survival of activated cells, and such disruptions also may contribute to CD4+ cell death.

HIV-1 replication can be induced in latently infected cells

by a number of stimuli, including coinfections with other viruses, such as cytomegalovirus (CMV) and herpes simplex virus, and a variety of cytokines, such as tumor necrosis factor (TNF)-α.[510, 533] Certain cytokines also have been found to have an HIV-suppressive effect. CD8+ lymphocytes from infected adults have been shown to produce soluble HIV-1–suppressive factors that have been identified as cytokines from the C-C chemokine subfamily called RANTES, MIP-1α, and MIP-1β.[126] In the presence of all three of these chemokines, replication of HIV-1, HIV-2, and SIV was suppressed in vitro; HTLV-I replication was not affected. The mechanism of this effect is unknown.

Degeneration of the germinal center follicular cell network and disruption of lymphoid architecture are associated with disease progression.[182, 509] Loss of follicular cell trapping of free virus permits viral release into the peripheral blood; destruction of lymphoid tissue results in impaired ability to mount an effective immune response against the virus, permitting increased viral replication and further destruction of lymphoid tissue. CD4+ cell replacement from lymphoid tissue becomes markedly diminished, accompanied by the decrease in CD4+ number and enhanced susceptibility to opportunistic infection characteristic of end-stage HIV-1 disease.

Apparent "resistance" to HIV-1 infection has been reported among some individuals who remain seronegative despite continued HIV-1 exposure.[123, 259, 263] An association with HLA class I and II haplotypes has been hypothesized.[643] HLA antigens derived from host cells are found on the HIV-1 envelope. Individuals with rare HLA haplotypes who have had repeated exposure to foreign antigens may show a strong allogenic immune response to HIV-1–associated HLAs that might block infection; alternatively, some forms of HLA class I proteins might process and present HIV-1 antigens more effectively than might others, allowing cytotoxic T lymphocytes in individuals with these alleles to block infection. Immunization with class I HLA antigen has been shown to protect macaques against SIV challenge.[111]

Unlike the cytopathic lentiviruses, the HTLVs are transforming retroviruses that are highly cell-associated. HTLV-I–infected cells express activation markers on the surface of infected cells, including increased IL-2 receptor p55 α chain expression, and spontaneously proliferate in the absence of exogenous antigens in vitro.[289] The presence of excessive receptors for IL-2, a known growth factor for T cells, may be linked to the development of the proliferative leukemic process of adult T-cell leukemia/lymphoma. In addition, HTLV-I–infected CD4+ cells have diminished function and secrete a variety of cytokines, and opportunistic infections may be seen in infected persons with and without evidence of malignancy. HTLV-II appears preferentially to infect CD8+, rather than CD4+, cells.[299]

ONCOVIRUSES: HUMAN T-CELL LYMPHOTROPIC VIRUS TYPES I AND II

Epidemiology

HTLV-I and HTLV-II are members of the *Oncovirinae* subfamily. Evaluation of the global distribution of these two viruses has been complicated by the considerable antigenic similarity between HTLV-I and HTLV-II (~60 per cent homology in nucleotide sequences). The initially developed ELISA and Western blot assays designed to detect HTLV were not able to discriminate between the presence of antibodies to HTLV-I and HTLV-II; DNA PCR was required to distinguish type-specific proviral sequences. Thus, early epidemiologic studies often were unable to distinguish between HTLV-I and HTLV-II infection. Second-generation assays use synthetic type-specific peptides that enable differentiation between HTLV-I and HTLV-II antibodies.[48, 562] More recent studies have been able to discriminate the epidemiologic distribution of the two viruses better.

HTLV-I is highly endemic in southwestern Japan, particularly on the islands of Kyushu, Shikoku, and Okinawa, where roughly 30 per cent of the adult population is seropositive.[289, 709] Geographic clustering of HTLV-I infection in southwestern Japan is observed, and marked variation may be seen within small geographic areas; this microclustering has been speculated to be due to the limited interchange, particularly intermarriage, between neighboring communities in Japan.[709]

Regions of moderate HTLV-I endemicity include areas of the Caribbean, including Jamaica, Trinidad, Barbados, and the West Indies.[43, 401, 465, 689] Parts of Africa also appear to have large reservoirs of HTLV-I infection; possible endemic areas have been identified within Gabon, Chad, Nigeria, Cameroon, Guinea, Zaire, and Ivory Coast.[108, 172, 676] Foci of HTLV-I infection also have been identified in Central and South America, including Panama, Brazil, Colombia, Venezuela, Surinam, Guyana, Ecuador, and Peru.[142, 465]

Genetically distinct variants of HTLV-I have been found among Melanesians in Papua New Guinea and the Solomon Islands and aboriginals in Australia.[30, 473, 711] HTLV-I strains from Japan, the Caribbean, Africa, and the Americas exhibit 97 per cent sequence similarities among envelope gene nucleotides, whereas the Australo-Melanesian variants have only 93 per cent sequence similarity with the other viruses and share nucleotide substitutions not found in HTLV-I from these other areas.[473]

In the United States, initial HTLV seroprevalence studies focused on blood donors and found a very low prevalence of infection. The immunoassays used in these early seroprevalence studies were not able to differentiate HTLV-I from HTLV-II. Seroprevalence among blood donors in the United States in the year after initiation of blood screening was 0.016 to 0.021 per cent. Females and blacks, Hispanics, and Asians were more likely to be seropositive than were males and whites.[87] During the same period, seropositivity among applicants for the U.S. Armed Forces was similarly relatively low but twice that observed among blood donors, that is, 0.41 per 1000.[563] Similar to the demographics observed for seropositive blood donors, the prevalence among black applicants was more than 30 times that among white applicants, and a disproportionate rate of seropositivity among female applicants was observed. Clusters of HTLV-I infection also have been reported among blacks in the southern and southeastern United States and immigrants from HTLV-I–endemic areas.[169, 185, 287, 693]

With the development of advanced immunoassays, differentiation of the epidemiology of HTLV-II infection from HTLV-I infection has been possible. In the United States, about half of HTLV-I/II–seropositive blood donations were found to be positive for HTLV-II by PCR; HTLV-II infection correlated with a history of intravenous drug use or sexual contact with a drug user, and HTLV-I infection correlated with birth of or sexual contact with a person from an HTLV-I–endemic area (Caribbean or Japan).[87] HTLV-II appears to be most prevalent in intravenous drug users in several different countries, and in the United States, HTLV-II accounts for the vast majority of HTLV infections among intravenous drug users.[108] In a study of HTLV-II and HIV seroprevalence among drug users from eight metropolitan areas of the United States, overall prevalence of HTLV-II alone was 15.1

per cent, 9.9 per cent for HIV-1 alone, and 3.3 per cent for dual HIV-1/HTLV-II infection; HTLV-II prevalence was higher in the Southwest and Midwest than Northeast, whereas HIV-1 prevalence was highest in the Northeast.[60] HTLV-II seroprevalence was highest in black and Hispanic persons, increased with age, and was higher in women than men in all age groups. The female predominance of HTLV-II infection may indicate more efficient sexual transmission of HTLV-II from men to women than vice versa; similar findings have been noted with HTLV-I. In persons attending sexually transmitted disease clinics in the United States, nearly two-thirds of HTLV infection is due to HTLV-II.[331]

Clusters of HTLV-II infection also have been identified among several non–drug-using Native American tribes in North and South America, including tribes in Panama, Brazil, New Mexico, and Florida.[276, 283, 374, 400] In Africa, HTLV-II seroprevalence appears to be relatively low; in one study, the prevalence of HTLV-II was 0.8 per cent in Ivory Coast, 0.05 per cent in Guinea, and 0.02 per cent in Senegal.[49]

Factors that influence HTLV-I seropositivity are age, race, sex, and geography. In endemic areas, prevalence in children is low but starts to increase during the teenage years; this age-related increase is more marked for females than males. By 40 to 50 years of age, women are significantly more likely to be infected than are men. This sex- and age-related pattern may be the result of more efficient male-to-female sexual transmission of HTLV-I among sexually active adults as well as a birth cohort effect (decrease in vertical and/or horizontal infection over successive birth cohorts).[637]

Modes of Transmission

Modes of HTLV-I/II transmission are similar to those of HIV-1: sexual contact, parenteral through blood transfusion or intravenous drug use, and perinatally, most often via breast milk. The efficiency of HTLV transmission appears significantly lower than that of HIV because HTLV is highly cell-associated, whereas HIV can be transmitted cell-free and cell-associated.

Sexual Transmission

Sexual transmission of HTLV-I is a significant source of HTLV-I acquisition among adults. Male-to-female sexual transmission appears to be more efficient than is female-to-male transmission.[709] Sexual transmission of HTLV-I from infected men to their wives in Japan increased with older age of the male partner and elevated HTLV-I antibody titer, suggesting that longer duration of infection and elevated viral load may be associated with increased transmissibility.[628] In Japan, rates of seropositivity also have been found to be higher in persons with a history of sexually transmitted diseases, suggesting that disruption of the genital mucosa and/or increase in leukocytes in genital secretions and semen may increase transmission risk.[470] In studies from several different countries, HTLV-I prevalence has been found to be elevated in female sex workers[159, 256, 470, 702]; lack of consistent condom use, duration of prostitution, older age, infection with *Chlamydia trachomatis* or syphilis, antibody to herpes simplex virus type 1, and concomitant HIV-1 infection were associated with elevated HTLV-I prevalence.[256, 470] Increased risk for HTLV-I seropositivity also has been observed among persons attending sexually transmitted disease clinics[223, 331, 470, 700]; in clinics in the United States, HTLV seropositivity ranged from 0.18 to 2.0 per cent.[331] Risk factors for HTLV-I infection among females included multiple sexual partners, bruising during sex, syphilis, and concomitant HIV infection, whereas for men, hepatitis B antigenemia, bruising during sex, older age of sexual activity onset, married status, and agricultural occupation were associated with increased risk.[223]

Sexual transmission of HTLV-II has been less well established than that of HTLV-I. Studies in non–drug-using native populations have shown a strong association between HTLV-II infection between spouses, and higher rates of sexually transmitted infections have been observed among HTLV-II–seropositive injection drug users, providing evidence that sexual transmission of HTLV-II does occur.[60, 595, 681, 682]

Homosexual men in endemic areas are at increased risk of HTLV-I acquisition, presumably through anal intercourse. In Trinidad, HTLV-I seropositivity was sixfold higher among homosexual men than the general population, and male-to-male sex was associated with elevated risk of seropositivity among men seen in sexually transmitted disease clinics in Baltimore, Maryland.[29, 700] The higher rate of HIV than HTLV infection among homosexual men in Trinidad is an indication of the higher efficiency of HIV transmission.

Perinatal Transmission

Perinatal transmission of HTLV-I is the major source of infection among children. Studies in Japan have shown that more than 90 per cent of HTLV-I–seropositive children have mothers who are seropositive themselves; overall, 20 to 25 per cent of children born to infected women become infected.[281, 319, 701] Transmission to the infant appears to occur predominantly post partum, reflected by infant seroconversion to seropositivity after loss of passively transferred maternal antibodies.

Substantial evidence supports that the majority of HTLV-I transmission occurs through breast feeding.[281] HTLV-I antigen has been detected in the breast milk of seropositive mothers, and HTLV-I proviral DNA has been identified by PCR in mononuclear cells from the breast milk of HTLV-I carrier women.[335, 468] In a marmoset animal model, transmission of HTLV-I has been shown by oral feeding of lymphocytes from the breast milk of HTLV-I–infected women.[336, 710] It has been hypothesized that lymphocyte-facilitated infection of gastrointestinal epithelial cells may be the mechanism for transmission.[717]

A number of variables have been associated with HTLV-I transmission risk, including maternal HTLV-I antibody type and titer, presence of maternal HTLV-I antigen in milk, older maternal age, and longer duration of breast feeding.[325, 403, 638, 701] Duration of breast feeding longer than 6 months appears to be associated with a threefold increased risk of transmission.[638, 701] In one study in Japan, no child who breast-fed for less than 6 months became infected, and in a study in Jamaica, children born to mothers with higher titers of HTLV-I antibody had delayed time to seroconversion, suggesting that passive transfer of maternal HTLV-I antibody may affect transmission timing and risk.[403, 636, 638] In an experimental rabbit model, passive immunization with HTLV-I hyperimmunoglobulin prevented milk-borne transmission of HTLV-I.[588] However, in some studies, higher levels of maternal antibody were associated with higher transmission risk, presumably because higher antibody levels may reflect higher viral load.[701] Thus, risk of breast milk transmission most likely is multifactorial, involving duration of exposure, amount and activation level of the virus, and presence of protective or enhancing specific and nonspecific immunity.

Transmission may be possible, albeit infrequent, during the in utero and/or intrapartum period. About 3 to 4 per cent of infants born to carrier mothers are infected despite bottle feeding, suggesting that intrauterine or intrapartum transmission may occur but with much lower efficiency than may transmission via breast milk.[327, 636] Restricted infection of human trophoblast cells by HTLV-I has been demonstrated in vitro.[388] HTLV-I has been identified in cord blood and placentas from HTLV-1–positive mothers by antigen detection and DNA PCR, although positive findings have not always correlated with eventual infection status of the infant[239, 327, 584]; in one study, none of seven children with positive cord blood were found to be infected during 2 to 4 years of follow-up, and cord blood was negative for HTLV-I DNA in nine formula-fed infants who were infected.[327]

HTLV-II also has been detected in the breast milk of carrier mothers, and mother-to-child transmission has been described in the presence of breast feeding.[277, 355, 356, 681] The rate of HTLV-II breast milk transmission described in the few small studies available (~14 per cent) is slightly lower than that found for HTLV-I (20 to 25 per cent). Like HTLV-I, HTLV-II appears to be transmitted infrequently in the absence of breast feeding.[242, 324, 670] Passive immunization with HTLV-II hyperimmunoglobulin in rabbits prevented blood-borne transmission of HTLV-II–infected cells.[454] Interestingly, only HTLV-II and not HTLV-I immunoglobulin were effective in preventing HTLV-II transmission, suggesting that despite some cross-reactivity on conventional ELISAs, there is minimal to no cross-neutralization between the viruses.

Parenteral Transmission

Parenteral transmission by transfusion and intravenous drug use is well documented. HTLV-I has been transmitted by transfusion of cellular components of blood, and transmission of HTLV-II by transfusion also has been recognized.[560] Comparative rates of transmission of HTLV-I, HLTV-II, and HIV-1 were evaluated retrospectively using a large repository of U.S. blood donor serum from the Transfusion Safety Study.[183] Consistent with a requirement for cell-cell contact for HTLV transmission and in contrast to HIV-1, HTLV-I and HTLV-II transmission only was observed with transfusion of cellular blood components. Infectivity appeared to decrease with increasing period of blood storage; no apparent transmission occurred from components stored more than 10 days, suggesting that the known decrease in ability of donor lymphocytes to be activated or proliferate with storage renders the cells noninfectious. The rates of transfusion-related transmission for HTLV-I and HTLV-II were similar, with approximately 27 per cent of recipients of blood components from seropositive donors becoming infected. In contrast, 89 per cent of recipients of HIV-1–positive blood were infected regardless of blood product component type, and no effect of storage on transmission risk was seen.

Screening of blood donors in the United States since 1988, as well as in other countries such as Japan, has reduced markedly transfusion-related transmission. However, in countries in which HTLV-I and HTLV-II screening of blood is not performed, transfusions provide an important source of infection. In a study among hospitalized children in Gabon, Africa, multiple blood transfusions secondary to complications of sickle-cell disease were as predominant a mode of HTLV-I transmission as perinatal transmission.[160] Similarly, in Martinique, the HTLV-I seroprevalence among patients with sickle-cell anemia was 10 per cent compared with 1 to 3 per cent among normal blood donors, and HTLV-I–seropositive patients had received more transfusions than had seronegative persons.[586]

HTLV-II infection in drug users has been associated with nonwhite race, older age, markers of prior hepatitis B virus infection, use of a specific needle-sharing practice called backloading, history of herpes simplex virus type 2 infection, and history of receiving money for sex.[60, 595, 682] Thus, HTLV-II infection among drug users appears to be associated with sexual contact as well as sharing contaminated injection equipment.

Environmental Cofactors

Descriptive studies have suggested that ecologic factors may influence the rate of seropositivity in a population. In Jamaica, residence at a low altitude in a tropical environment was associated with higher rates of seropositivity; similar findings have been observed in Colombia and the West Indies.[401, 437] A role for insect vectors, such as mosquitoes, for HTLV-I has been postulated because of the association of high seropositivity with some vector-transmitted parasitic diseases, such as filariasis in Japan, the aforementioned ecologic associations, and the decline in seroprevalence among persons who migrate from endemic to nonendemic areas.[287, 635] An epidemiologic association between HTLV-I antibodies and parasitic infection with *Strongyloides stercoralis* has been described in Japan and Jamaica.[565] It is possible that these vector associations may be the result of immunologic perturbations caused by exogenous pathogens that could cause lymphocyte activation and amplify the risk of HTLV infection. There is no evidence that retroviruses can replicate in arthropods, and any hypothesized insect-borne transmission would need to occur mechanically via mouth parts of biting insects that were contaminated with a significant amount of infected lymphocytes; such transmission, if it occurs, would be expected to be very unusual.[229] In other studies, the prevalence of antibodies to arboviruses was not significantly greater among HTLV-seropositive than HTLV-seronegative persons.[464]

Disease Associations

In adults, diseases associated with HTLV-I infection are malignancies and chronic degenerative neurologic syndromes. Pediatric manifestations of HTLV-I infection have been identified, and it now is recognized that exposure to HTLV-I early in life may be critical in the development of HTLV-I–associated diseases as adults, years to decades later. HTLV-I may be a prototype for other yet-to-be discovered retroviruses that predispose to diseases of long latency after exposure at birth or early in life.

Human T-Cell Lymphotropic Virus Type I

Adult T-Cell Leukemia and Other Malignancies

Adult T-cell leukemia/lymphoma (ATLL) was the first clinical disease to be linked with HTLV-I infection. This aggressive form of leukemia/lymphoma first was described in Japan prior to the discovery of HTLV-I. The disease is characterized by malignant skin involvement in 40 to 70 per cent of patients, lymphadenopathy, hypercalcemia, bone marrow involvement, and a uniformly fatal course, most often affecting adults between 40 and 60 years of age. Although an infectious etiology was postulated because of geographic clustering of ATLL in southern Japan, it was only after the discovery of HTLV-I in 1980 by Gallo and colleagues that a causal link was established between HTLV-I seropositivity and ATLL.[531]

There is a strong geographic correlation between HTLV-I–endemic areas and the occurrence of ATLL, best characterized in southern Japan, the West Indies, and South America and in migrants from HTLV-I–endemic areas. The incidence of ATLL in the United States is low, with cases primarily seen among immigrants from HTLV-I–endemic areas or among blacks in the southeastern United States, in whom endemic HTLV-I infection has been documented.[552] The male-to-female ratio is equal, and mean age of onset is between 40 and 60 years; the average age of ATLL onset is somewhat lower in patients from the Caribbean and Africa (43 years) than Japan (58 years).[709] The incubation period for ATLL appears to be as long as 20 to 30 years after infection with HTLV-I, and it is postulated that ATLL results from HTLV-I infection acquired during the first few years of life.[466] Only a minority (2 to 4 per cent in endemic areas) of HTLV-I–seropositive persons will develop ATLL.[108] It has been suggested that intermediate factors, such as host or oncogenic environmental stimuli, or both, may be involved in a multistep process leading to malignant transformation.[289]

ATLL has a broad clinical spectrum that can be classified into subtypes according to clinical and laboratory criteria.[108, 709] An asymptomatic HTLV-I carrier may experience a pre-ATLL state, associated with mild leukocytosis or the presence of abnormal lymphocytes with characteristic lobulated nuclei (flower cells) that are found to have monoclonal or oligoclonal HTLV-I provirus integrated into the cell genome. More than 50 per cent of such persons will experience resolution of the leukocytosis spontaneously. Acute ATLL is the rapidly aggressive form of leukemia/lymphoma that first was recognized in Japan, with characteristic cutaneous involvement, leukemia with circulating abnormal lymphocytes, generalized lymphadenopathy, hepatomegaly and/or splenomegaly, lytic bone lesions, hypercalcemia, and immunodeficiency leading to opportunistic infections. Smoldering ATLL is characterized by abnormal cells in the absence of leukocytosis and resembles mycosis fungoides, with an indolent clinical course, cutaneous involvement, and mild lymphadenopathy and/or splenomegaly. Chronic ATLL overlaps with cases of T-cell chronic lymphocytic leukemia and has an indolent clinical course and a moderate leukocytosis, with 0.5 to 3 per cent of circulating cells being malignant; cutaneous manifestations may be observed. Lymphoma-type ATLL overlaps with T-cell non-Hodgkin lymphoma and has prominent lymphadenopathy with the presence of monoclonally integrated HTLV-I in the malignant cells.

The pathogenesis of ATLL is not known. HTLV-I transforms normal CD4 lymphocytes in vitro, resulting in immortalization, high levels of IL-2 expression, and increased expression of the IL-2α chain receptor on the cell surface. Monoclonal HTLV-I provirus is found integrated into the DNA of the ATLL malignant cells. It has been theorized that the tax gene product of HTLV-I causes aberrant activation of host cellular genes and expression of IL-2 and IL-2α chain receptor in infected cells; these cells then may respond to IL-2 in an uncontrolled autocrine manner, leading to proliferation and malignancy.[709] It is not clear why some HTLV-I–infected individuals end up having ATLL or other HTLV-I–associated diseases; differences in host response to HTLV-I infection in part may determine the clinical course of disease.

Treatment regimens for ATLL remain unsatisfactory; high rates of relapse are seen with conventional chemotherapy treatment. Median survival with acute ATLL is less than 12 months, despite chemotherapy. Experimental therapies targeted at the postulated mechanism of pathogenesis are under evaluation, such as immunotherapy with toxin-conjugated monoclonal antibodies directed at the IL-2α chain receptor that is overexpressed on malignant cells.[686]

Other malignancies have been associated with HTLV-I infection, including multiple myeloma and B-cell chronic lymphocytic leukemia. It is thought that these malignancies may arise due to chronic antigenic stimulation of B cells by HTLV-I–infected T cells, resulting in uncontrolled B-cell expansion. In the Caribbean, HTLV-I has been associated with the development of T-cell non-Hodgkin lymphoma.[405] A single case of small-cell cancer of the lung with monoclonally integrated HTLV-I in the tumor has been reported. A pulmonary infiltrative syndrome resembling lymphoid pulmonary hyperplasia seen in HIV-1–infected children has been reported in patients with HTLV-I–associated myelopathy.[629]

Human T-Cell Lymphotropic Virus Type I–Associated Myelopathy

In 1985, a study in Martinique defined an association of HTLV-I seropositivity with a chronic myelopathy known as tropical spastic paraparesis (TSP).[251] Subsequently, a similar syndrome was described in Japan, where it was named HTLV-I–associated myelopathy (HAM).[498] Current terminology for this syndrome is HAM/TSP.

The disease usually has been reported from HTLV-I–endemic areas, including the Caribbean, southern Japan, equatorial Africa, Central and South America, Melanesia, and South Africa.[252] Sporadic cases have been described in nonendemic areas, usually in immigrants from endemic areas or their sexual contacts or recipients of blood transfusions (prior to HTLV blood screening). Estimates of incidence and prevalence are unreliable due to the insidious nature of the disease and lack of recognition of early symptoms by clinicians. In HTLV-I–seropositive persons in Japan, the prevalence of HAM/TSP reaches 68 per 100,000, with an incidence of 3.1 per 100,000 HTLV-I–infected persons per year.[252]

Case reports of HAM/TSP occurring after blood transfusion and the finding in Japan and Martinique that 13 to 20 per cent of HAM/TSP cases had a history of blood transfusion accelerated the decision of blood banks in the United States to screen for HTLV-I antibodies. In Japan, there was a 16 per cent decrease in the number of HAM/TSP cases in the 2 years after the initiation of blood screening.[497]

Although the mean onset of disease is in the fourth decade of life, incubation of this disease may be shorter than that of ATLL, as HAM/TSP has been reported to develop as early as 18 weeks after transfusion with contaminated blood.[258] Onset of symptoms is uncommon in persons younger than 20 years or older than 70 years of age. There is an excess of cases among women, with the male:female ratio being approximately 1:2.

The disorder is characterized by chronic progressive spastic paraparesis of the limbs, particularly the legs, mild sensory loss, painful paresthesias, and bladder and bowel sphincter impairments. Systemic nonneurologic symptoms suggestive of an autoimmune process also may occur, such as pulmonary aveolitis, uveitis, arthropathy, Sjögren syndrome, and vasculitis.[289] Progression is variable, and young age at onset has been associated with more rapid disease; 10 years after onset, 30 per cent of patients are bedridden and 45 per cent require crutches to walk.[252] Nonspecific lesions of the brain are observed with magnetic resonance imaging in as many as 75 per cent of patients, but there is no clear correlation of the lesions and symptoms. Multiple foci of increased T_2-signal intensity are found in periventricular matter, similar to the findings observed in patients with multiple sclerosis. However, cognitive impairment may be observed in multiple sclerosis and is not observed in HAM/TSP, and HTLV-I sequences have not been detected in the peripheral blood or central nervous systems of multiple sclerosis patients.[490]

Pathologically, there is macroscopic atrophy of the spinal cord, with changes consistent with a chronic inflammatory process of the spinal cord, particularly in the lower thoracic cord, and parenchymal damage of both white and gray matter. Although perivascular mononuclear cell infiltration in the brain may be seen, parenchymal damage of the central nervous system is rare.

Patients with HAM/TSP have higher HTLV-I antibody titers and higher levels of spontaneous lymphocyte proliferation than do asymptomatic seropositive and ATLL patients; HTLV-I antibodies may be found in the cerebrospinal fluid as well as in serum. A mild pleocytosis may be observed, and atypical cells containing HTLV-I proviral DNA may be found in about 3 to 15 per cent of circulating lymphocytes; unlike the monoclonal integration observed in ATLL, polyclonal integration of HTLV-I is observed.[252] Despite integration of virus, viral expression is low. High levels of HTLV-I cytotoxic CD8+ and CD4+ lymphocytes have been reported in the blood and cerebrospinal fluid of HAM/TSP patients. These findings have led to the hypothesis that patients with HAM/TSP demonstrate a heightened immune response against HTLV-I that could be involved in disease causation.

The pathogenesis of HAM/TSP is not known; one postulated mechanism is direct infection of central nervous system glial cells by HTLV-I, generating a direct cytotoxic immune response to the glial cell that results in demyelination.[289] However, there is no clear evidence that HTLV-I infects central nervous system cells. Alternatively, perivascular inflammatory infiltrates containing HTLV-I–infected T cells could activate cytotoxic CD8+ cells, with subsequent secretion of cytokines that might induce demyelination.[289] Another hypothesized mechanism is more indirect and involves HTLV-I–associated activation of autoreactive cells, which could lead to an autoimmune process that induces myelin destruction.

Similar to ATLL, no curative treatment has been developed. Symptomatic treatment includes measures to maintain muscle function and reduce spasticity. Corticosteroids may induce transient benefit in about 50 per cent of patients, and ZDV combined with α-interferon therapy has shown some promise.[271, 289]

Pediatric Manifestations

A clinical syndrome in children called infective dermatitis has been linked to perinatal HTLV-I infection.[354] The diagnostic features of infectious dermatitis are characterized by the acute onset of severe exudative eczema without preceding infantile eczema. This crusting eczema involves the scalp, eyelid margins, perinasal skin, retroauricular areas, axillae, and groin. The eczema often is accompanied by a generalized fine papular rash of the trunk and back, and a chronic nasal discharge in the absence of other causes of rhinitis may be seen. The age of onset usually is in the second to third year of life. The syndrome is a chronic, refractory condition often associated with recurrent bouts of infection with saprophytic *S. aureus* or beta-hemolytic streptococci, which require chronic antibiotic therapy to control.

Skin diseases ranging from infective dermatitis to cutaneous manifestations of ALT and other T-cell lymphomas, such as mycosis fungoides and Sézary syndrome, have been described in HTLV-I infection. In a rabbit model, infection with HTLV-I by intravenous inoculation was associated with the development of a generalized exfoliative papillary dermatitis characterized by T-cell infiltrates in the epidermis and epithelium of the hair follicle similar to that seen in cutaneous T-cell lymphoma.[611] HTLV-I envelope sequences were detected by DNA PCR in skin biopsy samples, and HTLV-I was isolated from cutaneous cultures of affected skin, indicating that the cutaneous manifestations may be a direct consequence of HTLV-I infection in the skin.

It is postulated that infective dermatitis represents an HTLV-I–associated immunodeficiency syndrome resulting from early life exposure to HTLV-I, primarily through mother-to-child transmission. Historically, some patients with this condition subsequently have developed ATL in adolescence, and in two cases, mothers may have died of ATL. The nature of the postulated immune defect is under research. A cross-sectional study of HTLV-I–seropositive and HTLV-I–seronegative Jamaican children 11 to 31 months of age showed that HTLV-I seropositivity was associated with an increase in CD4 cells expressing HLA-DR on their surface (a marker of T-cell activation) that was progressive and related to the duration of infection.[402] These findings appear to be an early marker for infection in children and may indicate an early perturbation in the immune system of infected children.

Other Disorders

Other data also suggest a role for HTLV-I in immunodeficiency. Perturbations in lymphokine and cytokine production have been observed with HTLV-I in vitro, most likely due to *tax*-mediated transactivation of various host-cell pathways. Spontaneous lymphocyte proliferation is seen in HAM/TSP and asymptomatic seropositive patients, and changes in T-cell subsets, reflecting an increase in activation markers, such as the IL-2 receptor, also are observed, supporting the concept that HTLV-I affects host immune regulation. *Pneumocystis carinii* pneumonia (PCP) and Norwegian scabies may develop in the absence of ATL, and infected patients also are more likely to acquire a number of infections, including tuberculosis, leprosy, and strongyloidiasis.

A number of autoimmune disorders have been associated with HTLV-I. In a study of 113 HTLV-I–infected patients in southern Florida, rheumatologic or autoimmune diseases were not uncommon, and some patients exhibited immune deficiencies in the absence of concomitant ATLL.[271] A large joint chronic oligoarthropathy associated with synovial proliferation has been described in seropositive persons; HTLV-I has been detected in synovial cells.[338] A chronic inflammatory arthropathy may be seen in HTLV-I transgenic mice.[306] An association of HTLV-I infection also has been reported with polymyositis and uveitis.[709] High levels of HTLV-I antibodies in serum and IgA antibodies in saliva have been associated with Sjögren syndrome in Japan.[647]

Because some of the geographic areas endemic for HTLV-I also are endemic for HIV-1, dual infection with both viruses may occur. Based on in vitro studies indicating that HTLV-I *tax* gene product can interact with the *tat* response element of the HIV-1 LTR and enhance HIV-1 replication, it has been proposed that dual infection might increase HIV-1 disease progression or increase the frequency of HTLV-I–associated diseases. In clinical studies, dual infection has been associated with elevated CD4+ lymphocyte number despite advanced symptoms of immunodeficiency.[219, 589] CD4+ number therefore may be an unreliable predictor of immunodeficiency in dually infected patients; HTLV-I may induce elevated CD4+ number through enhancing lymphocyte proliferation, but the function of these cells may be abnormal.

Human T-Cell Lymphotropic Virus Type II

HTLV-II first was identified in patients with hairy-cell leukemia, although subsequently it has become clear that most patients with hairy-cell leukemia are seronegative for HTLV-II. HTLV-II infection is widespread among intravenous drug users in the United States and Europe, and clusters of

HTLV-II seropositivity also have been found among Native Americans in South, Central, and North America.[695]

Like HTLV-I, HTLV-II can transform cells in vitro; interestingly, HTLV-II preferentially may infect CD8+ lymphocytes, whereas HTLV-I preferentially infects CD4+ lymphocytes.[695] This difference might lead to variations between the two viruses in disease consequences of infection.

Limited data are available regarding the association of clinical disease with HTLV-II infection. In contrast to the clear association of ATLL with HTLV-I infection, no convincing link of HTLV-II to malignancy has been observed. In an HTLV-II–endemic population of Native Americans in New Mexico, no apparent increase in the incidence of hairy-cell leukemia, mycosis fungoides, and chronic lymphocytic leukemia was observed over that observed in other ethnic groups.[283] HTLV-II has been isolated from patients with myeloneuropathies resembling HAM/TSP.[695] Patients with HIV-1 infection who have sensory peripheral polyneuropathy have been found to have a higher prevalence of HTLV-II coinfection, diagnosed by serology and DNA PCR, than have HIV-1–infected patients without neuropathy, suggesting that HTLV-II may be involved in the pathogenesis of the neuropathy.[719]

The natural history and clinical manifestations of HTLV-II need further delineation in the context of ongoing prospective natural history studies.

LENTIVIRUSES: HIV-1 AND HIV-2

HIV-1

Epidemiology of HIV-1 Infection: Women, Children, and Adolescents

The first pediatric case of AIDS was reported to the Centers for Disease Control and Prevention (CDC) in November 1982, 18 months after the first description of AIDS in adults. In the United States, more than 95 per cent of reported AIDS cases in children 0 to 4 years of age now are acquired perinatally. It is estimated that approximately 15,000 perinatally infected children were born in the United States between 1978 to 1993, more than half of whom were born since 1988.[153] Approximately 36 per cent of these children have developed AIDS, and 18 per cent have died. Additionally, an estimated 1630 newly infected infants are born each year.[153] HIV-1 infection already has had a significant impact on childhood mortality in the United States[118]; in 1992, HIV/AIDS was the seventh leading cause of death in all children 1 to 4 years of age and was the first and second leading case of death in Hispanic and black children in this age group in New York State.

Globally, the World Health Organization (WHO) estimates that 3.5 million women, most of child-bearing age, have been infected with HIV-1 and more than 1 million children have been infected, the vast majority through mother-to-child transmission. An estimated 3000 additional women become infected every day.[662] By the year 2000, WHO projects that as many as 5 to 10 million children will be infected, the majority in sub-Saharan Africa. HIV-1 has emerged as a leading contributor to childhood mortality worldwide; in areas in Africa with high HIV-1 seroprevalence among women, it is estimated that mortality among children younger than 5 years of age will increase by 33 to 75 per cent due to perinatal HIV-1 infection.[480] Thus, pediatric HIV-1 infection constitutes a significant global public health problem.

AIDS Surveillance and HIV-1 Classification Systems

The surveillance definition for AIDS in children younger than 13 years of age differs from that for adolescents and adults ($\geq$13 years of age), reflecting underlying differences in the natural history of HIV-1 infection of the immature neonatal immune system compared with the effect of infection on a more mature immune system. Expansion and revision of the pediatric case definition have occurred twice (1985 and 1987) in an attempt to encompass a broader spectrum of manifestations of HIV-1 infection in children by linking clinical symptomatology to serologic and laboratory findings. The current CDC definition of pediatric AIDS (Table 192–3) differs from that in adults in several important ways. Two specific entities, recurrent serious bacterial infection and lymphoid interstitial pneumonitis/pulmonary lymphoid hyperplasia (LIP/PLH), are unique AIDS-defining illnesses in children but not adults,[85] and pulmonary tuberculosis, recurrent pneumonia, and invasive cervical cancer have been added to an expanded AIDS surveillance definition for adults only.[93] In addition, the diagnosis of HIV-1 infection in children is subdivided by age, requiring virologic confirmation of infection status in seropositive infants younger than 18 months of age; seropositivity alone can confirm infection in children 18 months of age or older, as for adults[99] (Table 192–4). Finally, the AIDS case definition for adolescents and adults has been expanded to include a CD4+ lymphocyte count less than 200/mm^3 or less than 14 per cent as an AIDS-indicator condition.[93] However, because of the significant age-related changes in lymphocyte subsets during the first few years of life, CD4+ count has not been incorporated into the pediatric AIDS definition.

In recognition that the spectrum of HIV manifestations in children differs from that in adults and that a significant number of HIV-1–infected children may be symptomatic yet not have overt AIDS, a standard classification system for HIV-1 infection in children was developed in 1987[84] and subsequently modified in 1994.[99] In the current classification system, children are grouped into mutually exclusive categories based on three parameters: (1) infection status (exposed, infected, seroreverter), (2) clinical status (asymptomatic, mild, moderate, or severe signs and symptoms), and (3) immunologic status (age-related categories of no, moderate, or severe suppression) (Tables 192–5, 192–6, and 192–7). Reclassification to a less severe category does not occur, even if the child's clinical or immune status improves.

Epidemiology: AIDS Surveillance

Global surveillance for AIDS by WHO established that HIV-1 infection was distributed throughout the world by the end of the 1980s with more than 215,000 AIDS cases reported from more than 150 countries. The epidemic in North and Latin America, Western Europe, and Oceania was confined originally to homosexual men and intravenous drug users. However, with increased heterosexual spread of HIV-1 in these countries, the number of AIDS cases in women and children has mounted. In sub-Saharan Africa and the Caribbean, where AIDS has occurred predominantly in sexually active heterosexuals, more than one-half of AIDS cases occur in women and children.

In the United States, the incidence of AIDS is increasing more rapidly among women than men. Between 1985 and 1994, the proportion of AIDS cases among women increased nearly threefold, from 7 to 18 per cent.[101] For women with AIDS, HIV-1 acquisition through heterosexual contact (38 per cent of cases) has become as common as exposure through

TABLE 192–3. Pediatric (<13 Years of Age) AIDS Surveillance Definition: AIDS-Defining Conditions

AIDS-Defining Condition	Site	Comments
Bacterial Infections		
Recurrent, serious	Sepsis, meningitis, pneumonia, bone or joint infection or abscess of internal organ or body cavity (**excluding** otitis media, superficial skin or mucosal abscesses, and indwelling catheter–related infections)	Multiple/recurrent (≥2 within 2 years); must be culture-confirmed
Salmonella (nontyphoid)		Recurrent
Mycobacterium avium complex *Mycobacterium kansasii* *Mycobacterium,* other or unidentified species	Disseminated (at site other than or in addition to lungs, skin, or cervical or hilar lymph nodes)	Presumptive diagnosis permitted
Mycobacterium tuberculosis	Extrapulmonary or disseminated	
Fungal Infections		
Candidiasis	Esophagus Pulmonary (trachea/bronchi/lungs)	Presumptive diagnosis permitted
Cryptococcosis	Extrapulmonary	
Histoplasmosis	Disseminated (at site other than or in addition to lungs or cervical or hilar lymph nodes)	
Coccidioidomycosis	Disseminated (at site other than or in addition to lungs or cervical or hilar lymph nodes)	
Protozoal Infections		
Cryptosporidiosis or isosporiasis	Diarrhea	Persisting >1 month
Pneumocystis carinii	Pneumonia	Presumptive diagnosis permitted
Toxoplasmosis	Brain	Onset >1 month of age; presumptive diagnosis permitted
Viral Infections		
Cytomegalovirus	Retinitis or disease at site **other than** liver, spleen, or lymph nodes	Onset symptoms >1 month of age; presumptive diagnosis of retinitis with loss of vision permitted
Herpes simplex	Mucocutaneous; pulmonary (bronchitis or pneumonitis) or esophagitis	Ulcers persisting >1-month duration Onset symptoms >1 month of age
Papovavirus	Brain (progressive multifocal leukoencephalopathy)	
Cancers		
Kaposi sarcoma		Presumptive diagnosis permitted
Lymphoma	Primary, in brain; Burkitt (small, noncleaved cell); immunoblastic or large-cell; of B-cell or unknown immunologic phenotype	
Idiopathic Conditions		
Lymphoid interstitial pneumonitis/pulmonary lymphoid hyperplasia		Presumptive diagnosis permitted
Encephalopathy		At least one of the following progressive findings present for ≥2 months in absence of other etiology: 1) Failure to attain or loss of developmental milestones or loss of intellectual ability on standardized testing 2) Impaired brain growth (shown by serial head circumference measures or brain atrophy on CT or MRI) 3) Acquired symmetric motor deficit manifested by ≥2 of following: paresis, pathologic reflexes, ataxia, or gait disturbance
Wasting syndrome		Any of the following findings in absence of concurrent illness other than HIV: 1) Persistent weight loss >10% baseline 2) Downward crossing of ≥2 percentile lines on weight-for-age chart in child ≥1 year of age 3) <5 percentile on weight-for-height chart on two consecutive measure ≥30 days apart **plus** either • Chronic diarrhea (≥2 loose stools/day for ≥30 days) or • Documented fever (≥30 days, intermittent or constant)

CT, computed tomography; MRI, magnetic resonance imaging.

Modified from Centers for Disease Control: Revision of the CDC surveillance case definition for acquired immunodeficiency syndrome. M. M. W. R. *36*(No. 1–S):1–15, 1987.

TABLE 192–4. Requirements for Diagnosis of HIV-1 Infection in Children

Diagnosis: HIV-Infected

1. A child <18 months of age who is known to be HIV-1–seropositive or born to an HIV-infected mother **AND**:
   - has positive results on two separate determinations (excluding cord blood) from one or more of the following HIV detection tests:
   - HIV culture
   - HIV polymerase chain reaction
   - HIV p24 antigen

   OR
   - meets criteria for AIDs diagnosis based on the 1987 AIDS surveillance case definition
2. A child ≥18 months of age born to an HIV-1–infected mother or any child infected by blood, blood products, or other known modes of transmission (e.g., sexual contact) who:
   - is HIV-1–antibody–positive by repeatedly reactive enzyme immunoassay (EIA) and confirmatory test (e.g., Western blot, immunofluorescence assay [IFA])

   OR
   - meets any of the criteria in (1) above

Diagnosis: Perinatally Exposed

A child who does not meet the criteria above who:
- is HIV-1–seropositive by EIA and confirmatory test (e.g., Western blot, IFA) and is <18 months of age at the time of test;

OR
- has unknown antibody status but was born to a mother known to be infected with HIV-1

Diagnosis: Seroreverter

A child who is born to an HIV-1–infected mother and who:
- has been documented as HIV-1–antibody–negative (i.e., two or more negative EIA tests performed at 6 to 18 months of age or one negative EIA test after 18 months of age)

AND
- has had no other laboratory evidence of infection (has not had two positive viral detection tests, if performed)

AND
- has not had an AIDS-defining condition

Modified from Centers for Disease Control and Prevention: 1994 revised classification system for human immunodeficiency virus infection in children less than 13 years of age. M. M. W. R. *43*(No. RR-12):1–10, 1994.

TABLE 192–5. 1994 Revised Pediatric Classification System for HIV Infection in Children (<13 Years of Age)*

Immunologic Category	Clinical Category			
	N: No Signs/Symptoms	*A: Mild Signs/Symptoms*	*B: Moderate Signs/Symptoms*	*C: Severe Signs/Symptoms*
No suppression	N1	A1	B1	C1
Moderate	N2	A2	B2	C2
Severe	N3	A3	B3	C3

* Children whose HIV infection status is not confirmed are classified by using the above grid with a letter E (for perinatally exposed) placed before the appropriate classification code (e.g., EN2).

Modified from Centers for Disease Control and Prevention: 1994 revised classification system for human immunodeficiency virus infection in children less than 13 years of age. M. M. W. R. *43*(No. RR-12):1–10, 1994.

TABLE 192–6. 1994 Revised Pediatric HIV Classification System: Immunologic Axis Categories Based on Age-Specific CD4+ Lymphocyte Count and Per Cent

Immune Category	Age of Child					
	<12 mo		*1–5 yr*		*6–12 yr*	
	μL		μL		μL	
No suppression	≥1500	(≥25%)	≥1000	(≥25%)	≥500	(≥25%)
Moderate	750–1499	(15–24%)	500–999	(15–24%)	200–499	(15–24%)
Severe	<750	(<15%)	<500	(<15%)	<200	(<15%)

Modified from Centers for Disease Control and Prevention: 1994 revised classification system for human immunodeficiency virus infection in children less than 13 years of age. M. M. W. R. *43*(No. RR-12):1–10, 1994.

TABLE 192–7. 1994 Revised HIV Pediatric Classification System: Clinical Axis Categories

Category N: Not Symptomatic

Children who have no signs or symptoms considered to be the result of HIV infection or who have only one of the conditions listed in Category A

Category A: Mildly Symptomatic

Children with **two** or more of the conditions listed below but none of the conditions listed in Categories B and C

- Lymphadenopathy (≥0.5 cm at more than two sites; bilateral = one site)
- Hepatomegaly
- Splenomegaly
- Dermatitis
- Parotitis
- Recurrent or persistent upper respiratory infection, sinusitis, or otitis media

Category B: Moderately Symptomatic

Children who have symptomatic conditions other than those listed for Category A or C that are attributed to HIV infection

Examples of conditions in clinical Category B include but are not limited to:

- Anemia (<8 gm/dL), neutropenia (<1,000/mm³), or thrombocytopenia (<100,000/mm³) persisting ≥30 days
- Bacterial meningitis, pneumonia, or sepsis (single episode)
- Candidiasis, oropharyngeal (thrush) persisting (>2 months) in children >6 months of age
- Cardiomyopathy
- Cytomegalovirus infection, with onset before 1 month of age
- Diarrhea, recurrent or chronic
- Hepatitis
- Herpes simplex virus (HSV) stomatitis, recurrent (more than two episodes within 1 year)
- HSV bronchitis, pneumonitis, or esophagitis with onset before 1 month of age
- Herpes zoster (shingles) involving at least two distinct episodes or more than one dermatome
- Leiomyosarcoma
- Lymphoid interstitial pneumonia (LIP) or pulmonary lymphoid hyperplasia complex
- Nephropathy
- Nocardiosis
- Persistent fever (lasting >1 month)
- Toxoplasmosis, onset before 1 month of age
- Varicella, disseminated (complicated chickenpox)

Category C: Severely Symptomatic

Children who have any condition listed in the 1987 surveillance case definition for AIDS, with the exception of LIP (which is a Category B condition)

Modified from Centers for Disease Control and Prevention: 1994 revised classification system for human immunodeficiency virus infection in children less than 13 years of age. M. M. W. R. *43*(No. RR-12):1–10, 1994.

injecting drug use (39 per cent).[100] Among adolescent females with AIDS, heterosexual acquisition of HIV-1 is even more common, reported in more than 50 per cent of cases. The vast majority of women with AIDS are of child-bearing age, with a median age of 35 years. AIDS in women occurs predominantly among women of minority race/ethnicity, and minority women with AIDS are more likely than Caucasian women to have acquired infection heterosexually. Geographically, the AIDS epidemic among women initially was localized in urban epicenters. However, currently more than 25 per cent of women with AIDS are from nonurban and rural locales.[198]

Of the 476,899 AIDS cases reported to the CDC as of June 1995, 1.4 per cent have occurred in children younger than 13 years of age, 0.5 per cent in adolescents 13 to 19 years of age, and 3.7 per cent in young adults 20 to 24 years of age, the majority of whom were infected during their adolescent years.[100] Cases of pediatric AIDS have been reported from 49 states, although 63 per cent have been reported from four states and one territory—New York, Florida, New Jersey, California, and Puerto Rico. Perinatal transmission accounts for the vast majority of AIDS cases in children younger than 13 years of age; a substantial but dwindling minority have acquired infection from contaminated blood products (hemophilia/coagulation disorder, 3 per cent; receipt of blood transfusion, blood components, or tissue, 5 per cent), and in 2 per cent the mode of acquisition still is under investigation. Mirroring the epidemiology of AIDS in women, most children with AIDS are of minority race/ethnicity.

AIDS in the adolescent and young adult age group (<24 years of age) deserves special consideration. The relatively low number of reported AIDS cases in this age group fails to provide a true measure of the impact of HIV-1 infection on adolescents. Disease manifestations from HIV-1 infection acquired during adolescence will not be manifest for many years due to the long latency period from the time of infection to development of the end-stage disease of AIDS. Adolescents with AIDS are more likely than adults to be female and of minority race/ethnicity.[381] Acquisition of infection through heterosexual contact is most common for adolescent females, whereas for adolescent males, homosexual contact remains an important exposure category. Although most adolescent AIDS cases have been reported from inner-city areas, a significant minority of cases come from less urban areas with populations of less than 500,000.

Epidemiology: HIV-1 Surveillance

AIDS surveillance reports reflect the distribution of HIV-1 infection 7 to 10 years previously. To indicate the current magnitude and extent of HIV-1 infection more accurately, having information about HIV-1 seroprevalence is necessary. Such information has been obtained through analysis of data from special studies, localities with HIV-1 infection reporting, and anonymous HIV seroprevalence surveys.

HIV-1 seroprevalence among women seen in reproductive health clinics in 30 cities has ranged from 0 to 2.28 per cent, with rates of more than 1 per cent predominantly observed in clinics from the East Coast and Puerto Rico.[633] Infection rates were higher among black than Hispanic or white women (median rates of infection, 0.34, 0.11, and 0 per cent, respectively). Similar disproportionate clustering of HIV-1 infection among women of minority race/ethnicity was observed among women in the Army Reserve Corps (overall prevalence, 0.65 per 1000); other demographic risk factors for HIV-1 infection in women in the Army Reserve included residence in a low-income area or an area of high AIDS prevalence.[145] Estimates of HIV-1 seroprevalence among child-bearing women in the United States have been obtained by testing paper-absorbed newborn blood specimens routinely collected for metabolic screening for the presence of HIV-1 antibody.[288] The presence of HIV-1 antibody in the neonate reflects the infection status of the mother. From 1989 through 1993, the annual prevalence of HIV-1 infection among women giving birth remained relatively stable, ranging between 1.6 and 1.7 per 1000.[101] Distinct regional variations in seroprevalence were observed, with rates among child-bearing women in the Northeast decreasing over time from 4.1 to 3.4 per 1000, while rates in the South increased from 1.6 to 2.0 per 1000.[688] Based on these data, it is estimated that approximately 6500 HIV-1–infected women give birth annually in the United States; given a 20 to 30 per cent transmission rate, 1300 to 1950 newly infected infants may be born each year.

The prevalence of HIV-1 infection among adolescents has been studied in various subpopulations of youth. Overall HIV-1 seroprevalence rates have been 0.05 per cent or lower among youth who might be considered relatively low-risk, such as college students (0.04 per cent) and military recruits (0.03 per cent).[381] In these studies, higher seroprevalence rates were observed among adolescents from urban epicenters and racial/ethnic minorities. Among disadvantaged youth in the U.S. Job Corps, HIV-1 seroprevalence rates nearly 10 times higher were observed, with 0.3 per cent of applicants screened between 1988 and 1992 being seropositive.[139] A disproportionately high seroprevalence was observed in Job Corps applicants from the southeastern United States, particularly among women, consistent with spread of HIV-1 infection from urban to more rural areas. Seroprevalence was higher among youth of minority race/ethnicity and highest among black youth. HIV-1 seroprevalence among males appeared to decrease over time. In contrast, seroprevalence among females increased and exceeded that observed in men by 1990, indicating a shift in the HIV-1 epidemic to young women. Among pregnant adolescent women undergoing HIV-1 testing at a southern urban hospital, HIV-1 seroprevalence was 0.47 per cent.[383] Other studies of high-risk youth also have reported higher HIV-1 prevalence among adolescent minority females than males.[150, 499, 632, 696] Seroprevalence rates exceeding 5 per cent have been reported among some high-risk youth. Sites providing services to homeless/runaway youth have reported HIV-1 prevalence rates up to 7.3 per cent, and rates of 15.3 per cent were reported in adolescents with syphilis identified in adolescent and school-based health clinics in New York City.[9, 421] Characteristics of adolescents at particularly high risk of HIV-1 infection include minority race/ethnicity, particularly women; residence in inner-city urban areas with high general prevalence of HIV-1 infection; presence of other sexually transmitted diseases or pregnancy; out-of-school youth and runaways; and those practicing high-risk behavior, such as those using injecting drugs or young men having sex with men.

Globally, three broad geographic patterns of HIV-1 transmission have been described. Pattern I includes geographic areas such as North America and Western Europe. HIV-1 transmission in these areas began primarily among homosexual and bisexual men and injecting drug users. Subsequent spread among heterosexuals and perinatally to children followed more slowly. In pattern II countries, heterosexual transmission predominates. These countries contain the vast majority of infected persons and include Africa, the Caribbean, and some parts of South America. In these areas, the male:female ratio of AIDS cases approaches 1, and there is significant perinatal transmission. Pattern III constitutes those areas with emerging HIV-1 infection, such as Asia, the Middle East, and Eastern Europe. In these areas, rapid and successive spread among injecting drug users, commercial sex workers, and heterosexual men has occurred, with subsequent heterosexual transmission to women and, through perinatal transmission, children.

Modes of Transmission of HIV-1

Transmission of HIV-1 requires a quantity of virus sufficient to cause infection and a portal of entry that permits establishment of infection within host cells. HIV transmission occurs primarily (1) through sexual contact, (2) from mother to infant, and (3) through exposure to infected blood (such as transfusion, needle-sharing).

SEXUAL TRANSMISSION

The importance of sexual transmission of HIV-1 first was recognized among sexually active homosexual men, in whom the syndrome of AIDS initially was recognized. Male homosexual transmission continues to constitute a major source of HIV-1 infection, particularly in North America and parts of Latin America. Risk factors for acquisition of HIV-1 among homosexual men include receptive anal intercourse, multiple sexual partners, disease stage of the infected partner, the presence of ulcerative diseases (such as herpes simplex virus type 2), and lack of circumcision.[78] The likelihood of engaging in unsafe sexual practices may be highest among adolescent homosexual males, whose sexual identity is just becoming established and who may not appreciate what behaviors, including alcohol and other drug use, might put them at risk of HIV acquisition.

Worldwide, heterosexual transmission accounts for the vast majority of HIV-1 transmission. Compared with the efficiency of transmission by transfusion or perinatally, the efficiency of transmission via sexual contact is relatively low; the average estimated infectivity per sexual exposure is 0.3 per cent.[520] In studies that evaluated HIV-1 transmission in stable couples with a single infected partner, the efficiency of sexual transmission of HIV-1 from men to women was found to be significantly greater than from women to men.[216, 481, 503, 520] Several biologic factors may account for this difference. The cervicovaginal surface provides a more expansive area for viral contact than does the male genital tract, and contact with semen within the female genital tract is considerably longer than male genital contact with vaginal secretions. Additionally, HIV rapidly is inactivated at low pH. The ejaculation of semen, with pH 7.0 to 8.0, into the normally acid environment of the vagina (pH 4.0 to 5.0) modifies the female genital tract into a more favorable milieu for HIV survival.

The risk of sexual HIV-1 transmission may be modified by factors relating to the infected person, the virus, or the seronegative partner. The infectivity of the seropositive partner may be related to the stage of HIV disease and immunologic and virologic correlates of disease stage, such as CD4 count and level of cell-associated and cell-free virus. A number of studies have documented enhanced transmission risk from partners with advanced disease stage, as demonstrated by low CD4+ count or clinical AIDS.[457, 481, 482] These factors simply may be surrogates for higher genital viral load.[677] Sexually transmitted diseases could increase the infectivity of genital secretions; detection of HIV-1–infected cells in semen has been shown to be associated independently with the presence of urethritis and gonorrhea in infected men.[457] Immune response may play a role; sexual transmission was more common from persons with lower levels of cross-reactive V3 loop antibodies in one study.[224]

HIV-1 exhibits a high degree of genetic variability; different viral variants could vary in their ability to infect a new host. Virologic factors that have been associated with sexual transmission include nonsyncytia-inducing, macrophage-tropic phenotype[671] and viral subtype, with subtype E appearing to be more easily transmitted heterosexually than subtype B.[351, 414]

Host susceptibility to infection may be enhanced by the presence of genital ulcer disease or other sexually transmitted diseases, such as gonorrhea, chlamydia, and cervicitis.[82, 222, 434, 530, 587, 644] Lack of male circumcision has been associated with increased HIV-1 transmission in a number of studies.[174, 587, 597] Because macrophages and Langerhans cells are found in high concentrations in the foreskin, trapping of infected cells and free virus under the foreskin could provide more prolonged HIV exposure to susceptible cells.[348] Cervical ectopy, in which the simple columnar epithelium of the endocervix everts onto the normally more protective stratified squamous epithelium of the ectocervix, has been associated with increased transmission risk in some studies.[456] Cervical ectropion normally is present over as much as half of the ectocervix of adolescents, which could put them at greater risk for sexual acquisition of HIV. Use of oral contraceptives has been hypothesized to increase transmission risk due to increased rates of cervical ectropion, but studies have had conflicting results.[282, 323, 530] Use of intrauterine devices for contraception, intravaginal treatments, and douching have been associated with enhanced transmission risk in some studies, presumably due to inflammation causing an increase in susceptible cells in the genital tract.[149, 323, 612]

Other factors that have been associated with elevated risk of sexual transmission include heterosexual anal intercourse,[482, 502, 599] trauma/bleeding during sex and/or exposure to menstrual blood,[222, 398, 502, 599] number of sexual contacts with an infected person,[502] and multiple sex partners.[222, 398] Consistent use of condoms has been effective in reducing the risk of HIV-1 transmission in a large number of studies from different countries.[82, 173, 434, 502, 530]

PERINATAL TRANSMISSION

Transmission of HIV-1 from mother to child is the predominant source of HIV-1 acquisition in children. Early in the HIV-1 epidemic, the rate of perinatal transmission was estimated to be as high as 65 per cent. However, these early studies were performed prior to the availability of diagnostic tests for HIV-1 and therefore focused on infected women identified because of clinical symptoms or the prior birth of a child with AIDS.

Studies of more representative populations of HIV-1–infected women monitored prospectively have provided lower estimates of perinatal transmission rates. Intriguing differences have been observed between studies from industrialized countries, such as the United States and Europe, where transmission rates have ranged from 14 to 33 per cent, and some studies from the developing world, particularly Africa, where rates as high as 39 per cent have been reported (Table 192–8). The reasons for this variance are not defined yet but probably are multifactorial, including geographic variation in the prevalence of potential cofactors that could influence transmission, such as sexually transmitted diseases, chorioamnionitis, stage of maternal disease, nutritional deficiencies, breast feeding, and HIV-1 subtype.

Data support HIV transmission during both the antepartum and intrapartum periods, as well as postpartum via breast milk[444] (Table 192–9). Evidence for transmission in utero includes identification of HIV in placentas from HIV-1–infected women,[112, 378, 417] demonstration of in vitro HIV infection of placentally derived cells,[406, 524, 718] detection of HIV in fetal tissue obtained from abortuses as early as 8 weeks' gestation,[143, 360, 397, 407, 511, 617] and isolation of HIV from amniotic fluid cells and supernatant.[463, 680] In vitro studies have shown that fetal cells are highly susceptible to HIV infection; fetal thymic cells readily are infected with HIV, and cord blood macrophages are more susceptible than are adult macrophages to infection.[272, 574] Clinical stigmata consistent with infection occurring during the period of fetal organogenesis appear to be unusual with perinatally transmitted HIV-1. Although a craniofacial "AIDS embryopathy" consistent with HIV transmission early in utero transmission was described early in the HIV epidemic, subsequent studies have not confirmed this finding[199, 543]; these findings appear to be associated with maternal drug use during pregnancy rather than with HIV itself.

Current data suggest that the majority of transmission may occur during the intrapartum period. Clinical stigmata consistent with in utero transmission are infrequent. Intrauterine growth retardation appears to be uncommon with HIV infection; studies that have compared anthropomorphic parameters at birth in infants subsequently found to be HIV-1–infected with uninfected infants have not found significant differences, although a few studies have reported growth retardation confined to infected infants born at less than 35 weeks' gestation[41, 210, 240, 268, 298, 303, 371, 372, 382, 469] (see Table 192–8). Clinically, a bimodal distribution for onset of symptoms has been observed in perinatally infected children, with only a small proportion of infants (<30 per cent) having rapidly progressive disease presenting during the first year of life and the majority of infants not developing severe manifestations of HIV infection for several years, more consistent with acquisition of infection during the peripartum period.[42, 131, 209] A virologic pattern consistent with viral acquisition at birth has been observed in many infants, with negative viral studies at birth in 20 to 60 per cent of infants followed by viral production, which peaks at about 1 to 3 months of age.[8, 70, 164, 168, 337, 395, 426, 545] Serologic data also are consistent with most transmission occurring near birth, with only 20 to 48 per cent of infected infants having detectable HIV-1 IgA during the first week of life, rising to nearly 100 per cent by 3 to 6 months of age.[358, 412, 512, 544]

A number of studies have provided evidence that exposure of the infant's skin/mucous membranes to blood and secretions in the maternal genital tract during delivery plays an important role in transmission. Free virus as well as infected cells have been identified in cervicovaginal secretions of HIV-1–infected women, and some studies suggest that the concentration of HIV in genital secretions may be higher in pregnant than in nonpregnant infected women.[122, 278] Evaluation of the infection status of twins born to HIV-1–infected mothers has shown that the first-born has an almost threefold greater risk of infection than has the second-born, suggesting that relative exposure to birth canal secretions is important in transmission.[188] Consistent with this hypothesis is the finding that duration of membrane rupture is associated with

Text continued on page 2190

TABLE 192–8. Vertical HIV Transmission Rates: Review of Selected Studies

Site/Author/Reference/Year	Type of Study	Transmission Rate (No. Infants)	Length of Infant Follow-up	Definition of Infant Infection Status	Risk Factors for Transmission	Infant Outcome
United States						
Miami (Haitian)/ Hutto et al.[298] (1991)	Prospective	30% (82)	18 mo (median)	Infected: + culture Serial antibody titers Uninfected: − culture Declining antibody Normal CD4+ and immunoglobulins	Not associated: Breast feeding Mode of delivery	No difference in birth weight or gestational age in infected vs. uninfected infants
New York City/ Abrams et al.[1] (1995)	Prospective	24% (351)	>6 mo	Infected: ≥2 + PCR + antibody >15 mo AIDS-defining illness Symptoms and 1 + PCR Uninfected: ≥2 − PCR (1>6 mo) ≥1 − antibody tests No symptoms	Associated: Maternal AIDS CD4+ <500 Zidovudine (protective)	Higher rates of prematurity and intrauterine growth retardation in infected vs. uninfected infants
New York City/ Mayers et al.[420] (1991)	Prospective Case-control (33 HIV + ♀, 37 HIV − ♀)	21% (33)	24 mo (median)	Infected: Seropositive >15 mo AIDS ≥2 + culture/PCR Uninfected: Seronegative >15 mo	Associated: Symptoms	No difference in gestational age, birth weight, head circumference, or prematurity in infants born to HIV + vs. HIV − ♀ Seven seronegative infants had signs/symptoms of HIV
New York City/ Minkoff et al. (1995)[440]	Prospective	24% (127)	>15 mo	Infected: Seropositive ≥15 mo AIDS-defining illness + HIV-IgA × 2 at ≥6 mo Uninfected: No symptoms and either seronegative × 2 ≥6 mo or − HIV-IgA × 2 at ≥6 mo	Associated: Low CD4+ Duration of membrane rupture ≥4 hours	NS
Baltimore/Nair et al.[469] (1993)	Prospective	23% (134)	37–41 mo (mean)	Infected: CDC definition Uninfected: CDC definition	Associated (trend): Antenatal STD Chorioamnionitis Active illicit drug use Not associated: Mode of delivery	Birth weight <2500 g, small for gestational age, and 2 or more neonatal problems more likely in infected than uninfected infants Infected infants born ≤35 weeks' gestation more likely to have intrauterine growth retardation than infected infants born full-term
Atlanta/Nesheim et al.[475] (1994)	Prospective	17% (132)	35 mo (median)	Infected: Seropositive >18 mo + culture, PCR, p24 antigen ELISPOT Uninfected: No symptoms Seronegative >18 mo	Associated (trend): Injection drug use Not associated: Mode of delivery	No difference in birth weight, length, head circumference, or gestational age in infected vs. uninfected infants

Multinational/ Duliege et al.[188] (1995)	Retrospective Twin registry	20% (115 twin sets)	>15 mo	Infected: Seropositive >15 mo HIV-related disease Uninfected: Seronegative >12 mo No symptoms	Associated: First-born twin Vaginal delivery AIDS	Infected second-born twins with more rapid development of symptoms
Caribbean						
Haiti/Halsley et al.[268] (1990)	Prospective Case-control (308 HIV + ♀ 3360 HIV − ♀)	24% (230)	>12 mo	Infected: Seropositive >12 mo Excess mortality (13% excess at 3 mo) Uninfected: Seronegative >12 mo	Not associated: Breast feeding	Birth weight <2500 g, <37 weeks' gestation, and excess deaths more likely in infants born to HIV + ♀ vs. HIV − ♀ No difference in birth weight in infected vs. uninfected infants
Europe						
Italian Multicenter Collaborative/ Tovo et al.[659] (1996)	Registry	18.5% (975)	>18 mo	Infected: Seropositive >18 mo or ≥2 positive cultures Uninfected: Seronegative >18 mo No symptoms	Associated: Vaginal delivery Maternal symptoms Prematurity	No difference in birth weight in infected vs. uninfected infants
France/Mayaux et al.[419] (1995)	Prospective	20.2% (848)	>18 mo	Infected: Seropositive >18 mo AIDS-related death Uninfected: Seronegative >18 mo	Associated: Breast feeding p24 antigenemia Low CD4+ count High CD8+ per cent CDC stage III/IV Older age Not associated: Mode of delivery	NS
Sweden/Lindgren et al.[382] (1991)	Prospective and retrospective	31% (32)	>18 mo	Infected: Seropositive >18 mo + culture, p24 antigen Uninfected: Seronegative >18 mo − culture, p24 antigen No symptoms	Associated: Longer duration of HIV symptoms CD4+ <400/mm³ Vaginal delivery?	No difference in fetal growth or prematurity in infected vs. uninfected infants
Italy/Gabiano et al.[240] (1992)	Prospective	18–24% (551)	>15 mo	Infected: Seropositive >15 mo HIV-related death + culture, p24 antigen, PCR Uninfected: Seronegative >15 mo − culture, p24 antigen, PCR	Associated: Symptoms Breast feeding Female infant Not associated: Prematurity Mode of delivery	Decreased fetal growth in infants of symptomatic HIV + ♀ compared with HIV + ♀ without symptoms No increased rate of transmission to second-born of HIV + ♀ 6% seronegative infants had + viral studies No difference in birth weight or gestational age in infected vs. uninfected infants
European Collaborative Study[210, 214] (1992, 1994)	Prospective	14% (721)	>18 mo	Infected: ≥2 + cultures or p24 antigen Seropositive >18 mo AIDS HIV-related death Uninfected: Seronegative >18 mo − culture, p24 antigen	Associated: AIDS + p24 antigen CD4+ <700/mm³ Vaginal delivery Breast feeding? Obstetrical procedures?	No difference in congenital defects, prematurity, or birth weight in infected vs. uninfected infants

Table continued on following page

TABLE 192–8. Vertical HIV Transmission Rates: Review of Selected Studies *Continued*

Site/Author/Reference/Year	Type of Study	Transmission Rate (No. Infants)	Length of Infant Follow-up	Definition of Infant Infection Status	Risk Factors for Transmission	Infant Outcome
Asia						
India/Kumar et al.[350] (1995)	Prospective	48% (143)	>18 mo	Infected: Seropositive >18 mo + culture, p24 antigen; Uninfected: Seronegative >18 mo	Associated: Placental membrane inflammation; Prematurity; CDC stage III/IV; Low CD4+; Low birth weight	Low birth weight and prematurity more common in infected than in uninfected infants
Africa						
Kenya/Temmerman et al.[645, 646] (1994, 1995)	Prospective Case-control (315 HIV + ♀ 311 HIV − ♀)	31% (94)	>3 mo	Infected: + PCR; Uninfected: − PCR	Associated: Sexually transmitted disease; Chorioamnionitis; Low CD4+ count; Higher CD8+ count; Low CD4+/8+ ratio; Infant gender (female)	Prematurity and postpartum endometritis but not intrauterine growth retardation more likely in infants born to HIV + ♀ than HIV − ♀; No difference in birth weight and gestational age in infected vs. uninfected infants
Kenya/Datta et al.[152] (1994)	Prospective Case-control (323 HIV + ♀ 341 HIV − ♀)	42.8% (257)	>12 mo	Infected: Seropositive ≥12 mo; HIV-related death; Uninfected: Seronegative ≥12 mo	Associated: Marital status (married); Breast feeding: duration (≥15 mo); Not Associated: Disease stage (most were healthy); Mode of delivery	Low birth weight and death at <12 mo of age more likely in infant born to HIV + ♀ than HIV − ♀; No difference in birth weight in infected vs. uninfected infants
Zaire/Ryder et al.[581] (1989)	Prospective Case-control (466 HIV + ♀ 606 HIV − ♀)	39% (92)	>12 mo	Infected: + cord blood culture; Seropositive >12 mo; AIDS (WHO definition); Uninfected: Seronegative at 18 mo	Associated: CD4+ < 400/mm^3; Chorioamnionitis	Low birth weight, prematurity, and death more likely in infants born to HIV + ♀ than HIV − ♀

Zaire/St. Louis et al.[626] (1993)	Propective Case-control (324 HIV + ♀ 254 HIV − ♀)	26% (261)	>18 mo	Infected: ≥2 + culture or PCR Seropositive >15 mo Uninfected: Seronegative >15 mo All cultures/PCR −	Associated: + p24 antigen CD4+ >15% CD8+ ≥1800/mm³ Chorioamnionitis Fever ≥30 days Hb ≤0.85 gm/L? Preterm/postterm?	2.4% vs. 1.2% stillbirths in HIV + vs. HIV − ♀
Rwanda/Lepage et al.[371, 372] (1992, 1993)	Propective Case-control (215 HIV + ♀ 216 HIV − ♀)	25–26% (218)	>15 mo	Infected: Seropositive >15 mo HIV-related death AIDS Uninfected: Seronegative >15 mo Seronegative ≥9 mo plus no AIDS- or non-HIV–related death if lost to follow-up	Associated: CD4+/CD8+ <0.5 Not associated: Clinical status Mode of delivery STDs	Excess deaths in infants born to HIV + ♀ (11%) vs. HIV − ♀ Lower birth weight, length, and head circumference more likely in infected vs. uninfected infants
Rwanda/Bulterys et al.[67, 68] (1993, 1994)	Prospective Case-control (318 HIV + ♀ 309 HIV − ♀)	20–29% (162)	>12 mo	Infected: Seropositive >12 mo AIDS HIV-related death Uninfected: Seronegative >12 mo	Associated: ≥ three recent sex partners CD4+/CD8+ <0.5	Intrauterine growth retardation and placental weight more likely in infants born to HIV + ♀ vs. HIV − ♀ No difference in gestational age or neonatal deaths in infants born to HIV + ♀ vs. HIV − ♀
Tanzania/Bredberg-Raden et al.[55] (1995)	Prospective	21.7% (138)	NS	Infected: + PCR Uninfected: NS	Associated: CD4+ ≤20% β-2 microglobulin ≥2.0 + p24 antigen	NS
Zaire/Thea et al.[654] (1993)	Prospective Case-control (232 HIV + ♀ 188 HIV − ♀)	28% (192)	17 mo (mean)	Infected: NS Uninfected: NS	NS	Increased episodes of acute, recurrent, and persistent diarrhea and diarrhea-associated death in infected vs. uninfected infants

CDC, Centers for Disease Control and Prevention; STDs, sexually transmitted diseases; PCR, polymerase chain reaction; NS, not specified.
Modified from Mofenson, L. M.: Epidemiology and determinants of vertical HIV transmisstion. Semin. Pediatr. Infect. Dis. *5*:252–265, 1994.

TABLE 192–9. Timing of Perinatal Transmission

Intrauterine Transmission	Intrapartum Transmission	Postpartum Transmission (Breast Feeding)
HIV identified in placental tissue	HIV isolation from cervicovaginal secretions	HIV isolation from cellular and cell-free portions of breast milk
In vitro infection of placenta-derived cells	Intrapartum exposure to blood	Case reports of infants infected by breast feeding from mothers who become HIV-infected postpartum or from an infected "wet nurse"
HIV identified in fetal tissue, fetal blood samples, and amniotic fluid	Increased infection rates in first-born twin	Meta-analysis of pooled data indicates increased attributable risk of infection by breast feeding
Intrauterine growth retardation observed in some HIV-infected infants?	"Acute" primary infection virologic and immunologic pattern	
Positive viral studies in 20–60% of infected infants at birth	Negative viral studies at birth, followed by positive studies at first month of life in 40–80% of infected infants	
Bimodal onset of symptoms, with early onset (<12 months) in <30%	Bimodal onset of symptoms, with late onset (>12 mo) in >70%	
	HIV p24 antigen in cervicovaginal secretions associated with increased risk of infection	
	Association of duration membrane rupture with risk of infection	
AIDS embryopathy?	Possible protective effect of cesarean delivery	

Modified from Mofenson, L. M.: Epidemiology and determinants of vertical HIV transmission. Semin. Pediatr. Infect. Dis. *5*:252–265, 1994.

transmission risk[71, 357, 440] and the finding in some studies that cesarean delivery is associated with lower transmission than is vaginal delivery.[188, 193, 349, 445] Animal studies also have demonstrated that SIV infection can be established by an oral route in newborn monkeys.[23] Taken together, the accumulated clinical, serologic, and virologic data suggest that at least 40 per cent, and possibly as much as 80 per cent, of transmission may occur near to or during delivery.

HIV-1 also can be transmitted through breast milk, similar to other retroviruses. HIV has been identified in both the cell-free and cell-associated fractions of breast milk.[578] Prospective observational studies have shown a relatively high risk of HIV transmission from mothers who have primary HIV infection during the postpartum period while breast feeding, when the infant might be exposed to high levels of virus in the presence of little to no antiviral immune response[506]; a meta-analysis of several studies found a 29 per cent risk of HIV-1 transmission under such circumstances (95 per cent confidence interval, 16 to 42 per cent).[192] More controversy exists about the risk of transmission by breast milk from mothers with chronic infection during pregnancy. A meta-analysis suggested the attributable risk of transmission by breast milk in this situation to be 14 per cent (95 per cent confidence interval, 7 to 22 per cent)[192]; however, other studies have suggested that the risk may be as high as 32 or as low as 9 per cent.[152, 666] Given the availability of safe infant formula in industrialized countries such as the United States, it is recommended that HIV-1–infected women who live in such countries not breast feed. However, in the developing world, where provision of maternal antibodies against endemic pathogens via breast feeding may be important for infant health and unsanitary conditions make use of infant formula more risky, the benefit of breast feeding by an infected mother may outweigh the risk of HIV transmission. Under such circumstances, WHO recommends that infected women continue to breast feed their infants.[479, 666]

Risk for HIV transmission is likely to be multifactorial in nature. Improved understanding of transmission risk factors is important to enhance the development of targeted intervention strategies (Table 192–10). Maternal factors that have been shown to be associated with increased risk of perinatal transmission include advanced disease stage; general immunologic deterioration associated with low CD4+ lymphocyte count or per cent and elevated CD8+ lymphocyte number; low titers or affinity/avidity of maternal antibody to HIV-1 gp120 (V3 loop), gp41 and p24 proteins, although this is controversial; and low titers of maternal HIV-1–specific neutralizing antibody.[340, 419, 444] In one African study, deficiency of vitamin A was found to be associated with an increased risk of HIV-1 transmission[601]; vitamin A plays an important role in the maintenance of mucosal surfaces and immune response. The placenta may form an important protective barrier against intrauterine viral transmission. Conditions that perturb the integrity of the placenta have been associated with increased HIV-1 transmission risk in some studies, including the presence of chorioamnionitis, maternal illicit drug use, or smoking during pregnancy.[71, 566, 626]

Elevated maternal proviral and cell-free viral load, as measured by HIV coculture, p24 antigen (immune-dissociated), and DNA and RNA PCR, appears to be associated with increased transmission risk.[50, 178, 694] Monocyte-macrophage tropic viral phenotypes have been reported to be transmitted preferentially from mother to infant in some studies.[340, 492] Selective transmission of a single or limited number of minor maternal viral genotypic variants has been implied by some studies that have found a more homogeneous viral quasispecies in infected infants than in their mothers; others have reported transmission of more heterogeneous maternal variants as well.[59, 705] Selective transmission of a single viral variant escaping immune surveillance in the mother may be more important for transmission in utero, and multiple variants may be capable of intrapartum transmission. The presence of immune complex–dissociated p24 antigen and HIV-1–specific HIV IgA in third trimester maternal secretions was shown to be associated with increased transmission risk; the local production of secretory IgA in genital mucosa may reflect active local viral replication and high genital viral load. Consistent with an important role for exposure to genital secretions in transmission, some studies have found that longer duration of membrane rupture and vaginal delivery were associated with increased risk of transmission.

Possible genetic susceptibility to HIV has been suggested by some studies showing an association of certain HLA haplotypes with transmission risk.[317] A role of the newborn immune response to HIV exposure in averting transmission has been suggested by several studies purporting to detect HIV-specific cellular immune responses among 20 to 30 per cent of uninfected infants born to infected women.[125, 161, 575] Additionally, several investigators have reported the rare occurrence of apparent clearance of HIV-1 infection in perinatally exposed infants.[25, 64, 66, 478, 573]

The risk of HIV-1 transmission through breast milk has

TABLE 192–10. Potential Mediating Factors for Perinatal HIV Transmission and Potential Strategies for Intervention

Potential Mediating Factors	Potential Intervention Strategies
Maternal Factors	

• Advanced disease stage
• Low CD4+ count or per cent
• Elevated CD8+ count
• Low titers or avidity/affinity HIV-specific antibody
• Low HIV-specific cellular immunity?
• High viral load
• Viral genotype: selection of neutralization escape mutant?
• Viral phenotype: nonsyncytia-inducing; slow/low; macrophage tropic?
	Lower maternal viral load
	• Antiretroviral
	Boost maternal immune response
	• Passive immunization
	  • Polyclonal (HIVIG)
	  • Monoclonal
	• Active immunization
	• Passive-active immunization

Placental Factors	

• Differing CD4+ expression by placental cells
• Placental cell susceptibility to HIV infection
• Fc-mediated transfer of HIV-associated immune complexes?
• Breaks in placental barrier
  • Chorioamnionitis
  • Syphilis and other sexually transmitted diseases
  • Other etiologies (smoking, cocaine)
	Prevent viral attachment
	• Passive immunization
	• Other blockers (e.g., CD4-IgG)
	Restrict viral replication
	• Antiretroviral
	Prevention and treatment of cofactors
	• Chorioamnionitis
	• Sexually transmitted diseases
	• Smoking
	• Illicit drug use

Fetal Factors	
• Reduced functional immune competence • Fetal cell susceptibility to HIV infection • Genetic aspects (HLA haplotype)	**Prevent viral replication** • Antiretroviral **Boost immune response** • Passive immunization
Labor/Birth Canal Factors	
• Cervicovaginal viral load • Local HIV-specific immune response • Maternal-fetal micro/macrotransfusion of blood	**Lower viral load** • Antiretroviral • Vaginal viricide **Boost immune response** • Local passive or active immunization?
Obstetric Factors	
• Duration of membrane rupture • Mode of delivery • Invasive obstetric procedures/fetal monitoring	**Role of elective cesarean section** **Avoid invasive procedures**
Newborn Factors	
• Skin integrity • Gastric acid secretion low • Decreased functional immune responsiveness	**Avoid invasive procedures** **Lower viral load** • Antiretroviral **Boost immune response** • Passive immunization • Active immunization • Passive-active immunization
Breast Milk Factors	
• Cell-associated viral load • Cell-free viral load • Viral load in colostrum/early milk? • HIV-specific antibody • Nonspecific protection (e.g., glycosaminoglycan content)	**Avoid breast feeding if safe infant formula available** **Avoid breast feeding only of early breast milk?** **Lower viral load** • Antiretroviral **Boost immune response?** • Active immunization

HIVIG, hyperimmune HIV intravenous immunoglobulin.
From Mofenson, L. M.: Epidemiology and determinants of vertical HIV transmission. Semin. Pediatr. Infect. Dis. *5*:252–265, 1994.

been correlated with duration of breast feeding in some studies; time of exposure and infectivity of the milk also may play an important role. The high cellular content of colostrum and early milk suggests that such milk may pose a greater risk for HIV-1 transmission than may later milk. Cell-associated and cell-free HIV have been reported to be more common in early milk, obtained up to 7 days' postpartum, than in mature milk samples.[578] However, others have detected HIV in breast milk obtained as late as 12 months' postpartum. Higher levels of HIV-infected cells in breast milk have been associated with CD4+ cell depletion and severe vitamin A deficiency.[472] Human milk contains anti-HIV antibodies, and the presence of HIV-1 IgM and IgA in milk has been correlated with diminished risk of breast milk transmission in some studies but not others.[194, 668] Additionally, a glycosaminoglycan found in breast milk of infected and uninfected women has been shown to inhibit binding of gp120 to CD4+[476, 477]; this compound appears to be lowest in colostrum and highest in mature milk, and in one study its presence was found to correlate with protection against breast milk transmission.

Injection Drug Use

Injection drug use and sexual or perinatal transmission from injection drug users are responsible for 36 per cent of all AIDS cases in the United States and play a multifaceted role in the global spread of HIV-1 infection, with persons infected directly through drug use serving as a bridge to further spread of infection through sexual contact.[100] HIV-1 infection in injection drug users in the United States has been associated with minority race or ethnicity, residence in an HIV-1–endemic area, increased frequency and duration of drug injection, needle-sharing behavior, use of "shooting galleries," and other behaviors that increase the potential of blood exposure between users.[5] Needle sharing, the primary mechanism for HIV-1 transmission among injection drug users, appears to be associated with younger age, not completing high school, history of prior arrest, being on public assistance, and male-male sexual behavior; those sharing needles appear to inject drugs more frequently and are more likely to use cocaine.[404]

Globally, there is wide geographic variation in HIV-1 seroprevalence among drug users; in the United States, highest rates are seen in the Northeast.[10] This variation probably is multifactorial, including time of entry of HIV-1 into the injection drug user population, differences in the prevalence of behaviors that facilitate transmission (such as shooting galleries), and accessibility of drug treatment and HIV prevention programs, including availability of sterile injection equipment. A significant decrease in drug-related risky behavior and HIV-1 transmission among injection drug users has been associated with syringe and needle exchange programs in some localities.[170, 171, 690] Additionally, significant reductions in both drug and sexual risk behaviors and HIV-1 transmission have been demonstrated with comprehensive HIV risk reduction programs that have included drug treatment, availability of sterile needles, condom distribution, HIV risk reduction counseling, and voluntary testing.[170, 665]

Transmission from Blood Products/Organ Transplants

HIV-1 is transmitted efficiently by blood and blood products, presumably due to exposure to large amounts of infectious material. More than 90 to 95 per cent of HIV-1–infected blood transfusion recipients have become infected.[130, 184] Among recipients, age, gender, reason for transfusion, and underlying condition do not appear significantly to affect the risk of HIV-1 transmission. Infection appears to be more likely from infected donors in whom the blood donation occurred close to the onset of AIDS-related symptoms or who earlier had donated blood to recipients who became infected. This may be due to high viral load or a more virulent viral type in the donated blood. Lower infectivity may be associated with depletion of viable lymphocytes in the product being transfused; transfusion of washed red cells or prolonged storage of red cells from HIV-1–infected donors appeared to be associated with reduced (but not zero) infectivity in one report.[184] Neither albumin nor intravenous gamma globulin products have been associated with HIV-1 transmission.

The period of highest risk of blood product exposure to HIV-1 occurred between 1978 and April 1985, before the availability of HIV-1 antibody–screened blood products. Because there is significant variation between individuals in the time to development of HIV-related symptoms, HIV-1 testing should be offered to all persons who received transfusions prior to 1985. In an evaluation of a pediatric cohort who had been transfused prior to 1985 as neonates, 14 children with previously undiagnosed infection were identified, including 1 child who was asymptomatic 8 years after transfusion.[380]

Since the routine screening of all blood donations in the United States for HIV-1 antibody, there has been a dramatic decrease in transmission of HIV-1 from transfusions, with new transmissions almost exclusively originating from recently infected donors prior to the development of specific antibody (which may be detected with available antibody tests by approximately 25 days after infection). The risk of HIV-1 transmission through screened blood in the United States is very small, estimated at 1 in every 450,000 to 660,000 donations of screened blood.[353]

In the developing world, HIV-1 antibody screening of blood products often is not available and even if available, current antibody tests designed to detect HIV-1 subtype B may not detect other subtypes more common to Africa.[616] Transmission via transfusion is estimated to account for about 5 to 10 per cent of all infections in Africa.[232] The use of unscreened blood transfusions as a therapeutic modality along with reuse of unsterilized needles and intravenous catheters has resulted in major outbreaks of HIV-1 transmission in the newborn and pediatric populations in Africa, Russia, and Romania.[130, 232, 280]

Hemophiliacs received factor concentrates derived from large pools of plasma obtained from thousands of donors and thus were at high risk of HIV-1 exposure prior to antibody screening of blood. Risk of infection appears to be related directly to the amount of concentrate received and therefore is highest among those with the most severe clotting disorder. It is estimated that the prevalence of HIV-1 infection is 76 per cent in persons with severe factor VIII deficiency and 42 per cent in severe factor IX deficiency.[217] A small number of hemophiliacs (~6 per cent) who had repeated heavy exposure to potentially contaminated blood products have remained uninfected; in one study, the peripheral blood cells of such patients appeared to be less susceptible to HIV in vitro than did cells from healthy controls, implying that there may be some genetic component to HIV susceptibility.[365] Factor VIII/IX concentrates used for hemophiliacs have been heat-treated since 1984 and screened for HIV-1 antibodies since 1985, resulting in virtual elimination of new acquisition of HIV-1 infection through these products in this population.

Transmission of HIV-1 through organ transplantation has been rare but documented, as has transmission through artificial insemination.[16, 204] Since 1985, the Public Health Service has recommended that all donors of tissue and organ allografts be screened for HIV-1 prior to use. Because of the rare occurrence of HIV-1 transmission from organ donors who tested antibody-negative at the time of donation, it has been recommended that tissues from living donors, such as bone and semen, be preserved for 6 months and not used until the donor is tested again 6 months later and confirmed to be seronegative.[608]

Nosocomial Transmission

The risk of transmission via nosocomial percutaneous or mucous membrane exposure to HIV-1 is very low. The estimated risk for HIV infection after a single percutaneous exposure to HIV-infected blood is approximately 0.3 per cent (95 per cent confidence interval, 0.13 to 0.76 per cent) and 0.1 per cent (95 per cent confidence interval, 0.006 to 0.5 per cent) after mucous membrane exposure.[107, 275, 302] This contrasts with the 15 to 30 per cent risk of transmission from an infected mother to her infant and the 95 per cent estimated risk of acquiring infection after transfusion with infected blood. Although the risk of transmission from an infected patient to a health care worker is low, the number of health care workers who potentially are exposed is large. Therefore, prevention of percutaneous exposure of health care workers to blood-borne pathogens through proper use and disposal of sharps used for phlebotomy, use of barrier precautions such as gloves, and training about and incorporation of universal precautions into all health care settings is essential.[86]

Data from a number of investigations indicate that the risk of HIV-1 transmission from an infected health care worker to a patient is very small. Only one instance of such transmission has been substantiated; this occurred in a dental practice, and the mechanism of transmission has not been delineated clearly.[119] Studies of patients with potential exposure to HIV-1 from a number of infected health care workers who performed invasive procedures, such as gynecologic and oral surgery, have not documented any other such transmissions.[90, 307, 564]

Nosocomial infection from patient to patient due to inadequately disinfected or shared medical equipment in health care settings has been documented among children in Romania and Russia and dialysis patients in South America.[280, 674] Rare cases of transmission through apparent lapses in instrument hygiene also have been reported from countries with advanced systems of medical care, emphasizing the importance of adherence to recommendations for universal precautions.[455]

In a case-control study of health care workers with percutaneous exposure to blood, risk factors independently associated with risk of transmission included factors indicating exposure to larger quantities of blood, such as the presence of visible blood on the inoculating instrument; procedure involving a needle placed directly in a vein or artery; deep injury; and terminal illness in the source patient (presumably reflecting high viral load).[107] Postexposure use of ZDV appeared to have a protective effect (odds ratio, 0.2; 95 per cent confidence interval, 0.1 to 0.6).

Other

Multiple epidemiologic studies from the United States and Europe have evaluated the risk of transmission from casual household contact in the households of more than 1000 HIV-1–infected persons; no transmissions were observed in these studies.[607] Only eight cases of possible household transmission have been reported, six of which involved children.[83, 91, 95, 96, 226, 685] In four cases, HIV-1 transmission from an infected to previously uninfected child living in the household was observed; in three of these cases, genetic similarities between the donor and transmitted virus were seen. Two transmissions involved uninfected hemophiliacs who received consecutive home intravenous therapy with their infected siblings. Although the means of transmission is unknown, transmission via intravenous or percutaneous blood exposure is likely. In the third case of child-child transmission with genetic sequencing evidence, unrecognized exposure to blood was likely. A fourth report from Germany provided little information to judge its validity. In another instance, genetically related virus apparently was transmitted from an infected mother to her preschool-aged child. The child had contact with open eczemoid, bleeding skin lesions on the mother and shared toothbrushes, despite maternal gingival bleeding. The sixth pediatric case involved HIV-1 transmission from an infected child to its caregiver; extensive ungloved exposure to open sores on the child's skin provided probable viral exposure.

Oral exposure to semen has been linked to transmission among homosexual men but appears to be extremely uncommon.[78] No proven instances of transmission via oral-oral contact have been reported. HIV-genomic material has been identified in oral mucosal cells from saliva of infected persons.[546] However, infectious HIV rarely is isolated from saliva and, when found, is in small amounts[714]; additionally, saliva appears to contain substances that may have antiviral activity, similar to glycosoaminoglycans found in breast milk.[399, 477] The risk of HIV-1 transmission through exposure to saliva appears to be extremely low and would require saliva of unusually high infectivity to have contact with broken skin or mucosa. Transmission of HIV-1 by human bites, although biologically plausible, remains unlikely, and no well-documented cases of such transmission have been reported; no seroconversions have been observed in studies that prospectively have evaluated persons with such exposure.[557]

Diagnosis of HIV-1 Infection in Infants

Serologic diagnosis of HIV-1 infection in infancy is complicated by the presence of passively transferred maternal HIV-1 IgG antibody, which crosses the placenta to the fetus and may persist in the infant until 15 to 18 months of age. This long duration of maternal antibody persistence is due to the relatively high HIV-1 IgG antibody titers present in infected adults and the long half-life of IgG antibody (28 days).[614] Although HIV-1 antibody generally becomes undetectable in uninfected infants by about 10 to 13 months of age,[113, 209, 451, 505] occasionally it may remain detectable for as long as 18 months.[113, 555, 592] Therefore, the presence of HIV-1 IgG antibody is not reliably diagnostic of infection in the infant younger than 18 months of age, although it does identify an infected mother (see Table 192–4). Direct detection of the virus or its components through such virologic assays as HIV culture, immune-complex–dissociated p24 antigen, and DNA PCR has proved to be the most sensitive and specific diagnostic test. Immunodiagnostic strategies, although useful, have proved to be less sensitive for early diagnosis during the first few months of life.

Complicating diagnostic evaluations are issues relating to the timing of perinatal transmission. Using a variety of virologic detection tests, only 20 to 60 per cent of infants ultimately found to be infected have positive tests at birth or during the first few days of life.[444] However, by 1 to 6 months of age, the vast majority of infected infants can be detected. This is consistent with the hypothesis that most perinatal transmission occurs during or near the time of birth.

The sensitivity of HIV peripheral blood culture for diagnosis of perinatal infection has been evaluated by serial cultures in prospectively followed cohorts of children with perinatal exposure to HIV. In one study, culture sensitivity was only 24 per cent during the first week of life.[426] By 1 month of age, HIV culture identified nearly 90 per cent of infected children and was as sensitive for HIV diagnosis as were cultures obtained at later times. In another study, two negative cultures obtained after 1 month of age had a specificity of 99 to 100 per cent for identification of uninfected children.[342] Thus, HIV culture at 1 month of age appears to be highly sensitive and specific for the diagnosis of HIV infection but is time-consuming, is expensive, and requires extensive biohazard precautions; also, definitive results may not be available for 2 to 4 weeks.

Using gene amplification techniques, such as PCR, has the advantage of being able to detect very small amounts of viral nucleic acid (DNA or RNA). The sensitivity and specificity of PCR as an early diagnostic tool for the detection of proviral HIV-1 DNA have been evaluated by several investigators. In a meta-analysis combining data on 271 infected children from 16 studies from 12 centers, HIV-1 DNA was detected by PCR in an estimated 38 per cent of infected children tested on or within 24 hours of birth (90 per cent confidence interval, 29 to 46 per cent).[191] There was a rapid rise in sensitivity during the second week of life, with the detection of 93 per cent of infected infants by 14 days of age and 96 per cent by 28 days of age (90 per cent confidence interval, 89 to 98 per cent). False-positive tests have been reported, most commonly secondary to laboratory error due to carry-over of amplified product DNA from a previously analyzed sample. PCR also may be used to detect HIV-1 RNA. In one study evaluating the utility of RNA PCR for pediatric diagnosis, RNA PCR appeared to be slightly less sensitive than DNA PCR for early detection of infection.[207] HIV PCR can be performed reliably on filter paper dried blood spot samples, like those used for newborn screening for inborn errors of metabolism. Comparison of HIV DNA PCR performed on dried blood spots and corresponding venous blood samples showed 95 per cent sensitivity and 100 per cent specificity for dried blood spot testing.[81, 486] This method could facilitate sample collection and shipment in areas in which advanced technology may not be readily available.

Detection of HIV-1 p24 core antigen by EIA is limited by the complexing of antigen in the presence of high-titer HIV-1–specific antibodies (as often is the case in early infancy due to the presence of excess maternal IgG HIV-1 antibody), and p24 antigen has been found to be less sensitive than has HIV culture or PCR for early diagnosis of infection in infants.[15, 70] The sensitivity of this assay has been enhanced by the development of immune-complex–dissociated p24 antigen assays, which involve pretreatment of the sample with acid or heat to dissociate antigen-antibody immune complexes, freeing the antigen to react in the EIA.[436, 545, 591] However, although the p24 antigen and immune-complex–dissociated p24 antigen assays are rapid and less expensive than are HIV culture and PCR, comparative studies have found that even immune-complex–dissociated p24 antigen has lower sensitivity than have other methods for direct viral detection, and false-positive results have been reported using either antigen assay during the first few months of life.[69, 166, 300, 376]

Immunodiagnostic strategies for early detection of HIV-1 infection include quantitative analysis of HIV-1 IgG antibody indicating stable or rising titers over time[279, 451]; expanding Western blot band pattern or unique band reactivity in mono-antigen-based assays on serially tested serum[615]; demonstration of in vitro synthesis of HIV-1–specific antibody by peripheral blood lymphocytes[534]; detection of antibody-forming cells in infant blood[474]; and HIV-1–specific IgM and IgA antibody production.[592] HIV-1 IgA assays, generally using recombinant protein G absorption to remove nonspecific assay reactivity due to maternal IgG antibody present in the specimen, have been found to be relatively insensitive in infants younger than 3 months of age but provide a specific and fairly sensitive diagnostic tool for infants older than 3 months of age.[358, 387, 412, 512, 544] Similarly, most other immunodiagnostic tests appear to be most sensitive among children older than 3 to 6 months of age and therefore are not first-line tests for early diagnosis of HIV-1 in infancy.

Recommendations have been published for the diagnostic evaluation of HIV-1–exposed infants.[3, 707] Because 20 to 60 per cent of infected infants can be identified at birth, HIV culture or DNA PCR on a peripheral blood sample obtained during the first 48 hours of life is recommended. If negative, available data suggest that retesting be performed at 1 to 2 months of age[426] and, if negative, repeated at 4 to 6 months of age. A positive test at any time should be repeated to confirm the diagnosis. If HIV culture or PCR is not available, p24 antigen testing (preferably the immune-complex–dissociated p24 antigen assay) may be used for infants older than 1 month of age. To document that a child is uninfected, children with negative virologic evaluations at 6 months of age should have HIV-1 antibody status monitored through 18 months of age to substantiate HIV-1 antibody seroreversion to negative.

Natural History

In HIV-1–infected adults, estimates of the median time from infection to the development of clinical AIDS in the absence of antiretroviral therapy in homosexual men, transfusion recipients, and hemophiliacs cluster in the 7- to 10-year range.[6] Several studies have found that the risk of progression to AIDS among hemophiliacs appears to be related to age of infection, with children infected after infancy (>1 year of age) and adolescents having lower rates of progression than adults.[38, 218, 290, 494] These data suggest that there are as yet undefined factors operative in the mature but youthful immune system that result in improved response to HIV infection and survival.

In contrast, the immunologic and clinical response to HIV infection acquired while the immune system is immature may be poor. Acquisition of transfusion-related infection during the neonatal period is associated with more rapid disease progression than seen with acquisition at other ages; median time to AIDS among 297 patients with transfusion-acquired infection was 8 years for adults and 1.9 years for children younger than 5 years of age, most of whom acquired infection during the neonatal period.[433] Similarly, in a study of 111 HIV-1–infected children and adolescents from Bellevue Hospital in New York City, the median incubation period to AIDS was only 2 years in children with neonatal transfusion-acquired infection.[347] In the Italian Multicentre Study, disease progression was more rapid in children transfused in the neonatal period than in children with thalassemia or hemophilia, who presumably were infected in later childhood.[303] Thus, neonatal HIV infection, acquired at a time of immunologic naivete, appears to be associated with more rapid progression than does HIV infection acquired in later childhood.

Consistent with this hypothesis are studies that appear to indicate rapid progression to symptomatic disease in some infants with vertically acquired HIV-1 infection.[241, 596, 655] A bimodal distribution of disease progression in vertically infected infants has been described by a number of investigators from the United States, Europe, and Africa.[42, 131, 186, 189, 418] Early onset of symptoms at younger than 12 months of age with rapidly progressive disease and high mortality is observed in about 10 to 25 per cent of infected infants. The majority of children with vertical infection appear to have later onset of symptoms and a better prognosis, with median time to development of AIDS of more than 5 years and median survival of 6 to 9 years.[186, 214, 241, 305, 657] Early age of disease onset therefore appears to be a marker of poor prognosis.

It is postulated that children with early disease onset and rapid clinical course may have acquired HIV infection in utero, when infection of thymic or other immune progenitor cells could disrupt further maturation of the immune system, whereas those with slower progression may have acquired HIV infection during or near to birth, when the immune system is more competent.[65, 177, 528] The concept that disease progression may be related to time of perinatal HIV acquisition has some support from studies that compared disease progression rates between infants who acquired HIV infection by transfusion in the neonatal period and infants with vertically acquired infection (some proportion of whom presumably acquired infection in utero). In a community-based surveillance database in Los Angeles, California, children with perinatal HIV-1 infection developed symptomatic disease 2.5-fold more rapidly than did those who acquired infection via neonatal transfusion (median time to symptoms, 6.4 and 17.8 months, respectively).[235] Similar findings have been reported by others.[311, 347, 567] Overall survival also was longer for those with HIV-1 infection secondary to transfusion, primarily due to early mortality in the subset of children with perinatal infection who had early symptom onset (and who theoretically acquired infection in utero). Children with perinatal infection developing symptoms after 12 months of age (who theoretically acquired infection intrapartum) had a similar survival as those infected by neonatal transfusion. Additional data suggesting a relationship between time of transmission and disease progression have come from studies with prospective intensive virologic evaluation of infants from birth. Children with positive viral tests at birth demonstrated a more rapid increase in viral load, faster loss of CD4+ lymphocytes, and earlier onset of disease than did those children who were negative at birth but tested positive for HIV-1 after the first few weeks of life.[177]

However, other researchers have speculated that differences between infected children with rapid versus slow disease progression may be associated with factors other than or in addition to the timing of vertical transmission, such as the inherent virulence properties of the transmitted viral strain and/or initial viral burden[40, 658]; genetic factors, such as HLA genotype[317]; and the mother's and/or infant's cellular or humoral immune response.[389, 667]

Much of the early data on survival in children with perinatal HIV-1 infection were based on retrospective studies of children who met the criteria for CDC-defined AIDS and therefore were biased toward children with early presentation of disease. More recent reports suggest that the overall survival of infected children is longer than previously was thought, and reports of survival of vertically infected children into midadolescence have been published.[261, 305, 519] However, although a substantial number of children may survive beyond early childhood, the majority have demonstrated some manifestations of HIV disease, and long-term survival with nonprogression of disease appears to be uncommon.

In addition to age of symptom onset, certain disease symptom complexes appear to be associated with prognosis.[305, 528, 655, 657] Symptoms indicative of poor prognosis include development of opportunistic infections (especially PCP), encephalopathy, severe bacterial infections, anemia, and fever. Growth failure also has been associated with subsequent disease progression in some reports.[58, 431] In contrast, lymphoid interstitial pneumonitis, lymphadenopathy, hepatosplenomegaly, parotitis, skin disease, thrombocytopenia, and recurrent respiratory tract infections appear to be associated with milder disease and more prolonged survival.

In HIV-1–infected adults, virologic parameters have been correlated with disease outcome, and similar findings have been observed in infected children.[528] Disease progression in children has been associated with high levels of p24 antigen[17, 167, 177, 187]; rapid/high viral replication characteristics[167]; T-cell tropic virus[167]; proviral load as measured by HIV culture and/or DNA PCR[167, 177, 622]; and ZDV-resistant virus.[489, 620] In older children, transition from nonsyncytium-inducing to syncytium-inducing phenotype is correlated with low CD4+ lymphocyte count and ZDV resistance; however, in children younger than 1 year of age, disease progression has been observed with both phenotypes, suggesting that the immature immune system may be less able to contain HIV replication regardless of phenotype.[620]

Correlation of disease progression risk with CD4+ lymphocyte count in children is complicated by normal age-related changes in lymphocyte subsets during the first few years of life. Normative data for uninfected children indicate decline in CD4+ lymphocyte number and per cent over the first 6 years of life, and an age-related definition of immunosuppression has been developed.[165, 205, 211, 430, 684] Low age-related CD4+ lymphocyte number and per cent and rapid CD4+ cell decline have been correlated with disease progression in older infants and children.[75, 162, 189, 430] During the first year of life, CD4+ count appears to be less predictive, and opportunistic infections, such as PCP, have developed despite CD4+ counts in the normal range. Additional factors, such as immature CD4+ cell function and cellular immunity, may play an important role in the development of disease complications in the younger age group.

Disease progression risk has been correlated with other immunologic markers, including deficiency in T-helper cell function[570]; impaired in vitro lymphocyte proliferation[189]; low or absent titers of HIV-1–specific antibodies, including p24, syncytium inhibiting, neutralizing, and HIV-1–IgM antibodies[57, 187, 189, 279, 561, 667]; deficiency of HIV-specific cytotoxic T lymphocytes[396]; increased production of type 2 cytokines (IL-4 and IL-10)[679]; high IgE level[678, 679]; and elevated immunoglobulin levels.[162]

Additional laboratory markers that have been reported by some investigators to be correlated with disease progression risk in children include TNF[197]; β2-microglobulin and neopterin[179, 196, 605]; soluble CD8 level[605]; erythrocyte adenosine deaminase levels[507]; and serum vitamin A level.[144, 602]

Immunologic Manifestations of HIV-1 Infection in Children

The CD4+ lymphocyte, the target cell of HIV infection, plays a pivotal role in the complex interplay of the interlacing network of cells and soluble lymphokine mediators that constitute the immune response. The repercussions of CD4+ cell infection by HIV thus directly or indirectly affect all portions of the immune response and eventually result in global immunologic collapse. The developmental immaturity of the immune system and immunologic naivete of the neonate and young infant make the consequences of such defects more severe than in older children and adults.

B CELLS

Abnormalities in humoral immunity are common in children with HIV-1 infection and may precede the development of the more characteristic abnormalities in cell-mediated immunity. Defects in humoral immunity may result from primary B-cell abnormalities or reflect the indirect effects of immunodysregulation and cytokine abnormalities. B cells from HIV-1–infected children demonstrate polyclonal activation and increased spontaneous proliferation with hypersecretion of polyclonal immunoglobulins. Elevated levels of serum immunoglobulins (IgG, IgM, IgA, and/or IgD) are characteristic of HIV-1–infected children and appear very early in life, often before other laboratory abnormalities are noted. C1q-binding immune complexes along with classic complement pathway activation also may be found within the first 4 months of life in perinatally infected infants.[308] Abnormalities in IgG subclasses may be seen; IgG subclass 2 levels are decreased below the normal value for age in some patients.[568] Additionally, specific, antigen-triggered secretion of immunoglobulin is diminished significantly, which leads to impaired pathogen-specific antibody response. Abnormalities in both primary and secondary antibody response have been demonstrated to both T-cell–dependent antigens (e.g., diphtheria and tetanus toxoid) and T-cell–independent antigens (e.g., pneumococcal polysaccharide).[36] Poor in vitro mitogenic response to staphylococcal Cowan A, a specific B-cell mitogen, and to pokeweed mitogen, a T-cell–dependent B-cell mitogen, has been reported.[36] Thus, despite a chronic state of increased B-cell activation commonly evidenced by hypergammaglobulinemia, HIV-1–infected children functionally appear as if they were hypogammaglobulinemic with B cells unable to respond appropriately to specific antigenic stimulation. Compromise of the humoral immune system by HIV infection in infancy, at a time of immunologic naivete and a maturing but not yet functional immune system, may be particularly devastating and may account for the high frequency of severe bacterial infections seen in children.

T Cells

T-cell activation markers can be detected in HIV-1–infected infants as early as the first few months of life. Elevated levels of soluble CD8, a nonspecific measure of CD8+ cell activation, are increased substantially in infected infants even before a detectable increase in CD8+ lymphocytes is observed.[250] Both CD4+ and CD8+ lymphocytes from infected children show early phenotypic evidence of activation, including increases in the coexpression of HLA-DR and CD38 on CD4+ and CD8+ cells, loss of CD45RA+CD8+ cells, and increase in CD57+CD8+ cells.[529] It has been hypothesized that such immune system activation could lead to T-cell death by apoptosis.[364]

Impaired T-cell immunity, the hallmark of HIV infection in adults, also is seen in children, although commonly it is manifested later than B-cell dysfunction. Impairments include decreased in vivo and in vitro function of T cells as well as quantitative abnormalities of T cells. In vivo dysfunction of T cells is evidenced by anergy to delayed-type hypersensitivity skin testing; however, because the ability to respond to skin testing is age-related, negative skin tests in a young infant may not be informative.

Progressive decrease in CD4+ lymphocyte number is a characteristic finding in HIV-1–infected adults and children. Interpretation of lymphocyte subset quantitation among children must consider age as an important variable. Normal CD4 lymphocyte counts in healthy, uninfected infants are considerably higher than those observed in adults, with a subsequent decline to normal adult values over the first 6 years of life.

Prior to the loss of CD4+ lymphocytes, there is a sequential and progressive loss of CD4+ T-helper lymphocyte function, which has been assessed primarily by evaluating the in vitro ability of the patients' lymphocytes to produce IL-2 in response to specific antigens.[522, 603] The first T-helper functional loss is recall antigen response, followed by loss of T-helper response to allogenic HLA and lastly to phytohemagglutinin. This sequential loss has been correlated with disease progression in adults and in children. Loss of recall antigen response alone correlates with increased susceptibility to recurrent bacterial infections, whereas progressive loss of all three T-helper functional responses correlates with increased risk of opportunistic infections.[570]

CD4+ T-helper cell function can be divided into three interregulatory subpopulations that are defined on the basis of their associated cytokine profiles and functions. T-helper type 1 lymphocytes are associated with production of IL-2, IL-12, and interferon-γ and preferentially facilitate a cell-mediated immune response. T-helper type 2 lymphocytes are associated with production of IL-4, IL-5, IL-6, and IL-10 and preferentially facilitate T-cell–dependent humoral immune response. A clone of cells also can be found that produces a composite T-helper type 1/2 pattern; these cells are termed T-helper type 0. It has been hypothesized that a switch from a predominance of type 1 to a type 0 or 2 pattern of T-cell function might be associated with disease progression.[124, 309] Derangements in cytokine secretion have been observed in pediatric HIV-1 infection, although findings have not always been consistent. In some studies, HIV-1–infected children show diminished secretion of the T-helper type 1–associated cytokine, IL-2, compared with uninfected controls.[679] Lymphocytes from infected children show increased spontaneous secretion of IL-6, a T-helper type 2–associated cytokine, and TNF-α when compared with those from uninfected children, and the level of hypergammaglobulinemia correlates with IL-6 levels.[264, 553] These results are consistent with the hypothesis that there may be some imbalance in T-helper type 1 and 2 response to HIV infection. However, there have been discrepant results regarding T-helper type 2 cytokine IL-4 levels in infected children, with some reports showing an increase and others no difference from uninfected controls.[553, 679] One study reported augmented production of T-helper type 2 cytokines in symptomatic compared with asymptomatic children, but this needs further verification.[679]

HIV-specific cytotoxic T-lymphocyte (CTL) responses are detected uncommonly during the first few months of life in infected children and only inconsistently found after that, although precursor CTL function occasionally may be detected despite the absence of circulating, activated HIV-specific CTLs.[394, 424, 425] In contrast, infected adults develop HIV-specific CTLs soon after primary infection. The epitope specificity of the CTL response, the intensity of response, and the time that CTLs develop differ among infants.[7, 393] Additionally, the epitope specificity of CTLs may change in a single child over time. It has been proposed that HIV-specific CTLs may be associated with diminished disease progression; however, increase in viral load and decline in CD4+ count has been observed despite the presence of CTLs.[7, 393] A number of investigators have described finding transient HIV-specific CTLs among some uninfected infants born to HIV-1–infected women, suggesting that these uninfected infants had exposure to HIV and that the presence of a cell-mediated immune response may reflect protective immunity.[7, 125, 161] However, this phenomenon has not been detected by other researchers.[393, 424]

Other Immune Cells

In addition to T- and B-cell defects, functional defects in polymorphonuclear, monocyte, and natural killer cell function have been detected in infected children. Cells of the mononuclear phagocyte line are major target cells for HIV infection and are likely reservoirs of persistent virus in the body. Infection of monocytes may result in impaired capacity to present antigens to T cells and/or to produce cytokines. Neutrophil defects in chemotaxis in asymptomatic infected children and decreased bactericidal activity against *S. aureus* in asymptomatic and symptomatic children have been detected.[572] Decreased superoxide anion and hydrogen peroxide production by neutrophils and monocytes of infected children, deficient antibody-dependent cellular cytotoxicity polymorphonuclear function, and decreased natural killer cell activity also have been described.[47, 116, 547, 634]

Disease Manifestations

HIV disease manifestations in children predominantly reflect the consequences of infection acquired in the perinatal period, and the spectrum of clinical manifestations in children with perinatally acquired infection is distinct from that seen in adults or adolescents. In children with perinatal HIV-1 infection, early symptoms generally are nonspecific and distinguished only by their persistence and severity. Initial manifestations of HIV-related disease in children can be subtle and include failure to thrive, organomegaly and lymphadenopathy, persistent oral thrush, chronic or recurrent diarrhea, and recurrent fevers. HIV in both adults and children causes a multisystem disease. Infection can be asymptomatic, mild, moderate, or severe, and although the course of disease is heterogeneous in both the pediatric and adult population, ultimately progressive immune dysfunction with accompanying clinical deterioration may be expected.

INFECTIONS

The consequences of immunologic dysfunction, particularly in the humoral arm of the immune system, may be more pronounced in infected children than in adults. In adults, even if response to new antigens is diminished, preexisting memory cells provide some measure of immunity from common pathogens. However, if defective B-cell function occurs early in life, prior to the development of specific memory cells, recurrent and severe infection with otherwise common organisms may be seen.

Serious bacterial infections may be the first indication of perinatal HIV-1 infection. HIV-1–infected children have elevated rates of bacterial infection compared with age-matched peers; in one study, the rate of community-acquired invasive bacterial infections was three times higher among infected children.[14, 539] Bacteremia, often without a focus, is the most frequently reported serious infection[579]; other commonly reported serious infections include pneumonia, meningitis, urinary tract infection, cellulitis/abscess, septic arthritis, and gastroenteritis.[36, 346] Episodes of invasive bacterial disease may occur even in infected children with relatively normal CD4+ lymphocyte counts and probably are related to more subtle defects in T-helper cell function, such as loss of recall antigen response.[570] Often, the invading organisms are encapsulated bacterial pathogens commonly seen in childhood, such as *Streptococcus pneumoniae, Haemophilus influenzae, S. aureus,* and *Neisseria meningitidis*. Invasive pneumococcal disease particularly is common, with incidence rates as high as 11.3 per 100 child-years during the first 3 years of life, exceeding that observed among children with sickle-cell anemia.[220, 249] Less common pathogens also are seen, such as *Salmonella, Pseudomonas aeruginosa,* and other enterobacteria.[227, 569] Gram-positive organisms, such as *Staphylococcus epidermidis,* may be seen, most often in patients who are hospitalized with intravenous central lines or in patients who are neutropenic (either related to HIV infection or drugs).[571] A resurgence of *Mycobacterium tuberculosis* infection has been observed among HIV-1–infected adults. Tuberculosis in children reflects exposure to disease occurring primarily in adults, and an increase in tuberculosis cases among HIV-1–infected or HIV-exposed children born to HIV-1–infected women has been observed in the United States and Africa.[24, 117, 265] Less serious bacterial infections, such as chronic otitis media, sinusitis, urinary tract infections, and skin and soft tissue infections, also occur with increased frequency.[28, 447, 540] Atypical presentations of bacterial infections, such as pyomyositis, may be seen also.[550]

Common childhood viral infections may be problematic for these children, with increased likelihood of dissemination, severity, recurrence, and persistence. Severity may depend, in part, on the degree of existing immunologic compromise. Severe and fatal measles has been reported, which may be manifested without a typical rash and may occur despite a history of immunization.[345, 508] Primary varicella-zoster virus infection may be uncomplicated, especially in infected children who still are immunocompetent,[329] but also may be severe, disseminated, prolonged, or complicated by bacterial infections or varicella pneumonitis and may be fatal. Recurrent episodes of zoster and atypical, severe, and persistent cutaneous infection with varicella-zoster virus have been described, as well as the development of acyclovir-resistant virus.[316, 368, 369, 504] Herpes simplex virus infection may lead to recurrent and chronic ulcerative stomatitis with persistent viral shedding, or it may spread from the oropharynx to the esophagus or disseminate to other organ systems.[315] Active CMV infection may be found in up to 45 per cent of children with symptomatic HIV-1 infection.[237] The most common manifestations include retinitis and pneumonitis, which may occur in association with other pathogens, such as *P. carinii;* disseminated CMV can involve almost any organ system, and gastritis, colitis, adrenalitis, encephalitis, myelitis, bone marrow suppression, and even ureteritis and sinusitis have been described.[262, 461, 491, 521] CMV coinfection has been postulated as a possible cofactor in HIV disease progression.[140, 237] Epstein-Barr virus (EBV) seropositivity is common, with high titers to viral capsid and early antigen. The EBV genome has been found in lymph node, lung, and salivary gland tissue. A potential role of EBV in lymphoid interstitial pneumonitis (LIP), parotitis, leiomyosarcoma, and non-Hodgkin lymphoma has been postulated.[328, 423] Infection with common respiratory viruses, such as influenza, parainfluenza, adenovirus, and respiratory syncytial virus, may be associated with significantly prolonged viral shedding, in some cases for months.[333] Viral infections of the skin can be unusual and severe, including persistent molluscum contagiosum and severe anogenital warts (condylomata) refractory to therapy.[361]

As in HIV-1–infected adults, opportunistic infections with pathogens associated with defects in cell-mediated immunity may be seen in HIV-1–infected children. In adults, these infections generally represent reactivation of latent infection acquired earlier in life, often during childhood. Young children, lacking prior immunity to these organisms, may have a more fulminant course of disease when experiencing a primary infection. PCP is the most common opportunistic infection in children, seen in 37 to 40 per cent of all infected children and up to 65 per cent of children who develop AIDS in the first year of life.[253, 610] More than half of PCP cases occur among infected infants between the ages of 3 and 6 months; the estimated risk of acquiring PCP during the first year of life in perinatally infected infants is 7 to 20 per cent.[610] Onset typically is acute, often with a rapidly and fatal course in those younger than 1 year of age.[253] Degree of immunosuppression, as measured by age-adjusted CD4+ lymphocyte count or per cent, is predictive of PCP risk in adults and older infants and children but not in children younger than

TABLE 192–11. Recommendations for *Pneumocystis carinii* Pneumonia (PCP) Prophylaxis and CD4+ Monitoring for HIV-Exposed and HIV-Infected Children

Age/HIV Infection Status	PCP Prophylaxis	CD4+ Lymphocyte Monitoring
Birth to 4–6 weeks, HIV-exposed	No prophylaxis	1 month
4–6 weeks to 4 months, HIV-exposed	Prophylaxis	3 months
4–12 months		
HIV-infected or indeterminate	Prophylaxis	6, 9, and 12 months
HIV infection reasonably excluded*	No prophylaxis	None
1–5 years, HIV-infected	Prophylaxis if CD4+ count <500/mm³ or <15%	Every 3–4 months†
6–12 years, HIV-infected	Prophylaxis if CD4+ count <200/mm³ or <15%	Every 3–4 months†
Any age	Prophylaxis if prior episode of PCP	

*HIV infection reasonably can be excluded among children who have had two or more negative HIV virologic diagnostic tests (i.e., HIV culture or polymerase chain reaction), both of which were performed at ≥1 month of age and one of which was performed at ≥4 months of age OR two or more negative HIV-1 IgG antibody tests performed at >6 months of age among children with no clinical evidence of HIV disease.

†More frequent monitoring (e.g., monthly) is recommended for children whose CD4+ count or per cent is approaching the threshold at which prophylaxis is recommended.

Modified from Centers for Disease Control and Prevention: 1995 revised guidelines for prophylaxis against *Pneumocystis carinii* pneumonia for children infected with or perinatally exposed to human immunodeficiency virus. M. M. W. R. *44* (No. RR-4):1–11, 1995.

12 months of age, in whom PCP may occur at CD4+ levels above those indicative of severe immunosuppression.[609] Although PCP can be prevented effectively by chemoprophylaxis, the epidemiology of the disease indicates that early identification of HIV-1 exposure is crucial to enable prophylaxis to be initiated before 2 months of age, when PCP risk dramatically increases.[559, 609] Current prophylaxis guidelines recommend starting prophylaxis in all infants born to HIV-1–infected mothers beginning at 4 to 6 weeks of age, with subsequent discontinuation in children determined not to be infected and continuation for at least the first year of life in infected children[103] (see prophylaxis section and Tables 192–11 and 192–12).

Nontuberculous mycobacterial infection, particularly with *Mycobacterium avium-intracellulare* complex (MAC), is less common in infected children than in adults, occurring in 6 to 14 per cent of infected children overall, and is more common in transfusion- or hemophilia-associated than perinatal pediatric AIDS cases.[292, 293, 377] The incidence of MAC is highest among children with late-stage disease and severe immunosuppression, occurring primarily among children with a CD4+ lymphocyte count of less than 100/mm³. MAC can involve almost any organ system, and manifestations include asymptomatic bacteremia, localized infection, and disseminated disease with systemic symptoms, such as fever, night sweats, weight loss, abdominal pain, massive organomegaly, and bone marrow replacement resulting in anemia, neutropenia, and thrombocytopenia.[293, 377]

Oral candidiasis is the most common fungal infection seen in children; extension to the esophagus may occur in 20 per cent of pediatric AIDS patients with symptoms of poor appetite, weight loss, vomiting, and fever.[567] Disseminated candidiasis is uncommon, occurring primarily in late-stage patients associated with central venous catheter use.[370, 687] Other opportunistic fungal and parasitic infections, such as disseminated histoplasmosis, cryptococcosis, toxoplasmosis,

TABLE 192–12. Drug Regimens for *Pneumocystis carinii* Pneumonia (PCP) Prophylaxis for Children 4 Weeks of Age or Older

Drug	Dose	Schedule
Recommended Regimen		
Trimethoprim (TMP)–sulfamethoxazole (SMX)	150 mg TMP/m²/day with 750 mg SMX/m²/day administered orally	**Recommended Schedule:** • In divided doses twice a day three times per week on consecutive days (e.g., Monday–Tuesday–Wednesday) **Acceptable Alternative Schedules:** • As a **single daily dose** three times per week on consecutive days (e.g., Monday–Tuesday–Wednesday) • In divided doses twice a day administered **7 days per week** • In divided doses twice a day administered three times per week on **alternate days** (e.g., Monday–Wednesday–Friday)
Alternative Regimens if TMP-SMX Is Not Tolerated		
Dapsone	2 mg/kg (not to exceed 100 mg) administered orally	• As a single dose taken once daily
Aerosolized pentamidine* (children ≥5 years of age)	300 mg administered via Respirgard II inhaler	• Single monthly treatment

*If neither dapsone nor aerosolized pentamidine is tolerated, some clinicians use intravenous pentamidine, 4 mg/kg, administered every 2 or 4 weeks. Data regarding the pharmacokinetics of atovaquone in children currently are under study.

Modified from Centers for Disease Control and Prevention: 1995 revised guidelines for prophylaxis against *Pneumocystis carinii* pneumonia for children infected with or perinatally exposed to human immunodeficiency virus. M. M. W. R. *44* (No. RR-4):1–11, 1995.

and cryptosporidiosis, have been reported in children, although more rarely than in adolescents and adults.[37, 367, 442, 691] Endemic pathogens in the geographic region in which the child lives will determine the opportunistic organisms causing infections; for example, disseminated *Penicillium marneffei* infection has been reported among HIV-1–infected children in Thailand.[613]

A possible increase in the risk of cotransmission of other congenital infections has been reported for CMV, hepatitis C, toxoplasmosis, and Chagas' disease. This could occur due to high systemic levels of the opportunistic pathogen in immunocompromised pregnant women or placental disruption due to HIV, the pathogen, or both, facilitating cotransmission.[140, 236, 442, 500]

Respiratory Tract

Diseases of the upper and lower respiratory tract account for significant morbidity and mortality in pediatric HIV-1 infection. The influence of HIV on pulmonary immune defenses has not been well delineated. Alveolar macrophages can be infected by HIV.[77, 604] Infected macrophages could serve as a reservoir for HIV in the lung and produce cytokines causing inflammation that compromises lung function. Cytotoxic CD8+ lymphocytes produced in response to HIV infection could infiltrate the lung and impair pulmonary function. Additionally, HIV-induced abnormalities in macrophage or natural killer cell function could weaken the respiratory tract response to infecting organisms, resulting in more frequent and severe infections.

Upper respiratory tract disease related to HIV may occur early in the course of infection and includes recurrent and chronic otitis media.[540] Sinusitis in HIV-1–infected children is common and most often subacute and recurrent.[447] Lower respiratory tract disease can be divided into acute, usually infectious processes and chronic pulmonary disease of unknown etiology, including pulmonary lymphoid hyperplasia (PLH) and LIP.

Infectious pulmonary disease is common with a majority of HIV-1–infected children developing infectious pulmonary complications at some stage of their disease.[411, 452] The most common opportunistic infection seen in HIV-1–infected children is PCP. In adults, PCP often is due to reactivation of preexisting *P. carinii* infection, and an insidious onset of symptoms often is seen. In young children, PCP frequently is a primary infection with a more acute presentation, although a slower onset may be seen, particularly in older children. Chest radiographs initially may be normal but progress to a diffuse bilateral alveolar-interstitial disease picture. Definitive diagnosis is made by demonstration of pneumocysts in the lung via examination of induced sputum, bronchoalveolar lavage, or open lung biopsy.[77]

Bacterial pneumonias also are common in pediatric HIV-1 infection. Infection with encapsulated pyogenic bacteria predominates, particularly *S. pneumoniae*. HIV-1–infected children have been shown to have higher rates of mucosal colonization with pyogenic bacterial than have uninfected children, which may predispose to their high risk for lower tract bacterial infections.[146] Gram-negative pneumonia, including *P. aeruginosa*, also is seen and has a significant association with acute respiratory failure and an accompanying high mortality.[569] Mycobacterial infections may play an increasingly important role in pulmonary disease. A resurgence in *M. tuberculosis* infection in adults in the United States and throughout the world has been linked to coexisting HIV-1 infection. Extrapulmonary and miliary disease may be more frequent among HIV-1–infected children.[332] Pulmonary infection with nontuberculous mycobacteria, particularly MAC, occasionally may be seen, although disseminated disease is much more common.

A variety of other infectious agents may cause pulmonary disease in HIV-1–infected children, including such viruses as respiratory syncytial virus, measles, varicella, and CMV or other opportunistic pathogens, including *Aspergillus*, *Cryptococcus*, *Histoplasma*, and *Strongyloides*; concomitant infection with two or more agents may complicate diagnosis and treatment.[77, 129, 411]

Chronic pulmonary disease in HIV-1 infection is characterized by lymphoid infiltration of the lung. The lymphoid infiltrates are polyclonal, consisting of B and T lymphocytes; CD8+ T lymphocytes may predominate.[313] A spectrum of disease is observed, ranging from focal peribronchiolar infiltration of lymphocytes (PLH) to more diffuse infiltration involving the alveolar septa (LIP); because of overlap between these disorders histologically, they often are referred to as the PLH/LIP complex. Transformation to a paraneoplastic polyclonal polymorphic B-cell lymphoproliferative disorder and rarely into malignant lymphoma has been described.[648] PLH/LIP appears to be a distinctive marker for perinatally acquired HIV-1 infection and is an AIDS-defining illness for infected children.

The cause of PLH/LIP remains unknown. In sheep, infection with ovine lentivirus can induce an LIP similar to PLH/LIP in humans. Ovine lentivirus infects alveolar macrophages, and a correlation between severity of pulmonary disease and virus load in serum and alveolar macrophages is seen.[61] This supports the hypothesis that PLH/LIP may result from inflammation induced by HIV itself. Excessive local production of cytokines, recruitment of lymphocytes, particularly CD8+ lymphocytes, into the lung, and resultant further inflammation and tissue damage could occur in a self-perpetuating cycle. EBV coinfection also has been postulated as etiologic. EBV DNA has been found in lung biopsy specimens from children with LIP, and EBV viral capsid antigen titers typically are elevated.[577]

PLH/LIP is a chronic interstitial process associated with progressive alveolar-capillary block. Radiologically, persistent diffuse bilateral interstitial pulmonary infiltrates are seen, occasionally progressing to nodules, and hilar and paratracheal adenopathy may be present.[267] Clinically, there is an insidious onset of respiratory symptomatology with cough, mild-to-moderate hypoxia, and relatively normal auscultatory findings. With progressive disease, children may develop symptomatic hypoxia with accompanying digital clubbing. Definitive diagnosis is made by lung biopsy showing peribronchial and interstitial infiltrates of lymphocytes and plasma cells, although a presumptive diagnosis can be made when classic clinical and radiologic findings are present. There is no established therapy for PLH/LIP. PLH/LIP is considered an indication for antiretroviral therapy; if HIV is involved in the pathogenesis of PLH/LIP, it is possible that lung disease also may improve with these agents.[538] Because of the proposed inflammatory mechanism, corticosteriods have been used in some children and anecdotally have been reported to be associated with improvement, as has chloroquine.[80, 576] Use of cytokine inhibitors, such as the anti-TNF drug pentoxifylline, has not been studied in children to date.

Despite the chronic morbidity associated with PLH/LIP, children with this condition may constitute a distinct subgroup with a better prognosis than may children with other AIDS-defining conditions. They are more likely to have generalized adenopathy and salivary gland enlargement, and they tend to have highly elevated levels of serum IgG. They also tend to present with HIV-related symptomatology at an older age and have a more chronic course, often having a longer survival time and a lower prevalence of other opportunistic infections.[303, 577, 596]

Cardiovascular System

There is some controversy regarding the incidence of cardiac abnormalities in HIV-1–infected adults and children; cardiac manifestations have been reported in 6 to 73 per cent of infected adults and in 14 to 93 per cent of infected children.[90, 230, 384, 386, 596] This variation in reported incidence most likely is accounted for by differing methods of evaluation, differing definitions of cardiac disease, and referral bias (cardiac referral clinic vs. general HIV-1–infected population). Results from prospective studies of infected children that have included serial cardiac evaluation indicate that whereas clinically symptomatic cardiac disease may be relatively infrequent, subclinical disease is common.[385, 392] A wide range of manifestations have been described in children, including tachycardia; arrhythmias; progressive abnormalities of left ventricular structure and function, including hypertrophy, hypokinesis, depressed contractility, and dilation; dilated cardiomyopathy; congestive heart failure; pericardial effusion; pulmonary hypertension; lymphocytic pericarditis; nonbacterial endocarditis; and sudden death.[359] In one prospective cohort of 81 infected children, clinically significant chronic congestive heart failure was noted in 10 per cent and unexpected cardiorespiratory arrest in 9 per cent of children.[392] Clinically significant cardiomyopathy has been reported in 6.5 to 14 per cent of infected children from two large cohorts from the United States and Italy; in the Italian cohort, the presence of cardiomyopathy was associated with shorter survival.[305, 596, 657]

Although cardiac abnormalities may occur at any stage of HIV infection, they appear to be more frequent and severe in children with more advanced HIV disease. However, tachycardia, arrhythmia, and sudden cardiac arrest have been observed in children who were only mildly symptomatic, particularly in the presence of concomitant LIP.[392] The presence of HIV encephalopathy was a significant predictor of cardiac arrest, and coinfection with EBV significantly correlated with chronic congestive heart failure. Some experts recommend noninvasive cardiac evaluation on a yearly basis for asymptomatic infected children, with increased frequency if cardiac symptoms appear.[359, 392]

Pathologic findings include focal inflammatory changes and necrosis, lymphocytic infiltration, ventricular dilatation and hypertrophy, and nonspecific focal myocardial degeneration with cytoplasmic vacuolization and loss of myofibrils.[313] Although an infectious etiology for cardiac abnormalities rarely has been described, in most cases the heart disease is a primary cardiac abnormality with no definitive etiology. In some cases, HIV-1 DNA and RNA have been identified in heart tissue.[384]

The pathogenesis of the cardiac abnormalities probably is multifactorial. Factors that have received consideration include nutritional deficiencies, anemia, autoimmune phenomena, coinfections, cardiac injury from cytokines or some other substance induced by HIV infection, autonomic dysfunction, and toxicity from potentially cardiotoxic drugs, such as pentamidine, trimetrexate, ganciclovir, amphotericin B, and trimethoprim-sulfamethoxazole. The potential cardiotoxic effects of nucleoside analogues, particularly ZDV, are controversial. Although one prospective study in infected children found that ZDV administration was not associated with either a deterioration or improvement in cardiac function, another retrospective study found that the risk of developing cardiomyopathy was significantly greater in children who previously received ZDV compared with those who had never taken ZDV.[181, 385]

An arteriopathy in various organs has been reported in autopsy studies of children who died of AIDS.[46] Two types of lesions were identified: an inflammatory vasculitis seen in the brain and a fibrocalcific process associated with luminal narrowing in the elastic lamina and media of arteries in several organs, including the brain, lungs, thymus, kidneys, spleen, lymph nodes, and heart.[312] Luminal narrowing of small and medium-sized arteries in the heart and coronary artery aneurysm formation associated with myocardial infarction have been described, as well as cerebral artery aneurysm formation.[296]

Gastrointestinal Tract

Failure to thrive and growth failure are prominent findings among HIV-1–infected children. Growth failure has been shown to be associated with an elevated risk of mortality among perinatally infected children and hemophiliacs in the United States.[58, 431] Longitudinal assessment of growth in children born to infected mothers has shown that although anthropomorphic parameters are similar at birth in infected and uninfected children, infected children show small but significant abnormalities in growth very early in life.[215, 429, 583] Both weight and height velocity appear to be affected. These abnormalities are observed prior to the onset of HIV-related symptoms in most children, and their pathogenesis is not known. Factors that have been proposed include endocrine dysfunction, impaired gastrointestinal tract function, altered cytokine production, excessive energy expenditure, and poor oral intake. Experiments in transgenic mice demonstrated that expression of a nonreplicating HIV genome construct encoding envelope and regulatory genes was associated with postnatal growth failure; prenatal growth appeared to be normal.[234] This suggests that virally encoded products, independent of viral replication, may be involved in the pathogenesis of early growth retardation in infected children.

As HIV disease progresses, growth failure may become more profound due to the effect of recurrent opportunistic infections and complications of HIV disease on nutrient requirements, intake, or absorption. Micronutrient deficiency may be present before HIV-related symptoms appear and worsen with the onset of AIDS, further exacerbating existing immune defects.[517] Vitamin A is important for maintaining integrity of epithelial tissue and for immune function.[600] In Africa, vitamin A deficiency in HIV-1–infected pregnant women was associated with increased risk of perinatal HIV-1 transmission and higher mortality in the women themselves and their infants, and vitamin A supplementation of infected children has decreased infectious morbidity, particularly diarrhea.[144, 601, 602] Abnormalities in fat, protein, and carbohydrate (particularly lactose) absorption are detected in a majority of symptomatic infected children. These findings often are not associated with overt diarrhea, enteric infections, or degree of immunologic compromise.[304, 438, 715] In a study in Africa, diarrhea was significantly more frequent, severe, persistent, and recurrent among HIV-1–infected than uninfected children born to HIV-1–infected mothers and was associated with increased risk of mortality.[514, 654] However, enteric pathogens were found only in slightly more than half of infected children with diarrhea.

HIV has been shown to replicate in vitro within gastrointestinal tissue culture cell lines, identified in intestinal tissues by in situ hybridization, and fecal shedding of HIV-1 RNA in infected children has been demonstrated, particularly in children with diarrhea.[716] This implies that HIV may be replicating actively within epithelial cells or macrophages within the gastrointestinal tract and that HIV itself may play a role in diarrhea and/or malabsorption in which an infectious etiology can not be identified.

A number of infectious agents characteristically involve the gastrointestinal tract in children with AIDS, including bacteria (*Campylobacter, Salmonella, Shigella, Mycobacteria*), protozoa (*Giardia, Cryptosporidia, Isospora, Microsporidia, Blastocystis hominis*), viruses (CMV, rotavirus, adenovirus, astrovirus, calcivirus), and fungi (*Candida, Histoplasma*). Gastrointestinal infections may be localized (e.g., *Candida* esophagitis) or disseminated (e.g., CMV or *Mycobacteria* infection) and can involve any part of the gastrointestinal tract from pharynx to rectum. Small bowel bacterial overgrowth may be seen, as can *Clostridia difficile* colitis secondary to chronic antibiotic use.

A number of oral manifestations of pediatric HIV-1 infection have been described. Candidiasis is the most common oral manifestation of pediatric HIV-1 infection. Dental development may be delayed and dental caries more frequent in infected children; HIV-associated periodontal disease (atypical gingivitis and rapidly progressive periodontitis), common in infected adults, appears to be more unusual in children.[35, 664] Oral hairy leukoplakia and severe aphthous ulcers of the mouth and pharynx, although uncommon, have been reported in infected children.[35, 154]

Subclinical abnormalities in biochemical indices (serum amylase, lipase, trypsin) of pancreatic function may be seen in up to 30 per cent of symptomatic infected children and clinically symptomatic pancreatitis in about 17 per cent.[18, 439] Diverse etiologies have been identified, including therapeutic agents used for the treatment of HIV infection (e.g., parenteral pentamidine, dideoxyinosine, lamivudine) and, rarely, opportunistic infections.[76, 318] Increased risk of clinical pancreatitis has been correlated with the degree of immunosuppression, prior history of pancreatitis, and therapy with parenteral pentamidine, especially in patients with a CD4+ count less than 100/mm^3; coinfection with CMV was associated with more protracted episodes.[439] Elevated serum lipase was a more sensitive marker than was amylase for pancreatitis.

Hepatosplenomegaly accompanied by persistent, mild elevations in serum transaminase is not uncommon in HIV-1–infected children, although hepatic failure is rare. Hepatocellular injury and/or cholestasis may be caused by drugs used to treat complications of HIV, such as ZDV, didanosine (ddI), dapsone, trimethoprim-sulfamethoxazole, and ketoconazole. Chronic liver inflammation may be caused by known infectious agents, such as CMV, hepatitis B virus, hepatitis C virus, or atypical mycobacteria with progression to liver failure and portal hypertension. Additionally, a clinical syndrome of cholestasis and hepatitis of unknown etiology has been observed among some infants with perinatal HIV-1 infection who also have early immunologic dysfunction.[518] A histologic picture of chronic active hepatitis with lymphocytic infiltrates in the portal and lobular regions, giant-cell transformation of hepatocytes, and fatty degeneration may be seen, but no specific infectious agent has been identified. In one report of a child with cholestatic hepatitis, HIV-1 RNA and gp41 antigen were identified within cells in hepatic lobules, but others have not replicated this.[518]

Genitourinary Tract

Intermittent abnormalities on urinanalysis, such as transient proteinuria, are not uncommon among symptomatic infected children and probably are multifactorial in origin.[135] Clinically overt renal disease appears to be relatively infrequent, with rates from different prospective cohorts varying from 2 to 9 per cent.[301, 657] Although nephrotic syndrome rarely has been reported to be the presenting manifestation of HIV infection, renal disease appears to be most common among older, already symptomatic children.[135, 673] In a population-based comparison of the clinical course in children and adults after the diagnosis of AIDS, renal failure/insufficiency was observed in 3.7 per cent of infected adults compared with only 0.5 per cent of infected children (95 per cent confidence interval, 0.0 to 1.1 per cent).[661]

In adults, HIV nephropathy develops at all stages of HIV infection, progresses rapidly over weeks to renal failure, and histologically shows focal glomerulosclerosis. In contrast, in children, a wider range of histologic lesions has been identified, including mesangial hyperplasia, focal glomerulosclerosis, segmental necrotizing glomerulonephritis, and minimal change disease; tubuloreticular inclusions have been described within glomerular endothelial cells.[135, 301, 627] Although children with focal glomerulosclerosis appear to progress to renal failure, progression occurs more slowly than that observed in adults; in children with other histologic forms of nephropathy, progression to severe renal failure appears to be infrequent. Although the etiology of HIV-associated nephropathy is not known, some have hypothesized that it may be immunologically mediated.[135, 301]

Hematologic

Hematologic abnormalities found in HIV-1–infected children are similar to those observed in adults and tend to be more frequent and severe in advanced HIV disease. However, hematologic cytopenias occasionally may occur in asymptomatic HIV-1–infected infants and may be the only initial clinical manifestation of disease. These abnormalities may be the end result of a number of different processes, including bone marrow infiltration by infection or malignancy, adverse drug reactions, malnutrition, immune dysregulation, and HIV itself, and it may be difficult to differentiate primary HIV-associated hematologic abnormalities from those due to other causes. In addition to the CD4+ lymphopenia characteristic of AIDS, anemia, neutropenia, and thrombocytopenia all have been described in children with HIV-1 infection.[291]

Isolated thrombocytopenia can be the sole clinical manifestation of HIV-1 infection.[31, 558] Thrombocytopenia has been reported in 10 to 19 per cent of symptomatic HIV-1–infected children.[31] The risk for severe bleeding (the major concern being cerebral hemorrhage) appears to be higher in thrombocytopenia due to HIV, particularly in infected hemophiliacs. In many cases, an immune basis may be documented with elevated levels of antiplatelet antibodies and circulating immune complexes.[195, 558] Direct infection of megakaryocytes and platelets with HIV also has been reported, suggesting that antiretroviral therapy might have some utility in treating HIV-associated thrombocytopenia.[585, 720] Response to treatment with intravenous immunoglobulin (general immunoglobulin and antirhesus [Rh]-D immunoglobulin), steroids, and antiretroviral agents, such as ZDV and ddI has been reported.[31, 73, 255, 558] Splenectomy generally has been avoided due to concerns regarding increased risk of bacterial sepsis.

Neutropenia is relatively common in pediatric HIV-1 infection. Although immune neutropenia has been described, drug-induced neutropenia may be more common, particularly with certain antiretroviral agents (e.g., ZDV).[422] The use of cytokines, such as granulocyte–colony-stimulating factor, has been shown to improve neutropenia in HIV-1–infected children.

Anemia is frequent in HIV-1–infected children and may be due to a number of processes, including nutritional deficiencies (particularly iron and vitamin B_{12} deficiencies), chronic infection, immune-mediated processes, and antiretroviral or other therapies. In addition to treatment of underlying causes, such as iron deficiency, if endogenous erythropoietin levels are low, use of erythropoietin may decrease the need for transfusions and raise hemoglobin levels. Coagulation abnormalities in association with circulating anticoagulants also have been noted in several HIV-1–infected children.[72]

Nervous System

The prevalence of central nervous system disease in HIV-1 infection appears to be higher in children than in adults; AIDS dementia develops in 7 to 11 per cent of infected adults compared with the development of AIDS encephalopathy in 20 to 30 per cent of children with end-stage HIV disease.[441] Invasion of the central nervous system appears to occur very early in infection, evidenced by intra–blood-brain barrier synthesis of HIV-1–specific antibody and isolation of HIV from the cerebrospinal fluid near the time of seroconversion in both adults and children.[202, 286] HIV has been detected by in situ hybridization in fetal central nervous system tissue,[397] and immature human embryonic and early postnatal astrocytes appear to be infected preferentially by HIV in vitro when compared with adult human astrocytes, which do not appear to be infectable.[201, 471, 656] It is possible that the immature and developing nervous system of infants may be particularly vulnerable to infection by retroviruses.

Initial retrospective studies reported a high prevalence of encephalopathy in infected children, ranging from 60 to 90 per cent. These studies were problematic because of their retrospective nature, inclusion of children with preexisting neurologic abnormalities, inability to control for important confounding factors such as maternal drug use, use of different methods of assessment and definitions of abnormalities, and lack of an appropriate uninfected comparison group. More reliable estimates have come from prospective natural history studies with longitudinal standardized testing of both infected and uninfected children. These studies have shown significant and early delays in neurodevelopment in cohorts of children infected perinatally compared with uninfected children.[114, 244, 435, 458] However, some studies of children who acquired infection via blood products in which the children predominantly are asymptomatic have found only minimal differences, if any, in neurodevelopment compared with matched uninfected control children.[26, 128, 391, 485]

Stage of HIV disease has been correlated with the extent of neurodevelopmental and brain-imaging test abnormalities in infected children. In a cross-sectional, multicenter, active surveillance study in the United States (CDC-sponsored Pediatric Spectrum of Disease Consortium), HIV encephalopathy was diagnosed in 23 per cent of perinatally infected children with AIDS compared with 9.8 per cent of perinatally infected children overall.[390] In other perinatally infected cohorts in the United States, neurodevelopmental impairment appears to occur predominantly (although not exclusively) in children with severe HIV disease.[114, 485] Similarly, in the European Collaborative Study, neurologic abnormalities were present in 31 per cent of infected children in whom AIDS developed compared with none of the infected children with less severe symptoms and 1 per cent in uninfected control patients[208]; in a Rwandan cohort, neurologic manifestations were observed at 12 months of age in 87 per cent of infected infants with AIDS compared with 31 per cent of infected infants overall.[458] Computed tomographic brain scan abnormalities in both perinatally infected children and infected hemophiliacs also have been correlated with immune status and degree of p24 antigenemia.[63, 443]

The highest risk for development of overt encephalopathy appears to be the first year of life, with most cases diagnosed before the age of 3 years; in the CDC study, the median age of diagnosis was 19 months, and the estimated overall risk of HIV encephalopathy at 12 and 48 months of age was 4.0 and 13.9 per cent, respectively.[390] Children with encephalopathy also were more likely to have cardiomyopathy and more severe HIV disease than were children with other AIDS-defining conditions and had lower CD4+ lymphocyte counts during the first year of life and more hospitalizations. Median survival after diagnosis was only 20 months; other studies also have shown an elevated risk of mortality in children with encephalopathy.[596]

The characteristic clinical presentation seen in children is that of progressive encephalopathy with loss or plateau of developmental milestones and intellectual deterioration; impaired brain growth, manifested by acquired microcephaly or progressive loss of cerebral parenchymal volume on neuroimaging studies; and progressive motor dysfunction.[441] Motor development appears more likely to be affected early in HIV-related central nervous system disease. Gross motor retardation accounted for the principal difference between infected and uninfected children in Rwanda.[458] In a study that evaluated the independent contribution of HIV and prenatal drug exposure to central nervous system delay, HIV infection was associated with decreased motor performance, while prenatal drug exposure appeared to affect both motor and mental development significantly.[435] Other studies have shown that expressive language function is significantly more impaired than receptive early in the course of HIV central nervous system disease.[133, 706] Motor dysfunction may include weakness and bilateral pyramidal tract signs, including a spastic paraparesis. Extrapyramidal rigidity, gait ataxia, and pseudobulbar palsy with dysphagia are seen less commonly; seizures are relatively uncommon. Focal neurologic signs and symptoms are unusual and, if present, generally imply a coexistent pathologic process such as a tumor or, less frequently, an opportunistic infection. With progression of neurologic deterioration, marked apathy, weakness, and spasticity are seen with global loss of language and motor milestones. The encephalopathy may be episodic, with periods of deterioration followed by transiently stable plateaus. Rapidly progressive, subacute but progressive, and static encephalopathy courses have been described.[32]

Other less common neurologic manifestations seen in children include strokes,[513] spinal cord syndromes,[225] inflammatory myopathy,[441] progressive multifocal leukoencephalopathy,[33, 669] cerebral artery aneurysms,[296] and mass lesions, most frequently lymphomas of the central nervous system or, rarely, opportunistic infections such as CMV infection or toxoplasmosis.[515] Peripheral neuropathy of a variety of types, including Guillain-Barré syndrome, mononeuritis multiplex, inflammatory polyradiculopathy, sensory painful or ataxic neuropathy, and demyelinating polyneuropathy, has been described in adults; peripheral nervous system involvement in pediatric HIV-1 infection appears to be rare.[441, 549]

The clinical findings of central nervous system disease in infected children are consistent with a subcortical, diffuse white matter disease process, which is confirmed pathologically and radiologically. A characteristic calcific vasculopathy has been found in the brain with vascular and perivascular inflammatory changes in the small and medium-sized vessels of the basal ganglia and calcific plaques in vessel walls. Inflammatory infiltrates with microglial nodules, composed of microglia, mononuclear cells, astrocytes, lymphocytes, plasma cells, and multinucleated giant cells, have been observed, most often in the basal ganglia and pons. The multinucleated giant cells have been found to contain HIV genome and are most likely of macrophage origin. Associated abnormalities seen with computed tomography and magnetic resonance imaging include cerebral atrophy, ventricular enlargement, calcifications in the basal ganglia and periventricular white matter, and attenuation of signal intensity of the basal ganglia and deep white matter.[267] Electroencephalograms may show diffuse background slowing.

The mode of entry of HIV into the central nervous system is not known, but a number of mechanisms have been suggested, including direct invasion by virus via initial infection of blood-brain barrier microvascular endothelial cells; entry via HIV-infected monocyte/macrophages that cross the blood-brain barrier; and infection of perivascular microglial cells that phagocytize infected blood lymphocytes and migrate into brain tissue.[523, 532] The pathogenesis of the encephalopathy is unclear. Direct viral infection of glial or endothelial cells or astrocytes could cause demyelination, neuronal dysfunction, or disruption of the blood-brain barrier. An indirect neurotoxic effect of viral products, such as gp120 or tat, on neuronal cells causing direct damage of neural cells or competition with neurotransmitters also has been postulated; restricted viral replication within astrocytes with intracellular accumulation of early viral products has been reported.[45, 642] Another proposed mechanism has been by release of neurotoxic factors from infected brain macrophages, such as TNF-α, neopterin, cytokines, arachidonic acid metabolites, nitric oxide, or excitatory amino acids (e.g., quinolinic acid), impairing neuronal function or causing neuronal death, damaging myelin fibers, or interfering with important biochemical pathways, such as methylation and folate metabolism.[45, 62, 598, 631, 642, 713] It is likely that a combination of both direct and indirect factors eventually will be implicated in the causation of the encephalopathy because the extent of white matter destruction and severity of neurologic symptoms is out of proportion to the relatively small numbers of HIV-infected cells in the central nervous system.

ZDV therapy has been shown to improve neurodevelopmental assessments, neuroimaging studies, and neurologic symptoms in children.[441] The effect of other antiretroviral agents, some of which have poorer central nervous system penetration than does ZDV, on encephalopathy is under study. Other novel approaches are under study, including use of anti-inflammatory agents such as steroids and use of agents such as nimodipine, which block calcium channel receptors for excitatory amino acids (e.g., quinolinic acid agonist interaction with the *N*-methyl-D-aspartate receptor) or prevent calcium influx.[62, 625]

Skin

The skin is an immunologically active organ, containing cutaneous dendritic antigen-presenting cells (Langerhans cells) that interact with lymphocytes within the dermis. Although there is some controversy about the ability of skin dendritic cells to support productive infection in vivo,[34, 321] fusion of cutaneous dendritic cells with T cells to form syncytia that produce HIV has been shown in vitro,[535, 548] and HIV-1 DNA has been detected within epidermal Langerhans cells.[120] Alterations in antigen processing and impaired phagocytic function in the skin secondary to HIV infection could impair skin immunity and cause common skin conditions to present with a different appearance or an unusual course in HIV-1–infected patients and increase the likelihood of allergic skin reactions to drugs.

Dermatologic manifestations most often are related to infections, infestations, or allergic or neoplastic processes affecting the skin and are characterized by their increased severity, persistence, frequent recurrence, and poor responsiveness to standard therapies. In infected adults, it has been noted that the incidence of cutaneous disorders increases as immune function decreases, and the occurrence of some disorders appears to correlate with the CD4+ lymphocyte count; for example, seborrheic dermatitis occurs at relatively normal CD4+ counts, whereas molluscum contagiosum and resistant herpes simplex occur primarily when the CD4+ count is depressed significantly (<50 to 250 cells/mm³).[141, 699]

Bacterial, fungal, viral, and parasitic skin infections/infestations typical to childhood may be seen but may be more extensive in nature, recurrent or persistent, and recalcitrant to traditional therapy. Candidiasis is the most common mucocutaneous manifestation of pediatric HIV-1 infection, seen in up to 85 per cent of infected children, usually in the form of oral thrush or severe diaper dermatitis. Chronic fungal paronychia also is seen. A form of "chronic varicella zoster" infection has been described, with widespread skin lesions that may be nodular, hyperkeratotic, and ulcerative.[541] Atypical presentations of common diseases may be seen, such as the hyperinfestation state seen in "Norwegian scabies," or diffuse, severe molluscum contagiosum in atypical areas, such as the face.[641] Disseminated opportunistic infections, such as cryptococcosis and histoplasmosis, may give rise to skin manifestations. Bacillary angiomatosis (bacterial epithelioid angiomatosis) is a cutaneous vascular disorder seen primarily in infected adults consisting of firm violaceous to bright red papules and nodules that are caused by gram-negative bacilli of the *Rochalimaea* species that also cause cat-scratch disease. Visceral involvement, especially of the gastrointestinal tract, may be seen, and a pediatric case presenting as abdominal visceral granulomas has been reported.[699]

Seborrheic dermatitis is very common in infected children and adults, tending to be widespread, severe, and often recalcitrant to therapy. Atopic dermatitis and eczema also are increased in frequency and may be atypical in presentation and refractory to therapy. Psoriasis, reported to be found in up to 21 per cent of infected adults, appears to be more uncommon in infected children.[21] Occurrence of autoimmune cutaneous disorders, such as vitiligo, also may be increased with HIV-1 infection, and the incidence of cutaneous reactions to drugs, such as trimethoprim-sulfamethoxazole, dapsone, or aminopenicillins, also is increased in both infected adults and children.[141] In adults, acute (primary) HIV-1 infection may be associated with a maculopapular eruption and accompanying mononucleosis-like illness,[334] but this syndrome has not been described in perinatal HIV-1 infection.

Malignancies

In contrast to HIV-1 infection in adults, malignancies have been infrequent in children with HIV-1 infection. The incidence of malignancies may increase as the number of infected children increases and as the life expectancy of these children is prolonged through advances in supportive and antiretroviral therapy. Although the optimal treatment approach to cancer in such children remains to be defined, the presence of HIV infection does not necessarily appear to be predictive of a poor response to therapy.[450]

Kaposi sarcoma develops in 25 to 33 per cent of adults with AIDS, principally in homosexual men, and only rarely is reported in infected children. However, a study in Zambia documented an increase in the occurrence of Kaposi sarcoma among children, particularly among those younger than 5 years of age, since 1987.[22] Kaposi sarcoma was aggressive and fulminant among affected pediatric patients, more than 80 per cent of whom were HIV-1–seropositive. They presented with disseminated lymphoadenopathic disease as well as the more commonly recognized cutaneous manifestations.

In infected adults, the most frequent AIDS-related lymphoid neoplasm is B-cell non-Hodgkin lymphoma, seen in 3 to 4 per cent of AIDS patients. Lymphoid malignancies, mostly non-Hodgkin lymphoma, have been reported in a small number of HIV-1–infected children.[467] Involvement of the central nervous system has been observed in 40 to 68 per cent of cases, and lymphoma is the most common cause of focal mass lesions in pediatric HIV-1 infection.[467] A polyclonal polymorphic B-cell lymphoproliferative disorder with systemic involvement affecting the lung, lymph nodes, liver, kidney, spleen, and other tissues has been described[312]; however, progression of this disorder to malignant lymphoma is unclear. Other lymphoid neoplastic diseases reported in HIV-1–infected children include Hodgkin lymphoma, B-cell leukemia, and Burkitt lymphoma.[450]

Leiomyosarcoma, a previously rare smooth-muscle tumor in children, has been reported in an increasing number of HIV-1–infected children as well as in children after organ transplantation.[366, 423, 459] Soft tissue tumors now are the third most common malignancy found in HIV-1–infected children, following non-Hodgkin lymphoma and Kaposi sarcoma. EBV genome has been demonstrated within tumor cells by in situ hybridization, and although its role in malignant transformation is not yet defined, it is postulated that EBV could cause clonal expansion of EBV-infected smooth-muscle cells. EBV infection also has been linked to non-Hodgkin lymphoma in HIV-1–infected children.[328, 467]

Other unusual malignancies that have been reported in HIV-1–infected children include papillary carcinoma of the thyroid, rhabdomyosarcoma, and hepatocellular carcinoma.[176]

Other Clinical Manifestations

Endocrinologic function in HIV-1–infected children has been described incompletely. Although growth failure and short stature are common in HIV-1–infected children, an association with specific endocrinologic abnormalities has not been found. Growth hormone deficiency has been described among some HIV-1–infected children, as has deficiency in insulin growth factor-1 and somatomedin C levels, although results of testing have been heterogeneous and the correlation with growth failure uncertain.[314, 363, 415, 594] Some studies have shown subtle subclinical abnormalities in thyroid function suggestive of compensated hypothyroidism, while others have not.[44, 363, 373, 594] Mild abnormalities in thyroid function appeared to be more common in children with intercurrent severe illness or more advanced disease. Adrenal function appeared to be normal in the small number of children who have been tested, although subtle defects in steroidogenesis appeared to exist in some studies.[362, 363, 594] In a longitudinal study of HIV-1–infected and uninfected hemophiliac boys, linear growth retardation, reduced age-adjusted bone age, and delayed pubertal maturation were seen among infected boys.[248] However, serum testosterone levels did not differ between the two groups, and it was postulated that subtle differences in testosterone secretion pattern or in the concentration of sex-hormone binding globulins may exist.

Rheumatologic symptoms appear to be uncommon in infected children, and complaints of transient mild to moderate arthralgia and myalgia do not appear to exceed those reported in uninfected children.[593] Although evidence of immune dysregulation, such as hypergammaglobulinemia and circulating immune complexes, is common in infected children, autoimmune phenomena, such as positive rheumatoid factor or antinuclear antibody, are uncommon and do not correlate with symptoms.

HIV-1–associated salivary gland disease is characterized by enlargement of the major salivary glands, often with xerostomia; clinical enlargement is most frequent in the parotid glands. In children, persistent salivary gland enlargement or parotitis often is seen in association with LIP. It has been speculated that viruses, notably EBV and CMV, may play a role in salivary gland involvement; it does not appear that HIV plays a direct role in this disease manifestation.[590]

Retinitis in infected children most often is secondary to CMV, although the incidence appears to be much lower than in adults.[521] Varicella-zoster virus and, rarely, other opportunistic organisms also can cause retinal disease.[316] Perivasculitis of the retinal vessels not attributable to known viral disease also has been noted.[330] Asymptomatic peripheral retinal depigmentation has been associated temporally with ddI therapy in children.[697]

Treatment of HIV-1 Infection and Its Complications

General Management Issues

Treatment of pediatric HIV-1 infection requires a multidisciplinary team and a chronic disease–oriented approach. In addition to an infected child, there often are several HIV-1–infected family members. Therefore, optimal care of the infected child may require support and maintenance of an infected family unit. Routine pediatric health maintenance care especially is important in HIV-1–infected children to anticipate and avert any preventable assaults against their already fragile immune system. General supportive therapy should include nutritional guidance, appropriate developmental evaluation and intervention, educational supports, and pain management.[652]

Immunizations

Routine childhood immunizations are an important component of health care of infected children, for whom vaccine-preventable diseases can cause severe morbidity and mortality.[345, 493] It has been hypothesized that stimulation of the immune system by vaccines might enhance HIV expression; a transient increase in HIV RNA levels after vaccination has been reported by some investigators but not others.[712] The duration of maternally derived passive antibody protection against vaccine-preventable diseases may be shortened in infants born to HIV-1–infected women, due to low maternal antibody titers,[163] and routine childhood vaccines clinically appear safe when administered to infected children.[238, 432, 582] Impaired vaccine immunogenicity in HIV-1–infected children has been reported, which may be related to both loss of vaccine-induced antibody as well poor response to primary vaccination.[4, 19, 56, 109, 580] Immune status at the time of vaccination may correlate with immunogenicity, and poor responses have been observed in patients with rapidly progressive, more advanced disease and/or low CD4+ lymphocyte number.[175, 254, 320, 508, 672] This suggests that immunization early in the course of HIV infection may be more effective and emphasizes the importance of adherence to the routine childhood immunization schedule in HIV-1–exposed and infected children. Further studies will be necessary to determine if higher vaccine dosages or additional boosters would enhance vaccine responsiveness in infected children.

There are no contraindications to the use of killed vaccines (hepatitis B, diphtheria, tetanus, pertussis, *H. influenzae* type b, pneumococcal, and influenza vaccines) in infected children. Because of the potential severity of measles in HIV-1–infected children, live measles, mumps, and rubella vaccine also is recommended unless there is a contraindication. However, infected children with documented measles exposure should receive immunoglobulin prophylaxis, regardless of immunization history, due to their uncertain response to immunization. Inactivated poliovirus vaccine should be substituted for oral attenuated poliovirus vaccine, primarily because of concerns regarding postimmunization transmission of the excreted poliovirus to immunosuppressed, HIV-1–infected adults in the child's household. There currently are no safety or efficacy data available regarding use of the newly licensed live attenuated varicella vaccine in HIV-1–infected children; a phase I clinical trial is ongoing. Currently, HIV infection is considered a contraindication to varicella vaccine outside of clinical trials; zoster immunoglobulin should be given to infected children if there is close contact with a person with chickenpox or zoster.[132] Bacillus Calmette-Guerin vaccine, although recommended by WHO for infants born in countries in the developing world in which there is a high incidence of *M. tuberculosis* infection, is not recommended in the United States. An increase in mild to moderate complications of bacillus Calmette-Guerin immunization has been observed among some HIV-1–infected infants receiving vaccine.[487] However, disseminated bacillus Calmette-Guerin disease appears to be rare, supporting continued vaccine use in countries with high rates of tuberculosis where the benefits of vaccination outweigh the risks.[88]

Table 192–13 shows the immunization schedule for HIV-infected children in the United States; it is designed to deliver vaccine as early as possible but to limit the number of injections to two per visit.

TABLE 192–13. Immunization Schedule for HIV-Exposed and HIV-Infected Infants*

Age	Immunization (Dose No.)
Newborn	Hepatitis B (1)†
1 month	Hepatitis B (2)
2 months	Diphtheria-tetanus-pertussis (1) *Haemophilus influenzae* type b (1)
3 months	Enhanced inactivated polio vaccine (1)
4 months	Diphtheria-tetanus-pertussis (2) *Haemophilus influenzae* type b (2)
5 months	Enhanced inactivated polio vaccine (2)
6 months	Diphtheria-tetanus-pertussis (3) *Haemophilus influenzae* type b (3) Hepatitis B (3)
7 months	Influenza (1)§
8 months	Influenza (2)
12 months	*Haemophilus influenzae* type b (3 or 4)‡ Measles-mumps-rubella‖
15 months	Enhanced inactivated polio vaccine (3) Diphtheria-tetanus-acellular pertussis (4)¶
18 months	Diphtheria-tetanus-acellular pertussis (4)¶
24 months	Pneumococcal, 23 valent**

*This schedule differs from that for immunocompetent children in that (1) enhanced inactivated polio vaccine replaces oral polio vaccine, and the first two doses may be given at 3 and 5 months rather than at 2 and 4 months; (2) the second dose of hepatitis B vaccine is given at 1 month; and (3) influenza and pneumococcal vaccines are recommended. The schedule above is designed to provide vaccine to HIV-exposed and HIV-infected children as early as possible and to limit the number of injections to two a visit.

†Infants born to mothers who are positive for hepatitis B surface antigen also should receive hepatitis B immunoglobulin within 12 hours of birth in addition to hepatitis B vaccine.

‡The need for a third dose of *Haemophilus influenzae* type b vaccine depends on which formulation was used; regardless of whether the primary series requires two or three doses, a booster dose is required at 12 to 15 months of age.

¶Diphtheria-tetanus-acellular pertussis vaccine can be administered at 15 or 18 months of age.

§Primary immunization against influenza for children younger than 9 years of age requires two doses of vaccine, the first of which can be given as early as 6 months of age. Subsequent vaccination should be given annually before influenza season.

‖HIV-infected children who are exposed to measles should receive prophylactic immunoglobulin whether or not they have been given vaccine against measles.

**Some authorities recommend revaccination for HIV-infected children vaccinated 6 or more years previously.

Modified from Centers for Disease Control and Prevention: USPHS/IDSA guidelines for the prevention of opportunistic infections in persons infected with human immunodeficiency virus: A summary. M. M. W. R. *44* (No. RR-8):1–34, 1995.

Nutrition

Growth retardation may be evident in HIV-1–infected children as early as the first few months of life. Maintaining optimal nutrition in infected children, particularly those with symptomatic disease, poses a significant challenge. Nutritional status may be compromised by numerous complications of HIV disease due to decreased intake, malabsorption, and/or increased caloric requirements. Resultant malnutrition can compromise further the infected child's fragile immunologic and functional status. Studies have documented micronutrient deficiency among infected children at even early stages of infection,[517] and a trial showing reduced morbidity and mortality among HIV-1–infected children who received vitamin A supplementation illustrates the critical interaction of micronutrients and immune function.[144] Nutritional support is essential, and some children may require nasogastric feedings or parenteral hyperalimentation to achieve an adequate caloric and protein intake.[652]

Prophylaxis

Prompt recognition and treatment of infectious episodes is essential. After treatment, chronic suppressive secondary prophylaxis may be needed because infections often are persistent and recurrent in HIV disease. Infections with opportunistic organisms, such as *Candida,* particularly may be recalcitrant, and chronic oral antifungal agents, such as mycostatin or ketoconazole, are used commonly once symptomatic infection has occurred.

PCP is the most common opportunistic infection in children with perinatal HIV-1 infection; it occurs most commonly between 3 and 6 months of age, a time when definitive diagnosis of HIV-1 infection may not be made; and it often is acute in onset and associated with a poor prognosis.[610] Therefore, prophylaxis must begin very early in life to be effective and especially is critical during the first few months of life. Initial PCP prophylaxis recommendations for children were based upon age-adjusted CD4+ lymphocyte count thresholds.[89] However, data show that among infants younger than 12 months of age, CD4+ cell decline occurs very rapidly prior to the development of PCP and PCP may occur with CD4+ counts above the prophylaxis threshold.[609] Therefore, PCP prophylaxis recommendations for children were expanded in 1995[103] (see Table 192–11). Prophylaxis now is recommended for all infants born to HIV-1–infected women beginning at 4 to 6 weeks of age, regardless of CD4+ lymphocyte count. Prophylaxis should continue in all infected infants and those of indeterminate status until 12 months of age. Prophylaxis should be discontinued among infants in whom HIV-1 infection has been excluded on the basis of two or more negative viral diagnostic tests, both performed at 1 month of age or older and at least one of which is performed at 4 months of age or older. Because CD4+ count is a more reliable predictor of PCP risk in older children, after 12 months of age prophylaxis should be continued only in those children with documented HIV-1 infection who have CD4+ counts below the age-related threshold indicating severe immunosuppression or who have had a prior episode of PCP. The recommended prophylaxis regimen is oral trimethoprim-sulfamethoxazole three times weekly; alternative drugs include dapsone and aerosolized pentamidine[269, 495, 623] (see Table 192–12).

Two randomized, double-blind clinical trials have shown that infusions of 400 mg/kg of intravenous immunoglobulin every 28 days can reduce significantly the rate of serious and minor bacterial infections and hospitalizations in infected children with early-stage HIV infection as well as those with late-stage disease who are receiving ZDV.[619, 651] In children with early-stage disease, a decrease in viral infections and slowing of CD4+ cell decline also were observed.[446, 448] In the study of children with advanced disease, intravenous immunoglobulin efficacy appeared to be confined to those children not receiving trimethoprim-sulfamethoxazole, but this was not confirmed in children with earlier stage disease.[449] Intravenous immunoglobulin currently is recommended for children with evidence of humoral immune defects, including hypogammaglobulinemia, poor functional antibody development, and significant recurrent infections despite appropriate antimicrobial therapy.[707] Further studies are needed before it can be concluded that chemoprophylaxis with agents such as trimethoprim-sulfamethoxazole has efficacy equivalent to that observed with intravenous immunoglobulin.

Prophylaxis against MAC with rifabutin has been recommended for HIV-1–infected adults and adolescents with a CD4+ lymphocyte count less than 75/mm.[94, 105] Although disseminated MAC is less common in infected children than in adults, it appears to constitute a significant opportunistic pathogen in children with late-stage disease.[292, 293, 377] For children between the age of 6 and 12 years, a CD4+ count less than 75/mm^2 has been recommended as a reasonable threshold for initiation of prophylaxis.[105] Rifabutin, particularly when administered in higher doses, rarely has been associated with the development of acute uveitis in adults and in children.[190] There is not currently a pediatric formulation of rifabutin; for children older than 6 years of age, the adult dose of 300 mg daily may be used. For children younger than 6 years of age, a dose of 5 mg/kg daily has been used in pharmacokinetic studies.[105]

ANTIRETROVIRAL THERAPY

Because HIV integrates into the host genome, therapeutic strategies are complicated by potential host-cell toxicity and therefore attempt to target unique sequences in the HIV life cycle, such as viral attachment or reverse transcription (Table 192–14). Long-term and possibly lifelong therapy may be needed. The neurotropism and early central nervous system invasion of HIV in children require that therapeutic agents have adequate central nervous system penetration in addition to adequate serum levels. Ideally, drugs for HIV infection would have good oral bioavailability, penetrate the blood-brain barrier as well as other infected target organs, have limited side effects and toxicity, be easy to administer, and have low cost. It is unlikely that a single agent will be found with these characteristics. It is probable that synergistic combinations of drugs, ideally having different toxicity pro-

TABLE 192–14. HIV Replication Cycle Targets for Antiretroviral Interventions

Stage of HIV Replication Cycle	Potential Intervention	Examples of Antiretroviral Agents
Binding to host cell	Block receptor on host cell Block HIV envelope proteins	Recombinant CD4+ analogues Anti-HIV envelope antibody (passive and/or active immunization) Sulfated polysaccharides (e.g., dextran sulfate)
Entry into host cell and uncoating	Block fusion of HIV with cell membrane Block HIV uncoating	? Bicyclams
Transcription of HIV RNA to DNA	Reverse transcriptase inhibitors Nucleoside analogues	Dideoxynucleosides: Zidovudine (ZDV) Didanosine (ddI) Zalcitabine (ddC) Stavudine (d4T) Lamivudine (3TC) Acyclic nucleoside phosphonates: 9-(2-phosphonomethoxyethyl) adenine (PMEA, bis-POM-PMEA)
	Nonnucleoside inhibitors	Dipyridodiazepinone derivatives Nevirapine Delavirdine Atevirdine
RNA degradation	Inhibit HIV-specific RNase H	?
Integration of viral DNA into host DNA	Integrase inhibitor	Antisense oligonucleotides
Viral regulatory gene expression	Inhibitors of *tat/rev/nef*	Ro 5-3335 (Roche, anti-tat)
Transcription	Interfere with transcription of proviral DNA into viral mRNA	Antisense oligonucleotides
Translation	Interfere with translation of viral mRNA into proteins	Antisense oligonucleotides
Protease	Prevent cleavage of gag-pol polyproteins	Saquinavir Indinavir Ritonavir
Virion assembly	Glycosylation and myristoylation inhibitors	N-myristoyl transferase inhibitors Myristic acid analogues
Viral budding	Prevent viral budding from host cell membrane	Interferon-α Hypericin

files and lacking cross-resistance, will be needed in an effort to enhance efficacy in various organ systems, to permit reduction in drug toxicities, and to reduce the development of drug resistance. The use of immunomodulators to enhance the host's immune response against infection or to decrease antiretroviral drug toxicity also may play a role in the future.

The study, licensure, and use of antiretroviral agents in infants and children have lagged behind that in adults. As of early 1996, eight antiretroviral drugs have been approved for use in HIV-1–infected adults by the Food and Drug Administration (FDA): three nucleoside analogues as monotherapy, ZDV, ddI, and stavudine (d4T); two nucleoside analogues, zalcitabine (ddC) and lamivudine (3TC), for use in combination with ZDV; and three protease inhibitors, saquinavir (for use in combination with ZDV or other nucleoside analogues), ritonavir, and indinavir. Only ZDV, ddI, and 3TC have an approved pediatric indication from the FDA, although data from ongoing trials may permit approval of more agents in children in the near future.

Although criteria have been developed for initiation and modification of antiretroviral therapy in adults and children, the optimal indications for initiation and modification of therapy are in continual flux as the results from new clinical trials provide insight into novel therapeutic regimens with improved efficacy.[527, 707] Clinical trials of various drug combinations in HIV-1–infected adults provide some indication that combination therapy may confer virologic and immunologic advantages over monotherapy and more prolonged duration of benefit.

Nucleoside Analogues

Most antiretroviral agents evaluated to date have targeted the reverse transcription phase of the viral life cycle. Nucleoside analogue drugs have undergone most evaluation; these drugs include ZDV, ddI, ddC, d4T, and 3TC. The drugs are structurally similar prodrugs that require intracellular phosphorylation by host-cell kinases to their active 5′-triphosphate form. The active drug competes with endogenous triphosphate nucleotides for incorporation into proviral DNA synthesized by viral reverse transcriptase. Once incorporated, the triphosphate also acts as a chain terminator and prevents further elongation of the viral DNA chain. The drugs are incorporated more selectively into proviral rather than host-cell DNA because the affinity of the drugs for viral reverse transcriptase is much greater than for host-cell DNA polymerases. However, two mammalian DNA polymerases, DNA polymerase-γ, found in mitochondria, and DNA polymerase-β, have some affinity for the triphosphorylated nucleoside analogues; this may be the basis for some of the toxicities seen with nucleoside analogue drugs. Although similar in structure and mechanism of action, the drugs differ significantly in pharmacokinetics and intracellular phosphorylation pathways, which contribute to differences in patterns of toxicity.

Antiviral activity of all of these drugs when used as monotherapy appears to be time-limited, which probably is related to the emergence of drug-resistant virus.[203, 556] Amino acid substitutions in the viral reverse transcriptase due to mutations at specific points in the viral genome that encode for the enzyme mediate the development of nucleoside analogue resistance. Resistance to all the nucleoside analogues has been observed, and some cross-resistance between agents has been noted.

ZIDOVUDINE. Azido-2′,3-dideoxythymidine (ZDV) was approved by the FDA in 1987 for use in adults and adolescents older than 12 years of age and in May 1990 for use in pediatric patients 3 months to 12 years of age. ZDV has been associated with virologic, immunologic, and clinical benefit in children, including improvements in activity levels, weight gain, linear growth velocity, and neurocognitive function.[155, 427, 428, 526]

The drug is well absorbed orally but undergoes significant first-pass hepatic metabolism, resulting in bioavailability of about 65 per cent. Serum half-life is relatively short, about 1 hour, but the intracellular half-life of the active triphosphate drug is 3.3 hours. Metabolism primarily is hepatic and excretion renal. ZDV crosses the blood-brain barrier, with an average cerebrospinal fluid/plasma ratio of 0.6.

The recommended dose of ZDV in children 4 weeks of age or older is 180 mg/m^2 every 6 hours orally. However, a dose comparison trial in children with mild to moderate symptoms found that 90 mg/m^2 every 6 hours appears to be as efficacious as the higher dose.[54] Similar findings were seen in adults, in whom 500 mg/day of ZDV was equivalent in efficacy and substantially less toxic than was 1500 mg/day. Children with encephalopathy may benefit from the higher ZDV dose. ZDV pharmacokinetics in neonates differ from that in older children; serum half-life is longer and clearance lower.[52] For infants younger than 2 weeks of age, the recommended ZDV dose is 2 mg/kg orally every 6 hours, and for infants 2 to 4 weeks of age, 3 mg/kg orally every 6 hours.

The major toxicity of ZDV is hematologic, consisting of macrocytic anemia and neutropenia. These toxicities may be dose-limiting and exacerbated by concomitant use of other myelosuppressive drugs, such as trimethoprim-sulfamethoxazole or ganciclovir. If hematologic toxicity occurs, dose reduction and use of erythropoietin and/or granulocyte colony-stimulating factor may reduce ZDV-associated bone marrow toxicity without requiring drug discontinuation. ZDV has some affinity for mitochondrial DNA polymerase-γ, and mitochondrial DNA chain replication termination has been observed with ZDV in vitro,[379] raising concern of possible ZDV toxicity to mitochondria-rich organs, such as the heart, muscles, and liver. Although one study did not find a decrease in cardiac contractility associated with ZDV use in children,[385] in another, ZDV use was associated temporally with decreased left ventricular function and increased risk of cardiomyopathy.[181] Skeletal myopathy and a syndrome of fulminant hepatic failure associated with macrovesicular steatosis have been reported in a small number of adults receiving ZDV.[148, 624] Other reported adverse effects include nausea, vomiting, and headache.

ZDV resistance is associated with point mutations in the reverse transcriptase gene at codons 41, 67, 70, 215, and 219. Development of resistance may be associated with decreased drug efficacy and disease progression in children.[297, 489, 660] Stage of HIV disease, CD4+ lymphocyte count, and duration of therapy are related to development of resistance.

DIDANOSINE. ddI is a purine nucleoside analogue that is a prodrug for the active intracellular drug, dideoxyadenosine triphosphate. ddI was approved by the FDA in October 1991 for use in both adults and children with advanced HIV infection who are ZDV-intolerant or experience disease progression while receiving ZDV. In a dose-ranging phase I/II pediatric study, ddI provided clinical, immunologic, and virologic benefit in children with symptomatic HIV infection, with minimal hematologic toxicity.[27, 74] Despite ddI's lower cerebrospinal fluid penetration than ZDV's, improvement in neuropsychometric testing was observed in some patients, which correlated with ddI plasma concentration. Results of long-term follow-up of children receiving ddI for a median duration of almost 2 years showed that ddI appears to be safe, and clinical improvement, increase in CD4+ count, and decrease in p24 antigenemia persisted in some cases for several years.[460]

Bioavailablity of the drug is poor because the drug undergoes inactivation by rapid hydrolysis under acid conditions. Thus, the drug must be administered with antacids or in a buffered formulation and taken on an empty stomach at least 1 hour before or 2 hours after meals; significant interpatient variability in absorption is observed. The buffered formulation may interfere with the bioavailability of other drugs that require gastric acidity for optimal absorption, such as dapsone and ketoconazole; optimally, such drugs should be administered at least 2 hours prior to ddI. The plasma half-life of ddI is short, 0.5 hour, but the intracellular half-life of the active phosphorylated drug is more than 12 hours, permitting ddI to be administered on a less frequent basis than ZDV. About 40 per cent of the drug is cleared by renal mechanisms, and the remainder is metabolized by endogenous purine nucleoside catabolic pathways. The average cerebrospinal fluid/plasma ratio is 0.2.

The optimum dose of ddI in children has not been established yet, and in pediatric studies dosage has ranged from 60 to 540 mg/m^2 daily given in divided doses every 8 or 12 hours. The manufacturer recommends a starting ddI dose for children of 200 mg/m^2 daily, divided into two doses given orally every 12 hours.

ddI is less toxic to bone marrow progenitor cells than is ZDV, and hematologic toxicity is uncommon. Pancreatitis has been observed in about 7 per cent of children receiving ddI and appears to be dose-related; predisposing factors include prior history of pancreatitis, advanced disease, CD4+ lymphocyte count less than 50/mm^3, baseline elevation of serum transaminases, and concurrent administration of other drugs known to cause pancreatitis, such as pentamidine.[76] Peripheral neuropathy, seen in 13 to 34 per cent of infected adults receiving ddI, appears to be uncommon in children, occurring in less than 3 per cent. Asymptomatic peripheral retinal depigmentation has been observed in less than 5 per cent of children receiving ddI, is not associated with vision loss, and appears to reverse with discontinuation of therapy.[697] Diarrhea has been reported and may be more related to the antacid/buffer than to the drug itself. Elevation of liver enzymes has been reported with ddI therapy, and fulminant hepatitis rarely has been reported.[39, 352]

Mutations at codons 74, 184, and 135 of the reverse transcriptase gene are associated with ddI resistance. Development of the codon 74 mutation was associated with a greater decline in CD4+ count and higher viral burden in some studies in adults and children.[180, 344]

COMBINATION ZIDOVUDINE/DIDANOSINE THERAPY. A phase I/II study that evaluated combination ZDV/ddI therapy in children found potent antiviral activity, particularly in children without prior antiretroviral therapy, and no evidence for pharmacokinetic drug interactions or additive toxicity; however, marked interpatient variability in drug levels, particularly of ddI, was observed.[295, 462] A phase III randomized, double-blind trial (AIDS Clinical Trials Group [ACTG] protocol 152) compared initial therapy with ZDV alone (180 mg/m^2 every 6 hours) versus ddI alone (120 mg/m^2 every 12 hours) versus combination ZDV (120 mg/m^2 every 6 hours) and ddI (90 mg/m^2 every 12 hours) in symptomatic infected children. Children receiving either ddI monotherapy or ZDV/ddI combination therapy had significantly less disease progression and toxicity than did children receiving ZDV alone. No significant differences between ddI monotherapy and combination ZDV/ddI were observed in disease progression, survival, or toxicity.

ZALCITABINE. ddC was approved by the FDA in 1992 for use in combination with ZDV in HIV-1–infected adults with a CD4+ count less than 300/mm^3 and clinical or immunologic deterioration on ZDV monotherapy. A pediatric indication has not been approved yet. Initial studies of ddC monotherapy and of alternating ddC and ZDV therapy in pediatric patients showed increases in CD4 lymphocyte count and decrease in p24 antigenemia in some patients; however, IQ scores appeared to fall during ddC monotherapy.[525] Peripheral neuropathy, reported in 7 to 29 per cent of adults receiving ddC, was not observed in children in these studies, and there were no dose-limiting hematologic adverse effects, although neutropenia was observed. However, rashes and oral ulcerations were noted in more than 50 per cent of patients. Data from a clinical trial (ACTG 190) that is evaluating combination ddC/ZDV compared with ZDV monotherapy in stable, ZDV-experienced infected children should be available in 1996.

ddC is well absorbed, with an oral bioavailability of 54 to 87 per cent. Similar to that of ddI, ddC's plasma half-life is short, about 20 to 30 minutes, and ddC's passage into the cerebrospinal fluid is poorer and significantly less than that of ZDV. Intracellular half-life of the active triphosphate is 2.6 hours; elimination primarily is renal.

The optimum dose of ddC in children has not been defined. In a phase I study, ddC plasma concentrations were lower and drug half-life was shorter in children than adults given comparable doses, suggesting more rapid clearance of the drug in children.[110] Another pediatric clinical trial, ACTG 138, compared two doses of ddC (0.01 vs. 0.005 mg/kg given orally every 8 hours) for treatment of infected children with disease progression on ZDV monotherapy. Both doses appeared to be safe, and no difference in efficacy was observed between the higher and lower dose groups.[618] Although uncommon, peripheral neuropathy was observed in some children in this study.

Resistance to ddC has been observed and is associated with mutations in reverse transcriptase gene codons 65 and 184; cross-resistance with ddI and 3TC also has been reported. Alternating therapy of ddC and ZDV did not appear to prevent the emergence of ZDV resistance.[297]

STAVUDINE. d4T was approved by the FDA in 1994 for use in adults with intolerance or disease progression on other antiretroviral agents; a pediatric indication has not been approved yet. There is limited information about d4T in children. In a phase I/II dose-ranging trial (0.125 to 4 mg/kg daily in two divided doses) in symptomatic infected children, d4T was well tolerated, and there were no dose-related clinical or laboratory adverse events.[341] Improvement in growth was observed, and antiretroviral activity, measured by improvement in CD4+ count and decrease in p24 antigenemia, also was observed in some patients. Data from a clinical trial comparing monotherapy with d4T compared with ZDV (ACTG 240) should be available in 1996. The dose of d4T chosen for ACTG 240 is 2 mg/kg daily in two divided doses (1 mg/kg/dose).

d4T is acid-stable, and bioavailability exceeds 80 per cent; like other nucleoside analogues, the plasma half-life is short, about 1 hour. About 34 to 41 per cent of the drug is excreted unchanged in the urine, and the remainder is metabolized by nucleoside salvage pathways. The drug appears to penetrate the cerebrospinal fluid in comparable levels to that observed with ZDV, with cerebrospinal fluid levels between 20 and 70 per cent of serum concentration.

In adults, hematologic toxicity is uncommon. Peripheral neuropathy has been the major dose-limiting toxicity, occurring in 15 to 21 per cent of infected adults receiving d4T. Elevated hepatic transaminases were seen in about 11 per cent of recipients and pancreatitis reported in about 1 per cent.

As with other nucleosides, drug resistance has been observed and correlates with mutations in reverse transcriptase genome codons 50 and 75. Cross-resistance with ddI and ddC also has been reported; cross-resistance with ZDV appears to be less common.

LAMIVUDINE. 3TC was granted accelerated approval by the FDA in November 1995 for use in combination with ZDV for treatment of adults and for use in children (data on combination therapy in children were not available). In a phase I dose-ranging pharmacokinetic study of 3TC in children, 3TC was well tolerated and had antiretroviral activity,[527] and phase I/II trials of combination 3TC/ZDV in adults have shown sustained CD4+ increases and prolonged antiviral effect compared with monotherapy with either drug.[206] A phase III trial in children of combination 3TC and ZDV versus combination ddI/ZDV versus ddI monotherapy (ACTG 300) currently is ongoing.

The bioavailability of 3TC in children (~66 per cent) is somewhat less than in adults (~86 per cent). In children, systemic clearance also decreases with increasing age. The comparatively long plasma half-life of 2 hours in children (about 4 hours in adults) and an intracellular active triphosphate half-life of 10.5 to 15.5 hours permit twice-daily dosing. Excretion primarily is renal. In children, the nonsteady state mean cerebrospinal fluid:plasma ratio was 0.2. The recommended dose for children 3 months to 12 years of age is 8 mg/kg daily in two divided doses (4 mg/kg/dose).

3TC is less cytotoxic than the other nucleoside analogues and has little affinity for mitochondrial DNA polymerase-γ, suggesting that it may be less likely to induce the myopathy and peripheral neuropathy observed with other agents. Pancreatitis has been reported in a small number of pediatric patients with advanced HIV disease who received 3TC; whether the pancreatitis was related to the drug or the advanced stage of disease is unclear.

Nonnucleoside Reverse Transcriptase Inhibitors

The nonnucleoside reverse transcriptase inhibitors are a diverse group of structurally unrelated compounds that appear noncompetitively to inhibit viral reverse transcriptase by binding at a site distinct from the active site where the nucleoside analogues bind. These drugs appear to have a high degree of antiretroviral activity and minimal toxicity. However, resistance emerges very rapidly (within 1 to 2 weeks), accompanied by a rise in viral load and decline in CD4+ count. Therefore, the future of these agents primarily will be for use in combination with other agents; currently, no nonnucleoside reverse transcriptase inhibitor has received FDA approval. In pediatrics, the nonnucleoside reverse transcriptase inhibitor drug, nevirapine, is under evaluation in combination with ddI and ZDV/ddI for the treatment of children who have experienced disease progression while receiving antiretroviral agents (ACTG 245).

The major toxicity of nevirapine is rash. The incidence of rash has been diminished by starting with initial low drug doses, with subsequent dose increase after 2 weeks of lower-dose therapy. The rash generally is mild, but rare cases of life-threatening Stevens-Johnson syndrome have been observed.

Protease Inhibitors

HIV peptides are synthesized as large, single precursor polypeptides that are cleaved into individual biologically active structural proteins by the viral protease to produce infectious virions. A number of compounds have been designed to inhibit HIV protease; these compounds result in the production of immature viral particles that are noninfectious. In contrast to nucleoside analogues, the protease inhibitors do not require intracellular activation, and because the protease inhibitors act at a posttranslational step in viral replication, they should be active in chronically as well as acutely infected cells. The utility of these compounds has been limited by relative insolubility in aqueous solution, which results in suboptimal bioavailability, binding to plasma proteins with inhibition of drug intake into cells, difficulty in mass manufacturing of drug, and development of resistant viral strains. New agents with improved bioavailability are under development.

As of early 1996, three protease inhibitors have been approved by the FDA for therapy in adults: ritonavir (ABT-538, Norvir, Abbott Laboratories), indinavir (MK-639, Crixivan, Merck), and saquinavir (RO31-8959, Invirase, Hoffman-LaRoche). Phase I/II trials of monotherapy with these drugs in infected adults have shown impressive declines in viral load (1 to 2 log decreases in viral RNA copy number) and increases in CD4+ counts.[151, 339, 409, 675] However, with the development of resistance, increase in viral load and decrease in CD4+ count are observed.[134] Thus, the greatest utility of these agents will be in combination with other antiretroviral agents. In phase I/II trials in infected adults, a combination of saquinavir and ZDV was associated with greater CD4+ count response and more prolonged viral load declines (≥1.5 log) when compared with monotherapy with either agent.[339]

In November 1995, the FDA granted accelerated approval to saquinavir (Invirase) for use in combination with other licensed nucleoside analogue antiretroviral agents in infected adults, based on surrogate marker response to combination therapy, and in March 1996, ritonavir and indinavir were approved for infected adults. Phase III trials in adults evaluating clinical efficacy of various combination regimens are under way, and phase I/II clinical trials in children will begin soon.

Other Agents

Novel antiretroviral agents aimed at other steps in the viral life cycle are under development, and some are beginning phase I evaluation in infected adults.[156] Another approach to therapy has been to target factors associated with up-regulation of HIV replication in vivo; examples include pentoxifylline to reduce TNF-α levels and blockers of IL-6, an inflammatory cytokine.[527] Finally, enhancers of the immune response are under evaluation in infected adults and children, including therapy with certain cytokines, such as IL-2; hormones and growth factors, such as insulin growth factor 1 and growth hormone; active and passive immunization; and gene therapy.[527]

PREVENTION OF PEDIATRIC HIV-1 INFECTION

Prevention of HIV-1 infection in women clearly is critical to prevention of pediatric HIV-1 infection. HIV infection threatens the health of the woman herself, her sexual and needle-sharing partners, and all of her future children. Strategies in this area must concentrate on the treatment of injection drug use and the initiation and maintenance of safer sexual practices. Prevention of pediatric HIV-1 infection also entails the development of approaches to reduce the risk of perinatal transmission of HIV-1 from an already infected mother to her infant.

ACTG 076: Use of Zidovudine to Reduce Transmission

ACTG 076 was a randomized, double-blind, placebo-controlled clinical trial designed to evaluate the safety and efficacy of ZDV given to HIV-1–infected pregnant women and their newborns for the prevention of vertical transmission.[137] At the time the study was designed (1990), there was little information about the relative proportion of transmission occurring in utero versus intrapartum; therefore, the ZDV regimen was designed to target transmission that might occur during both periods to optimize potential success. Oral ZDV was administered to pregnant infected women, beginning at 14 to 34 weeks' gestation and continued throughout pregnancy, followed by intravenous infusion of ZDV during labor and oral administration of ZDV to the infant for 6 weeks after birth (Table 192–15). Because the trial was placebo-controlled, entry was limited to women with CD4+ counts above 200/mm^3 who had no clinical indication for antiretroviral therapy and had received no therapy during the current pregnancy.

A total of 477 HIV-1–infected pregnant women were enrolled between April 1991 and December 1993, and 409 gave birth to 415 live-born infants. There were no significant differences between the two study arms in maternal or obstetric characteristics that could alter transmission or in infant characteristics at birth. The study was stopped at the first interim efficacy analysis by the independent Data and Safety Monitoring Board because of a highly significant decrease in transmission observed with the ZDV regimen. At the time of the analysis, HIV infection status was known for 363 infants. Among 183 infants in the placebo group, 40 were infected, compared with only 13 of 180 infants in the ZDV group. The 18-month transmission rate, estimated by Kaplan-Meier analysis, was 25.5 per cent (95 per cent confidence interval, 18.4 to 32.5 per cent) in the placebo group compared with 8.3 per cent (95 per cent confidence interval, 3.9 to 12.8 per cent) in the ZDV group, corresponding to a 67.5 per cent reduction in the risk of vertical transmission ($p = 0.00006$).

The ZDV regimen was well tolerated by women and infants. The only short-term toxicity observed more frequently in the ZDV group was a mild transient anemia in infants that reached a nadir at 6 weeks of age and resolved by 12 weeks of age without requiring therapy. The incidence of minor and major congenital abnormalities was similar among infants in the placebo and ZDV groups, and no consistent pattern of defects was seen. Additional data on lack of teratogenicity with in utero ZDV exposure have come from the Antiviral Pregnancy Registry as well as observational studies.[53, 97, 221, 621]

Although the study did not assess the efficacy of ZDV

TABLE 192–15. Components of AIDS Clinical Trials Group Protocol 076 Zidovudine Regimen

Period of Drug Administration	Drug Dosage and Interval
Antepartum	100 mg of zidovudine (ZDV) given orally 5 times daily, beginning at 14–34 weeks' gestation and continued throughout pregnancy
Intrapartum	Intravenous infusion of ZDV, initiated with a loading dose of 2 mg/kg body weight over 1 hour, followed by continuous infusion of 1 mg/kg body weight per hour until delivery
Newborn	Oral administration to the newborn of ZDV syrup, 2 mg/kg body weight per dose given every 6 hours, beginning 8–12 hours after birth and continued for the first 6 weeks of life

among women with more advanced disease or those who had prior extensive ZDV therapy, in whom ZDV-resistant virus may be more likely, data from uncontrolled observational studies indicate that ZDV may be effective in reducing perinatal transmission even among women with advanced disease and a low CD4+ count.[53, 416] Additionally, the clinical trial could not evaluate the potential for long-term side effects of ZDV for infants or women; other protocols are providing follow-up of infants through age 21 years and women through 3 years postpartum. Extended follow-up on 333 uninfected infants from ACTG 076, all of whom were older than 15 months of age and some as old as 3 years of age, has shown no difference in growth, CD4+ count, or neurodevelopment between infants who had in utero exposure to ZDV compared with placebo.[138]

In August 1994, the U.S. Public Health Service published recommendations for use of ZDV to reduce the risk of perinatal HIV-1 transmission.[98] Because the data from the trial are only directly applicable to women with characteristics similar to those of the women in the study, recommendations need to be tailored to the individual woman's clinical situation. Recommendations for a series of clinical situations were provided to assist clinicians in assessing the appropriateness of the regimen for their patients (Table 192–16). Important considerations include gestational age of the pregnancy at the time of the woman's evaluation, her CD4+ lymphocyte count, clinical disease stage, and history of antiretroviral drug exposure.[136]

The trial results also had important implications for prenatal HIV counseling and testing. Unless a pregnant woman is aware of her HIV status, she cannot benefit from interventions to reduce perinatal transmission or therapy for herself. In 1995, the U.S. Public Health Service and the American Academy of Pediatrics recommended that routine HIV counseling and voluntary testing be provided to all pregnant women in the United States.[104, 542]

Other Interventions to Prevent Perinatal Transmission

A number of other perinatal intervention strategies are planned in the United States, Europe, Africa, and Thailand (Table 192–17). Several studies will evaluate the efficacy of modified, shortened ZDV regimens, while others will evaluate the use of short regimens of other antiretroviral drugs, such as combination ZDV/3TC or nevirapine. Passive immunization with hyperimmune HIV-1 immunoglobulin and active immunization of mothers and/or newborns with HIV-1 vaccines also are under evaluation. Interventions involving obstetrical factors include evaluation of virucidal cleansing of the birth canal before and during labor and cesarean versus vaginal delivery. In developing countries where nutritional deficiencies are common, micronutrient supplementation with vitamin A during pregnancy will be studied. Breast versus bottle feeding is being evaluated in a randomized trial in Kenya. Because these studies evaluate multiple strategies that are targeted at different times and mechanisms of potential vertical HIV transmission, their results should be complementary and provide important information regarding the timing and mechanisms of mother-to-child transmission and the design of future interventions.

HIV-2

HIV-2 is a lentivirus that has a morphology and life cycle that are similar to those of HIV-1, but it is antigenically distinct. The regulatory genes of HIV-2 differ from those of

TABLE 192–16. Use of Zidovudine to Reduce Perinatal HIV-1 Transmission: Clinical Scenarios and Recommendations

Clinical Scenario	Recommendation

Pregnant HIV-infected women
• with CD4+ T-lymphocyte counts ≥200/mm³,
• who are at 14–34 weeks' gestation,
• who have no clinical indication for ZDV, and
• who have no history of extensive (>6 months) prior antiretroviral therapy
	• The health care provider should recommend the full ACTG Protocol 076 regimen to all HIV-infected pregnant women in this category.
	• This recommendation should be presented to the pregnant woman in the context of a risk-benefit discussion:
	  • a reduced risk of transmission can be expected, but
	  • long-term adverse consequences of the regimen are not known.
	• The decision about this regimen should be made by the woman after discussion with her health care provider.

Pregnant HIV-infected women who • are at >34 weeks' gestation, • have no history of extensive (>6 months) prior antiretroviral therapy, and • do not require ZDV for their own health	• The health care provider should recommend the full ACTG Protocol 076 regimen in the context of a risk-benefit discussion with the pregnant woman. • The woman should be informed that ZDV therapy may be less effective than observed in ACTG Protocol 076 because the regimen is being initiated late in the third trimester.
Pregnant HIV-infected women • with CD4+ T-lymphocyte counts <200/mm³, • who are at 14–34 weeks' gestation, • who have no other clinical indication for ZDV, and • who have no history of extensive (>6 months) prior antiretroviral therapy	• The health care provider should recommend initiation of antenatal ZDV therapy to the woman for her own health benefit. • The intrapartum and neonatal components of the ACTG Protocol 076 regimen should be recommended until further information becomes available. • This recommendation should be presented in the context of a risk-benefit discussion with the pregnant woman.

Pregnant HIV-infected women who have a history of extensive (>6 months) ZDV therapy and/or other antiretroviral therapy before pregnancy	• Because data are insufficient to extrapolate the potential efficacy of the ACTG Protocol 076 regimen for this population of women, the health care provider should consider recommending the ACTG Protocol 076 regimen on a case-by-case basis after a discussion of the risks and benefits with the pregnant woman.
	• Issues to be discussed include
	  • her clinical and immunologic stability on ZDV therapy,
	  • the likelihood she is infected with a ZDV-resistant viral strain, and, if relevant,
	  • the reasons for her current use of an alternative antiretroviral agent (e.g., lack of response to or intolerance of ZDV therapy)
	• Consultation with experts in HIV infection may be warranted.
	• The health care provider should make the ACTG Protocol 076 regimen available to the woman, although its effectiveness may vary depending on her clinical status.

Pregnant HIV-infected women who have not received antepartum antiretroviral therapy and who are in labor	• For women with HIV infection who are in labor and who have not received the antepartum component of the ACTG Protocol 076 regimen (either because of lack of prenatal care or because they did not wish to receive antepartum therapy), the health care provider should discuss the benefits and potential risks of the intrapartum and neonatal components of the ACTG Protocol 076 regimen and offer ZDV therapy when the clinical situation permits.
Infants who are born to HIV-infected women who have received no intrapartum ZDV therapy	• If the clinical situation permits and if ZDV therapy can be initiated within 24 hours of birth, the health care provider should offer the ACTG Protocol 076 postpartum component of 6 weeks of neonatal ZDV therapy for the infant in the context of a risk-benefit discussion with the mother. • Data from animal prophylaxis studies indicate that if ZDV is administered, therapy should be initiated as soon as possible (within hours) after delivery. • If therapy cannot begin until the infant is >24 hours of age and the mother did not receive therapy during labor, no data support offering therapy to the infant.

ACTG, AIDS Clinical Trials Group; ZDV, zidovudine.

Modified from Centers for Disease Control and Prevention: Recommendations of the U.S. Public Health Service task force on the use of zidovudine to reduce perinatal transmission of human immunodeficiency virus. M. M. W. R. *43*(RR-11):1–20, 1994.

TABLE 192–17. Current Research Strategies to Reduce the Risk of Perinatal HIV Transmission

Type of Intervention	Targeted Period*	Agent Under Evaluation	Study Location, Current or Planned
Antiretroviral therapy	IU (late), IP, NB†	Various modifications of the ACTG Protocol 076 zidovudine regimen (including combination therapy regimens)	Ivory Coast, Thailand, Haiti, Uganda, World Health Organization multisite collaboration, United States
		Nevirapine‡	United States (phase I, ACTG Protocol 250)
Passive immunization	IU (multiple doses), NB	Hyperimmune HIV immunoglobulin	United States (ACTG Protocol 185)
	IU (single dose), NB		Uganda
	NB		Haiti
Active immunization	IU	Genentech MN rgp 120 vaccine‡ (to mothers)	United States (phase I, ACTG Protocol 235)
	NB	Genentech MN rgp 120 vaccine‡ and Biocene SF rgp 120 vaccine‡ (to newborns)	United States (phase I, ACTG Protocol 230)
Modified obstetric practices	IP	Cesarean vs. vaginal delivery	European Collaborative Group
	IP	Virucidal vaginal cleansing	
		Chlorhexidine vaginal washing	Malawi, Kenya
		Benzalkonium chloride suppositories	Ivory Coast (phase I)
Infant feeding practices	NB	Breast feeding vs. bottle feeding	Kenya
Micronutrient supplementation	IU	Vitamin A supplementation	Malawi, Tanzania, Zimbabwe, South Africa

*IU, intrauterine; IP, intrapartum; NB, newborn.
†Treatment regimens target all or combinations of these periods.
‡Use of trade names is for identification only and does not imply endorsement by the Public Health Service or the U.S. Department of Health and Human Services.
ACTG, AIDS Clinical Trials Group.
Modified from Rogers, M. F., Mofenson, L. M., Moseley, R. R.: Reducing the risk of perinatal HIV transmission through zidovudine therapy: Treatment recommendations and implications. J. Am. Med. Womens Assoc. *50*:78–93, 1995.

HIV-1; HIV-2 contains the vpx protein gene instead of the vpu protein gene of HIV-1. Genetic sequence homology between the two viruses is approximately 60 per cent for the *gag* and *pol* genes and only about 40 per cent for the *env* gene[488]; more similarity is seen between HIV-2 and monkey SIV, in which nucleic acid sequence homology between HIV-2 and SIV_{SM} and SIV_{MAC} strains is approximately 75 per cent.[408] Because of this antigenic variation, HIV-1 antibody screening EIA may not detect antibody to HIV-2, and combination screening tests containing antigens from both viruses have been developed and are in use in the United States for screening of blood donors. Additionally, confirmatory Western blot testing to detect HIV-2 requires the use of HIV-2–specific assays because not all samples from persons infected with HIV-2 will be positive on HIV-1 Western blot; some will test indeterminate or, rarely, negative.

HIV-2 is endemic in certain areas of western Africa, including Guinea-Bissau, Burkina Faso, the Gambia, Cape Verde, Senegal, and the Ivory Coast, and also in Angola and Mozambique in southern Africa.[408] Transmission is principally through heterosexual contact. The overall prevalence of HIV-2 in these areas is approximately 1 to 2 per cent, although seroprevalence of 8 per cent among pregnant women in Guinea-Bissau has been observed[650]; among high-risk groups such as urban commercial sex workers, HIV-2 prevalence rates of 15 to 64 per cent have been reported.[408] Although only limited distribution to other regions of the world has been observed, HIV-2–infected individuals have been identified in North America, South America, Europe, and India. Infected individuals generally have been immigrants from West Africa or their sexual contacts. In the United States, since implementation of combination HIV-1/HIV-2 screening of the blood supply in June 1992, only two new HIV-2–infected donors have been detected among an estimated 74 million blood donations.[102] Dual infection with HIV-1 and HIV-2, confirmed by PCR and culture, has been observed in areas that are endemic for both viruses.[246, 516]

HIV-2 shares CD4+ lymphocyte tropism and cytopathogenicity with HIV-1, and CD4+ cell depletion may be observed in persons infected with either virus. Some studies suggest that HIV-2 may be somewhat less cytotoxic to CD4+ cells in vitro. Different host cell proteins are required for stimulation of the transcriptional enhancer/promoter region of the HIV-2 LTR, and transcriptional up-regulation of HIV-2 may be disrupted more easily than that of HIV-1, perhaps accounting for differences in pathogenicity.[408] In most studies, the circulating viral load among HIV-2–infected persons appears to be considerably lower than that observed in HIV-1–infected persons of similar immune status, except possibly at the most advanced stages of HIV-2 disease.[157, 606, 640, 650] Higher levels of autologous neutralizing antibody also have been reported among HIV-2–infected than HIV-1–infected persons.[639] These findings suggest that HIV-2 strains may have low rates of viral replication and/or a reduced ability to mutate and escape the host immune response.

The modes of HIV-2 acquisition appear to be identical to those of HIV-1: heterosexual and homosexual intercourse, intravenous drug use, receipt of contaminated blood products, and perinatally. However, the infectivity of HIV-2 seems lower than that of HIV-1, and transmission of HIV-2 via sexual intercourse appears to be less than that observed with HIV-1.[322] Additionally, although immunodeficiency and AIDS may develop in HIV-2–infected persons, HIV-2 infection appears to be associated with slower immunologic deterioration, reduced rates of disease progression, and more favorable survival than does HIV-1 infection.[326, 408, 410, 698] However, infection with either virus appears to be associated with increased mortality when compared with seronegative persons.

Data from most studies of mother-infant pairs indicate that perinatal transmission of HIV-2 appears to be rare.[2, 245, 536, 650] In one large prospective study from the Ivory Coast, the risk of perinatal transmission from HIV-1–infected mothers was 21-fold greater than from HIV-2 infected mothers; transmission rates were 1.2 per cent from HIV-2–infected mothers compared with 24.7 per cent from HIV-1–infected mothers.[2] Transmission from women who are dually seropositive for HIV-1 and HIV-2 has been described; HIV-1 appears to be transmitted more efficiently than HIV-2, and transmission rates from dually infected women were similar to those from women infected with HIV-1 alone. Transmission of dual infection to the infant, although rare, has been described. In the Ivory Coast cohort, 19.0 per cent of dually infected women transmitted infection; of 11 infected infants, 10 were infected with HIV-1 alone and one was dually infected.[2] Infant mortality among infants born to HIV-1–infected or dually infected mothers was 2.6 to 4.2 times higher than that among infants born to HIV-2–infected mothers (mortality rates of 133, 82, and 32 per 1000, respectively).[157]

Similar to the clinical outcome of HIV-2 infection in infected adults, slower rates of disease progression and better survival have been observed among HIV-2–infected compared with HIV-1–infected or dually infected children, although survival of children infected with either virus was less than for noninfected children.[2, 157, 537] Despite generally slower progression in HIV-2–infected children, severe immunodeficiency and AIDS occurring early in life have been reported.[245, 453] It is possible that variations in replication and cytopathic characteristics between HIV-2 strains might be associated with differences in the progression rate in HIV-2–infected persons.

References

1. Abrams, E. J., Matheson, P. B., Thomas, P. A., et al.: Neonatal predictors of infection status and early death among 332 infants at risk of HIV-1 infection monitored prospectively from birth. Pediatrics *96*:451–458, 1995.
2. Adjorlolo-Johnson, G., De Cock, K. M., Ekpini, E., et al.: Prospective comparison of mother-to-child transmission of HIV-1 and HIV-2 in Abidjan, Ivory Coast. J. A. M. A. *272*:462–466, 1994.
3. Agency for Health Care Policy and Research: Evaluation and management of early HIV infection. U.S. Public Health Service, Washington, D.C., Publication Number *94*:0572, 1994.
4. Al-Attar, I., Reisman, J., Muehlmann, M., et al.: Decline of measles antibody titers after immunization in human immunodeficiency virus-infected children. Pediatr. Infect. Dis. J. *14*:149–150, 1995.
5. Alcabes, P., and Friedland, G.: Injection drug use and human immunodeficiency virus infection. Clin. Infect. Dis. *20*:1467–1479, 1995.
6. Alcabes, P., Munoz, A., Vlahov, D., et al.: Incubation period of human immunodeficiency virus infection. Epidemiol. Rev. *15*:303–318, 1993.
7. Aldhous, M. C., Watret, K. C., Mok, J. Y. Q., et al.: Cytotoxic T lymphocyte activity and CD8 subpopulations in children at risk of HIV infection. Clin. Exp. Immunol. *97*:61–67, 1994.
8. Alimenti, A., Luzuriaga, K., Stechenberg, B., et al.: Quantitation of HIV-1 in vertically-infected infants and children. J. Pediatr. *119*:225–229, 1991.
9. Allen, D. M., Lehman, J. S., Green, T. A., et al.: HIV infection among homeless adults and runaway youth, United States, 1989–1992. AIDS *8*:1593–1598, 1994.
10. Allen, D. M., Onorato, I. M., Green, T. A., et al.: HIV infection in intravenous drug users entering drug treatment, United States, 1988 to 1989. Am. J. Public Health *82*:541–546, 1992.
11. Ameisen, J. C.: Programmed cell death (apoptosis) and cell survival regulation: Relevance to AIDS and cancer. AIDS *8*:1197–1213, 1994.
12. Anderson, G. A., Guerena, M., and Dixon, C. M.: Human non-HIV retroviral infections. Infect. Med. *11*:545–549, 1994.
13. Anderson, S., Shugars, D., Swanstrom, R., et al.: Nef from primary isolates of human immunodeficiency virus type 1 suppresses surface CD4 expression in human and mouse T cells. J. Virol. *67*:4923–4931, 1993.
14. Andiman, W. A., Mezger, J., and Shapiro, E.: Invasive bacterial infections in children born to women infected with human immunodeficiency virus type 1. J. Pediatr. *124*:846–852, 1994.
15. Andiman, W. A., Silva, T. J., Shapiro, E. D., et al.: Predictive value of the human immunodeficiency virus 1 antigen test in children born to infected mothers. Pediatr. Infect. Dis. J. *11*:436–440, 1992.
16. Araneta, M. R., Mascola, L., Eller, A., et al.: HIV transmission through artificial donor insemination. J. A. M. A. *273*:854–858, 1995.
17. Arlievsky, N. Z., Pollack, H., Rigaud, M., et al.: Shortened survival in infants vertically infected with human immunodeficiency virus with elevated p24 antigenemia. J. Pediatr. *127*:538–543, 1995.
18. Arosio, A., Mezzi, G., Mariani, A., et al.: Pancreatic involvement in the HIV-positive paediatric population. AIDS *9*:654–656, 1995.
19. Arrazola, M. P., de Juanes, J. R., Ramos, J. T., et al.: Hepatitis B vaccination in infants of mothers infected with human immunodeficiency virus. J. Virol. *45*:339–341, 1995.
20. Artenstein, A. W., VanCott, T. C., Mascola, J. R., et al.: Dual infection with human immunodeficiency virus type 1 of distinct envelope subtypes in humans. J. Infect. Dis. *171*:805–810, 1995.
21. Ash, S., and Hewitt, C.: HIV-associated cutaneous disorders. Curr. Opinion Infect. Dis. *7*:195–201, 1994.
22. Athale, U. H., Patil, P. S., Chintu, C., et al.: Influence of HIV epidemic on the incidence of Kaposi's sarcoma in Zambian children. J. Acquir. Immune Defic. Syndr. *8*:96–100, 1995.
23. Baba, T. W., Koch, J., Mittler, E. S., et al.: Mucosal infection of neonatal rhesus monkeys with cell-free SIV. AIDS Res. Hum. Retrovir. *10*:351–357, 1994.
24. Bakshi, S. S., Alvarez, D., Hilfer, C. L., et al.: Tuberculosis in human immunodeficiency virus-infected children: A family infection. Am. J. Dis. Child. *147*:320–324, 1993.
25. Bakski, S. S., Tetali, S., Abrams, E. J., et al.: Repeatedly positive human immunodeficiency virus type 1 DNA polymerase chain reaction in human immunodeficiency virus-exposed seroreverting infants. Pediatr. Infect. Dis. J. *14*:658–662, 1995.
26. Bale, J. F., Contant, C. F., Garg, B., et al.: Neurologic history and examination results and their relationship to human immunodeficiency virus type 1 serostatus in hemophiliac subjects: Results from the Hemophilia Growth and Development Study. Pediatrics *91*:736–741, 1993.
27. Balis, F. M., Pizzo, P. A., Butler, K. M., et al.: Clinical pharmacology of 2′, 3′-dideoxyinosine in human immunodeficiency virus-infected children. J. Infect. Dis. *165*:99–104, 1992.
28. Barnett, E. D., Klein, J. O., Pelton, S. I., et al.: Otitis media in children born to human immunodeficiency virus-infected mothers. Pediatr. Infect. Dis. J. *11*:360–364, 1992.
29. Bartholomew, C., Saxinger, C., Clark, J. W., et al.: Transmission of HTLV-I and HIV among homosexuals in Trinidad. J. A. M. A. *257*:2604–2608, 1987.
30. Bastian, I., Gardner, J., Webb, D., et al.: Isolation of a strain of human T-lymphotropic virus type I from Australian aboriginals. J. Virol. *67*:843–851, 1993.
31. Beattie, R. M., Trounce, J. Q., Lyall, E. G. H., et al.: Early thrombocytopenia in HIV infection. Arch. Dis. Child. *67*:1093–1094, 1992.
32. Belman, A. L., Diamond, G., Dickson, D., et al.: Pediatric acquired immunodeficiency syndrome: Neurologic syndromes. Am. J. Dis. Child. *142*:29–35, 1988.
33. Berger, J. R., Scott, G., Albrecht, J., et al.: Progressive multifocal leukoencephalopathy in HIV-1–infected children. AIDS *6*:837–841, 1992.
34. Berger, R., Gartner, S., Rappersberger, K., et al.: Isolation of human immunodeficiency virus type 1 from human epidermis: Virus replication and transmission studies. J. Invest. Dermatol. *99*:271–277, 1992.
35. Berkowitz, R. J., Rakusan, T., McIlveen, L., et al.: Oral manifestations of pediatric HIV infection. Pediatr. AIDS HIV Infect. Fetus Adoles. *1*:49–52, 1990.
36. Bernstein, L. J., Krieger, B. Z., Novick, B., et al.: Bacterial infection in the acquired immunodeficiency syndrome of children. Pediatr. Infect. Dis. J. *4*:472–475, 1985.
37. Beyers, M., Feldman, S., and Edwards, J.: Disseminated histoplasmosis as the acquired immunodeficiency syndrome-defining illness in an infant. Pediatr. Infect. Dis. J. *11*:127–128, 1992.
38. Biggar, R. J., and the International Registry of Seroconverters: AIDS incubation in 1891 seroconverters from different exposure groups. AIDS *4*:1059–1066, 1990.
39. Blanche, S., Calvez, T., Rouzioux, C., et al.: Randomized study of two doses of didanosine in children infected with human immunodeficiency virus. J. Pediatr. *122*:966–973, 1993.
40. Blanche, S., Mayaux, M.-J., Rouzioux, C., et al.: Relation of the course of

HIV infection in children to the severity of the disease in their mothers at delivery. N. Engl. J. Med. 330:308–312, 1994.
41. Blanche, S., Rouzioux, C., Guihart Moscato, M.-L., et al.: A prospective study of infants born to women seropositive for human immunodeficiency virus type 1. N. Engl. J. Med. *320*:1643–1648, 1989.
42. Blanche, S., Tardieu, M., Duliege, A.-M., et al.: Longitudinal study of 94 symptomatic infants with perinatally acquired human immunodeficiency virus infection: Evidence for a bimodal expression of clinical and biological symptoms. Am. J. Dis. Child. *144*:1210–1215, 1990.
43. Blattner, W., Saxinger, C., Riedel, D., et al.: A study of HTLV-I and its associated risk factors in Trinidad and Tobago. J. Acquir. Immune Defic. Syndr. *90*:1102–1108, 1990.
44. Blethen, S. L., Nachman, S., and Chasalow, F. I.: Thyroid function in children with perinatally acquired antibodies to human immunodeficiency virus. J. Pediatr. Endocrinol. *7*:201–204, 1994.
45. Blumberg, B. M., Gelbard, H. A., and Epstein, L. G.: HIV-1 infection of the developing nervous system: Central role of astrocytes in pathogenesis. Virol. Res. *32*:253–267, 1994.
46. Bode, H., and Rudin, C.: Calcifying arteriopathy in the basal ganglia in human immunodeficiency virus-infection. Pediatr. Radiol. *25*:72–73, 1995.
47. Bonagura, V. R., Cunningham-Rundles, S. L., and Schuval, S.: Dysfunction of natural killer cells in human immunodeficiency virus-infected children with or without *Pneumocytsis carinii* pneumonia. J. Pediatr. *121*:195–201, 1992.
48. Bonis, J., Baillou, A., Barin, F., et al.: Discrimination between human T-cell lymphotropic virus type I and II (HTLV-I and HTLV-II) infections by using synthetic peptides representing an immunodominant region of the core protein (p19) of HTLV-I and HTLV-II. J. Clin. Microbiol. *31*:1481–1485, 1993.
49. Bonis, J., Verdier, M., Dumas, M., et al.: Low human T cell leukemia virus type II seroprevalence in Africa. J. Infect. Dis. *169*:225–227, 1994.
50. Borkowsky, W., Krasinski, K., Cao, Y., et al.: Correlation of perinatal transmission of human immunodeficiency virus type 1 with maternal viremia and lymphocyte phenotypes. J. Pediatr. *125*:345–351, 1994.
51. Bothe, K., Aguzzi, A., Lassmann, H., et al.: Progressive encephalopathy and myopathy in transgenic mice expressing human foamy virus genes. Science *253*:555–557, 1991.
52. Boucher, F. D., Modlin, J. F., Weller, S. et al.: Phase I evaluation of zidovudine administered to infants exposed at birth to the human immunodeficiency virus. J. Pediatr. *122*:137–144, 1993.
53. Boyer, P. J., Dillon, M., Navaie, M., et al.: Factors predictive of maternal-fetal transmission of HIV-1: Preliminary analysis of zidovudine given during pregnancy and/or delivery. J. A. M. A. *271*:1925–1930, 1994.
54. Brady, M. T., McGrath, N., Brouwers, P., et al.: Controlled trial of tolerance and efficacy of zidovudine at standard and low dose in children. Tenth International Conference on AIDS, August 1994, Yokohama, Japan, Abstract 268B.
55. Bredberg-Raden, U., Urassa, W., Urassa, E., et al.: Predictive markers for mother-to-child transmission in Dar es Salaam, Tanzania. J. Acquir. Immune Defic. Syndr. *8*:182–187, 1995.
56. Brena, A. E., Cooper, E. R., Cabral, H. J., et al.: Antibody response to measles and rubella vaccine by children with HIV infection. J. Acquir. Immune Defic. Syndr. *6*:1125–1129, 1993.
57. Brenner, T. J., Dahl, K. E., Olson, B., et al.: Relation between HIV-1 syncytium inhibition antibodies and clinical outcome in children. Lancet *337*:1001–1005, 1991.
58. Brettler, D. B., Forsberg, A., Bolivar, E., et al.: Growth failure as a prognostic indicator for progression to acquired immunodeficiency syndrome in children with hemophilia. J. Pediatr. *117*:584–588, 1990.
59. Briant, L., Wade, C. M., Puel, J., et al.: Analysis of envelope sequence variants suggests multiple mechanisms of mother-to-child transmission of human immunodeficiency virus type 1. J. Virol. *69*:3778–3788, 1995.
60. Briggs, N. C., Battjes, R. J., Cantor, K. P., et al.: Seroprevalence of human T cell lymphotropic virus type II infection, with or without human immunodeficiency virus type 1 coinfection, among US drug users. J. Infect. Dis. *172*:51–58, 1995.
61. Brodie, S. J., Marcom, K. A., Pearson, L. D., et al.: Effects of virus load in the pathogenesis of lentivirus-induced lymphoid interstitial pneumonia. J. Infect. Dis. *166*:531–541, 1992.
62. Brouwers, P., Heyes, M. P., Moss, H. A., et al.: Quinolinic acid in the cerebrospinal fluid of children with symptomatic human immunodeficiency virus type 1 disease: Relationship to clinical status and therapeutic response. J. Infect. Dis. *168*:1380–1386, 1993.
63. Brouwers, P., Tudor-Williams, G., DeCarli, C., et al.: Relation between stage of disease and neurobehavioral measures in children with symptomatic HIV disease. AIDS *9*:713–720, 1995.
64. Bryson, Y. J.: HIV clearance in infants: A continuing saga. AIDS *9*:1373–1375, 1995.
65. Bryson, Y. J., Luzuriaga, K., Sullivan, J. L., et al.: Proposed definition for in utero versus intrapartum transmission of HIV-1. N. Engl. J. Med. *327*:1246–1247, 1992.
66. Bryson, Y. J., Pang, S., Wei, L. S., et al.: Clearance of HIV infection in a perinatally infected infant. N. Engl. J. Med. *332*:833–838, 1995.
67. Bulterys, M., Chao, A., Dushimimana, A., et al.: Multiple sexual partners and mother-to-child transmission of HIV-1. AIDS *7*:1639–1645, 1993.
68. Bulterys, M., Chao, A., Munyemana, S., et al.: Maternal human immunodeficiency virus type 1 and intrauterine growth: A prospective cohort study in Butare, Rwanda. Pediatr. Infect. Dis. J. *13*:94–100, 1994.
69. Bulterys, M., Farzadegan, H., Chao, A., et al.: Diagnostic utility of immune-complex dissociated p24 antigen detection in perinatally acquired HIV-1 infection in Rwanda. J. Acquir. Immune Defic. Syndr. Hum. Retrovir. *10*:186–191, 1995.
70. Burgard, M., Mayauz, M-J., Blanche, S., et al.: The use of viral culture and p24 antigen testing to diagnose human immunodeficiency virus infection in neonates. N. Engl. J. Med. *327*:1192–1197, 1992.
71. Burns, D. N., Landesman, S., Muenz, L. R., et al.: Cigarette smoking, premature rupture of membranes and vertical transmission of HIV-1 among women with low CD4+ levels. J. Acquir. Immune Defic. Syndr. *7*:718–26, 1994.
72. Burns, E. R., Krieger, B., Bernstein, L., et al.: Acquired circulating anticoagulants in children with the acquired immunodeficiency syndrome. Pediatrics *82*:763–765, 1988.
73. Bussel, J. B., Graziano, J. N., Kimberly, R. P., et al.: Intravenous anti-D treatment of immune thrombocytopenic purpura: Analysis of efficacy, toxicity and mechanism of effect. Blood *77*:1884–1893, 1991.
74. Butler, K. M., Husson, R. N., Balis, F. M., et al.: Dideoxyinosine in children with symptomatic human immunodeficiency virus infection. N. Engl. J. Med. *324*:137–144, 1991.
75. Butler, K. M., Husson, R. N., Lewis, L. L, et al.: CD4 status and p24 antigenemia: Are they useful predictors of survival in HIV-infected children receiving antiretroviral therapy? Am. J. Dis. Child. *146*:932–936, 1992.
76. Butler, K. M., Venzon, D., Henry, N., et al.: Pancreatitis in human immunodeficiency virus-infected children receiving dideoxyinosine. Pediatrics *91*:747–751, 1993.
77. Bye, M. R.: Human immunodeficiency virus infections and the respiratory system in children. Pediatr. Pulmonol. *19*:231–242, 1995.
78. Caceres, C. F., and Griensven, G. J. P.: Male homosexual transmission of HIV-1. AIDS *8*:1051–1061, 1994.
79. Caliendo, A. M.: Laboratory methods for quantitating HIV RNA. AIDS Clin. Care *7*:89–93, 1995.
80. Campos, J. M. S., and Simonetti, J. P.: Treatment of lymphoid interstitial pneumonia with chloroquine. J. Pediatr. *122*:503, 1993.
81. Cassol, S., Butcher, A., Kinard, S., et al.: Rapid screening for early detection of mother-to-child transmission of human immunodeficiency virus type 1. J. Clin. Microbiol. *32*:2641–2645, 1994.
82. Celentano, D. D., Nelson, K. E., Suprasert, S., et al.: Risk factors for HIV-1 seroconversion among young men in northern Thailand. J. A. M. A. *275*:122–127, 1996.
83. Centers for Disease Control: Apparent transmission of human T-lymphotropic virus type III/lymphadenopathy-associated virus from a child to a mother providing healthcare. M. M. W. R. *35*:76–79, 1986.
84. Centers for Disease Control: Classification system for human immunodeficiency virus infection in children under 13 years of age. M. M. W. R. *36*:225–230, 235, 1987.
85. Centers for Disease Control: Revision of the CDC surveillance case definition for acquired immunodeficiency syndrome. M. M. W. R. *36*(Suppl.):1S–15S, 1987.
86. Centers for Disease Control: Guidelines for prevention of transmission of human immunodeficiency virus and hepatitis B virus to health care and public safety workers. M. M. W. R. *38*:1–37, 1989.
87. Centers for Disease Control: Human T-lymphocyte virus type I screening in volunteer blood donors: United States, 1989. M. M. W. R. *39*:915–924, 1990.
88. Centers for Disease Control: BCG vaccination and pediatric HIV infection: Rwanda, 1988–1990. M. M. W. R. *40*:833–836, 1991.
89. Centers for Disease Control: Guidelines for prophylaxis against *Pneumocystis carinii* pneumonia for children infected with human immunodeficiency virus. M. M. W. R. *40*(No.RR-2):1–13, 1991.
90. Centers for Disease Control: Recommendations for preventing transmission of human immunodeficiency virus and hepatitis B virus to patients during exposure-prone invasive procedures. M. M. W. R. *40*(RR-8):1–12, 1991.
91. Centers for Disease Control: HIV infection in two brothers receiving intravenous therapy for hemophilia. M. M. W. R. *41*:228–231, 1992.
92. Centers for Disease Control: Testing for antibodies to human immunodeficiency virus type 2 in the United States. M. M. W. R. *41*(No. RR-12):1–9, 1992.
93. Centers for Disease Control: 1993 revised classification system for HIV infection and expanded surveillance case definition for AIDS among adolescents and adults. M. M. W. R. *41*(RR-17):1–19, 1992.
94. Centers for Disease Control: Recommendations on prophylaxis and therapy for disseminated *Mycobacterium avium* complex for adults and adolescents infected with human immunodeficiency virus. M. M. W. R. *42*(RR-9):14–20, 1993.
95. Centers for Disease Control: HIV transmission between two adolescent brothers with hemophilia. M. M. W. R. *42*:948–951, 1993.
96. Centers for Disease Control: HIV virus transmission in household settings: U.S. M. M. W. R. *43*:347, 353–356, 1994.
97. Centers for Disease Control: Birth outcomes following zidovudine therapy in pregnant women. M. M. W. R. *43*:415–416, 1994.

98. Centers for Disease Control: Recommendations of the U.S. Public Health Service Task Force on the use of zidovudine to reduce perinatal transmission of human immunodeficiency virus. M. M. W. R. *43*(No. RR-11):1–20, 1994.
99. Centers for Disease Control: 1994 revised classification system for human immunodeficiency virus infection in children less than 13 years of age. M. M. W. R. *43*(No. RR-12):1–10, 1994.
100. Centers for Disease Control: HIV/AIDS surveillance report: June 1995 mid-year edition. *7*:1–34, 1995.
101. Centers for Disease Control: Update: AIDS among women—United States, 1994. M. M. W. R. *44*:81–84, 1995.
102. Centers for Disease Control: Update: HIV-2 infection among blood and plasma donors—United States, June 1992–June 1995. M. M. W. R. *44*:603–606, 1995.
103. Centers for Disease Control: 1995 revised guidelines for prophylaxis against *Pneumocystis carinii* pneumonia for children infected with or perinatally exposed to human immunodeficiency virus. M. M. W. R. *44*(RR-4):1–11, 1995.
104. Centers for Disease Control: U.S. Public Health Service recommendations for human immunodeficiency virus counseling and voluntary testing for pregnant women. M. M. W. R. *44*(No. RR-7):1–15, 1995.
105. Centers for Disease Control: USPHS/IDSA guidelines for the prevention of opportunistic infections in persons infected with human immunodeficiency virus: A summary. M. M. W. R. *44*(RR-8):1–34, 1995.
106. Centers for Disease Control: Update: Mortality attributable to HIV infection among persons aged 25–44 years—United States. M. M. W. R. *45*:121–125, 1996.
107. Centers for Disease Control: Case-control study of HIV seroconversion in health care workers after percutaneous exposure to HIV-infected blood: France, United Kingdom and United States, January 1988–August 1994. M. M. W. R. *44*:929–933, 1996.
108. Centers for Disease Control and Prevention and the U.S.P.H.S. Working Group: Guidelines for counseling persons infected with human T-lymphotropic virus type 1 (HTLV-I) and type II (HTLV-II). Ann. Intern. Med. *118*:448–454, 1993.
109. Chadwick, E. G., Chang, G., Decker, M. D., et al.: Serologic response to standard inactivated influenza vaccine in human immunodeficiency virus-infected children. Pediatr. Infect. Dis. J. *13*:206–211, 1994.
110. Chadwick, E. G., Nazareno, L. A., Nieuwenhuis, et al.: Phase I evaluation of zalcitabine administered to human immunodeficiency virus-infected children. J. Infect. Dis. *172*:1475–1479, 1995.
111. Chan, W. L., Rodgers, A., Grief, C., et al.: Immunization with class I histocompatibility leukocyte antigen can protect macaques against challenge infection with SIV_{mac}. AIDS 9:223–228, 1995.
112. Chandwani, S., Greco, M. A., Mittal, K., et al.: Pathology and human immunodeficiency virus expression in placentas of seropositive women. J. Infect. Dis. *163*:1134–1138, 1991.
113. Chantry, C. J., Cooper, E. R., Pelton, S. I., et al.: Seroreversion in human immunodeficiency virus-exposed but uninfected infants. Pediatr. Infect. Dis. J. *14*:382–387, 1995.
114. Chase, C., Vibbert, M., Pelton, S. I., et al.: Early neurodevelopmental growth in children with vertically transmitted human immunodeficiency virus infection. Arch. Pediatr. Adolesc. Med. *149*:850–855, 1995.
115. Chen, M. Y., Maldarelli, F., Karczewski, M., et al.: Human immunodeficiency virus type 1 vpu protein induces degradation of CD4 *in vitro*: The cytoplasmic domain of CD4 contributes to vpu sensitivity. J. Virol. *67*:3877–3884, 1993.
116. Chen, T. P., Roberts, R. L., Wu, K. G., et al.: Decreased superoxide anion and hydrogen peroxide production by neutrophils and monocytes in human immunodeficiency virus-infected children and adults. Pediatr. Res. *34*:544–550, 1993.
117. Chintu, C., Bhat, G., Luo, C., et al.: Seroprevalence of human immunodeficiency virus type 1 infection in Zambian children with tuberculosis. Pediatr. Infect. Dis. J. *12*:499–504, 1993.
118. Chu, S. Y., Buehler, J. W., Oxtoby, M. J., et al.: Impact of human immunodeficiency virus epidemic on mortality in children, United States. Pediatrics *87*:806–811, 1991.
119. Ciesielski, C., Marianos, D., Ou, C. Y., et al.: Transmission of human immunodeficiency virus in a dental practice. Ann. Intern. Med. *116*:798–805, 1992.
120. Cimarelli, A., Zambruno, G., Marconi, A., et al.: Quantitation by competitive PCR of HIV-1 proviral DNA in epidermal Langerhans cells of HIV-infected patients. J. Acquir. Immune Defic. Syndr. *7*:230–235, 1994.
121. Clements, J. E., and Zink, M. C.: Molecular biology and pathogenesis of animal lentivirus infection. Clin. Microbiol. Rev. *9*:100–117, 1996.
122. Clemetson, D. B., Moss, G. B., Willerford, D. M., et al.: Detection of HIV DNA in cervical and vaginal secretions: Prevalence and correlates among women in Nairobi, Kenya. J. A. M. A. *269*:2860–2864, 1993.
123. Clerci, M., Levin, J. M., Kessler, H. A., et al.: HIV-specific T-helper activity in seronegative health care workers exposed to contaminated blood. J. A. M. A. *271*:42–46, 1994.
124. Clerici, M., and Shearer, G. M.: A TH1-TH-2 switch is a critical step in the etiology of HIV infection. Immunol. Today *14*:107–122, 1993.
125. Clerici, M., Sison, A. V., Berzofsky, J. A., et al.: Cellular immune factors associated with mother-to-infant transmission of HIV. AIDS *7*:1427–1433, 1993.
126. Cocchi, F., DeVico, A. L., Garzino-Demo, A., et al.: Identification of RANTES, MIP-1α, and MIP-1β as the major HIV-suppressive factors produced by CD8+ T cells. Science *270*:1811–1815, 1995.
127. Cohen, J.: AIDS research: Differences in HIV strains may underlie disease patterns. Science *270*:30–31, 1995.
128. Cohen, S. E., Mundy, T., Karassik, B., et al.: Neuropsychological functioning in human immunodeficiency virus type 1 seropositive children infected through neonatal blood transfusion. Pediatrics *88*:58–68, 1991.
129. Cohen-Abbo, A., and Wright, P. F.: Complex etiology of pneumonia in infants perinatally infected with human immunodeficiency virus 1. Pediatr. Infect. Dis. J. *10*:545–547, 1991.
130. Colebunders, R., Ryder, R., Francis, H., et al.: Seroconversion rate, mortality and clinical manifestations associated with the receipt of a human immunodeficiency virus-infected blood transfusion in Kinshasa, Zaire. J. Infect. Dis. *164*:450–456, 1991.
131. Commenges, D., Alioum, A., Lepage, P., et al.: Estimating the incubation period of paediatric AIDS in Rwanda. AIDS *6*:1515–1520, 1992.
132. Committee on Infectious Diseases: Recommendations for the use of live attenuated varicella vaccine. Pediatrics *95*:791–796, 1995.
133. Condini, A., Axia, G., Cattelan, C., et al.: Development of language in 18–30 month-old HIV-1–infected but not ill children. AIDS *5*:735–739, 1991.
134. Condra, J. H., Schleif, W. A., Blahy, O. M., et al.: *In vivo* emergence of HIV-1 variants resistant to multiple protease inhibitors. Nature *374*:569–571, 1995.
135. Connor, E., Gupta, S., Joshi, V. et al.: Acquired immunodeficiency syndrome-associated renal disease in children. J. Pediatr. *113*:39–44, 1988.
136. Connor, E. M., and Mofenson, L. M.: Zidovudine for the reduction of perinatal human immunodeficiency virus transmission: Pediatric AIDS clinical trials group protocol 076: Results and treatment recommendations. Pediatr. Infect. Dis. J. *14*:536–541, 1995.
137. Connor, E. M., Sperling, R. S., Gelber, R., et al.: Reduction of maternal-infant transmission of human immunodeficiency virus type 1 with zidovudine treatment. N. Engl. J. Med. *331*:1173–1180, 1994.
138. Connor, E. M., Sperling, R., Shapiro, D., et al.: Long-term effect of zidovudine exposure among uninfected infants born to HIV-infected mothers in pediatric AIDS Clinical Trials Group Protocol 076. 35th Interscience Conference on Antimicrobial Agents and Chemotherapy, September 17–20, 1995, San Francisco, California, Abstract I1.
139. Conway, G. A., Epstein, M. R., Hayman, C. R., et al.: Trend in HIV prevalence among disadvantaged youth: Survey results from a national job training program, 1988 through 1992. J. A. M. A. *269*:1887–1889, 1993.
140. Cooper, E. R., Schwartz, T., Brena, A., et al.: Cytomegalovirus as a cofactor in transmission and progression of perinatal HIV infection. Pediatr. AIDS HIV Infect. Fetus Adolesc. *3*:302–307, 1992.
141. Coopman, S. A., Johnson, R. A., Platt, R., et al.: Cutaneous disease and drug reactions in HIV infection. N. Engl. J. Med. *328*:1670–1674, 1993.
142. Cortes, E., Dietels, R., Aboulafia, D. M., et al.: HIV-1, HIV-2 and HTLV-I infection in high-risk groups in Brazil. N. Engl. J. Med. *320*:953–958, 1989.
143. Courgnaud, V., Laure, F., Brossard, A., et al.: Frequent and early in utero HIV-1 infection. AIDS Res. Hum. Retroviruses *7*:337–341, 1991.
144. Coutsoudis, A., Bobat, R. A., Coovadia, H. M., et al.: The effects of vitamin A supplementation on the morbidity of children born to HIV-infected women. Am. J. Public Health *85*:1076–1081, 1995.
145. Cowen, D. N., Brundage, J. F., and Pomerantz, R. S.: HIV infection among women in the Army Reserve Components. J. Acquir. Immune Defic. Syndr. *7*:171–176, 1994.
146. Cruciani, M., Luzzati, R., Fioredda, F., et al.: Mucosal colonization by pyogenic bacteria among children with HIV infection. AIDS *7*:1533–1534, 1993.
147. Cullen, B. R., and Heitman, J.: Chaperoning a pathogen. Nature *372*:319–320, 1994.
148. Dalakas, M. C., Illa, I., Pezeshkpour, G. H., et al.: Mitochondrial myopathy caused by long-term zidovudine therapy. N. Engl. J. Med. *16*:1098–1105, 1990.
149. Dallabetta, G. A., Miotti, P. G., Chiphangwi, J., et al.: Traditional vaginal agents: Use and association with HIV infection in Malawian women. AIDS *9*:293–297, 1995.
150. D'Angelo, L., Getson, P. R., Luban, N. L. C., et al.: HIV infection in urban adolescents: Can we predict who is at risk? Pediatrics *88*:982–986, 1991.
151. Danner, S. A., Carr, A., Leonard, J. M., et al.: A short-term study of the safety, pharmacokinetics and efficacy of Ritonavir, an inhibitor of HIV-1 protease. N. Engl. J. Med. *333*:1528–1533, 1995.
152. Datta, P., Embree, J. E., Kreiss, J. K., et al.: Mother-to-child transmission of human immunodeficiency virus type 1: Report from the Nairobi Study. J. Infect. Dis. *170*:1134–1140, 1994.
153. Davis, S. F., Byers, R. H., Lindegren, M. L., et al.: Prevalence and incidence of vertically acquired HIV infection in the United States. J. A. M. A. *247*:952–955, 1995.
154. de Asis, M. L. B., Bernstein, L. J., and Schliozberg, J.: Treatment of resistant oral aphthous ulcers in children with acquired immunodeficiency syndrome. J. Pediatr. *127*:663–665, 1995.
155. DeCarli, C., Fugate, L., Falloon, J., et al.: Brain growth and cognitive

improvement in children with human immunodeficiency virus-induced encephalopathy after 6 months of continuous infusion zidovudine. J. Acquir. Immune Defic. 4:585–592, 1991.
156. De Clercq, E.: Antiviral therapy for human immunodeficiency virus infection. Clin. Microbiol. Rev. 8:200–239, 1995.
157. De Cock, K. M., Adjorlolo, G., Ekpini, E., et al.: Epidemiology and transmission of HIV-2: Why there is no HIV-2 pandemic. J. A. M. A. 270:2083–2086, 1993.
158. De Cock, K. M., Zadi, F., Adjorlolo, G., et al.: Retrospective study of maternal HIV-1 and HIV-2 infections and child survival in Abidjan, Côte d'Ivoire. Br. Med. J. 308:441–443, 1994.
159. Delaporte, E., Buve, A., Nzila, N., et al.: HTLV-I infection among prostitutes and pregnant women in Kinshasa, Zaire: How important is high-risk sexual behavior? J. Acquir. Immune Defic. Syndr. Human Retrovirol. 8:511–515, 1995.
160. Delaporte, E., Peeters, M., Bardy, J.-L., et al.: Blood transfusion as a major risk factor for HTLV-I infection among hospitalized children in Gabon (equatorial Africa). J. Acquir. Immune Defic. Syndr. 6:424–428, 1993.
161. De Maria, A., Cirillo, C., and Moretta, L.: Occurrence of human immunodeficiency virus type 1 (HIV-1)–specific cytolytic T cell activity in apparently uninfected children born to HIV-1–infected mothers. J. Infect. Dis. 170:1296–1299, 1994.
162. De Martino, M., Tovo, P.-A., Galli, L., et al.: Prognostic significance of immunologic changes in 675 infants perinatally exposed to human immunodeficiency virus. J. Pediatr. 119:702–709, 1991.
163. de Moraes-Pinto, M. I., Farhat, C. K., Carbonare, S. B., et al.: Maternally-acquired immunity in newborns from women infected by the human immunodeficiency virus. Acta. Paediatr. 82:1034–1038, 1993.
164. Denamur, E., Levine, M., Simon, F., et al.: Conversion of HIV-1 viral markers during the first few months of life in HIV-infected children born to seropositive women. AIDS 7:897–899, 1992.
165. Denny, T., Yogev, R., Gelman, R., et al.: Lymphocyte subsets in healthy children during the first 5 years of life. J. A. M. A. 267:1484–1488, 1992.
166. De Rossi, A., Ades, A. E., Mammano, F., et al.: Antigen detection, virus culture, polymerase chain reaction, and in vitro antibody production in the diagnosis of vertically-transmitted HIV-1 infection. AIDS 5:15–20, 1991.
167. De Rossi, A., Giaquinto, C., Ometto, L., et al.: Replication and tropism of human immunodeficiency virus type 1 as predictors of disease outcome in infants with vertically acquired infection. J. Pediatr. 123:929–936, 1993.
168. De Rossi, A., Ometto, L., Mammano, F., et al.: Time course of antigenemia and seroconversion in infants with vertically acquired HIV-1 infection. AIDS 7:1528–1529, 1993.
169. deShazo, R. D., Chadha, N., Morgan, J. E., et al.: Immunologic assessment of a cluster of asymptomatic HTLV-I–infected individuals in New Orleans. Am. J. Med. 86:65–69, 1989.
170. Des Jarlais, D. C., Coopanya, K., Vanichseni, S., et al.: AIDS risk reduction and reduced HIV seroconversion among injection drug users in Bangkok. Am. J. Public Health 84:452–455, 1994.
171. Des Jarlais, D. C., Friedman, S. R., Sotheran, J. L., et al.: Continuity and change within an HIV epidemic: Injecting drug users in New York City, 1984 through 1992. J. A. M. A. 271:121–127, 1994.
172. de Thé, G., Giordano, C., Gessain, A., et al.: Human retroviruses HTLV-I, HIV-1, and HIV-2 and neurological diseases in some equatorial areas of Africa. J. Acquir. Immune Defic. Syndr. 2:550–556, 1989.
173. de Vincenzi, I. for the European Study Group on Heterosexual Transmission of HIV: A longitudinal study of human immunodeficiency virus transmission by heterosexual partners. N. Engl. J. Med. 331:341–346, 1994.
174. de Vincenzi, I., and Mertens, T.: Male circumcision: A role in HIV prevention? AIDS 8:153–160, 1994.
175. Diamant, E. P., Schechter, C., Hodes, D. S., et al.: Immunogenicity of hepatitis B vaccine in human immunodeficiency virus-infected children. Pediatr. Infect. Dis. J. 12:877–878, 1993.
176. Diamond, F. B., Price, L. J., and Nelson, R. P.: Papillary carcinoma of the thyroid in a seven-year old HIV-positive child. Pediatr. AIDS HIV Infect. Fetus Adolesc. 5:232–235, 1994.
177. Dickover, R. E., Dillon, M., Gillette, S. G., et al.: Rapid increases in load of human immunodeficiency virus correlate with early disease progression and loss of CD4 cells in vertically infected infants. J. Infect. Dis. 170:1279–1284, 1994.
178. Dickover, R. E., Garratty, E. M., Horman, S. A., et al.: Identification of levels of maternal HIV-1 RNA associated with risk of perinatal transmission: Effect of maternal zidovudine treatment on viral load. J. A. M. A. 275:599–605, 1996.
179. Di Franco, M. J., Zaknun, D., Zaknun, J., et al.: A prospective study of the association of serum neopterin, β2-microglobulin and hepatitis B surface antigenemia with deaths in infants and children with HIV-1 disease. J. Acquir. Immune Defic. Syndr. 7:1079–1085, 1994.
180. Dimitrov, D. H., Hollinger, F. B., Baker, C. J., et al.: Study of human immunodeficiency virus resistance to 2', 3'-dideoxyinosine and zidovudine in sequential isolates from pediatric patients on long-term therapy. J. Infect. Dis. 167:818–823, 1993.
181. Domanski, M. J., Sloas, M. M., Follmann, D. A., et al.: Effect of zidovudine and didanosine treatment on heart function in children infected with human immunodeficiency virus. J. Pediatr. 127:137–146, 1995.
182. Donaldson, Y. K., Bell, J. E., Ironside, J. W., et al.: Redistribution of HIV outside the lymphoid system with onset of AIDS. Lancet 343:382–385, 1994.
183. Donegan, E., Lee, H., Operskalski, E. A., et al.: Transfusion transmission of retroviruses: Human T-lymphotropic virus types I and II compared with human immunodeficiency virus type 1. Transfusion 34:478–483, 1994.
184. Donegan, E., Stuart, M., Niland, J. C., et al.: Infection with human immunodeficiency virus type 1 (HIV-1) among recipients of antibody-positive blood donations. Ann. Intern. Med. 113:733–739, 1990.
185. Dosik, H., Goldstein, M. F., Poiesz, B. J., et al.: Seroprevalence of human T-lymphotropic virus in blacks from a selected central Brooklyn population. Cancer Invest. 12:289–295, 1994.
186. Downs, A. M., Salamina, G., and Ancelle-Park, R. A.: Incubation period of vertically acquired AIDS in Europe before widespread use of prophylactic therapies. J. Acquir. Immune Defic. Syndr. 9:297–304, 1995.
187. Duiculescu, D. C., Geffin, R. B., Scott, G. B., et al.: Clinical and immunological correlates of immune-complex–dissociated HIV-1 p24 antigen in HIV-1–infected children. J. Acquir. Immune Defic. Syndr. 7:807–815, 1994.
188. Duliege, A-M., Amos, C. I., Felton, S., et al.: Birth order, delivery route, and concordance in the transmission of human immunodeficiency virus type 1 from mothers to twins. J. Pediatr. 126:625–632, 1995.
189. Duliege, A-M., Messiah, A., Blanche, S., et al.: Natural history of human immunodeficiency virus type 1 infection in children: Prognostic value of laboratory tests on the bimodal progression of the disease. Pediatr. Infect. Dis. J. 11:630–635, 1992.
190. Dunn, A-M., Tizer, K., and Cervia, J. S.: Rifabutin-associated uveitis in a pediatric patient. Pediatr. Infect. Dis. J. 14:246–247, 1995.
191. Dunn, D. T., Brandt, C. D., Krivine, A., et al.: The sensitivity of HIV-1 DNA polymerase chain reaction in the neonatal period and the relative contributions of intra-uterine and intra-partum transmission. AIDS 9:F7–F11, 1995.
192. Dunn, D. T., Newell, M. L., Ades, A. E., et al.: Risk of human immunodeficiency virus type 1 transmission through breastfeeding. Lancet 340:585–588, 1992.
193. Dunn, D. T., Newell, M. L., Mayaux, M. J., et al.: Mode of delivery and vertical transmission of HIV-1: A review of prospective studies. J. Acquir. Immune Defic. Syndr. 7:1064–1066, 1994.
194. Duprat, C., Mohammed, Z., Datta, P., et al.: Human immunodeficiency virus type 1 IgA antibody in breast milk and serum. Pediatr. Infect. Dis. J. 13:603–608, 1994.
195. Ellaurie, M., Burns, E. R., Bernstein, L. J., et al.: Thrombocytopenia and human immunodeficiency virus in children. Pediatrics 82:905–908, 1988.
196. Ellaurie, M., Calvelli, T., and Rubinstein, A.: Neopterin concentrations in pediatric human immunodeficiency virus infection as predictor of disease activity. Pediatr. Infect. Dis. J. 11:286–289, 1992.
197. Ellaurie, M., and Rubinstein, A.: Tumor necrosis factor-α in pediatric HIV-1 infection. AIDS 6:1265–1268, 1992.
198. Ellerbrock, T. V., Bush, T. J., Chamberland, M. E., et al.: Epidemiology of women with AIDS in the United States, 1981 through 1990. J. A. M. A. 265:1971–1975, 1991.
199. Embree, J. E., Braddick, M., Datta, P., et al.: Lack of correlation of maternal human immunodeficiency virus infection with neonatal malformations. Pediatr. Infect. Dis. J. 8:700–704, 1989.
200. Embretson, J., Zupancic, M., Ribas, J. L., et al.: Massive covert infection of helper T lymphocytes and macrophages by HIV during the incubation period of AIDS. Nature 362:355–358, 1993.
201. Ensoli, F., Cafaro, A., Fiorelli, V., et al.: HIV-1 infection of primary human neuroblasts. Virology 210:221–225, 1995.
202. Epstein, L. G., Sharer, L. R., Oleske, J. M., et al.: Neurologic manifestations of human immunodeficiency virus infection in children. Pediatrics 78:678–687, 1986.
203. Erice, A., and Balfour, Jr., H. H.: Resistance of human immunodeficiency virus type 1 to antiretroviral agents: A review. Clin. Infect. Dis. 18:149–156, 1994.
204. Erice, A., Rhame, F. S., Heussner, R. C., et al.: Human immunodeficiency virus infection in patients with solid-organ transplants: Report of five cases and review. Rev. Infect. Dis. 13:537–547, 1991.
205. Erkeller-Yuksel, F. M., Deneys, V., Yuksel, B., et al.: Age-related changes in human blood lymphocyte subpopulations. J. Pediatr. 120:216–222, 1992.
206. Eron, J. J., Benoit, S. L., Jemsek, J., et al.: Treatment with lamivudine, zidovudine, or both in HIV-positive patients with 200 to 500 CD4 cells per cubic millimeter. N. Engl. J. Med. 333:1662–1669, 1995.
207. Escaich, S., Wallon, M., Baginski, I., et al.: Comparison of HIV detection by virus isolation in lymphocyte cultures and molecular amplification of HIV DNA and RNA by PCR in offspring of seropositive mothers. J. Acquir. Immune Defic. Syndr. 4:130–135, 1991.
208. European Collaborative Study: Neurologic signs in young children with human immunodeficiency virus infection. Pediatr. Infect. Dis. J. 9:402–406, 1990
209. European Collaborative Study: Children born to women with HIV-1 infection: Natural history and risk of transmission. Lancet 337:253–260, 1991.
210. European Collaborative Study: Risk factors for mother-to-child transmission of HIV-1. Lancet 339:1007–1012, 1992.
211. European Collaborative Study: Age-related standards for T lymphocyte

subsets based on uninfected children born to human immunodeficiency virus 1-infected women. Pediatr. Infect. Dis. J. *11*:1018–1026, 1992.
212. European Collaborative Study: Perinatal findings in children born to HIV-infected mothers. Br. J. Obstet. Gynecol. *101*:136–141, 1994.
213. European Collaborative Study: Caesarean section and risk of vertical transmission of HIV-1 infection. Lancet *343*:1464–1467, 1994.
214. European Collaborative Study: Natural history of vertically acquired human immunodeficiency virus-1 infection. Pediatrics *94*:815–819, 1994.
215. European Collaborative Study: Weight, height, and human immunodeficiency virus infection in young children of infected mothers. Pediatr. Infect. Dis. J. *14*:685–690, 1995.
216. European Study Group on Heterosexual Transmission of HIV: Comparison of female to male and male to female transmission of HIV in 563 stable couples. Br. Med. J. *304*:809–813, 1992.
217. Eyster, M. E.: Transfusion and coagulation factor-acquired human immunodeficiency virus infection. Pediatr. Infect. Dis. J. *10*:50–66, 1991.
218. Eyster, M. E., Rabkin, C. S., Hilgartner, M. W., et al.: Human immunodeficiency virus-related conditions in children and adults with hemophilia: Rates, relationship to CD4 counts and predictive value. Blood *81*:828–834, 1993.
219. Fantry, L., De Jonge, E., Auwaeter, P. G., et al.: Immunodeficiency and elevated CD4 T lymphocyte counts in two patients coinfected with human immunodeficiency virus and human lymphotropic virus type I. Clin. Infect. Dis. *21*:1466–1468, 1995.
220. Farley, J. J., King, J. C., Nair, P., et al.: Invasive pneumococcal disease among infected and uninfected children of mothers with human immunodeficiency virus infection. J. Pediatr. *124*:853–858, 1994.
221. Ferrazin, A., de Maria, A., Gotta, C., et al.: Zidovudine therapy of HIV-1 infection during pregnancy: Assessment of the effect on the newborns. J. Acquir. Immune Defic. Syndr. *6*:376–379, 1993.
222. Figueroa, J., Brathwaite, A., Morris, J., et al.: Rising HIV-1 prevalence among sexually transmitted disease clinic attenders in Jamaica: Traumatic sex and genital ulcers as risk factors. J. Acquir. Immune Defic. Syndr. *7*:310–316, 1994.
223. Figueroa, J. P., Morris, J., Brathwaite, A., et al.: Risk factors for HTLV-I among heterosexual STD clinic attenders. J. Acquir. Immune Defic. Syndr. Human Retrovir. *9*:81–88, 1995.
224. Fiore, J. R., Jansson, M., Scarlatti, G., et al.: Correlation between seroreactivity to HIV-1 V3 loop peptides and male-to-female heterosexual transmission. AIDS *7*:29–31, 1993.
225. Fiser, R. T., Hickerson, S. L., Sharp, G. B., et al.: Myelopathy as a presenting sign of acquired immunodeficiency syndrome. Pediatr. Infect. Dis. J. *14*:808–809, 1995.
226. Fitzgibbon, J. E., Gaur, S., Frenkel, L. D., et al.: Transmission from one child to another of HIV-1 with a zidovudine-resistance mutation. N. Engl. J. Med. *329*:1835–1841, 1993.
227. Flores, G., Stavola, J. J., and Noel, G. J.: Bacteremia due to *Pseudomonas aeruginosa* in children with AIDS. Clin. Infect. Dis. *16*:706–708, 1993.
228. Flugel, R. M.: Spumaviruses: A group of complex retroviruses. J. Acquir. Immune Defic. Syndr. *4*:739–750, 1991.
229. Foil, L. D., and Issel, C. J.: Transmission of retroviruses by arthropods. Annu. Rev. Entomol. *36*:355–381, 1991.
230. Fong, I. W., Howard, R., Elzawi, A., et al.: Cardiac involvement in human immunodeficiency virus-infected patients. J. Acquir. Immune Defic. Syndr. *6*:380–385, 1993.
231. Fordyce, E. J., Blum, S., Shum, R., et al.: The changing AIDS epidemic in New York City: A descriptive birth cohort analysis of AIDS incidence and age at diagnosis. AIDS *9*:605–610, 1995.
232. Foster, S., and Buve, A.: Benefits of HIV screening of blood transfusions in Zambia. Lancet *346*:225–227, 1995.
233. Franke, E. K., Yuan, H. E. H., and Luban, J.: Specific incorporation of cyclophilin A into HIV-1 virions. Nature *372*:359–362, 1995.
234. Franks, R. R., Ray, P. E., Babbott, C. C., et al.: Maternal-fetal interactions affect growth of human immunodeficiency virus type 1 transgenic mice. Pediatr. Res. *37*:56–63, 1995.
235. Frederick, T., Mascola, L., Eller, A., et al.: Progression of human immunodeficiency virus disease among infants and children infected perinatally with human immunodeficiency virus or through neonatal blood transfusion. Pediatr. Infect. Dis. J. *13*:1091–1097, 1994.
236. Freilij, H., Altcheh, J., and Muchinik, G.: Perinatal human immunodeficiency virus infection and congenital Chagas' disease. Pediatr. Infect. Dis. J. *14*:161–163, 1995.
237. Frenkel, L. M., Gaur, S., Tsolia, M., et al.: Cytomegalovirus infection in children with AIDS. Rev. Infect. Dis. *12*(Suppl. 7):S820–S826, 1990.
238. Frenkel, L. M., Nielsen, K., Garakian, A., et al.: A search for persistent measles, mumps and rubella vaccine virus in children with human immunodeficiency virus type 1 infection. Arch. Pediatr. Adolesc. Med. *148*:57–60, 1994.
239. Fujino, T., Fujiyoshi, T., Yashiki, S., et al.: HTLV-I transmission from mother to fetus via placenta. Lancet *340*:1157, 1992.
240. Gabiano, C., Tovo, P-A., de Martino, M., et al.: Mother-to-child transmission of human immunodeficiency virus type 1: Risk of infection and correlates of transmission. Pediatrics *90*:369–374, 1992.
241. Galli, L., de Martino, M., Tovo, P.-A., et al.: Onset of clinical signs in children with HIV-1 perinatal infection. AIDS *9*:455–461, 1995.
242. Gallo, D., Petru, A., Yeh, E. T., et al.: No evidence of perinatal transmission of HTLV-II. J. Acquir. Immune Defic. Syndr. *6*:1168–1170, 1993.
243. Gallo, R. C.: Human retroviruses: A decade of discovery and link with human disease. J. Infect. Dis. *164*:235–243, 1991.
244. Gay, C. L., Armstrong, F. D., Cohen, D., et al.: The effects of HIV on cognitive and motor development in children born to HIV-seropositive women with no reported drug use: Birth to 24 months. Pediatrics *96*:1078–1082, 1995.
245. Gayle, H. D., Gnaore, E., Adjorlolo, G., et al.: HIV-1 and HIV-2 infection in children in Abidjan, Cote d'Ivoire. J. Acquir. Immune Defic. Syndr. *5*:513–517, 1992.
246. George, J. R., Ou, C.-Y., Parekh, B., et al.: Prevalence of HIV-1 and HIV-2 mixed infections in Cote d'Ivoire. Lancet *340*:337–339, 1992.
247. Geraghty, R., and Panganiban, A.: Human immunodeficiency virus type 1 vpu has a CD4- and an envelope glycoprotein-independent function. J. Virol. *67*:4190–4194, 1993.
248. Gertner, J. M., Kaufman, F. R., Donfield, S. M., et al.: Delayed somatic growth and pubertal development in human immunodeficiency virus-infected hemophiliac boys: Hemophilia Growth and Development Study. J. Pediatr. *124*:896–902, 1994.
249. Gesner, M., Desiderio, D., Kim, M., et al.: *Streptococcus pneumoniae* in human immunodeficiency virus type 1-infected children. Pediatr. Infect. Dis. J. *13*:697–703, 1994.
250. Gesner, M., John, D. D., Krasinski, K., et al.: Increased soluble CD8 (sCD8) in human immunodeficiency virus 1-infected children in the first month and year of life. Pediatr. Infect. Dis. J. *13*:896–898, 1994.
251. Gessain, A., Barin, F., Vernant, J. C., et al.: Antibodies to human T-lymphotropic virus type-1 in patients with tropical spastic paraparesis. Lancet *2*:407–410, 1985.
252. Gessain, A., and Gout, O.: Chronic myelopathy associated with human T-lymphotropic virus type I (HTLV-I). Ann. Intern. Med. *117*:933–946, 1992.
253. Gibb, D. M., Davison, C. F., Holland, F. J., et al.: *Pneumocystis carinii* pneumonia in vertically acquired HIV infection in the British Isles. Arch. Dis. Child. *70*:241–244, 1994.
254. Gibb, D. M., Spoulou, V., Giacomelli, A., et al.: Antibody response to *Haemophilus influenzae* type b and *Streptococcus pneumoniae* vaccines in children with human immunodeficiency virus infection. Pediatr. Infect. Dis. J. *14*:129–135, 1995.
255. Glatt, A. E., and Anand, A.: Thrombocytopenia in patients infected with human immunodeficiency virus: Treatment update. Clin. Infect. Dis. *21*:415–423, 1995.
256. Gottuzzo, E., Sanchez, J., Escamilla, J., et al.: Human T cell lymphotropic virus type 1 infection among female sex workers in Peru. J. Infect. Dis. *169*:754–759, 1994.
257. Goudsmit, J.: The role of viral diversity in HIV pathogenesis. J. Acquir. Immune Defic. Syndr. Hum. Retrovirol. *10*(Suppl. 1):S15–S19, 1995.
258. Gout, O., Baulac, M., Gessain, A., et al.: Rapid development of myelopathy after HTLV-I infection acquired by transfusion during cardiac transplantation. N. Engl. J. Med. *322*:383–388, 1990.
259. Gozlan, M.: Update on HIV transmission and pathogenesis. Lancet *346*:1290, 1995.
260. Greene, W. C.: The molecular biology of human immunodeficiency virus type 1 infection. N. Engl. J. Med. *324*:308–317, 1991.
261. Grubman, S., Gross, E., Lerner-Weiss, N., et al.: Older children and adolescent living with perinatally acquired human immunodeficiency virus infection. Pediatrics *95*:657–663, 1995.
262. Gungor, T., Funk, M., Linde, R., et al.: Cytomegalovirus myelitis in perinatally acquired HIV. Arch. Dis. Child. *68*:399–401, 1993.
263. Gupta, P., Kingsley, L., Anderson, R., et al.: Low prevalence of HIV in high-risk seronegative homosexual men evidenced by virus culture and polymerase chain reaction. AIDS *6*:143–149, 1992.
264. Gurram, M., Chirmule, N., Wang, X.-P., et al.: Increased spontaneous secretion of interleukin 6 and tumor necrosis factor alpha by peripheral blood lymphocytes of human immunodeficiency virus-infected children. Pediatr. Infect. Dis. J. *13*:496–501, 1994
265. Gutman, L. T., Moye, J., Zimmer, B., et al.: Tuberculosis in human immunodeficiency virus-exposed or -infected United States children. Pediatr. Infect. Dis. J. *13*:963–968, 1994.
266. Hahn, B. H.: Viral genes and their products. *In* Broder, S., Merigan, T. C, Jr., and Bolongnesi, D. (eds.): Textbook of AIDS Medicine. Baltimore, Williams & Wilkins, 1994, pp. 21–43.
267. Haller, J. O., and Cohen, H. L.: Pediatric HIV infection: An imaging update. Pediatr. Radiol. *24*:224–230, 1994.
268. Halsey, N. A., Boulos, R., Holt, E., et al.: Transmission of HIV-1 infections from mothers to infants in Haiti: Impact on childhood mortality and malnutrition. J. A. M. A. *264*:1088–1092, 1990.
269. Hand, I. L., Wiznia, A. A., Porricolo, M., et al.: Aerosolized pentamidine for prophylaxis of *Pneumocystis carinii* pneumonia in infants with human immunodeficiency virus infection. Pediatr. Infect. Dis. J. *13*:100–104, 1994.
270. Harouse, J. M., Bhat, S., Spitalnik, S. L., et al.: Inhibition of entry of HIV-1 into neural cell lines by antibodies against galactosyl ceramide. Science *253*:320–323, 1991.
271. Harrington, W. J., Ucar, A., Gill, P., et al.: Clinical spectrum of HTLV-I in South Florida. J. Acquir. Immune Defic. Syndr. Hum. Retrovirol. *8*:466–473, 1995.

272. Hays. E. F., Uittenbogaart, C. H., Brewer, J. C., et al.: *In vitro* studies of HIV-1 expression in thymocytes from infants and children. AIDS *6*:265–272, 1992.
273. Heath, S. L., Tew, J. G., Tew, J. G., et al.: Follicular dendritic cells and human immunodeficiency virus infectivity. Nature *377*:740–743, 1995.
274. Heinzinger, N. K., Bukrinsky, M. I., Haggerty, S. A., et al.: The vpr protein of human immunodeficiency virus type 1 influences nuclear localization of viral nucleic acids in nondividing cells. Proc. Natl. Acad. Sci. U.S.A. *91*:7311–7315, 1994.
275. Henderson, D. K., Fahey, B. J., Willy, M., et al.: Risk for occupational transmission of human immunodeficiency virus type 1 (HIV-1) associated with clinical exposures: A prospective evaluation. Ann. Intern. Med. *113*:740–746, 1990.
276. Henine, W., Kaplan, J. E., Gracia, F., et al.: HTLV-II endemicity among Guyami Indians in Panama. N. Engl. J. Med. *324*:565, 1991.
277. Heneine, W., Woods, T., Green, D., et al.: Detection of HTLV-II in breast-milk of HTLV-II infected mothers. Lancet *340*:1157–1158, 1992.
278. Henin, Y., Mandelbrot, L., Henrion, R., et al.: Virus excretion in the cervicovaginal secretions of pregnant and nonpregnant HIV-infected women. J. Acquir. Immune Defic. Syndr. *6*:72–75, 1993.
279. Henrard, D., Fauvel, M., Samson, J., et al.: Ontogeny of the humoral immune response to human immunodeficiency virus type 1 in infants. J. Infect. Dis. *168*:288–291, 1993.
280. Heymann, D. L., and Piot, T.: The laboratory, epidemiology, nosocomial infection and HIV. AIDS *8*:705–706, 1994.
281. Hino, S., Yamaguchi, K., Katamine, S., et al.: Mother-to-child transmission of human T-cell leukemia virus type-I. Jpn. J. Cancer Res. *76*:474–480, 1985.
282. Hira, S. K., Kamanga, J., Macuacua, R., et al.: Oral contraceptive use and HIV infection. Int. J. STD AIDS *1*:447–448, 1990.
283. Hjelle, B., Mills, R., Swenson, S., et al.: Incidence of hairy cell leukemia, mycosis fungoides and chronic lymphocytic leukemia in first known HTLV-II–endemic population. J. Infect. Dis. *163*:435–440, 1991.
284. Hjelle, B., Scalf, R., and Swenson, S.: High frequency of human T-cell leukemia-lymphoma virus type II infection in New Mexico blood donors: Determination by sequence-specific oligonucleotide hybridization. Blood *76*:450–454, 1990.
285. Ho, D. D., Neumann, A. U., Perelson, A. S., et al.: Rapid turnover of plasma virions and CD4 lymphocytes in HIV-1 infection. Nature *373*:123–126, 1995.
286. Ho, D. D., Rota, T. R., Schooley, R. T., et al.: Isolation of HTLV-III from cerebrospinal fluid and neural tissues of patients with the acquired immunodeficiency syndrome. N. Engl. J. Med. *313*:1493–1497, 1985.
287. Ho, G. Y. F., Nomura, A. M. Y., Nelson, K., et al.: Declining seroprevalence and transmission of HTLV-I in Japanese families who immigrated to Hawaii. Am. J. Epidemiol. *134*:981–987, 1991.
288. Hoff, R., Beradrdi, V. P., Weiblen, B. J., et al.: Seroprevalence of human immunodeficiency virus among childbearing women: Estimation by testing samples of blood from newborns. N. Engl. J. Med. *318*:525–530, 1988.
289. Höllsberg, P., and Hafler, D. A.: Pathogenesis of diseases induced by human lymphotropic virus type I infection. N. Engl. J. Med. *328*:1173–1182, 1993
290. Holman, R. C., Gomperts, E. D., Jason, J. M., et al.: Age and human immunodeficiency virus infection in persons with hemophilia in California. Am. J. Public Health *80*:967–969, 1990.
291. Hoots, W. K., and O'Brien, N. C.: Hematologic manifestations of pediatric HIV infection. Semin. Pediatr. Infect. Dis. *1*:77–81, 1990.
292. Horsburgh, C. R., Caldwell, M. B., and Simonds, R. J.: Epidemiology of disseminated nontuberculous mycobacterial disease in children with acquired immunodeficiency syndrome. Pediatr. Infect. Dis. *12*:219–222, 1993.
293. Hoyt, L., Oleske, J., Holland, B., et al.: Nontuberculous mycobacteria in children with acquired immunodeficiency syndrome. Pediatr. Infect. Dis. J. *11*:354–360, 1992.
294. Hu, D. J., Dondero, T. J., Rayfield, M. A., et al.: The emerging genetic diversity of HIV: The importance of global surveillance for diagnostics, research and prevention. J. A. M. A. *275*:210–216, 1996.
295. Husson, R. N., Mueller, B. U., Farley, M., et al.: Zidovudine and didanosine combination therapy in children with human immunodeficiency virus infection. Pediatrics *93*:316–322, 1994.
296. Husson, R. N., Saini, R., Lewis, L. L., et al.: Cerebral artery aneurysms in children infected with human immunodeficiency virus. J. Pediatr. *121*:927–930, 1992.
297. Husson, R. N., Shirasaka, T., Butler, K. M., et al.: High level resistance to zidovudine but not to zalcitabine or didanosine in human immunodeficiency virus from children receiving antiretroviral therapy. J. Pediatr. *123*:9–16, 1993.
298. Hutto, C., Parks, W. P., Lai, S., et al.: A hospital-based prospective study of perinatal infection with human immunodeficiency virus type 1. J. Pediatr. *118*:347–353, 1991.
299. Ijichi, S., Ramundo, M. B., Takahashi, H., et al.: In vivo cellular tropism of human T cell leukemia virus type II. J. Exp. Med. *176*:293–296, 1992.
300. Ikeda, M. K., Andiman, W. A., Mezger, J. L., et al.: Quantitative leukoviremia and immune-complex–dissociated antigenemia as predictors of infection status in children born to mothers infected with human immunodeficiency virus type 1. J. Pediatr. *122*:524–531, 1993.
301. Ingulli, E., Tejani, A., Fikrig, S., et al.: Nephrotic syndrome associated with acquired immunodeficiency syndrome in children. J. Pediatr. *119*:710–716, 1991.
302. Ippiloto, G., Puro, V., and Decarli, G.: Italian Study Group on Occupational Risk of HIV Infection: The risk of occupational HIV infection in healthcare workers: Italian Multicenter Study. Arch. Int. Med. *153*:1451–1458, 1993.
303. Italian Multicentre Study: Epidemiology, clinical features and prognostic factors of pediatric HIV infection. Lancet *ii*:1043–1046, 1988.
304. Italian Paediatric Intestinal/HIV Study Group: Intestinal malabsorption of HIV-infected children: Relationship to diarrhoea, failure to thrive, enteric micro-organisms and immune impairment. AIDS *7*:1435–1440, 1993.
305. Italian Register for HIV Infection in Children: Features of children perinatally infected with HIV-1 surviving longer than 5 years. Lancet *343*:191–195, 1994.
306. Iwakura, Y., Tosu, M., Yoshida, E., et al.: Induction of inflammatory arthropathy resembling rheumatoid arthritis in mice transgenic for HTLV-I. Science *253*:1026–1028, 1991.
307. Jaffe, H. W., McCurdy, J. M., Kalish, M. L., et al.: Lack of HIV transmission in the practice of a dentist with AIDS. Ann. Intern. Med. *121*:855–859, 1994.
308. Jarvis, J. N., Taylor, H., and Iobidze, M.: Complement activation and immune complexes in early congenital HIV infection. J. Acquir. Immune Defic. Syndr. Hum. Retrovir. *8*:480–485, 1995.
309. Jason, J., Sleeper, L. A., Donfield, S. M., et al.: Evidence for a shift from type I lymphocyte pattern with HIV disease progression. J. Acquir. Immune Defic. Syndr. Hum. Retrovirol. *19*:471–476, 1995.
310. Johnson, M. A., and Cann, A. J.: Molecular determination of cell tropism of human immunodeficiency virus. Clin. Infect. Dis. *14*:747–755, 1992.
311. Jones, D. S., Byers, R. H., Bush, T. J., et al.: Epidemiology of transfusion-associated acquired immunodeficiency syndrome in children in the United States, 1981 through 1989. Pediatrics *89*:123–127, 1992.
312. Joshi, V. V., Oleske, J. M., and Connor, E. M.: Morphologic findings in children with acquired immunodeficiency syndrome: Pathogenesis and clinical implications. Pediatr. Pathol. *10*:155–164, 1990.
313. Joshi, V. V., Oleske, J. M., Minnefor, A. B., et al.: Pathologic pulmonary findings in children with the acquired immunodeficiency syndrome: A study of ten cases. Hum. Pathol. *16*:241–246, 1985.
314. Jospe, N., and Powell, K. R.: Growth hormone deficiency in an 8-year-old girl with human immunodeficiency virus infection. Pediatrics *86*:309–312, 1990.
315. Jue, S., and Whitley, R. J.: Herpesvirus infections in children with human immunodeficiency virus. *In* Pizzo, P. A., and Wilfert, C. M. (eds.): The Challenge of HIV Infection in Infants, Children and Adolescents. 2nd ed. Baltimore, Williams & Wilkins, 1994, pp. 345–363.
316. Jura, E., Chadwick, E. G., Josephs, S. H., et al.: Varicella-zoster virus infections in children infected with human immunodeficiency virus. Pediatr. Infect. Dis. J. *8*:586–590, 1989.
317. Just, J. J., Abrams, E., Louie, L. G., et al.: Influence of host genotype on progression to acquired immunodeficiency syndrome among children infected with human immunodeficiency virus type 1. Pediatrics *127*:544–549, 1995.
318. Kahn, E., Anderson, V. M., Greco, M. A., et al.: Pancreatic disorders in pediatric acquired immune deficiency syndrome. Hum. Pathol. *26*:765–770, 1995.
319. Kajiyama, W., Kashiwagi, S., Ikematsu, H., et al.: Intrafamilial transmission of adult T cell leukemia virus. J. Infect. Dis. *154*:851–857, 1986.
320. Kale, K. L., King, J. C., Farley, J. J., et al.: The immunogenicity of *Haemophilus influenzae* type b conjugate (HbOC) vaccine in human immunodeficiency virus-infected and uninfected infants. Pediatr. Infect. Dis. J. *14*:350–354, 1995.
321. Kalter, D. C., Greenhouse, J. J., Orenstein, J. M., et al.: Epidermal Langerhans cells are not principal reservoirs of virus in HIV disease. J. Immunol. *146*:3396–3404, 1991.
322. Kanki, P. J., Travers, K. U., MBoup, S., et al.: Slower heterosexual spread of HIV-2 than HIV-1. Lancet *343*:943–946, 1994.
323. Kapiga, S. H., Shao, J. F., Lwihula, G. K., et al.: Risk factors for HIV infection among women in Dar-es-Salaam, Tanzania. J. Acquir. Immune Defic. Syndr. *7*:301–309, 1994.
324. Kaplan, J. E., Abrams, E., Shaffer, N., et al.: Low risk of mother-to-child transmission of human T lymphotropic virus type II in non-breast fed infants. J. Infect. Dis. *166*:892–895, 1992.
325. Kashiwagi, S., Kajiyama, W., Hayashi, J., et al.: Antibody to p40tax protein of human T cell leukemia virus I and infectivity. J. Infect. Dis. *161*:426–429, 1990.
326. Kassim, S., Sassan-Morokro, M., Ackah, A., et al.: Two-year follow-up of persons with HIV-1– and HIV-2–associated pulmonary tuberculosis treated with short-course chemotherapy in West Africa. AIDS *9*:1185–1191, 1995.
327. Katamine, S., Moriuchi, R., Yamamoto, T., et al.: HTLV-I proviral DNA in umbilical cord blood of babies born to carrier mothers. Lancet *343*:1326–1327, 1994.

328. Katz, B. Z., Berkman, A. B., and Shapiro, E. D.: Serologic evidence of active Epstein-Barr virus infection in Epstein-Barr virus–associated lymphoproliferative disorders of children with acquired immunodeficiency syndrome. J. Pediatr. *120*:228–232, 1992.
329. Kelly, R., Mancao, M., Lee, F., et al.: Varicella in children with perinatally acquired human immunodeficiency virus infection. J. Pediatr. *124*:271–273, 1994.
330. Kestelyn, P., Lepage, P., and Van de Perre, P.: Perivasculitis of the retinal vessels as an important sign in children with AIDS-related complex. Am. J. Opthalmol. *100*:614–615, 1985.
331. Khabbaz, R. F., Onorato, I. M., Cannon, R. O., et al.: Seroprevalence of HTLV-I and HTLV-II among intravenous drug users and persons in clinics for sexually transmitted diseases. N. Engl. J. Med. *326*:375–380, 1992.
332. Khouri, Y. F., Mastrucci, M. T., Hutto, C., et al.: *Mycobacterium tuberculosis* in children with human immunodeficiency virus type 1 infection. Pediatr. Infect. Dis. J. *11*:950–955, 1992.
333. King, J. C., Burke, A. R., Clemens, J. D., et al.: Respiratory syncytial virus illness in human immunodeficiency virus- and noninfected children. Pediatr. Infect. Dis. J. *12*:733–739, 1993.
334. Kinloch-de Loes, S., de Saussure, P., Saurat, J.-H., et al.: Symptomatic primary infection due to human immunodeficiency virus type 1: Review of 31 cases. Clin. Infect. Dis. *17*:59–65, 1993.
335. Kinoshita, K., Hino, S., Amagasaki, T., et al.: Demonstration of adult T cell leukemia virus antigen in milk from three seropositive mothers. Jpn. J. Cancer Res. *75*:103–105, 1984.
336. Kinoshita, K., Yamanouchi, K., Ikeda, S., et al.: Oral infection of a common marmoset with human T cell leukemia virus type I (HTLV-I) by inoculating fresh human milk of HTLV-I carrier mothers. Jpn. J. Cancer Res. *76*:1147–1153, 1985.
337. Kirvine, A., Firtion, G., Cao, L., et al.: HIV replication during the first few weeks of life. Lancet *339*:1187–1189, 1992.
338. Kitajima, I., Yamamoto, K., Sato, K., et al.: Detection of human T cell lymphotropic virus type I proviral DNA and its gene expression in synovial cells in chronic inflammatory arthropathy. J. Clin. Invest. *88*:1315–1322, 1991.
339. Kitchen, V. S., Skinner, C., Ariyoshi, K., et al.: Safety and activity of saquinovir in HIV infection. Lancet *345*:952–955, 1995.
340. Kliks, S. C., Wara, D. W., Landers, D. V., et al.: Features of HIV-1 that could influence maternal-child transmission. J. A. M. A. *272*:467–474, 1994.
341. Kline, M. W., Dunkle, L. M., Church, J. A., et al.: A phase I/II evaluation of stavudine (d4T) in children with human immunodeficiency virus infection. Pediatrics *96*:247–252, 1995.
342. Kline, M. W., Lewis, D. E., Hollinger, B., et al.: A comparative study of human immunodeficiency virus culture, polymerase chain reaction and anti-human immunodeficiency virus immunoglobulin IgA antibody detection in the diagnosis during early infancy of vertically acquired human immunodeficiency virus infection. Pediatr. Infect. Dis. J. *13*:90–94, 1994.
343. Koot, M., Keet, I. P. M., Vos, A. H. V., et al.: Prognostic value of HIV-1 syncytium-inducing phenotype for rate of CD4+ cell depletion and progression to AIDS. Ann. Intern. Med. *118*:681–688, 1993.
344. Kozal, M. J., Kroodsma, K., Winters, M. A., et al.: Didanosine resistance in HIV-infected patients switched from zidovudine to didanosine monotherapy. Ann. Intern. Med. *121*:263–268, 1994.
345. Krasinski, K., and Borkowsky, W.: Measles and measles immunity in children infected with human immunodeficiency virus. J. A. M. A. *261*:2512–2516, 1989.
346. Krasinski, K., Borkowsy, W., and Bonk, S.: Bacterial infections in human immunodeficiency virus infected children. Pediatr. Infect. Dis. J. *7*:323–328, 1988.
347. Krasinski, K., Borkowsky, W., and Holzman, R. S.: Prognosis of human immunodeficiency virus infection in children and adolescents. Pediatr. Infect. Dis. J. *8*:216–220, 1989.
348. Kreiss, J. K., and Hopkins, S. G.: The association between circumcision status and human immunodeficiency virus infection among homosexual men. J. Infect. Dis. *168*:1404–1408, 1993.
349. Kuhn, L., Stein, Z. A., Thomas, P. A., et al.: Maternal-infant HIV transmission and circumstances of delivery. Am. J. Public Health *84*:1110–1115, 1994.
350. Kumer, R. M., Uduman, S. A., and Khurranna, A. K.: A prospective study of mother-to-infant HIV transmission in tribal women from India. J. Acquir. Immune Defic. Syndr. *9*:238–242, 1995.
351. Kunanusont, C., Foy, H. M., Kreiss, J. K., et al.: HIV-1 subtypes and male-to-female transmission in Thailand. Lancet *345*:1078–1083, 1995.
352. Lacaille, F., Ortigao, M. B., Debre, M., et al.: Hepatic toxicity associated with 2′-3′dideoxyinosine in children with AIDS. J. Pediatr. Gastroenterol. Nutr. *20*:287–290, 1995.
353. Lackritz, E. M., Satten, G. A., Aberle-Grasse, J., et al.: Estimated risk of transmission of human immunodeficiency virus by screened blood in the United States. N. Engl. J. Med. *333*:1721–1725, 1995.
354. LaGrenade, L., Hanchard, B., Fletcher, V., et al.: Infective dermatitis of Jamaican children: A marker for HTLV-I infection. Lancet *336*:1345–1347, 1990.
355. Lal, R. B., Gongora-Biachi, R. A., Pardi, D., et al.: Evidence for mother-to-child transmission of human T lymphotropic virus type II. J. Infect. Dis. *168*:586–591, 1993.
356. Lal, R. B., Owen, S. M., Segurado, A. A. C., et al.: Mother-to-child transmission of human T-lymphotropic virus type II (HTLV-II). Ann. Intern. Med. *120*:300–301, 1994.
357. Landesman, S. H., Kalish, L. A., Burns, D. N., et al.: Obstetrical factors and the transmission of human immunodeficiency virus type 1 from mother to child. N. Engl. J. Med. *334*:1617–1623, 1996.
358. Landesman, S., Weiblen, B., Mendez, H., et al.: Clinical utility of HIV-IgA immunoblot assay in the early diagnosis of perinatal HIV infection. J. A. M. A. *266*:3443–3446, 1991.
359. Lane-McAuliffe, E. M., and Lipshultz, S. E.: Cardiovascular manifestations of pediatric HIV infection. Nurs. Clin. North Am. *30*:291–316, 1995.
360. Langston, C., Lewis, D. E., Hammill, H. A., et al.: Excess intrauterine fetal demise associated with maternal human immunodeficiency virus infection. J. Infect. Dis. *172*:1451–1460, 1995.
361. Laraque, D.: Severe anogenital warts in a child with HIV infection. N. Engl. J. Med. *320*:1220–1221, 1989.
362. Laue, L., and Cutler, G. B.: The spectrum of growth and endocrine abnormalities in pediatric HIV infection. Pediatr. AIDS HIV Infect. Fetus Adoles. *5*:83–89, 1990.
363. Laue, L., Pizzo, P. A., Butler, K., et al.: Growth and neuroendocrine dysfunction in children with acquired immunodeficiency syndrome. J. Pediatr. *117*:541–545, 1990.
364. Lauener, R. P., Huttner, S., Buisson, M., et al.: T-cell death by apoptosis in vertically human immunodeficiency virus-infected children coincides with expansion of CD8+/Interleukin-2 Receptor-/HLA-DR+ T cells: Sign of a possible role for herpes viruses as cofactors. Blood *86*:1400–1407, 1995.
365. Lederman, M. M., Jackson, J. B., Kroner, B. L., et al.: Human immunodeficiency virus (HIV) type 1 infection status and *in vitro* susceptibility to HIV infection among high-risk HIV-1 seronegative hemophiliacs. J. Infect. Dis. *172*:228–231, 1995.
366. Lee, E. S., Locker, J., Nalesnik, M., et al.: The association of Epstein-Barr virus with smooth-muscle tumors occurring after organ transplantation. N. Engl. J. Med. *332*:19–25, 1995.
367. Leggiadro, R. J., Kline, M. W., and Hughes, W. T.: Extrapulmonary cryptococcoses in children with acquired immunodeficiency syndrome. Pediatr. Infect. Dis. J. *10*:658–662, 1991.
368. Leibovitz, E., Cooper, D., Giurgiutiu, D., et al.: Varicella-zoster virus infection in Romanian children infected with the human immunodeficiency virus. Pediatrics *92*:838–842, 1993.
369. Leibovitz, E., Kaul, A., Rigaud, M., et al.: Chronic varicella-zoster in a child infected with human immunodeficiency virus: Case report and review of the literature. Cutis *49*:27–31, 1992.
370. Leibovitz, E., Rigaud, M., Chandwani, S., et al.: Disseminated fungal infections in children infected with human immunodeficiency virus. Pediatr. Infect. Dis. J. *10*:888–894, 1991.
371. Lepage, P., Msellati, P., and Van de Perre, P.: Characteristics of newborns and HIV-1 infection in Rwanda. AIDS *6*:882–883, 1992.
372. Lepage, P., Van de Perre, P., Msellati, P., et al.: Mother-to-child transmission of human immunodeficiency virus type 1 and its determinants: A cohort study in Kigali, Rwanda. Am. J. Epidemiol. *137*:589–599, 1993.
373. Lepage, P., Van de Perre, P., Van Vliet, G., et al.: Clinical and endocrinologic manifestations in perinatally human immunodeficiency virus infected children aged 5 years or older. Am. J. Dis. Child. *145*:1248–1251, 1991.
374. Levine, P. H., Jacobson, S., Elliott, R., et al.: HTLV-II infection in Florida Indians. AIDS Res. Hum. Retroviruses *9*:123–127, 1993.
375. Levy, D., Fernandes, L., Williams, W., et al.: Induction of cell differentiation by human immunodeficiency virus 1 vpr. Cell *72*:541–550, 1993.
376. Lewis, D. E., Adu-Oppong, A., Hollinger, B., et al.: Sensitivity of immune complex-dissociated p24 antigen testing for early detection of human immunodeficiency virus infection in infants. Clin. Diagn. Labor Immunol. *2*:87–90, 1995.
377. Lewis, L. L., Butler, K. M., Husson, R. N., et al.: Defining the population of human immunodeficiency virus-infected children at risk for *Mycobacterium avium-intracellulare* infection. J. Pediatr. *121*:677–683, 1992.
378. Lewis, S. H., Reynolds-Kohler, C., Fox, H. E., et al.: HIV-1 in trophoblast and villous Hofbauer cells and haematological precursors in eight-week fetuses. Lancet *335*:565–568, 1990.
379. Lewis, W., Simpson, J. F., and Meyer, R. R.: Cardiac mitochondrial DNA polymerase-gamma is inhibited competitively and non-competitively by phosphorylated zidovudine. Circ. Res. *74*:344–348, 1994.
380. Lieb, L. E., Mundy, T. M., Goldfinger, D., et al.: Unrecognized human immunodeficiency virus type 1 infection in a cohort of transfused neonates: A retrospective investigation. Pediatrics *95*:717–721, 1995.
381. Lindegren, M. L., Hanson, C., Miller, K., et al.: Epidemiology of human immunodeficiency virus infection in adolescents, United States. Pediatr. Infect. Dis. J. *13*:525–535, 1994.
382. Lindgren, S., Anzen, B., Bohlin, A.-B., et al.: HIV and child-bearing: Clinical outcome and aspects of mother-to-infant transmission. AIDS *5*:1111–1116, 1991.
383. Lindsay, M. K., Johnson, N., Peterson, H. B., et al.: Human immunodeficiency virus infection among inner-city adolescent parturients undergo-

ing routine voluntary screening, July 1987 to March 1991. Am. J. Obstet. Gynecol. *167*:1096–1099, 1992.

384. Lipshultz, S. E., Fox, C. H., Perez-Atayde, A. R., et al.: Identification of human immunodeficiency virus-1 RNA and DNA in the heart of a child with cardiovascular abnormalities and congenital acquired immune deficiency syndrome. Am. J. Cardiol. *66*:246, 1990.
385. Lipshultz, S. E., Orav, E. J., Sanders, S. P., et al.: Cardiac structure and function in children with human immunodeficiency virus infection treated with zidovudine. N. Engl. J. Med. *18*:1260–1265, 1992.
386. Lipshultz, S. E., Orav, J., Sanders, S. P., et al.: Limitations of fractional shortening as an index of contractility in pediatric patients infected with human immunodeficiency virus. J. Pediatr. *125*:563–570, 1994.
387. Livingston, R. A., Hutton, N., Halsey, N. A., et al.: Human immunodeficiency virus-specific IgA in infants born to human immunodeficiency virus-seropositive women. Arch. Pediatr. Adoles. Med. *149*:503–507, 1995.
388. Liu, X. D., and Ebbesen, P.: *In vitro* HTLV-I transfer to human trophoblast cells: Implications for transplacental passage. J. Acquir. Immune Defic. Syndr. Hum. Retrovirol. *10*:263, 1995 (abstract).
389. Ljunggren, K., Moschese, V., Broliden, P. A., et al.: Antibodies mediating cellular cytotoxicity and neutralization correlate with a better clinical stage in children born to human immunodeficiency virus-infected mothers. J. Infect. Dis. *161*:198–202, 1990.
390. Lobato, M. N., Caldwell, M. B., Ng, P., et al.: Encephalopathy in children with perinatally-acquired human immunodeficiency virus infection. J. Pediatr. *126*:710–715, 1995.
391. Loveland, K. A., Stehbens, J., Contant, C., et al.: Hemophilia growth and development study: Baseline neurodevelopmental findings. J. Pediatr. Psychol. *19*:223–239, 1994.
392. Luginbuhl, L. M., Orav, J., McIntosh, K., et al.: Cardiac morbidity and related mortality in children with HIV infection. J. A. M. A. *269*:2869–2875, 1993.
393. Luzuriaga, K., Holmes, D., Hereema, A., et al.: HIV-1–specific cytotoxic T lymphocyte responses in the first year of life. J. Immunol. *154*:433–443, 1995.
394. Luzuriaga, K., Koup, R. A., Pikora, C. A., et al.: Deficient human immunodeficiency virus type 1-specific cytotoxic T cell responses in vertically infected children. J. Pediatr. *119*:230–236, 1991.
395. Luzuriaga, K., McQuilken, P., Alimenti, A., et al.: Early viremia and immune responses in vertical human immunodeficiency virus type 1 infection. J. Infect. Dis. *167*:1008–1013, 1993.
396. Luzuriaga, K., and Sullivan, J.: HIV-1–specific CTL in long-term survivors of vertical infection. Pediatr. Res. *33*:115A, 1993.
397. Lyman, W. D., Kress, Y., Kure, K., et al.: Detection of HIV in fetal central nervous system tissue. AIDS *4*:917–920, 1990.
398. Malamba, S. S., Wagner, H.-U., Maude, G., et al.: Risk factors for HIV-1 infection in adults in a rural Ugandan community: A case control study. AIDS *8*:253–257, 1994.
399. Malamud, D., Davis, C., Berthold, P., et al.: Human submandibular saliva aggregates HIV-1. AIDS Res. Hum. Retroviruses *9*:633–637, 1993.
400. Maloney, E. M., Biggar, R. J., Neel, J. V., et al.: Endemic human T cell lymphotropic virus type II infection among isolated Brazilian Amerindians. J. Infect. Dis. *166*:100–107, 1992.
401. Maloney, E. M., Murphy, E. L., Figueroa, J. P., et al.: Human T-lymphotropic virus type I (HTLV-I) seroprevalence in Jamaica. II. Geographic and ecologic determinants. Am. J. Epidemiol. *133*:1125–1134, 1991.
402. Maloney, E. M., Pate, E., Wiktor, S. Z., et al.: The relative distribution of T cell subsets is altered in Jamaican children infected with human T cell lymphotropic virus type I. J. Infect. Dis. *172*:867–870, 1995.
403. Maloney, E. M., Wiktor, S. Z., Pate, E. J., et al.: HTLV-I titers in children are associated with maternal titers. J. Acquir. Immune Defic. Syndr. Hum. Retrovirol *10*:259, 1995 (abstract).
404. Mandell, W., Vlahov, D., Latkin, C., et al.: Correlates of needle sharing among injection drug users. Am. J. Public Health *84*:920–923, 1994.
405. Manns, A., Cleghorn, F. R., Falk, R. T., et al.: Role of HTLV-I in development of non-Hodgkin lymphoma in Jamaica and Trinidad and Tobago. Lancet *342*:1447–1450, 1993.
406. Mano, H., and Cherman, J. C.: Replication of human immunodeficiency virus type 1 in primary cultured placental cells. Res. Virol. *142*:95–104, 1991.
407. Mano, H., and Sherman, J. C.: Fetal human immunodeficiency virus type 1 infection in different organs in the second trimester. AIDS Res. Hum. Retroviruses *7*:83–88, 1991.
408. Markovitz, D. M.: Infection with the human immunodeficiency virus type 2. Ann. Intern. Med. *118*:211–218, 1993.
409. Markowitz, M., Saag, M., Powderly, W. G., et al.: A preliminary study of Ritonavir, an inhibitor of HIV-1 protease, to treat HIV-1 infection. N. Engl. J. Med. *333*:1534–1539, 1995.
410. Marlink, R., Kanki, P., Thior, I., et al.: Reduced rate of disease development after HIV-2 infection as compared to HIV-1. Science *265*:1587–1590, 1994.
411. Marolda, J., Pace, B., Bonforte, R. J., et al.: Pulmonary manifestations of HIV infection in children. Pediatr. Pulmonol. *10*:231–235, 1991.
412. Martin, N. L., Levy, J. A., Legg, H., et al.: Detection of infection with human immunodeficiency virus (HIV) type 1 in infants by an anti-HIV immunoglobulin A assay using recombinant proteins. J. Pediatr. *118*:354–358, 1991.
413. Mascola, J. R., Louwagie, J., McCutchan, F. E., et al.: Two antigenically distinct subtypes of human immunodeficiency virus type 1: Viral genotype predicts neutralization serotype. J. Infect. Dis. *169*:48–54, 1994.
414. Mastro, T. D., Satten, G. A., Nopkesorn, T., et al.: Probability of female-to-male transmission of HIV-1 in Thailand. Lancet *343*:204–207, 1994.
415. Matarazzo, P., Palomba, E., Lala, R., et al.: Growth impairment, IGF 1 hyposecretion and thyroid dysfunction in children with perinatal HIV-1 infection. Acta. Pediatr. *83*:1029–1034, 1994.
416. Matheson, P. B., Abrams, E. J., Thomas, P. A., et al.: Efficacy of antenatal zidovudine in reducing perinatal transmission of human immunodeficiency virus type 1. J. Infect. Dis. *172*:353–358, 1995.
417. Mattern, C. F. T., Murray, K., Jensen, A., et al.: Localization of human immunodeficiency virus core antigen in term human placentas. Pediatrics *89*:207–209, 1992.
418. MaWhinney, S., Pagano, M., and Thomas, P.: Age at AIDS diagnosis for children with perinatally acquired HIV. J. Acquir. Immune Defic. Syndr. *6*:1139–1144, 1993.
419. Mayaux, M.-J., Blanche, S., Rouzioux, C., et al.: Maternal factors associated with perinatal HIV-1 transmission: The French Cohort Study: 7 years of follow-up observations. J. Acquir. Immune Defic. Syndr. *8*:188–194, 1995.
420. Mayers, M. M., Davenny, K., Schoenbaum, E. E., et al.: A prospective study of infants of human immunodeficiency virus seropositive and seronegative women with a history of intravenous drug use or of intravenous drug-using partners, in the Bronx, New York City. Pediatrics *88*:1248–1256, 1991.
421. McCabe, E., Jaffe, L. R., and Diaz, A.: Human immunodeficiency virus seropositivity in adolescents with syphilis. Pediatrics *92*:695–698, 1993.
422. McCance-Katz, E. F., Hoecker, J. L., and Vitale, N. B.: Severe neutropenia associated with anti-neutrophil antibody in a patient with the acquired immunodeficiency syndrome. Pediatr. Infect. Dis. J. *4*:417–418, 1987.
423. McClain, K. L., Leach, C. T., Jenson, H. B., et al.: Association of Epstein-Barr virus with leiomyosarcomas in young people with AIDS. N. Engl. J. Med. *332*:12–18, 1995.
424. McFarland, E. J., Curiel, T. J., Schoen, D. J., et al.: Cytotoxic T lymphocyte lines specific for human immunodeficiency virus type 1 gag and reverse transcriptase derived from a vertically infected child. J. Infect. Dis. *167*:719–723, 1993.
425. McFarland, E. J., Harding, P. A., Luckey, D., et al.: High frequency of gag- and env-specific cytotoxic T lymphocyte precursors in children with vertically acquired human immunodeficiency virus type 1 infection. J. Infect. Dis. *170*:766–774, 1994.
426. McIntosh, K., Pitt, J., Brambilla, D., et al.: Blood culture in the first 6 months of life for the diagnosis of vertically transmitted human immunodeficiency virus infection. J. Infect. Dis. *170*:996–1000, 1994.
427. McKinney, R. E., Maha, M. A., Connor, E. M., et al.: A multicenter trial of oral zidovudine in children with advanced human immunodeficiency virus disease. N. Engl. J. Med. *324*:1018–1025, 1991.
428. McKinney, R. E., Pizzo, P. A., Scott, G. B., et al.: Safety and tolerance of intermittent intravenous and oral zidovudine therapy in human immunodeficiency virus-infected pediatric patients. J. Pediatr. *116*:640–647, 1990.
429. McKinney, R. E., Robertson, J. W. R., and the Duke Pediatric AIDS Clinical Trials Unit: Effect of human immunodeficiency virus infection on the growth of young children. J. Pediatr. *123*:579–582, 1993.
430. McKinney, R. E., and Wilfert, C. M.: Lymphocyte subsets in children younger than 2 years old: Normal values in a population at risk for human immunodeficiency virus infection and diagnostic and prognostic application to infected children. Pediatr. Infect. Dis. *11*:639–644, 1992.
431. McKinney. R. E., Wilfert, C., and the AIDS Clinical Trials Group Protocol 043 Study Group: Growth as a prognostic indicator in children with human immunodeficiency virus infection treated with zidovudine. J. Pediatr. *125*:728–733, 1994.
432. McLaughlin, M., Thomas, P., Onorato, I., et al.: Live virus vaccines in human immunodeficiency virus-infected children: A retrospective survey. Pediatrics *82*:229–233, 1988.
433. Medley, G. F., Anderson, R. M., Cox, D. R., et al.: Incubation period of AIDS in patients infected via blood transfusion. Nature *328*:719–721, 1987.
434. Mehendale, S. M., Rodrigues, J. J., Brookmeyer, R. S., et al.: Incidence and predictors of human immunodeficiency virus type 1 seroconversion in patients attending sexually transmitted disease clinics in India. J. Infect. Dis. *172*:1486–1491, 1995.
435. Mellins, C. A., Levenson, R. L., Zawadzki, R., et al.: Effects of pediatric HIV infection and prenatal drug exposure on mental and psychomotor development. J. Pediatr. Psychol. *19*:617–628, 1994.
436. Miles, S. A., Balden, E., Magpantay, L., et al.: Rapid serologic testing with immune-complex–dissociated HIV p24 antigen for early detection of HIV infection in neonates. N. Engl. J. Med. *328*:297–302, 1993.
437. Miller, G. J., Lewis, L. L., Colman, S. M., et al.: Clustering of human T lymphotropic virus type I seropositivity in Monserrat, West Indies: Evidence for an environmental factor in transmission of the virus. J. Infect. Dis. *170*:44–50, 1994.
438. Miller, T. L., Orav, E. J., Martin, S. R., et al.: Malnutrition and carbohy-

drate malabsorption in children with vertically transmitted human immunodeficiency virus 1 infection. Gastroenterol *100*:1296–1302, 1991.
439. Miller, T. L., Winter, H. S., Luginbuhl, L. M., et al.: Pancreatitis in pediatric human immunodeficiency virus infection. J. Pediatr. *120*:223–227, 1992.
440. Minkoff, H., Burns, D. N., Landesman, S., et al.: The relationship of the duration of ruptured membranes to vertical transmission of human immunodeficiency virus. Am. J. Obstet. Gynecol. *173*:585–589, 1995.
441. Mintz, M.: Clinical comparison of adult and pediatric neuroAIDS. Adv. Neuroimmunol. *4*:207–221, 1994.
442. Mitchell, C. D., Erlich, S. S., Mastrucci, M. T., et al.: Congenital toxoplasmosis occurring in infants perinatally infected with human immunodeficiency virus type 1. Pediatr. Infect. Dis. J. *9*:512–518, 1990.
443. Mitchell, W. G., Nelson, M. D., Contant, C. F., et al.: Effects of human immunodeficiency virus and immune status on magnetic resonance imaging of the brain in hemophiliac subjects: Results from the Hemophilia Growth and Development Study. Pediatrics *91*:742–746, 1993.
444. Mofenson, L. M.: Epidemiology and determinants of vertical HIV transmission. Semin. Pediatr. Infect. Dis. *5*:252–265, 1994.
445. Mofenson, L. M.: A critical review of studies evaluating the relationship of mode of delivery to perinatal transmission of human immunodeficiency virus. Pediatr. Infect. Dis. J. *14*:169–177, 1995.
446. Mofenson, L. M., Bethel, J., Moye, J., et al.: Effect of intravenous immunoglobulin (IVIG) on CD4+ lymphocyte decline in HIV-infected children in a clinical trial of IVIG infection prophylaxis. J. Acquir. Immune Defic. Syndr. *6*:1103–1113, 1993.
447. Mofenson, L. M., Korelitz, J., Pelton, S., et al.: Sinusitis in children infected with human immunodeficiency virus: Clinical characteristics, risk factors and prophylaxis. Clin. Infect. Dis. *21*:1175–1181, 1995.
448. Mofenson, L. M., Moye, J., Bethel, J., et al.: Prophylactic immunoglobulin in HIV-infected children with CD4+ count of 0.2×10^9 or more: Effect on viral, opportunistic and bacterial infections. J. A. M. A. *268*:483–488, 1992.
449. Mofenson, L. M., Moye, J., Korelitz, J., et al.: Crossover of placebo patients to intravenous immunoglobulin confirms efficacy for prophylaxis of bacterial infections and reduction of hospitalizations in human immunodeficiency virus-infected children. Pediatr. Infect. Dis. J. *13*:477–484, 1994.
450. Montalvo, F. W., Casanova, R., and Clavell, L. A.: Treatment outcome in children with malignancies associated with human immunodeficiency virus infection. J. Pediatr. *116*:735–738, 1990.
451. Moodley, D., Bobat, R. A., Coutsoudis, A., et al.: Predicting perinatal human immunodeficiency virus infection by antibody patterns. Pediatr. Infect. Dis. J. *14*:850–852, 1995.
452. Moran, C. A., Suster, S., Pavlova, Z., et al.: The spectrum of pathological changes in the lung in children with the acquired immunodeficiency syndrome: An autopsy study of 36 cases. Hum. Pathol. *25*:877–882, 1994.
453. Morgan, G., Wilkins, H. A., Pepin, J., et al.: AIDS following mother-to-child transmission of HIV-2. AIDS *4*:879–882, 1990.
454. Morishita, N., Ishii, K., Tanaka, Y., et al.: Immunoglobulin prophylaxis against human T cell lymphotropic virus type II in rabbits. J. Infect. Dis. *169*:620–623, 1994.
455. Mortimer, P. P.: A lurking epidemic. Lancet *343*:368–370, 1994.
456. Moss, G. B., Clemetson, D., D'Costa, L., et al.: Association of cervical ectopy with heterosexual transmission of human immunodeficiency virus: Results of a study of couples in Nairobi, Kenya. J. Infect. Dis. 164:588–591, 1991.
457. Moss, G. B., Overbaugh, J., Welch, M., et al.: Human immunodeficiency virus DNA in urethral secretions of men: Association with gonococcal urethritis and CD4 cell depletion. J. Infect. Dis. *172*:1469–1474, 1995.
458. Msellati, P., Lepage, P., Hitimana, D.-G., et al.: Neurodevelopmental testing of children born to human immunodeficiency type 1 seropositive and seronegative mothers: A prospective cohort study in Kigali, Rwanda. Pediatrics *92*:843–848, 1993.
459. Mueller, B. U., Butler, K. A., Higham, M. C., et al.: Smooth muscle tumors in children with human immunodeficiency virus. Pediatrics *90*:460–463, 1992.
460. Mueller, B. U., Butler, K. M., Stocker, V. L., et al.: Clinical and pharmacokinetic evaluation of long-term therapy with didanosine in children with HIV infection. Pediatrics *94*:724–731, 1994.
461. Mueller, B. U., MacKay, K., Cheshire, L. B., et al.: Cytomegalovirus ureteritis as a cause of renal failure in a child infected with the human immunodeficiency virus. Clin. Infect. Dis. *20*:1040–1043, 1995.
462. Mueller, B. U., Pizzo, P. A., Farley, M., et al.: Pharmacokinetic evaluation of the combination of zidovudine and didanosine in children with human immunodeficiency virus infection. J. Pediatr. *125*:142–146, 1994.
463. Mundy, D. C., Schinazi, R. F., Gerver, A. R., et al.: Human immunodeficiency virus isolated from amniotic fluid. Lancet *ii*:459–460, 1987.
464. Murphy, E. L., Calisher, C. H., Figueroa, J. P., et al.: HTLV-I infection and arthropod vectors. N. Engl. J. Med. *320*:1146, 1989.
465. Murphy, E. L., Figueroa, J. P., Gibbs, W. N., et al.: Human T-lymphotropic virus type I (HTLV-I) seroprevalence in Jamaica. I. Demographic determinants. Am. J. Epidemiol. *133*:1114–1124, 1991.
466. Murphy, E. L., Hanchard, B., Figueroa, J. P., et al.: Modelling the risk of adult T-cell leukemia/lymphoma in persons infected with human T-lymphotropic virus type I. Int. J. Cancer *43*:250–252, 1989.
467. Nadal, D., Caduff, R., Frey, E., et al.: Non-Hodgkin's lymphoma in four children infected with the human immunodeficiency virus: Association with Epstein-Barr virus and treatment. Cancer *73*:224–230, 1994.
468. Nagamine, M., Nakashima, Y., Uemura, S., et al.: DNA amplification of human T lymphotropic virus type I (HTLV-I) proviral DNA in breast milk of HTLV-I carriers. J. Infect. Dis. *164*:1024–1025, 1991.
469. Nair, P., Alger, L., Hines, S., et al.: Maternal and neonatal characteristics associated with HIV infection in infants of seropositive women. J. Acquir. Immune Defic. Syndr. *6*:298–302, 1993.
470. Nakashima, K., Kashiwagi, S., Kajiyama, W., et al.: Sexual transmission of human T-lymphotropic virus type I among female prostitutes and among patients with sexually transmitted diseases in Fukuoka, Kyushu, Japan. Am. J. Epidemiol. *141*:305–311, 1995.
471. Nath, A., Hartloper, V., Furer, M., et al.: Infection of human fetal astrocytes with HIV-1: Viral tropism and the role of cell to cell contact in viral transmission. J. Neuropathol. Expt. Neurol. *54*:320–330, 1995.
472. Nduati, R. W., John, G. C., Richardson, B. A., et al.: Human immunodeficiency virus type 1-infected cells in breast milk: Association with immunosuppression and vitamin A deficiency. J. Infect. Dis. *172*:1461–1468, 1995.
473. Nerurkar, V. R., Song, K.-J., Bastian, I. B., et al.: Genotyping of human T cell lymphotropic virus type I using Australo-Melanesian topotype-specific oligonucleotide primer-based polymerase chain reaction: Insights into viral evolution and dissemination. J. Infect. Dis. *170*:1353–1360, 1994.
474. Nesheim, S., Lee, F., Sawyer, M., et al.: Diagnosis of human immunodeficiency virus infection by enzyme-linked immunospot assays in a prospectively followed cohort of infants of human immunodeficiency virus-seropositive women. Pediatr. Infect. Dis. J. *11*:635–639, 1992.
475. Nesheim, S., Lindsay, M., Sawyer, M. K., et al.: A prospective population-based study of HIV perinatal transmission. AIDS *8*:1293–1298, 1994.
476. Newburg, D. S., Linhardt, R., Ampofo, S. A., et al.: Human milk glycosaminoglycans inhibit HIV glycoprotein gp120 binding to its host cell CD4 receptor. J. Nutr. *125*:419–424, 1995.
477. Newburg, D. S., Viscidi, R. P., Ruff, A., et al.: A human milk factor inhibits binding of human immunodeficiency virus to the CD4 receptor. Pediatr. Res. *31*:22–28, 1992.
478. Newell, M.-L., Dunn, D., De Maria, A., et al.: Detection of virus in vertically exposed HIV-antibody negative children. Lancet *347*:213–215, 1996.
479. Nicoll, A., Newell, M.-L., Van Praag, E., et al.: Infant feeding policy and practice in the presence of HIV-1 infection. AIDS *9*:107–119, 1995.
480. Nicoll, A., Timaeus, I., Kigadye, R.-M., et al.: The impact of HIV-1 infection on mortality in children under 5 years of age in sub-Saharan Africa: A demographic and epidemiologic analysis. AIDS *8*:995–1005, 1994.
481. Nicolosi, A., Leite, M. L. C., Musicco, M., et al.: The efficiency of male-to-female and female-to-male sexual transmission of human immunodeficiency virus: A study of 730 stable couples. Epidemiology *5*:570–575, 1994.
482. Nicolosi, A., Musicco, M., Saracco, A., et al.: Risk factors for woman-to-man sexual transmission of the human immunodeficiency virus. J. Acquir. Immune Defic. Syndr. *7*:296–300, 1994.
483. Norkin, L. C.: Virus receptors: Implications for pathogenesis and design of antiviral agents. Clin. Microbiol. Rev. *8*:293–315, 1995.
484. Nowak, M. A.: AIDS pathogenesis: From models to viral dynamics in patients. J. Acquir. Immune Defic. Syndr. Hum. Retrovirol. *10*(Suppl. 1):S1–S5, 1995.
485. Nozyce, M., Hittleman, J., Muenz, L., et al.: Effect of perinatally acquired human immunodeficiency virus infection on neurodevelopment in children during the first two years of life. Pediatrics *94*:883–891, 1994.
486. Nyambi, P. N., Fransen, K., de Beenhouwer, H., et al.: Detection of human immunodeficiency virus type 1 (HIV-1) in heel prick blood on filter paper from children born to HIV-1 seropositive mothers. J. Clin. Microbiol. *32*:2858–2860, 1994.
487. O'Brien, K. L., Ruff, A. J., Louis, M. A., et al.: Bacillus Calmette-Guerin complications in children born to HIV-1 infected women with a review of the literature. Pediatrics *95*:414–418, 1995.
488. O'Brien, T. R., George, J. R., and Holmberg, S. D.: Human immunodeficiency virus type 2 infection in the United States: Epidemiology, diagnosis and public health implications. J. A. M. A. *267*:2775–2779, 1992.
489. Ogino, M. T., Dankner, W. M., and Spector, S. A.: Development and significance of zidovudine resistance in children infected with human immunodeficiency virus. J. Pediatr. *123*:1–8, 1993.
490. Oksenberg, J. R., Mantegazza, R., Kakai, K., et al.: HTLV-I sequences are not detected in peripheral blood genomic DNA or in brain cDNA of multiple sclerosis patients. Ann. Neurol. *28*:574–577, 1990.
491. Olivero, M. T., Nelson, R. P., Andrews, T., et al.: Cytomegalovirus sinus disease in a human immunodeficiency virus-infected child. Pediatr. Infect. Dis. J. *14*:629–630, 1995.
492. Ometto, L., Zanotto, C., Maccabruni, A., et al.: Viral phenotype and host-cell susceptibility to HIV-1 infection as risk factors for mother-to-child HIV-1 transmission. AIDS *9*:427–434, 1995.
493. Onorato, I. M., Markowitz, L. E., and Oxtoby, M. J.: Childhood immunization, vaccine-preventable diseases and infection with human immunodeficiency virus. Pediatr. Infect. Dis. J. *6*:588–595, 1988.
494. Operskalski, E. A., Stram, D. O., Lee, H., et al.: Human immunodeficiency virus type 1 infection: Relationship of risk group and age to rate of progression to AIDS. J. Infect. Dis. *172*:648–655, 1995.

495. Orcutt, T. A., Godwin, C. R., Pizzo, P. A., et al.: Aerosolized pentamidine: A well-tolerated mode of prophylaxis against *Pneumocystis carinii* pneumonia in older children with human immunodeficiency virus infection. Pediatr. Infect. Dis. J. *11*:290–294, 1992.
496. Orgino, M. T., Dankner, W. M., and Spector, S. A.: Development and significance of zidovudine resistance in children infected with human immunodeficiency virus. J. Pediatr. *123*:1–8, 1993.
497. Osame, M., Janssen, R., Kubota, H., et al.: Nationwide survey of HTLV-I–associated myelopathy in Japan: Association with blood transfusion. Ann. Neurol. *28*:50–56, 1990.
498. Osame, M., Usuku, K., Izumo, S., et al.: HTLV-I associated myelopathy, a new clinical entity. Lancet *1*:1031–1032, 1986.
499. Otten, M. W., Zaidi, A. A., Peterman, T. A., et al.: High rate of HIV seroconversion among patients attending urban sexually transmitted disease clinics. AIDS *8*:549–553, 1994.
500. Paccagnini, S., Principi, N., Massironi, E., et al.: Perinatal transmission and manifestation of hepatitis C virus infection in a high risk population. Pediatr. Infect. Dis. J. *14*:195–199, 1995.
501. Pachl, C., Todd, J. A., and Kern, D. G.: Rapid and precise quantification of HIV-1 RNA in plasma using a branched DNA signal amplification assay. J. Acquir. Immune Defic. Syndr. Hum. Retrovirol. *8*:446–454, 1995.
502. Padian, N. S., Shiboski, S. C., and Jewell, N. P.: The effect of number of exposures on the risk of heterosexual transmission. J. Infect. Dis. *161*:883–887, 1990.
503. Padian, N. S., Shiboski, S. C., and Jewell, N. P.: Female-to-male transmission of human immunodeficiency virus. J. A. M. A. *266*:1664–1667, 1991.
504. Pahwa, S., Biron, K., Lim, W., et al.: Continuous varicella-zoster infection associated with acyclovir resistance in a child with AIDS. J. A. M. A. *260*:2879–2882, 1988.
505. Palasanthiran, P., Robertson, P., Ziegler, J. B., et al.: Decay of transplacental human immunodeficiency virus type 1 antibodies in neonates and infants. J. Infect. Dis. *170*:1593–1596, 1994.
506. Palasanthiran, P., Ziegler, J. B., Stewart, G. J., et al.: Breast-feeding during primary maternal human immunodeficiency virus infection and risk of transmission from mother to infant. J. Infect. Dis. *167*:441–444, 1993.
507. Palomba, E., David, O., Boltri, A., et al.: Increased erythrocyte adenosine deaminase activity in children with perinatal human immunodeficiency virus infection. Pediatr. Infect. Dis. J. *8*:862–865, 1989.
508. Palumbo, P., Hoyt, L., Demasio, K., et al.: Population-based study of measles and measles immunization in human immunodeficiency virus-infected children. Pediatr. Infect. Dis. J. *11*:1008–1014, 1992.
509. Pantaleo, G., Cohen, O. J., Schwartzentruber, D. J., et al.: Pathologic insights from studies of lymphoid tissue from HIV-infected individuals. J. Acquir. Immune Defic. Syndr. Hum. Retrovirol. *10*(Suppl. 1):S6–S14, 1995.
510. Pantaleo, G., Graziosi, C., and Fauci, A. S.: Immunopathogenesis of human immunodeficiency virus infection. N. Engl. J. Med. *328*:327–335, 1993.
511. Papiernik, M., Brossard, Y., Mullinez, N., et al.: Thymic abnormalities in fetuses aborted from human immunodeficiency virus type 1 seropositive women. Pediatrics *89*:297–301, 1992.
512. Parekh, B. S, Shaffer, N., Coughlin, R., et al.: Human immunodeficiency virus 1-specific IgA capture enzyme immunoassay for early diagnosis of human immunodeficiency virus 1 infection in infants. Pediatr. Infect. Dis. J. *12*:908–913, 1993.
513. Park, Y. D., Belman, A. L., Kim, T.-S., et al.: Stroke in pediatric acquired immunodeficiency syndrome. Ann. Neurol. *28*:303–311, 1990.
514. Pavia, A. T., Long, E. G., Ryder, R. W., et al.: Diarrhea among African children born to human immunodeficiency virus 1-infected mothers: Clinical, microbiologic and epidemiologic features. Pediatr. Infect. Dis. J. *11*:996–1003, 1992.
515. Pavlakis, S. G., Frank, Y., Nocyze, M., et al.: Acquired immunodeficiency syndrome and the developing nervous system. Adv. Pediatr. *41*:427–451, 1994.
516. Peeters, M., Gersky-Damet, G.-M., Fransen, K., et al.: Virological and polymerase chain reaction studies of HIV-1/HIV-2 dual infections in Cote d'Ivoire. Lancet 340:339–340, 1992.
517. Periquet, B. A, Jammes, N. M., Lambert, W. E, et al.: Micronutrient levels in HIV-1–infected children. AIDS *9*:887–893, 1995.
518. Persaud, D., Bangaru, B., Breco, M. A., et al.: Cholestatic hepatitis in children infected with the human immunodeficiency virus. Pediatr. Infect. Dis. J. *12*:492–498, 1993.
519. Persaud, D., Chandwani, S., Rigaud, M., et al.: Delayed recognition of human immunodeficiency virus infection in preadolescent children. Pediatrics *90*:688–691, 1992.
520. Peterman, T. A., Stoneburner, R. L., Allen, J. R., et al.: Risk of human immunodeficiency virus transmission from heterosexual adults with transfusion-acquired infections. J. A. M. A. *259*:55–58, 1988.
521. Peters, M. J., Moeller, H. U., Russell-Eggitt, I., et al.: Cytomegalovirus retinitis in AIDS. Arch. Dis. Child. *72*:54–55, 1995.
522. Peterson, J., Church, J., Gomperts, E., et al.: Lymphocyte phenotype does not predict immune function in pediatric patients infected with human immunodeficiency virus type 1. J. Pediatr. *115*:944–948, 1989.
523. Peudenier, S., Hery, C., Montagnier, L., et al.: Human microglial cells: Characterization in cerebral tissue and in primary culture, and study of their susceptibility to HIV-1 infection. Ann. Neurol. *29*:152–161, 1991.
524. Phillips, D. M., and Tan, X.: HIV-1 infection of the trophoblast cell line BeWo: A study of virus uptake. AIDS Res. Hum. Retroviruses *8*:1683–1691, 1992.
525. Pizzo, P. A., Butler, K., Balis, F., et al.: Dideoxycytidine alone and in an alternating schedule with zidovudine in children with symptomatic human immunodeficiency virus infection. J. Pediatr. *117*:799–808, 1990.
526. Pizzo, P. A., Eddy, J., Falloon, J., et al.: Effect of continuous infusion of zidovudine (AZT) in children with symptomatic HIV infection. N. Engl. J. Med. *319*:889–896, 1988.
527. Pizzo, P. A., and Wilfert, C.: Antiretroviral therapy for infection due to human immunodeficiency virus in children. Clin. Infect. Dis. *19*:177–196, 1994.
528. Pizzo, P. A., Wilfert, C. M., and the Pediatric AIDS Siena Workshop II: Report of a Consensus Workshop, Siena, Italy, June 4–6, 1993: Markers and determinants of disease progression in children with HIV infection. J. Acquir. Immune Defic. Syndr. 8:30–44, 1995.
529. Plaeger-Marshall, S., Isacescu, V., O'Rourke, S., et al.: T cell activation in pediatric AIDS pathogenesis: Three-color immunophenotyping. Clin. Immunol. Immunopathol. *71*:19–26, 1994.
530. Plummer, F. A., Simonsen, J. N., Cameron, D. W., et al.: Cofactors in male-female sexual transmission of human immunodeficiency virus type 1. J. Infect. Dis. *163*:233–239, 1991.
531. Poiesz, B. J., Ruscetti, F. W., Gazdar, A. F., et al.: Detection and isolation of type C retrovirus particles from fresh and cultured lymphocytes of a patient with cutaneous T-cell lymphoma. Proc. Natl. Acad. Sci. U. S. A. *77*:7415–7419, 1980.
532. Poland, S. D., Rice, G. P. A., and Dekaban, G. A.: HIV-1 infection of human brain-derived microvascular endothelial cells in vitro. J. Acquir. Immune Defic. Syndr. *8*:437–445, 1995.
533. Poli, G., Pantaleo, G., and Fauci, A. S.: Immunopathogenesis of human immunodeficiency virus infection. Clin. Infect. Dis. *17*(Suppl. 1):S224–S229, 1993.
534. Pollack, H., Zhan, M. X., Ilmet-Moore, T., et al.: A novel detection assay for the early diagnosis of HIV-1 infected infants. J. Acquir. Immune Defic. Syndr. *6*:582–586, 1993.
535. Pope, M., Betjes, G. H., Romani, N., et al.: Conjugates of dendritic cells and memory T lymphocytes from skin facilitate productive infection with HIV-1. Cell *78*:389–398, 1994.
536. Poulson, A. G., Kvinesdal, B. B., Aaby, P., et al.: Lack of evidence of vertical transmission of human immunodeficiency virus type 2 in a sample of the general population in Bissau. J. Acquir. Immune Defic. Syndr. *5*:25–30, 1992.
537. Prazuck, T., Yameogo, J.-M. V., Heylinck, B., et al.: Mother-to-child transmission of human immunodeficiency virus type 1 and type 2 and dual infection: A cohort study in Banfora, Burkino Faso. Pediatr. Infect. Dis. J. *14*:940–947, 1995.
538. Principi, N., Marchisio, P., Massironi, E., et al.: Effect of zidovudine in HIV-infected children with lymphocytic interstitial pneumonitis. AIDS *5*:468–469, 1991.
539. Principi, N., Marchisio, P., Tornaghi, R., et al.: Occurrence of infections in children infected with human immunodeficiency virus. Pediatr. Infect. Dis. J. *10*:190–193, 1991.
540. Principi, N., Marchisio, P., Tornaghi, R., et al.: Acute otitis media in human immunodeficiency virus-infected children. Pediatrics *88*:566–571, 1991.
541. Prose, N. S.: Cutaneous manifestations of pediatric HIV infection. Pediatr. Dermatol. *9*:326–328, 1992.
542. Provisional Committee on Pediatric AIDS: Perinatal human immunodeficiency virus testing. Pediatrics *95*:303–307, 1995.
543. Qazi, Q. H., Shikh, T. M., Fikrig, D., et al.: Lack of evidence for craniofacial dysmorphism in perinatal human immunodeficiency virus infection. J. Pediatr. *112*:7–11, 1988.
544. Quinn, T. C., Kline, R. L., Halsey, N., et al.: Early diagnosis of perinatal HIV infection by detection of viral-specific IgA antibodies. J. A. M. A. *266*:3439–3442, 1991.
545. Quinn, T. C., Kline, R., Moss, M. W., et al.: Acid dissociation of immune complexes improves diagnostic utility of p24 antigen detection in perinatally acquired human immunodeficiency virus infection. J. Infect. Dis. *167*:1193–1196, 1993.
546. Qureshi, M. N., Barr, C. E., Seshamma, T., et al.: Infection of oral mucosal cells by human immunodeficiency virus type 1 in seropositive persons. J. Infect. Dis. *171*:190–193, 1995.
547. Radelli, L., Hu, C., Birindelli, S., et al.: Natural killer activity, tumor necrosis factor-α, and interferon-γ production in HIV-infected children at various stages of disease. Pediatr. AIDS HIV Infect. Fetus Adolesc. *6*:204–211, 1995.
548. Ramazzotti, E., Marconi, A., Re, M. C., et al.: *In vitro* infection of human epidermal Langerhans' cells with HIV-1. Immunology *85*:94–98, 1995.
549. Raphael, S. A., Price, M. L., Lischner, H. W., et al.: Inflammatory demyelinating polyneuropathy in a child with symptomatic HIV infection. J. Pediatr. *118*:242–245, 1991.
550. Raphael, S. A., Wolfson, B. J., Parker, P., et al.: Pyomyositis in a child with acquired immunodeficiency syndrome. Am. J. Dis. Child. *143*:779–781, 1989.

551. Ratner, L.: Molecular biology and pathogenesis of HIV infection. Curr. Opin. Infect. Dis. *6*:181–190, 1993.
552. Ratner, L., and Poiesz, B. J.: Leukemias associated with human T-cell lymphotropic virus type I in a non-endemic region. Medicine *67*:401–422, 1988.
553. Rautonen, J., Rautonen, N., Martin, N. L., et al.: Serum interleukin-6 concentrations are elevated and associated with elevated tumor necrosis factor-α and immunoglobulin G and A concentrations in children with HIV infection. AIDS *5*:1319–1325, 1991.
554. Reinhardt, P. P., Reinhardt, B., Lathey, J. L., et al.: Human cord blood mononuclear cells are preferentially infected by non-syncytium–inducing, macrophage-tropic human immunodeficiency virus type 1 isolates. J. Clin. Microbiol. *33*:292–297, 1995.
555. Report of a Consensus Workshop: Siena, Italy, January 17–18, 1992: Early diagnosis of HIV infection in infants. J. Acquir. Immune Defic. Syndr. *5*:1169–1178, 1992.
556. Richman, D. D.: Clinical significance of drug resistance in human immunodeficiency virus infection. Clin. Infect. Dis. *21*(Suppl. 2):S166–S169, 1995.
557. Richman, K. M., and Rickman, L. S.: The potential for transmission of human immunodeficiency virus through human bites. J. Acquir. Immune Defic. Syndr. *6*:402–406, 1993.
558. Rigaud, M., Leibovitz, E., Sin Quee, C., et al.: Thrombocytopenia in children infected with human immunodeficiency virus: Long-term follow-up and therapeutic considerations. J. Acquir. Immune Defic. Syndr. *5*:450–455, 1992.
559. Rigaud, M., Pollack, H., Leibovitz, E., et al.: Efficacy of primary chemoprophylaxis against *Pneumocystis carinii* pneumonia during the first year of life in infants infected with human immunodeficiency virus type 1. J. Pediatr. *125*:476–480, 1994.
560. Rios, M., Khabbaz, R. F., Kaplan, J. E., et al.: Transmission of human T cell lymphotropic (HTLV) type II by transfusion of HTLV-I screened blood products. J. Infect. Dis. *170*:206–210, 1994.
561. Robert-Guroff, M., Roilides, E., Muldoon, R., et al.: Human immunodeficiency virus (HIV) type 1 strain MN neutralizing antibody in HIV-infected children: Correlation with clinical status and prognostic value. J. Infect. Dis. *167*:538–546, 1993.
562. Roberts, B. D., Foung, S. K. H., Lipka, J. J., et al.: Evaluation of an immunoblot assay for serological confirmation and differentiation of human T-cell lymphotropic virus types I and II. J. Clin. Microbiol. *31*:260–264, 1993.
563. Roberts, C. R., Fipps, D. R., Brundage, J. F., et al.: Prevalence of human T-lymphotropic virus in civilian applicants for the United States Armed Forces. Am. J. Public Health *82*:70–73, 1992.
564. Roberts, L. M., Chamberland, M. E., Cleveland, J. L., et al.: Investigations of health care workers infected with HIV: The Centers for Disease Control and Prevention. Ann. Intern. Med. *122*:653–657, 1995.
565. Robinson, R. D., Lindo, J. F., Neva, F. A., et al.: Immunoepidemiologic studies of *Strongyloides stercoralis* and human T lymphotropic virus type I infections in Jamaica. J. Infect. Dis. *169*:692–696, 1994.
566. Rodriguez, E. M., Mofenson, L. M., Chang, B.-H., et al.: Association of maternal drug use during pregnancy with maternal HIV culture positivity and perinatal HIV transmission. AIDS *10*:273–282, 1996.
566a. Rogers, M. E., Mofenson, L. M., and Moseley, R. R.: Reducing the risk of perinatal HIV transmission through zidovudine therapy: Treatment recommendations and implications. J. Am. Med. Womens Assoc. 50:78–93. 1995.
567. Rogers, M. F., Thomas, P. A., Starcher, E. T., et al.: Acquired immunodeficiency syndrome in children: Report of the Centers for Disease Control national surveillance, 1982–1985. Pediatrics *79*:1008–1014, 1987.
568. Roilides, E., Black, C., Reimer, C., et al.: Dysbalances in immunoglobulin G subclasses in children infected with human immunodeficiency virus type 1. Pediatr. Infect. Dis. J. *10*:134–139, 1991.
569. Roilides, E., Butler, K. M., Husson, R. N., et al.: *Pseudomonas* infections in children with human immunodeficiency virus infection. Pediatr. Infect. Dis. J. *11*:547–553, 1992.
570. Roilides, E., Clerici, M., DePalma, L., et al.: Helper T-cell responses in children infected with human immunodeficiency virus type 1. J. Pediatr. *118*:724–730, 1991.
571. Roilides, E., Marshall, D., Venzon, D., et al.: Bacterial infections in human immunodeficiency virus type 1-infected children: The impact of central venous catheters and antiretroviral agents. Pediatr. Infect. Dis. J. *10*:813–819, 1991.
572. Roilides, E., Mertins, S., Eddy, J., et al.: Impairment of neutrophil chemotactic and bactericidal function in children infected with human immunodeficiency virus type 1 and partial reversal after in vitro exposure to granulocyte-macrophage colony-stimulating factor. J. Pediatr. *117*:531–540, 1990.
573. Roques, P. A., Gras, G., Parnet-Mathieu, F., et al.: Clearance of HIV infection in 12 perinatally infected children: Clinical, virologic and immunological data. AIDS *9*:F19–F26, 1995.
574. Rosenzweig, M., Clark, D. P., and Gaulton, G. N.: Selective thymocyte depletion in neonatal HIV-1 thymic infection. AIDS *7*:1601–1605, 1993.
575. Rowland-Jones, S. L., Nixon, D. F., Aldhous, M. C., et al.: HIV-specific cytotoxic T-cell activity in an HIV-exposed but uninfected infant. Lancet *341*:860–861, 1993.
576. Rubinstein, A., Berstein, L. J., Charytan, M., et al.: Corticosteroid treatment for pulmonary lymphoid hyperplasia in children with the acquired immunodeficiency syndrome. Pediatr. Pulmonol. *4*:13–17, 1988.
577. Rubinstein, A., Morecki, R., Silverman, B., et al.: Pulmonary disease in children with the acquired immunodeficiency syndrome and AIDS related complex. J. Pediatr. *108*:498–503, 1986.
578. Ruff, A. J., Coberly, J., Halsey, N. A., et al.: Prevalence of HIV-1 DNA and p24 antigen in breast milk and correlation with maternal factors. J. Acquir. Immune Defic. Syndr. *7*:68–73, 1994.
579. Ruiz-Contreras, J., Ramos, J. T., Hernandez-Sampelayo, T., et al.: Sepsis in children with human immunodeficiency virus infection. Pediatr. Infect. Dis. J. *14*:522–526, 1995.
580. Rutstein, R. M., Rudy, B., Codispoti, C., et al.: Response to hepatitis B immunization by infants exposed to HIV. AIDS *8*:1281–1284, 1994.
581. Ryder, R. W., Nsa, W., Hassig, S. E., et al.: Perinatal transmission of human immunodeficiency virus type 1 to infants of seropositive women in Zaire. N. Engl. J. Med. *320*:1637–1642, 1989.
582. Ryder, R. W., Oxtoby, M. J., Mvula, M., et al.: Safety and immunogenicity of bacille Calmette-Guerin, diphtheria-tetanus-pertussis, and oral polio vaccines in newborn children in Zaire infected with human immunodeficiency virus type 1. J. Pediatr. *122*:697–702, 1993.
583. Saavedra, J. M., Henderson, R. A., Paerman, J. A., et al.: Longitudinal assessment of growth in children born to mothers with human immunodeficiency virus infection. Arch. Pediatr. Adolesc. Med. *149*:497–502, 1995.
584. Saito, S., Furuki, K., Ando, Y., et al.: Identification of HTLV-I sequence in cord blood mononuclear cells of neonates born to HTLV-I antigen/antibody positive-mothers by polymerase chain reaction. Jpn. J. Cancer Res. *81*:890–895, 1990.
585. Sakaguchi, M., Sato, T., and Groopman, J. E.: Human immunodeficiency virus infection of megakaryotic cells. Blood *77*:481–485, 1991.
586. Sanhadji, K., Gessain, A., Chout, R., et al.: HTLV-I antibody and cell-mediated immunity status in sickle cell anemia. Clin. Immunol. Immunopathol. *43*:140–144, 1987.
587. Sassan-Morokro, M., Greenberg, A. E., Coulibaly, I.-M., et al.: High rates of sexual contact with female sex workers, sexually transmitted diseases, and condom neglect among HIV-infected and uninfected men with tuberculosis in Abidjan, Cote d'Ivoire. J. Acquir. Immune Defic. Syndr. Hum. Retrovirol. *11*:183–187, 1996.
588. Sawada, T., Iwahara, Y., Ishii, K., et al.: Immunoglobulin prophylaxis against milkborne transmission of human T cell leukemia virus type I in rabbits. J. Infect. Dis. *164*:1193–1196, 1991.
589. Schechter, M., Harrison, L. H., Halsey, N. A., et al.: Coinfection with human T-cell lymphotropic virus type I and HIV in Brazil. J. A. M. A. *271*:353–357, 1994.
590. Schiodt, M., Greenspan, D., Levy, J., et al.: Does HIV cause salivary gland disease? AIDS *3*:819–822, 1989.
591. Schupbach, J., Boni, J., Tomasik, Z., et al.: Sensitive detection and early prognostic significance of p24 antigen in heat-denatured plasma of human immunodeficiency virus type 1-infected infants. J. Infect. Dis. *170*:318–324, 1994.
592. Schupbach, J., Tomasik, Z., Jendis, J., et al.: IgG, IgM and IgA response to HIV in infants born to HIV-1 infected mothers. J. Acquir. Immune Defic. Syndr. *7*:421–427, 1994.
593. Schuval, S. J., Bonagura, V. R., and Ilowite, N. T.: Rheumatologic manifestations of pediatric human immunodeficiency virus infection. J. Rheumatol. *20*:1578–1582, 1993.
594. Schwartz, L. J., St. Louis, Y., Wu, R., et al.: Endocrine function in children with human immunodeficiency virus infection. Am. J. Dis. Child. *145*:330–333, 1991.
595. Schwebke, J., Calsyn, D., Shriver, K., et al.: Prevalence and epidemiologic correlates of human T cell lymphotropic virus infection among intravenous drug users. J. Infect. Dis. *169*:962–967, 1994.
596. Scott, G. B., Hutto, C., Makuch, R. W., et al.: Survival in children with perinatally acquired human immunodeficiency virus type 1 infection. N. Engl. J. Med. *321*:1791–1796, 1989.
597. Seed, J., Allen, S., Mertens, T., et al.: Male circumcision, sexually transmitted disease, and risk of HIV. J. Acquir. Immune Defic. Syndr. Hum. Retrovirol. *8*:83–90, 1995.
598. Sei, S., Saito, K., Stewart, S. K., et al.: Increased human immunodeficiency virus type 1 DNA content and quinolinic acid concentration in brain tissues from patients with HIV encephalopathy. J. Infect. Dis. *172*:638–647, 1995.
599. Seidlin, M., Vogler, M., Lee, E., et al.: Heterosexual transmission of HIV in a cohort of couples in New York City. AIDS *7*:1247–1254, 1993.
600. Semba, R. D.: Vitamin A, immunity and infection. Clin. Infect. Dis. *19*:489–499, 1994.
601. Semba, R. D., Miotti, P. G., Chiphangwi, J. D., et al.: Maternal vitamin A deficiency and mother-to-child transmission of HIV-1. Lancet *343*:1593–1597, 1994.
602. Semba, R. D., Miotti, P. G., Chiphangwi, J. D., et al.: Infant mortality and maternal vitamin A deficiency during human immunodeficiency virus infection. Clin. Infect. Dis. *21*:966–972, 1995.

603. Shearer, G. M., and Clerici, M.: Early T-helper cell defects in HIV infection. AIDS *5*:245–253, 1991.
604. Sierra-Madero, J. G., Toossi, Z., Hom, D. L., et al.: Relationship between load of virus in alveolar macrophages from human immunodeficiency virus type 1-infected persons, production of cytokines and clinical status. J. Infect. Dis. *169*:18–27, 1994.
605. Siller, L., Martin, N. L., Kostuchenko, P., et al.: Serum levels of soluble CD8, neopterin, β-2 microglobulin and p24 antigen as indicators of disease progression in children with AIDS on zidovudine therapy. AIDS *7*:369–373, 1993.
606. Simon, F., Matheron, S., Tamalet, C., et al.: Cellular and plasma viral load in patients infected with HIV-1. AIDS *11*:1411–1417, 1993.
607. Simonds, R. J., and Chanock, S.: Medical issues related to caring for HIV-infected children in and out of the home. Pediatr. Infect. Dis. J. *12*:845–852, 1993.
608. Simonds, R. J., Holmberg, S. D., Hurwitz, R. L., et al.: Transmission of human immunodeficiency virus type 1 from a seronegative organ and tissue donor. N. Engl. J. Med. *326*:726–732, 1992.
609. Simonds, R. J., Lindegren, M. L., Thomas, P., et al.: Prophylaxis against *Pneumocystis carinii* pneumonia among children with perinatally acquired HIV infection in the United States. N. Engl. J. Med. *332*:786–790, 1995.
610. Simonds, R. J., Oxtoby, M. J., Caldwell, M. B., et al.: *Pneumocystis carinii* pneumonia among U.S. children with perinatally acquired HIV infection. J. A. M. A. *270*:470–473, 1993.
611. Simpson, R. M., Leno, M., Hubbard, B. S., et al.: Cutaneous manifestations of human T cell leukemia virus type I infection in an experimental model. J. Infect. Dis. *173*:722–726, 1996.
612. Siraprapasiri, T., Thanprasertsuk, S., Rodklay, A., et al.: Risk factors for HIV among prostitutes in Chaingmai, Thailand. AIDS *5*:579–582, 1991.
613. Sirisanthana, V., and Sirisanthana, T.: Disseminated *Penicillium marneffei* infection in human immunodeficiency virus-infected children. Pediatr. Infect. Dis. J. *14*:935–940, 1995.
614. Sison, A. V., and Campos, J. M.: Laboratory methods for early detection of human immunodeficiency virus type 1 in newborns and infants. Clin. Microbiol. Rev. *5*:238–247, 1992.
615. Slade, H. B., Pica, R. V., and Pahwa, S. G.: Detection of HIV-specific antibodies in infancy by isoelectric focusing and affinity immunoblotting. J. Infect. Dis. *160*:126–130, 1989.
616. Sloand, E. M., Pitt, E., and Klein, H. G.: Safety of the blood supply. J. A. M. A. *274*:1368–1373, 1995.
617. Soiero, R., Rubinstein, A., Rashbaun, W. R., et al.: Frequency of human HIV-1 nucleic acid sequences in human fetal DNA. J. Infect. Dis. *166*:699–703, 1992.
618. Spector, S. A.: Pediatric antiretroviral choices. AIDS 4(Suppl. 3):S15–S18, 1994.
619. Spector, S. A., Gelber, R. D., McGrath, N., et al.: A controlled trial of intravenous immune globulin for the prevention of serious bacterial infections in children receiving zidovudine for advanced human immunodeficiency virus infection. N. Engl. J. Med. *331*:1181–1187, 1994.
620. Spencer, L. T., Ogino, M. T., Danker, W. M., et al.: Clinical significance of human immunodeficiency virus type 1 phenotypes in infected children. J. Infect. Dis. *169*:491–495, 1994.
621. Sperling, R. S., Stratton, P., O'Sullivan, M. J., et al.: A survey of zidovudine use in pregnant women with human immunodeficiency virus infection. N. Engl. J. Med. *326*:857–861, 1992.
622. Srugo, I., Brunell, P. A., Chelyapov, N. V., et al.: Virus burden in human immunodeficiency virus type 1-infected children: Relationship to disease status and effect of antiviral therapy. Pediatrics *87*:921–925, 1991.
623. Stavola, J. J., and Noel, G. J.: Efficacy and safety of dapsone prophylaxis against *Pneumocystis carinii* pneumonia in human immunodeficiency virus-infected children. Pediatr. Infect. Dis. J. *12*:644–647, 1993.
624. Stein, D.: A new syndrome of hepatomegaly with severe steatosis in HIV seropositive patients. AIDS Clin. Care *6*:17–20, 1994.
625. Stiehm, E. R., Bryson, Y. J., Frenkel, L. M., et al.: Prednisone improves human immunodeficiency virus encephalopathy in children. Pediatr. Infect. Dis. J. *11*:49–50, 1992.
626. St. Louis, M. E., Kamenga, M., Brown, C., et al.: Risk for perinatal HIV-1 transmission according to maternal immunologic, virologic and placental factors. J. A. M. A. *269*:2853–2859, 1993.
627. Strauss, J., Abitol, C., Zilleruelo, G., et al.: Renal disease in children with the acquired immunodeficiency syndrome. N. Engl. J. Med. *321*:625–630, 1989.
628. Stuver, S. O., Tachibana, N., Olayama, A., et al.: Heterosexual transmission of human T-cell leukemia/lymphoma virus type I among married couples in southwestern Japan: An initial report from the Miyazaki cohort study. J. Infect. Dis. *167*:57–63, 1993.
629. Sugimoto, M., Nakashima, H., Matsumoto, M., et al.: Pulmonary involvement in patients with HTLV-I–associated myelopathy: Increased soluble IL-2 receptors in bronchoalveolar lavage fluid. Am. Rev. Resp. Dis. *139*:1329–1335, 1989.
630. Sultan, J., Gaur, S., Sandhaus, L., et al.: Human immunodeficiency virus infection presenting as pancytopenia in an infant. Am. J. Pediatr. Hematol. Oncol. *16*:334–337, 1994.
631. Surtees, R., Hyland, K., and Smith, I.: Central-nervous-system methyl-group metabolism in children with neurologic complications of HIV infection. Lancet *335*:619–621, 1990.
632. Sweeney, P., Lindegren, M. L., Buehler, J. W., et al.: Teenagers at risk of human immunodeficiency virus type 1 infection: Results from seroprevalence surveys in the United States. Arch. Pediatr. Adolesc. Med. *149*:521–528, 1995.
633. Sweeney, P. A., Onorato, I. M., Allen, D. M., et al.: Sentinel surveillance of human immunodeficiency virus infection in women seeking reproductive health services in the United States, 1988–1989. Obstet. Gynecol. *79*:503–510, 1992.
634. Szelc, C. M., Mitcheltree, C., Roberts, R. L., et al.: Deficient polymorphonuclear cell and mononuclear cell antibody-dependent cellular cytotoxicity in pediatric and adult human immunodeficiency virus infection. J. Infect. Dis. *166*:486–493, 1992.
635. Tajima, K., Fujita, K., Tsukidate, S., et al.: Seroepidemiologic studies on the effects of filarial parasites on infestation of adult T-cell leukemia virus in the Goto Islands, Japan. Gann. *74*:188–191, 1983.
636. Tajima, K., Takezaki, T., Ito, M., et al.: Short-term breast feeding may reduce the risk of vertical transmission of HTLV-I. J. Acquir. Immune Defic. Syndr. Human Retrovirol. *10*:285, 1995 (abstract).
637. Takahashi, K., Tajima, K., Komoda, H., et al.: Incidence of human T lymphotropic virus type I seroconversion after age 40 among Japanese residents in an area where the virus is endemic. J. Infect. Dis. *171*:559–565, 1995.
638. Takahashi, K., Takezaki, T., Oki, T., et al.: Inhibitory effect of maternal antibody on mother-to-child transmission of human T-lymphotropic virus type I. Int. J. Cancer *49*:673–677, 1991.
639. Talalet, C., Simon, F., Dhiver, C., et al.: Autologous neutralizing antibodies and viral load in HIV-2–infected individuals. AIDS *9*:90–91, 1995.
640. Tamalet, C., Lafeuillade, A., Yahi, N., et al.: Comparison of viral burden and phenotype of HIV-1 isolates from lymph nodes and blood. AIDS *8*:1083–1088, 1994.
641. Tappero, J. W., Perkins, B. A., Wenger, J. D., et al.: Cutaneous manifestations of opportunistic infections in patients infected with human immunodeficiency virus. Clin. Microbiol. Rev. *8*:440–450, 1995.
642. Tardieu, M., and Janabi, N.: HIV-1 and the developing human nervous system: In vivo and in vitro aspects. Dev. Neurosci. *16*:137–144, 1994.
643. Taylor, R.: *In* focus: Histocompatibility antigens, protective immunity and HIV-1. J. N. I. H. Res. *6*:68–71, 1994.
644. Telzak, E. E., Chiasson, M. A., Bevier, P. J., et al.: HIV-1 seroconversion in patients with and without genital ulcer disease: A prospective study. Ann. Intern. Med. *119*:1181–1186, 1993.
645. Temmerman, M., Chomba, E. N., Ndinya-Achola, J., et al.: Maternal human immunodeficiency virus-1 infection and pregnancy outcome. Obstet. Gynecol. *83*:495–501, 1994.
646. Temmerman, M., Nyong'o, A, Bwayo, J., et al.: Risk factors for mother-to-child transmission of human immunodeficiency virus-1 infection. Am. J. Obstet. Gynecol. *172*:700–705, 1995.
647. Terada, K., Katamine, S., Eguchi, K., et al.: Prevalence of serum and salivary antibodies to HTLV-I in Sjögren's syndrome. Lancet *344*:1116–1119, 1994.
648. Teruya-Feldstein, J., Temeck, B. K., Sloas, M. M., et al.: Pulmonary malignant lymphoma of mucosa-associated lymphoid tissue (MALT) arising in a pediatric patient. Am. J. Surg. Pathol. *19*:357–363, 1995.
649. Thali, M., Bukovsky, A., Kondo, E., et al.: Functional association of cyclophilin A with HIV-1 virions. Nature *372*:363–365, 1994.
650. The HIV Infection in Newborns French Collaborative Study Group: Comparison of vertical human immunodeficiency virus type 2 and human immunodeficiency virus type 1 transmission in the French prospective cohort. Pediatr. Infect. Dis. J. *13*:502–506, 1994.
651. The National Institute of Child Health and Human Development Intravenous Immunoglobulin Study Group: Intravenous immune globulin for the prevention of bacterial infections in children with symptomatic human immunodeficiency virus infection. N. Engl. J. Med. *325*:73–80, 1991.
652. The Pediatric Supportive Care/Quality of Life Committee of NIAID's Pediatric ACTG: Enhancing supportive care and promoting quality of life: Clinical practice guidelines. Pediatr. AIDS HIV Infect. Fetus Adolesc. *6*:187–203, 1995.
653. The Working Group on Mother-to-Child Transmission of HIV: Rates of mother-to-child transmission of HIV-1 in Africa, America and Europe: Results from 13 perinatal studies. J. Acquir. Immune Defic. Syndr. *8*:506–510, 1995.
654. Thea, D. M., St. Louis, M. E., Atido, U., et al.: A prospective study of diarrhea and HIV-1 infection among 249 Zairian infants. N. Engl. J. Med. *329*:1696–1702, 1993.
655. Thomas, P., Singh, T., Williams, R., et al.: Trends in survival for children reported with maternally transmitted acquired immunodeficiency syndrome in New York City, 1982 to 1989. Pediatr. Infect. Dis. J. *11*:34–39, 1992.
656. Tornatore, C., Chandra, R., Berger, J. R., et al.: HIV-1 infection of subcortical astrocytes in the pediatric central nervous system. Neurology *44*:481–487, 1994.
657. Tovo, P.-A., de Martino, M., Gabiano, C., et al.: Prognostic factors and

survival in children with perinatal HIV-1 infection. Lancet *339*:1249–1253, 1992.

658. Tovo, P.-A., de Martino, M., Gabiano, C., et al.: AIDS appearance is associated with the velocity of disease progression in their mothers. J. Infect. Dis. *170*:806–807, 1994.
659. Tovo, P.-A., de Martino, M., Gabiano, C., et al.: Mode of delivery and gestational age influence perinatal HIV-1 transmission. J. Acquir. Immune Defic. Syndr. Human Retrovirol. *11*:88–94, 1996.
660. Tudor-Williams, G., St. Clair, M. H., McKinney, R. E., et al.: HIV-1 sensitivity to zidovudine and clinical outcome in children. Lancet *339*:15–19, 1992.
661. Turner, B. J., Eppes, S., McKee, L. J., et al.: A population-based comparison of the clinical course of children and adults with AIDS. AIDS *9*:65–72, 1995.
662. United Nations Development Programme: Young women: Silence, susceptibility and the HIV epidemic. Pediatr. AIDS HIV Infect. Fetus Adolesc. *5*:1–9, 1994.
663. Urnovitz, H. B., and Murphy, W. H.: Human endogenous retroviruses: Nature, occurrence and clinical implications in human disease. Clin. Microbiol. Rev. *9*:72–99, 1996.
664. Valdez, I. H., Pizzo, P. A., and Atkinson, J. C.: Oral health of pediatric AIDS patients: A hospital-based study. J. Dent. Child March–April:114–118, 1994.
665. van Ameijden, E. J. C., van den Hoek, A. J. A. R., and Coutinho, R. A.: Injecting risk behavior among drug users in Amsterdam, 1986 to 1992, and its relationship to AIDS prevention programs. Am. J. Public Health *84*:275–281, 1994.
666. Van de Perre, P.: Postnatal transmission of human immunodeficiency virus type 1: The breast-feeding dilemma. Am. J. Obstet. Gynecol. *173*:483–487, 1995.
667. Van de Perre, P., Lepage, P., Simonon, A., et al.: Biologic markers associated with prolonged survival in African children maternally infected by the human immunodeficiency virus type 1. AIDS Res. Hum. Retroviruses *8*:435–442, 1992.
668. Van de Perre, P., Simonon, A., Hitimana, D.-G., et al.: Infective and anti-infective properties of breastmilk from HIV-1–infected women. Lancet *341*:914–918, 1993.
669. Vandersteenhoven, J. J., Dbaibo, G., Boyko, O. B., et al.: Progressive multifocal leukoencephalopathy in pediatric acquired immunodeficiency syndrome. Pediatr. Infect. Dis. J. *11*:232–237, 1992.
670. Van Dyke, R. B., Heneine, W., Perrin, M. E., et al.: Mother-to-child transmission of human T-lymphotropic virus type II. J. Pediatr. *127*:924–928, 1995.
671. van't Wout, A. B., Kootstra, N. A., Mulder-Kampinga, G. A., et al.: Macrophage-tropic variants initiate human immunodeficiency virus type 1 infection after sexual, parenteral and vertical transmission. J. Clin. Invest. *94*:2060–2067, 1994.
672. Vardinon, N., Handsher, R., Burke, M., et al.: Poliovirus vaccination responses in HIV-infected patients: Correlation with T4 cell counts. J. Infect. Dis. *162*:238–241, 1990.
673. Vasishtha, S., Trachtman, H., Gauthier, B., et al.: Nephrotic syndrome as the initial manifestation of acquired immunodeficiency syndrome. J. Pediatr. *125*:1017, 1994.
674. Velandia, M., Fridkin, S. K., Cardenas, V., et al.: Transmission of HIV in dialysis centre. Lancet *345*:1417–1422, 1995.
675. Vella, S.: Update on HIV protease inhibitors. AIDS Clinical Care *7*:79–82, 1995.
676. Verdier, M., Denis, F., Sangare, A., et al.: Prevalence of antibody to human T cell leukemia virus type 1 (HTLV-1) in populations of Ivory Coast, Africa. J. Infect. Dis. *160*:363–370, 1989.
677. Vernazza, P. L., Eron, J. J., Cohen, M. S., et al.: Detection and biologic characterization of infectious HIV-1 in semen of seropositive men. AIDS *8*:1325–1329, 1994.
678. Vigano, A., Principi, N., Crupi, L., et al.: Elevation of IgE in HIV-infected children and its correlation with the progression of disease. J. Allergy Clin. Immunol. *95*:627–632, 1995.
679. Vigano, A., Principi, N., Villa, M. L., et al.: Immunologic characterization of children vertically infected with human immunodeficiency virus, with slow or rapid disease progression. J. Pediatr. *126*:368–374, 1995.
680. Viscarello, R. R., Cullen, M. T., DeGennaro, N. J., et al.: Fetal blood sampling in HIV-seropositive pregnancies before elective midtrimester termination of pregnancy. Am. J. Obstet. Gynecol. *167*:1075–1079, 1992.
681. Vitek, C. R., Gracia, F. I., Fiusti, R. A., et al.: Evidence for sexual and mother-to-child transmission of human T lymphotropic virus type II among Guaymi Indians, Panama. J. Infect. Dis. *171*:1022–1026, 1995.
682. Vlahov, D., Khabbaz, R. F., Cohn, S., et al.: Incidence and risk factors for human T-lymphotropic virus type II seroconversion among injecting drug users in Baltimore, Maryland, U.S.A. J. Acquir. Immune Defic. Syndr. Human Retrovirol. *9*:89–96, 1995.
683. von Schwedler, U., Song, J., Aiken, C., et al.: Vif is crucial for human immunodeficiency virus type 1 proviral DNA synthesis in infected cells. J. Virol. *67*:4945–4955, 1993.
684. Waecker, N. J., Ascher, D. P., Robb, M. L., et al.: Age-adjusted CD4+ lymphocyte parameters in healthy children at risk for infection with the human immunodeficiency virus. Clin. Infect. Dis. *17*:123–125, 1993.
685. Wahn, V., Kramer, H. H., Voit, T., et al.: Horizontal transmission of HIV infection between two siblings. Lancet *2*:694, 1986.
686. Waldmann, T. A.: Human T-cell lymphotropic virus type I-associated adult T-cell leukemia: The Joseph Goldberger Clinical Investigator Lecture. J. A. M. A. *273*:735–737, 1995.
687. Walsh, T. J., Gonzalez, C., Roilides, E., et al.: Fungemia in children infected with human immunodeficiency virus: New epidemiologic patterns, emerging pathogens, and improved outcome with antifungal therapy. Clin. Infect. Dis. *20*:900–906, 1995.
688. Wasser, S. C., Gwinn, M., and Fleming, P.: Urban-nonurban distribution of HIV infection in childbearing women in the United States. J. Acquir. Immune Defic. Syndr. *6*:1035–1042, 1993.
689. Wattel, E., Mariotti, M., Agis, F., et al.: Human T lymphotropic virus (HTLV) type I and II DNA amplification in HTLV-I/II-seropositive blood donors of the French West Indies. J. Infect. Dis. *165*:369–372, 1992.
690. Watters, J. K., Estilo, M. J., Clark, G. L., et al.: Syringe and needle exchange programs as HIV/AIDS prevention for injection drug users. J. A. M. A. *271*:115–120, 1994.
691. Weber, R., Sauer, B., Luthy, R., et al.: Intestinal coinfection with *Enterocytozoon bieneusi* and *Cryptosporidium* in a human immunodeficiency virus-infected child with chronic diarrhea. Clin. Infect. Dis. *17*:480–483, 1993.
692. Wei, Z., Ghosh, S. K., Taylor, M. E., et al.: Viral dynamics in human immunodeficiency virus type 1 infection. Nature *373*:117–122, 1995.
693. Weinberg, J. B., Spiegel, R. A., Blazey, D. L., et al.: Human T-cell lymphotropic virus I and adult T-cell leukemia: Report of a cluster in North Carolina. Am. J. Med. *95*:51–58, 1988.
694. Weiser, B., Nachman, S., Tropper, P., et al.: Quantitation of human immunodeficiency virus type 1 during pregnancy: Relationship of viral titer to mother-to-child transmission and stability of viral load. Proc. Natl. Acad. Sci. U.S.A. *91*:8031–8041, 1994.
695. Weiss, S. H.: The evolving epidemiology of human T-lymphotropic virus type II. J. Infect. Dis. *169*:1080–1083, 1994.
696. Wendell, D. A., Onorato, I. M., McCray, E., et al.: Youth at risk: Sex, drugs and human immunodeficiency virus. Am. J. Dis. Child. *146*:76–81, 1991.
697. Whitcup, S. M., Butler, K. M., Pizzo, P. A., et al.: Retinal lesions in children treated with dideoxyinosine. N. Engl. J. Med. *326*:1226–1227, 1992.
698. Whittle, H., Morris, J., Todd, T., et al.: HIV-2–infected patients survive longer than HIV-1–infected patients. AIDS *8*:1617–1620, 1994.
699. Whitworth, J. M., Janniger, C. K., Oleske, J. M., et al.: Cutaneous manifestations of childhood acquired immunodeficiency syndrome and human immunodeficiency virus infection. Cutis *55*:62–71, 1995.
700. Wiktor, S. Z., Cannon, R. O., Atkinson, W. L., et al.: Infection with human T lymphotropic virus types I and II in sexually transmitted disease clinics in Baltimore and New Orleans. J. Infect. Dis. *165*:920–924, 1992.
701. Wiktor, S. Z., Pate, E. J., Murphy, E. L., et al.: Mother-to-child transmission of human T-cell lymphotropic virus type I (HTLV-I) in Jamaica: Association with antibodies to envelope glycoprotein (gp46) epitopes. J. Acquir. Immune Defic. Syndr. *6*:1162–1167, 1993.
702. Wiktor, S. Z., Piot, P., Mann, J. M., et al.: Human T cell lymphotropic virus type I (HTLV-I) among female prostitutes in Kinshasa, Zaire. J. Infect. Dis. *161*:1073–1077, 1990.
703. Wilfert, C. M., Wilson, C., Luzuriaga, K., et al.: Pathogenesis of pediatric human immunodeficiency virus type 1 infection. J. Infect. Dis. *170*:286–292, 1994.
704. Wolinsky, S. M.: Retrovirology. Curr. Opin. Infect. Dis. *7*:65–71, 1994.
705. Wolinsky, S. M., Wike, C. M., Korber, B. T. M., et al.: Selective transmission of human immunodeficiency virus type-1 variant from mothers to infants. Science *255*:1134–1137, 1992.
706. Wolters, P. L., Brouwers, P., Moss, H. A., et al.: Differential receptive and expressive language functioning of children with symptomatic HIV disease and relation to CT scan brain abnormalities. Pediatrics *95*:112–119, 1995.
707. Working Group on Antiretroviral Therapy: National Pediatric HIV Resource Center: Antiretroviral therapy and medical management of the human immunodeficiency virus-infected child. Pediatr. Infect. Dis. J. *12*:513–522, 1993.
708. Wrin, T., Crawford, L., Sawyer, L., et al.: Neutralizing antibody responses to autologous and heterologous isolates of human immunodeficiency virus. J. Acquir. Immune Defic. Syndr. *7*:211–219, 1994.
709. Yamaguchi, K.: Human T-lymphotropic virus type I in Japan. Lancet *343*:213–216, 1994.
710. Yamanouchi, K., Kinoshita, K., Moriuchi, R., et al.: Oral transmission of human T cell leukemia virus type I into a common marmoset (*Callithrix jacchus*) as an experimental model for milk-borne transmission. Jpn. J. Cancer Res. *76*:481–487, 1985.
711. Yanagihara, R., Nerurkar, V. R., and Ajdukiewicz, A. B.: Comparison between strains of human T lymphotropic virus type 1 isolated from inhabitants of the Solomon Islands and Papua New Guinea. J. Infect. Dis. *164*:443–449, 1991.
712. Yerly, S., Wunderli, W., Wyler, C. A., et al.: Influenza immunization of HIV-1–infected patients does not increase viral load. AIDS *8*:1503–1504, 1994.

713. Yeung, M. C., Pulliam, L., and Lau, A. S.: The HIV envelope protein gp120 is toxic to human brain-cell cultures through the induction of interleukin-6 and tumor necrosis factor-α. AIDS *9*:137–143, 1995.
714. Yeung, S. C. H., Kazazi, F., Randle, C. G. M., et al.: Patients infected with human immunodeficiency virus type 1 have low levels of virus in saliva even in the presence of periodontal disease. J. Infect. Dis. *167*:803–809, 1993.
715. Yolken, R. H., Hart, W., Oung, I., et al.: Gastrointestinal dysfunction and disaccharide intolerance in children infected with human immunodeficiency virus. J. Pediatr. *118*:359–363, 1991.
716. Yolken, R. H., Li, S., Perman, J., et al.: Persistent diarrhea and fecal shedding of retroviral nucleic acids in children infected with human immunodeficiency virus. J. Infect. Dis. *164*:61–66, 1991.
717. Zacharopoulos, V. R., Perotti, M. E., and Phillips, D. M.: Lymphocyte-facilitated infection of epithelia by human T-cell lymphotropic virus type I. J. Virol. *66*:4601–4605, 1992.
718. Zacher, V., Spire, B., Norskov-Lauritsen, N., et al.: Cultured trophoblastic choriocarcinoma cells differentially express HIV-1 and cloned provirus. AIDS *5*:457–458, 1991.
719. Zehender, G., De Maddalena, C., Osio, M., et al.: High prevalence of human T cell lymphotropic virus type II infection in patients affected by human immunodeficiency type 1–associated predominantly sensory polyneuropathy. J. Infect. Dis. *172*:1595–1598, 1995.
720. Zucker-Franklin, D., Seremetis, S., and Zheng, Z. Y.: Internalization of human immunodeficiency virus type 1 and other retroviruses by megakaryocytes and platelets. Blood *75*:1920–1923, 1990.

S E C T I O N   E I G H T E E N

CHLAMYDIA

❏ ❏ ❏

193

CHLAMYDIA PNEUMONIA

Margaret R. Hammerschlag

The genus *Chlamydia* is a group of obligate intracellular parasites with a unique developmental cycle with morphologically distinct infectious and reproductive forms. All members of the genus have a gram-negative envelope without peptidoglycan, share a genus-specific lipopolysaccharide antigen, and utilize host adenosine triphosphate for the synthesis of chlamydial protein.[93] The chlamydial developmental cycle involves an infectious, metabolically inactive extracellular form (elementary body) and a noninfectious, metabolically active intracellular form (reticulate body). Elementary bodies, which are 200 to 400 mm in diameter, attach to the host cell by a process of electrostatic binding and are taken into the cell by endocytosis that does not depend on the microtubule system. Within the host cell, the elementary body remains within a membrane-lined phagosome. The phagosome does not fuse with the host cell lysosome. The elementary bodies then differentiate into reticulate bodies that undergo binary fission. After approximately 36 hours, the reticulate bodies differentiate into elementary bodies. At about 48 hours, release may occur by cytolysis or by a process of exocytosis or extrusion of the whole inclusion, leaving the host cell intact.

The genus now contains four species: *C. trachomatis*, *C. psittaci*, *C. pneumoniae* (TWAR strain), and *C. pecorum*.[40, 47] The first three species can cause infection in humans. *C. pecorum* was speciated off from *C. psittaci* and infects cattle and sheep; human infection as yet has not been described.[40] The routes of transmission, susceptible populations, and clinical presentations differ markedly for the three species that cause infection in humans (Table 193–1).

INFECTION DUE TO *C. TRACHOMATIS*

Epidemiology

C. trachomatis infection probably is the most prevalent sexually transmitted infection in the United States today.[22, 23] The Centers for Disease Control and Prevention estimates that the number of new *C. trachomatis* infections exceeds 4 million annually.[23] The prevalence of chlamydial infection is associated more weakly with socioeconomic status, urban or rural residence, and race or ethnicity than are gonorrhea and syphilis. The prevalence of *C. trachomatis* infection is consistently higher than 5 per cent among sexually active adolescent and young adult women attending outpatient clinics, regardless of the region of the country, location of the clinic (urban or rural), and the race or ethnicity of the population. Among sexually active adolescents, prevalences commonly exceed 10 per cent and may exceed 20 per cent.[60] Decreasing age at first intercourse and increasing age at marriage have contributed importantly to the higher prevalence of *C. trachomatis* infection. Infection with *C. trachomatis* tends to be asymptomatic and of long duration. If a pregnant woman has active infection during delivery, the infant may acquire the infection, developing either conjunctivitis or pneumonia. Rarely, children also may acquire chlamydial infection as a result of sexual abuse.

Infections in Infants (Table 193–2)

Pregnant women who have cervical infection with *C. trachomatis* can transmit the infection to their infants, who subsequently may develop neonatal conjunctivitis and pneumonia. Epidemiologic evidence strongly suggests that the infant acquires chlamydial infection from the mother during vaginal delivery.[38, 51, 56, 114] Infection after cesarean section is rare and usually occurs after early rupture of the amniotic membrane.[9] There is no evidence supporting postnatal acquisition from the mother or other family members. Approximately 50 to 75 per cent of infants born to infected women become in-

TABLE 193–1. Characteristics of Three *Chlamydia* Species

	C. trachomatis	*C. psittaci*	*C. pneumoniae*
Number of serovars	15	At least 4 avian serovars	1
% DNA homology to *C. pneumoniae*	<5	<10	94–100
Plasmid	Yes	Yes (rarely no)	No
Contains glycogen	Yes	No	No
Resistant to sulfonamides	No	Yes	Yes
Morphology of elementary body	Round	Round	Pear-shaped
Natural host	Humans	Birds, mammals	Humans
Population	Infants	Poultry workers, veterinarians, bird fanciers	All ages
Mode of transmission	Vertical (mother to baby)	Aerosol—animal-to-person	Aerosol—person-to-person
Estimated annual incidence of pneumonia in humans	10,000–15,000	150–200 reported to the Centers for Disease Control and Prevention	100,000

fected at one of more anatomic sites, including the conjunctiva, nasopharynx, rectum, and vagina.

Inclusion Conjunctivitis

C. trachomatis is the most frequent identifiable infectious cause of neonatal conjunctivitis and the major clinical manifestation of neonatal chlamydial infection. Approximately 30 to 50 per cent of infants born to *Chlamydia*-positive mothers develop conjunctivitis.[38, 51, 56, 114] Studies have identified *C. trachomatis* in 14 to 46 per cent of infants younger than 1 month of age presenting with conjunctivitis.[53, 54, 104, 106, 108, 112] The incubation period is 5 to 14 days after delivery or earlier if membranes have ruptured prematurely. At least 50 per cent of infants with chlamydial conjunctivitis also have nasopharyngeal infection.[6, 56] The presentation varies extremely, ranging from mild conjunctival injection with scant mucoid discharge to severe conjunctivitis with copious purulent discharge, chemosis, and pseudomembrane formation. The conjunctiva can be friable and may bleed when stroked with a swab. Chlamydial conjunctivitis needs to be differentiated from gonococcal ophthalmia in some infants, especially those born to mothers who did not receive any prenatal care, had gonorrhea during pregnancy, or abused drugs. Overlap in both incubation periods and presentation is possible.

Pneumonia

The nasopharynx is the most frequent site of perinatally acquired chlamydial infection.[52, 56] Approximately 70 per cent of infected infants have positive cultures at that site. The majority of these nasopharyngeal infections are asymptomatic and may persist for 3 years or more.[8, 56, 114] Chlamydial pneumonia develops in only about 30 per cent of infants with nasopharyngeal infection. In those who develop pneumonia, the presentation and clinical findings are characteristic.[6, 63] The children usually present between 4 and 12 weeks of age. A few cases have been reported presenting as early as 2 weeks of age, but no cases have been seen beyond 4 months of age. The infants frequently have a history of cough and congestion with an absence of fever. On physical examination the infant is tachypneic, and rales are heard on auscultation of the chest; wheezing is distinctly uncommon. There are no specific radiographic findings except hyperinflation.[6, 63] A review of chest films of 125 infants with chlamydial pneumonia revealed bilateral hyperinflation; diffuse infiltrates with a variety of radiographic patterns, including interstitial and reticulonodular; atelectasis; and bronchopneumonia.[103] Lobar consolidation and pleural effusions were not seen. Significant laboratory findings include peripheral eosinophilia (>300 cells/cm^3) and elevated serum immunoglobulins.[6, 63]

C. trachomatis rarely is isolated from the lungs of infants with chlamydial pneumonia, which led some to believe that an immune mechanism is involved in pathogenesis. Histopathologic studies have not revealed any characteristic features. Biopsy material has shown pleural congestion, near-total alveolar and partial bronchiolar mononuclear consolidation with occasional eosinophils, granular pneumocytes, and focal aggregations of neutrophils. Necrotic change in the bronchioles also is marked.[37] Follow-up studies have suggested that infantile chlamydial pneumonia may be associated with pulmonary function test abnormalities and respiratory tract symptoms 7 to 8 years after recovery from the acute illness.[122]

Infections at Other Sites

Infants born to *Chlamydia*-positive mothers also may become infected in the rectum and vagina.[114] Although infection at these sites appears to be totally asymptomatic, the infection may cause confusion if detected later. Schachter and associates[114] reported finding subclinical rectal and vaginal infection in 14 per cent of infants born to *Chlamydia*-positive women; some of these infants still were culture-positive at 18 months of age. Bell and colleagues[8] followed 22 infants born to women with culture-proven chlamydial infections and found that positive cultures were detected in these children as late as 28.5 months after birth. The longest duration of perinatally acquired infection occurred in the nasopharynx or oropharynx, 28.5 months, as mentioned previously. Nine infants had rectal or vaginal infections that persisted for slightly more than 12 months.

Infections in Older Children

C. trachomatis has not been associated with any specific clinical syndrome in older infants and children. Most attention to *C. trachomatis* infection in these children has concentrated on the relationship to sexual abuse. It has been suggested that the isolation of *C. trachomatis* from a rectal or genital site in children without prior sexual activity may be a marker of sexual abuse, although evidence for other modes of spread, such as through fomites, is lacking for this organism. As previously mentioned, perinatal maternal infant transmission resulting in vaginal or rectal infection has been documented with prolonged infection for periods of up to 3 years.[8, 114] This is an important and confounding variable.

Vaginal infection with *C. trachomatis* was reported uncom-

TABLE 193–2. Selected Studies of Perinatal Chlamydial Infection

	Prevalence of Maternal Genital Infection		Proportion of Infants Born to Infected Mothers Who Developed Chlamydial Infection				
Author, Year, City, Reference	***Total***	***No. Infected (%)***	***Total***	***Conjunctivitis***	***Pneumonia***	***Nasopharyngeal***	**Rectum/Vagina**
Frommell et al., 1979, Denver[38]	340	30 (8.8)	67	39%	11%	6%	NS*
Schachter et al., 1986, San Francisco[114]	5531	262 (4.7)	131	17.6%	16%	11.5%	14%
Hammerschlag et al., 1989, Brooklyn[59]	4357	341 (8)	45	15%	1%	4%	NS

*NS, not studied.

monly in prepubertal children before 1980. The possibility of sexual contact frequently was not even discussed. In 1981, Rettig and Nelson[105] reported concurrent or subsequent chlamydial infection in 9 of 33 episodes of gonorrhea (27 per cent) in a group of prepubertal children. However, *C. trachomatis* was not found in any of 31 children presenting with urethritis or vaginitis that was not gonococcal. No information was given about possible sexual activity.

Studies have identified rectogenital chlamydial infection in 2 to 13 per cent of sexually abused children when these children routinely were cultured for the organism. The majority of those with chlamydial infection were asymptomatic. In two early studies that had control groups, similar percentages of control patients also were infected.[57, 74] A subsequent larger study by Ingram and colleagues[75] found a stronger association between vaginal chlamydial infection and a history of sexual abuse, but not with pharyngeal infection, which was found in a similar number of controls. Rectal infection was detected in only 1 of 124 abused children.

In the setting of repeated abuse by a family member over long periods, development of infection would be difficult to demonstrate. The 1993 Sexually Transmitted Diseases Treatment Guidelines does not recommend that cultures for *C. trachomatis* be obtained routinely from the pharynx and urethra in children who are suspected victims of sexual abuse.[23] The major reasons were the low yield from the urethra, the tendency for longer persistence of perinatally acquired pharyngeal infection, and the potential confusion with *C. pneumoniae*.[5]

Although asymptomatic perinatally acquired nasopharyngeal infection with *C. trachomatis* may persist for at least 2 years, respiratory tract infection in older children and adults appears to be distinctly uncommon. The reasons for this are not clear. Studies of the interaction of *C. trachomatis* and alveolar macrophages from normal healthy adults have demonstrated that these cells kill both biovars of *C. trachomatis* efficiently.[94] *C. trachomatis* has been isolated from the pharynx of some adults, which apparently is related to certain sexual practices. These infections have been asymptomatic. Two earlier studies, based entirely on serology, suggested that *C. trachomatis* might be a cause of pharyngitis and community-acquired pneumonia in adults.[81, 82] Subsequent studies utilizing cultural methods did not confirm this.[44, 70] It appears that the original studies actually may have detected cross-reacting antibody to *C. pneumoniae.*

There are two specific situations in which *C. trachomatis* can cause pneumonia in older children or adults. One is in immunosuppressed persons. There have been several well-documented cases of pneumonia due to *C. trachomatis* in persons with leukemia, bone marrow transplant recipients, and those with AIDS.[77, 83, 86, 88] In all of these cases, *C. trachomatis* was isolated from biopsy specimens of lung tissue or bronchoalveolar lavage fluid. Several patients also had a serologic response that was diagnostic of acute *C. trachomatis* infection. Unfortunately, there was no characteristic clinical presentation. These adults had none of the findings that are characteristic of infantile chlamydial pneumonia.

There also have been several reports of pulmonary infection after exposure to *C. trachomatis* serovars L1 and L2 in the laboratory.[10] The infections probably were acquired by inhalation of aerosolized organisms. Clinically, these patients presented with high fever, night sweats, and cough and were found to have mediastinal lymphadenopathy, pneumonitis and splenomegaly, or both. In two cases, the diagnosis of lymphoma was considered seriously. These findings are not unexpected given the severity of lymphogranuloma venereum genital infection. Accidental exposure to aerosolized *C. trachomatis* trachoma biovar has not been associated with significant illness.

Diagnosis of *C. trachomatis* Infections

The "gold standard" remains isolation by culture of *C. trachomatis* from the conjunctiva, nasopharynx, vagina, or rectum. *Chlamydia* culture has been defined further by the Centers for Disease Control and Prevention as isolation of the organism in tissue culture and confirmation by microscopic identification of the characteristic inclusions by fluorescent antibody staining.[22] Several nonculture methods have Food and Drug Administration approval for diagnosis of chlamydial conjunctivitis. They include enzyme immunoassays, specifically Chlamydiazyme (Abbott Diagnostics, Chicago, IL), Pathfinder (Sanofi-Pasteur, Chaska, MN), and SureCell (Kodak, Rochester, NY), and direct fluorescent-antibody tests, including Syva MicroTrak (Genetic Systems, Seattle, WA) and Pathfinder (Sanofi-Pasteur, Chaska, MN). These tests appear to perform well with conjunctival specimens with sensitivities greater than or equal to 90 per cent and specificities greater than or equal to 95 per cent compared with culture.[53, 54, 104, 106] Unfortunately, the performance with nasopharyngeal specimens has not been as good, with sensitivities ranging from 33 to more than 90 per cent.[53, 54, 97, 106] The commercially available DNA probe, Pace II (GenProbe, San Diego, CA), has Food and Drug Administration approval only for cervical and urethral sites in adults, in whom its performance has been similar to that of most of the approved enzyme immunoassays available. It does not have approval for any site in children. The recently approved polymerase chain reaction assay, Amplicor (Roche Molecular Diagnostics, Nutley, NJ), has approval only for genital sites in adults. However, preliminary data suggest that polymerase chain reaction is equivalent to culture for detection of *C. trachomatis* in the conjunctiva and possibly superior to culture for detection of the organism in nasopharyngeal specimens.

Nonculture tests should never be used for rectal or vaginal sites in children or for any forensic purposes in adolescents or adults.[22] Use of these tests for vaginal and rectal specimens has been associated with a large number of false-positive results.[58, 102] Fecal material can give false-positive reactions with any enzyme immunoassay; none is approved for this site in adults. Common bowel organisms, including *Escherichia coli; Proteus* species; vaginal organisms, such as group B *Streptococcus* and *Gardnerella vaginalis;* and even some respiratory tract flora, such as group A *Streptococcus*, also can give positive reactions with enzyme immunoassays.[102] These types of tests are best for screening for genital infection in adolescents and adults in high-prevalence populations (prevalence of infection >7 per cent).[22] There are few reports on the performance of the DNA probe, but it appears to be equivalent to most available enzyme immunoassays, in terms of sensitivity and specificity, compared with culture for genital specimens. An enzyme immunoassay for respiratory tract specimens can lead to another problem. Because all of the available enzyme immunoassays use genus-specific antibodies, if used for respiratory tract specimens, these tests also detect *C. pneumoniae*.[5]

Prevention and Control

Because *C. trachomatis* infections are transmitted vertically from mother to infant during delivery, there are several possible options for intervention. One of the first to be considered was neonatal ocular prophylaxis. It generally has been assumed, based on the results of prospective studies of mother-to-infant transmission of *C. trachomatis*, that neonatal ocular prophylaxis with silver nitrate does not prevent the development of chlamydial conjunctivitis. Because erythromycin and tetracycline ophthalmic ointments also were approved and used for ocular prophylaxis, it was suggested that they also might be effective for prevention of chlamydial conjunctivitis.

In 1980, Hammerschlag and associates[55] in Seattle found that infants born to *Chlamydia*-positive women, 24 of whom received erythromycin, did not develop chlamydial conjunctivitis, compared with 33 per cent (12 of 36) of those who received silver nitrate drops. There was no effect on the incidence of nasopharyngeal infection or the subsequent development of chlamydial pneumonia. Subsequent studies have not confirmed this observation. A report by Bell and associates[7] found that erythromycin prophylaxis lacked efficacy compared with silver nitrate; the cumulative proportion of infants in whom chlamydial conjunctivitis developed was 25 per cent in each group. Both prophylactic preparations were used in the delivery room and given ad hoc as requested by the parents. The application of the preparations was delayed for as long as 1 hour after delivery in some infants.

A study by Laga and associates[84] in Nairobi, Kenya, compared tetracycline ointment with silver nitrate drops. In the infants born to women with cultures positive for *Chlamydia*, chlamydial ophthalmia developed in 10.1 per cent who received silver nitrate drops as prophylaxis and in 7.2 per cent who received tetracycline ointment. The authors initially concluded that both preparations were efficacious when compared with a historical cohort in which the disease developed in 31.3 per cent of the infants who did not receive prophylaxis and who were born to infected women. However, most of the infants in this study were followed only for the first 4 weeks of life, and the follow-up rate was less than 50 per cent. When Laga and associates examined a smaller group of infants who were followed for at least 6 months, 23 and 31 per cent of those who received silver nitrate and tetracycline, respectively, ultimately acquired an ocular infection with *C. trachomatis*. In 1989, Hammerschlag and associates[59] compared silver nitrate, erythromycin, and tetracycline as neonatal ocular prophylaxis in a large urban hospital in Brooklyn. The prophylaxis preparations were given within 30 minutes of birth. Chlamydial conjunctivitis developed in 20 per cent of infants (15 of 76) born to infected mothers who received silver nitrate drops, 14 per cent (13 of 92) who received erythromycin, and 11 per cent (7 of 62) who received tetracycline. There was no effect on the incidence of nasopharyngeal infection and pneumonia. A subsequent study from Taiwan compared silver nitrate, the two antibiotics, and no prophylaxis.[24] However, this study, in contrast with previous studies, did not follow specifically infants born to women with culture-documented chlamydial infection but followed all infants delivered during the period of the study, for 4 weeks, or when they developed conjunctivitis. Again, there was no difference in the incidence of neonatal chlamydial conjunctivitis among the four groups. The incidences of chlamydial conjunctivitis in the tetracycline, erythromycin, silver nitrate, and no prophylaxis groups were 1.3 per cent, 1.5 per cent, 1.7 per cent, and 1.6 per cent, respectively. *C. trachomatis* was diagnosed by a direct fluorescent antibody test rather than culture. No data were given as to the prevalence of maternal infection with *C. trachomatis* or *Neisseria gonorrhoeae*. Respiratory tract infection was not assessed.

A similar study from Kenya was reported by Isenberg and associates[76] comparing povidone-iodine, erythromycin ophthalmic ointment, and silver nitrate drops as neonatal ocular prophylaxis. Povidone-iodine was selected because in vitro it has a broad antibacterial spectrum; it also is antiviral and inexpensive compared with the other prophylaxis agents. As with the study from Taiwan, the pregnant women were not screened for *C. trachomatis* prenatally, and chlamydial conjunctivitis in the infants was diagnosed by a direct fluorescent-antibody test. Mothers were told to bring the infants back if conjunctivitis developed. Use of povidone-iodine appeared to result in a 50 per cent reduction in *C. trachomatis* conjunctivitis, compared with silver nitrate (5.5 per cent versus 10.5 per cent of infants), and an approximately 30 per cent reduction, compared with erythromycin (7.4 per cent). There was no difference in the proportions of infants who developed gonococcal ophthalmia. Because of the structure of the study, one cannot be sure if every infant who developed conjunctivitis returned to the clinic. Because the prevalence of chlamydial infection among the pregnant women in the population was unknown, the investigators did not know how many cases of chlamydial ophthalmia to expect. Use of povidone-iodine for neonatal ocular prophylaxis may be appropriate in some populations, mainly because of cost. It still would appear that neonatal ocular prophylaxis should be directed primarily toward preventing gonococcal ophthalmia because it is the agent that poses the greatest risk of eye injury.

The most effective method of control may be screening and treatment of pregnant women. This also would have the advantage of preventing chlamydial respiratory tract infection, including pneumonia infection of the vagina and rectum. Although the Centers for Disease Control and Prevention recommends four different treatment regimens (three erythromycin and one amoxicillin) for treatment of chlamydial infection in pregnant women, data on the efficacy of any of these regimens as well as the effects on infection in the infant are limited.[23] Unlike that of gonorrhea, treatment of *C. trachomatis* infection requires multiple-dose regimens, and tolerance and compliance are frequent problems.

In 1986, Schachter and associates[113] reported on the effect of the routine use of erythromycin for treating chlamydial infections in pregnancy on the outcome of infection in the infants. Treatment with erythromycin ethylsuccinate (400 mg four times a day for 7 days) was offered to 184 pregnant women with cervical chlamydial infection at 36 weeks' gestation. Thirty-two women refused treatment, and 24 of their infants were followed as controls. A large number of treated women were lost to follow-up. However, chlamydial infection developed in only 4 (7 per cent) of 59 infants of treated mothers compared with 12 (50 per cent) of the 24 infants of untreated mothers. Two published, controlled studies comparing erythromycin to amoxicillin for treatment of chlamydial infection in pregnant women have followed infants born to these women for the development of chlamydial infection.[1, 29] In both, the development of chlamydial conjunctivitis in the infants of treated women was reduced significantly compared with historical data (1 to 2 per cent versus 30 to 50 per cent).

Reasons for failure of maternal treatment to prevent infantile chlamydial infection include poor compliance and reinfection from an untreated sexual partner. Even with effective screening, some infected women will be missed, depending on the methods used. There also are women who do not seek prenatal care.

Treatment

Oral erythromycin suspension (ethylsuccinate or stearate) (50 mg/kg/day for 10 to 14 days) is the therapy of choice for the treatment of chlamydial conjunctivitis and pneumonia in infants. It provides better and faster resolution of the conjunctivitis as well as treats any concurrent nasopharyngeal infection, which prevents the development of pneumonia. Additional topical therapy is not needed. The efficacy of this regimen has been reported to range from 80 to 90 per cent; thus, as many as 20 per cent of infants may require another course of therapy.[56, 67, 98, 104] Erythromycin at the same dose for 2 to 3 weeks is the treatment of choice for pneumonia and does result in clinical improvement as well as elimination of the organism from the respiratory tract. Chlamydial infections in older children may be treated with oral erythromycin (50 mg/kg/day four times a day orally to a maximum of 2 g a day for 7 to 14 days). Children older than 8 years of age may be treated with tetracycline (25 to 50 mg/kg/day four times a day orally for 7 days). The new macrolide antibiotic, azithromycin, has been approved as single-dose treatment for uncomplicated chlamydial urethral and cervical infection in men and nonpregnant women.[23, 61]

INFECTION DUE TO *C. PSITTACI*

Human infection with *C. psittaci* probably first was described by Juergensen in 1874 or Ritter in 1876. Ritter described seven cases of an unusual pneumonia that appeared to be caused by parrots and finches that were caged in the study of his brother's home in Switzerland. After these reports, there were several outbreaks of a similar disease in Europe that established the association with an exposure to birds. The term *psittacosis* was coined by Morange in 1892 from the Greek word for parrots, *psittakos*.[2]

The Organism

C. psittaci is a diverse species that affects nonpsittacine birds and many mammalian species as well. The known host range includes 15 mammalian species and 130 avian species representing 10 orders.[2, 68] DNA homology among *C. psittaci*, *C. trachomatis*, and *C. pneumoniae* is only 5 to 10 per cent. *C. psittaci* also can be differentiated from *C. trachomatis* by a lack of glycogen in the inclusions, the morphologic features of the inclusions, and resistance to sulfonamides (see Table 193–1).[2]

The diversity of *C. psittaci* probably is a reflection of its wide host range. Strains of *C. psittaci* have been analyzed by patterns of pathogenicity, inclusion morphology in tissue culture, DNA restriction endonuclease analysis, and monoclonal antibodies, which indicate that there are nine mammalian serovars, seven avian serovars, and two koala biovars.[2, 68, 120] The mammalian strains differ greatly from avian strains in their antigenic characteristics. Two of the avian serovars, psittacine and turkey, are of major importance in the avian population of the United States. Each is associated with important host preferences and disease characteristics.

Strains of the turkey serovar all have been associated with a serious disease either in birds or human beings, with major epizootics in turkeys, often resulting in disease in humans. The psittacine serovar also has been associated with serious disease in humans; however, human involvement usually is limited to sporadic cases after exposure to pet birds or pigeons. However, the pathogenicity of each *C. psittaci* strain for humans is unknown.

Epidemiology

According to the most recent report from the Centers for Disease Control and Prevention, 1136 cases and 8 deaths from psittacosis were reported in the United States from 1975 to 1984.[20] Eighty-five per cent were associated with exposure to birds; 70 per cent of these reported cases were the result of exposure to caged pet birds. Those at highest risk of acquiring psittacosis included bird owners or fanciers and pet shop employees. Since 1984, there have been several major outbreaks of psittacosis in the United States in turkey processing plants, where approximately 300 persons were infected.[21, 66] Workers exposed to turkey viscera were at the highest risk of infection.[66]

Inhalation of infectious aerosols derived from feces, fecal dust, or secretions of *C. psittaci*–infected animals is believed to be the primary route of infection. The source birds can be infected asymptomatically or can show signs of infection such as anorexia, ruffled feathers, depression, and watery green droppings. Psittacosis frequently is a systemic infection in birds. The turkey strains can induce severe pericarditis. The gastrointestinal tract also is infected frequently. The psittacine serovar appears to be much less virulent in both turkeys and pigeons than in psittacine birds.[2]

Psittacosis is uncommon in children. In one large series from Australia of 135 cases over a 15-year period, the youngest patient was 17 years of age.[128] Children may be less likely to be exposed to birds. Bird keeping more commonly is a hobby of adults, and the parents are the ones who usually clean the cage of the family's pet bird. An outbreak of psittacosis involving two adolescents was reported from a small village in Scotland. The source of the infection appeared to be the local pet shop, which had taken delivery of four love birds, two of whom died shortly after arrival.[91] Another report describes a family outbreak during which three members of a family of nine persons contracted severe pneumonia.[14] A newly purchased cockatiel appeared to be the primary source, but person-to-person transmission was likely between 19-year-old twin brothers who shared a bedroom, one of whom had no direct contact with the bird. A retrospective review of the records of the Public Health Laboratory at Leeds, England, for cases with a fourfold rise in *Chlamydia* complement-fixation titers identified 219 patients over a 24-year period from 1965 to 1989.[30] The ages ranged from 9 months to 87 years; only five (2.2 per cent) of the patients were younger than 10 years of age, but only 34 of the total cases were felt to be psittacosis on review. All involved antecedent avian exposures, but the ages were not specified.

Clinical Manifestations

Infection with *C. psittaci* in humans may range from clinically inapparent to severe infection involving multiple organ systems as well as pneumonia. The mean incubation period is 15 days after exposure, and the range is 5 to 21 days. The onset usually is abrupt, with complaints of fever, cough, and headache. The fever is high and frequently associated with rigors and sweats. The headache can be so severe that meningitis can be considered a possibility; 33 per cent of the patients in the Australian series underwent lumbar punctures.[128] The cough usually is nonproductive.

Rales may be heard on auscultation. Chest radiographs usually are abnormal, with variable infiltrates. Pleural effusions also may be present.

Laboratory Findings

The white blood cell count usually is not elevated, but there may be a mild leukocytosis. Almost 50 per cent of the patients in the Australian series had abnormal liver function test results, including elevated levels of aspartate aminotransferase, alkaline phosphatase, and bilirubin.[128]

Diagnosis

Because of the varying clinical presentation, the diagnosis of psittacosis can be difficult. History of exposure to birds is important. However, as many as 20 per cent of patients with psittacosis may not have a history of contact with birds.[123] In the Australian series, 85 per cent of the patients had a history of recent bird contact; 71 per cent of these described a strong bird-contact history.[128] Only five patients had been exposed to poultry. Pneumonia due to *C. pneumoniae* also can have a similar clinical presentation.[45] Data from both Sweden and Denmark have suggested that a number of cases of "psittacosis" due to *C. pneumoniae* with no history of bird exposure probably have occurred, and the diagnosis has been established serologically with complement fixation.[39, 90] An outbreak of suspected psittacosis in a boys' boarding school in England was reported in 1984.[99] The outbreak involved 20 children, 13 to 18 years of age, and 4 adults. The illness was mild and characterized by pharyngitis and flu-like symptoms, including headache, fever, and cough. The diagnosis was made on the basis of serology (complement-fixation titers). No avian source was identified. The cases occurred over a 3-month period, suggesting person-to-person spread. A subsequent analysis of the sera suggested that the outbreak was due to *C. pneumoniae*.[100] Person-to-person spread is rare in psittacosis; the secondary cases tend to be severe.

Other infections that can produce the syndrome of pneumonia with high fever, unusually severe headache, and myalgia include *Mycoplasma pneumoniae* infection, tularemia, tuberculosis, fungal infections, legionnaires' disease, and various bacterial infections. Diagnosis of psittacosis in the human population is based primarily on clinical presentation, epidemiology, and serology. Culture of *C. psittaci* is not available outside of research laboratories.

The Centers for Disease Control and Prevention[20] has classified cases of psittacosis based on laboratory findings or exposures:

1. *Confirmed*—a clinical specimen yielding *C. psittaci* or compatible clinical illness and a fourfold rise in complement-fixation antibody titer
2. *Presumptive*—compatible clinical illness and a single serum sample titer of $\geq$1:32 or a stable antibody titer of $\geq$1:32 in two samples
3. *Suspect*—a case that does not meet the criteria in *1* or *2* but was associated with another case of avian chlamydiosis epornitic

Complement fixation is a genus-specific test; thus, infection due to *C. pneumoniae* can give titers of 1:32 or higher. Early treatment with tetracycline also may suppress the antibody response.

Although many laboratories can isolate *C. psittaci*, it is not a service provided routinely by most clinical microbiology laboratories. Recently, the Centers for Disease Control and Prevention reported using a modification of the microimmunofluorescence test for serodiagnosis of human psittacosis.[124] The 78 patients examined were diagnosed as having psittacosis on the basis of compatible clinical symptoms after exposure to sick birds. Conventional complement fixation was positive in 36 (46 per cent) of the patients. The microimmunofluorescence test detected diagnostic antibody responses in all the complement fixation–positive patients and in another 12 patients whose sera were negative or anticomplementary according to complement fixation. Seven other patients were felt to have *C. pneumoniae* infection because of their microimmunofluorescence antibody responses.

Several reports also have examined the use of nonculture methods, including direct fluorescent antibody, enzyme immunoassay, and polymerase chain reaction, for the direct identification of *C. psittaci* in clinical specimens. Oldach and associates[96] described two patients in whom psittacosis was diagnosed rapidly by direct fluorescent antibody staining of sputa with *Chlamydia* genus-specific monoclonal antibody. Chlamydial lipopolysaccharide antigen also was detected with a commercially available enzyme immunoassay kit. In one case, the diagnosis was confirmed by isolation of *C. psittaci* from sputum and a pharyngeal swab. Both patients had strong histories of exposure to sick birds. Microimmunofluorescence serology also was performed for both patients, and serologic cross-reactivity was observed between *C. psittaci*, *C. pneumoniae,* and *C. trachomatis* in the sera. *C. psittaci* also can be detected by two-step polymerase chain reaction, using primers directed against a portion of the major outer-membrane protein gene specific for *C. psittaci* and *C. pneumoniae* followed by amplification with primers targeted specifically at *C. pneumoniae*.[119] Tong and Sills[119] used this method to detect *C. psittaci* in sputum samples from four of eight patients with suspected psittacosis. Six of the sputum samples also were positive by *Chlamydia* genus enzyme immunoassay, and all were positive by direct fluorescent-antibody staining with an antilipopolysaccharide monoclonal antibody; two were culture-positive.

Treatment

The recommended treatment for psittacosis in adults and children older than 8 years of age is 500 mg of tetracycline every 6 hours, orally, for 7 to 10 days. Erythromycin (50 mg/kg/day up to 2 g/day for 7 to 10 days) also can be used. The experience in the Australian series[128] and anecdotal reports suggest that tetracycline may be more effective than erythromycin. Both patients reported by Oldach and associates[96] did not improve when placed initially on erythromycin; after doxycycline or tetracycline was added, both experienced defervescence within 48 hours.

Initial infection does not appear to be followed by long-term immunity. Reinfection and clinical disease can develop within 2 months of treatment; there are two well-documented cases of reinfection. A pet shop employee had two episodes of psittacosis 11 months apart. Each episode met the Centers for Disease Control and Prevention's confirmed case definition.[19]

INFECTION DUE TO *C. PNEUMONIAE*

The Organism

The first isolates of *C. pneumoniae* were obtained serendipitously during trachoma studies in the 1960s.[46] After the recovery of a similar isolate from the respiratory tract of a college student with pneumonia in Seattle, Grayston and colleagues[48] applied the designation TWAR after their first two isolates, TW-183 and AR-39. On the basis of inclusion morphology and staining characteristics in cell culture, TWAR was considered initially a *C. psittaci* strain. Subsequent analyses, however, have demonstrated that this organism is distinct from both *C. psittaci* and *C. trachomatis*. It is recognized as the third species of *Chlamydia*[46] (see Table 193–1). Ultrastructural studies have demonstrated a unique elementary body morphology distinct from *C. trachomatis* and *C.*

psittaci[25] (Fig. 193–1). However, some strains of *C. pneumoniae*, including IOL 207, have been found to have round elementary bodies.[18, 101] Thus, this may not be a consistent species characteristic. Restriction endonuclease pattern analysis and nucleic acid hybridization studies suggest a high degree of genetic relatedness (>95 per cent) among the *C. pneumoniae* isolates examined so far and less than 10 per cent homology with either *C. trachomatis* or *C. psittaci*.[17, 28, 47] Plasmids have not been detected in any isolate of *C. pneumoniae*.

Epidemiology

C. pneumoniae appears to be a primary human pathogen, and attempts to identify zoonotic reservoirs have been unsuccessful.[110] The mode of transmission remains uncertain but probably involves infected respiratory tract secretions. Acquisition of infection by droplet aerosol was described during a laboratory accident.[71] *C. pneumoniae* can remain viable on Formica counter tops for 30 hours and can survive small-particle aerosolization.[34, 117] Spread of *C. pneumoniae* within families and enclosed populations, such as military recruits, has been described.[60, 80, 126]

Several serologic surveys have documented rising chlamydial antibody prevalence rates in school age children that reach 30 to 45 per cent in adolescents.[12, 31, 111] With the advent of *C. pneumoniae*–specific serologic tests, it has become clear that this increasing prevalence of chlamydial antibody during childhood is attributable to *C. pneumoniae*.[15]

The proportion of community-acquired pneumonias asso-

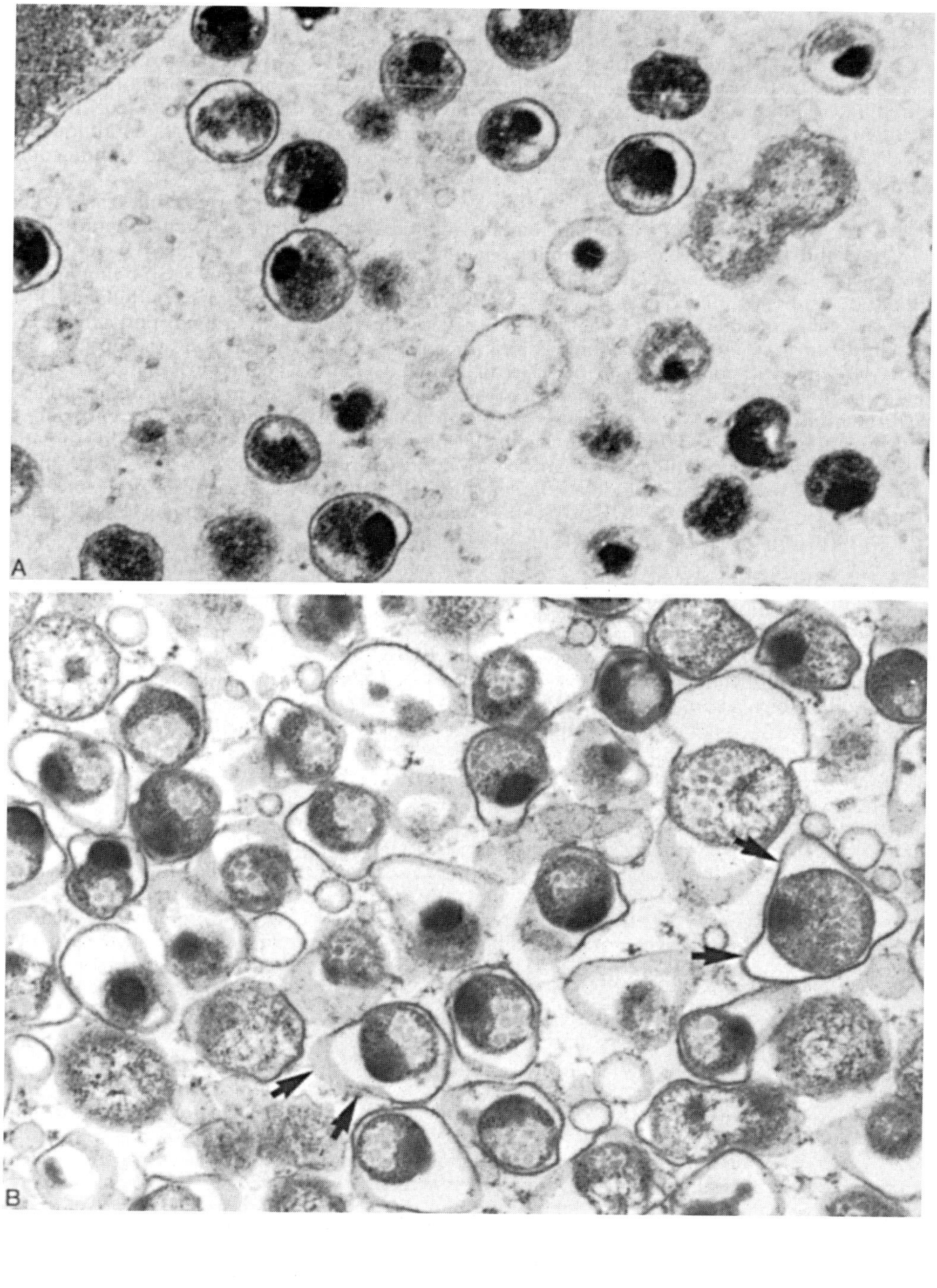

FIGURE 193–1. *Electron micrograph of* C. trachomatis *(A) and* C. pneumoniae *(B) inclusions demonstrating the elementary body (EB) morphology. The EBs of* C. pneumoniae *have a pear shape due to a loose periplasmic membrane (arrows), different from that of the typically round elementary bodies of* C. trachomatis *and* C. psittaci.

ciated with *C. pneumoniae* infection has ranged from 6 to 19 per cent, varying with geographic location and the age group examined.[13, 26, 35, 41, 43, 46, 49, 78, 109, 118] Several studies of the role of *C. pneumoniae* in lower respiratory tract infection in pediatric populations have found evidence of infection in 0 to more than 18 per cent (Table 193–3). Most of these studies have relied entirely on serology for diagnosis. Infection in children younger than 5 years of age has been rare in Seattle and Scandinavia[46]; however, in a study of Filipino children younger than 5 years of age presenting with lower respiratory tract infection, nearly 10 per cent had either acute or chronic antibody to *C. pneumoniae*.[109] In Brooklyn, the proportion of lower respiratory tract infections associated with *C. pneumoniae*, as determined by culture, increased from 9 per cent in children younger than 5 years of age to 19 per cent in children and adolescents 5 to 16 years of age.[26] Some studies that have utilized culture have found a poor correlation between culture and serology, especially in children. As part of a multicenter pneumonia treatment study in children 3 to 12 years of age, Block and associates[13] isolated *C. pneumoniae* from 34 (13.1 per cent) of the 260 children enrolled. Serologic evidence of acute infection was found in 48 (18.5 per cent), but only 8 (23 per cent) of the culture-positive children met the serologic criteria for acute infection.

In studies to date, acute infection with *C. pneumoniae* does not appear to vary by season. In Seattle and Scandinavia, cycles lasting several years have been described during which the incidence of new infection with *C. pneumoniae* waxed and waned.[45]

Prolonged culture positivity after acute infection lasting from several weeks to more than a year has been described.[26, 60, 126] Asymptomatic carriage occurs in 2 to 5 per cent of adults and children.[32, 45, 72] It is not known what role asymptomatic carriage plays in the epidemiology of *C. pneumoniae*, but it is possible that these persons may be a reservoir for spread of infection.

Clinical Manifestations

The spectrum of disease associated with *C. pneumoniae* is expanding. Most infections probably are mild or asymptomatic. Longitudinal serologic data obtained during an epidemic among military recruits in Finland suggest that only about 10 per cent of infections result in clinically apparent pneumonia.[80]

Initial reports emphasized mild atypical pneumonia clinically resembling that associated with *M. pneumoniae*.[48, 110] In several subsequent studies, however, pneumonia associated with *C. pneumoniae* clinically has been indistinguishable from other pneumonias.[13, 26, 46] Co-infection with other pathogens, especially *M. pneumoniae* and *Streptococcus pneumoniae*, can be frequent. Twenty per cent of the children in the multicenter pneumonia treatment study with positive *C. pneumoniae* cultures were co-infected with *M. pneumoniae*; they could not be distinguished from those children who were infected with either organism alone.[13] *C. pneumoniae* has been associated with severe illness and even death, although the role of preexisting chronic conditions as contributing factors in many of these patients is difficult to assess. In some cases, however, *C. pneumoniae* clearly appears to be implicated as a serious pathogen, even in the absence of underlying disease. *C. pneumoniae* was isolated from the respiratory tract and the pleural fluid of a previously healthy adolescent boy with severe pneumonia complicated by respiratory tract failure and pleural effusions[4] (Fig. 193–2).

The role of host factors remains to be determined. Although *C. pneumoniae* has been detected in bronchoalveolar lavage fluid from 10 per cent of a group of patients with AIDS and pneumonia, its clinical role in these patients is uncertain because most were coinfected with other well-recognized pathogens, such as *Pneumocystis carinii* and *Mycobacterium tuberculosis*.[3] Gaydos and colleagues[41] identified *C. pneumoniae* infection by polymerase chain reaction in 11 per cent of a group of immunocompromised adults with HIV infection, malignancies, and other immune disorders, including systemic lupus erythematosus, sarcoidosis, and common variable immunodeficiency. *C. pneumoniae* appeared to be responsible for 6 of 31 (19 per cent) episodes of acute chest syndrome in children with sickle-cell disease.[87] *C. pneumoniae* infection in these patients appeared to be associated with more severe hypoxia than did infection with *M. pneumoniae*.

C. pneumoniae also may act as an inflammatory trigger for asthma. There are several reports of patients with culture-documented *C. pneumoniae* infection who developed significant bronchospasm.[50, 60] One patient was diagnosed as having asthmatic bronchitis and was receiving systemic and topical steroids.[60] She did not improve until her chlamydial infection was treated. Hahn and associates[50] reported an association between serologic evidence of acute *C. pneumoniae* infection and wheezing in adults seen for lower respiratory tract illness. However, they were able to isolate the organism from only 1 of 365 patients. As part of a study in children, *C. pneumoniae* was isolated from 13 of 118 children (11 per cent) 5 to 15 years of age who were evaluated initially for either new or acute exacerbations of asthma.[32] Treatment of the infection appeared to result in both clinical improvement and improvement in pulmonary function test scores. Only five of the children with confirmed infection had detectable IgG antibody to *C. pneumoniae*. One child who did not comply with his antibiotic therapy was culture-positive on five occasions over a 3-month period. In addition, no anti–*C. pneumoniae* antibody was ever detected. However, specific anti–*C. pneumoniae* IgE was detected in 85.7 per cent of the culture-positive asthmatics, compared with 9 per cent of children

TABLE 193–3. Studies of *C. pneumoniae* Acute Lower Respiratory Tract Infection in Children

					No. of Positive Results/Tested (%)		
Investigators, Reference	**Year**	**Country**	**Age**	**No.**	***Culture***	***PCR***	***MIF***
Saikku et al.[109]	1988	Philippines	<5 y	220	ND	ND	14/220 (6.4)
Forgie et al.[35]	1991	Gambia	1–9 y	74	ND	ND	9/74 (12.1)
Yeung et al.[127]	1993	Canada	<6 m	86	ND	ND	0/86 (0)
Herrmann et al.[69]	1994	Sudan	<12 y	110	3/110 (2.7)	0/110 (0)	4/110 (3.6)
Jantos et al.[78]	1995	Germany	2 d–15 y	290	1/290 (0.3)	2/290 (0.7)	2/101 (2.0)
Block et al.[13]	1995	USA	3–12 y	260	34/260 (13.1)	ND	48/260 (18.5)

ND, not done; MIF, microimmunofluorescence; PCR, polymerase chain reaction.

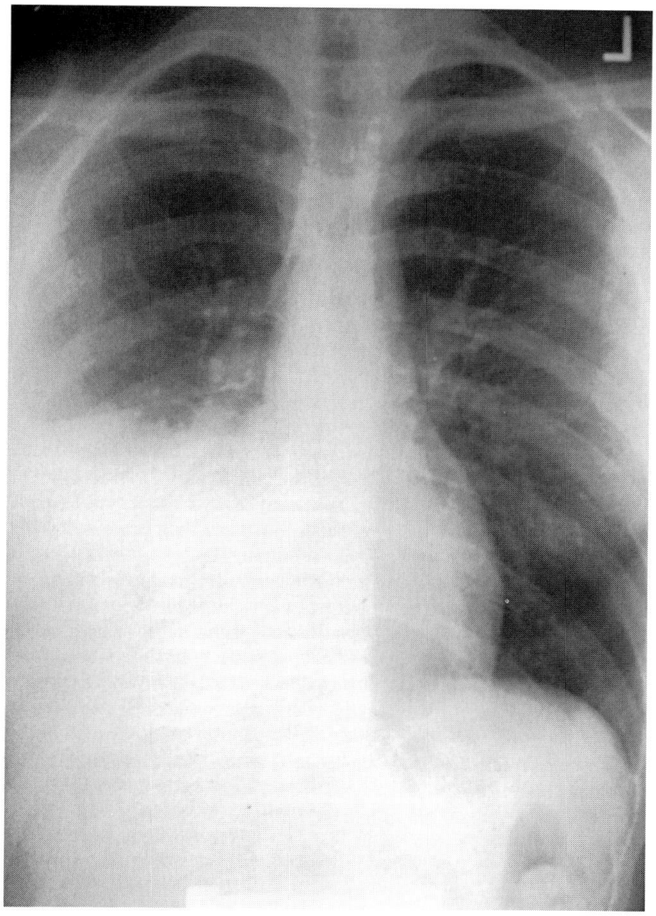

FIGURE 193–2. *Chest radiograph of a 19-year-old man with* C. pneumoniae *pneumonia demonstrating a right pleural effusion.* C. pneumoniae *was isolated from the pleural fluid.*

with *C. pneumoniae* pneumonia who were not wheezing.[33] This suggests that the bronchial reactivity seen with *C. pneumoniae* infection may be IgE-mediated. The potential of *C. pneumoniae* to cause prolonged, persistent infection may produce chronic inflammation and trigger bronchospasm in susceptible persons. *C. pneumoniae* has been demonstrated to induce in vitro ciliostasis in ciliated bronchial epithelial cells.[115] Animal studies also suggest that steroids can reactivate *C. pneumoniae* lung infection in mice.[85] Immune-mediated phenomena, including erythema nodosum and iritis, also have been described as complicating *C. pneumoniae* infection.[116, 125]

C. pneumoniae has been isolated from middle ear fluids of children and adults with otitis media.[95] There is one report of the isolation of the organism from a 47-year-old man with sinusitis.[65] Symptoms suggestive of sinus involvement are not uncommon in patients with upper respiratory tract infection associated with *C. pneumoniae.*

Diagnosis

A specific laboratory diagnosis of *C. pneumoniae* infection can be made by isolation of the organism from nasopharyngeal or throat swabs, sputa, or pleural fluid, if present. The nasopharynx appears to be the optimal site for isolation of the organism.[13] The relative yield from throat swabs and sputum is not known.

The isolation of *C. pneumoniae* requires culture in tissue; the organism cannot be propagated in cell-free media. Initial studies suggested that *C. pneumoniae* was difficult to isolate in tissue culture compared with *C. trachomatis.*[48] Originally, the same methods were used: HeLa or McCoy cells pretreated with dextran diethylaminoethyl. Multiple passages were needed, the inclusions were small and difficult to see, and, in general, the yield was poor. *C. pneumoniae* grows more readily in other cell lines derived from respiratory tract tissue, specifically HEp-2 and HL cells.[27, 107] Omission of pretreatment with dextran diethylaminoethyl results in much larger inclusions, and specimens need be passed only once. Culture with an initial inoculation and one passage should take 4 to 7 days.

Nasopharyngeal cultures can be obtained with Dacron-tipped, wire-shafted swabs. Specimens for culture should be placed in appropriate transport media, usually a sucrose-phosphate buffer with antibiotics and fetal calf serum, and stored immediately at 4° C for no longer than 24 hours. Viability decreases if specimens are held at room temperature. If the specimen cannot be processed within 24 hours, it should be frozen at −70° C until culture can be performed. After 72 hours of incubation, culture confirmation can be performed by staining with either a *C. pneumoniae* species-specific or a *Chlamydia* genus-specific (antilipopolysaccharide) fluorescein-conjugated monoclonal antibody.[89] Inclusions of *C. pneumoniae* do not contain glycogen and thus do not stain with iodine. Unfortunately, the availability of commercially produced *C. pneumoniae*–specific reagents is limited. If a genus-specific antibody is used, *C. pneumoniae* should be confirmed by differential staining with a specific *C. trachomatis* antibody; if the latter is negative, the isolate is either *C. pneumoniae* or *C. psittaci.* If there was no avian exposure, psittacosis would be highly unlikely.

Because isolation of *C. pneumoniae* was difficult and initially limited, more emphasis was placed on serologic diagnosis. However, performance of the microimmunofluorescence test also is limited to a small number of research laboratories. The microimmunofluorescence test was modified from the test used for *C. trachomatis* by using elementary bodies from TW 183 or other *C. pneumoniae* strains as the antigen. With the microimmunofluorescence test, one can detect IgG, IgM, and IgA antibodies. Grayston and colleagues[46] have proposed a set of criteria for serologic diagnosis of *C. pneumoniae* infection with the microimmunofluorescence test that is used by many laboratories and clinicians. For acute infection, the patient should have a fourfold rise in IgG titer, a single IgM titer of 1:16 or higher, or a single IgG titer of 1:512 or higher. Past or preexisting infection is defined as an IgG titer of 1:16 or higher but lower than 1:512. It was proposed further that the pattern of antibody response in primary infection differed from that seen in reinfection. In initial infection, the IgM response appears about 3 weeks after the onset of illness and the IgM response appears at 6 to 8 weeks. In reinfection, the IgM response may be absent and the IgG occurs earlier, within 1 to 2 weeks.[46] A fourfold titer rise or a titer 1:64 or higher with complement fixation also is felt to be diagnostic. Initially, Grayston and colleagues[49] found that less than one-third of hospitalized patients with suspected *C. pneumoniae* infection had detectable complement-fixation antibody. However, in a report of a small outbreak of *C. pneumoniae* infections among University of Washington students, all seven patients with pneumonia had complement-fixation titers of 1:64 or higher.[49] Complement fixation is genus-specific.

Because of the relatively long period until the development of a serologic response in primary infection, the antibody response may be missed if convalescent sera are obtained too soon (i.e., earlier than 3 weeks after the onset of illness). Use of paired sera also only affords a retrospective diagnosis, which is of little help in terms of deciding how to treat the patient. The criteria for use of a single serum sample have not been correlated with the results of culture and are based mainly on data from adults. The antibody response in acute infection may take longer than 3 months to develop. Acute, culture-documented infection also can occur without seroconversion, especially in children.[13, 26, 32] Only 28 per cent of the culture-positive children enrolled in the multicenter pneumonia treatment study had met the serologic criteria for acute infection; most had no detectable antibody by the microimmunofluorescence test, even after 3 months of follow-up.[13] However, the results of immunoblotting revealed that these children have antibody to a number of *C. pneumoniae* proteins but that less than 30 per cent react with the major outer-membrane protein, which is the antigen presented in the microimmunofluorescence test. Although the major outer-membrane protein has been demonstrated to be immunodominant in *C. trachomatis* infection, it does not appear to be immunodominant for *C. pneumoniae*.[11, 73]

Background rates of seropositivity also can be high in some populations. Hyman and associates,[72] as part of a study of asymptomatic *C. pneumoniae* infection among subjectively healthy adults in Brooklyn, found 81 per cent to have IgG or IgM titers of 1:16 or higher. Seventeen per cent had evidence of "acute infection" (IgG titer ≥1:512, IgM titer ≥1:16, or both). However, none of these persons was culture- or polymerase chain reaction–positive. Similar results were reported by Kern and associates[79] among healthy firefighters and policemen in Rhode Island. The specificity of the microimmunofluorescence IgM assay can be affected by the presence of rheumatoid factor. A study from the Netherlands found that there was an increased probability of false-positive results due to rheumatoid factor with increasing age.[121] Sera should be absorbed routinely before microimmunofluorescence IgM testing. Hyman and associates[72] absorbed all the IgM-positive sera; the titers did not change. Some IgG antibody may result from a heterotypic response to other chlamydial species because there are cross-reactions with the major outer-membrane protein between the three species as well as cross-reactions due to the genus lipopolysaccharide antigen. Moss and colleagues[92] reported that antibodies to *C. pneumoniae* and *C. psittaci* accounted for up to half of all chlamydial IgG-positive persons attending a clinic for sexually transmitted diseases. This point is reinforced by the observation that studies from the early 1980s suggesting that *C. trachomatis* was a cause of community-acquired pneumonia and pharyngitis in adults and children probably were detecting antibody to *C. pneumoniae* rather than *C. trachomatis*.[64, 81, 82]

Direct detection of *C. pneumoniae* elementary bodies in clinical specimens by fluorescent-antibody stains sometimes is possible but is insensitive and frequently nonspecific.[48] There also are no commercially available reagents that have been evaluated or approved for this purpose. All the currently available chlamydial enzyme immunoassays detect *C. pneumoniae* as well as *C. trachomatis* because they use polyclonal or genus-specific monoclonal antibodies. However, there are few data on the use of these assays in this setting, and data that are available also suggest that enzyme immunoassays are insensitive for detection of *C. pneumoniae* in respiratory tract specimens. Chirgwin and associates[26] obtained nasopharyngeal specimens from 91 patients with pneumonia for testing with Chlamydiazyme (Abbott Laboratories, Chicago). Although there were no false-positive results, the enzyme immunoassay detected only 2 of 15 patients (15 per cent) who were culture-positive for *C. pneumoniae*.

The number of *C. pneumoniae* organisms present in the respiratory tract of persons with pneumonia or other respiratory tract diseases is fewer than the number found in genital *C. trachomatis* infection. DNA amplification methods (e.g., polymerase chain reaction) appear to be the most promising technology in the development of a rapid, nonculture method for detection of *C. pneumoniae*. Although no kits are commercially available, several investigators have evaluated in-house polymerase chain reactions. In general, polymerase chain reaction appears to be at least as sensitive as culture for detecting *C. pneumoniae* in throat and nasopharyngeal specimens.[16, 42, 43]

Treatment

Chlamydia species are susceptible to tetracyclines, macrolides, and quinolones. *C. pneumoniae* and *C. psittaci* are resistant to sulfonamides.[62] To date, few published data have described the response of *C. pneumoniae* to antimicrobial therapy.[62] Most of the treatment studies of pneumonia caused by *C. pneumoniae* published so far have relied entirely on diagnosis by serology; thus, microbiologic efficacy could not be assessed. Anecdotal reports have suggested that prolonged courses, up to 3 weeks, of either tetracyclines or erythromycin may be needed to eradicate *C. pneumoniae* from the nasopharynx of adults with flu-like illness and pharyngitis.[60] One multicenter study compared erythromycin suspension with clarithromycin suspension, for 10 days, in children 3 to 12 years of age with radiographically proven pneumonia; both drugs were equally efficacious, eradicating the organism in 86 and 79 per cent of the children, respectively.[13] Preliminary data examining azithromycin in adults with pneumonia and bronchitis showed an eradication rate of 75 per cent.[62]

Based on these limited data, the following regimens for respiratory tract infection due to *C. pneumoniae* can be suggested: in adults, doxycycline, 100 mg twice a day for 14 to 21 days; tetracycline, 250 mg four times a day for 14 to 21 days; or azithromycin, 1.5 g over 5 days; for children, erythromycin suspension, 50 mg/kg/day for 10 to 14 days, or clarithromycin suspension, 15 mg/kg/day for 10 days. Some patients may require re-treatment.

References

1. Alary, M., Joly, J. R., Moutquin, J. M., et al.: Randomised comparison of amoxycillin and erythromycin in treatment of genital chlamydial infection in pregnancy. Lancet *344*:1461–1466, 1994.
2. Andersen, A. A., and Tappe, J. P.: Genetic, immunologic, and pathologic characterization of avian chlamydial strains. J. Am. Vet. Med. Assoc. *195*:1512–1526, 1989.
3. Augenbraun, M. H., Roblin, P. M., Chirgwin, K., et al.: Isolation of *Chlamydia pneumoniae* from the lungs of patients infected with the human immunodeficiency virus. J. Clin. Microbiol. *29*:401–402, 1990.
4. Augenbraun, M. H., Roblin, P. M., Mandel, L. J., et al.: *Chlamydia pneumoniae* pneumonia with pleural effusion: Diagnosis by culture. Am. J. Med. *91*:437–438, 1991.
5. Bauwens, J. E., Gibbons, M. S., Hubbard M. M., et al.: *Chlamydia pneumoniae* (strain TWAR) isolated from two symptom-free children during evaluation for possible sexual assault. J. Pediatr. *119*:591–593, 1991.
6. Beem, M. O., and Saxon, E. M.: Respiratory-tract colonization and a distinctive pneumonia syndrome in infants infected with *Chlamydia trachomatis*. N. Engl. J. Med. *296*:306–310, 1977.
7. Bell, T. A., Sandstrom, K. I., Gravett, M. G., et al.: Comparison of ophthalmic silver nitrate solution and erythromycin ointment for prevention of natally acquired *Chlamydia trachomatis*. Sex. Transm. Dis. *14*:195–200, 1987.
8. Bell, T. A., Stamm, W. E., Wang, S. A., et al.: Chronic *Chlamydia trachomatis* infections in infants. J. A. M. A., *267*:400–402, 1992.
9. Bell, T. A., Stamm, W. E., Kuo, C. C., et al.: Risk of perinatal transmission of *Chlamydia trachomatis* by mode of delivery. J. Infect. *29*:165–169, 1994.
10. Bernstein, D. I., Hubbard, T., Wenman, W. M., et al.: Mediastinal and supraclavicular lymphadenitis and pneumonitis due to *Chlamydia trachomatis* serovars L_1 and L_2. N. Engl. J. Med. *311*:1543–1546, 1984.
11. Black, C. M., Johnson, J. E., Farshy, C. E., et al.: Antigenic variation among strains of *Chlamydia pneumoniae*. J. Clin. Microbiol. *29*:1312–1316, 1991.

12. Black, S. B., Grossman, M., Cles, L., et al.: Serologic evidence of chlamydial infection in children. J. Pediatr. *98:*65–67, 1981.
13. Block, S., Hedrick, J., Hammerschlag, M. R., et al.: *Mycoplasma pneumoniae* and *Chlamydia pneumoniae* in pediatric community-acquired pneumonia: Comparative efficacy and safety of clarithromycin vs. erythromycin ethylsuccinate. J. Pediatr. Infect. Dis. *14:*471–477, 1995.
14. Bourke, S. J., Carrington, D., Frew, C. E., et al.: Serological cross-reactivity among chlamydial strains in a family outbreak of psittacosis. J. Infect. *19:*41–45, 1989.
15. Burney, P., Forsey, T., Darougar, S., et al.: The epidemiology of chlamydial infections in childhood: A serological investigation. Int. J. Epidemiol. *13:*491–495, 1984.
16. Campbell, L. A., Melgosa, M. P., Hamilton, D. J., et al.: Detection of *Chlamydia pneumoniae* by polymerase chain reaction. J. Clin. Microbiol. *30:*434–439, 1992.
17. Campbell, L. A., Kuo, C.-C., and Grayston, J. T.: Characterization of the new *Chlamydia* agent, TWAR, as a unique organism by restriction endonuclease analysis and DNA-DNA hybridization. J. Clin. Microbiol. *25:*1911–1916, 1987.
18. Carter, M. W., Sah, A. M., Treharne, J. D., et al.: Nucleotide sequence and taxonomic value of the major outer membrane protein gene of *Chlamydia pneumoniae* IOL-207. J. Gen. Microbiol. *137:*465–475, 1991.
19. Cartwright, K. A. V., Caul, E. O., and Lamb, R. W.: Symptomatic *Chlamydia psittaci* reinfection. Lancet *1:*1004, 1988.
20. Centers for Disease Control: Psittacosis surveillance 1975–1984. Atlanta, Centers for Disease Control, 1987, pp. 1–60.
21. Centers for Disease Control: Psittacosis at a turkey processing plant—North Carolina, 1989. M. M. W. R. *39:*460–469, 1990.
22. Centers for Disease Control: Recommendations for the prevention and management of *Chlamydia trachomatis* infections, 1993. M. M. W. R. *42:*No.RR-12, 1993.
23. Centers for Disease Control: 1993 Sexually Transmitted Diseases Treatment Guidelines. M. M. W. R. *42:*No.RR-14, 1993.
24. Chen, J. Y. Prophylaxis of ophthalmia neonatorum: Comparison of silver nitrate, tetracycline, erythromycin and no prophylaxis. J. Pediatr. Infect. Dis. *11:*1026–1030, 1992.
25. Chi, E. Y., Kuo, C.-C., and Grayston, J. T.: Unique ultrastructure in the elementary body of *Chlamydia* sp. strain TWAR. J. Bacteriol. *169:*3757–3763, 1987.
26. Chirgwin, K., Roblin, P. M., Gelling, M., et al.: Infection with *Chlamydia pneumoniae* in Brooklyn. J. Infect. Dis. *163:*757–761, 1961.
27. Cles, L. D., and Stamm, W. E.: Use of HL cells for improved isolation and passage of *Chlamydia pneumoniae.* J. Clin. Microbiol. *28:*938–940, 1990.
28. Cox, R. L., Kuo, C.-C., Grayston, J. T., et al.: Deoxyribonucleic acid relatedness of *Chlamydia* sp strain TWAR to *Chlamydia trachomatis* and *Chlamydia psittaci.* Int. J. System Bacteriol. *38:*265–268, 1988.
29. Crombleholme, W. R., Schachter, J., Grossman, M., et al.: Amoxicillin therapy for *Chlamydia trachomatis* in pregnancy. Obstet. Gynecol. *75:*752–756, 1990.
30. Crosse, B. A. Psittacosis: A clinical review. J. Infect. *21:*251–259, 1990.
31. Dwyer, R. S. C., Treharne, J. D., Jones, B. R., et al.: *Chlamydia* infection: Results of micro-immunofluorescence tests for the detection of type-specific antibody in certain chlamydial infections. Br. J. Vener. Dis. *48:*452–459, 1972.
32. Emre, U., Roblin, P. M., Gelling, M., et al.: The association of *Chlamydia pneumoniae* infection and reactive airway disease in children. Arch. Pediatr. Adolesc. Med. *148:*727–732, 1994.
33. Emre, U., Sokolovskaya, N., Roblin, P. M., et al.: Detection of anti-*Chlamydia pneumoniae* IgE in children with reactive airway disease. J. Infect. Dis. *172:*265–267, 1995.
34. Falsey, A. R., and Walsh, E. E. Transmission of *Chlamydia pneumoniae.* J. Infect. Dis. *168:*493–496, 1993.
35. Forgie, I. M., O'Neill, K. P., Lloyd-Evans, N., et al.: Etiology of acute lower respiratory tract infections in Gambian children. II. Acute lower respiratory tract infection in children ages one to nine years presenting at the hospital. J. Pediatr. Infect. Dis. *10:*42–47, 1991.
36. Fransen, L., Nsanze, H., Klauss, V., et al.: Ophthalmia neonatorum in Nairobi, Kenya: The roles of *Neisseria gonorrhoeae* and *Chlamydia trachomatis.* J. Infect. Dis. *153:*862–870, 1986.
37. Frommell, G. T., Bruhn, F. W., and Schwartzman, J. D.: Isolation of *Chlamydia trachomatis* from infant lung tissue. N. Engl. J. Med. *296:*1150–1152, 1977.
38. Frommell, G. T., Rothenberg, R., Wang, S. P., et al.: Chlamydial infection of mothers and their infants. J. Pediatr. *95:*28–32, 1979.
39. Fryden, A., Kihlstrom, E., Maller, R., et al.: A clinical and epidemiological study of "ornithosis" caused by *Chlamydia psittaci* and *Chlamydia pneumoniae* (strain TWAR). Scand. J. Infect. Dis. *21:*681–691, 1989.
40. Fukushi, H., Hirai, K. *Chlamydia pecorum*: The fourth species of genus *Chlamydia.* Microbiol. Immunol. *37:*516–522, 1993.
41. Gaydos, C. A., Fowler, C. L., Gill, V. J., et al.: Detection of *Chlamydia pneumoniae* by polymerase-chain reaction-enzyme immunoassay in an immunocompromised population. Clin. Infect. Dis. *17:*718–723, 1993.
42. Gaydos, C. A., Roblin, P. M., Hammerschlag, M. R., et al.: Diagnostic utility of PCR-enzyme immunoassay, culture and serology for detection of *Chlamydia pneumoniae* in symptomatic and asymptomatic patients. J. Clin. Microbiol. *32:*903–905, 1994.
43. Gaydos, C. A., Eiden, J. J., Oldach, D., et al.: Diagnosis of *Chlamydia pneumoniae* infection in patients with community-acquired pneumonia by polymerase chain reaction enzyme immunoassay. Clin. Infect. Dis. *19:*157–160, 1994.
44. Gerber, M. A., Ryan, R. W., Tilton, R. C., et al.: Role of *Chlamydia trachomatis* in acute pharyngitis in young adults. J. Clin. Microbiol. *20:*993–994, 1984.
45. Gnarpe, J., Gnarpe, H., and Sundelof, B.: Endemic prevalence of *Chlamydia pneumoniae* in subjectively healthy persons. Scand. J. Infect. Dis. *23:*387–388, 1991.
46. Grayston, J. T., Campbell, L. A., Kuo, C.-C., et al.: A new respiratory tract pathogen: *Chlamydia pneumoniae* strain TWAR. J. Infect. Dis. *161:*618–625, 1990.
47. Grayston, J. T., Kuo, C.-C., Campbell, L. A., et al.: *Chlamydia pneumoniae* sp. nov. for *Chlamydia* sp. strain TWAR. Int. J. System. Bacteriol. *39:*88–90, 1989.
48. Grayston, J. T., Kuo, C. C., Wang, S. P., et al.: A new *Chlamydia psittaci* strain, TWAR, isolated in acute respiratory tract infections. N. Engl. J. Med. *315:*161–168, 1986.
49. Grayston, J. T., Aldous, M. B., Easton, A., et al.: Evidence that *Chlamydia pneumoniae* causes pneumonia and bronchitis. J. Infect. Dis. *168:*1231–1235, 1993.
50. Hahn, D. L., Dodge, R. W., and Golubjatnikov, R.: Association of *Chlamydia pneumoniae* (strain TWAR) infection with wheezing, asthmatic bronchitis, and adult-onset asthma. J. A. M. A. *266:*225–230, 1991.
51. Hammerschlag, M. R.: *Chlamydia trachomatis* infections and pregnancy. *In* Reeve, P. (ed.): Chlamydial Infections. Heidelberg, Springer-Verlag, 1987, pp. 56–71.
52. Hammerschlag, M. R.: Chlamydial infections. J. Pediatr. *114:*727–734, 1989.
53. Hammerschlag, M. R., Roblin, P. M., Cummings, C., et al.: Comparison of enzyme immunoassay and culture for diagnosis of chlamydial conjunctivitis and respiratory infections in infants. J. Clin. Microbiol. *25:*2306–2308, 1987.
54. Hammerschlag, M. R., Roblin, P. M., Gelling, M., et al.: Comparison of two enzyme immunoassays to culture for diagnosis of chlamydial conjunctivitis and respiratory infections in infants. J. Clin. Microbiol. *28:*1725–1727, 1990.
55. Hammerschlag, M. R., Chandler, J. W., Alexander, E. R., et al.: Erythromycin ointment for ocular prophylaxis of neonatal chlamydial infection. J. A. M. A. *244:*2291, 1980.
56. Hammerschlag, M. R., Chandler, J. W., Alexander, E. R., et al.: Longitudinal studies on chlamydial infections in the first year of life. Pediatr. Infect. Dis. J. *1:*395–401, 1982.
57. Hammerschlag, M. R., Doraiswamy, B., Alexander, R., et al.: Are rectogenital chlamydial infections a marker of sexual abuse in children? Pediatr. Infect. Dis. J. *3:*100–104, 1984.
58. Hammerschlag, M. R., Rettig, P. J., and Shields, M. E.: False positive results with the use of chlamydial antigen detection tests in the evaluation of suspected sexual abuse in children. Pediatr. Infect. Dis. J. *7:*11–14, 1988.
59. Hammerschlag, M. R., Cummings, C., Roblin, P. M., et al.: Efficacy of neonatal ocular prophylaxis for the prevention of chlamydial and gonococcal conjunctivitis. N. Engl. J. Med. *320:*769–772, 1989.
60. Hammerschlag, M. R., Chirgwin, K., Roblin, P. M., et al.: Persistent infection with *Chlamydia pneumoniae* following acute respiratory illness. Clin. Infect. Dis. *14:*178–182, 1992.
61. Hammerschlag, M. R., Golden, N. H., Oh, M. K., et al.: Single dose of azithromycin for the treatment of genital chlamydial infections in adolescents. J. Pediatr. *122:*961–965, 1993.
62. Hammerschlag, M. R.: Antimicrobial susceptibility and therapy of infections caused by *Chlamydia pneumoniae.* Antimicrob. Agents Chemother. *38:*1873–1878, 1994.
63. Harrison, H. R., English, M. G., Lee, C. K., et al.: *Chlamydia trachomatis* infant pneumonitis: Comparison with matched controls and other infant pneumonitis. N. Engl. J. Med. *298:*702–708, 1978.
64. Harrison, H. R., Magder, L. S., Boyce, W. T, et al.: Acute *Chlamydia trachomatis* respiratory infection in childhood. Am. J. Dis. Child. *140:*1068–1072, 1986.
65. Hashigucci, K.: Isolation of *Chlamydia pneumoniae* from the maxillary sinus of a patient with purulent sinusitis. Clin. Infect. Dis. *15:*570–571, 1992.
66. Hedberg, K., White, K. E., Forfang, J. C., et al.: An outbreak of psittacosis in Minnesota turkey industry workers: Implications for modes of transmission and control. Am. J. Epidemiol. *130:*569–577, 1989.
67. Heggie, A. D., Jaffe, A. C., Stuard, L. A., et al.: Topical sulfacetamide vs oral erythromycin for neonatal chlamydial conjunctivitis. Am. J. Dis. Child. *139:*564–566, 1985.
68. Herring, A. J.: Typing *Chlamydia psittaci*: A review of methods and recent findings. Br. Vet. J. *149:*455–475, 1993.
69. Herrmann, S. B., Salih, M. A. M., Yousif, B. E., et al.: Chlamydial etiology of acute lower respiratory tract infections in children in the Sudan. Acta Paediatr. *83:*169–172, 1994.
70. Huss, H., Jungkind, D., Amadio, P., et al.: Frequency of *Chlamydia trachomatis* as the cause of pharyngitis. J. Clin. Microbiol. *22:*858–860, 1985.
71. Hyman, C. L., Augenbraun, M. H., Roblin, P. M., et al.: Asymptomatic

respiratory tract infection with *Chlamydia pneumoniae.* J. Clin. Microbiol. *29:*2082–2083, 1991.
72. Hyman, C. L., Roblin, P. M., Gaydos, C. A., et al.: Prevalence of asymptomatic nasopharyngeal carriage of *Chlamydia pneumoniae* in subjectively healthy adults: Assessment by polymerase chain reaction-enzyme immunoassay and culture. Clin. Infect. Dis. *20:*1174–1178, 1995.
73. Iijima, Y., Miyashita, N., Kishimoto, T., et al.: Characterization of *Chlamydia pneumoniae* species-specific proteins immunodominant in humans. J. Clin. Microbiol. *32:*583–588, 1994.
74. Ingram, D. L., Runyan, D. K., Collins, A. D., et al.: Vaginal *Chlamydia trachomatis* infection in children with sexual contact. Pediatr. Infect. Dis. *3:*97–99, 1984.
75. Ingram, D. L., White, S. T., Occhiuti, A. R., et al.: Childhood vaginal infections: Association of *Chlamydia trachomatis* with sexual contact. Pediatr. Infect. Dis. *5:*226–229, 1986.
76. Isenberg, S. J., Apt, L., and Wood, M.: A controlled trial of povidone-iodine as prophylaxis against ophthalmia neonatorum. N. Engl. J. Med. *332:*562–566, 1995.
77. Ito, J. I., Comess, K. A., Alexander, E. R., et al.: Pneumonia due to *Chlamydia trachomatis* in an immunocompromised adult. N. Engl. J. Med. *307:*95–98, 1982.
78. Jantos, C. A., Wienpahl, B., Schiefer, H. G., et al.: Infection with *Chlamydia pneumoniae* in infants and children with acute lower respiratory tract disease. Pediatr. Infect. Dis. J. *14:*117–122, 1995.
79. Kern, D. G., Neill, M. A., and Schachter, J.: A seroepidemiologic study of *Chlamydia pneumoniae* in Rhode Island. Chest *104:*208–213, 1993.
80. Kleemola, M., Saikku, P., Visakorpi, R., et al.: Epidemics of pneumonia caused by TWAR, a new *Chlamydia* organism, in military trainees in Finland. J. Infect. Dis. *157:*230–236, 1988.
81. Komaroff, A. L., Aronson, M. D., Pass, C. T., et al.: Serologic evidence of chlamydial and mycoplasmal pharyngitis in adults. Science *222:*927–928, 1983.
82. Komaroff, A. L., Aronson, M. D., and Schachter, J.: *Chlamydia trachomatis* infection in adults with community-acquired pneumonia. J. A. M. A. *245:*1319–1322, 1981.
83. Kroon, F. P., van't Wout, J. W., Weiland, H. T., et al.: *Chlamydia trachomatis* pneumonia in an HIV-seropositive patient. N. Engl. J. Med. *320:*806–807, 1989.
84. Laga, M., Plummer, F. A., Piot, P., et al.: Prophylaxis of gonococcal and chlamydial ophthalmia neonatorum. N. Engl. J. Med. *318:*653–657, 1988.
85. Malinverni, R., Kuo, C. C., Campbell, L. A., et al.: Reactivation of *Chlamydia pneumoniae* lung infection in mice by cortisone. J. Infect. Dis. *172:*593–595, 1995.
86. Meyers, J. D., Hackman, R. C., and Stamm, W. E.: *Chlamydia trachomatis* infection as a cause of pneumonia after human marrow transplantation. Transplantation *36:*130–134, 1983.
87. Miller, S. T., Hammerschlag, M. R., Chirgwin, K., et al.: The role of *Chlamydia pneumoniae* in acute chest syndrome of sickle cell disease. J. Pediatr. *118:*30–33, 1991.
88. Moncada, J. V., Schachter, J., and Wofsy, C.: Prevalence of *Chlamydia trachomatis* lung infection in patients with acquired immune deficiency syndrome. J. Clin. Microbiol. *23:*986, 1986.
89. Montalban, G. S., Roblin, P. M., and Hammerschlag, M. R.: Performance of three commercially available monoclonal reagents for confirmation of *Chlamydia pneumoniae* in cell culture. J. Clin. Microbiol. *32:*1406–1407, 1994.
90. Mordhorst, C. D., Wang, S.-P., Myhra, W., et al.: *Chlamydia pneumonia*, strain TWAR, infections in Denmark 1975–1987. *In* Bowie, W. R., et al. (eds.): Chlamydial Infections. Proceedings of the Seventh International Symposium on Human Chlamydial Infections. Cambridge, Cambridge University Press, 1990, pp. 418–421.
91. Morrison, W. M., Hutchinson, R. B., Thomason, J., et al.: An outbreak of psittacosis. Br. Soc. Study Infect. *91:*71–75, 1991.
92. Moss, T. R., Darougar, S., Woodland, R. M., et al.: Antibodies to chlamydia species in patients attending a genitourinary clinic and the impact of antibodies to *Chlamydia pneumoniae* and *Chlamydia psittaci* on the sensitivity and the specificity of *Chlamydia trachomatis* serology tests. Sex. Trans. Dis. *20:*61–65, 1993.
93. Moulder, J. W.: Interaction of chlamydiae and host cells in vitro. Am. Soc. Microbiol. *55:*143–190, 1991.
94. Nakajo, M. N., Roblin, P. M., Hammerschlag, M. R., et al.: Chlamydicidal activity of human alveolar macrophages. Infect. Immun. 58:3640–3644, 1990.
95. Ogawa, H., Hashiguchi, K., and Kazuyama, Y.: Recovery of *Chlamydia pneumoniae* in six patients with otitis media with effusion. J. Laryngol. Otol. *106:*490–492, 1992.
96. Oldach, D. W., Gaydos, C. A., Mundy, L. M., et al.: Rapid diagnosis of *Chlamydia psittaci* pneumonia. Clin. Infect. Dis. *17:*338–343, 1993.
97. Paisley, J. W., Lauer, B. A., Melinkovich, P., et al.: Rapid diagnosis of *Chlamydia trachomatis* pneumonia in infants by direct immunofluorescence microscopy of nasopharyngeal secretions. J. Pediatr. *109:*653–655, 1986.
98. Patamasucon, P., Rettig, P. J., Faust, K. L., et al.: Oral vs topical erythromycin therapies for chlamydial conjunctivitis. Am. J. Dis. Child. *136:*817–821, 1982.
99. Pether, J. V. S., Noah, N. D., Lau, Y. K., et al.: An outbreak of psittacosis in a boys' boarding school. J. Hyg. (Camb.) *92:*337–343, 1984.
100. Pether, J. V. S., Wang, S. P., and Grayston, J. T.: *Chlamydia pneumoniae*, strain TWAR, as the cause of an outbreak in a boys' school previously called psittacosis. Epidemiol. Infect. *103:*395–400, 1989.
101. Popov, V. L., Shatkin, A. A., Pankratova, V. N., et al.: Ultrastructure of *Chlamydia pneumoniae* in cell culture. FEMS Microbiol. Lett. *84:*129–134, 1991.
102. Porder, K., Sanchez, N., Roblin, P. M., et al.: Lack of specificity of chlamydiazyme for detection of vaginal chlamydial infection in prepubertal girls. Pediatr. Infect. Dis. J. *8:*358–360, 1989.
103. Radkowski, M. A., Kransler, J. K., Beem, M. O., et al.: *Chlamydia* pneumonia in infants: Radiography in 125 cases. Am. J. Roentgenol. *137:*703–706, 1981.
104. Rapoza, P. A., Quinn, T. C., Kiessling, L. A., et al.: Assessment of neonatal conjunctivitis with a direct immunofluorescent monoclonal antibody stain for *Chlamydia*. J. A. M. A. *255:*3369–3373, 1986.
105. Rettig, P. J., and Nelson, J. D.: Genital tract infection with *Chlamydia trachomatis* in prepubertal children. J. Pediatr. *99:*206–210, 1981.
106. Roblin, P. M., Hammerschlag, M. R., Cummings, C., et al.: Comparison of two rapid microscopic methods and culture for detection of *Chlamydia trachomatis* in ocular and nasopharyngeal specimens from infants. J. Clin. Microbiol. *27:*968–970, 1989.
107. Roblin, P. M., Dumornay, W., and Hammerschlag, M. R.: Use of HEp-2 cells for improved isolation and passage of *Chlamydia pneumoniae*. J. Clin. Microbiol. *30:*1968–1971, 1992.
108. Rowe, D. S., Aicardi, E. Z., Dawson, C. R., et al.: Purulent ocular discharge in neonates: Significance of *Chlamydia trachomatis*. Pediatrics *63:*628–632, 1979.
109. Saikku, P., Ruutu, P., Leinonen, M., et al.: Acute lower-respiratory-tract infection associated with chlamydial TWAR antibody in Filipino children. J. Infect. Dis. *158:*1095–1097, 1988.
110. Saikku, P., Wang, S. P., Kleemola, M., et al.: An epidemic of mild pneumonia due to an unusual *Chlamydia psittaci* strain. J. Infect. Dis. *151:*832–839, 1985.
111. San Joaquin, V. H., Rettig, P. J., Newton, J. Y., et al.: Prevalence of chlamydial antibodies in children. Am. J. Dis. Child. *136:*425–427, 1982.
112. Sandstrom, K. I., Bell, T. A., Chandler, J. W., et al.: Microbial causes of neonatal conjunctivitis. J. Pediatr. *105:*706–712, 1984.
113. Schachter, J., Sweet, R. L., Grossman, M., et al.: Experience with the routine use of erythromycin for chlamydial infections in pregnancy. N. Engl. J. Med. *314:*276–279, 1986.
114. Schachter, J., Grossman, M., Sweet, R. L., et al.: Prospective study of perinatal transmission of *Chlamydia trachomatis*. J. A. M. A. *255:*3374–3377, 1986.
115. Shemer, A. Y., and Lieberman, D.: *Chlamydia pneumoniae*-induced ciliostasis in ciliated bronchial epithelial cells. J. Infect. Dis. *171:*1274–1278, 1995.
116. Sundelof, B., Gnarpe, H., and Gnarpe, J.: An unusual manifestation of *Chlamydia pneumoniae* infection: Meningitis, hepatitis, iritis and atypical erythema nodosum. Scand. J. Infect. Dis. *25:*259–261, 1993.
117. Theunissen, H. J. H., Toom, N. A. L., Burggraaf, A., et al.: Influence of temperature and relative humidity on the survival of *Chlamydia pneumoniae* in aerosols. Am. Soc. Microbiol. *59:*2589–2593, 1993.
118. Thom, D. H., Grayston, T., Wang, S. P., et al.: *Chlamydia pneumoniae* strain TWAR, *Mycoplasma pneumoniae* and viral infections in acute respiratory disease in a university study health clinic population. Am. J. Epidemiol. *132:*248–256, 1990.
119. Tong, C. Y. W., and Sillis, M. Detection of *Chlamydia pneumoniae* and *Chlamydia psittaci* in sputum samples by PCR. J. Clin. Pathol. *46:*313–317, 1993.
120. Van Buuren, C. E., Dorrestein, G. M., and Van Dijk, J. E.: *Chlamydia psittaci* infections in birds: A review on the pathogenesis and histopathological features. Vet. Q. *16:*38–41, 1994.
121. Verkooyen, R. P., Hazenberg, M. A., Van Haaren, G. H., et al.: Age-related interference with *Chlamydia pneumoniae* microimmunofluorescence serology due to circulating rheumatoid factor. J. Clin. Microbiol. *30:*1287–1289, 1992.
122. Weiss, S. G., Newcomb, R. W., and Beem, M. O.: Pulmonary assessment of children after chlamydial pneumonia of infancy. J. Pediatr. *108:*659–664, 1986.
123. Williams, L. P.: Review of the epidemiology of chlamydiosis in the United States. J. Am. Vet. Med. Assoc. *195:*1518–1521, 1989.
124. Wong, K. H., Skelton, S. K., and Daugharty, H.: Utility of complement fixation and microimmunofluorescence assays for detecting serologic responses in patients with clinically diagnosed psittacosis. J. Clin. Microbiol. *32:*2417–2421, 1994.
125. Yamada, S., Tsumura, N., Nagaik, et al.: A child with iritis due to *Chlamydia pneumoniae* infection. J. Jpn. Assoc. Infect. Dis. *68:*1543–1547, 1994.
126. Yamazaki, T., Nakada, H., Sakurai, N., et al.: Transmission of *Chlamydia pneumoniae* in young children in a Japanese family. J. Infect. Dis. *162:*1390–1392, 1990.
127. Yeung, S. M., McLeod, K., Wang, S. P., et al.: Lack of evidence of *Chlamydia pneumoniae* infection in infants with acute lower respiratory tract disease. Eur. J. Clin. Microbiol. Infect. Dis. *12:*850–853, 1993.
128. Yung, A. P., and Grayson, M. L.: Psittacosis: A review of 135 cases. Med. J. Aust. *148:*228–233, 1988.

SECTION NINETEEN

RICKETTSIAL DISEASES

❑ ❑ ❑

194

Rickettsial Diseases

Morven S. Edwards and Ralph D. Feigin

The rickettsial diseases are caused by a family of microorganisms that have characteristics common to both bacteria and viruses. Rickettsiae depend on the intracellular milieu of animal cells for growth and reproduction; thus, they are considered by some to occupy a position between bacteria and viruses. The following properties, however, indicate their predominantly bacterial character: (1) they multiply by transverse binary fission, (2) they contain both DNA and RNA, (3) at least one species contains muramic acid, (4) they possess enzymes of the Krebs cycle, of electron transport, and of protein synthesis, (5) they are retained by a filter, and (6) their growth is inhibited by a variety of antibacterial agents. They resemble viruses mainly by the fact that they grow only within living cells.

These microorganisms have been named rickettsiae to honor Dr. H. T. Ricketts, who early in this century discovered and elaborated the cycle of the rickettsia causing Rocky Mountain spotted fever and who, in 1910, lost his life in Mexico after contracting typhus fever, which he was investigating.

The rickettsial diseases are grouped together because they possess the following common characteristics: (1) the etiologic agents are similar in size and shape, and all can be seen as coccobacillary forms under the light microscope, (2) they multiply intracellularly within certain cells of susceptible hosts, (3) the characteristic pathologic lesion is a widespread vasculitis of the small blood vessels except in Q fever, in which pneumonitis may be of equal importance, (4) all are acute infectious diseases characterized clinically by fever, headache, and a rash, with the exception of Q fever, which has no rash, and ehrlichiosis, which frequently has no rash, (5) in the early stages of the disease, all infections are susceptible to several of the broad-spectrum antibiotics, (6) all rickettsiae take on a characteristic red color when stained by the Gimenez method, (7) in all rickettsial infections, except Q fever, rickettsialpox, and ehrlichiosis, agglutinins are produced to the OX19, OX2, or OXK strains of the bacillus *Proteus vulgaris* (Weil-Felix reaction), and (8) all rickettsial organisms occur under natural conditions in either insects (lice and fleas) or arachnids (ticks and mites), and these arthropods are, in all cases except Q fever, the primary means by which these diseases are transmitted to humans.

All rickettsial organisms, except the heterogeneic strains of scrub typhus and *Ehrlichia,* produce complement-fixing antibodies. Data from complement fixation and, if available, Weil-Felix reactions, supplemented with the clinical and epidemiologic features of each individual patient, constitute definitive criteria for diagnosing each of the rickettsial diseases.

The immunity produced by any one of the rickettsial infections usually is of long duration against reinfection by the same etiologic agent. (Scrub typhus is an exception.)

There are four major groups of rickettsial diseases within the tribe Rickettsieae.[5] *Ehrlichia* is a genus within a separate rickettsial tribe, Ehrlichieae. With the exception of *Ehrlichia,* an infection by a rickettsia organism belonging to one of these four groups usually confers partial or complete immunity against an infection by any of the other rickettsiae belonging to the same group. In contrast, there is little or no cross-immunity among infections caused by rickettsiae belonging to different groups. As an exception, there is a minor degree of serologic cross-reaction between some rickettsiae of the typhus and spotted fever groups. In general, immunity after natural infection is more prolonged than that after immunization. Immunization, however, generally prevents mortality and has been used in specific populations.

A final general characteristic is that mammals and arthropods are natural hosts of rickettsiae. However, infection also can occur by an airborne route when infectious microorganisms gain access to conjunctival or respiratory surfaces. The airborne route appears to be a common mode of laboratory infections.

In all rickettsial infections, except louse-borne typhus, humans are only an incidental and accidental blind-end host and do not contribute to the survival of the rickettsial species. Rickettsial diseases vary enormously in severity, from benign, self-limited illnesses without mortality to some of the most fulminating infections known. A high index of suspicion, leading to prompt diagnosis and institution of appropriate therapy, is an important factor in enhancing the survival of the patient with rickettsial disease. Tables 194–1 and 194–2 summarize the epidemiologic and serologic characteristics of rickettsial diseases.

THE SPOTTED FEVERS

The spotted fevers are a group of infectious diseases caused by *Rickettsia rickettsii* and its antigenic variants. Because all are transmitted by ticks, they also are called tick typhuses.

Rocky Mountain spotted fever (RMSF) is by far the most severe and important disease in the spotted fever group; it occurs throughout the temperate zone of North America. An illness apparently identical to RMSF occurs in South America, where it is called São Paulo disease. Other less severe forms of tick typhus occur in Europe, Asia, Africa, and Australia; they are distinguished from each other by geographic location as well as by differences of the spotted fever rickettsiae that cause them.[42]

The spotted fever group of rickettsiae multiply not only in the cytoplasm but also fairly frequently in the nucleus of susceptible animal cells.[43] This is in contradistinction to other rickettsiae that grow exclusively in the cytoplasm.

Rocky Mountain Spotted Fever

This disease, caused by *R. rickettsii,* was recognized first in parts of Idaho and Montana at the turn of the century. For

TABLE 194–1. Important Epidemiologic Characteristics of Rickettsial Diseases

Disease	Agent	Epidemiologic Features: Geographic Occurrence	Epidemiologic Features: Usual Mode of Human Transmission	Reservoir
Typhus group				
Primary louse-borne typhus	*R. prowazekii*	Worldwide	Infected louse feces rubbed into broken skin or as aerosol to mucous membranes	Humans
Brill-Zinsser disease	*R. prowazekii*	Worldwide	Recrudescence months or years after primary attack of louse-borne typhus	
Murine typhus	*R. moosen**	Scattered pockets, worldwide	Flea bite	Rodents
Spotted fever group				
Rocky Mountain spotted fever	*R. rickettsii*	Western Hemisphere	Tick bite	Ticks/rodents
Tick typhuses (boutonneuse)	*R. conorii*†	Mediterranean, Caspian and Black Sea coastal regions, Africa, Southeast Asia	Tick bite	Ticks/rodents
Rickettsialpox	*R. adkari*	United States, Russia, Korea	Mite bite	Mites/mice
Scrub typhus	*R. tsutsugamushi*	Japan, Southeast Asia, West and Southwest Pacific	Mite bite	Mites/rodents
Q fever	*Coxiella burnetii*	Worldwide	Inhalation of infected particles from environment of infected animals	Ticks/mammals
Ehrlichiosis	*Ehrlichia chaffeensis*	Worldwide	Tick bite	Unknown
	E. equi‡	United States	Tick bite (presumed)	Unknown

*Also *Rickettsia typhi.*
†In addition, *Rickettsia australis* (Queensland tick typhus) in Australia, *Rickettsia siberia* (Siberian tick typhus) in North Asia, and *Rickettsia japonica* (Oriental spotted fever) in Japan are antigenically and geographically distinct entities.
‡Or a serologically closely related agent.

several decades, it was thought to be limited to the Rocky Mountain area; however, beginning in the 1930s, the disease began to be recognized in the eastern United States. It has been reported throughout all geographic areas of the United States. For a decade after the discovery of the broad-spectrum antibiotics around 1950, the incidence of RMSF declined in both the East and the West. However, beginning in the early 1960s, the incidence of RMSF soared exponentially, from fewer than 200 cases in 1960 to a peak of 1192 cases in 1981 (Fig. 194–1). However, since 1981, infection rates have waned considerably. There were 649 cases reported to the Centers for Disease Control and Prevention in 1990.[8]

Inexplicably, the incidence of RMSF in the Rocky Mountain area had begun a steady decline even before the broad-

TABLE 194–2. Complement-Fixation and Weil-Felix Reactions in Rickettsioses

Group	Disease	Rickettsial Complement Fixation (CF) Group Antigen Type: Typhus	RMSF	Q Fever	Weil-Felix (WF) Agglutination Proteus Strain: OX19	OX2	OXK
I	Primary louse-borne typhus	+ + +	±	0	+ + +	+	0
	Brill-Zinsser disease	+ + +	±	0	0 or +	0	0
	Murine typhus	+ + +	±	0	+ + +	+	0
II	Rocky Mountain spotted fever (RMSF)	±	+ + +	0	+ + +*	+ + +*	0
	Tick typhus	±	+ + +	0	+ + +*	+ + +*	0
	Rickettsialpox	±	+ + +	0	0	0	0
III	Scrub typhus	0	0	0	0	0	+ + +
IV	Q fever	0	0	+ + +	0	0	0

*In RMSF or tick typus, agglutinins to OX19, OX2, or both can be present in either high or low titer.
+ + +, Strong reactions 1:80 to 1:5120 in CF; 1:320 to 1:2560 in WF.
+, Relatively weaker reactions.
0, Negative at 1:5 dilution in CF; negative at 1:80 dilution in WF.
±, Cross-reactions between typhus and RMSF groups occur frequently.

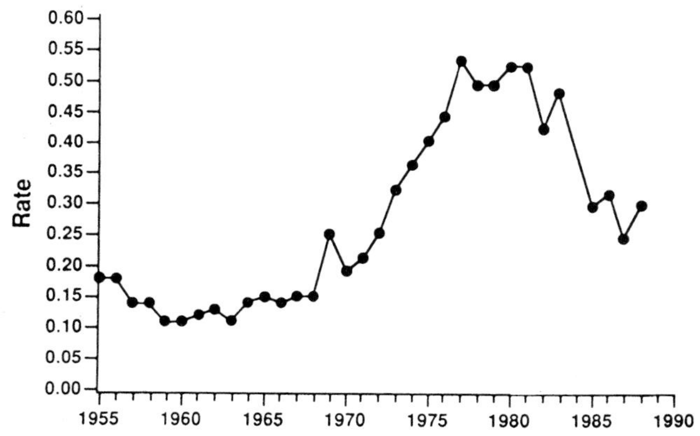

FIGURE 194–1. *Incidence of Rocky Mountain spotted fever by year in the United States (cases/100,000 population).*

spectrum antibiotic era in the 1950s; by 1988, fewer than 20 RMSF cases were reported in all the Rocky Mountain and Pacific Coast area. This trend has continued, and the major endemic regions include the South Atlantic and the West South Central regions (Fig. 194–2).

Today, RMSF is the most prevalent rickettsial disease in the United States and a growing infectious disease problem.

There are several reasons for pediatricians to have a special interest in RMSF. Nearly two-thirds of RMSF patients are younger than 15 years of age. Also, although both chloramphenicol and tetracyclines are highly effective against RMSF, the overall case-fatality rate is 3.9 per cent. Whereas this mortality can be attributed to various causes, a considerable number of deaths in children with RMSF can be attributed to failure to consider and diagnose this disorder at a time when an accurate diagnosis followed by proper therapy almost certainly would have been curative.

Etiology, Morphology, Growth, and Metabolism

R. rickettsii, the etiologic agent of RMSF, consists of small coccobacillary microorganisms measuring 0.3 to 0.5 μm in diameter and from 0.3 to 4 μm in length. They usually occur singly but also appear in strands. The most typical stained form is a diplobacillus with slightly pointed ends and a transparent band between the two bacilli. Electron microscopy reveals a two-layered cell wall and a cytoplasmic membrane. The chemical composition of rickettsiae is similar to that of gram-negative bacteria. Rickettsiae must penetrate into living cells in order to grow and multiply. They are grown most readily in the yolk sacs of embryonated eggs. Under special conditions, they also grow well in certain tissue-culture cells. Once inside, rickettsial cells multiply by transverse, binary fission.

The rickettsiae remain viable for several days in blood at +4° C (+39° F). Hence, an early specimen of blood from a suspected case of rickettsial disease can be held for a day or more in a refrigerator, pending isolation procedures.

The rickettsiae take on a characteristic red color when stained with the Gimenez stain. *R. rickettsii* organisms possess a soluble antigenic moiety that is shared with all their antigenic variants in the spotted fever group as well as with rickettsialpox. Living *R. rickettsii* organisms contain a toxin; when these organisms are injected intravenously, mice die within 6 to 12 hours, long before significant multiplication has occurred.

Epidemiology and Transmission

Because RMSF rickettsiae primarily are parasites of ticks, the epidemiology of the human disease is associated intimately with the biology of the ticks that transmit it. Disease may be acquired in the laboratory, and workers must comply with protective measures. RMSF has been transmitted by blood transfusion[51] and by the aerosol route.[22, 32]

The wood tick *(Dermacentor andersoni)* in the West, the dog tick *(Dermacentor variabilis)* in the East, and the Lone Star tick *(Amblyomma americanum)* in the Southwest are natural carriers and vectors of the disease. RMSF rickettsiae do not kill their arthropod hosts but are passed through unending generations of ticks transovarially. Congenitally acquired rickettsiae in tick eggs can persist through larval and nymphal stages and finally to the adult stage over a 2-year cycle;

FIGURE 194–2. *Reported cases of Rocky Mountain spotted fever by state in the United States in 1990.*

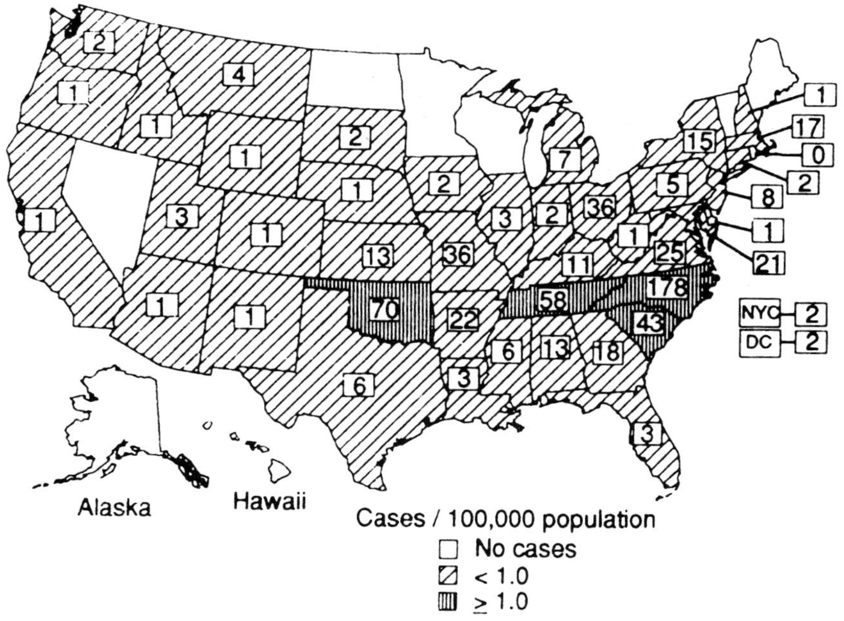

infected adults have been shown to survive for as long as 4 years without feeding.

The ticks require only three blood meals during a lifetime: just before molting from larva to nymph, again before molting from nymph to adult, and during copulation as adults before the female lays eggs. The larval and nymphal stages of the tick feed on a small mammal to proceed to the next stage. Adult females generally obtain their blood meal from a large domestic animal, such as a dog, sheep, or horse, and are the only stage of tick that feed on humans.

A study in Maryland and Virginia in the late 1960s showed that 15 different mammals, including field mice, and 18 types of birds can be intermediate hosts. Many small wild animals as well as dogs possess antibodies to RMSF, which indicates that they may be involved in promoting infection in the tick-mammal-tick cycle. Mammals act as the all-important blood-meal source for the ticks during their various metamorphoses. Still, the exact importance of these mammals in maintaining or increasing infections in the RMSF cycle is not clear because ticks themselves are reservoirs of the disease.[43]

Dogs long have been suspected of being an important link in the RMSF cycle in nature. Between 1975 and 1977 on Cape Cod, rickettsial strains were isolated for the first time from the blood of sick or dying dogs; the five rickettsial strains isolated appear to be related closely antigenically to or are identical to *R. rickettsii*, which causes RMSF disease in humans. In addition, rising titers of RMSF antibodies have been demonstrated in more than 30 clinically ill dogs. Dogs appear to be susceptible to virulent *R. rickettsii* organisms.

However, the epidemiology of RMSF in dogs is complicated by the fact that many dogs possess residual RMSF antibodies without any history of prior illness, and, at least on Cape Cod, less than 1 per cent of ticks examined appeared to be infected with rickettsial-like organisms.

Moreover, all but a few of these rickettsiae found in ticks appear to be distinct antigenically from the rickettsiae isolated from both sick dogs and humans. The data presently available do not clarify the role of dogs in the RMSF cycle. Dogs may be accidental hosts of RMSF rickettsiae much as humans are, they mechanically may transport ticks from infected tick islands to the proximity of humans, or they may play an important role in maintaining or increasing the reservoir of virulent *R. rickettsii* in nature.

The decline of RMSF in the West to fewer than 20 cases a year and its dramatic increase to more than 1000 cases annually in the East have been discussed; neither of these phenomena has been explained satisfactorily, although numerous hypotheses have been proposed.

Three additional prominent epidemiologic features of RMSF are (1) its seasonal character—most cases occur during the period of greatest tick activity from April to September, (2) the fact that about two-thirds of cases in the United States occur in children younger than 15 years of age,[43] and (3) its focal nature—relatively small areas in a state may account for a high percentage of that state's recorded RMSF cases; examples include (a) 89 per cent or more of all the cases of RMSF occurring in New York State are reported from Long Island, (b) Clermont County in Ohio reports approximately 10 per cent of all the Ohio cases of RMSF, and (c) Cape Cod and the offshore islands generally account for almost all of the cases reported in Massachusetts.

Pathogenesis

The primary pathologic lesion of RMSF is found in the vascular system after the bite of an infected tick. The rickettsiae multiply within the endothelial cells lining the small blood vessels and become widely disseminated by way of the blood stream. Rickettsiae can be demonstrated in both the cytoplasm and the nucleus of cells.[43] Focal areas of endothelial proliferation and perivascular mononuclear cell infiltration lead to thrombosis and leakage of red blood cells into the surrounding tissues. Numerous mechanisms for cellular injury have been postulated, including (1) injury to cell membranes due to penetration by multiple rickettsiae, followed by a crescendo of rickettsial release, (2) depletion of adenosine 5′-triphosphate by intracellular rickettsiae, which causes failure of the sodium pump and an influx of water, (3) competition by *R. rickettsii* for crucial metabolic substrates, and (4) damage to the cell by toxic products of rickettsial metabolism.[47, 50, 54]

Such vascular lesions appear to account for the more prominent clinical manifestations, such as rash, headache, and mental confusion, as well as terminal heart failure and shock. Vascular lesions can be found everywhere but are appreciated most readily in the skin, gonads, and adrenal glands. Parenchymatous inflammation accompanies the vasculitis in the heart and central nervous system. Interstitial myocarditis, patchy in distribution, can be demonstrated regularly in fatal cases. The location of the rickettsiae by immunofluorescence coincides with the patchy distribution of the myocarditis. Pathologic examination reveals interstitial edema and inflammation with relative preservation of myocardial fibers.[49] In the neural parenchyma itself, both mononuclear infiltrations and focal proliferative glial nodules usually are related topographically to inflamed blood vessels.[14] In the kidney, inflammation involves both vessels and interstitium in a majority of patients. Acute tubular necrosis occurs. In one study, immunofluorescence failed to demonstrate immune complex deposition, which suggests that the pathologic renal lesions in RMSF are not immune-mediated.[6] In the lung, rickettsial involvement of the pulmonary microcirculation results in interstitial pneumonia, as evidenced by alveolar septal congestion and interstitial edema, alveolar edema and hemorrhage with a fibrinous and mononuclear exudate, and interlobular septal edema. Organisms can be demonstrated in the pulmonary microcirculation by direct immunofluorescence, which indicates that the pathologic changes are due most likely to direct infection rather than to a circulating toxin. Hepatic lesions found to be statistically significant, compared with age- and sex-matched controls, were portal triaditis consisting of polymorphonuclear leukocytes and large mononuclear cells, portal vasculitis, sinusoidal leukocytosis, erythrophagocytosis by Kupffer cells, and increased hepatic weight. Again, via immunofluorescence microscopy, rickettsial organisms were demonstrated in portal blood vessels and sinusoidal lining cells.[21, 35]

More recent data add significantly to our understanding of the pathophysiology of this disease. Negative nitrogen balance may be extreme. Early in infection, this may be related to nitrogen excretion in the urine, but after several days, this is related to insufficient protein intake. Serum albumin concentration may be depressed as a result of the protein losses described before, hepatic dysfunction related to the disease process itself, and a leak of protein through the damaged endothelium of the blood vessel walls.

Profound hyponatremia is common. The studies of Liu and associates[29] and Kaplan and Feigin[24] suggest that this is related to several factors. These include (1) a shift in water from the intracellular to the extracellular spaces, (2) a loss of sodium via the urine, and (3) an exchange of sodium for potassium at the cellular level. Intracellular sodium increases slightly. Destruction of some cells results in increased serum concentrations of potassium and massive losses of potassium in the urine. Liu and associates[29] also found intracellular overhydration of the medulla oblongata and suggested that this may contribute to death in some of the patients who die a cerebral death. Plasma concentrations of aldosterone and antidiuretic hormone have been increased in some persons with this disease but have been normal in others.[24, 25, 39]

Clinical Manifestations[43]

Fever, headache, rash, toxicity, mental confusion, and myalgia are the major clinical features of RMSF.

The onset of the disease in humans, which usually occurs 2 to 8 days after an infected tick bite, may be either gradual or abrupt. The fever rises rapidly to 40° or 40.6° C (104° or 105° F). Although the pattern of fever may remain persistently high, a considerable number of patients show dramatic temperature oscillations of 1.8° to 2.8° C (35° to 37° F) over a few hours.

The rash of RMSF is an important pathognomonic feature of the disease, appearing by the second or third day in most patients; occasionally, it may be delayed until the sixth day or later. Characteristically, the initial lesions are small erythematous macules, which blanch on pressure. These lesions rapidly become maculopapular and petechial and later, in untreated patients, even confluently hemorrhagic. Rarely, they progress to massive skin necrosis.[17]

Usually, the rash appears first peripherally on the wrists and ankles, spreading within a few hours up the extremities to the trunk. An especially diagnostic feature of the rash of RMSF is its regular occurrence on the palms and soles. Eschars, which are characteristic of other rickettsial diseases, rarely have been reported with RMSF.[44] On occasion, RMSF may be "spotless" or "almost spotless."[40] The absence of a rash should not delay institution of appropriate therapy if the historical and clinical features suggest a diagnosis of RMSF.[16, 36]

The headache in adults and older children is characteristic. It is intense, persistent night and day, and intractable to all efforts at alleviation. However, young children may not complain of headaches. Toxicity is a salient feature of the disease. Signs of meningoencephalitis are common; the patient is restless, irritable, and apprehensive, and this stage may progress rapidly to mental confusion and delirium. The child may become comatose. Meningismus is not accompanied always by abnormalities in the cerebrospinal fluid. In fact, the cerebrospinal fluid generally is clear, with minor elevations of lymphocyte count ($<10/mm^3$). A case of eosinophilic meningitis caused by RMSF has been reported.[11] Grand mal or focal seizure may be noted. Cortical blindness and central deafness (transient or persistent) have been reported.[5] Other forms of neurologic involvement may include ataxia, spastic paralysis, and sixth nerve palsy. These signs and symptoms usually are short-lived but may persist beyond the period of hospitalization.[15, 43] RMSF exerts a mild but consistent effect on intellectual functioning.[17] This, in turn, suggests a higher probability of learning disability and corresponding difficulty with school performance in children who previously had RMSF.[57]

Cardiac involvement occurs frequently in RMSF. Close observation and evaluation with electrocardiogram, echocardiogram, and chest radiograph are indicated. Congestive heart failure and arrhythmias are common.[30]

Pulmonary involvement occurs in 10 to 40 per cent of reported cases and manifests itself as rales, abnormal chest radiograph, or abnormal arterial blood gas measurements. The chest radiograph may show focal infiltrates or pulmonary edema and cardiomegaly.[12, 31]

Myalgia or muscle tenderness is a common feature. Characteristically, the patient complains bitterly when the calf or thigh muscles are squeezed.

Ocular manifestations occur most commonly in the retina and include venous engorgement, retinal edema, papilledema, cotton-wool spots, retinal hemorrhages, and retinal artery occlusion. There has been one report of a patient with severe anterior segment uveitis and an iris nodule, presumed to be due to the widespread vasculitic process that occurs in RMSF.[13]

Other signs include edema of the extremities or face, stiff neck, and conjunctival suffusion. Enlargement of the spleen or liver is relatively infrequent, yet gastrointestinal symptoms and signs are common during the early course of RMSF. In one series of 131 patients, 56 per cent reported nausea or vomiting, 34 per cent reported abdominal pain, and 20 per cent reported diarrhea at the first presentation for medical care. Jaundice also has occurred with RMSF.[46]

As noted with other rickettsial diseases but not explained adequately, it appears that patients with glucose-6-phosphate dehydrogenase deficiency account for a disproportionate number of those who die of RMSF.[45]

Diagnosis

No laboratory test is available to establish quickly the diagnosis of RMSF early in the course of illness. Specific treatment must be initiated promptly; it is imperative that physicians recognize that they must make a clinical diagnosis based almost solely on symptoms, signs, and epidemiologic considerations. *R. rickettsii* may be identifiable by fluorescent or peroxidase-tagged antibody testing of a skin specimen obtained by biopsy.[52, 55] This may be a practical means of confirming the diagnosis during the early stages of illness before positive serologic reactions can be obtained. In one series, 9 of 17 cases of RMSF were diagnosed by immunofluorescence. There were no false-negative results in this series of patients. It should be recognized, however, that an experienced rickettsiologist usually is required to interpret the biopsy specimen and that false-negative results may occur. With optimal conditions, these tests are moderately sensitive ($\geq$70 per cent) and extremely specific (100 per cent).[1, 28] Significant serologic data rarely become available before the tenth to twelfth day of illness, by which time the majority of the 20 per cent of patients who will die if untreated are already moribund or dead.

A few laboratory data may give helpful clues to the diagnostician. For example, for the first 4 or 5 days after onset, the white blood cell count is normal or shows leukopenia (an uncommon feature of severe bacterial infections). As the disease progresses, secondary bacterial infections supervene, and leukocyte counts may rise to anywhere between 11,000 and 30,000 cells/mm^3.

Thrombocytopenia of varying severity develops in most cases, as with other severe infections.[37] Studies suggest that the adherence of platelets to the surface of *Rickettsia*-infected endothelial cells contributes to the reduction in the number of circulating platelets. Frequent monitoring for this development is critical because severe and unrecognized thrombocytopenia may lead to a fatal outcome, despite adequate specific antibiotic therapy.[41]

An additional hemostatic abnormality is the occurrence of an acquired coagulation inhibitor in association with RMSF. Acquired inhibitors also may accompany other infectious illnesses in children.[38]

Serologic tests are important, mainly in confirming a diagnosis of RMSF. Currently, many tests are considered confirmatory by Centers for Disease Control and Prevention. The Weil-Felix test is widely available and can be performed rapidly (in 3 to 5 minutes). It no longer is the preferred method of diagnosis because it lacks specificity as well as sensitivity.[1] The test depends on the fact that rickettsiae possess common antigens with certain strains of *Proteus* bacteria. Antibody to two *Proteus* strains, OX19 and OX2, either singly or together, shows rising titers during the second week of an untreated RMSF infection. In evaluating the Weil-Felix test results, it must be kept in mind that *Proteus* infections in humans are relatively common (particularly in the urinary tract), and, therefore, low-titered antibodies to *Proteus* OX strains of 1:20 to 1:80 often are found in normal human serum. Also, the test result can be positive in patients with leptospirosis, brucellosis, *Borrelia* infections, typhoid fever, and serious liver disease and occasionally during pregnancy.[58] However, a rising *Proteus* OX19 or OX2 titer or a titer of 1:160 or greater in a severely ill patient with symptoms and signs not unlike those of RMSF may be the only clue (and occasionally not too late to be lifesaving) to alert the physician not familiar with RMSF to start immediate specific therapy for RMSF if no other diagnosis is obvious.

The remaining available tests include complement fixation, microimmunofluorescence, indirect hemagglutination, latex agglutination, and microagglutination. The indirect-hemagglutination, microimmunofluorescence, and latex-agglutination tests are commercially available.[1] The highly specific complement-fixation and microagglutination tests lack sensitivity, and early treatment of RMSF delays the rise in antibody titer. The microimmunofluorescence test is the most specific and sensitive test available for confirming an infection with RMSF, but it is subject to observer bias.[4, 18, 19, 27, 33, 34, 53]

A microtiter enzyme-linked immunosorbent assay was developed to characterize the IgM and IgG response in RMSF. It is highly sensitive and accurate. However, as with other tests, the value of enzyme-linked immunosorbent assays in rapid diagnosis is limited because IgG and IgM seroconversion cannot be demonstrated until 6 days after the onset of illness. These tests may be useful in seroepidemiologic studies because they can detect antibody to rickettsiae at a single dilution of serum and in a single specimen collected at least 1 year after illness and they may be modified to establish a species-specific diagnosis.[9, 23]

Additionally, sera from patients with RMSF have a unique profile when analyzed by frequency-pulsed electron capture–gas liquid chromatography. Typical profiles could be detected as early as 1 day after onset of disease and before antibody could be detected. Establishing reliable frequency-pulsed electron capture–gas liquid chromatography tests could permit RMSF to be diagnosed earlier, leading to a reduction in fatalities.

A polymerase chain reaction assay has been developed that enables detection of specific sequences of DNA at the theoretic limit of one molecule and, therefore, one organism. A known pair of primers permits the detection of a common sequence found in the genome of *R. rickettsii*, *R. prowazekii*, and *R. typhi*. It is, therefore, a specific and useful screen and diagnostic tool for the most common rickettsial illnesses in the United States. The test can detect as few as 30 organisms per sample, takes approximately 48 hours to complete, and enables therapeutic intervention during the acute illness.[7]

The diagnosis of RMSF can be confirmed by isolating *R. rickettsii* in embryonated eggs or guinea pigs from blood drawn during the first week of illness before specific antibodies develop. However, serologic tests are so simple and regularly positive that the expensive, dangerous, and usually unavailable isolation techniques rarely are indicated.

With use of the specific complement-fixation or immunofluorescent test for diagnosis, extensive cross-reactions are observed between *R. rickettsii* and *R. conorii*. Differences in titers and less cross-reactivity with the murine typhus group make the distinction possible. If the geographic origin of infection is known or if the microimmunofluorescence/immunoglobulin, the rarely used immunofluorescence/immunoglobulin, or the indirect hemagglutination tests are utilized, the disease can be distinguished as RMSF or Mediterranean spotted fever.[19]

Differential Diagnosis

Measles and meningococcemia are the disorders for which RMSF is mistaken most frequently. However, a petechial rash that involves the palms and soles and spreads centripetally is unlike true or modified measles. A centripetally spreading rash may be seen, however, in the atypical measles syndrome. Thus, a careful history of prior measles immunization, particularly with killed vaccine, should be obtained. Meningococcemia can be a more difficult problem; early in both diseases, there may be a normal or low leukocyte count, signs of meningeal irritation, and a moderate pleocytosis in the cerebrospinal fluid. Inability to differentiate RMSF from meningococcemia definitively cannot be allowed to delay antimicrobial therapy because both diseases potentially are fulminating and fatal infections. Treatment should be initiated promptly with one of the tetracyclines or chloramphenicol as well as with penicillin G (as for meningococcal infection). When the diagnosis is certain, the inappropriate drug can be discontinued.

Other febrile illnesses that can be considered in the differential diagnosis include typhoid fever, leptospirosis, rubella, scarlet fever, disseminated gonococcal disease, infectious mononucleosis, secondary syphilis, rheumatic fever, enteroviral infections, immune thrombocytopenic purpura, thrombotic thrombocytopenic purpura, immune complex vasculitis, hypersensitivity reactions to drugs, murine typhus, rickettsialpox, recrudescent typhus, and sylvatic *R. prowazekii* infection that is enzootic in flying squirrels.[43]

Treatment

General Considerations for the Treatment of All Rickettsial Diseases

The rickettsial diseases, especially RMSF, louse-borne typhus, and scrub typhus, are potentially fatal infections for which specific therapy is available.

Adequate antibiotic treatment is highly effective, so patients who are treated during the first week of illness almost invariably improve promptly. On the other hand, if the disease is allowed to proceed into the second week untreated, even optimal therapy becomes progressively less effective.

Specific Treatment

Tetracyclines and chloramphenicol are the only antibiotics with proven efficacy and are highly effective when given early and in adequate dosage for the treatment of RMSF. Because rickettsial diseases—particularly RMSF—can be fulminant, prompt and optimal specific therapy is urgent. A maximally effective rickettsiostatic concentration of the antimicrobial should be attained in the blood and body fluids at the earliest possible moment.

Chloramphenicol may be given intravenously in a dose of 100 mg/kg/day up to a total daily dose of 3 g. This dose must be modified in the newborn period; RMSF, however, is rare during the first month of life. As the patients improve, treatment can be provided orally in a dose of 50 mg/kg/day in four divided doses.

Tetracycline is an important therapy for children diagnosed as having probable RMSF. Although tetracyclines generally should not be used in children who are younger than 9 years of age, the 1991 Report of the Committee on Infectious Diseases of the American Academy of Pediatrics allows for its use in this setting.[3] The rationale is several-fold: (1) staining of teeth by tetracycline apparently is dose-related, and it is unlikely in association with one or two short courses of therapy, (2) use of tetracycline obviates the concern of idiosyncratic aplastic anemic undertaken with use of chloramphenicol, (3) use of chloramphenicol mandates monitoring of serum chloramphenicol levels, which can be difficult logistically because it currently is employed so infrequently in pediatrics, and (4) tetracyclines also are the treatment of choice for ehrlichiosis, which can be confused clinically with RMSF.[2]

The use of doxycycline further may minimize the risk of tooth discoloration, possibly because it binds less to calcium. For children weighing less than 45 kg, the dosage is 2.2 mg/kg orally or intravenously twice daily on the first day of treatment and once or twice daily thereafter. Older children should receive 100 mg twice daily on the first day and once or twice daily thereafter.

When tetracyclines are provided, a dosage of 30 to 40 mg/kg/day may be given in four divided doses orally or 20 mg/kg/day intravenously may be given (maximum dose, 2 g/day). Treatment can be terminated 2 or 3 days after the temperature returns to normal for a full 24-hour period; however, a minimum of 10 days of therapy is recommended.[58] (For scrub typhus, sporadic late doses are given to prevent relapses.)

Penicillin and streptomycin have little or no effect against rickettsial infections and should be considered only when specifically indicated for secondary infections. The sulfonamides may have a harmful effect and are contraindicated.

The thrombocytopenia and blood-coagulation deficiencies that develop frequently in RMSF often signal the danger of disseminated intravascular coagulation. Prompt, adequate antimicrobial therapy is the first essential. Severe thrombocytopenia may be treated with concentrates of platelets prepared from freshly drawn blood.

Because of the widespread endothelial damage that occurs in severe rickettsial infections, a severely ill patient may be even more desperately ill than is apparent. Because both chloramphenicol and tetracycline are only rickettsiostatic, the host defenses of a severely ill patient are a major factor in recovery.

Supportive care of the patient cannot be overemphasized. Careful sequential evaluations of serum and urine electrolytes, renal function, and body weight are essential in helping to plan and guide fluid therapy. Hyponatremia most frequently is managed best by providing maintenance fluids (1500 mL/m^2/day) or by instituting modest fluid restriction. Administration of sodium-rich fluids generally precipitates cardiac decompensation and pulmonary edema without substantially raising the serum sodium concentration. Patients who are hypotensive and concomitantly hypoalbuminemic may be helped by administration of albumin (1 g/kg immediately). When clotting time is prolonged in patients without disseminated intravascular coagulation, administration of vitamin K (2 mg intramuscularly immediately) may be helpful. Marked anemia may require blood transfusion.

Workman and associates[56] have suggested that corticosteroid therapy was helpful in shortening the febrile period. This is not an unexpected outcome in persons receiving corticosteroids, but whether other specific therapeutic benefits accrue is not known.

Prognosis

Before the advent of specific therapy, the overall mortality rate from RMSF was approximately 25 per cent. Today, if appropriate antimicrobials are provided before the end of the first week of illness, recovery is the rule. Nevertheless, the overall mortality rate from RMSF in the United States still hovers between 5 and 7 per cent; death primarily occurs in patients in whom the diagnosis is delayed until the second week of illness. When death occurs (usually between the ninth and twelfth day of illness), vascular collapse, thrombocytopenia, and renal or heart failure, alone or in combination, are noted. Central nervous system involvement and disseminated intravascular clotting are common.

Complications are uncommon, especially if patients receive treatment. Bronchopneumonia may develop in seriously ill patients, and overzealous parenteral fluid administration may precipitate cardiac failure. The disease usually is mild in immunized persons. Solid immunity follows recovery from RMSF, even if therapy is begun as early as a day or two after onset.

Prevention

Two major preventive measures are effective: personal avoidance or reduction of tick contact and the use of killed vaccines.

Personal measures for reducing the amount of contact with ticks when in infected areas can be highly effective. Wearing pants tucked into boots and limiting access to the exposed skin to those areas around the neck and wrists allow frequent inspection for ticks reaching these areas. Frequent deticking particularly is valuable because infected ticks must be attached and feeding for 4 to 6 or more hours before they can transmit the disease. These facts should be emphasized in preventive education programs, particularly in geographic areas where the disease is endemic. Application of repellents, such as dimethyl phthalate, to the clothes and exposed parts of the body affords additional protection.

Killed vaccines have proved to be valuable in preventing deaths, although they do not always protect against acquiring the disease. The original vaccine was prepared in 1924 by Parker and Spence. They crushed ticks in phenol and injected a suspension of this product. Several years later, in 1938, a yolksac-derived vaccine was developed, the commercial distribution of which began in 1948. Neither vaccine conferred immunity in humans, and the latter vaccine subsequently was withdrawn from the market in the United States. More recently, a chicken embryo vaccine has been developed that may prove to be superior to the yolksac vaccine.[26] A study by Clements and associates[10] demonstrated that this vaccine was safe in the 52 volunteers vaccinated and that two doses of vaccine elicited low levels of antibodies to *R. rickettsii* in 50 per cent of the vaccinees.

Although the vaccination provided only partial protection against RMSF, it ameliorated the illness when it occurred.[10] Because an attack of RMSF imparts solid immunity, it has been suggested that vaccination with attenuated living strains of *R. rickettsii* or other live but less pathogenic rickettsiae would provide broader and more durable immunity than that provided by killed vaccines.[48] A cell culture vaccine was tested and failed to protect vaccinated volunteers when they were challenged.[43]

Control of ticks in the field with permethrin, a product with little toxicity for humans and other mammals but toxic to tick larvae and nymphs, is costly and not practical on a long-term basis.[20]

Mediterranean Spotted Fever

This disease first was described by Connor in 1910 and is a tick-borne infection caused by *R. conorii.* In September 1932, at the First International Congress of Mediterranean Hygiene, the name Mediterranean spotted fever was adopted. Other names given to this illness include boutonneuse fever, Kenya tick-bite fever, African tick typhus, India tick typhus, Israeli spotted fever, and Marseille fever. There has been a resurgence of this disease, especially in the Mediterranean countries, such as Spain, Italy, and Israel.[64, 67]

Epidemiology

R. conorii is an obligate, intracellular parasite of mites, which inoculate the microorganisms directly into the dermis during feeding. In the Mediterranean area, the vector is the brown dog tick, *Rhipicephalus sanguineus*, but other species of mites *(Hyalomma, Ixodes, Haemaphysalis)* may act as vectors in other geographic areas.[67]

Rickettsiae are widespread in ticks and can parasitize many organs, including the ovaries. The tendency of these parasites to invade not only the cytoplasm but also the nuclei of cells explains why they eventually may be transmitted transovarially. These vectors constitute a reservoir of infection. *R. conorii* can be identified in ticks by use of optical microscopy with Gimenez and Stamp stains or by immunofluorescence.

The epidemiologic pattern of Mediterranean spotted fever is determined by the biology of the tick, which results in a consistent seasonal peak that occurs from late June to mid-October. The natural cycle of the tick-borne rickettsiae may include dogs, wild rodents, and birds. Humans are introduced into the cycle accidentally and become a dead end in the transmission chain. Habitual contact with dogs appears to be the most common factor among people who acquire the infection. Occasionally, the disease develops after defleaing of a dog or from bites by ticks that are found on the ground.[71]

The exact prevalence of the disease is unknown. The incidence seems to be increasing, perhaps owing to an increase in the recognition of the infection, an increase in the number of dogs in urban areas, and possibly weather conditions, such as the serious droughts that have occurred in the Mediterranean region.[65]

Mediterranean spotted fever occurs in all age groups of both sexes. The incidence among certain occupational subgroups can be reduced through better standards of hygiene.[64]

Clinical Manifestations

The infecting bite passes unnoticed in most cases, and the incubation period varies from 6 to 10 days. The primary lesion, tache noire (black spot), was described and named by Pieri in 1925.[74] It develops at the site of the tick bite, is not painful, and rarely is pruritic. It becomes necrotic at its center, develops an eschar, and gives rise to enlargement of regional lymph glands. The initial lesion heals slowly and clears after 10 to 20 days without scarring. A discrete residual pigmentation can remain indefinitely.[60]

The tache noire is pathognomonic but not always present. Reported rates of incidence vary from 30 to 90 per cent. Multiple ulcers occasionally have been reported. The lesion appears to be the result of the combination of a substance secreted by the tick and another of rickettsial origin; it is not produced by a separate bite of an uninfected tick or by experimental inoculation of *R. conorii*. An inflammatory infiltrate, predominantly mononuclear, accumulates at the site of the tache noire and suggests the importance of T cell–mediated immunity in the local host defense.

The tache noire is localized predominantly on the head of children and on the legs of adults. Rickettsiae may be inoculated by scratching as well as via the conjunctival route.

The onset of disease usually is abrupt, with severe headache, malaise, and fever that reaches 39° to 40° C (102.2° to 104° F) within the first 2 or 3 days. The fever continues for 6 to 12 days, and antibiotics can shorten the febrile period. Generalized myalgias, especially of the leg muscles, are a prominent feature. Myositis can be demonstrated by electromyography and muscle biopsy, although these tests usually are unnecessary.[72]

The cutaneous features almost universally are present and are helpful diagnostically. The rash usually appears on the third, fourth, or fifth febrile day. The initial lesions are on the extremities; after 24 to 36 hours, the rash spreads to the trunk, neck, face, buttocks, palms, and soles. The first lesions are macular, pink, and irregularly defined and become maculopapular after a few hours. They generally measure 1 to 4 mm in diameter. The rash persists for 10 to 20 days after the remission of clinical symptoms. It may become purpuric or intensely pruritic, or it may be absent. A few patients develop atypical cutaneous manifestations, such as nodular lesions or maculoerythematous lesions, resembling the rash of murine typhus.[60, 64]

The cutaneous manifestations are due to the involvement of the vascular structures of the dermis. Rickettsemia during the incubation period probably seeds the endothelial cells of the capillaries, arterioles, and venules. The vasculitis produced is much like that seen in RMSF. The vasculitis gradually disappears during convalescence, and, as the maculopapules fade, a brown discoloration of the skin may be noticed.

Cardiovascular and respiratory changes are transient and nonspecific. Bradycardia is the most consistent finding, but other dysrhythmias have been reported. More seriously ill patients have developed pericarditis, heart failure, and myocarditis.

Phlebitis of the lower limbs is the main vascular complication. Venous thrombosis is a recognized complication, and pregnant patients particularly are prone to venous thrombosis. Pneumonitis, pleuritis, pleuropericarditis, and adult respiratory distress syndrome have been described in association with Mediterranean spotted fever.

In addition to the headache that is characteristic of rickettsial illnesses, varying degrees of impaired consciousness may occur. Rarely, stupor, delirium, convulsions, and transient hypoacusis may occur. Neurologic sequelae have been observed after rickettsial encephalitis.

Renal function is not altered in most cases, although nephritis with acute renal failure occasionally has been observed. The liver is palpable in one-third of patients, and the spleen may enlarge in 20 per cent of children. Tests of hepatic function reveal an increase in levels of serum transaminases in more than half of cases. Alkaline phosphatase levels are elevated in one-third of patients. Needle biopsy of the liver reveals foci of hepatocellular necrosis and a predominantly mononuclear reaction to the necrosis at sites of infection by *R. conorii*. The lesion differs from a true granuloma in that it is not an aggregate of epithelioid macrophages.[75]

A variety of other systemic symptoms may occur. Photophobia and bilateral conjunctivitis have been reported. Severe unilateral conjunctivitis suggests transmission of the disease via the conjunctival route. Uveitis, choroiditis, retinal artery occlusion, and neuroretinitis are uncommon ocular disturbances.[59, 63]

Hematologic abnormalities include isolated cases of autoimmune anemia and mixed cryoglobulinemia associated with Mediterranean spotted fever. Some studies report a high incidence of hypoproteinemia. There have been at least two reports of leukocytoclastic vasculitis secondary to infection with *R. conorii*.[62, 64]

On occasion, Mediterranean spotted fever may follow a malignant, rapidly fatal course, even in previously healthy children. The illness is consistent with a widespread vasculitis characterized by irreversible shock, encephalopathy, disseminated intravascular coagulopathy, and renal failure.[77]

Diagnosis

If biopsy is performed early in the course of disease, rickettsial organisms can be detected by immunofluorescence or by restriction fragment length polymorphism analysis of a polymerase chain reaction product from the tache noire.[76] *R. conorii* cannot be isolated from blood cultures by means of routine laboratory procedures. The clinical presentation, geographic location, and epidemiologic considerations help to establish the diagnosis. Laboratory diagnosis is an important adjunct and involves serologic identification of serum antibody.[70]

The Weil-Felix reaction relies on the antigenic cross-reactivity between certain *Proteus* species (OX19, OX2, and OXK) and rickettsiae. The test measures an agglutination reaction and is a nonspecific assay for serum antibody response. Single titers of 1:80 strongly support the diagnosis. However, results are variable, and there is a high rate of false-negative results. Antibodies appear on days 7 to 10 and peak during the third week of illness. Antibiotic therapy diminishes the immunologic response, and agglutination titers of greater than 1:640 rarely are reached.[71]

Complement-fixation, microagglutination, Western blot, and indirect immunofluorescence tests are available. Identification of specific IgM by immunofluorescence helps differentiate acute infection from a carrier state. Some patients with proven Mediterranean spotted fever treated early with antibiotics have normal IgM levels, however. One latex-agglutination test for detection of antibodies to *R. conorii* is both sensitive and specific. It is simpler and more rapid than microimmunofluorescence/immunoglobulin and can be performed in laboratories without specially trained personnel or sophisticated equipment.[61, 64, 68, 73]

Differential Diagnosis

Before the rash appears, differentiation of Mediterranean spotted fever from other acute infections is difficult. Even after appearance of the rash, the disease can be confused with measles, the rash of meningococcemia, toxicodermatosis, secondary syphilis, and leukocytoclastic angiitis. Other rickettsial diseases should be considered, especially in the absence of a tache noire. Cross-reactions among rickettsiae occur with the Weil-Felix reaction as well as with indirect immunofluorescence. Differentiation from typhoid fever is possible when agglutinins against antigens of typhoid or paratyphoid bacilli develop.

Treatment and Prevention

Mediterranean spotted fever generally runs a benign course, and fatalities are rare. Tetracycline is the drug of choice, and chloramphenicol is an acceptable alternative. Trimethoprim-sulfamethoxazole, ciprofloxacin, and erythromycin have been used, but treatment occasionally has failed. Recommended dosages for adolescents and adults are 2 g/day for tetracycline hydrochloride and 100 to 200 mg/day for doxycycline. The optimal duration of specific therapy has not been established definitively, and different antibiotic regimens ranging from single doses to treatment for up to 15 days have been reported.[66]

The major effective methods of control are concerned with avoidance of tick bites. Natural immunity occurs after infection, and specific antibodies have been shown to persist up to 4 years after acute illness. Effective vaccines are not available.[69]

Other Tick Typhus Fevers

Three other antigenically distinct diseases are Siberian tick typhus, Queensland tick typhus, and Oriental spotted fever. The etiologic agents share the same antigen with *R. rickettsii* but have distinguishing type-specific antigens demonstrated by complement-fixation and neutralization tests. Siberian tick typhus has been diagnosed throughout central Asia, Queensland tick typhus is found in eastern Australia, and Oriental spotted fever is found in Japan.[42]

Dogs are the principal mammalian reservoir; ticks also act as reservoirs by virtue of transovarial transmissions. Both of these diseases have similar clinical, pathologic, and epidemiologic patterns. They produce a mild disease, similar to that of Mediterranean spotted fever. As in RMSF, it has been suggested that patients with glucose-6-phosphate dehydrogenase deficiency are at risk for more severe complications from these diseases. This becomes an important factor in areas of the world with a high incidence of glucose-6-phosphate dehydrogenase deficiency.[78]

Treatment is similar to that for RMSF.

RICKETTSIALPOX

Rickettsialpox, first recognized in New York City in 1946, is a benign rickettsial infection caused by *R. akari,* an organism that is related antigenically to the spotted fever group.[85, 87, 96] Certain features of the disease that distinguish rickettsialpox include transmission by a mite, an eschar at the site of the infectious mite bite, a vesiculopapular rash, and the absence of Weil-Felix agglutinins.

The Organism

The etiologic agent *R. akari,* like that of RMSF, grows in the nucleus as well as in the cytoplasm of cells[81]; its soluble antigen cross-reacts with RMSF and the three other tick typhus rickettsiae, making it a bona fide member of the spotted fever group of organisms. However, its clinical, epidemiologic, and serologic features clearly set it apart from the other diseases of the spotted fever group.

Epidemiology and Transmission

Most cases of rickettsialpox in the United States have been reported from New York City. However, cases of rickettsialpox have been observed in a number of other cities in the northeastern United States, and what probably is the same disease has been described in Ukrainian and other former Soviet Union cities. In addition, a disease clinically consistent with rickettsialpox has been described in the Republic of South Africa; a typical strain of *R. akari* has been isolated from a field mouse in Korea. The number of reported cases has declined. It is unclear whether the incidence of the disease is decreasing or the disease simply is underreported. Sporadic periodic outbreaks of this disease are described.[79]

Whereas house mice are the natural hosts of the mite transmitting rickettsialpox in the United States, commensal rats have been shown to be infected in Russia, and wild rodents are suspected of carrying the disease in South Africa.

Rickettsialpox, therefore, may be much more prevalent worldwide than is reported, and its reservoir may extend to many other wild or domestic animals than those so far have been implicated.

The disease has a natural cycle between the mite vector *(Liponyssoides sanguineus)* and the house mouse *(Mus musculus)*. The mite passes the disease transovarially, so it is both reservoir and vector. Humans acquire infection when a depleted supply of mouse hosts caused by reduced food supplies, poison, disease, or trapping forces infected mites to seek an alternative host—people. The disease affects persons of all ages. Males and females are equally susceptible.[82, 83, 86, 87, 93]

Pathology

Because there is no mortality, no comprehensive pathologic study is available. Biopsy studies indicate thrombosis and necrosis of capillaries with mononuclear cell infiltration analogous to the angiitis of the other rickettsial diseases. A skin biopsy usually is unnecessary to confirm a diagnosis of rickettsialpox, although the histologic changes sufficiently are characteristic to aid in the diagnosis if a biopsy is performed.[79, 80] Organisms have not been demonstrated in skin biopsy specimens by light or electron microscopy, but they have been detected by direct fluorescent-antibody testing of eschars.[89]

Clinical Manifestations

The incubation period of rickettsialpox is 9 to 14 days but is difficult to determine precisely because most patients have continuous exposure to the vector in their home and usually are unaware of the mite bite.[95, 97]

Initially, a red papule develops at the site of the mite bite. This lesion slowly develops through a papulovesicle to become a black scab or eschar at about the time of onset of fever. Although the lesion most often is solitary, two eschars have been described in a number of cases.[81] Regional lymph nodes related to the primary eschar almost invariably are enlarged.

The fever is irregular, fluctuating between 37.8° and 39.5° C (100° and 103° F) and rarely lasts longer than 6 or 7 days. Usually, it is accompanied by the headache characteristic of rickettsial diseases. Rhinorrhea, cough, sore throat, nausea, vomiting, and abdominal pain have been reported.[81, 83, 91, 94]

The rash is the most remarkable aspect of the disease. It usually develops within several days of the onset of fever as scattered nonpruritic macules, which rapidly become firm maculopapules; within a day or two, vesicles develop on the summits of the papules. The lesions usually appear on the face, trunk, and extremities but also may be seen on the palms, soles, and mucous membranes. The number of lesions ranges from 5 or 6 to more than 100. The characteristic papulovesicles distributed so haphazardly on the body make the rickettsialpox rash similar in appearance to chickenpox rash in an adult.

Diagnosis

The diagnosis can be made serologically with either complement-fixation or immunofluorescent tests, with use of either RMSF or rickettsialpox antigens. Weil-Felix tests are useless because no *Proteus* agglutinins are produced.[88] Immunofluorescence of paraffin-embedded eschar material obtained by skin biopsy may be used to confirm diagnosis.[89] The major differential diagnostic problem is adult chickenpox. Infectious mononucleosis, gonococcemia, and infection with echovirus (types 9 and 16), coxsackievirus A (types 9 and 16), or coxsackievirus B (type 5) also should be considered.[80, 92, 93] Patients often give a history of having worked in basements or around incinerators or in similar areas that might be infested by house mice and their mites.

Treatment

Deaths have not been reported. Tetracycline is the drug of choice; chloramphenicol is an acceptable alternative.[79, 84] In infants and young children with mild illness, antibiotics may be withheld because the disease is self-limited.

TYPHUS GROUP

Three diseases—louse-borne typhus, Brill-Zinsser disease, and murine flea-borne typhus—make up the typhus group. Clinically and pathologically, these three illnesses are similar; epidemiologically, they are different and, hence, are described under separate headings.

Primary Louse-Borne Typhus Fever

Primary louse-borne typhus fever is an acute infectious disease transmitted to humans by the body louse. Louse-borne typhus has played a major role in the history of nations over the past five centuries. It undoubtedly has been more decisive than military campaigns, as Zinsser[116] has described convincingly in his book *Rats, Lice and History*.

Typhus fever occurs only in the presence of the lice, which multiply to astronomic numbers during periods of war, famine, and social upheaval. During the last century, epidemics occurred in Europe, Asia, Africa, and sporadically in the United States; the last recorded American epidemic occurred in Philadelphia in 1893. After World War I, more than 30 million people in Eastern Europe were infected with typhus fever, and an estimated 3 million died. During World War II, louse-borne typhus again infected millions in prison camps, the Eastern European combat zone, and North Africa. In the 1970s, tens of thousands of louse-borne typhus cases occurred in uncontrolled epidemics in Burundi and Rwanda in central Africa. In the 1980s, Ethiopia and Nigeria reported the greatest number of cases worldwide.[110]

Since 1976, at least 30 cases of disease due to *R. prowazekii* have been documented in the United States. These have occurred sporadically. The presumed source of infection is the flying squirrel *(Glaucomys volans)*.[100, 104, 108]

The Organism

The etiologic agent is *R. prowazekii*. Its morphologic features, growth, metabolism, toxin production, and staining characteristics are similar to those described for the rickettsiae of the spotted fever group. Antigenically, the organisms of louse-borne and flea-borne (murine) typhus form a separate group, although they show some minor antigenic crossover with the spotted fever group.

Epidemiology and Transmission

It has been assumed that the causative agent of epidemic typhus existed only in the human-louse-human cycle and that patients who had recovered from typhus constituted the reservoir of *R. prowazekii* in interepidemic periods. If this were the case, eradication of the epidemic typhus theoretically would be possible because few patients with Brill-Zinsser disease would be alive after long interepidemic periods. The findings of sporadic *R. prowazekii* infection, however, suggest that perpetuation of epidemic typhus is possible because it may persist in an animal reservoir.

The chain of typhus infection starts when *R. prowazekii* appears in a patient's blood during the acute febrile infection. A louse becomes infected during one of its frequent blood meals. After 5 to 10 days of incubation in the louse, large numbers of rickettsiae appear in the louse feces. Transmission of rickettsiae from an infected louse to a new host can occur by several mechanisms. Because a louse defecates as it feeds, infected feces can be rubbed into the louse bite wound. Additionally, dried louse feces also can gain access to the mucous membranes of the eye or respiratory tract. The epidemic spread of typhus throughout a community relates to temperature preferences of the louse. Lice prefer blood meals on humans with a normal temperature; hence, they tend to leave febrile patients (as well as the dead). Crowding during wars and famine makes transfer to new hosts easy.

Pathology

The pathologic process is similar to that described for the spotted fever group of diseases.

Clinical Manifestations

From 1 to 2 weeks after the bite of an infected louse, illness usually begins abruptly. The major clinical signs and symptoms are fever, headache, and a rash. Temperature usually rises rapidly to 40° C (104° F) or higher. In untreated patients, it remains at this level with minor fluctuations until death or recovery ensues. The rash usually appears on the trunk by the fourth to seventh day to spread peripherally to the extremities, usually sparing the face, palms, and soles. At first, the rash consists of macules that fade on pressure; they soon become fixed as maculopapules and later become petechial or hemorrhagic. A severe, intractable headache is characteristic. There are reports in the literature of typhus fever presenting as encephalitis, meningitis, or meningoencephalitis. Severe, untreated cases can progress to prostration, stupor, or delirium with terminal myocardial and renal failure. Complications are uncommon but can include gangrene, parotitis, otitis media, acute pericarditis, myocarditis, pericardial effusion, pleurisy, pleural effusion, and pneumonia.[103, 114, 115]

Diagnosis

The various factors concerned with the diagnosis of louse-borne typhus are analogous to those discussed for the diagnosis of RMSF, with a few differences. The rash of louse-borne typhus begins centrally on the trunk and spreads peripherally to the extremities, whereas the reverse is true for RMSF. Moreover, a rash on the palms and soles, common in RMSF, is rare in louse-borne typhus. Differentially, typhus usually occurs in epidemics under conditions of crowding and high louse populations.

On serologic examinations, the Weil-Felix reaction almost always is positive with the *Proteus* OX19 strain and less commonly with the OX2 strain. Complement-fixation and immunofluorescent tests technically are the same as with the spotted fevers; however, with louse-borne typhus, *R. prowazekii* strains are used as antigens. As noted in the section The Spotted Fevers, antigenic crossing between any of the members of the typhus and spotted fever groups of organisms is common.

An enzyme-linked immunosorbent assay and latex-agglutination test were evaluated and found to be sensitive and reproducible.[107] Owing to the antigenic cross-over between the typhus group of rickettsiae, work is being done to isolate the species-specific protein antigen of *R. prowazekii* for both immunodiagnosis and immunoprophylaxis.[102]

The most recent diagnostic tool is the polymerase chain reaction assay described earlier in the RMSF section. This test permits confirmation of rickettsial infection in 48 hours, allowing therapeutic intervention during the acute illness.[7]

Treatment

Treatment is analogous to that of the spotted fever group.

Prognosis

Case-fatality rates in untreated cases correlate with age. The rate of mortality, uncommon in children, is 10 per cent in young adults and may run as high as 60 to 70 per cent in those older than 50 years of age. Recovery from an attack gives rise to an enduring immunity. (For exceptions, see Brill-Zinsser Disease.)

Prevention

Two highly effective measures, vaccination and louse control, are available for controlling typhus epidemics. Potent killed vaccines produced from yolk sacs grown in chick embryos have proved highly effective in preventing mortality; these vaccines do not, however, regularly prevent infection. DDT and the newer insecticides lindane and malathion have proved highly effective in reducing louse infestation during typhus epidemics. The insecticides dusted into the clothes of louse-infested populations are effective in ridding the community of lice and curtailing louse-borne typhus epidemics.

Brill-Zinsser Disease[106]

Brill-Zinsser disease is a relapse or recrudescence of louse-borne typhus that occurs years after the primary attack. This relapsing form of typhus in many ways is analogous to a relapse of malaria. After a primary attack, the typhus rickettsiae remain dormant somewhere in the body, probably most commonly in cells of the reticuloendothelial system. Years later, they are reactivated by stress or some unknown factor to multiply and cause a second acute infection. Because of partial immunity remaining from the primary typhus attack, the recrudescent infection almost always is a milder, shorter, and less debilitating illness. The causative agent is the same as for primary louse-borne typhus; the symptoms, signs, and pathologic changes are similar to those described in the section Primary Louse-Borne Typhus Fever.

Tetracycline is the drug of choice. A single dose of doxycycline may lead to prompt resolution of clinical symptoms in selected cases.[111]

Murine Typhus[113]

Murine typhus is a disease of rats passed from rat to rat by the rat flea and only occasionally and accidentally transmitted to humans by an infected rat flea bite. The disease is worldwide and occurs primarily along coastal areas and around granaries where rats abound. During the first half of the twentieth century, it was highly prevalent along the Atlantic seaboard and Gulf Coast areas. Unlike other rickettsial infections, murine typhus often is acquired in cities—hence one of its names, urban fever.[99]

The Organism

The causative organism, *R. mooseri* (classified as *R. typhi* in *Bergey's Manual*) is similar to *R. prowazekii* in metabolism, growth, toxin production, and staining characteristics, although it is slightly smaller and more uniform in size. Because they possess a large common antigenic moiety, *R. mooseri* and *R. prowazekii* are classed together in one group. A new rickettsial agent, tentatively designated as the ELB agent, also has been identified as a cause of murine typhus.[112]

Epidemiology and Transmission[109]

Murine typhus usually is acquired by humans in the following manner. The rat flea, *Xenopsylla cheopis,* becomes infected when feeding on an acutely ill rat. The rickettsiae multiply in the flea without causing any ill effects, but the feces of the infected flea teem with rickettsiae for the rest of the flea's life. Rat fleas prefer to feed on rats but will feed on people if rats are not available. When an infected flea sucks blood, its dejecta is teeming with rickettsiae. If the flea bites a person, the infected feces may be rubbed into the bite wound or be transferred in a dried aerosol to the conjunctivae or respiratory tract. Humans obviously are not related to the maintenance of *R. mooseri* in nature. However, serologic and molecular analysis suggest that the cat flea, *Ctenocephalides felis,* which has a propensity to feed on humans, also may serve as a vector.[105] In California, sporadic cases have been related to transmission by fleas of *R. mooseri* from opossums to humans.[98]

In the early 1940s, 2000 to 5000 cases of murine typhus were reported annually in the United States. Most occurred in the southeastern and Gulf Coast states. Murine typhus is not reported in most states, and only 60 to 80 cases are reported annually. Approximately 80 per cent of the cases are reported from Texas.[101]

Pathology

The pathologic process is analogous to that described for the spotted fever group of organisms.

Clinical Manifestations

The incubation period ranges from 6 to 14 days. The symptoms and signs are similar to those of louse-borne typhus, the principal differences being that murine typhus is milder and shorter. The fever does not rise much above 39° C (102° F); it tends to be remittent and terminates after 9 to 13 days. The headache is less severe; the maculopapular rash is both less extensive and of shorter duration. Complications are uncommon, and the mortality rate is 1 per cent or less.

Diagnosis

The discussions of diagnosis of the spotted fever group and louse-borne typhus pertain in most respects to the diagnosis of murine typhus. There are a few differences. On serologic examination, the Weil-Felix responses of louse-borne and flea-borne typhus are almost identical. For the complement-fixation and immunofluorescent tests, *R. mooseri* antigens should be used to diagnose murine typhus. The isolation of species-specific (*R. mooseri*) protein antigens has been attempted to eliminate the problem of an antigenic cross-over in the typhus group. The most recent diagnostic tool is the polymerase chain reaction assay described in the RMSF section. This test permits confirmation of rickettsial infection in 48 hours and allows therapeutic intervention during the acute illness.[7]

Because the flea is the vector for murine typhus, epidemiologic considerations used by the physician to make a tentative diagnosis include studies of the patient's contacts with rats, fleas, or both. Because murine typhus is a mild illness and a rash may be evanescent, the disease may be confused with any disease that causes a fever of unknown origin in a patient who generally does not appear to be acutely ill.

Treatment

As with other rickettsial infections, tetracycline is the drug of choice. Chloramphenicol also may be used but has been associated with treatment failures and relapses.

Prevention

Limiting the size of rat populations is the principal factor in prevention and control of murine typhus. The first step is to scatter insecticides on rat runs to reduce the flea population. Rat populations then can be reduced by poisoning, trapping, and eliminating rat harborages and by rat-proofing buildings. Such preventive measures initiated in the coastal cities of the southeastern United States have reduced the incidence from more than 5000 cases immediately after World War II to only 60 to 80 cases per year. In recent years, approximately 80 per cent of those cases have been reported from Texas.[101]

TSUTSUGAMUSHI DISEASE (SCRUB TYPHUS)

Scrub typhus is an acute infectious disease of variable severity that is transmitted to humans by certain chiggers. The focus of the disease is restricted almost exclusively to a vast and roughly triangular area in the Southwest Pacific and in Southeast Asia. The points of the triangle are Japan, the Solomon Islands, and Pakistan. Patients who are seen with scrub typhus infection elsewhere almost certainly contracted their disease in this restricted triangle.

The Organism

The causative organism, *R. tsutsugamushi,* is distinguished by a remarkable antigenic heterogeneity. The marked strain differences of scrub typhus rickettsiae also appear to be related to the striking differences in severity of the disease in the same or different localities. This antigenic heterogeneity also has thwarted all efforts up to the present to develop an effective vaccine or a generally applicable specific serologic test. A slight modification of the Gimenez method is required to stain scrub typhus rickettsiae a bright red.

Epidemiology and Transmission

Trombiculid mites serve as both reservoirs and vectors, transmitting the rickettsiae to their own progeny via infected ova. They also possibly transmit the disease to small rodents on which they feed. Of the four stages of the trombiculid mites in nature, only one, the six-legged larval form, feeds on small mammals—or people who happen to camp in or traverse the soil locus where the mites breed and live. All other stages of the mite are spent in the soil, where they feed on organic matter.

Because of the prolonged persistence of *R. tsutsugamushi* in the human host, transplacentally acquired fetal infection is a possibility. Shirai and associates[129] examined paired mother-cord sera in an endemic area and found no serologic evidence of transplacental infection. Twenty-nine per cent of the mothers demonstrated serologic evidence of past infection; however, no mother was infected acutely at the time of the study.[128] Isolation of *R. tsutsugamushi* from the placenta has not been reported in humans. *Rickettsia* can be demonstrated in the placenta of experimentally infected mice, but no infection has been reported in their offspring.[129]

Pathology

The basic pathologic process of scrub typhus is a perivasculitis of the small blood vessels analogous to that of the other rickettsial diseases. In addition, an eschar or necrotic inflammatory lesion develops at the site of the mite bite, with consequent regional lymphadenopathy similar to rickettsialpox. General lymphadenopathy is common in scrub typhus but rare to absent in all other rickettsial diseases.

Clinical Manifestations

In more than 50 per cent of cases, an initial lesion develops into a necrotic eschar. Because mites frequently are acquired when people walk through the brush, the initial lesion commonly is on a lower limb; regional lymphadenopathy almost invariably accompanies the primary lesion. The incubation period is approximately 1 to 2 weeks, and it is about the time that the initial mite bite lesion and eschar are noted that the main characteristic features of the disease—fever, headache, rash, and general lymphadenopathy—develop. After regression of the eschar, a scar often remains and has been shown to persist for up to 25 years.[122]

A macular rash frequently appears on the trunk, for only a short time, between the fifth and eighth day of illness. Less commonly the rash persists, becomes maculopapular, and extends to the extremities. The general lymphadenopathy especially is prominent in the axilla, neck, and inguinal areas. Hepatosplenomegaly and conjunctival injection are common; deafness and tinnitus occur less commonly but are helpful diagnostic features when they do appear. Atypical pneumonia and overwhelming pneumonia resembling adult respiratory distress syndrome have been described.[118] Myocarditis and disseminated intravascular coagulation have been reported.[125] The severity of the clinical manifestations varies widely because there are several different strains of *R. tsutsugamushi.*

Diagnosis

The Weil-Felix OXK strain agglutination reaction may be the only serologic test available. It can aid in confirming (in early convalescence) a tentative diagnosis made during the acute phase of the disease when specific therapy can be lifesaving. However, only a few more than 50 per cent of scrub typhus patients develop OXK agglutinins. Moreover, it must be remembered that OXK agglutinins also are produced by relapsing fever.

Immunofluorescent tests are much more diagnostic and reliable. Unfortunately, because of the multiplicity of scrub strains, eight or more antigenic strains must be included in the sophisticated immunofluorescent tests for scrub typhus; these tests are available only in a few specialized laboratories. Brown and associates[117] demonstrated that the probability of a correct diagnosis of scrub typhus was 0.95 when a single serum specimen with an OXK titer greater than 1:320 and an immunofluorescent titer greater than 1:400 were obtained.

The antibody to *R. tsutsugamushi* measured by immunofluorescence is short-lived[128]; thus, the true incidence of scrub typhus in endemic areas is likely much greater than described initially. It is apparent that a high immunofluorescent titer may represent repeated infections. An indirect immunoperoxidase test now is available and is sensitive, specific, and reproducible. There is no cross-reactivity in testing against diseases other than scrub typhus. The indirect immunoperoxidase test is superior to the Weil-Felix and comparable with the immunofluorescent test in serodiagnosis of scrub typhus and seems to be a practical substitute for immunfluorescence.[119, 123]

A dot immunoassay utilizing nitrocellulose sheets, which strongly adsorb proteins and nucleic acids, also has been applied to the serodiagnosis of scrub typhus. No particular instruments are required for this procedure, and the results are interpreted easily by untrained personnel because the naked eye readily distinguishes the differences in color intensity between positive and negative reactions.[126, 132]

Diagnostic methods have been developed that allow identification of the rickettsial strain in infected patients. One of these uses strain-specific monoclonal antibodies in an inhibition enzyme-linked immunosorbent assay. In another, polymerase chain reaction with strain-specific primers appears to offer a method suitable for diagnosis in the acute stage of the illness.[120, 121]

Scrub typhus can be suspected when a patient gives a history of recent exposure in the geographic area where scrub typhus occurs. If, in addition, there is a local eschar, evanescent rash, and general and regional lymphadenopathy along with fever, headache, and conjunctival suffusion, the physician should be alerted to suspect scrub typhus; however, it cannot be differentiated certainly from dengue, leptospirosis, malaria, or typhoid fever. A trial of therapy with chloramphenicol or a tetracycline might be required.

Treatment

Both chloramphenicol and the tetracyclines are highly effective if given as described for the spotted fevers.

One study demonstrated that a single 200-mg dose of doxycycline was as effective as a 7-day course of tetracycline in treating patients with scrub typhus.[117] However, in this study, therapy was not instituted until day 10 of the disease. Immunity begins to develop only during the second week of the illness. Because both chloramphenicol and doxycycline are rickettsiostatic, scrub typhus patients treated in the first week of illness may require sporadic short courses of antibiotic therapy for preventing relapse.[130, 131]

Prognosis

Prognosis varies widely because there are significant differences in the severity of disease caused by different strains in different populations and in various geographic areas. Mortality rates in the pre-antibiotic era varied from 1 to 60 per cent. With the use of antimicrobials, fatalities are rare.

When treatment is begun early in scrub typhus, relapses as well as definite second attacks of the disease are common.[130] The wide heterogeneity of scrub typhus strains is believed to account for the frequent reinfections after scrub typhus infection; reinfections are rare to absent after other rickettsial diseases.

Prevention

Vector control involves impregnating clothing and smearing exposed skin surfaces with dimethyl or dibutyl phthalate.

Short-term vector control of camping grounds can be accomplished with cutting, burning, or bulldozing vegetation along with heavy spraying with insecticides, such as dieldrin or lindane.

Chemoprophylaxis is feasible for persons under high-risk exposure for short periods. Ley and associates[124] initially demonstrated that chloramphenicol was an effective prophylactic agent. However, it has been shown that doxycycline given in a dose of 200 mg once a week provides effective chemoprophylaxis of naturally transmitted scrub typhus if prophylaxis is started before exposure to infection and continued for 6 weeks after exposure.[127, 131] The potential hematologic complications of chloramphenicol coupled with the proven efficacy of doxycycline suggest that doxycycline now should be considered the antibiotic of choice for chemoprophylaxis of tsutsugamushi fever. No satisfactory vaccine has been produced.

Q FEVER

Q fever is an acute rickettsial infection of worldwide occurrence characterized in humans by fever, headache, and an associated pneumonitis in more than 50 per cent of cases. It is unique among the human rickettsial infections in that it primarily is a disease of animals transmitted to humans by inhalation of the agent rather than by an arthropod bite.

The Organism

The Q-fever rickettsia was discovered in the late 1930s independently by Burnet and Freeman in Australia and by Cox in the United States; the rickettsia has been named *Coxiella burnetii.* The organism is distinctive among rickettsiae in being highly resistant to heat, desiccation, and chemicals. Moreover, like *R. akari,* it fails to stimulate cross-reacting *Proteus* strain agglutinins (Weil-Felix reaction).

Epidemiology and Transmission

The epidemiology of Q fever differs markedly from that of the other rickettsiae. Q fever primarily is a zoonosis infecting cattle, sheep, goats, and rodents worldwide as well as marsupials in Australia and cats in Canada.[165, 179] Humans contract the disease when and where they come in contact with infected animals or materials contaminated by them.

In domestic livestock, the infection usually is inapparent and remains latent until some stress or physiologic alteration, such as parturition, leads to multiplication of the organism in the birth tissues and excretion of the rickettsiae in milk, urine, and feces.[156] At the time of parturition, placental tissues and fluids of sheep, cattle, and goats contaminate the ground; dried dust particles containing the markedly resistant organisms can be blown about and remain potential sources of infection for many months.

Epidemics of Q fever occur in abattoirs when infected (especially pregnant) animals are slaughtered, causing massive contamination of workers and creating aerosols that may be carried by air-conditioning systems to infect personnel far removed from the slaughtering area.[137] Sheep and cattle now are used commonly in research, which increases the possibility of laboratory-acquired infection. Several outbreaks of Q fever have been reported in research laboratories.[139, 140, 146, 157, 172] Q fever also is common in textile plants where bales of wool are processed, in tanneries, and in shearing camps, as well as among children in rural areas who are exposed at annual spring lambing time.[147]

Infection, in most cases, is believed to be by inhalation. Ticks are a negligible factor in passing the disease to humans but appear to be an important mode of transmission of the disease to small wild rodents and to some domestic animals. Chronic Q fever in pregnancy may involve the placenta. The use of a suppressive regimen that controls the mother's placentitis may contribute to the delivery of a healthy baby.[134] There have been at least two reports of confirmed cases of *C. burnetii* infection in a human fetus; however, no teratogenic effects have been reported. Human milk can serve as a source of infection in breast-fed babies.[169]

The prevalence of Q fever probably is underestimated. More than 40 per cent of persons with frequent contact with farm animals, such as goats, cattle, and sheep, were found to be seropositive for Q-fever antibodies. The disease has been diagnosed in an increasing number of children younger than 3 years of age and should be considered during a work-up for fever of unknown origin.[169]

Pathology

Mortality from the disease is rare, but the pathologic process has been well defined with use of both autopsy and biopsy specimens. *C. burnetii* has been demonstrated in lung macrophages at autopsy[178] and more recently in specimens obtained at transbronchoscopic lung biopsy and lobectomy.[151, 164] The abnormalities of liver function tests, as well as the common hepatosplenomegaly, suggest disease in these organs.[166] Liver biopsies demonstrate granulomatous changes with a dense fibrin ring surrounding a lipid vacuole. Rickettsial organisms are not found in these lesions, which are highly suggestive of but not pathognomonic for Q fever.[148, 163] Similar granulomas have been noted in bone marrow.[177] Valvular vegetations are seen when endocarditis complicates Q fever.[150] *Rickettsia* has been isolated from affected valves.[133, 154]

Clinical Manifestations[171]

After an incubation period of 9 to 20 days, the disease usually begins abruptly with chills, high fever, general malaise, myalgias, chest pain, and an intractable headache of the type characteristic of rickettsial diseases; however, there is no rash. Although physical findings in the chest are remarkably few, a radiograph reveals multiple round segmental opacities in more than 50 per cent of the patients. Other less common findings include pleural effusion, lobar consolidation, and linear atelectasis.[158, 160] Although pneumonitis is one of the primary characteristics of this disease, Q fever nonetheless is a systemic disease like the other rickettsioses. Hepatosplenomegaly is a frequent finding, along with abnormal liver function test results. Other reported findings include gastroenteritis and hemolytic anemia.[138, 155] The disease usually is mild and self-limited, lasting only 1 or 2 weeks. The overall mortality rate is approximately 1 per cent. Patients who develop chronic Q fever and endocarditis, however, have a mortality rate of 30 to 60 per cent.[175] Other reported complications include myocarditis, pericarditis, meningoencephalitis,[144] glomerulonephritis,[176] and inappropriate secretion of antidiuretic hormone.[136]

Diagnosis

Complement-fixation or immunofluorescent tests measuring anti–phase I and anti–phase II antibody are highly efficacious in diagnosing Q fever. IgM specific to *C. burnetii* measured by enzyme-linked immunosorbent assays, complement-fixation tests, and immunofluorescent tests has been shown to be useful for the confirmation of infection when a rising titer of complement-fixing antibody cannot be demonstrated because acute-phase blood samples are not available.[145, 149, 159] Anti–phase II antibody is present in early primary disease. Anti–phase I antibody is present in patients with chronic disease who have endocarditis or granulomatous hepatitis.[162]

Attempts to isolate the organism are both unnecessary and dangerous, predisposing laboratory personnel to infection. The polymerase chain reaction can be used on paraffin-embedded tissues; however, serology is a more convenient diagnostic tool.[167] Whereas clinical features of Q fever are not specific, careful evaluation of epidemiologic data can be valuable in suggesting a possible Q-fever diagnosis.

The often severe and puzzling cases of myocarditis, pericarditis, or endocarditis may develop months after the original infection. In such patients, serologic tests using Q-fever antigens may reveal extremely high Q-fever antibodies, thus providing a clue to the correct diagnosis.[142, 168]

An immunoenzymatic test for the detection of anti–*C. burnetii* IgG antibodies has been developed. It has proved to be more sensitive than the indirect fluorescent-antibody test for detecting low levels of antibody in persons who have not developed clinical disease. Whereas the indirect fluorescent-antibody test remains the test of choice for serologic diagnosis, the immunoenzymatic test is useful for seroepidemiologic surveys of Q fever.[170]

Treatment

The disease responds promptly to the tetracyclines, and relapses are rare. In vitro studies of the susceptibility of *C. burnetii* suggest that only tetracycline and chloramphenicol are effective in the therapy of Q fever.[161] Primary disease should be treated with tetracycline or chloramphenicol. There have been several reports of patients placed on erythromycin empirically who responded clinically and subsequently were shown to have Q fever.[141] The drug of choice, however, remains tetracycline. The most appropriate drug and duration of therapy for patients with endocarditis due to Q fever are unclear. Combination therapy that includes quinolones has been shown to be effective.[180] Tetracycline, chloramphenicol, lincomycin, rifampin, trimethoprim-sulfamethoxazole, and co-trimoxazole all have been used with varying degrees of success.[174, 175]

Prognosis

The overall mortality rate from uncomplicated Q fever is approximately 1 per cent. The vast majority of patients recover completely in a month or two with or without specific therapy, although antimicrobial therapy shortens the symptomatic period. In the rare instances of complications, such as myocarditis, pericarditis, and especially endocarditis, permanent disabilities and even fatal outcomes have been reported in 30 to 60 per cent of patients.[175]

It has been suggested that indirect fluorescent-antibody quantitative titers could aid in the prognosis of patients with Q fever. Particularly high IgM titers were found in cases of granulomatous hepatitis. IgA antibodies against phase I were found in cases of Q-fever endocarditis, although fatal cases have been shown to have few or no IgA antibodies, despite high IgG and IgM titers.[143]

Prevention

There are three Q-fever vaccine candidates available: phase I corpuscular untreated, soluble, and phase I corpuscular chloroform-methanol treated. Details concerning phase variation of *C. burnetii* as well as its genetic and antigenic stability must be worked out, but the outlook of Q-fever immunoprophylaxis certainly is promising.[152, 153]

The control of infected herds of economically valuable domestic animals has proved to be difficult. Effective controls have been stymied by the fact that the mild nature of the disease has failed to arouse public demand for controls. Hence, mild Q-fever infections continue to simmer in domestic animals, and epidemics of mild human disease appear sporadically. With the advent of antimicrobial therapy, morbidity from the disease has decreased further. This, in turn, additionally diminishes public pressure for developing preventive measures.

With the outbreaks of Q fever reported in research laboratories, specific control measures have been formulated. If possible, research laboratories utilizing sheep should be separated from other laboratories. If this is not possible, other control measures should be instituted, including the following: (1) Sheep should never be transported through a patient care area; ideally, any transport should be contained in a cart specifically designed to protect the environment from fomite and aerosol transmission. (2) All enclosed Q-fever biohazard areas should have an exhaust-air ventilation system. (3) Every investigator using sheep should register them as biohazards with the designated biosafety officer. (4) Protective clothing should be provided for use in and around sheep research and housing areas. (5) All personnel who come in contact with the sheep or sheep products should be identified and enrolled in a health education and medical surveillance program. The effectiveness of surveillance programs, including serologic monitoring, skin testing, and vaccination in susceptible laboratory personnel, is being investigated.[135, 173]

EHRLICHIOSIS

Two human tick-borne diseases caused by *Ehrlichia* species have been recognized in the United States since 1986. Both human monocytic ehrlichiosis (HME) and human granulocytic ehrlichiosis (HGE) are febrile illnesses characterized by headache, anorexia, and myalgias, often with associated leukopenia. Many patients have experienced tick attachment or bite within weeks before the onset of illness. Since the initial description of human illness by Maeda and associates in 1987,[205] a number of cases among children have been reported and the spectrum of infection has broadened considerably.

The Organisms

The members of the genus *Ehrlichia,* named after Paul Ehrlich, have been classified into three genogroups into which all previously recognized species fit.[181] One group is represented by *E. canis* and *E. chaffeensis,* the agent of HME. *E. canis* is the most extensively studied *Ehrlichia* organism because it was recognized as a cause of acute febrile illness in dogs in 1935. During the 1960s in Vietnam, the illness came to be known as tropical canine pancytopenia when a large number of trained military working dogs died with symptoms of anorexia, weight loss, and pancytopenia followed by fatal epistaxis.[218] *E. chaffeensis,* a name derived from Fort Chaffee, Arkansas, where the isolate originated, was identified in 1991 as the agent causing HME. The second group is represented by *E. sennetsu* and *E. risticii.* "Sennetsu fever" is a mononucleosis-like illness caused by *E. sennetsu* that is limited geographically to Japan and the Far East.[213] The third group is represented by *E. phagocytophilia,* a veterinary pathogen that infects neutrophils of sheep, cattle, and deer, and by *E. equi,* the agent of canine and equine granulocytic ehrlichiosis. The newly identified agent of HGE is closely related to *E. equi.*[191, 213]

Epidemiology and Transmission

Since the initial report of human illness, more than 400 cases of HME in adults and at least 20 cases in children have been described.[184–186, 190, 194, 201, 203, 204, 206, 207] Thirty states, primarily in the southeastern and south central areas of the country, have reported infection. Illness occurs in the months when ticks are prevalent, from March to October,[199] and approximately 80 per cent of the patients diagnosed with infection recall tick contact or bite within the 4 weeks before the onset of symptoms.

The Lone Star tick *Amblyoma americanum* is the putative principal vector of HME, although there may be alternative tick vectors, such as *Dermacentor,* in some geographic regions. The reservoir for HME has not been clarified, but deer and livestock are the preferred hosts of *A. americanum.* Proximity to a wildlife reserve served as a risk factor for HME in a recently reported cluster of cases.[216]

The initial reports of HGE were from the upper Midwestern states of Wisconsin and Minnesota. Infections also have been reported from Connecticut, New York, Maryland, and Florida. A tick bite frequently precedes illness, and bites of the deer tick *Ixodes scapularis* and the dog tick *D. variabilis* are the proposed vectors of infection. Because the predominant host of the deer tick, the white-tailed deer, has a wide geographic distribution, HGE may be more prevalent than currently is documented.[183, 188, 191, 202, 209, 212]

Pathogenesis and Pathology

The pathogenesis of ehrlichiosis is elucidated incompletely. Although capable of establishing infection in a number of organs and tissues, the primary target cell for HGE is the granulocyte and for HME is the macrophage. Granulomas of the bone marrow occur frequently in HME, suggesting that involvement of the reticuloendothelial system may be important in the pathogenesis.[192]

Ehrlichia enter the cytoplasm of host cells and multiply in phagosomes into elementary bodies. These individual *Ehrlichia* organisms multiply by binary fission into immature inclusions called initial bodies. Mature groups of elementary bodies form morulae that are released by rupture of the cell to reinitiate the infecting process.[205, 213]

Clinical Manifestations

The estimated incubation period for HME is 12 to 14 days. Like RMSF, HME is an acute febrile illness presenting with fever, headache, anorexia with or without vomiting, and myalgias (Table 194–3).[200, 210, 217] Rash, which may be macular, maculopapular, or petechial, is uncommon in adult infections. Among pediatric infections, rash appears to be common, with a distribution often including both trunk and extremities.

Meningitis as a manifestation of HME has been reported in three patients, including two children, with symptoms ranging from irritability and meningismus to obtundation with response only to painful stimuli.[184, 189, 201] Initial examination of cerebrospinal fluid has revealed pleocytosis ranging from approximately 50 to 1000 white blood cells, with a predominance of either neutrophils or lymphocytes; a range from 5 to 40 red blood cells; mildly elevated protein (85 to 120 mg/dL); and a normal to slightly low glucose value. Each of the three patients fully recovered.

The laboratory features of HME are shown in Table 194–3. One-half to two-thirds of adults and children have mild leukopenia and thrombocytopenia. One child had a documented decline in the white blood cell count from 13,000 to 1600 over a period of several hours.[195] Usually, thrombocytopenia is not associated with clinical bleeding; however, disseminated intravascular coagulopathy has been reported.[205] Elevations of aspartate aminotransferase, usually modest, peak at approximately 1 week into the illness, with values ranging from twice normal to several thousand. Other uncommon manifestations of illness include protracted fever,[215] elevation of renal function tests (occasionally of sufficient severity to require dialysis), hyponatremia, hypoalbuminemia, and toxic shock syndrome.[197] Persistent infection over a 2-month interval and infection complicating human immunodeficiency virus disease have been documented.[193, 208]

The clinical features of HGE are similar to those of HME, with fever, malaise, myalgia, and headache occurring consistently. Rash occurs in less than 10 per cent of cases. Morulae may be demonstrated in the cytoplasm of neutrophils but not of mononuclear cells. Leukopenia, generally mild, is a feature of illness in approximately one-half and thrombocytopenia in the majority of patients. As with HME, the level of serum aspartate aminotransferase is elevated in most cases (~90 per cent).[188, 191]

TABLE 194–3. Clinical and Laboratory Features of Adult and Pediatric Monocytic Ehrlichiosis

Feature*	Percentage of Cases Adult (N = 46)	Percentage of Cases Pediatric (N = 20)
Fever	96	100
Anorexia	76	78
Headache	80	100
Myalgia	74	67
Rash	20	65
Leukopenia†	61	72
Thrombocytopenia‡	52	78
Elevated aspartate aminotransferase§	76	83

*Some features not specified for all patients.
†Less than 4000 white blood cells/mm³.
‡Less than 150,000 platelets/mm³.
§More than 55 units/L.
NS, Not specified.

Diagnosis and Differential Diagnosis

The diagnosis of HME is established by documenting a fourfold increase in *E. chaffeensis* antibody titer (minimum titer, 64) or a single high serum-antibody titer ($\geq$128) in a patient with a clinically consistent history. The current recommendation for confirmation of HGE is a serologic reaction with a minimum titer of 80 or a fourfold rise in antibody titer to *E. equi* by the indirect fluorescent antibody test.[188, 191] Sera should be collected acutely and at 2 to 4 weeks after the onset of illness for serologic analysis.

Assays have been developed for the detection of both HME and HGE by polymerase chain reaction.[182, 183, 196] For HGE, the sensitivity of polymerase chain reaction depends on the quantity of infected neutrophils; for HME, the sensitivity of polymerase chain reaction is estimated at 80 to 87 per cent during the acute phase of infection. The specificity of the method is high.

In the initial reports of both HME and HGE, morula-like inclusions were demonstrated in the cytoplasm of peripheral white blood cells. These can be appreciated by light microscopy using Wright-stained smears. Immunohistochemical staining methods also may assist in diagnosis. The frequency with which morulae may be seen is unknown but for HME is estimated to be less than one-half of cases.

Human ehrlichiosis must be distinguished from other tick-borne diseases, especially RMSF. The illnesses are similar in that both have manifestations of diffuse vasculitis. Clinically, ehrlichiosis is less likely to be manifested by rash and more likely to have leukopenia or pancytopenia as a laboratory feature. The similarity of ehrlichiosis and RMSF is emphasized by two retrospective serosurveys in which approximately 10 per cent of specimens, from patients lacking the serologic criteria for diagnosis of RMSF, fulfilled the criteria for the diagnosis of ehrlichiosis.[204, 214] Other tick-borne illnesses, such as Lyme disease, babesiosis, Colorado tick fever, relapsing fever, and tularemia, should be included in the differential diagnosis.

Simultaneous HME and *Borrelia burgdorferi* infection has been described.[184] Whether this represents dual infection or is an instance of antigenic cross-reactivity is unknown. In children, Kawasaki syndrome may present with features mimicking ehrlichiosis; paired sera from a group of children with Kawasaki syndrome have failed to react with a panel of *Ehrlichia* antigens.[211]

Treatment

The treatment of choice for human ehrlichiosis is a tetracycline, such as doxycycline. The dosages are the same as those for spotted fevers. The in vitro susceptibility for *E. chaffeensis* has been established; it is susceptible only to doxycycline and rifampin and resistant to chloramphenicol. There are conflicting data concerning the clinical efficacy of chloramphenicol. Several children have been treated with chloramphenicol with apparent improvement, but there also have been reports of its ineffectiveness. Among hospitalized patients, those receiving tetracycline or chloramphenicol recovered significantly faster than those treated initially with other antibiotics. Mild clinical illness may resolve without specific antimicrobial treatment, although fever may be protracted.[199, 200, 210] However, human ehrlichiosis may have a fatal outcome. The risk/benefit ratio favors doxycycline as the treatment of choice based on current data.[187, 198]

Note: A portion of the material in this chapter originally was written by Edward S. Murray, now deceased.

References

General Characteristics

Murray, E. S.: The rickettsial diseases. *In* Conn, H. F., and Conn, R. R., Jr. (eds.): Current Diagnosis 5. Philadelphia, W. B. Saunders, 1977.

The Spotted Fevers

1. Abramson, J. S., and Givner, L. B.: Rocky Mountain spotted fever. Semin. Pediatr. Infect. Dis. *5:*131–136, 1994.
2. Abramson, J. S., and Givner, L. B.: Should tetracycline be contraindicated for therapy of presumed Rocky Mountain spotted fever in children less than 9 years of age? Pediatrics *86:*123–124, 1990.
3. American Academy of Pediatrics: Rocky Mountain spotted fever. *In* Peter G. (ed.): 1994 Red Book: Report of the Committee on Infectious Diseases. 23rd ed. Elk Grove Village, IL, American Academy of Pediatrics, 1994, p. 403.
4. Anacker, R. L., Philip, R. N., Thomas, L. A., et al.: Indirect hemagglutination test for detection of antibody to *Rickettsia rickettsii* in sera from humans and common laboratory animals. J. Clin. Microbiol. *10:*677–684, 1979.
5. Bell, W. E., and Lascari, A. D.: Rocky Mountain spotted fever. Neurology *20:*841–847, 1970.
6. Bradford, W. D., Croker, B. P., and Tisher, C. C.: Kidney lesion in Rocky Mountain spotted fever. Am. J. Pathol. *97:*381–392, 1979.
7. Carl, M., Tibbs C. W., Dobson, M. E., et al.: Diagnosis of acute typhus infections using the polymerase chain reaction. J. Infect. Dis. *161:*791–793, 1990.
8. Centers for Disease Control: Rocky Mountain spotted fever: United States, 1990. M. M. W. R. *40:*451–453, 459, 1991.
9. Clements, M. L., Dumler, J. S., Fiset, P., et al.: Serodiagnosis of Rocky Mountain spotted fever: Comparison of IgM and IgG enzyme linked immunosorbent assays and indirect fluorescent antibody test. J. Infect. Dis. *148:*876–880, 1983.
10. Clements, M. L., Wisseman, C. L., Woodward, T. E., et al.: Reactogenicity, immunogenicity, and efficacy of a chick embryo cell-derived vaccine for Rocky Mountain spotted fever. J. Infect. Dis. *148:*922–930, 1983.
11. Crennan, J. M., and VanScoy, R. E.: Eosinophilic meningitis caused by Rocky Mountain spotted fever. Am. J. Med. *80:*288–289, 1986.
12. Donohue, J.: Lower respiratory tract involvement in Rocky Mountain spotted fever. Arch. Intern. Med. *140:*223–227, 1980.
13. Duffey, R. J., and Hammer, M. E.: The ocular manifestations of Rocky Mountain spotted fever. Ann. Ophthalmol. *19:*301–306, 1987.
14. Feigin, R. D., Kissane, J. M., Eisenberg, C. S., et al.: Rocky Mountain spotted fever. Clin. Pediatr. *8:*331–343, 1969.
15. Gorman, R. J., Saxon, S., and Snead, O. C.: Neurologic sequelae of Rocky Mountain spotted fever. Pediatrics *67:*354–357, 1981.
16. Green, W. R., Walker, D. H., and Cain, B. G.: Fatal viscerotropic Rocky Mountain spotted fever. Am. J. Med. *64:*523–528, 1978.
17. Griffith, G. L., and Luce, E. A.: Massive skin necrosis in Rocky Mountain spotted fever. South. Med. J. *71:*1337–1340, 1978.
18. Hechemy, K. E., Raoult, D., Fox, J., et al.: Cross-reaction of immune sera from patients with rickettsial diseases. J. Med. Microbiol. *29:*199–202, 1989.
19. Hechemy, K. E., Stevens, R. W., Sasowski, S., et al.: Discrepancies in Weil-Felix and microimmunofluorescence test results for Rocky Mountain spotted fever. J. Clin. Microbiol. *9:*292–293, 1979.
20. Imperato, P. J.: Ticks, Lyme disease, and spotted fever. N. Y. State J. Med. *89:*313–314, 1989.
21. Jackson, M. D., Kirkman C., Bradford, W. D., et al.: Rocky Mountain spotted fever: Hepatic lesions in childhood cases. Pediatr. Pathol. *5:*379–388, 1986.
22. Johnson, V. E., III, and Kadull, P. J.: Rocky Mountain spotted fever acquired in a laboratory. N. Engl. J. Med. *277:*812, 1967.
23. Jones, D., Anderson, B., Olson, J., et. al.: Enzyme-linked immunosorbent assay for detection of human immunoglobulin G to lipopolysaccharide of spotted fever group rickettsiae. J. Clin. Microbiol. *31:*138–141, 1993.
24. Kaplan, S. L., and Feigin, R. D.: Personal communication, 1979.
25. Kaplowitz, L. G., and Robertson, G. L.: Hyponatremia in Rocky Mountain spotted fever: Role of antidiuretic hormone. Ann. Intern. Med. *98:*334–335, 1983.
26. Kenyon, R. H., and Pedersen, C. E., Jr.: Preparation of Rocky Mountain spotted fever vaccine suitable for human immunization. J. Clin. Microbiol. *1:*500–503, 1975.
27. Lackman, D. B., and Gerloff, R. K.: The effect of antibiotic therapy upon diagnostic serologic tests for Rocky Mountain spotted fever. Public Health Rep. *11:*97–99, 1952.
28. Linneman, C. C.: Skin biopsy in diagnosis of Rocky Mountain spotted fever. J. Pediatr. *96:*781–782, 1980.
29. Liu, C. T., Hilmas, D. E., Griffin, M. J., et al.: Alterations of body fluid compartments and distribution of tissue water and electrolytes in monkeys during Rocky Mountain spotted fever. J. Infect. Dis. *138:*42–48, 1978.
30. Marin-Garcia, J., and Barrett, F. F.: Myocardial function in Rocky Mountain spotted fever: Echocardiographic assessment. Am. J. Cardiol. *51:*341–343, 1983.

31. Martin, W., Chaplin, R. H., and Sheitzer, M. E.: The chest radiograph in Rocky Mountain spotted fever. A. J. R. Am. J. Roentgenol. *139:*889–893, 1982.
32. Oster, C. N., Burke, D. J., Kenyon, R. H., et al.: Laboratory acquired Rocky Mountain spotted fever. N. Engl. J. Med. *297:*859–863, 1977.
33. Philip, R. N., Casper, E. A., MacCormack, J. N., et al.: A comparison of serologic methods for diagnosis of Rocky Mountain spotted fever. Am. J. Epidemiol. *105:*56–67, 1976.
34. Philip, R. N., Casper, E. A., Ormsbee, R. A., et al.: Microimmunofluorescence test for the serological study of Rocky Mountain spotted fever and typhus. J. Clin. Microbiol. *3:*51–61, 1976.
35. Roggli, V. L., Keener, S., Bradford W. D., et al.: Pulmonary pathology of Rocky Mountain spotted fever in children. Pediatr. Pathol. *4:*47–57, 1985.
36. Roth, R. M., and Gleckman, R. A.: Human infections derived from dogs. Postgrad. Med. *77:*169–180, 1985.
37. Rubio, T., Riley, H. D., Jr., Nida, J. R., et al.: Thrombocytopenia in Rocky Mountain spotted fever. Am. J. Dis. Child. *116:*88–96, 1968.
38. Scimeca, P. G., Weinblatt, M. E., and Kochen, J. A.: Acquired coagulation inhibitor in association with Rocky Mountain spotted fever. Clin. Pediatr. *26:*459–463, 1987.
39. Sexton, D. J., and Clapp, J.: Inappropriate antidiuretic hormone secretion. Arch. Intern. Med. *137:*362–363, 1977.
40. Sexton, D. J., and Corey, G. R.: Rocky Mountain "spotless" and "almost spotless" fever: A wolf in sheep's clothing. Clin. Infect. Dis. *15:*439–448, 1992.
41. Silverman, D. J.: Adherence of platelets to human endothelial cells infected by *Rickettsia rickettsii.* J. Infect. Dis. *153:*694–700, 1986.
42. Uchida, T.: *Rickettsia japonica*, the etiologic agent of Oriental spotted fever. Microbiol. Immunol. *37:*91–102, 1993.
43. Walker, D. H.: Rocky Mountain spotted fever: A disease in need of microbiological concern. Clin. Microbiol. Rev. *2:*227–240, 1989.
44. Walker, D. H., Gay, R. M., and Valdes-Dapena, M.: The occurrence of eschars in Rocky Mountain spotted fever. J. Am. Acad. Dermatol. *4:*571–576, 1981.
45. Walker, D. H., Hawkins, H. K., and Hudson, P.: Rocky Mountain spotted fever: Idiopathic characteristics associated with glucose-6-phosphate dehydrogenase deficiency. Arch. Pathol. Lab. Med. *107:*121–125, 1983.
46. Walker, D. H., Henderson, F. W., and Hutchins, G. M.: Rocky Mountain spotted fever: Mimicry of appendicitis or acute surgical abdomen? Am. J. Dis. Child. *140:*742–744, 1986.
47. Walker, D. H., and Mattern, W. B.: Acute renal failure in Rocky Mountain spotted fever. Arch. Intern. Med. *139:*443–448, 1979.
48. Walker, D. H., Montenegro, M. R., Hegarty, B. C., et al.: Rocky Mountain spotted fever vaccine. South. Med. J. *77:*447–449, 1984.
49. Walker, D. H., Paletta, C. E., and Cain, B. G.: Pathogenesis of myocarditis in Rocky Mountain spotted fever. Arch. Pathol. Lab. Med. *104:*171–174, 1980.
50. Weiss, E.: Growth and physiology of rickettsiae. Bacterial Dis. *37:*259–283, 1973.
51. Wells, G. M., Woodward, T. E., Fiset, P., et al.: Rocky Mountain spotted fever caused by blood transfusion. J. A. M. A. *239:*2763–2765, 1978.
52. White, W. L., Patrick, J. D., and Miller, L. R.: Evaluation of immunoperoxidase techniques to detect *Rickettsia rickettsii* in fixed tissue specimens. Am. J. Clin. Pathol. *101:*747–752, 1994.
53. Wilfert, C. M., MacCormack, J. N., Kleeman, K., et al.: The prevalence of antibodies to *Rickettsia rickettsii* in an area endemic for Rocky Mountain spotted fever. J. Infect. Dis. *151:*823–831, 1985.
54. Wolbach, S. B.: Studies on Rocky Mountain spotted fever. J. Med. Res. *41:*1–198, 1919.
55. Woodward, T. E., Pedersen, C. E., Jr., Oster, C. N., et al.: Prompt confirmation of Rocky Mountain spotted fever: Identification of rickettsiae in skin tissues. J. Infect. Dis. *134:*297–305, 1976.
56. Workman, J. B., Hightower, J. A., Borges, F., et al.: Cortisone as an adjunct to chloramphenicol in treatment of Rocky Mountain spotted fever. N. Engl. J. Med. *246:*962, 1952.
57. Wright, L.: Intellectual sequelae of Rocky Mountain spotted fever. J. Abnorm. Psychol. *80:*315–316, 1972.
58. Zaki, M. H.: Selected tickborne infections: A review of Lyme disease, Rocky Mountain spotted fever, and babesiosis. N. Y. State J. Med. *89:*320–335, 1989.

Mediterranean Spotted Fever

59. Adan, A., Lopez-Soto, A., Moser, C., et al.: Use of steroids and heparin to treat retinal arterial occlusion in Mediterranean spotted fever. J. Infect. Dis. *151:*1139, 1988.
60. Anderson, J. A., Magnarelli, L. A., Burgdorfer, W., et al.: Importation into the United States from Africa of *Rhipicephalus simus* on a boutonneuse fever patient. Am. J. Trop. Med. Hyg. *30:*897–899, 1981.
61. De La Fuente, L., Anda, P., Rodriguez, I., et al.: Evaluation of a latex agglutination test for *Rickettsia conorii* antibodies in seropositive patients. J. Med. Microbiol. *28:*69–72, 1989.
62. DeMicco, C., Raoult, D., Benderitter, T., et al.: Immune complex vasculitis associated with Mediterranean spotted fever. J. Infect. *14:*163–165, 1987.
63. Diez Ruiz, A., Ramos Jimenez, A., Lopez Ruz, M. A., et al.: Boutonneuse fever transmitted by conjunctival inoculation. Klin. Wochenschr. *66:*1212–1213, 1988.
64. Font-Creus, B., Bella-Cueto, C., Tringali, G. R., et al.: Mediterranean spotted fever: A cooperative study of 227 cases. Rev. Infect. Dis. *7:*635–642, 1985.
65. Gross, E. M., Yagupsky, P., Torok, V., et al.: Resurgence of Mediterranean spotted fever. Lancet *2:*1107, 1982.
66. Gudiol, F., Pallares, R., Carratala, J., et al.: Randomized double-blind evaluation of ciprofloxacin and doxycycline for Mediterranean spotted fever. Antimicrob. Agents Chemother. *33:*987–988, 1989.
67. Harris, R. L., Kaplan, S. L., Bradshaw, M. W., et al.: Boutonneuse fever in American travelers. J. Infect. Dis. *153:*126–128, 1986.
68. Hechemy, K. E., Raoult, D., Eisemann, C., et al.: Detection of antibodies to *Rickettsia conorii* with latex agglutination test in patients with Mediterranean spotted fever. J. Infect. Dis. *153:*132–135, 1986.
69. Mansueto, S., Vitale, G., Bentinegna, M., et al.: Persistence of antibodies to *Rickettsia conorii* after an acute attack of boutonneuse fever. J. Infect. Dis. *151:*377, 1985.
70. Montenegro, M. R., Mansueto, S., Hegarty, B. C., et al.: The histology of "taches noires" of boutonneuse fever and demonstration of *Rickettsia conorii* in them by immunofluorescence. Virchows Arch. *900:*309–317, 1983.
71. Moraga, F. A., Martinez-Roig, A., Alonso J. L., et al.: Boutonneuse fever. Arch. Dis. Child. *57:*149–151, 1982.
72. San Jose, A., Bosch, J. A., Arderiu, A., et al.: Myositis due to *Rickettsia conorii* infection. Trans. R. Soc. Trop. Med. Hyg. *82:*346, 1988.
73. Teysseire, N., and Raoult, D.: Comparison of Western immunoblotting and microimmunofluorescence for diagnosis of Mediterranean spotted fever. J. Clin. Microbiol. *30:*455–460, 1992.
74. Walker, D. H., Occhino, C., Tringali, G. R., et al.: Pathogenesis of rickettsial eschars: The tache noire of boutonneuse fever. Hum. Pathol. *19:*1449–1454, 1988.
75. Walker, D. H., Staiti, A., Mansueto, S., et al.: Frequent occurrence of hepatic lesions in boutonneuse fever. Acta Trop. *43:*175–181, 1986.
76. Williams, W. J., Radulovic, S., Dasch, G. A., et al.: Identification of *Rickettsia conorii* infection by a polymerase chain reaction in a soldier returning from Somalia. Clin. Infect. Dis. *19:*93–99, 1994.
77. Yagupsky, P., and Wolach, B.: Fatal Israeli spotted fever in children. Clin. Infect. Dis. *17:*850–853, 1993.

Other Tick Typhus Fevers

78. Prias, M. A., Calia, G., Saba, F., et al.: Glucose-6-phosphate dehydrogenase deficiency in male patients with Mediterranean spotted fever in Sardinia. J. Infect. Dis. *147:*607–608, 1983.

Rickettsialpox

79. Brettman, C. R., Lewin, S., Holymein, R. S., et al.: Rickettsialpox: Report of an outbreak and a contemporary review. Medicine *60:*363–372, 1981.
80. Dolgopol, V. V.: Histologic changes in rickettsialpox. Am. J. Pathol. *24:*119, 1948.
81. Greenberg, M., and Pellitteri, O. J.: Rickettsialpox. Bull. N. Y. Acad. Med. *23:*338, 1947.
82. Greenberg, M., Pellitteri, O. J., and Jellison, W. L.: Rickettsialpox: A newly recognized rickettsial disease. III. Epidemiology. Am. J. Public Health *37:*860–868, 1947.
83. Greenberg, M., Pellitteri, O. J., Klein, I. F., et al.: Rickettsialpox: A newly recognized rickettsial disease. II. Clinical observation. J. A. M. A. *133:*901, 1947.
84. Grossman, E. R., Walchek, A., and Freedman, H.: Tetracyclines and permanent teeth: The relation between dose and tooth color. Pediatrics *47:*567, 1971.
85. Huebner, R. J., Jellison, W. L., and Armstrong, C.: Rickettsialpox: A newly recognized rickettsial disease. V. Recovery of *Rickettsia akari* from a house mouse *(Mus musculus).* Public Health Rep. *62:*777–780, 1947.
86. Huebner, R. J., Jellison, W. L., and Pomerantz, C.: Rickettsialpox: A newly recognized rickettsial disease. IV. Isolation of a rickettsia apparently identical with the causative agent of rickettsialpox from *Allodermanyssus sanguineus,* a rodent mite. Public Health Rep. *61:*1677–1682, 1946.
87. Huebner, R. J., Stamps, P., and Armstrong, C.: Rickettsialpox: A newly recognized rickettsial disease. I. Isolation of the etiologic agent. Public Health Rep. *61:*1605–1614, 1946.
88. Jacobson, J. M., Desmond, E. P., Kornblee, L. V., et al.: Positive Weil-Felix reactions in a case of rickettsialpox. Int. J. Dermatol. *28:*271–272, 1989.
89. Kass, E. M., Szaniawski, W. K., Levy, H., et. al.: Rickettsialpox in a New York City hospital, 1980 to 1989. N. Engl. J. Med. *331:*1612–1617, 1994.
90. Krinsky, W. L.: Does epizootic lymphocytic choriomeningitis prime the pump for epidemic rickettsialpox? Rev. Infect. Dis. *5:*1118–1119, 1983.
91. LaBocetta, A. C., Israel, H. L., Perri, A. M., et al.: Rickettsialpox: Report of four apparent cases in Pennsylvania. Am. J. Med. *13:*413, 1952.
92. Lerner, A. M., Klein, J. O., Cherry, J. D., et al.: New viral exanthems. N. Engl. J. Med. *269:*678, 736, 1963.
93. Murray, E. S., and Snyder, J. C.: Brill's Disease. II. Etiology. Am. J. Hyg. *53:*22, 1951.

94. Shankman, B.: Report of an outbreak of endemic febrile illness not identified, occurring in NYC. N. Y. State J. Med. *46*:2156, 1946.
95. Sleisinger, M. H., Murray, E. S., and Cohen, S.: Rickettsialpox case due to laboratory infection. Public Health Rep. *66*:311, 1951.
96. Sussman, L. N.: Kew Gardens' spotted fever. N. Y. Med. *2*:27, 1946.
97. Zdrodovskii, P. F., and Golinevich, E. H.: Vesicular and varioliform rickettsioses (rickettsialpox). *In* Zdrodovskii, P. F., and Golinevich, E. H. (eds.): The Rickettsial Diseases. New York, Pergamon Press, 1960, pp. 340–353.

Typhus Group

98. Adams, W. H., Emmons, R. W., and Brooks, J. E.: The changing ecology of murine (endemic) typhus in southern California. Am. J. Trop. Med. Hyg. *19*:311–318, 1970.
99. Brezina, R.: Diagnosis and control of rickettsial diseases. Acta Virol. *29*:338–349, 1985.
100. Current trends: Murine typhus. M. M. W. R. *31*:555–561, 1982.
101. Current trends: Outbreak of murine typhus: Texas. M. M. W. R. *32*:131–132, 1983.
102. Dasch, G. A.: Isolation of species-specific protein antigen of *Rickettsia typhi* and *Rickettsia prowazekii* for immunodiagnosis and immunoprophylaxis. J. Clin. Microbiol. *14*:333–341, 1981.
103. Diab, S. M., Araj, G. F., and French, F. F.: Cardiovascular and pulmonary complications of epidemic typhus. Trop. Geogr. Med. *41*:76–79, 1989.
104. Duma, R. J., Soneshine, D. E., Bozeman, F. M., et al.: Epidemic typhus in the United States associated with flying squirrels. J. A. M. A. *245*:2318–2323, 1981.
105. Dumler, J. S.: Murine typhus. Semin. Pediatr. Infect. Dis. *5*:137–142, 1994.
106. Gaon, J. A., and Murray, E. S.: The natural history of recrudescent typhus (Brill-Zinsser disease) in Bosnia. Bull. W. H. O. *35*:133–141, 1966.
107. Hechemy, K. E., Osterman, J. V., Eisemann, C. S., et al.: Detection of typhus antibodies by latex agglutination. J. Clin. Microbiol. *13*:214–220, 1981.
108. McDade, J. E., Shepard, C. C., Redus, M. A., et al.: Evidence of *Rickettsia prowazekii* infections in the United States. Am. J. Trop. Med. Hyg. *29*:277–284, 1980.
109. Older, J. J.: The epidemiology of murine typhus in Texas, 1969. J. A. M. A. *214*:2011–2017, 1970.
110. Perine, P. L., Chandler, B. P., Krause, D. K., et al.: A clinico-epidemiological study of epidemic typhus in Africa. Clin. Infect. Dis. *14*:1149–1158, 1992.
111. Perine, P. L., Krause, D. W., Awoke, S., et al.: Single-dose doxycycline treatment of louse-borne relapsing fever and epidemic typhus. Lancet *2*:742–744, 1974.
112. Schriefer, M. E., Sacci, J. B., Jr., and Dumler, J. S.: Identification of a novel rickettsial infection in a patient diagnosed with murine typhus. J. Clin. Microbiol. *32*:949–954, 1994.
113. White, P. C., Jr.: A brief historical review of murine typhus in Virginia and the United States. Va. Med. Monthly *94*:16–23, 1970.
114. Wolfman, D. E., Fenton, W., Jr., and Donald, P. J.: Typhus-induced facial necrosis. Otolaryngol. Head Neck Surg. *94*:390–393, 1986.
115. Woo, M. L., Leung, J. W., and French, G. L.: Rickettsial infection presenting as culture-negative meningitis. Postgrad. Med. J. *64*:614–616, 1988.
116. Zinsser, H.: Rats, Lice and History. New York, Blue Ribbon Books, 1943.

Scrub Typhus

117. Brown, G. W., Saunders, J. P., Singh, S., et al.: Single dose doxycycline therapy in scrub typhus. Trans. R. Soc. Trop. Med. Hyg. *72*:412–416, 1978.
118. Chayakul, P., Panich, V., and Silpapojakul, K.: Scrub typhus pneumonitis: An entity which is frequently missed. Q. J. Med. *68*:595–602, 1988.
119. Crum, J. W., Hanchaley, S., and Eamsila, C.: New paper enzyme-linked immunosorbent technique compared with microimmunofluorescence for detection of human serum antibodies to *Rickettsia tsutsugamushi*. J. Clin. Microbiol. *11*:584–588, 1980.
120. Furuya, Y., Yamamoto, S., Otu, M., et al.: Use of monoclonal antibodies against *Rickettsia tsutsugamushi* Kawasaki for serodiagnosis by enzyme-linked immunosorbent assay. J. Clin. Microbiol. *29*:340–345, 1991.
121. Furuya, Y., Yoshida, Y., Katayama, T., et al.: Serotype-specific amplification of *Rickettsia tsutsugamushi* DNA by nested polymerase chain reaction. J. Clin. Microbiol. *31*:1637–1640, 1993.
122. Jin-ju, W., Gui-zhong, T., and Shi-feng, S.: Study on *Leptotrombidium gaohuensis* sp. nov.: Newly discovered vectors of tsutsugamushi disease. Chin. Med. J. *100*:590–594, 1987.
123. Kelly, D. J., Wong, P. W., Gan, E., et al.: Comparative evaluation of the indirect immunoperoxidase test for the serodiagnosis of rickettsial disease. Am. J. Trop. Med. Hyg. *38*:400–406, 1988.
124. Ley, H. L., Jr., Diercks, F. H., Paterson, P. Y., et al.: Immunization against scrub typhus. IV. Living Karp vaccine and chemoprophylaxis in volunteers. Am. J. Hyg. *56*:303–312, 1952.
125. Ognibene, A. J., O'Leary, D. S., Czarnecki, S. W., et al.: Myocarditis and disseminated intravascular coagulation in scrub typhus. Am. J. Med. Sci. *262*:233–239, 1971.
126. Ohashi, N., Tamura, A., and Suto, T.: Immunoblotting analysis of anti-rickettsial antibodies produced in patients of tsutsugamushi disease. Microbiol. Immunol. *32*:1085–1092, 1988.
127. Olson, J. G., Bourgeois, A. L., Fang, R. C., et al.: Prevention of scrub typhus. Am. J. Trop. Med. Hyg. *29*:989–997, 1980.
128. Saunders, J. P., Brown, G. W., Shirai, A., et al.: The longevity of antibody to *Rickettsia tsutsugamushi* in patients with confirmed scrub typhus. Trans. R. Soc. Trop. Med. Hyg. *74*:253–257, 1980.
129. Shirai, A., Brown, G. W., Gan, E., et al.: *Rickettsia tsutsugamushi* antibody in mother cord pairs of sera. Jpn. J. Med. Sci. Biol. *34*:37–39, 1981.
130. Smadel, J. E., Bailey, C. A., and Diercks, F. H.: Chloramphenicol (chloromycetin) in the chemoprophylaxis of scrub typhus (tsutsugamushi disease). IV. Relapses of scrub typhus in treated volunteers and their prevention. Am. J. Hyg. *51*:229–241, 1950.
131. Twartz, J. C., Shirai, A., Selvaraju, G., et al.: Doxycycline prophylaxis for human scrub typhus. J. Infect. Dis. *146*:811–818, 1982.
132. Urakami, H., Yamamoto, S., Tsuruhar, T., et al.: Serodiagnosis of scrub typhus with antigens immobilized on nitrocellulose sheet. J. Clin. Microbiol. *27*:1841–1846, 1989.

Q Fever

133. Andrews, P. S., and Marmion, B. P.: Morbid anatomical and bacteriological findings in a patient with endocarditis. Br. Med. J. *1*:983, 1959.
134. Bental, T., Fejgin, M., Keysary, A., et al.: Chronic Q fever of pregnancy presenting as *Coxsiella burnetti* placentitis: Successful outcome following therapy with erythromycin and rifampin. Clin. Infect. Dis. *21*:1318–1321, 1995.
135. Bernard, K. W., Parham, G. L., Winkler, W. G., et al.: Q fever control measures: Recommendations for research facilities using sheep. Infect. Control *3*:461–464, 1982.
136. Biggs, B. A., Douglas, J. G., Grant, I. W., et al.: Prolonged Q fever associated with inappropriate secretion of antidiuretic hormone. J. Infect. *8*:61–63, 1984.
137. Brown, G. L., Colwell, D. L., and Hooper, W. L.: An outbreak of Q fever in Staffordshire. J. Hyg. (Camb.) *66*:649–655, 1968.
138. Cardellach, F., Font, J., Agusti, A. G., et al.: Q fever and hemolytic anemia. J. Infect. Dis. *148*:769, 1983.
139. Centers for Disease Control: Q fever at a university research center: California. M. M. W. R. *28*:333–334, 1979.
140. Curet, L. B., and Paust, J. C.: Transmission of Q fever from experimental sheep to laboratory personnel. Am. J. Obstet. Gynecol. *114*:566–568, 1972.
141. D'Angelo, L. J.: Q fever treated with erythromycin. Br. Med. J. *2*:305–306, 1979.
142. Diebel, R., Osterhout, G., and Culver, J.: Immune globulin to *Coxiella burnetii* in man determined by radioisotope precipitation technic. Am. J. Epidemiol. *90*:262–268, 1969.
143. Edlinger, E.: Immunofluorescence serology: A tool for prognosis of Q fever. Diagn. Microbiol. Infect. Dis. *3*:343–351, 1985.
144. Ferrante, M. A., and Dolan, M. J.: Q fever meningoencephalitis in a soldier returning from the Persian Gulf war. Clin. Infect. Dis. *16*:489–496, 1993.
145. Field, P. R., Hunt, J. G., and Murphy, A. M.: Detection and persistence of specific IgM antibody to *Coxiella burnetii* by enzyme-linked immunosorbent assay: A comparison with immunofluorescence and complement fixation tests. J. Infect. Dis. *148*:477–487, 1983.
146. Hall, C. J., Richmond, S. J., Caul, E. O., et al.: Laboratory outbreak of Q fever acquired from sheep. Lancet *1*:1004–1006, 1982.
147. Henderson, R. J.: Q fever and leptospirosis in the dairy farming community and allied workers of Worcestershire. J. Clin. Pathol. *22*:511–514, 1969.
148. Hofmann, C. E., and Heaton, J. W., Jr.: Q fever hepatitis: Clinical manifestations and pathological findings. Gastroenterology *83*:474–479, 1982.
149. Hunt, J. G., Field, P. R., and Murphy, A. M.: Immunoglobulin responses to *Coxiella burnetii* (Q fever): Single-serum diagnosis of acute infection using an immunofluorescence technique. Infect. Immun. *39*:977–981, 1983.
150. Hunter, W. H.: Some problems in Q fever infections in New South Wales. Med. J. Aust. *1*:900–904, 1968.
151. Janigan, D. T., and Maine, T. J.: An inflammatory pseudotumor of the lung in Q fever pneumonia. N. Engl. J. Med. *308*:86–88, 1983.
152. Kazar, J.: Immunity in Q fever. Acta Virol. *32*:358–368, 1988.
153. Kazar, J., and Rehacek, J.: Q fever vaccines: Present status and application in man. Zentralbl. Bakteriol. Mikrobiol. [A] *267*:74–78, 1987.
154. Kimbrough, R. C., III, Ormsbee, R. A., and Peacock, M. G.: Q fever endocarditis: A three and one-half year follow-up. *In* Burgdorfer, W., and Anacker, R. L. (eds.): Rickettsiae and Rickettsial Diseases. New York, Academic Press, 1981, pp. 125–132.
155. Lim, K. C., and Kang, J. Y.: Q fever presenting with gastroenteritis. Med. J. Aust. *1*:327, 1980.
156. Luoto, L., and Huebner, R. J.: Q fever studies in southern California. IX. Isolation of Q fever organisms from parturient placentas of naturally infected dairy cows. Public Health Rep. *65*:541–544, 1950.
157. Meiklejohn, G., Reimer, L. G., Graves, P. S., et al.: Cryptic epidemic of Q fever in a medical school. J. Infect. Dis. *144*:107–113, 1981.
158. Millar, J. K.: The chest film findings in Q fever: A series of 35 cases. Clin. Radiol. *29*:371–375, 1978.
159. Murphy, A. M., and Hunt, J. G.: Retrospective diagnosis of Q fever in a

country abattoir by the use of specific IgM globulin estimations. Med. J. Aust. *2*:326–327, 1981.
160. Murphy, P. P., and Richardson, S. G.: Q fever pneumonia presenting as an eosinophilic pleural effusion. Thorax *44*:228–229, 1989.
161. Ormsbee, R. A., Parker, H., and Pickens, E. C.: The comparative effectiveness of aureomycin, terramycin, chloramphenicol, erythromycin, and thiocymetin in suppressing experimental rickettsial infections in chick embryos. J. Infect. Dis. *96*:162, 1955.
162. Peacock, M. G., Philip, R. N., Wilhams, J. C., et al.: Serological evaluation of Q fever in humans: Enhanced phase I titers of immunoglobulin G and A are diagnostic for Q fever endocarditis. Infect. Immun. *41*:1089–1098, 1983.
163. Pellegrin, M., Delsol, G., Auvergnat, J. C., et al.: Granulomatous hepatitis in Q fever. Hum. Pathol. *11*:51–57, 1980.
164. Pierce, T. H., Tucht, S. C., Gorin, A. B., et al.: Q fever pneumonitis: Diagnosis by transbronchoscopic lung biopsy. West. J. Med. *130*:453–455, 1979.
165. Pinsky, R. L., Fishbein, D. B., Greene, C. R., et. al.: An outbreak of cat-associated Q fever in the United States. J. Infect. Dis. *164*:202-204, 1991.
166. Powell, O. W.: Liver involvement in Q fever. Aust. Ann. Med. *10*:52–58, 1961.
167. Raoult, D., and Marrie, T.: Q fever. Clin. Infect. Dis. *20*:489–496, 1995.
168. Raoult, D., Urvolgyi, J., Etienne, J., et al.: Diagnosis of endocarditis in acute Q fever by immunofluorescence serology. Acta Virol. *32*:70–74, 1988.
169. Richardus, J. H., Dumas, A. M., Huisman, J., et al.: Q fever in infancy: A review of 18 cases. Pediatr. Infect. Dis. *4*:369–373, 1985.
170. Roges, G., and Edlinger, E.: Immunoenzymatic test for Q fever. Diagn. Microbiol. Infect. Dis. *4*:125–132, 1986.
171. Ruiz-Contreras, J., Montero, R. G., Amador, J. T. R., et. al.: Q fever in children. Am. J. Dis. Child. *147*:300–302, 1993.
172. Schachter, J., Sung, M., and Meyer, K. F.: Potential danger of Q fever in a university hospital environment. J. Infect. Dis. *123*:301–304, 1971.
173. Simor, A. E., Bruntan, J. L., Salit, I. E., et al.: Q fever: Hazard from sheep used in research. Can. Med. Assoc. J. *130*:1013–1016, 1984.
174. Subramanya, N. I., Wright, J. S., and Kahn, M. A.: Failure of rifampin and co-trimoxazole in Q fever endocarditis. Br. Med. J. *285*:343–344, 1982.
175. Tobin, M. J., Cahill, N., Gearty, G., et al.: Q fever endocarditis. Am. J. Med. *72*:396–400, 1982.
176. Uff, J. S., and Evans, D. J.: Mesango-capillary glomerulonephritis associated with Q fever endocarditis. Histopathology *1*:463–472, 1977.
177. Voigt, J. J., Delsol, G., and Fabre, J.: Liver and bone marrow granulomas in Q fever. Gastroenterology *84*:887–888, 1983.
178. Whittick, J. W.: Necropsy findings in a case of Q fever in Britain. Br. Med. J. *1*:979–980, 1950.
179. Wisniewski, H. J., and Krumbiegel, E. R.: Epidemiological studies of Q fever in humans. Arch. Environ. Health *21*:66–70, 1970.
180. Yeaman, M. R., Roman, M. J., and Baca, O. G.: Antibiotic susceptibilities of two *Coxiella burnetti* isolates implicated in distinct clinical syndromes. Antimicrob. Agents Chemother. *33*:1052–1057, 1989.

EHRLICHIOSIS

181. Anderson, B. E., Dawson, J. E., Jones, D. C., et. al.: *Ehrlichia chaffeensis*, a new species associated with human ehrlichiosis. J. Clin. Microbiol. *29*:2838–2842, 1991.
182. Anderson, B. E., Sumner, J. W., Dawson, J. E., et al.: Detection of the etiologic agent of human ehrlichiosis by polymerase chain reaction. J. Clin. Microbiol. *30*:775–780, 1992.
183. Bakken, J. S., Dumler, J. S., Chen, S.-M., et al.: Human granulocytic ehrlichiosis in the upper midwest United States: A new species emerging? J. A. M. A. *272*:212–218, 1994.
184. Barton, L. L., Dawson, J. E., Letson, G. W., et al.: Simultaneous ehrlichiosis and Lyme disease. Pediatr. Infect. Dis. J. *9*:127–129, 1990.
185. Barton, L. L., and Foy, T. M.: *Ehrlichia canis* infection in a child. Pediatrics *4*:580–582, 1989.
186. Barton, L. L., Rathore, M. H., and Dawson, J. E.: Infection with *Ehrlichia* in childhood. J. Pediatr. *120*:998–1001, 1992.
187. Brouqui, P., and Raoult, D.: In vitro antibiotic susceptibility of the newly recognized agent of ehrlichiosis in humans, *Ehrlichia chaffeensis*. Antimicrob. Agents Chemother. *36*:2799–2803, 1992.
188. Centers for Disease Control and Prevention: Human granulocytic ehrlichiosis: New York, 1995. M. M. W. R. *44*:593–595, 1995.
189. Dimmitt, D. C., Fishbein, D. B., and Dawson, J. E.: Human ehrlichiosis associated with cerebrospinal fluid pleocytosis: A case report. Am. J. Med. *87*:677–678, 1989.
190. Doran, T. I., Parmley, R. T., Logas, P. C., et al.: Infection with *Ehrlichia canis* in a child. J. Pediatr. *114*:809–812, 1989.
191. Dumler, J. S., and Bakken, J. S. Ehrlichial diseases of humans: Emerging tick-borne infections. Clin. Infect. Dis. *20*:1102–1110, 1995.
192. Dumler, J. S., Dawson, J. E., and Walker, D. H.: Human ehrlichiosis: Hematopathology and immunohistologic detection of *Ehrlichia chaffeensis*. Hum. Pathol. *24*:391–396, 1993.
193. Dumler, J. S., Sutker, W. L., and Walker, D. H.: Persistent infection with *Ehrlichia chaffeensis*. Clin. Infect. Dis. *17*:903–905, 1993.
194. Edwards, M. S.: Ehrlichiosis in children. Semin. Pediatr. Infect. Dis. *5*:143–147, 1994.
195. Edwards, M. S., Jones, J. E., Leass, D. L., et al.: Childhood infection caused by *Ehrlichia canis* or a closely related organism. Pediatr. Infect. Dis. J. *7*:651–654, 1988.
196. Everett, E. D., Evans, K. A., Henry, R. B., et al.: Human ehrlichiosis in adults after tick exposure: Diagnosis using polymerase chain reaction. Ann. Intern. Med. *120*:730–735, 1994.
197. Fichtenbaum, C. J., Peterson, L. R., and Weil, G. J.: Ehrlichiosis presenting as a life-threatening illness with features of toxic shock syndrome. Am. J. Med. *95*:351–357, 1993.
198. Fishbein, D. B., Dawson, J. E., and Robinson, L. E.: Human ehrlichiosis in the United States, 1985 to 1990. Ann. Intern. Med. *120*:736–743, 1994.
199. Fishbein, D. B., Kemp, A., Dawson, J. E., et al.: Human ehrlichiosis: Prospective active surveillance in febrile hospitalized patients. J. Infect. Dis. *160*:803–809, 1989.
200. Fishbein, D. B., Sawyer, L. A., Holland, C. J., et al.: Unexplained febrile illnesses after exposure to ticks: Infection with an *Ehrlichia?* J. A. M. A. *257*:3100–3104, 1987.
201. Golden, S. E.: Aseptic meningitis associated with *Ehrlichia canis* infection. Pediatr. Infect. Dis. J. *8*:335–337, 1989.
202. Hardalo, C. J., Quagliarello, V., and Dumler, J. S.: Human granulocytic ehrlichiosis in Connecticut: Report of a fatal case. Clin. Infect. Dis. *21*:910–914, 1995.
203. Harkess, J. R., Ewing, S. A., Brumit, T., et al.: Ehrlichiosis in children. Pediatrics *87*:199–203, 1991.
204. Harkess, J. R., Ewing, S. A., Crutcher, J. M., et al.: Human ehrlichiosis in Oklahoma. J. Infect. Dis. *159*:576–579, 1989.
205. Maeda, K., Markowitz, N., Hawley, R. C., et al.: Human infection with *Ehrlichia canis*, a leukocytic rickettsia. N. Engl. J. Med. *316*:853–856, 1987.
206. Malpass, D. G., Heiman, H. S., and Sumaya, C. V.: Childhood ehrlichiosis: A case report and review of the literature. Int. Pediatr. *6*:354–358, 1991.
207. McDade, J. E.: Ehrlichiosis: A disease of animals and humans. J. Infect. Dis. *161*:609–617, 1990.
208. Paddock, C. D., Suchard, D. P., Grumbach, K. L., et al.: Brief report: Fatal seronegative ehrlichiosis in a patient with HIV infection. N. Engl. J. Med. *329*:1164–1167, 1993.
209. Pancholi, P., Kolbert, C. P., Mitchell, P. D., et al.: *Ixodes dammini* as a potential vector of human granulocytic ehrlichiosis. J. Infect. Dis. *172*:1007–1012, 1995.
210. Petersen, L. R., Sawyer, L. A., Fishbein, D. B., et al.: An outbreak of ehrlichiosis in members of an army reserve unit exposed to ticks. J. Infect. Dis. *159*:562–568, 1989.
211. Rauch, A. M.: Kawasaki syndrome: Review of new epidemiologic and laboratory developments. Pediatr. Infect. Dis. J. *6*:1016–1021, 1987.
212. Reed, K. D., Mitchell, P. D., Persing, D. H., et al.: Transmission of human granulocytic ehrlichiosis. J. A. M. A. *273*:23, 1995.
213. Ristic, M.: Pertinent characteristics of leukocyte rickettsiae of humans and animals. *In* Leive, L., Bonzentree, P. S., Morello, J. A., et al. (eds.): Microbiology 1986. Washington, D.C., American Society for Microbiology, 1986, pp. 182–187.
214. Rohrbach, B. W., Harkess, J. R., Ewing, S. A., et al.: Epidemiologic and clinical characteristics of persons with serologic evidence of *E. canis* infection. Am. J. Public Health *80*:442–445, 1990.
215. Roland, W. E., McDonald, G., Caldwell, C. W., et al.: Ehrlichiosis: A cause of prolonged fever. Clin. Infect. Dis. *20*:821–825, 1995.
216. Standaert, S. M., Dawson, J. E., Schaffner, W., et al.: Ehrlichiosis in a golf-oriented retirement community. N. Engl. J. Med. *333*:420–425, 1995.
217. Taylor, J. P., Betz, T. G., Fishbein, D. B., et al.: Serological evidence of possible human infection with *Ehrlichia* in Texas. J. Infect. Dis. *158*:217–220, 1988.
218. Walker, J. S., Rundquist, J. D., Taylor, R., et al.: Clinical and clinicopathologic findings in tropical canine pancytopenia. J. Am. Vet. Med. Assoc. *157*:43–55, 1970.

SECTION TWENTY

MYCOPLASMA

❑ ❑ ❑

195

MYCOPLASMA AND *UREAPLASMA* INFECTIONS

James D. Cherry

Mycoplasmas and ureaplasmas are the smallest free-living microorganisms; they are ubiquitous in nature. More than 92 species have been recovered from many animals, including human beings.[583] Of this group, 15 have been identified as human pathogens or as being part of the "normal" human flora, with *M. pneumoniae, M. hominis,* and *U. urealyticum* found to cause disease in children. A protean array of illness in children is due to infection with these organisms.

The generic name *Mycoplasma* is derived from Greek and Latin. *Myco* refers to the mycelial, or filamentous, characteristic, and *plasma* indicates the plasticity and pleomorphism of the organism.[572] *Urea* in *Ureaplasma* indicates the presence of urease in this genus.[199]

HISTORY

In 1898, Nocard and Roux[444] recovered the first *Mycoplasma* species from cattle with contagious pleuropneumonia. Shortly after the original discovery, many other mycoplasmas were recovered from several different animals.[239] These other mycoplasmas, which frequently were not associated with disease, originally were called pleuropneumonia-like organisms; this designation was abbreviated to PPLO. The term PPLO enjoyed general use until the early 1960s.

The first isolation of a mycoplasma from a human was reported in 1937 by Dienes and Edsall.[136] This organism, now recognized as *M. hominis,* was recovered from an abscessed Bartholin gland. In 1944, Eaton and colleagues[145] reported the recovery of an organism, originally called the Eaton agent, from persons ill with primary atypical pneumonia. The Eaton agent was considered to be a virus for many years, even though it was inhibited by streptomycin and chlortetracycline.[143, 144] In 1961, Marmion and Goodburn[382] noted that the Eaton agent was similar morphologically to pleuropneumonia-like organisms. In 1962, the organism now known as *M. pneumoniae* was cultivated on a cell-free agar medium and was shown in human volunteer studies to be the etiologic agent of primary atypical pneumonia.[83, 239]

In 1954, Shepard[518] reported the recovery of PPLOs with a distinctive small-colony characteristic from men with and without nongonococcal urethritis. These T strains (T for tiny), as they were called, now are classified as *U. urealyticum.* Several mycoplasmas have been noted to co-infect patients with HIV infections.[412]

CLASSIFICATION

Mycoplasma and *Ureaplasma* are the two genera of the family Mycoplasmataceae, in the order Mycoplasmatales, which belongs to the class Mollicutes.[199] Both *Mycoplasma* and *Ureaplasma* species require sterol for growth, have a genome with a molecular weight of about 4.5×10^8, and have nicotinamide adenine dinucleotide (NADH) oxidase localized in the cytoplasm. These species lack a cell wall, as do all organisms within the class Mollicutes.[266] Members of the genus *Mycoplasma* do not hydrolyze urea, whereas the three species within the genus *Ureaplasma* do.

There presently are 13 *Mycoplasma,* one *Ureaplasma,* and one *Acholeplasma* species that are part of the "normal" human mollicate flora.[77, 148, 199, 348, 578, 583] These organisms are listed by site of most common isolation and frequency of occurrence in Table 195–1. *M. salivarium* and *M. orale* commonly are part of the normal respiratory flora and have not been associated with illness in nonimmunocompromised persons. *M. hominis* and *U. urealyticum* also are recovered commonly from humans, and frequently they are related causally to illness.

M. buccale, M. faucium, M. primatum, A. laidlawii, and *M. lipophilum* are rarely isolated organisms and at present are not thought to cause disease in nonimmunocompromised humans. *M. genitalium* and *M. fermentans* have biologic and morphologic features that suggest they may be pathogenic in people, but their role in human genital disease has not been established.[567, 584] Persistent infections in blood, bones, joints, and kidneys with *M. fermentans, U. urealyticum, M. penetrans, M. pirum,* and *M. hominis* have occurred in patients with immunodeficiencies.[21, 410, 584] *M. pneumoniae* is a common cause of respiratory and other human illness.

TABLE 195–1. Mollicute Flora of Humans Listed by Site of Most Common Isolation and Prevalence[378, 348, 539, 578, 584, 586]

Organism	Prevalence
Respiratory tract	
Mycoplasma salvarium	Very common
Mycoplasma orale	Very common
Mycoplasma buccale	Rare
Mycoplasma faucium	Rare
Mycoplasma lipophilum	Rare
Mycoplasma pneumoniae	Common
Acholeplasma laidlawii	Rare
Genitourinary tract	
Mycoplasma hominis	Very common
Mycoplasma genitalium	Rare
Mycoplasma fermentans	Rare
Mycoplasma primatum	Rare
Mycoplasma spermatophilum	Rare
Mycoplasma penetrans	Rare
Ureaplasma urealyticum	Very common
Blood	
Mycoplasma pirum	Rare

MYCOPLASMA PNEUMONIAE

Properties

Morphology

Because mycoplasmas lack a cell wall, they all tend to be pleomorphic. Kammer and colleagues[296] studied (by scanning electron microscopy) the morphologic characteristics of *M. pneumoniae* organisms grown in broth medium and grouped their observations by days of incubation. From 0.3 to 2 days, the predominant morphologic feature consisted of 0.51 ± 0.011 μm symmetric round forms in tightly packed clusters. During the interval from day 2 to day 6, branched and straight filaments and bulbs were the predominant forms. The bulbous elements had a diameter of 0.25 ± 0.006 μ, and the filamentous forms were 0.19 ± 0.005 μm in diameter. The filaments were intertwined, and occasional round forms were observed. From day 6 to day 10, the organisms had a rounded shape but were asymmetric. Their diameter was 0.72 ± 0.027 μm, and they occurred in groups of three or four cells. Biberfeld and Biberfeld[33] noted that *M. pneumoniae* filamentous forms varied in length from 1 to 5 μm.

The ultrastructure of *M. pneumoniae,* as well as of all members of the family Mycoplasmataceae, is relatively simple, consisting of cell membrane and cytoplasm.[199, 588] In 7-day *M. pneumoniae* cultures, Domermuth and associates[138] noted the following characteristics: elementary bodies 105 × 120 nm in diameter; mature cells with a maximum diameter of 690 × 750 nm and an average diameter of 440 × 590 nm; asymmetry of limiting membrane; electron-dense lines outside the limiting membrane; and dense bodies as cytoplasmic inclusions.

Wilson and Collier[623] studied the ultrastructure of *M. pneumoniae* in hamster tracheal organ culture and noted filamentous organisms with trilaminar membranes; the cells were polymorphic, but each had a specialized terminal structure at the site of attachment to the organ culture. This terminal structure had a dense central core containing a denser central filament. Between the organism and the organ culture cell, fusion was not detected, but there was a loose network of fibrils between the two surfaces. The bodies of the mycoplasmas contained densely staining fibrillar material and cytoplasmic granules, both of which contained nucleic acids.

Motility and Multiplication

Bredt[55] studied *M. pneumoniae* motility and multiplication on a glass surface in liquid medium by phase contrast microscopy. It was observed that the organisms multiplied by binary fission; first, short filamentous structures were formed, which then separated into two cells. A growth cycle between two separations was about 3 hours. After division, the new cells moved by a gliding motion. The gliding speed has been noted to be about 0.2 to 0.5 μm/sec, but maximum speeds of 1.5 to 2.0 μm/sec have been observed.[477]

Composition

Mycoplasmas are composed of about 40 to 60 per cent protein, 10 to 20 per cent lipid, and a variable amount of carbohydrate. The *M. pneumoniae* genome is circular, double-stranded DNA with a contour length of 4.8 × 10^8 daltons.[416] The guanosine plus cytosine content of the DNA is 38.6 to 40.8 moles per cent.[46, 437, 565]

Growth Characteristics and Physical Properties[81, 239, 572, 588]

M. pneumoniae grows in *Mycoplasma* broth medium and on agar that is enriched with yeast extract and animal serum. *M. pneumoniae* ferments carbohydrates and requires sterol for growth. It grows under both anaerobic and aerobic conditions, but growth is more consistent when it is incubated in nitrogen and 5 per cent carbon dioxide. Compared with other mycoplasmas isolated from humans, *M. pneumoniae* grows relatively slowly, so that visible colony formation is rare in less than 1 week and may take 3 weeks or more. Repeated agar passage results in more rapid growth, so that laboratory strains produce colonies in 3 days.

M. pneumoniae colonies on agar generally appear different from the classic *Mycoplasma* "fried egg" look noted with other types recovered from humans. The *M. pneumoniae* colony is spherical and dense with a rough ("mulberry") surface.

M. pneumoniae has the following enzyme systems: $NADH_2$ oxidase, nicotinamide adenine dinucleotide phosphate $(NADPH)_2$ oxidase, lactic dehydrogenase, probably succinic dehydrogenase, and diaphorases.[239] In liquid medium, the following can be noted: acid color change in medium with added glucose and phenol red due to glucose metabolism, reduction of methylene blue in medium due to dehydrogenase activity, and reduction of 2-3-5 tetrazolium chloride to red formazan by dehydrogenase activity.[572]

On agar, *M. pneumoniae* hemolyzes erythrocytes in an agar overlay because of the liberation of peroxide. Erythrocytes and other cells adsorb to *M. pneumoniae* colonies, and organisms in suspension cause hemagglutination.

Mycoplasmas, including *M. pneumoniae,* are heat-sensitive. They have a half-life of less than 2 minutes at 50° C and lose viability within 1 week at room temperature.[588] They can be stored for several years at −20° C, but −70° C is optimal for long-term storage.

Mycoplasmas are resistant to osmotic environmental changes but are sensitive to detergents. They are inhibited by gold salts and antibiotics not directed against cell-wall synthesis.

Antigenic Composition

The following immunologic reactions have been noted in association with *M. pneumoniae*–host serum interactions: specific complement fixation; precipitation in gel; growth inhibition; indirect hemagglutination; metabolic inhibition; antigen-antibody union identified by immunofluorescence, enzyme-linked immunosorbent assay (ELISA), and radioimmunoassay; adherence inhibition assay; and nonspecific complement fixation (positive serologic test result for syphilis) and agglutination (cold and *Streptococcus* MG agglutinins).[68, 260, 273, 348, 473, 572] *M. pneumoniae* organisms have both membrane and cytoplasmic antigens.[162, 303] Two membrane antigens can be identified by immunodiffusion.[465] The major membrane antigen is found in the lipid fraction of the organism.[303] The antigens are glycolipids and are of major importance in complement fixation, metabolic inhibition, and mycoplasmacidal reactions.[65] The cytoplasmic (soluble) antigen, which also contains lipid, can be identified by complement fixation when the antigen is prepared by phenol extraction.

There are five principal protein antigens to which humans have an IgG immune response.[127, 197, 323, 479, 598] These five polypeptides have the following molecular masses: 170, 130, 90, 45, and 35 kd. The 170-kd antigen is the P1 protein. This protein is localized at the surface of the terminal organelle (terminal structure), is the major adhesin responsible for attachment, and is the cause of the gliding motility of the organism. Antibodies to the P1 protein inhibit hemadsorption and adherence to respiratory epithelium.[258, 259, 261, 272, 293, 324, 553] Dallo and associates[127, 128] have identified another adhesin-related 30-kd protein (P30 adhesin).

Membrane determinants of *M. pneumoniae* cross-react with the erythrocyte glycoprotein containing I antigen and the related sugar chain (F1)[242, 276]; pneumococcal serotypes 23 and 32[7]; and glycolipids of spinach, parsnips, carrots, and selected strains of *Staphylococcus aureus* and group A streptococci.[224, 304]

Animal Susceptibility

M. pneumoniae grows and causes pneumonia in hamsters and cotton rats and causes inapparent infection of the bronchial epithelium of chicken embryos.[473]

Epidemiology

Epidemic Pattern

In large urban areas, *M. pneumoniae* is endemic; infection and disease occur throughout the year. Foy and associates[180, 182] noted cultural or serologic evidence of *M. pneumoniae* infections in a Seattle prepaid medical care group during all seasons over an 11-year period. Similar endemicity has been noted in other studies.[409, 413, 443] In addition to the background endemic pattern, *M. pneumoniae* enjoys a cyclic epidemic pattern that is specific for a particular urban community. Epidemics have occurred at 3- to 7-year intervals.[152, 182, 291, 354, 443] Epidemics, which develop slowly, usually start in the fall and persist in the community for 12 to 30 months.

Incidence of Infection and Disease

In the past, illness due to *M. pneumoniae* in the general population was considered uncommon by most pediatricians and other physicians. Initial epidemiologic study was concerned mainly with the occurrence of pneumonia in closed populations, such as the military and boarding schools.[84, 409, 498, 550, 551, 595] During the last 30 years, many large studies in civilian populations, coupled with more sensitive serologic techniques, indicate that both infection and disease with *M. pneumoniae* are common.[4, 16, 18, 34, 62, 78, 117, 135, 140, 148, 164, 182, 186, 187, 189, 191, 193, 195, 211, 212, 215, 221, 255, 278, 286, 291, 354, 362, 413, 414, 443, 557]

Hornsleth[255] examined 367 serum samples collected from children hospitalized in Copenhagen from September 1963 to May 1965 for complement-fixing antibodies. He noted that 42 per cent of infants 6 to 11 months of age had demonstrable antibody; from 1 to 9 years of age, more than two-thirds of the children had antibody. Suhs and Feldman[557] noted a similar high prevalence of hemagglutinating-inhibiting antibody in the sera of Point Barrow, Alaska, residents, but only 5 per cent of serum samples from a children's home in Syracuse had measurable antibody.

Brunner and associates[62] noted serum antibody by the sensitive radioimmunoprecipitation test in 28 per cent of 7- to 12-month-old infants, 55 per cent of 13- to 24-month-old children, 67 per cent of 25- to 60-month-old children, and 97 per cent of persons older than 17 years of age. The high antibody prevalence noted in this study, as well as the findings in Copenhagen and Alaska, suggests an infection incidence rate of about 20 to 30 per cent per year in a susceptible population of young children. It is possible that the prevalent antibody noted at an early age in these studies is not due specifically to *M. pneumoniae* infection but is the result of exposure to the many cross-reacting antigens in nature.[7, 205, 304] However, studies by Fernald and colleagues,[164] in which infants and children in a day care center were monitored systemically, indicated a yearly infection rate of about 12 per cent.

Monto and colleagues,[413] in a large study involving 3243 persons, investigated the incidence of infection in six yearly cohort groups of children and adults. Infection was determined by significant rises in titer of complement-fixing antibody on three serum specimens collected during 1 year from each subject. The overall yearly infection rate was found to be 5.3 per cent. The highest rate (8.8 per cent) occurred in the 5- to 9-year-old group. Infants younger than 1 year of age had a rate of 2.8 per cent.

Brunner and associates[62] noted that geometric mean antibody titers tended to increase with increasing age, which suggested that the older children were being reinfected. Fernald and associates[164] noted that 5 of 22 children infected with *M. pneumoniae* in their investigation had reinfections during the 5-year observation period. In the study of Monto and associates,[413] 24.4 per cent of the 172 infections detected in subjects of all ages were reinfections. During a 12-year serologic surveillance period, Foy and associates[182] noted a great variation in incidence of *M. pneumoniae* infections; during the period from October 1965 to May 1966, only 0.2 per cent of 398 children had fourfold complement-fixation antibody titer rises, whereas during the May 1973 to May 1974 period, 35 per cent of 246 10- to 20-year-olds had serologic evidence of infection.

The incidence of disease due to *M. pneumoniae* depends on the endemic or epidemic prevalence of the organism in the community and is age-related. The incidence of *M. pneumoniae* by age for two epidemics and the surrounding endemic periods noted in Seattle by Foy and associates[182] is presented in Figure 195–1. The highest epidemic attack rate was 14 per 1000 children 5 to 9 years of age, and the highest endemic attack rate (4 per 1000) occurred in the same age group. Ten- to 14-year-old children had the second highest attack rate during both epidemic and endemic periods. The attack rate in children younger than 5 years of age was about twice that observed in young adults.

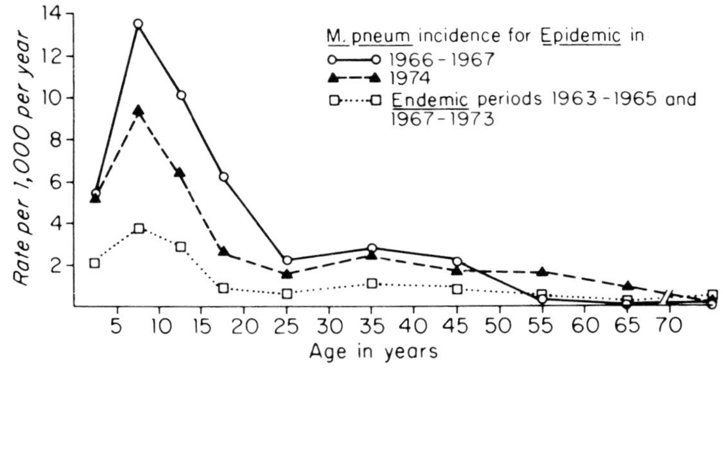

FIGURE 195–1. *Incidence of* Mycoplasma pneumoniae *pneumonia, by age, for two epidemics and the surrounding endemic periods in Seattle from 1963 to 1974. (From Foy, H. M., Kenny, G. E., Cooney, M. K., et al.: Long-term epidemiology of infections with* Mycoplasma pneumoniae. *J. Infect. Dis.* 139:681–687, 1979. *University of Chicago, publisher.)*

The ratio of symptomatic to asymptomatic infection has varied in different studies. In family studies, both Balassanian and Robbins[18] and Foy and associates[195] noted that only 15 per cent of infections were asymptomatic, whereas Saliba and associates[498] noted that 55 per cent of the residents of a boys' home had asymptomatic infection. Chanock and colleagues[84] observed that only 1 of 30 infections in Marine recruits was manifested as a clinically apparent pneumonia.

Incubation Period

The reported incubation period has varied from a mean of about 1 week in volunteer studies and point-source epidemics to 3 weeks in community outbreaks.[34, 117, 155, 193–195, 483, 501, 532, 583] In a volunteer study, Rifkind and colleagues[483] administered tissue culture–grown *M. pneumoniae* into the nose and posterior pharynx, in a concentration of 320 to 1280 EID_{50}, to 27 men with no demonstrable antibody. In this study, pneumonia occurred 9 to 12 days after inoculation, following 1 to 3 days of upper respiratory illness. In six volunteers, only upper respiratory illness occurred, and the incubation period varied from 4 to 9 days. In a similar study in which volunteers received 10^6 to 10^7 broth-grown organisms, the incubation period was 8 to 10 days.[533]

In an interesting common-source outbreak resulting from an intense 8-hour exposure at a party, the peak incubation period was 13 days, and the majority of cases occurred between day 11 and day 14.[155] In another probable point-source outbreak, which may have resulted from a room aerosol, the incubation period varied from 4 to 9 days.[501] In studies in families of case-to-case intervals, Foy and associates[195] noted a median incubation time of 23 days, with the majority of cases occurring between day 16 and day 25. In similar studies, Copps and colleagues[117] noted an average interval of 21 days, and Biberfeld and Sterner[34] found a modal value of 20 days. A point-source outbreak in a family unit was described in which all seven family members became ill 10 to 16 days after onset of symptoms in the index case.[305]

The longer incubation period in the family situation, compared with the volunteer studies and the point-source outbreaks, may be the result of larger inocula in the latter instances. An alternative explanation may be that in the community case-to-case situation, the index case may not transmit the organism effectively until symptoms have been manifest for a week or more.

Communicability

In contrast with other respiratory illnesses, such as measles and influenza, the spread of disease due to *M. pneumoniae* in both closed populations, such as military training units and boarding schools, and open communities usually is slow. For example, the introduction of influenza or measles into a family most often results in infection of all susceptible persons from the primary case. In contrast, the spread of *M. pneumoniae* through a family of six people likely would require three or four passages. Foy and associates[195] noted secondary attack rates in families of 64 per cent for children and 17 per cent for adults. Biberfeld and Sterner[34] noted secondary infection rates in families of 41 per cent and 84 per cent for adults and children, respectively. In contrast with family groups, the spread of *M. pneumoniae* in schools and other situations of brief exposure is low.[192, 193] In one Seattle elementary school, the infection rate was 18 per cent. Foy and colleagues[193] believe that neighborhood spread between playmates is more important than is school exposure in community *M. pneumoniae* transmission.

Transmission in families occurs during the acute phase of illness, and transmission by persons with asymptomatic infections has not been documented.[193]

Geography

The endemic and epidemic presence of *M. pneumoniae* has been demonstrated in urban areas in developed countries with temperate climates throughout the world.[34, 135, 158, 182, 193, 278, 354, 370, 380, 429, 443, 546] Serologic investigations in more remote areas, including both arctic and tropical zones, also indicate *M. pneumoniae* infection. Suhs and Feldman[557] found measurable antibody in the serum of 68 per cent of 169 persons in Point Barrow, and Golubjatnikov and associates,[215] in a study of children in a remote Mexican highland community, noted seropositivity in 16 per cent of 637 children. Serologic evidence of infection also has been noted in Cairo, Singapore, Hong Kong, the West Indies, and southern Africa.[79, 291] Incidence studies have not been performed in rural areas, but it seems likely that patterns of infection would be characterized by epidemic periods of a year or so and then complete absence of *M. pneumoniae* circulation for several years.

Sex

Although the results among studies have varied, the difference in the incidence of disease due to *M. pneumoniae* by sex is low. During the 11 years of study in Seattle, Foy and associates[182] noted that the rate of *M. pneumoniae* pneumonia was higher in females than in males in the 30- to 39-year age group (1.8 vs. 1.2 per 1000); in infants, boys were afflicted more often than girls, but otherwise the rates by sex for children virtually were identical. Jensen and associates[286] noted that pneumonia, otitis media, and nasopharyngitis in various combinations were more common in boys than in girls. Monto and colleagues[413] noted that boys younger than 5 years of age had more infections, but the reverse was true for children 5 to 14 years of age. In other studies involving all age groups, males have shown a slightly greater frequency of illness than have females.[380, 443] In the Seattle family studies, symptoms were more severe in boys than in girls.

Pathogenesis and Pathology

Sequence of Events in Infection

M. pneumoniae infection is acquired via the respiratory route from the respiratory secretions of an ill person infected with this agent. Spread can be by small-particle aerosols or large droplets of secretions that come in contact with the epithelial surface of the nasopharynx and perhaps the surfaces of the lower respiratory tract (trachea, bronchi, and bronchioles) as well. In volunteer studies, Couch[121] observed that the 50 per cent human infectious dose by small-particle aerosol was one colony-forming unit (nasal instillation required a dose that was 100 times greater).

Because epidemiologic data indicate the need for close and perhaps prolonged personal contact for infection transmission, it seems likely that small-particle aerosols rarely occur under natural conditions. After acquisition of the infectious agent, multiplication occurs extracellularly on mucous membrane surfaces. The incubation period, which varies from 4 days to more than 3 weeks, probably strongly depends on the size of the original inoculum. The extent of the respiratory infection increases during the incubation period, and organism shedding in respiratory secretions can be observed 2 to 8 days before clinical illness.[121] Initial symptoms of infection include headache, malaise, fever, sore throat, and cough;

evidence of lower respiratory tract disease is present within the succeeding 3 days.[135, 483] The method of extension of infection within the respiratory tract is unknown. It is possible that the extent of disease depends totally on the initial distribution of the infectious agent at the time of acquisition rather than spread of infection from a primary upper respiratory site.

After the onset of clinical symptoms, the concentration of *M. pneumoniae* in respiratory secretions peaks, remains high for about 1 week, and then persists for 4 to 6 weeks or more.[121, 135] Associated symptoms and signs in disease due to *M. pneumoniae* (meningitis, arthritis, hemolytic anemia, rash, pericarditis) suggest the possibility of frequent dissemination of the organism from the respiratory tract. Many reviews on the subject tend to discount the possibility of generalized *M. pneumoniae* infection and attribute the associated systemic clinical findings to immunologic events related to respiratory infection.[121, 135] However, there is little published evidence to indicate that the organism has been sought carefully in the blood and other sites of dissemination. In isolated instances, *M. pneumoniae* has been recovered from the blood, pericardial fluid, middle ear fluid, vesicular skin lesions, pleural fluid, kidney, brain, and cerebrospinal fluid.[3, 22, 177, 298, 318, 366, 369, 425, 428, 536] In addition, the observation of low cerebrospinal fluid glucose in *M. pneumoniae* meningoencephalitis suggests direct involvement by the organism.[315]

Pathology

Pathologic findings in *M. pneumoniae* disease of children have not been reported, and only minimal data from adults are available. However, a reasonable understanding of the pathologic process of *M. pneumoniae* disease can be constructed from studies in the hamster, various tracheal organ cultures, and human biopsy and postmortem material.[139, 292, 373, 401, 460, 575, 625] The primary damage in *M. pneumoniae* infection is to the epithelial lining of the mucosal surfaces of the respiratory tract. This damage has been observed on the surface of bronchi, bronchioles, and alveoli, and clinical symptoms in children suggest that similar pathologic changes occur in the trachea and the upper respiratory tract as well. Specifically conspicuous is the destruction of the ciliated epithelium of the bronchi and bronchioles. Because of mucosal desquamation and ulceration, the lumina contain considerable debris; added to this is an inflammatory exudate consisting of fibrin, mononuclear cells, and neutrophils. The alveolar spaces contain similar exudate and edema fluid.

The walls of the bronchi and bronchioles are thickened by edema and contain an infiltrate of macrophages, lymphocytes, and plasma cells. The alveoli walls also are thickened and contain lymphocytes, mononuclear cells, and erythrocytes. There is dilation of the septal capillaries. Edema and cellular infiltration extend into the interstitial spaces. Gross examination of the lungs reveals areas of hemorrhage and congestion. The pleura may contain patches of fibrinous exudate; pleural fluid may be present. The pneumonic areas may be discrete or widespread.

A biopsy specimen of a vesiculopustular skin lesion revealed an epidermis with mild acanthosis and marked edema that primarily was intracellular.[575] The papillary and upper reticular dermis contained neutrophils and round cells, and there were hemorrhagic foci within the upper corium and epidermis. The blister fluid contained plasma protein and neutrophils. Findings in other organs include mesenteric lymphadenitis, focal hepatic necrosis, follicular splenitis, acute myocarditis, and hemorrhagic encephalitis.

Immunologic Events

SPECIFIC ANTIBODY. A specific serum antibody response usually occurs after infection with *M. pneumoniae,* and this can be measured by many different serologic techniques: immunofluorescence, complement fixation, indirect hemagglutination, precipitation, growth inhibition, mycoplasmacidal antibody test, ELISA, radioimmunoassay, adherence inhibition assay, and radioimmunoprecipitation test.[62, 64, 65, 68, 141, 169, 240, 260, 273, 348, 359, 473, 508, 574] Complement-fixing antibodies occur early in *M. pneumoniae* disease, reach a peak titer in about 1 month, and then decline slowly over a variable period. Fluorescent-staining antibodies and antibody determined by ELISA have temporal patterns similar to that of complement-fixing antibodies. Growth-inhibiting antibodies appear later (2 to 3 weeks after the onset of illness), peak later, and persist longer than do complement-fixing antibodies. The initial serum immune response includes specific IgM, IgG, and IgA antibodies. After clinical illness and convalescence, specific antibody is located mainly in the IgG serum fraction. Occasionally, significant levels of IgM antibody persist for several months or years after infection.[30, 61, 150, 288] Antibody titer responses in infected children generally are of a lesser magnitude than are those in adults.[164] Asymptomatic infections in children may not be associated with a measurable serum antibody response. *M. pneumoniae*–specific IgE antibodies have been noted in the sera of patients with asthma, atopic dermatitis, or both.[580]

After infection, specific antibody also occurs in the nasal secretions and in the sputum.[31, 63] In volunteer studies, Brunner and colleagues[63] noted that 42 per cent and 73 per cent of the subjects had respective IgA nasal and sputum responses. Biberfeld and Sterner[32] noted specific antibody in 44 of 55 sputum specimens from patients with *M. pneumoniae* infections of the lower respiratory tract. They noted IgA antibody in all specimens tested, IgG antibody in 24 of 31 specimens, and IgM antibody in 13 of 27 specimens.

SPECIFIC CELL-MEDIATED IMMUNITY. Fernald and coworkers[165–167] have shown that lymphocytes from adults previously infected with *M. pneumoniae* undergo blast transformation when cultured in vitro in the presence of *M. pneumoniae* organisms. In age-related studies, it was noted that only one of nine children younger than 4 years of age with documented previous infection had evidence of specific cell-mediated immunity as measured by lymphocyte stimulation.[164] In contrast, 7 of 12 children older than 4 years of age and 87 per cent of an adult group had specific lymphocyte stimulation. This study suggests that specific cell-mediated immunity increases as a function of age and depends on repeated infections.

Martin and colleagues[384] found that leukocytes from volunteers with *M. pneumoniae* infections demonstrated chemotaxis in the presence of the organism, whereas leukocytes collected before infection did not. Patients infected with *M. pneumoniae* also respond with interferon-α in their blood and nasopharyngeal secretions early in infection and with interferon-γ during convalescence.[430, 431]

NONSPECIFIC RESPONSES. Antibodies to several diverse antigens occur during human infection with *M. pneumoniae.* The best known of these antibodies are cold agglutinins, and they are useful in diagnosis of *M. pneumoniae* pneumonia.[120, 159, 240, 278, 531] Cold agglutinins are directed against the I antigen of erythrocytes.[276, 353, 531] Most pneumonias in which serum cold agglutinins are noted are due to *M. pneumoniae.* Cold agglutinins are noted in the serum of about 75 per cent of patients with *M. pneumoniae* pneumonia. Their occurrence is less common in *M. pneumoniae* infections without pneumonia.[81]

Patients with *M. pneumoniae* also frequently develop antibodies to the MG strain of nonhemolytic streptococci[355] and occasionally to *M. genitalium*,[351] *M. hominis*,[504] *M. hyorhinis, M. orale, M. pulmonis, M. salivarium*, and *M. mycoides* var. *mycoides*, the etiologic agent of contagious pleuropneumonia of cattle.[340] Other heterologous antibodies noted in the serum of patients with *M. pneumoniae* infection include those to smooth muscle, mitotic spindle apparatus, brain, lung, liver, and Wasserman (WR) cardiolipin antigen.[28, 31, 350] In addition to these findings, Biberfeld and Norberg[29] noted immune complexes by the platelet aggregation technique in the sera of 16 of 39 patients with acute respiratory illness due to *M. pneumoniae.* Mizutani and Mizutani[405] demonstrated the presence of circulating immune complexes in most patients with pneumonia due to *M. pneumoniae.* The same investigators noted the presence of rheumatoid factor in the sera of patients with *M. pneumoniae* disease.[404]

Possible Mechanisms of Disease Production

Numerous studies have been performed in an attempt to understand the pathogenesis of respiratory disease due to mycoplasmas.[62, 92, 93, 95, 96, 106–108, 111, 113–116] Of particular interest in human *M. pneumoniae* infections is the apparent high prevalence of infection in infants, children, adolescents, and young adults but the frequently mild nature of disease in infants and young children compared with that in older patients. Some studies suggest that the more severe disease in the older patient is associated with reinfection and is mediated somewhat by immunologic responses.

Organ culture and animal studies indicate that damage at the site of primary infection—the respiratory epithelium—is the result of a close organism-cell attachment.[96, 114, 115, 262, 356, 357, 424, 471, 590] This attachment of organism to cell utilizes neuraminic acid receptors on the cells.[535] In an organ culture system with *M. mycoides* var. *capri*, ciliary damage was decreased when the cellular receptor sites were treated with receptor-destroying enzyme.[95] Lipman and associates[356, 357] noted that one attenuated *M. pneumoniae* strain had lost its ability to cytadsorb. The close association of organism and cell allows the transport of specific damaging material to the cell. Although the precise nature of this substance is not known, the available data suggest that it might be hydrogen peroxide. This is liberated by *M. pneumoniae* in vitro; in organ culture studies, peroxide has been shown to be the damaging factor in another *Mycoplasma* infection.[96, 357, 358] In cell culture, *M. pneumoniae* inhibits host-cell catalase activity.[9] This catalase activity inhibition enhances the toxicity of the hydrogen peroxide generated by the microorganism. *M. pneumoniae* also enters host cells and persists intracellularly for at least 7 days.[19]

Fernald and associates[164] have noted that specific cell-mediated immunity to *M. pneumoniae* as measured by lymphocyte transformation becomes more prevalent with increasing age, as does specific antibody. Their studies suggest that it may take more than one exposure to antigen to elicit both humoral and cellular responses. Fernald and Glezen,[165] in an inactivated *M. pneumoniae* vaccine trial in children, noted that many recipients developed lymphocyte sensitivity but not a humoral antibody response. Smith and associates,[533] in an inactivated vaccine trial in adults, noted that upon challenge infection, an exaggerated illness occurred in vaccinees who failed to develop humoral antibodies after immunization. These findings have led to the consideration that persistent specific cell-mediated responsiveness might contribute to the pulmonary process in *M. pneumoniae* infection. However, the incubation period of illness in adults and children is similar, which argues against the sensitization theory.[101]

Foy and associates[181] noted that complement-fixing antibodies remained elevated for 2 to 9 years after infections with pneumonia but fell quickly after the second year in persons with mild illness. Protection against reinfection was better in those who previously had pneumonia than in those with mild symptoms.

Clinical Manifestations

Pneumonia

Pneumonia is the most important clinical manifestation of *M. pneumoniae* infection, and this agent is responsible for 10 to 20 per cent of all cases of pneumonia.[104, 135, 189, 192, 196, 257, 396] As noted in Figure 195–1, the highest incidence of pneumonia due to *M. pneumoniae* in Seattle occurred in children 5 to 14 years of age. In a study in Chiba Prefecture, Japan, it was noted that the peak age of lower respiratory tract illness due to *M. pneumoniae* was 4 years.[426] Although it frequently is stated that *M. pneumoniae* pneumonia is rare in children younger than 5 years of age, in actuality the incidence in this group was found to be about twice that noted in young adults in Seattle. Pneumonia due to *M. pneumoniae* is less common in children younger than 2 years of age and rare in infants younger than 6 months of age. The apparent frequency of pneumonia due to *M. pneumoniae* is influenced by the relative occurrence of pneumonia due to other pathogens. During the first 5 years of life, *M. pneumoniae* is only one of many agents (e.g., respiratory syncytial virus, adenoviruses, parainfluenza viruses, influenza viruses, *Streptococcus pneumoniae, Haemophilus influenzae)* that cause pneumonia. During later childhood and adolescence, pneumonia resulting from infection with these other agents is rare; therefore, *M. pneumoniae* is the leading cause of pneumonia in these persons.

Because isolation rates of *M. pneumoniae* during both endemic and epidemic periods do not vary greatly by season as do those of common respiratory viruses, the proportion of patients with *M. pneumoniae* pneumonia increases during the summer months.

SYMPTOMS AND SIGNS. Since 1961, a large number of studies have indicated the frequencies of signs and symptoms in *M. pneumoniae* infections.[35, 36, 58, 89, 91, 104, 117, 152, 153, 158, 187, 196, 205, 234, 241, 267, 279, 375, 409, 421, 429, 496, 552] Unfortunately, many studies have involved only special populations such as the military, and, with few exceptions, community investigations have failed to indicate differences by age. In only three investigations have data regarding children been itemized separately.[58, 187, 552] In Table 195–2, the occurrence of symptoms and signs as compiled from eight studies in which both children and adults were included is presented. The hallmark of pneumonia due to *M. pneumoniae* is fever and cough. The onset of illness usually cannot be demarcated clearly, but malaise, fever, and headache are early complaints. Cough has its onset 3 to 5 days after the beginning of illness and initially is nonproductive. Foy and colleagues[192] and Biberfeld and colleagues[35] noted that 77 per cent and 100 per cent, respectively, of the respective patients that they studied had maximal temperatures greater than 38.9° C (102° F). Copps and associates[117] found that 58 per cent of the group that they evaluated had temperatures greater than 39.4° C (103° F) and 4 per cent had temperatures greater than 40.6° C (105° F).

The reporting of headache in association with *M. pneumoniae* pneumonia has varied considerably. Nakao and associates[429] noted this complaint in only 8 per cent of subjects, whereas Biberfeld and associates[35] and Foy and colleagues[192] reported it in two-thirds of those studied. Chills and sputum production are noted in about 50 per cent of ill patients.

TABLE 195–2. Frequency of Clinical Findings in Children and Adults with *Mycoplasma pneumoniae* Pneumonia

Finding	Frequency
Symptoms	
Fever	+ + + +
Cough	+ + + +
Malaise	+ + +
Headache	+ +
Sputum	+ +
Chills	+ +
Hoarseness	+
Earache	+
Coryza	+
Sore throat	+
Diarrhea	+
Nausea and/or vomiting	+
Chest pain	+
Signs	
Rales	+ + +
Pharyngitis	+ +
Lymphadenopathy	+
Conjunctivitis	±
Rash	±
Otitis media	±

Compiled from eight studies in which both children and adults were included: references 35, 36, 117, 192, 196, 279, 375, 429.
+ + + +, close to 100 per cent; + + +, 75 per cent; + +, 50 per cent; +, 25 per cent; ±, 0 to 10 per cent.

Again, great differences among investigations are noted, and these probably are related to the relative ages of the patients.

Coryza is unusual in *M. pneumoniae* pneumonia; therefore, its occurrence should suggest another etiologic agent for illness in a specific patient. In a study involving children exclusively, Stevens and colleagues[552] noted that coryza was more common in young children; as might be expected, they found productive cough more common in their older patients. Hoarseness, earache, sore throat, gastrointestinal complaints, and chest pain occur in about 25 per cent of patients.

On physical examination, about 75 per cent of patients have auscultatory evidence of pneumonia, and about one-half have pharyngitis. Remarkable lymphadenopathy, particularly with cervical involvement, is noted in about 25 per cent of patients. Twenty-one per cent of the patients studied by Foy and associates[192] had otitis media. In other studies, this manifestation was noted in about 5 to 10 per cent of cases. Conjunctivitis was reported in almost one-half of the patients reported by Fransen and associates.[196] In contrast, except for Jansson and associates,[279] who noted conjunctivitis in 3 per cent of their study group, this finding was not mentioned in the other reports. Similarly, rash was noted in 6 per cent, 11 per cent, and 17 per cent, respectively, in the studies in Minnesota, Wisconsin, and Seattle[117, 189, 375] but was not mentioned in the other studies.

The most common finding on chest auscultation is dry rales, but musical rales with expiration are noted occasionally. Rales usually persist for 2 weeks, and hearing them a month or more after disease onset is not unusual. Occasionally, patients have no auscultatory evidence of pulmonary disease throughout their illness, in spite of the presence of abnormalities on chest radiographs. During illness, cough becomes increasingly prominent; initially it is nonproductive, but later, in older children and adolescents, it may produce a frothy white sputum. The sputum also may appear purulent and contain blood. Cough persists for 3 to 4 weeks and persists long after nonrespiratory symptoms such as fever and headache have subsided.

In a study of 44 children with lower respiratory illnesses due to *M. pneumoniae,* Stevens and associates[552] noted the following frequencies of symptoms and signs: cough, 97 per cent; malaise, 82 per cent; vomiting, 40 per cent; abdominal pain, 35 per cent; headache, 32 per cent; skin rash, 20 per cent; fever greater than 38° C (greater than 100.4° F), 78 per cent; rales, 78 per cent; pharyngitis, 32 per cent; rhonchi, 30 per cent; bronchial breathing, 27 per cent; and otitis media, 27 per cent. Foy and coworkers[187] noted that chills and productive cough were more common in adults than in children and that temperatures tended to be higher in children.

In a large study involving 108 children with *M. pneumoniae* infections, wheezing occurred with the acute illness in 40 per cent.[496] When the children in this study were evaluated 3 years after their acute illnesses, they were found to have three indicators of lung function that had mean values significantly lower than in control children.

Few reports specifically described pneumonia due to *M. pneumoniae* in young children.[17, 97, 109, 195, 228, 426, 526, 552] However, a review of the case descriptions available indicates that illness, when it occurs, can be severe and relatively prolonged, compared with common viral and bacterial infections. Singer and DeVoe[526] reported a 3-year-old severely ill child who had a temperature of 39.4° C, a pulse of 150, and a respiratory rate of 40. Diffuse pulmonary involvement of the right upper lobe and lingular segments of the left lower lobe was observed by radiograph, although rales and altered breath sounds could not be heard. The patient's condition worsened over a 6-day period. At this time, specific therapy with erythromycin was instituted, and a slow recovery followed. The child had a normal white blood cell count, transiently elevated serum values of aspartate aminotransferase and alanine aminotransferase, and microscopic hematuria. Grix and Giammona[228] observed two 5-year-old children with extensive pneumonias, pleural effusions, and febrile periods of 10 and 16 days. Stevens and associates[552] reported a 5-year-old boy with a pulmonary consolidation and aseptic meningitis, and Clyde and Denny[109] described a 3-year-old boy with a "feathery infiltrate" in the right upper lung field who was asymptomatic. In a family study, Foy and colleagues[195] noted four children younger than 6 years of age. In one 4-year-old child, the pneumonia persisted for more than 1 month, and in this child's brother, the illness lasted about 2 weeks. I have seen a 4.5-year-old girl with scattered infiltrates throughout both lung fields with febrile illness of 14 days' duration.[97]

Severe and extensive pulmonary disease occurs occasionally in *M. pneumoniae* infections.[88, 90, 100, 118, 133, 172, 175, 228, 230, 346, 374, 400, 420, 428, 445, 460, 484, 520, 523, 525, 526, 538, 544] Massive lobar pneumonias occasionally are observed, and pleural effusions are fairly common.[16, 90, 99, 110, 133, 172, 175, 228, 363, 420, 427, 428, 445, 526, 544] The adult respiratory distress syndrome has been observed, and illness has suggested pulmonary embolism with infarction.[175, 525, 594] Chronic interstitial pulmonary fibrosis and fulminant fatal diffuse interstitial fibrosis have been noted in two adults with *M. pneumoniae* pneumonia, and a 20-year-old man developed localized bronchiectasis at the site of previous acute lung infection.[217, 293, 560] *M. pneumoniae* pneumonia generally is more severe in patients with preexisting cardiorespiratory problems, immunodeficiencies, and sickle-cell disease.[24, 100, 185, 201, 282, 400, 464, 520, 538]

Three patients, one adolescent and two adults, have been found to have lung abscesses in association with *M. pneumoniae* infections.[346, 523] The illnesses were characterized by productive cough and chest pain for 2 to 4 weeks. In one patient, clinical recovery and clearance of the pulmonary lesion were dramatic with tetracycline therapy; the other two patients received suboptimal therapy but eventually recovered. One 18-year-old boy with extensive consolidation of the right lower lung field had residual pleural scarring 8 months after the acute illness.[420]

A newborn with congenital pneumonia due to probable vertical transmission of *M. pneumoniae* has been reported.[592]

Clyde[104] reported factors that correlated with *M. pneumoniae* pneumonia in a study of 1139 subjects with community-acquired pneumonia. Positive factors were sore throat, headache, fever 37.8° C or higher and 38.9° C or higher, exanthem, family size of four or more, and ear infection. In the same study, pneumonia did not correlate with coryza, leukocytosis (15×10^9/L or more and 10×10^9/L or more), preexisting disease, recurrent pneumonia, hospitalization for treatment, and cigarette smoking.

Although recovery from *M. pneumoniae* pneumonia usually is complete, two studies suggest that persistent lung function abnormalities can occur after illness.[411, 496]

RADIOGRAPHY. Because the classic clinical entity, primary atypical pneumonia, has numerous causes but often is used as a synonym for *M. pneumoniae* pneumonia, there is much confusion about the spectrum of the radiographic appearance of the specific mycoplasmal infection. The radiographic pattern of primary atypical pneumonia is varied, but bilateral, diffuse, reticular infiltrates are common components.[364, 509, 529] Subsequent study indicates that the diffuse interstitial pattern is uncommon in *M. pneumoniae* infection and more often the result of infection with other agents such as viruses, fungi, and *Chlamydia*.[56, 204, 436, 475, 589]

Brolin and Wernstedt[56] carefully evaluated the radiographic findings in 56 patients with significant *M. pneumoniae* pneumonia; 21 of the patients were younger than 20 years of age. They noted the following distribution of different patterns: typical lobar pneumonia, 8 patients; predominantly alveolar but not total consolidation, 13; interstitial (either reticular or noduloreticular), 20; combination of lobar pneumonia and other alveolar involvement without total consolidation, 2; combination of lobar involvement and interstitial, 10; and combination of alveolar involvement without total consolidation and interstitial, 3. Alveolar patterns were more common in females; interstitial involvement was more frequent in males. Twenty-two per cent of patients had enlargement of the hilar or paratracheal lymph nodes, and 14 per cent had pleural effusion.

The persistence of radiographic changes is variable. Brolin and Wernstedt[56] noted that 13 per cent of their patients who underwent follow-up studies had abnormal findings more than 4 weeks after initial study. They noted that persistence tended to be longer in patients with alveolar disease, compared with those with interstitial patterns. The degree of clinical symptoms and pulmonary physical findings frequently correlates poorly with the apparent degree of involvement noted by radiograph. In many patients with significant symptoms, only minimal interstitial changes are observed. In other instances, patients with lobar pneumonias often have few clinical findings indicating pulmonary disease.

NONSPECIFIC LABORATORY DATA. The total leukocyte count in patients with pneumonia due to *M. pneumoniae* most often is normal, but variation is considerable.[36, 117, 152, 187, 192, 196, 278, 409, 552, 589] In a group of more than 250 children younger than 15 years of age, Foy and associates[187] noted that 30 per cent and 6 per cent had total leukocytes greater than 10,000 and 15,000 cells/mm^3, respectively. In a group of 45 children, Stevens and colleagues[552] observed leukocytosis in 33 per cent of patients and leukopenia in one patient. Sixty-seven per cent of the children had neutrophilia, and one patient had neutropenia. The increased percentage of band-form neutrophils in *M. pneumoniae* pneumonia is unusual.

The erythrocyte sedimentation rate is elevated in all cases,[36, 117, 278] and this elevation usually is marked. Biberfeld and colleagues[36] noted that 16 of 37 patients had erythrocyte sedimentation rate values of 50 mm/hr. Serologic tests for syphilis are found to be falsely positive on occasion, and serum cold agglutinins and antibodies to *Streptococcus* MG antigen are common.[30, 81, 84, 135] Results of the direct Coombs test frequently are positive, and elevated levels of serum IgM are noted.[30, 159] Urinalysis results usually are normal.

Respiratory Disease Other Than Pneumonia

COMMON COLD AND UNSPECIFIED UPPER RESPIRATORY ILLNESS. By strict definition (significant nasal symptoms, without pharyngitis, and with minimal fever), *M. pneumoniae* rarely causes the common cold. However, mild upper respiratory illness is noted frequently as the only manifestation of *M. pneumoniae* infection in children, adolescents, and young adults.[79, 119, 135, 140, 158, 160, 164, 192, 195, 253, 362, 409, 429, 439, 498] The frequency of unspecified upper respiratory tract illness as a manifestation of *M. pneumoniae* infection, compared with other manifestations resulting from infection with this agent, varies considerably among studies. Feizi[160] studied patients of a country practice in England and noted that 50 per cent of the patients presented with upper respiratory tract illness. Illness in these persons often was prolonged, however, lasting up to 7 to 10 weeks. In a review in Scotland, only 3 per cent of 596 *M. pneumoniae* infections were classified as upper respiratory tract symptoms. In studies of common respiratory illnesses of children in which viruses and other agents were sought, *M. pneumoniae* was noted in 2 to 5 per cent of the patients with upper respiratory tract illness.[79, 135, 362]

PHARYNGITIS AND NASOPHARYNGITIS. As noted in Table 195–2, pharyngitis is observed in about one-half of all patients with *M. pneumoniae* pneumonia. However, pharyngitis as the major manifestation of *M. pneumoniae* infection is less common. Parrott[462] noted that 12 per cent of children admitted to the hospital with severe "bronchitis—pharyngitis" had *M. pneumoniae* infections. Jensen and associates[286] observed the frequent occurrence of pharyngitis and otitis media in children infected with *M. pneumoniae.* In a study of 715 children and adolescents with pharyngitis, Glezen and colleagues[213] reported that 36.8 per cent had group A streptococcal infections and 3.1 per cent were infected with *M. pneumoniae.* When the *M. pneumoniae* infections were grouped by age, the peak (11.4 per cent) occurred in the 12- to 14-year group, and none was observed in children younger than 6 years of age. Five patients with *M. pneumoniae* infections had concomitant group A streptococcal infections, but the illnesses in these cases could not be distinguished clinically from those due to either agent alone. Cervical lymphadenopathy occurred in about 50 per cent of those infected, and the pharyngeal lesion was exudative in 43 per cent.

In a study involving 131 adult patients with pharyngitis, 10.6 per cent were found to have serologic evidence of *M. pneumoniae* infection.[319]

OTITIS MEDIA AND BULLOUS HEMORRHAGIC MYRINGITIS. Although the incidence has varied in different studies, otitis media is noted in about 5 per cent of children and adolescents with *M. pneumoniae* pneumonia. The role of *M. pneumoniae* as an etiologic agent in common acute otitis media in children is unclear. Halsted and associates[231] noted that 12 per cent of children with otitis media had serologic evidence of *M. pneumoniae* infection, but they were unable to recover the agent from middle ear fluid. In a study in which children were selected because of *M. pneumoniae* infection in a family member, 47 of 49 children with otitis media had *M. pneumoniae* infections.[286]

In a volunteer study, 13 of 52 subjects developed myringitis.[483] Findings usually were bilateral and associated with throbbing pain. The appearance of the tympanic membranes varied from mild injection to severe inflammation with edema. Hemorrhagic areas on the drum were noted in five subjects, and serous-appearing blebs containing blood were observed in two. Bullous myringitis also has been observed occasionally with natural *M. pneumoniae* infections.[58, 109, 192, 195, 375, 536] However, in one study of 148 children and adults with *M. pneumoniae* pneumonia, 27 (18 per cent) were found to have bullous myringitis.[375]

SINUSITIS. Although clinically recognized sinusitis has been reported rarely in patients with *M. pneumoniae* infection, Griffin and Klein[226] found radiographic evidence of sinusitis in about two-thirds of a group of Navy recruits with *M. pneumoniae* pneumonia. In general, the patients with sinusitis had more prolonged illnesses than did recruits without sinusitis. Savolainen and colleagues[506] noted that 11 of 310 patients with acute maxillary sinusitis had fourfold or greater rises in complement-fixing antibody to *M. pneumoniae.* In chronic suppurative maxillary sinusitis, cultures for *M. pneumoniae* have been performed, but no isolations have been observed.[27, 540]

ACUTE BRONCHITIS. Acute bronchitis characterized by fever, cough, and rhonchi with or without associated pharyngitis is a frequent manifestation of *M. pneumoniae* infection.[79, 80, 85, 153, 160, 253, 255, 429, 439, 462, 498] Of 40 patients with *M. pneumoniae* infections, Feizi[160] reported that 6 had bronchitis, 3 had upper respiratory tract illness plus bronchitis, and 1 had sinusitis plus bronchitis. In contrast with these findings, Hornsleth[255] noted that only 1 of 25 patients with *M. pneumoniae* infections had acute bronchitis. In the differential diagnosis of acute bronchitis, *M. pneumoniae* infection accounts for between 10 and 20 per cent of cases.[80, 85, 135, 153, 465]

CROUP. *M. pneumoniae* infection has been associated only occasionally with croup. Parrott[462] found no instances of *M. pneumoniae* infection in a large number of children with croup, and Chanock and Parrott[80] do not list this agent as an etiologic consideration in croup. In contrast, extensive studies in both Seattle and Chapel Hill have revealed that about 2 per cent of croup cases are associated with *M. pneumoniae* infection.[135, 186, 212, 363] Because no descriptions of clinical illness are available, it is reasonable to assume that croup due to *M. pneumoniae* infection generally is mild and without distinguishing characteristics.

BRONCHIOLITIS AND INFECTIOUS ASTHMA. About 5 per cent of cases of bronchiolitis are due to infection with *M. pneumoniae,* but the percentage varies among studies.[79, 80, 85, 135, 140, 186, 212, 363, 462] In two large studies, no instances of *M. pneumoniae*–associated bronchiolitis were described.[253, 255] *M. pneumoniae* also is a relatively common cause of asthmatic bronchitis and recurrent wheezing in the asthmatic child.[26, 254, 263] Horn and associates[254] noted that *M. pneumoniae* was isolated from 6.6 per cent of children with wheezy bronchitis, and Berkovich and associates[26] found *M. pneumoniae* infections in 7 of 33 episodes of wheezing in asthmatic children. Wheezing also occurs during *M. pneumoniae* pneumonia.[17, 496]

OTHER. Exacerbations of chronic obstructive pulmonary disease have been associated with *M. pneumoniae* infections.[94, 330, 397, 530, 618] However, Smith and associates[530] were unable to show increased susceptibility to infection in patients with chronic obstructive pulmonary disease compared with normal subjects. Illness suggestive of pertussis has been described in three children.[328, 552]

Exanthem and Enanthem

Exanthem as a manifestation of *M. pneumoniae* infection is common, but its incidence has varied considerably among different studies.[3, 71, 87, 90, 100, 117, 118, 152, 158, 178, 192, 194, 195, 216, 221, 230, 253, 278, 300, 328, 331, 332, 367, 369, 370, 375, 428, 429, 439, 493, 502, 545, 552, 556, 575, 589] In large studies involving children in which *M. pneumoniae* infections in a geographic area have been evaluated, the incidence of exanthem has varied from 3 to 33 per cent.[117, 158, 192, 195, 253, 278, 328, 370, 375, 429, 439, 545, 552] Foy and associates[192] noted skin rash in 17 per cent of 319 patients with *M. pneumoniae* pneumonia during a 5-year surveillance period. In a study involving only children, Stevens and colleagues[552] noted exanthem in 9 per cent of their patients. Copps and colleagues,[117] in a community outbreak in La Crosse, Wisconsin, found that 11 per cent of their pneumonia patients also had rash.

The cutaneous manifestations in *M. pneumoniae* infection are protean. Of most common occurrence is an erythematous maculopapular rash, which is most prominent on the trunk and back; the lesions may be discrete (rubelliform) or confluent (morbilliform). Although not the most common cutaneous manifestations of *M. pneumoniae* infection, erythema multiforme and Stevens-Johnson syndrome are the most often reported and the most serious.[16, 71, 90, 118, 158, 160, 194, 295, 300, 367, 369, 385, 439, 502, 522, 552, 556, 589]

In Table 195–3, the clinical findings in 29 well-documented cases of *M. pneumoniae* infection with exanthem are presented; in Table 195–4, the specific mucocutaneous findings in 20 of the 29 patients are itemized. Of the total group, all but 8 were males, and 24 of the 29 were younger than 20 years of age and 12 of the 20 were younger than 11 years of age. The duration of exanthem was greater than 7 days in all but 2 patients; all patients were febrile, and in 17 cases, the rash occurred during fever.

Fourteen patients had generalized ulcerative stomatitis, and seven had tonsillitis or pharyngitis. Severe conjunctivitis was observed in eight patients, and this manifestation was seen only in those with vesicular or bullous cutaneous lesions. All eight patients with severe conjunctivitis also had generalized ulcerative stomatitis. It is surprising that vesicular or bullous exanthems with oral and eye lesions (Stevens-Johnson syndrome) rarely occur in females.[16, 385, 552]

As noted in Table 195–3, 25 of the 29 patients had pneumonia. The occurrence of rash as the major manifestation of *M. pneumoniae* infection probably is rare. In a study of 112 patients with suspected infectious exanthems without pneumonia, Cherry and associates[98] could find none with *M. pneumoniae* infections. Foy and colleagues[195] noted a 2-year-old child with only skin rash, Stutman[556] reported a 15-year-old boy with Stevens-Johnson syndrome without pneumonia from whom the organism was recovered from a vesicular lesion, and Ruhrmann and Holthusen[493] observed frequent cases of mild erythema multiforme without pneumonia.

Many patients with *M. pneumoniae* infection and exanthem have a history of antibiotic administration before the development of rash; this observation suggests the possibility that the rash is drug-induced rather than from the infectious process. As noted in Table 195–3, 17 patients had received antibiotics before the rash appeared, and the exanthem was present before antibiotic therapy in 10. Whereas these data incriminate the infection as a cause of exanthem, the large number of occurrences in association with antibiotic administration raises the possibility that the antibiotic intensifies the dermosensitive potential of the infectious agent in a manner similar to that noted between Epstein-Barr virus and ampicillin in infectious mononucleosis. *M. pneumoniae* has been recovered from the blister fluid of two patients with erythema multiforme.[369]

TABLE 195–3. Selected Clinical Findings in 29 Patients with *Mycoplasma pneumoniae* Infection and Exanthem

Clinical Findings	No. of Patients
Predominant components of exanthem	
Erythematous macular	4
Erythematous maculopapular	14
Vesicular	14
Bullous	6
Petechial	1
Urticarial	2
Discrete lesions	11
Confluent lesions	7
Pruritic	6
Predominant distribution of exanthem	
Hands	9
Arms	20
Feet	8
Legs	19
Trunk	19
Face	11
Buttocks	9
Genitals	8
Duration of exanthem (days)	
<7	2
7–14	11
>14	10
Time of onset of exanthem	
Before fever	2
With fever	4
During fever	17
After fever	1
Antibiotics administered before exanthem	
Yes	17
No	10
Enanthem	
Generalized ulcerative stomatitis	14
Tonsillitis or pharyngitis	7
Conjunctivitis	
Severe	8
Mild	3
Pneumonia	
Yes	25
No	4

From Cherry, J. D.: Anemia and mucocutaneous lesions due to *Mycoplasma pneumoniae* infections. Clin. Infect. Dis. *17*(Suppl. 1):S47–S51, 1993. University of Chicago, Publisher.

Other unusual cutaneous manifestations include erythema nodosum, pityriasis rosea, varicella-like urticaria, and Cockade purpura.[90, 216, 221, 331, 428, 493, 511, 575]

Cardiac Manifestations

Cardiac involvement during *M. pneumoniae* infection generally is considered to be unusual.[86, 89, 157, 200, 221, 302, 306, 328, 345, 425, 442] However, studies of Pönkä[469] and Sands and associates[503] and survey data of Noah[443] and Assaad and Borecka[15] indicate that *M. pneumoniae* myocarditis and pericarditis are important causes of both morbidity and mortality. In a study of fatal viral and mycoplasmal infections, Assaad and Borecka[15] noted six cardiovascular deaths related to *M. pneumoniae* infection during a 9-year period. Noah[443] found that 1 per cent of 700 patients with *M. pneumoniae* infection had cardiac manifestations as the main clinical feature. Pönkä[469] published findings of a 7-year study involving 560 patients with serologic evidence of *M. pneumoniae* infection. In this group, 69 patients with cardiac manifestations were uncovered; of these 69 patients, 25 were selected who had carditis for which no causal agent other than *M. pneumoniae* could be incriminated. Pönkä[469] also reviewed the world literature and found a total of 33 other cases of carditis.

Of 25 cases carefully studied, 17 had respiratory symptoms before the diagnosis of carditis; 10 had radiologically confirmed pneumonia. All but four patients had fever. Of the 25 patients, 2 were younger than 10 years of age and 2 were in the 10- to 19-year age group. Of the 33 cases in the literature, 7 were 20 years of age or younger. Of this survey group, 25 of the 33 had respiratory illness, and in 19 it was recorded as pneumonia.

Of the 25 patients in Finland reviewed by Pönkä, 6 had pericarditis and the remainder had perimyocarditis. Antibiotic therapy in 11 patients did not appear to shorten the duration of illness or diminish the number of cardiac sequelae. At 16-month follow-up, 11 patients had persistent cardiac damage. Another interesting aspect of this study was the finding of *M. pneumoniae* complement-fixing antibody titer rises in five adults with myocardial infarcts.

Hematologic Manifestations

Severe hemolytic anemia has been reported on several occasions in association with *M. pneumoniae* infection.[87, 118, 157, 159, 171, 257, 306, 373, 485, 512, 552, 561] Most cases of *M. pneumoniae* hemolytic anemia have been associated with marked pulmonary involvement. Stevens-Johnson syndrome is a common associated finding, and myocarditis has been noted on two occasions.[118, 157, 160, 306, 552] In general, severity of illness correlates with high titers of cold agglutinins.

Hemolysis may be severe and acute, often with a 50 per cent reduction in hemoglobin concentration. In contrast with uncomplicated pulmonary disease, the leukocyte count in patients with hemolytic anemia frequently is elevated markedly with a predominance of neutrophils. Results of the direct Coombs test usually are positive. Clinical experience suggests that steroid administration in conjunction with proper antibiotic therapy may be beneficial in this illness. Boccardi and associates[44] observed one 7-year-old boy with hemolytic anemia and transitory paroxysmal cold hemoglobinuria.

Feizi[159] has demonstrated that clinically inapparent compensated hemolysis is common in association with *M. pneumoniae* pulmonary infections. Fiala and associates[171] noted that bone marrow suppression also contributed to anemia in a patient they studied. Ruhrmann and Holthusen[493] reported a hemorrhagic variant of erythema multiforme (Cockade purpura) similar to Henoch-Schönlein disease in *M. pneumoniae* infection; they also noted severe thrombocytopenia not associated with hemolytic anemia. Gill and Marrie[209] reported a 27-year-old man with hemophagocytosis during an *M. pneumoniae* infection.

Gastrointestinal Findings

NONSPECIFIC FINDINGS. About 25 per cent of patients with *M. pneumoniae* pneumonia have nausea, vomiting, diarrhea, or some combination thereof (see Table 195–2). Aside from these complaints, gastrointestinal problems in association with *M. pneumoniae* infections are rare. Stevens and associates[552] found that 15 per cent of a group of 44 children with infection had notable abdominal pain. Referred abdominal pain with pneumonia also has been observed.[160]

LIVER INVOLVEMENT. Liver involvement in *M. pneu-*

TABLE 195–4. Mucocutaneous Findings in 20 Patients with *Mycoplasma pneumoniae* Infection and Exanthem

Case	Reference	Age (yr)	Sex	Distinguishing Characteristic of Exanthem	Generalized Ulcerative Stomatitis	Severe Conjunctivitis
1	90	16	M	Fiery-red confluent maculopapular	0	0
2	90	17	F	Blotchy erythematous	0	0
3	97	4.5	F	Morbilliform	0	0
4	178	9	M	Erythematous maculopapular	+	0
5	178	8	M	Papulovesicular; "target" appearance	+	0
6	194	14	M	Symmetric macular and bullous	+	+
7	300	19	M	Erythematous maculopapular, vesicles; "iris" lesions	+	0
8	328	10	F	Macular and petechial	0	0
9	331	16	M	Varicella-like	+	+
10	589	8	M	Macular	+	0
11	589	6	M	Diagnosed as measles	0	0
12	367	16	M	Scattered vesicular; generalized	+	+
13	367	6	M	Vesicular; generalized	+	0
14	428	7	M	Urticarial	0	0
15	428	9	M	Maculopapular	0	0
16	502	10	M	Vesiculobullous and maculopapular	+	+
17	575	27	M	Vesiculopustular to papular; "pityriasis-like"	0	0
18	193	10	M	Vesiculobullous; generalized	+	0
19	332	5	M	Maculopapular	0	0
20	370	11	F	Papular; most marked on hands and feet	0	0

Modified from Cherry, J. D., Hurwitz, E. S., and Welliver, R. C.: *Mycoplasma pneumoniae* infections and exanthems. J. Pediatr. *87*:369–373, 1975. Used with permission.

moniae infection is surprisingly rare. Levine and Lerner[344] reported that mild increases in transaminases occur and that acute and chronic active hepatitis has been noted with respiratory symptoms and proven *M. pneumoniae* infection, but they provide no further information. MacLean[370] reported the case of a 13-year-old girl who initially had sore throat and then 9 days later showed clinical and laboratory evidence of hepatitis. Murray and associates[423] presented a case report of an adult with typical *M. pneumoniae* pneumonia in whom liver function and enzyme studies indicated hepatitis. Helms and colleagues[241] noted that 6 of 17 patients with *M. pneumoniae* pneumonia had elevated aspartate aminotransferase values. Enzyme changes have been noted in other case evaluations,[346, 375, 526] and hepatic necrosis has occurred.[373]

PANCREATITIS. In 1974, Mårdh and Ursing[378] reported six patients with respiratory illnesses, serologic evidence of *M. pneumoniae* infections, and pancreatitis. In four patients, pancreatic symptoms began 1 to 2 weeks after the onset of respiratory illness; in the other two patients, the pancreatitis was subclinical. Two patients developed diabetes, and one of them died. At postmortem examination, pneumonitis and pancreatitis were confirmed. In a study of pancreatitis, Leinikki and Pantzar[339] noted that sera from 18 of 56 patients had complement-fixing antibody titer rises to *M. pneumoniae.* Because none of the patients in this study had respiratory illness suggestive of *M. pneumoniae,* the investigators suggested that perhaps the antibody responses were not specific for *M. pneumoniae* infection but due to a cross-reacting infection or the result of autoantigens from pancreatic damage. Leinikki and associates[338] have done further studies; it is their belief that the antibody response is nonspecific, but their data neither confirm nor refute this assumption. In another study, Freeman and McMahon[198] also noted serologic evidence of *M. pneumoniae* infection in 33 per cent of patients with pancreatitis. Oderda and Kraut[448] reported a 22-month-old girl with pancreatitis and a complement-fixing antibody titer rise to *M. pneumoniae.* This child had no respiratory symptoms.

Arthritis

Mycoplasmas other than *M. pneumoniae* are a common cause of arthritis in animals other than human beings.[112, 277] In many instances, the animal diseases suggest human rheumatoid arthritis. Because of this, mycoplasmas have been searched for extensively in humans with this illness, but to date, no associations have been established. However, it is clear that *M. pneumoniae* infection occasionally is associated with joint manifestations.[25, 131, 201, 205, 245, 289, 328, 329, 378, 424, 432, 468, 495, 615] In a review of 1259 patients with *M. pneumoniae* infections, Pönkä[468] noted transient arthritis in 0.9 per cent. Two patients were reported to have Reiter syndrome. Hernandez and colleagues[245] reported seven instances of arthritis in 38 persons with *M. pneumoniae* respiratory disease. In one patient, the illness lasted 18 months and was associated with the development of rheumatoid factor.

Eighteen instances of illness suggestive of rheumatic fever have been described.[25, 102, 289, 329, 415, 425, 432, 615] In all 18 patients, large joints were involved; 15 patients had joint swelling or effusion, whereas 3 had only pain. Most patients had a history of preceding respiratory illness with sore throat, and 10 of 18 had radiographic evidence of pneumonia. The sedimentation rate was elevated in all patients in whom the test was performed. One child had an erythema marginatum–like rash as well as polyarthritis and fever.[415]

Neurologic Disease

Several large community and military studies of *M. pneumoniae* pneumonia and other respiratory illnesses are notable in that neurologic disease is not described.[84, 117, 152, 192, 278, 409, 421] However, other studies and particularly those more recently performed indicate a surprising spectrum of neurologic illness associated with *M. pneumoniae* infection.[1, 2, 10, 12, 14, 15, 18, 22, 34, 36, 105, 139, 142, 151, 154, 160, 176, 196, 214, 248, 249, 257, 270, 298, 307, 309, 315, 320, 321, 337, 352, 402, 417, 433, 439, 441, 443, 447, 448, 453, 466, 492, 519, 527, 545, 549, 552, 563, 590, 613, 618] The failure to find neurologic disease in the large studies mentioned probably was due not to its absence but to the orientation of the investigators; neurologic disease was not studied under the respiratory investigation protocols. In three large studies of *M. pneumoniae* illness involving 1856 cases, 2.6 to 4.8 per cent had neurologic illness.[439, 443, 466] Assaad and Borecka[15] noted five fatal *M. pneumoniae* infections in which central nervous system findings were the major clinical manifestations.

In 1973, Lerer and Kalavsky[343] reported 5 cases of neurologic disease associated with *M. pneumoniae* infection and analyzed 45 cases from the literature. They noted the following frequencies of specific clinical involvement: generalized encephalitis, 30 per cent; spinal nerve roots, 30 per cent; meningitis, 20 per cent; cranial nerves, 20 per cent; focal encephalitis, 16 per cent; cerebellum, 14 per cent; psychosis, 8 per cent; and spinal cord, 2 per cent. Combination involvement was noted in 36 per cent of the cases; in 79 per cent, there was a history of antecedent respiratory illness. Fifty-three per cent of the patients were 20 years of age or younger, and 15 per cent were younger than 10 years of age. Eighty per cent of the children and adolescents were males. The onset of neurologic disease occurred from 3 to 23 days after the onset of respiratory illness, with a mean value of 10 days. Five deaths were noted, and 22 per cent of the survivors had residual neurologic deficit.

In a review of 61 patients with *M. pneumoniae*–associated neurologic disease over a 24-year period in Helsinki, Finland, Koskiniemi[321] noted that 45 of the patients were children and that all of these children had encephalitis. Of the total group, 5 patients (8 per cent) died and 14 (23 per cent) had severe sequelae.

In other studies, aseptic meningitis is reported more frequently; other less common findings include poliomyelitis-like syndrome, bilateral sensorineural deafness, Reye syndrome, cerebral infarction, optic disk swelling, brain stem syndrome, transverse myelitis, psychosis, radiculopathy, brachial plexus neuropathy, Bell palsy, and Guillain-Barré syndrome.[10, 12, 139, 142, 214, 238, 248, 270, 307, 309, 315, 320, 352, 417, 441, 446, 461, 492, 519, 545, 552, 590, 613, 618] Klimek and associates[315] reported a 13-year-old boy with meningoencephalitis and transverse myelitis in association with low cerebrospinal fluid glucose values. Arthur and Margolis[14] noted at postmortem examination the appearance of *Mycoplasma*-like structures in granulomatous angiitis of the central nervous system in a 35-year-old man.

Mixed Infections

In many studies of *M. pneumoniae* infections, cultural or serologic evidence of concomitant or sequential infections with other infectious agents has been noted.[3, 18, 158, 161, 196, 213, 218, 225, 341, 353, 383, 408, 409, 435, 480, 541, 545, 546] In a large study of patients hospitalized with acute respiratory illness, Fransen and associates[196] found that 64 per cent of patients with complement-fixing antibody titer rises to *M. pneumoniae* also had antibody titer rises to viral, chlamydial, or bacterial agents. In this group, the most common concomitant infections were with parainfluenza viruses. The occurrence of mixed infection did not appear to have a pronounced effect on clinical manifestations; the only significant difference between patients with mixed infections and those with single *M. pneumoniae* infections was the more common occurrence of a high erythrocyte sedimentation rate in the former group. In several other large studies of disease due to *M. pneumoniae,* concomitant infections were common, but no evidence of synergistic or antagonistic roles of one agent for another was noted.[158, 213, 408, 545, 546] Renner and associates[480] found a lower than expected frequency of seropositivity to *M. pneumoniae* in 91 serum pairs with seroconversions to influenza A virus.

The observation by Grady and Gilfillan[218] that 81 per cent of patients with legionnaires' disease also had serologic evidence of *M. pneumoniae* infection is interesting. In the same study, 29 per cent of all cases seropositive for *M. pneumoniae* also were seropositive for the legionnaires' disease antigen. Similar studies done at the Centers for Disease Control and Prevention failed to find a similar rate of high copositivity in sera obtained in other legionnaires' disease epidemics. Another study found no serologic relationship between *M. pneumoniae* and *Legionella pneumophila.*[481] Severe bacterial disease has been noted occasionally after *M. pneumoniae* infection. Stadel and colleagues[541] noted *H. influenzae* pneumonia and bacteremia after a mild *M. pneumoniae* illness; Biberfeld and colleagues[35] reported staphylococcal septicemia in two cases of *M. pneumoniae* pneumonia, and Rykner and associates[495] recovered pneumococci from the pleural exudate of a patient with *M. pneumoniae* pneumonia.

Kleemola and Kayhty[313] found fourfold or greater increases in *M. pneumoniae* complement-fixing antibody titers in 40.7 per cent of 54 patients with bacterial meningitis. However, they felt that this antibody response was not due to specific *M. pneumoniae* infection but due to cross-reactive glycolipids resulting from the bacterial infections.[312, 313]

Lind and associates[352] noted that 4 of 19 patients with neurologic disease and *M. pneumoniae* infection had serologic evidence of concomitant viral infections.

Other Disease Associations

Foy and colleagues[195] noted that both ear involvement and pneumonia as manifestations of *M. pneumoniae* infection were more common in children with previous tonsillectomy. Putman and associates[474] found that in all but 3 of 31 patients with sarcoidosis, the serum complement-fixing antibody titer to *M. pneumoniae* was greater than or equal to 1:32, whereas in a similar-sized control group without sarcoidosis, only 2 persons had titers of 1:32 and none had higher titers. Other interesting observations include multiple birth defects in a newborn exposed to *M. pneumoniae* in utero,[51] a tubo-ovarian abscess in a young woman from whom *M. pneumoniae* in pure culture was isolated,[577] fever of unknown origin in a 32-year-old man,[325] glomerulonephritis in a few patients with pneumonia,[467] inappropriate secretion of antidiuretic hormone in a 6-year-old boy,[358] and optic disk swelling and iritis.[499]

Recurrent Disease

The findings in several investigations suggest that recurrent *M. pneumoniae* infections are frequent.[63, 165, 550] However, only relatively recently has it become clear that repeat infections can be associated with severe disease, such as pneumonia. In the Seattle studies, second attacks of pneumonia have been documented, and similar findings have been observed in England.[180, 183, 188, 253]

Diagnosis

Differential Diagnosis

Because the clinical manifestations of *M. pneumoniae* infections are protean and because infections in children and adolescents are common, this agent should be considered in the differential diagnosis of most infectious illnesses. Most important is its consideration in patients with pulmonary disease in whom illnesses due to viruses (particularly adenoviruses, parainfluenza viruses, influenza viruses), *Chlamydia psittaci, Chlamydia pneumoniae, Coxiella burnetii,* bacteria (particularly *S. pneumoniae, Bordetella pertussis, H. influenzae, Mycobacterium tuberculosis),* and fungi (particularly *Histoplasma capsulatum* and *Coccidioides immitis)* are the main differential possibilities. Because the clinical manifestations, including the radiographic appearance of the lungs, among the various differential possibilities frequently are similar, the following other factors are important: status of the host (normal or immunologically compromised), the environment (human, animal, or inanimate source), the age of the patient, the incubation period, and the season.

In otherwise healthy children, *M. pneumoniae* is a common cause of pneumonia in those older than 3 years of age and the leading cause of pneumonia in older children and adolescents. The lack of coryza sometimes is useful in differentiating pneumonia due to *M. pneumoniae* from that due to common viral agents, and the elevation of the white blood cell count with an increase in band-form neutrophils is evidence against a mycoplasmal etiologic agent. The occurrence of exanthem and, particularly, Stevens-Johnson syndrome should lead the physician to suspect *M. pneumoniae;* similarly, the occurrence of hemolytic anemia, joint manifestations, or neurologic signs and symptoms with pneumonia should make the physician strongly suspect *M. pneumoniae* as the etiologic agent. Because the pulmonary manifestations of *M. pneumoniae* infections are not always apparent clinically, the physician who is working up the unusual acute or subacute case (aseptic meningitis or other neurologic illness; exanthem; enanthem; hepatitis; pancreatitis; pericarditis, myocarditis, or both; and arthritis) would be wise to consider the possibility of *M. pneumoniae* as the etiologic agent and obtain appropriate chest radiographs as well as definitive cultures and serologic studies.

Specific Diagnosis

SERUM COLD AGGLUTININS. Although there is considerable confusion in the literature and by physicians in general regarding the diagnostic value of the serum cold agglutination test in *M. pneumoniae* infections, it is my opinion that when it is employed appropriately, the test is a simple and useful procedure. One cause for confusion was a report in 1966 in which only 1 of 28 children with positive cold agglutination titers actually had serologic evidence by complement fixation of *M. pneumoniae* infection.[558] However, this report can be criticized because the study population was composed of 444 children younger than 4 years of age and of this group, only 170 had pneumonia. Cold agglutinins are noted occasionally in the sera of patients of all ages with a variety of illnesses so that for useful results, their study should be restricted to patients likely to have *M. pneumoniae* lower respiratory tract disease.[90, 173, 205, 354] In various studies of pneumonia, serum cold agglutinins at a titer of greater than or equal to 1:32 were found in 50 to 90 per cent of patients with *M. pneumoniae* infection.[34, 81, 84, 196, 205, 278, 421, 552, 595] In general, the cold agglutinin response correlates directly with the severity of pulmonary involvement; patients with extensive lobar involvement nearly always have positive titers (^{3}1:32), whereas those with only minimal findings on radiographic study frequently have equivocal or negative titers. Positive cold agglutination titers have been observed in 18 per cent of adenoviral pneumonias in one study in a military population.[205] In general, the higher the cold agglutinin titer, the more likely a particular illness is due to *M. pneumoniae* infection.

A rapid screening test for cold agglutinins is available and useful.[203, 227] This test is performed by adding four drops of blood to a tube containing sodium citrate or other anticoagulant. The tube is placed in ice water (0° to 4° C) in a freezer for about 30 seconds and then examined immediately for coarse agglutination by tilting the tube on its side. On warming the tube, the agglutination should resolve, and it can be reproduced again by repeating the ice water cooling procedure.

SPECIFIC ANTIBODY DETERMINATIONS. Several specific antibody tests (growth inhibition, immunofluorescence, indirect hemagglutination, precipitation, mycoplasmacidal antibody, complement fixation, ELISA, adherence inhibition assay, radioimmunoassay, and radioimmunoprecipitation) can be used to measure serum antibodies to *M. pneumoniae,* but until relatively recently only the complement-fixation test was routinely available. A fourfold rise in complement-fixation antibody titer indicates acute *M. pneumoniae* infection. Because complement-fixation antibody in *M. pneumoniae* infections is of relatively short duration, the observation of a fourfold fall in titer also can be useful on occasion in assigning etiologic significance in a particular illness. High single titers (≥1:256) usually indicate recent infection but rarely can be used to relate an illness specifically with *M. pneumoniae.* Because *M. pneumoniae* infection is associated with a relatively long incubation period, antibody development is significant at the time of acute disease. Because of this, fourfold changes in titer can occur in a short interval (5 days) so that collection of two sera 5 to 7 days apart usually reveals a significant complement-fixation antibody titer rise.

In recent years, most diagnostic laboratories have replaced the complement-fixation test with commercial immunofluorescence or ELISA for the demonstration of antibodies to *M. pneumoniae* antigens.[5, 72, 146, 156, 174, 271, 316, 334, 418, 478, 524, 534, 576, 591] These tests, in addition to demonstrating antibody value rises in paired sera, can identify specific IgM and IgA antibodies in single serum samples. In general, when used by experienced laboratory personnel, both immunofluorescence and ELISA have sensitivities and specificities similar to the complement-fixation test for determining significant increases in antibody values in paired serum specimens. In addition, the demonstration of specific IgM or IgA antibody in a single serum sample suggests a recent infection. However, the specific IgM and IgA responses after infection may last for several months; therefore, the demonstration of these antibodies in a single serum may be misleading in regard to the diagnosis of specific illness. Because of this, in most instances, paired sera (5 to 14 days apart) should be examined to confirm a clinical diagnosis.

CULTURE. With proper media, experienced personnel have little difficulty in isolating *M. pneumoniae* from throat swabs of infected patients.[8, 587] However, because *M. pneumoniae* is relatively slow-growing, requiring more than 1 week of incubation in the majority of instances, culture is of less use in the diagnosis of the routine case than is serologic study. Cultures should be performed in all unusual situations; specifically, joint fluid, cerebrospinal fluid, pericardial fluid, and biopsy materials should be cultured. The modified SP-4 medium, which is more sensitive than are conventional mycoplasma culture media, coupled with the agar plate immunofluorescence identification procedure, may facilitate the cultural diagnosis of *M. pneumoniae.*[587]

DIRECT ANTIGEN DETECTION. Because *M. pneumoniae* culture is clinically impractical owing to the long time until organisms can be identified, the direct detection of antigen in respiratory secretions is an important priority. In 1987, a species-specific probe (Gen-Probe) that uses iodine 125-labeled complementary DNA, homologous to *M. pneumoniae* ribosomal RNA, became available.[235, 237, 311, 579] Clinical results with this probe have been variable. Hata and colleagues,[237] in a study in a pediatric population using throat swabs, noted a sensitivity of 76.7 per cent and a specificity of 91.7 per cent, compared with culture. Tilton and colleagues[579] found a sensitivity of 100 per cent and a specificity of 98 per cent in a study of sputum and throat cultures carried out in two hospital clinics in Connecticut. Kleemola and coworkers[311] also noted good sensitivity (95 per cent) and specificity (85 per cent) with sputum specimens in Army conscripts. In contrast with these results, Harris and associates[235] identified only 22 per cent of culture-positive patients with the Gen-Probe assay. This test is no longer available.[310]

Studies with indirect immunofluorescence and ELISA offer promise for antigen detection in clinical specimens.[247, 317]

A number of studies have indicated the usefulness of the polymerase chain reaction for the demonstration of specific *M. pneumoniae* DNA in nasopharyngeal, blood, and tissue specimens.[38, 67, 70, 132, 235, 265, 284, 294, 368, 434, 482, 596, 622] A number of different primers have been used to identify gene sequences of the PI cytoadhesin protein or 16 S ribosomal RNA gene sequences. Using culture plus serologic criteria as the comparative standard, several studies have shown excellent sensitivity and specificity.

Treatment

Antimicrobial Therapy

M. pneumoniae is sensitive in vitro to erythromycin, tetracyclines, chloramphenicol, clarithromycin, azithromycin, several aminoglycosides, and quinolones.[23, 135, 268, 269, 280, 377, 440, 528] It is resistant to all penicillins and for practical purposes to the cephalosporins. In spite of this demonstrated in vitro sensitivity of the organism, plus several studies that have shown clinical therapeutic effectiveness,[42, 81, 135, 192, 195, 205, 278, 308, 493, 510, 513, 528, 532] there is a common misconception among many physicians that antibiotic therapy is of little value in the treatment of illness due to *M. pneumoniae* infection. This idea had its origin before the present era, when many patients with viral pneumonia were given a diagnosis of primary atypical pneumonia and treated unsuccessfully with antibiotics.

In 1961, Kingston and associates[308] demonstrated the therapeutic effectiveness of demethylchlortetracycline in pneumonia due to *M. pneumoniae*. Since then, several other antibiotics have been studied carefully and also have been found to be effective against *M. pneumoniae* pneumonia.[81, 135, 192, 205, 278, 493, 513, 528, 532] The drugs of choice in pneumonia due to *M. pneumoniae* are either erythromycins or tetracyclines. Because of the adverse effects of tetracyclines on teeth, an erythromycin is the drug of choice in children. In *M. pneumoniae* pneumonia, the dose of erythromycin or tetracycline for children is 40 to 50 mg/kg/24 hours administered every 6 hours for a minimum of 10 days. For adolescents and adults, the dose is 2 g/24 hours. In general, the effectiveness of antibiotic therapy directly correlates with the severity of pneumonia and the elapsed time of illness before onset of therapy.

In all other clinical manifestations of *M. pneumoniae* infection except pneumonia (e.g., nonpulmonary respiratory infections, neurologic disease, Stevens-Johnson syndrome), antibiotic therapy has not been evaluated adequately. In general, it would appear that otitis media, pharyngitis, croup, and bronchiolitis are mild, self-limited illnesses that require no therapy. In more serious illness, such as Stevens-Johnson syndrome and neurologic disease, individual case studies indicate little evidence of therapeutic benefit with either erythromycin or tetracycline therapy. However, it is my opinion that, when diagnosed, most *M. pneumoniae* infections should be treated because there is little to lose and in vitro data suggest the possibility of efficacy. Jensen and colleagues[286] noted that prophylactic administration of oxytetracycline in family contacts prevented disease but not infection.

General Management

Children and adolescents with *M. pneumoniae* pneumonia should be discouraged from excessive physical activity during the acute illness and for a 2-week period during convalescence because clearance, as observed by radiography, is slow and lags behind apparent clinical well-being. Older children and adolescents should be advised of their contagiousness to others; this risk period exists as long as cough persists, even with successful antibiotic therapy.

Steroids have been used in the management of severe pulmonary disease, Stevens-Johnson syndrome, encephalitis, and hemolytic anemia. Although definitive data are lacking, several case studies suggest associated clinical benefit; steroids seem to be particularly useful in severe hemolytic anemia.

Prevention

Because of the marked and prolonged morbidity associated with *M. pneumoniae* infection, which particularly has been troublesome in the military, much effort has been directed toward the development of vaccines. In 1965, Jensen and associates[285] reported encouraging initial trials with an inactivated vaccine. In this study, 25 of 30 volunteers developed significant rises in *M. pneumoniae* growth-inhibiting antibody titers. Later challenge studies with the same vaccine indicated that 9 of 10 volunteers with serum antibody were protected, but illness more severe than that in the unvaccinated control group occurred in vaccinees who did not have an antibody response after initial immunization.[533] This altered reactivity upon challenge suggested a sensitization process perhaps similar to that observed with other inactivated antigen vaccines and indicated the need for caution in further trials.[123, 165] Other trials in both adults and children with inactivated vaccines have had varying degrees of success.[399, 407, 616]

A trial with a live attenuated vaccine (a temperature-sensitive mutant) gave encouraging results.[223] However, because further study of natural *M. pneumoniae* disease indicates that reinfection is common and because sensitization may play a role in pathogenesis, it seems prudent to proceed slowly in further vaccine trials in children.[164]

Because the degree of contagion of *M. pneumoniae* is relatively low, isolation methods should be effective in preventing disease spread. The studies of Jensen and associates[286] also indicate that in certain circumstances (in particular, high-risk subjects, such as patients with sickle-cell disease), prophylactic administration of antibiotics may be justified.

UREAPLASMA UREALYTICUM

Properties

Ureaplasmas (formerly T-strain mycoplasmas) are distinguished from all other members of the order Mycoplasmatales by their production of urease and their ability to hydrolyze urea.[515, 517] The genus *Ureaplasma* contains a single species (*U. urealyticum*) with 14 serovars.[349, 486, 614] The morphologic characteristics of *U. urealyticum* in young liquid medium cultures are similar to those of other mycoplasmas. There are round-ovoid elements approximately 330 nm in diameter with a range from 100 to 850 nm; rod-shaped and filamentous structures also occur, and the latter have a length of 2 μm and a width of 50 to 300 nm.[37, 515, 620] In clinical material, short, bacillary forms with monopointed ends are common. Organisms are surrounded by a single trilaminar membrane about 10 nm thick with pilus-like structures radiating from the surface. Multiplication occurs by a simple budding process and perhaps by binary fission.

On unbuffered standard *Mycoplasma* agars of pH 6.0, *U. urealyticum* colonies are small (20 to 30 μm) and circular, with irregular borders, and grow downward into the agar.[515] On buffered agar, *U. urealyticum* colonies are bigger and often have the "fried egg" appearance of typical large colony-forming mycoplasmas.[374]

Isolation of *U. urealyticum* from clinical material is facilitated by the demonstration of urease activity.[170, 516, 569] In liquid medium containing urea and phenol red, *U. urealyticum* growth results in ammonia production with resultant increase in the pH and color change. Subculture from broth to agar medium that contains urea and manganese sulfate yields dark brown ureaplasmal colonies.

Epidemiology

The main reservoirs of human strains of *U. urealyticum* are the genital tracts of adult men and women.[13, 191, 390, 391, 393, 569, 583, 590] Infants become colonized with *U. urealyticum* during passage through the birth canal of an infected woman.[190, 314, 336, 559] With ruptured membranes, the infant can be infected in utero.[314] *U. urealyticum* has been recovered from the following sites in newborn infants: throat, nose, genitourinary tract of girls, urine of boys, external auditory canals, umbilicus, and perineum. Not all infants of infected women become colonized, and neonatal colonization tends not to persist. In one study in which *U. urealyticum* was recovered from 38 per cent of girls and 6 per cent of boys at birth, follow-up over a 2-year period revealed a decreasing prevalence of colonization; at 2 years, none of the children had positive cultures.[191]

During prepubertal childhood, *U. urealyticum* only rarely is recovered from urine or genital specimens.[184, 336] After puberty, colonization is common and primarily is the result of sexual contact.[388, 391, 393] Colonization in adults is related directly to sexual activity. In population studies, isolation of *U. urealyticum* is rare from persons with no sexual experience but occurs in about 50 per cent of men and 75 per cent of women in whom sexual intercourse with three or more partners is reported.

Clinical Manifestations

Because *U. urealyticum* can be recovered with considerable frequency from the throat, eyes, and genitourinary tracts of babies and from the genitourinary tracts of postpubertal males and females who are well, it frequently has been difficult to establish cause and effect relations in disease. Studies suggest the following disease associations with *U. urealyticum* in human genitourinary and reproductive diseases: good to strong association with nongonococcal urethritis, prostatitis, and urethral syndrome; moderate association with epididymitis, involuntary infertility, repeated spontaneous abortion and stillbirth, chorioamnionitis, and low birth weight; weak association with urinary calculi, pyelonephritis, Reiter disease, and pelvic inflammatory disease; and no association with abscess of Bartholin gland, vaginitis, cervicitis, postabortal fever, and postpartum fever.[60, 76, 77, 149, 326, 327, 395, 547, 555, 568, 569, 581] The majority of illnesses related to or possibly related to *U. urealyticum* infection are not pediatric problems; only those of direct or indirect importance in pediatric and adolescent medicine are considered here.

Nongonococcal Urethritis

Nongonococcal urethritis is more common than gonococcal urethritis in men in most developed countries.[236, 275, 389, 599] About 40 per cent of the cases of nongonococcal urethritis are caused by *Chlamydia trachomatis,* and 20 to 30 per cent are the result of *U. urealyticum* infections.[47, 48, 122, 250, 390, 507] Clinical differentiation of disease due to *C. trachomatis* and *U. urealyticum* has not been studied, but nongonococcal and gonococcal urethritis have been evaluated comparatively.[233, 275, 335, 597]

The incubation period in nongonococcal urethritis is relatively long, with most cases occurring 10 to 20 days after exposure, whereas in gonorrhea, the period is shorter, usually less than 1 week.[233] The onset of symptoms in nongonococcal urethritis usually is more gradual than that associated with gonorrhea. Virtually all men with gonorrhea have urethral discharge, and most have both discharge and dysuria. In contrast, Jacobs and Kraus[275] found that only 38 per cent of men with nongonococcal urethritis had both dysuria and discharge. In the same study, 15 per cent of patients with nongonococcal urethritis had only dysuria, whereas only 2 per cent of those with gonococcal urethritis had a similar complaint. On examination, Handsfield[233] found the discharge in nongonococcal urethritis to be purulent in 36 per cent of his cases, nonpurulent in 9 per cent, and of an intermediate character in the remaining 55 per cent. In contrast, 73 per cent of patients with gonorrhea had purulent discharge, 27 per cent had intermediate discharge, and none had nonpurulent discharge. Because of the more gradual onset and the usually less severe symptoms, patients with nongonococcal urethritis are less prompt in seeking medical care than are patients with gonorrhea. Jacobs and Kraus[275] found that 76 per cent of patients with discharge and gonococcal infection came to the clinic within 4 days of onset, whereas only 43 per cent of similar nongonococcal urethritis patients visited the clinic within 4 days of disease onset. Without treatment, nongonococcal urethritis symptoms subside gradually in some patients over a 1- to 3-month period.[453]

After treatment of men with urethral gonorrhea with penicillin, ampicillin, or spectinomycin, urethritis recurs (postgonococcal urethritis) in many patients.[251] Studies of postgonococcal urethritis indicate an etiologic role for *C. trachomatis; U. urealyticum* probably is responsible for some cases.[455]

A 7.5-year-old sexually inactive boy with recurrent urethritis associated with *U. urealyticum* infection has been described.[514]

Low Birth Weight

In 1969, Klein and associates[314] found that *Mycoplasma* isolation was associated with low birth weight in a study of 221 newborns. Colonized babies (mainly with *U. urealyticum)* had a statistically lower mean birth weight (2605 g) than did babies in whom colonization was not detected (2952 g). In a second prospective study at the same center involving 484 pregnant women, it was noted that 28 per cent of babies with a birth weight of 2500 g or less were colonized by *U. urealyticum,* whereas only 5 per cent of those babies weighing more than 2500 g were colonized.[49] In this study, the association of *U. urealyticum* and low birth weight was not related to a shortened gestational period.

Since these early studies, at least 13 studies involving more than 7000 pregnant women have been conducted to evaluate the role of cervical ureaplasmal infection in prematurity.[6, 74, 150, 191, 490, 491] In several studies, an inverse correlation between vaginal colonization, cervical colonization, or both and premature birth has been observed. Alfa and coworkers[6] studied 108 full-term mothers and 104 preterm mothers in a tertiary care hospital and noted genital carriage rates of *U. urealyticum* of 25 per cent and 19.2 per cent, respectively. Acquisition of ureaplasmas in the respiratory tracts of the infants occurred significantly more frequently in the preterm group (8.5 per cent) than in the term infants (0.9 per cent). Newborns weighing 1500 g or less had a colonization rate of 19 per cent (5 of 26).

In spite of the apparent association between colonization with *U. urealyticum* and premature birth, a specific cause and effect relationship seems unlikely.[74, 151]

Chorioamnionitis

In a study of 249 puerperal women and their babies, Shurin and colleagues[521] noted on histologic examination of the placentas that *U. urealyticum* was recovered from 37.5 per cent of babies whose placentas showed chorioamnionitis and from only 19 per cent of those with normal placentas. In this study, no adverse effects could be attributed to either the placental lesions or the colonization of the babies. Some studies suggest that chorioamnionitis due to *U. urealyticum* is a cause of premature delivery.[74, 151, 246] Caspi and associates[73] reported a 32-year-old woman with amnionitis in whom *U. urealyticum* was recovered from the blood. After delivery, the same organism was recovered from the blood of one of the twin infants. *U. urealyticum* has been recovered from fetal tissues after abortion, stillbirth, and neonatal death.[137, 372, 489]

Neonatal Pneumonia

In a study of pneumonitis in early infancy, Stagno and associates[542] isolated *U. urealyticum* from the nasopharynx of 8 of 38 children (21 per cent) with pneumonia but from only 2 of 49 control children (4 per cent). Quinn and colleagues[476] noted fatal neonatal pneumonia resulting from an intrauterine infection with *U. urealyticum,* and more recently, Waites and associates[605] noted three neonates with pneumonia due to *U. urealyticum* associated with persistent pulmonary hypertension. Several recent studies indicate that *U. urealyticum* is a cause of acute respiratory distress and pneumonia in newborns.[66, 74, 449, 450, 458, 459, 600]

Chronic Lung Disease

Several large studies have found a significant association between *U. urealyticum* colonization of the respiratory tract in low-birth-weight infants and the development of bronchopulmonary dysplasia.[74, 75, 256, 290, 463, 500, 548, 608, 609, 612] It has been suggested that *U. urealyticum* is not a primary cause but that the organism might be the cause of undetected pneumonia that results in an increased requirement for supplemental oxygen.[75] The bronchopulmonary dysplasia is the result of oxygen toxicity due to the supplemental oxygen therapy. Recent studies support this hypothesis; *U. urealyticum* infection contributes to the development of bronchopulmonary dysplasia in some cases.[256, 290, 463, 548, 608, 609]

Neonatal Central Nervous System Infections

Garland and Murton[202] reported a 786-g newborn who developed meningitis due to *U. urealyticum* on day 10. The baby recovered after erythromycin and then chloramphenicol therapy. In a prospective study, Waites and coworkers[606] isolated *U. urealyticum* from the cerebrospinal fluid of eight infants who were being treated for meningitis or investigated for hydrocephalus. Six of these culture-positive babies had intraventricular hemorrhage, and hydrocephalus developed in three cases. In a second study, Waites and associates[604] studied an additional 318 infants in four suburban community hospitals and found 5 babies from whom *U. urealyticum* was recovered from the cerebrospinal fluid. Three of the five babies did not have pleocytosis, and they recovered without treatment. The fifth baby died secondary to a right frontal hemorrhage. In contrast with the findings of Waites and colleagues, Likitnukul and coworkers[347] cultured the cerebrospinal fluid and blood of 203 infants with suspected sepsis and failed to isolate *U. urealyticum.* Several recent studies have confirmed the association between *U. urealyticum* infection and meningitis.[74, 244, 451, 543, 600]

Sepsis

U. urealyticum has been recovered from the blood of newborns with pneumonia and meningitis.[70, 600]

Other Infections

U. urealyticum has been recovered from an abscess at the site of an internal fetal heart rate monitor.[232]

Diagnosis and Treatment

The demonstration of infection by *U. urealyticum* can be established easily by presently available culture techniques. However, assignment of disease causation is more difficult because of its ubiquitous presence in normal persons. In clinical practice, the most important differential consideration is between gonococcal infection and nongonococcal urethritis. Although the symptoms of the two illnesses frequently are different, there is enough overlap to make differential diagnosis without laboratory aid hazardous. Microscopic examination of a urethral specimen is essential. In most instances, the observation on Gram stain of gram-negative cell-associated diplococci is sufficient for a diagnosis of *Neisseria gonorrhoeae* infection. When smears reveal polymorphonuclear neutrophils without organisms suggestive of gonococci, a specific bacterial culture should be obtained. Because infection with multiple agents is common and postgonococcal urethritis is a frequent problem, it is advisable to study initial illnesses completely in adolescents with cultures for bacteria, *Chlamydia,* and *Ureaplasma. U. urealyticum* also can be detected by polymerase chain reaction.[39]

Patients with nongonococcal urethritis should be treated with tetracycline (40 mg/kg/24 hours every 6 hours; persons weighing more than 50 kg should receive 500 mg every 6 hours) for 10 days.[233, 252] *Chlamydia* and *Ureaplasma* also are sensitive to erythromycin, so this antibiotic is a useful alternative for those patients in whom tetracycline is contraindicated. With the adolescent patient, it is prudent to seek out and treat the sex partners whenever possible.

Upon diagnosis, *U. urealyticum* central nervous system and respiratory infections should be treated with erythromycin.[601, 602]

MYCOPLASMA HOMINIS

Properties

Three basic morphologic forms of *M. hominis* organisms have been observed by phase contrast microscopy: coccoidal cells 30 to 80 nm in diameter, diploforms and filamentous forms with a thickness of 30 to 40 nm, and forms with variable lengths reaching 40 μm or more.[43, 52, 54, 138] Bredt[53] studied newly isolated strains and noted that coccoid forms and ring- or disk-shaped cells were predominant; with some strains, filamentous forms of variable lengths also were noted. Multiplication occurs by binary fission, by fragmentation of filaments and rings, and by budding.[43, 487]

Anderson and Barile[11] studied the ultrastructure of *M. hominis* and noted considerable variability in the internal components. In some cells, there were ribosome-like granules in the cytoplasm and a more central area of net-like strands suggestive of a nucleus. Other cells had only irregular densities within the cytoplasm. In some instances, dense cytoplasmic bodies were observed; in other cells, vacuoles were seen.

On *Mycoplasma* agar, *M. hominis* colonies are about 200 to 300 μm in diameter and have the typical mycoplasma "fried egg" appearance.[569] *M. hominis* grows on ordinary blood agar and produces pinpoint nonhemolytic colonies. *M. hominis* metabolizes arginine to ammonia, so arginine-supplemented liquid medium with a pH indicator (phenol red) can be used for primary isolation. *M. hominis* can be identified specifically and differentiated from other human mycoplasmas that metabolize arginine by growth inhibition by specific antibody.

M. hominis has two cytoadhesins that are membrane proteins, which allows attachment to cells of the urogenital tract.[243] Attachment is to sulfated glycolipids of the host cells.[452]

Epidemiology

Like *U. urealyticum,* the main reservoirs of *M. hominis* are the genital tracts of adult men and women.[190, 387, 388, 391–392, 393, 569] Infants become colonized during passage through the birth canal, and this colonization tends not to persist. In a recent study of 208 women at delivery, *M. hominis* was recovered from cervicovaginal specimens in 11 per cent and the gastric secretions of 1 per cent of the newborns.[219] In prepubertal children, *M. hominis* only rarely is recovered from urine or genital specimens. Postpubertal genital tract colonization primarily results from sexual contact.

M. hominis can be recovered from the oral cavity of 1 to 5 per cent of normal adults.[539]

Clinical Manifestations

Studies suggest the following disease associations with *M. hominis* in human genitourinary and reproductive diseases: good to strong association with pyelonephritis, pelvic inflammatory disease, postabortal fever, and postpartum fever; moderate association with prostatitis, vaginitis, and cervicitis; weak association with abscess of Bartholin gland and low birth weight; and no association with nongonococcal urethritis, epididymitis, urinary calculi, Reiter disease, urethral syndrome, involuntary infertility, repeated spontaneous abortion and stillbirth, and chorioamnionitis.[41, 60, 76, 147, 149, 207, 229, 456, 457, 491, 547, 568, 569, 586] With the exception of pelvic inflammatory disease and complications of pregnancy, which occur in adolescents, the other disease associations reported do not involve pediatric patients.

Sacker and colleagues[497] reported a 5-day-old baby who had several abscess lesions in the supraclavicular area from which only *M. hominis* was recovered upon incision and drainage. Another newborn had submandibular lymphadenitis due to *M. hominis.*[470] Wound infections with *M. hominis* in neonates after cardiac surgery have been reported.[57, 342]

In three large studies in which cerebrospinal fluid was obtained in the work-up of suspected neonatal sepsis, *M. hominis* was recovered from the fluid in 23 of 387 patients.[593, 604, 606] Of the 23 with isolates, only 1 had cerebrospinal fluid findings indicative of meningitis. Several case reports of newborn babies with meningitis due to *M. hominis* have been reported.[45, 206, 208, 376] Cerebrospinal fluid examination reveals pleocytosis with the majority of cells being polymorphs, increased protein, and decreased glucose concentrations. Appropriate antibiotic therapy usually is delayed because the cerebrospinal fluid is not examined routinely for mycoplasmas. *M. hominis* has been recovered on two occasions from the cerebrospinal fluid of a 2.5-year-old girl with a ventriculoperitoneal shunt.[603] Because there were no complications from the infection and only minimal cerebrospinal fluid inflammation, no treatment was initiated. Three months later, the organism could not be isolated from the cerebrospinal fluid and the child was doing well.

M. hominis was recovered from the amniotic fluid in an instance in which the baby later died of respiratory distress syndrome.[59] Postmortem examination revealed interstitial pneumonia. A stillbirth attributed to an *M. hominis* infection acquired in utero has been reported.[398] Jones and Tobin[287] reported eight *M. hominis* eye infections in 250 newborns studied. In volunteer studies in adults, it was found that *M. hominis* could produce exudative pharyngitis.[419] Moffet and associates[406] isolated *M. hominis* from the throat of 1 of 174 infants and children with pharyngitis but made no similar isolation from a control group of children without pharyngitis. Neu and Ellner[438] recovered *M. hominis* from the throat of 1 child in a group of 56 with exudative pharyngitis. Other *M. hominis* infections include a scalp abscess as a complication of intrapartum monitoring,[210] a massive pericardial effusion in a newborn,[405] septicemia in a 10-month-old burned infant,[130] chronic multifocal osteomyelitis in an 8-year-old,[264] septicemia after heart surgery in a 5-year-old girl,[129] and exudative vaginitis in a 10-year-old girl.[607]

Diagnosis and Treatment

Illness due to *M. hominis* infection is rare in children. This organism should be considered an etiologic possibility in neonates with meningitis and with abscesses in whom routine cultures are negative. The possibility of *M. hominis* as an etiologic agent also should be considered in the adolescent girl with pelvic inflammatory disease.

M. hominis usually is sensitive to tetracycline, and this antibiotic is the drug of choice unless it is otherwise contraindicated.[50, 69, 554, 572, 573, 619] During the last decade, resistance of *M. hominis* to tetracyclines has increased.[125, 386] The organism also usually is sensitive to clindamycin, rifampicin, and chloramphenicol. In two cases of neonatal meningitis, treatment with chloramphenicol failed to eradicate the organism from the cerebrospinal fluid.[208, 394] Eradication was accomplished by doxycycline in one infant and clindamycin in the other. In contrast with *U. urealyticum* and *M. pneumoniae, M. hominis* is markedly resistant to erythromycin.

MYCOPLASMA FERMENTANS, MYCOPLASMA GENITALIUM, MYCOPLASMA PENETRANS, MYCOPLASMA PIRUM, AND AIDS-ASSOCIATED MYCOPLASMAL INFECTIONS

Mycoplasma fermentans

M. fermentans originally was isolated from the genital tract of men and women 45 years ago, but it has not been established as a cause of genitourinary disease.[494, 566, 583] This organism has been isolated from the blood of leukemia patients, from joint fluid of patients with arthritis, and from the blood and urine of patients with AIDS.[19, 40, 379, 412, 422, 621] In recent studies, *M. fermentans* has been identified by polymerase chain reaction in peripheral blood mononuclear cells and lymph nodes of HIV-infected patients.[238, 299, 323, 505] The organism also has been recovered from the blood of homosexual men without HIV infection.[299, 323, 371] *M. fermentans* has been identified in synovial fluid samples from 15 patients with inflammatory arthritis diseases, including rheumatoid arthritis.[537]

Mycoplasma genitalium

M. genitalium first was identified and reported in 1981.[564, 568, 583, 586] It was cultured from urethral swabs from two men with nongonococcal urethritis. The organism also has been recovered from the respiratory tract of patients with pneumonia who were participating in an *M. pneumoniae* vaccine trial.[20] Although this organism has biologic features that indicate its pathogenic potential and it has caused infection and disease in experimentally infected chimpanzees, its role in human disease has not been established clearly.[564, 583, 585] Using polymerase chain reaction, Jensen and associates[283] have presented evidence suggesting a causative role in some cases of nongonococcal urethritis. The organism also has been recovered in mixed culture with *M. pneumoniae* from the synovial fluid of a patient with pneumonia and subsequent polyarthritis.[582]

Mycoplasma penetrans

M. penetrans is a newly recognized species isolated from the urogenital tract of patients with AIDS.[360, 361] In a seroprevalence study, Wang and associates[611] found that 35.4 per cent of HIV-infected patients had antibody, whereas only 0.4 per cent of HIV-seronegative subjects had antibody. They subsequently noted a high prevalence of antibody to *M. penetrans* in the sera of homosexual men but not in the sera of other HIV transmission groups.[610] In a more recent study, Grau and colleagues[220] found that 18.2 per cent of HIV-infected patients had antibody to *M. penetrans*, whereas only 1.3 per cent of HIV-seronegative persons had antibody. *M. penetrans* antibody seroprevalence increased with progression of HIV-associated disease, and it was associated predominantly with homosexual practices in the HIV-infected patients. No pediatric data relating to *M. penetrans* seroprevalence are available.

Mycoplasma pirum

M. pirum originally was recovered from eukaryotic cell cultures, and its origin was traced to a human tumor cell line.[5, 134, 333] It has been recovered more recently from primary lymphocyte cells from AIDS patients.[40]

AIDS-Associated Mycoplasmal Infections

The frequent identification of *M. fermentans, M. pirum,* and *M. penetrans* infections in HIV-infected patients has led to the consideration that they may function as cofactors in the progression of HIV infection.[40, 412] Although these mycoplasmas have the capacity to invade cells and to be potent immunomodulators, their pathogenic role, if any, in association with HIV has not been determined yet.

MYCOPLASMA AND *UREAPLASMA* INFECTIONS IN IMMUNOCOMPROMISED PATIENTS

Patients with hypogammaglobulinemia are susceptible to severe persistent infections with *U. urealyticum, M. hominis, M. pneumoniae,* and *M. orale.*[179, 410, 472, 488] Clinical manifestations include osteomyelitis, arthritis, cellulitis, and chronic respiratory illness. The patients need to be treated for prolonged periods with high-dose intravenous immunoglobulin and antibiotics to which the specific agents are susceptible. Severe and persistent infections also have occurred in liver, kidney, and bone marrow transplant recipients, as well as in other immunocompromised patients.[103, 274, 297, 403, 464]

Yechouron and associates[624] reported a 64-year-old man with Hodgkin lymphoma who died of septicemia due to *M. arginini,* an animal pathogen.[624]

References

1. Abramovitz, P., Schvartzman, P., Harel, D., et al.: Direct invasion of the central nervous system by *Mycoplasma pneumoniae:* A report of two cases. J. Infect. Dis. *155:*487, 1987.
2. Agustin, E. T., Gill, V., and Cunha, B. A.: *Mycoplasma pneumoniae* meningoencephalitis complicated by diplopia. Heart Lung *23:*436–437, 1994.
3. Aiello, L. F., and Luby, J. P.: Concomitant *Mycoplasma* and adenovirus infection in a family. Am. J. Dis. Child. *128:*874–877, 1974.
4. Alexander, E. R., Foy, H. M., Kenny, G. E., et al.: Pneumonia due to *Mycoplasma pneumoniae:* Its incidence in the membership of a co-operative medical group. N. Engl. J. Med. *275:*131–136, 1966.
5. Alexander, T. S., Gray, L. D., Kraft, J. A., et al.: Performance of meridian immunocard *Mycoplasma* test in a multicenter clinical trial. J. Clin. Microbiol. *34:*1180–1183, 1996.
6. Alfa, M. J., Embree, J. E., Degagne, P., et al.: Transmission of *Ureaplasma urealyticum* from mothers to full and preterm infants. Pediatr. Infect. Dis. J. *14:*341–345, 1995.
7. Allen, P. Z., and Prescott, B.: Immunochemical studies on a *Mycoplasma pneumoniae* polysaccharide fraction: Cross-reactions with types 23 and 32 antipneumococcal rabbit sera. Infect. Immun. *20:*421–429, 1978.
8. Allen, V., Sueltmann, S., and Lawson, C.: Laboratory diagnosis of *Mycoplasma pneumoniae* in a public health laboratory. Health Lab. Sci. *4:*90–95, 1967.
9. Almagor, M., Yatziv, S., and Kahane, I.: Inhibition of host cell catalase by *Mycoplasma pneumoniae:* A possible mechanism for cell injury. Infect. Immun. *41:*251–256, 1983.
10. Al-Mateen, M., Gibbs, M., Dietrich, R., et al.: Encephalitis lethargica-like illness in a girl with mycoplasma infection. Neurology *38:*1155–1158, 1988.
11. Anderson, D. R., and Barile, M. F.: Ultrastructure of *Mycoplasma hominis.* J. Bacteriol. *90:*180–192, 1965.
12. Anikster, Y., Glustein, J. Z., Weill, M., et al.: Extrapulmonary manifestations of *Mycoplasma pneumoniae* infections. Israel J. Med. Sci. *30:*412–413, 1994.
13. Archer, J. F.: "T" strain *Mycoplasma* in the female urogenital tract. Br. J. Vener. Dis. *44:*232–234, 1968.
14. Arthur, G., and Margolis, G.: *Mycoplasma*-like structures in granulomatous angiitis of the central nervous system: Case reports with light and electron microscopic studies. Arch. Pathol. Lab. Med. *101:*382–387, 1977.
15. Assaad, F., and Borecka, I.: Nine-year study of WHO virus reports on fatal viral infections. Bull. W. H. O. *55:*445–453, 1977.
16. Azimi, P. H., Chase, P. A., and Petru, A. M.: Mycoplasmas: Their role in pediatric disease. Curr. Probl. Pediatr. *14:*1–46, 1984.
17. Azimi, P. H., and Koranyi, K. I.: *Mycoplasma pneumoniae* infections in a family. Clin. Pediatr. *16:*1138–1139, 1977.
18. Balassanian, N., and Robbins, F. C.: *Mycoplasma pneumoniae* infection in families. N. Engl. J. Med. *277:*719–725, 1967.
19. Baseman, J. B., Lange, M., Criscimagna, N. L., et al.: Interplay between mycoplasmas and host target cells. Microb. Pathog. *19:*105–116, 1995.
20. Baseman, J. B., Dallo, S. F., Tully, J. G., et al.: Isolation and characterization of *Mycoplasma genitalium* strains from the human respiratory tract. J. Clin. Microbiol. *26:*2266–2269, 1988.
21. Bauer, F. A., Wear, D. J., Angritt, P., Lo, S.-C.: *Mycoplasma fermentans* (incognitus strain) infection in the kidneys of patients with acquired immunodeficiency syndrome and associated nephropathy: A light microscopic immunohistochemical, and ultrastructural study. Hum. Pathol. *22:*63–69, 1991.
22. Bayer, A. S., Galpin, J. E., Theofilopoulos, A. N., et al.: Neurologic disease associated with *Mycoplasma pneumoniae* pneumonitis: Demonstration of viable *Mycoplasma pneumoniae* in cerebrospinal fluid and blood by radio-

isotopic and immunofluorescent tissue culture techniques. Ann. Intern. Med. *94*:15–20, 1981.
23. Bébéar, C., Dupon M., Renaudin, H., et al.: Potential improvements in therapeutic options for mycoplasmal respiratory infections. Clin. Infect. Dis. *17*(Suppl. 1):S202–S207, 1993.
24. Benisch, B. M., Fayemi, A., Gerber, M. A., et al.: Mycoplasmal pneumonia in a patient with rheumatic heart disease. Am. J. Clin. Pathol. *58*:343–348, 1972.
25. Berant, M., Cohen, N., and Wagner, Y.: *Mycoplasma pneumoniae* infection presenting as acute rheumatic fever. Helv. Paediatr. Acta *36*:567–572, 1981.
26. Berkovich, S., Millian, S. J., and Snyder, R. D.: The association of viral and *Mycoplasma* infections with recurrence of wheezing in the asthmatic child. Ann. Allergy *28*:43–49, 1970.
27. Bhattacharyya, T. K., Mehra, Y. N., and Agarwal, S. C.: Incidence of bacteria, L-form and mycoplasma in chronic sinusitis. Acta Otolaryngol. *74*:293–296, 1972.
28. Biberfeld, G., and Sterner, G.: Smooth muscle antibodies in *Mycoplasma pneumoniae* infection. Clin. Exp. Immunol. *24*:287–291, 1976.
29. Biberfeld, G., and Norberg, R.: Circulating immune complexes in *Mycoplasma pneumoniae* infection. J. Immunol. *112*:413–415, 1974.
30. Biberfeld, G.: Antibody responses in *Mycoplasma pneumoniae* infection in relation to serum immunoglobulins, especially IgM. Acta Pathol. Microbiol. Scand. [B] *79*:620–634, 1971.
31. Biberfeld, G.: Antibodies to brain and other tissues in cases of *Mycoplasma pneumoniae* infection. Clin. Exp. Immunol. *8*:319–333, 1971.
32. Biberfeld, G., and Sterner, G.: Antibodies in bronchial secretions following natural infection with *Mycoplasma pneumoniae*. Acta Pathol. Microbiol. Scand. [B] *79*:599–605, 1971.
33. Biberfeld, G., and Biberfeld, P.: Ultrastructural features of *Mycoplasma pneumoniae*. J. Bacteriol. *102*:855–861, 1970.
34. Biberfeld, G., and Sterner, G.: A study of *Mycoplasma pneumoniae* infections in families. Scand. J. Infect. Dis. *1*:39–46, 1969.
35. Biberfeld, G., Stenbeck, J., and Johnsson, T.: *Mycoplasma pneumoniae* infection in hospitalized patients with acute respiratory illness. Acta Pathol. Microbiol. Scand. *74*:287–300, 1968.
36. Biberfeld, G., Johnsson, T., and Jonsson, J.: Studies on *Mycoplasma pneumoniae* infection in Sweden. Acta Pathol. Microbiol. Scand. *63*:469–475, 1965.
37. Black, F. T., Birch-Andersen, A., and Freundt, E. A.: Morphology and ultrastructure of human T-mycoplasmas. J. Bacteriol. *111*:254–259, 1972.
38. Blackmore, T. K., Reznikov, M., and Gordon, D. L.: Clinical utility of the polymerase chain reaction to diagnose *Mycoplasma pneumoniae* infection. Pathology *27*:177–181, 1995.
39. Blanchard, A., Hentschel, J., Duffy, L., et al.: Detection of *Ureaplasma urealyticum* by polymerase chain reaction in the urogenital tract of adults, in amniotic fluid, and in the respiratory tract of newborns. Clin. Infect. Dis. *17*(Suppl. 1):S148–S153, 1993.
40. Blancard, A., and Montagnier, L.: AIDS-associated mycoplasmas. Ann. Rev. Microbiol. *48*:687–712, 1994.
41. Blanco, J. D., Gibbs, R. S., Malherbe, H., et al.: A controlled study of genital mycoplasmas in amniotic fluid from patients with intra-amniotic infection. J. Infect. Dis. *147*:650–653, 1983.
42. Block, S., Hedrick J., Hammerschlag, M. R., et al.: *Mycoplasma pneumoniae* and *Chlamydia pneumoniae* in pediatric community-acquired pneumonia: Comparative efficacy and safety of clarithromycin vs. erythromycin ethylsuccinate. Pediatr. Infect. Dis. J. *14*:471–477, 1995.
43. Boatman, E. S.: Morphology and ultrastructure of the mycoplasmatales. *In* Barile, M. F., and Razin, S. (eds.): The Mycoplasmas. Vol. 1. New York, Academic Press, 1979, pp. 63–102.
44. Boccardi, V., D'Annibali, S., DiNatale, G., et al.: *Mycoplasma pneumoniae* infection complicated by paroxysmal cold hemoglobinuria with anti-P specificity of biphasic hemolysin. Blut *34*:211–214, 1977.
45. Boe, O., Diderichsen, J., and Matre, R.: Isolation of *Mycoplasma hominis* from cerebrospinal fluid. Scand. J. Infect. Dis. *5*:285–288, 1973.
46. Bové, J. M.: Molecular features of mollicutes. Clin. Infect. Dis. *17*(Suppl. 1):S10–S31, 1993.
47. Bowie, W. R., Wang, S.-P., Alexander, E. R., et al.: Etiology of nongonococcal urethritis: Evidence for *Chlamydia trachomatis* and *Ureaplasma urealyticum*. J. Clin. Invest. *59*:735–742, 1977.
48. Bowie, W. R., Alexander, E. R., Floyd, J. F., et al.: Differential response of chlamydial and *Ureaplasma*-associated urethritis to sulphafurazole (sulfisoxazole) and aminocyclitols. Lancet *2*:1276–1278, 1976.
49. Braun, P., Lee, Y.-H., Klein, J. O., et al.: Birth weight and genital mycoplasmas in pregnancy. N. Engl. J. Med. *284*:167–171, 1971.
50. Braun, P., Klein, J. O., and Kass, E. H.: Susceptibility of genital mycoplasmas to antimicrobial agents. Appl. Microbiol. *19*:62–70, 1970.
51. Bray, P. F., and Hackett, T. N.: Multiple birth defects in a newborn exposed to *Mycoplasma pneumoniae* in utero. Am. J. Dis. Child. *130*:312–314, 1976.
52. Bredt, W., Heunert, H. H., Hofling, K. H., et al.: Microcinematographic studies of *Mycoplasma hominis* cells. J. Bacteriol. *113*:1223–1227, 1973.
53. Bredt, W.: Cellular morphology of newly isolated *Mycoplasma hominis* strains. J. Bacteriol. *105*:449–450, 1971.
54. Bredt, W.: Filamentous growth of some *Mycoplasma* species of man. Experientia *25*:1118–1119, 1969.
55. Bredt, W.: Motility and multiplication of *Mycoplasma pneumoniae*: A phase contrast study. Pathol. Microbiol. *32*:321–326, 1968.
56. Brolin, I., and Wernstedt, L.: Radiographic appearance of mycoplasmal pneumonia. Scand. J. Resp. Dis. *59*:179–189, 1978.
57. Brooker, R. J., Eason, J. D., and Solimano, A.: *Mycoplasma* surgical wound infection in a neonate. Pediatr. Infect. Dis. J. *13*:751–753, 1994.
58. Broome, C. V., LaVenture, M., Kaye, H. S., et al.: An explosive outbreak of *Mycoplasma pneumoniae* infection in a summer camp. Pediatrics *66*:884–888, 1980.
59. Brunell, P. A., Dische, R. M., and Walker, M. B.: *Mycoplasma*, amnionitis, and respiratory distress syndrome. J. A. M. A. *207*:2097–2099, 1969.
60. Brunner, H., Weidner, W., and Schiefer, H.-G.: Studies on the role of *Ureaplasma urealyticum* and *Mycoplasma hominis* in prostatitis. J. Infect. Dis. *147*:807–813, 1983.
61. Brunner, H., Schaeg, W., Bruck, U., et al.: Determination of IgG, IgM, and IgA antibodies to *Mycoplasma pneumoniae* by an indirect staphylococcal radioimmunoassay. Med. Microbiol. Immunol. *165*:29–41, 1978.
62. Brunner, H., Prescott, B., Greenberg, H., et al.: Unexpectedly high frequency of antibody to *Mycoplasma pneumoniae* in human sera as measured by sensitive techniques. J. Infect. Dis. *135*:524–530, 1977.
63. Brunner, H., Greenberg, H. B., James, W. D., et al.: Antibody to *Mycoplasma pneumoniae* in nasal secretions and sputa of experimentally infected human volunteers. Infect. Immun. *8*:612–620, 1973.
64. Brunner, H., Horswood, R. L., and Chanock, R. M.: More sensitive methods for detection of antibody to *Mycoplasma pneumoniae*. J. Infect. Dis. *127*(Suppl.):S52–S55, 1973.
65. Brunner, H., James, W. D., Horswood, R. L., et al.: Measurement of *Mycoplasma pneumoniae* mycoplasmacidal antibody in human serum. J. Immunol. *108*:1491–1498, 1972.
66. Brus, F., van Waarde, W. M., Schoots, C., et al.: Fatal ureaplasmal pneumonia and sepsis in a newborn infant. Eur. J. Pediatr. *150*:782–783, 1991.
67. Buck, G. E., O'Hara, L. C., and Summersgill, J. T.: Rapid, sensitive detection of *Mycoplasma pneumoniae* in simulated clinical specimens by DNA amplification. J. Clin. Microbiol. *30*:3280–3283, 1992.
68. Busolo, F., Tonin, E., and Meloni, G. A.: Enzyme-linked immunosorbent assay for serodiagnosis of *Mycoplasma pneumoniae* infections. J. Clin. Microbiol. *18*:432–435, 1983.
69. Bygdeman, S. M., and Märdh, P. A.: Antimicrobial susceptibility and susceptibility testing of *Mycoplasma hominis*: A review. Sex. Transm. Dis. *10*:366–370, 1983.
70. Cadieux, N., Lebel, P., and Brousseau, R.: Use of a triplex polymerase chain reaction for the detection and differentiation of *Mycoplasma pneumoniae* and *Mycoplasma genitalium* in the presence of human DNA. J. Gen. Microbiol. *139*:2431–2437, 1993.
71. Cannell, H., Churcher, G. M., and Milton-Thompson, G. J.: Stevens-Johnson syndrome associated with *Mycoplasma pneumoniae* infection. Br. J. Dermatol. *81*:196–199, 1969.
72. Carter, J. B.: Serologic diagnosis of *Mycoplasma pneumoniae* infection: Introduction of an indirect fluorescent antibody (IFA) procedure. Immunopathology *8*:1–7, 1984.
73. Caspi, E., Herczeg, E., Solomon, F., et al.: Amnionitis and T strain mycoplasmemia. Am. J. Obstet. Gynecol. *111*:1102–1106, 1971.
74. Cassell, G. H., Waites, K. B., Watson, H. L., et al.: *Ureaplasma urealyticum* intrauterine infection: Role in prematurity and disease in newborns. Clin. Microbiol. Rev. *6*:69–87, 1993.
75. Cassell, G. H., Crouse, D. T., Waites, K. B., et al.: Does *Ureaplasma urealyticum* cause respiratory disease in newborns? Pediatr. Infect. Dis. J. *7*:535–541, 1988.
76. Cassell, G. H., Davis, R. O., Waites, K. B., et al.: Isolation of *Mycoplasma hominis* and *Ureaplasma urealyticum* from amniotic fluid at 16–20 weeks of gestation: Potential effect on outcome of pregnancy. Sex. Transm. Dis. *10*:294–302, 1983.
77. Cassell, G. H., Younger, J. B., Brown, M. B., et al.: Microbiologic study of infertile women at the time of diagnostic laparoscopy: Association of *Ureaplasma urealyticum* with a defined subpopulation. N. Engl. J. Med. *308*:502–505, 1983.
78. Cassell, G. H., and Cole, B. C.: Mycoplasmas as agents of human disease. N. Engl. J. Med. *304*:80–89, 1981.
79. Chanock, R., Chambon, L., Chang, W., et al.: WHO respiratory disease survey in children: A serological study. Bull. W. H. O. *37*:363–369, 1967.
80. Chanock, R. M., and Parrott, R. H.: Acute respiratory disease in infancy and childhood: Present understanding and prospects for prevention. Pediatrics *36*:21–39, 1965.
81. Chanock, R. M.: *Mycoplasma* infections of man. N. Engl. J. Med. *273*:1199–1206, 1257–1264, 1965.
82. Chanock, R. M., Mufson, M. A., and Somerson, N. L.: Role of *Mycoplasma* (PPLO) in human respiratory disease. Am. Rev. Respir. Dis. *88*:218–231, 1963.
83. Chanock, R. M., Hayflick, L., and Barile, M. F.: Growth on artificial medium of an agent associated with atypical pneumonia and its identification as a PPLO. Proc. Natl. Acad. Sci. U. S. A. *48*:41–49, 1962.
84. Chanock, R. M., Mufson, M. A., Bloom, H. H., et al.: Eaton agent pneumonia. J. A. M. A. *175*:213–220, 1961.
85. Chanock, R. M., Cook, M. K., Fox, H. H., et al.: Serologic evidence of

infection with Eaton agent in lower respiratory illness in childhood. N. Engl. J. Med. *262*:648–654, 1960.
86. Chen, S.-C., Tsai, C. C., and Nouri, S.: Carditis associated with *Mycoplasma pneumoniae* infection. Am. J. Dis. Child. *140*:471–472, 1986.
87. Cherry, J. D.: Anemia and mucocutaneous lesions due to *Mycoplasma pneumoniae* infections. Clin. Infect. Dis. *17*(Suppl. 1):S47–S51, 1993.
88. Cherry, J. D.: *Mycoplasma* infections. *In* Shen, J. T. Y. (ed.): The Clinical Practice of Adolescent Medicine. New York, Appleton-Century-Crofts, 1980, pp. 80–93.
89. Cherry, J. D., and Welliver, R. C.: *Mycoplasma pneumoniae* infections of adults and children. West. J. Med. *125*:47–55, 1976.
90. Cherry, J. D., Hurwitz, E. S., and Welliver, R. C.: *Mycoplasma pneumoniae* infections and exanthems. J. Pediatr. *87*:369–373, 1975.
91. Cherry, J. D.: Newer respiratory viruses: Their role in respiratory illnesses of children. Adv. Pediatr. *20*:225–289, 1973.
92. Cherry, J. D., and Taylor-Robinson, D.: *Mycoplasma* pathogenicity studies in organ cultures. Ann. N. Y. Acad. Sci. *225*:290–303, 1973.
93. Cherry, J. D., and Taylor-Robinson, D.: Growth and pathogenicity studies of *Mycoplasma gallisepticum* in chicken tracheal organ cultures. J. Med. Microbiol. *4*:441–449, 1971.
94. Cherry, J. D., Taylor-Robinson, D., Willers, H., et al.: A search for mycoplasma infections in patients with chronic bronchitis. Thorax *26*:62–67, 1971.
95. Cherry, J. D., and Taylor-Robinson, D.: Peroxide production by mycoplasmas in chicken tracheal organ cultures. Nature *228*:1099–1100, 1970.
96. Cherry, J. D., and Taylor-Robinson, D.: Growth and pathogenesis of *Mycoplasma mycoides* var. *capri* in chicken embryo tracheal organ cultures. Infect. Immun. *2*:431–438, 1970.
97. Cherry, J. D.: Newer viral exanthems. Adv. Pediatr. *16*:233–286, 1969.
98. Cherry, J. D., Allen, V. D., and Sueltmann, S.: Search for *Mycoplasma pneumoniae* infection in patients with exanthem but without pneumonia. Arch. Environ. Health *16*:911–912, 1968.
99. Chester, A., Kane, J., and Garagusi, V.: *Mycoplasma* pneumonia with bilateral pleural effusions. Am. Rev. Respir. Dis. *112*:451–456, 1975.
100. Chusid, M. J., Lachman, B. S., and Lazerson, J.: Severe *Mycoplasma* pneumonia and vesicular eruption in SC hemoglobinopathy. J. Pediatr. *93*:449–451, 1978.
101. Cimolai, N., Mah, D. G., Taylor, G. P., et al.: Bases for the early immune response after rechallenge or component vaccination in an animal model of acute *Mycoplasma pneumoniae* pneumonitis. Vaccine *13*:305–309, 1995.
102. Cimolai, N., Malleson, P., Thomas, E., et al.: *Mycoplasma pneumoniae* associated arthropathy: Confirmation of the association by determination of the antipolypeptide IgM response. J. Rheumatol. *16*:1150–1152, 1989.
103. Clough, W., Cassell, G. H., Duffy, L. B., et al.: Septic arthritis and bacteremia due to *Mycoplasma* resistant to antimicrobial therapy in a patient with systemic lupus erythematosus. Clin. Infect. Dis. *15*:402–407, 1992.
104. Clyde, W. A., Jr.: Clinical overview of typical *Mycoplasma pneumoniae* infections. Clin. Infect. Dis. *17*(Suppl. 1):S32–S36, 1993.
105. Clyde, W. A.: Neurological syndromes and mycoplasmal infections. Arch. Neurol. *37*:65–66, 1980.
106. Clyde, W. A.: *Mycoplasma pneumoniae* infections of man. *In* Tully, J. G., and Whitcomb, R. F. (eds.): The Mycoplasmas. Vol. II. New York, Academic Press, 1979, pp. 275–306.
107. Clyde, W. A.: Immunopathology of experimental *Mycoplasma pneumoniae* disease. Infect. Immun. *4*:757–763, 1971.
108. Clyde, W. A.: An experimental model for human *Mycoplasma* disease. Yale J. Biol. Med. *40*:436–443, 1968.
109. Clyde, W. A., and Denny, F. W.: *Mycoplasma* infections in childhood. Pediatrics *40*:669–684, 1967.
110. Cockcroft, D. W., and Stilwell, G. A.: Lobar pneumonia caused by *Mycoplasma pneumoniae.* Can. Med. Assoc. J. *124*:1463–1468, 1981.
111. Cohen, G., and Somerson, N. L.: Glucose-dependent secretion and destruction of hydrogen peroxide by *Mycoplasma pneumoniae.* J. Bacteriol. *98*:547–551, 1969.
112. Cole, B. C., and Cassell, G. H.: *Mycoplasma* infections as models of chronic joint inflammation. Arthritis Rheum. *22*:1375–1381, 1979.
113. Collier, A. M., and Baseman, J. B.: Organ culture techniques with mycoplasmas. Ann. N. Y. Acad. Sci. *225*:277–289, 1973.
114. Collier, A. M., and Clyde, W. A.: Relationships between *Mycoplasma pneumoniae* and human respiratory epithelium. Infect. Immun. *3*:694–701, 1971.
115. Collier, A. M., Clyde, W. A., and Denny, F. W.: *Mycoplasma pneumoniae* in hamster tracheal organ culture: Immunofluorescent and electron microscopic studies. Proc. Soc. Exp. Biol. Med. *136*:569–573, 1971.
116. Collier, A. M., Clyde, W. A., and Denny, F. W.: Biologic effects of *Mycoplasma pneumoniae* and other mycoplasmas from man on hamster tracheal organ culture. Proc. Soc. Exp. Biol. Med. *132*:1153–1158, 1969.
117. Copps, S. C., Allen, V. D., Sueltmann, S., et al.: A community outbreak of *Mycoplasma* pneumonia. J. A. M. A. *204*:123–128, 1968.
118. Copps, S. C.: Primary atypical pneumonia: With hemolytic anemia and erythema multiforme. Clin. Pediatr. *3*:491–495, 1964.
119. Cordero, L., Cuadrado, R., Hall, C. B., et al.: Primary atypical pneumonia: An epidemic caused by *Mycoplasma pneumoniae.* J. Pediatr. *71*:1–12, 1967.
120. Costea, N., Yakulis, V. J., and Heller, P.: Inhibition of cold agglutinins (Anti-I) by *M. pneumoniae* antigens. Proc. Soc. Exp. Biol. Med. *139*:476–479, 1972.
121. Couch, R. B.: *Mycoplasma pneumoniae* (primary atypical pneumonia). *In* Mandell, G. L., Douglas, R. G., Jr., and Bennett, J. E. (eds.): Principles and Practice of Infectious Diseases. New York, John Wiley & Sons, 1980, pp. 1484–1498.
122. Coufalik, E. D., Taylor-Robinson, D., and Csonka, G. W.: Treatment of nongonococcal urethritis with rifampicin as a means of defining the role of *Ureaplasma urealyticum.* Br. J. Vener. Dis. *55*:36–43, 1979.
123. Craighead, J. E.: Report of a workshop: Disease accentuation after immunization with inactivated microbial vaccines. J. Infect. Dis. *131*:749–753, 1975.
124. Crouse, D. T., Odrezin, G. T., Cutter, G. R., et al.: Radiographic changes associated with tracheal isolation of *Ureaplasma urealyticum* from neonates. Clin. Infect. Dis. *17*(Suppl. 1):S122–S130, 1993.
125. Cummings, M. C., and McCormack, W. M.: Increase in resistance of *Mycoplasma hominis* to tetracyclines. Antimicrob. Agents Chemother. *34*:2297–2299, 1990.
126. Dajani, A. S., Clyde, W. A., and Denny, F. W.: Experimental infection with *Mycoplasma pneumoniae* (Eaton's agent). J. Exp. Med. *121*:1071–1086, 1965.
127. Dallo, S. F., Lazzell, A. L ., Chavoya, A., et al.: Biofunctional domains of the *Mycoplasma pneumoniae* P30 adhesin. Infect. Immun. *64*:2595–2601, 1996.
128. Dallo, S. F., Chavoya, A., and Baseman, J. B.: Characterization of the gene for a 30-kilodalton adhesin-related protein of *Mycoplasma pneumoniae.* Infect. Immun. *58*:4163–4165, 1990.
129. Dan, M., and Robertson, J.: *Mycoplasma hominis* septicemia after heart surgery. Am. J. Med. *84*:976–977, 1988.
130. Dan, M., Tyrrell, D. L. J., Stemke, G. W., et al.: *Mycoplasma hominis* septicemia in a burned infant. J. Pediatr. *99*:743–745, 1981.
131. Davis, C. P., Cochran, S., Lisse, J., et al.: Isolation of *Mycoplasma pneumoniae* from synovial fluid samples in a patient with pneumonia and polyarthritis. Arch. Intern. Med. *148*:969–970, 1988.
132. deBarbeyrac, B., Bernet-Poggi, C., Febrer, F., et al.: Detection of *Mycoplasma pneumoniae* and *Mycoplasma genitalium* in clinical samples by polymerase chain reaction. Clin. Infect. Dis. *17*(Suppl. 1):S83–S89, 1993.
133. Decancq, H. G., Jr., and Lee, F. A.: *Mycoplasma pneumoniae* pneumonia: Massive pulmonary involvement and pleural effusion. J. A. M. A. *194*:1010–1011, 1965.
134. Del Giudice, R. A., Tully, J. G., Rose, D. L., et al.: *Mycoplasma pirum* sp. nov., a terminal structured mollicute from cell cultures. Int. J. Syst. Bacteriol. *35*:285–291, 1985.
135. Denny, F. W., Clyde, W. A., and Glezen, W. P.: *Mycoplasma pneumoniae* disease: Clinical spectrum, pathophysiology, epidemiology, and control. J. Infect. Dis. *123*:74–92, 1971.
136. Dienes, L., and Edsall, J.: Observations on L-organisms of Klieneberger. Proc. Soc. Exp. Biol. Med. *36*:740–744, 1937.
137. Dische, M. R., Quinn, P. A., Czegledy-Nagy, E., et al.: Genital *Mycoplasma* infection. Intrauterine infection: Pathologic study of the fetus and placenta. Am. J. Clin. Pathol. *72*:167–174, 1979.
138. Domermuth, C. H., Nielsen, M. H., Freundt, E. A., et al.: Ultrastructure of *Mycoplasma* species. J. Bacteriol. *88*:727–744, 1964.
139. Dorff, B., and Lind, K.: Two fatal cases of meningoencephalitis associated with *Mycoplasma pneumoniae* infection. Scand. J. Infect. Dis. *8*:49–51, 1976.
140. Dowdle, W. R., Stewart, J. A., Heyward, J. T., et al.: *Mycoplasma pneumoniae* infections in a children's population: A five-year study. Am. J. Epidemiol. *85*:137–146, 1967.
141. Dowdle, W. R., and Robinson, R. Q.: An indirect hemagglutination test for diagnosis of *Mycoplasma pneumoniae* infections. Proc. Soc. Exp. Biol. Med. *116*:947–950, 1964.
142. Dowling, P. C., and Cook, S. D.: Role of infection in Guillain-Barré syndrome: Laboratory confirmation of herpesviruses in 41 cases. Ann. Neurol. *9*:44–55, 1981.
143. Eaton, M. D., and Liu, C.: Studies on sensitivity to streptomycin of the atypical pneumonia agent. J. Bacteriol. *74*:784–787, 1957.
144. Eaton, M. D.: Action of aureomycin and chloromycetin on the viruses of primary atypical pneumonia. Proc. Soc. Exp. Biol. Med. *73*:24–26, 1950.
145. Eaton, M. D., Meiklejohn, G., and van Herick, W.: Studies on the etiology of primary atypical pneumonia: A filterable agent transmissible to cotton rats, hamsters, and chick embryos. J. Exp. Med. *79*:649–668, 1944.
146. Echivarria, J. M., Leon, P., Balfagon, P., et al.: Diagnosis of *Mycoplasma pneumoniae* infection by microparticle agglutination and antibody-capture enzyme immunoassay. Eur. J. Clin. Microbiol. Infect. Dis. *9*:217–220, 1990.
147. Embree, J. E., Krause, V. W., and Embil, J. A.: *Mycoplasma hominis*: A placental pathogen? Sex. Transm. Dis. *10*:307–310, 1983.
148. Embree, J. E., and Embil, J. A.: Mycoplasmas in diseases of humans. Can. Med. Assoc. J. *123*:105–111, 1980.
149. Embree, J. E., Krause, V. W., Embil, J. A., et al.: Placental infection with *Mycoplasma hominis* and *Ureplasma urealyticum:* Clinical correlation. Obstet. Gynecol. *56*:475–481, 1980.
150. Emmons, J., Schluenderberg, A., and Cordero, L.: An aid to the rapid diagnosis of *Mycoplasma pneumoniae* infections. J. Infect. Dis. *119*:650–653, 1969.
151. Eschenbach, D. A.: *Ureaplasma urealyticum* and premature birth. Clin. Infect. Dis. *17*(Suppl. 1):S100–S106, 1993.

152. Evans, A. S., Allen, V., and Sueltmann, S.: *Mycoplasma pneumoniae* infections in University of Wisconsin students. Am. Rev. Respir. Dis. *96*:237–244, 1967.
153. Evans, A. S., and Brobst, M.: Bronchitis, pneumonitis and pneumonia in University of Wisconsin students. N. Engl. J. Med. *265*:401–409, 1961.
154. Evans, M. R. W., and Marshall, A. J.: Recovery from *Mycoplasma* meningoencephalitis, credited to penicillin allergy. Lancet *1*:1100, 1990.
155. Evatt, B. L., Dowdle, W. R., Johnson, McC., Jr., et al.: Epidemic *Mycoplasma* pneumonia. N. Engl. J. Med. *285*:374–377, 1971.
156. Fedorko, D. P., Emery, D. D., Franklin, S. M., et al.: Evaluation of a rapid enzyme immunoassay system for serologic diagnosis of *Mycoplasma pneumoniae* infection. Diagn. Microbiol. Infect. Dis. *23*:85–88, 1995.
157. Feizi, O., Grubb, C., Skinner, J. I., et al.: Primary atypical pneumoniae due to *Mycoplasma pneumoniae* complicated by haemorrhagic pleural effusion, haemolytic anaemia and myocarditis. Br. J. Clin. Pract. *27*:99–101, 1973.
158. Feizi, T., Maclean, H., Sommerville, R. G., et al.: Studies on an epidemic of respiratory disease caused by *Mycoplasma pneumoniae.* B. M. J. *1*:457–460, 1967.
159. Feizi, T.: Cold agglutinins, the direct Coombs' test and serum immunoglobulins in *Mycoplasma pneumoniae* infection. Ann. N. Y. Acad. Sci. *143*:801–812, 1967.
160. Feizi, T.: Syndromes associated with mycoplasmas. Postgrad. Med. J. *43*:106–108, 1967.
161. Fekety, F. R., Jr., Caldwell, J., Gump, D., et al.: Bacteria, viruses, and mycoplasmas in acute pneumonia in adults. Am. Rev. Respir. Dis. *104*:499–507, 1971.
162. Fernald, G. W.: Humoral and cellular immune reponses to mycoplasmas. *In* Tully, J. G., and Whitcomb, R. F. (eds.): The Mycoplasmas. Vol. II. New York, Academic Press, 1979, pp. 399–423.
163. Fernald, G. W., and Clyde, W. A., Jr.: Pulmonary immune mechanisms in *Mycoplasma pneumoniae* disease. *In* Kirkpatrick, C. H., and Reynolds, H. Y. (eds.): Immunologic and Infectious Reactions in the Lung. New York, Marcel Dekker, 1976, pp. 101–130.
164. Fernald, G. W., Collier, A. M., and Clyde, W. A.: Respiratory infections due to *Mycoplasma pneumoniae* in infants and children. Pediatrics *55*:327–335, 1975.
165. Fernald, G. W., and Glezen, W. P.: Humoral and cellular immune responses to an inactivated *Mycoplasma pneumoniae* vaccine in children. J. Infect. Dis. *127*:498–504, 1973.
166. Fernald, G. W.: Role of host response in *Mycoplasma pneumoniae* disease. J. Infect. Dis. *127*:S55–S58, 1973.
167. Fernald, G. W.: In vitro response of human lymphocytes to *Mycoplasma pneumoniae.* Infect. Immun. *5*:552–558, 1972.
168. Fernald, G. W., Clyde, W. A., and Bienenstock, J.: Immunoglobulin-containing cells in lungs of hamsters infected with *Mycoplasma pneumoniae.* J. Immunol. *108*:1400–1408, 1972.
169. Fernald, G. W., Clyde, W. A., and Denny, F. W.: Nature of the immune response to *Mycoplasma pneumoniae.* J. Immunol. *98*:1028–1038, 1967.
170. Fiacco, V., Miller, M. J., Carney, E., et al.: Comparison of media for isolation of *Ureaplasma urealyticum* and genital *Mycoplasma* species. J. Clin. Microbiol. *20*:862–865, 1984.
171. Fiala, M., Myhre, B. A., Chinh, L. T., et al.: Pathogenesis of anemia associated with *Mycoplasma pneumoniae.* Acta Haematol. *51*:297–301, 1974.
172. Fine, N. L., Smith, L. R., and Sheedy, P. F.: Frequency of pleural effusions in *Mycoplasma* and viral pneumonias. N. Engl. J. Med. *283*:790–793, 1970.
173. Finland, M., Peterson, O. L., Allen, H. E., et al.: Cold agglutinins. I. Occurrence of cold isohemagglutinins in various conditions. J. Clin. Invest. *24*:451–457, 1945.
174. Fischer, G. S., Sweimler, W. I., and Kleger, B.: Comparison of MYCOPLASM-ELISA with complement fixation test for measurement of antibodies to *Mycoplasma pneumoniae.* Diagn. Microbiol. Infect. Dis. *4*:139–145, 1986.
175. Fischman, R. A., Marschall, K. E., Kislak, J. W., et al.: Adult respiratory distress syndrome caused by *Mycoplasma pneumoniae.* Chest *74*:471–473, 1978.
176. Fisher, R. S., Clark, A. W., Wolinsky, J. S., et al.: Postinfectious leukoencephalitis complicating *Mycoplasma pneumoniae* infection. Arch. Neurol. *40*:109–113, 1983.
177. Fleischaur, P., Hube, U., Mertens, H., et al.: Nachweis von *Mycoplasma pneumoniae* in liquor bei akuter polyneuritis. Dtsch. Med. Wochenschr. *97*:678–682, 1972.
178. Fleming, P. C., Krieger, E., Turner, J. A. P., et al.: Febrile mucocutaneous syndrome with respiratory involvement, associated with isolation of *Mycoplasma pneumoniae.* Can. Med. Assoc. J. *97*:1458–1459, 1967.
179. Forgacs, P., Kundsin, R. B., Margles, S. W., et al.: A case of *Ureaplasma urealyticum* septic arthritis in a patient with hypogammaglobulinemia. Clin. Infect. Dis. *16*:293–294, 1993.
180. Foy, H. M.: Infections caused by *Mycoplasma pneumoniae* and possible carrier state in different populations of patients. Clin. Infect. Dis. *17*(Suppl. 1):S37–S46, 1993.
181. Foy, H. M., Kenny, G. E., Cooney, M. K., et al.: Naturally acquired immunity to pneumonia due to *Mycoplasma pneumoniae.* J. Infect. Dis. *147*:967–973, 1983.
182. Foy, H. M., Kenny, G. E., Cooney, M. K., et al.: Long-term epidemiology of infections with *Mycoplasma pneumoniae.* J. Infect. Dis. *139*:681–687, 1979.
183. Foy, H. M., Kenny, G. E., Sefi, R., et al.: Second attacks of pneumonia due to *Mycoplasma pneumoniae.* J. Infect. Dis. *135*:673–677, 1977.
184. Foy, H., Kenny, G., Bor, E., et al.: Prevalence of *Mycoplasma hominis* and *Ureaplasma urealyticum* (T strains) in urine of adolescents. J. Clin. Microbiol. *2*:226–230, 1975.
185. Foy, H. M., Ochs, H., and Davis, S. D.: *Mycoplasma pneumoniae* infections in patients with immunodeficiency syndromes: Report of four cases. J. Infect. Dis. *127*:388–393, 1973.
186. Foy, H. M., Cooney, M. K., Maletzky, A. J., et al.: Incidence and etiology of pneumonia, croup and bronchiolitis in preschool children belonging to a prepaid medical care group over a four-year period. Am. J. Epidemiol. *97*:80–92, 1973.
187. Foy, H. M., Cooney, M. K., McMahan, R., et al.: Viral and mycoplasmal pneumonia in a prepaid medical care group during an eight-year period. Am. J. Epidemiol. *97*:93–102, 1973.
188. Foy, H. M., Nugent, C. G., Kenny, G. E., et al.: Repeated *Mycoplasma pneumoniae* pneumonia after 4 and one half years. J. A. M. A. *216*:671–672, 1971.
189. Foy, H. M., Kenny, G. E., McMahan, R., et al.: *Mycoplasma pneumoniae* pneumonia in an urban area: Five years of surveillance. J. A. M. A. *214*:1666–1672, 1970.
190. Foy, H. M., Kenny, G. E., Wentworth, B. B., et al.: Isolation of *Mycoplasma hominis,* T-strains, and cytomegalovirus from the cervix of pregnant women. Am. J. Obstet. Gynecol. *106*:635–643, 1970.
191. Foy, H. M., Kenny, G. E., Levinsohn, E. M., et al.: Acquisition of mycoplasmata and T-strains during infancy. J. Infect. Dis. *121*:579–587, 1970.
192. Foy, H. M., Kenny, G. E., McMahan, R., et al.: *Mycoplasma pneumoniae* in the community. Am. J. Epidemiol. *93*:55–67, 1970.
193. Foy, H. M., and Alexander, E. R.: *Mycoplasma pneumoniae* infections in childhood. Adv. Pediatr. *16*:301–323, 1969.
194. Foy, H. M., Kenny, G. E., and Koler, J.: *Mycoplasma pneumoniae* in Stevens-Johnson's syndrome. Lancet *2*:550–551, 1966.
195. Foy, H. M., Grayston, J. T., Kenny, G. E., et al.: Epidemiology of *Mycoplasma pneumoniae* infection in families. J. A. M. A. *197*:859–866, 1966.
196. Fransen, H., Forsgren, M., Heigl, Z., et al.: Studies on *Mycoplasma pneumoniae* in patients hospitalized with acute respiratory illness. Scand. J. Infect. Dis. *1*:91–98, 1969.
197. Franzoso, G., Hu, P. C., Meloni, G. A., et al.: The immunodominant 90-kilodalton protein is localized on the terminal tip structure of *Mycoplasma pneumoniae.* Infect. Immun. *61*:1523–1530, 1993.
198. Freeman, R., and McMahon, M. J.: Acute pancreatitis and serological evidence of infection with *Mycoplasma pneumoniae.* Gut *19*:367–370, 1978.
199. Freundt, E. A., and Edward, D. G.: Classification and taxonomy. *In* Barile, M. F., and Razin, S. (eds.): The Mycoplasmas. Vol. I. New York, Academic Press, 1979, pp. 1–41.
200. Friedli, B., Renebey, F., and Rouge, J. C.: Complete heart block in a young child presumably due to *Mycoplasma pneumoniae* myocarditis. Acta Paediatr. Scand. *66*:385–388, 1977.
201. Ganick, D. J., Wolfson, J., Gilbert, E. F., et al.: *Mycoplasma* infection in the immunosuppressed leukemic patient. Arch. Pathol. Lab. Med. *104*:535–536, 1980.
202. Garland, S. M., and Murton, L. J.: Neonatal meningitis caused by *Ureaplasma urealyticum.* Pediatr. Infect. Dis. J. *6*:868–870, 1987.
203. Garrow, D. H.: A rapid test for the presence of increased cold agglutinins. B. M. J. *2*:206–208, 1958.
204. George, R. B., Weill, H., Rasch, J. R., et al.: Roentgenographic appearance of viral and mycoplasma pneumonias. Am. Rev. Respir. Dis. *96*:1144–1150, 1967.
205. George, R. B., Ziskind, M. M., Rasch, J. R., et al.: *Mycoplasma* and adenovirus pneumonias: Comparison with other atypical pneumonias in a military population. Ann. Intern. Med. *65*:931–942, 1966.
206. Gewitz, M., Dinwiddie, R., Rees, L., et al.: *Mycoplasma hominis:* A cause of neonatal meningitis. Arch. Dis. Child. *54*:231–239, 1979.
207. Gibbs, R. S., Blanco, J. D., St. Clair, P. J., et al.: *Mycoplasma hominis* and intrauterine infection in late pregnancy. Sex. Transm. Dis. *10*:303–306, 1983.
208. Gilbert, G. L., Law, F., and Macinnes, S. J.: Chronic *Mycoplasma hominis* infection complicating severe intraventricular hemorrhage, in a premature neonate. Pediatr. Infect. Dis. J. *7*:817–818, 1988.
209. Gill, K., and Marrie, T. J.: Hemophagocytosis secondary to *Mycoplasma pneumoniae* infection. Am. J. Med. *82*:668–670, 1987.
210. Glaser, J. B., Engelberg, M., and Hammerschlag, M.: Scalp abscess associated with *Mycoplasma hominis* infection complicating intrapartum monitoring. Pediatr. Infect. Dis. *2*:468–470, 1983.
211. Glezen, W. P., and Denny, F. W.: Epidemiology of acute lower respiratory disease in children. N. Engl. J. Med. *288*:498–504, 1973.
212. Glezen, W. P., Loda, F. A., Clyde, W. A., et al.: Epidemiologic patterns of acute lower respiratory disease of children in a pediatric group practice. J. Pediatr. *78*:397–406, 1971.
213. Glezen, W. P., Clyde, W. A., Senior, R. J., et al.: Group A streptococci, mycoplasmas, and viruses associated with acute pharyngitis. J. A. M. A. *202*:455–460, 1967.
214. Goldschmidt, B., Menonna, J., Fortunato, J., et al.: *Mycoplasma* antibody in Guillain-Barré syndrome and other neurological disorders. Ann. Neurol. *7*:108–112, 1980.

215. Golubjatnikov, R., Allen, V. D., Olmos-Blancarte, A. M. P., et al.: Serologic profile of children in a Mexican highland community: Prevalence of complement-fixing antibodies to *Mycoplasma pneumoniae,* respiratory syncytical virus and parainfluenza viruses. Am. J. Epidemiol. *101*:458–464, 1975.
216. Goodburn, G. M., Marmion, B. P., and Kendall, E. J. C.: Infection with Eaton's primary atypical pneumonia agent in England. Br. J. Med. *1*:1266–1270, 1963.
217. Goudie, B. M., Kerr, M. R., and Johnson, R. N.: *Mycoplasma* pneumonia complicated by bronchiectasis. J. Infect. *7*:151–152, 1983.
218. Grady, G. F., and Gilfillan, R. F.: Relation of *Mycoplasma pneumoniae* sero-reactivity, immunosuppression, and chronic disease to Legionnaires' disease: A twelve-month prospective study of sporadic cases in Massachusetts. Ann. Intern. Med. *90*:607–610, 1979.
219. Grattard, F., Soleihac, B., de Barbeyrac, B., et al.: Epidemiologic and molecular investigations of genital mycoplasmas from women and neonates at delivery. Pediatr. Infect. Dis. J. *14*:853–859, 1995.
220. Grau, O., Slizewicz, B., Tuppin, P., et al.: Association of *Mycoplasma penetrans* with human immunodeficiency virus infection. J. Infect. Dis. *172*:672–681, 1995.
221. Grayston, J. T., Alexander, E. R., Kenny, G. E., et al.: *Mycoplasma pneumoniae* infections: Clinical and epidemiologic studies. J. A. M. A. *191*:369–374, 1965.
222. Greenberg, H., Helms, C. M., Grizzard, M. B., et al.: Immunoprophylaxis of experimental *Mycoplasma pneumoniae* disease: Effect of route of administration on the immunogenicity and protective effect of inactivated *M. pneumoniae* vaccine. Infect. Immun. *16*:88–92, 1977.
223. Greenberg, H., Helms, C. M., Brunner, H., et al.: Asymptomatic infection of adult volunteers with a temperature sensitive mutant of *Mycoplasma pneumoniae.* Proc. Natl. Acad. Sci. U. S. A. *71*:4015–4019, 1974.
224. Greenberg, H., Prescott, B., Brunner, H., et al.: Sharing of glycolipid antigenic determinants by *Mycoplasma pneumoniae* vegetables and certain bacteria. *In* Proceedings of the Symposium on New Approaches for Inducing Natural Immunity to Pyogenic Organisms, Winter Park, Florida, 1973. Washington, D.C., U.S. Dept. HEW, No. (NIH) 74–553, 1973, pp. 151–156.
225. Greenstone, G.: Infectious mononucleosis complicated by pneumonia due to *Mycoplasma pneumoniae*: Report of two cases. J. Pediatr. *90*:492–493, 1977.
226. Griffin, J. P., and Klein, E. W.: Role of sinusitis in primary atypical pneumonia. Clin. Med. *78*:23–27, 1971.
227. Griffin, J. P.: Rapid screening for cold agglutinins in pneumonia. Ann. Intern. Med. *70*:701–705, 1969.
228. Grix, A., and Giammona, S. T.: Pneumonitis with pleural effusion in children due to *Mycoplasma pneumoniae.* Am. Rev. Respir. Dis. *109*:665–671, 1974.
229. Gump, D. W., Gibson, M., Ashikaga, T.: Lack of association between genital mycoplasmas and infertility. N. Engl. J. Med. *310*:937–941, 1984.
230. Gump, D. W., and Hawley, H. B.: Severe *Mycoplasma pneumoniae* pneumonia. Respiration *33*:475–486, 1976.
231. Halsted, C., Lepow, M. L., Balassanian, R., et al.: Otitis media: Clinical observations, microbiology and evaluation of therapy. Am. J. Dis. Child. *115*:542–551, 1968.
232. Hamrick, H. J., Mangum, M. E., and Katz, V. L.: *Ureaplasma urealyticum* abscess at site of an internal fetal heart rate monitor. Pediatr. Infect. Dis. J. *12*:410–411, 1993.
233. Handsfield, H. H.: Gonorrhea and nongonococcal urethritis. Med. Clin. North Am. *62*:925–943, 1978.
234. Hanukoglu, A., Hebroni, S., and Fried, D.: Pulmonary involvement in *Mycoplasma pneumoniae* infection in families. Infection *14*:3–8, 1986.
235. Harris, R., Marmion, B. P., Varkanis, G., et al.: Laboratory diagnosis of *Mycoplasma pneumoniae* infection. 2. Comparison of methods for the direct detection of specific antigen or nucleic acid sequences in respiratory exudates. Epidemiol. Infect. *101*:685–694, 1988.
236. Hart, G.: Sexually transmitted diseases. *In* Shen, J. T. Y. (ed.): The Clinical Practice of Adolescent Medicine. New York, Appleton-Century-Crofts, 1980, pp. 101–110.
237. Hata, D., Kuze, F., Mochizuki, Y., et al.: Evaluation of DNA probe test for rapid diagnosis of *Mycoplasma pneumoniae* infections. J. Pediatr. *116*:273–276, 1990.
238. Hawkins, R. E., Rickman, L. S., Vermund, S. H., et al.: Association of *Mycoplasma* and human immunodeficiency virus infection: Detection of amplified *Mycoplasma fermentans* DNA in blood. J. Infect. Dis. *165*:581–585, 1992.
239. Hayflick, L.: Fundamental biology of the class Mollicutes, order Mycoplasmatales. *In* Hayflick, L. (ed.): The Mycoplasmatales and the L-Phase of Bacteria. New York, Appleton-Century-Crofts, 1969, pp. 15–47.
240. Hayflick, L., and Chanock, R. M.: *Mycoplasma* species of man. Bacteriol. Rev. *29*:185–221, 1965.
241. Helms, C. M., Viner, J. P., Sturm, R. H., et al.: Comparative features of pneumococcal, mycoplasmal, and Legionnaires' disease pneumonias. Ann. Intern. Med. *90*:543–547, 1979.
242. Hengge, U. R., Kirschfink, M., Konig, A. L., et al.: Characterization of I/FI glycoprotein as a receptor for *Mycoplasma pneumoniae.* Infect. Immun. *60*:79–83, 1992.
243. Henrich, B., Feldmann, R. C., and Hadding, U.: Cytoadhesins of *Mycoplasma hominis.* Infect. Immun. *61*:2945–2951, 1993.
244. Hentschel, J., Abele-Horn, M., and Peters, J.: *Ureaplasma urealyticum* in the cerebrospinal fluid of a premature infant. Acta Paediatr. *82*:690–693, 1993.
245. Hernandez, L. A., Urquhart, G. E. D., and Dick, W. C.: *Mycoplasma pneumoniae* infection and arthritis in man. B. M. J. *2*:14–16, 1977.
246. Hillier, S. L., Martius, J., Krohn, M., et al.: A case-control study of chorioamnionic infection and histologic chorioamnionitis in prematurity. N. Engl. J. Med. *319*:972–978, 1988.
247. Hirai, Y., Shiode, J., Masayoshi, T., et al.: Application of an indirect immunofluorescence test for detection of *Mycoplasma pneumoniae* in respiratory exudates. J. Clin. Microbiol. *29*:2007–2012, 1991.
248. Hodges, G. R., Fass, R. J., and Saslaw, S.: Central nervous system disease associated with *Mycoplasma pneumoniae* infection. Arch. Intern. Med. *130*:277–282, 1972.
249. Hodges, G. R., and Perkins, R. L.: Landry-Guillain-Barré syndrome associated with *Mycoplasma pneumoniae* infection. J. A. M. A. *210*:2088–2090, 1969.
250. Holmes, K. K., Handsfield, H. H., Wang, S. P., et al.: Etiology of nongonococcal urethritis. N. Engl. J. Med. *292*:1199–1205, 1975.
251. Holmes, K. K., Johnson, D. W., Floyd, T. M., et al.: Studies of venereal disease. II. Observations on the incidence, etiology, and treatment of the postgonococcal urethritis syndrome. J. A. M. A. *202*:131–137, 1967.
252. Holmes, K. K., Johnson, D. W., and Floyd, T. M.: Studies of venereal disease. III. Double-blind comparison of tetracycline hydrochloride and placebo in treatment of nongonococcal urethritis. J. A. M. A. *202*:138–140, 1967.
253. Horn, M. E. C., Brain, E., Gregg, I., et al.: Respiratory viral infection in childhood: A survey in general practice, Roehampton 1967–1972. J. Hyg. (Camb.) *74*:157–168, 1975.
254. Horn, M. E. C., Brain, E. A., Gregg, I., et al.: Respiratory viral infection and wheezy bronchitis in childhood. Thorax *34*:23–28, 1969.
255. Hornsleth, A.: *Mycoplasma* pneumonia infection in infants and children in Copenhagen 1963–65: Incidence of complement-fixing antibodies in age groups 0–9 years. Acta Pathol. Microbiol. Scand. *69*:304–313, 1967.
256. Horowitz, S., Landau, D., Shinwell, E. S., et al.: Respiratory tract colonization with *Ureaplasma urealyticum* and bronchopulmonary dysplasia in neonates in southern Israel. Pediatr. Infect. Dis. J. *11*:847–851, 1992.
257. Hosker, H. S. R., Tam, J. S., Chan, C. H. S., et al.: *Mycoplasma pneumoniae* infection in Hong Kong: Clinical and epidemiological features during an epidemic. Respiration *60*:237–240, 1993.
258. Hu, P. C., Huang, C. H., Huang, Y. S., et al.: Demonstration of multiple antigenic determinants on *Mycoplasma pneumoniae* attachment protein by monoclonal antibodies. Infect. Immun. *50*:292–296, 1985.
259. Hu, P. C., Huang, C. H., Collier, A. M., et al.: Demonstration of antibodies to *Mycoplasma pneumoniae* attachment protein in human sera and respiratory secretions. Infect. Immun. *41*:437–439, 1983.
260. Hu, P. C., Powell, D. A., Albright, F., et al.: A solid-phase radioimmunoassay for detection of antibodies against *Mycoplasma pneumoniae.* J. Clin. Lab. Immunol. *11*:209–213, 1983.
261. Hu, P. C., Cole, R. M., Huang, Y. S., et al.: *Mycoplasma pneumoniae* infection: Role of a surface protein in the attachment organelle. Science *216*:313–315, 1982.
262. Hu, P., Collier, A. M., and Baseman, J. B.: Interaction of virulent *Mycoplasma pneumoniae* with hamster tracheal organ cultures. Infect. Immun. *14*:217–224, 1976.
263. Huhti, E., Mokka, T., Nikoskelainen, J., et al.: Association of viral and mycoplasma infections with exacerbations of asthma. Ann. Allergy *33*:145–149, 1974.
264. Hummell, D. S., Anderson, S. J., Wright, P. F., et al.: Chronic recurrent multifocal osteomyelitis: Are mycoplasmas involved? N. Engl. J. Med. *317*:510–511, 1987.
265. Ieven, M., Ursi, D., van Bever, H., et al.: Detection of *Mycoplasma pneumoniae* by two polymerase chain reactions and role of *M. pneumoniae* in acute respiratory tract infections in pediatric patients. J. Infect. Dis. *173*:1445–1452, 1996.
266. International Committee on Systematic Bacteriology, Subcommittee on the Taxonomy of Mollicutes: Proposal of minimal standards for descriptions of new species of the class *Mollicutes.* Int. J. Syst. Bacteriol. *29*:172–180, 1979.
267. Ionno, J. A., and Westfall, R. E.: *Mycoplasma pneumoniae* pneumonia: Clinical course and complications. Milit. Med. *135*:459–463, 1970.
268. Ishida, K., Kaku, M., Irifune, K., et al.: In vitro and in vivo activities of macrolides against *Mycoplasma pneumoniae.* Antimicrob. Agents Chemother. *38*:790–798, 1994.
269. Ishida, K., Kaku, M., Irifune, K., et al.: In vitro and in vivo activity of a new quinolone AM-1155 against *Mycoplasma pneumoniae.* J. Antimicrob. Chemother. 34:875–883, 1994.
270. Jachuck, S. J., Clark, F., Gardner-Thorpe, C., et al.: A brainstem syndrome associated with *Mycoplasma pneumoniae* infection: A report of two cases. Postgrad. Med. J. *51*:475–477, 1975.
271. Jacobs, E.: Serological diagnosis of *Mycoplasma pneumoniae* infections: A critical review of current procedures. Clin. Infect. Dis. *17*(Suppl. 1):S79–S82, 1993.
272. Jacobs, E., Rock, R., and Dalehite, L.: A B cell, T cell-linked epitope

located on the adhesin of *Mycoplasma pneumoniae.* Infect. Immun. *58*:2464–2469, 1990.

273. Jacobs, E., Schopperle, K., and Bredt, W.: Adherence inhibition assay: A specific serological test for detection of antibodies to *Mycoplasma pneumoniae.* Eur. J. Clin. Microbiol. *4*:113–118, 1985.
274. Jacobs, F., van de Stadt, J., Gelin, M., et al.: *Mycoplasma hominis* infection of perihepatic hematomas in a liver transplant recipient. Surgery *98*:98–100, 1992.
275. Jacobs, N. F., and Kraus, S. J.: Gonococcal and nongonococcal urethritis in men: Clinical and laboratory differentiation. Ann. Intern. Med. *82*:7–12, 1975.
276. Janney, F. A., Lee, L. T., and Howe, C.: Cold hemagglutinin cross-reactivity with *Mycoplasma pneumoniae.* Infect. Immun. *22*:29–33, 1978.
277. Jansson, E.: Mycoplasmas and arthritis. Scand. J. Rheumatol. *4*:39–42, 1975.
278. Jansson, E., von Essen, R., and Tuuri, S.: *Mycoplasma pneumoniae* pneumonia in Helsinki 1962–1970. Scand. J. Infect. Dis. *3*:51–54, 1971.
279. Jansson, E., Wager, O., Stenstrom, R., et al.: Studies on Eaton PPLO pneumonia. B. M. J. *1*:142–145, 1964.
280. Jao, R. L., and Finland, M.: Susceptibility of *Mycoplasma pneumoniae* to 21 antibiotics *in vitro.* Am. J. Med. Sci. *253*:639–650, 1967.
281. Jemski, J. V., Hetsko, C. M., Helms, C. M., et al.: Immunoprophylaxis of experimental *Mycoplasma pneumoniae* disease: Effect of aerosol particle size and site of deposition of *M. pneumoniae* on the pattern of respiratory infection, disease, and immunity in hamsters. Infect. Immun. *16*:93–98, 1977.
282. Jensen, J. S., Heilmann, C., and Valerius, N. H.: *Mycoplasma pneumoniae* infection in a child with AIDS. Clin. Infect. Dis. *19*:207, 1994.
283. Jensen, J. S., Orsum, R., Dohn, B., et al.: *Mycoplasma genitalium:* A cause of male urethritis? Genitourin. Med. *69*:265–269, 1993.
284. Jensen, J. S., Songergard-Andersen, J., Uldum, S. A., et al.: Detection of *Mycoplasma pneumoniae* in simulated clinical samples by polymerase chain reaction. APMIS *97*:1046–1048, 1989.
285. Jensen, K. E., Senterfit, L. B., and Chanock, R. M.: An inactivated *Mycoplasma pneumoniae* vaccine. J. A. M. A. *194*:248–252, 1965.
286. Jensen, K. J., Senterfit, L. B., Scully, W. E., et al.: *Mycoplasma pneumoniae* infections in children: An epidemiologic appraisal in families treated with oxytetracycline. Am. J. Epidemiol. *86*:419–432, 1967.
287. Jones, D. M., and Tobin, B.: Neonatal eye infections due to *Mycoplasma hominis.* B. M. J. *3*:467–468, 1968.
288. Jones, G. R., and Stewart, S. M.: A prospective study of the persistence of *Mycoplasma pneumoniae* antibody levels. Scott. Med. J. *19*:129–133, 1974.
289. Jones, M. C.: Arthritis and arthralgia in infection with *Mycoplasma pneumoniae.* Thorax *25*:748–750, 1970.
290. Jonsson, B., Karell, A.-C., Ringertz, S., et al.: Neonatal *Ureaplasma urealyticum* colonization and chronic lung disease. Acta Paediatr. *83*:927–930, 1994.
291. Joosting, A. C. C., Harwin, R. M., Coppin, A., et al.: A serological investigation of *Mycoplasma pneumoniae* infection on the Witwatersrand. S. Afr. Med. J. *50*:2134–2135, 1976.
292. Jordan, W. S., Jr., and Dingle, J. H.: *Mycoplasma pneumoniae* infections. *In* Dubos, R. J., and Hirsch, J. G. (eds.): Bacterial and Mycotic Infections of Man. Philadelphia, J. B. Lippincott, 1965, pp. 810–824.
293. Kahane, I., Tucker, S., Leith, D. K., et al.: Detection of the major adhesin P1 in triton shells of virulent *Mycoplasma pneumoniae.* Infect. Immun. *50*:944–946, 1985.
294. Kai, M., Kamiya, S., Yabe, H., et al.: Rapid detection of *Mycoplasma pneumoniae* in clinical samples by the polymerase chain reaction. J. Med. Microbiol. *38*:166–170, 1993.
295. Kalb, R. E., Grossman, M. E., and Neu, H. C.: Stevens-Johnson syndrome due to *Mycoplasma pneumoniae* in an adult. Am. J. Med. *79*:541–544, 1985.
296. Kammer, G. M., Pollack, J. D., and Klainer, A. S.: Scanning-beam electron microscopy of *Mycoplasma pneumoniae.* J. Bacteriol. *104*:499–502, 1970.
297. Kane, J. R., Shenep, J. L., Krance, R. A., et al.: Diffuse alveolar hemorrhage associated with *Mycoplasma hominis* respiratory tract infection in a bone marrow transplant recipient. Chest *105*:1891–1892, 1994.
298. Kasahara, I., Otsubo, Y., Yanase, T., et al.: Isolation and characterization of *Mycoplasma pneumoniae* from cerebrospinal fluid of a patient with pneumonia and meningoencephalitis. J. Infect. Dis. *152*:823–825, 1985.
299. Katseni, V. L., Gilroy, C. B., Ryait, B. K., et al.: *Mycoplasma fermentans* in individuals seropositive and seronegative for HIV-1. Lancet *341*:271–272, 1993.
300. Katz, H. I., Wooten, J. W., Davis, R. G., et al.: Stevens-Johnson syndrome: Report of a case associated with culturally proven *Mycoplasma pneumoniae* infection. J. A. M. A. *199*:504–506, 1967.
301. Kaufman, J. M., Cuvelier, C. A., and van der Straeten, M.: *Mycoplasma* pneumonia with fulminant evolution into diffuse interstitial fibrosis. Thorax *35*:140–144, 1980.
302. Kenney, R. T., Li, J. S., Clyde, W. A., Jr., et al.: Mycoplasmal pericarditis: Evidence of invasive disease. Clin. Infect. Dis. *17*(Suppl. 1):S58–S62, 1993.
303. Kenny, G. E.: Antigenic determinants. *In* Barile, M. F., and Razin, S. (eds.): The Mycoplasmas. Vol. I. New York, Academic Press, 1979, pp. 351–384.
304. Kenny, G. E., and Newton, R. M.: Close serological relationship between glycolipids of *Mycoplasma pneumoniae* and glycolipids of spinach. Ann. N. Y. Acad. Sci. *225*:54–61, 1973.
305. Khatib, R., and Schnarr, D.: Point-source outbreak of *Mycoplasma pneumoniae* infection in a family unit. J. Infect. Dis. *151*:186–187, 1985.
306. Khatib, R. E., and Lerner, A. M.: Myocarditis in *Mycoplasma pneumoniae* pneumonia: Occurrence with hemolytic anemia and extraordinary titers of cold isohemagglutinins. J. A. M. A. *231*:493–494, 1975.
307. Kidron, D., Barron, S. A., and Mazliah, J.: Mononeuritis multiplex with brachial plexus neuropathy coincident with *Mycoplasma pneumoniae* infection. Eur. Neurol. *29*:90–92, 1989.
308. Kingston, J. R., Chanock, R. M., Mufson, M. A., et al.: Eaton agent pneumonia. J. A. M. A. *176*:118–123, 1961.
309. Klar, A., Gross-Kieselstein, E., Hurvitz, H., et al.: Bilateral Bell's palsy due to *Mycoplasma pneumoniae* infection. Isr. J. Med. Sci. *21*:692–694, 1985.
310. Kleemola, M., Heiskanen-Kosma, T., Nohynek, H., et al.: Diagnostic efficacy of a *Mycoplasma pneumoniae* hybridization test in nasopharyngeal aspirates of children. Pediatr. Infect. Dis. J. *12*:344–345, 1993.
311. Kleemola, S. R. M., Karjalainen, J. E., and Raty, R. K. H.: Rapid diagnosis of *Mycoplasma pneumoniae* infection: Clinical evaluation of a commercial probe test. J. Infect. Dis. *162*:70–75, 1990.
312. Kleemola, M., Kayhty, H., and Raty, R.: Presence of antibodies to *Mycoplasma pneumoniae* in patients with bacterial meningitis: Reply. J. Infect. Dis. *148*:363–365, 1983.
313. Kleemola, M., and Kayhty, H.: Increase in titers of antibodies to *Mycoplasma pneumoniae* in patients with purulent meningitis. J. Infect. Dis. *146*:284–288, 1982.
314. Klein, J. O., Buckland, D., and Finland, M.: Colonization of newborn infants by mycoplasmas. N. Engl. J. Med. *280*:1025–1030, 1969.
315. Klimek, J. J., Russman, B. S., and Quintiliani, R.: *Mycoplasma pneumoniae* meningoencephalitis and transverse myelitis in association with low cerebrospinal fluid glucose. Pediatrics *58*:133–135, 1976.
316. Kok, T. W., Marmion, B. P., Varkanis, G., et al.: Laboratory diagnosis of *Mycoplasma pneumoniae* infection. 3. Detection of IgM antibodies to *M. pneumoniae* by a modified indirect haemagglutination test. Epidemiol. Infect. *103*:613–623, 1989.
317. Kok, T. W., Varkanis, G., Marmion, B. P., et al.: Laboratory diagnosis of *Mycoplasma pneumoniae* infection. 1. Direct detection of antigen in respiratory exudates by enzyme immunoassay. Epidemiol. Infect. *101*:669–684, 1988.
318. Koletsky, R. J., and Weinstein, A. J.: Fulminant *Mycoplasma pneumoniae* infection: Report of a fatal case, and a review of the literature. Am. Rev. Respir. Dis. *122*:491–496, 1980.
319. Komaroff, A. L., Aronson, M. D., Pass, T. M., et al.: Serologic evidence of chlamydial and mycoplasmas pharyngitis in adults. Science *222*:927–928, 1983.
320. Kopelman, P.: Raised mean cell volume and meningoencephalitis associated with *Mycoplasma pneumoniae* infection. B. M. J. *1*:881–882, 1977.
321. Koskiniemi, M.: CNS manifestations associated with *Mycoplasma pneumoniae* infections: Summary of cases at the University of Helsinki and review. Clin. Infect. Dis. *17*(Suppl. 1):S52–S57, 1993.
322. Kovacic, R., Launay, V., Tuppin, P., et al.: Search for the presence of six *Mycoplasma* species in peripheral blood mononuclear cells of subjects seropositive and seronegative for human immunodeficiency virus. J. Clin. Microbiol. *34*:1808–1810, 1996.
323. Krause, D. C.: *Mycoplasma pneumoniae* cytadherence: Unravelling the tie that binds. Mol. Microbiol. *20*:247–253, 1996.
324. Krause, D. C., and Baseman, J. B.: Inhibition of *Mycoplasma pneumoniae* hemadsorption and adherence to respiratory epithelium by antibodies to a membrane protein. Infect. Immun. *39*:1180–1186, 1983.
325. Kundsin, R. B., Driscoll, S. G., Monson, R. R., et al.: Association of *Ureaplasma urealyticum* in the placenta with perinatal morbidity and mortality. N. Engl. J. Med. *310*:941–945, 1984.
326. Kundsin, R. B., Driscoll, S. G., and Pelletier, P. A.: *Ureaplasma urealyticum* incriminated in perinatal morbidity and mortality. Science *213*:474–476, 1981.
327. Lam, K., and Bayer, A. S.: *Mycoplasma pneumoniae* as a cause of the "fever of unknown origin" syndrome. Arch. Intern. Med. *142*:2312–2313, 1982.
328. Lambert, H. P.: Infections caused by *Mycoplasma pneumoniae.* Br. J. Dis. Chest *63*:71–82, 1969.
329. Lambert, H. P.: Syndrome with joint manifestations in association with *Mycoplasma pneumoniae* infection. B. M. J. *3*:156–157, 1968.
330. Lambert, H. P.: Antibody to *Mycoplasma pneumoniae* in normal subjects and in patients with chronic bronchitis. J. Hyg. (Camb.) *66*:185–189, 1968.
331. Lascari, A. D., Garfunkel, J. M., and Mauro, D. J.: Varicella-like rash associated with *Mycoplasma* infection. Am. J. Dis. Child. *128*:254–255, 1974.
332. Leach, A., and Lewis, B. W.: Unusual *Mycoplasma pneumoniae.* B. M. J. *1*:185, 1969.
333. Leach, R. H., Hales, A., Furr, P. M., et al.: Problems in the identification of *Mycoplasma pirum* isolated from human lymphoblastoid cell cultures. FEMS Microbiol. Lett. *44*:293–297, 1987.
334. Lee, S. H., Charoenying, S., Brennan, T., et al.: Comparative studies of three serologic methods for the measurement of *Mycoplasma pneumoniae* antibodies. Am. J. Clin. Pathol. *92*:342–347, 1989.
335. Lee, Y. H., Rosner, B., Alpert, S., et al.: Clinical and microbiological investigation of men with urethritis. J. Infect. Dis. *138*:798–803, 1978.
336. Lee, Y. H., McCormack, W. M., Marcy, S. M., et al.: The genital mycoplas-

mas: Their role in disorders of reproduction and in pediatric infections. Pediatr. Clin. North Am. *21*:457–466, 1974.
337. Lehtokoski-Lehtiniemi, E., and Koskiniemi, M.-L.: *Mycoplasma pneumoniae* encephalitis: A severe entity in children. Pediatr. Infect. Dis. J. *8*:651–653, 1989.
338. Leinikki, P. O., Pantzar, P., and Tykka, H.: Immunoglobulin M antibody response against *Mycoplasma pneumoniae* lipid antigen in patients with acute pancreatitis. J. Clin. Microbiol. *8*:113–118, 1978.
339. Leinikki, P., and Pantzar, P.: Acute pancreatitis in *Mycoplasma pneumoniae* infections. B. M. J. *1*:554, 1973.
340. Lemcke, R. M., Shaw, E. J., and Marmion, B. P.: Related antigens in *Mycoplasma pneumoniae* and *Mycoplasma mycoides* var. *mycoides*. Aust. J. Exp. Biol. Med. Sci. *18*:761–770, 1965.
341. Lepow, M. L., Balassanian, N., Emmerich, J., et al.: Interrelationships of viral, mycoplasmal, and bacterial agents in uncomplicated pneumonia. Am. Rev. Respir. Dis. *97*:533–545, 1968.
342. Lequier, L., Robinson, J., and Vaudry, W.: Sternotomy infection with *Mycoplasma hominis* in a neonate. Pediatr. Infect. Dis. J. *14*:1010–1012, 1995.
343. Lerer, R. J., and Kalavsky, S. M.: Central nervous system disease associated with *Mycoplasma pneumoniae* infection: Report of five cases and review of the literature. Pediatrics *52*:658–667, 1973.
344. Levine, D. P., and Lerner, A. M.: The clinical spectrum of *Mycoplasma pneumoniae* infections. Med. Clin. North Am. *62*:961–978, 1978.
345. Lewes, D., Rainford, D. J., and Lane, W. F.: Symptomless myocarditis and myalgia in viral and *Mycoplasma pneumoniae* infections. Br. Heart J. *36*:924–932, 1974.
346. Lewis, J. E., and Sheptin, C.: Mycoplasmal pneumonia associated with abscess of the lung. Calif. Med. *117*:69–72, 1972.
347. Likitnukul, S., Kusmiesz, H., Nelson, J. D., et al.: Role of genital mycoplasmas in young infants with suspected sepsis. J. Pediatr. *109*:971–974, 1986.
348. Lin, J.-S. L.: Human mycoplasmal infections: Serologic observations. Rev. Infect. Dis. *7*:216–231, 1985.
349. Lin, J.-S. L., Kendrick, M. I., and Kass, E. H.: Serologic typing of human genital T-mycoplasmas by a complement-dependent mycoplasmacidal test. J. Infect. Dis. *126*:658–663, 1972.
350. Lind, K., Hoier-Madsen, M., and Wiik, S.: Autoantibodies to the mitotic spindle apparatus in *Mycoplasma pneumoniae* disease. Infect. Immun. *56*:714–715, 1988.
351. Lind, K., Lindhardt, B. O., Schutten, H. J., et al.: Serological cross-reactions between *Mycoplasma genitalium* and *Mycoplasma pneumoniae*. J. Clin. Microbiol. *20*:1036–1043, 1984.
352. Lind, K., Zoffmann, H., Larsen, S. O., et al.: *Mycoplasma pneumoniae* infection associated with infection of the central nervous system. Acta Med. Scand. *205*:325–332, 1979.
353. Lind, K.: Production of cold agglutinins in rabbits induced by *Mycoplasma pneumoniae, Listeria monocytogenes* or *Streptococcus* MG. Acta Pathol. Microbiol. Scand. [B] *81*:487–496, 1973.
354. Lind, K.: Incidence of *Mycoplasma pneumoniae* infection in Denmark from 1958 to 1969. Acta Pathol. Microbiol. Scand. [B] *79*:239–247, 1971.
355. Lind, K.: Immunological relationships between *Mycoplasma pneumoniae* and *Streptococcus* MG. Acta Pathol. Microbiol. Scand. *73*:237–244, 1968.
356. Lipman, R. P., and Clyde, W. A., Jr.: The interrelationship of virulence, cytadsorption, and peroxide formation in *Mycoplasma pneumoniae*. Proc. Soc. Exp. Med. Biol. *131*:1163–1167, 1969.
357. Lipman, R. P., Clyde, W. A., Jr., and Denny, F. W.: Characteristics of virulent, attenuated, and avirulent *Mycoplasma pneumoniae* strains. J. Bacteriol. *100*:1037–1043, 1969.
358. Little, T. M., and Dowdle, R. H.: *Mycoplasma* pneumonia with inappropriate secretion of antidiuretic hormone. B. M. J. *1*:571, 1975.
359. Liu, C., Eaton, M. D., and Heyl, J. T.: Studies on primary atypical pneumonia. II. Observations concerning the development and immunological characteristics of antibody in patients. J. Exp. Med. *109*:545–556, 1959.
360. Lo, S. C., Hayes, M. M., Tully, J. G., et al.: *Mycoplasma penetrans* sp. nov., from the urogenital tract of patients with AIDS. Int. J. Syst. Bacteriol. *42*:357–364, 1992.
361. Lo, S. C., Hayes, M. M., Wang, R. Y. H., et al. Newly discovered *Mycoplasma* isolated from patients infected with HIV. Lancet *388*:1415–1418, 1991.
362. Loda, F. A., Glezen, W. P., and Clyde, W. A., Jr.: Respiratory disease in group day care. Pediatrics *49*:428–437, 1972.
363. Loda, F. A., Clyde, W. A., Jr., Glezen, W. P., et al.: Studies on the role of viruses, bacteria, and *M. pneumoniae* as causes of lower respiratory tract infections in children. J. Pediatr. *72*:161–176, 1968.
364. Longcope, W. T.: Bronchopneumonia of an unknown etiology (Variety X). Bull. Johns Hopkins Hosp. *67*:268, 1940.
365. Loo, V. G., Richardson, S., and Quinn, P.: Isolation of *Mycoplasma pneumoniae* from pleural fluid. Diagn. Microbiol. Infect. Dis. *14*:443–445, 1991.
366. Lorber, J., Kalhan, S. C., and Mahgrefte, B.: Treatment of ventriculitis with gentamicin and cloxacillin in infants born with spina bifida. Arch. Dis. Child. *45*:178–185, 1970.
367. Ludlam, G. B., Bridges, J. B., and Benn, E. C.: Association of Stevens-Johnson syndrome with antibody for *Mycoplasma pneumoniae*. Lancet *1*:958–959, 1964.
368. Luneberg, E., Jensen, J. S., and Frosch, M.: Detection of *Mycoplasma pneumoniae* by polymerase chain reaction and nonradioactive hybridization in microtiter plates. J. Clin. Microbiol. *31*:1088–1094, 1993.
369. Lyell, A., Gordon, A. M., Dick, H. M., et al.: Mycoplasmas and erythema multiforme. Lancet *2*:1116–1118, 1967.
370. MacLean, D. W.: *Mycoplasma pneumoniae:* One year's experience in an urban practice. Scott. Med. J. *14*:312–320, 1969.
371. Macon, W. R., Lo, S.-C., Poiesz, B. J., et al.: Acquired immunodeficiency syndrome-like illness associated with systemic *Mycoplasma fermentans* infection in a human immunodeficiency-virus–negative homosexual man. Hum. Pathol. *24*:554–558, 1993.
372. Madan, E., Meyer, M. P., and Amortigui, A. J.: Isolation of genital mycoplasmas and *Chlamydia trachomatis* in stillborn and neonatal autopsy material. Arch. Pathol. Lab. Med. *112*:749–751, 1988.
373. Maisel, J. C., Babbitt, L. H., and John, T. J.: Fatal *Mycoplasma pneumoniae* infection with isolation of organisms from lung. J. A. M. A. *202*:287–290, 1967.
374. Manchee, R. J., and Taylor-Robinson, D.: Enhanced growth of T-strain mycoplasmas with *N*-2-hydroxy-ethylpiperazine-*N'*-2-ethanesulfonic acid buffer. J. Bacteriol. *100*:78–85, 1969.
375. Mansel, J. K., Rosenow, E. C., III., Smith, T. F., et al.: *Mycoplasma pneumoniae* pneumonia. Chest *95*:639–646, 1989.
376. Mårdh, P.-A.: *Mycoplasma hominis* infection of the central nervous system in newborn infants. Sex. Transm. Dis. *10*:331–334, 1983.
377. Mårdh, P.-A.: Human respiratory tract infections with mycoplasmas and their in vitro susceptibility to tetracyclines and some other antibiotics. Chemotherapy *21*(Suppl. 1):27–57, 1975.
378. Mårdh, P.-A., and Ursing, B.: The occurrence of acute pancreatitis in *Mycoplasma pneumoniae* infection. Scand. J. Infect. Dis. *6*:167–171, 1974.
379. Mårdh, P.-A., Nilsson, F. J., and Bjelle, A.: Mycoplasmas and bacteria in synovial fluid from patients with arthritis. Ann. Rheum. Dis. *32*:319–325, 1973.
380. Markham, J. G.: *Mycoplasma pneumoniae* infection in 1978. N. Z. Med. J. *90*:473–474, 1979.
381. Marmion, B. P., Williamson, J., Worswick, D. A., et al.: Experience with newer techniques for the laboratory detection of *Mycoplasma pneumoniae* infection: Adelaide, 1978–1992. Clin. Infect. Dis. *17*(Suppl. 1):S90–S99, 1993.
382. Marmion, B. P., and Goodburn, G. M.: Effect of an organic gold salt on Eaton's primary atypical pneumonia agent and other observations. Nature *189*:247–248, 1961.
383. Martelli, A.: Sulla reazione di fissazione del complemento per *Mycoplasma pneumoniae* nella diagnosi sierologica di affezioni respiratorie. G. Batteriol. Virol. Immunol. *65*:43–49, 1972.
384. Martin, E. R., Warr, G., Couch, R., et al.: Chemotaxis of human leukocytes: Responsiveness to *Mycoplasma pneumoniae*. J. Lab. Clin. Med. *81*:520–529, 1973.
385. McCormack, J. G.: *Mycoplasma pneumoniae* and the erythema multiforme Stevens-Johnson syndrome. J. Infect. *3*:32–36, 1981.
386. McCormack, W. M.: Susceptibility of mycoplasmas to antimicrobial agents: Clinical implications. Clin. Infect. Dis. *17*(Suppl. 1):S200–S201, 1993.
387. McCormack, W. M., Rosner, B., Alpert, S., et al.: Vaginal colonization with *Mycoplasma hominis* and *Ureaplasma urealyticum*. Sex. Transm. Dis. *13*:67–70, 1986.
388. McCormack, W. M.: Epidemiology of *Mycoplasma hominis*. Sex. Transm. Dis. *10*:261–262, 1983.
389. McCormack, W. M.: Common sexually transmitted diseases and their treatment. Bull. N. Y. Acad. Med. *54*:216–222, 1978.
390. McCormack, W. M., Braun, P., Lee, Y.-H., et al.: The genital mycoplasmas. N. Engl. J. Med. *288*:78–89, 1973.
391. McCormack, W. M., Lee, Y.-H., and Zinner, S. H.: Sexual experience and urethral colonization with genital mycoplasmas. Ann. Intern. Med. *78*:696–698, 1973.
392. McCormack, W. M., Rosner, B., and Lee, Y.-H.: Colonization with genital mycoplasmas in women. Am. J. Epidemiol. *97*:240–245, 1973.
393. McCormack, W. M., Almeida, P. C., Bailey, P. E., et al.: Sexual activity and vaginal colonization with genital mycoplasmas. J. A. M. A. *221*:1375–1377, 1972.
394. McDonald, J. C., and Moore, D. L.: *Mycoplasma hominis* meningitis in a premature infant. Pediatr. Infect. Dis. *7*:795–798, 1988.
395. McDonald, M. I., Lam, M. H., Birch, D. F., et al.: *Ureaplasma urealyticum* in patients with acute symptoms of urinary tract infection. J. Urol. *128*:517–519, 1982.
396. McIntosh, J. C., and Gutierrez, H. H.: Mycoplasmal infections: Epidemiology, immunology, diagnostic techniques, and therapeutic strategies. Immunol. Allergy Clin. North Am. *13*:43–57, 1993.
397. McNamara, M. J., Phillips, I. A., and Williams, O. B.: Viral and *Mycoplasma pneumoniae* infections in exacerbations of chronic lung disease. Am. Rev. Respir. Dis. *100*:19–24, 1969.
398. Meis, J. F., van Kuppeveld, F. J., Kremer, J. A., et al.: Fatal intrauterine infection associated with *Mycoplasma hominis*. Clin. Infect. Dis. *15*:753–754, 1992.
399. Metzgar, D. P., Woodhour, A. F., Vella, P. P., et al.: Respiratory virus vaccines. II. *Mycoplasma pneumoniae* (Eaton agent) vaccines. Am. Rev. Respir. Dis. *94*:1–9, 1966.

400. Meyers, B. R., and Hirschman, S. Z.: Fatal infections associated with *Mycoplasma pneumoniae:* Discussion of three cases with necropsy findings. Mt. Sinai J. Med. *39*:258–264, 1972.
401. Miller, T. C., Baman, S. I., and Albers, W. H.: Massive pericardial effusion due to *Mycoplasma hominis* in a newborn. Am. J. Dis. Child. *136*:271–272, 1982.
402. Mills, R. W., and Schoolfield, L.: Acute transverse myelitis associated with *Mycoplasma pneumoniae* infection: A case report and review of the literature. Pediatr. Infect. Dis. J. *11*:228–231, 1992.
403. Miranda, C., Carazo, C., Bañón, R., et al.: *Mycoplasma hominis* infection in three renal transplant patients. Diagn. Microbiol. Infect. Dis. *13*:329–331, 1990.
404. Mizutani, H., and Mizutani, H.: Circulating immune complexes in patients with mycoplasmal pneumonia. Am. Rev. Respir. Dis. *130*:627–629, 1984.
405. Mizutani, H., and Mizutani, H.: Immunologic responses in patients with *Mycoplasma pneumoniae* infections. Am. Rev. Respir. Dis. *127*:175–179, 1983.
406. Moffet, H. L., Siegel, A. C., and Doyle, H. K.: Nonstreptococcal pharyngitis. J. Pediatr. *73*:51–60, 1968.
407. Mogabgab, W. J.: Protective efficacy of killed *Mycoplasma pneumoniae* vaccine measured in large-scale studies in a military population. Am. Rev. Respir. Dis. *108*:899–908, 1973.
408. Mogabgab, W. J.: Beta-hemolytic streptococcal and concurrent infections in adults and children with respiratory disease, 1958 to 1969. Am. Rev. Respir. Dis. *102*:23–34, 1970.
409. Mogabgab, W. J.: *Mycoplasma pneumoniae* and adenovirus respiratory illnesses in military and university personnel, 1959–1966. Am. Rev. Respir. Dis. *97*:345–358, 1968.
410. Mohiuddin, A. A., Corren, J., Harbeck, R. J., et al.: *Ureaplasma urealyticum* chronic osteomyelitis in a patient with hypogammaglobulinemia. J. Allergy Clin. Immunol. *87*:104–107, 1991.
411. Mok, J. Y., Waugh, P. R., and Simpson, H.: *Mycoplasma pneumoniae* infection: A follow-up study of 50 children with respiratory illness. Arch. Dis. Child. *54*:506–511, 1979.
412. Montagnier, L., and Blanchard, A.: Mycoplasmas as cofactors in infection due to the human immunodeficiency virus. Clin. Infect. Dis. *17*(Suppl. 1):S309–S315, 1993.
413. Monto, A. S., Bryan, E. R., and Rhodes, L. M.: The Tecumseh study of respiratory illnesses. VII. Further observations on the occurrence of respiratory syncytial virus and *Mycoplasma pneumoniae* infections. Am. J. Epidemiol. *100*:458–468, 1975.
414. Monto, A. S., and Lim, S. K.: The Tecumseh study of respiratory illness. III. Incidence and periodicity of respiratory syncytial virus and *Mycoplasma pneumoniae* infections. Am. J. Epidemiol. *94*:290–301, 1971.
415. Moore, P., and Martland, T.: *Mycoplasma pneumoniae* infection mimicking acute rheumatic fever. Pediatr. Infect. Dis. J. *13*:81–82, 1994.
416. Morowitz, H. J., and Wallace, D. C.: Genome size and life cycle of the mycoplasma. Ann. N. Y. Acad. Sci. *225*:62–73, 1973.
417. Moskal, M. J., Kaylarian, V. H., and Doro, J. M.: Psychosis complicating *Mycoplasma pneumoniae* infection. Pediatr. Infect. Dis. *3*:63–66, 1984.
418. Moule, J. H., Caul, E. O., and Wreghitt, T. G.: The specific IgM response to *Mycoplasma pneumoniae* infection: Interpretation and application to early diagnosis. Epidemiol. Infect. *99*:685–692, 1987.
419. Mufson, M. A., Ludwig, W. M., Purcell, R. H., et al.: Exudative pharyngitis following experimental *Mycoplasma hominis* type 1 infection. J. A. M. A. *192*:1146–1152, 1965.
420. Mufson, M. A., Sanders, V., Wood, S. C., et al.: Primary atypical pneumonia due to *Mycoplasma pneumoniae* (Eaton agent): Report of a case with a residual pleural abnormality. N. Engl. J. Med. *268*:1109–1111, 1963.
421. Mufson, M. A., Manko, M. A., Kingston, J. R., et al.: Eaton agent pneumonia: Clinical features. J. A. M. A. *178*:369–374, 1961.
422. Murphy, W. H., Bullis, C., Dabich, L., et al.: Isolation of *Mycoplasma* from leukemic and nonleukemic patients. J. Natl. Cancer Inst. *45*:243–251, 1970.
423. Murray, H. W., Masur, H., Senterfit, L. B., et al.: The protean manifestations of *Mycoplasma pneumoniae* infection in adults. Am. J. Med. *58*:229–242, 1975.
424. Muse, K. E., Powell, D. A., and Collier, A. M.: *Mycoplasma pneumoniae* in hamster tracheal organ culture studied by scanning electron microscopy. Infect. Immun. *13*:229–237, 1976.
425. Naftalin, J. M., Wellisch, G., Kahana, Z., et al.: *Mycoplasma pneumoniae* septicemia. J. A. M. A. *228*:565, 1974.
426. Nagayama, Y., Sakurai, N., Yamamoto, K., et al.: Isolation of *Mycoplasma pneumoniae* from children with lower respiratory tract infections. J. Infect. Dis. *157*:911–917, 1988.
427. Nagayama, Y., Sakurai, N., Tamai, K., et al.: Isolation of *Mycoplasma pneumoniae* from pleural fluid and/or cerebrospinal fluid: Report of four cases. Scand. J. Infect. Dis. *19*:521–524, 1987.
428. Nakao, T., Orii, T., and Umetsu, M.: *Mycoplasma pneumoniae* pneumonia with pleural effusion, with special reference to isolation of *Mycoplasma pneumoniae* from pleural fluid. Tohoku J. Exp. Med. *104*:13–18, 1971.
429. Nakao, T., Umetsu, M., Watanabe, N., et al.: An outbreak of *Mycoplasma pneumoniae* infection in a community. Tohoku J. Exp. Med. *102*:23–31, 1970.
430. Nakayama, T., Sonoda, S., Urano, T., et al.: Interferon production during the course of *Mycoplasma pneumoniae* infection. Pediatr. Infect. Dis. J. *11*:72–77, 1992.
431. Nakayama, T., Urano, T., Osano, M., et al.: Alpha interferon in the sera of patients infected with *Mycoplasma pneumoniae.* J. Infect. Dis. *154*:904–906, 1986.
432. Naraqi, S., and Kabins, S. A.: *Mycoplasma pneumoniae* monoarticular arthritis. J. Pediatr. *83*:621–623, 1973.
433. Narita, M., Itakura, O., Matsuzono, Y., et al.: Analysis of mycoplasmal central nervous system involvement by polymerase chain reaction. Pediatr. Infect. Dis. J. *14*:236–237, 1995.
434. Narita, M., Matsuzono, Y., Itakura, O., et al.: Survey of mycoplasmal bacteremia detected in children by polymerase chain reaction. Clin. Infect. Dis. *23*:522–525, 1996.
435. Narita, M., Itakura, O., Matsuzono, Y., et al.: Analysis of mycoplasmal central nervous system involvement by polymerase chain reaction. Pediatr. Infect. Dis. *14*:236–237, 1995.
436. Nastro, J. A., Littner, M. R., Tashkin, D. P., et al.: Diffuse, pulmonary, interstitial infiltrate and mycoplasmal pneumonia. Am. Rev. Respir. Dis. *110*:659–662, 1974.
437. Neimark, H. C.: Division of mycoplasmas into subgroups. J. Gen. Microbiol. *63*:249–263, 1970.
438. Neu, H. C., and Ellner, P. D.: Role of *Mycoplasma* in exudative pharyngitis. N. Y. State J. Med. *69*:3026–3028, 1969.
439. News and Notes: Epidemiology: *Mycoplasma pneumoniae* 1977. B. M. J. *1*:726, 1978.
440. Niitu, Y., Hasegawa, S., Suetake, T., et al.: Resistance of *Mycoplasma pneumoniae* to erythromycin and other antibiotics. J. Pediatr. *76*:438–443, 1970.
441. Nishioka, K., Fujimoto, M., Date, R., et al.: Bilateral sensorineural deafness associated with *Mycoplasma pneumoniae* infection: The first case report. Hiroshima J. Med. Sci. *33*:585–589, 1984.
442. Nissen, M., McEniery, J., Delbridge, G., et al.: Acute hypertrophic cardiomyopathy possibly associated with *Mycoplasma pneumoniae* infection. Pediatr. Infect. Dis. J. *14*:74–75, 1995.
443. Noah, N. D.: *Mycoplasma pneumoniae* infection in the United Kingdom: 1967–73. B. M. J. *1*:544–546, 1974.
444. Nocard, E., and Roux, E. R.: Le microbe de la pleuro-pneumoniae. Ann. Inst. Pasteur (Paris) *12*:240–262, 1898.
445. Noriega, E. R., Simberkoff, M. S., Gilroy, F. J., et al.: Life-threatening *Mycoplasma pneumoniae* pneumonia. J. A. M. A. *229*:1471–1472, 1974.
446. Novelli, V. M., and Marshall, W. C.: Optic disc swelling and *Mycoplasma pneumoniae.* Pediatr. Infect. Dis. *3*:597, 1985.
447. Novelli, V. M., Matthew, D. J., and Dinwiddie, R. D.: Acute fulminant toxic encephalopathy associated with *Mycoplasma pneumoniae* infection. Pediatr. Infect. Dis. *4*:413–415, 1985.
448. Oderda, G., and Kraut, J. R.: Rising antibody titer to *Mycoplasma pneumoniae* in acute pancreatitis. Pediatrics *66*:305–306, 1980.
449. Ohlsson, A., Wang, E., and Vearncombe, M.: Leukocyte counts and colonization with *Ureaplasma urealyticum* in preterm neonates. Clin. Infect. Dis. *17*(Suppl. 1): S144–S147, 1993.
450. Ollikainen, J., Hiekkaniemi, H., Korppi, M., et al.: *Ureaplasma urealyticum* infection associated with acute respiratory insufficiency and death in premature infants. J. Pediatr. *122*:756–760, 1993.
451. Ollikainen, J., Hiekkaniemi, H., Korppi, M., et al.: *Ureaplasma urealyticum* cultured from brain tissue of preterm twins who died of intraventricular hemorrhage. Scand. J. Infect. Dis. *25*:529–531, 1993.
452. Olson, L. D., and Gilbert, A. A.: Characteristics of *Mycoplasma hominis* adhesion. J. Bacteriol. *175*:3224–3227, 1993.
453. Ong, E. L. C., Ellis, M. E., and Yuill, G. M.: Neurological complication of *Mycoplasma pneumoniae* infection. Resp. Med. *83*:441–442, 1989.
454. Oriel, J. D.: Treatment of nongonococcal urethritis. *In* Hobson, D., and Holmes, K. K. (eds.): Nongonococcal Urethritis and Related Infections. Washington, D.C., American Society for Microbiology, 1977, pp. 38–42.
455. Oriel, J. D., Ridgway, G. L., Reeve, P., et al.: The lack of effect of ampicillin plus probenecid given for genital infections with *Neisseria gonorrhoeae* on associated infections with *Chlamydia trachomatis.* J. Infect. Dis. *133*:568–571, 1976.
456. Paavonen, J., Miettinen, A., Stevens, C. E., et al.: *Mycoplasma hominis* in cervicitis and endometritis. Sex. Transm. Dis. *10*:276–280, 1983.
457. Paavonen, J., Miettinen, A., Stevens, C. E., et al.: *Mycoplasma hominis* in nonspecific vaginitis. Sex. Transm. Dis. *10*:271–275, 1983.
458. Panero, A., Pacifico, L., Rossi, N., et al.: *Ureaplasma urealyticum* as a cause of pneumonia in preterm infants: Analysis of the white cell response. Arch. Dis. Child. *73*:F37–F40, 1995.
459. Panero, A., Pacifico, L., Rossi, N., et al.: Elevated white blood cell counts associated with *Ureaplasma urealyticum* colonization in preterm neonates. Clin. Infect. Dis. *19*:980–981, 1994.
460. Parker, F., Jolliffe, L. S., and Finland, M.: Primary atypical pneumonia: Report of eight cases with autopsies. Arch. Pathol. *44*:581–608, 1947.
461. Parker, P., Puck, J., and Fernandez, F.: Cerebral infarction associated with *Mycoplasma pneumoniae.* Pediatrics *67*:373–375, 1981.
462. Parrott, R. H.: Viral respiratory tract illnesses in children. Bull. N. Y. Acad. Med. *39*:629–648, 1963.
463. Payne, N. R., Steinberg, S. S., Ackerman, P., et al.: New prospective

studies of the association of *Ureaplasma urealyticum* colonization and chronic lung disease. Clin. Infect. Dis. *17*(Suppl. 1):S117–S121, 1993.

464. Perez, C. R., and Leigh, M. W.: *Mycoplasma pneumoniae* as the causative agent for pneumonia in the immunocompromised host. Chest *100*:860–861, 1991.
465. Pollack, J. D., Somerson, N. L., and Senterfit, L. B.: Isolation, characterization, and immunogenicity of *Mycoplasma pneumoniae* membranes. Infect. Immun. *2*:326–329, 1970.
466. Pönkä, A.: Central nervous system manifestations associated with serologically verified *Mycoplasma pneumoniae* infection. Scand. J. Infect. Dis. *12*:175–184, 1980.
467. Pönkä, A.: The occurrence and clinical picture of serologically verified *Mycoplasma pneumoniae* infections with emphasis on central nervous system, cardiac and joint manifestations. Ann. Clin. Res. *11*(Suppl. 24):1–60, 1979.
468. Pönkä, A.: Arthritis associated with *Mycoplasma pneumoniae* infection. Scand. J. Rheumatol. *8*:27–32, 1979.
469. Pönkä, A.: Carditis associated with *Mycoplasma pneumoniae* infection. Acta Med. Scand. *206*:77–86, 1979.
470. Powell, D. A., Miller, K., and Clyde, W. A., Jr.: Submandibular adenitis in a newborn, caused by *Mycoplasma hominis*. Pediatrics *63*:798–799, 1979.
471. Powell, D. A., Hu, P. C., Wilson, M., et al.: Attachment of *Mycoplasma pneumoniae* to respiratory epithelium. Infect. Immun. *13*:959–966, 1976.
472. Puéchal, X., Hilliquin, P., Renoux, M., et al.: *Ureaplasma urealyticum* destructive septic polyarthritis revealing a common variable immunodeficiency. Arthritis Rheum. *38*:1524–1526, 1995.
473. Purcell, R. H., and Chanock, R. M.: Mycoplasmas of human origin. *In* Lennette, E. H. (ed.): Diagnostic Procedures for Viral and Rickettsial Infections. New York, American Public Health Association, 1969, pp. 786–825.
474. Putman, C. E., Baumgarten, A., and Gee, J. B. L.: The prevalence of mycoplasmal complement-fixing antibodies in sarcoidosis. Am. Rev. Respir. Dis. *111*:364–365, 1975.
475. Putman, C. E., Curtis, A. McB., Simeone, J. F., et al.: *Mycoplasma* pneumonia: Clinical and roentgenographic patterns. Am. J. Roentgenol. Radium Ther. Nucl. Med. *124*:417–422, 1975.
476. Quinn, P. A., Gillan, J. E., Markestad, T., et al.: Intrauterine infection with *Ureaplasma urealyticum* as a cause of fatal neonatal pneumonia. Pediatr. Infect. Dis. *4*:538–543, 1985.
477. Radestock, U., and Bredt, W.: Motility of *Mycoplasma pneumoniae*. J. Bacteriol. *129*:1495–1501, 1977.
478. Rastawicki, W., and Jagielski, M.: Enzyme-linked immunosorbent assay, complement fixation test and immunoelectroprecipitation test in the diagnosis of *Mycoplasma pneumoniae* infections: Comparative analysis. Zentralbl. Bakteriol. *283*:477–484, 1996.
479. Razin, S., and Jacobs, E.: *Mycoplasma* adhesion. J. Gen. Microbiol. *138*:407–422, 1992.
480. Renner, E. D., Helms, C. M., Johnson, W., et al.: Coinfections of *Mycoplasma pneumoniae* and *Legionella pneumophila* with influenza A virus. J. Clin. Microbiol. *17*:146–148, 1983.
481. Renner, E. D., Helms, C. M., Hall, N. H., et al.: Seroreactivity to *Mycoplasma pneumoniae* and *Legionella pneumophila*: Lack of a statistically significant relationship. J. Clin. Microbiol. *13*:1096–1098, 1981.
482. Reznikov, M., Blackmore, T. K., Finlay-Jones, J. J., et al.: Comparison of nasopharyngeal aspirates and throat swab specimens in a polymerase chain reaction-based test for *Mycoplasma pneumoniae*. Eur. J. Clin. Microbiol. Infect. Dis. *14*:58–62, 1995.
483. Rifkind, D., Chanock, R., Kravetz, H., et al.: Ear involvement (myringitis) and primary atypical pneumonia following inoculation of volunteers with Eaton agent. Am. Rev. Respir. Dis. *85*:479–489, 1962.
484. Roberts, J. E., and Isaacs, D.: Neurological and pulmonary complications of *Mycoplasma pneumoniae* infection in a preschool child. J. Infect. *12*:251–252, 1986.
485. Roberts-Thomson, I. C., Cottew, G. S., and Fraser, J. R. E.: *Mycoplasma* pneumonia with severe haemolytic anaemia. Med. J. Aust. *2*:1046–1047, 1973.
486. Robertson, J. A., and Stemke, G. W.: Expanded serotyping scheme for *Ureaplasma urealyticum* strains isolated from humans. J. Clin. Microbiol. *5*:873–878, 1982.
487. Robertson, J., Gonersall, M., and Gill, P.: *Mycoplasma hominis*: Growth, reproduction, and isolation of small viable cells. J. Bacteriol. *124*:1007–1018, 1975.
488. Roifman, C. M., Rao, C. P., Lederman, H. M., et al.: Increased susceptibility to *Mycoplasma* infection in patients with hypogammaglobulinemia. Am. J. Med. *80*:590–594, 1986.
489. Romano, N., Romano, F., and Carollo, F.: T-strains of *Mycoplasma* in bronchopneumonic lungs of an aborted fetus. N. Engl. J. Med. *285*:950–952, 1971.
490. Romero, R., Mazor, M., Oyarzun, E., et al.: Is genital colonization with *Mycoplasma hominis* or *Ureaplasma urealyticum* associated with prematurity/low birth weight? Obstet. Gynecol. *73*:532, 1989.
491. Ross, J. M., Furr, P. M., Taylor-Robinson, D., et al.: The effect of genital mycoplasmas on human fetal growth. Br. J. Obstet. Gynecol. *88*:749–755, 1981.
492. Rothstein, T. L., and Kenny, G. E.: Cranial neuropathy, myeloradiculopathy, and myositis: Complications of *Mycoplasma pneumoniae* infection. Arch. Neurol. *36*:476–477, 1979.
493. Ruhrmann, G., and Holthusen, W.: *Mycoplasma* infection and erythromycin therapy in childhood. Scott. Med. J. *22*:401–403, 1977.
494. Ruiter, M., and Wentholt, H. M. M.: A pleuropneumonia-like organism in primary fusospirochetal gangrene of the penis. J. Invest. Dermatol. *15*:301–304, 1950.
495. Rykner, G., Bonnafous, J., and Manigand, G.: Sérologie des infections à *Mycoplasma pneumoniae* par le test d'inhibition metabolique. Semin. Hôp. Paris *47*:1498, 1970.
496. Sabato, A. R., Martin, A. J., Marmion, B. P., et al.: *Mycoplasma pneumoniae:* Acute illness, antibiotics, and subsequent pulmonary function. Arch. Dis. Child. *59*:1034–1037, 1984.
497. Sacker, I., Walker, M., and Brunell, P. A.: Abscess in newborn infants caused by mycoplasma. Pediatrics *46*:303–304, 1970.
498. Saliba, G. S., Glezen, W. P., and Chin, T. D. Y.: *Mycoplasma pneumoniae* infection in a resident boys' home. Am. J. Epidemiol. *86*:408–418, 1967.
499. Salzman, M. B., Sood, S. K., Slavin, M. L., et al.: Ocular manifestations of *Mycoplasma pneumoniae* infection. Clin. Infect. Dis. *14*:1137–1139, 1992.
500. Sanchez, P. J., and Regan, J. A.: *Ureaplasma urealyticum* colonization and chronic lung disease in low birth weight infants. Pediatr. Infect. Dis. J. *7*:542–546, 1988.
501. Sande, M. A., Gadot, F., and Wenzel, R. P.: Point source epidemic of *Mycoplasma pneumoniae* infection in a prosthodontics laboratory. Am. Rev. Respir. Dis. *112*:213–217, 1975.
502. Sanders, D. Y., and Johnson, H. W.: Stevens-Johnson syndrome associated with *Mycoplasma pneumoniae* infection. Am. J. Dis. Child. *121*:243–245, 1971.
503. Sands, M. J., Jr., Satz, J. E., Turner, W. E., Jr., et al.: Pericarditis and perimyocarditis associated with active *Mycoplasma pneumoniae* infection. Ann. Intern. Med. *86*:544–548, 1977.
504. Sasaki, T., Bonissol, C., and Stoiljkovic, B.: Cross-reactive antibodies to mycoplasmas found in human sera by the enzyme-linked immunosorbent assay (ELISA). Microbiol. Immunol. *31*:521–530, 1987.
505. Sasaki, Y., Honda, M., Naitou, M., et al.: Detection of *Mycoplasma fermentans* DNA from lymph nodes of acquired immunodeficiency syndrome patients. Microb. Pathog. *17*:131–135, 1994.
506. Savolainen, S., Jousimies-Somer, H., Kleemola, M., et al.: Serological evidence of viral or *Mycoplasma pneumoniae* infection in acute maxillary sinusitis. Eur. J. Clin. Microbiol. Infect. Dis. *8*:131–135, 1989.
507. Schachter, J., Hanna, L., Hill, E. C., et al.: Are chlamydial infections the most prevalent venereal disease? J. A. M. A. *231*:1252–1255, 1975.
508. Schmidt, N. J., Lennette, E. H., Dennis, J., et al.: On the nature of complement-fixing antibodies to *Mycoplasma pneumoniae*. J. Immunol. *97*:95–99, 1966.
509. Schmitz, R. C.: Primary atypical pneumonia of unknown cause. Arch. Intern. Med. *75*:222–232, 1945.
510. Schönwald, S., Barsic, B., Klinar, I., et al.: Three-day azithromycin compared with ten-day roxithromycin treatment of atypical pneumonia. Scand. J. Infect. Dis. *26*:706–710, 1994.
511. Schulman, P., Piemonte, T. C., and Singh, B.: Acute renal failure, hemolytic anemia, and *Mycoplasma pneumoniae*. J. A. M. A. *244*:1823–1824, 1980.
512. Sequeira, W., Jones, E., and Bronson, D. M.: *Mycoplasma pneumoniae* infection with arthritis and a varicella-like eruption. J. A. M. A. *246*:1936–1937, 1981.
513. Shames, J. M., George, R. B., Holliday, W. B., et al.: Comparison of antibiotics in the treatment of mycoplasmal pneumonia. Arch. Intern. Med. *125*:680–684, 1970.
514. Shawn, D. H., Quinn, P. A., Prober, C., et al.: Recurrent urethritis associated with *Ureaplasma urealyticum* in a prepubertal boy. Pediatr. Infect. Dis. J. *6*:687–688, 1987.
515. Shepard, M. C., and Masover, G. K.: Special features of ureaplasmas. *In* Barile, M. F., and Razins, S. (eds.): The Mycoplasmas. Vol. I. New York, Academic Press, 1979, pp. 451–494.
516. Shepard, M. C., and Lunceford, C. D.: Differential agar medium (A7) for identification of *Ureaplasma urealyticum* (human T mycoplasmas) in primary cultures of clinical material. J. Clin. Microbiol. *3*:613–625, 1976.
517. Shepard, M. C., Lunceford, C. D., Ford, D. K., et al.: *Ureaplasma urealyticum* gen. nov. sp. nov.: Proposed nomenclature for the human T (T-strain) mycoplasmas. Int. J. Syst. Bacteriol. *24*:160–171, 1974.
518. Shepard, M. C.: The recovery of pleuropneumonia-like organisms from Negro men with and without nongonococcal urethritis. Am. J. Syph. *38*:113–124, 1954.
519. Sheth, R. D., Goulden, K. J., and Pryse-Phillips, W. E.: The focal encephalopathies associated with *Mycoplasma pneumoniae*. Can. J. Neurol. Sci. *20*:319–323, 1993.
520. Shulman, S. T., Bartlett, J., Clyde, W. A., Jr., et al.: The unusual severity of mycoplasmal pneumonia in children with sickle-cell disease. N. Engl. J. Med. *287*:164–167, 1972.
521. Shurin, P. A., Alpert, S. Rosner, B., et al.: Chorioamnionitis and colonization of the newborn infant with genital mycoplasmas. N. Engl. J. Med. *293*:5–8, 1975.
522. Sieber, O. F., John, T. J., Fulginiti, V. A., et al.: Stevens-Johnson syndrome associated with *Mycoplasma pneumoniae* infection. J. A. M. A. *200*:79–81, 1967.

523. Siegler, D. I. M.: Lung abscess associated with *Mycoplasma pneumoniae* infection. Br. J. Dis. Chest *67*:123–127, 1973.
524. Sillis, M.: The limitations of IgM assays in the serological diagnosis of *Mycoplasma pneumoniae* infections. J. Med. Microbiol. *33*:253–258, 1990.
525. Simmons, B. P., and Aber, R. C.: *Mycoplasma pneumoniae* pneumonia: Symptoms mimicking pulmonary embolism with infarction. J. A. M. A. *241*:1268–1269, 1979.
526. Singer, J. I., and DeVoe, W. M.: Severe *Mycoplasma pneumoniae* infection in otherwise healthy siblings. J. Pediatr. *95*:999–1001, 1979.
527. Skoldenberg, B.: Aseptic meningitis and meningoencephalitis in cold-agglutinin-positive infections. B. M. J. *1*:100–102, 1965.
528. Slotkin, R. I., Clyde, W. A., Jr., and Denny, R. W.: The effect of antibiotics on *Mycoplasma pneumoniae* in vitro and in vivo. Am. J. Epidemiol. *86*:225–237, 1967.
529. Smiley, D. F., Showacre, E., Lee, W., et al.: Acute interstitial pneumonitis: A new disease entity. J. A. M. A. *112*:1901, 1939.
530. Smith, C. B., Golden, C. A., Kanner, R. E., et al.: Association of viral and *Mycoplasma pneumoniae* infections with acute respiratory illness in patients with chronic obstructive pulmonary disease. Am. Rev. Respir. Dis. *121*:225–232, 1980.
531. Smith, C. B., McGinniss, M. H., and Schmidt, P. J.: Changes in erythrocyte I agglutinogen and anti-I agglutinins during *Mycoplasma pneumoniae* infection in man. J. Immunol. *99*:333–339, 1967.
532. Smith, C. B., Friedewald, W. T., and Chanock, R. M.: Shedding of *Mycoplasma pneumoniae* after tetracycline and erythromycin therapy. N. Engl. J. Med. *276*:1172–1175, 1967.
533. Smith, C. B., Friedewald, W. T., and Chanock, R. M.: Inactivated *Mycoplasma pneumoniae* vaccine: Evaluation in volunteers. J. A. M. A. *199*:353–358, 1967.
534. Smith, T. F.: *Mycoplasma pneumoniae* infections: Diagnosis based on immunofluorescence titer of IgG and IgM antibodies. Mayo Clin. Proc. *61*:830–831, 1986.
535. Sobeslavsky, O., Prescott, B., and Chanock, R. M.: Adsorption of *Mycoplasma pneumoniae* to neuraminic acid receptors of various cells and possible role in virulence. J. Bacteriol. *96*:695–705, 1968.
536. Sobeslavsky, O., Syrucek, L., Bruckova, M., et al.: The etiological role of *Mycoplasma pneumoniae* in otitis media in children. Pediatrics *35*:652–657, 1965.
537. Sohaeverbeke, T., Gilroy, C. B., Bébéar, C., et al.: *Mycoplasma fermentans* in joints of patients with rheumatoid arthritis and other joint disorders. Lancet *347*:1418, 1996.
538. Solanki, K. L., and Berdoff, R. L.: Severe mycoplasma pneumonia with pleural effusions in a patient with sickle cell-hemoglobin C (SC) disease: Case report and review of the literature. Am. J. Med. *66*:707–710, 1979.
539. Somerson, N. L., and Cole, B. C.: The *Mycoplasma* flora of human and nonhuman primates. *In* Tully, J. G., and Whitcomb, R. F. (eds.): The Mycoplasmas. Vol. II. New York, Academic Press, 1979, pp. 191–216.
540. Sprinkle, P. M.: Current status of mycoplasmatales and bacterial variants in chronic otolaryngologic disease. Laryngoscope *82*:737–747, 1972.
541. Stadel, B. V., Foy, H. M., Nuckolls, J. W., et al.: *Mycoplasma pneumoniae* infection followed by *Haemophilus influenzae* pneumonia and bacteremia. Am. Rev. Respir. Dis. *112*:131–133, 1975.
542. Stagno, S., Brasfield, D. M., Brown, M. B., et al.: Infant pneumonitis associated with cytomegalovirus, *Chlamydia, Pneumocystis,* and *Ureaplasma:* A prospective study. Pediatrics *68*:322–329, 1981.
543. Stahelin-Massik, J., Levy, F., Friderich, P., et al.: Meningitis caused by *Ureaplasma urealyticum* in a full term neonate. Pediatr. Infect. Dis. J. *13*:419–421, 1994.
544. Stallings, M. W., and Archer, S. B.: Atypical *Mycoplasma* pneumonia. Am. J. Dis. Child. *126*:837–838, 1973.
545. Stallman, N. D., Allan, B. C., and Wiemers, M. A.: Infection with *Mycoplasma pneumoniae:* Clinical and serological data on 286 patients. Med. J. Aust. *1*:340–343, 1976.
546. Stallman, N. D., and Allan, B. C.: A survey of antibodies to *Mycoplasma pneumoniae* in Queensland. Med. J. Aust. *1*:800–802, 1970.
547. Stamm, W. E., Running, K., Hale, J., et al.: Etiologic role of *Mycoplasma hominis* and *Ureaplasma urealyticum* in women with the acute urethral syndrome. Sex. Transm. Dis. *10*:318–322, 1983.
548. Stancombe, B. B., Walsh, W. F., Derdak, S., et al.: Induction of human neonatal pulmonary fibroblast cytokines by hyperoxia and *Ureaplasma urealyticum.* Clin. Infect. Dis. *17*(Suppl. 1):S154–S157, 1993.
549. Steele, J. C., Gladstone, R. M., Thanasophon, S., et al.: *Mycoplasma pneumoniae* as a determinant of the Guillain-Barré syndrome. Lancet *2*:710–714, 1969.
550. Steinberg, P., White, R. J., Fuld, S. L., et al.: Ecology of *Mycoplasma pneumoniae* infections in marine recruits at Parris Island, South Carolina. Am. J. Epidemiol. *89*:62–73, 1969.
551. Sterner, G., DeHevesy, G., Tunevall, G., et al.: Acute respiratory illness with *Mycoplasma pneumoniae:* An outbreak in a home for children. Acta Paediatr. Scand. *55*:280–286, 1966.
552. Stevens, D., Swift, P. G. F., Johnston, P. G. B., et al.: *Mycoplasma pneumoniae* infections in children. Arch. Dis. Child. *53*:38–42, 1978.
553. Stevens, M. K., and Krause, D. C.: Disulfide-linked protein associated with *Mycoplasma pneumoniae* cytadherence phase variation. Infect. Immun. *58*:3430–3433, 1990.
554. Stewart, S. M., Burnet, M. E. and Young, J. E.: In vitro sensitivity of strains of mycoplasmas from human sources to antibiotics and to sodium aurothiomalate and tylosin tartrate. J. Med. Microbiol. *2*:287–292, 1969.
555. Stray-Pedersen, B., Bruu, A. L., and Molne, K.: Infertility and uterine colonization with *Ureaplasma urealyticum.* Acta Obstet. Gynecol. Scand. *61*:21–24, 1982.
556. Stutman, H. R.: Stevens-Johnson syndrome and *Mycoplasma pneumoniae*: Evidence for cutaneous infection. J. Pediatr. *111*:845–847, 1987.
557. Suhs, R. H., and Feldman, H. A.: Serologic epidemiologic studies with *M. pneumoniae.* II. Prevalence of antibodies in several populations. Am. J. Epidemiol. *83*:357–365, 1966.
558. Sussman, S. J., Magoffin, R. L., Lennette, E. H., et al.: Cold agglutinins, Eaton agent, and respiratory infections of children. Pediatrics *38*:571–577, 1966.
559. Syrogiannopoulos, G. A., Kapatais-Zoumbos, K., Decavalas, G. O., et al.: *Ureaplasma urealyticum* colonization of full term infants: Perinatal acquisition and persistence during early infancy. Pediatr. Infect. Dis. J. *9*:236–240, 1990.
560. Tablan, O. C., and Reyes, M. P.: Chronic interstitial pulmonary fibrosis following *Mycoplasma pneumoniae* pneumonia. Am. J. Med. *79*:268–270, 1985.
561. Tanowitz, H. B., Robbins, N., and Leidich, N.: Hemolytic anemia: Associated with severe *Mycoplasma pneumoniae* pneumonia. N. Y. State J. Med. *78*:2231–2232, 1978.
562. Taylor, G., Taylor-Robinson, D., and Fernald, G. W.: Reduction in the severity of *Mycoplasma pneumoniae*-induced pneumonia in hamsters by immunosuppressive treatment with antithymocyte sera. J. Med. Microbiol. *7*:343–348, 1974.
563. Taylor, M. J., Burrow, G. N., Strauch, B., et al.: Meningoencephalitis associated with pneumonitis due to *Mycoplasma pneumoniae.* J. A. M. A. *199*:813–816, 1967.
564. Taylor-Robinson, D., Gilroy, C. B., and Hay, P. E.: Occurrence of *Mycoplasma genitalium* in different populations and its clinical significance. Clin. Infect. Dis. *17*(Suppl. 1):S66–S68, 1993.
565. Taylor-Robinson, D.: The Mycoplasmatales: *Mycoplasma, Ureaplasma, Acholeplasma, Spiroplasma* and *Anaeroplasma. In* Parker, M. T., and Duerden, B. I. (eds.): Principles of Bacteriology, Virology and Immunity. Vol. 2. Systemic Bacteriology. Philadelphia, B. C. Decker, 1990, pp. 664–681.
566. Taylor-Robinson, D.: Genital *Mycoplasma* infections. Clin. Lab. Med. *9*:501–523, 1989.
567. Taylor-Robinson, D.: *Mycoplasma* infections of the human urogenital tract with particular reference to nongonococcal urethritis. Ann. Microbiol. *135A*:129–134, 1984.
568. Taylor-Robinson, D., Tully, J. G., Furr, P. M., et al.: Urogenital *Mycoplasma* infections of man: A review with observations on a recently discovered *Mycoplasma.* Isr. J. Med. Sci. *17*:524–530, 1981.
569. Taylor-Robinson, D., and McCormack, W. M.: The genital mycoplasmas. N. Engl. J. Med. *302*:1003–1010, 1063–1067, 1980.
570. Taylor-Robinson, D., and Furr, P. M.: The distribution of T-mycoplasmas within and among various animal species. Ann. N. Y. Acad. Sci. *225*:108–117, 1973.
571. Taylor-Robinson, D., and Cherry, J. D.: A nonpathogenic mycoplasma inhibiting the effect of a pathogenic mycoplasma in organ culture. J. Med. Microbiol. *5*:291–298, 1972.
572. Taylor-Robinson, D.: The biology of mycoplasmas: Symposium on acute respiratory diseases. J. Clin. Pathol. *21*(Suppl. 2):38–51, 1968.
573. Taylor-Robinson, D.: Mycoplasmas of various hosts and their antibiotic sensitivities. Postgrad. Med. J. *43*(Suppl.):100–104, 1967.
574. Taylor-Robinson, D., Shirai, A., Sobeslavsky, O., et al.: Serologic response to *Mycoplasma pneumoniae* infection. II. Significance of antibody measured by different techniques. Am. J. Epidemiol. *84*:301–313, 1966.
575. Teisch, J. A., Shapiro, L., and Walzer, R. A.: Vesiculopustular eruption with *Mycoplasma* infection. J. A. M. A. *211*:1694–1697, 1970.
576. Thacker, W. L., and Talkington, D. F.: Comparison of two rapid commercial tests with complement fixation for serologic diagnosis of *Mycoplasma pneumoniae* infections. J. Clin. Microbiol. *33*:1212–1214, 1995.
577. Thomas, M., Jones, M., and Ray, S.: *Mycoplasma pneumoniae* in a tubo-ovarian abscess. Lancet *2*:774–775, 1975.
578. Thomsen, A. C.: Occurrence and pathogenicity of *Mycoplasma hominis* in the upper urinary tract: A review. Sex. Transm. Dis. *10*:323–326, 1983.
579. Tilton, R. C., Dias, F., Kidd, H., et al.: DNA probe versus culture for detection of *Mycoplasma pneumoniae* in clinical specimens. Diagn. Microbiol. Infect. Dis. *10*:109–112, 1988.
580. Tipirneni, P., Moore, B. S., Hyde, J. S., et al.: IgE antibodies to *Mycoplasma pneumoniae* in asthma and other atopic diseases. Ann. Allergy *45*:1–7, 1980.
581. Toth, A., Lesser, M. L., Brooks, C., et al.: Subsequent pregnancies among 161 couples treated for T-*Mycoplasma* genital-tract infection. N. Engl. J. Med. *308*:505–508, 1983.
582. Tully, J. G., Rose, D. L., Baseman, J. B., et al.: *Mycoplasma pneumoniae* and *Mycoplasma genitalium* mixture in synovial fluid isolate. J. Clin. Microbiol. *33*:1851–1855, 1995.
583. Tully, J. G.: Current status of the mollicute flora of humans. Clin. Infect. Dis. *17*(Suppl. 1):S2–S9, 1993.

584. Tully, J. G.: *Mycoplasma* flora of humans. Personal communication. Dec. 1, 1991.
585. Tully, J. G., Taylor-Robinson, D., Rose, D. L., et al.: Urogenital challenge of primate species with *Mycoplasma genitalium* and characteristics of infection induced in chimpanzees. J. Infect. Dis. *153*:1046–1054, 1986.
586. Tully, J. G., Taylor-Robinson, D., Rose, D. L., et al.: *Mycoplasma genitalium*, a new species from the human urogenital tract. Int. J. Syst. Bacteriol. *33*:387–396, 1983.
587. Tully, J. G., Rose, D. L., Whitcomb, R. F., et al.: Enhanced isolation of *Mycoplasma pneumoniae* from throat washings with a newly modified culture medium. J. Infect. Dis. *139*:478–482, 1979.
588. Tully, J. G.: Biology of the mycoplasmas. *In* McGarrity, G. J., Murphy, D. G., and Nichols, W. W. (eds.): *Mycoplasma* Infection of Cell Cultures. New York, Plenum, 1978, pp. 1–33.
589. Turner, J. A. P., Burchak, E. C., Bannatyne, R. M., et al.: The protean manifestations of *Mycoplasma* infections in childhood. Can. Med. Assoc. J. *99*:633–637, 1968.
590. Twomey, J. A., and Espir, M. L. E.: Neurological manifestations and *Mycoplasma pneumoniae* infection. B. M. J. *6194*:832–833, 1979.
591. Uldum, S. A., Jensen, J. S., Søndergård-Andersen, J., et al.: Enzyme immunoassay for detection of immunoglobulin M (IgM) and IgG antibodies to *Mycoplasma pneumoniae*. J. Clin. Microbiol. *30*:1198–1204, 1992.
592. Ursi, D., Ursi, J.-P., Ieven, M., et al.: Congenital pneumonia due to *Mycoplasma pneumoniae*. Arch. Dis. Child. *72*:F118–F120, 1995.
593. Valencia, G.B., Banzon, F., Cummings, M., et al.: *Mycoplasma hominis* and *Ureaplasma urealyticum* in neonates with suspected infection. Pediatr. Infect. Dis. J. *12*:571–573, 1993.
594. Van Bever, H. P., Van Doorn, J. W. D., and Demey, H. E.: Adult respiratory distress syndrome associated with *Mycoplasma pneumoniae* infection. Eur. J. Pediatr. *151*:227–228, 1992.
595. Van der Veen, J., and Van Nunen, C. J.: Role of *Mycoplasma pneumoniae* in acute respiratory disease in a military population. Am. J. Hyg. *78*:293–301, 1963.
596. Van Kuppeveld, F. J., Johansson, K. E., Galama, J. M., et al.: 16S rRNA based polymerase chain reaction compared with culture and serological methods for diagnosis of *Mycoplasma pneumoniae* infection. Eur. J. Clin. Microbiol. Infect. Dis. *13*:401–405, 1994.
597. Volk, J., and Kraus, S. J.: Nongonococcal urethritis: A venereal disease as prevalent as epidemic gonorrhea. Arch. Intern. Med. *134*:511–514, 1974.
598. Vu, A. C., Foy, H. M., Cartwright, F. D., et al.: The principal protein antigens of isolates of *Mycoplasma pneumoniae* as measured by levels of immunoglobulin G in human serum are stable in strains collected over a 10-year period. Infect. Immun. *55*:1830–1836, 1987.
599. Vulliemin, J. F.: Nongonococcal urethritis: Therapeutic considerations. Curr. Ther. Res. *26*:719–725, 1979.
600. Waites, K. B., Crouse, D. T., and Cassell, G. H.: Systemic neonatal infection due to *Ureaplasma urealyticum*. Clin. Infect. Dis. *17*(Suppl. 1):S131–S135, 1993.
601. Waites, K. B., Sims, P. J., Crouse, D. T., et al.: Serum concentrations of erythromycin after intravenous infusion in preterm neonates treated for *Ureaplasma urealyticum* infection. Pediatr. Infect. Dis. J. *13*:287–293, 1994.
602. Waites, K. B., Crouse, D. T., and Cassell, G. H.: Therapeutic considerations for *Ureaplasma urealyticum* infections in neonates. Clin. Infect. Dis. *17*(Suppl. 1):S208–S214, 1993.
603. Waites, K. B., Duffy, L. B., Baldus, K., et al.: Mycoplasmal infections of cerebrospinal fluid in children undergoing neurosurgery for hydrocephalus. Pediatr. Infect. Dis. J. *10*:952–953, 1991.
604. Waites, K. B., Duffy, L. B., Crouse, D. T., et al.: Mycoplasmal infections of cerebrospinal fluid in newborn infants from a community hospital population. Pediatr. Infect. Dis. J. *9*:241–245, 1990.
605. Waites, K. B., Crouse, D. T., Philips, J. B., III, et al.: Ureaplasmal pneumonia and sepsis associated with persistent pulmonary hypertension of the newborn. Pediatrics *83*:79–85, 1989.
606. Waites, K. B., Rudd, P. T., Crouse, D. T., et al.: Chronic *Ureaplasma urealyticum* and *Mycoplasma hominis* infections of central nervous system in preterm infants. Lancet *1*:17–21, 1988.
607. Waites, K. B., Brown, M. B., Stagno, S., et al.: Association of genital mycoplasmas with exudative vaginitis in a 10-year-old: A case of misdiagnosis. Pediatrics *71*:250–252, 1983.
608. Wang, E. E. L., Ohlsson, A., and Kellner, J. D.: Association of *Ureaplasma urealyticum* colonization with chronic lung disease of prematurity: Results of a metaanalysis. J. Pediatr. *127*:640–644, 1995.
609. Wang, E. E. L., Cassell, G. H., Sanchez, P. J., et al.: *Ureaplasma urealyticum* and chronic lung disease of prematurity: Critical appraisal of the literature on causation. Clin. Infect. Dis. *17*(Suppl. 1):S112–S116, 1993.
610. Wang, R. Y. H., Shih, J. W. K., Weiss, S. H., et al.: *Mycoplasma penetrans* infection in male homosexuals with AIDS: High seroprevalence and association with Kaposi's sarcoma. Clin. Infect. Dis. *17*:724–729, 1993.
611. Wang, R. Y. H., Shih, J. W. K., Grandinetti, T., et al.: High frequency of antibodies to *Mycoplasma penetrans* in HIV-infected patients. Lancet *340*:1312–1316, 1992.
612. Wang, E. E. L., Frayha, H., Watts, J., et al.: Role of *Ureaplasma urealyticum* and other pathogens in the development of chronic lung disease of prematurity. Pediatr. Infect. Dis. J. *7*:547–551, 1988.
613. Warren, P., Fischbein, C. Mascoli, N., et al.: Poliomyelitis-like syndrome caused by *Mycoplasma pneumoniae.* J. Pediatr. *93*:451–452, 1978.
614. Watson, H. L., Blalock, D. K., and Cassell, G. H.: Variable antigens of *Ureaplasma urealyticum* containing both serovar-specific and serovar-cross-reactive epitopes. Infect. Immun. *58*:3679–3688, 1990.
615. Weinstein, M. P., and Hall, C. B.: *Mycoplasma pneumoniae* infections associated with migratory polyarthritis. Am. J. Dis. Child. *127*:125–126, 1974.
616. Wenzel, R. P., Craven, R. B., Davies, J. A., et al.: Protective efficacy of an inactivated *Mycoplasma pneumoniae* vaccine. J. Infect. Dis. *136*(Suppl.): S204–S207, 1977.
617. Westerberg, S. C., Smith, C. B., and Renzetti, A. D.: *Mycoplasma* infections in patients with chronic obstructive pulmonary disease. J. Infect. Dis. *127*:491–497, 1973.
618. Westernfelder, G. O., Akey, T., Corwin, S. J., et al.: Acute transverse myelitis due to *Mycoplasma pneumoniae* infection. Arch. Neurol. *38*:317–318, 1981.
619. Westrom, L., and March, P. A.: The effect of antibiotic therapy on *Mycoplasma* in the female genital tract: In vitro and in vivo studies on the sensitivity of *Mycoplasma hominis* and T-mycoplasmas to tetracyclines and other antibiotics. Acta Obstet. Gynecol. Scand. *50*:25–31, 1971.
620. Whitescarver, J., and Furness, G.: T-mycoplasmas: A study of the morphology, ultrastructure and mode of division of some human strains. J. Med. Microbiol. *8*:349–355, 1975.
621. Williams, M. H., Brostoff, J., and Roitt, I. M.: Possible role of *Mycoplasma fermentans* in pathogenesis of rheumatoid arthritis. Lancet *2*:277–280, 1970.
622. Williamson, J., Marmion, B. P., Kok, T., et al.: Confirmation of fatal *Mycoplasma pneumoniae* infection by polymerase chain reaction detection of the adhesin gene in fixed lung tissue. J. Infect. Dis. *170*:1052–1053, 1994.
623. Wilson, M. H., and Collier, A. M.: Ultrastructural study of *Mycoplasma pneumoniae* in organ culture. J. Bacteriol. *125*:332–339, 1976.
624. Yechouron, A., Lefebvre, J., and Robson, H. G.: Fatal septicemia due to *Mycoplasma arginini:* A new human zoonosis. Clin. Infect. Dis. *15*:434–438, 1992.
625. Zinserling, A.: Peculiarities of lesions in viral and *Mycoplasma* infections of the respiratory tract. Virchows Arch. Pathol. Anat. *356*:259–273, 1972.

FUNGAL DISEASES

❑ ❑ ❑

196

CLASSIFICATION OF FUNGI

Dexter H. Howard and Heidi M. Kokkinos

The fungi are contained in a separate biologic kingdom called Fungi.[7] These organisms are divided into two groups on the basis of their basic growth pattern: yeast and molds. Yeasts are unicellular fungi that reproduce by budding or by fission. The molds are multicellular fungi that grow by means of filamentous threads called hyphae. Upon the hyphae are developed reproductive propagules.[2]

Fungi may reproduce sexually or asexually. The sexual form of growth is called the teleomorph, and the asexual form is called the anamorph. It is the sexual means of reproduction that forms the basis of the taxonomy of fungi. Each of the products of meiosis that result from sexual reproduction is housed in specialized structures called sexual spores. There are three types of sexual spores: zygospores, ascospores, and basidiospores, so named to indicate their particular method of formation. The phyla within the kingdom Fungi and the type of sexual spore formed are: (1) Zygomycota (zygospores), (2) Ascomycota (ascospores), (3) Basidiomycota (basidiospores), (4) Deuteromycota (sexual reproduction unknown), and (5) Mycophycophyta (ascospores or rarely basidiospores). The last named phylum contains the lichens and will not be considered further in this discussion.

Alternative taxónomic arrangements have been proposed. The phyla Ascomycota and Basidiomycota are united, in one scheme, into a single phylum: Dikaryomycota, which then is subdivided into the two initial phyla as subphyla Ascomycota and Basidiomycota.[5] There are details in life cycles of the two phyla (or subphyla) that make this combination arguably reasonable. Likewise, modern molecular techniques have allowed systematic decisions to be made independently from morphologic criteria, and the members of the form phylum Deuteromycota that do not produce sexual spores can be related to members of phyla that do. A discussion of the benefits (if any) of dropping the Deuteromycota as a formal taxonomic category was the topic of an international symposium held recently.[8]

A group of microorganisms with flagellated asexual spores were at one time considered to be fungi[1], although certain of their characteristics were divergent from more traditional representatives (true fungi), e.g., cellulose in the cell walls and motile asexual spores. These forms now are contained with a phylum, Oomycetes, in a separate kingdom, Protoctista. There is one rare human pathogen (*Pythium insidiosum*) and several important animal pathogens contained in the phylum Oomycetes.[6] Because of limited involvement in human disease, the taxonomy of the Oomycetes will not be included in this coverage.

The taxonomic scheme depicted is based on references 1, 5, 6, and 7. The original draft of the scheme appeared in reference 4 and has been modified in keeping with recent textbook treatments of the topic.[3, 6]

The basic taxonomic unit is the species, and it is grouped into hierarchal systems that include genera, families, orders, classes, and phyla. The delineation of the zoopathogen *Ajellomyces capsulatus*, the teleomorph of *Histoplasma capsulatum*, goes as follows:

- Kingdom: Fungi
  - Phylum: Ascomycota
    - Class: Ascomycetes
      - Order: Onygenales
        - Family: Onygenaceae
          - Genus: *Ajellomyces*
            - Species: *Ajellomyces capsulatus* (anamorph: *Histoplasma capsulatum*)

This consideration will include *only* those taxa known to contain medically important species. Those classes, orders, and families not known to contain such pathogens will be omitted. More detailed considerations can be had by consulting the references indicated.

- Kingdom: Fungi
  - Phylum: Zygomycota
    - Class: Zygomycetes
      - Order: Mucorales
        - Family: Mucoraceae
          - Genera: *Apophysomyces, Absidia, Mucor, Rhizomucor, Rhizopus*
        - Family: Cunninghamellaceae
          - Genus: *Cunninghamella*
        - Family: Mortierellaceae
          - Genus: *Mortierella*
        - Family: Saksenaeaceae
          - Genus: *Saksenaea*
        - Family: Syncephalastraceae
          - Genus: *Syncephalastrum*
        - Family: Thamnidiaceae
          - Genus: *Cokeromyces*
      - Order: Entomophthorales
        - Family: Basidiobolaceae
          - Genus: *Basidiobolus*
        - Family: Entomophthoraceae
          - Genus: *Conidiobolus*
  - Phylum: Ascomycota
    - Class: Hemiascomycetes
      - Order: Endomycetales
          - Genera: Teleomorphs of *Candida, Geotrichum,* etc.
    - Class: Ascomycetes
      - Order: Onygenales
          - Genera: Teleomorphs of dermatophytes *(Microsporum, Trichophyton), Histoplasma (H. capsulatum), Blastomyces (B. dermatitidis)*
      - Order: Eurotiales
          - Genera: Teleomorphs of *Aspergillus*

Order: Microascales
Genus: *Pseudallescheria (P. boydii, Scedosporium apiospermum)*
Order: Dothidiales
Genus: *Piedraia (P. hortae)*
Phylum: Basidiomycota
Class: Holobasidiomycetes (mushrooms)
Class: Heterobasidiomycetes
Order: Filobasidiales
Genera: Teleomorphs of some *Cryptococcus* species (e.g., *C. neoformans*), *Rhodotorula* species
Phylum: Deuteromycota (Fungi Imperfecti)
Form Class: Blastomycetes
Form Order: Cryptococcales
Form Genera: *Cryptococcus, Candida, Trichosporon, Rhodotorula*
Form Order: Coelomycetes
Form Genus: *Phoma*
Form Order: Hyphomycetes
Form Order: Moniliales
Form Family: Moniliaceae (conidia, hyphae hyaline)
Form Genera: *Coccidioides, Aspergillus, Penicillium, Acremonium, Fusarium, Sporothrix, Paracoccidioides,* etc.
Form Family: Dematiaceae (conidia, hyphae dark)
Form Genera: *Cladosporium, Bipolaris,* etc.

References

1. Alexopoulos, C. J., and Mims, C. W.: Introductory Mycology. 3rd ed. New York, John Wiley & Sons, 1979.
2. Baron, E. J., Chang, R. S., Howard, D. H., et al.: Medical Microbiology: A Short Course. New York, Wiley-Liss, 1984.
3. Crissey, J. T., Lang, H., and Parish, L. C.: Manual of Medical Mycology. Cambridge, Blackwell Science, 1995.
4. Howard, D. H.: An introduction to the taxonomy and nomenclature of zoopathogenic fungi. *In* Howard, D. H. (ed.): Fungi Pathogenic for Humans and Animals. Part A, Biology. New York, Marcel Dekker, 1983.
5. Kendrick, B.: The Fifth Kingdom. Waterloo, Canada, Mycologue Publications, 1985.
6. Kwon-Chung, K. J., and Bennett, J. E.: Medical Mycology. Philadelphia, Lea & Febiger, 1992.
7. Margulis, L., and Schwartz, K. V.: Five Kingdoms. 2nd ed. New York, W. H. Freeman, 1988.
8. Reynolds, D. R., and Taylor, J. W. (eds.): The Fungal Holomorph: Mitotic, Meiotic and Pleomorphic Speciation in Fungal Systematics. Oxon, United Kingdom, CAB International, 1993.

197

ASPERGILLUS INFECTIONS

Michael D. Blum and Bernhard L. Wiedermann

The term *Aspergillus* (Latin *aspergere,* to scatter), first coined by the Florentine botanist Micheli[103] in his *Nova Plantarum Genera* of 1729, referred to the perforated globe, or aspergillum, used to sprinkle holy water during religious ceremonies. Human disease first was described by Sluyter[149] in 1847 and reviewed by Virchow[163] in his classic paper of 1856. In 1897, Renon[125] reported an association of the disease with certain occupations, such as wig cleaning and pigeon handling. However, it was not until 1952 that the diverse clinical manifestations of aspergillosis were realized,[55] and only recently has the importance of *Aspergillus* infection in immunosuppressed patients been recognized. Systemic disseminated aspergillosis is a product of medical progress and the consequence of the widespread use of antibiotics and immunosuppressive agents in the modern age.

The genus *Aspergillus* includes more than 900 recognized species, of which only a small number have been documented to be pathogenic to the human host. *A. fumigatus* worldwide is the most common cause of human disease, although in some hospitals *A. flavus* has replaced *A. fumigatus* as the leading cause of disseminated aspergillosis in immunocompromised hosts. Other species reportedly associated with invasive human disease include *A. amstelodami, A. candidus, A. carneus, A. conicus, A. deflectus, A. fischeri, A. flavipes, A. glaucus, A. nidulans, A. niger, A. niveus, A. ochraceus, A. oryzae, A. parasiticus, A. restrictus, A. sydowi, A. terreus, A. ustus,* and *A. versicolor.*[124, 131] These species all exhibit thermotolerance, which may enhance pathogenicity in the human host.[131]

Fungi in the genus *Aspergillus* reproduce by means of asexual spores called conidia. In tissue preparation of clinical specimens, conidiophores usually are absent. Specimens characteristically show dichotomously branching, septate hyphae, which are suggestive but not specific for this genus. In culture, however, *Aspergillus* species are identified by characteristic colony appearance and by microscopic examination of the conidia and spore-bearing structures. For example, the major pathogenic species, *A. fumigatus,* is characterized by smoky, gray-green colonies; compact, columnar conidia; and phialides, which cover the upper half of flask-shaped vesicles. Mycologic characteristics of other *Aspergillus* species and techniques for preparation of fungal material have been well described.[48, 131]

Aspergillus species are known to produce a variety of mycotoxins in nonhuman hosts, including aflatoxin, ochratoxin, fungiclavine, and kojic acid. Whereas these toxins have not been isolated in the infected human host, several cases of acute aflatoxicosis have been reported secondary to contaminated foods.[29]

EPIDEMIOLOGY

Aspergillus species are ubiquitous worldwide, occurring in a variety of natural substrates, including grain, decaying vegetation, soil, and dung.[148] *Aspergillus* frequently is isolated from the air because spores are lightweight, resistant to desiccation, and easily dispersed. The fungus can be recovered from sputum for several days after exposure to a cloud of *Aspergillus* conidia.[131]

Inhalation of spores with an immune response has been described in regular smokers of contaminated marijuana cigarettes.[68] In addition, hospital outbreaks have been associated with airborne contamination secondary to bird droppings into air ducts,[81] road construction adjacent to hospital windows,[83] and hospital renovation.[172] Demolition of ducts and false ceilings close to a neonatal intensive care unit[76] and an adult hematology department[117] resulted in fatal pulmonary aspergillosis in immunocompromised patients. An outbreak of invasive aspergillosis in widely varying areas of one hospital was traced to construction activity in the central radiology suite.[56]

Control of such outbreaks has focused on the removal of immunosuppressed patients from construction sites, the equipment of rooms with high-efficiency air filters, and the use of laminar air-flow isolation.[8] Phenotypic methods, such as biotyping by the killer system, have permitted tracking of nosocomial outbreaks of aspergillosis.[41] However, genotypic methods, such as restriction fragment length polymorphism using random amplified polymorphic DNA probes, provide better discrimination among isolates in the outbreak setting.[25]

PATHOGENESIS

Phagocytic response, rather than antibody production, provides the primary host defense against *Aspergillus* infections. Because conidia are the inhaled particles that initiate infection, macrophages form the "front line" of defense by rapidly killing the fungus in the conidial stage. Neutrophils are involved only if the conidia escape the reticuloendothelial system and begin mycelial growth.[139]

Aspergillosis is relatively uncommon in patients with AIDS,[67] which implies a relative lack of importance of cell-mediated immunity in defense against this fungus. Invasive aspergillosis usually occurs in patients with advanced AIDS and has been considered to result from independent predisposing factors, such as neutropenia, corticosteroid therapy, or intravenous drug use.[147] Recently, however, HIV-infected children with age-adjusted CD4 lymphocyte counts less than 25 per cent of the normal median for age have been shown to have significant defects in the ability of neutrophils to damage nonopsonized hyphae of *A. fumigatus*.[132] Moreover, HIV-infected children manifested significantly decreased phagocytic activity of peripheral blood monocyte-derived macrophages compared with normal controls.[133] These host defects may account for the fact that, in some series of invasive aspergillosis in AIDS patients,[86] predisposing factors independent of HIV infection were present only in approximately 50 per cent of cases.

Aspergillus accounts for the vast majority of fungal infections in patients with chronic granulomatous disease[30] and on occasion may account for an unusual presentation of the disease.[142] The predisposition of patients with chronic granulomatous disease[171] or with selective defects in phagocytic killing[43, 112] underscores the importance of oxidative killing in the human host defenses against this disease.

With more severe immunosuppression, invasive aspergillosis can ensue. Predisposing factors include (1) corticosteroid treatment, (2) neutropenia, (3) cytotoxic chemotherapy, (4) broad-spectrum antimicrobial therapy, (5) acute leukemia in relapse, and (6) acute organ rejection.[129] Invasive aspergillosis in children also has been reported after influenza infection,[59, 78] subacute hepatic necrosis,[167] liver transplantation,[135] heart transplantation,[6] and bone marrow transplantation.[119] Invasive aspergillosis occurs in 4 to 8 per cent of patients after bone marrow transplantation and has been associated with delayed engraftment,[106] graft-versus-host disease,[102] and graft rejection.[98] Despite the absence of neutropenia, invasive aspergillosis was reported to occur in almost 2 per cent of one large series of liver transplantation patients and has been associated with the use of OKT3.[80]

Rare cases of fulminant aspergillosis have been described in normal hosts.[50] Aspergillosis is uncommon in the newborn period and usually presents as widely disseminated disease.[127] Predisposing factors include broad-spectrum antibiotics, corticosteroids, prematurity, and necrotizing enterocolitis.[143]

In immunosuppressed patients, *Aspergillus* tends to invade blood vessels, resulting in infarction, necrosis, and widespread hematogenous dissemination. Examination of affected organs reveals numerous septate hyphae with dichotomous branching as well as conidial heads when fungi are present in air-containing tissues.[95] In contrast, widespread dissemination secondary to vascular invasion is unusual in chronic granulomatous disease patients, who typically have isolated pneumonia with or without contiguous spread.[30] The unusual finding of diffuse nodular pneumonia in childhood may provide a clue for the diagnosis of chronic granulomatous disease and aspergillosis.[28]

Allergic reactions to *Aspergillus* may play a role in the pathologic process of this disease, as evidenced by patients with allergic bronchopulmonary aspergillosis. In this condition, patients with chronic respiratory diseases, such as asthma[128] or cystic fibrosis,[88] trap *A. fumigatus* in tenacious mucus, which results in an immune response and exacerbation of respiratory symptoms. Despite numerous luminal hyphae in the tissues, however, invasion of the bronchial wall and fungal dissemination have been reported rarely in the absence of other risk factors (e.g., indwelling catheters, hyperalimentation, corticosteroid therapy).[22, 27]

An immune response to trapped fungi also may result in allergic *Aspergillus* sinusitis, a chronic disease that tends to occur in young adults with a history of atopy, asthma, or nasal polyposis. Up to 30 per cent of patients may exhibit expansion or bony erosion of the involved sinus; invasion, however, has not been reported.[53]

CLINICAL MANIFESTATIONS

A variety of saprophytic and pathologic conditions have been attributed to species of *Aspergillus* (Table 197–1). Invasiveness appears to depend on the genetic and immune status of the host as well as the extent and duration of exposure to the spores. Disseminated aspergillosis, defined as infection of two or more noncontiguous organs, is the most severe form of clinical aspergillosis. Patients usually present with pulmonic disease and widespread organ involvement. The clinical features of invasive *Aspergillus* infections in a large pediatric hospital were reviewed recently.[165] The most common sites of *Aspergillus* infection in children are discussed in the following sections.

Ear and Sinus

Otomycosis, defined as fungal infection of the external ear canal, more commonly occurs in tropical and subtropical regions and particularly is prevalent among groups that regularly cover their ears with traditional garb.[115] It predominantly is a unilateral disease caused by *Aspergillus* or *Candida* species, often found in association with *Staphylococcus aureus, Pseudomonas, Proteus,* or other bacterial pathogens.[108] *Aspergillus* otomycosis, most commonly secondary to *A. niger,* produces a mass of black spores that start close to the tympanic membrane and spread outward to fill the ear canal. Disease in immunosuppressed patients rarely results in invasive otitis

TABLE 197–1. Clinical Spectrum of Aspergillosis in Children

Ear
Otitis externa
Invasive otitis externa
Paranasal sinuses
Indolent sinus aspergillosis
Aspergilloma
Invasive sinus aspergillosis
Eye
Traumatic keratitis
Postoperative endophthalmitis
Contiguous spread from paranasal sinuses
Lungs
Primary pulmonary aspergillosis
Hypersensitivity pneumonitis
Allergic bronchopulmonary aspergillosis
Mucoid impaction
Eosinophilic pneumonitis
Bronchocentric granulomatosis
Extrinsic allergic alveolitis
Aspergilloma
Invasive pulmonary aspergillosis
Central nervous system
Traumatic inoculation
Contiguous spread from paranasal sinuses
Disseminated disease
Bone
Traumatic osteomyelitis
Contiguous spread from lung or overlying skin
Skin and nails
Onychomycosis
Primary cutaneous aspergillosis
Contiguous spread from paranasal sinuses
Disseminated disease
Heart
Postoperative endocarditis
Isolated cardiac aspergillosis
Genitourinary tract
Ascending infection
Disseminated disease
Other
Splenic aspergillomas
Intraperitoneal aspergillosis

externa,[120] but in general, *Aspergillus* otomycosis is a localized, noninfiltrative process. Thorough removal of debris from the external canal and treatment directed against the underlying chronic otitis externa generally result in a good therapeutic response. Topical antifungal agents also have been successful.[115]

Aspergillus is the most common fungal infection of the nose and paranasal sinuses. It may present as an indolent case, aspergilloma, or fulminant disease. Indolent sinus aspergillosis may occur locally in the absence of predisposing factors, most commonly in warm, damp climates[7] or in association with dental disease or dental fillings.[82] Patients present with the typical manifestations of chronic sinusitis, including rhinorrhea, nasal obstruction, and sinus fullness. Radiographic studies usually indicate opacification without evidence of bone erosion. On occasion, patients with these symptoms present with a mass (aspergilloma) in the maxillary or ethmoid sinuses. Local surgery with drainage usually results in complete resolution in these cases of noninvasive sinus aspergillosis.

In contrast, invasive sinus aspergillosis, which generally occurs in immunosuppressed patients, may be fulminant, with early bone destruction, direct extension to the orbit and anterior cranial fossa, and widespread dissemination.[97] Infection usually progresses anteriorly, spreading from the nose to the facial skin and leaving a path of blackened, necrotic tissue destruction. This contrasts with the yellow-black, necrotic ulcerations of intraoral aspergillosis, which usually spread from the soft palate posteriorly.[40]

Fulminant aspergillosis secondary to primary infection of the paranasal sinuses occurs infrequently in children, generally in the setting of immunosuppression or neutropenia or after the administration of broad-spectrum antimicrobials.[12, 16] These children present with facial pain, swelling, and erythema; nasal crusting or ulceration is less common. Mortality is high in this group of patients. Because granulocytopenia may mask the signs and symptoms of sinus aspergillosis, aggressive attempts to diagnose this condition, using computed tomography (CT) and early biopsy, are necessary to reduce the high mortality rate associated with this entity. Characteristic CT findings include unilateral involvement of several sinuses; normal sinus cells between completely opacified cells; absence of air-fluid levels; and smooth, thickened sinus linings. In contrast with orbital cellulitis, bone destruction may be evident, but periosteal separation from the medial orbital wall does not occur typically.[26] Invasive *Aspergillus* sinusitis has been reported increasingly in bone marrow transplant[136] and AIDS[100] patients.

Eye

Involvement of the orbit and its contents most commonly presents as orbital aspergillosis secondary to local extension from the sinuses,[177] traumatic keratitis,[162] or postoperative endophthalmitis.[89] A case of *Aspergillus* endophthalmitis without any detectable cause has been described in an immunologically normal 1-month-old infant.[146] Rarely, patients with disseminated disease[37] or an occult focus of *Aspergillus* infection[152] present with endophthalmitis. In postmortem studies, approximately 8 per cent of patients with disseminated *Aspergillus* infections had evidence of ocular involvement.[96] Bilateral retinal infarction secondary to disseminated disease has been reported in a 10-month-old infant.[64]

Pulmonary

Pulmonary involvement occurs in approximately 90 per cent of *Aspergillus* infections, and in 70 per cent, it is the only site of infection (Fig. 197–1).[35] It is the most common site of invasive *Aspergillus* disease. Noninvasive pulmonary aspergillosis includes primary pulmonary aspergillosis, hypersensitivity reactions, and aspergilloma.

Noninvasive Pulmonary Aspergillosis

Primary pulmonary aspergillosis reportedly occurs in normal hosts without preexisting disease, although the existence of this entity has been questioned.[35] This rare disease, usually caused by inhalation of massive amounts of *A. fumigatus*, may be chronic and indolent or, on occasion, fulminant and fatal. Chest radiographs may show a variety of diffuse or localized cavitary or infiltrative processes.

The symptoms of allergic bronchopulmonary aspergillosis result from a host immune response to the fungus, which becomes trapped within the tenacious mucus of patients with asthma or cystic fibrosis. Diagnostic criteria have been well

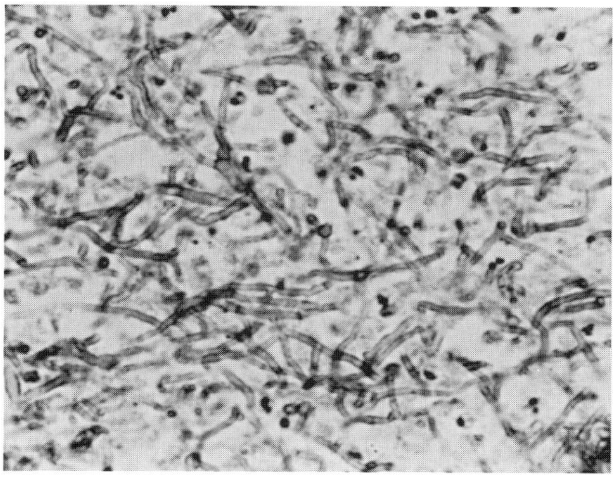

FIGURE 197–1. *Pulmonary aspergillosis illustrating septate hyphae and dichotomous branching. (H and E × 64.)*

described.[128] In addition, a subset of this population may develop mucoid impaction, bronchocentric granulomatosis, or eosinophilic pneumonia. Extrinsic allergic alveolitis represents a hypersensitivity lung reaction in normal hosts, secondary to heavy, primarily occupational exposure to *Aspergillus* spores.

Aspergilloma, usually secondary to *A. fumigatus,* represents the most frequent form of pulmonary aspergillosis. The pathologic lesion is a mycetoma, a ball of mycelia growing in a poorly drained lung space that communicates with the bronchial tree. Tuberculosis, especially in patients receiving a long course of antituberculous therapy, is the most common predisposing factor for the development of an aspergilloma, with an incidence ranging from 2 per cent of all tuberculosis patients[58] to almost 20 per cent of patients with residual cavities larger than 2.5 cm.[36] Other conditions predisposing to aspergilloma in children include bronchiectasis,[92] congenital heart disease,[46] congenital pulmonary cysts,[150] healed abscess cavities,[150] histoplasmosis,[144] sarcoidosis,[178] and invasive aspergillosis in immunosuppressed hosts.[101]

Clinical features of aspergilloma include hemoptysis, productive cough, clubbing, fever, and localizing sounds at the site of the lesion.[35] Hemoptysis on occasion may be massive and fatal.[72] The characteristic radiologic finding is an apical, pulmonary air meniscus sign,[159] that is, crescent-shaped air adjacent to an intracavitary body, with surrounding fibrocavitary changes. Diagnosis is confirmed by histologic examination and culture of a biopsy specimen; the presence of serum antibodies to *Aspergillus* and a positive sputum culture provide supportive evidence.[93] Treatment must be individualized,[34] with surgical resection generally recommended only for patients with severe hemoptysis.[62] Spontaneous resolution of pulmonary aspergillomas has been described in a few patients.[36]

Invasive Pulmonary Aspergillosis

Invasive pulmonary aspergillosis (Fig. 197–2) has become an increasingly important cause of morbidity and mortality in immunosuppressed patients with hematologic malignancies.[151] In one series,[179] 90 per cent of patients with invasive aspergillosis had underlying hematologic malignancy, with 70 per cent of patients having fewer than 500 granulocytes/mm^3. Invasive pulmonary aspergillosis after bone marrow transplantation has a particularly high mortality rate.[32]

Neutropenia is of paramount importance in this disease. In persistently febrile, neutropenic children receiving broad-spectrum antibiotics, approximately 50 per cent of new pulmonary infiltrates are due to fungal pneumonia, usually either *Candida* or *Aspergillus.*[31] Survival in these cases largely depends on recovery of the granulocyte count.

Invasive pulmonary aspergillosis most commonly presents as necrotizing bronchopneumonia or hemorrhagic infarction, although occasionally there are single or multiple abscesses,

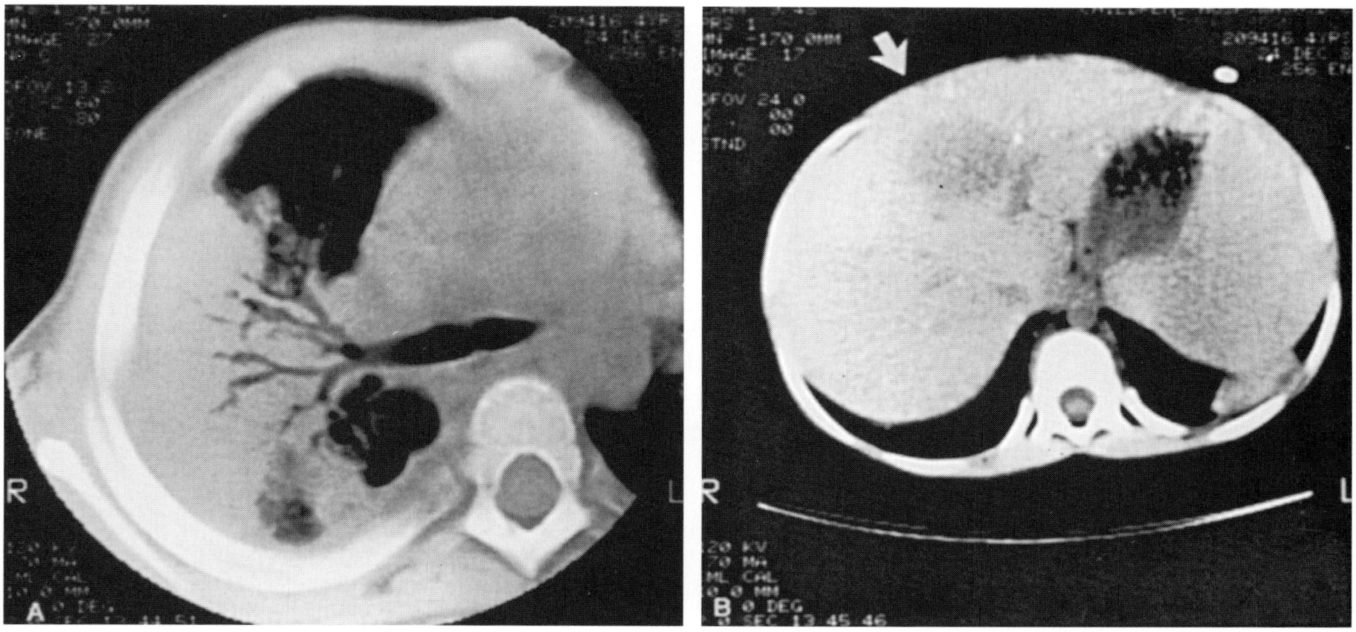

FIGURE 197–2. *Invasive aspergillosis in a 4-year-old boy with chronic granulomatous disease of childhood.* A, *Computed tomographic scan of the chest shows consolidation in the right lower lobe, with evidence of bronchiectasis.* B, *Computed tomographic scan of the upper abdomen shows involvement of the right lobe of the liver (arrow).*

granulomas, or lobar infiltrates. Positive surveillance nasal cultures for *Aspergillus* frequently precede the development of invasive pulmonary aspergillosis.[1]

The propensity for *Aspergillus* to invade blood vessels results in a variety of pulmonary manifestations of invasive disease, including focal necrosis, pulmonary infarction, and hemorrhagic consolidation. Several unusual variants in children have been reported. These include necrotizing bronchitis with pseudomembrane formation,[118] invasive tracheitis,[160] tracheoesophageal fistula,[69] and pleural aspergillosis.[70]

Clinical manifestations consist of fever, dyspnea, nonproductive cough, mild hemoptysis, and pleuritic chest pain, which especially may be prominent in patients with hemorrhagic pulmonary infarction. The diagnostic specificity of isolation of *Aspergillus* from the respiratory tract correlates directly with the degree of immunosuppression. Isolation of *A. fumigatus* or *A. flavus* from the respiratory tract of neutropenic, leukemic patients is highly suggestive of invasive pulmonary disease.[181] The lower specificity and sensitivity of sputum cultures in immunosuppressed, non-neutropenic patients, however, may warrant a more invasive diagnostic procedure. Histologic demonstration of parenchymal invasion of the lung by *Aspergillus* remains the gold standard of diagnosis.

As with the non–HIV-infected population, pulmonary aspergillosis in HIV-infected patients usually presents as cavitary upper lobe disease, focal alveolar infiltrates, or bilateral alveolar or interstitial infiltrates. However, there appear to be distinct differences.[104] Cavitary upper lobe disease disseminates only rarely whether patients are infected with HIV or not; however, hemoptysis is fatal more often in HIV-infected patients. Focal infiltrates can persist for months in HIV-infected patients, but they usually either progress or resolve spontaneously with recovery of granulocytes in leukemia or bone marrow transplant patients. The clinical manifestations of invasive tracheobronchitis due to *Aspergillus* in AIDS patients have been reviewed recently.[71]

Central Nervous System

Aspergillosis of the central nervous system may result from direct spread from the paranasal sinuses or, more commonly, from widespread dissemination in immunosuppressed patients. Unusual cases of inoculation of the brain through an unsuspected encephalocele[111] or rooster pecking[17] have been reported. Most cases are not recognized before the patient dies. In one study, cerebral aspergillosis was detected at autopsy in 20 per cent of liver transplantation patients.[23] Symptomatic patients generally present with focal neurologic signs secondary to hemorrhagic infarcts.[168] Invasion of the central nervous system by hyphal forms of *Aspergillus* results in CT findings consistent with vascular occlusion, infarct, and abscess formation.[176] Whereas nodular enhancing lesions secondary to caseating granulomas more commonly result from yeast forms, such as *Cryptococcus* or *Histoplasma*, cerebral[113] and cerebellar[138] aspergillomas have been described. Analysis of cerebrospinal fluid generally is not helpful in diagnosing aspergillosis of the central nervous system because infection of the meninges is relatively infrequent and usually not diffuse.[116, 168]

Aspergillus may invade the brain stem directly,[9] but involvement of the spinal cord invariably results from compression due to direct or hematogenous spread to the adjacent vertebral body.[42, 121]

Bone and Skin

Aspergillus osteomyelitis occurs predominantly in immunosuppressed patients, although traumatic tibial osteomyelitis has been reported in an immunologically normal adolescent.[33] In most cases, bone is invaded from a contiguous preexisting lesion in the lung or overlying skin. Spread from contiguous pneumonia most commonly occurs in patients with chronic granulomatous disease.[155] Radiologic findings generally are nonspecific, necessitating surgical biopsy and culture for confirmation of the diagnosis.

Aspergillus species were the most frequent fungi grown from superficial white onychomycosis in one series.[91] Skin involvement with *Aspergillus* usually is secondary to hematogenous dissemination or local spread in immunosuppressed patients. In fact, painless cutaneous induration and erythema of the face may be the earliest signs of fulminant sinus aspergillosis.[174] Primary cutaneous aspergillosis also presents in immunosuppressed patients. Usual environmental precipitants include intravenous armboards[94] or intravenous cannulas.[4] Lesions typically occur at the point of contact—that is, palm or foot for armboards, entry site for intravenous catheters. Lesions progress from erythematous or violaceous papules or plaques through a hemorrhagic bullous stage to a purpuric ulcer with central necrosis.[51] Infection occasionally invades the underlying tendons, necessitating widespread débridement.[66] Potassium hydroxide preparation and early skin biopsy may allow prompt diagnosis and treatment.[3] A recent review of cases of invasive aspergillosis in a large pediatric hospital, as well as reported cases in the literature, suggests that children present with cutaneous aspergillosis more commonly than previously was suspected.[165]

Heart

Aspergillus endocarditis, most commonly found in association with open heart surgery, is associated with a high mortality rate in adults and children.[10] Unlike *Candida* endocarditis, inoculation usually is airborne intraoperatively rather than catheter-related. Postmortem studies indicate more invasiveness than in candidal disease, with erosion through synthetic or natural tissue and widespread embolization.[169]

The cardinal features include persistent fever, evidence of embolic phenomena, and consumption coagulopathy after cardiac surgery. Peripheral blood cultures rarely are positive. Echocardiography may be useful in the detection of mycotic aneurysms, intracardiac vegetations, or intra-aortic vegetations.[73] Although diagnosis usually depends on the isolation of *Aspergillus* from surgical specimens, biopsy of an embolus may grow the fungus or demonstrate characteristic histopathologic features.[10]

Isolated cardiac aspergillosis has been reported in a child who underwent bone marrow transplantation for aplastic anemia.[65] Whereas *Aspergillus* infections most commonly extend from the endocardium outward, several cases of *Aspergillus* pericarditis from contiguous pleural foci have been described.[166]

Genitourinary Tract

Aspergillosis of the genitourinary tract results from hematogenous spread or ascending infection. The disease generally is more destructive than is candidal involvement of the kidney, with resultant large areas of thrombosis and necrosis of cortical and papillary tissue.[123] Clinical manifestations include fever, chills, and microhematuria. Unilateral flank pain may occur with ascending infection.[45] On occasion, an isolated unilateral *Aspergillus* cast of the renal pelvis develops and may be passed per urethrum. Although urinary mycetomas usually are due to *Candida* species, an aspergilloma in a leukemic child has been described during relapse.[90] Urine culture may be negative, despite almost total renal destruction.[45]

Other

Although they are less common than candidal abscesses, multiple splenic aspergillomas have been described in leukemic patients with no evidence of systemic involvement.[78] Fever may be the only presenting sign; left upper quadrant abdominal pain and splenomegaly occur in less than half of affected patients.[63] Intraperitoneal aspergillosis has been reported in children undergoing continuous cycling peritoneal dialysis.[77] Several children have experienced rupture of a mycotic aortic aneurysm secondary to invasive aspergillosis of the posterior mediastinum.[175] Involvement of the gastrointestinal tract, liver, thyroid, testis, and adrenal has been reported.[179]

DIAGNOSIS

Ideally, the diagnosis of aspergillosis should be based on (1) clinical and radiographic evidence of infection at a given site, (2) isolation and identification of *Aspergillus* in a high-quality specimen from that site, and (3) histologic identification of tissue invasion by a fungus with the same morphologic characteristics as the recovered agent. Potential diagnostic pitfalls include contamination of the clinical specimen, colonization of the site with noninvasive *Aspergillus* species, lack of specificity of fungal morphologic features in histologic samples, and confusion of a pathologic diagnosis with an etiologic diagnosis.[164]

Aspergillus species readily grow on almost all laboratory media. Because most species are inhibited by cycloheximide, only antibacterial antibiotics should be present in the isolation medium. Recommended media for primary isolation include Sabouraud dextrose agar, brain-heart infusion agar, 2 per cent malt extract agar, and potato-flakes agar.[129] Characteristic conidiophores usually are present within 48 hours of incubation at 37° C, the optimal growth temperature for most pathogenic species of *Aspergillus*.[131] Transfer of purified isolates to Czapek solution agar may facilitate species identification in individual cases.[48]

Respiratory specimens growing *Aspergillus* species may be misleading because uninfected persons may be colonized in the tracheobronchial tree.[101] However, the finding of two or more positive cultures of *A. flavus* or *A. fumigatus* is highly suggestive of pulmonary aspergillosis, particularly if the growth is heavy and free of other *Aspergillus* species.[157]

Blood cultures rarely are positive in disseminated aspergillosis.[179] The lack of specificity inherent in indirect sampling (e.g., sputum) and the potential morbidity associated with direct sampling have spawned efforts to detect early invasive disease by serologic means. IgG antibody to *Aspergillus* has been detected by immunodiffusion,[44] immunofluorescence,[140] and enzyme-linked immunosorbent assay (ELISA).[141] These techniques often fail to detect early invasive disease owing to a delay in antibody response or insufficient antibody production in immunosuppressed patients. In addition, an age-related increase in *Aspergillus* antibodies secondary to widespread environmental exposure limits the specificity of antibody detection.[140]

Significant work is ongoing to develop clinically useful antigen detection methods for *Aspergillus,* and this is a rapidly changing field. Attempts to detect *Aspergillus* antigen by ELISA,[114, 137, 153] radioimmunoassay,[173] or immunoblotting[180] have been more reliable for detecting early invasive disease but are not yet recommended for routine application.[13] Polymerase chain reaction techniques have not been as promising.[24] Techniques for antigen detection in invasive aspergillosis have been reviewed by Andriole.[5] Other noninvasive tests under study include the measurement of oxalic acid, a fermentation product of *Aspergillus,* in the bronchial lavage fluid of patients at risk for pulmonary aspergillosis.[15]

TREATMENT

Intravenous amphotericin B remains the drug of choice for invasive *Aspergillus* infection.[39] Early diagnosis and treatment with intravenous amphotericin B substantially improve the outcome in this disease.[2] The end-point of treatment generally is determined by the resolution of neutropenia or improvement after discontinuation of corticosteroids rather than by a total cumulative dose.[49]

Itraconazole, an oral triazole, has been approved by the Food and Drug Administration for the treatment of pulmonary and extrapulmonary aspergillosis in patients who are intolerant of or refractory to amphotericin B. Although efficacy has been shown in uncontrolled clinical trials,[61] relapse may be a problem in immunocompromised patients, despite long courses of therapy.[38] Itraconazole has been successful anecdotally in the treatment of invasive aspergillosis in patients with chronic granulomatous disease,[74, 109] and gamma-interferon may be a useful adjunct to therapy in this patient population.[18]

New antifungal agents are under development in an attempt to reduce the toxicity associated with amphotericin B. Liposomal amphotericin B has been administered to patients with progressive aspergillosis refractory to standard amphotericin B treatment, with particularly encouraging results in liver and sinus disease.[85] The Food and Drug Administration recently approved amphotericin B lipid complex for the treatment of aspergillosis in patients refractory to or intolerant of conventional amphotericin B therapy. Experience with use of both of these agents in children is growing.[74, 130] There appear to be fewer side effects associated with amphotericin B lipid complex than with conventional amphotericin B.[75] Semisynthetic pneumocandin analogs have shown promise in an experimental model of pulmonary aspergillosis when administered by either the parenteral or the aerosolized route.[79] Combination polyene-azole antifungal therapy also may hold promise for the future.[47, 154]

Administration of hematopoietic growth factors can play a role in the management of neutropenic patients with aspergillosis.[105] One group has proposed administration of elutriated monocytes, perhaps in conjunction with hematopoietic growth factors and gamma-interferon, as a future form of therapy.[134]

Surgical excision has been successful in the treatment of children with *Aspergillus* sinusitis,[122] cerebral mycetoma,[54] infected prosthetic valves,[10] and localized pulmonic infections.[145] Some have advocated early, complete resection of pulmonary lesions, combined with antifungal therapy, for the treatment of bone marrow transplant patients.[87] Surgical excision of a pulmonary aspergilloma usually is restricted to patients with severe hemoptysis and adequate pulmonary function for tolerating the procedure.[11, 62, 161] Selective bronchial artery embolization may be necessary before resection.[57] Intracavitary administration of antifungal agents may be an alternative to resection in localized pulmonic infections.[14, 52]

Surgical débridement is the mainstay of therapy for indolent sinus aspergillosis and is used in conjunction with antifungal therapy for invasive sinus aspergillosis. Surgical removal of infected tissue, combined with the administration of amphotericin B, is optimal for the treatment of *Aspergillus* endocarditis.[10] A combined medical and surgical approach was used successfully in a leukemic child with cerebral and sinus aspergillosis.[54] For most other sites of *Aspergillus* infection, surgical débridement seems to offer little advantage over medical therapy alone.

PREVENTION

Strategies to prevent invasive fungal infections in patients with neoplastic diseases have been reviewed.[21, 170] Attempts to reduce the exposure of immunosuppressed or neutropenic patients to *Aspergillus* spores are of paramount importance in the prevention of this disease.[126] High-risk patients should be isolated from areas of construction activity and placed in rooms equipped with high-efficiency particulate air filters. Ornamental plants and flowers should be removed from these rooms. Aerosolized copper-8-quinolinolate, a nontoxic antifungal powder, has been used for outbreak control.[110]

Because the toxicity of systemic amphotericin B precludes prophylactic use, several innovative approaches to antifungal prophylaxis have been initiated recently. Amphotericin B nasal spray may be effective in controlling respiratory and sinus colonization,[99] as well as the frequency of invasive disease,[60] in neutropenic patients. Also, aerosolized amphotericin B, delivered by a small-particle aerosol generator, has been studied for prophylactic use.[19, 20] Prophylactic itraconazole, with[156] or without[158] nasal amphotericin B, has been shown in preliminary studies to protect patients with prolonged granulocytopenia from fatal aspergillosis and also may be useful in patients with chronic granulomatous disease.[107] The clinical use of hematopoietic growth factors may provide the best prophylaxis in the future against *Aspergillus* infections.[105]

References

1. Aisner, J., Murillo, J., Schimpff, S. C., et al.: Invasive aspergillosis in acute leukemia: Correlation with nose cultures and antibiotic use. Ann. Intern. Med. *90*:4, 1979.
2. Aisner, J., Schimpff, S. C., and Wiernik, P. H.: Treatment of invasive aspergillosis: Relation of early diagnosis and treatment to response. Ann. Intern. Med. *86*:539, 1977.
3. Allen, U., Smith, C. R., and Prober, C. G.: The value of skin biopsies in febrile, neutropenic, immunocompromised children. Am. J. Dis. Child. *140*:459, 1986.
4. Allo, M. D., Miller, J., Townsend, T., et al.: Primary cutaneous aspergillosis associated with Hickman intravenous catheters. N. Engl. J. Med. *317*:1105, 1987.
5. Andriole, V. T.: Infections with *Aspergillus* species. Clin. Infect. Dis. *17*(Suppl. 2):S481, 1993.
6. Austin, J. M., Schulman, L. L., and Mastrobattista, J. D.: Pulmonary infection after cardiac transplantation: Clinical and radiologic correlations. Radiology *172*:259, 1989.
7. Bahadur, S., Kacker, S. K., D'Souza, B., et al.: Paranasal sinus aspergillosis. J. Laryngol. Otol. *97*:863, 1983.
8. Barnes, R. A., and Rogers, T. R.: Control of an outbreak of nosocomial aspergillosis by laminar air-flow isolation. J. Hosp. Infect. *14*:89, 1989.
9. Barrios, N., Tebbi, C. K., Rotstein, C., et al.: Brainstem invasion by *Aspergillus fumigatus* in a child with leukemia. N. Y. State J. Med. *88*:656, 1988.
10. Barst, R. J., Prince, A. S., and Neu, H. C.: *Aspergillus* endocarditis in children: Case report and review of the literature. Pediatrics *68*:73, 1981.
11. Battaglini, J. W., Murray, G. F., Keagy, B. A., et al.: Surgical management of symptomatic pulmonary aspergilloma. Ann. Thorac. Surg. *39*:512, 1985.
12. Baydala, L. T., Yanofsky, R., Akabutu, J., et al.: Aspergillosis of the nose and paranasal sinuses in immunocompromised children. Can. Med. Assoc. J. *138*:927, 1988.
13. Bennett, J. E.: Rapid diagnosis of candidiasis and aspergillosis. Rev. Infect. Dis. *9*:398, 1987.
14. Bennett, M. R., Weinbaum, D. L., and Fiehler, P. C.: Chronic necrotizing pulmonary aspergillosis treated by endobronchial amphotericin B. South. Med. J. *83*:829, 1990.
15. Benoit, G., Feuilhade de Chauvin, M., Cordonnier, C., et al.: Oxalic acid level in bronchoalveolar lavage fluid from patients with invasive pulmonary aspergillosis. Am. Rev. Respir. Dis. *132*:748, 1985.
16. Berkow, R. L., Weisman, S. J., Provisor, A. J., et al.: Invasive aspergillosis of paranasal tissues in children with malignancies. J. Pediatr. *103*:49, 1983.
17. Berkowitz, F. E., and Jacobs, D. W.: Fatal case of brain abscess caused by rooster pecking. Pediatr. Infect. Dis. J. *6*:941, 1987.
18. Bernhisel-Broadbent, J., Camargo, E. E., Jaffe, H.-S., et al.: Recombinant human interferon-γ as adjunct therapy for *Aspergillus* infection in a patient with chronic granulomatous disease. J. Infect. Dis. *163*:908, 1991.
19. Beyer, J., Barzen, G., Risse, G., et al.: Aerosol amphotericin B for prevention of invasive pulmonary aspergillosis. Antimicrob. Agents Chemother. *37*:1367, 1993.
20. Beyer, J., Schwartz, S., Barzen, G., et al.: Use of amphotericin B aerosols for the prevention of pulmonary aspergillosis. Infection *22*:143, 1994.
21. Beyer, J., Schwartz, S., Heinemann, V., et al.: Strategies in prevention of invasive pulmonary aspergillosis in immunosuppressed or neutropenic patients. Antimicrob. Agents Chemother. *38*:911, 1994.
22. Bhargava, V., Tomashefski, J. F., Jr., Stern, R. C., et al.: The pathology of fungal infection and colonization in patients with cystic fibrosis. Hum. Pathol. *20*:977, 1989.
23. Boon, A. P., Adams, D. H., and McMaster, P.: Cerebral aspergillosis in liver transplantation. J. Clin. Pathol. *43*:114, 1990.
24. Bretagne, S., Costa, J.-M., Marmorat-Khuong, M., et al.: Detection of *Aspergillus* species DNA in bronchoalveolar lavage samples by competitive PCR. J. Clin. Microbiol. *33*:1164, 1995.
25. Buffington, J., Reporter, R., Lasker, B. A., et al.: Investigation of an epidemic of invasive aspergillosis: Utility of molecular typing with the use of random amplified polymorphic DNA probes. Pediatr. Infect. Dis. J. *13*:386, 1994.
26. Centeno, R. S., Bentson, J. R., and Mancuso, A. A.: CT scanning in rhinocerebral mucormycosis and aspergillosis. Radiology *140*:383, 1981.
27. Chung, Y., Kraut, J. R., Stone, A. M., et al.: Disseminated aspergillosis in a patient with cystic fibrosis and allergic bronchopulmonary aspergillosis. Pediatr. Pulmonol. *17*:131, 1994.
28. Chusid, M. J., Sty, J. R., and Wells, R. G.: Pulmonary aspergillosis appearing as chronic nodular disease in chronic granulomatous disease. Pediatr. Radiol. *18*:232, 1988.
29. Ciegler, A., Burmeister, H. R., and Vesonder, R. F.: Poisonous fungi: Mycotoxins and mycotoxicoses. *In* Howard, D. H. (ed.): Fungi Pathogenic for Humans and Animals. Vol. 3, Part B. New York, Marcel Dekker, 1983, p. 413.
30. Cohen, M. S., Isturiz, R. E., Malech, H. L., et al.: Fungal infection in chronic granulomatous disease. Am. J. Med. *71*:59, 1981.
31. Commers, J. R., Robichaud, K. J., and Pizzo, P. A.: New pulmonary infiltrates in granulocytopenic cancer patients being treated with antibiotics. Pediatr. Infect. Dis. *3*:423, 1984.
32. Cordonnier, C., Bernaudin, J. F., Bierling, P., et al.: Pulmonary complications occurring after allogeneic bone marrow transplantation. Cancer *58*:1047, 1986.
33. Corrall, C. J., Merz, W. G., Rekedal, K., et al.: *Aspergillus* osteomyelitis in an immunocompetent adolescent: A case report and review of the literature. Pediatrics *70*:455, 1982.
34. Daly, R. C., Pairolero, P. C., Piehler, J. M., et al.: Pulmonary aspergilloma. J. Thorac. Cardiovasc. Surg. *92*:981, 1986.
35. Dar, M. A., Ahmad, M., Weinstein, A. J., et al.: Thoracic aspergillosis. Cleve. Clin. Q. *51*:615, 1984.
36. Davies, D. (Chairman): Aspergilloma and residual tuberculous cavities: The results of a resurvey. A report of the Research Committee of the British Thoracic and Tuberculosis Association. Tubercle *51*:227, 1970.
37. Demicco, D. D., Reichman, R. C., Violette, E. J., et al.: Disseminated aspergillosis presenting with endophthalmitis. Cancer *53*:1995, 1984.
38. Denning, D. W., Lee, J. Y., Hostetler, J. S., et al.: NIAID mycosis study group multicenter trial of oral itraconazole therapy for invasive aspergillosis. Am. J. Med. *97*:135, 1994.
39. Denning, D. W., and Stevens, D. A.: Antifungal and surgical treatment of invasive aspergillosis: Review of 2121 published cases. Rev. Infect. Dis. *12*:1147, 1990.
40. Dreizen, S., Bodey, G. P., McCredie, K. B., et al.: Orofacial aspergillosis in acute leukemia. Oral Surg. Oral Med. Oral Pathol. *59*:499, 1985.
41. Fanti, F., Conti, S., Campani, L., et al.: Studies on the epidemiology of *Aspergillus fumigatus* infections in a university hospital. Eur. J. Epidemiol. *5*:8, 1989.
42. Ferris, B., and Jones, C.: Paraplegia due to aspergillosis: Successful conservative treatment in two cases. J. Bone Joint Surg. Br. *67*:800, 1985.
43. Fietta, A., Sacchi, F., Mangiarotti, P., et al.: Defective phagocyte *Aspergillus* killing associated with recurrent pulmonary *Aspergillus* infections. Infection *12*:10, 1984.
44. Fisher, B. D., Armstrong, D., Yu, B., et al.: Invasive aspergillosis: Progress in early diagnosis and treatment. Am. J. Med. *71*:571, 1981.
45. Flechner, S. M., and McAninch, J. W.: Aspergillosis of the urinary tract: Ascending route of infection and evolving patterns of disease. J. Urol. *125*:598, 1981.
46. Flye, M. W., and Sealy, W. C.: Pulmonary aspergilloma: A report of its occurrence in two patients with cyanotic congenital heart disease. Ann. Thorac. Surg. *20*:196, 1975.
47. George, D., Kordick, D., Miniter, P., et al.: Combination therapy in experimental invasive aspergillosis. J. Infect. Dis. *168*:692, 1993.

48. Gray, L. D., and Roberts, G. D.: Laboratory diagnosis of systemic fungal diseases. Infect. Dis. Clin. North Am. *2*:779, 1988.
49. Graybill, J. R.: Therapeutic agents. Infect. Dis. Clin. North Am. *2*:805, 1988.
50. Greif, Z., Moscuna, M., Suprun, H., et al.: Fatal childhood pulmonary aspergillosis from contact with pigeons. Clin. Pediatr. *20*:357, 1981.
51. Grossman, M. E., Fithian, E. C., Behrens, C., et al.: Primary cutaneous aspergillosis in six leukemic children. J. Am. Acad. Dermatol. *12*:313, 1985.
52. Guleria, R., Gupta, D., and Jindal, S. K.: Treatment of pulmonary aspergilloma by endoscopic intracavitary instillation of ketoconazole. Chest *103*:1301, 1993.
53. Hartwick, R. W., and Batsakis, J. G.: Sinus aspergillosis and allergic fungal sinusitis. Ann. Otol. Rhinol. Laryngol. *100*:427, 1991.
54. Henze, G., Aldenhoff, P., Stephani, U., et al.: Successful treatment of pulmonary and cerebral aspergillosis in an immunosuppressed child. Eur. J. Pediatr. *138*:263, 1982.
55. Hinson, K. E., Moon, A. J., and Plummer, N. S.: Bronchopulmonary aspergillosis: A review and report of eight new cases. Thorax *7*:317, 1952.
56. Hopkins, C. C., Weber, D. J., and Rubin, R. H.: Invasive *Aspergillus* infection: Possible non-ward common source within the hospital environment. J. Hosp. Infect. *13*:19, 1989.
57. Hughes, C. F., Waugh, R., and Lindsay, D.: Surgery for pulmonary aspergilloma: Preoperative embolisation of the bronchial circulation. Thorax *41*:324, 1986.
58. Jain, S. K., Agrawal, R. L., and Agrawal, M.: *Aspergillus* infection in pulmonary tuberculosis. Indian J. Med. Sci. *36*:48, 1982.
59. Jariwalla, A. G., Smith, A. P., and Melville-Jones, G.: Necrotising aspergillosis complicating fulminating viral pneumonia. Thorax *35*:215, 1980.
60. Jeffery, G. M., Beard, M. E. J., Ikram, R. B., et al.: Intranasal amphotericin B reduces the frequency of invasive aspergillosis in neutropenic patients. Am. J. Med. *90*:685, 1991.
61. Jennings, T. S., and Hardin, T. C.: Treatment of aspergillosis with itraconazole. Ann. Pharmacol. *27*:1206, 1993.
62. Jewkes, J., Kay, P. H., Paneth, M., et al.: Pulmonary aspergilloma: Analysis of prognosis in relation to haemoptysis and survey of treatment. Thorax *38*:572, 1983.
63. Johnson, J. D., and Raff, M. J.: Fungal splenic abscess. Arch. Intern. Med. *144*:1987, 1984.
64. Johnson, R., and Rootman, J.: Bilateral retinal infarction in disseminated aspergillosis. Can. J. Ophthalmol. *17*:223, 1982.
65. Johnson, R. B., Wing, E. J., Miller, T. R., et al.: Isolated cardiac aspergillosis after bone marrow transplantation. Arch. Intern. Med. *147*:1942, 1987.
66. Jones, N. F., Conklin, W. T., and Albo, V. C.: Primary invasive aspergillosis of the hand. J. Hand Surg. *11*:425, 1986.
67. Joshi, V. V., Path, F. R., Oleske, J. M., et al.: Pathology of opportunistic infections in children with acquired immune deficiency syndrome. Pediatr. Pathol. *6*:145, 1986.
68. Kagen, S. L., Kurup, V. P., Sohnle, P. G., et al.: Marijuana smoking and fungal sensitization. J. Allergy Clin. Immunol. *71*:389, 1983.
69. Kapdushnik, J., Springer, C., Naparstek, E., et al.: Tracheoesophageal fistula induced by *Aspergillus* infection following bone marrow transplantation. Pediatr. Pulmonol. *17*:202, 1994.
70. Kearon, M. C., Power, J. T., Wood, A. E., et al.: Pleural aspergillosis in a 14-year-old boy. Thorax *42*:477, 1987.
71. Kemper, C. A., Hostetler, J. S., Follansbee, S. E., et al.: Ulcerative and plaque-like tracheobronchitis due to infection with *Aspergillus* in patients with AIDS. Clin. Infect. Dis. *17*:344, 1993.
72. Kibbler, C. C., Milkins, S. R., Bhamra, A., et al.: Apparent pulmonary mycetoma following invasive aspergillosis in neutropenic patients. Thorax *43*:108, 1988.
73. Kleiman, M. B.: Echocardiography in *Aspergillus* endocarditis. Pediatrics *69*:252, 1982.
74. Kline, M. W., Bocobo, F. C., Paul, M. E., et al.: Successful medical therapy of *Aspergillus* osteomyelitis of the spine in an 11-year-old boy with chronic granulomatous disease. Pediatrics *93*:830, 1995.
75. Kline, S., Larsen, T. A., Fieber, L., et al.: Limited toxicity of prolonged therapy with high doses of amphotericin B lipid complex. Clin. Infect. Dis. *21*:1154, 1995.
76. Krasinski, K., Holzman, R. S., Hanna, B., et al.: Nosocomial fungal infection during hospital renovation. Infect. Control *6*:278, 1985.
77. Kravitz, S. P., and Berry, P. L.: Successful treatment of *Aspergillus* peritonitis in a child undergoing continuous cycling peritoneal dialysis. Arch. Intern. Med. *146*:2061, 1986.
78. Kulkarni, R., Murray, D. L., Gupta, S., et al.: Multiple splenic aspergillomas in a patient with acute lymphoblastic leukemia. Am. J. Pediatr. Hematol. Oncol. *4*:141, 1982.
79. Kurtz, M. B., Bernard, E. M., Edwards, F. F., et al.: Aerosol and parenteral pneumocandins are effective in a rat model of pulmonary aspergillosis. Antimicrob. Agents Chemother. *39*:1784, 1995.
80. Kusne, S., Torre-Cisneros, J., Mañez, R., et al.: Factors associated with invasive lung aspergillosis and the significance of positive *Aspergillus* culture after liver transplantation. J. Infect. Dis. *166*:1379, 1992.
81. Kyriakides, G. K., Zinneman, H. H., Hall, W. H., et al.: Immunologic monitoring and aspergillosis in renal transplant patients. Am. J. Surg. *131*:246, 1976.
82. Legent, F., Billet, J., Beauvillain, C., et al.: The role of dental canal fillings in the development of Aspergillus sinusitis. Arch. Otorhinolaryngol. *246*:318, 1989.
83. Lentino, J. R., Rosenkranz, M. A., Michaels, J. A., et al.: Nosocomial aspergillosis: A retrospective review of airborne disease secondary to road construction and contaminated air conditioners. Am. J. Epidemiol. *116*:430, 1982.
84. Lewis, M., Kallenbach, J., Zaltzman, M., et al.: Invasive pulmonary aspergillosis complicating influenza A pneumonia in a previously healthy patient. Chest *87*:691, 1985.
85. Lopez-Berestein, G., Fainstein, V., Hopfer, R., et al.: Liposomal amphotericin B for the treatment of systemic fungal infections in patients with cancer: A preliminary study. J. Infect. Dis. *151*:704, 1985.
86. Lortholary, O., Meyohas, M.-C., Dupont, B., et al.: Invasive aspergillosis in patients with acquired immunodeficiency syndrome: Report of 33 cases. Am. J. Med. *95*:177, 1993.
87. Lupinetti, F. M., Behrendt, D. M., Giller, R. H., et al.: Pulmonary resection for fungal infection in children undergoing bone marrow transplantation. J. Thorac. Cardiovasc. Surg. *104*:684, 1992.
88. Maguire, S., Moriarty, P., Tempany, E., et al.: Unusual clustering of allergic bronchopulmonary aspergillosis in children with cystic fibrosis. Pediatrics *82*:835, 1988.
89. Mahajan, V. M.: Postoperative ocular infections: An analysis of laboratory data on 750 cases. Ann. Ophthalmol. *16*:847, 1984.
90. Marchand, R., Ahronheim, G. A., Patriquin, H., et al.: Aspergilloma of the renal pelvis in a leukemic child. Pediatr. Infect. Dis. J. *4*:103, 1985.
91. McAleer, R.: Fungal infections of the nails in western Australia. Mycopathologia *73*:115, 1981.
92. McCarthy, D. S., and Pepys, J.: Pulmonary aspergilloma: Clinical immunology. Clin. Allergy *3*:57, 1973.
93. McCarthy, G., FitzGerald, M. X., and Keelan, P.: The spectrum of pulmonary aspergillosis. Ir. J. Med. Sci. *157*:316, 1988.
94. McCarty, J. M., Flam, M. S., Pullen, G., et al.: Outbreak of primary cutaneous aspergillosis related to intravenous arm boards. J. Pediatr. *108*:721, 1986.
95. McDonald, G. S., and Crowe, P.: Clinicopathological patterns of invasive and superficial fungal infection. Ir. J. Med. Sci. *157*:185, 1988.
96. McDonnell, P. J., McDonnell, J. M., Brown, R. H., et al.: Ocular involvement in patients with fungal infections. Ophthalmology *92*:706, 1985.
97. McGill, T. J., Simpson, G., and Healy, G. B.: Fulminant aspergillosis of the nose and paranasal sinuses: A new clinical entity. Laryngoscope *90*:748, 1980.
98. McWhinney, P. H. M., Kibbler, C. C., Hamon, M. D., et al.: Progress in the diagnosis and management of aspergillosis in bone marrow transplantation: 13 years' experience. Clin. Infect. Dis. *17*:397, 1993.
99. Meunier, F.: Prevention of mycoses in immunocompromised patients. Rev. Infect. Dis. *9*:408, 1987.
100. Meyer, R. D., Gaultier, C. R., Yamashita, J. T., et al.: Fungal sinusitis in patients with AIDS: Report of 4 cases and review of the literature. Medicine *73*:69, 1994.
101. Meyer, R. D., Young, L. S., Armstrong, D., et al.: Aspergillosis complicating neoplastic disease. Am. J. Med. *54*:6, 1973.
102. Meyers, J. D.: Fungal infections in bone marrow transplant patients. Semin. Oncol. *17*(Suppl. 6):10, 1990.
103. Micheli, P.: Nova Plantarum Genera juxta Tournefortii Methodum Disposita. Florentiae, Paperinii, 1729.
104. Miller, W. T., Sais, G. J., Frank, I., et al.: Pulmonary aspergillosis in patients with AIDS. Chest *105*:37, 1994.
105. Milliken, S. T., and Powles, R. L.: Antifungal prophylaxis in bone marrow transplantation. Rev. Infect. Dis. *12*:S374, 1990.
106. Morrison, V. A., Haake, R. J., and Weisdorf, D. J.: Non-candidal fungal infections after bone marrow transplantation: Risk factors and outcome. Am. J. Med. *96*:497, 1994.
107. Mouy, R., Veber, F., Blanche, S., et al.: Long-term itraconazole prophylaxis against *Aspergillus* infections in thirty-two patients with chronic granulomatous disease. J. Pediatr. *125*:998, 1994.
108. Mugliston, T., and O'Donoghue, G.: Otomycosis: A continuing problem. J. Laryngol. Otol. *99*:327, 1985.
109. Neijens, H. J., Frenkel, J., de Muinck Keizer-Schrama, S. M., et al.: Invasive *Aspergillus* infection in chronic granulomatous disease: Treatment with itraconazole. J. Pediatr. *115*:1016, 1989.
110. Opal, S. M., Asp, A. A., Cannady, P. B., Jr., et al.: Efficacy of infection control measures during a nosocomial outbreak of disseminated aspergillosis associated with hospital construction. J. Infect. Dis. *153*:634, 1986.
111. Ouammou, A., el Ouanzazi, A., Belghmaidi, M., et al.: Cerebral aspergillosis and encephalomeningocele. Childs Nerv. Syst. *2*:216, 1986.
112. Pagani, A., Spalla, R., Ferrari, F. A., et al.: Defective *Aspergillus* killing by neutrophil leucocytes in a case of systemic aspergillosis. Clin. Exp. Immunol. *43*:201, 1981.
113. Partridge, B. M., and Chin, A. T.: Cerebral aspergilloma. Postgrad. Med. J. *57*:439, 1981.
114. Patterson, T. F., Miniter, P., Patterson, J. E., et al.: *Aspergillus* antigen detection in the diagnosis of invasive aspergillosis. J. Infect. Dis. *171*:1553, 1995.
115. Paulose, K. O., Al Khalifa, S., Shenoy, P., et al.: Mycotic infection of the ear (otomycosis): A prospective study. J. Laryngol. Otol. *103*:30, 1989.

116. Peacock, J. E., McGinnis, M. R., and Cohen, M. S.: Persistent neutrophilic meningitis: Report of four cases and review of the literature. Medicine *63*:379, 1984.
117. Perraud, M., Piens, M. A., Nicoloyannis, N., et al.: Invasive nosocomial pulmonary aspergillosis: Risk factors and hospital building works. Epidemiol. Infect. *99*:407, 1987.
118. Pervez, N. K., Kleinerman, J., Kattan, M., et al.: Pseudomembranous necrotizing bronchial aspergillosis. Am. Rev. Respir. Dis. *131*:961, 1985.
119. Peterson, P. K., McGlave, P., Ramsay, N. K., et al.: A prospective study of infectious diseases following bone marrow transplantation: Emergence of *Aspergillus* and cytomegalovirus as the major causes of mortality. Infect. Control *4*:81, 1983.
120. Phillips, P., Bryce, G., Shepherd, J., et al.: Invasive external otitis caused by *Aspergillus*. Rev. Infect. Dis. *12*:277, 1990.
121. Polatty, R. C., Cooper, K. R., and Kerkering, T. M.: Spinal cord compression due to an aspergilloma. South. Med. J. *77*:645, 1984.
122. Quiney, R. E., Rogers, M. J., Davidson, R. N., et al.: Craniofacial resection for extensive paranasal sinus aspergilloma. J. Laryngol. Otol. *102*:1172, 1988.
123. Raghavan, R., Date, A., and Bhaktaviziam, A.: Fungal and nocardial infections of the kidney. Histopathology *11*:9, 1987.
124. Raper, K. B., and Fennell, D. I.: The Genus *Aspergillus*. Baltimore, Williams & Wilkins, 1965.
125. Renon, L.: Etude sur l'Aspergillose chez les Animaux et chez l'Homme. Paris, Masson et Cie, 1897.
126. Rhame, F. S., Streifel, A. J., Kersey, J. H., Jr., et al.: Extrinsic risk factors for pneumonia in the patient at high risk of infection. Am. J. Med. *76*(5A):42, 1984.
127. Rhine, W. D., Arvin, A. M., and Stevenson, D. K.: Neonatal aspergillosis. Clin. Pediatr. *25*:400, 1986.
128. Ricketti, A. J., Greenberger, P. A., Mintzer, R. A., et al.: Allergic bronchopulmonary aspergillosis. Chest *86*:773, 1984.
129. Rinaldi, M. G.: Invasive aspergillosis. Rev. Infect. Dis. *5*:1061, 1983.
130. Ringden, O., and Tollemar, J.: Liposomal amphotericin B (AmBisone®) treatment of invasive fungal infections in immunocompromised children. Mycoses *36*:187, 1993.
131. Rippon, J. W.: Medical Mycology. 3rd ed. Philadelphia, W. B. Saunders, 1988.
132. Roilides, E., Holmes, A., Blake, C., et al.: Impairment of neutrophil antifungal activity against hyphae of *Aspergillus fumigatus* in children infected with human immunodeficiency virus. J. Infect. Dis. *167*:905, 1993.
133. Roilides, E., Holmes, A., Blake, C., et al.: Defective antifungal activity of monocyte-derived macrophages from human immunodeficiency virus-infected children against *Aspergillus fumigatus*. J. Infect. Dis. *168*:1562, 1993.
134. Roilides, E., Holmes, A., Blake, C., et al.: Antifungal activity of elutriated human monocytes against *Aspergillus fumigatus* hyphae: Enhancement by granulocyte-macrophage colony-stimulating factor and interferon-gamma. J. Infect. Dis. *170*:894, 1994.
135. Rossi, G., Tortorano, A. M., Viviani, M. A., et al.: *Aspergillus fumigatus* infections in liver transplant patients. Transplant. Proc. *21*:2268, 1989.
136. Saah, D., Raverman, E., Drakos, P. E., et al.: Rhinocerebral aspergillosis in patients undergoing bone marrow transplantation. Ann. Otol. Rhinol. Laryngol. *103*:306, 1994.
137. Sabetta, J. R., Miniter, P., and Andriole, V. T.: The diagnosis of invasive aspergillosis by an enzyme-linked immunosorbent assay for circulating antigen. J. Infect. Dis. *152*:946, 1985.
138. Salmon, M. A.: Aspergilloma of the cerebellum. J. R. Soc. Med. *76*:611, 1983.
139. Schaffner, A., Douglas, H., and Braude, A.: Selective protection against conidia by mononuclear and against mycelia by polymorphonuclear phagocytes in resistance to *Aspergillus*. J. Clin. Invest. *69*:617, 1982.
140. Schonheyder, H., and Andersen, P.: An indirect immunofluorescence study of antibodies to *Aspergillus fumigatus* in sera from children and adults without aspergillosis. Sabouraudia *20*:41, 1982.
141. Schonheyder, H., and Andersen, P.: IgG antibodies to purified *Aspergillus fumigatus* determined by enzyme-linked immunosorbent assay. Int. Arch. Allergy Appl. Immunol. *74*:262, 1984.
142. Schoumacher, R. A., Tiller, R. E., and Berkow, R. L.: Invasive pulmonary aspergillosis in an infant: An unusual presentation of chronic granulomatous disease. Pediatr. Infect. Dis. J. *6*:215, 1987.
143. Schwartz, D. A., Jacquette, M., and Chawla, H. S.: Disseminated neonatal aspergillosis: Report of a fatal case and analysis of risk factors. Pediatr. Infect. Dis. J. *7*:349, 1988.
144. Schwartz, J., Baum, G. L., and Straub, M.: Cavitary histoplasmosis complicated by fungus ball. Am. J. Med. *31*:692, 1961.
145. Shamberger, R. C., Weinstein, H. J., Grier, H. E., et al.: The surgical management of fungal pulmonary infections in children with acute myelogenous leukemia. J. Pediatr. Surg. *20*:840, 1985.
146. Sihota, R., Agarwal, H. C., Grover, A. K., et al.: *Aspergillus* endophthalmitis. Br. J. Ophthalmol. *71*:611, 1987.
147. Singh, N., Yu, V. L., and Rihs, J. D.: Invasive aspergillosis in AIDS. South. Med. J. *84*:822, 1991.
148. Sinski, J. T.: The epidemiology of aspergillosis. *In* Al-Doory, Y. (ed.): The Epidemiology of Human Mycotic Disease. Springfield, Charles C Thomas, 1975, pp. 210–226.
149. Sluyter, T.: De Vegetabilibus Organismi Animalis Parasitis ac de novo Epiphyto Pityriasi Versicolore Obvio (Diss.). Berlin, G. Schade, 1847.
150. Solit, R. W., McKeown, J. J., and Smullens, S.: The surgical implications of intracavitary mycetomas (fungus balls). J. Thorac. Cardiovasc. Surg. *62*:411, 1971.
151. Spearing, R. L., Pamphilon, D. H., and Prentice, A. G.: Pulmonary aspergillosis in immunosuppressed patients with hematologic malignancies. Q. J. Med. *59*:611, 1986.
152. Stenson, S., Brookner, A., and Rosenthal, S.: Bilateral endogenous necrotizing scleritis due to *Aspergillus oryzae*. Ann. Ophthalmol. *14*:67, 1982.
153. Stynen, D., Goris, A., Sarfati, J., et al.: A new sensitive sandwich enzyme-linked immunosorbent assay to detect galactofuran in patients with invasive aspergillosis. J. Clin. Microbiol. *33*:497, 1995.
154. Sugar, A. M.: Use of amphotericin B with azole antifungal drugs: What are we doing? Antimicrob. Agents Chemother. *39*:1907, 1995.
155. Tack, K. J., Rhame, F. S., Brown, B., et al.: *Aspergillus* osteomyelitis: Report of four cases and review of the literature. Am. J. Med. *73*:295, 1982.
156. Todeschini, G., Murari, C., Bonesi, R., et al.: Oral itraconazole plus nasal amphotericin B for prophylaxis of invasive aspergillosis in patients with hematologic malignancies. Eur. J. Clin. Microbiol. Infect. Dis. *12*:614, 1993.
157. Treger, T. R., Visscher, D. W., Bartlett, M. S., et al.: Diagnosis of pulmonary infection caused by *Aspergillus*: Usefulness of respiratory cultures. J. Infect. Dis. *152*:572, 1985.
158. Tricot, G., Joosten, E., Boogaerts, M. A., et al.: Ketoconazole vs. itraconazole for antifungal prophylaxis in patients with severe granulocytopenia: Preliminary results of two nonrandomized studies. Rev. Infect. Dis. *9*:S94, 1987.
159. Tuncel, E.: Pulmonary air meniscus sign. Respiration *46*:139, 1984.
160. Vail, C. M., and Chiles, C.: Invasive pulmonary aspergillosis: Radiologic evidence of tracheal involvement. Radiology *165*:745, 1987.
161. Varkey, B., and Rose, H. D.: Pulmonary aspergilloma: A rational approach to treatment. Am. J. Med. *61*:626, 1976.
162. Venugopal, P. L., Venugopal, T. L., Gomathi, A., et al.: Mycotic keratitis in Madras. Indian J. Pathol. Microbiol. *32*:190, 1989.
163. Virchow, R.: Beitrage zur lehre von den beim menschen vorkommenden pflanzlichen parasiten. Arch. Pathol. Anat. Physiol. Klin. Med. *9*:557, 1856.
164. Walker, D. H., and McGinnis, M. R.: Opportunistic fungal infection: What the clinician, pathologist, and mycologist can accomplish if they work together. Clin. Lab. Med. *2*:407, 1982.
165. Walmsley, S., Devi, S., King, S., et al.: Invasive *Aspergillus* infections in a pediatric hospital: A ten-year review. Pediatr. Infect. Dis. J. *12*:673, 1993.
166. Walsh, T. J., and Bulkley, B. H.: *Aspergillus* pericarditis: Clinical and pathologic features in the immunocompromised patient. Cancer *49*:48, 1982.
167. Walsh, T. J., and Hamilton, S. R.: Disseminated aspergillosis complicating hepatic failure. Arch. Intern. Med. *143*:1189, 1983.
168. Walsh, T. J., Hier, D. B., and Caplan, L. R.: Aspergillosis of the central nervous system: Clinicopathological analysis of 17 patients. Ann. Neurol. *18*:574, 1985.
169. Walsh, T. J., Hutchins, G. M., Bulkley, B. H., et al.: Fungal infections of the heart: Analysis of 51 autopsy cases. Am. J. Cardiol. *45*:357, 1980.
170. Walsh, T. J., and Lee, J. W.: Prevention of invasive fungal infections in patients with neoplastic diseases. Clin. Infect. Dis. *17*(Suppl. 2):S468, 1993.
171. Washburn, R. G., Gallin, J. I., and Bennett, J. E.: Oxidative killing of *Aspergillus fumigatus* proceeds by parallel myeloperoxidase-dependent and -independent pathways. Infect. Immun. *55*:2088, 1987.
172. Weems, J. J., Jr., Davis, B. J., Tablan, O. C., et al.: Construction activity: An independent risk factor for invasive aspergillosis and zygomycosis in patients with hematologic malignancy. Infect. Control *8*:71, 1987.
173. Weiner, M. H., Talbot, G. H., Gerson, S. L., et al.: Antigen detection in the diagnosis of invasive aspergillosis. Ann. Intern. Med. *99*:777, 1983.
174. Weingarten, J. S., Crockett, D. M., and Lusk, R. P.: Fulminant aspergillosis: Early cutaneous manifestations and the disease process in the immunocompromised host. Otolaryngol. Head Neck Surg. *97*:495, 1987.
175. Wells, W. J., Fox, A. H., Theodore, P. R., et al.: Aspergillosis of the posterior mediastinum. Ann. Thorac. Surg. *57*:1240, 1994.
176. Whelan, M. A., Stern, J., and de Napoli, R. A.: The computed tomographic spectrum of intracranial mycosis: Correlation with histopathology. Radiology *141*:703, 1981.
177. Whitehurst, F. O., and Liston, T. E.: Orbital aspergillosis: Report of a case in a child. J. Pediatr. Ophthalmol. Strabismus *18*:50, 1981.
178. Wollschlager, C., and Khan, F.: Aspergillomas complicating sarcoidosis. Chest *86*:585, 1984.
179. Young, R. C., Bennett, J. E., Vogel, C. L., et al.: Aspergillosis: The spectrum of disease in 98 patients. Medicine *49*:147, 1970.
180. Yu, B., Niki, Y., and Armstrong, D.: Use of immunoblotting to detect *Aspergillus fumigatus* antigen in sera and urines of rats with experimental invasive aspergillosis. J. Clin. Microbiol. *28*:1575, 1990.
181. Yu, V. L., Muder, R. R., and Poorsattar, A.: Significance of isolation of *Aspergillus* from the respiratory tract in diagnosis of invasive pulmonary aspergillosis. Am. J. Med. *81*:249, 1986.

198

Blastomycosis

Gordon E. Schutze

Blastomyces dermatitidis is a dimorphic fungus responsible for a systemic disease characterized by granulomatous and suppurative lesions. Illness occurs when fungal spores are inhaled into the lungs and undergo transition into an invasive yeast phase. Once in the yeast phase, these organisms may not be cleared by the bronchopulmonary phagocytes and may proliferate prior to the development of immunity. The infection may be halted and resolved by the host at this point, or progression of the infection leading to localized pulmonary involvement or extrapulmonary disease may occur. Such dissemination results in the involvement of other organs, most notably the skin and bones. Although the highest prevalence of disease with this organism is in North America, blastomycosis has been documented to occur worldwide.

Gilchrist and Stokes[18, 19] were the first to describe blastomycosis in the late 1890s. Over the next decade, the heightened awareness of the disease by the medical community produced reports from various regions of the United States, with most cases occurring in the Chicago area.[43] Because of this, blastomycosis became known as Chicago disease or Gilchrist disease. A widely accepted concept during these early studies was that two forms of the disease existed (cutaneous and systemic) and that each represented a different portal of entry by the organism. It was not until many years later that Schwarz and Baum[48] established the fact that blastomycosis was a primary pulmonary process and that the cutaneous manifestations were secondary to dissemination from the lung. More recently, blastomycosis became known as North American blastomycosis due to an erroneous belief that the disease was limited to North America, but because this disease now is recognized as having a worldwide distribution, it is known at present as blastomycosis.

THE ORGANISM

B. dermatitidis is the causative agent of blastomycosis. The organism has two forms: a sexual form (teleomorphic or perfect state) and an asexual form (anamorphic or imperfect state). The sexual form of the fungus is named *Ajellomyces dermatitidis*, whereas the asexual form actually is *B. dermatitidis*. The asexual stage exhibits dimorphism, during which the fungus grows as a yeast form at body temperature and as a mycelial form at room temperature. At 37° C, the yeast form appears as a large round organism (6 to 15 μm in diameter) with a thick wall that can produce a single bud (Fig. 198–1). This bud is connected characteristically to the parent yeast by a wide base of attachment and usually will equal the size of the parent prior to detachment. At 25° to 30° C on laboratory medium, *B. dermatitidis* grows as a white to gray-brown mold (mycelia) with a delicate, silky appearance. Microscopically, the mold is characterized by filamentous colonies composed of thin, uniform septate hyphae (1 to 2 μm in width) that produce conidiophores that branch at right angles to the main hyphal segment. The solitary conidia (spores), which are located at the end of the conidiophores, are small (2 to 10 μm in diameter) and may be oval or pyriform (pear shaped). These conidia are similar to the microconidia of *Histoplasma capsulatum*, but the conidia of *B. dermatitidis* do not form tuberculate macroconidia as do those of *Histoplasma*. The appearance of the mycelia of *B. dermatitidis* is not pathogenic for the organism, and the definitive identification depends on the conversion of the organism to the yeast form by culture at 37° C.

ECOLOGY AND EPIDEMIOLOGY

There is a paucity of data concerning the ecology and epidemiology of this disease. Without data concerning the ecology of the organism, knowledge about the epidemiology of disease caused by this organism is derived from studies of sporadic cases. Although significant data concerning the epidemiology of the disease have been gathered with such studies, gaps in our knowledge will become clarified when the ecology of the agent is defined better. Because *B. dermatitidis* cannot be recovered easily from nature and an adequate skin test antigen is not available for conducted population surveys, the present knowledge of this disease is based on case reports of sporadic infections as well as outbreaks of human and canine disease.

The natural reservoir of *B. dermatitidis* is not defined as precisely as those for the causes of the other systemic mycoses (e.g., bird droppings, *H. capsulatum*), but it is assumed that this organism has its reservoir in a similar habitat as the other dimorphic fungi. *B. dermatitidis* appears to be a soil saprophyte and presumably exists in the mycelial form in nature. The organism probably thrives in a location that is high in organic material, abundant in moisture, has an acid pH, and even may be enriched with animal excreta.[29] The yeast and mycelial phases of the organism appear to disappear rapidly when placed in the soil, whereas the conidia can survive for several weeks.[34] Desiccation of such an area with the subsequent disturbance of the site results in an infectious aerosol of mycelial fragments and conidia. Conidia

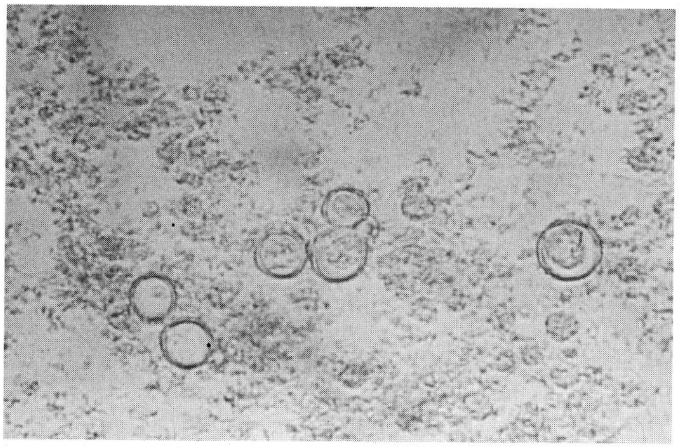

FIGURE 198–1. *A wet preparation demonstrating the spherical shape of* Blastomyces dermatitidis.

also may be released from the mycelia on the soil or from decaying material when wetted or disturbed.[25, 27]

Speculation on the natural source of this organism began shortly after it was recognized. Several investigators have noted an association between water and *B. dermatitidis.* Denton and Di Salvo[14] were able to recover the organism in 10 of 356 samples along 1 mile of road by the Savannah River. Furcolow and associates[17] published an extensive review of canine and human blastomycosis over a prolonged period (1885–1968) and found a high incidence of disease south of the Ohio River and east of the Mississippi River. Additionally, at least five human outbreaks of blastomycosis have occurred along river banks.[8, 28, 29, 53] The exact role of the water, however, currently is not understood.

Blastomycosis has been reported to occur worldwide, but many of these reported cases have not withstood scrutiny. Unequivocal cases of blastomycosis from South America have not been described in the last four decades. Isolated cases have been reported from England, Switzerland, and Poland, whereas sporadic infections have been found in the Middle East and India. The majority of cases, however, are reported from the eastern half of North America (east of the 100th meridian), with a smaller number of cases scattered throughout Africa.[1]

All age groups of patients are susceptible to blastomycosis. The age distribution varies with each series of cases published based upon the population examined. The majority of patients are between the ages of 20 and 70 years, whereas only 3 to 11 per cent of reported cases occur in patients younger than 20 years of age.[17, 35] Two patients who were 3 weeks of age or younger have been reported.[33, 55] Exceptions to this age spectrum occur in outbreaks in which cases in children can predominate. Although some studies in adults have demonstrated that there is a predominance of males infected with *B. dermatitidis,* previous studies in children and adolescents have not demonstrated such a trend.[31, 42, 51, 58] Case rates for blastomycosis have been described to be highest for African American patients, but it generally is speculated that the racial difference in case rates reflects the population in the community of the endemic region. The age, sex, and race distributions of children with blastomycosis appear, therefore, to be a matter of exposure and not susceptibility of the individual.

Dogs appear to be as susceptible to *B. dermatitidis* as humans. Because of this, canine blastomycosis has become a surrogate marker for human blastomycosis. The incidence and prevalence of canine blastomycosis have been studied extensively to supplement our knowledge about the geographic distribution of the disease. Menges and associates[36] were among the first to conclude that humans and dogs acquire their infections from the same source and that there is no evidence of passive transmission of illness from dog to human or vice versa.

PATHOGENESIS AND PATHOLOGY

Five methods of *B. dermatitidis* transmission have been described: inhalation, accidental inoculation, dog bites, conjugal transmission, and intrauterine transmission. By far the most common portal of entry into the body is through the lungs. It was not until the work of Schwartz and Baum[48] in the early 1950s that it was recognized that *B. dermatitidis* was inhaled from the environment and resulted in a subclinical or mild respiratory illness. In the majority of situations, disease at other body sites is the result of hematogenous spread from the lungs, even if not recognized clinically. Primary cutaneous blastomycosis has occurred secondary to accidental needle inoculation, often to a veterinarian or pathologist or via dog bites.[20, 30] Person-to-person spread of blastomycosis does not occur, except in certain situations. There has been one well-recognized case of conjugal transmission and two of intrauterine transmission to neonates.[10, 33, 55]

Blastomycosis begins with the inhalation of the conidia of *B. dermatitidis* into the lungs followed by an inflammatory response with neutrophils and macrophages. The majority of conidia are killed easily by these phagocytes, but those that succeed in changing into the yeast form are more resistant to phagocytosis. The large size of the yeast forms and the resistance to the oxidative mechanisms of killing used by the phagocytes make the yeast form more difficult to kill. Over the next 4 to 8 weeks, the unphagocytosed yeast forms will proliferate and patients may be asymptomatic or complain of an influenza-like illness, with fever, arthralgia, myalgia, a productive cough, and pleuritic chest pain.[46] The infection may be halted by the host at this stage, or progression of the infection leading to localized pulmonary and extrapulmonary disease may occur.

Subclinical cases of blastomycosis probably occur more commonly than symptomatic ones.[54] The high amount of asymptomatic infections supports the theory that healthy individuals are fairly resistant to infection. The exact mechanism of both natural and acquired resistance to infection is not understood. Natural resistance is thought to be mediated by neutrophils, monocytes, and alveolar macrophages. Human neutrophils phagocytize the conidia of *B. dermatitidis* rapidly and effectively, and within 2 hours 90 per cent of the conidia are located intracellularly,[16] whereas the yeast forms moderately are resistant to killing by neutrophils. Human alveolar macrophages have phase transition–associated fungicidal and fungistatic activities by irreversibly blocking conidial phase transition to the yeast form or reversibly inhibiting phase transition by causing the accumulation of unusual intermediate forms.[52]

Only recently have we been able to characterize features of acquired resistance in blastomycosis. It appears that there is no relationship between the presence of specific antibody against *B. dermatitidis* and the development of resistance to disease. Specific cellular immunity, however, appears to occur in all patients infected with this organism. Antigen-specific T cells are stimulated to produce lymphokines (e.g., interferon-γ) that activate macrophages, resulting in enhanced fungicidal activity.[3]

CLINICAL MANIFESTATIONS

Pulmonary Disease

Approximately 50 per cent of infected children will develop symptomatic illness. The majority of these illnesses will present as an acute or chronic pulmonary process. Patients with acute pulmonary blastomycosis present with symptoms similar to those of an acute bacterial process. Cough (which may be productive), fever, malaise, and chest pain are the most common complaints from patients.[42] In many instances, patients may respond initially to routine antimicrobial therapy, only to have their constitutional symptoms return at a later date. Unlike adults, whose disease may take years to progress to a chronic pulmonary process, children's disease rarely progresses longer than 6 months without the return of symptoms.[58]

A mass effect, fibronodular patterns, and consolidation are common findings on chest radiography with blastomycosis in adults.[6, 12] There is little information on commonly encountered chest radiographic patterns in children, but extensive

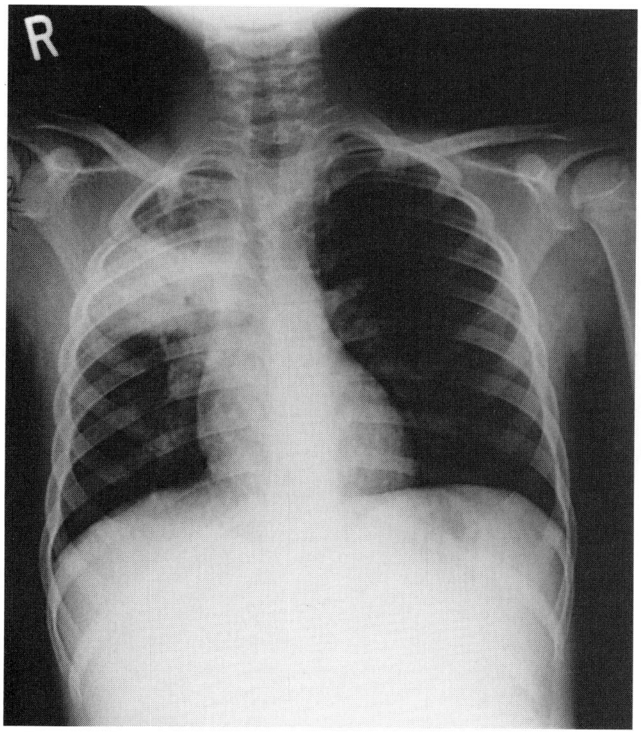

FIGURE 198–2. *Chest radiograph of a right upper lobe infiltrate due to* Blastomyces dermatitidis.

consolidation of the involved lobes appears to be the most common finding among children.[7, 31, 42, 47] Consolidation has been described to involve all lobes of the lung and may be multilobar or bilateral. Multiple small cavitary lesions, pleural effusions, hilar adenopathy, and nodular infiltrates also have been described. Mass lesions, which are common in adults, frequently are not demonstrated in children. This probably is due to the fact that mass lesions more commonly are associated with chronic disease, whereas lobar consolidations are more consistent with acute disease. The consolidation demonstrated on chest radiography may mimic that of an acute bacterial process (Fig. 198–2), whereas chronic chest abnormalities associated with blastomycosis (e.g., mass lesions, cavitary lesions) may be confused with tuberculosis or neoplasms. Mass lesions, consolidation, air bronchograms, nodular infiltrates, and satellite lesions commonly are described findings in adults with pulmonary blastomycosis who have undergone computed tomography of the chest.[56] Computed tomographic findings in children have been limited to consolidation, pulmonary abscess, and paratracheal adenopathy (Fig. 198–3).[47]

Disseminated Disease

Although the numbers are small, it appears that disseminated disease is present in 50 to 80 per cent of children diagnosed with blastomycosis.[47, 51, 58] The most common site involved with disseminated disease in children is the bones (Fig. 198–4). Although long bones (e.g., tibia, humerus), ribs, and vertebrae are involved most frequently, almost any bone is vulnerable. Skin disease has been described in children, but the classic verrucous lesions seen in adults usually do not occur. Pustular or ulcerative lesions may be demonstrated but usually occur in children as a result of underlying bony

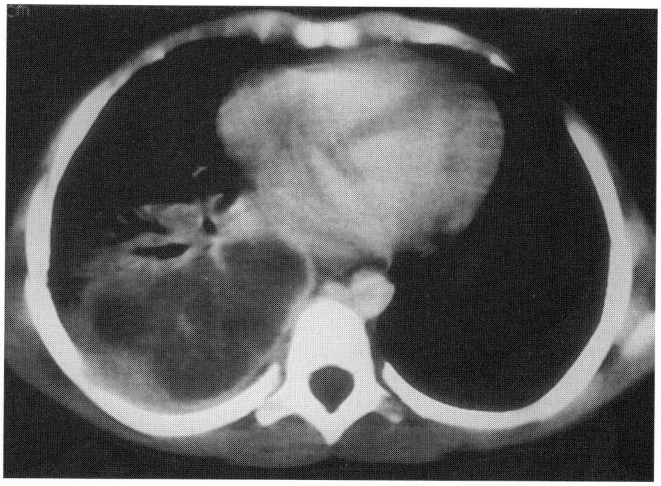

FIGURE 198–3. *Computed tomographic scan of the chest revealing consolidation and abscess formation in the right lower lobe of the lung.*

involvement (Fig. 198–5). Skin lesions involving the sun-exposed areas of the body (e.g., nose, ears) also may be seen (Fig. 198–6). Other areas of involvement that have been described include the liver, spleen, heart, lymph nodes, psoas muscle, kidney, middle ear, and the central nervous system.[22, 24, 58]

Disease in Immunocompromised Patients

Information concerning infections with *B. dermatitidis* in immunocompromised children is lacking, and there are only limited data concerning blastomycosis in immunocompromised adults.[41, 49, 57] Unlike other fungi (e.g., *H. capsulatum, Cryptococcus neoformans*), there have been only a small number of patients with AIDS who have become infected with this agent. This probably is due to less exposure of many patients with AIDS to the endemic regions of the organism. Pulmonary involvement is the most common manifestation of disease in immunocompromised patients, but adult respiratory distress syndrome is encountered more frequently than with immunologically normal hosts. Multiple organ and central nervous system involvement in these patients is relatively common, compared with that in the normal host. Increased mortality rates (30 to 54 per cent) have been described, with a large proportion of patients who die of other causes having evidence of persistent blastomycosis at the time of death. Many issues regarding therapy for this group

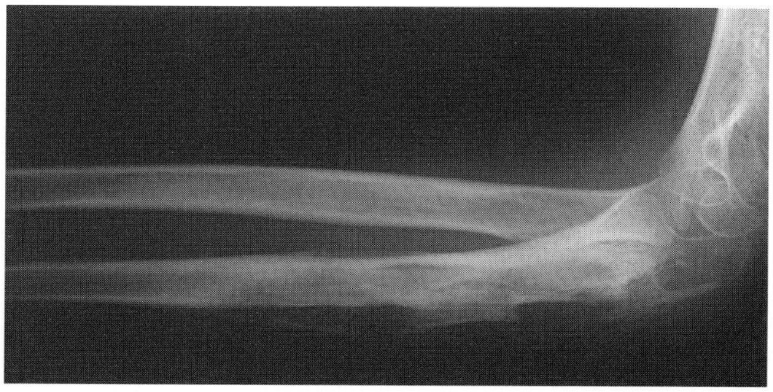

FIGURE 198–4. *Bony destruction of the ulna with blastomycosis.*

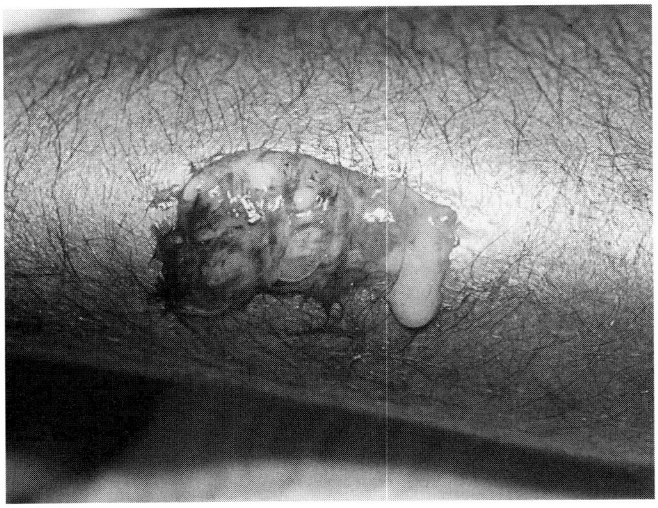

FIGURE 198–5. *Purulent wound drainage overlying a region of osteomyelitis with blastomycosis.*

of patients are not understood. Lifetime suppressive therapy appears to be indicated for this group of patients.

Disease During Pregnancy

The prenatal diagnosis of blastomycosis in pregnant women has been well documented.[9, 13, 21, 23, 32, 38] Of the seven women described to date, three had evidence of disseminated disease, three had pulmonary disease alone, and the remaining patient developed adult respiratory distress syndrome and required ventilatory support and early cesarean section. These seven pregnancies culminated in the birth of eight infants, which included one set of twins. None of the infants were found to be infected at birth, nor did they develop signs or symptoms consistent with blastomycosis at a later date. The placentas of the three women with disseminated disease and the woman with adult respiratory distress syndrome were examined for evidence of *B. dermatitidis*. Only the mother with adult respiratory distress syndrome demonstrated organisms in the placenta.[32] The organisms were located on the maternal as well as the fetal side of the placenta.

Neonatal Disease

Two neonates who presented with an acute onset of respiratory distress within 3 weeks after birth and were diagnosed with pulmonary blastomycosis have been described.[33, 55] Both infants died of their illness, and abnormalities on autopsy were limited to the lungs. One mother was noted to have lesions consistent with blastomycosis on her face and thigh,[33] whereas the second mother was noted to have a lesion on her right lower extremity.[55] Only one mother allowed an extensive physical examination to be performed, and her genital examination was unremarkable; the second mother denied having genital lesions. The second mother refused any therapy for her blastomycosis and 2.5 years later died with a disseminated illness due to *B. dermatitidis*. On autopsy, her uterus and both ovaries had multiple abscesses, with the left ovary being almost entirely unrecognizable secondary to chronic infection.[59] The pathophysiology of neonatal disease is not understood entirely. Although certainly because the pathologic changes due to *B. dermatitidis* were limited to the lungs in these neonates, this illness could have been due to aspiration of vaginal secretions that were colonized with this organism at birth. Autopsy findings of the second mother, however, certainly raise the question of transplacental passage of the organism.

DIAGNOSIS

Because there is no clinical syndrome that is characteristic of blastomycosis, the unequivocal diagnosis requires the isolation of the organism from a clinical specimen. A presumptive diagnosis can be made when the characteristic yeast is visualized in respiratory secretions, purulent material, or histopathologic sections. For patients with pulmonary disease, respiratory secretions can be obtained through sputum production, bronchoscopy with bronchoalveolar lavage, or open lung biopsy. Sputum samples more commonly are helpful in the older patient; such specimens are difficult to obtain in young children. Likewise, obtaining adequate specimens with the use of bronchoscopy and bronchoalveolar lavage in young children has been demonstrated to be problematic. The need for open lung biopsy in patients with pulmonary blastomycosis after negative results from flexible bronchoscopy with bronchoalveolar lavage demonstrates the technical limitations of this procedure in the pediatric population.[47] Bronchial brushings and bronchoscopic-directed biopsy would improve recovery of the organism but are technically

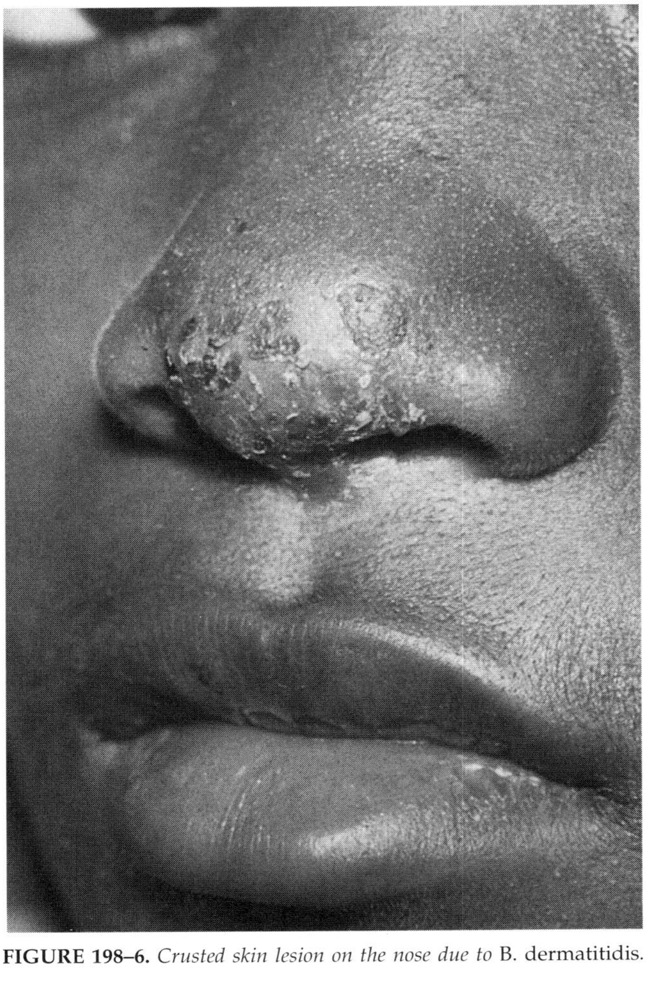

FIGURE 198–6. *Crusted skin lesion on the nose due to* B. dermatitidis.

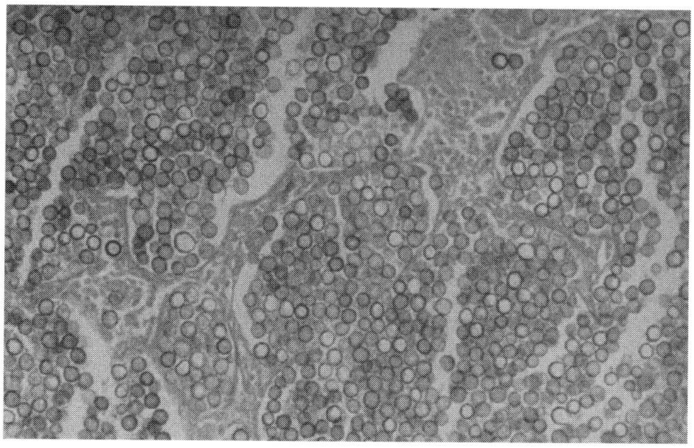

FIGURE 198–7. *Overwhelming infection with* B. dermatitidis *demonstrated in lung tissue with a silver stain.*

difficult to perform in the younger patient at this time. Based upon the difficulty of establishing the diagnosis of pulmonary blastomycosis in young patients, it is recommended that children and adolescents who are suspected of having blastomycosis undergo lung biopsy if sputum and bronchoscopy examination are nondiagnostic.[47]

Respiratory or purulent wound secretions can be examined under light microscopy by wet preparations with or without the use of potassium hydroxide in order to visualize the characteristic yeast forms. Other staining techniques, such as the calcofluor white stain, can be useful for specimens when the number of organisms in the specimen is limited. The Gomori methenamine silver stain or the periodic acid–Schiff stain may be useful for histopathologic specimens (Fig. 198–7). The presence of pyogranulomas in a pathologic specimen should alert one to the diagnosis of blastomycosis, but organisms may be difficult to locate with the use of the hematoxylin and eosin stains; in such instances, the Gomori methenamine silver or periodic acid–Schiff stain may be helpful. Specimens collected for culture should be placed on a culture medium, which will ensure the recovery of all clinically significant fungi. A more enriched agar, such as Sabouraud agar with brain-heart infusion, is essential for the recovery of such organisms as *B. dermatitidis*. Specimens potentially contaminated with bacteria or other fungal agents should be placed on an additional agar containing antimicrobial agents (e.g., chloramphenicol, cycloheximide) to inhibit the growth of these contaminants.

In some situations, however, isolation attempts are unsuccessful and alternative laboratory tests may be used. Most currently available serologic tests are performed by complement fixation, immunodiffusion, or enzyme immunoassay using a yeast-phase antigen (A antigen). These assays have been most useful as epidemiologic tools, not for the clinical diagnosis of disease, due to the cross-reactivity with antigens of other fungi (e.g., *H. capsulatum)* that results in poor sensitivity and specificity. The most sensitive of these tests is the commercially available enzyme immunoassay.[4] However, a 120-kDa protein that reacts with antibodies to *Blastomyces* has been identified.[26] This surface protein, designated WI-1, has been demonstrated to be a key antigenic target of humoral and cellular responses during infection. In a study comparing WI-1 and A antigen, WI-1 was found to be more reactive and specific for the binding of serum antibodies to *Blastomyces*.[27] Preliminary testing using WI-1 as a target in a radioimmunoassay demonstrated that 93 per cent of 27 patients with blastomycosis had positive serology within 60 days of diagnosis and that only 5 per cent of 84 patients from whom the fungus was not identified were positive.[50] Because such testing using the WI-1 antigen currently is not available clinically, the role of serology is limited. If serology is used, the most accurate method for testing is the enzyme immunoassay.

TREATMENT

Before the availability of antifungal medications, the mortality rate associated with blastomycosis usually exceeded 60 per cent. After the introduction of effective medications for the treatment of blastomycosis, all patients received therapy when the diagnosis was established. The concept has been challenged due to the toxicity of amphotericin B and the recognition that self-limited cases of pulmonary blastomycosis exist.[45] Since the advent of safe and effective oral medications for the treatment of blastomycosis in adults, this controversy has lessened. In children, however, in whom up to 80 per cent with blastomycosis have disseminated disease, the decision to withhold therapy for pneumonia due to blastomycosis must be made very cautiously. If a culture diagnosis of blastomycosis is established after the patient has made a spontaneous recovery without therapy, the use of antifungal therapy might be questioned. If therapy is withheld, patients must be followed carefully for months or even years for evidence of reactivation or dissemination of disease. Accidental introductions of blastomycosis into the skin through needle punctures or bite wounds usually can be treated locally with vigorous cleaning with tincture of iodine, an iodophor, or chlorhexidine.

Much of the therapy currently available for the treatment of blastomycosis in adults is based upon the use of the newer oral azole antifungal agents (ketoconazole, fluconazole, itraconazole), but there is a lack of data on pharmacokinetics, safety, and efficacy of these medications in children. Another obstacle to the widespread use of these drugs in children is the lack of commercially prepared oral liquid preparations (ketoconazole, itraconazole) for those patients unable to take tablets or capsules. Although ketoconazole can be formulated as a liquid preparation with a short shelf life (7 days), clinicians often resort to crushing tablets and instructing parents in the art of disguising medications to ensure their delivery. The delivery of medications in such a fashion may reduce efficacy and compliance because these preparations are neither well tolerated nor standardized.

The use of ketoconazole (400 to 800 mg/day for 6 months) for blastomycosis in adults has demonstrated cure rates of up to 89 per cent.[5] However, little is known about the use of ketoconazole for blastomycosis in children. The recommended dose of ketoconazole for children established for the treatment of infections with *Candida* is 5 to 10 mg/kg/day given as a once-daily dose,[11] which would approximate the 400 to 800 mg suggested for blastomycosis based upon a 70-kg individual. Recently, however, it was demonstrated that when such a dose was used in five children with blastomycosis, two had relapse (one associated with noncompliance) and two had progression of their disease. The one patient who was cured also underwent a lobectomy, which would have eliminated the area of a large number of organisms.[47] Until more data become available, it would appear that ketoconazole is not effective for the treatment of blastomycosis at the currently suggested doses for pediatric patients.

Fluconazole has been demonstrated to be effective against blastomycosis in 65 per cent of adults at a dose of 200 to 400 mg daily.[40] A treatment failure of 30 per cent was observed in the high-dose (400 mg/day) group, which included the youngest patient in the study. The investigators concluded that fluconazole was moderately effective against blastomycosis in adults and that its efficacy was similar to that of ketoconazole. There are no data available for the treatment of blastomycosis with fluconazole in patients younger than 18 years of age. Because of this, fluconazole does not have a role in the therapy of blastomycosis in the pediatric patient.

Itraconazole (200 to 400 mg/day) for 6 months now is the recommended therapy of choice for acute non–life-threatening blastomycosis in adults.[15, 44] There currently are no accepted recommendations for doses of itraconazole in pediatric patients, but in low birth weight infants and patients with chronic granulomatous disease, doses of 5 to 10 mg/kg daily have been used safely and effectively.[2, 37, 39] There have been limited published data on the use of itraconazole for blastomycosis in the pediatric patient. One review used itraconazole (5 to 7 mg/kg/day; maximum, 200 mg/day) to treat four pediatric patients with blastomycosis.[47] Two patients were treated successfully with itraconazole after an initial treatment failure with a previous antifungal regimen. A third patient's initial trial with itraconazole for his pulmonary blastomycosis failed, despite directly observed therapy. This patient had undetectable itraconazole levels in the serum, presumably due to drug-drug interactions between primidone and itraconazole. The fourth patient completed a 6-month course of itraconazole for her pulmonary blastomycosis without relapse. Although limited because of extremely small numbers of patients studied, itraconazole appears to be superior to ketoconazole or fluconazole for the treatment of blastomycosis in children. The exact dose required, however, has not been established.

The agent with the greatest proven success for the treatment of blastomycosis in pediatric patients remains amphotericin B.[42, 47, 51, 58] A total course of 25 to 30 mg/kg approaches a 100 per cent cure rate. Because there are no comparative trials evaluating amphotericin B and itraconazole for the treatment of blastomycosis in the pediatric patient, itraconazole should be used cautiously in this age group. Therefore, for pediatric patients with osteomyelitis or disseminated and/or life-threatening disease due to blastomycosis, a full course of amphotericin B (25 to 30 mg/kg) is recommended. Neonates and pregnant and immunocompromised patients should be treated in a similar manner. For patients with pulmonary blastomycosis, if an oral agent is used alone or in sequential therapy with amphotericin B, that agent should be itraconazole. Due to the unpredictable nature of drug interactions, however, any patient receiving itraconazole with other medications that may interact with itraconazole should be followed closely and have documentation of adequate serum levels. Close follow-up of these patients for identification of those with progression or relapse of their disease is mandatory. If patients do not have a clinical response within 2 to 4 weeks, if adequate serum levels are not obtainable, or if clinical deterioration is documented, amphotericin B should be substituted for itraconazole for the treatment of blastomycosis.

Surgery, other than for the establishment of the diagnosis, has a limited role in the therapy of blastomycosis. Surgery is indicated for the drainage of large abscesses or for the removal of devitalized tissue in the occasional patient with osteomyelitis who is responding poorly to therapy. Surgery should never be considered curative and always should be performed in association with appropriate antifungal therapy. The duration of therapy should not be shortened just because the patient has undergone surgical resection of the involved area.

Isolation of patients with pulmonary disease due to blastomycosis is not required, because the person-to-person contact spread of this disease has never been attributed to respiratory secretions. Furthermore, no special precautions are required of those patients with open wounds due to blastomycosis.

References

1. Baily, G. G., Robertson, V. J., Neill, P., et al.: Blastomycosis in Africa: Clinical features, diagnosis, and treatment. Rev. Infect. Dis. *13*:1005–1008, 1991.
2. Bhandari, V., and Narang, A.: Oral itraconazole therapy for disseminated candidiasis in low birth weight infants. J. Pediatr. *120*:330, 1992.
3. Bradsher, R. W., Balk, R. A., and Jacobs, R. F.: Growth inhibition of *Blastomyces dermatitidis* in alveolar and peripheral macrophages from patients with blastomycosis. Am. Rev. Respir. Dis. *135*:412–417, 1987.
4. Bradsher, R. W., and Pappas, P. G.: Detection of specific antibodies in human blastomycosis by enzyme immunoassay. South. Med. J. *88*:1256–1259, 1995.
5. Bradsher, R. W., Rice, D. C., and Abernathy, R. S.: Ketoconazole therapy for endemic blastomycosis. Ann. Intern. Med. *103*:872–879, 1985.
6. Brown, L. R., Swenson, S. J., Van Scoy, R. E., et al.: Roentgenologic features of pulmonary blastomycosis. Mayo Clin. Proc. *66*:29–38, 1991.
7. Chesney, J. C., Gourley, G. R., Peters, M. E., et al.: Pulmonary blastomycosis in children: Amphotericin B therapy and a review. Am. J. Dis. Child. *133*:1134–1139, 1979.
8. Cockerill, F. R., III, Roberts, G. D., Rosenblatt, J. E., et al.: Epidemic of pulmonary blastomycosis (Namekagon fever) in Wisconsin canoeists. Chest *86*:688–692, 1984.
9. Cohen, I.: Absence of congenital infection and teratogenesis in three children born to mothers with blastomycosis and treated with amphoterecin B during pregnancy. Pediatr. Infect. Dis. J. *6*:76–77, 1987.
10. Craig, M. W., Davey, W. N., and Green, R. A.: Conjugal blastomycosis. Am. Rev. Respir. Dis. *102*:86–90, 1970.
11. Cross, J. T., Jr., Hickerson, S. L., and Yamauchi, T.: Antifungal drugs. Pediatr. Rev. *16*:123–129, 1995.
12. Cush, R., Light, R. W., and George, R. B.: Clinical and roentgenographic manifestations of acute and chronic blastomycosis. Chest *69*:345–349, 1976.
13. Daniel, L., and Salit, I. E.: Blastomycosis during pregnancy. Can. Med. Assoc. J. *131*:759–761, 1984.
14. Denton, J. F., and Di Salvo A, F.: Isolation of *Blastomyces dermatitidis* from natural sites at Augusta, Georgia. Am. J. Trop. Med. Hyg. *13*:716–722, 1964.
15. Dismukes, W. E., Bradsher, R. W., Jr., and Cloud, G. C. et al.: Itraconazole therapy for blastomycosis and histoplasmosis. Am. J. Med. *93*:489–497, 1992.
16. Drutz, D. J., and Frey, C. L.: Intracellular and extracellular defenses of human phagocytes against *Blastomyces dermatitidis* conidia and yeasts. J. Lab. Clin. Med. *105*:737–750, 1985.
17. Furcolow, M. L., Chick, E. W., Busey, J. F., et al.: Prevalence and incidence studies of human and canine blastomycosis. I. Cases in the United States, 1885–1968. Am. Rev. Respir. Dis. *102*:60–67, 1970.
18. Gilchrist, T. C.: A case of blastomycetic dermatitis in man. Johns Hopkins Hosp. Rep. *1*:269–283, 1896.
19. Gilchrist, T. C., and Stokes, W. R.: The presence of an *Oidium* in the tissues of a case of pseudo-lupus vulgaris: Preliminary report. Johns Hopkins Hosp. Bull. *7*:129–133, 1896.
20. Gnann, J. W., Jr., Bressler, G. S., Bodet, C. A., et al.: Human blastomycosis after a dog bite. Ann. Intern. Med. *98*:48–49, 1983.
21. Hager, H., Welt, S. I., Cardasis, J. P., et al.: Disseminated blastomycosis in a pregnant woman successfully treated with amphoterecin B: A case report. J. Reprod. Med. *33*:485–488, 1988.
22. Hughes, W. T., Franco, S., and Oh, M. H. K.: Systemic blastomycosis in childhood: Case report and review. Clin. Pediatr. *8*:597–601, 1969.
23. Ismail, M. A., and Lerner, S. A.: Disseminated blastomycosis in a pregnant woman: Review of amphoterecin B usage during pregnancy. Am. Rev. Respir. Dis. *126*:350–353, 1982.
24. Istorico, L. J., Sanders, M., Jacobs, R. F., et al.: Otitis media due to blastomycosis: Report of two cases. Clin. Infect. Dis. *14*:355–358, 1992.
25. Kitchen, M. S., Reiber, C. D., and Eastin, G. B.: An urban epidemic of North American blastomycosis. Am. Rev. Respir. Dis. *115*:1063–1066, 1977.
26. Klein, B. S., and Jones, J. M.: Isolation, purification, and radiolabeling of a novel 120-kD surface protein on *Blastomyces dermatitidis* yeasts to detect antibody in infected patients. J. Clin. Invest. *85*:152–161, 1990.
27. Klein, B. S., and Jones, J. M.: Purification and characterization of the major antigen WI-1 from *Blastomyces dermatitidis* yeasts and immunological comparison with A antigen. Infect. Immun. *62*:3890–3900, 1994.
28. Klein, B. S., Vergeront, J. M., Di Salvo, A. F., et al.: Two outbreaks of blastomycosis along rivers in Wisconsin: Isolation of *Blastomyces dermatitidis* from riverbank soil and evidence of its transmission along waterways. Am. Rev. Respir. Dis. *136*:1333–1338, 1987.
29. Klein, B. S., Vergeront, J. M., Weeks, R. J., et al.: Isolation of *Blastomycosis dermatitidis* in soil associated with a large outbreak of blastomycosis in Wisconsin. N. Engl. J. Med. *314*:529–534, 1986.
30. Larson, D. M., Eckman, M. R., Alber, R. L., et al.: Primary cutaneous

(inoculation) blastomycosis: An occupational hazard to pathologists. Am. J. Clin. Pathol. *79*:253–255, 1983.
31. Laskey, W. K., and Sarosi, G. A.: Blastomycosis in children. Pediatrics *65*:111–114, 1980.
32. MacDonald, D., and Alguire, P. C.: Adult respiratory distress syndrome due to blastomycosis during pregnancy. Chest *98*:1527–1528, 1990.
33. Maxson, S., Miller, S. F., Tryka, A. F., et al.: Perinatal blastomycosis: A review. Pediatr. Infect. Dis. J. *11*:760–763, 1992.
34. McDonough, E. S., Van Prooien, R., and Lewis, A. L.: Lysis of *Blastomyces dermatitidis* yeast phase cells in natural soil. Am. J. Epidemiol. *81*:86–94, 1965.
35. Menges, R. W., Doto, I. L., and Weeks, R. J.: Epidemiologic studies of blastomycosis in Arkansas. Arch. Environ. Health *18*:956–971, 1969.
36. Menges, R. W., Furcolow, M. L., Selby, L. A. et al.: Clinical and epidemiologic studies on seventy-nine canine blastomycosis cases in Arkansas. Am. J. Epidemiol. *81*:164–179, 1965.
37. Mouy, R., Veber, F., Blanche, S., et al.: Long-term itraconazole prophylaxis against *Aspergillus* infection in thirty-two patients with chronic granulomatous disease. J. Pediatr. *125*:998–1003, 1994.
38. Neiberg, A. D., Mavromatis, F., Dyke, J., et al.: *Blastomyces dermatitidis* treated during pregnancy: Report of a case. Am. J. Obstet. Gynecol. *128*:911–912, 1977.
39. Neijens, H. J., Frenkel, J., de Muinck Keizer-Schrama, S. M. P. F., et al.: Invasive *Aspergillus* infection in chronic granulomatous disease: Treatment with itraconazole. J. Pediatr. *115*:1016–1019, 1989.
40. Pappas, P. G., Bradsher, R. W., Chapman, S. W., et al.: Treatment of blastomycosis with fluconazole: A pilot study. Clin. Infect. Dis. *20*:267–271, 1995.
41. Pappas, P. G., Threlkeld, M. G., Bedsole, G. D., et al.: Blastomycosis in immunocompromised patients. Medicine *72*:311–325, 1993.
42. Powell, D. A., and Schuit, K. E.: Acute pulmonary blastomycosis in children: Clinical course and follow-up. Pediatrics *63*:736–740, 1979.
43. Ricketts, H. T.: Oidiomycosis (blastomycosis) of the skin and its fungi. J. Med. Res. *6*:373–547, 1901.
44. Sarosi, G. A., and Davies, S. F.: Therapy for fungal infections. Mayo Clin. Proc. *69*:1111–1117, 1994.
45. Sarosi, G. A., Davies, S. F., and Phillips, J. R.: Self-limited blastomycosis: A report of 39 cases. Semin. Respir. Infect. *1*:40–44, 1986.
46. Sarosi, G. A., Hammerman, K. J., Tosh, F. E., et al.: Clinical features of acute pulmonary blastomycosis. N. Engl. J. Med. *290*:540–543, 1974.
47. Schutze, G. E., Hickerson, S. L., Fortin, E. M., et al.: Blastomycosis in children. Clin. Infect. Dis. *22*:496–502, 1996.
48. Schwarz, J., and Baum, G. L.: Blastomycosis. Am. J. Clin. Pathol. *21*:999–1029, 1951.
49. Serody, J. S., Mill, M. R., Detterbeck, F. C., et al.: Blastomycosis in transplant recipients: Report of a case and review. Clin. Infect. Dis. *16*:54–58, 1993.
50. Soufleris, A. J., Klein, B. S., Courtney, B. T., et al.: Utility of anti-WI-1 serological testing in the diagnosis of blastomycosis in Wisconsin residents. Clin. Infect. Dis. *19*:87–92, 1994.
51. Steele, R. W., and Abernathy, R. S.: Systemic blastomycosis in children. Pediatr. Infect. Dis. J. *2*:304–307, 1983.
52. Sugar, A. M., Picard, M., Wagner, R., et al.: Interactions between human bronchoalveolar macrophages and *Blastomyces dermatitidis* conidia: Demonstration of fungicidal and fungistatic effects. J. Infect. Dis. *171*:1559–1562, 1995.
53. Tosh, F. E., Hammerman, K. J., Weeks, R. J., et al.: A common source epidemic of North American blastomycosis. Am. Rev. Respir. Dis. *109*:525–529, 1974.
54. Vaaler, A. K., Bradsher, R. W., and Davies, S. F.: Evidence of subclinical blastomycosis in forestry workers in northern Minnesota and northern Wisconsin. Am. J. Med. *89*:470–476, 1990.
55. Watts, E. A., Gard, P. D., and Tuthill, S. W.: First reported case of intrauterine transmission of blastomycosis. Pediatr. Infect. Dis. J. *2*:308–310, 1983.
56. Winer-Muram, H. T., Beals, D. H., and Cole, F. H., Jr.: Blastomycosis of the lung: CT features. Radiology *182*:829–832, 1992.
57. Witzig, R. S., Hoadley, D. J., Greer, D. L., et al.: Blastomycosis and human immunodeficiency virus: Three new cases and review. South. Med. J. *87*:715–719, 1994.
58. Yogev, R., and Davis, T.: Blastomycosis in children: A review of the literature. Mycopathologia *68*:139–143, 1979.
59. Young, L., and Schutze, G. E.: Perinatal blastomycosis: The rest of the story. Pediatr. Infect. Dis. J. *14*:83, 1995.

199

CANDIDIASIS

Walter T. Hughes and Patricia M. Flynn

Candidiasis is a "white plague" of the immunocompromised host. Clinical expression of the disease implies debility, ranging in magnitude from the weak neonate to the individual with a profound congenital or acquired immunodeficiency disorder. For some 2000 years after Hippocrates described thrush in the mouths of babes, the infection was viewed as an annoying and insignificant superficial disease. It is only within the past century that candidiasis of deep organs has been recognized. Since the 1960s, certain important therapeutic and diagnostic advances in medicine have affected host defenses and microbial ecology to the extent that these ubiquitous yeasts have gained prominence as pathogens of the first order with capabilities of producing life-threatening disease. Fortunately, in ordinary circumstances, the totally healthy person has little need to fear the malady.

THE ORGANISM

Members of the genus *Candida* characteristically are round to oval vegetative cells possessing the ability to produce pseudohyphae (chains of elongated yeast forms) under certain conditions and the inability to develop ascospores (spores within a parent cell). They often are classified as Fungi Imperfecti (Deuteromycetes). The taxonomy of yeasts is far from complete. The recent suggestion that the genus *Torulopsis* be reclassified as *Candida* is reasonable, but this concept is not yet in general use. From the clinical standpoint, the infections caused by these two genera best can be discussed separately. The earlier terms *Monilia* and *Oidium* are obsolete and no longer applied to the genus *Candida.*

The Latin word *candidus* means "dazzling white" and appropriately applies to the appearance of the thallus (colony). *Candida* species form round, well-demarcated, smooth, glistening, and creamy-white colonies on culture media. The yeast form of *Candida* is round to oval, measures 2 to 6 μm in diameter, and reproduces by budding. It does not possess a capsule, a feature that easily differentiates it from species of *Cryptococcus.* It is a dimorphic yeast in that it may, under appropriate conditions, exist as a yeast form (blastospore) or a pseudohyphal form. Some cells may produce septated cylindrical extensions from the blastospore. This phenomenon is called a germ tube and can be provoked by the incubation of *Candida* blastospores in human serum. Laboratories have taken advantage of this characteristic to provide quick (tentative) identification of a yeast such as *C. albicans.* The majority of *C. albicans* strains undergo chlamydospore formation under controlled stressful conditions. This feature is sufficiently unique to *C. albicans* for use as a diagnostic test. However, a few other yeasts, such as *C. tropicalis,* may develop chlamydospores. The utilization of carbohydrate

TABLE 199–1. Diseases and Compromising Factors That Predispose to Candidiasis

Category	Selected References	Category	Selected References
Infancy	Baley et al., 1984[7]	Tranquilizers	Pollack et al., 1964[137]
	Baley et al., 1988[8]	Antibiotics	Winner and Hurley, 1964[172]
	Stamos et al., 1995[159]		Odds, 1979[128]; Seelig, 1966[150]
	Botas et al., 1995[20]		Smits et al., 1966[155]
	Leibovitz et al., 1992[103]		Caruso, 1964[25]; Fitzpatrick and Topley, 1966[47]
	Ward et al., 1983[168]		Lehner and Ward, 1970[100]
	Fiax, 1984,[42] 1992[43]		Lehner and Ward, 1970[100]
	Johnson et al., 1984[81]		Toala et al., 1970[164]
	Odds, 1979[128]		
	Klein et al., 1972[92]		
	Taschdjian and Kozinin, 1957[162]		
	Winner and Hurley, 1964[173]		
Pregnancy	Stanley et al., 1972[160]	Corticosteroids	Bernhardt et al., 1972[13]
	Pederson, 1964[132]		Lehner and Ward, 1970[100]
	Bland et al., 1937[15]		Zegarelli and Kutscher, 1964[176]
Hypovitaminosis A	Montes et al., 1973[122]		Godfrey et al., 1974[58]
Malnutrition	Barbhaiya, 1966[10]	Oral contraceptives	Bourg, 1964[21]
Iron-deficiency anemia	Fletcher et al., 1975[48]		Walsh et al., 1968[167]
Burns	Macmillan et al., 1972[107]		Diddle et al., 1969[32]
Trauma	Mailbach and Kligman, 1962[108]	Intravascular catheters and hyperalimentation	Freeman et al., 1972[53]
	Dixon et al., 1969[33]		Glew et al., 1975[57]
Diabetes mellitus	Hesseltine, 1955[102]		Henderson et al., 1981[64]
	Sonck and Somersalo, 1963[158]		Solomon et al., 1984[157]
Addison disease	Podolsky and Ferguson, 1970[137]		Michel et al., 1979[118]
	Hung et al., 1963[74]		Hughes, 1982[70]
			Toala et al., 1970[164]
Cushing syndrome	Giombetti et al., 1971[56]	Urinary catheters	Bernhardt et al., 1972[13]
Hypothyroidism	Odds, 1979[128]		Schönebeck, 1972[148]
Hypoparathyroidism	Odds, 1979[128]		Fisher et al., 1982[46]
	Hung et al., 1963[74]		Toala et al., 1970[164]
Polyendocrinopathy	Ahonen et al., 1990[1]		
	Anttila, et al., 1994[3]		
Malignancy	Boggs et al., 1961[19]; Bodey, 1966[16]	X-irradiation	Chen and Webster, 1974[26]
		Surgery	Bernhardt et al., 1972[13]
	Schumacher et al., 1964[149]		Gaines and Remington, 1972[54]
			Richards et al., 1972[142]
	Richet et al., 1991[143]		
	Hughes, 1971[69]; Young et al., 1974[175]	Organ transplantation	Wingard et al., 1991[171]
	Robbins et al., 1974[144]		Atkinson et al., 1979[6]
	Kostiala et al., 1982[94]		Goodrich et al., 1991[60]
	Hughes, 1982[70]		Lipton et al., 1984[106]
			Clift, 1984[28]
	Bodey, 1984[17]	Congenital immune deficiency disorders	Edwards et al., 1978[38]
	Maksymiuk et al., 1984[109]	AIDS	Gottlieb et al., 1981[61]

substrates varies sufficiently among *Candida* species to serve as a biochemical basis for identification. By determining the utilization of selected carbohydrates as carbon sources in the presence of oxygen (assimilation) and in the absence of oxygen (fermentation), profiles have been established for the purpose of speciation. The majority of medically important *Candida* species cannot utilize potassium nitrate as a sole source of nitrogen, although *C. utilis* is an exception.

More than 150 species of *Candida* have been described, but only a portion of these are considered to be of medical importance; however, it is reasonable to expect that others eventually will be associated with disease in the immunocompromised host. *C. albicans* by far is the most frequent species causing disease in humans. Of considerable concern has been the observation from several sources that disease caused by non-*albicans* species is increasing in prevalence. These include *C. tropicalis, C. pseudotropicalis, C. paratropicalis, C. krusei, C. guilliermondi, C. parapsilosis, C. lusitaniae, C. rugosa,* and *C. stellatoidea.*

Host Susceptibility

An axiom that most simply expresses the host-parasite relationship of *Candida* species and humans can be formulated as follows: extent of disease equals number of organisms times virulence, divided by host resistance. Knowledge accrued to date suggests that there is little strain-to-strain variation in virulence of *C. albicans,* as well as other *Candida* species, although *C. albicans* usually is more virulent than other species. Compared with organisms that cause disease in the immunocompetent host, *Candida* species possess relatively low virulence factors. Thus, for establishment of a disease state, (1) the host resistance mechanisms must be impaired, (2) the number of organisms to which the host is exposed must be high, or (3) a combination of these is required.

The importance of the number of organisms to which the host is challenged should not be minimized. For example, a healthy adult volunteer experimentally ingested a suspension of *C. albicans* in the enormous amount of 80 g (more than 10^{12} organisms). Within 3 hours he was febrile, and *C. albicans* was cultured from blood and urine samples.[97] In practice, the number of organisms to which the patient is exposed usually is not known, and because virulence is rather constant, the predominant determinant for disease is the extent of impairment to normal host defenses. As might be expected, no single defect in the immune response can account for increased susceptibility to infection. However, in one specific form of the disease, chronic mucocutaneous candidiasis, defects in cell-mediated immunity have been well established. Here, the most consistent abnormality involves subnormal production of lymphokines by T cells in response to *Candida* antigens.[90]

Studies of responses of the immunocompetent host to *Candida* species suggest that eventually all components of the immune system respond to the microbe. Receptor sites on buccal and vaginal epithelial cells permit adherence of the yeast.[88] Lysozyme (muramidase) causes agglutination and killing of *C. albicans*.[112] Secretory and humoral anti-*Candida* IgA antibodies are generated.[121] Also, specific anti-*Candida* IgE antibodies are demonstrable.[115] Most normal adults have circulating IgG antibodies to *Candida* antigens.[169] Transient IgM antibody response occurs with the infection.[169] IgG antibodies effectively opsonize *C. albicans*. The organism activates the alternative complement pathway.[163] Polymorphonuclear leukocytes,[31] monocytes, and eosinophils[101, 102] ingest and kill *Candida*. A polysaccharide component of *C. albicans* can induce the formation of suppressor lymphocytes,[135] and mitogen-stimulated lymphocytes produce a lymphokine that kills the organism.[37] Unsaturated lactoferrin has antifungal activity that can be reversed with iron, an essential element for *Candida* growth.[91] The normal skin is resistant to colonization and infection with *Candida* species. Also, the ecology of the microbial flora of the skin and mucosal surfaces is an important defense system against *Candida* species.

The underlying diseases and immunocompromising factors that have been associated with increased susceptibility to candidiasis are noted in Table 199–1. A detailed review of disorders that predispose to candidiasis has been prepared by Odds.[128]

EPIDEMIOLOGY

Candida species of medical importance have a rather restricted distribution in nature and are found primarily in association with humans and other warm-blooded animals.[128] Even when *C. albicans* has been isolated from soil, foliage, or the atmosphere, it has been at sites where human or animal contamination was probable. *C. stellatoidea* has been isolated only from humans. From 1980 to 1989, the rates of disseminated candidiasis increased 11 times (from 0.013 to 0.15 case per 1000 admissions to United States hospitals).[45] During the 1990s, the rate of fungal liver infection (largely *Candida)* in 731 bone marrow transplantation patients has been 9 per cent.[146]

In considering colonization rates for *Candida* in persons without candidiasis, a distinction must be made between healthy infants and children and those who are hospitalized or suffering from an illness. Also, colonization varies with topographic sites. The frequency of *C. albicans* in isolates as determined in selected studies is given in Table 199–2.

C. albicans organisms, and in some instances other *Candida* species, have been isolated from monkeys, chimpanzees, baboons, gorillas, cats, dogs, goats, horses, pigs, sheep, cattle, mice, rats, rabbits, chickens, ducks, turkeys, pigeons, parrots, seagulls, sparrows, and other animals.[128]

The transmission of *Candida* under usual circumstances seems to require direct approximation of a colonized site with a susceptible mucous membrane or skin surface. Oral and cutaneous infections in the neonate are acquired from the infected vaginal mucosa during passage of the infant through the birth canal.[95, 123] Transmission between the breast

TABLE 199–2. Colonization Rates for *Candida albicans* in Persons without Evidence of Candidiasis

Site and Category	Number Studied	Patients with *C. albicans* (%)	Reference
Mouth			
Healthy children (5–18 yr)	503	5.4	Clayton and Noble, 1966[27]
Hospitalized children	200	46.0*	Marks et al., 1975[102]
Normal infants	68	17.6	Dixon et al., 1969[33]
Infants with skin lesions	117	30.6	Dixon et al., 1969[33]
Feces			
Healthy children (school age)	743	12.2	Pan and Pan, 1964[130]
Hospitalized children	86	16.3	Pan and Pan, 1964[130]
Normal infants	69	23.2	Pederson, 1969[133]
Infants with skin lesions	117	41.9	Dixon et al., 1969[33]
Skin			
Normal children	31	0.0	Hughes and Kim, 1973[73]
Fingers, normal children	407	0.6	Clayton and Noble, 1966[27]
Children, chronic leg disorders	86	3.5	Hughes and Kim, 1973[73]
Breast, women in labor	259	0.4	Gillespie et al., 1960[55]
Vagina			
Obstetric patients	1194	27.6	Hurley, 1966[75]
Obstetric patients	6629	21.8	Hurley et al., 1973[76]
Nonpregnant patients	81	24.7	Mardh et al., 1971[111]

*Includes all yeast isolates.

and infant's oral mucosa may result from breast feeding.[59] Intrauterine infection of the fetus is rare and has been attributed to ascending infection from the vagina of the mother, although transplacental transmission may be a possible route for infection.[36] Midgley and Clayton[120] readily were able to culture *C. albicans* from the air of rooms housing patients with cutaneous candidiasis. The significance of airborne transmission has not been established. Studies on infant-to-infant transmission of *Candida* in hospital nurseries indicate that cross-infection is uncommon and that segregation of infected infants with thrush has little impact on infection rates.[63, 96] However, recent epidemiologic studies using restriction-enzyme analyses have demonstrated that the organism may be acquired from the environment or from staff members in bone marrow transplant and neonatal intensive care units.[14, 147, 175]

Nosocomial candidiasis has been reported with increased frequency in recent years.[22, 125] Information from the National Nosocomial Infection Surveillance system during 1980 to 1990 noted a fivefold overall increase in the incidence of nosocomial blood stream infections.[9] A case-controlled study in nonleukemic, hospitalized patients identified seven risk factors for candidemia: (1) a central line, (2) a bladder catheter, (3) two or more antibiotics, (4) azotemia, (5) transfer from another hospital to a tertiary hospital, (6) diarrhea, and (7) candiduria.[22] New typing procedures for differentiating isolates of *C. albicans* with the use of DNA restriction-enzyme fragment analysis offer promise for more powerful epidemiologic studies.[50, 161]

PATHOGENESIS AND PATHOLOGY

The initial step in colonization is the adherence of *Candida* blastospores to the mucosal or dermal epithelial cells. Before, during, or after invasion, the filamentous or pseudohyphal form of the organism develops. This transformation may be related to the resistance factors or microenvironmental conditions of the host tissue.[40] As the infection is established, the cascade of events mentioned in the section on host susceptibility ensues, depending on the capabilities and the immunocompetence of the host. Invasion of the mucous membrane results in the formation of an adherent pseudomembrane composed of epithelial cells, leukocytes, keratin, and food debris associated with both blastospore and pseudohyphal forms of *Candida*. Especially in the intestinal tract, mucosal lesions progress to sharply demarcated ulcers, with a base of granulation tissue covered by a fibrinous exudate and granulocytes intermixed with the organisms. Dissemination of *Candida* to deep visceral organs likely is by hematogenous routes. One can deduce that the portal of entry for systemic infection primarily is from mucous membrane lesions. With systemic disease, the kidneys, lungs, liver, brain, and spleen are affected most frequently, although all organs of the body have been involved. With systemic disease, a pyogenic response occurs with microabscess formation. Granulomatous reactions can occur but are infrequent.

Recent studies have helped to elucidate the pathogenic mechanism of systemic candidiasis. Toxic components of *Candida* have been isolated by Iwata and Yamamoto[78] and others. This "canditoxin" is acutely toxic to mice. Glycoproteins isolated from *C. albicans* by these investigators may act to release histamine, which accounts for some of the clinical manifestations of the disease.

CLINICAL TYPES

Although *Candida* species may cause disease at any body site from scalp to toenail, certain areas are affected more frequently than are others. Also, the site and extent of the infection often serve as indicators of the immunocompetence of the host. For example, a healthy-appearing infant with oral thrush or cutaneous candidiasis of the diaper area usually has no underlying immunodeficiency disorder, whereas the patient with chronic mucocutaneous candidiasis or systemic candidiasis likely has a significant underlying abnormality. A topographic classification of candidiasis provides the most useful approach to the clinical features of the disease.

Oropharyngeal Candidiasis

Three patterns of oropharyngeal candidiasis have been described.

Thrush (Acute Pseudomembranous Candidiasis)

This is the most common type of candidiasis in infants and children. The lesions become visible as superficial strands or patches of pearly-white material on the mucosal surface, resembling curds of milk. These lesions may become confluent to form an adherent pseudomembrane composed of desquamated epithelial cells, leukocytes, keratin, necrotic tissue, and food deposits.[35] Blastospore and pseudohyphal forms are abundant, although these organisms rarely penetrate deeper than the stratum corneum. The subepithelial tissues may be involved, with edema and microabscesses. Removal of the pseudomembrane leaves a denuded erythematous lesion. In mild cases, the lesions are not painful. The most frequently involved sites are the buccal mucosa, dorsum, and lateral areas of the tongue, gingivae, and pharynx. *C. albicans* by far is the most frequent cause of thrush.

Acute Atrophic Candidiasis (Glossitis)

This lesion occurs as a result of antibiotic therapy and is manifested by erosions of the oral mucosa and depapillation of the dorsum of the tongue. The white pseudomembranous lesions are minimal or absent. The tongue appears smooth and erythematous. Glossodynia (painful tongue) is a frequent complaint. This lesion is believed to evolve from the effects of broad-spectrum, rarely narrow-spectrum, oral antibiotics on the bacterial flora of the mouth. The lesions and symptoms usually resolve after the discontinuation of antibiotics.

Angular Cheilosis (Perlèche)

This lesion is characterized by fissuring, erythema, and pain at the corners of the mouth. Perlèche results from habitual licking at the corners of the mouth, which provides a site for infection with *Candida*. The lesions may become granular, with shiny erythematous erosions and desquamation of the epithelium surrounded by hyperkeratosis.

Two additional *Candida* lesions of the mouth, leukoplakia and chronic atrophic candidiasis, are seen in adults but rarely in children.

Esophageal Candidiasis

The most frequent symptom of esophageal candidiasis is dysphagia. Pain may be experienced with swallowing or as a persistent retrosternal, paravertebral, intrascapular, or subscapular annoyance.[165] Nausea and vomiting may occur. Hematemesis and melena are rare. Approximately half of these patients have thrush.[151] Many patients experience no symptoms from esophageal candidiasis. In the immunocompromised host, concomitant infection with herpes simplex virus as well as bacteria may occur.[37] The site most frequently affected with *Candida* is the inferior one-third of the esophagus, although any area may be involved. Endoscopy reveals thrush-like lesions on an erythematous and friable mucosa. An esophagram with barium typically shows ulcerations of the mucosa, which produces a cobblestone-like pattern. In advanced lesions, edema and inflammation may result in tumor-like lesions or strictures. Perforation of the esophagus and fistulae may be found.

Gastrointestinal Candidiasis

The true incidence of gastric and intestinal candidiasis is not known. Cases that have been documented adequately have been associated with an underlying abnormality. Gastric lesions have been found predominantly in patients with peptic ulcers or malignancies and after gastric resection. Abdominal pain and weight loss have been noted in such cases.[165]

The association of clinical manifestations and intestinal candidiasis must be approached with caution. Whereas diarrhea and abdominal pain have been reported, substantiation of cause and effect is lacking. Kumar and colleagues[98] attributed the cause of diarrhea to *Candida* in 15 of 592 Indiana infants with diarrhea. They were of the opinion that the finding of pseudohyphal forms in fecal specimens was of diagnostic importance. A recent review of the literature concluded that the available data show a strong correlation between cessation of diarrhea in patients with *Candida* species in their stools and treatment with an antifungal drug compared with those not so treated.[104]

In 109 children with cancer and systemic candidiasis (deep organ involvement) studied ante mortem and at autopsy, *Candida* lesions were found in the esophagus in 49, stomach in 40, small intestine in 37, and colon in 48. Signs and symptoms could not be attributed accurately to these lesions.[69] More than 30 cases of biliary and gall bladder candidiasis have been reported.[126]

Peritoneal Candidiasis

Peritonitis caused by *Candida* species may occur as a complication of peritoneal dialysis or intestinal surgery or with bowel perforation. The typical signs for peritonitis may be absent.[77] Abdominal distention, fever, and vomiting may occur in some cases. Candidal infection of the peritoneal cavity tends to remain localized, and dissemination to other organs is uncommon.[12, 79, 156] Clinical features of fungal peritonitis cannot be differentiated from bacterial peritonitis, except by Gram stain and culture of peritoneal fluid.[39]

Candidiasis of the Urinary Tract

Candida may cause infections of the kidney, bladder, ureter, and urethra. The presence of *Candida* in voided urine is not uncommon in the immunocompromised host, in those receiving antibiotics, or in those with an indwelling catheter. There are no data to show that greater than or equal to 100,000 colonies of *Candida* species per milliliter of urine is more indicative of urinary tract infection than are lower counts.[128] The symptoms of urinary tract candidiasis are similar to those that occur with bacterial infections at respective sites.[44] Lesions similar to oral thrush may be seen by cystoscopy on the bladder mucosa with cystitis. Renal microabscesses, papillary necrosis, calyceal distortion, perinephritic abscesses, and obstructive lesions from a fungus ball may be caused by *Candida*. In 26 cases with candidiasis and candiduria at the Mayo Clinic, 23 (88 per cent) had urinary tract abnormalities.[2]

Vaginal Candidiasis

Vaginitis due to *C. albicans* is common and does not imply necessarily a serious underlying disease. Pruritus and vaginal discharge are the most frequent symptoms. The discharge is white and creamy or watery; the vaginal mucosa is erythematous, with typical lesions of thrush. Skin of the perineum may be involved, with intertriginous papular or ulcerative lesions.

Respiratory Tract Candidiasis

Candida may affect the respiratory tract in three ways: by colonization of the mucous membrane, by invasive infiltration of deeper tissues, and by an allergic response to the antigens. Any site may be involved. A distinct syndrome of extensive oral candidiasis and hoarseness has been described in patients undergoing immunosuppression therapy for cancer or HIV infection. In these children, discrete plaques can be visualized on the vocal cords by laryngoscopy.[99, 145]

Candidiasis limited to the bronchi is rare and is associated more frequently with pulmonary and systemic disease. Pulmonary candidiasis with invasion of the parenchyma may present as localized or diffuse pneumonia, nodular lesions, abscesses, or empyema.[61, 128, 173] Fever and tachypnea are frequent symptoms, and a definitive diagnosis requires an invasive procedure, such as an open lung biopsy, to demonstrate the organism in tissue.

Pulmonary allergy is not well defined, but several studies suggest that the entity exists. *C. albicans* has provoked asthmatic attacks in atopic persons.[84] Both polysaccharide and protein extracts of *C. albicans* have induced respiratory reactions.

Bone, Joint, and Muscle Candidiasis

Candida arthritis has been reported in patients ranging in age from newborns to elderly adults. In the majority of cases, the infection has been associated with systemic candidiasis. The knee has been the joint most frequently affected. Joints may be infected by direct inoculation, in association with osteomyelitis, or from hematogenous spread. Nonsystemic candidal infection after prosthetic arthroplasty has been reported in 10 cases.[30]

Candida osteomyelitis of the spine, wrist, femur, scapula, costochondral junction, humerus, mandible, ribs, and sternum has been reported.[38, 128] More than 22 cases of arthritis and osteomyelitis have been reported in infants younger than 14 weeks of age. Typically, the lesion is a fusiform swelling of the lower extremity and is warm to the touch; radiographs reveal osteolysis and cortical bone erosion.[168] Candidal infection of muscle has been described, in which pain has been the localized symptom.[3]

Cardiac Candidiasis

Candida species may invade the endocardium, myocardium, and pericardium. The clinical manifestations of *Can-*

dida endocarditis are similar to those found with subacute bacterial endocarditis. Unlike bacterial endocarditis, blood cultures frequently are sterile with the fungal infection. In a review of 319 cases of fungal endocarditis, *Candida* accounted for 67 per cent of cases.[116] Of 109 children with systemic candidiasis, 28 had cardiac lesions.[70] Whereas 5 (18 per cent) of the 28 children with carditis had indwelling central venous catheters, only 3 (3.7 per cent) of the 81 without cardiac involvement had catheters. Furthermore, an increase in the incidence of *Candida* carditis was related temporally to the introduction of central venous catheters into the clinical management of cancer patients. The valves most commonly involved are the aortic and mitral; however, infection of all areas of the heart has been described. Lesions of carditis include colonization and invasion of the endocardium with yeast and pseudohyphal forms, emboli occluding major arteries, necrosis, and microabscess formation. Nonspecific electrocardiographic changes with myocarditis include supraventricular arrhythmias, QRS changes, and marked T-wave changes.[52] Rarely, valvular lesions of *Candida* endocarditis may be discernible by two-dimensional echocardiography.

Central Nervous System Candidiasis

Primary candidiasis of the brain and meninges is rare, whereas the central nervous system (CNS) frequently is involved in disseminated candidiasis. In a review of 29,659 autopsies, Vorreith[166] found 7 (0.023 per cent) cases with CNS candidiasis; 5 of these also had other organs infected. Nearly a decade later, Parker and associates[131] reported the rate of 0.3 per cent of CNS candidiasis in 2040 autopsies. In recent studies of systemic candidiasis, one-fourth[70] to one-half[106] have had CNS involvement. It seems likely that the prevalence of CNS candidiasis is increasing and that, in almost all cases, other organs also are involved.

The neuropathologic lesions include macroabscesses and microabscesses, noncaseating granulomata, diffuse glial nodules, vasculitis, thrombosis, meningitis, ependymitis, mycotic aneurysm, densely packed balls of pseudohyphae, demyelination, and transverse myelitis.[106]

The clinical features are not well defined; they range from signs and symptoms of meningeal inflammation or encephalitis to no discernible CNS abnormality. With meningeal involvement, no more than half of patients have cerebrospinal fluid pleocytosis or hypoglycorrhachia. If present, the organisms can be visualized with Gram stain. Computed axial tomography often helps in revealing rather typical, well-demarcated, abscess-like lesions of the brain. The frequent concomitant occurrence of cardiac and CNS candidiasis dictates the need to evaluate patients for both lesions when one is found.

Ophthalmic Candidiasis

Candida keratitis may follow minor trauma but more frequently follows as a secondary invader of keratitis of other causes when topical antibiotics and corticosteroids are used.[177] In recent years, *Candida* endophthalmitis as a component of systemic candidiasis has been established clearly as a clinical entity—so much so that in any patient suspected of having systemic candidiasis, a careful examination of the retina is mandatory. The typical lesions are white, cottonlike, chorioretinal abnormalities that may extend to the vitreous. They often resemble a colony of *Candida* growing on blood agar. Color photographs of these lesions are provided in the paper by Fishman and colleagues.[46] Pain, blurred vision, "spots before the eyes," scotomata, and photophobia have been associated with the infection.

Candida endophthalmitis has been found frequently in patients receiving intravenous hyperalimentation. In a prospective study, Montgomerie and Edwards[124] found lesions in 5 of 25 such patients, and Henderson and associates[64] reported that 13 (9 per cent) of 131 postoperative patients receiving hyperalimentation developed the lesion. In a careful study of 10 low-birth-weight infants with systemic candidiasis, 4 had retinal lesions.[7] It seems wise routinely to monitor patients in these high-risk categories with careful ophthalmoscopic examination. Retinal infections may occur in other immunocompromised patients with systemic candidiasis. Some experimental evidence suggests that such lesions may not be discernible readily in severely neutropenic patients, possibly because of the lack of inflammatory response.[65]

Cutaneous Candidiasis

The primary cutaneous infections due to *Candida* are described in Chapter 70.

Acute Disseminated (Systemic) Candidiasis

Disseminated candidiasis may involve any tissue of the body, but in most cases the infection is predominant in two or three organs. The term disseminated is used to designate disease in which deep organs of the body are infected with *Candida*. The portal of entry usually is lesions of the gastrointestinal tract or oral mucosa or skin puncture sites, and organisms are disseminated by the hematogenous route to the tissues of one or more organs. Transient "candidemia" may occur without discernible foci of infection. In severely immunocompromised patients, however, the majority with candidemia have disseminated disease.[175] The most frequent sites of infection in patients with disseminated candidiasis include the lungs, kidneys, liver, spleen, and brain. The clinical manifestations depend on the sites involved and the extent of involvement. The aforementioned descriptions of topographic infections apply to organs involved with disseminated candidiasis. Infants with the disseminated disease appear clinically similar to those with sepsis due to other organisms.

Those with underlying conditions who are more likely to have disseminated candidiasis include cancer patients, recipients of organ transplants, debilitated premature infants, patients with indwelling central venous catheters and hyperalimentation lines, and patients with immunodeficiency disorders who have undergone complicated major surgery.

Two clinical manifestations of disseminated candidiasis strongly indicate this infection. One of these is the ocular lesions of *Candida* endophthalmitis described earlier; the other is a maculopapular rash. The skin lesions have been found in patients with hematologic malignancies. In one study, 10 (13 per cent) of 77 patients with disseminated candidiasis and cancer had cutaneous lesions.[18, 85] Typically, the discrete, firm, erythematous papules measure 0.5 to 1.0 cm in diameter. A nodular center often is surrounded by an erythematous halo. The rash may be generalized, and biopsy specimens show yeast and pseudohyphal forms.

Mycotic cervical lymphadenitis after oral mucositis and neutropenia has been observed in children with cancer and may herald systemic candidiasis.[152] In recent years, disseminated candidiasis has become more prevalent in low-birth-weight infants who require intensive care management. In the study by Baley and associates,[7] the infants had one or more of the following clinical abnormalities: respiratory deterioration, abdominal distention, melena, carbohydrate intolerance, hypotension, candiduria, endophthalmitis, meningitis, skin abscesses, temperature instability, or erythematous rash. The mean age at time of diagnosis was 1 month. In other cases, carditis, arthritis, and osteomyelitis have occurred.[81] *C. albicans* is the most frequent cause, but other *Candida* species also may cause the infection.

Of the organ transplant recipients, those undergoing bone marrow transplantation are at greatest risk for disseminated candidiasis. In an autopsy study of 266 bone marrow transplant recipients, 23 had disseminated candidiasis.[28] The incidence was higher in those with aplastic anemia (17.5 per cent) than in those with hematologic malignancies (5.9 per cent).

A study of 109 children with disseminated candidiasis and cancer provides some insight into the clinical features of the infection.[70] These cases were evaluated for 2 months before death, and clinical manifestation was compared with autopsy findings. Fever, granulocytopenia, relapse of the malignancy, and therapy with antibiotics and immunosuppressive drugs made up the clinical profile in about 90 per cent of the cases. The major organs involved, in order of highest frequency, were the lungs, spleen, kidney, liver, heart, and brain. In 88 per cent of these cases, more than one organ was involved, excluding the gastrointestinal tract, many of which were not apparent from clinical evaluation. For example, in half the patients with *Candida* infection of the pulmonary parenchyma, the lesions were not detectable by radiographs made within the last 10 days of life, whereas 93 per cent of the pulmonary lesions were grossly visible at autopsy. Renal and hepatic function tests were normal in half the patients with candidiasis of these organs. Candiduria was not a dependable indicator of systemic or renal disease. *Candida* carditis was more frequent in patients with indwelling central venous catheters.

Despite frequent sampling with antemortem blood cultures (1032 specimens), only 17 per cent of patients yielded the organism. However, 93 per cent of these children were colonized at one or more sites with *Candida* species. Recent studies have shown an increased incidence of hematogenous candidiasis in pediatric patients who are colonized at multiple sites compared with those who are not colonized.[113, 114] It is important to note that candidiasis was the cause of death in only 15 per cent of cases. This statistic underscores the need for thorough and repeated evaluation of patients with systemic candidiasis for concomitant infections, especially those of bacterial origin. Other studies have noted similar findings.[109]

DIAGNOSIS

The diagnosis of candidiasis basically requires the association of clinical observations with laboratory tests for the isolation and identification of the organism. In some types of candidiasis, a biopsy may be required to demonstrate the causative organism in diseased tissue.

Direct microscopic examination of materials swabbed or scraped from surface lesions, fluids aspirated from closed lesions, or imprints from biopsy specimens may help to quickly establish a diagnosis. Specimens from surface lesions can be mounted in 10 to 20 per cent potassium hydroxide to reveal the ovoid budding yeast cells approximately 3 to 7 μm in diameter, pseudohyphae, or both. The organisms stain well with periodic acid–Schiff, Gomori methenamine silver nitrate, toluidine blue, or Gram stains. Even typical organisms only tentatively can be identified as *Candida*. In some preparations, it may be difficult to differentiate *Aspergillus, Trichosporon,* and *Geotrichum* species from *Candida.*

In biopsy specimens, the early tissue reaction is acute suppurative inflammation that may progress to granulomatous inflammation. Microabscess formation is frequent. Both yeast and pseudohyphae are found in the diseased tissue.

Candida species may be cultured on Sabouraud dextrose media. If specimens are likely to be contaminated with bacteria, chloramphenicol should be incorporated into the media. Cycloheximide, sometimes included in media to prevent saprophytic fungal overgrowth, should not be used because it may inhibit some strains of *Candida.* Blood culture bottles should be vented for optimal growth, although some strains may grow anaerobically. A radiometric blood culture system was found to provide earlier identification of *Candida* and other yeasts than is obtained with the more standard methods.[68] The lysis-centrifugation (Isolator) blood culture method also is reported to improve detection of *Candida* species compared with standard methods.[62, 89] On solid media, *Candida* species appear as white or cream-colored colonies that are moist and pasty with well-demarcated borders. In contrast with most other species, *C. albicans* produces germ tubes when suspended in human serum, or serum from certain lower animals, for a period of 1 to 4 hours. Biochemical fermentation and assimilation tests serve specifically to identify *Candida* species.

Many serologic tests for antibody to *Candida* have been studied, but, to date, none has proved useful for the specific diagnosis of candidiasis. In recent years, attention has been directed to the detection of antigenic components and metabolic products of *Candida* in blood and other body fluids of patients with systemic forms of candidiasis. Techniques such as precipitation, agglutination, enzyme-linked immunosorbent assay, counterimmunoelectrophoresis, gas-liquid chromatography, and radioimmunoassay have been applied. Techniques for the detection of mannan,[105, 170] cytoplasmic antigen,[4] and D-arabinitol[87] offer promise but have not been perfected for general application in the diagnosis of candidiasis of deep organs. Most recently, preliminary studies of polymerase chain reaction have proven successful in identifying clinical specimens with *Candida.*[23, 67]

A definitive diagnosis of deep-organ or disseminated candidiasis is difficult to establish. Cultivation of *Candida* from otherwise sterile body fluids (blood, spinal fluid, bone marrow) with compatible clinical features in an immunocompromised patient, in whom other causes of infection have been excluded, warrants the diagnosis. Computed axial tomography scans especially are helpful in recognizing involvement of the liver, spleen, kidneys, or brain. Lesions at these sites sufficiently are characteristic for a presumptive diagnosis.[11] In patients with hematologic malignancies requiring frequent bone marrow examination, routine cultures of the marrow occasionally reveal *Candida* species of clinical significance.[69]

TREATMENT AND PREVENTION

Several drugs are available for the treatment of candidiasis. Selection of the appropriate drug, or drug combination, depends on the location and extent of infection. Anti-*Candida* drugs in general use include nystatin, clotrimazole, gentian violet, amphotericin B, flucytosine, miconazole, fluconazole, and ketoconazole.[29] Itraconazole is effective in vitro but has not been studied adequately in patients. See Chapter 70 for discussion of the treatment of cutaneous candidiasis.

Oropharyngeal candidiasis usually responds to the administration of nystatin oral suspension, 200,000 U every 4 to 6 hours for at least 1 week or longer. The suspension is swished in the mouth for 5 minutes or longer and then swallowed. In infants and patients not able to retain the drug in the mouth, the dose should be given at least six times daily. Clotrimazole also is effective and is given as a 10-mg dissolvable tablet five or six times daily. The tablet is held in the mouth until it is dissolved completely.[174] Alternatively, a vaginal suppository of nystatin, 100,000 units every 4 hours, may be held in the mouth until it is dissolved.[35] Gentian violet as a 0.5 or 1.0 per cent solution swabbed onto the buccal mucosa twice daily is moderately effective but causes irritation and ulceration of the mucosa with prolonged use. Ketoconazole, 200 mg/m^2/day given orally in two doses for 2 weeks, causes regression of lesions in about three-fourths of patients, but culturable organisms remain in approximately 60 per cent of patients with oral thrush.[72] Fluconazole suspension given as a 6-mg/kg dose followed by a single daily dose of 3 mg/kg for 13 days has proved superior to nystatin for the treatment of oropharyngeal candidiasis in immunocompromised children, including those undergoing cancer therapy or with HIV infection.[49] Severe cases of oral candidiasis, especially in granulocytopenic patients, may benefit from short courses of amphotericin B, 0.5 mg/kg/day intravenously for 3 to 5 days. With bottle- or breast-fed and thumb-sucking infants, these respective sites may be colonized with *Candida;* nystatin cream applied four to six times daily to the skin areas and boiling of bottle nipples (or using disposable nipples) are important techniques in management. Avoidance of antibacterial drugs also is desirable.

Vaginal candidiasis is treated equally well with clotrimazole, miconazole, or nystatin suppositories. Butoconazole cream also is effective.[66] Oral fluconazole in a single dose of 150 mg successfully treats vaginal candidiasis in adults.[127, 134]

Esophageal, gastric, and intestinal candidiasis can be treated as described for oral candidiasis, with the exception of gentian violet. Patients with mild cases may respond to oral nystatin or clotrimazole. In moderately severe and severe cases of esophageal candidiasis, fluconazole or intravenous amphotericin B should be administered to the patient because this site is prone to complications of stricture, secondary infection, and perforation. If the patient does not have an indwelling catheter and the infection is due to susceptible *C. albicans* (minimal inhibitory concentration $<$1.25 μg/mL), flucytosine, 150 mg/kg/day in four divided doses, is recommended. A course of 2 weeks' treatment usually is adequate, but the treatment should be shortened or extended on the basis of clinical response and immunocompetence of the host. An alternative to amphotericin B is oral ketoconazole or intravenous miconazole. These drugs are less toxic than is amphotericin B, although less experience has been accumulated in their use for esophageal candidiasis.[165]

Candida cystitis, without renal or systemic involvement, can be treated with flucytosine orally, bladder irrigation with amphotericin B, or a combination of these drugs.[51, 166] Isolated candiduria has been treated successfully with short courses of intravenous amphotericin B (less than 10 days) in cases in which the therapy mentioned earlier was not successful.[93] With an indwelling catheter, continuous or intermittent irrigation with a solution of 50 μg/mL of amphotericin B in sterile water should be used.[149] The duration of treatment required can be determined by cultured monitoring of urine samples. In patients with renal candidiasis and in those in whom disseminated infection is suspected, intravenous amphotericin B with flucytosine (if the strain is susceptible) provides the most effective treatment, and 4 to 6 weeks of therapy usually is required.

Patients with systemic candidiasis, as well as those with *Candida* ophthalmitis, endocarditis, meningitis, or pneumonitis, must be treated with amphotericin B intravenously for at least 1 month. Because some synergy may exist with amphotericin B and flucytosine,[117] this combination is recommended for all patients as optimal therapy. The studies of Smego and associates[154] show that the combination especially is important in the treatment of *Candida* meningitis. Amphotericin B penetrates into the spinal fluid poorly, whereas effective spinal fluid levels of flucytosine easily are achievable. Patients should be maintained on 0.5 to 1.0 mg/kg/day of amphotericin B as a daily infusion over 4 to 6 hours and 150 mg/kg/day of flucytosine orally in four equally divided doses. Treatment should be continued for at least 1 month and for longer in complicated cases. Antibiotics and immunosuppressive drugs should be avoided if possible.

Butler and associates[24] treated neonates with systemic candidiasis successfully using amphotericin B alone. If it was associated with a central intravascular catheter, the candidemia was treated with a total course dose of 10 to 15 mg/kg amphotericin B and removal of the device. Similar success with short courses of intravenous amphotericin B (7 to 14 days after sterilization of blood) has been reported after removal of infection-associated devices.[34] For severe, disseminated candidiasis, a total course dose of 25 to 30 mg/kg was used.

Systemic candidiasis treated with intravenous miconazole is followed by recovery in only 20[17] to 37 per cent[83] of patients. In a comparative study of ketoconazole and amphotericin B in the treatment of serious *Candida* infections, the response rate was 45 per cent with amphotericin B and 24 per cent with ketoconazole.[44]

In febrile, granulocytopenic ($<$500 granulocytes/mm^3) cancer patients with no causative agent identified and whose infections fail to respond to broad-spectrum antibiotics within a week or so, the likelihood of systemic fungal infection is sufficient (about 30 per cent of cases) to warrant consideration of empiric amphotericin B therapy.[71, 136] A study of 206 adults with neutropenia and candidemia randomized to receive amphotericin B or fluconazole showed that the treatments were successful in 79 per cent and 70 per cent of the patients, respectively ($p = 0.22$).[141] The use of colony-stimulating factors has not been studied adequately in such patients but may offer promise in management.

Of considerable concern is the report by Powderly and associates,[139] showing that some *Candida* species isolated from severely immunocompromised patients with systemic candidiasis were resistant to the usual concentrations of amphotericin B attainable in vivo. All episodes of candidemia due to isolates with minimal inhibitory concentrations greater than 0.8 μg/mL of amphotericin B were fatal, whereas one-half of those with minimal inhibitory concentrations of 0.8 μg/mL and less recovered. A more recent study by Rex and associates,[140] using the National Committee for Clinical Laboratory Standards method, failed to demonstrate that the results of in vitro susceptibility testing for amphotericin B and fluconazole predicted outcome of therapy for patients with candidemia.

Attempts to prevent *Candida* infection have not proved highly successful. Perhaps efforts to minimize the factors that predispose to candidiasis are the most productive. Several studies have evaluated the administration of antifungal drugs prophylactically to patients at high risk for the infection; generally, the results have not provided clear-cut directions. Ketoconazole has been compared with nystatin in patients with granulocytopenia. One study[82] reported ketoconazole to be somewhat more advantageous than nystatin; another study found them equally effective. However, fungal infections occurred during the use of either of the drugs.[118]

The most convincing study, prospective and with double-blind control, showed clotrimazole troches (10 mg three times a day) to be effective in preventing oral candidiasis in renal transplant recipients.[129] However, the recent study by Wingard and associates[171] shows the complexity of prophylaxis. In their study, fluconazole prophylaxis in bone marrow transplant recipients led to a reduction in disseminated *C. albicans* and *C. tropicalis* infections but a sevenfold increase in *C. krusei* infections. Winston and associates,[173] in a placebo-controlled study, were not able to show a reduction in invasive fungal infections, mortality, or the use of amphotericin B with fluconazole prophylaxis in leukemic patients. A similar study by Slavin and associates,[153] in bone marrow transplantation, showed a significant reduction of systemic fungal infection when fluconazole prophylaxis was used.

References

1. Ahonen, P., Myllärniemi, S., Sipila, I., et al.: Clinical variation of autoimmune polyendocrinopathy-candidiasis-ectodermal dystrophy (APECED) in a series of 68 patients. N. Engl. J. Med. *322*:1829, 1990.
2. Ang, B. S. P., Telenti, A., King, B., et al.: Candidemia from a urinary tract source: Microbiological aspects and clinical significance. Clin. Infect. Dis. *17*:662, 1993.
3. Anttila, V.-J., Ruutu, P., Bondestam, S., et al.: Hepatosplenic yeast infection in patients with acute leukemia: A diagnostic problem. Clin. Infect. Dis. *18*:979, 1994.
4. Araj, G. F., Hopfer, R. L., Chestnut, S., et al.: Diagnostic value of the enzyme-linked immunoadsorbent assay for detection of *Candida albicans* cytoplasmic antigen in sera of cancer patients. J. Clin. Microbiol. *16*:46, 1982.
5. Arena, F. P., Perlin, M., and Brahman, H.: Fever, rash and myalgias of disseminated candidiasis during antifungal therapy. Arch. Intern. Med. *141*:1233, 1981.
6. Atkinson, K., Storb, R., Prentice, R. L., et al.: Analysis of late infections in 89 long-term survivors of bone marrow transplantation. Blood *53*:720, 1979.
7. Baley, J. E., Kliegman, R. M., and Faranoff, A. A.: Disseminated fungal infection in very low-birth-weight infants: Clinical manifestations and epidemiology. Pediatrics *73*:144, 1984.
8. Baley, J. E., and Silverman, R. A.: Systemic candidiasis: Cutaneous manifestations in low birth weight infants. Pediatrics *82*:211, 1988.
9. Banerjee, S. N., Emori, T. G., and Culver, D. H.: Secular trends in nosocomial primary bloodstream infection in the United States, 1980–1989. Am. J. Med. *91*(Suppl. 3B):86S, 1991.
10. Barbhaiya, H. C.: Antifungal prophylaxis during antibiotic therapy. Indian J. Med. Sci. *20*:145, 1966.
11. Bartley, D. L., Hughes, W. T., Parvey, L. S., et al.: Computed tomography of hepatic and splenic fungal abscesses in leukemic children. Pediatr. Infect. Dis. *1*:317, 1982.
12. Bayer, A. S., Blumenkrantz, M. J., Montgomerie, J. Z., et al.: *Candida* peritonitis: Report of 22 cases and review of the English literature. Am. J. Med. *61*:832, 1976.
13. Bernhardt, H. E., Orlando, J. C., Benfield, J. R., et al.: Disseminated candidiasis in surgical patients. Surg. Gynecol. Obstet. *134*:819, 1972.
14. Betremieux, P., Chevrier, S., Quindos, G., et al.: Use of DNA fingerprinting and biotyping methods to study a *Candida albicans* outbreak in a neonatal intensive care unit. Pediatr. Infect. Dis. J. *13*:899, 1994.
15. Bland, P. B., Rakoff, A. E., and Pincus, I. J.: Experimental vaginal and cutaneous moniliasis: Clinical and laboratory study of certain monilias associated with vaginal, oral and cutaneous thrush. Arch. Dermatol. Syph. *36*:760, 1937.
16. Bodey, G. P.: Fungal infections complicating acute leukemia. J. Chronic Dis. *19*:667, 1966.
17. Bodey, G. P.: Candidiasis in cancer patients. Am. J. Med. *77*:13, 1984.
18. Bodey, G. P., and Luna, M.: Skin lesions associated with disseminated candidiasis. J. A. M. A. *229*:1466, 1974.
19. Boggs, D. R., Williams, A. F., and Howell, A.: Thrush in malignant neoplastic disease. Arch. Intern. Med. *107*:354, 1961.
20. Botas, C. M., Kurlat, I., Young, S. M., et al.: Disseminated candidal infections and intravenous hydrocortisone in preterm infants. Pediatrics *95*:883, 1995.
21. Bourg, R.: Les candidiases vaginales ont-elles une incidence hormonale? Bull. Acad. R. Med. Belge *7*:699, 1964.
22. Bross, J., Talbot, G. H., Maislin, G., et al.: Risk factors for nosocomial candidemia: A case-control study in adults without leukemia. Am. J. Med. *87*:614, 1989.
23. Burgener-Kairuz, P., Zuber, J. P., Jaunin, P., et al.: Rapid detection and identification of *Candida albicans* and *Torulopsis (Candida) glabrata* in clinical specimens by species-specific nested PCR amplification of a cytochrome P-450 lanosterol-alpha-demethylase (L1A1) gene fragment. J. Clin. Microbiol. *32*:1902, 1994.
24. Butler, K. M., Rench, M. A., and Baker, C. J.: Amphotericin B as a single agent in the treatment of systemic candidiasis in neonates. Pediatr. Infect. Dis. *9*:51, 1990.
25. Caruso, L. J.: Vaginal moniliasis after tetracycline therapy. Am. J. Obstet. Gynecol. *90*:374, 1964.
26. Chen, T. Y., and Webster, J. H.: Oral monilia study on patients with head and neck cancer during radiotherapy. Cancer *34*:246, 1974.
27. Clayton, Y. M., and Noble, W. C.: Observations on the epidemiology of *Candida albicans*. J. Clin. Pathol. *19*:76, 1966.
28. Clift, R. A.: Candidiasis in the transplant patient. Am. J. Med. *77*:34, 1984.
29. Como, J. A., and Dismukes, W. E.: Oral azole drugs as systemic antifungal therapy. N. Engl. J. Med. *330*:263, 1994.
30. Darouiche, R. O., Hamill, R. J., Musher, D. M., et al.: Periprosthetic candidal infections following arthroplasty. Rev. Infect. Dis. *11*:89, 1989.
31. Diamond, R. D., Krzesicki, R., and Wellington, J.: Damage to pseudohyphal forms of *Candida albicans* by neutrophils in the absence of serum in vitro. J. Clin. Invest. *61*:349, 1978.
32. Diddle, A. W., Gardner, W. H., Williamson, P. J., et al.: Oral contraceptive medication and vulvovaginal candidiasis. Obstet. Gynecol. *34*:373, 1969.
33. Dixon, P. N., Warin, R. P., and English, M. P.: Role of *Candida albicans* infection in napkin rashes. B. M. J. *2*:23, 1969.
34. Donowitz, L. G., and Hendley, J. O.: Short-course amphotericin B therapy for candidemia in pediatric patients. Pediatrics *95*:888, 1995.
35. Dreizen, S.: Oral candidiasis. Am. J. Med. *77*:28, 1984.
36. Dvorak, A. M., and Gavaller, B.: Congenital systemic candidiasis. N. Engl. J. Med. *274*:540, 1966.
37. Edwards, J. E.: *Candida* species. *In* Mandell, G. L., Douglas, R. G., and Bennett, J. E. (eds.): Principles and Practice of Infectious Diseases. 2nd ed. New York, John Wiley & Sons, 1985, pp. 1435–1447.
38. Edwards, J. E., Lehrer, R. I., Stiehm, E. R., et al.: Severe candidal infections: Clinical perspective, immune defense mechanisms, and current concepts of therapy. Am. J. Med. *89*:91, 1978.
39. Eisenberg, E. S., Leviton, I., and Soeiro, R.: Fungal peritonitis in patients receiving peritoneal dialysis: Experience with 11 patients and review of the literature. Rev. Infect. Dis. *8*:309, 1986.
40. Epstein, J. B., Truelove, E. L., and Izutzu, K. T.: Oral candidiasis: Pathogenesis and host defense. Rev. Infect. Dis. *6*:96, 1984.
41. Fainstein, V., Elting, L., McCredie, K., et al.: Ketoconazole versus amphotericin B in the treatment of antibiotic resistance foci in neutropenic cancer patients. 23rd Interscience Conference on Antimicrobial Agents and Chemotherapy, 1983, p. 265. Abstract 979.
42. Fiax, R. G.: Systemic *Candida* infections in infants in intensive care nurseries: High incidence of central nervous system involvement. J. Pediatr. *105*:616, 1984.
43. Fiax, R. G.: Invasive neonatal candidiasis: Comparison of *albicans* and *parapsilosis* infection. Pediatr. Infect. Dis. J. *11*:88, 1992.
44. Fisher, J. F., Chew, W. H., Shadomy, S., et al.: Urinary tract infection due to *Candida albicans*. Rev. Infect. Dis. *4*:1107, 1982.
45. Fisher-Hoch, S. P., and Hutwagner, L.: Opportunistic candidiases: An epidemic of the 1980s. Clin. Infect. Dis. *21*:897, 1995.
46. Fishman, L. S., Griffin, J. R., Sapico, F. L., et al.: Hematogenous *Candida* endophthalmitis: A complication of candidemia. N. Engl. J. Med. *286*:675, 1972.
47. Fitzpatrick, J. J., and Topley, H. E.: Ampicillin therapy and *Candida* outgrowth. Am. J. Med. Sci. *252*:310, 1966.
48. Fletcher, J., Mather, J., Lewis, M. J., et al.: Mouth lesions in iron-deficiency anemia: Relationship to *Candida albicans* in saliva and the impairment of lymphocyte transformation. J. Infect. Dis. *131*:44, 1975.
49. Flynn, P. M., Cunningham, C. K., Kerkering, T., et al.: Oropharyngeal candidiasis in immunocompromised children: A randomized, multicenter, study of orally administered fluconazole suspension versus nystatin. J. Pediatr. *127*:322, 1995.
50. Fox, B. C., Mobley, H. L. T., and Wade, J. C.: The use of a DNA probe for epidemiological studies of candidiasis in immunocompromised hosts. J. Infect. Dis. *159*:488, 1989.
51. Fan-Haward, P., O'Donovan, C., Smith, S. M., et al.: Oral fluconazole versus amphotericin B bladder irrigation for treatment of candidal funguria. Clin. Infect. Dis. *21*:960, 1995.
52. Franklin, W. G., Simon, A. B., and Sodeman, T. M.: *Candida* myocarditis without valvulitis. Am. J. Cardiol. *38*:924, 1976.
53. Freeman, J. B., Lemire, A., and Maclean, L. D.: Intravenous alimentation and septicemia. Surg. Gynecol. Obstet. *135*:708, 1972.
54. Gaines, J. D., and Remington, J. S.: Disseminated candidiasis in the surgical patient. Surgery *72*:730, 1972.
55. Gillespie, H. L., Inmon, W. B., and Slater, V.: Incidence of *Candida* in the vagina during pregnancy: Study utilizing the Pagano-Levin culture medium. Obstet. Gynecol. *16*:185, 1960.
56. Giombetti, R., Hagstrom, J. W. C., Landey, S., et al.: Cushing's syndrome in infancy: A case complicated by monilial endocarditis. Am. J. Dis. Child. *122*:264, 1971.
57. Glew, R. H., Buckley, H. R., Rosen, H. M., et al.: Value of prospective

Candida precipitins in fungemia in patients with hyperalimentation. Surg. Forum 26:113, 1975.

58. Godfrey, S., Hambleton, G., and König, P.: Steroid aerosols and candidiasis. B. M. J. 2:387, 1974.
59. Gonzalez-Ochoa, A., and Dominiguez, L.: Algunas observaciones epidimiologicas y patogenicas sobre la moniliasis oral del recien nacido. Rev. Inst. Salub. Enprm. Trop. 17:1, 1957.
60. Goodrich, J. M., Reed, E. C., Mori, M., et al.: Clinical features and analysis of risk factors for invasive candidal infection after marrow transplantation. J. Infect. Dis. 164:731, 1991.
61. Gottlieb, M. S., Schroff, R., Schauber, H. M., et al.: *Pneumocystis carinii* pneumonia and mucosal candidiasis in previously healthy homosexual men. N. Engl. J. Med. 305:1425, 1981.
62. Guerra-Romero, L., Edson, R. S., Cockerill, F. R., III, et al.: Comparison of DuPont Isolator and Roche Septi-Chek for detection of fungemia. J. Clin. Microbiol. 25:1623, 1987.
63. Harris, L. J.: Further observations on a simple procedure to eliminate thrush from hospital nurseries. Am. J. Obstet. Gynecol. 80:30, 1959.
64. Henderson, D. K., Edwards, J. E., and Montgomerie, J. Z.: Hematogenous *Candida* endophthalmitis in patients receiving parenteral hyperalimentation fluids. J. Infect. Dis. 143:655, 1981.
65. Henderson, D. K., Edwards, J. E., Jr., Ishida, K., et al.: Experimental hematogenous *Candida* endophthalmitis diagnostic approaches. Infect. Immun. 23:858, 1979.
66. Hesseltine, H. C.: Specific therapy for vaginal mycosis. Am. J. Obstet. Gynecol. 70:403, 1955.
67. Holmes, A. R., Cannon, R. D., Shepherd, M. G., et al.: Detection of *Candida albicans* and other yeasts in blood by PCR. J. Clin. Microbiol. 32:228, 1994.
68. Hopfer, R. L., Orengo, A., Chestnut, S., et al.: Radiometric detection of yeasts in blood cultures of cancer patients. J. Clin. Microbiol. 12:329, 1980.
69. Hughes, W. T.: Leukemia monitoring with fungal bone marrow cultures. J. A. M. A. 218:441, 1971.
70. Hughes, W. T.: Systemic candidiasis: A study of 109 fatal cases. Pediatr. Infect. Dis. 1:11, 1982.
71. Hughes, W. T., Armstrong, D., Bodey, G. P., et al.: Guidelines for the use of antimicrobial agents in neutropenic patients with unexplained fever. J. Infect. Dis. 161:381, 1990.
72. Hughes, W. T., Bartley, D. L., Patterson, G. G., et al.: Ketoconazole and candidiasis: A controlled study. J. Infect. Dis. 147:1060, 1983.
73. Hughes, W. T., and Kim, H. K.: Mycoflora in cystic fibrosis: Some ecologic aspects of *Pseudomonas aeruginosa* and *Candida albicans*. Mycopathol. Mycol. Appl. 50:261, 1973.
74. Hung, W., Migeon, C. J., and Parrott, R. H.: Possible autoimmune basis for Addison's disease in three siblings, one with idiopathic hypoparathyroidism, pernicious anemia and superficial moniliasis. N. Engl. J. Med. 269:65–68, 1963.
75. Hurley, R.: Pathogenicity of genus *Candida*. *In* Weiner, H. I., and Hurley, R. (eds.): Symposium on *Candida* Infections. London, Livingstone, 1966, pp. 13–25.
76. Hurley, R., Leask, B. G. S., Faktor, J. A., et al.: Incidence and distribution of yeast species and *Trichomonas vaginalis* in the vagina of pregnant women. J. Obstet. Gynaecol. Br. Commonw. 80:252, 1973.
77. Hurwich, B. J.: Monilial peritonitis. Arch. Intern. Med. 117:405, 1966.
78. Iwata, K., and Yamamoto, Y.: Glycoprotein toxins produced by *Candida albicans*. *In* The Black and White Yeasts. Proceedings of the Fourth International Conference on the Mycoses, Pan American Health Organizations Scientific Publ. No. 356. Washington, D.C., 1978, pp. 246–257.
79. Jacobs, L. G., Skidmore, E. A., Cardoso, L. A., and Ziv, F.: Bladder irrigation with amphotericin B for treatment of fungal urinary tract infections. Clin. Infect. Dis. 18:313, 1994.
80. Johnson, D. E., Conroy, M. M., Foker, J. E., et al.: *Candida* peritonitis in the newborn infant. J. Pediatr. 97:298, 1980.
81. Johnson, D. E., Thompson, T. R., Green, T. P., et al.: Systemic candidiasis in very low-birth-weight infants (<1500 grams). Pediatrics 73:138, 1984.
82. Jones, P. G., Kauffman, C. A., McAuliffe, L., et al.: Ketoconazole vs. nystatin for prevention of fungal infections in neutropenic patients. 23rd Interscience Conference on Antimicrobial Agents and Chemotherapy, 1983, p. 265. Abstract 982.
83. Jordan, W. M., Bodey, G. P., Rodriguez, V., et al.: Miconazole therapy for the treatment of fungal infections in cancer patients. Antimicrob. Agents Chemother. 16:792, 1979.
84. Kabe, J., Aoki, Y., Ishizaki, T., et al.: Relationship of dermal and pulmonary sensitivity to extracts of *Candida albicans*. Am. Rev. Respir. Dis. 104:348, 1971.
85. Kaidbey, K. H., and Kurban, A. K.: Unusual granuloma of the skin seen in Lebanon. Acta Derm. Venereol. 51:225, 1971.
86. Kan, V. L.: Polymerase chain reaction for the diagnosis of candidemia. J. Infect. Dis. 168:779, 1993.
87. Kiehn, T. E., Bernard, E. M., Gold, J. W. M., et al.: Candidiasis detection by gas-liquid chromatography of d-arabinitol, a fungal metabolite, in human serum. Science 206:577, 1979.
88. King, R. D., Lee, J. C., and Morris, A. L.: Adherence of *Candida albicans* and other *Candida* species to mucosal epithelial cells. Infect. Immun. 27:667, 1980.
89. Kirkley, B. A., Easley, K. A., and Washington, J. A.: Controlled clinical evaluation of Isolator and EXP aerobic blood systems for detection of bloodstream infections. J. Clin. Microbiol. 32:1547, 1994.
90. Kirkpatrick, C. H.: Host factors in defense against fungal infections. Am. J. Med. 77:1, 1984.
91. Kirkpatrick, C. H., Green, I., Rich, R. R., et al.: Inhibition of growth of *Candida albicans* by iron-insaturated lactoferrin: Relation to host defense mechanisms in chronic mucocutaneous candidiasis. J. Infect. Dis. 124:539, 1971.
92. Klein, J. D., Yamauchi, T., and Horlick, S. P.: Neonatal candidiasis, meningitis, and arthritis: Observation and a review of the literature. J. Pediatr. 81:31, 1972.
93. Kohn, D. B., Uehling, D. T., Peters, M. E., et al.: Short-course amphotericin B therapy for isolated candiduria in children. J. Pediatr. 110:310, 1987.
94. Kostiala, I., Kostiala, A. A., Kahanpää, A., et al.: Acute fungal stomatitis in patients with hematologic malignancies: Quantity and species of fungi. J. Infect. Dis. 146:101, 1982.
95. Kozinin, P. J., Taschdjian, C. L., and Wiener, H.: Incidence and pathogenesis of neonatal candidiasis. Pediatrics 21:421, 1958.
96. Kozinin, P. J., Wiener, H., Taschdjian, C. L., et al.: Is isolation of infants with thrush necessary? J. A. M. A. 170:1172, 1959.
97. Krause, W., Matheis, H., and Wulf, K.: Fungaemia and funguria after oral administration of *Candida albicans*. Lancet 1:598, 1969.
98. Kumar, V., Chandrasekaran, R., and Kumar, L.: *Candida* diarrhea. Lancet 1:752, 1976.
99. Lawson, R., Bodey, G., and Luna, M.: Case report: *Candida* infection presenting as laryngitis. Am. J. Med. Sci. 280:173, 1980.
100. Lehner, T., and Ward, R. G.: Iatrogenic oral candidiasis. Br. J. Dermatol. 83:161, 1970.
101. Lehrer, R. I.: Measurement of candidal activity of specific leukocyte types in mixed cell population. II. Normal and chronic granulomatous disease eosinophils. Infect. Immun. 3:800, 1971.
102. Lehrer, R. I.: The fungicidal mechanisms of human monocytes. I. Evidence for myeloperoxidase-linked and myeloperoxidase-independent candidicidal mechanisms. J. Clin. Invest. 53:338, 1975.
103. Leibovitz, E., Juster-Reicher, A., Amitai, M., et al.: Systemic candidal infections associated with use of peripheral venous catheters in neonates: A 9-year experience. Clin. Infect. Dis. 14:485, 1992.
104. Levine, J., Dykoski, R. K., and Janoff, E. N.: *Candida*-associated diarrhea: A syndrome in search of credibility. Clin. Infect. Dis. 21:881, 1995.
105. Lew, M. A., Siber, G. R., Donahue, D. M., et al.: Enhanced detection with enzyme-linked immunosorbent assay of *Candida* marrow in antibody-containing serum after heat extraction. J. Infect. Dis. 145:45, 1982.
106. Lipton, S. A., Hickey, W. F., Morris, J. H., et al.: Candidal infection in the central nervous system. Am. J. Med. 76:101, 1984.
107. Macmillan, B. G., Law, E. J., and Holder, I. A.: Experience with *Candida* infections in the burn patient. Arch. Surg. 104:509, 1972.
108. Mailbach, H. I., and Kligman, A. M.: The biology of experimental human cutaneous moniliasis *(Candida albicans)*. Arch. Dermatol. 85:233, 1962.
109. Maksymiuk, A. W., Thongprasert, S., Hopfer, R., et al.: Systemic candidiasis in cancer patients. Am. J. Med. 77:20, 1984.
110. Mardh, P. A., Stormy, N., and Weström, L.: Mycoplasma and vaginal cytology. Acta Cytol. 15:310, 1971.
111. Marks, M. I., Marks, S., and Brazean, M.: Yeast colonization in hospitalized and nonhospitalized children. J. Pediatr. 87:524, 1975.
112. Marquis, G., Montplaisir, S., Gargon, S., et al.: Fungitoxicity of muramidase: Ultrastructural damage to *Candida albicans*. Lab. Invest. 46:627, 1982.
113. Martino, P., Girmenia, C., Micozzi, A., et al.: Prospective study of *Candida* colonization, use of empiric amphotericin B and development of invasive mycosis in neutropenic patients. Eur. J. Clin. Microbiol. Infect. Dis. 13:797, 1994.
114. Martino, P., Girmenia, C., Vendetti, M., et al.: *Candida* colonization and systemic infection in neutropenic patients: A retrospective study. Cancer 64:2030, 1989.
115. Mathur, S. J., Goust, E. O., Horger, E. O., III, et al.: Immunoglobulin E anti-*Candida* antibodies and candidiasis. Infect. Immun. 18:257, 1977.
116. McLeod, R., and Remington, J. S.: Postoperative fungal endocarditis. *In* Duma, R. J. (ed.): Infections of Prosthetic Heart Valves and Vascular Grafts: Prevention, Diagnosis and Treatment. Baltimore, University Park Press, 1977, p. 163.
117. Medoff, G., Comfort, M., and Kobayashi, G. S.: Synergistic action of amphotericin B and 5-fluorocytosine against yeast-like organisms. Proc. Soc. Exp. Biol. Med. 138:571, 1971.
118. Meunier-Carpentier, F., Cruciani, M., and Klastersky, J.: Oral prophylaxis with miconazole or ketoconazole of invasive fungal disease in neutropenic cancer patients. Eur. J. Cancer Clin. Oncol. 19:43, 1983.
119. Michel, L., McMichan, J. C., and Bachy, J. L.: Microbial colonization of indwelling central nervous catheter: Statistical evaluation of potential contaminating factors. Am. J. Surg. 137:745, 1979.
120. Midgley, G., and Clayton, Y. M.: Distribution of dermatophytes and *Candida* spores in the environment. Br. J. Dermatol. 86:69, 1972.
121. Milne, J. D., and Warnock, D. W.: Antibodies to *Candida albicans* in human cervicovaginal secretions. Br. J. Vener. Dis. 53:375, 1977.
122. Montes, L. F., Krumdieck, C., and Cornwell, P. E.: Hypovitaminosis A in patients with mucocutaneous candidiasis. J. Infect. Dis. 128:227, 1973.

123. Montes, L. F., Pittilo, R. F., Hunt, D., et al.: Microbial flora of infant's skin. Arch. Dermatol. *103*:400, 1971.
124. Montgomerie, J. Z., and Edwards, J. E., Jr.: Association of infection due to *Candida albicans* with intravenous hyperalimentation. J. Infect. Dis. *137*:197, 1978.
125. Moro, M. L., Maffei, C., Manso, E., et al.: Nosocomial outbreak of systemic candidiasis associated with parenteral nutrition. Infect. Control Hosp. Epidemiol. *11*:27, 1990.
126. Morris, A. B., Sands, M. L., Shiraki, M., et al.: Gallbladder and biliary tract candidiasis: Nine cases and review. Rev. Infect. Dis. *12*:483, 1990.
127. Multicentre Study Group: Treatment of vaginal candidiasis with a single oral dose of fluconazole. Eur. J. Clin. Microbiol. Infect. Dis. *7*:364, 1988.
128. Odds, F. C.: *Candida* and Candidiasis. Baltimore, University Park Press, 1979, p. 382.
129. Owens, N. J., Nightinggale, C. H., Schweizer, R. T., et al.: Prophylaxis of oral candidiasis with clotrimazole troches. Arch. Intern. Med. *144*:290, 1984.
130. Pan, N. C., and Pan, I.-H.: Prevalence rate of *Candida* species in stool of children in Taipei. J. Formosan Med. Assoc. *63*:396, 1964.
131. Parker, J. C., McClosky, J. J., Solanki, K. V., et al.: Candidiasis: The most common postmortem cerebral mycosis in an endemic fungal area. Surg. Neurol. *6*:123, 1976.
132. Pederson, G. T.: Yeasts isolated from the throat, rectum, and vagina in 60 women examined during pregnancy and ½ to 1 year after labour. Acta Obstet. Gynaecol. Scand. *6*(Suppl. 42):47, 1964.
133. Pederson, G. T.: Yeast flora in mother and child: A mycological-clinical study of women followed up during pregnancy, the puerperium and 5–12 months after delivery, and their children on the 7th day of life and at the age of 5–12 months. Nord. Med. *81*:207, 1969.
134. Perry, C. M., Whittington, R., and McTavish, D.: Fluconazole: An update of its antimicrobial activity, pharmacokinetic properties, and therapeutic use in vaginal candidiasis. Drugs *49*:984, 1995.
135. Piccolella, E., Lombardi, G., and Morelli, R.: Generation of suppressor cells in the response of human lymphocytes to a polysaccharide from Candida albicans. J. Immunol. *126*:2151, 1981.
136. Pizzo, P. A., Robichand, K. J., Gill, F. A., et al.: Empiric antibiotics and antifungal therapy for cancer patients with prolonged fever and granulocytopenia. Am. J. Med. *72*:101, 1982.
137. Podolsky, S., and Ferguson, B. D.: Fatal systemic candidiasis following treatment of Addison's crisis in a juvenile diabetic. Diabetes *19*:438, 1970.
138. Pollack, B., Buck, I. F., and Kalmins, L.: An oral syndrome complicating psychopharmacotherapy: Study II. Am. J. Psychiatry *121*:384, 1964.
139. Powderly, W. G., Kobayaski, G. S., Herzig, G. P., et al.: Amphotericin B-resistant yeast infection in severely immunocompromised patients. Am. J. Med. *84*:826, 1988.
140. Rex, J. H., Bennett, J. E., Sugar, A. M., et al.: Intravascular catheter exchange and duration of candidemia. Clin. Infect. Dis. *21*:994, 1995.
141. Rex, J. H., Bennett, J. E., Sugar, A. M., et al.: A randomized trial comparing fluconazole with amphotericin B for the treatment of candidemia in patients without neutropenia. N. Engl. J. Med. *331*:1325, 1994.
142. Richards, K. E., Pierson, C. L., Bucciarelli, L., et al.: Monilial sepsis in the surgical patient. Surg. Clin. North Am. *52*:1399, 1972.
143. Richet, H. M., Andremont, A., Tancrede, C., et al.: Risk factors for candidemia in patients with acute lymphocytic leukemia. Rev. Infect. Dis. *13*:211, 1991.
144. Robbins, J. S., Mittemeyer, B. T., and Borski, A. A.: Primary renal candidiasis masking transitional-cell carcinoma. Urology *4*:332, 1974.
145. Roig, P., Carrasco, R., Salavert, M., et al.: Laringitis candidiascia e infeccion por VIH: Descripcion de cuatro casos. Rev. Clin. Esp. *191*:261, 1992.
146. Rossetti, F., Brawner, D. L., Bowden, R. et al.: Fungal liver infection in marrow transplant recipients: Prevalence at autopsy, predisposing factors, and clinical features. Clin. Infect. Dis. *20*:8801, 1995.
147. Sanchez, V., Vazquez, J. A., Barth-Jones, D., et al.: Nosocomial acquisition of *Candida parapsilosis:* An epidemiologic study. Am. J. Med. *94*:577, 1993.
148. Schönebeck, J.: Asymptomatic candiduria prognosis, complications and some other considerations. Scand. J. Urol. Nephrol. *6*:136, 1972.
149. Schumacher, H. R., Ginns, D. A., and Warren, W.: Fungus infection complicating leukemia. Am. J. Med. Sci. *247*:313, 1964.
150. Seelig, M. S.: Mechanisms by which antibiotics increase the incidence and severity of candidiasis and alter the immunological defense. Bacteriol. Rev. *30*:442, 1966.
151. Sheft, D. J., and Shrago, G.: Esophageal moniliasis, the spectrum of the disease. J. A. M. A. *213*:1859, 1970.
152. Shenep, J. L., Kalwinsky, D. K., Feldman, S., et al.: Mycotic cervical lymphadenitis following oral mucositis in children with leukemia. J. Pediatr. *106*:243, 1985.
153. Slavin, M. A., Osborne, B., Adams, R., et al.: Efficacy and safety of fluconazole prophylaxis for fungal infections after marrow transplantation: A prospective randomized, double-blind study. J. Infect. Dis. *171*:1545, 1995.
154. Smego, R. A., Perfect, J. R., and Durack, D. T.: Combined therapy with amphotericin B and 5-flucytosine for *Candida* meningitis. Rev. Infect. Dis. *6*:791, 1984.
155. Smits, B. J., Prior, A. P., and Arablaster, P. G.: Incidence of *Candida* in hospital in-patients and the effects of antibiotic therapy. B. M. J. *1*:208, 1966.
156. Solomkin, J. S., Flohr, A. B., Quie, P. G., et al.: The role of *Candida* in intraperitoneal infections. Surgery *88*:524, 1980.
157. Solomon, S. L., Khabbaz, R. F., Parker, R. H., et al.: An outbreak of *Candida parapsilosis* bloodstream infection in patients with parenteral nutrition. J. Infect. Dis. *149*:98, 1984.
158. Sonck, C. E., and Somersalo, O.: The yeast flora of the anogenital region in diabetic girls. Arch. Dermatol. *88*:846, 1963.
159. Stamos, J. K., and Rowley, A. H.: Candidemia in a pediatric population. Clin. Infect. Dis. *20*:571, 1995.
160. Stanley, V. C., Hurley, R., and Carrol, C. J.: Distribution and significance of *Candida* precipitins in sera from pregnant women. J. Med. Microbiol. *5*:313, 1972.
161. Stevens, D. A., Odds, F. C., and Scherer, S.: Application of DNA typing methods to *Candida albicans* epidemiology and correlations with phenotype. Rev. Infect. Dis. *12*:258, 1990.
162. Taschdjian, C. L., and Kozinin, P. J.: Laboratory and clinical studies on candidiasis in the newborn infant. J. Pediatr. *50*:426, 1957.
163. Thong, Y. H., and Ferrante, A.: Alternative pathway of complement activation by *Candida albicans.* Aust. N. Z. J. Med. *8*:620, 1978.
164. Toala, P., Schroeder, S. A., Raly, A. K., et al.: *Candida* at Boston City Hospital. Arch. Intern. Med. *136*:983, 1970.
165. Trier, J. S., and Bjorkman, D. J.: Esophageal, gastric, and intestinal candidiasis. Am. J. Med. *77*:39, 1984.
166. Vorreith, M.: Mycotic encephalitis. Acta Neuropathol. (Berlin) *11*:55, 1968.
167. Walsh, H., Hilderbrandt, R. J., and Prystowsky, H.: Oral progestational agents as a cause of *Candida* vaginitis. Am. J. Obstet. Gynecol. *101*:991, 1968.
168. Ward, R. M., Sattler, F. R., and Dalton, A. S.: Assessment of antifungal therapy in an 800-gram infant with candidal arthritis and osteomyelitis. Pediatrics *72*:234, 1983.
169. Warnock, D. W., Milne, J. D., and Fielding, A. W.: Immunoglobulin classes of human serum antibodies in vaginal candidiasis. Mycopathologia *63*:173, 1978.
170. Wiener, M. H., and Yount, W. J.: Mannan antigenemia in the diagnosis of invasive *Candida* infections. J. Clin. Invest. *58*:1045, 1976.
171. Wingard, J. R., Merz, W. G., Rinaldi, M. G., et al.: Increase in *Candida krusei* infections among patients with bone marrow transplantation and neutropenia treated prophylactically with fluconazole. N. Engl. J. Med. *325*:1274–1277, 1991.
172. Winner, H. I., and Hurley, R.: *Candida albicans.* London, Churchill, 1964, pp. 62–75.
173. Winston, D. J., Chandrasekar, P. H., Lazarus, H. M., et al.: Fluconazole prophylaxis of fungal infections in patients with acute leukemia. Ann. Intern. Med. *118*:495, 1993.
174. Yap, B.-S., and Bodey, G. P.: Oropharyngeal candidiasis treated with a troche form of clotrimazole. Arch. Intern. Med. *139*:646, 1979.
175. Young, R. C., Bennett, J. E., Geelhoed, G. W., et al.: Fungemia with compromised host resistance: A survey of 70 cases. Ann. Intern. Med. *80*:605, 1974.
176. Zegarelli, E. V., and Kutscher, A. H.: Oral moniliasis following intraoral topical corticosteroid therapy. J. Oral Ther. *1*:304, 1964.
177. Zimmerman, L. E.: Keratomycosis. Surv. Ophthalmol. *8*:1, 1963.

200

COCCIDIOIDOMYCOSIS

Ziad M. Shehab

Coccidioidomycosis is an infection caused by a dimorphic fungus: *Coccidioides immitis.* The primary pulmonary infection produced by this organism usually is self-limited, but disseminated and fatal disease may occur. In the United States, coccidioidomycosis is an endemic disease of the southwestern states and results in 100,000 infections per year.[55] In other parts of the United States, it also is seen in individuals who have traveled or lived in the Southwest.[145] The disease is endemic in other areas of the Western Hemisphere, most notably in certain countries in South and Central America and in northern Mexico.[112] With population growth in the endemic areas of the Southwest and increased population mobility, it is likely that clinicians in nonendemic parts of the country will encounter this disease, particularly in its more severe or disseminated forms.

The history[34, 49] of coccidioidomycosis exemplifies the process of chance, insight, and careful scientific study as it applies to the acquisition of medical knowledge. Coccidioidal granuloma, a form of disseminated coccidioidomycosis, first was described by Posadas in 1892 in Argentina. The disease was thought initially to be a form of skin tumor. Rixford and Gilchrist associated it with what they thought was a protozoon resembling coccidia and named it *Coccidioides.* They divided it into two species: *immitis* and *pyogenes.* Ophüls and Moffitt, in 1900, were the first to attribute coccidioidal granuloma to the fungus *C. immitis.* Although earlier investigators had noted fungal growth on cultures from pathologic specimens, they dismissed these organisms as contaminants. Between 1900 and 1936, numerous reports of coccidioidal granuloma appeared in the medical literature, but the association between coccidioidal granuloma and acute pulmonary infection remained unrecognized. In 1936, Gifford and associates[61] and Dickson[40] were responsible for the concept that *C. immitis* could cause either a primary or a secondary type of illness. The primary form previously had been known in California as San Joaquin fever or valley fever.

In the period that followed, the epidemiology of the disease[138, 142] and ecology of the organism[45, 96] were studied carefully by many investigators, led by the efforts of Dr. Charles Smith. Many different forms of therapy were tried for the disseminated disease during this era, but none proved satisfactory.[49] In 1957, amphotericin B became available, and the prognosis associated with the disseminated form of the disease improved. Since 1970, the major efforts of investigators have been to develop more successful, less toxic modes of therapy and a means of disease prevention.

As with many pathogenic fungi, the life cycle of *C. immitis* demonstrates two distinct phases: a saprophytic, or vegetative, phase and a parasitic phase. In nature and on most laboratory media, the organism grows as a mycelium with branching, septate hyphae. After 5 to 7 days, the aerial mycelia show development of rectangular spores (arthrospores, arthroconidia) separated by empty nonviable cells (Fig. 200–1). At this stage, the hyphae become fragile, and the arthroconidia, measuring 2 to 8 μm in diameter, easily become airborne. Because of their size, they can reach the alveolar spaces of the lung when inhaled.

Upon gaining access to the tissues of the mammalian host, the arthroconidia begin the parasitic phase of the life cycle. They enlarge and develop into spherules over about 48 hours by undergoing internal segmentation containing endospores that are 2 to 5 μm in size. The spherules (Fig. 200–2) are round, double-walled structures, 20 to 100 μm in diameter. The endospores are released into the surrounding tissues by rupture of the spherule wall. They, in turn, may grow into mature spherules by maturation of the endospores in vivo to spherules repeating the tissue phase of the life cycle of the organism. Alternatively, when the spherule ruptures, releasing the endospores into the environment, hyphal formation can occur and the cycle thus is repeated in nature.[79]

C. immitis grows on laboratory media relatively easily, producing colonies that become visible in 3 to 4 days, representing the mycelial phase of the fungus. They appear as flat, smooth, and gray colonies, from which spicules may project in some, whereas others have the look of a velvety membrane. The colonies appear as tufts in the second week and then develop cobweb-like aerial hyphae. Pigmentation may be seen after 2 weeks and is observed best as a brownish undersurface. Variability in colony morphology can be significant, but only one species of *C. immitis* is recognized currently. Identification is accomplished by inoculation of the mycelia into laboratory animals and demonstration of the

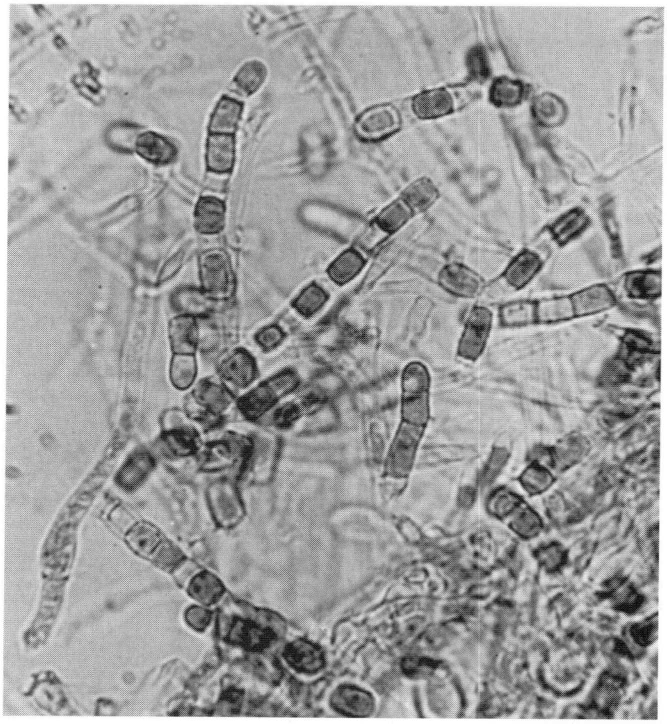

FIGURE 200–1. *Mycelial form of* Coccidioides immitis. *Arthroconidia are separated by vacuolated cells. (From Davis, B. D., Delbecco, R., Eisen, H. W., et al.: Microbiology: Including Immunology and Molecular Genetics. 3rd ed. Hagerstown, Harper & Row, 1980.)*

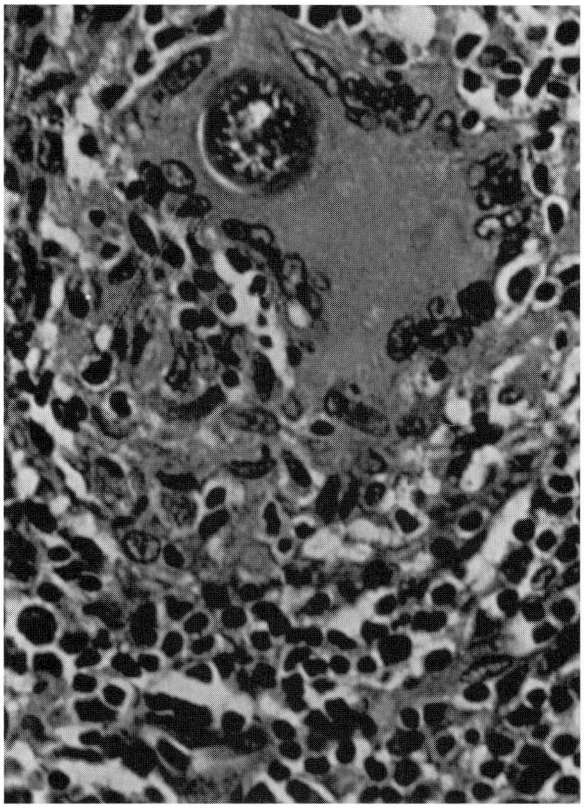

FIGURE 200–2. *Coccidioidal granuloma showing a multinucleated giant cell containing a spherule filled with endospores. The adjacent field contains lymphocytes and plasma cells.*

conversion of the fungus to the spherule phase. However, reliable techniques showing in vitro conversion to the spherule stage, demonstration of specific exoantigens, or identification of the organism by genetic probes have been developed and obviate the need for animal inoculation.[33, 111, 146, 150]

EPIDEMIOLOGY

Coccidioidomycosis is endemic in the Western Hemisphere between 40 degrees of latitude north and south. In the United States, these areas lie in the southwestern states, especially in western Texas, New Mexico, Arizona, and California. The areas in which coccidioidomycosis is prevalent generally correspond to the lower Sonoran life zone.[99, 112] This life zone is characterized by an arid to semiarid climate, with hot summers and relatively short winters with limited rainfall and few freezes. Most of the fungal growth occurs during the rainy season in alkaline soil and at low altitude, conditions that favor the growth of the creosote bush that often coexists with *C. immitis*.[45] The fungus is found in the soil to a depth of 20 cm, especially in the walls of rodent burrows, and is isolated infrequently from surface soil during hot, dry weather[45] or in soils rich with other organisms.[96] Environmental conditions in endemic regions apparently inhibit growth of competitive organisms.[45] A variety of animals, including rodents, cattle, sheep, and dogs, have been shown to develop naturally acquired infection.[47] Arthroconidia become airborne during wind storms[53] or by disruption of soil by construction work and farming. Prolonged droughts followed by heavy rains also have resulted in an increase in cases, such as occurred in California in 1992 and 1993.[6] Archeologic excavations and digging by children in soil containing the organism have been reported to result in local outbreaks.[125, 152, 163, 167] In addition, transmission has been reported to occur by contaminated fomites, such as dusty clothing and farm products.[1, 130] Because of the ease by which arthroconidia become airborne, the organism is dangerous to laboratory personnel. Epidemics have resulted from inadvertent opening of a single culture plate.[83, 94]

Primary coccidioidal infection occurs most frequently in summer and fall,[138, 139] when arthroconidia are more likely to become dispersed because of the dry weather. However, the number of cases observed is greater after a winter with heavy rainfall, presumably because the wet environment promotes greater hyphal growth.[45, 112]

Susceptibility to primary coccidioidal infection is unaffected by age, sex, or racial background.[49] Estimates of infection rates in endemic areas are based on the risk of infection in children and have declined. Reactivity to skin test antigens that used to be 55 per cent in elementary school children and 68 per cent in high school students in Kern County, California, in 1939, had decreased markedly to 8 per cent and 24 per cent, respectively, by 1964.[91] Similarly, the annual risk has been estimated to be down to between 2 and 4 per cent in college students in Tucson, Arizona.[88] Incidence rates are higher in older male children, in rural areas, during wind storms, and for those with occupational exposure.[127, 129, 138] In contrast with susceptibility to primary infection, the frequency of dissemination varies considerably, being higher in infants,[24, 26, 80, 135] Filipinos, Hispanics, and blacks.[53, 61, 74] Filipinos have 170 times and blacks 10 times the incidence of dissemination in non-Hispanic whites. However, some of this increased risk may reflect environmental exposure to high inocula of *C. immitis*.[5] Immunosuppressed hosts also are at increased risk for dissemination. In particular, patients with active coccidioidomycosis and HIV infection are at greatly increased risk of developing severe pulmonary disease and disseminated infection.[52, 56]

The tissue phase of the infection is the spherule that is not infectious. Although mycelial growth can be found in cavities when carefully searched for, there is no evidence of person-to-person spread of *C. immitis*,[50, 123, 165] except in special situations in which the fungus is allowed to revert to its airborne form, such as growth from wound drainage on a plaster cast.[44] Patients with coccidioidomycosis do not require isolation, even when draining wounds are present. In such circumstances, dressings should be changed frequently to prevent growth of the fungus and the formation of arthroconidia.

Once limited to the lower Sonoran life zone, the disease cannot be ignored throughout the country because more cases are seen everywhere because of the ease and frequency of travel, increased population in endemic areas, and reactivation of infection in immunocompromised hosts, including transplant recipients and patients with AIDS. In these patients, delays in diagnosis can be fatal, and rapid recognition of the diagnosis and prompt institution of appropriate therapy mandate timely and accurate diagnosis.

PATHOGENESIS AND PATHOLOGY

Acquisition of *C. immitis* infection usually is via the respiratory tract. It is surmised that most human infections may result from exposure to only a single spore (Fig. 200–3).[55] Rarely, direct cutaneous inoculation may occur by puncture of the skin with a contaminated object.[64, 73, 108, 110] Growth of the organism stimulates an intense inflammatory response,[151]

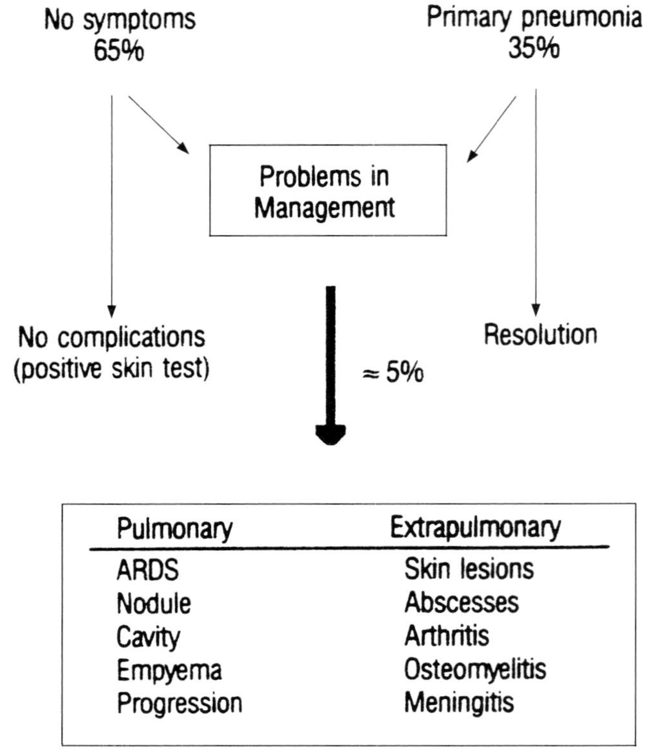

FIGURE 200–3. *Clinical spectrum of coccidioidomycosis. ARDS, adult respiratory distress syndrome. (From Galgiani, J. N.: Coccidioidomycosis. Reprinted by permission of the Western Journal of Medicine, 159:153–171, 1993.)*

and in most patients the infection remains localized to the lung and hilar nodes. In a minority of patients, clinically significant extrapulmonary dissemination occurs by way of lymphatics or the blood stream.

The initial inflammatory response of acute pulmonary coccidioidomycosis predominantly is a polymorphonuclear leukocyte reaction, possibly related to a chemotactic effect of endospores or complement activation from other *C. immitis* antigens. Tissue necrosis, spherules, and a few mononuclear cells are present at this stage of the disease, but epithelial giant cells are infrequent. This bronchopneumonic process can occur in any lobe of the lung. The inflammatory response, however, is ineffective because neutrophils do not show any killing of coccidioidal forms at any stage of growth of the organism. Although this response may slow the progress of the infection temporarily, it ultimately cannot arrest the disease process.[55] Killing has been demonstrated with natural killer cells and mononuclear leukocytes. A number of studies have demonstrated the importance of T cells in controlling the infection as evidenced by delayed cutaneous hypersensitivity, peripheral lymphocyte transformation, and the production of interferon-γ.[55] Dermal hypersensitivity correlates well with other measures of peripheral blood lymphocyte responsiveness, such as lymphocyte transformation and cytokine production.[2] As the disease progresses, cell-mediated immune defenses become defective, possibly as a result of antigen overload, suppressor cells, immune complexes, or fungal immunosuppressive substances, resulting in an ineffective response by type 2 helper cells.[148]

Disseminated coccidioidomycosis resembles progressive tuberculosis of childhood by its spread, which usually occurs within weeks or months after the initial infection. However, endogenous reactivation of treated primary disease may occur, particularly among children receiving immunosuppressive therapy[38, 107] or among those with HIV infection.[17, 56]

Extrapulmonary spread may occur anywhere in the body, but lesions are most frequent in bone, soft tissue, lymph nodes, and the meninges.[75] Bone lesions resemble chronic osteomyelitis (Fig. 200–4). Infection of the brain substance is rare, but meningitis is common and frequently localizes in the basilar area.[14, 74]

The pathologic findings of fatal coccidioidomycosis have been reviewed extensively.[75] The tissue reaction in disseminated disease predominantly is granulomatous but can be accompanied by elements of acute inflammation. Typically, the granulomatous lesions contain abundant giant cells and histiocytes. Caseous necrosis is common, and spherules usually can be identified lying freely and within macrophages (see Fig. 200–2). Fibrous tissue may surround areas of inflammation, but calcification is infrequent. Autopsy studies in patients with coccidioidomycosis and AIDS show poor granulomatous responses and larger numbers of organisms in lung tissue than those seen in non-AIDS patients.[65]

Most cases of disseminated coccidioidal infection in the first months of life have been associated with heavy exposure to dust, with these infants apparently acquiring their infection by the respiratory route.[26, 80] Nearly all the reported infants in this age group have had severe disease,[24, 26, 80, 154] but primary infection sometimes may go unrecognized.[26] Although women who develop coccidioidomycosis late in pregnancy may be at increased risk of disseminated disease,[160] with a few exceptions[131] infants nearly always are born free of infection.[27, 28, 136, 158] In several patients with apparent perinatal transmission, the mothers had coccidioidal endometritis, and infected amniotic fluid was the most likely source of their infants' infections.[11, 133, 144]

Dissemination of coccidioidomycosis is more frequent in

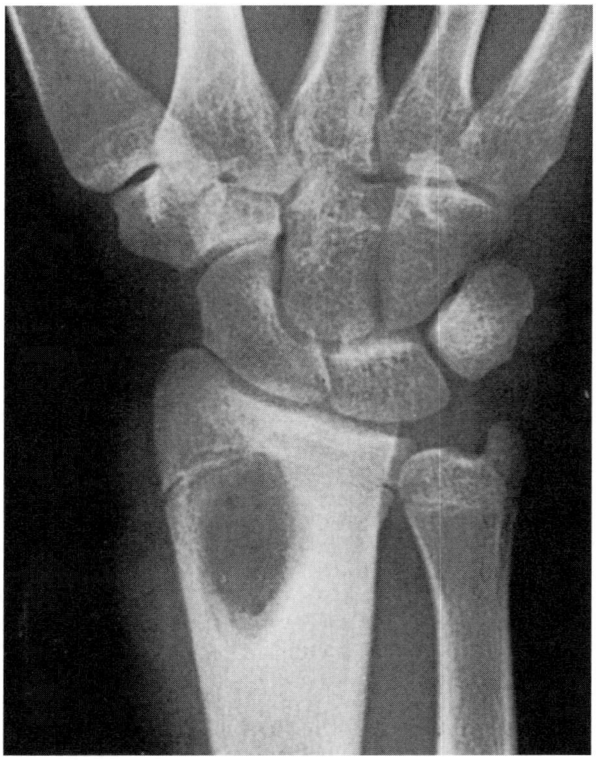

FIGURE 200–4. *Osteomyelitis in a 14-year-old boy with disseminated coccidioidomycosis. An osteolytic lesion involves the distal radius.*

immunosuppressed patients who have resided in an endemic area,[38, 98, 107] but immunologic abnormalities have not been detected in other groups, such as Filipinos, who also are at high risk for disseminated disease. Once dissemination occurs, the patient's cell-mediated immunity frequently is impaired,[20, 31, 143] especially if extensive infection is present.[9, 141] Dissemination can occur in patients who have a selective lack of response to coccidioidal antigens as evidenced by negative skin test results to coccidioidin and spherulin and who do not have evidence of generalized anergy. In vitro measurements of lymphocyte reactivity (transformation) to phytohemagglutinin or to specific cell-wall antigens of *C. immitis* also are depressed.[9, 29–31, 37] In contrast, patients with disseminated disease with positive skin test results usually have normal in vitro lymphocyte responses that are similar to those found in healthy persons who have recovered from primary infection.[31, 36, 109, 170] Furthermore, patients recovered from severe disseminated disease may show return of specific and nonspecific cell-mediated immunity.[9, 20, 49, 143] Infected children demonstrate immunologic findings similar to those described in adults but have not been as well studied.

CLINICAL MANIFESTATIONS

Primary Infection

The clinical features of acute coccidioidomycosis in children are thought to be similar to the manifestations observed in adults.[140] Studies in Air Force personnel indicate that infection is subclinical or indistinguishable from a mild upper respiratory tract infection in 60 per cent of nonimmunocompromised hosts.[140, 143] In the remaining 40 per cent, the severity varies from insignificant flu-like illness lasting 1 to 2 days to severe lower respiratory illness with lobar pneumonia, pleural effusions, and, occasionally, pericarditis.[47, 49, 55, 120, 137] Occasionally, the disease may mimic bacterial pneumonia and sepsis.[95] The most common form of symptomatic infection is a subacute, self-limited pulmonary illness, but some patients will experience more complicated pulmonary infections or even extrapulmonary disease. The latter patients are those who are most likely to be seen by physicians outside of the endemic areas, and these patients may require extensive work-ups and delays in diagnosis if coccidioidomycosis is not considered.

The usual incubation period is 10 to 16 days but may range from less than a week to almost a month.[49] In young adults, fatigue (77 per cent), cough (64 per cent), chest pain (53 per cent), and dyspnea (17 per cent) are the most common symptoms. Fever was present in 46 per cent, with arthralgia, myalgia, and headaches being reported in 22 per cent each.[97, 153] In infants, stridor rarely may be present as a result of primary infection of subglottic tissue.[60, 69] Chest pain sometimes is severe and usually is pleuritic.[153] It may be followed by vague chest pain that persists for several months.[43, 49, 55] Transient skin rashes probably are more frequent in children than they are in adults and are observed in slightly more than one half of symptomatic children.[73, 127] Two types of rashes are seen, based on time of presentation and immune status. Those present early in the illness are erythematous and maculopapular.[49, 73, 163, 167] They vary in severity, ranging from diffuse eruptions resembling measles or scarlet fever to more common and less extensive processes localized to the lower trunk and thighs.[49, 73] In a few patients, urticarial lesions may be present.[163]

Erythema nodosum and erythema multiforme appear somewhat later in the course of illness, usually after the third day to as late as 3 weeks.[49, 138] Erythema nodosum correlates with the development of cell-mediated immunity and is associated with a low incidence of dissemination.[43, 49, 138] This symptom complex may occur in other diseases, including acute histoplasmosis[104] and group A beta-hemolytic streptococcal infections. However, its presence in a child residing in some endemic areas, such as the San Joaquin Valley, nearly always signifies acute coccidioidal infection. For unknown reasons, erythema nodosum occurs less frequently in infected children inhabiting other endemic areas, such as Tucson.[127] The condition is self-limited, usually resolving within a few days to several weeks. Erythema nodosum occurs two to four times more frequently in adult females than in adult males, but this difference is not apparent in childhood infection.[138] The rash is infrequent in blacks, Hispanics, and Filipinos. Erythema multiforme for some reason is more common in children.

Acute arthritis or arthralgia is an additional hypersensitivity manifestation, and occasionally one or both accompany primary coccidioidal infection. Because these findings usually are transient and do not signify dissemination, it is presumed that spherules are not present in the involved joints at this stage of the disease.[43]

The radiographic appearance of primary coccidioidomycosis is not specific.[10, 23, 68, 127] Bronchopneumonic infiltrates are the most frequent finding and often are associated with hilar lymphadenopathy. Segmental or lobar consolidation and nodular or patchy pulmonary infiltrates also can occur. Small pleural effusions or pleuropericardial reactions also occur frequently (Fig. 200–5) and usually are sterile.[93] These radiographic findings resolve in 90 to 95 per cent of symptomatic cases, albeit slowly in some, and usually do not necessitate specific therapy.

In a minority of patients, cavitation, nodule formation, bronchiectasis, or calcification may develop at the site of the pulmonic infiltrate.[12, 18] The cavities usually are thin-walled and asymptomatic and rarely require surgical therapy. Many resolve spontaneously[89] but result nonetheless in the need for prolonged care and convalescence. Rarely, the cavities lead to the development of an empyema or a bronchopleural fistula. These complications are a lot more likely in patients with immunosuppression or diabetes.[81]

Nodules and thin-walled cavities develop in 5 per cent of patients with coccidioidal pneumonia.[148] These lesions are well circumscribed, typically single, and less than 6 cm in

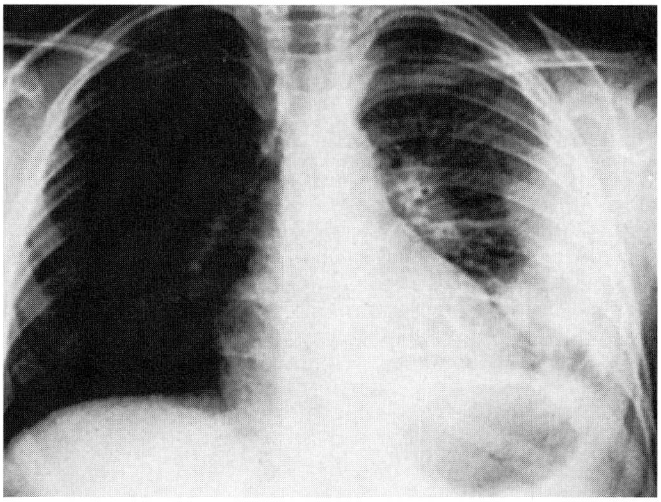

FIGURE 200–5. *Chest radiograph of a patient with acute pulmonary coccidioidomycosis showing pulmonary infiltrates, extensive pleural fluid, and enlargement of the left hilum.*

diameter. In most patients, these lesions are asymptomatic. In adults, these nodules may be confused with carcinoma of the lung, thus requiring excision or diagnostic fine-needle aspiration.[41]

In neonates, the constellation of radiographic findings of focal consolidation with diffuse nodular densities associated with nonspecific symptoms and minimal clinical evidence of respiratory tract infection has been described but is not specific for coccidioidomycosis at this age.[11, 23] Chorioretinitis as a manifestation of systemic disease also has been reported.[62]

In contrast with primary pulmonary infection, primary cutaneous coccidioidomycosis is uncommon.[64, 108, 110] Most cases have been reported in laboratory workers,[83] but this form of infection also is recognized in children.[108] The lesion of primary cutaneous disease resembles a chancre and is associated with regional lymphadenitis. In adults, usually only mild constitutional symptoms are present, and the process spontaneously resolves within 2 to 3 months. However, in children, progressive and prolonged infection may be more common; antifungal therapy may be necessary.[108, 166]

The manifestations of primary coccidioidal disease thus are varied, and no constellation of symptoms and signs is specific enough, making the use of specific laboratory tests a requirement for diagnosis.

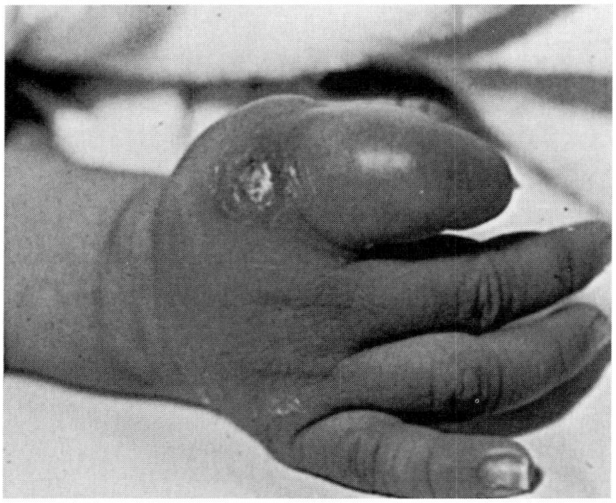

FIGURE 200–6. *Swelling and chronic draining sinus over the proximal phalanx of the index finger. The infant has disseminated coccidioidomycosis with involvement of the underlying bone.*

Disseminated Coccidioidomycosis

Except in very young children, dissemination appears to be less frequent in pediatric patients than in adults (0.5 per cent), although this view has been questioned.[85, 135, 137] Spread of infection usually becomes apparent within a few weeks to a few months after the initial infection and is heralded by persistent fever, toxicity, and insidious development of lesions outside the chest. An occasional patient develops disseminated disease after an asymptomatic primary infection.[32, 48, 85] Disseminated disease can manifest with involvement of the larynx.[15]

Skin Disease

The most common cutaneous manifestation of disseminated coccidioidomycosis is verrucous granuloma that characteristically is located at the nasolabial fold.[49, 73] These lesions may heal or may continue to progress. The lesions mimic those due to other fungi, tuberculosis, actinomycetes, and syphilis. The subcutaneous tissues also may be involved and result in large "cold" abscesses and the development of sinus tracts leading to chronic ulcers.[43]

Bone and Joint Disease

Invasion of bone by *C. immitis* results in chronic osteomyelitis,[13, 15, 82] which may drain into soft tissue (Fig. 200–6) and form fistulas to the overlying skin.[32] The bones most frequently infected are the vertebrae, tibia, metatarsals, skull, and metacarpals. The lesions are present in a single bone in 60 per cent of the cases; two bones are involved in 20 per cent and three in another 10 per cent. Radiographically, the lesions typically are lytic (see Fig. 200–4). Vertebral osteomyelitis is characterized by involvement of all parts of the vertebra with relative sparing of the disk.[43] Meningitis is a serious concern with vertebral osteomyelitis.

Meningitis

Meningitis may be the sole site of extrapulmonary disease, particularly in whites, but it also occurs as part of widespread dissemination.[14, 72, 87, 134] It may present acutely with the primary infection or appear up to 6 months later. The most common symptoms are headache, sluggishness, ataxia, and vomiting. The child often lacks signs of meningeal irritation and sometimes presents with signs of focal neurologic deficits. The pathology is that of granulomatous and suppurative basilar meningitis, with frequent presence of parenchymal involvement with granulomas and abscesses of the spinal cord and brain.[106] Vasculitic complications with infarction and stroke-like findings have been described and may be abrupt in onset.[164] The cerebrospinal fluid formula usually reveals moderate pleocytosis with mononuclear cell predominance, low cerebrospinal fluid glucose, and an elevated protein level.[21, 72, 134] The presence of eosinophilic pleocytosis in the cerebrospinal fluid is common in coccidioidal meningitis but is of no prognostic value.[124] The cerebrospinal fluid culture often is negative for the fungus, whereas cerebrospinal fluid antibody often is detectable.[21] The diagnosis is confirmed by a positive cerebrospinal fluid culture, serology, or both. These findings are typical for the lumbosacral cerebrospinal fluid; there is, however, considerable variation in the cell count, chemistry, and antibody content of fluid obtained from the ventricles, cisterna magna, or lumbosacral space,[63, 72, 134] with the latter exhibiting the more severe changes. Evidence is supported by a positive serum serologic result or culture of *C. immitis* from a nonpulmonary site. Prior to the availability of amphotericin B, coccidioidal meningitis uniformly was fatal and the average length of survival in children was 5.5 months. Death with coccidioidal meningitis now is a relatively rare event.

Genital Coccidioidomycosis

Like tuberculosis, coccidioidomycosis can involve the pelvic organs. Early studies had indicated an alarming risk of dissemination and death in women who acquired coccidioidomycosis, especially during the third trimester of pregnancy.[119] In a population-based study, Wack and colleagues[160] showed that coccidioidomycosis occurs infrequently during pregnancy but remains associated with serious complications when the disease develops in the third trimester or soon after delivery. Coccidioiduria may be a silent manifestation of disseminated disease.[118]

Coccidioidomycosis in the Immunocompromised Host

Conditions that result in immune suppression, particularly T-lymphocyte dysfunction, such as those present in patients with lymphoma or bone marrow or solid organ transplantation, predispose to more fulminant forms of coccidioidomycosis.[25, 70, 128] Solid organ transplantation patients are at the highest risk in the first year after transplantation, especially during their primary infection. Dissemination also can occur late as a result of reactivation of old infection. Lymphopenia is an important risk factor for dissemination. Cell-mediated immunity probably is the most important host factor in controlling coccidioidal infection. Therefore, it is not surprising that patients infected with HIV are at a greatly increased risk for developing severe forms of pulmonary coccidioidomycosis[52] and extrapulmonary diseases, including meningitis. In HIV-infected patients, active coccidioidomycosis may represent recrudescence of old healed disease.[17] However, coccidioidomycosis in most of these patients probably represents a primary infection.[56] In coccidioidomycosis-endemic areas, the risk of dissemination is highest in those with HIV infection acquired from intravenous drug use or blood transfusion.[84] A CD4 count of less than 250/μL is associated significantly with the development of active disease.[3] The clinical manifestations vary, ranging from minimal systemic symptoms without a pulmonary focus to severe cough and dyspnea associated with diffuse pulmonary disease and a radiographic pattern showing a discretely nodular appearance resembling *Pneumocystis carinii* infection. The severity of presentation is correlated inversely with CD4 counts, and severe disease is most common in patients with CD4 counts of less than 200/μL.[56] Even with appropriate antifungal therapy, the prognosis of HIV-infected patients with depressed CD4 counts who develop diffuse pulmonary coccidioidomycosis is poor, with a mortality rate of 70 per cent.[52, 56] HIV-infected patients also may present with evidence of extrapulmonary dissemination. Patients who have documented extrapulmonary dissemination in association with positive serologic tests for HIV are regarded as sufficiently immunoincompetent to be classified as having AIDS.[22] It is important to note that many HIV-infected patients who have positive serologic results without evidence of active disease go on to develop active coccidioidomycosis over time[8] and may be candidates for therapy.

DIAGNOSIS

In endemic areas where there is awareness of the disease, the diagnosis of coccidioidomycosis usually is established readily by obtaining appropriate laboratory studies. In other locations, the diagnosis is not considered unless a travel history is obtained. It should be remembered that cases have occurred even after brief exposure in an endemic area. Primary pulmonary coccidioidomycosis resembles other lower respiratory illnesses, including those caused by viruses, bacteria, mycoplasma, *Mycobacterium tuberculosis,* and other fungi (e.g., *Histoplasma).*

The hematologic findings in primary coccidioidal infection consist of elevation of the erythrocyte sedimentation rate, leukocytosis, and frequently eosinophilia.[49, 137] Marked eosinophilia may be a clue that dissemination has occurred.[71] Specific diagnosis usually is based on the results of skin tests, serologic reactions, and sputum examination.

Culture and Identification of the Fungus

The organism is detected readily by direct examination and culture from purulent material. The yield from other sources, such as pleural fluid, blood, and gastric aspirates, is somewhat lower. Only about one-third of spinal fluid samples are culture-positive, and direct examination of the cerebrospinal fluid almost always yields negative results.[72, 134] Detection of the fungus from the blood is uncommon and is associated with severe forms of disseminated disease.[4]

In severe pulmonary or disseminated disease, microscopic examination of bronchopulmonary lavage specimens, exudates, or biopsy specimens is diagnostic if typical spherules containing endospores are seen. Hematoxylin and eosin–stained sections can be used to demonstrate spherules but are used mainly to show the inflammatory process. The periodic acid–Schiff stain is useful for demonstrating the spherule contents (Fig. 200–7), whereas methenamine silver stains highlight the wall of the spherule. Cytologic examination of sputa is more sensitive than are potassium hydroxide stains.[161]

In HIV-infected patients who present with pulmonary infiltrates, coccidioidal spherules may be identified in bronchopulmonary lavage specimens by the same methenamine silver stain used to identify *P. carinii.* Indeed, in areas endemic for coccidioidomycosis, the possibility of concomitant pulmonary infections with both *C. immitis* and *P. carinii* or other pathogens should be kept in mind in this patient group.[56, 100] Cytologic examination of bronchial wash or bronchoalveolar fluid is diagnostic in only about one-third of persons with or without HIV infection and is less sensitive than is culture.[41] With the rare exception of persons with primary cutaneous infection, the finding of spherules in tissues outside the thoracic cavity is evidence that the patient has disseminated disease. For this reason, biopsy may be useful for establishing a diagnosis, particularly in patients with borderline or low complement-fixation antibody titers. Cultures of *C. immitis*

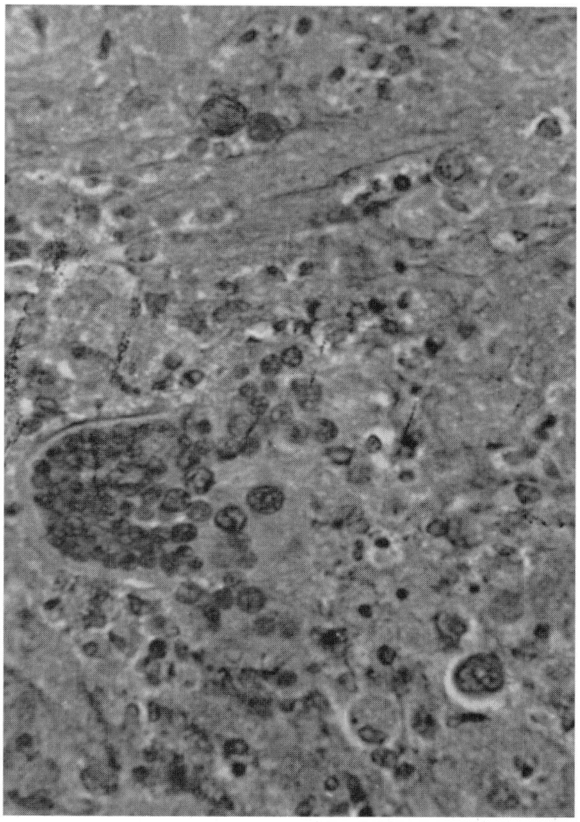

FIGURE 200–7. *A spherule that recently has ruptured and is in the process of releasing endospores.*

from body fluids, sputum, or exudates can be performed on most laboratory media. If *C. immitis* is suspected, the use of mycologic media containing cycloheximide can be helpful. The handling of the cultures is hazardous and requires special biosafety precautions.[83] Once a nonpigmented mold is grown, final identification requires conversion of the mycelial phase to the spherule stage. This is accomplished by animal inoculation or by the use of special media.[150] A more rapid detection method is the detection of specific exoantigens of the fungus in the culture media.[33, 146] Genetic probes now are available and allow for rapid and specific identification of *C. immitis*.[111]

Skin Test

The clinical usefulness of skin testing in patients suspected of having coccidioidomycosis has been reviewed. Two antigenic preparations derived from lysates of either the mycelial phase (coccidioidin)[126] or spherule phase (spherulin) are used clinically to elicit delayed hypersensitivity.[149] A positive skin test result to either preparation means that the patient has had infection at some time.[73, 131] The skin test results become positive 2 to 21 days after the onset of symptoms, usually before the serologic results have become positive. By the second week of illness, a negative skin test result would be unusual in primary coccidioidomycosis (<10 per cent).[143] However, a negative skin test result 1 month after the onset of symptoms frequently suggests latent dissemination or that the disease may disseminate later.[49, 137, 143]

The skin test is applied intradermally, and the presence of 5 mm or more of induration at 48 hours is interpreted as a positive result. The standard dose of coccidioidin is a dilution of 1:100; with spherulin, 0.1 mL of a solution containing 2.8 μg is applied. In patients with erythema nodosum, it is wise to initiate skin testing with a 10-fold dilution of these preparations to avoid severe local and systemic reactions. There is a low level of cross-reactivity with antigens from *Histoplasma capsulatum* or *Blastomyces dermatitidis*. However, skin testing does not induce delayed hypersensitivity[126] or serum antibody responses to coccidioidin[137] but may induce cross-reacting antibodies to histoplasmin.[117]

The skin test may be unreliable in immunosuppressed patients in whom a delayed hypersensitivity response may be impossible.

In a child who is a long-time resident of an endemic area, a positive skin test result is not helpful in the diagnosis of acute infection unless it is shown that the patient's skin test previously was negative. The greatest usefulness of the skin test is in population surveys for obtaining prevalence data and as a measure of cellular immunity, a factor in prognosis.

Serologic Studies

Figure 200–8 illustrates the serologic and skin test responses of symptomatic patients with primary coccidioidomycosis. The initial antibody response to coccidioidal infection predominantly is in the IgM fraction and is responsible for the positive precipitin test result that accompanies primary infection.[116, 132] These responses can be measured by tube precipitins, latex agglutination, enzyme immunoassay, or immunodiffusion methods.[117] Fifty per cent of patients yield positive results in the first week, and 90 per cent show precipitins within 2 to 3 weeks.[142] Thereafter, antibody reversion occurs, and by 5 months, only 10 per cent of patients with uncomplicated infection yield positive results.[142] Serum precipitins may persist in some patients with disseminated infection or may reappear with reactivation of infection. Precipitating IgM antibody detected by the tube precipitin assay or by immunodiffusion usually indicates acute infection.[142] In contrast with that seen with complement fixation, the magnitude of the precipitating antibody titer does not correlate with an increased risk of dissemination.[141] Occasionally, IgM antibody has been detected in cord blood of newborns whose mothers had detectable antibody. These infants did not have any evidence of infection on follow-up.[117] Latex agglutination is sensitive, rapid, and easy to perform but frequently yields false-positive reactions,[114, 117] and positive results should be confirmed by a second method. It also gives false-positive results in spinal fluids and in diluted sera and should not be used for these specimens.[115]

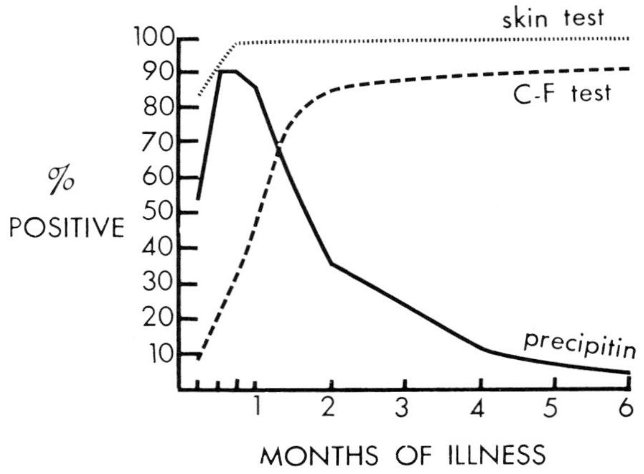

FIGURE 200–8. *Immunologic reactions in symptomatic primary coccidioidomycosis, relating time of appearance and duration to the frequency of positive reactions. (Based on Smith, C. E., Beard, R. R., Rosenberger, H. G., et al.: Effect of season and dust control on coccidioidomycosis. J. A. M. A. 132:833–838, 1946.)*

Serum IgG antibodies that fix complement usually appear later and last 6 to 8 months.[117] They are more common in more symptomatic infections and are detected in 50 to 90 per cent by 3 months after the onset of symptoms. At least 90 per cent of persons show a positive IgM or IgG response after symptomatic primary infections. The two main methods of detection of these antibodies are immunodiffusion and complement fixation.[117, 162] The two assays correlate well,[77] and immunodiffusion particularly is useful for the detection of antibody in patients whose sera are anticomplementary.[117]

Immunodiffusion yields few false-positive results and can detect early asymptomatic infection in persons infected with HIV.[8] This method seems to be slightly more sensitive than does complement fixation in detecting early infections.[86]

More recently, enzyme immunoassay has become available. This assay compares well with more traditional assays (complement fixation, immunodiffusion, latex agglutination) and does not suffer from the subjectivity required to interpret the other assays.[54, 102] The IgG enzyme immunoassay has a sensitivity of 92 per cent, whereas the IgM assay has a sensitivity of 77 per cent. When both assays are combined, the sensitivity is excellent,[86, 102] but the test suffers from false-positive results in patients with blastomycosis or suspected noncoccidioidal pulmonary illness.[86]

Antibodies measured by complement fixation are slower to develop and primarily are in the IgG fraction.[116, 117] Usually, they are not detected in serum samples obtained during the first week of infection, and their rise may occur as late as 3 months after onset of symptoms.[76, 142]

The magnitude of the complement-fixation antibody response correlates closely with the severity of infection and the likelihood of dissemination.[142] Although the antibody titer cannot be used as the sole indicator of dissemination, titers in most laboratories of 1:32 or greater are highly suggestive of extrapulmonary spread of infection[77, 142]; 61 per cent of these patients have a titer of at least 1:16, whereas 95 to 100 per cent of those without dissemination have a titer lower than 1:16. The titer of complement-fixation antibody parallels disease activity and is useful in following the progress of patients with disseminated disease. A few patients, especially those with extensive pulmonary involvement and pleural effusion, develop high titers without other clinical evidence of dissemination.[93] Conversely, some patients with dissemination, particularly those with single lesions in skin, bone, or meninges, have lower titers.

Some patients with immunodeficiency disease, in particular HIV infection, may have extensive disease with low or undetectable antibody levels[6, 52, 117] and negative skin test results to coccidioidal and other antigens.[56] Bone marrow transplant recipients may yield no serologic or skin test response before or shortly after bone marrow transplantation and may require aggressive attempts at culturing the fungus for diagnosis.[128] Some patients with HIV infection may have persistently positive serologic test results in the absence of any clinical disease. These patients are at high risk for active coccidioidomycosis and should be treated early.[8]

The complement-fixation antibody is detectable in the cerebrospinal fluid of 70 per cent of patients at the time of diagnosis of coccidioidal meningitis and eventually becomes detectable in all. The antibody measured is not a reflection of serum levels but rather is thought to indicate specific immunoglobulin biosynthesis by cells residing within or contiguous to the central nervous system. Occasionally, patients with vertebral osteomyelitis or epidural abscesses yield low complement-fixation titers in the cerebrospinal fluid without other evidence of meningeal involvement.

TREATMENT

Primary Infection

In more than 90 per cent of children, primary coccidioidomycosis is a self-limited illness, and antifungal therapy is not needed. In some children with severe primary disease, therapy with antifungal antibiotics may be justified to either abbreviate the period of morbidity or to lessen the chance of dissemination in those with an elevated complement-fixation titer.

Treatment is recommended for patients with continuous fever for more than 1 month, with extensive or progressive pulmonary disease, with severe prostration, with negative skin test results, with debilitation, who are pregnant women or are infants who have primary infection, who are receiving immunosuppressive therapy, and who are HIV-infected. Children from high-risk populations, such as Filipinos, or those with diseases that would be aggravated by coccidioidomycosis also should be treated. Treatment also should be considered for those with exposure to large inocula because of the increased risk of complications in these patients. The majority of other patients with primary disease do not have these indications for therapy but may have a number of minor criteria that adversely affect the course of illness. Seropositive asymptomatic patients with HIV infection also should be treated because of the high risk of dissemination in this population.

Because some of these patients may benefit from rapid improvement in symptoms, amphotericin B often is used as the initial drug of choice, followed by therapy with oral azoles. In adults, the usual cumulative dose is at least 1 g of amphotericin B.[59] For others, a trial of a month to a year of oral azoles may be indicated.[55]

Disseminated Disease

Nonmeningeal Dissemination

Patients with disseminated disease who have clinically apparent lesions outside of the thoracic cavity almost always should receive antifungal therapy; the agent of choice in fulminant infections is amphotericin B.

Treatment is indicated for patients with extrapulmonary dissemination. The classic therapy consists of amphotericin B administered initially at 1 to 1.5 mg/kg/day and then tapered to 1 to 1.5 mg/kg/day three times a week.[42] The usual total dose in adults is 1 to 2.5 g. In children, the maximal dose has not been defined because children tolerate amphotericin B better than adults do.[169] Local instillation or irrigation of abscesses and cavities with amphotericin B or other antifungal agents may be beneficial but has not been studied systematically.[13, 82] Amphotericin lipid-complexed preparations offer the possibility of administering higher doses with less toxicity; their role in the treatment of coccidioidomycosis remains to be defined and needs further study.

The total dose of amphotericin B depends on the patient's age and severity of disease; it ranges from 7.5 mg/kg in mild disease of older children to 100 mg/kg in patients with severe, protracted illness. Most patients, however, respond to between 15 and 45 mg/kg, with total dose and duration of therapy determined by the patient's response.

General clinical improvement, lowering of complement-fixation titers, and conversion to negative culture are favorable signs. These should be evaluated periodically, especially before therapy is discontinued.

The azoles have been tested extensively in this form of the disease. There have not been any comparative studies of ketoconazole, itraconazole, and fluconazole. In general, these drugs offer equivalent levels of efficacy, with response rates of about 50 to 60 per cent but also significant relapse rates after discontinuation of therapy.[55] As with other azoles,[58] the relapse rate after discontinuation of fluconazole therapy was 37 per cent, including a 50 per cent relapse rate for bone and joint infections.[19] Ketoconazole has the advantage of being significantly less costly than are the other two azoles; it is associated, however, with more gastrointestinal discomfort and may impair testosterone secretion and adrenal steroid synthesis without causing an adrenal crisis.[16, 122, 147] Itraconazole and ketoconazole have important drug interactions, most notably with cyclosporine and diphenylhydantoin.[66] In general, the azoles are used for a few months after resolution of symptoms or for at least a year of therapy.

Surgical therapy seldom is required in patients with primary disease, but therapeutic thoracentesis may be indicated rarely when pneumonitis is complicated by large pleural effusions.[93] Surgery also is necessary when pericardial involvement is complicated by tamponade. Patients with persistent coccidioidal cavities (>1 year) may require lobectomy, especially if the lesions are symptomatic.[101] Coccidioidal lymphadenopathy occasionally requires excision. In general, bone and joint disease requires a combined surgical and medical approach. Coccidioidal arthritis typically responds poorly to systemic therapy, and synovectomy may aid in the control of symptoms.[13, 121, 168] When surgical procedures are performed, a course of systemic therapy in the perioperative period is advisable to prevent further spread of disease.[51] Osteomyelitis optimally is dealt with by curetting and draining the involved bone with the addition of amphotericin B therapy or sometimes fluconazole.[13, 19, 35] Within endemic areas, it may be useful to screen HIV-infected patients serologically using immunodiffusion or complement fixation at a frequency of once every 6 months in order to identify active cases early. Consideration should be given to offering antifungal prophylaxis to such persons.[103] It is unclear whether such prophylaxis is effective, and the potential for drug resistance should be weighed.

Meningeal Disease

Amphotericin therapy of coccidioidal meningitis has been associated with a marked improvement in survival.[46, 87, 90] However, this treatment needs to include prolonged intrathecal therapy via lumbar, ventricular, or cisternal administration. This therapy is associated with significant side effects that include arachnoiditis headache, nausea, vomiting, chills and fever, arachnoiditis, and, occasionally, paralysis, seizures, and coma. These symptoms of arachnoiditis may be indistinguishable from those of microbiologic relapses.[72] Ketoconazole has been used with some success in meningitis but also is associated with a high relapse rate[39]; in high doses (1200 mg daily in adults, 15 to 23 mg/kg/day in children), therapy has been successful, but such doses tend to be tolerated poorly in adults.[55, 67, 72, 134]

Studies using 400 mg of fluconazole or itraconazole in the treatment of meningitis without concurrent use of amphotericin B show good results, with response rates of about 80 per cent.[57, 155–157] Many patients who do not show improvement on this regimen demonstrate clinical improvement when the dose is increased to 800 mg. Patients generally respond clinically within 1 to 2 months, although abnormalities of the cerebrospinal fluid may persist in some patients for a prolonged period. When therapy has been stopped, increases in cerebrospinal fluid cell count or complement-fixation antibody titer may be the only indications of reactivation of meningeal disease and signify a need to intensify therapy.[43]

Significant attention should be paid to cerebrospinal fluid flow dynamics because almost all children with coccidioidal meningitis develop obstructive hydrocephalus, which requires ventriculoperitoneal shunting and rarely a second shunt to drain a "trapped" fourth ventricle.[72, 134] Hence, the advantage of such a drug as fluconazole, which can be given systemically, obviates the problems of impaired cerebrospinal fluid flow faced when intrathecal or intraventricular therapy is used.

Recent studies have indicated that the relapse rate after discontinuation of azole therapy is high. Eleven of 14 (78 per cent) persons treated with azoles (ketoconazole, itraconazole, or fluconazole) for periods ranging from 8 to 101 months for coccidioidal meningitis had a relapse of disseminated coccidioidomycosis within 0.5 to 30 months after therapy was stopped. There were no clinical or laboratory predictors of patients at risk for a relapse. The data thus indicate that moderately prolonged azole therapy for coccidioidal meningitis suppresses but does not eradicate the infection, suggesting the need for prolonged if not lifelong therapy.[39, 148]

PROGNOSIS

Primary pulmonary coccidioidal infection usually is self-limited, with complete recovery in 1 to 3 weeks. In a small proportion of cases, localized complications of the primary infection, such as pleural effusion or pericarditis, prolong the clinical course. Dissemination is rare in whites and is less likely in patients with positive skin test results. Until the late 1950s, there was no effective therapy for the more severe forms of coccidioidomycosis, and the mortality rate of patients with disseminated disease was approximately 50 per cent.[49] The mortality rate of patients with multiple sites of dissemination and those with coccidioidal meningitis approached 100 per cent.[46, 159] Presently, therapy with amphotericin B or azoles may cure some of these patients, and in many others prolongs useful life. Certain forms of disseminated infection, such as joint involvement, particularly are resistant to systemic therapy and may persist for many years without other signs of dissemination. For patients with HIV infection, therapy of disseminated coccidioidomycosis usually is not curative, and lifelong suppressive therapy with intermittent doses of amphotericin B or oral therapy with ketoconazole or fluconazole may be required to prevent relapses.[105] Some experts even advise use of lifelong suppressive therapy for HIV-infected patients with uncomplicated pulmonary coccidioidomycosis.

PREVENTION

A killed vaccine has been prepared from spherules and is efficacious in experimental animals.[78, 92] In trials conducted in adult humans, the vaccine was tolerated reasonably well but did not result in significant decreases in attack rates or severity of disease.[113] Live attenuated strains of *C. immitis* also are highly immunogenic in experimental animals, but viable organisms tend to persist in the immunized host. Furthermore, the strains are unstable, reverting to their virulent form after several passages in animals. For these reasons, there is no effective means currently available for prevention of human coccidioidomycosis.

Other efforts at prevention have been aimed at dust control and eradication of the organisms from the soil.[139] Whether or not these measures are effective is unproved, and in rural areas they are costly and impractical. Immunosuppressed children with negative skin test results should be advised not to engage in field activities or organized excursions into areas highly endemic for coccidioidomycosis.[152, 163]

References

1. Albert, B. L., and Sellers, T. F., Jr.: Coccidioidomycosis from fomites. Arch. Intern. Med. *112*:253–261, 1963.
2. Ampel, N. M., Bejarano, G. C., Salas, S. D., et al.: In vitro assessment of cellular immunity in human coccidioidomycosis: Relationship between dermal hypersensitivity, lymphocyte transformation, and lymphokine production by peripheral blood mononuclear cells from healthy adults. J. Infect. Dis. *165*:710–715, 1992.
3. Ampel, N. M., Dols, C. L., and Galgiani, J. N.: Coccidioidomycosis during human immunodeficiency virus infection: Results of a prospective study in a coccidioidal endemic area. Am. J. Med. *94*:235–240, 1993.
4. Ampel, N. M., Ryan, K. J., Carry, P. J., et al.: Fungemia due to *Coccidioides immitis:* An analysis of 16 episodes in 15 patients and a review of the literature. Medicine *65*:312–321, 1986.
5. Ampel, N. M., Wieden, M. A., and Galgiani, J. N.: Coccidioidomycosis: Clinical update. Rev. Infect. Dis. *11*:897–911, 1989.
6. Anonymous: Coccidioidomycosis: United States, 1991–1992. M. M. W. R. *42*:21–24, 1993.
7. Antoniskis, D., Larsen, R. A., Akil, B., et al.: Seronegative disseminated coccidioidomycosis in patients with HIV infection. AIDS *4*:691–693, 1990.
8. Arguinchona, H. L., Ampel, N. M., Dols, C. L., et al.: Persistent coccidioidal seropositivity without clinical evidence of active coccidioidomycosis in patients with human immunodeficiency virus. Clin. Infect. Dis. *20*:1281–1285, 1995
9. Barbee, R. A., and Hicks, M. J.: Clinical usefulness of lymphocyte transformation in patients with coccidioidomycosis. Chest *93*:1003–1007, 1988.
10. Batra, P.: Pulmonary coccidioidomycosis. J. Thorac. Imag. *7*:29–38, 1992.
11. Bernstein, D. I., Tipton, J. R., Schott, S. F., et al.: Coccidioidomycosis in a neonate: Maternal-infant transmission. J. Pediatr. *99*:752–754, 1981.

12. Birsner, J. W.: The roentgen aspects of five hundred cases of pulmonary coccidioidomycosis. Am. J. Roentgenol. Rad. Ther. *72*:556–573, 1954.
13. Bisla, R. S., and Taber, T. H., Jr.: Coccidioidomycosis of bone and joints. Clin. Orthop. *121*:196–204, 1976.
14. Bouza, E., Dreyer, J. S., Hewitt, W. L., et al.: Coccidioidal meningitis: An analysis of thirty-one cases and review of the literature. Medicine *60*:139–172, 1981.
15. Boyle, J. O., Coulthard, S. W., and Mandel, R. M.: Laryngeal involvement in disseminated coccidioidomycosis. Arch. Otolaryngol. Head Neck Surg. *117*:433–438, 1991.
16. Britton, H., Shehab, Z., Lightner, E., et al.: Adrenal response in children receiving high doses of ketoconazole for coccidioidomycosis. J. Pediatr. *112*:488–492, 1988.
17. Bronnimann, D. A., Adam, R. D., Galgiani, J. N., et al.: Coccidioidomycosis in acquired immune deficiency syndrome. Ann. Intern. Med. *106*:372–379, 1987.
18. Castellino, R. A., and Blank, N.: Pulmonary coccidioidomycosis: The wide spectrum of roentgenographic manifestations. Calif. Med. *109*:41–49, 1969.
19. Catanzaro, A., Galgiani, J. N., Levine, B. E., et al.: Fluconazole in the treatment of chronic pulmonary and nonmeningeal disseminated coccidioidomycosis: NIAID Mycoses Study Group. Am. J. Med. *98*:249–256, 1995.
20. Catanzaro, A., Spitler, L. E., and Moser, K. M.: Cellular immune response in coccidioidomycosis. Cell. Immunol. *15*:360–371, 1975.
21. Caudill, R. G., Smith, C. E., and Reinarz, J. A.: Coccidioidal meningitis: A diagnostic challenge. Am. J. Med. *49*:360–365, 1970.
22. Centers for Disease Control: Revision of the CDC surveillance case definition of acquired immunodeficiency syndrome. M. M. W. R. *36*(Suppl. 1):S3–S15, 1987.
23. Child, D. C., Newell, J. D., Bjelland, J. C., et al.: Radiographic findings of pulmonary coccidioidomycosis in neonates and infants. A. J. R. Am. J. Roentgenol. *145*:261–263, 1985.
24. Christian, J. R., Sarre, S. G., Peers, J. H., et al.: Pulmonary coccidioidomycosis in a twenty-one-day-old infant. Am. J. Dis. Child. *92*:66–73, 1956.
25. Cohen, I. M., Galgiani, J. N., Potter, D., et al.: Coccidioidomycosis in renal replacement therapy. Arch. Intern. Med. *142*:489–494, 1982.
26. Cohen, R.: Coccidioidomycosis: Case studies in children. Arch. Pediatr. *66*:241–265, 1949.
27. Cohen, R.: Placental *Coccidioides*: Proof that congenital *Coccidioides* is nonexistent. Arch. Pediatr. *68*:59–66, 1951.
28. Cohen, R., and Burnip, R.: Coccidioidin skin testing during pregnancy and in infants and children. Calif. Med. *72*:31–33, 1950.
29. Cox, R. A.: Cross-reactivity between antigens of *Coccidioides immitis, Histoplasma capsulatum,* and *Blastomyces dermatitidis* in lymphocyte transformation assays. Infect. Immun. *25*:932–938, 1979.
30. Cox, R. A., Brummer, E., and Lecara, G.: In vitro lymphocyte responses of coccidioidin skin test–positive and –negative persons to coccidioidin, spherulin, and a *Coccidioides* cell wall antigen. Infect. Immun. *15*:751–755, 1977.
31. Cox, R. A., Vivas, J. R., Gross, A., et al.: In vivo and in vitro cell-mediated responses in coccidioidomycosis: Immunologic responses of persons with primary, asymptomatic infections. Am. Rev. Respir. Dis. *114*:937–943, 1976.
31a. Davis, B. D., Delbecco, R., Eisen, H. W., et al.: Microbiology: Including Immunology and Molecular Genetics. 3rd ed. Hagerstown, Harper & Row, 1980.
32. Dennis, J. L., and Hansen, A. E.: Coccidioidomycosis in children. Pediatrics *14*:481–494, 1954.
33. Denys, G. A., Newman, M. A., and Standard, P. G.: Evaluation of a commercial exoantigen test system for the rapid identification of systemic fungal pathogens. Am. J. Clin. Pathol. *79*:379–381, 1983.
34. Deresinski, S. C.: History of coccidioidomycosis: Dust to dust. *In* Stevens, D. A. (ed.): Coccidioidomycosis: A Text. New York, Plenum Medical, 1980, pp. 1–20.
35. Deresinski, S. C.: Coccidioidomycosis of bone and joints. *In* Stevens, D. A. (ed.): Coccidioidomycosis: A Text. New York, Plenum Medical, 1980, pp. 195–224.
36. Deresinski, S. C., Applegate, R. J., Levine, H. B., et al.: Cellular immunity to *Coccidioides immitis:* In vitro lymphocyte response to spherules, arthrospores, and endospores. Cell. Immunol. *32*:110–119, 1977.
37. Deresinski, S. C., Levine, H. B., and Stevens, D. A.: Soluble antigens of mycelia and spherules in the in vitro detection of immunity to *Coccidioides immitis*. Infect. Immun. *10*:700–704, 1974.
38. Deresinski, S. C., and Stevens, D. A.: Coccidioidomycosis in compromised hosts. Medicine *54*:377–395, 1974.
39. Dewsnup, D. H., Galgiani, J. N., Graybill, J. R., et al.: Is it ever safe to stop azole therapy for *Coccidioides immitis* meningitis? Ann. Intern. Med. *124*:305–310, 1996.
40. Dickson, E. C.: "Valley fever" of the San Joaquin Valley and fungus. Calif. West. Med. *47*:151–155, 1937.
41. DiTomasso, J. P., Ampel, N. M., Sobonya, R. E., et al.: Bronchoscopic diagnosis of pulmonary coccidioidomycosis: Comparison of cytology, culture, and transbronchial biopsy. Diagn. Microbiol. Infect. Dis. *18*:83–87, 1994.
42. Drutz, D. J.: Amphotericin B in the treatment of coccidioidomycosis. Drugs *26*:337–346, 1983.
43. Drutz, D. J., and Catanzaro, A.: Coccidioidomycosis. Am. Rev. Respir. Dis. *117*:559–585, 727–771, 1978.
44. Eckmann, B. H., Schaefer, G. L., and Huppert, M.: Bedside interhuman transmission of coccidioidomycosis via growth on fomites: An epidemic involving six persons. Am. Rev. Respir. Dis. *89*:175–185, 1964.
45. Egeberg, R. O., and Ely, A. F.: *Coccidioides immitis* in the soil of the southern San Joaquin Valley. Am. J. Med. Sci. *23*:151–154, 1956.
46. Einstein, H. E., Holemann, C. W., Sandidge, L. L., et al.: Coccidioidal meningitis: The use of amphotericin B in treatment. Calif. Med. *94*:339–343, 1961.
47. Emmons, C. W.: Isolation of *Coccidioides* from soil and rodents. Public Health Rep. *57*:109–111, 1942.
48. Feigin, R. D., Shackelford, P. G., Lins, R. D., et al.: Subcutaneous abscess due to *Coccidioides immitis*. Am. J. Dis. Child. *124*:734–735, 1972.
49. Fiese, M. J.: Coccidioidomycosis. Springfield, Charles C Thomas, 1958.
50. Fiese, M. J., Cheu, S., and Sorensen, R. H.: Mycelial forms of *Coccidioides immitis* in sputum and tissues of the human host. Ann. Intern. Med. *43*:255–270, 1955.
51. Findlay, F. M., and Melick, D. W.: Treatment of cavitary coccidioidomycosis. *In* Ajello, L. (ed.): Coccidioidomycosis. Tucson, University of Arizona Press, 1967, pp. 79–83.
52. Fish, D. G., Ampel, N. M., Galgiani, J. N., et al.: Coccidioidomycosis during human immunodeficiency virus infection: A review of 77 patients. Medicine *69*:384–391, 1990.
53. Flynn, N. M., Hoeprich, P. D., Kawachi, M. M., et al.: An unusual outbreak of windborne coccidioidomycosis. N. Engl. J. Med. *301*:358–361, 1979.
54. Gade, W., Ledman, D. W., Wethington, R., et al.: Serological responses to various *Coccidioides* antigen preparations in a new enzyme immunoassay. J. Clin. Microbiol. *30*:1907–1912, 1992.
55. Galgiani, J. N.: Coccidioidomycosis. West. J. Med. *159*:153–171, 1993.
56. Galgiani, J. N., and Ampel, N. M.: Coccidioidomycosis in human immunodeficiency virus-infected patients. J. Infect. Dis. *162*:1165–1169, 1990.
57. Galgiani, J. N., Catanzaro, A., Cloud, G. A., et al.: Fluconazole therapy for coccidioidal meningitis: The NIAID-Mycoses Study Group. Ann. Intern. Med. *119*:28–35, 1993.
58. Galgiani, J. N., Stevens, D. A., Graybill, J. R., et al.: Ketoconazole therapy of progressive coccidioidomycosis: Comparison of 400 and 800 mg doses and observations at higher doses. Am. J. Med. *84*:603–608, 1988.
59. Gallis, H. A., Drew, R. H., and Pickard, W. W.: Amphotericin B: 30 years of clinical experience. Rev. Infect. Dis. *12*:308–329, 1990.
60. Gardner, S., Seilheimer, D., Catlin, F., et al.: Subglottic coccidioidomycosis presenting with persistent stridor. Pediatrics *66*:623–625, 1980.
61. Gifford, M. A., Buss, W. I. C., and Duds, R. J.: Data on *Coccidioides* fungus infection, Kern County, 1900–1936. *In* Kern County Health Department Annual Report. 1936–1937, pp. 39–54.
62. Golden, S. E., Morgan, C. M., Bartley, D. L., et al.: Disseminated coccidioidomycosis with chorioretinitis in early infancy. Pediatr. Infect. Dis. *5*:272–274, 1986.
63. Goldstein, E., Winship, M. J., and Pappagianis, D.: Ventricular fluid and the management of coccidioidal meningitis. Ann. Intern. Med. *77*:243–246, 1972.
64. Goodman, D. H., and Schabarum, B.: Primary cutaneous coccidioidomycosis: Visible classic demonstration of delayed hypersensitivity. Ann. Intern. Med. *59*:84–90, 1963.
65. Graham, A. R., Sobonya, R. E., Bronnimann, D. A., et al.: Quantitative pathology of coccidioidomycosis in acquired immunodeficiency syndrome. Hum. Pathol. *19*:800–806, 1988.
66. Graybill, J. R.: Treatment of coccidioidomycosis. Curr. Top. Med. Mycol. *5*:151–179, 1993.
67. Graybill, J. R., Stevens, D. A., Galgiani, J. N., et al.: Ketoconazole treatment of coccidioidal meningitis. Ann. N. Y. Acad. Sci. *544*:488–496, 1988.
68. Greendyke, W. H., Resnick, D. L., and Harvey, W. C.: The varied roentgen manifestations of primary coccidioidomycosis. Am. J. Roentgenol. Radium Ther. Nucl. Med. *109*:491–499, 1970.
69. Hajare, S., Rakusan, T. A., Kalia, A., et al.: Laryngeal coccidioidomycosis causing airway obstruction. Pediatr. Infect. Dis. *8*:54–56, 1989.
70. Hall, K. A., Sethi, G. K., Rosado, L. J., et al.: Coccidioidomycosis and heart transplantation. J. Heart Lung Transplant. *12*:525–526, 1993.
71. Harley, W. B., and Blaser, M. J.: Disseminated coccidioidomycosis associated with extreme eosinophilia. Clin. Infect. Dis. *18*:627–629, 1994.
72. Harrison, H. R., Galgiani, J. N., Sprunger, L., et al.: Amphotericin B and imidazole therapy for coccidioidal meningitis in children. Pediatr. Infect. Dis. *2*:216–221, 1983.
73. Hobbs, E. R.: Coccidioidomycosis. Dermatol. Clin. *7*:227–239, 1989.
74. Huntington, R. W., Jr.: Morphology and racial distribution of fatal coccidioidomycosis: Report of a 10-year autopsy series in an endemic area. J. A. M. A. *169*:115–118, 1959.
75. Huntington, R. W.: Pathology of coccidioidomycosis. *In* Stevens, D. A. (ed.): Coccidioidomycosis: A Text. New York, Plenum Medical, 1980, pp. 113–132.
76. Huppert, M.: Serology of coccidioidomycosis. Mycopathol. Mycol. Appl. *41*:107–113, 1970.
77. Huppert, M., and Bailey, J. W.: The use of immunodiffusion tests in coccidioidomycosis. I. The accuracy and reproducibility of the immunodiffusion test which correlates with complement fixation. Am. J. Clin. Pathol. *44*:364–373, 1965.
78. Huppert, M., Levine, H. B., Sun, S. H., et al.: Resistance of vaccinated

mice to typical and atypical strains of *Coccidioides immitis.* J. Bacteriol. *94*:924–927, 1967.
79. Huppert, M., and Sun, S. H.: Overview of mycology, and the mycology of *Coccidioides immitis. In* Stevens, D. A. (ed.): Coccidioidomycosis: A Text. New York, Plenum Medical, 1980, pp. 21–46.
80. Hyatt, H. W., Sr.: Coccidioidomycosis in a 3-week-old infant. Am. J. Dis. Child. *105*:93–98, 1963.
81. Hyde, L.: Coccidioidal pulmonary cavitation. Dis. Chest *54*(Suppl. 1):273–277, 1968.
82. Iger, M.: Coccidioidal osteomyelitis. *In* Ajello, L. (ed.): Coccidioidomycosis. Miami, Symposia Specialists, 1977, pp. 177–190.
83. Johnson, J. E., III, Perry, J. E., Fekety, F. R., et al.: Laboratory-acquired coccidioidomycosis: A report of 210 cases. Ann. Intern. Med. *60*:941–956, 1964.
84. Jones, J. L., Fleming, P. L., Ciesielski, C. A., et al.: Coccidioidomycosis among patients with AIDS in the United States. J. Infect. Dis. *171*:961–966, 1995.
85. Kafka, J. A., and Catanzaro, A. T.: Disseminated coccidioidomycosis in children. J. Pediatr. *98*:355–361, 1981.
86. Kaufman, L., Sekhon, A. S., Moledina, N., et al.: Comparative evaluation of commercial Premier EIA and microimmunodiffusion and complement fixation tests for *Coccidioides immitis* antibodies. J. Clin. Microbiol. *33*:618–619, 1995.
87. Kelly, P. C.: Coccidioidal meningitis. *In* Stevens, D. A. (ed.): Coccidioidomycosis: A Text. New York, Plenum Medical, 1980, pp. 163–193.
88. Kerrick, S. S., Lundergan, L. L., and Galgiani, J. N.: Coccidioidomycosis at a university health service. Am. Rev. Respir. Dis. *131*:100–102, 1985.
89. Knoper, S. R., and Galgiani, J. N.: Coccidioidomycosis. Infect. Dis. Clin. North Am. *2*:861–875, 1988.
90. Labadie, E. L., and Hamilton, R. H.: Survival improvement in coccidioidal meningitis by high-dose intrathecal amphotericin B. Arch. Intern. Med. *146*:2013–2018, 1986.
91. Larwood, T.: Further drop in Kern County coccidioidin reactivity. Transactions of the Ninth Annual Coccidioidomycosis Conference. Los Angeles and Oakland, California Thoracic Society, 1964, pp. 8–9.
92. Levine, H. B., Pappagianis, D., and Cobb, J. M.: Development of vaccines for coccidioidomycosis. Mycopathol. Mycol. Appl. *41*:177–185, 1970.
93. Lonky, S. A., Catanzaro, A., Moser, K. M., et al.: Acute coccidioidal pleural effusion. Am. Rev. Respir. Dis. *114*:681–688, 1976.
94. Looney, J. M., and Stein, T.: Coccidioidomycosis: The hazards involved in diagnostic procedures, with report of a case. N. Engl. J. Med. *242*:77–82, 1950.
95. Lopez, A. M., Williams, P. L., and Ampel, N. M.: Acute pulmonary coccidioidomycosis mimicking bacterial pneumonia and septic shock: A report of two cases. Am. J. Med. *95*:236–239, 1993.
96. Lubarsky, R., and Plunkett, O. A.: Some ecologic studies of *Coccidioides immitis* in soil. *In* Sternberg, T. H., and Newcomer, V. D. (eds.): Therapy of Fungus Diseases, an International Symposium. Boston, Little, Brown, 1955, pp. 308–310.
97. Lundergan, L. L., Kerrick, S. S., and Galgiani, J. N.: Coccidioidomycosis at a university outpatient clinic: A clinical description. *In* Einstein, H. E., and Catanzaro, A. (eds.): Coccidioidomycosis. Proceedings of the Fourth International Conference. Washington D.C., National Foundation for Infectious Diseases, 1985, pp. 47–54.
98. MacDonald, N., Steinhoff, M. C., and Powell, K. R.: Review of coccidioidomycosis in immunocompromised children. Am. J. Dis. Child. *135*:553–556, 1981.
99. Maddy, K. T.: Observations on *Coccidioides immitis* found growing naturally in soil. Ariz. Med. *22*:281–288, 1965.
100. Mahaffey, K. W., Hippenmeyer, C. L., Mandel, R., et al.: Unrecognized coccidioidomycosis complicating *Pneumocystis carinii* pneumonia in patients infected with the human immunodeficiency virus and treated with corticosteroids: A report of two cases. Arch. Intern. Med. *153*:1496–1498, 1993.
101. Marks, T. S., Spence, W. F., and Baisch, B. F.: Limited resection for pulmonary coccidioidomycosis. *In* Ajello, L. (ed.): Coccidioidomycosis. Tucson, University of Arizona Press, 1967, pp. 73–78.
102. Martins, T. B., Jaskowski, T. D., Mouritsen, C. L., et al.: Comparison of commercially available enzyme immunoassay with traditional serological tests for detection of antibodies to *Coccidioides immitis*. J. Clin. Microbiol. *33*:940–943, 1995.
103. McNeil, M. M., and Ampel, N. M.: Coccidioidomycosis in patients infected with human immunodeficiency virus: Prevention issues and priorities. Clin. Infect. Dis. *21*:S111–S113, 1995.
104. Medeiros, A. A., Marty, S. D., Tosh, F. E., et al.: Erythema nodosum and erythema multiforme as clinical manifestations of histoplasmosis in a community outbreak. N. Engl. J. Med. *274*:415–420, 1966.
105. Minamoto, G., and Armstrong, D.: Fungal infections in AIDS: Histoplasmosis and coccidioidomycosis. Infect. Dis. Clin. North Am. *2*:447–456, 1988.
106. Mischel, P. S., and Vinters, H. V.: Coccidioidomycosis of the central nervous system: Neuropathological and vasculopathic manifestations and clinical correlates. Clin. Infect. Dis. *20*:400–405, 1995.
107. Murphy, S. M., Drash, A. L., and Donnelly, W. H.: Disseminated coccidioidomycosis associated with immunosuppressive therapy following renal transplantation. Pediatrics *48*:144–145, 1971.
108. O'Brien, J. J., and Gilsdorf, J. R.: Primary cutaneous coccidioidomycosis in childhood. Pediatr. Infect. Dis. *5*:485–486, 1986.
109. Opelz, G., and Scheer, M. I.: Cutaneous sensitivity and in vitro responsiveness of lymphocytes in patients with disseminated coccidioidomycosis. J. Infect. Dis. *132*:250–255, 1975.
110. Overholt, E. L., and Hornick, R. B.: Primary cutaneous coccidioidomycosis. Arch. Intern. Med. *114*:149–153, 1964.
111. Padhye, A. A., Smith, G., Standard, P. G., et al.: Comparative evaluation of chemiluminescent DNA probe assays and exoantigen tests for rapid identification of *Blastomyces dermatitidis* and *Coccidioides immitis*. J. Clin. Microbiol. *32*:867–870, 1994.
112. Pappagianis, D.: Epidemiology of coccidioidomycosis. Curr. Top. Med. Mycol. *2*:199–238, 1988.
113. Pappagianis, D.: Evaluation of the protective efficacy of the killed *Coccidioides immitis* spherule vaccine in humans: The Valley Fever Vaccine Study Group. Am. Rev. Respir. Dis. *148*:656–660, 1993.
114. Pappagianis, D., and Kobayashi, G. S.: Approaches to the physiology of *Coccidioides immitis*. Ann. N. Y. Acad. Sci. *89*:109–121, 1960.
115. Pappagianis, D., Krasnow, R. I., and Beall, S.: False-positive reactions of cerebrospinal fluid and diluted sera with the coccidioidal latex agglutination test. Am. J. Clin. Pathol. *66*:916–921, 1976.
116. Pappagianis, D., Lindsey, N. J., Smith, C. E., et al.: Antibodies in human coccidioidomycosis: Immunoelectrophoretic properties. Proc. Soc. Exp. Biol. Med. *118*:118–122, 1965.
117. Pappagianis. D., and Zimmer, D. L.: Serology of coccidioidomycosis. Clin. Microbiol. Rev. *3*:247–268, 1990.
118. Petersen, E. A., Friedman, B. A., Crowder, E. D., et al.: Coccidioiduria: Clinical significance. Ann. Intern. Med. *85*:34–38, 1976.
119. Peterson, C. M., Schuppert, K., Kelly, P. C., et al.: Coccidioidomycosis and pregnancy. Obstet. Gynecol. Surv. *48*:149–156, 1993.
120. Pinckney, L., and Parker, B. R.: Primary coccidioidomycosis in children presenting with massive pleural effusion. A. J. R. Am. J. Roentgenol. *130*:247–249, 1978.
121. Pollock, S. F., Morris, J. M., and Murray, W. R.: Coccidioidal synovitis of the knee. J. Bone Joint Surg. [Am.] *49*:1397–1407, 1967.
122. Pont, A., Williams, P. L., Azhar, S., et al.: Ketoconazole blocks testosterone synthesis. Arch. Intern. Med. *142*:2137–2140, 1982.
123. Puckett, T. F.: Hyphae of *Coccidioides immitis* in tissues of the human host. Am. Rev. Tuberc. *70*:320–327, 1954.
124. Ragland, A. S., Arsura, E., Ismail, Y., et al.: Eosinophilic pleocytosis in coccidioidal meningitis: Frequency and significance. Am. J. Med. *95*:254–257, 1993.
125. Ramras, D. G., Walch, H. A., Murray, J. P., et al.: An epidemic of coccidioidomycosis in the Pacific Beach area of San Diego. Am. Rev. Respir. Dis. *101*:975–978, 1970.
126. Rapaport, F. T., Lawrence, H. S., Millar, J. W., et al.: The immunologic properties of coccidioidin as a skin test reagent in man. J. Immunol. *84*:368–373, 1960.
127. Richardson, H. B., Jr., Anderson, J. A., and McKay, B. M.: Acute pulmonary coccidioidomycosis in children. J. Pediatr. *70*:376–382, 1967.
128. Riley, D. K., Galgiani, J. N., O'Donnell, M., et al.: Coccidioidomycosis in bone marrow transplant recipients. Transplantation *56*:1531–1533, 1993.
129. Roberts, P. L., and Lisciandro, R. C.: A community epidemic of coccidioidomycosis. Am. Rev. Respir. Dis. *96*:766–772, 1967.
130. Rothman, P. E., Graw, R. G., and Harris, J. C.: Coccidioidomycosis: Possible fomite transmission: A review and report of a case. Am. J. Dis. Child. *118*:792–801, 1969.
131. Sarosi, G. A., Catanzaro, A., Daniel, T. M., et al.: Clinical usefulness of skin testing in histoplasmosis, coccidioidomycosis, and blastomycosis. Am. Rev. Respir. Dis. *138*:1081–1082, 1988.
132. Sawaki, Y., Huppert, M., Bailey, J. W., et al.: Patterns of human antibody reactions in coccidioidomycosis. J. Bacteriol. *91*:422–427, 1966.
133. Shafai, T.: Neonatal coccidioidomycosis in premature twins. Am. J. Dis. Child. *132*:634, 1978.
134. Shehab, Z. M., Britton, H., and Dunn, J. H.: Imidazole therapy of coccidioidal meningitis in children. Pediatr. Infect. Dis. J. *7*:40–44, 1988.
135. Sievers, M. L.: Disseminated coccidioidomycosis among southwestern American Indians. Am. Rev. Respir. Dis. *109*:602–612, 1974.
136. Smale, L. E., and Waechter, K. G.: Dissemination of coccidioidomycosis in pregnancy. Am. J. Obstet. Gynecol. *107*:356–361, 1970.
137. Smith, C. E.: Coccidioidomycosis. Pediatr. Clin. North Am. *2*:109–125, 1955.
138. Smith, C. E.: Epidemiology of acute coccidioidomycosis with erythema nodosum ("San Joaquin" or "Valley Fever"). Am. J. Public Health *30*:600–611, 1940.
139. Smith, C. E., Beard, R. R., Rosenberger, H. G., et al.: Effect of season and dust control on coccidioidomycosis. J. A. M. A. *132*:833–838, 1946.
140. Smith, C. E., Beard, R. R., Whiting, E. G., et al.: Varieties of coccidioidal infection in relation to the epidemiology and control of the diseases. Am. J. Public Health *36*:1394–1402, 1946.
141. Smith, C. E., Saito, M. T., Beard, R. R., et al.: Serological tests in the diagnosis and prognosis of coccidioidomycosis. Am. J. Hyg. *52*:1–21, 1950.

142. Smith, C. E., Saito, M. T., and Simons, S. A.: Pattern of 39,500 serologic tests in coccidioidomycosis. J. A. M. A. *160*:546–552, 1956.
143. Smith, C. E., Whiting, E. G., Baker, E. E., et al.: The use of coccidioidin. Am. Rev. Tuberc. *57*:330–360, 1948.
144. Spark, R. P.: Does transplacental spread of coccidioidomycosis occur? Arch. Pathol. Lab. Med. 105:347–350, 1981.
145. Standaert, S. M., Schaffner, W., Galgiani, J. N., et al.: Coccidioidomycosis among visitors to a *Coccidioides immitis*–endemic area: An outbreak in a military reserve unit. J. Infect. Dis. *171*:1672–1675, 1995.
146. Standard, P. G., and Kaufman, L.: Immunological procedure for the rapid and specific identification of *Coccidioides immitis* cultures. J. Clin. Microbiol. *5*:149–153, 1977.
147. Stevens, D. A.: Ketoconazole metamorphosis: An antimicrobial becomes an endocrine drug. Ann. Intern. Med. *145*:813–815, 1985.
148. Stevens, D. A.: Coccidioidomycosis. N. Engl. J. Med. *332*:1077–1082, 1995.
149. Stevens, D. A., Levine, H. B., Ten Eyck, D. R., et al.: Dermal sensitivity to different doses of spherulin and coccidioidin. Chest *65*:530–533, 1974.
150. Sun, S. H., Huppert, M., and Vukovich, K. R.: Rapid in vitro conversion and identification of *Coccidioides immitis*. J. Clin. Microbiol. *3*:186–190, 1976.
151. Tarbet, J. E., and Breslau, A. M.: Histochemical investigation of the spherule of *Coccidioides immitis* in relation to host reactions. J. Infect. Dis. *92*:183–190, 1953.
152. Teel, K. W., Yow, M. D., and Williams, T. W., Jr.: A localized outbreak of coccidioidomycosis in southern Texas. J. Pediatr. *77*:65–73, 1970.
153. Tom, P. F., Long, T. J., and Fitzpatrick, S. B.: Coccidioidomycosis in adolescents presenting as chest pain. J. Adolesc. Health Care *8*:365–371, 1987.
154. Townsend, T. E., and McKey, R. W.: Coccidioidomycosis in infants. Am. J. Dis. Child. *86*:51–53, 1953.
155. Tucker, R. M., Denning, D. W., Dupont, B., et al.: Itraconazole therapy for chronic coccidioidal meningitis. Ann. Intern. Med. *112*:108–112, 1990.
156. Tucker, R. M., Galgiani, J. N., Denning, D. W., et al.: Treatment of coccidioidal meningitis with fluconazole. Rev. Infect. Dis. *12*:S380–S389, 1990.
157. Tucker, R. M., Williams, P. L., Arathoon, E. G., et al.: Pharmacokinetics of fluconazole in cerebrospinal fluid and serum in human coccidioidal meningitis. Antimicrob. Agents Chemother. *32*:369–373, 1988.
158. Vaughan, J. E., and Ramirez, H.: Coccidioidomycosis as a complication of pregnancy. Calif. Med. *74*:121–125, 1951.
159. Vincent, T., Galgiani, J. N., Huppert, M., et al.: The natural history of coccidioidal meningitis: VA-Armed Forces cooperative studies, 1955–1958. Clin. Infect. Dis. *16*:247–254, 1993.
160. Wack, E. E., Ampel, N. M., Galgiani, J. N., et al.: Coccidioidomycosis during pregnancy: An analysis of ten cases among 47,120 pregnancies. Chest *94*:376–379, 1988.
161. Warlick, M. A., Quan, S. F., and Sobonya, R. E.: Rapid diagnosis of pulmonary coccidioidomycosis: Cytologic v. potassium hydroxide preparations. Arch. Intern. Med. *143*:723–725, 1983.
162. Weiden, M. A., Galgiani, J. N., and Pappagianis, D.: Comparison of immunodiffusion techniques with standard complement fixation assay for quantitation of coccidioidal antibodies. J. Clin. Microbiol. *18*:529–534, 1983.
163. Werner, S. B., Pappagianis, D., Heindl, I., et al.: An epidemic of coccidioidomycosis among archeology students in northern California. N. Engl. J. Med. *28*:507–512, 1972.
164. Williams, P. L., Johnson, R., Pappagianis, D., et al.: Vasculitic and encephalitic complications associated with *Coccidioides immitis* infection of the central nervous system in humans: Report of 10 cases and review. Clin. Infect. Dis. *14*:673–682, 1992.
165. Winn, R. E., Johnson, R., Galgiani, J. N., et al.: Cavitary coccidioidomycosis with fungus ball formation: Diagnosis by fiberoptic bronchoscopy with coexistence of hyphae and spherules. Chest *105*:412–416, 1994.
166. Winn, W. A.: Primary cutaneous coccidioidomycosis. Arch. Dermatol. *9*:221–228, 1965.
167. Winn, W. A., Levine, H. B., Broderick, J. E., et al.: A localized epidemic of coccidioidal infection: Primary coccidioidomycosis occurring in a group of ten children infected in a backyard playground in the San Joaquin Valley of California. N. Engl. J. Med. *268*:867–870, 1963.
168. Winter, W. G., Jr., Larson, R. K., Honeggar, M. M., et al.: Coccidioidal arthritis and its treatment: 1975. J. Bone Joint Surg. [Am.] *57*:1152–1157, 1975.
169. Ziering, W. H., and Rockas, H. R.: Coccidioidomycosis: Long-term treatment with amphotericin B of disseminated disease in a three-month-old baby. Am. J. Dis. Child. *108*:454–459, 1964.
170. Zweiman, B., Pappagianis, D., Mailbach, H., et al.: Coccidioidin delayed hypersensitivity: Skin test and in vitro lymphocyte reactivities. J. Immunol. *102*:1284–1289, 1969.

201

PARACOCCIDIOIDOMYCOSIS

Angela Restrepo-Moreno

Paracoccidioidomycosis, formerly South American blastomycosis, generally is a progressive chronic disease that preferentially involves the lungs, skin, mucous membranes, adrenals, and reticuloendothelial system. Benign, self-limited infections also have been documented in rare cases. The mycosis is limited geographically to various Latin American countries.[24, 25, 36, 52]

The disease was described originally by Lutz[25] in Brazil in 1908 and initially observed in children in 1911 by Montenegro (cited in reference 47).

THE ORGANISM

Paracoccidioides brasiliensis is the etiologic agent of this disease. It is an imperfect, dimorphic fungus that grows as a mold at room temperature and as a yeast at 37° C. In the mycelial phase, growth is slow (approximately 3 to 4 weeks); the colony is white to tan and compact, with short aerial mycelia. Microscopically thin, septated hyphae and chlamydospores usually are seen, but under special conditions (natural substrates, media with reduced carbohydrate content), arthroconidia and aleurioconidia also are produced.[9, 32] The small size of these conidia makes them compatible with alveolar deposition; furthermore, such conidia have been shown to be infectious.[41]

The mycelial phase is not distinctive, and subcultures at 37° C are required for complete identification. At 37° C, *P. brasiliensis* produces soft, wrinkled, cream-colored colonies that are well developed in about 10 days. Microscopically, the most characteristic feature is the presence of multiple budding yeast cells; the parent cell produces various peripheral buds and acquires the appearance of a pilot's wheel. Single buds and short chains also are produced, but they are not diagnostic. Cells are variable in size (2 to 40 μm) and have a thick cell wall and internal vacuoles. This phase of growth is identical to the one observed in tissues and pathologic materials.[2, 25, 32, 55] The organism cannot be stained readily with most bacterial or hematologic stains. *P. brasiliensis* is aerobic and, in its mycelial phase, grows well in the regular mycologic media to which antibiotics and cycloheximide have been added in order to reduce growth of bacteria and saprophytic fungi.[2, 25, 32, 55]

TRANSMISSION

Paracoccidioidomycosis is not a contagious disease.[33, 58] Although person-to-person transmission has not been confirmed, skin-test studies with paracoccidioidin have shown a significantly higher rate of positive reactions in the wives of patients with this disease.[30] Epidemic outbreaks have not been reported, and only a few cases in family members have been documented.[58, 62, 75] Culture-proven infection in animals has been reported only in armadillos that must have acquired the infection from the natural reservoir of the fungus.[49] Unfortunately, the reservoir has not been identified clearly; soil has been incriminated, but the number of isolations is small. The fungus requires high humidity and may grow well beside sources of water.[62] Paracoccidioidomycosis was thought, and still is by some, to be acquired by trauma; however, clinical and experimental data indicate that infection is acquired most commonly by inhalation.[28, 33, 53]

EPIDEMIOLOGY

Age

More than 70 per cent of the patients are 30 years of age or older. The proportion of reported cases in children is small: 2.1 per cent in the first decade of life.[4, 18, 35] One of the largest series of children with paracoccidioidomycosis was that reported by Castro and del Negro,[18] who found only 70 (3.6 per cent) patients 14 years of age or younger in a 30-year period among 1899 patients with this disease seen at the Hospital das Clinicas in São Paulo, Brazil. In 1992, Barbosa[4] reviewed 30 cases in children younger than 12 years of age who were diagnosed in central Brazil. A total of 143 published reports of paracoccidioidomycosis in children younger than 14 years of age were found in a literature search.[4, 5, 7, 10, 14, 18, 28, 34, 35, 54, 56, 66–70, 73] Londero and Melo[35] compiled the records of 106 children with the mycosis, including those formerly analyzed by Castro and del Negro.[18] This series plus a more recent compilation[35] revealed that the disease is more frequent in individuals 12 to 17 years of age. These data, in conjunction with the information in Table 201–1, indicate a tendency toward an increase in the number of cases with age. The relative paucity of children with this mycosis in comparison with the figures reported in adults, close to 10,000 cases,[4] may be explained, in part, by the long incubation period characteristic of the mycosis or by the establishment of latent foci that may become apparent clinically many years after initial exposure.[30, 36, 37] Benard and associates[6] believe that the association with different age groups is related to the epidemiology of paracoccidioidomycosis because in the endemic areas, children become exposed to the fungus at an early age. In this group of patients, appropriate defenses usually curtail development of the mycosis. This is not the case in malnourished children; the youngest malnourished children have the highest risk of acquiring the disease.[4, 6]

TABLE 201–1. Age and Sex Distribution in 143 Children with Paracoccidioidomycosis

	Age (Yr)		Total by Sex (%)
	4–9	*10–14*	
Sex			
Males	31	53	84 (58.7)
Females	24	35	59 (41.2)
Totals by age (%)	55 (38.4)	88 (61.5)	143 (100)

Data from references 4, 5, 14, 18, 34, 58, 67, and 69.

Sex

Adult males are afflicted with much greater frequency than females (ratio 14:1).[33, 52] In children, however, the disease affects males and females in equal proportions.[4, 18, 35, 64] In the two series of cases described by Londero and associates,[34, 35] which included children up to 14 years of age, there was a slight predominance of males in the older group (Table 201–1). These findings suggest that the sex hormones, the hormone-dependent immunologic factors, or both play a role in determining the outcome of the host-parasite interaction.[22, 48, 63] It has been shown that in vitro estrogens inhibit mycelium-to-yeast transition of *P. brasiliensis*.[60, 63]

Occupation and Race

Almost half the reported cases in adults occur in individuals whose occupations require extensive exposure to the soil.[24, 52, 75] Adult residents of areas in which paracoccidioidomycosis is endemic generally develop disease that is less severe than that seen in immigrants or in persons who migrate to highly endemic settings. These people often develop disseminated infection, much like the juveniles do.[6, 24, 25, 36]

Geographical Distribution

Paracoccidioidomycosis is restricted to Latin America, from Mexico to Argentina; some countries within this area (Chile and some of the Caribbean Islands), however, are free of the disorder. In endemic countries, the disease is not distributed evenly; the majority of cases are found in individuals living in the tropical and subtropical forests.[62, 75] The endemic area is centered in Brazil; 6000 of the 10,000 patients reported to date were natives of this country.[4] Although paracoccidioidomycosis has been reported in patients not living in endemic areas, prior residence in Latin America has been documented in every case.[1] In some of these patients, the interval between residence in the endemic area and clinical manifestations of the disease has been 10 to 40 years.[1, 58] Within endemic areas, 10 to 50 per cent of healthy individuals react to the intradermal administration of paracoccidioidin, suggesting previous contact or subclinical infection with this fungus.[11, 38, 47] In spite of its apparently restricted ecological niche, the habitat of the etiologic agent has not been determined precisely.[62]

PATHOGENESIS AND PATHOLOGY

The initial stages of the host-parasite interaction are unknown due to our inability to detect the precise moment when infection occurs.[24, 38, 53] In the past, traumatic implantation of the fungal propagules in the skin and mucosae was thought to cause primary lesions, whereas other manifestations were regarded as secondary. However, based on the study of many cases, including autopsies, pulmonary lesions are considered to be primary, with the infection taking place by inhalation of fungal particles.[14, 23, 28, 53] It appears that, in most cases, the initial pulmonary infection does not cause undue symptoms.[2, 33, 37, 38, 62] Furthermore, the primary infection can remain latent for many years and may give rise, by endogenous reactivation, to overt disease.[1] In young people, the initial lung infection may pass unnoticed but is followed by prompt dissemination to other organs and tissues. In adults, the mycosis evolves slowly (the chronic form), lung pathology is frequent, and the lesions are unifocal or multifocal. Pathology is restricted to the lungs in some of these

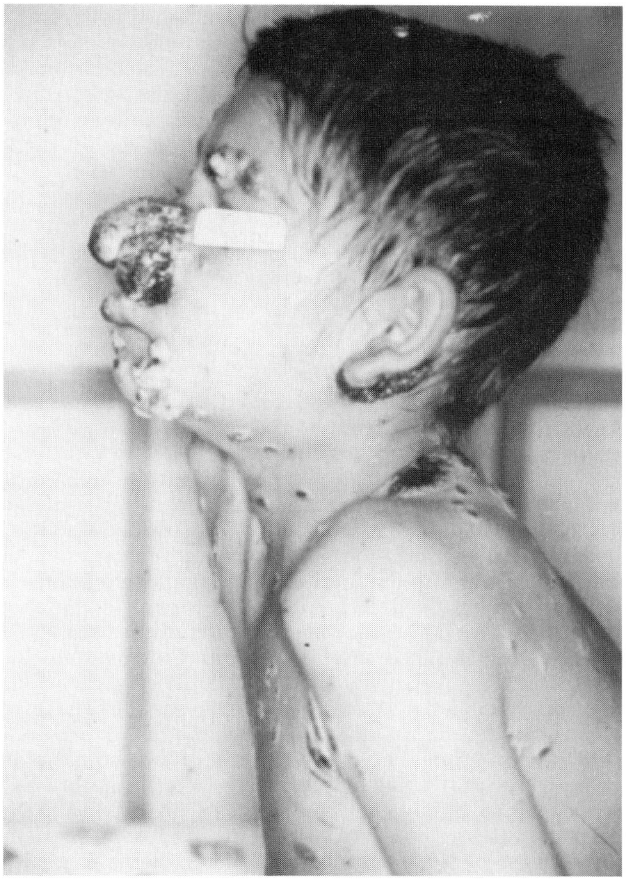

FIGURE 201–1. *Multiple cutaneous lesions in a child with disseminated paracoccidioidomycosis.*

patients, but, in the majority, other organs also are afflicted. Paracoccidioidomycosis involves, preferentially and in order of importance, the lungs, the reticuloendothelial system, the mucous membranes, the skin, and the adrenals. Any organ or system, however, may be affected.[2, 10, 24, 32, 36, 43, 52] After appropriate therapy, residual lesions, mostly fibrotic, become established.[23, 28, 43, 47]

In children, the disease is acute or subacute and progressive (the juvenile form).[3, 5, 10, 18, 35, 69] The time of onset of symptoms is variable, from less than 2 to 24 months.[4] In such patients, paracoccidiodiomycosis is a severe, systemic disorder that involves preferentially the reticuloendothelial system to such an extent that authors consider it as the hallmark of the process.[4, 5, 20, 36, 47]

Pulmonary lesions may be pneumonic, fibrotic, fibrocaseous, or cavitary. Emphysematous areas of lung, pleural thickening, and enlarged hilar and mediastinal lymph nodes also can be observed. Right ventricular hypertrophy may be found in cases of long duration.[2, 59, 76]

In children and adolescents, the pulmonary component commonly goes unnoticed both clinically and radiologically; only a minor proportion of the cases reported (14 per cent) have had lung problems.[14, 34, 35] However, this problem may be more apparent than real because the weight of the extrapulmonary lesions tends to minimize the less-intense respiratory manifestations. Underdiagnosis and confusion with tuberculosis are frequent.[35, 36, 54, 56, 61, 65] A careful search of pulmonary samples, including induced sputum, will reveal the characteristic *P. brasiliensis* yeast cells.[35, 54, 56, 62, 65] New diagnostic methods, such as gallium imaging, allow detection of incipient or small lesions that are not revealed in the plain radiograph.[12]

Mucosal lesions may be infiltrative, ulcerated, or nodular and usually have a granulomatous aspect. The base of the ulcerated lesions is covered by small abscesses (the mulberry-like lesions). The lesions may be warty, vegetating, covered by heavy crusts and infiltrative, or granulomatous.[2, 47, 59, 71]

In children, mucosal and skin pathologies are rather uncommon (20 to 25 per cent). Both in adults and children, skin lesions are polymorphic and may appear as abscess-like nodules, acneiform lesions, crust-covered ulcerations, and draining sinuses (Fig. 201–1). In the latter patients, skin lesions usually are in the same stage of development, indicating their hematogenous origin.[69] Reports of septic shock due to septicemia by *P. brasiliensis* show that the fungus can be blood-borne.[3]

The reticuloendothelial system is the target organ in both children and young adults. Lymph node involvement is a frequent autopsy finding and occurs in 65 per cent of all cases.[2, 10, 47, 68] Half of the patients, especially those with the juvenile form, present with clinically hypertrophied lymph nodes. Lymph nodes vary in size, number, consistency, and location; with time, they liquefy, forming abscesses or fistulas (Fig. 201–2). Masses of lymph nodes may be palpated, especially in the abdomen, where they cause enlargement. The spleen and liver are involved very frequently in children and young adults (80 per cent). Splenic lesions are nodular or miliary. Gross hepatic lesions may not be apparent, but histopathologic examination regularly reveals fungal invasion.[2–5, 10, 35, 47, 64, 69]

The adrenals often are involved in patients with the chronic form of the mycoses, many of whom suffer from adrenal insufficiency. They contain multiple, granulomatous foci, and diffuse necrosis may be seen in the most severe cases. Hyperplasia of the adrenal glands is the rule.[2]

Histologically, granuloma formation is the rule, except in juvenile patients with disseminated disease.[2, 22, 48] The granulomatous inflammation is associated with a mixed pyogenic component, especially in the case of ulcerated skin lesions or ruptured lymph nodes. In the granulomas, abundant epithelial cells, Langhans or foreign-body giant cells, plasmocytes,

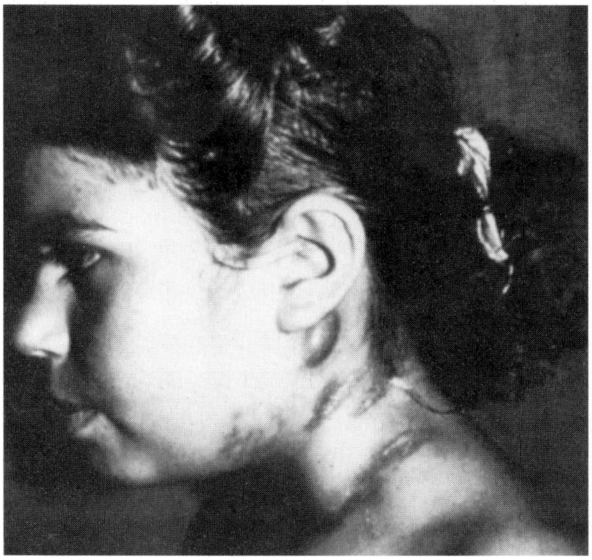

FIGURE 201–2. *Enlarged lymph nodes with draining sinuses in a patient with paracoccidioidomycosis.*

and lymphocytes are seen; often, phagocytosis of the yeast cells can be observed. There may be caseation and central necrosis. In the juvenile disseminated disease, the inflammatory reaction is diffuse, with an abundance of both mononuclear and fungal cells but with sparse granuloma formation.[2, 6, 18, 59] Skin and mucous membrane lesions usually exhibit pseudoepitheliomatous hyperplasia and intraepithelial microabscesses.[2, 6, 10, 48, 68]

Tissue reactions are nonspecific; thus, diagnosis depends upon finding *P. brasiliensis*. If the parasite is abundant, it may be identified by hematoxylin and eosin stains. Special fungal stains (Grocott silver methenamine), however, always should be employed, especially when granulomas are examined. The typical multiple budding yeast cell must be found to establish a diagnosis. The presence of fungal cells of different sizes (2 to 40 μm) suggests the presence of *P. brasiliensis*. In some cases, short chains and cells with single buds also are observed, and, in these patients, differentiation of *P. brasiliensis* from *Cryptococcus neoformans, Blastomyces dermatitidis*, and even *Histoplasma capsulatum* must be made. When disease is chronic, most of the fungal cells are found inside the macrophages, but free yeast cells predominate in disseminated cases. Internalized yeast cells exhibit altered morphology.[2, 10, 32, 48, 68]

In paracoccidioidomycosis, the host-parasite interaction is complex, and both arms of the immune system play important roles.[5, 6, 9, 16, 22, 47, 48] Patients with the mycosis have no deficiency in antibody production; on the other hand, there is a polyclonal activation of the humoral system with high serum concentrations of specific IgG isotypes and IgE.[5, 6, 13, 70, 72] Antibodies exert opsonic activity that is potentiated by the complement system; furthermore, they facilitate elimination of antigens.[16, 22] Nonetheless, high antibody titers correlate with disseminated disease.[5, 13, 22]

In untreated patients, characterization of cellular immunity has revealed an imbalance in the mononuclear cell subsets, with elevated numbers of monocyte/null cells, a low helper-to-suppressor ratio, and reduction of both the percentage of total T cells and of the helper/inducer subset.[22, 23, 48] In this mycosis, there is a generalized depression of cell-mediated immunity, whose intensity parallels the severity of the infectious process.[9, 16, 20, 48] Marked down-regulation of the suppressor-cell circuit can be induced by *P. brasiliensis* antigens.[22, 48] Studies have revealed the pivotal role of interleukin-4 secretion in discriminating between the functional subsets of both CD4 and CD8 T-cell populations, as it suppresses the beneficial effect of other cytokines, such as interferon-γ.[49] Experimentally, it has been shown that mice infected with *P. brasiliensis* treated with an azole drug and subjected to the effects of both anti–interleukin-4 and anti–interferon-γ recovered more efficiently than did other animals.[31] This particular study also revealed that improvement parallels the decrease of IgE antibodies.[31] As in severe cases, eosinophilia is manifested regularly; this abnormality has been linked to an increase in the production of interleukin-5.[70]

Macrophages activated by cytokines represent the most important single host defense mechanism against *P. brasiliensis*. It has been shown that intracellular killing of *P. brasiliensis* yeast cells and conidia occurs only when previous activation has taken place.[9] In general, there is adequate correlation between active cellular immune responses and restriction of fungal growth in tissues.[9, 22, 48]

Benard and associates[5, 6] studied the immune responses of five young patients with paracoccidioidomycosis and found that peripheral blood lymphocytes failed to respond to several mitogens (concanavalin, pokeweed, candidin), as well as to paracoccidioidin. They postulated that a highly stimulated B-cell compartment (high antibody titers, hyperglobulinemia) would result in a break of the normal balance between the T-helper 1 (dominant cellular immune responses) and the T-helper 2 (predominance of humoral patterns) cellular modes. The latter would be present in patients with severe paracoccidioidomycosis who experience marked immunosuppression. If therapy proves successful, the patient would regain the T-helper 1 response mode with ensuing remission.[5, 6]

It has been shown that the immunodepression occurring in paracoccidioidomycosis has other consequences, manifested by the appearence of other microbial infections with further decline of the health status of the patient.[69]

CLINICAL MANIFESTATIONS

Previously, paracoccidioidomycosis was classified as one of four forms: mucocutaneous, lymphatic, visceral, or mixed.[2, 32] The disease is, however, quite polymorphic, and more than one organ system is affected at a particular time. Thus, topographic classification is unrealistic. Preferentially, the disease should be classified as determined by Franco and associates.[23] This classification takes into consideration not only the organs affected but also the immune condition of the host. The infection is categorized as a subclinical form and the overt process subdivided as acute-subacute or chronic disease. The former pattern is noted in children and young adults. According to the severity of the process, these patients are assigned to two subgroups: severe and moderate. These patients are at greater risk than those exhibiting the chronic disease. The chronic progressive form of paracoccidioidomycosis (the adult type) may produce localized pulmonary disease or may be disseminated from its primary foci. Disseminated disease is characterized by involvement of the skin, mucosa, reticuloendothelial system, adrenal glands, and, less frequently, the gastrointestinal tract, genitourinary tract, bones, and central nervous system. The chronic form can be mild, moderate, or severe.[23]

Patients with acute or subacute disease develop signs and symptoms of a wasting process. Fever, malaise, listlessness, weight loss, and emaciation are recorded frequently. The severity of these symptoms is proportional to the degree of organ involvement. The clinical characteristics of paracoccidioidomycosis in 72 children younger than 14 years of age, whose records were complete, are shown in Table 201–2. In this series, hepato- and/or splenomegaly was the predominant sign (81.9 per cent) and, in more than half of the patients, abdominal enlargement was accompanied by other abdominal complaints. Signs and symptoms of an acute abdomen were present in some cases as masses constituted by adjacent lymphadenopathies, produced intestinal occlusion, blockage of lymphatic drainage, and later on, ascites.[2, 4] Diarrhea and vomiting also were very frequent (56.9 per cent). Mesenteric lymphatic status causes enteric mucosal edema, accompanied by abnormal intestinal absorption. These consequences of the primary fungal process adversely affect the health status of the patient.[5, 69] The newer imaging procedures (computed tomography, magnetic resonance imaging) are helpful in determining the extent and nature of abdominal involvement.[4, 5, 54]

Hypertrophy of the lymph nodes is observed regularly (45.8 per cent). Cervical, inguinal, or mesenteric lymphadenopathy can be detected in almost every case.[2, 4, 18, 35, 36] Paracoccidioidomycosis is a disease of the reticuloendothelial system that damages the organs of the system as a result of severe macrophage dysfunction.[4] In rare cases, overwhelming fungemia occurs and secondary pathology develops in bone, skin, subcutaneous tissues, kidney, brain, and other organs.[3, 4, 10, 28, 29, 50, 53, 58, 59, 64]

TABLE 201–2. Clinical Findings in Children with Paracoccidioidomycosis

Signs and Symptoms	No. of Children with Organic Involvement (%)
Fever	53 (73.6)
Weight loss	43 (59.7)
Abdominal complaints and/or enlargement	37 (51.4)
Diarrhea/vomiting	41 (56.9)
Hepato- and/or splenomegaly	59 (81.9)
Enlarged lymph nodes	33 (45.8)
Bone and joint problems	25 (34.7)
Skin lesions	18 (25.0)
Mucosal lesions	18 (25.0)
Lungs*	16 (22.2)
Others†	11 (15.2)

*Lung radiographs were obtained in less than 50 per cent of the cases.

†Other sites involved were the central nervous system, retina, kidney, subcutaneous tissues, adrenal glands, tongue, and tonsils.

Data from references 3, 4, 5, 14, 18, 33, 34, 54, 59, 66, 69, and 73.

Bone damage (osteomyelitis, fractures) and articular problems also were important components (34.7 per cent) of disseminated disease, especially in younger children. Skin and mucosal lesions were noted in 25 per cent of the cases, with a tendecy toward higher frequency with increasing age.[4, 29, 30, 35, 36, 54, 69, 73]

Lung abnormalities were recorded in a smaller proportion of cases. However, even in the absence of clinical and radiological involvement, colonization of the lung by *P. brasiliensis* can be demonstrated by direct examination and by culture.[59, 61] When chest radiographs were abnormal, enlarged hilar lymph nodes and miliary infiltrates predominated.[14, 35, 54, 56, 59, 67]

Placental involvement in a pregnant female has been reported.[8] Although the placenta was infected with the fungus, there was no transmission to the offspring.

Anemia, an increased erythrocyte sedimentation rate, severe hypoalbuminemia, and hypergammaglobulinemia with high IgG serum concentrations are found regularly.[4, 5, 24, 69, 70] Eosinophilia as well as elevated IgE antibody titers have been detected in severely compromised children.[70] In some patients, no antibodies are detectable, possibly because of the formation of antigen-antibody complexes.[13, 27, 44]

There have been some reports of the presence of paracoccidioidomycosis in patients with AIDS, although none in children.[40] The mycosis also has been diagnosed occasionally in other patients whose immune function may be depressed.[40] It is of interest, however, that the incidence of this mycosis has not been increased as a consequence of AIDS or iatrogenic immunosuppression.

In the chronic, progressive, adult form of paracoccidioidomycosis, signs and symptoms differ substantially from those found in children. Descriptions of the disease in adults are beyond the scope of this text but are referenced.[2, 24, 25, 32, 33, 37, 43, 52, 59, 71]

DIAGNOSIS

Disseminated or pulmonary paracoccidioidomycosis can be confused with tuberculosis, histoplasmosis, leukemia, malignancies, or Hodgkin disease. When the skin or mucous membranes are affected, paracoccidioidomycosis must be differentiated from histoplasmosis, leishmaniasis, leprosy, syphilis, lupus erythematosus, and a variety of malignancies. In children, acute abdominal syndrome, intestinal obstruction, osteomyelitis, and rheumatic fever also are important in the differential diagnoses of this disorder.[2, 10, 18, 24, 32, 34, 48, 52, 69, 76]

Specific diagnosis depends upon laboratory confirmation. Histopathologic study of biopsy materials is one of the best methods for establishing the diagnosis. Although the hemotoxylin and eosin stain is acceptable, precise identification is facilitated by the special fungal stain (Grocott silver methenamine).[2, 10, 47, 68] Experimental studies indicate that immunohistochemical detection of specific glycoproteins by means of monoclonal antibodies is a valuable procedure.[26]

In the mycology laboratory, *P. brasiliensis* can be observed by direct (potassium hydroxide) preparation. When multiple samples of carefully collected specimens are examined, diagnosis can be made in 85 to 95 per cent of cases by direct examination.[17, 32]

Cultures should be obtained to support the diagnosis and to establish the viability of the fungus. They are not always positive, however, because the presence of other microorganisms in the samples makes isolation difficult. *P. brasiliensis* is a slow-growing microorganism that can be overgrown readily by bacteria, yeasts (especially *Candida*), and contaminant molds. Isolation should be attempted by the concomitant use of modified Sabouraud agar and yeast extract agar plus antibiotics and cycloheximide (incubated at room temperature) and brain-heart infusion agar plus blood and antibiotics (without cycloheximide) and Kelly hemoglobin agar (incubated at 37° C). Cultures should be observed for 4 weeks; classification can be accomplished only in the yeast phase.[17, 25, 32, 58]

Serologic procedures are extremely valuable for both diagnosis and follow-up of patients. Agar gel immunodiffusion (ID) and complement fixation (CF) have been employed most often, but such techniques as immunoelectrophoresis, indirect immunofluorescence, enzyme-linked immunosorbent assays, and the newer dot immunobinding and Western blotting all have been utilized.[9, 13, 45, 72] Some of the newer tests have employed purified antigens, such as glycoprotein 43, which are well characterized and more specific. ID and CF that employ antigens derived from the yeast phase can detect between 85 and 95 per cent of active cases. Titers are highest and the number of precipitin bands greatest in the most severe cases. Cross-reactions between patient sera and *Histoplasma* antigens occur but with insufficient frequency to invalidate the test.[15, 17, 21] ID is very simple and specific. Three precipitin bands, two of which are specific for *P. brasiliensis*, have been identified.[15, 17, 21]

CF also has prognostic value. When CF and ID are nonreactive on two successive occasions at least 3 months apart, treatment can be discontinued. If positive CF titers persist at a low level, prognosis also appears to be good.[17, 21, 50, 74]

Developments in the detection in patients' sera of specific fungal antigens are being introduced.[27, 44, 45] They will allow a more precise diagnosis in disseminated childhood and adult disease, in which antibodies are undetectable because of their coupling to excess antigen. Follow-up studies also may benefit from antigen detection.[27, 44, 45]

The skin test with paracoccidioidin is negative in 30 to 50 per cent of individuals when they are tested initially.[4, 5] Conversely, a positive skin test indicates previous contact with the fungus but not necessarily active disease. When histoplasmin skin-test material is used, cross-reactions have been verified.[32, 65] When the skin test with paracoccidioidin is negative and the patient is treated, the skin test may become positive and the patient has a good prognosis.[43, 51, 65]

TREATMENT

Paracoccidioidomycosis is the only fungal disease that can be treated successfully with sulfa drugs. Until 1958, when amphotericin B was introduced, no other treatment was available. Both sulfa and amphotericin B are fungistatic; thus, an adequate humoral and cellular immune response is required to control the mycosis. Cellular immunity, however, may be impaired in a large number of patients because of malnutrition or the disease process itself.[4, 5, 48] Supportive therapy, therefore, is imperative. Bed rest, adequate nutrition, correction of anemia, and treatment of other concomitant infections are essential.[43, 57] In children, sulfadiazine can be provided orally at a daily dose of 60 to 100 mg/kg divided in four to six equal parts; in adults, maximum daily doses of 4 g can be used. After clinical and serologic improvement, the dosage can be cut in half. Slow-acting sulfa drugs (sulfamethoxypyridazine or sulfadimethoxine) also can be provided, but the maximum adult daily dose is 1 g. Treatment should be provided for 3 to 5 years; the precise duration of therapy is dictated by the clinical and serologic response of the patient to treatment. Water intake should be encouraged during therapy.[4, 42] The importance of continuous treatment must be emphasized because relapses occur if the drug is not taken regularly. Moreover, if the drug is interrupted prematurely, the patient's isolate may become resistant to sulfonamides.[57] Sulfonamides can be used in ambulatory patients with mild or moderately severe disease. They also can be used for patients who have been treated initially with amphotericin B.[39, 42] Brazilian physicians frequently employ trimethoprim-sulfamethoxazole (80 mg of trimethoprim and 400 mg of sulfamethoxazole per tablet) given at a dose of two tablets and administered orally at 12-hour intervals. Children should be given half the dose given to adults.[4, 42] Duration of this type of treatment varies in each case but usually lasts for 6 months. It is recommended that serum concentrations of sulfonamides be obtained when this drug is used. Serum concentrations of sulfonamides should not exceed 50 μm per mL. The advent of imidazole drugs has decreased the use of sulfa drugs.[29, 42, 50, 51, 57]

Amphotericin B is quite effective, but it should be reserved for severely disseminated cases.[5, 39, 42] It also could be used in patients who relapse during the course of or after treatment with sulfonamide. The effectiveness of therapy with azoles has curtailed the need for more aggressive regimens. Amphotericin B should be provided as described in Chapter 200. More than one course of therapy may be required in some patients.

Some investigators have suggested a combined amphotericin B–sulfonamide treatment. A total cumulative dose in adults of amphotericin B of 1 to 1.2 g followed by sulfa drugs, given as indicated previously, usually is sufficient.[4, 5, 42] With this drug combination, clinical improvement can be achieved in about 75 per cent of patients; about 10 per cent do not respond as well, and the remainder die during treatment. Relapses are expected in about 10 to 15 per cent of optimally treated patients.

The use of oral ketoconazole has improved the prognosis of the progressive forms of this disease greatly.[42, 51, 57, 65] Lesions clear at the same rate with ketoconazole and with amphotericin B, but compared with sulfonamide therapy, less time is required to ensure a sustained remission (6 months versus 3 to 5 years). Ketoconazole is not as toxic as amphotericin B and does not require parenteral administration. Adults have been treated with 200 to 400 mg once daily for periods of 6 to 12 months with no problems and have shown a lower relapse rate (10 per cent).[42, 51, 57, 65]

The role of ketoconazole in childhood paracoccioidomycosis remains controversial because relatively few children have been treated. The results available to date suggest that the drug is effective. When careful observation during therapy is possible, children may be treated with ketoconazole administered at doses varying from 5 to 8 mg/kg/day, in accordance with the manufacturer's indications. Ketoconazole also is available as a suspension (20 mg/mL), and it has been shown that this formulation is absorbed from the gastrointestinal tract. Children treated with ketoconazole should be monitored for changes in liver enzymes.[39, 42, 52] In adults, liver toxicity as well as gonadal changes also should be evaluated, especially during prolonged therapy.[39, 42]

Ketoconazole no longer is considered the choice therapy due to its side effects and numerous drug interactions When the new imidazole derivatives for oral administration (itraconazole, fluconazole) became available, they were tested in patients with paracoccidioidomycosis. Today, more experience has been gained with itraconazole, albeit the number of juvenile patients treated thus far still is small.[43, 50, 51] This triazole is more potent and less toxic than ketoconazole and is equally as or even more effective than the parent compound. It is administered in 100-mg capsules that should be given with a meal. One to two capsules—depending on the severity of the fungal process—taken daily for 6 months have been shown to be effective in reducing all active lesions; the large majority (98 per cent) of the patients, including children and young adults, respond.[42, 50, 51, 54, 57, 74] Posttherapy observations indicate a low proportion of relapses (2.1 per cent). Side effects have been few and include transient elevation of hepatic enzymes.[42, 50, 74] At present, this new triazole is the preferred drug for the treatment of paracoccidioidomycosis in the majority of the patients. This drug is costly and may be unaffordable by patients of low socioeconomic status.[42, 74]

Fluconazole is not as effective in this disorder; higher doses, up to 600 mg/day, and longer treatment periods are required. Recrudescence and relapse of disease occur more frequently than when itraconazole is used.[5, 42, 51] Fluconazole may be useful in severely ill patients who must be treated intravenously.[42, 51]

PROGNOSIS

Paracoccidioidomycosis is considered to be progressive in most cases and fatal if left untreated. However, residual lesions have been observed in a few persons with no known history of active mycotic infection.[2, 33, 53] Prognosis depends upon the status of the patient at the time of diagnosis. Children and young adults in whom fungemia has taken place and who have multiple organ involvement do not respond well to therapy. In less disseminated cases, the response to treatment depends upon the severity of disease at the time of diagnosis. The fatality rate in young patients is about 25 per cent. In the adult group, cumulative death rates also are high, but these patients have a greater chance of survival because of the chronic nature of the disease process. Once specific treatment is instituted, lesions regress promptly; skin lesions may heal completely in 2 to 4 weeks. Complete remission is possible in 20 to 25 per cent of patients with chronic disease.[24, 42] Imidazoles have improved the prognosis for patients with mycosis greatly, as shown by the decrease in positive mycologic tests during and after therapy (Fig. 201–3).[42, 74]

Complications vary, and, like prognosis, their occurrence depends upon the extent of fungal invasion. Intestinal obstruction, jaundice, or both that result from enlarged mesenteric lymph nodes may be noted. Lymph nodes may suppurate, and fistulas can develop. Dysphagia and dysphonia, edema of the glottis, dyspnea, and emphysema can be observed. Sequelae are not as common in children as in adults. In the former group, scarring and fibrosis of the affected nodes and residual pulmonary fibrosis have been noted.[2, 35] In general, fibrosis is the cause of serious problems in persons

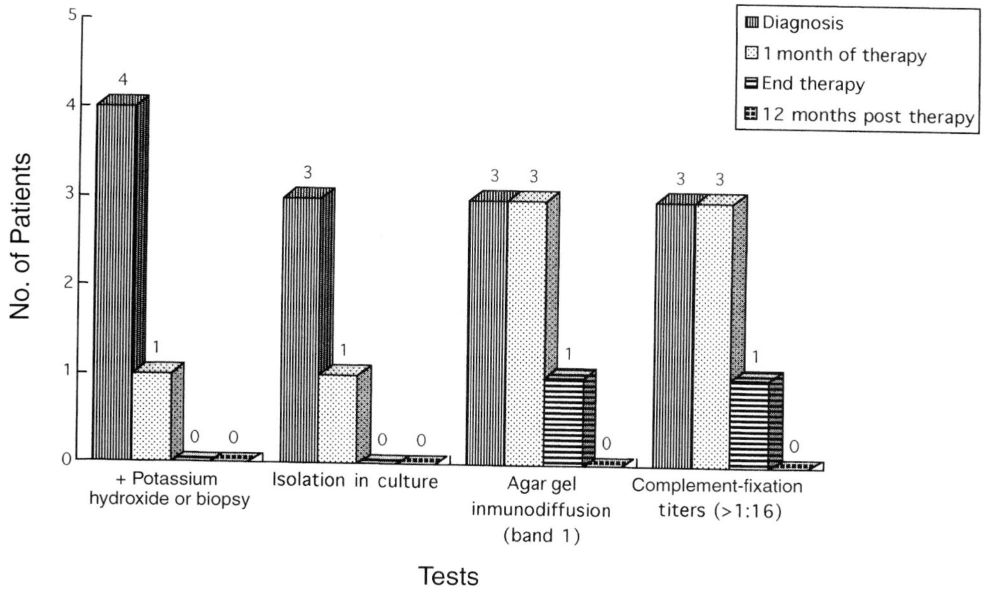

FIGURE 201–3. *Results of mycologic tests in four patients with juvenile paracoccidioidomycosis treated with azole drugs.*

who respond to therapy. In spite of the newer, very effective therapies, these sequelae preclude, in many cases, complete restoration of patients to their previous state of health.[43, 50, 74]

References

1. Ajello, L., and Polonelli, L.: Imported paracoccidioidomycosis: A public health problem in non-endemic areas. Eur. J. Epidemiol. 1:160–165, 1985.
2. Angulo, A., and Pollak, L.: Paracoccidioidomycosis. *In* Baker, R. D. (ed.): The Pathologic Anatomy of the Mycoses: Human Infections with Fungi, Actinomycetes and Algae. Berlin, Springer Verlag, 1971, pp. 507–576.
3. Azulay, R. D., Velloso, M. B., Suguimoto, S. Y., et al.: Acute disseminated paracoccidioidomycosis. Int. J. Dermatol. *27*:510–511, 1988.
4. Barbosa, G. L. Paracoccidioidimicose na crianca. Rev. Pat. Trop. (Brazil) *21*:269–383, 1992.
5. Benard, G., Orri, N. W., Marques, H. H. S., et al.: Severe acute paracoccidioidomycosis in children. Pediatr. Infect. Dis. *13*:510–515, 1994.
6. Benard, G., Neves, C. P., Gryschek, R. C. B., et al.: Severe juvenile type of paracoccidioidomycosis in an adult. J. Med. Vet. Mycol. *33*:67–71, 1995.
7. Bittencourt, A. L., Andrade, J. A. F., and Cendon, S. P.: Paracoccidioidomycosis in a 4-year-old boy. Mycopathologia *93*:55–59, 1986.
8. Blotta, M. H. S., Altermani, A. M., Amaral, E., et al.: Placental involvement in paracoccidioidomycosis. J. Med. Vet. Mycol. *31*:249–257, 1993.
9. Brummer, E., Castañeda, E., Restrepo, A.: Paracoccidioidomycosis: An update. Clin. Microbiol. Rev. *6*:89–117, 1993.
10. Brass, K.: Observaciones sobre la anatomia patológica, patogénesis y evolución de la paracoccidioidom. Mycopathologia *37*:119–138, 1969.
11. Cadavid, D., and Restrepo, A.: Factors associated with *Paracoccidiodes brasiliensis* infection among permanent residents of 3 endemic areas in Colombia. Epidemiol. Infect. *111*:121–133, 1993.
12. Calegari, J. M. M., Salinas, L. F. G., Gomes, E. F., et al.: Acompanhemento terapêutico da paracoccidioidomicose por imagens com ^{67}Ga. Arq. Brasil. Med. *68*:381–385, 1994.
13. Camargo, Z. P., and Cano, L. E.: Humoral immunity. *In* Franco, M., Lacaz, C. S., Restrepo, A., et al. (eds.): Paracoccidioidomycosis. Boca Raton, CRC Press, 1994, pp. 187–202.
14. Campos, E. P., Bertoli, J. C., and Barbosa, K. S.: Linfonodo pulmonar na paracoccidioidomicose aguda infantil. Rev. Soc. Brasil. Med. Trop. *25*:195–200, 1992.
15. Cano, L. E., and Restrepo, A.: Predictive value of serologic tests in the diagnosis and follow-up of patients with paracoccidioidomycosis. Rev. Inst. Med. Trop. São Paulo *29*:276–283, 1987.
16. Cano, L. E., Singer-Vermes, L. M., Vaz, C. A. C., et al.: Pulmonary paracoccidioidomycosis in resistant and susceptible mice: Relationship among progression of infection, bronchoalveolar cell activation, cellular immune responses and specific isotype patterns. Infect. Immun. *63*:1777–1783, 1995.
17. Castillo, N., Ordõnez, N., López, S, et al.: Paracoccidioidomicosis. Diagnóstico por el laboratorio de 333 casos. Biomédica *14*:230–239, 1994.
18. Castro, R. M., and del Negro, G.: Particularidades clinicas da paracoccidioidomicose na crianca. Rev. Hosp. Clin. Fac. Med. São Paulo *31*:194–198, 1976.
19. Colombo, A. L., Fa ical, S., and Katar, L. E.: Systemic evaluation of the adrenocortical function in patients with paracoccidioidomycosis. Mycopathologia *127*:89–94, 1994.
20. del Negro, G., Lacaz, C. S., Zamith, V. A., et al.: General clinical aspects: Polar forms of paracoccidioidomycosis, the disease in childhood. *In* Franco, M., Lacaz, C. S., Restrepo, A., et al. (eds.): Paracoccidioidomycosis. Boca Raton, CRC Press, 1994, pp. 225–232.
21. del Negro, G. M. B., Garcia, N. M., Rodriguez, E. G., et al.: The sensitivity, specificity and efficiency values of some serological tests used in the diagnosis of paracoccidoidomycosis. Rev. Inst. Med. Trop. São Paulo *33*:277–280, 1991.
22. Franco, M. F.: Host-parasite relationship in paracoccidioidomycosis. J. Med. Vet. Mycol. *25*:5–18, 1987.
23. Franco, M., Montenegro, M. R., Mendes, R. P., et al.: Paracoccidioidomycosis: A recently proposed classification of its clinical forms. Rev. Soc. Brasil. Med. Trop. *20*:129–132, 1987.
24. Franco, M., Mendes, R. P., Moscardi-Bacchi, M. M., et al.: Paracoccidioidomycosis. Bailliere's Clin. Trop. Med. Comm. Dis. *4*:185–220, 1989.
25. Franco, M., Lacaz, C. S., Restrepo, A., et al. (eds.): Paracoccidioidomycosis. Boca Raton, CRC Press, 1994.
26. Figueroa, J. L., Hamilton, A., Allen, M., et al.: Immunohistochemical detection of a novel 22- to 25-Da glycoprotein of *Paracoccidioides brasiliensis* in biopsy materials and partial characterization by using species-specific monoclonal antibodies. J. Clin. Microbiol. *32*:1566–1574, 1994.
27. Garcia, N. M., Del Negro, G. M. B., Martins, H. P., et al.: Detection of paracoccidioidomycosis circulating antigen by the immunoelectrophoresis immunodiffusion technique. Rev. Inst. Med. Trop. São Paulo *29*:327–328, 1987.
28. Giraldo, R., Restrepo, A., Gutierrez, F., et al.: Pathogenesis of paracoccidioidomycosis: A model based on the study of 46 patients. Mycopathologia *58*:63–70, 1976.
29. Gonzalez, A., and Naranjo, M. S.: Micosis sistémicas severas y su tratamiento con derivados imidazólicos. Medicina UPB (Colombia) *6*:47–55, 1987.
30. Greer, D. L., and Restrepo, A.: Epidemiology of paracoccidioidomycosis. *In* Al Doory, Y. (ed.): The Epidemiology of Human Mycotic Diseases. Springfield, Charles C Thomas, 1975, p. 117.
31 Hostetler, J. S., Brummer, E., Coffman, R. L., et al.: Effect of anti-IL4, interferon gamma and an antifungal triazole (Sch-42427) in paracoccidioidomycosis: Correlation of IgE levels with outcome. Clin. Exp. Immunol. *94*:11–16, 1993.
32. Lacaz, C. S., Porto, E., and Martins, J. E. C.: Paracoccidioidomicose. *In* Lacaz, C. S, Porto, E., and Martins, J. E. C. (eds.): Micologia Medica. 4th ed. São Paulo, Sarvier Publishers, 1991, pp. 248–261.
33. Londero, A. T.: Paracoccidioidomicose: Patogenia, formas clinicas, manifestacões pulmonares e diagnostico. J. Pneumol. (Brazil) *12*:41–57, 1986.
34. Londero, A. T., Goncalves, A. J. R., Cruz, M. L. S., et al.: Paracoccidioidomicose disseminada "infanto-juvenil" em adolescentes. Arq. Bras. Med. *61*:5–12, 1987.
35. Londero, A. T., and Melo, I. S.: Paracoccidioidomycosis in childhood: A critical review. Mycopathologia *82*:49–55, 1983.
36. Londero, A. T., and Melo, I. S.: Paracoccidioidomicose. J. Brasil Med. (JBM) *55*:96–111, 1988.
37. Lopez, R., and Restrepo, A.: Spontaneous regression of pulmonary paracoccidioidomycosis. Mycopathologia *83*:187–189, 1984.

38. Marques, S. A., Franco, M. F., and Mendes, R. P., et al.: Some epidemiological aspects of paracoccidioidomycosis in Botucatu endemic area, State of São Paulo, Brazil. Rev. Inst. Med. Trop. Šao Paulo *25*:87–92, 1983.
39. Marques, S. A., Dillon, N. L., Franco, M. F., et al.: Paracoccidioidomycosis: A comparative study of the evolutionary serologic, clinical and radiologic results for patients treated with ketoconazole or amphotericin B plus sulfonamides. Mycopathologia *89*:19–25, 1985.
40. Marques, S. A., and Shikanai-Yasuda, M. A.: Paracoccidioidomycosis associated to immunosuppression, AIDS, and Cancer. *In* Franco, M., Lacaz, C. S., Restrepo, A., et al. (eds.): Paracoccidioidomycosis. Boca Raton, CRC Press, 1994, pp. 393–405.
41. McEwen, J. G., Bedoya, V., Patiño, M. M., et al.: Experimental paracoccidioidomycosis induced by the inhalation of conidia. J. Med. Vet. Mycol. *25*:165–175, 1987.
42. Mendes, R. P., Negroni, R., and Arechavala, A.: Treatment and control of cure. *In* Franco, M, Lacaz, C. S., Restrepo, A., et al. (eds.): Paracoccidioidomycosis. Boca Raton, CRC Press, 1994, pp. 373–392.
43. Mendes, R. P.: The gamut of clinical manifestations. *In* Franco, M., Lacaz, C. S., Restrepo, A., et al. (eds.): Paracoccidioidomycosis. Boca Raton, CRC Press, 1994, pp. 233–258.
44. Mendes-Giannini, M. J. S., Bueno, J. P., Shikanai, M. A., et al.: Detection of the 43000 molecular-weight glycoprotein in sera of patients with paracoccidioidomycosis. J. Clin. Microbiol. *27:* 2842–2845, 1989.
45. Mendes-Gianinni, M. J. S., del Negro, G. B., and Siquiera, A. M.: Serodiagnosis. *In* Franco, M., Lacaz, C. S., Restrepo, A., et al. (eds.): Paracoccidioidomycosis. Boca Raton, CRC Press, 1994, pp. 345–365.
46. Montenegro, B.: Blastomicose. Arch. Soc. Med. Cirug. (São Paulo) *2*:324–332, 1911.
47. Montenegro, M. R., and Franco, M.: Pathology. *In* Franco, M., Lacaz, C. S., Restrepo, A., et al. (eds.): Paracoccidioidomycosis. Boca Raton, CRC Press, 1994, pp. 131–150.
48. Musatti, C. C., Peracoli, M. T. S., Soares, M. V. C., et al.: Cell-mediated immunity in paracoccidioidomycosis. *In* Franco, M., Lacaz, C. S., Restrepo, A., et al. (eds.): Paracoccidioidomycosis. Boca Raton, CRC Press, 1994, pp. 175–202.
49. Naiff, R. D., Ferreira, L. C. L., Barret, T. V., et al.: Enzootic paracoccidioidomycosis in armadillos *(Dasypus novemcinctus)* in Para State, Brazil. Rev. Inst. Med. Trop. São Paulo *28*:19–27, 1986.
50. Naranjo, M. S., Trujillo, M., Múnera, M. I., et al.: Treatment of paracoccidioidomycosis with itraconazole. J. Med. Vet. Mycol. *28*:67–76, 1990.
51. Negroni, R., and Arechavala, A.: Itraconazole: Pharmacokinetics and Indications. Arch. Med. Res. *24*:387–393, 1993.
52. Negroni, R.: Paracoccidioidomycosis (South American blastomycosis, Lutz mycosis). Int. J. Dermatol. 12:847–859, 1993.
53. Negroni, R.: Pathogenesis. *In* Franco, M., Lacaz, C. S., Restrepo, A., et al. (eds.): Paracoccidioidomycosis. Boca Raton, CRC Press, 1994, pp. 203–212.
54. Ochoa, M. T., Franco, L., and Restrepo, A.: Características de la paracoccidioidomicosis infantil: Informe de 4 casos. Medicina U. P. B. *10*:97–108, 1991.
55. Queiroz-Telles, F.: *Paracoccidioides brasiliensis:* Ultrastructural findings. *In* Franco, M., Lacaz, C. S., Restrepo, A., et al. (eds.): Paracoccidioidomycosis. Boca Raton, CRC Press, 1994, pp. 27–48.
56. Ramos, C. D., Londero, A. T., and Gal, M. C. L.: Pulmonary paracoccidioidomycosis in a 9-year-old girl. Mycopathologia *74*:15–18, 1981.
57. Restrepo, A.: Paracoccidioidomycosis. *In* Jacobs, P. H., and Nall, L. (eds.): Antifungal Drug Therapy: A Complete Guide for the Practitioner. New York, Marcel Dekker, 1990, pp. 181–205.
58. Restrepo, A., and Greer, D. L.: Paracoccidioidomycosis. *In* Di Salvo, A. (ed.): Occupational Mycoses. Philadelphia, Lea & Febiger, 1983, p. 43.
59. Restrepo, A., Robledo, M., Giraldo, R., et al.: The gamut of paracoccidioidomycosis. Am. J. Med. *61*:33–42, 1976.
60. Restrepo, A., Salazar, M. E., Cano, L. E., et al.: Estrogens inhibit mycelium to yeast transformation in the fungus *Paracoccidioides brasiliensis:* Implications for resistance of females to paracoccidioidomycosis. Infect. Immun. *46*:346–353, 1984.
61. Restrepo, A., Trujillo, M., and Gómez, I.: Innapparent lung involvement in patients with the subacute juvenile type of paracoccidioidomycosis. Rev. Inst. Med. Trop. São Paulo *31*:18, 1989.
62. Restrepo, A.: Ecology of *Paracoccidioides brasiliensis. In* Franco, M., Lacaz, C. S., Restrepo, A., et al. (eds.): Paracoccidioidomycosis. Boca Raton, CRC Press, l994, pp. 121–130.
63. Restrepo, A., Clemmons, K. V., Salazar, M. E., et al.: Hormonal influences in paracoccidioidomycosis. Clin. Infect. Dis. (Suppl.), in press.
64. Rios-Goncalves, A. J., Rozenbaum, R., Londero, A. T., et al.: Apresentação incomum da paracoccidioidomicose disseminada "tipo juvenil." Arq. Brasil. Med. 66:335–337, 1992.
65. Robledo, M. A., Gomez, I., Gutiérrez, F., et al.: Evaluación a largo plazo de pacientes con paracoccidioidomicosis tratados con ketoconazol. Acta Med. Col. *10*:155–169, 1985.
66. Rodriguez, C., and Peñate, F. M.: La paracoccidioidomicosis brasilienses en Venezuela: Estudio de 120 casos, observaciones clinicas. Gac. Med. Caracas *74*:101–140, 1966.
67. Rosario-Filho, N. A., Telles-Filho, F. O., Costa, O., et al.: Paracoccidioidomycosis in children with different skeletal involvement. Rev. Inst. Med. Trop. São Paulo *27*:337–340, 1985.
68. Salfelder, K., Doehnert, G., and Doehnert, H. R.: Paracoccidioidomycosis: Anatomic study with complete autopsies. Virchows Arch. Pathol. Anat. Physiol. *348*:51–76, 1969.
69. Shikanai-Yasuda, M. A., Segurado, A. A. C., Pinto, W. P., et al.: Immunodeficiency secondary to juvenile paracoccidioidomycosis. Mycopathologia *120*:23–28, 1992.
70. Shikanai-Yasuda, M. A., Higaki, Y., Uip, D. E., et al.: Comprometimiento da medula ossea e eosinofilia na paracoccidiodiomicose. Rev. Inst. Med. Trop. São Paulo *34*:85–90, 1992.
71. Sposto M. R., Mendes-Giannini, M. J. S., Moraes, R. A., et al.: Paracoccidioidomycosis manifesting as oral lesions: Clinical, cytological and serological investigation. J. Oral Pathol. Med. *23*:85–87, 1994.
72. Taborda, C. P., and Camargo, Z. P.: Diagnosis of paracoccidioidomycosis by dot immunobinding assay for antibody detection using the purified and specific antigen gp43. J. Clin. Microbiol. *32*:554–556, 1994.
73. Terra, G. M. F., Rios-Goncalves, A., Londero, A. T., et al.: Paracoccidioidomicose em criancas. Arq. Brasil. Med. *8*:65–68, 1991.
74. Tobón, A. M., Gómez, I., Franco, L., et al.: Seguimiento post-terapia en pacientes con paracoccidioidomicosis tratados con itraconazol. Rev. Colombiana Neumol. *7*:74–78, 1995.
75. Wanke, B., and Londero, A. T.: Epidemiology and paracoccidioidomycosis infection. *In* Franco, M., Lacaz, C. S., Restrepo, A., et al. (eds.): Paracoccidioidomycosis. Boca Raton, CRC Press, 1994, pp. 109–120.
76. Valle, A. C. F., Guimaraes, R. R., Lopes, D. J., et al.: Aspectos radiológicos torácicos na paracoccidioidomicose. Rev. Inst. Med. Trop. São Paulo *34*:107–115, 1992.

202

CRYPTOCOCCOSIS

Walter T. Hughes

Cryptococcosis is a life-threatening systemic fungal infection caused by the monomorphic yeast *Cryptococcus neoformans*. Historically, the disease has been referred to as torulosis, European blastomycosis, and Busse-Buschke disease. Both the organism and the disease it causes were discovered independently a century ago. In 1894, Busse, a German pathologist, found the yeast in the tibial lesion of a 31-year-old woman who later died of systemic infection under the medical care of Buschke, her physician. Meanwhile, in 1895, Sanfelice, an Italian, had cultured for the first time the encapsulated yeast *Saccharomyces* (later *Cryptococcus*) *neoformans* from peach juice. Sanfelice pointed out the similarity of the isolates from Busse's case and from the peach juice. The first case in which *C. neoformans* was recognized as the cause of meningitis was reported in 1914 by Verse, although other cases in retrospect had been described earlier.

Cryptococcosis involves predominantly the central nervous system, lungs, skin, and bones, but other organs also have been affected. Although most cases are in immunocompromised patients, the systemic disease also may occur in seemingly immunocompetent individuals.

THE ORGANISM

Cryptococcosis is caused by *C. neoformans*, 1 of 19 species of the genus *Cryptococcus*. Only rarely do other species of *Cryptococcus* cause disease. *C. neoformans* is an encapsulated yeast varying in size from 4 to 8 μm or more in diameter. Two varieties of *neoformans* have been identified. Variety *neoformans* in the telemorphic state is designated *Filobasidiella neoformans* variety *neoformans* and has two serotypes, A and D. Variety *gattii*, also *Filobasidiella neoformans* variety *gattii*, has two serotypes, B and C.

C. neoformans replicates by budding. As budding occurs, a long, slender neck between the parent and daughter cells may be seen. A feature of all *C. neoformans* strains is the mucopolysaccharide capsule surrounding the cell wall. This capsule may vary from a size up to twice the diameter of the yeast to a barely detectable thickness. The presence of this capsule is useful for identification of the genus and may be recognized with the use of a mucicarmine stain or with negative staining using India ink. The Fontana-Masson stain is useful in the identification of *C. neoformans* in fixed tissues. This stain detects melanin precursors in the cell wall and differentiates *C. neoformans* from other yeasts.[27]

C. neoformans forms smooth, mucoid colonies on solid media. Initially cream-colored, the colonies become dry and tan, pinkish, or yellow with aging. The fungus produces urease, is nonfermative, and utilizes several carbohydrates. Species of the genus are separated with carbohydrate assimilation tests and potassium nitrate. The organism grows at 37° C, is lactose-negative, and does not produce pseudomycelia on cornmeal agar. It does not grow well at room temperature (25° C). The development of DNA probes for hybridization with RNA of organisms appears promising for rapid and sensitive methods for the identification of *C. neoformans*.[15] Growth on agar containing L-canavanine, glycine, and thymol-blue indicator serves to differentiate serotypes B and C from A and D. Color change occurs with B and C but not with A and D serotypes.[23]

EPIDEMIOLOGY

Cryptococcosis occurs worldwide as a sporadic infection but not in epidemics. *C. neoformans* is found in soil, especially in sites enriched with avian guano. Although pigeons have been associated with cryptococcosis, the organism resides in the feces and the birds are not infected. Serotypes A and D of *C. neoformans* are found worldwide and usually associated with pigeon excreta, whereas serotypes B and C more often are located in tropical and subtropical countries. *C. neoformans* variety *gattii* (serotype B) has been found to flourish in the environment of the river red gum tree (*Eucalyptus camaldulensis*).[10, 20] Naturally acquired infections occur in lower mammals, especially cats. Neither animal-to-man nor man-to-man infections have been reported.[11] One study shows a higher rate of delayed hypersensitivity skin test reactions to cryptococcal antigen in normal people with heavy exposure to pigeons than those without such exposure.[29] It is believed cryptococcal infection is acquired by inhalation of the yeast into the lungs from a soil reservoir. From the lungs, hematogenous dissemination may occur. Systemic infection may occur in otherwise normal individuals, but most cases of cryptococcosis occur in immunosuppressed individuals. Some of the underlying immunosuppressive conditions include leukemia, lymphoma, Hodgkin disease, lupus erythematosus, Cushing syndrome, sarcoidosis, organ transplantation, chronic mucocutaneous candidiasis, congenital immunodeficiency disorders, and AIDS. The AIDS epidemic has become a major factor in the increased prevalence of cryptococcosis since 1980.[7] It is estimated that cryptococcosis occurs in about 8 per cent of AIDS patients in the United States.[17] In adults with AIDS, cryptococcal meningitis is most frequent in blacks, Haitians, and intravenous drug users.

There is no explanation for the higher rate of cryptococcosis in males than in females.

Cryptococcosis seems to occur less frequently in children than in adults. A Brazilian study[39] found 4 cases of cryptococcosis among 170 HIV-infected children. Of 100 adult patients studied post mortem, 8 had cryptococcal infection.[4]

PATHOPHYSIOLOGY

Considerable evidence suggests *C. neoformans* becomes airborne from soil or dried pigeon excreta. These organisms, or fomites, usually measure less than 2 μm in diameter and therefore are of a size that easily can reach the lung parenchyma through the airways of the lower respiratory tract.[28, 32, 34] After inhalation, the yeast becomes deposited in the alveolar spaces, where replication may or may not occur and where alveolar macrophages and the primary immune response attempt to protect the host from invasion.

The variety of *C. neoformans* may be a factor in the pathology of the infection. Some studies show that infection with *C. neoformans* variety *gattii* (serotypes B and C) more often is associated with immunocompetent individuals with cerebral mass lesions (with or without hydrocephalus) and pulmonary lesions than is infection with *C. neoformans* variety *neoformans*.[25] However, the histopathologic features are indistinguishable.

After inhalation of the yeast, localized pulmonary infection may occur, although this may not be evident clinically at the time of and after hematogenous dissemination. Early lesions are characterized by collections of encapsulated yeasts surrounded by a gelatinous-like material. Granulomatous and chronic inflammatory reactions occur after the acute infection. Four basic patterns of reaction are seen in the lung: one or more peripheral granulomas, granulomatous pneumonia with intra-alveolar organisms and varying degrees of inflammatory response, diffuse invasion of organisms within alveolar capillaries and interstitial tissues with little or no inflammation, and massive intra-alveolar and intravascular organisms.[22]

Studies in the experimental rat show that *C. neoformans* penetrates the lung parenchyma shortly after infection (2 hours). Immunocompetent rats control the infection effectively with minimal extrapulmonary spread and low levels of the capsular glucuronoxylomannan, and that macrophage activation plays a key role in limiting infection to the lung.[14]

The lesions of the brain and meninges are different from those of the lung. Typically, cyst-like lesions, especially of the cerebral cortex, are seen. These represent masses of yeast forms and little, if any, inflammatory reaction. When an inflammatory response is seen, macrophages predominate and *C. neoformans* may be found in the cytoplasm of these cells. Granulomatous lesions are uncommon in the brain. The meninges may be thickened with the gelatinous polysaccharide of the yeast capsule.[12]

Bone lesions may be found in 5 per cent or more of cases

of extrapulmonary cryptococcosis. Here, acute and chronic inflammation occurs, often associated with giant cells and granulomata.[1] Other sites of dissemination include skin, joints, eye, urinary tract, adrenal, liver, lymph nodes, sinuses, gastrointestinal tract, and the female reproductive system.

The capsular polysaccharide of *C. neoformans* is predominantly glucuronoxylomannan. This material elicits an antibody and is the determinant for the yeast's serotype. It does not, in the purified state, elicit a delayed hypersensitivity reaction. Whole-cell organisms as well as protein-containing fractions will elicit a delayed hypersensitivity reaction.

Impaired cell-mediated immunity of the host is a major determinant in the infection and progression of this infection. Furthermore, evidence suggests that, during the infection, cryptococcosis affects some specific components of cell-mediated immunity.[6] Athymic (nude) mice and T-cell–depleted mice are highly susceptible to cryptococcal infection. When normal mice are inoculated with *C. neoformans,* a response of CD4+ and CD8+ T lymphocytes limits the infection and prevents dissemination.[24] *C. neoformans* undergoes attachment, ingestion, and digestion by phagocytes when provided antibody and complement. Some evidence suggests that the organism's polysaccharide capsule may impair phagocytosis and killing and that administration of monoclonal antibodies to the capsular polysaccharide may be protective.[26]

CLINICAL MANIFESTATIONS

One of the most comprehensive studies of the clinical features of cryptococcosis is the publication of 171 well-documented cases of both immunocompromised and immunocompetent patients.[33] This report studied all cases from 24 health care institutions in Brazil over a period of 30 years. Of the 171 cases, only 3 patients (1.8 per cent) were 10 years of age or younger and only 10 patients (5.8 per cent) were younger than 20 years of age. Of these 10 patients, 2 had AIDS, 2 had other causes of immunocompromise, and 6 were not immunocompromised. The central nervous system was involved in 76 per cent of the 171 patients, with similar rates for the immunocompetent and immunosuppressed with or without AIDS. Disseminated cryptococcosis occurred in 92 per cent of patients and pulmonary cryptococcosis in 8 per cent.

Central Nervous System Involvement

Headache and fever are the most common symptoms. Nausea and vomiting occur in one-half of the cases. Stiff neck is seen in 75 per cent of those who are not immunocompromised and in only 33 per cent of those with AIDS. Other less frequent manifestations include alteration of consciousness, impaired mental function, cranial nerve lesions, visual deficits, papilledema, seizures, diplopia, focal neurologic deficits, photophobia, and abnormal cerebellar signs.[33] The duration of symptoms prior to diagnosis varies from less than a week to as long as 18 months.

Pulmonary Involvement

Primary pulmonary cryptococcosis has not been well described in children because most cases of this infection are disseminated at the time of diagnosis. Based on studies in adults,[3] about one-third of the cases are asymptomatic in the immunocompetent host. About one-half the patients have cough or chest pain, and lesser percentages have sputum production (32 per cent), weight loss (26 per cent), fever (26 per cent), and hemophysis (18 per cent). In the immunocompromised host, the onset may be more severe and the course more rapid.[24]

Cutaneous Lesions

A variety of skin lesions have been described due to *C. neoformans,* including ulcers, nodules, vesicles, abscesses, papules, cellulitis, acneiform plaques, and purpuric and sinus tracts. Thus, histologic examination and culture are essential to identify specifically the cryptococcal skin lesion.

Extrapulmonary Cryptococcosis in Immunocompromised Infants and Children

The extent of knowledge about cryptococcosis in infants and children is reflected by reports and reviews.[18, 19] Since 1966, only 22 non-AIDS immunosuppressed children and 13 children with AIDS and extrapulmonary cryptococcosis have been reported. Aspects of these cases are summarized in Table 202–1.

DIAGNOSIS

The diagnosis is established by the demonstration of *C. neoformans* during the disease state. This may be done by direct examination using India ink preparations for cerebrospinal fluid, urine, or sputum specimens or mucicarmine and Mason-Fontana silver stains for histologic examinations; by isolation in culture; and by the detection of cryptococcal antigen. With cryptococcal meningitis, the India ink preparation will reveal the yeast in 77 to 94 per cent of cases; the culture will yield the organism in 87 to 100 per cent and the cryptococcal antigen test will be positive in 83 to 100 per cent of cases. The leukocyte count of the cerebrospinal fluid may be normal or increased to low levels rarely exceeding 100 cells/mm^3, and the glucose will be less than 50 mg/dL in 65 to 75 per cent of the patients.[33]

A high yield from cultures is influenced by the collection and processing of specimens. The methods suggested by Kwon-Chung and Bennett[17] are optional. For the initial culture, Sabouraud agar and niger seed agar medium are used and cultures are maintained at 30 to 32° C (not 37° or 25° C). The sediment from centrifuged cerebrospinal fluid or urine specimens is spread on several plates or slants. Alternatively, 2 to 5 mL of cerebrospinal fluid can be inoculated into Sabouraud broth and incubated on a shaker. Cycloheximide should not be used because it may inhibit the growth of *C. neoformans*. Blood should be cultured by the lysis-centrifugation procedure (Isolator tube).[38] Evidence of growth may be as early as 3 days, but cultures should be held for 3 to 4 weeks before being considered sterile.

Detection of cryptococcal antigen in cerebrospinal fluid, serum, and urine offers a highly sensitive and specific diagnostic tool. Latex agglutination utilizes hyperimmune rabbit immunoglobulin anti–*C. neoformans* antibodies bound to latex particles. Titers of 1:4 and greater suggest cryptococcal infection. Commercial kits detect as little as 10 ng of cryptococcal antigen and have a sensitivity rate of about 95 per cent in experienced hands. Enzyme immunoassays use monoclonal or polyclonal antibody to detect antigen. Comparison studies show close agreement between latex agglutination and enzyme immunoassays.[13] Both latex agglutination and enzyme immunoassay kits are commercially available.

TABLE 202–1. Extrapulmonary Cryptococcosis in Immunosuppressed Infants and Children Reported Since 1966

Clinical Type	Chronic Cutaneous Candidiasis n=4	Systemic Lupus Erythematosis n=6	Acute Lymphoblastic Leukemia n=9	AIDS n=13	Other* n=3
Years of Age: Range (Mean)	*3–14 (10)*	*8–17 (12)*	*3–17 (13)*	*2–17 (8)*	*½–10 (5)*
Meningitis	3	3	4	8	
Meningitis + cutaneous			1		
Disseminated + meningitis					1
Disseminated	1	1	1	1	
Cryptococcemia			1	4	2
Cryptococcemia + meningitis		1			
Peritonitis		1			
Cutaneous only			2		

*Hyperimmunoglobulin E, severe combined immunodeficiency syndrome, renal transplant.
Data from Leggiadro, R. J., Barrett, F. F., and Hughes, W. T.: Extrapulmonary cryptococcosis in immunosuppressed infants and children. Pediatr. Infect. Dis. J. *11*:43–47, 1992; and Leggiadro, R. J., Kline, M. W., and Hughes, W. T.: Extrapulmonary cryptococcosis in children with acquired immunodeficiey syndrome. Pediatr. Infect. Dis. J. *10*:658–662, 1991.

The antigen-detection test (CALAS, Meridian Diagnostics, Cincinnati, OH) has been applied to the diagnosis of pulmonary cryptococcosis.[21] In 41 patients suspected of having pulmonary cryptococcosis, 8 were proved to have *C. neoformans* infection by culture and histology. The transthoracic needle aspirate was positive for cryptococcal antigen in all 8 cases, and only 1 of the 33 patients without cryptococcosis had a false-positive test.

Polymerase chain reaction amplification of *C. neoformans* DNA is being developed, but this technique probably will have the greatest application to epidemiologic investigations because the antigen tests are adequate for diagnostic purposes and can be done quickly in most hospital laboratories.

TREATMENT

Three factors must be considered in guiding the treatment of cryptococcosis: (1) the underlying disease (none, AIDS, or non-AIDS immunocompromise); (2) extent of infection (pulmonary or extrapulmonary with and without neural involvement); and (3) choice of drugs.

Most investigators agree that a 6- to 10-week course of treatment usually is adequate for systemic cryptococcosis in immunocompetent individuals and with some patients who are immunocompromised for a limited period. However, AIDS patients require continuation of antifungal drugs indefinitely because of the high recurrence rate of cryptococcosis. As for the extent of infection, some immunocompetent patients with pulmonary cryptococcosis have recovered without antifungal therapy. However, cases must be evaluated individually as to the wisdom of this approach. Several years ago, the choice of a drug for treatment was simple because amphotericin B was the only drug with efficacy. Now several drugs are available with therapeutic efficacy, including flucytosine, fluconazole, itraconazole, miconazole, and ketoconazole.

Reliable in vitro susceptibility tests to predict the in vivo efficacy are desirable, but such tests are not sufficiently standardized and applicable to general hospital laboratories at this time. However, of all the fungi causing serious human infection, *C. neoformans* seems to hold great promise for such testing. Velez and associates[40] found a positive correlation between the minimum inhibitory concentration determined

TABLE 202–2. Basic Information for Amphotericin B and Flucytosine Treatment for Cryptococcal Meningitis

Category	Amphotericin	Flucytosine
Dose	0.5 mg/kg/day or 1 mg/kg every other day	100 mg/kg/day
Route	Intravenous, single dose over 2–6 hours	Oral, in four divided doses
Peak plasma concentration	0.5–2.0 μg/mL (dose of 0.5 mg/kg/day)	30–40 μg/mL (2-g dose)
Protein binding	≥90%	2–4%
Volume of distribution	Neonate = 1.5–9.4 L per kg Child = 0.4–8.3 L per kg Adult = 4.0 L per kg	Approximates total body water
Central nervous system distribution	Poor	60–90% of serum level
Elimination	Renal = 40% over 7 days Biliary = minimal Dialysis = poorly dialyzable	Renal = >90%
Major adverse effects	Hypokalemia, renal impairment, anemia, thrombophlebitis, cardiac arrhythmias	Anemia, leukopenia, thrombocytopenia, rash, confusion. Greatest when serum levels >100 μg/mL

TABLE 202–3. Azole Alternatives for the Treatment of Cryptococcosis

Category	Fluconazole	Itraconazole†
Dose	3–6 mg/kg/day* Adults = 200–400 mg/day	Child* 3–16 years of age = 100 mg/day Adults = 200–400 mg/day
Route	Intravenous or oral; once daily	Oral: once or twice daily
Peak plasma concentration	4.5 to 8 μg/mL	0.234 μg/mL
Protein binding	11%	99%
Volume of distribution (Vol_D)	0.7 to 1.0 L/kg	796 L (adult)
Central nervous system distribution	54–85% serum level	<10% of serum level
Half-life (normal renal function)	14–20 hours	64 hours (steady state)
Elimination: (renal excretion biliary)	>80%	0.03%
(biliary excretion)	Small	3–18%
Major adverse effects	Nausea, vomiting, diarrhea, rash, increase in serum aminotransferase levels	Nausea, vomiting, rash, hypertension, increase in serum aminotransferase

*No pediatric dose has been established; dose estimate.
†No Food and Drug Administration approval for cryptococcosis in pediatric use.

in vitro for *C. neoformans* and in vivo responses of murine cryptococcal meningitis treated with fluconazole.

Antifungal Drugs for Cryptococcosis

Amphotericin B plus oral flucytosine is the treatment of choice for cryptococcal meningitis in critically ill patients with mental obtundation and high spinal fluid titers of cryptococcal antigen. However, the use of flucytosine in less critically ill patients is controversial but probably is not essential for the treatment of most such cases.

Amphotericin B is indicated for the initial therapy of all cases of cryptococcosis. Essentially all strains are susceptible to this drug. A dose of 0.5 mg/kg/day intravenously over a period of 2 to 6 hours usually is adequate. Once the patient has shown a favorable clinical response, the dosage scheme of 1.0 mg/kg (double the daily dose) given every other day may be considered. The main advantage of this latter regimen is convenience and adaptability to outpatient use. There are three main drawbacks to amphotericin B therapy: toxicity, poor perfusion into cerebrospinal fluid, and the requirement for intravenous administration. Knowledge of the drug and experience in its use are real factors in successful therapy. Key points to keep in mind are summarized in Table 202–2.

Several studies have evaluated amphotericin B alone and in combination with flucytosine,[2, 8, 31] with results tending to favor the combination but without overwhelming differences. Special caution should be given to patients with impaired renal function because of delayed clearance and increased toxicity. Adverse effects are increased in frequency and severity when serum concentrations exceed 100 ng/mL. In centers where serum concentrations of flucytosine cannot be monitored, it probably is advisable to omit flucytosine from the therapy of patients with impaired renal function.

Several studies in adults with cryptococcal meningitis have shown fluconazole alone to be effective.[9, 37] Another approach used in AIDS patients is initial therapy with amphotericin B and maintenance therapy with oral fluconazole. Fluconazole has not been evaluated in children with severe cryptococcal infection.

Itraconazole has been effective in some patients with cryptococcosis.[5, 36] This drug has not been approved by the Food and Drug Administration for use in children or for the treatment of cryptococcosis. However, it might be considered as an alternative drug in some cases, keeping in mind the poor penetration to cerebrospinal fluid (Table 202–3).

Patients with AIDS should be kept on lifelong maintenance therapy, usually with fluconazole or weekly doses of amphotericin B.

Other therapy includes the occasional need for a ventricular shunt for hydrocephalus or corticosteroids for cerebral edema.

PROGNOSIS

Based on the reports of extrapulmonary cryptococcosis in immunosuppressed infants and children, the prognosis for severe systemic cryptococcosis is reasonably good. Of the 13 children with AIDS and cryptococcosis,[19] 2 untreated patients died and 10 of the 11 treated patients had a clinical response to amphotericin B with or without flucytosine, although 7 of the 10 had died of human immunodeficiency virus infection at the time of the report. Of the 15 non-AIDS but immunosuppressed patients reviewed by Leggiadro and associates,[18] responses also were favorable but difficult to evaluate clearly because of other diseases and complications.

The cryptococcal antigen titer in cerebrospinal fluid and serum has been used as a guide to therapeutic response in patients with meningitis due to *C. neoformans*. In non-AIDS patients, high titers of cryptococcal antigen in serum and cerebrospinal fluid at baseline were correlated with higher mortality during therapy.[2, 6] A study of AIDS-associated meningitis showed no correlation between outcome and antigen titer.[31] However, during therapy for acute meningitis, an unchanged or increased titer of antigen in cerebrospinal fluid correlated with clinical and microbiologic failure to respond to treatment.

References

1. Behrman, R. E., Masci, J. R., and Nicholas, P.: Cryptococcal skeletal infections: Case report and review. Rev. Infect. Dis. *12*:181–190, 1990.
2. Bennett, J. E., Dismukes, W. E., Duma, R. J., et al.: A comparison of amphotericin B alone and combined with flucytosine in the treatment of cryptococcal meningitis. N. Engl. J. Med. *301*:126–131, 1979.
3. Campbell, G. D.: Primary pulmonary cryptococcosis. Am. Rev. Respir. Dis. *94*:236–243, 1966.
4. Climent, C., DeVinatea, M. L., Lasala, G., et al.: Geographical pathology profile of AIDS in Puerto Rico: The first decade. Mod. Pathol. *7*:647–651, 1994.
5. De Gans, G., Portegies, P., Tiessens, G., et al.: Itraconazole compared with amphotericin B plus flucytosine in AIDS patients with cryptococcal meningitis. AIDS *6*:185, 1992.

6. Diamond, R. D., and Bennett, J. E.: Prognostic factors in cryptococcal meningitis: A study in 111 cases. Ann. Intern. Med. *80*:176–181, 1974.
7. Dismukes, W. E.: Cryptococcal meningitis in patients with AIDS. J. Infect. Dis. *157*:624–628, 1988.
8. Dismukes, W. E., Cloud, G., Gallis, H. A., et al.: Treatment of cryptococcal meningitis with combination amphotericin B and flucytosine for four as compared with six weeks. N. Engl. J. Med. *317*:334–341, 1987.
9. Dupont, B. and Drouhet, E.: Cryptococcal meningitis and fluconazole. Ann. Intern. Med. *106*:778, 1987.
10. Ellis, D. H., and Pfeiffer, T. J.: Natural habitat of *Cryptococcus neoformans gatii*. J. Clin. Microbiol. *28*:1642–1644, 1990.
11. Faggi, E., Gargani, G., Pizzirani, C., et al.: Cryptococcosis in domestic mammals. Mycoses *36*:165–170, 1993.
12. Fetter, B. F., Klintworth, G. K., and Henry, W. S.: Mycoses of the central nervous system. Baltimore, Williams & Wilkins, 1976, p. 100.
13. Frank, U. K., Nishimura, S. L., Li, N. C., et al.: Evaluation of an enzyme immunoassay for detection of cryptococcal capsular polysaccharide antigen in serum and cerebrospinal fluid. J. Clin. Microbiol. *31*:97–101, 1993.
14. Goldman, D., Lee, S. C., and Casadevall, A.: Pathogenesis of pulmonary *Cryptococcus neoformans* infection in the rat. Infect. Immun. *62*:4755–4761, 1994.
15. Huffnagle, K. E., and Gander, R. M.: Evaluation of Gen-Probe's *Histoplasma capsulatum* and *Cryptococcus neoformans* AccuProbes. J. Clin. Microbiol. *31*:419–421, 1993.
16. Kovacs, J. A., Kovacs, A. A., Polis, M., et al.: Cryptococcosis in the acquired immunodeficiency syndrome. Ann. Intern. Med. *103*:533–538, 1985.
17. Kwon-Chung, K. J., and Bennett, J. E.: Medical Mycology. Philadelphia, Lea & Febiger, 1992.
18. Leggiadro, R. J., Barrett, F. F., and Hughes, W. T.: Extrapulmonary cryptococcosis in immunosuppressed infants and children. Pediatr. Infect. Dis. J. *11*:43–47, 1992.
19. Leggiadro, R. J., Kline, M. W., and Hughes, W. T.: Extrapulmonary cryptococcosis in children with acquired immunodeficiency syndrome. Pediatr. Infect. Dis. J. *10*:658–662, 1991.
20. Levitz, S. M.: The ecology of *Cryptococcus neoformans* and the epidemiology of cryptococcosis. J. Infect. Dis. *13*:1163–1169, 1991.
21. Liaw, Y. S., Yang, P. C., Yu, C. V., et al.: Direct determination of cryptococcal antigen in transthoracic needle aspirates for diagnosis of pulmonary cryptococcosis. J. Clin. Microbiol. *33*:1588–1591, 1995.
22. McDonnell, J. M., and Hutchins, G. M.: Pulmonary cryptococcosis. Hum. Pathol. *16*:121–128, 1985.
23. Min, K. H., and Kwon-Chung, K. J.: The biochemical basis for the distribution between the two *Cryptococcus neoformans* varieties with CGB medium. Centralbl. Bakteriol. *261*:481, 1986.
24. Mitchell, T. G., and Perfect, J. R.: Cryptococcosis in the era of AIDS: 100 years after the discovery of *Cryptococcus neoformans*. Clin. Microbiol. Rev. *8*:515, 1995.
25. Mitchell, D. H., Sorrell, T. C., Allworth, A. M., et al.: Cryptococcal disease of the CNS in immunocompromised hosts: Influence of cryptococcal variety on clinical manifestations and outcome. Clin. Infect. Dis. *20*:611–616, 1995.
26. Mukherjee, S., Lee, S., Mukherjee, J., et al.: Monoclonal antibodies to *Cryptococcus neoformans* capsular polysaccharide modify the course of intravenous infection in mice. Infect. Immun. *62*:1079–1088, 1994.
27. Murray, P. R., Baron, E. J., Pfaller, M. A., et al.: Manual of Clinical Microbiology. 6th ed. Washington, D.C., ASM Press, 1995.
28. Neilson, J. B., Fromtling, R. A., and Bulmer, G. S.: *Cryptococcus neoformans*: Size range of infectious particles from aerosolized soil. Infect. Immun. *17*:634–638, 1977.
29. Newberry, W. M., Walter, J. E., Chandler, J. W., et al.: Epidemiologic study *Cryptococcus neoformans*. Ann. Intern. Med. *67*:724–732, 1967.
30. Powderly, W. G.: Therapy for cryptococcal meningitis in patients with AIDS. Clin. Infect. Dis. *140*(Suppl. 1):554–559, 1992.
31. Powderly, W. G., Cloud, G. A., Dismukes, W. E., et al.: Measurement of cryptococcal antigen in serum and cerebrospinal fluid: Value in the management of AIDS-associated cryptococcal meningitis. Clin. Infect. Dis. *18*:789–792, 1994.
32. Powell, K. E., Dahl, B. A., Weeks, R. J., et al.: Airborne *Cryptococcus neoformans:* Particles from pigeon excreta compatible with alveolar deposition. J. Infect. Dis. *125*:412, 1972.
33. Rosenbaum, R., and Goncalves, A. J. R.: Clinical epidemiological study of 171 cases of cryptococcosis. Clin. Infect. Dis. *18*:369–380, 1994.
34. Ruiz, A., and Blumer, G. S.: Particle size of airborne *Cryptococcus neoformans* in a tower. Appl. Environ. Microbiol. *41*:1225, 1981.
35. Saag, M. S., Powderly, W. G., Cloud, G. A., et al.: Comparison of amphotericin B with fluconazole in the treatment of acute AIDS-associated cryptococcal meningitis. N. Engl. J. Med. *326*:83–89, 1992.
36. Sharkey, P. K., Rinaldi, M. G., Dunn, J. F., et al.: High-dose itraconazole in the treatment of severe mycoses. Antimicrob. Agents Chemother. *35*:707–713, 1991.
37. Stern, J. J., Hartman, B. J., Sharkey, P., et al.: Oral fluconazole therapy for patients with acquired immunodeficiency syndrome and cryptococcosis: Experience with 22 patients. Am. J. Med. *85*:477–480, 1988.
38. Tarrand, J. J., Guillot, C., Wenglar, M., et al.: Clinical comparison of the resin-containing BACTEC 26 Plus and the Isolator 10 blood culturing systems. J. Clin. Microbiol. *29*:2245–2249, 1991.
39. Valada, M. G., Nunes, C., Jacob, C. M., et al.: Cryptococcosis in HIV-infected children. International Conference on AIDS *10*:254 (Abstract No. PB0446) Aug. 7–12, 1994.
40. Velez, J. D., Allendoefer, R., Luther, M., et al.: Correlation of in vitro azole susceptibility with in vivo response in a murine model of cryptococcal meningitis. J. Infect. Dis. *168*:508–510, 1993.

203

HISTOPLASMOSIS

Bernhard L. Wiedermann

Histoplasmosis is the most common pulmonary and systemic mycosis of humans. Infections occur worldwide, and approximately 500,000 Americans are exposed to the etiologic agent, *Histoplasma capsulatum,* each year.[188] Of these, an estimated 55,000 to 200,000 infected individuals become symptomatic, and 1500 to 4000 require hospitalization.[122]

H. capsulatum first was described in 1906 by Samuel Darling, a pathologist in the Panama Canal Zone.[33] After studying the histopathology of autopsy specimens obtained from a man with a chronic, wasting illness, he discovered an organism he believed to be an encapsulated plasmodium residing within histiocytes. The illness caused by this new pathogen was named reticuloendothelial cytomycosis.[119] In 1932, Dodd and Tompkins[40] demonstrated intracellular *H. capsulatum* in the peripheral blood smear of a febrile child, and DeMonbreum[37] subsequently grew the organism from this same child and correctly classified the organism as a fungus. Christie and Peterson,[30] in 1944, developed histoplasmin and, after subcutaneous inoculation, demonstrated a positive cutaneous reaction in a child with histoplasmosis.

In 1945, Parson and Zarafonetis[135] characterized the disease as rare and usually fatal after studying 71 patients with disseminated histoplasmosis, but Christie and Peterson[30] soon demonstrated histoplasmosis to be a common disease of humans. They attributed histoplasmosis to the large numbers of patients noted with radiographic evidence of pulmonary calcifications but nonreactive tuberculin skin tests. Further characterization of the natural habitat and potential means of acquisition of the fungus occurred in the late 1940s and early 1950s with demonstration of the organism in soil and air samples.[1, 46, 189]

THE ORGANISM

H. capsulatum is a thermally dimorphic, saprophytic fungus of the class Ascomycetes, family Gymnoascaceae, subdivision

Ascomycotina. There are five different serotypes of the organism, and avirulent strains with different cell wall compositions also have been identified.[92, 98] The sexual forms for *H. capsulatum* include the + and − types. Ninety per cent of infections are caused by the − type. The perfect sexual form of the organism is *Emmonsiella capsulata.*[101]

At temperatures of 25° to 30° C, the fungus grows as a white to brown mold. Microscopically, mycelia, microconidia (1 to 5 μm), and macroconidia (8 to 16 μm, forming characteristic trabeculated spores) are seen (Fig. 203–1). It grows slowly, requiring 1 to 2 weeks for laboratory strains and as long as 8 to 12 weeks from clinical specimens. At temperatures of 37° C on artificial media containing cystine and cysteine, the mold transforms to the yeast form.[122] The small, heaped, pasty colonies appear microscopically as ovoid, budding yeasts (1 to 3 μm × 3 to 5 μm) with rare pseudohyphae.[122, 132]

In its natural habitat, the soil, *H. capsulatum* exists as mycelia and spores. It survives best in moist soil (95 to 100 per cent humidity) with temperatures 37° C or higher and can be found as deep as 1 m below the soil surface.[184, 188] The fungus also has a predilection for bird droppings and bat guano, apparently using the uric acid in the excreta as a nitrogen source.[109] If present in either soil or bird droppings, *H. capsulatum* can remain viable for many years.[209]

A variant of *H. capsulatum, H. capsulatum* variety *duboisii*, has been described across central and western Africa. This forms a larger yeast of 7 to 15 μm, which microscopically resembles *Blastomyces dermatitidis.*[132]

EPIDEMIOLOGY

Edwards and colleagues[44] described the geographic distribution of *H. capsulatum* in the United States by performing histoplasmin skin testing on 275,558 Navy recruits between 1958 and 1965. The highest concentration of the fungus is found in the Ohio–Mississippi–Missouri, the St. Lawrence, and the Rio Grande River valleys.[122] More than 50 per cent of adults in the Ohio–Mississippi River valleys are skin test–positive.[25] Blackbird roosts, pigeon roosts, chicken houses, caves, attics, old buildings, and hollow trees all have been found to harbor the organism, and activities that involve these types of sites have been implicated in the acquisition of histoplasmosis.[144] Birds do not become infected because of their high body temperature, but bat infection with *H. capsulatum* is described.[45] No human-to-human or animal-to-human transmission has been documented, although a single episode of an infection in an infant has occurred after exposure to feathers from a pillow.[22]

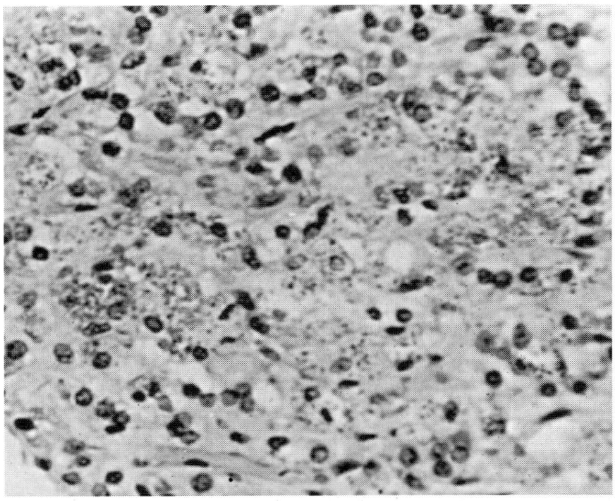

FIGURE 203–1. *Culture of* Histoplasma capsulatum *from sputum illustrating tuberculate macroaleuriospores and microaleuriospores. (Lactophenol cotton blue × 52.)*

Numerous histoplasmosis outbreaks have been documented and offer some means of assessing the spread of the disease. One large outbreak in Indianapolis, Indiana, involved exposure of 100,000 persons within a 400 square mile area and lasted nearly 1 year.[204] Symptomatic cases were found in 435 individuals (including 49 younger than 15 years of age), and 46 of these developed disseminated disease. Teenagers and young adults (15 to 34 years of age) were more likely to become infected than were other age groups, and there was an equal sexual distribution of cases prior to puberty. Males predominated in a 3:1 ratio in older individuals.

PATHOPHYSIOLOGY

In experimental animals, acute pulmonary histoplasmosis can develop after inhalation of microconidia or mycelial fragments.[6] Due to their small size, microconidia are believed to travel to the smaller airways more easily than macroconidia and, therefore, are more virulent. Within 2 to 3 days after inhalation, the spores germinate within the bronchioles into yeast forms. In the first week, there is an initial neutrophilic response that is replaced by helper lymphocytes and macrophages by the second week. The yeasts are phagocytosed by macrophages, but killing does not occur. Instead, asexual budding occurs within the phagosomes, and the organisms can spread via lymphatics to the reticuloendothelial system. Macrophages from HIV-infected individuals can ingest yeasts bound to the cell membrane, but binding ability itself is poor.[29] Normal human neutrophils can phagocytose yeast cells, and fungistatic activity resides within azurophil granules.[19, 130]

The incubation period and the ability of the organisms to proliferate are dependent on the previous immune status of the host and the inhaled inoculum size.[65] The incubation period seems to vary inversely with the degree of immunity in the host. In a highly immune host after inhalation of a heavy inoculum, the incubation period is about 3 to 5 days, whereas in the nonimmune child, the period typically is 12 to 16 days but may extend as long as 24 days.[65] Also, because infants are likely to demonstrate little native immunity, they are more likely than adults or previously infected individuals to develop a symptomatic illness after exposure.[65]

In large pulmonary lesions, central necrosis may develop, and dissemination occurs rarely, largely dependent on host factors. Cellular immune mechanisms develop 10 to 21 days after exposure that largely are responsible for containment of the infection.[173] Healing generally occurs over the next 2 to 4 months, and calcification usually develops. This latter process seems to be age-dependent, with calcification occurring within months in children to as long as 10 years in adults.[65] Splenic calcifications often accompany pulmonary calcifications.[169]

Early in the course of histoplasmosis, cellular immunity appears to be suppressed.[140] In the mouse model, *H. capsulatum* infection is associated with generation of T-suppressor cell activity, which depresses T-cell–dependent antibody production as well as delayed-type hypersensitivity, mitogen-induced lymphocyte transformation, and cytotoxic activity.[5] T-cell immunity develops approximately 10 to 21 days after exposure, and splenic T-suppressor cell numbers decrease while T-helper cells rise. Natural killer cells appear to have a role in the control of extracellular fungus.[189]

Humoral immunity also is important in the pathogenesis of histoplasmosis. High antibody titers in patients with histoplasmosis correlate with a poor cellular response as measured by suppressed delayed-type hypersensitivity and blast transformation.[173] It is hypothesized that antibody may bind to the fungus and, therefore, mask key antigenic determinants, which makes them inaccessible to T-cell stimulation. Immune complexes also may stimulate T-suppressor cells.[173] Patients with chronic relapsing forms of disseminated histoplasmosis show impaired lymphocyte proliferation to mitogen stimulus during active disease but revert to normal mitogen responses during periods of remission.[138]

PATHOLOGY

Histoplasmosis typically results in a localized mononuclear cell infiltrate that may develop into tuberculoid granulomata with multinucleated giant cells.[65] Blood vessels may show necrotizing granulomatous vasculitis.[115] Organisms may be seen in tissue and within macrophages with many different stains, but the Gomori methenamine silver and periodic acid–Schiff stains are most useful, particularly if granulomatous lesions are present.[132] In disseminated disease, there is a diffuse distribution of infected macrophages throughout the reticuloendothelial system.[67] Intracellular organisms may be seen, but there is little tissue reaction.[65] Eventually, all lesions undergo caseation necrosis, and fibrosis or calcification can be present.[115]

CLINICAL MANIFESTATIONS

Approximately 95 per cent of *H. capsulatum* infections are asymptomatic, and typically the only sequelae seen are the delayed-type hypersensitivity and calcifications. Inoculum size is an important determinant of symptoms; only 1 per cent of individuals develop symptoms after low inoculum exposure, and 50 to 100 per cent become ill with heavy exposure.[188] When symptomatic disease develops, a myriad of clinical syndromes is possible (Table 203–1). The severity of disease, including mortality, is greatest at the extremes of age. A 20-year, retrospective study in Tennessee of children with symptomatic histoplasmosis detected 35 cases.[21] Ages ranged from 7 months to 16 years (mean, 5.9 years), and 24 were boys. Twenty-nine children had pulmonary or mediastinal infection, five had disseminated disease, and one had cutaneous histoplasmosis.

TABLE 203–1. Clinical Manifestations of Pediatric Histoplasmosis

- Asymptomatic infection
- Pulmonary disease
  - Acute (mild, moderate, severe forms)
  - Mediastinal adenopathy
  - Obstruction (mediastinal structures)
  - Mediastinal fibrosis
  - Pericarditis
  - Chronic disease with cavitation
- Primary cutaneous infection
- Disseminated infection
  - Acute
  - Subacute
  - Chronic
- Presumed ocular histoplasmosis

Pulmonary Histoplasmosis

The pulmonary manifestations of *H. capsulatum* infection represent the most common symptomatic form of histoplasmosis. Acute pulmonary histoplasmosis usually is heralded by the onset of fever and headache; two-thirds of patients develop chills, cough, and chest pain.[65] Nausea, vomiting, diarrhea, asthenia, weight loss, myalgia, and fatigue also may be seen. About 80 per cent of affected individuals have mild disease, which consists of mainly upper respiratory symptoms along with low-grade fever and chest pain.[188] The typical course lasts 1 to 5 days. Moderate disease consists of cough, chest pain, dyspnea, and hoarseness with higher temperatures and lasts 5 to 15 days. Severe disease has additional manifestations of fatigue, night sweats, weight loss, and fever of 102° to 106° F lasting 10 to 21 days.[65] Hepatosplenomegaly and erythema nodosum also may be present.[65, 108] Pleural effusions are uncommon in children with histoplasmosis. Acute migratory polyarthritis has been reported and is presumed to be an immune-mediated manifestation of histoplasmosis.[31]

Histoplasmosis often can present as asymptomatic mediastinal masses, and biopsy may be necessary if serologic studies fail to exclude malignancy, primarily lymphoma.[56, 186, 215] Pediatric series of mediastinal masses reveal rates of 1 to 57 per cent with histoplasmosis as the etiology.[16, 56, 186, 215] This large discrepancy probably is explained best by the geographic location of the study, with higher rates reported from endemic areas, or by the possibility that some series may have included individuals involved in outbreaks of histoplasmosis.

Complications resulting from acute pulmonary histoplasmosis occur uncommonly and usually are caused by involvement of lymphatic tissue in the thoracic cavity. Increasing lymph node size may cause bronchial, tracheal, esophageal, or vascular obstruction.[42, 136, 153, 214] Broncholithiasis may occur with lithoptysis.[10] Esophageal complications can be manifested by fistula formation and motility disturbances. Children are more susceptible to tracheobronchial compression due to encroachment by enlarged azygous lymph nodes.[59] The risk of contiguous structure involvement with such mediastinal granulomas is related to thickness of the capsule rather than to overall size of the node.[65]

Acute pericarditis can develop from contiguous inflamed lymph nodes.[217] Granulomatous pericarditis develops when there is penetration of the pericardium, whereas fibrinous pericarditis is produced by adjacent inflammation without penetration.[65] About one-fourth of patients present with symptoms of tamponade.[189] Pericardial fluid typically is bloody.[189] Constrictive pericarditis develops in 15 per cent of these patients.

Mediastinal fibrosis is a late complication of pulmonary disease, which can cause stenosis or obstruction of mediastinal structures, such as the superior vena cava, tracheobronchial tree, pulmonary artery, or esophagus.[112] Likewise, pulmonary "histoplasmomas" may enlarge over a period of 10 to 15 years and cause symptoms of a mass lesion.[68]

Chronic pulmonary histoplasmosis with subsequent cavitary formation may develop, although this is uncommon in children. Acute cavitation occurred in a 10-year-old boy without previous chronic obstructive lung disease.[8] Individuals with chronic lung disease are at higher risk for this complication and often present with low-grade fever, productive cough, weakness, and fatigue.[66]

Primary Cutaneous Histoplasmosis

Cutaneous histoplasmosis can develop after primary inoculation of skin or mucocutaneous structures, such as the conjunctiva.[163, 179] Although the disease generally remains localized, spread to contiguous structures and dissemination can occur.

Disseminated Histoplasmosis

Disseminated histoplasmosis is defined as the presence of extrapulmonary disease (other than cutaneous histoplasmosis) determined by culture or histopathology. Disseminated histoplasmosis in the normal host usually reflects exogenous primary infection or reinfection. In contrast, endogenous infection (reactivation) can result in dissemination in immunocompromised hosts. The most common sites involved in disseminated histoplasmosis include the spleen, liver, lymph nodes, adrenal glands, gastrointestinal tract, and bone marrow.[25] Less commonly, the central nervous system, kidney, and heart are affected; vaginal and penile ulcers, soft tissue nodules, recurrent panniculitis, carpal tunnel syndrome, osteomyelitis and arthritis, enteropathies, immune hemolytic anemia, and epididymitis all have occurred.[85, 90, 96, 134, 147, 155, 163, 170, 187] One child with a symptom complex of cervical lymphadenopathy, cerebrospinal fluid pleocytosis, arthritis, and interstitial nephritis has been reported.[187]

Immunosuppressed individuals, particularly oncology patients, patients receiving immunosuppressive therapy, dialysis patients, intravenous drug users, patients with AIDS, hyposplenic patients, and infants, as well as histiocytosis X, systemic lupus erythematosus, diabetes mellitus, sarcoidosis, chronic mucocutaneous candidiasis, and hyper-IgM syndrome patients are at risk for dissemination.[50, 80, 89, 114, 121, 122, 150, 175, 188, 189, 206] However, up to 20 per cent of cases of disseminated histoplasmosis occur in presumably healthy individuals. Unlike other opportunistic infectious syndromes that tend to occur in cancer patients in relapse with neutropenia, disseminated histoplasmosis can occur during either remission or relapse.[81]

Disseminated disease presents as acute, subacute, or chronic infection.[67] The acute form is seen predominantly in infants with overwhelming involvement of the reticuloendothelial system by yeast forms.[84] Temperatures are high (101° to 105° F), and gastrointestinal symptoms are common. In the later stages, an interstitial pneumonitis with cough and tachypnea may develop. Hepatosplenomegaly and intra-abdominal lymphadenopathy are common, but only one-third have peripheral lymphadenopathy. Anemia, granulocytopenia, and thrombocytopenia may be prominent.[67, 104] A similar clinical picture can develop in the older patient with chronic disseminated disease who undergoes immunosuppressive therapy.

A subacute form of disseminated infection also is seen, but only one-third of these individuals are in the pediatric age range.[67] Predominant symptoms are nonspecific; fever, malaise, and weight loss are common. In three-fourths of adult patients, a focal lesion, such as intestinal ulceration, adrenal insufficiency, endocarditis, or meningitis, is recognized. Oropharyngeal ulcers can be seen in one-fourth of patients, and hepatosplenomegaly may be present.

Chronic disseminated histoplasmosis is seen almost exclusively in adults.[67] Oropharyngeal ulcers are accompanied by chronic, mild, intermittent constitutional symptoms. A chronic relapsing disseminated form of the disease has been described in two younger patients, 9 and 20 years of age, with chronic mucocutaneous candidiasis.[50]

Adrenal involvement in disseminated histoplasmosis is of special concern. In 80 to 90 per cent of autopsied adult cases with disseminated disease, adrenal infection was present.[67] In another study, 54 per cent showed adrenal disease, half of which had some degree of adrenal insufficiency and 15 per cent of which had frank Addison disease.[165] In general, physicians treating patients with adrenal enlargement or Addison disease should include histoplasmosis as a consideration in the differential diagnosis, and individuals with disseminated histoplasmosis should have an evaluation of their adrenal function (Fig. 203–2).

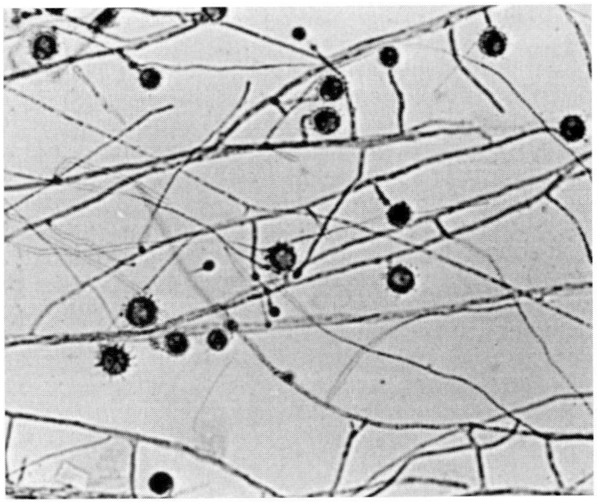

FIGURE 203–2. *Histoplasmosis of adrenal illustrating histiocytic response with numerous cells of* Histoplasma capsulatum *within the cytoplasm. (H and E × 52.)*

When histoplasmal gastrointestinal infection occurs in disseminated disease, fever and pulmonary symptoms are uncommon. Gastrointestinal symptoms predominate, and the clinical course may resemble granulomatous ileitis in the one-third of patients with involvement of the terminal ileum.[23]

Central nervous system involvement, usually in the form of meningitis, is seen in 10 to 30 per cent of patients with disseminated infection.[156, 160, 165] It is suspected ante mortem in only 40 per cent of cases.[86] A chronic, progressive infection of the central nervous system was reported in a child.[154] Cardiac disease generally is typical of fungal endocarditis with large valvular vegetations and a high rate of embolic phenomena.[61]

Presumed Ocular Histoplasmosis Syndrome

H. capsulatum has been identified in the fundi of patients with either disseminated histoplasmosis or solitary chorioretinal granulomata.[161] They appear as scattered, yellow, well-circumscribed, choroidal lesions. There are macular subretinal neovascular membranes present with or without hemorrhage. Peripapillary atrophy is present with an absence of inflammatory changes in the vitreous or anterior chambers. Histoplasmin reactivity usually is present, but the clinical syndrome also likely occurs in disorders other than histoplasmosis via immune-mediated mechanisms.

Histoplasmosis and AIDS

In 1987, the diagnostic criteria for AIDS were expanded to include disseminated histoplasmosis in the presence of HIV infection. In 1988, less than 0.5 per cent of AIDS patients had disseminated disease.[69] As in the general population, it is most common in endemic areas, where as many as 21 to 53 per cent of AIDS patients show evidence of active histoplasmosis.[14, 205, 206] It is recognized increasingly in HIV-infected children; one center in Arkansas reported histoplasmosis as the AIDS-defining illness in 8 per cent of their perinatal population.[162] However, it also can be seen in individuals in nonendemic areas.[157] Thus, in the AIDS patient with fever, weight loss, and hepatosplenomegaly or respiratory symptoms, disseminated histoplasmosis should be suspected.[158] Studies have suggested that AIDS patients may be infected with less virulent, temperature-sensitive variants of *H. capsulatum*.[167]

Common clinical findings in addition to those seen in other hosts include an interstitial pulmonary infiltrate in half the cases and central nervous system involvement including brain microabscesses, chorioretinitis, and cutaneous lesions.[4, 14, 83, 116, 158, 205] One-third of AIDS patients with disseminated histoplasmosis may follow a fulminant course similar to that of gram-negative sepsis with evidence of disseminated intravascular coagulation, adult respiratory distress syndrome, encephalopathy, and acute renal failure.[205] Extensive gastrointestinal involvement also may be seen.[74] Up to one-third may have concurrent tuberculosis.

Illness Due to Infection with *Histoplasma capsulatum* variety *duboisii*

The clinical presentation of illness due to infection with *H. capsulatum* variety *duboisii* is similar to that of chronic disseminated histoplasmosis.[32, 113, 210] Focal lesions are seen more commonly in bones (usually femur, ribs, or skull) or skin (cutaneous or subcutaneous). The lungs, gastrointestinal tract, liver, spleen, and lymph nodes rarely are involved.

Radiologic Findings

Approximately 75 per cent of pediatric histoplasmin skin test converters have normal chest radiographs on evaluation.[208] Also, the same percentage of individuals with acute pulmonary histoplasmosis, both primary infection and reinfection, present with a normal chest radiograph; the remainder tend to show small infiltrates. These infiltrates usually are 2 to 5 mm in diameter, up to 10 to 15 mm, in the basilar portions of the lungs (Fig. 203–3). Hilar nodes may be enlarged and eventually can calcify. In infants and young children, clusters of small infiltrates occasionally may coalesce into a larger (10 cm) bronchopneumonic lesion, and some patients may develop 2- to 3-cm coin lesions with areas of central necrosis, termed "histoplasmomas."[65] Pleural effusions may be seen in 10 per cent of adults with acute histoplasmosis.[204]

Heavy pulmonary inoculations can produce three characteristic radiologic patterns.[65] Individuals from nonendemic areas may show patchy infiltrates initially, which over time will be replaced by "buckshot" calcifications. These infil-

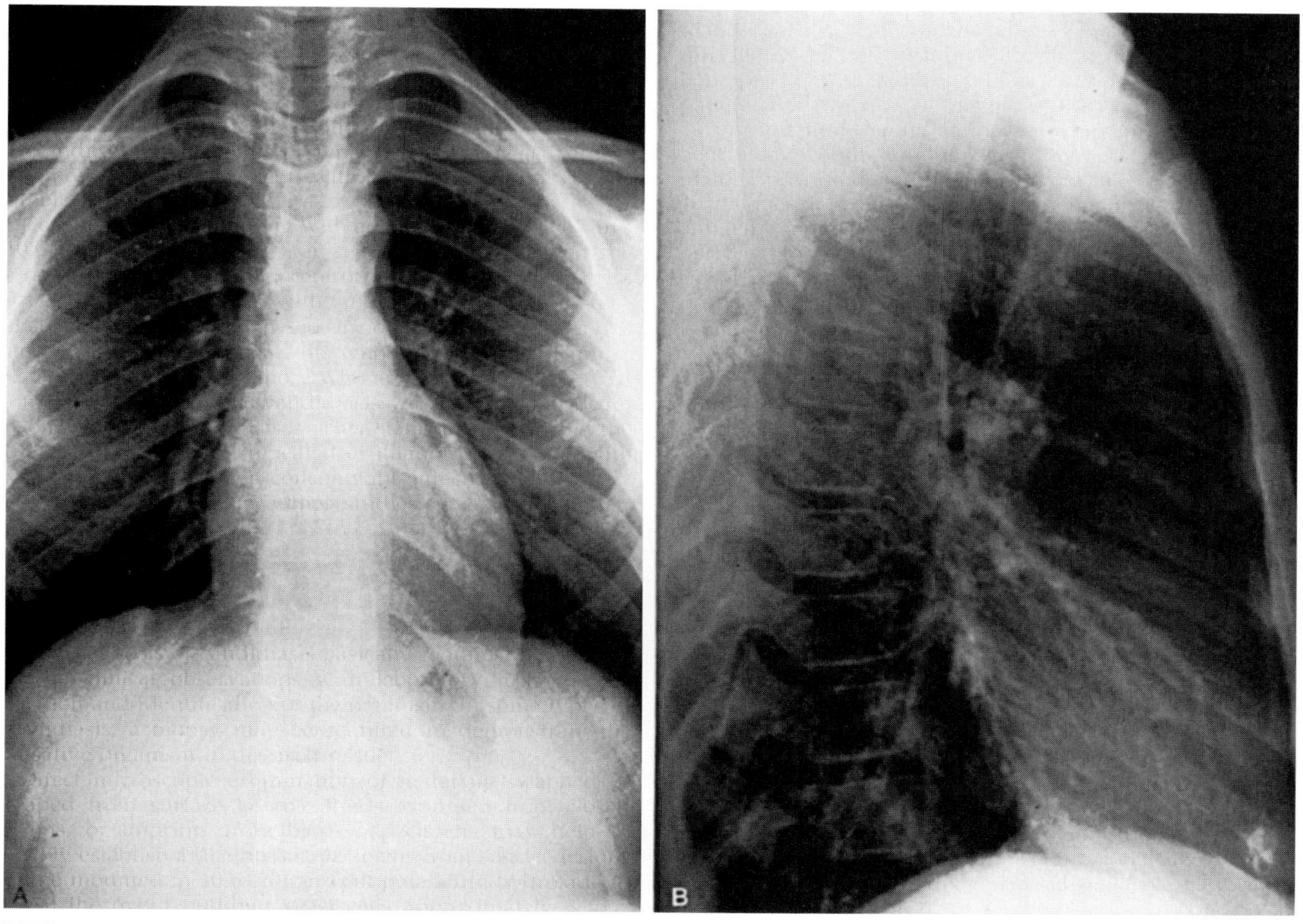

FIGURE 203–3. *Chest radiograph of an asymptomatic boy showing in the right lower lobe a calcification overlying the diaphragm between ribs 10 and 11 in the posteroanterior view* (A) *and overlying the apex of the heart in the lateral view* (B). *These films also demonstrated punctate calcifications overlying the spleen and right axilla (not shown).*

trates are thought to represent a hypersensitivity phenomenon. The second and most common infiltrate is smaller and nodular in appearance, as shown in Figure 203–4. This form is seen in individuals from both endemic and nonendemic areas. Finally, a diffuse miliary pattern may be seen, usually in a patient with a high level of immunity.

Calcifications typically appear to be very regular with a surrounding halo and may be seen in both the liver and spleen in addition to the respiratory tract.[133] As stated previously, calcification can develop more rapidly in children than in adults.

In acute disseminated histoplasmosis, the chest radiograph shows evidence of infection in only one-fourth of patients, characterized by diffuse interstitial infiltrates in one-fourth of those with abnormal roentgenograms. In contrast, patients with subacute disseminated disease seldom show interstitial pneumonitis. Abdominal computed tomographic scanning or sonography may show evidence of adrenal enlargement with disseminated disease.[111, 213] Patients with chronic pulmonary histoplasmosis characteristically have a single lesion on chest radiograph, although up to one-third may have multiple lesions.[24]

DIAGNOSIS

The various methods for diagnosing histoplasmosis are listed in the sections that follow (Table 203–2). The utility of each of these methods varies with the clinical presentation of the patient, and no single method is highly reliable in all settings.

Histologic Demonstration of Organisms

It often is difficult to find *H. capsulatum* in tissue specimens. In tissue, *H. capsulatum* can appear to be similar to *Leishmania, Toxoplasma, Pneumocystis carinii, Nosema,* small variants of *Cryptococcus, Blastomyces,* and *Torulopsis.* Numerous staining strategies exist.[115]

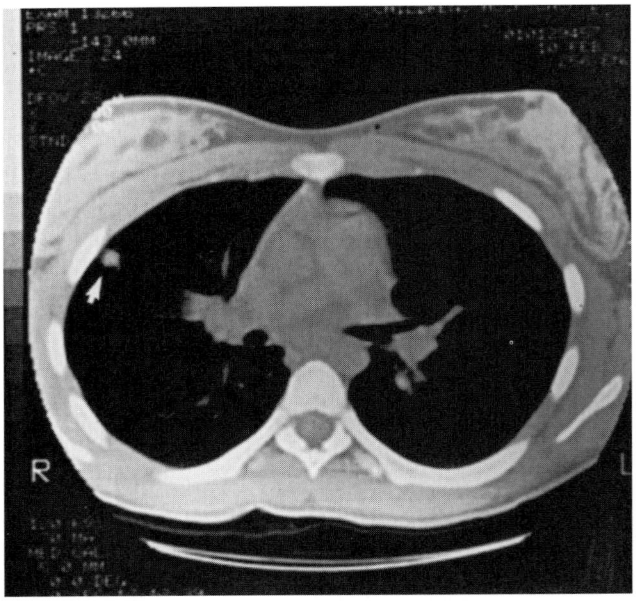

FIGURE 203–4. *Computed tomographic view of the chest of a teenage girl from Tennessee complaining of right arm pain with swimming. A nodular density is seen in the periphery of the right lung field (arrow), and the right hilum is enlarged slightly. Serologic tests and needle biopsy of the lesion were nondiagnostic, but excisional biopsy showed necrotizing granulomata with numerous histoplasmal yeast forms.*

TABLE 203–2. Serologic and Culture Positivity in Pediatric Histoplasmosis

	Culture (Any Site)	Serology	
		CF-Y	*ID*
Asymptomatic infection	− − −	+ +	+ + +
Acute self-limited infection	+	+ + +	+ + +
Acute disseminated infection	+ + + +	+ + +	+ + + +

− − − is less than 10 per cent of cases positive; + is 10 to 25 per cent; + + is 26 to 50 per cent; + + + is 51 to 75 per cent; + + + + is greater than 75 per cent. See text for detailed information.

CF-Y, complement fixation with yeast-phase antigen; ID, immunodiffusion.

Wright, Giemsa, and periodic acid–Schiff stains all have utility in the identification of fungal elements.[115, 122] Hematoxylin and eosin staining may demonstrate a false capsule around the organism; this actually represents the cytoplasm shrinking away from the cell wall.[111] Yeasts may be found in calcified lesions.[118] Gomori methenamine silver stain is the most sensitive reagent for demonstrating *H. capsulatum,* and it has the additional advantage that calcification artifacts dissolve during the staining procedure.[132] This may permit easier identification of organisms in tuberculoid granulomata.[12] In mediastinal fibrosis, the presence of nonviable yeast forms makes visualization with either periodic acid–Schiff or Gomori methenamine silver stains difficult, but a 90-minute stain with silver nitrate may be helpful.[115]

Examination of peripheral blood smears for histoplasmosis may be helpful in immunocompromised patients. In one study of 16 AIDS patients, 5 had blood smears positive for the fungus by Wright-Giemsa staining. Bone marrow examination also can be rewarding in this patient population.[83]

Limited experience exists with an immunoperoxidase *Histoplasma* antibody stain that can be used with tissue specimens.[97] In one study of patients with mediastinal fibrosis or mediastinal granuloma, antigen staining showed the presence of yeasts in 4 of 22 (18.2 per cent) patients.[38]

Culture

Specimens for culture of *Histoplasma* should be plated on (1) Sabouraud dextrose agar without antibiotics at 25° to 30° C; (2) Sabourand dextrose agar with antibiotics (cycloheximide and either chloramphenicol and gentamicin or penicillin and streptomycin) at 25° to 30° C; (3) brain-heart infusion agar with 5 per cent sheep's blood and antibiotics at 25° to 30° C; or (4) brain-heart infusion agar with 5 per cent sheep's blood without antibiotics at 37° C.[122] The brain-heart infusion media probably are best suited for rapid growth of *Histoplasma.* Other more selective media are available but probably are not needed for routine use. Plates should be kept for at least 12 weeks before being considered negative, although most isolates grow in 3 to 4 weeks.[198]

Sensitivity of culture is dependent on the source of the specimen and the extent of the illness. Common sites for recovery of *H. capsulatum* include the lower respiratory tract, blood, bone marrow, cerebrospinal fluid, liver, spleen, skin lesions, and synovium.[3]

In acute, self-limited histoplasmosis, less than 10 per cent of patients have a positive culture from any site. With increasing use of the lysis-centrifugation technique for blood cultures, this recovery rate may improve slightly. Two cases of acute, self-limited pulmonary histoplasmosis demonstrated positive blood cultures after the use of this technique.[139] This particularly is important to consider because the presence of a positive blood culture cannot be considered as the sole criterion for diagnosis of disseminated histoplasmosis, and a decision to treat a patient with histoplasmosis should not be based on this finding alone.

In other forms of pulmonary histoplasmosis, sputum may be a reliable site for the recovery of the organism, particularly in cavitary disease, in which positive cultures have been reported in up to 70 per cent of patients.[66] Sensitivity of sputum culture may be increased with multiple sampling.[196] Cultures of extrapulmonary sites rarely are positive in chronic pulmonary disease.[207]

Bronchoscopy with bronchoalveolar lavage may be particularly helpful in patients with pulmonary disease. In a study of bronchoscopy in 71 adults, bronchoalveolar lavage was positive in only 4 per cent of individuals with a single pulmonary nodule, but this increased to 55 per cent in the remainder of the patient group. The highest yield of 88 per cent (7/8) was seen in patients with infiltrates or cavitary disease.[148] Bronchoscopy did not appear to be helpful in evaluating patients with adenopathy, chronic pleural effusion, or bronchopleural fistulas.

In disseminated histoplasmosis, sensitivity for positive culture from any site is 88 per cent; bone marrow has the highest yield of 75 per cent positivity.[160, 189] Urine and sputum were positive 40 to 70 per cent and 60 per cent of the time, respectively.[165] Use of the lysis-centrifugation system for blood culture has shortened the time for identification of a positive culture from approximately 16 days to 9 days.[11] As the disease evolves from acute to subacute and chronic disseminated states, the rates of positive lysis-centrifugation cultures from peripheral blood fall from nearly always (acute) to 50 per cent (subacute) to virtually never in chronic patients.[111] Radiometric mycobacterial broth blood cultures also may yield *H. capsulatum*, particularly in AIDS patients.[120]

In histoplasma meningitis, cerebrospinal fluid cultures have been reported positive in 25 to 50 per cent of individuals, requiring 2 to 4 weeks for growth.[86, 165] In patients with mediastinal granuloma and fibrosis, cultures were positive in only 3.8 to 10 per cent.[38, 112]

Antibody and Antigen Detection

The serologic methods used most commonly for the diagnosis of histoplasmosis are immunodiffusion (ID) and complement fixation (CF). CF serology is more sensitive than ID is and becomes positive 2 to 4 weeks sooner, approximately 4 to 6 weeks after infection in most cases.[189] However, ID remains positive longer than CF does after resolution of symptoms. In those patients with a positive CF, 25 per cent have a negative ID result, but less than 1 per cent of those with a positive ID have a negative CF.[34]

Serologic testing for detecting disseminated disease in relatively immunocompetent hosts is good with approximately 70 per cent sensitivity using CF.[69] However, in immunosuppressed patients, the positivity rate is only 50 per cent for disseminated disease.[35, 92]

Skin testing can cause elevations of both CF and ID antibody titers for up to 3 months after histoplasmin inoculation.[122] This occurs in approximately 12 to 27 per cent of individuals with a positive skin test and is most pronounced with the mycelial phase antigen of CF (CF-M).[3, 20, 91] However, the yeast-phase antigen (CF-Y) also may increase from negative to 1:32 after skin testing.[78, 94]

Cross-reactivity with other fungal antigens is a problem with both CF and ID serology, most commonly involving blastomycosis, coccidioidomycosis, and paracoccidioidomycosis.[198] However, this also can be seen with candidiasis, tuberculosis, aspergillosis, and cryptococcosis.[115, 198] In *H. capsulatum* testing, cross-reactivity especially is true with blastomycosis, with which titers of 1:8 to 1:16 can be seen.[93] Cross-reactivity also is seen not uncommonly in patients with chronic cavitary tuberculosis, but simultaneous infection with tuberculous and fungal pathogens can occur.[55] Also, some variability in quality of commercial reagents has been reported to cause false-negative results.[105] The more specific ID may be helpful in interpreting a positive CF where cross-reactivity is a concern, but ID may show false positivity in up to 25 to 50 per cent of other fungal infections.[198]

Complement Fixation

CF utilizes sensitized sheep red blood cells, histoplasmin antigen, and killed *H. capsulatum* yeast cells.[122] After exposure in acute pulmonary histoplasmosis, the titer may become positive in up to 6 per cent of individuals at 3 weeks and 73 per cent and 77 per cent at 4 and 6 weeks, respectively.[34, 198] With resolution of infection, the titer drops to 1:8 to 1:16 within 4 to 6 months and less than 1:8 by 9 months. Reported sensitivities for a single titer range from 70 to 95 per cent and depend on the definition or cut-off for considering a result positive. However, one report showed that 12 of 28 patients with non-*Histoplasma* febrile pneumonias had CF titers greater than or equal to 1:32.[178]

The presence of a fourfold rise between acute and convalescent sera is the best evidence of recent infection. Both the individual yeast (CF-Y) and mycelial (CF-M) phases can be measured. The CF-Y is more sensitive than the CF-M for recent or active infection and particularly may be useful in endemic areas, where background CF serologic positivity typically is 5 to 15 per cent of the adult population but may range as high as 30 per cent.[62, 65, 111] In a series of 11 children with acute pulmonary histoplasmosis, CF-Y was greater than or equal to 1:32 in 9 children, but CF-M was greater than or equal to 1:32 in only 3 children.[215]

The height of the titer does not correlate with disease severity, but individuals with more severe localized disease are more likely to be seropositive.[188] For example, in severe acute histoplasmosis, seropositivity approached 90 to 100 per cent in one study. In moderate, mild, and asymptomatic disease, the seropositivity fell to 86 per cent, 75 per cent, and 18 per cent, respectively.[103] Twenty-five per cent of patients with acute histoplasmosis have CF titers that could be termed borderline positive, between 1:8 and 1:16.[34] Titers greater than or equal to 1:32 are less likely to be falsely positive or residual from prior infection.

CF results vary by disease state. In chronic pulmonary histoplasmosis, the CF titer is negative in 25 per cent of individuals and greater than or equal to 1:32 in about 50 per cent.[66] In children with mediastinal masses, 67 per cent of those with histoplasmosis have CF titers greater than or equal to 1:32, and 75 per cent of patients with chronic cavitary disease have similar titers.[56]

Histoplasma meningitis can pose a special serologic problem. Both CF and ID can be positive in cerebrospinal fluid, but up to one-half of patients with other chronic fungal meningitides may show false-positive results.[145, 197] Cerebrospinal fluid CF-M antibody appears to be the most sensitive and specific test for this indication. In one study, there were no false-positive cerebrospinal fluid CF-M titers in patients with cryptococcal meningitis, but CF-Y falsely was positive in 5 of the 18 patients.[197] Individuals with fibrosing mediastinitis or mediastinal granuloma generally have negative or very low levels of CF antibody.[188] Serology in AIDS patients generally has not been helpful, although one study reported five of seven patients positive by CF.[205]

Immunodiffusion

ID is used to detect precipitin bands formed by reaction between a patient's serum and the histoplasmin antigen in agarose gel.[122] It is more specific than CF, approaching 99 per cent.[199] There are two distinct precipitin bands seen with ID: the M and H bands. The M band appears soon after infection and is present in 25 per cent by the fourth week of infection and in 50 to 86 per cent by the sixth week.[7, 34, 142] It can persist for 18 to 36 months after recovery but eventually disappears. For this reason, in contrast to CF, ID serology is positive in less than 1 per cent of individuals from an endemic area.[62] The H band is present infrequently in patients with histoplasmosis. It appears transiently and, therefore, denotes active infection.[65] It is not detected typically in children with histoplasmosis.[187]

In patients with active pulmonary histoplasmosis, between one-half and three-fourths have an M band present alone, but the H band is seen in only 10 to 20 per cent of acute infections.[3, 71, 93, 199] Only 10 per cent of individuals have both M and H bands present, a finding that is most specific for active disease.[3] For patients with disseminated disease, in contrast, both bands are present in 25 per cent of individuals.[3] The M band has been detected in 52 per cent and 57 per cent of patients with chronic pulmonary and disseminated disease, respectively.[71] In a small study of patients with AIDS and histoplasmosis, four of seven patients had M bands detected, and two had an H band.[205] Because it is more specific, ID can be of value for the confirmation of a diagnosis of histoplasmosis in patients with histoplasma CF titers in the borderline 1:8 to 1:16 range.[185]

Antibody Detection by Radioimmunoassay

Antibody detection with radioimmunoassay (RIA) can allow for earlier detection of cases, compared with the use of conventional serology alone, and can be determined for antibody to both histoplasmin and yeast antigen.[142] In one study, RIA sensitivity was 52 per cent at 3 weeks after exposure, compared with 6 per cent for CF and 0 per cent for ID.[198] The detection rate for RIA increases to 93 per cent at 6 weeks.[34] Among patients with nonhistoplasmal pulmonary disease who live in endemic areas, antibody determined by RIA for IgG alone, IgM alone, and combined titers is elevated in 27 per cent, 10 per cent, and 5 per cent of patients, respectively.[201]

The main drawback to antibody measurement by RIA is the cross-reactivity with other infections, which occurs in as high as 50 per cent of cases of other fungal infections and tuberculosis.[198] Cross-reactivity in one study of patients with bacterial, mycobacterial, and viral disease was 28 per cent overall for detection of histoplasma IgM. In patients with other fungal infections, the false-positive rate was 49 per cent for RIA IgM, compared with 18 per cent and 5 per cent for the CF and ID methodologies, respectively.

Antibody Detection by Enzyme Immunoassay

Enzyme immunoassay, another method for detection of histoplasma antibody, may be a more sensitive method than CF or ID. In 12 patients with either chronic pulmonary or disseminated histoplasmosis, the sensitivity was 100 per cent.[102] Because enzyme immunoassay is adapted more readily to the hospital laboratory than is RIA, this method of antibody measurement may come into widespread use. However, to date, the use of enzyme immunoassay to detect antigen has not achieved the level of sensitivity attained with RIA.[220]

Antigen Detection by Radioimmunoassay

RIA with either histoplasmin or yeast antigen may be performed on any body fluid to detect either antigen or antibody. One key advantage of the RIA method for antigen detection is the ability to monitor response to therapy.[202] With successful treatment or spontaneous recovery, the RIA becomes negative. With relapse, antigen detected by RIA becomes positive again.

In one study in which both urine and serum were obtained from infected patients, antigen detection by RIA was positive in the urine of 20 and in the serum of 11 of 22 episodes of disseminated disease.[202] In sarcoid-like disease and in acute diffuse pulmonary histoplasmosis, detection rates are about 50 per cent. However, other forms of histoplasmosis have lower levels of antigen detection. In acute self-limited disease, 19 per cent (6/32) were antigen-positive, and only 6 per cent (2/32) of patients with cavitary disease had detectable antigen. In general, urine is more likely to yield a positive result than serum is. Specificity is good; in 295 controls, all sera and urines were negative for antigen. In an outbreak of histoplasmosis involving 195 patients, polysaccharide antigen testing detected 92 per cent, 21 per cent, and 39 per cent of patients with disseminated, chronic pulmonary, and self-limited forms of disease, respectively.[211] In 26 children with histoplasmosis, retrospective urinary antigen testing was positive in all.[51] Most (85 per cent) had disseminated disease. A decline in urinary antigen concentrations was seen in all 12 patients available for study who received amphotericin B treatment.

In patients with AIDS and histoplasmosis, urine and serum antigen testing by RIA has been helpful to diagnose infection, monitor response to therapy, and detect relapses.[191–193] It also has been used to test bronchoalveolar lavage fluid in this patient population.[194]

Antigen detection by RIA in cerebrospinal fluid can be helpful.[199, 203] In one study, 5 of 12 patients had detectable antigen, and in another study of 11 patients with chronic meningeal histoplasmosis, 9 were positive. There was one false-positive result in an individual with coccidioidal meningitis. Antibody detection in cerebrospinal fluid is less useful; although IgG antibody can be detected, the false-positive rate approached 50 per cent.

Skin Testing

Skin testing is performed using histoplasmin antigen prepared from mycelial-phase culture filtrate. After intradermal administration, an area of induration greater than or equal to 5 mm at 48 hours is considered to be a positive result.[122] Skin test reactivity usually becomes positive within 2 to 4 weeks after infection.[54] By 12 years of age, 80 per cent of children in an endemic area may have a reactive histoplasmin skin test.[188] False-positive skin tests have been seen with both blastomycosis and coccidioidomycosis.[44]

After resolution of active disease, cutaneous reactivity may diminish over time but persists indefinitely in most individuals. In an early study, Zeidberg and associates[218] demonstrated that 15 to 20 per cent of individuals previously skin test–positive became negative within 2 years. Others have shown waxing and waning skin test reactivity over time, which suggests recurrent episodes of infection. Later follow-up showed that most became positive eventually, and other experience has demonstrated skin test reactivity to remain for 10 or more years in 80 per cent of infected persons.[65, 188]

In chronic pulmonary disease, including cavitary disease, the skin test is positive in three-fourths of patients.[54] In contrast, individuals with disseminated disease seldom have positive results.[2] The problem of serologic boosting by skin testing has limited its diagnostic use, although it has been suggested that utilization of a histoplasmin yeast-phase antigen may not cause a CF booster effect.[2] Overall, the histoplasmin skin test shows little diagnostic utility, particularly in individuals from endemic areas.[65]

TREATMENT

The majority of individuals with histoplasmosis recover spontaneously and do not require specific therapy.[65] Bed rest often is recommended for symptomatic acute histoplasmosis.[79] However, individuals with complicated disease may require treatment. The mainstay of therapy is antifungal agents, primarily itraconazole for mild disease and amphotericin B for more severely infected patients.

Medical

Indications for antifungal therapy include patients with chronic pulmonary histoplasmosis with progression of lesions or persistence of cavitation, disseminated histoplasmosis, acute pulmonary histoplasmosis complicated by the adult respiratory distress syndrome, cutaneous fistulas, and mediastinal granuloma with symptomatic obstruction.[66, 171, 188] Other clinical manifestations may require treatment in special circumstances.

For individuals with severe disease, regardless of type of infection, amphotericin B remains the drug of choice.[65, 67] It usually is given in doses of 0.5 to 1.0 mg/kg/day until a total dosage of 30 to 35 mg/kg has been administered.[41, 65] However, shorter courses of therapy may be appropriate. Amphotericin B first was used in infants with disseminated disease in 1959, and subsequent experience showed good clinical responses with shorter courses of therapy.[104, 107] Fosson and Wheeler[52] reported cures in five infants (only two with microbiologic confirmation) with an initial dose of 0.25 mg/kg on the first day and 0.5 mg/kg on the second day, followed by 1 mg/kg for 7 to 11 days. In other experiences, 19 of 20 individuals treated with amphotericin B recovered, but 3 of the 19 had recurrences.[81] Newer experience with azole compounds suggests that "step-down" therapy with ketoconazole or itraconazole after 1 or 2 weeks of amphotericin B may be appropriate.

Ketoconazole has demonstrated efficacy in the treatment of histoplasmosis. Response rates for ketoconazole in immunocompetent patients are good (70 to 100 per cent), but poor results have been found in immunosuppressed patients.[127, 181] Slama[164] administered 200 mg of ketoconazole daily to 10 adults with disseminated disease; all 7 who had no known underlying disease were cured, whereas the 3 whose treatment failed had an underlying malignancy. Ketoconazole also has been used for therapy in immunocompetent patients with histoplasmal endocarditis and for central nervous system infection, although cerebrospinal fluid penetration is poor.[18, 49, 64, 124] In a multicenter, prospective study of 54 adults with chronic cavitary disease (23 patients), localized infection (15), or disseminated disease (16), ketoconazole was given as either 400 or 800 mg orally on a daily basis.[124] Efficacy in the low-dose group was 77 per cent (24/31) versus 43 per cent in the high-dose group. Side effects were more frequent in the high-dose group. Another group documented poor response to therapy with ketoconazole in chronic cavitary histoplasmosis.[149] Although there is little published experience with ketoconazole use for histoplasmosis in the pediatric population, a daily dose of 6 mg/kg is likely to be safe and effective.

Clearly, ketoconazole therapy is preferable to amphotericin B for histoplasmosis in selected patients because of the ease of oral administration and the overall lower incidence of side effects. However, ketoconazole use is not entirely safe. Gastrointestinal absorption is impaired in those in achlorhydric states, such as in postgastrectomy patients or in individuals receiving antacids or H_2-blockers, and, therefore, levels are unpredictable.[117, 177, 183] Also, ketoconazole is fungistatic rather than fungicidal, and it penetrates poorly into the cerebrospinal fluid and peritoneal cavity.[15, 49, 70, 123] The primary side effects include hepatotoxicity (hepatitis in 1 in 10,000 to 15,000 patients) and endocrinologic problems.[77, 82, 106] The latter instance includes gynecomastia in male recipients, impotence, decrease in libido due to interference with testosterone synthesis in the adrenals and testes, and a blunting of the adrenocorticotropic hormone stimulation of the adrenal glands.[36, 146, 180] This latter condition particularly can be problematic in AIDS and other immunocompromised patients who may have adrenal involvement with histoplasmosis, cytomegalovirus infection, or other opportunistic infections.[9, 72] Ketoconazole also can interfere with the metabolism of other drugs, such as isoniazid, rifampin, phenytoin, and cyclosporine, and care is required if they are to be used concomitantly.[18, 66, 88]

Itraconazole, an oral triazole antifungal agent first synthesized in 1980, is more active in vitro against *H. capsulatum* than is ketoconazole.[47, 58, 76, 166, 182] Patients have responded more quickly to itraconazole therapy than to ketoconazole; in adults given 100 mg orally on a daily basis, 16 of 17 showed either cure or improvement in one study.[75, 125] Those who were treated successfully received 50 mg of itraconazole daily for 6 months. In a study in Argentina, 32 adult patients (29 with chronic disseminated disease, 2 with chronic pulmonary disease, and 1 with subacute disseminated illness) were treated with 100 mg daily for 2 months followed by 50 mg daily for 4 months.[126] Twenty-nine were cured, 2 improved, and 1 was not evaluable. There were no relapses in the 23-month follow-up period.

Subsequent studies of itraconazole in histoplasmosis have cemented its role as the drug of choice for all mild forms of histoplasmosis that require therapy. In a large multicenter trial in adults receiving 200 to 400 mg daily for a median of 9 months, the overall cure rate was 81 per cent.[39] In the subgroup of patients with chronic pulmonary disease, a group very difficult to cure, the success rate was 65 per cent (13/20). Side effects were relatively minimal; 29 per cent of patients treated for histoplasmosis or blastomycosis had some adverse effects, most commonly nausea, vomiting, or diarrhea.[39] Unlike the azoles, triazole compounds do not appear to produce ill effects in the endocrine system.[126]

Itraconazole also has been shown to be effective in the treatment of histoplasmosis in patients with AIDS. Negroni and colleagues[128] treated 27 adults with disseminated disease, and 23 responded to a 6-month course of therapy. In a larger trial, 50 of 59 evaluable patients responded to a 3-month course of therapy.[200] Although these were uncontrolled trials, the reponses compare favorably with historical controls treated with amphotericin B. Still, amphotericin B remains the drug of choice for initial therapy for moderate to severe disease in these patients. Itraconazole also appears to have a promising role in the treatment of renal transplant patients with disseminated disease, but because of poor cerebrospinal fluid penetration, it should not be used for the treatment of central nervous system disease.[143]

All AIDS patients appear to require indefinite suppressive therapy to prevent relapse of histoplasmosis.[84, 190, 205] Itraconazole, ketoconazole, and fluconazole may be useful as suppressive therapy after an initial treatment course with standard agents. Ketoconazole given as a dose of 400 mg daily for an indefinite period seems helpful for suppression, similar to a regimen of once-weekly amphotericin B administration.[188] However, in one study, 3 of 11 AIDS patients relapsed while receiving ketoconazole prophylaxis.[69] This may have been caused in part by the relative achlorhydria seen in AIDS patients, which reduces ketoconazole absorption. Itraconazole also has been effective in preventing relapse in this patient population. Forty-two adult patients in one study were treated initially with amphotericin B for a period of 4 to 12 weeks, followed by 400 mg daily of itraconzole.[195] With a median follow-up of approximately 2 years, there were only two relapses, both in patients not receiving therapy due to noncompliance or withdrawal from the study. Preliminary results of fluconazole as initial therapy for histoplasmosis in humans have not been encouraging, but one study showed efficacy in preventing relapse in AIDS patients when used at a dose of at least 200 mg/day.[57, 131]

Other promising experimental therapy has been seen with liposome-encapsulated amphotericin B and with the methyl ester of amphotericin B.[28, 110, 129, 174] This latter compound is produced through methyl esterification of the single free carboxyl group of amphotericin B, making it water-soluble. Little toxicity is noted, and peak concentrations are seen that are 10-fold higher than are those achieved with amphotericin B.[13] A report of the use of amphotericin B methyl ester in an elderly man with disseminated histoplasmosis demonstrated his ability to tolerate up to 150 mg/kg total dose without adverse effects after suffering severe toxicities during prior amphotericin B therapy.[129]

Corticosteroid therapy may be helpful in the rare patient with adult respiratory distress syndrome complicating histoplasmosis, and these agents also appeared to be beneficial in a child with tracheal obstruction and respiratory compromise.[73, 87, 176, 216] Steroids, if used, always should be given in conjunction with antifungal therapy.

Surgical

Surgical treatment is needed occasionally for selected individuals with histoplasmosis. In a surgical experience from St. Louis, Missouri, 94 patients 10 to 40 years of age were evaluated from 1975 to 1984.[59] The most common reason for evaluation was obstruction of thoracic structures due to enlarged mediastinal masses. Seventy-five patients eventually underwent surgery or endoscopy to relieve obstruction of the pulmonary artery, superior vena cava, bronchus, or esophagus. Recurrent pneumonia, tracheoesophageal fistula, hemoptysis, and broncholithiasis were other indications for surgical management.[59, 99, 219]

Attempts at total excision of soft caseous nodes can lead to damage of contiguous structures, and it is preferable simply to unroof and evacuate debris from such lesions, which leaves the invasive portion of the capsule intact.[48, 59, 141, 212] Once calcification has occurred in fibrosing mediastinitis, surgical repair is not feasible.[115] Prophylactic excision of large mediastinal nodes cannot be supported because this therapy has not been shown to prevent fibrosis, and patients with large mediastinal lymph nodes who otherwise are asymptomatic may never progress to develop mediastinal fibrosis.[188]

PROGNOSIS

As stated previously, most cases of acute histoplasmosis result in asymptomatic calcification of lymph nodes and the development of skin test conversion to histoplasmin. Disease severity and mortality are greatest in the age extremes and in the immunocompromised host.[122]

Little information is available regarding long-term outcome in acute pulmonary histoplasmosis, but one study examined pulmonary function testing for almost 2 years in a mother and her six children who developed acute histoplasmosis after cleaning a chicken coop.[100] A researcher also became infected and was studied. One child had respiratory failure with severe hypoxemia during the acute episode but recovered after treatment with amphotericin B. Initial pulmonary function studies showed mild diminution in most of the patients, which included both obstructive and restrictive patterns as well as impaired diffusion of carbon monoxide. By 6 months after infection, all obstructive components had normalized, and the restrictive patterns became normal by the tenth month. There also was a defect in carbon monoxide diffusion, which persisted in three of the patients for the 22-month duration of follow-up. The child with respiratory failure remained hypoxemic at 22 months.

In untreated acute disseminated histoplasmosis, death occurs in 83 to 93 per cent of patients within 3 months.[53, 115, 159] Subacute disseminated disease runs a more prolonged course but still demonstrates a high mortality.[67] However, the use of amphotericin B therapy has dropped the mortality rate in disseminated disease to 7 to 23 per cent.[151, 159, 160] Patients who receive less than 30 mg/kg of amphotericin B (if this agent is used as the sole treatment) are more prone to relapse (5 to 23 per cent), which usually occurs within 1 year of discontinuation of treatment.[159, 160] In chronic pulmonary histoplasmosis, mortality is 21 per cent, and recurrence can be seen as long as 6 months after treatment in up to one-fifth of individuals.[24, 172] Late relapses occur rarely.[17, 159]

With treatment, most patients with histoplasmosis show some improvement within 1 to 2 weeks.[160] Conditions to be considered when response is slow or relapse occurs include insufficient dose of the antifungal agent, concurrent immunosuppressive drug administration, endocarditis, infection of vascular grafts and mycotic aneurysms, chronic meningitis, presence of adrenal insufficiency, and presence of concomitant immunodeficiency, such as AIDS.[17, 138, 188]

PREVENTION

Prevention of infection with *H. capsulatum* is limited to the manipulation of environmental factors, which can be difficult when the source of an outbreak cannot be pinpointed. Formaldehyde spraying of areas associated with avian-borne *H. capsulatum* is thought to be helpful.[27] However, this method probably is ineffective in bat caves because the bats, as opposed to avian hosts, themselves are infected with the fungus and recontaminate the environment.[26] A recombinant protein vaccine made from cloned sequences of DNA coding for *H. capsulatum* cell wall glycoprotein was protective in a mouse model of pulmonary disease.[63]

Acknowledgment

The author wishes to acknowledge the invaluable assistance of Dr. Brad Leissa in preparing the previous edition of this chapter.

References

1. Ajello, L., and Zeidberg, L. D.: Isolation of *Histoplasma capsulatum* and *Allescheria boydii* from soil. Science *113*:662, 1951.
2. American Thoracic Society: Clinical usefulness of skin testing in histoplasmosis, coccidioidomycosis and blastomycosis. Am. Rev. Respir. Dis. *138*:1081–1082, 1988.
3. American Thoracic Society: Medical Section of the American Lung Association: Laboratory diagnosis of mycotic and specific fungal infections. Am. Rev. Respir. Dis. *132*:1373–1379, 1985.
4. Anders, K. H., Guerra, W. F., Tomiyasu, U., et al.: The neuropathology of AIDS: UCLA experience and review. Am. J. Pathol. *124*:537–558, 1986.
5. Artz, R. P, and Bullock, W. E.: Immunoregulatory responses in experimental disseminated histoplasmosis: Depression of T-cell-dependent and T-cell-effector responses by activation of splenic suppressor cells. Infect. Immun. *23*:893–902, 1979.
6. Baughman, R. P., Kim, C. K., Vinegar, A., et al.: The pathogenesis of experimental pulmonary histoplasmosis: Correlative studies of histopathology, bronchoalveolar lavage, and respiratory function. Am. Rev. Respir. Dis. *134*:771–776, 1986.
7. Bauman, D. S., and Smith, C. D.: Comparison of immunodiffusion and complement fixation tests in the diagnosis of histoplasmosis. J. Clin. Microbiol. *2*:77–80, 1975.
8. Bennish, M., Radkowski, M. A., and Rippon, J. W.: Cavitation in acute histoplasmosis. Chest *84*:496–497, 1983.
9. Best, T. R., Jenkins, J. K., and Murphy, F. Y., et al.: Persistent adrenal insufficiency secondary to low-dose ketoconazole therapy. Am. J. Med. *82*:676–680, 1987.
10. Bhagavan, B. S., Rao, D. R. G., and Weinberg, T.: Histoplasmosis producing broncholithiasis. Arch. Pathol. *91*:577–579, 1971.
11. Bille, J., Stockman, L., Roberts, G. D., et al.: Evaluation of a lysis-centrifugation system for recovery of yeasts and filamentous fungi from blood. J. Clin. Microbiol. *18*:469–471, 1983.
12. Binford, C., and Dooley, J.: Histoplasmosis. *In* Binford, C., and Connors, D. (eds.): Pathology of Tropical and Extraordinary Diseases. Washington, D.C., Armed Forces Institute of Pathology, 1976, p. 578.
13. Bonner, D. P., Terwari, R. P., and Solotorovsky, M., et al.: Comparative chemotherapeutic activity of amphotericin B and amphotericin B methyl ester. Antimicrob. Agents Chemother. *7*:724–729, 1975.
14. Bonner, J. R., Alexander, W. J., Dismukes, W. E., et al.: Disseminated histoplasmosis in patients with the acquired immune deficiency syndrome. Arch. Intern. Med. *144*:2178–2181, 1984.
15. Borgers, M.: Mechanism of action of antifungal drugs, with special reference to the imidazole derivatives. Rev. Infect. Dis. *2*:520–534, 1980.
16. Bower, R. J., and Kiesewetter, W. B.: Mediastinal masses in infants and children. Arch. Surg. *112*:1003–1009, 1977.
17. Bradsher, R. W., Alford, R. H., Hawkins, S. S., et al.: Conditions associated with relapse of amphotericin B–treated disseminated histoplasmosis. Johns Hopkins Med. J. *150*:127–131, 1982.
18. Brass, C., Galgiani, J. N., Blaschke, T. F., et al.: Disposition of ketoconazole, an oral antifungal, in humans. Antimicrob. Agents Chemother. *21*:151–158, 1982.
19. Brummer, E., Kurita, N., Yosihida, S., et al: Fungistatic activity of human neutrophils against *Histoplasma capsulatum*: Correlation with phagocytosis. J. Infect. Dis. *164*:158–162, 1991.
20. Buechner, H. A., Seabury, J. H., Campbell, C. C., et al.: The current status of serologic, immunologic and skin tests in the diagnosis of pulmonary mycoses. Chest *63*:259, 1973.
21. Butler, J. C., Heller, R., and Wright, P. F.: Histoplasmosis during childhood. South Med. J. *87*:476–480, 1994.
22. Campbell, C. C., Hill, G. B., and Falgout, B. T.: *Histoplasma capsulatum* isolated from feather pillow associated with histoplasmosis in an infant. Science *136*:1050, 1962.
23. Cappell, M. S., Mandell, W., Grimes, M. M., et al.: Gastrointestinal histoplasmosis. Dig. Dis. Sci. *33*:353–360, 1988.
24. Case records of the Massachusetts General Hospital: Weekly clinicopathological exercises. Case 49-1988. A 40-year-old man with a persistent nodular density in the left lower lobe. N. Engl. J. Med. *319*:1530–1537, 1988.
25. Case records of the Massachusetts General Hospital: Weekly clinicopathological exercises. Case 24-1984. Pancytopenia and fever in a renal-transplant recipient. N. Engl. J. Med. *310*:1584–1594, 1984.
26. Centers for Disease Control: Cave-associated histoplasmosis: Costa Rica. M. M. W. R. *37*:312, 1988.
27. Centers for Disease Control: Histoplasmosis control: Decontamination of bird roosts, chicken houses, and other point sources. Atlanta, U.S. Department of Health, Education, and Welfare, Public Health Service, 1979. HEW Publication No. (CDC) 80-8380.
28. Chance, M. L., and New, R. R. C.: Enhancement of efficacy of antifungal agents by entrapment inside liposomes. *In* Trinci, A. P. J., and Ryley, J. F. (eds.): Mode of Action of Antifungals. British Mycological Society Symposium 9. Cambridge, Cambridge University Press, 1984, p. 377.
29. Chaturvedi, S., Frame, P., and Newman, S. L.: Macrophages from human immunodeficiency virus–positive persons are defective in host defense against *Histoplasma capsulatum*. J. Infect. Dis. *171*:320–327, 1995.
30. Christie, A., and Peterson, J. C.: Pulmonary calcification in negative reactors to tuberculin. Am. J. Public Health *35*:1131, 1945.
31. Class, R. N., and Cascio, F. S.: Histoplasmosis presenting as acute polyarthritis. N. Engl. J. Med. *287*:1133–1134, 1972.
32. Cockshott, W. P., and Lucas, A. O.: Histoplasmosis duboisii. Q. J. Med. *133*:223, 1964.
33. Darling, S. T.: A protozoan general infection producing pseudo tubercles in the lungs and focal necrosis in the liver, spleen, and lymph nodes. J. A. M. A. *46*:1283, 1906.
34. Davies, S. F.: Serodiagnosis of histoplasmosis. Semin. Respir. Infect. *1*:9–15, 1986.
35. Davies, S. F., Khan, M., and Sarosi, G. A.: Disseminated histoplasmosis in immunologically suppressed patients: Occurrence in a non-endemic area. Am. J. Med. *64*:98–100, 1978.
36. DeFelice, R., Johnson, D. G., and Galgiani, J. N.: Gynecomastia with ketoconazole. Antimicrob. Agents Chemother. *19*:1073–1074, 1981.
37. DeMonbreum, W. A.: The cultivation and cultural characteristics of Darling's *H. capsulatum*. Am. J. Trop. Med. *14*:93, 1934.
38. Dines, D. E., Payne, W. S., Bernatz, P. E., et al.: Mediastinal granuloma and fibrosing mediastinitis. Chest *75*:320–324, 1979.
39. Dismukes, W. E., Bradsher, Jr., R. W., Cloud, G. C., et al.: Itraconazole therapy for blastomycosis and histoplasmosis. Am. J. Med. *93*:489–497, 1992.
40. Dodd, K., and Tompkins, E.: Case of histoplasmosis of Darling in an infant. Am. J. Trop. Med. *14*:127, 1934.
41. Drutz, D. J., Spickard, A., Rogers, D. E., et al.: Treatment of disseminated mycotic infections. Am. J. Med. *45*:405–418, 1968.
42. Dukes, R. J., Strimian, V., Dines, D. E., et al.: Esophageal involvement with mediastinal granuloma. J. A. M. A. *236*:2313–2315, 1976.
43. Edwards, L. B., Acquaviva, F. A., Livesay, V. T., et al.: An atlas of sensitivity to tuberculin, PPD-B, and histoplasmin in the United States. Am. Rev. Respir. Dis. *99*(Suppl.):1–132, 1969.
44. Edwards, L. B., Acquaviva, F. A., and Livesay, V. T.: Further observations on histoplasmin sensitivity in the United States. Am. J. Epidemiol. *98*:315–325, 1973.
45. Emmons, C. W., Klite, P. D., Baer, G. M., et al.: Isolation of *Histoplasma capsulatum* from bats in the United States. Am. J. Epidemiol. *84*:103–109, 1966.
46. Emmons, C. W., Morlan, H. B., and Hill, E. L.: Isolation of *Histoplasma capsulatum* from soil. Public Health Rep. *64*:892, 1949.
47. Epsinel-Ingroff, A., Shadomy, S., and Gebhardt, R. J.: In vitro studies with R 51,211. Antimicrob. Agents Chemother. *26*:5–9, 1984.
48. Ferguson, T. B., and Burford, T. H.: Mediastinal granuloma: A 15-year experience. Ann. Thorac. Surg. *1*:125, 1965.
49. Fibbe, W. E., Van Der Meer, J. W. M., Thompson, J., et al.: CSF concentrations of ketoconazole. J. Antimicrob. Chemother. *6*:681, 1980.
50. Flynn, P. M., Barrett, F. F., and Herrod, H. G.: Disseminated histoplasmosis in two patients with chronic mucocutaneous candidiasis. Pediatr. Infect. Dis. *6*:691–693, 1987.
51. Fojtasek, M. F., Kleiman, M. B., Connolly-Stringfield, P., et al.: The *Histoplasma capsulatum* antigen assay in disseminated histoplasmosis in children. Pediatr. Infect. Dis. J. *13*:801–805, 1994.
52. Fosson, A. R., and Wheeler, W. E.: Short-term amphotericin B treatment of severe childhood histoplasmosis. J. Pediatr. *86*:32–36, 1975.
53. Furcolow, M. L.: Comparison of treated and untreated severe histoplasmosis. J. A. M. A. *183*:121, 1963.
54. Furcolow, M. L.: Tests of immunity in histoplasmosis. N. Engl. J. Med. *268*:357, 1963.
55. Furcolow, M. L., Schubert, J., Tosh, F. E., et al.: Serologic evidence of histoplasmosis in sanatoriums in the U.S. J. A. M. A. *180*:109, 1962.
56. Gaebler, J. W., Kleiman, M. B., Cohen, M., et al.: Differentiation of lymphoma from histoplasmosis in children with mediastinal masses. J. Pediatr. *104*:706–709, 1984.
57. Galgiani, J. N.: Fluconazole, a new antifungal agent. Ann. Intern. Med. *113*:177–179, 1990.
58. Ganer, A., Arathoon E., and Stevens, D. A.: Initial experience in therapy for progressive mycoses with itraconazole, the first clinically studied triazole. Rev. Infect. Dis. *9*(Suppl. 1):S77–S86, 1987.
59. Garrett, H. E., Jr., and Roper, C. L.: Surgical intervention in histoplasmosis. Ann. Thorac. Surg. *42*:711–722, 1986.
60. Gass, M., and Kobayashi, G. S.: Histoplasmosis: An illustrative case with unusual vaginal and joint involvement. Arch. Dermatol. *100*:724–727, 1969.
61. Gaynes, R. P., Gardner, P., and Causey, W.: Prosthetic valve endocarditis caused by *Histoplasma capsulatum*. Arch. Intern. Med. *141*:1533–1537, 1981.
62. George, R. B., and Lambert, R. S.: Significance of serum antibodies to *Histoplasma capsulatum* in endemic areas. South. Med. J. *77*:161–163, 1984.
63. Gomez, F. J., Allendoerfer, R., and Deepe, G. S., Jr.: Vaccination with recombinant heat shock protein 60 from *Histoplasma capsulatum* protects mice against pulmonary histoplasmosis. Infect. Immun. *63*:2587–2595, 1995.
64. Goodpasture, H. C., Hershberger, R. E., Barnett, A. M., et al.: Treatment of central nervous system infection with ketoconazole. Arch. Intern. Med. *145*:879–880, 1985.

65. Goodwin, R. A., Loyd, J. E., and Des Prez, R. M.: Histoplasmosis in normal hosts. Medicine *60*:231–266, 1981.
66. Goodwin, R. A., Owens, F. T., Snell, J. D., et al.: Chronic pulmonary histoplasmosis. Medicine *55*:413–452, 1976.
67. Goodwin, R. A., Shapiro, J. L., Thurman, G. H., et al.: Disseminated histoplasmosis: Clinical and pathologic correlation. Medicine *59*:1–33, 1980.
68. Goodwin, R. A., and Snell, J. D., Jr.: The enlarging histoplasmoma: Concept of tumor-like phenomenon encompassing the tuberculoma and coccidioidoma. Am. Rev. Respir. Dis. *100*:1–12, 1969.
69. Graybill, J. R.: Histoplasmosis and AIDS. J. Infect. Dis. *158*:623–626, 1988.
70. Graybill, J. R., and Drutz, D. J.: Ketoconazole: A major innovation for treatment of fungal disease. Ann. Intern. Med. *93*:921–923, 1980.
71. Graybill, J. R., Patino, M. M., Gomez, A. M., et al.: Detection of histoplasmal antigens in mice undergoing experimental pulmonary histoplasmosis. Am. Rev. Respir. Dis. *132*:752–756, 1985.
72. Greene, L. W., Cole, W., Greene, J. B., et al.: Adrenal insufficiency as a complication of the acquired immunodeficiency syndrome. Ann. Intern. Med. *101*:497–498, 1984.
73. Greenwood, M. F., and Holland, P.: Tracheal obstruction secondary to *Histoplasma* mediastinal granuloma. Chest *62*:642–643, 1972.
74. Haggerty, C. M., Britton, M. C., Dorman, J. M., et al.: Gastrointestinal histoplasmosis in the acquired immune deficiency syndrome. West. J. Med. *143*:244–246, 1985.
75. Hay, R. J., Dupont, B., and Graybill, J. R.: First international symposium on itraconazole: A summary. Rev. Infect. Dis. *9*(Suppl. 1):S1–S152, 1987.
76. Heeres, J., Backx, L. J. J., and Van Custem, J.: Antimycotic azoles. 7. Synthesis and antifungal properties of a series of novel triazol-3-ones. J. Med. Chem. *27*:894–900, 1984.
77. Heiberg, J. K., and Svejaard, E.: Toxic hepatitis during ketoconazole therapy. Br. Med. J. *283*:825–826, 1981.
78. Heusinkveld, R., Tosh, F., and Newberry, W.: Antibody response to the histoplasmin skin test. Am. Rev. Respir. Dis. *96*:1069–1071, 1967.
79. Horton, G. E., Larkin, J. C., and Phillips, S.: Acute pulmonary histoplasmosis. South. Med. J. *52*:912, 1959.
80. Hostoffer, R. W., Berger, M., Clark, H. T., et al.: Disseminated *Histoplasma capsulatum* in a patient with hyper IgM immunodeficiency. Pediatrics *94*:234–236, 1994.
81. Hughes, W. T.: Hematogenous histoplasmosis in the immunocompromised child. J. Pediatr. *105*:569–575, 1984.
82. Janssen, P. A. J., and Symoens, J. E.: Hepatic reactions during ketoconazole treatment. Am. J. Med. *74*(1B):80–82, 1983.
83. Johnson, P. C., Khardori, N., Butt, F., et al.: Progressive disseminated histoplasmosis in patients with acquired immunodeficiency syndrome. Am. J. Med. *85*:152–158, 1988.
84. Johnson, P. C., Sarosi, G. A., and Septimus, E. J.: Progressive disseminated histoplasmosis in patients with the acquired immunodeficiency syndrome: A report of 12 cases and a literature review. Semin. Respir. Infect. *1*:1–8, 1986.
85. Jones, R. C., and Goodwin, R. A.: Histoplasmosis of the bone. Am. J. Med. *70*:864–866, 1981.
86. Karalakulasingam, R., Arora, K. K., Adams, G., et al.: Meningoencephalitis caused by *Histoplasma capsulatum*. Arch. Intern. Med. *136*:217–220, 1983.
87. Kataria, Y. P., Campbell, P. B., and Burlingham, B. T.: Acute pulmonary histoplasmosis presenting as adult respiratory distress syndrome: Effect of therapy on clinical and laboratory features. South. Med. J. *74*:534–537, 1981.
88. Katzir, D., and Blaschke, T. F.: The cyclosporine-ketoconazole interaction. Hosp. Ther. *15*:99, 1990.
89. Kauffman, C. A., Israel, M. S., Smith, J. W., et al.: Histoplasmosis in immunosuppressed patients. Am. J. Med. *64*:923–932, 1978.
90. Kauffman, C. A., Slama, T. G., and Wheat, L. J.: *Histoplasma capsulatum* epididymitis. J. Urol. *125*:434–435, 1981.
91. Kaufman, L.: Serological tests for histoplasmosis: Their use and interpretation. *In* Ajello, L., Chick, E. W., and Furcolow, M. L. (eds.): Histoplasmosis. Proceedings of the Second National Conference. Springfield, IL, Charles C Thomas, 1971, p. 321.
92. Kaufman, L., and Blumer, S.: Occurrence of serotypes among *Histoplasma capsulatum* strains. J. Bacteriol. *91*:1434, 1966.
93. Kaufman, L., and Reiss, E.: Serodiagnosis of fungal diseases. *In* Lennette, E. H., Balows, A., Hausler, W. J., Jr., et al. (eds.): Manual of Clinical Microbiology. 4th ed. Washington, D.C., American Society of Microbiology, 1985, p. 924.
94. Kaufman, L., Terry, R. T., Schubert, J. H., et al.: Effect of a single histoplasmin skin test on the serological diagnosis of histoplasmosis. J. Bacteriol. *94*:798, 1967.
95. Keller, F. G., and Kurtzberg, J.: Disseminated histoplasmosis: A cause of infection-associated hemophagocytic syndrome. Am. J. Pediatr. Hematol. Oncol. *16*:368–371, 1994.
96. King, R. W., and Kraikitpanitch, S.: Subcutaneous nodules caused by *Histoplasma capsulatum*. Ann. Intern. Med. *86*:586–587, 1977.
97. Klatt, E. C., Cosgrove, M., and Meyer, P. R.: Rapid diagnosis of disseminated histoplasmosis in tissues. Arch. Pathol. Lab. Med. *110*:1173–1175, 1986.
98. Klimpel, K. R., and Goldman, W. E.: Isolation and characterization of spontaneous avirulent variants of *Histoplasma capsulatum*. Infect. Immun. *55*:528–533, 1987.
99. Knight, P. J., Mulne, A. F., and Vassay, L. E.: When is lymph node biopsy indicated in children with enlarged peripheral nodes? Pediatrics *69*:391–396, 1982.
100. Kritski, A. L., Lemle, A., de Souza, G. R. M., et al.: Pulmonary function changes in the acute stage of histoplasmosis, with follow-up: An analysis of eight cases. Chest *97*:1244–1245, 1990.
101. Kwong-Chung, K. J.: Sexual stage of *Histoplasma capsulatum*. Science *175*:326, 1972.
102. Lambert, R. S., and George, R. B.: Evaluation of enzyme immunoassay as a rapid screening test for histoplasmosis and blastomycosis. Am. Rev. Respir. Dis. *136*:316–319, 1987.
103. Larrabee, W. F., Ajello, L., and Kaufman, L.: An epidemic of histoplasmosis on the isthmus of Panama. Am. J. Trop. Med. Hyg. *27*:281–283, 1977.
104. Leggiadro, R. J., Barrett, F. F., and Hughes, W. T.: Disseminated histoplasmosis of infancy. Pediatr. Infect. Dis. *7*:799–805, 1988.
105. Leland, D. S., Zimmerman, S. E., Cunningham E. B., et al.: Variability in commercial histoplasma complement fixation antigens. J. Clin. Microbiol. *29*:1723–1724, 1991.
106. Lewis, J. H., Zimmerman, H. J., Benson, G. D., et al.: Hepatic injury associated with ketoconazole therapy: Analysis of 33 cases. Gastroenterology *86*:503–513, 1984.
107. Little, J., Bruce, J., Andrews, H., et al.: Treatment of disseminated infantile histoplasmosis with amphotericin B. Pediatrics *24*:1, 1959.
108. Little, J. A., and Steigman, A. J.: Erythema nodosum in primary histoplasmosis. J. A. M. A. *173*:875, 1960.
109. Lockwood, G. F., and Garrison, R. G.: The possible role of uric acid in the ecology of *Histoplasma capsulatum*. Mycopathologia *35*:377–388, 1968.
110. Lopez-Berenstein, G., Fainstein, V., Hopfer, R., et al.: Liposomal amphotericin B for the treatment of systemic fungal infections in patients with cancer: A preliminary study. J. Infect. Dis. *151*:704–710, 1985.
111. Loyd, J. E., Des Prez, R. M., and Goodwin, R. A., Jr.: *Histoplasma capsulatum*. *In* Mandell, G. L., Douglas, R. G., Jr., and Bennett, J. E. (eds.): Principles and Practice of Infectious Diseases. 3rd ed. New York, Churchill Livingstone, 1990, p. 1989.
112. Loyd, J. E., Tillman, B. F., Atkinson, J. B., et al.: Mediastinal fibrosis complicating histoplasmosis. Medicine *67*:295–310, 1988.
113. Lucas, A. O.: Cutaneous manifestations of African histoplasmosis. Br. J. Dermatol. *82*:435–447, 1970.
114. Ma, K. W.: Disseminated histoplasmosis in dialysis patients. Clin. Nephrol. *24*:155–157, 1985.
115. Macher, A.: Histoplasmosis and blastomycosis. Med. Clin. North Am. *64*:447–459, 1980.
116. Macher, A., Rodrigues, M. M., Kaplan, W., et al.: Disseminated bilateral chorioretinitis due to *Histoplasma capsulatum* in a patient with acquired immunodeficiency syndrome. Ophthalmology *92*:1159–1164, 1985.
117. Mannisto, P. T., Mantyla, R., Nykanen, S., et al.: Impairing effect of food on ketoconazole absorption. Antimicrob. Agents Chemother. *21*:730–733, 1982.
118. Mashburn, J. D., Dawson, D. F., and Young, J. M.: Pulmonary calcifications and histoplasmosis. Am. Rev. Respir. Dis. *84*:208, 1961.
119. Meleney, H. E.: Histoplasmosis (reticulo-endothelial cytomycosis): A review with mention of 13 unpublished cases. Am. J. Trop. Med. *20*:603, 1940.
120. Merz, W. G., Kodsy, S., and Merz, C. S.: Recovery of *Histoplasma capsulatum* from blood in a commercial radiometric mycobacterium medium. J. Clin. Microbiol. *30*:237–239, 1992.
121. Miller, C. R., and Grossmann, H.: Disseminated histoplasmosis in chronic mucocutaneous candidiasis. Pediatr. Radiol. *23*:104–105, 1993.
122. Mitchell, T. G.: Systemic mycoses. *In* Joklik, W. K., Willett, H. P., and Amos, D. B. (eds.): Zinsser Microbiology. 14th ed. Norwalk, CT, Appleton-Century-Crofts, 1984, p. 1138.
123. Morford, D. W.: Disseminated histoplasmosis in dialysis patients. Clin. Nephrol. *25*:273, 1986.
124. National Institute of Allergy and Infectious Diseases Mycoses Study Group, Birmingham, Alabama, and Bethesda, Maryland: Treatment of blastomycosis and histoplasmosis with ketoconazole. Ann. Intern. Med. *103*:861–872, 1985.
125. Negroni, R., Palmieri, O., Koren, F., et al.: Oral treatment of paracoccidioidomycosis and histoplasmosis with itraconazole in humans. Rev. Infect. Dis. *9*(Suppl. 1):S47–S50, 1987.
126. Negroni, R., Robles, A. M., Arechavala, A., et al.: Itraconazole in human histoplasmosis. Mycoses *32*:123–130, 1989.
127. Negroni, R., Robles, A. M., Arechavala, A., et al.: Ketoconazole in the treatment of paracoccidioidomycosis and histoplasmosis. Rev. Infect. Dis. *2*:643–649, 1980.
128. Negroni, R., Taborda, A., Robles, A. M., et al.: Itraconazole in the treatment of histoplasmosis associated with AIDS. Mycoses *35*:281–287, 1992.
129. Neihart, R. E., Hinthorn, D. R., Hoeprich, P. D., et al.: Successful treatment of progressive disseminated histoplasmosis with amphotericin B methyl ester. Diagn. Microbiol. Infect. Dis. *12*:17–19, 1989.
130. Newman, S. L., Gootee, L., and Gabay, J. E.: Human neutrophil-mediated

fungistasis against *Histoplasma capsulatum*: Localization of fungistatic activity to the azurophil granules. J. Clin. Invest. 92:624–631, 1993.
131. Norris, S., Wheat, J., McKinsey, D., et al.: Prevention of relapse of histoplasmosis with fluconazole in patients with the acquired immunodeficiency syndrome. Am. J. Med. *96*:504–508, 1994.
132. O'Hara, M.: Histopathologic diagnosis of fungal diseases. Infect. Control *7*:78–84, 1986.
133. Okudiara, M., Straub, M., and Schwarz, J.: The etiology of discrete splenic and hepatic calcifications in an endemic area of histoplasmosis. Am. J. Pathol. *39*:599, 1961.
134. Orchard, J. L., Luparello, F., and Brunskill, D.: Malabsorption syndrome occurring in the course of disseminated histoplasmosis. Am. J. Med. *66*:331–336, 1979.
135. Parsons, R. J., and Zarafonetis, C. J. D.: Histoplasmosis in man: Report of 7 cases and a review of 71 cases. Arch. Intern. Med. *75*:1, 1945.
136. Pate, J. W., and Hammon, J.: Superior vena cava syndrome due to histoplasmosis in children. Ann. Surg. *166*:778, 1965.
137. Patrick, C. C., Flynn, P. M., Henwick, S., et al.: Disseminated histoplasmosis presenting as a cystic duct obstruction. Pediatr. Infect. Dis. J. *11*:593–594, 1992.
138. Paya, C. V., Hermans, P. E., Van Scoy, R. E., et al.: Repeatedly relapsing disseminated histoplasmosis: Clinical observations during long-term follow-up. J. Infect. Dis. *156*:308–312, 1987.
139. Paya, C. V., Roberts, G. D., and Cockerill, F. R.: Transient fungemia in acute pulmonary histoplasmosis: Detection by new blood-culturing techniques. J. Infect. Dis. *156*:313–315, 1987.
140. Payan, D. G., Wheat, L. J., Brahmi, Z., et al.: Changes in immunoregulatory lymphocyte populations in patients with histoplasmosis. J. Clin. Immunol. *4*:98–107, 1984.
141. Peabody, J. W., Jr., Brown, R. B., Davis, E. W., et al.: Surgical implications of mediastinal granulomas. Am. Surg. *25*:357, 1959.
142. Penn, R. L., Lambert, R. S., and George, R. B.: Invasive fungal infections: The use of serologic tests in diagnosis and management. Arch. Intern. Med. *143*:1215–1220, 1983.
143. Phillips, P., Fetchick, R., Weisman, I., et al.: Tolerance to and efficacy of itraconazole in treatment of systemic mycoses: Preliminary results. Rev. Infect. Dis. *9*(Suppl. 1):S87–S93, 1987.
144. Pladson, T. R., Stiles, M. A., and Kuritsky, J. N.: Pulmonary histoplasmosis: A possible risk in people who cut decayed wood. Chest *86*:435–438, 1984.
145. Plouffe, J. F., and Fass, R. J.: *Histoplasma* meningitis: Diagnostic value of cerebrospinal fluid serology. Ann. Intern. Med. *92*:189–191, 1980.
146. Pont, A., Graybill, J. R., Craven, P. C., et al.: High-dose ketoconazole therapy and adrenal and testicular function in humans. Arch. Intern. Med. *144*:2150–2153, 1984.
147. Pottage, J. C., Trenholme, G. M., Aronson, I. K., et al.: Panniculitis with histoplasmosis and alpha-1-antitrypsin deficiency. Am. J. Med. *75*:150–153, 1983.
148. Prechter, G. C., and Prakash, U. B.: Bronchoscopy in the diagnosis of pulmonary histoplasmosis. Chest *95*:1033–1036, 1989.
149. Quinones, C. A., Reuben, A. G., Hamill, R. J., et al.: Chronic cavitary histoplasmosis: Failure of oral treatment with ketoconazole. Chest *95*:914–916, 1989.
150. Racela, L. S., Papasian, C. J., Watanabe, I., et al.: Systemic talc granulomatosis associated with disseminated histoplasmosis in a drug abuser. Arch. Pathol. Lab. Med. *112*:557–560, 1988.
151. Reddy, P., Gorelick, D. F., Brasher, C. A., et al.: Progressive disseminated histoplasmosis as seen in adults. Am. J. Med. *48*:629–636, 1970.
152. Rescorla, F. J., Kleiman, M. B., and Grosfeld, J. L.: Obstruction of the common bile duct in histoplasmosis. Pediatr. Infect. Dis. J. *13*:1017–1019, 1994.
153. Riggs, W., and Nelson, P.: The roentgenographic findings in infantile and childhood histoplasmosis. A. J. R. Am. J. Roentgenol. *97*:181, 1966.
154. Rivera, I. V., Curless, R. G., Indacochea, F. J., et al.: Chronic progressive CNS histoplasmosis presenting in childhood: Response to fluconazole therapy. Pediatr. Neurol. *8*:151–153, 1992.
155. Rosenthal, J., Brandt, K. D., Wheat, L. J., et al.: Rheumatologic manifestations of histoplasmosis in the recent Indianapolis epidemic. Arthritis Rheum. *26*:1065–1070, 1983.
156. Rubin, H., Furcolow, M. L., and Yates, J. L.: The course and prognosis of histoplasmosis. Am. J. Med. *27*:278, 1959.
157. Salzman, S. H., Smith, R. L., and Aranda, C. P.: Histoplasmosis in patients at risk for the acquired immunodeficiency syndrome in a nonendemic setting. Chest *93*:916–921, 1988.
158. Sarosi, G. A., Johnson, P. C.: Disseminated histoplasmosis in patients infected wiht human immunodeficiency virus. Clin. Infect. Dis. *14*(Suppl. 1):S60–S67, 1992.
159. Sarosi, G. A., Voth, D. W., Dahl, B. A., et al.: Disseminated histoplasmosis: Results of long-term follow-up. Ann. Intern. Med. *75*:511–516, 1971.
160. Sathapatayavongs, B., Batteiger, B. E., Wheat, L. J., et al.: Clinical and laboratory features of disseminated histoplasmosis during two large urban outbreaks. Medicine *62*:263–270, 1983.
161. Schlaegel, T. F.: Update on ocular histoplasmosis. Ophthalmol. Clin. *23*:1, 1983.
162. Schutze, G. E., Tucker, N. C., and Jacobs, R. F.: Histoplasmosis and perinatal human immunodeficiency virus. Pediatr. Infect. Dis. J. *11*:501–502, 1992.
163. Sills, M., Schwartz, A., and Weg, J. G.: Conjugal histoplasmosis: A consequence of progressive dissemination in the index case after steroid therapy. Ann. Intern. Med. *79*:221–224, 1973.
164. Slama, T. G.: Treatment of disseminated and progressive cavitary histoplasmosis with ketoconazole. Am. J. Med. *74*(1B):70–73, 1983.
165. Smith, J. W., and Utz, J. P.: Progressive disseminated histoplasmosis. Ann. Intern. Med. *76*:557–565, 1972.
166. Sobel, J. D., and Muller, G.: Comparison of itraconazole and ketoconazole in the treatment of experimental candidal vaginitis. Antimicrob. Agents Chemother. *26*:266–267, 1984.
167. Spitzer, E. D., Keath, E. J., Travis, S. J., et al.: Temperature-sensitive variants of *Histoplasma capsulatum* isolated from patients with acquired immunodeficiency syndrome. J. Infect. Dis. *162*:258–261, 1990.
168. Steele, C. J., and Kleiman, M. B.: Disseminated histoplasmosis, hypercalcemia and failure to thrive. Pediatr. Infect. Dis. J. *13*:421–422, 1994.
169. Straub, M., and Schwarz, J.: Healed primary complex in histoplasmosis. Am. J. Clin. Pathol. *25*:727, 1955.
170. Strayer, D. S., Gutwein, M. B., Herbold, D., et al.: Histoplasmosis presenting as the carpal tunnel syndrome. Am. J. Surg. *141*:286–288, 1981.
171. Sutliff, W. D.: Histoplasmosis cooperative study 4. Amphotericin B dosage for chronic pulmonary histoplasmosis. Am. Rev. Respir. Dis. *105*:60–67, 1972.
172. Sutliff, W. D., Andrews, C. E., Jones, E., et al.: Histoplasmosis cooperative study. Am. Rev. Respir. Dis. *89*:641, 1964.
173. Taylor, M. L., Diaz, S., Gonzalez, P. A., et al.: Relationship between pathogenesis and immune regulation mechanisms in histoplasmosis: A hypothetical approach. Rev. Infect. Dis. *6*:775–782, 1984.
174. Taylor, R. L., Williams, D. M., Craven, P. C., et al.: Amphotericin B in liposomes: A novel therapy for histoplasmosis. Am. Rev. Respir. Dis. *125*:610–611, 1982.
175. Tebib, J. G., Piens, M. A., Guillaux, M., et al.: Sarcoidosis possibly predisposing to disseminated histoplasmosis. Thorax *43*:73–74, 1988.
176. Tegeris, A. S., and Smith, D. T.: Acute disseminated pulmonary histoplasmosis treated with cortisone and MRID-112. Ann. Intern. Med. *48*:1414, 1958.
177. Terrell, C. L., and Hermans, P. E.: Antifungal agents used for deep seated mycotic infections. Mayo Clin. Proc. *62*:1116–1128, 1987.
178. Terry, P. B., Rosenow, E. C., and Roberts, G. D.: False-positive complement fixation serology in histoplasmosis. J. A. M. A. *238*:2453–2456, 1978.
179. Tesh, R. B., and Schneidau, J. C., Jr.: Primary cutaneous histoplasmosis. N. Engl. J. Med. *275*:597, 1966.
180. Tucker, W. S., Jr., Snell, B. B., Island, D. P., et al.: Reversible adrenal insufficiency induced by ketoconazole. J. A. M. A. *253*:2413–2414, 1985.
181. Utz, J. P.: Chemotherapy of the systemic mycoses. Med. Clin. North Am. *66*:221–233, 1982.
182. Van Cauteren, H., Heykants, J., De Coster, R., et al.: Itraconazole: Pharmacologic studies in animals and humans. Rev. Infect. Dis. *9*(Suppl. 1):S43–S46, 1987.
183. Van Der Meer, J. W. M., Keuning, J. J., Scheigground, H. W., et al.: The influence of gastric acidity on the bio-availability of ketoconazole. J. Antimicrob. Chemother. *6*:552–554, 1980.
184. Vandiviere, H. M., Goodman, N. L., Melvin, I. G., et al.: Histoplasmosis in Kentucky: Can it be prevented? J. KY Med. Assoc. *79*:719–726, 1981.
185. Ward, J. I., Weeks, M., Allen, D., et al.: Acute histoplasmosis: Clinical, epidemiologic and serologic findings of an outbreak associated with exposure to a fallen tree. Am. J. Med. *66*:587–595, 1979.
186. Weber, T. R., Grosfeld, J. L., Kleiman, M. B., et al.: Surgical implications of endemic histoplasmosis in children. J. Pediatr. Surg. *18*:486–491, 1983.
187. Weinberg, G. A., Kleiman, M. B., Grosfeld, J. L., et al.: Unusual manifestations of histoplasmosis in childhood. Pediatrics *72*:99–105, 1983.
188. Wheat, L. J.: Histoplasmosis. Infect. Dis. Clin. North Am. *2*:841, 1988.
189. Wheat, L. J.: Diagnosis and management of histoplasmosis. Eur. J. Clin. Microbiol. Infect. Dis. *8*:480, 1989.
190. Wheat, L. J., and Butkus-Small, C.: Disseminated histoplasmosis in the acquired immune deficiency syndrome. Arch. Intern. Med. *144*:2147–2149, 1984.
191. Wheat, L. J., Connolly-Stringfield, P., Blair, R., et al.: Histoplasmosis relapse in patients with AIDS: Detection using *Histoplasma capsulatum* variety *capsulatum* antigen levels. Ann. Intern. Med. *115*:936–941, 1991.
192. Wheat, L. J., Connolly-Stringfield, P., Blair, R., et al.: Effect of successful treatment with amphotericin B on *Histoplasma capsulatum* variety *capsulatum* polysaccharide antigen levels in patients with AIDS and histoplasmosis. Am. J. Med. *92*:153–160, 1992.
193. Wheat, L. J., Connolly-Stringfield, P., Kohler, R. B., et al.: *Histoplasma capsulatum* polysaccharide antigen detection in diagnosis and management of disseminated histoplasmosis in patients with acquired immunodeficiency syndrome. Am. J. Med. *87*:396–400, 1989.
194. Wheat, L. J., Connolly-Stringfield, P., Williams, B., et al.: Diagnosis of histoplasmosis in patients with the acquired immunodeficiency syndrome by detection of *Histoplasma capsulatum* polysaccharide antigen in bronchoalveolar lavage fluid. Am. Rev. Respir. Dis. *145*:1421–1424, 1992.
195. Wheat, L. J., Hafner, R., Wulfsohn, M., et al.: Prevention of relapse of

histoplasmosis with itraconazole in patients with the acquired immunodeficiency syndrome. Ann. Intern. Med. *118*:610–616, 1993.
196. Wheat, L. J., and French, M. L. V.: Diagnosis of histoplasmosis (in response to letter). Ann. Intern. Med. *98*:260, 1983.
197. Wheat, L. J., French, M. L., Batteiger, B., et al.: Cerebrospinal fluid *Histoplasma* antibodies in central nervous system histoplasmosis. Arch. Intern. Med. *145*:1237, 1985.
198. Wheat, L. J., French, M. L. V., Kamel, S., et al.: Evaluation of cross-reactions in *Histoplasma capsulatum* serologic tests. J. Clin. Microbiol. *23*:493–499, 1986.
199. Wheat, L. J., French, M. L. V., Kohler, R. B., et al.: The diagnostic laboratory tests for histoplasmosis. Ann. Intern. Med. *97*:680–685, 1982.
200. Wheat, J., Hafner, R., Korzun, A. H., et al.: Itraconazole treatment of disseminated histoplasmosis in patients with the acquired immunodeficiency syndrome. Am. J. Med. *98*:336–342, 1995.
201. Wheat, L. J., Kohler, R. B., French, M. L. V., et al.: Immunoglobulin M and G histoplasma antibody response in histoplasmosis. Am. Rev. Respir. Dis. *128*:65–70, 1982.
202. Wheat, L. J., Kohler, R. B., and Tewari, R. P.: Diagnosis of disseminated histoplasmosis by detection of *Histoplasma capsulatum* in serum and urine specimens. N. Engl. J. Med. *314*:83–88, 1986.
203. Wheat, L. J., Kohler, R. B., Tewari, R. P., et al.: Significance of *Histoplasma* antigen in the cerebrospinal fluid of patients with meningitis. Arch. Intern. Med. *149*:302–304, 1989.
204. Wheat, L. J., Slama, T. G., Eitzen, H. E., et al.: A large urban outbreak of histoplasmosis: Clinical features. Ann. Intern. Med. *94*:331–337, 1981.
205. Wheat, L. J., Slama, T. G., and Zeckel, M. L.: Histoplasmosis in the acquired immune deficiency syndrome. Am. J. Med. *78*:203–210, 1985.
206. Wheat, L. J., and Small, C. B.: Disseminated histoplasmosis in the acquired immunodeficiency syndrome. Arch. Intern. Med. *144*:2147–2149, 1984.
207. Wheat, L. J., Wass, J., Norton, J., et al.: Cavitary histoplasmosis occurring during two large urban outbreaks: Analysis of clinical, epidemiologic, roentgenographic, and laboratory features. Medicine *63*:201–209, 1984.
208. Whitehouse, W. M., Davey, W. M., Engelke, O. K., et al.: Roentgen findings in histoplasmin-positive school children. J. Mich. Med. Soc. *58*:1266, 1959.
209. Wilcox, K. R., Waisbren, B. A., and Martin, J.: The Walworth, Wisconsin, epidemic of histoplasmosis. Ann. Intern. Med. *49*:338, 1958.
210. Williams, A. O., Lawson, E. A., and Lucas, A. O.: African histoplasmosis due to *Histoplasma duboisii*. Arch. Pathol. *87*:306–318, 1969.
211. Williams, B., Fojtasek, M., Connolly-Stringfield, P., et al.: Diagnosis of histoplasmosis by antigen detection during an outbreak in Indianapolis, Ind. Arch. Pathol. Lab. Med. *118*:1205–1208, 1994.
212. Williams, K. R., and Burford, T. H.: Surgical treatment of granulomatous paratracheal lymphadenopathy. J. Thorac. Cardiovasc. Surg. *48*:13, 1964.
213. Wilson, D. A., Nguyen, C. L., and Tytle T. L., et al.: Sonography of the adrenal glands in chronic disseminated histoplasmosis. J. Ultrasound Med. *5*:69–73, 1986.
214. Woods, L. P.: Mediastinal granuloma causing tracheal compression in a 4-year-old child. Surgery *58*:448, 1965.
215. Woods, W. G., Singher, L. J., Krivit, W., et al.: Histoplasmosis simulating lymphoma in children. J. Pediatr. Surg. *14*:423–425, 1979.
216. Wynne, J. W., and Olsen, G. N.: Acute histoplasmosis presenting as the adult respiratory distress syndrome. Chest *66*:158–161, 1974.
217. Young, E. J., Vainrub, B., and Musher, D. M.: Pericarditis due to histoplasmosis. J. A. M. A. *240*:1750–1751, 1978.
218. Zeidberg, L. D., Dillon, A., and Gass, R. S.: Some factors in the epidemiology of histoplasmin sensitivity in Williamson County, Tennessee. Am. J. Public Health *41*:80, 1951.
219. Zeiss, J., Woldenberg, L. S., Morgan, R. et al.: Pulmonary histoplasmoma presenting as massive hemoptysis. Pediatr. Infect. Dis. *6*:689–691, 1987.
220. Zimmerman, S. E., Stringfield, P. C., Wheat, L. J., et al.: Comparison of sandwich solid-phase radioimmunoassay and two enzyme-linked immunosorbent assays for detection of *Histoplasma capsulatum* polysaccharide antigen. J. Infect. Dis. *160*:678–685, 1989.

204

SPOROTRICHOSIS

Bernhard L. Wiedermann

Sporotrichosis is an infection caused by the fungus *Sporothrix schenckii* that is manifested most commonly as an ulcerating nodule at a site of local trauma, with spread along regional lymphatic channels. Infection of other tissues or widespread dissemination is rare but does occur. It is a relatively uncommon problem in children, but young adults seem to be infected more frequently, presumably owing to more frequent exposure to soil, plants, and decaying vegetable matter that harbor the organism. The disease first was described by a medical student, Benjamin Schenck, in 1898, and most of what is known about the clinical syndrome has been learned from study of large outbreaks, particularly one occurring in gold miners near Johannesburg, South Africa, in the early 1940s.[60, 69]

THE ORGANISM

S. schenckii is a dimorphic fungus found principally in decaying vegetable matter or plant debris, even though it does not appear to be a plant pathogen. It grows well on most culture media and is resistant to cycloheximide. Preferred culture media are Sabouraud glucose agar and blood agar, incubated at 25° to 27° C. Most isolates grow readily from clinical material within 3 to 5 days, although there are occasional reports of slow growth, and cultures should be held at least 4 weeks before being called negative. Incubation on blood agar at higher temperatures (37° C) allows growth of the yeast phase, which is necessary for specific identification of the organism in culture.[57]

EPIDEMIOLOGY

Most cases of sporotrichosis are reported from Central and South America, especially from Mexico and Brazil, and cases in the United States seem to cluster in the Midwest, particularly along the Mississippi and Missouri River areas.[28, 52] Disease in humans usually results from inoculation of minor wounds by debris containing *S. schenckii,* and thus gardeners and nursery workers, forestry workers, miners, and other persons exposed to contaminated plant materials are at higher risk of acquiring the disease.[9, 13] Laboratory personnel working with the organism have become infected after needle-stick injuries.[68] The large South African epidemic in the gold mines of Transvaal probably resulted from the miners' brushing against rotting timbers in the mines, and a cluster of cases after a brick-throwing incident in Florida was traced to *S. schenckii* in the packing straw of the bricks.[59, 69] Pulmonary disease may result from inhalation of spores.[52] Uncommonly, transmission of disease from animals, particularly domestic cats with cutaneous disease, or from family members occurs.[20, 24, 25, 55] In South America, armadillo hunters are at risk for developing sporotrichosis, but it has been shown to be acquired from the decaying plant debris in armadillo nests rather than from the animals themselves.[46] DNA typing of isolates can be useful in outbreak investigations.[12]

PATHOGENESIS AND PATHOLOGY

As indicated, the most common mode of acquisition of sporotrichosis is by inoculation of the organism into skin structures, although disease also may develop from inhalation of spores of the organism. The incubation period varies highly, commonly ranging from 7 to 30 days after cutaneous inoculation, but it may be as long as 6 months.[57] The disease usually remains relatively localized: of the 2825 cases of sporotrichosis in the Transvaal mine epidemic, none had systemic spread.[69]

S. schenckii, like other yeasts, appears to bind specifically to the glycosphingolipid lactosylceramide, which is present on the cell surface of animal cells.[36] This may be one mechanism by which the organism establishes a foothold in the host. Cell-mediated immune responses probably are important for containment of infection. One study documented intact responses in patients with cutaneous forms of the disease, whereas patients with systemic sporotrichosis had impaired cell-mediated immunity.[51] This study is supported by the observation that systemic disease tends to occur in persons with underlying diseases that alter cell-mediated immunity.

Histopathologic examination of primary cutaneous lesions usually reveals changes in the epithelium, with hyperkeratosis, parakeratosis, and pseudoepitheliomatous hyperplasia. Intraepidermal microabscesses may be seen as well. In more established lesions, the pathologic process involves the dermis and below, with inflammatory infiltrate extending perivascularly.[44] The classic lesion on microscopic examination is a granuloma with an asteroid body at the center, although this picture is not pathognomonic for sporotrichosis. The asteroid body is an antigen-antibody complex deposited on the surface of the organism.[43] Unfortunately, it often is difficult to demonstrate fungi in tissue sections, even with special staining techniques, because of the paucity of organisms in tissue. They may be seen on Gram stain as gram-positive but irregularly staining bodies, sometimes as cigar-shaped 3- to 5-μm yeast forms. Periodic acid–Schiff and silver stains probably are better suited for detection of fungi in tissue sections.[44, 57] Immunohistochemical staining techniques may prove superior to standard methods.[47, 50]

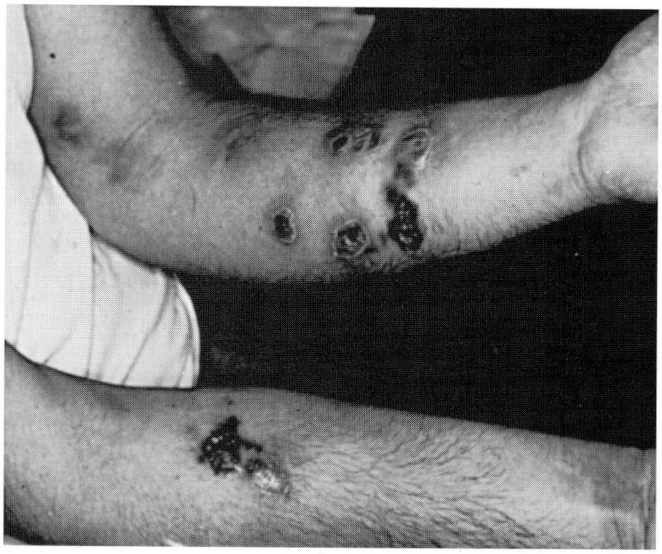

FIGURE 204–1. *Cutaneous lymphatic sporotrichosis of both arms. Note the characteristic involvement of lymphatics that drain the sites of the primary lesions. (Courtesy of G. Medoff and G. S. Kobayashi.)*

CLINICAL MANIFESTATIONS

Sporotrichosis can occur in both cutaneous and extracutaneous forms, with the cutaneous varieties accounting for approximately 80 per cent of all cases.[57] These categories can be broken down further into the organ system involved (Table 204–1).

Cutaneous Sporotrichosis

Cutaneous disease with *S. schenckii* can be either lymphocutaneous or fixed cutaneous, with the fixed cutaneous form being much less frequent. In lymphocutaneous cases, the initial lesion appears as a firm, slightly tender subcutaneous nodule. This progresses along local lymphatic channels, with multiple nodules appearing. The lesions typically enlarge and then may ulcerate and suppurate (Fig. 204–1). Untreated, they may heal slowly over months or persist, and recurrences are common. Differential diagnosis includes cutaneous nocardiosis, atypical mycobacterial disease, leishmaniasis, rosacea, syphilis, and pyoderma gangrenosum, as well as cutaneous manifestations of other fungal diseases.[17, 38, 67, 75]

The fixed cutaneous form of the disease is just as the name implies, with no evidence of lymphatic spread. The primary lesions are identical to those seen in the lymphocutaneous form. Although it has been suggested that sporotrichosis in childhood is more likely to appear in the fixed cutaneous form, compared with adults, this has not been borne out in prior studies. Table 204–2 shows results from five reports of series of cases of sporotrichosis in childhood. The 76 per cent rate for the lymphocutaneous form does not seem to differ much from the 90 per cent figure quoted for adults, particularly when one takes into account that the earlier pediatric studies were reports of small numbers of cases and may have resulted from selection bias.

Extracutaneous Sporotrichosis

Sporotrichosis occurring in extracutaneous sites either may be localized (related to an unusual area of trauma) or may

TABLE 204–1. Clinical Forms of Sporotrichosis[1, 30, 31, 40, 52, 58]

Cutaneous	Extracutaneous
Lymphocutaneous	Osteoarticular
Fixed cutaneous	Pulmonary
	Muscular
	Ocular
	Genitourinary
	Central nervous system

TABLE 204–2. Summary of 37 Cases of Pediatric Sporotrichosis[10, 15, 27, 45, 48]

Duration of symptoms before diagnosis	3–10 weeks
Lymphatic involvement	28/37*
Culture-positive	29/34
Relapse after therapy	1/21

*Numerator is number of patients positive; denominator is number of patients tested.

represent disseminated disease. In the absence of trauma, the presence of extracutaneous sporotrichosis should raise suspicion of disseminated disease and consideration of immunodeficiency states. Overall, infection of bones and joints is the most common form of extracutaneous disease.[73] Sporotrichal arthritis usually is an indolent and slowly progressive disease that may occur with or without cutaneous or lymphatic disease, which suggests a hematogenous route of infection for most cases. Diagnosis generally requires synovial biopsy with culture for demonstrating the organism.[61, 73] Two studies showed diagnostic delays averaging 17 and 25 months, respectively, from the onset of symptoms.[4, 14] Sporotrichal osteomyelitis usually occurs with concomitant arthritis, but isolated bone involvement has been recorded. Lytic lesions and periosteal changes are noted most frequently.[29, 73]

Pulmonary sporotrichosis is unusual with cases of disseminated disease and probably develops after inhalation of spores, as with primary pulmonary histoplasmosis.[52] The presence of cavitary lesions in the upper lobes often leads to a diagnosis of tuberculosis, and fungal culture of sputum, bronchoscopic specimens, lung tissue, or gastric aspirate usually is needed for diagnosis.[21, 52, 71] Pleural involvement is uncommon (3 of 47 cases in one review), and complications such as massive hemoptysis are rare.[22, 32, 52]

Sporotrichosis has been found to involve virtually every organ system in the body as part of disseminated disease.[73] Most commonly, underlying immunodeficiency states, such as diabetes, prolonged steroid therapy, alcoholism, and AIDS, are present.[1, 23, 30, 33, 40, 66, 73] Fungemia in the absence of disseminated disease has been documented in one otherwise healthy adult with a lysis-centrifugation blood culture system.[39] Interestingly, dissemination in patients with neoplasia is uncommon.

DIAGNOSIS

A high index of suspicion is necessary to make the diagnosis of sporotrichosis. In the largest outbreak in the United States, which occurred in 1988 among horticulturists and forestry workers, only 15 per cent of cases were diagnosed at the time of initial presentation to a physician.[11] Culture is the gold standard for diagnosis of sporotrichosis. Although organisms occasionally are seen on pathologic specimens, the yield is low enough to make biopsy unnecessary. If the diagnosis is suspected, scrapings of cutaneous lesions for culture should be sufficient to establish the diagnosis.[57]

Serodiagnosis has been explored in recent years. A skin test antigen has been available for many years but, as with the histoplasmin skin test for histoplasmosis, it is useful mainly as an epidemiologic tool. Immunoprecipitation or commercially available slide latex agglutination can be useful when material for culture is difficult to obtain or cultures are negative, such as with sporotrichal meningitis.[18, 62] Similarly, an enzyme-linked immunosorbent assay has been utilized for diagnosis. Antibody titers in cerebrospinal fluid tend to fall with successful therapy, and such tests might prove useful for monitoring response to therapy.[62] Western blotting has been used to detect sporotrichal antibody.[63] Using a crude antigen preparation, Scott and Muchmore[63] determined that detection of antibody to three antigens, 32, 40, and 70 kDa, seems to be both sensitive and specific for diagnosis of active sporotrichosis. Furthermore, patients with extracutaneous disease seemed to form antibody to a greater number of *S. schenckii* organisms than did those with cutaneous disease. Further studies of the immune response in sporotrichosis should enable development of better serodiagnostic tests than those that now are routinely available.

TREATMENT AND PROGNOSIS

Sporotrichosis may resolve spontaneously, but treatment is indicated in most circumstances.[3, 53] Heat applied to the site of cutaneous disease has been reported anecdotally to cause resolution of lesions in patients in whom medical therapy was contraindicated.[26, 58, 70] One prospective study demonstrated good results utilizing benzene pocket warmers for heat therapy of facial lesions in children.[34] Surgical removal of infected skin and soft tissue has been utilized, but skin grafting may be required.[7] This form of treatment usually is unnecessary with the availability of medical management, except possibly for some cases of pulmonary infection (particularly if it is confined to one lobe) and other extracutaneous disease.[14, 29, 52]

A saturated solution of potassium iodide, a proteolytic agent whose mechanism of action in sporotrichosis is unclear,[42] can be utilized for uncomplicated sporotrichosis. The in vitro growth of *S. schenckii* is not inhibited appreciably by iodide, but free iodine has a marked inhibitory effect on growth.[72] It is possible that the small amount of free iodine in a saturated solution of potassium iodide is sufficient to cause resolution of disease. The pediatric dosage of a saturated solution of potassium iodide is somewhat empiric, but it usually is given three times daily in juice or milk, starting at a low dose (e.g., 1 to 2 drops per year of age) and increasing the dose over several days to a maximum of 30 to 40 drops per dose.[10, 45, 48] For younger children, lower dosages may be acceptable.[45, 54] Treatment is continued until a few weeks after all lesions have resolved. Adverse reactions, such as salivary gland swelling, excessive lacrimation or salivation, nausea, vomiting, and abdominal pain, may resolve with temporary cessation of therapy followed by reinstitution at a lower dosage.

Itraconazole, an oral azole derivative, is the drug of choice for treatment of both cutaneous and extracutaneous forms of sporotrichosis.[6, 37, 65] Restrepo and colleagues[56] showed clinical cures in all 17 patients with cutaneous forms of sporotrichosis treated with itraconazole (100 mg daily), with no major side effects. However, Borelli[5] reported a treatment failure in a patient treated with 100 mg a day who subsequently responded when the dose was increased to 200 mg a day. Systemic disease also has been treated with itraconazole with favorable clinical responses, although all information is from cases in adults.[2, 41, 49, 65, 74]

Intravenous amphotericin B remains the drug of choice for patients with disseminated or severe sporotrichosis.[73] Duration of therapy in children has not been studied but probably should require 30 mg/kg as a total dose. Occasionally, intra-articular amphotericin B is used for sporotrichal arthritis if response to other therapy is poor.[19] Amphotericin B therapy in patients with pulmonary sporotrichosis is less effective than in other forms of sporotrichosis, which has prompted many clinicians to use a combined medical-surgical approach,[52] which should be re-evaluated as further experience with itraconazole is gained. Amphotericin B appears to be effective for sporotrichal meningitis when it is given early in the course of the disease, but adjunctive therapy with flucytosine or rifampin might be helpful.[62] Itraconazole also may have a role in meningitis.[37] Fluconazole, an imidazole compound with good cerebrospinal fluid penetration, has poor in vitro activity against *S. schenckii.*

S. schenckii does not appear to be particularly susceptible to ketoconazole in vitro, and clinical experience with ketoconazole treatment of sporotrichosis has been mixed.[8, 16, 64] It is possible that relatively large doses of ketoconazole are needed to produce a good clinical response. Terbinafine, an allylamine, cured five adults with cutaneous sporotrichosis, but further experience with this agent is needed.[35]

Prognosis for cutaneous forms of disease is excellent, but the extracutaneous forms are associated with significant morbidity and mortality, in part related to the underlying conditions predisposing these persons to disseminated disease. Many cases of osteoarticular disease result in permanent disability.[14]

PREVENTION

The key to prevention of sporotrichosis is the elimination of exposure to the organism, particularly with regard to skin surfaces and mucous membranes. Usually, this can be accomplished by the use of protective clothing during high-risk procedures, such as working with sphagnum moss or other decaying, moist plant material.[9, 11] Nursery workers should be educated about the hazards and early signs of sporotrichosis, and physicians and veterinarians should be aware of the uncommon circumstances of spread of the infection from family members and domestic cats. The epidemic in the Transvaal gold mines was stopped when timbers in the mine shafts were sprayed with a fungicide.[69] Although reporting of individual cases of sporotrichosis is not required in the United States, reporting of clusters of cases can aid epidemiologic investigations and stop the spread of the disease.

References

1. Agger, W. A., Caplan, R. H., and Maki, D. G.: Ocular sporotrichosis mimicking mucormycosis in a diabetic. Ann. Ophthalmol. *10*:767, 1978.
2. Baker, J. H., Goodpasture, H. C., Kuhns, H. R., Jr., et al.: Fungemia caused by an amphotericin B–resistant isolate of *Sporothrix schenckii:* Successful treatment with itraconazole. Arch. Pathol. Lab. Med. *113*:1279, 1989.
3. Bargman, H. B.: Sporotrichosis of the nose with spontaneous cure. Can. Med. Assoc. J. *124*:1027, 1981.
4. Bayer, A. S., Scott, V. J., and Guz, C. B.: Fungal arthritis. III. Sporotrichal arthritis. Semin. Arthritis Rheum. *9*:66, 1979.
5. Borelli, D.: A clinical trial of itraconazole in the treatment of deep mycoses and leishmaniasis. Rev. Infect. Dis. *9*(Suppl. 1):S57, 1987.
6. Breeling, J. L., and Weinstein, L.: Pulmonary sporotrichosis treated with itraconazole. Chest *103*:313, 1993.
7. Bullpitt, P., and Weedon, D.: Sporotrichosis: A review of 39 cases. Pathology *10*:249, 1978.
8. Calhoun, D. L., Waskin, H., White, M. P., et al.: Treatment of systemic sporotrichosis with ketoconazole. Rev. Infect. Dis. *13*:47, 1991.
9. Centers for Disease Control: Multistate outbreak of sporotrichosis in seedling handlers, 1988. M. M. W. R. *37*:652, 1988.
10. Chandler, J. W., Jr., Kriel, R. L., and Tosh, F. E.: Childhood sporotrichosis. Am. J. Dis. Child. *115*:368, 1968.
11. Coles, F. B., Schuchat, A., Hibbs, J. R., et al.: A multistate outbreak of sporotrichosis associated with sphagnum moss. Am. J. Epidemiol. *136*:475, 1992.
12. Cooper, C. R., Jr., Breslin, B. J., Dixon, D. M., et al.: DNA typing of isolates associated with the 1988 sporotrichosis epidemic. J. Clin. Microbiol. *30*:1631, 1992.
13. Cote, T. R., Kasten, M. J., and England, A. C., III: Sporotrichosis in association with Arbor Day activities. N. Engl. J. Med. *319*:1290, 1988.
14. Crout, J. E., Brewer, N. S., and Tompkins, R. B.: Sporotrichosis arthritis: Clinical features in seven patients. Ann. Intern. Med. *86*:294, 1977.
15. Dahl, B. A., Silberfarb, P. M., Sarosi, G. A., et al.: Sporotrichosis in children: Report of an epidemic. J. A. M. A. *215*:1980, 1971.
16. Dall, L., and Salzman, G.: Treatment of pulmonary sporotrichosis with ketoconazole. Rev. Infect. Dis. *9*:795, 1987.
17. Day, T. W., Gibson, G. H., and Guin, J. D.: Rosacea-like sporotrichosis. Cutis *33*:549, 1984.
18. de Albornoz, M. B., Villanueva, E., and de Torres, E. D.: Application of immunoprecipitation techniques to the diagnosis of cutaneous and extracutaneous forms of sporotrichosis. Mycopathologia *85*:177, 1984.
19. Downs, N. J., Hinthorn, D. R., Mhatre, V. R., et al.: Intra-articular amphotericin B treatment of *Sporothrix schenckii* arthritis. Arch. Intern. Med. *149*:954, 1989.
20. Dunstan, R. W., Langham, R. F., Reimann, K. A., et al.: Feline sporotrichosis: A report of five cases with transmission to humans. J. Am. Acad. Dermatol. *15*:37, 1986.
21. England, D. M., and Hochholzer, L.: *Sporothrix* infection of the lung without cutaneous disease: Primary pulmonary sporotrichosis. Arch. Pathol. Lab. Med. *111*:298, 1987.
22. Fields, C. L., Ossorio, M. A., and Roy, T. M.: Empyema associated with pulmonary sporotrichosis. South. Med. J. *82*:910, 1989.
23. Fitzpatrick, J. E., and Eubanks, S.: Acquired immunodeficiency syndrome presenting as disseminated cutaneous sporotrichosis. Int. J. Dermatol. *27*:406, 1988.
24. Frean, J. A., Isaacson, M., Miller, G. B., et al.: Sporotrichosis following a rodent bite: A case report. Mycopathologia *116*:5, 1991.
25. Frumkin, A., and Tesserand, M. E.: Sporotrichosis in a father and son. J. Am. Acad. Dermatol. *20*:964, 1989.
26. Galiana, J., and Conti-Diaz, I. A.: Healing effects of heat and a rubefacient on nine cases of sporotrichosis. Sabouraudia *3*:64, 1963.
27. Gluckman, I.: Sporotrichosis in children. S. Afr. Med. J. *39*:991, 1965.
28. Goncalves, A. P.: Geopathology of sporotrichosis. Int. J. Dermatol. *12*:115, 1973.
29. Govender, S., Rasool, M. N., and Ngcelwane, M.: Osseous sporotrichosis. J. Infect. *19*:273, 1989.
30. Gullberg, R. M., Quintanilla, A., Levin, M. L., et al.: Sporotrichosis: Recurrent cutaneous, articular, and central nervous system infection in a renal transplant recipient. Rev. Infect. Dis. *9*:369, 1987.
31. Halverson, P. B., Lahiri, S., Wojno, W. C., et al.: Sporotrichal arthritis presenting as granulomatous myositis. Arthritis Rheum. *28*:1425, 1985.
32. Haponik, E. F., Hill, M. K., and Craighead, C. C.: Case report: Pulmonary sporotrichosis with massive hemoptysis. Am. J. Med. Sci. *297*:251, 1989.
33. Heller, H. M., and Fuhrer, J.: Disseminated sporotrichosis in patients with AIDS: Case report and review of the literature. AIDS *5*:1243, 1991.
34. Hiruma, M., Kawada, A., Noguchi, H., et al.: Hyperthermic treatment of sporotrichosis: Experimental use of infrared and far infrared rays. Mycoses *35*:293, 1992.
35. Hull, P. R., and Vismer, H. F.: Treatment of cutaneous sporotrichosis with terbinafine. Br. J. Dermatol. *126*(Suppl. 39):51, 1992.
36. Jimenez-Lucho, V., Ginsburg, V., and Krivan, H. C.: *Cryptococcus neoformans, Candida albicans,* and other fungi bind specifically to the glycosphingolipid lactosylceramide (GalB1-4GlcB1–1Cer), a possible adhesion receptor for yeasts. Infect. Immun. *58*:2085, 1990.
37. Kauffman, C. A.: Old and new therapies for sporotrichosis. Clin. Infect. Dis. *21*:981, 1995.
38. Kibbi, A.-G., Karam, P. G., and Kurban, A. K.: Sporotrichoid leishmaniasis in patients from Saudi Arabia: Clinical and histologic features. J. Am. Acad. Dermatol. *17*:759, 1987.
39. Kosinski, R. M., Axelrod, P., Rex, J. H., et al.: *Sporothrix schenckii* fungemia without disseminated sporotrichosis. J. Clin. Microbiol. *30*:501, 1992.
40. Kurosawa, A., Pollock, S. C., Collins, M. P., et al.: *Sporothrix schenckii* endophthalmitis in a patient with human immunodeficiency virus infection. Arch. Ophthalmol. *106*:376, 1988.
41. Lavalle, P., Suchil, P., De Ovando, F., et al.: Itraconazole for deep mycoses: Preliminary experience in Mexico. Rev. Infect. Dis. *9*(Suppl. 1):S64, 1987.
42. Lieberman, J., and Kurnick, N. B.: Induction of proteolysis within purulent sputum by iodides. Clin. Res. *11*:81, 1963.
43. Lurie, H. I.: Histopathology of sporotrichosis: Notes on the nature of the asteroid body. Arch. Pathol. *75*:93, 1963.
44. Lurie, H. I., and Still, W. J. S.: The "capsule" of *Sporotrichum schenckii* and the evolution of the asteroid body: A light and electron microscopic study. Sabouraudia *7*:64–70, 1969.
45. Lynch, P. J., and Botero, F.: Sporotrichosis in children. Am. J. Dis. Child. *122*:325, 1971.
46. Mackinnon, J. E., Conti-Diaz, I. A., Gezuele, E., et al.: Isolation of *Sporothrix schenckii* from nature and considerations on its pathogenicity and ecology. Sabouraudia *7*:38, 1969.
47. Marques, M. E. A., Coelho, K. I. R., Sotto, M. N., et al.: Comparison between histochemical and immunohistochemical methods for diagnosis of sporotrichosis. J. Clin. Pathol. *45*:1089, 1992.
48. Orr, E. R., and Riley, H. D., Jr.: Sporotrichosis in childhood: Report of ten cases. J. Pediatr. *78*:951, 1971.
49. Oscherwitz, S. L., and Rinaldi, M. G.: Disseminated sporotrichosis in a patient infected with human immunodeficiency virus. Clin. Infect. Dis. *15*:568, 1992.
50. Padhye, A. A., Kaufman, L., Durry, E., et al.: Fatal pulmonary sporotrichosis caused by *Sporothrix schenckii* var. *luriei* in India. J. Clin. Microbiol. *30*:2492, 1992.
51. Plourre, J. F., Jr., Silva, J., Jr., Fekety, R., et al.: Cell-mediated immune responses in sporotrichosis. J. Infect. Dis. *139*:152, 1979.
52. Pluss, J. L., and Opal, S. M.: Pulmonary sporotrichosis: Review of treatment and outcome. Medicine *65*:143:1986.
53. Pueringer, R. J., Iber, C., Deike, M. A., et al.: Spontaneous remission of extensive pulmonary sporotrichosis. Ann. Intern. Med. *104*:366, 1986.
54. Rafal, E. S., and Rasmussen, J. E.: An unusual presentation of fixed cutaneous sporotrichosis: A case report and review of the literature. J. Am. Acad. Dermatol. *25*(5 Pt. 2):928, 1991.
55. Reed, K. D., Moore, F. M., Geiger, G. E., et al.: Zoonotic transmission of sporotrichosis: Case report and review. Clin. Infect. Dis. *16*:384, 1993.
56. Restrepo, A., Robledo, J., Gomez, I., et al.: Itraconazole therapy in lymphangitic and cutaneous sporotrichosis. Arch. Dermatol. *122*:413, 1986.

57. Rippon, J. W.: Medical Mycology: The Pathogenic Fungi and the Pathogenic Actinomycetes. 3rd ed. Philadelphia, W. B. Saunders, 1988.
58. Romig, D. A., Voth, D. W., and Liu, C.: Facial sporotrichosis during pregnancy: A therapeutic dilemma. Arch. Intern. Med. *130*:910, 1972.
59. Sanders, E.: Cutaneous sporotrichosis: Beer, bricks, and bumps. Arch. Intern. Med. *127*:482, 1971.
60. Schenck, R. B.: On refractory subcutaneous abscesses caused by a fungus possibly related to sporotricha. Bull. Johns Hopkins Hosp. *9*:286, 1898.
61. Schwartz, D. A.: *Sporothrix* tenosynovitis: Differential diagnosis of granulomatous inflammatory disease of the joints. J. Rheumatol. *16*:550, 1989.
62. Scott, E. N., Kaufman, L., Brown, A. C., et al.: Serologic studies in the diagnosis and management of meningitis due to *Sporothrix schenckii*. N. Engl. J. Med. *317*:935, 1987.
63. Scott, E. N., and Muchmore, H. G.: Immunoblot analysis of antibody responses to *Sporothrix schenckii*. J. Clin. Microbiol. *27*:300, 1989.
64. Shadomy, S., White, S. C., Yu, H. P., et al.: Treatment of systemic mycoses with ketoconazole: In vitro susceptibilities of clinical isolates of systemic and pathogenic fungi to ketoconazole. J. Infect. Dis. *152*:1249, 1985.
65. Sharkey-Mathis, P. K., Kauffman, C. A., Graybill, J. R., et al.: Treatment of sporotrichosis with itraconazole. Am. J. Med. *95*:279, 1993.
66. Shaw, J. C., Levinson, W., and Montanaro, A.: Sporotrichosis in the acquired immunodeficiency syndrome. J. Am. Acad. Dermatol. *21*:1145, 1989.
67. Spiers, E. M., Hendrick, S. J., Jorizzo, J. L., et al.: Sporotrichosis masquerading as pyoderma gangrenosum. Arch. Dermatol. *122*:691, 1988.
68. Thompson, D. W., and Kaplan, W.: Laboratory-acquired sporotrichosis. Sabouraudia *15*:167, 1977.
69. Transvaal Mine Medical Officers' Association: Sporotrichosis infection on mines of the Witwatersrand: A symposium. Johannesburg, Transvaal Chamber of Mines, 1947.
70. Trejos, A., and Ramirez, O.: Local heat in the treatment of sporotrichosis. Mycopathol. Mycol. Appl. *30*:47, 1966.
71. Velji, A. M., Hoeprich, P. D., and Slovak, R.: Multifocal systemic sporotrichosis with lobar pulmonary involvement. Scand. J. Infect. Dis. *20*:565, 1988.
72. Wada, R.: Studies on mode of action of potassium iodide upon sporotrichosis. Mycopathol. Mycol. Appl. *34*:97, 1968.
73. Wilson, D. E., Mann, J. J., Bennett, J. E., et al.: Clinical features of extracutaneous sporotrichosis. Medicine *46*:265, 1967.
74. Winn, R. E., Anderson, J., Piper, J., et al.: Systemic sporotrichosis treated with itraconazole. Clin. Infect. Dis. *17*:210, 1993.
75. Wlodaver, C. G., Tolomeo, T., and Benear, J. B., II: Primary cutaneous nocardiosis mimicking sporotrichosis. Arch. Dermatol. *124*:659, 1988.

205

ZYGOMYCOSIS

Bernhard L. Wiedermann

Zygomycosis is the preferred nomenclature for infectious syndromes, previously called phycomycosis or mucormycosis, caused by fungi of the class Zygomycetes. The designation phycomycosis refers to a now outdated taxonomic scheme, but references to mucormycosis still occur in the literature and probably still are useful. However, this term could mislead because the clinical syndromes caused by members of Zygomycetes include organisms from the order Entomophthorales as well as those in the order Mucorales. Although members of Entomophthorales tend to produce disease in normal hosts that is markedly different from the classic mucormycosis seen in immunocompromised patients, this distinction is becoming blurred and has resulted in adoption of the taxonomically proper term zygomycosis. Some authors use the term entomophthoromycosis for the more indolent clinical syndromes caused by members of this order. In this chapter, zygomycosis refers to infections caused by any of the organisms in the class Zygomycetes; mucormycosis and entomophthoromycosis are used to describe disease due to members of the two pathogenic orders of the Zygomycetes.

Human disease consistent with zygomycosis probably first was described by Kurchenmeister in 1855, but the first English language description of the disease did not appear until Gregory and associates[29] described rhinocerebral disease in three diabetics in 1943. Since that description, it has become clear that zygomycosis encompasses a relatively uncommon but frequently fatal group of diseases occurring predominantly in immunocompromised hosts, particularly those with diabetes mellitus or impairment of neutrophil function, as well as a syndrome of relatively limited infection of skin and soft tissue in normal persons caused by fungi in the order Entomophthorales.[42, 72, 73]

THE ORGANISMS

Members of Zygomycetes are ubiquitous in nature and have perhaps a wider impact on humans as plant pathogens causing fruit decay than they do as human and animal pathogens.[7, 73] The class consists of two orders, Mucorales and Entomophthorales, each containing several species reported to cause disease in humans (Table 205–1). They grow readily on common laboratory media but are inhibited by cycloheximide.[2] With members of Mucorales, on solid agar plates one sees rapid growth of woolly colonies, often with spores seen as tiny dark dots to the naked eye. Hyphae characteristically are large (10 to 30 μm in diameter), nonseptate, and often twisted or ribbon-like. The lack of septation and the tendency of hyphae to branch at right angles usually serve to distinguish them from *Aspergillus* species, which are septate and smaller and branch at acute angles.[2] Genera usually are differentiated from one another by examination of mycelia. Speciation of members of Zygomycetes often is difficult.

TABLE 205–1. Fungi Causing Zygomycosis in Humans

Order Mucorales
Family Mucoraceae
Absidia corymbifera, A. ramosa[47, 84]
Apophysomyces elegans[16, 98]
Mucor indicus, M. ranosissimus, M. circinelloides, M. hiemalis[41, 68, 90]
Rhizomucor pusillus[97]
Rhizopus arrhizus, R. oryzae, R. rhizopodiformis[19, 27, 96]
Family Cunninghamellaceae
Cunninghamella bertholletiae[56, 70, 71, 89]
Family Choanophoraceae
Cokermyces recurvatus[5]
Family Saksenaeaceae
Saksenaea vasiformis[66, 69]
Order Entomophthorales
Family Entomophthoraceae
Conidiobolus coronatus, C. incongruus[31, 55, 57, 83]
Family Basidiobolaceae
Basidiobolus ranarum[21, 79]

For members of Entomophthorales, growth also occurs readily on solid media but appears as flat, gray or pale yellow waxy colonies with velvety white mycelia on the surface.[2, 73] The hyphae often are septate, and differentiation between genera and among species is based on morphologic characteristics of cultured organisms.

EPIDEMIOLOGY

All members of Zygomycetes are ubiquitous in nature and are found in all parts of the world, regardless of climate or other factors. Many are animal pathogens. Members of Mucorales are present in soil and occasionally are isolated from the hospital environment.[41, 93, 95] However, studies have suggested a relationship between hospital construction activity and development of zygomycosis in immunocompromised hosts.[41, 74, 95] *Rhizopus* species frequently are found in moldy bread and fruits.[73] Members of Entomophthorales commonly are found in feces of reptiles and other animals as well as in decaying vegetable matter. Some are insect pathogens.[73]

The ubiquitous nature of these organisms coupled with the paucity of human disease is strong evidence for their relative saprophytic characteristics. Most human disease due to members of Mucorales is concentrated in North America, perhaps because of a concentration of seriously immunocompromised hosts.[7] *Rhizopus, Rhizomucor,* and *Absidia* are the most common genera encountered in clinical medicine. On the other hand, infections caused by the Entomophthorales genera *Basidiobolus* and *Conidiobolus* occur predominantly in Africa, India, and the Far East, although a few cases have been acquired in North and South America.[73] Typically, *Basidiobolus* infections are seen in young children and adolescents with superficial infections of the trunk or extremities, whereas *Conidiobolus* tends to infect rhinofacial areas of young adult males.[50]

MUCORMYCOSIS

Pathogenesis and Pathology

Mucormycosis usually is acquired by humans after inhalation of spores, and the organisms may colonize the sinuses and nasopharynx of some persons.[73] Occasionally, mucormycosis results from cutaneous inoculation of spores, as has occurred with contaminated elastic adhesive tape, and disseminates from the cutaneous or subcutaneous site.[19, 27] Person-to-person transmission has not been documented. The key to production of disease, however, is the immune status of the host. The neutrophil appears to be the primary component of the immune response against these organisms and may serve to prevent germination of inhaled spores.[20] Diabetes mellitus, and in particular diabetic ketoacidosis, is the most common underlying disease in patients with mucormycosis.[40, 72] Other underlying diseases accompanied by acidosis, such as uremia or sepsis, also may predispose to mucormycosis.[46, 72] Other predisposing illnesses, some of which are accompanied by acidosis, are listed in Table 205–2. Important by its absence is AIDS, which of course predominantly is a lymphocytic disorder. Zygomycosis reported in patients with AIDS tends to occur in intravenous drug users and may reflect this risk factor more than the immunodeficiency itself.[56, 81] Disease may follow a less fulminant course in AIDS patients compared with other immunocompromised populations.[8] It is perhaps further evidence of the low virulence of these organisms that mucormycosis still is an uncommon disease, even though many of the illnesses in Table 205–2 are common.

TABLE 205–2. Underlying Diseases Commonly Associated with Increased Risk of Mucormycosis

Diabetes mellitus[11, 40, 65]	Intravenous drug use[56]
Neutropenia or neutrophil dysfunction[40]	Organ transplantation[30, 84, 90, 101]
Malignancy[40, 52, 65]	Trauma or surgery[3, 22, 28, 47, 66]
Malnutrition[58]	Burn patients[16, 48]
Deferoxamine therapy[30, 71, 78, 99]	Corticosteroid therapy[52]
	Methylmalonicaciduria[45]

Serum from persons with diabetic ketoacidosis does not inhibit the growth of *Rhizopus,* but serum from those same persons after treatment of the ketoacidosis does show inhibitory properties similar to normal human serum.[12, 25] Furthermore, iron may play a key role in lowering host defenses, as demonstrated by the tendency for deferoxamine therapy to result in progression of both natural and experimental mucormycosis.[18, 30, 71, 78] This phenomenon seems to be common, particularly in patients undergoing hemodialysis.[9, 99] Studies in experimental animals suggest that deferoxamine may serve as a siderophore for *Rhizopus* species, with resultant increased fungal growth and increased mortality in a guinea pig model.[17] However, in vitro data conflict on the exact effects of iron or deferoxamine on promoting the growth of members of Mucorales.[60] Much remains to be understood about the pathogenesis of mucormycosis, and a unifying concept will have to incorporate the effects of steroids, acidosis, and iron on host neutrophils and macrophages in failing to suppress fungal replication.

The hallmark of histologic examination of mucormycosis is vascular invasion with resultant thrombosis and tissue necrosis and accompanying acute and chronic inflammation.[58, 65, 73] Most of the clinical findings of progressive disease can be related to these effects on blood vessels. Septic emboli may affect all parts of the body. In the rhinocerebral form of the disease, disease may progress along nerve roots during intracranial spread. Although relatively sparse, hyphal forms may be seen in tissue on routine hematoxylin and eosin staining more than with silver or other special fungal stains (Fig. 205–1).[73]

Clinical Manifestations

The clinical forms of mucormycosis are considered best by type of organ system involvement (Table 205–3).

Acute Rhinocerebral Mucormycosis

This form of mucormycosis most commonly occurs in the setting of diabetic ketoacidosis and has a high mortality rate.[42, 49, 80] Initially, there may be a history of pain, swelling, or tenderness of the face, with proptosis, headache, and altered mental status appearing as the infection progresses. Bloody or necrotic lesions may appear at the nasal turbinates or palate, but soon symptoms of central nervous system

TABLE 205–3. Clinical Forms of Mucormycosis

Rhinocerebral	Gastrointestinal
Cutaneous	Disseminated
Pulmonary	Miscellaneous

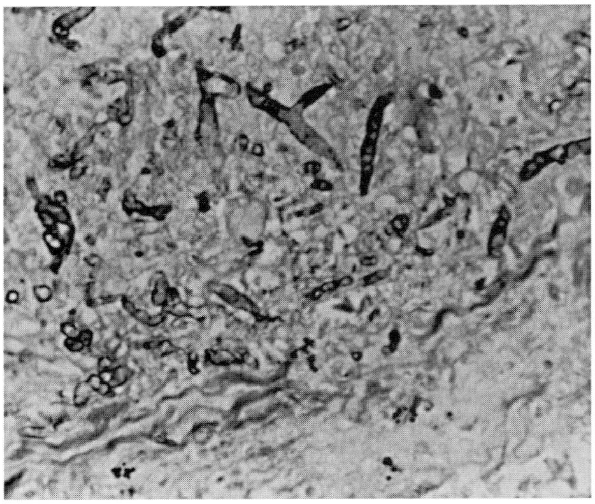

FIGURE 205–1. *Zygomycosis caused by* Rhizopus. *Observe the varied morphologic features of the coenocytic hyphae and large size. (H and E × 64.)*

involvement predominate. The function of cranial nerves II, III, IV, and VI becomes impaired, and cranial nerves I, V, and VII also are involved commonly. Thrombosis of the cavernous sinus or internal carotid artery is a feared complication.

Cutaneous Mucormycosis

Cutaneous mucormycosis occurs occasionally, usually at the site of trauma, burns, or invasive procedures in immunocompromised hosts.[16, 39, 85, 97] Of 25 patients with mucormycosis treated over a recent 14-year period, 10 had cutaneous infections.[1] Several cases of mucormycotic cellulitis due to contaminated elastic adhesive bandages occurred in the 1970s, and later other dressings were implicated.[27, 96] Some affected persons have developed locally aggressive or disseminated disease. In general, the lesions varied morphologically initially, but local progression was devastating in some cases. Overall, cutaneous mucormycosis either may appear as a relatively indolent, local infection with ulceration or may cause gangrenous cellulitis with local and distant extension.[76] This latter complication seems to be more common in burn wound infections and in immunocompromised hosts, including premature infants.[3, 48]

In addition to primary inoculation of zygomycosis in cutaneous or subcutaneous sites, nodular skin lesions resulting from hematogenous spread also may occur.[39] Often, a diagnosis of disseminated disease is made possible by appearance of skin lesions that then are biopsied. Blood cultures generally are negative, but this form of cutaneous disease is an indication of widespread dissemination and is associated with poor outcome, regardless of therapy.[72, 73]

Pulmonary Mucormycosis

Pulmonary disease due to mucormycosis is most common in the setting of disseminated infection, but it also is well described as an isolated phenomenon.[51, 52, 65, 70, 84, 101] Mucormycotic pneumonia typically develops in the severely immunocompromised patient, such as patients with malignancy and neutropenia, but also has occurred in juvenile diabetics and in a normal host.[14, 30, 62] Affected persons usually are febrile and have hemoptysis. Massive pulmonary hemorrhage may result from vascular erosion. Radiographic appearance may vary from a nonspecific infiltrate to cavity formation. Pleural involvement is uncommon. Rarely, fungus balls have been noted.[65] The disease usually is fulminant but may be milder in hosts with less severe immune compromise.

Gastrointestinal Mucormycosis

Gastrointestinal involvement probably results from ingestion of fungal spores, either from the environment or from colonized upper airways. Occasionally, hematogenous or direct extension routes result in intestinal tract involvement. Malnutrition, prematurity, uremia, and underlying gastrointestinal disease such as typhoid fever or amebiasis are predisposing factors.[43, 53, 54, 58] All sites along the intestinal tract can be involved, with the stomach and colon being most common.[58] Nonspecific abdominal pain with hematemesis, hematochezia, or melena may occur. Premature infants may experience necrotizing enterocolitis, with or without pneumatosis intestinalis.[86, 100] Dissemination to other sites may occur by hematogenous routes. Perforation after bowel wall necrosis is not uncommon. Diagnosis usually is made at autopsy.

Disseminated Mucormycosis

Disseminated mucormycosis not surprisingly occurs in the most severely immunocompromised patients and most commonly is an autopsy diagnosis.[34, 88] Clinical findings are nonspecific, and a high index of suspicion and readily accessible tissue for biopsy are needed for diagnosis. The pulmonary system is affected most commonly, followed by the central nervous system, but virtually any organ can be involved. A subacute form of disseminated disease with a protracted but fatal course has been reported.[61] The combination of severe immune compromise and subtle clinical findings makes this form of mucormycosis the most difficult to treat.

Miscellaneous Forms of Mucormycosis

There are a variety of case reports of mucormycosis involving isolated areas of the body. Thus, mucormycotic endocarditis, myocarditis, meningitis, brain abscess, peritonitis, Budd-Chiari syndrome, osteomyelitis, arthritis, myositis, endophthalmitis, pyelonephritis, and cystitis all have been reported.[5, 10, 11, 22, 24, 47, 64, 66, 67, 82, 87] Common to these disease manifestations is some type of local trauma, either accidental or surgical, that results in a ready access site for fungal organisms to invade. Outcome varies highly and depends on the underlying condition of the host as well as the extent of disease.

Diagnosis

Diagnosis of mucormycosis can be difficult. As mentioned previously, blood cultures usually are negative, even in the presence of hematogenous dissemination. Growth of an organism from the respiratory tract or wound also is not proof of infection because these fungi may colonize body surfaces.[73] The gold standard of diagnosis is tissue biopsy showing characteristic hyphal forms invading tissue. It also is likely that specimens obtained via skinny needle biopsy or bronchoalveolar lavage reflect mucormycosis accurately.[44, 75] Although this type of information alone does not permit absolute identification of the organism involved (growth in culture is needed for speciation), it is sufficient to diagnose infection by a member of Mucorales.

Work continues on other methods of diagnosis. Although

many members of Mucorales have antigenic cross-reactivity, detection of specific antibodies in patients with mucormycosis has been somewhat disappointing. A comparison of immunodiffusion with enzyme-linked immunosorbent assays for antibody to antigens of *Rhizopus arrhizus* and *Rhizomucor pusillus* in 46 patients with zygomycosis (43 with infections due to members of Mucorales) showed relatively poor sensitivity and specificity. With 43 control cases of aspergillosis, candidiasis, cryptococcosis, and pseudallescheriasis, sensitivity was only 66 per cent and 81 per cent for immunodiffusion and enzyme immunoassay, respectively.[38] False positivity in patients with aspergillosis and candidiasis was encountered. Part of the problem with antibody detection may result from the poor immune responses seen in patients with mucormycosis, and it is possible that antigen detection methods may be more rewarding for diagnosis.

Treatment

Mucormycosis is too rare to allow accurate assessment of effects of specific therapeutic regimens. Therefore, most treatment recommendations have resulted from anecdotal experiences rather than controlled trials. In an infectious syndrome occurring predominantly in immunocompromised hosts, it is essential to attempt to correct or improve the underlying disease as much as possible. In the case of mucormycosis, this would include aggressive correction of hyperglycemia and acidosis in diabetics, discontinuation of deferoxamine therapy in those receiving this drug, and decreasing doses of or discontinuing immunosuppressive therapy, such as cancer chemotherapy, corticosteroids, and cyclosporine. The role of white blood cell transfusions in ameliorating the neutropenic state has not been addressed critically in mucormycosis.

Standard medical therapy is amphotericin B, given at maximal dosages of 1 to 1.5 mg/kg/day, based on the individual's tolerance of side effects.[4] The most seriously diseased patients are given a total of at least 30 mg/kg. There are some reports of cure with shorter duration of therapy, which should be reserved for well-localized disease in relatively normal hosts, in combination with surgical débridement.[77] Amphotericin B lipid complex has been used successfully in at least two pediatric patients.[92]

Christenson and colleagues[13] reported a diabetic child with mucormycotic pneumonia treated with a combination of amphotericin B and rifampin in whom clinical improvement appeared to coincide with addition of the rifampin. In vitro susceptibility testing of the clinical isolate *(Rhizopus oryzae)* as well as other strains suggested evidence of synergy. The child's serum fungistatic activity increased when rifampin was added to the amphotericin B therapy. Flucytosine sometimes has been used in combination with amphotericin B.[15, 59] Ketoconazole was used, perhaps successfully, to treat one patient with mucormycosis, but in general these organisms are resistant to the azole compounds.[6, 26] These studies certainly suggest the need for further work on combination drug therapy for these situations.

Most authorities agree that aggressive surgical débridement, when possible, is a necessary complement to medical therapy.[28, 32, 62] All necrotic-appearing tissue should be removed, and often patients require repeated surgical procedures for removal of devitalized tissue. Surgical débridement alone may be sufficient to cure localized cutaneous disease.[69]

Hyperbaric oxygen therapy has been used for some of these patients in an attempt to limit the extent of gangrene and tissue necrosis.[23, 28] In one retrospective study, two of six patients receiving hyperbaric oxygen, along with standard medical and surgical therapy, died, compared with four deaths in seven patients not receiving hyperbaric oxygen.[23] Hyperbaric oxygen therapy was successful, in combination with liposomal amphotericin B and interferon-γ, in one patient with trauma-associated mucormycosis.[63] Although this might appear promising, the number of patients evaluated with this form of treatment is much too small to permit any firm conclusions on benefit.

Prognosis and Prevention

As indicated throughout this section, mucormycosis is a serious disease occurring largely in immunocompromised hosts that results in a high mortality rate. However, there is some evidence for improved prognosis. In one study of 33 cases over a 44-year period, there was a shift in the 1970s from a predominantly postmortem diagnosis to a predominantly premortem diagnosis.[65] Furthermore, survival increased from 6 to 73 per cent during this time. It is likely that more aggressive means of diagnosis and treatment plus the availability of amphotericin B accounted for this shift. Still, survival is tied most closely to the extent of the infection and the severity of the underlying immunocompromised state, and not all reports suggest improvement in outcome. In Kline's[40] review of mucormycosis at one large children's center, only 1 of 15 confirmed patients survived, but only 3 of the 15 were diagnosed prior to death. An overall survival rate of approximately 50 per cent in cases diagnosed prior to death seems reasonably accurate.[72] Any improvement in prognosis over the next few years likely will result from a heightened index of suspicion of the disease in the appropriate clinical settings, combined with continued aggressive means of diagnosis and medical and surgical treatment.

Prevention of mucormycosis can be addressed in three areas. First, control of underlying disease such as diabetes can limit the risks of developing disease. Second, use of less immunosuppressive drugs for transplantations and other conditions will help, as will lessening the degree of neutropenia during treatment of malignancies. Finally, patients at risk should be shielded from situations in which they are likely to encounter the organisms (e.g., at construction sites, around decaying plant matter) or by the use of nonsterile dressings over wound sites. Hospitals can exercise caution in exposure of immunocompromised patients to construction activity within the hospital and use filtering systems to prevent transmission of spores by the airborne route.

ENTOMOPHTHOROMYCOSIS

Pathogenesis and Pathology

Entomophthoromycosis presumably develops via inhalation of spores to cause sinus disease or cutaneous inoculation to cause cutaneous or subcutaneous infection. However, the exact mechanisms are unclear, and no specific animal model has been developed. The organisms are of extremely low virulence, as manifested by the rarity of these infections, even though the fungi are ubiquitous. Although discrete clinical syndromes have been assigned to the two genera causing disease, this distinction is artificial, and it should be recognized that either group could cause either form of entomophthoromycosis or even a syndrome more suggestive of mucormycosis.[79, 91, 94]

Histopathologic examination of affected tissues shows some similarities to mucormycosis. Areas of acute and chronic inflammation are found in association with broad hyphal elements that may or may not display septations. The hyphae are more visible with hematoxylin and eosin staining than with more specific fungal stains.[73] However, the tendency for vascular invasion typical of mucormycosis does not occur with entomophthoromycosis, and necrosis is uncommon. Instead, a so-called Splendore-Hoeppli phenomenon likely consisting of hyphae surrounded by eosinophilic material in a stellate pattern occurs.[73] However, this feature is not pathognomonic of entomophthoromycosis and has been seen in cases of mucormycosis.

Clinical Manifestations

Chronic Rhinofacial Zygomycosis

Chronic rhinofacial zygomycosis, also called entomophthoromycosis conidiobolae because most infections are caused by *Conidiobolus coronatus,* is an indolent subcutaneous infection involving the face.[31, 55, 57] Typically, bilateral intranasal swelling eventually progresses to invasion of the sinuses and soft tissue swelling of the face, unaccompanied by fever or pain. Symptoms commonly persist for weeks or months, but deep-tissue progression is unlikely.

Chronic Subcutaneous Zygomycosis

This syndrome, also known as entomophthoromycosis basidiobolae, is similar to chronic rhinofacial disease with the exception that the lesions usually are on the trunk or extremities. The etiologic agent is *Basidiobolus ranarum.* Painless subcutaneous nodules may progress to invade deeper soft tissues, and massive soft tissue swelling may develop. Facial infection similar to chronic rhinofacial zygomycosis also may occur.[21] With rare exceptions, most cases are slowly progressive.[35, 73]

Diagnosis

Entomophthoromycosis often can be diagnosed presumptively on the basis of clinical presentation and geographic origin of the patient, but usually biopsy is required.[50, 73] Recent work on serodiagnosis by immunodiffusion has been promising.[33, 37] Onchocerciasis, filariasis, and Burkitt lymphoma sometimes are in the differential diagnosis.[35, 50]

Treatment

Evaluation of therapy for this group of diseases is difficult because of occasional reports of spontaneous resolution. Many agents have been tried with varying success. Taylor and colleagues[83] treated a young man with rhinofacial disease with amphotericin B, corticosteroids, miconazole, and multiple surgical procedures before noting resolution some months after any therapy had been given. They performed susceptibility testing, which showed minimal inhibitory effects of amphotericin B and no benefit of adding flucytosine or rifampin. Miconazole, ketoconazole, and potassium iodide did not have impressive in vitro activity in their assay.

Other anecdotal reports of efficacy of trimethoprim-sulfamethoxazole or ketoconazole raise hopes for effective therapy but must be tempered by the fact that small numbers of patients have been treated.[31, 83] Currently, there is no "drug of choice" for this condition, although some type of medical therapy seems indicated for all cases. The role of surgery is less in this group of disorders than for mucormycosis, but patients with well-circumscribed areas, such as nodular lesions, may benefit from surgical excision. Even so, it is not uncommon for such patients to have recurrence of disease after surgery.[83]

Prognosis and Prevention

Mortality due to the entomophthoromycoses is unlikely, but morbidity and disfigurement are common. The efficacy of medical and surgical therapy is unclear, but probably all patients should receive attempts at treatment because the natural history of the disease is one of slow progression. Specific means for disease prevention are not available because so little is known about factors predisposing to these chronic zygomycotic syndromes.

References

1. Adam, R. D., Hunter G., DiTomasso, J., et al.: Mucormycosis: Emerging prominence of cutaneous infections. Clin. Infect. Dis. *19*:67, 1994.
2. American Thoracic Society: Laboratory diagnosis of mycotic and specific fungal infections. Am. Rev. Respir. Dis. *132*:1373, 1985.
3. Arisoy, A. E., Arisoy, E. S., Correa-Calderon, A., et al.: *Rhizopus* necrotizing cellulitis in a preterm infant: A case report and review of the literature. Pediatr. Infect. Dis. J. *12*:1029, 1993.
4. Armstrong, D.: Problems in management of opportunistic fungal diseases. Rev. Infect. Dis. *11*(Suppl. 7):S1591, 1989.
5. Axelrod, P., Kwon-Chung, K. J., Frawley, P., et al.: Chronic cystitis due to *Cokermyces recurvatus:* A case report. J. Infect. Dis. *155*:1062, 1987.
6. Barnert, J., Behr, W., and Reich, H.: An amphotericin B–resistant case of rhinocerebral mucormycosis. Infection *13*:134, 1985.
7. Benbow, E. W., and Stoddart, R. W.: Systemic zygomycosis. Postgrad. Med. J. *62*:985, 1986.
8. Blatt, S. P., Lucey, D. R., DeHoff, D., et al.: Rhinocerebral zygomycosis in a patient with AIDS. J. Infect. Dis. *164*:215, 1991.
9. Boelaert, J. R., Fenves, A. Z., and Coburn, J. W.: Mucormycosis among patients on dialysis. N. Engl. J. Med. *321*:190, 1989.
10. Branton, M. H., Johnson, S. C., Brooke, J. D., et al.: Peritonitis due to *Rhizopus* in a patient undergoing continuous ambulatory peritoneal dialysis. Rev. Infect. Dis. *13*:19, 1990.
11. Case Records of the Massachusetts General Hospital (Case 36–1988). N. Engl. J. Med. *319*:629, 1988.
12. Chinn, R. Y. W., and Diamond, R. D.: Generation of chemotactic factors by *Rhizopus oryzae* in the presence and absence of serum: Relationship to hyphal damage mediated by human neutrophils and effects of hyperglycemia and ketoacidosis. Infect. Immun. *38*:1123, 1982.
13. Christenson, J. C., Shalit, I., Welch, D. F., et al.: Synergistic action of amphotericin B and rifampin against *Rhizopus* species. Antimicrob. Agents Chemother. *31*:1775, 1987.
14. Cohen-Abbo, A., Bozeman, P. M., and Patrick, C. C.: *Cunninghamella* infections: Review and report of two cases of *Cunninghamella* pneumonia in immunocompromised children. Clin. Infect. Dis. *17*:173, 1993.
15. Cook, B. A., White, C. B., Blaney, S. M., et al.: Survival after isolated cerebral mucormycosis. Am. J. Pediatr. Hematol. Oncol. *11*:330, 1989.
16. Cooter, R. D., Lim, I. S., Ellis, D. H., et al.: Burn wound zygomycosis caused by *Apophysomyces elegans.* J. Clin. Microbiol. *28*:2151, 1990.
17. Cutsem, J. V., and Boelaert, J. R.: Effects of deferoxamine, feroxamine and iron on experimental mucormycosis (zygomycosis). Kidney Int. *36*:1061, 1989.
18. Daly, A. L., Velazquez, L. A., Bradley, S. F., et al.: Mucormycosis: Association with deferoxamine therapy. Am. J. Med. *87*:468, 1989.
19. Dennis, J. E., Rhodes, K. H., Cooney, D. R., et al.: Nosocomial *Rhizopus* infection (zygomycosis) in children. J. Pediatr. *96*:824, 1980.
20. Diamond, R. D., Krzesicki, R., Epstein, B., et al.: Damage to hyphal forms of fungi by human leukocytes in vitro: A possible host defense mechanism against aspergillosis and mucormycosis. Am. J. Pathol. *91*:313, 1978.
21. Dworzack, D. L., Pollock, A. S., Hodges, G. R., et al.: Zygomycosis of the maxillary sinus and palate caused by *Basidiobolus haptosporus.* Arch. Intern. Med. *138*:1274, 1978.
22. Fergie, J. E., Fitzwater, D. S., Einstein, P., et al.: *Mucor* peritonitis associated with acute periotoneal dialysis. Pediatr. Infect. Dis. J. *11*:498, 1992.
23. Ferguson, B. J., Mitchell, T. G., Moon, R., et al.: Adjunctive hyperbaric oxygen for treatment of rhinocerebral mucormycosis. Rev. Infect. Dis. *10*:551, 1988.
24. Fong, K. M., Seneviratne, E. M. E., and McCormack, J. G.: Mucor cerebral

abscess associated with intravenous drug use. Aust. N. Z. J. Med. *20*:74, 1990.

25. Gale, G. R., and Welch, A.: Studies of opportunistic fungi. I. Inhibition of *R. oryzae* by human serum. Am. J. Med. Sci. *45*:604, 1971.
26. Galgiani, J. N.: Fluconazole, a new antifungal agent. Ann. Intern. Med. *113*:177, 1990.
27. Gartenberg, G., Bottone, E. J., Keusch, G. T., et al.: Hospital-acquired mucormycosis *(Rhizopus rhizopodiformis)* of skin and subcutaneous tissue: Epidemiology, mycology and treatment. N. Engl. J. Med. *299*:1115, 1978.
28. Gordon, G., Indeck, M., Bross, J., et al.: Injury from silage wagon accident complicated by mucormycosis. J. Trauma *28*:866, 1988.
29. Gregory, J. E., Golden, A., and Haymaker, W.: Mucormycosis of the central nervous system: A report of three cases. Bull. Johns Hopkins Hosp. *73*:405, 1943.
30. Hamdy, N. A. T., Andrew, S. M., Shortland, J. R., et al.: Fatal cardiac zygomycosis in a renal transplant patient treated with desferrioxamine. Nephrol. Dial. Transplant *4*:911, 1989.
31. Herstoff, J. K., Bogaars, H., and McDonald, C. J.: Rhinophycomycosis entomophthorae. Arch. Dermatol. *114*:1674, 1978.
32. Hsu, J., Clayman, J. A., and Geha, A. S.: Survival of a recipient of renal transplantation after pulmonary phycomycosis. Ann. Thorac. Surg. *47*:617, 1989.
33. Imwidthaya, P., and Srimuang, S.: Immunodiffusion test for diagnosing basidiobolomycosis. Mycopathologia *118*:127, 1992.
34. Ingram, C. W., Sennesh, J., Cooper, J. N., et al.: Disseminated zygomycosis: Report of four cases and review. Rev. Infect. Dis. *11*:741, 1989.
35. Jelliffe, D. B., Burkitt, D., O'Conor, G. T., et al.: Subcutaneous phycomycosis in an East African child. J. Pediatr. *59*:124, 1961.
36. Johnson, G. M., and Baldwin, J. J.: Pulmonary mucormycosis and juvenile diabetes. Am. J. Dis. Child. *135*:567, 1981.
37. Kaufman, L., Mendoza, L., and Standard, P. G.: Immunodiffusion test for serodiagnosing subcutaneous zygomycosis. J. Clin. Microbiol. *28*:1887, 1990.
38. Kaufman, L., Turner, L. F., and McLaughlin, D. W.: Indirect enzyme-linked immunosorbent assay for zygomycosis. J. Clin. Microbiol. *27*:1979, 1989.
39. Khardori, N., Hayat, S., Rolston, K., et al.: Cutaneous *Rhizopus* and *Aspergillus* infections in five patients with cancer. Arch. Dermatol. *125*:952, 1989.
40. Kline, M. W.: Mucormycosis in children: Review of the literature and report of cases. Pediatr. Infect. Dis. *4*:672, 1985.
41. Krasinski, E., Holzman, R. S., Hanna, B., et al.: Nosocomial fungal infection during hospital renovation. Infect. Control *6*:278, 1985.
42. Lehrer, R. I., Howard, D. H., Sypherd, P. S., et al.: Mucormycosis. Ann. Intern. Med. *93*:93, 1980.
43. Levinson, S. E., and Isaacson, C.: Spontaneous perforation of the colon in the newborn infant. Arch. Dis. Child. *35*:378, 1960.
44. Levy, S. A., Schmitt, K. W., and Kaufman, L.: Systemic zygomycosis diagnosed by fine needle aspiration and confirmed with enzyme immunoassay. Chest *90*:146, 1986.
45. Lewis, L. L., Hawkins, H. K., and Edwards, M. S.: Disseminated mucormycosis in an infant with methylmalonicaciduria. Pediatr. Infect. Dis. J. *9*:851, 1990.
46. Lloyd, T. R., and Bolte, R. G.: Rhinocerebral mucormycosis in an infant with streptococcal sepsis and purpura fulminans. Pediatr. Infect. Dis. *5*:575, 1986.
47. Mackenzie, D. W. R., Soothill, J. F., and Millar, J. H. D.: Meningitis caused by *Absidia corymbifera*. J. Infect. *17*:241, 1988.
48. Majeski, J. A., and MacMillan, B. G.: Fatal systemic mycotic infections in the burned child. J. Trauma *17*:320, 1977.
49. Maniglia, A. J., Mintz, D. H., and Novak, S.: Cephalic phycomycosis: A report of eight cases. Laryngoscope *92*:755, 1982.
50. Manson-Bahr, P. E. C., and Bell, D. R.: Manson's Tropical Diseases. 19th ed. London, Balliere Tindall, 1987.
51. Medoff, G., and Kobayashi, G. S.: Pulmonary mucormycosis. N. Engl. J. Med. *286*:86, 1972.
52. Meyer, R. D., Rosen, P., and Armstrong, D.: Phycomycosis complicating leukemia and lymphoma. Ann. Intern. Med. *77*:871, 1972.
53. Michalak, D. M., Cooney, D. R., Rhodes, K. H., et al.: Gastrointestinal mucormycoses in infants and children: A cause of gangrenous intestinal cellulitis and perforation. J. Pediatr. Surg. *15*:320, 1980.
54. Mooney, J. E., and Wanger, A.: Mucormycosis of the gastrointestinal tract in children: Report of a case and review of the literature. Pediatr. Infect. Dis. J. *12*:872, 1993.
55. Moretz, M. L., Grist, W. J., and Sewell, C. W.: Zygomycosis presenting as nasal polyps in a healthy child. Arch. Otolaryngol. Head Neck Surg. *113*:550, 1987.
56. Mostaza, J. M., Barbado, F. J., Fernandez-Martin, J., et al.: Cutaneoarticular mucormycosis due to *Cunninghamella bertholletiae* in a patient with AIDS. Rev. Infect. Dis. *11*:316, 1989.
57. Nathan, M. D., Keller, A. P., Jr., Lerner, C. J., et al.: Entomophthorales infection of the maxillofacial region. Laryngoscope *92*:767, 1982.
58. Neame, P., and Raynor, D.: Mucormycosis: A report of twenty-two cases. Arch. Pathol. *70*:261, 1960.
59. Ng, P. C., and Dear, P. R. F.: Phycomycotic abscesses in a preterm infant. Arch. Dis. Child. *64*:862, 1989.
60. Niimi, O., Kokan, A., and Kashiwagi, N.: Effect of deferoxamine mesylate on the growth of Mucorales. Nephron *53*:281, 1989.
61. Nolan, R. L., Carter, R. R., III, Griffith, J. E., et al.: Case report: Subacute disseminated mucormycosis in a diabetic male. Am. J. Med. Sci. *298*:252, 1989.
62. Ochi, J. W., Harris, J. P., Feldman, J. I., et al.: Rhinocerebral mucormycosis: Results of aggressive surgical debridement and amphotericin B. Laryngoscope *98*:1339, 1988.
63. Okhuysen, P. C., Rex, J. H., Kapusta, M., et al.: Successful treatment of extensive posttraumatic soft-tissue and renal infections due to *Apophysomyces elegans*. Clin. Infect. Dis. *19*:329, 1994.
64. Orgel, I. K., and Cohen, K. L.: Postoperative zygomycetes endophthalmitis. Ophthalmic Surg. *20*:584, 1989.
65. Parfrey, N. A.: Improved diagnosis and prognosis of mucormycosis: A clinicopathologic study of 33 cases. Medicine *65*:113, 1986.
66. Pierce, P. F., Wood, M. B., Roberts, G. D., et al.: *Saksenaea vasiformis* osteomyelitis. J. Clin. Microbiol. *25*:933, 1987.
67. Polo, J. R., Luno, J., Menarguez, C., et al.: Peritoneal mucormycosis in a patient receiving continuous ambulatory peritoneal dialysis. Am. J. Kidney Dis. *13*:237, 1989.
68. Prevoo, R. L., Starink, T. M., and de Haan, P.: Primary cutaneous mucormycosis in a healthy young girl: Report of a case cased by *Mucor hiemalis* Wehmer. J. Am. Acad. Dermatol. *24*(5 Pt. 2):882, 1991.
69. Pritchard, R. C., Muir, D. B., Archer, K. H., et al.: Subcutaneous zygomycosis due to *Saksenaea vasiformis* in an infant. Med. J. Aust. *145*:630, 1986.
70. Reed, A. E., Body, B. A., Austin, M. B., et al.: *Cunninghamella bertholletiae* and *Pneumocystis carinii* pneumonia as a fatal complication of chronic lymphocytic leukemia. Hum. Pathol. *19*:1470, 1988.
71. Rex, J. H., Ginsberg, A. M., Fries, L. F., et al.: *Cunninghamella bertholletiae* infection associated with deferoxamine therapy. Rev. Infect. Dis. *10*:1187, 1988.
72. Rinaldi, M. G.: Zygomycosis. Infect. Dis. Clin. North Am. *3*:19, 1989.
73. Rippon, J. W.: Medical Mycology: The Pathogenic Fungi and the Pathogenic Actinomycetes. 3rd ed. Philadelphia, W. B. Saunders, 1988.
74. Rosen, P. P., and Sternberg, S. S.: Decreased frequency of aspergillosis and mucormycosis. N. Engl. J. Med. *295*:1319, 1976.
75. Rozich, J., Oxendine, D., Heffner, J., et al.: Pulmonary zygomycosis: A cause of positive lung scan diagnosed by bronchoalveolar lavage. Chest *95*:238, 1989.
76. Ryan, M. E., and Ochs, J.: Primary cutaneous mucormycosis: Superficial and gangrenous infections. Pediatr. Infect. Dis. *1*:110, 1982.
77. Ryan-Poirier, K., Eiseman, R. M., Beaty, J. H., et al.: Post-traumatic cutaneous mucormycosis in diabetes mellitus: Short-term antifungal therapy. Clin. Pediatr. *27*:609, 1988.
78. Sane, A., Manzi, S., Perfect, J., et al.: Deferoxamine treatment as a risk factor for zygomycete infection. J. Infect. Dis. *159*:151, 1989.
79. Schmidt, J. H., Howard, R. J., Chen, J. L., et al.: First culture proven gastrointestinal entomophthoromycosis in the United States: A case report and review of the literature. Mycopathologia *95*:101, 1986.
80. Schwartz, J. N., Donnelly, E. H., and Klintworth, G. K.: Ocular and orbital phycomycosis. Surv. Ophthalmol. *22*:3, 1977.
81. Smith, A. G., Bustamante, C. I., and Gilmor, G. D.: Zygomycosis (absidiomycosis) in an AIDS patient. Mycopathologia *105*:7, 1989.
82. Stave, G. M., Heimberger, T., and Kerkering, T. M.: Zygomycosis of the basal ganglia in intravenous drug users. Am. J. Med. *86*:115, 1989.
83. Taylor, G. D., Sekhon, A. S., Tyrrell, D. L. J., et al.: Rhinofacial zygomycosis caused by *Conidiobolus coronatus:* A case report including in vitro sensitivity to antimycotic agents. Am. J. Trop. Med. Hyg. *36*:398, 1982.
84. Tazelaar, H. D., Baird, A. M., Mill, M., et al.: Bronchocentric mycosis occurring in transplant recipients. Chest *96*:92, 1989.
85. Umbert, I. J., and Su, W. P. D.: Cutaneous mucormycosis. J. Am. Acad. Dermatol. *21*:1232, 1989.
86. Vadeboncoeur, C., Walton, J. M., Raisen, J., et al.: Gastrointestinal mucormycosis causing an acute abdomen in the immunocompromised pediatric patient: Three cases. J. Pediatr. Surg. *29*:1248, 1994.
87. Vallaeys, J. H., Praet, M. M., Roels, H. J., et al.: The Budd-Chiari syndrome caused by a zygomycete: A new pathogenesis of hepatic vein thrombosis. Arch. Pathol. Lab. Med. *113*:1171, 1989.
88. Varricchio, F., Reyes, M. G., and Wilks, A.: Undiagnosed mucormycosis in infants. Pediatr. Infect. Dis. J. *8*:660, 1989.
89. Ventura, G. J., Kantarjian, H. M., Anaissie, E., et al.: Pneumonia with *Cunninghamella* species in patients with hematologic malignancies: A case report and review of the literature. Cancer *58*:1534, 1986.
90. Wajszczuk, C. P., Dummer, J. S., Ho, M., et al.: Fungal infections in liver transplant recipients. Transplantation *40*:347, 1985.
91. Walker, S. D., Clark, R. V., King, C. T., et al: Fatal disseminated *Conidiobolus coronatus* infection in a renal transplant patient. Am. J. Clin. Pathol. *98*:559, 1992.
92. Walsh, T. J., Hiemenz, J. W., Seibel, N., et al.: Amphotericin B lipid complex in the treatment of 228 cases of invasive mycosis. 34th ICAAC, Orlando, 1994, poster M69.
93. Walsh, T. J., and Pizzo, P. A.: Nosocomial fungal infections: A classification for hospital-acquired fungal infections and mycoses arising from endogenous flora or reactivation. Ann. Rev. Microbiol. *42*:517, 1988.

94. Walsh, T. J., Renshaw, G., Andrews, J., et al: Invasive zygomycosis due to *Conidiobolus incongruus*. Clin. Infect. Dis. *19*:423, 1994.
95. Weems, J. J., Jr., Davis, B. J., Tablan, O. C., et al.: Construction activity: An independent risk factor for invasive aspergillosis and zygomycosis in patients with hematologic malignancy. Infect. Control *8*:71–75, 1987.
96. White, C. B., Barcia, P. J., and Bass, J. W.: Neonatal zygomycotic necrotizing cellulitis. Pediatrics *78*:100, 1986.
97. Wickline, C. L., Cornitius, T. G., and Butler, T.: Cellulitis caused by *Rhizomucor pusillus* in a diabetic patient receiving continuous insulin infusion pump therapy. South. Med. J. *82*:1432, 1989.
98. Wieden, M. A., Steinbronn, K. K., Padhye, A. A., et al.: Zygomycosis caused by *Apophysomyces elegans*. J. Clin. Microbiol. 22:522, 1985.
99. Windus, D. W., Stokes, T. J., Julian, B. A., et al.: Fatal *Rhizopus* infections in hemodialysis patients receiving deferoxamine. Ann. Intern. Med. *107*:678, 1987.
100. Woodward, A., McTigue, C., Hogg, G., et al.: Mucormycosis of the neonatal gut: A "new" disease or a variant of necrotizing enterocolitis. J. Pediatr. Surg. *27*:737, 1992.
101. Zeluff, B. J.: Fungal pneumonia in transplant recipients. Semin. Respir. Infect. *5*:80, 1990.

206

Miscellaneous Mycoses

John W. Rippon

Numerous reports of soilborne and airborne fungi as etiologic agents for a variety of diseases have appeared during the past 70 years. Most of the common fungal pathogens are slow growing and often difficult to isolate. Soil and air contaminants, however, grow rapidly and frequently are isolated from patients with infectious diseases; for the most part, they are not responsible for disease in the patient from whom they have been recovered. Yet rarely, an organism not normally encountered as a pathogen may cause disease. It must be noted that strain variation in fungi is great, and mutations may occur that impart pathogenic potential to otherwise harmless organisms. Thus, isolates of soil-inhabiting species of *Penicillium, Acremonium, Alternaria,* and *Aspergillus* that normally do not grow at 37° C have been isolated from sick patients and found to be thermo-tolerant.

With the increase in the numbers of immunosuppressed patients, patients on cytotoxins, organ transplant patients, and others, the incidence of infections caused by "saprophytic" fungi has increased. The list of these rarely encountered agents has grown so long that two new disease categories have been defined to encompass these infections. Hyalohyphomycosis refers to infection by a mycelial fungus that has colorless cell walls as seen in tissue infected by the fungus in sections not stained specifically for fungi (i.e., hematoxylin and eosin–stained sections). The agents in this category include *Penicillium* species, *Acremonium* species, and others; about 40 agents have been listed so far. This category does not include infection by *Aspergillus* species or *Pseudallescheria boydii* because infection by these agents is so common as to warrant a separate category for each one. Mycelial fungi whose cell walls contain melanin are dark brown or black; they are called dematiaceous fungi. Infection by these fungi is called phaeohyphomycosis. In hematoxylin and eosin–stained sections, the mycelium will be gold-brown because of the melanin. *Alternaria, Exophiala,* and 40 other species are in this category (Tables 206–1 and 206–2).

There are at least three major situations in which these normally saprophytic organisms may be involved in a disease. The first and most common is when the organism acts as an opportunist. The use of immunosuppressive drugs, cytotoxins, and steroids greatly has increased the list of "opportunistic species." By lowering the natural defenses of a patient, fungi of low virulence may be able to colonize and invade. This occurs most frequently in individuals with inborn errors of the immune system or in those in whom the natural barrier imposed by the skin or mucous membranes has been bypassed (e.g., after surgery, with indwelling catheters, use of unsterile material by drug abusers, intrathecal injections, hemodialysis). Thus, we have such reports as a mushroom growing on a mitral valve after open heart surgery, *Scopulariopsis* granulomata developing in the lung after injection of crude opium, and many more fascinating cases.

Colonization of injured or debilitated tissue also may occur. Generally, this has been the predisposing situation in reports of *Alternaria* infection of the nose after submucous resection, *Fusarium* colonization of burned skin, chronic *Mucor* in the injured foot of a diabetic, and *Pseudallescheria* of the knee after an auto accident. These three situations—opportunism, barrier break, and colonizing of debilitated tissue—account for the vast majority of cases of "miscellaneous mycoses." Rarely, a case will occur in which no detectable predisposing factor is found; the patient appears otherwise normal. Such cases include *Mycocentrospora acerina* (a plant pathogen) infection of the face, *Aureobasidium* (a soil saprophyte) involvement of the skin, and granulomata of the lung containing *Beauvaria bassiana,* a pathogen of insects.

In this chapter, infection caused by unusual or uncommon agents of mycoses is discussed.

Pseudallescheriasis

HISTORY

Allescheria boydii was described by Shear[40] in 1922 as the etiologic agent of pedal mycetoma in a patient in West Texas.[7] The agent defined by Shear was a homothallic ascomycete that produced cleistothecia containing ascospores. In addition, it also produced two types of asexual conidiophores: byssoid (simple) and coremias. Several years earlier, however, Saccardo[37] had delineated an asexual hyphomycete isolated from a mycetoma of another patient.[43] The fungus had been isolated in 1909, and Saccardo's diagnosis[37] and a complete description of the pathologic process by Radaeli[33] appeared in 1911. For many years afterward, the imperfect phase name, *Monosporium apiospermum,* appeared in the literature as a frequently isolated agent of mycetoma.

The connection between the two fungi was demonstrated unequivocally by Emmons[14] in 1944. He worked with a culture of *M. apiospermum* from the first Canadian case of mycetoma[12] and noted that in continuous transfer, sclerotia began to appear and finally fertile ascocarps with ascospores. Thus, the two fungi were appreciated to be two phases of one species.

TABLE 206–1. Currently Known Agents of Hyalohyphomycosis of Animals and Man

Acremonium	*Microascus*
A. alabamensis	*M. cinereus*
A. kiliense	*Myriodontium*
A. potroni	*M. keratinophylum*
A. roseo-griseum	*Paecilomyces*
A. falciforme	*P. fumoso-roseus*
A. strictum	*P. lilacinum*
Anxiopsis	*P. marquandii*
A. fulvescens	*P. variotii*
A. sterocaria	*P. javanicus*
Arthrographis	*Penicillium*
A. kalrae	*P. chrysogenum*
Beauvaria	*P. glaucum?*
B. alba	*P. citrinum*
B. bassiana	*P. commune*
Chrysosporium	*P. expansum*
Chrysosporium sp.	*P. spinulosum*
Coprinus	*P. marneffei* (as a schizo-yeast and mycelium in tissue)
C. cinereus	*Schizophylum*
C. delicatulus	*S. commune*
Cylindrocarpon	*Scopulariopsis*
C. lichenicola	*S. acremonium*
C. vaginae	*S. brevicaulis*
Fusarium	*Scytalidium*
F. chlamydosporum	*S. hyalinum*
F. dimerum	*Trichoderma*
F. moniliforme	*T. viride*
F. simifectum	*Tritrachium*
F. oxysporum	*T. oryzae*
F. solani	*Volutella*
F. roseum	*V. cinerscens*
Lecythophora	
L. hoffmani	
L. mutabilis	

From Rippon, J. W.: Medical Mycology: The Pathogenic Fungi and the Pathogenic Actinomycetes. 3rd ed. Philadelphia, W. B. Saunders, 1988.

As is the case with several other fungi, the anamorph (asexual) and teleomorph (sexual) phases were discovered and described at different times. The teleomorph phase is more important taxonomically because the fungus can be related to other genera and species. However, the use of the anamorph phase name may continue (International Code of Botanical Nomenclature), particularly when production of the sexual structures is a rare event. The sexual and asexual phases simply are different methods of reproduction for different purposes and usually are a response to some environmental factor. These phases have nothing to do with the ability to cause disease,[22] which is a characteristic of the species itself and not related to a specific reproductive phase.

The taxonomy of this organism particularly has been confusing. The names for both phases have been changed. McGinnis and colleagues[25] showed that both *Allescheria* and the proposed name *Petriellidium* are invalid as teleomorph designations and that an older genus name, *Pseudallescheria,* first proposed by Negroni and colleagues,[30] is the correct genus. *P. boydii* is the valid taxon of the organism. The genus *Monosporium* was deemed invalid by Hughes,[20] which left the species without a taxonomic home. However, Cooke and Kahler[9] found an adequate description of this imperfect phase, and the correct epithet is *Scedosporium apiospermum.* A second species, *Scedosporium inflatum,* has been described and has been isolated from several cases of infection in children after trauma as well as from horses, dogs, and other animals.[34]

What appears to be historically the first case of human infection and, indeed, the first isolation of this fungus was published in 1889. A fungus was isolated from a case of chronic otitis of a child described in a volume by Siebenmann on fungus infections of the ear.[41] The description given is of the coremial or synnematous state of *P. boydii* and is called *Verticillium graphii.* Apparently, Bezold had isolated it three times between 1870 and 1879 from the ears of children. Belding and Umanzio[4] in 1935 also described the isolation of a new species of *Monosporium* in a patient with an ear infection. Reinterpretation of their work suggests that the organism falls within the limitation of the anamorph state of *P. boydii.* Benham and Georg[6] in 1948 described a case of granulomatous meningitis due to *P. boydii.* There was no underlying disease in this patient, but the patient had received spinal anesthesia a month before the onset of symptoms.

The first reported cases of pulmonary disease appear to be those of Creitz and Harris[10] and Drouhet[13] in 1955. In the former, the patient had chronic bronchitis and emphysema that did not respond to months of multiple antibiotic therapy. In the latter, no clinical details were given. About 80 cases of pulmonary infection have been recorded,[3] plus a few cases of meningitis, systemic mycosis,[3] mycotic keratitis, endophthalmitis, prostatitis, and chronic otitis. Many of these infections have occurred in children.[34]

TABLE 206–2. Phaeohyphomycosis

Alternaria alternata	*E. rostratum* (a)
A. chartarum	*E. longirostratum*
A. dianthicoia	*Fonsecaea pedrosoi* (a, c)
A. infectoria	*Moniliella suaveolens* (a)
A. stemphyloides	*Mycocentrospora acerina*
A. tenuissima	*Oidiodendron cerealis*
Alternaria species (a)	*Peyroneliaea (Phoma) glomerata* (a)
Anthopsis deltoidea	*Phaeosciero dermatiodes* (a)
Arnium ieporinum	*Phialophora bubakii*
Aureobasidium pullulans (a)	*P. parasitica*
Bipolaris howaiiensis (c)	*P. repens*
B. australiensis	*P. richardsiae*
B. spicifera (a)	*P. verrucosa* (c)
Chaetoconidum species	*Phialemonium abovatum* (c)
Chawtonium funicolum	*Phoma cruris-hominis*
C. globosum	*P. eupyrena*
Cladosporium cladosporoides	*P. herbarum* (a)
C. devriesil	*P. hiibernica*
C. elatum	*P. cava* (a)
C. oxysporum	*Phyllosticta (Phyllostictina) citracarpa*
C. sphaerospermum	*Pseudomicrodochium suttonii* (a)
C. carrionii	*Rhamichioridum schulzeri*
Curvularia geniculata	*Sarcinomyces phaeomuriformis*
C. junato (c)	*Scolecobasidium humicola* (a)
C. pallescens (c)	*S. tshawytschae* (a)
Dactytaria (Ochroconis) gallopava (a, c)	*Scytalidium lignicola*
Exophiala jeanselmei (a, c)	*Trichomaris invadens* (a)
E. moniliae (a)	*Ulocladium chartarum*
E. pisciphila (a)	*Wangiella dermatitidis* (a, c)
E. salmonis (a)	*Xylohypha (Cladosporium) bantiana* (a, c)
E. spinifera	
Exserohilum mcginnisii	

From Rippon, J. W.: Medical Mycology: The Pathogenic Fungi and the Pathogenic Actinomycetes. 3rd ed. Philadelphia, W. B. Saunders, 1988. (a, animal infection; c, cerebral involvement).

ETIOLOGY, ECOLOGY, AND DISTRIBUTION

S. apiospermum has been isolated numerous times from cases of mycetoma in various parts of the world. Many colonial variants have been described subsequently as new species; these include *V. graphii, Aleurisma apiospermum, Indiella americana, Glenospora clapieri,* and *Acromoniella lutei.*[25, 34] These all appear to be variants of the same species, and at present there is only one recognized etiologic agent: *P. boydii* and its anamorph *S. apiospermum.*

P. boydii appears to have a worldwide distribution. The first isolation from the soil was recorded by Ajello.[1] This was accomplished by injection of soil into mice in search for *Histoplasma capsulatum.* Since then, it has been found by direct spraying of soil from Ohio on plates, from polluted streams and sewage sludge in Ohio,[9] from tide-washed ocean coast in California, from marine soil in Bombay, from farm soils in Maharashtra,[11] from heated soils in India, and from manure of poultry and cattle by Rippon and Carmichael[35] and Bell.[5]

Infections in children most often follow aspiration of stagnant water, mud, farm animal detritus, or sewage or occur after trauma.[34]

To these records of the saprophytic occurrence of *P. boydii* can be added the more numerous publications of its isolation from clinical situations. The first records of infection due to the fungus are ear infections in Switzerland[41] and mycetoma in Italy.[33] It is the agent recovered most commonly from patients with mycetoma in the United States,[1, 35] Canada,[12] and other temperate regions of the world. Mahgoub and Murray[26] have suggested that rainfall is a more important climatic factor than is temperature. The presence of *P. boydii* in soil may not correlate with its isolation from pathologic material. It is isolated frequently from a variety of saprophytic environments in India, but it is isolated very rarely from clinical material in that country[32] and only on occasion from a mycetoma. This discrepancy may be related to differences in the pathogenic potential of different strains and the geographic distribution of those strains.[22]

Mycetoma due to *P. boydii* is more frequent in men than in women (ratio, 3 to 5:1) and more common in rural than in urban areas. The greatest number of cases occur in those 20 to 40 years of age. Other clinical syndromes caused by *P. boydii* usually are associated with the use of immunosuppressive drugs, underlying disease, trauma, or barrier breaks. Almost all recorded patients with otitis media associated with *P. boydii* have been children. No predisposing factors have been noted except previous otitis media of bacterial origin.

CLINICAL DISEASE

The clinical manifestations of infection by *P. boydii* are quite varied. Although at least 99 per cent of such infections are mycetomas, the remainder have included infections of the eye, ear, central nervous system, internal organs, and, more commonly, the lungs.

Mycetoma

The most common clinical condition involving *P. boydii* is mycetoma. The symptoms essentially are the same for this organism as for other agents of eumycotic mycetoma. The usual history is that of trauma or a puncture wound to the feet, legs, arms, or hands.[18] There is some evidence that, after initial implantation, the organism remains quiescent for some time; possibly another insult to the area in order to manifest symptoms or time to adapt to the host is required. When the primary lesion does develop, it is a locally invasive, indolent, tumor-like process or a small, painless, subcutaneous swelling. This gradually enlarges and softens to become phlegmonous. It ruptures to the surface, forming sinus tracts, then burrows into the deeper tissue to produce swelling and distortion of the tissues. *P. boydii* invades subcutaneous tissues and ligaments primarily, but tendons, muscle, and bone are spared. The burrowing follows fascial planes and incites suppuration and abscess formation that drain through the sinus tracts. The tracts may remain open for long periods, heal, and then reopen. The drainage, when expressed, contains numerous small particles or grains representing microcolonies of the organism.[34]

The grains formed by *P. boydii* are large (up to 2 mm), white to yellowish, soft to firm, and round to lobulated (Fig. 206–1). The hyphae are broad (up to 5 μm), septate, and intertwined and show numerous swollen cells (15 to 20 μm in diameter). These are called intercalary chlamydoconidia. There is no cementing substance between the hyphae composing the grain. In tissue sections, the grains are seen to be in the lumen of the sinus tract. This often is filled with a pyogenic infiltrate, and large accumulations of neutrophils in all stages of degeneration are seen clinging to the grain.

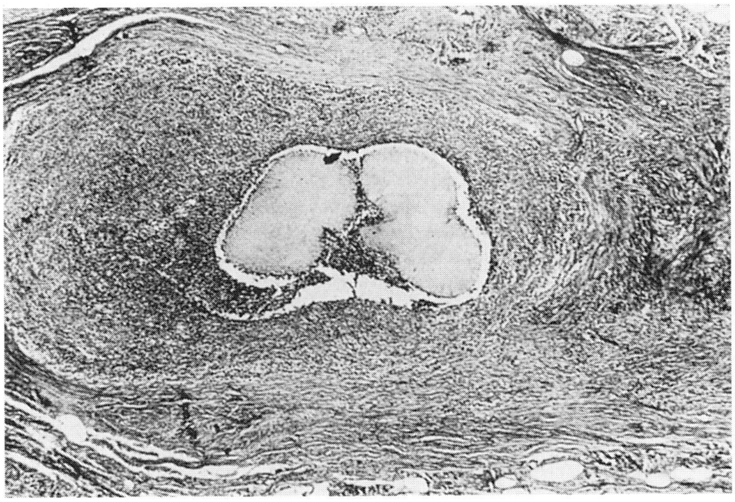

FIGURE 206–1. *Large grain of* Pseudallescheria boydii *in sinus tract of mycetoma. Extensive fibrosis is seen in the periphery of the tract, and the tract is filled with a mixed granulomatous and pyogenic infiltrate. (H and E × 100.) (Courtesy of Centers for Disease Control and Prevention.)*

Immediately around this abscess is an area of dense fibrosis and granulation tissue that is rich in capillaries, epithelial cells, macrophages, and multinucleated giant cells. White grain mycetoma of such histologic character can be caused by six or more different species of fungi. These include *Aspergillus, Fusarium,* and *Acremonium* species.

In uncomplicated mycetoma, there usually are no other constitutional disturbances. Pyrexia may develop if there is secondary bacterial infection; otherwise, there are no other symptoms. The lesions of mycetoma associated with *P. boydii* seldom, if ever, heal spontaneously. The disease may be chronic and continue for 40 or 50 years. Unlike some agents of mycetoma, dissemination of *P. boydii* to other parts of the body essentially is unknown. However, in 1961, isolation of the fungus in inguinal lymph glands in a case of far-advanced mycetoma was reported.[34]

The medical management of eumycotic mycetomas in general has been unrewarding. The organism essentially is resistant to all systemically useful agents, such as 2-hydroxystilbamidine, potassium iodide, 5-fluorocytosine, and amphotericin B. Nielsen[31] found only three strains of *P. boydii* inhibited by 2 μg/mL of amphotericin B at 48 hours. Ernest and Rippon[15] described an isolate that was resistant to 50 μg/mL at 48 hours. Miconazole has been found to inhibit *P. boydii* at concentrations of 0.25 μg/mL. With a blood level of 1 μg/mL achievable after an intravenous dose of 9 mg/kg, the medical treatment of such infections in the future looks promising. In a series of various types of *P. boydii* infections, Stevens[42] found marked efficacy and even clinical cure with the use of miconazole. In some infections, however, relapse occurred. Ketoconazole appears to be inactive in the treatment of *P. boydii* infections, although a few cases that have been treated successfully have been reported. At present, there is no antimycotic agent of choice for *P. boydii* infections.

A far more successful approach to eumycotic mycetoma has been surgical. This is not difficult if the lesion is small and localized. A relapse rate of 80 per cent has been reported after inadequate surgical removal.[26] The margin of tumor in eumycotic mycetoma is encapsulated, which aids in the isolation of the lesion and its removal. In advanced cases, amputation is the only successful treatment. In most cases of mycetoma of the foot, the heel is uninvolved and the calcaneum and talus are unaffected. Thus, the fore part of the foot can be removed with complete arthrodesis and union of tibia, fibula, and calcaneum. The stump is capable of bearing a load at its end. More advanced cases may require below-the-knee amputation. Lesions in areas in which radical surgery is countermanded are more difficult to treat. Simple curettage of as much of the tissue as possible has some value.

Mycetoma caused by *P. boydii* in areas other than the feet is quite rare.[18] By definition, a designation of mycetoma requires tumefaction, sinus tract formation, and grains. Thus, so-called mycetomas of the brain, lung, and other organs are described erroneously. In one case described by Rippon and Carmichael,[35] there was a mixed infection of *Actinomyces israelii* and *P. boydii* in a mycetoma involving the parotid. Serologic, cultural, and histopathologic confirmations were obtained.

Pulmonary Pseudallescheriasis

The most commonly encountered site of infection due to *P. boydii* other than from mycetoma is the lung and upper respiratory tract.[3, 34]

Bronchial colonization has occurred in several cases.[35] In one case, *P. boydii* was seen in direct examination of sputum. The patient was receiving prednisone for rheumatoid arthritis and had coughing, wheezing, and pulmonary congestion. Prednisone was stopped, and the condition cleared. Steroids were started again, and the disease reappeared. When prednisone was discontinued again, the symptoms disappeared. This patient had symptoms and signs similar to those seen in patients with allergic bronchopulmonary aspergillosis and had IgG antibodies to *P. boydii.*

Pulmonary colonization by far is the most common manifestation of pseudallescheriasis of the lung. Creitz and Harris[10] were the first to describe this condition. Their patient had a cavity subsequent to a pyogenic abscess that was invaded secondarily by *P. boydii.* The organism was recovered from sputum, and in long-term follow-up, the fungus again was recovered from bilateral upper lobe cavities. Lutwick and associates[24] noted a preformed cavity in all but one of 14 recorded cases. Mycelial strands within a cyst in the lung have been found. Similar findings were noted by Travis and coworkers[44] in a patient with sarcoidosis. Ropes of mycelium (plectenchyma) and conidia have been found in large residual cavities in a case of healed tuberculosis.[2] The predisposing conditions noted most often are sarcoid and tuberculosis.

The histologic findings are similar to those seen in secondary invasion by *Aspergillus* species. There are fungal abscesses partially walled off by granulation tissue. The surrounding parenchyma often is necrotic. In bronchial cysts colonized by *P. boydii,* the squamous epithelial lining may show some degree of nuclear atypia. Unless conidiophores and conidia are seen in the specimen, it is not possible to distinguish the mycelium of *Aspergillus* species from that of *P. boydii* or other hyphomycete opportunists. Both may coexist in the same infection. Culture and serologic analysis are necessary for confirmation of the etiologic agent.

Transient colonization of the lower respiratory tract may give rise to *P. boydii* pneumonia. This has occurred during the course of a bacterial pneumonia[28] or during steroid therapy.[24] In one patient with pneumonia, death followed acute neurologic decompensation. *P. boydii* was isolated from necrotic lesions of the brain and thyroid. This patient, a child, had aspirated pond water after falling from a bicycle.[34]

True fungus ball formation has been considered several times[2] but has been confirmed only a few times.[35] In one confirmed case, a classic fungus ball of the aspergilloma type formed in a pulmonary cavity after resolution of a sarcoid lesion (Fig. 206–2). On histologic examination, concentric rings of compact mycelial growth were seen, and conidiation occurred on the periphery of the mass (Fig. 206–3). Invasive pulmonary disease is a rarely reported manifestation of infection due to *P. boydii.*[24] Again, the morphologic character of the organism in tissue is indistinguishable from that of *Aspergillus* species.

Localized pulmonary lesions have been treated surgically with success.[19] The use of amphotericin B as treatment has been unrewarding, and most strains of the fungus are resistant to the drug. Miconazole has had clinical trials in pulmonary disease with some success; other cases have relapsed.[42]

Meningitis and Systemic Infections

The first case of *P. boydii* infection of the central nervous system was reported by Benham and Georg.[6] The patient developed progressive meningoencephalitis 1 month after spinal anesthesia. Ten of 13 cultures of cerebrospinal fluid were positive for *P. boydii.* Ovoid bodies were seen in the fluid, possibly representing conidia. Eight months after onset of symptoms, the patient died. At autopsy, granulomatous meningitis was present, covering the cord, brain stem, and cerebellum. A report of extradural infection of the thoracic

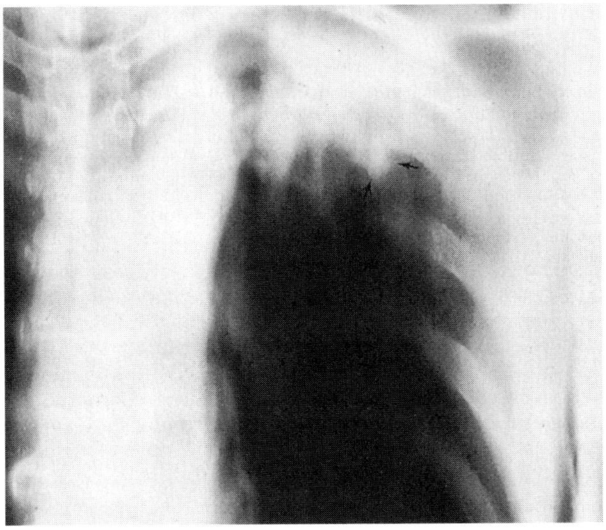

FIGURE 206–2. *Fungus ball caused by* Pseudallescheria boydii. *Tomogram of lung in which several cavities are present. A spherical mass compatible with a fungoma is present in one (arrows) at the level of the aortic arch. (From Rippon, J. W., and Carmichael, J. W.: Petriellidiosis [allescheriosis]: Four unusual cases and review of literature. Mycopathologia* 58:117–124, 1976.)

spine was identified histologically.[39] A well-documented report of systemic infection has appeared.[36] The patient had proliferative glomerulonephritis and died of renal failure. She had been treated with azathioprine and steroids. At postmortem examination, *P. boydii* was found in the thyroid and brain. Recently, more anecdotal reports of systemic infection have appeared. These involve patients receiving immunosuppressive therapy or subsequent to massive aspiration pneumonia. Endocarditis after implantation of prosthetic heart valves also has been reported.[34] Prostatitis caused by this fungus is another rare condition.[27]

Trauma

A case of joint infection due to *P. boydii* has been described after trauma to the head and lacerations of the face, elbows, and knees from an auto accident.[24] The patient's right knee became swollen and erythematous, and *P. boydii* was isolated from aspirated fluid. The knee was irrigated for a month with amphotericin B, but cultures remained positive. Synovectomy and menisectomy were performed with resolution of the condition. Mycelium was noted in the surgical specimen, but culture was negative. Other cases have followed injury in football and soccer playing as well as penetrating wounds.[34]

Mycotic Keratitis and Endophthalmitis

Mycotic keratitis is an infection of the cornea of the eye and usually is the result of secondary fungal colonization of a lesion resulting from some previous trauma or insult. *P. boydii* has been recovered in several such cases.[34] In general, the infection is preceded by an abrasion or herpetic infection; frequently, the use of steroids is noted. Scrapings from the lesions reveal hyphal masses; sometimes conidiophores and conidia are seen. Treatment by irrigation with amphotericin B usually has not been successful. Green and colleagues[17] showed that during subconjunctival or intravenous therapy in experimental rabbit keratitis, the drug was detectable in the aqueous but not the vitreous humor. In cases of fungal keratitis, irrigation with nystatin[15] or pimaricin has been successful. Pimaricin now is considered the drug of choice.[34]

Endophthalmitis caused by *P. boydii* also has been reported.[16, 34] In one case, it responded to topical amphotericin B (4 mg/mL every 2 hours for 6 weeks), whereas in the other,[34] *P. boydii* grew from cultures of vitreous fluid despite instillation of 5 μg of amphotericin B into the vitreous cavity. A vitrectomy was performed, and *P. boydii* also grew from cultures of the tissue. Miconazole therapy was begun, followed by enucleation of the eye. At this time, cultures of the tissue were negative.

Otomycosis

Chronic mycotic otitis has been reported repeatedly. Several fungi may be isolated concomitantly from patients with otomycosis. Generally, there is bacterial otitis externa, and fungi may become secondary invaders. Most commonly, the fungi involved are *Aspergillus niger* and *Aspergillus fumigatus*. Persistent colonization of the external ear canal was noted by Rippon and Carmichael,[35] who described hyphal strands in a swab specimen taken from a chronic discharge of the ear of a boy. Most cases of otomycosis involving *P. boydii* have occurred in children.

IMMUNOLOGY AND SEROLOGY

P. boydii apparently is unable to produce an infection in an uncompromised host except after a barrier break or traumatic

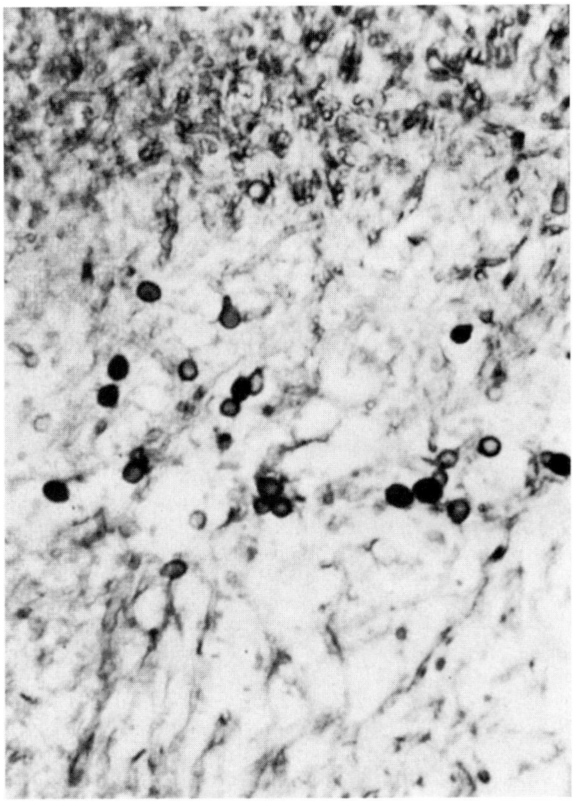

FIGURE 206–3. Pseudallescheria boydii *fungus ball. Periphery of fungus ball, showing characteristic dark staining conidia of the* Scedosporium *type. The spores are* 5 × 7 μm. *(GMS × 100.) (From Rippon, J. W., and Carmichael, J. W. Petriellidiosis [allescheriosis]: Four unusual cases and review of literature. Mycopathologia* 58:117–124, 1976.)

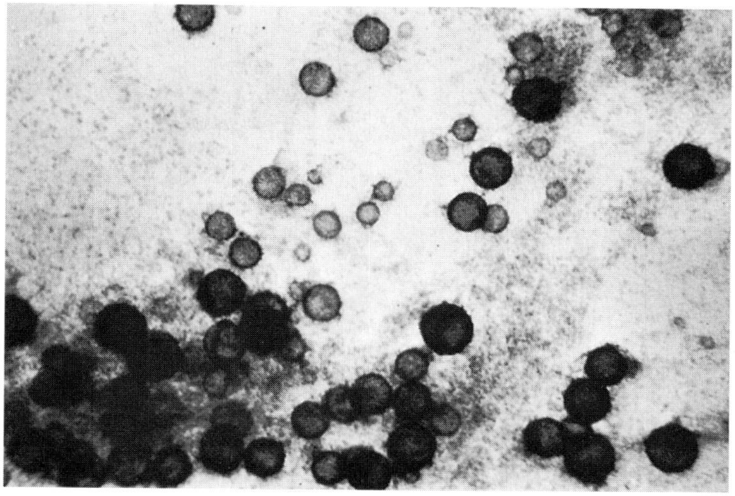

FIGURE 206–4. Pseudallescheria boydii. *Masses of thick-walled black cleistothecia produced in culture. (Unstained × 5.) (From Ernest, T., and Rippon, J. W.: Corneal ulcer due to* Allescheria boydii. *Am. J. Ophthal. 62:1202–1204, 1966.)*

implantation with mycetoma formation. In the compromised host, it is encountered rarely, compared with the more virulent opportunists (e.g., aspergillosis, zygomycosis). This also has been demonstrated in experimental infections. Benham and Georg[6] were unable to produce meningitis in rabbits with an isolate that came from a patient with meningitis.

Serologic procedures have become standard in the diagnosis and prognostic evaluation of the various forms of *P. boydii* infections.[21, 29] They particularly are useful when cultural confirmation is lacking. Attempts to develop complement fixation have been unsuccessful, but immunodiffusion appears to be a reliable procedure.[23] Precipitin bands have been found in cases of mycetoma, bronchial colonization, fungoma, mixed mycetoma, and bovine abortion.[34]

An immunologically specific carbohydrate antigen (antigen I) was isolated from culture filtrates of several strains of *P. boydii.*[23] Such antigens can be used in cases of possible fungus colonization when the etiologic agent is unknown. Crude culture filtrates also appear to be specific and do not cross-react with *Aspergillus* or *Candida* antigens. These are adequate for simple serologic screening procedures.

MYCOLOGY

The type species of the teleomorph stage was described by Shear[40] in 1922 as *A. boydii.* However, the genus later was found to be invalid, as was the proposed genus *Petriellidium.* An older genus, *Pseudallescheria,* now is considered valid.[25]

As Shear[40] noted, *P. boydii* had two asexual methods of conidiation. He called the simple unbranched conidiophore (byssoid) ending in a single large conidiospore *Cephalosporium.* Conidiophores cemented together (coremia or synnema) ending in a conidia were designated *Dendrostilbella.* Neither of these names is considered correct. Different strains of the organism produce three reproductive propagule types in varying quantities. Thus, a long list of names has evolved over the years. The name *M. apiospermum* of Saccardo[37, 38] has been the one used most widely, but the genus now is considered invalid.[20] A description of another conidial state of the organism was deemed adequate and the organism transferred to the genus *Scedosporium.*[8] Thus, the etiologic agent is *P. boydii* (Shear) in its teleomorph state.[26, 32] It is in the class Ascomycetae, order Microascales, family Microascaceae. The anamorph or asexual form is *S. apiospermum.*[37]

The fungus grows readily and rapidly on most laboratory media. However, it is inhibited by cycloheximide found in many primary isolation agars. On rich media such as Sabouraud agar, the cleistothecia may not be formed. It sometimes requires repeated transfer on deficient media (such as oatmeal, potato dextrose, or water agar) to induce ascocarp formation.

Colonies on oatmeal agar have a growth rate of 4 to 5 mm per 24 hours at 25° C. The colony initially is white, becomes a house-mouse gray, and sometimes may have a rosy hue in some areas. Ascocarps (cleistothecia) are spherical, nonostiolate (closed), 140 to 200 μm in diameter, and usually submerged (Fig. 206–4). The cells consist of yellow-to-brown, thick-walled hyphae that are 2 to 3 μm in diameter. The wall of the fruiting body is 4 to 6 μm thick and composed of two to three layers of meandrous interwoven filaments, which gives a polygonal appearance when it is viewed from above. The asci nearly are spherical, 12 to 18 × 9 to 13 μm, and evanescent. They contain eight ascospores that are ellipsoidal, symmetric or somewhat flattened, and straw-colored, and they have two germ pores. They are 6 to 6.5 × 3.5 to 4 μm in diameter.

Two types of asexual conidia are produced. The first (*Scedosporium*-type) consists of conidia broadly clavate or ovoid, rounded above and attenuated or truncate at the base, with a distinct brown wall (Fig. 206–5). They are 6 to 12 × 3.5 to 6 μm in diameter. They usually are single and borne terminally or laterally on solitary conidiophores. Annel-

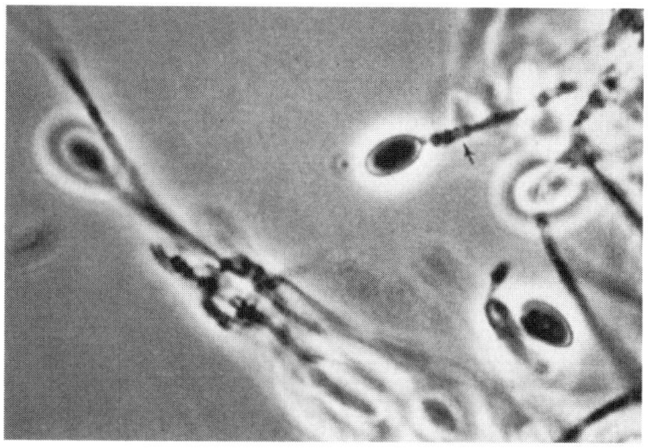

FIGURE 206–5. Pseudallescheria boydii. *Asexual conidia of* Scedosporium *type. As each succeeding conidia is produced, it leaves a ring (arrow) at the terminus of the conidiophore. These rings are called annelations. (× 1320.) (Courtesy of J. W. Carmichael.)*

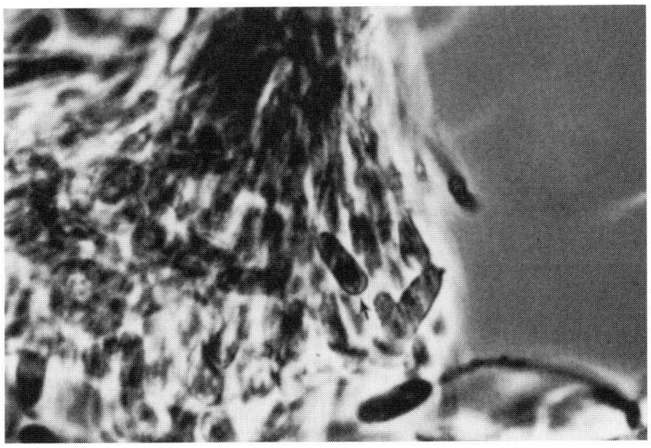

FIGURE 206–6. Pseudallescheria boydii. *Asexual conidia of* Graphium *type (coremia). The conidiophores are cemented together (top) with their ends free, giving a brushlike effect. The ends produce cylindric conidia (arrow).*

lations are observed behind the conidia. The second type of conidiation (*Graphium*-type) consists of smaller conidia (5 to 7 × 2 to 3 μm), clavate or cylindric with a truncate base, that are hyaline. These are borne on short sympodulae or elongating conidiophores that are cemented together to form a synnemata or coremia (Fig. 206–6). The conidia may form a globular mass after abstriction. This form of conidiation is seen infrequently in most cultures, but in a few it is the dominant conidia type.

References

1. Ajello, L.: The isolation of *Allescheria boydii* Shear, an etiologic agent of mycetomas from soil. Am. J. Trop. Med. Hyg. *1*:227–238, 1952.
2. Alture-Werber, E., Edberg, S. C., and Singer, J. M.: Pulmonary infection with *Allescheria boydii.* Am. J. Clin. Pathol. *66*:1019–1024, 1976.
3. Arnett, J. C., and Hatch, H. B.: Pulmonary allescheriasis: Report of a case and review of the literature. Arch. Intern. Med. *135*:1250–1253, 1975.
4. Belding, D. L., and Umanzio, C. B.: A new species of the genus *Monosporium* associated with chronic otomycosis. Am. J. Pathol. *11*:856–857, 1935.
5. Bell, R. G.: The development in beef cattle manure of *Petriellidium boydii,* a potential pathogen for man and cattle. Can. J. Microbiol. *22*:552–556, 1976.
6. Benham, R. W., and Georg, L. K.: *Allescheria boydii,* causative agent in a case of meningitis. J. Invest. Dermatol. *10*:99–110, 1948.
7. Boyd, M. F., and Crutchfield, E. D.: A contribution to the study of mycetoma in North America. Am. J. Trop. Med. *1*:215–289, 1921.
8. Castellani, A.: Fungi and fungous diseases. Arch. Dermatol. *16*:423, 1927.
9. Cooke, W. B., and Kahler, P. W.: Isolation of potentially pathogenic fungi from polluted water and sewage. Public Health Rep. *70*:689–694, 1955.
10. Creitz, S., and Harris, H. W.: Isolation of *Allescheria boydii* from sputum. Am. Rev. Tuberc. *71*:126–130, 1955.
11. Dabrowa, N., Landau, J. W., and Newcomer, V. D.: A survey of tide-washed coastal areas of Southern California for fungi potentially pathogenic to man. Mycopathologia *24*:137, 1964.
12. Dowding, E. S.: *Monosporium apiospermum,* a fungus causing Madura foot in Canada. Can. Med. Assoc. J. *33*:128–132, 1935.
13. Drouhet, M.: The status of fungal diseases in France. *In* Therapy of Fungus Diseases, an International Symposium. Boston, Little, Brown, 1955, pp. 43–53.
14. Emmons, C. W.: *Allescheria boydii* and *Monosporium apiospermum.* Mycologia *36*:188–193, 1944.
15. Ernest, T., and Rippon, J. W.: Corneal ulcer due to *Allescheria boydii.* Am. J. Ophthalmol. *62*:1202–1204, 1966.
16. Glassman, M. I., Henkind, P., and Alture-Werber, E.: *Monosporium apiospermum* endophthalmitis. Am. J. Ophthalmol. *76*:821–824, 1973.
17. Green, W. R., Bennett, J. E., and Goos, R. D.: Ocular penetration of amphotericin B. Arch. Ophthalmol. *73*:769–775, 1965.
18. Greither, A., and Itani, Z.: Mycetome provoque par *Allescheria boydii.* Bull. Soc. Francaise Dermatol. Syph. *81*:263, 1974.
19. Hainer, J. W., Ostrow, J. H., and Mackenzie, D. W. R.: Pulmonary monosporosis. Chest *66*:601–603, 1974.
20. Hughes, S. J.: Revisiones hyphomycetum aliquot cum appendice de nominilus rejiciendis. Can. J. Bot. *36*:727–836, 1958.
21. Knudtson, W. U., Wohlgemuth, K., Kirkbride, C. A., et al.: Mycologic, serologic and histologic findings in bovine abortion associated with *Allescheria boydii.* Sabouraudia *12*:81–86, 1974.
22. Lupan, D. M., and Cazin, J.: Pathogenicity of *Allescheria boydii* for mice. Infect. Immun. *8*:743–751, 1973.
23. Lupan, D. M., and Cazin, J.: Serological diagnosis of petriellidiosis (allescheriosis). I. Isolation and characterization of soluble antigens from *Allescheria boydii* and *Monosporium apiospermum.* Mycopathologia *58*:31–38, 1976.
24. Lutwick, L. I., Galgiani, J. N., Johnson, R. H., et al.: Visceral fungal infections due to *Petriellidium boydii (Allescheria boydii).* Am. J. Med. *61*:632–640, 1976.
25. McGinnis, M. R., Padhye, A. A., and Ajello, A.: *Pseudallescheria* Negroni et Fischer and its later synonym *Petriellidium* Mallock, 1970. Mycotaxon *14*:94–103, 1982.
26. Mahgoub, E. S., and Murray, I. G.: Mycetoma. London, W. Heinemann Medical Books, 1973, p. 10.
27. Meyer, E., and Harrold, R. D.: *Allescheria boydii* isolated from a patient with chronic prostatitis. Am. J. Pathol. *35*:155–159, 1961.
28. Misra, S. P., Shende, G. Y., Yerwadekar, S. N., et al.: *Allescheria boydii* and *Emmonsia ciferrina* isolated from patients with chronic pulmonary infections. Hindustan Antibiot. Bull. *9*:99–103, 1966.
29. Murray, I. G., and Mahgoub, E. S.: Further studies in the diagnosis of mycetoma by double diffusion in agar. Sabouraudia *6*:106–110, 1968.
30. Negroni, P., Hermann, H. H., and Fisher, I.: Artritis aguda purulenta producida por el Ascomycete *Pseudallescheria shearii* n.g. n. sp. Pensa Med. Argentina *30*:2389–2399, 1943.
31. Nielsen, H. S.: Effects of amphotericin B in vitro on perfect and imperfect strains of *Allescheria boydii.* Appl. Microbiol. *15*:86–91, 1967.
32. Padhye, A. A., and Thirumalachar, M. J.: Distribution of *Allescheria boydii* Shear in soil of Maharashtra State. Hindustan Antibiot. Bull. *10*:200–201, 1968.
33. Radaeli, Fr.: Micosi del piede da *Monosporium apiospermum.* Lo Sperimentale *65*:f. 4, 1911.
34. Rippon, J. W.: Medical Mycology: The Pathogenic Fungi and the Pathogenic Actinomycetes. 3rd ed. Philadelphia, W. B. Saunders, 1988.
35. Rippon, J. W., and Carmichael, J. W.: Petriellidiosis (allescheriosis): Four unusual cases and review of literature. Mycopathologia *58*:117–124, 1976.
36. Rosen, F. J., Deck, J. H., and Rewcastle, N. B.: *Allescheria boydii:* Unique systemic dissemination to thyroid and brain. Can. Med. Assoc. J. *93*:1125–1127, 1955.
37. Saccardo, P. A.: In notae mycologicae. Series XIII. Ann. Mycologici *9*:254–255, 1911.
38. Saccardo, P. A., and Sydow, P.: Sylloge Fungorum *14*:464, 1899.
39. Selby, E.: Pachymeningitis secondary to *Allescheria boydii.* J. Neurosurg. *36*:225–227, 1972.
40. Shear, C. L.: Life history of an undescribed ascomycete isolated from granular mycetoma of man. Mycologia *14*:239–243, 1922.
41. Siebenmann, F.: Die Schimmelmykosen des menschlichen Ohnes. Wiesbaden, J. F. Bergmann, 1899, p. 95.
42. Stevens, D. A.: Miconazole in the treatment of fungal infections. Am. Rev. Respir. Dis. *116*:801–806, 1977.
43. Tarozzi, R.: Ric. anatomopat. bact. e sperim. sopra un caso di actinomicosi del piede. Arch. Sc. Med. *33,* n.25, 1909.
44. Travis, R. E., Urich, E. W., and Phillips, S.: Pulmonary allescheriasis. Ann. Intern. Med. *54*:141–152, 1961.

Cutaneous, Visceral, and Cerebral Chromoblastomycosis and Phaeohyphomycosis

Aside from the immunology of dermatophyte infections, no topic in medical mycology has evoked as much controversy as the nomenclature and taxonomy of infections due to dematiaceous ("dark") fungi. Chromoblastomycosis was the oldest standard term for the clinical entity consisting of verrucous, keloid-like growths on the legs and feet containing brown, planate, dividing "yeast" cells. As time went on, other types of lesions were encountered in which brown mycelial elements were found instead of the "yeasts." "Blasto" was dropped from the name, and the term *chromo*- (referring to the pigmented hyphae) *-mycosis* with various modifications has appeared in the literature. Chromoblastomycosis has been revived as the designation for the clinical entity consisting of verrucous keloid-like growths.

The term *phaeohyphomycosis* was proposed by Ajello and colleagues[1–3] in defining a disease caused by a new species of *Phialophora*. In this case, the organism as seen in tissue was composed of brown, septate, branching mycelium instead of the planate, dividing sclerotic cells or "yeast" bodies of typical verrucous chromoblastomycosis, which is a common disease of the tropics caused by several species of *Phialophora* and *Cladosporium*. In a later paper, Ajello[1] emphasized that phaeohyphomycosis was a designation of convenience to cover certain rarely encountered infections. These infections are due to a number of dematiaceous species. The common denominator is the appearance in tissue of brown (phaeo), branched, septate mycelium, which may be distorted and contain various swollen cells, cyst-like bodies, chlamyconidia- and arthroconidia-like cells, and cells in chains. In the past few years, many cases have been described in which species of the genera *Alternaria, Phoma, Cladosporium, Cercospora, Bipolaris, Curvularia, Exophiala, Phialophora,* and so on have been isolated. In many of these cases, this was the first and only isolation of the organism from a disease process. In some, the species was new. Previously, most such diseases had been called infections by dematiaceous fungi, or a few reports were detailed as phaeosporotrichosis by Mariat and colleagues.[22]

In this section, all such cases have been designated as cases of phaeohyphomycosis. In this are grouped reports of cutaneous, visceral, and cerebral diseases that have in common an agent that appears in tissue as some sort of brown hyphae or cells. Chromoblastomycosis is separated out and includes the commonly encountered disease entity in which the organism has the appearance of planate, dividing, sclerotic "yeast" cells. This conservative approach is used because the same species that regularly elicits chromoblastomycosis also may be involved in cerebral or opportunistic systemic disease in which it appears simply as brown, distorted hyphae.

CHROMOBLASTOMYCOSIS

The clinical entity correctly called chromoblastomycosis is characterized by keloid-like hyperplastic areas of the dermis and epidermis that form warty growths or pedunculated cauliflower-like tumors at the site of traumatic implantation of the etiologic fungus (Fig. 206–7). It also is called verrucous dermatitis, and several cases of malignant transformation have been reported in chronic disease.[25] The only verified etiologic agents are *Phialophora verrucosa, Fonsecaea pedrosoi, Fonsecaea compactum,* and *Cladosporium carrioni.* All have the same morphologic features in tissue: planate dividing sclerotic cells ("copper pennies," "Medlar bodies") with brown cell walls, which readily are visible with hematoxylin and eosin stain. The lesions are hyperplastic, granulomatous (foreign body giant cells) severe acanthosis, with microabscesses containing the fungal sclerotic cells. In culture, they all grow as dark hyphae without a yeast phase. *P. verrucosa* produces only conidia from vase-like phialides; *C. carrioni,* only branching chains of conidia; and *Fonsecaea* species, a variety of conidial types.

Surgical excision and flucytosine and itraconazole[25] are used in treatment. Dissemination of the fungus to the brain has been reported.

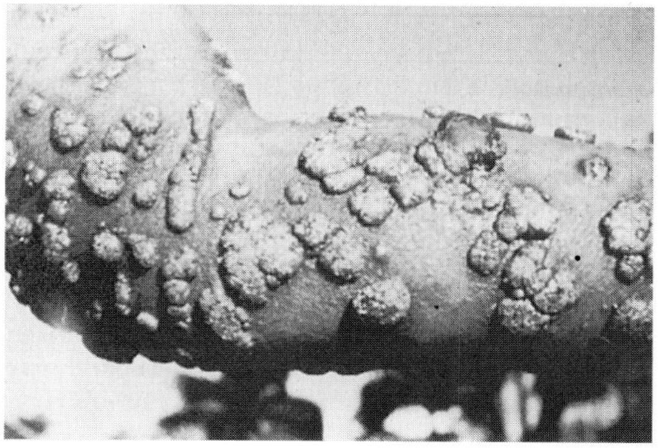

FIGURE 206–7. *Chromoblastomycosis. The warty-like growth of epidermis and dermis is the result of traumatic implantation of the etiologic agent with subsequent autoinoculation from scratching. The agent was* Fonsecaea pedrosoi.

PHAEOHYPHOMYCOSIS (Table 206–2)

Species of the genus *Alternaria* are very common members of the soil flora, and many cause disease in plants. They also are very common allergens, particularly in the spring and fall in the temperate parts of the world, and are important agents that may trigger the onset of asthma and chronic bronchitis. *Alternaria* species also are isolated commonly from the air and from the skin, where they represent an incidental finding and are considered contaminants. In a few patients, however, they may cause opportunistic infections.[6, 12, 19]

In 1976, Pedersen and colleagues[25a] reviewed the literature and found 10 cases of cutaneous disease to which they added 2. Of these, only six had histologic examination and thus could be considered unequivocal. Papules, pustules, and ulcers have been noted most commonly on the cheeks, hands, forearms, legs, and nose.

On histologic examination, the Pedersen team found that lesions consisted of microabscesses containing neutrophils and some lymphocytes.[25a] Septate hyphae were seen, 3 to 5 μm in diameter, in the stratum corneum and invading the stratum spinosum. The dermis showed some inflammatory changes with capillary dilatation and perivascular infiltrate. Sometimes a granulomatous response has been noted with numerous histiocytes and some giant cells. Thus, the histologic appearance varies considerably, probably a reflection of the immune status of the patient. Young mycelium was noted to be hyaline, whereas mature mycelium often was brown in sections stained with hematoxylin and eosin.

Only three cases of subcutaneous alternariosis have been noted. The first occurred in a young woman in Chicago who had a submucous resection and rhinoplasty.[27] When the packing was removed, it was noted that an erythematous ulcerative process was in progress in the upper turbinates. On biopsy, broad, septate, branching hyphae were seen. Cultures of the biopsy material revealed many colonies of *Alternaria alternata.* Precipitins to *Alternaria* antigen were found in the serum. Surgical débridement was performed, and a course of amphotericin B was given. The lesions regressed. Two years later, the lesions reappeared.

A second case occurred in a patient with acute myelogenous leukemia. During an episode of severe granulocytopenia, black mucosa was noted over the middle turbinate. Culture and biopsy were performed. *Alternaria* was recovered, and septate hyphae were seen in biopsy (Fig. 206–8*A*). With return of granulocytes and a short course of amphotericin B therapy, the lesion resolved. Disease of the mucosa over the turbinates also was described in a third case. Dematia-

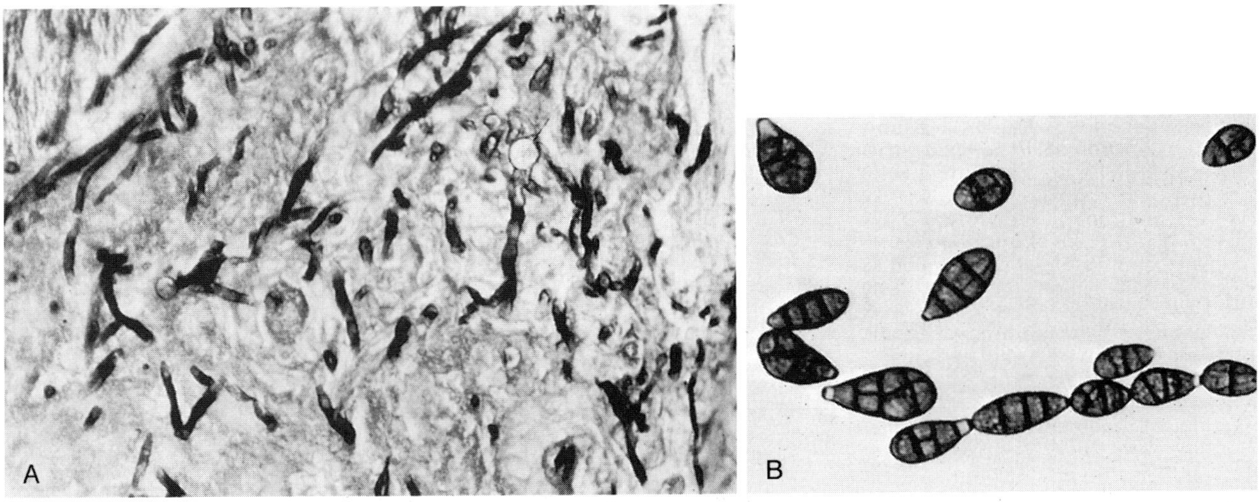

FIGURE 206–8. A, Alternaria, *an example of phaeohyphomycosis. Biopsy of middle turbinate; septate mycelial strands and cyst-like cells (chlamydoconidia) are seen in subcutaneous tissue. Necrosis and a small amount of pyogenic type of cell infiltrate were seen in tissue section. (GMS × 500.)* B, Alternaria *species muriform conicia (porospores) that have both longitudinal and transverse septation and are produced in chains. (× 100.) (Courtesy of J. Gallup.)*

ceous hyphae were seen in histologic section, and *A. alternata* was recovered in culture.

Reddy and associates[26] have produced lesions in the scarified skin of rabbits, and precipitins developed in the rabbit sera.

Alternaria species are identified easily in the laboratory. The colony grows rapidly (10 mm/day) and develops mycelium close to the agar, which is grayish at first and then becomes black with a gray periphery. The texture is loose, even, and fur-like. The reverse of the colony is black. In old colonies, tufts of cottony white and gray mycelium are seen. Under the microscope, large muriform conidia (longitudinal and transverse septation) are produced in chains from simple conidiophores (see Fig. 206–8*B*). The mycelium and conidia are dark. The conidial chain is produced by budding of the terminal cell of the conidia beneath it (acrepetal), and there is a dark spot at the point of attachment. Branched chains of conidia also are seen.[13]

Phialophora parasitica was isolated from the subcutaneous tissue of a kidney transplant patient on immunosuppressive therapy.[3] Irregular, branching hyphae were seen in tissue (Fig. 206–9). On agar, the organism produces a gray-brown colony. On microscopic examination, it forms phialides that extrude ovoid to ellipsoid phialospores.

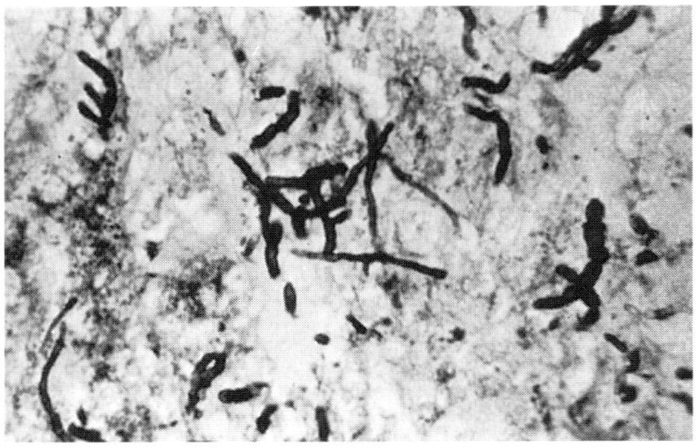

FIGURE 206–9. *Systemic phaeohyphomycosis. Irregular branching septate hyphae in tissue due to* Phialophora parasitica. *(GMS × 500.) (From Ajello, L., Georg, L. K., Steigbigel, R. T., et al.: A case of phaeohyphomycosis caused by a new species of* Phialophora. *Mycologia 66:490–498, 1974.)*

Wangiella dermatitidis has been isolated from small papillomatous lesions on the skin that fused and became smooth, granulated, ulcer-like eruptions.[14] Short chains of irregular cells were seen in tissue section. The disease was cured by application of tar-sulfur ointment. The organism also has been found in disseminated infections,[17] brain abscesses,[28] and a subcutaneous abscess.[29] In the last case, histologic examination of a biopsy revealed elongate, distorted mycelium.

The organism is glabrous, moist, and yeast-like on initial isolation. It is covered gradually by olive-gray aerial mycelium. Annelophores are produced. The organism is quite susceptible to amphotericin B (0.195 μg/mL) and nystatin (0.78 units/mL).[16, 29]

Exophiala jeanselmei has been isolated from several patients with dermal cysts, mycetoma, and systemic infections. These cysts result from puncture wounds, usually from thorns. The organism forms brown, round cells and distorted mycelium in tissue. It also has been found as an opportunist in a patient receiving steroids.[15]

The organism is moist, dark, glabrous, and yeast-like on initial isolation. Later, the colony is covered by olive-gray mycelium. Long, thin annelophores are produced as well as peg-like sterigmata that bud off blastospores. These tend to accumulate in clusters. The organism clears tyrosine agar and does not grow at 40° C, separating it from *W. dermatitidis.*

Phialophora richardsiae is a common, lignicolous, wood-decay fungus isolated once from a subcutaneous cyst. In the central necrotic area, dark hyphal strands and rounded cells were found. It grows as a tufted, woolly, brownish-gray colony with concentric zonations. The phialides have a conspicuous saucer-like flaring lip and ovoid phialospores.[24]

Exophiala spinifera was recovered from a subcutaneous granuloma where it existed as rounded cells and short, brown hyphae.[3] It grows slowly as a black, glabrous, yeast-like colony. It may remain yeast-like almost indefinitely. Apicular and simple or branched annelophores are produced; they are at right angles to the mycelium (spine-like) (Fig. 206–10).

Phialophora repens was recovered from a patient with a subcutaneous abscess.[23] The patient was immunosuppressed during the course of treatment for lepromatous leprosy. In tissue, granulomata were seen, which contained brown to hyaline hyphal elements, some of which were aggregated

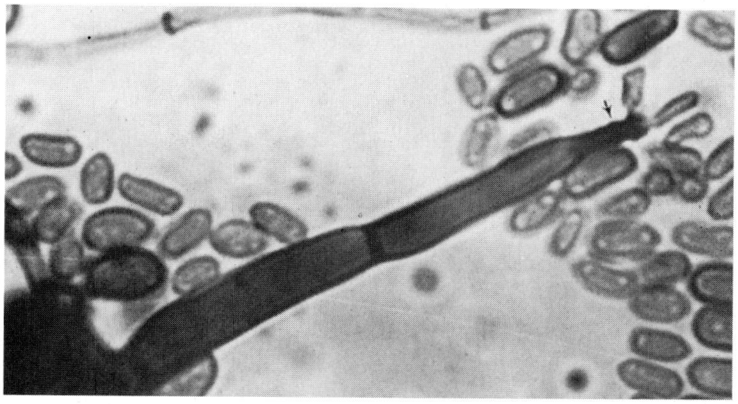

FIGURE 206–10. Exophila spinifera. *In culture, spine-like annellophores are produced. At the growing tip, rings (annellations) are laid down by each successive conidium that is produced (arrow). (× 1300.) (Courtesy of Dante Borelli.)*

into masses of 20 to 110 μm. These were small and not embedded in sinus tracts or surrounded by eosinophilic material; thus, they would not be classed as a mycetoma.

The colonies are light to dark brown and tufted. Phialophores are produced singly or in tufts and are 10 to 15 μm long, tapering from 2 to 4 μm in diameter at the base to 1 to 1.5 μm at the tip. A short collarette is present. The conidia are hyaline, curved, or cylindric, 1.3 to 2.8 × 2.5 to 8 μm, and accumulated in masses at the apex of the phialophore.

Xylohypha bantiana, also called *Cladosporium trichoides,* has been recovered from 60 patients with cerebritis.[5, 8] The lesions are single or multiple. Multiple lesions suggest hematogeneous spread from a focal infection elsewhere. They consist of encapsulated abscesses with masses of brown hyphal strands, chlamydospore-like cells, and beaded (moniliform) cells of arthroconidia-like morphology. Concurrently, on occasion, small lesions have been found in the lungs, the skin of the abdomen, or the ear. Often the affected patients are debilitated or on steroid therapy.[10] *Cladosporium trichoides* also has been recovered from lesions of the skin and subcutaneous tissue.[9]

The organism grows moderately rapidly, producing a spreading, folded, olive-gray to olive-brown colony. Conidiophores are produced that bud off long-branched flexuous chains of elongate conidia (2 to 3 × 4 to 7 μm). *Fonsecaea pedrosoi* and *Phialophora verrucosa,* agents of classic verrucous chromoblastomycosis, also have caused disseminated infections with involvement of the brain.

Phoma hibernica has been recovered from previously injured skin.[4] In this case, the patient had recurring lesions on the lower leg that had been treated with steroids, coal tar, and grenz rays. A granuloma developed in the treated area. On histologic examination, hyphal elements were seen in tissue. Young and colleagues[30] described a subcutaneous abscess in which brown-tinged hyphae and short chains of rounded cells were found. They were unable to classify the organism to the species level.

Phoma cava has been isolated from an infection of the hair of a child and from facial lesions of two children.[27] *Phoma* species produce a moderately fast-growing colony (35 mm in 8 days) that is tufted pink and black and overgrown by loose, grayish, mycelium-producing, large, black-walled pycnidia, 200 to 300 μm in diameter. These are flask shaped. If crushed, they are seen to contain masses of hyaline conidia.

Cercospora apii, a parasite of celery *(Apium graveolens),* has been recovered only once from a human infection.[7] Lie-kien and Tjoei[20] repeatedly isolated a fungus identified as *C. apii* from chronic destructive verrucous lesions on the face of a young Indonesian boy (Fig. 206–11). The lesion appeared many years earlier as a nodule on the cheek. Eleven biopsies were taken over a period of several years. There was no lymphadenopathy or fever, and no underlying disease was detected. In the granulomatous lesions, septate brown mycelium was seen, 4 to 8 μm in diameter. The patient died several years later with destruction of the nose, palate, eyelids, and cheeks. The isolate has been redescribed as *Mycocentrospora acerina.*

The fungus grew at 30° C but not at 37° C. The colony was olive-gray. Irregular conidiophores produced terminal conidia in series. Initially, they were small and single celled (4 to 6 μm); as the conidiophore matured, the conidia were multicellular (26 × 120 μm). Morphologically, the organism resembles *Dactylaria* and *Diplorhinotrichum.*

Bipolaris hawaiiensis is a dematiaceous soil fungus of wide geographic distribution. It has been isolated once in a fatal case of meningoencephalitis in a patient who had unsus-

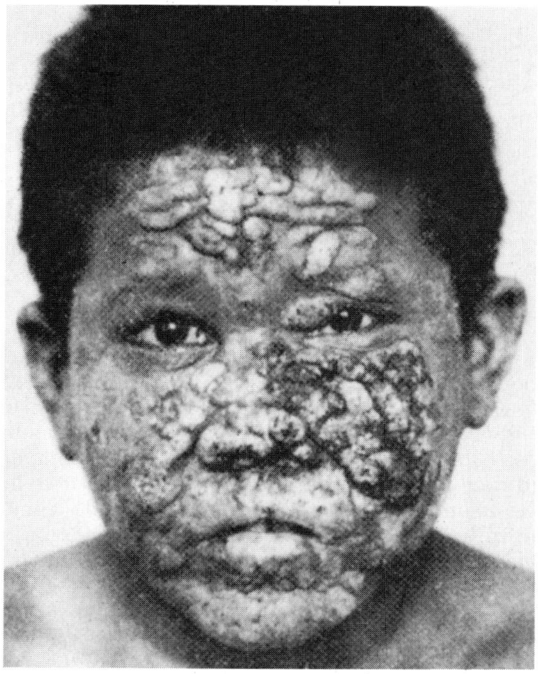

FIGURE 206–11. *Phaeohyphomycosis. Numerous granulomatous lesions due to* Cercospora apii, *now renamed* Mycocentrospora aurina. *(From Lie-kien, J., and Tjoei, N. I.: A new verrucous mycosis caused by* Cercospora apii. *Arch. Dermatol. 75:864–870, 1957. Copyright 1957, American Medical Association.)*

pected lymphosarcoma.[15] Brown septate mycelium was found in several areas of the brain. In areas of vasculitis, there were numerous giant cells and distorted, swollen, bizarre hyphal elements. The colony is a cottony, blackish-brown mold. The conidia are thick walled and transversely septate. They resemble the conidia of *Helminthosporium* and *Drechslera,* but, as noted by Ellis,[13] because of the acrepetalous succession of porospores produced sympodially on an extending conidiophore, they now are grouped as *Bipolaris.*

Helminthosporium species are common dematiaceous fungi of the soil. Some species cause banana rot, corn leaf blight, and so on. They frequently are isolated from sputum and skin as contaminants. Dolan and associates[11] reported two cases of *Helminthosporium* infection. Both patients had chronic pulmonary disease, with purulent sputum, hemoptysis, and fever. Multiple cavities and abscesses were found in the lungs. These contained histiocytes, lymphocytes, plasma cells, and granulocytes. Light brown, septate, branching mycelium was seen in tissue and found in bronchi, bronchioles, and alveoli. In modern taxonomy, these various isolates would be included in the genus *Bipolaris* or *Exserohilum.*

Helminthosporium produces a fast-growing, cottony, gray-black colony (40 mm in 5 days). The long, rounded conidia, 10 μm, are brown and thick walled, with several transverse septations, and are produced as porospores from knobby, branched conidiophores.

Curvularia geniculata, a common member of soil and air flora, has been isolated from a patient with endocarditis.[18] Brown, septate hyphae were found in the vegetations, and at autopsy, mycotic emboli were found in the left renal and anterior iliac arteries. Mycotic infarcts also were found in the heart, kidney, spleen, thyroid, and brain.

The fungus grows rapidly, producing a velvety, silver-gray, cottony mycelium. Abundant conidia are produced that are curved slightly and three-celled (the center cell being larger) with dark brown walls. This fungus and several other soil organisms are encountered frequently in mycotic keratitis. *Curvularia lunata* has been isolated from mycetoma and from onychomycosis.

Chaetocladium was isolated from a lesion of the ankle and subcutaneous nodules on the knee in a 16-year-old male. The boy was receiving immunosuppressive therapy after a renal allograft. The initial lesion developed at the site of an injury that broke the skin. This patient also had an infection due to an acid-fast bacillus and cryptococcosis.[21]

The thermophilic pathogen of chickens and turkeys, *Ochcroconis (Dactylaria) gallopavum,* was reported in a brain abscess in a man with malignant lyphoma.[29] Septate, branching, light brown hyphae were seen in tissue.

References

1. Ajello, L.: Phaeohyphomycosis: Definition and etiology. *In* Mycoses. Washington, D.C., Pan American Health Organization, Scientific Publication No. 304, 1976, pp. 126–133.
2. Ajello, L., McGinnis, M. R., and Camper, J.: An outbreak of phaeohyphomycosis in rainbow trout caused by *Scolecobasidium humicula.* Mycopathologia *62*:15–22, 1977.
3. Ajello, L., Georg, L. K., Steigbigel, R. T., et al.: A case of phaeohyphomycosis caused by a new species of *Phialophora.* Mycologia *66*:490–498, 1974.
4. Bakerspigel, A.: The isolation of *Phoma hibernica* from a lesion on the leg. Sabouraudia *7*:261–264, 1970.
5. Binford, C. H., and Thompson, R. K.: Mycotic abscess due to *Cladosporium trichoides,* a new species. Am. J. Clin. Pathol. *22*:535–542, 1952.
6. Botticher, W. W.: *Alternaria* as a possible human pathogen. Sabouraudia *4*:256–258, 1966.
7. Chupp, C.: The possible infection of the human body with *Cercospora apii.* Mycologia *49*:773–774, 1957.
8. Crichlow, D. K., Enrile, F. T., and Memon, M. Y.: Cerebellar abscess due to *Cladosporium trichoides (bantianum).* Am. J. Clin. Pathol. *60*:416–421, 1973.
9. Desai, S. C., and Bhatikar, M. L.: Cerebral chromoblastomycosis due to *Cladosporium trichoides*: Parts I and II. Neurology (Bombay) *14*:1–18, 1966.
10. Di Salvo, A. F., and Chew, W. H.: *Phialophora gougerotii,* an opportunistic fungus in a patient treated with steroids. Sabouraudia *6*:241–245, 1968.
11. Dolan, C. T., Weed, L. A., and Dines, F.: Bronchopulmonary helminthosporosis. Am. J. Clin. Pathol. *53*:235–242, 1970.
12. Dooley, J. R.: Case for diagnosis: Phaeosporotrichosis. Milit. Med. *138*:807, 827, 1973.
13. Ellis, M. B.: Dematiaceous Hyphomycetes. Kew, England, Commonwealth Mycological Institute, 1971.
14. Emmons, C. W., and Lie-kien, J.: *Basidiobolus* and *Cercospora* from human infections. Mycologia *49*:1–10, 1957.
15. Fuste, F. J., Ajello, L., Threlkeld, R., et al.: *Drechslera hawaiiensis:* Causative agent of a fatal fungal meningoencephalitis. Sabouraudia *11*:59–63, 1973.
16. Jen, T. M., and Lin, W. H.: Studies on the morphology of *Phialophora dermatitidis* isolated in China and its susceptibility to amphotericin B and mycostatin. J. Formosan Med. Assoc. *73*:671–680, 1973.
17. Jotisankasa, V., and Nielsen, H. S.: *Phialophora dermatitidis:* Its morphology and biology. Sabouraudia *8*:98–107, 1970.
18. Kaufman, S. M.: *Curvularia geniculata* endocarditis following cardiac surgery. Am. J. Clin. Pathol. *56*:466–470, 1971.
19. Kawaski, H., Kagi, M. A., and Nishimura, N.: A case of cutaneous alternariosis. Jpn. J. Med. Mycol. *11*:218, 1970.
20. Lie-kien, J., and Tjoei, N. I.: A new verrucous mycosis caused by *Cercospora apii.* Arch. Dermatol. *75*:864–870, 1957.
21. Lomvardias, S., and Madge, G. E.: *Chaetocladium* and atypical acid-fast bacilli in skin ulcers. Arch. Dermatol. *106*:875–876, 1972.
22. Mariat, F., Segretain, G., Destombos, P., et al.: Kyste souscutene mycosique (phaeosporotrichose) á *Phialophora gougerotii* (Matruchot 1910) Borelli 1955 observé au Senegal. Sabouraudia *5*:209–219, 1967.
23. Meyers, W. M., Dooley, R. J., and Chung, K. T.: Mycotic granuloma caused by *Phialophora repens.* Am. J. Clin. Pathol. *64*:545–551, 1975.
24. Nielsen, H. S., and Conant, N. F.: A new human pathogenic *Phialophora.* Sabouraudia *6*:228–231, 1968.
25. Paul, C., Dupont, B., Pialoux, G., et al.: Chromoblastomycosis with malignant transformation and cutaneous synovial secondary localization. The potential therapeutic role of itraconazole. J. Med. Vet. Mycol. *29*:313–316, 1991.

25a. Pedersen, N. B., Mardh, P. A., Hallberg, T., et al.: Cutaneous alternariosis. Br. J. Dermatol. *94*:201–209, 1976.

26. Reddy, B. D., Kelley, D. C., Miocha, H. C., et al.: Pathogenicity of *Alternaria alternata* and its antibody production in experimental animals. Mycopathologia *54*:385–390, 1974.
27. Rippon, J. W.: Medical Mycology: The Pathogenic Fungi and the Pathogenic Actinomycetes. 3rd ed. Philadelphia, W. B. Saunders, 1988, pp. 276–324.
28. Shimazona, Y., Kiminori, I., and Otsuka, R.: Brain abscess due to *Hormodendrum dermatitidis* (Kano) Conant 1953. Folia Psychiatr. Neurol. Jpn. *17*:80–96, 1963.
29. Sides, E. H., Benson, J. D., and Padhye, A. A.: Phaeohyphomycosis brain abscess due to *Ochroconis gallopavum* in a patient with malignant lymphoma of a large cell type. J. Med. Vet. Mycol. *29*:317–322, 1991.
30. Young, N. A., Kwon Chung, K. J., and Freeman, F.: Subcutaneous abscess caused by a *Phoma* sp. resembling *Pyrenochaeta romeroi.* Am. J. Clin. Pathol. *59*:810–816, 1973.

Basidiomycosis

Basidiomycetes, which include rusts, smuts, and mushrooms, are very common in nature but seldom associated with human disease. However, Kwon-Chung[7] showed that *Cryptococcus neoformans* was the imperfect yeast form of Basidiomycota, the sexual stage of which is *Filobasidiella neoformans.* This is in the order Aphyllophorales and thus is related to the bracken fungi. Aside from allergic reactions, particularly to the bran spores of corn smut,[13] very few basidiomycetes have been recovered from a human disease process, and even fewer have been identified unequivocally as the responsible agent.

Cutaneous lesions and granulomatous meningitis due to basidiomycetes have been described.[8, 9] The most commonly encountered basidiomycete associated with human disease is *Schizophyllum commune.* This common fleshy fungus grows as a fan-shaped mushroom from dead tree trunks, organic debris, and even thatched roofs of houses.

Kligman[6] isolated the fungus from a patient with onychomycosis. Scrapings of the nails revealed fungus with large hyphae and clumps of mycelium resembling the grains of actinomycosis. Specimens of the nails were cultured on several agar plates. Six weeks later, it was found that sporophores typical of *S. commune* had developed in all cultures. A 24-year-old male had symptoms of "atypical meningitis," described as "dullness of mind and some irregular modulations of alpha waves."[1] A lumbar puncture was performed, and *S. commune* was recovered. In another case, Ciferri and colleagues[2] recovered *S. commune* on three separate occasions from sputum of a patient with chronic lung disease. Mycelial strands were observed on direct examination of the sputum. A well-documented case of palatal infection was reported by Restrepo and associates[10] in a 4-month-old girl with ulceration and perforation of the hard palate. A biopsy revealed mycelium in the tissue. The mycelium had evident clamp connections and thus was identifiable as a basidiomycete. Amphotericin B was given in a dose of 0.25 mg/kg (total dose was 200 mg over 3 months). The lesion regressed, and the patient was discharged. On histologic examination, a chronic inflammatory and granulomatous response was seen in the submucosa. Necrosis was not evident, but foreign body giant cells were observed. Two cultures made 10 days apart grew *S. commune.*

Another mushroom genus isolated from human material is that of *Coprinus.* In 1954, Emmons[4] reported the repeated isolation of *Coprinus micaceus* from sputa of a patient. Mycelia were seen on direct examination of the specimens. *Coprinus* also has been reported as a cause of endocarditis.[3, 12]

Experimental infections using basidiomycetes have been attempted several times.[5, 10, 11] Salfelder and associates[11] inoculated a variety of basidiomycetes (*Polyporus sanguineus, Polyporus versicolor, Lenzites trabea, Schizophyllum commune,* a telephoraceae, *Poria* species, *Daedalea* species, *Fomes* species, and one unidentified) into mice.[11] Granulomata were formed, and the fungi could be recovered from tissue. *S. commune* elicited lesions in the skin.

References

1. Chavez Batista, A., Maia, J. A., and Singer, R.: Basidioneuromycosis in man. Sociedade de Biologia de Pernambuco Pub. No. 42. Annals *3*:52–60, 1955.
2. Ciferri, R., Chavez Batista, A., and Campos, S.: Isolation of *Schizophyllum commune* from a sputum. Atti. Inst. Botanica Laboratorio Criptogamico Univ. de Pavia *14*(1–3):118–120, 1956.
3. DeVries, G. A., Kemp, R. F. O., and Speller, D. C. E.: Endocarditis caused by *Coprinus delicatulus.* Compte Rendus de Commun. V. Congress. Paris, ISHAM, 1971, pp. 185–186.
4. Emmons, C.: Isolation of myxotrichum and gymnoascus from lungs of animals. Mycologia *46*:334–338, 1954.
5. Greer, D. L., and Bolanos, B.: Pathogenic potential of *Schizophyllum commune* isolated from a human case. Sabouraudia *12*:233–244, 1974.
6. Kligman, A. M.: A basidiomycete probably causing onychomycosis. J. Invest. Dermatol. *14*:67–70, 1950.
7. Kwon-Chung, K. J.: Morphogenesis of *Filobasidiella neoformans,* the sexual state of *Cryptococcus neoformans.* Mycologia *68*:821–833, 1976. A new species of *Filobasidiella,* the sexual state of *Cryptococcus neoformans* B and C serotypes. Mycologia *68*:943–946, 1976.
8. Moore, M., Russell, W. O., and Sachs, E.: Chronic leptomeningitis and ependymitis caused by an *Ustilago,* probably *U. zeae* (corn smut). Am. J. Pathol. *22*:761–773, 1946.
9. Preininger, T.: Durch maisbrand *(Ustilago maydis)* bedingte dermatomykose. Arch. Dermatol. Syph. *176*:109, 1937.
10. Restrepo, A., Greer, D. L., Robledo, M., et al.: Ulceration of the palate caused by a basidiomycete, *Schizophyllum commune.* Sabouraudia *9*:201–204, 1971.
11. Salfelder, K., de Roman, A. R., de Mendolovici, M., et al.: Inoculation of basidiomycetes into mice: Tissue reaction and survival of fungi in tissue. Mykosen *18*:417–424, 1975.
12. Speller, D. C. E., and MacIver, A. G.: Endocarditis caused by a *Coprinus* species: A fungus of the toadstool group. J. Med. Microbiol. *4*:370–374, 1971.
13. Wittich, F. W.: Further observations on allergy to smuts. Lancet *59*:382, 1939.

Adiospiromycosis

HISTORY

Adiospiromycosis refers to the in vivo development, without replication, of adioconidia from the inhaled aleurioconidia of species of the fungal genus *Chrysosporium.* Adiospore, or more properly adiaconidia, signifies the enlargement without replication of a fungal conidia under the influence of elevated temperature. Adiospiromycosis is the term used to indicate this development within an animal tissue.

The disease first was described in 1942 as occurring in desert rodents (*Perognathus* species and *Dipodomys merriami*) in Arizona.[7] The new fungus was called *Haplosporangium parvum* because of its resemblance to *Haplosporangium bisporale.* It later was determined to be a new genus and species, *Emmonsia parva,* by Ciferri and Montemartini[2] in 1959. A second species was described in 1960 as *Emmonsia crescens.*[8] The diameter of the adiospores of this species ranged up to 400 μm. This species was found to be very prevalent and worldwide in distribution.[9, 14] At present, the accepted names for the agents are *Chrysosporium parvum* and *Chrysosporium parvum* variety *crescens.*

About a dozen human infections have been described.[3, 4, 10, 11, 13, 15, 16] In general, these infections have been noted incidentally, but in a few cases involving children, the disease was quite severe. In one 11-year-old boy, functional impairment of the lung was present[10, 15]; in a 10-year-old boy, treatment was required, which consisted of inhalation of "mycophetin" (1 million units/24 hours), an aerosol containing nystatin, and amphotericin B for 10 days.[11]

ETIOLOGY, ECOLOGY, AND DISTRIBUTION

To date, only two agents have been identified that produce adioconidia in animal tissue: *E. parva* and *E. crescens* (*C. parvum* and *C. parvum* variety *crescens,* respectively). Both species are similar morphologically to species of the genus *Chrysosporium*[1] and now are classified in that genus. Other *Chrysosporium* species are unable to produce adioconidia under the influence of temperature. Some authors speculate that adiospores may serve for dissemination of the species[5, 10a] (Fig. 206–12).

CLINICAL DISEASE AND PATHOLOGY

Naturally occurring adiospiromycosis is restricted to the lungs. The conidia do not migrate, replicate, or disseminate, so lesions are found only in the endobronchial or alveolar spaces. When the initial inhaled dose is very large, enough tissue damage may be elicited so that conidia may end in intravascular spaces and be carried to other organs. Phagocytosis with dispersal to tracheal lymph nodes also could occur.[10]

When only a few conidia are present, little cellular response is evoked.[16] A few mononuclear cells are found in the area of the developing conidia. In time, a granuloma may be formed. A heavy dose of inhaled conidia evokes an alveolitis and pyogenic response, followed by granulomatosis.[7] In the original observations by Emmons and Ashburn,[7] adioconidia and spherules of *C. immitis* were found in the same granulomata.

In natural infections, the adioconidia of *C. parvum* are 10 to 13 μm in diameter. They are surrounded by mononuclear cells without other host reaction.

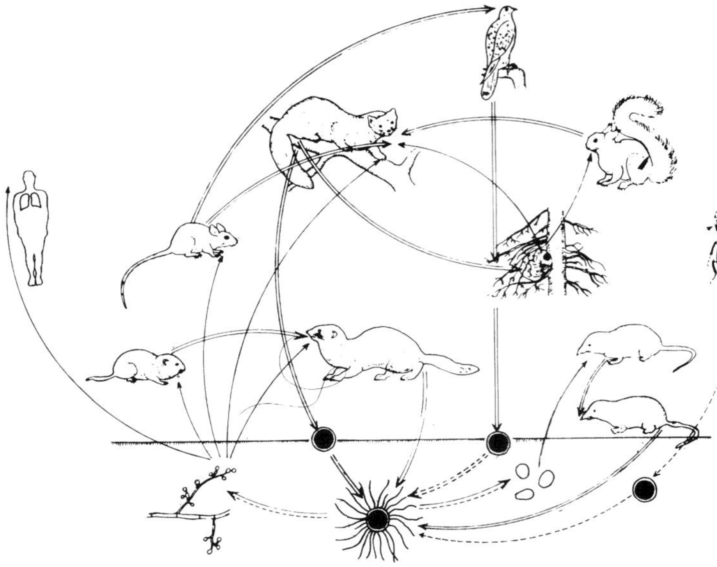

FIGURE 206–12. *Circulation of the fungus* Chrysosporium parvum *variety* crescens *in nature. Double solid lines with the arrow represent the circulation of the adiosporic stage in the predator food chain. The single solid line represents circulation of the mycelial stage and airborne aleuriospores. Dashed lines indicate other possible cycles. (From Krivanec, K., and Otcnasek, M.: Importance of free-living mustelid carnivores in circulation of adiospiromycosis. Mycopathologia 60:139–144, 1977.)*

C. parvum variety *crescens* in natural infections may attain a diameter of 220 μm[8] (Fig. 206–13). The conidia are surrounded by a few histiocytes and the compressed cells of the alveoli. In human infections when adioconidia are an incidental finding, a single conidium usually is found in the center of a tuberculoid granuloma. Such cases have been associated with some other lung disease, for example, cystic disease, tuberculosis, aspergillosis, hypertension, atheromatosis, silicosis, or metastasizing cancer. Rarely, the inhalation of large numbers of conidia has led to hundreds of thousands of adiospores that produce severe pulmonary disease.

MYCOLOGY

The taxonomy of the etiologic agent of adiospiromycosis is unsettled. In culture, the organism produces asexual conidia (aleurioconidia) of the *Chrysosporium* type. These conidia are similar to those produced by *Blastomyces dermatitidis, Paracoccidioides brasiliensis,* and numerous species of the genus *Chrysosporium.*[12] The genus *Emmonsia* was created to accommodate the two types of isolates that produce adioconidia. *E. crescens* and *E. parva* differ only in the size and nuclear number of the conidia within tissue. *E. parva* and *E. crescens* probably are one species and preferably are designated *C. parvum* and *C. parvum* variety *crescens.*[1]

Both strains vary considerably in colonial morphology. On peptone agar, they begin as a small, glabrous, whitish colony often tufted with white aerial hyphae. A diameter of 5 cm is reached by 2 weeks. The color varies from pinkish-brown and tan to dirty-white and yellowish.

On microscopic examination, the hyphae are septate and branching with a diameter of 0.5 to 2 μm. Numerous aleurioconidia are produced on conidiophores that arise at right angles to undifferentiated hyphae.[6] These conidia are spherical, although slightly flattened at the vertical axis, and are 3 to 3.5 μm in diameter. They may be covered with fine spines. Secondary and tertiary conidia may arise from these primary conidia by germination and production of short conidiophores. The conidia of variety *crescens* are reported to be somewhat larger (>4.5 μm) and more ovoid.

When placed on agar at 37° C, aleurioconidia or hyphal elements of *C. parvum* enlarge to adioconidia of 10 to 25 μm. Most of the hyphae disintegrate. If aleurioconidia are introduced into mice, uninucleate adioconidia greater than 40 μm will develop. If the same is done to aleurioconidia of *C. parvum* variety *crescens* in vitro, multinucleate adioconidia of 200 to 700 μm are produced. When in vivo in mice, a

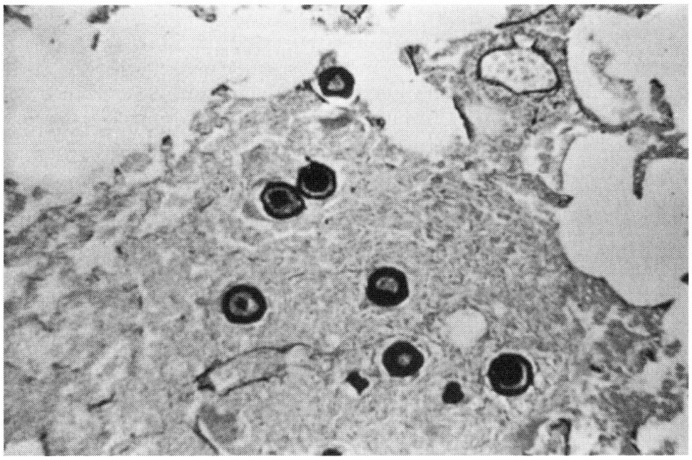

FIGURE 206–13. *Adiospiromycosis. Section of rat lung, which contains large vacuolated spherules surrounded by granulomata. (GMS × 60.)*

diameter of 400 to 600 μm is attained. If adiospores produced at 37° C are incubated at 25° C, numerous mycelial elements will germinate from them.

References

1. Carmichael, J. W.: *Chrysosporium* and some other aleurosporic hyphomycetes. Can. J. Bot. *40*:1137–1173, 1962.
2. Ciferri, R., and Montemartini, A.: Taxonomy of *Haplosporangium parvum*. Mycopathologia *10*:303–316, 1959.
3. Cueva, J. A., and Little, M. D.: *Emmonsia crescens* infection (adiaspiromycosis) in man in Honduras. Am. J. Trop. Med. *20*:282–287, 1971.
4. Doby-Dubois, M., Chevrel, M. L., Doby, J. M., et al.: Premier cas humain d'adiospiromycose par *Emmonsia crescens*. Bull. Soc. Pathol. Exot. *57*:240–244, 1964.
5. Dvorak, J., Otcenasek, M., and Rosicky, B.: Conception on the circulation of *Emmonsia crescens* Emmons and Jellison 1900 in nature. Folia Parsitol. (Praha) *13*:150–157, 1966.
6. Emmons, C. W.: Budding in *Emmonsia crescens*. Mycologia *56*:415–419, 1964.
7. Emmons, C. W., and Ashburn, L. L.: The isolation of *Haplosporangium parvum* sp. and *Coccidioides immitis* from wild rodents. U.S. Public Health Rep. *57*:1715–1727, 1942.
8. Emmons, C. W., and Jellison, W. L.: *Emmonsia crescens* sp. nov. and adiospiromycosis (haplomycosis) in mammals. Ann. N. Y. Acad. Sci. *89*(Art. 1):91–101, 1960.
9. Jellison, W. L., and Vinson, J. W.: The distribution of *Emmonsia crescens* in Europe. Mycologia *53*:524–535, 1961.
10. Kodousek, R., and Vojtek, V.: Systemic pulmonary adiospiromycosis caused by *E. crescens*. Cas. Lek. Cesk. *109*:923–924, 1970.
10a. Krivanec, K., and Otcnasek, M.: Importance of free-living mustelid carnivores in circulation of adiospiromycosis. Mycopathologia *60*:139–144, 1977.
11. Leshchenko, V. M., and Sheklakov, N. D.: Adiaspromikoz (English abstract). Vestn. Dermatol. Venerol. *6*:46–52, 1974.
12. Padhye, A. A., and Carmichael, J. W.: *Emmonsia brasiliensis* and *Emmonsia ciferrina* are *Chrysoporium pruinosum*. Mycologia *60*:445–447, 1968.
13. Salfelder, K., Fingerland, A., de Mendelovici, M., et al.: Two cases of adiospiromycosis. Beitr. Pathol. *148*:94–100, 1973.
14. Taylor, R. L., and Cavanaugh, D. C.: Adiospiromycosis in small mammals of Viet Nam. Mycologia *60*:450–451, 1968.
15. Vojtek, V., Kodousek, R., Fingerland, A., et al.: L'adiospiromycose pulmonaire chez enfant de II ans. J. Franc. Med. Chirurg. Thorac. *26*:383–388, 1972.
16. Watts, J. C., Callaway, C. S., Chandler, F. W., et al.: Human pulmonary adiospiromycosis. Arch. Pathol. *99*:11–15, 1975.

Rhinosporidiosis

Rhinosporidiosis is an infection of the mucocutaneous tissue caused by an organism given the name *Rhinosporidium seeberi*. The organism has not been cultivated or classified satisfactorily, but presumably it is a fungus. The disease that results is characterized by the production of polyps, tumors, papillomas, or wart-like vegetative growth that is hyperplastic, highly vascularized, friable, and sessile or pedunculated. The sites involved most frequently are the nose and conjunctiva. Infection of the nose is common in damp tropical climates, whereas conjunctivitis is more common in dry, dusty areas. Infection of the anus, penis, vagina, ears, pharynx, and larynx may occur. The disease first was described independently in Tennessee, India, and Argentina.[3, 10, 14, 17, 20]

ETIOLOGY, ECOLOGY, AND DISTRIBUTION

To date, all efforts to cultivate *R. seeberi* have failed. From time to time, reports are made of its replication in vitro, but these lack substantiation.[5, 15]

Clustering of cases seems to occur, and in many epidemiologic studies, an association with immersion in stagnant pools or streams of fresh water was noted. Study of a group of sand workers found that those who dove into the water to recover the sand had a high rate of infection. In contrast, those who worked on the banks had an attack rate that was normal for the area.

When the world literature was reviewed in 1964 by Karunaratne,[7] 2000 cases had been recorded. Of these, 88 per cent were from India and Ceylon. Allen and Dave[2] reported 60 cases in an 18-month period in India. South America, particularly Brazil[11] and Argentina,[12] also had endemic areas. About 40 reports came from the United States. The nose was involved in half of these cases and the conjunctiva in the remainder. Most of the cases of conjunctival involvement occurred in Texas or the Southwest.[13] Cases have been reported in Canada, Mexico,[4] Europe, Russia, Iran, Ghana, South Africa, and Kenya and sporadically throughout most of the world.

Although the age of patients has ranged from 3 to 90 years, the age bracket in most cases was 20 to 40 years. The lesions develop very slowly and without symptoms or distress; thus, most infections probably begin in childhood. Infection also has been noted in many animal species.[19]

CLINICAL DISEASE

The exact mechanism of infection is not known, but it appears that some initial injury to the nose or conjunctiva may predispose to invasion. The most common site of infection is the mucous membrane of the septum, inferior turbinate, and floor of the nasal cavity. The only symptom apparent for years is the feeling that a foreign body is present. In time, the lesion may grow (Fig. 206–14) and change from sessile to pedunculated (Fig. 206–15). The lesions are bright to dark red, highly vascularized, and friable and contain numerous whitish, macroscopically visible spherules. Lesions often are spleen-like in appearance. As growth continues, the mass may hang down from the meatus of the nose and have the appearance of a ripe fig. Weights up to 20 g have been recorded. Mucous secretions may be voluminous, and because the lesions are friable, these may be blood stained.

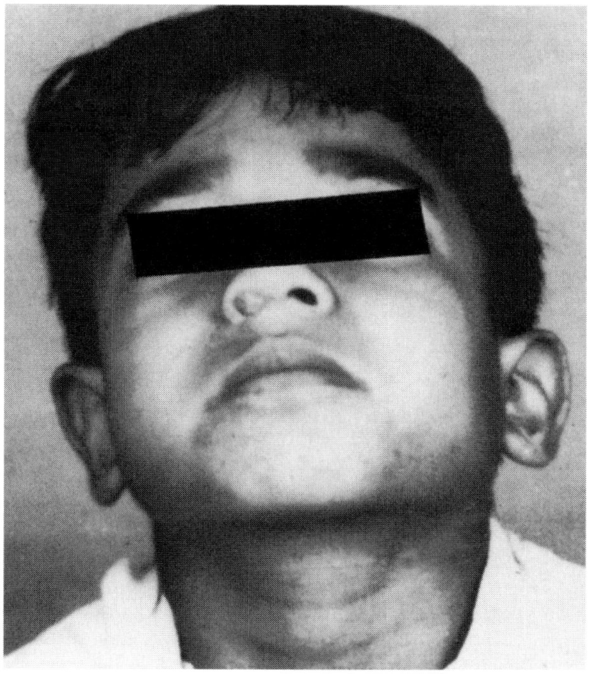

FIGURE 206–14. *Rhinosporidiosis. Polyp developing in nose. (Courtesy of S. Banerjee.)*

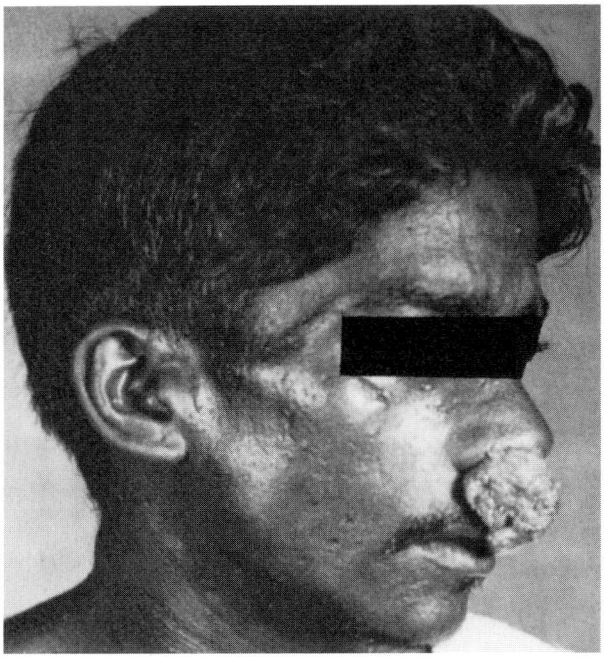

FIGURE 206–15. *Rhinosporidiosis. Pedunculated polypoid tumor. (Courtesy of C. Satyanarayana.)*

Infection in other areas develops similarly. If the conjunctiva is involved (most often the palpebral), the lesions grow and conform to the anatomic space. Pedunculated lesions hanging out of the penis, vagina, and rectum are reported.[8] Autoinoculation from scratching has led to involvement of the skin, although this is rare. A significant number of cases involve the larynx,[9] pharynx, uvula, and bronchi. Enlarging lesions may lead to interference with breathing or swallowing. A case in which spherules occurred in the brain, lung, skin, and muscle (by hematogenous dissemination) has been reported.[1]

The gross appearance of lesions is similar to that of ordinary nasal polyps. However, in rhinosporidiosis, the tissue is dense and mucous cysts are absent. In histologic sections, it can be seen that the layers of transitional epithelium often are invaginated, and flask-shaped cysts are formed. These contain leukocytes, spores, and mucinous material. Mature sporangia lie near the thinned epithelial borders (Fig. 206–16*A*). The cellular infiltrate consists of plasma cells, lymphocytes, histiocytes, and neutrophils. The mature spores are released through a pore from the mature spherule (see Fig. 206–16*B*). These course across the surface and lodge in tissue. The spore now enlarges to 6 to 10 μm, the "trophic" stage. This grows to 50 μm, and nuclear divisions begin. At maximum size (250 to 350 μm), as many as 16,000 endospores may be present.

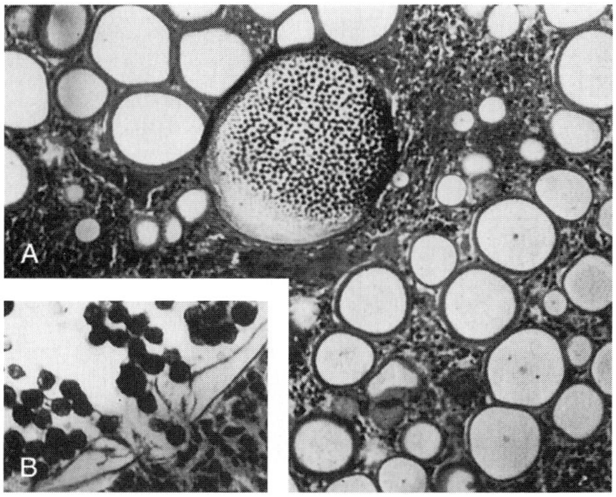

FIGURE 206–16. *Rhinosporidiosis.* A, *Spherule with maturing endospores among immature spherules.* B, *Extrusion of spores through micropyle. (GMS × 200.) (From Londero, A. T., Santos, M. N., and Freitas, C. J.: Animal rhinosporidiosis in Brazil. Mycopathologia 60:171–173, 1977.)*

The spherules of *R. seeberi* are seen easily in sections stained with hematoxylin and eosin. These also are stained by the Gomori methenamine silver, Gridley, and periodic acid–Schiff methods. Early trophic cysts lack chitin and are not stained by periodic acid–Schiff or Gridley but are demonstrable by Gomori methenamine silver stain. The inner cellulose-like material of the spherule is stained by mucicarmine; this is the only medically important fungus, except the capsule of *Cryptococcus neoformans,* to stain distinctly by this method.

The only successful treatment has been surgical removal of the infected tissue. This is carried out with use of a hot or cold snare for avoidance of spreading infection to adjacent tissue.[6, 16] Recurrences are common, and copious bleeding, secondary bacterial infection, and fatal sepsis are hazards of treatment.

MYCOLOGY

R. seeberi[18] has not been grown in culture.

References

1. Agrawal, S. K., Sharma, D., and Shrivastava, J. B.: Generalized rhinosporidiosis with visceral involvement: Report of a case. Arch. Dermatol. *80*:22–26, 1959.
2. Allen, F. R., and Dave, M.: Treatment of rhinosporidiosis in man based on sixty cases. Ind. Med. Gaz. *71*:376–395, 1936.
3. Ashworth, J. H.: On *Rhinosporidium seeberi* (Wernicke 1903) with special reference to its sporulation and affinities. Trans. R. Soc. Edinburgh *53*:301–342, 1923.
4. Gonzalez-Mendoza, A.: Rhinosporidiosis en Mexico revision de la literatura nacional y comentarios epidemiologicos a propositio de la observation de dos neuvos cases. Bol. Soc. Mex. Mic. *9*:149–153, 1975.
5. Grover, S.: *Rhinosporidium seeberi:* A preliminary study of the morphology and life cycle. Sabouraudia *7*:249–251, 1970.
6. Kameswaran, S.: Surgery in rhinosporidiosis: Experience with 293 cases. Int. Surg. *46*:602–605, 1966.
7. Karunaratne, W. A. E.: Rhinosporidiose in Man. London, University of London, The Atheone Press, 1973.
8. Kutty, M. K., and Unni, P. N.: Rhinosporidiosis of the urethra: A case report. Trop. Geogr. Med. *21*:338–340, 1969.
9. Lasser, A., and Smith, H. W.: Rhinosporidiosis. Arch. Otolaryngol. *102*:308–310, 1976.
9a. Londero, A. T., Santos, M. N., and Freitas, C. J.: Animal rhinosporidiosis in Brazil. Mycopathologia *60*:171–173, 1977.
10. Minchin, E. A., and Fanthum, H. B.: *Rhinosporidium kinealyi* n.g.n. gp.: A new sporozoan from the mucous membrane of the septum nasi of man. J. Microbiol. Sci. *49*:521–532, 1905.
11. Moses, J. S., Balachandran, C., Singh, B., et al.: *Rhinosporidum seeberi*: Light phase contrast, fluorescent and scanning electron microscopic study. Mycopathologia *114*:17–20, 1991.
12. Nino, F. L., and Friere, R. S.: Exienciade un faco endemico de rhinosporidiosis en la provencia del Choco. V. Estudio de nuevas observaciones y consideraciones finales. Mycopathologia *24*:92–102, 1964.
13. Norman, W. B.: Rhinosporidiosis in Texas. Arch. Otolaryngol. *72*:361–363, 1960.
14. O'Kinealy, F.: Localized psorospermosis of the mucous membrane of the septum nasi. Proc. Laryngol. Soc. London *10*:109–112, 1903.
15. Rao, S. N.: *Rhinosporidium seeberi*: A histochemical study. Indian J. Exp. Biol. *4*:10–14, 1966.

16. Satyanarayana, C.: Rhinosporidiosis. *In* Rob, C., and Smith, R. (eds.): Clinical Surgery. London, Butterworth, 1966.
17. Seeber, G. R.: Un nuevo esporozuario parasito del hombre: Dos casos en contrades eu polipos nasales. Tesis Univ. Nat. de Buenos Aires, 1900.
18. Seeber, G. R.: *Rhinosporidium kinealyi* et *Rhinosporidium seeberi*. Une question de priorté. Buenos Aires, 1912.
19. Stuart, B. P., and Malley, N. O.: Rhinosporidiosis in a dog. J. Am. Vet. Med. Assoc. *167*:941–942, 1975.
20. Wright, J.: A nasal sporozoon, *Rhinosporidium kinealyi*. N. Y. Med. J. *86*:1149–1153, 1907.

Geotrichosis

This is a very rare opportunistic infection caused by the yeast-like hyphomycete *Geotrichum candidum.* The organism is ubiquitous and may be found in the soil or air or as part of the normal human flora. For many years, hundreds of reports have been published linking the organism to a variety of diseases. Unfortunately, in the great majority of such cases, the pathogenic role of the fungus was not substantiated, and its delineation from *Candida albicans* or *Trichosporon beigelii* often is confused.

Bennett[1] in 1842 recovered the organism from a superinfection of an old cavity of tuberculous origin and differentiated it from *Candida.* There probably are no more than three dozen cases of well-documented geotrichosis in the world literature.[8]

ETIOLOGY, ECOLOGY, AND DISTRIBUTION

G. candidum first was isolated from decaying leaves in 1809. The concept of the genus has gone through many changes over the years, and several species have been named.[3, 7]

It is one of the most ubiquitous fungal organisms in the world and may be recovered from feces, vaginal secretions, saliva, swabs of normal skin, and bronchial secretions. It also is recovered regularly from cottage cheese, dairy products, ripe fruits, and pickle brine. Because it is omnipresent, it is very difficult to establish its role as the etiologic agent of disease.

CLINICAL DISEASE

Pulmonary Geotrichosis

Approximately 24 reports of pulmonary geotrichosis have appeared.[5, 8] Most of these were superinfections of preexisting

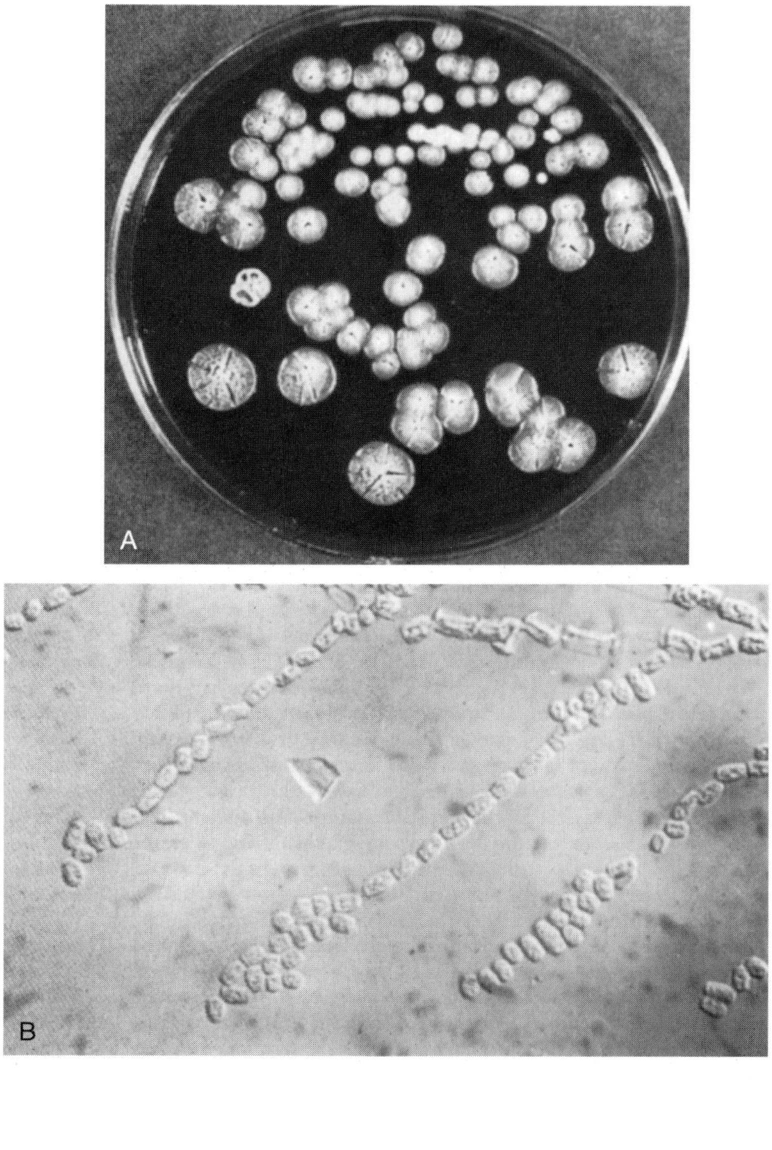

FIGURE 206–17. Geotrichum candidum. A, *Colonies on blood agar.* B, *Fragmentation of mycelium into arthrospores. (Courtesy of S. McMillen.)*

cavitary disease due to tuberculosis or sarcoidosis. There usually is little or no fever or sputum production. If sputum is produced, it is light gray, thick, and mucoid. The chest radiograph may show patchy or dense infiltrates, and fine rales may be heard.[10] The infection usually is chronic, and serious disease is rare. It may be treated with amphotericin B.[8]

Bronchial Geotrichosis

This is an endobronchial infection not involving the lungs. Patchy peribronchial thickenings are seen on radiograph. Medium to coarse rales are heard. Other symptoms include chronic cough and gelatinous sputum, but there is no fever. Organisms are visible on direct examination of sputum.[8, 11]

Oral lesions have been recorded that are identical to the lesions of thrush. Sometimes there is an overgrowth of *Geotrichum* on lesions of chronic candidiasis.[8] A case of gastrointestinal overgrowth was associated with glutamic acid therapy.[9] Symptoms of enterocolitis disappeared with cessation of this therapy. Colonization of soft tissue after a skin graft has been noted.[6]

PATHOLOGY

In a case of disseminated geotrichosis occurring as an opportunistic infection in a patient with carcinoma of the colon, lesions were found throughout the body.[4] Infection of the colonic mucosa adjacent to the carcinoma was considered the point of entry for the organism. The lesions appeared as necrotic foci in the heart, lungs, and spleen. On microscopic examination, suppuration and necrosis were present. Organisms resembling *Geotrichum* were seen.

The arthrospores are 4 to 8 μm in diameter, have square to rounded ends, and may be seen to bud. However, these buds develop into septate mycelium; true blastospore formation is not found. Arthrospores are seen in sputum, pus, or lesions by direct examination of specimens.

MYCOLOGY

Geotrichum grows as a dry, mealy, white to cream-colored colony at 25° C. At 37° C, growth is very slow and subsurface (Fig. 206–17*A*). The mycelium breaks up into chains of arthroconidia 4 to 8 μm (see Fig. 206–17*B*), and spherical cells (chlamydoconidia) from 4 to 10 μm also are found. Sugars are not fermented, but a number of carbohydrates are assimilated. The perfect stage has been described.[2]

References

1. Bennett, J. H.: On the parasitic fungi found growing in living animals. Trans. R. Soc. Edinburgh *15*:277–298, 1842.
2. Butler, E. E., and Petersen, L. J.: *Endomyces geotrichum*, a perfect state of *Geotrichum candidum*. Mycologia *64*:365–375, 1971.
3. Carmichael, J. W.: *Geotrichum candidum*. Mycologia *49*:820–829, 1957.
4. Chang, W. W. L., and Buerger, I. L.: Disseminated geotrichosis: Case report. Arch. Intern. Med. *113*:356–360, 1964.
5. Fishbach, R. S., White, M. L., and Finegold, S. M.: Bronchopulmonary geotrichosis. Am. Rev. Respir. Dis. *108*:1388–1392, 1973.
6. Goldman, S., and Lipscomb, R. R.: *Geotrichum* tumefaction of the hand. J. Bone Joint Surg. *51*:587–590, 1969.
7. Gueho, E., and Bussiere, J.: Methode d'identification biochimique de champignons filamenteaux arthrospores apportenant au genre *Geotrichum* link ex pers. Ann. Microbiol. (Paris) *126*:483–500, 1975.
8. Morenz, S.: Geotrichosis. *In* Baker, R. D. (ed.): Handbuch der Speziellen Pathologischen Anatomie. Vol. 3. Berlin, Springer-Verlag, 1971.
9. Neagoe, G., and Neagoe, M.: Enterokolitis durch *Geotrichum candidum* nach therapie mit glutaminsäure. Dtsch. Z. Verdau Stoffwechselkr. *27*:205–208, 1967.
10. Ross, J. D., and Reid, K. D. G.: Bronchopulmonary geotrichosis with severe asthma. Br. Med. J. *1*:1400–1402, 1966.
11. Webster, B. H.: Bronchopulmonary geotrichosis: A review of four cases. Dis. Chest *35*:273–281, 1959.

Protothecosis

Protothecosis is a rare infection caused by species of the achloric alga genus *Prototheca*. The organisms are ubiquitous in nature and may be recovered as a contaminant from clinical material.[2, 6]

In 1952, Lerche[8] reported a case of bovine mastitis due to *P. zopfii*. Twelve years later, the first human infection was recorded in Sierra Leone.[4, 5] It was seen in a rice farmer in a condition similar to mossy foot.[4] Originally designated a new species, *P. subgwema*, the organism, since has been identified as *P. wickerhamii*.[1] A femoral lymph gland also contained the organism. Since then, about 60 more cases have been recorded. Most of these were cutaneous or subcutaneous infections. The most common site of infection is the olecranon process,[12] with a few reports of involvement of the legs,[7, 11] forehead,[3, 9] face,[10] and arms.[16] Systemic disease has been reported,[3] and several cases of opportunistic infection are known. Disease has been noted in dogs, deer, and cattle.[15]

The cutaneous lesions usually are rugose papules with raised edges.[5] They slowly advance, with scar formation and fibrosis developing in the center. Dome-shaped verrucous growths[9] (Fig. 206–18) or confluent papules forming a plaque also have been described.[9, 17] Tissue reaction as seen on histologic examination may reveal minimal cellular response, chronic granulomatous inflammation,[3, 9] or mixed acute and chronic granulomatous inflammation[9, 10, 12] with eosinophils.[4, 9]

In the reported case of systemic disease,[3] *P. wickerhamii* was isolated from scrapings of the forehead, peritoneal nodules, nose biopsy, and blood culture (Fig. 206–19). Cell-mediated immunity was depressed in the patient. Other cases of opportunistic infection have been documented.[7, 16]

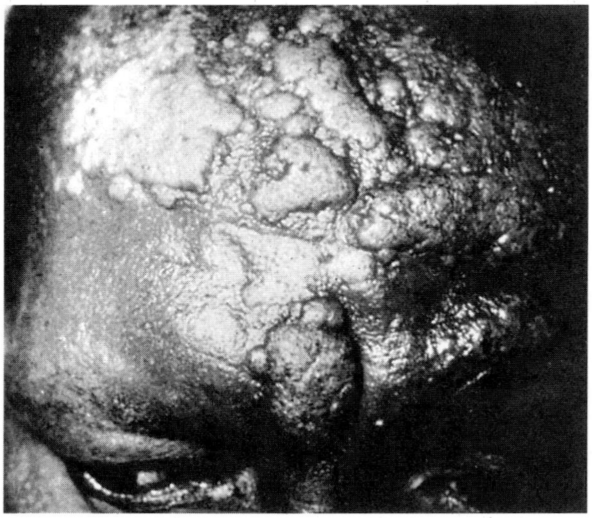

FIGURE 206–18. *Protothecosis. Lesions on forehead and scalp. (From Mars, P. W., Rabson, A. R., Rippey, J. J., et al.: Cutaneous protothecosis. Br. J. Dermatol. 85:76–84, 1971.)*

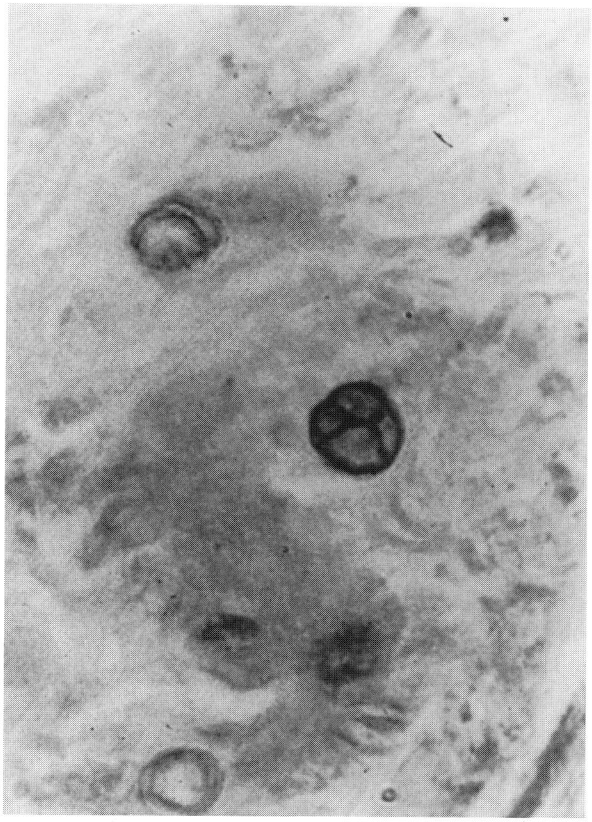

FIGURE 206–19. Prototheca wickerhamii *in cutaneous tissue. (PAS × 400.) (Courtesy of L. Ajello.)*

The organisms are identified readily in tissue. They are large (8 to 20 μm in diameter), nonbudding, round to elliptical cells. As they mature, the round cells (theca) will contain a number of autospores (similar to the process in *Chlorella*) and have a morula (raspberry-like) appearance. They stain by the periodic acid–Schiff or Gomori methenamine silver method.

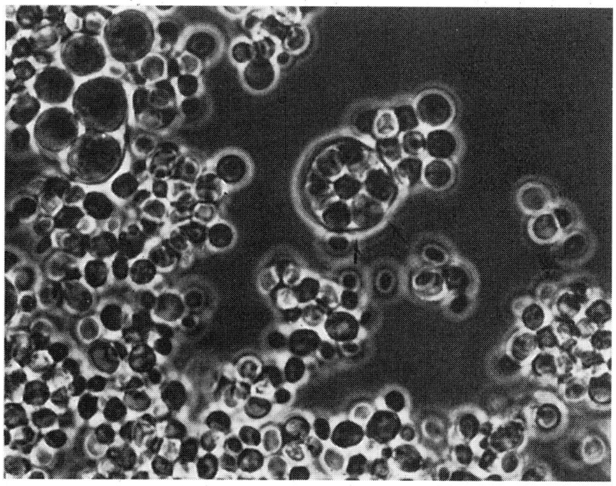

FIGURE 206–20. Prototheca wickerhamii *in various stages of development from culture. A mature theca and autospores are indicated by the arrows. (Courtesy of M. Feo.)*

Treatment regimens have included surgery and various antibiotics. If the cutaneous lesions are small, surgical excision is curative. Extensive lesions require medical management. The several species of *Prototheca* are reported to be sensitive to amphotericin B and nystatin at static levels of 1.25 to 3 μg/mL and cidal levels of 5 μg/mL, up to 12.5 μg/mL.[3, 10, 14] Davies and associates[4] reported that their isolate was sensitive to 5 to 10 μg/mL of pentamidine, but treatment with this drug failed. Successful treatment with low-dosage (6.6 mg over 5 weeks) amphotericin B has been reported.[3, 9, 17] Transfer factor was added to the regimen in two cases.[3, 17] The organism is resistant to flucytosine, griseofulvin, rifampin, miconazole, and tetracycline[10, 15] but is sensitive to 1 μg/mL of polymyxin B.

P. zopfii and *P. wickerhamii* both grow as moist, cream-colored colonies at 25° C. Optimal growth occurs at 30° C. The cells vary from 8 to 24 × 10 to 26 μm in size for *P. zopfii* to 8 to 13 × 10 to 16 μm for *P. wickerhamii. P. wickerhamii* has more autospores (as many as 50 per theca).

Multiplication occurs by single or multiple nuclear divisions, followed by cytoplasmic cleavage and spore formation (Fig. 206–20). At first there are two to eight uninucleate daughter cells within the theca, with subsequent divisions to 20 to 50 autocells. These increase in size and cause the wall of the mother cell to burst, freeing the daughter cells.[1]

A selective medium for the isolation of *Prototheca* has been formulated by Pore.[13]

P. filamenta has been recovered from athlete's foot infection, but it was not incriminated as a cause of the infection.[16] It has been transferred to a new genus, *Fissuracella,* by Pore and colleagues[14] and redesignated a yeast. It has been isolated from scrotal dermatoses *(Trichosporon inkin),* skin lesions, and bone marrow.

References

1. Arnold, P., and Ahearn, D. G.: The systemics of the genus *Prototheca* with a description of a new species, *P. filamenta.* Mycologia *64*:265–276, 1972.
2. Ashford, B. K., Ciferri, R., and Dalman, M. L.: A new species of *Prototheca* and a variety of some isolated from human intestine. Arch. Protisten. *70*:619–638, 1930.
3. Cox, G. E., Wilson, J. D., and Brown, P.: Protothecosis, a case of disseminated algal infection. Lancet *2*:379–382, 1974.
4. Davies, R. R., Spencer, H., and Wakelin, P. O.: A case of human protothecosis. Trans. R. Soc. Trop. Med. Hyg. *58*:448–451, 1964.
5. Davies, R. R., and Wilkinson, J. L.: Human protothecosis: Supplementary studies. Ann. Trop. Med. Parasitol. *61*:112–115, 1967.
6. Feo, M.: Cinco cepas de prototheca de origen humano. Mycopathologia *46*:53–59, 1972.
7. Klintworth, G. K., Fetter, B. F., and Nielsen, J. S.: Protothecosis, an algal infection in man. J. Med. Microbiol. *1*:211–216, 1968.
8. Lerche, M.: Einen durch algen nervorgerufene mastitis der kuh. Berl. Münch. Med. Wochenschr. *65*:64–69, 1952.
9. Mars, P. W., Rabson, A. R., Rippey, J. J., et al.: Cutaneous protothecosis. Br. J. Dermatol. *85*:76–84, 1971.
10. Mayhall, C. G., Miller, C. W., Eisen, A. Z., et al.: Cutaneous protothecosis: Successful treatment with amphotericin B. Arch. Dermatol. *112*:1749–1752, 1976.
11. Nabrai, H., and Mehregan, A. H.: Cutaneous protothecosis: Report of a case from Iran. J. Cutan. Pathol. *1*:180–185, 1974.
12. Nosanchuk, J. S., and Greenberg, R. D.: Protothecosis of the olecranon bursa caused by a chloric algae. Am. J. Clin. Pathol. *59*:567–573, 1973.
13. Pore, S.: Selective medium for isolation of *Prototheca.* Appl. Microbiol. *26*:648–649, 1973.
14. Pore, R. S., D'Amato, R. F., and Ajello, L.: *Fissuracella* gen. nov., a new taxon for *Prototheca filamenta.* Sabouraudia *15*:69–78, 1977.
15. Segel, E., Padhye, A. A., and Ajello, L.: Susceptibility of *Prototheca* species to antifungal agents. Antimicrob. Agents Chemother. *10*:75–79, 1976.
16. Sudman, M. S.: Protothecosis: A critical review. Am. J. Clin. Pathol. *61*:10–19, 1974.
17. Wolfe, I. D., Sacks, H. G., Samorodin, C. S., et al.: Cutaneous protothecosis in a patient receiving immunosuppressive therapy. Arch. Dermatol. *112*:829–832, 1976.

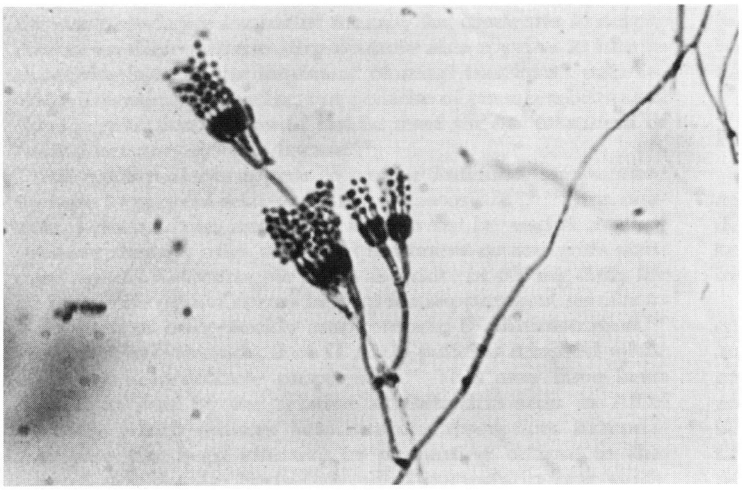

FIGURE 206–21. Penicillium *species conidiophore showing asymmetric branching, giving rise to metulae that bear phialide sterigmata. These produce a chain of conidia.*

Penicilliosis

Documented infections by members of the genus *Penicillium* are very rare. After inhalation, the conidia of *Penicillium* remain viable for long periods. They can be isolated repeatedly from sputum samples of patients after exposure to conidia-containing dust. This probably accounts for most of the reports of bronchopulmonary penicilliosis.[4, 7, 10, 11, 13–16, 18, 20–25] In personal experience, three cases of "pulmonary penicilliosis" were traced to an inadequately sterilized bronchial brush. Isolation of contaminants or transient colonization probably led to the description of *Penicillium* causation of mycetoma,[19] otomycosis,[26] and mycotic keratitis.

The ubiquity of *Penicillium* species and the ease of isolation from a variety of human material has led to a long list of human "penicillioses." In surveying sputum from several hundred normal patients, Comstock and colleagues[3] recovered *Penicillium* species in 80 per cent of specimens. It has been recovered in blood cultures from compromised patients receiving intravenous therapy[27] and regularly from intestinal[6] and vaginal cultures. The frequency of isolation from vaginal cultures has led to association with a syndrome called endometritis mycotica.[17] There is no evidence that *Penicillium* species or any other fungus or yeast is responsible for this disease entity. In well-documented cases of vaginal candidiasis, other fungi, including *Penicillium* species, often are isolated as contaminants (Fig. 206–21).

In two cases, *Penicillium* species (*P. citrinum* and *P. glaucum*) have been recovered as a voided "bolus" in urinary tract infections. In both reports, colonization of the bladder occurred after trauma and stasis,[2, 9] and these "infections" resolved spontaneously.

Huang and Harris[11] described a systemic mycosis as a terminal event in an acute blast crisis in a patient with leukemia. Radiating, septate, dichotomously branching mycelium and conglomerates of crystals were seen in necrotic lesions of the lung. Hyphae also were found in thrombotic and hemorrhagic infarcts of the right superior frontal gyrus. *P. commune* was isolated from cultures taken of lung tissue. A "blue dot" dermatophyte-like disease of the scalp was reported by Leavell and associates.[12] *Penicillium* species and *Aureobasidium pullulans* were recovered from several cultures.

An infection that unequivocally was due to *Penicillium* was described in 1973 by DiSalvo and colleagues[5] (Fig. 206–22). At 25° C, the fungus, named *P. marneffei*, grows as a wrinkled, folded, grayish colony produced with a reddish-stained mycelium and gray-green conidia. A diffusable, brownish to cerise pigment is produced. The conidiophores are of the asymmetrica divaricata type. The phialides are 9 to 11 μm in size, and the smooth globose conidia are 2 μm in diameter.[1] At 37° C, the organism grows as a whitish, glabrous, yeast-

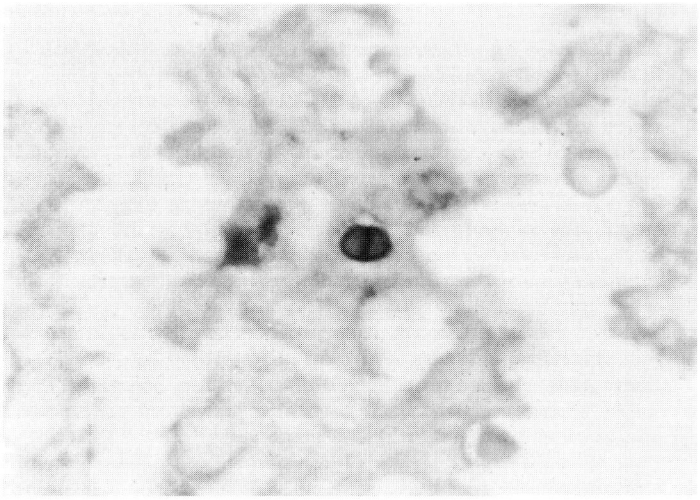

FIGURE 206–22. Penicillium marneffei *planate dividing yeast-like cell from liver biopsy of patient. (× 440.) (From DiSalvo, A. F., Fickling, A., and Ajello, L.: Infection caused by* Penicillium marneffei. *Am. J. Clin. Pathol. 60:259–263, 1973.)*

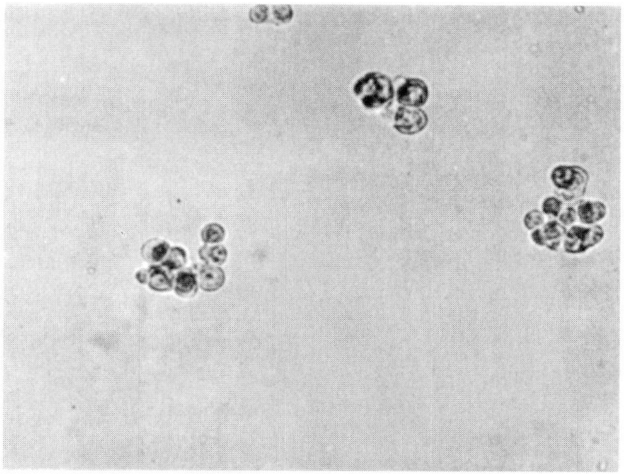

FIGURE 206–23. Penicillium *species in forced yeast phase grow at 37° C. It is able to cause systemic disease in mice in this form. (From Rippon, J. W., Conway, T. P., and Domes, A. L.: Pathogenic potential of* Aspergillus *and* Penicillium *species. J. Infect. Dis. 115:27–32, 1965.)*

like colony. The cells are 4 to 5 μm in diameter and replicate by planate division. The internal structure is similar to that of *Histoplasma* and *Blastomyces* yeast cells.[5, 8] The morphologic appearance was identical to that described in the animal infection.

Penicillium species can be grown as a yeast at 37° C. (Fig. 206–23). In this form, the organism can produce systemic disease in experimentally infected mice.[19]

References

1. Capponi, M., Sareau, P., and Segretain, G.: Penicilliose de rhizomys sinesis. Bull. Soc. Pathol. Exot. *49*:418–421, 1956.
2. Chute, A. L.: An infection of the bladder with *Penicillium glaucum.* Boston Med. Surg. J. *164*:420–422, 1911.
3. Comstock, G. W., Palmer, C. E., Stone, R. W., et al.: Fungi in the sputum of normal men. Mycopathologia *54*:55–62, 1974.
4. Delore, P., Condet, J., Lambert, R., et al.: Un cas de mycose bronchique avec localizations muscularies septicemiques. Presse Med. *63*:1580–1582, 1955.
5. DiSalvo, A. F., Fickling, A., and Ajello, L.: Infection caused by *Penicillium marneffei.* Am. J. Clin. Pathol. *60*:259–263, 1973.
6. Emami, M., Hohsenine, H., and Parvine, N.: Recherche sur les champignons de l'appareil digestif des jeunes gens. Med. Trop. *35*:407–410, 1975.
7. Garreton, U. E.: Un caso de bronquitis micotica a *Penicillium.* Ann. Med. Concepcion *2*:103–105, 1945.
8. Garrison, R. G., and Boyd, K. S.: Dimorphism of *Penicillium marneffei* as observed by electron microscope. Can. J. Microbiol. *19*:1305–1309, 1973.
9. Gilliam, J. S., Jr., and Vest, S. A.: *Penicillium* infection of the urinary tract. J. Urol. *65*:484–489, 1951.
10. Giordano, M.: Un caso di micosi polmonare de *Penicillium glaucum.* Ann. Med. Roma *2*:912–917, 1918.
11. Huang, S. N., and Harris, L. S.: Acute disseminated penicilliosis. Am. J. Clin. Pathol. *39*:167–174, 1963.
12. Leavell, U. W., Tucker, E. B., and Muelling, R.: Blue dot infection of the scalp in two brothers. J. Kentucky Med. Assoc. *64*:1107–1110, 1966.
13. Maddoux, G. L., Mohr, J. A., and Muchmore, H. G.: Pulmonary penicilliosis: A case presentation and review of the literature. J. Oklahoma State Med. Assoc. *65*:418–421, 1972.
14. Mantrelli, C., and Negri, G.: Ricerche spermentali sull' agente eziologico di' un micetoma a grani negri *(Penicillium mycetogenum)* n. f. G. Acad. Med. Torino *21*:161–167, 1955.
15. Nino, F. L.: Broncomicosis penicilliar. Semena Med. *2*:1015–1020, 1932.
16. Nussbaum, R., and Benedek, T.: Pneumono mycosis penicillima eine gewerbe krankheit zum kapitel der lungengeschwülte. Beitr. Klin. Tuberk. *67*:756–770, 1927.
17. Ostrzensk, A.: Endometritis mycotica-rozpoz-nawanie i syniki leczenica. Ginekol. Pol. *45*:1113–1116, 1974.
18. Polyanskiy, L. N.: A case of otogenic abscess of the temporal lobe of the brain produced by *Penicillium.* Zhur. Ush. Nos. Gorl. Bolez. *15*:138–140, 1938.
19. Rippon, J. W., Conway, T. P., and Domes, A. L.: Pathogenic potential of *Aspergillus* and *Penicillium* species. J. Infect. Dis. *115*:27–32, 1965.
20. da Silva Lacaz, C.: Consideragoes sobre um caso di peniciliose pulmonar. Hospital Rio de Janeiro *15*:327–339, 1939.
21. Segretain, G.: *Penicillium marneffei* n. sp., agent d'une mycose du systeme reticuloendothelial. Mycopathologia *11*:327–353, 1959.
22. Segretain, G.: Description d'une nouvelle espece de Penicillium: *Penicillium marneffei* n. sp. Bull. Soc. Mycol. France *75*:414–416, 1959.
23. Segretain, G.: Some new or infrequent fungous pathogens. *In* Dalldorf, G. (ed.): Fungi and Fungous Diseases. Springfield, IL, Charles C Thomas, 1962.
24. Talice, R. V., and Mackinnon, J. E.: *Penicillium bertai* (I) n.sp., agent d'une mycose bronchopulmonaire de' l'homme. Ann. Parasitol. *7*:97–106, 1929.
25. Virchow, R.: Beitraege zur lehre von den beim menschen verkommenden pflanzlichen parasiten. Arch. Pathol. Anat. *9*:557–593, 1856.
26. Wolf, F.: Relation of various fungi to otomycosis. Arch. Otolaryngol. *46*:361–374, 1947.
27. Young, R. C., Bennett, J. E., Geelhoed, G. W., et al.: Fungemia with compromised host resistance: A study of 70 cases. Ann. Intern. Med. *80*:605–612, 1974.

Hyalohyphomycosis

As noted in the introductory text, more and more species of fungi are being isolated from human disease processes, particularly opportunistic infection (see Table 206–1). To simplify nomenclature, such rarely encountered entities should be included in the general category of hyalohyphomycosis. Hyalohyphomycosis is a fungus infection in which mycelium is seen in tissue sections.

Scopulariopsis brevicaulis is a very common soil organism. It produces an annelid 3 to 4 × 8 to 20 μm in size that tapers to the fertile tip, which is swollen just below the point of conidium formation. The conidia are large, 6 to 9 μm in diameter, and top shaped, with verrucous, tuberculate, or warty projections. Long chains are formed. The colony grows rapidly and produces masses of conidia. This fungus is seen occasionally as a secondary invader in onycholytic onychomycosis.[13, 18] In such nails, hyphae 2 to 10 μm in diameter may be found. Other diseases ascribed to the organism are ulcerating granulomata and granulomatous inflammation of the tendon sheath and muscle.[12, 16] Many strains of *S. brevicaulis* have been shown to be pathogenic for mice.[7]

Scopulariopsis brumptii has been recovered from multiple granulomata in the lung of a patient who had injected himself with a crude opium preparation.[8] The organism did not reproduce in tissue but remained viable and incited an antibody response (Fig. 206–24).

Beauvaria bassiana was shown to be the cause of muscardine in silkworms. This was the first demonstration of the microbial origin of a disease process and preceded the works of Koch and Pasteur by many years. It is a commonly encountered soil organism and is known to be pathogenic for beetles and tortoises.[6] The only human case is that of Freour and associates,[5] who described a patient with ulcerative cervical lymphadenopathy. A pulmonary cavity was noted on chest radiograph. On surgical removal, mycelia were demonstrated in tissue, and *B. bassiana* (called *B. tayeaui*) was isolated.

B. bassiana grows as a whitish, fluffy to powdery colony. The conidiophores are simple or branched and, starting from a bulbous base, taper to a slender, conidia-bearing portion. The spore-bearing tip grows sympodially, producing a zigzag configuration. The conidia are single, small, and round.

Acremonium (Cephalosporium) is a common soil and sewage hyalohyphomycete. Its colony is white, yellowish, pinkish, gray, or brick colored. At first it is glabrous, and the organisms are budding and yeast-like. Later, mycelia are produced that are single stranded or funiculose. Simple phialide conidiophores produce a series of one-celled globose, ovoid, or cylindric conidia. These may mass at the top of the conidio-

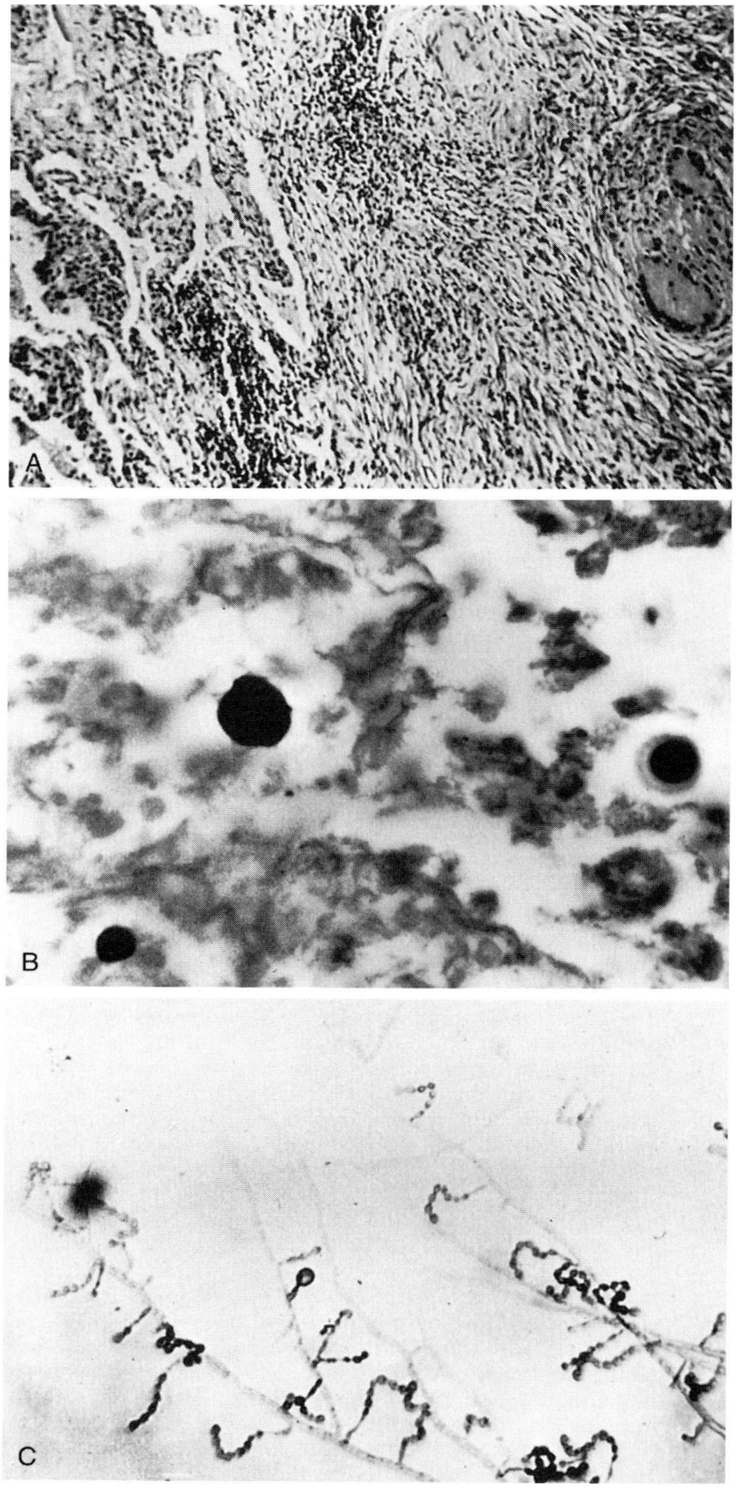

FIGURE 206–24. Scopulariopsis brumptii. A, *Granuloma with foreign body giant cells. (H and E × 100.)* B, *Various-sized spores of fungus within granuloma. (GMS × 500.)* C, *Culture mount in which can be observed chains of small conidia arising from annellophores and large sessile aleuriospore of the same size as seen in the pulmonary granulomata. (From Grieble, H., Rippon, J. W., Maliwan, N., et al.:* Scopulariopsis *and hypersensitivity pneumonitis in an addict. Ann. Intern. Med. 83:326–329, 1976.)*

phore, forming a head or cephalus. Some species of *Acremonium (A. falciforme, A. kiliense,* and *A. recifei)* are isolated from cases of mycetoma. Species of the genus are encountered regularly as causes of mycotic keratitis and as a secondary invader in onychomycosis. Others are the source of the cephalosporins and cephalins. Only rarely has systemic disease been ascribed to the genus *Acremonium.* In one case, a midline granuloma with eroding destruction of the hard palate and involvement of the maxilla and mandible was described.[2] Hyphae were seen in tissue sections, and an *Acremonium* was isolated. Meningitis due to *Acremonium* has been described after a spinal anesthetic.[4] An *Acremonium* species also has been isolated from sputum, resected lung, and the skin of patients with burns.[3, 15]

Fusarium species are very common soil organisms and important plant pathogens. They are encountered frequently in patients with mycotic keratitis, particularly in southern Florida. Pulmonary infections and disseminated opportunistic infection also have been recorded.[19, 20] As with other invasive hyalohyphomycetes, it is not possible to distinguish these several fungi in tissue section from invasive aspergillosis. In culture they grow rapidly, producing a spreading fluffy colony that is pink, white, yellow, purple, or green. The conidiophores are grouped into sporodochia or are single.

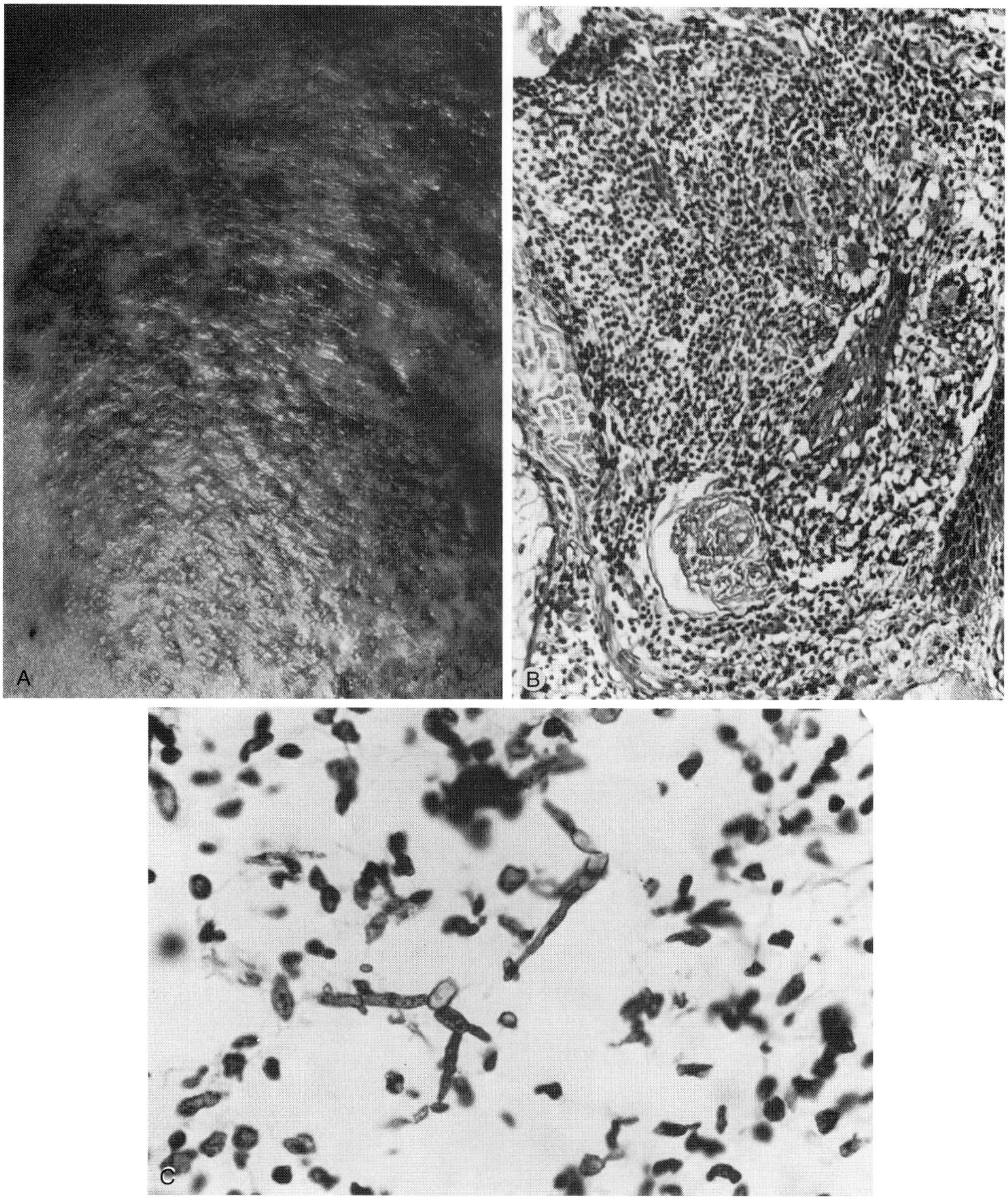

FIGURE 206–25. Paecilomyces lilacinum. A, *Erythematous scaly plaques on left cheek of 20-year-old woman.* B, *Chronic granulomatous response composed of lymphocytes, epithelioid cells, and giant cells in upper dermis. (H and E × 100.)* C, *Septate mycelial units in tissue section. (PAS × 800.) (From Takayasu, S., Agaki, M., and Shimzu, Y.: Deep mycosis caused by* P. lilacinum. *Arch. Dermatol.* 113:1687–1690, 1977. *Copyright 1977, American Medical Association.)*

Conidia are produced from phialides on the conidiophores or directly on fertile hyphae. Conidia are single but mass to form balls. The conidia vary in size from 1 to 20 μm and are single or multiple celled, round, cylindric, or, more frequently, crescent shaped. The crescent shape is the characteristic spore. Small, round microspores and chlamydoconidia also are produced.

Most well-documented cases of human *Fusarium* infections occur in the skin of patients with burns.[9, 14] In one case, a 2-year-old girl had second- and third-degree burns over 60 per cent of her body.[1] After a stormy course, the patient died. At autopsy, both kidneys were found to be studded with abscesses, as were the heart and brain. *Fusarium* was isolated from skin and renal abscesses.

Paecilomyces is another common soil hyalohyphomycete. Species of this genus have been recovered from patients with mycotic keratitis and endophthalmitis. *Paecilomyces* resemble *Penicillium* species in colony type and conidiation but do not produce greenish-blue colors. The colonies grow rapidly, are fluffy, and in color are buff, greenish-gold, or lilac. The conidiophores are simple to branched septate and usually hyaline. The phialides are produced singly or verticillate on conidiophores or directly from hyphae. They have a bulbous base and taper abruptly to form a long narrow tube. Conidia are produced in long unbranched chains that reflex away from the axis of the conidiophore. The conidia are ovate to lemon-shaped or cylindric, and they are smooth or rough. Aleurioconidia and chlamydoconidia are produced by some species.

Infection has been described in various animal species.[6, 7, 10, 11] The only human case reported to date occurred in a patient who died after developing endocarditis subsequent to a valve replacement.[17] At autopsy, fungal elements (1.5 to 3 μm) were seen within thrombi in the mitral valve and in an iliac embolus. Tuberculoma-like lesions were seen in vessels near the embolus, which were characterized by caseous necrosis and epithelioid and giant cells. *Paecilomyces varioti* was recovered from the valves. Figure 206–25 shows aspects of a case of *Paecilomyces lilacinum* infection.[16a]

References

1. Abramowsky, C. R., Quinn, D., Bradford, W. D., et al.: Systemic infection by *Fusarium* in a burned child: The emergence of a saprophytic strain. J. Pediatr. *84*:561–564, 1974.
2. Cowen, D. E., Dines, D. E., Chessen, J., et al.: *Cephalosporium* midline granuloma. Ann. Intern. Med. *62*:791–795, 1965.
3. Craddock, D. R., and McDonald, P. J.: Pulmonary mycetoma and its surgical management. Med. J. Aust. *2*:1477–1480, 1972.
4. Drouhet, E., Martin, L., Segretain, G., et al.: Mycose meningocérébrale à *Cephalosporium*. Presse Med. *31*:1809–1814, 1965.
5. Freour, P., Lahourcade, M., and Chomy, P.: Une mycose nouvelle: Étude clinique et mycologique d'une localisation pulmonaire de "Beauveria." Bull. Soc. Med. Hop. Paris *117*:197–206, 1966.
6. Georg, L. K., Williamson, W. M., Tilden, E. B., et al.: Mycotic pulmonary disease of captive giant tortoises due to *Beauvaria bassiana* and *Paecilomyces fumoso-roseus*. Sabouraudia 2:80–86, 1962.
7. Gonzalez-Ochoa, A., and Dallaly Castillo, E.: Frequencia de *Scopulariopsis brevicaulis* en muestras de suelos en cuevas y minas del pais. Rev. Inst. Salubr. Enferm. Trop. (Mex.) *20*:247–252, 1960.
8. Grieble, H., Rippon, J. W., Maliwan, N., et al.: *Scopulariopsis* and hypersensitivity pneumonitis in an addict. Ann. Intern. Med. *83*:326–329, 1976.
9. Holzegal, K., and Kempf, H. F.: *Fusarium* mykose und der haut eines verbrannten. Dermatol. Wochenschr. *150*:651–658, 1964.
10. Hoven, E., and McKenzie, R. A.: Suspected paecilomycosis in a dog. Aust. Vet. J. *50*:368–369, 1974.
11. Jang, S. S., Biberstein, E. L., Slauson, D. O., et al.: Paecilomycosis in a dog. J. Am. Vet. Med. Assoc. *159*:1775–1779, 1971.
12. Markley, A. J., Philpott, O. S., and Weidman, F. D.: Deep scopulariopsis of ulcerating granuloma type confirmed by culture and animal inoculation. Arch. Dermatol. *33*:627–641, 1936.
13. Padhye, A. A., and Sekhon, A. S.: Dermatophytoses in Alberta (1959–1971). Can. J. Public Health *64*:180–184, 1973.
14. Peterson, J. E., and Baker, J. J.: An isolate of *Fusarium roseum* from human burns. Mycologia *51*:453–456, 1959.
15. Sander, K., and Schonborn, C.: Schimmelpilzinfektion der haut bei asgedehnter berbrennung. Dtsch. Gesundheits. *28*:125–128, 1973.
16. Sekhon, A. S., Willans, D. J., and Harvey, J. H.: Deep scopulariopsis: A case report and sensitivity studies. J. Clin. Pathol. *27*:837–843, 1974.

16a. Takayasu, S., Agaki, M., and Shimzu, Y.: Deep mycosis caused by *P. lilacinum*. Arch. Dermatol. *113*:1687–1690, 1977.

17. Uys, C. J., Don, P. A., Schrire, V., et al.: Endocarditis following cardiac surgery due to the fungus *Paecilomyces*. S. Afr. Med. J. *37*:1276–1280, 1963.
18. Wolfringer, A., and Percebois, G.: Données sur l'onyxis causé de *Scopulariopsis brevicaulis* (à propos de 6 cas). Ann. Med. Nancy *15*:215–218, 1976.
19. Young, C. N., and Meyers, A. M.: Opportunistic fungal infection by *Fusarium oxysporum* in a renal transplant patient. Sabouraudia *17*:219–223, 1979.
20. Young, N. A., Kwon-Chung, K. J., Kubota, T. T., et al.: Disseminated infection by *Fusarium moniliforme* during treatment for malignant lymphoma. J. Clin. Microbiol. *7*:589–594, 1978.

S E C T I O N   T W E N T Y - T W O

PARASITIC DISEASES

❑ ❑ ❑

207

CLASSIFICATION/NOMENCLATURE OF HUMAN PARASITES

Lynne S. Garcia

Although common names frequently are used to describe parasitic organisms, these names may represent different parasites in different parts of the world. In order to eliminate these problems, a binomial system of nomenclature is used in which the scientific name consists of the genus and species. These names generally are of Greek or Latin origin. In certain publications, the scientific name often is followed by the name of the individual who originally named the parasite. The date of naming also may be provided. If the name of the individual is in parentheses, it means that the person used a generic name no longer considered to be correct.

On the basis of life histories and morphologic characteristics, systems of classification have been developed to indicate the relationship among the various parasite species. Closely related species are placed in the same genus, related genera in the same family, related families in the same order, related orders in the same class, and related classes in the same phylum, one of the major categories in the animal kingdom. As one progresses up the classification schema, each category becomes more broad; however, each category still has characteristics in common.

Parasites of humans are classified in five major divisions. These include the Protozoa (amebae, flagellates, ciliates, sporozoans, coccidia, microsporidia), the Platyhelminthes or flatworms (cestodes, trematodes), the Acanthocephala or thorny-headed worms, the Nematoda or roundworms, and the Arthropoda (insects, spiders, mites, ticks, and so on). Although these categories appear to be well defined, there often is considerable confusion in attempting to classify parasitic organisms. One of the primary reasons is the lack of known specimens. Some organisms recovered from humans are very rare; thus, there is difficulty in determining morphologic and physiologic variation among such groups. Type specimens must be deposited for study before a legitimate species name can be given. Even when certain parasites are numerous, they may represent strains or races of the same species with slightly different characteristics.

Generally, reproductive mechanisms are a valid concept in determining species definitions, but there are so many exceptions within parasite groups that it is difficult to take into consideration things like sexual reproduction, parthenogenesis, and asexual reproduction. Another difficulty in species recognition is the ability and tendency of the organisms to alter their morphologic forms according to age, host, or nutrition, which often results in several names for the same organism. An additional problem involves alternation of parasitic and free-living phases in the life cycle. These organisms may be very different and difficult to recognize as belonging to the same species. In spite of these difficulties, newer, more sophisticated molecular methods of grouping organisms of-

TABLE 207–1. Human Vector-Borne Infections

Infection (Disease)	Causative Agent	Vector (Common Name)
Protozoal		
Malaria	*Plasmodium* species	Mosquitoes
Leishmaniasis	*Leishmania* species	Sandflies
Chagas disease	*Trypanosoma cruzi*	Triatomid bugs
East African trypanosomiasis	*T. brucei rhodesiense*	Tsetse flies
West African trypanosomiasis	*T. brucei gambiense*	Tsetse flies
Babesiosis	*Babesia* species	Ticks
Helminthic		
Filariasis	*Wuchereria bancrofti*	Mosquitoes
Filariasis	*Brugia malayi*	Mosquitoes
Filariasis	*Dirofilaria* species	Mosquitoes
Filariasis	*Mansonella perstans*	Biting midges
Filariasis	*M. streptocerca*	Biting midges
Filariasis	*M. ozzardi*	Biting midges
Onchocerciasis	*Onchocerca volvulus*	Black flies
Loiasis	*Loa loa*	Deer flies
Dog tapeworm infection	*Dipylidium caninum*	Dog louse, flea, human flea
Rat tapeworm infection	*Hymenolepis diminuta*	Rat flea, beetles, grain beetles
Dwarf tapeworm	*H. nana*	Grain beetles (rare)

TABLE 207–2. Medically Important Arthropods

Local or Systemic Problems	Vector (Common Name)	Local or Systemic Problems	Vector (Common Name)
Skin reaction to bites	Sucking lice Bedbugs Kissing bugs Biting midges Sandflies Black flies Mosquitoes Deer flies Tsetse flies Soft ticks Hard ticks	Painful sting, potential anaphylaxis	Honeybees Bumblebees Wasps, hornets, yellow jackets Fire ants Scorpions
Painful bite	Horseflies Fire ants Centipedes	Dermatitis, ulcerations	Fleas
Intense itching	Human itch mites Chiggers	Nodular ulceration with subsequent secondary infection	Chigoe flea
		Blistering of skin after contact with adult beetles	Blister beetles
		Bite, usually painless, delayed systemic reaction	Black widow spiders
		Initial blister followed by extensive necrosis and slow healing	Brown recluse spiders South American brown spiders

ten have confirmed taxonomic conclusions reached hundreds of years before by experienced taxonomists.

As investigators continue in parasitic genetics, immunology, and biochemistry, the species designation will be defined more clearly. Originally, these species designations were determined primarily by morphologic differences—thus, a phenotypic approach. With use of highly sophisticated molecular techniques, the approach will continue to be more genotypic.

Although there are gaps in our knowledge concerning classification of all human parasites, the binomial system has allowed the classification of 1.5 million species of organisms in the animal kingdom such that all published information can be retrieved, regardless of the language spoken. The difficulty for the clinician arises when one considers the rapid increase in information concerning microbiology during the past few years and changing considerations such as the role of immunosuppression in the host-parasite interaction.

The classification of parasites is presented in tabular form. Although certain species designations may be somewhat controversial, this classification scheme is designed to provide some order and meaning to a widely divergent group of organisms. No attempt has been made to include every possible organism, but only those that are considered to be clinically relevant in the context of human parasitology. The main groups that are presented include protozoa, nematodes (roundworms), cestodes (tapeworms), and trematodes (flukes). Some relevant information on arthropods is presented in Tables 207–1 and 207–2. It is hoped this information will provide some insight into the parasite groupings, thus leading to a better understanding of parasitic infections and the appropriate diagnostic and clinical approach.

I. PROTOZOA

1. *(Amebae)—Intestinal*

These organisms are characterized by having pseudopods (motility) and trophozoite and cyst stages in the life cycle. There are some exceptions in which a cyst form has not been identified. Amebae usually are acquired by humans via fecal-oral transmission or mouth-to-mouth contact (Entamoeba gingivalis).

Current Name
*Entamoeba histolytica**
*Entamoeba dispar**
Entamoeba hartmanni†
Entamoeba coli

**Entamoeba histolytica* is being used to designate pathogenic zymodemes (strains), whereas *E. dispar* now is being used to designate nonpathogenic zymodemes (strains). However, unless trophozoites containing ingested red blood cells (*E. histolytica*) are seen, the two organisms cannot be differentiated on the basis of morphology. Because the differences in pathogenicity are genetic and not just phenotypic, the decision to treat is one that must be left to the physician. Reports of finding organisms in the genus *Entamoeba* in patient specimens must continue to be reported to state and county Departments of Public Health (follow your particular state reporting regulations).

†*Entamoeba hartmanni* is nonpathogenic and is totally different from *E. histolytica*. "Small race *Entamoeba histolytica*" is incorrect and should not be used at any time to designate *E. hartmanni*.

Current Name
Entamoeba polecki
Entamoeba gingivalis
Endolimax nana
Iodamoeba bütschlii
Blastocystis hominis

2. *(Flagellates)—Intestinal*
These organisms move by means of flagella and are considered to be acquired by fecal-oral transmission. With the exception of Dientamoeba fragilis *(internal flagella) and those in the genus* Trichomonas, *they have both the trophozoite and cyst stages in the life cycle. Neither* D. fragilis *nor* Trichomonas *species have a cyst stage.*

Current Name
*Giardia lamblia**
Chilomastix mesnili
Dientamoeba fragilis
Trichomonas hominis
Trichomonas tenax
Enteromonas hominis
Retortamonas intestinalis

3. *(Ciliates)—Intestinal*
These organisms, which move by means of cilia, are acquired by humans through fecal-oral transmission. They have both the trophozoite and cyst forms in the life cycle.

Current Name
Balantidium coli

4. *(Coccidia, Microsporidia)—Intestinal*
These organisms are acquired by humans by ingestion of various meats or through fecal-oral transmission via contaminated food and/or water.

Current Name
Coccidia
Cryptosporidium parvum
Cyclospora cayetanensis
Isospora belli
Sarcocystis hominis
Sarcocystis suihominis
Sarcocystis bovihominis
Sarcocystis "lindermanni"
Microsporidia
Enterocytozoon bieneusi
Encephalitozoon intestinalis†

5. *(Amebae, Flagellates)—Other Body Sites*
The amebae are pathogenic, free-living organisms that may be associated with warm, fresh-water areas. They have been found in the central nervous system, the eye, and other sites. Trichomonas vaginalis *usually is acquired by sexual transmission. This particular flagellate is found in the genitourinary system.*

*Although some individuals have changed the species designation for the genus *Giardia* to *G. intestinalis* or *G. duodenalis*, there is no general agreement. Therefore, for this listing, we will retain the name *Giardia lamblia*.

†Formerly called *Septata intestinalis*.

Current Name
Amebae
Naegleria fowleri
Acanthamoeba species
Hartmanella species
Balamuthia mandrillaris (Leptomyxid ameba)
Flagellates
Trichomonas vaginalis

6. *(Coccidia, Microsporidia, Undecided Classification)—Other Body Sites*
These organisms particularly are important in the compromised patient. They also may infect many individuals who have no apparent symptoms. On the basis of several RNA studies, Pneumocystis carinii *is linked more closely to the fungi. However, for the present, it will continue to be listed here.*

Current Name
Coccidia
Toxoplasma gondii
Sarcocystis "lindermanni"
Microsporidia
Nosema connori
Vittaforma corneae
Pleistophora
Trachipleistophora hominis
Encephalitozoon hellem
Encephalitozoon cuniculi
*Encephalitozoon intestinalis**
Enterocytozoon bieneusi†
"Microsporidium"‡
Undecided Classification
Pneumocystis carinii§

7. *(Sporozoa, Flagellates)—Blood and Tissues*
All of these organisms are arthropod-borne. Diagnosis may be somewhat more difficult than that of the intestinal protozoa, particularly if automated blood differential systems are used. The leishmania have undergone extensive revisions in classification. However, from a clinical perspective, recovery and identification of the organisms still are related to body site. Recovery of the organisms is limited to the site of the lesion in infections other than those caused by the Leishmania donovani *complex (visceral leishmaniasis).*

Current Name
Sporozoa (Malaria, Babesiosis)
Malaria
Plasmodium vivax
Plasmodium ovale
Plasmodium malariae
Plasmodium falciparum

*Formerly called *Septata intestinalis.*
†*Enterocytozoon bieneusi* has been recovered from sites other than the intestinal tract (findings confirmed in 1996 and 1997).
‡This designation is not a true genus, but a "catch-all" for those organisms that have not been (or may never be) identified to the genus and/or species levels.
§*Pneumocystis carinii* now has been reclassified with the fungi.

Current Name
Babesiosis
Babesia species
Flagellates (Leishmaniasis, Trypanosomiasis)
Leishmaniasis
Leishmania tropica complex (cutaneous leishmaniasis)
Leishmania mexicana complex (cutaneous leishmaniasis)
Leishmania braziliensis complex (mucocutaneous leishmaniasis)
Leishmania donovani complex (visceral leishmaniasis)
Trypanosomiasis
Trypanosoma brucei gambiense (West African trypanosomiasis)
Trypanosoma brucei rhodesiense (East African trypanosomiasis)
Trypanosoma cruzi (South American trypanosomiasis)
Trypanosoma rangeli

II. NEMATODES

1. *Intestinal*

   These organisms normally are acquired by egg ingestion or skin penetration of larval forms from the soil.

Current Name
Ascaris lumbricoides
Enterobius vermicularis (pinworm)
Ancylostoma duodenale (Old World hookworm)
Necator americanus (New World hookworm)
Strongyloides stercoralis
Trichostrongylus species
Trichuris trichiura (whipworm)
Capillaria philippinensis

2. *Tissue*

   For the most part, these organisms rarely are seen within the United States; however, the first three are more important.

Current Name
Trichinella spiralis
Toxocara canis or *T. cati* (visceral or ocular larva migrans)
Ancylostoma braziliense or *A. caninum* (cutaneous larva migrans)
Dracunculus medinensis
Angiostrongylus cantonensis
Angiostrongylus costaricensis
Gnathostoma spinigerum
Anisakiasis (larvae from salt-water fish)
Anisakis species
Phocanema species
Contracaecum species
Capillaria hepatica
Thelazia species

3. *(Filarial Worms)—Blood, Body Fluids, Skin*

   These organisms also are arthropod-borne. The adult worms tend to live in the tissues or lymphatics. Diagnosis is made on the basis of the recovery and identification of the larval worms (microfilariae) in the blood, other body fluids, or skin. Elephantiasis may be associated with some of the organisms listed.

Current Name
Wuchereria bancrofti
Brugia malayi
Loa loa

Current Name
Onchocerca volvulus
Mansonella ozzardi
Mansonella streptocerca
Mansonella perstans
Dirofilaria immitis ("coin" lesion in the lung) Dog heartworm
Dirofilaria species (may be found in subcutaneous nodules)

III. CESTODES

1. *Intestinal*

   The adult form of these organisms is acquired by humans through ingestion of the larval forms contained in poorly cooked or raw meats or fresh-water fish. In the case of Dipylidium caninum, *infection is acquired by the accidental ingestion of dog fleas. Both* Hymenolepis nana *and* H. diminuta *are transmitted via ingestion of certain arthropods (fleas, beetles). Also,* H. nana *can be transmitted through egg ingestion (life cycle can bypass the intermediate beetle host). The human can serve as both the intermediate and definitive hosts in* H. nana *and* T. solium *infections.*

Current Name
Diphyllobothrium latum (broad, fish tapeworm)
Dipylidium caninum (dog tapeworm)
Hymenolepis nana (dwarf tapeworm)
Hymenolepis diminuta (rat tapeworm)
Taenia solium (pork tapeworm)
Taenia saginata (beef tapeworm)

2. *(Larval Forms)—Tissue*

   The ingestion of certain tapeworm eggs or accidental contact with certain larval forms can lead to the following diseases.

Current Name
Taenia solium (cysticercosis)
Echinococcus granulosus (hydatid disease)
Echinococcus multilocularis (alveolar hydatid disease)
Multiceps multiceps (Coenurus disease)
Diphyllobothrium species (sparganosis)
Spirometra mansonoides (sparganosis)

IV. TREMATODES

1. *Intestinal*

   These infections are uncommon within the United States.

Current Name
Fasciolopsis buski (giant intestinal fluke)
Echinostoma ilocanum
Heterophyes heterophyes
Metagonimus yokogawai

2. *Liver, Lung*

   These organisms are not seen commonly within the United States; however, some Southeast Asian refugees do harbor some of these parasites.

Current Name
Clonorchis (Opisthorchis) sinensis (Chinese liver fluke)
Opisthorchis viverrini
Fasciola hepatica (sheep liver fluke)
Paragonimus westermani (lung fluke)
Paragonimus species

Current Name

3. *Blood*

The schistosomes are acquired by skin penetration by the cercarial forms that are released from fresh-water snails. Although they are not endemic within the United States, occasionally patients are seen who may have these infections.

Current Name
Schistosoma mansoni
Schistosoma haematobium
Schistosoma japonicum
Schistosoma intercalatum
Schistosoma mekongi

V. ARTHROPODS

See Tables 207–1 and 207–2.

Bibliography

1. Beaver, C. B., Jung, R. C., and Cupp, E. W.: Clinical Parasitology. Philadelphia, Lea & Febiger, 1984, 825 pp.
2. Bryan, R. T., Cali, A., Owen, R. L., et al.: Microsporidia: Opportunistic pathogens in patients with AIDS. *In* Sun, T. (ed.): Progress in Clinical Parasitology. Vol. II. New York, Field & Wood Medical Publishers (distributed by W.W. Norton), 1991.
3. Edman, J. C., Kovacs, J. A., Masur, H., et al.: Ribosomal RNA sequence shows *Pneumocystis carinii* to be a member of the fungi. Nature *334*:519–522, 1988.
4. Garcia, L. S., and Bruckner, D. A.: Diagnostic Medical Parasitology. 3rd ed. Washington, D.C., American Society for Microbiology, 1997, 937 pp.
5. Hartskeerl, R. A., Van Gool, T., Schuitema, A. R. J., et al.: Genetic and immunological characterization of the microsporidian *Septata intestinalis* Cali, Kotler, and Orenstein, 1993: Reclassification to *Encephalitozoon intestinalis*. Parasitology *110*:277–285, 1995.
6. Levine, N. D.: Veterinary Parasitology. Minneapolis, Burgess Publishing, 1978, 236 pp.
7. Molina, J. M., Oksenhendler, E., Beauvais, B., et al.: Disseminated microsporidiosis due to *Septata intestinalis* in patients with AIDS: Clinical features and response to albendazole therapy. J. Infect. Dis. *171*:245–249, 1995.
8. Murray, P. R., Baron, E. J., Pfaller, M. A., et al. (eds.): Manual of Clinical Microbiology. 6th ed. Washington, D.C., American Society for Microbiology, 1995, 1482 pp.
9. Ortega, Y., Sterling, C. R., Gilman, R. H., et al.: *Cyclospora* species: A new protozoan pathogen of humans. N. Engl. J. Med. *328*:1308–1312, 1993.
10. Pape, J. W., Verdier, R. I., Boncy, M., et al.: *Cyclospora* infection in adults infected with HIV: Clinical manifestations, treatment, and prophylaxis. Ann. Intern. Med. *121*:654–657, 1994.
11. Stringer, S. L., Hudson, K., Blase, M. A., et al.: Sequence from ribosomal RNA of *Pneumocystis carinii* compared to those of four fungi suggests an ascomycetous affinity. J. Protozool. *36*:14S–16S, 1989.
12. Zierdt, C. H.: *Blastocystis hominis*: Past and future. Clin. Microbiol. Rev. *4*:61–79, 1991.

❑ ❑ ❑

SUBSECTION ONE

PROTOZOA

Amebae

208

AMEBIASIS

Peter J. Hotez and Alan D. Strickland

Amebiasis is a major infectious diarrheal disease among children living in the developing countries of the tropics as well as those who emigrate from these areas to the United States. The frequencey of amebiasis in less developed countries is high. For instance, approximately 10 to 20 per cent of Mexican children harbor amoeba, and up to 5 per cent of their episodes of acute diarrhea are due to amebiasis.[70] More than half of all patients treated for amebiasis in a hospital in Lagos, Nigeria, were children younger than 10 years of age.[70] As in many other parasitic diseases, infants and toddlers with amebiasis often will present with clinical features of their disease that usually are not found in adults, including a fulminating variant of amebic colitis.[30, 38, 65]

Amebiasis is caused by either *Entamoeba histolytica*, a protozoan named for the pathologic evidence of "lysis" of tissues, or *Entamoeba dispar*, which is identical morphologically but so far has been implicated only as a cause of an asymptomatic carrier state.[87] The first demonstration of the organism in human tissues was made by W. D. Lambl in 1859 in the postmortem examination of the colon of a child who died as a result of having excess diarrhea.[15, 71] No correlation of the organism with the disease was made until 1875, when Losch, in St. Petersburg, Russia, found the organism at autopsy in the colon of a woodcutter. Losch induced diarrhea and ulcerations in a dog given feces from the patient.[56] He did not, however, think that there was a connection between the organism and the disease. The first patient described in the United States was a physician treated by William Osler for an amebic liver abscess in 1890.[71] Councilman and Lafleur further described the organism and the disease in 1891.[22, 40] Further investigation of the disease was delayed until a better understanding of the life cycle of *E. histolytica* could be obtained.[26] Within the last 10 years, the application of modern molecular biology techniques to the study of *E. histolytica* and *E. dispar* has resulted in an explosion of information about the mechanisms of virulence, pathogenicity, and immune responses to these organisms.[87, 92]

ETIOLOGY

Studies using molecular (DNA and RNA) and immunologic (monoclonal antibodies) probes demonstrate the existence of two distinct species of the genus *Entamoeba*, which are identical morphologically.[13, 16, 20, 24, 66, 75, 114] *E. histolytica* is the pathogenic species having the capacity to invade tissue and cause symptomatic disease, whereas *E. dispar* (as well as *E. histolytica*) is associated with the asymptomatic carrier state.[87] Morphologically distinct members of the genus *Entamoeba*, such as *Entamoeba coli* and *Entamoeba hartmanni*, also are nonpathogenic.

Members of the genus *Entamoeba* (protozoan organisms belonging to the subphylum Sarcodina) have both trophozoite and cyst forms. The cysts of *E. histolytica* and *E. dispar* are almost spherical, being surrounded by a cell wall composed of chitin. The cysts may have one to four nuclei, although quadrinucleate cysts are most typical. This feature allows differentiation from *E. coli*, which usually has six to eight nuclei in the cysts and may have as many as 32 nuclei.[72] Cysts of *E. histolytica* are 5 to 20 μm in diameter (average, 12 μm) and have a greenish tint in the unstained condition.[59] Young cysts contain chromatoid bodies, which are composed of ribosome particles in crystalline arrays.[12] The cysts of *E. hartmanni* appear identical to those of *E. histolytica* except for having a smaller size of 4 to 10 μm. *E. histolytica* cysts will survive for days in the dried state at 30° C or for months at 0° to 4° C. They may be killed by temperatures above 50° C for 5 minutes.[40] They are completely resistant to the concentrations of chlorine used in water supplies but may be killed with hyperchlorination or with iodine solutions.[59, 72] They are filtered out of water supplies that pass through a sand filtration phase. They resist acids well.

When these quadrinucleate cysts are ingested, they resist the acid pH of the stomach and ultimately excyst in the alkaline environment of the bowel. The process of excystation results in the release of four trophozoites that divide by binary fission to produce eight trophozoites. The usual trophozoites have a diameter of 25 μm with a range between 10 and 60 μm.[26, 87] They have a single nucleus that is 3 to 5 μm in diameter containing fine peripheral chromatin with a slightly eccentric karyosome. There is a granular endoplasm that typically contains vacuoles in which bacteria and debris can be seen. Some glycogen is present and can be stained with periodic acid–Schiff. Mitochondria, Golgi membranes, and rough endoplasmic reticulum are absent.[36] The presence of ingested erythrocytes is a characteristic feature of *E. histolytica* but not *E. dispar*.[87] Movement is accomplished by extension of clear pseudopodia. Replication is by binary fission. These protozoa live in the colon of humans and other mammals. Trophozoites die quickly outside the body and are quite sensitive to acid—they generally are not considered to be infective.[36] When cooled (as when feces are expelled and gradually cool from body temperature) or stimulated by as yet undefined luminal conditions, the trophozoites form cysts that can remain viable for weeks to months upon excretion.[87]

Trophozoites of *E. coli* are 15 to 50 μm, have much more sluggish motility than *E. histolytica*, and have blunt pseudopodia rather than the sharp, finger-like pseudopodia of *E. histolytica*. Trophozoites of *E. hartmanni* are 4 to 14 μm and have much less glycogen than *E. histolytica*.[26]

EPIDEMIOLOGY

Amebiasis is worldwide in distribution. Estimates indicate that about 500 million people are carrying either *E. dispar* or *E. histolytica*, that 50 million people each year will have active disease, and that there are between 50,000 and 100,000 deaths per year due to the organism.[80, 86, 123] Generally speaking, asymptomatic *E. dispar* infection is about 10-fold more common than *E. histolytica* infection, and symptomatic invasive amebiasis develops in only about 10 per cent of *E. histolytica*–infected individuals.[87] Thus, only about 1 per cent of patients found to harbor *Entamoeba* by stool microscopy will develop clinically apparent amebiasis.

The prevalence of *Entamoeba* infection varies from an estimated 5 per cent of the population in the United States to as much as 50 per cent of the population of certain underdeveloped parts of Africa and Indochina and in areas of South and Central America.[15, 26, 86] High rates of invasive disease occur among Mexican Americans who are recent immigrants to the United States. Most immigrants who develop amebic liver abscess from *E. histolytica* infection usually will present within 5 months from the time of entry into their new country.[50] Other high-risk groups in the United States include institutionalized populations[74] and, at one time, the gay male populations of New York City and San Francisco.[63, 106, 113] The prevalence of *Entamoeba* infection among gay men has decreased in recent years as a consequence of safer sex practices.[25] Small children serve as sources of infection for entire families. Cases of severe disease and fatality have been recorded in contacts of humans who have asymptomatic infections.[26] The age distribution is reported as a bimodal one with a peak incidence between 2 and 3 years of age (with a case fatality rate of 20 per cent) and another peak after 40 years of age (with a case fatality rate of 69 per cent).[53]

PATHOGENESIS AND PATHOLOGY

Clinical amebiasis occurs when trophozoites invade the colonic tissue. This process is initiated when the trophozoite adheres to the mucins lining the surface of the large bowel,[40, 72, 86] followed by enzymatic destruction of the basement membrane of the mucosa and its underlying tissue. Host inflammatory responses also contribute to the destruction of tissue.

In the relatively anaerobic environment of the colon, the 10- to 20-μm trophozoites of *E. histolytica* are found to attach themselves to bacteria actively through a surface receptor that can be blocked by mannose.[68] *Escherichia coli* is highly favored for attack by *E. histolytica*, which rapidly lyses the bacteria and ingests them. These trophozoites also may attach to the interglandular region of the intestinal mucosa[36, 40, 72, 86] or to colonic mucus.[18] The adherence to the mucus and the intestinal wall is associated with a 260-kDa amebic adherence lectin, consisting of 170-kDa and 35-kDa subunits.[77, 88] The 170-kDa subunit is the functional component that binds to galactose and consists of a short cytoplasmic domain, a transmembrane domain, and a large extracellular portion that is cysteine-rich.[9, 18, 19, 23, 76, 77, 90, 115] The 170-kDa subunit of the amebic lectin protects the parasite by blocking the assembly of host complement components onto its surface.[14] The cysteine-rich component of the 170-kDa lectin is immunogenic and has been shown to be effective in animals as a potential subunit vaccine target.[19]

Lectin-mediated adherence by the trophozoite is a prerequisite for the subsequent lysis of target interglandular intestinal cells. Target cell lysis is a complex process requiring the presence of calcium[91] and several parasite-derived virulence factors, including a calcium-dependent phospholipase,[55, 89] a target cell ionophore,[52] and a hemolysin.[43] Thus, cytolysis of the target cell is completed extracellularly by the trophozoite. The killed cells then can be engulfed with intact cell membrane, or the cytoplasm and the nucleus can be ingested through a broken membrane.[36, 62] The nucleus of the target cell loses its membrane even before ingestion and no longer stains in the usual electron-dense manner.

Invasion of the mucosa then may occur, but many factors are involved in instituting this invasion. The presence and adherence of bacteria often are required for invasiveness.[53, 62, 68] Parasite-derived hydrolytic enzymes greatly contribute to the destruction of cells and the surrounding extracellular matrix. These include several types of proteases[47, 70, 93, 95, 107] and glycosidases.[118, 125] The former has been shown to participate in parasite-mediated immune evasion by degrading IgA molecules and mimicking the activity of certain complement components.[48]

A vigorous infiltration by neutrophils and other inflammatory cells occurs in response to trophozoite invasion.[36, 62, 86, 87, 96] The host polymorphonuclear response greatly contributes to the destruction of host tissues. The 170-kDa lectin of *E. histolytica* attaches the trophozoite to polymorphonuclear neutrophils, peripheral blood mononuclear cells, monocytes, and monocyte-derived macrophages.[86, 117] Neutrophils are killed and lysed similarly to intestinal cells. However, cytolysis of neutrophils releases some substance or substances that are locally effective in augmenting the cytolytic efficacy of virulent *E. histolytica,* thus making the inflammatory response increase the damage rather than contain the infection.[103] Invading trophozoites release substances that have not been characterized but strongly attract more neutrophils to the invading *E. histolytica* and allow these neutrophils to be killed as well.[98] Thus, the immune response to the initial infection with *E. histolytica* often is not effective, and there are few viable neutrophils found in the material left behind the active infection. Nevertheless, cell-mediated immunity has an important role in limiting the extent of invasive amebiasis and in protecting the host from a recurrence.[87, 92] The major cell-mediated effector mechanisms include trophozoite killing by activated macrophages and $CD8^+$ cytotoxic lymphocytes.[98–103] Cytokines such as tumor necrosis factor and interferon-γ contribute to immunocompetent cell activation. Humoral antibodies produced during a primary infection have been shown to protect against further infection and cause further damage to the host. One IgG antibody was found to be cytotoxic to *E. histolytica* in a manner independent of the complement system.[105] Another antibody has been found to be a liver autoantibody.[27] Numerous other antibodies have been noted, but their significance in most cases awaits further study.[44, 49, 112, 116]

The initial lesions of clinical amebiasis often are small interglandular ulcers with a diameter of approximately 1 mm. These extend only to the muscularis mucosa.[15, 62] The margins may be hyperemic, and there is slight edema of the surrounding mucosa. *E. histolytica* organisms seen in these ulcers will stain quite well with periodic acid–Schiff.[79] Bleeding and friability are not prominent at this stage, although proctoscopic examination may find mucus coming from these ulcers with abundant amebas present.

The next stage of intestinal disease is the production of deeper ulcers. These "buttonhole" ulcers may be as large as 1 cm in diameter and may extend into the submucosa.[15, 79] The ulcer often extends laterally under normal-appearing mucosa forming a characteristic "flask shape." Occasional perforation through the serosa with resultant peritonitis or pneumoperitoneum is found.[111] Extensive necrosis may be present, but there usually is very little inflammation. Rarely, a pseudomembranous colitis may develop.[29] The edema is more intense, but the mucosa between ulcers is relatively normal in contrast to the marked inflammatory response seen in bacterial enteritis. When ulceration is more extensive, the edema surrounding the ulcers becomes confluent and the mucosa appears gelatinous. In young children, this can progress to a fulminant necrotizing colitis associated with transmural necrosis. The pathologic events associated with this phenomenon are not understood. Rarely, there is an inflammatory response resulting in granulation tissue with a fibrous outer wall.[72] This is given the name ameboma. Occasionally, an ameboma fills a significant portion of the lumen, which causes stricture or obstruction. Other complications of intestinal amebiasis result from direct extension of the ulcers. This may result in cutaneous involvement of the perianal area or lesions of the penis, vulva, vagina, or cervix.[3, 72] Cutaneous and ophthalmologic amebiasis also are caused by fecal contamination of the face.[64]

Amebas disseminate to the liver in as many as 50 per cent of patients with fulminant amebiasis.[3, 4] Dissemination to other organs directly from the intestine probably does not occur, but dissemination from the liver to lung, heart, brain, spleen, scapula, larynx, stomach, and aorta has been described.[15] Amebic abscess of the liver occurs more often in adult males than in females by a ratio of 16 to 1 but occurs equally often in prepubertal children of both sexes.[4, 15] Abscesses are more common in adults but occur in children as young as 4 months of age.[69] These abscesses vary from microscopic lesions to massive necrosis of as much as 90 per cent of the liver. Fever, right upper quadrant pain, and the presence of serum antibodies to ameba point to hepatic amebic abscess.[86] The abscesses usually are free of bacterial contamination and have little inflammatory component. Examination of the fluid from such an abscess frequently reveals a reddish "anchovy paste" fluid that rarely may appear white or green. The fluid is acidic, with a pH ranging from 5.2 to 6.7.[85] Amebas are found in the walls of the abscess and only rarely in the fluid of the abscess. The walls are composed of a thin connective-tissue capsule. The right lobe of the liver is involved with amebic liver abscess approximately six times as often as the left lobe. Abscesses in the right lobe can perforate and cause disease below the diaphragm or in the thoracic cavity. Abscesses in the left lobe can lead to pericardial effusions, which therefore are less common than pleural effusions.[37, 42]

Pleural effusions can remain loculated or lead to cutaneous fistulas or to bronchopleural fistulas. Drainage from these fistulas is acidic, in contrast to the neutral secretions in the normal lung. Seeding of the cardiac valves and of the brain has been described.[15] Cerebral abscesses have the same microscopic findings as liver abscesses, with a thin capsule of connective tissue surrounding a fluid with little or no associated inflammatory response.

CLINICAL MANIFESTATIONS

Intestinal Amebiasis

ASYMPTOMATIC INTRALUMINAL AMEBIASIS. The most common type of amebic infestation is an asymptomatic cyst passing carrier state. All *E. dispar* infections and up to 90 per cent of *E. histolytica* infections are asymptomatic, presenting only with *Entamoeba* cysts in the feces.[34, 80] Some investigators have suggested that stools of these individuals generally will be more liquid than in individuals without trophozoites.[26] Furthermore, no longitudinal studies have been conducted to determine whether *E. dispar* or asymptomatic *E. histolytica* infections cause intermittent episodes of diarrhea or contribute to malnutrition and physical growth impairment of children.

ACUTE AMEBIC COLITIS. Amebic dysentery is the most common form of symptomatic invasive amebiasis. Seventy per cent of patients have a gradual onset of symptoms over 3 or 4 weeks after infestation, with increasingly severe diarrhea as the primary complaint. Occasionally, the onset may be acute or may be delayed for several months after infestation. The diarrhea is associated with pain in virtually 100 per cent of children. Pain may be of such severity that an acute abdomen is suspected.[3, 10, 45, 79] The stools contain blood and mucus in virtually all cases.[3, 79] Fever occurs in less than half of the patients. Abdominal distention and dehydration occur in less than 10 per cent of patients. In young children, intussusception, perforation and peritonitis, or necrotizing colitis may develop rapidly.[10, 45, 111]

AMEBOMA. This is an unusual presentation of intestinal amebiasis occurring in less than 1 per cent of patients with amebic colitis. These patients present with an abdominal mass that gives an "apple-core" appearance on radiographs, which can mimic colonic carcinoma.

Extraintestinal Amebiasis

AMEBIC LIVER ABSCESS. The second most frequent presentation of invasive amebiasis is an amebic liver abscess, which occurs in 1 to 7 per cent of children with invasive amebiasis[15, 69, 97] and 10 to 50 per cent of adults with invasive intestinal amebiasis.[4, 15] However, less than 30 per cent of patients with amebic liver abscess have active diarrhea at any time before presentation. Symptoms of amebic liver abscess in adults include upper abdominal pain in 77 per cent of patients, fever in 90 per cent, hepatomegaly with tenderness in 93 per cent, and poor right diaphragmatic excursion in 58 per cent. Jaundice occurs in 12 per cent of patients.[51, 84, 97] Occasionally, pain is reported in the right shoulder or the right side of the chest.

In childhood, abdominal pain is reported infrequently with amebic liver abscess.[38, 65] More commonly, high fever, abdominal distention, irritability, and tachypnea are noted. Some of these children are admitted to the hospital as having a fever of unknown origin. Hepatomegaly is frequent, but elicitation of hepatic tenderness is not well documented. In one report, four of five children younger than 5 years of age died with amebic liver abscesses because the diagnosis was not suspected.[51] Death usually results from rupture of the liver abscess into the peritoneum, thorax, or pericardium but may follow extensive hepatic damage and liver failure.[4, 84]

METASTATIC AMEBIASIS. Extra-abdominal amebiasis presumably follows direct extension from liver abscesses rather than direct dissemination from the intestine.[4, 15] Thoracic amebiasis is the most common type of extra-abdominal amebiasis and occurs in about 10 per cent of patients with amebic liver abscess.[15, 42] Symptoms depend on the type of involvement. Empyema, bronchohepatic fistulas, or extension of a pleuropulmonary abscess into the pericardium may occur. Pericardial amebiasis is the next most common form of extraintestinal involvement and may result from rupture of a liver abscess in the left lobe of the liver into the pericardium or via extension of the right-sided pleural amebiasis.[15, 28, 32, 37] It is estimated to occur in 3 per cent of patients with hepatic abscesses.[32] It presents as acute pericarditis with tamponade and, occasionally, as pneumopericardium.[28] Amebic liver abscess in the left lobe also may rupture directly into the left chest.[61]

Cerebral amebic abscesses were found in 8 per cent of patients with amebic infections discovered at autopsy in one study.[54] In other studies, lower rates of only 0.66 to 4.7 per cent of patients with amebic liver abscess having brain abscesses were reported.[41] Patients with cerebral amebiasis frequently are so ill from the intestinal, liver, and possibly lung involvement that neurologic signs are not always assessed easily. However, in 18 patients with proven cerebral amebiasis, initial neurologic examination was normal in 13, and only 1 later developed seizures.

Other foci of infection are quite rare, but amebic rectovesical fistula formation and involvement of pharynx, heart, aorta, and scapula have been reported. Cutaneous extension is an extremely painful rare complication.[15, 72]

DIAGNOSIS

As many as 40 per cent of adults with amebiasis and an even greater percentage of children escape diagnosis because this disease is not included as a diagnostic consideration. The diagnosis of amebiasis should be considered in any child who is passing bloody stools or stools with mucus; any child with an hepatic abscess; and any febrile child with right upper quadrant pain, abdominal distention, or tachypnea.[51, 65]

MICROSCOPIC DIAGNOSIS. The investigation of a child for amebiasis should include examination of three stools by wet mount (within 1 to 2 hours of stool passage) and by fixation in formalin and polyvinyl alcohol for permanent stains and concentration.[40, 72, 110] Multiple examinations often are necessary because the cysts are shed only intermittently. The stools should not be contaminated with water and urine (because these destroy trophozoites) or with interfering substances such as barium, laxatives, antibiotics, and soapsuds enemas.[72, 87] Saline does not destroy the trophozoites. A single, formed stool reveals amebic cysts by these techniques in 30 to 50 per cent of infected individuals.[40, 72] Examination of three stools, taken at daily intervals, will diagnose 60 to 70 per cent of patients with amebic colitis and 40 to 50 per cent of patients with amebic hepatic abscesses. The polyvinyl alcohol preserves trophozoites well, and the formalin allows good preservation and concentration of the cysts.[72] Staining with periodic acid–Schiff highlights the trophozoite forms, and the trichrome stain provides definition of intracellular characteristics of both trophozoites and cysts. It is important to be certain that any organisms seen are *E. histolytica* (or *E. dispar*) rather than the nonpathogenic *E. coli* or *E. hartmanni*. A negative stool examination should not preclude further work-up if no other explanation of the patient's symptoms has been found by this stage.

LABORATORY, SEROLOGIC, AND MOLECULAR DIAGNOSTIC TESTS. Most patients with amebic colitis will have occult blood in their feces—this often is a useful and inexpensive screening test.[87] A majority of the patients with amebic liver abscess will have a leukocytosis and an elevated alkaline phosphatase. In contrast, liver transaminases often are not elevated.

Serologic studies also can be helpful in the diagnosis of invasive amebiasis, whereas asymptomatic infections with *E. dispar* usually do not elicit a measurable serologic response. Moreover, the absence of serum antibodies to *E. histolytica* after 1 week of symptoms is evidence against the diagnosis of invasive amebiasis.[1, 87, 109] Gel diffusion (both agar gel diffusion and cellulose acetate diffusion), counterimmunoelectrophoresis, indirect hemagglutination, the indirect immunofluorescent test, and enzyme-linked immunosorbent assay are currently available tests.[6, 31, 72, 104, 110, 127] Indirect immunofluorescent and indirect hemagglutination titers persist for years after an infection, which makes them less useful in endemic areas.[72, 110] Counterimmunoelectrophoresis and gel diffusion will often revert to negative within months. Purified recombinant parasite antigens have been used in serologic tests for amebic liver abscesses and to distinguish between acute and convalescent infections.[1, 87] Enzyme-linked immunosorbent assays using genetically engineered polypeptides will likely become an important new tool for the diagnosis of invasive amebiasis.[112]

Newer molecular diagnostic tools ultimately may allow the clinician to distinguish the nonpathogenic *E. dispar* species from *E. histolytica*. These include enzyme-linked immunosorbent assays, which employ monoclonal antibodies developed against pathogen-specific epitopes,[1, 39, 94, 112] and the polymerase chain reaction, which uses species-specific oligonucleotides to differentiate *E. histolytica* from *E. dispar* in stool samples.[2]

RADIOGRAPHIC STUDIES. Radiologic imaging has become helpful in the diagnosis of extraintestinal amebiasis. Ultrasonography, computed tomography (CT), and magnetic resonance imaging (MRI) all have been shown to be helpful in demonstrating extracolonic amebiasis in the liver, paracecal masses, the brain, and other sites.[81–83, 121, 122] These modalities also improve the precision with which needle aspirations of these abscesses can be done.[122] At present, there appears to be no advantage in CT or MRI over sonography of the liver. The majority of patients with amebic liver abscess have a single abscess in the right lobe of the liver, although multiple lesions also can occur.[5] Chest radiographs show elevation of the right diaphragm in 56 per cent of patients with hepatic abscess.[4] The diagnosis of cerebral amebiasis requires careful neurologic evaluation and radiographic evaluation with either CT or MRI.[15, 41, 54] Because of the risk of perforation, barium studies are relatively contraindicated for patients with amebic colitis.

BIOPSY STUDIES. The colonic and rectal mucosa in amebic colitis usually reveals ulcerations with a diameter of 1 to 10 mm. Amebic trophozoites often are at the periphery of these necrotic areas, which can be sampled through a biopsy specimen taken during sigmoidoscopy or colonoscopy.[35, 40, 122] Because of the potential for perforation, colonoscopy should be undertaken with caution.

Amebic trophozoites are found near the capsule of amebic liver abscesses. In instances when a clinical diagnosis of amebic liver abscess is in doubt, needle aspiration of the liver abscess under CT or ultrasound guidance can be performed. This procedure has associated risks, including bleeding, peritoneal spillage of trophozoites, secondary superinfection, and accidental rupture of an echinococcal cyst.[87, 92]

DIFFERENTIAL DIAGNOSIS

Invasive amebic colitis may resemble ulcerative colitis, Crohn disease of the colon (inflammatory bowel disease), bacillary dysentery, or tuberculous colitis.[11, 17, 29, 40] Stool examinations, colonoscopic examination with biopsies, and serologic examination should be able to differentiate these diseases. Histologic examination of involved colonic mucosa should differentiate amebic colitis, with its relative lack of inflammation and rare granulation tissue, from the inflammatory responses seen in ulcerative colitis, bacillary dysentery, and Crohn disease of the colon. Tuberculous colitis and Crohn disease are more likely to show granuloma formation than amebiasis. Ileocecal or small bowel involvement as seen on barium studies would suggest Crohn disease or tuberculosis of the gastrointestinal tract rather than amebiasis. Tuberculous colitis usually is associated with pulmonary tuberculosis and with a strong reaction to tuberculin skin testing. In some cases, it may not be possible to differentiate between invasive amebic colitis and inflammatory bowel disease. If a patient with this differential diagnosis is placed on corticosteroids and deteriorates, the corticosteroids should be stopped and repeat investigation for amebiasis performed.[17, 65, 72]

Amebic liver abscess must be differentiated from pyogenic abscesses and neoplastic lesions. Total leukocyte counts and cultures of blood may help to differentiate pyogenic and amebic abscesses. However, many children with pyogenic liver abscesses have negative blood cultures. Often, both amebic and pyogenic liver abscesses will show similar features on CT and MRI. Occasionally, nuclear imaging with gallium is helpful because, unlike a pyogenic abscess, there are very few neutrophils contained within the amebic liver abscess (in this instance, the term amebic liver abscess is a misnomer).[87, 92] Hence, gallium scanning of an amebic liver abscess may reveal a cold spot, possibly with a bright rim. Several investigators recommend a trial with an appropriate drug for amebic abscess for 3 or 4 days while serologic and culture results are awaited.[65, 126] Patients with amebic liver abscess should respond to treatment in this length of time by becoming afebrile. No change in liver size or the size of the abscess should be noted in this time, because resolution of the abscess usually takes 2 months to several years.[5, 81, 82, 108, 124] Neoplastic lesions frequently can be proved to be solid masses by ultrasound examination. A history of weight loss without symptoms of dysentery or presence of *E. histolytica* in the stool suggests neoplastic disease.

COMPLICATIONS

Complications of amebiasis may be prevented by early diagnosis and treatment with appropriate agents.[41, 65] When complications occur, the prognosis generally is poor.

Invasive intestinal amebiasis has been associated most commonly with perforation and peritonitis.[7, 10, 45, 65, 111, 120] This apparently is an end result of "necrotizing" or "toxic" amebic colitis. In children, perforation may be heralded by the appearance of an acute abdomen or pneumoperitoneum, with rapid progression to death, presumably from sepsis.[7, 65, 120] Surgical resection and therapy for endotoxic shock improve the prognosis.[120] This complication is not rare and accounts for more than 30 per cent of the deaths from amebiasis in childhood.[11, 46] Massive intestinal hemorrhage causes about 3 per cent of deaths from amebiasis. Intussusception occasionally occurs and can be reduced with gentle barium enema. Multiple colonic strictures also can occur and cause obstructive symptoms. Fistulas to other organs or to the skin may develop.

Liver abscesses and their resultant complications account for about 40 per cent of the deaths from amebiasis.[46] Liver abscess also was found in 13 per cent of patients with amebiasis who had postmortem examinations. Liver abscess with rupture into the abdomen was present in 8 per cent of patients who died with amebiasis. Rupture of a liver abscess into the right pleural space was found in 12 per cent of amebic deaths.[46] Bacterial superinfection is found in 10 per cent of cases of pleural amebiasis.[42] In cases free of bacterial contamination, the fluid has few inflammatory cells and an acidic pH. Amebic pericarditis or pneumopericardium occurs rarely and is found in only 1 per cent of patients whose death was caused by amebiasis.[28, 32, 37, 46] The fluid is similar to that found in the pleural space. A cerebral abscess was found in 4 per cent of patients with amebiasis who died.[46] It has been reported in fewer than 10 children, only 1 of whom survived.[8, 15, 41, 54] Other complications include infections of the retroperitoneal space, stomach, spleen, esophagus, and duodenum.[54]

PREVENTION

Prevention of amebiasis requires sanitation, health education, early treatment of cases, and adequate surveillance and control programs.[87, 92] Because the only known mode of infection is ingestion of matter contaminated with cysts of *E. histolytica*, their removal through the disposal of human feces and water sterilization is essential. The cysts can be removed adequately from drinking water by sand filtration, hyperchlorination, or boiling.[59, 72] However, this still allows spread via raw fruits or vegetables contaminated with cysts. Infected food handlers are a major source of transmission. Travelers can avoid infection by avoiding unpeeled fruits and vegetables and drinking only boiled, bottled, or disinfected (iodination with tetraglycine hydroperiodide) water.[92] Early treatment of patients with intraluminal amebiasis also is important because asymptomatic individuals excrete up to 15 million cysts per day, which can survive in water for several weeks and often are resistant to the levels of chlorination used commonly for water purification.[67]

Therapy that targets individuals with *E. histolytica* but not *E. dispar* infections may become possible over the next few years as molecular diagnostic techniques improve.

TREATMENT

Intestinal Amebiasis

ASYMPTOMATIC INTRALUMINAL AMEBIASIS. Treatment of asymptomatic cyst passers is controversial. Many authors suggest that such treatment is mandatory because these individuals serve as a source of infection for other individuals and themselves may become symptomatic with a change in the intracolonic environment.[63, 67, 113] Other authors suggest that asymptomatic individuals not be treated, because the medications have severe toxicities, amebiasis is so widespread, and some individuals rid themselves of the disease with no therapy.[113] This controversy most likely will disappear once diagnostic methods that distinguish between *E. histolytica* and *E. dispar* infections become more widely available to clinicians. Until this time, it is most prudent to treat all children. Controversies surrounding the treatment of amebiasis during pregnancy will not be addressed here.

The three intraluminal agents most widely used to treat asymptomatic intraluminal amebiasis are iodoquinol, diloxanide furoate, and paromomycin. Each has a high rate of success for eradication of cyst passage.[57, 58]

Iodoquinol, or diiodohydroxyquin, is a poorly absorbed amebicidal agent with side effects of abdominal pain, nausea, vomiting, and diarrhea in the usual doses.[3, 57–60, 126] A small fraction is absorbed and can cause skin rashes or, through deiodination, thyroid function test abnormalities. In very large doses for prolonged periods, it has been reported to cause optic neuritis, optic atrophy, and peripheral neuropathy. It is not useful for extraintestinal amebiasis. The dosage of iodoquinol (Yodoxin) is 30 to 40 mg/kg/day to a maximum of 1950 mg in three divided oral doses for 20 days.

Diloxanide furoate (Furamide) is a poorly absorbed agent that is quite active only against intraluminal amebiasis but treats symptomatic as well as asymptomatic disease.[31, 60, 126] Cure rates have been more than 90 per cent with a 10-day oral course of diloxanide furoate at 20 mg/kg/day in three divided doses (maximum dose of 1500 mg/day).[57, 58, 73] It has few side effects; marked flatulence is the main problem. It is available through the Centers for Disease Control and Prevention by calling the CDC Drug Service (tel. 404-639-3670).

Paromomycin is a nonabsorbable aminoglycoside that is active against both the cyst and trophozoite stages. High cure rates have been reported with a 7-day oral dose of paromomycin at 25 to 35 mg/kg/day in three divided doses.

ACUTE AMEBIC COLITIS. Metronidazole is an imidazole compound that is available as a well-absorbed oral agent or as an intravenous medication.[3, 4, 21, 60, 79, 87, 92, 126] It is the most effective amebicide for treatment of amebic colitis and works by exploiting the anaerobic metabolism of the organism. By undergoing reduction and reacting with nucleic acids, metronidazole causes some mutagenicity and carcinogenicity in mice and hamsters, but no genetic disturbances have been found in humans.[60] Other side effects include nausea, headaches, a metallic taste of the saliva, dizziness, abdominal pain, glossitis, stomatitis, and diarrhea. Rarely, seizures or neuropathy occurs. It has an effect similar to that of disulfiram when taken while the patient consumes ethanol.[60] The oral dosage is 35 to 50 mg/kg/day (to a maximum of 2250 mg/day) in three divided doses for 10 days for severe intestinal or extraintestinal amebiasis. Cure rates for extraintestinal amebiasis are excellent, but one-third of patients with intraluminal amebiasis treated with metronidazole alone will have a relapse.[126] Therefore, treatment should be followed by an intraluminal agent, usually iodoquinol. Related imidazoles such as tinidazole and ornidazole, which are not marketed in the United States, may prove to be tolerated better than metronidazole.

Emetine and its derivative dehydroemetine are tissue-active amebicides derived from an ipecac alkaloid that inhibits protein synthesis.[60, 126] They have many side effects. Very common problems include diarrhea, vomiting, precordial chest pain, arrhythmias, electrocardiographic changes of inverted T waves and prolonged Q-T intervals, and tachycardia (especially if the patient is ambulatory). Emetine is cleared by renal excretion and still can be detected in urine up to 2 months after cessation of treatment; therefore, side effects may continue after stopping the emetine. Given the apparent success of the imidazoles for the treatment of amebiasis, it is anticipated that the use of emetine and dehydroemetine for intestinal amebiasis will continue to decrease.

Agents such as metronidazole that are active against invasive and extraintestinal amebiasis are well absorbed and do not necessarily stay in the lumen long enough to have an effect on intestinal amebiasis. Thus, these agents should be used in conjunction with a luminal agent either simultaneously or with the luminal agent used after the tissue-active agent.

Extraintestinal Amebiasis

AMEBIC LIVER ABSCESS AND METATSTATIC AMEBIASIS. Extraintestinal and severe intestinal amebiasis must be treated with the tissue-active agents. Metronidazole (35 to 50 mg/kg/day in three divided doses for 10 days) is the preferred drug because it is both quite effective and relatively free of serious side effects.[3, 4, 60, 87, 92, 126] It is effective for extraintestinal amebiasis in any location, although amebic brain abscesses usually are not treated successfully by any medications. Most patients with amebic liver abscess respond to metronidazole within 72 hours. As for amebic colitis, follow-up therapy with a luminal agent is very important because of the high rates of asymptomatic intestinal colonization in patients with amebic liver abscess.

If metronidazole cannot be used, a combination of chloroquine with either emetine or dehydroemetine is necessary, but side effects are a problem.

Because extraintestinal amebiasis begins most commonly with a hepatic abscess that ruptures into the abdomen, the right side of the chest, the pericardium, or the left side of the chest (from the left lobe of the liver), the issue of draining the hepatic abscess or the site of rupture must be considered.[46] Draining is indicated for (1) cysts greater than 12 cm in size that are in danger of rupture, (2) failure to respond to medical therapy, (3) a left lobe abscess that might predispose to pericardial rupture, (4) initial diagnosis to exclude pyogenic liver abscess, or (5) a ruptured abscess.[87, 119]

PROGNOSIS

Available statistics sugest that there are 500 million people infected with *E. histolytica* in the world. Invasive disease develops in 50 million people each year, and there are 50,000 to 100,000 deaths per year from the invasive disease.[80, 86, 87] This gives a case-fatality ratio of between 1:500 and 1:1000 diagnosed cases. However, among patients with illness severe enough to require hospitalization, the case-fatality ratio is higher. One small study in children reported a 9 per cent mortality rate and a 27 per cent morbidity rate.[65]

Bowel necrosis or perforation is the cause of death from purely intestinal amebiasis, and early surgical intervention can lower the mortality rate from these complications from 100 to 28 per cent.[120] Amebic liver abscess has a case-fatality rate of 10 to 15 per cent in combined figures of adults and children.[51, 69, 84] The mortality rate when pleural involvement is noted is 14 per cent.[42, 51] Amebic pericarditis has a case-fatality rate of 40 per cent.[37] Cerebral amebiasis has a case-fatality rate of 96 per cent.

References

1. Abd-Alla, M., Jackson, T. F. H. G., Gathirim, V., et al.: Differentiation of pathogenic from nonpathogenic *Entamoeba histolytica* infection by detection of galactose-inhibitable adherence protein antigen in sera and feces. J. Clin. Microbiol. *31*:2845–2850, 1993.
2. Acuna-Soto, R., Samuelson, J., De Girolami, P., et al: Application of the polymerase chain reaction to the epidemiology of pathogenic and nonpathogenic *Entamoeba histolytica*. Am. J. Trop. Med. Hyg. *48*:58–70, 1993.
3. Adams, E. B., and MacLeod, I. N.: Invasive amebiasis. I. Amebic dysentery and its complications. Medicine *56*:315–323, 1977.
4. Adams, E. B., and MacLeod, I. N.: Invasive amebiasis. II. Amebic liver abscess and its complications. Medicine *56*:325–334, 1977.
5. Ahmed, L., Salama, Z. A., El Rooby, A., et al.: Ultrasonographic resolution time for amebic liver abscess. Am. J. Trop. Med. Hyg. *41*:406–410, 1989.
6. Ambroise-Thomas, P., and Truong, T. K.: Fluorescent antibody test in amebiasis: Clinical applications. Am. J. Trop. Med. Hyg. *21*:907–911, 1972.
7. Azar, H., Nazarian, I., and Sadrieh, M.: A study of cause of death in patients with fulminant amebic colitis. Am. J. Proctol. *28*:80–84, 1977.
8. Bachy, A.: Cerebral abscesses in amebiasis. J. Pediatr. *88*:364–365, 1976.
9. Bailey, G. B., Nudelman, E. D., Day, D. B., et al.: Specificity of glycosphingolipid recognition by *Entamoeba histolytica* trophozoites. Infect. Immun. *58*:43–47, 1990.
10. Balikian, J. P., Bitar, J. G., Rishani, K. K., et al.: Fulminant necrotizing amebic colitis in children. Am. J. Proctol. *28*:69–73, 1977.
11. Balikian, J. P., Uthman, S. M., and Kabakian, H. A.: Tuberculous colitis. Am. J. Proctol. *28*:75–79, 1977.
12. Barker, D. C.: Differentiation of *Entamoeba*. Patterns of nucleic acids and ribosomes during encystation and excystation. *In* Van den Bossche H. (ed.): Biochemistry of Parasites and Host-Parasite Relationships. Amsterdam, Elsevier Biomedical, 1976, p. 253.
13. Bhattacharya, S., Bhattacharya, A., Diamond, L. S., et al.: Circular DNA of *Entamoeba histolytica* encodes ribosomal RNA. J. Protozool. *36*:455–458, 1989.
14. Braga, L. L., Ninomiya, H., McCoy, J. J., et al. Inhibition of the complement membrane attack complex by the galactose-specific adhesion of *Entamoeba histolytica*. J. Clin. Invest. *90*:1131–1137, 1992.
15. Brandt, H., and Tamayo, R. P.: Pathology of human amebiasis. Hum. Pathol. *1*:351–385, 1970.
16. Burch D. J., Li, E., Reed, S., et al.: Isolation of a strain-specific *Entamoeba histolytica* cDNA clone. J. Clin. Microbiol. *29*:297–302, 1991.
17. Case records of the Massachusetts General Hospital: Weekly clinicopathological exercises: Case 32–1977. N. Engl. J. Med. *297*:322–330, 1977.
18. Chadee, K., Petri, W. A., Jr., Innes, D. J., et al.: Rat and human colonic mucins bind and inhibit adherence lectin of *Entamoeba histolytica*. J. Clin. Invest. *80*:1245–1254, 1987.
19. Chu-Jing, G. S., Kain, K. C., Abd-Alla, M., et al.: A recombinant cysteine-rich section of the *Entamoeba histolytica* galactose-inhibitable lectin is efficacious as a subunit vaccine in the gerbil model of amebic liver abscess. J. Infect. Dis. *171*:645–651, 1995.
20. Clark, C. G., and Diamond, L. S.: Ribosomal RNA genes of "pathogenic" *Entamoeba histolytica* are distinct. Mol. Biochem. Parasitol. *49*:297–302, 1991.
21. Cohen, H. G., and Reynolds, T. B.: Comparison of metronidazole and chloroquine for the treatment of amoebic liver abscess. Gastroenterology *69*:35–41, 1975.
22. Councilman, W. T., and Lafleur, H. A.: Amoebic dysentery. Johns Hopkins Hosp. Rep. *2*:395–548, 1891.
23. DeMeester, F., Shaw, E., Scholze, H., et al.: Specific labeling of cysteine proteinases in pathogenic and nonpathogenic *Entamoeba histolytica*. Infect. Immun. *58*:1396–1401, 1990.
24. Diamond, L. S., and Clark, C. G.: A redescription of *Entamoeba histolytica* Schaudinn. 1903 (Emended Walker, 1911) separating it from *Entamoeba dispar* (Brumpt, 1925). J. Eukaryotic Microbiol. *40*:340–344, 1993.
25. Druckman, D. A., and Quinn, T. C.: *Entamoeba histolytica* infection in homosexual men. *In* Ravdin, J. I. (ed.): Amebiasis: Human Infection by *Entamoeba histolytica*. New York, Churchill Livingstone, 1988, pp. 563–571.
26. Elsdon-Dew, R.: The epidemiology of amoebiasis. Adv. Parasitol. *6*:1–62, 1968.
27. Faubert, G. M., Meerovitch, E., and McLaughlin, J.: The presence of liver auto-antibodies induced by *Entamoeba histolytica* in the sera from both naturally infected humans and immunized rabbits. Am. J. Trop. Med. Hyg. *27*:892–895, 1978.
28. Freeman, A. L., and Bhoola, K. D.: Pneumopericardium complicating amoebic liver abscess: A case report. S. Afr. Med. J. *50*:551–553, 1976.
29. Friedrich, I. A., Korsten, M. A., and Gottfried, E. B.: Necrotizing amebic colitis with pseudomembrane formation. Am. J. Gastroenterol. *74*:529–531, 1980.
30. Fuchs, G., Ruiz-Palacios, G., and Pickering, L.K.: Amebiasis in the pediatric population. *In* Ravdin J. I. (ed.): Amebiasis: Human Infection by *Entamoeba histolytica*. New York, Churchill Livingstone, 1988, pp. 594–613.
31. Gandhi, B. M., Irshad, M., Acharya, S. K., et al.: Amebic liver abscess and circulating immune complexes of *Entamoeba histolytica* proteins. Am. J. Trop. Med. Hyg. *39*:440–444, 1988.
32. Ganesan, T. K., and Kandaswamy, S.: Amebic pericarditis. Chest *67*:112–113, 1975.
33. Garfinkel, L. I., Giladi, M., Huber, M., et al.: DNA probes specific for *Entamoeba histolytica* possessing pathogenic and nonpathogenic zymodemes. Infect. Immun. *57*:926–931, 1989.
34. Gathiram, V., and Jackson, T. F. H. G.: A longitudinal study of asymptomatic carriers of pathogenic zymodemes of *Entamoeba histolytica*. S. Afr. Med. J. *72*:669–672, 1987.
35. Gilman, R., Islam, M., Paschi, S., et al.: Comparison of conventional and immunofluorescent techniques for the detection of *Entamoeba histolytica* in rectal biopsies. Gastroenterology *78*:435–439, 1980.
36. Griffin, J. L.: Human amebic dysentery: Electron microscopy of *Entamoeba histolytica* contacting, ingesting, and digesting inflammatory cells. Am. J. Trop. Med. Hyg. *21*:895–906, 1972.
37. Guimaraes, A. C., Vinhaes, L. A., Filho, A. S., et al.: Acute suppurative amebic pericarditis. Am. J. Cardiol. *34*:103–106, 1974.
38. Haffar, A., Boland, J., and Edwards, M. S.: Amebic liver abscess in children. Pediatr. Infect. Dis. *1*:322–327, 1982.
39. Haque, R., Kress, K., Wood, S., et al.: Diagnosis of pathogenic *Entamoeba histolytica* infection using a stool ELISA based on monoclonal antibodies to the galactose-specific adhesin. J. Infect. Dis. *167*:247–249, 1993.
40. Harries, J.: Amoebiasis: A review. J. R. Soc. Med. *75*:190–197, 1982.
41. Hughes, F. B., Faehnle, S. T., and Simon, J. L.: Multiple cerebral abscesses complicating hepatopulmonary amebiasis. J. Pediatr. *86*:95–96, 1979.
42. Ibarra-Perez, C., and Selman-Lama, M.: Diagnosis and treatment of amebic "empyema": Report of eighty-eight cases. Am. J. Surg. *134*:283–287, 1977.
43. Jansson, A., Gillin, F., Kagardt, U., et al.: Coding of hemolysins within the ribosomal RNA repeat on a plasmid in *Entamoeba histolytica*. Science *263*:144–1443, 1994.
44. Joyce, M. P., and Ravdin, J. I.: Antigens of *Entamoeba histolytica* recognized by immune sera from liver abscess patients. Am. J. Trop. Med. Hyg. *38*:74–80, 1988.
45. Kala, P. C., Sharma, G. C., and Haldia, K. N.: Fulminating amoebic colitis with multiple perforations. Am. J. Proctol. *28*:31–34, 1977.
46. Kean, B. H., Gilmore, H. R., Jr., and Van Stone, W. W.: Fatal amebiasis:

Report of 148 fatal cases from the Armed Forces Institutes of Pathology. Ann. Intern. Med. *44*:831–843, 1956.
47. Keene, W. E., Petitt, M. G., Allen, S., et al.: The major neutral proteinase of *Entamoeba histolytica*. J. Exp. Med. *163*:536–549, 1986.
48. Kelsall, B. L., and Ravdin, J. I.: Proteolytic degradation of human IgA by *Entamoeba histolytica*. J. Infect. Dis. *168*:1319–1322, 1993.
49. Kettis, A. A., Thorstensson, R., and Utter, G.: Antigenicity of *Entamoeba histolytica* strain NIH 200: A survey of clinically relevant antigenic components. Am. J. Trop. Med. Hyg. *32*:512–522, 1983.
50. Knobloch J., and Mannweiler D.: Development and persistence of antibodies to *Entamoeba histolytica* in patients with amebic liver abscess: analysis of 216 cases. Am. J. Trop. Med. Hyg. *32*:727–732, 1983.
51. Lamont, A. C., and Wicks, A. C. B.: Amoebic liver abscess in Rhodesian Africans. Trans. R. Soc. Trop. Med. Hyg. *70*:302–305, 1976.
52. Leippe, M., Tannich, E., Nickel, R., et al.: Primary and secondary structure of the pore-forming protein produced by *Entamoeba histolytica*. EMBO J. *11*:3501–3506, 1992.
53. Leitch, G. J.: Intestinal lumen and mucosal microclimate H+ and NH3 concentrations as factors in the etiology of experimental amebiasis. Am. J. Trop. Med. Hyg. *38*:480–486, 1988.
54. Lombardo, L., Alonso, P., Arroyo, L. S., et al.: Cerebral amebiasis: Report of 17 cases. J. Neurosurg. *21*:704–709, 1964.
55. Long-Krug, S. A., Hysmith, R. M., Fischer, K. J., et al.: The phospholipase A enzymes of *Entamoeba histolytica*: Description and subcellular localization. J. Infect. Dis. *152*:536–541, 1985.
56. Losch, F.: Massenhafte entwicklung von amoben in dickdarm. Virchows Arch. [A] *65*:196–211, 1975.
57. McAuley, J. B., Herwaldt, B. L., Stokes, S. L., et al.: Diloxanide furoate for treating asymptomatic *Entamoeba histolytica* cyst passers: 14 years' experience in the United States. Clin. Infect. Dis. *15*:464–468, 1992.
58. McAuley, J. B., and Juranek, D. D.: Luminal agents in the treatment of amebiasis. Clin. Infect. Dis. *14*:1161–1162, 1992.
59. Mahmoud, A. A. F., and Warren, K. S.: Algorithms in the diagnosis and management of exotic diseases. XVII. Amebiasis. J. Infect. Dis. *134*:639–643, 1976.
60. Mandell, W. F., and Neu, H. C.: Parasitic infections: Therapeutic considerations. Med. Clin. North Am. *72*:669–690, 1988.
61. Markwalder, K.: Left-side pleuropulmonary amoebiasis: A case report from Chad. Trans. R. Soc. Trop. Med. Hyg. *75*:308–309, 1981.
62. Martinez-Palomo, A., Tsutsumi, V., Anaya-Velazquez, F., et al.: Ultrastructure of experimental intestinal invasive amebiasis. Am. J. Trop. Med. Hyg. *41*:273–279, 1989.
63. Mathews, H. M., Moss, D. M., Healy, G. R., et al.: Isoenzyme analysis of *Entamoeba histolytica* isolated from homosexual men. J. Infect. Dis. *153*:793–795, 1986.
64. Mendoza, J. B., and Barba, E. J. R.: Cutaneous amebiasis of the face: A case report. Am. J. Trop. Med. Hyg. *35*:69–71, 1986.
65. Merritt, R. J., Coughlin, E., Thomas, D. W., et al.: Spectrum of amebiasis in children. Am. J. Dis. Child. *136*:785–789, 1982.
66. Mirelman, D., Bracha, R., Rozenblatt, S., et al.: Repetitive DNA elements characteristic of pathogenic *Entamoeba histolytica* strains can also be detected after polymerase chain reaction in a cloned nonpathogenic strain. Infect. Immun. *58*:1660–1663, 1990.
67. Mirelman, D., DeMeester, F., Stolarsky, T., et al.: Effects of covalently bound silica-nitroimidazole drug particles on *Entamoeba histolytica*. J. Infect. Dis. *159*:303–309, 1989.
68. Mirelman, D., Feingold, C., Wexler, A., et al.: Interactions between *Entamoeba histolytica*, bacteria and intestinal cells. Ciba Found. Symp. *99*:2–30, 1983.
69. Moorthy, B., Mehta, S., Mitra, S. K., et al.: Amoebic liver abscess in a four-month-old infant. Aust. Paediatr. J. *13*:53–55, 1977.
70. Munoz, O.: Clinical spectrum of amebiasis in children. *In* Kretschmer, R. R. (ed.): Amebiasis: Infection and Disease by *Entamoeba histolytica*. Boca Raton, CRC Press, 1990, pp. 209–220.
71. Osler, W.: On the *Amoeba coli* in dysentery and in dysenteric liver abscess. Johns Hopkins Hosp. Bull. *1*:53–54, 1890.
72. Patterson, M., and Schoppe, L. E.: The presentation of amoebiasis. Med. Clin. North Am. *66*:689–705, 1982.
73. Pehrson, P., and Bengtsson, E.: Treatment of non-invasive amoebiasis: A comparison between tinidazole alone and in combination with diloxanide furoate. Trans. R. Soc. Trop. Med. Hyg. *77*:845–846, 1983.
74. Petri, W. A., and Ravdin, J. I.: Amebiasis in institutionalized populations. *In* Ravdin, J. I. (ed.): Amebiasis: Human Infection by *Entamoeba histolytica*. New York, Churchill Livingstone, 1988.
75. Petri, W. A., Jr., Jackson, T. F. H. G., Gathiram, V., et al.: Pathogenic and nonpathogenic strains of *Entamoeba histolytica* can be differentiated by monoclonal antibodies to the galactose-specific adherence lectin. Infect. Immun. *58*:1802–1806, 1990.
76. Petri, W. A., Jr., Smith, R. D., Schlesinger, P. H., et al.: Isolation of the galactose-binding lectin that mediates the in vitro adherence of *Entamoeba histolytica*. J. Clin. Invest. *80*:1238–1244, 1987.
77. Petri, W. A., Jr., Chapman, M. D., Snodgrass, T., et al.: Subunit structure of the galactose and N-acetyl galactosamine-inhibitable adherence lectin of *Entamoeba histolytica*. J. Biol. Chem. *264*:3007–3012, 1989.
78. Pittman, F. E., El-Hashimi, W. K., and Pittman, J. C.: Studies of human amebiasis. I. Clinical and laboratory findings in eight cases of acute amebic colitis. Gastroenterology *65*:581–587, 1973.
79. Pittman, F. E., El-Hashimi, W. K., and Pittman, J. C.: Studies of human amebiasis. II. Light and electron microscopic observations of colonic mucosa and exudate in acute amebic colitis. Gastroenterology *65*:588–603, 1973.
80. Prevention and Control of Intestinal Parasitic Infections. World Health Organization Technical Report *749*:1–80, 1987.
81. Radin, D. R, Ralls, P. W., Colletti, P. M., et al.: CT of amebic liver abscess. A. J. R. Am. J. Roentgenol. *150*:1297–1301, 1988.
82. Ralls, P. W., Henley, D. S., Colletti, P. M., et al.: Amebic liver abscess: MR imaging. Radiology *165*:801–804, 1987.
83. Ralls, P. W., Quinn, M. F., Boswell, W. D., et al.: Patterns of resolution in successfully treated hepatic amebic abscess: Sonographic evaluation. Radiology *149*:541–543, 1983.
84. Ramachandran, S., Goonatillake, H. D., and Induruwa, P. A. C.: Syndromes in amoebic liver abscess. Br. J. Surg. *63*:220–225, 1976.
85. Ramachandran, S., Induruwa, P. A. C., and Perera, M. V. F.: pH of amoebic liver pus. Trans. R. Soc. Trop. Med. Hyg. *70*:159–160, 1976.
86. Ravdin, J. I.: *Entamoeba histolytica:* From adherence to enteropathy. J. Infect. Dis. *159*:420–429, 1989.
87. Ravdin, J. I.: Amebiasis. Clin. Infect. Dis. 20:1453–1466, 1995
88. Ravdin, J. I., and Guerrant, R. L.: Role of adherence in cytopathogenic mechanisms of *Entamoeba histolytica*. J. Clin. Invest. *68*:1305–1313, 1981.
89. Ravdin, J. I., Murphy, C. F., Guerrant, R. L., et al.: Effect of calcium and phospholipase A antagonists on the cytopathogenicity of *Entamoeba histolytica*. J. Infect. Dis. *152*:542–549, 1985.
90. Ravdin, J. I., Murphy, C. F., Salata, R. A., et al.: N-acetyl-D-galactosamine-inhibitable adherence lectin of *Entamoeba histolytica*. I. Partial purification and relation to amoebic virulence in vitro. J. Infect. Dis. *151*:804–815, 1985.
91. Ravdin, J. I., Moreau, F., Sullivan, J. A., et al.: The relationship of free intracellular calcium ions to the cytolytic activity of *Entamoeba histolytica*. Infect. Immun. *56*:1505–1512, 1988.
92. Reed, S. L., and Ravdin J. I.: Amebiasis. *In* Blaser, M. J., Smith P. D., Ravdin, J. I., et al. (eds.): Infections of the Gastrointestinal Tract. New York, Raven Press, 1995, pp. 1065–1080.
93. Reed, S. L., Keene, W. E., McKerrow, J. H., et al.: Cleavage of C3 by a neutral cysteine proteinase of *Entamoeba histolytica*. J. Immunol. *143*:189–195, 1989.
94. Reed, S. L., Flores, B. M., Batzer, M. A., et al: Molecular and cellular characterization of the 29-kDa peripheral membrane protein of *Entamoeba histolytica*: Differentiation between pathogenic and nonpathogenic isolates. Infect. Immun. *60*:542–549, 1992.
95. Reed, S., Bouvier, J., Pollack, A. S., et al.: Cloning of a virulence factor of *Entamoeba histolytica*. J. Clin. Invest. *91*:1532–1540, 1993.
96. Rodriguez, M. A., and Orozco, E.: Isolation and characterization of phagocytosis- and virulence-deficient mutants of *Entamoeba histolytica*. J. Infect. Dis. *154*:27–32, 1986.
97. Rustgi, A. K., and Richter, J. M.: Pyogenic and amebic liver abscess. Med. Clin. North Am. *73*:847–858, 1989.
98. Salata, R. A., Ahmed, P., and Ravdin, J. I.: Chemoattractant activity of *Entamoeba histolytica* for human polymorphonuclear neutrophils. J. Parasitol. *75*:644–646, 1989.
99. Salata, R. A., Martinez-Palomo, A., Murray, H. W., et al.: Patients treated for amebic liver abscess develop cell-mediated immune responses effective in vitro against *Entamoeba histolytica*. J. Immunol. *136*:2633–2639, 1986.
100. Salata, R. A., Murray, H. W., Rubin, B. Y., et al.: The role of gamma interferon in the generation of human macrophages and T lymphocytes cytotoxic for *Entamoeba histolytica*. Am. J. Trop. Med. Hyg. *37*:72–78, 1987.
101. Salata, R. A., Pearson, R. D., and Ravdin, J. I.: Interaction of human leukocytes and *Entamoeba histolytica*. Killing of virulent amebae by the activated macrophage. J. Clin. Invest. *76*:491–499, 1985.
102. Salata, R. A., and Ravdin, J. I.: N-acetyl-D-galactosamine-inhibitable adherence lectin of *Entamoeba histolytica*. II. Mitogenic activity for human lymphocytes. J. Infect. Dis. *151*:816–822, 1985.
103. Salata, R. A., and Ravdin, J. I.: The interaction of human neutrophils and *Entamoeba histolytica* increases cytopathogenicity for liver cell monolayers. J. Infect. Dis. *154*:19–26, 1986.
104. Sathar, M. A., Bredenkamp, B. L., Gathiram, V., et al.: Detection of *Entamoeba histolytica* immunoglobulins G and M to plasma membrane antigen by enzyme-linked immunosorbent assay. J. Clin. Microbiol. *28*:332–335, 1990.
105. Saxena, A., Chugh, S., and Vinayak, V. K.: Elucidation of cellular population and nature of anti-amoebic antibodies in cytotoxicity to *Entamoeba histolytica* (NIH:200). J. Parasitol. *72*:434–438, 1986.
106. Schmerin, M. J., Gelstron, A., and Jones, T. C.: Amebiasis: An increasing problem among homosexuals in New York City. J. A. M. A. *238*:1386–1387, 1977.
107. Schulte, W., and Scholze, H.: Action of the major protease from *Entamoeba histolytica* on proteins of the extracellular matrix. J. Protozool. *36*:538–543, 1989.
108. Sheen, I. S., Chien, C. S. C., Lin, D. Y., et al.: Resolution of liver abscesses: Comparison of pyogenic and amebic liver abscesses. Am. J. Trop. Med. Hyg. *40*:384–389, 1989.

109. Shetty, N., Das, P., Pal, S. C., et al.: Observations on the interpretation of amoebic serology in endemic areas. J. Trop. Med. Hyg. *91*:222–227, 1988.
110. Shetty, N., and Prabhu, T.: Evaluation of faecal preservation and staining methods in the diagnosis of acute amoebiasis and giardiasis. J. Clin. Pathol. *41*:694–699, 1988.
111. Sotela-Avila, C., Kline, M., Silberstein, M. J., et al.: Bloody diarrhea and pneumoperitoneum in a 10-month-old girl. J. Pediatr. *113*:1098–1104, 1988.
112. Stanley S. L., Jackson, T. F. H. G., Reed, S. L., et al.: Serodiagnosis of invasive amebiasis using a recombinant *Entamoeba histolytica* protein. J. A. M. A. 266:1984–1986, 1991.
113. Takeuchi, T., Okuzawa, E., Nozaki, T., et al.: High seropositivity of Japanese homosexual men for amebic infection. J. Infect. Dis. *159*:808, 1989.
114. Tannich, E., Horstmann, R. D., Knobloch, J., et al.: Genomic DNA differences between pathogenic and nonpathogenic *Entamoeba histolytica*. Proc. Natl. Acad. Sci. U. S. A. *86*:5118–5122, 1989.
115. Tannich, E., Ebert, F., and Horstmann, R. D.: Primary structure of the 170-kDa surface lectin of pathogenic *Entamoeba histolytica*. Proc. Natl. Acad. Sci. U. S. A. *88*:1849–1853, 1991.
116. Torian, B. E., Reed, S. L., Flores, B. M., et al.: Serologic response to the 96,000-Da surface antigen of pathogenic *Entamoeba histolytica*. J. Infect. Dis. *159*:794–797, 1989.
117. Torian, B. E., Reed, S. L., Flores, B. M., et al.: The 96-kilodalton antigen as an integral membrane protein in pathogenic *Entamoeba histolytica*: Potential differences in pathogenic and nonpathogenic isolates. Infect. Immun. *58*:753–760, 1990.
118. Udezulu, I. A., and Leitch, G. J.: A membrane-associated neuraminidase in *Entamoeba histolytica* trophozoites. Infect. Immun. *36*:795–801, 1981.
119. vanSonnenberg, E., Mueller, P. R., Schiffman, H. R., et al.: Intrahepatic amebic abscess: Indications for and results of percutaneous catheter drainage. Radiology *156*:631–635, 1985.
120. Vargas, M., and Pena, A.: Toxic amoebic colitis and amoebic colon perforation in children: An improved prognosis. J. Pediatr. Surg. *11*:223–225, 1976.
121. Vicary, F. R., Cusick, G., Shirley, I. M., et al.: Ultrasound and amoebic liver abscess. Br. J. Surg. *64*:113–114, 1977.
122. Walsh, T. J., Berkman, W., Brown, N. L., et al.: Cytopathologic diagnosis of extracolonic amebiasis. Acta Cytol. *27*:671–675, 1983.
123. Wanke, C., Butler, T., and Islam, M.: Epidemiologic and clinical features of invasive amebiasis in Bangladesh: A case-control comparison with other diarrheal diseases and postmortem findings. Am. J. Trop. Med. Hyg. *38*:335–341, 1988.
124. Watt, G., Padre, L. P., Adapon, B., et al.: Nonresolution of an amebic liver abscess after parasitologic cure. Am. J. Trop. Med. Hyg. *35*:501–504, 1986.
125. Werries, E., Nebinger, P., and Franz, A.: Degradation of biogene oligosaccharides by beta-N-acetylglucosaminidase secreted by *Entamoeba histolytica*. Mol. Biochem. Parasitol. *7*:127–140, 1983.
126. Wolfe, M. S.: The treatment of intestinal protozoan infections. Med. Clin. North Am. *66*:707–720, 1982.
127. Yang, J., and Kennedy, M. T.: Evaluation of enzyme-linked immunosorbent assay for the serodiagnosis of amebiasis. J. Clin. Microbiol. *10*:778–785, 1979.

209

BLASTOCYSTIS HOMINIS INFECTION

Peter J. Hotez

Blastocystis hominis is a protist that inhabits the gastrointestinal tract of humans and possibly other animals. Although new information about the molecular and cell biology of this organism has been acquired over the last 10 years, there still is considerable controversy regarding its true taxonomy and life cycle.[4, 26] The pathogenicity of *B. hominis* and its ability to cause gastrointestinal illness in humans are equally controversial.[10, 13, 16, 23, 24]

ETIOLOGY AND PATHOGENESIS

Since its discovery in the early part of the 20th century by Alexeieff and then Brumpt,[1, 6] *B. hominis* has been assigned to many different phyla in both animal and plant kingdoms. Early on, it was identified by various workers as vegetable material, a yeast, a fungus, or a protozoan. Although the organism was identified as a protozoan parasite in 1967, its subphylum status bounced between the Sporozoa and the Sarcodina.[4] Nucleic acid sequencing data now suggest that *B. hominis* does not belong to either category but instead probably comprises its own group more closely related to the ameboflagellates belonging to a new proposed subphylum called Blastocysta.[4, 11, 12] Additional molecular taxonomic data suggest that the intraspecific variation between stocks of *B. hominis* is sufficiently different to warrant at least two separate species assignments for the organism.[5] This observation ultimately may have a bearing on the current controversies surrounding the pathogenicity of the organism.

Ultrastructural information gathered from light and electron microscopy on organisms obtained from in vitro culture and from fresh fecal material indicates the existence of several different parasite forms, including cyst forms, ameboid forms, and the so-called granular, avacuolar, and vacuolar forms.[4] The *B. hominis* vacuolar cell is the most distinctive and appears as a thin peripheral band of cytoplasm surrounding a large membrane-enclosed central vacuole.[4] The central vacuole may have a storage function. Although *B. hominis* is believed to have predominantly anaerobic metabolism, structures that look like mitochondria have been identified on transmission electron microscopy. It has been proposed that the *Blastocystis* mitochondria may function only in lipid biosynthesis and not oxidative phosphorylation.[4, 26] Alternatively, what appears to be a *Blastocystis* mitochondrion on electron microscopy actually may be a hydrogenosome.[4]

Several highly speculative life cycles of *B. hominis* have been proposed.[4, 12] The infective stage probably is a dormant cyst form, which undergoes excystation in response to host gastric acid and intestinal enzymes. Excystation may result in the release of avacuolar forms that can undergo facultative transformation to either an ameboid or a multivacuolar form. The multivacuolar form, in turn, either may encyst to an infective stage or coalesce to the vacuolar form.[4] These stages are believed to predominate in the large intestine, although organisms also have been recovered from duodenal aspirates. Which, if any, of these life cycle stages invade tissue or cause disease is not known. Acquisition of knowledge in this area has been hampered by lack of a suitable animal model, although infection of gnotobiotic guinea pigs with this organism was reported to result in mild intestinal hyperemia and superficial invasion of *B. hominis* into the mucosa of the cecum. Nonspecific inflammation (infiltration of lymphocytes and plasmocytes) and edema of the colonic mucosa have been seen during sigmoidoscopy with biopsy in some patients.[4] Thus far, no serologic antibody response to the organism has been demonstrated.[7] The possibility remains that *B. hominis* is entirely commensal in humans. The epidemiologic association between infection and disease is reviewed next.

EPIDEMIOLOGY AND CLINICAL MANIFESTATIONS

B. hominis has a worldwide distribution in both tropical and temperate regions, with up to 54 per cent infection rates among some populations.[2–4, 8, 9, 18, 19, 22, 25] High rates of infection also have been reported in individuals with a recent history of travel,[21] with exposure to pets or farm animals,[8] and living in institutionalized settings.[4] In many of these individuals, however, *B. hominis* probably is a commensal parasite. Although *B. hominis* is common in preschool and schoolchildren,[18–20] children overall do not appear to be at increased risk for infection.[4]

The majority of studies investigating the association between *B. hominis* infection and disease are based primarily on clinical laboratory isolates of the organism in patients exhibiting gastrointestinal symptoms. Common clinical complaints include abdominal discomfort, bloating, cramping, diarrhea, and vomiting.[2] Weight loss associated with a protein-losing enteropathy also has been described. Infective arthritis also has been reported.[14] Because *B. hominis* commonly is found in both symptomatic and asymptomatic individuals, some investigators have proposed that only very heavy infections result in disease.[15, 17, 23] Many of these reports are not controlled, however. Shlim and colleagues[23] conducted a large prospective controlled study among a population of expatriates and tourists in Katmandu, Nepal, who were at high risk for traveler's diarrhea. They concluded that *B. hominis* in high concentrations was not associated with diarrhea and the presence of higher concentrations of the organism in stool was not associated with more severe symptoms.[23] In a subsequent editorial, several design features were cited that may "weaken the authors' conclusions."[13] At least four other prospective trials have been conducted, with one supporting *B. hominis* as a cause of diarrhea, one arguing against it, and two others that were inconclusive.[21] The confusion may be resolved partly by the identification of separate human "demes" of *Blastocystis*,[5, 12] which might lead to improved molecular diagnostic techniques for distinguishing pathogenic from nonpathogenic species. This situation is somewhat analogous to the morphologically identical species of *Entamoeba* (*E. histolytica* and *E. dispar*), only one of which causes colitis.

DIAGNOSIS

Light microscopy of wet preparations of fresh or concentrated stool usually will identify *B. hominis*. Staining of preparations with iodine or trichome also is of some benefit. Many laboratories will attempt to identify the characteristic vacuolar forms, which actually may be underrepresented in clinical material.[4] Under these circumstances, the services of an experienced technologist are required to identify the less distinctive multivacuolar forms in the feces. Organisms also can be recovered from biopsy material obtained during sigmoidoscopy and colonoscopy.

TREATMENT

Given the controversy surrounding the pathogenicity of *B. hominis*, it is prudent to refrain from treating asymptomatic immunocompetent individuals. In individuals who have gastrointestinal illness and in whom other pathogens have been excluded, it may be reasonable to administer a course of antiprotozoal chemotherapy. Some investigators have reported symptomatic improvement in patients receiving either metronidazole or tinidazole.[4, 9] Using an in vitro assay that employed metabolic labeling, the drugs emetine, satranidazole, furazolidone, and quinacrine were superior in activity to either metronidazole or tinidazole.[4] The authors caution, however, that the in vitro assay does not take into account the pharmacokinetic properties of the drugs.

References

1. Alexeieff, A.: Sur la nutre des formations dites "kystes de *Trichomonas intestinalis*." Comptes Rendus des Seances de la Societe de Biologies *71*:296–298, 1911.
2. Al-Tawil, Y. S., Gilger, M. A., Gopalakrishna, G. S., et al.: Invasive *Blastocystis hominis* infection in a child. Arch. Pediatr. Adolesc. Med. *148*:882–885, 1994.
3. Ashford, R. W., and Atkinson, E. A.: Epidemiology of *Blastocystis hominis* infection in Papua New Guinea: Age-prevalence and associations with other parasites. Ann. Trop. Med. Parasitol. *86*:129–136, 1992.
4. Boreham, P. F. L., and Stenzel, D. J.: Blastocystis in humans and animals: Morphology, biology, and epizootiology. Adv. Parasitol. *32*:1–70, 1993.
5. Boreham, P. F., Upcroft, J. A., and Dunn, L. A.: Protein and DNA evidence for two demes of *Blastocystis hominis* from humans. Int. J. Parasitol. *22*:49–53, 1992.
6. Brumpt, E.: *Blastocystis hominis* n. sp. et formes voisines. Bull. Soc. Pathol. Exot. Filiales *5*:725–730, 1912.
7. Chen, J., Vaudry, W. L., Kowalewska, K., and Wenman, W.: Lack of serum immune response to *Blastocystis hominis*. Lancet *1*:1021, 1987.
8. Doyle, P. W., Helgason, M. M., Mathias, R. G. and Proctor, E. M.: Epidemiology and pathogenecity of *Blastocystis hominis*. J. Clin. Microbiol. *28*:116–121, 1990.
9. El Masry, N. A., Bassily, S., and Farid, Z.: *Blastocystis hominis*: Clinical and therapeutic aspects. Trans. R. Soc. Trop. Med. Hyg. *82*:173, 1988.
10. Garcia, L. S., Bruckner, D. A., and Clancy, M. N.: Clinical relevance of *Blastocystis hominis*. Lancet *1*:1233–1234, 1984.
11. Jiang, J.-H., and He, J.-G.: Taxonomic status of *Blastocystis hominis*. Parasitol. Today *9*:2–3, 1993.
12. Johnson, A. M., Thanous, A., Boreham, P. F. L., and Baverstock, P. R.: *Blastocystis hominis*: Phylogenetic affinities determined by rRNA sequence comparison. Exp. Parasitol. *68*:283–288, 1989.
13. Keystone, J. S.: Editorial: *Blastocystis hominis* and traveler's diarrhea. Clin. Infect. Dis. *21*:102–103, 1995.
14. Lee, M. G., Rawlins, S. C., Didier, M., et al.: Infective arthritis due to *Blastocystis hominis*. Ann. Rheum. Dis. *49*:192–193, 1990.
15. Logar, J., Andlovic, A., and Poljsak-Prijatel, M.: Incidence of *Blastocystis hominis* in patients with diarrhoea. J. Infect. *28*:151–154, 1994.
16. Markell, E. K.: Editorial: Is there any reason to continue treating *Blastocystis* infections? Clin. Infect. Dis. *21*:104–105, 1995.
17. Markell, E. K., and Udkow, M. P.: *Blastocystis hominis*: Pathogen or fellow traveler? Am. J. Trop. Med. Hyg. *35*:1023–1026, 1986.
18. Nimri, L. F.: Evidence of an epidemic of *Blastocystis hominis* infections in preschool children in northern Jordan. J. Clin. Microbiol. *31*:2706–2708, 1993.
19. Nimri, L. F., and Batchoun, R.: Intestinal colonization of symptomatic and asymptomatic schoolchildren with *Blastocystis hominis*. J. Clin. Microbiol. *32*:2865–2866, 1994.
20. O'Gorman, M. A., Orenstein, S. R., Proujansky, R., et al.: Prevalence and characteristics of *Blastocystis hominis* infection in children. Clin. Pediatr. *32*:91–96, 1993.
21. Patterson, J. E., Patterson, T. F., Edberg, S. C., et al.: The traveler with *Blastocystis hominis*: Experience from a traveler's clinic and review. Infect. Dis. Clin. Pract. *1*:28–32, 1992.
22. Senay, H., and MacPherson, D.: *Blastocystis hominis*: Epidemiology and natural history. J. Infect. Dis. *162*:987–990, 1990.
23. Shlim, D. R., Hoge, C. W., Rajah, R., et al.: Is *Blastocystis hominis* a cause of diarrhea in travelers? A prospective controlled study in Nepal. Clin. Infect. Dis. *21*:97–101, 1995.
24. Udkow, M. P., and Markell, E. K.: *Blastocystis hominis*: Prevalence in asymptomatic versus symptomatic hosts. J. Infect. Dis. *168*:242–244, 1993.
25. Zierdt, C. H.: *Blastocystis hominis*, a protozoan parasite and intestinal pathogen of human beings. Clin. Microbiol. Newslett. *5*:57–59, 1983.
26. Zierdt, C. H.: *Blastocystis hominis*: Past and future. Clin. Microbiol. Rev. *4*:61–79, 1992.

210

ENTAMOEBA COLI INFECTION

Peter J. Hotez

Until recently, *Entamoeba coli* (*E. coli*) was considered to be entirely nonpathogenic and was of interest to the clinician only because of its morphologic similarities to *Entamoeba histolytica* that might result in misdiagnosis. In 1991, however, several case reports from northern Europe appeared that implicated *E. coli* as a possible cause of infectious diarrhea.[2, 7] Two cases of *E. coli*–associated diarrhea have been described in children.[2]

ETIOLOGY AND PATHOGENESIS

E. coli, like other members of the genus *Entamoeba*, has both trophozoite and cyst forms. The trophozoite is similar in size to *E. histolytica* (15 to 50 μm) but has a more sluggish motility with short pseudopodia.[4] The cytoplasm is described as being "granular," "coarse," or "frothy" and contains numerous bacteria, yeasts, and other food materials.[4, 6] Occasionally, red blood cells are seen in the cytoplasm, but they are not nearly as common as in pathogenic strains of *E. histolytica*. During passage through the colon, the trophozoite will round up and synthesize a chitin-containing cyst wall. *E. coli* cysts measure 10 to 35 μm and usually contain 8 to 16 nuclei, although 32 nuclei are seen on occasion.

Transmission of *E. coli* infection occurs via the fecal-oral route in the same manner as *E. histolytica* infection. Upon cyst ingestion, the total number of excysting trophozoites usually is less than eight.[4] The *E. coli* trophozoites colonize the lumen of the large intestine. Very little is known about the events by which *E. coli* trophozoites occasionally will cause human gastrointestinal illness. It is presumed that even with a pathogenic *E. coli* strain, the invasive potential of this organism is not nearly as great as *E. histolytica* because diarrheal disease in *E. coli*–infected patients is not associated with dysentery or accompanied by a leukocytosis or elevated serum IgA.[7]

EPIDEMIOLOGY AND CLINICAL MANIFESTATIONS

E. coli is worldwide in distribution, although it is more common in warmer climates and in some populations of homosexual men.[4, 5] In 1991, Wahlgren[7] described eight patients from Sweden with mild or persistent diarrhea who harbored *E. coli*. Prior to specific antiamebic chemotherapy, all eight patients had their stools examined repeatedly by (1) light microscopy, to exclude other protozoa and helminths; (2) electron microscopy, to exclude the presence of some pathogenic viruses; and (3) both aerobic and anaerobic culture, to exclude pathogenic bacteria. These patients typically complained of a long history of loose but not watery stools (without blood or mucus), flatulence, and colicky pain. One patient was a parasitology laboratory technician who had symptoms for more than 15 years. Every patient responded to specific antiamebic chemotherapy.[7] Two children with similar symptoms who also responded to antiamebic chemotherapy subsequently were described from Ireland.[2]

DIAGNOSIS AND TREATMENT

E. coli sometimes is difficult to distinguish from *E. histolytica*, particularly because the nuclear structures of their trophozoite stages are similar.[3] There are some differences, however, including the karyosome, which is eccentric in *E. coli* but central in *E. histolytica,* and the cytoplasm, which is coarse and seldom contains red blood cells in *E. coli*, in contrast to *E. histolytica*.[3] The differences between the cyst stages of *E. coli* and *E. histolytica* (and *Entamoeba dispar*) are more apparent. For example, the *E. coli* cyst typically will have two to four times more nuclei than those in *E. histolytica*. The *E. coli* cyst has been reported to become more refractive during fixation, so that it often is visualized better in a wet preparation.[4]

Generally speaking, *E. coli* still is regarded by most investigators as a commensal organism. However, in patients with persistent diarrhea whose diagnostic fecal evaluation reveals only the presence of *E. coli*, it is reasonable to administer a course of specific antiamebic therapy.[1] All of the Swedish patients were reported to respond to a 10-day course of diloxanide furoate in a dose of 500 mg three times daily.[7] Children also may respond to an equivalent pediatric dose of 20 mg/kg/day in three divided doses for 10 days. As of 1994, diloxanide furoate was available in the United States from the Centers for Disease Control and Prevention Drug Service. Alternatively, two children from Ireland (where diloxanide furoate was not available) were treated successfully for *E. coli*–associated diarrhea with metronidazole.[2]

References

1. Cooperstock, M., DuPont, H. L., Corrado, M. L., et al.: Evaluation of new anti-infective drugs for the treatment of diarrhea caused by *Entamoeba histolytica*. Clin. Infect. Dis. *15*(Suppl. 1):S254–S258, 1992.
2. Corcoran, G. D., O'Connell, B., Gilleece, A., and Mulvihill, T. E.: *Entamoeba coli* as possible cause of diarrhea. Lancet *338*:254, 1991.
3. Despommier, D. D., Gwadz, R. W., and Hotez, P. J.: Parasitic Diseases. 3rd ed. New York, Springer-Verlag, 1995, pp. 232–233.
4. Garcia, L. S., and Bruckner, D. A.: Diagnostic Medical Parasitology. 2nd ed. Washington, D.C., American Society for Microbiology, 1992, pp. 18–20.
5. Jokipii, L., Sargeaunt, P. G., and Jokipii, A. M. M.: Coincidence of deficient delayed hypersensitivity and intestinal protozoa in homosexual men. Scand. J. Infect. Dis. *21*:563–571, 1989.
6. Proctor, E. M.: Laboratory diagnosis of amebiasis. Clin. Lab. Med. *11*:829–859, 1991.
7. Wahlgren, M.: *Entamoeba coli* as cause of diarrhoea? Lancet *337*:675, 1991.

211

GIARDIASIS

James P. Keating

Giardiasis is a diarrheal illness caused by a flagellated protozoa, *Giardia lamblia*, which was studied and sketched by the seventeenth-century haberdasher and microscopist Leeuwenhoek. After rediscovery by Lambl in 1859, the organism was considered, arguably, a human pathogen during the first half of the twentieth century. Doubts concerning its pathogenicity were dispelled by epidemiologic studies of the acute form of the illness in a series of single-point outbreaks beginning with the Aspen, Colorado, episode.[14] Now a reportable disease in most states, giardiasis is the most common protozoal illness afflicting the citizens of this country.

CLASSIFICATION

The genus *Giardia* belongs to the phylum Protozoa superclass Mastigophora, and family Hexamitidae and is kin to the plasmodia and trichomonads. The belief that *Giardia* is host-specific led to a large number of species (e.g., *G. bovis, G. canis, G. cati, G. muris*); it now is thought that one or two species (*G. duodenalis* and *G. muris*) are responsible for infection of most mammalian species, a belief that is based on observations of human-animal cross-transmission.[5, 12, 19, 22] Now that *Giardia* can be cultured axenically (1970), it is likely that the true number of species will be delineated.

MORPHOLOGY

The trophozoite (Fig. 211–1) usually is seen in preparations of duodenal mucus or freshly passed diarrheal stools. It is a pear-shaped disk approximately 15 μm in length and 5 to 15 μm in width. Paired nuclei, each containing a large central karyosome, produce a "bespectacled" appearance. Organelle details visible in stained specimens include the eight flagellae, longitudinal rods (axostyles), and transverse bars (parabasal bodies).

The cyst, the most common form seen in stool, is ovoid, is smaller (10 to 12 μm long × 5 to 10 μm wide), and contains two to four nuclei and remnants of the organelles.

Scanning electron microscopy[15] has demonstrated a "carpeting" of the duodenal mucosal surface by large numbers of trophozoites, which provides support for Veghelyi's[26] hypothesis that *Giardia* poses a physical barrier between the intestinal lumen and the absorptive surface of the enterocyte. The ventral surface of the organism is dominated by a spiral organelle ("the sucking disk"), which appears to interdigitate with the microvilli of the intestinal brush border, leaving an impression when the *Giardia* is removed. The dorsal surface is pitted and lacks the elaborate microtubular lamellae of the ventral surface, which suggests that the enterocyte, not the intestinal lumen, is the source of nutrients for the organism.

PATHOLOGY AND PATHOGENESIS

Rare reports of trophozoites in the biliary tree, trachea, and colon continue to appear, but the organism's exclusive target appears to be the proximal small bowel. After ingestion of infected material, excystation occurs in the stomach. Reproducing by binary fission, the trophozoite colonizes the duodenum, attaching to the mucosal surface near the base of the villi. In symptomatic patients, the histologic appearance of the mucosa often is normal, but histologic changes, including reduction in villus height, increase in lamina propria inflammatory cells, and, rarely, penetration of the epithelium by trophozoites, can be seen. Enterocyte production and crypt-to-villus migration of enterocytes are increased.

Suggested mechanisms of the diarrhea and other symptoms include (1) physical barrier impeding nutrient absorption, (2) disruption of the unstirred layer and removal of microvilli at the brush border, (3) elaboration of a soluble toxin, (4) disruption of intraluminal events necessary for fat absorption, and (5) competition for nutrients.

TRANSMISSION AND EPIDEMIOLOGY

Person-to-person transmission is the most common mechanism of infection. The infection is spread by the fecal-oral route, shared toys, and oral-anal sexual acts. Infection may occur after ingestion of 10 cysts, contained in a few micrograms of feces. Cysts will remain viable for 3 months in moist environments and resist chlorination sufficient for killing coliforms and bacterial pathogens.

Drinking water has been implicated repeatedly as a source of outbreaks. In some instances, the water has been obtained from mountain streams contaminated by fecal matter from

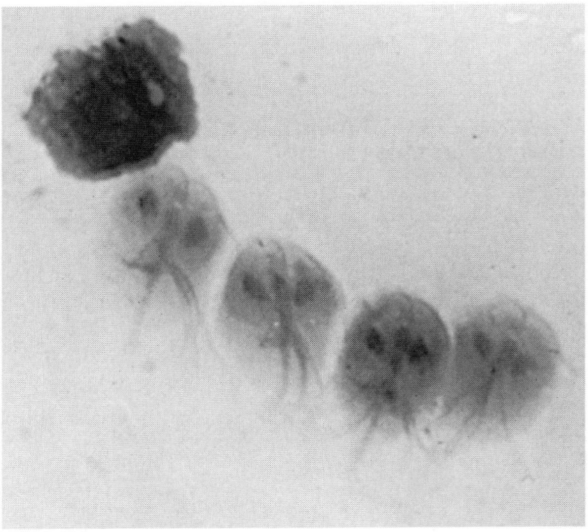

FIGURE 211–1. *Four* Giardia lamblia *trophozoites (and an ink mark) from a mucosal imprint made from a jejunal biopsy of a 2-year-old boy. The nuclei, flagella, and longitudinal axostyles are seen. In the organism on the far left, a transverse parabasal body stains darkly.*

TABLE 211–1. Symptoms During Two Epidemics of Giardiasis

Symptoms	Percentage of Persons with Stated Symptoms	
	Aspen[14]	*St. Petersburg*[2]
Diarrhea	93	92
Weight loss	73	62
Abdominal cramps	77	61
Abdominal distention	62	42
Nausea	59	60
Vomiting	NS	29
Fever	NS	17

NS, not stated in original report.

beaver or other wildlife. The 1966 Aspen outbreak[14] was attributed to sewerage contamination of the municipal water supply. The importance of flocculation and filtration in water treatment became apparent when the Rome, New York, municipal water treatment failed in 1975; more than 300 persons had confirmed giardiasis, and 1 in 10 of the general population suffered from a *Giardia*-like illness. Samples of the tap water caused giardiasis in pathogen-free dogs.[22]

Swimming pool–centered outbreaks[18] have resulted when fecal accidents involving diapered or handicapped, and infected, children occur in inadequately chlorinated water. Investigators estimated that proper chlorination will eliminate the cysts over 50 minutes and advised pool managers to clean the pool for that length of time after such accidents.[10]

Food-borne outbreaks of giardiasis are rare.[8] In three carefully studied episodes, the food involved (salmon, noodle salad, tacos) was contaminated by a bare-handed preparer of a meal.

CLINICAL MANIFESTATIONS

Diarrhea is the most consistent complaint, although it can be overshadowed by behavioral changes, growth arrest, chronic abdominal pain, or fecal incontinence in a given patient. The stools can be watery but more often are thick and formless, large in volume, and odiferous. When chronic infection begins early in life, the child's mother may not consider the stools abnormal.

In the Normal Host

The symptoms of acute giardiasis were similar in the Aspen[14] and St. Petersburg, Russia,[2] outbreaks (Table 211–1). Those infected were adult travelers who apparently had no prior exposure, which appears to impart some protection. In this form of the illness, the incubation time was 15 to 30 days, and symptoms persisted for 10 to 100 days. The average weight loss was 3 to 4 kg; the recurrence rate was 25 per cent. The frequency of physical findings, laboratory abnormalities, or secondary spread was not established.

Clinical investigations of sporadic cases, presumably biased toward those that are more severe, have yielded evidence of malabsorption of fat, lactose, vitamin B_{12}, and xylose; protein-losing enteropathy, irritable bowel syndrome, lymphoma, dysentery, ulcerative colitis, Crohn disease, gastrointestinal allergy, cystic fibrosis, celiac disease, and depression have been diagnosed incorrectly in patients eventually found to have giardiasis.

In Children

Many infants and children infected with *Giardia* are asymptomatic[17] or have symptoms that are not caused by the organism. In a population with a high prevalence of asymptomatic infection, the most determined efforts, including a trial of therapy, may fail to establish a causal relationship between *Giardia* and a given symptom.

Although a spectrum of illness is presumed to exist, reports have focused on the most severely affected children. The syndrome of chronic malabsorption that was described in 1938[26] has gained broad acceptance.[3] Symptoms may commence at any age, although most of the reported patients have been toddlers. Protuberance of the abdomen, spindly extremities, and retardation of growth are the most constant signs; peripheral or generalized edema and pallor may occur. Anemia usually is hypochromic and microcytic. Eosinophilia is rare in otherwise healthy individuals with giardiasis; when it is present, a second condition (e.g., *Toxocara* infection) must be considered. Increased stool fat excretion, decreased serum carotene, abnormal xylose absorption, and "malabsorption pattern" on radiologic study are common but neither specific nor necessary to the diagnosis.

There are no incidence figures for chronic giardiasis. Burke,[3] in Kentucky, considers it second only to cystic fibrosis as a cause of childhood steatorrhea. In Scotland, where the prevalence of celiac disease is high, giardiasis was the second most common diagnosis made in a study of 93 patients referred for evaluation of the symptoms of malabsorption.[4] In selected populations, chronic giardiasis may be as common as the acute illness.[6] The usual course of giardiasis is self-limiting; the host determinants of chronic giardiasis are unknown. Until more accurate and less invasive methods are developed to separate asymptomatic carriage from chronic illness, the most convincing evidence for the causal role of *Giardia* is the reversal of signs and symptoms with treatment.

Reinfection appears to be common when the the patient remains in an endemic environment. Ninety-eight per cent of successfully treated Peruvian children, remaining in their neighborhoods, were reinfected within 6 months. Immigration to a developed world environment is associated with a decrease in prevalence from the high values seen in the Third World (20 to 40 per cent) to the much lower rates (2 to 4 per cent) common in countries with highly developed water purification and sewage treatment.

In the Vulnerable Host

In 1965, Hermans and associates[9] called attention to the association of hypogammaglobulinemia, nodular lymphoid hyperplasia of the small intestine, chronic diarrhea, and giardiasis. Since then, our understanding and classification of the immunodeficiency diseases have changed, and there is little question that patients with hypogammaglobulinemia, absence of plasma cells in the intestinal lamina propria, and AIDS (HIV) are susceptible to chronic giardiasis. Individuals suffering from X-linked agammaglobulinemia,[16] selective IgA deficiency, and Wiskott-Aldrich and Nezelof syndromes seem to be less susceptible. Treatment of giardiasis in hypogammaglobulinemic patients may reduce gastrointestinal symptoms markedly, but recurrence is common. Whereas the habitat of the organism suggests a defect in secretory or surface defense mechanisms, a complete understanding of the special relationship of *Giardia* and altered host defenses has not been achieved; phagocytosis of trophozoites by sensitized mucosal macrophages has been observed in experimental models. Villus injury ("hypogammaglobulinemic sprue") and chronic diarrhea are major problems for immune-deficient patients, and *Giardia* is not always the cause. If symptoms are relieved by therapy directed to *Giardia*, it often is necessary to continue or repeat the treatment for long periods.

Chronic pancreatitis, achlorhydria, gastrectomy, and cystic fibrosis may increase susceptibility to *Giardia* infection.[20]

DIAGNOSIS

Physicians should consider giardiasis in any patient who has unexplained diarrhea for 7 or more days. The likelihood of giardiasis is increased if (1) the child or a sibling attends a day care center,[1] (2) the patient or family member traveled to an endemic area (e.g., Rocky Mountains,[28] St. Petersburg) within a month prior to the onset of symptoms, (3) the family has emigrated recently from an area of high prevalence, (4) an adolescent is engaged in male homosexual practices,[13] or (5) the patient swam or played in inadequately filtered water, especially wading or waterslide pools where very young children play in untreated or inadequately treated surface water.

The diagnosis usually is established by microscopic examination of feces. Trophozoites are found in wet-mounted preparations of fresh diarrheal stools stained with Lugol iodine, but identification of cysts in specimens collected in perservatives and later concentrated in the laboratory is the more common method. A single stool ova and parasite examination identifies the presence of *Giardia* or other protozoal parasites in 92 per cent of those infected; the traditional practice of ordering three such examinations in patients with diarrhea should be employed only in selected patients. In some patients, cyst excretion is inconstant and unpredictable, and several specimens, obtained on different days, may be needed to demonstrate the organism. However, if clinical concern is high and the first fecal examination is negative, the use of other diagnostic methods often is preferable to further ova and parasite studies.

Use of a weighted string, swallowed in a gelatin capsule (Entero-Test),[25] is a method of sampling duodenal mucus and may provide a prompt answer when giardiasis is strongly suspected. The handling of specimens obtained in this fashion has not been standardized, but the sensitivity of the test is presumed by some authors to be greater than that of stool examinations.[11] The test may be a safe and economical alternative to esophagogastroduodenoscopy for some patients, but superficial linear abrasions of the mucosa at the gastroesophageal junction have been seen on endoscopic examination after the string has been pulled out; patients with esophageal varices or coagulopathies should be excluded. In some patients, the line cannot be withdrawn owing to extreme resistance, and the patient must swallow the entire string, an apparently harmless event.

Duodenal biopsy, currently obtained most frequently by esophagogastroduodenoscopy, is believed to be the most sensitive method of diagnosis[11] but also is the most expensive (approximately $1000, including sedation and processing of specimens) and invasive and should be reserved for patients whose fecal ova and parasite study is negative and who have persisting symptoms requiring clarification. *Giardia* trophozoites can be difficult to see in fixed sections. Transferring the trophozoite-rich mucus to a glass slide by touching it to the fresh biopsy specimen or rolling the specimen on the slide ("mucousal impression" or "touch cytology")[29] and staining with Giemsa or trichrome before microscopic examination are believed to increase the sensitivity of biopsy by as much as 50 per cent (see Fig. 211–1). Trophozoite and flagellar movements can be observed in fresh specimens mixed with saline, but the value of such observations is unclear; fixed and stained specimens are preferred in clinical practice. Endoscopy and biopsy seldom are carried out solely to establish the diagnosis of giardiasis, making useful cost comparisons with other methods of diagnosis difficult. Usually, peptic disease, *Helicobacter* pyloridis, celiac disease, cryptosporidiosis, and other specific and nonspecific enteropathies are under consideration in addition to giardiasis. If the clinician strongly suspects giardiasis but is unable to or chooses not to attempt to confirm the diagnosis, a trial of therapy often is successful; this approach is least satisfactory when the patient has been ill for some time and alternative diagnoses (e.g., malignancy, depression) are serious concerns.

Assays for fecal antigens of cysts and trophozoites increasingly are employed when diagnostic interest is restricted to *Giardia*. These tests are more sensitive than the microscopic examination of feces.

Serum antibodies to *Giardia* antigens are useful in epidemiologic and pathophysiologic studies.[27] IgG and IgA antibodies to trophozoite antigens are detectable in 68 per cent of newly infected individuals when a serum specimen is obtained 4 weeks after the onset of symptoms, with an even lower yield from earlier sampling. The utility of these antibodies as a diagnostic test is limited by their late appearance in the course of the clinical illness and low sensitivity. If the antibodies are employed where populations (e.g., in developing countries) have a high rate of seropositivity, the positive predictive value (disease+/test+) is likely to be very low.

There are few critical comparative studies of the methods of diagnosis; each has its place in current practice.

TREATMENT

When treatment is indicated, quinacrine (Atabrine) can be given orally in a dosage of 6 mg/kg/day for 10 days.[7] The adult dosage is 100 mg three times daily; the daily dose should not exceed 300 mg. Side effects include gastrointestinal upset, dermatitis, yellow discoloration of the skin (one-third of young children),[7, 23] and toxic psychosis. The only manufacturer of quinacrine ceased production and sale of the medication in 1995.

Furazolidone (Furoxone) is provided in a suspension containing 50 mg/15 mL and as 100-mg tablets. The dosage is 8 mg/kg/day for 10 days; children older than 5 years of age are given 25 to 50 mg four times daily. Infants younger than 1 month of age should not be given furazolidone because hemolytic anemia due to glutathione instability may occur. Errors in dosing and resultant treatment failure may occur because the concentration (50 mg/15 mL) is unlike many other pediatric medications, which usually provide the appropriate dose in 5-mL quantities.

Metronidazole (Flagyl), 250 mg thrice daily, is recommended in adults; a dose of 10 to 15 mg/kg/day has been recommended for children. This drug has been found to be mutagenic and carcinogenic in bacteria and animal species, and it should not be used in women during their child-bearing period.

Metronidazole and quinacrine have a disulfiram-like effect and should be avoided in children receiving ethanol-containing medications (e.g., elixir, digoxin). All three medications may cause vomiting; none is good-tasting or disguised easily. Neither metronidazole nor quinacrine is commercially available in a liquid; a method for making a suspension of quinacrine has been described by Craft and colleagues.[7]

A 10 to 20 per cent rate of symptom recurrence can be expected after completion of therapy; re-treatment usually is successful.

If infection persists despite repeated treatment, reinfection from the environment or an immune defect should be considered. Standard therapy frequently is unsuccessful in children with chronic diarrhea and malnutrition; a repeat course of therapy after nutritional rehabilitation should be considered.[24]

References

1. Black, R. D., Dykes, A. C., Sinclair, S. P., et al.: Giardiasis in day-care centers: Evidence of person-to-person transmission. Pediatrics *60*:486–491, 1977.
2. Brodsky, R. E., Spencer, H. C., and Schultz, M. G.: Giardiasis in American travelers to the Soviet Union. J. Infect. Dis. *130*:139, 1974.
3. Burke, J. A.: Giardiasis in childhood. Am. J. Dis. Child. *129*:1304–1310, 1975.
4. Carswell, F., Gibson, A. A. M., and McAllister, T. A.: Giardiasis and coeliac disease. Arch. Dis. Child. *48*:414–418, 1973.
5. Centers for Disease Control: M. M. W. R. *26*:31, 1977.
6. Chester, A. C., MacMurray, F. G., Restifo, M. D., et al.: Giardiasis as a chronic disease. Dig. Dis. Sci. *30*:215–218, 1985.
7. Craft, J. C., Murphy, T., and Nelson, D.: Furazolidone and quinacrine: Comparative study of therapy for giardiasis in children. Am. J. Dis. Child. *135*:164–166, 1981.
8. Grabowski, D. J., Tiggs, K. J., Hall, J. D., et al.: Common-source outbreak of giardiasis: New Mexico. M. M. W. R. *38*:405–407, 1989.
9. Hermans, P. E., Huizenga, K. A., Hoffman, H. N., et al.: Dysgammaglobulinemia associated with nodular lymphoid hyperplasia of the small intestine. Am. J. Med. *40*:78–89, 1965.
10. Jarroll, E. L., Bingham, A. K., and Meyer, E. A.: Effect of chlorine on *Giardia lamblia* cyst viability. Appl. Environ. Microbiol. *41*:483–487, 1981.
11. Kamath, K. R., and Marugasu, R.: A comparative study of four methods for detecting *Giardia lamblia* in children with diarrheal disease and malabsorption. Gastroenterology *66*:16–21, 1974.
12. Marcus, L. C.: Gastrointestinal diseases. *In* Gellis, S. S. (ed.): Year Book of Pediatrics, 1977. Chicago, Year Book Medical Publishers, 1977, p. 105.
13. Meyers, J. D., Kuharic, H. A., and Holmes, K. K.: *Giardia lamblia* in homosexual men. Br. J. Vener. Dis. *53*:54–55, 1977.
14. Moore, G. T., Cross, W. M., McGuire, D., et al.: Epidemic giardiasis at a ski resort. N. Engl. J. Med. *281*:402–407, 1969.
15. Mueller, J. C., Jones, A. L., and Brandborg, L. L.: Scanning electron microscopy: Observation in human giardiasis; and Erlandsen, S. L.: Scanning electron microscopy of intestinal giardiasis: Lesions of the microvillous border of villus epithelial cells produced by trophozoites of *Giardia*. *In* Proceedings of the Workshop on Advances in Biomedical Applications of the SEM. Chicago, ITT Research Institute, 1974.
16. Ochs, H. D., Ament, M. E., and Davis, S. D.: Giardiasis with malabsorption in X-linked agammaglobulinemia. N. Engl. J. Med. *287*:341–342, 1972.
17. Pickering, L. K., Woodward, W. E., DuPont, H. L., et al.: Occurrence of *Giardia* in day care centers. J. Pediatr. *104*:522–526, 1984.
18. Porter, J. D., Ragazzoni, H. P., Buchanon, J. D., et al.: *Giardia* transmission in a swimming pool. Am. J. Public Health *78*:659–662, 1988.
19. Rendtorff, R. C., and Holt, C. J.: The experimental transmission of human intestinal protozoan parasites. Am. J. Hyg. *60*:327–338, 1954.
20. Roberts, D. M., Craft, J. C., and Mather, F. J.: Prevalence of giardiasis in patients with cystic fibrosis. J. Pediatr. *112*:555–559, 1988.
21. Saha, T., and Ghosh, T. K.: Invasion of small intestinal mucosa by *Giardia lamblia* in man. Gastroenterology *72*:402–405, 1977.
22. Shaw, P. K., Brodsky, R. E., Lyman, D. O., et al.: A community outbreak of giardiasis with evidence of transmission by a municipal water supply. Ann. Intern. Med. *87*:426–432, 1977.
23. Sokol, R. J., Lichtenstein, P. K., and Farrell, M. K.: Quinacrine hydrochloride-induced yellow discoloration of the skin in children. Pediatrics *69*:232–233, 1982.
24. Sullivan, P. B., Marsh, M. N., Phillips, M. B., et al.: Prevalence and treatment of giardiasis in chronic diarrhea and malnutrition. Arch. Dis. Child. *65*:304–306, 1990.
25. Thomas, G. E., Goldsmid, J. M., and Wicks, A. C. B.: Use of the Entero-Test duodenal capsule in the diagnosis of giardiasis. S. Afr. Med. *48*:2218–2220, 1974.
26. Veghelyi, P.: Giardiasis in children. Am. J. Dis. Child. *56*:1231–1239, 1938.
27. Visvesvara, G. S., Smith, P. D., Healy, G. R., et al.: An immunofluorescence test to detect serum antibodies to *Giardia lamblia*. Ann. Intern. Med. *93*:802–805, 1986.
28. Wright, R. A., Spencer, H. C., Brodsky, R. E., et al.: Giardiasis in Colorado: An epidemiologic study. Am. J. Epidemiol. *105*:330–336, 1977.
29. Yardley, J. H., Takano, J., and Hendris, T. R.: Epithelial and other mucosal lesions of the jejunum in giardiasis: Jejunal biopsy studies. Bull. Johns Hopkins Hosp. *115*:389–406, 1964.

212

DIENTAMOEBA FRAGILIS INFECTION

Lisa M. Frenkel

Dientamoeba fragilis is a protozoan that may inhabit the human gastrointestinal tract. In 1918, *D. fragilis* was recognized as a distinct species by Jepps and Dobell,[26] who believed it to be a rare intestinal commensal. In unpreserved feces, the morphologic characteristics of *D. fragilis* do not persist, which most likely accounts for its perceived rarity in some surveys. Careful studies using preserved fecal specimens have found an association between *D. fragilis* infection and acute and chronic gastrointestinal symptoms, which has led to the acceptance of its role as a pathogen.

THE ORGANISM

D. fragilis, unlike most other intestinal protozoa, has no known cyst form. The trophozoite initially was classified in the genus *Endamoeba.* The similarity of *D. fragilis* to flagellates, specifically to *Histomonas meleagridis,* the cause of "blackhead" enterohepatitis in fowl, was noted on careful examination under the light microscope.[12] *H. meleagridis* is a flagellate when it is found in the cecum of fowl, and its flagella are lost when it invades tissues.[12] *D. fragilis* in the binucleate form resembles the tissue form of *Histomonas.*[12] However, *D. fragilis* has not been found to invade tissues. Antigenic and ultrastructural relatedness to *Histomonas* has been based on fluorescent antibody and electron microscopic studies, respectively.[9, 13] *D. fragilis* was reclassified in 1974 by Honigberg as a nonflagellate trichomonad of the order Trichomonadida, family Monocercomonadidae, subfamily Dientamoebinae, and genus *Dientamoeba.*[6, 15]

D. fragilis infects the mucosal crypts of the large intestine in close proximity to mucosal epithelium from the cecum to the rectum. The organism varies in size from 3 to 18 μm in diameter, but it usually is 7 to 12 μm. The pseudopodia of *D. fragilis* have a delicate, leaf-like appearance and serrated margins.[25] This protozoan is seen to move actively in fresh feces but quickly becomes rounded after standing. *D. fragilis* is relatively easy to isolate and grow in vitro in media containing solid rice starch.[12] Cultures should be maintained at 37° to 38° C (98.6° to 100.4° F) because the organism rounds up and stops moving and feeding at lower temperatures. *D. fragilis* will thrive in temperatures up to 41° C (105.8° F). This organism feeds on bacteria and starch grains and will ingest human red blood cells. *D. fragilis* reproduces by binary fission.[12] Although the organisms are found most commonly in the binucleate form, about 20 per cent are in the uninucleate form, and a few are multinucleate.[25, 26, 29, 60, 63] Each nucleus contains a large, fragmented (four to eight granules) karyosome surrounded by a clear zone with no peripheral chromatin and a fine nuclear membrane.[26, 62] Occasionally, some aberrant forms may be found. These forms usually are uninucleate and may be as large as 20 μm; they do not reproduce. Humans appear to be the natural host of *D. fragilis. D. fragilis* infection has been reported in two simian species.[12] Multiple attempts to infect other animals have been unsuccessful thus far.

EPIDEMIOLOGY AND TRANSMISSION

D. fragilis was thought to be uncommon until improved techniques for preserving the organism were utilized.[18, 21, 50] The trophozoites of *D. fragilis* have been noted to be quite sensitive to an aerobic environment.[9] They die and disintegrate within 1 hour in an isotonic salt solution at room temperature; when smeared on slides, they round up and become granular within 15 minutes during microscopic examination at room temperature and low humidity.[9]

D. fragilis has been reported worldwide, with a prevalence in selected populations of 1.4 to 38 per cent.[2–4, 7, 9, 14, 30, 32, 34, 35, 38, 42, 45, 47, 55–57, 60, 61, 66] Higher prevalence rates, from 19 to 69 per cent, have been reported in people in various crowded living situations, such as institutionalized persons and communal groups,[4, 34, 36, 37, 57] and in persons traveling outside the United States.[30, 46, 54]

The mode of transmission of *D. fragilis* is unknown; however, two mechanisms have been postulated. It is hypothesized that *D. fragilis* is transmitted in the eggs of *Enterobius vermicularis* (pinworm) in a manner similar to the transmission of *H. meleagridis* in the eggs of the avian nematode *Heterakis gallinae*.[5, 12, 58, 61] In support of this theory, a number of investigators have noted a high frequency of concomitant infection with *D. fragilis* and *E. vermicularis*.[5, 12, 20, 58] Ockert[39] provided the most convincing support for this theory when, by ingesting eggs of *E. vermicularis*, which he had washed with water and exposed to pepsin and hydrochloric acid, he became infected with both *E. vermicularis* and *D. fragilis*. Others noting a high rate of concomitant infection of *D. fragilis* and organisms known to be transmitted by the fecal-oral route suggest this mode of transmission.[32, 34, 37, 61]

CLINICAL MANIFESTATIONS

Gastrointestinal and less frequently systemic symptoms have been reported to occur in association with *D. fragilis* in the fecal specimens of children and adults.[8, 19, 20, 22–28, 36, 37, 40, 43, 46, 53, 54, 56, 59, 60, 63, 67] Symptomatic infections vary from 15 to 85 per cent of infected individuals.[27, 31, 32, 36, 46, 52–54, 66] Both acute watery diarrhea and a chronic recurrent abdominal pain syndrome have been associated with *D. fragilis* in children and adults.[11, 22–28, 36–38, 40, 43–46, 51–54, 56, 59, 60, 67]

Persons with acute diarrhea also have reported abdominal pain, anorexia, nausea, vomiting, and, less frequently, fever, weight loss, headache, malaise, fatigue, irritability, and weakness.[11, 22, 27, 28, 43, 52, 53, 63, 67] The stools have been described as greenish-brown, mushy or sticky with a foul odor, and at times bloody and with mucus.[27, 28] Abdominal tenderness has been found commonly on physical examination.[27, 53]

D. fragilis is associated most frequently with chronic abdominal pain (Table 212–1),[35, 52, 53] which may persist for months to years.[22, 63] The pain commonly is described as dull, achy, crampy, or colicky and usually is located in the lower abdominal quadrants.[50, 53, 63] Complaints of flatulence, fatigue, and alternating diarrhea and constipation are not uncommon in persons with *D. fragilis* infections.[26, 53] Laboratory and radiologic studies usually are normal.[27] Eosinophilia, not usually seen with protozoal infections, occasionally has been reported in infected children and adults, most commonly in association with chronic symptoms.[52, 53]

DIAGNOSIS

A high index of suspicion is important for the diagnosis of *D. fragilis* infection. Infection with this organism should be considered when abdominal pain and/or diarrhea persists beyond 1 week, particularly if the child lives in an institution, has lived or traveled to a location where sanitary practices are poor, or is infected with pinworms.

Investigation for *D. fragilis* infection should include the collection of at least three stool specimens immediately placed in a stool preservative such as polyvinyl alcohol for

TABLE 212–1. Clinical Findings in Patients with *Dientamoeba fragilis* Infection (% Occurrence)

Symptom	Patients Submitting O & P Specimens to Laboratory		Semicommunal Group Members*		Yang and Scholten[66]	
	Children	*Adults*	*Children*	*Adults*	*Observed*	*Literature Review*
Diarrhea	51	68	10	8	58.4	42.5
Abdominal pain	60	78	43	54	53.7	46.7
Anorexia	31	20	11	27	1.2	5.4
Nausea and vomiting	17	42	11	19	3.9	20.4
Weight loss	26	6.6	—	—	3.5	10.4
Flatulence	—	16	23	54	5.9	19.9
Constipation	14	6	2	15	2.4	6.5
Fatigue and irritability	29	24	—	54	5.9	13.4
Urticaria and pruritus	6	12	—	—	6.7	0
Eosinophilia	34	35	—	—	5.1	4.3
Number of patients	35	50	44	33	255	186

*References 36, 53–54.
From Millet, V., Spencer, M. J., Chapin, M. R., et al.: Dig. Dis. Sci. *28*:335–339, 1983.

allowing the morphologic characteristics of the delicate trophozoite to be retained.[50] Diagnosis also can be made by permanent stained smear of a fresh or purged fecal specimen.[5, 21, 60] Three fecal specimens properly collected and stained will lead to the identification of this intestinal protozoan in 70 to 93 per cent of infected individuals.[24, 49] Stool specimens should be collected on alternate days because *D. fragilis* has been observed to be excreted in a cyclic pattern.[11] Stool samples should be collected before radiologic studies with barium because barium interferes with detection of the protozoa.[17] Other medications interfering with parasite identification include antibiotics, mineral oil, antimalarial agents, antiprotozoan agents, nonabsorbable diarrheal preparations, and bismuth.[17] These substances may interfere with the detection of parasites for as long as 3 weeks.[17] After arrival in the laboratory, stool specimens are processed with the use of formalin-ether sedimentation concentration technique and stained with either iron hematoxylin or trichrome and examined by qualified and experienced individuals for the proper identification of *D. fragilis*.[16, 41] Garcia and associates[17, 18] reported that 92.2 per cent of *D. fragilis* trophozoites were determined solely on the basis of the trichrome-stained smear. Diagnostic characteristics of *D. fragilis* on a permanently stained smear include a high percentage of binucleate trophozoites and nuclei without peripheral chromatin but with four to eight chromatin granules in a central mass.[10, 15] Detection of *D. fragilis* by indirect immunofluorescence[8] or by culture[48] appears promising in limited investigations. No serologic test is available for diagnosis.

TREATMENT

Several different agents have been used in the treatment of *D. fragilis* infection. However, owing to the lack of clinical studies, all therapy is considered investigational by the U.S. Food and Drug Administration. At present, three drugs are recommended for the treatment of *D. fragilis* infection: iodoquinol, tetracycline, and paromomycin.[1, 31, 33] Metronidazole also may be effective in the treatment of *D. fragilis*.[8, 153] Iodoquinol, 650 mg three times a day for 10 to 21 days, is recommended for adults and 40 mg/kg/day divided three times a day for children. The tablets should be taken with meals. Side effects include abdominal discomfort, diarrhea, anal irritation and pruritus, headache, and dysesthesias of the hands and feet. Paromomycin in a dosage of 25 to 30 mg/kg/day in divided doses for 7 days may be more effective than iodoquinol.[65] Adverse reactions to paromomycin include nausea, abdominal cramps, and diarrhea. It is absorbed poorly after oral administration and, unfortunately, no longer is available in syrup form in the United States. Alternative therapies are tetracycline hydrochloride, 500 mg four times daily for 10 days, and doxycycline, 100 mg twice daily for 10 days. Tetracycline should be given on an empty stomach because food and dairy products may interfere with absorption of the drug. Tetracycline should not be given to children younger than 9 years of age because it may accumulate and cause discoloration of the teeth. Stool specimens should be reexamined 3 to 4 weeks after therapy to determine whether the parasite was eliminated successfully.

References

1. Abromowicz, M. (ed.): Drugs for parasite infections. Med. Lett. Drugs Ther. *24*:5–12, 1982.
2. Boe, J.: The occurrence of human intestinal protozoa in Norway. Acta Med. Scand. *113*:321–328, 1943.
3. Bruckner, D. A., Garcia, L. S., and Voge, M.: Intestinal parasites in Los Angeles, California. Am. J. Med. Technol. *45*:1020–1022, 1979.
4. Brug, S. L.: Observation on *Dientamoeba fragilis*. Ann. Trop. Med. Parasitol. *30*:441–452, 1936.
5. Burrows, R. B., and Swerdlow, H. A.: *Enterobius vermicularis*: A probable vector of *Dientamoeba fragilis*. Am. J. Trop. Med. Hyg. *5*:256–264, 1956.
6. Camp, R. R., Mattern, C. F. T., and Honigberg, B. M.: Study of *Dientamoeba fragilis*, Jepps and Dobell. I. Electron microscopic observations of the binucleate stages. II. Taxonomic position and revision of genus. J. Protozool. *21*:69–82, 1974.
7. Centers for Disease Control: Intestinal parasite surveillance: Annual summary 1978. Atlanta, Georgia, U.S. Public Health Service, 1979.
8. Chan, F. T. H., Guan, M. X., Mackinzie, A. M. R., et al.: Susceptibility testing of *Dientamoeba fragilis* ATCC 30948 with iodoquinol, paromymycin, tetracycline, and metroidazole. Antimicrob. Agents Chemother. *38*:1157–1160, 1994.
9. Chang, M.: Parasitization of the parasite. J. A. M. A. *223*:1510, 1973.
10. Committee on Education, American Society of Parasitologists: Procedure suggested for use in the examination of clinical specimens for parasitic infection. J. Parasitol. *63*:959–960, 1977.
11. Desser, S. S., and Yang, Y. J.: *Dientamoeba fragilis* in idiopathic gastrointestinal disorders. Can. Med. Assoc. J. *114*:290–293, 1976.
12. Dobell, C: Researches on the intestinal protozoa of monkeys and man. X. The life-history of *Dientamoeba fragilis*: Observations, experiments, and speculations. Parasitology *32*:417–461, 1940.
13. Dwyer, D. M.: *Trichomonas, Histomonas, Dientamoeba* and *Entamoeba*. I. Quantitative fluorescent antibody methods. J. Protozool. *19*:316–325, 1972.
14. Fantham, H. B., and Porter, A.: Some entozoa of man as seen in Canada and South Africa. Can. Med. Assoc. J. *34*:414–421, 1936.
15. Faust, E. C., Beaver, P. C., and Jung R. C.: Animal Agents and Vectors of Human Disease. 4th ed. Philadelphia, Lea & Febiger, 1975.
16. Finegold, S. M., Martin, W. J., and Scott, E. G.: Bailey and Scott's Diagnostic Microbiology. 5th ed. St. Louis, C. V. Mosby, 1978.
17. Garcia, L. S., and Ash, L. R.: Diagnostic Parasitology. St. Louis, C. V. Mosby, 1975, pp. 9–20.
18. Garcia, L. S., Brewer, T. C., and Bruckner, D. A.: A comparison of the formalin-ether concentration and trichrome-stained smear methods for the recovery and identification of intestinal protozoa. Am. J. Med. Technol. *45*:932–935, 1979.
19. Gittings, J. C., and Waltz, A. D.: *Dientamoeba fragilis*. Am. J. Dis. Child. *34*:543–546, 1927.
20. Grendon, J. H., Di Giacomo, R. F., and Frost, F. J.: Descriptive features of *Dientamoeba fragilis* infections. J. Trop. Med. Hyg. *98*:309–315, 1995.
21. Goldman, M., and Brooke, M. M.: Protozoans in stools unpreserved and preserved in PVA-fixative. Public Health Rep. *68*:703, 1953.
22. Hakansson, E. G.: *Dientamoeba fragilis*, some further observations. Am J. Trop. Med. Hyg. *16*:175–183, 1936.
23. Hakansson, E. G.: *Dientamoeba fragilis*, some further observations. Am. J. Trop. Med. Hyg. *17*:349–352, 1937.
24. Hiatt, R. A., Markell, E. K., and Ng, E.: How many stool examinations are necessary to detect pathogenic intestinal protozoa? Am. J. Trop. Med. Hyg. *53*:36–39, 1995.
25. Hood, M.: Diarrhea caused by *Dientamoeba fragilis*. J. Lab. Clin. Med. *25*:914–918, 1940.
26. Jepps, M. W., and Dobell, C.: *Dientamoeba fragilis*, NDN>SP>, a new intestinal amoeba from man. Parasitology *10*:352–367, 1918.
27. Kean, B. H., and Malloch, C. L.: The neglected amoeba: *Dientamoeba fragilis*. A report of 100 pure infections. Am. J. Dig. Dis. *11*:735–744, 1966.
28. Knoll, E. W., and Howell, K. M.: Studies on *Dientamoeba fragilis*: Its incidence and possible pathogenicity. Am. J. Clin. Pathol. *15*:178–183, 1945.
29. Kudo, R.: Observation on *Dientamoeba fragilis*. Am. J. Trop. Med. Hyg. *6*:299–305, 1926.
30. Mackie, T. T., Larsh, J. E., Jr., and Mackie, J. W.: A survey of intestinal parasitic infections in the Dominican Republic. Am. J. Trop. Med. *31*:825–832, 1951.
31. Markell, E. K., and Voge, M.: Parasitology. 6th ed. Philadelphia, W. B. Saunders, 1986, pp. 63–65.
32. McQuay, R. M.: Parasitologic studies in a group of furloughed missionaries. I. Intestinal protozoa. Am. J. Trop. Med. Hyg. *16*:154–160, 1967.
33. The Medical Letter on Drugs and Therapeutics: Drugs for parasitic infections. Med. Lett. Drugs Ther. *34*:17–26, 1992.
34. Melvin, D. M., and Brooke, M. M.: Parasitologic surveys on Indian reservations in Montana, South Dakota, New Mexico, Arizona and Wisconsin. Am. J. Trop. Med. Hyg. *11*:765–772, 1962.
35. Miller, M. J.: The intestinal protozoa of man in midwestern Canada. J. Parasitol. *25*:355–357, 1939.
36. Millet, V. E., Spencer, M. J., Chapin, M. R., et al.: *Dientamoeba fragilis*, a protozoan parasite in adult members of a semicommunal group. Dig. Dis. Sci. *28*:335–339, 1983.
37. Millet, V. E., Spencer, M. J., Chapin, M. R., et al.: Intestinal protozoan infection in a semicommunal group. Am. J. Trop. Med. Hyg. *32*:54–60, 1983.
38. Naimen, H. L., Sekla, L., and Albritton, W. L.: Giardiasis and other parasitic infections in a Manitoba residential school of the mentally retarded. Can. Med. Assoc. J. *122*:185–188, 1980.
39. Ockert, G.: Zur epidemiologie von *Dientamoeba fragilis*. II. Mitteilung: Ver-

suche über die übertragung der art mit enterobius-eiern. J. Hyg. Epidemiol. Immunol. *16*:222–225, 1972.
40. Oxner, R. B., Paltridge, G. P., Chapman, B. A., et al.: *Dientamoeba fragilis*: A bowel pathogen? N. Z. Med. J. *100*:64–65, 1987.
41. Parasitology Subcommittee/Microbiology Section of Scientific Assembly, American Society of Medical Technology: Recommended procedures for the examination of clinical specimens submitted for the diagnosis of parasitic infections. Am. J. Med. Technol. *44*:1101–1106, 1978.
42. Porter, A.: Remarks on intestinal parasites in Montreal and the relation of *Entamoeba histolytica* to colitis. Can. Med. Assoc. J. *30*:134–137, 1934.
43. Robertson, A.: Note on a case infected with *Dientamoeba fragilis*: Jepps and Dobell. Am. J. Trop. Med. Hyg. *1923*:26–243, 1917.
44. Rothman, M. D., and Epstein, H. J.: Clinical symptoms associated with the so-called nonpathogenic amoeba. J. A. M. A. *116*:694–700, 1941.
45. Ruebush, T. K., Juranek, D. D., and Brodsky, R. E.: Diagnoses of intestinal parasites by state and territorial public health laboratories, 1976. J. Infect. Dis. *138*:114–117, 1978.
46. Sapero, J. J.: Clinical studies in nondysenteric intestinal amebiasis. Am. J. Trop. Med. Hyg. *19*:497–514, 1939.
47. Saunders, L. G.: A survey of helminth and protozoan incidence in man and dogs at Fort Chipewyan, Alberta. J. Parasitol. *35*:31–34, 1949.
48. Sawangjaroen, N., Luke, R., and Prociv, P.: Diagnosis by faecal culture of *Dientamoeba fragilis* infections in Australian patients with diarrhoea. Trans. R. Soc. Trop. Med. Hyg. *87*:163–165, 1993.
49. Sawitz, W. G., and Faust, E. C.: The probability of detecting intestinal protozoa by successive stool examinations. Am. J. Trop. Hyg. *22*:131–136, 1942.
50. Scholten, T. H., and Yang, J.: Evaluation of unpreserved and preserved stools for the detection of intestinal parasites. Am. J. Clin. Pathol. *62*:563–567, 1974.
51. Spencer, M.: *Dientamoeba fragilis. In* Feigin, R. D., and Cherry, J. D. (eds.): Textbook of Pediatric Infectious Diseases. 2nd ed. Philadelphia, W. B. Saunders, 1987, p. 2024.
52. Spencer, M. J., Chapin, M. R., and Garcia, L. S.: *Dientamoeba fragilis,* a gastrointestinal protozoan parasite in adults. Am. J. Gastroenterol. *70*:565–569, 1982.
53. Spencer, M. J., Garcia, L. S., and Chapin, M. R.: *Dientamoeba fragilis,* an intestinal pathogen in children? Am. J. Dis. Child. *133*:390–393, 1979.
54. Spencer, M. J., Millet, V. E., and Garcia, L. S.: Parasitic infections in a pediatric population. Pediatr. Infect. Dis. *2*:110–113, 1983.
55. Stein, B., and Talis, B.: The prevalence of *Dientamoeba fragilis* in Tel Aviv and its surroundings. Res. Council Israel *8E*:55, 1959.
56. Steinitz, H., Talis, B., and Stein, B.: *Entamoeba histolytica* and *Dientamoeba fragilis* and the syndrome of chronic recurrent intestinal amoebiasis in Israel. Digestion *3*:146–153, 1970.
57. Svennson, R. M.: A survey of human intestinal protozoa in Sweden and Finland. Parasitology *20*:237–249, 1928.
58. Swerdlow, M. A., and Burrows, R. B.: *Dientamoeba fragilis*: An intestinal pathogen. J. A. M. A. *158*:176–178, 1955.
59. Taliafero, W. H., and Becker, E. R.: A note on the human intestinal amoeba, *Dientamoeba fragilis.* Am. J. Hyg. *4*:71–74, 1924.
60. Thompson, J. G.: *Dientamoeba fragilis,* Jepps and Dobell, 1917: A case of human infection in England. J. Trop. Med. Hyg. *26*:135–136, 1923.
61. Weiner, D., Brooke, M. M., and Witkow, A.: Investigation of parasitic infections in the central area of Philadelphia. Am. J. Trop. Med. Hyg. *8*:625–629, 1959.
62. Wenrich, D. H.: Studies on *Dientamoeba fragilis* (protozoa). I. Observations with special reference to nuclear structure. J. Parasitol. *22*:76–83, 1936.
63. Wenrich, D. H.: Studies on *Dientamoeba fragilis* (protozoa). II. Report on unusual morphology in one case with suggestions as to pathogenicity. J. Parasitol. *23*:183–196, 1937.
64. Wenrich, D. H., Stabler, R. M., and Arnett, J. H.: *Entamoeba histolytica* and other intestinal protozoa in 1,060 college freshmen. Am. J. Trop. Med. Hyg. *15*:331–345, 1935.
65. Wolfe, M. S.: *In* Strickland, G. (ed.): Hunter's Tropical Medicine. Philadelphia, W. B. Saunders, 1991, p. 580.
66. Yang, J., and Scholten, T.: *Dientamoeba fragilis*: A review with notes on its epidemiology, pathogenicity, mode of transmission and diagnosis. Am. J. Trop. Med. Hyg. *26*:16–22, 1977.
67. Yoeli, M.: A report on intestinal disorders accompanied by large number of *Dientamoeba fragilis.* Trop. Med. Hyg. *58*:38–41, 1955.

213

TRICHOMONAS INFECTIONS

Joan S. Purcell and Mariam R. Chacko

Trichomonas species are found in both animals and humans. The most widely studied member of this species is *Trichomonas vaginalis* because it is the trichomonad most relevant to human disease. Donne first described *T. vaginalis* in 1836 as motile microorganisms in the purulent frothy leukorrhea of women presenting with vaginal discharge and genital irritation.[16] Epidemiologic information concerning *Trichomonas* infection is most detailed in the adult population; nevertheless, studies that document the epidemiology of *T. vaginalis* in children and adolescents are available.[9, 11, 17, 20, 21, 23, 25, 31, 33, 34, 43, 44, 46, 49, 55]

BACTERIOLOGY

Trichomonads are acellular flagellated protozoans. The Trichomonadidae family is characterized as mononucleate with an axial organelle with an undulating membrane.[57] *Trichomonas* genus comprises those organelles with three to four anterior flagella and an undulating membrane composed of the posterior flagella posteriorly.[57] In animals, the three important pathogenic species of *Trichomonas* are *Trichomonas gallinae, Trichomonas gallinorum,* and *Trichomonas foetus.*[57] In humans, there are five species of *Trichomonas,* including *Trichomonas tenax, Trichomonas ardin delteili, Trichomonas faecalis, Trichomonas hominis,* and *T. vaginalis.*[57]

T. vaginalis is the most clinically relevant human trichomonad. The structure consists of four anterior flagella and a posterior flagellum incorporated into the undulating membrane. *T. vaginalis* can survive but cannot multiply at room temperature.[57]

T. tenax resembles the morphology of *T. vaginalis* but is smaller. *T. hominis* can survive for up to 7 hours at room temperature and can multiply; in contrast, *T. vaginalis* cannot multiply at room temperature.[57]

T. hominis has five anterior flagella and a trailing posterior flagellum. *T. hominis* can survive and multiply at room temperature. Only *T. hominis* can survive in media without serum and in feces for up to 24 hours.[57]

PATHOGENESIS

Virulence factors associated with *T. vaginalis* infection have been defined. The identified virulence factors include adherence, contact-independent factors, hemolysis, and host macromolecule acquisition. Epithelial cell adherence is dependent on an intact cytoskeleton and *Trichomonas* protein ligands and proteases, which are necessary to activate adherence molecules.[12] Cell-contact–independent factors include pH variability and cell-detaching factor, which in vitro inhibit reorganizing of cells infected with *T. vaginalis. T. vaginalis* produces lactic acid and acetic acids as a byproduct of glucose metabolism.[12] These acids lower the pH, which is cytotoxic to epithelial cells. Another metabolic byproduct of *T. vaginalis* is cell-detaching factor, which has a cytopathic effect on epithelial cells and increases subepithelial vascularity, producing the clinical sign of "strawberry cervix."[12] The activity of cell-detaching factor is optimal at pH 5.0 or greater. Hemolysis is seen only in the presence of live trichomonads. Cysteine proteases appear to be important for hemolysis because introduction of their inhibitors in vitro eliminates hemolysis by *T. vaginalis*.[12, 26] Addition of metronidazole reduces levels of hemolysis by 50 per cent.[12] Hemolytic activity of *T. vaginalis* is temperature-dependent, with maximal hemolysis at 37° C. Hemolysis is inhibited with separation of trichomonads from erythrocytes by a 3-μm filter, suggesting a contact-dependent mechanism.[12] As a parasite, *T. vaginalis* is dependent on host macromolecules for nutrition, including plasma proteins and lactoferrin.

The host responds to *T. vaginalis* infection at the cellular level with polymorphonuclear cells and lymphocyte activity. *T. vaginalis* secretes proteases that are chemotactic to polymorphonuclear leukocytes with resultant phagocytosis and killing of the trichomonad by oxidative mechanisms.[12] *T. vaginalis* secretions are mitogenic to lymphocytes, which serve to enhance phagocytosis by polymorphonuclear cells, and may suppress host immune response if large numbers of suppressor lymphocytes are activated. Clinically, gender differences to *T. vaginalis* infection exist. Women largely are symptomatic, whereas only a small minority of men have symptoms with *T. vaginalis* infection, many of whom undergo spontaneous cure. Estrogen levels in females directly correlate with infection at peak estradiol levels. In an early study of premenarchal vaginitis in children 3 months to 9 years of age, *T. vaginalis* infection accounted for only 2.8 to 4.4 per cent of vaginitis in the unestrogenized vagina, compared with 50 per cent of infections in the fully estrogenized vaginas of patients nearing puberty.[20] Male animals treated with estrogens had an increased susceptibility to infection.[38] *T. vaginalis* demonstrates increased adherence in the presence of estradiol in vitro. In asymptomatic males infected with *T. vaginalis,* the prostate gland serves as a reservoir. Men may remain asymptomatic due to the concentration of zinc salts in prostatic fluid, which is cytocidal for trichomonads.[28] In vitro, testosterone decreases the growth of *T. vaginalis* as well.[18]

In the host, trichomonads may serve as a vector for bacteria and viruses, as demonstrated by the high co-infection rate with *T. vaginalis* and human papillomavirus. Whereas bacteria contaminate trichomonads externally, it is believed that trichomonads ingest virus-infected cells and destroy them, leaving the active virus intact.[21] *T. vaginalis* has been implicated in the etiology of pelvic inflammatory disease via ascension from the vagina to the fallopian tubes. Studies in vitro have demonstrated *Escherichia coli* strains, a part of the normal vaginal flora, intimately attached to trichomonads via glycoprotein strands.[26] Trichomonads contaminated with bacteria serve as a vector for the bacteria to produce pelvic infection upon reaching the uterus, fallopian tubes, or peritoneum.[26] In contrast, vaginal colonization with *Lactobacillus* species was thought to inhibit trichomonal invasion by lowering vaginal pH. In a study of 336 African women 15 to 49 years of age, 199 of whom were pregnant, 31 per cent were culture-positive for *T. vaginalis*, whereas only 40 per cent of the patients tested positive for *Lactobacillus*. Although the rate of *Lactobacillus* colonization in these African women was low, the high rate of *T. vaginalis* infection was not related to the absence of *Lactobacillus*. Thus, trichomonads may not alter the vaginal flora substantially.[39]

There is a spectrum of disease severity in patients infected with *T. vaginalis*. Some patients are asymptomatic, but others experience severe symptomatic inflammation and discomfort. The virulence of *T. vaginalis* isolates vary; whether this variance is due to host response or inherent properties of the parasite is unknown. There is evidence, however, that dramatic heterogenity exists on the surface of the parasite, leading to antigenic diversity among different isolates of *T. vaginalis*. In one study, prominent immunogens absent on the surface of *T. vaginalis* isolates led to enhanced ability of the parasite to cause cytoadherence-dependent killing of HeLa cells in monolayer cultures. In addition, only those adherent parasites possessed adhesins, which directly affected the parasites' cytoadherence and cytotoxicity.[1] The cysteine proteases of *T. vaginalis* may be responsible for the cytoadherence, nutrient acquisition, and cytotoxicity of *T. vaginalis*. These proteinases are shed during the life cycle and growth of *T. vaginalis*. One hundred per cent of the sera from women infected with *T. vaginalis* but none from normal uninfected women possessed IgG to numerous trichomonad cysteine proteinases. This serum antiproteinase antibody disappeared after effective treatment of the infection.[2]

IMMUNOLOGY

The interaction between *T. vaginalis* and host immunoglobulins is not clear. In women infected with *T. vaginalis*, specific local antibodies, IgG and IgA, are seen in vaginal secretions. IgA may serve to increase opsonization of the parasite by IgG, resulting in enhanced phagocytosis. IgG specific for *Trichomonas* cysteine proteases and surface proteins is seen, but it does not help rid the host of infection.[2] *T. vaginalis* synthesizes high-molecular-weight proteins with variable surface expression.[3] Of samples obtained from women infected with *T. vaginalis*, 70 per cent of vaginal washes and 80 per cent of vaginal mucous samples had IgG to a specific *T. vaginalis* surface protein immunogen with a molecular mass of 230,000 daltons (P230). In contrast, no antibody to P230 was detected in uninfected women or in detergent extract depleted of P230, suggesting a highly specific antibody.[3] Clinically, this may account for the lack of resistance to repeated *Trichomonas* infections and variable host antibody titers in infected persons.

EPIDEMIOLOGY

T. gallinae infects the digestive tract of pigeons; *T. gallinorum* infects the ceca of chickens and the ceca and liver of turkeys; and *T. foetus* infects the genital tract of cattle, resulting in balanitis in bulls and pyometria, abortion, and sterility in cows.[57]

In humans, there are four species of *Trichomonas*, the most important of which is *T. vaginalis,* which is found in the human vagina, urethra, and prostate. *T. vaginalis* can be inoculated into the vagina; however, inoculation experiments with *T. vaginalis* in the mouth and intestines failed to establish infection in these sites.[57] *T. tenax* is found in the mouth, whereas *T. hominis, T. ardin delteili,* and *T. faecalis* are found in the bowel. *T. tenax* is found in approximately 5 per cent of patients with *T. vaginalis*.[57] *T. hominis* can infect humans and a variety of animals. The incidence of *T. hominis* in humans is between 0.4 and 3.5 per cent and is associated with gastroenteric dysentery.[57] *T. hominis* is found only rarely in the stools of patients who concordantly have *T. vaginalis*.[57] Each of the trichomonads is specific to its location in the host and does not establish infection in sites outside of the aforementioned locations. With the exception of *T. vaginalis,* all of the trichomonads found in humans are part of the normal flora and are nonpathogenic.[57] In addition, *T. tenax* and *T. hominis* are not found in the vagina, eliminating confusion in infection with *T. vaginalis*.[46]

T. vaginalis infection may be the sexually transmitted disease encountered most commonly, with an estimated 180 million cases worldwide. The prevalence of *T. vaginalis* urogenital infection varies from 5 to 65 per cent in different studies. Many of the studies of urogenital trichomoniasis are biased due to lack of random sampling, variance in the sensitivity and specificity of the diagnostic tests employed, and sample selection, often from sexually transmitted disease clinics.[36] One of the reasons for the high prevalence of *T. vaginalis* infection is its rate of asymptomatic carriage; thus, reliance on clinical symptoms alone will cause a practitioner to miss up to 80 per cent of infections.[42]

T. vaginalis has been associated with newborn and infant infections, presumably from contamination upon passage through the infected birth canal.[49] Most of the cases reported have involved premature infant females. Vertical transmission of the organism occurs as the infant passes through the infected maternal birth canal.

T. vaginalis in the prepubertal or nonsexually active female must raise suspicion of sexual abuse and prompt an evaluation for other sexually transmitted diseases.[17, 43, 57] In a study of 409 children suspected of having been sexually abused, 4 children, 10 to 12 years of age, were diagnosed with *T. vaginalis* on wet-mount examination of vaginal secretions. This study may underrepresent cases of *T. vaginalis* in patients suspected of having been sexually abused because a saline wet-mount preparation was available in only 18 of the 409 children studied.[56] *T. vaginalis* most commonly is seen in postmenarchal sexually active females; however, *T. vaginalis* vaginitis is seen occasionally in children.[21] One study of 54 premenarchal females (median age, 5.8 years) with vulvovaginitis failed to identify *T. vaginalis*.[44] Lang[34] identified *T. vaginalis* in 3.6 per cent of 9- to 12-year-old girls. In adolescents, the prevalence of *T. vaginalis* is between 5.5 and 34 per cent.[23]

Trichomonal infections can be found in both males and females, although the incidence in females is greater. It is found in all age groups, from neonates to adults.[42] The incidence of *T. vaginalis* infection is between 10 and 25 per cent of sexually active females worldwide. In males attending a sexually transmitted disease clinic, the prevalence of *T. vaginalis* was 22 per cent among sexual contacts of females with trichomoniasis and 6 per cent among homosexual males attending the same clinic.[27] *T. vaginalis* was found in 58 per cent of 85 black males, 16 to 22 years of age, who currently were sexually active.[48] Sixty-nine per cent previously had a sexually transmitted disease. *T. vaginalis* was more prevalent than gonorrhea, chlamydial infection, condyloma acuminatum, and pediculosis.

The rate of infection with *T. vaginalis* is increased in black females, as well as in females with other sexually transmitted diseases. The rate of *T. vaginalis* infection also is increased in females with gonococcal cervicitis, with a vaginal pH shift above 4.5, and who are pregnant and may be increased around menarche and after menopause.[15, 41, 57] Trichomoniasis does not appear to have a seasonal pattern of infection.[36] Urogenital trichomoniasis is seen more commonly in inner-city patients and among patients in the 20- to 30-year-old age group.[36] Infection with *T. vaginalis* increases in direct relationship with the number of sexual partners and in an inverse relationship with monthly episodes of coitus. Oral contraceptives diminish the rate of infection with *T. vaginalis*, compared with an intrauterine device or tubal ligation.[36] Use of nonoxynol 9 spermicidal cream was not related significantly to a decrease in *Trichomonas* infection.[4] In another study of 226 women attending a sexually transmitted disease clinic, trichomonal infection was noted in 44 per cent of the patients.[41] There was no association between patient age, frequency of coitus, date of most recent coitus, day of menstrual cycle, antibiotic use, contraceptive methods, or symptoms of discharge or pruritus.[41] Other risk factors for females may involve a change in the normal vaginal flora, with overgrowth of *Gardnerella vaginalis*, *Bacteroides*, or *Peptostreptococcus*. These bacteria may serve as sources of nutrients for trichomonads, thus allowing the trichomonads to thrive. In males, sexual contact with a female infected with *T. vaginalis*, nongonoccal urethritis, or nongonoccal nonchlamydial urethritis was associated with increased risk of infection with *T. vaginalis*.[30] In trichomoniasis, lactobacilli are absent from the vagina. This promotes alkalinity of the vaginal pH, thereby enhancing the overgrowth of anaerobes and trichomonads.[52] Another study carried out in Africa failed to demonstrate a significant role for *Lactobacillus* in patients with *T. vaginalis* infection.[14, 39]

T. vaginalis usually is sexually transmitted in adolescents and adults. Large numbers of trichomonads are found in the prostatic secretions of husbands of women with recurrent *T. vaginalis* infection. In a clinic for patients with sexually transmitted diseases, 60 per cent of husbands of women who were suffering from chronic, repeated *T. vaginitis* infection were culture-positive for *T. vaginalis*, compared with 8 per cent in a control group of male patients attending the same clinic.[55] These data support the concept of sexual transmission of *T. vaginalis*.

Nonsexual transmission of *T. vaginalis* has been reported. In rural India, a point prevalence survey on random samples of juvenile and adolescent females complaining of leukorrhea revealed that 76 per cent were infected with *T. vaginalis*. Of those who were infected, 38 per cent were younger than 12 years of age. In this study, poor genital hygiene and underwear use were correlated with a higher incidence of infection. In studying the epidemiology and risk factors for transmission of *T. vaginalis* other than sexual intercourse, a significantly higher risk occurred for those females who washed or bathed in tanks or rivers compared with those who used pipe or well water. Thus, in the tropics, nonsexual transmission may account for infection with *T. vaginalis* in juvenile and adolescent females.[11] *T. vaginalis* can survive on toilet seats for up to 1 hour, on wet clothes for 3 hours, for 30 minutes in fresh water, for 2 or 3 days in warm mineral water, and for hours in urine. Thus, it is possible for the transmission of *Trichomonas* to occur via fomites (washcloths, towels), particularly when people are living together in crowded, confined spaces.[43]

CLINICAL MANIFESTATIONS

The vagina of the infant may serve as a reservoir of infection that goes unnoticed until the infant presents 5 to 6 weeks after birth with fever. Motile trichomonads and pyuria are seen on examination of the urine. Symptoms resolve upon treatment with metronidazole.[49] Premenarchal children present with diffuse bubbly leukorrhea and pruritus.[34] Vaginitis with a purulent foul-smelling discharge is the most common presentation of infection with *T. vaginalis* in females; in some patients, trichomonads may be found in the urine initially, with development of frank signs of vaginitis 7 to 28 days later.[25]

As many as 50 per cent of females and 90 per cent of males infected with *T. vaginalis* will be asymptomatic.[54] When one controls for co-infection with other organisms, *T. vaginalis* infection is associated significantly with purulent discharge, vulvar itching, colpitis macularis ("strawberry cervix"), and vaginal and vulvar erythema. The sensitivity of the other signs and symptoms of *Trichomonas* vaginitis is low. These include vaginal burning, dysuria, urinary frequency, dyspareunia, frothy discharge, and cervical friability.[22] Although frothy leukorrhea was associated most frequently with *Trichomonas* infection, 29 per cent of the patients with frothy discharge in one study did not have *Trichomonas* infection.[22] The strawberry cervix was pathognomonic of *T. vaginalis* infection, but it was noted in only 2 to 3 per cent of patients. Thus, one cannot depend upon this finding to establish a clinical diagnosis of *T. vaginalis* vaginitis in most patients.[15] A diagnosis of *Trichomonas* infection should be entertained in any female presenting with vaginal discharge.

Trichomonads may ascend the fallopian tubes and, if contaminated with bacteria, can produce the syndrome of pelvic inflammatory disease.[9, 26] In males, *T. vaginalis* may present as symptomatic urethritis with dysuria secondary to urethral inflammation and discharge. On examination, the discharge often is not visualized. When a discharge is present, it is clear to cloudy but not grossly purulent. On microscopy, numerous inflammatory cells are seen.[27, 32] *T. vaginalis* also may be a cause of chronic nonbacterial prostatitis and present as chronic prostatitis resistant to standard therapy.[24, 32] *T. vaginalis* also has been reported to be an etiologic agent of epididymitis in males presenting with purulent urethral discharge and scrotal swelling with enlargement of the epididymis.[15] Although rare, *T. vaginalis* has been reported to infect the median raphe of the penis.[51]

DIAGNOSIS

Clinical Examination

In females, the presence of frothy purulent discharge, vulvar/vaginal erythema, and strawberry cervix should suggest *Trichomonas* infection. Males tend to be asymptomatic or, if symptomatic, have purulent urethral discharge and urethral inflammation. Eighty per cent of infections will be missed if the physician relies on clinical examination alone.[16, 52]

Wet-Mount Examination

The diagnosis of trichomoniasis in women is made commonly by wet-mount examination of vaginal secretions. Wet preparations are obtained by swabbing the lateral and anterior vaginal fornices to attain vaginal epithelial cells; the secretions are placed into normal saline and mounted on a slide. This method also may be used to obtain urethral specimens in the male. These preparations are easy to prepare and the method is cost-effective, but its sensitivity is low (51 per cent).[16] In addition, the validity of the result is dependent on the technical skill of the examiner and the rapidity with which the specimen is examined; cooling greatly affects the motility of the trichomonads, which may hinder identification.[31]

Papanicolaou Smear

Papanicolaou smears are unreliable in the diagnosis of trichomoniasis in women because *T. vaginalis* does not always appear in its typical pear-shaped morphology after fixation on the slide. Rather, it may appear to be more rounded, similar to a polymorphonuclear leukocyte. The sensitivity of Papanicolaou smears for diagnosing *Trichomonas* in culture-proven infection is as low as 56 per cent.[29] In a study of 1199 women, 37 per cent would have been diagnosed falsely with *T. vaginalis* infection based on Papanicolaou smear results. In a second study, 44 per cent of patients with culture-proven *T. vaginalis* infection would not have been diagnosed based on negative Papanicolaou smear findings.[45]

Staining Techniques

Acridine orange is a compound that differentially stains DNA (yellow-green) and RNA (bright red). *T. vaginalis* stains brick-red with an oval, yellow-green nucleus. The flagellae do not stain. Unfixed smears are kept at room temperature for up to 24 hours; fixed slides may be kept for up to 5 days. Acridine orange stains may permit a rapid, accurate diagnosis of *T. vaginalis* infection. The diagnosis can be confirmed by other diagnostic methods in 93 per cent of cases.[40] Acridine orange staining appears to be at least as sensitive as wet-mount examination.[6]

Culture

Diagnosis of *T. vaginalis* by culture has been considered the gold standard. The secretions are collected from the vagina or urethra with a cotton-tipped swab and placed directly on the culture media. Cultures of cervical specimens show 99 per cent concordance with vaginal cultures for *Trichomonas*. Nevertheless, 8 per cent of vaginal infections with positive vaginal cultures would be missed if only cervical specimens were obtained.[7] Several culture media, including Diamond, modified Diamond, Feinberg-Whittington, Kupferberg, and Lash medium, are available. The reformulated media currently prepared commercially are Diamond, Kupferberg, and Lash media.[50] These media contain antibiotics to inhibit bacterial overgrowth and may contain either yeast extract, horse or sheep serum, or both.[50] Cultures are observed for 7 days by placing a drop of sediment from the culture tube and performing a wet-mount examination. In a study of 200 females cultured simultaneously on modified Diamond and Feinberg-Whittington media, there was no difference in results obtained with the two culture media. No differences were demonstrated with different collection techniques, such as vaginal irrigation or swab collection. Culture of *T. vaginalis* on these media detected fewer than 10 trichomonads. Cultures were not affected by douching in the previous 24 hours. In contrast, the sensitivity of wet-mount preparation decreased from 57 to 22 per cent after douching.[16] Limitations of culture include the failure of culture media to support growth of trichomonads in some cases by culture day 7. Growth in culture media also is inoculum-dependent; less sensitive media require higher inocula of trichomonads.[50] The sensitivity of culture in wet-mount–positive cases is higher than in wet-mount–negative cases, 91 to 96 per cent compared with 86 to 89 per cent.[29] The ability to detect infection increases with duplicate cultures, with a sensitivity reaching 98 per cent in one study.[29] In males, prostatic massage prior to specimen collection and culture of both urethral samples and urinary sediment have a sensitivity of 94 to 98 per cent.[30, 48]

The plastic envelope or pouch method is a simplified method of culture that is selective for *T. vaginalis*. Vaginal secretions are placed into a dry medium that has been reconstituted with distilled water. The solution is contained in pouches with separate chambers that are mixed easily for culture. Subsequently, the upper chamber is placed on a slide mount and is viewed for motile trichomonads. Both wet-mount and immediate examination of the envelope for motile trichomonads had a sensitivity of 66 per cent compared with traditional culture (sensitivity, 89 to 91 per cent) and the envelope or pouch culture (sensitivity, 89 to 97 per cent). The pouch or envelope method is more convenient to use than wet-mount plus traditional culture. In addition, these methods have equivalent sensitivity for diagnosing *T. vaginalis* infection and are relatively inexpensive.[5, 13] Furthermore, the pouch culture method allows direct daily visualization without sampling or opening the pouches.[13]

Direct Fluorescent Antibody Staining

The sensitivity of direct fluorescent antibody (DFA) staining approaches 86 per cent compared with culture and is not related to the number of trichomonads seen on wet-mount examination. The sensitivity of DFA staining is superior to that of wet-mount examination or acridine orange staining in females who have *T. vaginalis* infection and comparable with that of these techniques in females infected with multiple organisms.[6, 29] Interpretation of DFA staining may be accomplished in less than 1 hour.[29] In a study of high-risk males who underwent prostatic massage prior to specimen collection, DFA staining on urethral samples had a sensitivity of 63 per cent.[48]

A monoclonal-based enzyme-linked immunosorbent assay (ELISA) was developed using a monoclonal antibody specific for a 65-kDa surface polypeptide of *T. vaginalis.* Polyclonal rabbit anti–*T. vaginalis* antibody labeled with horseradish peroxidase was used as the probe. In a limited study of 36 females, this ELISA had a sensitivity of 89 per cent and a specificity of 97 per cent.[35]

Other Rapid Diagnostic Tests

Synthetic oligonucleotide probes are rapid, semiautomated commercial systems and are more sensitive than wet-mount examination for the diagnosis of *T. vaginalis* infection (83 versus 67 per cent) when the results of these two methods are compared with true-positive results obtained on Diamond culture medium. The advantage of this method compared with culture is reflected in the brief processing time (i.e., 40 minutes compared with 3 to 7 days for culture).[8, 47] In addition, probes are specific for the organism and do not cross-react with bacteria, viruses, protozoa, fungi, or human nucleic acids.[47]

TREATMENT

Metronidazole is the treatment of choice for *T. vaginalis* infection and is the only drug available for treatment of trichomoniasis in the United States currently. Worldwide, other drugs used for trichomoniasis include nifuratel, nimorazole, tinidazole, ornidazole, secnidazole, and carnidazole. Despite the availability of these other drugs worldwide, metronidazole remains the standard treatment for trichomoniasis. Metronidazole enters the trichomonad via passive diffusion, where its nitro group is reduced to a cytotoxic intermediate that reacts with DNA, resulting in cell death. Metronidazole is 93 to 95 per cent bioavailable and, after oral administration, peak serum levels are attained in 1 to 3 hours and a steady state in 2 to 3 days. Metronidazole is metabolized by the liver, and only 20 per cent is protein bound; thus, the drug is distributed well in the body.[37] Side effects reported with metronidazole use include nausea, vomiting, anorexia, a metallic taste, headache, dizziness, and darkening of the urine. Urticaria, reversible peripheral neuropathy, seizures, and ataxia have been reported with intravenous use. The side effects tend to be dose-related and self-limited.[37] In a study of 1199 females with *T. vaginalis* infection treated with metronidazole, only 4 to 5 per cent experienced symptoms of nausea, coated tongue, dryness of the mouth, anorexia, or diarrhea. All symptoms disappeared within a few days of treatment completion, and in only one case was treatment discontinued due to side effects. In addition, relative and absolute leukopenia was not observed in these subjects. Of note, metronidazole enhances or reactivates the growth of *Candida albicans* in the vagina.[45] Metronidazole may potentiate the actions of anticonvulsants and warfarin. A significant disulfiram-like effect is produced when the drug is combined with moderate alcohol intake.[37] Alcohol should be avoided during and for 48 hours after completion of a course of therapy with metronidazole.

T. vaginalis infection should be treated to relieve symptoms, to prevent further transmission of disease, and to prevent chronic inflammation of Bartholin and Skene glands.[54] In males, chronic infection may lead to prostatitis or urethral stricture.[54] Adolescent and adult males who are asymptomatic may harbor *T. vaginalis* in their prostatic secretions, thus reinfecting their partners. Therefore, male partners of females infected with *T. vaginalis* should be treated.[55]

The treatment of *T. vaginalis* is metronidazole, 2 g orally in a single dose or 500 mg twice daily for 7 days in adolescents and adults. Each regimen is 95 per cent effective.[10] Some strains of *T. vaginalis* have reduced susceptibility to metronidazole. If the infection fails to respond to either of the above regimens, it should be re-treated with metronidazole 500 mg twice daily for 7 days.[10] If treatment failure continues, the patient can be treated with 2 g of metronidazole once daily for 3 to 5 days.[10] Metronidazole is contraindicated in the first trimester of pregnancy due to possible teratogenic effects on the fetus. It may be used safely after the first trimester.[10] The breast-fed infant consumes approximately 1 per cent of a single 2-g oral dose of metronidazole; therefore, infants of mothers who are breast feeding and who are treated with a single dose of metronidazole for trichomoniasis should be removed from the breast for at least 24 hours after treatment.[37]

In children with infections of the genital organs, local therapy with metronidazole is preferred due to fewer systemic side effects. Cotton-tipped swabs saturated with metronidazole are introduced into the hymen and applied locally. In multifocal infections, genital infections that fail to respond to local therapy, and infections in newborn or infant boys, oral therapy with metronidazole is given[33] (Table 213–1). Before administration of oral or intravenous metronidazole therapy in children, baseline hematologic, renal, and liver function tests should be obtained to follow changes as therapy continues. Resolution of signs and symptoms of infection indicates a response to treatment. Eradication of *T. vaginalis* should be

TABLE 213–1. Dosing of Metronidazole in Children

		Metronidazole Administered (mg)	
Age (yr)	Weight (kg)	*Orally**	*Locally†*
0–1	10	150	10
1–6	20.5	250	50
7–12	40	500	150
>12	>40	500–1000	250–500

*Oral dose = one-third of the total dose administered every 8 hours for 5–10 days.

†Local dose = total dose administered intravaginally once daily or half the total dose administered twice daily for 5–10 days.

Adapted from Kurnatowska, A., and Komorowska, A.: Urogenital trichomoniasis in children. *In* Honigberg, B. M. (ed.): Trichomonads Parasitic in Humans. New York, Springer-Verlag, 1989, p. 268.

confirmed by wet mount or culture (if available) 3 to 5 days after completion of treatment in children.[33]

PROGNOSIS

If untreated, *T. vaginalis* can lead to chronic inflammation of Bartholin and Skene glands in the female and to prostatitis and urethritis with urethral stricture formation in the male.[53] Complete resolution of symptoms and eradication of *T. vaginalis* usually are noted when treatment is provided promptly.

References

1. Alderete, J. F.: Alternating phenotypic expression of two classes of *Trichomonas vaginalis* surface markers. Rev. Infect. Dis. *10*:S408–S412, 1988.
2. Alderete, J. F., Newton, E., Dennis, C., et al.: Antibody in sera of patients infected with *Trichomonas vaginalis* is to trichomonad proteinases. Genitourin. Med. *67*:331–334, 1991.
3. Alderete, J. F., Newton, E., Dennis, C., et al.: Vaginal antibody of patients with trichomoniasis is to a prominent surface immunogen of *Trichomonas vaginalis*. Genitourin. Med. *67*:220–225, 1991.
4. Barbone, F., Austin, H., Louv, W. C., et al.: A follow-up study of methods of contraception, sexual activity, and rates of trichomoniasis, candidiasis, and bacterial vaginosis. Am. J. Obstet. Gynecol. *163*:510–514, 1990.
5. Beal, C., Goldsmith, R., Kotby, M., et al.: The plastic envelope method: A simplified technique for culture diagnosis of trichomoniasis. J. Clin. Microbiol. *30*:2265–2268, 1992.
6. Bickley, L. S., Krisher, K. K., Punsalang, A., Jr., et al.: Comparison of direct fluorescent antibody, acridine orange, wet mount, and culture for detection of *Trichomonas vaginalis* in women attending a public sexually transmitted diseases clinic. Sex. Transm. Dis. *16*:127–131, 1989.
7. Boeke, A. J. P., Dekker, J. H., and Peerbooms, P. G. H.: A comparison of yield from cervix versus vagina for culturing *Candida albicans* and *Trichomonas vaginalis*. Genitourin. Med. *69*:41–43, 1993.
8. Briselden, A. M., and Hillier, S. L.: Evaluation of affirm VP microbial identification test for *Gardnerella vaginalis* and *Trichomonas vaginalis*. J. Clin. Microbiol. *32*:148–152, 1994.
9. Cates, W., Jr., and Rauh, J. L.: Adolescents and sexually transmitted diseases: An expanding problem. J. Adolesc. Health Care *6*:257–261, 1985.
10. Centers for Disease Control and Prevention: 1993 sexually transmitted disease treatment guidelines. M. M. W. R. *42*(No. RR-14):70–71, 1993.
11. Charles, S. X.: Epidemiology of *Trichomonas vaginalis* in rural adolescent and juvenile children. J. Trop. Pediatr. *37*:90, 1991.
12. Dailey, D. C., Chang, T., and Alderete, J. F.: Characterization of *Trichomonas vaginalis* hemolysis. Parasitology *101*:171–175, 1990.
13. Draper, D., Parker, R., Patterson, E., et al.: Detection of *Trichomonas vaginalis* in pregnant women with the InPouch TV Culture System. J. Clin. Microbiol. *31*:1016–1018, 1993.
14. Ekwempu, C. C., Lawande, R. V., and Egler, L. J.: Microbial flora of the lower genital tract of women in labour in Zaria, Nigeria. J. Clin. Pathol. *34*:82–83, 1981.
15. Fisher, I., and Morton, R. S.: Epididymitis due to *Trichomonas vaginalis*. Br. J. Vener. Dis. *45*:252–253, 1969.
16. Fouts, A. C., and Kraus, S. J.: *Trichomonas vaginalis*: Reevaluation of its clinical presentation and laboratory diagnosis. J. Infect. Dis. *141*:137–143, 1980.
17. Frau, L. M., and Alexander, E. R.: Public health implications of sexually transmitted diseases in pediatric practice. Pediatr. Infect. Dis. *4*:453–467, 1985.
18. Garber, G. E., Lemchuk-Favel, L. T., and Rousseau, G.: Effect of estradiol on cell detaching factor of *Trichomonas vaginalis*. Clin. Microbiol. *29*:1847–1849, 1991.
19. Graves, A., and Gardner, W. A., Jr.: Pathogenicity of *Trichomonas vaginalis*. Clin. Obstet. Gynecol. *36*:145–152, 1993.
20. Gray, L. A., and Kotcher, E.: Vulvovaginitis in childhood. Clin. Obstet. Gynecol. *3*:165–174, 1960.
21. Hammerschlag, M. R., Alpert, S., Rosner, I., et al.: Microbiology of the vagina in children: Normal and potentially pathogenic organisms. Pediatrics *62*:57–62, 1978.
22. Hanssen, P. W., Krieger, J. N., et al.: Clinical manifestations of vaginal trichomoniasis. J. A. M. A. *261*:571–576, 1989.
23. Hardy, P. H., Hardy, J. B., Nell, E. E., et al.: Prevalence of six sexually transmitted disease agents among pregnant inner-city adolescents and pregnancy outcome. Lancet *2*:333–337, 1984.
24. Ireton, R. C., and Berger, R. E.: Prostatitis and epididymitis. Urol. Clin. North Am. *11*:87–88, 1984.
25. Jones, J. G., Yamauchi, T., and Lambert, B.: *Trichomonas vaginalis* infestation in sexually abused girls. Am. J. Dis. Child. *139*:846–847, 1985.
26. Keith, L. G., Berger, G. S., Edelman, D. A., et al.: On the causation of pelvic inflammatory disease. Am. J. Obstet. Gynecol. *149*:215–224, 1983.
27. Krieger, J. N., Jenny, C., Verdon, M., et al.: Clinical manifestations of trichomoniasis in men. Ann. Intern. Med. *118*:844–849, 1993.
28. Krieger, J. N., and Rein, M. F.: Zinc sensitivity of *Trichomonas vaginalis*: In vitro studies and clinical implications. J. Infect. Dis. *146*:341–345, 1982.
29. Krieger, J. N., Tam, M. R., Stevens, C. E., et al.: Diagnosis of trichomoniasis: Comparison of conventional wet-mount examination with cytologic studies, cultures, and monoclonal antibody staining of direct specimens. J. A. M. A. *259*:1223–1227, 1988.
30. Krieger, J. N., Verdon, M., Siegel, N., et al.: Risk assessment and laboratory diagnosis of *Trichomoniasis* in men. J. Infect. Dis. *166*:1362–1366, 1992.
31. Krowchuk, D. P., Anglin, T. M., and Kumar, M. L.: Rapid diagnosis of common sexually transmitted diseases in adolescents: A review. Pediatr. Dermatol. *6*:278–279, 1989.
32. Kuberski, T.: *Trichomonas vaginalis* associated with nongonococcal urethritis and prostatitis. Sex. Transm. Dis. *7*:135–136, 1980.
33. Kurnatowska, A., and Komorowska, A.: Urogenital trichomoniasis in children. *In* Honigberg, B. M. (ed.): Trichomonads Parasitic in Humans. New York, Springer-Verlag, 1989, pp. 246–273.
34. Lang, W. R.: Premenarchal vaginitis. Obstet. Gynecol. *13*:723–729, 1959.
35. Lisi, P. J., Dondero, R. S., Kwiatkoski, D., et al.: Monoclonal-antibody–based enzyme-link immunosorbent assay for *Trichomonas vaginalis*. J. Clin. Microbiol. *26*:1684–1686, 1988.
36. Lossick, J.: Epidemiology of urogenital trichomoniasis. *In* Honigberg, B. M. (ed.): Trichomonads Parasitic in Humans. New York, Springer-Verlag, 1989, pp. 311–323.
37. Lossick, J.: Therapy of urogenital trichomoniasis. *In* Honigberg, B. M. (ed.): Trichomonads Parasitic in Humans. New York, Springer-Verlag, 1989, pp. 324–341.
38. Martinotti, M. G., Musso, T., and Savoia, D.: Influence of gender in pathogenesis of trichomoniaisis in congenitally athymic (nude) mice. Genitourin. Med. *64*:18–21, 1988.
39. Mason, P. R., Mac Callum, M. J., and Poynter, B.: Association of *Trichomonas vaginalis* with other microorganisms. Lancet *1*:1067, 1982.
40. Mason, P. R., Super, H., and Fripp, P. J.: Comparison of four techniques for the routine diagnosis of *Trichomonas vaginalis* infection. J. Clin. Pathol. *29*:154–157, 1976.
41. McLellan, R., Spence, M. R., Brockman, M., et al.: The clinical diagnosis of trichomoniasis. Obstet. Gynecol. *60*:30–34, 1982.
42. Moldwin, R. M.: Sexually transmitted protozoal infections. Urol. Clin. North Am. *19*:93–96, 1992.
43. Neinstein, L. S., Goldenring, J., and Carpenter, S.: Nonsexual transmission of sexually transmitted diseases: An infrequent occurrence. Pediatrics *74*:71–72, 1984.
44. Paradise, J. E., Campos, J. M., Friedman, H. M., et al.: Vulvovaginitis in premenarchal girls: Clinical features and diagnostic evaluation. Pediatrics *70*:193–198, 1982.
45. Perl, G. A.: Errors in the diagnosis of *Trichomonas vaginalis* infection as observed among 1199 patients. Obstet. Gynecol. *39*:7–9, 1972.
46. Ross, J. D. C., and Scott, G. R.: *Trichomonas vaginalis* infection in prepubertal girls. Med. Sci. Law *33*:82–85, 1993.
47. Rubino, S., Muresu, R., Rappelli, P., et al.: Molecular probe for identification of *Trichomona vaginalis*. J. Clin. Microbiol. *29*:702, 1991.
48. Saxena, S. B., and Jenkins, R. R: Prevalence of *Trichomonas vaginalis* in men at high risk for sexually transmitted diseases. Sex. Transm. Dis. *18*:138–142, 1991.
49. Schares, T., Machtinger, S., D'Harlingue, A. E., et al.: *Trichomonas vaginalis* urinary tract infection in an infant. Pediatr. Infect. Dis. *1*:340–341, 1982.
50. Schmid, G. P., Matheny, L. C., Zaidi, A. A., et al.: Evaluation of six media for the growth of *Trichomonas vaginalis* from vaginal secretions. J. Clin. Microbiol. *6*:1230–1233, 1989.
51. Sowmini, C. N., Vijayalakshmi, K., Chellamuthiah, C., et al.: Infections of the median raphe of the penis: Report of three cases. Br. J. Vener. Dis. *49*:469–474, 1972.
52. Spence, M. R., Hollander, D. H., Smith, J., et al.: The clinical and laboratory diagnosis of *Trichomonas vaginalis* infection. Sex. Transm. Dis. *7*:168–171, 1980.
53. Spiegel, C: Microflora associated with *Trichomonas vaginalis* and vaccination against vaginal trichomoniasis. *In* Honigberg, B. M. (ed.): Trichomonads Parasitic in Humans. New York, Springer-Verlag, 1989, pp. 213–224.
54. Thomason, J. L., and Gelbart, S. M.: *Trichomonas vaginalis*. Obstet. Gynecol. *74*:536–540, 1989.
55. Watt, L., and Jennison, R. F.: Incidence of *Trichomonas vaginalis* in marital partners. Br. J. Vener. Dis. *36*:163–166, 1960.
56. White, S. T., Loda, F. A., Ingram, D. L., et al.: Sexually transmitted diseases in sexually abused children. Pediatrics *72*:16–21, 1983.
57. Wilcox, R. R.: Epidemiological aspects of human trichomoniasis. Br. J. Vener. Dis. *36*:167–174, 1960.

Bibliography

Honigberg, B. M.: Trichomonads Parasitic in Humans. New York, Springer-Verlag, 1989.

214

Balantidium coli Infection

Peter J. Hotez

Balantidium coli is the largest protozoan parasite and the only ciliate to infect humans.[6, 9, 15] The organism has a worldwide distribution, but it is found more commonly in the less developed nations of the tropics. Because pigs are a principal animal reservoir, most human infections have been reported in tropical regions where swine have close contact with humans, such as in the islands of the South Pacific (including Papua New Guinea) and Central and South America.[10] Balantidiasis occurs in areas where other swine-associated parasitic zoonoses (e.g., taeniasis, trichinellosis, ascariasis) also are prevalent, although infection with *B. coli* still is rare. Fewer than 1000 cases of human balantidiasis are reported in the literature.[9] The organism first was described in 1857 by P. H. Malmsten, who observed the ciliates from two patients in Sweden.[3]

ETIOLOGY AND PATHOGENESIS

The organism has both trophozoite and cyst stages. The trophozoite is a large, pear-shaped organism covered with cilia. Estimates of size range between 50 to 100 μm in length and 40 to 70 μm in width.[6] This relatively enormous protozoan organism typically can be seen by light microscopy using only low-power magnification.[6] Subcellular organelles such as a cytostome and many large vacuoles containing bacteria and debris are visualized under higher magnification. Like many other ciliates, *B. coli* trophozoites have a macronucleus and a micronucleus. The trophozoites colonize the large intestine, where ultimately they round up and secrete a cyst wall as they pass down the lumen. The cysts measure from 50 to 70 μm and also contain a macronucleus and a micronucleus. The cyst stages can survive in the outside environment and are infectious to a wide range of animals, including humans (discussed later).

Frequently, *B. coli* does not invade human tissues and therefore does not cause clinical disease. Under conditions that are not understood well, however, *B. coli* also has the potential for highly aggressive tissue invasion and destruction. It is not clear whether the invasive potential of *B. coli* results from parasite virulence, compromised host defenses, or some combination of these two factors. The observation that invasive disease is more common in debilitated patients and in patients with polyparasitism suggests that host defenses have an important role in limiting *B. coli* tissue destruction.[1, 9]

When parasite invasion occurs, it begins in the colonic mucosa, where ulcerations and secondary microabscesses can result. Extensive tissue damage in the cecum and appendix results in clinical presentations of typhlitis and appendicitis, respectively.[4, 5, 9] Histopathologic examination of these tissues reveals flask-shaped ulcerations and necrosis with an extensive inflammatory infiltrate made up predominantly of polymorphonuclear leukocytes.[4, 9] *B. coli* probably creates mucosal ulcerations through the release of histolytic enzymes similar to those described from *Entamoeba histolytica*.[12] Ulcerations can lead to hemorrhage or even colonic perforation. There is a report of a second type of histopathology wherein patients harboring *B. coli* develop inflammatory polyposis of the rectum and sigmoid colon.[8]

When tissue invasion is extensive, the organism can metastasize to extraintestinal sites and cause hepatic and pulmonary involvement. Polymorphonuclear inflammatory cell infiltration results in abscesses at these sites.[3, 5, 8] Most patients with metastatic balantidiasis have recognizable defects in host defenses.[8]

EPIDEMIOLOGY

As noted earlier, human balantidiasis has a worldwide distribution, but epidemic foci have reported from the swine-producing areas of Papua New Guinea, Micronesia, the Seychelles Islands, and Central and South America.[3, 10, 13] Incidence rates can be high among swine farmers and slaughterhouse workers. It is believed that the potential for human *B. coli* infections is high in areas of poor hygiene where there is extensive contact between humans and pigs. A notorious outbreak of human balantidiasis occurred after a devastating typhoon on the Pacific islands of Truk caused widespread contamination of ground and surface water supplies with pig feces.[13] A number of other animals also can serve potentially as reservoir hosts, including nonhuman primates, guinea pigs, horses, cattle, and rats.[3] *B. coli* also colonizes many great apes, including baboons, orangutans, chimpanzees, and gorillas, and clinical balantidiasis has been reported from these primates when they are maintained in captivity.[9] Human epidemics also have been described in institutional settings, especially where crowding mixes with low levels of personal hygiene.[13] In these instances, human-to-human spread has been postulated.

CLINICAL MANIFESTATIONS

Asymptomatic Infection

The majority of infections are asymptomatic or cause occasional loose stools. This situation probably accounts for up to 85 per cent of patients harboring *B. coli*.[9] Asymptomatic infection may be more common in children than in adults.[14]

Diarrhea

The next most frequent presentation of *B. coli* infections is patients who have intermittent diarrhea, abdominal pain, and weight loss.[14] Sometimes, discrete ulcerations can be observed during sigmoidoscopy.[9] A subset of these persons develop invasive disease subsequently.

Invasive Colonic Balantidiasis

The hallmark of *Balantidium* colitis is dysentery with bloody and mucous stools, colonic tenderness, leukocytosis, and fever. Sigmoidoscopy and colonoscopy of these patients reveal ulcerations and mucosal granuloma formation.[1, 9, 11, 13] Involvement of the large intestine can be diffuse, although in some cases right-sided colonic lesions predominate. Right-sided colonic lesions can progress to typhlitis or appendicitis.[4, 5, 9] Transmural involvement of the colon frequently results in intestinal obstruction, hemorrhage, and balantidial peritonitis. Colonic perforation is an ominous complication that is associated with extremely high mortality.[9]

Metastatic Balantidiasis

Highly invasive balantidiasis leading to metastatic disease of the mesenteric lymph nodes, liver, and lung is a rare complication that can occur in malnourished, debilitated, and immunocompromised patients.

DIAGNOSIS

Stools from patients harboring *B. coli* have been described as having a "pig-pen" odor.[14] The examination of wet preparations of fresh or concentrated stools usually demonstrates cyst and trophozoite forms of *B. coli.* Cilia motility and rapid rotary motion of the trophozoites sometimes can be appreciated under low-power magnification. Because the organism takes up heavy concentrations of dye, stained preparations typically do not reveal internal structures or even cilia.[6] These large organisms can be confused with helminth ova, especially on stained preparations.[6] As an adjunct to direct fecal examinations, sigmoidoscopy can demonstrate ulcerations from which abundant trophozoites may be obtained for diagnosis.[14]

TREATMENT

For the treatment of intestinal balantidiasis, a number of chemotherapeutic regimens have been tried, usually with some improvement. In many cases, however, the parasite is not eradicated.[9] For children older than 8 years of age, tetracycline (40 mg/kg/day in four doses for 10 days [maximum, 2 g/day]) is the treatment of choice. Tetracycline is considered to be investigational for this condition by the U.S. Food and Drug Administration. Also considered investigational for balantidiasis are the drugs iodoquinol (40 mg/kg/day in three doses for 20 days) and metronidazole (35 to 50 mg/kg/day in three doses for 5 days).[2, 7] Alternative chemotherapeutic agents that have been tried with varying degrees of success include paromomycin and chloroquine.[9] Surgical intervention often is required for gastrointestinal invasive complications of *B. coli,* such as typhlitis, appendicitis, and peritonitis.

References

1. Arean, V. M., and Koppisch, E: Balantidiasis. A review and report of cases. Am. J. Pathol. *32*:1089–1116, 1956.
2. Beasley, J. W., and Walzer, P. D.: Ineffectiveness of metronidazole in treatment of *Balantidium coli* infections. Trans. R. Soc. Trop. Med. Hyg. *66*:519, 1972.
3. Despommier, D. D., Gwadz, R. W., and Hotez, P. J.: Parasitic Diseases. 3rd ed. New York, Springer-Verlag, 1995, pp. 159–160.
4. Dodd, L. G.: *Balantidium coli* infestation as a cause of acute appendicitis. J. Infect. Dis. *163*:1392, 1991.
5. Dorfman, S., Rangel, O., and Bravo, L. G.: Balantidiasis: Report of a fatal case with appendicular and pulmonary involvement. Trans. R. Soc. Trop. Med. Hyg. *78*:833–834, 1984.
6. Garcia, L. S., and Bruckner, D. A.: Diagnostic Medical Parasitology. 2nd ed. Washington, D.C., American Society for Microbiology, 1993, pp. 44–46.
7. Garcia-Laverde, A., and DeBonilla, L.: Clinical trials with metronidazole in human balantidiasis. Am. J. Trop. Med. Hyg. *24*:781–783, 1975.
8. Ladas, S. D., Savva, S., Frydas, A., et al.: Invasive balantidiasis presented as chronic colitis and lung involvement. Dig. Dis. Sci. *34*:1621–1623, 1989.
9. Lee, R. V., Prowten, A. W., Anthone, S., et al.: Typhlitis due to *Balantidium coli* in captive lowland gorillas. Rev. Infect. Dis. *12*:1052–1059, 1990.
10. Radford, A. J.: Balantidiasis in Papua New Guinea. Med. J. Aust. *1*:238–241, 1971.
11. Swartzwelder, J. C.: Balantidiasis. Am. J. Dig. Dis. *17*:173–179, 1950.
12. Tempelis, C. H., and Lysenko, M. G.: The production of a hyaluronidase by *B. coli*. Exp. Parasitol. *6*:31–36, 1957.
13. Walzer, P. D., Judson, F. N., Murphy, K. B., et al.: Balantidiasis outbreak in Truk. Am. J. Trop. Med. Hyg. *22*:33–41, 1973.
14. Woody, N. C., and Woody, H. B.: Balantidiasis in infancy: Review of literature and report of a case. J. Pediatr. *56*:485–489, 1960.
15. Young, M. D.: Balantidiasis. J. A. M. A. *113*:580–584, 1939.

Coccidia, Inicnosporidia (Intestinal)

215

CRYPTOSPORIDIOSIS, *CYCLOSPORA* INFECTION, ISOSPORIASIS, AND MICROSPORIDIOSIS

Jane T. Atkins, Enrique Caceres, and Thomas G. Cleary

The enteric coccidian parasites *(Cryptosporidium, Cyclospora,* and *Isospora)* and microsporidia are obligate intracellular protozoans that now are known to cause gastrointestinal disease in both immunocompetent and immunocompromised humans.[223, 250] *Sarcocystis,* another coccidian organism that may use humans as intermediate hosts, rarely causes disease. These pathogens virtually were unknown before the HIV epidemic. In the immunocompetent host, these enteric coccidian parasites typically cause an illness that is short lived, but in the immunodeficient host, they cause prolonged life-threatening diarrheal illness as well as extraintestinal disease.

CRYPTOSPORIDIOSIS

Cryptosporidium is a coccidian protozoan that infects the gastric and respiratory epithelium of vertebrates.[64, 89] It first was identified in the gastric glands of laboratory mice by Tyzzer[283] in 1907 and for decades was considered to be nonpathogenic. In 1955, Slavin[265] associated *Cryptosporidium* with enteritis in turkeys, and in 1971 it was recognized as a significant cause of diarrhea in calves.[222] However, it was not until 1976 that the first human cases of cryptosporidiosis were reported.[190, 212] Prior to 1982, fewer than 10 cases of human cryptosporidiosis were reported in the literature.[89] With the advent of the AIDS epidemic, *Cryptosporidium* has emerged as a significant human pathogen and now is recognized as one of the most common causes of diarrheal disease in the immunocompetent as well as the immunocompromised host.[64, 105]

Microbiology

Cryptosporidium species are ubiquitous, small (2 to 6 μm), obligate, intracellular parasites that infect the microvilli of the gastrointestinal and respiratory tracts of vertebrates.[61, 64] They are related to *Toxoplasma, Isospora, Plasmodium, Eimeria,* and *Sarcocystis*. The taxonomic classification of *Cryptosporidium, Isospora, Cyclospora*, and *Sarcocystis* is summarized in Figure 215–1. *Cryptosporidium* and *Plasmodium* species belong to the same order (Eucoccidiorida) but are in a different suborder. *Cryptosporidium* species, *Toxoplasma gondii, Isospora belli, Eimeria* species, and *Sarcocystis* species share the same suborder Eimeriorina and are considered true coccidia.[64]

It initially was assumed that *Cryptosporidium*, like other coccidia, was host-specific. Thus, cryptosporidia were speciated according to the animal that they infected.[64, 89] However, cross-transmission studies revealed that there is little or no host specificity for species.[77, 89, 284] In 1984, Levine[159] consolidated the 21-named species into four. Currently, six species of the genus *Cryptosporidium* are recognized. They are *C. nasorum*, which infects fish, *C. serpentis*, which infects reptiles, *C. baileyi* and *C. meleagrides*, which infect birds, and *C. muris* and *C. parvum*, which infect mammals. *C. parvum*[273] is responsible for virtually all documented cases of cryptosporidiosis in humans.[292]

Life Cycle

The life cycle of *Cryptosporidium* is monoxenous—that is, the entire life cycle is completed in a single host. Similar to other true coccidia, the life cycle of *Cryptosporidium* is characterized by six major developmental stages: (1) excystation, release of infective sporozoites, (2) merogamy, asexual multiplication in the host, (3) gametogony, the formation of

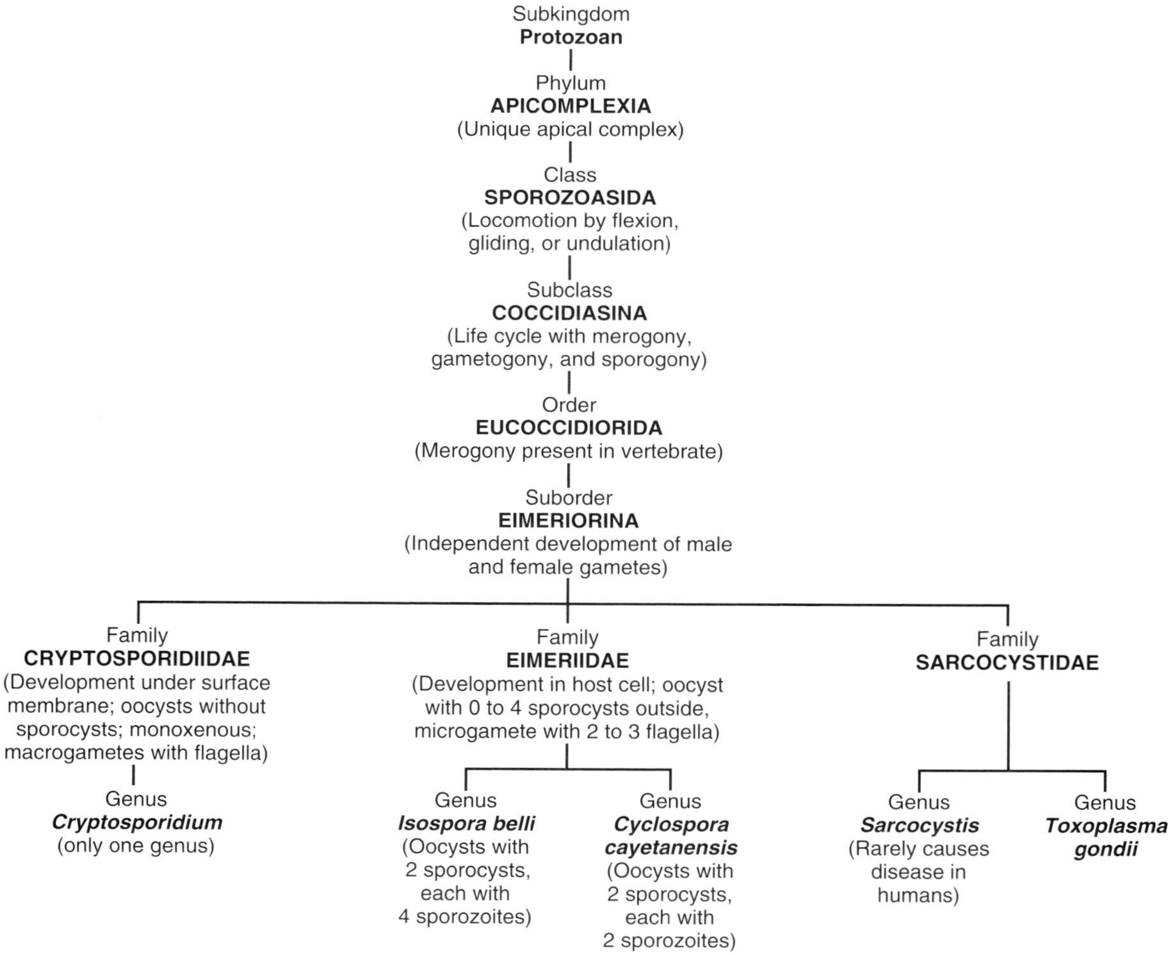

FIGURE 215–1. *Taxonomic classification of* Cryptosporidium, Isospora, Cyclospora, *and* Sarcocystis.

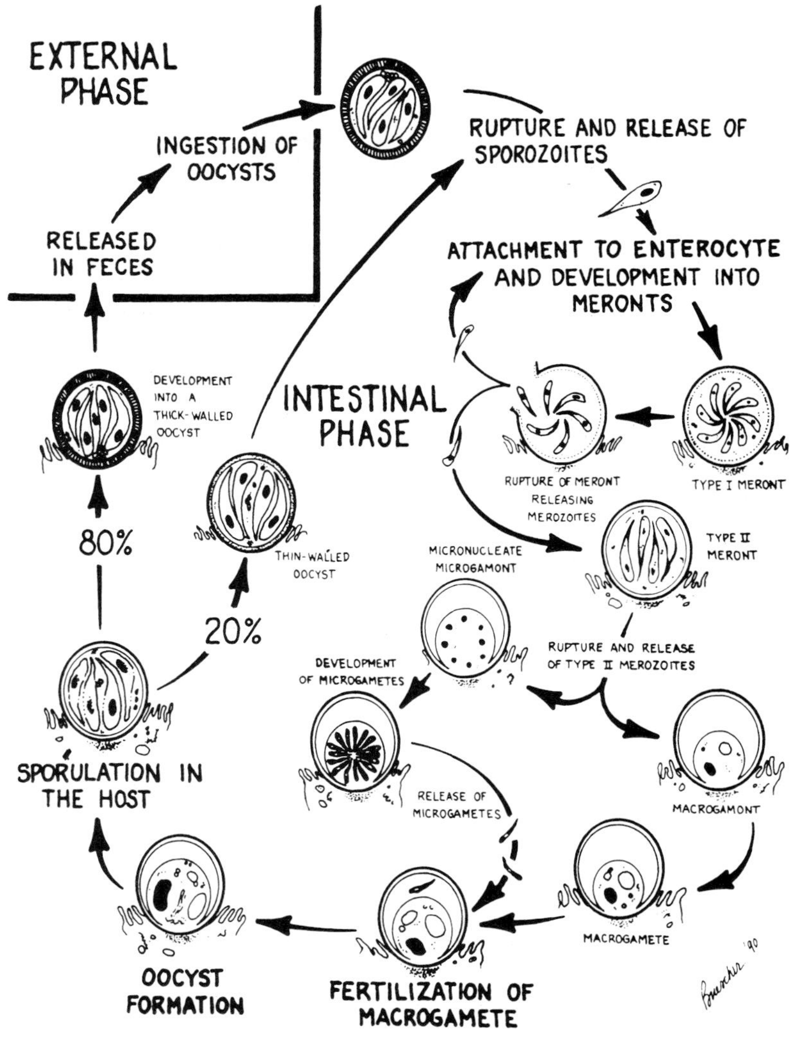

FIGURE 215–2. *Life cycle of* Cryptosporidium.

the microgametocytes and macrogametocytes, (4) fertilization, the union of microgametocyte and macrogametocyte, (5) oocyst formation, and (6) sporogony, the formation of infectious sporozoites within the oocyst wall.[58, 64, 65]

The life cycle of *Cryptosporidium* is summarized in Figure 215–2.

In humans, the life cycle begins with the ingestion or possibly the inhalation of the thick-walled oocyst from the environment. Excystation occurs in the small intestines, resulting in the release of four nonflagellated sporozoites that penetrate into the microvilli of enterocytes by a flexing and twisting motion.[64] For most coccidia, excystation requires pancreatic enzymes, reducing conditions, and bile salt. Excystation of *Cryptosporidium* sporozoites can occur in an aqueous solution without these conditions, although excystation is optimal in the presence of trypsin and sodium taurocholate. The ability of *Cryptosporidium* to excyst without much stimulation may explain why it infects extraintestinal sites.[284] Once excystation has occurred, the sporozoite indents and invaginates the enterocyte surface in a glove-like manner to form a parasitiferous vacuole that is confined to the microvillous region. At the base of the parasitiferous vacuole is the "feeder organelle" (Fig. 215–3*A*). This organelle is formed at the attachment site by complex folding of the parasite membrane and serves as a source of sustenance.[175]

The sporozoite differentiates into a spherical, uninucleated trophozoite that undergoes merogony (asexual replication) to form the type I meront. The mature type I meront contains six to eight merozoites (Fig. 215–3*B*) that are released into the intestinal lumen and invade new uninfected microvilli either to develop into more type I meronts (autoinfection) or to differentiate into type II meronts. The mature type II meront releases four merozoites that invade uninfected microvilli and undergo gametogony (sexual multiplication) to form either microgametocytes or macrogametocytes. The fourth developmental stage (fertilization) occurs when free microgametes make contact with the parasitiferous membrane covering the female macrogamete and penetrate into the macrogamete. The fertilized macrogametocyte matures into an oocyst that undergoes sporogony, thus completing the life cycle.[58, 64, 65] Approximately 80 per cent of the oocysts are released into the environment in the feces as dense, thick-walled cysts. The remaining 20 per cent develop into thin-walled cysts that sporulate within the intestinal tract and autoinfect the host.[66] The presence of two autoinfective stages (type I meront and thin-walled oocyst) in the life cycle of

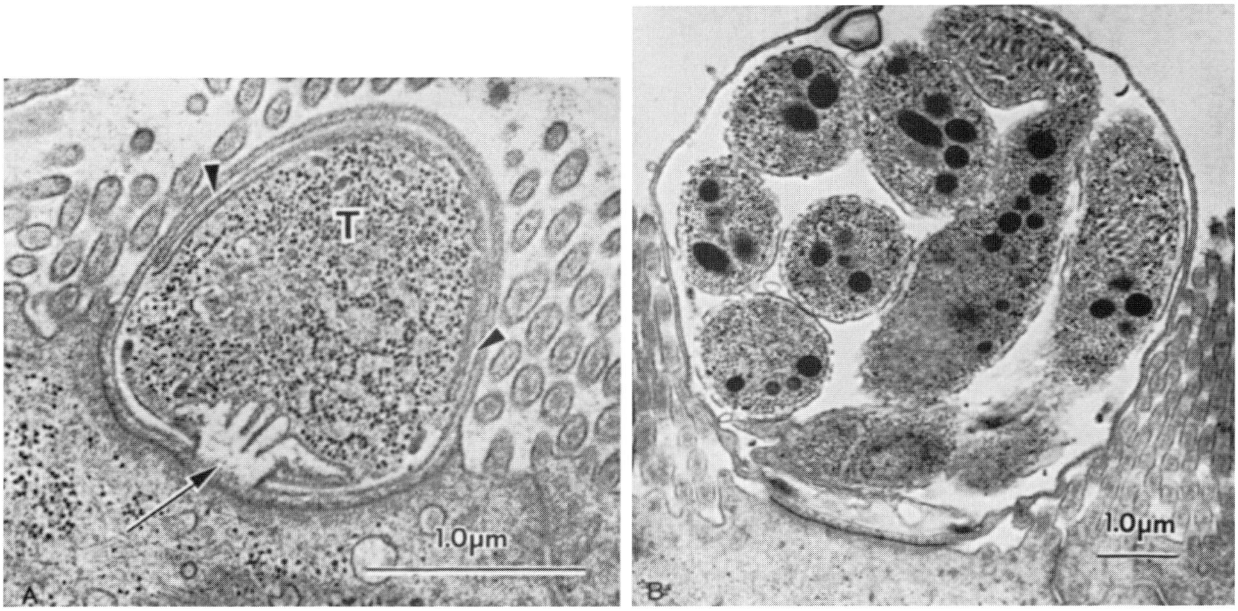

FIGURE 215–3. *Intestinal biopsy of a patient with AIDS infected with* Cryptosporidium. A, *Transmission electron micrograph of a trophozoite (T) within a parasitophorous vacuole. A space (arrowheads) separates the outer double membrane of the infected host intestinal cell from the inner double membrane surrounding the trophozoite. The "feeder organelle" (arrow) lies just above the dense attachment zone.* B, *Transmission electron micrograph of a type 1 meront, containing portions of seven merozoites within the parasitophorous vacuole.*

Cryptosporidium may explain why severe infection can result after ingestion of small numbers of oocysts and why immunocompromised hosts can develop persistent, life-threatening illness.[64]

Epidemiology

Cryptosporidium is distributed worldwide.[58, 64, 330] Prevalence rates in general are higher in developing countries than in industrialized countries. This observation reflects the unsanitary living conditions that promote the person-to-person spread of this highly contagious parasite. Prevalence of *Cryptosporidium* in the stool has been reported to be 1 to 3 per cent in industrialized countries of North America and Europe; in undeveloped countries it ranges from 5 per cent in Asia to 10 per cent in Africa.[64] The seroprevalence of antibodies to *Cryptosporidium* in industrialized regions of North America and Europe ranges from 25 to 35 per cent and is as high as 64 per cent in developing countries of South America.[39, 64, 124, 287] Travelers to endemic areas are at risk for acquiring cryptosporidiosis.[288]

Cryptosporidium has been reported more commonly in children than in adults. In India, the prevalence rate for children is 5.5 to 9.8 per cent[71, 181]; in Liberia, it is 5.9 per cent[133]; and in Guatemala, it is 5.4 to 11.6 per cent.[22, 60] The prevalence of asymptomatic infection with *Cryptosporidium* among children younger than 5 years of age varies with geographic location and is estimated to be less than 0.5 per cent.[301] However, Pettoello-Mantovani and colleagues[228] recently reported a high prevalence of asymptomatic infection with *Cryptosporidium* among children from Naples, Italy (6.4 per cent in immunocompetent children and 22 per cent in immunodeficient children). Young children in the day care setting are at a high risk for acquiring infection.[56, 80] Outbreaks of cryptosporidiosis in child care centers have been reported from the United States,[3, 44, 53, 125, 214, 264, 274, 278, 279] Great Britain,[118] Australia,[59, 90] France,[30] Portugal,[191] Chile,[210, 316] and South Africa.[303]

Seasonal variation has been noted in some geographic locations. In tropical climates, the incidence of cryptosporidiosis is higher during the warm, humid months,[166, 180, 227, 259, 313] whereas in temperate climates, a late summer/early fall peak is observed.[173, 196, 203, 281, 323] In the United States, investigators have not observed a consistent seasonal variation.[14, 135, 145, 286, 323] However, day care outbreaks of cryptosporidiosis in the United States occur most often in the late summer and early autumn.[56]

Transmission

Person-to-person transmission through the fecal-oral route is the principal mechanism of transmission of *Cryptosporidium.* Airborne transmission has been suggested but has not been proved.[21, 132] Secondary spread of *C. parvum* has been reported in the day care setting,[56, 118] among household contacts,[62, 211] and in the hospital setting.[52, 82, 151, 179, 206, 208] The estimated median infective dose is 132 organisms, but as few as 30 organisms can cause infection in a susceptible host.[84] The incubation period of cryptosporidiosis in humans has been estimated to be 2 to 14 days.[58, 146]

During the acute diarrheal illness, large quantities of oocysts are excreted in the stool and are highly infectious. Smaller quantities of oocysts are excreted with asymptomatic infections and during the convalescent phase.[3, 53] Asymptomatic shedding of the oocyst may continue for up to 5 weeks after an acute episode of diarrhea.[274] Transmission to contacts can occur even when low quantities of oocysts are excreted.[3, 53] Fomites may play a role in transmission of *Cryptosporidium,* especially in the day care setting, where fecal contamination is common.[3, 56, 294]

Cryptosporidium is a resilient organism. It is not known how long the oocysts remain viable once they are excreted in the natural environment. In the laboratory, oocysts suspended in calf feces are viable for at least 2 days on a dried wooden surface at room temperature.[6] Freezing at $-20°$ C for 72 hours[240] and heating to 45° to 55° C for 20 minutes[5, 88] reduce the infectivity. An aqueous suspension of oocysts can be rendered noninfectious by exposure to 72.4° C for 1 minute, 64.2° C for greater than 2 minutes,[91] or ultraviolet light for at least 150 minutes.[164] The parasite is resistant to disinfectants, including 3 per cent hypochlorite, sodium hydroxide, iodophors, cresylic acid, benzalkonium chloride, and 5 per cent formaldehyde, that commonly are used by hospitals and day care centers. It is sensitive to prolonged exposure to 70 to 100 per cent bleach, 5 to 10 per cent ammonia, and 10 per cent formaldehyde.[7, 8, 36]

Infected water is a major source of transmission of *Cryptosporidium.* Water-borne outbreaks of cryptosporidiosis have occurred in association with contaminated water from artesian wells,[70] surface water,[99, 173] swimming pools,[47, 49, 144, 184, 272] and filtered public drinking water.[124, 147, 237] *Cryptosporidium* has been found in treated water that meets the standard requirements for water purification, including filtration and chlorination.[70, 99, 124] The largest water-borne outbreak of cryptosporidiosis due to a contaminated public water supply occurred in Milwaukee, Wisconsin, in the Spring of 1993; it is estimated that more than 400,000 persons were infected.[169]

A wide variety of vertebrates are infected with *Cryptosporidium,* including fish, reptiles, birds, and mammals (e.g., horses, sheep, cows, primates, domestic dogs and cats).[7, 31, 78, 90, 136, 139, 174, 197, 284] Farmers and animal handlers are at increased risk for infection. However, zoonotic transmission is not as common as person-to-person and water-borne spread.[4, 67, 85, 235, 284] Transmission of *Cryptosporidium* from invertebrates is rare. There is a single report of *Cryptosporidium* detected in the gut of a common cockroach *(Periplaneta americana)* that was suspected to be the source of infection in a Peruvian child.[327, 328]

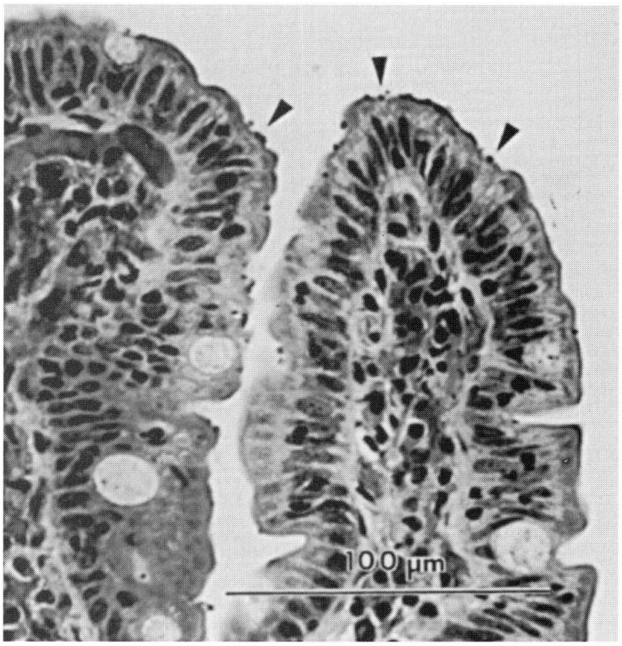

FIGURE 215–4. *Spherical, darkly stained cryptosporidia (arrows) embedded in surfaces of jejunal villi from a boy with chronic diarrhea and congenital immunoglobulin deficiency. Light micrograph. (From Heyworth, M. F., and Owen, R. L.: Gastrointestinal aspects of the acquired immunodeficiency syndrome. Surv. Dig. Dis. 3:197, 1985, with permission from S. Karger A. G., Basel, Switzerland.)*

Pathogenesis and Immunology

The precise mechanism of human cryptosporidiosis has not been determined. The proximal small bowel is the primary site of infection.[41, 77, 284] In the immunocompromised patient, the entire intestinal tract from the oropharynx to the rectum may be infected. Histopathologic findings (Fig. 215–4) of cryptosporidiosis include patchy infection of the intestinal mucosa with mild to moderate villous atrophy, crypt hyperplasia, and mononuclear and polymorphonuclear cell infiltration of the lamina propria.[209] The different stages in the life cycle of the parasite can be visualized with electron microscopy (see Fig. 215–3). In animals, there is an association between the extent of intestinal damage and clinical symptoms; however, this has not been demonstrated in humans.[284] The profuse, watery diarrhea suggests a toxin-mediated process. However, an enterotoxin has not been identified. Recently, a protein with hemolytic activity (HemA) and its corresponding gene were identified in *C. parvum.* The peptide sequence of this hemolytic protein was similar to that of *Escherichia coli* O157 plasmid-encoded hemolysin. It is speculated that this hemolysin may play a role in the formation of the parasitiferous vacuole and feeding organelle.[270]

Both humoral and cell-mediated immunity appear to be necessary in the host defense against *C. parvum.* The importance of cell-mediated immunity is suggested by chronic disease that is seen in AIDS; the relevance of humoral immunity is suggested by the observation that patients with hypogammaglobulinemia may have severe disease.[157, 166] Specific IgG, IgA, IgM, IgE, and secretory IgA antibodies can be measured by indirect fluorescent antibody and enzyme-linked immunosorbent assays, but the significance of these antibodies is not clear.[35, 39, 57, 63, 287, 288] High levels of specific serum and secretory antibodies have been observed in AIDS patients with protracted diarrhea, suggesting that a specific antibody response alone is not sufficient to control this infection.[57]

Gomez Morales and colleagues[111] noted an antigen-specific in vitro proliferation of the peripheral blood mononuclear cells from patients who were sensitized to *C. parvum.* They also found that the supernatant of the peripheral blood mononuclear cells from the immunocompetent persons contained interleukin 10 and interferon-τ after exposed to *C. parvum* and that levels of interferon-τ were significantly higher in persons who recovered from cryptosporidiosis. Children have much lower levels of interferon-τ than do adults; patients with AIDS also had impaired production of interferon-τ. This may explain why some children and adults with AIDS have a more severe course with cryptosporidiosis.[111]

Clinical Manifestations

The clinical spectrum of disease caused by *Cryptosporidium* is broad and depends on the immunologic status of the host. In the immunocompetent host, *Cryptosporidium* infection usually is manifested by intestinal symptoms, whereas in immunodeficient patients, there may be intestinal or extraintestinal involvement. Regardless of the immunologic status of the patient, diarrhea is the most common clinical presentation of cryptosporidiosis. In the immunocompetent patient, the onset of diarrhea is abrupt and the illness usually is self-limited, lasting several days to 2 weeks.[149] In contrast, in the AIDS patient, the onset of diarrhea is insidious and can last months, resulting in severe wasting that is life-threatening. Although intestinal cryptosporidiosis in patients with AIDS usually results in severe diarrhea, asymptomatic infection and spontaneous resolution of diarrhea have been reported in HIV-infected patients.[140, 327]

Intestinal cryptosporidiosis is characterized by a profuse, watery (cholera-like) diarrhea indistinguishable from that associated with other enteric coccidian parasites. Massive fluid loss is common. In patients with AIDS, the average fluid loss is 3 to 6 liters per day but can be 17 to 20 liters per day and 70 stools per day.[43] The stools rarely contain blood and fecal leukocytes; mucus occasionally is seen.[105] Charcot-Leyden crystals are not present. Other less common clinical findings include low-grade fever (<39° C), crampy abdominal pain, flatulence, nausea, and vomiting.[121, 270] In addition, flu-like symptoms, such as myalgia, malaise, headache, and anorexia, occasionally occur. Weight loss is a common finding in both immunocompetent and immunosuppressed hosts.[64, 105]

In developing countries, infants and toddlers may develop severe diarrhea,[38, 177] resulting in failure to thrive or contributing to malnutrition.[121, 138, 156, 170, 281] Malnourished children tend to have a protracted course and shed oocysts longer. They often require hospitalization for parenteral therapy and may have a fatal outcome.[25, 139, 156, 170, 281]

Other immunodeficient states besides AIDS and malnutrition have been associated with infection with *Cryptosporidium.* These conditions include cancer,[160, 189, 190, 198, 215, 276] hypogammaglobulinemia,[157, 266] severe combined immune deficiency,[152] bone marrow[52, 150] and renal transplantation,[243, 315] and concurrent viral infections, such as measles[75] and cytomegalovirus infection.[314] The severity and duration of illness generally depend on the degree of immune deficiency. In patients receiving immunosuppressive therapy, the diarrhea resolved with discontinuation of chemotherapy.[190, 198, 315] In the immunodeficient patient, extraintestinal involvement may occur in the respiratory tract, biliary tract, or pancreas.

Respiratory *Cryptosporidium* infection causes cough, shortness of breath, wheezing, croup, and hoarseness.[28, 64, 95, 119, 134, 150, 152, 168, 199, 205] *Cryptosporidium* has been reported as a cause of laryngobronchitis in children.[119] Not all patients have concurrent intestinal cryptosporidiosis. The oocysts can be identified in the sputum, bronchoalveolar lavage, tracheal aspirates, and lung biopsy and brush biopsy specimens.[65] *Cryptosporidium* has been identified as the only pathogen or as a co-infecting agent with cytomegalovirus, *Pneumocystis carinii,* and *Mycobacterium* species.[229]

Cryptosporidiosis of the biliary tract usually presents as acalculous cholecystitis and less frequently as sclerosing cholangitis and hepatitis.[18, 24, 114, 116, 176, 230, 253, 293] Signs and symptoms associated with biliary cryptosporidiosis include fever, nonradiating right upper quadrant pain, jaundice, nausea, vomiting, and diarrhea.[18, 64, 280] Elevation of the bilirubin, alkaline phosphatase, and transaminases may occur.[18, 64, 280, 293] HIV-infected patients with CD4 counts of less than 50/mm^3 are predisposed to develop biliary cryptosporidiosis.[293] Radiographic findings include dilation of extrahepatic and intrahepatic ducts, thickening of the wall of the gall bladder and extrahepatic ducts, pericholecystic fluid, and stenosis of the distal extrahepatic duct.[18, 280] Concomitant infection with cytomegalovirus can occur and frequently is associated with intrahepatic duct irregularities.[18, 129, 148, 280] The definitive diagnosis of biliary cryptosporidiosis is made by biopsy and demonstration of the various stages of *Cryptosporidium* in the biliary tree in a patient with compatible symptoms and abnormal radiographic results.[64, 293]

Pancreatitis is an uncommon manifestation of cryptosporidiosis but has been reported in both adults and children infected with HIV.[37, 114, 123, 129, 148, 152, 200, 280] Pancreatitis may occur concurrently with cholecystitis.[129, 148, 280] *Cryptosporidium* oocysts have been identified in the pancreatic duct, usually near the head of the pancreas.[152, 280] The associated ductal

TABLE 215–1. Diagnostic Characteristics of Enteric Coccidian Protozoa and Microsporidia

Organism	Characteristics of Oocyst	Specimen	Recommended Diagnostic Procedure	Comments
Cryptosporidium	Spherical 4–6 μm; oocyst is sporulated when passed in stool; sporulated oocyst contains 4 sporozoites	Stool	Direct microscopy Modified acid-fast stain Monoclonal antibody stain	Concentration methods enhance recovery, especially when the stool is formed; fluorescence with auramine rhodamine
		Intestinal biopsy	Histopathology Electron microscopy	
Isospora belli	Oval 20–30 μm × 10–19 μm; oocyst is unsporulated when passed in stool; sporulated oocyst contains 2 sporoblasts, each with 2 sporozoites	Stool	Direct microscopy Modified acid-fast stain	Oocyst excreted intermittently; concentration method enhances recovery; variable fluorescence with auramine rhodamine
		Intestinal biopsy	Histopathology Electron microscopy	
Cyclospora cayetanensis	Spherical 8–10 μm; oocyst is unsporulated when passed in stool; sporulated oocyst contains 2 sporoblasts, each with 4 sporozoites	Stool	Direct microscopy Modified acid-fast stain	Concentration method enhances the recovery; bright blue autofluorescence under ultraviolet light
		Intestinal biopsy	Histopathology Electron microscopy	
Microsporidia	Spores with internal extrusion apparatus; variable size depends on species: 0.7–3.0 μm × 1.5–5.0 μm	Stool and body fluids	Chromotrope stain Chemofluorescent stain Giemsa stain Electron microscopy	Light microscopy of stool and tissue is sensitive when performed by someone with experience; electron microscopy is required to confirm diagnosis
		Intestinal biopsy	Histopathology Electron microscopy	

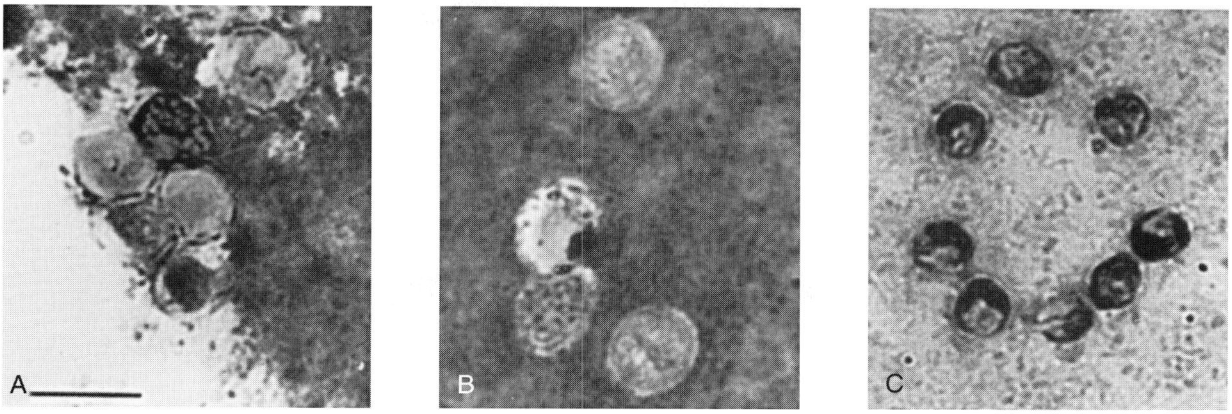

FIGURE 215–5. *Modified acid-fast stain of* Cyclospora *species* (A), Cryptosporidium muris (B), *and* Cryptosporidium parvum (C). *Bar* = *10 μM. (From Ortega, Y. R., Sterling, C. R., Gilman, R. H., et al.:* Cyclospora *species: A new protozoan pathogen of humans. N. Engl. J. Med. 328:1308–1312, 1993. Copyright 1993, Massachusetts Medical Society.)*

epithelium usually is transformed to hyperplastic squamous metaplasia.[280]

Diagnosis

Intestinal cryptosporidiosis usually is diagnosed by examination of the stool for oocysts. The oocyst of *Cryptosporidium* readily is distinguished from the oocyst of other enteric coccidian parasites by its size and by the presence of four mature sporozoites (Table 215–1 and Figs. 215–5 and 215–6). In acute cryptosporidiosis, oocysts are excreted in high concentration and can be seen in direct preparations. Several special stain methods have been explored, including auramine-rhodamine, auramine-carbofuchsin, dimethyl sulfoxide stain, Giemsa stain, safranin-methylene blue stain, analine-carbolmethyl violet, and acridine orange.[64, 93, 127, 171, 195, 204] However, the modified acid-fast stain is the most reliable and is used by most clinical laboratories.[40, 93, 171] The stains that are used routinely to detect other intestinal parasites (trichrome and iron hematoxylin) do not detect *Cryptosporidium*. Monoclonal immunofluorescent stain and enzyme-linked immunosorbent assay for detection of *Cryptosporidium* in the stool are available and are highly sensitive and specific.[1, 10, 100, 101, 104, 186, 217, 244, 247, 275]

Most clinical laboratories do not screen for *Cryptosporidium* routinely; therefore, one specifically must request testing. Concentration techniques enhance the recovery of the parasite from the stool, especially when formed stools are examined.[64, 188, 303, 305] Several concentration methods have been employed with varying degrees of success, including flotation methods (Sheather sugar solution, zinc sulfate, or saturated sodium chloride) and sedimentation methods (formalin-ethyl acetate and formalin-ether). Some investigators feel that the Sheather sucrose is superior to the sedimentation methods, whereas others report no difference in the two methods.[64, 188, 204, 305] Weber and colleagues[306] reported improved recovery of *Cryptosporidium* oocysts using a modified concentration technique that combines sedimentation and flotation methods.[306]

Serologic tests for *Cryptosporidium* (immunofluorescent antibody assays or enzyme-linked immunosorbent assays)[35, 39, 290]

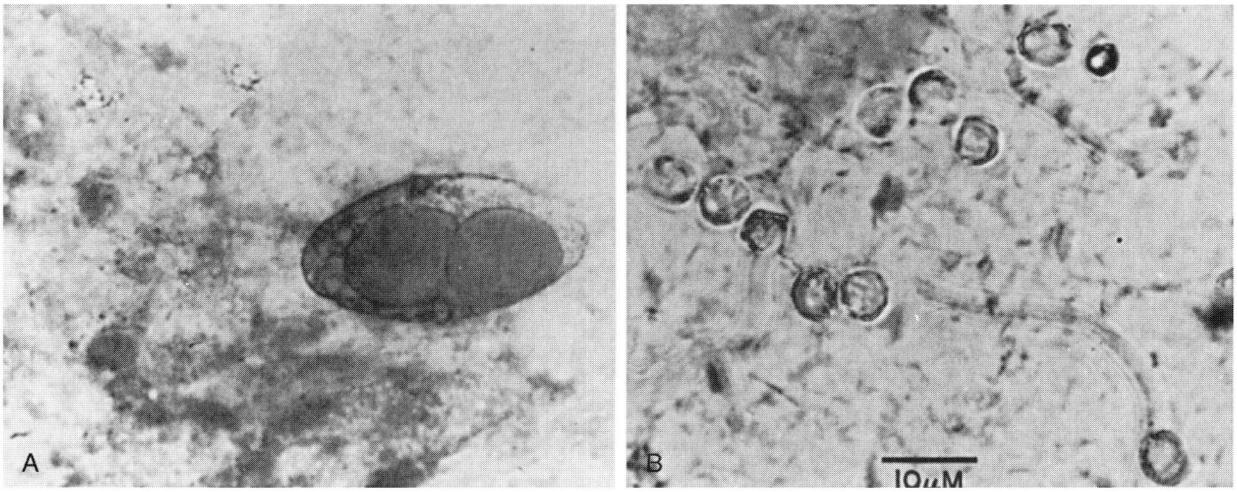

FIGURE 215–6. *Unconcentrated fresh stool sample from two patients with AIDS, stained with modified Kinyoun stain.* Isospora belli (A) *and* Cryptosporidium (B). *Note the difference in size and shape of the two coccidian parasites;* Isospora *averages 25 × 15 μm and contains two sporoblasts, whereas* Cryptosporidium *averages about 5 μm in diameter. (From DeHovitz, J. A., Pape, J. W., Boncy, M., et al.: Clinical manifestations and therapy of* Isospora belli *infection in patients with the acquired immunodeficiency syndrome. N. Engl. J. Med. 315:87–90, 1986. Copyright 1986, Massachusetts Medical Society.)*

have been developed but are of limited value for the diagnosis of acute illness.[5, 39] These tests are useful to study the epidemiology or seroprevalence of *Cryptosporidium*.[287–290]

Biopsy of the intestine usually is not necessary for the diagnosis of intestinal infection. However, identifying the various stages of the life cycle of *Cryptosporidium* in the tissue is helpful for the diagnosis of extraintestinal disease. The parasite can be visualized using light microscopy staining with hematoxylin and eosin stain or electron microscopy[65, 66, 110] (see Figs. 215–3 and 215–4). Indirect immunofluorescent antibody stains using *Cryptosporidium*-specific monoclonal antibodies also have been utilized.[163]

Treatment and Prevention

In the immunocompetent host, the illness is self-limited and antimicrobial therapy is not necessary. However, in the immunocompromised host, especially patients with AIDS, the management of intestinal cryptosporidiosis is problematic. Fluid losses can be excessive; thus, rehydration with oral or intravenous fluid is an essential part of the management.

More than 100 therapeutic agents have been investigated in humans or animals with variable success. Agents targeted at reducing diarrheal symptoms include peptidomimetics and antimotility drugs. Antimicrobials and passive immunotherapy have been used to try to kill or eliminate the pathogen.[236]

The peptidomimetic agents, octreotide and vapreotide, are synthetic analogues of somatostatin. The mechanism of action of these compounds is inhibition of secretion of gastrointestinal hormones to enhance electrolyte and water absorption and decrease jejunal transit time.[84, 115] Octreotide also may act to inhibit HIV-induced activation of vasoactive intestinal peptide receptors in the gut.[246] Octreotide has been used to manage other causes of secretory diarrhea successfully.[207] Both octreotide[42, 51, 86, 155, 161, 242] and vapreotide[108, 113] have been used to treat HIV patients with chronic intestinal cryptosporidiosis. They have had limited success in reducing the symptoms. Adverse effects of octreotide include inhibition of gall bladder emptying and pancreatic secretion, resulting in cholelithiasis and pancreatitis.[113, 194] These agents do not eradicate the pathogen. Antimotility agents, such as loperamide and opiates, control the diarrhea but, like the peptidomimetic agents, do not eradicate the parasite.[93, 239]

Several antiprotozoan agents have been studied. Initial reports using the macrolide antibiotic spiramycin were encouraging.[133, 206, 233, 249] However, a subsequent placebo-controlled study conducted by the AIDS Clinical Trial Group revealed that spiramycin was no better than placebo.[239, 321] In animal studies, the newer macrolide antibiotics, azithromycin and clarithromycin, are promising.[37, 237] Azithromycin was used successfully to treat two children with cancer who had severe diarrhea due to *Cryptosporidium*.[299] Preliminary data from a controlled trial of azithromycin for cryptosporidiosis in adult AIDS patients revealed a significant decrease in oocyst shedding and a trend toward decreased stool frequency and weight loss.[269]

Paromomycin is a poorly absorbed aminoglycoside that is used to treat intestinal amebiasis. In vitro, it has excellent activity against *Cryptosporidium*.[34, 178] Several anecdotal reports and uncontrolled trials have indicated that paromomycin may be an effective agent against *Cryptosporidium* in HIV-infected patients.[9, 20, 50, 91, 112, 252, 302] In the only double-blind, placebo-controlled study, paromomycin resulted in improved clinical and parasitologic parameters in patients with AIDS and CD4 counts of less than 100.[319] Unfortunately, paromomycin does not eradicate oocysts or result in resolution of symptoms consistently. The response to paromomycin appears to be dose-related and depends on the degree of immunosuppression.[20] The typical adult dose is 1 to 2 g per day administered every 6 hours.[236] Doses of 50 to 100 mg/kg/day are required in some adults. Duration of therapy has been variable, and maintenance therapy often has been required to prevent relapse.[20, 236] Paromomycin is considered to be first-line therapy for cryptosporidiosis.[20, 236]

Other antiprotozoan agents that have been investigated include atovaquone,[241] diclazuril,[55, 192] and latrazuril[120] (an analogue of diclazuril). In vivo studies of atovaquone using the severe combined immunodeficient mouse model yielded inconclusive results.[241] Atovaquone has not been tested in humans. Diclazuril is an agent used to treat coccidian infections in veterinary medicine; anecdotal reports have shown variable efficacy in AIDS patients.[55, 192] The results of a phase I trial of latrazuril are not encouraging. Fifty per cent of the 14 evaluable AIDS patients had a favorable response.[120]

In vitro and in vivo studies in the BALB/c mice model suggest that paromomycin combined with clarithromycin or 14-OH clarithromycin is synergistic.[34] Human trials are planned using paromomycin combined with clarithromycin as well as azithromycin. Preliminary studies of agents that block the autoinfection cycle by inhibiting aminopeptidase activity, resulting in inhibition of excystation, are encouraging.[216]

There are several anecdotal reports on the successful use of hyperimmune bovine colostrum in immunodeficient patients.[251, 260, 284, 285, 291] The only published double-blind, placebo-controlled study using hyperimmune bovine colostrum reported a significant reduction in oocyst shedding in the treated patients. However, this study was flawed because there was a significant difference between the treated and control groups with respect to parasite load, clinical symptoms, and antiretroviral therapy.[213]

Bovine transfer factor is a purified bovine lymphocyte extract. It was beneficial in five of eight patients with cryptosporidiosis.[165] A controlled trial using a bovine dialyzable leukocyte extract resulted in weight gain in six of seven patients and eradication of oocysts in five. When the five control patients subsequently were given the bovine dialyzable leukocyte extract, symptoms improved in two and oocysts were eradicated in two. Overall, the clinical response was favorable in 10 of 12 patients who received the bovine dialyzable leukocyte extract.[187] Orally administered human immunoglobulin appeared to be helpful in a child with leukemia and chronic cryptosporidiosis.[26, 27]

Because adequate therapy is lacking, prevention is paramount, especially for the immunocompromised host. Prevention should be aimed at reducing potential exposure to the infectious oocysts in contaminated water, feces, soil, animals, or other humans. In the hospital or child care setting, hand washing is the single most important measure to prevent the spread of any enteric pathogen. In the hospital setting, enteric precautions (hand washing, wearing gloves, and wearing gowns if soiling is likely) are important measures to prevent nosocomial spread. Contaminated equipment, such as endoscopes and bronchoscopes, should be autoclaved.

Control of water-borne transmission of cryptosporidiosis is a major public health concern. This issue is complicated by the ability of *Cryptosporidium* to escape the filtration system used by most public water facilities and its resistance to chlorination. In 1994, after the massive outbreak in Milwaukee, the Centers for Disease Control and Prevention convened a panel of experts to address the issue of water-borne transmission of *Cryptosporidium*.[48] It recommended that during outbreak situations, immunocompromised patients boil tap water for 1 minute, use a submicron personal-use filtration system to remove particles of 1 μm or less in diameter, or use bottled water prepared by distillation or reverse osmotic filtration. In nonoutbreak situations, no special measures are recommended. However, it may be prudent to employ the outbreak measures outlined earlier for severely immunosuppressed patients routinely.[48]

CYCLOSPORA INFECTION

C. cayetanensis is a coccidian parasite that infects the gastrointestinal tract of both immunocompetent and immunocompromised patients.[226, 326] This organism was described in feces from humans without enteritis as early as 1979.[12] The first documented cases of diarrheal disease attributed to *Cyclospora* were reported in 1986 in four immunocompetent patients who had traveled from the United States to either Haiti or Mexico.[268] At that time, it was referred to as an unsporulated, coccidian body or a fungal spore. It was not until 1993 that this protozoan officially was designated *Cyclospora*.[11, 220, 221] Before the mid-1980s, reports of diarrheal illness caused by *Cyclospora* were rare. With the advent of the AIDS epidemic, this organism has gained increasing recognition as an enteric pathogen.[226, 326]

Microbiology

Cyclospora is a round to ovoid, variable acid-fast organism that measures 8 to 10 μm in diameter[220] (see Fig. 215–5). It also has been referred to as a *Cyanobacterium*-like body, a blue-green algae, a coccidian-like body, *Cryptosporidium*-like, or big *Cryptosporidium*.[12, 17, 45, 131, 220, 221, 232, 261, 271] In 1993, Ortega and associates[220, 221] assigned this organism to the family Eimeriidae and the genus *Cyclospora* and proposed the name *C. cayetanensis* for the species that infects humans. This classification was based on its sporulation characteristics, and the name was derived from the institution where the original research was performed (Universidad Peruana Cayetano Heredia in Lima, Peru).[325]

Cyclospora, like *Isospora* (also a member of the family Eimeriidae), sporulates exogenously and has two sporocysts per oocyst. It differs from *Isospora* in that *Cyclospora* has two sporozoites per sporocyst, whereas *Isospora* has four sporozoites per sporocyst. *Cyclospora* species are ubiquitous, infecting a variety of animals, including vipers, moles, rodents, and myriapods. Humans are the only known host of *C. cayetanensis*. Organisms resembling *C. cayetanensis* have been found in the stool of chimpanzees living in Uganda.[326] The complete life cycle of *C. cayetanensis* has not been elucidated.

Epidemiology

The true prevalence of this organism is not known. A majority of the fecal isolates have been obtained from residents of developing countries or from travelers returning from developing countries.[130, 220, 221, 232, 261] It appears to be endemic in Haiti, Nepal, and Peru.[130, 221, 232, 261] Seasonal variation has been reported. In Nepal, most cases occurred between May and August, corresponding to the rainy season.[130] In Peru, the peak is between April and June, during the fall.[221] Little is known about the transmission of *Cyclospora*. Water-borne outbreaks have been reported in Chicago and in Nepal.[45, 325] One author speculated that uncooked meat may be a source of infection; however, this has not been substantiated by other investigators.[11] Asymptomatic carriage of *Cyclospora* has been reported.[17, 232] These carriers may act as reservoirs for infection.

Clinical Manifestations

Cyclospora causes disease in both immunocompetent and immunocompromised patients.[221, 226, 232, 261, 325] The incubation period has not been established. In the Chicago outbreak, cases occurred 1 to 7 days after the suspected contamination of the water supply.[45] In the immunocompetent host, diarrheal symptoms may last up to 7 weeks and may be remitting.[325] Resolution of symptoms usually correlates with disappearance of the organism from the stool.[130, 226] However, asymptomatic excretion of cysts has been reported.[17, 232] In the immunocompromised host, the duration of diarrhea is highly variable, ranging from a few days to several months; in most cases, it is protracted.

The illness is characterized by abrupt onset of watery diarrhea. Flu-like symptoms, including malaise, myalgia, and anorexia, also occur.[49, 325] Fever is reported in approximately 25 per cent.[45, 261, 325] Vomiting may occur but is less common than diarrhea. Weight loss occurs in both immunocompetent and immunocompromised patients.[130, 268, 326] In HIV-infected patients, *Cyclospora* causes symptoms that are indistinguishable from those of *Cryptosporidium* and *Isospora* infection.[325] Recently, biliary disease was reported in two AIDS patients infected with *Cyclospora*. These patients had clinical and radiographic evidence of biliary disease and did not have evidence of infection with other pathogens. Both patients had acalculous cholecystitis that was responsive to therapy with trimethoprim-sulfamethoxazole.[262]

Diagnosis

Cyclospora, unlike *Cryptosporidium*, can be visualized by light microscopy after formol-ether concentration of the stool. In fresh stool, the oocysts are unsporulated. They appear as refractile spherical bodies measuring 8 to 10 μm with a central greenish morula that contains six to nine refractile globules.[220] Safranin staining enhances the outline of the membrane but does not stain internal structures. The sensitivity of the wet mount is 75 per cent.[225] Oocysts exhibit bright blue autofluorescence when exposed to ultraviolet light. Staining is variable with modified Ziehl-Neelsen stain[221] (see Fig. 215–5). Fluorescence with auramine rhodamine staining enhances the visualization of internal structures, but this stain usually is weak and irregular. *Cyclospora* is not visualized by Gram, Giemsa, Grocott-Gomori silver, Lugol-iodine, periodic acid–Schiff, or hematoxylin and eosin staining.[226, 325]

Treatment

The disease appears to be self-limited in the immunocompetent host. In a small, uncontrolled study, therapy with trimethoprim-sulfamethoxazole appeared to be beneficial, resulting in resolution of symptoms and reduction in the length of shedding of oocysts from 9 to 1.3 days.[172] In a recent placebo-controlled trial among travelers to Nepal, trimethoprim-sulfamethoxazole for 7 days eradicated *Cyclospora* from the stool in 96 per cent of the patients.[130] In contrast, 88 per cent of the placebo group still had detectable *Cyclospora* in the stool at the end of 7 days. Eradication of the organism correlated with resolution of symptoms. In one study, patients with *Cyclospora* did not improve when treated with empiric therapy (norfloxacin, tinidazole, quinacrine, nalidixic acid, and diloxanide furoate[261]) that was aimed at other enteric pathogens. Prophylaxis with trimethoprim-sulfamethoxazole 3 days a week appears to prevent recurrent episodes in HIV-infected patients.[225]

ISOSPORIASIS

I. belli is another enteric coccidian parasite that closely is related to *Toxoplasma, Cryptosporidium, Sarcocystis,* and *Cyclospora* (see Fig. 215–1). There are numerous species of *Isospora* that infect reptiles, birds, and mammals. However, *I. belli* is the only species that infects humans. *Isospora,* like the other enteric coccidian parasites, causes a self-limited diarrheal illness in the immunocompetent host and a prolonged diarrheal illness in the immunocompromised host. The first reported cases of human isosporiasis were in 1915.[318, 324] Like the other enteric coccidian diseases, isosporiasis was reported infrequently before the AIDS epidemic.

Microbiology and Life Cycle

I. belli is a monoxenous coccidian parasite that most closely is related to *Cyclospora.*[141] The mature oocyst of *I. belli* is oval-shaped, measuring 10 to 20 μm × 20 to 33 μm, and has a translucent thin wall that contains two round sporoblasts, each with four crescent-shaped sporozoites[54] (see Fig. 215–6). Infection follows the ingestion of the mature sporulated oocyst. Excystation occurs in the proximal small intestine, resulting in the release of sporozoites that invade the enterocytes of distal duodenum and proximal jejunum and develop into trophozoites. The trophozoites reproduce asexually to form merozoites. The merozoites undergo asexual replication (schizogony or merogony) or sexual replication (gametogony) that results in the production of the immature unsporulated oocyst. This latter form is excreted in the stool and requires 12 to 48 hours to mature into the infectious form, the sporulated oocyst.[26]

Epidemiology and Transmission

The true prevalence of *I. belli* is not known. It is more common in tropical and subtropical regions.[87] It is endemic in Africa, Southeast Asia, and South America. In North America, it has been implicated as a cause of diarrhea among institutionalized patients.[143] It also has been implicated as a cause of traveler's diarrhea.[107, 258] Before the AIDS pandemic, *Isospora* was an uncommon cause of diarrhea, even in endemic regions. Between 1976 and 1980, *Isospora* oocysts were detected in 0.17 per cent of the stool specimens from 1139 refugees from Southeast Asia.[26] In 1973, De Oliviera and colleagues[76] studied 45,012 stool specimens and reported a prevalence of 0.36 per cent among patients from Brazil. *Isospora* is found in 3 to 18 per cent of AIDS patients from developing countries and less than 0.2 per cent of AIDS patients from the United States and Europe.[137, 224, 270] In Haiti, *Isospora* accounts for 15 per cent of chronic diarrhea in patients with AIDS.[74]

It generally is accepted that humans are the only host of *I. belli* and that there are no animal reservoirs. However, organisms resembling *I. belli* have been identified in the stool of dogs.[106] Transmission is by the fecal-oral route. Sexual transmission of *Isospora* also has been suggested.[96] Infection occurs by ingestion of oocysts in fecally contaminated food or water or from environmental surfaces.[96, 226, 270] The incubation period is believed to be 3 to 14 days.[26, 126] The infectious dose has not been established. In one investigation, a single volunteer developed symptoms after ingesting 3000 organisms and failed to develop symptoms with a second challenge.[183] If untreated, the organism is shed in the stool for 11 to 120 days.[126] The oocysts of *I. belli* are highly resistant to commonly used disinfectants and may remain viable for months in a cool, moist environment.

Pathogenesis and Immunology

The pathologic findings with isosporiasis are nonspecific. The histopathologic changes include shortening of the villi, hypertrophy of the crypts, and infiltration of the lamina propria with plasma cells, lymphocytes, polymorphonuclear leukocytes, and eosinophils.[26, 29, 54, 224, 282] All stages of the life cycle have been identified within the villous epithelium (Fig. 215–7) and always are enclosed within a parasitiferous vessel.[29, 224, 282] Extracellular merozoites are rare in the intestinal lumen or in the lamina propria.[54]

Isosporiasis is characterized by massive fluid loss suggestive of toxin-mediated hypersecretion. However, an enterotoxin has not been identified.[224] The pathophysiology of isosporiasis is not defined. Cell-mediated immunity appears to be important in the pathogenesis of villous changes. Activated T cells are mitogenic to enterocytes, resulting in crypt hyperplasia, which in turn leads to villous atrophy. Local T-cell activation results in the release of lymphokines, increased intraepithelial lymphocytes, and increased expression of HLA-DR antigens on the enterocytes of the villi and crypts. Intestinal mast cells also may play a role in the pathogenesis by releasing a collagen-IV protease.[32]

Clinical Manifestations

The clinical presentation is indistinguishable from that of other enteric coccidian parasites. The spectrum of disease ranges from asymptomatic infection to severe, protracted, life-threatening diarrhea. Immunocompetent patients usually have a self-limited illness that spontaneously resolves over several weeks.[224, 270, 322] Intractable diarrhea has been reported in infants.[162] Patients with AIDS, alpha-chain disease, lymphoblastic leukemia, and human T-cell lymphotropic virus type 1–related T-cell leukemia are predisposed to life-threat-

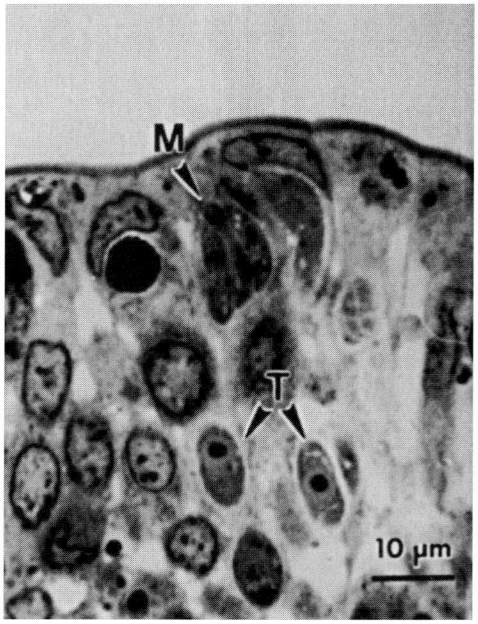

FIGURE 215–7. Isospora *infecting the jejunum of a patient with severe diarrhea. Trophozoites (T) divide within enterocytes by schizogony to form merozoites (M). (From Garica, L. S., Owen, R. L., and Current, W. L.: Isosporiasis.* In *Balows, A., Hausler, W. J., Jr., Ohashi, M., and Turano, A. (eds.): The Laboratory Diagnosis of Infectious Diseases: Principles and Practice. Vol. 1. New York, Springer-Verlag, 1988, pp. 897–903.)*

ening illness.[245] In these patients, the onset of illness is insidious and is associated with nonspecific symptoms, such as low-grade fever, headache, malaise, myalgia, and anorexia.[74, 224] Nausea, vomiting, and diffuse crampy abdominal pain also are present. The stool is watery and may contain mucus but does not contain blood or leukocytes. Chronic intermittent diarrhea with a mean duration of 7.9 months (range, 2 to 26 months) is the major clinical manifestation.[226] Dehydration occurs in 70 per cent of patients and requires intravenous fluids in 10 per cent of patients. The average daily fluid loss is 2 liters, with some patients losing up to 20 liters.[224] Malabsorption, steatorrhea, severe weight loss (>10 per cent of body weight), and lactose intolerance have been reported.[29, 74, 282, 320] Charcot-Leyden crystals are a common finding in the stool. Peripheral eosinophilia occurs in more than 50 per cent of patients.[142, 226] Nonspecific radiographic findings include prominent mucosal folds, thickening of the intestinal wall, and disordered motility.[270]

Biliary disease and extraintestinal manifestations of *I. belli* are rare but have been reported in patients with AIDS.[32, 193, 236] The organism has been identified in tracheobronchial, mediastinal, and mesenteric lymph nodes, the spleen, and the liver.[193, 236] Acalculous cholecystitis has been reported in a single patient.[16]

Diagnosis

The diagnosis is made by identifying the oocyst in the stools or by visualizing the parasite in biopsy specimens of the small intestine.[26, 226, 270] Like *Cryptosporidium, Isospora* can be detected in the stool by using modified acid-fast or auramine-rhodamine stain. However, unlike *Cryptosporidium, Isospora* can be detected readily in the stool by direct wet preparation. Organisms are sparse; thus, concentration techniques, such as zinc sulfate, hypertonic sodium chloride, formalin-ether sedimentation, and Sheather sucrose solution, are used to enhance recovery.[224, 270] *Isospora* oocysts are distinguished easily from *Cryptosporidium* oocysts. They are oval, contain one to two sporoblasts, and are 10 times larger than *Cryptosporidium* oocysts. In comparison, *Cryptosporidium* oocysts are round, contain four sporozoites, and measure 2 to 5 μm in diameter (see Fig. 215–6). The sensitivity and specificity of the different methods for detection of *Isospora* in stool are not known.[224] It is possible to detect the parasite by biopsy and not visualize oocysts in the stool.[29] The parasite usually is found in the proximal small bowel (Fig. 215–8). However, in AIDS patients, it can be found in both small and large intestine.

Treatment

In stark contrast with *Cryptosporidium, Isospora* is responsive to antimicrobial therapy. The treatment of choice is trimethoprim-sulfamethoxazole given four times a day for 10 days.[74, 226, 270, 320] Pyramethamine-sulfadiazine (Fansidar) is an alternative agent. For the sulfonamide allergic patient, data suggest that either metronidazole[96] or pyramethamine[316] is effective. Patients generally respond within 2 days of initiating therapy. Unfortunately, 50 per cent of AIDS patients have recurrent isosporiasis.[74, 226] Therefore, prophylaxis with trimethoprim-sulfamethoxazole three times a week or sulfadoxine-pyrimethamine (500 mg/25 mg) once a week is necessary to prevent relapse.[226] Weiss and colleagues[316] reported that prophylaxis with pyrimethamine alone was successful in two AIDS patients and that this may be an alternative drug for the sulfonamide-allergic patient.

MICROSPORIDIOSIS

Microsporidiosis is caused by an extensive group of obligate intracellular, phylogenetically ancient, protozoan parasites that affect vertebrate and invertebrate animals.[15, 308] In humans, microsporidia first were detected from cerebrospinal fluid in 1959 in Japan in a child with seizures.[184] This infection has been reported infrequently in normal hosts. The number of cases described has increased since 1985, after the recognition of diarrhea and wasting syndrome in AIDS patients. The pathogenic role in other immunocompromised persons remains to be studied, as well as the mode of transmission and the sources of infection. The broad range of clinical manifestations includes keratoconjunctivitis, sinopulmonary infections, myositis, cholecystitis, hepatitis, and disseminated infections with tubulointerstitial nephritis.[308]

Microbiology

Microsporidia, a nontaxonomic nomenclature, refers to a group of protozoan parasites belonging to the phylum Microspora that are characterized by the presence in the spore stage of an extrusion apparatus with a polar tubule that allows the transfer of protoplasmic material into the host cell.[256, 308] More than 100 microsporidial genera and 1000 species infect animals. Only four genera have been described in humans: *Enterocytozoon, Encephalitozoon, Nosema,* and *Pleistophora.* Unclassified microsporidia have been grouped under the term *Microsporidium.* In the HIV era, three new species were described: *Enterocytozoon bienusi, Encephalitozoon hellem,* and *Encephalitozoon (Septata) intestinalis.*[218] The classification of the organisms traditionally has been based on morphologic characteristics of the stages of the parasite. However, recent advances in differentiation are based on phenotypic (protein antigenic patterns) and genotypic characteristics based on polymerase chain reaction techniques, small subunit ribosomal RNA patterns, and restriction fragment length polymorphism.[72, 122, 254, 277, 300] These studies have allowed the reclassification of the genus *Septata* into the previously known *Encephalitozoon.*[72] *E. hellem,* a new species isolated from patients with AIDS, is differentiated from *Encephalitozoon cuniculi* only by antigenic and molecular analysis.[202, 248] A final taxonomic classification may develop after more precise molecular analysis.[308]

These spore-forming unicellular organisms are true eukaryotes, but the lack of mitochondria and the small rRNA and ribosomes resemble those of prokaryotes. The asexual life cycle in the host cell is divided into two phases: the merogonic, or proliferative vegetative phase, and the sporogonic phase that results in production of mature spores.[256] Intracellular stages proliferate by binary or multiple fission appearing as multinucleated elements that can be in direct contact with the cell cytoplasm (e.g., *E. bienusi, Nosema* species) or engulfed in a parasitiferous vacuole *(Encephalitozoon* species). In the case of *E. intestinalis,* septa are formed by a fibrillar structure.[308] The spore consists of a surrounding protective three-layered wall and an internal infective nucleated material that is injected into the host cell by extrusion of a coiled polar tubule attached to an anchoring disk. The average size of the vegetative stages ranges from 2 to 6 μm × 1 to 3 μm, and the average size of the spores ranges from 0.7 × 1.64 μm *(E. bienusi)* to 3 × 5 μm *(Nosema oculorum).*

Cell culture systems are available for a few species, including *Nosema corneum, E. hellem,* and *E. intestinalis.*[72, 122, 201, 257, 296, 310] These isolated organisms are useful for the development of specific antisera that may allow differentiation of the microsporidial species.

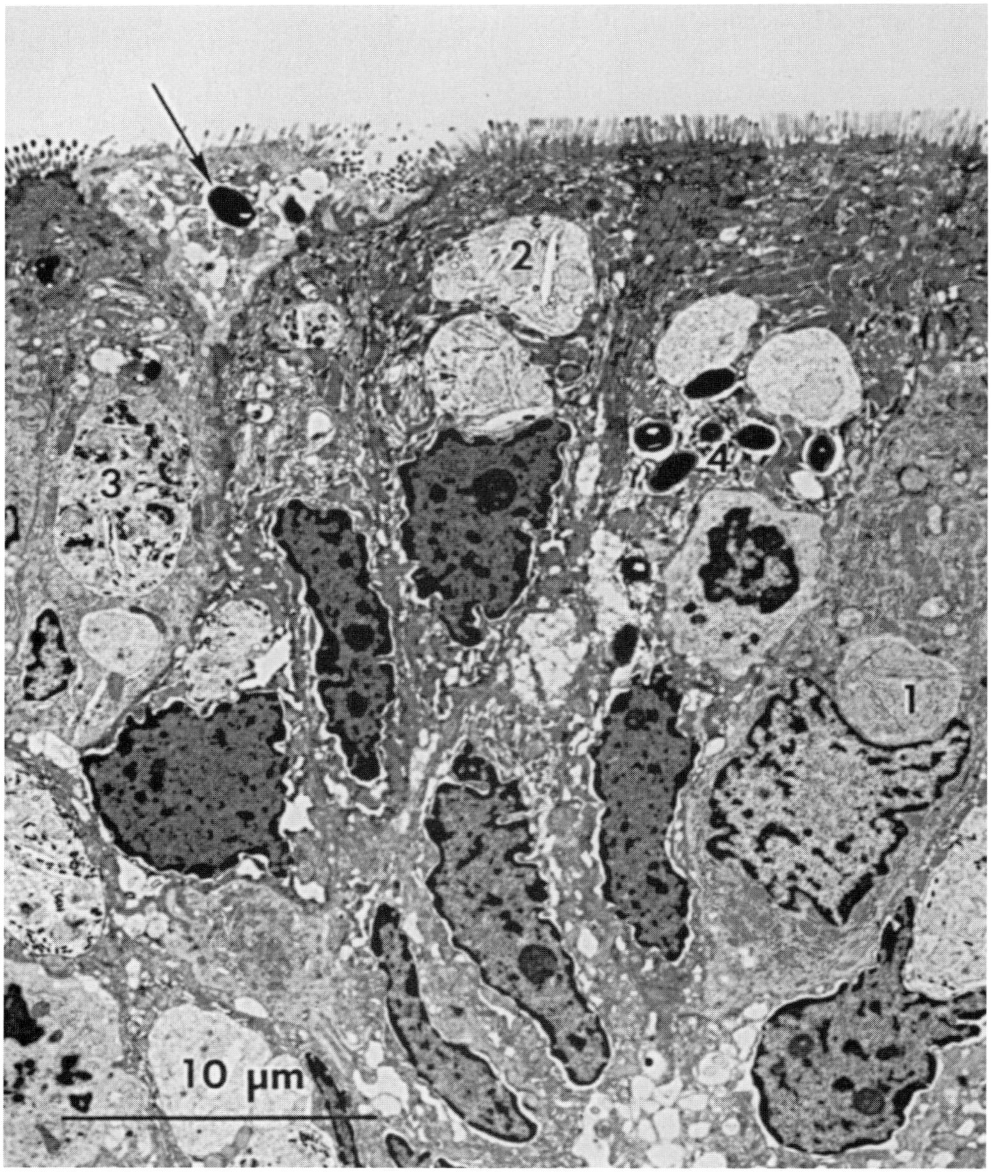

FIGURE 215–8. *Jejunal biopsy from a patient with AIDS and severe diarrhea. Various developmental stages of the intestinal microsporidian* Enterocytozoon *infect almost every enterocyte. Stages include proliferative plasmodia (1), early sporogonial plasmodia (2), late sporogonial plasmodia (3), and mature spores (4). Spore (arrow) within a necrotic enterocyte, which appears ready to slough into the lumen. (Reproduced from Cali, A., and Owen, R. L.: Intracellular development of* Enterocytozoon*: A unique microsporidian found in the intestine of AIDS patients. J. Protozool. 37:145, 1990, with permission from the Society of Protozoologists.)*

Epidemiology

Precise data about the incidence, relevant reservoirs, source of infection, and mode of transmission are not defined. Symptomatic cases have been documented in non-AIDS patients, and half of them had evidence of altered immune status.[117, 304] Only two cases of self-limited diarrhea have been reported in apparently normal hosts.[94, 304] In HIV-infected patients, about 25 to 50 per cent of cases of chronic diarrhea of undetermined etiology or roughly 15 per cent of total cases of diarrhea may be caused by these organisms.[23, 154, 202, 297, 298] The percentages have varied, depending on the population studied and diagnostic techniques employed. Young homosexual or bisexual adults usually are affected,[13, 92, 234, 277] but severely immunosuppressed children with congenital HIV can be affected.[311] *E. bienusi* has been the most prevalent microsporidium and is found mainly in persons with CD4 counts of less than 100/mm^3.[79, 92] Asymptomatic infection and persistent carriage in immunosuppressed patients have been reported.[234]

Microsporidia are ubiquitous in nature, and some of the species infecting humans (e.g., *E. cuniculi*) are present in domestic animals, such as dogs. However, no specific role of animal reservoirs is known.[69] There are no reports of outbreaks due to contamination of water or food. An aerosol route of infection for bronchopulmonary infection with species such as *Encephalitozoon* that are not found in the gut is supported by histopathologic findings in the bronchial tract.[310] Direct contact with conjunctival mucosa is postulated to be the source of ocular infections.[219] Serologic surveys using *E. cuniculi* antigens have found antibodies in multiple population groups, but they likely represent cross-reactivity with either various microsporidia species or other organisms.[256] *Nosema* species is the only member of this group not reported in AIDS patients; rather, it has been described as a disseminated infection in children with athymic aplasia and as local keratitis in normal hosts with or without previous trauma.[257, 308] *Pleistophora* species may present as myositis infiltrating muscle fibers and may cause atrophy and degeneration.[158]

Co-infection with other opportunistic agents, including cytomegalovirus, *Mycobacterium avium intracellular,* and *Cryptosporidium* and other parasites, has been reported in 5 to 60 per cent of cases.[13, 97, 154, 202, 218, 234] Unsuspected *Cryptosporidium* infection may be found in up to 20 per cent of patients with microsporidia.[103]

Pathogenesis and Pathology

The mechanism of disease in humans is unknown.[308] Latent asymptomatic infection or acute disease has not been described fully in humans. With the exception of local ocular disease, the parasite proliferates when immunologic defenses, especially cell-mediated immunity, are defective.

E. bienusi almost always is limited to the intestinal and biliary tract; it has a preference for enterocytes in the small intestine. It produces a limited inflammatory reaction and abnormalities of the villi[92] but rarely invades the lamina propria.[309] Exceptionally, respiratory epithelia may be infected. *E. intestinalis* can reach the submucosa; its presence in kidneys and lower airways presumably results from systemic dissemination.[81, 201] Mucosal injury, characterized by partial villus atrophy and crypt hyperplasia, correlates with xylose malabsorption and decreased activities of mucosal disaccharidases.[153] Other types of encephalitozoonosis, including infection with *E. cuniculi* and *E. hellem,* have a greater potential of dissemination.[254] *E. cuniculi* was the first microsporidium reported in children with seizures,[19, 182] hepatitis, peritonitis, and disseminated infection. Recently, it has been found in conjunctival and sinopulmonary infections associated with colonization of the intestinal tract.[98] The portal of entry for the organism in these cases is uncertain. *E. hellem* may involve the urinary tract, bronchial epithelium, and conjunctiva.[254] In sections of corneal scrapings, the cytoplasm of superficial epithelial cells contains vacuoles with the granular organisms, causing minimal nuclear distortion.[33]

Clinical Manifestations

Intestinal and Biliary Tract Microsporidiosis

Chronic diarrhea and wasting syndrome are associated with microsporidial infection, particularly with *E. bienusi* and *E. intestinalis,* in severely immunodeficient HIV-infected patients (CD4 cell count <50 to $100/mm^3$).[13, 202, 277] In some cases, microsporidiosis is the AIDS-defining opportunistic infection.[185, 218] The usual presentation is afebrile, loose to watery, nonbloody, nonmucoid diarrhea, with 3 to 20 bowel movements per day, worsened by food intake and associated with progressive weight loss, malabsorption, and anorexia.[13, 219] Absorption of fat, D-xylose, and zinc is abnormal.[13, 202] Persistent or intermittent symptoms may lead to severe cachexia by a combination of decreased intake and malabsorption.[277] Half of patients have abdominal pain; some complain of nausea and vomiting.[218] Affected children may suffer from failure to thrive, chronic diarrhea, and intermittent abdominal pain.[311] There are sporadic reports of *E. bienusi* and *E. intestinalis* causing self-limited diarrhea, with diffuse abdominal pain and nausea, in immunocompetent persons.[94, 304]

Patients with cholangitis and acalculous cholecystitis present with right upper quadrant abdominal pain. Imaging studies may reveal dilatation of intrahepatic and common bile ducts or irregularities of the bile duct and gall bladder wall. The AIDS cholangiopathy is similar to that associated with cytomegalovirus and cryptosporidial infection.[231]

Ocular Infection

Immunocompetent patients with histologically confirmed ocular infection with *M. ceylonensis* and *M. africanum* as well as *Nosema* species (*N. corneum* and *N. oculorum*) have been reported.[68, 257, 308] The infection may be associated with previous trauma and lead to progressive decrease in visual acuity secondary to severe corneal stroma disruption or corneal ulcer. *Encephalitozoon* species, in particular *E. hellem,* are a cause of keratoconjunctivitis or scleritis in HIV-infected patients, presenting with conjunctival inflammation, photophobia, blurred vision, a foreign body sensation, decreased visual acuity, and punctate epithelial keratopathy.[219, 255] The lesion usually is bilateral and not associated with ocular trauma. Occasionally, the ocular involvement is accompanied by evidence of disseminated infection.[117]

Systemic Microsporidiosis

HIV-positive patients may present with disseminated systemic infection. Both *Encephalitozoon* species (*E. cuniculi* and *E. hellem*) have been associated with tubulointerstitial nephritis, ureteritis, cystitis, conjunctivitis, and colonization or infection of the respiratory tract; these findings may occur in the absence of gastrointestinal symptoms.[72, 117, 300, 304, 310] Flank pain, hematuria, and dysuria are symptoms of the urinary tract involvement, and progressive nonproductive cough, wheezing, and pleuritic pain are seen with lower respiratory involvement. Disseminated *E. cuniculi* infection including the intestinal tract has been reported.[98] *E. intestinalis* infection usually is limited to the intestinal tract, although systemic manifestations with urinary tract involvement (interstitial nephritis) and sinopulmonary dissemination may follow invasion of the intestinal lamina propria.[81, 117, 201]

There is recent serologic evidence (enzyme immunoassay and counter immunoelectrophoresis) that *E. intestinalis* causes central nervous system infection characterized by severe headache and seizures in HIV-infected patients.[298] Disseminated *Nosema conorii* infection has been described with chronic diarrhea, fever, and weight loss in an immunodeficient athymic child; the parasite was found in the myocardium, diaphragm, kidney tubules, liver, and lungs.[256]

Severely immunosuppressed hosts may develop myositis (caused by *Pleistophora* species) with nonspecific symptoms of generalized muscle weakness or myalgias and elevated creatinine phosphokinase. Muscle biopsy provides the definitive diagnosis.[159] Sinusitis with mucopurulent nasal discharge or lower respiratory tract involvement with bronchiolitis, pneumonia, and respiratory failure has been described with *E. bienusi* and *Encephalitozoon* species.[309] The source of the organism is unknown and may represent primary respiratory acquisition or secondary dissemination from other mucosal surfaces.

Diagnosis

A definitive diagnosis is made by direct morphologic demonstration of organisms in stools, body fluids (duodenal aspirate, bile, bronchoalveolar lavage, nasal secretion, urine, conjunctival smear), or tissue sections[117, 201, 202, 308, 310]; microsporidia sometimes can be cultured.[201] Light microscopy is reliable, although the small size and staining properties of the microsporidia make recognition difficult. Electron microscopy usually is necessary to define the ultrastructural features of the different genera. Immunologic, molecular, antigenic, and biochemical analysis of isolated organisms can be used if ultrastructure does not allow differentiation among similar species.[72, 122, 254, 310]

Weber chromotrope-based stain,[307] with modifications[248] that allow better resolution from the background, has shown good sensitivity and specificity for the analysis of unconcentrated stool samples and other body fluids, including urine.[13, 73, 79, 81, 117, 310, 312] Under oil immersion, the pinkish-red spore wall of the microsporidia must be differentiated morphologically from some yeast elements and bacteria.[277] Uvitex 2B[73, 295, 297] and Calcofluor White[167] are useful, but fungi can give false-positive results.[79] Giemsa stain appears less satisfactory for stool analysis.[277] It is not clear whether intermittent shedding occurs, so multiple stool samples are needed for detection.[15, 202] Acid-fast staining has been attempted with some success in the cytologic examination of centrifuged fluids.[231]

Recognition of microsporidia by light microscopy[153, 202, 309] in paraffin-embedded tissue sections has been reported with routine techniques, including hematoxylin and eosin,[219, 254] tissue Gram,[219, 254, 277] periodic acid–Schiff, silver,[92] and Giemsa stains.[238, 277] The accuracy of each technique is related to the intensity of infection[297] and to the level of training of the person performing the analysis. The spores often are on the surface of the villi; the multinucleated sporogonial stage appears as a collection of granules easily confused with cytoplasmic organelles.[218, 219] Some workers prefer touch preparations of small intestine stained with Giemsa.[15, 202, 263] The histologic examination of ultrathin plastic sections stained with toluidine blue or methylene blue azure II fuchsin stain may increase the sensitivity.[219, 277] Differentiation of the spores by the immunofluorescent assay may allow species identification.[10, 103, 255, 307, 310] Monoclonal antibodies produced against isolated microsporidia may allow specification in cytologic and histologic analysis.[2, 300] Cross-reactivity of *Encephalitozoon* antisera has been used in the diagnosis of *E. bienusi* infection in stool and intestinal biopsy tissue.[2, 329] In ocular microsporidiosis, conjunctival and corneal scrapings or biopsy prepared with Giemsa and other routine histologic stains can be used for diagnosis.[33, 219] Less invasive conjunctival swabs may be positive with the same stains as are used for stool samples.[201, 310]

Electron microscopy of stools, body fluids, and tissue sections[117, 201, 219, 231, 234, 277, 309] is considered the gold standard for confirmation of infection; it allows the evaluation of the multiple stages of the parasite in tissues. The sensitivity may be lower than with other techniques for the detection of spores in stool and urine specimens.[69] Successful isolation of *Encephalitozoon* species, *N. corneum,* and *E. intestinalis* is possible using several cell lines.[72, 122, 201, 257, 296, 310]

Serologic tests were available first for *E. cuniculi* infections.[19] The sensitivity and specificity are unknown, and cross-reactivity is likely. Presumed *E. intestinalis* infection has been diagnosed in AIDS patients by enzyme-linked immunosorbent assay and counter immunoelectrophoresis and techniques.[298] Polymerase chain reaction testing of intestinal biopsies may be a useful diagnostic approach for *E. bienusi* infection in HIV patients[97] and for species differentiation in disseminated disease.[72, 300, 310]

Treatment

Studies of the treatment of microsporidiosis are limited; blinded placebo-controlled trials have not been performed. Albendazole may be useful for infections due to *E. intestinalis* and other *Encephalitozoon* species.[13, 81, 92, 201, 312] It is not clear whether intestinal *E. bienusi* infection responds to albendazole.[23] Treatment with albendazole may lead to improvement of the diarrhea without eradication of the spores in the stool specimens obtained; diarrhea eventually may recur.[201, 202, 312] Albendazole is administered to adults at 200 to 400 mg twice daily. Preliminary reports of responses with metronidazole and octreotide are controversial.[202, 263, 277] Stool volume and frequency are reduced on a low-fat, low-residue diet.[13]

References

1. Aarnaes, S. L., Blanding, J., Speier, S., et al.: Comparison of the ProSpecT and Color Vue enzyme-linked immunoassay for the detection of *Cryptosporidium* in stool specimens. Diagn. Microbiol. Infect. Dis. *19*:221–225, 1994.
2. Aldras, A. M., Orenstein, J. M., Kotler, D. P., et al.: Detection of microsporidia by indirect immunofluorescence antibody test using polyclonal and monoclonal antibodies. J. Clin. Microbiol. *32*:608–612, 1994.
3. Alpert, G., Bell, L. M., Kirkpatrick, C. E., et al.: Outbreak of cryptosporidiosis in a day care center. Pediatrics *77*:152–157, 1986.
4. Anderson, B. C., Donndelinger, T., Wilkins, R. M., et al.: Cryptosporidiosis in a veterinary student. J. Am. Vet. Med. Assoc. *180*:408–409, 1982.
5. Anderson, B. C.: Moist heat inactivation of *Cryptosporidium* sp. Am. J. Public Health *75*:1433–1434, 1985.
6. Anderson, B. C.: Effects of drying on the infectivity of cryptosporidia-laden calf feces for 3- to 7-day-old mice. Am. J. Vet. Res. *47*:2272–2273, 1986.
7. Angus, K. W.: Cryptosporidiosis in man, domestic animals, and birds: A review. J. R. Soc. Med. *76*:62–70, 1983.
8. Angus, K. W., Sherwood, D., Hutchinson, G., et al.: Evaluation of the effect of two aldehyde-based disinfectants on the infectivity of fecal cryptosporidia for mice. Res. Vet. Sci. *33*:379–381, 1982.
9. Armitage, K., Flanigan, T. Carey, J., et al.: Treatment of cryptosporidiosis with paromomycin: A report of five cases. Arch. Intern. Med. *152*:2497–2499, 1992.
10. Arrowood, M. J., and Sterling, C. R.: Comparison of conventional staining methods and monoclonal antibody-based methods for *Cryptosporidium* oocyst detection. J. Clin. Microbiol. *27*:1490–1495, 1989.
11. Ashford, R. W.: Occurrence of an undescribed coccidian in man in Papua New Guinea. Ann. Trop. Med. Parasitol. *73*:497–500, 1979.
12. Ashford, R. W., Warhurst, D. C., and Reid, G. D. F.: Human infections with *Cyanobacterium*-like bodies. Lancet *341*:1034, 1993.
13. Asmuth, D. M., DeGirolami, P. C., Federman, M., et al.: Clinical features of microsporidiosis in patients with AIDS. Clin. Infect. Dis. *18*:819–825, 1994.
14. Baxby, D., and Hart, C. A.: The incidence of cryptosporidiosis: A two-year prospective survey in a children's hospital. J. Hyg. *96*:107–111, 1986.
15. Beauvais, B., Sarfati, C., Molina, J. M., et al.: Comparative evaluation of five diagnostic methods for demonstrating microsporidia in stool and intestinal biopsy specimens. Ann. Trop. Med. Parasitol. *87*:99–102, 1993.
16. Benator, D. A., French, A. L., Beaudet, L. M., et al.: *Isospora belli* infection associated with acalculous cholecystitis in a patient with AIDS. Ann. Intern. Med. *121*:663–664, 1994
17. Bendell, R.P., Lucas S., Moody A., et al.: Diarrhoea associated with *Cyanobacterium*-like bodies: A new coccidian enteritis in man. Lancet. *341*:590–592, 1993.
18. Benhamou, Y., Caumes E., Gerosa Y., et al.: AIDS-related cholangiopathy: Critical analysis of a prospective series of 26 patients. Dig. Dis. Sci. *38*:1113–1118, 1993.
19. Bergquist, N. R. G., Stintzing, L., Smedman, T., et al.: Diagnosis of encephalitozoonosis in man by serological tests. B. M. J. *288*:902, 1984.
20. Bissuel, F., Cotte, L., Rabodonirina, M., et al.: Paromomycin: An effective treatment for cryptosporidial diarrhea in patients with AIDS. Clin. Infect. Dis. *18*:447–449, 1994.
21. Blagburn, B. L., and Current, W. L.: Accidental infection of a researcher with human *Cryptosporidium*. J. Infect. Dis. *148*:772–773, 1983.
22. Blanco, R. A., and Samayoa, J. C.: Diarrhea and *Cryptosporidium* in Guatemala. Bol. Med. Hosp. Infant. Mex. *45*:139–143, 1988.
23. Blanshard, C., Ellis, D. S., Tovey, D. G., et al.: Treatment of intestinal microsporidiosis with albendazole in patients with AIDS. AIDS *6*:311–313, 1992.
24. Blumberg, R. S., Kelsey, P., Perrone, T., et al.: Cytomegalovirus and *Cryptosporidium* associated with acalculous gangrenous cholecystitis. Am. J. Med. *76*:1118–1123, 1984.
25. Bogaerts, J., Lepage, P., Rouvroy, D., et al.: *Cryptosporidium* spp. a frequent cause of diarrhea in central Africa. J. Clin. Microbiol. *20*:874–876, 1984.
26. Bonnin, A., Dei-Cas, E., and Camerlynck, P.: *Cryptosporidium* and *Isospora*. *In* Myint, S., and Cann, A. (eds.): Molecular and Cell Biology of Opportunistic Infections in AIDS. London, Chapman and Hall, 1992, pp. 139–161.
27. Borowitz, S. M., and Saulsbury, F. T.: Treatment of chronic cryptosporidiosis with orally administered human serum immune globin. J. Pediatr. *119*:593–595, 1991.
28. Brady, E., Margolis M. L., and Korzeniowski, O. M.: Pulmonary cryptosporidiosis in acquired immune deficiency syndrome. J. A. M. A. *252*:89–90, 1984.
29. Brandborg, L. L., Goldberg, S. B., and Briedenbach, W. C.: Human coccidiosis, a possible cause of malabsorption: The life cycle in a small bowel

mucosal biopsy as a diagnostic feature. N. Engl. J. Med. *283*:1306–1313, 1970.
30. Bretagne, S., Jacovella, J., Breuil, J., et al.: Cryptosporidiosis in children: Outbreaks and sporadic cases. Ann. Pediatr. *37*:381–386, 1990.
31. Brownstein, D. G., Strandberg, J. D., Montali, R. J., et al.: *Cryptosporidium* in snakes with hypertrophic gastritis. Vet. Pathol. *14*:606–617, 1977.
32. Buret, A., Gall, D. G., Nation, P. N., et al.: Intestinal protozoa and epithelia cell kinetics, structure and function. Parasitol. Today *6*:375–380, 1990.
33. Cali, A., Meisler, D. M., Rutherford, I., et al.: Corneal microsporidiosis in a patient with AIDS. Am. J. Trop. Med. Hyg. *44*:463–468, 1991.
34. Cama, V., Ortega, Y., Marshall M., et al.: In vitro and in vivo anti-cryptosporidiosis activities of paromomycin, clarithromycin, and 14-OH clarithromycin. Abstracts of the 35th Interscience Chemotherapy and Antimicrobial Agents Conference. Abstract No. E43, 1995, pp. 93.
35. Campbell, P. N., and Current, W. L.: Demonstration of serum antibodies to *Cryptosporidium* sp. in normal and immunodeficient humans with confirmed infections. J. Clin. Microbiol. *18*:165–169, 1983.
36. Campbell, I., Tzipori, S., Hutchinson, G., et al.: Effect of disinfectants on survival of *Cryptosporidium* oocyst. Vet. Rec. *111*:414–415, 1982.
37. Cappell, M. S., and Hassan, T.: Pancreatic disease in AIDS: A review. J. Clin. Gastroenterol. *17*:254–263, 1993.
38. Carter, M. J., and Anziinlt, T.: *Cryptosporidium:* An important cause of gastrointestinal disease in immunocompetent patients. N. Z. Med. J. *99*:101–103, 1986.
39. Casemore, D. P.: The antibody response to *Cryptosporidium:* Development of a serological test and its use in a study of immunologically normal persons. J. Infect. Dis. *14*:125–134, 1987.
40. Casemore, D. P., and Roberts, C.: Guidelines for the screening for *Cryptosporidium* in stools: Report of a joint working group. J. Clin. Pathol. *46*:2–4, 1993.
41. Casemore, D. P., Sands, R. L., and Curry, A.: *Cryptosporidium* species a "new" human pathogen. J. Clin. Pathol. *38*:1321–1336, 1985.
42. Cello J. P., Grendell, J. H., Basuk, P., et al.: Effect of octreotide on refractory AIDS-associated diarrhea: A prospective, multicenter clinical trial. Ann. Intern. Med. *115*:705–710, 1991.
43. Centers for Disease Control: Cryptosporidiosis: An assessment of chemotherapy of males with acquired immunodeficiency syndrome (AIDS). M. M. W. R. *31*:589–592, 1982.
44. Centers for Disease Control: Cryptosporidiosis among children attending day-care centers: Georgia, Pennsylvania, Michigan, California, New Mexico. M. M. W. R. *33*:599–601, 1984.
45. Centers for Disease Control: Outbreak of diarrheal illness associated with *Cyanobacteria* (blue-green algae)-like bodies: Chicago and Nepal, 1989 and 1990. M. M. W. R. *40*:325–327, 1991.
46. Centers for Disease Control: Microsporidian keratoconjunctivitis in patients with AIDS. M. M. W. R. *39*:188, 1990.
47. Centers for Disease Control and Prevention: Cryptosporidiosis infections associated with swimming pools: Dane County, Wisconsin, 1993. M. M. W. R. *43*:561–563, 1994.
48. Centers for Disease Control and Prevention: Assessing the public health threat associated with waterborne cryptosporidiosis: Report of a Workshop. M. M. W. R. *44*(RR6):1–16, 1995.
49. Chiodini, P. L.: A "new" parasite: Human infection with *Cyclospora cayetanensis*. Trans. R. Soc. Trop. Med. Hyg. *88*:369–371, 1994.
50. Clezy, K., Gold J., Blaze, J., et al.: Paromomycin for the treatment of cryptosporidial diarrhea in AIDS patients. AIDS *5*:1146–1147, 1991.
51. Clotet, B., Sirera, G., Cofan, F., et al.: Efficacy of the somatostatin analogue (SMS–201–995), Sandostatin, for cryptosporidial diarrhoea in patients with AIDS. AIDS *3*:857–858, 1989.
52. Collier, A. C., Miller, R. A., and Meyers, J. D.: Cryptosporidiosis after marrow transplantation, person to person transmission and treatment with spiramycin. Ann. Intern. Med. *101*:205–206, 1984.
53. Combee, C. L., Collinge, M. L., and Britt, E. M.: Cryptosporidiosis in a hospital-associated day care center. Pediatr. Infect. Dis. *5*:528–532, 1986.
54. Comin, C. E., and Santucci, M.: Submicroscopic profile of *Isospora belli* enteritis in a patient with acquired immune deficiency syndrome. Ultrastruct. Pathol. *18*:437–482, 1994.
55. Connolly, G. M., Youle, M., and Gazzard, B. G.: Diclazuril in the treatment of severe cryptosporidial diarrhoea in AIDS patients. AIDS *4*:700–701, 1990.
56. Cordell, R. L., and Addiss, D. G.: Cryptosporidiosis in child care setting: A review of the literature and recommendation for prevention and control. Pediatr. Infect. Dis. J. *13*:310–317, 1994.
57. Cozon, G., Biron, F., Jeannin, M., et al.: Secretory IgA antibodies to *Cryptosporidium parvum* in AIDs patients with chronic cryptosporidiosis. J. Infect. Dis. *169*:696–699, 1994.
58. Crawford, F. G., and Vermund, S. H.: Human cryptosporidiosis. C. R. C. Crit. Rev. Microbiol. *16*:113–159, 1988.
59. Cruickshank, R., Ashdown, L., and Croese, J.: Human cryptosporidiosis in north Queensland. Aust. N. Z. J. Med. *18*:582–586, 1988.
60. Cruz, J. R., Cano, F., Caceres P., et al.: Infection and diarrhea caused by *Cryptosporidium* spp among Guatemalan infants. J. Clin. Microbiol. *26*:88–91, 1988.
61. Current, W. L.: *Cryptosporidium:* Its biology and potential for environmental transmission. C. R. C. Crit. Rev. Environ. Control *17*:21–51, 1986.
62. Current, W. L.: *Cryptosporidium parvum:* Household transmission. Ann. Intern. Med. *120*:518–519, 1994.
63. Current, W. L., and Bick, P. H.: Immunobiology of *Cryptosporidium* spp. Pathol. Immunopathol. Res. *8*:141–160, 1989.
64. Current, W. L., and Garcia L. S.: Cryptosporidiosis. Clin. Microbiol. Rev. *4*:325–358, 1991.
65. Current, W. L., and Garcia L. S.: Cryptosporidiosis. Clin. Lab. Med. *11*:873–895, 1991.
66. Current, W. L., and Reese, N. C.: A comparison of endogenous development of three isolates of *Cryptosporidium* in suckling mice. J. Protozool. *33*:98–108, 1986.
67. Current, W. L., Reese, N. C., Ernst, J. V., et al.: Human cryptosporidiosis in immunocompetent and immunodeficient persons: Studies of an outbreak and experimental transmission. N. Engl. J. Med. *308*:1252–1257, 1983.
68. Current, W. L., Upton, S. J., and Haynes, T. B.: The life cycle of *Cryptosporidium baileyi* n. sp. (Apicocomplexa: Cryptosporidiidae) infecting chickens. J. Protozool. *33*:289–296, 1986.
69. Curry, A., and Canning, E. U.: Human microsporidiosis. J. Infect. *27*:229–236, 1993.
70. D'Antonio, R. G., Win, R. E., Taylor, J. P., et al.: A waterborne outbreak of cryptosporidiosis in normal hosts. Ann. Intern. Med. *103*:886–888, 1985.
71. Das, P., Sengupta, K., Dutta, P., et al.: Significance of *Cryptosporidium* as an aetiologic agent of acute diarrhoea in Calcutta: A hospital base study. J. Trop. Med. Hyg. *96*:124–127, 1993.
72. De Groote, M. A., Visvesvara, G., Wilson, M. L., et al.: Polymerase chain reaction and culture confirmation of disseminated *Encephalitozoon cuniculi* in patients with AIDS: Successful therapy with albendazole. J. Infect. Dis. *171*:1375–1378, 1995.
73. DeGirolami, P. C., Ezratty, C. R., Desai, G., et al.: Diagnosis of intestinal microsporidiosis by examination of stool and duodenal aspirate with Weber's modified trichrome and uvitex 2B stains. J. Clin. Microbiol. *33*:805–810, 1995.
74. DeHovitz, J. A., Pape, J. W., Boncy, M., et al.: Clinical manifestations and therapy of *Isospora belli* infection in patients with the acquired immunodeficiency syndrome. N. Engl. J. Med. *315*:87–90, 1986.
75. DeMol, P., Mukashuma, S., Bogaerts, J., et al.: *Cryptosporidium* related to measles diarrhea in Rwanda. Lancet *2*:42–43, 1884.
76. De Oliveira, G. S., Barboso, W., and Dasilva, A. L.: Isosporose humana em Goias. Rev. Pat. Trop. 387–395, 1973.
77. DeRycke, J., Bernard, S., Laporte, J., et al.: Prevalence of various enteropathogens in the feces of diarrheic and healthy calves. Ann. Rech. Vet. *17*:159–168, 1986.
78. Dhillon, A. S., Thacker, H. L., Dietzel, A. V., et al.: Respiratory cryptosporidiosis in broiler chickens. Avian Dis. *25*:747–751, 1981.
79. Didier, E. S., Orenstein, J. M., Aldras, A., et al.: Comparison of three staining methods for detecting microsporidia in fluids. J. Clin. Microbiol. *33*:3138–3145, 1995.
80. Diers, J., and McCallister, G. L.: Occurrence of *Cryptosporidium* in home day care centers in west central Colorado. J. Parasitol. *75*:637–638, 1989.
81. Dore, G. J., Marriott, D. J., Hing, M. C., et al.: Disseminated microsporidiosis due to *Septata intestinalis* in nine patients infected with the human immunodeficiency virus: Response to therapy with albendazole. Clin. Infect. Dis. *21*:70–76, 1995.
82. Dryjanski, J., Gold, J. W., Ritchie, M. T., et al.: Cryptosporidiosis: Case report in a health team worker. Am. J. Med. *80*:751–752, 1986.
83. Dueno, M. I., Bai, J. C., Santangelo, W. C., et al.: Effects of somatostatin analog on water and electrolyte transport and transit time in human small bowel. Dig. Dis. Sci. *32*:1092–1096, 1987.
84. DuPont, H. L., Chappell, C. L., Sterling, C. R., et al.: The infectivity of *Cryptosporidium parvum* in healthy volunteers. N. Engl. J. Med. *332*:855–859, 1995.
85. Fang, G., Aruajo, V., and Guerrant, R. L.: Enteric infections associated with exposure to animals and animal products. Infect. Dis. Clin. North Am. *5*:681–701, 1991.
86. Fanning, M., Monte, M., Sutherland, L. R., et al.: Pilot study of Sandostatin (octreotide) therapy of refractory HIV-associated diarrhea. Dig. Dis. Sci. *36*:476–480, 1991.
87. Faust, E. C., Giraldo, L. E., Caicedo, G., et al.: Human isosporosis in the Western hemisphere. Am. J. Med. *10*:343–349, 1983.
88. Fayer, R.: Effects of high temperature on infectivity of *Cryptosporidium parvum* oocyst in water. Appl. Environ. Microbiol. *60*:2732–2735, 1994.
89. Fayer, R., and Ungar, B. L. P.: *Cryptosporidium* spp. and cryptosporidiosis. Microbiol. Rev. *50*:458–483, 1986.
90. Ferson, M. J., and Young, L. C.: *Cryptosporidium* and coxsackievirus B5 causing epidemic diarrhoea in a child care center. Med. J. Aust. *156*:813, 1992.
91. Fichtenbaum, C. J., Ritchie, D. J., and Powderly, W. G.: Use of paromomycin for treatment of cryptosporidiosis in patients with AIDS. Clin. Infect. Dis. *16*:290–300, 1993.
92. Field, A. S., Hing, M. C., Miliken, S. T., et al.: Microsporidia in the small intestine of HIV-infected patients: A new diagnostic technique and a new species. Med. J. Aust. *158*:390–394, 1993.
93. Flanigan, T. P., and Soave, R.: Cryptosporidiosis. Prog. Clin. Parasitol. *3*:1–20, 1993.

94. Flepp, M., Sauer, B., Luthy, R., et al.: Human microsporidiosis in HIV seronegative, immunocompetent patients. Abstracts of the 35th Interscience Chemotherapy and Antimicrobial Agents Conference. Abstract No. LM25, 1995, p. 331.
95. Forgacs, P., Tarchis, A., Ma, P., et al.: Intestinal and bronchial cryptosporidiosis in an immunodeficient homosexual man. Ann. Intern. Med. *99*:793–794, 1983.
96. Forthal, D. N., and Guest, S. S.: *Isospora belli* enteritis in three homosexual men. Am. J. Trop. Med. Hyg. *33*:1060–1064, 1984.
97. Franzen, C., Muller, A., Hegener, P., et al.: Detection of microsporidia in intestinal biopsies of HIV infected patients by polymerase chain reaction. Abstracts of the 35th Interscience Chemotherapy and Antimicrobial Agents Conference. Abstract No. D102, 1995, p. 84.
98. Franzen, C., Schwartz, D., Visvesvara, G., et al.: Disseminated antibody confirmed *Encephalitozoon cuniculi* infection with asymptomatic involvement of the gastrointestinal tract in a patient with AIDS. Abstracts of the 35th Interscience Chemotherapy and Antimicrobial Agents Conference. Abstract No. LM97, 1995, p. 344.
99. Gallaher, M. M., Herndon, J. L., Nims, L. J., et al.: Cryptosporidiosis and surface water. Am. J. Public Health *79*:39–42, 1989.
100. Garcia, L. S., Brewer, T. C., and Bruckner, D. A.: Incidence of *Cryptosporidium* in all patients submitting stool specimens for ova and parasites examination: Monoclonal antibody IFA method. Diagn. Microbiol. Infect. Dis. *11*:25–27, 1988.
101. Garcia, L. S., Brewer, T. C., and Bruckner, D. A.: Fluorescent detection of *Cryptosporidium* oocyst in human fecal specimens by using monoclonal antibodies. J. Clin. Microbiol. *25*:119–121, 1987.
102. Garcia, L. S., Owen, R. L., and Current W. L.: Isosporiasis. *In* Balows, A., Hausler, W. J., Jr., Ohashi, M., and Turano, A. (eds.): The Laboratory Diagnosis of Infectious Diseases: Principles and Practice. Vol. 1. New York, Springer-Verlag, 1988, pp. 897–903.
103. Garcia, L. S., Shimizu, R. Y., and Bruckner, D. A.: Detection of microsporidial spores in fecal specimens from patients diagnosed with cryptosporidiosis. J. Clin. Microbiol. *32*:1739–1741, 1994.
104. Garza, D., Hopfer, R. L., Eichelberger, C., et al.: Fecal staining for screening *Cryptosporidium* oocysts. J. Med. Technol. *1*:560–563, 1984.
105. Gellin, B. G., and Soave, R.: Coccidian infections in AIDS. Med. Clin. North Am. *76*:205–234, 1992.
106. Giraldo, L. E., Faust, E. C., Bonfante, R., et al.: Diagnostic findings from parasitological examination of excreta of dogs, human beings, and a hog collected in the streets of Ward Siloe, Cali, Colombia. J. Parasitol. *45*:46, 1959.
107. Girard, D. E., and Keefe, E. B.: *Isospora* and travelers diarrhea. Ann. Intern. Med. *106*:908, 1987.
108. Girard, P. M., Goldschmidt, E., Vittecoq, D., et al.: Vapreotide, a somatostatin analogue, in cryptosporidiosis and other AIDS-related diarrheal diseases. AIDS *6*:715–718, 1992.
109. Glaser, C. A., Angulo, F. J., and Rooney, J. A.: Animal-associated opportunistic infections among persons infected with the human immunodeficiency virus. Clin. Infect. Dis. *18*:14–24, 1994.
110. Goebel, E., and Brandler, U.: Ultrastructure of microgametogenesis, microgametes, and gametogomy of *Cryptosporidium* sp. in the intestine of mice. Prostistologica *18*:331–334, 1982.
111. Gomez Morales, M. A., Ausiello, C. M., Urbani, F., et al.: Crude extract and recombinant protein of *Cryptosporidium parvum* oocysts induce proliferation of human peripheral blood mononuclear cells in vitro. J. Infect. Dis. *172*:211–216, 1995.
112. Goodgame, R. W., Genta, R. M., White, A. C., et al.: Intensity of infection in AIDS-associated cryptosporidiosis. J. Infect. Dis. *167*:704–709, 1993.
113. Gradon, J. D., Schulman, R. H., Chapnick, E. K., et al.: Octreotide-induced acute pancreatitis in a patient with acquired immonodeficiency syndrome. South. Med. J. *84*:1410–1411, 1991.
114. Gross, T. L., Wheat, J., Bartlett, M., et al.: AIDS and multiple system involvement with *Cryptosporidium*. Am. J. Gastroenterol. *81*:456–458, 1986.
115. Grossman, I., and Simon, D.: Potential gastrointestinal uses of somatostatin and its synthetic analogue octreotide. Am. J. Gastroenterol. *85*:1061–1072, 1990.
116. Guarda, L. A., Stein, S. A., Cleary, K. A., et al.: Human cryptosporidiosis in the acquired immune deficiency syndrome. Arch. Pathol. Lab. Med. *107*:562–566, 1983.
117. Gunnarson, G., Hurlbut, D., DeGirolami, P. C., et al.: Multiorgan microsporidiosis: Report of five cases and review. Clin. Infect. Dis. *21*:37–44, 1995.
118. Hannah, J., and Riordan, T.: Case to case spread of cryptosporidiosis evidence from a day nursery outbreak. Public Health *102*:539–544, 1988.
119. Harari, M. D., West, B., and Dwyer, B.: *Cryptosporidium* as a cause of laryngotracheitis in an infant. Lancet *1*:1207, 1986.
120. Harris, M., Deutsch, G., MacLean, D., et al.: A phase I study of letrazuril in AIDS-related cryptosporidiosis. AIDS *8*:1109–1113, 1994.
121. Hart, C. A., Baxby, D., and Blundell, N.: Gastroenteritis due to *Cryptosporidium:* A prospective survey in a children's hospital. J. Infect. *9*:264–270, 1984.
122. Hartskeerl, R. A., Van Gool, T., Schuitema, A. R., et al.: Genetic and immunological characterization of the microsporidian *Septata intestinalis* Cali, Kotler and Orenstein, 1993: Reclassification to *Encephalitozoon intestinalis*. Parasitology *110*:277–285, 1995.
123. Hawkins, S. P., Thomas, R. P., and Teasdale, C.: Acute pancreatitis: A new finding in *Cryptosporidium* enteritis. B. M. J. *294*:483–484, 1987.
124. Hayes, E. B., Matte, T. D., O'Brien, T. R., et al.: Large community outbreak of cryptosporidiosis due to contamination of a filtered public water supply. N. Engl. J. Med. *320*:1372–1376, 1989.
125. Heijbel, H., Slaine, K., Seigel, B., et al.: Outbreak of diarrhea in a day care center with spread to household members: The role of *Cryptosporidium.* Pediatr. Infect. Dis. J. *6*:532–535, 1987.
126. Henderson, A. E., Gillespie, G. W., Kaplan, P., et al.: The human *Isospora.* Am. J. Hyg. *78*:302–309, 1963.
127. Henricksen, S. A., and Pohlenz, J. F. L.: Staining of *Cryptosporidium* by a modified Ziehl-Neelsen technique. Acta Vet. Scand. *22*:594–596, 1981.
128. Heyworth, M. F., and Owen R. L.: Gastrointestinal aspects of the acquired immunodeficiency syndrome. Surv. Dig. Dis. *3*:197–209, 1985.
129. Hinnant, K., Swartz, A., Rotterdam, H., et al.: Cytomegaloviral and cryptosporidial cholecystitis in two patients with AIDS. Am. J. Surg. Pathol. *13*:57–60, 1989.
130. Hoge, C. W., Shlim, D. R., Ghimire, M., et al.: Placebo-controlled trial of co-trimoxazole for *Cyclospora* infection among travellers and foreign residents in Nepal. Lancet *345*:691–693, 1995.
131. Hoge, C. W., Shlim, D. R., and Rajah, R.: Epidemiology of diarrhoeal illness associated with coccidian-like organism among travellers and foreign residents in Nepal. Lancet *341*:1175–1179, 1993.
132. Hojlyng, N., Holten-Anderson, W., and Jepsen, S.: Cryptosporidiosis: A case of airborne transmission. Lancet *2*:271–272, 1987.
133. Hojlyng, N., Molbak, K., and Jepsen, S.: *Cryptosporidium* spp., a frequent cause of diarrhea in Liberian children. J. Clin. Microbiol. *23*:1109–1113, 1986.
134. Hojlyng, N., and Jensen, B. N.: Respiratory cryptosporidiosis in HIV-positive patients. Lancet *2*:590–591, 1988.
135. Holley, H. P., Jr., and Dover, C.: *Cryptosporidium:* A common cause of parasitic diarrhea in otherwise healthy individuals. J. Infect. Dis. *153*:365–368, 1986.
136. Hoover, D. M., Hoerr, F. J., Carlton, W. W., et al.: Enteric cryptosporidiosis in a naso tang. *Naso lituratus* Block and Schneider. J. Fish Dis. *4*:425–428, 1981.
137. Hunter, G., Bagshawe, A. F., Baboo, K. S., et al.: Intestinal parasites in Zambian patients with AIDS. Trans. R. Soc. Trop. Med. Hyg. *86*:543–545, 1992.
138. Iseki, M.: *Cryptosporidium felis* sp. n. (Protozoa: Eimeriorina) from the domestic cat. Jpn. J. Parasitol. *28*:285–307, 1979.
139. Issacs, D., Hunt, G. H., Phillips, A. D., et al.: Cryptosporidiosis in immunocompetent children. J. Clin. Pathol. *38*:78–81, 1985.
140. Janoff, E. N., Limas C., and Gebhard, R. L.: Cryptosporidial carriage without symptoms in the acquired immunodeficiency syndrome (AIDS). Ann. Intern. Med. *112*:75–76, 1990.
141. Jarpa, A.: Isosporosis humana. Bol. Chileno Parasitol. *12*:31, 1957.
142. Jarpa Gana, A.: Coccidiosis humana. Biologica *39*:3–26, 1966.
143. Jeffrey, G. M.: Epidemiologic considerations of isosporiasis in a school for mental defective children. Ann. J. Hyg. *67*:251–255, 1958.
144. Joce, R. E., Bruce, J., Kiely, D., et al.: An outbreak of cryptosporidiosis associated with a swimming pool. Epidemiol. Infect. *107*:497–508, 1991.
145. Jokipii, A., Hemila, M., and Jokipii, L.: Prospective study of acquisition of *Cryptosporidium, Giardia lamblia,* and gastrointestinal illness. Lancet *2*:487–489, 1985.
146. Jokipii, L., and Jokipii, A. M.: Timing of symptoms and oocyst excretion in human cryptosporidiosis. N. Engl. J. Med. *315*:1643–1647, 1987.
147. Joseph, C., Hamilton, G., O'Connor M., et al.: Cryptosporidiosis in the Isle of Thanet: An outbreak associated with local drinking water. Epidemiol. Infect. *107*:509–519, 1991.
148. Kahn, D. G., Garfinkle, J. M., Klonoff, D. C., et al.: Cryptosporidial and cytomegalovirus hepatitis and cholecystitis. Arch. Pathol. Lab. Med. *111*:879–881, 1987.
149. Keren, G., Barzilia A., Barzilay, Z., et al.: Life-threatening cryptosporidiosis in immunocompetent infants. Eur. J. Pediatr. *146*:187–189, 1987.
150. Kibbler, C. C., Smith, A., Hamilton-Dutoit, S. J., et al.: Pulmonary cryptosporidiosis occurring in a bone marrow transplant patient. Scand. J. Infect. *19*:581–584, 1987.
151. Koch, K. J., Phillips, D. J., Aber, R. C., et al.: Cryptosporidiosis in hospital personnel: Evidence for person-to-person transmission. Ann. Intern. Med. *102*:593–596, 1985.
152. Kocoshis, S. A., Cibull, M. L., Davis, T. E., et al.: Intestinal and pulmonary cryptosporidiosis in an infant with severe combined immune deficiency. J. Pediatr. Gastroenterol. Nutr. *3*:149–157, 1984.
153. Kotler, D. P., Giang, T. T., Garro, M. L., et al.: Light microscopic diagnosis of microsporidiosis in patients with AIDS. Am. J. Gastroenterol. *89*:540–544, 1994.
154. Kotler, D. P., and Orenstein, J. M.: Prevalence of intestinal microsporidiosis in HIV-infected individuals referred for gastroenterological evaluation. Am. J. Gastroenterol. *89*:1998–2002, 1994.
155. Kreinik, G., Burstein, O., and Landor, M., et al.: Successful management of intractable cryptosporidiosis diarrhea with intravenous octreotide, a somatostatin analogue. AIDS *5*:765–767, 1991.

156. Lahdevirta, J., Jokipii, A. M. M., Sammalkorpi, K., et al.: Perinatal infection with *Cryptosporidium* and failure to thrive. Lancet 1:48–49, 1987.
157. Lasser, K. H., Lewin, K. J., and Ryning, F. W.: Cryptosporidial enteritis in a patient with congenital hypogammaglobulinemia. Hum. Pathol. *10*:234–240, 1979.
158. Ledford, D. K., Overman, M. D., Gonzalvo, A., et al.: Microsporidiosis myositis in a patient with acquired immunodeficiency syndrome. Ann. Intern. Med. *102*:628–630, 1985.
159. Levine, N. D.: Taxonomy and review of the coccidian genus *Cryptosporidium* (Protozoa, Apicocomplexa). J. Protozool. *31*:94–98, 1984.
160. Lewis, I. S., Hart, C. A., and Baxby, D.: Diarrhea due to *Cryptosporidium* in acute lymphoblastic leukemia. Arch. Dis. Child. *60*:60–62, 1985.
161. Liberti, A., Bisogno, A., and Izzo, E.: Octreotide treatment of secretory and cryptosporidial diarrhea with acquired immunodeficiency syndrome (AIDS): Clinical evaluation. J. Chemother. *4*:303–305, 1992.
162. Liebman, W. M., Thaler, M. M., DeLorimier, A., et al.: Intractable diarrhea of infancy due to intestinal coccidiosis. Gastroenterology *78*:579–584, 1980.
163. Loose, J. H., Sedergran D. J., and Cooper, H. S.: Identification of *Cryptosporidium* in paraffin-embedded tissue sections with the use of a monoclonal antibody. Am. J. Clin. Pathol. *91*:206–209, 1989.
164. Lorenzo-Lorenzo, M. J., Ares-Mazas, M. E., Villacorta-Martinez de Maturana, I., et al.: Effect of ultraviolet disinfection of drinking water on the viability of *Cryptosporidium parvum* oocysts. J. Parasitol. *79*:67–70, 1994.
165. Louie, E., Barkowsky, W., and Klesius, P. H.: Treatment of cryptosporidiosis with oral bovine transfer factor. Clin. Immunol. Immunopathol. *44*:329–334, 1987.
166. Loureiro, E. C., Linhares, A. da C., and Mata, L.: Acute diarrhoea associated with *Cryptosporidium* sp. in Belem, Brazil (preliminary report). Rev. Inst. Med. Trop. Sao Paulo *28*:138–140, 1986.
167. Luna, V. A., Stewart, B. K., Bergeron, D. L., et al.: Use of the fluorochrome calcofluor white in the screening of stool specimens for spores of microsporidia. Am. J. Clin. Pathol. *103*:656–659, 1995.
168. Ma, P., Villanueva, T. G., Kaufman, D., et al.: Respiratory cryptosporidiosis in the acquired immunodeficiency syndrome. J. A. M. A. *252*:1298–1301, 1984.
169. Mac Kenzie, W. R., Hoxie, N. J., Proctor, M. E., et al.: A massive outbreak in Milwaukee of *Cryptosporidium* infection transmitted through the public water supply. N. Engl. J. Med. *331*:161–167, 1994.
170. MacFarlane, D. E., and Horner-Bryce, J.: Cryptosporidiosis in well nourished and malnourished children. Acta Paediatr. Scand. *76*:474–477, 1987.
171. MacPherson, D. W., and McQueen, R.: Cryptosporidiosis: Multiattribute evaluation of six diagnostic methods. J. Clin. Microbiol. *31*:193–202, 1993.
172. Madico, G., Gilman, R., Miranda, E., et al.: Treatment of *Cyclospora* infections with co-trimoxazole. Lancet *342*:122–123, 1993.
173. Madore, M. S., Rose, J. B., Gerba, C. P., et al.: Occurrence of *Cryptosporidium* oocysts in sewage effluents and select surface waters. J. Parasitol. *73*:702–705, 1983.
174. Mann, E. D., Sekla, L. H., Nayer, G. P., et al.: Infection with *Cryptosporidium* spp. in humans and cattle in Manitoba. Can. J. Vet. Res. *50*:174–148, 1986.
175. Marcial, M. A., and Madara, J. L.: *Cryptosporidium*: Cellular localization, structural analysis of absorptive cell-parasite membrane-membrane interactions in guinea pigs, and suggestion of protozoan transport by M cells. Gastroenterology *90*:583–594, 1986.
176. Margulis, S. J., Honig, C. L., Soave, R., et al.: Biliary tract obstruction in the acquired immunodeficiency syndrome. Ann. Intern. Med. *105*:207–210, 1986.
177. Marshall, A. R., Al-Jumaili, I. J., Fenwick, G. A., et al.: Cryptosporidiosis in patients in a large teaching hospital. J. Clin. Microbiol. *25*:172–173, 1987.
178. Marshall, R. J., and Flanigan, T. P.: Paromomycin inhibits *Cryptosporidium* infection of a human enterocyte line. J. Infect. Dis. *165*:772–774, 1992.
179. Martino, P., Gentile, G., Caprioli, A., et al.: Hospital acquired cryptosporidiosis in a bone marrow transplantation unit. J. Infect. Dis. *158*:647–648, 1988.
180. Mata, L., Bolanos, H., Pezarro, D., et al.: Cryptosporidiosis in children from some highland Costa Rican rural and urban areas. Am. J. Trop. Med. Hyg. *33*:24–29, 1984.
181. Mathan, M., Venkatesan, S., George, R., et al.: *Cryptosporidium* and diarrhoea in southern Indian children. Lancet *2*:1172–1175, 1985.
182. Matsubayashi, H., Koike, T., Mikata, T., et al.: A case of *Encephalitozoon*-like body infection in man. Arch. Pathol. *67*:181–187, 1959.
183. Matsubayashi, H., and Nozawa, T.: Experimental infection of *Isospora hominis* in man. Am. J. Trop. Hyg. *2*:633–637, 1948.
184. McAnulty, J. M., Flemming, D. W., and Gonzalez, A. H.: A community-wide outbreak of cryptosporidiosis associated with swimming in a wave pool. J. A. M. A. *272*:1597–1600, 1994.
185. McDougall, R. J., Tandy, M. W., Boreham, R. E., et al.: Incidental finding of microsporidian parasite from an AIDS patient. J. Clin. Microbiol. *31*:436–439, 1993.
186. McLaughlin J., Casemore D. P., Harrison, T. G., et al.: Identification of *Cryptosporidium* oocyst by monoclonal antibody. Lancet *1*:51, 1987.
187. McMeeking, A., Borkowsky, W., Klesius, P. H., et al.: A controlled trial of bovine dialyzable leukocyte extract for cryptosporidiosis in patients with AIDS. J. Infect. Dis. *161*:108–112, 1990.
188. McNabb, S. J. N., Hensel, D. M., Welch, D. F., et al.: Comparison of sedimentation and flotation techniques for identification of *Cryptosporidium* sp. oocysts in a large outbreak of human diarrhea. J. Clin. Microbiol. *22*:587–589, 1985.
189. Mead, G. M., Sweetenham, J. W., Ewins D. L., et al.: Intestinal cryptosporidiosis: A complication of cancer treatment. Cancer Treat. Rep. *70*:769–770, 1986.
190. Meisel, J. L., Perera, D. R., Meligro, B. S., et al.: Overwhelming watery diarrhoea associated with a *Cryptosporidium* in an immunosuppressed patient. Gastroenterology *70*:1156–1160, 1976.
191. Melo Cristino, J. A. G., Carvalho, M. I. P., and Salgado, M. J.: An outbreak of cryptosporidiosis in a hospital day-care center. Epidemiol. Infect. *101*:355–359, 1988.
192. Menichetti, F., Moretti, M. V., Marroni, M., et al.: Diclazuril for cryptosporidiosis in AIDS. Am. J. Med. *90*:271–272, 1991.
193. Michiels, J. F., Hofman P., Bernard, E., et. al.: Intestinal and extraintestinal *Isospora belli* infection in an AIDS patient. Pathol. Res. Pract. *190*:1089–1093, 1994.
194. Michielsen, P. P., Fierens, H., and Van Maercke, Y. M.: Drug-induced gallbladder disease: Incidence, aetiology and management. Drug Safety *7*:32–45, 1992.
195. Milacek, P., and Vitovec, J.: Differential staining of cryptosporidia beaniline-carbolmethyl violet and tartarzine in smears of feces and scrapping of intestinal mucosa. Folia Parasitol. *32*:50, 1985.
196. Miller, N. M., and VanDen, E. S.: Seasonal prevalence of *Cryptosporidium* associated diarrhea in young children. S. Afr. Med. J. *70*:636–637, 1986.
197. Miller, R. A., Bronsdon, M. A., and Morton, W. R.: Experimental cryptosporidiosis in a primate model. J. Infect. Dis. *161*:312–315, 1990.
198. Miller, R. A., Holmberg, R. E., and Clausen, C. R.: Life-threatening diarrhea caused by *Cryptosporidium* in a child undergoing therapy for acute lymphocytic leukemia. J. Pediatr. *103*:256–259, 1983.
199. Miller, R. A., Wasserheit, J. N., Kerihara, J., et al.: Detection of *Cryptosporidium* oocysts in sputum during screening for *Mycobacterium*. J. Clin. Microbiol. *20*:1191–1193, 1984.
200. Miller, T. L., Winter, H. S., Luginbuhl L. M., et al.: Pancreatitis in pediatric human immunodeficiency virus infection. J. Pediatr. *120*:223–227, 1992.
201. Molina, J. M., Oksenhendler, E., Beauvais, B., et al.: Disseminated microsporidiosis due to *Septata intestinalis* in patients with AIDS: Clinical features and response to albendazole therapy. J. Infect. Dis. *171*:245–249, 1995.
202. Molina, J. M., Sarfati, C., Beauvais, B., et al.: Intestinal microsporidiosis in human immunodeficiency virus–infected patients with chronic unexplained diarrhea: Prevalence and clinical and biological features. J. Infect. Dis. *167*:217–221, 1993.
203. Montessori, G. A., and Bischoff, L.: Cryptosporidiosis cause of summer diarrhea in children. Can. Med. Assoc. J. *132*:1285, 1985.
204. Moodley, D., Jackson, T. F. H. G., Gathiram, B., et al.: A comparative assessment of commonly employed staining procedures for the diagnosis of cryptosporidiosis. S. Afr. Med. J. *79*:314–317, 1991.
205. Moore, J. A., and Frenkel, J. K.: Respiratory and enteric cryptosporidiosis in humans. Arch. Pathol. Lab. Med. *115*:1160–1162, 1991.
206. Moskovitz, B. L., Stanton, T. L., and Kusmierek, J. J. E.: Spiramycin therapy for cryptosporidial diarrhea in immunocompromised patients. J. Antimicrob. Agents Chemother. *22*(Suppl. B):189–191, 1988.
207. Mozzell, E. J., Woltering, E. A., and O'Dorisio, T. M.: Non-endocrine applications of somatostatin and octreotide acetate: Facts and flights of fancy. Dis. Month *12*:754–810, 1991.
208. Navarrett, S., Stetler, H. C., Avila, C., et al.: An outbreak of *Cryptosporidium* diarrhea in a pediatric hospital. Pediatr. Infect. Dis. J. *10*:248–250, 1991.
209. Navin, T. R., and Juranek, D. D.: Cryptosporidiosis: Clinical, epidemiological, and parasitological review. Rev. Infect. Dis. *6*:313–327, 1984.
210. Neira, P., Tardio, M. T., Carabelli, M., et al.: Cryptosporidiosis in the V region of Chile. III. Study of malnourished patients, 1985–1887. Bol. Chil. Parasitol. *44*:34–36, 1989.
211. Newman, R. D., Zu, S. X., Wuhib, T., et al.: Household epidemiology of *Cryptosporidium parvum* infection in an urban community in northeast Brazil. Ann. Intern. Med. *120*:500–505, 1994.
212. Nime, F. A., Burek, J. D., Page, D. L., et al.: Acute enterocolitis in a human being infected with the protozoan *Cryptosporidium*. Gastroenterology *70*:592–598, 1976.
213. Nord, J., Ma, P., and DiJohn, D.: Treatment with bovine hyperimmune colostrum of cryptosporidial diarrhea in AIDS patients. AIDS *4*:581–584, 1990.
214. Nwanyanwu, O. C., Baird, J. N., and Reeve, G. R.: Cryptosporidiosis in a day care center. Tex. Med. *85*:40–43, 1989.
215. Oh, S. H., Jaffe, N., Fainstein, V., et al.: Cryptosporidiosis and anticancer therapy. J. Pediatr. *104*:963–964, 1984.
216. Okhuysen, P. C., Chakravarthy. S., Chappell, C. L., et al.: Alpha-aminoboronic acid, inhibitors of *C. parvum* aminopeptidase, prevent *in vitro* excystation. Abstracts of the 35th Interscience Chemotherapy and Antimicrobial Agents Conference. Abstract No. B56, 1995, p. 36.
217. Ongerth, J. E., and Stibbs, H. H.: Identification of *Cryptosporidium* oocysts in river water. Appl. Environ. Microbiol. *53*:672–676, 1987.
218. Orenstein, J. M.: Microsporidiosis in the acquired immunodeficiency syndrome. J. Parasitol. *77*:843–863, 1991.

219. Orenstein, J. M., Chiang, J., Steinberg, W., et al.: Intestinal microsporidiosis as a cause of diarrhea in human immunodeficiency virus-infected patients: A report of 20 cases. Hum. Pathol. *21*:475–481, 1990.
220. Ortega, Y. R., Gilman R. H., and Sterling, C. R.: A new coccidian parasite (Apicomplexa: Eimeridae) from humans. J. Parasitol. *80*:625–629, 1993.
221. Ortega, Y. R., Sterling C. R., Gilman, R. H., et al.: *Cyclospora* species: A new protozoan pathogen of humans. N. Engl. J. Med. *328*:1308–1312, 1993.
222. Panciera, R. J., Thomassen, R. W., and Garner, F. M.: Cryptosporidial infection in a calf. Vet. Pathol. *8*:479–484, 1971.
223. Panosian, C. B.: Parasitic diarrhea. Infect. Dis. Clin. North Am. *2*:685–703, 1988.
224. Pape, J. W., and Johnson, W. D., Jr.: *Isospora belli* Infections. *In* Sun, T. (ed.): Progress in Clinical Parasitology. Vol. 2. New York, Field and Wood, 1991, pp. 119–127.
225. Pape, J. W., Verdier, R., Boney, M., et al.: *Cyclospora* infection in adults infected with HIV: Clinical manifestations, treatment, and prophylaxis. Ann. Intern. Med. *121*:654–657, 1994.
226. Pape, J. W., Verdier, R., and Johnson, W. D.: Treatment and prophylaxis of *Isospora belli* infection in patients with the acquired immunodeficiency syndrome. N. Engl. J. Med. *320*:1044–1047, 1989.
227. Perez-Schael, I., Boher, Y., Mata, L., et al.: Cryptosporidiosis in Venezuelan children with acute diarrhea. Am. J. Trop. Med. Hyg. *34*:721–722, 1985.
228. Pettoello-Mantovani, M., Di Martino, L., Dettori, G., et al.: Asymptomatic carriage of intestinal *Cryptosporidium* in immunocompetent and immunodeficient children: A prospective study. Pediatr. Infect. Dis. J. *14*:1042–1047, 1995.
229. Pilla, A. M., Rybak, M. J., and Chandrasekar, P. H.: Spiramycin in the treatment of cryptosporidiosis. Pharmacotherapy *7*:188–190, 1987.
230. Pitlik, S., Fainstein V., Rios, A., et al.: Cryptosporidial cholecystitis. N. Engl. J. Med. *308*:967, 1983.
231. Pol, S., Romana, C. A., and Richard, S.: Microsporidia infection in patients with the human immunodeficiency virus and unexplained cholangitis. N. Engl. J. Med. *328*:95–99, 1993.
232. Pollok, R. C., Bendell, R. P., Moody, A., et al.: Traveller's diarrhoea associated with *Cyanobacterium*-like bodies. Lancet *340*:556–557, 1992.
233. Portnoy, D., Whiteside, M. E., Buckley, E., et al.: Treatment of intestinal cryptosporidiosis with spiramycin. Ann. Intern. Med. *101*:202–204, 1984.
234. Rabeneck, L., Gyorkey, F., Genta, R. M., et al.: The role of microsporidia in the pathogenesis of HIV-related chronic diarrhea. Ann. Intern. Med. *119*:895–899, 1993.
235. Rahaman, A. S. M. H., Sanyal, S. C., Al-Mahmud, K. A., et al.: Cryptosporidiosis in calves and their handlers in Bangladesh. Lancet 2:221, 1984.
236. Restrepo, C., Macher, A. M., and Radany, E. H.: Disseminated extraintestinal isosporiasis in a patient with acquired immunodeficiency syndrome. Am. J. Clin. Pathol. *87*:536–542, 1987.
237. Richardson, A. J., Frankenberg, R. A., Buck, A. C., et al.: An outbreak of waterborne cryptosporidiosis in Swindon and Oxfordshire. Epidemiol. Infect. *107*:485–495, 1991.
238. Rijpstra, A. C., Canning, E. U., van Ketel, R. J., et al.: Use of light microscopy to diagnose small intestinal microsporidiosis in patients with AIDS. J. Infect. Dis. *157*:827–831, 1988.
239. Ritchie, D. J., and Becker, E. S.: Update on the management of intestinal cryptosporidiosis in AIDS. Ann. Pharmacother. *28*:767–778, 1994.
240. Robertson, L. J., Campbell, A. T., and Smith, H. V.: Survival of *Cryptosporidium parvum* oocysts under various environmental pressures. Appl. Environ. Microbiol. *58*:3494–3500, 1992.
241. Rohlman, V. C., Kuhls, T. L., Mosier, D. A., et al.: Therapy with atovaquone for *Cryptosporidium parvum* in neonatal severe combined immunodeficiency mice. J. Infect. Dis. *168*:258–260, 1993.
242. Romeu, J., Miro, J. M., Sirera, G., et al.: Efficacy of octreotide in the management of chronic diarrhoea in AIDS. AIDS *5*:1495–1499, 1991.
243. Roncoroni, A. J., Gomez, M. A., Mera, J., et al.: *Cryptosporidium* infection in renal transplant patients. J. Infect. Dis. *160*:559, 1989.
244. Rosenblatt, J. E, and Sloan, L. M.: Evaluation of an enzyme-linked immunosorbent assay for detection of *Cryptosporidium* spp. in stool specimens. J. Clin. Microbiol. *31*:1468–1471, 1993.
245. Rotterdam, H., and Tsang, P.: Gastrointestinal disease in the immunocompromised patient. Hum. Pathol. *25*:1123–1140, 1994.
246. Ruff, M. R., Martin, B. M., Ginns, E. I., et. al.: CD4 receptor binding peptides that block HIV infectivity cause human monocyte chemotaxis relationship to human monocyte chemotaxis. FEBS Lett. *211*:17–22, 1987.
247. Rusnak, J., Hadfield, T. L., Rhodes, M., et al.: Detection of *Cryptosporidium* oocysts in human fecal specimens by an indirect immunofluorescence assay with monoclonal antibodies. J. Clin. Microbiol. *27*:1135–1136, 1989.
248. Ryan, N. J., Sutherland, G., Coughlan, K., et al.: A new trichrome-blue stain for detection of microsporidial species in urine, stool and nasopharyngeal specimens. J. Clin. Microbiol. *31*:3264–3269, 1993.
249. Saez-Llorens, X., Odio, C. M., Umana, M. A., et al.: Spiramycin vs. placebo for treatment of acute diarrhea caused by *Cryptosporidium*. Pediatr. Infect. Dis. J. *8*:136–140, 1989.
250. Sallon, S., Deckelbaum, R. J., Schmid, I. I., et al.: *Cryptosporidium*, malnutrition, and chronic diarrhea in children. Am. J. Dis. Child. *142*:312–315, 1988.
251. Saxon, A., and Weinstein, W.: Oral administration of bovine colostrum anti-cryptosporidia antibody failed to alter the course of human cryptosporidiosis. J. Parasitol. *73*:413–415, 1987.
252. Scaglia, M., Atzori, C., Marchetti, M., et al.: Effectiveness of aminosidine (Paromomycin) sulfate in chronic *Cryptosporidium* diarrhea in AIDS patients: An open, uncontrolled, prospective, clinical trial. J. Infect. Dis. *170*:1349–1350, 1994.
253. Schneiderman, D. J., Cello J. P., and Laing, F. C.: Papillary stenosis and sclerosing cholangitis in the acquired immunodeficiency syndrome. Ann. Intern. Med. *106*:546–549, 1987.
254. Schwartz, D. A., Bryan, R. T., Hewan-Lowe, K. O., et al.: Disseminated microsporidiosis *(Encephalitozoon hellem)* and acquired immunodeficiency syndrome: Autopsy evidence for respiratory acquisition. Arch. Pathol. Lab. Med. *116*:660–668, 1992.
255. Schwartz, D. A., Visvesvara, G. S., Diesenhouse, M. C., et al.: Pathologic features and immunofluorescent antibody demonstration of ocular microsporidiosis *(Encephalitozoon hellem)* in seven patients with acquired immunodeficiency syndrome. Am. J. Ophthalmol. *115*:285–292, 1993.
256. Shadduck, J. A., and Greeley, E.: Microsporidia and human infections. Clin. Microbiol. Rev. *2*:158–165, 1989.
257. Shadduck, J. A., Meccoli, R. A., Davis, R., et al.: Isolation of microsporidia from a human patient. J. Infect. Dis. *162*:773–776, 1990.
258. Shaffer, N., and Moore, L.: Chronic travelers' diarrhea in a normal host due to *Isospora belli*. J. Infect. Dis. *3*:596–597, 1989.
259. Shahid, N. S., Rahman, A. S., Anderson, B. C., et al.: Cryptosporidiosis in Bangladesh. B. M. J. *290*:114–115, 1985.
260. Sheild, J., Melville C., Novelli, V., et al.: Bovine colostrum immunoglobulin concentrate for cryptosporidiosis in AIDS. Arch. Dis. Child. *69*:451–453, 1993.
261. Shlim, D. R., Cohen, M. T., Easton, M., et al.: An alga-like organism associated with an outbreak of prolonged diarrhea among foreigners in Nepal. Am. J. Trop. Med. Hyg. *45*:383–389, 1991.
262. Sifuentes-Osornio, J., Porras-Cortes, G., and Bendall, R. P.: *Cyclospora cayetanensis* infection in patients with and without AIDS: Biliary disease as another clinical manifestation. Clin. Infect. Dis. *21*:1092–1097, 1995.
263. Simon, D., Weiss, L. M., Tanowitz, H. B., et al.: Light microscopic diagnosis of human microsporidiosis and variable response to octreotide. Gastroenterology *100*:271–273, 1991.
264. Skeel, M. R., Sokolow, R., Hubbard, C. V., et al.: *Cryptosporidium* infection in Oregon public health clinic patients 1985–88: The value of statewide laboratory surveillance. Am. J. Public Health. *80*:305–308, 1990.
265. Slavin, D.: *Cryptosporidium meleagridis* (sp. nov.). J. Comp. Pathol. *65*:262–266, 1955.
266. Sloper, K. S., Dourmashkin, R. R., Bird, R. B., et al.: Chronic malabsorption due to cryptosporidiosis in a child with immunoglobulin deficiency. Gut *23*:80–82, 1982.
267. Smitskamp, H., and Dey-Muller, E.: Geographic distribution and clinical significance of human coccidiosis. Trop. Geogr. Med. *18*:133–136, 1966.
268. Soave, R., Dubey, J. P., Ramos, L. L., et al.: A new intestinal pathogen? Clin. Res. *34*:533A, 1986.
269. Soave, R., Havlir, D., Lancaster, D., et al.: Azithromycin therapy of AIDS-related cryptosporidial diarrhea: A multi-center, placebo-controlled, double-blinded study. Abstracts of the 33rd Interscience Chemotherapy and Antimicrobial Agents Conference. Abstract No. 405, 1993.
270. Soave, R., and Johnson, W. D.: *Cryptosporidium* and *Isospora belli* infections. J. Infect. Dis. *157*:225–229, 1988.
271. Soave, R., and Johnson, W. D.: *Cyclospora:* Cqnquest of an emerging pathogen. Lancet *345*:667–668, 1995.
272. Sorvillo, F. J., Fujioda, K., Nahlen, B., et al.: Swimming-associated cryptosporidiosis. Am. J. Public Health *82*:742–744, 1992.
273. Steele, M. I., Kuhls, T. L., Nida, K, et al.: A *Cryptosporidium parvum* genomic region encoding hemolytic activity. Infect. Immun. *63*:3840–3845, 1995.
274. Stehr-Green, J. K., McCaig, L., and Ramsen, H. M.: Shedding of oocysts in immunocompetent individuals infected with *Cryptosporidium*. Am. J. Trop. Med. Hyg. *36*:338–342, 1987.
275. Sterling, C. R., and Arrowood, M.: Detection of *Cryptosporidium* species infections using direct immunofluorescent assay. Pediatr. Infect. Dis. J. *5*:S139–S142, 1986.
276. Stine, K. C., Harris, J. A., Lindsey, N. J., et al.: Spontaneous remission of cryptosporidiosis in a child with acute lymphoblastic leukemia. Clin. Pediatr. *24*:722–724, 1985.
277. Sun, T., Kaplan, M. H., Teichberg, S., et al.: Intestinal microsporidiosis: Report of five cases. Ann. Clin. Lab. Sci. *24*:521–532, 1994.
278. Tangermann, R. H., Gordon, S., Wiesner, P., et al.: An outbreak of cryptosporidiosis in a day-care center in Georgia. Am. J. Epidemiol. *133*:471–476, 1991.
279. Taylor, J. P., Perdue, J. N., Dingley, D., et al.: Cryptosporidiosis outbreak in a day-care center. Am. J. Dis. Child. *139*:1023–1025, 1985.
280. Teixidor, H. S., Godwin, T. A., and Ramirez, E. A.: Cryptosporidiosis of the bilary tract. Radiology *180*:51–56, 1991.
281. Thomson, M. A., Benson, J. W., and Wright, P. A.: Two-year study of *Cryptosporidium* infection. Arch. Dis. Child. *62*:559–563, 1987.
282. Trier, J. S., Moxey, P. C., Schimmel, E. M., et al.: Chronic intestinal coccidiosis in man: Intestinal morphology and response to treatment. Gastroenterology *66*:923–925, 1974.

283. Tyzzer, E. E.: A sporozoan found in the peptic glands of the common mouse. Proc. Soc. Exp. Biol. Med. *5*:12–13, 1907.
284. Tzipori, S.: Cryptosporidiosis in animals and humans. Microbiol. Rev. *47*:84, 1983.
285. Tzipori, S., Roberton, D., and Chapman, C.: Remission of diarrhea due to cryptosporidiosis in an immunodeficient child with hyperimmune bovine colostrum. B. M. J. *293*:1276–1277, 1986.
286. Tzipori, S., Smith, M., Birch, C., et al.: Cryptosporidiosis in hospital patients with gastroenteritis. Am. J. Trop. Med. Hyg. *32*:931–934, 1983.
287. Ungar, B. L. P., Gilman, R. H., Lanata, C. F., et al.: Seroepidemiology of *Cryptosporidium* infection in two Latin American populations. J. Infect. Dis. *157*:551–556, 1988.
288. Ungar, B. L. P., Mulligan, M., and Nutman, T. B.: Serologic evidence of *Cryptosporidium* infection in US volunteers before and during Peace Corps service in Africa. Arch. Intern. Med. *149*:894–897, 1989.
289. Ungar, B. L. P., and Nash, T. E.: Quantification of specific antibody response to *Cryptosporidium* antigens by laser densitometry. Infect. Immun. *53*:124–128, 1986.
290. Ungar, B. L. P., Soave, R., Fayer, R., et al.: Enzyme immunoassay detection of immunoglobulin M and G antibodies to *Cryptosporidium* in immunocompetent and immunocompromised persons. J. Infect. Dis. *153*:570–578, 1986.
291. Ungar, B. L. P., Ward, D. S., Fayer, R., et al.: Cessation of *Cryptosporidium* associated diarrhea in an acquired immunodeficiency syndrome patient after treatment with hyperimmune bovine colostrum. Gastroenterology *98*:486–489, 1990.
292. Upton, S. J., and Current, W. L.: The species of *Cryptosporidium* (Apicocomplexa: Cryptosporidiidae) infecting mammals. J. Parasitol. *71*:625–629, 1985.
293. Vakil, N. B., Schwartz, S. M., Buggy, B. P., et al.: Biliary cryptosporidiosis in HIV-infected people after the waterborne outbreak of cryptosporidiosis in Milwaukee. N. Engl. J. Med. *334*:19–23, 1996.
294. Van, R., Morrow, A. L., Reves, R. R., et al.: Environmental contamination in child day-care centers. Am. J. Epidemiol. *133*:460–470, 1991.
295. Van Gool, T., Canning, E. U., and Dankert, J.: An improved practical and sensitive technique for the detection of microsporidian spores in stool samples. Trans. R. Soc. Trop. Med. *88*:189–190, 1994.
296. Van Gool, T., Canning, E. U., Gilis, H., et al.: *Septata intestinalis* frequently isolated from stool of AIDS patients with a new cultivation method. Parasitology *109*:281–289, 1994.
297. Van Gool, T., Snijders, F., Reiss, P., et al.: Diagnosis of intestinal and disseminated microsporidial infections in patients with HIV by a new rapid fluorescence technique. J. Clin. Pathol. *46*:694–699, 1993.
298. Van Gool, T., Vetter, J. C., Van Dam, A. P., et al.: Serological diagnosis of *Septata intestinalis* infections. Abstracts of the 35th Interscience Chemotherapy and Antimicrobial Agents Conference. Abstract No. D79, 1995, p. 80.
299. Vargas, S. L., Shenep, J. L., Flynn, P. M., et al.: Azithromycin for treatment of severe *Cryptosporidium* diarrhea in two children with cancer. J. Pediatr. *123*:154–156, 1993.
300. Visvesvara, G. S., Leitch, G. J., Da Silva, A. J., et al.: Polyclonal and monoclonal antibody and PCR-amplified small-subunit rRNA identification of a microsporidian, *Encephalitozoon hellem,* isolated from an AIDS patient with disseminated infection. J. Clin. Microbiol. *32*:2760–2768, 1994.
301. Vuorio, A. F., Jokipii, A. M. M., and Jokipii, L.: *Cryptosporidium* in asymptomatic children. Rev. Infect. Dis. *13*:261–264, 1991.
302. Wallace, W. R., Nguyen, M. T., and Newton, J. A., Jr.: Use of paromomycin for the treatment of cryptosporidiosis in patients with AIDS. Clin. Infect Dis. *17*:1070–1071, 1993.
303. Walters, I. N., Miller, N. M., Van den Ende, J., et al.: Outbreak of cryptosporidiosis among children attending a day-care center in Durban. S. Afr. Med. J. *74*:496–499, 1988.
304. Weber, R., and Bryan, R. T.: Microsporidial infections in immunodeficient and immunocompetent patients. Clin. Infect. Dis. *19*:517–521, 1994.
305. Weber, R., Bryan, R. T., Bishop, H. S., et al.: Threshold of detection of *Cryptosporidium* oocyst in human stool specimens: Evidence for low sensitivity of current diagnostic methods. J. Clin. Microbiol. *29*:1323–1327, 1991.
306. Weber, R., Bryan, R. T., and Juranek D. D.: Improved stool concentration procedures for the detection of *Cryptosporidium* oocyst in fecal specimens. J. Clin. Microbiol. *30*:2869–2873, 1992.
307. Weber, R., Bryan, R. T., Owen, R. L., et al.: Improved light microscopical detection of microsporidia spores in stool and duodenal aspirates. N. Engl. J. Med. *326*:161–166, 1992.
308. Weber, R., Bryan, R. T., Schwartz, D. A., et al.: Human microsporidial infections. Clin. Microbiol. Rev. *7*:426–461, 1994.
309. Weber, R., Kuster, H., Keller, R., et al.: Pulmonary and intestinal microsporidiosis in a patient with the acquired immunodeficiency syndrome. Am. Rev. Respir. Dis. *146*:1603–1605, 1992.
310. Weber, R., Kuster, H., Visvesvara, G. S., et al.: Disseminated microsporidiosis due to *Encephalitozoon hellem:* Pulmonary colonization, microhematuria, and mild conjunctivitis in a patient with AIDS. Clin. Infect. Dis. *17*:415–419, 1993.
311. Weber, R., Sauer, B., Luthy, R., et al.: Intestinal coinfection with *Enterocytozoon bieneusi* and *Cryptosporidium* in a human immunodeficiency virus-infected child with chronic diarrhea. Clin. Infect. Dis. *17*:480–483, 1993.
312. Weber, R., Sauer, B., Spycher, M. A., et al.: Detection of *Septata intestinalis* in stool specimens and coprodiagnostic monitoring of successful treatment with albendazole. Clin. Infect. Dis. *19*:342–345, 1994.
313. Weikel, C. S., Johnson, L. I., DeSousa, M. A., et al.: Cryptosporidiosis in northeastern Brazil: Association with sporadic diarrhea. J. Infect. Dis. *151*:963–965, 1985.
314. Weinstein, L., Edelstein, S. M., Madura, J. L., et al.: Intestinal cryptosporidiosis complicated by disseminating cytomegalovirus infection. Gastroenterology *81*:584–591, 1981.
315. Weisburger, W. R., Hutcheon, D. F., Yardley, J. H., et al.: Cryptosporidiosis in an immunosuppressed renal-transplant recipient with IgA deficiency. Am. J. Clin. Pathol. *72*:473–478, 1979.
316. Weiss, L. M., Perlman, D. C., Sherman, J., et al.: *Isospora belli* infection: Treatment with pyrimethamine. Ann. Intern. Med. *109*:474–475, 1988.
317. Weitz, J. C., Tassara, O. R., and Mercado, R.: Cryptosporidiosis in Chilean children. Trans. R. Soc. Trop. Med. Hyg. *82*:335, 1988.
318. Wenyon, C. M.: Observations on the common intestinal protozoa of men: Their diagnosis and pathogenicity. Lancet *2*:1173, 1915.
319. White, A. C., Chappell, C. L., Hayat, C. S., et al.: Paromomycin for cryptosporidiosis in AIDS: A prospective double-blind trial. J. Infect. Dis. *170*:419–424, 1994.
320. Whiteside, M. E., Barkin, J. S., and May, R. G.: Enteric coccidiosis among patients with the acquired immunodeficiency syndrome. Am. J. Trop. Med. Hyg. *33*:1065–1072, 1984.
321. Wittenberg, D. F., Miller, N. M., and Van den Ende, J.: Spiramycin is not effective in treating *Cryptosporidium* diarrhea in infants: Results of a double-blind randomized trial. J. Infect. Dis. *159*:131–132, 1989.
322. Wittner, M., Tanowitz, H. B., and Weiss, L. M.: Parasitic infections in AIDS patients: Cryptosporidiosis, isosporiasis, microsporidiosis, cyclosporiasis. Infect. Dis. Clin. North Am. *7*:569–586, 1993.
323. Wolfson, J. S., Richter, J. M., Waldron, M. A., et al.: Cryptosporidiosis in immunocompetent patients. N. Engl. J. Med. *312*:1278–1282, 1985.
324. Woodcock, H. M.: Notes on the protozoan parasites in the excreta. Addendum to Ledingham, J. C. G., and Penfold, W. J.: Recent bacteriological experiences with typhoidal disease and dysentery. B. M. J. *2*:709, 1915.
325. Wurtz, R.: *Cyclospora:* A newly identified intestinal pathogen of humans. Clin. Infect. Dis. *18*:620–623, 1994.
326. Wurtz, R. M., Kocka, F. E., Peters, C. S., et al.: Clinical characteristics of seven cases of diarrhea associated with a novel acid-fast organism in stool. Clin. Infect. Dis. *16*:136–138, 1993.
327. Zar, F., Geiseler, P. J., and Brown, V. A.: Asymptomatic carriage of *Cryptosporidium* in the stool of a patient with acquired immunodeficiency syndrome. J. Infect. Dis. J. *151*:195, 1985.
328. Zerpa, R., and Huicho L.: Childhood cryptosporidial diarrhea associated with identification of *Cryptosporidium* sp. in the cockroach *Periplaneta americana.* Pediatr. Infect. Dis. *13*:546–548, 1994.
329. Zierdt, C. H., Gill, V. J., and Zierdt, W. S.: Detection of microsporidian spores in clinical samples by indirect fluorescent-antibody assay using whole-cell antisera to *Encephalitozoon cuniculi* and *Encephalitozoon hellem.* J. Clin. Microbiol. *31*:3071–3074, 1993.
330. Zu, S. X., and Guerrant, R. L.: Cryptosporidiosis. J. Trop. Med. *39*:132–135, 1993.

216

BABESIOSIS

Peter J. Krause

The first reference to babesiosis may have been in the Bible, where a widespread murrain or plague in cattle and other domestic animals is described in Exodus, Chapter 9, Verse 3: *"Behold, the hand of the Lord is upon thy cattle which is in the field, upon the horses, upon the asses, upon the camels, upon the oxen, and upon the sheep: there shall be a very grievous murrain."* The word "murrain" still is used to describe redwater fever, a form of babesiosis found in cattle in parts of Ireland.[20] Although babesiosis long has been recognized as an important disease in livestock, having a significant economic impact in many parts of the world, the first human case was not described until 1957.[28, 95]

Babesiosis is a disease caused by an intraerythrocytic protozoon that is transmitted by ticks and has many clinical features similar to those of malaria. The parasite first was described in animals in 1888 by Babes.[4] In 1893, it became the first microorganism shown to be transmitted by arthropods when Smith and Kilbourne[98] identified a tick as the vector for a species of babesiosis *(Babesia bigemina)* in Texas cattle. Since the initial report of babesiosis in humans, more than 300 clinical cases have been described, including 5 in children.[15, 21, 23, 60, 64, 93, 111] There is evidence that the disease is more common in both children and adults than these cases would suggest and is occurring more frequently than in the past.[21, 48, 49, 64] Over the past 30 years, the epidemiology of the disease has changed from a few isolated cases to the establishment of endemic areas on the islands off the southern New England coast, eastern Long Island, and Wisconsin and reports from a wide geographic range in North America and Europe.

EPIDEMIOLOGY

Worldwide, there are more than 70 species in the genus *Babesia* that infect a wide variety of wild and domestic animals. For example, *B. bigemina, B. bovis, B. divergens,* and *B. major* are found in cattle; *B. equi* in horses; *B. canis* in dogs; *B. felis* in cats; and *B. microti* in rodents.[56] It previously had been thought that each species was host-specific, but now it is recognized that the host range of some species is quite broad.[35, 55, 56, 101, 108] There has been some confusion in taxonomy because the identification of different *Babesia* species has been based largely on morphology and the vertebrate host.[38] Most *Babesia* species are small (1.0 to 5.0 μm in length) and pear-shaped, round, or oval.[55] Two *Babesia* species have been found to cause disease in humans: *B. microti* in North America and *B. divergens* in Europe.

Human babesiosis is a zoonotic disease with transmission by a tick vector from an infected animal reservoir (Fig. 216–1). Humans are a rare and terminal host for *Babesia* species, which depend on other species for survival. The primary reservoir for *B. microti* in eastern North America is the white-footed mouse *(Peromyscus leucopus)*, but the parasite also has been found in shrews, chipmunks, voles, and rats.[35, 101, 107] As many as two-thirds of *P. leucopus* have been found to be parasitemic in endemic areas.[102] *Babesia* species are transmitted by hard-bodied (ixodid) ticks. The primary vector in the northeastern United States is *Ixodes dammini*, which is the same tick that transmits *Borrelia burgdorferi*, the etiologic agent of Lyme disease.[43, 99, 100, 102–104] *I. dammini* ticks may be infected simultaneously with *B. burgdorferi* and *B. microti*.[61, 72] Furthermore, there is both clinical and serologic evidence of the simultaneous occurrence of Lyme disease and babesiosis.[5, 48, 49, 51, 58] There are three active stages in the life cycle of *I. dammini:* larva, nymph, and adult. Each takes a blood meal from a vertebrate host in order to mature to the next stage. Ingested babesial organisms infect intestinal tissue of the tick and subsequently travel to the salivary glands, from which they may be introduced into a new vertebrate host.[73] The *Babesia* species are transmitted to the subsequent tick stage (transstadial passage). In some species of ticks, such as *B. bigemina,* the organisms may invade the ovaries and pass transovarially to the larvae. In late summer, newly hatched larvae ingest the parasite with a blood meal from an infected rodent and maintain the parasite to the nymphal stage. Nymphs transmit the *Babesia* species to rodents in late spring and summer of the following year.[101, 102] Larvae, nymphs, and adults can feed on humans, but the nymph is the primary vector.[73] All active tick stages also feed on the white-tailed deer *(Odocoileus virginianus),* which is an important host for the tick but is not a reservoir for *B. microti*.[74, 102] An increase in the deer population over the past few decades is thought to be a major factor in the spread of *I. dammini* and the resulting increase in human cases.[33, 102, 103] Domestic animals such as the dog may carry the adult *I. dammini* but do not appear to be important hosts for the tick and are not infected with *B. microti*.[89, 100]

Most human cases of babesiosis occur in the summer. In areas where human *B. microti* infections have been reported, the tick, rodents, and deer are in close proximity to humans.[101, 105] *B. microti* has been identified in rodent populations in several parts of the United States,[2, 3, 83, 101] and human cases have been reported in Connecticut, Massachusetts, Rhode Island, New York, Minnesota, and Wisconsin.[15, 21, 83, 105] Human babesiosis caused by organisms that morphologically are distinct from *B. microti* has been reported in California, Georgia, and Mexico, although the precise species in these cases have not been identified.[36, 69, 92] Moderately severe illness caused by a new babesia-like organism, designated *WA1*, has been reported in adults living in Washington state and California.[71, 76] WA1 morphologically is indistinguishable from *B. microti* but antigenically and genotypically distinct.[71, 76] A case of human babesiosis due to *B. divergens* was described in Missouri.[37] In Europe, *B. divergens* infections are believed to be transmitted by the cattle tick *I. ricinus*.[38] Human cases have been reported in the former Yugoslavia, France, Ireland, Great Britain, and the former Soviet Union.[26, 27] An absence of clinical cases of babesiosis in the tropics may be due to cross-immunity from other endemic protozoal diseases.[45] Rarely, babesiosis is acquired through blood transfusions.[31, 42, 59, 97, 111] Whole blood, frozen erythrocytes, and platelets have been implicated. The incubation period in these cases appears to be 6 to 9 weeks. Transplacen-

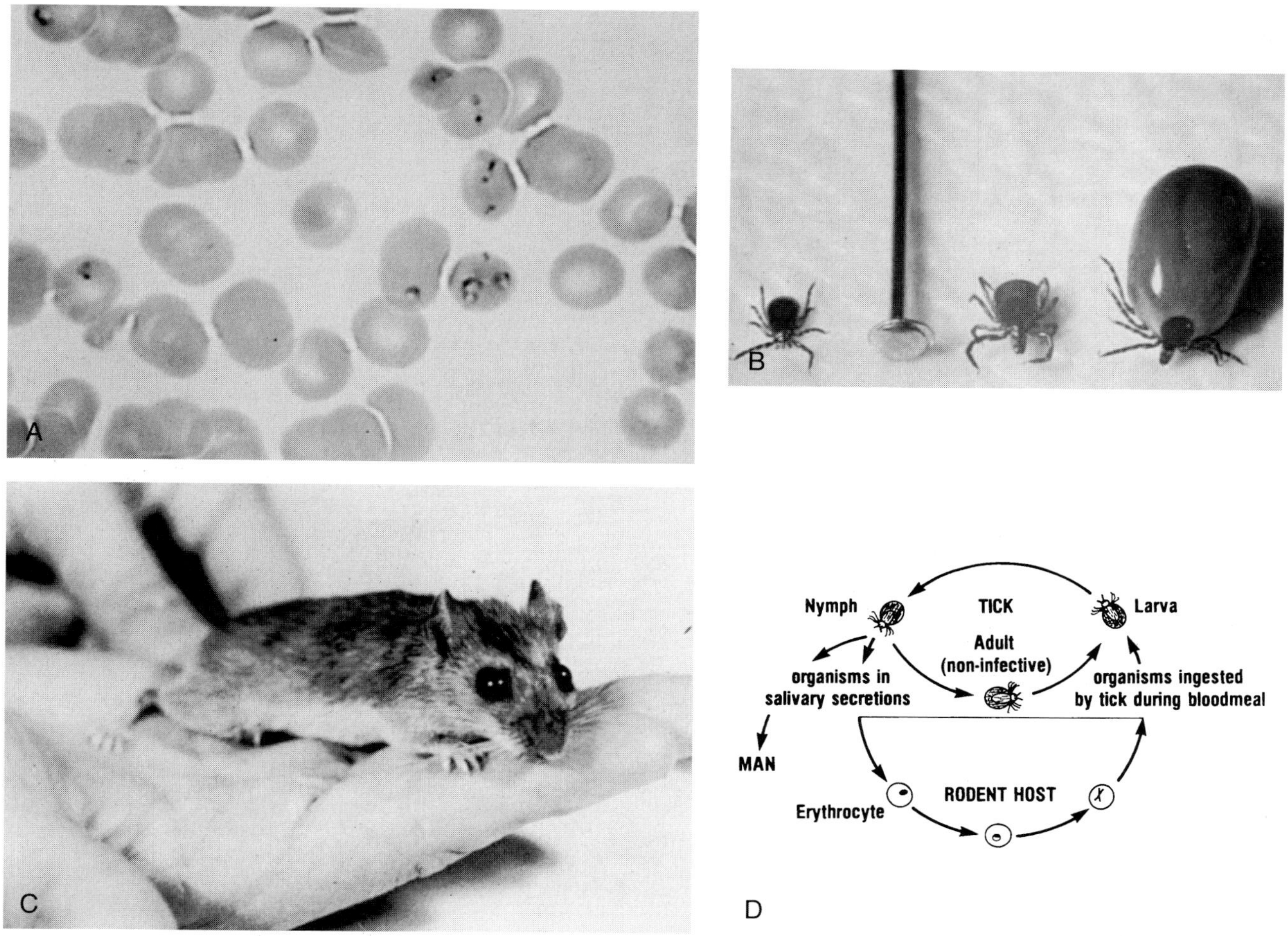

FIGURE 216–1. *Life cycle of* Babesia microti. A, *Ring forms of* B. microti *in human blood film (× 1000).* B, Ixodes dammini *ticks and a common pin. The ticks are an adult male, an adult female, and an engorged female. (Courtesy of Mike Frigione, Pfizer, Inc.)* C, *White-footed mouse* (Peromyscus leucopus). D, *Life cycle of* B. microti. *(Modified from Ruebush, T. K., II: Babesiosis.* In *Strickland, G. T. [ed.]: Hunter's Tropical Medicine. Philadelphia, W. B. Saunders, 1984.)*

tal/perinatal transmission of babesiosis also has been described.[23]

PATHOGENESIS AND PATHOLOGY

Our understanding of the pathogenesis and pathology of babesiosis in humans is incomplete and is based in large part on information gathered from studies of babesiosis in other animals. *Babesia* species are intraerythrocytic protozoa, and extracellular forms are seen only in heavily parasitized cases.[1, 106] Jack and Ward[41] have presented data suggesting that *B. rodhani* gains entry into the erythrocyte by activation of the alternative complement pathway. They found that the C3b receptor plays a key role in modification of the parasite or red cell, allowing penetration of the parasite into the cell. Rudzinska and colleagues[46, 81, 82] have studied the life cycle of *B. microti* in erythrocytes using electron microscopy. After adhesion and entry into the erythrocyte, the organism multiplies by asexual budding into two to four daughter cells, or merozoites. Unlike *Plasmodium* species merozoites, which are released from the erythrocytes all at once (synchrony), *Babesia* species merozoites are released at varying intervals. New erythrocytes then are infected, and the cycle is repeated. It is not known whether the initial merozoite release leads to destruction of the host erythrocyte, but there is alteration of the erythrocyte membrane and eventual lysis.[81, 106] Erythrocyte lysis is responsible for many of the clinical manifestations and complications of the disease, including fever, hemolytic anemia, jaundice, hemoglobinemia, hemoglobinuria, and renal insufficiency. The absence of synchrony decreases the possibility of massive hemolysis and may explain why patients heavily parasitized with *Babesia* species may be less ill than those with *Plasmodium* species.[106] Ischemia and necrosis result from obstruction of blood vessels by parasitized erythrocytes, which may result in hepatomegaly and hepatic dysfunction, splenomegaly, and cerebral abnormalities.[20, 79, 85] Such clinical manifestations as hypotension, vascular congestion, and anoxia also may result from the activation of fibronectin, kallikreins, and complement.[22, 113, 114]

A number of immune mechanisms limit the severity of babesial infections, but immunity is incomplete because parasitemia may exist for months to years in animals and as long as 10 months in humans after recovery from the initial illness.[12] Furthermore, reinfection may occur, although it is uncommon. Age is an important factor in host defense against babesial disease in both animals and humans. The majority of clinically apparent cases have occurred in adults 40 to 60 years of age, yet serologic surveys indicate that children and persons 20 to 40 years of age equally are susceptible to infection and presumably are exposed to ticks to the same extent.[49, 83, 89] Four of the five pediatric cases reported have been in neonates.[23, 60, 93, 111] It has been postulated that the increased severity of babesiosis observed in the elderly and in neonates may have been the result of impaired splenic function because the spleen plays a critical role in protection against *Babesia* species.[13, 23, 93, 111, 113] The spleen is thought to protect against babesial infections by (1) removing parasites from infected erythrocytes through a process known as "pitting," (2) ingestion of parasites by reticuloendothelial cells and mononuclear phagocytes, and (3) production of antibabesial antibody.[13, 19, 22, 113] It long has been known that splenectomized animals have more severe babesiosis than do animals with intact spleens. Furthermore, animals that have recovered from babesiosis and have had negative blood smears have developed parasitemia again after splenectomy.[57, 90] Most fatal cases of babesiosis in humans have occurred in splenectomized individuals, although asplenia does not result always in death or even severe illness.[11, 80] Other host defense mechanisms that may help limit babesial infection include antibody[13, 43]; complement[8, 113]; a soluble nonantibody factor[18]; macrophages; and macrophage products such as tumor necrosis factor,[22, 113] B lymphocytes,[63] T lymphocytes,[13, 63, 87, 112] and polymorphonuclear leukocytes.[94]

CLINICAL MANIFESTATIONS

The clinical manifestations of babesiosis range from subclinical illness to fulminating disease resulting in death. Overt signs and symptoms begin after an incubation period of 1 to 6 weeks from the beginning of tick feeding.[89] The unengorged *I. dammini* nymph is about 2 mm in length, and there often is no recollection of a tick bite. In most cases, there is a gradual onset of malaise, anorexia, and fatigue followed by intermittent temperature to as high as 40° C (104° F) and one or more of the following: chills, sweats, myalgia, arthralgia, nausea, and vomiting.[1, 27, 60, 83, 88, 89, 105] Less commonly noted are emotional lability and depression, hyperesthesia, headache, sore throat, abdominal pain, conjunctival injection, photophobia, weight loss, and nonproductive cough.[47, 85, 105, 106] Unlike other tick-borne illnesses, such as Lyme disease, Rocky Mountain spotted fever, or tularemia, rash seldom is noted.[21] Ecchymoses and petechiae have been described.[47, 106] Erythema chronicum migrans has been noted in patients with babesiosis,[5] but it is likely these patients had Lyme disease as well.

The findings on physical examination generally are minimal, often consisting only of fever.[1, 36, 88, 105] Mild splenomegaly, hepatomegaly, or both are noted occasionally.[85, 111] Slight pharyngeal erythema, jaundice, and retinopathy with splinter hemorrhages and retinal infarcts also have been reported.[47, 60, 68] Several abnormal laboratory findings in patients with babesiosis reflect the invasion and subsequent lysis of erythrocytes by the parasite.[47, 60, 83, 85] There is mild to moderately severe hemolytic anemia, with an elevated reticulocyte count. Elevated liver function tests occur in about half the patients.[83] The leukocyte count is normal to slightly decreased, with a "left shift." Thrombocytopenia may occur.[85] The erythrocyte sedimentation rate is elevated. Proteinuria and an elevated blood urea nitrogen and creatinine also may be noted.[47, 60, 85] The illness usually lasts for a few weeks to several months, with prolonged recovery of up to 18 months.[1, 5, 85, 88, 105] Parasitemia may continue even after the patient feels well. It has been demonstrated in humans for as long as 10 months, and relapse of illness as noted with malaria has been described 8 months after the initial episode.[9, 12]

Some patients, especially those with *B. divergens* infection or prior splenectomy, suffer a more severe form of the disease consisting of fulminant illness lasting about a week and ending in death or a prolonged convalescence.[27, 47, 58, 68, 106] Signs and symptoms include high fever, hemolytic anemia, hemoglobinemia and hemoglobinuria, jaundice, ecchymoses, petechiae, congestive heart failure, pulmonary edema, renal failure, adult respiratory distress syndrome, and coma.[29, 30, 47, 105, 106, 110] Patients with babesiosis who are coinfected with Lyme disease also have more severe illness than those with babesiosis alone.[32, 58] Coinfected patients usually experience moderate to severe acute illness often followed by persistent fatigue. Between 10 and 66 per cent of patients with antibody to *B. burgdorferi* also have been found to have antibody to *B. microti*.[7, 48, 49]

Inapparent infection also may occur. Data from seven serosurveys suggest that this may be the most common form of the disease. In a survey on Nantucket Island in Massachusetts, 2 per cent of 577 random blood samples and 7.5 per cent of 133 blood samples from patients with a history of tick bite or fever had *B. microti* indirect immunofluorescent antibody (IFA) titers of 1:64 or greater.[88] A survey of adults living on Shelter Island, New York, showed that 6 of 136 (4.4 per cent) and 7 of 102 (6.9 per cent) had *B. microti* IFA antibody at titers of 1:64 or greater.[24] In a survey of Massachusetts blood donors, 29 of 779 (37 per cent) from Cape Cod had *B. microti* IFA antibody titers of 1:16 compared with 7 of 148 (4.7 per cent) from metropolitan Boston.[75] In a serosurvey in Connecticut, 72 of 735 (9.5 per cent) residents who were seropositive for *B. burgdorferi* had positive *B. microti* IFA antibody titers of 1:64 compared with 8 of 299 (2.7 per cent) seronegative for *B. burgdorferi*.[48] Serosurveys in Mexico, Nigeria, and Taiwan also demonstrated high *B. microti* seroprevalence rates in comparison with the number of indigenous reported cases of babesiosis.[40, 54, 69]

DIAGNOSIS

Specific diagnosis of babesiosis is made by microscopic identification of the organism by Giemsa or Wright stains of thick or thin blood smears and by detection of babesial antibodies by one of several serologic tests. *Babesia* species are round, oval, or pear-shaped and have a blue cytoplasm with a red chromatin. The ring form is most common and is very similar to the rings of *Plasmodium falciparum*.[34] *Babesia* species can be distinguished from *Plasmodium* species by (1) the absence of pigment, which is present in older trophozoites of *Plasmodium* species, (2) the absence of schizonts and gametocytes, (3) the absence of synchronous stages within the erythrocytes, and (4) the presence of the infrequently noted tetrad or Maltese cross forms, in which four compact masses, each containing nuclear material, are joined by strands of cytoplasm.[34] Multiple thick and thin blood smears should be examined because only a few erythrocytes are infected in the early stage of the illness when most people seek medical attention.[34] New rapid automated differential blood analyzers may fail to distinguish erythrocytic inclusions.[11] In thick smears, the *Babesia* organism appears as a tiny red to purple nucleus with a thin tail of light blue cytoplasm. Maximum erythrocyte infection is approximately 10 per cent in normal hosts but up to 85 per cent in asplenic individuals.[105] Usually less than 1 per cent of erythrocytes are parasitized early in the course of the illness, and the laboratory investigation of possible babesiosis should include more than an examination of blood smears.

Numerous serologic tests have been developed to detect babesial antibodies. Of the commonly used serologic tests, the IFA assay is the most reliable.[16, 48, 85] The IFA test is simpler, cheaper, and more rapid than the complement-fixation test. Both IgG and IgM IFA antibodies can be detected.[51] During the acute phase of the illness, titers usually exceed 1:1024 but decline to 1:64 or less within 8 to 12 months. Thus, a babesial IFA titer of 1:1024 or greater usually signifies active or recent infection.[16, 85] Although cross-reactions occur to different *Babesia* species and *Plasmodium* species with the IFA test, these titers almost always are low (1:16 or fewer).[16, 17] The problem of cross-reactivity with *Plasmodium* species is minimized in areas where there is no indigenous malaria. Enzyme-linked immunosorbent assays for detection of *B. divergens* and *B. major* have been found to be superior to complement fixation and IFA procedures.[10, 77, 108]

In cases in which the presence of *Babesia* species is suspected but not demonstrated by blood smears or antibody studies, blood from the patient can be injected by the intravenous or intraperitoneal route into small laboratory animals such as hamsters or gerbils. If present in the patient, *B. microti* usually appears in the blood of the inoculated animal within 2 to 4 weeks.[6] DNA probes and polymerase chain reaction for the detection of *Babesia* species are useful new diagnostic techniques.[69, 77]

PREVENTION AND TREATMENT

The current therapy of choice for babesiosis is the combination of clindamycin (20 mg/kg/day in children; in adults, 300 to 600 mg every 6 hours given intravenously or orally) and quinine (25 mg/kg/day in children; in adults, 650 mg every 6 to 8 hours) taken for 7 to 10 days.[14, 29] This combination was used initially in the first reported case of babesiosis in a child, an 8-week-old who contracted babesiosis from a blood transfusion.[111] Initially, she was thought to have malaria. Clindamycin and quinine were given after failure with chloroquine. Her favorable outcome suggested the prospective use of this combination in adults. A number of children and adults subsequently have been treated with clindamycin and quinine with prompt clearing of parasitemia and resolution of clinical signs and symptoms.[14, 15, 23, 60, 93, 105] Chloroquine has been used to treat babesiosis because of the occasional misdiagnosis of babesiosis as *P. falciparum* infection. Although chloroquine may give some symptomatic relief of fever and myalgia by its anti-inflammatory action, it often fails to clear parasitemia in guinea pigs and humans and is not recommended.[14, 65] Other antimalarial drugs, such as quinacrine, primaquine, pyrimethamine, pyrimethamine-sulfadoxine, sulfadiazine, and tetracycline, have no effect on parasitemia in animals. Pentamidine isothionate has been found to decrease fever and parasitemia, but the organisms are not eradicated and the drug has proved to be ineffective in animals and humans.[25] Diminazene aceturate was effective in clearing parasitemia and clinical symptoms in one patient, but he developed Guillain-Barré syndrome during recovery, possibly as a result of receiving the drug.[90] Pentamidine and trimethoprim-sulfamethoxazole were used successfully to treat a case of *B. divergens* infection in France.[77] Atovaquone has been found to be effective for treatment of babesiosis in hamsters and offers promise for use in humans because of its excellent safety record.[39] Exchange blood transfusions have been used successfully in splenectomized patients with life-threatening *Babesia* species infections.[12, 42, 106] This can decrease the degree of parasitemia rapidly and remove toxic byproducts of babesial infections but should be used only in the most severe infections.

Prevention of babesiosis can be accomplished by avoiding areas in May through September where ticks, deer, and mice are known to thrive. It especially is important for asplenic individuals in endemic areas to avoid tall grass and brush where ticks may abound. Use of clothing that covers the lower part of the body and that is sprayed or impregnated with diethyltoluamide, dimethyl phthalate, or permethrin (Permanone) is recommended for those who travel in the foliage of endemic areas.[20, 96] A search for ticks on people and pets should be carried out and the ticks removed as soon as possible.[20] The latter is accomplished best by removal with tweezers by grasping the mouth parts without squeezing the body of the tick.[21, 67] Attempts to reduce the tick, mouse, or deer populations in endemic areas are less effective.[62, 96, 103] It has been recommended that prospective blood donors who reside in endemic areas and who present with a history of fever within the preceding 1 to 2 months be excluded from giving blood in order to prevent transfusion-related cases.[84] Effective *B. bovis* and *B. bigemina* vaccines have been developed for use in cattle, but there is no *B. microti* vaccine.[66, 115]

Babesiosis is a new zoonosis that has been reported in North America *(B. microti)* and Europe *(B. divergens)*. It commonly presents as a mild clinical infection, and it is likely that the incidence in the United States and throughout the rest of the world is greater than presently recognized. The clinical symptoms of babesiosis usually are nonspecific, and detection of the organism in blood smears often is difficult. Although fatalities have been reported in splenectomized individuals and in those with *B. divergens* infections, complete recovery with antibabesial chemotherapy is the rule.

Acknowledgments

I am indebted to the following people who helped with this manuscript: Andrew Spielman, Sc.D., Raymond W. Ryan, Ph.D., and Sam R. Telford, III, Sc.D.

References

1. Anderson, A. E., Cassaday, P. B., and Healy, G. R.: Babesiosis in man: Sixth documented case. Am. J. Clin. Pathol. *62*:612–618, 1974.
2. Anderson, J. F., and Magnarelli, L. A.: Spirochetes in *Ixodes dammini* and *Babesia microti* on Prudence Island, Rhode Island. J. Infect. Dis. *148*:1124, 1983.
3. Anderson, J. F., Magnarelli, L. A., and Kurz, J.: Intraerythrocytic parasites in rodent populations of Connecticut: *Babesia* and *Grahamella* species. J. Parasitol. *65*:599–604, 1979.
4. Babes, V.: Sur l'hemoglubinurie bacterienne boeuf. Compt. Rend. Acad. Sci. *107*:692–694, 1888.
5. Benach, J. L., and Hibicht, G. S.: Clinical characteristics of human babesiosis. J. Infect. Dis. *144*:481, 1981.
6. Benach, J. L., White, D. J., and McGovern, J. P.: Babesiosis in Long Island: Host-parasite relationship of rodent- and human-derived *Babesia microti* isolates in hamsters. Am. J. Trop. Med. Hyg. *27*:1073–1078, 1978.
7. Benach, J. L., Coleman, J. L., Habicht, G. S., et al.: Serological evidence for simultaneous occurrences of Lyme disease and babesiosis. J. Infect. Dis. *152*:473–477, 1985.
8. Benach, J. L. Mabicht, G. S. and Manburger, M. I.: Immunoresponsiveness in acute babesiosis in humans. J. Infect. Dis. *146*:369–380, 1982.
9. Benezra, D., Brown, A. E., Polsky, B., et al.: Babesiosis and infection with human immunodeficiency virus (HIV). Ann. Intern. Med. *107*:944, 1987.
10. Bidwell, D. E., Turp, P., Joyner, L. P., et al.: Comparisons of serologic tests for *Babesia* in British cattle. Vet. Rec. *103*:446–449, 1978.
11. Bruckner, D. A., Garcia, L. S., Shimizu, R. Y., et al.: Babesiosis: Problems in diagnosis using autoanalyzers. Am. J. Clin. Pathol. *83*:320–321, 1985.
12. Cahill, K. M., Benach, J. L., Reich, L. M., et al.: Red cell exchange: Treatment of babesiosis in a splenectomized patient. Transfusion *21*:193–198, 1981.
13. Carson, C. A., and Phillips, R. S.: Immunologic response of the vertebrate host to *Babesia*. *In* Ristic, M., and Kreier, J. P. (eds.): Babesiosis. New York, Academic Press, 1981, pp. 411–443.
14. Centers for Disease Control: Clindamycin and quinine treatment tor *Babesia microti* infections. M. M. W. R. *32*:65–72, 1983.
15. Centers for Disease Control: Babesiosis—Connecticut. M. M. W. R. *38*:649–650, 1989.
16. Chisholm, E. S., Ruebush, T. K., II, Sulzer, A. J., et al.: *Babesia microti*

infection in man: Evaluation of an indirect immunofluorescent antibody test. Am. J. Trop. Med. Hyg. *27*:14–19, 1978.
17. Chisholm, E. S., Sulzer, A. J., and Ruebush, T. K.: Indirect immunofluorescence test for human *Babesia microti* infection: Antigenic specificity. Am. J. Trop. Med. Hyg. *35*:921–925, 1986.
18. Clark, I. A., Wills, E. J., Richmond, J. E., et al.: Immunity to intraerythrocytic protozoa. Lancet *2*:1128–1129, 1973.
19. Cullen, J. M., and Levine, J. F.: Pathology of experimental *Babesia microti* infection in the Syrian hamster. Lab. Animal Sci. *37*:640–643, 1987.
20. Dammin, G. J.: Babesiosis. *In* Weinstein, L., and Fields, B. N. (eds.): Seminars in Infectious Disease. New York, Stratton, 1978, pp. 169–199.
21. Dammin, G. J., Spielman, A., Benach, J. L., et al.: The rising incidence of clinical *Babesia microti* infection. Hum. Pathol. *12*:398–400, 1981.
22. DeVos, A. J., Dalgliesh, R. J., and Callow, L. L.: Babesia. *In* Soulsby, E. J. L. (ed.): Immune Responses in Parasitic Infections: Immunology, Immunopathology, and Immunoprophylaxis. Vol. 3. Boca Raton, CRC Press, 1987, pp. 183–222.
23. Esernio-Jenssen, D., Scimeca, P. G., Benach, J. L., et al.: Transplacental/perinatal babesiosis. J. Pediatr. *110*:570–572, 1987.
24. Filstein, M. R., Benach, J. L., White, D. J., et al.: Serosurvey for human babesiosis in New York. J. Infect. Dis. *141*:518–521, 1980.
25. Francioli, P. B., Keithly, J. S., Jones, T. C., et al.: Response of babesiosis to pentamidine therapy. Ann. Intern. Med. *94*:326–330, 1981.
26. Garnham, P. C. C.: Human babesiosis: European aspects. Trans. R. Soc. Trop. Med. Hyg. *74*:153–155, 1980.
27. Garnham, P. C. C., Donelly, J., Hoogstraal, H., et al.: Human babesiosis in Ireland: Further observations and the medical significance of this infection. Br. Med. J. *4*:768–770, 1969.
28. Gibbons, W. J.: Diseases of Cattle. 2nd ed. Wheaton, IL, Veterinary Publications, 1963, pp. 665–673.
29. Golightly, L. M., Hirschhorn, L. R., and Weller, P. F.: Fever and headache in a splenectomized woman. Rev. Infect. Dis. *11*:629–637, 1989.
30. Gordon, S., Cordon, R. A., Mazdzer, E. J., et al.: Adult respiratory distress syndrome in babesiosis. Chest *86*:633–634, 1984.
31. Grabowski, E. F., Giardina, P. J. V., Goldberg, D., et al.: Babesiosis transmitted by a transfusion of frozen-thawed blood. Ann. Intern. Med. *96*:466–467, 1982.
32. Grunwaldt, E., Barbour, A. G., and Benach, J. L.: Simultaneous occurrence of babesiosis and Lyme disease. N. Engl. J. Med. *308*:1166, 1983.
33. Healy, G.: The impact of cultural and environmental changes on the epidemiology and control of human babesiosis. Trans. R. Soc. Trop. Med. Hyg. *83*(Suppl.):35–38, 1989.
34. Healy, G. R., and Ruebush, T. K., II: Morphology of *Babesia microti* in human blood smears. Am. J. Clin. Pathol. *73*:107–109, 1980.
35. Healy, G. R., Spielman, A., and Gleason, N.: Human babesiosis: Reservoir of infection on Nantucket Island. Science *192*:479–480, 1976.
36. Healy, G. R., Walzer, P. D., and Sulzer, A. J.: A case of asymptomatic babesiosis in Georgia. Am. J. Trop. Med. Hyg. *25*:376–378, 1976.
37. Herwald, B. L., Persing, D. H., Précigont, E. A., et al.: A fatal case of babesiosis in Missouri: Identification of another piroplasm that infects humans. Ann. Intern. Med. *124*:643–650, 1996.
38. Hoare, C. A.: Comparative aspects of human babesiosis. Trans. R. Soc. Trop. Med. Hyg. *74*:143–148, 1980.
39. Hughes, W. T., and Oz, H. S.: Successful prevention and treatment of babesiosis with atovaquone. J. Infect. Dis. *172*:1042–1046, 1995.
40. Hsu, N. H., and Cross, J. H.: Serologic survey for human babesiosis on Taiwan. J. Formosan Med. Assoc. *76*:950–954, 1977.
41. Jack, R. M., and Ward, P. A.: *Babesia rodhaini* interactions with complement: Relationship to parasitic entry into red cells. J. Immunol. *124*:1566–1573, 1980.
42. Jacoby, G. A., Hunt, J. V., Kosinski, K. S., et al.: Treatment of transfusion-transmitted babesiosis by exchange transfusion. N. Engl. J. Med. *303*:1098–1100, 1980.
43. James, M. A.: Immunology of *Babesia* infections. *In* Ristic, M., Ambroise-Thomas, P., and Kreier, J. (eds.): Malaria and Babesiosis: Research Findings and Control Measures. Dordrecht, Martinus Nijhoff Publishers, 1984, pp. 53–63.
44. Johnson, R. C., Schmid, G. P., Hyde, F. W., et al.: *Borrelia burgdorferi*: Etiologic agent of Lyme disease. Int. J. Syst. Bacteriol. *34*:496–497, 1984.
45. Kakoma, I., and Ristic, M.: Pathogenesis of babesiosis. *In* Ristic, M., Ambroise-Thomas, P., and Kreier, J. (eds.): Malaria and Babesiosis: Research Findings and Control Measures. Dordrecht, Martinus Nijhoff Publishers, 1984, pp. 85–93.
46. Karakashian, S. J., Rudzinska, M. A., Spielman, A., et al.: Primary and secondary ookinetes of *Babesia microti* in the larval and nymphal stages of the tick *Ixodes dammini*. Can. J. Zool. *64*:328–339, 1986.
47. Kennedy, C. C.: Human babesiosis: Summary of a case in Ireland. Trans. R. Soc. Trop. Med. Hyg. *74*:156, 1980.
48. Krause, P. J., Telford, S. R., Ryan, R., et al.: Geographical and temporal distribution of babesial infection in Connecticut. J. Clin. Microbiol. *29*:1–4, 1991.
49. Krause, P. J., Telford, S. R., Pollack R. J., et al.: Babesiosis: An underdiagnosed disease of children. Pediatrics *89*: 1045–1048, 1992.
50. Krause, P. J., Telford, S. R., Ryan, R., et al.: Diagnosis of babesiosis: Evaluation of a serologic test for the detection of *Babesia microti* antibody. J. Infect. Dis. *169*:923–926, 1994.
51. Krause, P. J., Telford, S. R., Spielman, A., et al.: Concurrent Lyme disease and babesiosis: Evidence for increased severity and duration of illness. J. A. M. A. *275*:1657–1660, 1996.
52. Krause, P. J., Ryan, R., Telford, S. R., et al.: Efficacy of immunoglobulin M serodiagnostic test for rapid diagnosis of acute babesiosis. J. Clin. Microbiol. *34*:2014–2016, 1996.
53. Krause, P. J., Telford, S. R., Spielman, A., et al.: Comparison of PCR with blood smear and inoculation of small animals for diagnosis of *Babesia microti* parasitemia. J. Clin. Microbiol. *34*:2791–2794, 1996.
54. Leeflang, P., Oomen, J. M. V., Zwart, D., et al.: The prevalence of *Babesia* antibody in Nigerians. Int. J. Parasitol. *6*:159–161, 1976.
55. Levine, N. D: Protozoan Parasites of Domestic Animals and of Man. Minneapolis, Burgess Publishing Company, 1966, pp. 292–293.
56. Levine, N. D.: Taxonomy of the piroplasms. Trans. Am. Micros. Soc. *90*:2–33, 1971.
57. Lykins, J. D., Ristic, M., and Weisiger, R. M.: *Babesia microti*: Pathogenesis of parasite of human origin in the hamster. Exp. Parasitol. *37*:388–397, 1975.
58. Marcus, L. C., Steere, A. C., Duray, P. H., et al.: Fatal pancarditis in a patient with coexistent Lyme disease and babesiosis: Demonstration of spirochetes in the myocardium. Ann. Intern. Med. *103*:374–376, 1985.
59. Marcus, L. C., Valigorsky, J. M., Fanning, W. L., et al.: A case report of transfusion-induced babesiosis. J. A. M. A. *248*:465–467, 1982.
60. Mathewson, H. O., Anderson. A. E., and Hazard, G. W.: Self-limited babesiosis in a splenectomized child. Pediatr. Infect. Dis *3*:148–149, 1984.
61. Mather, T. N., Telford, S. R., Moore, S. I., et al.: *Borrelia burgdorferi* and *Babesia microti*: Efficiency of transmission from reservoirs to vector ticks (*Ixodes dammini*). Exp. Parasit. *70*:55–61, 1990.
62. Mather, T. N., Ribeiro, J. M. C., and Spielman, A.: Lyme disease and babesiosis: Acaridice focused on potentially infected ticks. Am. J. Trop. Med. Hyg. *36*:609–614, 1987.
63. Meeusen, E., Lloyd, S., and Soulsby, E. J. L.: *Babesia microti* in mice: Adoptive transfer of immunity with serum and cells. Aust. J. Exp. Biol. Med. Sci. *62*:551–566, 1984.
64. Meldrum, S. C., Birkhead G. S., White D. J., et al.: Human babesiosis in New York state: An epidemiological description of 136 cases. Clin. Infect. Dis. *15*: 1019–1023, 1992.
65. Miller, L. H., Neva, F. A., and Gill, F.: Failure of chloroquine in human babesiosis (*Babesia microti*): Case report and chemotherapeutic trials in hamsters. Ann. Intern. Med. *88*:200–202, 1978.
66. Montenegro-James, S.: Immunoprophylactic control of bovine babesiosis: Role of exoantigens of *Babesia*. Trans. R. Soc. Trop. Med. Hyg. *83*(Suppl.):85–94, 1989.
67. Needham, G. R.: Evaluation of five popular methods for tick removal. Pediatrics *75*:997–1002, 1985.
68. Ortiz, J. M., and Eagle, R. C., Jr.: Ocular findings in human babesiosis (Nantucket fever). Am. J. Ophthalmol. *93*:307–311, 1982.
69. Osorno, B. M., Vega, C., Ristic, M., et al.: Isolation of *Babesia* spp. from asymptomatic human beings. Vet. Parasitol. *2*:111–120, 1976.
70. Persing, D. H., Mathiesen, D., Marshall, W. F., et al.: Detection of *Babesia microti* by polymerase chain reaction. J. Clin. Microbiol. *30*:2097–2103, 1992.
71. Persing, D. H., Herwaldt, B. L., Glaser C., et al.: Infection with a *Babesia*-like organism in northern California. N. Engl. J. Med. *332*:298–303, 1995.
72. Piesman, J., Hicks, T. C., Sinsky, R. J., et al.: Simultaneous transmission of *Borrelia burgdorferi* and *Babesia microti* by individual nymphal *Ixodes dammini* ticks. J. Clin. Microbiol. *25*:2012–2013, 1987.
73. Piesman, J., and Spielman, A.: Human babesiosis on Nantucket Island: Prevalence of *Babesia microti* in ticks. Am. J. Trop. Med. Hyg. *29*:742–746, 1980.
74. Piesman, J., Spielman, A., Etkind, P., et al.: Role of deer in the epizootiology of *Babesia microti* in Massachusetts, U.S.A. J. Med. Entomol. *15*:537–540, 1979.
75. Popovsky, M. A., Lindbert, L. E., Syrek, A. L., et al.: Prevalence of *Babesia* antibody in a selected blood donor population. Transfusion *28*:59–61, 1987.
76. Quick, R. E., Herwaldt, B. L., Thomford, J. W., et al.: Babesiosis in Washington State: A new species of *Babesia*? Ann. Intern. Med. *119*:284–290, 1993.
77. Raoult, D., Soulayrol, L., Toga, B., et al.: Babesiosis, pentamidine, and cotrimoxazole. Ann. Intern. Med. *107*:944, 1987.
78. Reiter, I., and Weiland, G.: Recently developed methods for the detection of babesial infections. Trans. R. Soc. Trop. Med. Hyg. *83*(Suppl.):21–23, 1989.
79. Riek, R. F.: Babesiosis. *In* Weinman, D., and Ristic, M. (eds.): Infectious Blood Diseases of Man and Animals. Vol. 2. New York, Academic Press, 1968, pp. 219–268.
80. Rosner, F., Zarrabi, M. H., Benach, J. L., et al.: Babesiosis in splenectomized adults: Review of 22 reported cases. Am. J. Med. *76*:696–701, 1984.
81. Rudzinska, M. A.: Morphological aspects of host-cell-parasite relationships in babesiosis. *In* Ristic, M., and Kreier, J. P. (eds.): Babesiosis. Academic Press, New York, 1981, pp. 87–141.
82. Rudzinska, M. A., Spielman, A., Lewengrub, S., et al.: Sexuality in piro-

plasms as revealed by electron microscopy in *Babesia microti*. Proc. Natl. Acad. Sci. U. S. A. *80*:2966–2970, 1983.
83. Ruebush, T. K., II: Human babesiosis in North America. Trans. R. Soc. Trop. Med. Hyg. *74*:149–152, 1980.
84. Ruebush, T. K., II: Babesiosis. *In* Strickland, G. T. (ed.): Hunter's Tropical Medicine. Philadelphia, W. B. Saunders Co., 1984, pp. 608–611.
85. Ruebush, T. K., II, Cassaday, P. B., Marsh, H. J., et al.: Human babesiosis on Nantucket Island: Clinical features. Ann. Intern. Med. *86*:6–9, 1977.
86. Ruebush, T. K., II, Chisholm, E. S., Sulzer, A. J., et al.: Development and persistence of antibody in persons infected with *Babesia microti*. Am. J. Trop. Med. Hyg. *30*:291–292, 1981.
87. Ruebush, M. J., and Hanson, W. L.: Thymus dependence of resistance to infection with *Babesia microti* of human origin in mice. Am. J. Trop. Med. Hyg. *29*:507–515, 1980.
88. Ruebush, T. K., II, Juranek, D. D., Chisholm, E. S., et al.: Human babesiosis on Nantucket Island: Evidence for self-limited and subclinical infections. N. Engl. J. Med. *297*:825–827, 1977.
89. Ruebush, T. K., II, Juranek, D. D., Spielman. A., et al.: Epidemiology of human babesiosis on Nantucket Island. Am. J. Trop. Med. Hyg. *30*:937–941, 1981.
90. Ruebush, T. K., II, Piesman, J., Collins, W. E., et al.: Tick transmission of *Babesia microti* to rhesus monkeys *(Macaca mulatta)*. Am. J. Trop. Med. Hyg. *30*:555–559, 1981.
91. Ruebush, T. K., II, Rubin, R. H., Wolpow, E. R., et al.: Neurologic complications following the treatment of human *Babesia microti* infection with diminazene aceturate. Am. J. Trop. Med. Hyg. *28*:184–189, 1979.
92. Scholtens, R. G., Braff, E. H., Healy, G. R., et al.: A case of babesiosis in man in the United States. Am. J. Trop. Med. Hyg. *17*:810–813, 1968.
93. Scimeca, P.G., Weinblatt, M. E., Schonfeld, G., et al.: Babesiosis in two infants from eastern Long Island, N.Y. Am. J. Dis. Child. *140*:971, 1986.
94. Simpson, C. F.: Phagocytosis of *Babesia canis* by neutrophils in the peripheral circulation. Am. J. Vet. Res. *35*:701–704, 1974.
95. Skrabalo, A., and Deanovic, A.: Piroplasmosis in man: Report on a case. Doc. Med. Geogr. Trop. *9*:11–16, 1957.
96. Smith, R. D., Kakoma, I.: A reappraisal of vector control strategies for babesiosis. Trans. R. Soc. Trop. Med. Hyg. *83*(Suppl.):43–52, 1989.
97. Smith, R. P., Evans, A. T., Popovsky, M., et al.: Transfusion-acquired babesiosis and failure of antibiotic treatment. J. A. M. A. *256*:2726–2727, 1986.
98. Smith, T., and Kilbourne, F. L.: Investigation into the nature, causation, and prevention of southern cattle fever. U. S. Dept. Agr. Bur. Anim. Indust. Bull. *1*:1–301, 1893.
99. Spielman, A.: Human babesiosis on Nantucket Island: Transmission by nymphal *Ixodes* ticks. Am. J. Trop. Med. Hyg. *25*:784–787, 1976.
100. Spielman, A., Clifford, C. M., Piesman, J., et al.: Human babesiosis on Nantucket Island, U.S.A.: Description of the vector, *Ixodes (Ixodes) dammini*, n. sp. (Acarina: Ixodidae). J. Med. Entomol. *15*:218–234, 1979.
101. Spielman, A., Etkind, P., Piesman, J., et al.: Reservoir hosts of human babesiosis on Nantucket Island. Am. J. Trop. Med. Hyg. 30:560–565, 1981.
102. Spielman, A., Wilson, M. L., Levine. J. F., et al.: Ecology of *Ixodes dammini*-borne human babesiosis and Lyme disease. Ann. Rev. Entomol. *30*:439–460, 1985.
103. Spielman, A.: Lyme disease and human babesiosis: Evidence incriminating vector and reservoir hosts. *In* Englund, P. T., and Sher, A. (eds.): The Biology of Parasitism. New York, Alan R. Liss, 1988, pp. 147–165.
104. Steere, A. C., and Malawista, S. E.: Cases of Lyme disease in the United States: Locations correlated with distribution of *Ixodes dammini*. Ann. Intern. Med. *91*:730–733, 1979.
105. Steketee, R. W., Eckman, M. R., Burgess, E. C., et al.: Babesiosis in Wisconsin: A new focus of disease transmission. J. A. M. A. *253*:2675–2678, 1985.
106. Sun, T., Tenenbaum, M. J., Greenspan, J., et al.: Morphologic and clinical observations in human infection with *Babesia microti*. J. Infect. Dis. *148*:239–248, 1983.
107. Telford, S. R., Mather T. N., Adler G. H., et al.: Short-tailed shrews as resevoirs of the agent of Lyme disease and human babesiosis. J. Parasitol. *76*:681–683, 1990.
108. Telford, S. R., Gorenflot, A. Brasseur P., et al.: Babesial infections in man and wildlife. *In* Kreirer, J. P., and Baker, J. R. (eds.): Parasitic Protozoa. 2nd ed. San Diego, Academic Press, 1991.
109. Todorovic, R. A., and Carson, C. A.: Methods for measuring the immunological response to *Babesia*. *In* Ristic, M., and Kreier, J. P. (eds.): Babesiosis. New York, Academic Press, 1981, pp. 381–410.
110. William, H.: Human babesiosis. Trans. R. Soc. Trop. Med. Hyg. *74*:157, 1980.
111. Wittner, M., Rowin, K. S., Tanowitz, H. B., et al.: Successful chemotherapy of transfusion babesiosis. Ann. Intern. Med. *96*:601–604, 1982.
112. Wolf, R. E.: Effects of antilymphocyte serum and splenectomy on resistance to *Babesia microti* infection in hamsters. Clin. Immunol. Immunopathol. *2*:381–394, 1974.
113. Wright, I. G., Goodger, B. V., Buffington, G. D., et al.: Immunopathophysiology of babesial infections. Trans. R. Soc. Trop. Med. Hyg. *83*(Suppl.):11–13, 1989.
114. Wright, I. G., and Mahoney, D. F.: The activation of kallikrein in acute *Babesia argentina* infections of splenectomized calves. Z. Parasitenkd. *43*:271–278, 1974.
115. Wright, I. G., Mirre, G. B., Rode-Bramanis, K., et al.: Protective vaccination against virulent *Babesia bovis* with a low-molecular-weight antigen. Infect. Immun. *48*:109–113, 1985.

217

MALARIA*

Coy D. Fitch

Malaria is a febrile disease caused by the asexual reproduction of protozoan parasites in erythrocytes. Its characteristic chills and fever have been known since antiquity.[34, 63] An effective antimalarial agent (cinchona bark) was introduced into Europe from South America by the Jesuits more than three centuries ago,[47] and an outline of the life cycle of the parasites in humans and mosquitoes was completed several decades ago.[132] Yet despite this knowledge and determined efforts to eradicate the disease by mosquito control and other measures, malaria not only persists but has re-emerged in some countries in which it previously had been under control.[26, 75] It is a real threat to at least 40 per cent of the world's population and is a major cause of infant death. Most of the deaths occur in children between 1 and 5 years of age.[9, 65, 151]

Editors' Note: We appreciate the contributions to this chapter and the editorial assistance of Dr. Philip R. Fischer, Associate Chief, Division of General Pediatrics, Department of Pediatrics, University of Utah School of Medicine, Salt Lake City.

The modern history of malaria began late in the nineteenth century as the parasites were identified and their complicated life cycle (Fig. 217–1) was appreciated.[94] Malaria parasites were discovered in human erythrocytes in 1880 by Laveran, a military physician working in Constantine, Algeria. Early descriptions of these parasites are recorded in monographs by Laveran,[80] Marchiafava and Bignami,[95] and Mannaberg.[93] Laveran observed both the asexual forms (merozoites, trophozoites, schizonts) and gametocytes, and he witnessed exflagellation of the microgametocyte to produce microgametes (spermatozoa). The significance of exflagellation was not appreciated, however, until MacCallum,[88] while a medical student in 1897 at Johns Hopkins University, observed fertilization of the macrogamete to form a zygote.

We now know that fertilization occurs in the stomach of the mosquito within a few minutes after ingestion of a blood meal containing gametocytes and that the zygote develops into a motile ookinete, which penetrates an intestinal cell to form an oocyst. When the oocyst matures, it ruptures and

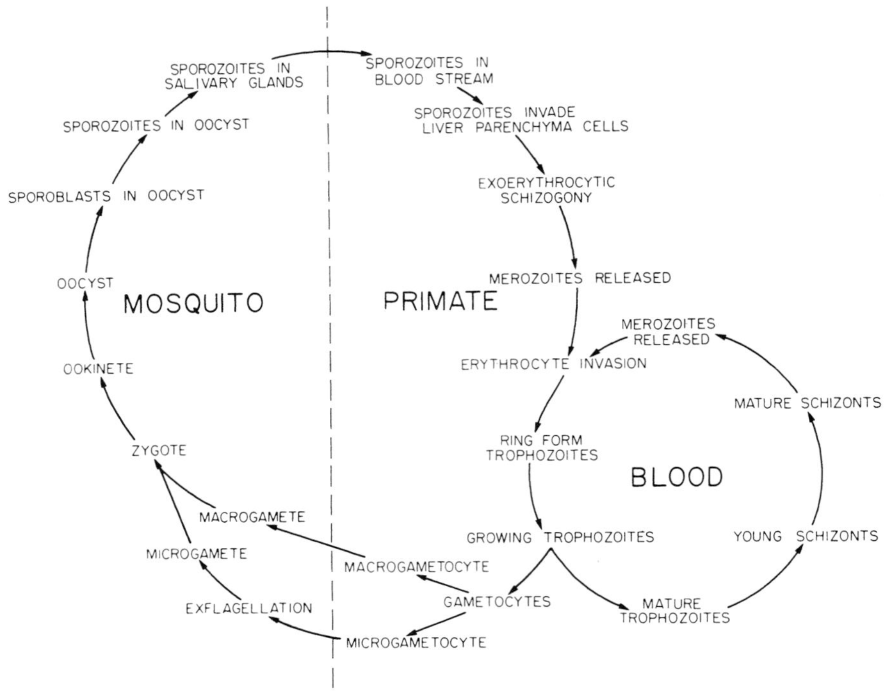

FIGURE 217–1. *Life cycle of malaria parasites. (From Coatney, G. R., Collins, W. E., Warren, M., et al.: The Primate Malarias. Bethesda, MD, U.S. Department of Health and Human Services, National Institutes of Health, National Institute of Allergy and Infectious Diseases, 1971.)*

releases its progeny of sporozoites to migrate to the salivary glands of the mosquitoes, whence they can be injected into people. Ross, another military physician, first observed the oocysts of *Plasmodium falciparum* in the stomach wall of anopheline mosquitoes in India in 1897.[123, 124]

The outline of the life cycle finally was completed in 1948 when Shortt and Garnham[132] announced the discovery of exoerythrocytic parasites in the liver of monkeys infected with *Plasmodium cynomolgi,* a malaria parasite of nonhuman primates. Exoerythrocytic schizogony subsequently has been observed for each of the malaria parasites of humans.[34, 63]

It is no accident that the two people who have won Nobel prizes for work on malaria, Laveran and Ross, were military physicians. Malaria always has been and remains a threat to the military. In the twentieth century, the necessity for coping with malaria during wartime spurred malaria research in general and, in particular, the search for new antimalarial drugs. Thus, when Germany was denied quinine in World War I, a search for synthetic antimalarial drugs eventually led to the use of chloroquine, the keystone of modern antimalarial therapy.[33, 65] Much of the research on malaria in recent years was stimulated by the realization that chloroquine resistance in *P. falciparum* is becoming widespread.[104, 149, 155] In order to find alternatives to quinine and chloroquine, hundreds of thousands of compounds have been screened for antimalarial activity in the current United States Army program, which has given us mefloquine,[8, 140] as well as other potentially useful drugs.[21, 72] Extensive research to produce a vaccine to prevent malaria also is in progress.[71, 107]

THE MALARIA PARASITES OF HUMANS

Four species of malaria parasites belonging to the genus *Plasmodium* commonly are responsible for disease in humans: *P. falciparum, P. vivax, P. malariae,* and *P. ovale.* The morphologic characteristics of these parasites in various stages of development in erythrocytes are shown and discussed later in connection with the diagnosis of malaria. Detailed descriptions of the parasites and discussions of their taxonomy and evolution are given by Garnham,[63] by Coatney and associates,[34] and by Escalante and associates.[53]

In addition to the four species commonly found in humans, approximately another 100 species of malaria parasites have been identified in other animals.[63] Some of the species infecting nonhuman primates are transmissible to humans by mosquitoes,[37] and there is one report of a naturally acquired human infection with *P. knowlesi,*[28] a parasite of nonhuman primates. Likewise, certain nonhuman primates can be infected with the malaria parasites of humans. The chimpanzee is a natural host for *P. malariae*[63]; another nonhuman primate, the owl monkey (*Aotus trivirgatus*), has been used extensively since 1967 as an experimental host for human malaria parasites.[64, 128] The risk of nonhuman primates serving as reservoirs of malaria generally is assumed to be small but, nevertheless, real.

The four species of malaria parasites infecting people are similar enough to be considered as a group for a discussion of their biologic characteristics. In each, human infection is initiated by injection of sporozoites from the bite of an infected anopheline mosquito.[34, 63] These sporozoites fail to recognize erythrocytes and, within a few minutes, preferentially select liver parenchymal cells for infection. In the liver, nuclear division occurs as the exoerythrocytic schizont develops. Eventually, thousands of merozoites are produced.[18] At maturity, the exoerythrocytic schizont ruptures to release these merozoites, which now are capable of infecting erythrocytes. The length of time required for exoerythrocytic schizogony usually is on the order of 1 to 3 weeks, but it may be prolonged to several months in some strains of *P. vivax.* Furthermore, the exoerythrocytic stages of *P. vivax* and *P. ovale,* but not of *P. falciparum,* may persist for months or years and can be responsible for relapses long after the erythrocytic stages have been eradicated by the host response or by treatment with antimalarial drugs. Whether the exoerythrocytic stages of *P. malariae* persist in the liver after the initial cycle still is uncertain.[34] Descriptions of exoerythrocytic schizogony may be found in a review by Bray[18] and in books by Garnham[63] and by Coatney and associates.[34]

The extracellular merozoite initiates an infection by recognizing and attaching to the erythrocyte surface. There is evidence that this process involves an interaction between lectin-like polypeptides belonging to the parasite and erythrocyte receptors.[67, 102] A requirement for an interaction between specific surface molecules probably explains why merozoites recognize and infect only erythrocytes and why some parasites, such as *P. vivax,* are obligate parasites of immature erythrocytes.[34, 63] After initial contact is made between the apical end of the parasite and the erythrocyte[12, 49, 91, 133] and after ligands and other materials are released from paired organelles (rhoptrics) and small dense bodies (micronemes and microspheres), there is widespread deformation of the erythrocyte surface, and a process of invagination begins that eventually engulfs the parasite.[49] As the process of entry is completed, the surface coat is lost and the parasite is enclosed in a parasitophorous vacuole, the membrane of which contains the lipids but not the protein cytoskeleton of the host erythrocyte.[12, 147] Although the molecular details of the process of attachment and engulfment of the parasite are unknown, clearly it is specific and highly specialized.

After the merozoite enters the erythrocyte and begins to develop, it is called a trophozoite until nuclear division begins; thereafter, it is called a schizont. Besides the nucleus, the trophozoite possesses the intracellular organelles needed for growth and reproduction, including rough and smooth endoplasmic reticulum, ribosomes, a poorly developed Golgi apparatus, and an organelle with a double membrane that is thought to be analogous to a mitochondrion.[1] In addition, there is a cytostome, through which the parasite ingests host cytoplasm by a process that involves the formation of acidic vesicles (food vacuoles). These vacuoles contain a cysteine protease with an acidic pH optimum and the ability to digest hemoglobin and release amino acids required by the parasite for growth and development.[111] Hemoglobin digestion, however, also releases ferriprotoporphyrin IX (heme), which is toxic to the parasite. To avoid toxicity, the parasite polymerizes ferriprotoporphyrin IX to form an insoluble, dark-brown pigment (hemozoin) and stores it in the food vacuole.[31, 111, 135] This pigment is a visible product of metabolism that eventually is dumped into the circulation when the host erythrocyte ruptures.

Most of the energy of the parasite is derived from anaerobic glycolysis,[143] and most of the other metabolic requirements apparently are supplied by host cytoplasm. Some nutrients, however, including para-aminobenzoic acid,[11, 92] certain vitamins, and a few amino acids, may be obtained from the circulation of the host. As culture systems for malaria parasites are perfected, it should be possible to define these requirements more accurately.[68, 139] For obtaining nutrients from outside the erythrocyte, it has been proposed that malaria parasites open "metabolic windows" in the erythrocyte membrane.[17, 52] Parasitized erythrocytes incorporate parasite antigens into the host membrane, and they exhibit prominent membrane changes that could provide a structural basis for metabolic windows. These changes include caveola-vesicle complexes along the erythrocyte membrane[2] and excrescences on the erythrocyte surface.[1]

At the completion of schizogony, the erythrocyte ruptures and releases its contents, including merozoites, malaria pigment, and other material that has accumulated during schizogony. The merozoites now infect other erythrocytes to repeat the cycle. When enough erythrocytes become infected to permit detection on blood films, the infection is said to be patent. Erythrocytic schizogony requires approximately 48 hours for *P. falciparum, P. vivax,* and *P. ovale* and 72 hours for *P. malariae.* After one or more erythrocytic cycles, some of the merozoites develop into micro- and macrogametocytes.[34, 63] The nature of the signal for differentiation into sexual forms is not known.

TRANSMISSION

Malaria is transmitted from person to person in nature through the interposition of a female anopheline mosquito, which serves as the vector and host for sexual reproduction of the parasite.[88, 123] Hybridization of parasites of the same species can and does occur during the process of fertilization in the stomach of the mosquito.[145] After fertilization, the zygote develops into a motile ookinete that encysts in the midgut of the mosquito and undergoes meiotic division.[13] Then, as the oocyst develops, there is repeated mitotic division to produce sporoblasts (sporogony). At maturity, the oocyst may contain as many as 10,000 haploid sporozoites, each one of which presumably is capable of initiating an infection.[118] The length of sporogony varies, depending on the species of malaria parasite, the mosquito, and the environmental conditions, such as temperature and humidity, but it is on the order of a week or two.[34, 63] For completion of the cycle illustrated in Figure 217–1, the oocyst ruptures and the sporozoites find their way to the salivary glands, after which they can be injected into people by the bite of the mosquito.

Malaria can be transmitted directly from one person to another by the passage of blood containing erythrocytic parasites. In this case, the sexual part of the life cycle, as well as exoerythrocytic schizogony, is bypassed. Direct transmission of malaria thus may occur accidentally with blood transfusion and with the sharing of contaminated paraphernalia used for the injection of drugs by addicts. Direct transmission of malaria by passage of blood across the placenta also occurs and should be considered as the possible etiology of fever in any infant whose mother has a history of exposure to malaria.[3, 38] The placenta is a site relatively privileged for erythrocytic schizogony, especially of *P. falciparum.*[84, 85]

Because of the modes of transmission of malaria, patients with the disease do not require isolation from other people. Precautions should be taken, however, to prevent exposure to mosquitoes and to preclude the passage of infected blood. In particular, prospective blood donors should be asked if they have a history of malaria or of exposure to malaria. The problem of transfusion malaria has been reviewed comprehensively by Bruce-Chwatt.[20]

The geographic distribution and certain other characteristics of more than 50 species of anopheline mosquitoes known to serve as vectors of malaria have been tabulated by Young.[154] In the United States, *Anopheles freeborni,* which is prevalent in the western states, and *Anopheles quadrimaculatus,* which is prevalent in the eastern states, are known to be good vectors of malaria. Other potential vectors are distributed widely throughout the temperate and tropical areas of the world. Fortunately, the presence of a vector is not sufficient to perpetuate malaria. With urbanization and deliberate attempts to control mosquito populations, malaria has receded from most temperate zones.

EPIDEMIOLOGY

It is estimated that there are 300 to 500 million malarial infections annually.[9] *P. falciparum* and *P. vivax* are the most prevalent species of malaria parasites in humans and are distributed widely in Southeast Asia, Africa, and Central and South America. *P. malariae* is less prevalent than *P. vivax* or

P. falciparum, although it commonly is found in Southeast Asia and tropical Africa and occasionally in other areas. *P. ovale* occurs in tropical Africa, most commonly on the west coast. Other than in Central America and in parts of the Middle East, chloroquine-resistant *P. falciparum* is present almost everywhere malaria is transmitted.[25] Chloroquine-resistant strains of *P. vivax* also have been identified. For the international traveler, the World Health Organization periodically publishes in the *Weekly Epidemiological Record* a country-by-country listing of the risk of malaria. Current information on malaria in the United States may be found in the *Morbidity and Mortality Weekly Report* and the *Malaria Surveillance Annual Summary* published by the Centers for Disease Control and Prevention. Although rare, transmission of malaria can occur outside of endemic areas. Of interest, malaria has been transmitted in suburban and urban areas of the United States.[82]

PATHOGENESIS AND PATHOLOGY

During erythrocytic schizogony, the peripheral circulation receives malaria pigment and other parasite byproducts as well as erythrocyte membranes and intracellular contents. Malaria pigment itself may be toxic, and it serves as a conspicuous marker of the release of foreign products.

Macrophages in the circulation and throughout the reticuloendothelial system take up the pigment, causing a leaden-gray staining of most tissues and organs of the body. Except for malaria pigment, the putative toxins introduced into the circulation by schizogony are not well characterized. Purified malaria pigment has been shown to release tumor necrosis factor, other cytokines, and presumably other pyrogens from macrophages,[115, 131] and it is reasonable to suppose that other malaria products could do likewise. Furthermore, some of these products apparently activate the coagulation cascade[42] and cause diffuse intravascular coagulation, which may contribute to the pathology and morbidity of malaria. A detailed description of the pathogenesis of malaria has been published by White and Ho.[150] Detailed descriptions of the pathology of malaria have been described by Maegraith[90] and by Edington and Gilles.[51]

Although it is probable that malaria pigment and possibly other toxins released during schizogeny account for the common, nonfatal, febrile illness characteristic of malaria, additional pathophysiologic mechanisms are involved in the severe morbidity and mortality produced by *P. falciparum*. When these parasites infect erythrocytes, the infected cells attract uninfected erythrocytes to aggregate around them in rosettes, and they also adhere to venular endothelium.[117, 150] As a result, small vessels in the brain and other tissues may become occluded. Presumably, it is the plugging of venules that largely is responsible for severe and fatal disease. The biochemical basis for the rosetting and cytoadherence induced by *P. falciparum* is under intensive investigation. Upregulation of intercellular molecular adhesion molecules may be involved.[117]

One of the severe illnesses caused by *P. falciparum* is cerebral malaria.[96, 127, 150] In this illness, the brain has a gray color from the malaria pigment, and it may be edematous and hyperemic. Small petechial hemorrhages are scattered through the white matter and may extend into the spinal cord. On microscopic examination, many of the small and medium vessels are filled with parasitized erythrocytes, and fibrin clot may be present. There may be a cellular reaction in the perivascular spaces involving glial cells and sometimes lymphocytes and plasma cells. In addition, there may be extensive perivascular hemorrhage. Vascular involvement is not limited to the brain but may be found in the heart, gastrointestinal tract, or anywhere else in the body[150] and may be responsible for diverse clinical presentations of malaria.

Because schizogony causes the destruction of erythrocytes, anemia is an expected feature of malaria. The severity of the anemia, however, may be out of proportion to the degree of parasitemia, indicating an abnormality of erythrocytes other than those hosting parasites.[156] It is possible that a malarial toxin causes malfunction of erythrocytes. In addition, dyserythropoiesis occurs in some patients with malaria and may contribute to the anemia.[150] The role of autoantibodies to erythocytes in causing the anemia is unclear.

A special subcategory of the hemolytic anemia of malaria is blackwater fever. This is one of the pernicious forms of malaria due to *P. falciparum.* It is characterized by massive intravascular hemolysis, hemoglobinuria, acute renal failure due to tubular necrosis, and high mortality. There long has been a suspicion that treatment with quinine may provoke blackwater fever.[51] Mefloquine and halofantrine also may provoke intravascular hemolysis.[141]

In addition to developing anemia, patients who die of malaria always show prominent changes in the reticuloendothelial system, and they may have involvement of any organ system. The spleen is enlarged, congested, and pigmented and occasionally ruptures. In it, there are parasites in abundance in macrophages; phagocytosis of erythrocytes, both infected and uninfected, is common. With chronic malaria, reticular hyperplasia with a vast increase in macrophages occurs. Of particular interest is the tropical splenomegaly syndrome or hyperreactive malarial splenomegaly[150] in chronic malaria. It is associated with high serum levels of IgM and malarial antibodies and probably represents an unusual immunologic response to chronic malaria.[142] Rearrangements of the immunoglobulin gene may occur in certain hyperreactive malarial splenomegaly patients, raising the possibility that clonal lymphoproliferation in these patients may evolve into a malignant lymphoproliferative disorder.[16]

The liver also enlarges in patients with malaria, and the Kupffer cells, like other cells in the reticuloendothelial system, participate in the phagocytic response. Consequently, the liver is chocolate-red to slate-gray or black. With chronic malaria, there is diffuse periportal infiltration with mononuclear cells, which progresses with repeated attacks of malaria. Hepatomegaly with mononuclear cell infiltration is part of the tropical splenomegaly syndrome. Centrilobular necrosis occurs in those patients who have been in shock.

In addition to being stained with malaria pigment, the kidney may be involved with either of two pathologic processes: acute tubular necrosis[134] or an immune complex, membranoproliferative glomerulonephritis.[73, 142] Acute tubular necrosis may occur in association with the massive hemolysis and hemoglobinuria of blackwater fever, but it also may occur in the absence of hemolysis, apparently from reduction in blood flow due to hypovolemia and hyperviscosity of the blood.[134, 137] Glomerulonephritis occurs both with *P. falciparum* and with *P. malariae* infections. *P. falciparum* produces only a transient nephritis. *P. malariae* may cause chronic glomerulonephritis and the nephrotic syndrome.

Many of the later consequences of malaria can be attributed to the immune response mounted by the host.[7, 142] This response includes autoantibodies as well as antibodies to parasite antigens. Concentrations of IgG and IgM especially are high in patients from areas where malaria is prevalent and there is a high incidence of rheumatoid factor–like antiglobulins, antinuclear antibodies, heterophile antibodies, and antibodies to autologous erythrocytes. The occurrence of these antibodies is accompanied by a decrease in serum complement concentrations. As previously mentioned, this immune response plays a role in the anemia, hyperreactive malarial splenomegaly (tropical splenomegaly syndrome), hepatomegaly, and renal disease associated with malaria. Immunosuppression also occurs with malaria[98] and has led to the hypothesis that malaria may predispose its victims to other diseases, such as Burkitt lymphoma.[23, 105]

CLINICAL MANIFESTATIONS

The early symptoms of malaria coincide with the maturation and rupture of erythrocytic schizonts. Exoerythrocytic schizogony does not produce symptoms. If there is only one brood of parasites developing synchronously in the blood, the patient has paroxysms of chills and fever with characteristic periodicities of 48 hours (tertian) for *P. vivax, P. ovale,* and *P. falciparum* and of 72 hours (quartan) for *P. malariae.* Unfortunately, early in the course of the infections, when the diagnosis should be made, there may be more than one brood of parasites developing asynchronously, and fever may occur daily (quotidian). Indeed, almost any type of fever pattern is possible, particularly with *P. falciparum* infections, and the physician should not wait for a characteristic pattern before considering the diagnosis of malaria.

The various clinical forms that malaria takes are well described in case reports in the monograph by Marchiafava and Bignami.[95] A more recent, detailed discussion of the clinical manifestations of malaria by Young[154] serves as the basis for the following description of the malarial attack.

The typical attack starts with a chill of a few minutes to an hour in duration and is accompanied by tachycardia and often by nausea, vomiting, and frequent micturition. Within the hour, the temperature rises to 40° to 41.1° C (104° to 106° F), ending the chill with a feeling of warmth that soon becomes intense heat. By this time, a severe headache usually is present, and there may be mild delirium, epigastric discomfort, and more nausea and vomiting. A profuse diaphoresis then follows as the fever subsides. Now the patient may sleep. Upon awakening, the patient may feel well, except for being tired. The diaphoretic stage lasts 2 to 3 hours, and the total duration of the paroxysm is on the order of 10 hours. Such a typical paroxysm of chills and fever is more apt to occur with *P. vivax* or *P. ovale* infection than with *P. falciparum* or *P. malariae* infection.

In association with the chills and fever, there may be postural hypotension, herpes labialis, anemia, hepatosplenomegaly, jaundice, hypoglycemia, and laboratory evidence of liver disease. During a paroxysm, leukocytosis may occur. Between paroxysms, leukopenia is the rule, and thrombocytopenia is common.

The disease produced by *P. vivax* and *P. ovale* is self-limited, with parasitemia lasting from several days to 3 months after the initial attack. This persistent parasitemia is responsible for short-term relapses (recrudescences) of malaria. Without appropriate treatment, exoerythrocytic parasites persist in liver parenchymal cells and may be responsible for long-term relapses (recurrences) at intervals varying from a few weeks to 9 months. Relapses of *P. vivax* may occur for as long as 3 or 4 years. *P. ovale* produces a milder disease, and relapses occur less often and rarely for more than a year. *P. malariae* likewise causes a relatively mild disease, except for the nephropathy, but is notable for its ability to persist for many years, perhaps as long as 50 years, apparently as an erythrocytic infection.[34]

Outside of endemic areas, congenital malaria may present with fever, anemia, and splenomegaly during the first months of life, and diagnosis sometimes is delayed.[74] In endemic areas, it is difficult to differentiate congenitally acquired malaria from mosquito-acquired malaria in children after the first 10 days of life, but as many as 29 per cent of newborns have been found to be parasitemic at birth.[81] Congenital malaria has been associated with fever and death during the first days of life.[108]

In contrast to infections with the other three species, a *P. falciparum* infection in a nonimmune patient always should be considered a life-threatening disease. This parasite can reach very high densities in the circulation, and because there may be little pattern to the fever and chills it provokes, it may be mistaken for influenza or a variety of other infectious diseases. If not treated promptly, patients with *P. falciparum* infection may deteriorate within a matter of hours and die.[43, 95, 154] Patients may experience severe delirium, coma, extreme hyperpyrexia, or convulsions (cerebral malaria); hemoglobinuria and acute renal failure (blackwater fever); hepatic failure (bilious remittent fever); extensive vascular involvement of the gastrointestinal tract accompanied by nausea, vomiting, acute diarrhea, and profound prostration (algid malaria); or an acute respiratory distress syndrome.[19]

The mortality rate for these pernicious forms of *P. falciparum* malaria may be as high as 50 per cent. If the disease is recognized and treated appropriately early in its course, the mortality rate is less that 0.5 per cent.[146] The exoerythrocytic states of *P. falciparum* do not persist in the liver, so there is no true recurrences of this disease; there may be recrudescences, however, because low-grade erythrocytic infections may persist for as long as 3 months.[34]

DIAGNOSIS

Because the characteristic periodicity of chills and fever may not be present at the beginning of the first attack of malaria in the nonimmune patient, malaria may mimic other febrile diseases.[10, 62, 69, 77, 119, 146, 153] Consequently, malaria should be suspected whenever the patient has fever, chills, splenomegaly, anemia, respiratory distress, or a decreased level of consciousness. It should be given very careful consideration if one or more of the aforementioned signs is present and there is a positive geographic history (i.e., travel or residence in an area endemic for malaria) or if there is a history of recent blood transfusion or intravenous drug use. An algorithm to aid in the diagnosis of malaria has been prepared by Butler, Warren, and Mahmoud.[24]

In malaria-endemic areas, malaria is a common cause of fever. Laboratory confirmation of parasitemia, however, is not always readily available, and delayed diagnosis can increase the risk of a poor outcome. Thus, national policies often have advocated antimalarial therapy for all febrile children. Efforts have been made better to identify and select children who actually need antimalarial treatment on the basis of clinical presentation. During the rainy season in Niger, children with high fever of short duration without other obvious cause of the fever were most likely to have malaria.[125] In Malawi, identifying splenomegaly and pallor was helpful both in identifying children with malaria and in avoiding overtreatment of children without parasitemia.[120]

In areas where malaria is common, it also is important to be able to identify patients at risk of poor outcomes from plasmodial infection. In two studies of African children with malaria, impaired consciousness and respiratory distress at the time of presentation were independently predictive of fatal outcomes.[96, 144]

The definitive diagnosis of malaria is made by examination of thick and thin blood films. The thick film makes it possible to find parasites when they are present in small numbers, whereas the thin film is most useful for determination of the species of parasite. The thin film is prepared in the same way as for an ordinary differential white blood cell count. The thick film is prepared at approximately 10 times the thickness of the thin film by placing a drop of blood on a glass slide and spreading it over an area of approximately 1 cm by use of the corner of another slide. Giemsa is the preferred stain, but the parasites can be recognized in films stained with Wright stain. If Wright stain is to be used, the thick film should be decolorized by dipping it into distilled water.

Except for infections with *P. falciparum,* the parasitemia of malaria rarely exceeds 1 or 2 per cent, that is, infection of 1 or 2 per cent of circulating erythrocytes. With *P. falciparum* infections, the parasitemia may reach 60 per cent or more. Because the parasitemia may be low and may fluctuate, a diagnosis of malaria may require examination of blood films taken at several different times during the day or the use of a method to concentrate parasitized erythrocytes, such as selectively lysing nonparasitized erythrocytes with saponin.[113] The latter method allows detection of parasitemias as low as 0.00001 per cent. Also available is a rapid, sensitive, and accurate dipstick antigen capture assay for the diagnosis of malaria due to *P. falciparum*.[44] It is based on the fact that these parasites produce a soluble histidine-rich protein that is present in blood during parasitemia and for a few days thereafter. Another specific and sensitive diagnostic test based on the polymerase chain reaction is available but is technically more challenging than the dipstick test.[86, 110] Indirect immunofluorescence and hemagglutination tests are available and have been widely applied in epidemiologic studies.[36, 46, 152]

The appearance of malaria parasites in thin blood films is shown in Figures 217–2 through 217–5, courtesy of Coatney and associates.[34] *P. vivax* (see Fig. 217–2) usually selects a reticulocyte to infect, and, consequently, it is found in large polychromatophilic erythrocytes. The parasite first is seen as a ring trophozoite, which grows and becomes actively ameboid before it begins schizogony. The rapid movement of the trophozoite of this species is responsible for its name, *vivax.* As schizogony proceeds, pigment accumulates, and the infected erythrocyte becomes decolorized and stippled with blue-staining dots, Schüffner dots, which correspond to the caveola-vesicle complexes seen by electron microscopy.[2] These dots are of diagnostic importance, although they are not present invariably. During schizogony, as many as 24 merozoites may be produced. The usual number of merozoites per schizont is 16. The gametocytes are rounded and compact.

Except for subtle differences, the erythrocytic stages of *P. ovale* (see Fig. 217–3) have the same appearance as those of *P. vivax.* In *P. ovale* infections, the host cell not only is enlarged and marked by Schüffner dots but also frequently is oval with fimbriated edges. This group of features is an artifact associated with low humidity during preparation of the films, but it has some value as a diagnostic aid. Also, the pigment has a darker color, and there are fewer merozoites per schizont during the primary attack—8 instead of 16. It may be extremely difficult to distinguish *P. ovale* from *P. vivax,* but failure does not make a significant difference clinically because both species cause a benign tertian type of malaria and both are treated in the same way at the present. *P. ovale* is established as a separate species by the characteristics of its oocysts and exoerythrocytic schizonts and by cross-immunity studies.

P. falciparum (see Fig. 217–4) infects erythrocytes of all ages, so it often is found in erythrocytes of normal size and color. It differs from *P. vivax* and *P. ovale* by having smaller, more delicate ring forms, which may be found at the very edge of the erythrocyte as appliqué or accolé forms, and by the absence of Schüffner dots. Instead of Schüffner dots, infected erythrocytes may have a stippled appearance when appropriately stained because of the presence of blotches, known as *Maurer clefts* (not shown in the figure). During schizogony, the parasitized erythrocytes generally are sequestered from the peripheral circulation, with the result that schizonts are scarce in blood films, except in very severe infections. The number of merozoites produced by a schizont varies from 8 to 30, with the usual number being 16. The most distinctive feature of *P. falciparum* is the sausage shape of its gametocytes. They appear in the circulation approximately 10 days after the appearance of the asexual forms, whereas in the other three species, gametocytes appear at about the same time as asexual forms.

The erythrocytic stages of *P. malariae* are shown in Figure 217–5. This parasite can be distinguished from *P. vivax* and *P. ovale* because it infects mature erythrocytes and does not produce Schüffner dots. The growing trophozoite fills much of the space in the erythrocyte, and it assumes various shapes. For example, band forms, in which the trophozoite is stretched across the erythrocyte, occur with enough frequency to have some diagnostic value. On the average, 8 merozoites are produced by each schizont, with a range of 6 to 12. The merozoites are placed symmetrically in the mature schizont to give the appearance of a rosette or "daisy head." In addition to the appearance of the trophozoites and schizonts, *P. malariae* can be distinguished from *P. falciparum* by its mature gametocytes, which are round and completely fill the host cell.

INNATE AND ACQUIRED RESISTANCE

The most dramatic example of innate resistance to malaria in humans is the lack of susceptibility of West Africans and many American blacks to *P. vivax.* In fact, whenever a West African harbors a parasite resembling *P. vivax,* the parasite usually will prove to be *P. ovale.* An explanation for this high degree of resistance to *P. vivax* was provided by Miller and his associates.[101–103] They showed that the resistant individuals are negative for Duffy blood group determinants, in contrast to susceptible individuals who are Duffy blood group–positive. Furthermore, they showed in vitro that *P. vivax* and *P. knowlesi,* a parasite of nonhuman primates, invade Duffy-positive but not Duffy-negative human erythrocytes and that proteolytic digestion of Duffy-positive erythrocytes rendered them resistant to invasion. These findings indicate that a Duffy blood group determinant, or something closely linked to it, is a receptor that the merozoite must recognize before it can initiate an infection of an erythrocyte.

There also is reason to believe that certain erythrocyte cytoplasmic factors confer an innate resistance to malaria. Of this group of factors, sickle-cell anemia, beta-thalassemia, and glucose-6-phosphate dehydrogenase deficiency have received the most consideration.[4, 87, 101] Evidence suggests that the hemoglobin of these variant erythrocytes may be denatured preferentially by malaria parasites, releasing a toxic form of heme (ferriprotoporphyrin IX)[59] that has antimalarial properties.[112] These variant erythrocytes have a genetic basis, and their geographic distribution correlates well with present or past areas of endemic malaria. It is noteworthy that it is individuals who are heterozygous for these traits who have a significant advantage either because the homozygous individual has severe disease from the genetic abnormality or because resistance to malaria is not manifested in the homozygous cell.

Text continued on page 2447

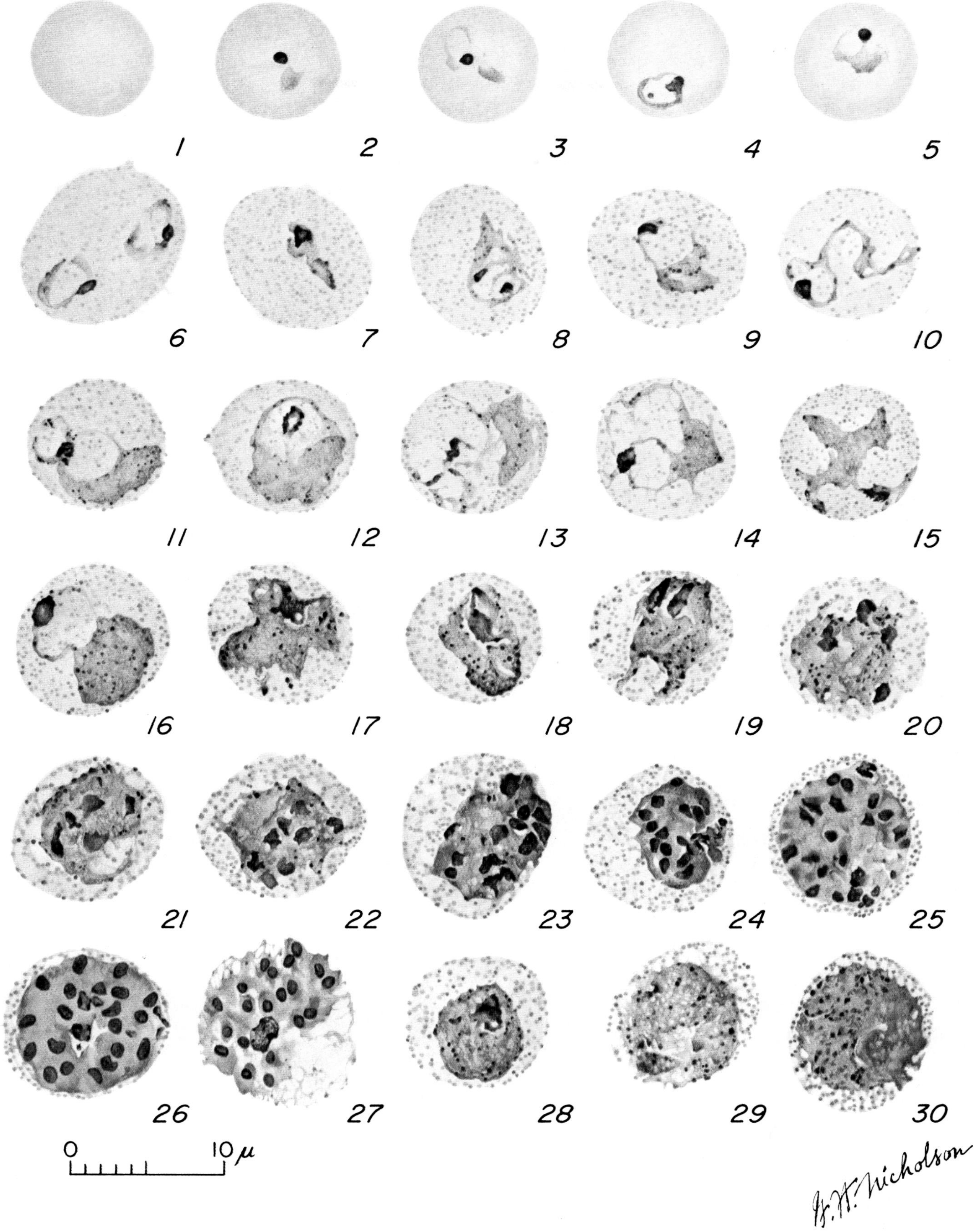

FIGURE 217–2. Plasmodium vivax. *1, Normal erythrocyte; 2–5, young trophozoites; 6–16, growing trophozoites; 17, 18, mature trophozoites; 19–21, early schizonts; 22, 23, developing schizonts; 24–27, nearly mature and mature schizonts; 28, 29, nearly mature and mature macrogametocytes; 30, mature microgametocyte. (From Coatney, G. R., Collins, W. E., Warren, M., et al.: The Primate Malarias. Bethesda, MD, U.S. Department of Health and Human Services, National Institutes of Health, National Institute of Allergy and Infectious Diseases, 1971.)*

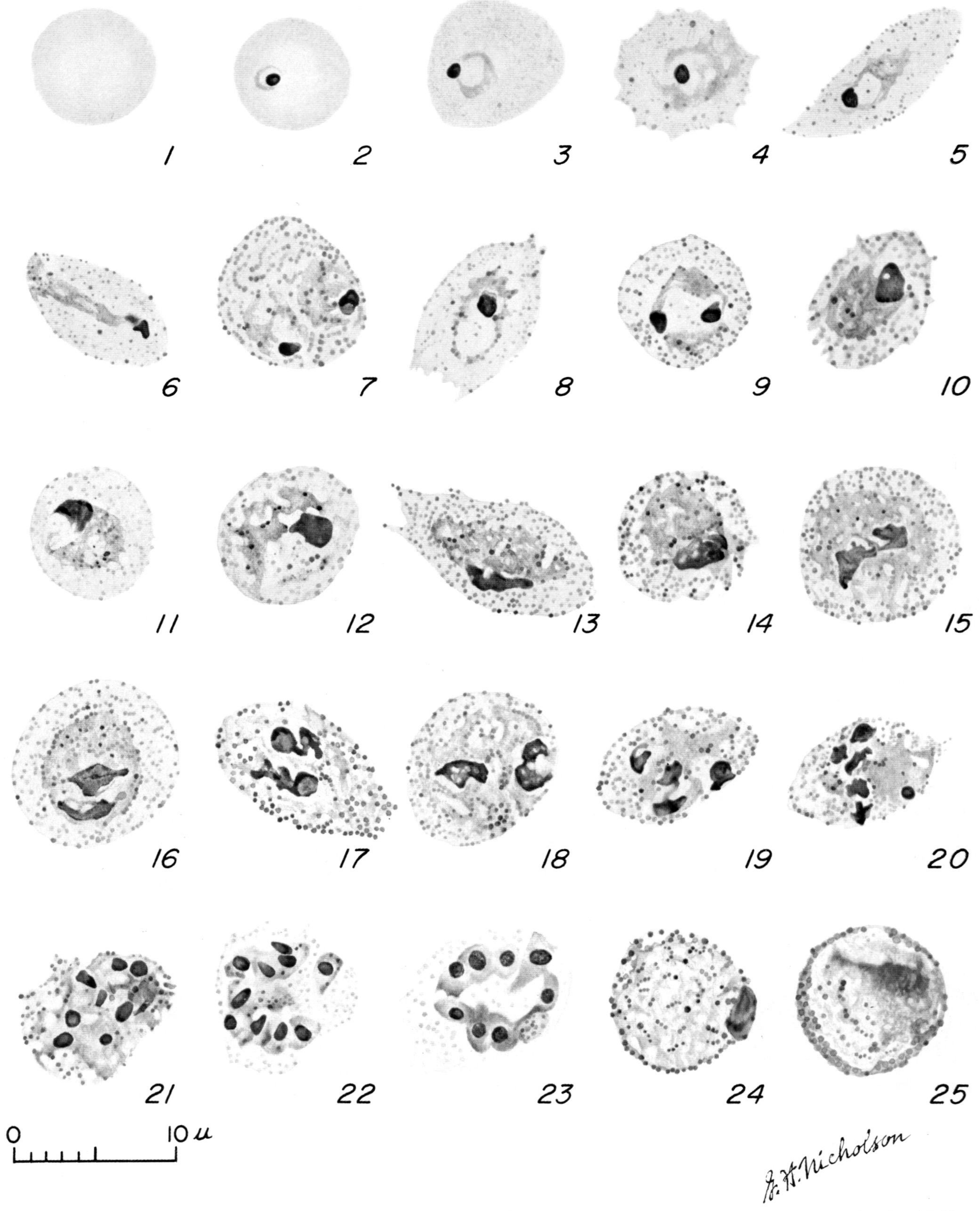

FIGURE 217–3. Plasmodium ovale. *1, Normal erythrocyte; 2–5, young trophozoites; 6–16, growing trophozoites; 13–15, mature trophozoites; 16–22, developing schizonts; 23, mature schizont; 24, adult macrogametocyte; 25, adult macrogametocyte. (From Coatney, G. R., Collins, W. E., Warren, M., et al.: The Primate Malarias. Bethesda, MD, U.S. Department of Health and Human Services, National Institutes of Health, National Institute of Allergy and Infectious Diseases, 1971.)*

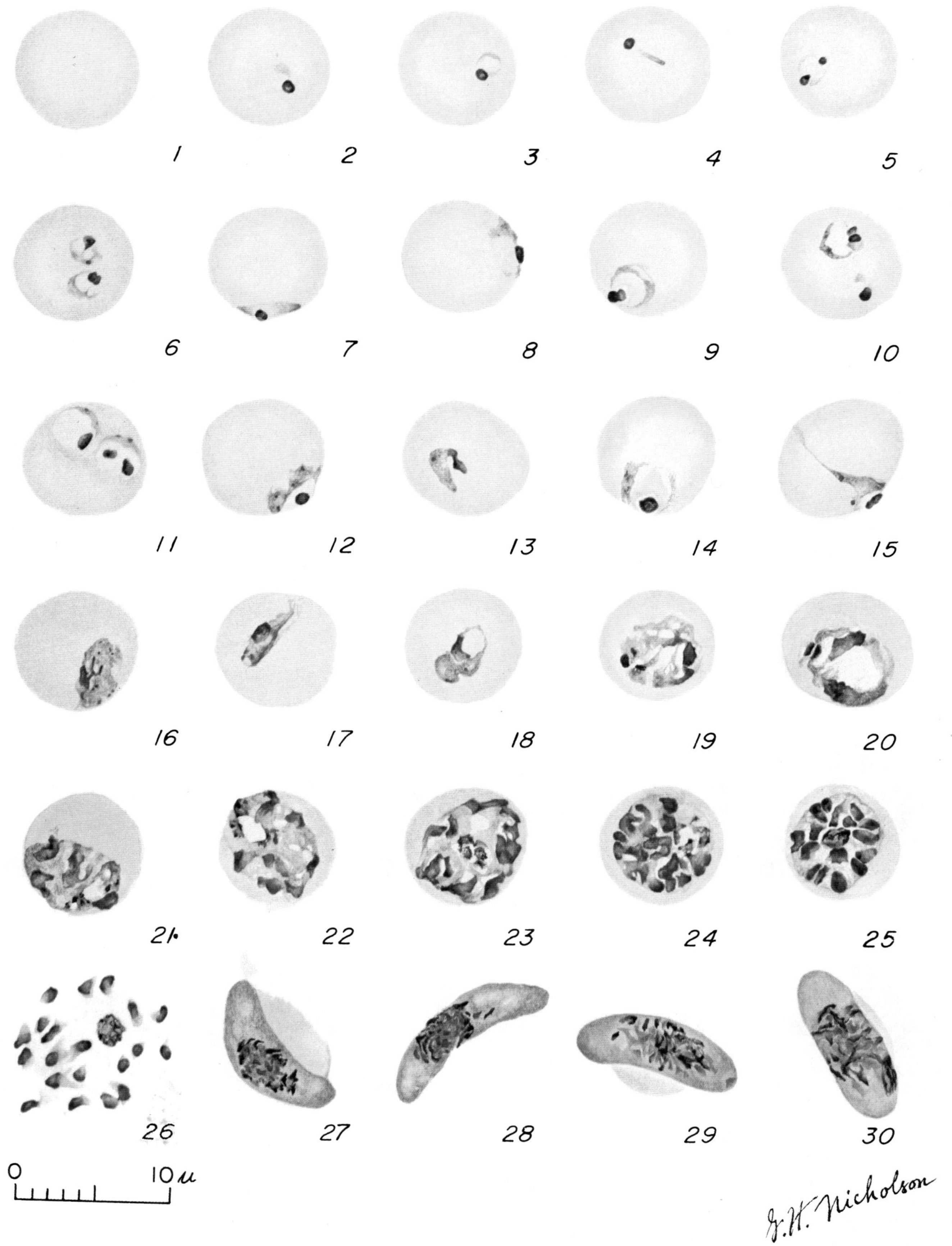

FIGURE 217–4. Plasmodium falciparum. *1, Normal erythrocyte; 2–11, young trophozoites; 12–15, growing trophozoites; 16–18, mature trophozoites; 19–22, developing schizonts; 23–26, nearly mature and mature schizonts; 27, 28, mature macrogametocytes; 29, 30, mature microgametocytes. (From Coatney, G. R., Collins, W. E., Warren, M., et al.: The Primate Malarias. Bethesda, MD, U.S. Department of Health and Human Services, National Institutes of Health, National Institute of Allergy and Infectious Diseases, 1971.)*

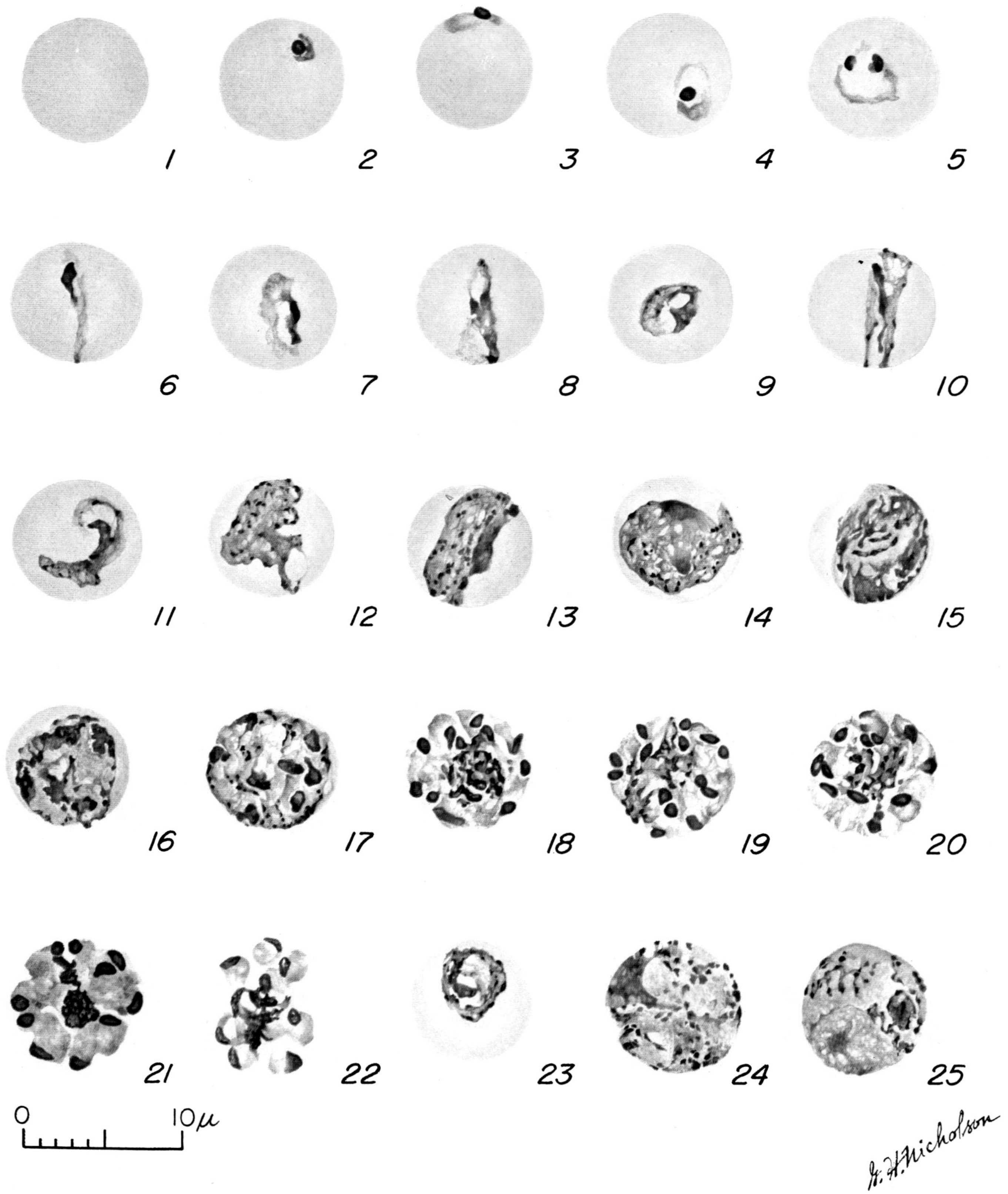

FIGURE 217–5. Plasmodium malariae. *1, Normal erythrocyte; 2–5, young trophozoites; 6–11, growing trophozoites; 12, 13, nearly mature and mature trophozoites; 14–20, developing schizonts; 21, 22, mature schizonts; 23, developing gametocyte; 24, mature macrogametocyte; 25, mature microgametocyte. (From Coatney, G. R., Collins, W. E., Warren, M., et al.: The Primate Malarias. Bethesda, MD, U.S. Department of Health and Human Services, National Institutes of Health, National Institute of Allergy and Infectious Diseases, 1971.)*

Another important participant in innate resistance to malaria is cellular immunity, which may involve the imposition of an oxidant stress by activated macrophages.[5, 32] Splenectomy will cause recrudescence of subpatent human malaria infections and often will render innately resistant animals susceptible to experimental malaria. The loss of this resistance factor must be remembered when splenectomy is necessary in patients who may be subject to malaria.

Unfortunately, there is little cross-immunity between species of malaria parasites.[99] In fact, immunity is relatively specific to the strain of infecting parasites. Thus, after a patient develops immunity to one strain of parasites, there may be partial or complete resistance to that strain, but there will be only partial protection at best from other strains of parasites of the same species. Except for *P. malariae,* there are many strains within each species. Moreover, in certain cases of malaria in animals, it is possible to demonstrate that a single strain of parasite varies its antigens to evade the immune response.[35]

Acquired resistance to malaria involves primarily the immune response. Malaria infection provokes large increases in concentrations of IgG and IgM in the blood, and some of the antibodies in these classes, probably IgG, are protective against merozoites, preventing them from invading erythrocytes. Some of the antibodies also probably promote phagocytosis of erythrocytes containing maturing schizonts.[7] Maternally derived humoral antibodies are important in protecting infants during their first few months of life.[85]

In endemic areas where children frequently are exposed to mosquitoes transmitting malaria, acquired immunity develops gradually.[29] With repeated infection, for a given level of parasitemia, clinical symptoms and signs are reduced. Eventually, asymptomatic parasitemia may be noted. Severe, potentially fatal malaria usually is confined to the first 5 years of life in these areas.[70] In areas of sporadic malaria transmission or in cases of individuals leaving endemic areas, acquired immunity is not persistent, and severe disease may be seen at any age.

Finally, it should be mentioned that the nutritional state of the host affects parasitemia. Malnutrition may suppress parasitemia, and refeeding may be associated with an increase in parasitemia.[106] Presumably, this phenomenon reflects nutritional needs of the parasite that must be supplied by the diet. In animal malarias, insufficient dietary para-aminobenzoic acid[92] and vitamin E[50] have been shown to suppress parasitemia. The apparent requirement of malaria parasites for vitamin E can be accentuated by feeding diets rich in polyunsaturated fatty acids.[83]

CHEMOTHERAPY AND CHEMOPROPHYLAXIS

Antimalarial Drugs

The drugs in current use may be divided into seven therapeutic classes: (1) quinine, quinidine, mefloquine, halofantrine, and related drugs; (2) chloroquine, amodiaquine, and other 4-amino-quinoline derivatives; (3) pyrimethamine, proguanil, and related drugs; (4) sulfonamides; (5) primaquine; (6) artemisinin and its derivatives; and (7) a miscellaneous group including certain antibiotics and experimental agents.

Drugs in the first two classes have certain features in common. They are effective as blood schizontocides, and they are gametocidal except in infections with *P. falciparum.* They are ineffective as tissue schizontocides and in the treatment of persistent exorythrocytic parasites in the liver.[116] They induce a prompt remission of the symptoms of malaria, usually eliminating fever within a day, and they compete for a common mechanism for uptake by parasitized erythrocytes.[56] Nevertheless, these two classes of drugs apparently have different modes of action. The class represented by chloroquine reduces heme polymerization to hemozoin and causes some to accumulate as ferriprotoporphyrin IX in parasitized erythrocytes, whereas the class represented by quinine does not.[31]

Because malaria parasites normally release large amounts of heme by degrading hemoglobin[111] and because ferriprotoporphyrin IX and chloroquine–ferriprotoporphyrin IX complexes are toxic for malaria parasites,[58, 60, 112] reduction of heme polymerization probably is the basis for the antimalarial action of chloroquine and other drugs in its class.[31] Current evidence indicates that ferriprotoporphyrin IX and drug–ferriprotoporphyrin IX complexes[30] may be toxic because of an interaction with membrane phospholipids[48, 59] or because they inhibit parasite proteases.[111] Mefloquine but not chloroquine binds with high affinity to phospholipids in the absence of heme.[27] This direct interaction with phospholipids may explain the superiority of mefloquine and other hydrophobic agents, such as quinine, quinidine, and halofantrine, in the treatment of chloroquine-resistant *P. falciparum* infections.[57, 72, 130]

Chloroquine resistance is associated with reduced accumulation of the drug in parasitized erythrocytes. This observation originally was made by Macomber and associates[89] in a rodent malaria due to *P. berghei* and was confirmed with the use of owl monkey erythrocytes infected with *P. falciparum.*[55] The reduced accumulation of chloroquine may be attributable in part to inaccessibility of heme[59, 61] and in part to enhanced export of chloroquine from erythrocytes infected with chloroquine-resistant parasites.[78] Verapamil and other amphipathic agents can block the enhanced export of chloroquine and thereby reverse chloroquine resistance in culture systems in vitro.[78, 97] This interesting phenomenon has not found clinical application yet, however, and there is concern that it might potentiate chloroquine toxicity for the host.

Pyrimethamine and related drugs and sulfonamides have their greatest utility in the treatment and chemoprophylaxis of chloroquine-resistant *P. falciparum.*[21, 43] Neither class approaches the ideal as an antimalarial agent for two reasons: neither relieves the symptoms of malaria very promptly, and they both rapidly induce resistance under laboratory and field conditions.[116, 129] The class of drugs represented by pyrimethamine and proguanil acts by inhibiting tetrahydrofolate dehydrogenase. The sulfonamides are metabolic antagonists of para-aminobenzoic acid in malaria parasites,[92] as in bacteria. Because these two classes of drugs show synergism when used together, they commonly are combined to treat malaria. They are effective against the erythrocytic stages of malaria but not against the exoerythrocytic stages. Malaria parasites develop resistance to pyrimethamine and related drugs by changing their tetrahydrofolate dehydrogenase; they produce more enzyme with less affinity for the drugs.[54] The mechanism of resistance to sulfonamides still is unknown.

Primaquine is an 8-aminoquinoline derivative that is effective against all stages of the malaria parasite, although toxicity precludes its use as a drug against the blood stages.[116] It is the drug of choice as a tissue schizontocide for treatment of the exoerythrocytic stages of malaria,[43, 77, 116] although its mechanism of action has not been elucidated. Resistance to primaquine has not become a problem, despite the fact that the dose required to treat some strains of *P. vivax* is twice the usual dose.[116]

Artemisinin is an experimental drug that is effective against chloroquine-resistant *P. falciparum.*[76] It is a sesquiterpene lactone bearing a peroxide group, which was isolated from *Artemisia annua L* by scientists in the People's Republic of China. A crude extract of *Artemisia annua L* has been in use in Chinese traditional medicine for 2000 years for treatment of fever.[76] Its mode of action may involve an oxidant stress.[100] Artemisinin is the first member of a presumably novel class of antimalarial drugs. Semisynthetic drugs related to artemisinin are under development.[14, 66]

Certain antibiotics, including erythromycin, tetracycline, lincomycin derivatives, and fluoroquinolines, have antimalarial activity, but they are not superior to the other drugs in our armamentarium, and they are not recommended commonly for the treatment of malaria.[21, 43]

The toxicity of the various antimalarial drugs is low. Chloroquine, quinine, halofantrine, and related drugs may cause cardiac arrhythmias, and they are more toxic for children than for adults. In addition, chloroquine may cause pruritus in black people.[109] When used chronically, chloroquine may cause retinal degeneration, but it is estimated that the total dose must exceed 100 g.[21] Quinine and quinidine cause the syndrome of cinchonism, which consists of tinnitus, headache, visual disturbances, and nausea and may include severe gastrointestinal, neurologic, and cardiovascular symptoms. Quinine and quinidine also may cause hypoglycemia. Primaquine causes oxidative hemolysis of glucose-6-phosphate dehydrogenase–deficient erythrocytes; pyrimethamine, by inhibiting the reduction of folic acid, can produce megaloblastic anemia, and the sulfonamides can cause the Stevens-Johnson syndrome or a serum sickness–like syndrome. In the doses ordinarily employed for the treatment of malaria, these toxic effects are unusual, except for the oxidative hemolysis provoked by primaquine in susceptible individuals.

Comprehensive reviews of chemotherapy and drug resistance in malaria and of the chemistry and pharmacology of antimalarial drugs are available.[21, 116, 126, 136, 138, 148]

Treatment Schedules

Unless the patient is suspected of having an infection with chloroquine-resistant parasites, the initial treatment of malaria in a nonimmune patient is the same, regardless of the species of parasite involved. Chloroquine in the form of a phosphate or sulfate salt is the drug of choice. Ordinarily, it is given in four doses spread over a 3-day period to achieve a total dose of 25 mg of the base per kilogram of body weight (a 500-mg chloroquine phosphate tablet provides approximately 300 mg of chloroquine base). The first two doses are given 6 hours apart on the first day, and a single dose is given on each of the next 2 days. The recommended total dose of chloroquine for older children and adults is 1.5 g of the base distributed as follows: 600 mg in the first dose, 300 mg 6 hours after the first dose, and 300 mg on each of the next 2 days. Amodiaquine is as effective as chloroquine on a weight basis.

If chloroquine-resistant *P. falciparum* is suspected, quinine, mefloquine, and halofantrine are the drugs of choice because of their ability to relieve the symptoms of malaria rapidly. The dose of quinine sulfate is 25 mg of the salt per kilogram of body weight daily for 7 to 10 days. The daily dose of quinine sulfate usually is divided into three parts to be taken orally after meals. For older children and adults, the maximum recommended dose of quinine sulfate is 650 mg of the salt three times daily for 7 to 10 days. The therapeutic dose of mefloquine is 15 mg of the base per kilogram of body weight as a single dose. The maximum dose of mefloquine is 1250 mg.[114] The therapeutic dose of halofantrine is 8 mg of the base per kilogram of body weight every 6 hours for three doses.[22] For nonimmune patients, halofantrine is given in the same amount again after 7 days. In addition to quinine, mefloquine, or halofantrine, pyrimethamine in combination with a sulfonamide should be used. Fansidar, a combination of 25 mg of pyrimethamine and 500 mg of sulfadoxine, is available for this purpose. For the treatment of malaria with a single dose of Fansidar, 2 to 3 tablets are recommended for adults, 2 tablets for children 9 to 14 years of age, 1 tablet for children 4 to 8 years of age, ½ tablet for children 1 to 3 years of age, and ¼ tablet for infants.

Although they are not approved for use in the United States, artemisinin and some of its derivatives are effective in the treatment of malaria due to parasites that are resistant to chloroquine and mefloquine. One of the derivatives, artesunate, is available in oral, rectal, and parenteral formulations.[14] Treatment regimens for artesunate still are being evaluated.[14] In addition, pyronaridine, an acridine derivative, has been studied in adults[122] and eventually may find a place in the treatment of chloroquine-resistant malaria.

When the patient is gravely ill and can not retain medication taken by mouth, quinine and quinidine intravenously are the drugs of choice. They are the drugs of choice even for malarial hemoglobinuria unless the patient has a prior history of blackwater fever associated with the use of quinine, in which case parenteral chloroquine may be used. Intravenous use of quinine and quinidine carries a significant risk and can be justified only in emergencies. The usual dose of quinine intravenously is 30 mg of the base per kilogram of body weight per day. For a 25-kg patient, therefore, 300 mg of quinine dihydrochloride (which provides approximately 250 mg of the base) is diluted to 200 mL or more with a dextrose-containing solution and administered as a slow intravenous drip over a period of 4 hours. This dose may be repeated at 8-hour intervals if it still is not possible to use the oral route. More aggressive therapy has been used in the intensive care unit setting.[41] The patient should be monitored for hypoglycemia, hypotension, and cardiac arrhythmias and for neurologic toxic effects, such as twitching, confusion, delirium, convulsions, and coma. If these signs occur or if clinical deterioration occurs during the infusion, it probably is best to discontinue the infusion when 5 mg of quinine base per kilogram has been given. As soon as possible, oral treatment should be started, even if it is necessary to use a stomach tube.

In addition to treatment with quinine, the various complications of malaria should be treated appropriately as they arise. For example, anticonvulsant agents should be used for the convulsions of cerebral malaria; peritoneal dialysis or hemodialysis may be required for acute renal failure.[45]

In the case of a patient with severe malaria acquired in an area where chloroquine resistance is not prevalent or if there is a history of repeated attacks of blackwater fever after treatment with quinine, chloroquine intramuscularly is the next treatment of choice. It may be given in a dose of 3.5 mg of the base per kilogram of body weight intramuscularly every 6 hours.[151] The total daily dose of chloroquine intramuscularly should not exceed 10 mg per kilogram, especially in infants and children, in whom overdosage may produce respiratory depression, cardiovascular collapse, shock, convulsions, and death. Chloroquine also may be given as a continuous infusion of 0.83 mg of the base per kilogram of body weight per hour for as long as 30 hours.[151] If there is reason to believe that blackwater fever is due to chloroquine-resistant *P. falciparum*, Fansidar should be added to the treatment regimen.

For completely eliminating the parasites of *P. vivax*, *P. ovale*, and possibly *P. malariae* from the body, that is, to achieve a radical cure, it is necessary to use a drug that is effective against the exoerythrocytic parasites in the liver. For this purpose, primaquine phosphate is the drug of choice. It is given in a daily dose of 0.3 mg of the base (or 0.5 mg of the salt) per kilogram of body weight for 14 days. For older children and adults, the dose of primaquine is 15 mg of the base (26.5 mg of the salt) daily for 14 days. Patients receiving this drug must be observed for evidence of hemolytic anemia. Primaquine is not necessary in the treatment of malaria due to *P. falciparum* because the exoerythrocytic stages of this parasite do not persist in the liver.

Chemoprophylaxis

Chloroquine continues to be the safest and probably the most effective antimalarial drug for prophylaxis, but its use will not ensure protection from chloroquine-resistant *P. falciparum*. As a prophylactic agent, chloroquine generally is used as a single weekly dose of 5 mg of the base per kilogram of body weight, not to exceed 300 mg, beginning 1 week before travel and continuing for 4 weeks after leaving the malarious area. Some authorities recommend that a single therapeutic dose of Fansidar also be available to the traveler when chloroquine prophylaxis is used. The Fansidar could be used if symptoms of malaria develop and medical help is not available immediately.[79] Because of the risk of serious toxic skin reactions from Fansidar, it no longer is used as a prophylactic agent. Mefloquine is available for travelers to areas where chloroquine resistance is prevalent. It is taken as a single weekly dose of 3 to 6 mg per kilogram of body weight not to exceed 250 mg, beginning 1 week before travel and continuing for 4 weeks after leaving the malarious area.[114] Mefloquine is not recommended for children weighing less than 15 kg, for pregnant women during the first trimester, for patients taking beta blockers, for people with a history of epilepsy or psychiatric disorders, or for people who need to have fine coordination or spatial discrimination. Another option for areas with chloroquine-resistant malaria is to use weekly chloroquine and daily proguanil (approximately 3 mg/kg). Older children also could use daily doxycycline (approximately 1.5 mg/kg in children older than 8 years of age) as chemoprophylaxis. Recommendations for malarial prophylaxis may change rapidly, and travelers to areas where malaria is endemic should seek up-to-date advice from a public health department or travel clinic. The traveler also should receive advice on how to avoid mosquito bites.

Late onset of malaria due to the exoerythrocytic development of *P. vivax* or *P. ovale* can be prevented if primaquine is added to the regimen for chemoprophylaxis.[15, 21] For this purpose, tablets containing 300 mg of chloroquine base and 45 mg of primaquine base are commercially available and may be used for older children and adults instead of chloroquine alone in the weekly regimen. Alternatively, primaquine may be administered after the individual returns from an area in which malaria is endemic, with the same 14-day schedule as for the treatment of malaria.

PREVENTION

In theory, it should be possible to interrupt the transmission of malaria either by eliminating it from the human host or the mosquito or by eliminating the mosquito.[124] Although mass chemoprophylaxis has been tried, it carries the risk of inducing drug resistance. Thus, the mainstay of the malaria eradication program sponsored by the World Health Organization has been the control of mosquito populations.[75] Despite the success of this program in controlling the disease in approximately 80 per cent of the areas in which malaria originally was endemic, it has not been possible to implement mosquito control in many tropical areas, or the measures have not been successful. Nevertheless, from the standpoint of an individual, it should be remembered that malaria can be avoided by avoiding mosquitoes. For this reason, appropriate clothing should be worn to minimize exposure of the skin to mosquitoes, outdoor activities should be minimized during the evening and night hours, insect repellents should be used, and the person should sleep in a properly screened building or under mosquito netting. The use of permethrin-impregnated bednets has been effective in decreasing childhood mortality in endemic areas, but programs to make such bednets available to the population may be prohibitively expensive.[40]

Because neither mass chemoprophylaxis nor currently available measures for mosquito control promise to eradicate malaria in the near future, the possibility of vaccination against malaria continues to attract interest.[71, 107, 121] No suitable vaccine is on the immediate horizon, but field trials of a candidate vaccine are being conducted.[6, 39] This vaccine, Spf66, seemed to be somewhat less effective in Gambian[39] than in Tanzanian[6] children.

References

1. Aikawa, M.: *Plasmodium*: The fine structure of malaria parasites. Exp. Parasitol. *30*:284–320, 1971.
2. Aikawa, M., Miller, L. H., and Rabbege, J.: Caveola-vesicle complexes in the plasmalemma of erythrocytes infected by *Plasmodium vivax* and *P. cynomolgi*. Am. J. Pathol. *79*:285–294, 1975.
3. Akindele, J. A., Sowunmi, A., and Abohweyere, A. E.: Congenital malaria in a hyperendemic area: A preliminary study. Ann. Trop. Ped. *13*:273–276, 1993.
4. Allison, A. C.: Protection afforded by sickle-cell trait against subtertian malaria infection. Br. Med. J. *1*:290–294, 1954.
5. Allison, A. C., and Eugui, E. M.: The role of cell-mediated immune responses in resistance to malaria, with special reference to oxidant stress. Ann. Rev. Immunol. *1*:361–392, 1983.
6. Alonso, P. L., Smith, T., Schellenberg, J. R., et al.: Randomized trial of efficacy of Spf66 vaccine against *Plasmodium falciparum* malaria in children in southern Tanzania. Lancet *344*:1175–1181, 1994.
7. Anonymous: Developments in malaria immunology. WHO Technical Reports Series, No. 579, 1975.
8. Anonymous: Development of mefloquine as an antimalarial drug. Bull. W. H. O. *61*:169–178, 1983.
9. Anonymous: World malaria situation in 1992, Part I. Weekly Epidemiol. Rec. *69*:309-314, 1994.
10. Asch, A. J.: Malaria at the Hospital for Sick Children, Toronto. Can. Med. Assoc. J. *115*:405–406, 1976.
11. Ball, E. G., Anfinsen, C. B., Geiman, Q. M., et al.: In vitro growth and multiplication of the malaria parasite, *Plasmodium knowlesi*. Science *101*:542–544, 1945.
12. Bannister, L. H., and Dlazewski, A. R.: The ultrastructure of red cell invasion in malaria infections: A review. Blood Cells *16*:257–292, 1990.
13. Bano, L.: A cytological study of the early oocysts of seven species of *Plasmodium* and the occurrence of postzygotic meiosis. Parasitology *49*:559–585, 1959.
14. Barradell, L. B., and Fitton, A.: Artensunate: A review of its pharmacology and therapeutic efficacy in the treatment of malaria. Drugs *50*:714–741, 1995.
15. Barrett-Connor, E.: Chemoprophylaxis of malaria for travelers. Ann. Intern. Med. *81*:219–224, 1974.
16. Bates, I., Bedu-Addo, G., Bevan, D. H., et al.: Use of immunoglobulin rearrangements to show clonal lymphoproliferation in hyper-reactive malarial splenomegaly. Lancet *337*:505–507, 1991.
17. Bodammer, J. E., and Bahr, G. F.: The initiation of a "metabolic window" in the surface of host erythrocytes by *Plasmodium berghei* NYU-2. Lab. Invest. *28*:708–718, 1973.
18. Bray, R. S.: The exoerythrocytic phase of malaria parasites. Int. Rev. Trop. Med. *2*:41–74, 1963.
19. Brooks, M. H., Kiel, F. W., Sheehy, T. W., et al.: Acute pulmonary edema in falciparum malaria: A clinicopathological correlation. N. Engl. J. Med. *279*:732–737, 1968.
20. Bruce-Chwatt, L. J.: Transfusion malaria. Bull. W. H. O. *50*:337–346, 1974.
21. Bruce-Chwatt, L. J. (ed.): Chemotherapy of Malaria. 2nd ed. Geneva, World Health Organization, 1981.

22. Bryson, M. H., and Goa, K. L.: Halofantrine: A review of its antimalarial activity, pharmacokinetic properties and therapeutic potential. Drugs *43*:236–258, 1992.
23. Burkitt, D. P.: Etiology of Burkitt's lymphoma: An alternative hypothesis to a vectored virus. J. Natl. Cancer Inst. *42*:19–28, 1969.
24. Butler, T., Warren, K. S., and Mahmoud, A. A. F.: Algorithms in the diagnosis of exotic diseases. XIII. Malaria. J. Infect. Dis. *133*:721–726, 1976.
25. Centers for Disease Control and Prevention: Health Information for International Travel. Washington, D.C., U. S. Department of Health and Human Services, 1995.
26. Chapin, G., and Wasserstrom, R.: Agriculture production and malaria resurgence in Central America and India. Nature *293*:181–185, 1981.
27. Chevli, R., and Fitch, C. D.: The antimalarial drug mefloquine binds to membrane phospholipids. Antimicrob. Agents Chemother. *21*:581–586, 1982.
28. Chin, W., Contacos, P. G., Coatney, G. R., et al.: A naturally acquired quotidian-type malaria in man transferable to monkeys. Science *149*:865, 1965.
29. Chongsuphajaisiddhi, T.: Malaria. *In* Stanfield, P., Brueton, M., Chan, M., et al. (eds.): Diseases of Children in the Subtropics and Tropics. 4th ed. London, Edward Arnold, 1991, pp. 657–674.
30. Chou, A. C., Chevli, R., and Fitch, C. D.: Ferriprotoporphyrin IX fulfills the criteria for identification as the chloroquine receptor of malaria parasites. Biochemistry *19*:1543–1549, 1980.
31. Chou, A. C., and Fitch, C. D.: Control of heme polymerase by chloroquine and other quinoline derivatives. Biochem. Biophys. Res. Commun. *195*:422–427, 1993.
32. Clark, I. A., and Hunt, N. H.: Evidence for reactive oxygen intermediates causing hemolysis and parasite death in malaria. Infect. Immun. *39*:1–6, 1983.
33. Coatney, G. R.: Pitfalls in a discovery: The chronicle of chloroquine. Am. J. Trop. Med. Hyg. *12*:121–128, 1963.
34. Coatney, G. R., Collins, W. E., Warren, M., et al.: The Primate Malarias. Bethesda, MD, U.S. Department of Health, Education and Welfare, National Institutes of Health, National Institute of Allergy and Infectious Diseases, 1971.
35. Cohen, S., Butcher, G. A., and Mitchell, G. H.: Mechanisms of immunity to malaria. Bull. W. H. O. *50*:251–257, 1974.
36. Collins, W. E., and Skinner, J. C.: The indirect fluorescent antibody test for malaria. Am. J. Trop. Med. Hyg. *21*:690–695, 1972.
37. Contacos, P. G.: Primate malarias: Man and monkeys. J. Wildl. Dis. *6*:323–328, 1970.
38. Covell, G.: Congenital malaria. Trop. Dis. Bull. *47*:1147–1167, 1950.
39. D'Alessandro, U., Leach, A., Drakeley, C. J., et al.: Efficacy trial of malaria vaccine Spf66 in Gambian infants. Lancet *346*:462–467, 1995.
40. D'Alessandro, U., Olaleye, B. O., McGuire, W., et al.: Mortality and morbidity from malaria in Gambian children after introduction of an impregnated bednet programme. Lancet *345*:479–483, 1995.
41. Davis, T. M. E., Supanaranond, W., Pukrittayakamee, S., et al.: A safe and effective consecutive-infusion regimen for rapid quinine loading in severe falciparum malaria. J. Infect. Dis. *161*:1305–1308, 1990.
42. Dennis, L. H., Eichelberger, J. W., Inman, M. M., et al.: Depletion of coagulation factors in drug-resistant *Plasmodium falciparum* malaria. Blood *29*:713–721, 1967.
43. Desjardins, R. E., Doberstyn, E. B., and Wernsdorfer, W. H.: The treatment and prophylaxis of malaria. *In* Wernsdorfer, W. H., and McGregor, I. (eds.): Malaria: Principles and Practice. Edinburgh, Churchill Livingstone, 1988, pp. 827–864.
44. Dietze, R., Perkins, M., Boulos, M., et al.: The diagnosis of *Plasmodium falciparum* infection using a new antigen detection system. Am. J. Trop. Med. Hyg. *52*:45–49, 1995.
45. Donadio, J. V., Whelton, A., and Kazyak, L.: Quinine therapy and peritoneal dialysis in acute renal failure complicating malarial haemoglobinuria. Lancet *1*:375–379, 1968.
46. Draper, C. C., Voller, A., and Carpenter, R. G.: The epidemiologic interpretation of serologic data in malaria. Am. J. Trop. Med. Hyg. *21*:696–703, 1972.
47. Duran-Reynals, M. L.: The Fever Bark Tree: The Pageant of Quinine. Garden City, NY, Doubleday and Company, 1946.
48. Dutta, P., and Fitch, C. D.: Diverse membrane-active agents modify the hemolytic response to ferriprotoporphyrin IX. J. Pharmacol. Exp. Therap. *225*:729–734, 1983.
49. Dvorak, J. A., Miller, L. H., Whitehouse, W. C., et al.: Invasion of erythrocytes by malaria parasites. Science *187*:748–749, 1975.
50. Eaton, J. W., Eckman, J. R., Berger, E., et al.: Suppression of malaria infections by oxidant-sensitive host erythrocytes. Nature *264*:758–760, 1976.
51. Edington, G. M., and Gilles, H. M.: Pathology in the Tropics. Baltimore, Williams & Wilkins, 1969, pp. 9–31, 404–407.
52. Elford, B. C., Cowman, G. M., and Ferguson, D. J. P.: Parasite-regulated membrane transport processes and metabolic control in malaria-infected erythrocytes. Biochem. J. *308*:361–374, 1995.
53. Escalante, A. A., Barrio, E., and Ayala, F. J.: Evolutionary origin of human and primate malarias: Evidence from the circumsporozoite protein gene. Mol. Biol. Eval. *12*:616–626, 1995.
54. Ferone, R.: Dihydrofolate reductase from pyrimethamine-resistant *Plasmodium berghei*. J. Biol. Chem. *245*:850–854, 1970.
55. Fitch, C. D.: *Plasmodium falciparum* in owl monkeys: Drug resistance and chloroquine binding capacity. Science *169*:289–290, 1970.
56. Fitch, C. D.: Chloroquine resistance in malaria: Drug binding and cross resistance patterns. Proc. Helminthol. Soc. Wash. *39*:265–271, 1972.
57. Fitch, C. D.: Chloroquine-resistant *Plasmodium falciparum:* Difference in handling ^{14}C-amodiaquine and ^{14}C-chloroquine. Antimicrob. Agents Chemother. *3*:545–548, 1973.
58. Fitch, C. D.: Mode of action of antimalarial drugs. *In* Malaria and the Red Cell. London, Pitman Medical (Ciba Found. Symp. 94), 1983, pp. 222–232.
59. Fitch, C. D.: Ferriprotoporphyrin IX: Role in chloroquine susceptibility and resistance in malaria. *In* Eaton, J. W., Meshnick, S. R., and Brewer, G. J. (eds.): Malaria and the Red Cell 2. New York, Alan R. Liss, 1989, pp. 45–62.
60. Fitch, C. D., Chevli, R., Banyal, H. S., et al.: Lysis of *Plasmodium falciparum* by ferriprotoporphyrin IX and a chloroquine-ferriprotoporphyrin IX complex. Antimicrob. Agents Chemother. *21*:819–822, 1982.
61. Fitch, C. D., Chevli, R., and Gonzalez, Y.: Chloroquine accumulation by erythrocytes: A latent capability. Life Sci. *14*:2441–2446, 1974.
62. Freedman, D. O.: Imported malaria: Here to stay. Am. J. Med. *93*:239–242, 1992.
63. Garnham, P. C. C.: Malaria Parasites and Other Haemosporidia. Oxford, Blackwell Scientific Publications, 1966.
64. Geiman, Q. M., and Meagher, M. J.: Susceptibility of a New World monkey to *Plasmodium falciparum* from man. Nature *215*:437–439, 1967.
65. Gilles, H. M.: Malaria: An overview. J. Infect. *18*:11–23, 1989.
66. Gutteridge, W. E.: Antimalarial drugs currently in development. J. R. Soc. Med. *82*(Suppl. 17):63–66, 1989.
67. Hadley, T. J., Klotz, F. W., Pasvol, G., et al.: Falciparum malaria parasites invade erythrocytes that lack glycophorin A and B (M^k M^k). Strain differences indicate receptor heterogeneity and two pathways for invasion. J. Clin. Invest. *80*:1190–1193, 1987.
68. Haynes, J. D., Diggs, C. L., Hines, F. A., et al.: Culture of human malaria parasites: *Plasmodium falciparum*. Nature *263*:767–769, 1976.
69. Heineman, H. S.: The clinical syndrome of malaria in the United States: A current review of diagnosis and treatment for American physicians. Arch. Intern. Med. *129*:607–616, 1972.
70. Hendrickse, R. G.: Malaria. *In* Hendrickse, R. G., Barr, D. G. D., and Matthews, T. S. (eds.): Paediatrics in the Tropics. London, Blackwell Scientific Publications, 1991, pp. 695–710.
71. Holder, A. A.: Developments with anti-malarial vaccines. Ann. N. Y. Acad. Sci. *700*:7–21, 1993.
72. Horton, R. J.: Introduction of halofantrine for malaria treatment. Parasitol. Today *4*:238–239, 1988.
73. Houba, V.: Immunopathology of nephropathies associated with malaria. Bull. W. H. O. *52*:199–207, 1975.
74. Hulbert, T. V.: Congenital malaria in the United States: Report of a case and review. Clin. Infect. Dis. *14*:922–926, 1992.
75. Jeffrey, G. M.: Malaria control in the twentieth century. Am. J. Trop. Med. Hyg. *25*:361–371, 1976.
76. Jiang, J.-B., Guo, X.-B., Li, G.-Q., et al.: Antimalarial activity of mefloquine and qinghaosu. Lancet *1*:285–288, 1982.
77. Katz, M.: Medical progress: Parasitic infections. J. Pediatr. *87*:165–178, 1975.
78. Krogstad, D. J., Gluzman, I. Y., Kyle, D. E., et al.: Efflux of chloroquine from *Plasmodium falciparum:* Mechanism of chloroquine resistance. Science *238*:1283–1285, 1987.
79. Krogstad, D. J., and Herwaldt, B. L.: Chemoprophylaxis and treatment of malaria. N. Engl. J. Med. *319*:1538–1540, 1988.
80. Laveran, A.: Paludism. London, The New Sydenham Society, 1893. (Translated by J. W. Martin.)
81. Larkin, G. L., and Thuma, P. E.: Congenital malaria in a hyperendemic area. Am. J. Trop. Med. Hyg. *45*:587–592, 1991.
82. Layton, M., Parise, M. E., Campbell, C. C., et al.: Mosquito-transmitted malaria in New York City, 1993. Lancet *346*:729–731, 1995.
83. Levander, O. A., Ager, A. L., Morris, V. C., et al.: Menhaden-fish oil in a vitamin E–deficient diet: Protection against chloroquine-resistant malaria in mice. Am. J. Clin. Nutr. *50*:1237–1239, 1989.
84. Lewis, R., Lauersen, N. H., and Birnbaum, S.: Malaria associated with pregnancy. Obstet. Gynecol. *42*:696–700, 1973.
85. Logie, D. E., McGregor, I. A., Rowe, D. S., et al.: Plasma immunoglobulin concentrations in mothers and newborn children with special reference to placental malaria: Studies in the Gambia, Nigeria, and Switzerland. Bull. W. H. O. *49*:547–554, 1973.
86. Long, G. W., Fries, L., Watt, G. H., et al.: Polymerase chain reaction amplification from *Plasmodium falciparum* on dried blood spots. Am. J. Trop. Med. Hyg. *52*:344–346, 1995.
87. Luzzatto, L.: Genetic factors in malaria. Bull. W. H. O. *50*:195–202, 1974.
88. MacCallum, W. G.: On the flagellated form of the malaria parasite. Lancet *2*:1240–1241, 1897.
89. Macomber, P. B., O'Brien, R. L., and Hahn, F. E.: Chloroquine: Physiological basis of drug resistance in *Plasmodium berghei*. Science *152*:1374–1375, 1966.

90. Maegraith, B. G.: Malaria. *In* Spencer, H. (ed.): Tropical Pathology. Berlin, Springer-Verlag, 1973, pp. 319–349.
91. Magowa, C., Coppel, R. L., Lau, A. D. T., et al.: Role of the *Plasmodium falciparum* mature-parasite infected erythrocytes surface antigen (MESA/PfEMP-2) in malaria infection of erythrocytes. Blood *86*:3196–3204, 1995.
92. Maier, J., and Riley, E.: Inhibition of antimalarial action of sulfonamides by *p*-aminobenzoic acid. Proc. Soc. Exp. Biol. Med. *50:*152–154, 1942.
93. Mannaberg, J.: The Malaria Parasites: A Description Based upon Observations Made by the Author and by Other Observers. London, The New Sydenham Society, 1894. (Translated by R. W. Felkin.)
94. Manson-Bahr, P.: The story of malaria: The drama and the actors. Int. Rev. Trop. Med. *2:*329–390, 1963.
95. Marchiafava, E., and Bignami, A.: On Summer-Autumn Malaria Fevers. London, The New Sydenham Society, 1894. (Translated by J. H. Thompson.)
96. Marsh, K., Forster, D., Waruiru, C., et al.: Indicators of life-threatening malaria in African children. N. Engl. J. Med. *332*:1399–1404, 1995.
97. Martin, S. K., Oduola, A. M. J., and Milhous, W. R.: Reversal of chloroquine resistance in *Plasmodium falciparum* by verapamil. Science *235*:899–901, 1987.
98. McBride, J. S., Micklem, H. S., and Ure, J. M.: Immunosuppression in murine malaria. I. Response to type III pneumococcal polysaccharide. Immunology *32*:635–644, 1977.
99. McGregor, I. A.: Immunity to plasmodial infections: Consideration of factors relevant to malaria in man. Int. Rev. Trop. Med. *4:*1–52, 1971.
100. Meshnick, S. R., Tsang, T. W., Lin, F. B., et al.: Activated oxygen mediates the antimalarial activity of qinghaosu. *In* Eaton, J. W., Meshnick, S. R., and Brewer, G. J. (eds.): Malaria and the Red Cell 2. New York, Alan R. Liss, 1989, pp. 95–104.
101. Miller, L. H., and Carter, R.: Innate resistance in malaria. Exp. Parasitol. *40:*132–146, 1976.
102. Miller, L. H., Haynes, J. D., McAuliffe, F. M., et al.: Evidence for differences in erythrocyte surface receptors for the malaria parasites, *Plasmodium falciparum* and *Plasmodium knowlesi*. J. Exp. Med. *146:*277–281, 1977.
103. Miller, L. H., Mason, S. J., Clyde, D. F., et al.: The resistance factor to *Plasmodium vivax* in blacks: The Duffy–blood-group genotype, Fy Fy. N. Engl. J. Med. *295:*302–304, 1976.
104. Moore, D. V., and Lanier, J. E.: Observations on two *Plasmodium falciparum* infections with abnormal response to chloroquine. Am. J. Trop. Med. Hyg. *10:*5–9, 1961.
105. Morrow, R. H., Gutensohn, N., and Smith, P. G.: Epstein-Barr virus–malaria interaction models for Burkitt's lymphoma: Implications for preventive trials. Cancer Res. *36:*667–669, 1976.
106. Murray, M. J., Murray, N. J., Murray, A. B., et al.: Refeeding: Malaria and hyperferraemia. Lancet *1:*653–654, 1975.
107. Nussenzweiz, R. S., and Long, C. A.: Malaria vaccines: Multiple targets. Science *265*:1381–1383, 1994.
108. Nyirjesy, P., Kavasya, T., Axelrod, P., et al.: Malaria during pregnancy: Neonatal morbidity and mortality and the efficacy of chloroquine chemoprophylaxis. Clin. Infect. Dis. *16*:127–132, 1993.
109. Olatunde, I. A.: Chloroquine concentrations in the skin of rabbits and man. Br. J. Pharmacol. *43:*335–340, 1971.
110. Oliveira, D. A., Holloway, B. P., Durigon, E. L., et al.: Polymerase chain reaction and a liquid-phase nonisotopic hybridization for species-specific and sensitive detection of malaria infection. Am. J. Trop. Med. Hyg.: *52*:139–144, 1995.
111. Olliaro, P. L., and Goldberg, D. E.: The *Plasmodium* digestive vacuole: Metabolic headquarters and choice drug target. Parasitol. Today *11*:294–297, 1995.
112. Orjih, A. U., Banyal, H. S., Chevli, R., et al.: Hemin lyses malaria parasites. Science *214*:667–669, 1981.
113. Orjih, A. U., Saponin haemolysis for increasing concentration of *Plasmodium falciparum* infected erythrocytes. Lancet *343*:295, 1994.
114. Palmer, K. J., Holliday, S. M., and Brogden, R. N.: Mefloquine: A review of its antimalarial activity, pharmacokinetic properties and therapeutic efficacy. Drugs *45*:430–475, 1993.
115. Pichyangkul, S., Saengkrai, P., and Webster, H. K.: *Plasmodium falciparum* pigment induces monocytes to release high levels of tumor necrosis factor–α and interleukin-1-β. Am. J. Trop. Med. Hyg. *51*:430–435, 1994.
116. Peters, W.: Chemotherapy and Drug Resistance in Malaria. London, Academic Press, 1970.
117. Prada, J., Graninge, W., Lehman, L. G., et al.: Up-regulation of ICAM-1, Il-1 and reactive oxygen intermediates (ROI) by exogenous antigens from *Plasmodium falciparum* parasites *in vitro* and of SICAM-1 in the acute phase of malaria. J. Chemother. *7*:424–426, 1995.
118. Pringle, G.: A count of the merozoites in an oocyst of *Plasmodium falciparum*. Trans. R. Soc. Trop. Med. Hyg. *59:*289–290, 1965.
119. Ransome-kuti, O.: Malaria in childhood. Adv. Pediatr. *19:*319–340, 1972.
120. Redd, S. C., Kazembe, P. N., Luby, S. P., et al.: Clinical algorithm for treatment of *Plasmodium falciparum* malaria in children. Lancet *347*:223–227, 1996.
121. Richards, W. H. G., Mitchell, G. H., Butcher, G. A., et al.: Merozoite vaccination of rhesus monkeys against *Plasmodium knowlesi* malaria: Immunity to sporozoite (mosquito-transmitted) challenge. Parasitology *74:*191–198, 1977.
122. Ringwald, P., Bickii, J., and Basco, L.: Randomised trial of pyronaridine versus chloroquine for acute uncomplicated falciparum malaria in Africa. Lancet *347*:24–28, 1996.
123. Ross, R.: The Prevention of Malaria. London, John Murray, 1911.
124. Ross, R.: On some peculiar pigmented cells found in two mosquitoes fed on malaria blood. Br. Med. J. *2:*1786–1788, 1897.
125. Rougemont, A., Breslow, N., Brenner, E., et al.: Epidemiological basis for clinical diagnosis of childhood malaria in endemic zone in West Africa. Lancet *338*:1292–1295, 1991.
126. Rozman, R. S.: Chemotherapy of malaria. Annu. Rev. Pharmacol. *13:*127–152, 1973.
127. Schmid, A. H.: Cerebral malaria. Eur. Neurol. *12:*197–208, 1974.
128. Schmidt, L. H.: Infections with *Plasmodium falciparum* and *Plasmodium vivax* in the owl monkey: Model systems for basic biological and chemotherapeutic studies. Trans. R. Soc. Trop. Med. Hyg. *67:*446–474, 1973.
129. Schmidt, L. H.: Chemotherapy of the drug-resistant malarias. Annu. Rev. Microbiol. *23:*427–454, 1969.
130. Schmidt, L. H., Vaughan, D., Mueller, D., et al.: Activities of various 4-aminoquinolines against infections with chloroquine-resistant strains of *Plasmodium falciparum*. Antimicrob. Agents Chemother. *11:*826–843, 1977.
131. Sherry, B. A., Alava, G., Tracey, K. J., et al.: Malaria-specific metabolite hemozoin mediates the release of several potent and endogenous pyrogens (TNF, MIP-1, and MIP-1) *in vitro*, and altered thermoregulation *in vivo*. J. Inflamm. *45*:85–96, 1995.
132. Shortt, H. E., and Garnham, P. C. C.: Pre-erythrocytic stage in mammalian malaria parasites. Nature *161:*126, 1948.
133. Sim, B. K., Chitnis, C. E., Wasniowska, K., et al.: Receptor and ligand domains for invasion of erythrocytes by *Plasmodium falciparum*. Science *264*:1941–1944, 1994.
134. Sitprija, V., Vongsthongsri, M., Poshyachinda, V., et al.: Renal failure in malaria: A pathophysiologic study. Nephron *18:*277–287, 1977.
135. Slater, A. F. G., and Cerami, A.: Inhibition by chloroquine of a novel haem polymerase enzyme activity in malaria trophozoites. Nature *355*:167–169, 1992.
136. Steck, E. A.: The chemotherapy of protozoan diseases. Washington, D.C., Division of Medicinal Chemistry, Walter Reed Army Institute of Research, 1971, pp. 23.1–23.376.
137. Stone, W. J., Hanchett, J. E., and Knepshield, J. H.: Acute renal insufficiency due to *falciparum* malaria. Arch. Intern. Med. *129:*620–628, 1972.
138. Thompson, P. E., and Werbel, L. M.: Antimalarial Agents: Chemistry and Pharmacology. New York, Academic Press, 1972.
139. Trager, W., and Jensen, J. B.: Human malaria parasites in continuous culture. Science *193:*673–675, 1976.
140. Trenholme, G. M., Williams, R. L., Desjardins, R. E., et al.: Mefloquine (WR 142, 490) in the treatment of human malaria. Science *190:*792–794, 1975.
141. Vachon, F., Fajac, I., Gachot, B., et al.: Halofantrine and acute intravascular hemolysis. Lancet *340*:909–910, 1992.
142. Voller, A.: Immunopathology of malaria. Bull. W. H. O. *50:*177–186, 1974.
143. Von Brand, T.: Biochemistry of Parasites. 2nd ed. New York, Academic Press, 1973, pp. 89–170.
144. Waller, D., Krishna, S., Crawley, J., et al.: Clinical features and outcome of severe malaria in Gambian children. Clin. Infect. Dis. *21*:577–587, 1995.
145. Walliker, D., Carter, R., and Sanderson, A.: Genetic studies on *Plasmodium chabaudi:* Recombination between enzyme markers. Parasitology *70:*19–24, 1975.
146. Walzer, P. D., Gibson, J. J., and Schultz, M. G.: Malaria fatalities in the United States. Am. J. Trop. Med. Hyg. *23:*328–333, 1974.
147. Ward, G. E., Miller, L. H., and Dvorak, J. A.: The origin of parasitophorous vacuole membrane lipids in malaria-infected erythrocytes. J. Cell. Sci. *106*:237–248, 1993.
148. Warhurst, D. C.: Chemotherapeutic agents and malaria research. Symp. Br. Soc. Parasitol. *11:*1–28, 1973.
149. Wernsdorfer, W. H.: Epidemiology of drug resistance in malaria. Acta. Trop. *56*:143–156, 1994.
150. White, N. J., and Ho, M.: The pathophysiology of malaria. Adv. Parasitol. *31*:83–173, 1992.
151. White, N. J., Miller, K. D., Churchill, F. C., et al.: Chloroquine treatment of severe malaria in children. N. Engl. J. Med. *319:*1493–1500, 1988.
152. Wilson, M., Fife, E. H., Jr., Mathews, H. M., et al.: Comparison of the complement fixation, indirect immunofluorescence, and indirect hemagglutinin tests for malaria. Am. J. Trop. Med. Hyg. *24:*755–759, 1975.
153. Winters, R. A., and Murray, H. W.: The mime revisited: Fifteen more years of experience at a New York City teaching hospital. Am. J. Med. *93*:243–246, 1992.
154. Young, M. D.: Malaria. *In* Hunter, G. W., Swartzwelder, J. C., and Clyde, D. F. (eds.): Tropical Medicine. 5th ed. Philadelphia, W. B. Saunders, 1976, pp. 353–396.
155. Young, M. D., and Moore, D. V.: Chloroquine resistance in *Plasmodium falciparum*. Am. J. Trop. Med. Hyg. *10:*317–320, 1961.
156. Zuckerman, A.: Current status of the immunology of malaria and of the antigenic analysis of plasmodia. Bull. W. H. O. *40:*55–66, 1969.

218

LEISHMANIASIS

Murray Wittner

Leishmaniasis consists of a diverse group of diseases that may affect the viscera, skin, and/or mucous membranes with a wide spectrum of clinical activity caused by obligate intracellular hemoflagellates of the genus *Leishmania*. The infections are transmitted by several genera and species of phlebotomine sandflies. Three major clinical syndromes usually are recognized: visceral, cutaneous, and mucocutaneous leishmaniasis. In each type of disease, macrophages of the reticuloendothelial system are parasitized.

The clinical manifestations of leishmaniasis appear to depend upon a complex set of factors, including tropism and virulence of the parasite strain, as well as the susceptibility of the host that may be determined genetically. Cell-mediated immune mechanisms appear to be the major factors in modulating these diseases.

Each species of *Leishmania* has well-recognized clinical variants that seem to cause similar disease patterns in the same host species. Thus, in the case of visceral leishmaniasis (kala-azar), *L. donovani, L. chagasi,* and *L. infantum* invade cells of the reticuloendothelium of viscera, resulting in the enlargement of these organs and profound anemia; the disease is progressive and, if untreated, usually is fatal. In cutaneous disease, *L. tropica* (with some notable exceptions), *L. major,* and *L. mexicana* usually are restricted to reticuloendothelial cells of the skin and generally are self-limited, healing spontaneously. Similarly, *L. braziliensis* invades the reticuloendothelial cells of the skin, although it may metastasize to the mucous membranes of the nose, mouth, and pharynx, resulting in serious disfigurement, if not death. Recent observations have shown that some strains of *L. tropica* may cause visceral disease.

THE ORGANISM

In the vertebrate host, the various species of *Leishmania* are obligate intracellular parasites that exist only in the amastigote stage. The species that infect humans usually are indistinguishable from one another morphologically at both the light microscopic and ultrastructural levels. The organisms are round to oval bodies about 2 to 4 μm in diameter and possess a single nucleus and kinetoplast; they lack a free flagellum. The amastigotes are engulfed by macrophages and reside within the parasitophorous vacuole of the macrophage host. In this environment, they multiply by binary fission, eventually destroying the host cell. They subsequently are phagocytized, and the process occurs repeatedly. There is no evidence that *Leishmania* species actively penetrate host cells, as has been reported for *Trypanosoma cruzi*.

When the vector, a female sandfly, feeds on an infected person, it may ingest an infected cell from blood or tissue. The amastigotes are liberated in the fly's midgut, and within a few hours, transformation to the promastigote occurs. These are elongated flagellates, 15 to 25 μm long by 1.5 to 3.5 μm wide, with an anterior, free flagellum that measures about 15 to 28 μm in length. Binary fission then begins, and large numbers of promastigotes are produced that gradually move forward to the pharynx, buccal cavity, and mouth parts. At 8 to 20 days, depending on temperature and the species of sandfly, the mouth parts of the fly may be blocked partially or completely by huge numbers of promastigotes. These organisms may be dislodged into the bite wound when the fly next takes a blood meal.

Transmission is believed to occur also by contamination of the bite wound. Once they have been inoculated, many of the promastigotes do not survive because mammalian tissue fluids contain cytolytic substances. Those organisms that are phagocytized transform to amastigotes and initiate replication. The organisms can be seen readily in tissues or smears by light microscopy, especially with Giemsa or Wright stain, with which the nucleus and kinetoplast stain bright red and the cytoplasm stains pale blue. In Novey, McNeal, Nicolle (NNN) culture medium at 24° C, the organisms grow readily, assuming the promastigote or insect form.

At present, the taxonomic status of *Leishmania* remains unclear. Both specific and subspecific designations generally have been arrived at by the clinical syndrome caused by an isolate in a particular geographic area. However, these characteristics are imprecise and unreliable. Recently, various molecular biologic techniques have been employed to characterize the strains and species of clinical isolates: endonuclease restriction studies of the kinetoplast DNA (K-DNA), buoyant density of the K-DNA and mitochondrial DNA (M-DNA) on cesium chloride, leishmanial isozyme patterns, monoclonal antibody specificity, and exoantigen secretor 4 factor serotyping.

VISCERAL LEISHMANIASIS

Visceral leishmaniasis is caused by various organisms in the *L. donovani* species complex, although recently, strains of *L. tropica* from the Middle East have been found to cause this syndrome.

Visceral leishmaniasis, or kala-azar, is found in a broad belt that extends from the Straits of Gibraltar across the Mediterranean through Asia to the east coast of China, at a latitude of between 30 and 48 degrees north. It is transmitted by various sandfly vectors, although occasionally congenital and blood-borne infections also occur. It has been reported from 47 countries, although the Sudan and India account for more than half the cases. In the Western Hemisphere, it is found in Brazil, northern Argentina, Paraguay, Venezuela, Colombia, Guatemala, and Mexico. Kala-azar appears to exist in at least three epidemiologic forms:

1. A Mediterranean type of visceral leishmaniasis, with a canine reservoir, in which young children (1 to 4 years of age) are infected, and dogs, foxes, or feral animals are the reservoirs (*L. infantum*). This type extends from the Mediterranean littoral through central Asia into China; it also is present in parts of South America (*L. chagasi*), where foxes and dogs are reservoir hosts. In Brazil, young males most often are infected.

2. An Indian type (*L. donovani*) of visceral leishmaniasis, with a human reservoir, in which the disease predominates in Indian children between 5 and 15 years of age; humans are the only known reservoir. Although sought, evidence of

natural infection in dogs has not been found. Rodent reservoirs have not been looked for to any degree.

3. An African type of visceral leishmaniasis in which rodents are the reservoir hosts. The Nile rat in the Sudan and probably the gerbil in Kenya are the reservoirs. In Kenya, it has been noted that kala-azar often is related to old or eroded termite mounds where young males often congregate (Fig. 218–1).

Pathology

The principal pathologic lesions are the result of reticuloendothelial cell hyperplasia, especially in the spleen and liver. Later, bone marrow and lymph nodes are filled with infected macrophages, and a concomitant leukopenia and anemia develop. Similarly, the kidneys may be filled with the infected macrophages, and invasion of the submucosa and mucosa of the digestive tract, especially in the duodenum and jejunum, results in hypertrophic congested and edematous villi. Small ulcerations and hemorrhages may occur. The spleen gradually enlarges, sometimes assuming enormous proportions, eventually extending into the pelvis. Splenic infarcts are seen commonly. The capsule is thickened, and more deeply the sinuses are dilated. It is common to see erythrophagocytosis by histiocytes, and the anemia so typical of kala-azar, in part, may be the result of such sequestration of red cells. Kupffer cells of the liver, filled with amastigotes, are swollen and hyperplastic, and centrilobular necrosis or fatty infiltration of the hepatic parenchyma often is observed. In late-stage or chronic disease, increased hepatic fibrosis may give a nodular cirrhotic appearance. Lymphadenopathy, especially of the mesenteric glands, reveals large numbers of parasite-filled macrophages and is an early finding. The bone marrow often is filled with parasitized histiocytes, which replace the normal marrow elements, resulting in a myelophthistic anemia.

The immunologic response to kala-azar infection imperfectly is understood. At the bite wound, a small, pea-sized, dermal lesion may form, i.e., a leishmanioma; the parasites, initially localized in dermal macrophages, disseminate within the macrophages to the spleen, liver, bone marrow, and lymph nodes.

The outcome of an infection appears to depend on the interaction of the host's ability to raise a suitable cell-mediated immune response and the virulence of the invading organism. Experimentally, resistance in mice appears to be determined by a single autosomal gene. It has been shown that in experimental infections, disease is controlled by the Th_1 subset of CD4+ T cells and appears to be related to the production of cytokines, such as interferon-γ, interleukin-2, and tumor necrosis factor–β. However, the genetics of resistance in humans remains undefined.

If the infection is not eliminated by the host's cellular immune response, it then becomes clinically evident. Lymphocytogenesis and histiocytogenesis occur within the affected organs, with resultant hepatosplenomegaly and lymphadenopathy. Polyclonal B-cell activation occurs, causing hyperglobulinemia. This outpouring of humoral antibodies, chiefly IgG and largely nonspecific, is not protective, may exceed 5 g/dL, and may represent more than half the total serum proteins of the patient. Those specific antibodies that are produced during active disease have diagnostic significance. Fluorescent antibody, enzyme-linked immunosorbent assay (ELISA), indirect hemagglutination, and complement-fixation tests are reasonably reliable diagnostic procedures.

Resistance to kala-azar essentially is absent once the infection has become evident clinically. However, after chemotherapeutic cure, acquired immunity emerges; delayed hypersensitivity as demonstrated by the Montenegro (leishmanin) skin test (see later) also becomes evident. Moreover, hypergammaglobulinemia abates concomitant with chemical cure and the appearance of delayed hypersensitivity. Usually, immunity to visceral leishmaniasis is complete and long-lasting after chemotherapeutic cure. However, relapse as seen in post–kala-azar dermal leishmaniasis (see later) is characterized by delayed hypersensitivity, dermal localization of parasites, and moderate hypergammaglobulinemia. It is of interest that whereas macrophage activation has resulted in enhanced phagocytosis of parasites, macrophages remain unable to eliminate parasites. The appearance of dermal delayed hypersensitivity at the time acquired immunity appears suggests that cell-mediated immunity plays an important role in protection. Further work on this aspect of visceral leishmaniasis is needed.

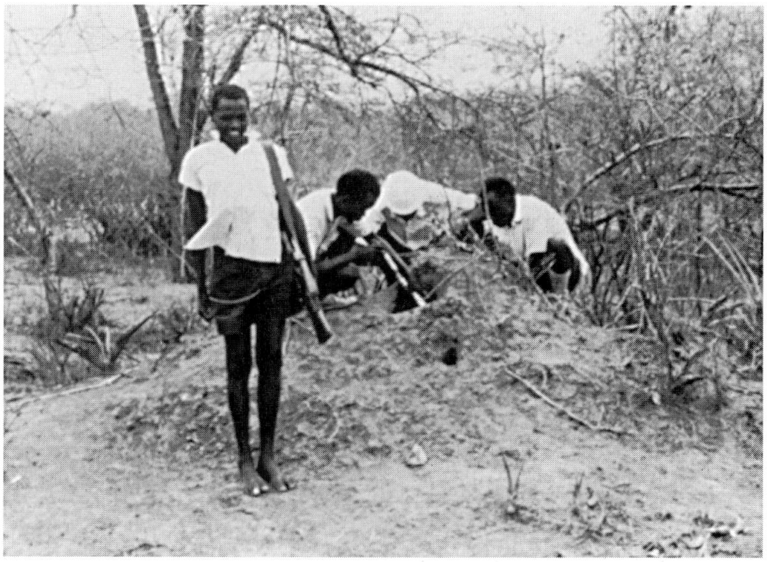

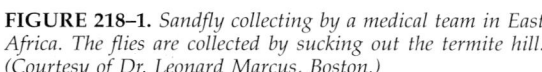

FIGURE 218–1. *Sandfly collecting by a medical team in East Africa. The flies are collected by sucking out the termite hill. (Courtesy of Dr. Leonard Marcus, Boston.)*

Clinical Manifestations

The clinical prepatent period varies widely—from 6 weeks to 6 months—but has been reported to be as early as 10 to 14 days and as long as 10 years. A primary skin nodule infrequently is seen, although in African leishmaniasis, it is a more regular feature. Infantile kala-azar (*L. infantum*) may begin either suddenly with high fevers and vomiting or insidiously with irregular daily fever, anorexia, weight loss, lassitude, and pallor. When fever is present, double daily spikes are a characteristic sign, the fever reaching 40° to 40.6° C. The spleen gradually enlarges, so that by the end of the first month, it usually can be palpated readily. If the symptoms continue unabated, the spleen may extend to the umbilicus or even into the pelvis. Diarrhea or frank dysentery is not unusual, and blood sometimes is observed. A general bleeding diathesis often becomes evident shortly before death. After several months, if the disease is untreated, patients usually die.

In less fulminating cases, the clinical course is more protracted, usually ending fatally after a year or two. In older age groups, the disease tends to assume a more chronic course, with marked emaciation, brittle hair, massive splenomegaly, lymphadenopathy, and a dusky slate-gray complexion. Hyperglobulinemia, leukopenia, and anemia typically are found. As a result of the child's general debility, death often results from such intercurrent infections as pneumonia, amebic or bacillary dysentery, malaria, or cancrum oris in more than 90 per cent of cases.

Cutaneous manifestations of kala-azar frequently are encountered. Especially in India, the dark-gray appearance of the skin has given rise to the name kala-azar (black sickness).

In some cases of treated visceral leishmaniasis, a skin condition termed post–kala-azar dermal leishmaniasis may ensue if all parasites are not eradicated. In Indian leishmaniasis, this complication is encountered in about 12 to 17 per cent of cases and often appears several years after therapy. In African disease, it is much less common, often occurring during therapy in about 2 to 3 per cent of cases, and heals spontaneously in a few months. The lesions are characterized by the appearance of hypopigmented, erythematous, or nodular lesions of the skin of the face, chest, neck, and buttocks. At times, the nodular lesions of the face may resemble lepromatous leprosy. The lesions are believed to represent a modified form of *L. donovani* infection in which the parasites no longer invade the viscera and are localized to the skin. These lesions seem to be related to the host's immune response; this change to dermal tropism is said to coincide with recovery from visceral disease and to disappear with relapse.

Pancytopenia is not unusual. Characteristically, anemia always is evident, with hemoglobin levels below 8 g/dL. Red cell survival is shortened as a result of several possible factors, including a Coombs-positive hemolytic anemia and hypersplenism. Leukopenia of 2000 to 3000 cells/mm^3 typically is found with neutropenia, relative lymphocytosis, an almost total absence of eosinophils, and thrombocytopenia. Serum albumin usually is less than 3 g/dL, and globulin levels (mostly IgG) often are greater than 5 g/dL.

Recently, kala-azar has been reported as an important opportunistic infection in patients infected with HIV-1 and who were not known to have had *Leishmania* infection previously. These patients appear to have a more severe and fulminant form of kala-azar. In this regard, inapparent *Leishmania* infection may become evident after immunosuppression for various reasons, such as chemotherapy for malignant disease. The diagnosis may be particularly difficult inasmuch as the presentation often is atypical, with low-grade fever, fatigue, cough, and gastrointestinal complaints. Similar, atypical visceral disease caused by *L. tropica* was seen in individuals who participated in Operation Desert Storm in the Persian Gulf.

Diagnosis

Visceral leishmaniasis is diagnosed by finding the organism in stained smears of spleen aspirate, peripheral blood, or bone marrow. In Indian kala-azar, the parasites may be found regularly in peripheral blood monocytes (i.e., buffy coat), but in African and Mediterranean forms, they may be difficult to find by this technique. Blood and marrow cultures grown on NNN medium or in Schneider insect medium with 15 to 20 per cent fetal calf serum are most useful. Splenic puncture, bone marrow aspiration, and liver biopsy usually are the most rewarding procedures, although they are not without serious hazard in individuals with a bleeding diathesis. In some hands, splenic rather than bone marrow aspiration has been the most rewarding procedure. Contraindications include a soft or diffluent, acutely enlarging spleen. Patients with low platelets and/or prolonged prothrombin time should not have the needle biopsy procedure. In children younger than 5 years of age, splenic aspiration should be performed only by a fully experienced physician.

Spleen and bone marrow aspirates should be placed in culture medium and smeared on slides, and saline-diluted aspirates should be inoculated into the peritoneal cavity of hamsters (Fig. 218–2).

Nonspecific tests reflecting the markedly elevated serum globulins, such as the formol gel and Sia water tests, are helpful in acute disease and are performed readily in the field. Antileishmanial antibodies usually are present and can be used to aid in the diagnosis. The fluorescent antibody test is highly specific, as are the indirect hemagglutination and gel diffusion tests. The complement-fixation test, however, is positive in only 65 to 70 per cent of cases. Sera from patients with visceral leishmaniasis are known to give false-positive results when patients who may have antibodies to *T. cruzi* are present, so that in the Western Hemisphere it may be necessary to absorb out these antibodies. It is important to recognize that fluorescent antibody titers usually fall after complete cure, so that a negative titer often is regarded as a sign of successful therapy. ELISA has been a very useful diagnostic modality, especially in large-scale epidemiologic studies, because of its specificity and sensitivity. DNA-DNA hybridization tests, so-called dot-blot techniques, are being tested and promise exquisite specificity and sensitivity for the diagnosis of leishmaniasis. A positive serologic test can occur as a result of past or subclinical inapparent infection.

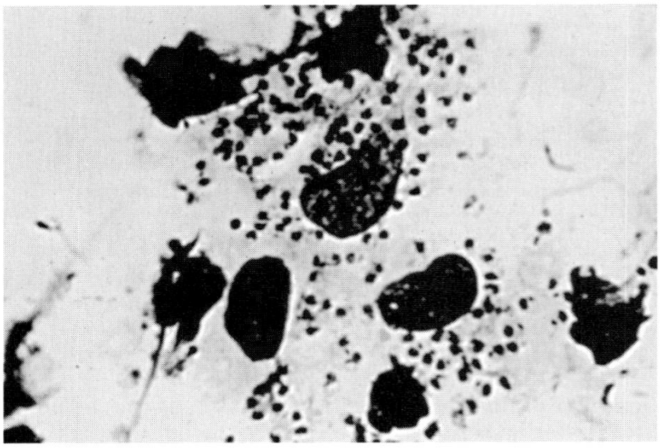

FIGURE 218–2. Leishmania donovani *in liver touch preparation. Original magnification,* × *288.*

The usual tests may be negative in patients with HIV disease or *L. tropica* infection or in otherwise profoundly immunocompromised patients. Recently, however, two genomic fragments encoding portions of a single 210-kDa *L. tropica* protein have proved useful for the diagnosis of viscerotropic *L. tropica* infection in Desert Storm patients.

The leishmanin or Montenegro skin test, like the lepromin or tuberculin skin tests, is a measure of delayed hypersensitivity to leishmanial antigen. It consists of 10^6 phenol-killed, culture-grown promastigotes in 1 mL of 0.5 per cent phenol in saline. The test is performed like the tuberculin test, that is, 0.1 mL is injected intradermally. A positive result is a palpable area of induration at least 5 mm in diameter in 48 to 72 hours. The leishmanin test can be positive in cutaneous or visceral leishmaniasis; therefore, results must be evaluated carefully. In visceral leishmaniasis, the test remains negative throughout the period of active disease. Once chemotherapeutic control begins to occur and immunocompetent lymphocytes are able to respond, the test begins to turn positive. Thus, recovery from kala-azar is characterized by the development of cell-mediated immunity. The change from a negative to positive leishmanin test in visceral leishmaniasis is regarded as an important prognostic sign that the patient is developing or has developed protective immunity. Because a number of reports have appeared recently noting positive leishmanin tests in individuals who have had no history of visceral leishmaniasis, it has been postulated that many individuals in an endemic area may become immune by prior inapparent infection.

Prognosis

Untreated visceral leishmaniasis is fatal in 75 to 85 per cent of infantile and 90 per cent of adult cases. Properly treated at an early stage, it can be cured in 85 to 95 per cent of cases. The prognosis for patients who develop pancytopenia or bleeding diatheses or who fail to develop a delayed hypersensitivity skin reaction usually is poor.

Treatment

Kala-azar usually responds to treatment with pentavalent antimonials, such as stibogluconate sodium (Pentostam, Triostam), which is the usual drug of choice in the United States. The pediatric and adult dose is 20 mg/kg daily, administered intramuscularly or intravenously for 28 days. Treatment can be repeated. In areas where leishmanial parasites may have developed relative resistance to pentavalent antimonials, such as India and East Africa, it may be necessary to extend therapy for more than 4 weeks. Side effects include nausea, vomiting, urticaria, nonspecific electrocardiographic changes, and bradycardia. In antimony-resistant patients, most often encountered in Africa, pentamidine isethionate (Lomidine) is an alternative. It is given intramuscularly every third or fourth day, 2 to 4 mg/kg for up to 15 doses, depending on the side effects, such as hypotension, vomiting, and blood dyscrasias. Pentamidine occasionally may exacerbate diabetes mellitus or precipitate latent diabetes. Shock and liver and renal damage have been reported. Amphotericin B can be used instead of pentamidine, administered up to 1.5 mg/kg on alternate days by slow intravenous drip in 5 per cent glucose. The total adult dose is 2 g. (For a detailed discussion of amphotericin B, see Chapter 234.)

All patients should be hospitalized for therapy; supportive and corrective measures should be instituted in the event of other infections. An occasional patient may be encountered who may require splenectomy in order to relieve the profound hypersplenism and the resulting anemia. Response to therapy often can be assessed by the return of the patient's temperature to normal, a brisk reticulocytosis, a gradual reduction in spleen size, and the reappearance of eosinophils on the peripheral blood smear.

Recently, allopurinol has been used with pentavalent antimonials to treat cases of visceral leishmaniasis that did not respond to pentavalent antimonials alone. Several recent reports suggest that recombinant interferon-γ is helpful, along with pentavalent antimonial drugs, for successful therapy of this disease. Aminosidine, 15 mg/kg/day intravenuously or intramuscularly, has been used with some success. It is the equivalent of paromomycin but is not available in the United States.

Because it is difficult to assess whether a cure has been achieved, it is essential that patients be followed at 6-month intervals for up to 2 years. Fluorescent antibody titers should be absent by the end of 1 year and complement fixation by 6 to 8 months.

If post–kala-azar dermal leishmaniasis occurs, treatment should be reinstituted.

Prevention

There are many aspects to the control of visceral leishmaniasis. Sandflies (*Phlebotomus* and *Lutzomyia*) can be eliminated readily by residual spraying. Because sandflies ordinarily do not fly very high, sleeping quarters should be above ground levels. Animal reservoirs, such as infected dogs and rodents, should be destroyed. Early therapy will prevent family and neighborhood transmission.

OLD WORLD CUTANEOUS LEISHMANIASIS

Definition and Epidemiology

Old World cutaneous leishmaniasis is caused by *L. major* (rural), *L. tropica* (urban), and *L. aethiopica*. It is found throughout the Middle East; along the Mediterranean basin and islands; and in East and West Africa, India, and southwestern Asia. In humans, infection by *L. tropica* usually produces self-limited skin ulcers in which intracellular (amastigote) parasites can be found situated in macrophages in and about the lesions. These protozoan hemoflagellates almost never visceralize in humans. However, several recent reports described *L. tropica* isolates from patients with visceral leishmaniasis (see Visceral Leishmaniasis). In many areas, dogs or rodents are found naturally infected and are believed to be the natural reservoirs of infection. As with visceral leishmaniasis, various *Phlebotomus* species of sandflies transmit the infection, although contact transmission is possible and is the basis of the long-time practice in middle and central Asia of immunizing inoculations, that is, "vaccination," to prevent possible disfigurement by a natural infection (Fig. 218–3).

Old World leishmaniasis, or Oriental sore (Delhi boil, Aleppo button), often is classified into "wet" and "dry" types. The wet or rural form is caused by *L. major* and is found chiefly in various rodents on the edge of deserts. The dry or urban type is anthropronotic preponderantly, caused by *L. tropica*, and transmitted by phlebotomine species that frequently feed on humans and dogs. The dry or urban form of Oriental sore is characterized by a long incubation period, long duration of active infection, and large numbers of parasites in the dermis. In contrast, the moist or rural type has a relatively short incubation period, with rapid healing and

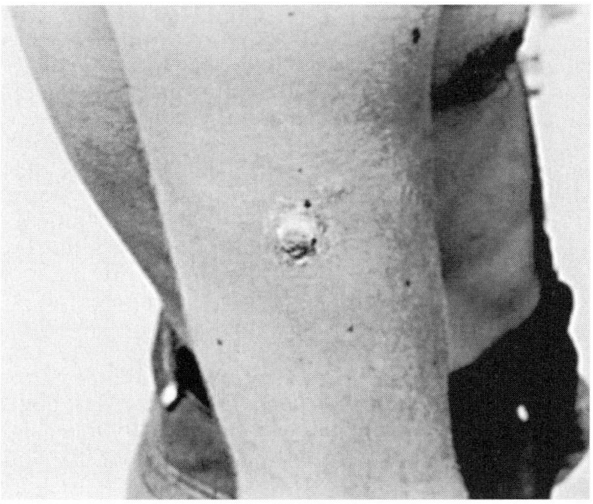

FIGURE 218–3. Leishmania tropica. *Immunization by induced lesion. (From a nonprofit cooperative endeavor by numerous colleagues under the editorship of Dr. Herman Zaiman, New York.)*

few parasites in the skin. *L. aethiopica* is restricted to the mountain valleys of the Rift Valley of Ethiopia and Kenya, where the rock and tree hyraxes are infected regularly. Humans become infected when they intrude in these areas. This form of cutaneous leishmaniasis usually is self-limiting, although in a small number of individuals (ratio, 1:100,000), nonhealing diffuse cutaneous disease has been reported.

Pathology

At the site of the bite wound, promastigotes are engulfed by histiocytes, in which they multiply repeatedly. The histiocytes are destroyed, and amastigotes are released into the tissues, where the process is repeated. Lymphocytic and plasma cell infiltration along with histiocytic hyperplasia becomes evident. In some lesions, epithelioid and giant cells may be seen. Early, there is hypertrophy of the stratum corneum and hyperplasia of dermal papillae. Usually, this is followed by necrosis of the area due to capillary obstruction and endothelial proliferation, so that the epithelium overlying the center of the lesion becomes necrotic and is sloughed, forming a characteristic ulcer. Secondary neutrophil infiltration then is noted. At this point, there is a depressed ulcer with a raised indurated border and a base of friable granulation tissue. Amastigotes usually are intracellular, although during the period of necrosis, organisms may be seen outside cells but not dividing.

In *L. tropica,* the development of the lesion may take weeks to months, and there are relatively few lymphocytes and plasma cells and large numbers of parasites in nests of macrophages. In *L. major* infections, the onset is rapid, with an outpouring of lymphocytes and plasma cells; parasites sometimes are difficult to find. In some cases, extensive satellite lesions form in the proximity of the primary lesion so that local spread often is seen. The pathologic reaction may be florid, with marked pseudoepitheliomatous hyperplasia that can be mistaken for carcinoma. Secondary bacterial infection may complicate the lesion and delay healing. Once the ulcer heals, however, usually by fibrosis, the patient has long-lasting immunity.

Several forms of cutaneous leishmaniasis have been described and seem to be associated with the ability of the patient to develop cell-mediated immune mechanisms. Whether these mechanisms directly are responsible for protection in humans still is not certain. Thus, in a small number of patients, the inability to mount a suitable cell-mediated immune reaction is associated with specific anergy to leishmanin and an indolent nonhealing lesion. This condition is known as diffuse cutaneous leishmaniasis (DCL, or leishmaniasis tegumentaria diffusa). Characteristically, lesions in DCL are filled with large, parasite-containing histiocytes, and there is an absence of lymphocytes. Recent studies of DCL from the Dominican Republic suggest that immune suppression plays an important role in this form of the disease.

At the other extreme, there is a small group of patients whose cell-mediated immune response to infection with leishmanial organisms is exaggerated markedly, so that lesions heal by scarring. At the edge of the scar, however, new lesions appear, so the disease seems to extend from the margins. Eventually, damage may be rather extensive. On histologic examination, there are many lymphocytes, plasma cells, epithelioid cells, and large multinucleated giant cells. Organisms are difficult to locate but sometimes can be cultured from these lesions. This form of cutaneous leishmaniasis is called leishmaniasis recidivans. Patients exhibit marked delayed hypersensitivity to leishmanin. The studies of Turk and Bryceson[17] have provided the concept that cutaneous leishmaniasis may be a spectrum of diseases analogous to leprosy. They regard DCL at one end of the spectrum, representing anergy, and leishmaniasis recidivans at the other, representing marked allergy, with ordinary Oriental sore as the center in which there is balance.

Clinical Manifestations

The disease usually begins with the appearance of a pruritic, red, vesicular papule that appears weeks to months after the bite of a sandfly. The papule gradually enlarges, often measuring 1 to 2 cm in diameter. When the surface of the papule dries, it encrusts and drops off, revealing a shallow ulcer. The ulcer may or may not enlarge progressively and characteristically has raised, sharp, indurated margins. Healing usually takes place in 3 to 18 months, often leaving an obvious hypo- or hyperpigmented depressed scar. It is not uncommon, however, for single or multiple papules to heal directly without extensive ulceration. If the lesions do not become infected secondarily, there usually are no complications.

Diagnosis

Microscopic examination of Giemsa or Wright stain smears of tissue obtained from non-necrotic areas of the ulcer or from the base should be performed. Aspiration and culture of tissue fluid taken from the ulcer margin can be rewarding. Biopsy material taken from the edge of the ulcer should be examined histologically, as should small fragments macerated in saline and inoculated into NNN medium or Schneider's insect medium, together with penicillin and streptomycin. Clinically, the lesions often are characteristic, so that the diagnosis should be suspected in a patient who has visited an endemic area.

Although the leishmanin test usually is positive in patients with ulcerated lesions, the material is not readily available in the United States. However, a positive leishmanin skin test may help distinguish a variety of skin lesions, such as syphilis, tropical phagedenic ulcer, yaws, tuberculosis, and various fungal diseases. The indirect fluorescent antibody test or direct agglutination test may be positive in this infection, although often at low titers and therefore of little value.

Treatment

Uncomplicated *L. tropica* lesions usually respond well to chemotherapy or to conservative management. Because Old World cutaneous leishmaniasis usually remains a local lesion, if the ulcer is not disfiguring and appears to be healing, it is not unreasonable to permit the lesion to heal spontaneously. Systemic therapy with Pentostam (see Visceral Leishmaniasis) is very satisfactory in most cases. Recent reports have indicated limited success in treating skin lesions with heat. It generally was necessary to raise the intralesional temperature to 40° to 42° C for 12 hours per day in order to obtain a satisfactory result. Recently, recombinant interferon-γ was reported to accelerate healing in this disease. Various parenteral, topical, and oral agents have been been used, but the data are anecdotal and/or conflicting. Thus, allopurinol and various imidazoles (e.g., ketoconazole, itraconazole) have been used and appear to have limited antileishmanial activity. Recently, an ointment containing paromomycin (aminosidine) and methylbenzethonium chloride has been reported to show some promise in treating cutaneous lesions.

Prevention

Residual spraying for sandflies, eradication of reservoir hosts, and vaccination procedures have reduced and limited this disease in many areas of the Middle East and central Asia. Because of the indolent nature of the healing with vaccination, this practice has been discontinued in Israel.

AMERICAN CUTANEOUS LEISHMANIASIS

The epidemiology and etiology of American cutaneous leishmaniasis have become extremely complex subjects. In South and Central America, it is evident that there are many varieties of leishmaniasis, the mucocutaneous form, or espundia, being but one of these. In contrast to Old World cutaneous leishmaniasis, American cutaneous disease is tied closely to the forests of South and Central America, and each variety has its own distinct epidemiologic, pathologic, and clinical picture. Whether it is justified to indicate each of the clinical types of American cutaneous leishmaniasis by a separate species of *Leishmania* is not clear. With regard to the American cutaneous forms, two main groups of organisms are distinguished: the *L. mexicana* and *L. braziliensis* complexes (Figs. 218–4, 218–5, and 218–6). The former are characterized by growing rapidly in culture medium and in hamsters, and the latter are organisms that grow slowly in culture and hamsters.

Leishmania mexicana Complex

1. *L. (mexicana) mexicana* is transmitted by species of sandflies of the genus *Lutzomyia* and *Psychodopygus*. There are many rodent reservoir hosts. This species is found in Mexico, Guatemala, and Belize. It causes mild infection, often a single cutaneous lesion that is self-limited, or persistent chronic ear lesions. It causes Chiclero ulcer. There has been one recorded case of DCL. This species probably is the cause of the occasional cases of cutaneous leishmaniasis in the southern United States.
2. *L. (mexicana) amazonensis* is found along the Amazon basin and in Trinidad. It rarely infects humans but is transmitted by various species of *Lutzomyia* in rodents. In humans, it causes a mild and self-limited skin lesion. Occasionally, patients reportedly develop DCL.

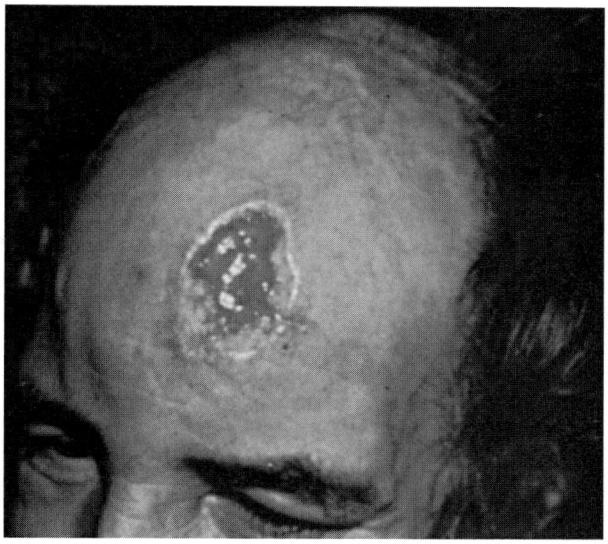

FIGURE 218–4. *Healing cutaneous leishmaniasis in a patient from Venezuela.*

Leishmania braziliensis Complex

1. *L. (braziliensis) braziliensis* is transmitted by various species of *Lutzomyia* and *Psychodopygus* in Brazil and in the forest areas east of the Andes. This is the "prototype" of American or mucocutaneous leishmaniasis, or espundia. It may cause destructive ulcerative lesions of the naso-oropharynx as a result of early or late metastases from a more superficial site.
2. *L. (braziliensis) guyanesis* is transmitted by species of *Lutzomyia* and *Psychodopygus* in Guyana, Surinam, Brazil, and Venezuela. It causes single or multiple spreading cutaneous ulcers over many parts of the body. It is believed to metastasize along lymphatics but does not visceralize. It sometimes spreads to the naso-oropharynx, causing mucosal disease. It sometimes is referred to as pian bois, or forest yaws.
3. *L. (braziliensis) panamensis* is transmitted by species of

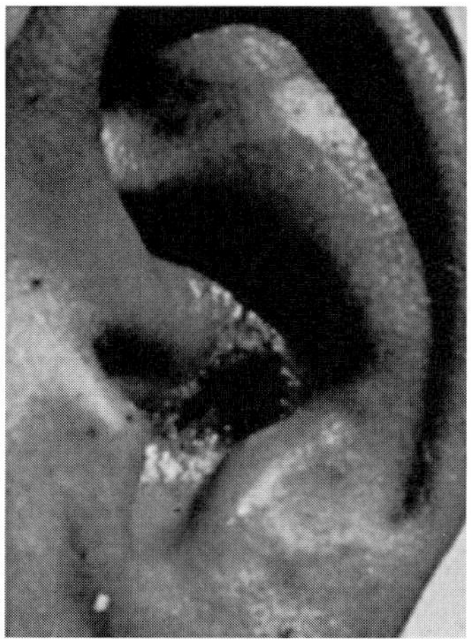

FIGURE 218–5. *Chiclero ulcer* Leishmania (mexicana) mexicana. *A typical chronic lesion of the external ear. These never metastasize.*

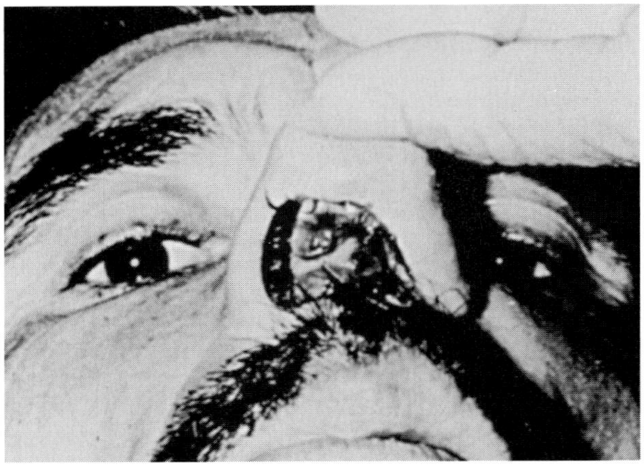

FIGURE 218–6. *Mucocutaneous leishmaniasis* Leishmania (braziliensis) braziliensis. *The entire nasal septum has been eroded. Few organisms could be found by smear or biopsy; however, promastigote forms were cultured from the lesion.*

Lutzomyia and *Psychodopygus* in Panama and possibly farther north and south. It may cause single to several superficial ulcers and may metastasize along the lymphatics may metastasize to the naso-oropharynx.

4. *L. (braziliensis) peruviana* is seen in Peru on the western slopes of the Andes to an altitude of 3000 meters. It causes a single or a few self-healing ulcers. There is no oronasopharyngeal spread. Often, it is referred to as uta. Dogs are regarded as the reservoir hosts.

In mucocutaneous leishmaniasis as represented by espundia, it is estimated that nasal involvement may occur in as many as 80 per cent of infections and that up to 30 per cent of these eventually may mutilate the mucous membranes of the mouth, nose, palate, larynx, and trachea. These cases often are fatal because of the intervening sepsis. Lesions of the mucous membranes often arise several years to decades after a cutaneous ulcer has healed. Once mucous membrane involvement occurs, the infection may be difficult to eradicate by chemotherapy.

Diagnosis

The discussion of Old World cutaneous leishmaniasis includes the various methods for diagnosis. In mucocutaneous disease, the fluorescent antibody test using amastigote antigen is most useful, being positive in 75 to 85 per cent of cases, with declining titers after therapeutic cure. A direct agglutination test employing promastigotes also is used frequently, as is ELISA. Recently, a DNA-DNA hybridization or dot-blot test has been used that is highly sensitive and species-specific in tissue or biopsy specimens. Isozyme analysis of isolated organisms currently is being used to help identify the species causing the infection.

Treatment

As in Old World cutaneous leishmaniasis, treatment for most lesions will succeed if pentavalent antimonials are employed. Because it is believed that prompt and adequate therapy for primary cutaneous lesions may reduce the risk of subsequent metastatic disease in potentially mucocutaneous infections, pentavalent antimony should be used. If lesions should prove to be unresponsive to antimony therapy, amphotericin B should be tried. Relapses with this form of leishmaniasis are not uncommon and must be treated again. Pentavalent antimonials are moderately effective in mild mucosal disease but often are unsatisfactory in cases of severe mucosal involvement. Leishmaniasis tegumentaria diffusa (DCL) should be treated with Pentostam; when there are relapses, amphotericin B should be used next, inasmuch as this disease usually is refractory to further antimony therapy. Pentamidine also has been used with limited success when lesions have proved to be resistant to antimony compounds. Pentavalent antimony–resistant cutaneous disease, such as leishmania recidivans, has been treated with limited success with ketoconazole, 400 to 600 mg daily for 4 weeks.

Prevention

This is an extremely difficult disease to prevent because it is a forest disease. It can be avoided only by sleeping in tents under fine-mesh netting, wearing long-sleeved clothing, and employing insect repellents.

Bibliography

1. Ashford, R. W., Desjeux, P., and deRaadt, P.: Estimation of population at risk of infection and number of cases of leishmaniasis. Parasitol. Today *8*:104, 1992.
2. Arnot, D. E., and Barker, D. C.: Biochemical identification of cutaneous leishmaniasis by analysis of kinetoplast DNA. II. Sequence homologies in *Leishmania* kDNA. Mol. Biochem. Parasitol. *3*:47–56, 1981.
3. Blackwell, J., Pratt, D. M., and Shaw, J.: Molecular biology of *Leishmania.* Parasitol. Today *2*:45–53, 1986.
4. Badaro, R., Jones T. C., and Carvalho, E. M.: New perspectives on a subclinical form of visceral leishmaniasis. J. Infect. Dis. *154*:1003–1011, 1986.
5. Berman, J. D.: Chemotherapy for leishmaniasis: Biochemical mechanisms, clinical efficacy, and future strategies. Rev. Infect. Dis. *10*:560–586, 1988.
6. Carvalho, E. M., Teixeira, R. S., and Johnson, W. D., Jr.: Cell-mediated immunity in American visceral leishmaniasis reversible immunosuppression during acute infection. Infect. Immun. *33*:498–500, 1981.
7. Chulay, J. D., and Bryceson, A. D. M.: Quantitation of amastigotes of *Leishmania donovani* in smears of splenic aspirates from patients with visceral leishmaniasis. Am. J. Trop. Med. Hyg. *32*:475–479, 1983.
8. Convit, J., Pinardi, M. E., and Rondon, A. J.: Diffuse cutaneous leishmaniasis: A disease due to an immunologic defect of the host. Trans. R. Soc. Trop. Med. Hyg. *66*:603–610, 1972.
9. Dillon, D. C., Day, C. H., Whittle, J. A., et al.: Characterization of a *Leishmania tropica* antigen that detects immune responses in Desert Storm viscerotropic leishmaniasis patients. Proc. Natl. Acad. Sci. U. S. A. *92*:7981–7985, 1995.
10. Grimaldi, G., Jr., and Tesh, R. B.: Leishmaniasis of the New World: Current concepts and implications for future research. Clin. Microbiol. Rev. *6*:230–250, 1993.
11. Herwaldt, B. L., and Berman, J. D.: Recommendations for treating leishmaniasis with sodium stibogluconate (Pentostam) and review of pertinent clinical studies. Am. J. Trop. Med. Hyg. *46*:296–306, 1992.
12. Magill, A. J., Grogl, M., Gasser, R. A., et al.: Visceral infection caused by *Leishmania tropica* in veterans of Operation Desert Storm. N. Engl. J. Med. *328*:1383–1387, 1993.
13. Medrano, F. J., Hernandez-Quero, J., Jimenez, E., et al.: Visceral leishmaniasis in HIV-1-infected individuals: A common opportunistic infection in Spain? AIDS *6*:1499–1503, 1992.
14. Sampio, S., Castro, M. R., Dillon, N. L., et al.: Treatment of mucocutaneous leishmaniasis with amphotericin B: Report of 70 cases. Int. J. Dermatol. *10*:179–181, 1971.
15. Shaw, J. J., and Lainson, R.: Ecology and epidemiology: New World. *In* Peters, W., and Killick-Kendrick, R. (eds.): The Leishmaniases in Biology and Medicine. Vol. I. London, Academic Press, 1987, pp. 78–87.
16. Shaw, P. K., Quigg, L. T., Allain, D. S., et al.: Autochthonous dermal leishmaniasis in Texas. Am. J. Trop. Med. Hyg. *25*:788–796, 1976.
17. Turk, J. L., and Bryceson, A. D.: Immunological phenomenon in leprosy and related diseases. Adv. Immunol. *13*:209–266, 1971.
18. Weigle, K. A., de Davalaos, M., Heredia, P., et al.: Diagnosis of cutaneous and mucocutaneous leishmaniasis in Columbia: A comparison of seven methods. Am. J. Trop. Med. Hyg. *36*:489–496, 1987.

219

TRYPANOSOMIASIS

Murray Wittner

AMERICAN TRYPANOSOMIASIS

American trypanosomiasis, or Chagas disease, is caused by the protozoan hemoflagellate *Trypanosoma cruzi*, which first was discovered by Carlos Chagas in 1911 in the blood of a seriously ill, wasted Brazilian child suffering from fever, lymphadenopathy, and anemia. The disease, transmitted by reduviid bugs, is limited to the Western Hemisphere, being prevalent in South and Central America and Mexico. There have been several autochthonous and laboratory-acquired cases reported from the United States in recent years. Chagas disease in some endemic areas represents the most important cause of heart disease and may cause serious chronic digestive tract pathology.

The Organism

T. cruzi is a pleomorphic, spindle-shaped organism whose size is quite variable, depending upon the strain. In a series of mensural studies, it was shown that the length of the blood forms (trypomastigote) in humans may vary widely, from 11.7 to 30.4 μm (means of 16.3 to 21.8 μm), including a free anterior flagellum of 2.0 to 11.2 μm. In about 75 to 80 per cent of blood forms, the cell assumes a C or S shape, with the nucleus just anterior to the middle of the cell. The undulating membrane is small and originates from a very large posterior DNA-containing kinetoplast that often bulges the cell surface (Fig. 219–1).

T. cruzi undergoes an obligatory developmental and reproductive cycle in the alimentary tract of reduviid or triatomine bugs when ingested with a blood meal. The entire cycle takes place in the lumen of the gut over a 6- to 15-day period, depending upon whether the bug is in its larval stage (6 or 7 days) or nymphal and adult stages (10 to 15 days). Within a few hours after taking an infective blood meal, short, spindle-shaped forms, lacking a free flagellum, can be found in the insect's foregut. These forms develop into small epimastigote forms that continue to divide, giving rise to large (35 to 40 μm) epimastigotes, so that by the third or fourth day after the blood meal, these organisms can be found attached to the rectal epithelium. By about the fifth day, the epimastigotes have begun to round up and gradually develop into short, stout trypomastigotes, which then proceed to elongate, and by the seventh and eighth days become the long, slender (17 to 22 μm), infective, metacyclic trypomastigotes. These forms do not divide again but are passed out with the feces some time after the blood meal. There may be 3000 to 4000 organisms per microliter of excreta.

Despite the long-maintained controversy that infection occurs via the insect bite, it now is well established that transmission occurs by means of infected insect excreta and metacyclic forms readily negotiate mucosa, conjunctiva, and abraded or otherwise broken skin (puncture site). Thus, extensive experimental evidence has demonstrated clearly that infection is by contamination rather than by insect inoculation.

Once the infective metacyclic trypomastigotes traverse the skin, they invade and multiply locally in many cell types, having transformed into intracellular amastigote forms. In the ensuing several weeks, during which time there have been repeated cycles of multiplication, cell destruction, and cell reinvasion, flagellates enter the blood stream as trypomastigotes and the infection becomes disseminated, predominantly to muscle cells, which become infected and in which multiplication is sustained. Polymorphism of the blood forms has been studied and is believed to represent various physiologic states of the organism. Suffice it to say, broad, stumpy forms are believed to be capable only of developing further in the insect vector, whereas the long, slender forms are able to invade vertebrate cells but not develop in invertebrate hosts. Additional evidence for this concept is suggested by the observation that reduviids that fed upon vertebrates infected with predominantly long, slender blood forms failed to become infected.

Epidemiology

Chagas disease in man extends from Mexico to Chile and Argentina. Only the Caribbean Islands, Belize, Surinam, and Guyana are reported to be free of this infection. Few autochthonous U.S. cases have been documented, despite the presence of infected vectors. It has been difficult to estimate the number of persons infected with *T. cruzi*, but various estimates are about 50 thousand deaths and about 10 to 20 million individuals at risk. Most workers believe these fig-

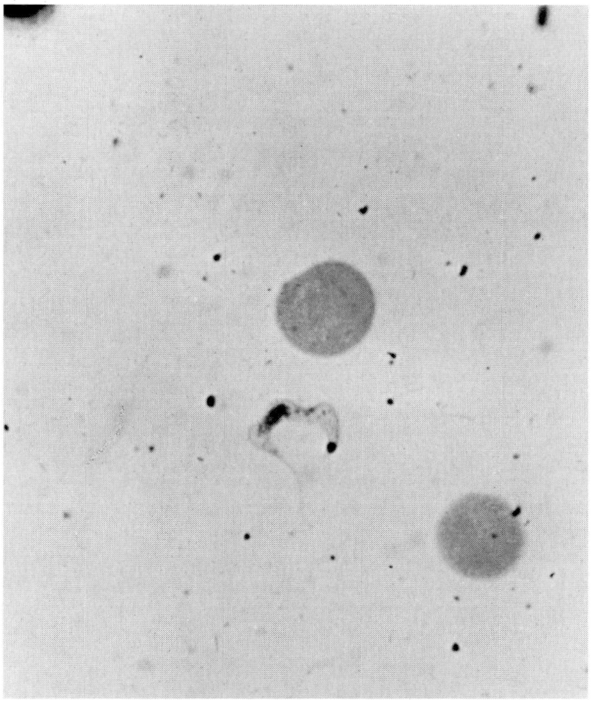

FIGURE 219–1. Trypanosoma cruzi *trypomastigote forms in a blood smear. Note the large posterior kinetoplast. (Original magnification × 288.)*

ures far too conservative. The reduviid vectors are found from the southern part of the United States to southern Argentina and Chile.

Although many species of triatomine bugs have been found to harbor *T. cruzi* naturally, only about 12 are important epidemiologically. Generally, triatomines are found in rural wooded areas closely associated with feral animal species; humans intervene only occasionally. Thus, this infection usually is a zoonosis. However, a number of species have become more or less adapted to houses, where they may live in cracks; on roofs, walls, and floors; and beneath little-moved objects. Other triatomine species have developed regular visiting habits to human dwellings but have not taken up residence as yet. The triatomine insects have been categorized according to their present relationship to human dwellings as follows: (1) those that after centuries of human contact have become well-adapted to human dwellings and essentially are anthropocentric; (2) those insects that are in the process of adapting to human habitation but still prefer and maintain natural forest ecotopes; (3) those bugs that remain closely associated with wild animals but on occasion, in nymph form, have been found within human dwellings; (4) those bugs that also essentially are wild but on occasion, in adult form, may be found in or around a dwelling (they do not seem to do well in this environment); and (5) those wild insects not reported in association with human habitation at all.

Although Chagas disease always has been associated with rural areas and low socioeconomic groups, some species of *Triatoma* have been reported to have adapted to areas undergoing urbanization, such as Guayaquil, Ecuador, and Recife and Salvador in Brazil. Various suitable hosts, such as the opossum, that often live close to humans may provide the transition between wild and domestic infection. It frequently is observed that domestic animals, such as pigs, cattle, goats, and sheep, are kept in close contact with the domicile and that triatomines closely associated with these animals can be carried into the home.

Weather conditions clearly modify the distribution and transmission of Chagas disease because at temperatures below 15° C, *T. cruzi* fails to develop at all in *Triatoma infestans*, and between 15° and 22° C, no metacyclic forms are produced; at 36° to 37° C, epimastigotes and trypomastigotes are scarce. The optimum temperature is reported to be between 23° and 27° C. In many countries where the seasons are delineated clearly, there is a definite increase of acute disease in spring and summer. Although insect transmission is the usual means of infection, congenital transmission is well known, and as early as 1911, Chagas first suggested this means of transmission. This manner of infection has been demonstrated experimentally in dogs and guinea pigs; more recently in lower primates, placentitis and abortion have been reported. Similarly, in humans in endemic areas, *T. cruzi* has been shown to be an important cause of abortion, placentitis, and congenital infection associated with prematurity. The overall incidence of congenital Chagas disease was 2 per cent in 500 deliveries, and when mothers had Chagas disease, the incidence was 10.5 per cent.

The possibility of transmission by maternal milk is suggested by observations of organisms in lactating mice. Similar observations have been made in other experimental animals. Transmission by organ transplantation and especially blood transfusion remains an important factor in endemic areas, where it has been reported that among more than 50,000 blood donors in Buenos Aires, Argentina, almost 6 per cent had a positive serology; in Brazil 15 per cent and in Venezuela 3 per cent were positive. The problem is compounded when one considers that in stored refrigerated blood, blood forms can live for weeks without losing their infectivity. Moreover, it currently is believed that once an individual has acquired an infection, organisms always are present in the tissues and very small numbers of trypomastigotes are present in the blood either intermittently or continuously. If looked for, organisms usually can be demonstrated by blood culture techniques or xenodiagnosis.

Ingestion of infected mice by cats or cannibalism among rodents has been shown to transmit the infection successfully. Furthermore, several recent reports indicate the acquisition of infection by humans from infected meat. It is not clear, however, how important these routes of infection might be in maintaining the disease in nature or in humans. It is of some interest that these same means of transmission may have appeared in Maryland when several raccoons were found infected with *T. cruzi* but no insect vector could be found.

There are a large number of feral and domestic reservoirs of *T. cruzi*. Various species of the opossum are regarded as among the most important sylvatic reservoirs. In some areas, armadillos have been implicated. In the United States, the wood rat, raccoon, armadillo, and opossum are important feral hosts. Nevertheless, the reason Chagas disease is so scarce in the United States is not clear. Various suggestions, including low strain virulence and adverse vector feeding habits, have been advocated. Dogs and cats, especially in Brazil and Chile, have been shown to have a high index of infection and are believed to represent important domestic reservoirs.

Pathogenesis and Pathology

Once metacyclic trypomastigotes traverse the skin or mucous membrane, they may be phagocytized by tissue macrophages or actively penetrate other cells (Figs. 219–2 and 219–3). Within the cell, trypomastigotes rapidly transform into rounded amastigotes and division begins (Fig. 219–4). In vitro studies suggest that those parasites within macrophage vacuoles are killed soon by hydrogen peroxide if the parasite is unable to escape the vacuole and reach the cytoplasm where they reproduce. Within these cells large numbers of amastigotes are formed, and within a few days the greatly distended cell ruptures, freeing trypomastigotes and amastigotes into the tissues. These actively invade fresh cells, and the process is repeated. A nodular swelling or chagoma develops at the site of entry (Fig. 219–5). This area soon is

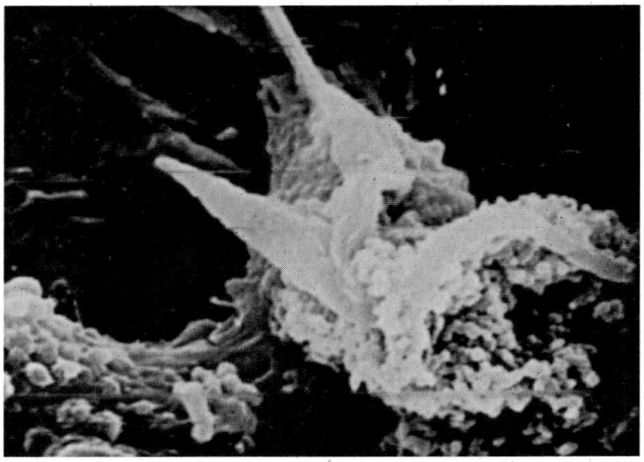

FIGURE 219–2. Trypanosoma cruzi *being phagocytized by a mouse peritoneal macrophage. (Scanning electron micrograph × 6000.)*

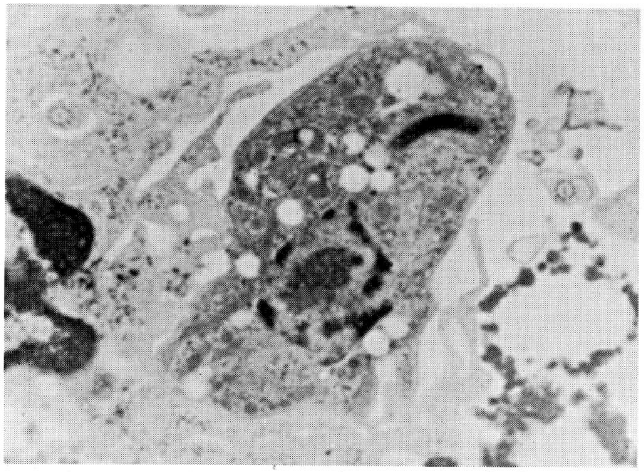

FIGURE 219–3. Trypanosoma cruzi *being phagocytized by a mouse peritoneal macrophage. (Transmission electron micrograph × 7000.)*

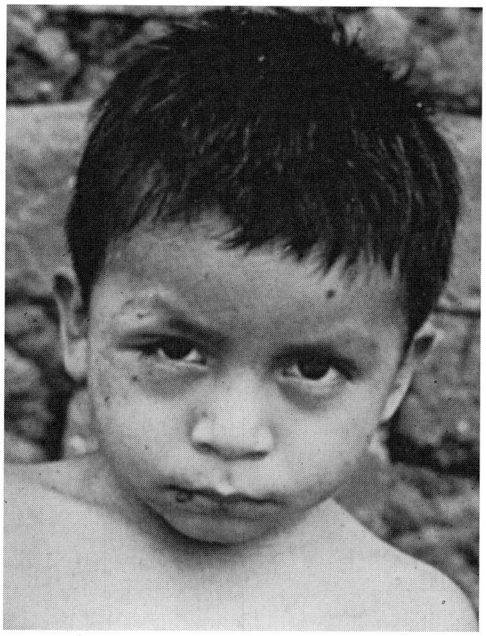

FIGURE 219–5. *Chagas disease. Chagoma on the mucocutaneous junction of the lip and moderate unilateral periorbital edema are present. (From a nonprofit cooperative endeavor by numerous colleagues under the editorship of Dr. Herman Zaiman, New York.)*

infiltrated with macrophages surrounded by lymphocytes, eosinophils, and polymorphonuclear neutrophils. The process spreads to the regional lymph nodes, where focal lymphadenitis becomes evident. Shortly thereafter, blood forms appear and disseminate throughout the body. The acute pathologic process is related to the invasion and subsequent destruction of cells by the replicating intracellular parasites. Associated with these areas of cellular destruction is a marked host inflammatory reaction characterized by local accumulation of polymorphonuclear leukocytes, lymphocytes, and plasma cells. No tissue is spared, but cardiac and skeletal muscle, particularly, and reticuloendothelial and neuroglial cells most often are affected. The myocardium reveals focal myonecrosis, contraction band necrosis, interstitial fibrosis, and lymphocytic infiltration. Interspersed among the degenerating fibers is a marked mixed inflammatory cell exudate, which with time becomes predominantly mononuclear. The course of the acute infection can be quite variable, with severe tissue destruction, or the infection can be silent, with little or no obvious pathology. Nevertheless, the parasites have entered various cells of the body successfully and have formed pseudocysts, each containing hundreds to thousands of amastigotes (Fig. 219–6). Those who recover from the acute episode, including those who have had an inapparent infection, probably harbor these intracellular parasites for the rest of their lives.

In the chronic stage of Chagas disease, the heart usually is enlarged. The chambers may be dilated, and one often may find an apical left ventricular aneurysm, which rarely rup-

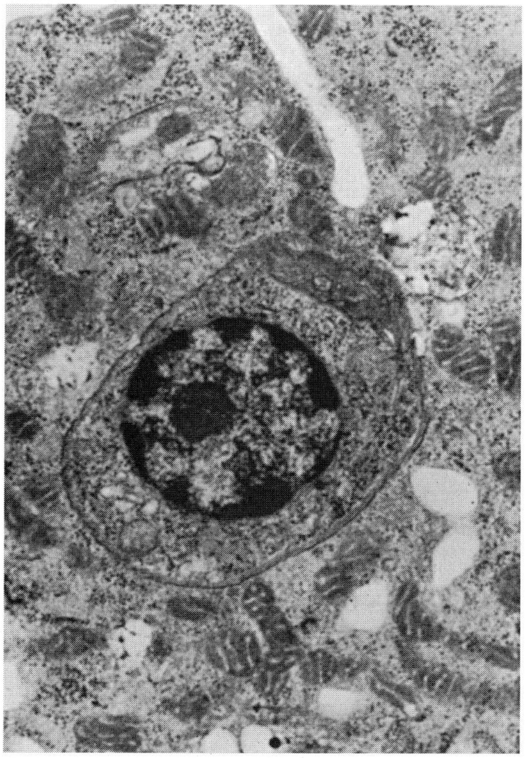

FIGURE 219–4. Trypanosoma cruzi *amastigote forms in the cytoplasm of a macrophage. (Transmission electron micrograph × 7000.)*

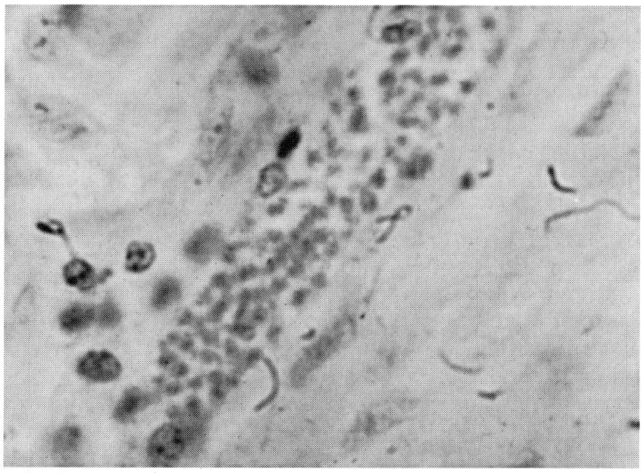

FIGURE 219–6. Trypanosoma cruzi *amastigote forms in cardiac muscle. (Original magnification × 288.)*

tures. Mural thrombi, especially of the right atrium and apex of the left ventricle, are seen commonly. These may cause widespread embolization, especially to the brain, lungs, spleen, and kidneys. The myocardium often reveals diffuse fibrosis with small numbers of mononuclear cells scattered throughout, and in from 60 to 70 per cent of patients it may be quite difficult to find parasites in the myocardium. The pathogenesis of chronic chagasic cardiomyopathy is poorly understood. Autoimmunity, alterations in the autonomic nervous system, and injury to the coronary microvasculature have been suggested as important factors.

Lesions of the digestive tract have been studied carefully. Destruction of more than 95 per cent of the ganglion cells of the myenteric plexus in the esophagus and similar pathology in the colon leading to megaesophagus and megacolon have been demonstrated. In experimental studies, destruction of ganglionic cells of both heart and digestive tract largely is the result of parasitic destruction during the acute phase of the disease. How early neuronal destruction may contribute to the development of congestive cardiomyopathy currently is under active study.

During acute Chagas disease, high titers of complement-fixing, hemagglutinating, and precipitating antibodies can be detected, which also is the time the largest number of parasites is in the blood. At this period, most of the antibody is IgM. Later, in the latent and chronic stages, antibodies predominantly are in the IgG and IgA class. Thus far, antigenic variation, as seen in African trypanosomiasis, does not seem to occur in *T. cruzi* infection. In experimental rodent infection, humoral immunity seems to modify infection, but the precise role of antibodies has not been elucidated. Moreover, there is experimental evidence that cell-mediated immunity plays an important role in protection against *T. cruzi* infection and interferon (IFN)-γ serves to up-regulate macrophage killing. Administration of antilymphocyte serum and neonatal thymectomy results in increased parasitemia and death. Presently, the role of immunity in Chagas disease is undergoing intensive investigation.

Clinical Manifestations

Clinical Chagas disease can be viewed best as having three phases: acute, latent, and chronic.

Seroepidemiologic studies indicate that the vast majority of individuals infected with *T. cruzi* fail to develop overt or clinically recognizable disease and that estimates of up to 99 per cent of those infected have inapparent or subclinical infection. The vast majority of those who develop clinical disease are infants, who are rather helpless in warding off the bite of triatomes, or "kissing-bugs," as well as other young children up to 10 years of age.

After a clinical prepatent period of about 7 to 14 days, acute clinical symptoms may begin with anorexia, lassitude, headache, and intermittent or remitting fevers of 38° to 40.5° C (100.4° to 104.9° F). In young infants, swelling and edema of the Bichât fat-pad may make feeding painful and unrewarding. Locally, or near the site of initial infection, a characteristic unilateral painless palpebral edema, often with conjunctivitis, may be recognized. This so-called Romaña's sign, when present in the endemic area (25 to 30 per cent of patients), is highly suggestive of early acute Chagas disease. However, the edema may be generalized only to be mistaken for nephrotic syndrome, or swelling of the preauricular region may be so severe as to suggest mumps. Generalized lymphadenopathy, moderate hepatosplenomegaly, vomiting, and diarrhea as well as signs of meningeal irritation commonly are encountered. Skin lesions can vary from a generalized maculopapular or morbilliform eruption to urticaria. Neurologic symptoms, found more often in younger infants than in older patients, include focal to generalized seizures. Signs and symptoms of cardiac involvement are seen in almost every patient if sought for carefully. Tachycardia, unrelated to fever (perhaps due to destruction of cardiac sympathetic ganglia), cardiac enlargement, or a gallop rhythm associated with cardiac failure may be noted. Evidence of myocarditis frequently can be found and in the vast majority of patients is mild. The electrocardiogram may show sinus tachycardia, prolongation of the PR interval, low-voltage QRS, and primary T-wave change. The early development of cardiac arrhythmias, such as premature ventricular contractions, atrial fibrillation, partial or complete A-V block, and progressive congestive failure, does not bode well for the patient. Examination of the blood during this phase often will reveal actively swimming trypomastigote forms, leukocytosis with a relative lymphocytosis, an elevated erythrocyte sedimentation rate, and an increase in serum globulins.

Although the vast majority of patients recover, apparently without sequelae, 5 to 10 per cent may die, usually of severe myocarditis. Young infants, however, often die of severe meningoencephalitis.

As the acute stage subsides in 8 to 12 weeks, fewer and fewer parasites can be found in the peripheral blood, antibodies are evident, and as the disease enters the latent period, organisms may be found by special techniques described later.

In its acute stage, congenital Chagas disease often resembles the acquired disease. The onset may be at birth or a few months later, with the infant presenting with hepatosplenomegaly, mild to severe anemia, jaundice, edema, widespread petechiae, tremors, and convulsions. At this time, erythroblastosis fetalis, congenital toxoplasmosis, cytomegalovirus infection, and herpes simplex virus infection can confound the diagnosis. Edema is similar to that found in the acquired disease, and although frank meningoencephalitis has been observed, it is more likely to be silent. Prognosis of meningoencephalitis in congenital disease is better than in the acquired form of disease. Examination of the cerebrospinal fluid often reveals *T. cruzi*. Necrotic and hemorrhagic lesions of the oral mucosa and skin are thought to represent hematogenously disseminated chagomas. Digestive tract lesions manifested by dysphagia may appear early and can cause early death of the patient by aspiration.

The latent phase of clinical Chagas disease represents that period between the infection and the onset of chronic signs and symptoms. The duration of this period spans 10 to 40 years, and in the overwhelming majority of cases, overt clinical disease never occurs, despite the fact that in asymptomatic individuals organisms often can be isolated by culture techniques. Long-term, large-scale, follow-up studies are necessary to ascertain the outcome of latent infection. These currently are being done in Brazil.

Chronic chagasic cardiopathy is the most frequent manifestation of chronic Chagas disease. Digestive tract disorders are seen much less frequently.

Commonly, mild to severe congestive failure is the first sign of chagasic heart disease. Cardiomegaly with radiographic evidence of an enlarged globular heart shadow with clear lung fields is seen frequently. Signs of right-sided heart failure are observed more commonly than those of left-sided. Heart sounds may be distant, and murmurs of functional mitral and tricuspid insufficiency sometimes are heard. In the endemic area, the electrocardiogram abnormalities may be suggestive of chagasic cardiopathy. Premature ventricular contractions and right bundle branch block occur in up to 50 per cent of cases; A-V block of varying degree occurs in about 30 per cent of cases; complete A-V block is much less common, and left bundle branch block is not characteristic. The presence of right bundle branch block with anterior fascicular block is highly suggestive of chagasic heart disease, which has been reported in both teenagers and young adults.

Once heart failure occurs, it usually is intractable and difficult to treat. Death often is associated with a fatal arrhythmia or due to embolism of a thrombus typically found in the left ventricle or right atrium.

Megaesophagus and megacolon are the result of destruction of the ganglion cells of the myenteric plexus. Although these usually are not fatal complications, except in congenital disease, the marked dilatations of the colon and esophagus are most distressing. Almost any hollow viscus can be involved, but esophageal and colonic disease is encountered most frequently. Dysphagia, regurgitation with retrosternal burning, singultus, and paroxysmal night coughs, presumably due to aspiration while sleeping, are associated with megaesophagus; chronic constipation, long-term fecal retention, impaction, and volvulus are seen with megacolon.

In some regions, it is not unusual for patients with digestive disease to have symptomatic chagasic heart disease as well. There is wide geographic variation in the prevalence of cardiac and gastrointestinal disease. In Panama, Venezuela, and Colombia, "megas" almost never are encountered, whereas in parts of Brazil, both forms of Chagas disease may be seen in the same individual. Patients iatrogenically immunosuppressed or patients with AIDS may have reactivation of acute disease.

Patients with latent or chronic Chagas disease can develop reactivated acute disease when immunosuppressed by chemotherapy or if they have HIV-1 disease. In these patients, central nervous system lesions present in computed axial tomographic scans are indistinguishable from those of central nervous system toxoplasmosis.

Diagnosis and Treatment

Definitive diagnosis depends upon the demonstration of the parasite in the blood or tissues. It must be emphasized that examination of the peripheral blood is of value only during the initial acute disease (6 to 12 weeks) or during chronic exacerbation. Animal inoculation with the patient's blood often will aid in the diagnosis. In chronic stages, it often is useful to take 30 to 50 mL of the patient's blood and inoculate a large number of cultures in order to obtain a positive diagnosis. Liver biopsy, bone marrow aspiration, or splenic puncture often will provide the answer. At times, xenodiagnosis may be the only means by which organisms can be found. In this technique, laboratory-reared reduviid bugs are permitted to feed on the patient or his fresh blood; subsequently, the bugs are allowed to feed on uninfected guinea pigs. The latter are examined for trypomastigotes after about 45 days.

Serologic tests can be useful during various stages of the disease. The precipitin test may be positive during the acute episode, whereas complement fixation (Machado-Guerreiro test) is useful for diagnosis of chronic disease. The fluorescent antibody and indirect hemagglutination tests are valuable tools for the diagnosis of Chagas disease. However, patients with leishmaniasis, malaria, collagen vascular disease, and syphilis may give false-positive reactions.

In congenital disease, an indirect immunofluorescence test utilizing anti-IgM may demonstrate acute congenital disease. Recently, polymerase chain reaction (PCR) has been used to aid in the diagnosis of both acute and chronic disease. Examination of the blood by PCR can be extremely sensitive and specific; theoretically, a single trypomastigote can be detected by this method. In addition to serologic and morphologic diagnosis of Chagas disease, clinical diagnosis rests upon a history that the patient lives or once lived in an endemic area and that the cardiac or digestive tract lesions are compatible with Chagas disease.

During the chronic stage, serologic methods may be the only means to arrive at a diagnosis. Thus, PCR, the indirect fluorescent antibody test, enzyme-linked immunosorbent assay, complement fixation, and the direct agglutination test may be useful.

In evaluating the patient with chagasic heart disease, rheumatic heart disease, arteriosclerotic heart disease, and other idiopathic myocardiopathies must be considered. As previously mentioned, congenital Chagas disease must be differentiated from erythroblastosis fetalis, toxoplasmosis, cytomegalovirus infection, and herpes simplex virus infection.

There is no uniformly effective drug for the treatment of Chagas disease. Nifurtimox (Lampit) has been used extensively with limited success. In some regions, the drug has had a high failure rate. It appears to reduce the period of the acute disease and to reduce mortality associated with meningoencephalitis and myocarditis. The period of parasitemia is shortened. It is believed by some researchers that if treatment is instituted early in the acute disease, nifurtimox may cure patients with acute *T. cruzi* infection inasmuch as they fail to develop antibodies to *T. cruzi*. Whether these individuals then are at risk to develop chronic Chagas disease at a later time is unknown. Nifurtimox has been most effective in Chile and Argentina but less so in Brazil.

There is no evidence that nifurtimox is useful in the treatment of chronic Chagas disease, although some workers treat chronic chagasic cardiomyopathy with prolonged courses of nifurtimox or benznidazole. The former is available in the United States from the Parasitic Drug Service of the Centers for Disease Control and Prevention in Atlanta, Georgia. It is supplied in 30- and 120-mg tablets. The usual dose for adults is 8 to 10 mg/kg body weight/day. For adolescents (11 to 16 years of age), it is 12.5 to 15 mg/kg/day, and for children (1 to 10 years of age), it is 15 to 20 mg/kg/day. It is given in four divided doses daily for 90 to 120 days. There are many untoward reactions to this drug. These include abdominal pain, nausea, vomiting, anorexia, restlessness, disorientation, insomnia, twitching, paresthesia, polyneuritis, and seizures. Skin reactions also are seen.

Another drug similar to nifurtimox, benznidazole, has had limited clinical use. It appears to have similar efficacy. Some researchers believe it is tolerated better, with less adverse reaction. It is used extensively in Brazil at 5 mg/kg/day for 30 to 120 days. Bone marrow depression and peripheral neuritis have limited its use.

Recently, a child who contracted transfusion-associated Chagas disease and a laboratory worker with acute disease were treated with nifurtimox and recombinant interferon-γ. Experimental data suggest that interferon-γ may be a useful adjunct in treatment by activating macrophage killing.

Patients with chronic chagasic cardiomyopathy may be helped for a varying period by implanting a cardiac pacemaker, but the congestive failure usually is refractory to the usual cardiac glycosides and vasoactive drugs.

Megacolon usually is treated by dietary fiber, laxatives, and enemas. When these fail, surgical resection may be required. Megaesophagus usually is amenable to therapy by a combination of diet and dilation of the esophagastric region. In more severe disease, various surgical procedures have been used with variable success to relieve the symptoms of achalasia.

Prevention

Regular insecticide spraying programs with benzene hexachloride could reduce the transmission of the infection, at least around domiciles. Proper screening and improved housing for those in endemic areas also would serve to reduce transmission. Careful screening of blood donors would help prevent transfusion transmission in endemic areas. The development of a chemoprophylactic agent or vaccine holds out the best hope for prevention and subsequent eradication of Chagas disease.

Transfusion-acquired disease is a major public health problem in endemic areas. Treatment of the blood with gentian violet inactivates the parasite. Transfusion-acquired infection has been reported in the United States also. Because there is no effective rapid means to detect the parasite, it has been suggested that persons from endemic areas be rejected as blood donors.

AFRICAN TRYPANOSOMIASIS

African sleeping sickness is caused by two variants of hemoflagellate protozoans: *Trypanosoma brucei gambiense,* the cause of West African or Gambian sleeping sickness, and *T. brucei rhodesiense,* the cause of East African or Rhodesian disease. Although these parasites produce similar diseases, the Gambian form usually is chronic and evolves slowly, often over many years, ending fatally if untreated, whereas the Rhodesian form is characterized by being acute, usually killing the host in a matter of weeks or months. These diseases exist wherever the various species of *Glossina,* the tsetse fly, are found.

The Organism

T. brucei gambiense and *rhodesiense* are pleomorphic flagellates varying from 15 to 30 μm in length by 1.5 to 3.5 μm in breadth. In Giemsa-stained blood smears, they may appear long and slender with an undulating membrane and free anterior flagellum or short and broad without a free anterior flagellum. There are no intracellular forms. At various stages of disease, trypomastigote forms may be found in the peripheral blood, lymphatics, lymph nodes, cerebrospinal fluid, and neural tissue. Thus, although the two subspecies morphologically are indistinguishable, they seem to maintain separate biologic characteristics, especially with regard to virulence in cross-inoculation experiments. Outside of humans there is no important reservoir host for *T. brucei gambiense,* whereas *T. brucei rhodesiense* is found naturally infecting wild game animals.

Within the insect vector, the tsetse fly, trypomastigote forms ingested with a blood meal settle in the posterior portion of the midgut, where they multiply by binary fission for about 7 to 10 days. The slender trypomastigotes then migrate anteriorly to the foregut, where they remain for the next 2 to 3 weeks. They next move further forward and finally enter the salivary glands, in which they transform into epimastigote forms, that is, forms in which the kinetoplast has migrated just anterior to the nucleus, and continue to replicate. After several cycles of division, they transform into infective metacyclic trypomastigote forms, which are the small, broad or "stumpy" forms that lack a free anterior flagellum. When next feeding, the infective tsetse fly may inoculate into the bite wound upwards of several thousands of these infective trypomastigotes. The entire dipteran cycle spans a period of 15 to 35 days.

Within the human host, trypomastigotes multiply by binary fission in blood, lymph, and extracellular spaces. The central nervous system eventually is invaded, at which time multiplication continues unabated.

Transmission by blood transfusion, hypodermic needle, or other insects may occur. Congenital transmission has been reported.

Epidemiology

Human African sleeping sickness is restricted to those areas south of the Sahara where the annual rainfall exceeds 500 mm (20 inches) because the larval stages of the tsetse fly are vulnerable to desiccation. There are at least 20,000 new cases annually of African sleeping sickness and about 50 million people at risk. In 1986, there were 10,500 cases in Zaire alone. The Gambian form occurs mainly in the western portion of tropical Africa, with focal incursions eastward north of Lake Victoria into the Sudan. *Glossina palpalis* is the main tsetse fly vector, although other related species, such as *G. tachinoides* and *G. fuscipes,* also are implicated. The Rhodesian form is found in the southeastern portion of Africa.

Although *T. brucei gambiense* can infect various mammals, humans appear to be more susceptible and maintain high enough parasitemias to maintain the fly-human-fly cycle. The prolonged chronicity of Gambian disease with infectious individuals continually exposed to tsetse flies undoubtedly helps to sustain the disease. Asymptomatic carriers of the infection also may be an important factor in maintaining the disease in a community. Furthermore, it has been reported that among the important factors that may limit Gambian infection to humans is the transient and low parasitemia that results from an infective tsetse fly bite in mammals, usually ungulates. Thus, it has been observed that Gambian disease usually is maintained only when there is a close and repeated relationship between humans and tsetse flies. The practical result of all this is that West African sleeping sickness is maintained by those members of the *G. palpalis* group of tsetse flies that utilize and/or prefer human blood almost exclusively. Experimentally, domestic animals, such as pigs and goats, can maintain infection with *T. brucei gambiense.* It is not clear if this observation is of epidemiologic significance.

In contrast to Gambian disease, *T. brucei rhodesiense* infection usually is maintained in wild mammals. Therefore, the fly-human-fly cycle tends to be unimportant inasmuch as the acute nature of the disease usually quickly removes acutely ill humans as an infective source. However, the intervention of wild game animals, in whom the disease tends to be less acute and whose blood appears to be more attractive, seems to have relegated humans to an occasional or facultative host for *T. brucei rhodesiense.* The *G. morsitans* group of tsetse flies that inhabit the relatively dry East African savannah readily feed upon wild ungulates, especially the bush-buck, *Tragelaphus scriptus,* and the hartebeest, *Alcelaphus buselaphus.* On occasion, Rhodesian disease may reach epidemic proportions, and at these times direct human-fly-human cycles may intervene.

Although all age groups are susceptible to infection, the factors that influence human prevalence rest more on occupational exposure to suitable tsetse flies, as well as the flies' breeding and feeding habits. Thus, although young adult males are found most frequently to be infected, during epidemics, when all age groups are infected, mechanical transmission is said to occur. Tourists on camera safaris possibly are at risk.

Pathogenesis and Pathology

The metacyclic infective trypomastigote forms are inoculated by the tsetse fly into the skin, where they multiply at the inoculation site. A characteristic, hard, sometimes painful, chancre is formed. By about the tenth day, long slender forms are found in the blood stream and lymphatics, and for the next several days, their numbers increase logarithmically. Soon thereafter, the organisms nearly disappear from the blood stream as a result of immune lysis, only to reappear again. The interval between waves of parasitemia may vary from 1 to 8 days, with clinical symptoms accompanying each bout of parasitemia. This can be accounted for by the highly developed antigenic variation strategy of the parasite. Thus, the trypomastigote is covered with a variable surface glycoprotein (VSG), and with each peak of parasitemia there is a predominant variable antigen type (VAT) displayed by the organism. The specific antibody response to this coat protein (VSG) leads to the destruction of those parasites that display the predominant VAT or homotype. There are a number of heterotypes within each population of parasites, one of which becomes the next homotype, which is not recognized by the host's immune system. The parasite in each successive wave of parasitemia bears a different VAT. A single trypomastigote may contain up to 1000 genes, each encoding for a specific VSG. Each successive parasitemic wave represents a new antigenic variant, which has emerged to elude the host's antibody response to the previous antigen.

As a result of successive waves of immune lysis and parasitemia, a marked early humoral antibody response, predominantly involving 19S IgM, is seen regularly. These macroglobulins contain not only antitrypanosomal antibodies, which are directed against the surface antigens, but a variety of other antibodies, such as heterophile and rheumatoid factor. It has been shown experimentally that because of polyclonal B-cell activation, many antibodies are produced to a wide variety of antigens, including brain-specific autoantibodies directed against myelin basic protein, gangliosides, and cerebrosides. Circulating immune complexes have been reported regularly and may be responsible for the glomerulonephritis, hypocomplementemia, and hemolytic anemia that often accompany acute and chronic disease. Cell-mediated immunity also is important in African trypanosomiasis.

The main pathologic lesions involve especially the posterior cervical, submaxillary, supraclavicular, and mesenteric lymph nodes and the central nervous system. The lymphatic tissue usually reveals generalized hyperplasia with diffuse proliferation of lymphocytes. Later, the nodes may become small and fibrotic; however, they initially markedly are hemorrhagic, containing large numbers of trypomastigotes.

The central nervous system remains normal until invaded by organisms, but then a progressive chronic leptomeningitis develops. The brain becomes edematous, and there is prominent perivascular cuffing by glial cells, lymphocytes, and plasma cells. When the latter become vacuolated with pyknotic nuclei, they often are referred to as the morula cells of Mott and Marshalko. Organisms often can be found in the brain tissue in proximity to vessels and also may be found in the cerebrospinal fluid. Glomerulonephritis, myocarditis, pericardial effusion, pulmonary edema, and a hypoplastic bone marrow with an associated anemia may be seen. The pathogenesis of the neuropsychiatric manifestations are not understood. Recent experimental studies suggest that changes in the levels of brain neurotransmitters, deposition of immune complexes, and alteration in prostaglandin and cytokine production may, in part, account for these behavioral changes.

Clinical Manifestations

Clinical manifestations of *T. brucei gambiense* and *T. brucei rhodesiense* disease are similar, except that Rhodesian infection is a more fulminant, acute disease that may run its course in several weeks to 6 to 9 months, whereas Gambian infection may last for years. Typically, the incubation period in Rhodesian infection is brief (3 to 21 days), whereas the onset of symptoms with Gambian infection may be delayed from several weeks or for years. About a week after infection and at the site of the tsetse fly bite, a hard and painful chancre sometimes appears, lasting several weeks. During the early stages when recurrent bouts of fever may be the only symptom, the blood and lymphatics primarily are involved and infection often is mistaken for malaria, especially if a chancre is not obvious or a history of exposure to tsetse flies is not obtained. The period of intermittent fevers may last for months to years with Gambian infection. During this time, persistent headache and tachycardia often are encountered. In whites, a circinate erythematous rash or erythema multiforme sometimes is noted. Fever abates gradually. In many patients, characteristic posterior cervical lymphadenopathy becomes evident (Winterbottom's sign). The nodes are nontender, reaching about a centimeter in diameter. They tend to become small and fibrotic in about 6 months.

Untreated patients with Gambian disease often develop signs of central nervous system invasion. Initial signs and symptoms of neurologic involvement can be difficult to assess. These may consist of alterations of behavior and/or personality that eventually may manifest as a severe psychosis. Severe headache, loss of nocturnal sleep, and a feeling of impending doom typically are described. Next, there may be progressive mental deterioration, and with unrelenting deterioration, patients become incapable of caring for themselves. Tremors, especially of the tongue, hands, or feet, and generalized or focal convulsive episodes may occur. Almost any neurologic psychiatric manifestation can be seen, and with progressive mental deterioration, patients finally lapse into a coma and die. During the final period of the disease, patients often die of such intercurrent infections as bacterial pneumonia, amebiasis, and malaria. Wasting and malnutrition are a large component of the progressive deterioration of these patients. Sleeping sickness can be a difficult disease for early diagnosis in young children. It usually is found only after a child presents with obtundation, seizures, or psychomotor retardation.

Diagnosis

Definitive diagnosis only can be made by finding trypanosomes in blood and bone marrow smears, in lymph node aspirates in early or acute disease, and in cerebrospinal fluid in late or chronic disease. It is essential to employ both thick and thin smears, as well as to examine the buffy coat from 10 to 20 mL of citrated whole blood or the sediment from 5 mL of centrifuged cerebrospinal fluid. Culture and/or animal inoculation sometimes is the only successful means of obtaining a diagnosis. In advanced central nervous system disease, lymphocytosis and elevated IgM are characteristic of the cerebrospinal fluid.

Serologic diagnosis of African trypanosomiasis usually depends upon detection of high levels of nonspecific serum IgM. The detection of specific antibody by the indirect immunofluorescent technique is helpful, especially when the serum is tested with trypanosomes of the homologous human species. Using direct agglutination and a microscale version of the enzyme-linked immunosorbent assay is highly reliable method for specific diagnosis of trypanosomiasis.

The differential diagnosis of African trypanosomiasis spans a wide spectrum of diseases, but chronic relapsing fevers associated with enlarged cervical lymph nodes in an individual who has been to Africa are suggestive. As indicated earlier, it is not unusual to consider such diseases as malaria, syphilis, Hodgkin disease, visceral leishmaniasis, and leprosy. Later, encephalitis of other etiologies must be excluded. An important diagnostic feature is the frequent finding of a markedly elevated erythrocyte sedimentation rate, which is a reflection of the markedly increased serum macroglobulins.

Prognosis

If therapy is initiated prior to significant central nervous system involvement, the outcome usually is favorable. Untreated infection often ends fatally.

Treatment

Early African trypanosomiasis yields more readily to therapy than disease in the late chronic stage. Prior to central nervous system disease, suramin (Naphuride, Antrypol), which does not cross the blood-brain barrier, may be used. Although it is of low toxicity, suramin is excreted almost entirely by the kidneys and may cause renal damage. Therefore, urinalysis should be done the day after each dose of suramin to assure that there is no evidence of renal damage. Therapy must be discontinued if albuminuria and/or granular casts appear. The drug is dissolved in 10 mL of sterile distilled water. The initial test dose in an adult is 100 to 200 mg intravenously; then 1 g is administered intravenously on days 1, 3, 7, 14, and 21. The pediatric dose is 20 mg/kg administered on the same schedule. Even though suramin does not cross the blood-brain barrier, intrathecal administration should not be attempted. Suramin is believed to be a lysosomotropic agent, and at 10 to 100 μm/mL, concentrations known to inhibit infectivity, suramin has been shown to inhibit adenosine triphosphatase.

Recent reports have indicated that DFMO (eflornithine) is highly effective in the treatment of West African trypanosomiasis. It is an inhibitor of ornithine decarboxylase and is highly effective against both the hemolymphatic and central nervous system stages of *T. brucei gambiense* infection. However, its effectiveness against *T. brucei rhodesiense* infection is variable. Efficacy in children has not been determined. A 3-year-old with *T. brucei gambiense* infection in the central nervous system stage was treated successfully. The recommended dose is 400 mg/kg/day for 14 days followed by 300 mg/kg/day for an additional 30 days. Side effects include anemia, thrombocytopenia, diarrhea, and seizures; these are short-lived and reversible.

Pentamidine is an effective alternative drug for the treatment of early African trypanosomiasis. It is given as an intramuscular injection of 4 mg/kg of the base daily for 10 days or every other day extended over 20 days. The pediatric dose is the same as that for the adult. Pentamidine is dissolved in no more than 3 mL of water. The course may be repeated 1 week after completion of the first. Patients should receive this drug while lying down because transient hypotensive episodes, palpitations, and vertigo are not uncommon. It is contraindicated in renal disease.

In chronic or late stage disease with central nervous system involvement, melarsoprol (Mel B, Arsobal) may be used. Melarsoprol is a combination of the trivalent arsenical melarsen oxide and British antilewisite and is administered in the hospital as a 5 per cent solution in propylene oxide. The recommended adult dose is 2 to 3.6 mg/kg/day intravenously on 3 consecutive days and after 1 week, 3.6 mg/kg/day intravenously for 3 consecutive days. Therapy is repeated after 10 to 21 days. The pediatric dose is 18 to 25 mg/kg total dose administered over a 1-month period. The initial dose is 0.36 mg/kg intravenously increasing gradually to a maximum of 3.6 mg/kg. The injections are given every 1 to 5 days, depending on the patient's reaction. Usually, a total of 9 to 10 doses is given. Neither renal nor optic nerve toxicity is observed with this drug, but arsenic toxicity can be a problem. In weak or debilitated patients, it often is recommended that therapy begin with 18 mg of melarsoprol and the dose incrementally increased. Prior treatment with suramin usually is advocated for frail or debilitated patients. Patients with late-stage disease treated with Mel B may develop fatal posttreatment reactive encephalopathy. Alternatively, DFMO may be used to treat central nervous system Gambian disease. Congenital trypanosomiasis has been treated successfully.

Prophylaxis

Chemoprophylaxis with suramin, 0.3 to 0.7 g intravenously every 2 to 3 months, has been advocated and is reported to be highly effective. The development of a vaccine is being worked on actively in many laboratories throughout the world but has been hampered by antigenic variation. Attempts to make vaccines with x-irradiated or low-virulence strains only resulted in variant-specific protection.

Prevention

With few exceptions, control of the vector has proved to be a difficult task and has reduced but not eliminated the tsetse fly. Prevention of tsetse fly bites and chemoprophylaxis may be the best means of eliminating the disease from an area.

Bibliography

1. Adams, J. H., Haller, L., Boa, F. Y., et al.: Human African trypanosomiasis (*T. b. gambiense*): A study of 16 fatal cases of sleeping sickness with some observations on acute reactive encephalopathy. Neuropathol. Appl. Neurobiol. *12*:81–94, 1986.
2. Amole, B., Sharpless, N., Wittner, M., et al.: Neurochemical measurements in the brains of mice infected with *Trypanosoma brucei brucei* (TREU 667) Ann. Trop. Med. Parasitol. *83*:225–232, 1989.
3. Azogue, E., LaFuente, C., and Darras, C.: Congenital Chagas' disease in Bolivia: Epidemiological aspects and pathological findings. Trans. R. Soc. Trop. Med. Hyg. *79*:176–180, 1985.
4. Bacchi, C, J., and McCann, P. P.: Parasitic protozoa and polyamines. *In* McCann, P. P., Pegg, A. E., and Sjoerdsma, A. (eds.): Inhibition of Polyamine Metabolism: Biological Significance and Basis for New Therapies. New York, Academic Press, 1987, p. 317.
5. Bittencourt, A. L.: Congenital Chagas' disease. Am. J. Dis. Child. *130*:97–103, 1976.
6. Bittencourt, A. L., Vieira, G. O., Tavares, H. C., et al.: Esophageal involvement in congenital Chagas' disease: Report of a case with megaesophagus. Am. J. Trop. Med. Hyg. *33*:30–33, 1984.
7. Borst, P.: Molecular genetics of antigenic variation. Immunol. Today *7*:A29–A33, 1991.
8. Buyst, H.: Sleeping sickness in children. Ann. Soc. Belg. Med. Trop. *57*:201–212, 1977.
9. Doua, F., Boa, F. Y., Schechter, P. F., et al.: Treatment of human late stage gambiense trypanosomiasis with alpha-difluoromethylornithine (eflornithine): Efficacy and tolerance in 14 cases in Cote d'Ivoire. Am. J. Trop. Med. Hyg. *37*:525–533, 1987.
10. Factor, S. M., Cho, S., Wittner, M., et al.: Abnormalities of the coronary microcirculaion in acute murine Chagas' disease. Am. J. Trop. Med. Hyg. *34*:246–253, 1985.
11. Grant, I. H., Gold, J. W. M., Wittner, M., et al.: Transfusion associated acute Chagas' disease acquired in the United States. Ann. Intern. Med. *111*:849–851, 1989.

12. Greenwood, B. M., and Whittle, H. C.: The pathogenesis of sleeping sickness. Trans. R. Soc. Trop. Med. Hyg. *74*:716–725, 1980.
13. Kirchhoff, L. V.: American trypanosomiasis (Chagas' disease): A tropical disease now in the United States. N. Engl. J. Med. *329*:639–644, 1993.
14. Maguire, J. H., Hoff, R., Sherlock, I., et al.: Cardiac morbidity and mortality due to Chagas' disease: Prospective electrocardiographic study of a Brazilian community. Circulation *75*:1140–1145, 1987.
15. Oliviero, J. S.: A natural human model of intrinsic heart nervous system denervation: Chagas' cardiomyopathy. Am. Heart J. *110*:1092–1098, 1985.
16. Reed, S. G.: In vivo administration of recombinant IFN-gamma induces macrophage activation and prevents acute disease, immune suppression, and death in experimental *Trypanosoma cruzi* infections. J. Immunol. *140*:4342–4347, 1988.
17. Tanowitz, H. B., Kirchhoff, L. V., Simon, D., et al.: Chagas' disease. Clin. Microbiol. Rev. *5*:400–419, 1992.
18. Wery, M., Mulumba, P. M., Lambert, P. H., et al.: Hematologic manifestations, diagnosis and immunopathology of African trypanosomiasis. Semin. Hematol. *19*:83–92, 1982.

220

NAEGLERIA, ACANTHAMOEBA, AND LEPTOMYXID AMEBA

James S. Seidel

Potentially pathogenic free-living amebae of the genera *Acanthamoeba* and *Naegleria* and the newly recognized pathogenic leptomyxid ameba of the order Leptomyxida can produce disease in humans and animals. *Naegleria* is capable of producing a fatal fulminant primary meningoencephalitis, and *Acanthamoeba* and leptomyxid ameba (*Balamuthia* species) can produce a protracted granulomatous amebic encephalitis. Contact lens wearers also may contract *Acanthamoeba* keratitis.

Although small free-living amebae occasionally were seen in stool specimens, they were considered harmless until 1957, when they were found to cause cytotoxic changes in green monkey tissue cultures.[32] Amebae were isolated from the brains of mice and monkeys who died of meningoencephalitis after intracerebral injection with tissue-culture fluid. These isolates were instilled intranasally into mice, who also died of hemorrhagic meningoencephalitis.[17] Experimental infections with *Acanthamoeba* produced fulminant disease that killed animals in 4 to 7 days.[16, 18] The first human cases were reported in 1965 in Australia by Fowler and Carter[25] and in 1966 in Florida by Butt,[10] who named the disease primary amebic meningoencephalitis. The infection subsequently has been reported worldwide.[40, 51, 66, 69]

A few cases of granulomatous amebic encephalitis due to a leptomyxid ameba that is thought to be of the genus *Balamuthia* have been described in the literature.[2, 34, 61] Most patients have been immunosuppressed, very young, or old.[26]

EPIDEMIOLOGY

Free-living amebae have a worldwide distribution and can be recovered from warm, natural bodies of water, including hot springs, quarries, lakes, rivers, improperly treated swimming pools and spas, moist soil, puddles, air conditioners, and other containers where stagnant water may collect.[13, 14, 36] Granulomatous encephalitis and disseminated disease have occurred in immunosuppressed patients with AIDS and cancer and after bone marrow transplantation.[3, 32, 46, 56] Patients who acquire *Naegleria* usually have a history of bathing in a warm body of water. Infections are more common in the spring and summer. Acquisition of *Acanthamoeba* and leptomyxid ameba probably occurs from contact with or inhalation of contaminated water or soil. Patients usually are debilitated or immunocompromised but may not have any history or indication of immunosuppression. Keratitis occurs from contaminated cleaning solutions for lens care and has been reported from hard and soft lens wearers.

THE ORGANISMS

Amebae are not obligate parasites of humans, and the exact host factors that allow for parasitic invasion to occur are not well understood. Factors that contribute to virulence include the immune status of the host and the virulence properties of the organism, such as adherence, complement resistance, cytopathic enzymes, and migration ability.[11, 37, 60] The genera *Naegleria* and *Acanthamoeba* as well as an ameba from the order Leptomyxida have been isolated from humans. The classification of these organisms has been described by Page[48] and Chang.[15]

Acanthamoeba is found as a trophozoite and cyst (Fig. 220–1). The trophozoite has multiple pseudopods with explosive movement of stellate extrusions of the cytoplasm and very little progressive motility. The cyst is smaller and has two distinct thick walls: an inner polyhedral or stellate cyst and an outer wall with an irregular shape. Both forms may be found in tissue[5, 53] (see Fig. 220–1). The species implicated in human disease include *A. culbertsoni, A. polyphaga, A. castellani,* and *A. astronyxis.*

Only the trophozoite of *Naegleria* is found in tissue or the cerebrospinal fluid. The organism is 10 to 20 μm in size and has a large central nuclear karyosome. Progressive slow motility of the pseudopods may be noted on a warm saline preparation or in the cerebrospinal fluid (Fig. 220–2). The organism also may exist in a flagellate form when exposed to certain environmental conditions, such as instillation into fresh warm water (Fig. 220–3). Small cysts with a single outer wall rarely are seen.

The leptomyxid ameba, *Balamuthia,* is found in stagnant water and may be transmitted like *Acanthamoeba.* It may be seen in tissue as a trophozoite or cyst. The trophozoites are similar to those of *Acanthamoeba* (Fig. 220–4). The cyst may appear to have a double cyst wall similar to that of *Acanthamoeba;* however, on electron microscopy the cyst has three walls (see Fig. 220–1).

There is some evidence that *Acanthamoeba* may serve as a reservoir for *Legionella pneumophila*. Amebae isolated from sites of water collection in a hospital were found to have

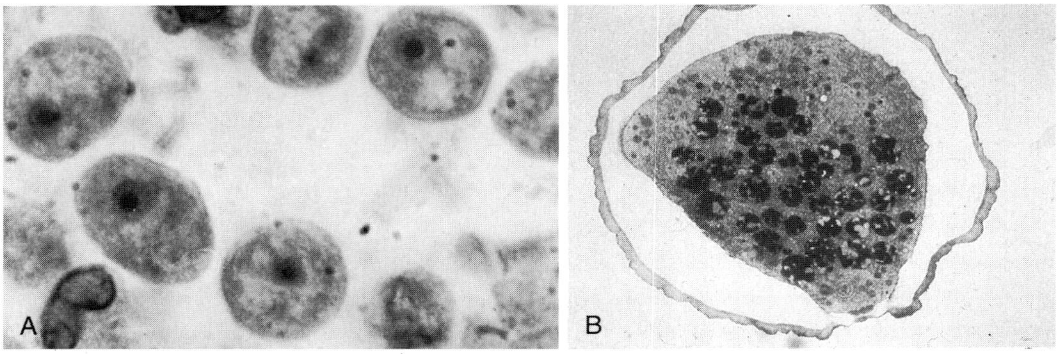

FIGURE 220–1. A, *Trophozoite of* Acanthamoeba. B, *Cyst of* Acanthamoeba. *(Scanning electron micrograph.) (*A *from Jager, B. V., and Stamm, W. P.: Brain abscesses caused by free-living amoeba probably of the genus* Hartmannella *living in a patient with Hodgkin disease. Lancet 2:1343–1345, 1972. © The Lancet Ltd., 1972.)*

phagocytized the bacterial organisms. *Haemophilus influenzae* also may cohabitate with amebae, which supply necessary growth factors for the bacteria. Thus, these potentially pathogenic amebae may serve as a vector for both of these organisms within the respiratory tract.[1, 67]

CLINICAL MANIFESTATIONS

Naegleria fowleri

Infections with *Naegleria fowleri* occur in patients 5 to 15 days after bathing or swimming in warm, untreated water. Most people who have contracted the disease have been young, healthy individuals in their first, second, or third decades of life.[52] The exact factors responsible for disease in some individuals are unknown. Although many individuals may be exposed to contaminated water, very few will develop an illness.[30] Invasive disease may be due to predisposing factors, such as the immune status of the host, or predisposing pathology, such as inflammation or trauma to the respiratory tract. Strain differences in the amebae also may play a role in the pathobiology of infection.

The prodrome usually is nonspecific and may consist of headache, fever, nausea, vomiting, and malaise. This may progress rapidly to meningitis with nuchal rigidity, abnormal reflexes, papilledema, seizures, and altered level of consciousness. Death may occur rapidly unless there are early diagnosis and treatment. There are no distinguishing characteristics of this disease to separate it from fulminant bacterial meningitis, except for the history of recent exposure to a warm body of water. Laboratory data are not helpful in distinguishing it from bacterial disease, except for the presence of amebae in the cerebrospinal fluid.

Acanthamoeba

Acanthamoeba has been associated with primary amebic meningoencephalitis, granulomatous amebic encephalitis, and other infections. The organism has been isolated from chronic otitis media, skin, lungs, and patients with keratitis.[38, 46, 66] Those who contract granulomatous encephalitis usually are very young, old, debilitated, immunosuppressed, or chronically ill.[47] The course of the disease is indolent, with acute, subacute, or chronic symptoms, including headache, nausea, vomiting, fever, somnolence, seizures, aphasia, hemiparesis, behavioral changes, and a clinical picture of encephalitis.[20] In some cases, the signs and symptoms resemble a tumor or space-occupying lesion of the brain.[31] Patients initially may present with a chronic skin lesion that is culture-negative for bacteria and fungi. The lesion may be vesicular and pustular and increase in size until there is a large area of nodular indurated tissue with superficial ulcerations. Amebae are found in the skin and may serve as a nidus for later invasion of the central nervous system.[28] Organisms also

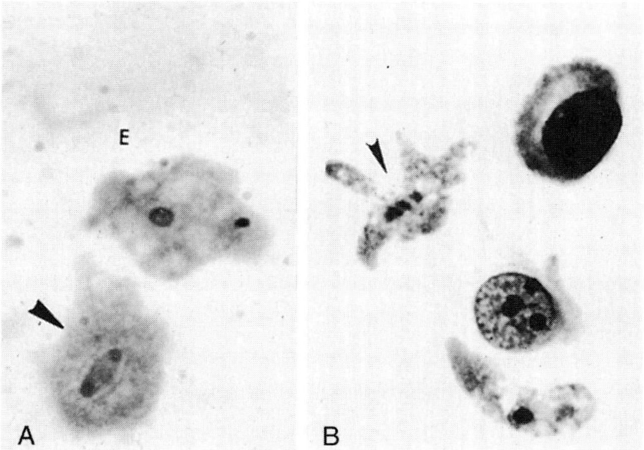

FIGURE 220–2. A *and* B, *Trophozoites of* Naegleria.

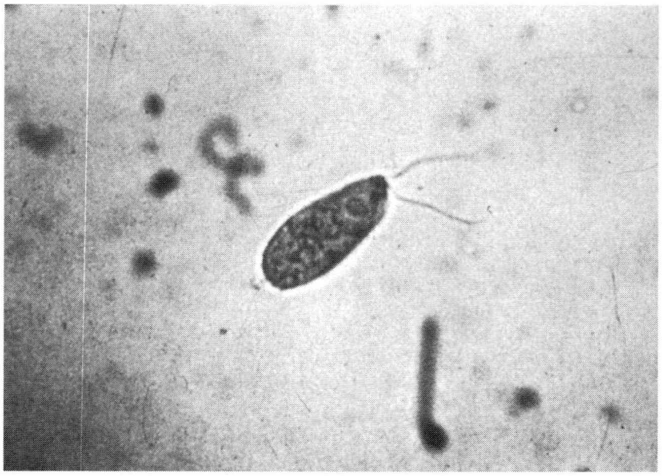

FIGURE 220–3. *Flagellate form of* Naegleria fowleri.

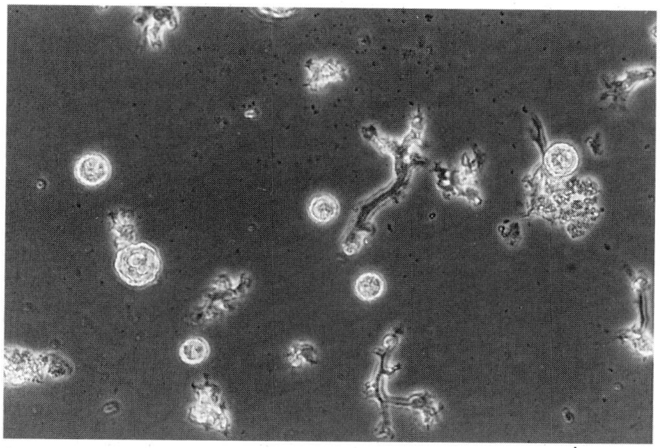

FIGURE 220–4. *Cyst and trophozoite of* Balamuthia mandillaris. *(Courtesy of Govinda S. Visvesvara, Centers for Disease Control and Prevention.)*

have been recovered from cases of osteomyelitis, lung, and sinuses.[27, 38, 42]

Most patients who contract *Acanthamoeba* keratitis are healthy individuals who wear contact lenses. All types of lenses have been implicated in infection, including disposable soft and extended-wear lenses. All contact lenses contain water, which serves as a medium for oxygen exchange. The water content of soft lenses is 50 to 75 per cent. Contact lenses thus can absorb pathogens, including bacteria and ameba, from cleaning solutions, carrying cases, hands, and water.[4, 11] When the lens comes in contact with contaminated water, amebae quickly adhere to the lens surface. If there is corneal trauma, the organisms invade the corneal tissue and produce infection[35] (Fig. 220–5). Persons who do not wear contact lenses also may be infected if they have corneal trauma and come in contact with contaminated water. The nidus for infection is most likely trauma to the cornea, but it also may be related to infection with herpesvirus or bacterial conjunctivitis. Symptoms may appear rapidly or after several weeks. Patients usually complain of a unilateral red eye, a foreign body sensation, tearing, photophobia, or severe pain. Often, the diagnosis is made in persons with keratitis who fail to respond to usual antibacterial therapy. The disease may progress rapidly if not recognized and treated, and a deeply penetrating keratitis may lead to loss of the cornea. In addition, the infection has been associated with the complications of iritis, cataracts, hypopyon, glaucoma, scleritis, and penetrating keratitis.[6]

Leptomyxid Ameba

There are no distinguishing clinical features of chronic granulomatous encephalitis caused by leptomyxid ameba. Patients may or may not be immunosuppressed or chronically ill and will present with headache, meningismus, nausea, vomiting, seizures, and focal neurologic signs. Neuroimaging studies may show a hyperdense, space-occupying lesion that can be confused with a brain abscess or tumor. Multiple areas of the brain may be involved, which mimic fungal and bacterial abscesses in patients with HIV infection. Tissue biopsy and electron microscopy may be necessary to diagnose infection. The infection may be indolent or progressive and usually results in death.

PATHOLOGY

Most cases of primary amebic meningoencephalitis involve the cerebellum and the cerebral cortex. The tissue generally is soft, friable, and edematous with evidence of hemorrhage and necrosis. Uncal herniation may be evident. A purulent exudate may be seen on the brain surface, which particularly may be prominent over the sulci and basal cisternae; the olfactory bulbs may be necrotic (Fig. 220–6). The spinal cord often is involved with a necrotizing hemorrhagic myelitis. Microscopic examination of the tissue shows an acute menin-

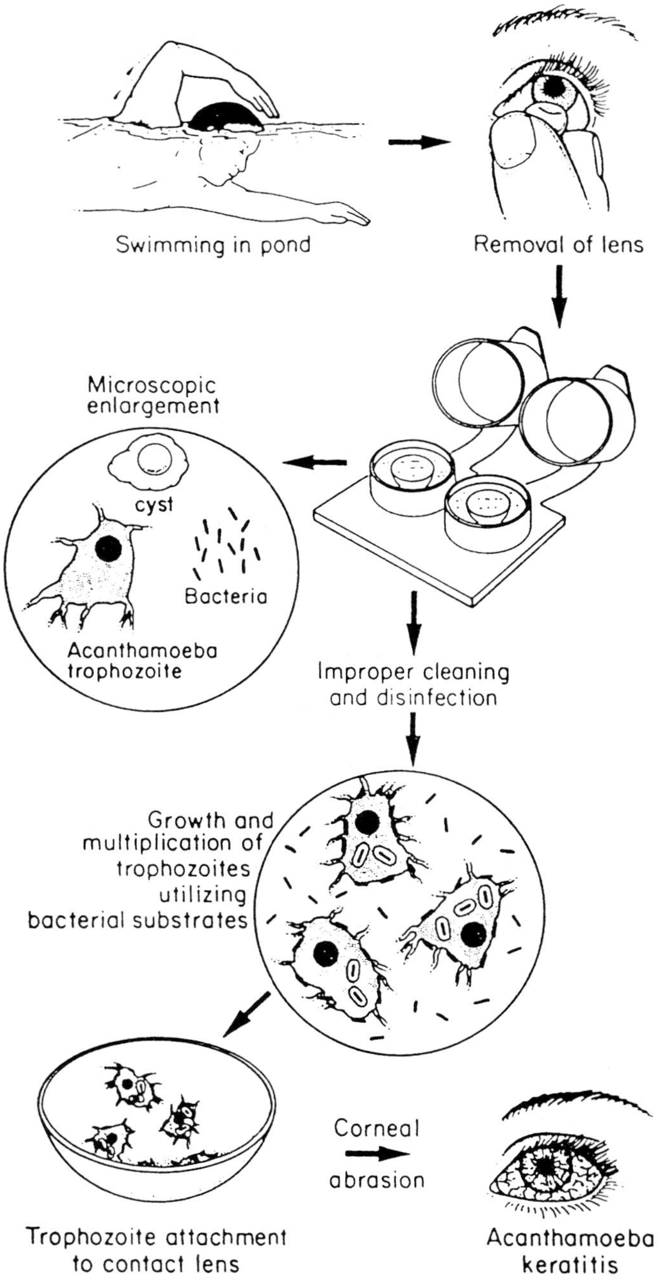

FIGURE 220–5. *Proposed mechanism for* Acanthamoeba *keratitis. Bacterial contaminants in the water on the lens support the growth of the ameba, leading to an increased number of invading organisms. The organisms adhere to the contact lens and enter the tissue through the damaged cornea, resulting in keratitis.*

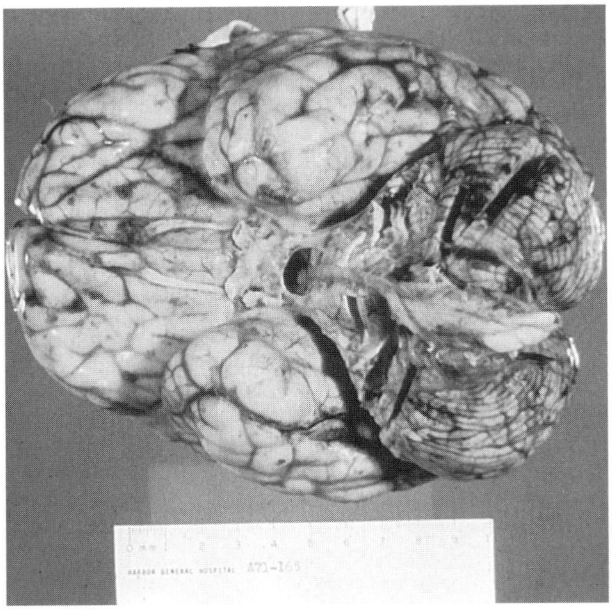

FIGURE 220–6. *Brain from a fatal case of* Naegleria *meningoencephalitis. Note the areas of necrosis on the basalar surface of the brain.*

geal and encephalitic inflammatory exudate of mononuclear and polymorphonuclear leukocytes that is prominent in the areas of the basal cistern, sulci, and sylvian fissures. The exudate may widen the Virchow-Robin spaces and extend into the cortex.[43]

Lesions of the brain, lung, eyes, and skin can be associated with infection with *Acanthamoeba.* The cerebral hemispheres have a mild focal edema with areas of necrosis and hemorrhage. There is narrowing of the sulci and flattening of the gyri in areas of active infection. Other areas of the cerebral cortex may appear normal. The central nervous system lesions are associated with a chronic granulomatous reaction, with collections of macrophages and necrotic foci in the walls of the arteries and arterioles, all of which suggest an angiitis. The lesions may resemble brain abscesses. Both cysts and trophozoites are seen within the brain tissue. Amebae may be seen in groups with little or no surrounding inflammatory reaction.[41] Trophozoites and cysts may be seen in the alveoli accompanied by a mononuclear cellular infiltrate. Skin lesions may be nodular and ulcerative, with subcutaneous inflammation and abscess formation. Cysts and trophozoites are seen within the affected tissue.[41] A similar reaction may be seen in ulcerations of the cornea.[63]

LABORATORY DIAGNOSIS

Routine laboratory tests do not distinguish amebic infection of the central nervous system from other causes of meningoencephalitis. The white blood cell count usually is elevated, with a preponderance of neutrophils and bands. Serum electrolyte analysis may be normal or show evidence of inappropriate secretion of antidiuretic hormone. Analysis of the cerebrospinal fluid reveals an elevated protein level with a normal or low glucose level and a pleocytosis with a high count of white and red blood cells.

Direct Microscopic Identification

Naegleria may be identified on wet mount of cerebrospinal fluid by their morphology and motility. The cerebrospinal fluid should be kept warm before it is examined and should not be refrigerated. The cerebrospinal fluid should be placed directly on a slide with a coverslip or first gently centrifuged at 150 × *g* for 5 minutes. The supernatant should be placed on a slide and covered with a No. 1 coverslip. Small (8- to 20-μm) trophozoites with progressive motility can be seen.[44] The cytoplasm may appear granular, and the nucleus is large and has a dense central karyosome (Fig. 220–7). It should be noted that activated macrophages often extrude pseudopods and may be mistaken for amebae. The supernatant also can be fixed for electron microscopy or dried on slides for staining. To ensure that the organism adheres to the slide, a drop of cerebrospinal fluid should be placed in polyvinyl alcohol and smeared onto a slide. As an alternative method, a gelatin-coated glass slide may be used, or the dried specimen may be fixed with several drops of warmed Schaudinn solution. Wright, Giemsa, and trichrome stains may be used to stain the organism for identification. Tissue should be processed rapidly, fixed, and stained with hematoxylin and eosin. Gram stain is not useful in making the diagnosis because it often fails to stain the nuclear structure. The ultrastructure of the organism is well described, and material can be processed for electron microscopy by placing it in chilled 2.5 per cent glutaraldehyde. The trophozoite shows an irregular cell border and a distinct polar orientation, with one end of the cell characterized by a uniformly appearing blunt or rounded pseudopod. The cell contains numerous vacuoles and a large nucleus with a prominent, dense central nucleolus. There are numerous ribosomes and food vacuoles and occasional mitochondria that may or may not be dumbbell shaped.[30, 43]

Corneal scrapings may be stained with calcofluor white, which gives a fluorescence to the cysts of *Acanthamoeba.*[70] Indirect fluorescent antibody staining also may be performed for *Acanthamoeba* and *Naegleria.*

Culture of *Naegleria* and *Acanthamoeba*

Naegleria may be cultured from cerebrospinal fluid and tissue. The cerebrospinal fluid should be centrifuged at 2 × *g* for 10 minutes. The supernatant should be removed and placed on a non-nutrient agar plate that has been covered with a suspension of *Escherichia coli* or *Enterobacter aerogenes.*[55]

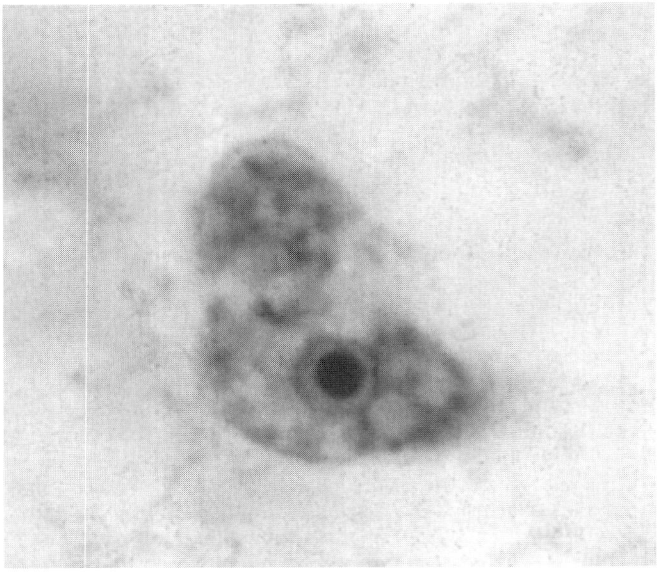

FIGURE 220–7. *Trichrome stain of a trophozoite of* Naegleria fowleri.

Tissue that has been ground up in a sterile fashion may be planted on the same type of agar plate. Amebae will feed on the bacterial lawn and be isolated easily. *Acanthamoeba* can be cultured in a similar manner. A culture amplification technique for recovery of *Acanthamoeba* from corneal scrapings has been described.[11] Transformation of the cyst form in culture occurs after a few days, when the nutrient bacteria are not prevalent. Axenic cultures techniques have been described by Nelson. Material also may be placed in monolayer cell cultures of monkey kidney, MRC human embryonic lung cells, and HeLa cells.[44, 53, 64] Transformation to the flagellate form may be accomplished by dropping the organisms into distilled water for several hours.

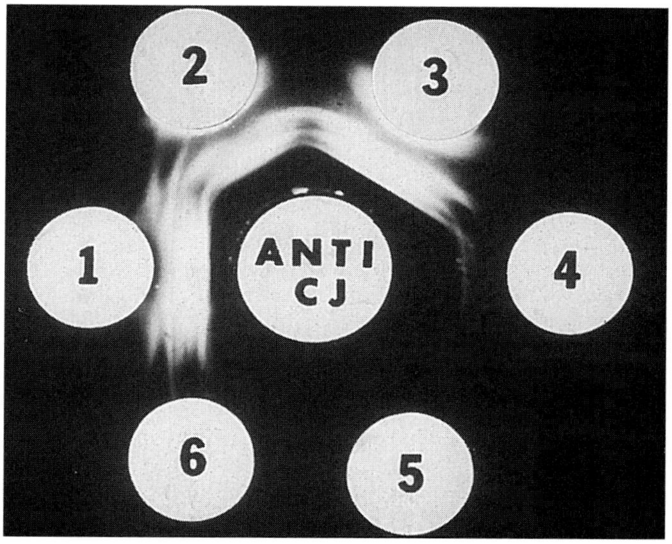

FIGURE 220–9. *Gel diffusion pattern showing interaction between anti-CJ serum and the following amebae: (1) CJ strain of* Naegleria fowleri, *(2) HBSW pathogenic strain of* N. fowleri, *(3) HBC-1 California strain of* N. fowleri, *(4) and (5) EG strain of* N. gruberi *(nonpathogenic), (6) normal saline. (Courtesy of G. S. Visvesvara, Centers for Disease Control and Prevention.)*

Serology

Routine commercial tests are not available. However, the Centers for Disease Control and Prevention will perform an indirect immunofluorescent antibody and immunoperoxidase test on the organism.

Antigenic and Isoenzyme Analysis

Organisms can be classified by antigenic analysis by the use of gel diffusion, immunoelectrophoresis, immunofluorescence, and immunoblot assays (Figs. 220–8 and 220–9). Ameba also may be processed for isoenzyme analysis, which can distinguish the genera and species of the ameba.[24, 44, 64, 65]

TREATMENT

Naegleria Meningoencephalitis

Meningoencephalitis caused by free-living amebae is a medical emergency. Only a few patients have survived, and treatment regimens have varied.[9, 49] Strain differences and host immunity probably play a role in the pathogenicity of the organism. Pathogenic strains of the organism are resistant to complement-mediated cell damage. In addition, early diagnosis and institution of therapy may have played a role in the handful of patients who have been treated successfully.

Several drugs have been shown to be active against *Naegleria* in vitro.[21] These include amphotericin B, miconazole, and rifamycin.[12, 33, 59, 68] Synergism between drugs also has been demonstrated in vitro with tetracycline and amphotericin B and amphotericin B and miconazole.[53, 59] Antagonism between the two latter drugs has been shown against *Candida albicans*.[50]

Therapy has included high-dose intravenous amphotericin B at 1 mg/kg/day to 1.5 mg/kg/day alone or in combination with other drugs, including miconazole, rifampin, sulfa drugs, and tetracycline.[39] In addition, intrathecal amphotericin was used in one patient. Intrathecal drugs given via a cisternal reservoir have resulted in cerebral hypertension and death.

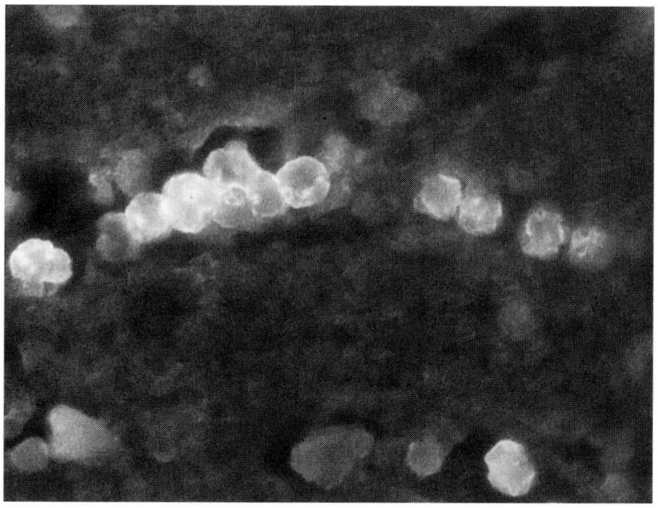

FIGURE 220–8. *Indirect fluorescent antibody of* Naegleria fowleri. *(Courtesy of Govinda S. Visvesvara, Centers for Disease Control and Prevention.)*

Acanthamoeba Infection of the Central Nervous System

Acanthamoeba infection of the central nervous system is difficult to treat because of the presence of cysts in tissue that are relatively resistant to chemotherapeutic agents. Immunosuppressed patients with disseminated disease have a poor prognosis. Both the necrotizing acute meningoencephalitis and chronic granulomatous disease may respond to sulfadiazine and other sulfa drugs. However, the effects of therapy are inconsistent, and death often ensues in spite of therapy. Recovery from infection of the central nervous system has been reported after treatment with chloramphenicol and co-trimoxazole.[54] An immunosuppressed patient was treated successfully with intravenous pentamidine isethionate, topical chlorhexidine, and 2 per cent ketoconazole cream, followed by oral itraconazole.[57]

Acanthamoeba Keratitis

Medical treatment of keratitis has been inconsistent, and chemotherapy often is combined with surgical treatment.

Cures have been reported with the use of 0.1 per cent propamidine isethionate, a combination of chlorhexidine and propamidine, or propamidine, neomycin, and polyhexamethylene biguanide, or propamidine isethionate, neomycin sulfate, and co-trimoxazole.[2, 8, 19, 29, 62, 71] Recently, a large number of patients were treated successfully with 0.02 per cent topical polyhexamethylene biguanide.[22] Penetrating keratoplasty has been combined successfully with medical therapy to control infections that were severe or resistant to therapy.[7, 23] Topical or systemic corticosteroid therapy is contraindicated and results in severe complications.[58] Successful therapy for keratitis depends on early diagnosis and rapid intensive medical and/or surgical therapy directed at killing the cysts in the tissue, removing infected tissue, and preventing secondary bacterial infections.

Leptomyxid Ameba

Treatment for leptomyxid ameba infection has not been investigated. Because it resembles *Acanthamoeba* so closely, sulfa drugs may have some effect on the organism.

References

1. Allen, S. D., Place, D. A., and Culbertson C. G.: In vitro interaction of *Acanthamoeba* and *Haemophilus influenzae*. J. Protozool. *37*:48A–49A, 1990.
2. Alpuche-Arnada, C., and Santos Preciado, J. I.: Infeccion del sistema nervioso central de origen oscuro: Meningoencefalitis ambiana. Bol. Med. Hosp. Infect. Mex. *46*:581, 1989.
3. Andrelini, P., Przepiorka, D., Luna, M, et al.: *Acanthamoeba* meningoencephalitis after bone marrow transplantation. Bone Marrow Transplant. *14*:450–461, 1994.
4. Asbell, P. A.: *Acanthamoeba* keratitis: There and back again. Mount Sinai Med. J. *60*:279–282, 1993.
5. Ash, L. R., and Orihel, T. C.: Atlas of Human Parasitology. 3rd ed. Chicago, American Society of Clinical Pathologists, 1990.
6. Auran, J. D., Starr, M. B., and Jakobiec, F. A.: *Acanthamoeba* keratitis: A review of the literature. Cornea *6*:2–26, 1987.
7. Bacon, A. S., Frazer, D. G., Dart, J. K., et al.: A review of 72 consecutive cases of *Acanthamoeba* keratitis. Eye *7*:719–725, 1993.
8. Brasseur, G., Favennec, L., Perrine D., et al.: Successful treatment of *Acanthamoeba* keratitis by hexamindine. Cornea *13*:459–462, 1994.
9. Brown, R. L.: Successful treatment of primary amebic meningoencephalitis. Arch. Int. Med. *151*:1201–1202, 1991.
10. Butt, C. G.: Primary meningoencephalitis. N. Engl. J. Med. *274*:1473–1476, 1966.
11. Buttone, E. J.: Free-living amebas of the genera *Acanthamoeba* and *Naegleria*: An overview of basic microbiologic correlates. Mount Sinai Med. J. *60*:260–269, 1993.
12. Carter, R. F.: Sensitivity to amphotericin B of a *Naegleria* species isolated from a case of primary amebic meningoencephalitis. J. Clin. Pathol. *22*:472–474, 1969.
13. Centers for Disease Control: Primary amebic meningoencephalitis: North Carolina, 1991. M. M. W. R. *41*:437–440, 1992.
14. Cerva, L., Novak, K., and Culbertson, C. G.: An outbreak of acute fatal amebic meningoencephalitis. Am. J. Epidemiol. *88*:336–344, 1968.
15. Chang, S. L.: Small free-living amebas: Cultivation, quantitation, identification, classification, pathogenesis, and resistance. Curr. Top. Comp. Pathobiol. *1*:201–254, 1971.
16. Culbertson, C. G., Ensminger, P. W. and Overton, W. M.: The isolation of additional strains of pathogenic *Hartmannella* sp.: Proposed culture method for application of biological material. Am. J. Pathol. *35*:383–387, 1965.
17. Culbertson, C. G., Smith, J. W., Cohen, H. K., et al.: Experimental infection of mice and monkeys by *Acanthamoeba*. Am. J. Pathol. *35*:185–197, 1959.
18. Culbertson, C. G, Smith, J. W., and Minner, J. D.: *Acanthamoeba* observation on animal pathogenicity. Science *127*:1506, 1958.
19. D'Aversa, G., Stern, G. A., and Driebe, W. T., Jr.: Diagnosis and successful medical treatment of *Acanthamoeba* keratitis. Arch. Opthalmol. *113*:1120–1123, 1995.
20. Di Gregorio, C., Rivasi, F., Mongiardo, N. et al.: *Acanthamoeba* meningoencephalitis in a patient with acquired immunodeficiency syndrome. Arch. Pathol. Lab. Med. *116*:1363–1365, 1992.
21. Duma, R. J., and Finley, R.: In vitro susceptibility of pathogenic *Naegleria* and *Acanthamoeba* species to a variety of chemotherapeutic agents. Antimicrob. Agents Chemother. *10*:370–376, 1976.
22. Elder, M. J., and Dart, K.: Chemotherapy for *Acanthamoeba* keratitis. Lancet *345*:791–792, 1995.
23. Ficker, L. A., Kirkness, C., and Wright, P.: Prognosis for keratoplasty in *Acanthamoeba* keratitis. Ophthalmalogy *100*:105–110, 1993.
24. Flores, B. M., Garcia, C. A., Stamm, W. E., et al.: Differentiation of *Naegleria fowleri* from *Acanthamoeba* species by using monoclonal antibodies and flow cytometry. J. Clin. Microbiol. *28*:1999–2002, 1990.
25. Fowler, M. and Carter, R. F.: Acute pyogenic meningitis probably due to *Acanthamoeba* sp.: A preliminary report. Br. Med. J. *2*:740–742, 1965.
26. Friedland, L. R., Rapheal, S. A., Deutsch, E. S. et al.: Disseminated *Acanthamoeba* infection in a child with symptomatic human immunodeficiency virus infection. Pediatr. Infect. Dis. J. *11*:404–407, 1993.
27. Gonzalez, M. D., Gould, E., Dickinson, G., et al.: Acquired immunodeficiency syndrome associated with *Acanthamoeba* and other opportunistic organisms. Arch. Pathol. Lab. Med. *110*:749–751, 1986.
28. Gutierrez, Y.: Diagnostic Pathology of Parasitic Infections with Clinical Correlations. Philadelphia, Lea & Febiger, 1990.
29. Hay, J., Kirkness, C. M., Seal, D. V., et al.: Drug resistance and *Acanthamoeba* keratitis: The quest for alternative antiprotozoal chemotherapy. Eye *8*:555–563, 1994.
30. Hecht, R. H. and Cohen, A. H.: Primary amebic meningoencephalitis in California. West J. Med. *117*:69–73, 1972.
31. Jaeger, B. V., and Stamm, W. P.: Brain abscesses caused by a free-living amoeba, probably of the genus *Hartmannella* in a patient with Hodgkin's disease. Lancet *2*:1342–1345, 1972.
32. Jahnes, W. G., Fullmer H. M., and Li, C. P.: Free-living amoebae as contaminants in monkey tissue culture. Proc. Soc. Exp. Biol. Med. *96*:484–488, 1957.
33. Jamison, A.: The effects of clotrimazole on *Naegleria fowleri*. J. Clin. Pathol. *28*:446, 1975.
34. Jarmillo-Rodriguez, Y., Chavez-Macias, L. G., Olvera-Rabich, J. E., et al.: Encefalitis por una nueva amiba di vida libre, probablemente *Leptomyxid*. Patologia *27*:137–141, 1989.
35. John, T., Desai, D., and Sahm, D.: Adherence of *Acanthamoeba castellani* cysts and trophozoites to unworn soft contact lenses. Am. J. Ophthalmol. *108*:658–664, 1989.
36. John, D. T., and Howard, M. J.: Seasonal distribution of pathogenic free-living amebae in Oklahoma waters. Parasitol. Res. *81*:193–201, 1995.
37. Kilvington, S., and Beeching, J.: Identification and epidemiological typing of *Naegleria fowleri* with DNA probes. Appl. Environ. Microbiol. *61*:2071–2078, 1995.
38. Lengy, J., Jakovljevich, R., and Talis, B.: Recovery of hartmannelloid amoeba from purulent ear discharge. Trop. Dis. Bull. *68*:818–819, 1971.
39. Loschiavo, F., Ventura-Spangolo, T., Sessa, E., et al.: Acute primary meningoencephalitis from entamoeba *Naegleria fowleri*: Report of a clinical case with a favorable outcome. Acta. Neurol. *15*:330–340, 1993.
40. Ma, P., Visvesvara, G. S., Martinez, A. J., et al.: *Naegleria* and *Acanthamoeba* infection. Rev. Infect. Dis. *12*:490–513, 1990.
41. Martinez, A. J.: Free living amebas: Infection of the central nervous system. Mount Sinai J. Med. *60*:271–278, 1993.
42. Martinez, A. J.: Free Living Amebas: Natural History, Prevention, Diagnosis, Pathology and Treatment of Disease. Boca Raton, FL, CRC Press, 1985.
43. Martinez, A. J., dos Santos Neto, J. G., Nelson, E. C., et al.: Primary amebic meningoencephalitis. Pathol. Ann. *2*:225–250, 1977.
44. Martinez, A. J., and Visvesvara, G. S.: Laboratory diagnosis of pathogenic free-living amoebas: *Naegleria, Acanthamoeba* and Leptomyxida. Clin. Lab. Med. *11*:861–872, 1991.
45. Moore, M. B., and McCulley, J. P.: Acanthamoeba keratitis associated with contact lenses: Six consecutive cases of successful management. Br. J. Ophthalmol. *73*:271–275, 1989.
46. Newsome, A. L., Curtis, F. T., and Culbertson C. G., et al.: Identification of *Acanthamoeba* in broncholalveolar lavage specimens. Diagn. Cytopathol. *8*:231–134, 1992.
47. Ofori-Kwakye, S. K., Sidebottom, D. G., Herbert, J., et al.: Granulomatous brain tumor caused by *Acanthamoeba*: Case report. J. Neurosurg. *64*:505–509, 1986.
48. Page, F. C.: Taxonomic criteria for limax amebae with descriptions of three new species of *Hartmanella* and three of *Vahlkampfia*. J. Protozool. *14*:449–521, 1967.
49. Poungvarfian, N., and Jariya, P. L.: The fifth nonlethal case of primary amoebic meningoencephalitis. J. Med. Assoc. Thai. *74*:112–115, 1991.
50. Schacter, L. P., Owellen R. J., Rathbun, H. K., et al.: Antagonism between miconazole and amphotericin B. Lancet *2*:318, 1976.
51. Schoeman, C. J., van der Vyver, A. E., and Visvesvara, G. S.: Primary amoebic meningo-encephalitis in southern Africa. J. Infect. *26*:211–214, 1993.
52. Seidel, J. S.: Primary amebic meningoencephalitis. Pediatr. Clin. North Am. *32*:881–892, 1985.
53. Seidel, J. S., Harmatz, P., Visvesvara, G. S., et al.: Successful treatment of primary amebic meningoencephalitis. N. Eng. J. Med. *30*:346–348, 1982.
54. Sharma, P. P., Gupta, P., Murali, M. V., et al.: Primary meningoencephalitis caused by *Acanthamoeba* successfully treated with cotrimoxazole. Indian Pediatr. *30*:1219–1222, 1993.
55. Singh, B. N.: Pathogenic and Non-Pathogenic Amoebae. New York, John Wiley & Sons, 1975.
56. Sison, J. P., Kemper, C. A., Loveless, M., et al.: Disseminated *Acanthamoeba* infection in patients with AIDS: Case reports and review. Clin. Infect. Dis. *20*:1207–1216, 1995.

57. Slater, C. A., Sickel, J. Z., Visvesvara, G. S., et al.: Brief report: Successful treatment of disseminated *Acanthamoeba* infection in an immunocompromised patient. N. Engl. J. Med. *331*:85–87, 1994.
58. Stern, G. A., and Buttross, M.: Use of corticosteroids in combination with antimicrobial drugs in the treatment of infectious corneal disease. Ophthalmology *98*:847–853, 1991.
59. Thong, Y. H., Rowan-Kelly, B., Shephard, C., et al.: Growth inhibition of *Naegleria fowleri* by tetracycline, rifamycin, and miconazole. Lancet 2:876, 1977.
60. Toney, D. M., and Marciano-Cabral, F.: Modulation of complement resistance and virulence of *Naegleria fowleri* amoebae by alterations in growth media. J. Eukaryot. Microbiol. *41*:337–343, 1994.
61. Valenzuela, G., Lopez-Corella, E., DeJonckheere, J. F.: Primary amoebic meningoencephalitis in a young male from northwestern Mexico. Trans. R. Soc. Trop. Med. Hyg. *78*:558–559, 1984.
62. Varga, J. H., Wolff, T. C., Jensen, H. G., et al.: Combined treatment of *Acanthamoeba* keratitis with propamidine, neomycin, and polyhexamethylene biguanide. Am. J. Ophthalmol. *115*:466–470, 1993.
63. Visvesvara, G. S., Jones, D. B., and Robinson, N. M.: Isolation, identification and biologic characterization of *Acanthamoeba polyphaga* from a human eye. Am. J. Trop. Med. Hyg. *24*:784–790, 1975.
64. Visvesvara, G. S., Mirra, S. S., Brandt, F. H., et al.: Isolation of two strains of *Acanthamoeba castellani* from human tissue and their pathogenicity and isoenzyme profiles. J. Clin. Microbiol. *18*:1405–1409, 1983.
65. Visvesvara, G. S., Peralta, M. J., Brandt, F. H., et al.: Production of monoclonal antibodies to *Naegleria fowleri*, agent of primary amebic meningoencephalitis. J. Clin. Microbiol. *25*:1629–1631, 1987.
66. Visvesvara, G. S., and Stehr-Green, J. K.: Epidemiology of free-living ameba infections. J. Protozool. *37*:25S–33S, 1990.
67. Wadowsky, R. M., Butler, L. J., Cook, M. K., et al.: Growth-supporting activity for *Legionella pneumophilia* in tap water cultures and implication of Hartmannellid amoebae as growth factors. Appl. Environ. Microbiol. *54*:2677–2682, 1988.
68. Wang, A., Kay, R., Poon, W. S., et al.: Successful treatment of amoebic meningoencephalitis in a Chinese living in Hong Kong. Clin. Neurol. Neurosurg. *95*:249–252, 1993.
69. Willaert, E.: Primary amoebic meningoencephalitis: A selected bibliography and tabular survey of cases. Ann. Soc. Belg. Med. Trop. *54*:429–440, 1974.
70. Wilhelmus, K. R., Osato, M. S., Font, R. L., et al.: Rapid diagnosis of *Acanthamoeba* keratitis using calcofluor white. Arch. Opthalmol. *104*:1309–1321, 1986.
71. Wright, E., Warhurst, D., and Jones, B. R.: *Acanthamoeba* keratitis successfully treated medically. Br. J. Ophthalmol. *69*:778–782, 1985.

221

TOXOPLASMOSIS

Kenneth M. Boyer, Jack S. Remington, and Rima L. McLeod

Toxoplasma gondii is an obligate intracellular protozoan parasite (phylum Apicomplexa, class Sporozoasida, order Eucoccidiida). Infection may be clinically inapparent or result in disease. Disease produced by *T. gondii* is called toxoplasmosis. This parasite first was observed in 1908 by Nicolle and Manceaux[99, 100] in mononuclear cells in the spleen and liver of a North African rodent, the gundi *(Ctenodactylus gundi)*. The organism soon was identified as a cause of disease in other animals,[128] and in 1923, Janku[61] first recognized a case in a human. He described a parasite found in the retina of an infant; it was recognized later by Levaditi[73] as *Toxoplasma*.

In 1937, Wolf and Cowen[136] reported a case of congenital granulomatous encephalitis that they considered to be due to an "encephalitozoon." Sabin,[110] who previously had encountered *T. gondii* in guinea pigs, made the correct diagnosis. The discovery of *Toxoplasma* as a cause of disease acquired later in life has been credited to Pinkerton and Weinman,[104] who in 1940 described a generalized fatal illness due to this organism in a young man. In retrospect, a case of acquired toxoplasmosis had been reported in 1908 by Darling.[31] In 1948, Sabin and Feldman[111] described a serologic test, the dye test, that allowed numerous investigators to study epidemiologic and clinical aspects of toxoplasmosis and to define the spectrum of disease in humans. It was not until 1969, some 60 years after discovery of the parasite, that Frenkel and colleagues[42, 46, 48] established that *Toxoplasma* was a coccidian protozoan and that its definitive host was the cat.

THE ORGANISM AND ITS TRANSMISSION

T. gondii exists in three forms, or stages: the proliferative stage, or *tachyzoite*; a tissue cyst that contains *bradyzoites*; and an oocyst, within which *sporozoites* develop. The cat family is the definitive host of the organism. The tachyzoite and tissue cyst occur in extraintestinal tissues of cats but also are seen in other mammalian and avian hosts. The oocyst is formed during the intestinal epithelial stage of infection, exclusively in members of the cat family. Each stage of the organism has antigens in common with the other stages and also unique antigens. A number of these antigens have been cloned, sequenced, and localized to microanatomic structures.[89]

The tachyzoite form (Fig. 21–1*A, B,* and *C*) is crescent-shaped or oval, measuring approximately 3 μm × 7 μm, and is seen during the acute stage of infection. It stains well with Wright or Giemsa stain. Ultrastructural features include the apical complex of microtubules and rings, secretory organelles called rhoptries, and a chloroplast-like structure with its own unique DNA.[19] Tachyzoites can invade all mammalian cells except perhaps non-nucleated red blood cells. They cannot withstand freezing and thawing, desiccation, or brief exposure to gastric or duodenal digestive juices. After penetration, the tachyzoite multiplies by endodyogeny, ultimately causing disruption of the cell.

The bradyzoite form (see Fig. 221–1*D, E,* and *F*) is capable of persisting in encysted form in all tissues, resulting in a chronic (latent) infection for the entire life span of the infected host. Cysts are demonstrable in tissues as early as the first week of infection and vary in size from approximately 10 to 100 μm. They have an argyrophilic wall but stand out most clearly from surrounding tissue when stained with periodic acid–Schiff stain. There usually is no inflammatory reaction around cysts. Because this form may persist for many years in the tissues of clinically normal children and adults, its demonstration in histologic sections does not signify recent infection necessarily. Peptic or tryptic digestive fluids immediately disrupt the cyst wall, but the liberated bradyzoites (which resemble the tachyzoite form under light microscopy) can survive in these fluids for several hours, which allows time for invasion of local cells. The cyst is

The authors acknowledge the contribution of Christopher B. Wilson, M.D., to this chapter in the previous edition of this text.

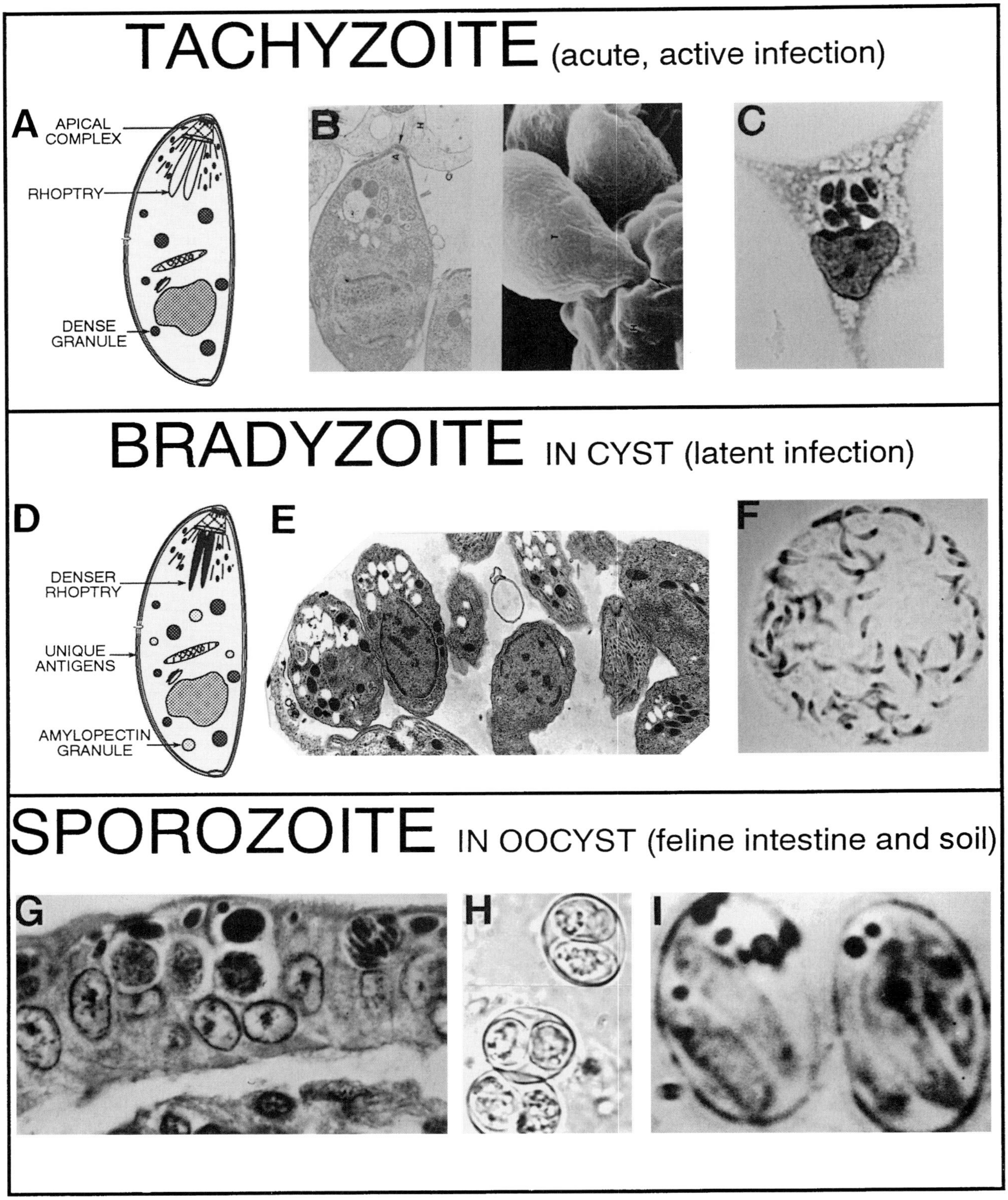

FIGURE 221–1. *Stages of* Toxoplasma gondii. A, *Schematic diagram of tachyzoite.* B, *Transmission and scanning electron micrographs of tachyzoite invading a host cell.* C, *Light micrograph of tachyzoites replicating within a parasitiferous vacuole in the host cell cytoplasm.* D, *Schematic diagram of bradyzoite.* E, *Transmission electron micrograph of cyst containing bradyzoite (arrow indicates amylopectin granules).* F, *Light micrograph of cyst containing bradyzoites.* G, *Development of oocysts in cat intestine.* H, *Oocysts in lumen of cat intestine.* I, *Sporulating oocysts that contain sporozoites. (From Boyer, K. M., and McLeod, R. L.:* Toxoplasma gondii *[Toxoplasmosis].* In *Long, S. S., Pickering, L. K., and Prober, C. G. [eds.]: Principles and Practice of Pediatric Infectious Diseases. New York, Churchill Livingstone, 1997, p. 1423.)*

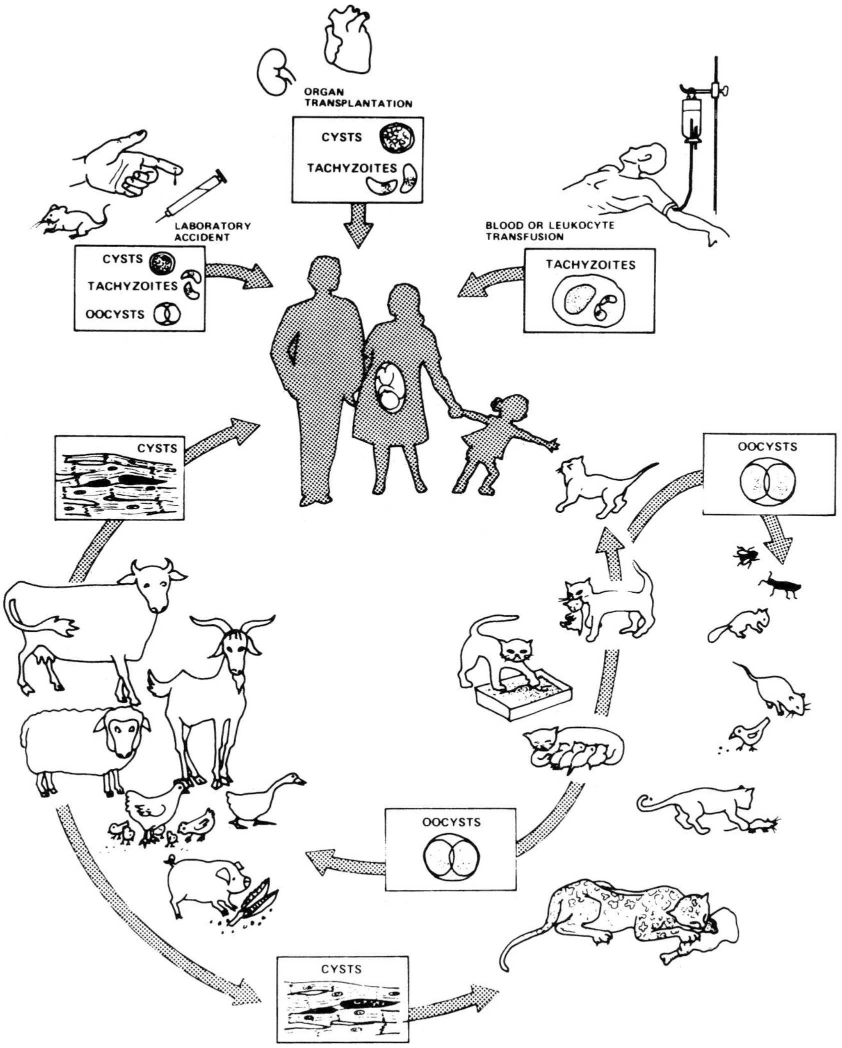

FIGURE 221–2. *Life cycle of* Toxoplasma gondii. *Cats are definitive hosts. Humans and other mammals are intermediate hosts. (From Remington, J. S., and McLeod, R.: Toxoplasmosis.* In *Braude, A. I. [ed.]: International Textbook of Medicine. Vol. II. Medical Microbiology and Infectious Disease. Philadelphia, W. B. Saunders, 1981, p. 1818.)*

destroyed by heating to 66° C, by freezing (below −20° C) and thawing, and by desiccation. It can survive for some months at refrigeration temperatures (4° C) if it is in tissue. Therefore, infection in humans may be acquired by eating inadequately cooked meat that contains cysts (Fig. 221–2). In carnivorous animals, infection may be acquired by eating raw meat or prey species that contain encysted organisms.

The oocyst form (see Fig. 221–1*G*, *H*, and *I*) is found only in the feces of members of the cat family, the definitive host for *Toxoplasma,* and is the result of gametogony and schizogony, which occur in the intestinal epithelium.[60] The oocyst is ovoid and approximately 10 μm × 12 μm. Infected cats may shed as many as 10 million oocysts each day, which may be excreted for up to 3 weeks after primary (acute) infection but rarely thereafter. Excreted oocysts become infectious only after they undergo sporulation (eight sporozoites form in each oocyst); this occurs from 1 to 21 days (most commonly 2 to 8 days) after excretion, depending on temperature and the availability of oxygen. The oocyst is far more resistant than the other life cycle forms and can survive for months in water and for a year or more in moist soil. Ingestion of sporulated oocysts transmits the infection. This fact suggests that the oocyst plays a major role in transmission by the fecal-oral route in animal reservoirs and, by inadvertent ingestion, in humans.

The genome of *T. gondii* consists of 8×10^7 base pairs, distributed among 12 chromosomes. Much of the genome has been sequenced, and a genetic linkage map has been constructed.[63, 67, 117] The factors that regulate stage conversion from tachyzoite to bradyzoite are beginning to be defined.[89]

EPIDEMIOLOGY

Acquired Infection

Infection with *Toxoplasma* is common in humans. The incidence of toxoplasmosis in the United States probably is decreasing at present, although data are relatively limited.[119] This decline may relate in part to widespread public awareness of the "dangers of kitty litter" for women who are pregnant. People appear to be less informed about the potential for disease transmission from raw or undercooked meat. However, the common practice of freezing commercial meats before releasing them for sale, combined with the use of home freezers, also may be having a beneficial effect.[119] Estimates are that about 8 per cent of commercial beef, 20 per cent of commercial pork, and 25 per cent of commercial lamb contains encysted *Toxoplasma* bradyzoites.[106]

In the United States, the prevalence of seropositivity has been determined from studies of military recruits and surveys in major cities. In the early 1960s, the overall prevalence in military recruits was 14 per cent, with the lowest rates in the Mountain (3 per cent) and Pacific (8 per cent) states and the highest rates in the Northeastern (20 per cent) and East South Central (19 per cent) states.[119] A more recent study showed a similar geographic distribution but consistently lower prevalences.[119] Urban studies in U.S. women of child-bearing age have yielded variable rates: Denver, 3 per cent; Palo Alto, 10 per cent; Chicago, 12 per cent; Boston, 14 per cent; and Birmingham, 30 per cent.[106] Internationally, rates also are variable: Thailand, 3 per cent; Australia, 23 per cent; Japan, 6 per cent; United Kingdom, 35 per cent; Poland, 36 per cent; Belgium, 53 per cent; Tahiti, 77 per cent; and France, 87 per cent.[106] In part, the prevalence of infection is determined by climate: colder regions and those that are hot and dry or at high altitudes have lower rates of human infection than are noted in warmer, more moist areas.

The cat is central in the parasite's life cycle. Humans and other mammals are intermediate hosts. If infected tissue (e.g., a mouse) is consumed by a susceptible cat, the sexual cycle is induced in the cat intestine; oocysts are excreted and are infectious for mammals and birds in which the life cycle (tachyzoites and cysts) is perpetuated. Cats shed oocysts for only brief durations (days to weeks) but in extremely large numbers ($>10^7$/day). A cat is more likely to acquire infection if it is an outdoor cat or a predator or is fed fresh, uncooked table scraps. Humans come in contact with cat excrement either directly (e.g., emptying the litter pan) or by more insidious means (e.g., cleaning a horse stall, weeding the garden, playing in a sandbox). Meat for human consumption may serve as a source of infection if it is eaten raw or undercooked. Again, accidental ingestion may occur under circumstances that are unsuspected. Examples include an Amish farm wife preparing sausage, a couple consuming steak tartare in an expensive restaurant, and a rancher butchering a deer.[79]

Common-source outbreaks of acute acquired *Toxoplasma* infection have been documented. In some instances, unique and clear-cut sources have been documented to be highly likely, such as exposure to aerosolized cat excrement in a riding stable[126] or consumption of unpasteurized goat milk.[112] In other circumstances, extensive investigations have failed to yield convincing answers.[78, 116] Because of the possibility of common-source exposure, however, the families of patients with acute acquired infection should be evaluated for subclinical infection.[76]

Accidental self-inoculation with a needle contaminated with *Toxoplasma* has resulted in a number of acquired infections in laboratory workers. Infections also have been ascribed to blood transfusions and organ transplantation.[45]

Congenital Infection

Congenital infection is considered to occur, with rare exceptions, only when *primary* maternal infection with *Toxoplasma* occurs.[36, 106] The only two well-documented exceptions to this rule have occurred in immunodeficient pregnant women.[93, 106] In a large series of more than 800 carefully studied women who had given birth to congenitally infected children, however, not a single case of congenital infection occurred in subsequent pregnancies.[106] It also is believed generally that only acute infection beginning *during* pregnancy can lead to congenital infection. Although there are a few well-documented instances of biopsy-proven lymphadenopathic toxoplasmosis occurring 2 months *prior to* conception that resulted in congenitally infected babies,[128] this pattern of occurrence also appears to be extremely rare.[50]

The prevalence of congenital toxoplasmosis in a population, therefore, is determined by the risk of a woman's experiencing primary infection while she is pregnant. This risk depends in turn on three factors: the age-specific incidence of primary infection during child-bearing years, the age distribution of pregnant women in the population, and the fetal transmission rate in primary infection. A theoretic analysis based on these three factors by Frenkel,[46] assuming a child-bearing age group of 20 to 29 years and an overall fetal transmission rate of 40 per cent, showed that maximum risk occurs when the age-specific incidence rate in a population is 3 to 5 per cent per year, which corresponds to prevalences of seropositivity of 50 to 80 per cent in women of child-bearing age. In such a population, the predicted prevalence of congenital toxoplasmosis would be 4.4 to 4.6 per 1000 pregnancies. At higher age-specific incidences, rates of congenital toxoplasmosis would be lower because nearly all pregnant women already would be infected chronically. At lower incidences, rates would be lower, but because of less frequent exposure.

Studies in the early 1970s revealed prevalences of congenital toxoplasmosis in the United States of approximately 2 per 1000 births.[1, 9, 68, 106] The only prospective data currently available in the United States are derived from the screening of approximately 600,000 newborns in Massachusetts and New Hampshire using the IgM enzyme-linked immunosorbent assay (ELISA) as applied to filter paper blood samples.[54] The prevalence of infection identifiable at birth in this more recent study was approximately 1 in 12,000. The limitations of the testing method (small serum volumes, a test that yields positive results in only 75 per cent of cases) undoubtedly make this estimate a conservative one, but it supports the notion that prevalence has declined in recent years.

PATHOLOGY

After intracellular multiplication at the site of entry, tachyzoites are disseminated in the blood and may invade all organs and tissues. Severity of the infection probably is the result of strain virulence and host susceptibility rather than of tissue tropisms of certain strains. Proliferation of tachyzoites results in death of invaded cells and eventually in small necrotic foci surrounded by intense cellular reaction. With recovery, cysts without an inflammatory response around them may persist in brain, bone marrow, lymph nodes, liver, spleen, and lung and in skeletal, heart, and smooth muscle.[45–47]

In active infection of the central nervous system, *Toxoplasma*-filled cells are scattered throughout the gray matter, producing diffuse meningoencephalitis with miliary microglial nodules and foci of perivascular inflammation.[21] Large lesions may mimic cerebral tumor. Areas of basal ganglial and periventricular inflammation may calcify in the fetus.[40, 102] Obstruction of the aqueduct of Sylvius or the foramen of Monro may result in hydrocephalus in congenital infection.

Enlarged lymph nodes in acute acquired toxoplasmosis show characteristic pathologic changes that may warrant a presumptive diagnosis.[41, 128] These changes include reactive follicular hyperplasia, epithelioid histiocytes encroaching on and blurring the margins of germinal centers, and distention of subcapsular and trabecular sinuses by monocytoid cells. Tachyzoites and cysts are seen rarely.[41]

In the eye, active chorioretinitis begins in the retina with severe inflammation and necrosis and exudation into the vitreous. Single or multiple foci occur, and secondary involvement of the choroid always is present. Both tachyzoites and cysts have been found in these lesions.[11, 12]

In immunocompromised hosts, widespread necrotizing lesions may be seen in heart, muscle, brain, and other organs. These lesions, particularly involving the central nervous system, have been found frequently with reactivation of toxoplasmosis in patients with AIDS.[74]

IMMUNOLOGY

Cell-mediated immune responses are the major immunologic mechanisms that prevent reactivation of *T. gondii* in the chronically infected normal host.[20, 30] A number of effector mechanisms contribute to protection in murine models and human infection: CD8+ cytotoxic T lymphocytes, CD4+ T lymphocytes, monocyte oxidative mechanisms, production of gamma interferon by natural killer cells, and activation of macrophages by gamma interferon and tumor necrosis factor alpha.[52, 55, 64, 66, 117, 123] Killing the parasite within activated macrophages is associated with intracellular production of nitric oxide. Interleukin-2 and -12 enhance host resistance to *T. gondii*; interleukin-10 impairs the ability of macrophages to kill the parasite.[51]

In murine models, there is evidence for genetic determination of host resistance to infection.[13, 14, 85] The presence of the DQ3 allele appears to be associated with toxoplasmic encephalitis in patients with AIDS and hydrocephalus in infants with congenital toxoplasmosis.[14] Successful immunization of mice[15] and sheep[16] with *T. gondii* components raises the possibility of developing a human vaccine.[62, 86]

CLINICAL SYNDROMES

The disease in children may be considered in three categories: postnatally acquired, congenital, and ocular (which may be congenital or acquired). Clinically apparent infection in older children may be acquired recently or due to reactivation of latent congenital or postnatally acquired infection. Both congenital and acquired infections usually are subclinical, but congenital infection ultimately leads to serious sequelae in most cases.

Acute Acquired Toxoplasmosis

Acquired *Toxoplasma* infection most often is asymptomatic. It most frequently goes unrecognized; only 10 to 15 per cent of infected persons have clinical symptoms and signs. However, in certain recent outbreaks related to infection by oocysts, more than half of the infected patients have been symptomatic.[126] The most common presentations are lymphadenopathy and fatigue without fever.[81] The nodes are discrete and may or may not be tender. They do not suppurate. The groups of nodes most commonly involved are cervical, suboccipital, supraclavicular, axillary, and inguinal. Adenopathy may be localized or involve multiple areas, including retroperitoneal and mesenteric nodes. Uncommonly, the lymphadenopathy is accompanied by fever, malaise, fatigue, sore throat, and myalgia, a picture that closely simulates that of infectious mononucleosis but without serologic evidence of acute Epstein-Barr virus infection. The differential diagnosis of the lymphadenopathy often includes lymphoma. Chorioretinitis may develop, but it does not occur commonly.[78, 95] The liver may be involved, and liver function tests may reflect hepatocellular damage. In persons with normal immunologic function and without severe underlying disease, the infection usually is self-limited and rarely requires treatment.

In contrast, more severe and frequently fulminant infections are seen in patients receiving immunosuppressive therapy, in those who have disease of the bone marrow or reticuloendothelial system, in patients with agammaglobulinemia, in recipients of bone marrow transplants, and in those with AIDS.[33, 74, 109, 127] Encephalitis and rarely pneumonitis and myocarditis are the most important localized forms that may be encountered in immunocompromised patients. In toxoplasmic encephalitis, the predominant neurologic symptoms are headache, disorientation, and drowsiness. Presentations may simulate aseptic meningitis or a mass lesion. In view of the variety of clinical manifestations of central nervous system involvement, it is important to consider toxoplasmosis whenever there is evidence of acute central nervous system disease.

Congenital Toxoplasmosis

Congenital infection most often is the result of an asymptomatic acute infection in the mother.[44] In a small proportion of cases, spontaneous abortion, prematurity, or stillbirth may result. Congenital toxoplasmosis has a wide spectrum of clinical manifestations but most often is subclinical in the newborn infant. When clinically apparent, it may mimic other diseases of the newborn. Fever, hydrocephalus or microcephaly, hepatosplenomegaly, jaundice, convulsions, chorioretinitis (usually bilateral), cerebral calcifications, and abnormal cerebrospinal fluid (markedly increased protein and mononuclear pleocytosis) are considered the classic features of congenital toxoplasmosis.[40, 91] These manifestations were common in an early series of patients reported by Eichenwald (Table 221–1).[43] The case-fatality rate was 12 per cent. In survivors in this series, sequelae included mental retardation in 86 per cent; convulsions, spasticity, and palsies in almost 75 per cent; and severely impaired vision in 60 per cent.[43] Other occasional findings included rash (maculopapular, petechial, or both), myocarditis, pneumonitis and respiratory distress, hearing defects, an erythroblastosis-like picture, thrombocytopenia, lymphocytosis, monocytosis, and nephrotic syndrome. It now is known that these signs are most typical of the severe form of the infection in the absence of treatment.

The often subclinical nature of congenital toxoplasmosis in the newborn is seen in a French prospective study of 154 mothers who had acquired *Toxoplasma* infection during pregnancy and who did not receive treatment.[36] Nine pregnancies (6 per cent) ended in stillbirth, and 85 (55 per cent) resulted in the birth of infected liveborn infants. Of those liveborn infants who were infected, 64 (75 per cent) had subclinical infections, 14 (16 per cent) had mild disease, and only 7 (8 per cent) had clinically obvious severe disease.[36, 106]

The risk of transmission to the fetus varies significantly with the trimester of gestation during which the mother becomes infected. For untreated women, it is approximately 25 per cent in the first trimester, 54 per cent in the second trimester, and 65 per cent in the third trimester; these are minimum estimates that are derived from placental-isolation studies.[36] In contrast, the severity of clinical disease in congenitally infected infants is related inversely to the gestational age at the time of primary maternal infection. In two studies from France,[25, 36] severe disease or fetal/neonatal death occurred in approximately 40 to 79 per cent of infants born to mothers with first-trimester infection, 15 to 18 per cent with second-trimester infection, and 0 to 3 per cent with third-trimester infection.

TABLE 221–1. Signs and Symptoms Occurring Before Diagnosis or During the Course of Untreated Acute Congenital Toxoplasmosis in 152 Infants and 101 of These Same Patients After 4 Years or More of Follow-up[a]

Signs and Symptoms	Frequency of Occurrence in Patients With: *Neurologic Disease*[b]	*Generalized Disease*[c]
Infants	N = 108	N = 44
Chorioretinitis	102 (94)	29 (66)
Abnormal spinal fluid	59 (55)	37 (84)
Anemia	55 (51)	34 (77)
Jaundice	31 (29)	35 (80)
Splenomegaly	23 (21)	40 (90)
Convulsions	54 (50)	8 (18)
Fever	27 (25)	34 (77)
Intracranial calcification	54 (50)	2 (4)
Hepatomegaly	18 (17)	34 (77)
Lymphadenopathy	18 (17)	30 (68)
Vomiting	17 (16)	21 (48)
Hydrocephalus	30 (28)	0 (0)
Diarrhea	7 (6)	11 (25)
Pneumonitis	0 (0)	18 (41)
Microcephalus	14 (13)	0 (0)
Eosinophilia	6 (4)	8 (18)
Rash	1 (1)	11 (25)
Abnormal bleeding	3 (3)	8 (18)
Hypothermia	2 (2)	9 (20)
Cataracts	5 (5)	0 (0)
Glaucoma	2 (2)	0 (0)
Optic atrophy	2 (2)	0 (0)
Microphthalmia	2 (2)	0 (0)
Children 4 years of age or older	N = 70	N = 31
Mental retardation	62 (89)	25 (81)
Convulsions	58 (83)	24 (77)
Spasticity and palsies	53 (76)	18 (58)
Severely impaired vision	48 (69)	13 (42)
Hydrocephalus or microcephalus	31 (44)	2 (6)
Deafness	12 (17)	3 (10)
Normal	6 (9)	5 (16)

[a]Data indicate numbers of patients, with percentages in parentheses.
[b]Patients with central nervous system diseases in the first year of life.
[c]Patients with non-neurologic diseases during the first 2 months of life.
Modified from Eichenwald, H. G.: A study of congenital toxoplasmosis, with particular emphasis on clinical manifestations, sequelae, and therapy. *In* Siim, J. C. (ed.): Human Toxoplasmosis. Copenhagen, Munksgaard, 1960, p. 44.

Another French prospective study of 210 congenitally infected infants born to mothers who were identified to have primary infection acquired during pregnancy revealed significant morbidity in 94 newborns.[25] Overall, 2 cases (0.9 per cent) were fatal, 21 cases (10.9 per cent) were severe, and 71 cases (33.8 per cent) were mild; 116 cases were asymptomatic. It should be noted that approximately 40 to 45 per cent of the mothers in this study had been treated with spiramycin during pregnancy. These observations confirm that most congenital infections are subclinical at birth. Obvious presentations are relatively infrequent. In the same study by Couvreur and associates,[25] 116 infants were thought initially not to be infected on the basis of a routine newborn physical examination. On more intensive examination, however, 39 (34 per cent) of them had one or more abnormalities. Twenty-two (19 per cent) had abnormal cerebrospinal fluid on lumbar puncture, 17 (15 per cent) had chorioretinitis on indirect ophthalmoscopic examination, and 10 (9 per cent) had intracranial calcifications on head radiographs or computed tomography. Guerina and colleagues[54] made remarkably similar observations in the congenitally infected newborns they identified in New England by heelstick blood sampling.

Some infected children without overt disease as neonates may escape serious sequelae of the infection, whereas most develop chorioretinitis, strabismus, blindness, hydrocephalus or microcephaly, cerebral calcifications, developmental delay, epilepsy, or deafness months or even years later. Three studies provide data that define the incidence of these late sequelae.

In a study from Paris,[71] 26,402 apparently healthy infants were checked routinely for serologic evidence of *Toxoplasma* infection at 10 months of age. Fifty-one of these infants had positive serologic results for *Toxoplasma*, indicating congenital infection. None had been treated for *Toxoplasma* infection in infancy. Of the 51, 5 were found to have chorioretinal scars by ophthalmologic examination, and another 4 had developed chorioretinal lesions by 4 years of age, the longest period of follow-up. Some eventually lost functional vision in one eye. Three had intracranial calcifications.

Similarly, in a study from Holland in which a cohort of 1821 pregnant women were screened serologically, 12 congenitally infected infants were detected and 11 of these were followed for 20 years.[68, 69] Of the 11, 5 were treated as neonates for 1 month only and 6 were not. Of the five treated infants, four had eye disease as neonates and one had parasites in the cerebrospinal fluid, which prompted therapy. Nine of these 11 (82 per cent) had chorioretinal scars by 20 years of age and 4, including 2 who initially were normal, had severe visual impairment or blindness in one eye. Onset of disease leading to blindness developed as late as 18 years of age. No neurologic or cognitive sequelae were observed.

The results in this prospective study are similar to those previously reported by Wilson and associates[135] from Alabama in a retrospective analysis of patients from the United States. In this analysis, 11 of 13 congenitally infected children (85 per cent) who had no signs of disease on detailed examination in the newborn period developed sequelae over a mean period of follow-up of 8.3 years. Sequelae included chorioretinal lesions in 11 children (75 per cent), severe neurologic disability in 1 child (8 per cent), and mental retardation in 2 children (15 per cent). Sequelae first were noted at ages ranging from 1 month to 9 years. These 13 children were detected either as a result of routine screening of cord serum for IgM antibodies to *Toxoplasma*,[8] because acute *Toxoplasma* infection was diagnosed in the mother,[2] or as a result of nonspecific findings in the neonatal period (2 were small for gestational age, and 1 had transient borderline thrombocytopenia).

That treatment may decrease the frequency or severity of sequelae is suggested by the Alabama and Paris studies, in which only untreated infants developed chorioretinitis between 10 months and 4 years of age. Taken together, these data indicate that most congenitally infected children who receive no or relatively brief treatment, including those with inapparent infection as neonates, suffer untoward sequelae during childhood. Current treatment regimens—prolonged for at least 1 year and often initiated before birth—appear to be associated with substantially less frequent and severe sequelae (see Treatment).

Congenital toxoplasmosis may mimic or coexist with infection with other organisms. It must be differentiated from other perinatal infections due to cytomegalovirus (CMV), herpes simplex virus, rubella virus, *Treponema pallidum* (syphilis), HIV-1, and certain bacteria (e.g., *Listeria*). Herpesvirus and CMV infections, syphilis, and rubella may cause chorioretinitis; CMV and HIV-1 may cause encephalopathies associated with cerebral calcifications. Degenerative encephalopathies and storage diseases presenting in older children also may resemble congenital toxoplasmosis.

A number of infants or preschool children with coexisting HIV infection and toxoplasmosis have been reported.[92, 93] In at least six of these patients, both HIV and *Toxoplasma* infection appeared to have been acquired in utero. Of these six cases, all but one had clinical evidence of central nervous system disease, and in most this was associated with other findings common in congenital infection. These findings included hepatosplenomegaly, fever, and chorioretinitis and were evident at birth (one infant) or developed by 4 months of age. Two of the other infants remained asymptomatic, one of whom was treated for *Toxoplasma* infection and one of whom was not. One additional infant who acquired HIV infection at 18 months of age from a blood transfusion died at 5 years of age of toxoplasmic encephalitis. The findings in this patient resembled those in adults with AIDS and toxoplasmic encephalitis.[74]

Ocular Toxoplasmosis

In active congenital toxoplasmosis, retinal lesions usually are bilateral.[91] In older children, chorioretinitis may involve only one eye and may be the only manifestation of congenital toxoplasmosis. Toxoplasmic chorioretinitis, even in older children and adults, usually is considered to be the result of congenital infection.[95] In some studies, *Toxoplasma* infection has accounted for as many as 5 per cent of severe visual impairments in children.[65] Active lesions on the fundus appear as white or yellowish foci with elevated, edematous margins surrounded by a zone of hyperemia (Fig. 221–3). Cells and fibrinous exudate in the vitreous may obscure the fundus. Older lesions appear as glial scars, and in areas in which the retina has been destroyed, the choroid and sclera are visible. Around the depigmented areas, there is deposition of pigment from the destroyed retina. The position of the lesion may be macular, juxtapapillary, or peripheral.

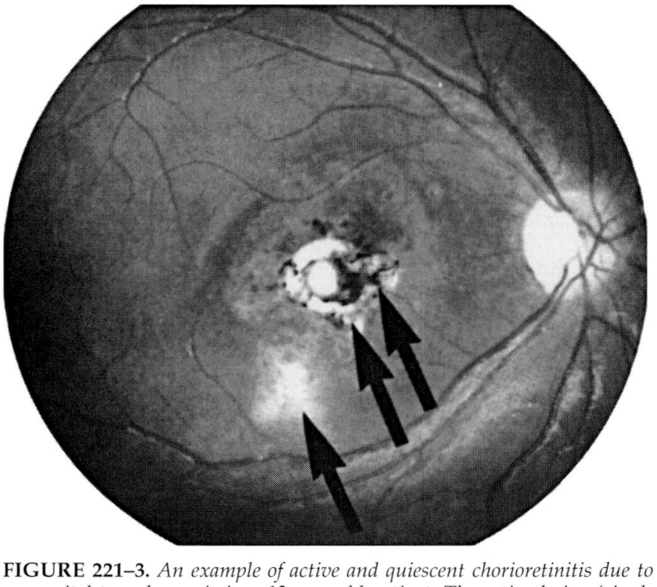

FIGURE 221–3. *An example of active and quiescent chorioretinitis due to congenital toxoplasmosis in a 12-year-old patient. The active lesion (single arrow) satellites an old chorioretinal scar (two arrows). (From Mets, M., Holfels, E., Boyer, K. M., et al.: Eye manifestations of congenital toxoplasmosis. Am. J. Ophthalmol. 122:309–324, 1996. Ophthalmic Publishing Co., publisher.)*

The patient may present with marked loss of central vision (due to a perimacular lesion), with hazy vision (due to accumulated exudate), or with "floaters" (due to reactivation of peripheral foci). Neonates or infants with toxoplasmic eye disease may present with microphthalmia, small cornea, posterior cortical cataract, anisometropia, strabismus, and nystagmus.[91] Strabismus and nystagmus in a child of any age should raise the possibility of congenital toxoplasmosis. The appearance of lesions in the fundus is not specific for toxoplasmosis. Similar lesions may occur with other less common granulomatous diseases in the eye, such as toxocariasis, cat-scratch disease, and tuberculosis. Chorioretinitis may be recurrent, most commonly with reactivation at the margins of preexisting lesions.

LABORATORY DIAGNOSIS

Acute infection can be diagnosed by isolation of *T. gondii* from blood or body fluids; demonstration of tachyzoites in histologic sections of tissue or cytologic preparations of body fluids; characteristic lymph node histology; demonstration of *Toxoplasma* cysts in placenta, fetus, or neonate; detection of the *Toxoplasma* genome by polymerase chain reaction in body fluids; and characteristic serologic test results. Each of these methods is discussed; serologic tests are emphasized because they are the most common way to establish the diagnosis (Table 221–2).

Serologic Methods

Measurements of IgG Antibody

The most useful tests for detection of IgG antibodies to *Toxoplasma* include the Sabin Feldman dye test,[111] the indirect immunofluorescent antibody (IFA) test, agglutination tests, and ELISA. Titers in the ELISA are expressed in different terms for different commercial kits, thereby precluding a discussion of IgG ELISA titers per se in relation to diagnosis of the acute infection.[39, 129] In these tests, IgG antibodies appear within the first week of primary infection and reach peak titers (usually 1:500 or greater) within 1 to 2 months; detectable titers usually persist for life. Although the dye test is the most reliable, it is available only in a few reference laboratories. The IFA test and ELISA are the most widely available and, when properly performed, yield results similar to those obtained in the dye test; however, many laboratories use commercially available kits that are not consistently reliable. Some sera that contain antinuclear antibodies yield false-positive IFA results. The direct agglutination tests that currently are available use formalin-fixed tachyzoites or antigen-coated latex particles, are simple to perform, and are accurate.[119]

Other tests vary in their reliability. Indirect hemagglutination is widely available, but the results frequently are negative in newborns with congenital infection.[131] It should *not* be used for screening pregnant women because detectable titer rises are delayed, compared with the rises detected by ELISA and the dye, IFA, and agglutination tests.

Meaningful interpretation of changes in titer on sequential sera requires that assays on each sample be performed in the same run by a reliable laboratory.

Measurements of IgM Antibody

IgM antibodies are detected most commonly by IgM-IFA, IgM-immunosorbent agglutination assay (ISAGA), or IgM-

TABLE 221–2. Guidelines for Interpretation of Serologic Tests for Toxoplasmosis[a]

Test	Positive Titer	Titer in Congenital Infection (Infant) or Acute Infection (Older Child, Adult)	Titer in Chronic Infection	Duration of Elevation of Titer
IgG				
Sabin-Feldman dye test	Undiluted	NC, S OCA, 1:4 to ≥1:1,000 (usual)	1 : 4 to 1 : 2,000	Years
Direct agglutination	≥1 : 20	NC, S OCA, rises slowly from negative to low to high titer (1 : 512)	Stable (≥1 : 1,000) or slowly decreasing titer	≥1 year
Indirect fluorescent IgG antibody	≥1 : 10	NC, S OCA, ≥1:1,000	1 : 8 to 1 : 2,000	Years
Indirect hemagglutination	≥1 : 16	NC, S OCA, ≥1:1,000	1 : 16 to 1 : 256	Years
Complement fixation	≥1 : 4	NC, S OCA, varies among laboratories	Negative to 1 : 8	Years
IgM				
Indirect fluorescent IgM antibody	≥1 : 10, adults	OCA, ≥1:80 (use only for OCA, not NC)	Negative to 1 : 20	Weeks to months, occasionally years
Double sandwich IgM EIA	≥0.2, newborn, fetus ≥1.7, older children, adults	NC, ≥0.2 OCA, ≥1.7	Negative to 1.7 (OCA)	Can be ≥1 year
Immunosorbent test for IgM	≥3, infant 8, adult	NC, ≥3 OCA, >8	Negative to 1	Unknown, can be ≥1 year
IgA				
IgA, EIA	≥1.0, infants ≥1.4, adults	NC, ≥1.0 OCA, >1.4	Negative to <1.0 Negative to ≤1.3	Weeks to months, occasionally longer
IgE				
IgE, EIA	≥1.9 infants and adults	NC and OCA, ≥1.9	Negative	Weeks to months, occasionally longer
Immunosorbent test for IgE	≥4 infants and adults	NC and OCA, ≥4	Negative	Weeks to months, occasionally longer
AC/HS	See reference 29	See reference 29	See reference 29	Usually <9 months
PCR (amniotic fluid; CSF)	Positive	Positive	Negative	Only when *Toxoplasma* DNA present during active infection

NC, titer in newborn with congenital infection; OCA, titer in older child or adult with acute, acquired infection; S, usually the same as the mother; EIA, enzyme immunosorbent; AC/HS, differential agglutinin test; PCR, polymerase chain reaction; CSF, cerebrospinal fluid.

[a]Values are those of one reference laboratory; each laboratory must provide its own standards and interpretation of results in each clinical setting.

Modified from McLeod, R., and Remington, J. S.: Toxoplasmosis. *In* Braunwald, E., Isselbacher, K. J., Petersdorf, R. G., et al. (eds.): Harrison's Principles of Internal Medicine. New York, McGraw-Hill, 1987, p. 795. With permission from The McGraw-Hill Companies.

ELISA. IgM antibodies appear in the first week of primary infection and peak within 1 month. Depending on the sensitivity of the method used, IgM antibodies may be demonstrable for from 2 to 3 months to 1 year or longer. IgM-ELISA and IgM-ISAGA are much more sensitive than IgM-IFA is. Absence of IgM-ELISA or IgM-ISAGA antibodies in an immunologically normal older child (older than 1 year of age) or adult essentially rules out a recently acquired infection. A negative IgM-IFA result is not as sensitive in ruling out recently acquired infection. Ninety-three per cent of sera that were negative in IgM-IFA and obtained from adults who recently had acquired toxoplasmosis were strongly positive in IgM-ELISA.[98] IgM-IFA detects specific IgM antibody in only 25 per cent of infants with proven congenital infection, whereas IgM-ELISA detects antibody in approximately 75 per cent of such cases.[98] The presence of rheumatoid factor or of antinuclear antibodies may cause false-positive results in IgM-IFA.[2]

The "double-sandwich" IgM-ELISA avoids both the false-positive results due to the presence of rheumatoid factor, which the infant can produce in utero, and the false-negative results due to competition from high levels of maternal IgG antibody that occur in IgM-IFA.[97] Also, false-positive results in IgM-IFA due to antinuclear antibodies are not found in IgM-ELISA.[2, 96]

ISAGAs are used widely in Europe. Like IgM-ELISA, they capture IgM on a solid surface, detect specific IgM, and involve adding whole formalin-fixed organisms or *Toxoplasma* antigen–coated latex particles.[38, 105] These assays are commercially available and give results comparable with those of IgM-ELISA, are simpler to perform, and do not require expensive equipment.

Measurements of IgA and IgE Antibodies

Demonstration of IgA and IgE antibodies in the fetus or newborn infant by ELISA and ISAGA appears to be at least comparable in sensitivity for diagnosis of congenital *Toxoplasma* infection to demonstration of IgM antibody.[32, 121, 137] The IgA test also appears to be more sensitive than the IgM test for detection of acquired infection. Specificity remains an issue. Neither ELISA nor ISAGA, therefore, has superceded the IgM test for diagnosis of the acquired infection. However, IgA and IgE antibodies have somewhat longer persistence than IgM and therefore may be useful in subacute illness or when IgM titers are low.

Differential Agglutination

Acetone and formulin-fixed *T. gondii* tachyzoites may yield differing agglutination titers depending on the acuity of infection. This test based on this phenomenon is called the AC/HS differential agglutination test.[29] In general, a disproportionately high agglutination titer with acetone-fixed organisms suggests acute infection; a disproportionately high titer with formalin-fixed organisms suggests chronic infection. Interpretative norms for this test have been established.[29] This test, combined with the dye test, IgM-ELISA, IgA-ELISA, IgE-ELISA, and IgE-ISAGA, constitutes a "toxoplasmic serologic profile" that permits the most accurate evaluation of infection acuity in the pregnant woman[94, 138] and often can resolve inconclusive or discrepant results obtained in a hospital or commercial laboratory.

Nonserologic Methods

Nonserologic methods are used less commonly for diagnosis of *Toxoplasma* infection because they are not widely available and because they require tissue specimens.

Isolation of the Organism

Isolation of *Toxoplasma* from blood or body fluids (e.g., cerebrospinal fluid) establishes that the infection is acute. In the case of the neonate, isolation from the placenta or the infant's tissues is sufficient to diagnose congenital *Toxoplasma* infection. Isolation from the placenta usually (about 90 per cent), but not always, is associated with congenital infection.[106] Isolation of *Toxoplasma* from tissues of older children or adults, however, may reflect only the presence of latent infection (cyst form). The organism may be isolated by inoculation of body fluids, leukocytes, or tissue specimens into the peritoneal cavities of mice or into tissue cultures. Specimens should be processed and inoculated immediately; however, tissue and blood may be stored at 4° C overnight. Freezing and thawing or formalin treatment kills the organism. Definitive diagnosis by isolation of *Toxoplasma* from tissues usually takes 4 to 6 weeks by mouse inoculation; tissue culture is less sensitive for recovering *Toxoplasma,* but results are available sooner.

Histology

Demonstration of tachyzoites, but not cysts, in tissue sections or smears of body fluids (e.g., cerebrospinal fluid) establishes a diagnosis of acute infection. The organism may be difficult to see with routine stains. The peroxidase-antiperoxidase technique is exquisitely sensitive and has been used with a high degree of sensitivity and specificity to demonstrate the organism in the central nervous system of patients with AIDS.[21] In older children and adults, the histopathologic changes in toxoplasmic lymphadenitis sufficiently are distinctive to enable pathologists to make a presumptive diagnosis of acute acquired toxoplasmosis (see Pathology).[41, 128] Histologic demonstration of cysts establishes that a patient has *Toxoplasma* infection, but they are diagnostic of toxoplasmosis only in the placenta, fetus, or newborn infant.

Antigen-Specific Lymphocyte Transformation

Lymphocyte transformation in response to *Toxoplasma* antigens is a specific and sensitive indicator of prior *Toxoplasma* infection in adults and has been used successfully to diagnose congenital *Toxoplasma* infection in infants 2 months of age or older.[84, 122, 133] Lymphocyte transformation often is absent in the newborn period, particularly in more severely affected infants, a reflection of specific immune tolerance.[84, 88]

Polymerase Chain Reaction

Amplification of the B1 genome of *T. gondii* DNA by polymerase chain reaction permits detection of the parasite in body fluids or tissue, such as cerebrospinal fluid, amniotic fluids, or lymph nodes.[53, 56, 128] Experience with the test in France, where it was studied along with the results of percutaneous umbilical blood sampling in 339 pregnant women, indicates close to 100 per cent sensitivity and specificity for the diagnosis of intrauterine infection.[56] In view of the considerably lower risk of amniocentesis compared with percutaneous umbilical blood sampling and the fact that amniocentesis potentially can be performed earlier in gestation, this diagnostic procedure appears to be a major advance in prenatal diagnosis.

Diagnosis in Specific Clinical Situations

Acute Acquired Toxoplasmosis

If IgM or IgG antibody is not detectable, the diagnosis of acute *Toxoplasma* infection in the immunocompetent child virtually is excluded. The diagnosis of recently acquired infection is confirmed if there is seroconversion from a negative to a positive titer or if there is a serial fourfold rise in titer to high levels when sera drawn at 3-week intervals are run in parallel. A single high titer in any test is not diagnostic. A dye test or IFA titer of 1:500 or greater in the presence of a high IgM antibody titer probably is diagnostic of recent acute infection. The absence of IgM antibodies in IgM-ELISA or IgM-ISAGA essentially excludes the diagnosis of acute infection. In contrast, absence of IgM antibodies in IgM-IFA does not mean necessarily that the infection is not acute; in one series, 25 per cent of results in adults with acute infection were negative in IgM-IFA.[98]

Toxoplasma *Infection in the Immunodeficient Child*

Serologic tests should be performed to identify persons who are at risk of acquiring toxoplasmosis, such as organ transplant recipients and bone marrow transplant patients. The available serologic tests may be inadequate to detect acute active infection in some immunodeficient patients because their antibody response may be abnormal. This especially is true in bone marrow transplant recipients.[34] Experience in the Palo Alto, California, reference laboratory has revealed that acute infection may be present in patients with AIDS and in bone marrow transplant recipients without any demonstrable IgM antibody and in some immunocompromised patients who have little or no IgG antibody. In AIDS patients with active *Toxoplasma* infection, antibody titers in the modified direct agglutination test[39] clearly may be elevated in the presence of low or undetectable titers in the dye test or IFA.[80] These and other immunodeficient patients can present with progressive, lethal toxoplasmosis. In almost all of the cases, encephalitis, brain abscesses, or both are the predominant findings; hepatic involvement, pneumonitis, and myocarditis may be present. In these patients, a high index of suspicion is necessary, and immunoperoxidase staining of appropriate biopsy specimens often is required for diagnosis. For the special problem of interpretation of IgM and IgG antibody rises in organ transplant recipients, the reader is referred to the article by Luft and colleagues.[75]

Toxoplasma Infection in the Pregnant Woman

Toxoplasma infection acquired during pregnancy is associated with clinical signs (e.g., lymphadenopathy) in only 10 to 15 per cent of patients. The fetus, however, is at risk of contracting the infection whether or not the mother is symptomatic. To detect acute infection in the pregnant woman in the absence of a routine screening program in which serologic tests are performed periodically throughout pregnancy, a suitable test for IgM antibody (IgM-ELISA or IgM-ISAGA) should be performed if other serologic tests are positive at any titer. If a suitable IgM antibody test is unavailable and the original serum contains IgG antibodies, the IgG antibody test should be repeated in 3 weeks, in parallel with the original serum, to determine if the titer is stable or rising. If the IgM-ELISA or IgM-ISAGA result is negative and if the IgG antibody titer is stable and less than 1:500, no further evaluation is necessary. Because IgG titers usually stabilize at high levels (e.g., dye test or IFA titer ≥1:500) 6 to 8 weeks or longer after acquisition of the infection, if the dye test or IFA titer is less than or equal to 1:500 and stable (regardless of IgM antibody titer), infection was acquired at least 4 weeks and probably more than 8 weeks prior to the time the serum was obtained. However, in the United States, it is common for an asymptomatic woman to be evaluated for the first time more than 8 weeks after conception. If her dye test or IFA titer is greater than or equal to 1:500, her IgM-ELISA or IgM-ISAGA result is negative, and no significant rise in titer in any test can be demonstrated, it almost is certain that her infection was acquired prior to conception. In women with elevated IgM titers or rising IgG test titers, it is possible that infection was acquired during pregnancy. A complete toxoplasmic serologic profile[94] in a reference serologic laboratory is recommended to settle the question.

Fetal Diagnosis

As noted earlier, severe disease almost always is associated with primary maternal infection in the first or second trimester of pregnancy, but only 25 and 54 per cent, respectively, of such cases result in fetal infection. These rates may be reduced by half by maternal treatment with spiramycin. Identification of cases in which the fetus already is infected permits a parental decision to terminate the pregnancy or to treat the fetal infection more aggressively with pyrimethamine-sulfadiazine.

Studies by workers in Paris have established an approach that allows definitive diagnosis and treatment of fetal infection in utero.[27, 37, 56] These workers initially sought to establish the diagnosis of fetal infection at 20 to 29 weeks of gestation by isolation of *Toxoplasma* from amniotic fluid or from fetal blood obtained by percutaneous umbilical blood sampling, using the sensitive mouse inoculation method. Prenatal diagnosis was attempted in 746 pregnancies in which primary *Toxoplasma* infection was acquired near the time of conception or before the twenty-sixth week of gestation. In 39 of these pregnancies, fetal infection was diagnosed in utero. *Toxoplasma* was isolated from fetal blood alone in 12 cases, from amniotic fluid alone in 7 cases, and from both in 15 cases for a total of 34. *Toxoplasma*-specific IgM antibodies were detected in fetal blood in only nine cases using the highly sensitive ISAGA, and none was positive before 24 weeks of gestation. By follow-up examination up until 3 months post partum or by examination of aborted fetal tissue, a total of 42 cases were proved to have been infected. Thus, these workers were able successfully to detect 39 (92 per cent) of 42 cases of fetal infection occurring before the twenty-sixth week of gestation; there were no false-positive diagnoses. These workers subsequently have extended their series and have reported that a definitive diagnosis of infection was established in utero in 80 (90 per cent) of 89 cases in which the fetus was infected.[57] These results may not be reproduced easily by others for various reasons: the ability to detect maternal infection soon after it occurred because of monthly monitoring for new maternal infections, sampling of fetal blood and amniotic fluid on more than one occasion, the use of optimal laboratory methods and conditions, and experience in these procedures.

With the use of polymerase chain reaction to amplify the B1 gene of *Toxoplasma* in amniotic fluid obtained after 18 weeks of gestation, these same investigators now have been able to achieve sensitivity and specificity for the diagnosis of fetal infection that both approach 100 per cent.[56] Sensitivity and specificity for this test as specimens currently are processed and handled in the United States, however, remain to be determined.

Most of the mothers in these French studies had received treatment with spiramycin soon after primary maternal infection was diagnosed. In contrast with its beneficial effect on maternal-to-fetal transmission, spiramycin appears not to decrease the severity of fetal infection once it has been established. Thus, the impetus for detecting fetal infection in early to middle gestation is to allow for intervention either to terminate the pregnancy or to treat the fetus more aggressively. In the extended series of 89 infected fetuses reported by Hohlfeld and colleagues,[57] 34 pregnancies were terminated at the requests of the parents. In each of these cases, which were selected either for detectable central nervous system disease on ultrasound examination or for onset of maternal infection before 12 weeks of gestation, brain necrosis was found on examination of tissue. These data indicate the value of specifically identifying those fetuses that truly are infected and at high risk for severe disease because selective termination of these pregnancies allowed the successful completion of the majority of pregnancies in which fetal infection did not occur. In addition to the 34 terminated pregnancies with proved fetal infection, 52 pregnancies with 55 offspring were carried to term. In these 52, 43 had fetal infection proved prenatally, and 9 additional offspring were found to be infected by postnatal examination. In the 43 pregnancies in which prenatal diagnosis of fetal infection was established, more aggressive therapy with pyrimethamine and a sulfonamide compound was given in the latter part of pregnancy. This treatment appeared to decrease the number of parasites, as indicated by an approximate 50 per cent reduction in the fraction of placentas from which *Toxoplasma* was isolated at delivery compared with cases in which no treatment or spiramycin alone was given.

Regarding clinical outcome, the authors interpreted their data to indicate that such treatment decreased the incidence of severe disease.[57] However, this conclusion was based on a retrospective comparison with a group of historical controls in which information regarding fetal deaths and pregnancy terminations was not available. Because pregnancies with proven or probable severe fetal infection were terminated selectively at the parents' request, it is not possible to conclude with certainty that the outcome of the infants born to mothers with first-trimester infection was improved by the more aggressive therapy; the outcome of those born to mothers with second-trimester infection appears to have been improved.[132] It would be desirable to have data from studies in which the effects of such therapy are compared directly in a randomized, concurrent study; such studies, however, are unlikely to be performed. Nevertheless, these studies have established the utility of an aggressive approach to prenatal diagnosis in allowing an accurate, early diagnosis of fetal infection. If the fetus is infected and affected, as determined by ultrasonography, a decision for selective termination of pregnancy can be made rationally. Aggressive therapy with pyrimethamine-sulfadiazine may be offered in cases in which termination is not considered desirable, and it may improve outcome.

Diagnosis of Congenital Toxoplasmosis After Birth

A thorough clinical and laboratory evaluation is necessary to evaluate fully the existence and extent of congenital toxoplasmosis in a newborn (Table 221–3). Demonstration of IgM, IgA, or IgE antibody in an infant's blood or cerebrospinal fluid at any time is diagnostic of congenital infection if contamination by maternal blood reasonably can be excluded. Specimens obtained after 10 days of age are more reliable in this regard. If the much less sensitive IgM-IFA is used, the presence of antinuclear antibody and rheumatoid factor also must be excluded. As mentioned earlier, the detection rate of congenitally infected infants is 25 per cent for IgM-IFA and 75 per cent for IgM-ELISA and IgM-ISAGA. (Data are insufficient for prediction of how often IgA and IgE antibodies are detected.) IgM antibodies may be demonstrable in the first few days of life or may appear at varying times after birth.

If *Toxoplasma* is not isolated and IgM, IgA, or IgE antibodies are not detected, follow-up serologic testing is the only means of establishing the diagnosis. Maternally transmitted IgG antibodies may persist for 6 to 12 months or longer, depending on the original titer. The higher the original titer, the longer maternal antibody is detectable in the infant. Thus, the presence of IgG antibody at even 8 to 12 months of age does not prove necessarily that the infant is infected. Synthesis of IgG *Toxoplasma* antibody usually is demonstrable by the third month of life if the infant is not treated; it may be delayed until the sixth or ninth month if the infant is treated. At the time the infant begins to synthesize IgG antibody, infection may be documented by computing the specific "antibody load," that is, the ratio of specific serum antibody titer to the level of serum IgG in the infant.[106] In the absence of infection, the antibody load decreases in the second or third month as the infant begins to produce IgG that does not contain specific *Toxoplasma* antibodies. In the presence of *Toxoplasma* infection, the infant produces specific antibodies, and thus the antibody load remains the same or increases.

TABLE 221–3. Evaluation of Neonate When Serology of Mother, or Illness of Neonate, Indicates That Diagnosis of Congenital Toxoplasmosis Is Suspected or Likely

In addition to a careful general examination, the baby is examined by the following:

Clinical evaluation and nonspecific tests
- A pediatric ophthalmologist
- A pediatric neurologist
- Brain CT
- Blood tests
  - Complete blood cell count with differential and platelet counts
  - Serum total IgM, IgG, IgA, and albumin
  - Serum alanine aminotransferase, total and direct bilirubin
  - CSF cell count, glucose, protein, and total IgG

Toxoplasma gondii–*specific tests*
- Newborn serum analyzed for antibody detected by Sabin-Feldman dye test, IgM-ISAGA, IgA-EIA, IgE-EIA/ISAGA (0.5 mL serum to *Toxoplasma* Serology Laboratory, Palo Alto Medical Foundation, 860 Bryant Street, Palo Alto, CA 94301, 415-326-8120)
- Newborn blood for inoculation into mice (1–2 mL clotted whole blood in red-topped tube to *Toxoplasma* Serology Laboratory, address above)
- Lumbar puncture: CSF dye test and IgM-EIA (0.5 mL CSF to *Toxoplasma* Serology Laboratory, address above); consider PCR (1 mL frozen CSF to *Toxoplasma* Serology Laboratory, address above)
- Sterile placental tissue (100 g in saline, from fetal side near insertion of cord, no formalin) to *Toxoplasma* Serology Laboratory for subinoculation (address above)
- Maternal serum analyzed for antibody detected by dye test, IgM-EIA, IgA-EIA, IgE-EIA/ISAGA, and AC/HS

CT, computed tomography; CSF, cerebrospinal fluid; EIA, enzyme immunoassay; ISAGA, immunosorbent test for IgM; PCR, polymerase chain reaction; AC/HS, differential agglutination test.

Modified from McLeod, R., Wisner, J., and Boyer, K.: Toxoplasmosis. *In* Krugman, S., Katz, S. L., and Gershon, A. A. (eds.): Infectious Diseases of Children. St. Louis, Mosby Year Book, 1992, p. 539.

Ocular Toxoplasmosis

Toxoplasma has been estimated to cause 35 per cent of the cases of chorioretinitis in the United States and central and Western Europe.[113] Acquired toxoplasmosis usually is not accompanied by chorioretinitis. It is thought that most cases result from congenital infection that does not become clinically apparent until reactivation occurs. This is most common in adolescence. Although the presence of chorioretinitis should prompt a search for *Toxoplasma* infection, proof that *Toxoplasma* caused the eye disease often is lacking. The titer of antibody in the serum does not correlate necessarily with the presence of active lesions in the fundus. In fact, low titers of IgG antibody are the usual finding in patients with reactivation *Toxoplasma* chorioretinitis. IgM antibodies usually are absent.

Toxoplasma probably is excluded as a cause of chorioretinitis if the results of serologic tests are negative in undiluted serum. If retinal lesions are characteristic and serologic test results are positive, the diagnosis is likely. If the retinal lesions are atypical and the serologic test results are positive, the diagnosis of *Toxoplasma* chorioretinitis is less certain because of the increasing prevalence of *Toxoplasma* antibodies with age in the normal population. Finding *Toxoplasma* antibodies in the child's mother supports the possibility of congenital infection, as does detection of intracranial calcification on computed tomographic examination of the patient. Demonstration of local antibody production in aqueous humor obtained by paracentesis of the anterior chamber can be used to establish the diagnosis of *Toxoplasma* chorioretinitis in equivocal cases.[106] However, the risk of this procedure in a situation of threatened vision, when weighed against the relatively low risk of a short course of treatment, is such that it seldom is performed.

TREATMENT

The need for therapy and the duration of therapy are determined by the nature and severity of the clinical illness and by the immune status of the infected patient. Antibody titers are not useful indicators of therapeutic response, and an increasing antibody titer soon after discontinuation of therapy ("serologic rebound") is not an indication of therapeutic failure. Specific therapy acts primarily against the tachyzoite form; currently available drugs do not eradicate the encysted form. Close, longitudinal follow-up and supportive interventions are extremely important contributors to therapeutic success.

Therapeutic Agents

The therapeutic agents used, their dosages, and indications for their use in the management of toxoplasmosis are included in Table 221–4 and are discussed next.

Spiramycin

This macrolide has been used extensively in Europe to reduce transmission of the infection from an acutely infected mother to the fetus in utero.[22] It is concentrated in the placenta and is reported to reduce transmission by 50 to 60 per cent. It reduces the ability to isolate the organism from placentas of definitively infected newborns from 95 to 80 per cent.[24] It is less effective than pyrimethamine-sulfadiazine in the treatment of congenital infection and toxoplasmic encephalitis.[24, 35, 114, 115] Toxoplasmic encephalitis has developed in patients ingesting spiramycin and then has been treated effectively with pyrimethamine-sulfadiazine. Toxicities include allergic manifestations, gastrointestinal intolerance, and paresthesias. Spiramycin does not appear to treat manifestations of *T. gondii* infection in the fetus in utero.[24, 35, 57, 114] it formerly was used in alternate-month regimens with pyrimethamine and sulfadiazine for treatment of congenital toxoplasmosis in France.[106] Spiramycin is not approved by the U.S. Food and Drug Administration but may be obtained with compassionate clearance by calling 301-827-4420. The manufacturer (Rhone-Poulenc) may be contacted at 610-454-5399.

Pyrimethamine

Pyrimethamine has been demonstrated to be effective against *T. gondii* in vitro,[87, 90] in animal models,[49] and in human infections.[26, 28, 49, 77, 90, 138] When used in conjunction with sulfadiazine, synergy can be demonstrated. Pyrimethamine pharmacokinetics have been studied in infants and adults.[88] Pyrimethamine is metabolized in the liver, and its pharmacokinetics are not altered by renal insufficiency but are affected by concomitantly administered drugs (e.g., phenobarbital). Pyrimethamine toxicities include reversible marrow suppression (most commonly) and allergy. Aplastic anemia, hepatotoxicity, and various allergic manifestations (including Stevens-Johnson syndrome) also have been listed as toxicities of this medication. Pyrimethamine always should be administered in conjunction with leukovorin (i.e., folinic acid) because human cells can use folinic acid for the synthesis of their nucleic acids, but *T. gondii* cannot.[88]

Leukovorin

Leukovorin always is administered during treatment with pyrimethamine. Increased doses of leukovorin are used in the event of marrow suppression. Because of the long half-life of pyrimethamine, continuation of leukovorin therapy for 1 week after discontinuing pyrimethamine is recommended.

Sulfadiazine, Sulfamerazine, and Sulfamethazine

These three sulfonamides (known as triple sulfa when used in combination) are the most active of the sulfonamides against *T. gondii* and are synergistic with pyrimethamine in their activity against *T. gondii*. Of the three, only sulfadiazine currently is available in the United States. All other sulfonamides are less active in vitro.[87] They are excreted by the kidney, and dosage must be adjusted for patients with renal insufficiency. Toxicities include allergy, marrow suppression, and both hepatic and renal toxicity. Pharmacokinetics in infants have been studied.[106]

Clindamycin

Although the effect of clindamycin is delayed, it does have an effect in vitro against *T. gondii* with prolonged time in culture.[103] It has been demonstrated to be effective in murine models as well. It has been found to be comparable in efficacy to sulfadiazine for treatment of toxoplasmic encephalitis in adult AIDS patients when used in a combined high-dose regimen with pyrimethamine.[28, 77] It should be noted that high-dosage pyrimethamine also is effective alone and that this was not compared directly with the other two regimens in the latter study.

Other Antimicrobial Agents

A number of other antimicrobial agents have been demonstrated to be effective in vitro or in animal models either against tachyzoites or encysted bradyzoites,[3–6, 58, 59] but their role, if any, in the treatment of human disease remains to be defined. Atovoquone (5-hydroxy-naphthoquinone), for example, was effective against bradyzoites within cysts in vitro.[59] Unfortunately, however, 40 per cent of AIDS patients developed relapse of their toxoplasmic encephalitis while being treated with this antimicrobial agent. Other antimicrobial agents with effect on *T. gondii* in vitro or in vivo include cycloguanil,[58] artemisinin,[58] pyrimethamine-sulfadoxine (Fansidar),[87] rifabutin,[6a] trovafloxacin,[65a] and the newer macrolides clarithromycin, azithromycin, and roxithromycin.[3, 5, 6]

Because the activity of sulfamethoxazole is less than that of sulfadiazine, trimethoprim-sulfamethoxazole has been considered less effective as a treatment for toxoplasmosis. However, a number of investigators successfully have used this combination to treat toxoplasmic encephalitis in adults with AIDS. Doses of trimethoprim-sulfamethoxazole, as used to prevent *Pneumocystis carinii* pneumonia in the context of HIV infection, also may prevent episodes of reactivated toxoplasmosis.[17] Pyrimethamine combined with sulfadoxine, despite its lower in vitro activity than that of pyrimethamine-sulfadiazine, also has been used in Europe to treat reactivated and congenital infection.[9a]

Therapy in Specific Clinical Settings

Acquired Toxoplasmosis

Most immunologically normal patients with the lymphadenopathic form of toxoplasmosis do not require specific treatment. Indications for treatment in these cases are the presence of severe and persistent symptoms or damage to vital organs. Because of the high incidence of severe morbidity and of mortality in immunocompromised patients, toxoplasmosis should be treated in this population. Most immunocompromised patients in whom the diagnosis is established ante mortem improve when specific therapy is administered. The

TABLE 221–4. Treatment of Toxoplasmosis

Manifestation of Infection	Medication	Dosage	Duration of Therapy
Pregnant women with acute toxoplasmosis First 18 weeks of gestation or until term if fetus not infected	Spiramycin[a]	1 g q8h without food	Until fetal infection is documented or excluded at 18–20 weeks; if documented, has been used in France in alternate months with pyrimethamine, sulfadiazine, and leukovorin until term[b]
Pregnant women with fetal infection confirmed after 17th week of gestation or if maternal infection acquired in last few weeks of gestation (after amniocentesis and PCR to determine if there is *Toxoplasma* infection in the fetus)	Pyrimethamine	Loading dose: 100 mg/day in 2 divided doses for 2 days then 50 mg/day	Until term (leukovorin is continued 1 week after pyrimethamine is discontinued)
	Sulfadiazine	Loading dose: 75 mg/kg/day in 2 divided doses (maximum, 4 g/day) for 2 days, then 100 mg/kg/day in 2 divided doses (maximum, 4 g/day)	
	Leukovorin (folinic acid)	5–20 mg daily[c]	
Congenital *Toxoplasma* infection in infants	Pyrimethamine[d]	Loading dose: 2 mg/kg/day for 2 days, then 1 mg/kg/day for 2 or 6 months,[f] then this dose every Monday, Wednesday, and Friday	1 year[e] (leukovorin is continued 1 week after pyrimethamine is discontinued)[e]
	Sulfadiazine[d]	100 mg/kg/day in 2 divided doses	
	Leukovorin[d]	5–10 mg 3 times weekly[c]	
CSF protein ≥1 g/dL or active chorioretinitis that threatens vision	Corticosteroids (prednisone)	1 mg/kg/day in 2 divided doses[g]	Until resolution of elevated CSF protein level or active chorioretinitis
Active chorioretinitis in older children	Pyrimethamine	Loading dose: 2 mg/kg/day (maximum, 50 mg) for 2 days, then maintenance, 1 mg/kg/day (maximum, 25 mg)	Usually 1–2 weeks beyond resolution of signs and symptoms (leukovorin is continued 1 week after pyrimethamine is discontinued)
	Sulfadiazine	Loading dose: 75 mg/kg, then maintenance, 50 mg/kg q12h	
	Leukovorin	5–20 mg 3 times weekly[c]	
	Corticosteroids	1 mg/kg/day in 2 divided doses[g]	Until resolution[g]
Immunologically normal children			
Lymphadenopathy	No therapy		
Significant organ damage that is life-threatening	Pyrimethamine	Same as above for "active chorioretinitis in older children," no corticosteroids	Usually 4–6 weeks or 2 weeks beyond resolution of signs and symptoms
	Sulfadiazine		
	Leukovorin		
Immunocompromised children			
Non-AIDS	Pyrimethamine	Same as above for "active chorioretinitis in older children," no corticosteroids	Usually 4–6 weeks beyond complete resolution of signs and symptoms
	Sulfadiazine		
	Leukovorin		
AIDS	Pyrimethamine	Same as above for "active chorioretinitis in older children," no corticosteroids	Lifetime
	Sulfadiazine		
	Leukovorin		
	Clindamycin has been used in place of sulfadiazine	Reported trials for adults, but not infants and children	

PCR, polymerase chain reaction; CSF, cerebrospinal fluid.

[a] Available only by request from the Food and Drug Administration, telephone 301-443-5680.

[b] The only studies are those of Daffos et al.[27] However, because Daffos and his colleagues found pyrimethamine-sulfadiazine therapy to be superior to spiramycin for treatment of the fetus, continuous therapy with pyrimethamine, sulfadiazine, and leukovorin should be considered in the third trimester.

[c] Adjusted for megaloblastic anemia, granulocytopenia, or thrombocytopenia; blood counts, including platelets, should be monitored as described in text.

[d] Optimal dosage, feasibility, and toxicity currently being evaluated or planned in ongoing Chicago-based National Collaborative Treatment Trial, telephone 312-791-4152.

[e] In infants with AIDS. The duration of therapy is unknown. See discussion under section on congenital toxoplasmosis and AIDS.

[f] These two regimens currently are being compared in a randomized National Collaborative Treatment Trial. Data are not available to determine which, if either, is superior. Both regimens appear to be feasible and relatively safe.

[g] Corticosteroids should be continued until signs of inflammation (high CSF protein ≥1 g/dL) or active chorioretinitis that threatens vision have subsided; dosage then can be tapered and discontinued; use only with pyrimethamine, sulfadiazine, and leukovorin.

Modified from McLeod, R., Wisner, J., and Boyer, K.: Toxoplasmosis. *In* Krugman, S., Katz, S. L., and Gershon, A. A. (eds.): Infectious Diseases of Children. St. Louis, Mosby Year Book, 1992, pp. 541–542.

major problem lies in making the diagnosis early enough to institute treatment.

The optimal duration of specific therapy for toxoplasmosis is unknown. Patients who appear to be immunologically normal but who have severe and persistent symptoms or damage to vital organs should receive specific therapy for 2 to 6 weeks until symptoms resolve. In the immunocompromised patient, therapy should continue at least 4 to 6 weeks beyond complete resolution of all signs and symptoms of active disease. Careful follow-up of these patients is imperative because relapse may occur, requiring prompt reinstitution of therapy. In patients with AIDS who develop toxoplasmosis, lifelong suppressive therapy with pyrimethamine-sulfadiazine or pyrimethamine-clindamycin should be used.

The Pregnant Woman

Treatment of the acutely infected woman during pregnancy may prevent transmission of the infection to the fetus. The rationale for such treatment is derived from the observation that the lag period between the onset of maternal infection and infection in the fetus may be significant. Data from France,[35, 36] where women were treated with spiramycin, and from Austria[7, 8] and Germany,[70] where women were treated with pyrimethamine and sulfonamides, indicate that the incidence of congenital infection in the offspring of mothers treated during gestation is at least 50 per cent less than that in the offspring of untreated mothers. None of these studies was controlled rigidly. Despite this, results in the large numbers of women studied by the group from France (154 untreated and 388 treated patients) strongly suggest that intrauterine treatment does reduce transmission of maternal infection to the fetus.[36, 106]

It should be emphasized that spiramycin treatment of pregnant women with recently acquired primary infection should be instituted empirically, in the hope of preventing spread of infection to the fetus. Once fetal infection has occurred, it appears that maternal treatment with spiramycin does not alter the evolution and severity of disease in the fetus. This is why evaluation of the potentially exposed fetus by polymerase chain reaction amplification of amniotic fluid permits informed decisions about pregnancy termination or treatment of the fetus in utero with pyrimethamine-sulfadiazine.

Congenital Infection

POSTNATAL TREATMENT. Data regarding the efficacy of postnatal treatment of infants with congenital *Toxoplasma* infection are becoming available. Uncontrolled studies in humans and controlled studies in experimental animals[106] have been interpreted as indicating beneficial effects of postnatal treatment on the development of sequelae both in symptomatic and asymptomatic infants with congenital *Toxoplasma* infection. The controlled National Collaborative Treatment Trial now is in progress in Chicago. This study seeks to define optimal therapeutic regimens. Physicians treating patients with congenital *Toxoplasma* infection who are younger than 2.5 months of age may wish to contact this multidisciplinary group regarding potential enrollment of their patients in that study (312-791-4152).

Outcomes to date from the National Collaborative Treatment Trial substantially are better for most, but not all, infants treated from the neonatal period for 12 months with pyrimethamine-sulfadiazine and leukovorin, compared with historical controls receiving no or short-course therapy.[82] Signs of active infection resolve within weeks of initiation of treatment. In substantial numbers of children, the appearance of brain computed tomographic scans has improved remarkably (Fig. 221–4). Cerebral calcifications have diminished in size or resolved for most such treated children.[102] In conjunction with this improvement in brain computed tomographic scans, cognitive function has been in the normal range for 69 per cent of such treated children.[108, 124] This is in striking contrast with the 86 per cent of children with "men-

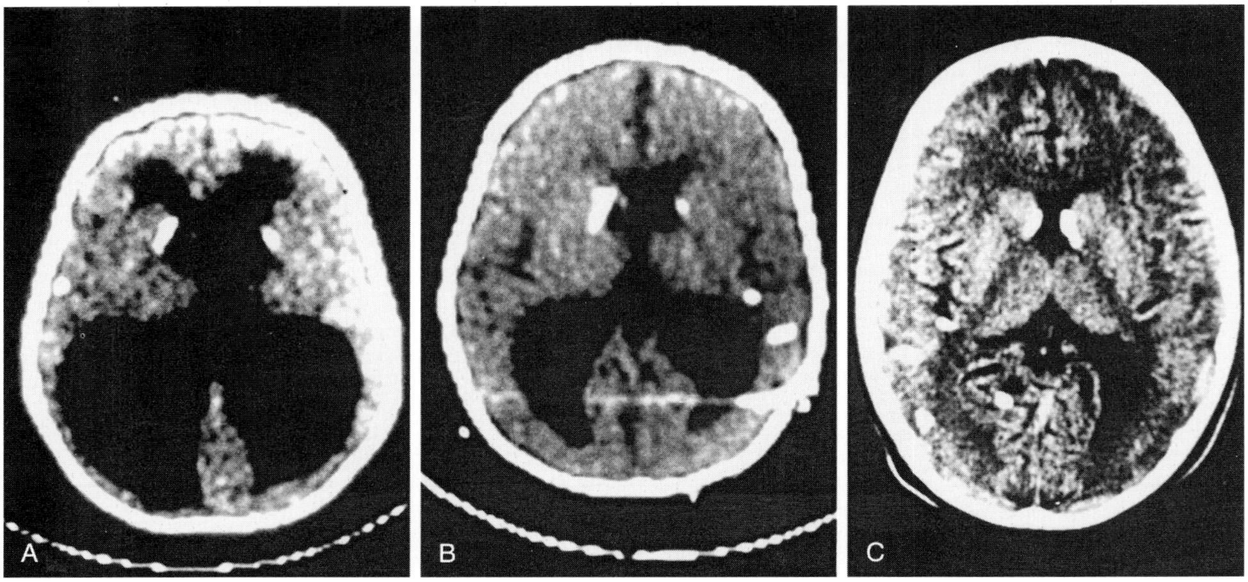

FIGURE 221–4. *An example of hydrocephalus and intracranial calcifications in a treated patient with congenital toxoplasmosis.* A, *Computed tomograph at 3 months of age showing hydrocephalus due to aqueductal stenosis (before shunting) with cortical and periventricular basal ganglion calcifications.* B, *Computed tomograph at 4 months of age after shunt placement.* C, *Computed tomograph at 8 years of age. Stanford-Binet IQ was about 100 at 3 and 6 years of age. (From McAuley, J. B., Boyer, K. M., Patel, D., et al.: Early and longitudinal evaluations of treated infants and children and untreated historical patients with congenital toxoplasmosis: The Chicago Collaborative Treatment Trial. Clin. Infect. Dis. 18:38–72, 1994. University of Chicago, publisher.)*

tal retardation" in the Eichenwald series noted earlier (see Table 221–1).[43] There has been no significant diminution of cognitive function over time, and most treated children are functioning well in regular school classrooms. Although the number of children compared is limited, for a small subset of these children, measures of cognitive function appear to be less than for siblings. No sensorineural hearing loss has been ascribable to congenital toxoplasmosis in the treated children.[83] Despite the much improved neurologic outlook for most of these children, a subset of children with significant irreversible neurologic damage already present in the perinatal period have manifested profound developmental delays, motor impairment, and seizures. For the most part, these were children with hydrocephalus, high cerebrospinal fluid protein (>1 g/dL), minimal improvement of brain computed tomographic scans after shunting, and often substantial delays in shunt placement or needed revision for shunt failure or other intercurrent medical problems.[124] This experience emphasizes the importance of recognizing hydrocephalus and managing it aggressively.

Although treatment during the first year of life arrests all signs of active disease, results in normal cognitive and motor outcome for most children, and may result in resolution of seizures without recurrence for some treated children, currently available drugs do not eradicate all cysts containing bradyzoites. This is apparent because in most children, serologic titers of *T. gondii*–specific antibodies rebound in the 3 to 4 months after treatment.[79] To date, new retinal lesions have occurred in 7 of 54 children in the National Collaborative Treatment Trial during 3 to 10 years' follow-up after the 1-year course of treatment.[91] These active lesions have responded to brief courses of treatment with pyrimethamine, sulfadiazine, and leukovorin without subsequent loss of visual acuity. Although the follow-up durations are shorter, this contrasts with the almost uniform eventual occurrence of retinal lesions in studies of untreated or briefly treated children.[23, 43, 68, 69, 135] We recommend that infected children undergo retinal examinations each month for 3 months after discontinuing treatment around their first birthday, then each 3 months until they are old enough to describe visual symptoms accurately, and then every 6 months. Also, an ophthalmologic evaluation should be performed promptly for any acute visual signs or symptoms that may be related to recrudescence of congenital ocular toxoplasmosis.[91]

SEQUENTIAL FETAL AND POSTNATAL TREATMENT. Hohlfeld and colleagues[27, 57] have described outcome for patients treated in utero with continuing treatment during the first year of life. As noted earlier, however, pregnancies in which fetuses had obvious manifestations on ultrasound examination and most pregnancies with definite first trimester infection were terminated.

Nonetheless, it is remarkable that when this French method of initiating aggressive treatment of fetuses in utero was applied, retinal disease was reported in only 3 of 50 such infants followed to 2 years of age. This contrasts with the presence of retinal or neurologic involvement in 50 per cent of asymptomatic newborns detected by serologic screening in Massachusetts[54] and in 75 per cent of children whose pediatricians referred them to our National Collaborative Treatment Trial for treatment in the perinatal period.[91] A prospective, carefully controlled study (as part of the National Collaborative Study) directly to compare outcome for infants detected and treated in utero, as detected by systematic neonatal screening and detected by pediatricians in the neonatal period and then referred, is under way. It is noteworthy that outcome of pregnancies with infection acquired in the first trimester after in utero treatment also has been reported to be favorable in another study[10] in which only those pregnancies in which the fetus had hydrocephalus were terminated.

Although a rare occurrence compared with adults with AIDS, the number of children with toxoplasmosis and coexistent HIV infection or AIDS appears to be increasing.[92] The majority of these children have had congenital toxoplasmosis; most have been symptomatic. For such children, therapy with pyrimethamine and sulfadiazine plus folinic acid is recommended in the doses described in Table 221–4. In adults, it is necessary to administer maintenance therapy to prevent relapse after toxoplasmic encephalitis, and it seems appropriate also to recommend lifelong therapy for children with dual HIV and congenital *Toxoplasma* infection. Zidovudine antagonizes the toxoplasmacidal effect of pyrimethamine and its in vitro synergy with sulfonamide. It is unknown whether this effect occurs in vivo.[72] Consultation regarding dually infected children is available from Dr. Charles Mitchell in Miami (305-547-6676).

Ocular Toxoplasmosis

Prompt initiation of specific treatment in active ocular toxoplasmosis is mandatory in order to preserve vision. Inflammatory reactions in the vitreous frequently are a major pathogenetic phenomenon in patients with active disease, and in such cases, corticosteroids in addition to specific anti-*Toxoplasma* therapy are strongly recommended.[101] Their use also is recommended for cases of retinochoroiditis involving the macula, maculopapillary bundle, or optic nerve. The initial daily dosage of prednisone is 1 mg/kg orally to a maximum of 75 mg in 24 hours. The equivalent dosage of another corticosteroid may be given. The dosage of corticosteroid may be reduced gradually when the lesion appears to be well demarcated and pigmentation has begun. Some have used systemic or intraocular clindamycin to treat patients in whom use of corticosteroid and pyrimethamine plus sulfadiazine has failed[125]; its efficacy has not been proved in humans.

PREVENTION

Congenital infection may be avoided by preventing the occurrence of primary *Toxoplasma* infection during pregnancy.[82, 138] It is the responsibility of all physicians caring for pregnant women at risk to inform them of the specific hygienic measures (Table 221–5) for avoiding *Toxoplasma* infection. Similar measures are useful for prevention of acquired infection in other settings as well. The ability of a 10-minute education program, offered as part of prenatal care, to reduce the risk of acquiring *Toxoplasma* infection by modifying behavior of pregnant women in regard to cats, food, and personal hygiene has been demonstrated.[18] Pamphlets that describe methods to prevent toxoplasmosis in pregnant women are available from the March of Dimes (312-435-4007), from Abbott Diagnostics (800-323-9100), and on the Internet (http://www.iit.edu/~toxo/pamphlet).

Once primary maternal infection has occurred, there are several problems inherent in the secondary prevention of congenital toxoplasmosis by therapeutic abortion or by treatment of the pregnant woman. Because 80 to 90 per cent of women with primary *Toxoplasma* infection are asymptomatic, most primary infections are overlooked unless sequential serologic testing is performed routinely in pregnant women. The cost-effectiveness of routine screening in the prevention of congenital toxoplasmosis is clear in European countries where screening is mandated by law.[36] In countries with lower incidence, cost-efficiency has not been proved.[107] In the

TABLE 221–5. Prevention of *Toxoplasma* Infection

Prevention of Acquired Infection (Primary Prevention)
Cook meat to >150° F (>66° C), smoke it, or cure it in brine.
Wash fruits and vegetables before consumption.
Avoid touching mucous membranes of mouth and eyes while handling uncooked meat or unwashed fruits or vegetables.
Wash hands and kitchen surfaces thoroughly after contact with raw meat or unwashed fruits or vegetables.
Prevent access of flies, cockroaches, and other coprophagic insects to fruits and vegetables.
Avoid contact with materials that potentially are contaminated with cat feces, such as cat litter boxes, or wear gloves when handling such materials and when gardening.
Disinfect cat litter box for 5 minutes with nearly boiling water.
Prevention of Congenital Infection (Secondary Prevention)
Identify women at risk by serologic testing.
Treatment during pregnancy results in approximately 50 per cent reduction in incidence of infection in infants.
Therapeutic abortion prevents birth of infected infant: considered only in cases of women who acquired infection in first or second trimester.

Adapted from Remington, J. S., and Wilson, C. B.: Toxoplasmosis. *In* Kass, E. H., and Platt, R. (eds.): Current Therapy in Infectious Disease, 1983–1984. Philadelphia, B. C. Decker, 1983, pp. 149–153.

absence of such data, physicians may choose to screen patients on an individual basis.[134] If screening is undertaken, a reliable serologic test for IgG antibodies (see Laboratory Diagnosis) should be performed prior to conception or as soon as possible thereafter and then repeated every 2 to 3 months until the time of delivery. Serologic test results that suggest acquisition of primary infection during pregnancy should be confirmed by a reference laboratory. Decisions regarding treatment or therapeutic abortion should be based on a consideration of whether the fetus is infected or affected, as determined by amniocentesis and ultrasonography.

References

1. Alford, C. A., Jr., Stagno, S., and Reynolds, D. W.: Congenital toxoplasmosis: Clinical, laboratory and therapeutic considerations, with special reference to subclinical disease. Bull. N.Y. Acad. Med. *50*:160, 1974.
2. Araujo, F. G., Barnett, E. V., Gentry, L. O., et al.: False positive anti-*Toxoplasma* fluorescent antibody tests in patients with antinuclear antibodies. Appl. Microbiol. *22*:270, 1971.
3. Araujo, F. G., Guptill D. R., and Remington, J. S.: Azithromycin, a macrolide antibiotic with potent activity against *Toxoplasma gondii.* Antimicrob. Agents Chemother. *32*:755–757, 1988.
4. Araujo, F. L., Lin, T., and Remington, J. S.: The activity of atovaquone (566C80) in murine toxoplasmosis is markedly augmented when used in combination with pyrimethamine or sulfadiazine. J. Infect. Dis. *167*:494–497, 1993.
5. Araujo, F., Prokocimer, P., and Remington, J.: Clarithromycin-minocycline is synergistic in a murine model of toxoplasmosis. J. Infect. Dis. *165*:788, 1992.
6. Araujo, F., and Remington, J.: Recent advances in the search for new drugs for treatment of toxoplasmosis. Int. J. Antimicrob. Agents *1*:153–164, 1992.

6a. Araujo, F. G., Slifer, T., and Remington, J. S.: Rifabutin is active in murine models of toxoplasmosis. Antimicrob. Agents Chemother. *38*:570–575, 1994.

7. Aspock, H.: Prevention of congenital toxoplasmosis by serological surveillance during pregnancy: Current strategies and future perspectives. *In* Marget, W., Lang, W., and Gabler-Sandberger, E. (eds.): Parasitic Infections, Immunology, Mycotic Infections, General Topics. Vol. 3. Muenchen, Medizin Verlag, 1986, pp. 69–72.
8. Aspock, H., Flamm, H., and Pilcher, O.: Die *Toxoplasmose*-überwachung während der schwangerschaft 10-jahre erfahrungen in Österreich. Mitt. Oesterr. Ges. Trophenmed. Parasitol. *8*:105–113, 1986.
9. Beach, P. G.: Prevalence of antibodies to *Toxoplasma gondii* in pregnant women in Oregon. J. Infect. Dis. *140*:780, 1979.

9a. Berger, R., Merkel, S., and Rudin, C.: Toxoplasmosis and pregnancy: Findings from umbilical cord blood screening in 30,000 newborn infants. Schweiz. Med. Wochenschr. *125*:1168–1173, 1995.

10. Berrebi, A., Kobuch, W. E., Bessieres, M. H., et al.: Termination of pregnancy for maternal toxoplasmosis. Lancet *344*:36–38, 1994.
11. Boyer, K. M., and McLeod, R.: *Toxoplasma gondii* (Toxoplasmosis). *In* Long, S. S., Pickering, L. K., and Prober, C. G. (eds.): Principles and Practice of Pediatric Infectious Diseases. New York, Churchill Livingston, 1997, pp. 1421–1448.
12. Brezin, A. P., Kasner, L., Thulliez, P., et al.: Ocular toxoplasmosis in the fetus: Immunohistochemistry analysis and DNA amplification. Retina *14*:19026, 1994.
13. Brown, C. R., Estes, R. G., Bechmann, E., et al.: Definitive identification of a toxoplasmosis resistance gene. Res. Immunol. Ann. Inst. Pasteur. *144*:61–66, 1993.
14. Brown, C., and McLeod, R: Class I MHC genes and CDA^{+}T cells determine cyst number in *Toxoplasma gondii* infection. J. Immunol. *145*:3438–3441, 1990.
15. Bülow, R., and Boothroyd, J. C.: Protection of mice from fatal *Toxoplasma gondii* infection by immunization with p30 antigen in liposomes. J. Immunol. *147*:3496–3500, 1991.
16. Buxton, D.: Toxoplasmosis: The first commercial vaccine. Parasitol. Today *9*:335–337, 1993.
17. Carr, A., Tindall, B., Brew, B. J., et al.: Low-dose trimethoprim-sulfamethoxazole prophylaxis for toxoplasmic encephalitis in patients with AIDS. Ann. Intern. Med. *117*:106–111, 1992.
18. Carter, A. O., Gelmon, S. B., Wells, G. A., et al.: The effectiveness of a prenatal education programme for the prevention of congenital toxoplasmosis. Epidemiol. Infect. *103*:539–545, 1989.
19. Cesbron-Delau, M. F.: Dense-granule organelles of *Toxoplasma gondii*: Their role in the host-parasite relationship. Parasitol. Today *10*:293–296, 1994.
20. Cesbrons, M. F., Dubremetz, J. F., and Sher, A. (eds.): The immunobiology of toxoplasmosis. Res. Immunol. Ann. Inst. Pasteur *144*:7–8, 1993.
21. Conley, F. K., Jenkins, H. T., and Remington, J. S.: *Toxoplasma gondii* infection of the central nervous system. Hum. Pathol. *12*:690, 1981.
22. Couvreur, J., and Desmonts, G.: Congenital and maternal toxoplasmosis: A review of 300 congenital cases. Dev. Med. Child. Neurol. *4*:519–530, 1962.
23. Couvreur, J., Desmonts, G., and Aron-Rosa, D.: Le pronostic oculaire de la toxoplasmosis congenital: Role du traitement. Ann. Pediatr. *31*:855–858, 1994.
24. Couvreur, J., Desmonts, G., and Thulliez, P.: Prophylaxis of congenital toxoplasmosis: Effect of spiramycin on placental infection. J. Antimicrob. Chemother. *22*:193–200, 1988.
25. Couvreur, J., Desmonts, G., Tournier, G., et al.: Etude d'une serie homogene de 210 cas de toxoplasmose congenitale chez des nourrissons ages de 0 a 11 mois et depistes de facon prospective. Ann. Pediatr. *31*:815, 1984.
26. Couvreur, J., Thulliez, P., Daffos, F., et al.: Foetopathie toxoplasmique: Traitment in utero par l'association pyrimethamine-sulfamides. Arch. Fr. Pediatr. *48*:397–403, 1991.
27. Daffos, F., Forestier, F., Capella-Pavlovsky, et al.: Prenatal management of 746 pregnancies at risk for congenital toxoplasmosis. N. Engl. J. Med. *318*:271–275, 1988.
28. Dannemann, B., McCutchan, J. A., Israelski, D., et al.: Treatment of toxoplasmic encephalitis in patients with AIDS: A randomized trial comparing pyrimethamine plus clindamycin to pyrimethamine plus sulfonamides. Ann. Intern. Med. *116*:33–43, 1992.
29. Dannemann, B. R., Vaughan, W. C., Thulliez, P., et al.: The differential agglutination test for diagnosis of recently acquired infection with *Toxoplasma gondii.* J. Clin. Microbiol. *28*:1928–1933, 1990.
30. Darcy, F., and Santoro, F.: Toxoplasmosis. *In* Kierszenbaum, F. (ed.): Parasitic Infections and the Immune System. San Diego, Academic Press, 1994, pp. 163–190.
31. Darling, S. T.: Sarcosporidiosis: With report of a case in man. Proc. Canal Zone Med. Assoc. *1*:141, 1908.
32. Decoster, A., Darcy, F., Caron, A., et al.: IgA antibodies against P30 as markers of congenital and acute toxoplasmosis. Lancet *2*:1104, 1988.
33. Derouin, F., Devergie, A., and Auber, P.: Toxoplasmosis in bone marrow-transplant precipients: Report of seven cases and review. Clin. Infect. Dis. *15*:267–270, 1992.
34. Derouin, F., Gluckman, E., Beauvais, B., et al.: *Toxoplasma* infection after human allogeneic bone marrow transplantation: Clinical and serological study of 80 patients. Bone Marrow Transplant. *1*:67, 1986.
35. Desmonts, G., and Couvreur, J.: Congenital toxoplasmosis: A prospective study of 378 pregnancies. N. Engl. J. Med. *290*:1110, 1974.
36. Desmonts, G., and Couvreur, J.: Congenital toxoplasmosis: A prospective study of the offspring of 54 women who acquired toxoplasmosis during pregnancy: Pathophysiology of congenital disease. *In* Thalhammer, O., Baumgarten, K., and Pollak, A. (eds.): Perinatal Medicine. Sixth European Congress, Vienna, 1978. Stuttgart, Georg Thieme, 1979.
37. Desmonts, G., Daffos, F., Forestier, F., et al.: Prenatal diagnosis of congenital toxoplasmosis. Lancet *1*:500, 1985.
38. Desmonts, G., Naot, Y., and Remington, J. S.: Immunoglobulin M-immu-

nosorbent agglutination assay for diagnosis of infectious disease: Diagnosis of acute congenital and acquired *Toxoplasma* infections. J. Clin. Microbiol. *14*:486, 1981.
39. Desmonts, G., and Remington, J. S.: Direct agglutination test for diagnosis of *Toxoplasma* infection: Method for increasing sensitivity and specificity. J. Clin. Microbiol. *11*:562, 1980.
40. Diebler, C., Dussler, A., and Dulac, O.: Congenital toxoplasmosis: Clinical and neuroradiological evaluation of the cerebral lesions. Neuroradiology *27*:125–130, 1985.
41. Dorfman, R. F., and Remington, J. S.: Value of lymph node biopsy in the diagnosis of acute acquired toxoplasmosis. N. Engl. J. Med. *289*:878, 1973.
42. Dubey, J. P., Miller, N. L., and Frenkel, J. K.: The *Toxoplasma gondii* oocyst from cat feces. J. Exp. Med. *132*:636–662, 1970.
43. Eichenwald, H. G.: A study of congenital toxoplasmosis. *In* Siim, J. C. (ed.): Human Toxoplasmosis. Copenhagen, Munksgaard, 1960, pp. 41–49.
44. Featherstone, H.: A Difference in the Family. New York, Penguin, 1987.
45. Frenkel, J. K.: Toxoplasmosis. *In* Marcial-Rojas, R. A. (ed.): Pathology of Protozal and Helminthic Diseases. Baltimore, Williams & Wilkins, 1971, pp. 254–290.
46. Frenkel, J. K.: Toxoplasmosis: A parasite life cycle, pathology, and immunology. *In* Hammond, D. M. (ed.): The Coccidian. Baltimore, University Park Press, 1973, pp. 343–410.
47. Frenkel, J. K.: Pathology and pathogenesis of congenital toxoplasmosis. Bull. N. Y. Acad. Med. 50:182–191, 1974.
48. Frenkel, J., Dubey, J. P., and Miller, N. L.: *Toxoplasma gondii* in cats: Fecal stage identified as coccidian oocysts. Science *167*:893–896, 1970.
49. Frenkel, J. K., Weber, R. W., and Lunde, M. N.: Acute toxoplasmosis: Effective treatment with pyrimethamine, sulfadiazine, leucovorin calcium and yeast. J. A. M. A. *173*:1471–1476, 1960.
50. Garcia, A. G. P.: Congenital toxoplasmosis in two successive sibs. Arch. Dis. Child. *43*:705–709, 1979.
51. Gazzinelli, R. T., Hayashi, S., Wysocka, M., et al.: Role of IL-12 in the initiation of cell-mediated immunity by *Toxoplasma gondii* and its regulation by IL-10 and nitric oxide. J. Eukar. Microbiol. *41*:9S, 1994.
52. Gazzinelli, R. T., Oswald, I. P., James, S. L., et al.: IL-10 inhibits parasite killing and nitrogen oxide production by IFN-γ-activated macrophages: IL-10 prevents IFN-γ from inducing activity against *T. gondii* and increasing production of RNIs by murine macrophages. J. Immunol. *148*:1792–1796, 1992.
53. Grover, C. M., Thulliez, P., Remington, J. S., et al.: Rapid prenatal diagnosis of congenital *Toxoplasma* infection using polymerase chain reaction and amniotic fluid. J. Clin. Microbiol. *28*:2297, 1990.
54. Guerina, N. G., Hsu, H.-W., Meissner, H. C., et al.: Neonatal serologic screening and early treatment for congenital *Toxoplasma gondii* infection. N. Engl. J. Med. *33*:1858–1863, 1994.
55. Hakim, F. T., Gazzinelli, R. T., Denkers, E., et al.: $CD8^+$ T cells from mice vaccinated against *Toxoplasma gondii* are cytotoxic for parasite-infected or antigent pulsed host cells. J. Immunol. *147*:3955, 1991.
56. Hohlfeld, P., Daffos, T., Costa, J. M., et al.: Prenatal diagnosis of congenital toxoplasmosis with a polymerase-chain reaction test on amniotic fluid. N. Engl. J. Med. *331*:695–699, 1994.
57. Hohlfeld, P., Daffos, F., Thulliez, P., et al.: Fetal toxoplasmosis: Outcome of pregnancy and infant follow-up after in utero treatment. J. Pediatr. *115*:765–769, 1989.
58. Holfels, E., McAuley, J., Mack, D., et al.: In vitro effects of artemisinin ether, cycloguanil hydrochloride (alone and in combination with sulfadiazine), quinine sulfate, mefloquine, primaquine phosophate, trifluoperazine hydrochloride, and verapamil on *Toxoplasma gondii.* Antimicrob. Agents Chemother. *38*:1392–1396, 1994.
59. Huskinson-Mark, J., Araujo, F. G., and Remington, J. S.: Evaluation of the effect of drugs on the cyst form of *Toxoplasma gondii.* J. Infect. Dis. *164*:170–177, 1991.
60. Hutchison, W. M., Dunachie, J. F., Siim, J. C., et al.: Coccidian-like nature of *Toxoplasma gondii.* B. M. J. *1*:142, 1970.
61. Janku, J.: Pathogenesa a pathologicka anatomie tak nazveneho vrozeneho kolobomu slute skvrny v oku normalne velikem a mikrophthalmickem s nalezem parazitu v sitnici. Cas. Lek. Cesk. *60*:1021, 1923.
62. Johnson, A., McLeod, R., Cesbron-Delauw, M. F., et al.: Vaccine Development and Technology to Prevent Toxoplasmosis. Fontevraud, France, WHO Working Group, 1992, p. 1.
63. Joiner, K. A., and Dubremetz, J. F.: *Toxoplasma gondii:* A protozoan for the nineties. Infect. Immun. *61*:1169–1172, 1993.
64. Kasper, L. H., Khan, I. A., Ely, K. H., et al.: Antigen-specific (P30) mouse $CD8^+$ T cells are cytotoxic against *Toxoplasma gondii*-infected peritoneal macrophages. J. Immunol. *148*:1493, 1992.
65. Kazdan, J. J., McCulloch, J. C., and Crawford, J. S.: Uveitis in children. Can. Med. Assoc. J. *96*:385, 1967.
65a. Khan, A. A., Slifer, T., Araujo, F. G., et al.: Trovafloxacin is active against *Toxoplasma gondii.* Antimicrob. Agents Chemother. *40*:1855–1859, 1996.
66. Khan, I. A., Ely, K. H., and Kasper, L. H.: A purified parasite antigen (p30) mediates CD8+ T cell immunity against fatal *Toxoplasma gondii* infection in mice. J. Immunol. *147*:3501–3506, 1991.
67. Kim, K., Soldati, D., and Boothroyd, J. C.: Gene replacement in *Toxoplasma gondii* with chloramphenicol acetyltransferase as selectable marker. Science *262*:911–914, 1993.
68. Koppe, J. G., Kloosterman, G. J., deRoever-Bonnet, H. et al.: Toxoplasmosis and pregnancy, with a long-term follow-up of the children. Eur. J. Obstet. Gynecol. Reprod. Biol. *413*:101–110, 1974.
69. Koppe, J. G., Loewer-Sieger, D. H., and de Roever-Bonnet, H.: Results of 20-year follow-up of congenital toxoplasmosis. Lancet *1*:254–256, 1986.
70. Kräubig, H.: Preventive behandlung der konatalen *Toxoplasmose. In* Kirchoff, H., and Kräubig, H. (eds.): *Toxoplasmose:* Praktische Fragen und Ergebnisse. Stuttgart, Georg Thieme Verlag, 1966.
71. Labadie, M. D., and Hazemann, J. J.: Apport des bilans de sante de l'enfant pour le depistage et l'etude epidemiologique de la toxoplasmose congenitale. Ann. Pediatr. *31*:823, 1984.
72. Leport, C., Chakroun, M., Matheron, S., et al.: Zidovudine efficacy and tolerance in 32 patients with cerebral toxoplasmosis in the acquired immunodeficiency syndrome. Presse Med. *17*:1813–1814, 1988.
73. Levaditi, C.: Au sujet de certaines protozooses hereditaires humaines a localisations oculaires et nerveuses. C. R. Soc. Biol. *98*:297, 1928.
74. Luft, B. J., Conley, F., and Remington, J. S.: Outbreak of central-nervous-system toxoplasmosis in Western Europe and North America. Lancet *1*:781, 1983.
75. Luft, B. J., Naot, Y., Araujo, F. G., et al.: Primary and reactivated *Toxoplasma* infection in patients with cardiac transplants: Clinical spectrum and problems in diagnosis in a defined population. Ann. Intern. Med. *99*:27, 1983.
76. Luft, B. J., and Remington, J. S.: Acute *Toxoplasma* infection among family members of patients with acute lymphadenopathic toxoplasmosis. Arch. Intern. Med. *144*:53, 1984.
77. Luft, B. J., and Remington, J. S.: Toxoplasmic encephalitis in AIDS. Clin. Infect. Dis. *15*:211–222, 1992.
78. Masur, H., Jones, T. C., Lempert, J. A., et al.: Outbreak of toxoplasmosis in a family and documentation of acquired retinochoroiditis. Am. J. Med. *64*:396, 1978.
79. McAuley, J. B., Boyer, K. M., Patel, D., et al.: Early and longitudinal evaluations of treated infants and children and untreated historical patients with congenital toxoplasmosis: The Chicago Collaborative Treatment Trial. Clin. Infect. Dis. *18*:38–72, 1994.
80. McCabe, R., Gibbons, D., Brooks, R. G., et al.: Agglutination test for diagnosis of toxoplasmosis in AIDS. Lancet *2*:680, 1983.
81. McCabe, R. E., Brooks, R. G., Dorfman, R. F., et al.: Clinical spectrum in 107 cases of toxoplasmic lymphadenopathy. Rev. Infect. Dis. *9*:754, 1987.
82. McCabe, R. E., and Remington, J. S.: Toxoplasmosis: The time has come. N. Engl. J. Med. *318*:313–315, 1988.
83. McGee, T., Wolters, C., Stein, L., et al.: Absence of sensorineural hearing abnormalities in treated infants with congenital toxoplasmosis. Otolaryngol. Head Neck Surg. *106*:75–80, 1992.
84. McLeod, R., Beem, M. O., and Estes, R. G.: Lymphocyte anergy specific to *Toxoplasma gondii* antigens in a baby with congenital toxoplasmosis. J. Clin. Lab. Immunol. *17*:149, 1985.
85. McLeod, R., Brown, C., and Mack, D.: Immunogenetics inflence outcome of *Toxoplasma gondii* infection. J. Immunol. *142*:3247–3255, 1989.
86. McLeod, R., Frenkel, J. K., Estes, R. G., et al.: Subcutaneous and intestinal vaccination with tachyzoites of *Toxoplasma gondii* and acquisition of immunity to peroral and congenital *Toxoplasma* challenge. J. Immunol. *140*:1632–1637, 1988.
87. McLeod, R., and Mack, D.: A new micromethod to study effects of antimicrobial agents of *Toxoplasma gondii:* Comparison of sulfdoxone and sulfadiazine and study of clindamycin, metronidazole, and cyclosporin A. Antimicrob. Agents Chemother. *26*:26–30, 1984.
88. McLeod, R., Mack, D. G., Boyer, K. M., et al.: Phenotypes and functions of lymphocytes in congenital toxoplasmosis. J. Lab. Clin. Med. *116*:623–635, 1990.
89. McLeod, R., Mack, D., and Brown, C.: New advances in cellular and molecular biology of *Toxoplasma gondii.* Exp. Parasitol. *72*:109–121, 1991.
90. McLeod, R., Mack, D., Foss, R., et al.: Levels of pyrimethamine in sera and cerebrospinal and ventricular fluids from infants treated for congenital toxoplasmosis. Antimicrob. Agents Chemother. *36*:1040–1048, 1992.
90a. McLeod, R., and Remington, J. S.: Toxoplasmosis. *In* Braunwald, E., Isselbacher, K. J., Petersdorf, R. G., et al. (eds.): Harrison's Principles of Internal Medicine. New York, McGraw-Hill, 1987, p. 795.
90b. McLeod, R., Wisner, J., and Boyer, K.: Toxoplasmosis. *In* Krugman, S., Katz, S. L., and Gershon, A. A. (eds.): Infectious Diseases of Children. St. Louis, Mosby Year Book, 1992, pp. 539–542.
91. Mets, M. B., Holfels, E. M., Boyer, K. M., et al.: Eye manifestations of congenital toxoplasmosis. Am. J. Ophthalmol. *122*:309–324, 1996.
92. Miller, M. J., and Remington, J. S.: Toxoplasmosis in infants and children with HIV infection or AIDS. *In* Pizzo, P. A., and Wilfert, C. M. (eds.): Pediatric AIDS: The Challenge of HIV Infection in Infants, Children and Adolescents. Baltimore, Williams & Wilkins, 1990, pp. 299–307.
93. Mitchell, C. D., Erlich, S. S., Mastrucci, M. T., et al.: Congenital toxoplasmosis occurring in three infants perinatally infected with the human immunodeficiency virus (HIV-1). Pediatr. Infect. Dis. J. *9*:512, 1990.
94. Montoya, J. G., and Remington, J. S.: Studies on the serodiagnosis of toxoplasmic lymphadenitis. Clin. Infect. Dis. *20*:781–789, 1995.
95. Montoya, J. G., and Remington, J. S.: Toxoplasmic chorioretinitis in the setting of acute acquired toxoplasmosis. Clin. Infect. Dis. *23*:277–282, 1996.
96. Naot, Y., Barnett, E. V., and Remington, J. S.: Method for avoiding false

positive results occurring in immunoglobulin M enzyme-linked immunosorbent assays due to presence of both rheumatoid factor and antinuclear antibodies. J. Clin. Microbiol. *14*:73, 1981.
97. Naot, Y., Desmonts, G., and Remington, J. S.: IgM enzyme-linked immunosorbent assay test for the diagnosis of congenital *Toxoplasma* infection. J. Pediatr. *98*:32, 1981.
98. Naot, Y., and Remington, J. S.: An enzyme-linked immunosorbent assay for detection of IgM antibodies to *Toxoplasma gondii:* Use for diagnosis of acute acquired toxoplasmosis. J. Infect. Dis. *142*:757, 1981.
99. Nicolle, C., and Manceaux, L.: Sur une infection à corps de Leishman (ou organisme voisins) du gondi. C. R. Acad. Sci. *147*:763, 1908.
100. Nicolle, C., and Manceaux, L.: Sur une protozoaire nouveau du gondi. C. R. Acad. Sci. *148*:369, 1909.
101. O'Connor, G. R.: Manifestations and management of ocular toxoplasmosis. Bull. N. Y. Acad. Med. *50*:192, 1974.
102. Patel, D. V., Hofels, E., Vogel, N., et al.: Resolution of intracerebral calcifications in children with treated congenital toxoplasmosis. Radiology *199*:433–440, 1996.
103. Pfefferkorn, E. R., Nothnagel, R. F., and Borotz, S. E.: Parasiticidal effect of clindamycin on *Toxoplasma gondii* grown in cultured cells and selection of a drug-resistant mutant. Antimicrob. Agents Chemother. *36*:1091–1096, 1992.
104. Pinkerton, H., and Weinman, D.: *Toxoplasma* infection in man. Arch. Pathol. *30*:374, 1940.
105. Remington, J., Eimstad, W., and Araujo, F.: Detection of immunoglobulin M antibodies with antigen-tagged latex particles in an immunosorbent assay. J. Clin. Microbiol. *17*:939, 1983.
105a. Remington, J. S., and McLeod, R.: Toxoplasmosis. *In* Braude, A. I. (ed.): International Textbook of Medicine. Vol. II. Medical Microbiology and Infectious Disease. Philadelphia, W. B. Saunders, 1981, p. 1818.
106. Remington, J. S., McLeod, R., and Desmonts, G.: Toxoplasmosis. *In* Remington, J. S., and Klein, J. O. (eds.): Infectious Diseases of the Fetus and Newborn. 4th ed. Philadelphia, W. B. Saunders, 1995, pp. 140–263.
106a. Remington, J. S., and Wilson, C. B.: Toxoplasmosis. *In* Kass, E. H., and Platt, R. (eds.): Current Therapy in Infectious Disease: 1983–1984. Philadelphia, B. C. Decker, 1983, pp. 149–153.
107. Roberts, T., and Frenkel, J. K.: Estimating income losses and other preventable costs caused by congenital toxoplasmosis in people in the United States. J. A. M. A. *2*:249–257, 1990.
108. Roizen, N., Swisher, C., Stein, M. A., et al.: Neurologic and developmental function in treated congenital toxoplasmosis. Pediatrics *95*:11–20, 1995.
109. Ruskin, J., and Remington, J. S.: Toxoplasmosis in the compromised host. Ann. Intern. Med. *84*:193, 1976.
110. Sabin, A. B.: Toxoplasmic encephalitis in children. J. A. M. A. *116*:801–807, 1941.
111. Sabin, A. B., and Feldman, H. A.: Dyes as microchemical indicators of a new immunity phenomenon affecting a protozoon parasite *(Toxoplasma)*. Science *108*:660, 1948.
112. Sacks, J. J., Roberto, R. R., and Brooks, N. F.: Toxoplasmosis infection associated with raw goat's milk. J. A. M. A. *248*:1728, 1982.
113. Schlaegel, T. F.: Ocular Toxoplasmosis and Pars Planitis. New York, Grune & Stratton, 1978.
114. Schoondermark-Van de Ven, E., Galama, J., Camps, W., et al.: Pharmacokinetic of spiramycin in the rhesus monkey: Transplacental passage and distribution in tissue in the fetus. Antimicrob. Agents Chemother. *38*:1922–1929, 1994.
115. Schoondermark-Van de Ven, E., Melchers, W., Camps, W., et al.: Effectiveness of spiramycin for treatment of congenital *Toxoplasma gondii* infection in rhesus monkeys. Antimicrob. Agents Chemother. *38*:1930–1936, 1994.
116. Shenep, J. L., Barenkamp, S. J., Brammeier, S. A., et al.: An outbreak of toxoplasmosis on an Illinois farm. Pediatr. Infect. Dis. *3*:518, 1984.
117. Sher, A., Oswald, I. P., Hieny, S., et al.: *Toxoplasma gondii* induces a T-independent IFN-γ response in natural killer cells that requires both adherent accessory cells and tumor necrosis factor-α. J. Immunol. *150*:3982–3989, 1993.
118. Sibley, L. D., Pfefferkorn, E. R., and Boothroyd, J. C.: Development of genetic systems for *Toxoplasma gondii*. Parasitol. Today *9*:392–395, 1993.
119. Smith, K. L., Wilson, M., Hightower, A. L., et al.: Prevalence of *Toxoplasma gondii* antibodies in U. S. military recruits in 1989: Comparison with data published in 1965. Clin. Infect. Dis. *23*:1182–1183, 1996.
120. Splendore, A.: Un nuovo protozoa parassita dei conigli: Incontrato nelle lesioni anatomiche d'una malattia che ricorda in molti punti il Kalaazar dell'uomo. Rev. Soc. Sci. *3*:109, 1908.
121. Stepick-Biek, P., Thulliez, P., Araujo, F. G., et al.: IgA antibodies for diagnosis of acute congenital and acquired toxoplasmosis. J. Infect. Dis. *162*:270, 1990.
122. Stray-Pedersen, B.: Infants potentially at risk for congenital toxoplasmosis: A prospective study. Am. J. Dis. Child. *134*:638, 1980.
123. Suzuki, Y., Orellana, M. A., Schreiber, R. D., et al.: Interferon γ: The major mediator of resistance against *Toxoplasma gondii.* Science *240*:516, 1988.
124. Swisher, C. N., Boyer, K., and McLeod, R.: Congenital toxoplasmosis. *In* Bodenstein, J. B. (ed.): Seminars in Pediatric Neurology. Vol. 1. Philadelphia, W. B. Saunders, 1994.
125. Tabbara, K., and O'Connor, R.: Treatment of ocular toxoplasmosis with clindamycin and sulfadiazine. Ophthalmology *87*:129, 1980.
126. Teutsch, S. M., Juranek, D. D., Sulzer, A., et al.: Epidemic toxoplasmosis associated with infected cats. N. Engl. J. Med. *300*:695, 1979.
127. Vietzke, W. M., Gelderman, A. H., Grimley, P. M., et al.: Toxoplasmosis complicating malignancy. Cancer *21*:816, 1968.
128. Vogel, N., Kirisits, M., Michael, E., et al.: Congenital toxoplasmosis transmitted from an immunologically competent mother infected before conception. Clin. Infect. Dis. *23*:1055–1060, 1996.
129. Walls, K. W., and Remington, J. S.: Evaluation of a commercial latex agglutination method for toxoplasmosis. Diagn. Microbiol. Infect. Dis. *1*:265, 1983.
130. Weiss, L. M., Harris, C., Berger, M., et al.: Pyrimethamine concentrations in serum and cerebrospinal fluid during treatment of acute *Toxoplasma* encephalitis in patients with AIDS. J. Infect. Dis. *157*:580–583, 1988.
131. Welch, P. C., Masur, H., Jones, T. C., et al.: Serologic diagnosis of acute lymphadenopathic toxoplasmosis. J. Infect. Dis. *142*:256, 1981.
132. Wilson, C. B.: Treatment of congenital toxoplasmosis during pregnancy. J. Pediatr. *116*:1003–1004, 1990.
133. Wilson, C. B., Desmonts, G., Couvreur, J., et al.: Lymphocyte transformation in the diagnosis of congenital *Toxoplasma* infection. N. Engl. J. Med. *302*:785, 1980.
134. Wilson, C. B., and Remington, J. S.: What can be done to prevent congenital toxoplasmosis? Am. J. Obstet. Gynecol. *138*:357, 1980.
135. Wilson, C. B., Remington, J. S., Stagno, S., et al.: Development of adverse sequelae in children born with subclinical congenital *Toxoplasma* infection. Pediatrics *66*:767, 1980.
136. Wolf, A., and Cowen, D.: Granulomatous encephalomyelitis due to an encephalitozoon (encephalitozoic encephalomyelitis): A new protozoan disease of man. Bull. Neurol. Inst. N. Y. *6*:307, 1937.
137. Wong, S. Y., Hajdu, M. P., Ramirez, R., et al.: The role of specific immunoglubulin E in the diagnosis of acute *Toxoplasma* infection and toxoplasmosis. J. Clin. Microbiol. *31*:2952–2959, 1993.
138. Wong, S. Y., and Remington, J. S.: Toxoplasmosis in pregnancy. Clin. Infect. Dis. *18*:853–862, 1994.

222

PNEUMOCYSTIS CARINII PNEUMONIA

Walter T. Hughes and Donald C. Anderson

Pneumocystis carinii pneumonia (PCP) is an opportunistic infection of increasing importance to pediatricians. A marked increase in the prevalence of this disorder in the United States over the past decade has paralleled therapeutic advances in the management of immunologic and neoplastic diseases, resulting in longer survival of children with these underlying disorders. Since 1980, the infection has occurred in epidemic proportions in association with AIDS.

THE ORGANISM

As early as 1909, Chagas[16] identified what he interpreted as the spherical and sickle-shaped forms of the parasite *Trypanosoma cruzi* in the lungs of experimentally infected guinea pigs. The same organism was identified later by Carini[14] and others[151] in animals and human patients with trypanosome infections. In 1912, Delanoe and Delanoe[24] identified this parasite in the lungs of rats and guinea pigs not infected with trypanosomes and proposed an independent genus of *P. carinii.* These and other investigators, including Chagas, subsequently demonstrated that this agent was not related to the trypanosome.[39]

Attempts have been made to find a taxonomic place for *P. carinii.* Studies of DNA sequences coding for ribosomal RNA have shown that *P. carinii* has greater homology with certain fungi than with certain protozoa.[31] Unlike the dihydrofolate reductase of protozoa, the *P. carinii* enzyme is not a bifunctional polypeptide with thymidylate synthetase.[30] The cyst wall contains chitin and β-1,3-glucan, which are common components of fungal cell walls but also are found in certain protozoa and algae.[94, 150a] However, unlike fungi, the cyst wall does not contain ergosterol or the characteristic protein elongation factor 3.[69] The antifungal drugs amphotericin B, ketoconazole, nystatin, 5-flucytosine, and miconazole have no effect against PCP, whereas the drugs with demonstrated anti–*P. carinii* activity also are anti-protozoan drugs: pentamidine *(Leishmania donovani* and *Trypanosoma gambiense),* trimethoprim-sulfamethoxazole *(Isospora belli),* and pyrimethamine-sulfadiazine *(Toxoplasma gondii* and *Plasmodium falciparum).* Although a fixed taxonomic position for *P. carinii* is desirable, it is more important to elucidate the biologic characteristics of the organism in achieving effective and safe therapy. Molecular probes for the detection and study of *P. carinii*[149] and the identification of *P. carinii* chromosomes and mapping of genes[84, 92] offer promise for further elucidation of this organism.

Three developmental forms of this organism have been identified by light microscopy: cysts, "sporozoites," and "trophozoites." Cysts occur in lung tissue or respiratory secretions as spherical or crescent-shaped structures approximately 5 μm in diameter (Figs. 222–1 and 222–2). They may contain as many as eight oval bodies or sporozoites, 1 to 2 μm in diameter. A third extracystic pleomorphic structure, called a trophozoite, varying in size from 2 to 5 μm in diameter, is identified in association with cysts. Ultrastructural morphologic features identified by electron microscopy and scanning electron microscopy are well described in the literature.[12, 114, 117, 158]

Pifer and associates[114] reported successful though limited propagation of *P. carinii* in vitro in primary chick epithelial lung cells. Subsequently, propagation of *P. carinii* has been reported with Vero, Chang liver, and MRC-5 cells,[82] as well as WI-38[3] and A-549 cell lines.[22]

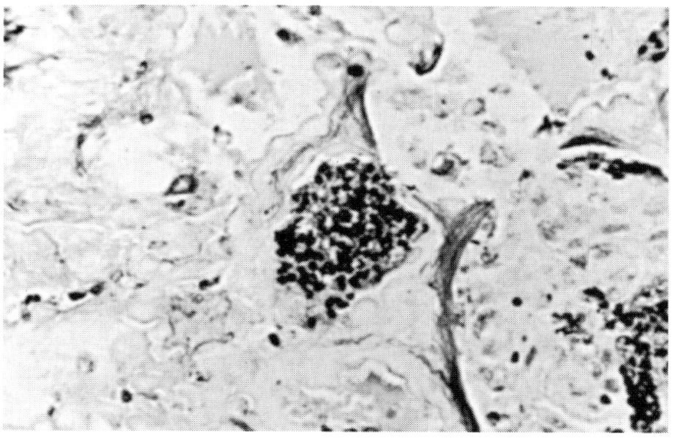

FIGURE 222–1. *Typical cyst forms demonstrated by Gomori silver methenamine stain of lung tissue obtained by open lung biopsy from a 20-month-old child with severe combined immunodeficiency disease. (× 100.)*

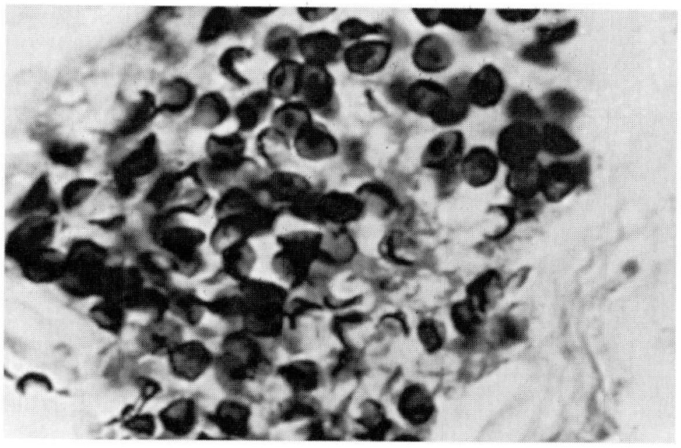

FIGURE 222–2. *Same as Figure 222–1. (× 1000.)*

TRANSMISSION AND EPIDEMIOLOGY

The mode of transmission in humans and the natural habitat of *P. carinii* largely remain unknown. This organism has been recognized in many wild and laboratory animal species over a wide geographic distribution. An association between animal reservoirs and human infection has not been established. Animal-to-animal transmission by the airborne route has been demonstrated in laboratory rats.[49, 52] Furthermore, DNA sequences identical to those of *P. carinii* have been detected in ambient air.[148]

Before and during World War II, epidemics of interstitial plasma cell pneumonitis secondary to *P. carinii* were recognized in debilitated and premature infants throughout European institutions and nursing homes.[6, 129] In 1942, Van der Meer and Brug[144] identified *P. carinii* in the lungs of humans with interstitial plasma cell pneumonitis. Subsequent studies confirmed this organism as the cause of the pneumonitis. The interruption of outbreaks by the introduction of strict isolation of affected patients within these institutions suggests the probable importance of person-to-person spread of disease within that setting.[132]

In the United States, PCP was not reported until 1956.[23] In contrast with the early European patterns, American cases largely have been sporadic and have occurred almost exclusively in children with impaired host defenses.[109] A limited number of outbreaks of PCP within families[154] or among closely associated groups of hospitalized cancer patients have been reported, further suggesting the importance of contagion in the spread of this disease.[7, 127, 128, 137]

Autopsy studies have demonstrated the occasional occurrence of *Pneumocystis* organisms in lungs of patients without evidence of underlying host defense disorders or pulmonary disease.[86] Furthermore, autopsy studies have demonstrated that inapparent (asymptomatic) infection occurs frequently in cancer patients or other immunocompromised populations.[111, 157] An extensive review of autopsies at St. Jude Children's Research Center (1962 to 1969) demonstrated the occurrence of inapparent *Pneumocystis* infection in 4.7 per cent of pediatric cancer patients, compared with 0.1 per cent of children who died without malignant disease.[111] The epidemiologic importance of these asymptomatic carriers in the transmission of *Pneumocystis* disease is unknown. Organisms are detected frequently in sputum, pharyngeal secretions, and tracheal aspirates of symptomatic patients.[48] Cysts have been shown to survive in dried lung specimens maintained at room temperature for several months.[62] These observations, in addition to the almost universal localization of disease within the lungs of affected patients, suggest that infection probably results from inhalation of the organism. In view of this possibility, respiratory isolation of symptomatic patients should be maintained to prevent exposure to other highly susceptible patients. No data support the isolation of such patients from otherwise healthy persons.

Asymptomatic *P. carinii* infection is highly prevalent in humans. Serologic studies have shown that more than 90 per cent of adults have antibody to *P. carinii* and that about 75 per cent had acquired *P. carinii* antibody before 4 years of age.[79, 97, 110, 115]

Persons infected with HIV-1 are at a remarkably high risk for *P. carinii* pneumonitis. The pneumonitis was diagnosed in 1080 (39 per cent) of the 2786 pediatric AIDS patients reported to the Centers for Disease Control and Prevention (CDC) through 1990.[158] Approximately 75 per cent of adults with AIDS acquire the pneumonitis. Among children with AIDS, *P. carinii* pneumonitis may occur at any age, but most frequently it is found between the ages of 3 and 6 months.[78, 133, 135]

Although intrauterine transmission of *P. carinii* has been documented in one stillborn infant and has been implicated in three siblings with no demonstrable immunologic abnormalities who developed infection in the neonatal period,[4] the paucity of such cases does not support the epidemiologic importance of this mode of transmission. Of the infants of eight women with AIDS and PCP during pregnancies, only one infant had evidence of *P. carinii* infection.[50, 103] Studies in severe combined immunodeficiency mice have failed to demonstrate transplacental passage of this organism.[66]

PATHOGENESIS

That *P. carinii* is an organism of low pathogenicity is clearly emphasized by the rare occurrence of infections in intact hosts. Despite widespread occurrence in the lungs of healthy laboratory animals, it rarely causes pulmonary disease unless experimentally provoked.

Before the AIDS epidemic, *Pneumocystis* pneumonia occurred almost exclusively in patients with primary immunologic disorders or in those receiving immunosuppressive treatment for oncologic disease or organ transplantation.[25, 41, 111, 146, 153] Of 194 cases reported to the CDC between 1967 and 1970, 29 occurred in infants younger than 1 year of age, 83 per cent of whom had primary immunodeficiency disorders. In contrast, acute lymphocytic leukemia was the most common underlying disease in children older than 1 year of age.[153] Of 1251 children with malignancies at the St. Jude Research Hospital (1962 to 1971), PCP occurred in 51 (4.1 per cent). In that series, the incidence of infection in 872 children with leukemia, Hodgkin disease, neuroblastoma, reticulum cell sarcoma, and Letterer-Siwe disease was 5.8 per cent, whereas in 379 patients with other types of neoplasia and 1669 children without malignant disease, *P. carinii* infection was not encountered.[62]

Within populations of cancer patients, *P. carinii* infection occurs more commonly in persons with generalized lymphoproliferative malignancy than in those with solid tumors.[9, 136] The extent of malignant disease and the intensity of chemotherapy or radiotherapy provided are associated with an increased risk for the development of *Pneumocystis* infections.[53, 111, 136] In children with acute lymphocyte leukemia, mediastinal involvement or radiation of the mediastinum, or both, also is associated with an increased incidence of *Pneumocystis* pneumonia.[53]

The European outbreaks of PCP in debilitated infants, in addition to the well-known association of malnutrition and impaired resistance to a variety of infectious disorders, suggest the possible importance of malnutrition as an additional host determinant for the development of *P. carinii* infections.[63, 69, 70, 131]

Pneumocystis pneumonia has been reported in congenital and acquired hypogammaglobulinemia, severe combined immunodeficiency disease, partial immunodeficiency disease, and secondary immunodeficiency states. Only one patient with a pure T-cell deficiency (DiGeorge syndrome) has been reported with an associated *Pneumocystis* infection.[25]

No characteristic pattern of serum immunoglobulin abnormality has been demonstrated. Low levels of IgG were the most consistent finding in two reported series of children with immunodeficiency disease.[9, 153] In contrast, normal or elevated levels of IgG were documented in 70 per cent of leukemic children with PCP. Administration of serum immunoglobulin to infected children with these disorders usually provided no therapeutic benefit.[153] The role of IgA antibody in host defense against *P. carinii* probably is not of major importance because secretory IgA levels are normal in most affected patients and those with immunodeficiency states characterized by IgA deficits are not unduly susceptible.[9, 153]

The development of specific antibodies to *P. carinii* in infected patients has been inconsistent. During the course of "epidemic" disease in malnourished infants, IgM values frequently increase markedly, with variable changes in IgG and IgA values. IgG antibody concentrations increase in serum 4 to 6 weeks after infection and are thought to provide permanent immunity in those infants.[77] In selected instances, specific antibody responses (IgG, IgA, and IgM) have been demonstrated in normal persons who have been associated closely with infected patients.[9, 96] The development of specific immunoglobulins (IgG and IgM) in two patients with lymphoreticular malignancies who recovered from PCP further emphasizes the probable importance of humoral immunity in determining the outcome of infection.[9]

Utilizing immunofluorescent staining techniques, Brzosko and colleagues[8] demonstrated IgG and IgM antibody with smaller amounts of IgA antibody and β-1-C globulin deposits on the surface of *Pneumocystis* organisms within alveoli of infants with "epidemic" *Pneumocystis* pneumonia. Late in the course of their disease, less immunoglobulin was present within alveoli, whereas increased numbers of plasma cells and alveolar macrophages containing fluorescent material were identified. It appears possible that specific antibody fixes complement (β-1-C globulin) on the surface of *Pneumocystis* organisms, allowing subsequent phagocytosis by alveolar macrophages.[8]

The importance of impaired cellular immune responses in patients with PCP is evident. The ability of corticosteroids to induce *P. carinii* infection in laboratory animals, the occurrence of PCP in AIDS patients and in at least one patient with a pure T-cell deficiency disease,[25] and the occurrence of PCP in malnourished hosts with significantly impaired cellular immune responses[63, 69, 85, 131] provide indirect evidence of the potential importance of cellular immunity in protecting the host against this opportunist. Because corticosteroids, cytotoxic agents, and malnutrition variably depress both humoral and cellular immune mechanisms as well as nonspecific immune responses (inflammation),[9, 19, 113] no absolute statement can be made regarding the relative importance of each defense mechanism. Strong evidence has implicated the importance of T-lymphocyte competence in the pathogenesis of PCP. Experimental studies in rats demonstrated the provocation of the pneumonitis after the administration of cyclosporine.[65] This compound specifically affects T-cell–mediated immune responses related to impairment of interleukin-2 production and receptor site inhibition and has no direct effect on other components of the immune system. Especially convincing is the remarkable susceptibility of AIDS patients to PCP. In this syndrome, the host compromise is limited primarily to impaired T-cell functions, and at least 50 per cent of affected patients acquire PCP.[15]

In infants, children, and adults with AIDS, the quantity of peripheral blood CD4 (T4) T-helper lymphocytes serves as a useful predictor of *P. carinii* pneumonitis. As the CD4 lymphocyte count decreases, the risk for *P. carinii* pneumonitis increases. In the adult, a CD4 cell count less than $200/mm^3$ is highly predictive of impending *P. carinii* pneumonitis. Because infants and children have relatively higher total lymphocyte counts, the absolute CD4 cell counts are higher than that in the adult. Therefore, the threshold for risk for *P. carinii* is age-related. Estimates indicate that risk for *P. carinii* pneumonitis in AIDS patients warrants consideration of chemoprophylaxis if the CD4 lymphocyte counts are less than $750/mm^3$ in those 12 to 23 months of age, less than $500/mm^3$ in children 24 months to 5 years of age, and less than $200/mm^3$ for those 6 years of age or older.[78]

With any of the underlying causes of immunocompromise, patients recovering from *P. carinii* pneumonitis remain at high risk for recurrent episodes.

For infants younger than 1 year of age, the CD4 lymphocyte count is less predictive of the PCP risk and cannot be relied on for decisions about prophylaxis.[33, 134] However, most PCP episodes occur after the CD4 lymphocyte count decreases below 1500 $cells/mm^3$ during the first year of life.

There is some evidence to suggest that *P. carinii* pneumonitis may occur in immunocompetent infants in the United States.[140] In a prospective study of 67 infants 2 to 12 weeks of age with pneumonitis in Birmingham, Alabama, 10 were found to have serologic evidence of this infection. In 1 of the 10 babies, the diagnosis was proved by lung biopsy. Additional studies are needed for assessment of the true incidence of this pneumonitis in otherwise healthy infants.

PATHOLOGY

P. carinii infections are unique, in that the pathologic findings, with rare exceptions, are limited to the lungs even in fatal cases. In the infantile "epidemic" form of disease, essentially all alveoli contain large numbers of organisms. Extensive interstitial plasma cell infiltrates distend alveolar walls from 5 to 20 times their normal thickness, and almost no intra-alveolar fibrinous exudate is noted.[28, 48] In the childhood and adult forms of PCP, the histogenesis has been described in three stages.[48, 62, 117] An initial stage is characterized by the presence of cysts and trophozoites attached by fibronectin to alveolar walls.[116] No septal inflammatory or cellular response is evident, and no clinical disease is associated with this stage. A second stage, which may or may not be associated with clinical signs and symptoms, is characterized by desquamation of alveolar cells and an increase in the number of cysts within alveolar macrophages. Tumor necrosis factor may be a major mediator involved in the killing of *P. carinii* by activated alveolar macrophages and may be induced by oxidative stresses in the alveoli.[112] The final stage is typified by extensive reactive and desquamative alveolitis manifested by marked cytoplasmic vacuolization of macrophages, mononuclear and plasma cell infiltrates within alveolar septa, and clusters of organisms located predominantly within macrophages in the lumen of alveoli. The histopathology of this final stage definitely is associated with clinical manifestations of pneumonitis.[117] In rare instances, *P. carinii* organisms have been detected in lymph nodes, spleen, liver, retina, bone marrow, gastrointestinal tract, pancreas, heart, adrenals, and peripheral blood.[45, 118, 141] A fatal case of disseminated *P. carinii* infection occurring in a 13-month-old infant with thymic alymphoplasia has been reported.[118]

CLINICAL MANIFESTATIONS

The natural course of *P. carinii* infections in children varies highly and depends primarily on the status of host defenses in individual patients. The onset may be insidious, with a clinical course of 3 or more weeks, or fulminant and rapidly progressive over a few days.

The clinical course of infantile epidemic pneumocystosis is typified in the premature, debilitated, or marasmic infant between 2 and 6 months of age. These patients often have chronic diarrhea and weight loss prior to the development of respiratory symptoms. Characteristically, the onset is insidious, with progression of cough, tachypnea, and respiratory distress over a 1- to 4-week interval. Fever is either absent or low-grade in most cases.[29]

Symptoms in immunosuppressed children or adults without AIDS may be more abrupt in onset and more rapidly progressive than in the infantile epidemic cases. Even with these patients, the course also varies highly.[9, 41, 48, 62, 120, 153] The mortality rate is approximately 100 per cent in untreated cases, reflecting the overall severity of the disease in immunocompromised patients.[48] In cases in children and adults, in contrast with infantile cases, fever generally is present and high-grade. It often precedes the onset of nonproductive cough, tachypnea, and severe dyspnea. Fever, tachypnea, and the radiographic appearance of pulmonary infiltrates, in that sequence, from 1 to 21 days prior to diagnosis, occurred in a group of children with malignancy.[62] In half of those patients, signs and symptoms occurred within 5 days prior to initiation of treatment. In a select group of 10 untreated patients, the extent of fever, respiratory distress, and radiographic abnormalities varied from mild to severe. Pulmonary infiltrates were apparent 1 to 13 days before death, and the total course of infection ranged from 4 to 21 days.

The time of onset of clinical disease in non-AIDS, high-risk patients is unpredictable but often occurs after the discontinuance or reduction in dose of corticosteroid therapy. Rifkind and coworkers[122] noted the clinical onset of infection in transplant patients when prednisone dosage was reduced below 1 mg/kg body weight/24 hours. In another series, 9 of 46 patients developed PCP while steroids were being reduced.[9] However, it is possible that the relationship is to the duration of corticosteroid therapy rather than to the withdrawal or reduction in dosage. A patient with severe combined immunodeficiency disease who received a bone marrow transplant subsequently developed fulminant PCP when apparent immunologic reconstitution had taken place.[9] A similar case in Houston occurred in a child with severe combined immunodeficiency disease who was the recipient of a thymic epithelial explant. This patient became clinically well, and evidence of engraftment and return of normal immunologic function was documented by in vitro studies approximately 6 weeks after the transplant. At that time, he developed fulminant PCP, determined by open lung biopsy (see Figs. 222–1 and 222–2). These observations imply that the development of clinical disease depends in part on normal inflammatory responses, which may be impaired somewhat as a result of the patient's underlying disease, the therapeutic regimen, or both.

Infants and children with AIDS usually are acutely ill at the time of onset with *P. carinii* pneumonitis, with fever (79 per cent), cough (86 per cent), dyspnea (88 per cent), tachypnea (88 per cent), and an alveolar-arterial oxygen gradient greater than 30 mm Hg (95 per cent). The median length of survival after the diagnosis of *P. carinii* pneumonitis was only 2 months in the study by Connor and associates.[20]

In children and adults both with and without AIDS, physical examination at the time of initial presentation may reveal tachypnea; nasal flaring; and intercostal, subcostal, or supracostal retractions. An ashen color or cyanosis may be present or may develop rapidly. Auscultation of the chest frequently is characterized by a conspicuous absence of adventitious sounds despite rapid (80 to 100/minute), shallow respirations. Scattered rales, rhonchi, or wheezes most often are detected later in the clinical course as resolution occurs. Aside from variable temperature elevation, few other physical abnormalities are noted, except those referable to pulmonary disease or secondary to the patient's underlying disease or treatment.[9, 48, 62, 153]

A variety of radiographic abnormalities have been observed in documented cases of isolated PCP.[11, 13, 21, 26, 35, 38, 104, 119, 147, 156] These variations partly result from observations at different stages in the course of disease. Bilateral diffuse parenchymal infiltrates (Fig. 222–3) are most common, but no pattern is specific enough to either exclude or confirm a consideration of *P. carinii* disease. Although initially a reticulogranular interstitial process, *Pneumocystis* pneumonitis progresses to a predominantly alveolar process with coalescence and air bronchogram formation. Late in the course of the disease, lung fields may opacify completely.[26, 35] Hilar adenopathy and pleural effusion are not characteristic unless they are a result of an underlying disorder. During treatment, radiographs show gradual clearing after a variable latent period, during which they may appear worse. Residual interstitial fibrosis occurs in a small percentage of patients.[156] Unusual radiographic findings, including an asymmetric distribution, consolidated lobar infiltrates,[11, 21, 35] pneumothorax and pneumomediastinum,[13] localized parenchymal nodular densities,[21, 26] and pleural effusion,[35] have been documented. One investigator noted the occurrence of at least one "atypical" radiographic finding in 56 per cent of 30 cases of PCP.[26]

DIAGNOSIS

Characteristic clinical features are not specific enough to differentiate PCP from other opportunistic pulmonary infections in highly susceptible pediatric patients. Furthermore, mixed infections with viral, bacterial, fungal, or parasitic agents along with *P. carinii* have been documented.[9, 42, 81, 127, 142, 143] Implicit in these observations is the importance and urgency of establishing a definitive diagnosis prior to institution of specific therapy. An etiologic diagnosis can be ascertained only by the demonstration of *P. carinii* organisms in lung tissue or respiratory secretions.

A variety of techniques have been utilized to obtain suitable materials for diagnostic purposes. Although specimens obtained by noninvasive methods from sputum[36, 90] or pharyngeal,[32] tracheal,[83] or gastric[18] secretions occasionally reveal *P. carinii* in infected patients, these sources are not sufficiently reliable to exclude the diagnosis if organisms are not identified.[48] Bronchopulmonary lavage,[27, 48] endobronchial brush biopsy,[34, 121] and transbronchial lung biopsy[46, 73] have been utilized successfully to establish a diagnosis of PCP in adult patients. Limited experience and significant morbidity associated with these procedures in pediatric patients do not justify their routine use in children.

Invasive techniques, including open lung biopsy, closed needle biopsy, and percutaneous needle aspiration, are the most reliable methods for confirming a diagnosis.[48, 81, 99, 124, 152] Open lung biopsy provides the most reliable specimen from which identification of the organism, as well as the extent of the infection, can be ascertained. Its chief disadvantage is the need for general anesthesia. A closed needle biopsy procedure is less reliable in providing adequate tissue and is associated with significantly greater morbidity than open thoracotomy.[74] Percutaneous needle aspiration has proved to be a relatively reliable and safe procedure in selected centers.[48, 75] Bronchoalveolar lavage has been safe and successful, especially in AIDS patients, in whom organisms are in great abundance. Bye and colleagues[10] used bronchoalveolar lavage in infants as young as 2 months of age. Specimens thus obtained can be processed rapidly and stained utilizing a method not adaptable to biopsy sections.[74] The optimal procedure used in obtaining a specimen depends on many factors, including the clinical status of the patient, the facilities available, and the preferential experience of the patient's physician. Regardless of the procedure selected, of critical importance is the avoidance of undue delay in establishing a diagnosis before the patient's condition deteriorates sufficiently to preclude any definitive diagnostic procedure.

For diagnostic purposes, the methenamine silver nitrate method of Gomori[43] and the less widely used but more rapid

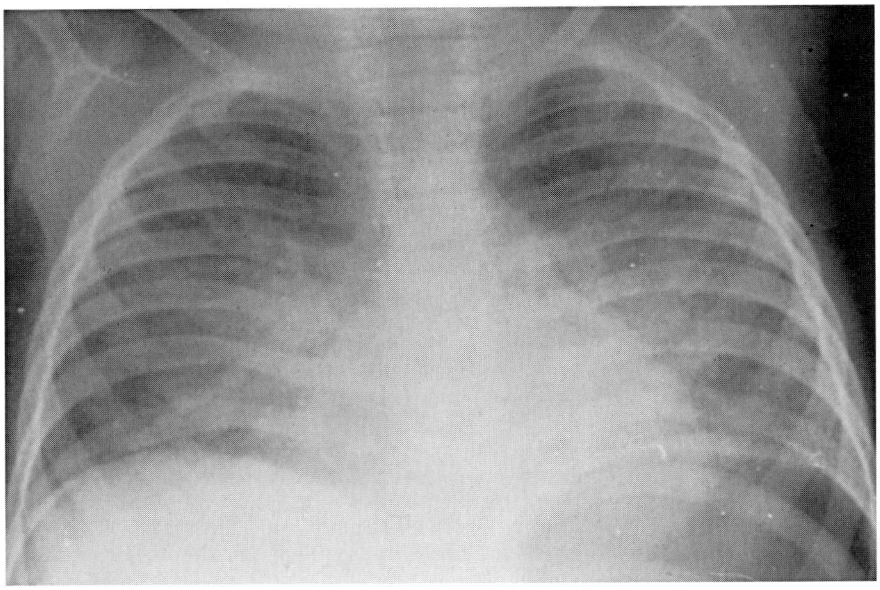

FIGURE 222–3. *Typical diffuse interstitial infiltrates seen in a 20-month-old child with severe combined immunodeficiency disease at the time of presentation with clinical* Pneumocystis carinii *pneumonitis.*

toluidine blue O stain[17] are most useful for demonstrating cyst forms in tissue sections, aspirates, or imprints. Because the Gomori stain as modified by Grocott[44] requires approximately 4 hours for processing, a rapid methenamine silver nitrate procedure is utilized by some investigators and can be adapted to lung tissue aspirates but not to tissue sections.[139] For more detailed morphologic study of intracystic sporozoites and trophozoites, polychrome stains, including Giemsa, Wright, Gram, and methylene blue stains, are more suitable.[75] In tissue sections, the Gomori stain in combination with hematoxylin and eosin stain allows study of both the organism and host tissue.[55] An immunofluorescent monoclonal antibody technique has become commercially available (Meridian Diagnostics, Cincinnati, Ohio). This technique has no definite advantage over the more conventional methods, although one report describes slightly higher detection rates of *P. carinii* in sputum samples by the immunofluorescence method.[79, 80]

Serologic methods, including complement fixation, immunofluorescence,[106] enzyme-linked immunosorbent assay, and latex agglutination,[5] have been developed but generally are not useful for diagnostic purposes.[72] A lack of specificity or sensitivity inherent in the procedures themselves, in addition to the likelihood of impaired immune responses in affected patients, precludes interpretation of results in most cases. Antibody responses in infected patients with primary or secondary immune deficiency states, as well as those of healthy populations, have not been established clearly. Because it is possible that *P. carinii* is prevalent in a latent state in the general population, detection of specific antibody in selected patients may well be of no diagnostic value.[55]

A method for the detection of *P. carinii* antigenemia by counterimmunoelectrophoresis was described in 1978.[115] Although this study indicated promise for use as a diagnostic test, subsequent studies have yielded conflicting results.[93, 98] In one of these studies, more than 60 per cent of bone marrow transplant recipients with viral or idiopathic pneumonia had demonstrable antigenemia.[98] Another controlled study of patients with AIDS found the test to be inadequate as a diagnostic test for *P. carinii* pneumonitis.[93]

Several investigators[91, 108, 130, 148, 150] have amplified *P. carinii* DNA by polymerase chain reaction as a molecular diagnostic method. At this time, it remains a research tool and is not applicable to clinical practice.

Hematologic studies are of no diagnostic value primarily because of baseline abnormalities, reflecting the underlying disease of afflicted patients. Eosinophilia has been reported in isolated cases but usually is not present.[72] Depressed serum total protein and albumin values frequently are noted, reflecting the poor nutritional status of representative patients.[63] Lactic dehydrogenase activity is increased, but this is not a specific reaction for PCP and is of little diagnostic benefit.

PROGNOSIS, TREATMENT, AND PREVENTION

Prior to the availability of specific therapeutic agents, the overall prognosis of patients with PCP was poor. Despite supportive care, almost all infected patients with underlying neoplastic or immunodeficiency disorders died, whereas up to 50 per cent of affected infants in the European epidemics died as a result of this pulmonary infection.[47, 87, 100] To control the European epidemics, Ivády and Páldy[67] first suggested the use of pentamidine isethionate, a diamidine with previously demonstrated antifungal and antiprotozoal activity.[71, 145] Use of this therapeutic agent in infants over the next several years resulted in a dramatic reduction of the mortality rate from 50 per cent to 3.5 per cent.[68, 74]

Pentamidine became available to investigators in the United States through the CDC in 1967. Over the next 3 years, 163 children and adults with documented PCP were treated with pentamidine, of whom 43 per cent recovered.[152, 155] However, of 404 patients to whom the drug was administered for suspected or documented *P. carinii* infection, 189 (47 per cent) experienced significant toxic manifestations. Toxicity ranged from localized reaction at injection sites (18 per cent) to systemic effects, including impaired renal function (24 per cent), liver toxicity (10 per cent), hypoglycemia (6 per cent), hematologic abnormalities (4 per cent), hypotension (10 per cent), and hypocalcemia (1 per cent).[152] Although pentamidine was effective treatment for this disorder, the high incidence of toxicity emphasized the need for an alternative therapeutic agent. Before about 1982, essentially all administration of pentamidine was by the intramuscular route. With the AIDS epidemic, it soon became apparent that the drug could be given intravenously, which reduced the incidence of injection site reactions but with little change in other adverse effects.

Early animal studies[37] and limited investigations in human patients[127] suggested that a combination of pyrimethamine and sulfadiazine might be effective in the treatment of PCP. When a somewhat similar combination of trimethoprim and sulfamethoxazole (co-trimoxazole) became available, it also was investigated as an agent of potential therapeutic value in this disorder.[54] Initial studies in infected rats demonstrated therapeutic efficacy equal to that of pentamidine, as well as successful prevention of pneumocystic infection.[61] The efficacy of co-trimoxazole was demonstrated in the treatment of PCP complicating childhood leukemia. A controlled, randomized study involving 50 leukemic children with PCP was reported. Overall recovery rates of 75 per cent for pentamidine and 77 per cent for co-trimoxazole suggest that these drugs are equally effective in the treatment of PCP in this patient population. Of great importance was the fact that no significant toxicity secondary to co-trimoxazole therapy was observed in this investigation.[55] Subsequent studies have confirmed the efficacy of this drug combination in the treatment of the pneumonitis.[51] At present, trimethoprim-sulfamethoxazole appears to be the drug of choice for the treatment and prevention of PCP. The therapeutic dosage is 20 mg of trimethoprim and 100 mg of sulfamethoxazole per kilogram per day orally in four equally divided doses. The intravenous dose is 15 mg of trimethoprim and 75 mg of sulfamethoxazole per kilogram per day in four doses.

Patients with AIDS have a remarkably high rate of adverse reactions to co-trimoxazole[10] as well as pentamidine. Those who cannot take co-trimoxazole should be treated with intravenous pentamidine given as a single daily dose in the amount of 4.0 mg/kg.

Several other promising drugs are in various stages of clinical evaluation, although none has been investigated systematically in children. Those with evidence of efficacy include trimethoprim-dapsone,[56, 89] pyrimethamine and sulfadoxine,[76, 125] trimetrexate,[1] clindamycin and primaquine,[126] and atovaquone.[57, 60] Animal studies show that the combination of erythromycin-sulfisoxazole has strong anti–*P. carinii* activity through a synergistic mechanism.[58]

Studies in adults with AIDS and *P. carinii* pneumonitis suggest that the administration of corticosteroids early in the course of moderately severe pneumonitis reduces the occurrence of respiratory failure and improves oxygenation.[105] More limited studies of this supportive therapy have been reported in children.

P. carinii pneumonitis effectively can be prevented by che-

TABLE 222–1. Recommendations for *Pneumocystis carinii* Pneumonia Prophylaxis and CD4+ Monitoring for HIV-Exposed Infants and HIV-Infected Children, by Age and HIV Infection Status

Age/HIV Infection Status	PCP Prophylaxis	CD4+ Monitoring
Birth to 4–6 wk, HIV-exposed	No prophylaxis	1 mo
4–6 wk to 4 mo, HIV-exposed	Prophylaxis	3 mo
4–12 mo		
HIV-infected or indeterminate	Prophylaxis	6, 9, and 12 mo
HIV infection reasonably excluded*	No prophylaxis	None
1–5 yr, HIV-infected	Prophylaxis if: CD4+ count is <500 cells/μL or CD4+ percentage is <15%‡	Every 3–4 mo†
6–12 yr, HIV-infected	Prophylaxis if: CD4+ count is <200 cells/μL or CD4+ percentage is <15%¶	Every 3–4 mo†

*HIV infection reasonably can be excluded among children who have had two or more negative HIV diagnostic tests (i.e., HIV culture or PCR), both of which are performed at ≥1 mo of age and one of which is performed at ≥4 mo of age, or two or more negative HIV IgG antibody tests performed at >6 mo of age among children who have no clinical evidence of HIV disease.

†More frequent monitoring (e.g., monthly) is recommended for children whose CD4+ counts or percentages are approaching the threshold at which prophylaxis is recommended.

‡Children 1–2 yr of age who were receiving PCP prophylaxis and had a CD4+ count of <750 cells/μL or percentage of <15% at <12 mo of age should continue prophylaxis.

¶Prophylaxis should be considered on a case-by-case basis for children who might otherwise be at risk for PCP, such as children with rapidly declining CD4+ counts or percentages or children with Category C conditions.[133] Children who have had PCP should receive lifelong PCP prophylaxis.

From Centers for Disease Control and Prevention: 1995 revised guidelines for prophylaxis against *Pneumocystis carinii* pneumonia for children infected with or perinatally exposed to human immunodeficiency virus. M. M. W. R. *44*(RR-4):1–10, 1995.

moprophylaxis with co-trimoxazole when given in the dosage of 150 mg of trimethoprim and 750 mg of sulfamethoxazole per square meter daily[59] or only 3 days a week.[64] *P. carinii* pneumonitis can be prevented in more than 95 per cent of patients at high risk for the disease. Patients in high-risk groups, such as those with cancer or congenital immunodeficiency disorders and organ transplant recipients, should be placed on a chemoprophylaxis regimen throughout the risk period. Generally, the patients within these categories who are the most severely immunosuppressed are the ones who require prophylaxis.

Revised guidelines for *P. carinii* prophylaxis in infants and children with AIDS have been proposed by an expert committee.[15] Because of the high risk for PCP during the first year of life, often before the HIV infection is recognized,[133, 134] all infants born of HIV-infected women should be started on PCP prophylaxis at 4 to 6 weeks of age, regardless of the CD4 lymphocyte cell counts. The use of chemoprophylaxis in this age group has been highly effective in HIV-infected infants.[123] Once infants are shown not to be infected with HIV, the prophylaxis may be stopped. Also, at 1 year of age and subsequently, the use of chemoprophylaxis is based on the CD4 lymphocyte count and other AIDS-defining features (Table 222–1). Co-trimoxazole given 3 days per week is the preferred drug. For those unable to take co-trimoxazole, dapsone (2.0 mg/kg/day) is suggested.[40, 101] An alternative to dapsone is aerosolized pentamidine (300 mg via Respirgard II inhaler monthly).[102] The dosage for aerosolized pentamidine is that described for adults.[88, 101] Studies in adults show that daily doses of dapsone[95] or one dose of dapsone per week is effective prophylaxis.[52] Table 222–1 summarizes the approach to selection of patients at risk.

Although the currently available anti–*P. carinii* drugs effectively may prevent activation of the latent infection, they do not eradicate the organism. Thus, patients are protected from the pneumonitis only while receiving chemoprophylaxis and become susceptible again when the drugs are discontinued.

References

1. Allegra, C. J., Chabner, B. A., Tuazon C. U., et al.: Trimetrexate for the treatment of *P. carinii* pneumonia in patients with the acquired immunodeficiency syndrome. N. Engl. J. Med. *317*:978–985, 1987.
2. Barone, S. R., Auito, L. T., and Krilov, L. R.: Increased survival of young infants with *Pneumocystis carinii* pneumonia and acute respiratory failure with early steroid administration. Clin. Infect. Dis. *19*:212–213, 1994.
3. Bartlett, M. S., Verbanac, P. A., and Smith, J. W.: Cultivation of *Pneumocystis carinii* with WI-38 cells. J. Clin. Microbiol. *10*:796–799, 1979.
4. Bazaz, G. R., Manfredi, O. L., Howard, P. G., et al.: *Pneumocystis carinii* pneumonia in three full-term siblings. J. Pediatr. *76*:767–773, 1970.
5. Benaz, P. J.: À propos du diagnostic immunologique des affections à *Pneumocystis carinii.* Le test d'agglutination au latex. Bull. Soc. Pathol. Exot. *66*:32–42, 1973.
6. Bommer, W.: Die interstitielle plasmacelluläre pneumoniae und *Pneumocystis carinii.* Ergeb. Mikrobiol. *38*:116–122, 1964.
7. Brazinsky, J. H., and Phillips, J. E.: Pneumocystis pneumonia transmission between patients with lymphoma. J. A. M. A. *209*:1527–1529, 1969.
8. Brzosko, W. J., Madalinski, K., Krawczynski, K., et al.: Immunohistochemistry in studies on the pathogenesis of Pneumocystis pneumonia in infants. Ann. N. Y. Acad. Sci. *177*:156–171, 1971.
9. Burke, B. A., and Good, R. A.: *Pneumocystis carinii* infection. Medicine *52*:23–51, 1973.
10. Bye, M. R., Bernstein, L. J., Glaser, J., et al.: *P. carinii* pneumonia in young children with AIDS. Pediatr. Pulmonal. *9*:251–253, 1990.
11. Byrd, R. B., and Horn, B. R.: Infection due to *Pneumocystis carinii* simulating lobar bacterial pneumonia. Chest *70*:91–92, 1976.
12. Campbell, W. G., Jr.: Ultrastructure of pneumocystis in human lung: Life cycle in human pneumocystosis. Arch. Pathol. *93*:312–329, 1972.
13. Capitanio, M. A., and Kirkpatrick, J. A., Jr.: *Pneumocystis carinii* pneumonia. A. J. R. Am. J. Roentgenol. *97*:174–177, 1966.
14. Carini, A.: Formas de eschizogonia do trypanosoma Lewisii. Soc. Med. Cir. Sao Paulo, 16 Aout 1910, in Bulletin de l'Institut Pasteur *9*:937–939, 1911.
15. Centers for Disease Control and Prevention: 1995 revised guidelines for prophylaxis against *Pneumocystis carinii* pneumonia for children infected with or perinatally exposed to human immunodeficiency virus. M. M. W. R. *44*:1–10, 1995.
16. Chagas, C.: Nova trypanomiazaia humana. Mem. Inst. Oswaldo Cruz *1*:159, 1909.
17. Chalvardjian, A. M., and Growe, L. A.: A new procedure for the identification of *Pneumocystis carinii* in tissue sections and smears. J. Clin. Pathol. *16*:383–384, 1963.
18. Chan, H., Pifer, L., Hughes, W. T., et al.: Comparison of gastric contents to pulmonary aspirates for the cytologic diagnosis of *Pneumocystis carinii* pneumonia. J. Pediatr. *90*:243–244, 1977.
19. Chandra, R. K.: Immunocompetence in under-nutrition. J. Pediatr. *81*:1194–1200, 1972.
20. Conner, E., Bagarazzi, M., McSherry, G., et al.: Clinical and laboratory correlates of *P. carinii* pneumonia in children infected with HIV. J. A. M. A. *265*:1693–1697, 1991.
21. Cross, A. S., and Steigbigel, R. T.: *Pneumocystis carinii* pneumonia presenting as localized nodular densities. N. Engl. J. Med. *291*:831–832, 1974.
22. Cushion, M. T., and Walzer, P. D.: Growth and serial passage of *Pneumocystis carinii* in the A549 cell line. Infect. Immun. *44*:245–251, 1984.

23. Dauzier, G., Willis, T., and Barnet, R.: *Pneumocystis carinii* in an infant. Am. J. Clin. Pathol. *26*:787–793, 1956.
24. Delanoe, P., and Delanoe, M.: Sur les rapports des kystes de carinii du pneumon des rats avec le trypanosoma Lewisii. C. R. Acad. Sci. *155*:658, 1912.
25. DiGeorge, A. M.: Congenital absence of the thymus and its immunologic consequences: Occurrence with congenital hypoparathyroidism. *In* Good, R. A., and Bergsma, D. (eds.): Immunologic Deficiency Diseases in Man. Birth Defects, Original Article Series *4*:116–122, 1968.
26. Doppman, J. L., Geelhoed, G. W., and DeVita, V. T.: Atypical radiographic features in *Pneumocystis carinii* pneumonia. Radiology *114*:39–44, 1975.
27. Drew, W. L., Finley, T. N., Mintz, L., et al.: Diagnosis of *Pneumocystis carinii* pneumonia by bronchopulmonary lavage. J. A. M. A. *23*:713–715, 1974.
28. Dutz, W., Post, C., and Kohout, E.: Pneumocystosis: Cancer and therapy. 13th International Congress of Pediatrics, Vienna, 1971.
29. Dutz, W.: *Pneumocystis carinii* pneumonia. Pathol. Annu. *5*:309–341, 1970.
30. Edman, J. C., Edman, U., Cao, M., et al.: Isolation and expression of the *P. carinii* dihydrofolate reductase gene. Proc. Natl. Acad. Sci. U. S. A. *86*:8625–8629, 1989.
31. Edman, J. C., Kovacs, J. A., Masur, H., et al.: Ribosomal RNA sequence shows *P. carinii* to be a member of the fungi. Nature *334*:519–522, 1988.
32. Erchol, J. E., Williams, L. P., and Murgham, P. P.: *Pneumocystis carinii* in hypopharyngeal material. N. Engl. J. Med. *267*:926–928, 1962.
33. European Collaborative Study Group: CD_4 T cell count as predictor of Pneumocystis carinii pneumonia in children born to mothers infected with HIV. B. M. J. *308*:437–440, 1994.
34. Finley, R., Kieff, E., Thompson, S., et al.: Bronchial brushing in the diagnosis of pulmonary disease in patients at risk for opportunistic infection. Am. Rev. Respir. Dis. *109*:379–387, 1974.
35. Forest, J. V.: Radiographic findings in *Pneumocystis carinii* pneumonia. Radiology *103*:539–544, 1972.
36. Fortuny, I. E., Tempero, K. F., and Amsden, T. W.: *Pneumocystis carinii* pneumonia diagnosed from sputum and successfully treated with pentamidine isethionate. Cancer *26*:911–913, 1970.
37. Frenkel, J. K., Good, J. T., and Schulata, J. A.: Latent pneumocystis infection of rats: Relapse and chemotherapy. Lab. Invest. *15*:1559–1577, 1966.
38. Friedman, B. A., Wenglin, B. D., Hyland, R. N., et al.: Roentgenographically atypical *Pneumocystis carinii* pneumonia. Am. Rev. Respir. Dis. *111*:89–93, 1975.
39. Gajdusek, D. C.: *Pneumocystis carinii*: Etiologic agent of interstitial plasma cell pneumonia of premature and young infants. Pediatrics *19*:543–565, 1957.
40. Gatti, G., Loy, A., Casazza, R., et al.: Pharmacokinetics of dapsone in human immunodeficiency virus-infected children. Antimicrob. Agents Chemother. *39*:1101–1106, 1995.
41. Giebink, G. S., Sholler, L., Keenan, T. P., et al.: *Pneumocystis carinii* pneumonia in two Vietnamese refugee infants. Pediatrics *58*:115–118, 1976.
42. Gilbert, C. F., Fordham, C. C., and Benson, W. R.: Death resulting from pneumocystis pneumonia in an adult. Arch. Intern. Med. *112*:56–60, 1963.
43. Gomori, G. A.: New histochemical tests for glycogen and mucin. Am. J. Clin. Pathol. *10*:177–179, 1946.
44. Grocott, R. G.: A stain for fungi in tissue sections and smears. Am. J. Clin. Pathol. *25*:975–979, 1955.
45. Henderson, D. W., Humeniuk, V., Meadows, R., et al.: *Pneumocystis carinii* pneumonia with vascular and lymph nodal involvement. Pathology *6*:235–241, 1974.
46. Hodgkin, J. E., Anderson, H. A., and Rosenow, E. C.: Diagnosis of *Pneumocystis carinii* pneumonia by transbronchoscopic lung biopsy. Chest *64*:551–554, 1973.
47. Hughes, W. T.: Treatment of *Pneumocystis carinii* pneumonitis. N. Engl. J. Med. *295*:726–727, 1976.
48. Hughes, W. T.: Current status of laboratory diagnosis of *Pneumocystis carinii* pneumonitis. CRC Crit. Rev. Clin. Lab. Sci. *6*:145–170, 1975.
49. Hughes, W. T.: Natural mode of acquisition for de novo infection with *Pneumocystis carinii*. J. Infect. Dis. *145*:842–848, 1982.
50. Hughes, W. T.: *Pneumocystis carinii* infections in monthers, infants and non-AIDS elderly adults. *In* Sattler, F., and Walzer, P. (eds.): Bailliére's Clinical Infectious Diseases *2*:1–10, 1995.
51. Hughes, W. T.: Trimethoprim-sulfamethoxazole therapy for *Pneumocystis carinii* pneumonitis in children. Rev. Infect. Dis. *4*:602–607, 1982.
52. Hughes, W. T., Bartley, D. L., and Smith, B. M.: A natural source of infection due to *Pneumocystis carinii*. J. Infect. Dis. *147*:595, 1983.
53. Hughes, W. T., Feldman, S., Aur, R. J., et al.: Intensity of immunosuppressive therapy and the incidence of *Pneumocystis carinii* pneumonitis. Cancer *36*:2004–2009, 1975.
54. Hughes, W. T., Feldman, S., and Sanyal, S. K.: Treatment of *Pneumocystis carinii* pneumonitis with trimethoprim-sulfamethoxazole. Can. Med. Assoc. J. *112*:47S–50S, 1975.
55. Hughes, W. T., Feldman, S., and Chaudhary, S., et al.: Comparison of pentamidine isethionate and trimethoprim-sulfamethoxazole in the treatment of *Pneumocystis carinii* pneumonitis. J. Pediatr. *92*:285–291, 1978.
56. Hughes, W. T., Kennedy, W., Dugdale, M., et al.: Prevention of *P. carinii* pneumonitis in AIDS patients with weekly dapsone. Lancet *2*:1066, 1990.
57. Hughes, W. T., Kennedy, W., Shenep, J. L., et al.: Safety and pharmacokinetics of 566C80, a hydroxynaphthoquinone with anti–*P. carinii* activity: A phase I study in human immunodeficiency virus-infected men. J. Infect. Dis. *163*:843–848, 1991.
58. Hughes, W. T., and Killmar, J. T.: Synergistic anti–*P. carinii* effects of erythromycin and sulfisoxazole. J. Acquir. Immune Defic. Syndr. *4*:532–537, 1991.
59. Hughes, W. T., Kuhn, S., Chaudhary, S., et al.: Successful chemoprophylaxis for *Pneumocystis carinii* pneumonitis. N. Engl. J. Med. *297*:1419–1426, 1977.
60. Hughes, W. T., Leoung, G., Kramer, F., et al.: Comparison of atovaquone (566C80) with trimethoprim-sulfamethoxazole to treat *Pneumocystis carinii* pneumonia in patients with AIDS. N. Engl. J. Med. *328*:1521–1527, 1993.
61. Hughes, W. T., McNabb, P. C., and Makres, T. D.: Efficacy of trimethoprim and sulfamethoxazole in the prevention and treatment of *Pneumocystis carinii* pneumonitis. Antimicrob. Agents Chemother. *5*:289–293, 1974.
62. Hughes, W. T., Price, R. A., Kim, H., et al.: *Pneumocystis carinii* pneumonitis in children with malignancies. J. Pediatr. *82*:404–415, 1973.
63. Hughes, W. T., Price, R. A., Sisko, F., et al.: Protein-calorie malnutrition: A host determinant for *Pneumocystis carinii* infection. Am. J. Dis. Child. *128*:44–52, 1974.
64. Hughes, W. T., Rivera, G. K., Schell, M. J., et al.: Successful intermittent chemoprophylaxis for *Pneumocystis carinii* pneumonitis. N. Engl. J. Med. *316*:1627–1632, 1987.
65. Hughes, W. T., and Smith, B.: Provocation of *Pneumocystis carinii* by cyclosporin A. J. Infect. Dis. *145*:767, 1982.
66. Ito, M., Tsugane, T., Kobayashi, K., et al.: Study on placental transmission of *Pneumocystis carnii* in mice using immunodeficient SCID mice as a new animal model. J. Protozool. *38*:218S–219S, 1991.
67. Ivády, G., and Páldy, L.: A new form of treatment for interstitial plasma-cell pneumonia in premature infants with pentavalent antimony and aromatic diamidines. Monatsschr. Kinderheilk. *106*:10–14, 1958.
68. Ivády, G., Páldy, L., Koltay, M., et al.: *Pneumocystis carinii* pneumonia. Lancet *1*:616–617, 1967.
69. Jackson, H. C., Colthurst, D., Hancock, V., et al.: No detection of characteristic fungal protein elongation factor EF-3 in *P. carinii*. J. Infect. Dis. *163*:675–677, 1991.
70. James, J. W.: Longitudinal study of the morbidity of diarrheal and respiratory infections in malnourished children. Am. J. Clin. Nutr. *25*:690–694, 1972.
71. Jonchere, H.: Treatment of the blood-lymph stage of human trypanosomiasis with diamidines in French West Africa. Bull. Soc. Pathol. Exot. *44*:603–612, 1951.
72. Jose, D. G., Gatti, R. A., and Good, R. A.: Eosinophilia with *Pneumocystis carinii* pneumonia and immune deficiency syndromes. J. Pediatr. *79*:748–754, 1971.
73. Joyner, L. R., and Scheinhorn, D. J.: Transbronchial forceps lung biopsy through the fiberoptic bronchoscope. Chest *65*:532–535, 1975.
74. Kilman, J. W., Clatworthy, H. W., Hering, J., et al.: Open lung biopsy compared with needle biopsy in infants and children. J. Pediatr. Surg. *9*:347–353, 1974.
75. Kim, H. K., and Hughes, W. T.: Comparison of methods for identification of *Pneumocystis carinii* in pulmonary aspirates. Am. J. Clin. Pathol. *60*:462–466, 1973.
76. Kirby, H. B., Kenamore, B., and Guckian, J. G.: *Pneumocystis carinii* pneumonia treated with pyrimethamine and sulfadiazine. Ann. Intern. Med. *75*:505–509, 1971.
77. Koltay, M., and Illyes, M.: A study of immunoglobulins in the blood serum of infants with interstitial plasma cellular pneumonia. Acta Paediatr. Scand. *55*:489–496, 1966.
78. Kovacs, A., Frederick, T., Church, J., et al.: CD_4 T-lymphocyte counts and *P. carinii* pneumonia in pediatric HIV infection. J. A. M. A. *265*:1698–1703, 1991.
79. Kovacs, J. A., Halpern, J. L., Swan, J. C., et al.: Identification of antigens and antibodies specific for *P. carinii*. J. Infect. Dis. *140*:2023–2025, 1988.
80. Kovacs, J. A., Ng, V., Masur, H., et al.: Diagnosis of *P. carinii*: Improved detection in sputum using monoclonal antibodies. N. Engl. J. Med. *318*:589–593, 1988.
81. Kramer, R. I., Cirone, V. C., and Moore, H.: Interstitial pneumonia due to *Pneumocystis carinii* and cytomegalic inclusion disease and hypogammaglobulinemia occurring simultaneously in an infant. Pediatrics *29*:816–819, 1962.
82. Latorre, C. R., Sulzer, A. J., and Norman, L. G.: Serial propagation of *Pneumocystis carinii* in cell line cultures. Appl. Environ. Microbiol. *33*:1204–1206, 1977.
83. Lau, W. K., Young, L. S., and Remington, J. S.: *Pneumocystis carinii* pneumonia: Diagnosis by examination of pulmonary secretions. J. A. M. A. *236*:2399–2402, 1976.
84. Lau, W. K., and Young, L. S.: Trimethoprim-sulfamethoxazole treatment of *Pneumocystis carinii* in adults. N. Engl. J. Med. *295*:716–718, 1976.
85. Law, D. I., Dudrick, S. J., and Abdou, N. I.: Immunocompetence of patients with protein-calorie malnutrition. Ann. Intern. Med. *79*:545–550, 1973.
86. LeClair, R. A.: *Pneumocystis carinii* and interstitial plasma cell pneumonia: A review. Am. Rev. Respir. Dis. *96*:1131–1136, 1967.

87. LeClair, R. A.: Descriptive epidemiology of interstitial pneumocystic pneumonia. Am. Rev. Respir. Dis. *99*:542–547, 1969.
88. Leoung, G. S., Feigal, D. W., Montgomery, A. B., et al.: Aerosolized pentamidine for prophylaxis against *P. carinii* pneumonia. N. Engl. J. Med. *323*:669–675, 1990.
89. Leoung, G. S., Mills, J., Hopewell, P. C., et al.: Dapsone-trimethoprim for *P. carinii* pneumonia in acquired immunodeficiency syndrome. Ann. Intern. Med. *105*:45–48, 1988.
90. Lim, S. K., Eveland, W. C., and Porter, R. J.: Direct fluorescent-antibody method for the diagnosis of *Pneumocystis carinii* pneumonitis from sputa or tracheal aspirates from humans. Appl. Microbiol. *27*:144–149, 1974.
91. Lipschik, G. Y., Gill, V. J., Lundgren, J. D., et al.: Improved diagnosis of *Pneumocystis carinii* infection by polymerase chain reaction on induced sputum and blood. Lancet *340*:203–206, 1992.
92. Lundgren, B., Cotton, R., Lundgren, J. D., et al.: Identification of *P. carinii* chromosomes and mapping of five genes. Infect. Immun. *58*:1705–1710, 1990.
93. Maddison, S. E., Wall, K. W., Haverkos, H. W., et al.: Evaluation of serologic tests for *Pneumocystis carinii* antibody and antigenemia in patients with acquired immunodeficiency syndrome. Diagn. Microbiol. Infect. Dis. *2*:69–73, 1984.
94. Matsumoto, Y., Matsuda, S., and Jegoshi, T.: Yeast glucan in cyst wall of *P. carinii*. J. Protozol. *36*:21–22(S), 1989.
95. Metroka, C. E., Jacobus, D., and Lewis, N.: Successful chemoprophylaxis for *Pneumocystis* with dapsone or bactrim. Proceedings of the 5th International Conference on AIDS, Montreal, 1989.
96. Meuwissen, J. H. E., Brzosko, W. J., Nowoslawski, A., et al.: Diagnosis of *Pneumocystis carinii* pneumonia in the presence of immunological deficiency. Lancet *1*:1124, 1970.
97. Meuwissen, J. H. E., Tauber, I., Leeuwenberg, A. D., et al.: Parasitologic and serologic observations of infection with *P. carinii* in humans. J. Infect. Dis. *136*:43–48, 1977.
98. Meyers, J. D., Pifer, L. L., Sale, G. E., et al.: The value of *Pneumocystis carinii* antibody and antigen detection for diagnosis of *Pneumocystis carinii* pneumonia after marrow transplantation. Am. Rev. Respir. Dis. *120*:1283–1287, 1979.
99. Michaelis, L. L., Leight, G. S., Powell, R. D., et al.: *Pneumocystis* pneumonia: The importance of early open lung biopsy. Ann. Surg. *183*:301–306, 1976.
100. Minielly, J. A., Mills, S. D., and Holley, K. E.: *Pneumocystis carinii* pneumonia. Can. Med. Assoc. J. *100*:846–854, 1969.
101. Mirochnick, M., Michaels, M., Clarke, D., et al.: Pharmacokinetics of dapsone in children. J. Pediatr. *122*:806–809, 1993.
102. Montaner, J. S. G., Lawson, L. M., Gervais, A., et al.: Aerosolized pentamidine for the prevention of AIDS-related *Pneumocystis carinii* pneumonia: Results of the Canadian Cooperative Trial. Am. Rev. Respir. Dis. *141*:A268, 1990.
103. Morlier, E., Pouchot, J., Boss, P., et al.: Maternal-fetal transmission of *Pneumocystis carnii* in human immunodeficiency virus infection. N. Engl. J. Med. *332*:825, 1995.
104. Munk, J.: The radiologic differentiation between acute diffuse interstitial pneumonia and pulmonary interstitial oedema in infancy and early childhood. Br. J. Radiol. *47*:752–757, 1974.
105. National Institutes of Health—University of California Expert Panel for Corticosteroids as Adjunctive Therapy for *Pneumocystis* Pneumonia: Consensus statement on the use of corticosteroids as adjunctive therapy for *Pneumocystis* pneumonia in the acquired immunodeficiency syndrome. N. Engl. J. Med. *323*:1500–1504, 1990.
106. Norman, L., and Kagan, I. G.: A preliminary report of an indirect fluorescent-antibody test for detecting antibodies to cysts of *Pneumocystis carinii* in human sera. Am. J. Clin. Pathol. *58*:170–176, 1972.
107. Ognibene, F. P., Shelhamer, J., Gill, V., et al.: The diagnosis of *Pneumocystis carinii* pneumonia in patients with the acquired immunodeficiency syndrome using subsegmental bronchoalveolar lavage. Am. Rev. Respir. Dis. *129*:929–932, 1984.
108. Olsson, M., Elvin, K., Lofdahl, S., et al.: Detection of *Pneumocystis carinii* DNA in sputum and bronchoalveolar lavage samples by polymerase chain reaction. J. Clin. Microbiol. *32*:221–226, 1993.
109. Patterson, J. H., Lindsay, I. L., Edwards, E. S., et al.: *Pneumocystis carinii* pneumonia and altered host resistance: Treatment of one patient with pentamidine isethionate. Pediatrics *38*:388–392, 1966.
110. Peglow, S. L., Smulian, A. G., Linke, M. J., et al.: Serologic responses to *Pneumocystis carinii* antigens in health and disease. J. Infect. Dis. *161*:296–306, 1990.
111. Perera, D. R., Western, K. A., Johnson, H. D., et al.: *Pneumocystis carinii* pneumonia in a hospital for children: Epidemiologic aspects. J. A. M. A. *214*:1074–1078, 1970.
112. Pesanti, E. L.: Interaction of cytokines and alveolar cells with *Pneumocystis carinii* in vitro. J. Infect. Dis. *163*:611–616, 1991.
113. Pickering, L. K., Anderson, D. C., Choi, S., et al.: Leukocyte function in children with malignancies. Cancer *35*:1365–1371, 1974.
114. Pifer, L. L., Hughes, W. T., and Murphy, M. J.: Propagation of *Pneumocystis carinii in vitro.* Pediatr. Res. *11*:305–316, 1977.
115. Pifer, L. L., Hughes, W. T., Stagno, S., et al.: *Pneumocystis carinii* infection: Evidence for high prevalence in normal and immunosuppressed children. Pediatrics *61*:35–41, 1978.
116. Pottratz, S. T., and Martin, W. J., II: Role of fibronectin in *Pneumocystis carinii* attachment of cultured lung cells. J. Clin. Invest. *85*:351–356, 1990.
117. Price, R. A., and Hughes, W. T.: Histopathology of *Pneumocystis carinii* infestation and infection in malignant disease. Hum. Pathol. *5*:737–752, 1974.
118. Rahimi, S. A.: Disseminated *Pneumocystis carinii* in thymic alymphoplasia. Arch. Pathol. *97*:162–165, 1974.
119. Reed, J. C., and Maxwell, J. E.: The airbronchogram in interstitial disease of the lungs. Radiology *116*:1–8, 1975.
120. Remington, J. S., and Anderson, S. E.: Diagnosis and treatment of pneumocystosis and toxoplasmosis in the immunosuppressed host. Transplant. Proc. *5*:1263–1270, 1973.
121. Repsher, L. H., Schröter, G., and Hammond, W. S.: Diagnosis of *Pneumocystis carinii* pneumonitis by means of endobronchial brush biopsy. N. Engl. J. Med. *287*:340–341, 1972.
122. Rifkind, D., Starzl, T. E., Marchioro, T. Z., et al.: Transplantation pneumonia. J. A. M. A. *189*:808–821, 1964.
123. Rigaud, M., Pollack, H., Leibovitz, E., et al.: Efficacy of primary chemoprophylaxis against *Pneumocystis carinii* pneumonia during the first year of life in infants infected with human immunodeficiency virus type 1. J. Pediatr. *125*:476–480, 1994.
124. Rosen, P. R., Martini, R., and Armstrong, D.: *Pneumocystis carinii* pneumonia. Am. J. Med. *58*:794–802, 1975.
125. Ruf, B., and Phole, H. D.: Pyrimethamine-sulfadoxine (Fansidar) in primary and secondary chemoprophylaxis of *Pneumocystis carinii* pneumonia. Am. Rev. Respir. Dis. *141*:A154, 1990.
126. Ruf, B., Rohde, I., and Pohle, H. D.: Efficacy of clindamycin/primaquine vs treatment of *Pneumocystis carinii* pneumonia. Am. Rev. Respir. Dis. *141*:A154, 1990.
127. Ruskin, J., and Remington, J. S.: The compromised host and infection. I. *Pneumocystis carinii* pneumonia. J. A. M. A. *202*:1070–1074, 1967.
128. Ruskin, J., and Remington, J. S.: *Pneumocystis carinii* infection in the immunosuppressed host. Antimicrob. Agents Chemother. *7*:70–76, 1967.
129. Salfelder, K., and Schwarz, V.: Pneumocystosis. Am. J. Dis. Child. *114*:693–699, 1967.
130. Schluger, N., Godwin, T., Sepkowitz, K., et al.: Application of DNA amplification to pneumocystosis: Presence of serum *Pneumocystis carinii* DNA during human and experimentally induced pneumonia. J. Exp. Med. *176*:1327–1333, 1992.
131. Scrimshaw, N. S.: Synergism of malnutrition and infection. J. A. M. A. *212*:1685–1691, 1970.
132. Sheldon, W.: Pulmonary *Pneumocystis carinii* infection. J. Pediatr. *61*:780–791, 1962.
133. Simonds, R. J., Hughes, W. T., Feinberg, J., et al.: Preventing *Pneumocystis carinii* pneumonia in persons infected with human immunodeficiency virus. Clin. Infect. Dis. *21*(Suppl. 1):544–548, 1995.
134. Simonds, R. J., Lindegren, M. L., Thomas, P., et al.: Prophylaxis against *Pneumocystis carnii* pneumonia among children with perinatally acquired HIV infection in the United States. N. Engl. J. Med. *332*:786–790, 1995.
135. Simonds, R. J., Oxtoby, M. J., Caldwell, M. B., et al.: *Pneumocystis carinii* pneumonia among U.S. children with perinatally acquired HIV infection. J. A. M. A. *270*:470–473, 1993.
136. Simone, J. V., Aur, R. J., Hustu, H. O., et al.: Acute lymphocyte leukemia in children. Cancer *36*:770–774, 1975.
137. Singer, C., Armstrong, D., and Rosen, P. P.: *Pneumocystis carinii* pneumonia: A cluster of eleven cases. Ann. Intern. Med. *82*:772–777, 1975.
138. Sleasman, J. W., Hemenway, C., Klein, A. S., et al.: Corticosteroids improve survival of children with AIDS and *Pneumocystis carinii* pneumonia. Am. J. Dis. Child. *147*:30–34, 1993.
139. Smith, J. W., and Hughes, W. T.: A rapid staining technique for *Pneumocystis carinii.* J. Clin. Pathol. *25*:269–271, 1972.
140. Stagno, S., Pifer, L. L., Hughes, W. T., et al.: *Pneumocystis carinii* pneumonitis in young immunosuppressed infants. Pediatrics *66*:56–62, 1980.
141. Telzak, E. E., Cote, R. J., Gold, J. W. M., et al.: Extrapulmonary *Pneumocystis carinii* infections. Rev. Infect. Dis. *12*:380–386, 1990.
142. Theologides, A., Pflueger, O. H., and Kennedy, B. J.: Toxoplasmosis and *Pneumocystis carinii* pneumonitis. Minn. Med. *52*:737–742, 1969.
143. Tokumitsu, S., and Sajaki, T.: An autopsy case of generalized cytomegalic inclusion disease associated with *Pneumocystis carinii* pneumonia. Kumamoto Med. J. *28*:105–110, 1975.
144. Van der Meer, G., and Brug, S. L.: Infection par pneumocystis chez l'homme et chez les animaux. Ann. Soc. Belge Med. Trop. *22*:301, 1942.
145. VanHoof, L., Herrard, C., and Peel, E.: Pentamidine in the prevention and treatment of trypanosomiasis. Trans. R. Soc. Trop. Med. Hyg. *37*:271–280, 1944.
146. Vereerstraeten, P., Dekoster, J. P., Vereerstraeten, J., et al.: Pulmonary infections after kidney transplantation. Proc. Eur. Dial. Transplant. Assoc. *11*:300–307, 1975.
147. Vessal, K., Post, C., and Dutz, W.: Roentgenologic changes in infantile *Pneumocystis carinii* pneumonia. Am. J. Roentgenol. Radium Ther. Nucl. Med. *120*:254–260, 1974.
148. Wakefield, A. E.: Detection of DNA sequences identical to *Pneumocystis carinii* in samples of ambient air. J. Euk. Microbiol. *41*:116(S), 1994.

149. Wakefield, A. E., Banerji, S., Pixley, F. J. et al.: Molecular probes for the detection of *Pneumocystis carinii.* Trans. R. Soc. Trop. Med. Hyg. *84*(Suppl. 1):17–18, 1990.
150. Wakefield, A. E., Guiver, L., Miller, R. M., et al.: DNA amplification on induced sputum samples for diagnosis of *Pneumocystis carinii* pneumonia. Lancet *337*:1378–1379, 1993.
150a. Walker, A. N., Garner, R. E., and Horst, M. N.: Immunocytochemical detection of chitin in *Pneumocystis carinii.* Infect. Immun. *58*:412–415, 1990.
151. Walker, C. L.: The schizogony of *Trypanosoma evansi* in the spleen of the vertebrate host. Philip. J. Sci. *7*:53–63, 1912.
152. Walzer, P., Perl, D. P., Krogstad, D. J., et al.: *Pneumocystis carinii* pneumonia in the United States. Ann. Intern. Med. *80*:83–93, 1974.
153. Walzer, P. D., Schultz, M. G., Western, K. A., et al.: *Pneumocystis carinii* pneumonia and primary immune deficiency diseases of infancy and childhood. J. Pediatr. *82*:416–422, 1973.
154. Watanabe, J. M., Chinchinian, J., Weitz, C., et al.: *Pneumocystis carinii* pneumonia in a family. J. A. M. A. *193*:685–686, 1965.
155. Western, K. A., Perera, D. R., and Schultz, M. G.: Pentamidine isethionate in the treatment of *Pneumocystis carinii* pneumonia. Ann. Intern. Med. *73*:695–699, 1970.
156. Whitcomb, M. E., Schwarz, M. I., and Charles, M. A.: Interstitial fibrosis after *Pneumocystis carinii* pneumonia. Ann. Intern. Med. *73*:761–764, 1970.
157. Winder, F. G., and Rooney, S. A.: *Pneumocystis carinii* in lungs of adults at autopsy. Am. Rev. Respir. Dis. *97*:935–937, 1968.
158. Yoshida, Y., Matsumoto, Y., Yamada, M., et al.: *Pneumocystis carinii* electron microscopic investigation on the interaction of trophozoite and alveolar lining cell. Zentralbl. Hyg. Umweltmed. *256*:390–399, 1984.

SUBSECTION TWO

NEMATODES

223

PARASITIC NEMATODE INFECTIONS

Michael Katz and Peter J. Hotez

INTESTINAL NEMATODES

The three major intestinal nematodes of children, *Ascaris lumbricoides, Trichuris trichiura,* and the hookworms, together have a substantial impact on the health and well-being of children living in the less developed nations of the world. This "unholy trinity" of parasites deprives hundreds of millions of young children of their full intellectual and growth potential. Building on studies from the early part of this century,[9, 10] extensive new data from many different geographic regions confirm that chronic intestinal nematode infections during childhood suppress both cognitive and intellectual development[4–6] and impair physical growth and fitness.[2, 11–13] Because many of these detrimental effects are reversible upon elimination of nematodes from the intestinal tract with anthelminthic drugs,[12, 13] several investigators and international relief agencies have advocated the administration of benzimidazole anthelminthics as a cornerstone of public health programs directed at school age children.[1, 7] However, because reinfection with *A. lumbricoides*, *T. trichiura,* and hookworms usually occurs within 6 months after anthelminthic treatment in highly endemic areas,[33] this strategy probably is not a practical means of control unless the drugs are used frequently. Some have pointed to the use of genetically engineered anti-helminth vaccines as one possible solution to the problem of worm reinfection and disease during childhood.[3]

In addition to the chronic effects seen when children harbor large numbers of intestinal nematodes, new information points to the increasing recognition of unique neonatal and infantile syndromes that may result from vertical transmission of the infective stages of some intestinal nematodes, probably in colostrum and breast milk.[8] The best documented example of vertical transmission in infants results in the "swollen belly syndrome" caused by *Strongyloides fuelleborni,* although other perinatal nematode infections probably also occur (discussed later). Finally, children experience significant morbidity during zoonotic transmission of the infective stages of intestinal nematodes of companion animals, such as dogs and cats. The resultant aberrant migrations of these foreign nematode larvae (visceral larva migrans) have become a major pediatric public health problem in the large urban areas of the United States and Europe.

Ascaris lumbricoides

Ascariasis is among the most prevalent infections in the world. In the classic analysis of its prevalence, Stoll[30] calculated that there were more than 600 million cases in the world. In view of the fact that population has increased geometrically but sanitary conditions have not improved substantially, it readily can be assumed that no fewer than 1 billion infections exist currently in the world. Accurate estimates based on 1,477,742 fecal examinations indicate that more than 500 million cases of ascariasis occur in China alone![34] In parts of Africa, the average rate of infection is in the range of 95 per cent and in Central and South America in the range of 45 per cent. In the rural Southern communities of the United States, surveys conducted entirely or predominantly among children have shown prevalence rates of 20 to 67 per cent.[15]

Ascaris infection, when relatively light, usually is inapparent until the patient passes a worm through the rectum. In heavy infections, there may be constitutional symptoms during the early phase and intestinal malabsorption and even obstruction in the later phase. The infection is acquired by ingestion of the infective eggs, which hatch in the upper part of the small intestine, freeing the larvae. The larvae penetrate the intestinal wall, reach venules or lymphatics, and pass through the portal circulation to the liver, the right side of the heart, and the lungs.

In the lungs, the larvae break out of the capillaries and begin ascending through the respiratory radicles until they reach the glottis, and then, passing over the epiglottis, they enter the esophagus and are carried down to the small intestine, where they mature and become adult worms. The adult female *Ascaris* produces huge numbers of eggs, possibly as many as 200,000 a day. To ensure adequate quantities of egg-requiring cholesterol, the parasite sequesters oxygen through a specially modified hemoglobin; the oxygen then is used for cholesterol biosynthesis.[27] The entire cycle, beginning with the infective eggs and resulting in ovipositing females, lasts approximately 2 months. Infection is maintained in the community by deposition of human stools in the soil, permitting embryonated eggs to develop to the infective stage. This takes approximately 2 weeks. The high prevalence of infection results not only from deficient sanitary facilities for disposal of human excreta but also from the deliberate use of human feces as fertilizer.

Epidemiology

Ascaris is a ubiquitous parasite that is present in both temperate and tropical zones, but its highest prevalence is in warm countries where sanitation is deficient. All ages are affected by the parasite; young children, who are exposed more often to the contaminated soil, are affected most frequently. These children usually harbor greater numbers of adult worms in their intestine than do adults living under similar conditions.[11–13, 19] This predisposition to "worminess" in childhood also may have a genetic or immunologic basis. Because *Ascaris* is extremely hardy and relatively resistant to extremes of temperature, it is common to find high rates of ascariasis in impoverished urban environments (e.g., Guatemala City, Mexico City), including those in some temperate zones, where the eggs can survive the ordinary freezing temperatures of winter months. The eggs also are resistant to chemical disinfectants and are not destroyed readily by sewage treatment. In some areas, pigs may serve as a reservoir for zoonotic *Ascaris* infection.[14]

Pathophysiology

During the migratory phase of the infection, the larvae evoke an inflammatory response associated with eosinophilic infiltration. *Ascaris* antigens—the so-called ABA-1 allergen—released during the molting of larvae evoke an immune response, and specific antibodies of the IgG class have been detected; they form the basis of complement fixation and precipitin tests.[16, 28] Little is known about the IgA response to this infection. The primary defense mechanism most probably is of the cellular immune type in association with humoral immunity; in experimental animals infected with various nematodes, rejection of the worms by sensitized hosts has been reported.

During the intestinal stage of the infection, symptoms derive primarily from the physical presence of the worms in the gut, through aberrant migration into other lumina, or through perforation into the peritoneum. Moreover, *Ascaris* secretes peptides that block the action of pancreatic digestive enzymes (trypsin, chymotrypsin, elastase)[20, 23]—as a protective mechanism for its own survival—which may play a role in parasite-associated malabsorption. It is unknown whether malabsorption of nutrients, or even malnutrition at all, is the basis of *Ascaris*-associated physical growth retardation during childhood, but chronic moderate and heavy *Ascaris* infections during childhood adversely affect physical growth and development.[2, 11–13, 19, 29]

Clinical Presentation

The degree of disease induced by the migratory phase of *Ascaris* relates directly to the number of larvae migrating simultaneously. In light infections, this phase is unrecognized. Heavy infection, as for example that induced in himself by Koino,[25] who swallowed 2000 infected eggs, may cause severe pneumonitis.

In the lumen of the intestine, ascarid worms may become matted together and form a bolus large enough to cause intestinal obstruction. The incidence of this complication has been estimated as 2 per 1000 infected children per year.[15] When recognized early, the obstruction can be treated with medical management, but in many cases surgical intervention is mandatory.

Less common complications are perforation of the intestine and hepatobiliary and pancreatic ascariasis resulting from blockage of the bile duct and pancreatic duct, respectively. Patients thus afflicted can present with cholecystitis, acute cholangitis, "biliary colic," acute pancreatitis, or hepatic abscess.[24] Certain irritants, such as halogenated hydrocarbons (e.g., carbon tetrachloride and tetrachloroethylene, used in the past to treat certain hookworm infections), and elevation of body temperature have been known to precipitate aberrant migrations.

Whatever the mechanism of interference by *Ascaris* with growth or nutrition, treatment with anthelmintics leads to substantial "catch-up" growth of the previously parasitized children.[2, 11–13, 19, 29] Ascariasis of pregnant women leads to intrauterine growth retardation.[32]

The majority of people with light infections rarely are symptomatic (such persons become aware of the parasites by passage of the adult worms in the stool or through regurgitating and vomiting of the adult worms), although it has been conjectured that even these persons may exhibit subtle deficits in cognitive and intellectual development.[5, 6]

Several cases of neonatal ascariasis have been described in the literature.[17, 18] The mode of acquisition of these infections is not known, but canine and feline ascarid infections commonly are acquired by a transplacental route, suggesting the possibility that this also may occur in humans.

Differential and Specific Diagnoses

Differential diagnosis of pneumonia caused by *Ascaris* suggests a parasitic etiology because of the peripheral eosinophilia. However, any nematode with the migratory phase through the lungs can mimic this infection. *Ascaris* must be considered as a cause of intestinal obstruction in any geographic locale where its prevalence is high.

The diagnosis of intestinal ascariasis is established by identification of the characteristic ascarid eggs through microscopic examination of the stool. Serologic tests are of limited value. The simpler tests are subject to cross-reactions; the more complicated ones are laborious and require sophisticated laboratory facilities. They stand in contrast with the simplicity of the stool examination. Among these, radioimmunoprecipitation offers some opportunity for the assessment of the intensity of the infection.[21] Detection of *Ascaris* metabolites in the urine by gas-liquid chromatography also correlates with the worm burden.[22]

Hepatobiliary and pancreatic ascariases are suspected in heavily infected children who present with signs of biliary obstruction as noted earlier. Ultrasonography and endoscopic retrograde cholangiopancreatography are useful adjunct diagnostic procedures for these patients.[24]

Treatment

For an ordinary *Ascaris* infection, mebendazole, administered at a fixed dose of 100 mg twice daily for 3 days, is effective. The disadvantage of this drug is that it requires several doses.[31] Another benzimidazole, albendazole, offers no real advantage over mebendazole, except that it may be effective in a single dose.[26, 29] As an alternative drug, pyrantel pamoate, administered as a single dose of 11 mg/kg, not to exceed 1 g, is extremely effective. Neither benzimidazole nor pyrantel pamoate "officially" has been tested in children younger than 2 years of age. Therefore, all of the printed statements caution against the use of these drugs in the younger age group. Nevertheless, these drugs do not seem to act differently in this younger age group than they do in older children or adults, and widespread use overseas indicates that the benzimidazoles probably are safe.[91] However, because of their potential for embryotoxicity, judicious use of these drugs in young children is warranted. In cases of intestinal obstruction, piperazine citrate may be effective because this drug paralyzes the myoneural junction of the *Ascaris* and may result in relaxation of the matted bolus of worms. It is antagonistic to pyrantel pamoate, and therefore these two drugs should not be given together.

Management of intestinal obstruction or hepatobiliary ascariasis often is surgical. For some patients, biliary decompression may be performed with endoscopic retrograde cholangiopancreatography.[24]

Prognosis

Prognosis is excellent in the great majority of cases of ascariasis. In cases of the complications of obstruction or perforation, prognosis depends entirely on the speed of recognition and therapy.

Prevention

The infection could be eliminated entirely through proper disposal of human excreta. Unfortunately, as an isolated means of improvement of health in the world, this has never been successful. Elimination of *Ascaris* from a community or a substantial reduction in the incidence of this infection usually follows a general improvement in the standard of living. Periodic community-wide therapy with anthelmintics has been effective in reducing worm burden as a short-term strategy. In the absence of aggressive sanitation and other control measures, however, reinfection often occurs within 6 months after treatment.[33]

Trichuris trichiura

Trichuriasis has a prevalence approximating that of the other major intestinal nematode infections, or some 800 million cases in the world,[35] but the infection usually is asymptomatic because in the majority of cases it is light. However, children with so-called asymptomatic light infections may have impaired deficits in cognition.[44]

The infection is acquired by ingestion of embryonated eggs, which are picked up from the soil on hands or through contaminated food. The eggs hatch in the upper part of the small intestine, and the liberated larvae penetrate the villi. Unlike the larvae of *Ascaris, Trichuris* larvae do not undergo extraintestinal migration but remain in situ for approximately 1 week, when they begin a progressive descent into the cecum and the colon. They mature there, and the attenuated anterior end of the adult worm embeds itself in the colonic mucosa. Creation of syncytial tunnels (derived from the columnar epithelium of the colon) is facilitated by the release of a parasite-derived, pore-forming protein.[38] It is from these colonic mucosal tunnels that the parasites derive their nourishment. The entire cycle from the ingestion of embryonated ova to the development of sexually mature adults takes approximately 2 months. Persistence of the infection in a community depends on continual contamination of the soil with human feces.

Epidemiology

These parasites are most common in the tropical regions but also are found in the subtropical areas, such as the southern states of the United States. The distribution of this worm closely parallels that of *Ascaris*. Also, as in the case of *Ascaris*, children with trichuriasis usually harbor greater numbers of worms than do adults living under similar conditions.[35, 36] Consequently, children suffer greater morbidity from trichuriasis than do adults. The mechanistic basis of added worminess in children is unknown, although it has been observed that *Trichuris* infections are *aggregated*, so that a minority of children suffer from particularly heavy infections. These heavily infected children appear to have genetic or immunologic predisposition to *Trichuris* infection.[35, 36] Children also are the major source of *Trichuris* eggs in the environment, which when deposited in the soil become infective in about 1 month and remain viable for several months. They are killed by exposure to temperatures in excess of 40° C within 1 hour. Freezing temperatures below −8° C also destroy these eggs. Like ascarid eggs, they are relatively resistant to chemical disinfectants.

Pathophysiology

At the site of attachment, the adult worm elicits the characteristic changes in the colonic mucosa as noted earlier. Inflammatory cells also are at these sites, but these do not appear to account for the clinical resemblance of trichuriasis to some forms of inflammatory bowel disease.[35, 42] Like many other intestinal worms, *Trichuris* is expelled through the action of the host's immune system. This results from a combined effect of antibody and lymphoid cells.[45] The regulation of *Trichuris* populations in the gut has been attributed to a carefully orchestrated balance of host-derived cytokines.[39] Although anemia has been attributed to trichuriasis,[40] the amount of blood loss caused by this parasite is much less than hookworm-associated blood loss and is not sufficient to account for anemia.[41] One possibility is that *Trichuris* anemia results from chronic inflammation, similar to the anemia of inflammatory bowel disease.[35, 36]

Clinical Presentation

Two major disease syndromes are caused by heavy *Trichuris* infections during childhood.[35–36] The *Trichuris* dysentery syndrome (TDS) is associated with severe diarrhea with blood and mucus. Children with TDS are anemic and frequently manifest growth retardation and failure to thrive.[37] Infants and toddlers with TDS are at risk for developing protracted tenesmus, which leads to rectal prolapse. *Trichuris* colitis is a more chronic manifestation of moderate to heavy infection and presents as a form of inflammatory bowel disease similar to what happens in Crohn disease or ulcerative colitis. Children with this form of colitis also can have chronic malnutrition and short stature. Moderately and heavily infected (and possibly even lightly infected) children are at risk for deficits in cognition and intellectual development.[44]

Differential and Specific Diagnoses

Diagnosis is established by the identification of the characteristic barrel-shaped eggs through microscopic examination of the stool. Heavily infected children with TDS clinically may resemble children with amebic or bacillary dysentery. Children with *Trichuris* colitis may have manifestations that resemble other forms of inflammatory bowel disease. However, the erythrocyte sedimentation rate is not elevated in children with *Trichuris* colitis.

Treatment

In the past, when relatively noxious or toxic drugs had to be used, only patients with heavy infections were treated. Currently, any patient with this infection can be treated by the administration of mebendazole, 100 mg twice daily for 3 days.[43] There is no need to adjust the dose to the weight of the patient because the drug is not well absorbed from the gastrointestinal tract. Albendazole is a suitable alternative. As noted earlier, the safety of the benzimidazoles in young children has not been established in a study approved by the U.S. Food and Drug Administration. As an alternative, the drug oxantel is effective for the treatment of trichuriasis. In some countries, oxantel is formulated with pyrantel pamoate.[35]

Prevention

As in the case of other nematodes, sanitary disposal of the excreta—but more important, improvement in the standard of living—tends to reduce the incidence of infection. Frequent mass treatments with mebendazole reduce the worm burden in a community.

Hookworms

Hookworm infection is one of the most important childhood infections in the developing world, with an estimated prevalence of 1 billion cases. Hookworms exert their pathogenic effect by causing intestinal blood loss, which leads to iron-deficiency anemia. Considering the average blood loss induced by each worm, the average number of worms per infected individual, and the prevalence, it can be estimated that these parasites are responsible for a daily loss of more than 1 million liters of blood in the world. Because loss of blood represents loss of erythrocytes *and* plasma, heavy infections, especially in malnourished populations, also contribute to malnutrition. Two major species of hookworms infect human intestine: *Ancylostoma duodenale* and *Necator americanus*. Of the two, *A. duodenale* is the more virulent species, causing greater blood loss and morbidity, which leads to iron-deficiency anemia and hypoproteinemia.[49] Two other members of the genus *Ancylostoma, A. ceylonicum* and the dog hookworm, *A. caninum*,[53] are much less frequent causes of intestinal pathology in humans.[49]

The infection is acquired either by exposure of skin to the moist soil infested with the larvae of these worms *(A. duodenale* and *N. americanus)* or by ingestion of the infective larvae *(A. duodenale* only). The most propitious circumstances for the infection are shady areas and sandy or loam soil. Infection is particularly likely early in the morning when the ground is moist with dew or after a rainfall. After the larvae enter the host, they initiate a developmental program that continues until they enter the intestine.[3, 47, 51] Larvae that enter through the skin are carried by venous circulation to the right side of the heart and there follow the route described for *Ascaris*, whereas larvae that are ingested may develop entirely within the gastrointestinal tract.

Upon reaching the small intestine, the larvae mature to adult worms, which become attached with their mouth parts to the intestinal mucosa. The worms sustain themselves by releasing hydrolytic enzymes that degrade the intestinal mucosa and then feeding on cellular and connective tissue debris.[49–51] During this process, capillaries and arterioles are eroded and lacerated, resulting in blood extravasation. The adult worms also ingest the blood. An anticoagulant that blocks the activity of host factor Xa facilitates blood flow and is responsible for continued bleeding from the original site after the worm has moved to a new one.[46] The entire cycle from penetration of the skin or larval ingestion to the development of mature worms usually takes approximately 6 to 8 weeks. At that time, hookworm eggs appear in the feces. However, *A. duodenale* larvae also may undergo a period of developmental arrest, which lasts weeks or months within the human host. Thus, intestinal ancylostomiasis can occur for up to a year (and possibly longer) after initial exposure to infective larvae.[55] It has been conjectured that the reservoir of arrested *A. duodenale* larvae enters the mammary glands and breast milk.[55] This sequence of events may account for cases of infantile ancylostomiasis noted in Africa, India, and China.[48] Humans are the major reservoir of these organisms, and this infection is maintained by continual contamination of soil by human feces.

Epidemiology

Although in ancient times these parasites had a worldwide distribution, they currently are most prevalent in the tropical and subtropical zones and can be found in the temperate climates only in isolated areas. *A. duodenale* predominates in many parts of the Indian subcontinent and China.[3] Estimates based on the examination of 1,477,742 fecal samples indicate that almost 200 million cases occur in China alone.[34] *A. duodenale* also is a major parasite in Egypt and other parts of the Mediterranean region, Africa, and possibly even focal areas of South America. *N. americanus* is the prevailing species in the Western Hemisphere, most of Africa, Southeast Asia, Indonesia, parts of Australia, and certain islands of the Pacific. This differential distribution is not absolute, and small numbers of either parasite are present where the other predominates. Mixed infections with both species are extremely common. *A. ceylonicum* occurs in focally endemic areas of southern Asia,[49] whereas the dog hookworm *A. caninum* has been described as a cause of human eosinophilic enteritis in Australia and possibly elsewhere.[53]

Larvae survive in the soil for 6 weeks. They are destroyed by drying, freezing temperatures, and heat in excess of 45° C. Hookworm infection occurs in areas of high agricultural intensity and is not found frequently in urban areas, where *Ascaris* and *Trichuris* might predominate. Because shade and moisture are essential for survival at the infective larval stage, it is not surprising to find high rates of hookworm infection among families that harvest tea in India and Bangladesh, mulberry leaves (for the silkworm industry) in eastern China, sweet potatoes and corn in western China, coffee and bananas in Central and South America, and rubber in Africa.

Like other intestinal nematode infections, hookworm infections usually are aggregated such that the majority of persons harbor light worm burdens, whereas a substantial minority harbor moderate or heavy infections.[56] Even after specific anthelminthic chemotherapy, the moderately and heavily infected persons appear to be predisposed toward reacquiring heavy infections.[56] Predisposition to hookworm infection may have a genetic or immunologic basis.

Pathophysiology

During the migratory phase of the infection, the larvae evoke an inflammatory response, associated with eosinophilic infiltration. Immune responses to the infection have been difficult to study in humans, but in an animal model, the dog infected with *A. caninum* can be rendered immune to challenge infections by repeated dosing with the infective larvae. This observation has provided a means of producing a live attenuated larval vaccine in the laboratory but one that is not suitable for humans. Reproduction of this larval vaccine effect by employing specifically genetically engineered polypeptides is in progress.[3, 51]

The major source of injury to the host is the loss of blood. A single *A. duodenale* organism is responsible for the loss of approximately 0.2 mL of blood per day, and an *N. americanus* organism is responsible for 0.02 mL. Rarely, massive bleeding has been reported.[52] Iron-deficiency anemia results when iron loss exceeds the host's iron reserves. Hookworms may affect cognitive development because iron is important for the development of dopaminergic neurons and for the biosynthesis of some neurotransmitters. Heavy infections result in the characteristic features of severe iron deficiency. Protein loss further contributes to malnutrition. The problem of malabsorption in hookworm infection is moot. Although it has been demonstrated in patients infected with these parasites, it appears to be a secondary effect, due to hypoproteinemia, which can be corrected by a high-protein diet without deworming of the patient.[54]

Clinical Presentation

Penetration by the larvae causes pruritus, proportional in intensity to the number of infecting larvae. The "ground itch," or "dew itch," or pruritus of the soles after walking in the morning dew is an example. The symptoms result from a hypersensitivity reaction.

The acute intestinal phase, in heavy infections, is characterized by abdominal pain, diarrhea, nausea, and anorexia.[57] After the acute phase abates, well-nourished persons with relatively light infections have no symptoms and no evidence of anemia or malnutrition. At the other extreme, heavily infected, malnourished children can have hemoglobin as low as 2 g/dL and edema due to hypoproteinemia. Infants with severe ancylostomiasis present with failure to thrive, profound pallor, and melena.[48]

Deficits in physical and intellectual growth resulting from chronic hookworm infection in childhood have been reported since the early part of this century.[9, 10] Some recovery has been described after specific anthelminthic therapy or iron supplementation, although some deficits occurring in infancy may be irreversible.

Differential and Specific Diagnoses

As in the case of ascariasis, differential diagnosis of pneumonia suggests parasitic etiology because of peripheral eosinophilia. Anemia is caused by blood loss; therefore, it must be distinguished from all other causes of intestinal loss of blood. In the developing countries, where severe hookworm anemia is common, the probability of the rarer causes of intestinal blood loss, such as Meckel diverticulum, polyps, and so on, is low. The opposite holds true for the regions where hookworm infections are light or infrequent.

Diagnosis is established by the identification of the characteristic eggs through microscopic examination of the stool. The eggs of *A. duodenale* and *N. americanus* cannot be distinguished easily from each other, but the worms can through direct examination of the infective larvae or adults. Therefore, one must assume that it is one or the other species on the basis of geographic origin of the patient. Although this decision is not of paramount importance, it does have some therapeutic implications, including the possibility that arrested larvae of *A. duodenale* will become reactivated and either repopulate the intestine sometime after treatment or enter the breast milk during or after parturition.

Treatment

For *N. americanus* infection, the drug of choice is pyrantel pamoate, given as a single dose of 11 mg/kg, not to exceed 1 g. Mebendazole (100 mg twice daily for 3 days) is equally effective but has the disadvantage that it must be given over time. *A. duodenale* infection, on the other hand, is more likely to be eradicated by mebendazole than by pyrantel pamoate; therefore, mebendazole is considered the drug of choice. Albendazole is a suitable alternative. In areas endemic for ancylostomiasis, the health provider should be aware of the potential for arrested tissue larvae for repopulating the intestine or entering breast milk and infecting infants during the perinatal period. Iron supplementation and transfusion are occasional important adjunctive therapies for pediatric hookworm infections.

Prevention

As in all cases of nematode infections transmitted through soil, sanitary control of the disposal of excreta would eliminate the infection entirely. Unfortunately, this has not been feasible in most of the world. The popular recommendation to wear shoes is naive because the most virulent species of hookworm, *A. duodenale,* is orally infective and because large segments of human populations go barefoot for economic and cultural reasons. Moreover, contact with infested soil through any segment of skin results in infection. Because infants often are placed on the soil and toddlers play in it, protection of the soles of the feet is inconsequential. Studies to investigate the possibility of vaccination against hookworm infection are in progress.[3, 51]

Enterobius vermicularis

Pinworm infection (enterobiasis), or oxyuriasis (the older term), is the most common of all human helminth infections and one that particularly is common in North America and Europe.[60] The majority of infected persons are children, and the infection is found in all socioeconomic classes. It is acquired by ingestion of the infective eggs that are picked up on the perianal skin, in the air, or on bedclothes and underwear. Swallowed eggs, transmitted to the mouth by the fingers or through inhalation, hatch in the duodenum, and the liberated larvae undergo additional maturational steps in the small intestine before reaching the cecum. There, the sexually mature worms copulate and then proceed to the rectum and eventually to the perianal skin, where the gravid females lay eggs. The eggs become infective within 2 to 4 hours after deposition. The entire cycle from the ingestion of the egg to the egg-laying phase of the gravid female is 4 to 6 weeks. Rarely, there is retrograde infection, in which eggs hatch on the anal mucosa and the larvae migrate up the bowel and mature to adult worms. Although enterobiasis is a human infection, anthropoid apes can be infected experimentally.

Epidemiology

The infection is worldwide in distribution, and children are infected most frequently. Communal living, especially assembling in school gymnasia and living in crowded households, promotes the infection. Adults tend to be infected through their contact with children; therefore, parents and teachers are the most vulnerable. Orphanages and day care centers frequently are affected.[60]

Pathophysiology

No intestinal reactions occur during the migratory phase, and, in view of the fact that there is no tissue migration, there is no eosinophilia of the order seen with some of the other nematodes. Occasionally, hypersensitive persons may experience a slight increase of eosinophils. The deposited ova induce pruritus on the perianal skin. There is no evidence that some persons are more susceptible than others to this infection.

Enterobius occasionally has been found in the vermiform appendix removed at surgery. Its causal relationship to appendicitis has not been established, but some evidence points to the possibility that this worm induces granuloma formation and, therefore, may cause obstruction of this vestigial structure.[58]

When the adult gravid female migrates along the perineal skin into the vagina, it may cause vulvitis as a reaction to the eggs deposited in that region. Some investigators speculate that migrating pinworms may introduce bacteria into the lower urinary tract, resulting in urinary tract infections.[63] Other aberrant infections, such as those causing hepatic granuloma, are rarer.[62]

Clinical Presentation

Pruritus is the most common symptom; its intensity varies from mild itching to acute, intractable pain. Secondary cellulitis also may occur in severely pruritic cases.[61] Vaginal discharge and vulval itching are symptoms in those rare cases in which a worm has migrated into the vagina. Insomnia, restlessness, irritability, loss of appetite, loss of weight, and grinding of teeth all have been reported anecdotally in persons with pinworm infections, but there is no evidence that any of them are related causally to the *Enterobius* infection. Enuresis also has been blamed on the pinworm, but one epidemiologic study failed to determine the causality.[64]

Specific Diagnosis

Enterobius vermicularis eggs are identified readily on a low-power microscopic observation of transparent adhesive tape previously applied to the perianal skin and then affixed to a microscope slide.

Treatment

Pyrantel pamoate, administered as a single dose of 11 mg/kg, not to exceed 1 g, is effective. Single-dose therapy with 100 mg of mebendazole is equally effective. With the current availability of these two highly effective drugs, intensive laundering of underwear and bed clothing, recommended in the older literature, is no longer necessary. It is advisable, however, to treat all members of the household because they all must be presumed to be infected. Re-treatment in 2 or 3 weeks to destroy any adult worms that have hatched from the eggs swallowed at the time of initial therapy may be necessary, although there is evidence that mebendazole, in contrast with pyrantel, removes young larvae as well as adult worms.[59] Neither drug destroys the eggs.

One of the most important aspects of management of this infection is reassurance that its ubiquity virtually precludes its effective eradication. Therefore, reinfection can be anticipated by any family infected with pinworms because of the high prevalence of this worm in the community. It also is important to reassure families that the presence of pinworms does not suggest poor hygienic standards in the family.

Strongyloides stercoralis and *Strongyloides fuelleborni*

Strongyloides stercoralis and *Strongyloides fuelleborni* infections are among the most virulent helminthic pathogens of humans, although they are much less prevalent than *Ascaris* or hookworm. *S. stercoralis* has the unusual ability to cause autoinfection, which can lead to hyperinfection and disseminated infection in immunocompromised hosts.[68, 70, 72–77, 83, 84] *S. fuelleborni* causes an aggressive infantile protein-losing enteropathy that leads to ascites and high mortality.[65, 66]

S. stercoralis infection is acquired by exposure of the skin to infective larvae in the soil, much as in the case of hookworm infection. Similar circumstances that promote survival of the hookworm larvae in the soil (i.e., moisture, sandy or loam soil, and shade) promote survival of *Strongyloides*. Larvae penetrate skin, facilitated by a potent histolytic protease that they secrete.[67, 80] From the moment of penetration of the skin to the arrival of the worms in the intestine, the cycle commonly is believed to be similar to that of hookworm, although experimental evidence suggests that *S. stercoralis* also may explore routes of migration that bypass the lungs.[86] Within the intestine, the small adult worms do not attach to the mucosa as do hookworms but instead lie embedded in its folds. The cycle from skin penetration to the development of mature worms in the intestine is approximately 28 days. There are no parasitic adult male worms to fertilize the eggs. Instead, the mature eggs develop by parthenogenesis. Also unlike those of other parasitic nematodes, these eggs usually are not found in the feces but instead embryonate within the intestine and develop into larvae, which are deposited in the soil with human stool. These so-called rhabditiform larvae must molt before they become infective.

This cycle has two variations. One permits the development of nonparasitic male and female adults in the soil, which can maintain infestation of the soil for a certain period; this free-living phase sometimes is called the heterogonic life cycle. The second variation has much greater clinical relevance. Under certain conditions that are still not well defined, the rhabditiform larvae molt to new infective larvae while still in the intestine. These new infective larvae can penetrate the intestine and set up a new cycle, commonly called autoinfection, or the autoinfective cycle.[75] In this fashion, this nematode, unlike most other intestinal nematodes of humans, actually can increase in number without reinfection from the outside world. This phenomenon also is responsible for the persistence of this infection for decades in an untreated host.[77] When host defenses are impaired (discussed later), *S. stercoralis* can undergo multiple rounds of autoinfection, which leads to the production of thousands or even hundreds of thousands of adult parasites in the intestine. This phenomenon is known as hyperinfection.[68, 72, 76, 83] One possible consequence of hyperinfection is disseminated infection, in which larval and adult worms are identified at extraintestinal sites.

S. fuelleborni larvae are passed on to infants by their ingestion in breast milk.[65, 69] Transmammary infection by nematode larvae is an extremely common route of transmission in nonhuman nematode infections,[8] and although it has not been well studied, probably also is common in humans.

Epidemiology

S. stercoralis infection has a worldwide distribution, but it is most prevalent in the tropical and subtropical regions. In North America, strongyloidiasis is focally endemic in some parts of Appalachia[70] and is common among Southeast Asian immigrants.[78] In one study, 76.6 per cent of Kampuchean immigrants and 55.6 per cent of Laotian immigrants were seropositive for *S. stercoralis* infection.[78] Strongyloidiasis also is endemic in Jamaica and presumably elsewhere in the Caribbean.[84] Because of the possibility of autoinfection and, by extension, infection through contamination of skin by infested feces, strongyloidiasis is highly prevalent in mental hospitals, prisons, and homes for retarded children. Dogs and anthropoid apes may serve as animal reservoir hosts for *S. stercoralis. S. fuelleborni* infection is endemic in Papua New Guinea and parts of sub-Saharan Africa.[65, 66]

Pathophysiology

During the migratory phase of the infection, the larvae of *S. stercoralis* evoke an inflammatory response associated with eosinophilic infiltration. The adult phase in the intestine, even in moderate infections, may be associated with an inflammatory reaction, sufficient to be symptomatic. There is evidence that *Strongyloides* induces a malabsorption syndrome, which has been treated effectively by deworming.[70, 82] It is of interest that this form of malabsorption involves steatorrhea, but D-xylose absorption is normal. The explanation for this dissociation is not available, but at least one speculation suggests that malabsorption is caused by edema of the lamina propria caused by the release of histamine from mast cells.[82] Young children with *S. stercoralis*–induced malabsorption experience growth stunting and failure to thrive.[70]

The deficits in host defense that promote hyperinfection and disseminated strongyloidiasis are not well understood. Although cell-mediated immune deficits, such as those occurring in immunosuppression, organ transplantation, severe malnutrition, and cytotoxic chemotherapy for neoplasms and collagen-vascular diseases, are associated with this phenomenon, certain established deficits in cell-mediated immunity, such as those in HIV infection, do not trigger hyperinfection necessarily.[75] It has been suggested that patients receiving large doses of corticosteroids particularly are susceptible to hyperinfection because the corticosteroids themselves function as direct signals or ligands for the parasite to undergo autoinfection.[75] It is interesting that patients in Japan and Jamaica with human T-cell lymphotropic virus type I appear to be at high risk for opportunistic strongyloidiasis,[73] possibly because of a specific deficit in their effector IgE immune responses.[84]

The pathogenesis of the marked protein-losing enteropathy that leads to ascites in the swollen belly syndrome of *S. fuelleborni* infection has not been established.

Clinical Presentation

During the migratory phase of larval strongyloidiasis, patients can develop pneumonitis associated with eosinophilia. Larval migration through the skin can result in larva currens. Although the majority of patients harboring *S. stercoralis* in their intestine are asymptomatic, those with moderate or heavy infections classically have intense diarrhea productive of watery, mucous stool. There may be periods of alternating diarrhea and constipation. Anorexia and cachexia, which lead to failure to thrive and other deficits in physical growth, are common features of pediatric strongyloidiasis.[70]

In disseminated strongyloidiasis due to the hyperinfective cycle, larvae may invade all tissues, including the central nervous system. Moreover, because the larvae penetrate the intestine, they may carry with them enteric flora and cause sepsis or meningoencephalitis.[68] Although diarrhea is the most commonly recognized consequence of *Strongyloides* infection, it is the hyperinfective cycle that has the greatest portent for immunosuppressed patients.

Infants with *S. fuelleborni* infection may manifest the swollen belly syndrome with marked abdominal ascites and pleural effusions that can be fatal.

Differential and Specific Diagnoses

Strongyloides pneumonitis can resemble the clinical manifestations of lung migrations of other nematode parasites, such as *Ascaris* and hookworm. Differential diagnosis of the diarrhea must include causes of chronic diarrheal disease. However, in view of its association with marked eosinophilia, diarrhea due to *Strongyloides* ought not to be confused with diarrhea due to the enteric bacteria or the pathogenic protozoa. Likewise, the noninfectious causes of diarrhea, such as regional enteritis and ulcerative colitis, are not likely.

The diagnosis is established by identification of the characteristic larvae during microscopic examination of the stool. This is not easy because rhabditiform larvae usually are not produced in abundance. Specific stool concentration techniques are available to increase the sensitivity of fecal examination, although they are not as effective as amplifying the heterogonic life cycle by the Baermann technique or looking for characteristic larval tracks on nutrient agar plates.[87] The stools of all immunosuppressed persons, including those given corticosteroids for any reason, who have ever been in a region where *Strongyloides* is found must be examined to rule out this infection. If the routine stool examination results are negative, the stool should be processed as outlined earlier. In addition, examination of duodenal contents can be attempted, either by an aspiration or by the string test (Enterotest). This, however, only divulges contents of the duodenum and can miss the larvae in the lower small intestine. An enzyme-linked immunosorbent assay looking for *Strongyloides*-specific antibodies is available on a research basis.[78, 84]

Children with the swollen belly syndrome from *S. fuelleborni* infection shed eggs in their feces rather than larvae. Large numbers of eggs are common in clinical cases.

Treatment

The drug of choice for both *S. stercoralis* and *S. fuelleborni* infections is thiabendazole, administered at a dose of 50 mg/kg/24 hours, divided into two equal doses on each of 2 successive days. In disseminated strongyloidiasis, thiabendazole should be continued for at least 5 days. Thiabendazole still is considered by the Food and Drug Administration to be an investigational drug for this condition. Nevertheless, it is an effective drug with a cure rate in nondisseminated infections approaching 100 per cent.[71] The drug is not without side effects, most frequently nausea, vomiting, and vertigo. Rarely, it induces leukopenia, skin rashes, and even Stevens-Johnson syndrome. Because the drug is detoxified in the liver, its dose may have to be reduced for patients with liver failure. In case of only partial removal of the worms, the therapy may be repeated. Treatment with ivermectin gives a cure rate of 80 per cent.[79, 81] Its application as routine therapy must await further studies. Because the mortality rate of patients with disseminated strongyloidiasis remains high despite thiabendazole therapy, it is not uncommon to add ivermectin to the treatment regimen. No published studies indicate whether this practice is effective. Because secondary bacterial complications, such as sepsis and meningitis, are common with disseminated strongyloidiasis, judicious use of broad-spectrum antimicrobial agents often is indicated for this condition. As an additional supportive measure, patients on high-dose therapy with corticosteroids with hyperinfective strongyloidiasis probably benefit from steroid taper. Curiously, transplant patients receiving cyclosporine may benefit from some of the direct helminthotoxic properties of this compound.[85]

Prognosis

Prognosis is excellent in patients who do not have disseminated infection and who are treated promptly. Unrecognized disseminated infection can be lethal.

Prevention

Proper disposal of human excreta reduces substantially the prevalence of strongyloidiasis in any community. In closed institutions, where control of direct spread is unlikely, identification and treatment of the infected persons are the only feasible controls.[74]

ABERRANT INFECTIONS WITH INTESTINAL NEMATODES

Toxocara canis

As indicated in the previous sections, the life cycles of the intestinal nematodes are adjusted precisely through evolutionary selection. In many instances, only one host in which the cycle can be completed is parasitized by the nematode. Infections of an unnatural host, in most cases, lead to complete failure of development and cause no disease. In a few instances, an infection may be established but the cycle is not completed. Under such circumstances, the process of aberrant migration of the larvae may be more pathogenic than the steps in the natural cycle.

One of the most dramatic examples of an aberrant infection is that with *Toxocara canis,* called visceral larva migrans. This roundworm causes intestinal infection in the dog, in which its cycle resembles that of *A. lumbricoides* in humans. People become infected by *Toxocara* through the ingestion of an embryonated egg, much as in the human infection with *Ascaris.* Larvae hatch in the small intestine, penetrate the villi, and begin a migration that takes them through every organ and tissue of the body. Because they cannot mature, the larvae tend to migrate for months, until they are overcome by the inflammatory reaction of the host and die. Although larvae of other toxocarids, such as *Toxocara cati* and *Toxascaris leonina,* have been suggested as possible causes of visceral larva migrans, they probably are much less important as zoonotic pathogens in humans.

Epidemiology

Prevalence of toxocariasis is difficult to assess because of the failure of diagnosis in many cases. The disease has been reported from many parts of the world, and it can be assumed that it is found wherever humans and dogs coexist. Young children often come into contact with *T. canis* eggs while playing in sandboxes and on playgrounds that were contaminated by a family pet.[98, 99, 101] The level of contamination of public areas also is difficult to ascertain. In several studies, the presence of the ova was reported in 5 to 25 per cent of soil samples obtained, and surveys of dogs in urban communities have shown frequent infection, particularly in puppies, which almost universally are infected with *T. canis* (canine infection occurs transplacentally).[88, 95] The seroprevalence of toxocariasis in the United States is high, and the parasite should be considered an emerging pathogen in some urban areas. Among some groups of socioeconomically disadvantaged black children, the seroprevalence is as high as 30 per cent.[98, 104] High rates have been described in some institutional settings.[100] Major risk factors for acquiring toxocariasis include having a litter of puppies in the home and the habit of geophagia.[102] The latter risk factor probably accounts for an observed association between toxocariasis and elevated lead levels.[102]

The incidence of a positive skin test for toxocariasis statistically is associated with poliomyelitis.[108] No direct causal relationship exists; it is possible that the circumstances leading to ingestion of *Toxocara* ova also are conducive to ingestion of poliomyelitis virus. Likewise, seizures are correlated with seropositivity for *Toxocara* antibodies, but a causal relationship has not been established.[89] Some investigators have postulated that toxocariasis may be an important cause of so-called idiopathic seizures in young children.[98]

Pathophysiology

The entire infection is restricted to the migratory phase and therefore represents an "exaggeration" of the symptoms found during the early phases of *A. lumbricoides* infection. Symptoms are protean and depend on which organ or tissue is infected. For unknown reasons, visceral migration through the liver, lungs, and brain is more common in toddlers and children younger than 5 years of age, whereas older children tend to have ocular involvement almost exclusively.[98, 99, 101] Thus, there is epidemiologic evidence that this infection produces two distinct syndromes, visceral and ocular, because involvement of one tends to occur in the absence of the other.[97] Visceral migration elicits eosinophilic granuloma formation in the target organs leading to hepatitis, pneumonitis, or cerebritis. Larval migration in the retina leads to ocular larva migrans, which includes granuloma formation in the retina.[90, 94, 106] The lesion so resembles retinoblastoma that often it is confused with it. Endophthalmitis[94] or papillitis[93] also may develop. Invasion of other organs and tissues induces granuloma formation there.

Clinical Presentation

Visceral larva migrans typically presents in a young child with symptoms and signs of a multisystem disease, associated with fever, hepatosplenomegaly, lung infiltrates accompanied by wheezing, a high degree of eosinophilia (approaching 80 per cent), and elevation of the immunoglobulins, particularly of the IgM class.[96, 99, 101, 102] Seizures and neuropsychiatric disturbances also are common. In one case report, the child's major neurologic manifestation was a static encephalopathy.[96]

In contrast, ocular larva migrans presents with unilateral vision deficit and, sometimes, strabismus. Ophthalmologic examination frequently reveals one or more posterior poles or peripheral pole granulomas.[94, 101, 106] More global eye inflammation also can occur (discussed earlier). Children with ocular involvement usually present with few, if any, systemic manifestations. Often, no laboratory abnormalities are detected.

Differential and Specific Diagnoses

Visceral larva migrans must be distinguished from the migratory phase of the other nematode infections. Because of hepatosplenomegaly and hypereosinophilia, eosinophilic leukemia occasionally has been suspected, but it can be ruled out readily by bone marrow examination.

T. canis larvae can be identified in tissues, as, for example, in liver biopsy, but the diagnostic yield is low. Therefore, one must resort to indirect means, recognizing that a multisystem disease with elevation of IgM and hypereosinophilia fits the diagnostic criteria. An enzyme-linked immunosorbent assay test available at the Centers for Disease Control and Prevention is highly specific and diagnostic.[101, 104, 105]

Ocular larva migrans usually is diagnosed by an experienced ophthalmologist who recognizes the characteristic granulomas and larval tracks on retinal examination. Presumably because of minimal antigen presentation by a few migrating larvae in the eye, there often is no measurable immune response in this condition. For this reason, the enzyme-linked immunosorbent assay often is not reliable for making the diagnosis of ocular larva migrans.[98, 101, 102, 104, 105]

Treatment

Traditionally, treatment for visceral larva migrans primarily was symptomatic, especially because much of the morbidity is associated with immunopathologic responses against dying parasites. In the 1960s, thiabendazole and diethylcarbamazine were determined to be effective against the migrating larvae.[103] Since then, new agents of the benzimidazole class have been claimed to be equally effective but associated with fewer drug toxicities.[99] In a comparative study with thiabendazole, the drug albendazole (10 mg/kg/day in two divided doses for 5 days) was shown to be well tolerated and less toxic.[107] Another benzimidazole, mebendazole, also may be effective when given in doses high enough to achieve significant extraintestinal levels.[91] Although anecdotal experience with albendazole and mebendazole overseas suggests that these drugs are safe in children,[92] the large doses required for treatment of larva migrans may be associated with hepatic and other toxicities (including embryotoxicities) and therefore have not been approved for this purpose.

Treatment of ocular larva migrans often requires surgical management, particularly in cases associated with tractional retinal detachment.[94, 106] Specific anthelminthic adjunct chemotherapy appears to be of benefit in some cases.[94, 99, 106]

Prognosis

Except for the patients in whom blindness develops as a consequence of retinal damage and a rare fatal case resulting from the intensity of the acute clinical reaction, the vast majority of patients recover. However, the recovery phase may be slow, lasting up to 2 years.

Prevention

Theoretically, the disease can be prevented by elimination of dog feces from the human environment, but in practice this is no less difficult than control of human excrement disposal.

Other Aberrant Infections with Intestinal Nematodes

Baylisascaris procyonis, a parasite of raccoons, also can cause visceral larva migrans. *Baylisascaris* infection occurs when humans accidentally ingest parasite eggs that are shed in barn lofts and attics accessible to raccoons.[101, 116, 118] In at least one reported human case, the infection was fatal in an infant.[116] Like the infection caused by *Toxocara, Baylisascaris* larvae within aberrant hosts cannot complete their cycle and continue their aimless migration through the tissues of these hosts. The lesions caused by the larvae are eosinophilic granulomas, which tend to be concentrated in the central nervous system, resulting in eosinophilic meningitis. Neither the frequency nor the range of severity of this infection in humans is known. Most human cases have been diagnosed at autopsy. Currently, there is no literature on specific anthelminthic chemotherapy.

Other, less severe aberrant infections of importance to humans are those caused by the dog hookworm, primarily *Ancylostoma braziliense,* but also *A. caninum* and *Uncinaria stenocephala.*[49, 114, 115, 126] Infection with the larvae of *A. braziliense* and *U. stenocephala* cannot be completed, and they remain viable and migrate in the skin (usually between the epidermis and dermis)—hence the terms cutaneous larva migrans and creeping eruption. Failure of these zoonotic hookworms to complete entry through the human skin may reflect differences in their released hydrolytic enzymes.[114, 115] Infection is acquired in the same fashion as that of the human hookworms. Children who expose their whole bodies to the contaminated soil may be infected at any site. Adults are most likely to develop infection in the lower extremities, but plumbers in the tropics, who often must crawl beneath houses, acquire infection on the elbows and knees. The interval from exposure to first symptoms is approximately 2 weeks; papules 2 mm in diameter then begin to appear on the skin. Behind them usually are serpiginous, erythematous, intracutaneous tunnels. The entire area itches intensely. Left untreated, cutaneous larva migrans tends to last 2 months. Thiabendazole or albendazole is effective when administered orally. Topical therapy with 15 per cent aqueous suspension of thiabendazole was successful in one reported series. Forty-seven of 50 patients achieved permanent cure in 2 weeks, and 2 more patients were cured after a third week.[129] Placebo-treated patients were used as controls in this study. In contrast with skin penetration of zoonotic hookworms, oral ingestion of the dog hookworm *A. caninum* results in an eosinophilic enteritis syndrome, which is discussed in the section on hookworm infection.

Rarer aberrant infections include those caused by various species of *Trichostrongylus, Oesophagostomum, Angiostrongylus, Capillaria,* and *Anisakis. Trichostrongylus* is a common parasite of many mammals, and it has been found in the small intestine of humans, mainly in Asia, Africa, and Australia. Ingestion of larvae leads to the development of adult worms in the small intestine. Whether this leads to any disease remains a moot point because infections tend to be mild and usually are associated with other helminth infections.[113] *Oesophagostomum bifurcum* is a common nematode of subhuman primates in Africa and has been reported to be a relatively common intestinal nematode that causes nodular disease of the intestines in humans living in West Africa.[120, 123] Human oesophagostomiasis has been treated successfully with pyrantel pamoate.[120]

Land snails and slugs serve as the intermediate hosts for *Angiostrongylus* species. *Angiostrongylus cantonensis* is a cause of eosinophilic meningitis throughout East Asia and Hawaii[111, 119, 124, 125]; *Angiostrongylus costaricensis* is a cause of mesenteric arteritis and abdominal pain in Central and South America and among Latin American immigrants to the United States.[117] The rat serves as the natural host of these parasites, which live either in the lung *(A. cantonensis)* or mesenteric arteries *(A. costaricensis).* The rat eats the infected mollusks and thus ingests the larvae, which migrate to their final destination. People who ingest either the mollusks or food contaminated by the mollusks develop an incomplete infection. *A. cantonensis* infection usually is limited to the central nervous system, occurring as eosinophilic meningitis.[111, 119, 124, 125] Signs and symptoms include meningismus, severe headache, paresthesias, and, less commonly, cranial nerve palsies. No specific treatment is available (although the anthelminthics thiabendazole and ivermectin are effective in some experimental animal models[111]), but the disease is self-limited, lasting no more than 2 weeks. Symptomatic relief has been reported with the use of prednisone. In contrast, *A. costaricensis* infection typically presents with abdominal or right iliac fossa pain, fever, and eosinophilia. Children with this condition may be diagnosed as having appendicitis or Meckel diverticulum.[117] High doses of mebendazole have been tried as a treatment for this condition.

Capillaria philippinensis is a common parasite of water fowl in the Philippines.[110] The mode of transmission of this parasite to people is unknown, but human cases have been reported in which as many as 40,000 adult worms were found embedded in the crypts of the small intestine. *C. philippinensis,* like *S. stercoralis,* can undergo autoinfection and hyperinfection in humans.[110] There is no associated inflammatory reaction, but flattening of villi, loss of epithelial surface, and severe malabsorption have been reported.[110, 112, 128] In one series of 1000 cases of *C. philippinensis* infections, a mortality rate of 10 per cent was reported.[112] Thiabendazole may be effective in shortening the course of the infection,[128] although albendazole more recently has become the treatment of choice.[110] Another member of the genus, *Capillaria hepatica,* a rare zoonosis of humans, has been known to disseminate to the lungs, liver, and other viscera.[122]

Anisakis species are nematode parasites of marine mammals, with fish being the intermediate hosts. When the infective larvae of the parasite are ingested as a result of eating raw or poorly cooked fish, they may become embedded in the gastric mucosa and cause eosinophilic granuloma.[50, 109, 121, 127, 130, 131] In adults, it may resemble carcinoma of the stomach both clinically and radiographically. Human anisakiasis occurs with considerable frequency in Japan, where raw marine fish are eaten commonly, and in Holland, where lightly pickled herring is considered a delicacy.

FILARIAL PARASITES

Except for rare instances of zoonotic *Brugia* infections,[132, 137] the filarial worms parasitizing humans affect people within the geographic area almost entirely limited by the two Tropics. Although accurate data are lacking, the latest World Health Organization estimates suggest that 400 million people are infected with one or more filarial worms. The various human parasites in this category have certain characteristics in common. They are all spread by vectors, and the adults invade and occupy the lymphatics, skin, connective tissue, or blood. They produce live embryos, called microfilariae, which enter the blood stream or skin, where they can survive for weeks or even years without further development. The range of diseases caused by these worms is wide; some produce no symptoms, and others can be responsible for severe clinical disorders.

The life cycles of the filarial worms are similar in that infections are acquired through an insect bite, during which transmission of microfilariae is accomplished by transference of the infective larvae onto the skin of the host from the mouthparts of the insect. The larvae then enter the wound in the skin and make their way to the respective tissue, where they mature into adult worms. The adults mate and produce live larvae, which migrate to the blood through the walls of the lymphatics or through the thoracic duct. They are ingested by blood-sucking insects, in which they undergo metamorphosis through two larval stages until they reach the third, infective stage. The interval from the infective bite to the appearance of microfilariae in the blood of the host can be as long as 6 months.

The host develops immunologic responses to the filarial infections, which can be used for immunodiagnosis. More significant, these immunologic host inflammatory responses themselves elicit pathology. Indeed, some of the most dramatic clinical manifestations of human filarial infections (e.g., elephantiasis, river blindness) usually result from immunopathologic-mediated damage occurring over a period of years. For that reason, these sequelae are not common in children.

Lymphatic Filariasis: *Wuchereria bancrofti* and *Brugia* Species

Epidemiology

Wuchereria bancrofti is prevalent primarily between the two Tropics but also is encountered north of the Tropic of Cancer in Africa. As many as 400 million people may suffer from lymphatic filariasis caused by this parasite. In each of its geographic locales, it has a specific anopheline or culicine mosquito vector. In the Caribbean area, South America, Asia, East and West Africa, and New Guinea, the microfilariae of this worm exhibit nocturnal periodicity; in the South Pacific, their periodicity is diurnal. *W. bancrofti* has no animal hosts.

Brugia malayi occurs in India, Malaysia, and other parts of Southeast Asia. Some strains of *B. malayi* are associated with animal reservoirs, as are some other members of the genus *Brugia,* such as *Brugia timori.* In the United States, zoonotic *Brugia* infections caused by *Brugia beaveri* and *Brugia lepori* have been reported in humans.[132, 137]

Pathophysiology

The initial host response is that of inflammation around dead and dying adult worms in the lymphatics, resulting in lymphangitis, which leads eventually to the enlargement of the affected lymph nodes, then hyperplasia, epithelioid granulomas, and eventual fibrosis. It develops with a characteristic, painful, cord-like swelling, associated with a reddish streak on the overlying skin. This usually is associated with a systemic reaction of fever, headache, and general malaise. Inflammatory reactions of other tissues, such as testes and synovial membranes, also occur occasionally. The obstruction also may lead to chyluria and chylous diarrhea. In the majority of infected persons, the response is not severe enough to cause clinical disease. This especially is true of children because the clinical manifestations are a result of years of repeated infections. The microfilariae themselves apparently are harmless.

Clinical Presentation

Children living in endemic areas often develop asymptomatic microfilaremia. It is believed that with repeated exposure these children will later, as adolescents or young adults, begin to have occasional episodes of acute lymphangitis with some systemic manifestations. These "filarial fevers" often are accompanied by headache, malaise, and myalgias.[134] Benign lymphedema has been described in a few patients in the United States with zoonotic *Brugia* infections.[132, 137]

Clinical lymphatic filariasis results in lymphatic blockage through fibrosis, causing lymphedema proximal to the obstruction. This leads to the development of classic elephantiasis of the scrotum or labia majora and lower extremities.

Chronic, recurrent pneumonitis associated with wheezing, cough, chest pain, pulmonary infiltrations, and hypereosinophilia is a hypersensitivity reaction caused by the migration of microfilariae through the lungs. This condition, known as tropical pulmonary eosinophilia, is common among young adult males living in parts of the Indian subcontinent.[135]

Differential and Specific Diagnoses

Differential diagnosis of lymphatic obstruction in children should rule out other more likely conditions before focusing on filariasis. In older children and adults, familial lymphedema (Milroy disease) can mimic filariasis.

Diagnosis only becomes definitive with the identification of the characteristic microfilariae in the blood. In view of the circadian periodicity of the appearance of large numbers of larvae in the blood, a specimen should be collected at the appropriate time. It need not be examined immediately but may be placed in a large volume of formalin for subsequent concentration and staining. It also is possible to provoke the migration of microfilariae into the peripheral circulation at other times by administering diethylcarbamazine. Immunodiagnostic tests that measure either specific antibody or even filarial antigen are under development.[133, 134]

Treatment

There is a need for new agents that would be effective against the adult filarial worm and at the same time elicit minimal immunopathologic damage.[138] Currently, the major drugs employed are effective mainly in eradicating the microfilariae. Although diethylcarbamazine remains the standard drug, ivermectin—currently classified as an experimental drug—may be better therapy. Side effects of specific antifilarial therapy include allergic and febrile reactions, which may be caused by the release of worm antigens rather than by the drug itself. These systemic manifestations can be treated symptomatically with antihistamines or corticosteroids.

Ivermectin has the advantage over diethylcarbamazine because only a single oral dose is required. It also may be more effective than diethylcarbamazine. A double-blind, randomized clinical trial comparing this new drug with the older one showed that it cleared microfilariae of all 26 men treated, in contrast with a cure rate of 79 per cent (11 of 14 patients) with diethylcarbamazine.[136]

The difficulty in management of filariasis by drugs is that late symptoms, such as elephantiasis, do not abate. The main usefulness of chemotherapy is in cases recognized early, before the anatomic abnormalities develop. The latter can be treated surgically if they are disfiguring or if they interfere with normal life.

Prevention

Prevention depends on vector control, which has been less than satisfactory, primarily because of the difficulties of the development of effective insecticides that also would be nontoxic to the rest of the environment. Periodic massive treatment with diethylcarbamazine of populations at risk has merit, especially because there is no known animal reservoir (with the sole exception in Malaya) for this infection.

Loa loa

Loa loa infection is limited to a small area of western and central Africa and is spread by the *Chrysops* flies. Periodicity in the *Loa loa* microfilariae is diurnal. The parasites elicit a number of allergic inflammatory responses that are most evident in expatriates.[140–142] These persons develop high eosinophilia and recurrent angioedema, which when localized develop into painful, pruritic, subcutaneous swellings, known as Calabar swellings, which appear on the extremities and the face. Rarely, some cases of lymphatic obstruction of the lower extremities and hydroceles have been reported.

The most dramatic manifestation of this infection is an occasional appearance of a migrating *Loa loa* adult under the conjunctiva of the eye. It does not damage the eye and can be removed surgically. Treatment with diethylcarbamazine, as indicated earlier, effectively destroys the adults, but reactions may be more intense than in the therapy of *Wuchereria* and *Brugia* infections.[139] Coadministration of corticosteroids often is required during treatment. Allergic encephalopathy has been described in patients receiving diethylcarbamazine.[139] Ivermectin appears to elicit fewer allergic symptoms during treatment and generally may be less toxic.

Onchocerca volvulus

Onchocerca volvulus infection is acquired through the bite of the *Simulium* fly, which tends to breed along the rivers and streams (hence the name of the disease: river blindness).

Epidemiology

The disease is limited to Africa, Central America, and northern parts of South America. In view of human dependence on water and the establishment of settlements along the rivers, the frequency of infections tends to be high in the areas where *Simulium* prevails. The development of hydroelectric power, based on construction of large dams, has increased the breeding sites of *Simulium* and hence has increased the incidence of *Onchocerca* infection.

Pathophysiology

Larvae deposited by the *Simulium* bite remain in the subcutaneous tissue and develop there into adult worms. Adult worms tend to become coiled, and worms of both sexes become enveloped by fibrous tissues and form nodules within which they reproduce. The larvae produced by the fertilized females invade the skin, where they remain until they are picked up by a *Simulium* bite or they die some 30 months later. In addition to the skin, the microfilariae penetrate the eye and affect every layer from the conjunctiva to the optic nerve. In African onchocerciasis, chorioretinitis and optic atrophy are common; in the Central American disease, iritis is the primary lesion.

The probability of the development of the eye disease relates to the location of the adult worms. When the nodules are situated about the head, the eye lesions are common; when they are in the lower parts of the body, the eye lesions are less frequent. In Africa, the nodules tend to be distributed primarily in the lower parts of the body, but because of the high prevalence of the infection, onchocercal blindness is common. In Central America, the lesions tend to be on the upper part of the body.

Clinical Presentation

The appearance of the skin nodules and the presence of live microfilariae within the eye (readily seen with an ophthalmoscope) are the manifestations of early and intermediate disease. Later the eye involvement includes keratitis, iridocyclitis, chorioretinitis, and eventual blindness. The microfilariae in the skin cause an inflammatory reaction, which includes acute pruritus and chronic changes, such as edema, hypertrophy, and reddish hyperpigmentation (peau d'orange).

Differential and Specific Diagnoses

Because the skin invasion is associated with itching, the pruritus of onchocercal infections must be differentiated from contact dermatitis, prickly heat, and insect bites.

Onchocerciasis is identified by examination of a skin snip. Examination of sectioned and stained tissue or stained impression smear reveals microfilariae.

Treatment

Surgical removal of all the visible nodules may extirpate radically the source of new microfilariae, which invade the eye. Chemotherapy with ivermectin is the treatment of choice. Ivermectin also can be used in mass treatment to interrupt transmission by the vector and thus to control the incidence of this infection.[143, 144] The older drug, diethylcarbamazine, has no role in the treatment of onchocerciasis because of its highly pathogenic side effects.

Prevention

Vector control, periodic treatment of the infected persons, and surgical removal of skin lesions by roving teams of physicians and other health care workers currently are the only means of prevention, but their success is limited.

Mansonella perstans and *Mansonella ozzardi*

Neither *Mansonella perstans* nor *Mansonella ozzardi* is known to cause significant human pathology, but the microfilariae present in the blood must be distinguished morphologically from those of the other more pathogenic filariae. *M. ozzardi* is found throughout the Caribbean (especially Haiti) and Central America. It has been suggested as a cause of chronic arthritis in these regions. *M. perstans* also is found in Africa, where it has been identified as a cause of painless nodules in the conjunctiva and secondary eyelid swelling. For that reason, it sometimes is called the Kampala or Ugandan eye worm.[145]

Dirofilaria immitis

Dirofilaria immitis is a filarial worm commonly found in dogs, in which it occupies the right ventricle of the heart. It produces microfilariae, which circulate in blood and are transmitted to new animals through the bite of culicine mosquitoes. Fewer than 100 cases of human infection have been reported, none of them in children. Most human hosts infected with *Dirofilaria* were asymptomatic, but those who had symptoms complained of chest pains, wheezing, and cough. All of the infected persons had coin lesions detected on pulmonary radiographs.[146, 147] It is possible that lesions in the pediatric age group have been missed because they might have been considered to represent a Ghon complex.

Human infection probably is transmitted through the mosquito bite, but this has not been established. As with visceral larva migrans, the microfilariae of *D. immitis* cannot complete their cycle in humans. No microfilariae of this worm have ever been demonstrated in human peripheral blood. All patients evaluated for pulmonary dirofilariasis have had mild peripheral eosinophilia, usually not exceeding 10 per cent. Because the radiographic picture is not diagnostic and in view of the potential seriousness of a coin lesion,[146] the lesion must be examined histologically. If a worm is found, the diagnosis of dirofilariasis can be made; if it is not found, the diagnosis still is tenable. In the presence of eosinophilia and pneumonitis, however, a whole range of other diagnostic possibilities must be considered, including eosinophilic pneumonia, polyarteritis nodosa, Wegener granulomatosis, and histiocytosis X. No treatment is necessary for this infection of humans.

Dracunculus medinensis

Infection by *Dracunculus medinensis* also is limited largely to the tropics. The adult female worm lies in the subcutaneous tissue and can extend over a length of 50 to 120 cm. There is no information about the fate of the male. The adult lives for up to 18 months. At the end of the first year of infection, the adult female migrates to the subcutaneous tissues, where it produces an indurated papule, which tends to vesiculate and ulcerate. When the surface of the ulcer comes in contact with water, the worm discharges motile larvae. These are, in turn, ingested by a crustacean, *Cyclops*, in which they undergo additional maturation and development. Humans become infected by swallowing the *Cyclops* in drinking water. The larvae then penetrate through the gut into the subcutaneous tissue by a route not yet fully understood. Multiple infections are common. In Nigeria, this disease has been reported to cause 25 per cent absenteeism in school children.[149] Secondary bacterial infections leading to cellulitis are common, as are secondary arthritis and contractures that can lead to permanent disability.[149]

Stagnant water is necessary for the maintenance of the infection, which therefore tends to be infrequent where running water and properly constructed wells are available. Diagnosis is established readily by the observation of the emerging larvae from a cutaneous ulcer. Moreover, the outline of the worm can be seen readily under the skin.

The classic treatment of this infection involves incision of the skin and tying the end of the worm to a small piece of wood. By daily turning of the wood, it is possible to extract the worm over a period of several weeks. This is an unsatisfactory therapy, often resulting in failure of complete extraction. If the worm tears, it releases into the subcutaneous tissues larvae that provoke intense inflammatory reaction and skin sloughing. It is far better to continue exposing the protruding end of the worm to water, so that larvae can be extruded completely before forcible extraction is attempted.

Treatment with chemotherapeutic agents, such as niridazole, metronidazole, thiabendazole, and mebendazole, is controversial. Some investigators report that treatment with these agents helps to decrease inflammation and facilitate removal of the worm.

Because filtering of the drinking water effectively would prevent this infection, there is optimism that this parasite can be eradicated through appropriate control measures.[148–150]

References

INTESTINAL NEMATODES

1. Bundy, D. A. P.: New initiatives in the control of helminths. Trans. R. Soc. Trop. Med. Hyg. *84*:467–468, 1990.
2. Hall, A.: Intestinal worms and the growth of children. Trans. R. Soc. Trop. Med. Hyg. *87*:241–242, 1993.
3. Hotez, P. J., and Pritchard, D. I.: Hookworm infection. Sci. Am. *272*:68–75, 1995.
4. Kvalsvig, J. D., Cooppan, R. M., and Connolly, K. J.: The effects of parasite

infections on cognitive processes in children. Ann. Trop. Med. Parasitol. *85*:551–568, 1991.
5. Nokes, C., Cooper, E. S., Robinson, B. A., et al.: Geohelminth infection and academic assessment in Jamaican children. Trans. R. Soc. Trop. Med. Hyg. *85*:272–273, 1991.
6. Nokes, C., Grantham-McGregor, S. M., Sawyer, A. W., et al.: Parasitic helminth infection and cognitive function in school children. Proc. R. Soc. Lond. B. 77–81, 1992.
7. Savioli L., Bundy, D., and Tomkins, A.: Intestinal parasitic infections: A soluble public health problem. Trans. R. Soc. Trop. Med. Hyg. *86*:353–354, 1992.
8. Shoop, W. L.: Vertical transmission of helminths: Hypobiosis and amphiparatenesis. Parasitol. Today *7*:51–54, 1991.
9. Smillie, W. G., and Augustine, D. L.: Hookworm infestation: The effect of varying intensities on the physical condition of school children. Am. J. Dis. Child. *31*:151–168, 1926.
10. Smillie, W. G., and Spencer, C. R.: Mental retardation in school children infested with hookworms. J. Educ. Psychol. *17*:314–321, 1926.
11. Stephenson, L. S.: Helminth parasites, a major factor in malnutrition. World Health Forum *15*:169–172, 1994.
12. Stephenson, L. S., Latham, M. C., Kinoti, S. N., et al.: Improvements in physical fitness of Kenyan schoolboys infected with hookworm, *Trichuris trichiura*, and *Ascaris lumbricoides* following a single dose of albendazole. Trans. R. Soc. Trop. Med. Hyg. *84*:277–282, 1990.
13. Stephenson, L. S., Latham, M. C., Kurz, K. M., et al.: Treatment with a single dose of albendazole improves growth of Kenyan schoolchildren with hookworm, *Trichuris trichiura*, and *Ascaris lumbricoides* infections. Am. J. Trop. Med. Hyg. *41*:78–87, 1989.

Ascaris lumbricoides

14. Anderson, T. J. C.: *Ascaris* infections in humans from North America: Molecular evidence for cross-infection. Parasitology *110*:215–219, 1995.
15. Blumenthal, D. S., and Schultz, M. G.: Incidence of intestinal obstruction in children infected with *Ascaris lumbricoides*. Am. J. Trop. Med. Hyg. *24*:801–805, 1975.
16. Christie, J. F., Dunbar, B., Davidson, I., et al.: N-terminal amino acid sequence identity between a major allergen of *Ascaris lumbricoides* and *Ascaris suum*, and MHC-restricted IgE responses to it. Immunology *69*:596–602, 1990.
17. Chu, W. G., Chen, P. M., Huang, C. C., et al.: Neonatal ascariasis. J. Pediatr. *81*:783–785, 1972.
18. Costa-Macedo, L. M., and Rey, L.: *Ascaris lumbricoides* in neonate: Evidence of congenital transmission of intestinal nematodes. Rev. Inst. Med. Trop. São Paulo *32*:351–354, 1990.
19. Crompton, D. W. T.: Ascariasis and childhood malnutrition. Trans. R. Soc. Trop. Med. Hyg. *86*:577–579, 1992.
20. Grasberger, B. L., Clore, G. M., and Gronenborn, A. M.: High resolution structure of *Ascaris* trypsin inhibitor in solution: Direct evidence for a pH-induced conformational transition in the reactive site. Structure *2*:669–678, 1994.
21. Hall, A., and Romanova, T.: *Ascaris lumbricoides*: Detecting its metabolites in the urine of the infected people using gas-liquid chromatography. Exp. Parasitol. *70*:35–42, 1990.
22. Haswell-Elkins, M. R., Kennedy, M. W., Maizels, R. M., et al.: Detection of *Ascaris* metabolites in the urine by gas-liquid chromatography also correlates with the worm burden. Parasite Immunol. *11*:615–627, 1989.
23. Huang, K., Strynadka, N. C., Bernard, V. D., et al.: The molecular structure of the complex of *Ascaris* chymotrypsin/elastase inhibitor with porcine elastase. Structure *2*:679–689, 1994.
24. Khuroo, M. S., Zargar S. A., and Mahajan, R.: Hepatobiliary and pancreatic ascariasis in India. Lancet *335*:1503–1506, 1990.
25. Koino, S.: Experimental infections on human body with ascarides. Jpn. Med. World *2*:317–320, 1922.
26. Pamba, H. O., Bwibo, N. O., Chunge, C. N., et al.: A study of the efficacy and safety of albendazole (Zentel) in the treatment of intestinal helminthiasis in Kenyan children less than 2 years of age. East Afr. Med. J. *66*:197–202, 1989.
27. Sherman, D. R., Guinn, B., Perdok, M. M., et al.: Components of sterol biosynthesis assembled on the oxygen-avid hemoglobin of *Ascaris*. Science *258*:1930–1932, 1992.
28. Spence, H. J., Moore, J., Brass, A., et al.: A cDNA encoding repeating units of the ABA-1 allergen of *Ascaris*. Mol. Biochem. Parasitol. *57*:339–344, 1993.
29. Stephenson, L. S., Latham, M. C., Kurz, K. M., et al.: Treatment with a single dose of albendazole improves growth of Kenyan schoolchildren with hookworm, *Trichuris trichiura*, and *Ascaris lumbricoides* infections. Am. J. Trop. Med. Hyg. *41*:78–87, 1989.
30. Stoll, N. R.: This wormy world. J. Parasitol. *33*:1–18, 1947.
31. Tankhiwalle, S. R., Kukade, A. L., Sarmah, H. C., et al.: Single dose therapy of ascariasis: A randomized comparison of mebendazole and pyrantel. J. Commun. Dis. *21*:71–74, 1989.
32. Villar, J., Klebanoff, M., and Kestler, E.: The effect on fetal growth of protozoan and helminthic infection during pregnancy. Obstet. Gynecol. *74*:915–929, 1989.
33. Albomico, M., Smith, P. G., Ercole, E., et al.: Rate of reinfection with intestinal nematodes after treatment of children with mebendazole or albendazole in a highly endemic area. Trans. R. Soc. Trop. Med. Hyg. *89*:538–541, 1995.
34. Xu L., Jian Z., Yu S., et al.: Nationwide survey of the distribution of human parasites in China: Infection with parasite species in human population. Chin. J. Parasitol. Parasitic Dis. *13*:1–7, 1995.

Trichuris trichiura

35. Bundy, D. A. P., and Cooper, E. S.: *Trichuris* and trichuriasis in humans. Adv. Parasitol. *28*:107–173, 1989.
36. Cooper E. S., and Bundy, D. A. P.: *Trichuris* is not trivial. Parasitol. Today *4*:301–305, 1988.
37. Cooper, E., Bundy, D., MacDonald, T., et al.: Growth suppression in the *Trichuris* dysentery syndrome. Eur. J. Clin. Nutr. *44*:285–291, 1990.
38. Drake, L., Korchev, Y., Bashford, L., et al.: The major secreted product of the whipworm *Trichuris* is a pore-forming protein. Proc. R. Soc. Lond. B. *257*:255–261, 1994.
39. Else, K. J., Finkelman, F. D., Maliszewski, C. R., et al.: Cytokine-mediated regulation of chronic intestinal helminth infection. J. Exp. Med. *179*:347–351, 1994.
40. Layrisse, M., Aparcedo, L., Martinez Torres, C., et al.: Blood loss due to infection with *Trichuris trichiura*. Am. J. Trop. Med. Hyg. *16*:613–616, 1967.
41. Lotero, M., Tripathy, K., and Bolanos, O.: Gastrointestinal blood loss in *Trichuris* infection. Am. J. Trop. Med. Hyg. *23*:1203–1207, 1974.
42. MacDonald, T. T., Choy, M. Y., Spencer, J., et al.: Histopathology of the caecum in children with *Trichuris* dysentery syndrome. J. Clin. Pathol. *44*:194–199, 1991.
43. Maqbool, S., Lawrence, D., and Katz, M.: Treatment of trichuriasis with a new drug, mebendazole. J. Pediatr. *86*:463–465, 1975.
44. Simeon, D. T., Grantham-McGregor, S. M., and Wong, M. S.: *Trichuris trichiura* infection and cognition in children: Results of a randomized clinical trial. Parasitology *110*:457–464, 1995.
45. Wakelin, D., and Gelby, R. G.: Immune expulsion of *Trichuris muris* from resistant mice: Suppression by irradiation and restoration by transfer of lymphoid cells. Parasitology *72*:41–50, 1976.

Hookworms

46. Cappello, M., Vlasuk, G. P., Bergum, P. W., et al.: *Ancylostoma caninum* anticoagulant peptide (AcAP): A novel hookworm-derived inhibitor of human coagulation factor Xa. Proc. Natl. Acad. Sci. U. S. A. *92*:6152–6156, 1995.
47. Hawdon, J. M., Jones, B., Perregaux, M., et al.: *Ancylostoma caninum*: Resumption of hookworm larval feeding coincides with metalloprotease release. Exp. Parasitol. *80*:205–211, 1995.
48. Hotez, P. J.: Hookworm disease in children. Pediatr. Infect. Dis. J. *8*:516–520, 1989.
49. Hotez, P. J.: Human hookworm infection. *In* Farthing, M. J. G., Keusch, G. T. and Wakelin, D. (eds.): Enteric Infection 2. Intestinal Helminths. London, Chapman and Hall, 1995, pp. 129–150.
50. Hotez, P. J., Cappello, M., Hawdon, J., et al.: Hyaluronidases from the gastrointestinal invasive nematodes *Ancylostoma caninum* and *Anisakis simplex:* their function in the pathogenesis of human zoonoses. J. Infect. Dis. *170*:918–926, 1994.
51. Hotez, P., Hawdon, J., Cappello, M. et al: Molecular approaches to vaccinating against disease. Pediatr. Res. *40*:515–521, 1996.
52. Naik, S. R., Mitra, S. K., and Mehta, S.: Massive intestinal hemorrhage due to infection with *Ancylostoma duodenale*. J. Trop. Med. Hyg. *79*:2–4, 1976.
53. Prociv, P., and Croese, J.: Human eosinophilic enteritis caused by dog hookworm, *Ancylostoma caninum*. Lancet *335*:1299–1302, 1990.
54. Saraya, A. K., and Tandon, B. N.: Hookworm anemia and intestinal malabsorption associated with hookworm infestation. Prog. Drug Res. *19*:108–118, 1975.
55. Schad, G. A.: Hypobiosis and related phenomena in hookworm infection. *In* Hookworm Disease, Current Status and Future Directions. London, Taylor and Francis, 1990, pp. 71–88.
56. Schad, G. A., and Anderson, R. M.: Predisposition to hookworm infection. Science *228*:1537–1540, 1985.
57. Takafuji, E. T., Kelley, P. W., Thompson, N. J. et al.: An outbreak of hookworm infection following a military deployment to Grenada. Abstract No. 33. Proceedings of the 33rd Annual Meeting of the American Society of Tropical Medicine and Hygiene, December, 1984.

Enterobius vermicularis

58. Bhaskaran, C. S., Devi, E. S., and Rao, K. V.: *Enterobius vermicularis* and vermiform appendix. J. Indian Med. Assoc. *64*:334–336, 1975.
59. Cho, S.-Y., Hong, S.-T., Kang, S.-Y., et al.: Morphological observation of *Enterobius vermicularis* expelled by various anthelminthics. Korean J. Parasitol. *19*:18–26, 1981.
60. Crawford, F. G., and Vermund, S. H.: Parasitic infections in day care centers. Pediatr. Infect. Dis. J. *6*:744–749, 1987.

61. Mattia, A. R.: Perianal mass and recurrent and cellulitis due to *Enterobius vermicularis*. Am. J. Trop. Med. Hyg. *47*:811–815, 1992.
62. Mondou, E. N., and Gnepp, D. R.: Hepatic granuloma resulting from *Enterobius vermicularis*. Am. J. Clin. Pathol. *91*:97–100, 1989.
63. Simon, R. D.: Pinworm infestation and urinary tract infection in young girls. Am. J. Dis. Child. *128*:21–22, 1974.
64. Weller, T. H., and Gorenson, C. W.: Enterobiasis: Its incidence and symptomatology in a group of 505 children. N. Engl. J. Med. *224*:143–146, 1941.

Strongyloides stercoralis and *Strongyloides fuelleborni*

65. Ashford, R. W., Vince, J. D., Gratten, M. J., et al.: *Strongyloides* infection associated with acute infantile disease in Papua New Guinea. Trans. R. Soc. Trop. Med. Hyg. *72*:554, 1978.
66. Barnish, G., and Ashford, R. W.: *Strongyloides cf. fuelleborni* and hookworm in Papua New Guinea: Patterns of infection within the community. Trans. R. Soc. Trop. Med. Hyg. *83*:684–689, 1989.
67. Brindley, P. J., Gam, A. A., McKerrow, J. H., and Neva, et al.: Ss40: The zinc endopeptidase secreted by infective larvae of *Strongyloides stercoralis*. Exp. Parasitol. *80*:1–7, 1995.
68. Brown, H. W., and Perna, V. P.: An overwhelming *Strongyloides* infection. J. A. M. A. *168*:1648–1651, 1958.
69. Brown, R. C., and Girardeau, M. H. F.: Transmammary passage of *Strongyloides* sp. larvae in the human host. Am. J. Trop. Med. Hyg. *26*:215–219, 1977.
70. Burke, J. A.: Strongyloidiasis in childhood. Am. J. Dis. Child. *132*:1130–1136, 1978.
71. Campbell, W. C., and Cuckler, A.: Thiabendazole in the treatment and control of parasitic infection in man. Tex. Rep. Biol. Med. *27*:665–692, 1964.
72. DeVault, G. A., King, J. W., Rohr, M. S., et al.: Opportunistic infections with *Strongyloides stercoralis* in renal transplantation. Rev. Infect. Dis. *12*:653–671, 1990.
73. Dixon, A. C., Yanaghihara, E. T., Kwock, D. W., et al.: Strongyloidiasis associated with human T-cell lymphotropic virus type 1 infection in a nonendemic area. West. J. Med. *151*:410–413, 1989.
74. Genta, R. M.: Global prevalence of strongyloidiasis: Critical review with epidemiologic insights into the prevention of disseminated disease. Rev. Infect. Dis. *11*:755–767, 1989.
75. Genta, R. M.: Dysregulation of strongyloidiasis: A new hypothesis. Clin. Microbiol. Rev. *5*:345–355, 1992.
76. Genta, R. M., Miles, P., and Fields, K.: Opportunistic *Strongyloides stercoralis* infection in lymphoma patients: Report of a case and review of the literature. Cancer *63*:1407–1411, 1989.
77. Gill, G. V., and Bell, D. R.: Longstanding tropical infections amongst former war prisoners of the Japanese. Lancet *1*:958–959, 1982.
78. Gyorkos, T. W., Genta, R. M., Viens, P., et al.: Seroepidemiology of *Strongyloides* infection in the southeast Asian refugee population in Canada. Am. J. Epidemiol. *132*:257–264, 1990.
79. Lyagoubi, M., Datry, A., Mayorga, R. et al.: Chronic persistent strongyloidiasis cured by ivermectin. Trans. R. Soc. Trop. Med. Hyg. *86*:541, 1992.
80. McKerrow, J. H., Brindley, P., Brown, M., et al.: *Strongyloides stercoralis*: Identification of a protease that facilitates penetration of skin by the infective larvae. Exp. Parasitol. *70*:134–143, 1990.
81. Naquira, C., Jimenez, G., Guerra, J. G., et al.: Ivermectin for human strongyloidiasis and other intestinal helminths. Am. J. Trop. Med. Hyg. *40*:304–309, 1989.
82. O'Brien, W.: Intestinal malabsorption in acute infection with *Strongyloides stercoralis*. Trans. R. Soc. Trop. Med. Hyg. *69*:69–77, 1975.
83. Purtillo, D. T., Meyers, W. M., and Connor, D. H.: Fatal strongyloidiasis in immunosuppressed patients. Am. J. Med. *56*:488–493, 1974.
84. Robinson, R. D., Lindo, J. F., Neva, F. A., et al.: Immunoepidemiologic studies of *Strongyloides stercoralis* and human T lymphotropic virus type I infections in Jamaica. J. Infect. Dis. *169*:692–696, 1994.
85. Schad, G. A.: Cyclosporine may eliminate the threat of overwhelming strongyloidiasis in immunosuppressed patients. J. Infect. Dis. *153*:178, 1986.
86. Schad, G. A., Aikens, L. M., and Smith, G.: *Strongyloides stercoralis*: Is there a canonical migratory route through the host? J. Parasitol. *75*:740–749, 1989.
87. Sukhavat, K., Morakote, N., Chaiwong, P., et al.: Comparative efficacy of four methods for the detection of *Strongyloides stercoralis* in human stool specimens. Ann. Trop. Med. Parasitol. *88*:95–96, 1994.

ABERRANT INFECTIONS WITH INTESTINAL NEMATODES

Toxocara canis

88. Anonymous: Editorial: The public health significance of canine ascarid infections. Vet. Rec. *99*:37–38, 1976.
89. Arpino, C., Gattinara, G. C., Piergili, D., et al.: Toxocara infection and epilepsy in children: A case-control study. Epilepsia *31*:33–36, 1990.
90. Ashton, N.: Larval granulomatosis of the retina due to *Toxocara*. Br. J. Ophthalmol. *44*:129–148, 1960.
91. Bekhti, A.: Mebendazole in toxocariasis. Ann. Intern. Med. *100*:463, 1984.
92. Biddulph, J.: Mebendazole and albendazole for infants. Pediatr. Infect. Dis. J. *9*:373, 1990.
93. Bird, A. C., Smith, J. L., and Curtin, V. T.: Nematode optic neuritis. Am. J. Ophthalmol. *69*:72–77, 1970.
94. Dinning, W. J., Gillespie, S. H., Cooling, R. J., et al.: Toxocariasis: A practical approach to management of ocular disease. Eye *2*:580–582, 1988.
95. Douglas, J. R., and Baker, N. F.: Some host-parasite relationships of canine helminths. *In* McCauley, J. E. (ed.): Host-Parasite Relationships. Proc. 26th Annual Biol. Colloq. Corvallis, Oregon State University Press, 1966, pp. 97–115.
96. Fortenberry, J. D., Kenney, R. D., and Younger, J.: Visceral larva migrans producing static encephalopathy in an infant. Pediatr. Infect. Dis. J. *10*:403–406, 1991.
97. Glickman, L. T., and Schantz, P. M.: Epidemiology and pathogenesis of zoonotic toxocariasis. Epidemiol. Rev. *10*:143–148, 1982.
98. Hotez, P. J.: Visceral and ocular larva migrans. Semin. Neurol. *13*:175–179, 1993.
99. Hotez, P. J.: *Toxocara canis*. *In* Burg, F. D., Ingelfinger, J. R., et al. (eds.): Gellis and Kagan's Current Pediatric Therapy. 15th ed. Philadelphia, W. B. Saunders, 1996.
100. Huminer, D., Symon, K., Groskopf, I., et al.: Seroepidemiologic study of toxocariasis and strongyloidiasis in institutionalized mentally retarded adults. Am. J. Trop. Med. Hyg. *46*:278–281, 1992.
101. Kazacos, K. R.: Visceral and ocular larva migrans. Semin. Vet. Med. Surg. (Small Animal) *6*:227–235, 1991.
102. Marmor, M., Glickman, L., Shofer, F., et al.: *Toxocara canis* infection of children: Epidemiologic and neuropsychologic findings. Am. J. Public Health *77*:554–559, 1987.
103. Nelson, J. D., McConnel, T. H., and Moore, D. V.: Thiabendazole therapy of visceral larva migrans: A case report. Am. J. Trop. Med. Hyg. *15*:930–933, 1966.
104. Schantz, P. M.: *Toxocara* larva migrans now. Am. J. Trop. Med. Hyg. *41*(Suppl.):21–34, 1989.
105. Schantz, P. M., Meyer, D., and Glickman, L. T.: Clinical, serologic, and epidemiologic characteristics of ocular toxocariasis. Am. J. Trop. Med. Hyg. *28*:24–28, 1979.
106. Small, K. W., McCuen, B. W., De Juan, E., et al.: Surgical management of retinal retraction caused by toxocariasis. Am. J. Ophthalmol. *108*:10–14, 1989.
107. Sturchler, D., Schubarth, P., Fualzata, M., et al.: Thiabendazole vs. albendazole in treatment of toxocariasis. A clinical study. Ann. Trop. Med. Parasitol. *83*:473–478, 1989.
108. Woodruff, A. W., Bisseru, B., and Bowe, J. C.: Infection with animal helminths as a factor in causing poliomyelitis and epilepsy. B. M. J. *5503*:1576–1579, 1966.

Other Aberrant Infections with Intestinal Nematodes

109. Chitwood, M.: Nematodes of medical significance found in market fish. Am. J. Trop. Med. Hyg. *19*:599–602, 1970.
110. Cross, J.: Intestinal capillariasis. Clin. Microbiol. Rev. *5*:120–129, 1992.
111. Cuckler, A. C., Egerton, J. R., and Alicata, J. E.: Therapeutic effect of thiabendazole on *Angiostrongylus cantonensis* infections in rats. J. Parasitol. *51*:392–396, 1965.
112. Dauz, V., Cabrera, B. D., and Cancas, B.: Human intestinal capillariasis: I. Clinical features. Acta Med. Philipp. *4*:72–83, 1967.
113. Ghadirian, E., and Arfaa, F.: Present status of trichostrongyliasis in Iran. Am. J. Trop. Med. Hyg. *24*:935–941, 1975.
114. Hotez, P. J., Haggerty, J., Hawdon, J., et al.: Infective *Ancylostoma* hookworm larval metalloproteases and their possible functions in tissue invasion and ecdysis. Infect. Immun. *58*:3883–3892, 1990.
115. Hotez, P. J., Narasimhan, S., Haggerty, J., et al.: Hyaluronidase from *Ancylostoma* hookworm larvae and its function as a virulence factor in cutaneous larva migrans. Infect. Immun. *60*:1018–1023, 1992.
116. Huff, D. S., Neaffie, R. C., Binder, M. J., et al.: The first fatal *Baylisascaris* infection in humans: An infant with eosinophilic meningoencephalitis. Pediatr. Pathol. *2*:1–20, 1984.
117. Hurlbert, T. V., Larsen, R. A., and Chandrasoma, P. T.: Abdominal angiostrongyliasis mimicking acute appendicitis and Meckel's diverticulum: Report of a case in the United States and review. Clin. Infect. Dis. *14*:836–840, 1992.
118. Kazacos, K. R., and Boyce, W. M.: *Baylisascaris* larva migrans. J. Am. Vet. Med. Assoc. *195*:894–903, 1990.
119. Koo, J., Pien, F., and Kliks, M. M.: *Angiostrongylus (Parastrongylus)* eosinophilic meningitis. Rev. Infect. Dis. *10*:1155–1162.
120. Krepel, H. P., and Polderman, A. M.: Egg production of *Oesophagostomum bifurcum*, a locally common parasite of humans in Togo. Am. J. Trop. Med. Hyg. *46*:469–472, 1992.
121. McKerrow, J. H., Sakanari, J. A., and Deardorff, T. L.: Revenge of the "sushi parasite." N. Engl. J. Med. *319*:1228–1229, 1988.
122. Otto, G. I., Berthrong, M., Appleby, R. E., et al.: Eosinophilia and hepatomegaly due to *Capillaria hepatica* infection. Bull. Johns Hopkins Hosp. *94*:319–336, 1954.
123. Polderman, A. M., Kepel, H. P., Baeta, S., et al: Oesophagostomiasis, a

common infection of man in northern Togo and Ghana. Am. J. Trop. Med. Hyg. *44*:336–344, 1991.
124. Rosen, L., Chappel, R., Laquer, G. L., et al.: Eosinophilic meningoencephalitis caused by a metastrongyloid lungworm of rats. J. A. M. A. *179*:620–624, 1962.
125. Rosen, L., Loisen, G., Laigret, J., et al.: Studies of eosinophilic meningitis. III. Epidemiologic and clinical observations on Pacific islands and the possible etiologic role of *Angiostrongylus cantonensis*. Am. J. Epidemiol. *85*:17–24, 1967.
126. Schad, G. A.: Hookworms: Pets to humans. Ann. Intern. Med. *120*:434–435, 1994.
127. Schantz, P. M.: The dangers of eating raw fish. N. Engl. J. Med. *320*:1143–1145, 1989.
128. Whalen, G. E., Rosenberg, E. B., Strickland, G. T., et al.: Intestinal capillariasis: A new disease in man. Lancet *1*:13–16, 1969.
129. Whitting, D. A.: The successful treatment of creeping eruption with topical thiabendazole. S. Afr. Med. J. *50*:253–255, 1976.
130. Wittner, M., Turner, J. W., and Jacquette, G.: Eustrongylidiasis: A parasitic infection acquired by eating sushi. N. Engl. J. Med. *320*:1124–1126, 1989.
131. Yoshimura, H., Akao, N., Kondo, K., et al.: Clinicopathological studies on larval anisakiasis, with special reference to the report of extragastrointestinal anisakiasis. Jpn. J. Parasitol. *28*:347–354, 1979.

FILARIAL PARASITES

Lymphatic Filariasis: *Wuchereria bancrofti* and *Brugia* Species

132. Baird, J. K., Alpert, L. I., and Friedman, R.: North American brugian filariasis: Report of nine infections of humans. Am. J. Trop. Med. Hyg. *35*:1205, 1986.
133. Grove, D. I., Cabrera, B. D., Valeza, F. S., et al.: Sensitivity and specificity of skin reactivity to *Brugia malayi* and *Dirofilaria immitis* antigens in bancroftian and Malayan filariasis in the Philippines. Am. J. Trop. Med. Hyg. *26*:220–229, 1977.
134. Nanduri, J., and Kazura, J. W.: Clinical and laboratory aspects of filariasis. Clin. Microbiol. Rev. *2*:39–60, 1986.
135. Ottesen, E. A., and Nutman, T. B.: Tropical pulmonary eosinophilia. Annu. Rev. Med. *43*:417–424, 1992.
136. Ottesen, E. A., Vijayasekaran, V., Kumaraswami, V., et al.: A controlled trial of ivermectin and diethylcarbamazine in lymphatic filariasis. N. Engl. J. Med. *322*:1113–1117, 1990.
137. Simmons, C. F., Jr., Winter, H. S., Berde, C., et al.: Zoonotic filariasis with lymphedema in an immunodeficient infant. N. Engl. J. Med. *310*:1243–1245, 1984.
138. Vande, W. A. A.: Chemotherapy of filariases. Parasitol. Today *7*:194–199, 1991.

Loa loa

139. Carme, B., Boulesteix, J., Boutes, H., et al.: Five cases of encephalitis during treatment of loiasis with diethylcarbamazine. Am. J. Trop. Med. Hyg. *44*:684–690, 1991.
140. Kilon, A. D., Massoughbodji, A., Sadeler, B. C., et al.: Loiasis in endemic and nonendemic populations: Immunologically mediated differences in clinical presentation. J. Infect. Dis. *163*:1318–1325, 1991.
141. Nutman, T. B., Reese, W., Poindexter, R. W., et al.: Immunologic correlates of the hyperresponsive syndrome of loiasis. J. Infect. Dis. *157*:544–550, 1988.
142. Olness, K., Franciosi, R. A., and Johnson, M. M.: Loiasis in an expatriate American child: Diagnostic and treatment difficulties. Pediatrics *80*:943, 1987.

Onchocerca volvulus

143. Taylor, H. R., and Greene, B. M.: The status of ivermectin in the treatment of human onchocerciasis. Am. J. Trop. Med. Hyg. *41*:460–466, 1989.
144. Taylor, H. R., Pacque, M., Munoz, B., et al.: Impact of mass treatment of onchocerciasis with ivermectin on the transmission of infection. Science *250*:116–118, 1990.

Mansonella* and *Mansonella ozzardi perstans

145. Baird, J. K., Neafie, R. C., and Connor, D. H.: Nodules in the conjunctiva, bung-eye, and bulge-eye in Africa caused by *Mansonella perstans*. Am. J. Trop. Med. Hyg. *38*:553–557, 1988.

Dirofilaria immitis

146. Bloc, T., Glynn, T., and Hinshaw, M.: Human pulmonary dirofilariasis. Indiana Med. *83*:24–27, 1990.
147. Dayal, Y., and Neafie, R. C.: Human pulmonary dirofilariasis: A case report and review of the literature. Am. Rev. Respir. Dis. *112*:437–443, 1975.

Drancunculus medinensis

148. Hopkins, D. R., and Ruiz-Tiben, E.: Strategies for dracunculiasis eradication. Bull. W. H. O. *69*:533–540, 1991.
149. Ilegbodu, V. A., Oladele, K. O., Wise, R. A., et al.: Impact of guinea worm disease on children in Nigeria. Am. J. Trop. Med. Hyg. *35*:962–964, 1986.
150. M. M. W. R: Update: Dracunculiasis eradication—Ghana and Nigeria, 1990. M. M. W. R. *40*:245–247, 1991.

❑ ❑ ❑

SUBSECTION THREE

CESTODES

224

CESTODES

Jerrold A. Turner

The adult forms of tapeworms (cestodes) share common characteristics. They possess a specialized attachment organ called the scolex, which may have sucking grooves *(Diphyllobothrium, Spirometra)* or four circular suckers, as in the other medically important genera. In addition to having circular suckers, the scoleces of some species have hooks, which assist in attaching to the mucosa of the definitive hosts. The body of the adult worm is ribbon-like and has no gastrointestinal tract or internal cavity. An undifferentiated neck region, situated immediately behind the scolex, is an area of great metabolic activity and growth. The remainder of the worm is differentiated into segments or proglottids. Each proglottid develops both male and female reproductive organs as it matures. The proglottids become increasingly mature the more distal they are to the neck region. Usually the terminal proglottids are gravid and contain egg-filled uteri. The eggs of *Diphyllobothrium* and *Spirometra* require an aquatic environment, and larval development involves at least two intermediate hosts. The other species of tapeworm considered here parasitize their intermediate hosts when the eggs are ingested. In *Hymenolepis nana* infection, humans may serve as both definitive and intermediate hosts.

In certain circumstances, humans may be accidental intermediate hosts for tapeworms. Major examples of this phenomenon are cysticercosis, hydatid disease (echinococcosis), coenurosis, and sparganosis.

TAENIASIS SAGINATA (*TAENIA SAGINATA* INFECTION, BEEF TAPEWORM INFECTION)

Goez, in 1782, first recognized *T. saginata* as a separate species. In 1861, Leuckart defined the relationship between the adult worms and the larval forms found in cattle.

T. saginata is synonymous with *Taeniarhynchus saginatus*. Variations of morphology have led to the designation of species such as *T. confusa*, *T. hominis*, and *T. africana*. The validity of these species has been questioned, and *T. saginata* generally is used as an inclusive term.[100]

The Organism

The scolex of *T. saginata* measures 1 to 2 mm in diameter and has four cup-shaped muscular suckers but bears no hooks. The length of the parasite usually varies from 4 to 10 m but may reach 25 m. The size of the proglottids depends on their stage of development and their state of muscular relaxation. Gravid proglottids are 16 to 20 mm in length and 5 to 7 mm in width. The linear, central uterine stem has 12 to 30 main lateral branches on each side. The eggs measure 30 to 40 μm in diameter. The six-hooked embryo is surrounded by a brownish, radially striated embryophore.

When eggs of *T. saginata* are ingested by an intermediate host, they hatch and the embryo burrows through the intestinal mucosa, gaining access to the circulation. After lodging in capillaries in various locations in the body of the intermediate host, the embryo develops into the larval cysticercus or bladder worm. This cystic, ovoid structure measures 7 to 10 mm by 4 to 6 mm and contains an invaginated scolex.

Domestic bovine animals are the principal intermediate hosts, but infections have been found in reindeer and a variety of wild African herbivorous animals.[78] Humans are the only definitive host. Although there have been rare reports of human cysticercosis caused by *T. saginata* cysticerci, the diagnosis usually is questionable.

Transmission

Completion of the life cycle of *T. saginata* requires transmission of the infection to the intermediate host and subsequently to humans. Contamination of pastures or feed lots with human feces or untreated sewage is the initial step. *Taenia* eggs ingested by cattle hatch in the intestine and develop into cysticerci in the tissues. When raw or rare beef containing viable cysticerci is eaten by humans, the scolex evaginates from the cysticercus and attaches to the intestinal wall, and development of the adult tapeworm begins. Gravid proglottids appear 84 to 120 days after infection is acquired.[78, 92] Infection may persist for the life of the human host. In most geographic areas, parasitization with more than a single worm is noted in less than 1 per cent of infections, but in highly endemic areas multiple infection may be found in more than 60 per cent.[78]

Ova may be shed within the intestinal lumen by detached gravid proglottids, but dissemination of eggs more commonly occurs when single gravid proglottids actively migrate from the anus or out of the fecal mass. As these muscular proglottids crawl about, eggs are expressed from the anterior margin. Each proglottid contains about 80,000 eggs. Egg survival is optimal in a moist, cool environment. Although *T. saginata* eggs may survive for 1 to 3 months, they are rendered noninfectious rapidly under dry conditions.

Information on the longevity of cysticerci in cattle indicates a wide variability, which may depend on the strains of the parasite and the genetics and age of the host, as well as other factors. Viable cysticerci have been recovered from cattle several years after infection.

The ova of *T. solium* and *T. saginata* are not distinguishable on morphologic grounds. Although *T. saginata* eggs are not a hazard to humans, *T. solium* eggs can hatch within the intestine and cause cysticercosis. Therefore, until the diagnosis of *T. saginata* infection is confirmed by examination of proglottids, the patient should not be involved in food handling or preparation and should take extra care with personal hygiene and the disposition of underclothing.

Epidemiology

A review of taeniasis published in 1972[78] indicated the inadequacy of epidemiologic data from nearly all sources. In general, prevalence rates for human infections were below 1 per cent in all but the highly endemic areas. In the former Soviet Union, the areas of the Caucasus and the South-Central Asian republics had prevalence rates ranging from 7 to 45 per cent. Cattle-raising areas of Africa, excluding Egypt and South Africa, report rates above 10 per cent. A review of the prevalence of taeniasis in 1982 showed no significant changes.[77] Although the incidence of taeniasis in the United States is low, transmission does occur. The incidence of cysticercosis in cattle has been noted to be 20 times greater in California than in other states.[86]

Pathogenesis and Pathology

Little is known of the pathology or pathogenesis of intestinal taeniasis. Speculation as to local mucosal trauma, irritation, the production of toxic substances, or the induction of clinically significant hypersensitivity has scant documentation. Rare, ectopic localization of worms or proglottids may stimulate local inflammatory reactions. Infections in the middle ear, nasopharynx, and an abdominal mass have been reported. Proglottids have been recovered from the uterine cavity, and acute appendicitis has been attributed to wandering proglottids on many occasions. It is not clear whether the appendiceal inflammation is a direct result of obstruction and irritation caused by proglottids or whether the presence of the parasite merely is a coincidental finding.

Clinical Manifestations

The most common complaint is the discomfort and embarrassment caused by the migration of gravid proglottids from the anus. The patient's awareness of the infection frequently causes a preoccupation with gastrointestinal function. A summary of eight studies of *T. saginata* infection[78] revealed abdominal pain, nausea, weakness, and loss of weight as the most common symptoms recorded. Alterations in appetite and bowel habits were reported inconsistently.

Severe symptoms especially are likely in infants, who may develop vomiting, diarrhea, fever, weight loss, and irritability.

Intestinal obstruction or the occurrence of symptoms related to ectopic localization of proglottids is extremely rare.

Although taeniasis usually is not associated with significant eosinophilia, one study of four patients showed transient eosinophilia that sometimes exceeded 30 per cent between the sixth and ninth week after the initial infection. At the time the patients first began passing proglottids, the eosinophilia had returned to normal or near normal.[46] Another series of observations showed a syndrome of marked eosinophilia and severe colicky abdominal pain, which occurred about 1 month prior to the passage of *Taenia* proglottids.[7]

A single experimental infection noted symptoms of nausea, headache, and disturbed sleep at about the time gravid proglottids appeared in the stool 84 days after infection. There was an increase in eosinophils of 10.5 per cent and an increase in lymphocytes of 13 per cent.[92]

Diagnosis

The scolex of *T. saginata* lacks hooks and may be differentiated easily from the scolex of *T. solium*, which bears a row of hooks. However, the scolex usually is not recovered, even after successful treatment. Eggs of *T. saginata* and *T. solium* morphologically are similar but may be distinguished by use of the Ziehl-Neelsen stain.[18] *T. saginata* eggs retain the stain, whereas eggs of *T. solium* are negative. DNA probes have been shown to be highly sensitive and specific in differentiating the two species of *Taenia* eggs.[21, 43]

Eggs may be seen on routine fecal wet mounts, but the likelihood of detection is enhanced by concentration methods. Cellulose tape swabs applied to the anal and perianal skin, as used for the diagnosis of *Enterobius* infection, have been found to be even more efficient than fecal concentration.[65, 95]

Examination of the gravid proglottid is the usual method used to diagnose *T. saginata* infection. The patient or parents are instructed to collect proglottids in a vial of saline and deliver the specimen to the laboratory as soon as possible. Fixatives such as alcohol or formalin tend to make the proglottids rigid and opaque. The proglottid should be compressed between two microscope slides. If the uterus contains enough ova, it is relatively easy to count the main branches of the uterine stem. The visibility of the uterus may be enhanced by inserting a fine intradermal needle in the midportion of the proglottid and injecting a small amount of India ink. Counts of 13 or fewer branches on one side of the stem are considered diagnostic for *T. solium*. If the count is 14 or greater, the species is designated *T. saginata*. Because of morphologic variations, this method has been criticized, particularly when the decision is based on gravid proglottids with counts in the range of 12 to 15. Analysis of many specimens of *Taenia*, identified by scolex, showed that mature proglottids with fully developed sex organs could be differentiated by several characteristics.[79] The most prominent features are a vaginal sphincter seen only in *T. saginata* and a third ovarian lobe that is present only in *T. solium*. To define these and other features, the proglottids require painstaking staining and clearing as well as examination by a skilled parasitologist. DNA probes have been used successfully to distinguish between *T. saginata* and *T. solium* proglottid fragments.[54] Polymerase chain reaction techniques have been developed that can be applied to fecal diagnosis.[51] Investigators claim that polymerase chain reaction can detect a single egg and differentiate between species.[51]

Although there have been many attempts to develop diagnostic serologic tests and skin sensitivity tests for taeniasis, the antigens have not been sensitive or specific enough to be useful clinically. Dot enzyme-linked immunosorbent assay (ELISA) dipsticks have been developed that can detect antigens from the genus *Taenia* in stools.[2]

Occasionally, the larger portions of the worm may appear as ribbon-like defects in the barium column during contrast studies of the gastrointestinal tract. It rarely may be seen on plain films of the abdomen as a linear density in a gas-filled loop of bowel.

Treatment

The drug of choice is praziquantel. This pyrazinoisoquinoline derivative is supplied as 600-mg, film-coated, scored tablets that easily are broken into 150-mg quarters. Praziquantel is administered in a single dose of 5 to 10 mg/kg. It is not recommended in pregnancy, and its safety in children younger than 4 years of age has not been established. Lactating mothers should avoid nursing for 72 hours after treatment. Praziquantel must be administered with caution to patients at risk for neurocysticercosis (see later).

Paromomycin has been used as an alternative. This nonabsorbable aminoglycoside is supplied in 250-mg capsules. It is administered in a dosage of 11 mg/kg every 15 minutes for four doses (maximum total dose of 4 g). Side effects of paromomycin are common and usually consist of nausea, abdominal pain, and diarrhea. Neither praziquantel nor paromomycin has been approved by the U.S. Food and Drug Administration for the treatment of tapeworm infections. Therefore, the use of these drugs for this indication would be investigational.

Albendazole, a benzimidazole compound that has been approved for use in the United States for cysticercosis and hydatid disease, also has an effect on *Taenia* infections but requires further evaluation.[26] The same caution would apply, as with praziquantel, in treating patients who may have neurocysticercosis.

Quinacrine, used in the past for taeniasis, required multiple purges and frequently was associated with vomiting. It has been replaced by praziquantel. Niclosamide, a safe and effective taeniacidal drug, is approved for use in the United States but has been withdrawn from the market by the manufacturer.

After treatment, the patient is requested to watch for proglottids. Proglottids may be seen for up to 3 days after treatment. Proglottids or ova found 7 days after treatment indicate treatment failure, and the patient should be instructed to return for treatment. Four months after treatment, fecal examination should be performed for ova and proglottids.

Prognosis

T. saginata infections are of little clinical significance except for the rare complications of ectopic location of the worm or intestinal obstruction. Symptoms, when present, may be annoying but do not alter health significantly. Treatment is highly effective.

Prevention

Meat inspection is effective in detecting all but light infections. Cooking beef to a temperature of 56° C kills cysticerci. Education of workers in the cattle-raising industry, coupled with detection and prompt treatment of human infection, may reduce transmission.

Mass examinations and mass treatment have been helpful

in decreasing the prevalence of infection in endemic areas of the former Soviet Union; however, this is not feasible economically in many developing countries that have high prevalence rates.

ASIAN TAENIASIS

A tapeworm resembling *T. saginata* has been described from specimens recovered in Taiwan, China, Korea, Indonesia, the Philippines, and Malaysia. This organism possesses a prominent protuberance in the center of the scolex called a rostellum. There are 16 to 21 uterine branches on each side of the uterine stem in the gravid proglottids. This is similar to the gravid proglottids of *T. saginata*. The cysticercus contains a scolex with a rostellum and rudimentary hooks. The outer surface of the cysticercus is covered with wart-like protuberances. Pigs are the most common and important intermediate hosts, but cattle, goats, monkeys, and wild boar also may be infected. The cysticerci are found in the livers of the intermediate hosts. Most human infections have been reported from areas where raw or undercooked pork is eaten. An experimental infection demonstrated a period of 76 days between ingestion of the cysticercus and the appearance of gravid proglottids.[37] Although the species designation *T. asiatica* has been proposed,[38] genetic studies suggest that this organism is a subspecies or strain of *T. saginata*.[15]

TAENIASIS SOLIUM (*TAENIA SOLIUM* INFECTION, PORK TAPEWORM INFECTION, CYSTICERCOSIS)

The life cycle of *T. solium* is similar to that of *T. saginata*. The pig is the intermediate host, and infection is acquired by the ingestion of inadequately cooked pork. The tapeworm is not as large as *T. saginata* and rarely exceeds 7 m in length. The gravid proglottids are less motile than those of *T. saginata* and usually are passed in the feces.

T. solium infection is rare in the United States, but it is common in Mexico, Central and South America, parts of Africa, India, Korea, Thailand, and other Southeast Asian countries.

The diagnosis has been discussed in a previous section.

Clinical manifestations are similar to or perhaps even less prominent than those of *T. saginata* infections.

T. solium assumes its medical importance because people can be intermediate as well as definitive hosts. Cysticercosis is the name given to human infection with the larval stage of *T. solium*. Autopsy studies in heavily infected areas such as Mexico show that approximately 3.5 per cent of the population have cysticercosis. Cysticercosis affects both sexes equally and first may be manifest in infancy. Human cysticercosis has been reviewed in detail.[16, 43, 108]

Cysticercosis usually is acquired by ingestion of eggs of *T. solium* in food or drink contaminated with human feces. Persons harboring an adult worm also are a potential danger to themselves, in that eggs can be introduced from the anus to the mouth (external autoinfection) or possibly by regurgitation of gravid proglottids into the stomach during vomiting. Only 20 per cent of patients with cysticercosis have a history of intestinal tapeworm, but patients with such a history are more likely to have many cysticerci.[34]

Embryos are liberated from eggs in the intestine, enter the blood stream, and are carried to distant sites. Any tissue may be affected. The most common are brain, subcutaneous tissue, muscle, and eye. Full maturation of the cyst takes 3 to 4 months; the size of the mature cyst varies from 2 to 4 mm to 2 cm in diameter. In tissue other than brain, the cysticercus is enveloped in a fibrous capsule, where it may survive for 3 to 6 years or longer. After the death of the parasite, calcification begins in the scolex and later may be seen in the cyst wall as well. Radiographically detectable calcifications are rare in muscle until at least 4 years after muscle invasion. Eye cysts, often subretinal, may lead to blindness as a consequence of retinal detachment or inflammatory changes.

Neurocysticercosis involving the brain has the potential for causing the most serious complications. Cysticerci can be found in the subarachnoid spaces or ventricles, embedded in brain parenchyma, or clustered at the base of the brain. In the last location, they may grow in the subarachnoid space in grape-like clusters, the "racemose cyst." The vesicles of this form of the organism lack a demonstrable scolex. They often obstruct the flow of spinal fluid with their membranes. Living cysticerci usually evoke little host response and rarely produce signs of nervous system disease unless present in large numbers or located in critical areas. The host reaction depends on the viability of the cyst. Young intact cysts induce little reaction. A granulomatous reaction occurs around dead or dying cysts, presumably reflecting the release of antigen or toxin after the loss of cyst integrity. Approximately 20 per cent of cerebral cysts eventually calcify. An excellent review of neurocysticercosis has been published.[10]

The clinical picture of neurocysticercosis is a consequence of the size, number, location, and age of the cysts. There may be transient myalgia, fever, and eosinophilia at the time of larval invasion, but this stage usually is unrecognized. Cysticerci, which localize in subcutaneous tissue, cause firm, mobile nodules that range in size from a few millimeters to several centimeters in diameter. The average size is 1 to 2 cm. These nodules usually are nontender and are found on the extremities and trunk more often than on the face. A review of the English language literature on subcutaneous cysticercosis has been published.[108]

Central nervous system symptoms often appear 5 to 7 years after probable infection; latencies as short as 6 months and as long as 30 years have occurred.[34] Almost any combination of neurologic symptoms can be seen. Relatively few or single cysts often present as a space-occupying lesion; in endemic areas, such as Mexico, up to one-quarter of all suspected brain tumors prove to be cysticerci. Single or usually multiple cysts also may cause cerebral swelling with papilledema and other signs of increased intracranial pressure or simulate a psychotic illness with delirium or hallucinations. This syndrome particularly is common in children.[61] Cysts at the base of the brain may cause signs and symptoms of intermittent or permanent hydrocephalus or acute or chronic meningitis. Subarachnoid cysts in this area have been implicated as a cause of vasculitis resulting in ischemic infarcts.[27] Intraventricular cysts also may cause hydrocephalus. The most common symptom, occurring separately or in combination with any of the aforementioned presentations, is epilepsy. Seizures, generalized or focal motor, occur in the majority of cases and may be the only symptom in up to one-third. In a series of 238 patients with cysticercosis in California, 56 per cent presented with seizures and 21 per cent with increased intracranial pressure.[84] Spinal cord involvement occurs in 1 to 5 per cent of cases of neurocysticercosis. Symptoms usually are caused by extramedullary compression of the spinal cord or by arachnoiditis. Intramedullary cyst formation is rare.

The prognosis of neurocysticercosis varies highly. Less than 10 per cent of patients with cerebral lesions die, usually within the first 5 to 10 years of illness. Many more are incapacitated with seizures or deterioration of higher cerebral functions. The clinical course often is characterized by spontaneous partial or complete remissions followed by one or more exacerbations. Usually, seizures become less frequent over time, so that the patient gradually may improve after several years. One series of 52 children with parenchymal cysts showed complete resolution of the lesions or residual punctate calcification within 2 to 9 months of observation. Sixty per cent of the children were weaned successfully from anticonvulsants with no recurrence of seizures.[68]

Peripheral blood eosinophil and white cell counts typically are normal, as is the erythrocyte sedimentation rate. With meningeal involvement, the cerebrospinal fluid usually is under increased pressure and shows pleocytosis. Typically, there is a moderate increase in protein. In approximately half the patients, the spinal fluid glucose is low, in some cases very low (in the range of 5 mg per cent). The spinal fluid findings and clinical picture readily are confused with tuberculous or bacterial meningitis. Eosinophilia of the cerebrospinal fluid may be helpful when present, but it is seen in less than half of cases of neurocysticercosis.

Skull radiographs showing spherical calcification of the 1- to 2-mm scolex, surrounded by a partially or totally calcified cyst 7 to 12 mm in diameter, are diagnostic. Old cysts are shrunken and less spherical. Computed tomography may be diagnostic when multiple cysts or typical calcifications are seen. Magnetic resonance imaging is superior to computed tomography for noncalcified cysts, especially in the diagnosis of ventricular and cisternal cysts and cysts near the base of the brain.

Serologic tests are available, but results have been variable. An enzyme-linked immunoelectrotransfer blot assay using purified glycoprotein antigen was found to be 98 per cent sensitive and 100 per cent specific in human cysticercosis.[97] Unfortunately, this test often yields negative results in patients with a single intracerebral lesion, and 75 per cent of children present with single lesions.[88] The test is used on serum. Testing of cerebrospinal fluid offers no advantage.[88] Serum specimens for enzyme-linked immunoelectrotransfer blot assay are submitted to state public health department laboratories, which forward them to the Centers for Disease Control and Prevention, where the test is performed.

Treatment

Praziquantel is an antiparasitic drug that is approved for use in the United States for schistosomiasis and certain liver fluke infections. It is active against cysticerci. Clinical trials have shown that treatment with praziquantel often causes lesions to disappear. It has been administered in a dose of 50 mg/kg of body weight daily divided into three equal doses for 15 days. The death of the parasites during drug therapy causes an inflammatory response. Side effects occur in 80 per cent or more of patients and may be more intense in those patients with greater numbers of cysts. Side effects include fever, headache, nausea, vomiting, seizures, and increased intracranial pressure. Cerebral infarction has been reported as a result of praziquantel treatment.[107] Reduction in the frequency and severity of side effects can be accomplished by using corticosteroids. However, concomitant corticosteroid use may lower the blood level of praziquantel by as much as 50 per cent and reduce its efficacy. Praziquantel levels also are reduced by concomitant use of phenytoin or carbamazepine. Cimetidine, conversely, raises praziquantel levels.

A benzimidazole compound, albendazole, also kills cysticerci. Albendazole appears more effective than praziquantel in resolving intraparenchymal cysts.[90] The standard course of albendazole has been 15 mg/kg of body weight per day divided into two or three doses given for 8 to 28 days and repeated if necessary. A course of 3 days of treatment at that dosage has been effective.[1] Drug therapy is much less effective in ventricular and subarachnoid cysts. However, albendazole appears to be superior to praziquantel in these locations. Side effects with albendazole are similar in frequency and degree to those with praziquantel and probably result from the host reaction to the death of the parasite. Dexamethasone administration may increase plasma levels of albendazole. American authorities recommend pretreating the patients with corticosteroids and continuing this during therapy with albendazole or praziquantel.[4] Mexican investigators feel that steroids should be reserved to treat only severe side effects as they occur during the course of treatment.[30]

There is no definitive agreement on the indications for drug therapy of neurocysticercosis.[28, 59] It is of no benefit when all of the cysticerci are calcified. Chemotherapy has been contraindicated with ocular involvement, but reports of favorable responses in ocular cysticercosis call for a reassessment.[63] The treatment of extraparenchymal neurocysticercosis has been reviewed.[9] No conclusions could be reached about the indications for medical treatment, but cases resolved or improved after drug treatment of both subarachnoid and intraventricular cysts.[9]

Other investigators state that drug treatment should be reserved for cystic parenchymal lesions that show no enhancement or surrounding edema on computed tomography. Enhancement and edema signify that inflammation is occurring around a dying parasite and that spontaneous resolution or calcification can be expected. The rapid and spontaneous resolution of parenchymal cysts in the absence of treatment in children[68] indicates that a conservative approach seems appropriate in most of these infections. However, some authorities believe that aggressive medical therapy is indicated to minimize residual calcification and, possibly, to reduce the persistence of seizures.[31] Should drug therapy be used, patients should be observed carefully for a prolonged period because of the occasional development or progression of hydrocephalus.

A study often cited by proponents of drug treatment of neurocysticercosis found that medically treated patients with either enhancing or nonenhancing lesions had significantly fewer seizures than untreated controls with similar lesions.[99] However, another study found that treated patients had a high frequency of neurologic sequelae when compared with untreated controls.[90] It is clear from the latter report that all patients with increased intracranial pressure are at significant risk when treated medically with either praziquantel or albendazole.

Surgical intervention is undergoing reassessment as reports of successful medical treatment of conditions such as intraventricular cysts and giant subarachnoid cysts are published.[29, 31] However, surgical placement of ventricular shunts may be a life-saving procedure in cases of progressive intracranial hypertension. In cases of increased intracranial pressure, shunt placement should precede medical therapy.[31]

Even though the yield is low, patients with cysticercosis always should be investigated for infection with the adult *T. solium*. In some circumstances, examination of family members or close contacts for *T. solium* infection is warranted.

Treatment of infection with adult *T. solium* is identical to that recommended for *T. saginata*; however, the patient should be made aware of a theoretic risk of cysticercosis if niclosamide, praziquantel, or paromomycin is used. This risk is based on the possibility that the gravid proglottids will liberate infective eggs within the intestine as a result of the treatment and that these eggs could be exposed to conditions that would induce hatching. This phenomenon has never been documented in humans, and the risk, if it exists, must be small. Some authorities recommend a mild purgative after specific treatment. It is doubtful that this is necessary or advantageous.[80]

Adequate cooking of pork prevents infection with adult tapeworms, and protection of food and drink from contamination with human feces should prevent cysticercosis.

DIPHYLLOBOTHRIASIS (*DIPHYLLOBOTHRIUM LATUM* INFECTION, FISH TAPEWORM INFECTION)

Diphyllobothriasis occurs in humans in areas where raw, pickled, or lightly smoked freshwater fish are eaten frequently. The prevalence of infection increases with age in endemic areas. Nonspecific gastrointestinal complaints may occur. Megaloblastic anemia is common in infected persons from certain geographic areas.

D. latum first was described in 1592 from specimens found in Switzerland. The life cycle was not known completely until the development of larval stages in copepods was demonstrated in 1917.

Several species of *Diphyllobothrium* have been reported from humans. A review of the taxonomy of the genus has led to the designation of *D. latum* of humans as a prototype for a complex of latum-like worms of the genus *Diphyllobothrium*.[102] Several of these species primarily are parasites of fish-eating birds, marine mammals, bears, dogs, and foxes. Humans, who coexist in the endemic areas, may be infected incidentally.[24]

Dibothriocephalus latus is a synonym of *D. latum* that some authors prefer.

The Organism

The scolex of *D. latum* possesses two deep grooves rather than discrete suckers. The entire worm may be as long as 15 m. The gravid proglottids have a characteristic rosette-shaped central uterus. Eggs measure 55 to 61 μm by 37 to 56 μm and have light brown, operculated shells. The eggs are shed in an unembryonated state from a uterine pore into the fecal stream. Development of six-hooked embryos within the eggs takes place in fresh water. The ciliated embryos hatch from the eggs and must be ingested by copepods in order to develop further. The larval stages found in copepods then develop into more advanced stages in muscles of fish that feed on the infected crustaceans. As the smaller fish are eaten by larger species, the larvae parasitize the muscles of the new host. Eventually, the larvae are found in fish that are sources of food for humans, such as species of pike, perch, turbot, lake trout, and white fish. The forms found in fish are called plerocercoid larvae or spargana. They are whitish, ribbon-like worms approximately 5 cm in length.

Transmission

Plerocercoid larvae are infectious for humans when they are ingested in fish, fish liver, or roe that have not been treated adequately by heat, freezing, or chemical agents.

The cycle of infection is perpetuated by the discharge of untreated sewage into freshwater lakes and streams.

Some fish-eating mammals also may serve as definitive hosts for *D. latum* and maintain the cycle of infection in the absence of humans. Because *D. latum* requires intermediate hosts, direct transmission is impossible and no techniques of isolation or special precautions are required for infected patients.

Epidemiology

The prevalence of infection increases with age in endemic areas. However, infections have been reported in children younger than 1 year of age.[103] The disease is worldwide in distribution, but areas of endemicity are associated with cultures in which people traditionally eat roe or freshwater fish raw, lightly salted, or pickled without cooking. The infection occurs frequently in the Baltic countries and the adjacent areas of the former Soviet Union; South America; Scandinavia; Switzerland and adjacent lake regions of Italy, France, and Germany; the Danube River delta; the lake areas of the northern United States; Canada; and the river deltas of Alaska. There is a report of human infection in Cuba.[14] Prevalence rates in Finland have fallen from 70 per cent to less than 2 per cent. In one study in northern Canada, 83 per cent of Eskimos older than 2 years of age were infected with *D. latum*.[6]

In Japan, *D. nihonkaiense* is transmitted to humans by ingestion of salmonid fish. In the far eastern part of the former Soviet Union, *D. klebanovskii* is acquired from Pacific salmon.

In 1980, a small outbreak of diphyllobothriasis in southern California was associated with eating fresh salmon. Several cases were linked to the raw fish dish, sushi.[81] The complication of megaloblastic anemia in *D. latum* infection is rare outside of Finland and the former Soviet Union, where it may occur in 2 per cent of tapeworm carriers.[74]

Pathology and Pathogenesis

Little is known about the direct effects of parasitization, with the exception of megaloblastic anemia.[3, 5] The following factors may be significant: (1) The strains of *D. latum* found in Finland, where anemia occurs, absorb seven times more vitamin B_{12} than do strains from North America, where anemia has not been reported. (2) There is interference with vitamin B_{12} absorption in nonanemic carriers, as well as in those with anemia. Deficient stores of B_{12} plus the B_{12} malabsorption may contribute to the anemic state. (3) Dietary intake of B_{12} may be low in anemic patients. Oral B_{12} has been shown to cause a reticulocytosis in the presence of the worm. (4) Worms found in anemic patients take up more of an oral dose of B_{12} than do worms in asymptomatic carriers, and worms are attached more proximally in the small intestine in anemic patients. (5) Secretion of intrinsic factor is reduced in anemic patients.

Clinical Manifestations

Most infections are asymptomatic, but patients may notice proglottids or chains of segments in their stools. In Finland, comparison of nonanemic infected patients with uninfected controls revealed an increase in the symptoms of fatigue, weakness, craving for salt, lack of well-being, dizziness, and numbness of the extremities that were reported by the infected group.[82]

Significant gastrointestinal symptoms occur infrequently. However, an experimental infection with seven larvae produced nausea, severe periumbilical pain, and marked weight loss.[91] Episodes of intestinal obstruction associated with the vomiting of masses of tapeworms have been reported.[103] Eosinophilia is uncommon.

Megaloblastic anemia caused by *D. latum* infection is extremely rare outside of Finland and neighboring endemic areas. Usually, it is seen in patients older than 50 years of age, but it has been reported in children as young as 9 years of age. The symptoms are identical to those seen in pernicious anemia, and neurologic involvement is not uncommon.

Diagnosis

Identification of the characteristic eggs or proglottids provides the diagnosis. The parasite produces nearly one million eggs per day, and ova usually are detected easily by fecal examination.

Treatment and Prevention

Treatment using the regimen noted for *T. saginata* is highly effective. Tapeworm anemia is reversible by treating the infection but should be supplemented initially with vitamin B_{12}.

The disease may be prevented by treating fish products with freezing or adequate cooking.

SPARGANOSIS (*SPIROMETRA* SPECIES INFECTION)

In 1854, the term *sparganum* was applied originally to the second-stage larvae of diphyllobothriid tapeworms whose adult forms were unknown. Human infection with these larvae is called sparganosis.

The Organism

Evidence indicates that the amorphous, thin, ribbon-like spargana recovered from human infections belong to the genus *Spirometra*. The adult tapeworms are found in dogs, cats, raccoons, and a variety of wild carnivores. Eggs passed in the feces of these definitive hosts hatch in fresh water. The embryo that emerges from the egg is ingested by a copepod, a common freshwater crustacean, where it undergoes larval development. When the infected copepod is ingested by a second intermediate host, the larva develops into a sparganum. There is a wide range of second intermediate hosts, which include amphibians, reptiles, birds, and mammals. Rodents, foxes, humans, and other primates also have been infected with spargana. When the second intermediate host is eaten by the definitive host, the sparganum attaches to the intestinal mucosa and develops into the adult tapeworm.

Little is known about the species of diphyllobothriid larvae found in humans. Because there are no distinguishing morphologic features of spargana, they must be fed to definitive hosts such as dogs and cats, and the adult worms must be recovered for study. Because this rarely is possible, the designation of species found in humans is based largely on epidemiologic relationships to species described in local animals. The species found in Africa, Asia, Europe, and South America usually is called *S. mansoni* or *S. erinacei*, and the species infecting humans in the United States is called *S. mansonoides*.

A rare form of sparganosis that buds, branches, and multiplies asexually to massive numbers in humans is called sparganum proliferum. It may be an aberrant or mutant form, or it may be the result of viral infection of a sparganum.[16] Adult forms of sparganum proliferum are unknown.

Transmission

In parts of Asia, it is common practice to apply poultices of amphibian or reptile flesh to wounds or sores. This is an apparent source for contact sparganosis when the spargana migrate from the poultice into human tissues. This probably is the most common cause of ocular sparganosis. Experimental infections of monkeys easily are induced by feeding them copepods containing the first larval stages. Human sparganosis in the United States often is associated with drinking well water or untreated surface water that could contain the minute copepods. Transmission by ingestion of raw or inadequately cooked flesh of second intermediate hosts has been proved experimentally in humans.[109] Animal sources that have been incriminated in human infections are snakes, frogs, chickens, and pigs. Larval stages from crushed copepods can penetrate the unbroken skin. Even though human infection has been induced in this manner, it seems an unlikely natural mode of transmission.

Epidemiology

Human infections are uncommon. In the United States, almost all of the reports have come from the southern or southeastern states and Puerto Rico or were reported in persons who had been in those areas. The only report of infection in a child in the United States came from southern California.[23] Reports of human infection have come from China, Southeast Asia, Japan, India, Indonesia, the Philippines, Australia, Africa, Italy, South America, and the former Soviet Union.

The rare sparganum proliferum infections have been reported in Japan, the United States, and South America.

Pathology, Pathogenesis, and Clinical Manifestations

The larva penetrates tissue either on contact, as in the poultice application, or through the intestinal mucosa. Ocular sparganosis, usually acquired by contact, may involve conjunctival, retro-orbital, or palpebral tissues, causing conjunctivitis, periorbital and palpebral edema, exophthalmos, chemosis, and corneal ulcerations. Subcutaneous sparganosis is the most common form of the infection, with the trunk frequently involved. The lesion usually is nodular. Tenderness and inflammation may be absent, intermittent, or constant. Some lesions are migratory. The lesions have variable inflammatory responses.[98] Eosinophils may or may not be present. Some infections have had an associated peripheral eosinophilia, but this is not a constant finding. Other less common sites for spargana are the extremities, head, muscles, spermatic cord, jejunum, colon, urethra, bladder, and pulmonary artery. The rare cerebral sparganosis usually causes seizures but may be associated with a variety of neurologic manifestations.[20]

The disease caused by sparganum proliferum consists of a progressive replacement of the host tissues by the multiplying organisms. The patient may survive many years until the parasites impair the function of a vital organ. The initial evidence of proliferative sparganosis often is the expression of a sparganum from a skin lesion. Eleven cases reported from the world literature were reviewed in 1990.[73]

Diagnosis

The diagnosis may be suspected in persons with typical subcutaneous lesions and a suggestive epidemiologic background. Usually, however, the diagnosis is made during surgical removal of a painful or cosmetically disturbing lump without anticipating the parasitic etiology. The spargana vary considerably in width and length. They usually are several centimeters in length, whitish, and opaque, and they may show the grooved indentations on the anterior end that are the precursors of the bothria or suckers of the adult worm. Cross-section of the parasite reveals the calcareous corpuscles seen in cestodes. Small portions of spargana are difficult to distinguish grossly or microscopically from cysticerci and other less common larval cestodes. Computed tomography may yield characteristic findings in cerebral sparganosis.[20] An enzyme-linked immunosorbent assay (ELISA) for serum and cerebrospinal fluid antibody appears useful.[17] A sparganum-specific protein also has been used in an ELISA for the diagnosis of other forms of sparganosis.[75]

Treatment

Surgical removal is the only known form of therapy. Mebendazole and praziquantel have been tried in one case of proliferative sparganosis.[71] Although the patient improved while on mebendazole, motile parasites still were present and new lesions were developing. Severe reactions to praziquantel caused cessation of treatment.

Prevention

Filtration of water prevents the ingestion of copepods from wells or ponds. Proper cooking of meat eliminates second intermediate hosts as sources of infection. Educational efforts should be made to warn of the dangers of applying raw flesh poultices in areas where that is a cultural practice.

DIPYLIDIASIS (*DIPYLIDIUM CANINUM* INFECTION, DOG TAPEWORM INFECTION)

D. caninum, the common tapeworm of dogs and cats, also infects infants and young children. Transmission occurs through accidental ingestion of infected fleas. Variable gastrointestinal symptoms may develop, or the patients may be asymptomatic.

D. caninum was described first by Linnaeus in 1758, but it had been recorded from a human infection by a student of Linnaeus in 1751. The life cycle was described fully in 1916.

The Organism

D. caninum adult worms have a scolex with four cup-shaped suckers and a central protrusible structure, the rostellum, which bears one to seven rows of small hooks. The worm ranges from 10 to 70 cm in length. The gravid proglottids resemble cucumber seeds in size and shape. The proglottids have two pairs of sex organs, and a genital pore opens on each lateral margin. The eggs measure 35 to 65 μm in diameter and appear in packets of 5 to 30 enclosed in a membrane. The gravid proglottids are excreted in the feces or migrate actively from the anus. The eggs are liberated as the proglottid disintegrates. Several species of flea serve as intermediate hosts. The larval flea ingests the egg of *D. caninum*. Development of the tapeworm's larval stages takes place as the flea metamorphoses into an adult. When the flea is ingested by the definitive host, the adult worm develops in the small intestine.

Transmission

Humans acquire the infection by the accidental ingestion of infected fleas. Dogs may transfer infective larvae to humans by licking after nipping at fleas. Because of the motility of the proglottids, eggs may be disseminated widely in the environment of animal hosts. Fleas are so ubiquitous that transmission to the intermediate host is accomplished readily.

Epidemiology

Infection of dogs and cats occurs throughout the world. *D. caninum* also has been found in foxes, jackals, hyenas, dingoes, and a variety of wild felids. Considering the close relationship between children and their pets, the opportunity for infection appears to be great. Reports of dipylidiasis in humans in the United States, however, are uncommon.[53] It generally is agreed that human infections are far more frequent than the reports indicate.

Clinical Manifestations

Although the incubation period in humans is unknown, infection has been seen in infants 5 weeks of age.

Frequently, the only evidence of infection is the finding of proglottids in the stool or in an infant's diapers. Varying degrees of abdominal pain, diarrhea, irritability, and pruritus have been recorded in symptomatic children.

Diagnosis, Prognosis, and Treatment

The characteristic proglottids must be differentiated from other parasites. A frequent error is to assume, from the parents' description, that small, motile proglottids that migrate from the anus are pinworms. Proglottids also may be mistaken for fly larvae.

Examination of stool specimens may be spuriously negative because the proglottids tend to migrate from the fecal mass and disintegrate on the walls of the specimen container.

The infection has not been associated with serious symptoms, and response to treatment with praziquantel as used in *T. saginata* infection is excellent.

Prevention

Infected dogs and cats should be treated. Flea control requires the use of appropriate insecticides on the pets. In addition, particular attention must be given to carpets and areas where the pets sleep because these are the sites of development of the larval fleas. Aerosol insecticides specifically made for flea control are useful for large areas.

HYMENOLEPIASIS (*HYMENOLEPIS NANA* INFECTION, DWARF TAPEWORM INFECTION)

Infection with *H. nana*, the dwarf tapeworm, occurs throughout the world and probably is maintained by direct fecal-oral transmission from person to person, although insects may serve as intermediate hosts. Infection may be asymptomatic, but gastrointestinal, neurologic, and allergic symptoms have been reported. Treatment with praziquantel is successful.

The Organism

H. nana first was reported from rodents in 1845. A human case was discovered at autopsy in 1851. In 1892, the development of adult worms from the ingestion of eggs was proved experimentally. It was not until 1928 that insects were shown to be effective intermediate hosts for the parasite.

There is controversy about the identity of *H. nana* found in humans and the morphologically identical organisms found in rodents. The rodent strains often are called *H. fraterna* or *H. nana* variety *fraterna*.

Adult worms of *H. nana* measure only 5 to 45 mm in length and are less than 1 mm in maximum width. The tiny scolex has four cup-shaped suckers and a protrusible rostellum with a circle of 20 to 30 small hooks. Gravid proglottids disintegrate within the intestine, and eggs are found in the feces. The eggs measure from 30 to 50 μm in diameter and contain a six-hooked embryo within two envelopes. The space between the two envelopes contains filaments that extend from two small polar protrusions on the inner envelope. Insect intermediate hosts develop larval stages after ingestion of the eggs. If the definitive host ingests eggs, larval stages develop in the intestinal villi in 4 to 5 days, then break into the lumen and develop into adult worms. Ova appear in the feces 2 to 4 weeks after infection.

Transmission

Human infection is acquired most commonly by ingestion of eggs from feces of infected persons. Humans serve as both intermediate and definitive hosts in this direct cycle. Transmission via this route is enhanced by poor hygienic habits, overcrowding, lack of running water, and any other factor that fosters fecal-oral transmission.

The rodent strains of *H. nana* are infectious for humans, and food contaminated by rodent feces is a possible source of infection. Pet rodents, such as rats, mice, and hamsters, often are infected, and close contact, as in playful fondling, could result in transmission by contaminated hands.

Ingestion of insect intermediate hosts accidentally or in infested food also may cause infection. This mode of infection may be common in rodents but probably is infrequent in people.

Adequate information on the duration of infection in humans is lacking. Eggs may be produced for periods longer than 1 year, but the possibility of recurrent autoinfection obscures the observation of the duration of the initial infection.

Internal autoinfection may occur when ova from gravid proglottids are exposed to appropriate conditions within the intestinal lumen. Hatching occurs and the embryos penetrate the mucosa, undergo larval development, and eventually emerge as adult worms.

Although there is little information concerning immunity to *H. nana* infection in humans, rodent experiments indicate that the larval stages occurring in the intestinal villi stimulate an immune response, which probably predominantly is T-cell–dependent.[64] Serum from infected animals also has been shown to protect uninfected mice from challenge infections.[33] Antibody has been demonstrated in infected humans.[49]

Epidemiology

H. nana is a common parasite of rats and mice throughout the world. Prevalence of infection in commercially supplied hamsters has been reported at 44 per cent.[89] Monkeys and chimpanzees rarely are infected. Flour beetles, meal worms, fleas, and cockroaches may serve as intermediate hosts.

The distribution of infection in humans is worldwide, with an increased prevalence in some urban areas.[44] Surveys have shown certain areas to have a high level of endemicity: Sicily has shown rates of 46 per cent; 34 per cent of schoolchildren in Algeria were infected; and the former southern Soviet Union had rates of 26 per cent. Children between the ages of 4 and 10 years have the highest prevalence rates, and infections tend to affect several members of a family. Prevalence also is high in institutionalized children.

Pathology and Pathogenesis

Little is known of the pathogenesis and pathology of *H. nana* infection in humans. Local reactions consisting of mucosal inflammation or atrophy may occur at the site of attachment of the adult worms in the small intestine.

The larval stage of *H. nana* is a cyst-like structure about 250 μm in diameter and called a cysticercoid. In mice deprived of T cells, these larval stages may develop in an aberrant manner and produce multiple fluid-filled cysts several millimeters in diameter. These cysts spread from the intestinal villi to lymphatics, liver, and lung.[64] A patient with Hodgkin disease undergoing radiation therapy and receiving immunosuppressive drugs developed a disseminated larval cestode infection thought to be caused by sparganum proliferum. It now is felt that this represented aberrant *H. nana* larvae.[64] A 13-year-old Egyptian female with filariasis and a history of taking corticosteroids had dissemination of larval stages that were seen in her venous blood sample.[87]

Clinical Manifestations

A wide variety of symptoms have been ascribed to *H. nana* infection, but well-controlled clinical studies are lacking. In a series of 43 patients with *H. nana* infection reported from South America, these symptoms were noted in order of decreasing frequency: restlessness, irritability, diarrhea, abdominal pain, restless sleep, and anal and nasal pruritus.[35] Eosinophilia above 5 per cent was noted in one-third of these patients. In contrast, neither diarrhea nor eosinophilia was correlated with the presence of *H. nana* infection in an extensive epidemiologic study in western Pakistan.[17]

Symptoms reported from various series of infected cases include anorexia or increase in appetite, nausea, vomiting, pains in extremities, dizziness, and headache.

A study of 10 children in Thailand showed that worm burdens of 3000 or more were associated with abdominal pain, diarrhea or loose stools, malnutrition, growth retardation, and lethargy. Children with fewer than 100 worms appeared normal but had occasional soft stools.[22]

One peculiar case of ectopic localization of *H. nana* was reported from Japan. An adult worm containing eggs was found in a mass on the chest wall of an elderly woman.[69]

Nervous system involvement, with the production of seizures, has received much attention in the former Soviet Union. This is considered to result from *H. nana* infection and occurs most frequently in children between the ages of 7 and 15 years.[50]

General experience suggests that patients either lack symptoms or present with nonspecific gastrointestinal complaints.

Diagnosis

The detection of the characteristic eggs in fecal examination by direct saline wet mounts or by concentration techniques usually is not difficult. However, a single examination not always is adequate to rule out infection.

Treatment

Praziquantel and paromomycin are effective in treating *H. nana* infections. Because of the lack of action on the larval stages in the intestinal villi, paromomycin must be given in courses over a 7-day period. Praziquantel, however, is effective in a single dose. When praziquantel or paromomycin is used for *H. nana* infections in the United States, it is considered investigational. Paromomycin is given in a dosage of 45 mg/kg in a single dose daily for 7 days. Praziquantel is given in a single dose of 25 mg/kg. Because praziquantel is effective in a single dose, patient compliance can be expected to be better than in the 7-day course.

A series of fecal examinations 3 to 4 weeks after the completion of treatment is necessary to assess the effectiveness of therapy. Family members should be examined and treated if they are infected.

Prognosis

H. nana infection is not serious and responds well to appropriate treatment. Metastatic larval forms of *H. nana* are rare.[12, 64] The susceptibility of patients with impaired T-cell function, such as those with acquired immunodeficiency syndrome, has not been determined.

Prevention

Transmission of *H. nana* infections largely could be eliminated if proper methods of personal hygiene and disposal of human waste could be invoked throughout the world.

Infected food handlers always should be treated and followed to ensure that treatment has been successful. Stored food should be protected from rodents and insects.

ECHINOCOCCOSIS (*ECHINOCOCCUS* SPECIES INFECTION, HYDATID DISEASE)

Humans may be infected with larval stages of several species of *Echinococcus*. The larvae most frequently develop in the liver but may develop in many different tissues. Humans acquire the infection by ingestion of ova from feces of carnivorous definitive hosts. The disease in humans and intermediate hosts often is called hydatid disease. It also may be designated according to the morphology of the larval stages: unilocular echinococcosis caused by *E. granulosus*, multilocular or alveolar echinococcosis caused by *E. multilocularis*, and polycystic echinococcosis caused by *E. vogeli*.

Excellent recent reviews of echinococcosis are available.[57, 93, 96]

The Organism

The life cycles of the three major species of *Echinococcus* are similar, but the geographic distribution, types of hosts, and morphology of the parasites differ significantly. *E. granulosus* is the most common species found in human infections. There are two major strains. The adult tapeworms of the domestic or pastoral strain most often are found in dogs. Sheep are the usual hosts for the larval stages. The sylvatic strain involves wolves, moose, and reindeer. The adult tapeworm is only 3 to 8 mm long and has two to five segments. Dogs often are hosts to thousands of adult worms. When the eggs are ingested by the intermediate hosts, by ungulates such as sheep, or by humans, the eggs hatch in the intestine and the embryos burrow through the intestinal wall and gain access to the portal circulation. Many embryos are destroyed, but those that survive may develop in many tissues, most commonly in the liver or lung, where they become the cystic larval structures called hydatid cysts. The cyst is composed of an outer laminated, acellular membrane that is lined by the thin, cellular germinal membrane. Spherical structures, called brood capsules, grow from the germinal membrane. Within the brood capsules, the protoscoleces develop. These structures contain suckers and hooks and become the scoleces of adult worms when they are eaten by dogs. Compression from the growth of the cyst produces a "pericyst" of compact host tissue around its exterior. Older cysts may have smaller cysts develop within the cyst cavity, so-called "daughter cysts."

E. multilocularis typically involves foxes as definitive hosts and rodents as intermediate hosts. In human infections, the larval parasite grows by progressive external budding in liver tissue. The laminated membrane and host pericyst are thin. The larval mass slowly enlarges, replacing liver tissue much as a malignancy does. The larvae may invade contiguous structures and rarely metastasize. *E. vogeli* is a parasite of bush dogs and feral dogs in South America. The common intermediate host is a rodent. When humans are infected, the germinal membrane grows externally to form additional cysts and develops septa within the original cyst. This is the "polycystic" variety of hydatid disease. *E. oligarthrus* is a fourth species that is an extremely rare cause of disease in humans. The definitive hosts are wild felids, such as pumas and jaguars. Pacas, agoutis, and spiny rats serve as intermediate hosts. Most infections occur in Central and South America.

Transmission

Humans acquire unilocular hydatid disease by ingestion of food or drink contaminated with feces from infected definitive hosts, usually dogs. Close contact with dogs can result in infections because tapeworm eggs can be found on the dog's perianal hair, muzzle, and paws. Flies and other insects may disseminate the eggs from dogs' feces. In Lebanon, the high prevalence rate of infection in shoemakers was thought to be related to the practice of tanning leather with a mixture of water and dog feces.

Alveolar hydatid disease most often is acquired by exposure to foxes, although dogs, cats, and coyotes have been infected. Fur traders and hunters may be exposed by skinning foxes or by handling the fur. Sled dogs have been implicated as sources of infection in Arctic villages.

Polycystic hydatid disease caused by *E. vogeli* is rare. Transmission is thought to occur from infected hunting dogs.[25]

Epidemiology

The domestic strain of *E. granulosus* is found worldwide in areas of sheep raising. The custom of feeding sheep viscera to sheep dogs maintains foci of infection. In the United States, Basques in central California, Mormon ranchers in Utah, and Native Americans in Arizona and New Mexico have been infected. The disease is endemic in the sheep-raising areas of South America, Australia, the Mediterranean basin, and the former Soviet Union. One of the highest morbidity rates is seen in rural Africans in Kenya and Uganda, where they live in close association with their dogs. The sylvatic form of *E. granulosus* infection is found in parts of the Western Hemisphere. In Alaska and Canada, human infection usually is limited to Eskimos and Native Americans who have working dogs that are fed on moose and reindeer viscera. The strain found in this region often presents as giant pulmonary cysts. The course of infection usually is benign.[41, 60] Sylvatic *E. granulosus* also can be found in northern Scandinavia and the former Soviet Union, but human infection is uncommon.

Alveolar hydatid disease is found only in the Northern Hemisphere, where it is common in a cycle involving arctic foxes and rodents. Infection in animals extends into the northern portion of many Midwestern states in the United States. The first human case of alveolar hydatid disease in the contiguous United States was diagnosed in Minnesota in 1977. The disease is endemic in large areas of the former Soviet Union, and human cases have been reported from northern Japan and from Switzerland and adjacent European countries.

Polycystic hydatid disease is limited to South and Central America, where it is a rare infection in humans.

Pathogenesis and Pathology

In unilocular hydatid disease, the development of disease is related to compression or displacement of host tissue. Cyst growth is variable but probably averages about 1 cm in diameter per year. Rates up to 4 to 5 cm per year have been reported.[57] The cyst may exceed 35 cm in diameter in the abdominal cavity. When there is rupture or leakage of a cyst, an allergic reaction caused by the antigenic cyst contents usually occurs. Cysts may calcify after many years, and this usually signifies the death of the parasite. Hydatid cysts may form foci for secondary bacterial infection.

In alveolar hydatid disease, there is a slow replacement of liver tissue by the parasite, which may continue for as long as 30 years. The central area becomes a necrotic, pus-containing cavity. The margins of the lesion are indefinite. Microscopic examination shows multiple vesicles of different sizes advancing into normal hepatic tissue. The vesicles rarely contain protoscoleces. Metastatic lesions to brain, lung, and mediastinum occur in 2 per cent of infections, and invasion of organs contiguous to the liver occurs in 15 per cent.

Polycystic hydatid disease shows multiple vesicles and cysts, which measure from a few millimeters to several centimeters in diameter. Protoscoleces usually are abundant within blood capsules.

Clinical Manifestations

Most patients with *E. granulosus* infection have a single unilocular cyst, but in 15 to 30 per cent of patients, multiple unilocular cysts, usually but not always in a single organ system, are seen. Approximately one in five children with a pulmonary cyst also has a concurrent liver cyst. In adults and children, 10 per cent of hydatids are found neither in the liver nor in the lung but in some other tissue. The northern sylvatic strain of *E. granulosus* found in Canada and Alaska characteristically produces pulmonary cysts. Hydatid cysts have been reported in all organs, most notably in the eye, brain, spleen, heart, endocrine glands, bone, and genitourinary tract. Central nervous system hydatid disease is much more common in children than in adults.[19] Bone cysts, which may be seen in preschool children, are most common in vertebral and long bones. Unlike cysts in other sites, bone hydatids characteristically are multilocular and contain little fluid. Eye, bone, and brain cysts typically are small when discovered, whereas cysts in other sites may exceed 35 cm in diameter when detected. Cysts grow about 1 to 5 cm in diameter each year. Serious morbidity is the consequence of enlargement, secondary infection, or a cyst rupture. Some children with hydatid disease also show retarded growth patterns.[66] Infection of hydatid cysts and leakage or rupture with hypotension, urticaria, and eosinophilia are relatively uncommon complications of hydatid disease.

Symptoms are caused most often by pressure produced by an expanding cyst; its location determines the clinical presentation. Fever, cough, chest pain, and hemoptysis are common symptoms of patients with pulmonary hydatids. Up to one-third of pulmonary cysts rupture into the pleural space or into a bronchus. In the latter case, the patient may describe "coughing up grape skins." Symptomatic intrahepatic cysts cause constant or intermittent right upper quadrant pain or jaundice. From 5 to 15 per cent of adults with hepatic hydatid have rupture of the cyst into the biliary tract, simulating choledocholithiasis and ascending cholangitis with fever, pain, and jaundice; this complication is rare during childhood.[58] Bone cysts are seen with bone pain or as a pathologic fracture. Vertebral hydatid disease causes spinal cord and radicular compression signs and symptoms; severe pain on palpation over the affected spine is characteristic. Fifty to 75 per cent of intracranial hydatids are seen in children.[39] Increased intracranial pressure with headache and vomiting is a common presentation. Seizures also can occur.

Symptoms of alveolar hydatid disease most often occur in older adults but have been reported in children as young as 5 years of age. The most common finding is hepatomegaly, often tender to palpation. Abdominal masses continuous with the liver also are common. Jaundice occurs in about 20 per cent of infections.

Polycystic hydatid disease is rare and also is manifested in adults. The clinical picture may resemble cirrhosis, hepatic tumor or abscess, or intra-abdominal tumor. Hepatomegaly, abdominal masses, and jaundice are frequent presenting signs.

Diagnosis

The diagnosis usually is suspected on the basis of clinical or radiologic findings plus the history of residence in an endemic area. Physical examination rarely is definitive. Only half of patients with hepatic hydatids have abnormal liver function tests. Eosinophilia more often is absent than present, although serum IgE levels characteristically are elevated.[32] On occasion, scoleces of the parasite can be identified in vomitus, stool, urine, or sputum when the cyst has ruptured spontaneously, but usually the parasite is not seen until surgery.

The initial suspicion of unilocular hydatid disease often is based on radiographic findings. An unruptured pulmonary hydatid has a sharply demarcated smooth border, is round or oval, has a homogeneous cannonball appearance, and sometimes is surrounded by a layer of atelectatic lung.[8, 52] There may be pericystic emphysema around the bronchiole when the cyst is about to rupture. After the cyst has ruptured into a bronchus, a crescent-shaped air layer may be seen that virtually is diagnostic. In addition to the arc of air between the parasite and the host cyst wall, there also may be air in the cyst lumen. The membrane of a collapsed cyst floating on the surface of the fluid in a ruptured hydatid has a characteristic "water lily" appearance.

Radiographically apparent cyst wall calcification occurs only in liver or spleen cysts and usually takes more than 20 years to develop; thus, it rarely is helpful for diagnosis in children. Cysts usually are seen easily and measured with

TABLE 224–1. Less Common Tapeworms That Can Infect Humans

	Scolex	Approximate Length/Width	Proglottids	Eggs	Geographic Distribution	Intermediate Hosts	Transmission	Clinical Manifestations
Hymenolepis diminuta (rat tapeworm)	Four small suckers, no hooks	10–60 cm/ 4 mm max.	2.5 mm wide by 0.75 mm in length; usually not seen in feces	60–85 μm in diameter; embryo separated from egg shell by large space	Worldwide in rats and mice; human infections are uncommon but most frequent in children	Rat and mouse fleas; flour and grain beetles	Accidental ingestion of insect intermediate host, usually in uncooked or precooked cereal	Frequently asymptomatic; may have anorexia, nausea, vomiting, weight loss, abdominal pain, or diarrhea
Bertiella species	Four ovoid suckers, no hooks	26–45 cm/ 6 mm max.	6 mm wide by 0.75 mm in length; usually found in feces in chains of 10 or more	46–50 μm in diameter; irregularly ovoid; embryo envelope possesses a bicornuate protrusion	Found in primates worldwide; human infections are rare (less than 50 cases); usually in children in close contact with pet monkey or other primate	Oribatid mites	Accidental ingestion of mite; usually history of close contact with pet monkey	Usually asymptomatic; nonspecific gastrointestinal complaints have been reported
Raillietina species	Four suckers with tiny hooks; rostellum with double row of 80 or more hooks	Up to 12 m/ 3 mm	Resemble rice grains and appear motile in feces; contain egg capsules with several eggs in each capsule	Numbers of eggs included in capsule depend on species	Usually in infants and young children; found in South America (Ecuador is endemic), Philippines,	Unknown, probably insects	Unknown	Reports from Ecuador[37] list nausea, vomiting, sialorrhea, flatulence, colic, diarrhea, nervous disorders, tachycardia,

					Japan, Taiwan, Thailand, Indonesia, and Tahiti			arrhythmia, syncope, anemia, and eosinophilia; asymptomatic infections also have been described
Inermicapsifer madagascariensis	Four suckers, no hooks	Up to 42 cm/2.6 mm	"Rice grains," similar to *Raillietina,* are passed in feces; eggs in capsules in gravid segments	Six or more eggs per capsule; 35–50 μm in diameter	Usually found in children younger than 6 years of age; reported from Africa, also from Venezuela, Malaya, Thailand, and Philippines; more than 100 cases reported from Cuba	Unknown	Unknown	Not adequately described; probably asymptomatic
Mesocestoides species	Four suckers with slit-like openings	40 cm/2 mm (variable with species)	Passed in feces; bead-like; 1.5 mm wide by 2.5 mm in length; eggs located in a mass in the parauterine organ	Oval; approximately 20–26 μm in maximum diameter	Rare in humans; several infections in adults in Japan; few cases in children from United States and Africa; single case in Korea	Life cycle incompletely known; second intermediate hosts are birds, reptiles, frogs, and rodents	Probably ingestion of raw flesh of second intermediate hosts; Japanese cases associated with ingestion of raw reptile viscera and blood	Abdominal pain and severe diarrhea reported in Japanese adults; children have been asymptomatic

computed tomography. Ultrasound techniques can be used to differentiate fluid-filled cysts from solid tumors. Septa or daughter cysts, when present, produce echoes that are highly characteristic of hydatid cysts. Angiography is said to show a characteristic halo effect around the cyst in some cases. Bone cysts typically produce radiolucencies without periosteal reaction.

Needling of cysts for diagnosis has been considered to be extremely dangerous because leakage of hydatid fluid can induce anaphylactic shock. The percutaneous route has been used for both diagnosis and treatment with few untoward events.

The Casoni skin test, which basically is injection of hydatid fluid into the dermis, yields an erythematous papule in less than 60 minutes in 50 to 80 per cent of patients. False-negative and false-positive results occur in up to 30 per cent. Serologic tests, such as ELISA, indirect hemagglutination, and fluorescent antibody tests, may be negative in 10 to 50 per cent of patients with cystic hydatid disease. False-negative results seem to be more common in patients with pulmonary hydatids and in children. Tests using arc number 5 as determined by immunoelectrophoresis were thought to be sensitive and highly specific, but cross-reactions have occurred in cysticercosis. The use of an ELISA together with an immunoblot or arc 5 test seems to have the highest yield.[57] No serologic test now available rules out the diagnosis of cystic hydatid disease. A highly sensitive and specific ELISA for alveolar hydatid disease has been developed using a species-specific fraction (Em_2) of whole organism extract.[62] The identification of another epitope (Em_{18}) may provide a method for determining the activity of the infection.[56]

Often, the diagnosis of alveolar hydatid disease is based first on an abdominal radiograph showing scattered large areas of amorphous calcification containing 2- to 4-mm radiolucent areas surrounded by calcium.[94] The degree of liver invasion at surgery often is found to be much more extensive than the calcified area.

In the absence of a characteristic radiologic finding, the diagnosis frequently is missed preoperatively. The diagnosis is confirmed at surgery by the demonstration of the characteristic laminated membrane by periodic acid–Schiff staining or the presence of protoscoleces or hooklets.

Treatment and Prognosis

In most cases, surgery is considered to be the treatment of choice for echinococcosis. However, studies employing medical therapy call this traditional statement into question. Medical therapy is discussed later. The sylvatic strains of *E. granulosus* from Alaska and Canada do not produce anaphylaxis upon rupture, and pulmonary cysts spontaneously resolve after evacuating into bronchi. Thoroughly calcified cysts in older persons rarely require treatment. Surgical success depends on the size and location of cysts and the skill of the surgeon. In unilocular disease, rupture of cyst contents at the time of surgery carries an immediate risk of anaphylaxis and a delayed risk of disseminated echinococcosis. The latter, relatively uncommon even after a spillage, is a greatly feared complication. As a consequence, multiple surgical techniques are directed toward preventing spillage of viable cyst contents during surgery for hepatic cysts. These include injection of hypertonic saline, alcohol, or cetrimide into the cyst. There is increasing agreement that the hazards of injecting scolecidal substances into the cyst outweigh unproven benefits. Opinions differ as to the optimal type of surgical procedure for hepatic cysts. Some surgeons prefer to sterilize and evacuate the cyst contents, refill the cyst with normal saline, and leave it in place. Other techniques are oriented toward obliterating the large residual cavity after a cyst has been removed or emptied. Percutaneous cyst drainage followed by alcohol or hypertonic saline injection and reaspiration has been carried out with success.[11, 45] Currently, this technique only is recommended for inoperable lesions or when a patient refuses surgery. Reviews of surgical management are available.[36, 48, 70, 76, 83]

In general, the surgical mortality rate is 3 to 5 per cent, including multilocular cysts and reoperations. In some areas, one in five patients requires reoperation. Serologic and skin tests may remain positive for at least 10 years after successful surgery; a falling titer suggests cure, but a persistent elevated titer does not equal recurrence necessarily.

Mebendazole was the first benzimidazole to be tried in hydatid disease. Extremely high doses had to be used because the drug is absorbed poorly from the gastrointestinal tract. The results were inconsistent. Albendazole now has replaced mebendazole. It is well absorbed and diffuses into the cysts in effective concentrations. Levels of the active albendazole metabolite are increased with concomitant administration of cimetidine. The usual approach to the administration of albendazole is to give variable numbers of courses depending on individual responses. Each course is 28 days in length and is followed by a 14-day rest period. In adults, albendazole is given at a total dose of 800 mg daily divided into two doses. If a response to albendazole is not evident after three courses of treatment, subsequent courses are unlikely to be beneficial. A randomized, controlled study of albendazole in uncomplicated hepatic hydatid disease in adults concluded that 10 mg/kg/day for 3 months, without rest periods, was highly effective and should be tried before surgical intervention.[47] Other trials of albendazole also have shown beneficial effects in many, but not all, cases of hydatid disease.[72, 105] In children, the dose of albendazole is 15 mg/kg/day for 28 days and is repeated as necessary. Albendazole may cause reversible liver function abnormalities, transient leukopenia, and alopecia. Severe hepatotoxicity associated with jaundice has been reported in up to 5 per cent of patients treated. Liver function tests should be monitored closely. Albendazole also is useful in inoperable cases of hydatid disease, and it may be used before or after surgery to reduce the risk of intraoperative dissemination and recurrence. Favorable response to albendazole has been reported in both alveolar and polycystic hydatid disease.[67, 106] Information on current drug therapy in hydatid disease may be obtained from the Centers for Disease Control and Prevention in Atlanta.

The prognosis of hydatid disease varies widely. Hepatic cysts may undergo spontaneous death and calcification in up to one-fourth of cases. Up to two-thirds of symptomatic patients without intervention die. The survivors usually experience the spontaneous rupture and spontaneous evacuation of the cyst into a hollow viscus.

Untreated alveolar hydatid disease has a mortality rate exceeding 90 per cent within 10 years of diagnosis. More than 70 per cent of patients have lesions that are unresectable at the time of diagnosis. In some cases, a partial hepatectomy or hepatic lobectomy can remove all of the multilocular cyst and still preserve enough organ function to sustain life. To eradicate the infection, all invaded tissue and a margin of normal tissue must be resected en bloc. Liver transplantation has been useful both as a curative approach in selected patients and as palliation in incurable disease.[96] Chemotherapy with albendazole probably should be used as an adjunct to surgery. In inoperable patients, chemotherapy may arrest the progression of the disease and possibly, in some, bring about a cure.[106]

Prevention

Prevention of the disease requires elimination of the infection in dogs by using suitable veterinary taeniacides. Proper disposal of carcasses and entrails on ranges and from slaughterhouses prevents dogs from gaining access to them. The dog-sheep cycle is interrupted most easily; other cycles may be impossible to control. The effectiveness of dog control combined with educational efforts is demonstrated best in Iceland. The disease initially was found in 22 per cent of the population and now has been eradicated. Those who have contact with dogs that feed on carcasses of large deer should be warned against contamination of hands, food, or drink with dog feces. The hazards of exposure to wild foxes and dogs in the Arctic regions also must be made known.

COENUROSIS (COENURIASIS, *TAENIA [MULTICEPS]* SPECIES INFECTION)

Several species of *Taenia* have a larval stage called a coenurus, which consists of a cystic membranous structure up to 6 cm in diameter from which multiple scoleces bud internally or externally. Because of this unique larval morphology, the parasite was given the species name *multiceps*. Currently, the preferred genus name is *Taenia* because of the morphology of the adult worms and the inability to justify genus designation based solely on the form of larvae.[40] Many publications still refer to the genus as *Multiceps*. The relationships of various species of coenurus-producing *Taenia (Multiceps)* are defined inadequately. The following species generally are accepted for purposes of discussion.

The adult tapeworm of *T. (M.) multiceps* is found in dogs, and the larval stages occur in herbivores, such as sheep, cattle, goats, and horses. These larvae often develop in the central nervous system and produce a condition known as gid or staggers in sheep. Because sheep infection has not been found in the United States for more than 60 years, it is thought that this species is an unlikely candidate for the forms of human coenurosis in this area. In sheep-raising areas of Europe and Asia, the infection still is endemic in animals.

T. (M.) serialis adult worms also are found in dogs and other canids, but common intermediate hosts are rabbits, hares, and rodents. The coenurus develops in subcutaneous and intramuscular tissues. In experimental infections in rodents, central nervous system involvement has been demonstrated. *T. serialis* has been reported from the United States, Canada, France, and Africa.

T. (M.) brauni is the name given to tapeworms of dogs, jackals, foxes, and genets found in tropical Africa. The larvae develop in gerbils and other rodents.

Humans are a rare accidental host for the larval stages of these worms. The disease is called coenurosis or coenuriasis. Fewer than 100 human infections have been recorded. Most infections are from Africa, with many in children. It nearly is impossible to give a species designation based solely on the morphology of organisms recovered from human tissue. It is presumed that the infection is acquired by the ingestion of eggs excreted by the definitive hosts, usually dogs. Because of the subcutaneous and subconjunctival location of cysts in infections in tropical Africa, it has been suggested that direct contact of the eggs on skin or the conjunctiva is a mode of transmission.

The clinical manifestations of coenurosis are related to the location of the parasite. Central nervous system involvement produces a spectrum of illness that resembles that of cysticercosis (discussed earlier), including meningeal reactions. Larvae have been seen in subconjunctival and subretinal tissues, extraocular muscles, anterior chamber, and vitreous. Subcutaneous and intramuscular lesions are most common in the abdomen and chest wall.

The definitive diagnosis is made by the demonstration of the characteristic morphology of the larva recovered at surgery. The multiple scoleces that bud from the delicate cyst membrane have double rows of hooklets of typical shape, size, and number. In instances in which no scoleces are found, it is impossible to differentiate a coenurus from the racemose cysticercus of *T. solium*. Radiographic studies, such as computed tomography, are useful in cerebral coenurosis but do not differentiate the parasite from other cystic lesions.

Treatment is surgical. Mortality in cerebral disease is high. Organisms in other locations, with the exception of subretinal lesions, easily are removed. Praziquantel has been used successfully to treat sheep with cerebral coenurosis.[101] A combination of praziquantel and corticosteroid was administered to a patient with a subretinal coenurus, causing the death of the parasite, which resulted in a severe inflammatory reaction, retinal detachment, and permanent loss of vision.[55] A patient with subarachnoid coenurosis received praziquantel, but the details of her response, other than awakening and speaking, were not reported.[85] An unreported patient with intramuscular coenurosis was given a single dose of praziquantel and developed a marked inflammatory reaction. Praziquantel should be used with great caution, if at all, in cases of human coenurosis.

Although the exact mode of infection in humans has not been identified, it is prudent to avoid close contact with dogs and dog excreta, which are the most likely sources of infection.

OTHER, LESS COMMON TAPEWORMS

Table 224–1 summarizes data concerning the less common tapeworms that may infect humans. The recommended treatment for these infections is praziquantel, as used in *T. saginata* infection.

References

1. Alarcon, F., Escalante, L., Duēnas, G., et al.: Neurocysticercosis: Short course of treatment with albendazole. Arch. Neurol. *46*:1231–1236, 1989.
2. Allan, J. C., Mencos, F., Garcia-Noval, J., et al.: Dipstick dot ELISA for the detection of *Taenia* coproantigens in humans. Parasitolology *107*:79–85, 1993.
3. Anonymous: Anaemia and the fish tapeworm. Lancet *1*:292, 1977.
4. Anonymous: Drugs for parasitic infections. Medical Letter on Drugs and Therapeutics *32*:23–32, 1990.
5. Anonymous: Pathogenesis of tapeworm anaemia. Br. Med. J. *2*:1028, 1976.
6. Arh, I.: Fish tapeworm in Eskimos in the Port Harrison area, Canada. Can. J. Public Health *51*:268–271, 1960.
7. Auche, Y., Bernard, J. P., and Faivre, J.: Grandes eosinophilies sanguines et taeniasis. Arch. Fr. Mal. App. Diag. *60*:491–492, 1971.
8. Aytac, A., Yurdakul, Y., Ikizler, C., et al.: Pulmonary hydatid disease: Report of 100 patients. Ann. Thorac. Surg. *23*:145–151, 1977.
9. Bandres, J. C., White, A. C., Samo, T., et al.: Extraparenchymal neurocysticercosis: Report of five cases and review of management. Clin. Infect. Dis. *15*:799–811, 1992.
10. Barry, M., and Kaldjian, L. C.: Neurocysticercosis. Semin. Neurol. *13*:131–143, 1993.
11. Bastid, C., Azar, C., Doyer, M., et al.: Percutaneous treatment of hydatid cysts under sonographic guidance. Dig. Dis. Sci. *39*:1576–1580, 1994.
12. Beaver, P. C., and Rolon, F. A.: Proliferating larval cestode in man in Paraguay: A case report and review of the literature. Am. J. Trop. Med. Hyg. *30*:625–637, 1981.
13. Botero, D., Tanowitz, H. B., Weiss, L. M., et al.: Taeniasis and cysticercosis. Infect. Dis. Clin. North Am. *7*:683–697, 1993.
14. Bouza Suarez, M., Hormilla Manso, G., Dumenigo Ripoll, B., et al.: The first certain case of *Diphyllobothrium latum* in Cuba. Rev. Cubana Med. Trop. *42*:9–12, 1990.
15. Bowles, J., and McManus, D. P.: Genetic characterization of the Asian *Taenia*, a newly described taeniid cestode of humans. Am. J. Trop. Med. Hyg. *50*:33–44, 1994.
16. Buergett, C. D., Greiner, E. C., and Senior, D. F.: Proliferative sparganosis in a cat. J. Parasitol. *70*:121–125, 1984.

17. Buscher, H. N., and Haley, A. J.: Epidemiology of *Hymenolepis nana* infections of Punjabi villagers in West Pakistan. Am. J. Trop. Med. Hyg. *21*:42–49, 1972.
18. Capron, A., and Rose, F.: Sur la constitution des oeufs d'helminthes. II. L'alcolo-acido-resistance chez les cestodes. Difference de colorabilite par le Ziehl des embryophores de *Taenia saginata* et *Taenia solium*. Bull. Soc. Pathol. Exot. *55*:765–767, 1962.
19. Carrea, R., Dowling, E., Jr., and Guevara, J. A.: Surgical treatment of hydatid cysts of the central nervous system in the pediatric age (Dowling's techniques). Child's Brain *1*:4–21, 1975.
20. Chang, K. H., Chi, J. G., Cho, S. Y., et al.: Cerebral sparganosis: Analysis of 34 cases with emphasis on CT features. Neuroradiology *34*:1–8, 1992.
21. Chapman, A., Vallejo, V., Mossie, K. G., et al.: Isolation and characterization of species-specific DNA probes from *Taenia solium* and *Taenia saginata* and their use in an egg detection assay. J. Clin. Microbiol. *33*:1283–1288, 1995.
22. Chitchang, S., Piamjinda, T., Yodmani, B., et al.: Relationship between severity of the symptom and the number of *Hymenolepis nana* after treatment. J. Med. Assoc. Thailand *68*:423–426, 1985.
23. Corrall, C. J., II, and Appel, B. L.: Sparganosis: A clinical and pathologic observation of the first observed case in a child. Pediatr. Infect. Dis. *J.* *6*:481–485, 1987.
24. Curtis, M. A., and Bylund, G.: Diphyllobothriasis: Fish tapeworm disease in the circumpolar north. Arct. Med. Res. *50*:18–24, 1991.
25. D'Alessandro, A., Rausch, R. L., Cuello, C., et al.: *Echinococcus vogeli* in man, with a review of polycystic hydatid disease in Colombia and neighboring countries. Am. J. Trop. Med. Hyg. *28*:303–317, 1979.
26. de Kaminsky, R. G.: Albendazole treatment in human taeniasis. Trans. Roy. Soc. Trop. Med. Hyg. *85*:648–650, 1991.
27. Del Brutto, O. H.: Cysticercosis and cerebrovascular disease: A review. J. Neurol. Neurosurg. Psych. *55*:252–254, 1992.
28. Del Brutto, O. H.: Medical treatment of cysticercosis: Effective. Arch. Neurol. *52*:102–104, 1995.
29. Del Brutto, O. H., and Sotelo, J.: Albendazole therapy for subarachnoid and interventricular cysticercosis: Case report. J. Neurosurg. *72*:816–817, 1990.
30. Del Brutto, O. H., and Sotelo, J.: Neurocysticercosis: An update. Rev. Infect. Dis. *10*:1075–1087, 1988.
31. Del Brutto, O. H., Sotelo, J., and Roman, G. C.: Therapy for neurocysticercosis: A reappraisal. Clin. Infect. Dis. *17*:730–735, 1993.
32. Dessaint, J. P., Bout, D., Wattre, P., et al.: Quantitative determination of specific IgE antibodies to *Echinococcus granulosus* and IgE levels in sera from patients with hydatid disease. Immunology *29*:813–823, 1975.
33. Di Conza, J. J.: Protective action of passively transferred immune serum and immunoglobulin fractions against tissue invasive stages of the dwarf tapeworm *Hymenolepis nana*. Exp. Parasitol. *25*:368–375, 1969.
34. Dixon, H. B., and Lipscomb, F. M.: Cysticercosis: An analysis and follow-up of 450 cases. Med. Res. Spec. Rep. (Lond.) *299*:1–58, 1961.
35. Donckaster, R., and Habibe, O.: Contribucion al estudio de la infeccion por *Hymenolepis nana*: Sintomalogia y eosinophilia relativa. Bol. Chil. Parasitol. *13*:9–11, 1958.
36. Elburjo, M., and Gani, E. A.: Surgical management of pulmonary hydatid cysts in children. Thorax *50*:396–398, 1995.
37. Eom, K. S., and Rim, H. J.: Experimental human infection with Asian *Taenia saginata* metacestodes obtained from naturally infected Korean domestic pigs. Kisaengchunghak Chapchi *30*:21–24, 1992.
38. Eom, K. S., and Rim, H. J.: Morphologic descriptions of *Taenia asiatica* sp. N. Korean J. Parasitol. *31*:1–6, 1993.
39. Ersahin, Y., Mutluer, S., and Guzelbag, E.: Intracranial hydatid cysts in children. Neurosurgery *33*:219–224, 1993.
40. Esch, G. W., and Self, J. T.: A critical study of the taxonomy of *Taenia pisiformis* Bloch 1780; *Multiceps multiceps* (Leske, 1780); and *Hydatigera taeniaeformis* Batsch, 1786. J. Parasitol. *51*:932–937, 1965.
41. Finlay, J. C., and Speert, D. P.: Sylvatic hydatid disease in children: Case reports and review of endemic *Echinococcus granulosus* infection in Canada and Alaska. Pediatr. Infect. Dis. J. *11*:322–326, 1992.
42. Flisser, A.: Taeniasis and cysticercosis due to *Taenia solium*. Prog. Clin. Parasitol. *4*:77–116, 1994.
43. Flisser, A., Reid, A., Garcia-Zepeda, E., et al.: Specific detection of *Taenia saginata* eggs by DNA hybridisation. Lancet 2:1429–1430, 1988.
44. Foresi, C.: Indagini sulla epidemiologia della imenolepiasi in Italia (Nota 1[a]). Arch. Ital. Sci. Med. Trop. *48*:251–262, 1967.
45. Gargouri, M., Ben Amor, N., Ben Chehida, F., et al.: Percutaneous treatment of hydatid cysts (*Echinococcus granulosus*). Cardiovasc. Intervent. Radiol. *13*:169–173, 1990.
46. Garin, J. P., and Mojon, M.: L'eosinophilie sanguine au cours du taeniasis a *T. saginata*. Lyon Med. *228*:339–343, 1972.
47. Gil-Grande, L. A., Rodriguez-Caabeiro, F., Prieto, J. G., et al.: Randomised controlled trial of efficacy of albendazole in intra-abdominal hydatid disease. Lancet *342*:1269–1272, 1993.
48. Golematis, B. C., and Peveretos, P. J.: Hepatic hydatid disease: Current surgical treatment. Mt. Sinai J. Med. *62*:71–76, 1995.
49. Gomez-Priego, A., Godinez-Hana, A. L., and Gutierrez-Quiroz, M.: Detection of serum antibodies in human *Hymenolepis* infection by enzyme immunoassay. Trans. R. Soc. Trop. Med. Hyg. *85*:645–647, 1991.
50. Gordadze, G. N., and Gigitashvilli, M. S.: Epileptoid fits provoked by *Hymenolepis nana*. Med. Parazit. (Moskva) *28*:430–434, 1959.
51. Gottstein, B., Deplazes, P., Tanner, I., et al.: Diagnostic indentification of *Taenia saginata* with the polymerase chain reaction. Trans. R. Soc. Trop. Med. Hyg. *85*:248–249, 1991.
52. Grunebaum, M.: Radiological manifestations of lung echinococcosis in children. Pediatr. Radiol. *3*:65–69, 1975.
53. Hamrick, H. J., Drake, W. R., Jr., Jones, H. M., et al.: Two cases of dipylidiasis (dog tapeworm infection) in children: Update on an old problem. Pediatrics *72*:114–117, 1983.
54. Harrison, L. J., Delgado, J., and Parkhouse, R. M.: Differential diagnosis of *Taenia saginata* and *Taenia solium* with DNA probes. Parasitology *100*:459–461, 1990.
55. Ibechukwu, B. I., and Onwukeme, K. E.: Intraocular coenurosis: A case report. Br. J. Ophthal. *75*:430–431, 1991.
56. Ito, A., Schantz, P. M., and Wilson, J. F.: Em18, a new serodiagnostic marker for differentiation of active and inactive cases of alveolar hydatid disease. Am. J. Trop. Med. Hyg. *52*:41–44, 1995.
57. Kammerer, W. S., and Schantz, P. M.: Echinococcal disease. Infect. Dis. Clin. North Am. *7*:605–618, 1993.
58. Kattan, Y. B.: Intrabiliary rupture of hydatid cyst of the liver. Ann. R. Coll. Surg. Engl. *59*:108–114, 1977.
59. Kramer, L. D.: Medical treatment of cysticercosis: Ineffective. Arch. Neurol. *52*:101–102, 1995.
60. Lamy, A. L., Cameron, B. H., LeBlanc, J. G., et al.: Giant hydatid cysts in the Canadian northwest: Outcome of conservative treatment in three children. J. Pediatr. Surg. *28*:1140–1143, 1993.
61. Lang, E., and Vinas, F.: Cysticercosis of the brain. Surg. Clin. North Am. *38*:887–896, 1958.
62. Lanier, A. P., Trujillo, D. E., Schantz, P. M., et al.: Comparison of serologic tests for the diagnosis and follow-up of alveolar hydatid disease. Am. J. Trop. Med. Hyg. *37*:609–615, 1987.
63. Lozano, D., and Barbosa, S.: Tratamiento con albendazole de la cisticercosis intraocular. Revista Mexicana de Oftalmologia *64*:15–28, 1990.
64. Lucas, S. B., Hassounah, O. A., Doeuhoff, M., et al.: Aberrant form of *Hymenolepis nana*: Possible opportunistic infection in immunosuppressed patients. Lancet *2*:1372–1373, 1979.
65. Mazzoti, L.: Presencia de huevecillos de *Taenia* en la region perianal. Rev. Inst. Salubr. Enferm. Trop. Mex. *5*:153–155, 1944.
66. McIntyre, A.: Hydatid disease in children in South Australia. Med. J. Aust. *1*:1064–1065, 1971.
67. Meneghelli, U. G., Martinelli, A. L., Bellucci, A. D., et al.: Polycystic hydatid disease (*Echinococcus vogeli*): Treatment with albendazole. Ann. Trop. Med. Parasitol. *86*:151–156, 1992.
68. Mitchell, W. G., and Crawford, T. O.: Intraparenchymal cerebral cysticercosis in children: Diagnosis and treatment. Pediatrics *82*:76–82, 1988.
69. Mori, Y., Shirayama, T., Agui, T., et al.: A case of chest wall tumor brought on by *Hymenolepis nana*. Bull. Osaka Med. Sch. *13*:52–54, 1967.
70. Morris, D. L., and Richards, K. S.: Hydatid Disease: Current Medical and Surgical Management. Oxford, Butterworth-Heinemann, 1992.
71. Moulinier, R., Martinez, E., Torres, J., et al.: Human proliferative sparganosis in Venezuela: Report of a case. Am. J. Trop. Med. Hyg. *31*:358–363, 1982.
72. Nahmias, J., Goldsmith, R., Soibelman, M., et al.: Three- to 7-year follow-up after albendazole treatment of 68 patients with cystic echinococcosis (hydatid disease). Ann. Trop. Med. Parasitol. *88*:295–304, 1994.
73. Nakamura, T., Hara, M., Matsuoka, M., et al.: Human proliferative sparganosis. Am. J. Clin. Pathol. *94*:224–228, 1990.
74. Nyberg, W., Grasbeck, R., Saarni, M., et al.: Serum vitamin B_{12} levels and incidence of tapeworm anemia in a population heavily infected with *Diphyllobothrium latum*. J. Lab. Clin. Med. *57*:240–246, 1961.
75. Oh, S. J., Chi, J. G., and Lee, S. E.: Eosinophilic cystitis caused by vesical sparganosis: A case report. J. Urol. *149*:581–583, 1993.
76. Ozcelik, C., Inci, I, Toprak, M., et al.: Surgical treatment of pulmonary hydatidosis in children: Experience in 92 patients. J. Pediatr. Surg. *29*:392–395, 1994.
77. Pawlowski, Z. S.: Taeniasis and cysticercosis. *In* Steele, J. H. (ed.): CRC Handbook Series in Zoonoses: Parasitic Zoonoses, Vol. 1. Boca Raton, CRC Press, 1982, pp. 313–348.
78. Pawlowski, Z., and Schultz, M. G.: Taeniasis and cysticercosis *(Taenia saginata)*. Adv. Parasitol. *10*:269–343, 1972.
79. Proctor, E. M.: Identification of tapeworms. S. Afr. Med. J. *46*:234–238, 1972.
80. Richards, F., Jr., and Schantz, P. M.: Treatment of *Taenia solium* infections. Lancet *1*:1264–1265, 1985.
81. Ruttenber, A. J., Weniger, B. G., Sorvillo, F., et al.: Diphyllobothriasis associated with salmon consumption in Pacific Coast states. Am. J. Trop. Med. Hyg. *33*:455–459, 1984.
82. Saarni, M., Nyberg, W., Grasbeck, R., et al.: Symptoms in carriers of *Diphyllobothrium latum*. Acta Med. Scand. *173*:147–154, 1963.
83. Safioleas, M., Misiakos, E., Manti, C., et al.: Diagnostic evaluation and surgical management of hydatid disease of the liver. World J. Surg. *18*:859–865, 1994.
84. Scharf, D.: Neurocysticercosis: Two hundred thirty-eight cases from a California hospital. Arch. Neurol. *45*:777–780, 1988.

85. Schellhas, K. P., and Norris, A. G.: Disseminated human subarachnoid coenurosis: Computed tomographic appearance. Am. J. Neuroradiol. *6*:638–640, 1985.
86. Schultz, M. G., Hermos, J. A., and Steele, J. A.: Epidemiology of beef tapeworm in the United States. Public Health Rep. *85*:169–176, 1970.
87. Sidky, H. A., Hassan, Z. A., Hassan, R. R., et al.: Disseminated *Hymenolepis nana* in blood of a filarial patient. J. Egypt. Soc. Parasitol. *17*:155–159, 1987.
88. St. Geme, J. W., III, Maldonado, Y. A., Enzmann, D., et al.: Consensus: Diagnosis and management of neurocysticercosis in children. Pediatr. Infect. Dis. J. *12*:455–461, 1993.
89. Stone, W. B., and Manwell, R. D.: Potential helminth infections in humans from pet or laboratory mice and hamsters. Public Health Rep. *81*:647–653, 1966.
90. Takayanagui, O. M., and Jardim, E.: Therapy for neurocysticercosis: Comparison between albendazole and praziquantel. Arch. Neurol. *49*:290–294, 1992.
91. Tarassov, V.: De L'immunite envers le bothriocephale *Diphyllobothrium latum* (L.). Ann. Parasitol. Hum. Comp. *15*:524–528, 1937.
92. Tesfa-Yohannes, T. M.: Observations on self-induced *Taenia saginata* infection. Ethiop. Med. J. *28*:91–93, 1990.
93. Thompson, R. C. A., and Lymbery, A. J. (eds.): *Echinococcus* and Hydatid Disease. The University of Arizona Press, 1995, p. 477.
94. Thompson, W. M., Chisholm, D. P., and Tank, R.: Plain film roentgenographic findings in alveolar hydatid disease: *Echinococcus multilocularis*. A. J. R. Radium. Ther. Nucl. Med. *116*:345–358, 1972.
95. Thornton, H., and Goldsmid, J. M.: Cellophane tape as an aid to the detection of *Taenia saginata* eggs. Cent. Afr. J. Med. *19*:149–151, 1973.
96. Tornieporth, N. G., and Disko, R.: Alveolar hydatid disease (*Echinococcus multilocularis*): Review and update. Prog. Clin. Parasitol. *4*:55–76, 1994.
97. Tsang, V. C., Brand, J. A., and Boyer, A. E.: An enzyme-linked immunoelectrotransfer blot assay and glycoprotein antigens for diagnosing human cysticercosis *(Taenia solium)*. J. Infect. Dis. *159*:50–59, 1989.
98. Tsou, M. H., and Huang, T. W.: Pathology of subcutaneous sparganosis: Report of two cases. J. Formos. Med. Assoc. *92*:649–653, 1993.
99. Vazquez, V., and Sotelo, J.: The course of seizures after treatment for cerebral cysticercosis. N. Engl. J. Med. *327*:696–701, 1992.
100. Verster, A.: A taxonomic revision of the genus *Taenia* Linnaeus, 1758. Onderstepoort J. Vet. Res. *36*:3–58, 1969.
101. Verster, A., and Tustin, R. C.: Treatment of the larval stage of *Taenia multiceps* with praziquantel. J. S. Afr. Vet. Assoc. *53*:107–108, 1982.
102. Vik, R.: The genus *Diphyllobothrium*: An example of the interdependence of systematics and experimental biology. Exp. Parasitol. *15*:361–380, 1964.
103. von Bonsdorff, B.: In which part of the intestinal canal is the fish tapeworm found? Acta Med. Scand. *129*:142–144, 1947.
104. Webbe, G.: Human cysticercosis: Parasitology, pathology, clinical manifestations and available treatment. Pharmacol. Ther. *64*:175–200, 1994.
105. Wen, H., Zou, P. F., Yang, W. G., et al.: Albendazole chemotherapy for human cystic and alveolar *echinococcosis* in north-western China. Trans. R. Soc. Trop. Med. Hyg. *88*:340–343, 1994.
106. Wilson, J. F., Rausch, R. L., McMahon, B. J., et al.: Parasiticidal effect of chemotherapy in alveolar hydatid disease: Review of experience with mebendazole and albendazole in Alaskan Eskimos. Clin. Infect. Dis. *15*:234–249, 1992.
107. Woo, El, Yu, L., and Huang, C. Y.: Cerebral infarct precipitated by praziquantel in neurocysticercosis: A cautionary note. Trop. Geogr. Med. *40*:143–146, 1988.
108. Wortman, P. D.: Subcutaneous cysticercosis. J. Am. Acad. Dermatol. *25*:409–414, 1991.
109. Yokogawa, S., and Kobayashi, H.: On the species of *Diphyllobothrium mansoni* sensu lato and the infectious mode of human sparganosis. Far Eastern Association of Tropical Medicine. Transactions of the Eighth Congress. Bangkok, 1930, *2*:215–226, 1932.

❑ ❑ ❑

SUBSECTION FOUR

TREMATODES

225

TREMATODES

Jerrold A. Turner

The class of flatworms called trematodes or flukes contains several important species that cause infections in humans. Although schistosomes are trematodes, major differences in their morphology, biology, and clinical aspects require that they be considered separately. Trematodes other than schistosomes all have common characteristics. The adult worm usually is flat and leaf-shaped, and it possesses an oral and ventral sucker and a bifurcated, blind-ended gastrointestinal tract. It is hermaphroditic and produces operculated eggs. The operculum, a lid-like structure at one end of the egg, covers the opening through which a ciliated larva will hatch. Depending on the species of fluke, the snail intermediate host is infected either by direct penetration by the ciliated larva or by ingestion of the unhatched egg. Complex larval development and multiplication occur within the snail host, ultimately producing large numbers of larvae called cercariae. In most trematode life cycles, the cercariae emerge from aquatic snails and swim about until they attach to the appropriate second intermediate host, which may be fish, crustaceans, mollusks, or aquatic vegetation, depending on the species of fluke. After attachment, the larvae secrete a protective cyst wall and become infectious for the definitive hosts. It is estimated that more than 40 million people have foodborne trematode infections.[1] Many of the medically important flukes have a relatively wide range of definitive hosts. Fluke infections usually are diagnosed by demonstration of the characteristic ova. Advances in the identification of specific antigens and the use of enzyme-linked immunosorbent assays, immunoblotting techniques, DNA probes, and polymerase chain reaction may produce tests that especially are valuable in the diagnosis of lung and liver flukes.

FASCIOLOPSIASIS

The Organism

The adult form of *Fasciolopsis buski,* the giant intestinal fluke, measures up to 7.5 cm in length and attaches to the mucosa of the proximal small intestine. It begins producing eggs about 3 months after infection. The adult worm has a life span of about 6 months.[18] The eggs are excreted in the stool. The oval eggs of *Fasciolopsis* measure approximately 130 to 140 μm in length by 80 to 85 μm in breadth. A single parasite may excrete 25,000 eggs daily. After several weeks in fresh water, the ciliated larvae hatch from the eggs and penetrate snails, where they undergo further larval development. Cercariae emerge from the snail about 1 to 2 months later and encyst on a wide variety of aquatic vegetation.

Transmission

The infective larvae are encysted on aquatic plants, which, if ingested raw, cause infection. Water chestnuts, caltrop, and water bamboo are common sources of infection. Water chestnuts often are peeled with the teeth, fostering the ingestion of larvae attached to the outer coat of the nut.

Epidemiology

Fasciolopsiasis occurs most commonly in China, Southeast Asia, Bangladesh, and Assam State in India. Human infection has been reported in many other areas of India and the Far East, but the prevalence appears relatively low. A common reservoir host in many areas is the domestic pig. The level of infection in the human population correlates with the practice of cultivating edible aquatic vegetation in ponds that are fertilized with human feces. Infection rates often are highest among school children.

Pathology and Pathogenesis

The parasites usually are found in the duodenum and jejunum but have been reported, in heavy infections, to involve the stomach, ileum, and colon. The intestinal mucosa may develop inflammation, ulceration, and small abscesses where the parasites are attached. Increased mucus secretion and minimal bleeding may occur. Intestinal obstruction may develop in massive infections. There is no satisfactory explanation for the systemic effects of fasciolopsiasis. The edema and ascites that occur in severe infections have been attributed to toxic metabolites of the parasite or to a reaction to parasite allergens. Protein-losing enteropathy and malabsorption associated with hypoalbuminemia also have been suggested as possible causes.[18] Children with heavy infections particularly appear to be vulnerable to the systemic manifestations.

Clinical Manifestations

Usually, but not always, the severity of symptoms is correlated with numbers of parasites. Epigastric pains resembling "hunger pains" or peptic ulcer disease and relieved by food intake have been reported as early as 30 days after exposure. Diarrhea and abdominal pain may be intermittent and may occur separately or simultaneously. In heavy infections, nausea and vomiting may develop. Facial edema, anasarca, and ascites are encountered in advanced, severe infections. Eosinophilia with counts greater than 30 per cent are not uncommon. Neutropenia may be noted.

In endemic areas, it is not unusual for a child to have multiple intestinal parasites and a borderline nutritional status. Fasciolopsiasis adds an additional burden to the host defense mechanisms and may be responsible, in concert with the other stresses, for significant morbidity.

Diagnosis

The eggs of *Fasciolopsis* are demonstrated easily by routine fecal examination, but they virtually are indistinguishable from those of the liver fluke, *Fasciola hepatica,* and the echinostomes. Epidemiologic information, such as travel history and exposure to sources of infection, may be helpful in determining the diagnosis. Because of the short life span of the adult worm, anyone who has been absent from an endemic area for longer than 9 months is not likely to have persisting infection with *Fasciolopsis.* Therefore, eggs present in the stool would be attributable to the longer-lived *Fasciola.*

Treatment and Prognosis

Praziquantel, 25 mg/kg/dose given three times in 1 day, is effective and has few side effects. Although praziquantel has been approved by the U.S. Food and Drug Administration for use in clonorchiasis and opisthorchiasis, it is considered investigational for *Fasciolopsis* infections.

Infections treated early and most light infections, even when untreated, have an excellent prognosis. Heavy infections in children, especially when complicated by intestinal obstruction, edema, or concomitant secondary infections, have a much graver prognosis.

Prevention

Fasciolopsiasis is prevented easily by cooking aquatic vegetation or by immersing the plants or nuts briefly in boiling water. The use of human feces as fertilizer in aqua culture is a major cause of human infection, and this practice should be discouraged. Successful efforts in health education appear to have reduced the transmission of this parasite in some endemic areas.

HETEROPHYIASIS

More than 10 different species of the family Heterophyidae have been reported to cause human infections. Except for two species, *Heterophyes heterophyes* and *Metagonimus yokogawai,* these infections are relatively uncommon and are incidental to the prevalence in other mammals and birds.

The Organisms

H. heterophyes and *M. yokogawai* adult worms attach to the mucosa of the small intestine. The parasites are only 1 to 2.5 mm long and less than 1 mm wide. They often burrow deeply into the mucosa. The eggs measure 26 to 30 μm in length and 15 to 17 μm in width. The eggs of the two species essentially are identical and also resemble eggs of *Opisthorchis (Clonorchis)* species. Careful study of egg size and shape has not provided a definitive method for differentiating these species.[4] Eggs excreted in the stool are embryonated fully. The snail intermediate host becomes infected by ingesting the trematode egg. After multiplication in the snail, cercariae emerge and encyst under the scales or in the skin or flesh of a variety of fresh-water fish. After ingestion by the definitive host, the metacercariae are freed from their cysts and develop into adults in as little as 5 days.

Transmission and Epidemiology

Humans acquire the infection by eating fresh-water fish that is raw, inadequately cooked, pickled, or salted.

Heterophyiasis occurs worldwide. Areas of endemic human infection are Southeast Asia, the Middle East, China, Japan, Taiwan, the Philippines, and parts of the former Soviet Union. Many reservoir hosts, such as dogs, cats, and fish-eating birds, may play an important role in maintenance of infection in some endemic areas. Detailed lists of distribution and hosts of heterophyid species are available.[25]

Pathology and Pathogenesis

The small heterophyid flukes may produce superficial inflammation and erosion at the sites of mucosal attachment.

When the mucosa is penetrated, eggs may be deposited in the tissues, producing granulomatous lesions that contain eosinophils. Eggs may gain access to intestinal capillaries or lymphatics and embolize to distant sites. The myocardium, brain, spinal cord, liver, lungs, and spleen have been involved. The complications of embolic heterophyiasis particularly appear to be frequent in the Philippines, where heart disease often is attributed to heterophyiasis. The embolized eggs produce a granulomatous response, eventually producing fibrosis in the affected tissues.

Clinical Manifestations

Light infections without ectopic egg deposition usually are asymptomatic, although eosinophilia may be found. In heavier infections, abdominal pain, often suggestive of peptic ulcer disease, is common. Intermittent diarrhea may occur. Seizures may result from eggs carried to the brain. Congestive heart failure or arrhythmias may follow cardiac involvement.

Diagnosis

Routine fecal examinations demonstrate eggs, but differentiation of *Opisthorchis* from *Clonorchis* eggs is difficult. Eggs recovered from biliary drainage or from persons who have been out of endemic areas for more than 2 years can be assumed to be those of *Opisthorchis* or *Clonorchis*.[18] The heterophyid worms have a relatively short life span compared with that of the liver flukes.

Treatment and Prognosis

Praziquantel as used in fasciolopsiasis (discussed earlier) or the drug niclosamide is effective.

With the exception of the complication of egg emboli to distant organs, the prognosis is excellent.

Prevention

If fresh-water fish were cooked adequately, heterophyiasis would disappear from the human population. Unfortunately, it is not an easy task to change human behavior or cultural traditions. Education concerning sources of infection and the need to prevent feeding raw fish to dogs and cats may reduce the prevalence of the disease.

PARAGONIMIASIS

Paragonimus westermani is the species of lung fluke that causes most human infections. Several other species have been recovered from humans and in some instances have been found in distinct endemic foci.

The Organism

The adult forms of *Paragonimus* measure about 15 mm long by about 6 mm wide. They are nearly as thick as they are wide. The worms are located in the lungs. Eggs measuring 80 to 118 μm by 48 to 60 μm are discharged into the bronchi and are either expectorated or swallowed and excreted in the feces. The larva hatches from the egg after at least 2 weeks of development in water. The free-swimming larva penetrates the snail intermediate host and undergoes development and multiplication for several weeks. Cercariae emerge and encyst in the tissues of freshwater crabs and crayfish. When the flesh of these second intermediate hosts is ingested by humans or reservoir hosts, the larvae penetrate the wall of the intestine and migrate through or around the diaphragm to reach the lungs. In some instances, the worms may lodge in ectopic sites within the abdomen, in subcutaneous tissue, or in the central nervous system. The worms usually are found singly or in pairs within a capsule or cyst of reactive host tissue. About 2 to 3 months is required from the time of ingestion until the worms fully are mature. In most infections, the worms die within 10 years; however, there are records of the production of eggs for 20 years after leaving the endemic area.

Transmission and Epidemiology

The infection is acquired by eating fresh-water crabs or crayfish that are raw, inadequately cooked, salted, pickled, or soaked in wine. Cooked foods may be contaminated with viable larvae from the hands, utensils, or cutting boards used in the preparation of crabs or crayfish.

Cats, civet cats, wild felids, foxes, wolves, dogs, pigs, and mongooses are significant reservoir hosts for *P. westermani*. Infection in humans is endemic in China, Taiwan, Korea, Japan, eastern India, Sri Lanka, Southeast Asia, Indonesia, and some areas of the former Soviet Union.

More than 10 different species of *Paragonimus* affect humans. In many areas, the distribution of these species often overlaps that of *P. westermani*. Significant foci of human infection with other species occur in West Africa and the Congo Valley, Mexico, South America, China, and Japan. The potential exists for transmission of paragonimiasis in the United States, as is exemplified by a single case report of infection probably acquired in Missouri.[16]

The distribution and epidemiology of the various species of *Paragonimus* were reviewed in 1995.[1]

Pathology and Pathogenesis

After penetration of the pleura, the worms locate near larger bronchioles or bronchi, where an exudate of neutrophils and eosinophils forms around them. In time, the area about the parasite organizes into a fibrotic wall, which may be thin or several millimeters thick. The cysts usually measure 1 to 2 cm in diameter and often are filled with a brownish material that probably contains hematin. The cyst often opens to a bronchiole or bronchus, which provides a route for discharge of the eggs into the sputum. Secondary bacterial infection of the cysts or chronic bronchitis, bronchiectasis, and pneumonia are complications of the disease.

Cerebral paragonimiasis results when the parasites migrate into the brain. The theory that the parasites travel to the brain via the jugular foramina has not been confirmed. All areas of the brain and meninges are susceptible to invasion. The parasites and the eggs cause areas of central necrosis and granuloma formation with dense collagenous walls surrounded by lymphocytes, plasma cells, eosinophils, and Charcot-Leyden crystals. The lesions vary in size, may be several centimeters in diameter, and may appear cystic. Eventually, the wall may calcify. Spinal cord lesions are similar. Other sites at which worms may cause cysts or abscesses are the intestinal wall, mesentery, peritoneal cavity, liver, diaphragm, myocardium, and subcutaneous tissue.

Clinical Manifestations

The migration of the worms from the intestinal tract to the lungs usually causes no symptoms, but diarrhea, abdominal pain, and urticaria may occur in the first 3 weeks after exposure. These symptoms may be followed closely by chest discomfort, cough, dyspnea, fever, and night sweats.

The established pulmonary infection often is asymptomatic, but frequently there is a chronic cough that is productive of mucoid, rust-colored, or blood-streaked sputum. Hemoptysis usually is intermittent and occasionally may be severe. Eosinophilia is common in the early stages of infection but may return to normal over a period of many months or years.

Complications of pneumothorax, pleural effusion, empyema, and pneumonia occur more often in association with heavy infections.

Cerebral paragonimiasis occurs in less than 1 per cent of infections but results in serious morbidity and often death.[13]

Cerebral involvement is more common in children, with more than half of the infections occurring before 10 years of age. This form of paragonimiasis may present as a mass lesion, a seizure disorder, meningitis, or a cerebrovascular accident. Seizures often begin as the focal motor type but progress to generalized seizures as the disease worsens. Visual disturbances, headache, and elevation of cerebrospinal fluid pressure are common. There may be a pleocytosis with eosinophilia in the cerebrospinal fluid.

The variety of neurologic manifestations depends on the number, location, and size of the lesions. Spinal cord lesions often are extradural and mimic mass lesions caused by tumors or infection.

Cutaneous paragonimiasis is manifested by the appearance of subcutaneous nodules, which may be fixed or migratory. In China, species of *Paragonimus* found in the northern region often cause subcutaneous, migratory lesions associated with fever and eosinophilia. Worms recovered from these lesions are immature.

Diagnosis

In light pulmonary infections, normal results on chest radiographs are not unusual. However, radiographic abnormalities may develop as the worms enter the lungs. Initially, the chest film shows basilar pneumonic infiltrates that are poorly defined. These areas become better demonstrated as cysts or nodules within a few weeks. There may be some initial pleural reaction, usually at the base of the lung, which may be associated with effusion. Although the nodules and cysts of the chronic stage of infection may occur in any area of the lung, including the apices, they tend to localize in the periphery of the middle and lower lung fields. A common radiographic diagnostic feature is the "ring shadow." This finding represents the circular or oval thin-walled cyst with a crescent-shaped opacity along one side.

Cerebral paragonimiasis may be seen as an avascular mass on computerized axial tomography. In long-standing cerebral infections, the cyst-like structures may calcify and may be seen as a cluster of "soap bubbles." The individual oval or spherical bubbles may measure from 2 to 40 mm in diameter, and a cluster of these structures may extend 10 cm.

Pulmonary paragonimiasis is diagnosed definitively by finding the characteristic eggs in sputum or stool. Several immunodiagnostic tests have been developed, and they appear especially useful in infections in which eggs are not demonstrated easily, such as in cerebral paragonimiasis.[26] Intradermal testing cannot distinguish between past and current infections, but it has been useful in epidemiologic studies.

Pulmonary paragonimiasis often is mistaken for tuberculosis. A careful history may provide information about travel and food habits that point to the correct diagnosis.

Treatment and Prognosis

Praziquantel, 25 mg/kg/dose, is given three times a day for 2 days. In the United States, the drug is considered investigational when used for this purpose. Bithionol is an alternative drug, which is available in the United States through the Centers for Disease Control and Prevention in Atlanta. Bithionol is given in single doses of 30 to 50 mg/kg on alternate days for a total of 10 to 15 doses. Side effects are much more common with bithionol than with praziquantel.

The prognosis is good in most pulmonary infections, even if untreated, although symptoms may persist for many years. Treatment effectively resolves pulmonary lesions and symptoms. The prognosis for central nervous system involvement depends on the location and extent of the lesions but usually is grave.

Prevention

The key in prevention is education of the population in endemic areas concerning the source of infection. Crabs and crayfish, prepared in a manner that transmits paragonimiasis, are delicacies in many parts of the world. Changing attitudes about food habits is no easy task, but it is doubtful that even mass treatment and improved sanitation completely would prevent human infections because of animal reservoirs.

FASCIOLIASIS

Fascioliasis is caused by the sheep liver fluke, *F. hepatica. Fasciola gigantica* is a closely related liver fluke that has a more limited geographic distribution and much less frequently is reported as a cause of infection in humans.

The Organism

The adult of *F. hepatica* measures up to 30 mm in length and 13 mm in width. The surface has scale-like spines, and the anterior portion of the worm is cone-shaped. The worms reside in the bile ducts, and eggs appear in the bile and eventually are excreted in the feces. Eggs measure about 130 μm in length and up to 90 μm in width. The eggs are indistinguishable from those of *F. buski*. After incubation in water for several days, the ciliated larva hatches from the egg and swims about in search of the snail intermediate host. The larva penetrates the snail and undergoes a complex cycle of asexual multiplication. Cercariae, which are the final stage of this asexual cycle, leave the snail and encyst on fresh water vegetation, often watercress. These encysted metacercariae initiate infection when the mammalian host ingests the raw aquatic vegetation or drinks water contaminated with metacercariae. The metacercariae excyst in the intestine, penetrate the intestinal wall, and migrate in the peritoneal cavity to the liver. The developing worms penetrate the liver capsule and burrow through the parenchyma to the bile ducts. The adult worms feed on liver cells and duct epithelium.

Transmission and Epidemiology

Ingestion of infected raw watercress is the most frequent cause of infection in humans. Water from ponds or marshes with infected vegetation may contain metacercariae. Infections occur in humans who have no history of eating watercress but have ingested water from sources that potentially are infected. The distribution of fascioliasis is worldwide, with the highest numbers of infected humans reported from Peru, Bolivia, Ecuador, Egypt, Iran, France, and Portugal. Autochthonous cases in the United States are rare. Sheep, goats, and cattle serve as the most common reservoir hosts, but many mammals are susceptible to infection. A detailed review of the epidemiology of fascioliasis has been published.[2] *F. gigantica* infections predominantly are infections in cattle. Human infection with *F. gigantica* occurs in Africa, the former Soviet Union, Vietnam, Hawaii, and Iraq.

Pathology and Pathogenesis

Significant damage to liver tissues occurs as the juvenile worms migrate through the liver tissue to the bile ducts. Linear necrotic lesions containing eosinophils form as the worms progress through the liver parenchyma. Flukes that die before reaching the bile ducts may produce necrotic cavities that eventually evolve into fibrous scar tissue. Adult worms in the bile ducts cause inflammation and adenomatous changes in biliary epithelium. Ductal and periductal fibrosis occurs. The gallbladder and extrahepatic ducts may be invaded and undergo similar inflammatory and fibrotic reactions. Adult worms may migrate back into liver parenchyma through eroded biliary epithelium and cause abscess formation.

Heavy infections often are associated with anemia, which is attributed partially to blood loss from the biliary tract.

Juvenile flukes that fail to find their way into the liver may wander about, causing ectopic fascioliasis. They may appear in the intestine, pancreas, subcutaneous tissue, brain, eye, and other locations.

Clinical Manifestations

The first symptoms of fascioliasis occur about 4 to 6 weeks after infection, but this varies widely, depending on host response and numbers of parasites. The acute stage of infection occurs during the migration of worms in the liver. Children often have severe symptoms of right upper quadrant or generalized abdominal pain, tender hepatomegaly, fever, anemia, and eosinophilia. These symptoms may be accompanied by sweating, dizziness, wheezing, and urticaria. This stage may last 1 to 3 months. The chronic form of the disease is less well defined and includes a variety of symptoms related to the biliary system. These symptoms frequently are identical to the symptoms of gallbladder disease, cholangitis, and pancreatitis caused by nonparasitic conditions. Patients often endure years of biliary tract symptoms before the diagnosis of fascioliasis is considered.

Chronic infection with *F. hepatica* also may be asymptomatic but often is associated with eosinophilia.

Diagnosis

Routine stool examination using a formalin–ethyl acetate concentration technique should reveal ova of *Fasciola* in established infections. The problem of differentiating *Fasciolopsis* and *Fasciola* eggs was discussed in the section on fasciolopsiasis. False-positive stool examinations may occur when the patient ingests infected liver. Keeping the patient on a diet free of liver for 3 days prior to the collection of the stool specimen eliminates this unusual possibility.

Because ova are not produced until about 4 months after infection (range, 3 to 18 months), diagnosis of fascioliasis during the acute stage of liver migration must rely on a combination of clinical findings, imaging studies, and immunologic tests. Obtaining a history of eating raw watercress or drinking surface water from an area that may be contaminated by domestic animals is helpful. The syndrome of fever, hepatomegaly, and eosinophilia is consistent with the diagnosis. Radiologic imaging of the liver may demonstrate findings of tract-like small abscesses, subcapsular lesions, and slow evolution of the lesions on follow-up examinations.[11] Computed tomography detects parenchymal lesions, and ultrasonography effectively evaluates the biliary tract and gallbladder. A variety of immunologic tests have been developed. An enzyme-linked immunosorbent assay using excretory-secretory products from adult worms has been useful in detecting serum antibodies without cross-reactivity with other trematode infections.[6, 7, 20] Serologic tests also should be useful in the diagnosis of ectopic fascioliasis.

Chronic fascioliasis may be detected during radiologic studies of the biliary tract or gallbladder. Adult worms may be seen on ultrasonography or appear as curvilinear lucent areas in the contrast medium at cholangiography.

Treatment and Prognosis

Unlike the other trematode infections, fascioliasis is relatively resistant to praziquantel. Treatment with bithionol is effective; however, this drug is available for experimental use only and must be obtained from the Centers for Disease Control and Prevention. It usually is administered in a dose of 30 mg/kg given either daily for 5 days or on alternate days for a total of five doses.[1, 8] More intense courses of 30 to 50 mg/kg on alternate days for 10 to 15 doses also have been recommended. Triclabendazole, which has been used successfully in veterinary medicine, currently is undergoing evaluation by the World Health Organization for the treatment of fascioliasis. A case report and review of the use of triclabendazole in humans conclude that it is the drug of choice in this condition.[14] It is given in the dosage of 10 mg/kg/day divided into two doses. The doses are given after meals and separated by 6 to 8 hours.[1] Triclabendazole is effective against both migrating worms and established infections.

Children with severe acute infections have been treated with 5 to 10 mg of prednisone prior to using specific fasciolicidal drugs.[9]

Heavy infections in children may be fatal during the acute stage of the disease. However, most resolve to become chronic or, possibly, asymptomatic. The variable reaction of the human host and the numbers of parasites determine the outcome. In heavy infections, hepatic damage may be significant, with fibrotic scarring or abscess formation. Chronic or recurrent biliary tract problems are common.

Prevention

Watercress grown for human consumption should be protected from human and animal fecal contamination. Animal fascioliasis can be targeted for chemotherapeutic control, and efforts can be made to control the snail intermediate hosts with molluscicides. Efforts should be made to educate the population at risk regarding the dangers of raw watercress harvested from unprotected waters.

CLONORCHIASIS AND OPISTHORCHIASIS

Three similar trematodes of the genus *Opisthorchis* infect the bile ducts of humans. Although the name *Opisthorchis sinensis* is proper parasitologically, this organism more commonly is called *Clonorchis sinensis,* and the name of the infection, clonorchiasis, is well entrenched in the clinical literature. This organism also is called the Chinese or Oriental liver fluke. *Opisthorchis viverrini* and *Opisthorchis felineus* have similar life cycles and produce similar lesions and illnesses in humans.

The Organisms

The adult flukes measure from 4 to 20 mm in length by 2 to 3 mm in breadth. They are found in the intrahepatic biliary ducts. The small operculate eggs, similar to those of the heterophyid flukes, appear in the bile and are excreted in the feces. The snail intermediate host ingests the embryonated egg, and free-swimming cercariae emerge from the snail about 6 to 8 weeks later. The cercariae encyst under the scales and in the flesh of a variety of fresh-water fish. When the raw, inadequately cooked, or pickled fish is eaten, the larvae excyst and migrate to the intrahepatic bile ducts, usually through the ampulla of Vater and the common duct. The worms probably survive for as long as 30 years.

Transmission and Epidemiology

The ingestion of raw, inadequately cooked, or pickled fresh-water fish that have encysted larvae in their tissues initiates infection.

C. sinensis is endemic in China, Japan, Korea, Taiwan, and Vietnam. High prevalence rates in Hong Kong are attributed to the importation of fish from mainland China. Natural reservoir hosts are cats, dogs, pigs, and rats.

O. viverrini is fairly localized to northern areas of Thailand, where a dish prepared from chopped raw fish, called koi pla, frequently is eaten. Cats, civet cats, dogs, and other fish-eating mammals serve as reservoirs. In China and other Asian countries, edible fish often are raised in ponds that are fertilized with human feces, providing perfect conditions for the entire life cycle of the parasite.

O. felineus is endemic in central Siberia and in eastern and southeastern Europe. Cats, dogs, and foxes serve as major reservoirs. Human infection is limited to those groups that habitually consume raw, dried, or freshly salted fish or fish lightly pickled in garlic juice. Sporadic infections with *O. felineus* have been reported from several Asian countries.

The distribution of infection of all species in human infections depends on the eating habits of the population. In most areas, the prevalence is higher in older persons, but in Thailand, even infants are infected.

Pathology and Pathogenesis

The epithelium of infected bile ducts reacts with desquamation, adenomatous hyperplasia, and metaplasia of goblet cells accompanied by an increase in mucus production. This is thought to be caused by mechanical damage from the flukes' suckers and from metabolites of the worms. Ductal dilatation and bile stasis probably increase susceptibility to bacterial cholangitis. Inflammation of the bile duct wall usually indicates secondary infection.[5] Chronic infections may show considerable periductal fibrosis, but this does not progress to portal cirrhosis.[5] The presence of the parasites in addition to other factors appears to make the host susceptible to cholangiocarcinoma. Experiments in hamsters show that a nitrosamine carcinogen combined with *O. viverrini* infection induces cholangiocarcinoma, but infection alone or carcinogen alone does not.[23] An extensive analysis of available data concerning cancer and liver flukes concludes that infection with *O. viverrini* is carcinogenic to humans, and infection with *C. sinensis* probably is carcinogenic to humans.[3] There were not enough data to determine the status of *O. viverrini* infections. *O. viverrini* infections frequently involve the gallbladder. Complications may include cholecystitis and gallstone formation. The parasites often are found in the pancreatic ducts, where reactions of the epithelium are similar to those in the bile duct. Pancreatitis occurs infrequently in these liver fluke infections and usually is mild.

Clinical Manifestations

The intensity of infection probably correlates with the occurrence of symptoms. Light and moderate infections in endemic areas appear asymptomatic. Patients with heavy infections may complain of right upper quadrant abdominal pain, weakness, or malaise and have significant hepatic enlargement.[24] Studies of patients with chronic clonorchiasis who have left the endemic areas failed to find significant symptoms or any evidence of liver dysfunction associated with the infection.[17, 22] However, clonorchiasis has been found in most cases of pancreatitis among Chinese immigrants.[1] An uncontrolled study of patients with *O. viverrini* infections in Thailand showed general improvement in well-being after treatment.[19] Symptoms of abdominal distress and epigastric pain declined significantly.

Acute infections, with fever, malaise, anorexia, diarrhea, tender hepatomegaly, and eosinophilia, have been reported. These symptoms may develop in heavy infections 10 to 26 days after ingestion of the larvae. The eosinophilia of acute infection gradually decreases and, in chronic infection, disappears.[17]

Complications probably are more likely in heavy infections. Relapsing cholangitis, cholecystitis, bilirubin gallstones, pancreatitis, and cholangiocarcinoma may occur in association with infection.[12]

Diagnosis

Symptoms of acute infections may develop 3 to 4 weeks before eggs appear in the stool. Suspicion of the diagnosis may be based on epidemiologic information. Serologic tests would be helpful in this situation, but these are not readily available in the United States. In chronic infections, eggs should be evident in routine fecal examinations. Filtration of fluid obtained at duodenal intubation is claimed to be diagnostically more sensitive than examination of two fecal specimens.[10] A monoclonal antibody–based enzyme-linked immunosorbent assay has been developed for the demonstration of *O. viverrini* antigen in fecal specimens. This test appears to be specific and highly sensitive.[21]

Cholangiography often shows multiple cystic dilatations of the ducts. A combination of large cystic dilatations and small cystic ectasias or mulberry-like dilatations is considered diagnostic. The flukes may be evident as linear lucencies in the cholangiogram.

The eggs of *O. viverrini* and *C. sinensis* virtually are identical. *O. felineus* is reported as having a narrower egg, as determined by the ratio of length to width. It is difficult to differentiate between the eggs of these species of liver flukes and the eggs of the small heterophyid flukes. Fortunately, treatment with praziquantel is identical for all of these parasites.

Treatment and Prognosis

These liver fluke infections respond well to treatment with praziquantel, 25 mg/kg per dose, given three times in a single day. Side effects of headache and dizziness are common. Although untreated light and moderate infections appear asymptomatic and may have little, if any, clinical significance, the availability of a safe, easily administered drug makes treatment seem appropriate, especially for those who have left endemic areas. Treatment also may decrease the risk of cholangiocarcinoma that may accompany the infection. Albendazole also has been found to be effective in clonorchiasis.[21] Praziquantel and albendazole have been shown to be an effective combination.[15] In addition to the successful elimination of clonorchiasis, the albendazole component also is effective in several other intestinal roundworm infections. Effective treatment has reversed the biliary tract abnormalities in *O. viverrini* infections and would be expected to have a similar salutary effect in clonorchiasis and *O. felineus* infections.

The prognosis of heavy infections depends on the complications. Superimposed bacterial infections are the most common cause of morbidity and mortality.

Prevention

Education of the population at risk about the consumption of raw fish in its various forms—dried, pickled, salted, or smoked—is about the only hope for reducing prevalence in humans. There is a large reservoir in domestic and wild animals; therefore, attempts to reduce human infection by mass treatment are unlikely to succeed. Prohibiting the fertilization of fish ponds with raw human sewage might reduce transmission.

LESS COMMON TREMATODE INFECTIONS

Table 225–1 summarizes information about some of the less common trematodes that may infect humans. All have snails as the first intermediate host, and the diagnosis is made by the identification of eggs on fecal examination. Infections with trematodes listed in this table probably are treated effectively with praziquantel, 25 mg/kg/dose given three times daily for 1 day. *Nanophyetus salmincola* infection

TABLE 225–1. Less Common Trematodes That Can Infect Humans

	Location in Human	Adult Length/ Width (mm)	Eggs Length/ Width (μm)	Geographic Distribution	Second Intermediate Hosts	Reservoir Hosts	Transmission	Clinical Manifestations
Nanophyetus salmincola	Intestine	1.1/0.5	60–80/34–50	Pacific coast of Canada and Northwest U.S. and Siberia	Salmonid fish	Dog, coyote, fox, skunk, mink, lynx, and others	Ingestion of raw, undercooked, or lightly smoked salmon or trout	Diarrhea, abdominal discomfort, nausea, vomiting, eosinophilia
Dicrocoelium dendriticum	Bile ducts	15/2.5	38–45/22–30	Widespread in animals. Sporadic human cases from Europe, the former Soviet Union, Middle East, South America, China, and elsewhere	Ant	Sheep, cattle, and many other ruminants	Accidental ingestion of ants contaminating food	Information is inadequate. Abdominal pain, nausea, diarrhea, constipation, and eosinophilia are reported. Spurious infection from eating infected liver
Echinostomes—Several genera and many species	Small intestines	Wide range, up to 22/2.2. Collar of spines around oral sucker	Usually greater than 100 μm in length. Depends on species. Resembles *Fasciolopsis* and *Fasciola* eggs	Southeast Asia, Indonesia, Japan, Taiwan, Philippines, and sporadic cases elsewhere	Snails, clams, tadpoles, fish	Waterfowl and other birds, rats, dogs, muskrats, cats, and pigs	Ingestion of uncooked snails, clams, tadpoles, and fish	Scant information. Diarrhea, constipation, abdominal cramps, and eosinophilia. Light infections are asymptomatic
Gastrodiscoides hominis	Cecum and ascending colon	5–8/5–14. Pear shape, large disk-shaped posterior	150/60–70. Greenish-brown, tapered at both ends	Common in Assam, India. Sporadic in Vietnam, Philippines, the former Soviet Union, and other areas	Unknown, possibly aquatic vegetation	Pigs	Unknown, possibly ingestion of raw vegetation	Mucous diarrhea

responds to a regimen of 60 mg/kg divided into three doses given in a single day.

References

1. Anonymous: Control of foodborne trematode infections. Report of a WHO Study Group. WHO Tech. Rep. Ser. *849*:1–157, 1995.
2. Anonymous: Fascioliasis. Wkly. Epidemiol. Rec. *67*:326–329, 1992.
3. Anonymous: Schistosomes, liver flukes and *Helicobacter pylori*. IARC Monogr. Eval. Carcinog. Risks Hum. *61*:1–241, 1994.
4. Ditrich, O., Giboda, M., Scholz, T., et al.: Comparative morphology of eggs of the Haplorchiinae (Trematoda: Heterophyidae) and some other medically important heterophyid and opisthorchiid flukes. Folia Parasitologica *39*:123–132, 1992.
5. Dooley, J. R., and Neafie, R. C.: *In* Binford, C. H., and Connor, D. H. (eds.): Pathology of Tropical and Extraordinary Diseases. Vol. 2. Washington, D. C., Armed Forces Institute of Pathology, 1976, pp. 509–516.
6. Espino, A. M., Dumenigo, B. E., Fernandez, R., et al.: Immunodiagnosis of human fascioliasis by enzyme-linked immunosorbent assay using excretory-secretory products. Am. J. Trop. Med. Hyg. *37*:605–608, 1987.
7. Espino, A. M., and Finlay, C. M.: Sandwich enzyme-linked immunosorbent assay for detection of excretory-secretory antigens in humans with fascioliasis. J. Clin. Microbiol. *32*:190–193, 1994.
8. Farag, H. F., Salem, A., el-Hifni, S. A., et al.: Bithionol (Bitin) treatment in established fascioliasis in Egyptians. J. Trop. Med. Hyg. *91*:240–244, 1988.
9. Farid, Z., Mansour, N., Kamal, M., et al.: The treatment of acute *Fasciola hepatica* infection in children. Trop. Geogr. Med. *42*:95–96, 1990.
10. Feldmeier, H., and Horstmann, R. D.: Filtration of duodenal fluid for the diagnosis of opisthorchiasis. Ann. Trop. Med. Parasitol. *75*:462–465, 1981.
11. Han, J. K., Choi, B. I., Cho, J. M., et al.: Radiological findings of human fascioliasis. Abdom. Imaging *18*:261–264, 1993.
12. Kurathong, S., Lerdverasirikul, P., Wongpaitoon, V., et al.: *Opisthorchis viverrini* infection and cholangiocarcinoma: A prospective case-controlled study. Gastroenterology *89*:151–156, 1985.
13. Kusner, D. J., and King, C. H.: Cerebral paragonimiasis. Semin. Neurol. *13*:201–208, 1993.
14. Laird, P. P., and Boray, J. C.: Human fascioliasis successfully treated with triclabendazole. Aust. N. Z. J. Med. *22*:45–47, 1992.
15. Li, S., He, G., Lu, Z., et al.: Efficacy of praziquantel combined with albendazole in the treatment of clonorchiasis. Chung-Kuo Chi Sheng Chung Hsueh Yu Chi Sheng Chung Ping Tsa Chih *13*:61–63, 1995.
16. Mariano, E. G., Borja, S. R., and Vruno, M. J.: A human infection with *Paragonimus kellicotti* (lung fluke) in the United States. Am. J. Clin. Pathol. *86*:685–687, 1986.
17. Markell, E. K.: Laboratory findings in chronic clonorchiasis. Am. J. Trop. Med. Hyg. *15*:510–515, 1966.
18. Markell, E. K., and Goldsmith, R.: *In* Strickland, G. T. (ed.): Hunter's Tropical Medicine. 6th ed. Philadelphia, W. B. Saunders, 1984, pp. 743–754.
19. Pungpak, S., Chalermrut, K., Harinasuta, T., et al.: *Opisthorchis viverrini* infection in Thailand: Symptoms and signs of infection: A population-based study. Trans. R. Soc. Trop. Med. Hyg. *88*:561–564, 1994.
20. Shaheen, H., al Khafif, M., Farag, R. M., et al.: Serodifferentiation of human fascioliasis from schistosomiasis. Trop. Geogr. Med. *46*:326–327, 1994.
21. Sirisinha, S., Chawengkirttikul, R., Haswell-Elkins, M. R., et al.: Evaluation of the monoclonal antibody-based enzyme-linked immunosorbent assay for the diagnosis of *Opisthorchis viverrini* infection in an endemic area. Am. J. Trop. Med. Hyg. *52*:521–524, 1995.
22. Strauss, W. G.: Clinical manifestations of clonorchiasis: A controlled study of 105 cases. Am. J. Trop. Med. Hyg. *11*:625–630, 1962.
23. Thamavit, W., Bhamarapravati, N., Sahaphong, S., et al.: Effects of dimethylnitrosamine on induction of cholangiocarcinoma in *Opisthorchis viverrini*–infected Syrian golden hamsters. Cancer Res. *38*:4634–4639, 1978.
24. Upatham, E. S., Viyanant, V., Kurathong, S., et al.: Morbidity in relation to intensity of infection in *Opisthorchis viverrini*: Study of a community in Khon Kaen, Thailand. Am. J. Trop. Med. Hyg. *31*:1156–1163, 1982.
25. Velasquez, C. C.: Heterophyidiasis. *In* Steele, J. H. (ed.): CRC Handbook Series in Zoonoses. Vol. 3. Boca Raton, FL, CRC Press, 1982, pp. 99–107.
26. Zhang, Z., Zhang, Y., Zhiming, S., et al.: Diagnosis of active *Paragonimus westermani* infections with a monoclonal antibody–based antigen detection assay. Am. J. Trop. Med. Hyg. *49*:329–334, 1993.

❑ ❑ ❑

SUBSECTION FIVE

ARTHROPODS

226

ARTHROPODS

Sheldon L. Kaplan

TICKS

Hard (family Ixodidae) and soft (family Argasidae) ticks are of medical importance primarily for their role as vectors in the transmission of infectious agents to people (Table 226–1). Ticks serve as both vectors and reservoirs for many rickettsiae, which actually can be identified in the tick hemolymph by fluorescent technique.

Tick bites may result in a local reaction that appears to be mediated by complement. These bites may persist and develop into a so-called tick bite granuloma. Systemic reactions such as fever, chills, nausea, vomiting, abdominal pain, and headache can be associated with tick bites.

Tick Paralysis

Tick paralysis is a neurologic syndrome characterized chiefly by an ascending flaccid paralysis in association with the attachment of certain species of ticks. This illness has been reported more frequently in children, especially between 2 and 5 years of age, than in adults. Numerous genera of ticks are known to be associated with tick paralysis. In North America, *Dermacentor andersoni* (wood tick) and *Dermacentor variabilis* (dog tick) are the primary species responsible for tick paralysis.[19] In Australia, ticks implicated most commonly are *Ixodes holocyclus* and *Ixodes cornatus*. Adult female and male as well as immature ticks have been implicated in this nervous system disorder. Most cases of tick paralysis in the United States occur in the west and southeast regions.

Pathogenesis

Tick paralysis is thought to be caused by a neurotoxin (holocyclotoxin) released by pregnant female ticks at the site of attachment. The neurotoxin is a protein that has temperature-dependent activity.[5] The exact mechanism and location of the toxin's action are not known but may include decreased entry of calcium into motor-nerve terminals or interference with presynaptic excitation-secretion coupling, which

TABLE 226–1. Human Infectious Diseases for Which Ticks Are a Vector

Disease	Agent
Relapsing fever	*Borrelia duttonii*
Q fever	*Coxiella burnetii*
Tularemia	*Francisella tularensis*
Queensland tick typhus	*Rickettsia australis*
Fièvre boutonneuse	*R. conorii*
Rocky Mountain spotted fever	*R. rickettsii*
Asian tick typhus	*R. sibirica*
Colorado tick fever	Arbovirus
Encephalitis	Arbovirus
Lyme disease	*Borrelia burgdorferi*
Human monocytic ehrlichiosis	*Ehrlichia chaffeensis*
Human granulocytic ehrlichiosis	*Ehrlichia* species
Babesiosis	*Babesia microti*

leads to a reduction of acetylcholine release at the motor end-plate.

Investigations in children with tick paralysis have implicated primarily peripheral nerve dysfunction, because their nerve conduction velocities were diminished somewhat.[13, 27] Compound muscle action potentials that are abnormally low or low-normal in amplitude when the patient has maximal neurologic deficits are reversed rapidly once the tick is removed.[19] Swift and Ignacio[27] postulate that the major effect of the toxin is to prevent depolarization in the terminal portions of the motor neurons.

Clinical Manifestations

The symptoms of tick paralysis usually occur within 1 to 2 days after the tick attaches but may appear earlier. The syndrome progresses in two stages. Initially, the patient demonstrates ataxia and areflexia. Sensory changes may or may not be present in the affected extremities. If the tick remains attached, the syndrome progresses to a gradual ascending flaccid paralysis that ultimately may involve the trunk, upper extremities, tongue, and pharynx. If the paralysis involves the cranial nerves, the patient may have changes in voice and have difficulty in swallowing and handling secretions. Nystagmus, strabismus, and convulsions may occur as well.[13] Respiratory compromise leads to stupor and ultimately to death. Throughout this course, the patient usually is afebrile or only mildly febrile.

Routine laboratory tests are not helpful in establishing diagnosis. The white blood cell count, urine analysis, cerebrospinal fluid, and erythrocyte sedimentation rate usually are normal.

Diagnosis

The diagnosis of tick paralysis can be established when the patient shows the typical clinical picture and improves when a tick is removed. The differential diagnosis of tick paralysis includes Guillain-Barré syndrome, poliomyelitis, myelitis, spinal cord neoplasm, syringomyelia, porphyria, and botulism.

Treatment

The earlier the tick is removed in the course of the syndrome, the more promptly the syndrome will clear. Recovery is complete within 1 to 5 days. Intensive supportive care is required if the patient has cranial nerve dysfunction. Ineffective ventilation and ensuing respiratory failure require assisted ventilation.

MYIASIS

Myiasis is the invasion of a host's tissues by the larval stage (maggot) of nonbiting flies. These larvae can invade either previously traumatized skin or intact skin.

Etiology

The true flies of the order Diptera undergo metamorphosis in four stages: the egg, larva, pupa, and adult. Some larvae of the suborder Cyclorrhapha have adapted to a parasitic relationship with humans to different degrees. Some are classified as obligate, facultative, or accidental parasites in humans. In each case, the larval stage of the fly is able to invade the tissues of the host and progress in the stages of metamorphosis.

Epidemiology

The occurrence of human myiasis has been linked to humid and warm climates that favor the breeding of flies. Epizootics in livestock, marginal housing, poor refuse disposal, and undernutrition also are important factors in the development of human myiasis.[21] In the United States, myiasis has been reported from flies both native to North America and from the larvae of flies acquired during foreign travel. More than 50 species of flies have been reported to cause human myiasis.

Pathogenesis

The pathogenesis of human myiasis differs with the degree of parasitic adaptation of each fly. *Dermatobia hominis* (the human botfly) utilizes a bloodsucking insect as a vector to deposit its eggs on a warm-blooded host. The larvae emerge from the eggs and then penetrate the host's skin, frequently utilizing the puncture site of the carrier insect. The larvae develop within the dermal layer of skin, which leads to a boil-like swelling. During this period, the human host develops clinical symptoms. *D. hominis* and *Cochliomyia hominivorax*, the primary screwworm, are examples causing obligate myiasis.[21] *C. hominivorax* can be responsible for aural or nasal myiasis.

The genus *Sarcophaga* (flesh flies) is capable of causing facultative myiasis. The adult fly is attracted to wounds or ulcers containing purulent and necrotic material. The adult fly deposits eggs in the open wound where the larvae hatch.

Accidental myiasis can occur when humans ingest eggs or larvae and the larvae remain in the intestinal tract. Genitourinary myiasis is thought to occur by the deposition of eggs around the external urethral orifice. The larvae then may migrate into and up the urethra.

Clinical Manifestations

The lesions of cutaneous myiasis generally are located over the exposed area of the body. Early in the course of cutaneous myiasis, pruritus is the predominant symptom. As the larvae grow after the first week of infestation, a serous exudate may drain from the penetrating site. At this point, pain and pruritus are prominent symptoms and the lesion appears as a small furuncle (furuncular myiasis). Tissue destruction by the larvae may continue, and secondary bacterial infection can occur. *Staphylococcus aureus* and group A streptococci, as well as gram-negative organisms, have been isolated from infected cutaneous myiasis wounds.

Abdominal pain, diarrhea, and anal bleeding are the symptoms of intestinal myiasis, which is self-limited and may last

2 to 6 weeks. Larvae within the genitourinary tract may lead to proteinuria, dysuria, hematuria, and pyuria. Nasal myiasis can extend into bone, sinus cavities, and even the meninges.[1] Aural myiasis has been described in a child without underlying pathology.[6] Ophthalmomyiasis is characterized by an acute catarrhal conjunctivitis.[7] Penetration into the brain has been associated with intracerebral hematomas.[18]

Diagnosis

A careful history of travel, occupation, and exposure is necessary for diagnosis when the physician is confronted with unusual skin lesions that are pruritic and have not resolved with usual local care.[12, 17] Myiasis is confirmed if larvae are demonstrated within the wound. A parasitologist or entomologist may be able to identify the species of larvae responsible.

Treatment

The removal of the larvae is necessary in any of the forms of myiasis. Endoscopic removal of nasal infestation is recommended. Surgical intervention may be required to expose the larvae in the wound. Forceps are used to pick out the larvae; the application of 5 per cent chloroform in olive oil may facilitate removal. Occlusive coverings of the wound opening are helpful in extruding *Dermatobia* larvae because this maneuver diminishes the oxygen supply to the larvae. A thick layer of petroleum jelly (Vaseline) effectively interrupts air flow to larvae. Local or systemic antibiotics may be required if secondary bacterial infection is present.

The prevention of human myiasis requires good wound care, adequate personal hygiene, screening to protect against flies, and the prevention of myiasis in domestic animals.

MITES

Mites are classified in the same order (Acarina) as ticks and also can be vectors for infectious agents. The house mite, *Liponyssoides sanguineus*, is the vector for the rickettsialpox agent. Chiggers, which are larvae of mites (family Trombiculidae), transmit to humans the agent responsible for scrub typhus, *Rickettsia tsutsugamushi*.

Sarcoptes scabiei is the burrowing itch mite associated with human scabies. This infestation appears to have an increased incidence in 15-year cycles.[26] Scabies are transmitted person-to-person through direct and usually prolonged contact. Clothing and bed items are felt to be less important in the transmission of the *Sarcoptes* mite. Epidemic outbreaks of scabies have been reported in hospitals and other institutions where people were living closely together and especially where poor sanitation predominated.[3]

The scabies mite burrows into the stratum corneum layer of skin, and a superficial tunnel is created. The gravid female mite deposits eggs and fecal masses (scybala) within this tunnel. The wastes and other antigenic products of the mites lead to pathologic changes within the epidermis.

Papulovesicular scabies is characterized by perivascular lymphohistiocytic infiltrates with eosinophils. The papillary dermis is edematous. The histologic appearance of nodular scabies is one of a dense, superficial, and deep perivascular lymphohistiocytic infiltrate with many plasma cells and eosinophils. Various vascular changes also may be apparent. Norwegian scabies (crusted scabies) is distinguished by numerous mites that are found in histologic sections of the stratum corneum, and hyperkeratosis is noted.[9] This form of scabies occurs most commonly in debilitated individuals, such as institutionalized retarded children or immunosuppressed children, including children with HIV infection.

Scabies is characterized by moderate to severe pruritus that starts several weeks to months after infestation, at which time the host has become hypersensitive to the mite or its products. A papular or vesicular eruption with pustules and linear burrows occurs and classically involves the webs between the fingers, flexures of the arms, axillae, and genital regions. In infants and children, scabies may occur over the palms, soles, head, and neck. Eczematous or bullous lesions also can be present.[2] In infants and children, scabies often is not suspected because of the atypical skin lesions that result from vigorous scratching and secondary infections.[15] Acute glomerulonephritis may be associated with pyoderma in scabies. A careful history may reveal that other family members or child caretakers have pruritus and skin lesions consistent with scabies. It frequently is helpful to examine the skin of family members for signs of scabies. Norwegian scabies may present not with the typical pruritic papules but rather with a nonspecific hyperkeratosis that may be generalized or localized to the hands or feet.[8]

The diagnosis of scabies can be overlooked easily and should be considered when the physician is faced with an unusual papular or bullous rash. The differential diagnosis of scabies in children includes impetigo, atopic eczema, seborrheic or contact dermatitis, psoriasis, histiocytosis, and chickenpox.[15, 16] The diagnosis can be confirmed by finding the mites, eggs, or scybala in a mineral oil preparation from the scrapings of an early burrow or papule, although this commonly is unrewarding.[19] In some cases, a variety of biopsy techniques can be useful.[4]

The management of scabies involves the application of a topical scabicide to all areas of skin (except the face) and subsequent removal in 8 to 24 hours, depending on the product applied. Effective scabicides are gamma benzene hexachloride (lindane), permethrin 5 per cent, and 10 per cent crotamiton. Antibiotics may be necessary if secondary bacterial infection is present. Articles of clothing and bed sheets should be washed in hot water at the end of therapy. There is some evidence that gamma benzene hexachloride may not be safe for use in infants and young children because of transcutaneous absorption and subsequent adverse central nervous system effects.[15, 20] These adverse effects possibly may be prevented by a careful explanation of the application and removal of lindane after 8 to 12 hours.[8, 14] The agent of choice for infants and young children is permethrin topical cream, which can be applied to the entire head, neck, and body of the infant.[15] Ivermectin has proved to be highly efficacious as an oral therapy of scabies in a single dose for otherwise healthy or HIV-infected adults.[22] It is not approved for use in children. All family members should be treated simultaneously.[24] Pruritus often persists for some time after successful treatment with a scabicide and may be relieved by oral antihistamine or mild to moderate topical steroids.[4, 24] In hospitalized patients, contact isolation is recommended to lessen the potential for nosocomial transmission.

PEDICULOSIS

Arthropods of the order Anoplura (sucking lice) are important as vectors of rickettsial or spirochetal illnesses. The body louse *Pediculus humanus humanus* is the vector for epidemic typhus *(Rickettsia prowazekii)*, trench fever *(Rochalimaea quintana)*, and louse-borne relapsing fever *(Borrelia recurrentis)*. The body louse, head louse *(Pediculus humanus capitus)*, and crab louse *(Phthirus pubis)* all are capable of human infestation.

SPIDERS

Species of the genus *Loxosceles* are the spiders predominantly responsible for necrotic arachnidism in the United States. The dermonecrotic factor of the brown recluse spider venom appears to be sphingomyelinase, a phospholipase.[29] The necrosis due to the venom is dependent on neutrophils, but the neutrophils are not activated by the venom itself. Rather, the venom is a potent stimulus for the inflammatory response of endothelial cells, which in turn activates the polymorphonuclear neutrophils to cause tissue destruction.[23] The bites of the brown recluse spider can produce a broad spectrum of clinical response that varies from self-limited urticaria to severe necrosis with considerable systemic symptoms.[10] Disseminated intravascular coagulation, multiorgan failure, and death have been reported in children.[11, 28] Careful supportive care is required if symptoms are severe. Systemic corticosteroid therapy may be of some benefit if the patient has systemic symptoms. Dapsone, an inhibitor of neutrophil function, appears to decrease the development of wound complications and subsequent need for surgical excision.[25]

References

1. Badia, L., and Lund, V.: Vile bodies: An endoscopic approach to nasal myiasis. J. Laryngol. Otol. *108*:1083–1085, 1994.
2. Bean, S. F.: Bullous scabies. J. A. M. A. *230*:878, 1974.
3. Bernstein, B., and Mihan, R.: Hospital epidemic of scabies. J. Pediatr. *83*:1086–1087, 1973.
4. Burgess, I.: *Sarcoptes scabiei* and scabies. Adv. Parasitol. *35*:235–292, 1994.
5. Cooper, B. J., and Spence, I.: Temperature-dependent inhibition of evoked acetylcholine release in tick paralysis. Nature *263*:693–695, 1976.
6. Cunningham, D. G., and Zonga, J. R.: Myiasis of the external auditory canal. J. Pediatr. *84*:856–858, 1974.
7. Elgart, M. L.: Flies and myiasis. Dermatol. Clin. *8*:237–244, 1990.
8. Elgart, M. L.: Scabies. Dermatol. Clin. *8*:253–263, 1990.
9. Fernandez, N., Torres, A., and Ackerman, A. B.: Pathologic findings in human scabies. Arch. Dermatol. *113*:320–324, 1977.
10. Gendron, B. P.: *Loxosceles reclusa* envenomation. Am. J. Emerg. Med. *8*:51–54, 1990.
11. Ginsburg, C. M., and Weinberg, A. G.: Hemolytic anemia and multiorgan failure associated with localized cutaneous lesion. J. Pediatr. *112*:496–499, 1988.
12. Guillozet, N.: Diagnosing myiasis. J. A. M. A. *244*:698–699, 1980.
13. Haller, J. S., and Fabara, J. A.: Tick paralysis: Case report with emphasis on neurological toxicity. Am. J. Dis. Child. *124*:915–917, 1972.
14. Honig, P. J.: Bites and parasites. Pediatr. Clin. North Am. *30*:563–581, 1983.
15. Hurwitz, S.: Clinical Pediatric Dermatology. 2nd ed. Philadelphia, W. B. Saunders, 1993, pp. 405–412.
16. Hurwitz, S.: Scabies in babies. Am. J. Dis. Child. *126*:226–228, 1973.
17. Iannini, P. B., Brandt, D., and La Force, F. M.: Furuncular myiasis. J. A. M. A. *233*:1375–1376, 1975.
18. Kalelioglu, M., Akturk, G., Akturk, F., et al.: Intracerebral myiasis from *Hypoderma bovis* larva in a child. J. Neurosurg. *71*:929–931, 1989.
19. Kincaid, J. C.: Tick bite paralysis. Semin. Neurol. *10*:32–34, 1990.
20. Lee, B., and Croth, P.: Scabies: Transcutaneous poisoning during treatment. Pediatrics *59*:643, 1977.
21. Macias, E. G., Graham, A. J., Green, M., et al.: Cutaneous myiasis in South Texas. N. Engl. J. Med. *289*:1239–1241, 1973.
22. Meinking, T. L., Taplin, D., Hermida, J. L., et al.: The treatment of scabies with ivermectin. N. Engl. J. Med. *333*:26–30, 1995.
23. Patel, K. D., Modur, V., Zimmerman, G. A., et al.: The necrotic venom of the brown recluse spider induces dysregulated endothelial cell-dependent neutrophil activation: Differential induction of GM-CSF, IL-8, and E-selectin expression. J. Clin. Invest. *94*:631–642, 1994.
24. Rasmussen, J. E.: Scabies. Pediatr. Rev. *15*:110–114, 1994.
25. Rees, R. S., Altenbern, D. P., Lynch, J. B., et al.: Brown recluse spider bites: A comparison of early surgical excision versus dapsone and delayed surgical excision. Ann. Surg. *202*:659–663, 1985.
26. Shaw, P. K., and Juranek, D. D.: Recent trends in scabies in the United States. J. Infect. Dis. *134*:414–416, 1976.
27. Swift, T. R., and Ignacio, O. J.: Tick paralysis: Electrophysiologic studies. Neurology *25*:1130–1133, 1975.
28. Vorse, H., Seccareccio, P., Woodruff, K., et al.: Disseminated intravascular coagulopathy following fatal brown spider bite. J. Pediatr. *80*:1035–1037, 1972.
29. Wilson, D. C., and King, L. E., Jr.: Spiders and spider bites. Dermatol. Clin. *8*:272–286, 1990.

HEALTH INFORMATION FOR INTERNATIONAL TRAVEL

❑ ❑ ❑

227

HEALTH INFORMATION FOR INTERNATIONAL TRAVEL

Margaret A. Tipple and Rosamond Dewart

Americans increasingly are a nation of travelers, both for business and for pleasure. It is estimated that, in 1994, approximately 15 million Americans traveled to Europe, 4.4 million to East Asia and the Pacific, 300,000 to Africa, 270,000 to South Asia, and 240,000 to the Middle East.[14]

As travel to developing countries increases, American travelers are at risk for illness or injury from a variety of infectious agents and environmental hazards that are rare in the United States. Infectious diseases have been of most concern and therefore the most studied. It is reported that up to 55 per cent of travelers of all ages to high-risk areas suffer gastrointestinal illness during leisure travel lasting up to 14 days. More exotic infections (e.g., malaria) are uncommon but can have serious consequences when appropriate treatment is delayed or unavailable.[3, 10, 12] In adult travelers to developing countries, injuries and complications from preexisting medical conditions actually are more common causes of serious morbidity and mortality than are infectious diseases.[11, 12] Little information is available on either the number of children traveling and living abroad or the health problems they encounter as a result of travel.

The pediatrician or other health care professional responsible for providing travel health information to children faces several challenges: (1) the limited data on travel-related illness in children forces development of guidelines and recommendations on an empiric basis, (2) some vaccines (e.g., yellow fever vaccine) and medications (e.g., drugs for malaria prophylaxis) rarely are prescribed for children in the United States, so few physicians have enough experience to be comfortable with their use, (3) health information for international travel is an evolving "industry," and locating reliable, current information may seem complicated and time-consuming, and (4) parents may leave health-related travel preparations until just before departure, limiting opportunities for counseling and making immunizations especially problematic.

PRETRAVEL EVALUATION: ROLES OF THE PARENT AND THE HEALTH CARE PROVIDER

The parent, the child (if old enough), and the health care provider each has a vital role in preparing a child for international travel. Ideally, such preparation would start several weeks before travel, particularly if the itinerary is complicated, the trip is a long one (>1 month), or the trip includes destinations in tropical or developing countries.

With some assistance from the health care provider, the parents can obtain most of the health information required. Current information is widely available in the public sector and can be obtained as the parent researches other aspects of the trip. The additional advantage to the parent is that he or she becomes familiar with the health issues that are important not only to the child but also to the rest of the family during travel.

The health care provider may offer suggestions to the parents as to where to look for travel-related health information and should review carefully the material collected by the parent. The health care provider then can use the materials collected by the parent, other published materials (e.g., Advisory Committee on Immunization Practices [ACIP] guidelines for specific vaccines and package inserts for medications), and the child's medical record to determine what the child actually requires before the trip.

The Parent's Role: Gathering Information

The first task for the parent is to develop a detailed itinerary and description of the trip, which includes:

1. A list of all the countries to be visited, in the order of travel, with approximate dates of travel. This is important because some countries have requirements (e.g., proof of yellow fever vaccination) for travelers arriving from certain other countries.
2. The purpose, duration, locations, and expected activities within each country. The short-term traveler to an urban area, even in a developing country, encounters different conditions than the person who stays for a long period in local housing in a rural part of the same country. The long-term visitor to a rural area may require additional immunizations (e.g., typhoid, rabies) or malaria prophylaxis not routinely recommended for the tourist in an urban or resort area.
3. Information on the terrain, elevation above sea level, and climate/weather likely to be encountered at the time of year travel is planned (e.g., high and low daily temperatures, rainy vs. dry season).

If the parent cannot answer some of these questions, he or she should do so before specific health information is sought. Country-specific travel guides are a good source of information on climate, living conditions, quality of food and water, and commonly encountered health problems. For families preparing to live overseas, employers, sponsors, or colleagues who have returned recently from the area can provide information on local conditions, especially housing (e.g., air conditioning, screens, need for mosquito nets) and local medical resources (e.g., hospitals, emergency care facilities).

Once the general questions about the trip are answered, the parent can seek more specific health information. The whole area of health information and recommendations for international travel is evolving rapidly, and health conditions can vary over time, even at a familiar destination, so the following activities are recommended before each trip:

1. *Seek health information while obtaining trip documents.* Ask travel agents, tour organizers, embassies, or consulates of the countries to be visited. Some countries have certain requirements (e.g., immunizations) for all travelers entering the country to protect residents of that country from imported diseases. Inquire as to required medical documents. Ask whether any immunizations or laboratory tests are required (e.g., yellow fever vaccine may be required for travelers from an infected area). HIV antibody testing may be required by some countries for long-term visitors (usually those planning to stay more than 3 months). One should be aware that the information provided sometimes is incomplete and occasionally inaccurate, so it should be checked against another source.

2. *Read country-specific guidebooks.* Most have some information on recommended immunizations, need for malaria prophylaxis, and quality of food and water. Most also have general information for travelers with infants and children (e.g., likely availability of infant formula and disposable diapers).

3. *Consult travel health books available at a public library or bookstore or recommended by the child's physician.* Be sure they are current (published within the last 1 to 2 years). Virtually all have recommendations for medicines and supplies to carry, ways to prevent insect bites, and guidelines for choosing safe food and water. Some are intended to be carried along during the trip and include descriptions of most of the health problems that could be encountered in a developing area, with lists of signs, symptoms, and recommendations for treatment. Some have guidelines for travelers with chronic medical conditions (e.g., diabetes, pulmonary disease). Some have extensive information for travelers with children. Content, style, and emphasis vary considerably among these books, so it may be useful to read more than one.

4. Consult Health Information for International Travel (HIIT) documents prepared by the World Health Organization (WHO) or the Centers for Disease Control and Prevention (CDC).[2, 13] The CDC has several publications and services for travelers. A book entitled *Health Information for International Travel* is published yearly. It contains current immunization recommendations and requirements, recommendations for malaria prophylaxis, and information on infectious disease risks for each region of the world. The CDC also has region-specific health information, available by telephone (404-332-4559) and by fax (404-332-4565). Both services are available 24 hours a day and are updated regularly.

5. Consult the Internet, an increasingly useful source of health information for travelers. Documents from the CDC, including *Health Information for International Travel,* and current immunization recommendations are available on the World Wide Web (www) URL http://www.cdc.gov. The WHO Internet location can be accessed from the CDC www site. Other individuals and institutions also are making travelers' health information available on the Internet. These can be located with one of the search tools readily available on the Internet, using such key words as "travel" and "health."

The Health Care Provider's Role

Assuming that the parent has followed the sequence suggested, the physician's job is fairly straightforward, with the help of a few additional references. The physician should do the following:

1. Review the child's medical record. Ensure that routine immunizations are current or that contraindications are documented. Note chronic or recurring medical problems and allergies to medications.
2. Review the trip itinerary and additional information on local conditions at the destination prepared by the parent.
3. Review materials that the parent may have obtained on immunizations and preventive measures from the CDC, WHO, or other verifiable sources (they strongly should have been encouraged to do so).
4. Consult additional information sources as needed. These fall into five general categories:
   a. Published guidelines. Both the CDC and WHO publish health information books for international travel.[2, 13] These books contain current information on disease risks, recommended immunizations, and prophylactic/preventive measures (e.g., malaria prophylaxis). They are updated yearly, readily available, and relatively inexpensive. The CDC's *Health Information for International Travel* may be purchased for a nominal fee from the Superintendent of Documents, United States Government Printing Office, Washington, DC 20402 (202-512-1800). The CDC publication is supplemented by "Blue Sheets" and Advisory Memoranda. The Blue Sheets are published biweekly and update material contained in the book. Advisory Memoranda are published when outbreaks occur and provide additional information on vaccinations, other prevention measures, and travel restrictions. Subscriptions to both the Blue Sheets and Advisory Memoranda may be obtained at no cost for physicians by calling 404-332-4559. The American Academy of Pediatrics Report of the Committee on Infectious Diseases (Red Book)[9] also contains information on a variety of infectious diseases and vaccines. The ACIP also publishes immunization guidelines.[1, 4, 6]
   b. Commercially available compact disk–read only memory (CD-ROM) or diskette-based programs for personal computers. All contain information similar to that found in the published guidelines cited earlier. Some are available by subscription, with regular updates. Some are packaged with printed materials (e.g., guidelines for selecting safe food and water) suitable for distribution to patients. Information on these programs can be found in *The Journal of Travel Medicine,* published quarterly by Decker Periodicals, Hamilton, Ontario, Canada (905-522-7017).
   c. Voice and fax information system. The CDC maintains a voice and fax information system based on the CDC printed materials listed earlier. These are updated as needed to provide current information on new vaccine recommendations and outbreaks of illness that may be of concern to travelers to a specific region. The telephone number for the voice information is 404-332-4559, and the fax information system number is 404-332-4565.
   d. The Internet. Among other "Health Alerts," documents that include information on outbreaks can be

found at URL http://www.cdc.gov. It is important to note that although there is a wealth of information available through the Internet, the quality of this information varies.

e. Infectious disease or travel medicine consultants. The sources cited should be enough for the preparation of most children for travel to most destinations. However, it may be necessary to refer the child with complex medical problems, allergies, or other conditions to a pediatric infectious disease specialist with experience in tropical diseases or travel medicine. Most U.S. travel clinics are geared to adult travelers, but some may have sufficient pediatric experience to do pediatric travel consultations. Children with anemia, heart disease, and pulmonary disease may be at risk for complications from hypoxia during flight.[7, 8] If a child needs supplemental oxygen, the airline must be contacted, because travelers generally are not allowed to bring their own oxygen tanks and equipment aboard. Some airlines require that such patients be evaluated by physicians chosen by the airline before they can travel. Consult the airline with which the family will travel for further information.

5. Determine, based on the itinerary, the child's medical history, and review of the cited references, which vaccines and medications (e.g., malaria prophylaxis) are indicated. Ensure that routine (i.e., ACIP-recommended) immunizations are current; then consider the additional immunizations (e.g., meningococcal, Japanese encephalitis, rabies, yellow fever) recommended for the specific itinerary. Consult the CDC guidelines for possible contraindications (age, allergies). As a final check for dosage, indications, and precautions, read the manufacturer's package insert or *Physician's Desk Reference* (PDR). Most vaccines can be given in any physician's office or clinic. Yellow fever vaccine use is restricted, but most communities have at least one provider who can administer the vaccine and certify receipt of the vaccine on the required official immunization record (the International Certificate of Vaccination [ICV]). Information on yellow fever vaccine providers usually can be obtained by calling the local health department. If malaria prophylaxis is indicated, review the CDC guidelines or the "Red Book" for appropriate drugs and dosages; then consult the manufacturer's package insert or PDR for further information before writing the prescription. Most pharmacies do not stock mefloquine routinely, so several days may be needed to obtain the drug.

6. Consider other prevention measures. Depending on the itinerary, duration of the trip, and the child's medical history, it may be appropriate to:
   a. Recommend dental and eye examinations, if there is a history of problems or the travel will be of long duration.
   b. Perform a tuberculin skin test, preferably a Mantoux test, as a baseline if the child will have prolonged travel or residence in an area of high prevalence of tuberculosis. If the family will reside in such an area, discuss with parents the possible need to screen household help for tuberculosis before employing them.
   c. Review all regularly used prescription and over-the-counter medications. If possible, have the parents carry enough of each medication for the entire trip. Counsel parents that many medications available only by prescription in the United States are easily available elsewhere but that dosages and quality may not be comparable. Antibiotics and other drugs (e.g., cough suppressants) often are available as combination preparations. These should be avoided.
   d. Prescribe medications, as appropriate, for use in case of illness during the trip. These might include antibiotics for use in case of traveler's diarrhea or recurrent otitis media. Provide written instructions for use.
   e. Review contents of the family's travel medicine kit (e.g., first-aid materials, antipyretics, antidiarrheals). Ensure that written instructions and medication dosages for various members of the family are included.
   f. Prescribe oral rehydration salts or provide instructions for use of locally available fluids for management of diarrhea.[5] Instructions should be tailored to the age and weight of the child. If oral rehydration salts are not available locally, they can be obtained from Jianas Bothers Packaging Company (816-421-2880).
   g. Review food and water precautions. Discuss the need for adequate fluids in hot climates.
   h. Remind the parent and child that mosquitoes can carry a variety of diseases other than malaria. Review use of insect repellents, mosquito nets, long-sleeved clothing, and other preventive measures.
   i. Counsel teenage travelers and their parents regarding the risks of HIV infection and other sexually transmitted diseases.
   j. Remind parents that child seats and automobiles with seat belts are not universally available. Travel agents, airlines, and rental car companies can provide more information, but parents may wish to take child seats with them.
   k. Review indications for sun screen.
   l. Review precautions for swimming in fresh water (e.g., risk of schistosomiasis in travelers to endemic areas in the Caribbean, South America, Africa, and Asia).
   m. Recommend that parents review their medical insurance coverage. Not all policies cover medical care outside of the United States.
   n. Recommend that parents carry with them telephone numbers for the U.S. embassy/consulates in their destination countries. U.S. embassies do not provide medical care but usually can recommend local medical facilities for emergency care. Travelers are responsible for costs of medical care.

7. Finally, assure the parents and the child that travel is to be enjoyed and that with the reasonable precautions outlined earlier, serious illness and injury are uncommon.

References

1. Centers for Disease Control and Prevention: General recommendations on immunization: Recommendations of the Advisory Committee on Immunization Practices (ACIP). M. M. W. R. *43*(RR-1):1–38, 1994.
2. Centers for Disease Control and Prevention: Health Information for International Travel 1994. Atlanta, U. S. Department of Health and Human Services (Publication No. 93-8280), 1994.
3. Centers for Disease Control and Prevention: Malaria surveillance—United States, 1992. CDC Surveillance Summaries, October 20, 1995. M. M. W. R. *44*(SS-5):1–17, 1995.
4. Centers for Disease Control and Prevention: Recommendations of the Advisory Committee on Immunization Practices (ACIP): Use of vaccines and immune globulins in persons with altered immunocompetence. M. M. W. R. *42*(RR-4):1–18, 1993.
5. Centers for Disease Control: The management of acute diarrhea in children: Oral rehydration, maintenance, and nutritional therapy. M. M. W. R. *41*(RR-16):1–38, 1992.
6. Centers for Disease Control: Update on adult immunization: Recommendations of the Immunization Practices Advisory Committee (ACIP). M. M. W. R. *40*(RR-12):1–94, 1991.
7. Gong, H.: Air travel and oxygen therapy in cardiopulmonary patients. Chest *101*:1104–1113, 1992.

8. Gong, H., Mark, J. A. L., and Cowan, M. N.: Preflight medical screenings of patients. Chest *104*:788–794, 1993.
9. Peter, G. (ed.): 1994 Red Book: Report of the Committee on Infectious Diseases. 23rd ed. Elk Grove Village, IL, American Academy of Pediatrics, 1994.
10. Schwartz, I. K.: Prevention of malaria. Infect. Dis. Clin. North Am. *6*:313–331, 1992.
11. Steffen, R.: Health risks for short-term travelers. *In* Lobel, H., Haworth, J., and Bradley, D. J. (eds.): Travel Medicine: Proceedings of the First Conference on International Travel Medicine, Zurich, Switzerland, April 5–8, 1988. New York, Springer-Verlag, 1989.
12. Steffen, R.: Travel medicine: Prevention based on epidemiological data. Trans. R. Soc. Trop. Med. Hyg. *85*:156–162, 1991.
13. World Health Organization: International travel and health: Vaccination requirements and health advice: Situation as of 1 January, 1995. Geneva, World Health Organization, 1995.
14. World Tourism Organization: Tourism market trends: World 1985–1994. Madrid, World Tourism Organization, 1995.

PART

4

INFECTION CONTROL

SECTION TWENTY-FOUR

HOSPITAL CONTROL OF INFECTIONS

❏ ❏ ❏

228

NOSOCOMIAL INFECTIONS

W. Charles Huskins and Donald A. Goldmann

Nosocomial infections generally have been defined as infections that develop in hospitalized patients and were neither present nor incubating at admission.[48, 145] The term *nosocomial* originates from the Greek words *nosos* (disease) and *komeion* (to take care of).[388] In light of this etymology, a more inclusive definition would be infections that occur as a consequence of medical care, regardless of whether or not they arise during hospitalization. This definition would include a surgical site infection that occurred after an outpatient surgical procedure or a case of varicella acquired during an emergency room visit. Infections in hospital personnel caused by microorganisms acquired in the hospital also may be considered nosocomial infections. This expanded view of nosocomial infections fits well with recent trends in medicine that have placed increased emphasis on outpatient care, more comprehensive assessment of outcomes of medical care, and the risk of occupational diseases facing medical personnel.

In some cases, it may be difficult to determine whether an infection is a consequence of medical care. Infections with long or variable incubation periods, such as hepatitis B or late-onset prosthetic valve endocarditis, may manifest themselves long after medical procedures, raising doubt regarding their causation. Infections in immunocompromised patients occurring during hospitalization, such as *Pneumocystis carinii* pneumonia, often are perceived as attributable to the patients' underlying risk of infection and previous colonization, rather than as a result of hospital care.

Despite these ambiguities, defining nosocomial infections as infections resulting from medical care makes sense because it identifies the population at risk. The study of infections that occur in persons exposed to medical care affords us the opportunity to understand better the mechanisms involved in causing these infections and to design interventions that can prevent them. This chapter discusses the general epidemiology of nosocomial infections (including those that are introduced into the hospital from the community); infections related to invasive devices, procedures, and treatments; and infections in special populations. Programmatic approaches to the prevention and control of nosocomial infections are discussed in Chapter 229.

HISTORICAL ASPECTS

The history of nosocomial infections and their control is linked tightly to developments in institutional medical care. Two recent publications describe this history in considerable detail.[234, 388] Unfortunately, historical data regarding nosocomial infections in children are relatively limited. Nonetheless, there is ample evidence that efforts to study and prevent infection among hospitalized children have contributed significantly to the development of nosocomial infection control and prevention efforts in general.

Hospitals in Europe during the Middle Ages and the Renaissance were notorious for their overcrowding and unsanitary conditions, and one can imagine that children suffered greatly from the epidemics of contagious diseases that spread through hospitals during this period. By the 18th and 19th centuries, sketchy information regarding the impact of nosocomial infections in pediatric patients began to emerge. These data, summarized at a report presented in a landmark seminar regarding nosocomial infections in pediatric patients at the Sixth Northern Pediatric Congress in Stockholm in 1934,[136] provide dramatic evidence that nosocomial infections were the cause of considerable morbidity and mortality in hospitalized children.

Semmelweis' classic studies of puerperal fever in the Vienna Lying-In Hospital in the mid-1800s provide insights into the etiology of infections in newborn infants, not just their afflicted mothers.[389] Semmelweis noted that rates of mortality in infants born to women in the First Division of the hospital (the division where medical students who had come from the autopsy table cared for women in labor) were several-fold higher than those in infants born to women on the Second Division of the hospital (the division where midwives cared for women in labor). In support of his theories regarding the infectious etiology of puerperal fever, he noted that rates of infant mortality closely paralleled rates of maternal mortality from puerperal fever and that autopsy findings were remarkably similar in infants and mothers.

The opening of wards and entire hospitals designated for the treatment of patients with infectious diseases in the early 20th century stimulated interest in the study of "cross-infection" with measles, chickenpox, scarlet fever, whooping cough, diphtheria, and invasive meningococcal disease.[388] The potential for cross-infection with classic contagious diseases on pediatric wards, especially wards caring for infants, was well recognized in the leading hospitals of the day and stimulated a number of interventions to minimize this problem. Quarantine areas for new admissions, confinement of each child in an individual cubicle, cohorting of patients admitted during community epidemics, the use of masks by persons caring for patients, exclusion of visitors, and strict control of the health of nurses and physicians caring for the patients were employed to minimize the spread of contagious diseases.[44, 53, 183, 248, 259] Some hospitals even used closed cubicles with outside exhaust of air for patients with measles or varicella.[183] Analysis of the effectiveness of these interventions contributed to improved understanding of how these contagious diseases are spread in hospitals.

Undoubtedly because of this vigilance, the first systematic surveys of nosocomial infections in pediatric patients in hospitals in Europe and the United States published in the 1930s and 1940s demonstrated that nosocomial spread of the classic contagious diseases occurred but was relatively uncommon.[183, 248, 284, 333, 444] However, nosocomial respiratory infections of various types were encountered frequently; gastrointestinal and skin infections also were relatively common.[183, 248, 284, 444]

Although nosocomial infections caused by beta-hemolytic streptococci have been a scourge of obstetric and surgical wards for centuries, advances in diagnostic microbiology and serotyping of streptococci in the mid-1900s led to greater appreciation of the etiologic role of these organisms in nosocomial scarlet fever; postpartum infections; postoperative infections; and secondary infections in patients with burns, measles, and influenza.[376, 388] The decline of these organisms as major nosocomial pathogens coincided with the introduction of antibiotic therapy in the 1940s and 1950s.[376]

Outbreaks of *Staphylococcus aureus* infection in hospitalized newborn infants had been documented in late 1800s and early 1900s,[61, 218] but the pandemic of *S. aureus* infections that plagued hospitals in the 1950s and 1960s drew special attention to the impact of nosocomial infections caused by this organism. Outbreaks of staphylococcal disease particularly were devastating in newborn nurseries, where epidemics caused by specific phage types caused substantial morbidity and mortality.[376, 382]

This serious nosocomial staphylococcal infection problem spawned more comprehensive efforts to document the impact and consequences of nosocomial infections and served as the impetus to develop organized infection control programs, particularly in Great Britain (with its tradition of infection control sisters) and North America. A year-long study of nosocomial infections in pediatric patients at the Hospital for Sick Children in Toronto was conducted in 1959.[364–366] The cumulative incidence of nosocomial infection was 6.5 per cent; respiratory and gastrointestinal infections occurred most commonly. *S. aureus* caused infection in only 2.6 per cent of patients overall but accounted for the vast majority of surgical-site infections. Even this early study recognized the important consequences of nosocomial infection, reporting that nosocomial infections caused 16 deaths and 2070 extra hospital days.

In 1970, a nosocomial infection surveillance and control program was established at Children's Hospital in Boston, and data were reported to the nascent National Nosocomial Infections Study at the Centers for Disease Control.[139] The cumulative incidence of infection was 4.6 per cent. *S. aureus* was the most common pathogen, but more than 60 per cent of the pathogens were gram-negative bacilli, including *Pseudomonas aeruginosa*, *Escherichia coli*, *Klebsiella* species, *Enterobacter* species, *Proteus* species, and *Serratia* species. It should be noted that study of the epidemiology of specific nosocomial pathogens in this period was hampered because few clinical laboratories then performed extensive speciation. Moreover, the detection of nosocomial viral infections was hindered by the limited availability of suitable diagnostic techniques. The Children's Hospital study emphasized the association of nosocomial infections with exposure to invasive devices and procedures (e.g., surgical site infections in patients undergoing surgery, urinary tract infections in patients with indwelling urinary catheters, blood stream infections and septic phlebitis associated with intravascular catheters, central nervous system infections associated with ventriculoatrial and ventriculoperitoneal cerebrospinal fluid shunts). The introduction of intensive care units (ICUs) for newborn infants and children in the 1970s and early 1980s accelerated these trends.[160, 187, 193, 266]

Advances in viral diagnostics in the 1970s led to greater appreciation of the importance of viruses as a significant cause of nosocomial infections, particularly in pediatric patients.[432, 449] Nosocomial spread of respiratory and gastrointestinal viruses, especially respiratory syncytial virus (RSV) and rotavirus, was found to be a severe problem in pediatric wards.[104, 176, 293, 369, 452]

The past 20 years have witnessed the re-emergence and predominance of gram-positive organisms, including coagulase-negative staphylococci, *S. aureus*, enterococci, and, to a lesser extent, streptococci, as nosocomial pathogens.[127, 202] Bacteria have become increasingly resistant to available antibiotics; methicillin-resistant *S. aureus*, vancomycin-resistant enterococci, and gram-negative bacilli producing extended-spectrum β-lactamases have been especially troublesome.[299, 353, 430] As increasing numbers of severely ill and immunosuppressed children have been cared for in hospitals, there has been a dramatic increase in the incidence of fungal infections, especially infections due to *Candida* and *Aspergillus*.[127, 202] The risk of nosocomial infections caused by blood-borne pathogens, such as HIV, hepatitis B virus, and hepatitis C virus, among patients as well as health care workers has been recognized.[14, 43, 151, 152, 327]

In summary, the history of nosocomial infections in children is tied closely to the progress of medicine itself. New therapies and invasive procedures have had the unwanted side effect of increased nosocomial infection risk. Longer survival from conditions formerly causing early death and increasing numbers of immunocompromised children have resulted in a growing population of children with impaired host defenses who are at increased risk of infections. The selective pressure of widespread use of new, broad-spectrum antimicrobial agents has resulted in the development of previously unknown forms of antimicrobial resistance and the emergence of fungi as serious nosocomial pathogens.

GENERAL EPIDEMIOLOGY OF NOSOCOMIAL INFECTIONS

Perhaps more than any other area of infectious disease epidemiology, the method used to study the epidemiology of nosocomial infections itself has been subjected to intense investigation and validation. This section describes the epidemiology of nosocomial infections in pediatric patients in general terms, highlighting important methodologic issues. The epidemiology of specific nosocomial infections and pathogens is discussed in later sections.

Rates of Nosocomial Infection

A number of hospital surveys have examined rates of nosocomial infections in pediatric patients in the modern era.[86, 127, 139, 202, 286, 364–366, 449] These surveys have been useful in documenting the nature and frequency of nosocomial infections and in illustrating trends in infections caused by various pathogens (see Historical Aspects). However, it is difficult to evaluate and compare the infection rates in these studies because of important methodologic differences. The types of nosocomial infections studied and the definitions used to identify these infections have varied considerably. The sensitivity of the case-finding techniques employed and the vigor with which viral infections have been sought and confirmed have varied greatly. In most cases, there has been insufficient adjustment for length of hospitalization, case mix,

TABLE 228–1. Overall Median Nosocomial Infection Rates by Service in National Nosocomial Infections Surveillance System Hospitals

Service	Infections/ 100 Discharges	Infections/ 1000 Patient Days
Medicine	3.5	5.7
Oncology	5.1	8.1
Burn	14.9	11.9
Cardiac surgery	9.8	13.8
Orthopedics	3.9	5.8
Ophthalmology	0.0	0.0
Obstetrics	0.9	5.0
Pediatrics	0.4	0.9
Newborn intensive care unit	14.0	9.9
Normal newborn nursery	0.4	1.1

Data are from 1986 to 1990.

severity of illness, and exposure to invasive devices and procedures that increase the risk of nosocomial infection.

Many, but not all, of these methodologic concerns are alleviated by examining rates of nosocomial infection in pediatric patients provided by the National Nosocomial Infections Surveillance (NNIS) System coordinated by the Hospital Infections Program at the Centers for Disease Control and Prevention (CDC). As of 1993, 163 United States acute-care hospitals actively were reporting data regarding the incidence of nosocomial infections to the NNIS system.[377] Participating hospitals follow NNIS system methods, which include the use of published definitions of nosocomial infections,[145] standardized coding of data, structured data collection sheets, and a microcomputer surveillance software program specifically designed for the NNIS system.[116] Case-finding methods are not specified in the NNIS method, although the vast majority of hospitals identify nosocomial infections by reviewing microbiology result reports and patient charts.[116] However, post-discharge surveillance varies highly, and the NNIS method has not been validated independently as yet.

Table 228–1 contains overall infection rates by service for NNIS hospitals from 1986 to 1990. The cumulative incidence of nosocomial infections (number of nosocomial infections per 100 discharges) for pediatric services and normal newborn nurseries is lower than for most other services. Newborn ICUs, on the other hand, have a comparatively high cumulative incidence of infection, rivaling that of burn services.

Length of hospitalization is an important factor in assessing rates of nosocomial infection because the cumulative probability that an individual will experience at least one nosocomial infection increases with increasing exposure to the hospital. To minimize the effect of differences in length of hospitalization, rates of nosocomial infection are expressed as an incidence density (the number of nosocomial infections per 1000 patient-days). Table 228–1 also contains the incidence density of nosocomial infections by service for NNIS hospitals. When expressed as an incidence density, the frequency of nosocomial infections in newborn ICUs is not as striking compared with other services. This is likely the result of the adjustment for length of hospitalization, which can be long for premature infants and severely ill full-term infants.

Other factors increase the risk of nosocomial infection, and additional adjustment of infection rates is necessary to reflect these risks accurately. The invasive devices that are a routine part of modern hospital care especially are important risk factors. Central venous catheters increase the risk of blood stream infection, mechanical ventilation increases the risk of pneumonia, and indwelling urinary catheters increase the risk of urinary tract infection. To adjust for exposure (as well as the duration of exposure) to these devices, infection rates can be expressed as the number of infections among persons exposed to the device per 1000 days of device exposure. Table 228–2 contains data regarding the device-associated incidence density of blood stream infection, pneumonia, and urinary tract infection for adult and pediatric ICUs in NNIS hospitals.[305] Table 228–3 contains data regarding device-associated incidence density of blood stream infections and pneumonia stratified by birth weight for newborn ICUs in NNIS hospitals.[305] These data show that the pooled mean rate of blood stream infection is higher in pediatric ICUs and newborn ICUs, particularly for lower birth weight categories, than in adult ICUs (except for burn ICUs). Conversely, the pooled mean rate of pneumonia is substantially lower in pediatric ICUs and newborn ICUs than in adult ICUs. The pooled mean rate of urinary tract infections in pediatric ICUs is slightly lower than in adult ICUs.

The risk of nosocomial infection also varies with individual patient characteristics and the nature and severity of patients' underlying diseases. Simple systems for classifying severity of illness have existed for decades, such as the system proposed by McCabe and Jackson[280] and the American Society of Anesthesiologists Physical Status Classification (ASA score).[216] Recently, methods for quantifying severity of illness

TABLE 228–2. Pooled Means of Device-Associated Infection Rates by Type of Intensive Care Unit (ICU) in National Nosocomial Infections Surveillance System Hospitals

	Pooled Means		
Type of ICU	*Central Line–Associated Blood Stream Infection/1000 Central Line Days*	*Ventilator-Associated Pneumonia/1000 Ventilator Days*	*Catheter-Associated Urinary Tract Infection/1000 Urinary Catheter Days*
Adult ICUs			
Coronary	5.0	9.8	8.6
Medical	6.7	9.6	9.3
Medical/surgical	4.9	12.7	6.1
Surgical	5.5	15.4	6.0
Burn	15.6	22.2	7.6
Pediatric ICUs	8.0	6.0	5.6

Data are from January 1990 to April 1995.

Modified from National Nosocomial Infections Surveillance System: National Nosocomial Infection Surveillance (NNIS) semi-annual report, May 1995. Am. J. Infect. Control *23*:377–385, 1995.

TABLE 228–3. Pooled Means of Device-Associated Infection Rates by Birth Weight Category in Newborn Intensive Care Units in National Nosocomial Infections Surveillance System Hospitals

	Pooled Means	
Birth Weight Category	*Central or Umbilical Intravascular Catheter–Associated Blood Stream Infection/ 1000 Central or Umbilical Line Days*	*Ventilator-Associated Pneumonia/1000 Ventilator Days*
≤1000 g	12.9	4.8
1001–1500 g	8.3	4.6
1501–2500 g	6.3	3.9
>2500 g	4.9	3.0

Data are from January 1992 to May 1995.

Modified from National Nosocomial Infections Surveillance System: National Nosocomial Infections Surveillance (NNIS) semi-annual report, May 1995. Am. J. Infect. Control *23*:377–385, 1995.

have become considerably more numerous and complex.[164] Progress has been made in the development and application of valid measures to quantify severity of illness in pediatric patients, although this process has lagged behind that for adult patients.

The Physiologic Stability Index (PSI) was developed and validated as a severity-of-illness measure for pediatric ICU patients.[469] The Pediatric Risk of Mortality (PRISM) score provided a streamlined scoring system by reducing the number of variables in the PSI through regression analysis and weighting of physiologic variables in order to reflect their contribution to the risk of mortality better.[329] Although the utility of PRISM in estimating mortality risk has been validated extensively, only one study has examined PRISM scores as a predictor of nosocomial infection in pediatric ICU patients.[330] In this study, the cumulative incidence of nosocomial infection in patients with PRISM scores of 10 or greater was threefold higher than that in patients with PRISM scores of less than 10 (10.8 per cent vs. 3.4 per cent, $p < 0.001$). When only patients with ICU stays of 7 days or more were analyzed, a PRISM score of 10 or greater still was associated significantly with increased risk of nosocomial infection, indicating that the risk of infection was not merely a reflection of longer ICU stays among sicker patients. However, rates of infection reported in this study were not adjusted for device exposure. Consequently, it is not clear whether the increased risk of infection in patients with PRISM scores of 10 or greater was attributable to increased severity of illness alone or to specific therapeutic factors, such as more frequent use of central vascular catheters, urinary catheters, and mechanical ventilation.

The NNIS system collects information on severity of illness in ICU patients using its own qualitative classification of physiologic stability.[116] However, the validity of this measure has not been established. The NNIS system has not incorporated its physiologic stability index, or any other measure of severity of illness, as an adjuster for nosocomial infection rates in pediatric ICU patients in its published reports.[305]

The association between birth weight and risk of nosocomial infection in newborn ICU patients is well recognized.[131, 187] For this reason, the NNIS system stratifies data regarding nosocomial infections in newborn ICUs into four birth weight strata: less than or equal to 1000 g, 1001 to 1500 g, 1501 to 2500 g, and greater than 2500 g. Table 228–3 displays the device-associated incidence density of blood stream infections and pneumonia for these birth weight strata.[305] There is a progressive and marked increase in rates of blood stream infection in sequentially lower birth weight categories, such that the rate of infection in infants less than or equal to 1000 g is two and a half times the rate in infants greater than 2500 g. Higher rates of pneumonia also occur in lower birth weight categories, but this trend is much less marked than for blood stream infections.

Figure 228–1 displays the device-associated incidence density of blood stream infection stratified by birth weight category in newborn ICUs in NNIS hospitals.[148] As can be seen in this figure, blood stream infection rates among newborn ICUs vary widely, even within specific birth weight strata.[148] Birth weight also is an insufficient adjustment to explain variation in mortality rates among newborn ICUs.[168] These variations may be attributable to differences in practice style or quality of care but also could be due to the failure of birth weight or device exposure to adjust fully for severity of illness. Several measures of severity of illness in newborn ICU patients have been developed in order to adjust for disease severity and facilitate more valid comparisons of the outcomes of care among newborn ICUs.[163, 355, 356, 426] One of these measures, the Score for Neonatal Acute Physiology (SNAP), was shown to be a strong predictor of nosocomial coagulase-negative staphylococcal bacteremia among very low birth weight (<1500 g) infants, even after adjustment for duration of stay in the newborn ICU and birth weight.[162] However, rates of infection in this study were not adjusted for exposure to central or umbilical lines, and information regarding other significant risk factors, such as administration of lipid emulsions,[130] was not available.

Ideally, rates of nosocomial infections should be adjusted simultaneously for several important risk factors yet remain simple enough to interpret and apply in practice. Developed by analysis of 4 years of surgical-site infection data reported to the NNIS system, the surgical-site infection risk index is an example of this type of composite risk adjustment.[93] This risk index is calculated by counting one point for each of the following three risk factors: a preoperative ASA score of 3, 4, or 5; an operation classified as either contaminated or dirty-infected; and an operation with a duration of more than T hours, where T depends on the operative procedure performed.[93] As seen in Table 228–4, this risk index provides a much better assessment of risk than traditional wound classification alone. Composite risk indexes for other specific nosocomial infections have not been developed yet.

TABLE 228–4. Surgical-Site Infection Rates* by Traditional Wound Classification and Risk Index†

	Risk Index†				
Wound Classification	*0*	*1*	*2*	*3*	*Cumulative*
Clean	1.0	2.3	5.4	—	2.1
Clean-contaminated	2.1	4.0	9.5	—	3.3
Contaminated	—	3.4	6.8	13.2	6.4
Dirty-infected	—	3.1	8.1	12.8	7.1
Cumulative	1.5	2.9	6.8	13.0	

*Surgical-site infections per 100 operative procedures.

†Calculated by counting one point for each of the following three risk factors: a preoperative ASA score of 3, 4, or 5; an operation classified as either contaminated or dirty-infected; and an operation with a duration of more than T hours (T is the 75th percentile for the duration of surgery rounded to the nearest hour for procedures included in the NNIS database; see reference below).

Modified from Culver, D. H., Horan, T. C., Gaynes, R. P., et al.: Surgical wound infection rates by wound class, operative procedure, and patient risk index. Am. J. Med. *91*:152S–157S, 1991.

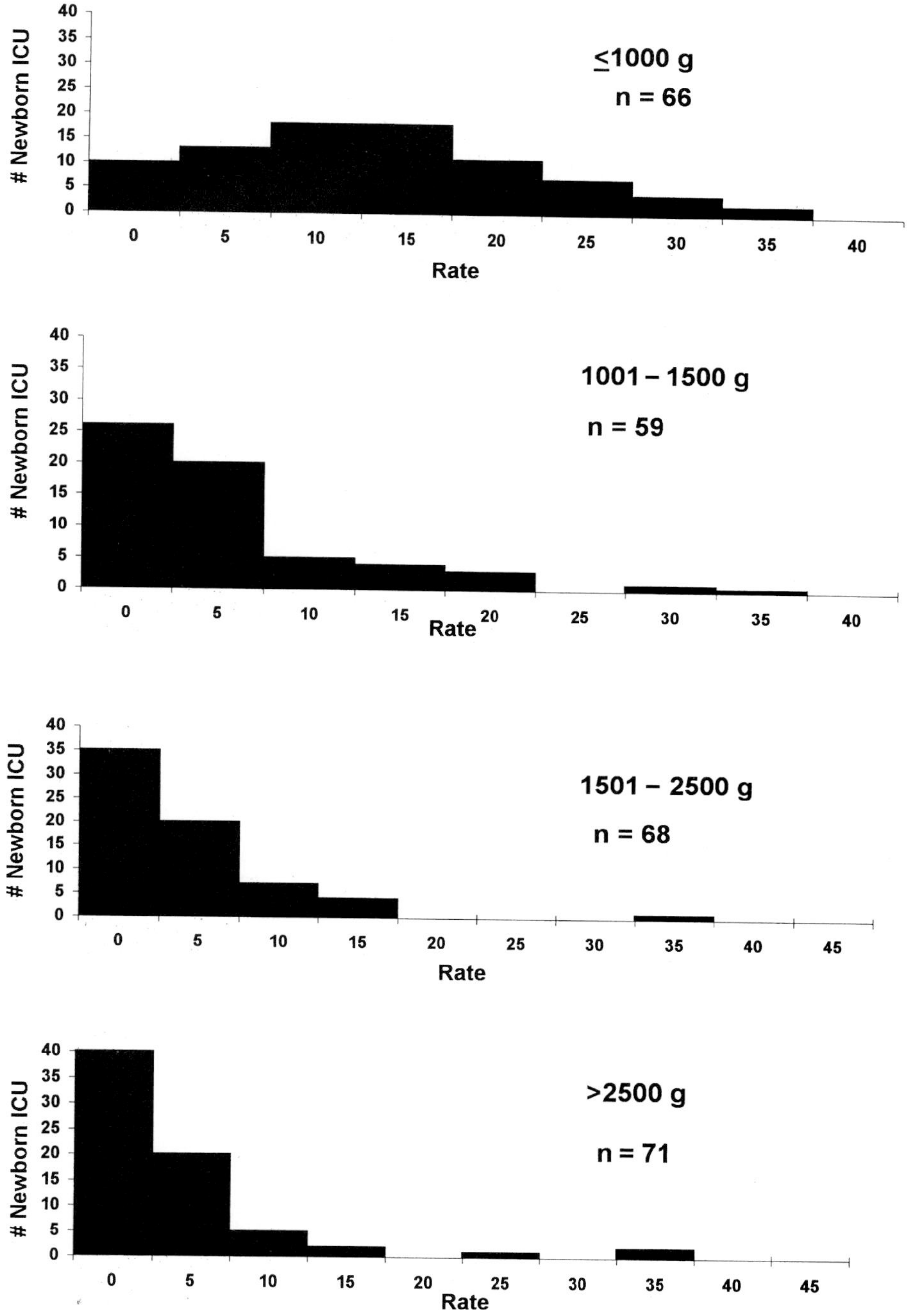

FIGURE 228–1. *Central or umbilical intravascular catheter–associated blood stream infection (BSI) rates by birth weight category for newborn intensive care units (ICU) in National Nosocomial Infections Surveillance System hospitals. Data for >2500 g and 1501–2500 g birth weight categories are from October 1986 to September 1994; data for 1001–1500 g and ≤1000 g birth weight categories are from January 1992 to September 1994. Rate = the number of central or umbilical intravascular catheter–associated BSI per 1000 central or umbilical catheter days. (Modified from Gaynes, R. P., Edwards, J. R., Jarvis, W. R., et al.: Nosocomial infections among neonates in high-risk nurseries in the United States. Pediatrics 98:357–361, 1996.)*

In summary, the method for providing meaningful rates of nosocomial infection has advanced remarkably in the past decade, primarily through refinements in appropriate adjustment for important risk factors. Incorporating adjustment for severity of illness into routine surveillance and reporting mechanisms and further development of composite risk indices for specific infections remain challenges for the future.

Sites of Nosocomial Infection

Table 228–5 contains data regarding the major site distribution of nosocomial infections by service in NNIS hospitals.[117] The site distribution of nosocomial infections among children and newborns differs substantially from that among adults. Blood stream infections account for a considerably greater proportion of nosocomial infections in children and newborns than in adults. Conversely, urinary tract infections and, to a lesser extent, pneumonia and surgical-site infections account for lower proportions of infections in children and newborns.

Some of these differences are due to differences in exposure to invasive devices, but others are not. For example, urinary catheters are used much less commonly in children and newborns, decreasing the risk of urinary tract infections.[305] On the other hand, central lines are used at comparable or lower rates in children and newborns than in adults,[305] so the greater proportion of blood stream infections in children and newborns cannot be explained by device exposure.

TABLE 228–5. Site Distribution of Major Nosocomial Infections by Service in National Nosocomial Infections Surveillance System Hospitals

All Services	Blood Stream	Pneumonia	Urinary Tract	Surgical Site	Other
Adult					
General surgery	9.5	16.4	30.2	24.5	19.4
Medical	14.8	17.0	42.1	2.3	23.8
Pediatric	29.7	12.7	12.7	6.1	38.8
Newborn	36.1	14.9	4.2	1.8	43.1

Data are from 1990 to 1992.
Modified from Emori, T. G., and Gaynes, R. P.: An overview of nosocomial infections, including the role of the microbiology laboratory. Clin. Microbiol. Rev. *6*:428–442, 1993.

Indeed, as discussed previously (see Rates of Infection), rates of blood stream infections adjusted for device exposure are higher in children and newborns.[305] Utilization of mechanical ventilation also is an inadequate explanation for the relative infrequency of pneumonia (see Rates of Infection). Other factors playing a role in these differences are discussed in greater detail in other portions of this chapter (see Nosocomial Infections Related to Invasive Devices, Procedures, and Treatments and Nosocomial Infections in Special Populations).

Infections at sites other than the four major sites listed in Table 228–5 account for a substantial proportion of infections in children and newborns. Upper respiratory tract infections, gastrointestinal infections, and skin and soft tissue infections particularly are common.[127, 449] These infections are discussed in detail in other portions of this chapter (see Nosocomial Infections Due to Spread of Infections Common in the Community).

Nosocomial Pathogens

Table 228–6 contains data regarding the distribution of pathogens for major sites of nosocomial infections in NNIS hospitals.[117] *S. aureus*, coagulase-negative staphylococci, *Enterococcus* species, and a variety of gram-negative bacilli are responsible for the vast majority of nosocomial infections in hospitalized patients. Pathogens responsible for specific nosocomial infections in pediatric patients are discussed in more detail in other portions of this chapter (see Nosocomial Infections Due to Spread of Infections Common in the Community; Nosocomial Infections Related to Invasive Devices,

TABLE 228–6. Pathogen Distribution for Major Sites of Nosocomial Infection in National Nosocomial Infections Surveillance System Hospitals*

	Percentage of All Isolates					
Pathogen	*All Sites (N = 70,411)*	*Blood Stream Infection (N = 9444)*	*Pneumonia (N = 8891)*	*Urinary Tract Infection (N = 25,371)*	*Surgical Site Infection (N = 11,724)*	*Other Infection (N = 14,981)*
Gram-positive bacteria						
Staphylococcus aureus	12	16	20	2	19	17
Coagulase-negative *Staphylococcus*	11	31	2	4	14	14
Enterococcus species	10	9	2	16	12	5
Group B streptococci	1	2	1	1	1	1
Group D streptococci	1	1	0	2	2	1
Other *Streptococcus* species	2	4	1	1	3	2
Other gram-positive aerobes	1	1	0	0	2	1
Gram-positive anerobes	4	1	0	0	1	19
Gram-negative bacteria						
Escherichia coli	12	5	4	25	8	4
Pseudomonas aeruginosa	9	3	16	11	8	6
Enterobacter species	6	4	11	5	7	4
Klebsiella pneumoniae	5	4	7	7	3	3
Other *Klebsiella* species	1	1	2	1	1	1
Proteus mirabilis	3	1	2	5	3	2
Acinetobacter species	1	2	4	1	1	1
Serratia marcescens	1	1	3	1	1	1
Citrobacter species	1	1	1	2	1	1
Other Enterobacteriaceae aerobes	1	0	1	1	1	1
Other non-Enterobacteriaceae aerobes	1	1	4	0	1	2
Bacillus fragilis	1	1	0	0	2	0
Haemophilus influenzae	1	0	5	0	0	2
Fungi						
Candida albicans	5	5	5	8	3	5
Other *Candida* species	2	3	1	2	1	1
Other fungi	2	1	1	3	0	1
Viruses	1	0	1	0	0	2

Data are from 1990 to 1992.
*Pathogens that constituted <1% of isolates from all sites are not listed.
Modified from Emori, T. G., and Gaynes, R. P.: An overview of nosocomial infections, including the role of the microbiology laboratory. Clin. Microbiol. Rev. *6*:428–442, 1993.

Procedures, and Treatments; and Nosocomial Infections in Special Populations).

Several general trends in the microbial etiology of nosocomial infections that are relevant for pediatric patients as well as adult patients should be emphasized. Infections due to coagulase-negative staphylococci have increased dramatically in the past decade and a half, almost entirely as a result of an increase in the frequency of blood stream infections caused by these microorganisms.[381] This trend particularly is impressive in newborns,[305] which is explained at least in part by the increased survival of very low birth weight infants with long hospital stays and their dependence on intravascular catheters and parenteral nutrition. Several studies using molecular epidemiologic techniques indicate that specific strains of coagulase-negative staphylococci may become endemic in newborn ICUs and may be transmitted via the hands of caregivers.[197, 260, 318] The frequency of *Candida* species, especially *Candida albicans*, has increased for all major sites of infection[381]; infections caused by these fungi have had a great effect on immunocompromised children and premature infants.[36, 102, 203] The frequency of infections caused by *S. aureus*, *Enterococcus* species, *P. aeruginosa*, and *Enterobacter* species has increased slightly.[381]

More alarming is the dramatic increase in antimicrobial resistance. Following general trends in NNIS hospitals,[314] the incidence of methicillin-resistant *S. aureus* increased progressively in children's hospitals in the 1980s.[205] Outbreaks of methicillin-resistant *S. aureus* in children and newborns have been reported,[311, 348, 352, 357] and methicillin-resistant *S. aureus* has become endemic in some institutions.[351, 362] Only a few institutions have had substantial success in controlling or eradicating this microorganism.[111, 170, 348, 396, 415] Resistance to non–β-lactam agents, such as quinolones, erythromycin, clindamycin, trimethoprim-sulfamethoxazole, and rifampin, also is increasing among *S. aureus* isolates.[299] Vancomycin resistance has not been documented in clinical isolates of *S. aureus* yet, although low-level resistance to teicoplanin has been reported from France.[465]

Methicillin resistance among coagulase-negative staphylococci has exceeded that in *S. aureus* and is found in more than 60 per cent of hospital isolates (>80 per cent in the authors' institution).[381] Resistance to glycopeptides, particularly resistance to teicoplanin, has been reported in various species of coagulase-negative staphylococci from a variety of countries, including the United States.[465]

Resistance among enterococci has become a particularly alarming problem, especially given the increasing frequency of nosocomial infections caused by these organisms. Enterococci intrinsically are resistant to many antimicrobial agents, including all cephalosporins, clindamycin, and trimethoprim-sulfamethoxazole.[353] However, acquired resistance has made many enterococcal infections essentially impossible to treat effectively with commercially available compounds.[353] Enterococci, especially *Enterococcus faecium*, always have been relatively resistant to penicillin, but high-level resistance due to mutations in penicillin-binding proteins now is relatively common.[353] High-level resistance to aminoglycosides emerged in the 1970s and became widespread in the 1980s.[353] Enterococci resistant to both streptomycin and gentamicin are resistant to the synergistic activity of all known antimicrobial combinations.[353] Penicillin resistance due to β-lactamase production in conjunction with high-level gentamicin resistance also has been reported.[350, 450] As alarming as these trends were, the explosion in the number of enterococcal isolates with resistance to vancomycin in the early 1990s was astounding.[68, 465] From 1989 to 1993, the percentage of enterococcal isolates resistant to vancomycin reported to the NNIS system rose from 0.3 per cent to more than 7 per cent.[68] Vancomycin-resistant enterococci have caused infections in pediatric patients, although most isolates have been obtained from colonized children.[41, 42, 255, 367]

The serious problem of antimicrobial resistance among gram-negative bacilli has been recognized for decades. Aminoglycoside resistance has been widespread for years.[420] The introduction and use of third-generation cephalosporins were followed by the emergence and dissemination of gram-negative rods with inducible and constitutive expression of chromosomally encoded cephalosporinases.[420] In the late 1980s and early 1990s, plasmid-borne, extended-spectrum β-lactamases capable of inactivating third-generation cephalosporins were identified in gram-negative rods around the world, including *Klebsiella* species, *Enterobacter* species, *E. coli*, *Citrobacter* species, *Morganella morganii*, and *P. aeruginosa*.[200] These pathogens, which generally carry genes for resistance to aminoglycosides and other front-line antibiotics on their plasmids, have caused a number of outbreaks,[49, 290, 306, 315, 354] one involving pediatric oncology patients,[306] and have become widespread in the United States.[57, 213, 371] Resistance to imipenem and fluoroquinolones also is a growing problem,[88, 147] and other gram-negative bacilli, such as *Acinetobacter* species and *Stenotrophomonas (Xanthomonas) maltophilia*,[235, 258, 380, 429, 439] have intrinsic and acquired resistance to numerous agents.

Interactions Between Hosts and Pathogens

Generally, newborns begin life devoid of microbial flora but quickly become colonized with a broad array of microorganisms. The vast majority of these microorganisms do not produce disease unless their human host's natural defenses against infection are compromised. In contrast, exposure to microbial pathogens may lead to infection, unless the host has specific immunity to these microorganisms. In hospitalized children, weakened host defenses, coupled with the aggressive medical care required to sustain critically ill children, tend to be more important factors than the pathogenic potential of the specific microorganisms that happen to be circulating in the institution at any given moment.

Neonates are at particular risk for infection due to the relative immaturity of their immune systems, especially if they are born prematurely. A full review of the deficits in newborn immune function is beyond the scope of this chapter, but a few of the most important problems deserve emphasis.[247] Infants born before approximately 28 weeks of gestation do not have the benefit of transplacentally acquired maternal antibody, and even more mature newborns lack specific antibodies to many of the pathogens they can expect to encounter early in life. The alternative pathway of complement activation is designed to protect the host in the absence of specific antibody but may not function adequately against newborn pathogens. Neonates have limited neutrophil reserves, which may be exhausted quickly in the face of aggressive pathogens. In addition, neutrophil migration is decreased and phagocytosis is less effective. Not surprisingly, opsonophagocytosis is compromised by the combination of inadequate specific antibody; suboptimal complement activation; and qualitative defects in neutrophil recruitment, migration, and function. Immature cellular immunity also compromises the response of neonates to viral and other intracellular pathogens. Moreover, the neonate's lack of an established normal bacterial flora provides no natural "colonization resistance" against pathogens entering the upper respiratory or alimentary tracts, and the fragile skin of premature infants is less resistant to trauma and the resulting microbial invasion.

Even after their immune system has matured and they are

capable of mounting their own vigorous immune response to infection, infants and young children remain susceptible to communicable diseases that may be spread in hospitals, such as varicella, measles, and parvovirus infection, if they lack specific immunity. Some pathogens, such as RSV, provoke such a limited immune response that infants become susceptible again a short time after infection. Others, such as influenza virus, change their antigenic presentation so rapidly that immunity acquired in one year is of limited value in the next.

Underlying diseases, especially those that compromise the immune system, predispose the host to infections caused by a wide array of microorganisms that ordinarily do not cause disease in normal hosts. For instance, granulocytopenic children particularly are susceptible to filamentous fungal infections, such as invasive pulmonary aspergillosis, that rarely affect other children.[441] Immunocompromised children also may suffer more severe consequences from infections that would be relatively trivial in normal hosts. For example, RSV and adenovirus may cause prolonged lower respiratory tract infection or even fatal pneumonia in transplant patients; rotavirus and cryptosporidia may cause chronic diarrhea in children with AIDS. Pathogens that remain well localized in normal hosts may disseminate widely in compromised children (e.g., disseminated candidiasis in granulocytopenic children).

Medical treatment also has an important impact on the risk of infection. Common features of modern medical care include the use of intravascular catheters and infusions, indwelling urinary catheters, and mechanical ventilation. Many pediatric patients require much more sophisticated care, including invasive hemodynamic monitoring, extracorporeal membrane oxygenation, intensive chemotherapy, bone marrow and solid organ transplantation, hemodialysis, plasmapheresis, or intracranial pressure monitoring. Aggressive surgical procedures, such as reconstructive surgery and sophisticated cardiovascular surgery, not only are performed more frequently but are performed on children at a very young age. Antibiotics that are used liberally in critically ill children predispose to colonization and infection with antimicrobial-resistant bacteria or fungi.

Although there is considerable knowledge about the host factors that influence the risk of nosocomial infection, substantially less is known about the properties of specific microorganisms that render them more or less pathogenic in hospitalized patients. For the most part, it remains a mystery why some microorganisms do not disseminate widely in a hospital while others do and why some microorganisms colonize many patients but produce few infections while others cause devastating epidemics of disease. Why, for example, did the *S. aureus* phage type 80/81 cause a worldwide pandemic of staphylococcal disease, especially in nurseries, while other phage types had a much more limited range, appeared to disseminate less readily in hospital wards, and produced serious infections less frequently?[376]

Contemporary laboratory techniques gradually are unraveling the pathogenic properties of specific microorganisms. For example, coagulase-negative staphylococci produce a capsular polysaccharide that facilitates adherence to prosthetic materials and "slime" that protects them from clearance by host defense mechanisms.[225] *Citrobacter diversus* elaborates a surface protein that contributes to its propensity to produce destructive meningitis and cerebral abscesses.[223, 224] *E. coli* with the K1 capsular serotype are more likely to invade the meninges[201]; group A streptococci that produce an exuberant hyaluronic acid capsule are more likely to evade opsonophagocytosis[454]; and *E. coli* that produce P pili, are hemolytic, and have specific capsular serotypes and colicin types are more likely to produce urinary tract infections.[209] Nonetheless, we are a long way from understanding the factors that govern the ecology and pathogenic potential of most nosocomial microorganisms.

Modes of Transmission of Nosocomial Infections

Modes of transmission are the general mechanisms involved in the transfer of microorganisms from the reservoirs where they live and replicate to susceptible hosts. Table 228–7 lists the important modes of transmission. Examples of specific nosocomial infections are listed, including the relevant reservoirs, sources, and modes of transmission of microorganisms causing these infections. Because reservoirs often cannot be eliminated, strategies must be designed to interrupt modes of transmission. These strategies are discussed in detail in Chapter 229.

There are three basic types of airborne transmission: dissemination of droplet nuclei, "shedding" of skin squames (or "rafts") by colonized or infected individuals, and aerosolization of fungal spores. Droplet nuclei are small particles (<5 μm) generated by the desiccation of larger droplets expelled by coughing, sneezing, or speaking such letters as "T" or "P" forcefully. Because they are extremely light, droplet nuclei can travel over long distances on air currents. If ventilation is poor and the microorganisms in the droplet nuclei are hardy, these infectious particles may remain suspended in the air of enclosed spaces for relatively long periods in concentrations sufficient to cause infection, even if the index patient no longer is present. Because they are so small, droplet nuclei can remain suspended in inhaled air, evading the mechanical host defenses of the upper respiratory tract, and reach the lungs. Classic diseases spread by respiratory droplet nuclei include measles, tuberculosis, and, under certain circumstances, influenza and varicella.[158] Legionnaires' disease may be spread by small aerosolized droplets generated by such devices as cooling towers, shower heads, and even bed pan cleaners.[422]

Certain persons are heavy "shedders" of skin squames contaminated by staphylococci or, more rarely, group A streptococci and other skin microorganisms (e.g., *Rhodococcus)*.[376] Shedders may have obvious dermatitis or a clinical infection but often are asymptomatic. Shedders have been implicated in outbreaks of infection, especially in operating rooms, but the vast majority of personnel who are colonized with potential pathogens do not dispense large numbers of bacteria and do not pose a threat to patients.[376]

Spores of filamentous fungi, such as *Aspergillus* and *Zygomycetes,* are ubiquitous in the environment, especially where there is decaying organic matter and moisture. Their small size (<3 μm) and aerodynamic shape permit dispersion over long distances and facilitate penetration of hospital air handling systems and the respiratory tract of susceptible persons.[158]

Aerosolization of other organisms, such as *Coxiella burnetii*, can occur in hospitals under special circumstances. For example, Q fever broke out among personnel when sheep were transported through the corridor of a university hospital for a research study.[287]

Contact transmission is the principal mode of transmission for most nosocomial infections.[158] Direct contact transmission involves physical contact between a person harboring the microorganism, such as a caregiver with a staphylococcal infection on his or her hand, and the host. Indirect contact transmission involves transfer of microorganisms via an intermediary person or object. The hands of caregivers are the

TABLE 228–7. Modes of Transmission with Examples of Specific Nosocomial Infections and the Reservoirs and Sources Involved in the Transmission of These Infections

Mode of Transmission	Nosocomial Infection	Reservoir	Source
Airborne	Measles, varicella,* pulmonary tuberculosis	Infected persons	Airborne droplet nuclei
Contact			
Direct	Neonatal staphylococcal skin infection	Infected/colonized caregiver	Drainage from infected wound on the hand of a caregiver
Indirect	Respiratory syncytial virus infection	Infected persons	Hands of caregivers, fomites
	Infection with antimicrobial-resistant bacteria	Infected/colonized persons	Hands of caregivers, fomites
Droplet	Pertussis, invasive meningococcal disease, group A streptococcal infection	Infected/colonized persons	Large respiratory droplets
Endogenous (autoinfection)†	Coagulase-negative staphylococcal bacteremia associated with a central venous line	Skin at the site of the catheter insertion	Intravascular catheter
	Escherichia coli urinary tract infection associated with an indwelling urinary catheter	Periurethral skin and mucous membranes	Indwelling urinary catheter
Common vehicle	Gram-negative bacteremia associated with intravenous infusion	Liquid substances in the environment	Intrinsically or extrinsically contaminated intravenous fluids
	Posttransfusion infection with blood-borne pathogen (HIV, hepatitis B virus, hepatitis C virus, cytomegalovirus)	Infected persons	Blood products from infected donors
	Salmonellosis	Infected/colonized persons	Contaminated food
Vector	Enteric infection	Infected persons or infectious material	Flies, Pharaoh's ants

*Varicella-zoster virus may be transmitted by airborne, direct contact, and droplet contact transmission.
†See text.

most common source for indirect contact transmission, but fomites also are important for certain pathogens (e.g., gram-positive cocci, *Clostridium difficile,* and RSV).[158] Droplet contact transmission involves transfer of microorganisms by large respiratory droplets, such as those generated by coughing or sneezing, that typically travel no further than 3 feet before settling. Important nosocomial pathogens spread by this route include *Bordetella pertussis, Neisseria meningitidis,* and group A streptococci.[158]

Endogenous infection (or autoinfection) is caused by a patient's own flora.[158] These generally harmless commensals cause disease when the patient's host defenses are compromised by severe underlying disease, immunosuppressive therapy, or invasive devices and procedures. Microorganisms that produce endogenous infections are not always part of a patient's normal flora that he or she brought into the hospital from the community. Commonly, these microorganisms are transferred from other patients via the hands of caregivers and become part of a patient's colonizing endogenous flora.[158] Consequently, these infections can be considered as a special case of contact transmission.

Common vehicle (common source) transmission involves the widespread dissemination of a microorganism to many persons via a contaminated item or substance. Many outbreaks of infection in hospitals have been caused by nonenteric, gram-negative bacilli, such as *Burkholderia cepacia* or *P. aeruginosa,* that thrive in medications, solutions, or wet equipment and relatively are resistant to antimicrobial preservatives, antiseptics, and disinfectants.[158] Vector transmission of microorganisms, either on (extrinsic) or within (intrinsic) insects, is rare in hospitals. Extrinsic vector transmission of enteric pathogens may occur when these microorganisms are transported on the legs of flies, roaches, or ants.[31, 77, 128] Intrinsic vector transmission, such as transmission of malaria or dengue, involves more than physical transfer because a portion of the life cycle of the microorganism is completed in the vector. Although intrinsic vector transmission in the hospital is possible theoretically, to the authors' knowledge there are no reported cases.

Some infections may be spread by more than one mode of transmission. For example, varicella-zoster virus may be spread by airborne and direct contact transmission.

Consequences and Costs of Nosocomial Infections

Valid, well-controlled studies of the consequences and costs of nosocomial infections in pediatric patients are limited. This is due in part to difficulty in determining whether the consequences or costs are attributable directly to the nosocomial infection. In order to attribute a consequence to nosocomial infection, there must be careful matching of infected and noninfected patients by such criteria as age, sex, presence of underlying conditions, severity of illness, operative procedures, and length of stay, or appropriate statistical analyses to control for potential confounding factors must be performed.

Pediatric studies that have made an effort rigorously to measure attributable risk suggest that nosocomial infections have a substantial adverse effect on hospitalized children. For example, Valenti and colleagues[432] matched infected and noninfected patients by age, sex, underlying illness, and time of year of admission and found that nosocomial infections increased the length of stay by an average of 9 days. Patients infected with RSV and influenza virus had average increases in length of stay of 6 and 5 days, respectively.[432] Appropriately designed cohort studies of coagulase-negative staphylococcal bacteremia in newborn ICUs (including adjustment for birth weight and severity of illness) have found increased length of stay (approximately 14 days), increased antibiotic use, and increased hospital charges (about $25,000) but no increased mortality from this infection.[129, 162]

Controlled studies performed in hospitalized adult patient populations also indicate that the consequences and cost of nosocomial infections are substantial. For instance, nosocomial blood stream infections in adult surgical ICU patients were estimated to have an attributable mortality rate of 35 per cent, to prolong length of stay in the ICU by 8 days, to prolong the overall hospital stay by 24 days, and to cost $40,000 per survivor.[325] Studies of blood stream infections due to specific pathogens, such as *Candida* and *Enterococcus*,[238, 455] have revealed comparably significant adverse outcomes. A study of pneumonia in mechanically ventilated patients estimated that the attributable mortality rate of this infection was 27 per cent and that it prolonged the ICU stay by 13 days.[119] A study of surgical-site infection was estimated to increase the length of hospital stay by an average of 8 days and resulted in average extra hospital costs of more than £1000.[83]

Acknowledging the methodologic difficulties inherent in determining the consequences of nosocomial infections, published estimates of the general burden of nosocomial infections in U.S. hospitals help to illustrate the magnitude of the problem.[276] Nosocomial infections are estimated to prolong hospital stay an average of 4 days and result in average extra hospital costs of $2100 per infection.[276] These infections are estimated to cause 19,000 deaths directly and to contribute to another 58,000 deaths each year.[276] Counting only the 19,000 direct causes of death, nosocomial infections rank just below the tenth leading cause of death in the United States.[276]

NOSOCOMIAL INFECTIONS DUE TO SPREAD OF INFECTIONS COMMON IN THE COMMUNITY

Nosocomial infections that result from the in-hospital transmission of infections common in the community are a major concern for all facilities providing health care to children. Several principles regarding the general epidemiology of these infections, modified from those initially published by Hall[171] in relation to the epidemiology of nosocomial respiratory viruses, can be summarized as follows. First, their appearance and spread in the wards parallel closely the disease activity in the community. Second, significant exposure to these pathogens generally results in infection in any host that lacks specific immunity; consequently, a susceptible child is at risk, regardless of the nature or severity of his or her underlying disease or specific medical treatment. Third, these infections often are more severe in hospitalized patients who have underlying diseases (e.g., pulmonary or cardiac disease) or who are immunocompromised. Fourth, children hospitalized as a result of the community-acquired infections are the most important reservoir for microorganisms causing these infections, but mildly symptomatic or asymptomatically colonized children and adult caregivers also may be important reservoirs in some cases (e.g., RSV infection, pertussis). Fifth, prevention depends primarily on the timely implementation of and compliance with isolation precautions specifically designed to interrupt transmission of the microorganisms involved. In some infections, other interventions also are indicated, such as antimicrobial therapy to reduce the risk of transmission from children with pertussis and passive immunization with varicella-zoster immunoglobulin to protect high-risk persons exposed to varicella. Finally, unless postdischarge surveillance is performed, reports of the frequency of these infections are likely to be gross underestimations, especially given recent trends toward shorter lengths of hospital stay, because many of these infections may be in the incubation period at the time of discharge and manifest themselves only after the child returns home.

Respiratory Infections

Respiratory Syncytial Viruses

RSV by far is the most common nosocomial respiratory virus infection, especially among children in the first 2 years of life.[127, 161, 171, 432, 449] Community outbreaks occur every year in the fall or winter, although their precise timing, intensity, and duration may vary.[161] As illustrated by a study in Rochester, New York, RSV infection may account for a substantial number of hospital admissions in children younger than 2 years of age during epidemic periods, resulting in high rates of nosocomial transmission of RSV not only to other patients but also to caregivers.[176] Attack rates tend to be high because immunity after infection is short-lived and because inoculation of virus into the nose or eyes reliably leads to infection.[173] Moreover, RSV survives for relatively long periods in the environment, and infected children excrete high titers of virus in their copious secretions, ensuring substantial environmental contamination.[175] Not surprisingly, duration of hospitalization (and thus the duration of potential exposure) correlates strongly with the risk of infection because there is a greater opportunity for direct or indirect contact transmission to occur.[176] Outbreaks in newborn ICUs have been reported, some in association with other viruses.[177, 288, 404, 431, 461] Low birth weight and mechanical ventilation were important risk factors for infection and mortality in these outbreaks.[177, 431] Nosocomial RSV infections in patients who have underlying cardiac or pulmonary disease or are immunocompromised can result in severe, protracted disease.[161, 178, 261, 326]

Scrupulous attention to hand washing and the use of barriers (gloves and gowns) when touching patients or their immediate inanimate environment can reduce markedly the transmission of RSV.[240] Goggles, masks, or both may be effective in reducing the RSV attack rate in personnel,[3, 138] which in turn can reduce transmission of virus in patients, but these control measures have not achieved wide popularity, perhaps because of cost and inconvenience. Covering only the nose and mouth with a mask probably is not effective.[174] Some investigators have demonstrated that cohorting infected patients, combined with the use of barriers, can reduce the spread of RSV.[228, 264] However, it is not clear whether cohorting by clinical symptoms alone is effective or whether all admitted patients must be screened for RSV infection to identify children with minimal symptoms who may be excreting the virus. Moreover, the added value of strict cohorting, which may be expensive or difficult to implement, as opposed to the rigorous use of barrier technique, has not been demonstrated.

Treatment of RSV infection with ribavirin reduces shedding of RSV, which may decrease the potential for nosocomial transmission.[161] RSV immunoglobulin has shown promise in preventing or reducing the severity of RSV infection in high-risk patients and may have an effect on reducing the potential of nosocomial transmission as well.[188] Development of vaccines against RSV is under way and may lead to more effective prevention strategies in the future.[246]

Nosocomial infections due to parainfluenza virus are similar to those due to RSV in their epidemiology and prevention, although they tend to be more common in the spring and fall than in the winter.[161]

Nosocomial influenza is a common cause of intercurrent fever in hospitalized children during epidemic periods.[172] Explosive outbreaks among patients and hospital staffs have occurred.[161] Although the modes of transmission of influenza have not been defined completely, direct, indirect, and droplet contact are likely to be most important in the hospitals. Rapid spread of infection in some confined populations suggests that airborne transmission also can occur.[161, 301] In addition to the precautions described for RSV, masks should be worn during close contact. The need for isolation rooms with negative air pressure relative to hallways has not been established; however, a recently published guideline encourages use of these rooms.[422] If this is not feasible, placement of a patient in a private room without special air handling and cohorting of patients with proven influenza are alternatives.[422]

Annual influenza vaccination of high-risk persons and hospital staff members limits the potential for large outbreaks of influenza if the vaccination both is offered at the appropriate time and is accepted by patients and staff.[422] Rimantadine can be used for prophylaxis of high-risk patients in confined populations during outbreaks of influenza A.[422]

Nosocomial adenovirus infections occur sporadically throughout the year; however, outbreaks of respiratory infection and pharyngoconjunctival fever are well described.[125, 302, 323, 332, 399, 417, 453] Outbreaks in ICUs have been associated with severe disease and substantial mortality.[399, 453] Children undergoing liver transplantation also are at high risk for severe disease and death in the immediate posttransplantation period.[292] In addition to direct and indirect contact, adenovirus may be spread by droplet contact, necessitating the use of masks during close contact.

Nosocomial rhinovirus infections generally are mild, and outbreaks of infection have not been associated with substantial morbidity.[161] The mode of transmission of rhinovirus infection still is controversial. Some studies suggest direct and indirect contact transmission as the primary mode of transmission; others suggest droplet contact may be more important.[189] Hand washing is sufficient as a control measure.

Pertussis

Outbreaks of pertussis in hospitals and chronic care institutions are well documented.[126, 230, 253, 393, 411, 424, 433] The role of adults in spreading pertussis to hospitalized children emphasized in several of these reports is consistent with the greater general appreciation of adults in the transmission of *B. pertussis* to children.[79, 230, 253, 433]

Prevention of nosocomial pertussis has focused on the appropriate isolation of children in whom the infection is suspected, use of masks to prevent droplet contact transmission, antimicrobial treatment of confirmed cases to minimize the potential for transmission, and prophylactic treatment of exposed persons. Evaluation and treatment of hospital staff members presenting with symptoms suggesting pertussis (upper respiratory tract infection with severe, prolonged cough) have been important components of the control of nosocomial pertussis.

The aggressive steps taken to control nosocomial spread of pertussis during a community-wide epidemic of pertussis in Cincinnati in 1993 are noteworthy because they demonstrate the beneficial impact but relatively high cost of an aggressive approach.[80] During this epidemic, 102 patients were hospitalized with pertussis and pertussis was diagnosed in 87 hospital staff members on clinical or microbiologic grounds. Fifteen strict control measures were implemented to prevent transmission within the hospital, including prompt investigation of all suspected cases among patients and staff, appropriate isolation of proven and suspected cases among patients, furloughs for all staff members with suspected pertussis until they had completed 5 days of antimicrobial therapy, and antimicrobial therapy for all close contacts of confirmed cases. There was only one case of nosocomial pertussis—an infant who was infected by a symptomatic nurse later confirmed to be culture-positive. Among 274 culture-confirmed cases in the community, only 2 were linked epidemiologically to hospital staff members with pertussis. These measures cost more than $85,000.

With the development of acellular pertussis vaccines, boosting immunity among the hospital staff may be a cost-effective intervention in the future. Acellular vaccine was used as an adjunctive control measure in a recent hospital outbreak of pertussis.[393] The vaccine was tolerated reasonably well, but no efficacy data were reported.

Gastrointestinal Infections

Gastrointestinal Viruses

Rotavirus is the most common cause of endemic and epidemic nosocomial gastrointestinal virus infection among hospitalized children and newborns.[78, 127, 161, 236, 341, 360, 432, 442, 449] Risk of infection is associated closely with the length of hospitalization.[85, 103] Infection usually is self-limited, although prolonged diarrhea may occur in immunocompromised patients.[161] One study associated an outbreak of necrotizing enterocolitis in a newborn nursery with concurrent rotavirus infection,[363] although the etiology of necrotizing enterocolitis remains controversial.

Patients infected with rotavirus in the hospital or community may shed the virus in their stool for many days after symptomatic infection.[458] Asymptomatically infected patients also may shed virus.[85, 458] Together, these patients constitute a substantial reservoir of virus that may be transmitted easily to other patients. In addition, rotavirus can be transferred via hands and can survive for extended periods on environmental surfaces.[18, 378] Clearly, the primary mode of transmission is indirect contact via the contaminated hands of caregivers, and the scrupulous use of barriers (gowns and gloves), hand washing, and appropriate disinfection of environmental surfaces is critical. An experimental study suggests that rotavirus infection also can be spread by the respiratory route,[335] further complicating control efforts.

A variety of other gastrointestinal viruses also have been documented to cause endemic and epidemic nosocomial infections, including enteric adenoviruses,[226] Norwalk-like viruses,[408] calicivirus,[409] and astrovirus.[231]

Clostridium difficile

Although toxin-producing *C. difficile* is a well-recognized cause of antimicrobial-associated diarrhea in adults, studies of the role of this organism as a cause of nosocomial diarrhea in hospitalized children and infants have been limited.

Toxin-producing *C. difficile* frequently can be found in the stools of neonates and young infants.[322] Because *C. difficile* seldom is found in the stool of healthy women and because clusters of colonized infants often can be detected in nurseries,[322] it can be presumed that nosocomial, as opposed to vertical, transmission plays a role in the acquisition of this microorganism by neonates. However, it appears that *C. difficile* rarely produces disease in newborns or infants in the first few months of life.[322]

Symptomatic *C. difficile* infection clearly occurs in older children, almost always in association with antimicrobial therapy. Two outbreaks in pediatric oncology units have been reported.[54, 63] Investigation of the molecular epidemiology of one of these outbreaks using polymerase chain reaction ribotyping revealed that a small number of strains were responsible for the majority of the cases.[63] Given that *C. difficile* is a significant cause of nosocomial diarrhea in adults,[281] it is reasonable to assume that it is common among hospitalized children as well. In fact, an ongoing epidemiologic investigation of nosocomial diarrhea caused by *C. difficile* in Children's Hospital has revealed that it is both common and increasing in frequency (unpublished observations).

C. difficile can be found on the hands of personnel and in the patient's immediate environment,[281] where *C. difficile* spores can survive for prolonged periods and are relatively resistant to disinfectants. Therefore, direct or indirect contact is responsible for the spread of this microorganism from patient to patient. Barriers (gowns and gloves) and hand washing may reduce transmission. Vigorous environmental cleaning probably is important and certainly is prudent, although the use of specific disinfecting agents in preventing transmission has not been well defined. However, because asymptomatic carriage of this microorganism is more common than symptomatic disease and excretion often continues for long periods,[281] the impact of these interventions may be limited somewhat, unless all patients are screened and precautions are used for colonized patients—an expensive and usually impractical approach. The use of oral metronidazole in asymptomatic patients is not effective in eliminating carriage; oral vancomycin may reduce carriage temporarily, but recrudescence of carriage and reinfection are common.[210]

Other Bacteria

Bacterial pathogens are rare causes of endemic nosocomial diarrhea in United States hospitals.[112] Consequently, in the absence of an outbreak, the yield of routine stool cultures in the evaluation of nosocomial diarrhea is extremely low. One study examining the utility of various diagnostic studies for the evaluation of nosocomial diarrhea in a pediatric hospital found that stool cultures were the most commonly ordered test, yet no bacterial pathogens were identified in any of 195 stool cultures ordered.[51]

Outbreaks of nosocomial salmonellosis have been documented throughout the world, although they are reported more commonly from developing countries.[166, 179, 217, 267, 300, 317, 373, 400, 414, 467] Neonates particularly are susceptible to infection by *Salmonella* species, and invasive disease, such as bacteremia, meningitis, and osteomyelitis, is common.[166, 179, 217, 267, 400, 414, 467] Transmission occurs through a variety of means, including contaminated food, direct contact between patients, and indirect contact transmission via contaminated hands or instruments.

Outbreaks of nosocomial shigellosis are much less common. Only one hospital outbreak has been reported in the United States,[34] although shigellosis can be a major problem in institutions caring for disabled children.[26, 113] A study in a hospital in Kenya cultured *Shigella* species from the stools of 2.5 per cent of patients with nosocomial diarrhea.[317] *Shigella* is transmitted easily by direct or indirect contact, and only a small inoculum is required to establish infection.[112]

Nosocomial cholera has been documented in developing countries.[291, 370] One of these reports is notable because it provides evidence that nosocomial acquisition of *Vibrio cholerae* by children who were discharged to home before becoming symptomatic was instrumental in initiating and sustaining an outbreak of cholera in the surrounding community.[291] The mechanism involved in nosocomial transmission of cholera in these studies is not clear, but direct or indirect contact transmission, as opposed to transmission via contaminated water, was suspected.

Other bacterial pathogens have caused outbreaks of diarrhea, including *Campylobacter* species,[60, 190, 214, 435] *Yersinia* species,[62, 346] and various types of *E. coli*.[150, 390]

Protozoa

Nosocomial infections due to protozoa appear to be rare. An outbreak of cryptosporidiosis was reported from a pediatric hospital in Mexico.[307] The index case was a patient with AIDS who had chronic diarrhea due to infection with *Cryptosporidium.* Although giardiasis is a common cause of diarrhea in institutionalized children,[425] infections in hospitalized children or neonates have not been reported. Given the large number of severely immunocompromised children in United States hospitals and the relative ease of transmitting protozoa by direct or indirect transmission in families and day care centers, it is somewhat surprising that nosocomial gastroenteritis due to *Giardia, Cryptosporidium, Microsporidium,* and other intestinal protozoa has not been reported more frequently.

Varicella-Zoster Virus

Outbreaks of nosocomial varicella in hospitals have been documented in numerous reports.[135, 167, 242, 383] These reports demonstrate conclusively that varicella can be transmitted by the airborne route, although spread via direct and droplet contact may be more efficient. In these outbreaks, secondary infections occurred in patients who had no face-to-face contact with the index patients and who were separated from the index patient by considerable physical distances (in some cases more than 30 meters).[167, 242] Air flow studies indicated that air in the rooms of index patients flowed into the hallway and into other rooms of susceptible and subsequently infected patients.[167, 242] In one report, air flowed through an open window in the index patient's room, traveled along the exterior of the building, and entered other patient rooms via through-the-wall ventilation units.[242] The majority of secondary infections in each of these outbreaks occurred in patients who had been discharged and were detected only by telephone contact or home visit.[167, 242] Several susceptible hospital staff members also were infected.

These clinical observations of airborne spread of varicella-zoster virus are supported by a study that used polymerase chain reaction to detect airborne virus in hospital rooms of patients with active varicella-zoster virus infection.[379] Varicella-zoster virus was detected in air samples collected 1.2 to 5.5 meters from patients' beds for 1 to 6 days after the onset of rash. Varicella-zoster virus DNA also could be detected in some air samples obtained in the hallway just outside the patient's negative pressure isolation rooms.

Nosocomial transmission of varicella can be minimized if infected patients are cared for in single rooms with separate exhaust systems and negative air pressure relative to the hallway.[12] Because infected persons are infectious for 24 to 48 hours before distinctive symptoms and signs appear, prompt recognition and isolation of patients and visitors who may be in the contagious phase of varicella also are critical. A simple series of screening questions can help identify these persons (see Chapter 229). Barriers to prevent direct and indirect contact transmission (gloves and gowns) can reduce the nosocomial spread of this infection dramatically. In addition, caregivers who are not immune to varicella either should wear a mask to enter the room of patients with confirmed or probable varicella or should avoid caring for such patients, if possible. Varicella-zoster immunoglobulin can prevent infection or mitigate the consequences of infection in high-risk, exposed, susceptible persons if administered within 96 hours, but preferably within 48 hours, of exposure.[10] Intravenous acyclovir should be administered to these persons to limit the replication of virus if infection develops.[10] Hospitalized exposed children should remain in isolation from day 8 to day 21 after exposure; if varicella-zoster immunoglobulin is administered, isolation should be continued until day 28 after exposure.[10] Management of exposed health care workers is discussed in Chapter 229.

It is hoped that the recent licensure of a varicella-zoster virus vaccine will diminish the risk of nosocomial varicella by reducing the number of children hospitalized as a consequence of this disease and by limiting the pool of susceptible children in hospital wards (see Chapter 229).

Cytomegalovirus

Perhaps no issue is the subject of as much concern and misinformation among health care workers as the risk of nosocomial cytomegalovirus (CMV) infection. Concern among caregivers undoubtedly has been heightened by reports of CMV infection among day care center staff members. Day care centers provide optimal conditions for CMV transmission because many children are excreting CMV in their saliva or urine and there are abundant opportunities for sustained contact with contaminated secretions. However, even in this setting, transmission of CMV to susceptible care providers occurs slowly.[2] This reflects the relative inefficiency of direct or indirect contact transmission of CMV, a virus that is inactivated easily by soaps, detergents, and disinfectants and is not stable on environmental surfaces for long periods.[2]

In hospitals, the risk to staff members appears to be negligible. A meta-analysis of a number of studies that have examined the risk of CMV among pediatric nurses indicates that the rate of CMV infection in this population is comparable to that in control populations (persons of comparable age and sex who are not nurses).[2] A subanalysis of these data suggests that nursery nurses may have a slightly higher rate of infection than do control populations.[2] However, studies of CMV infection in nursery nurses using restriction-enzyme analysis of CMV isolates have shown that the nurses did not acquire CMV from the infants in their care[2] and presumably contracted their infections from children in their own households through sexual contact or from other community sources.

In conclusion, few, if any, data suggest that nosocomial transmission of CMV is a significant risk to health care workers. Given the frequency of asymptomatic CMV excretion in children (for example, approximately 1 per cent of newborns excrete the virus), health care workers should assume that individual children may be excreting virus and should practice hand washing and use standard precautions (see Chapter 229) as a part of routine patient care. Additional interventions are not indicated, and pregnant staff members need not be given special assignments.

Two restriction-enzyme studies have documented probable patient-to-patient spread of CMV in a newborn ICU and a chronic care unit.[101, 407] In both situations, the infected children had been in close proximity and were cared for by common caregivers for extended periods.

Herpes Simplex Virus

Nosocomial transmission of herpes simplex virus type 1 to newborn infants has been confirmed through restriction-enzyme analysis.[180, 251, 374, 434] The mode of transmission is not clear in all of these cases. Direct contact with a hospital worker with herpes labialis was implicated in one case.[434] In the other cases, indirect contact transmission from one infected infant to another is most likely, although direct contact transmission from an asymptomatic parent or caregiver cannot be ruled out.[180, 251, 374] Nosocomial herpes simplex virus infections among health care workers, patients, and family members also have been described in ICUs.[1, 321] Herpetic whitlow is a common manifestation in nurses, presumably as a result of direct transmission during suctioning of oral and respiratory secretions from infected patients.[1] The risk associated with this procedure is substantial, given recent data indicating that herpes simplex virus commonly is found in mucosal and orofacial cultures obtained from intubated patients, including those without obvious lesions.[182] When present, lesions often are atypical in appearance and commonly are found in the distribution of tape used to secure endotracheal tubes.[182] Substantial risk of transmission also is present in immunocompromised patients, in whom reactivation of latent herpes simplex virus infection is common.[443, 464] The use of standard precautions (see Chapter 229), particularly the use of gloves during contact with oral and respiratory secretions and hand washing, prevents transmission of herpes simplex virus.

Surveys of nosocomial infections in pediatric wards indicate that nosocomial herpes simplex virus infections are uncommon.[127, 432, 449] When documented, these infections usually are attributed to reactivation of preexisting endogenous infection rather than primary infection.[432] However, as with ICU patients, subclinical infection in other hospitalized children may be more common than presently is recognized.

Measles, Mumps, and Rubella Viruses

Transmission of measles in health care facilities is uncommon but can serve as a nidus for community-wide infection.[283, 340, 359] Nosocomial infection may be initiated by unrecognized introduction of measles in patients from the immediate community or visitors or immigrants from foreign countries. Conversely, patients who acquire measles in the hospital can serve as a nidus for spread of infection in the community when they return to their homes. Two reported outbreaks particularly are instructive.

During a community outbreak in Los Angeles in 1988, six children with unrecognized measles were hospitalized, resulting in exposure of 107 other hospitalized children and 24 hospital staff members.[359] Nosocomial measles developed in four patients, one of whom died from measles-related pneumonia, and four hospital staff members, two of whom required hospitalization for pneumonia. One of the patients who had been exposed to measles in this hospital subsequently was admitted to another hospital, exposing eight additional patients before isolation precautions were instituted. In an outbreak of measles in two counties in Florida, transmission of measles in the hospital was linked directly to the initiation and propagation of the outbreak in the community.[340] In one of the involved hospitals, inadequate isolation of patients with measles and failure to vaccinate or passively immunize exposed, susceptible persons contributed to transmission.[340]

National statistics indicate that nosocomial measles accounts for a small but increasing proportion of all measles cases (from 0.7 per cent in 1980 to 1982 to 2.9 per cent in 1983 to 1984 to 3.5 per cent in 1985 to 1989).[19, 98] Moreover, measles also may be transmitted in health care facilities, such as emergency rooms and medical clinics, not just in inpatient hospital wards.[98, 121, 199] Investigation of every reported case of measles in Oklahoma in 1981 to 1985 found that 27 per cent of cases were associated with nosocomial transmission in medical offices and clinics and an additional 18 per cent of cases were secondary cases resulting from exposure to nosocomially infected persons.[199] Another survey of measles cases during outbreaks in Los Angeles and Houston found that exposure to emergency rooms was a substantial risk factor for infection.[121]

Measles is transmitted by airborne droplet nuclei, as is demonstrated by a report of an outbreak in a pediatrician's office.[349] Four susceptible children visiting the office on the same day as the index child subsequently developed measles, even though none of these children had face to face contact with the index child or was even in the same room at the same time. Three children visited the office 60 to 75 minutes after the index case had left.

Prevention of nosocomial measles hinges on the prompt recognition of infected or potentially infected patients and placement of these patients in isolation rooms with negative air pressure relative to the hallway.[144] Prophylactic vaccination of exposed susceptible persons within 3 days of the exposure reliably prevents measles, whereas administration of immunoglobulin within 3 days attenuates disease but does not guarantee that the exposed person will not develop contagious infection.[9] To avoid outbreaks of nosocomial measles among health care workers, it is recommended that health care facilities require new employees involved in patient care to provide evidence of immunity or appropriate vaccination or to receive vaccination with either measles vaccine or measles, mumps, and rubella vaccine as a condition of employment (see Chapter 229).[229] Persons born before 1957 generally are considered to be immune to measles because childhood measles was widespread at the time, but occasional cases have developed in this age group during hospital outbreaks.[387]

Outbreaks of nosocomial mumps and rubella have been reported less commonly than nosocomial measles.[191, 328, 416, 456] The primary concern with regard to nosocomial spread of both of these infections relates to potential complications in health care workers. Mumps orchitis in adult males can cause sterility; rubella in pregnant staff members can result in fetal infection and the congenital rubella syndrome. Information regarding the transmission of both of these viruses is limited, but transmission probably occurs primarily via droplet contact. Masks should be worn during close contact with infected patients.[144] Patients with congenital rubella syndrome may excrete large amounts of virus in their urine and respiratory secretions, and excretion of virus in the urine may persist for months or even years. Consequently, gowns and gloves should be worn for contact with these patients for the first year of life, unless nasopharyngeal and urine cultures are negative by 3 months of age.[144] There is no known effective postexposure prophylaxis for exposed persons. As with prevention of nosocomial measles, it is recommended that health care facilities require new employees involved in patient care to provide evidence of immunity or appropriate vaccination or to receive vaccination with measles, mumps, and rubella vaccine as a condition of employment (see Chapter 229).[229]

Parvovirus B19

Parvovirus B19 causes the relatively benign syndrome of erythema infectiosum (occasionally accompanied by arthritis, particularly in older children and adults), acute aplastic crisis in children with hemaglobinopathies, and chronic infection and anemia in immunocompromised children. Recent reports suggest an association with vasculitis and other immunologically mediated diseases.[124, 466] An experimental study of acute parvovirus B19 infection in normal adults detected virus in respiratory secretions in three of four patients during a period of viremia and systemic symptoms 6 to 13 days after inoculation.[16] Detectable virus in respiratory secretions disappeared as viremia and systemic symptoms diminished, and virus was not demonstrable in respiratory secretions when rash, arthralgias, and arthritis developed several days later.[16] Recognition of the wide spectrum of disease caused by parvovirus, coupled with well-documented nosocomial outbreaks of infection, has fueled efforts to understand the transmission and control of this virus in hospitals.[35, 118, 324]

Two outbreaks of nosocomial parvovirus B19 infection occurred among hospital staff members after exposure to adolescents with sickle-cell disease and aplastic crisis.[35] Both outbreaks were recognized when nurses developed symptoms and signs consistent with erythema infectiosum. Of the 40 health care workers who were exposed to the two index cases, 8 (20 per cent) had evidence of past infection and were not susceptible; 12 (38 per cent) of the remaining 32 susceptible health care workers showed evidence of infection by serologic testing, and all but 1 had symptomatic disease. None of the infected persons was pregnant, and no other complications were reported. All but one of the infected persons were nurses, and all but two had contact with an index case in the first several days of hospitalization when titers of virus in the blood stream and respiratory secretions of patients with aplastic crisis would have been highest. A play therapist was infected after infection control measures had been instituted during the second outbreak, apparently as a consequence of spending less than 5 minutes in the isolation room of one of the patients. She did not wear a mask or have any physical contact with the patient. No community outbreak of erythema infectiosum was noted at the time of these outbreaks.

In another outbreak of parvovirus B19 infection in a children's ward, two nurses developed infection on the same day.[324] It is not clear whether they acquired their infection from an undetected case in the hospital or in the community, but they apparently transmitted parvovirus to a number of hospital staff members and patients. In all, infection occurred in 10 of 30 (33 per cent) exposed, susceptible staff members and to 2 of 9 (22 per cent) exposed, susceptible immunocompromised patients. All but one of the infected staff members were symptomatic, but neither of the two infected immunocompromised patients developed symptoms, perhaps because they were given prophylactic immunoglobulin when the outbreak first was recognized.

In another hospital, 10 susceptible health care workers had substantial exposure to an immunocompromised patient with pure red blood cell aplasia and chronic parvovirus B19. None developed infection, even though no isolation precautions were instituted for the first 3½ weeks of hospitalization.[227]

From these studies, it is apparent that parvovirus B19 infection can be transmitted by acutely infected patients, probably as a result of the high levels of virus in their blood and in their respiratory sections. The likelihood of transmission from chronically infected, immunocompromised patients is unknown, but it appears from the just-described report that these patients are not highly infectious. The mode of transmission also is not clear but probably involves direct or indirect contact with respiratory secretions or droplet contact transmission. Therefore, gloves and gowns should be worn during contact with infected patients or fomites contaminated with respiratory secretions, and a mask should be worn during close contact.[144] The discussed play therapist who acquired parvovirus despite her lack of close contact with an infected patient has led to concern about possible airborne transmission, but the need for use of isolation rooms with negative air pressure has not been established and currently is not recommended.[144]

Limited data in one of the outbreaks described earlier suggest that standard immunoglobulin preparations may be useful in mitigating the consequences of infection in high-risk, exposed, susceptible contacts.[324] However, data are insufficient to recommend the routine use of immunoglobulin for postexposure prophylaxis.

Hepatitis A Virus

Although nosocomial outbreaks of hepatitis A are uncommon, this pathogen can cause major epidemics before infection is detected and contained. The largest outbreak of hepatitis A resulted from blood transfusion from a single donor who was viremic but had not developed symptomatic disease yet; 11 newborns received contaminated transfusions, and there were 55 secondary cases in two hospitals.[310] Other transfusion outbreaks have been described,[23, 222] as well as outbreaks traced to asymptomatic excretion by an infected child[109] and vertical transmission from mother to infant.[445]

Because children, particularly newborns and young infants, usually have subclinical infection, outbreaks usually are detected only when secondary symptomatic infections develop in adult caregivers.[23, 109, 222, 310, 445] Given the long incubation period for this infection, there is ample opportunity for transmission of virus to caregivers and other hospitalized children before secondary symptomatic cases are recognized. Secondary cases among hospitalized children and their young siblings usually are asymptomatic, facilitating amplification of the outbreak both in the hospital and in the community through successive cycles of infection and transmission. Direct contact is responsible for transmission of the virus from infected children to caregivers; indirect contact generally is responsible for transmission of the virus from one child to another in the hospital setting.

Given this epidemiology, the control of a nosocomial hepatitis A outbreak is difficult and usually requires the assistance of the local health department, especially if nonhospitalized contacts or more than one institution is involved. To limit the potential for indirect contact transmission, hospitalized infected children should be cohorted. Hand washing and use of barrier precautions should be emphasized to prevent direct-contact transmission to caregivers and indirect-contact transmission to other children.[144] These precautions should be maintained for the duration of hospitalization in children younger than 3 years of age and for 2 weeks in children 3 to 14 years of age.[144] Older children hospitalized with symptomatic disease have rapidly decreasing titers of virus in their stool by the time they become symptomatic and are not very contagious at this point. Nevertheless, barrier precautions should be used for 7 days.[144]

Immunoglobulin should be administered to all exposed, susceptible persons.[8] Symptomatic health care providers should be furloughed until 1 week after the onset of symptomatic infection or until all susceptible persons have received immunoglobulin.[8] Tracing of contacts is necessary to prevent additional secondary cases. The role of the newly licensed hepatitis A vaccine in the control of outbreaks of hepatitis A has yet to be determined.

Enteroviruses

A number of outbreaks of nosocomial enterovirus have been reported, most occurring in newborn nurseries.[186, 208, 221, 343] In most cases, adult caregivers infected in the community transmitted the virus to one or more hospitalized children through direct contact, with subsequent indirect contact transmission from one child to another. In one nursery outbreak, the virus was introduced by a perinatally infected child.[343] Newborns with severe underlying illness were more likely to be infected, presumably because the prolonged and intensive care these infants required provided more opportunities for transmission.[221, 343] Nosocomial enterovirus infections in newborn infants can be severe—even fatal—but mild and subclinical illnesses also may occur.[296, 343] The presence of maternally derived antibody may play a role in limiting the severity of disease in some infants.[296, 343]

Surveys of nosocomial infections in pediatric wards indicate that nosocomial enterovirus infections are uncommon,[127, 432, 449] yet the potential for nosocomial transmission of these viruses is substantial. Large community outbreaks of echovirus and coxsackievirus infections occur predictably every summer and fall. Because virus is excreted in stool for long periods, a large number of hospitalized children and caregivers certainly are excreting virus during these periods. Detection of nosocomial infection may be compromised because viral cultures may not be readily available, some enteroviruses are difficult to cultivate in tissue culture, and infection may not become manifest until after discharge.

Like hepatitis A virus, enteroviruses are picornaviruses, and the principles described for the control of nosocomial hepatitis A virus infections can be applied to the control of nosocomial enterovirus infection, particularly in nurseries. Accordingly, hand washing and barrier precautions are of paramount importance, and cohorting of infected infants is prudent.[144] The upper respiratory tract may be involved in acute enteroviral infection, but most authorities do not recommend the use of masks during the care of infected patients.[144] These same principles should be applied to confirmed or suspected enteroviral infections in children, especially young diapered children, although the need for cohorting is debatable and may not be feasible during summer and fall epidemics. The efficacy of immunoglobulin as prophylaxis for persons exposed during the course of an outbreak is unclear, but it may be helpful if the preparation used has significant titers of antibody to the outbreak strain, especially in newborn infants who are at risk for severe disease.

Tuberculosis

Nosocomial transmission of tuberculosis is an age-old concern, but this issue has been brought to the forefront again by outbreaks of multidrug-resistant *Mycobacterium tuberculosis* among adult patients and health care workers in several hospitals in New York and Florida.[32, 87, 206] Nosocomial tuberculosis in hospitals caring for pediatric patients occurs almost exclusively as a result of transmission of *M. tuberculosis* from infected adults—parents, visitors, and health care workers—to other children and adults and has yet to involve multi-drug-resistant *M. tuberculosis*.[24, 149, 413, 446] Probable transmission from infected children to adult caregivers has been described.[342] Transmission from children to other children or adults is exceedingly uncommon, presumably because children infrequently have cavitary disease and consequently have fewer tubercle bacilli in their endobronchial secretions and because young children do not tend to generate aerosols of airborne droplet nuclei.[410] Whether children with AIDS or other diseases that severely compromise the immune system will turn out to be more contagious has not been evaluated.

The risk of nosocomial tuberculosis in adult hospitals has been minimized by prompt recognition and treatment of pulmonary tuberculosis and adequate isolation of infectious patients in rooms with negative air pressure relative to the hallway.[45, 70, 418, 451] If rooms with appropriate ventilation are unavailable, alternative engineering solutions, such as well-placed and -maintained ultraviolet lights, may be useful.[70, 303] Personnel entering the rooms of infected patients should wear respiratory protection devices. Particulate respirators with a National Institute for Occupational Safety and Health certification of N95 or better satisfy the CDC specifications for these devices.[70, 304] These devices must be fit-tested on the individuals using them according to the standards of the Occupational Safety and Health Administration.[70] Prompt identification of tuberculosis in parents, visitors, and health care workers in hospitals caring for pediatric patients is an integral part of reducing the risk of nosocomial tuberculosis.

Invasive Bacterial Infections

Nosocomial transmission of *Neisseria meningitidis* appears to be rare and has been demonstrated in hospitalized patients only when the index patient has meningococcal pneumonia,[84, 361] an uncommon clinical presentation of disease in children. Other situations in which nosocomial transmission has occurred have involved special circumstances. For instance, a mother became infected after nursing her infant who was hospitalized with meningococcemia,[273] and several microbiology laboratory workers developed fatal disease after working with cultures of this microorganism.[64] Hospital personnel caring for patients, on the other hand, appear to be at minimal risk unless they have extensive face-to-face contact and fail to wear a mask.

Nosocomial transmission of *Haemophilus influenzae* and *Streptococcus pneumoniae* also has been regarded as a rare phenomenon but may be more common than previously recognized. A few reports from the 1980s documented transmission of *H. influenzae* type B among pediatric patients,[25, 29] and cases among elderly adults and even hospital staff members were reported in the late 1980s and early 1990s.[195, 282, 319, 403] Presumably, widespread immunization of infants with *H. influenzae* type B conjugate vaccine will reduce greatly the risk of nosocomial transmission of this microorganism in pediatric patients. A number of outbreaks of nosocomial infection due to nonencapsulated *H. influenzae* in elderly patients and hospital staff members also have been reported recently.[13, 195] Nosocomial infection with penicillin-resistant *S. pneumoniae* has been a well-documented problem among hospitalized children in South Africa for many years,[134] but outbreaks in hospitalized adults recently have been seen in other countries.[274, 294] A recent case report in a pediatric patient is a likely portent of future difficulties with penicillin-resistant *S. pneumoniae* in United States hospitals.[95]

The microorganisms described are spread by droplet contact transmission, and it is unclear why nosocomial transmission in medical settings is not more common. Masks should be worn by health care workers during the care of patients with suspected invasive meningococcal disease until the patient has completed 24 hours of parenteral antimicrobial therapy.[144] In the past, the use of masks during care of patients with infections caused by *H. influenzae* type B varied in many hospitals. However, a recent CDC guideline recommends use of masks to prevent droplet contact transmission from patients infected with *H. influenzae* until the patient has completed 24 hours of parenteral antimicrobial therapy.[144] The guideline does not recommend the use of a mask when caring for patients with *S. pneumoniae* or even penicillin-resistant *S. pneumoniae*,[144] perhaps because nosocomial transmission of this microorganism has not been a problem in the United States. However, given the reports of nosocomial transmission of *S. pneumoniae* discussed earlier, the authors recommend using masks when caring for patients with infections caused by penicillin-resistant *S. pneumoniae*. Antimicrobial prophylaxis should be administered to persons with close, unprotected contact with patients infected with *N. meningitidis* but is not recommended for exposure to patients infected with *H. influenzae* or *S. pneumoniae* unless an outbreak clearly is in progress.

Ectoparasites

Scabies and pediculosis are common infections in children, and incidental diagnosis of these infections among hospitalized children is not uncommon. A large number of outbreaks of scabies have been reported from a variety of health care institutions.[244] The presence of crusted scabies, which is associated with defects in cellular immunity, including HIV infection, increases the risk of transmission because of the large number of mites in these lesions.[244] Although nosocomial transmission of pediculosis is possible, the direct or indirect contact necessary to spread this infection (i.e., head-to-head contact or sharing of combs) is less likely in medical settings than at home.

Intestinal Helminths

Person-to-person transmission of four intestinal helminths, *Enterobius vermicularis* (pinworm), *Strongyloides stercoralis, Hymenolepsis nana,* and *Taenia solium,* is possible because these microorganisms do not require an intermediate host and because the eggs or larvae excreted in the stool are infectious.[245] However, evidence of nosocomial transmission of these microorganisms is limited.[245]

Other Infections

A variety of unusual, potentially fatal infections may be transmitted nosocomially. International air travel has increased the mobility of the world's population, making it possible for persons to travel long distances during the incubation period of these infections. A high index of suspicion and prompt institution of appropriate isolation precautions are necessary to reduce the risk of nosocomial transmission.

As graphically demonstrated by the well-publicized outbreak of Ebola virus infection in Zaire in 1995, viral hemorrhagic fevers can cause serious outbreaks among hospitalized patients and health care workers.[75] Transmission of Ebola virus by reuse of contaminated needles and close contact with infectious body fluids contributed to a previous outbreak of Ebola virus involving a hospital in Sudan in the 1970s.[28] Lassa, Crimean-Congo, and Marburg viruses also have been spread in hospitals.[215, 298, 402, 419] The bulk of evidence suggests that airborne transmission of these viruses does not occur in clinical settings, although there is insufficient epidemiologic data to exclude this possibility.[74] At present, the CDC recommends the use of negative-pressure isolation rooms for hospitalized patients, protective respirators similar to those used by persons caring for patients with active pulmonary tuberculosis, and barrier techniques.[74]

Anecdotal, unpublished reports have described the nosocomial spread of dengue virus by mosquitoes. Nosocomial transmission of hantavirus has not been reported but is possible theoretically. Rabies has been transmitted by corneal transplants,[15] but spread via contact with infected patients has not been reported.

The potential for nosocomial transmission of diphtheria has been emphasized by the recent large outbreak of this disease in Russia and Ukraine. Diphtheria acquired during travel to these regions has been reported in U.S. citizens, and imported cases have been documented in other European countries.[73] An imported case of diphtheria in a child from Haiti resulted in exposure of a large number of hospital contacts in Florida. Secondary cases were reported among household contacts but not among hospital contacts.[122] Health care workers should wear masks during the care of patients with pharyngeal diphtheria. Investigation and prophylaxis of contacts should be pursued aggressively.[122]

Plague is endemic in portions of the western United States and in other countries. No person-to-person transmission of plague has been identified in the United States for more than a half century,[91] but a recent outbreak in India illustrates the potential for importation of plague to other countries.[69, 72] Droplet contact transmission of *Yersinia pestis* is well documented from persons with pulmonary involvement. Health care workers should wear masks during the care of patients with signs or symptoms of pulmonary involvement. Tetracycline can be used for prophylaxis of contacts.[91]

NOSOCOMIAL INFECTIONS RELATED TO INVASIVE DEVICES, PROCEDURES, AND TREATMENTS

Infections Related to Intravascular Catheters and Infusions

Local infections related to the use of intravascular catheters include infection at the site where the catheter exits the skin (exit-site infection), infection along the subcutaneous track of a tunneled catheter (tunnel infection), and infection in the subcutaneous pocket containing an implanted catheter (pocket infection).[76] Phlebitis is a common local complication related to the use of intravascular catheters but usually is caused by chemical or mechanical irritation as opposed to infection and is less common in children than in adults.[141]

Systemic infections related to the use of intravascular catheters include blood stream infections occurring as a result of microbial colonization of the catheter (catheter-related blood stream infection) and contamination of fluids or medications infused through the catheter (infusate-related blood stream infection).[76] Endocarditis, septic thrombophlebitis, and infection at other body sites as a result of hematogenous seeding (e.g., meningitis, pyelonephritis, hepatic or splenic abscesses, osteomyelitis, septic arthritis, endophthalmitis) are serious complications of blood stream infection.

The risk of endemic local and systemic infections associated with intravascular catheters varies by the type of catheter in use. Percutaneously inserted peripheral intravenous catheters, especially catheters made with modern pliant, nonthrombogenic materials, are associated with a low rate of local infection in children, and blood stream infections are rare.[141, 142] Rates of local and blood stream infection also are low in newborn infants,[140] but infusion of lipid emulsions through these catheters significantly increases the risk of blood stream infection with coagulase-negative staphylococci and probably *Candida*.[59, 130] Peripheral arterial catheters generally also have a low rate of endemic local and systemic infectious complications; two reports studying more than 400 arterial catheters did not identify any catheter-related blood stream infections.[110, 137]

The vast majority of endemic catheter-related blood stream infections in pediatric patients are associated with central venous catheters.[204] As shown in Tables 228–2 and 228–3, rates of blood stream infection associated with central venous catheters in pediatric ICUs and central and umbilical intravascular catheters in newborn ICUs are higher than rates in adult ICUs in United States hospitals participating in the NNIS system.[305] Rates of infection among low birth weight infants (<1500 g) in newborn ICUs are higher than among any other ICU population, except among patients in ICUs caring exclusively for patients with severe burns.[305] These data do not distinguish rates of infection associated with specific catheter types, nor do they distinguish which catheter is the source of the infection in patients with multiple catheters.

Comparisons of blood stream infection rates associated with different types of central venous catheters in pediatric patients are confounded by a number of factors.[457] Patient populations in whom these catheters are used have diverse underlying diseases (e.g., cancer, cystic fibrosis, prematurity, short bowel syndrome, AIDS) with widely variant intrinsic risk of blood stream infection. Even among pediatric oncology patients, risk varies considerably with the type of cancer and the intensity of chemotherapy,[198] and younger children have a higher risk of infection, even when the underlying disease and the type of catheter utilized are similar.[198, 468] Use of the catheter for multiple purposes and infusion of lipid emulsions also increases the risk of infection.[219]

With these caveats, a recent review suggests that rates of blood stream infection are lower in totally implanted (0.1 to 0.7 infections/1000 catheter-days) than tunneled (0.4 to 7.8 infections/1000 catheter-days) catheters.[457] This conclusion is supported by several studies directly comparing rates of infection between these two types of catheters.[233, 295, 391, 468] These studies demonstrated lower rates of infection with implanted catheters, although differences were not statistically significant in every report.

Rates of blood stream infection associated with percutaneously inserted central venous catheters in pediatric and newborn ICU patients appear to be at least several times higher (6 to 10 infections/1000 catheter-days) than rates associated with either tunneled or implanted catheters.[196, 412] Rates of infection associated with hemodialysis catheters have not been reported in pediatric patients, although rates of infection associated with the use of these catheters in adults are higher than for any type of central venous catheter.[76] Rates of infection associated with intracardiac catheters used in pediatric patients after open heart surgery have not been reported. The use of midline and peripherally inserted central venous catheters is increasing in newborn ICUs, pediatric ICUs, and pediatric wards, but there are few data regarding rates of infection associated with these catheters. A recent study of umbilical catheters in neonates found that blood stream infection occurred in 5 per cent of neonates with umbilical artery catheters and 3 per cent of neonates with umbilical venous catheters (rates of infections per 1000 catheter-days were not reported).[237]

In contrast with endemic infections, which are associated closely with the type of catheter used, epidemics of blood stream infection generally are related to other factors.[33] Improperly disinfected pressure transducers are the most common cause of epidemics of blood stream infection.[33] Use of disposable domes may reduce but do not obviate this risk. Microorganisms contaminating the transducer head may be transferred to the dome and the infusion system by the hands of staff members who manipulate these components of the apparatus during setup, calibration, and blood drawing.[33] Detailed investigation of practices often is necessary to identify and eliminate causes of blood stream infection outbreaks, as illustrated by an outbreak of candidemia in a newborn ICU related to retrograde administration of medications into intravenous tubing.[394]

The principal risk factors for catheter-related nosocomial blood stream infection in adult patients have been identified.[268] Heavy colonization of the skin at the catheter exit site is an important risk factor for colonization of the external surface of catheters of all types and is correlated with increased risk of blood stream infection.[268] Colonization of the catheter hub also is an important risk factor for blood stream infection, especially disease occurring late in the course of central venous catheterization.[100, 250] Other risk factors related to central venous catheters include longer duration of insertion (>3 days), insertion in the internal jugular vein as opposed to the subclavian vein, use of catheters with multiple lumens as opposed to single lumens, and the presence of a mural or atrial thrombus.[76, 268, 337]

Unfortunately, information regarding risk factors in children and newborn infants is far more limited than in adults. Two studies of peripheral intravenous catheters in pediatric patients found that the likelihood of colonization of the external surface of the catheter was slightly greater with increasing duration of insertion, but blood stream infections were extremely uncommon, even in patients with colonized catheters.[141, 142] A study of catheter colonization in newborn ICU patients found that duration of insertion greater than 3 days was a significant risk factor for colonization of peripheral intravenous catheters and umbilical catheters.[92] A similar trend was seen with central venous catheters in this patient population, although the number of catheters studied was limited and no conclusions could be drawn with regard to the risk of blood stream infection.[92] Current information is not sufficient to state whether the site of insertion of central venous catheters affects the risk of infection, although one study in pediatric ICU patients found similar rates of infection between catheters inserted in the femoral vein and catheters inserted into veins at other sites.[412] As in adult patients, there is a higher risk of infection with the use of larger catheters (i.e., multiple lumen vs. single lumen catheters).[81] Finally, a series of studies of coagulase-negative staphylococcal blood stream infection in patients in newborn ICUs found that length of stay, birth weight, and administration of lipid emulsions were significant risk factors for infection.[130, 131] No studies in children or newborn infants have examined colonization of the catheter hub.

Microorganisms associated with catheter-related blood stream infections in patients of all ages in United States hospitals participating in the NNIS system are displayed in Table 228–6.[117] Nearly a third of infections are caused by coagulase-negative staphylococci. Other gram-positive bacteria, including *S. aureus*, *Enterococcus* species, and various streptococci, account for another third of infections. One-quarter of infections are due to gram-negative bacteria, including *E. coli*, *P. aeruginosa*, *Klebsiella pneumoniae*, *Enterobacter* species, *Acinetobacter* species, *Serratia marcescens*, *Citrobacter* species, and other aerobic gram-negative bacilli. *C. albicans*, other *Candida* species, and other fungi together cause approximately 10 per cent of infections. Atypical mycobacteria are occasional causes of blood stream infection.[278] Recent data from the NNIS system regarding microorganisms causing blood stream infection in newborn ICUs reveal a similar distribution; however, coagulase-negative staphylococci account for an even greater percentage (51 per cent) of isolates in this population.[148] NNIS data regarding the distribution of microorganisms causing blood stream infection in general pediatric and pediatric ICU patients have not been published.

Mechanisms involved in the pathogenesis of infections associated with intravascular catheters and infusions are depicted in Figure 228–2. A large number of studies, including studies utilizing molecular typing of isolates, have demonstrated that most infections arise from microorganisms colonizing the skin at the insertion site that migrate along the external surface of the catheter through its subcutaneous tract and into the blood vessel.[76, 268, 289] Colonization of the interior surface of the catheter occurs via contamination of the catheter hub.[76, 268] The relative contributions of these two mechanisms may depend on the duration of catheterization.[339] Detailed microbiologic studies and scanning electron microscopy have demonstrated that colonization of the external surface predominated in the first 10 days after insertion, whereas colonization of the internal surface increased with the length of catheterization and was significantly more common in catheters in place for more than 30 days. Microorganisms on the hands of health care workers can contaminate the catheter, the insertion site, or the hub during insertion and maintenance of the infusion system.

A variety of microbial and host factors play a role in the pathogenesis of blood stream infections. For example, capsular polysaccharide adhesin enhances the ability of coagulase-negative staphylococci to adhere to prosthetic materials.[225] Biofilm composed of host proteins and microbial exopolysaccharide (i.e., "slime") coats the external and internal catheter surfaces soon after insertion and may enhance the ability of microorganisms to persist on catheter surfaces and evade host defenses.[225] Slime production is common among coagulase-negative staphylococci[225]; recent data suggest that *Candida* species also may produce slime, particularly in the presence of glucose-containing fluids.[52]

Catheter materials may be important in catheter colonization and infection. Catheters made of polyvinyl chloride or polyethylene are less resistant to colonization in vitro than catheters made of Teflon, silicon elastomer, or polyurethane.[76] Trauma to blood vessels is more likely with the use of stiff plastics (e.g., polyvinyl chloride) than newer plastic materials (Teflon, silicon elastomer, or polyurethane), predisposing to phlebitis and infection. Other factors, such as surface irregularities and the thrombogenicity of catheter material, also may play a role.[76]

Other mechanisms involved in the pathogenesis of these infections are depicted in Figure 228–2. Contaminated intravenous infusions,[270, 394] medications,[37, 269] blood products,[67] and hemodynamic monitoring systems[33] have resulted in serious outbreaks of infection. Purposeful contamination of infusates as a form of child abuse also has been reported.[254] The frequency of hematogenous seeding of the catheter from a distant site of infection is unknown but is likely to be low.

Clinical and culture criteria for the diagnosis of infections related to intravascular catheters and infusions developed by

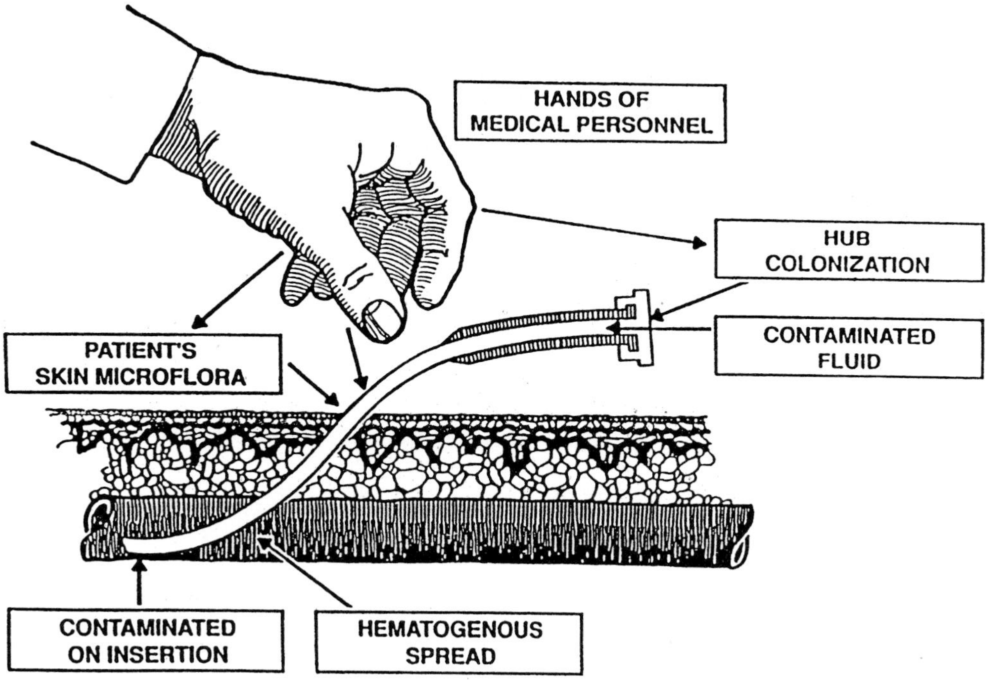

FIGURE 228–2. *Mechanisms involved in the pathogenesis of infections associated with intravascular catheters and infusions. (From Pearson, M. L., and Hospital Infection Control Practices Advisory Committee: Guideline for prevention of intravascular device–related infections. Infect. Control Hosp. Epidemiol. 17:438–473, 1996.*

the CDC and the Hospital Infection Control Practices Advisory Committee (HICPAC) are listed in Table 228–8.[76] Definitions used by the NNIS system are similar but do not define separate local infections specifically and include two subcategories of blood stream infection (laboratory-confirmed blood stream infection and clinical sepsis).[145]

Potential blood stream infections should be evaluated with at least two blood cultures, including at least one blood culture drawn by venipuncture, before the institution of antimicrobial therapy. If possible, the catheter should be removed using aseptic technique and cultured to determine whether it is colonized. Central venous catheters should be changed over a wire or removed and cultured. The semiquantitative roll-plate culture technique is the best-accepted and most widely available method.[272] More than 15 colony-forming units (cfu) is regarded as evidence of colonization of the external surface of the catheter but does not predict risk of blood stream infection reliably; more than 100 cfu has greater positive predictive value for blood stream infection.[272] However, this technique does not detect colonization of the catheter hub or the intraluminal surface. Quantitative culture of the catheter tip, which includes flushing the catheter with liquid culture media and sonication of the catheter, is the most sensitive technique and detects colonization of both the external and internal surfaces.[338, 395] However, this technique is more time-consuming and is not available universally. Because these techniques require removal of the catheter, some investigators have attempted to diagnose catheter-associated blood stream infection by comparing quantitative blood cultures of paired specimens, one specimen drawn through the catheter and the other drawn by venipuncture. In a small study of children with tunneled catheters, a 10-fold higher concentration in the catheter specimen or a concentration of greater than 2000 cfu/mL in the catheter specimen was predictive of catheter-related blood stream infection.[347] In another study of infants and young children, an acridine orange stain of blood drawn through a central venous catheter had 87 per cent sensitivity and 94 per cent specificity for the diagnosis of catheter-related blood stream infection compared with quantitative blood cultures drawn from the catheter and from venipuncture.[368] An advantage of this test is that it can be completed in approximately 1 hour. Further studies are required to investigate the cost-effectiveness of this technique. Buffy coat Gram stain of a blood sample drawn from the catheter may reveal yeast forms in some patients with candidemia. If the catheter is removed, Gram

TABLE 228–8. Diagnostic Criteria for Infections Related to Intravascular Catheters and Infusions

Infection	Diagnostic Criteria
Exit-site infection	Erythema, tenderness, and induration or purulence within 2 cm of the skin at the exit site of the catheter
Tunnel infection	Erythema, tenderness, and induration in the tissues overlying the catheter and >2 cm from the exit site
Pocket infection	Erythema, tenderness, and induration or necrosis of the tissues over the reservoir of a totally implantable device or purulent exudate in the subcutaneous pocket containing the reservoir
Catheter-related blood stream infection	Isolation of the same microorganism (i.e., identical species and antibiogram) from a semiquantitative or quantitative culture of a catheter segment and from the blood (preferably drawn from a peripheral vein) of a patient with accompanying clinical symptoms of a blood stream infection and no other apparent source of infection
Infusate-related blood stream infection	Isolation of the same microorganism (i.e., identical species and antibiogram) from infusate and from separate percutaneous blood cultures, with no other identifiable source of infection

Modified from Pearson, M. L., and Hospital Infection Control Practices Advisory Committee: Guideline for prevention of intravascular device–related infections. Infect. Control Hosp. Epidemiol. *17*:438–473, 1996.

staining of adherent material also may facilitate rapid diagnosis.

In practice, several difficulties arise in the diagnosis of nosocomial blood stream infections. Physicians' designation of microorganisms isolated from blood cultures as pathogens or contaminants may be confounded by the patient's age and underlying condition and the presence of an intravascular catheter, particularly a central venous catheter. For example, in a study performed in the authors' institution, physicians were more likely to interpret the coagulase-negative staphylococci in blood cultures drawn from very low birth weight infants as clinically significant.[132]

The terminology used to describe the clinical manifestations of blood stream infection in pediatric patients requires standardization. Consensus definitions of the systemic inflammatory response syndrome (a condition arising from a variety of processes, including blood stream infection), sepsis, severe sepsis, and septic shock in adult patients have been published.[47] An epidemiologic study of these conditions found that blood stream infections occurred in 17 per cent of patients with sepsis, 25 per cent of patients with severe sepsis, and 69 per cent of patients with septic shock.[345] Although the pathophysiology and management of sepsis in pediatric patients also have been reviewed,[372] precise definitions of sepsis in children and newborn infants have not been promulgated and validated. The definition of blood stream infection used by the NNIS system lists clinical criteria for sepsis, including criteria for use in children younger than 12 months of age, but the sensitivity and specificity of these criteria have not been examined.

In many instances, culture information is not sufficient to satisfy the diagnostic criteria in Table 228–8. Obtaining cultures by venipuncture is difficult in young children, and clinicians may be reluctant to obtain blood for more than one culture in low birth weight infants. Given the potential complications associated with reinsertion of a new catheter and the fact that many catheter-related blood stream infections can be treated with the catheter in place, central venous catheters often are not removed for culture. Finally, unless infusate-related blood stream infection is suspected, obtaining cultures of intravenous fluids or medications often is overlooked.

Empiric antimicrobial therapy for suspected blood stream infection while awaiting culture results should be based on local knowledge of the relative frequency and susceptibility patterns of nosocomial pathogens. In most situations, empiric therapy should include an agent effective against gram-positive bacteria, such as oxacillin or vancomycin, and an agent effective against most gram-negative bacteria, such as an aminoglycoside, a third-generation cephalosporin, or aztreonam. In the authors' institution, gentamicin is used routinely instead of a third-generation cephalosporin or aztreonam because of its generally equivalent activity against gram-negative rods, its synergy with β-lactams and vancomycin against susceptible *Enterococcus* species, and its lower cost. Unless renal toxicity or ototoxicity is a major concern, we limit the use of third-generation cephalosporins and aztreonam for empiric therapy to reduce the emergence of resistance to these agents. Empiric use of two agents with activity against gram-negative rods (e.g., a third-generation cephalosporin and gentamicin) is appropriate in a severely ill patient when infection with a resistant gram-negative rod is suspected. Empiric antifungal therapy is initiated only in rare situations when suspicion of fungemia is high (i.e., a severely ill patient heavily colonized with *Candida* species already receiving broad-spectrum antimicrobial therapy). Once culture information is available, the treatment regimen can be tailored accordingly or discontinued if no infection is identified.

The role of thrombolytic agents in the treatment of catheter-related blood stream infection has not been defined. Two noncontrolled studies reported good responses to treatment of catheter-related blood stream infections using a combination of antimicrobial therapy and low-dose urokinase.[212, 386] However, a small, randomized, controlled study found no benefit from the combination of urokinase and antimicrobial therapy.[232] This trial was stopped early because of a lack of evidence of increased treatment efficacy with urokinase and because several patients receiving urokinase experienced fever, chills, and hypotension during infusion.[232]

There is substantial evidence that the vast majority of uncomplicated blood stream infections associated with central venous catheters can be treated effectively without removing the catheter.[457] However, treatment of catheter-associated fungemia without removal of the catheter has a relatively low success rate and may be associated with higher mortality as well as other complications.[94] Strong consideration also should be given to removing catheters associated with difficult-to-treat bacteria, such as antimicrobial-resistant enterococci or gram-negative rods. In the authors' experience, in situ treatment is not as likely to be successful with implanted catheters, but few published data specifically address this issue. Percutaneously inserted central venous catheters may be changed over a wire and the catheter tip sent for culture.[76] If the culture of the tip is negative, the replacement catheter can be left in place.[76] If the culture of the tip is positive, the replacement catheter should be removed and a new catheter inserted at a new site.[76] Catheters should be removed immediately if there is evidence of embolic phenomena, septic thrombophlebitis, or endocarditis or if the patient is hemodynamically unstable.

There are few data regarding the optimal duration of therapy of blood stream infections if the catheter remains in place, but experience suggests that 14 days usually is adequate. Short courses of therapy are appropriate if the catheter is removed, especially for uncomplicated infections caused by relatively less virulent pathogens, such as coagulase-negative staphylococci.

Persistently positive blood cultures, despite antimicrobial therapy, or recrudescence of infection after therapy is complete should prompt removal of the catheter. However, preliminary results of an alternative treatment approach, the "antibiotic lock technique," have been reported recently.[207] In this study, patients with catheter-related blood stream infection who had responded to antimicrobial therapy clinically but who had persistently positive blood cultures drawn through a central venous catheter (and negative blood cultures drawn by venipuncture) were treated with infusion of 3 to 4 mL of antibiotic solution into the catheter lumen every 12 hours for 10 to 14 days. No additional antimicrobial therapy was given. Ten of 12 episodes of infection caused by a variety of microorganisms were cured without removal of the catheter. The need to remove catheters from patients with persistent fever but no positive culture results and no evidence of infection at another site is controversial and should be dealt with case by case.

Some success has been reported in the treatment of uncomplicated exit-site infections with the catheter in place.[278, 457] A trial of a combination of local therapy and systemic antimicrobial treatment is warranted before a decision to remove the catheter is made. In contrast, treatment outcomes of tunnel or pocket infections generally are poor if the catheter is left in place.[278, 457]

A guideline for the prevention of infections related to intravascular catheters and infusions has been developed by the CDC and the HICPAC.[76] Several critical aspects of the prevention of these infections are emphasized in the following paragraphs.

Intravascular catheters and infusions should be used only when necessary, and caregivers should monitor catheterized patients closely for signs of local and systemic infection. Interventions directed at minimizing contamination of the catheter during insertion include use of an effective skin antiseptic (chlorhexidine-based agents appear more effective than agents based on povidone-iodine or alcohol)[140, 271] and use of full sterile barrier precautions during insertion of central venous catheters.[336]

Routine application of topical antimicrobials to the catheter exit site has not been supported by most studies,[76] although a European trial suggested that mupirocin applied to the site at the time of insertion and at the time of dressing changes might be effective.[192] Exit-site patches impregnated with chlorhexidine have not been evaluated adequately. Transparent semipermeable dressings facilitate inspection of the catheter site. However, some studies suggest that they may increase microbial proliferation at the site of insertion and predispose to blood stream infection; other studies have shown no difference in colonization of the site or infection rates in comparison to gauze and tape dressings.[76] Despite the controversy, transparent dressings, often combined with a small piece of gauze at the site of insertion to absorb moisture, are in widespread use. Central venous catheters impregnated with antimicrobials and silver-impregnated subcutaneous catheter cuffs have shown promise in adult studies,[76] but they have not been evaluated in pediatrics. Studies of the use of "prophylactic" vancomycin added to intravenous fluids and flush solutions to prevent infections by vancomycin-sensitive microorganisms have shown conflicting results,[344, 406] and the impact of this type of intervention on the emergence of vancomycin-resistant pathogens has not been assessed.

Manipulation of the catheter and infusion sets should be minimized, and these sets should be maintained as closed systems whenever possible. When manipulation is necessary, hand washing and aseptic technique should be practiced. Infusion sets used for standard intravenous fluid administration need not be changed more frequently than every 72 hours.[76] If parenteral nutrition or blood products are administered, infusion sets should be changed at least every 24 hours.[76]

The apparatus for hemodynamic monitoring should be maintained as a closed system, and manipulations of this system should be minimized.[76] When manipulation is necessary, hand washing and aseptic technique should be practiced. Disposable domes and transducers used for hemodynamic monitoring should be changed every 96 hours.[76] Reused transducers should be reprocessed appropriately between uses.[76]

Stopcocks are common components of intravenous infusion and hemodynamic monitoring systems and are used as portals for injection of medications, infusion of fluids (e.g., parenteral nutrition), and collection of blood samples. These devices can become contaminated during use, although their role in blood stream infections is not well studied.[76] Manipulation of these devices should be minimized, and the access port should be disinfected before it is entered.

Infections Related to Respiratory Therapy

The vast majority of nosocomial pneumonias are caused by bacteria and are associated with mechanical ventilation. Pneumonia also can be caused by respiratory viruses, but these infections are caused by intrahospital transmission of common community infections rather than by exposure to medical devices or ICUs (see Nosocomial Infections Due to Spread of Infections Common in the Community, Respiratory Infections). *Legionella* and filamentous fungi also cause pneumonia, but these infections occur almost exclusively in immunocompromised patients and are related to inhalation of contaminated aerosols or fungal spores, not respiratory therapy (see Nosocomial Infections in Special Populations, Immunocompromised Children).

Tables 228–2 and 228–3 display rates of pneumonia associated with mechanical ventilation in pediatric ICUs and newborn ICUs in U.S. hospitals participating in the NNIS system.[305] Rates of pneumonia are considerably lower in pediatric and newborn ICUs than in adult ICUs.[305] The rate of infection was even lower (0.9 pneumonias/1000 ventilator-days) in a 2-year study of the incidence of ventilator associated pneumonia in two pediatric ICUs in the authors' institution (a multidisciplinary ICU and a cardiology/cardiovascular surgery ICU).[153] Differences in the definition of pneumonia are likely to account, at least in part, for lower rates of infection reported from the authors' institution. For example, the NNIS system definition of pneumonia includes viral causes of pneumonia, whereas the authors' study examined only bacterial infections (discussed later). In general, discrepancies in rates of pneumonia among studies using differing definitions must be interpreted cautiously. No pediatric studies have been performed using even more rigorous criteria for pneumonia, such as a threshold concentration of bacteria on quantitative cultures obtained by bronchoscopy using a protected brush or bronchoalveolar lavage.

Nosocomial pneumonia related to the use of equipment generating contaminated mists has not been reported recently in pediatric patients, although a number of outbreaks caused by "water bacteria" (e.g., *Flavobacterium meningosepticum*, *P. aeruginosa*, *Achromobacter* species) in pediatric patients in the 1950s and 1960s were linked to the use of centrifugal, Venturi, and ultrasonic mechanical nebulizers.[297] Such devices can aerosolize droplets that are small enough to reach the distal airways, so contamination of their fluid reservoirs is extremely hazardous. Large-volume mechanical nebulizers largely have been replaced by heated humidifiers. These devices are considerably less dangerous because they do not generate small-particle aerosols and are less prone to heavy contamination because heating the reservoir retards the growth of most potential pathogens. Mist tents used today for patients with bronchiolitis and croup do have mechanical nebulizers, but they generate larger particles that are deposited in the environment, mouth, and pharynx and generally do not reach the lower respiratory tract. Nonetheless, an effective cleaning and disinfection program is required to minimize the likelihood of infection.

On the other hand, small-volume, hand-held nebulizers used commonly for inhalation therapy in pediatric patients are designed intentionally to generate particles small enough to reach the distal airways, and the potential for nosocomial pneumonia related to the use of these devices is underappreciated by most caregivers. An outbreak of *Legionella* pneumonia caused by contaminated medication administered using small-volume nebulizers has been reported.[277] In addition, the small-volume medication nebulizers used in conjunction with mechanical ventilators can become contaminated by bacteria colonizing the ventilator circuit and thus generate bacteria-laden aerosols.[90]

Mechanical ventilation is a major risk factor not only for nosocomial pneumonia but for sinusitis and otitis media because the nasotracheal tube interferes with normal drainage of the ostia of the sinuses and the eustachian tube.[38, 165] Detection of these infections requires a high index of suspicion because they often are "silent," with little in the way of symptoms other than fever.

Risk factors for pneumonia in adults have been summarized in a recent review.[422] This review groups risk factors into several categories: (1) host factors, such as chronic pulmonary disease and immunosuppression, that increase general susceptibility to pneumonia; (2) factors that enhance bacterial colonization of the oropharynx and stomach with pathogenic bacteria, such as severe underlying disease, administration of antimicrobials, and, possibly, agents that raise gastric pH (e.g., antacids, H2 blockers); (3) factors that increase the likelihood of reflux of gastric contents and aspiration into the lower airway, such as depressed mental status, supine positioning, nasogastric tubes, and enteral feeding; (4) conditions that require prolonged ventilation and hence increase potential exposure to contaminated respiratory equipment and contact with contaminated hands of caregivers; and (5) factors that hinder adequate pulmonary toilet, such as thoracic or abdominal surgery and immobilization.[422] There are no comparable studies in patients in pediatric and newborn ICUs, but it is likely that at least some of these risk factors are important in children as well.

Microorganisms associated with nosocomial pneumonia in patients of all ages in U.S. hospitals participating in the NNIS system are displayed in Table 228–6.[117] Not reflected in this table is the fact that the majority of pneumonias are polymicrobial and often include both gram-positive and gram-negative bacteria.[422] More than half of the bacterial isolates are gram-negative bacilli, with *P. aeruginosa, Enterobacter* species, and *Klebsiella* species accounting for approximately two-thirds of gram-negative isolates. *S. aureus* is the major gram-positive pathogen. *S. pneumoniae* and *H. influenzae* have been recognized increasingly as causes of nosocomial pneumonia in adults.[422] *Moraxella catarrhalis* is an occasional pathogen in mechanically ventilated patients in the authors' institution. Anaerobic bacteria are implicated uncommonly as a cause of pneumonia,[422] but they may play a role in some polymicrobial infections, especially when pneumonia is caused by aspiration. Although *C. albicans* and other *Candida* species are isolated in some cases, they rarely, if ever, are the primary cause of nosocomial pneumonia. Limited data suggest that this distribution of microorganisms is similar in ventilator-associated pneumonia in pediatric ICU patients,[30] but there are no data from patients in newborn ICUs. The distribution of microorganisms causing sinusitis and otitis media in nasotracheally intubated patients is similar to that of pneumonia, although anaerobic bacteria may play a greater role.

The pathogenesis of ventilator-associated pneumonia is complex but can be reduced to two general mechanisms: aspiration of microorganisms colonizing the stomach and oropharynx and inhalation of contaminated aerosols.[422] Aspiration is responsible for most endemic pneumonias, whereas inhalation of contaminated aerosols tends to occur in the context of common source outbreaks of infection.

A variety of factors facilitate colonization of the oropharynx and upper respiratory tract with pathogenic bacteria. Adherence of gram-negative organisms to mucosal cells is enhanced in severely ill or debilitated patients by exposure of epithelial bacterial receptors and by changes in the amount and character of respiratory secretions.[422] Bacterial factors, such as the presence of pili in *P. aeruginosa*, also play a role.[422] Antimicrobial therapy reduces the concentration of normal flora, reducing "colonization resistance" and allowing antimicrobial-resistant nosocomial microorganisms to gain a foothold. Bacteria may reach the pharynx via the hands of caregivers or from contaminated equipment or aerosols, or they may be regurgitated into the pharynx from the stomach. Normal gastric pH prevents heavy contamination of stomach contents, but bacteria proliferate to high levels when stomach acid is neutralized by antacids or H2 blockers.[422] Although the role of these agents in fostering gastric colonization is supported by most studies, the degree to which they are associated with an increased risk of nosocomial pneumonia is less clear.[422] Factors that increase the reflux of gastric contents into the upper airway, such as bolus enteral feedings, nasogastric tubes, and supine position, probably increase the risk substantially but have not been studied intensively.

Regardless of how nosocomial microorganisms reach the upper respiratory tract, contaminated secretions can be aspirated into the lower respiratory tract of mechanically ventilated patients during changes in position or deflation of the endotracheal tube cuff. Uncuffed endotracheal tubes are used in the majority of pediatric patients, so there is a constant potential for aspiration.

Pneumonia associated with inhalation of contaminated aerosols is much less common than that associated with colonization of the oropharynx and aspiration.[422] As noted previously, such infections are likely to be caused by *P. aeruginosa*, *Legionella*, and a variety of other nonenteric gram-negative bacilli that can survive and proliferate in medications and solutions used in respiratory therapy.[422]

Once microorganisms have entered the lower airway, the status of normal defense mechanisms is extremely important in determining whether infection results. Diseases that compromise the mucociliary clearance system (e.g., cystic fibrosis, chronic lung disease) and the ability of the immune system to contain and inactivate these microorganisms (e.g., chemotherapy, HIV infection) increase the risk of infection dramatically.

Methods used to diagnose community-acquired pneumonia, such as auscultation of the chest, examination of sputum, and a chest radiograph, are helpful but much less precise tools for the diagnosis of nosocomial pneumonia in mechanically ventilated patients. Auscultation often is hindered by sounds of the ventilation system itself. Furthermore, a variety of underlying pulmonary diseases (e.g., bronchopulmonary dysplasia, adult respiratory distress syndrome, cystic fibrosis) and conditions (e.g., fluid overload) may produce sounds indistinguishable from those present in pneumonia. Cultures of tracheal aspirates may be misleading because the endotracheal tube often is colonized with potential pathogens, especially in patients ventilated more than a few days.[154] A Gram stain of the tracheal aspirate can assess semiquantitatively both the number of neutrophils and the number and type of microbial flora, but localized irritation or superficial infection of the trachea related to the endotracheal tube may produce purulent secretions that are laden with bacteria on Gram stain. Finally, the presence of new radiographic findings consistent with pneumonia may be extraordinarily difficult to assess in patients with underlying lung disease or patients recovering from thoracic or complicated cardiac surgery.

A variety of techniques to improve the diagnosis of nosocomial pneumonia in mechanically ventilated patients have been tested recently. Bronchoscopic techniques (e.g., quantitative culture of protected brush specimens, bronchoalveolar lavage, and protected bronchoalveolar lavage) offer greater sensitivity and specificity compared with traditional clinical and laboratory diagnostic criteria in adult patients.[422] However, these tests are invasive, are difficult to perform safely in severely ill patients, and are difficult to interpret in patients who have been treated with antimicrobial agents. Furthermore, bronchoscopes necessary to perform these procedures are too large for use in small children and newborns. Blind catheterization of the distal airway to obtain specimens for Gram stain and quantitative culture of the endotracheal aspirate is more practical than bronchoscopic techniques.[422] In a study of blind catheterization of the distal airway in a pediatric ICU, positive cultures were correlated strongly with the independent diagnosis of bacterial nosocomial pneumonia using specific clinical, laboratory, and radiographic criteria.[30] However, cultures also were positive in nearly a third of patients with noninfectious pulmonary infiltrates.

Future study may lead to better diagnostic methods, but at present the diagnosis of ventilator-associated nosocomial pneumonia in pediatric patients still depends on a constellation of clinical, laboratory, and radiographic criteria. The authors' institution uses the following definition: a new or worsening infiltrate on chest radiograph compatible with pneumonia (by the pediatric radiologist's report) after more than 48 hours of mechanical ventilation, purulent tracheobronchial secretions (described as tan, beige, yellow, or green in the hospital record or showing moderate or abundant numbers of neutrophils per high-power field on Gram stain), and growth of a pathogen in moderate or abundant amounts from an endotracheal aspirate culture. Other definitions for use in pediatric patients also have been published.[30, 145] Viral pneumonias require demonstration of the pathogen by direct detection, culture, or serology.

Evaluation of fever in a mechanically ventilated patient should include examination for otitis media. If an etiology of the fever is not established, consideration should be given to radiographic studies of the sinuses (e.g., sinus films or a computed tomographic scan), especially if the child has a nasotracheal tube. If otitis media or sinusitis is diagnosed, tympanocentesis or a tap of the sinuses for culture should be considered to guide antimicrobial therapy.

Empiric antimicrobial therapy of nosocomial pneumonia in the mechanically ventilated patient should be guided by the Gram stain of the endotracheal aspirate. Once culture information is available, the treatment regimen can be tailored accordingly or discontinued if no infection is identified. Prolonged treatment of patients in whom the diagnosis is questionable should be avoided because this often leads to endotracheal colonization with antimicrobial-resistant bacteria. Treatment duration has not been studied. The authors usually treat uncomplicated cases with approximately 10 days of therapy. If a necrotizing gram-negative pneumonia is diagnosed (rare in pediatric patients), therapy should be administered for at least 14 days.

In nasotracheally intubated patients with otitis media or sinusitis, the nasotracheal tube should be changed to an orotracheal tube. Short-term treatment with a decongestant and lavage of the sinuses (often performed at the time of the sinus tap) may aid the treatment of sinusitis. Treatment of these infections also has not been studied extensively, but the authors generally use approximately 10 days of therapy for otitis media; extensive sinusitis warrants at least 14 days of therapy.

The CDC and the HICPAC have developed a comprehensive guideline for the prevention of nosocomial pneumonia.[422] Key features of this guideline are emphasized in the following paragraphs.

Mechanical ventilation should be used only when necessary, and caregivers should monitor ventilated patients carefully for signs of pneumonia, otitis media, and sinusitis. Prevention of cross-colonization with "hospital flora," especially antimicrobial-resistant bacteria, should be stressed. Hand washing and use of gloves during contact with respiratory secretions or objects or surfaces contaminated with respiratory secretions are important, especially in busy ICUs caring for many sick patients. Suctioning should be performed gently using a sterile, single-use catheter, and sterile fluids should be used to loosen secretions and clear the suction catheter. Data are insufficient to recommend sterile versus clean, nonsterile gloves or multi-use, closed-system suction catheters versus single-use, open-system catheters.

Endotracheal tubes and ventilator circuits become contaminated with the patient's own oropharyngeal flora quickly, and repeatedly changing this equipment does not reduce the risk of infection. Ventilator circuits and humidifiers should be changed no more frequently than every 48 hours. The maximum "permissible" period of use has not been established.[422] Care should be taken to prevent condensate that collects in the ventilator tubing from draining into the endotracheal tube because this fluid can be contaminated with a large number of microorganisms. Tubing should be maintained in a dependent position relative to the endotracheal tube, and condensate should be discarded routinely. The effect of various innovations, such as traps to collect condensate, bacterial filters, hygroscopic condenser-humidifiers, and heat exchange humidifiers, on the risk of pneumonia has not been determined.

Large-volume mechanical nebulizers should not be used unless they are cleaned scrupulously and reprocessed daily. Only sterile water should be used in these devices. Small, hand-held medication nebulizers should be rinsed with sterile water and allowed to air dry between uses. These devices should be reprocessed before use in another patient. Only sterile, aseptically dispensed medications should be used in these devices. Other respiratory therapy equipment should be reprocessed between patients.

Development and application of effective procedures for reprocessing of all reused respiratory therapy and ventilator equipment have played a major role in reducing the risk of serious gram-negative pneumonia. Items that have direct or indirect contact with the mucous membranes or respiratory secretions should be cleaned thoroughly and either sterilized or disinfected in a manner consistent with high-level disinfection.[422]

Many issues related to prevention of oropharyngeal or gastric colonization, reflux of gastric contents, and aspiration remain unresolved. Several procedures to prevent reflux of gastric contents during enteral feeding, such as elevating the head of the bed, avoiding rapid infusion of large fluid volumes, and avoiding external pressure on the stomach, are simple to implement and probably helpful. Use of continuous versus intermittent bolus feedings and use of duodenal versus gastric placement of the feeding tube have not been studied in sufficient detail. If a regimen to prevent gastric stress ulcers is needed, it is prudent to use agents that do not elevate gastric pH (e.g., sucralfate), but it is not clear whether this actually reduces the incidence of nosocomial pneumonia. Finally, the effectiveness of selective decontamination of the digestive tract has been debated extensively, but large, double-blind, placebo-controlled trials in adults have not demonstrated an overall benefit.[146, 181] Cost and concern regarding the emergence of resistant bacteria also have discouraged widespread use.

Infections Related to Instrumentation of the Urinary Tract

Urinary tract infections are the most common nosocomial infection in hospitalized adults, accounting for approximately 40 per cent of all infections in this group.[169] In contrast, urinary tract infections constitute a much smaller proportion (10 per cent or less) of nosocomial infections in hospitalized children.[127, 202, 449] This difference can be explained in part by differences in urinary tract catheterization in these two populations. Data from the NNIS system indicate that indwelling urinary catheters are utilized about half as frequently in pediatric ICUs as they are in adult ICUs.[305] Indwelling urinary catheters are used infrequently in newborn ICU patients. On the other hand, the infectious risk associated with the use of indwelling urinary catheters is similar in adults and children. As shown in Table 228–2, rates of urinary tract infection associated with indwelling urinary catheters are only slightly lower in pediatric ICUs than in adult ICUs in U.S. hospitals participating in the NNIS system.[305]

Several studies have examined the descriptive epidemiology of urinary tract infections in pediatric patients.[97, 256, 257] In a prospective cohort study, catheterized patients were identified and followed prospectively for symptoms and signs of urinary tract infection (in which case a urinalysis and culture were performed); weekly urinalyses and urine cultures were performed, regardless of symptoms.[257] Nosocomial urinary tract infections in noncatheterized patients also were studied. Urinary tract infections were detected in 11 per cent of all catheterized patients, including 11 per cent of those in whom only indwelling catheterization was used, 9 per cent with both indwelling and intermittent catheterization, and 12 per cent with intermittent catheterization alone. The incidence density of infection was not reported. The median duration of catheterization preceding infection was 7 days (range, 2 to 77 days). Three quarters of the infections identified were symptomatic. No definite cases of secondary bacteremia were detected.

Additional information regarding the spectrum of nosocomial urinary tract infections in this study was provided by combining data from catheterized and noncatheterized patients.[257] Catheterization and female sex were identified as risk factors for urinary tract infection: 77 per cent of all infections occurred in catheterized patients, and 75 per cent of all infections occurred in females. The vast majority of infections in noncatheterized patients occurred in the newborn ICU and the preschool age ward. A wide range of underlying diagnoses were reported, but neurologic, renal, oncologic, orthopedic, or trauma-related diagnoses accounted for 50 per cent of cases.

There are no published data regarding rates of urinary tract infection associated with different types of indwelling catheters (e.g., urethral, suprapubic, ureteral, nephrostomy) in pediatric patients. In the authors' experience, infection (or at least bacteriuria or candiduria) is common in catheters that remain in place for long periods (i.e., more than 1 to 2 weeks), regardless of the type of catheter used. Data regarding the incidence of infection after cystoscopy, renal transplantation, or other types of urinary tract instrumentation in pediatric patients are not available. In the authors' experience, infections are uncommon after cystoscopy alone or urologic surgery in which preexisting infection or bacteriuria is not present and long-term use of indwelling catheters is not necessary. Bacteriuria and urinary tract infection appear to be more common among patients undergoing renal transplantation, although it is difficult to determine whether this is due to the use of urinary catheters in this population or inherent risks of the transplantation procedure itself.

Although no outbreaks of nosocomial urinary tract infection in pediatric patients have been reported, outbreaks in adult patients in the 1970s and 1980s were attributed to contamination of the urine-collecting system by nosocomial pathogens on the hands of hospital personnel, contaminated drainage pans and measuring containers, and use of inadequate or contaminated antiseptics.[56] Several outbreaks demonstrated that use of urinary catheters contributed to the emergence of antimicrobial resistance among gram-negative bacilli.[56] Antibiotics excreted in the urine provide selective pressure for the emergence of resistant populations of bacteria colonizing urine collection systems, and the large numbers of different types of bacteria present in these systems facilitate the transfer of resistant plasmids between species.[56]

Microorganisms associated with urinary tract infections in patients of all ages in U.S. hospitals participating in the NNIS system are displayed in Table 228–6.[117] One-quarter of infections are caused by *E. coli* alone, and another third are caused by various other gram-negative bacteria. *Enterococcus* species and various *Candida* species account for 16 per cent and 10 per cent of infections, respectively. The distribution of microorganisms in pediatric studies is similar,[97, 256, 257] except that the percentage of urinary tract infections attributed to coagulase-negative infections in newborn ICU patients has been reported to exceed 30 per cent.[97, 256]

Microbial colonization of the urine is the first step in the pathogenesis of urinary tract infection. A number of studies in catheterized adults have correlated microorganisms colonizing the urethral meatus with those most frequently causing infection.[56] These microorganisms can be carried into the bladder during catheter insertion, or, more commonly, once the catheter is in place they can migrate along the external surface of the catheter into the bladder. The shorter length of the urethra in females has been suggested as an explanation for their increased risk of infection. However, meatal colonization with pathogenic microorganisms, which also is more common in females, also may be important.[56] Distention of the urethra by the catheter, obstruction of periurethral glands, adherence of pathogenic microbes to the uroepithelium and the external surface of the catheter, and formation of a biofilm composed of host proteins and microbial exopolysaccharide on the external surface of the catheter all play a role in initiating infection, although the relative contributions of each of these factors is poorly understood.[56]

Microorganisms also may be introduced into the bladder from exogenous reservoirs. Although modern catheters and urine-collecting systems are "closed" systems, microorganisms may be introduced into the interior of the system at three points: the junction between the urinary catheter and the collecting system, the port used to aspirate urine specimens and irrigate the catheter, and the drainage spigot attached to the collection container. Some urinary catheters are fused to the collection system during manufacture, eliminating the possibility of junction disconnection, but such catheters are not in widespread use. Improper technique in the use of the aspiration/irrigation port or the spigot also may result in contamination of the interior surfaces of the system. Once microorganisms gain access to the interior of the catheter or collecting system, they can multiply quickly, reaching concentrations in the collection container exceeding 10^5 cfu/mL of urine in a matter of a few days. Encrustations on the interior surface of the system may serve as sites for microbial attachment and proliferation. Movement of microorganisms into the bladder is facilitated by obstruction of urine flow and reflux of urine into the bladder (i.e., raising the collection system above the level of the bladder), but many gram-negative bacteria are motile and can "swim" upstream, even if the system is maintained properly.

Microorganisms that reach the bladder multiply in the small, but persistent, reservoir of urine that is not drained completely by the catheter.[56] Infection (i.e., symptoms and signs of tissue invasion) is not an inevitable result of colonization of the bladder, and many chronically catheterized patients go for long periods with gross urine colonization but no clinical evidence of infection. Because many young children have vesicoureteral reflux, ascending infection involving the kidneys is a significant concern, but the epidemiologic studies discussed earlier have not demonstrated pyelonephritis and secondary bacteremia to be common problems.

The diagnosis of a nosocomial urinary tract infection depends heavily on the result of a quantitative urine culture. Urine specimens from noncatheterized patients should be obtained aseptically using one of three techniques: midstream clean-catch collection, "straight" catheterization of the bladder, or suprapubic aspiration. Cultures of urine specimens obtained from external bag collectors are of dubious value because they are contaminated frequently. Specimens from patients with indwelling urinary catheters should be obtained from the aspiration port because urine collected from the collection container may reflect colonization of this reservoir rather than infection.

Although diagnostic criteria for catheter-associated urinary tract infection vary, several definitions established for surveillance purposes generally are well accepted.[145] Symptomatic urinary tract infection is defined as the presence of symptoms or signs of infection (e.g., fever, urgency, frequency, dysuria, suprapubic tenderness) and a quantitative urine culture with more than 10^5 cfu/mL of urine of no more than two different species. Asymptomatic bacteriuria or candiduria (also called asymptomatic urinary tract infection in some studies, including the cohort study discussed earlier[257]) is defined as the absence of symptoms or signs of infection and a quantitative urine culture with more than 10^5 cfu/mL of urine of no more than two different species.[145] The diagnosis of asymptomatic bacteriuria is complicated by the fact that approximately 5 per cent of healthy school age and adolescent girls in the community have asymptomatic bacteriuria that may be detected only after hospitalization. A urinalysis showing evidence of pyuria (e.g., dipstick positive for leukocyte esterase or $\geq$10 white blood cells/mm^3 of urine) or nitrate provides corroborating evidence of infection, and a Gram stain of an unspun urine specimen is useful in guiding initial treatment decisions. However, it should be noted that patients with indwelling catheters and low-level bacteriuria ($<10^5$ cfu/mL of urine) tend to progress to frank bacteriuria with greater than or equal to 10^5 cfu/mL of urine within a few days if antibiotics are not administered.

The diagnosis of symptomatic urinary tract infection in patients with urinary catheters often is complicated by the fact that these patients do not manifest symptoms, such as urgency, frequency, and dysuria, and the assessment of abdominal pain and tenderness may be difficult in newborns and severely ill children in ICUs. Consequently, fever is the most commonly identified sign of infection in these patients, emphasizing the importance of a quantitative urine culture in the evaluation of a new fever in a hospitalized child.

Therapy for nosocomial urinary tract infection is similar to that for community-acquired infection, although parenteral therapy usually is used initially until secondary bacteremia is excluded. Empiric therapy should be based on knowledge of the relative frequency and susceptibility patterns of nosocomial pathogens in a given hospital. In the authors' institution, ampicillin and gentamicin is the most commonly used parenteral regimen for empiric therapy. If renal toxicity from the use of an aminoglycoside is a serious concern, use of trimethoprim-sulfamethoxazole, a third-generation cephalosporin, aztreonam, or a quinolone in older children is appropriate. If the Gram stain reveals only gram-negative bacilli, gentamicin alone is used because enterococcal infection is unlikely. If the Gram stain reveals only yeast, antifungal therapy (e.g., bladder irrigation with amphotericin, oral or parenteral fluconazole, parenteral amphotericin) is initiated instead. Once culture information is available, the treatment regimen can be tailored accordingly or discontinued if no infection is identified. Whenever possible, indwelling urinary catheters should be removed. Cases of asymptomatic bacteriuria (or asymptomatic candiduria) often resolve with removal of the catheter alone.

There are few data regarding the appropriate duration of therapy for nosocomial urinary tract infections. Although simple community-acquired cystitis in older children and adolescents often can be treated successfully with 1 to 3 days of oral therapy, it is prudent to treat uncomplicated hospital-acquired urinary tract infections for at least 7 days. If the infection is uncomplicated and the child has responded to therapy, oral therapy can be used to complete the course. Even pyelonephritis may be treated with oral agents if the pathogen is susceptible, but therapy should be extended to at least 14 days. Secondary bacteremia usually is treated parenterally. Treatment of asymptomatic candiduria with a short course (i.e., 5 days) of therapy is sufficient, but infection is likely to recur unless the catheter is removed. Likewise, infections involving nephrostomy or suprapubic catheters often recur if these catheters must remain in place. In cases in which nephrostomy tubes must be used for extended periods, the authors often use suppressive antimicrobial therapy after treatment is completed. Although there is a risk of secondary infection with resistant bacteria or yeast with this approach, this has not proved to be a significant problem.

The prospective cohort study discussed previously examined the consequences of nosocomial urinary tract infection during the 6 months after infection.[257] Four patients (7.8 per cent) suffered relapses, and one patient (2 per cent) suffered a reinfection. There were no deaths, and no additional complications were identified. The need for evaluation of vesicoureteral reflux or anatomic abnormalities of the kidney or urine-collecting system after a nosocomial urinary tract infection in infants or young children has not been evaluated. The authors do not perform these studies routinely if the infection appears to be related to a urinary catheter.

The CDC developed a comprehensive guideline for the prevention of nosocomial urinary tract infections in the mid-1980s.[462] Key features of the prevention of these infections are emphasized in the following paragraph.

Reducing unnecessary use of urinary catheters is the most effective preventative measure. Davies and colleagues[97] reduced the rate of nosocomial urinary tract infection in a pediatric ICU by 90 per cent over an 8-month period simply by instituting a policy whereby nurses automatically removed urinary catheters from patients after 48 to 72 hours unless a physician indicated that continued catheterization was necessary. Urinary catheters should be inserted by trained personnel using a careful aseptic technique after the meatus has been cleansed and an effective antiseptic (e.g., povidone-iodine) has been applied to the meatus and surrounding skin.[462] Contamination of the interior surfaces of the catheter and collection system can be minimized by maintaining a closed system (i.e., avoiding disruption of the connection between the catheter and the collection system), disinfecting the aspiration/irrigation port before accessing this port, and minimizing contamination of the spigot on the collection container.[462] The collecting system should be examined regularly to ensure that urine flow is not impeded, and care should be taken always to maintain the collection system in a dependent position relative to the bladder to prevent reflux of urine.[462] Treatment of preexisting urinary tract infection is important, especially among patients with underlying renal, urologic, or neurologic disease, in whom these infections are common.[462] Systemic antibiotics are effective in preventing urinary tract infection for short periods (5 days or less)[56]; however, routine use of antibiotics for this purpose is likely to facilitate the emergence of resistant pathogens. A wide variety of other interventions have been studied, most with limited or variable benefit.[56] Manufacturers continue to attempt to design a catheter that will resist adherence of microorganisms, minimize urethral trauma, or both. However, trials of these catheters have not been conclusive with regard to optimal characteristics of catheter design, and no studies in pediatric patients have been performed.

Infections Related to Surgical Procedures

Patients undergoing surgical procedures are at risk for a variety of nosocomial infections. A 1-year study of more than 600 pediatric patients undergoing surgical procedures found that surgical-site infection was the most common nosocomial infection after surgery, occurring in 3.5 per cent of patients.[40] Blood stream infection occurred in 2.3 per cent of patients, with one-half of these infections occurring in patients whose surgical procedure was insertion of a tunneled central venous catheter. Other reported infections included pneumonia (1.6 per cent), urinary tract infection (0.8 per cent), gastrointestinal infection due to rotavirus (0.3 per cent), and necrotizing enterocolitis (0.2 per cent). A report of nosocomial infections in pediatric patients undergoing cardiovascular surgery found that surgical-site infection and bacteremia accounted for 28 per cent and 27 per cent of all infections, respectively.[331]

Data from the handful of reports that have described the epidemiology of surgical site infections in general pediatric surgery patients are displayed in Table 228–9.[39, 96, 99, 106, 263, 392] These studies were performed in pediatric referral hospitals using prospective case-finding methods and definitions of surgical-site infections that are identical or similar to published criteria.[5, 460] Outpatient surgery was excluded in studies performed in the United States[39, 99]; studies in other countries did not state specifically whether these patients were included in their reports.[96, 106, 392] Postdischarge follow-up is a critical aspect of surveillance because 20 to 70 per cent of surgical-site infections may not be detected until after the patient has been discharged.[427] Follow-up methods have included direct observation by the investigators[39, 392] and a questionnaire mailed to surgeons 1 month after the surgery.[99]

As can be seen in Table 228–9, wound class was a powerful predictor of the likelihood of surgical-site infection in these studies. This is expected because wound classification was devised to predict the degree of microbial contamination of the wound and, consequently, the risk of infection.[5] Rates of infection by wound class in adult patients from U.S. hospitals participating in the NNIS system also are displayed in Table 228–9 and show similar, although less dramatic, step-ups in the risk of infection with increasing contamination of the wound. Infection rates vary considerably within wound class categories among the pediatric studies, suggesting that other factors must affect strongly the risk of infection. In fact, this has been well demonstrated in adult patients. A composite risk index developed through the analysis of data from the NNIS system, which includes measures of severity of illness (the ASA score) and duration of surgery in addition to wound class, is a much better predictor of surgical-site infection risk than wound class alone (see Table 228–4).[93]

The studies listed in Table 228–9 identified other specific risk factors for surgical-site infection in pediatric patients. Longer duration of surgery has been identified consistently as an important risk factor.[40, 96, 99, 106] This variable was identified as the strongest independent predictor of infection in the only study to employ logistic regression analysis.[99]

Several studies have found higher rates of infection in young children, especially neonates,[106, 263, 392] but others have not.[39, 99] Other identified risk factors have included prolonged preoperative hospital stay,[96, 99, 106] emergency surgery,[39, 106] longer length of incision,[96, 106] and the presence of underlying diseases.[39] The experience of the surgeon (i.e., resident vs.

TABLE 228–9. Cumulative Incidence of Surgical-Site Infection Rates by Wound Class* in Pediatric and Adult Patients

Ref.	Location	Year(s) of Study	Age Group	No. of Patients	Cumulative Incidence of Surgical-Site Infection by Wound Class (%)				
					Clean	*Clean-Contaminated*	*Contaminated*	*Dirty-Infected*	*Overall*
105	England	1973	Overall	329	3.5	16.0	37.5†	—	13.7
			Neonates	65	18.5	45.0	55.6†	—	38.4
			1 mo–1 y	54	16.0	20.0	33.3†	—	24.1
			1–5 y	73	2.5	33.3	44.4†	—	19.2
			>5 y	137	5.6	15.8	72.7†	—	12.4
98	United States	1980–1981	Overall	1045	3.1	7.8	16.7	9.7	4.2
389	India	NS	Overall	1325	1.8	5.8	27.0†	—	5.4
			Neonates	160	5.3	21.2	42.9†	—	13.8
			1 mo–1 y	326	2.4	3.9	33.3†	—	6.7
			1–5 y	396	1.0	5.0	25.5†	—	3.8
			>5 y	443	0.5	3.2	17.1†	—	2.9
95	England	1974–1987	Neonates	1094	11.1	20.9	20.5†	—	18.0
40	United States	1986–1988	Overall	676	1.0	2.9	7.9	6.3	2.5
			Neonates	137	—	—	—	—	0.7
			1 mo–1 y	197	—	—	—	—	4.1
			>1 y	342	—	—	—	—	2.3
261	England	NS	Neonates	143	3.9	11.3		16.7†	9.1
92	United States‡	1987–1990	Adults	84,691	2.1	3.3	6.4	7.1	

*Wound class as defined in Altemeier, W. A., Burke, J. F., and Sandusky, W. R. (eds.): Manual on Control of Infection in Surgical Patients. 2nd ed. Philadelphia, J. B. Lippincott, 1984.

†Combined contaminated and dirty-infected categories.

‡Data from U.S. hospitals participating in the NNIS system; modified from Culver, D. H., Horan, T. C., Gaynes, R. P., et al.: Surgical wound infection rates by wound class, operative procedure, and patient risk index. Am. J. Med. *91*:152S–157S, 1991.

Abbreviation: NS = not stated in the report.

attending surgeon) performing the surgery was not found to be a risk of infection in any of these studies.

Two types of surgical procedures—cardiovascular procedures and neurosurgical procedures—are discussed in the following paragraphs because of the particularly serious nature of surgical-site infections associated with these procedures.

A study of more than 300 children undergoing cardiovascular surgery found an infection rate of 7.1 per cent.[331] Surprisingly, infection rates in this study were lower among patients undergoing open heart surgery with cardiopulmonary bypass (6.7 per cent) than among patients undergoing closed heart surgery without bypass (8.1 per cent), but this difference was not statistically significant. Infection rates were higher among patients in whom the sternum was left open after surgery (27.6 per cent in patients with open sternums vs. 5.0 per cent in patients with closed sternums, $p < 0.001$) and among patients with higher PRISM scores (10.7 per cent in patients with PRISM scores ≥ 10 vs. 2.3 per cent in patients with PRISM scores < 10, $p < 0.01$). It is not clear from the data presented in this study whether an open sternum after surgery was an independent risk factor for infection or whether the increased risk of infection in patients with open sternums was attributable entirely or in part to increased severity of illness (i.e., higher PRISM score).

Rates of infection after cerebrospinal fluid shunting procedures vary widely, but many studies are dated, report rates of infection related to ventriculoatrial and ventriculoperitoneal shunts, involve small numbers of patients, or do not incorporate perioperative antimicrobial prophylaxis into the regimen of care routinely.[470] The largest pediatric series, a series of more than 500 patients undergoing ventriculoperitoneal shunting procedures performed in the late 1970s and early 1980s, the vast majority of whom received perioperative antimicrobial prophylaxis, reported an infection rate of 11 per cent.[313] Rates of infection were higher among patients with myelomeningocele and patients who had undergone previous shunting procedures. One-half of the infections occurred in the 2 weeks after surgery and were not associated commonly with simultaneous incisional infection.

Microorganisms associated with surgical-site infections in patients of all ages in U.S. hospitals participating in the NNIS system are displayed in Table 228–6.[117] Gram-positive cocci account for approximately one-half of the isolates. *S. aureus* is the most common isolate, but coagulase-negative staphylococci and *Enterococcus* species also are common. Gram-negative bacilli of various types make up another 40 per cent of isolates. *Bacteroides fragilis* and other anaerobic bacteria are isolated uncommonly, but it is unclear how frequently anaerobic cultures were performed. *C. albicans* and other *Candida* species are isolated from a minority (4 per cent) of surgical-site infections. This distribution of microorganisms is similar in the several studies of surgical-site infection in general pediatric surgery patients cited previously.[40, 96, 392] Studies of pediatric cardiovascular surgery patients have described a similar distribution of microorganisms.[115, 331] Gram-positive bacteria more commonly are the cause of cerebrospinal fluid shunt infections. In the large study cited previously, gram-positive bacteria accounted for three-fourths of the infections; coagulase-negative staphylococci were the cause of 40 per cent of the infections.[313]

The pathogenesis of surgical-site infection relates to the degree of microbial contamination of the wound, the condition of the host (both resistance to infection and the ability to heal the wound), and the conduct of the procedure itself. Microbial contamination of the surgical site occurs almost exclusively during the time the incision is open. This is likely to be the reason that longer duration of surgery is associated with increased risk of infection, although longer procedures also may reflect other factors that influence risk (i.e., complexity of the surgery, skill of the surgeon, care in dissection). If the incision is closed primarily, subsequent contamination of the site from external sources (i.e., use of contaminated antiseptics or dressings) is uncommon. The vast majority of the microorganisms contaminating open wounds are endogenous (i.e., microorganisms colonizing the skin and respiratory, gastrointestinal, and genitourinary tracts). Infrequent outbreaks of surgical-site infection caused by *S. aureus*, group A streptococci, and group C streptococci have been traced to personnel in the operating room (but not necessarily participating in the surgery itself) who are heavy shedders of these microorganisms, usually as a result of rectal, vaginal, or nasal carriage.[159, 358, 376] The inanimate environment of the operating room (e.g., walls, floors, other surfaces, surgical instruments) is a rare source of microorganisms causing surgical-site infections.[21] Postoperative hematogenous seeding of the surgical site can occur but is uncommon.

Host factors, such as underlying diseases (e.g., malignancy, uremia), the competence of the immune system, and nutritional status, are likely to be important, but the nature and degree to which these factors affect the risk of infection are not well described.

Even with careful skin preparation in clean surgery, small numbers of microorganisms are present at the surgical site of virtually every procedure, and careful surgical technique is necessary to avoid conditions that favor the growth of these microorganisms in the postoperative period. Damaged and devascularized tissue created by rough tissue handling and overuse of electrocautery is less resistant to infection.[5] Hematomas and seromas, which provide optimal growth conditions for bacteria, may develop if dead spaces are not obliterated or if hemostasis is inadequate.[5] Low-pressure suction drains are indicated to facilitate drainage of blood and secretions and to facilitate adherence of tissues and surfaces and promote wound healing.[5] To the extent that they accomplish this goal, surgical drains are useful. However, unnecessary use of drains should be avoided because they provide a portal of entry for microorganisms and may inhibit healing.

Consensus criteria for surgical-site infections developed through the collaborative efforts of the CDC, surgeons, and infection control professionals have been published.[194] Surgical-site infections are subcategorized into superficial incisional infections (involving the skin or subcutaneous tissues), deep incisional infections (involving the muscle or fascia), and organ/space infections (involving visceral organs or deep body spaces or cavities). For the most part, these criteria rely on observations made by direct inspection of the surgical site. Cultures of wound drainage are useful to determine the microbial etiology of the infection, but these criteria rely on the results of wound cultures only when wound drainage is not clearly purulent (i.e., serosanguineous drainage must be culture-positive for it to be considered as evidence of an infection). Stitch abscesses are not considered surgical-site infections.

Principles of the treatment of surgical-site infections are described elsewhere.[5] Significant fluid collections, especially collections of purulent material, should be drained. In some cases, fluid collections may be inaccessible or an attempt at drainage may compromise the patient seriously. In these cases, antimicrobial therapy alone may be successful in resolving the infection, although therapy needs to be chosen carefully to ensure adequate penetration into the area and to minimize the potential for emergence of antimicrobial resistance. Clinical response must be monitored closely. Devitalized tissue should be débrided, and any tension, pressure, or obstruction in the area should be relieved to allow adequate blood flow and drainage. Foreign bodies should be removed. For instance, cerebrospinal fluid shunt infections are unlikely to resolve without shunt removal.[470] In some special cases, antimicrobial therapy successfully can suppress infection with foreign bodies in place during postoperative healing (i.e., plates and screws to stabilize bones during healing after orthopedic procedures). However, removal of these devices generally is necessary to achieve complete cure. Systemic antimicrobial therapy should be prescribed for serious infections, but many superficial infections resolve with local care and application of topical antimicrobial agents.

A guideline developed by the CDC for the prevention of surgical-site infections is available,[143] as are other detailed references.[5, 463] The focus of the following paragraphs is on prevention measures that have the common goal of minimizing microbial contamination of the surgical site.

Preoperative interventions have a major effect on the nature and degree of microbial contamination of the surgical site. It is prudent to minimize preoperative hospitalization[143] because hospitalized patients are more likely to become colonized with "hospital flora" (e.g., methicillin-resistant staphylococci). Treatment of preexisting infections is important because microorganisms causing these infections may contaminate the surgical site,[143] but unnecessary therapy should be avoided because it increases the likelihood of colonization with antimicrobial-resistant microorganisms.

Preoperative bathing using an agent with antimicrobial activity is a logical prevention measure; however, several studies in adult general surgery patients have failed to demonstrate any benefit.[463] A comparative study of chlorhexidine versus iodophor shampoos before neurosurgical procedures in children demonstrated that chlorhexidine shampoos reduced the number of microorganisms on the scalp before surgery and the frequency of wound contamination; however, the number of patients studied was not sufficient to demonstrate any effect on infection rates.[241]

Although removing hair appears to provide a "cleaner" operative site, shaving the skin, especially when performed the day before surgery, has the paradoxical effect of increasing skin colonization by liberating resident skin flora from deeper skin structures and causing microscopic skin trauma that facilitates the growth of bacteria. If hair removal is necessary, hair should be clipped instead of shaved.[143] If shaving is necessary, it should be done immediately before surgery.[143]

Appropriately administered perioperative antimicrobial prophylaxis eradicates or at least retards the growth of bacteria that gain access to the surgical site. Numerous studies have examined the effectiveness of perioperative antimicrobial prophylaxis for various surgical procedures performed on adults, but few studies have been performed with pediatric patients. Consequently, recommendations regarding perioperative antimicrobial prophylaxis for pediatric surgery largely follow regimens recommended for use in adults.[7, 17] Prophylaxis should be administered within the 2 hours preceding the time of the surgical incision.[82] If prophylaxis is administered outside of this 2-hour window, effectiveness is diminished greatly; administration more than 6 hours after the incision essentially has no effect.[82] If the surgical procedure is prolonged, another dose should be administered after two half-lives of administered agent have elapsed (e.g., 4 to 6 hours for cefazolin). Additional doses in the postoperative period are unnecessary. Ensuring appropriate use and timing of perioperative antimicrobial prophylaxis is an important quality-of-care issue (see Chapter 229); likewise, ensuring that prophylaxis is not used unnecessarily is important for cost containment.

A variety of intraoperative practices and procedures are intended to prevent microbial contamination of the surgical site. However, the effectiveness of many of these measures either is minimal or has not been studied rigorously. Cleaning the skin and applying an antiseptic (e.g., alcohols, iodophors, chlorhexidine) reduce the number of viable bacteria at the surgical site.[239] The surgical hand scrub performed by members of the operative team using an effective antiseptic (e.g., alcohols, iodophors, chlorhexidine) reduces the number of bacteria on the hands and the potential for contamination of the surgical site through visible or microscopic breaks in surgical gloves.[239] Barriers worn by the surgical team (e.g., masks, caps, gowns) are a logical part of operating room practice and provide protection for the operative team against exposure to blood and body fluids, but there is little evidence that they substantially affect the risk of surgical-site infection.[463] Traffic and activity in the operating room increase the bacterial count in the air, and it is reasonable to keep the number of persons and movement to a minimum, although the effect on the risk of infection is likely to be minimal. Bacterial counts in the air also can be minimized by regularly servicing the operating room ventilation system and by maintaining adequate ventilation parameters (15 air changes with 3 changes of outside air per hour).[463] Laminar air flow and ultraviolet lights can decrease bacterial counts in the air to low levels, but their effectiveness in reducing the incidence of infections remains controversial.

Proper surgical technique also is important in the prevention of surgical-site infections, as discussed previously. A number of studies have demonstrated that confidential feedback of surgeon-specific rates of infection to individual surgeons reduces rates of infection.[427] This approach has been endorsed by the CDC, surgeons, and infection control professionals as a means by which individual surgeons may examine their own rates of infection and adjust their operative techniques accordingly.[427]

Infections Related to the Administration of Blood Products

The infectious risks associated with the administration of blood products have been summarized in a comprehensive review.[401] Blood-borne infections in health care personnel as a consequence of exposures that occur in the workplace are discussed in Chapter 229.

The blood supply in the United States now is safer than ever because of procedures to minimize infectious risks during blood donation and preparation of blood products. Prospective donors are provided written information on possible risk factors for blood-borne infections to encourage self-deferral of donation.[401] A face-to-face interview, a limited examination, and additional opportunities for self-deferral are provided.[401] This screening process alone is estimated to reduce the risk of transmission of HIV from a blood transfusion by 40 to 80 times.[105]

In addition to exclusion of persons with identified behavioral risk factors, persons who have lived in or have traveled to areas of the world where transfusion-transmissible infections are common are excluded from donation. For example, persons who have lived in areas of the world where malaria is prevalent are excluded from donation for a period of 3 years. This approach effectively has minimized transfusion-acquired malaria in the United States.[401] The need to exclude donors who have lived in rural areas of Latin America where Chagas disease is common is being considered in areas of the country with substantial immigrant populations.[401]

Donated blood is tested routinely for the following laboratory markers of infection: HIV-1 antibody, HIV-2 antibody, hepatitis B surface antigen (HBsAg), hepatitis B core antibody (HBcAb), hepatitis C antibody, human T-cell lymphotropic virus (HTLV)-I/II antibody, and nontreponemal antibody.[401] Serum alanine aminotransferase levels have been performed as an indirect screening test for donors with non-A, non-B hepatitis; however, a recent National Institutes of Health Consensus Panel has recommended discontinuation of this procedure because specific testing for hepatitis C now is available.[309]

Despite these measures, transfusion of blood containing infectious agents continues to occur because of "window" periods between the time of infection in the donor and the time that indirect markers of infection are detectable. The likelihood of transmission after transfusion of infected blood is high (80 to 90 per cent) for HIV-1, hepatitis B virus, and hepatitis C virus but is lower (20 to 30 per cent) for HTLV-I/II.[401] The risk of infection from a single unit of screened blood presently is estimated at 1:40,000 to 1:400,000 for HIV-1,[401] 1:200,000 for hepatitis B virus,[66] 1:3300 for hepatitis C virus (using a first-generation antibody assay),[107] and 1:70,000 for HTLV-I/II.[308] The estimated risk for hepatitis C virus infection undoubtedly has been reduced significantly by the availability of second-generation antibody assays.

Improvements in diagnostic tests may reduce window periods and the risks associated with administration of blood products. The window period for HIV-1 seroconversion is approximately 6 to 8 weeks using standard enzyme immunosorbent assays (EIAs). Newer EIAs appear to able to reduce the window period to approximately 4 weeks.[58] Direct virus-detection assays, such as p24 antigen tests and polymerase chain reaction for HIV RNA, can reduce the window period by another 6 to 10 days.[58] The usefulness of these newer tests presently is under evaluation.[401] Second-generation EIAs have reduced dramatically the window period for hepatitis C virus seroconversion, now estimated at about 4 weeks, and improved the sensitivity of this test in general.[401] Some patients recovering from acute, uncomplicated hepatitis B virus infection may have a window period when HBsAg, a direct marker of infection present early in the infection, disappears but hepatitis B surface antibody is not detectable yet.[401] Antibody to hepatitis core antigen (HBcAb) often is present during this period. For this reason, continued use of an assay for HBcAb is recommended.[309]

The incidence of blood stream infection as a result of bacterial contamination of blood products is not well defined but is estimated to be substantially higher than the incidence of transfusion-associated infection with HIV or hepatitis B virus.[440] A variety of skin flora, including coagulase-negative staphylococci, *S. aureus,* and dipththeroids, have been found to contaminate blood products, particularly platelet concentrates.[440] *Yersinia enterocolitica* blood stream infections have occurred in association with the administration of contaminated transfusions of red blood cells, presumably as a result of unrecognized bacteremia in the donors.[67] Half of the donors recalled a history of diarrhea within 30 days of donation. The particular propensity of this microorganism to grow at reduced temperatures is the likely explanation for this outbreak. Units of red blood cells should be inspected visually for darkening that can occur as a result of hemolysis and reduced oxygen content related to contamination.[401] Transfusion-associated syphilis is extremely rare because of the screening of donated blood and the fact that spirochetes do not survive in refrigerated, citrate-anticoagulated blood for longer than 72 hours.[401]

Transfusion-associated CMV infection is uncommon, despite the fact that most blood donors are positive for antibody to CMV.[401] Transfusion-acquired infection with CMV is mild or asymptomatic in most immunocompetent hosts but may be severe in CMV antibody–negative immunocompromised recipients and newborns.[401] Superinfection with a new strain of CMV in CMV antibody–positive immunocompromised persons has been described.[401] Risk of infection is confined to transfusion of cellular components and can be reduced dramatically by procedures that ensure depletion of white blood cells, either by filtration or additional centrifugation of red blood cells or platelets.[401] Transfusion of blood products from CMV antibody–negative donors is another strategy to prevent transmission to high-risk recipients.

Hepatitis A virus may be transmitted by transfusion from donors who are viremic but who have not manifested clinical features of infection yet. Transfusion-associated infection has been reported primarily in relation to hepatitis A virus outbreaks in newborn nurseries and ICUs (see Nosocomial Infections Due to Spread of Infections Common in the Community, Hepatitis A Virus).

Immigration of persons from rural areas of Central and South America, where infection with the protozoan *Trypanosoma cruzi* (the etiologic agent of Chagas disease) is common, has raised concern regarding the potential for transfusion-associated infection caused by this agent in the United States.[385, 401] Transfusion-associated infections are well described in other countries, and several cases have been reported in the United States and Canada.[385] This organism survives well in blood and in components frozen or stored for 21 days at 4° C.[401] The risk for this infection is highest where immigrant populations are substantial, particularly southern California and Texas. Predonation screening to eliminate persons from endemic areas as donors may be helpful. Tests for screening donated blood for antibody against *T. cruzi* also are available.

New infectious threats related to transfusion of blood products continue to arise. In 1994, cases of hepatitis C virus infection were associated with the receipt of a contaminated intravenous immunoglobulin preparation from a specific manufacturer.[71] Manufacturing processes for intravenous immunoglobulin have been modified subsequently to include solvent-detergent treatment, which is designed to inactivate contaminating viruses.[20] However, there presently is concern about the possibility of parvovirus contamination of clotting factors[243] and the potential for HIV variants, which are not detected by current antibody assays, to contaminate the blood supply.[108]

Nosocomial infection with blood-borne pathogens also may occur through means other than transfusion with blood products. Indirect transmission of hepatitis B virus has been demonstrated to result from inadequately disinfected instruments, such as a device used for fingerstick glucose measurements,[327] and is a well-documented problem for both patients and health care workers in hemodialysis units.[123] For this reason, most dialysis units physically separate HbsAg-positive patients from uninfected patients.[123] Hepatitis B vaccine is encouraged strongly for all dialysis patients and health care workers in dialysis units.[123] The risk of hepatitis C virus transmission through indirect transmission is not clear at present, although studies in hemodialysis units suggest that hepatitis C virus transmission may occur in this setting.[123] HIV transmission has been documented in a dialysis center in South America as the result of inadequate disinfection procedures[437] and in other countries as the result of reusing needles.[46] A possible case of HIV transmission in a pediatric ward in the United States has been reported, although extensive investigation failed to reveal a source of the infection.[43]

Infections Related to Endoscopy

Few systematic, prospective studies of infection after endoscopy have been performed, and there essentially are no data regarding rates of infection specifically in children. In general, however, infectious complications after endoscopy are uncommon,[22, 275, 405] especially given the large number of procedures performed.

Endoscopy-related infections may be from exogenous (i.e., contamination of the endoscope) or endogenous (i.e., transfer of microorganisms from one body site to another during the procedure) sources.[22, 275] Exogenous infections have been reported more frequently.[22, 275, 405] Improper cleaning and disinfection procedures may result in transmission of microorganisms from one patient to another,[405] and even conscientious reprocessing may be foiled by the complicated design of many endoscopes.[405] Exogenous infections also can be caused by the contamination of endoscopes during reprocessing itself. Even apparently sophisticated, automated reprocessing machines are not immune to this problem, as evidenced by some reports.[6, 65, 405] An outbreak of pseudoinfection (i.e., exogenous contamination of culture specimens) from contaminated endoscopes also has been described.[65]

The most common endogenous infection is transient bacteremia, which can occur after instrumentation of the gastrointestinal, respiratory, or genitourinary tracts.[22, 275] Most patients do not develop clinical symptoms, but endocarditis has been reported.[22, 275] Cholangitis is a significant complication of endoscopic retrograde cholangiopancreatography, especially when there is biliary tract obstruction.[22, 275] Pneumonia after bronchoscopy, wound infection and perforation of the intestine associated with operative endoscopy (e.g., cholecystectomy), and joint infection after arthroscopy also have been reported.[22]

A summary of published reports found that *Salmonella* species and *P. aeruginosa* were the most common etiologic agents present after gastrointestinal endoscopy.[405] Infection due to other gram-negative enteric bacilli (e.g., *Klebsiella* species, *Enterobacter* species, and *S. marcescens*), enterococci, and *Helicobacter pylori* also occurs.[405] *M. tuberculosis,* atypical mycobacteria, and *P. aeruginosa* were the most commonly reported causes of pneumonia present after bronchoscopy.[405] One case of hepatitis B virus transmission via gastrointestinal endoscopy has been described.[405]

Proper reprocessing procedures are critical for the prevention of exogenous infection after endoscopic procedures. Reprocessing requirements vary according to the intended use of the endoscope (i.e., entry into sterile tissues or cavities vs. contact only with mucous membranes), tolerance of the equipment to various reprocessing methods (i.e., steam sterilization, immersion in liquid disinfectants/sterilants, or both), and the specified turnaround time. Detailed reviews of reprocessing procedures have been published recently.[22, 275, 405]

Antimicrobial prophylaxis for endoscopy is controversial. At a minimum, it is prudent to administer appropriate antimicrobial prophylaxis to patients at risk for endocarditis during procedures with a potential for transient bacteremia (e.g., procedures involving instrumentation of the gastrointestinal, respiratory, and genitourinary tracts), during endoscopic retrograde cholangiopancreatography, and during cystoscopy performed in the presence of probable or confirmed bacteriuria.[22]

NOSOCOMIAL INFECTIONS IN SPECIAL POPULATIONS

Newborn Infants

Healthy newborns are thrust into the world quickly, becoming colonized with microorganisms derived from their mothers and the immediate environment within several days. Predominant colonizers are coagulase-negative staphylococci on the skin and umbilicus and in the nose and alpha-hemolytic streptococci in the mouth. Colonization of the gastrointestinal tract is more complex: lactobacilli predominate in breast-fed babies, whereas more "adult" flora composed of *Bacteroides* species, other anaerobes, and *E. coli* colonize formula-fed babies.[155] These commensals help resist colonization with pathogenic microorganisms. Because pathogens can spread quickly in crowded nurseries, rooming-in and early discharge reduce the potential for transmission to normal newborns. However, early discharge also makes it more difficult to detect significant problems when they occur. For instance, the incubation period for *S. aureus* infection generally is longer than a newborn's stay in the hospital, and significant outbreaks can escape detection unless an aggressive reporting system is established.[185, 262]

Premature and full-term infants requiring care in newborn ICUs face a far different fate. Colonization of these infants is delayed substantially, perhaps because of limited contact with their mothers, delayed enteral feeding, and administration of parenteral antimicrobial agents.[155] When colonization does occur, it is with markedly different microorganisms. Coagulase-negative staphylococci colonize the skin, umbilicus, and nose of these infants as well[155]; however, recent molecular typing studies have demonstrated that particular strains of coagulase-negative staphylococci can persist in newborn ICUs over extended periods, being transmitted on the hands of caregivers and causing blood stream infection in some infants.[197, 260, 318] *S. aureus* may colonize a variety of sites, particularly the umbilicus and nose.[155] Although lactobacilli and anaerobes still colonize the gut, aerobic gram-negative bacilli, including *E. coli, Klebsiella* species, *Enterobacter* species, *P. aeruginosa, S. marcescens,* and *Citrobacter* species, account for a much larger proportion of the intestinal flora than in normal newborns.[155] Antimicrobial-resistant strains of these bacteria are a particular problem in many newborn ICUs. Because these bacteria can reach concentrations in the stool of 10^6 to 10^8 cfu/g, it is not surprising that the hands of caregivers are contaminated easily, providing an important route of nosocomial transmission. *Enterococcus* and *Candida* can become established on the skin and umbilicus and in the gut,[155] again because of contamination of the hands of caregivers and selection pressure imposed by treatment with antimicrobial agents. Unfortunately, the medical devices that help sustain these infants, such as intravascular catheters and mechanical ventilation, provide portals of entry for these microorganisms to invade sterile sites and cause infection (see Nosocomial Infections Related to Invasive Devices, Procedures, and Treatments).

Hand washing, preferably with an agent with antimicrobial activity, is the most effective intervention to prevent spread of pathogenic microorganisms. However, the hands of some staff members may remain colonized with these microorganisms for prolonged periods, despite scrupulous hand washing.[155] Other general recommendations regarding the prevention of nosocomial infections in normal nurseries and newborn ICUs have been published, including recommendations regarding the design of facilities, staffing, and procedures.[133, 157]

Several novel approaches have been tested for their effectiveness in preventing nosocomial infection in high-risk infants. A number of investigators purposefully colonized infants in newborn ICUs with nonpathogenic microorganisms in order to "interfere" with colonization by potential pathogens.[157] Some of these studies have demonstrated favorable results, but the consequences of this intervention have not been studied sufficiently and the practice has not gained wide acceptance.

Several well-designed trials have examined the effectiveness of intravenous immunoglobulin in preventing nosocomial infection in premature infants[27, 120, 220, 265, 448]; however, only one trial demonstrated any benefit in reducing overall nosocomial infection rates.[27] A recent evaluation of the opsonic activity of commercially available standard intravenous immunoglobulin preparations demonstrated a large degree of variability in opsonic activity against common neonatal pathogens among lots produced by various manufacturers.[447] Individual lots also demonstrated variable levels of opsonic activity against different pathogens.[447] This variability appeared to be a function of the donor pool rather than the manufacturing method.[447] It remains to be seen whether intravenous preparations with known pathogen-specific antibody content may be effective in reducing nosocomial infections with specific agents.

Preceding sections have described a variety of microorganisms generally regarded as community pathogens that often cause outbreaks of nosocomial infection in nurseries and newborn ICUs, including RSV and other respiratory viruses, rotavirus, *Salmonella* and other enteric bacterial pathogens, herpes simplex virus, CMV, hepatitis A virus, and enteroviruses. Specific interventions to prevent these infections have been discussed previously (see Nosocomial Infections Due to Spread of Infections Common in the Community).

Other important pathogens in normal newborn nurseries and newborn ICUs are highlighted in the following paragraphs.

S. aureus remains a significant pathogen in newborn infants, although not nearly to the degree it was in the 1950s and 1960s. Staphylococcal skin and soft tissue infections, including superficial skin infections, mastitis, and omphalitis, are the most common infections; severe staphylococcal pneumonia now is rare.[376] Because newborns are not colonized with this organism at birth, it must be transmitted to them postnatally. Direct contact with colonized caregivers is the predominant mode of transmission.[376] Indirect contact transmission from infected or colonized infants and droplet contact transmission from infants with coexisting viral respiratory tract infection (so-called "cloud babies") are uncommon.[376] Colonization of the skin, nose, and umbilicus precedes infection, but rates of colonization correlate poorly with rates of infection. Typically, the number of colonized infants far exceeds the number of infected infants[376]; conversely, outbreaks of staphylococcal infection can occur in nurseries with low colonization rates.[376] For this reason and because of cost considerations, surveillance cultures to detect colonized infants are not recommended except under outbreak conditions.

Barrier precautions (e.g., gloves, gowns) and hand washing are effective means of preventing transmission of *S. aureus* from heavily colonized or infected infants. The use of hexachlorophene (3 per cent) for bathing is effective in reducing colonization,[157] but this agent was found to cause cystic degenerative changes in the white matter of premature infants,[334, 397, 398] although there was no evidence that this agent posed a hazard to full-term infants. A warning against use of hexachlorophene was issued by the Food and Drug Administration in 1972. The use of this agent for infant bathing remains an option during outbreaks of *S. aureus* infection, although it should be diluted by 1:4 or 1:5 in water and should not be used for bathing very low birth weight infants.[157] Chlorhexidine is a reasonable alternative because it has good antistaphylococcal activity and studies in neonates have demonstrated negligible absorption after bathing or cord care and no recognized toxicity.[4, 89, 211] Use of iodophors may cause adsorption of iodine, and alcohols may cause chemical burns, so these agents should not be used for bathing. A variety of agents have been used for cord care, including triple dye (an aqueous mixture of brilliant green, proflavine hemisulfate, and crystal violet), alcohol, bacitracin, chlorhexidine, and mupirocin, although extensive efficacy and safety data are not available for any of these compounds.[157]

Fifty to seventy-five per cent of women with group B streptococcal vaginal colonization transmit this microorganism to their newborn infants, although only 1 to 2 per cent of colonized infants become infected. The CDC defines these and other infections transmitted via the birth canal as nosocomial infections.[145, 148] The logic behind this designation has not been stated explicitly, but because these infections occur after an event (i.e., delivery) usually associated with medical care, it is reasonable to consider them nosocomial infections. However, the impact of conventional infection control interventions on early-onset (i.e., within the first 7 days of life) invasive group B streptococcal infection is likely to be limited. Selected intrapartum prophylaxis of women colonized with group B streptococci who have risk factors for infection is far more effective intervention to reduce infection rates in newborns.[11] It is important to note that group B streptococci can be associated with nosocomial infection, not just perinatal infection. Outbreaks of group B streptococcal infection due to indirect contact transmission in nurseries have been well documented.[114, 156, 312]

Citrobacter diversus has been responsible for a number of outbreaks of nosocomial infection in newborn infants.[249, 316, 459] Although most infants colonized with this microorganism do not develop clinical disease, infection almost always results in meningitis due to the particular neurotropism of this bacteria (see General Epidemiology of Nosocomial Infections, Interactions Between Hosts and Pathogens) and usually is accompanied by formation of one or more brain abscesses. Outbreaks of infection caused by these bacteria may occur sporadically over an extended period.[249, 316, 459] Transmission of these bacteria on the hands of caregivers has been implicated in several of these outbreaks.[316, 459] On the other hand, molecular techniques have demonstrated that *C. diversus* also can be acquired perinatally by vertical transmission.[184]

Immunocompromised Children

The greatest nosocomial infection threats to immunocompromised children are those discussed previously (see Nosocomial Infections Due to Spread of Infections Common in the Community and Nosocomial Infections Related to Invasive Devices, Procedures, and Treatments). However, several issues regarding the epidemiology and prevention of nosocomial infections in these high-risk patients deserve additional comment.

Candida species and other yeasts (e.g., *Malassezia furfur, Candida glabrata, Trichosporon belgii)* are significant nosocomial pathogens in immunocompromised children because these hosts have impaired host defenses and because they often require invasive devices (such as central venous catheters), parenteral nutrition, and broad-spectrum antimicrobial therapy. The spectrum of disease includes superficial infection (e.g., mucocutaneous candidiasis), blood stream infection associated with central venous catheters, and disseminated infection (e.g., meningitis, hepatosplenic infection, renal infection, ophthalmitis). Granulocytopenia greatly increases the risk of disseminated disease.[203] Although generally regarded as endogenous flora, molecular epidemiologic studies have demonstrated that specific *Candida* strains can be acquired within the hospital by indirect contact transmission.[375, 436] Hand washing and use of standard precautions (see Chapter

229) when caring for high-risk patients are likely to be helpful in reducing nosocomial transmission of *Candida* species.

Herpes simplex virus and varicella-zoster virus also are common causes of infection in hospitalized immunocompromised patients; however, reactivation of a preexisting latent infection is more frequent than primary infection. Development of a lymphoproliferative disorder secondary to reactivation of Epstein-Barr virus is a significant complication of solid-organ transplantation (particularly liver, heart, and heart/lung transplants) and T-cell–depleted allogeneic bone marrow transplants. Primary nosocomial CMV infection is a particular problem in allogeneic bone marrow or solid-organ transplant patients because the scarcity of suitable donors does not allow selection of CMV-negative donors for CMV-negative recipients. Prophylaxis to prevent disease in immunocompromised patients related to herpesviruses is discussed in detail in other chapters.

Nosocomial respiratory virus infections can be severe and prolonged in patients with profoundly compromised immune systems (see Nosocomial Infections Due to Spread of Infections Common in the Community). A number of outbreaks of nosocomial multidrug-resistant tuberculosis in adult patients with HIV infection have been reported,[32, 87] although this has not proved to be a significant problem among HIV-infected children thus far.

Although far less common, *Legionella* and filamentous fungi cause serious, potentially lethal disease in immunocompromised children.[50, 441] The principal reservoir for *Legionella* is the hospital water supply, particularly aging systems with large dead spaces.[422] Contaminated aerosols generated by shower heads, faucet aerators, and even bed pan cleaners may lead to nosocomial disease.[422] Decontamination of the water supply is a difficult and expensive endeavor. The most cost-effective approach among those described in the CDC/HICPAC guideline for prevention of nosocomial pneumonia has not been determined.[422]

Spores of *Aspergillus* and other filamentous fungi virtually are ubiquitous wherever there is decaying organic matter or moisture. Airborne spores may enter the hospital through inadequate air filtration systems and open windows or doors. Spores also may originate from within the hospital (e.g., air ducts, wet wood or plaster, fireproofing materials, soil of plants, pepper). Hospital construction may release clouds of fungal spores, and, once in the hospital, spores can survive indefinitely in dust.

Patients with prolonged severe neutropenia, such as bone marrow transplant patients, are at serious risk for invasive pulmonary aspergillosis and should be cared for in environments that are protected from contamination by fungal spores as much as possible. The following characteristics are recommended in the CDC/HICPAC guideline for prevention of nosocomial pneumonia: (1) filtration of incoming air using central or point-of-use high-efficiency particulate air filters that are 99.97 per cent efficient in filtering 0.3 μm-sized particles, (2) directed room airflow from the intake on one side of the room, across the patient, and out through the exhaust on the opposite side of the room, (3) positive room-air pressure relative to the corridor, (4) well-sealed rooms, (5) high rates of room-air changes (≥12 per hour).[422] The effectiveness of protected environments using laminar airflow (a bank of high-efficiency particulate air filters along an entire wall pumping air at a uniform velocity across the patient and out the door of the room, achieving room-air exchange rates of 100 to 400 changes per hour) in reducing the incidence of invasive pulmonary aspergillosis in bone marrow transplant patients has been demonstrated.[422] However, these systems are expensive to install and maintain. The effectiveness of less expensive alternatives that do not achieve laminar airflow but conform to the recommendations listed earlier has not been studied sufficiently.[422]

Children with Burns

Rates of nosocomial infections in patients with burns are among the highest for any group of hospitalized patients (see Tables 228–1 and 228–2). Information regarding the epidemiology of nosocomial infections in pediatric burn patients is limited to a single retrospective case review,[384] which found a cumulative incidence of nosocomial infection of 14 per cent among 224 pediatric patients in two burn units over a 7½-year period. The surprisingly low infection rate and low mortality rate (only one death was caused by nosocomial infection) may be attributable to the limited number of patients with extensive burns in these units (only 8 per cent had full-thickness burns involving 20 per cent of body surface area). Burn wound infection, urinary tract infection, pneumonia, and blood stream infection each accounted for approximately one-fifth of all infections. Patients with full-thickness burn involving 20 per cent or more of body surface area were more likely to develop a burn wound infection, and patients with smoke inhalation injury were more likely to develop pneumonia. The vast majority of urinary tract infections were associated with the use of indwelling urinary catheters. Blood stream infections and local catheter insertion site infections were associated with the use of central venous catheters. In an older study of viral infections in pediatric burn patients, CMV infection was relatively common, perhaps in part because of transfusion-related infection.[252] Isolation of herpes simplex virus from pharyngeal and perioral cultures also was common, but clinical symptoms were infrequent.

Interventions to reduce the incidence of nosocomial infections in burn patients include use of barrier techniques to reduce cross-colonization of patients, prevention of cross-colonization during hydrotherapy treatments, use of topical antibiotics to retard growth of microorganisms in the burn wound, appropriate use of systemic antibiotics, and early excision and closure of the burn wound.[279] Care of high-risk patients in single-bed isolation rooms (as opposed to beds on open wards) appears to reduce the risk of infection,[285] although this intervention has not been subjected to a controlled trial. A recent study outlined an effective program for the control of methicillin-resistant *S. aureus* in a pediatric burn unit that also may be applicable to the control of other antimicrobial-resistant microorganisms.[396]

Children with Cystic Fibrosis

Epidemiologic and molecular typing studies have demonstrated person-to-person transmission of *B. (Pseudomonas) cepacia* among children with cystic fibrosis.[421] This finding, coupled with the association of *B. cepacia* colonization and a rapid decline in pulmonary function in some cystic fibrosis patients,[423] has fueled debate regarding the risk of nosocomial transmission of pulmonary pathogens in these patients. Data suggest that person-to-person transmission of *B. cepacia* may occur after close and prolonged contact,[421] direct hand contact,[320] and contact with contaminated respiratory therapy equipment.[55] However, the frequency of transmission in hospitals, the exact mechanisms involved in transmission, and the effectiveness of various prevention measures still are unresolved. The relevance of these findings to the transmission of other pulmonary pathogens in children with cystic fibrosis, including multidrug-resistant *P. aeruginosa*, *S. (Xan-*

thomonas) maltophilia, atypical mycobacteria, and methicillin-resistant *S. aureus*, also is unclear.

Segregation of persons with cystic fibrosis who are colonized with *B. cepacia* from those who are not colonized may reduce the risk of transmission.[428] However, this intervention logistically may be difficult to apply and, in the opinion of some, unnecessarily stigmatizes colonized patients. The recently published CDC/HICPAC guideline for isolation precautions in hospitals advises against placing colonized and noncolonized patients in the same room and suggests that noncolonized persons with cystic fibrosis may elect to wear a mask when within 3 feet of a colonized person.[144]

In an effort to prevent transmission of potential pathogens among cystic fibrosis patients without classifying them into specific groups, the authors' institution has developed a policy that applies to all cystic fibrosis patients regardless of their colonization status. Patients are educated to avoid contact with mucous membranes or any items contaminated with respiratory secretions from other cystic fibrosis patients; to avoid coming within an arm's length (<3 feet) of other cystic fibrosis patients; and to "smile, wink, or wave" greetings to other patients, rather than shake hands, hug, or kiss. Patients also are instructed to wash their hands with an antimicrobial soap after contact with their own respiratory secretions or items contaminated with their respiratory secretions. Cystic fibrosis patients (except members of the same household) are not allowed to be roommates.

Children in Long-Term Care Facilities

Preceding sections have described a variety of microorganisms that have caused disease in long-term care facilities for children, including various viral infections and enteric pathogens. Specific interventions to prevent these infections were discussed earlier (see Nosocomial Infections Due to Spread of Infections Common in the Community).

A prospective, longitudinal study of nosocomial infections in a pediatric long-term care facility illustrates the spectrum of endemic nosocomial infections in this population.[438] The cumulative incidence of infection was 40 per cent among the more than 400 patients cared for in this facility over a 2-year period. Upper respiratory tract infections and urinary tract infections accounted for 37 and 31 per cent of infections, respectively. Nearly 80 per cent of the urinary tract infections occurred in a small group of patients with neural tube defects or neuromuscular disorders, but the study did not differentiate between symptomatic infections and asymptomatic bacteriuria. The rate of infection among children exposed to indwelling or intermittent catheterization also was not reported. Upper and lower respiratory tract infections were common among young children with tracheostomies. Skin infections accounted for 16 per cent of infections, but the specific percentage of decubitus ulcers was not reported. Gastrointestinal infections were remarkably uncommon (4 per cent of all nosocomial infections).

Prevention of nosocomial infections in this population rests primarily on hand washing, proper care of patients with indwelling devices (e.g., tracheostomies) or who require invasive procedures (e.g., bladder catheterization), prevention of decubitus ulcers, age-appropriate immunization (including yearly influenza vaccine, hepatitis B vaccine, and, depending on local epidemiologic conditions, hepatitis A vaccine), and early detection and control of outbreaks of infection.

References

1. Adams, G., Stover, B. H., Keenlyside, R. A., et al.: Nosocomial herpetic infections in a pediatric intensive care unit. Am. J. Epidemiol. *113*:126–132, 1981.
2. Adler, S. P.: Hospital transmission of cytomegalovirus. Infect. Agents Dis. *1*:43–49, 1992.
3. Agah, R., Cherry, J. D., Garakian, A. J., et al.: Respiratory syncytial virus (RSV) infection rate in personnel caring for children with RSV infections: Routine isolation procedure vs routine procedure supplemented by use of masks and goggles. Am. J. Dis. Child. *141*:695–697, 1987.
4. Aggett, P. J., Cooper, L. V., Ellis, S. H., et al.: Percutaneous absorption of chlorhexidine in neonatal cord care. Arch. Dis. Child. *56*:878–880, 1981.
5. Altemeier, W. A., Burke, J. F., and Sandusky, W. R. (eds.): Manual on Control of Infection in Surgical Patients. 2nd ed. Philadelphia, J. B. Lippincott, 1984.
6. Alvarado, C. J., Stolz, S. M., and Maki, D. G.: Nosocomial infections from contaminated endoscopes: A flawed automated endoscope washer: An investigation using molecular epidemiology. Am. J. Med. *91*:272S–280S, 1991.
7. American Academy of Pediatrics: Antimicrobial prophylaxis in pediatric surgery patients. *In* Peter G (ed.): 1994 Red Book: Report of the Committee on Infectious Diseases. 23rd ed. Elk Grove, American Academy of Pediatrics, 1994, pp. 535–539.
8. American Academy of Pediatrics: Hepatitis A. *In* Peter, G. (ed.): 1994 Red Book: Report of the Committee on Infectious Diseases. 23rd ed. Elk Grove, American Academy of Pediatrics, 1994, pp. 221–224.
9. American Academy of Pediatrics: Measles. *In* Peter, G. (ed.): 1994 Red Book: Report of the Committee on Infectious Diseases. 23rd ed. Elk Grove, American Academy of Pediatrics, 1994, pp. 308–323.
10. American Academy of Pediatrics: Varicella-zoster infections. *In* Peter, G. (ed.): 1994 Red Book: Report of the Committee on Infectious Diseases. 23rd ed. Elk Grove, American Academy of Pediatrics, 1994, pp. 510–517.
11. American Academy of Pediatrics Committee on Infectious Diseases and Committee on Fetus and Newborn: Guidelines for prevention of group B streptococcal (GBS) infection by chemoprophylaxis. Pediatrics *90*:775–778, 1992.
12. Anderson, J. D., Bonner, M., Scheifele, D. W., et al.: Lack of nosocomial spread of varicella in a pediatric hospital with negative pressure ventilated patient rooms. Infect. Control *6*:120–121, 1985.
13. Anderson, J. R., Smith, M. D., Kibbler, C. C., et al.: A nosocomial outbreak due to non-encapsulated *Haemophilus influenzae*: Analysis of plasmids coding for antibiotic resistance. J. Hosp. Infect. *27*:17–27, 1994.
14. Anderson, L. J.: Major trends in nosocomial viral infections. Am. J. Med. *91*:107S–111S, 1991.
15. Anderson, L. J., Williams, L., Jr., Layde, J. B., et al.: Nosocomial rabies: Investigation of contacts of human rabies cases associated with a corneal transplant. Am. J. Public Health *74*:370–372, 1984.
16. Anderson, M. J., Higgins, P. G., Davis, L. R., et al.: Experimental parvoviral infection in humans. J. Infect. Dis. *152*:257–265, 1985.
17. Anonymous: Antimicrobial prophylaxis in surgery. Med. Lett. Drugs Ther. *35*:91–93, 1993.
18. Ansari, S. A., Sattar, S. A., Springthorpe, V. S., et al.: Rotavirus survival on human hands and transfer of infectious virus to animate and nonporous inanimate surfaces. J. Clin. Microbiol. *26*:1513–1518, 1988.
19. Atkinson, W. L., Markowitz, L. E., Adams, N. C., et al.: Transmission of measles in medical settings: United States, 1985–1989. Am. J. Med. *91*:320S–324S, 1991.
20. AuBuchon, J. P., and Birkmeyer, J. D.: Safety and cost-effectiveness of solvent-detergent–treated plasma: In search of a zero-risk blood supply. J. A. M. A. *272*:1210–1214, 1994.
21. Ayliffe, G. A.: Role of the environment of the operating suite in surgical wound infection. Rev. Infect. Dis. *13*:S800–S804, 1991.
22. Ayliffe, G. A.: Nosocomial infections associated with endoscopy. *In* Mayhall, C. G. (ed.): Hospital Epidemiology and Infection Control. Baltimore, Williams & Wilkins, 1995, pp. 680–693.
23. Azimi, P. H., Roberto, R. R., Guralnik, J., et al.: Transfusion-acquired hepatitis A in a premature infant with secondary nosocomial spread in an intensive care nursery. Am. J. Dis. Child. *140*:23–27, 1986.
24. Aznar, J., Safi, H., Romero, J., et al.: Nosocomial transmission of tuberculosis infection in pediatrics wards. Pediatr. Infect. Dis. J. *14*:44–48, 1995.
25. Bachrach, S.: An outbreak of *Haemophilus influenzae* type b bacteraemia in an intermediate care hospital for children. J. Hosp. Infect. *11*:121–126, 1988.
26. Bachrach, S. J.: Successful treatment of an institutional outbreak of shigellosis. Clin. Pediatr. *20*:127–131, 1981.
27. Baker, C. J., Melish, M. E., Hall, R. T., et al.: Intravenous immune globulin for the prevention of nosocomial infection in low-birth-weight neonates. N. Engl. J. Med. *327*:213–219, 1992.
28. Baron, R. C., McCormick, J. B., and Zubeir, O. A.: Ebola virus disease in southern Sudan: Hospital dissemination and intrafamilial spread. Bull. W. H. O. *61*:997–1003, 1983.
29. Barton, L. L., Granoff, D. M., and Barenkamp, S. J.: Nosocomial spread of *Haemophilus influenzae* type b infection documented by outer membrane protein subtype analysis. J. Pediatr. *102*:820–824, 1983.
30. Barzilay, Z., Mandel, M., Keren, G., et al.: Nosocomial bacterial pneumonia in ventilated children: Clinical significance of culture-positive peripheral bronchial aspirates. J. Pediatr. *112*:421–424, 1988.
31. Beatson, S. H.: Pharaoh's ants as pathogen vectors in hospitals. Lancet *1*:425–427, 1972.

32. Beck-Sague, C., Dooley, S. W., Hutton, M.D., et al.: Hospital outbreak of multidrug-resistant *Mycobacterium tuberculosis* infections: Factors in transmission to staff and HIV-infected patients. J. A. M. A. *268*:1280–1286, 1992.
33. Beck-Sague, C. M., and Jarvis, W. R.: Epidemic bloodstream infections associated with pressure transducers: A persistent problem. Infect. Control Hosp. Epidemiol. *10*:54–59, 1989.
34. Beers, L. M., Burke, T. L., and Martin, D. B.: Shigellosis occurring in newborn nursery staff. Infect. Control Hosp. Epidemiol. *10*:147–149, 1989.
35. Bell, L. M., Naides, S. J., Stoffman, P., et al.: Human parvovirus B19 infection among hospital staff members after contact with infected patients. N. Engl. J. Med. *321*:485–491, 1989.
36. Bendel, C. M., and Hostetter, M. K.: Systemic candidiasis and other fungal infections in the newborn. Semin. Pediatr. Infect. Dis. *5*:35–41, 1994.
37. Bennett, S. N., McNeil, M. M., Bland, L. A., et al.: Postoperative infections traced to contamination of an intravenous anesthetic, propofol. N. Engl. J. Med. *333*:147–154, 1995.
38. Berman, S. A., Balkany, T. J., and Simmons, M. A.: Otitis media in the neonatal intensive care unit. Pediatrics *62*:198–201, 1978.
39. Bhattacharyya, N., and Kosloske, A. M.: Postoperative wound infection in pediatric surgical patients: A study of 676 infants and children. J. Pediatr. Surg. *25*:125–129, 1990.
40. Bhattacharyya, N., Kosloske, A. M., and Macarthur, C.: Nosocomial infection in pediatric surgical patients: A study of 608 infants and children. J. Pediatr. Surg. *28*:338–343, 1993.
41. Bingen, E., Lambert-Zechovsky, N., Mariani-Kurkdjian, P., et al.: Bacteremia caused by a vancomycin-resistant *Enterococcus*. Pediatr. Infect. Dis. J. *8*:475–476, 1989.
42. Bingen, E. H., Denamur, E., Lambert-Zechovsky, N. Y., et al.: Evidence for the genetic unrelatedness of nosocomial vancomycin-resistant *Enterococcus faecium* strains in a pediatric hospital. J. Clin. Microbiol. *29*:1888–1892, 1991.
43. Blank, S., Simonds, R. J., Weisfuse, I., et al.: Possible nosocomial transmission of HIV. Lancet *344*:512–514, 1994.
44. Blatt, M. L.: Cross-infection: Its prevention in a children's hospital. Illinois Med. J. *70*:483–487, 1936.
45. Blumberg, H. M., Watkins, D. L., Berschling, J. D., et al.: Preventing the nosocomial transmission of tuberculosis. Ann. Intern. Med. *122*:658–663, 1995.
46. Bobkov, A., Garaev, M. M., Rzhaninova, A., et al.: Molecular epidemiology of HIV-1 in the former Soviet Union: Analysis of env V3 sequences and their correlation with epidemiologic data. AIDS *8*:619–624, 1994.
47. Bone, R. C., Balk, R. A., Cerra, F. B., et al.: Definitions for sepsis and organ failure and guidelines for the use of innovative therapies in sepsis. Chest *101*:1644–1655, 1992.
48. Brachman, P. S.: Epidemiology of nosocomial infections. *In* Bennett, J. V., and Brachman, P. S. (eds.): Hospital Infections. Boston, Little Brown, 1992, pp. 3–15.
49. Bradford, P. A., Cherubin, C. E., Idemyor, V., et al.: Multiply resistant *Klebsiella pneumoniae* strains from two Chicago hospitals: Identification of the extended-spectrum TEM-12 and TEM-10 ceftazidime-hydrolyzing beta-lactamases in a single isolate. Antimicrob. Agents Chemother. *38*:761–766, 1994.
50. Brady, M. T.: Nosocomial legionnaires disease in a children's hospital. J. Pediatr. *115*:46–50, 1989.
51. Brady, M. T, Pacini, D. L., Budde, C. T, et al.: Diagnostic studies of nosocomial diarrhea in children: Assessing their use and value. Am. J. Infect. Control *17*:77–82, 1989.
52. Branchini, M. L., Pfaller, M. A., Rhine-Chalberg, J., et al.: Genotypic variation and slime production among blood and catheter isolates of *Candida parapsilosis*. J. Clin. Microbiol. *32*:452–456, 1994.
53. Brennemann, J.: The infant ward. Am. J. Dis. Child. *43*:577–584, 1932.
54. Brunetto, A. L., Pearson, A. D., Craft, A. W., et al.: *Clostridium difficile* in an oncology unit. Arch. Dis. Child. *63*:979–981, 1988.
55. Burdge, D. R., Nakielna, E. M., and Noble, M. A.: Case-control and vector studies of nosocomial acquisition of *Pseudomonas cepacia* in adult patients with cystic fibrosis. Infect. Control Hosp. Epidemiol. *14*:127–130, 1993.
56. Burke, J. P., and Riley, D. K.: Nosocomial urinary tract infections. *In* Mayhall, C. G. (ed.): Hospital Epidemiology and Infection Control. Baltimore, Williams & Wilkins, 1995, pp. 139–153.
57. Burwen, D. R., Banerjee, S. N., Gaynes, R. P., et al.: Ceftazidime resistance among selected nosocomial gram-negative bacilli in the United States. J. Infect. Dis. *170*:1622–1625, 1994.
58. Busch, M. P., Lee, L. L., Satten, G. A., et al.: Time course of detection of viral and serologic markers preceding human immunodeficiency virus type 1 seroconversion: Implications for screening of blood and tissue donors. Transfusion *35*:91–97, 1995.
59. Butler, K. M., and Baker, C. J.: *Candida*: An increasingly important pathogen in the nursery. Pediatr. Clin. North Am. *35*:543–563, 1988.
60. Butzler, J. P., and Goossens, H.: *Campylobacter jejuni* infection as a hospital problem: An overview. J. Hosp. Infect. *11*:374–377, 1988.
61. Call, E. L.: An epidemic of pemphigus neonatorum. Am. J. Obstet. *50*:473–477, 1904.
62. Cannon, C. G., and Linnemann, C., Jr.: *Yersinia enterocolitica* infections in hospitalized patients: The problem of hospital-acquired infections. Infect. Control Hosp. Epidemiol. *13*:139–143, 1992.
63. Cartwright, C. P., Stock, F., Beekmann, S. E., et al.: PCR amplification of rRNA intergenic spacer regions as a method for epidemiologic typing of *Clostridium difficile*. J. Clin. Microbiol. *33*:184–187, 1995.
64. Centers for Disease Control: Laboratory-acquired meningococcemia: California and Massachusetts. M. M. W. R. *40*:46–47, 55, 1991.
65. Centers for Disease Control: Nosocomial infection and pseudoinfection from contaminated endoscopes and bronchoscopes: Wisconsin and Missouri. M. M. W. R. *40*:675–678, 1991.
66. Centers for Disease Control: Public Health Service inter-agency guidelines for screening donors of blood, plasma, organs, tissues, and semen for evidence of hepatitis B and hepatitis C. M. M. W. R. *40*:1–17, 1991.
67. Centers for Disease Control: Update: *Yersinia enterocolitica* bacteremia and endotoxin shock associated with red blood cell transfusions: United States, 1991. M. M. W. R. *40*:176–178, 1991.
68. Centers for Disease Control and Prevention: Nosocomial enterococci resistant to vancomycin: United States, 1989–1993. M. M. W. R. *42*:597–599, 1993.
69. Centers for Disease Control and Prevention: Detection of notifiable diseases through surveillance for imported plague: New York, September–October 1994. M. M. W. R. *43*:805–807, 1994.
70. Centers for Disease Control and Prevention: Guidelines for preventing the transmission of *Mycobacterium tuberculosis* in health care facilities, 1994. M. M. W. R. *44*:1–132, 1994.
71. Centers for Disease Control and Prevention: Outbreak of hepatitis C associated with intravenous immunoglobulin administration: United States, October 1993–June 1994. M. M. W. R. *43*:505–509, 1994.
72. Centers for Disease Control and Prevention: Update: Human plague: India, 1994. M. M. W. R. *43*:722–723, 1994.
73. Centers for Disease Control and Prevention: Diphtheria acquired by U.S. citizens in the Russian Federation and Ukraine: 1994. M. M. W. R. *44*:237, 243–234, 1995.
74. Centers for Disease Control and Prevention: Management of patients with suspected viral hemorrhagic fever: United States. M. M. W. R. *44*:475–479, 1995.
75. Centers for Disease Control and Prevention: Viral haemorrhagic fever in Zaire: Update. Commun. Dis. Rep. Wkly. *5*:93, 1995.
76. Pearsen, M. L., and Hospital Infection Control Practices Advisory Committee: Guideline for prevention of intravascular device–related infections. Infect. Control Hosp. Epidemiol. *17*:438–473, 1996.
77. Chadee, D. D., and Le Maitre, A.: Ants: Potential mechanical vectors of hospital infections in Trinidad. Trans. R. Soc. Trop. Med. Hyg. *84*:297, 1990.
78. Chapin, M., Yatabe, J., and Cherry, J. D.: An outbreak of rotavirus gastroenteritis on a pediatric unit. Am. J. Infect. Control *11*:88–91, 1983.
79. Cherry, J. D.: Nosocomial pertussis in the nineties. Infect. Control Hosp. Epidemiol. *16*:553–555, 1995.
80. Christie, C. D. C., Glover, A. M., Willke, M. J., et al.: Containment of pertussis in the regional pediatric hospital during the Greater Cincinnati epidemic of 1993. Infect. Control Hosp. Epidemiol. *16*:556–563, 1995.
81. Clark-Christoff, N., Watters, V. A., Sparks, W., et al.: Use of triple-lumen subclavian catheters for administration of total parenteral nutrition. J. Parenter. Enter. Nutr. *16*:403–407, 1992.
82. Classen, D. C., Evans, R. S., Pestotnik, S. L., et al.: The timing of prophylactic administration of antibiotics and the risk of surgical-wound infection. N. Engl. J. Med. *326*:281–286, 1992.
83. Coello, R., Glenister, H., Fereres, J., et al.: The cost of infection in surgical patients: A case-control study. J. Hosp. Infect. *25*:239–250, 1993.
84. Cohen, M. S., Steere, A. C., Baltimore, R., et al.: Possible nosocomial transmission of group Y *Neisseria meningitidis* among oncology patients. Ann. Intern. Med. *91*:7–12, 1979.
85. Cone, R., Mohan, K., Thouless, M., et al.: Nosocomial transmission of rotavirus infection. Pediatr. Infect. Dis. J. *7*:103–109, 1988.
86. Cooper, R. G., and Sumner, C.: Hospital infection data from a children's hospital. Med. J. Aust. *2*:1110–1113, 1970.
87. Coronado, V. G., Beck-Sague, C. M., Hutton, M. D., et al.: Transmission of multidrug-resistant *Mycobacterium tuberculosis* among persons with human immunodeficiency virus infection in an urban hospital: Epidemiologic and restriction fragment length polymorphism analysis. J. Infect. Dis. *168*:1052–1055, 1993.
88. Coronado, V. G., Edwards, J. R., Culver, D. H., et al.: Ciprofloxacin resistance among nosocomial *Pseudomonas aeruginosa* and *Staphylococcus aureus* in the United States. Infect. Control Hosp. Epidemiol. *16*:71–75, 1995.
89. Cowen, J., Ellis, S. H., and McAinsh, J.: Absorption of chlorhexidine from the intact skin of newborn infants. Arch. Dis. Child. *54*:379–383, 1979.
90. Craven, D. E., Lichtenberg, D. A., Goularte, T. A., et al.: Contaminated medication nebulizers in mechanical ventilator circuits: Source of bacterial aerosols. Am. J. Med. *77*:834–838, 1984.
91. Craven, R. B., and Barnes, A. M.: Plague and tularemia. Infect. Dis. Clin. North Am. *5*:165–175, 1991.
92. Cronin, W. A., Germanson, T. P., and Donowitz, L. G.: Intravascular catheter colonization and related bloodstream infection in critically ill neonates. Infect. Control Hosp. Epidemiol. *11*:301–308, 1990.
93. Culver, D. H., Horan, T. C., Gaynes, R. P., et al.: Surgical wound infection

rates by wound class, operative procedure, and patient risk index. Am. J. Med. *91*:152S–157S, 1991.

94. Dato, V. M., and Dajani, A. S.: Candidemia in children with central venous catheters: Role of catheter removal and amphotericin B therapy. Pediatr. Infect. Dis. J. *9*:309–314, 1990.
95. Daum, R. S., Nachman, J. P., Leitch, C. D., et al.: Nosocomial epiglottitis associated with penicillin- and cephalosporin-resistant *Streptococcus pneumoniae* bacteremia. J. Clin. Microbiol. *32*:246–248, 1994.
96. Davenport, M., and Doig, C. M.: Wound infection in pediatric surgery: A study in 1,094 neonates. J. Pediatr. Surg. *28*:26–30, 1993.
97. Davies, H. D., Jones, E. L., Sheng, R. Y., et al.: Nosocomial urinary tract infections at a pediatric hospital. Pediatr. Infect. Dis. J. *11*:349–354, 1992.
98. Davis, R. M., Orenstein, W. A., Frank, J., Jr., et al.: Transmission of measles in medical settings, 1980 through 1984. J. A. M. A. *255*:1295–1298, 1986.
99. Davis, S. D., Sobocinski, K., Hoffman, R. G., et al.: Postoperative wound infections in a children's hospital. Pediatr. Infect. Dis. J. *3*:114–116, 1984.
100. de Cicco, M., Panarello, G., Chiaradia, V., et al.: Source and route of microbial colonisation of parenteral nutrition catheters. Lancet *2*:1258–1261, 1989.
101. Demmler, G. J., Yow, M. D., Spector, S. A., et al.: Nosocomial cytomegalovirus infections within two hospitals caring for infants and children. J. Infect. Dis. *156*:9–16, 1987.
102. DeMuri, G. P., and Hostetter, M. K.: Resistance to antifungal agents. Pediatr. Clin. North Am. *42*:665–685, 1995.
103. Dennehy, P. H., and Peter, G.: Risk factors associated with nosocomial rotavirus infection. Am. J. Dis. Child. *139*:935–939, 1985.
104. Ditchburn, R. K., McQuillin, J., Gardner, P. S., et al.: Respiratory syncytial virus in hospital cross-infection. B. M. J. *3*:671–673, 1971.
105. Dodd, R. Y.: The risk of transfusion-transmitted infection. N. Engl. J. Med. *327*:419–421, 1992.
106. Doig, C. M., and Wilkinson, A. W.: Wound infection in a children's hospital. Br. J. Surg. *63*:647–650, 1976.
107. Donahue, J. G., Munoz, A., Ness, P. M., et al.: The declining risk of post-transfusion hepatitis C virus infection. N. Engl. J. Med. *327*:369–373, 1992.
108. Dondero, T. J., Hu, D. J., and George, J. R.: HIV-1 variants: Yet another challenge to public health. Lancet *343*:1376, 1994.
109. Drusin, L. M., Sohmer, M., Groshen, S. L., et al.: Nosocomial hepatitis A infection in a paediatric intensive care unit. Arch. Dis. Child. *62*:690–695, 1987.
110. Ducharme, F. M., Gauthier, M., Lacroix, J., et al.: Incidence of infection related to arterial catheterization in children: A prospective study. Crit. Care Med. *16*:272–276, 1988.
111. Dunkle, L. M., Naqvi, S. H., McCallum, R., et al.: Eradication of epidemic methicillin-gentamicin–resistant *Staphylococcus aureus* in an intensive care nursery. Am. J. Med. *70*:455–458, 1981.
112. DuPont, H. L.: Nosocomial salmonellosis and shigellosis. Infect. Control Hosp. Epidemiol. *12*:707–709, 1991.
113. DuPont, H. L., Gangarosa, E. J., Reller, L. B., et al.: Shigellosis in custodial institutions. Am. J. Epidemiol. *92*:172–179, 1970.
114. Easmon, C. S., Hastings, M. J., Clare, A. J., et al.: Nosocomial transmission of group B streptococci. B. M. J. *283*:459–461, 1981.
115. Edwards, M. S., and Baker, C. J.: Median sternotomy wound infections in children. Pediatr. Infect. Dis. *2*:105–109, 1983.
116. Emori, T. G., Culver, D. H., Horan, T. C., et al.: National nosocomial infections surveillance system (NNIS): Description of surveillance methods. Am. J. Infect. Control *19*:19–35, 1991.
117. Emori, T. G., and Gaynes, R. P.: An overview of nosocomial infections, including the role of the microbiology laboratory. Clin. Microbiol. Rev. *6*:428–442, 1993.
118. Evans, J. P. M., Rossiter, M. A., Kumaran, T. O., et al.: Human parvovirus aplasia: Case due to cross infection in a ward. B. M. J. *288*:681, 1984.
119. Fagon, J. Y., Chastre, J., Hance, A. J., et al.: Nosocomial pneumonia in ventilated patients: A cohort study evaluating attributable mortality and hospital stay. Am. J. Med. *94*:281–288, 1993.
120. Fanaroff, A. A., Korones, S. B., Wright, L. L., et al.: A controlled trial of intravenous immune globulin to reduce nosocomial infections in very low-birth-weight infants. N. Engl. J. Med. *330*:1107–1113, 1994.
121. Farizo, K. M., Stehr-Green, P. A., Simpson, D. M., et al.: Pediatric emergency room visits: A risk factor for acquiring measles. Pediatrics *87*:74–79, 1991.
122. Farizo, K. M., Strebel, P. M., Chen, R. T., et al.: Fatal respiratory disease due to *Corynebacterium diphtheriae*: Case report and review of guidelines for management, investigation, and control. Clin. Infect. Dis. *16*:59–68, 1993.
123. Favero, M. S., Alter, M. J., and Bland, L. A.: Nosocomial infections associated with hemodialysis. *In* Mayhall, C. G. (ed.): Hospital Epidemiology and Infection Control. Baltimore, Williams & Wilkins, 1995, pp. 693–714.
124. Finkel, T. H., Torok, T. J., Ferguson, P. J., et al.: Chronic parvovirus B19 infection and systemic necrotising vasculitis: Opportunistic infection or aetiological agent? Lancet *343*:1255–1258, 1994.
125. Finn, A., Anday, E., and Talbot, G. H.: An epidemic of adenovirus 7a infection in a neonatal nursery: Course, morbidity, and management. Infect. Control. Hosp. Epidemiol. *9*:398–404, 1988.
126. Fisher, M. C., Long, S. S., McGowan, K. L., et al.: Outbreak of pertussis in a residential facility for handicapped people. J. Pediatr. *114*:934–939, 1989.
127. Ford-Jones, E. L., Mindorff, C. M., Langley, J. M., et al.: Epidemiologic study of 4684 hospital-acquired infections in pediatric patients. Pediatr. Infect. Dis. J. *8*:668–675, 1989.
128. Fotedar, R., Banerjee, U., Singh, S., et al.: The housefly (*Musca domestica*) as a carrier of pathogenic microorganisms in a hospital environment. J. Hosp. Infect. *20*:209–215, 1992.
129. Freeman, J., Epstein, M. F., Smith, N. E., et al.: Extra hospital stay and antibiotic usage with nosocomial coagulase-negative staphylococcal bacteremia in two neonatal intensive care unit populations. Am. J. Dis. Child. *144*:324–329, 1990.
130. Freeman, J., Goldmann, D. A., Smith, N. E., et al.: Association of intravenous lipid emulsion and coagulase-negative staphylococcal bacteremia in neonatal intensive care units. N. Engl. J. Med. *323*:301–308, 1990.
131. Freeman, J., Platt, R., Epstein, M. F., et al.: Birth weight and length of stay as determinants of nosocomial coagulase-negative staphylococcal bacteremia in neonatal intensive care unit populations: Potential for confounding. Am. J. Epidemiol. *132*:1130–1140, 1990.
132. Freeman, J., Platt, R., Sidebottom, D. G., et al.: Coagulase-negative staphylococcal bacteremia in the changing neonatal intensive care unit population: Is there an epidemic? J. A. M. A. *258*:2548–2552, 1987.
133. Freeman, R. K., Poland, R. L., Hauth, J. C., et al. (eds.): Guidelines for Perinatal Care. Elk Grove, American Academy of Pediatrics, 1992.
134. Friedland, I. R., and Klugman, K. P.: Antibiotic-resistant pneumococcal disease in South African children. Am. J. Dis. Child. *146*:920–923, 1992.
135. Friedman, C. A., Temple, D. M., Robbins, K. K., et al.: Outbreak and control of varicella in a neonatal intensive care unit. Pediatr. Infect. Dis. J. *13*:152–154, 1994.
136. Frölich, T.: Infections nosocomiales dans les crèches et hôpitaux pour enfants. Acta Pediatr. *17*:18–23, 1935.
137. Furfaro, S., Gauthier, M., Lacroix, J., et al.: Arterial catheter-related infections in children: A 1-year cohort analysis. Am. J. Dis. Child. *145*:1037–1043, 1991.
138. Gala, C. L., Hall, C. B., Schnabel, K. C., et al.: The use of eye-nose goggles to control nosocomial respiratory syncytial virus infection. J. A. M. A. *256*:2706–2708, 1986.
139. Gardner, P., and Carles, D. G.: Infections acquired in a pediatric hospital. J. Pediatr. *81*:1205–1210, 1972.
140. Garland, J. S., Buck, R. K., Maloney, P., et al.: Comparison of 10% povidone-iodine and 0.5% chlorhexidine gluconate for the prevention of peripheral intravenous catheter colonization in neonates: A prospective trial. Pediatr. Infect. Dis. J. *14*:510–516, 1995.
141. Garland, J. S., Dunne, W. M., Jr., Havens, P., et al.: Peripheral intravenous catheter complications in critically ill children: A prospective study. Pediatrics *89*:1145–1150, 1992.
142. Garland, J. S., Nelson, D. B., Cheah, T., et al.: Infectious complications during peripheral intravenous therapy with Teflon catheters: A prospective study. Pediatr. Infect. Dis. J. *6*:918–921, 1987.
143. Garner, J. S.: CDC guideline for prevention of surgical wound infections, 1985. Infect. Control *7*:193–200, 1986.
144. Garner, J. S., and Hospital Infection Control Practices Advisory Committee: Guideline for isolation precautions in hospitals. Infect. Control Hosp. Epidemiol. *17*:53–80, 1996.
145. Garner, J. S., Jarvis, W. R., Emori, T. G., et al.: CDC definitions for nosocomial infections, 1988. Am. J. Infect. Control *16*:128–140, 1988.
146. Gastinne, H., Wolff, M., Delatour, F., et al.: A controlled trial in intensive care units of selective decontamination of the digestive tract with nonabsorbable antibiotics. N. Engl. J. Med. *326*:594–599, 1992.
147. Gaynes, R. P., and Culver, D. H.: Resistance to imipenem among selected gram-negative bacilli in the United States. Infect. Control Hosp. Epidemiol. *13*:10–14, 1992.
148. Gaynes, R. P., Edwards, J. R., Jarvis, W. R., et al.: Nosocomial infections among neonates in high-risk nurseries in the United States. Pediatrics *98*:357–361, 1996.
149. George, R. H., Gully, P. R., Gill, O. N., et al.: An outbreak of tuberculosis in a children's hospital. J. Hosp. Infect. *8*:129–142, 1986.
150. Gerards, L. J., Hennekam, R. C., von Dijk, W. C., et al.: An outbreak of gastroenteritis due to *Escherichia coli* 0142:H6 in a neonatal department. J. Hosp. Infect. *5*:283–288, 1984.
151. Gerberding, J. L.: Management of occupational exposures to blood-borne viruses. N. Engl. J. Med. *332*:444–451, 1995.
152. Gerst, P. H., Fildes, J. J., Rosario, P. G., et al.: Risks of human immunodeficiency virus infection to patients and healthcare personnel. Crit. Care Med. *18*:1440–1448, 1990.
153. Giardina, R., Hsu, H., Kirkpatrick, J., et al.: Ventilator-associated nosocomial bacterial pneumonia in pediatric ICUs. Abstract No. 122. Second Annual Meeting of the Society for Hospital Epidemiology of America, Baltimore, 1992.
154. Golden, S. E., Shehab, Z. M., Bjelland, J. C., et al.: Microbiology of endotracheal aspirates in intubated pediatric intensive care unit patients: Correlations with radiographic findings. Pediatr. Infect. Dis. J. *6*:665–669, 1987.
155. Goldmann, D. A.: Bacterial colonization and infection in the neonate. Am. J. Med. *70*:417–422, 1981.
156. Goldmann, D. A.: Strategies for preventing neonatal group B streptococcal disease. Infect. Control *7*:137–139, 143, 1986.

157. Goldmann, D. A.: Prevention and management of neonatal infections. Infect. Dis. Clin. North Am. *3*:779–813, 1989.
158. Goldmann, D. A.: Transmission of infectious diseases in children. Pediatr. Rev. *13*:283–292, 1992.
159. Goldmann, D. A., and Breton, S. J.: Group C streptococcal surgical wound infections transmitted by an anorectal and nasal carrier. Pediatrics *61*:235–237, 1978.
160. Goldmann, D. A., Durbin, W., Jr., and Freeman, J.: Nosocomial infections in a neonatal intensive care unit. J. Infect. Dis. *144*:449–459, 1981.
161. Graman, P. S., and Hall, C. B.: Epidemiology and control of nosocomial viral infections. Infect. Dis. Clin. North Am. *3*:815–841, 1989.
162. Gray, J. E., Richardson, D. K., McCormick, M. C., et al.: Coagulase-negative staphylococcal bacteremia among very low birth weight infants: Relation to admission illness severity, resource use, and outcome. Pediatrics *95*:225–230, 1995.
163. Gray, J. E., Richardson, D. K., McCormick, M. C., et al.: Neonatal therapeutic intervention scoring system: A therapy-based severity-of-illness index. Pediatrics *90*:561–567, 1992.
164. Gross, P. A.: Use of severity of illness indices in hospital epidemiology and infection control. *In* Mayhall, C. G. (ed.): Hospital Epidemiology and Infection Control. Baltimore, Williams & Wilkins, 1995, pp. 90–104.
165. Guerin, J. M., Lustman, C., Meyer, P., et al.: Nosocomial sinusitis in pediatric intensive care patients. Crit. Care Med. *18*:902, 1990.
166. Gupta, P., Ramachandran, V. G., Sharma, P. P., et al.: *Salmonella senftenberg* septicemia: A nursery outbreak. Indian Pediatr. *30*:514–516, 1993.
167. Gustafson, T. L., Lavely, G. B., Brawner, E., Jr., et al.: An outbreak of airborne nosocomial varicella. Pediatrics *70*:550–556, 1982.
168. Hack, M., Horbar, J. D., Malloy, M. H., et al.: Very low birth weight outcomes of the National Institute of Child Health and Human Development Neonatal Network. Pediatrics *87*:587–597, 1991.
169. Haley, R. W., Culver, D. H., White, J. W., et al.: The nationwide nosocomial infection rate: A new need for vital statistics. Am. J. Epidemiol. *121*:159–167, 1985.
170. Haley, R. W., Cushion, N. B., Tenover, F. C., et al.: Eradication of endemic methicillin-resistant *Staphylococcus aureus* infections from a neonatal intensive care unit. J. Infect. Dis. *171*:614–624, 1995.
171. Hall, C. B.: Nosocomial viral respiratory infections: Perennial weeds on pediatric wards. Am. J. Med. *70*:670–676, 1981.
172. Hall, C. B., and Douglas, R., Jr.: Nosocomial influenza infection as a cause of intercurrent fevers in infants. Pediatrics *55*:673–677, 1975.
173. Hall, C. B., and Douglas, R., Jr.: Modes of transmission of respiratory syncytial virus. J. Pediatr. *99*:100–103, 1981.
174. Hall, C. B., and Douglas, R., Jr.: Nosocomial respiratory syncytial viral infections: Should gowns and masks be used? Am. J. Dis. Child. *135*:512–515, 1981.
175. Hall, C. B., Douglas Jr., R., and Geiman, J. M.: Possible transmission by fomites of respiratory syncytial virus. J. Infect. Dis. *141*:98–102, 1980.
176. Hall, C. B., Douglas, R., Jr., Geiman, J. M., et al.: Nosocomial respiratory syncytial virus infections. N. Engl. J. Med. *293*:1343–1346, 1975.
177. Hall, C. B., Kopelman, A. E., Douglas, R., Jr., et al.: Neonatal respiratory syncytial virus infection. N. Engl. J. Med. *300*:393–396, 1979.
178. Hall, C. B., Powell, K. R., MacDonald, N. E., et al.: Respiratory syncytial viral infection in children with compromised immune function. N. Engl. J. Med. *315*:77–81, 1986.
179. Hammami, A., Arlet, G., Ben Redjeb, S., et al.: Nosocomial outbreak of acute gastroenteritis in a neonatal intensive care unit in Tunisia caused by multiply drug-resistant *Salmonella wien* producing SHV-2 beta-lactamase. Eur. J. Clin. Microbiol. Infect. Dis. *10*:641–646, 1991.
180. Hammerberg, O., Watts, J., Chernesky, M., et al.: An outbreak of herpes simplex virus type 1 in an intensive care nursery. Pediatr. Infect. Dis. *2*:290–294, 1983.
181. Hammond, J. M., Potgieter, P. D., Saunders, G. L., et al.: Double-blind study of selective decontamination of the digestive tract in intensive care. Lancet *340*:5–9, 1992.
182. Hanley, P. J., Conaway, M. M., Halstead, D. C., et al.: Nosocomial herpes simplex virus infection associated with oral endotracheal intubation. Am. J. Infect. Control *21*:310–316, 1993.
183. Harries, E. H. R.: Infection and its control in children's wards. Lancet *2*:173–178, 1935.
184. Harvey, B. S., Koeuth, T., Versalovic, J., et al.: Vertical transmission of *Citrobacter diversus* documented by DNA fingerprinting. Infect. Control Hosp. Epidemiol. *16*:564–569, 1995.
185. Hedberg, K., Ristinen, T. L., Soler, J. T., et al.: Outbreak of erythromycin-resistant staphylococcal conjunctivitis in a newborn nursery. Pediatr. Infect. Dis. J. *9*:268–273, 1990.
186. Helin, I., Widell, A., Borulf, S., et al.: Outbreak of coxsackievirus A-14 meningitis among newborns in a maternity hospital ward. Acta Paediatr. Scand. *76*:234–238, 1987.
187. Hemming, V. G., Overall, J., Jr., and Britt, M. R.: Nosocomial infections in a newborn intensive-care unit: Results of forty-one months of surveillance. N. Engl. J. Med. *294*:1310–1316, 1976.
188. Hemming, V. G., Prince, G. A., Groothuis, J. R., et al.: Hyperimmune globulins in prevention and treatment of respiratory syncytial virus infections. Clin. Microbiol. Rev. *8*:22–33, 1995.
189. Hendley, J. O., and Gwaltney, J. M., Jr.: Mechanisms of transmission of rhinovirus infections. Epidemiol. Rev. *10*:243–258, 1988.
190. Hershkowici, S., Barak, M., Cohen, A., et al.: An outbreak of *Campylobacter jejuni* infection in a neonatal intensive care unit. J. Hosp. Infect. *9*:54–59, 1987.
191. Heseltine, P. N., Ripper, M., and Wohlford, P.: Nosocomial rubella: Consequences of an outbreak and efficacy of a mandatory immunization program. Infect. Control *6*:371–374, 1985.
192. Hill, R. L., Fisher, A. P., Ware, R. J., et al.: Mupirocin for the reduction of colonization of internal jugular cannulae: A randomized controlled trial. J. Hosp. Infect. *15*:311–321, 1990.
193. Hoogkamp-Korstanje, J. A., Cats, B., Senders, R. C., et al.: Analysis of bacterial infections in a neonatal intensive care unit. J. Hosp. Infect. *3*:275–284, 1982.
194. Horan, T. C., Gaynes, R. P., Martone, W. J., et al.: CDC definitions of nosocomial surgical site infections, 1992: A modification of CDC definitions of surgical wound infections. Am. J. Infect. Control *20*:271–274, 1992.
195. Howard, A. J.: Nosocomial spread of *Haemophilus influenzae*. J. Hosp. Infect. *19*:1–3, 1991.
196. Hruszkewycz, V., Holtrop, P. C., Batton, D. G., et al.: Complications associated with central venous catheters inserted in critically ill neonates. Infect. Control Hosp. Epidemiol. *12*:544–548, 1991.
197. Huebner, J., Pier, G. B., Maslow, J. N., et al.: Endemic nosocomial transmission of *Staphylococcus epidermidis* bacteremia isolates in a neonatal intensive care unit over 10 years. J. Infect. Dis. *169*:526–531, 1994.
198. Ingram, J., Weitzman, S., Greenberg, M. L., et al.: Complications of indwelling venous access lines in the pediatric hematology patient: A prospective comparison of external venous catheters and subcutaneous ports. Am. J. Pediatr. Hematol. Oncol. *13*:130–136, 1991.
199. Istre, G. R., McKee, P. A., West, G. R., et al.: Measles spread in medical settings: An important focus of disease transmission? Pediatrics *79*:356–358, 1987.
200. Jacoby, G. A., and Medeiros, A. A.: More extended-spectrum beta-lactamases. Antimicrob. Agents Chemother. *35*:1697–1704, 1991.
201. Jann, K., and Jann, B.: Capsules of *Escherichia coli*, expression and biological significance. Can. J. Microbiol. *38*:705–710, 1992.
202. Jarvis, W. R.: Epidemiology of nosocomial infections in pediatric patients. Pediatr. Infect. Dis. J. *6*:344–351, 1987.
203. Jarvis, W. R.: Epidemiology of nosocomial fungal infections, with emphasis on *Candida* species. Clin. Infect. Dis. *20*:1526–1530, 1995.
204. Jarvis, W. R., Edwards, J. R., Culver, D. H., et al.: Nosocomial infection rates in adult and pediatric intensive care units in the United States. Am. J. Med. *91*:185S–191S, 1991.
205. Jarvis, W. R., Thornsberry, C., Boyce, J., et al.: Methicillin-resistant *Staphylococcus aureus* at children's hospitals in the United States. Pediatr. Infect. Dis. J. *4*:651–655, 1985.
206. Jereb, J. A., Klevens, R. M., Privett, T. D., et al.: Tuberculosis in health care workers at a hospital with an outbreak of multidrug-resistant *Mycobacterium tuberculosis*. Arch. Intern. Med. *155*:854–859, 1995.
207. Johnson, D. C., Johnson, F. L., and Goldman, S.: Preliminary results treating persistent central venous catheter infections with the antibiotic lock technique in pediatric patients. Pediatr. Infect. Dis. J. *13*:930–931, 1994.
208. Johnson, I., Hammond, G. W., and Verma, M. R.: Nosocomial coxsackie B4 virus infections in two chronic-care pediatric neurological wards. J. Infect. Dis. *151*:1153–1156, 1985.
209. Johnson, J. R.: Virulence factors in *Escherichia coli* urinary tract infection. Clin. Microbiol. Rev. *4*:80–128, 1991.
210. Johnson, S., Homann, S. R., Bettin, K. M., et al.: Treatment of asymptomatic *Clostridium difficile* carriers (fecal excretors) with vancomycin or metronidazole: A randomized, placebo-controlled trial. Ann. Intern. Med. *117*:297–302, 1992.
211. Johnsson, J., Seeberg, S., and Kjellmer, I.: Blood concentrations of chlorhexidine in neonates undergoing routine cord care with 4% chlorhexidine gluconate solution. Acta Paediatr. Scand. *76*:675–676, 1987.
212. Jones, G. R., Konsler, G. K., Dunaway, R. P., et al.: Prospective analysis of urokinase in the treatment of catheter sepsis in pediatric hematology-oncology patients. J. Pediatr. Surg. *28*:350–355, 1993.
213. Jones, R. N., Kehrberg, E. N., Erwin, M. E., et al.: Prevalence of important pathogens and antimicrobial activity of parenteral drugs at numerous medical centers in the United States. I. Study on the threat of emerging resistances: Real or perceived? Diagn. Microbiol. Infect. Dis. *19*:203–215, 1994.
214. Karmali, M. A., Norrish, B., Lior, H., et al.: *Campylobacter* enterocolitis in a neonatal nursery. J. Infect. Dis. *149*:874–877, 1984.
215. Keane, E., and Gilles, H. M.: Lassa fever in Panguma Hospital, Sierra Leone, 1973–6. B. M. J. *1*:1399–1402, 1977.
216. Keats, A. S.: The ASA classification of physical status: A recapitulation. Anesthesiology *49*:233–236, 1978.
217. Khan, M. A., Abdur-Rab, M., Israr, N., et al.: Transmission of *Salmonella worthington* by oropharyngeal suction in hospital neonatal unit. Pediatr. Infect. Dis. J. *10*:668–672, 1991.
218. Kilham, E. B.: An epidemic of pemphigus neonatorum. Am. J. Obstet. *22*:1039–1044, 1889.

219. King, D. R., Komer, M., Hoffman, J., et al.: Broviac catheter sepsis: The natural history of an iatrogenic infection. J. Pediatr. Surg. *20*:728–733, 1985.
220. Kinney, J., Mundorf, L., Gleason, C., et al.: Efficacy and pharmacokinetics of intravenous immune globulin administration to high-risk neonates. Am. J. Dis. Child. *145*:1233–1238, 1991.
221. Kinney, J. S., McCray, E., Kaplan, J. E., et al:. Risk factors associated with echovirus 11 infection in a hospital nursery. Pediatr. Infect. Dis. *5*:192–197, 1986.
222. Klein, B. S., Michaels, J. A., Rytel, M. W., et al.: Nosocomial hepatitis A: A multinursery outbreak in Wisconsin. J. A. M. A. *252*:2716–2721, 1984.
223. Kline, M. W., Kaplan, S. L., Hawkins, E. P., et al.: Pathogenesis of brain abscess formation in an infant rat model of *Citrobacter diversus* bacteremia and meningitis. J. Infect. Dis. *157*:106–112, 1988.
224. Kline, M. W., Mason, E. O., Jr., and Kaplan, S. L.: Characterization of *Citrobacter diversus* strains causing neonatal meningitis. J. Infect. Dis. *157*:101–105, 1988.
225. Kloos, W. E., and Bannerman, T. L.: Update on clinical significance of coagulase-negative staphylococci. Clin. Microbiol. Rev. *7*:117–140, 1994.
226. Kotloff, K. L., Losonsky, G. A., Morris, J., Jr., et al.: Enteric adenovirus infection and childhood diarrhea: An epidemiologic study in three clinical settings. Pediatrics *84*:219–225, 1989.
227. Koziol, D. E., Kurtzman, G., Ayub, J., et al.: Nosocomial human parvovirus B19 infection: Lack of transmission from a chronically infected patient to hospital staff. Infect. Control Hosp. Epidemiol. *13*:343–348, 1992.
228. Krasinski, K., LaCouture, R., Holzman, R. S., et al.: Screening for respiratory syncytial virus and assignment to a cohort at admission to reduce nosocomial transmission. J. Pediatr. *116*:894–898, 1990.
229. Krause, P. J., Gross, P. A., Barrett, T. L., et al.: Quality standard for assurance of measles immunity among health care workers. Infect. Control Hosp. Epidemiol. *15*:193–199, 1994.
230. Kurt, T. L., Yeager, A. S., Guenette, S., et al.: Spread of pertussis by hospital staff. J. A. M. A. *221*:264–267, 1972.
231. Kurtz, J. B., Lee, T. W., and Pickering, D.: Astrovirus associated gastroenteritis in a children's ward. J. Clin. Pathol. *30*:948–952, 1977.
232. La Quaglia, M. P., Caldwell, C., Lucas, A., et al.: A prospective randomized double-blind trial of bolus urokinase in the treatment of established Hickman catheter sepsis in children. J. Pediatr. Surg. *29*:742–745, 1994.
233. La Quaglia, M. P., Lucas, A., Thaler, H. T., et al.: A prospective analysis of vascular access device-related infections in children. J. Pediatr. Surg. *27*:840–842, 1992.
234. LaForce, F. M.: The control of infections in hospitals: 1750 to 1950. *In* Wenzel, R. P. (ed.): Prevention and Control of Nosocomial Infections. Baltimore, Williams & Wilkins, 1993, pp. 1–12.
235. Laing, F. P., Ramotar, K., Read, R. R., et al.: Molecular epidemiology of *Xanthomonas maltophilia* colonization and infection in the hospital environment. J. Clin. Microbiol. *33*:513–518, 1995.
236. Lam, B. C., Tam, J., Ng, M. H., et al.: Nosocomial gastroenteritis in paediatric patients. J. Hosp. Infect. *14*:351–355, 1989.
237. Landers, S., Moise, A. A., Fraley, J. K., et al.: Factors associated with umbilical catheter-related sepsis in neonates. Am. J. Dis. Child. *145*:675–680, 1991.
238. Landry, S. L., Kaiser, D. L., and Wenzel, R. P.: Hospital stay and mortality attributed to nosocomial enterococcal bacteremia: A controlled study. Am. J. Infect. Control *17*:323–329, 1989.
239. Larson, E.: Guideline for use of topical antimicrobial agents. Am. J. Infect. Control *16*:253–266, 1988.
240. Leclair, J. M., Freeman, J., Sullivan, B. F., et al.: Prevention of nosocomial respiratory syncytial virus infections through compliance with glove and gown isolation precautions. N. Engl. J. Med. *317*:329–334, 1987.
241. Leclair, J. M., Winston, K. R., Sullivan, B. F., et al.: Effect of preoperative shampoos with chlorhexidine or iodophor on emergence of resident scalp flora in neurosurgery. Infect. Control *9*:8–12, 1988.
242. Leclair, J. M., Zaia, J. A., Levin, M. J., et al.: Airborne transmission of chickenpox in a hospital. N. Engl. J. Med. *302*:450–453, 1980.
243. Lefrere, J. J., Mariotti, M., and Thauvin, M.: B19 parvovirus DNA in solvent/detergent-treated anti-haemophilia concentrates. Lancet *343*:211–212, 1994.
244. Lettau, L. A.: Nosocomial transmission and infection control aspects of parasitic and ectoparasitic diseases. Part III. Ectoparasites/summary and conclusions. Infect. Control Hosp. Epidemiol. *12*:179–185, 1991.
245. Lettau, L. A.: Nosocomial transmission and infection control aspects of parasitic and ectoparasitic diseases. Part I. Introduction/enteric parasites. Infect. Control. Hosp. Epidemiol. *12*:59–65, 1991.
246. Levin, M. J.: Treatment and prevention options for respiratory syncytial virus infections. J. Pediatr. *124*:S22–S27, 1994.
247. Lewis, C. B., and Wilson, C. B.: Developmental immunology and role of host defenses in neonatal susceptibility to infection. *In* Remington, J. S., and Klein, J. O. (eds.): Infectious Diseases of the Fetus and Newborn Infant. 4th ed. Philadelphia, W. B. Saunders, 1995, pp. 20–95.
248. Lichtenstein, A.: Nosocomial infections in children's hospitals and institutions: Our means for combating these infections. Acta Paediatr. *17*:36–49, 1935.
249. Lin, F. C., Devoe, W. F., Morrison, C., et al.: Outbreak of neonatal *Citrobacter diversus* meningitis in a suburban hospital. Pediatr. Infect. Dis. J. *6*:50–55, 1987.
250. Linares, J., Sitges-Serra, A., Garau, J., et al.: Pathogenesis of catheter sepsis: A prospective study with quantitative and semiquantitative cultures of catheter hub and segments. J. Clin. Microbiol. *21*:357–360, 1985.
251. Linnemann, C. C., Jr., Buchman, T. G., Light, I. J., et al.: Transmission of herpes-simplex virus type 1 in a nursery for the newborn: Identification of viral isolates by D.N.A. "fingerprinting". Lancet *1*:964–966, 1978.
252. Linnemann, C. C., and MacMillan, B. G.: Viral infections in pediatric burn patients. Am. J. Dis. Child. *135*:750–753, 1981.
253. Linnemann, C. C., Jr., Ramundo, N., Perlstein, P. H., et al.: Use of pertussis vaccine in an epidemic involving hospital staff. Lancet *2*:540–543, 1975.
254. Liston, T. E., Levine, P. L., and Anderson, C.: Polymicrobial bacteremia due to Polle syndrome: The child abuse variant of Munchausen by proxy. Pediatrics *72*:211–213, 1983.
255. Livingston, R. A., Froggatt, J. W., McLaughlin, J. M., et al.: Vancomycin-resistant enterococci: Infection and colonization within a children's center. Pediatr. Res. *29*:178A, 1991.
256. Lohr, J. A., Donowitz, L. G., and Sadler, J. E.: Hospital-acquired urinary tract infection. Pediatrics *83*:193–199, 1989.
257. Lohr, J. A., Downs, S. M., Dudley, S., et al.: Hospital-acquired urinary tract infections in the pediatric patient: A prospective study. Pediatr. Infect. Dis. J. *13*:8–12, 1994.
258. Lortholary, O., Fagon, J. Y., Hoi, A. B., et al.: Nosocomial acquisition of multiresistant *Acinetobacter baumannii*: Risk factors and prognosis. Clin. Infect. Dis. *20*:790–796, 1995.
259. Lövegren, E.: Infection risks in nursing institutions for infants and young children and measures for their prevention. Acta Paediatr. *17*:50–55, 1935.
260. Lyytikainen, O., Saxen, H., Ryhanen, R., et al.: Persistence of a multiresistant clone of *Staphylococcus epidermidis* in a neonatal intensive-care unit for a four-year period. Clin. Infect. Dis. *20*:24–29, 1995.
261. MacDonald, N. E., Hall, C. B., Suffin, S. C., et al.: Respiratory syncytial viral infection in infants with congenital heart disease. N. Engl. J. Med. *307*:397–400, 1982.
262. Mackenzie, A., Johnson, W., Heyes, B., et al.: A prolonged outbreak of exfoliative toxin A–producing *Staphylococcus aureus* in a newborn nursery. Diagn. Microbiol. Infect. Dis. *21*:69–75, 1995.
263. Madden, N. P., Levinsky, R. J., Bayston, R., et al.: Surgery, sepsis, and nonspecific immune function in neonates. J. Pediatr. Surg. *24*:562–566, 1989.
264. Madge, P., Paton, J. Y., McColl, J. H., et al.: Prospective controlled study of four infection-control procedures to prevent nosocomial infection with respiratory syncytial virus. Lancet *340*:1079–1083, 1992.
265. Magny, J. F., Bremard-Oury, C., Brault, D., et al.: Intravenous immunoglobulin therapy for prevention of infection in high-risk premature infants: Report of a multicenter, double-blind study. Pediatrics *88*:437–443, 1991.
266. Maguire, G. C., Nordin, J., Myers, M. G., et al.: Infections acquired by young infants. Am. J. Dis. Child. *135*:693–698, 1981.
267. Mahajan, R., Mathur, M., Kumar, A., et al.: Nosocomial outbreak of *Salmonella typhimurium* infection in a nursery intensive care unit (NICU) and paediatric ward. J. Clin. Commun. Dis. *27*:10–14, 1995.
268. Maki, D. G.: Infections due to infusion therapy. *In* Bennett, J. V., and Brachman, P. S. (eds.): Hospital Infections. Boston, Little Brown, 1992, pp. 849–898.
269. Maki, D. G., Klein, B. S., McCormick, R. D., et al.: Nosocomial *Pseudomonas pickettii* bacteremias traced to narcotic tampering: A case for selective drug screening of health care personnel. J. A. M. A. *265*:981–986, 1991.
270. Maki, D. G., Rhame, F. S., Mackel, D. C., et al.: Nationwide epidemic of septicemia caused by contaminated intravenous products. I. Epidemiologic and clinical features. Am. J. Med. *60*:471–485, 1976.
271. Maki, D. G., Ringer, M., and Alvarado, C. J.: Prospective randomised trial of povidone-iodine, alcohol, and chlorhexidine for prevention of infection associated with central venous and arterial catheters. Lancet *338*:339–343, 1991.
272. Maki, D. G., Weise, C. E., and Sarafin, H. W.: A semiquantitative culture method for identifying intravenous-catheter–related infection. N. Engl. J. Med. *296*:1305–1309, 1977.
273. Malhotra, V. L., Prakash, K., and Lakshmy, A.: Hospital-acquired meningococcaemia. J. Hosp. Infect. *18*:332, 1991.
274. Mandigers, C. M., Diepersloot, R. J., Dessens, M., et al.: A hospital outbreak of penicillin-resistant pneumococci in The Netherlands. Eur. Respir. J. *7*:1635–1639, 1994.
275. Martin, M. A., Reichelderfer, M., and Association for Professionals in Infection Control and Epidemiology Inc, et al.: APIC guidelines for infection prevention and control in flexible endoscopy. Am. J. Infect. Control *22*:19–38, 1994.
276. Martone, R. W., Jarvis, W. R., Culver, D. H., et al.: Incidence and nature of endemic and epidemic nosocomial infections. *In* Bennett, J. V., and Brachman, P. S. (eds.): Hospital Infections. Boston, Little, Brown, 1992, pp. 182–205.
277. Mastro, T. D., Fields, B. S., Breiman, R. F., et al.: Nosocomial Legionnaires' disease and use of medication nebulizers. J. Infect. Dis. *163*:667–671, 1991.
278. Mayhall, C. G.: Diagnosis and management of infections of implantable devices used for prolonged venous access. Curr. Clin. Top. Infect. Dis. *12*:83–110, 1992.
279. Mayhall, C. G.: Nosocomial burn wound infections. *In* Mayhall, C. G.

(ed.): Hospital Epidemiology and Infection Control. Baltimore, Williams & Wilkins, 1995, pp. 225–236.
280. McCabe, W. R., and Jackson, G. G.: Gram-negative bacteremia. I. Etiology and ecology. Arch. Intern. Med. *110*:847–853, 1962.
281. McFarland, L. V., Mulligan, M. E., Kwok, R. Y., et al.: Nosocomial acquisition of *Clostridium difficile* infection. N. Engl. J. Med. *320*:204–210, 1989.
282. McGechie, P. B.: Nosocomial bacteraemia in hospital staff caused by *Haemophilus influenzae* type b. J. Hosp. Infect. *21*:159–160, 1992.
283. McGrath, D., Swanson, R., Weems, S., et al.: Analysis of a measles outbreak in Kent County, Michigan, in 1990. Pediatr. Infect. Dis. J. *11*:385–389, 1992.
284. McKhann, C. F., Steeger, A., and Long, A. P.: Hospital infections: A survey of the problem. Am. J. Dis. Child. *55*:579–599, 1938.
285. McManus, A. T., Mason, A., Jr., McManus, W. F., et al.: A decade of reduced gram-negative infections and mortality associated with improved isolation of burned patients. Arch. Surg. *129*:1306–1309, 1994.
286. McNamara, M. J., Hill, M. C., Balows, A., et al.: A study of the bacteriologic patterns of hospital infections. Ann. Intern. Med. *66*:480–488, 1967.
287. Meiklejohn, G., Reimer, L. G., Graves, P. S., et al.: Cryptic epidemic of Q fever in a medical school. J. Infect. Dis. *144*:107–113, 1981.
288. Meissner, H. C., Murray, S. A., Kiernan, M. A., et al.: A simultaneous outbreak of respiratory syncytial virus and parainfluenza virus type 3 in a newborn nursery. J. Pediatr. *104*:680–684, 1984.
289. Mermel, L. A., McCormick, R. D., Springman, S. R., et al.: The pathogenesis and epidemiology of catheter-related infection with pulmonary artery Swan-Ganz catheters: A prospective study utilizing molecular subtyping. Am. J. Med. *91*:197S–205S, 1991.
290. Meyer, K. S., Urban, C., Eagan, J. A., et al.: Nosocomial outbreak of *Klebsiella* infection resistant to late-generation cephalosporins. Ann. Intern. Med. *119*:353–358, 1993.
291. Mhalu, F. S., Mtango, F. D., and Msengi, A. E.: Hospital outbreaks of cholera transmitted through close person-to-person contact. Lancet *2*:82–84, 1984.
292. Michaels, M. G., Green, M., Wald, E. R., et al.: Adenovirus infection in pediatric liver transplant recipients. J. Infect. Dis. *165*:170–174, 1992.
293. Middleton, P. J., Szymanski, M. T., and Petric, M.: Viruses associated with acute gastroenteritis in young children. Am. J. Dis. Child. *131*:733–737, 1977.
294. Millar, M. R., Brown, N. M., Tobin, G. W., et al.: Outbreak of infection with penicillin-resistant *Streptococcus pneumoniae* in a hospital for the elderly. J. Hosp. Infect. *27*:99–104, 1994.
295. Mirro, J., Jr., Rao, B. N., Kumar, M., et al.: A comparison of placement techniques and complications of externalized catheters and implantable port use in children with cancer. J. Pediatr. Surg. *25*:120–124, 1990.
296. Modlin, J. F.: Perinatal echovirus and group B coxsackievirus infections. Clin. Perinatol. *15*:233–246, 1988.
297. Moffet, H. L., and Allan, D.: Colonization of infants exposed to bacterially contaminated mists. Am. J. Dis. Child. *114*:21–25, 1967.
298. Monath, T. P., Mertens, P. E., Patton, R., et al.: A hospital epidemic of Lassa fever in Zorzor, Liberia, March–April 1972. Am. J. Trop. Med. Hyg. *22*:773–779, 1973.
299. Moreira, B. M., and Daum, R. S.: Antimicrobial resistance in staphylococci. Pediatr. Clin. North Am. *42*:619–648, 1995.
300. Morosini, M. I., Canton, R., Martinez-Beltran, J., et al.: New extended-spectrum TEM-type beta-lactamase from *Salmonella enterica* subsp. *enterica* isolated in a nosocomial outbreak. Antimicrob. Agents Chemother. *39*:458–461, 1995.
301. Moser, M. R., Bender, T. R., Margolis, H. S., et al.: An outbreak of influenza aboard a commercial airliner. Am. J. Epidemiol. *110*:1–6, 1979.
302. Nakayama, M., Miyazaki, C., Ueda, K., et al.: Pharyngoconjunctival fever caused by adenovirus type 11. Pediatr. Infect. Dis. J. *11*:6–9, 1992.
303. Nardell, E. A.: Interrupting transmission from patients with unsuspected tuberculosis: A unique role for upper-room ultraviolet air disinfection. Am. J. Infect. Control *23*:156–164, 1995.
304. National Institute for Occupational Safety and Health, Centers for Disease Control and Prevention, Public Health Service, et al.: Respiratory protective devices: Final rules and notice. Federal Register *60*:30336–30404, 1995.
305. National Nosocomial Infections Surveillance System: National Nosocomial Infection Surveillance (NNIS) semi-annual report, May 1995. Am. J. Infect. Control *23*:377–385, 1995.
306. Naumovski, L., Quinn, J. P., Miyashiro, D., et al.: Outbreak of ceftazidime resistance due to a novel extended-spectrum beta-lactamase in isolates from cancer patients. Antimicrob. Agents Chemother. *36*:1991–1996, 1992.
307. Navarrete, S., Stetler, H. C., Avila, C., et al.: An outbreak of *Cryptosporidium* diarrhea in a pediatric hospital. Pediatr. Infect. Dis. J. *10*:248–250, 1991.
308. Nelson, K. E., Donahue, J. G., Munoz, A., et al.: Transmission of retroviruses from seronegative donors by transfusion during cardiac surgery: A multicenter study of HIV-1 and HTLV-I/II infections. Ann. Intern. Med. *117*:554–559, 1992.
309. NIH Conference Development Panel on Infectious Disease Testing for Blood Transfusions: Infectious disease testing for blood transfusions. J. A. M. A. *274*:1374–1379, 1995.
310. Noble, R. C., Kane, M. A., Reeves, S. A., et al.: Posttransfusion hepatitis A in a neonatal intensive care unit. J. A. M. A. *252*:2711–2715, 1984.
311. Noel, G. J., Kreiswirth, B. N., Edelson, P. J., et al.: Multiple methicillin-resistant *Staphylococcus aureus* strains as a cause for a single outbreak of severe disease in hospitalized neonates. Pediatr. Infect. Dis. J. *11*:184–188, 1992.
312. Noya, F. J., Rench, M. A., Metzger, T. G., et al.: Unusual occurrence of an epidemic of type Ib/c group B streptococcal sepsis in a neonatal intensive care unit. J. Infect. Dis. *155*:1135–1144, 1987.
313. Odio, C., McCracken, G. H., Jr., and Nelson, J. D.: CSF shunt infections in pediatrics: A seven-year experience. Am. J. Dis. Child. *138*:1103–1108, 1984.
314. Panlilio, A. L., Culver, D. H., Gaynes, R. P., et al.: Methicillin-resistant *Staphylococcus aureus* in U.S. hospitals, 1975–1991. Infect. Control Hosp. Epidemiol. *13*:582–586, 1992.
315. Papanicolaou, G. A., Medeiros, A. A., and Jacoby, G. A.: Novel plasmid-mediated beta-lactamase (MIR-1) conferring resistance to oxyimino- and alpha-methoxy beta-lactams in clinical isolates of *Klebsiella pneumoniae*. Antimicrob. Agents Chemother. *34*:2200–2209, 1990.
316. Parry, M. F., Hutchinson, J. H., Brown, N. A., et al.: Gram-negative sepsis in neonates: A nursery outbreak due to hand carriage of *Citrobacter diversus*. Pediatrics *65*:1105–1109, 1980.
317. Paton, S., Nicolle, L., Mwongera, M., et al.: *Salmonella* and *Shigella* gastroenteritis at a public teaching hospital in Nairobi, Kenya. Infect. Control Hosp. Epidemiol. *12*:710–717, 1991.
318. Patrick, C. H., John, J. F., Levkoff, A. H., et al.: Relatedness of strains of methicillin-resistant coagulase-negative *Staphylococcus* colonizing hospital personnel and producing bacteremias in a neonatal intensive care unit. Pediatr. Infect. Dis. J. *11*:935–940, 1992.
319. Patterson, J. E., Madden, G. M., Krisiunas, E. P., et al.: A nosocomial outbreak of ampicillin-resistant *Haemophilus influenzae* type b in a geriatric unit. J. Infect. Dis. *157*:1002–1007, 1988.
320. Pegues, D. A., Schidlow, D. V., Tablan, O. C., et al.: Possible nosocomial transmission of *Pseudomonas cepacia* in patients with cystic fibrosis. Arch. Pediatr. Adolesc. Med. *148*:805–812, 1994.
321. Perl, T. M., Haugen, T. H., Pfaller, M. A., et al.: Transmission of herpes simplex virus type 1 infection in an intensive care unit. Ann. Intern. Med. *117*:584–586, 1992.
322. Pickering, L. K., Guerrant, R. L., and Cleary, T. G.: Microorganisms responsible for neonatal diarrhea. *In* Remington, J. S., and Klein, J. O. (eds.): Infectious Diseases of the Fetus & Newborn Infant. 4th ed. Philadelphia, W. B. Saunders, 1995, pp. 1142–1195.
323. Piedra, P. A., Kasel, J. A., Norton, H. J., et al.: Description of an adenovirus type 8 outbreak in hospitalized neonates born prematurely. Pediatr. Infect. Dis. J. *11*:460–465, 1992.
324. Pillay, D., Patou, G., Hurt, S., et al.: Parvovirus B19 outbreak in a children's ward. Lancet *339*:107–109, 1992.
325. Pittet, D., Tarara, D., and Wenzel, R. P.: Nosocomial bloodstream infection in critically ill patients: Excess length of stay, extra costs, and attributable mortality. J. A. M. A. *271*:1598–1601, 1994.
326. Pohl, C., Green, M., Wald, E. R., et al.: Respiratory syncytial virus infections in pediatric liver transplant recipients. J. Infect. Dis. *165*:166–169, 1992.
327. Polish, L. B., Shapiro, C. N., Bauer, F., et al.: Nosocomial transmission of hepatitis B virus associated with the use of a spring-loaded finger-stick device. N. Engl. J. Med. *326*:721–725, 1992.
328. Polk, B. F., White, J. A., DeGirolami, P. C., et al.: An outbreak of rubella among hospital personnel. N. Engl. J. Med. *303*:541–545, 1980.
329. Pollack, M. M., Ruttimann, U. E., and Getson, P. R.: Pediatric risk of mortality (PRISM) score. Crit. Care Med. *16*:1110–1116, 1988.
330. Pollock, E., Ford-Jones, E. L., Corey, M., et al.: Use of the Pediatric Risk of Mortality Score to predict nosocomial infection in a pediatric intensive care unit. Crit. Care Med. *19*:160–165, 1991.
331. Pollock, E. M., Ford-Jones, E. L., Rebeyka, I., et al.: Early nosocomial infections in pediatric cardiovascular surgery patients. Crit. Care Med. *18*:378–384, 1990.
332. Porter, J. D., Teter, M., Traister, V., et al.: Outbreak of adenoviral infections in a long-term paediatric facility, New Jersey, 1986/87. J. Hosp. Infect. *18*:201–210, 1991.
333. Poulsen, V.: Über das heutige auftreten der nosocomialen infektionen auf kinderkrankenhäusern, insbesondere in bezug auf dei häufigkeit und die infektionswege. Acta Pediatr. *17*:25–35, 1935.
334. Powell, H., Swarner, O., Gluck, L., et al.: Hexachlorophene myelinopathy in premature infants. J. Pediatr. *82*:976–981, 1973.
335. Prince, D. S., Astry, C., Vonderfecht, S., et al.: Aerosol transmission of experimental rotavirus infection. Pediatr. Infect. Dis. *5*:218–222, 1986.
336. Raad, I. I., Hohn, D. C., Gilbreath, B. J., et al.: Prevention of central venous catheter-related infections by using maximal sterile barrier precautions during insertion. Infect. Control Hosp. Epidemiol. *15*:231–238, 1994.
337. Raad, I. I., Luna, M., Khalil, S. A., et al.: The relationship between the thrombotic and infectious complications of central venous catheters. J. A. M. A. *271*:1014–1016, 1994.
338. Raad, I. I., Sabbagh, M. F., Rand, K. H., et al.: Quantitative tip culture methods and the diagnosis of central venous catheter-related infections. Diagn. Microbiol. Infect. Dis. *15*:13–20, 1992.
339. Raad, I. I., Costerton, W., Sabharwal, U., et al.: Ultrastructural analysis of

indwelling vascular catheters: A quantitative relationship between luminal colonization and duration of placement. J. Infect. Dis. *168*:400–407, 1993.

340. Raad, I. I., Sherertz, R. J., Rains, C. S., et al.: The importance of nosocomial transmission of measles in the propagation of a community outbreak. Infect. Control Hosp. Epidemiol. *10*:161–166, 1989.
341. Raad, I. I., Sherertz, R. J., Russell, B. A., et al.: Uncontrolled nosocomial rotavirus transmission during a community outbreak. Am. J. Infect. Control *18*:24–28, 1990.
342. Rabalais, G., Adams, G., and Stover, B.: PPD skin test conversion in health-care workers after exposure to *Mycobacterium tuberculosis* infection in infants. Lancet *338*:826, 1991.
343. Rabkin, C. S., Telzak, E. E., Ho, M. S., et al.: Outbreak of echovirus 11 infection in hospitalized neonates. Pediatr. Infect. Dis. J. *7*:186–190, 1988.
344. Rackoff, W. R., Weiman, M., Jakobowski, D., et al.: A randomized, controlled trial of the efficacy of a heparin and vancomycin solution in preventing central venous catheter infections in children. J. Pediatr. *127*:147–151, 1995.
345. Rangel-Frausto, M. S., Pittet, D., Costigan, M., et al.: The natural history of the systemic inflammatory response syndrome (SIRS): A prospective study. J. A. M. A. *273*:117–123, 1995.
346. Ratnam, S., Mercer, E., Picco, B., et al.: A nosocomial outbreak of diarrheal disease due to *Yersinia enterocolitica* serotype 0:5, biotype 1. J. Infect. Dis. *145*:242–247, 1982.
347. Raucher, H. S., Hyatt, A. C., Barzilai, A., et al.: Quantitative blood cultures in the evaluation of septicemia in children with Broviac catheters. J. Pediatr. *104*:29–33, 1984.
348. Reboli, A. C., John, J., Jr., and Levkoff, A. H.: Epidemic methicillin-gentamicin–resistant *Staphylococcus aureus* in a neonatal intensive care unit. Am. J. Dis. Child. *143*:34–39, 1989.
349. Remington, P. L., Hall, W. N., Davis, I. H., et al.: Airborne transmission of measles in a physician's office. J. A. M. A. *253*:1574–1577, 1985.
350. Rhinehart, E., Smith, N. E., Wennersten, C., et al.: Rapid dissemination of beta-lactamase–producing, aminoglycoside-resistant *Enterococcus faecalis* among patients and staff on an infant-toddler surgical ward. N. Engl. J. Med. *323*:1814–1818, 1990.
351. Ribner, B. S.: Endemic, multiply resistant *Staphylococcus aureus* in a pediatric population: Clinical description and risk factors. Am. J. Dis. Child. *141*:1183–1187, 1987.
352. Ribner, B. S., Landry, M. N., Kidd, K., et al.: Outbreak of multiply resistant *Staphylococcus aureus* in a pediatric intensive care unit after consolidation with a surgical intensive care unit. Am. J. Infect. Control *17*:244–249, 1989.
353. Rice, L. B., and Shlaes, D. M.: Vancomycin resistance in the enterococcus: Relevance in pediatrics. Pediatr. Clin. North Am. *42*:601–618, 1995.
354. Rice, L. B., Willey, S. H., Papanicolaou, G. A., et al.: Outbreak of ceftazidime resistance caused by extended-spectrum beta-lactamases at a Massachusetts chronic-care facility. Antimicrob. Agents Chemother. *34*:2193–2199, 1990.
355. Richardson, D. K., Gray, J. E., McCormick, M. C., et al.: Score for Neonatal Acute Physiology: A physiologic severity index for neonatal intensive care. Pediatrics *91*:617–623, 1993.
356. Richardson, D. K., Phibbs, C. S., Gray, J. E., et al.: Birth weight and illness severity: Independent predictors of neonatal mortality. Pediatrics *91*:969–975, 1993.
357. Richardson, J. F., Quoraishi, A. H., Francis, B. J., et al.: Beta-lactamase–negative, methicillin-resistant *Staphylococcus aureus* in a newborn nursery: Report of an outbreak and laboratory investigations. J. Hosp. Infect. *16*:109–121, 1990.
358. Richman, D. D., Breton, S. J., and Goldman, D. A.: Scarlet fever and group A streptococcal surgical wound infection traced to an anal carrier. J. Pediatr. *90*:387–390, 1977.
359. Rivera, M. E., Mason, W. H., Ross, L. A., et al.: Nosocomial measles infection in a pediatric hospital during a community-wide epidemic. J. Pediatr. *119*:183–186, 1991.
360. Rodriguez, W. J., Kim, H. W., Brandt, C. D., et al.: Rotavirus: A cause of nosocomial infection in the nursery. J. Pediatr. *101*:274–277, 1982.
361. Rose, H. D., Lenz, I. E., and Sheth, N. K.: Meningococcal pneumonia: A source of nosocomial infection. Arch. Intern. Med. *141*:575–577, 1981.
362. Rosenfeld, C. R., Laptook, A. R., and Jeffery, J.: Limited effectiveness of triple dye in preventing colonization with methicillin-resistant *Staphylococcus aureus* in a special care nursery. Pediatr. Infect. Dis. J. *9*:290–291, 1990.
363. Rotbart, H. A., Levin, M. J., Yolken, R. H., et al.: An outbreak of rotavirus-associated neonatal necrotizing enterocolitis. J. Pediatr. *103*:454–459, 1983.
364. Roy, T. E., McDonald, S., Patrick, M. L., et al.: A survey of hospital infection in a pediatric hospital. Part I. Description of hospital, organization of survey, population studied and some general findings. Can. Med. Assoc. J. *87*:531–538, 1962.
365. Roy, T. E., McDonald, S., Patrick, M. L., et al.: A survey of hospital infection in a pediatric hospital. Part II. The distribution of hospital infections in different areas of the hospital, postoperative wound infections and the consequences of infection. Can. Med. Assoc. J. *87*:592–599, 1962.
366. Roy, T. E., McDonald, S., Patrick, M. L., et al.: A survey of hospital infection in a pediatric hospital. Part III. Staphylococcal infections, notes on antibiotic sensitivity of the staphylococci from postoperative wound and other infections, discussion and summary. Can. Med. Assoc. J. *87*:656–660, 1962.
367. Rubin, L. G., Tucci, V., Cercenado, E., et al.: Vancomycin-resistant *Enterococcus faecium* in hospitalized children. Infect. Control Hosp. Epidemiol. *13*:700–705, 1992.
368. Rushforth, J. A., Hoy, C. M., Kite, P., et al.: Rapid diagnosis of central venous catheter sepsis. Lancet *342*:402–403, 1993.
369. Ryder, R. W., McGowan, J. E., Hatch, M. H., et al.: Reovirus-like agent as a cause of nosocomial diarrhea in infants. J. Pediatr. *90*:698–702, 1977.
370. Ryder, R. W., Rahman, A. S., Alim, A. R., et al.: An outbreak of nosocomial cholera in a rural Bangladesh hospital. J. Hosp. Infect. *8*:275–282, 1986.
371. Sader, H. S., Pfaller, M. A., and Jones, R. N.: Prevalence of important pathogens and the antimicrobial activity of parenteral drugs at numerous medical centers in the United States. II. Study of the intra- and interlaboratory dissemination of extended-spectrum beta-lactamase-producing Enterobacteriaceae. Diagn. Microbiol. Infect. Dis. *20*:203–208, 1994.
372. Saez-Llorens, X., and McCracken, G. H., Jr.: Sepsis syndrome and septic shock in pediatrics: Current concepts of terminology, pathophysiology, and management. J. Pediatr. *123*:497–508, 1993.
373. Saha, M. R., Sircar, B. K., Dutta, P., et al.: Occurrence of multi-resistant *Salmonella typhimurium* infection in a pediatric hospital at Calcutta. Indian Pediatr. *29*:307–311, 1992.
374. Sakaoka, H., Saheki, Y., Uzuki, K., et al.: Two outbreaks of herpes simplex virus type 1 nosocomial infection among newborns. J. Clin. Microbiol. *24*:36–40, 1986.
375. Sanchez, V., Vazquez, J. A., Barth-Jones, D., et al.: Epidemiology of nosocomial acquisition of *Candida lusitaniae*. J. Clin. Microbiol. *30*:3005–3008, 1992.
376. Sands, K., and Goldmann, D. A.: Epidemiology of *Staphylococcus aureus* and group A streptococci. *In* Bennett, J. V., and Brachman, P. S. (eds.): Hospital Infections. 4th ed. Boston, Little, Brown, (in press).
377. Sartor, C., Edwards, J. R., Gaynes, R. P., et al.: Evolution of hospital participation in the National Nosocomial Infection Surveillance (NNIS) System, 1986 to 1993. Am. J. Infect. Control *23*:364–368, 1995.
378. Sattar, S. A., Lloyd-Evans, N., Springthorpe, V. S., et al.: Institutional outbreaks of rotavirus diarrhoea: Potential role of fomites and environmental surfaces as vehicles for virus transmission. J. Hyg. *96*:277–289, 1986.
379. Sawyer, M. H, Chamberlin, C. J., Wu, Y. N., et al.: Detection of varicella-zoster virus DNA in air samples from hospital rooms. J. Infect. Dis. *169*:91–94, 1994.
380. Scerpella, E. G., Wanger, A. R., Armitige, L., et al.: Nosocomial outbreak caused by a multiresistant clone of *Acinetobacter baumannii*: Results of the case-control and molecular epidemiologic investigations. Infect. Control Hosp. Epidemiol. *16*:92–97, 1995.
381. Schaberg, D. R., Culver, D. H., and Gaynes, R. P.: Major trends in the microbial etiology of nosocomial infection. Am. J. Med. *91*:72S–75S, 1991.
382. Schaffer, T. E., Sylvester, R. F., Jr., and Baldwin, J. N.: Staphylococcal infections in newborn infants. II. Report of 19 epidemics caused by an identical strain of *Staphylococcus pyogenes*. Am. J. Public Health *47*:990–1008, 1957.
383. Scheifele, D., and Bonner, M.: Airborne transmission of chickenpox. N. Engl. J. Med. *303*:281–282, 1980.
384. Schlager, T., Sadler, J., Weber, D., et al.: Hospital-acquired infections in pediatric burn patients. South. Med. J. *87*:481–484, 1994.
385. Schmunis, G. A.: *Trypanosoma cruzi*, the etiologic agent of Chagas' disease: Status in the blood supply in endemic and nonendemic countries. Transfusion *31*:547–557, 1991.
386. Schuman, E. S., Winters, V., Gross, G. F., et al.: Management of Hickman catheter sepsis. Am. J. Surg. *149*:627–628, 1985.
387. Schwarcz, S., McCaw, B., and Fukushima, P.: Prevalence of measles susceptibility in hospital staff: Evidence to support expanding the recommendations of the Immunization Practices Advisory Committee. Arch. Intern. Med. *152*:1481–1483, 1992.
388. Selwyn, S.: Hospital infection: The first 2500 years. J. Hosp. Infect. *18*:5–64, 1991.
389. Semmelweis, I. F.: The Etiology, the Concept and the Prophylaxis of Childbed Fever. Birmingham, Classics of Medicine Library, 1981.
390. Senerwa, D., Olsvik, O., Mutanda, L. N., et al.: Enteropathogenic *Escherichia coli* serotype O111:HNT isolated from preterm neonates in Nairobi, Kenya. J. Clin. Microbiol. *27*:1307–1311, 1989.
391. Severien, C., and Nelson, J. D.: Frequency of infections associated with implanted systems vs cuffed, tunneled Silastic venous catheters in patients with acute leukemia. Am. J. Dis. Child. *145*:1433–1438, 1991.
392. Sharma, L. K., and Sharma, P. K.: Postoperative wound infection in a pediatric surgical service. J. Pediatr. Surg. *21*:889–891, 1986.
393. Shefer, A., Dales, L., Nelson, M., et al.: Use and safety of acellular pertussis vaccine among adult hospital staff during an outbreak of pertussis. J. Infect. Dis. *171*:1053–1056, 1995.
394. Sherertz, R. J., Gledhill, K. S., Hampton, K. D., et al.: Outbreak of *Candida* bloodstream infections associated with retrograde medication administration in a neonatal intensive care unit. J. Pediatr. *120*:455–461, 1992.
395. Sherertz, R. J., Raad, I. I., Belani, A., et al.: Three-year experience with

sonicated vascular catheter cultures in a clinical microbiology laboratory. J. Clin. Microbiol. *28*:76–82, 1990.
396. Sheridan, R. L., Weber, J., Benjamin, J., et al.: Control of methicillin-resistant *Staphylococcus aureus* in a pediatric burn unit. Am. J. Infect. Control *22*:340–345, 1994.
397. Shuman, R. M., Leech, R. W., and Alvord, E. C., Jr.: Neurotoxicity of hexachlorophene in the human. I. A clinicopathologic study of 248 children. Pediatrics *54*:689–695, 1974.
398. Shuman, R. M., Leech, R. W., Alvord, E. C., Jr.: Neurotoxicity of hexachlorophene in humans. II. A clinicopathological study of 46 premature infants. Arch. Neurol. *32*:320–325, 1975.
399. Singh-Naz, N., Brown, M., and Ganeshananthan, M.: Nosocomial adenovirus infection: Molecular epidemiology of an outbreak. Pediatr. Infect. Dis. J. *12*:922–925, 1993.
400. Sirinavin, S., Hotrakitya, S., Suprasongsin, C., et al.: An outbreak of *Salmonella urbana* infection in neonatal nurseries. J. Hosp. Infect. *18*:231–238, 1991.
401. Sloand, E. M., Pitt, E., and Klein, H. G.: Safety of the blood supply. J. A. M. A. *274*:1374–1379, 1995.
402. Smith, D. H., Johnson, B. K., Isaacson, M., et al.: Marburg-virus disease in Kenya. Lancet *1*:816–820, 1982.
403. Smith, P. F., Stricof, R. L., Shayegani, M., et al.: Cluster of *Haemophilus influenzae* type b infections in adults. J. A. M. A. *260*:1446–1449, 1988.
404. Snydman, D. R., Greer, C., Meissner, H. C., et al.: Prevention of nosocomial transmission of respiratory syncytial virus in a newborn nursery. Infect. Control Hosp. Epidemiol. *9*:105–108, 1988.
405. Spach, D. H., Silverstein, F. E., and Stamm, W. E.: Transmission of infection by gastrointestinal endoscopy and bronchoscopy. Ann. Intern. Med. *118*:117–128, 1993.
406. Spafford, P. S., Sinkin, R. A., Cox, C., et al.: Prevention of central venous catheter-related coagulase-negative staphylococcal sepsis in neonates. J. Pediatr. *125*:259–263, 1994.
407. Spector, S. A.: Transmission of cytomegalovirus among infants in hospital documented by restriction-endonuclease-digestion analyses. Lancet *1*:378–381, 1983.
408. Spender, Q. W., Lewis, D., and Price, E. H.: Norwalk-like viruses: Study of an outbreak. Arch. Dis. Child. *61*:142–147, 1986.
409. Spratt, H. C., Marks, M. I., Gomersall, M., et al.: Nosocomial infantile gastroenteritis associated with minirotavirus and calicivirus. J. Pediatr. *93*:922–926, 1978.
410. Starke, J. R.: Tuberculosis in children. Curr. Opin. Pediatr. *7*:268–277, 1995.
411. Steketee, R. W., Burstyn, D. G., Wassilak, S. G., et al.: A comparison of laboratory and clinical methods for diagnosing pertussis in an outbreak in a facility for the developmentally disabled. J. Infect. Dis. *157*:441–449, 1988.
412. Stenzel, J. P., Green, T. P., Fuhrman, B. P., et al.: Percutaneous femoral venous catheterizations: A prospective study of complications. J. Pediatr. *114*:411–415, 1989.
413. Stewart, C. J.: Tuberculosis infection in a paediatric department. B. M. J. *1*:30–32, 1976.
414. Stone, A., Shaffer, M., and Sautter, R. L.: *Salmonella poona* infection and surveillance in a neonatal nursery. Am. J. Infect. Control *21*:270–273, 1993.
415. Stover, B. H., Duff, A., Adams, G., et al.: Emergence and control of methicillin-resistant *Staphylococcus aureus* in a children's hospital and pediatric long-term care facility. Am. J. Infect. Control *20*:248–255, 1992.
416. Strassburg, M. A., Imagawa, D. T., Fannin, S. L., et al.: Rubella outbreak among hospital employees. Obstet. Gynecol. *57*:283–288, 1981.
417. Straube, R. C., Thompson, M. A., Van Dyke, R. B., et al.: Adenovirus type 7b in a children's hospital. J. Infect. Dis. *147*:814–819, 1983.
418. Stroud, L. A., Tokars, J. I., Grieco, M. H., et al.: Evaluation of infection control measures in preventing the nosocomial transmission of multidrug-resistant *Mycobacterium tuberculosis* in a New York City hospital. Infect. Control Hosp. Epidemiol. *16*:141–147, 1995.
419. Suleiman, M. N., Muscat-Baron, J. M., Harries, J. R., et al.: Congo/Crimean haemorrhagic fever in Dubai: An outbreak at the Rashid Hospital. Lancet *2*:939–941, 1980.
420. Swartz, M. N.: Hospital-acquired infections: Diseases with increasingly limited therapies. Proc. Natl. Acad. Sci. U. S. A. *91*:2420–2427, 1994.
421. Tablan, O. C.: Nosocomially acquired *Pseudomonas cepacia* infection in patients with cystic fibrosis. Infect. Control Hosp. Epidemiol. *14*:124–126, 1993.
422. Tablan, O. C., Anderson, L. J., Arden, N. H., et al.: Guideline for prevention of nosocomial pneumonia. Infect. Control Hosp. Epidemiol. *15*:587–627, 1994.
423. Tablan, O. C., Chorba, T. L., Schidlow, D. V., et al.: *Pseudomonas cepacia* colonization in patients with cystic fibrosis: Risk factors and clinical outcome. J. Pediatr. *107*:382–387, 1985.
424. Tanaka, Y., Fujinaga, K., Goto, A., et al.: Outbreak of pertussis in a residential facility for handicapped people. Dev. Biol. Stand. *73*:329–332, 1991.
425. Thacker, S. B., Kimball, A. M., Wolfe, M., et al.: Parasitic disease control in a residential facility for the mentally retarded: Failure of selected isolation procedures. Am. J. Public Health *71*:303–305, 1981.
426. The International Neonatal Network: The CRIB (clinical risk index for babies) score: A tool for assessing initial neonatal risk and comparing performance of neonatal intensive care units. Lancet *342*:193–198, 1993.
427. The Society for Hospital Epidemiology of America, the Association for Practitioners in Infection Control, the Centers for Disease Control, et al.: Consensus paper on the surveillance of surgical wound infections. Infect. Control Hosp. Epidemiol. *13*:599–605, 1992.
428. Thomassen, M. J., Demko, C. A., Doershuk, C. F., et al.: *Pseudomonas cepacia*: Decrease in colonization in patients with cystic fibrosis. Am. Rev. Respir. Dis. *134*:669–671, 1986.
429. Tilley, P. A., and Roberts, F. J.: Bacteremia with *Acinetobacter* species: Risk factors and prognosis in different clinical settings. Clin. Infect. Dis. *18*:896–900, 1994.
430. Toltzis, P., and Blumer, J. L.: Antibiotic-resistant gram-negative bacteria in the critical care setting. Pediatr. Clin. North Am. *42*:687–702, 1995.
431. Valenti, W. M., Clarke, T. A., Hall, C. B., et al.: Concurrent outbreaks of rhinovirus and respiratory syncytial virus in an intensive care nursery: Epidemiology and associated risk factors. J. Pediatr. *100*:722–726, 1982.
432. Valenti, W. M., Menegus, M. A., Hall, C. B., et al.: Nosocomial viral infections. I. Epidemiology and significance. Infect. Control *1*:33–37, 1980.
433. Valenti, W. M., Pincus, P. H., and Messner, M. K.: Nosocomial pertussis: Possible spread by a hospital visitor. Am. J. Dis. Child. *134*:520–521, 1980.
435. van Dijk, W. C., and van der Straaten, P. J.: An outbreak of *Campylobacter jejuni* infection in a neonatal intensive care unit. J. Hosp. Infect. *11*:91–92, 1988.
434. Van Dyke, R. B., and Spector, S. A.: Transmission of herpes simplex virus type 1 to a newborn infant during endotracheal suctioning for meconium aspiration. Pediatr. Infect. Dis. *3*:153–156, 1984.
436. Vazquez, J. A., Sanchez, V., Dmuchowski, C., et al.: Nosocomial acquisition of *Candida albicans*: An epidemiologic study. J. Infect. Dis. *168*:195–201, 1993.
437. Velandia, M., Fridkin, S. K., Cardenas, V., et al.: Transmission of HIV in dialysis centre. Lancet *345*:1417–1422, 1995.
438. Vermaat, J. H., Rosebrugh, E., Ford-Jones, E. L., et al.: An epidemiologic study of nosocomial infections in a pediatric long-term care facility. Am. J. Infect. Control *21*:183–188, 1993.
439. Villarino, M. E., Stevens, L. E., Schable, B., et al.: Risk factors for epidemic *Xanthomonas maltophilia* infection/colonization in intensive care unit patients. Infect. Control Hosp. Epidemiol. *13*:201–206, 1992.
440. Wagner, S. J., Friedman, L. I., and Dodd, R. Y.: Transfusion-associated bacterial sepsis. Clin. Microbiol. Rev. *7*:290–302, 1994.
441. Walmsley, S., Devi, S., King, S., et al.: Invasive *Aspergillus* infections in a pediatric hospital: A ten-year review. Pediatr. Infect. Dis. J. *12*:673–682, 1993.
442. Walther, F. J., Bruggeman, C., and Daniels-Bosman, M. S.: Rotavirus infections in high-risk neonates. J. Hosp. Infect. *5*:438–443, 1984.
443. Wasserman, R., August, C. S., and Plotkin, S. A.: Viral infections in pediatric bone marrow transplant patients. Pediatr. Infect. Dis. J. *7*:109–115, 1988.
444. Watkins, A. G., and Lewis-Fanning, E.: Incidence of cross-infection in children's wards. B. M. J. *2*:616–619, 1949.
445. Watson, J. C., Fleming, D. W., Borella, A. J., et al.: Vertical transmission of hepatitis A resulting in an outbreak in a neonatal intensive care unit. J. Infect. Dis. *167*:567–571, 1993.
446. Weinstein, J. W., Barrett, C. R., Baltimore, R. S., et al.: Nosocomial transmission of tuberculosis from a hospital visitor on a pediatrics ward. Pediatr. Infect. Dis. J. *14*:232–234, 1995.
447. Weisman, L. E., Cruess, D. F., and Fischer, G. W.: Opsonic activity of commercially available standard intravenous immunoglobulin preparations. Pediatr. Infect. Dis. J. *13*:1122–1125, 1994.
448. Weisman, L. E., Stoll, B. J., Kueser, T. J., et al.: Intravenous immune globulin prophylaxis of late-onset sepsis in premature neonates. J. Pediatr. *125*:922–930, 1994.
449. Welliver, R. C., and McLaughlin, S.: Unique epidemiology of nosocomial infection in a children's hospital. Am. J. Dis. Child. *138*:131–135, 1984.
450. Wells, V. D., Wong, E. S., Murray, B. E., et al.: Infections due to beta-lactamase–producing, high-level gentamicin-resistant *Enterococcus faecalis*. Ann. Intern. Med. *116*:285–292, 1992.
451. Wenger, P. N., Otten, J., Breeden, A., et al.: Control of nosocomial transmission of multidrug-resistant *Mycobacterium tuberculosis* among health-care workers and HIV-infected patients. Lancet *345*:235–240, 1995.
452. Wenzel, R. P., Deal, E. C., and Hendley, J. O.: Hospital-acquired viral respiratory illness on a pediatric ward. Pediatrics *60*:367–371, 1977.
453. Wesley, A. G., Pather, M., and Tait, D.: Nosocomial adenovirus infection in a paediatric respiratory unit. J. Hosp. Infect. *25*:183–190, 1993.
454. Wessels, M. R., Moses, A. E., Goldberg, J. B., et al.: Hyaluronic acid capsule is a virulence factor for mucoid group A streptococci. Proc. Natl. Acad. Sci. U. S. A. *88*:8317–8321, 1991.
455. Wey, S. B., Mori, M., Pfaller, M. A., et al.: Hospital-acquired candidemia: The attributable mortality and excess length of stay. Arch. Intern. Med. *148*:2642–2645, 1988.
456. Wharton, M., Cochi, S. L., Hutcheson, R. H., et al.: Mumps transmission in hospitals. Arch. Intern. Med. *150*:47–49, 1990.
457. Wiener, E. S.: Catheter sepsis: The central venous line Achilles' heel. Semin. Pediatr. Surg. *4*:207–214, 1995.

458. Wilde, J., Yolken, R., Willoughby, R., et al.: Improved detection of rotavirus shedding by polymerase chain reaction. Lancet *337*:323–326, 1991.
459. Williams, W. W., Mariano, J., Spurrier, M., et al.: Nosocomial meningitis due to *Citrobacter diversus* in neonates: New aspects of the epidemiology. J. Infect. Dis. *150*:229–235, 1984.
460. Wilson, A. P., Weavill, C., Burridge, J., et al.: The use of the wound scoring method "ASEPSIS" in postoperative wound surveillance. J. Hosp. Infect. *16*:297–309, 1990.
461. Wilson, C. W., Stevenson, D. K., and Arvin, A. M.: A concurrent epidemic of respiratory syncytial virus and echovirus 7 infections in an intensive care nursery. Pediatr. Infect. Dis. J. *8*:24–29, 1989.
462. Wong, E. S.: Guideline for prevention of catheter-associated urinary tract infections. Am. J. Infect. Control *11*:28–36, 1983.
463. Wong, E. S.: Surgical site infections. *In* Mayhall, C. G. (ed.): Hospital Epidemiology and Infection Control. Baltimore, Williams & Wilkins, 1995, pp. 154–175.
464. Wood, D. J., and Corbitt, G.: Viral infections in childhood leukemia. J. Infect. Dis. *152*:266–273, 1985.
465. Woodford, N., Johnson, A. P., Morrison, D., et al.: Current perspectives on glycopeptide resistance. Clin. Microbiol. Rev. *8*:585–615, 1995.
466. Woolf, A. D., and Cohen, B. J.: Parvovirus B19 and chronic arthritis: Causal or casual association? Ann. Rheum. Dis. *54*:535–536, 1995.
467. Wu, S. X., and Tang, Y.: Molecular epidemiologic study of an outbreak of *Salmonella typhimurium* infection at a newborn nursery. Chin. Med. J. *106*:423–427, 1993.
468. Wurzel, C. L., Halom, K., Feldman, J. G., et al.: Infection rates of Broviac-Hickman catheters and implantable venous devices. Am. J. Dis. Child. *142*:536–540, 1988.
469. Yeh, T. S., Pollack, M. M., Ruttimann, U. E., et al.: Validation of a physiologic stability index for use in critically ill infants and children. Pediatr. Res. *18*:445–451, 1984.
470. Yogev, R.: Cerebrospinal fluid shunt infections: A personal view. Pediatr. Infect. Dis. *4*:113–118, 1985.

229

Prevention and Control of Nosocomial Infections in Hospitalized Children

W. Charles Huskins and Donald A. Goldmann

The history of formal hospital programs to prevent and control nosocomial infections generally is traced to the organized efforts of hospitals in Great Britain and North America to control the pandemic of *Staphylococcus aureus* infections in the 1950s and early 1960s. However, programs to study and control the nosocomial spread of contagious diseases were well established in pediatric hospitals in several European countries and North America even in the mid-1930s.[8, 9, 53, 70, 71, 77] In the past half century, the scope and complexity of these hospital infection prevention and control programs have expanded dramatically. Hospitals today are populated by increasing numbers of severely ill children with compromised host defenses. Advances in medical care and technology have improved the survival and prognosis of these vulnerable patients, but this progress has gone hand in hand with an increased risk of nosocomial infection from an ever-expanding spectrum of microbial pathogens. The small but significant risk of infection among medical professionals providing care to hospitalized children always has been present but is recognized more openly today.

This chapter highlights key elements of a comprehensive program to prevent and control nosocomial infections in pediatric patients and health care workers. A description of how to develop, implement, and maintain an effective program is beyond the scope of this chapter, and the reader is referred to several excellent and authoritative references on this topic.[4, 29, 75, 102] Specific nosocomial infections are discussed in Chapter 228.

EXTERNAL ORGANIZATIONS INFLUENCING HOSPITAL INFECTION PREVENTION AND CONTROL PROGRAMS

The nature and activity of the large number of external organizations that have significant influence on hospital infection prevention and control programs in the United States are described elsewhere.[76] A discussion of a few of the most influential of these organizations follows.

The Hospital Infections Program (HIP), a part of the Centers for Disease Control and Prevention's (CDC's) National Center for Infectious Diseases, has a major role in providing information and guidance to hospital infection control programs as well as conducting its own investigations. The HIP has the single largest experience in nosocomial infection outbreak investigation and can provide assistance to individual hospitals.[57] In general, hospitals requesting HIP assistance must do so through their state health department.

Coordinated by the HIP, the National Nosocomial Infection Surveillance (NNIS) System collects data on the incidence of nosocomial infections in more than 150 U.S. hospitals.[32, 92] Participation in the NNIS System is voluntary; consequently, data reported by the NNIS System do not necessarily represent the universe of U.S. hospitals. Nonetheless, these data are useful in detecting and describing broad-based trends in the incidence and microbial etiology of nosocomial infections in the United States. In addition, the NNIS System regularly reports several key device-associated, exposure-adjusted infection rates (e.g., number of central venous catheter infections per 1000 central venous catheter days), device utilization rates in intensive care units (e.g., number of central venous catheters used per 100 patients), and risk-adjusted surgical site infection rates for specific operative procedures.[81] Although comparisons of infection rates among hospitals still are hampered by incomplete adjustment for severity of illness, hospitals analyzing their performance relative to these benchmarks may identify areas for improvement.[80]

The Hospital Infection Control Practices Advisory Committee (HICPAC) was established in 1991 to provide advice and guidance to the HIP and the CDC regarding the practice of hospital infection control and strategies for surveillance, prevention, and control of nosocomial infections in U.S. hospitals. HICPAC issues evidence-based guidelines for infection control, and several of these guidelines have been published recently.[38, 56, 84a, 96]

A large number of professional and trade associations also

develop recommendations and guidelines related to infection control. Most prominent among these are the Society of Healthcare Epidemiology of America (SHEA) and the Association for Professionals in Infection Control and Epidemiology (APIC).

Over the past several decades, the Joint Commission on Accreditation of Healthcare Organizations (JCAHO), a private, not-for-profit organization, has had a major influence on the structure and activity of hospital infection prevention and control programs.[84] JCAHO standards regarding these programs have evolved significantly over the past several years consistent with the JCAHO's Agenda for Change, an initiative to place greater emphasis on organizational performance regarding processes that significantly affect patient care.[84] One of the goals of this effort is to develop indicators that can be used not only to track organizational performance, but also to facilitate comparisons of quality of care (benchmarking) among hospitals. Candidate indicators are being solicited and reviewed for possible application in hospitals as a part of the accreditation process.

Current JCAHO accreditation standards reflect movement away from assessment of the structural elements of an infection control program, such as the existence of an infection control committee, toward integration of nosocomial infection prevention and control into the everyday activities of the hospital as a whole.[59] A primer for preparing for a JCAHO inspection has been published recently.[82]

Responding to the hazards of occupational exposure to blood-borne pathogens and tuberculosis, the U.S. Department of Labor's Occupational Safety and Health Administration (OSHA) has issued regulations that have had a major impact on the structure and activity of hospital infection prevention and control activities. In 1991, OSHA issued its regulations regarding blood-borne pathogens, "Occupational Exposure to Bloodborne Pathogens: Final Rule," mandating specific exposure prevention strategies, health care worker education, evaluation and management of exposures, voluntary hepatitis B vaccination at no cost to employees, and detailed record-keeping.[83] OSHA currently is in the process of developing regulations regarding occupational exposure to *Mycobacterium tuberculosis* that are proving to be even more controversial, particularly in regard to the type and use of masks worn by health care workers caring for patients with possible or confirmed active pulmonary or laryngeal tuberculosis (see Policies and Procedures, Occupational Health).[26] Hospital infection prevention and control programs and other hospital departments (e.g., occupational health, safety) have spent an enormous amount of time trying to interpret and comply with these regulations.

INTEGRATION OF HOSPITAL INFECTION PREVENTION AND CONTROL AND QUALITY IMPROVEMENT EFFORTS

Many hospitals have implemented continuous quality improvement (CQI) initiatives (also called total quality management [TQM]) as a means for improving the quality of hospital care.[6, 24, 25, 64] Some individuals involved in hospital infection prevention and control programs have led this effort because they know how to apply epidemiologic principles to the collection, analysis, and interpretation of data and they have extensive experience in improving systems of hospital care—both central components of the CQI approach. Systems of care that affect the risk of nosocomial infections typically are complex and involve personnel from many departments. Infection control personnel do not "own" any of these systems. Therefore, they must assist others in using epidemiologically valid methods to study and improve systems of care critical for nosocomial infection prevention. This section illustrates how epidemiologic studies and systems improvement can be integrated into an overall CQI effort.

A system of care can be analyzed in terms of its structure (i.e., essential facilities, equipment, supplies, personnel, and organizational networks), processes (i.e., the relationships and interactions between structural elements), and outcomes (i.e., nosocomial infection rates or mortality rates, the cost of nosocomial infections, patient satisfaction).[28] The systems of care critical for the prevention of surgical site infection provide an excellent illustration of this conceptual model.

Structural elements important for the prevention of surgical-site infections are well described (e.g., presence of skilled surgeons, a program for surveillance and feedback of surgical site infection rates to surgeons, guidelines for perioperative antimicrobial prophylaxis, effective sterilization methods for surgical instruments, adequately designed and equipped operating rooms),[108] although not all of the individual contributions of each of these elements have been confirmed by rigorous experimental trials. Processes important in the prevention of surgical-wound infection (e.g., methods of preoperative hair removal, procedures for preparation of the skin at the site of the incision, the timing of perioperative antimicrobial prophylaxis) have been studied extensively.[108] Methods for collecting data regarding surgical-site infections and calculating risk-adjusted rates of surgical-site infection for specific surgical procedures are well described as a result of decades of methodologic investigation.[22, 97]

Epidemiologic studies (e.g., experimental clinical trials, cohort studies, case-control studies, population-based studies) have defined the impact of various structures and processes on surgical-site infection rates. For example, many clinical trials have examined the effectiveness of various regimens for perioperative antimicrobial prophylaxis in the prevention of surgical-site infections. Based on these studies, guidelines for perioperative antimicrobial prophylaxis have been developed.[1, 61] Yet several studies have shown that utilization of perioperative prophylaxis is less than optimal.[23, 31, 94] Currier and colleagues[23] found that only 60 per cent of patients with indications for prophylaxis actually received it; conversely, prophylaxis was administered to 41 per cent of patients with no indication. Prophylaxis often is continued for excessively long periods (>2 days).[23, 31, 94] A recent cohort study demonstrated the critical importance of the timing of perioperative antimicrobial prophylaxis in the prevention of surgical-site infections. Classen and colleagues[20] demonstrated that the effectiveness of prophylaxis was maximized only if it was administered during a 2-hour window period before the start of the procedure; prophylaxis administered before or after this period was much less effective, and prophylaxis administered 6 or more hours after the start of the procedure essentially had no effect. Nearly 40 per cent of patients in this study did not receive prophylaxis within this critical window period.[20]

CQI is suited ideally to address multidisciplinary, interdepartmental systems problems, such as timely administration of perioperative antimicrobial prophylaxis. With the help of personnel (e.g., surgeons, nurses, pharmacists, anesthesiologists) intimately involved in this system, the reasons that patients do not receive prophylaxis at the appropriate time can be examined and the system for ordering, dispensing, delivering, and administrating prophylactic agents can be streamlined. A comprehensive guide to assist hospitals in using CQI to improve utilization of antimicrobial agents and prevent and control the emergence and dissemination of antimicrobial resistant microorganisms has been published.[42]

ORGANIZATION OF THE HOSPITAL INFECTION CONTROL PROGRAM

The Study on the Efficacy of Nosocomial Infection Control (SENIC) Project conducted in U.S. hospitals in the mid-1970s found that hospitals with a trained, effective infection control physician, one infection control nurse per 250 acute care hospital beds, and a system for reporting surgical-site infection rates to surgeons could reduce their nosocomial infection rates by 32 per cent compared with hospitals with no infection control program.[50] However, because relatively few hospitals had implemented these maximally effective programs, only 6 per cent of the theoretically preventable infections nationwide were, in fact, prevented. A repeat survey of a sample of the participating hospitals in 1983 found that the percentage of hospitals with one infection control nurse per 250 acute care hospital beds had increased from 22 per cent to 57 per cent; however, the percentage with a physician trained in infection control remained low (15 per cent), and the percentage of hospitals performing surgical-site infection surveillance and reporting these rates to surgeons actually decreased.[51] The percentage of preventable infections that were avoided had risen to 9 per cent. Apart from this landmark study, there has been little objective evaluation of the efficacy of various components of infection control programs.

Nonetheless, a large amount of practical experience has guided the development of hospital infection control programs. The programs have a clear mandate and well-defined responsibilities (often described in the hospital bylaws), a direct line of reporting to the hospital administration, and a staff that fosters collegial and mutually respectful relationships with clinicians and other health care professionals.

Infection control committees are an almost universal component of hospital infection prevention and control programs in the United States, in part because of past JCAHO accreditation requirements and the management and operational style of U.S. hospitals. A recently published paper provides practical advice on the composition of the infection control committee and on increasing the productivity and value of committee meetings.[105]

It is clear from the SENIC Project, as well as from practical experience, that physicians provide valuable input into the hospital infection prevention and control program.[47, 50] The SENIC Project found that a physician was at least the nominal leader of these programs in the majority of U.S. hospitals; the vast majority of large hospitals and hospitals affiliated with medical schools had programs with physician leaders.[47] In programs in which the physician is not the leader of the program, consultative input from a physician often is available. The term *hospital epidemiologist* has been used to describe the leader of the hospital infection control program. The SENIC project indicated that, at least in the mid-1970s, this group was heterogeneous with regard to clinical background, previous training in infection control, and level of time commitment to the program.[47] Larger hospitals and hospitals affiliated with medical schools were more likely to have physicians with infectious diseases training as their hospital epidemiologists.[47] A repeat survey performed in 1983 indicated that the percentage of hospital epidemiologists with training in infectious diseases had increased in teaching hospitals and that an increasing number received compensation for this role but that the percentage who had specific infection control training was unchanged (25 per cent).[49] More recently, training in hospital infection prevention and control has become a requirement for accreditation of infectious diseases training programs, and the CDC, SHEA, and the American Hospital Association (AHA) have sponsored biannual intensive training courses for hospital epidemiologists.

As described by Haley[49] in 1987, the essential roles of a hospital epidemiologist are to (1) develop specific, focused surveillance objectives, (2) design surveillance reports relevant to clinicians, (3) interpret surveillance results to physicians, (4) investigate outbreaks, (5) guide the infection control committee in making policies, and (6) collaborate with the infection control practitioner. Wenzel[103] recently described his views on various practical aspects of serving in this position.

The rationale for an expanded role for the hospital epidemiologist, and indeed for hospital epidemiology as a discipline, has been the subject of considerable discussion for several years.[41, 44, 65, 100, 101, 103] In addition to hospital infection prevention and control, some hospital epidemiologists have become involved in CQI programs; utilization, monitoring, and control of antimicrobials; product evaluation; technology assessment; and occupational health. The ranks of hospital epidemiologists who have embraced this expanded role appear to be increasing rapidly, in part as a response to administrative consolidation in hospitals and the evolving standards of the JCAHO.

It is equally clear, both from the SENIC Project and from practical experience, that trained infection control professionals are critical to the effectiveness of the program.[50] The development of the profession of infection control and applied epidemiology in the field of health care has been advanced by the establishment of a professional society (APIC),[89] publication of a training curriculum,[5, 95] and the institution of a certification test in 1983.[86] Defined by a survey of these persons in 1982 and updated in 1987, the roles of these persons are to (1) develop policies and procedures for patient care and nonpatient care departments, (2) identify and isolate patients with transmissible infectious diseases and provide advice regarding the management of exposed persons, (3) develop surveillance strategies, (4) collect, analyze, and report data regarding the frequency of nosocomial infections, (5) conduct outbreak investigations, (6) interpret microbiologic information in relation to hospital infection prevention and control, (7) evaluate and select agents for hand washing and products used for antisepsis, disinfection, and sterilization, (8) evaluate the infectious risks of new products and develop interventions to minimize this risk, (9) provide education for hospital personnel regarding issues related to hospital infection prevention and control, (10) develop policies and procedures for prevention and management of occupationally related infectious diseases, (11) serve as a liaison for external agencies regarding hospital infection prevention and control, (12) communicate with clinicians and the hospital administration regarding pertinent issues, and (13) manage the program.[66, 93]

With this long list of responsibilities, the question as to what constitutes an adequate number of program staff members frequently is asked and hotly debated. The SENIC Project provided a benchmark of one infection control professional per 250 acute care hospital beds[50]; however, optimal staffing should be guided by programmatic responsibilities and institutional requirements in individual hospitals.

The hospital infection prevention and control program should maintain close relationships with the microbiology laboratory and the information services department. Review of microbiology results should be a routine part of the surveillance of nosocomial infections (see later). Laboratory results also can serve as an "early warning system" for the identification of patients infected or colonized with epidemiologically important microorganisms. A list of critical microbiology results (e.g., vancomycin-resistant enterococci) that should prompt immediate notification of infection control staff should be established and reviewed regularly. Microbiology laboratory leadership and infection control should establish guidelines for saving isolates that may be needed for further testing. For example, it is prudent to save blood culture isolates, unusual isolates, and highly resistant strains so that genotyping can be performed at a later date if indicated epidemiologically. Computerization of results can be enormously helpful by facilitating nosocomial infection surveillance (see later), flagging patients who are colonized with antimicrobial-resistant microorganisms and tracking these patients automatically so that they can be recognized immediately if they are readmitted to the hospital later, and generating summaries of antimicrobial resistance patterns of nosocomial isolates.

SURVEILLANCE STRATEGIES

Surveillance of nosocomial infections is necessary to understand the specific nosocomial infection problems of individual hospitals. Surveillance data can focus prevention and control efforts on the highest-risk patients and provide a means of evaluating the effectiveness of these interventions. By establishing endemic rates of nosocomial infections, surveillance also facilitates detection of outbreaks. For these reasons, surveillance traditionally has been regarded as an essential component of a hospital infection prevention and control program, a view that was validated by the SENIC Project.[50]

Prevalence surveys often are used by hospitals when initiating surveillance programs to gain a global perspective of their nosocomial infection problem quickly. These surveys also can be used to validate the sensitivity and specificity of ongoing surveillance. For hospitals that focus surveillance efforts on high-risk patients, periodic prevalence surveys can provide reassurance that previously low-risk populations or low-priority problems have not become more problematic. In general, however, surveillance systems that measure the incidence of nosocomial infections provide a more detailed assessment of infection risk and are much more likely to detect outbreaks.

Hospital-wide surveillance, frequently performed by programs in the 1970s and 1980s, largely has been abandoned because of the substantial time commitment required for data collection, although some hospitals have developed computerized systems for case finding that have improved the efficiency of this approach considerably.[10, 33] Most hospitals currently favor focused (or targeted) surveillance, which concentrates on specific high-risk groups (e.g., patients in intensive care units, surgical patients), specific sites of infection (e.g., blood stream, surgical site), or specific pathogens (e.g., respiratory virus, toxin-producing *Clostridium difficile,* multidrug-resistant microorganisms). This approach is designed to maximize the efficiency of surveillance and to focus on particularly problematic infections or pathogens. Haley[48] has advocated a refinement of focused surveillance that he calls surveillance-by-objective. This approach ensures that surveillance supports specific programmatic goals, providing concrete measures of success. It is suited only for mature surveillance programs that have a clear understanding of their priorities and are confident of their capacity to detect outbreaks through means other than ongoing analysis of endemic infection rates. Hospitals with advanced CQI programs will find this data-driven approach to advancing institutional priorities familiar.

A surveillance plan for an individual hospital may incorporate various types of surveillance. For example, in the authors' hospital, the surveillance plan includes surveillance for (1) infections of all types in patients in the newborn intensive care unit, (2) laboratory-confirmed blood stream infections in all patients, (3) surgical-site infections in patients undergoing cardiovascular surgery, (4) respiratory virus infections (respiratory syncytial virus, influenza A and B viruses, parainfluenza type 3 virus) and gastrointestinal virus infections (rotavirus) in all patients during the peak season for community infection caused by these viruses (November through April), (5) toxin-producing *C. difficile* in all patients, (6) gram-negative rods resistant to third-generation cephalosporins or aminoglycosides, methicillin-resistant *S. aureus,* enterococci with high-level gentamicin resistance, and vancomycin-resistant enterococci in all patients, and (7) infections caused by airborne filamentous fungi in all patients. Detection of key antimicrobial-resistant pathogens is facilitated by performing periodic surveillance cultures on the highest-risk patient populations.

A written plan for surveillance activity should be reviewed yearly and modified as necessary. For each surveillance component, the plan should include a description of (1) the rationale for surveillance, (2) the target population, (3) infection definitions, (4) case-finding methods, (5) the source of denominators used for rate calculations, (6) collection of additional data regarding risk factors, (7) calculation of infection rates (including stratification by risk factors, if planned), (8) the frequency of reporting to specific target groups (e.g., clinicians, infection control committee, hospital leadership), and (9) the estimated time commitment of staff for data collection, analysis, and reporting.

When choosing a particular surveillance strategy, it is important to consider its sensitivity and specificity. For example, self-reporting by clinicians notoriously is insensitive, and surveillance that relies on microbiology culture results alone is likely to be both insensitive and nonspecific. The research regarding case-finding methods is considerable.[39, 85] In general, active, concurrent case finding—that is, active searching for cases by trained persons—should be used. The gold standard for case finding includes bedside examination, interviews with ward staff members, review of the patient charts and all kardexes, and verification of all related microbiologic information by a trained surveyor.[35] However, few programs have the staff for this labor-intensive effort. Many programs rely on positive microbiology culture reports as a starting point for the investigation of infections, such as blood stream infections, for which cultures are obtained routinely with subsequent review of patient charts to confirm or refute the presence of a nosocomial infection. Nosocomial infections that are not evaluated with microbiology cultures are, of course, missed by this approach. Surgical-site infections, on the other hand, are investigated by first reviewing the patient's chart, interviewing staff, examining the patient, or performing a combination thereof. Prescription of antimicrobial agents has been used to identify postpartum infections and surgical-site infections in adults,[54, 109] but the usefulness of this approach for identifying nosocomial infections in pediatric patients has not been examined.

Decentralized surveillance methods that allow persons other than infection control staff members (e.g., a bedside nurse) to identify possibly infected patients, whose records subsequently are reviewed by a trained infection control professional, also have been developed. Such systems depend on clear identification criteria, such as signs or symptoms of infection (e.g., fever), significant risk factors for infection (e.g., invasive devices or procedures), and treatment with antimicrobial agents, as well as a simple record-keeping document (e.g., a checksheet) that is completed reliably. For example, an infection control sentinel sheet system (ICSSS), used at the Hospital for Sick Children in Toronto, Canada, was highly sensitive (>90 per cent), although not very specific, for detecting nosocomial infections.[34] Surveillance in the pediatric intensive care unit in this hospital required only 20 minutes of an infection control professional's time each day.

Surveillance performed by review of information accessible by a desktop computer is a reality in some hospitals today. The most sophisticated computer systems can link bedside information with data from the clinical laboratories, radiology, the pharmacy, and other sources.[10, 19, 33] When coupled with artificial intelligence programs, such systems can screen efficiently for patients likely to have a nosocomial infection.[10, 19, 33]

Calculations of infection rates should include appropriate adjustments whenever possible (see Chapter 228). The simplest technique merely is to adjust for exposure to a particular device or procedure (e.g., number of blood stream infections per 100 patients with central venous catheters). Adjustment for the duration of exposure to the hospital (e.g., number of infections per 1000 patient-days) or device exposure (e.g., number of blood stream infections per 1000 central venous catheter days) is more useful if the necessary denominator data can be obtained. Surgical-site infections should be stratified by wound class and preferably by the surgical-site infection risk index.[22] Some investigators have adjusted infection rates using sophisticated severity of illness scoring systems, such as Acute Physiology, Age, Chronic Health Evaluation (APACHE), Pediatric Risk of Mortality (PRISM), and Score for Neonatal Acute Physiology (SNAP),[43, 45, 87] but this type of adjustment has yet to become routine in surveillance data analysis. Infection rates in newborn intensive care units can be adjusted by birth weight category,[81] although this adjustment alone does not adequately adjust for severity of illness (see Chapter 228).

Feedback of infection rates to clinicians should be performed regularly using an easy-to-understand format. Graphic displays of data are most effective. For example, rates of specific infections can be reported on a run chart, distributions of microorganisms can be displayed as a pie chart, and resistance to key antimicrobials can be displayed in a table with trends noted by up-pointing or down-pointing arrows. Surveillance data also should be used to target areas for further investigation, additional staff education, and specific interventions. High-priority nosocomial infection problems should be addressed by a systematic approach to problem-solving as discussed earlier (see Integration of Hospital Infection Prevention and Control and Quality Improvement Efforts).

Surveillance and reporting of communicable infections to state departments of health is a duty retained by some hospital infection prevention and control programs, although others delegate this responsibility primarily to the microbiology laboratory.

OUTBREAK INVESTIGATION

It is estimated that a community hospital can expect to experience at least one nosocomial infection outbreak per year[52]; teaching hospitals can expect to experience several outbreaks every year.[104] Because outbreaks of nosocomial infections often are associated with significant patient morbidity and mortality, clusters of infection should be investigated promptly. A single, highly unusual infection, such as a post-operative group A streptococcal infection, is sufficient cause for an investigation. Clusters of nosocomial infections caused by an uncommon microorganism, a common microorganism with an unusual antimicrobial susceptibility pattern, or a series of infections at the same anatomic site (e.g., an outbreak of diarrhea) also are obvious indications for an investigation. However, some outbreaks are more difficult to recognize because they occur intermittently, involve multiple microorganisms, or involve infection at various anatomic sites.

TABLE 229–1. Approach to the Investigation of Clusters of Nosocomial Infections

1. Confirm the diagnosis.
2. Make a case definition.
3. Search for additional cases.
4. Plot the epidemic curve.
5. Compare pre-epidemic rates to current rates using statistical tests to prove that an epidemic exists.
6. Perform a literature review.
7. Open lines of communication with leaders of relevant departments, the microbiology laboratory, and the hospital administration.
8. Keep detailed records of events and conversations.
9. Review charts of all cases and compile a line listing of relevant information.
10. Formulate a hypothesis about a likely reservoir and mode of transmission.
11. Institute temporary control measures.
12. Perform a case-control study to develop epidemiologic evidence to support or refute the hypotheses.
13. Update control measures.
14. Document the reservoir and mode of transmission microbiologically. Confirm the relatedness of isolates using molecular genotyping techniques if necessary.
15. Document the efficacy of control measures.
16. Write a report and distribute it to the appropriate persons.
17. Change policies and procedures if necessary.

A guide to the investigation of a cluster of nosocomial infections is described in Table 229–1; detailed discussions of the methodology for outbreak investigation also are found in other references.[27, 110] The large number of published outbreak investigations is an invaluable resource because they often provide insight into potential causes of the outbreak.[57] For example, an outbreak caused by *Stenotrophomonas (Xanthomonas) maltophilia*, *Burkholderia (Pseudomonas) cepacia*, or *Pseudomonas* species should suggest the possibility of a common-source outbreak due to a contaminated solution or medication or an inadequately disinfected piece of equipment. On the other hand, it is hazardous to jump to conclusions regarding the cause of a particular cluster of infections based on the results of a prior investigation. Careful investigation is necessary to establish or refute epidemiologic links between cases and potential causes.

Molecular genotyping techniques are a valuable adjunct to outbreak investigation and largely have replaced older phenotyping techniques, such as phage typing and colicin typing.[7, 58] Despite rapid advances in recent years, gold-standard techniques do not exist for all microorganisms, and testing generally is not available outside of academic medical centers. Genotyping is most useful when it is applied to test a hypothesis about the relatedness of various isolates established during the course of a thorough outbreak investigation utilizing traditional epidemiologic methods (cohort or case-control studies).

POLICIES AND PROCEDURES

Policies and procedures are necessary to optimize and standardize hospital routines and patient care practices. Certain generic policies and procedures apply to all departments, such as those for hand washing, isolation precautions, prevention of transmission of infectious diseases from and to visitors and health care workers, reprocessing of reusable patient care items, and disposal of medical waste. Other policies and procedures should be tailored to the potential infection risks relevant to specific departmental activities. Numerous guidelines have been published that can help hospitals develop policies and procedures.[15, 18, 37, 38, 56, 68, 83, 84a, 90, 96, 107]

As shown by numerous studies documenting poor compliance with policies for hand washing and isolation precautions,[67] compliance with policies and procedures often is less than optimal. Unfortunately, few studies have attempted to elucidate the reasons for noncompliance or to investigate methods for modifying staff behavior.[67, 106] To have any chance of improving performance in such critical aspects of infection prevention, hospital and departmental leaders must make compliance an organizational priority.[42, 67, 69] Staff members responsible for implementation should be included in the process of developing policies and procedures to ensure that the resulting documents are workable, as well as to develop their sense of ownership and responsibility for successful implementation and sustained compliance. Staff education is important but not sufficient in and of itself. Prompt feedback of data concerning key outcome and process measures also is critical in motivating staff members, and barriers to improvement must be identified and removed.[42, 67, 69] For example, clinicians cannot be expected to comply with an isolation precaution policy if gloves are not available or are located inconveniently. Additional investigation into engineering solutions, cognitive approaches, behavioral modification, and training strategies also is needed.

Hand Washing

Proper hand washing decreases the transmission or reduces carriage of potential nosocomial pathogens by the contaminated hands of health care workers.[68] Surprisingly, however, evidence that hand washing directly leads to lower nosocomial infection rates is limited.[21, 67] Nonetheless, hand washing is regarded widely as the quintessential prevention measure.

Indications and procedures for hand washing are reviewed in detail in a recent APIC guideline.[68] In general, hands should be washed before and after patient contact; after contact with body fluids and substances, mucous membranes, nonintact skin, and objects that are likely to be contaminated; before performing invasive procedures; and after removing gloves (see Isolation Precautions). Many health care professionals fail to appreciate the importance of hand washing after removing gloves. Gloves have been demonstrated to have macroscopic and microscopic holes that may lead to hand contamination,[62] and hands may be contaminated in the process of removing soiled gloves.

Hand washing with plain (bland) soap and water mechanically removes organic material and transient flora from the hands but does not reduce necessarily counts of microorganisms on the hands, especially counts of resident (colonizing) flora.[68] Frequent hand washing actually may increase microbial counts by increasing shedding of microorganisms in desquamated epithelium.[68] Recent data suggest that plain soap does not eliminate reliably transient carriage of antimicrobial-resistant microorganisms, such as vancomycin-resistant enterococci.[98] Various topical antimicrobial agents substantially reduce hand counts of transient and resident flora (by 90 per cent or more) through their bactericidal and bacteriostatic effects.[68] Certain topical antimicrobial agents used for hand washing (e.g., iodophors, triclosan, chlorhexidine gluconate) also have persistent residual antimicrobial activity.[68] The specific indications for choosing hand washing agents with antimicrobial activity instead of plain soap have not been defined clearly, but some general recommendations can be made. Plain soap and water are sufficient for hand washing in most hospital settings.[68] However, it is prudent to use agents with antimicrobial activity before performing an invasive procedure.[68] Agents with residual activity particularly are useful during long surgical procedures in which persistent suppression of skin flora on the glove hands may be advantageous.[68] Use of these agents also should be considered when caring for high-risk patients (e.g., patients in intensive care units, immunocompromised patients) or in special situations (e.g., outbreaks, settings in which antimicrobial-resistant microorganisms are a particular concern). An adequate means of drying the hands after hand washing is necessary (e.g., paper towels, single-use hand towels). A variety of waterless hand washing agents with antimicrobial activity is useful when hand washing facilities and supplies are limited or when hand washing at a sink is inconvenient.[68] Alcohol combined with emollients makes a waterless hand washing agent that rapidly kills transient and colonizing hand flora and is inexpensive and generally well accepted by personnel.

Isolation Precautions

Proper utilization of isolation precautions is important for all hospitals but especially is critical in hospitals caring for pediatric patients. Children hospitalized as the result of infections acquired in the community account for a substantial proportion of pediatric admissions, and nosocomial transmission of these infections to other susceptible patients is a significant problem (see Chapter 228). Effective use of appropriate isolation precautions markedly reduces nosocomial transmission of these agents.[2, 69]

A CDC/HICPAC guideline describes the evolution of isolation practices in the United States and describes a new system of isolation precautions for hospitals.[38] The objectives of this new isolation system are to adopt the best components of existing systems and use terminology that is self-explanatory and avoids confusion with previously used terms. Most importantly, HICPAC has endeavored to create a system that is as simple and user-friendly as possible. The guideline contains two tiers of precautions, Standard Precautions and Transmission-Based Precautions, that are described next in greater detail.[38]

Standard Precautions

Standard Precautions synthesize elements of two previous precautions systems: Universal Precautions (UP) and Body Substance Isolation (BSI). UP was a strategy developed in 1985, largely in response to the HIV epidemic, to protect health care workers from exposure to blood-borne pathogens, including HIV and hepatitis B virus.[11, 12] Because many persons requiring health care may have unrecognized infection with a blood-borne pathogen, UP was to be used during the care of all patients to prevent health care workers from exposure to blood and other specific body fluids potentially contaminated with a blood-borne pathogen. BSI was developed in 1987 with the intention of providing a simpler, easy-to-use alternative to the isolation precautions systems in use at that time.[72] BSI was similar to UP in that it was to be used during the care of all patients; however, it differed from UP in that it advocated use of barriers to prevent contact by health workers with all moist body substances and mucous membranes, not just blood and body fluids potentially contaminated by blood-borne pathogens. BSI was designed not only to protect health care workers from blood-borne pathogens, but also to prevent cross-infection due to hand contamination while caring for patients who may have undetected colonization with a nosocomial pathogen. The advantages and disadvantages of these two systems and the confusion regarding the interpretation and implementation of these systems by health care workers are described in detail in the CDC/HICPAC guideline.[38]

Standard Precautions represent a new system that combines the goals of protecting health care workers from blood-borne pathogens and protecting health care workers and patients from transmission of microorganisms from moist body substances.[38] Standard Precautions apply to all patients at all times regardless of their diagnosis or presumed infection status.[38] Standard Precautions apply to any planned or potential contact with (1) blood, (2) all body fluids, secretions, and excretions, except sweat, regardless of whether they contain visible blood, (3) nonintact skin, and (4) mucous membranes.[38] Table 229–2 lists the components of Standard Precautions.

It should be noted that OSHA's blood-borne pathogens standard includes prevention measures embodied in UP (see Occupational Health).[83] The prevention measures included in Standard Precautions comply with the provisions of the OSHA standard.

Transmission-Based Precautions

Other precautions are needed to prevent transmission of contagious diseases (e.g., varicella, measles, tuberculosis, pertussis) and other epidemiologically important microorganisms (e.g., multidrug-resistant microorganisms, toxin-producing *C. difficile)* from infected or colonized patients. Transmission-Based Precautions are designed to provide the necessary measures, in addition to those already specified by Standard Precautions, to interrupt known modes of transmission of these microorganisms (see Chapter 228).[38] There are three types of Transmission-Based Precautions: Airborne, Droplet, and Contact.

Airborne Precautions (Table 229–3) are designed to prevent transmission of microorganisms spread by droplet nuclei (e.g., measles, varicella, tuberculosis), which can be carried on air currents over substantial distances.[38] Special air handling and ventilation are required.[38] Droplet Precautions (see Table 229–3) are designed to prevent transmission of microorganisms spread by large respiratory droplets that only travel short distances (<3 feet) before settling.[38] Special air handling and ventilation are not required. Contact Precautions (see Table 229–3) are designed to prevent transmission of microorganisms spread by direct and indirect contact.[38] Some infections are spread by more than one mode of transmission, so precautions systems may need to be combined for these infections (e.g., varicella requires Airborne Precautions and Contact Precautions). Patients infected or colonized with more than one microorganism also may require a combination of precautions systems (e.g., a patient with active pulmonary tuberculosis and *C. difficile* enterocolitis requires Airborne Precautions and Contact Precautions).

Table 229–4 lists clinical syndromes and conditions warranting empiric use of Transmission-Based Precautions, in addition to Standard Precautions, to prevent transmission of epidemiologically important pathogens until infection with these microorganisms is excluded.[38] To ensure that appropriate empiric precautions are implemented promptly, hospitals must have systems in place to evaluate patients for these infections as a part of their routine preadmission and admission care. Table 229–5 lists the type and duration of Transmission-Based Precautions, to be used in addition to Standard Precautions, for specific clinical syndromes and infectious agents. Only agents requiring one or more of the three Transmission-Based Precautions are listed.

The CDC/HICPAC guideline recommends only Standard Precautions for infections caused by penicillin-resistant *Streptococcus pneumoniae*. Based on reports of nosocomial transmission of penicillin-resistant *S. pneumoniae* in hospitals outside the United States and the possibility that these infections were spread by droplet transmission,[36, 73, 78] the authors recommend use of Droplet Precautions until 24 hours of effective antimicrobial therapy have been completed. The CDC/HICPAC guideline recommends Droplet Precautions for patients requiring isolation for parvovirus B19 infection. Because of an outbreak report where airborne transmission may have occurred,[3] the authors use Airborne Precautions in their hospital.

Visitors

Visitors with communicable diseases inadvertently can expose hospitalized patients and health care workers, unless procedures to identify and exclude them are in place. Varicella, measles, and tuberculosis are the most problematic infections because these diseases are spread by airborne transmission, enabling infected visitors to expose a large number of persons in a short time. In addition, visitors with pertussis, viral respiratory and gastrointestinal infections, parvovirus B19 infection, rubella, and mumps can pose a significant hazard to patients and health care workers with whom they have close contact.

Procedures to identify potentially infected visitors can be targeted toward visiting children because they are the most likely persons to be infected with these agents. At the authors' hospital, parents or guardians of all visiting children younger than 12 years of age are asked to complete a questionnaire at the hospital's reception desk. The questionnaire asks a set of screening questions regarding the presence of fever, rash, and respiratory and gastrointestinal symptoms in the visiting child, as well as any recent exposure to children with chicken pox, measles, or whooping cough. Children without any significant symptoms or exposures are allowed to visit with no restrictions and are given a green dinosaur sticker to wear on their clothing. Children with a history of fever or vomiting in the past 24 hours or an upper respiratory tract infection in the past week are allowed to visit with restrictions and are given a yellow dinosaur sticker. The yellow sticker alerts the nurse on the ward to reinforce the need for restrictions and to assess the potential for transmission in more detail. A guideline for parents details the restrictions for various symptoms, which generally include avoiding close contact (<3 feet) with any patient; no visits to the activity room; and no sharing of food, drinks, or toys. Children with upper respiratory tract infections are not allowed to visit children with congenital heart disease, bronchopulmonary dysplasia, cellular immunodeficiency, or other conditions that predispose to severe infection with respiratory viruses. Children with significant exposures to chickenpox, measles, or whooping cough who may be in the incubation period of the disease are not allowed to visit the hospital. The stickers are dated for 1 day, and this process is repeated each day the child visits the hospital. This procedure does not guarantee that a child is not in the incubation phase of a contagious disease at the time of his or her visit—varicella is an obvious example—but it has proved to be both well accepted and useful in limiting potential exposures.

TABLE 229–2. Standard Precautions*

A. Hand washing

Wash hands after touching blood, body fluids, secretions, excretions, and contaminated items, whether or not gloves are worn.

Wash hands immediately after gloves are removed, between patient contacts, and when otherwise indicated to avoid transfer of microorganisms to other patients or environments.

It may be necessary to wash hands between tasks and procedures on the same patient to prevent cross-contamination of different body sites.

Use a plain (nonantimicrobial) soap for routine hand washing.

Use an antimicrobial agent or a waterless antiseptic agent for specific circumstances (e.g., control of outbreaks or hyperendemic infections), as defined by the infection control program. (See Table 229–4, Contact Precautions, for additional recommendations on using antimicrobial and antiseptic agents.)

B. Gloves

Wear gloves (clean nonsterile gloves are adequate) when touching blood, body fluids, secretions, excretions, and contaminated items.

Put on clean gloves just before touching mucous membranes and nonintact skin.

Change gloves between tasks and procedures on the same patient after contact with material that may contain a high concentration of microorganisms.

Remove gloves promptly after use, before touching noncontaminated items and environmental surfaces, and before going to another patient and wash hands immediately to avoid transfer of microorganisms to other patients or environments.

C. Mask, eye protection, and face shield

Wear a mask and eye protection or a face shield to protect mucous membranes of the eyes, nose, and mouth during procedures and patient care activities that are likely to generate splashes or sprays of blood, body fluids, secretions, and excretions.

D. Gown

Wear a gown (a clean, nonsterile gown is adequate) to protect skin and prevent soiling of clothing during procedures and patient care activities that are likely to generate splashes or sprays of blood, body fluids, secretions, or excretions.

Select a gown that is appropriate for the activity and amount of fluid likely to be encountered.

Remove a soiled gown as promptly as possible and wash hands to avoid transfer of microorganisms to other patients or environments.

E. Patient care equipment

Handle used patient care equipment soiled with blood, body fluids, secretions, and excretions in a manner that prevents skin and mucous membrane exposures, contamination of clothing, and transfer of microorganisms to other patients and environments.

Ensure that reusable equipment is not used for the care of another patient until it has been cleaned and reprocessed appropriately.

Ensure that single-use items are discarded properly.

F. Environmental control

Ensure that the hospital has adequate procedures for the routine care, cleaning, and disinfection of environmental surfaces, beds, bedrails, bedside equipment, and other frequently touched surfaces and ensure that these procedures are followed.

G. Linen

Handle, transport, and process used linen soiled with blood, body fluids, secretions, and excretions in a manner that prevents skin and mucous membrane exposures and contamination of clothing and that avoids transfer of microorganisms to other patients and environments.

H. Occupational health and blood-borne pathogens

Take care to prevent injuries when using needles, scalpels, and other sharp instruments or devices; when handling sharp instruments after procedures; when cleaning used instruments; and when disposing of used needles.

Never recap used needles or otherwise manipulate them using both hands or any other technique that involves directing the point of a needle toward any part of the body; rather, use either a one-handed "scoop" technique or a mechanical device designed for holding the needle sheath.

Do not remove used needles from disposable syringes by hand and do not bend, break, or otherwise manipulate used needles by hand.

Place used disposable needles and syringes, scalpel blades, and other sharp items in appropriate puncture-resistant containers, which are located as close as practical to the area in which the items were used, and place reusable syringes and needles in a puncture-resistant container for transport to the reprocessing area.

Use mouth pieces, resuscitation bags, or other ventilation devices as an alternative to mouth-to-mouth resuscitation methods in areas where the need for resuscitation is predictable.

I. Patient placement

Place a patient who contaminates the environment or who does not (or cannot be expected to) assist in maintaining appropriate hygiene or environmental control in a private room.

If a private room is not available, consult with infection control professionals regarding patient placement or other alternatives.

*Standard Precautions apply to all patients regardless of their diagnosis or presumed infection status. Standard precautions apply to any planned or potential contact with (1) blood, (2) all body fluid secretions and excretions except sweat, regardless of whether they contain visible blood, (3) nonintact skin, and (4) mucous membranes.

From Garner, J. S., and Hospital Infection Control Practices Advisory Committee: Guideline for isolation precautions in hospitals. Infect. Control Hosp. Epidemiol. *17*:53–80, 1996.

TABLE 229–3. Transmission-Based Precautions*

Airborne Precautions

A. Patient placement

Place the patient in a private room that has (1) monitored negative air pressure in relation to the surrounding areas, (2) 6 to 12 air changes per hour, and (3) appropriate discharge of air outdoors or monitored high-efficiency filtration of room air before the air is circulated to other areas in the hospital.

Keep the room door closed and the patient in the room.

When a private room is not available, place the patient in a room with a patient who has active infection with the same microorganism but with no other infection, unless otherwise recommended.

When a private room is not available and cohorting is not desirable, consultation with infection control professionals is advised before patient placement.

B. Respiratory protection

Wear respiratory protection when entering the room of a patient with known or suspected infectious pulmonary tuberculosis.

Susceptible persons should not enter the room of patients known or suspected to have measles (rubella) or varicella (chickenpox) if other immune caregivers are available.

If susceptible persons must enter the room of a patient known or suspected to have measles or varicella, they should wear respiratory protection.

Persons immune to measles or varicella need not wear respiratory protection.

C. Patient transport

Limit the movement and transport of the patient from the room to essential purposes only.

If transport or movement is necessary, minimize the patient's dispersal of droplet nuclei by placing a surgical mask on the patient, if possible.

D. Additional precautions for preventing transmission of tuberculosis

Consult the Centers for Disease Control and Prevention "Guidelines for Preventing the Transmission of Tuberculosis in Health Care Facilities" for additional prevention strategies.[15]

Droplet Precautions

A. Patient placement

Place the patient in a private room.

When a private room is not available, place the patient in a room with a patient or patients who have active infection with the same microorganism but with no other infection.

When a private room is not available and cohorting is not achievable, maintain spatial separation of at least 3 feet between the infected patient and other patients and visitors.

Special air handling and ventilation are not necessary, and the door may remain open.

B. Mask

Wear a mask when working within 3 feet of the patient. (Logistically, some hospitals may want to implement the wearing of a mask to enter the room.)

C. Patient transport

Limit the movement and transport of the patient from the room to essential purposes only.

If transport or movement is necessary, minimize patient dispersal of droplets by placing a surgical mask on the patient, if possible.

Contact Precautions

A. Patient placement

Place the patient in a private room.

When a private room is not available, place the patient in a room with a patient or patients who have active infection with the same microorganism but with no other infection.

When a private room is not available and cohorting is not achievable, consider the epidemiology of the microorganism and the patient population when determining patient placement; consultation with infection control professionals is advised before patient placement.

B. Gloves

Wear gloves (clean nonsterile gloves are adequate) when entering the room.

During the course of providing care for a patient, change gloves after having contact with infective material that may contain high concentrations of microorganisms (fecal material and wound drainage).

Remove gloves before leaving the patient's environment and wash hands immediately with an antimicrobial agent or a waterless antiseptic agent.

After glove removal and hand washing, ensure that hands do not touch potentially contaminated environmental surfaces or items in the patient's room to avoid transfer of microorganisms to other patients or environments.

C. Gown

Wear a gown (a clean, nonsterile gown is adequate) when entering the room if you anticipate that your clothing will have substantial contact with the patient, environmental surfaces, or items in the patient's room or if the patient is incontinent or has diarrhea, an ileostomy, a colostomy, or wound drainage not contained by a dressing.

Remove the gown before leaving the patient's environment.

After gown removal, ensure that clothing does not contact potentially contaminated environmental surfaces to avoid transfer of microorganisms to other patients or environments.

D. Patient transport

Limit the movement and transport of the patient from the room to essential purposes only.

If the patient is transported out of the room, ensure that precautions are maintained to minimize the risk of transmission of microorganisms to other patients and contamination of environmental surfaces or equipment.

E. Patient care equipment

When possible, dedicate the use of noncritical patient care equipment to a single patient (or a cohort of patients infected or colonized with the pathogen requiring precautions) to avoid sharing between patients.

If the use of common equipment or items is unavoidable, then adequately clean and disinfect them before use for another patient.

F. Additional precautions for preventing the spread of vancomycin resistance

Consult the Hospital Infection Control Practices Advisory Committee report on preventing the spread of vancomycin resistance for additional prevention strategies.[56]

*Transmission-Based Precautions are followed, when indicated, in addition to Standard Precautions.

From Garner, J. S., and Hospital Infection Control Practices Advisory Committee: Guideline for isolation precautions in hospitals. Infect. Control Hosp. Epidemiol. *17*:53–80, 1996.

TABLE 229–4. Clinical Syndromes or Conditions Warranting Empiric Use of Transmission-Based Precautions to Prevent Transmission of Epidemiologically Important Pathogens Until Infection with These Microorganisms Is Excluded*

Clinical Syndrome or Condition†	Potential Pathogens‡	Empiric Precautions
Diarrhea		
Acute diarrhea with a likely infectious cause in an incontinent or diapered patient	Enteric pathogens§	Contact
Diarrhea with a history of recent antibiotic use	*Clostridium difficile*	Contact
Meningitis	*Neisseria meningitidis*	Droplet
Rash or exanthems, generalized, etiology unknown		
Petechial/ecchymotic with fever	*Neisseria meningitidis*	Droplet
Vesicular	Varicella	Airborne and contact
Maculopapular with coryza and fever	Rubeola (measles)	Airborne
Respiratory infections		
Cough/fever/upper lobe pulmonary infiltrate in an HIV-negative patient or a patient at low risk for HIV infection	*Mycobacterium tuberculosis*	Airborne
Cough/fever/pulmonary infiltrate in any lung location in an HIV-infected patient or a patient at high risk for HIV infection	*Mycobacterium tuberculosis*	Airborne
Paroxysmal or severe persistent cough during periods of pertussis activity	*Bordetella pertussis*	Droplet
Respiratory infections, particularly bronchiolitis and croup, in infants and young children	Respiratory syncytial or parainfluenza virus	Contact
Risk of multidrug-resistant microorganisms		
History of infection or colonization with multidrug-resistant organisms¶	Resistant bacteria	Contact
Skin, wound, or urinary tract infection in a patient with recent hospital or long-term care in a facility where multidrug-resistant organisms are prevalent	Resistant bacteria	Contact
Skin or wound infection		
Abscess or draining wound that cannot be covered	*Staphylococcus aureus*, group A *Streptococcus*	Contact

*Infection control professionals are encouraged to modify or adapt this table according to local conditions. To ensure that appropriate empiric precautions are implemented always, hospitals must have systems in place to evaluate patients routinely according to these criteria as a part of their preadmission and admission care.

†Patients with the syndromes or conditions listed may present with atypical signs or symptoms (e.g., pertussis in neonates and adults may not be associated with paroxysmal or severe cough). The clinician's index of suspicion should be guided by the prevalence of specific conditions in the community, as well as clinical judgment.

‡The microorganisms listed are not intended to represent the complete, or even the most likely, diagnosis but rather possible etiologic agents that require precautions in addition to standard precautions until they can be ruled out.

§These pathogens include enterohemorrhagic *Escherichia coli* O157:H7, *Shigella*, hepatitis A virus, and rotavirus.

¶Resistant bacteria judged by the infection control program, based on current state, regional, or national recommendations, to be of special clinical or epidemiological significance.

From Garner, J. S., and Hospital Infection Control Practices Advisory Committee: Guideline for isolation precautions in hospitals. Infect. Control Hosp. Epidemiol. *17*:53–80, 1996.

Occupational Health

Health care workers require protection from the significant infectious risks inherent in patient care; conversely, patients and other health care workers need to be protected from exposure to health care workers with communicable diseases. Integrating management and prevention strategies to accomplish these two goals requires close collaboration between hospital infection prevention and control programs and occupational health departments.

Evaluation of Ill Health Care Workers

Hospital staff and volunteers with symptoms such as persistent fever, conjunctivitis, skin lesions or rashes, diarrhea, and persistent cough should be evaluated for the presence of a contagious disease. Possible cases of varicella, herpes zoster on an exposed area of the body, herpetic whitlow, adenoviral conjunctivitis, measles, mumps, rubella, pertussis, staphylococcal skin infection, enteric infection in a food service worker, and active pulmonary tuberculosis should be investigated promptly and confirmed with laboratory tests if necessary. Although many health care workers choose to have these problems evaluated by their primary care provider, occupational health departments have an interest in completing these assessments, especially if there is a question of whether the condition was acquired in the workplace, requires a furlough from work, or may have exposed patients or other health care workers. Infection control staff can provide assistance in these evaluations as needed and should be kept abreast of the results.

Postexposure Evaluation and Management of Health Care Workers

A structured approach to the assessment and management of exposures of health care workers to patients with infectious diseases is critical to provide postexposure prophylaxis promptly, if indicated, and allay anxiety while avoiding unnecessary interventions and loss of work days. The first step is to develop criteria for assessing the nature of the exposure because many reported encounters are not significant. Some exposures (e.g., varicella, hepatitis B) may require an assessment of the susceptibility of the health care worker to infection, and procedures should describe the indications for laboratory tests as well as the interpretation of results. Postexposure prophylaxis regimens are discussed in Chapter 228 and later. Finally, counseling regarding the risks and consequences of the exposure is an important component of this service.

Postexposure evaluation and management of varicella, blood-borne pathogens, and tuberculosis are highlighted later because they are a common focal point for interactions between the hospital infection prevention and control program and the occupational health department.

Exposure to varicella is common in hospitals caring for pediatric patients. Fortunately, the vast majority of hospital staff members have protective immunity.[30] A previous history of varicella is a reliable indicator of immunity, and most health care workers without a past history of varicella have serologic evidence of immunity.[30] Nonetheless, some health care workers are susceptible to varicella, particularly workers born and raised in tropical and subtropical countries. Some hospitals perform serologic tests for antibody to varicella-zoster virus in workers without a history of varicella at the time of hire in order to identify these persons prospectively; others perform this test only if a worker is exposed. Susceptible workers who are exposed to varicella either inside or outside the hospital usually are furloughed beginning 8 to 10 days after their initial exposure until 21 days after their last exposure (until 28 days if they received varicella-zoster immunoglobulin), unless they become infected and recover sooner. Alternative strategies to allow these persons to continue to work with specific safeguards may reduce the number of lost work days substantially but may result in preventable secondary exposures of patients and other hospital workers.[46, 60] Administration of varicella-zoster immunoglobulin should be considered for high-risk persons (pregnant and immunocompromised persons); some physicians advocate varicella-zoster immunoglobulin for all exposed, susceptible adults because of the potential severity of varicella in this population. Acyclovir may decrease the severity of the disease if started as soon as infection is noted. The recent licensure of a varicella vaccine should provide a way to actively immunize susceptible persons. Guidelines for the administration of this vaccine to health care workers and postvaccination serologic testing have been formulated.[18]

The OSHA blood-borne pathogens standard requires hospitals to test the source patient for evidence of a blood-borne infection, when consent can be obtained, and to provide postexposure prophylaxis in accordance with CDC recommendations.[13, 14, 83] Significant exposures are defined as percutaneous, mucous membrane, or nonintact skin exposure to blood, other potentially infectious body fluids (cerebrospinal fluid, pericardial fluid, pleural fluid, peritoneal fluid, synovial fluid, amniotic fluid, semen, cervical/vaginal secretions), tissue, or visibly bloody fluids, excretions, or secretions.[14]

Summary risk estimates are helpful in counseling persons who have suffered an exposure, although a number of factors may affect the risk of infection in an individual case (e.g., level of viremia in the source patient, amount of blood involved in the exposure, the nature of the exposure). Hepatitis B by far is the most infectious of the blood-borne viruses, probably because titers of virus in the blood are higher for hepatitis B than for other agents.[40] The risk of hepatitis B virus infection after a percutaneous exposure to blood is estimated to be 2 to 40 per cent, with greater risk associated with the presence of hepatitis B e antigen in the source patient.[40] The risk of hepatitis B virus infection after mucous membrane or nonintact skin exposures is not well quantified, but infection clearly can occur.[40] The risk of HIV infection after percutaneous exposure to blood from an infected person is estimated to be 0.2 per cent (confidence interval, 0.1 to 0.5).[40] Infection after mucous membrane exposure has been reported anecdotally but is considered much less likely.[40] The risk of hepatitis C virus infection after percutaneous exposure is not well quantified (estimated at 3 to 10 per cent), and infection after mucous membrane exposure has not been documented.[40]

Recommendations for hepatitis B prophylaxis after percutaneous or mucous membrane exposures are listed in Table 229–6.[13] There is no known effective prophylaxis for hepatitis C virus infection.

The efficacy of antiretroviral chemoprophylaxis after occupational exposure to HIV has not been established. Nonetheless, as summarized in a recent publication,[56a] several lines of evidence indicate that chemoprophylaxis may be effective in preventing infection. A retrospective case-control study of 31 health care workers with HIV seroconversion after a documented percutaneous exposure to HIV-infected blood and 679 seronegative controls with similar exposures suggested that postexposure prophylaxis with zidovudine had a protective effect.[18a] In this study, independent risk factors for infection were a deep injury, visible blood on the device causing the injury, a procedure involving a needle placed directly in a vein or artery, and terminal illness in the source patient. Although the unadjusted risk of infection among persons receiving zidovudine was not different significantly between cases (seroconverters) and controls, multiple regression analysis revealed a significantly lower adjusted risk of infection (i.e., a risk that adjusts for the effect of other independent risk factors) in persons who received zidovudine (adjusted odds ratio = 0.2; confidence interval, 0.1 to 0.6). Additional evidence of the potential efficacy of chemoprophylaxis includes studies that have demonstrated the effectiveness of zidovudine in reducing the rate of vertical transmission of HIV from mother to infant, prevention of experimental infection in laboratory animals, and the profound inhibitory effect of combination antiretroviral therapy on HIV replication in HIV-infected individuals.[56a]

The use of chemoprophylaxis in uninfected health care workers who have been exposed to HIV must balance carefully the risk of infection associated with a particular exposure, the effectiveness of various combinations of antiretroviral agents in inhibiting viral replication, and the potential adverse effects of the individual agents included in a particular regimen. Provisional recommendations for chemoprophylaxis after occupational exposure to HIV developed by a U.S. interagency governmental working group were published in 1996.[18a] However, information regarding the efficacy and adverse effects of antiretroviral agents is evolving rapidly, and updates of these recommendations can be expected in the future.

Persons exposed to active pulmonary tuberculosis should be evaluated by purified protein derivative (PPD) skin testing if they do not have a history of PPD reactivity. A skin test should be administered after the exposure and, if the results are negative, 12 weeks later.[15] Skin test "converters" and persons with signs of active tuberculosis should be treated as indicated.[15] All skin tests should be placed and interpreted by trained personnel according to the CDC guideline.[15]

Because exposure to tuberculosis may be unrecognized, hospitals should require health care workers to undergo periodic PPD skin testing.[15] Persons who do not have a history of prior PPD reactivity and who do not have a documented negative PPD result within the preceding 12 months should undergo a baseline PPD skin test employing the two-step method in order to detect the booster phenomena that could be misinterpreted as a skin test conversion.[15] Thereafter, persons can be screened using a single PPD skin test, with the

TABLE 229–5. Type and Duration of Transmission-Based Precautions Needed for Selected Infections and Conditions

Infection/Condition	Precautions: *Type*	*Duration*
Abscess, draining (no dressing or dressing does not contain drainage adequately)	C	DI
Adenovirus infection in infants and young children	D, C	DI
Bordetella pertussis (see Pertussis)		
Campylobacter species (see Gastroenteritis, *Campylobacter* species)		
Cellulitis, uncontrolled drainage	C	DI
Chickenpox (varicella)	A, C	F[1]
Chickenpox (varicella) exposure	A, F[2]	F[2]
Cholera (see Gastroenteritis, *Vibrio cholerae*)		
Clostridium difficile	C	DI
Congenital rubella	C	F[3]
Conjunctivitis, acute viral (acute hemorrhagic)	C	DI
Decubitus ulcer, infected (no dressing or dressing does not contain drainage adequately)	C	DI
Diphtheria		
Cutaneous	C	CN, F[4]
Pharyngeal	D	CN, F[4]
Ebola viral hemorrhagic fever	C, F[5]	DI
Enterococcus species (see Multidrug-resistant organisms, infection, or colonization if epidemiologically significant or vancomycin-resistant)		
Enterocolitis, *Clostridium difficile*	C	DI
Enteroviral infections in infants and young children	C	DI
Epiglottitis due to *Haemophilus influenzae*	D	U[24 hrs]
Furunculosis, staphylococcal, in infants and young children	C	DI
Gastroenteritis		
Campylobacter species	C, F[6]	DI
Vibrio cholerae (cholera)	C, F[6]	DI
Clostridium difficile	C	DI
Cryptosporidium species	C, F[6]	DI
Escherichia coli		
Enterohemorrhagic O157:H7	C, F[6]	DI
Other species	C, F[6]	DI
Giardia lamblia	C, F[6]	DI
Rotavirus	C, F[6]	DI
Salmonella species (including *Salmonella typhi*)	C, F[6]	DI
Shigella species	C, F[6]	DI
Vibrio parahaemolyticus	C, F[6]	DI
Viral, other than rotavirus	C, F[6]	DI
Yersinia enterocolitica	C, F[6]	DI
German measles (rubella; see also Congenital rubella)	D	F[7]
Giardiasis (see Gastroenteritis, *Giardia lamblia*)		
Haemophilus influenzae	D	U[24 hrs]
Hand, foot, and mouth disease (see Enteroviral infections)		
Hemorrhagic fevers (e.g., Lassa, Ebola, Marburg)	C, F[5]	DI
Hepatitis A in diapered or incontinent patients	C	F[8]
Herpes simplex		
Neonatal infection	C	DI
Neonatal exposure	C, F[9]	DI
Mucocutaneous, disseminated or primary, severe	C	DI
Herpes zoster (varicella-zoster) disseminated or localized in immunocompromised patients	A, C, F[10]	DI
Impetigo	C	U[24 hrs]
Influenza	D, F[11]	DI
Lassa fever	C, F[5]	DI
Lice (pediculosis)	C	U[24 hrs]
Marburg virus disease	C, F[5]	DI
Measles (rubeola), all presentations	A	DI
Meningitis		
Enterovirus, known or suspected in infants and young children	C	DI
Haemophilus influenzae, known or suspected	D	U[24 hrs]
Neisseria meningitidis, known or suspected	D	U[24 hrs]
Streptococcus pneumoniae, penicillin-resistant, known or suspected	D, F[12]	U[24 hrs]
Meningococcemia (meningococcal sepsis)	D	U[24 hrs]
Multidrug-resistant organisms, infection, or colonization[13]		
Gastrointestinal	C	CN
Respiratory	C	CN
Skin, wound, or burn	C	CN
Mumps (infectious parotitis)	D	F[14]
Mycobacterium tuberculosis (see Tuberculosis)		
Neisseria meningitidis	D	U[24 hrs]
Mycoplasma pneumoniae (see Pneumonia, *Mycoplasma*)		
Parainfluenza virus infection, respiratory, in infants and young children	C	DI
Parvovirus B19 infection	A or D, F[15]	F[16]
Pediculosis (lice)	C	U[24 hrs]
Pertussis (whooping cough)	D	F[17]
Plague, pneumonic	D	U[72 hrs]
Pneumococcemia (pneumococcal sepsis), penicillin-resistant	D[12]	U[24 hrs]

TABLE 229–5. Type and Duration of Transmission-Based Precautions Needed for Selected Infections and Conditions *Continued*

Infection/Condition	Precautions Type	Precautions Duration
Pneumonia		
Adenovirus	D, C	DI
Haemophilus influenzae in infants and children (any age)	D	U[24 hrs]
Neisseria meningitidis	D	U[24 hrs]
Mycoplasma pneumoniae (primary atypical pneumonia)	D	DI
Streptococcus, group A, in infants and young children	D	U[24 hrs]
Streptococcus pneumoniae, penicillin-resistant	D, F[12]	U[24 hrs]
Viral, in infants and young children (see Respiratory infectious disease, acute)		
Respiratory infectious disease, acute (if not covered elsewhere), in infants and young children	C	DI
Respiratory syncytial virus infection in infants and young children and immunocompromised adults	C	DI
Rotavirus infection (see Gastroenteritis, Rotavirus)		
Rubella (German measles; see also Congenital rubella)	D	F[7]
Rubeola (measles)	A	DI
Salmonellosis (see Gastroenteritis, *Salmonella* species)		
Scabies	C	U[24 hrs]
Shigellosis (see Gastroenteritis, *Shigella* species)		
Staphylococcal disease (*Staphylococcus aureus*)		
Skin, wound, or burn, major (no dressing or dressing does not contain drainage adequately)	C	DI
Streptococcal disease (group A *Streptococcus*)		
Skin, wound, or burn, major (no dressing or dressing does not contain drainage adequately)	C	U[24 hrs]
Pharyngitis in infants and young children	D	U[24 hrs]
Pneumonia in infants and young children	D	U[24 hrs]
Scarlet fever in infants and younger children	D	U[24 hrs]
Streptococcus pneumoniae, penicillin-resistant	D, F[12]	U[24 hrs]
Tuberculosis, pulmonary or laryngeal, confirmed or suspected	A	F[17]
Varicella (chickenpox)	A, C	F[1]
Varicella (chickenpox) exposure	A, F[2]	F[2]
Vibrio cholerae (see Gastroenteritis, Cholera)		
Vibrio parahaemolyticus (see Gastroenteritis, *Vibrio parahaemolyticus*)		
Whooping cough	D	F[18]
Wounds infections, major, (no dressing or dressing does not contain drainage adequately)	C	DI
Yersinia enterocolitica infection (see Gastroenteritis, *Yersinia enterocolitica*)		

Abbreviations: A, airborne; C, contact; D, droplet; CN, until antimicrobial agents are discontinued and culture-negative; DI, duration of illness (with wound lesions, DI means until they stop draining); U, until time specified in hours (hrs) after initiation of effective therapy; F, see footnote number.

Standard Precautions apply to all patients at all times in addition to the specified transmission-based precautions.

[1]Maintain precautions until all lesions are crusted.

[2]Place exposed, susceptible patients on Airborne Precautions beginning 8 days after exposure and continuing until 21 days after the last exposure (up to 28 days if varicella-zoster immunoglobulin has been given).

[3]Place infant on Contact Precautions during any admission until 1 year of age, unless nasopharyngeal and urine cultures are negative for virus after 3 months of age.

[4]Until two cultures taken at least 24 hours apart are negative.

[5]Call state health department and Centers for Disease Control and Prevention for specific advice about management of a suspected case.

[6]Use Contact Precautions for diapered or incontinent children and any child younger than 6 years of age for the duration of the illness.

[7]Until 7 days after the onset of the rash.

[8]Maintain precautions in infants and children younger than 3 years of age for the duration of the hospitalization; in children 3 to 14 years of age, until 2 weeks after onset of symptoms; and in others, until 1 week after the onset of symptoms.

[9]For infants delivered vaginally or by cesarean section and if the mother has active infection and membranes have been ruptured for more than 4 to 6 hours.

[10]Persons susceptible to varicella also are at risk for developing varicella when exposed to patients with herpes zoster lesions; therefore, susceptible persons should not enter the room if other immune caregivers are available.

[11]The "Guideline for Prevention of Nosocomial Pneumonia"[96] recommends surveillance, vaccination, antiviral agents, and use of private rooms with negative air pressure as much as feasible for patients in whom influenza is suspected or diagnosed. Many hospitals encounter logistic difficulties and physical plant limitations when admitting multiple patients with suspected influenza during community outbreaks. If sufficient private rooms are unavailable, consider cohorting patients or, at the very least, avoid room sharing with high-risk patients. See "Guideline for Prevention of Nosocomial Pneumonia"[96] for additional prevention and control strategies.

[12]The Centers for Disease Control and Prevention/Hospital Infection Control Practices Advisory Committee (CDC/HICPAC) guideline recommends only standard precautions for infections caused by penicillin-resistant *Streptococcus pneumoniae.* Based on reports of nosocomial transmission of penicillin-resistant *S. pneumoniae* in hospitals outside the United States and the possibility that these infections were spread by droplet transmission,[36, 73, 78] the authors recommend the use of Droplet Precautions until 24 hours of effective antimicrobial therapy have been completed.

[13]Resistant bacteria judged by the infection control program, based on current state, regional, or national recommendations, to be of special clinical or epidemiological significance.

[14]For 9 days after onset of parotid swelling.

[15]The CDC/HICPAC guideline recommends the use of Droplet Precautions. Based on an outbreak report where airborne transmission may have occurred,[3] the authors use Airborne Precautions in their hospital.

[16]Maintain precautions for duration of hospitalization when chronic disease occurs in an immunodeficient patient. For patients with transient aplastic crisis or red blood cell crisis, maintain precautions for 7 days.

[17]Maintain precautions until 5 days after patient is placed on effective therapy.

[18]Discontinue precautions only when a tuberculosis patient is on effective therapy, is improving clinically, and has three consecutive negative sputum smears collected on different days or when tuberculosis is ruled out. Also see the Centers for Disease Control and Prevention's "Guideline for Preventing the Transmission of Tuberculosis in Health Care Facilities."[15]

Modified from Garner, J. S., and Hospital Infection Control Practices Advisory Committee: Guideline for isolation precautions in hospitals. Infect. Control Hosp. Epidemiol. *17*:53–80, 1996.

TABLE 229–6. Recommendations for Hepatitis B Prophylaxis After Percutaneous or Mucous Membrane Exposure

Exposed Person	Treatment When Source Is Found to Be: HBsAg-Positive	HBsAg-Negative	Not Tested or Unknown
Unvaccinated	HBIG* × 1; initiate and complete HBV† series	Initiate and complete HBV† series	Initiate and complete HBV† series
Previously vaccinated			
Known responder with adequate anti-HBs level§ in past 24 months	No testing and no intervention	No testing and no intervention	No testing and no intervention
Known responder with no anti-HBs level in past 24 months	Test exposed for anti-HBs: If adequate,§ no treatment If inadequate, HBV† booster dose	No treatment	No treatment
Known nonresponder	HBIG* × 2 or HBIG* × 1 plus 1 dose of HBV†	No treatment	
Response unknown	Test exposed for anti-HBs: If adequate,§ no treatment If inadequate,§ HBIG* × 1 plus HBV† booster dose	No treatment	Test exposed for anti-HBs: If adequate,§ no treatment If inadequate,§ HBV† booster dose

Abbreviations: HBsAg, hepatitis B surface antigen; HBIG, hepatitis B immunoglobulin; HBV, hepatitis B vaccine; anti-HBs, antibody to hepatitis B surface antigen.

*The HBIG dose is 0.06 mL/kg intramuscularly.

†HBV dosing requirements vary according to the manufacturer, the age of the recipient, and other factors (persons undergoing dialysis and immunocompromised persons require higher doses); follow the manufacter's dosing recommendations.

§An adequate anti-HBs level is ≥10 mIU/mL.

Modified from Centers for Disease Control: Protection against viral hepatitis: Recommendations of the Immunization Practices Advisory Committee (ACIP). M. M. W. R. *39*:1–26,1990.

frequency of testing dictated by the risk of exposure.[15] Persons with a history of prior PPD reactivity should be assessed periodically for evidence of active disease.[15] To ensure compliance, many hospitals currently require periodic skin tests as a prerequisite for reappointment of physicians or continuing employment of other hospital staff.

Prevention of Occupationally Acquired Infections in Health Care Workers

Because vaccination against infectious diseases is a highly cost-effective prevention strategy, hospitals should offer vaccinations free of charge. Vaccination against measles is so effective that ensuring immunity to measles (either as the result of immunity or vaccination) among hospital staff is regarded as an appropriate quality-of-care indicator for occupational health programs.[63] Because the combined measles, mumps, and rubella vaccine readily is available, immunity against mumps and rubella can be ensured analogously. Influenza vaccination of health care workers is recommended by the Immunization Practices Advisory Committee.[17] However, acceptance of this vaccine by health care workers often is poor.[99] Consequently, occupational health departments need to consider aggressive and innovative strategies to encourage annual influenza vaccination. Given the significant occupational risk of hepatitis B virus infection in hospitals, hepatitis B vaccination should be offered routinely to health care workers. The OSHA blood-borne pathogens standard requires hospitals to offer hepatitis B vaccination free of charge; workers who do not wish to be vaccinated must sign a specific "informed refusal." Other vaccine advances, such as the development of acellular pertussis vaccine and the licensure of a varicella vaccine, offer the hope that hospitals soon may be able to eliminate or at least drastically reduce occupational acquisition of these diseases as well.

In addition to hepatitis B vaccination, the OSHA blood-borne pathogens standard mandates other specific prevention measures, including (1) the development of an exposure control plan that identifies employees with occupational risk of exposure to blood-borne pathogens, (2) annual training for these persons regarding the risk of blood-borne infection and prevention measures, (3) provision of personal protective clothing and equipment, (4) work practice controls, including equipment and procedures for the safe handling and disposal of sharps, and (5) procedures for identification, transportation, storage, and disposal of contaminated items and waste.[83]

The CDC's "Guidelines for Preventing the Transmission of *Mycobacterium tuberculosis* in Health Care Facilities, 1994" emphasizes a hierarchy of prevention and control measures.[15] The first level is made up of administrative controls, including (1) developing and implementing effective written policies and protocols to ensure the rapid identification, isolation, diagnostic evaluation, and treatment of persons likely to have tuberculosis, (2) implementing effective work practices among health care workers (e.g., using and correctly wearing respiratory protection, keeping doors to isolation rooms closed), (3) educating, training, and counseling health care workers about tuberculosis, and (4) screening health care workers for *M. tuberculosis* infection and disease. The second level is the use of engineering controls to eliminate or reduce the concentration of droplet nuclei (e.g., controlling the amount, direction, and exhaust of ventilation systems; high-efficiency particulate air filtration or ultraviolet irradiation). Because it is not possible to eliminate infectious droplet nuclei in some areas of the hospital (e.g., patient isolation rooms, treatment rooms where cough-inducing procedures are performed), the third level involves the use of personal respiratory protection devices by health care workers to prevent the inhalation of droplet nuclei. Particulate respirators with a National Institute for Occupational Safety and Health certification of N95 or better satisfy the CDC specifications for these devices.[15, 79] These devices must be fit-tested on the individuals using them according to OSHA standards.[15] The nature of future OSHA regulations regarding the specifications for engineering controls, such as ventilation and filtration requirements, and personal respiratory protection devices is not clear at present.

Reprocessing of Reusable Patient Care Items

A large number of nosocomial infection outbreaks have been related to the use of contaminated equipment. Consequently, hospital infection prevention and control programs must work closely with all hospital departments, reprocessing reusable patient care items to ensure proper selection, implementation, and quality monitoring of reprocessing methods. An APIC guideline discusses the characteristics and efficacy of various classes of disinfectants and provides recommendations for methods used to reprocess specific patient care items.[90]

Regulated Medical Waste

Regulated medical waste refers to waste that has at least the potential to transmit infectious agents to humans. However, it is important to recognize that infections resulting from exposure to regulated medical waste (other than those related to percutaneous exposures within hospitals) have not been documented.[91] Moreover, waste from hospitals accounts for 1 per cent or less of the total municipal waste generated annually and has been demonstrated to have a lower microbial burden than common household waste.[91]

Nonetheless, a variety of national, state, and local regulations pertain to the identification, packaging, transport, storage, and disposal of regulated medical waste.[88] A full discussion of this topic is beyond the scope of this chapter, but hospital infection prevention and control programs can provide valuable input into the design of rational approaches to complying with these regulations. Because the management of regulated medical waste is considerably more expensive than that of traditional waste, ensuring proper sorting of regulated medical waste from nonregulated hospital waste can result in considerable cost savings.

EDUCATION AND TRAINING OF HEALTH CARE WORKERS

Providing education and training in both general principles and specific aspects of hospital infection prevention and control is one of the primary responsibilities of program staff. Program staff in many hospitals are responsible for providing training regarding the risks of blood-borne pathogens and prevention measures mandated by OSHA. Program staff members need to be familiar with principles of adult learning, assessing the educational needs of the audience, defining learning objectives, determining optimal instructional formats, using effective teaching and communication skills, and weighing the merits of various educational tools.[55]

ANTIBIOTIC UTILIZATION AND ANTIMICROBIAL-RESISTANT MICROORGANISMS

The rapid emergence of pathogens resistant to multiple antimicrobial agents (e.g., vancomycin-resistant enterococci, gram-negative bacteria producing extended-spectrum β-lactamases) and the widespread dissemination of these resistant microorganisms constitute an unprecedented crisis for hospitals worldwide.[42] The mechanisms involved in the emergence and spread of antimicrobial resistance are complex but are facilitated no doubt by intense selection pressure caused by overuse and misuse of antimicrobial agents in hospitals, particularly newer broad-spectrum agents. Dissemination of resistant strains is facilitated by poor compliance with hand washing and isolation precautions procedures.

Solutions to this problem are complex and require a multidisciplinary, systems-oriented approach, catalyzed and supported by hospital leadership.[42] In 1994, a workshop sponsored by the National Foundation for Infectious Diseases, the HIP, and the CDC developed strategic goals related to improving the use of antimicrobial agents and reducing the transmission of antimicrobial-resistant microorganisms in hospitals (Table 229–7).[42] Outcome and process measure-

TABLE 229–7. Strategic Goals Related to the Use of Antimicrobial Agents and the Transmission of Antimicrobial-Resistant Microorganisms in Hospitals

Strategies to Optimize the Use of Prophylactic, Empiric, and Therapeutic Use of Antimicrobial Agents

1. Optimize antimicrobial prophylaxis for operative prophylaxis
2. Optimize the choice and duration of empiric antimicrobial therapy
3. Improve antimicrobial prescribing practices by educational and administrative means
4. Establish a system to monitor and provide feedback on the occurrence and effect of antimicrobial resistance
5. Define and implement institutional or health care system delivery guidelines for important types of antimicrobial use

Strategies for Detecting, Reporting, and Preventing Transmission of Antimicrobial-Resistant Microorganisms

1. Develop a system to recognize and promptly report significant changes and trends in antimicrobial resistance to hospital and physician leaders; medical, nursing, infection control, and pharmacy staffs; and others who need to know
2. Develop a system for rapid detection and reporting of resistant microorganisms in individual patients to appropriate personnel (caregivers and infection control staff) and for rapid response by caregivers
3. Increase adherence to policies and procedures, especially hand hygiene, barrier precautions, and environmental control measures
4. Incorporate the detection, prevention, and control of antimicrobial resistance into institutional strategic goals and provide required resources (e.g., by providing adequate facilities and resources for hand washing, isolation, and environmental hygiene; funding ongoing monitoring and data collection, including infection control/hospital epidemiology and quality improvement in the planning process; and setting managerial goals and accountability for reductions in colonization and infection with resistant microorganisms)
5. Develop a plan for identifying, transferring, discharging, and readmitting patients colonized with specified antimicrobial-resistant microorganisms*

*Each hospital should specify a list of problematic pathogens, such as methicillin-resistant *Staphylococcus aureus,* vancomycin-resistant and high-level gentamicin-resistant enterococci, and gram-negative bacilli resistant to third-generation cephalosporins and aminoglycosides.

From Goldmann, D. A., Weinstein, R. A., Wenzel, R. P., et al.: Strategies to prevent and control the emergence and spread of antimicrobial-resistant microorganisms in hospitals: A challenge to hospital leadership. J. A. M. A. *275*:234–240, 1996.

ments useful in gauging progress toward these strategic goals, as well as potential barriers to success and effective countermeasures, are described in the workshop report.[42] Other recommendations for improving the use of antimicrobial agents in hospitals and preventing the spread of particular antimicrobial-resistant microorganisms also are available.[56, 74]

PRODUCT EVALUATION

A large number of new medical products are introduced to the health care market every year. Although some of these products have the potential to reduce infectious risks, data to substantiate the safety and efficacy claims of manufacturers often are limited. Many devices marketed to hospitals caring for children have never been tested in children. Because these products often are substantially more expensive than existing products, there must be a compelling rationale for their use. Hospital infection prevention and control staff members can provide valuable assistance to hospital committees evaluating new products and, in some cases, can design and conduct appropriate clinical trials.

References

1. American Academy of Pediatrics: Antimicrobial prophylaxis in pediatric surgery patients. *In* Peter, G. (ed.): 1994 Red Book: Report of the Committee on Infectious Diseases. 23rd ed. Elk Grove, American Academy of Pediatrics, 1994, pp. 535–539.
2. Anderson, J. D., Bonner, M., Scheifele, D. W., et al.: Lack of nosocomial spread of varicella in a pediatric hospital with negative pressure ventilated patient rooms. Infect. Control *6*:120–121, 1985.
3. Bell, L. M., Naides, S. J., Stoffman, P., et al.: Human parvovirus B19 infection among hospital staff members after contact with infected patients. N. Engl. J. Med. *321*:485–491, 1989.
4. Bennett, J. V., and Brachman, P. S. (eds.): Hospital Infections. 3rd ed. Boston, Little, Brown, 1992.
5. Berg, R. (ed.): The APIC Curriculum for Infection Control Practice. Dubuque, Kendall/Hunt Publishing, 1988.
6. Berwick, D. M.: Continuous improvement as an ideal in health care. N. Engl. J. Med. *320*:53–56, 1989.
7. Bingen, E.: Applications of molecular methods to epidemiologic investigations of nosocomial infections in a pediatric hospital. Infect. Control Hosp. Epidemiol. *15*:488–493, 1994.
8. Blatt, M. L.: Cross-infection: Its prevention in a children's hospital. Ill. Med. J. *70*:483–487, 1936.
9. Brennemann, J.: The infant ward. Am. J. Dis. Child. *43*:577–584, 1932.
10. Broderick, A., Mori, M., Nettleman, M. D., et al.: Nosocomial infections: Validation of surveillance and computer modeling to identify patients at risk. Am. J. Epidemiol. *131*:734–742, 1990.
11. Centers for Disease Control: Recommendations for preventing transmission of infection with human T-lymphotropic virus type III/lymphadenopathy-associated virus in the workplace. M. M. W. R. *34*:681–686, 1985.
12. Centers for Disease Control: Recommendations for prevention of HIV transmission in health-care settings. M. M. W. R. 36:1S–18S, 1987.
13. Centers for Disease Control: Protection against viral hepatitis: Recommendations of the Immunization Practices Advisory Committee (ACIP). M. M. W. R. *39*:1–26, 1990.
14. Centers for Disease Control: Public Health Service statement on management of occupational exposure to human immunodeficiency virus, including considerations regarding zidovudine postexposure use. M. M. W. R. *39*:1–14, 1990.
15. Centers for Disease Control and Prevention: Guidelines for preventing the transmission of *Mycobacterium tuberculosis* in health care facilities, 1994. M. M. W. R. *44*:1-132, 1994.
16. Centers for Disease Control and Prevention: Case-control study of HIV seroconversion in health care workers after percutaneous exposure to HIV-infected blood: France, United Kingdom, and United States, January 1988–August 1994. M. M. W. R. *44*:929–933, 1995.
17. Centers for Disease Control and Prevention: Prevention and control of influenza: Recommendations of the Advisory Committee on Immunization Practices (ACIP). M. M. W. R. *44*:1-22, 1995.
18. Centers for Disease Control and Prevention: Prevention of varicella: Recommendations of the Advisory Committee on Immunization Practices (ACIP). M. M. W. R. *45*(No. RR-11):1–36, 1996.

18a. Centers for Disease Control and Prevention: Update: Provisional Public Health Service recommendations for chemoprophylaxis after occupational exposure to HIV. M. M. W. R. *45*:468–472, 1996.

19. Classen, D. C.: Information management in infectious diseases: Survival of the fittest. Clin. Infect. Dis. *19*:902–909, 1994.
20. Classen, D. C., Evans, R. S., Pestonik, S. L., et al.: The timing of prophylactic administration of antibiotics and the risk of surgical-wound infection. N. Engl. J. Med. *326*:281–286, 1992.
21. Conly, J. M., Hill, S., Ross, J., et al.: Handwashing practices in an intensive care unit: The effects of an educational program and its relationship to infection rates. Am. J. Infect. Control *17*:330–339, 1989.
22. Culver, D. H., Horan, T. C., Gaynes, R. P., et al.: Surgical wound infection rates by wound class, operative procedure, and patient risk index: National Nosocomial Infections Surveillance System. Am. J. Med. *91*:152S–157S, 1991.
23. Currier, J. S., Campbell, H., Platt, R., et al.: Perioperative antimicrobial prophylaxis in middle Tennessee, 1989–1990. Rev. Infect. Dis. *13*:S874–S878, 1991.
24. Decker, M. D.: The application of continuous quality improvement to healthcare. Infect. Control Hosp. Epidemiol. *13*:226–229, 1992.
25. Decker, M. D.: Continuous quality improvement. Infect. Control Hosp. Epidemiol. *13*:165–169, 1992.
26. Decker, M. D., and Schaffner, W.: Tuberculosis control in the hospital: Compliance with OSHA requirements. *In* Mayhall, C. G. (ed.): Hospital Epidemiology and Infection Control. Baltimore, Williams & Wilkins, 1995, pp. 850–859.
27. Doebbeling, B. N.: Epidemics: Identification and management. *In* Wenzel, R. P. (ed.): Prevention and Control of Nosocomial Infections. 2nd ed. Baltimore, Williams & Wilkins, 1993, pp. 177–206.
28. Donabedian, A.: Contributions of epidemiology to quality assessment and monitoring. Infect. Control Hosp. Epidemiol. *11*:117-121, 1990.
29. Donowitz, L. G. (ed.): Hospital-Acquired Infection in the Pediatric Patient. Baltimore, Williams & Wilkins, 1988.
30. Donowitz, L. G., Hunt, E. H., Pugh, V. G., et al.: Comparison of historical and serologic immunity to varicella-zoster virus in 373 hospital employees. Am. J. Infect. Control *15*:212–214, 1987.
31. Durbin, W., Jr., Lapidas, B., and Goldmann, D. A.: Improved antibiotic usage following introduction of a novel prescription system. J. A. M. A. *246*:1796–1800, 1981.
32. Emori, T. G., Culver, D. H., Horan, T. C., et al.: National nosocomial infections surveillance system (NNIS): Description of surveillance methods. Am. J. Infect. Control *19*:19–35, 1991.
33. Evans, R. S., Burke, J. P., Classen, D. C., et al.: Computerized identification of patients at high risk for hospital-acquired infection. Am. J. Infect. Control *20*:4–10, 1992.
34. Ford-Jones, E. L., Mindorff, C. M., Pollock, E., et al.: Evaluation of a new method of detection of nosocomial infection in the pediatric intensive care unit: The Infection Control Sentinel Sheet System. Infect. Control Hosp. Epidemiol. *10*:515–520, 1989.
35. Freeman, J., and McGowan, J. E., Jr.: Methodologic issues in hospital epidemiology. I. Rates, case-finding and interpretation. Rev. Infect. Dis. *3*:658–667, 1981.
36. Friedland, I. R., and Klugman, K. P.: Antibiotic-resistant pneumococcal disease in South African children. Am. J. Dis. Child. *146*:920–923, 1992.
37. Garner, J. S.: CDC guideline for prevention of surgical wound infections, 1985. Infect. Control *7*:193–200, 1986.
38. Garner, J. S., and Hospital Infection Control Practices Advisory Committee: Guideline for isolation precautions in hospitals. Infect. Control Hosp. Epidemiol. 17:53–80, 1996.
39. Gaynes, R. P., and Horan, T. C.: Surveillance of nosocomial infections. *In* Mayhall, C. G. (ed.): Hospital Epidemiology and Infection Control. Baltimore, Williams & Wilkins, 1995, pp. 1017–1031.
40. Gerberding, J. L.: Management of occupational exposures to blood-borne viruses. N. Engl. J. Med. *332*:444–451, 1995.
41. Goldmann, D. A.: Contemporary challenges for hospital epidemiology. Am. J. Med. *91*:8S–15S, 1991.
42. Goldmann, D. A., Weinstein, R. A., Wenzel, R. P., et al.: Strategies to prevent and control the emergence and spread of antimicrobial-resistant microorganisms in hospitals: A challenge to hospital leadership. J. A. M. A. *275*:234–240, 1996.
43. Gray, J. E., Richardson, D. K., McCormick, M.C., et al.: Coagulase-negative staphylococcal bacteremia among very low birth weight infants: Relation to admission illness severity, resource use, and outcome. Pediatrics *95*:225–230, 1995.
44. Gross, P. A.: The future of the hospital epidemiologist in the 1990s. Infect. Control Hosp. Epidemiol. *16:179*–182, 1995.
45. Gross, P. A.: Use of severity of illness indices in hospital epidemiology and infection control. *In* Mayhall, C. G. (ed.): Hospital Epidemiology and Infection Control. Baltimore, Williams & Wilkins, 1995, pp. 90–104.
46. Haiduven, D. J., Hench, C. P., and Stevens, D. A.: Postexposure varicella management of nonimmune personnel: An alternative approach. Infect. Control Hosp. Epidemiol. *15*:329–334, 1994.
47. Haley, R. W.: The "hospital epidemiologist" in U.S. hospitals, 1976–1977: A description of the head of the infection surveillance and control program: Report from the SENIC Project. Infect. Control *1*:21–32, 1980.
48. Haley, R. W.: Surveillance by objective: A new priority-directed approach

to the control of nosocomial infections. Am. J. Infect. Control *13*:78–89, 1985.
49. Haley, R. W.: The role of infectious disease physicians in hospital infection control. Bull. N. Y. Acad. Med. *63*:597–604, 1987.
50. Haley, R. W., Culver D. H., White, J. W., et al.: The efficacy of infection surveillance and control programs in preventing nosocomial infections in US hospitals. Am. J. Epidemiol. *121*:182–205, 1985.
51. Haley, R. W., Morgan, W. M., Culver, D. H., et al.: Update from the SENIC project: Hospital infection control: Recent progress and opportunities under prospective payment. Am. J. Infect. Control *13*:97–108, 1985.
52. Haley, R. W., Tenney, J. H., Lindsey, J. D., et al.: How frequent are outbreaks of nosocomial infection in community hospitals? Infect. Control *6*:233–236, 1985.
53. Harries, E. H. R.: Infection and its control in children's wards. Lancet *2*:173–178, 1935.
54. Hirschhorn, L. R., Currier, J. S., and Platt, R.: Electronic surveillance of antibiotic exposure and coded discharge diagnoses as indicators of postoperative infection and other quality assurance measures. Infect. Control Hosp. Epidemiol. *14*:21–28, 1993.
55. Hoffmann, K. K., and Clontz, E. P.: Education of health care workers in the prevention of nosocomial infections. *In* Mayhall, C. G. (ed.): Hospital Epidemiology and Infection Control. Baltimore, Williams & Wilkins, 1995, pp. 1086–1094.
56. Hospital Infection Control Practices Advisory Committee: Recommendations for preventing the spread of vancomycin resistance. Infect. Control Hosp. Epidemiol. *16*:105–113, 1995.
56a. Ippolito, G., Puro, V., Petrosilo, N., et al.: Prevention, Management, and Chemoprophylaxis of Occupational Exposure to HIV. Charlottesville, International Health Care Worker Safety Center, University of Virginia, 1997.
57. Jarvis, W. R.: Nosocomial outbreaks: The Centers for Disease Control's Hospital Infections Program experience, 1980–1990. Am. J. Med. *91*:101S–106S, 1991.
58. Jarvis, W. R.: Usefulness of molecular epidemiology for outbreak investigations. Infect. Control. Hosp. Epidemiol. *15*:500–503, 1994.
59. Joint Commission on Accreditation of Healthcare Organizations: Surveillance, Prevention, and Control of Infection: 1996 Comprehensive Accreditation Manual for Hospitals. Chicago, Joint Commission on Accreditation of Healthcare Organizations, 1995, pp. 449–466.
60. Josephson, A., Karanfil, L., and Gombert, M. E.: Strategies for the management of varicella-susceptible healthcare workers after a known exposure. Infect. Control Hosp. Epidemiol. *11*:309–313, 1990.
61. Kaiser, A. B.: Antimicrobial prophylaxis in surgery. N. Engl. J. Med. *315*:1129–1138, 1986.
62. Korniewicz, D. M., Kirwin, M., Cresci, K., et al.: Leakage of latex and vinyl exam gloves in high and low risk clinical settings. Am. Ind. Hyg. Assoc. J. *54*:22–26, 1993.
63. Krause, P. J., Gross, P. A., Barrett, T. L., et al.: Quality standard for assurance of measles immunity among health care workers. Infect. Control. Hosp. Epidemiol. *15*:193–199, 1994.
64. Kritchevsky, S. B., and Simmons, B. P.: Continuous quality improvement: Concepts and applications for physician care. J. A. M. A. *266*:1817–1823, 1991.
65. Kunin, C. M.: The future of hospital epidemiology. Infect. Control Hosp. Epidemiol. *10*:276–279, 1989.
66. Larson, E., Eisenberg, R., and Soule, B. M.: Validating the certification process for infection control practice. Am. J. Infect. Control *16*:198–205, 1988.
67. Larson, E., and Kretzer, E. K.: Compliance with handwashing and barrier precautions. J. Hosp. Infect. *30*:88–106, 1995.
68. Larson, E. L., and 1992, 1993, 1994, APIC Guidelines Committee, Association for Professionals in Infection Control and Epidemiology, Inc.: APIC guideline for handwashing and hand antisepsis in health care settings. Am. J. Infect. Control *23*:251–269, 1995.
69. Leclair, J. M., Freeman, J., Sullivan, B. F., et al.: Prevention of nosocomial respiratory syncytial virus infections through compliance with glove and gown isolation precautions. N. Engl. J. Med. *317*:329–334, 1987.
70. Lichtenstein, A.: Nosocomical infections in children's hospitals and institutions: Our means for combating these infections. Acta Paediatr. *17*:36–49, 1935.
71. Lövegren, E.: Infection risks in nursing institutions for infants and young children and measures for their prevention. Acta Paediatr. *17*:50–55, 1935.
72. Lynch, P., Jackson, M. M., Cummings, M. J., et al.: Rethinking the role of isolation practices in the prevention of nosocomial infections. Ann. Intern. Med. *107*:243–246, 1987.
73. Mandigers, C. M., Diepersloot, R. J., Dessens, M., et al.: A hospital outbreak of penicillin-resistant pneumococci in The Netherlands. Eur. Respir. J. *7*:1635–1639, 1994.
74. Marr, J. J., Moffet, H. L., and Kunin, C. M.: Guidelines for improving the use of antimicrobial agents in hospitals: A statement by the Infectious Diseases Society of America. J. Infect. Dis. *157*:869–876, 1988.
75. Mayhall, C. G. (ed.): Hospital Epidemiology and Infection Control. Baltimore, Williams & Wilkins, 1995.
76. McDonald, L. L., and Pugliese, G.: Regulatory, accreditation, and professional agencies influencing infection control programs. *In* Wenzel, R. P. (ed.): Prevention and Control of Nosocomial Infections. Baltimore, Williams & Wilkins, 1993, pp. 58–69.
77. McKhann, C. F., Steeger, A., and Long, A. P.: Hospital infections: A survey of the problem. Am. J. Dis. Child. *55*:579–599, 1938.
78. Millar, M. R., Brown, N. M., Tobin, G. W., et al.: Outbreak of infection with penicillin-resistant *Streptococcus pneumoniae* in a hospital for the elderly. J. Hosp. Infect. *27*:99–104, 1994.
79. National Institute for Occupational Safety and Health, Centers for Disease Control and Prevention, Public Health Service, et al.: Respiratory protective devices: Final rules and notice. Fed. Reg. *60*:30336–30404, 1995.
80. National Nosocomial Infections Surveillance System: Nosocomial infection rates for interhospital comparison: Limitations and possible solutions: A report from the National Nosocomial Infections Surveillance (NNIS) System. Infect. Control Hosp. Epidemiol. *12*:609–621, 1991.
81. National Nosocomial Infections Surveillance System: National Nosocomial Infection Surveillance (NNIS) semi-annual report, May 1995. Am. J. Infect. Control *23*:377–385, 1995.
82. Nettleman, M. D.: Preparing for and surviving a JCAHO inspection. Infect. Control Hosp. Epidemiol. *16*:236–239, 1995.
83. Occupational Safety and Health Administration, Department of Labor: Occupational exposure to bloodborne pathogens: Final rule. Fed. Reg. *56*:64175–64182, 1991.
84. Patterson, C. H.: Joint Commission on Accreditation of Healthcare Organizations. Infect. Control Hosp. Epidemiol. *16*:36–42, 1995.
84a. Pearson, M. L., and Hospital Infection Control Practices Committee: Guideline for prevention of intravascular device–related infections. Infect. Control Hosp. Epidemiol. *17*:438–473, 1996.
85. Perl, T. M.: Surveillance, reporting, and the use of computers. *In* Wenzel, R. P. (ed.): Prevention and Control and Nosocomial Infections. 2nd ed. Baltimore, Williams & Wilkins, 1993, pp. 139–176.
86. Pirwitz, S.: The Certification Board of Infection Control, Inc. Infect. Control Hosp. Epidemiol. *16*:518–521, 1995.
87. Pollock, E., Ford-Jones, E. L., Corey, M., et al.: Use of the Pediatric Risk of Mortality score to predict nosocomial infection in a pediatric intensive care unit. Crit. Care Med. *19*:160–165, 1991.
88. Reinhardt, P. A., Gordon, J. G., and Alvarado, C. J.: Medical waste management. *In* Mayhall, C. G. (ed.): Hospital Epidemiology and Infection Control. Baltimore, Williams & Wilkins, 1995, pp. 1099–1108.
89. Russell, B.: The Association for Professionals in Infection Control and Epidemiology, Inc. Infect. Control Hosp. Epidemiol. *16*:522–525, 1995.
90. Rutala, W. A., 1994, 1995, 1996 APIC Guidelines Committee, and Association for Professionals in Infection Control and Epidemiology, Inc.: APIC guideline for selection and use of disinfectants. Am. J. Infect. Control *24*:313–342, 1996.
91. Rutala, W. A., and Weber, D. J.: Infectious waste: Mismatch between science and policy. N. Engl. J. Med. *325*:578–582, 1991.
92. Sartor, C., Edwards, J. R., Gaynes, R. P., et al.: Evolution of hospital participation in the National Nosocomial Infection Surveillance (NNIS) System, 1986 to 1993. Am. J. Infect. Control *23*:364–368, 1995.
93. Shannon, R., McArthur, B. J., Weinstein, S., et al.: A national task analysis of infection control practitioners, 1982. Part two: Tasks, knowledge, and abilities for practice. Am. J. Infect. Control *12*:187–196, 1984.
94. Shapiro, M., Townsend, T. R., Rosner, B., et al.: Use of antimicrobial drugs in general hospitals: Patterns of prophylaxis. N. Engl. J. Med. *301*:351–355, 1979.
95. Soule, B. M. (ed.): The APIC Curriculum for Infection Control Practice. Dubuque, Kendall/Hunt Publishing, 1983.
96. Tablan, O. C., Anderson, L. J., Arden, N. H., et al.: Guideline for prevention of nosocomial pneumonia. Infect. Control Hosp. Epidemiol. *15*:587–627, 1994.
97. The Society for Hospital Epidemiology of America, the Association for Practitioners in Infection Control, the Centers for Disease Control, et al.: Consensus paper on the surveillance of surgical wound infections. Infect. Control Hosp. Epidemiol. *13*:599–605, 1992.
98. Wade, J. J., Desai, N., and Casewell, M. W.: Hygienic hand disinfection for the removal of epidemic vancomycin-resistant *Enterococcus faecium* and gentamicin-resistant *Enterobacter cloacae*. J. Hosp. Infect. *18*:211–218, 1991.
99. Watanakunakorn, C., Ellis, G., and Gemmel, D.: Attitude of healthcare personnel regarding influenza immunization. Infect. Control Hosp. Epidemiol. *14*:17–20, 1993.
100. Wenzel, R. P.: Expanding roles of hospital epidemiology: Quality assurance. Infect. Control Hosp. Epidemiol. *10*:255–256, 1989.
101. Wenzel, R. P.: Instituting health care reform and preserving quality: Role of the hospital epidemiologist. Clin. Infect. Dis. *17*:831–834, 1993.
102. Wenzel, R. P. (ed.): Prevention and Control of Nosocomial Infections. 2nd ed. Baltimore, Williams & Wilkins, 1993.
103. Wenzel, R. P.: The hospital epidemiologist: Practical ideas. Infect. Control Hosp. Epidemiol. *16*:166–169, 1995.
104. Wenzel, R. P., Thompson, R. L., Landry, S. M., et al.: Hospital-acquired infections in intensive care unit patients: An overview with emphasis on epidemics. Infect. Control *4*:371–375, 1983.
105. Wiblin, R. T., and Wenzel, R. P.: The infection control committee. Infect. Control Hosp. Epidemiol. *17*:44–46, 1996.
106. Williams, C. O., Campbell, S., Henry, K., et al.: Variables influencing worker compliance with universal precautions in the emergency department. Am. J. Infect. Control *22*:138–148, 1994.

107. Wong, E. S.: Guideline for prevention of catheter-associated urinary tract infections. Am. J. Infect. Control *11*:28–36, 1983.
108. Wong, E. S.: Surgical site infections. *In* Mayhall, C. G. (ed.): Hospital Epidemiology and Infection Control. Baltimore, Williams & Wilkins, 1995, pp. 154–175.
109. Yokoe, D. S., and Platt, R.: Surveillance for surgical site infections: The uses of antibiotic exposure. Infect. Control Hosp. Epidemiol. *15*:717–723, 1994.
110. Zaza, S., and Jarvis, W. R.: Investigation of outbreaks. *In* Mayhall, C. G. (ed.): Hospital Epidemiology and Infection Control. Baltimore, Williams & Wilkins, 1995, pp. 105–113.

PART 5

THERAPEUTICS

230

FUNDAMENTALS OF PHARMACOKINETICS, ANTI-INFECTIVE PHARMACODYNAMICS, AND THERAPEUTIC DRUG MONITORING

Christine A. Lindsay and John A. Bosso

Therapeutic drug monitoring is based on the concept that the pharmacologic response of many drugs, be it therapeutic or toxic, correlates better with the concentration of drug in some body fluid or tissue than with the administered dose. The dose of most drugs correlates somewhat with the intensity of pharmacologic effects, but, due to interpatient and intrapatient variation in the pharmacokinetics (absorption, distribution, metabolism, and excretion) of drugs, this relationship may vary widely. Therefore, standard dosages may not produce always predictable drug concentrations or effects.

For certain drugs, studies in patients have provided information on the plasma concentration range that is effective and safe in treating specific diseases (i.e., within this range, the desired effects of the drug occur without side effects). Below this range, the therapeutic benefits are not realized; above it, toxicity may occur. There are no absolute boundaries that separate subtherapeutic, therapeutic, and toxic drug concentrations for a given drug. Furthermore, many therapeutic ranges have been established in studies in which assays that quantify total drug concentrations were used. Because pharmacologic effect only can be caused by free (that unbound to plasma protein or tissue) drug, conditions that alter this free fraction of drug may be associated with apparent alterations in a drug's pharmacodynamics. Variability in a patient's response thus may be influenced by both pharmacodynamic (concentration-effect relationship) and pharmacokinetic (drug concentrations over time, in relation to dosage administration) factors. Individual differences in drug metabolism, elimination, and absorption will affect therapeutic response. It is known that certain drug metabolic pathways (e.g., *N*-acetylation) are under genetic control.[1] The resultant variation in drug metabolism may yield different drug dose-concentration relationships ultimately causing quantitatively different responses to the same drug dose administered to two members of the "normal" population. *Pharmacogenetics* is the term used to describe hereditary variations in response to drugs.[2] In fact, most well-known examples of pharmacogenetic variation can be explained by clinical expression of pharmacokinetic differences based upon genetically controlled metabolic pathways. In addition, disease states that alter certain physiologic functions (e.g., renal function) can change a drug's pharmacodynamics, usually by influencing its pharmacokinetics.

Determination of drug concentrations in body fluids with the intent of optimizing a patient's pharmacotherapy is known as therapeutic drug monitoring (TDM). The goals of TDM are the optimization of therapeutic drug benefits and the minimization of toxic drug effects. An obvious requirement of TDM is a reliable drug assay. There are several criteria that such an assay must meet. First, the assay method must be specific, accurate, and precise for the intended range of drug concentrations. That is, it must distinguish the drug from naturally occurring substances in the biologic matrix (usually serum, plasma, or urine), the target drug's inactive metabolites, and other medications that may have been administered to the patient. Results from the assay must be reproducible (adequate precision). An adequate assay also should provide for quantitation of active metabolites if such metabolites make a significant contribution to the overall pharmacologic effect. The second criterion necessary for successful TDM is the establishment of a relationship between the drug concentration and its pharmacologic effect. Third, information on the absorption, distribution, metabolism, and rate of elimination must be available. These pharmacokinetic variables aid in the determination of the sample collection time and the clinical interpretation of drug concentrations and provide the means for adjusting dosage regimens based upon the patient's measured drug concentrations.

Measuring drug concentrations is time consuming and expensive. Therefore, before routine monitoring of drug concentrations can be justified, the indications for doing so must be considered carefully. The general indications for drug concentration monitoring are as follows:

1. Wide interpatient or intrapatient variation in drug concentrations from a given dose. An example would be the aminoglycoside antibiotics for which wide interpatient variation in drug disposition has been described. This type of variation particularly can be important in children, in whom differences in body weight, extracellular fluid volumes, and elimination rates are great.
2. The relationship between drug dose (or amount in the body) and the amount of drug eliminated per unit time is nonlinear (i.e., zero-order, Michaelis-Menton, or saturation pharmacokinetics). With such drugs, the elimination rate may vary with dose, yielding disproportionate changes in concentration as dose is adjusted.
3. A narrow therapeutic index (i.e., when therapeutic concentrations/doses are close to toxic concentrations/doses, as with aminoglycoside antibiotics).
4. The desired pharmacologic effects cannot be assessed readily by other simple means (e.g., defervescence of fever or other signs/symptoms of infection), or the usual response is hidden (e.g., negative cultures in a clinically septic patient).
5. Symptoms occur that might be the result of toxicity or undertreatment of the underlying disease and can be confirmed or ruled out by determining drug concentrations.
6. Prognosis and management are related to blood concentrations after acute overdose (e.g., acetaminophen, barbiturates, ethanol).
7. Gastrointestinal, hepatic, or renal disease is present, causing possible alterations in drug absorption, distribution, metabolism, and/or excretion.
8. A patient is being supported by an extracorporeal circuit (such as with continuous renal replacement therapies or extracorporeal membrane oxygenation) or with dialysis, and drug removal is anticipated or suspected.
9. A drug-drug or drug-food interaction is suspected and

can be confirmed or ruled out by determining drug concentrations.

10. During clinical trials of experimental drugs being performed to establish therapeutic and toxic ranges and/or elucidate the drug pharmacokinetics.

Again, it is an obvious requirement that the relationship between drug concentration in a readily sampled body fluid and pharmacologic effect must be established before TDM is a viable clinical tool. Nonetheless, it must be recognized that such relationships are not absolute and other methods of patient assessment should be used, when possible. With a number of drugs, measurement of the plasma concentration is invaluable, but it is no substitute for careful clinical assessment of the patient's response. A plasma concentration that falls outside the established therapeutic range may not warrant a dosage adjustment if, on clinical grounds, a patient has shown satisfactory response to therapy without evidence of toxicity. Therapeutic ranges should be considered as applicable to most patients most of the time. Exceptions occur with regular frequency, and the clinician must be aware of this possibility.

PHARMACOKINETIC PRINCIPLES

When a therapeutic range for a drug is established, knowledge of the drug's disposition in the body may be used to design dosage regimens to achieve the desired concentrations. Pharmacokinetics defines the relationship between the dose administered and the concentration of drug reached in the plasma at any given time relative to the time of administration. A basic knowledge of pharmacokinetic principles is needed to order and interpret drug concentrations properly and calculate dosage regimens based on the concentrations obtained. Without an understanding of these principles, drug concentration monitoring can be ineffective, needlessly can waste time and money, and possibly can be harmful to the patient. Useful basic definitions and terms follow, although the reader must be aware that only very rudimentary concepts and mathematical relationships are presented in this chapter. The interested reader is referred to one or more of several excellent texts/workbooks on the topic that provide a much more thorough grounding in the discipline.[3–5]

Bioavailability

The bioavailability of a drug is defined as the percentage of the dose reaching the systemic circulation as unchanged drug after administration by any route. It is assumed that a drug administered intravenously is 100 per cent bioavailable, and bioavailability observed with other routes of elimination is described in relation to that standard. As an example, oral bioavailability is a reflection of the fraction of an oral dose that reaches the systemic circulation, compared with an equivalent intravenous dose. It generally is determined by comparing the areas under the serum or plasma concentration versus time curves (AUC) observed after administration of the same size dose (i.e., $AUC_{po}/AUC_{iv} \cdot 100$ = relative bioavailability). Any two routes of administration can be compared to obtain a relative bioavailability, although that relative to intravenous administration may be most meaningful.

Bioavailability is accounted for in pharmacokinetic computations by multiplying the dose (quantity) administered by a bioavailability factor (F). The bioavailability of intravenously administered drugs is assumed to be 100 per cent, and therefore the bioavailability factor is 1. When drugs are administered by other routes, the bioavailability factor may be (and often is) less than 1. For example, with orally administered drugs, absorption may be incomplete. One common example of alterations in oral antimicrobial drug absorption is the administration of drugs with or without meals. Many antibiotics have enhanced drug absorption when given on an empty stomach because the acidity produced by the presence of food will impair drug absorption (e.g., penicillins). However, certain antibiotics require the presence of food for greater bioavailability (e.g., itraconazole, oral ganciclovir). In addition, certain drug preparations are not considered necessarily to be bioequivalent. For example, cefuroxime axetil tablets and suspension, although both given orally, cannot be substituted on a milligram-per-milligram basis because different amounts of drug are absorbed in adults from the two preparations. Furthermore, with drugs that effectively are extracted by the liver, a large amount may be removed as the splanchnic blood perfuses the hepatic sinusoids. This is known as the first-pass effect, reflecting hepatic clearance of drug during the "first passage" of drug-containing blood through the liver en route to the system circulation. Most important for extensively metabolized drugs, the first-pass effect (and thus bioavailability) may be altered by conditions that affect splanchnic blood flow or plasma protein concentrations (generally speaking, only unbound drug can diffuse into hepatocytes and undergo metabolism). It is important to recognize that equivalent bioavailability for two routes of administration or dosage forms does not imply that other pharmacokinetic parameters are identical. For example, although the dose of an antibiotic administered intramuscularly may exhibit bioavailability equivalent to that with intravenous administration, the maximum concentration and/or the time at which that maximum concentration is observed (after dosage administration) usually is different for the two routes.

The amount of drug absorbed or drug that enters the systemic circulation also will be affected by the salt form (S) of the drug. The salt form of a drug is important to consider, especially when the drug is measured in the plasma as the base or when doses are being converted from one form to the other. Phenytoin sodium is a good example. Intravenous phenytoin is supplied as phenytoin sodium, which is equivalent to 92 per cent phenytoin base. Therefore, the salt factor is .92. Phenytoin capsules also are phenytoin sodium; however, the suspension and chewable tablets are phenytoin base. To convert from intravenous phenytoin sodium to oral phenytoin suspension, the intravenous dose would need to be multiplied by 0.92 in order to determine an equivalent oral phenytoin base dose.

Rectal drug absorption exhibits similar phenomena. The inferior and middle hemorrhoidal veins bypass the hepatic portal circulation and drain directly into the inferior vena cava. However, the superior hemorrhoidal vein drains directly into the hepatic portal system, and therefore first-pass metabolism is possible. Variations in the absorption of drug via the rectal route may be attributed to the site from which the drug is absorbed. If a drug is placed high in the rectum, it may undergo first-pass metabolism. On the other hand, a drug placed lower in the rectum may have a more immediate pharmacologic effect.

Drug Distribution Principles

Once they reach the systemic circulation, drugs travel throughout the body and may find access to extravascular sites depending on their molecular size, degree of ionization at physiologic pH, and water solubility (versus lipophilicity). Those drugs with small size (true for most antibiotics), low ionization, and high lipophilicity tend to distribute beyond the vascular system. In the blood stream, drugs often are bound, at least to some extent, to plasma proteins. Again, depending on chemical characteristics, drugs may find their way into various tissues where they may reside in tissue water, bind to tissue, or reach intracellular sites.

Volume of Distribution

The apparent volume of distribution (Vd) of a drug relates the amount of drug in the body to the concentration (C) of drug in the blood or plasma. This term has no exact physiologic meaning but reflects the theoretic volume that would be needed to account for all the drug in the body based upon a blood concentration. That is, it indicates the extent rather than the site of distribution. A small volume of distribution suggests that the drug is retained largely within the vascular compartment (e.g., gentamicin, which has an average volume of distribution of 0.25 L/kg in adults, 0.35 L/kg in children, and 0.5 L/kg in neonates). Larger volumes of distribution imply distribution beyond the vascular system and throughout the total body water or perhaps sequestration in certain tissues. An example would be vancomycin, which has a mean volume of distribution of approximately 0.7 to 0.9 L/kg in adults and children. Apparent volume of distribution may be calculated after a bolus dose by dividing the drug dose by the plasma concentration of the drug immediately after drug administration (at time 0; C_0) if one assumes instantaneous distribution:

$$Vd = \frac{\text{Dose}}{C_0} \qquad (1)$$

The limitation of this method of estimation is that anti-infective agents seldom are administered by bolus injection and distribution is not instantaneous, even with a drug with distribution limited to the intravascular space. When drugs are distributed beyond the intravascular space and well-perfused organs/tissues (see discussion of compartmental models later), calculation of other volume terms is possible. In such cases, the previous term reflects the apparent distribution volume before the completion of drug distribution (after a dose) and is referred to as the apparent volume of the central compartment or the initial volume of distribution. The apparent volume of distribution at steady state reflects the entire distribution volume.

Plasma Protein Binding

Unless otherwise noted, the plasma concentration of a drug is the total amount of drug (i.e., drug bound to plasma proteins plus the drug that is unbound or "free") in the plasma. Drugs are bound to plasma proteins to various extents. Acidic and neutral drugs generally are bound to albumin, whereas basic drugs may be bound to alpha_1 acid glycoprotein. It generally is assumed that plasma protein binding is important, from a pharmacokinetic or pharmacodynamic standpoint, when it is extensive. To illustrate, consider the case of ceftriaxone, a drug that is 95 per cent bound to plasma protein. If one were to decrease the binding by a mere 2.5 per cent (i.e., from 95 to 92.5 per cent), the free (pharmacologically active) amount would be increased by 50 per cent (from 5 to 7.5 per cent). Thus, small changes in plasma protein binding of extensively bound drugs can have profound therapeutic or toxic consequences. Because only the unbound portion is active pharmacologically, the concentration may be only an indirect reflection of the concentration of active drug available at the site of action. A number of disease states or conditions are associated with decreased plasma proteins (renal failure, hepatic cirrhosis, hepatitis, thermal injury, malnutrition, and stress or trauma) or with decreased binding of drugs to plasma proteins due to competition from naturally occurring organic substances (hyperbilirubinemia, uremia). Alpha_1 acid glycoprotein is known to rise in short- and long-term inflammation, malignancy, stress, and various hematologic conditions. Qualitative changes in protein binding also may occur. It is important to realize that the usual concentration-effect relationships (i.e., the therapeutic range) may be altered when plasma protein binding is altered. Thus, signs of drug toxicity or absence of the expected therapeutic effect may occur even though drug concentrations are within the normal therapeutic range. Therefore, when interpreting plasma drug concentrations, altered protein binding and the possibility of altered free fractions of the drug must be considered.

Compartmental Distribution

When the time course of drug concentrations in the blood is measured after a dose is administered, several patterns can emerge that suggest different patterns of distribution in the body. Classically, one plots the natural logarithm (ln) of drug concentration versus time, which, in many cases, yields a straight line (Fig. 230–1*A*) with a negative slope equal to the drug's elimination rate constant. The plot illustrated in Figure 230–1*A* simulates a drug being administered in a manner to produce instantaneous, complete delivery to the blood stream (as with an intravenous bolus "push") and assumes instantaneous distribution in the blood stream and highly perfused organs or tissues. From a conceptual standpoint, drugs given by this method of administration act as if the body were a single fluid compartment. It is assumed that the drug is confined to that particular compartment and that elimination takes place only from that compartment (Fig. 230–2*A*). This is referred to as a one-compartment model. A graphical representation of plasma drug concentrations over time for a drug administered orally, intramuscularly, or by a short intravenous infusion in a one-compartment model is illustrated in Figure 230–1*B*. In either case, the exponent describing the slope of the declining part of the natural logarithm of drug concentration versus time line equals the elimination rate constant.

When the declining section of the natural logarithm of drug concentration versus time curve is biexponential (see Fig. 230–1*C*), distribution beyond the vascular system and highly perfused organs is likely. Distribution of such a drug is depicted in Figure 230–2*B*. The compartment into which the drug is administered/absorbed and from which it is eliminated from the body is referred to as the central compartment. During the first phase of drug concentration decline, drug not only is being eliminated from the body but also is being removed from the central compartment to a second compartment. Nonetheless, the exponent describing the slope of that part of the line customarily is referred to as the distribution rate constant, although it obviously is a hybrid constant reflecting both elimination and distribution rates. In the case of such a two-compartment model, the second compartment usually is referred to as the peripheral compartment and is assumed to be composed of less well-perfused organs/tissues or "third spaces," such as ascitic fluid. Again, the exponent describing the slope of the second part of the declining concentration versus time line equals the elimination rate constant and sometimes is referred to as the terminal elimination rate constant. It is desirable to identify the compartmental model that best describes the disposi-

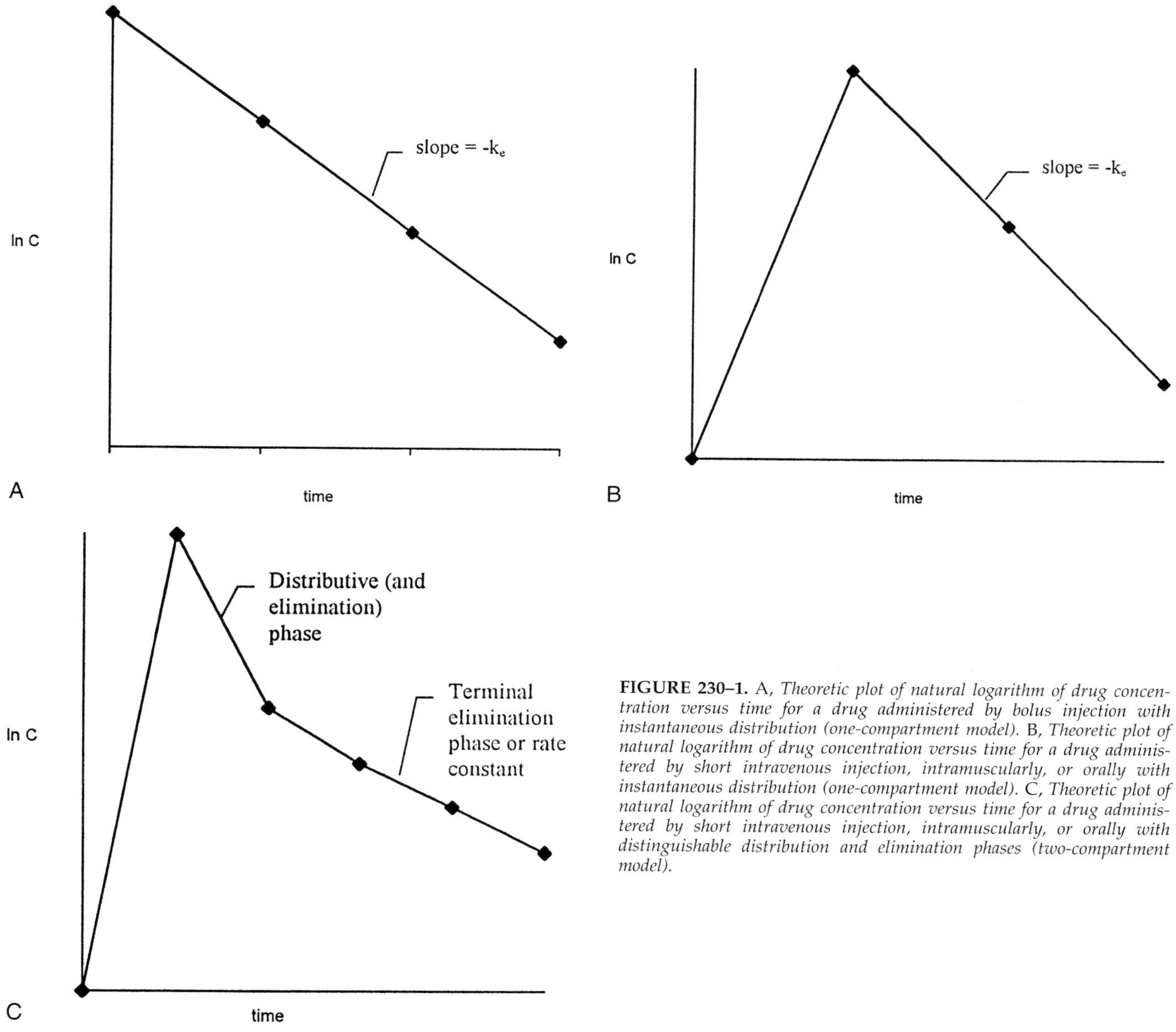

FIGURE 230–1. A, *Theoretic plot of natural logarithm of drug concentration versus time for a drug administered by bolus injection with instantaneous distribution (one-compartment model).* B, *Theoretic plot of natural logarithm of drug concentration versus time for a drug administered by short intravenous injection, intramuscularly, or orally with instantaneous distribution (one-compartment model).* C, *Theoretic plot of natural logarithm of drug concentration versus time for a drug administered by short intravenous injection, intramuscularly, or orally with distinguishable distribution and elimination phases (two-compartment model).*

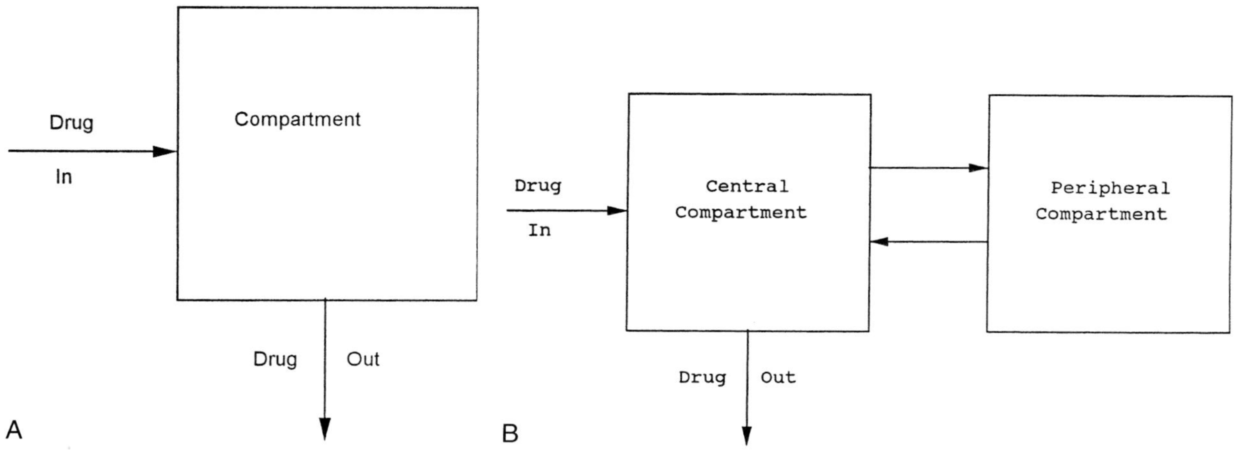

FIGURE 230–2. A, *Schematic of one-compartment model with drug administered or absorbed into and eliminated from the compartment.* B, *Schematic of a two-compartment model illustrating drug administration or absorption into the central compartment, drug passage between central and peripheral compartments, and elimination from the central compartment.*

tion of a drug, such that an accurate mathematical relationship could be derived, allowing for precise dosage adjustment. The number of exponents needed to describe the elimination line of the natural logarithm of drug concentration versus time is equivalent to the number of compartments in the conceptual/mathematical model that best describes drug disposition. The disposition of aminoglycosides and vancomycin is described most accurately by multicompartment models. As one would expect, the mathematical expressions needed to describe or predict concentrations at a given time after a dose become more complex, requiring sophisticated computer software for analysis, as the number of exponents describing elimination is increased.

To simplify clinical pharmacokinetic calculations/manipulations, clinicians "assume" a one-compartment model, even though it is known that a multicompartment model may be more accurate. Such "conveniences" are possible when little error is introduced by the false assumption. However, it still is important to be aware of the true model because this should be taken into account for proper blood sampling.

Half-life and Elimination Rate Constant

A drug's half-life ($t_{1/2}$) is the time it takes for the plasma concentration to fall by one-half. As described earlier, a plot of the natural logarithm of drug concentration versus time (see Fig. 230–1*A*) frequently yields a straight line, the slope of which is the elimination rate constant. The half-life is related to the elimination rate constant (k_e). Specifically:

$$t_{1/2} = 0.693/k_e \tag{2}$$

Just as 50 per cent of the drug will be eliminated in one half-life, 75 per cent will be eliminated in two half-lives, 87.5 per cent will be eliminated in three half-lives, and so on. Thus, almost all of the drug will be eliminated in about five half-lives, which is important to remember when estimating the time to total drug elimination after the last dose. This same half-life principle will guide in the estimation of when steady state will be reached once a dosing regimen has commenced. Steady state is the condition reached when drug being delivered into the sampling compartment per unit time is equal to the amount of drug being eliminated from that same compartment per unit time. This is a critical principle because commonly cited therapeutic drug concentrations or ranges relate to steady-state conditions.

Clearance

Clearance is one of the more important pharmacokinetic parameters. Simply put, it describes the volume of blood from which drug totally is removed per unit of time. It accounts for drug loss from the body and is a representation of the ability of the body to eliminate a drug. In a one-compartment model with first-order elimination, it is the product of the volume of distribution and the elimination rate constant:

$$Cl = Vd \times k_e \tag{3}$$

Total drug clearance from the body may be the sum of two of more clearance components. For example, a drug may be cleared from the body by the kidneys as well as by nonrenal mechanisms. Thus, renal clearance and nonrenal clearance could be described. In this case, total body clearance (Cl_T) is equal to the sum of renal clearance (CL_R) and nonrenal clearance (CL_{NR}). Organ clearance is a function of blood flow to that organ and the extraction ratio:

$$Cl_{organ} = Q \times E \tag{4}$$

where Q is blood flow (volume per time) and E is the extraction ratio. Extraction ratio is determined by dividing the difference in drug concentrations between blood entering and leaving the organ by the drug concentration in blood entering the organ:

$$E = \frac{C_{in} - C_{out}}{C_{in}} \tag{5}$$

BASIC PHARMACOKINETIC CALCULATIONS

It is the aim of clinical pharmacokinetics to design safe and effective dosage regimens. Such techniques particularly are useful when a drug's blood concentrations in relation to dose otherwise are unpredictable due to interpatient or disease-induced variability. Pharmacokinetic calculations for drugs that exhibit linear pharmacokinetics are more straightforward because the elimination rate constant does not change as the dosage is changed. Once a patient's elimination rate constant and volume of distribution are known, it is relatively simple to adjust doses and intervals to achieve desired serum concentrations. For the purposes of the following discussion, a "peak" concentration is defined as the plasma concentration obtained a fixed period of time after the end of the drug infusion, and a "trough" is defined as a concentration obtained immediately prior to the next maintenance dose. Peaks and troughs are not the same as maximum and minimum plasma concentrations. They completely are dependent upon the sampling time in relationship to the given dose.

Derivation of the basic pharmacokinetic equations is beyond the scope of this chapter, and thus, only the final, clinically useful equations are presented with examples. Only one-compartment equations are utilized because these are more clinically relevant and are, more often than not, more accurate in determining a patient's pharmacokinetic parameters to design a dosage regimen. Again, the reader is referred to texts in the area for a broader grounding and coverage of advanced concepts.[3, 4]

First-Order Pharmacokinetics

Multiple, Short Intravenous Infusions

Most intravenous antibiotics are administered using this method, i.e., gentamicin 40 mg infused over 30 minutes every 8 hours. In order to adjust doses and intervals, two basic parameters must be calculated: the volume of distribution and the elimination rate constant. These parameters are determined using measured serum concentrations from the patient. For example, when a patient is started on aminoglycoside therapy and serum concentrations are determined at at least two different times after a dose at steady state, the parameters readily can be calculated. Not only can new doses be calculated, but also one can determine the time when certain concentrations will be achieved after a dose or, conversely, what concentration will be achieved at any given time, as follows:

$$C_t = C_0 \times e^{-ket} \tag{6}$$

where C_t is concentration at time t (after dose is administered), C_0 is the concentration immediately after the dose, and k_e is the elimination rate constant. This relationship also can be used to determine a concentration (at any point in time after a dose) when another concentration (the patient's elimination rate constant) and the time between the two concentrations are known.

EXAMPLE 1. A 20-kg child is given 50 mg of gentamicin every 8 hours. The third dose is given at 1600 hours, and a peak is obtained at 1700 hours (6 mg/L). The elimination rate constant is known to be 0.198 hour^{-1}. What is the predicted plasma concentration at 2400 hours? (Answer: Using Equation 6, where C_0 = 6 mg/L, k_e = 0.198 hour^{-1}, and t = 7 hours, the predicted concentration at 2400 hours is 1.5 mg/L.)

If two concentrations (e.g., a peak and a trough) are known and the time that has elapsed between these concentrations is known (t_2-t_1, where t_1 is the time after the dose at which the peak concentration is measured and t_2 is the time after the dose at which the trough is measured), the elimination rate constant can be calculated as follows:

$$k_e = \frac{\ln \dfrac{(\text{peak})}{(\text{trough})}}{t_2 - t_1} \qquad (7)$$

EXAMPLE 2. A 30-kg child is given 300 mg of vancomycin every 6 hours. A peak is obtained after the third dose at 1700 hours (30 mg/L), and a trough is obtained after the third dose at 2100 hours (7.5 mg/L). What is the elimination rate constant? What is the half-life? (Answer: Using Equation 7, where peak = 30 mg/L, trough = 7.5 mg/L, t_2 = 2100 hours, and t_1 = 1700 hours, the elimination rate constant is 0.347 hour^{-1}. Using Equation 2, the half-life is 2 hours.) It should be obvious that what is being calculated in Equation 7 is the slope of the concentration versus time line (change in Y axis divided by relative change in X axis). The reader should note that these and the following equations all utilize this value (k_e). It therefore should be evident that its accurate determination is vital.

The maximum serum concentration occurring at steady state after completion of a short intravenous infusion for a drug for which the disposition is described adequately by a one-compartment model may be calculated as follows:

$$C_{max_{ss}} = \frac{k_0}{Vd \times k_e} \frac{(1 - e^{-k_e t})}{(1 - e^{-k_e \tau})} \qquad (8a)$$

where k_o is infusion rate, t is time of infusion, and τ is the dosage interval. This equation not only provides for accumulation of drug concentrations to steady state but also accounts for drug elimination during the infusion. The equation is rearranged easily to solve for volume of distribution. After calculating the patient's volume of distribution and elimination rate constant, the maximum serum or plasma concentration (occurring at the end of the infusion) can be calculated for a given dose or the necessary dose to produce a desired maximum concentration can be derived, depending on the situation. The expression for minimum concentration at steady state is:

$$C_{min_{ss}} = \frac{k_0 (1 - e^{-k_e t})}{Vd \times k_e (1 - e^{-k_e \tau})} e^{-k_e t'} \qquad (8b)$$

where t′ is the time difference between C_{max} and C_{min} and all other terms are as defined previously.

EXAMPLE 3. Calculate the volume of distribution for the child in Equation 1 when the gentamicin is infused over 30 minutes. (Answer: Using Equation 8a, where K_0 = 100 mg/hour, k_e = 0.198 hour$^{-1,}$ t = 0.5 hour, τ = 8 hours, and $C_{max\ ss}$ = 6 mg/L, Vd is 9.98 L or 0.5 L/kg.)

It must be stressed that the term $C_{max\ ss}$ is, mathematically, the maximum concentration occurring immediately at the end of dosage infusion, assuming instantaneous distribution (one-compartment model). As discussed earlier, a drug's disposition often is assumed to be described adequately by a one-compartment model, even though it technically is more accurate to utilize a multicompartment model. This obviously is done for clinical convenience, but one must be cognizant of the assumptions being made and the relative error introduced into the calculation. Accounting for such an error is well illustrated by examining the normal process for adjusting dosages in patients being treated with aminoglycoside antibiotics.

Aminoglycoside pharmacokinetics are described better by a two-compartment model, but clinicians often assume that use of a one-compartment model is clinically adequate. A two-compartment model is more appropriate because distribution is not complete by the end of a normal 30-minute infusion. This is accounted for in a relatively simple way. Customarily, one waits for at least 30 minutes after completion of the drug infusion to determine the first drug concentration (often referred to as the "peak" concentration). When the elimination rate constant is calculated in this manner, it is based on two concentrations from the terminal elimination phase of the concentration versus time plot. The determination of the elimination rate constant now is more accurate, and subsequent pharmacokinetic calculations assuming a one-compartment model will be valid. If the first concentration was determined at a time before distribution was complete, an incorrect slope (k_e) would have been determined and all subsequent calculations would be affected adversely by that error.

In the previous scenario, the patient's pharmacokinetic parameters were determined based upon clinically derived drug concentrations and then subsequently utilized to calculate other values leading to a dosage change. At times, such as when first starting therapy, drug concentrations are not available and the clinician has reasons not to use the "usual" dose (e.g., in the face of renal impairment). In such cases, the same calculations can be made, based on Equation 8, but using population parameters of the volume of distribution and the elimination rate constant. These values must be obtained from the relevant literature describing the drug's pharmacokinetics in similar patients.[6] Once therapy has commenced and drug concentrations have been measured, it is possible to determine the patient's own pharmacokinetic parameters and, if necessary, determine an appropriate dosage adjustment.

Loading Dose

At times, it is desirable to reach the therapeutic or steady-state drug concentration as quickly as possible for a rapid therapeutic effect. It should be remembered that it will take about five drug half-lives to reach steady state and that this could be a considerable period for a drug with a long half-life. In such cases, giving a loading dose, which is intended to produce the desired therapeutic concentration almost immediately, may be appropriate. Fortunately, determination of a loading dose for a drug eliminated by first-order pharmacokinetics and well described by a one-compartment model is straightforward. In the case of a bolus injection, the loading dose would be calculated as follows:

$$\text{Loading dose} = C \times Vd \qquad (9)$$

where C is the concentration immediately after the dose (with instantaneous distribution). Loading doses for antibiotics have been suggested for premature infants and neonates due to immature renal function and larger volumes of distribution and for patients in renal failure who have prolonged drug elimination. The purpose is to achieve therapeutic concentrations with the first dose so as not to prolong the attainment of adequate therapy. When loading doses are given, the plasma concentrations are higher versus when the loading dose is not given. However, no study has shown improved patient outcome as a result of given a loading dose. The rate at which a loading dose can be given depends on several factors: (1) drug toxicity (i.e., relationship between concentration and signs of toxicity), (2) site of drug action (i.e., in plasma or in tissue), (3) rate of equilibration of the drug into various body compartments, and (4) degree of plasma protein binding.

EXAMPLE 4. A 10-kg infant is to be started on amikacin for documented gram-negative sepsis and renal failure. The physician wishes to give a loading dose for the first dose and then measure plasma concentrations at 1 and 8 hours after the dose to determine the elimination rate constant. The physician wishes to obtain a plasma concentration of 20 mg/L with the loading dose, and the population volume of distribution for this child is 0.4 L/kg. What is the estimated loading dose? (Answer: Using Equation 9, where C = 20 mg/L and Vd = 0.4 L/kg × 10 kg, the loading dose would be 80 mg of amikacin.)

Mean Steady-State Concentration

The concept of an average steady-state concentration particularly may be useful when dealing with a drug with a long half-life. In such a case, maximum and minimum (or peak and trough) blood concentrations do not vary widely from one another. The mean steady state concentration ($\overline{C}ss$) may be described conveniently by the following relationship:

$$\overline{C}ss = \frac{F \times D}{Vd \times k_e \times \tau} \qquad (10)$$

where F signifies the bioavailability factor (equals 1 with an intravenously administered drug), D is dose, τ is dosage interval, and other terms are as defined previously.

Constant-Infusion Dosing

Calculations involving drugs given by constant infusion particularly are simple. This especially is true when one can assume that the elimination rate constant and volume of distribution are not changing (as with first-order elimination). Prior to reaching steady state, serum concentrations with a constant infusion at any point in time after starting the infusion are described as follows:

$$C_t = \frac{k_0}{Vd \times k_e}(1 - e^{-k_e t}) \qquad (11)$$

where t is the time since starting the infusion and all other terms are as defined previously. Once steady state is achieved, this relationship simplifies to:

$$C = \frac{k_0}{Vd \times k_e} \qquad (12)$$

Note that, at steady state, the concentration and infusion rate are directly proportional and that if the volume of distribution and elimination rate constant are constant, any change in the infusion rate will produce a proportional change in concentration.

If a bolus is given at the time the infusion is started, it will contribute to the time to achieve steady state. This is because the drug from the bolus is being cleared from the body at the same rate the drug from the infusion is accumulating in the body. In one half-life, 50 per cent of the bolus will have been eliminated, but 50 per cent of the infusion will have accumulated, theoretically resulting in 100 per cent of steady state being achieved. The contribution of both the bolus and the infusion can be calculated at each time point to determine that steady state has indeed been achieved. This underscores the potential importance of giving a bolus of drug not only when starting infusions but also when adjusting infusion rates, because it again will take about five half-lives to achieve steady state with infusion rate changes.

Zero-Order Pharmacokinetics

As noted, most drugs exhibit first-order or linear elimination pharmacokinetics. First-order elimination occurs when the amount of drug eliminated from the body is directly proportional (linear) to the amount of drug in the body or dose. In other words, changing the dose does not change the half-life, and thus the fraction of a drug in the body eliminated over a given time remains constant. This concept is different from zero-order elimination, in which the amount of drug eliminated per unit of time is constant, regardless of the amount of drug in the body. This suggests an upper limit to the rate at which a zero-order drug can be eliminated. This type of drug elimination is founded in the capacity of the enzyme system responsible for drug metabolism. Once the enzyme system is saturated (i.e., operating at full capacity), the maximum amount of drug that can be eliminated per unit of time is reached. Once this occurs, a small increase in dose can result in a large increase in plasma concentration. Because virtually all drug biotransformation, renal tubular secretion, and certain biliary secretion processes involve enzyme or carrier systems, these systems are capable of being saturated if enough drug is administered, resulting in zero-order kinetics.

In terms of pharmacokinetic calculations, accounting for zero-order pharmacokinetics is more complex. The mathematical relationship describing the elimination rate of a drug undergoing zero-order elimination is as follows:

$$k_e = \frac{V_{max} \times C}{K_{max} \times C} \qquad (13)$$

where V_{max} is the maximum rate of the elimination process, C is drug concentration, and K_{max} is the drug concentration when the rate of elimination is one-half of its maximum. One would need to determine the patient's maximum rate of the elimination process and drug concentration when the rate of elimination is one-half of its maximum to determine the elimination rate constant at any observed drug concentration in order to make dosage calculations. This often requires the determination of steady-state concentrations at a fixed time relative to dose at two different dosages. Thus, many clinicians can make small dosage adjustments of applicable drugs (e.g., phenytoin, aspirin) and perform frequent blood concentration monitoring rather than attempt mathematically to derive dosage changes. Fortunately, almost all anti-infective agents are eliminated according to first-order pharmacokinetics.

PEDIATRIC PHARMACOKINETIC DIFFERENCES

Pharmacokinetics in children often varies from that in adults. The underlying physiologic differences accounting for the different pharmacokinetics are most pronounced in newborns. It is beyond the scope of this chapter to provide a detailed discussion, but basic differences merit review. The reader is referred to more complete discussions of this issue elsewhere.[7, 8]

The pharmacokinetic parameters absorption, distribution, metabolism, and excretion may be different in infants and children than in adults. Gastrointestinal absorption of drugs may vary due to differences in gastric pH, gastric emptying time, intestinal transit time, digestive enzyme activity, and specialized intestinal transport. Percutaneous absorption of drugs may be greater in infants due to the higher surface area to body weight ratio and the decreased thickness of the stratum corneum. Intramuscular absorption of drugs also may vary in neonates. Drug distribution should be expected to vary, especially in the newborn, due to differences in relative body composition, with a much higher percentage of body weight being made up of water. Tissue binding may vary because the tissue mass of various organs changes with age. Protein binding often is less in neonates because of lower amounts of alpha$_1$ acid glycoprotein and potential hypoproteinemia. Metabolism and excretion take place at lesser rates in the newborn. Phase I and phase II metabolic reactions are decreased in capacity due to lower concentrations of relevant enzymes. Both glomerular filtration and tubular secretion of drugs by the kidney occur at lower rates. Thus, age-dependent alterations in drug pharmacokinetics and ultimately pharmacodynamics are observed commonly. If these differences are not appreciated, needless drug toxicity or ineffective therapy may result.

PRINCIPLES OF BLOOD SAMPLING

In order to obtain useful drug concentrations, a plan for plasma sampling must consider the route of administration, dosage form, dosing schedule, and pharmacokinetic variables of the drug. Proper interpretation of the drug concentrations can be made only if the dose, dosage form, administration times, and sampling time are documented accurately. Without this correct information, the drug concentrations obtained can be useless or even dangerously misleading. It also is imperative that blood samples be handled appropriately prior to analysis. For example, the in vitro inactivation of aminoglycosides by extended-spectrum penicillins (e.g., ticarcillin) is a well-known phenomenon.[9]

The timing of the sample must be as close to steady state as possible to access the efficacy of the current dosage regimen. Knowing that it takes four half-lives to reach 93 per cent of steady state and that the usually defined therapeutic ranges are based on steady state concentrations provides the rationale for waiting until three to five half-lives have elapsed after starting drug therapy (or changing dose) before determining drug concentrations. This is not a hard-and-fast rule, however, and it may be appropriate to determine concentrations prior to achieving steady-state conditions, for example, in cases of possible drug toxicity. A patient's elimination rate constant and volume of distribution can be calculated from concentrations determined even after the first dose, and, using the first-order equations presented earlier, one can predict the eventual concentrations that will be achieved at steady state. The important assumption used here is that the drug exhibits first-order elimination and a one-compartment model.

When drawing blood for pharmacokinetic purposes, the two plasma samples should be drawn at least 1.5 half-lives apart to ensure an accurate estimate of half-life for the patient. Furthermore, it is critical that the first sample be obtained after distribution is complete. It is commonplace in clinical practice to obtain blood for determination of trough concentrations prior to a dose and blood for determination of peak concentrations after that same dose. This is acceptable once steady-state conditions have been achieved because, under those conditions, all peaks are the same and the same is true for troughs. However, it is important to recognize that the other assumption being made is that the dosing interval always is the same (an unlikely scenario in most hospitals). Although small variations in dosage interval would not be expected to produce large errors in such calculations, large variations would.

The timing of the sample also must take into consideration the time of the dose, the route of administration, and the nature of the desired drug concentration (maximum, mean, or minimum). Enough time must be allowed for a drug to distribute from the plasma compartment to its site of action, which may be in the tissues of a specific organ. Again, recommended drug concentrations quoted in the literature are those observed after distribution (if applicable) is complete. If a drug concentration is obtained prior to completion of this distribution phase, it may be significantly higher than expected and an incorrect adjustment in dosage might be made. For most intravenously administered drugs, a sample taken at least 1 hour after the infusion is complete will avoid the initial distribution phase. For most drugs administered orally, the distribution phase will be shorter than the absorption phase, so that blood sampling may be done at any time after absorption is complete, usually 1 to 2 hours. It also is important to be cognizant of the definitions used in the literature or by clinicians for desired concentrations. For example, conventional wisdom for therapeutic aminoglycoside concentrations (gentamicin or tobramycin) would suggest a "peak" of 5 to 10 μg/mL with conventional every-8-hour dosing. However, a review of the underlying literature reveals that "peak," in this case, refers to the plasma concentration observed 1 hour after the completion of a half-hour dosage infusion. This obviously is not the highest concentration that will occur in such a patient. More importantly, it is not the same as the maximum concentration occurring immediately at the end of dosage infusion, as described in Equation 8a. One must be very careful, therefore, in defining terms and conditions being used in pharmacokinetic calculations and decision making.

Care must be taken not to obtain the blood sample for determination of drug concentration from the same intravenous catheter through which the drug is administered. Even if the catheter is "flushed," enough drug still may be present to contaminate the sample, causing a falsely elevated plasma concentration measurement. However, because limited venous access is a common problem in pediatric patients, one often has to resort to flushing a common catheter. In such cases, the line should be irrigated with a volume at least equal to the capacity of the intravenous extension tubing and catheter.

INTERPRETATION OF PLASMA DRUG CONCENTRATIONS

To interpret plasma drug concentrations, one must take into account all available clinical information. Therapeutic ranges have been established for many drugs, but these are average values to guide dosing and may not apply to all patient situations. Some examples of commonly used anti-infective therapeutic ranges are presented in Table 230–1. Again, the reader must be aware that even though the ranges are presented in terms of "peaks" and "troughs," these values should not be confused with the maximum and minimum concentrations that can be derived mathematically or perhaps measured in the patient's blood (see Equations 8a and 8b). For example, the highest-occurring blood concentration for an intravenously administered drug does not occur

TABLE 230–1. Therapeutic Drug Monitoring Guidelines for Anti-infective Agents

Drug	Optimal Sampling Times at Steady State	Optimal Plasma Concentration* Range (μg/mL)
Amikacin	Peak: 30 minutes after the end of a 30-minute infusion Trough: Immediately prior to the next maintenance dose	Peak: 20–30 Trough: <10
Chloramphenicol	Peak: 2 hours after the end of a 30-minute infusion or 2 hours after an oral dose Trough: Immediately prior to the next maintenance dose	Peak: 10–25 Trough: 5–15
Flucytosine	Peak: 2 hours after a dose Trough: Immediately prior to the next maintenance dose	Peak: <100 Trough: >25
Ganciclovir†	Peak: 1 hour after the end of a 1-hour infusion or 1 hour after an oral dose Trough: Immediately prior to the next maintenance dose	Peak: 4.7–10 Trough: 0.2–1
Gentamicin *(not for once-daily dosing)*	Peak: 30 minutes after the end of a 30-minute infusion Trough: Immediately prior to the next maintenance dose	Peak: 5–12 Trough: <2
Tobramycin *(not for once-daily dosing)*	Peak: 30 minutes after the end of a 30-minute infusion Trough: Immediately prior to the next maintenance dose	Peak: 5–12 Trough: <2
Vancomycin	Peak: 1 hour after the end of a 1-hour infusion or 30 minutes after the end of a 2-hour infusion Trough: Immediately prior to the next maintenance dose	Peak: 25–40 Trough: <10

*"Peaks" presented are not true maximum concentrations.
†Limited data in children. No data on oral dosing in children.

half an hour after completion of the infusion (when blood for "peaks" often are drawn) but, instead, immediately after completion of the infusion. Therefore, it sometimes is necessary to extrapolate, using Equation 6, to determine a concentration at some time other than when patient values were measured.

Many factors affect a patient's response to a given concentration of drug at its site of action. Some patients with a seemingly "subtherapeutic" or "toxic" drug concentration may experience an adequate therapeutic effect or be free of significant toxicity, respectively. Other patients may develop tolerance to a drug after prolonged administration and will require maintenance at a concentration higher than the normal therapeutic limit. Therapeutic ranges of plasma drug concentrations may need to be redefined if synergistic or antagonistic drugs are administered at the same time. Changes in drug protein binding or the existence of pharmacologically active metabolites also must be considered in any interpretation of plasma drug concentrations. It can not be overemphasized that recommended therapeutic ranges of drugs are only guidelines for dosing. Patient condition and clinical response also must be considered in the evaluation and management of each patient's pharmacotherapy.

Unexpectedly high or low drug concentrations observed in some patients can be caused by several physiologic factors or by system errors. In the case of the latter, for example, a "high" concentration may be the result of failing to wait for distribution to be complete prior to sampling. In addition, one always must consider that an inappropriate dosage might have been given due to an incorrect drug order, misinterpretation of an order, or an error in administration. Malabsorption of an orally administered drug in a patient with decreased gastrointestinal motility due to surgery, concomitant drug therapy, or disease can result in reduced concentrations. Changes in bioavailability can occur when drug formulations are changed, yielding unexpected changes in plasma drug concentrations.

When many drugs are being administered concurrently to the critically ill patient, the possibility of drug-drug interactions always must be considered. The concentration of one or both of the drugs in question can be affected, and the change in concentration can be either an increase or a decrease. Altered plasma drug concentrations can be a result of modification of intestinal absorption of one drug by another, competition for plasma protein binding sites, altered peripheral compartments such as that observed with ascites, or changes in hepatic metabolism and/or renal excretion of one or both of the drugs. Drugs given intravenously also may be incompatible when mixed together (chemically inactivating one or both), with or without an obvious physical reaction taking place.

Presence of renal or hepatic disease can decrease the elimination or metabolism of many drugs to varying degrees. Ignoring changes in these organ functions can lead to accumulation of drug with potentially fatal results. If a critically ill patient is known to have renal or hepatic insufficiency, a sampling strategy along with a plan for interpretation of the plasma concentrations is needed prior to giving the drug in order to prevent overdosing and maximize drug therapy.

The effects of altered protein binding must be considered in the interpretation of concentrations of any drugs that demonstrate significant binding. In disease states with decreased plasma protein or decreased binding of drugs to plasma, drugs that usually are highly protein-bound (greater than 90 per cent) have a larger per cent of unbound drug in the plasma. As a result, a greater pharmacologic effect can be expected for a given concentration of total drug in the plasma (which more commonly is measured and reported by laboratories), and a lower total drug concentration than normal will be needed to obtain the desired therapeutic effect without significant toxicity.

Once plasma drug concentrations have been obtained and interpreted, a decision must be made as to whether the dose and dosing interval are appropriate. If a change in dosage is needed, it often can be accomplished by making a change in the maintenance dose proportional to the change in steady-state plasma concentration desired, if the drug is eliminated by first-order pharmacokinetics. For example, if a "peak" plasma concentration of gentamicin is 4.5 μg/mL in a patient receiving 40 mg intravenously every 8 hours, an initial dose increase of 25 per cent (to 50 mg intravenously every 8 hours) would raise the plasma concentration to approximately 5.6 μg/mL. In critical situations in which a more exact calculation of dosage is needed, a set of plasma drug concentrations can be used to determine individual pharmacokinetic parameters (volume of distribution and elimination rate constant) that then can be used for a more precise estimate of that patient's drug dosing regimen using the methods described earlier. Patients with an abnormally large volume of distribution from ascites or another "third space" often will require larger doses to achieve optimal plasma concentrations. At the same time, such patients may not require dosing as frequently as in other children due to concomitant renal or hepatic impairment. Taking the time to calculate these simple pharmacokinetic parameters not only will assist in optimizing therapy in a timely manner, but also will minimize the number of plasma samples required and therefore reduce the overall cost of therapy.

BASIC PHARMACODYNAMICS

Although pharmacokinetics describes the time course of drug concentrations in relation to dose/dosage regimen, pharmacodynamics describes the concentration-effect relationship, which is time-independent. A combination of the two allows a description of drug effect over time. Such knowledge should be the basis for the design of drug dosing regimens in humans. These relationships have been explored for antibiotics, and it is known that β-lactam antibiotics are time-dependent in their antibacterial activity and drugs that inhibit protein or nucleic acid synthesis (e.g., aminoglycosides) are concentration-dependent in their antibacterial action.[10, 11] These properties suggest that maintaining β-lactam concentrations at or above the minimum inhibitory concentration (MIC) of the infecting organism should optimize antibacterial effect. At the same time, it would appear that maximizing the peak concentration of an aminoglycoside or a fluoroquinolone (or the area under the plasma concentration versus time curve) would maximize its antibacterial effect. Peak concentrations also may be important in preventing the emergence of resistance through selection of resistant mutants in the infecting bacterial population. Elucidation of these principles has led to the current interest and growing practices of administering β-lactams by constant infusion and administering aminoglycosides once daily.[12–15] Although such properties appear to be consistent across a given class of antibiotics, relevant differences within a class are more elusive. Another pharmacodynamic phenomenon that merits discussion is the post-antibiotic effect. This effect can be considered the continued suppression of bacterial growth after antibiotic concentrations have fallen below the MIC for the organism.[16] It typically is seen, in vitro, with inhibitors of protein synthesis (e.g., aminoglycosides) but not with β-lactams.

To date, most published pharmacodynamic-pharmacokinetic information has been generated in in vitro pharmacodynamic models or in animals. A neutropenic murine thigh or lung infection model has been utilized extensively, and resultant publications represent what are considered classic works in this area.[17–19] In the neutropenic murine infection model, antibiotic effect has been reflected as the change in numbers of infecting bacteria in infected tissue (reduction in colony-forming units with antibiotic treatment) or as protective dose (survival). Optimal dosage regimen principles have been characterized by fitting such data to the sigmoidal dose-effect (Emax) mathematical model.[11] Furthermore, major dosage properties or pharmacokinetic-pharmacodynamic characteristics (e.g., time the antibiotic concentration exceeds the MIC of the infecting organism) that relate to maximum antibacterial action have been identified by correlating them to effect through univariate and step-wise multilinear regression analysis. These studies clearly have demonstrated the importance of time above the MIC for β-lactams and of peak MIC (or AUC MIC) for aminoglycosides. The validity (to human infection) of such work has been demonstrated, to a limited extent, in clinical studies involving β-lactams,[18–20] aminoglycosides,[2–22] and quinolones.[23]

It would seem intuitive that one should try to take advantage of these pharmacodynamic phenomena or properties in the design of therapeutic dosage regimens in patients. Use of the pharmacokinetic principles reviewed earlier in this chapter can optimize such parameters as peak concentration MIC, AUC MIC, and/or time above MIC. The existence of a post-antibiotic effect also could be factored into the design of a dosage regimen. Although addressing these considerations in clinical practice may appear to be in its infancy, the wide acceptance of once-daily dosing of aminoglycosides in adult populations may be viewed as a common application taking advantage of both the importance of peak MIC and the potential for postantibiotic effect.

References

1. Relling, M. V.: Polymorphic drug metabolism. Clin. Pharmacol. *8*:852–863, 1989.
2. Gibaldi, M.: Pharmacogenetics. Ann. Pharmacother. *26*:121–126, 255–261, 1992.
3. Evans, W. E., Schentag, J. J., and Jusko, W. J. (eds.): Applied Pharmacokinetics. Principles of Therapeutic Drug Monitoring. 3rd ed. Vancouver, WA, Applied Therapeutics, 1992.
4. Rowland, M., and Tozer, T. N.: Clinical pharmacokinetics: Concepts and applications. 3rd ed. Media, PA, Williams & Wilkins, 1995.
5. DiPiro, J. T., Blouin, R. A., Pruemer, J. M., et al.: Concepts in Clinical Pharmacokinetics: A Self-Instructional Course. Bethesda, MD, American Society of Hospital Pharmacists, 1988.
6. Murphy, J. E. (ed.): Clinical Pharmacokinetics Pocket Reference. Bethesda, MD, American Society of Hospital Pharmacists, 1993.
7. Routledge, P. A.: Pharmacokinetics in children. J. Antimicrob. Chemother. *34*(Suppl. A):19–24, 1994.
8. Reed, M. D., and Blumer, J. L.: Therapeutic drug monitoring in the pediatric intensive care unit. Pediatr. Clin. North Am. *42*:1227–1243, 1994.
9. Riff, L. J., and Thomason, J. L.: Comparative aminoglycoside inactivation by β-lactam antibiotics: Effect of a cephalosporin and six penicillins on five aminoglycosides. J. Antibiot. *35*:850, 1982.
10. Vogelman, B., Gudmundsson, S., Leggett, J., et al.: Correlation of antimicrobial pharmacokinetic parameters with therapeutic efficacy in an animal model. J. Infect. Dis. *158*:831–847, 1988.
11. Leggett, J. E., Fantin, B., Ebert, S., et al.: Comparative antibiotic dose-effect relations at several dosing intervals in murine pneumonitis and thigh-infection models. J. Infect. Dis. *159*:281–292, 1989.
12. Craig, W. A., and Ebert, S. C.: Continuous infusion of β-lactam antibiotics. Antimicrob. Agents Chemother. *36*:2577–2583, 1992.
13. Gilbert, D. N.: Once-daily aminoglycoside therapy. Antimicrob. Agents Chemother. *35*:399–405, 1991.
14. Nicolau, D. P., Freeman, C. D., Belliveau, P. P., et al.: Experience with a once-daily aminoglycoside program administered to 2,184 adult patients. Antimicrob. Agents Chemother. *39*:650–655, 1995.
15. Munckhof, W. J., Grayson, M. L., and Turnidge, J. D.: A meta-analysis of studies on the safety and efficacy of aminoglycosides given either once daily or as divided doses. J. Antimicrob. Chemother. *37*:645–663, 1996.
16. Vogelman, B., and Craig, W. A.: Postantibiotic effects. J. Antimicrob. Chemother. *15*(Suppl. A):37–46, 1985.
17. Leggett, J. E., Ebert, S., Fantin, B., et al.: Comparative dose-effect relations at several dosing intervals for beta-lactam, aminoglycoside and quinolone antibiotics against gram-negative bacilli in murine thigh-infection and pneumonitis models. Scand. J. Infect. Dis. *74*:179–184, 1991.

18. Schentag, J. J, Reitberg, R. P, and Cumbo, T. J.: Cefmenoxime efficacy, safety, and pharmacokinetics in critical care patients with nosocomial pneumonia. Am. J. Med. 77(Suppl. 6A):34–42, 1984.
19. Bodey, G. P., Ketchel, S. J., and Rodriquez, V.: A randomized study of carbenicillin plus cefamandole or tobramycin in the treatment of febrile episodes in cancer patients. Am. J. Med. 67:608–616, 1979.
20. Drusano, G. L.: Role of pharmacokinetics in the outcome of infections. Antimicrob. Agents Chemother. 32:289–297, 1988.
21. Noone, P. T., Parsons, M. C., Pattison, J. R., et al.: Experience in monitoring gentamicin therapy during treatment of serious gram-negative sepsis. Br. Med. J. 1:477–481, 1974.
22. Moore, R. D., Lietman, P. S., and Smith, C. R.: Clinical response to aminoglycoside therapy: Importance of the ratio of peak concentration to minimal inhibitory concentration. J. Infect. Dis. 155:93–99, 1987.
23. Peloquin, C. A., Cumbo, T. J., Nix, D. E., et al.: Intravenous ciprofloxacin in patients with nosocomial lower respiratory tract infections: Impact of plasma concentrations, organism MIC, and clinical condition on bacterial eradication. Arch. Intern. Med. 149:2269–2273, 1989.

231

ANTIBACTERIAL THERAPEUTIC AGENTS

Sheila M. Hickey and George H. McCracken, Jr.

This review of the use of antimicrobial agents is divided into two sections: (1) the clinical pharmacology of currently available drugs and (2) the various aspects of administration of antimicrobial agents to infants and children. The second section includes dosage schedules and routes, prophylactic uses of antimicrobial agents, considerations in writing orders and prescriptions, and other aspects of administration. Drugs of value in treatment of disease caused by viruses, fungi, mycobacteria, and parasites are discussed in other chapters dealing with these pathogens. Only antimicrobial agents approved for use in infants and children by the Food and Drug Administration (FDA) are discussed.

CLINICAL PHARMACOLOGY

The antimicrobial agents of value in treatment of infectious diseases in infants and children may be classified into five groups:

1. The β-lactams, including the penicillins, the cephalosporins, and the carbacephems
2. The glycopeptides (i.e., vancomycin)
3. The aminoglycosides
4. The macrolides, including erythromycin, clarithromycin, and azithromycin
5. Miscellaneous antibacterial agents, including the sulfonamides, chloramphenicol, clindamycin, and the tetracyclines

The following properties that govern the use of each group of drugs in infants and children are considered: mechanism of action, mechanisms of resistance, in vitro efficacy, therapeutic uses, available preparations, and side effects and toxicity.

β-Lactams

Biochemical Structure

The β-lactams are a large group of compounds that have in common a four-membered β-lactam ring. The subclasses of β-lactams differ from one another with regard to their side chains and the presence of other ring structures: the penicillins contain a five-membered thiazolidine α-ring fused to the β-lactam ring,[90] the cephalosporins have a six-membered dihydrothiazine instead of the five-membered thiazolidine ring, and the carbacephems have a methylene group replacing the sulfur atom in the dihydrothiazine ring of the cephalosporin nucleus. The β-lactam ring is essential for antibacterial activity, whereas the side chains influence the pharmacologic properties of the β-lactam and the spectrum of antibacterial activity.

Mechanism of Action

The exact mechanism of action of the β-lactams remains elusive. Previously, it was thought that binding of the β-lactam to a bacterial cell membrane–associated enzyme (transpeptidase) blocked the terminal step in synthesis of the peptidoglycan layer of the bacterial cell wall. Cell death would ensue because the weakened cell wall could not withstand the osmotic and mechanical pressure resulting from a growing bacterium.[193, 195] Recent evidence suggests that it is a more complex process involving inhibition of cell wall synthesis and activation of endogenous autolytic systems.[194, 196] The known targets of β-lactams are enzymes, called penicillin-binding proteins (PBPs), that are vital for cell division, cell shape, and structural integrity. Because the specific PBPs within each bacterial species and the affinity of each β-lactam antibiotic for a particular PBP differ, some β-lactams have better activity than others against a particular bacteria. The various β-lactam antibiotics can have different morphologic effects on the same bacterial species; this is thought to be related to specific functions of the PBP to which the β-lactam binds.[180] Some bacteria have a deficiency in the system of autolytic enzymes resulting in inhibition but not killing of the bacteria by a β-lactam that otherwise would be bactericidal. This phenomenon is called tolerance and is demonstrated in vitro by a minimum inhibitory concentration (MIC) in the susceptible range and a minimum bacterial concentration (MBC)/MIC ratio of ≥ 32.[74]

β-Lactam antibiotics are bactericidal against most susceptible bacteria. The nature of bactericidal activity has been described as concentration-independent and time-dependent, compared with the concentration-dependent bactericidal activity of aminoglycosides.[50, 100, 201] Bactericidal activity is believed to be optimal when the concentration of β-lactam antibiotic at the site of infection is 4 to 10 times greater than that of the MIC (MBC) of the infecting organism. The rapidity and the extent of killing are not increased when concentrations exceed that ratio. A more important determinant of bactericidal activity for β-lactams is the length of time during the dosing interval that the concentration of antibiotic exceeds the MIC or MBC for the infecting organism.

Mechanisms of Resistance

Bacteria can acquire resistance to an antibiotic by at least three mechanisms: (1) alteration in the antimicrobial target, (2) decreased uptake of the antibiotic, and (3) production of an enzyme that inactivates the antibiotic.[138] With respect to β-lactam antibiotics, this involves alterations in the PBPs leading to a decreased affinity for the β-lactam, decreased permeability of the bacterial cell wall resulting in diminished amounts of the β-lactam reaching the PBPs, or production of β-lactamases that hydrolyze the β-lactam ring. Hydrolysis of the β-lactam is the mechanism that is most significant clinically. Gram-positive bacteria excrete their β-lactamases outside the cell wall, whereas the β-lactamases of gram-negative bacteria remain in the periplasmic space. The spectrum of BLA activity involves narrow-spectrum penicillinases that preferentially hydrolyze penicillins; broad-spectrum β-lactamases that hydrolyze penicillins and cephalosporins equally well; cephalosporinases that preferentially hydrolyze cephalosporins and are resistant to inhibition by clavulanic acid; extended-spectrum β-lactamases that hydrolyze first-, second-, and third-generation cephalosporins but are susceptible to inhibition by clavulanic acid; and carbapenemases that inactivate all β-lactams, including imipenem-cilastatin.[27]

Penicillins

Although first discovered by Fleming in the late 1920s, penicillin G was not available for general use in the United States for another 20 years. Since that time, numerous semisynthetic penicillins have been developed. The penicillins can be classified into four groups based on their antimicrobial activity, with some overlap (Table 231–1). The spectrum of activity among the compounds within each group usually is similar to the major differences related to pharmacologic properties (Table 231–2).

Specific Agents

PENICILLIN G AND PENICILLIN V. Despite the more than 50 years that penicillin G has been in use, some bacteria continue to be exquisitely susceptible. Resistant strains of *Streptococcus pyogenes* (group A *Streptococcus*) and *Streptococcus agalactiae* (group B *Streptococcus*) have not emerged. Penicillin G remains the drug of choice for treatment of disease caused by a wide variety of microorganisms (Table 231–3).

The mechanism by which most bacteria have acquired resistance to penicillin G is that of β-lactamase production; resistance caused by altered PBPs is less common. The great majority of strains of *Staphylococcus aureus* and *Staphylococcus epidermidis* produce penicillinase. *Neisseria gonorrhoeae* was thought to be uniformly susceptible to penicillin G, but some strains that produce a β-lactamase and are highly resistant to penicillin G have been identified, first in the Far East and later in military personnel and their contacts in the United States. Although there is geographic variation in the prevalence of penicillinase-producing strains of *Haemophilus influenzae,* recent surveillance studies estimate that approximately 30 per cent of type b and 15 per cent of nontypable strains are penicillin-resistant.[87] The majority of *Moraxella catarrhalis* isolates produce β-lactamase. Penicillinase or cephalosporinase production is the most common cause of β-lactam resistance in gram-negative anaerobes, including *Bacteroides* species.[143] Although uncommon, strains of *Neisseria meningitidis* resistant to penicillin because of altered PBPs and because of β-lactamase production have been reported from Spain and from South Africa and Britain, respectively.

Of most recent concern are reports of disease caused by strains of *Streptococcus pneumoniae* resistant to penicillin G resulting from altered PBPs.[23] The first documented clinical case of infection caused by penicillin-resistant pneumococcus was reported in 1967 from Australia. Recently, resistant pneumococcal infections have been seen worldwide, with most cases occurring in Spain, South Africa, Hungary, and the Far

TABLE 231–1. Classification Scheme for Penicillins

Generic Name	Trade Name	Route
Natural penicillins		
Penicillin G	Many	PO, IM, IV
Penicillin V	Many	PO
Aminopenicillins		
Ampicillin	Many	PO, IM, IV
Amoxicillin	Many	PO
Amoxicillin/clavulanic acid	Augmentin	PO
Ampicillin/sulbactam*	Unasyn	IM, IV
Penicillinase-resistant penicillins		
Cloxacillin	Cloxapen, Tegopen	PO
Dicloxacillin	Dycill, Dynapen, Pathocil	PO
Methicillin	Celbenin, Staphcillin	IM, IV
Nafcillin	Nafcil, Nallpen, Unipen	IM, IV, PO
Oxacillin	Bactocill, Prostaphlin	IM, IV, PO
Extended-spectrum penicillins		
Carbenicillin	Geocillin	PO
Ticarcillin	Ticar	IM, IV
Ticarcillin/clavulanic acid*	Timentin	IV
Mezlocillin	Mezlin	IM, IV
Piperacillin*	Pipracil	IM, IV
Piperacillin/tazobactam*	Zosyn	IV

*Safety and efficacy have not been established for children younger than 12 years of age.
IM, intramuscularly; IV, intravenously; PO, orally.
Modified from *USP DI®, Volume I, Information for the Health Care Professional.* Copyright 1996, The USP Convention, Inc. Permission granted.

TABLE 231–2. Pharmacokinetics of Penicillins

Antibiotic	Oral Absorption (%)	Protein Binding (%)	Metabolized (%)	Urinary Recovery* (%)	Approximate Half-Life† (hours)
Natural penicillins					
Penicillin G	15–30	60	20	20/60–90	0.5–0.7
Penicillin V	60–73	80	55	20–40	0.5–1
Aminopenicillins					
Ampicillin	35–50	20	10	40–45/75–90	1–1.5
Amoxicillin	75–90	20	10	60–75	1
Penicillinase-resistant penicillins					
Cloxacillin	50	95	20	30–60	0.5–1
Dicloxacillin	37–50	95–98	10	50–70	0.5–1
Methicillin		40	10	60–80	0.3–1
Nafcillin	Erratic	90	60–70	11–30	0.5–1.5
Oxacillin	30–35	90–94	45	55–60	0.4–0.7
Extended-spectrum penicillins					
Carbenicillin indanyl	30	50	0–2	36	1.0–1.5
Ticarcillin		45–60	15	60–80	1.0–1.2
Mezlocillin		16–42	20–30	55–60	0.8–1.1
Piperacillin		16	20–30	60–80	0.6–1.2

*Urinary recovery after oral/parenteral administration.
†With normal renal function.
Modified from *USP DI®, Volume I, Information for the Health Care Professional.* Copyright 1996, The USP Convention, Inc. Permission granted.

East. In the United States, the percentage of pneumococci resistant to penicillin varies geographically and ranges from 4 to 48 per cent.[112] Many strains of penicillin-resistant pneumococci, especially those with an MIC greater than or equal to 2 μg/mL, also are resistant to other commonly used antibiotics, such as trimethoprim-sulfamethoxazole (TMP-SMX), erythromycin, chloramphenicol, clindamycin, and, occasionally, third-generation cephalosporins. Although there have been reports of patients developing penicillin-resistant pneumococcal meningitis while receiving vancomycin for pneumococcal sepsis,[33] no treatment failures have been documented when the appropriate dosage of vancomycin has been administered.

Several oral and parenteral forms of penicillin G are available. Choice of preparation for the patient is based on the pattern of antimicrobial activity, including the peak and duration of activity in serum and tissues, and factors that reflect the absorption, distribution, and excretion of the drug. These characteristics of the penicillins are as follows:

1. Aqueous (water-soluble) penicillin G produces high peak concentrations of antibacterial activity in serum within 30 minutes after intramuscular administration but is excreted rapidly; thus, the concentration in serum is low within 2 to 4 hours. If aqueous penicillin G is given by the intravenous route, the peak is higher and earlier and the duration of antibacterial activity in serum is shorter (approximately 2 hours). Aqueous penicillin G, given intramuscularly or intravenously, is used for severe disease, such as meningitis, pneumonia, and endocarditis. In such cases, the drug should be given at frequent intervals, usually every 4 hours, until the infection has been controlled.

2. Procaine penicillin G given intramuscularly produces lower concentrations of serum antibacterial activity (approximately 10 to 30 per cent of the peak concentration achieved by the same dosage of the aqueous form), but activity persists in serum for as long as 12 hours. Intramuscular administration of procaine penicillin G should be reserved for patients with mild to moderate disease who cannot tolerate oral preparations.

3. Benzathine penicillin G given intramuscularly is a repository preparation providing low concentrations of serum activity (approximately 1 to 2 per cent of the peak concentration achieved by the same dosage of the aqueous form). After administration of this drug, concentrations of penicillin activity are measurable in serum for 3 weeks or more and in urine for several months. Pain at the site of injection is the major deterrent to widespread use of this unique antibiotic. Combination of the benzathine and procaine salts (900,000 and 300,000 units, respectively) is less painful and is comparable in efficacy with benzathine alone (1,200,000 units) for treatment of streptococcal pharyngitis.[12] Benzathine penicillin G is appropriate only for highly sensitive organisms present in tissues that are well vascularized so that the drug can diffuse readily to the site of infection. Thus, benzathine penicillin G is suitable for treatment of children with group A

TABLE 231–3. Microorganisms for Which Penicillin G Is the Drug of Choice

- *Streptococcus* groups A, B, C, D, G; viridans group, anaerobic strains
- *Streptococcus pneumoniae**
- *Staphylococcus aureus*†
- *Neisseria meningitidis*
- *Neisseria gonorrhoeae*†
- *Treponema pallidum*
- *Leptospira* species
- *Bacillus anthracis*
- *Clostridium* species
- *Corynebacterium diphtheriae*
- *Pasteurella multocida*
- *Spirillum minus*
- *Streptobacillus moniliformis*
- *Actinomyces israelii*

*Only those without altered penicillin-binding proteins.
†Strains that do not produce β-lactamase.

streptococcal pharyngitis or impetigo and for prophylaxis of streptococcal infection in children who have had rheumatic carditis. Current recommendations of the Centers for Disease Control and Prevention (CDC)[31] for management of syphilis include use of benzathine penicillin G for primary, secondary, and early latent syphilis (< 1 year's duration). Benzathine penicillin G also is recommended for infants with suspected congenital syphilis who do not meet criteria for therapy with a 10-day course of aqueous or procaine penicillin G but whose follow-up cannot be ensured.

4. Oral preparations of buffered penicillin G and phenoxymethyl penicillin (penicillin V) are absorbed well from the gastrointestinal tract. The peak concentration of serum activity of penicillin V is approximately 40 per cent and that of buffered penicillin G approximately 20 per cent of the concentration achieved by the same dosage of aqueous penicillin G administered intramuscularly. Therefore, oral penicillins may be satisfactory for treatment of mild to moderately severe infections caused by susceptible organisms. Penicillin V and penicillin G have equivalent activity in vitro against gram-positive cocci, but penicillin V is less active than penicillin G against *N. meningitidis, N. gonorrhoeae,* and *H. influenzae.*[90]

All penicillins are excreted by both glomerular filtration and tubular secretion. The concomitant use of probenecid, a drug that blocks tubular secretion of organic acids, with a penicillin can produce higher peak and more sustained concentrations of antimicrobial activity. Dosages and dosing intervals may need adjustment when administering penicillins to persons with altered renal function.

PENICILLINASE-RESISTANT PENICILLINS. The semisynthetic penicillinase-resistant penicillins were developed in response to the emergence of penicillinase-producing staphylococci. The acyl side chain, by means of steric hindrance, prevents hydrolysis of the β-lactam ring by penicillinases.

Most strains of *S. aureus* produce penicillinase, regardless of whether the infection is nosocomial or community-acquired. Thus, the penicillinase-resistant penicillins are the drugs of choice for initial management of patients with suspected staphylococcal disease. With the exception of methicillin, these agents are active against streptococci and can be used for empiric treatment of infections commonly caused by both staphylococci and streptococci. Because these agents are less active than penicillin G against streptococci, however, penicillin G should be used instead of these agents if streptococci alone are isolated from culture. Penicillinase-resistant penicillins have no activity against gram-negative bacteria or enterococci.[110]

Methicillin was the first penicillinase-resistant penicillin to be introduced and is available in parenteral form only. Oxacillin and nafcillin are available in both parenteral and oral preparations and have greater in vitro activity against gram-positive cocci than does methicillin. Cloxacillin and dicloxacillin are available in oral forms only and are absorbed more efficiently from the gastrointestinal tract than are the other oral drugs. Differences among these five penicillins include routes of elimination, degree of binding to proteins and of degradation by β-lactamases, and in vitro susceptibility[135]; however, all are effective for treatment of staphylococcal disease, and clinical studies have shown them to be equivalent when used in appropriate dosage schedules.

Disease caused by methicillin-resistant staphylococci was reported shortly after introduction of the drug. Resistance is caused by alterations in the PBPs rather than by β-lactamase production.[32] The *mecA* gene, a transposon integrated into the chromosome, encodes for a new PBP (2a), which has a low affinity for β-lactams, resulting in resistance to all currently available β-lactam antibiotics, including penicillinase-resistance penicillins, cephalosporins, and carbapenems. Many of these methicillin-resistant strains also are resistant to other antimicrobial agents whose mechanism of action is unrelated to PBPs, including the macrolides and clindamycin, fusidic acid, some aminoglycosides, and sulfonamides. This resistance can be plasmid-mediated or chromosomal.[107]

Coagulase-negative staphylococci, including *S. epidermidis,* are residents of the normal microbial flora of the skin and are occasional contaminants of body fluid cultures. These organisms can be pathogens in certain settings, such as in neonates, or in infections of prosthetic devices, such as heart valves or cerebrospinal fluid shunts. Most strains of coagulase-negative staphylococci produce a penicillinase that inactivates penicillin G, penicillin V, and ampicillin, and many strains have an altered PBP (2a) leading to methicillin resistance. These methicillin-resistant, coagulase-negative staphylococci also frequently are resistant to cephalosporins, erythromycin, and clindamycin. Vancomycin is the drug of choice for disease known or suspected to be caused by methicillin-resistant *S. aureus* or *S. epidermidis.*

AMINOPENICILLINS. The aminopenicillins are semisynthetic β-lactam antibiotics formed by the addition of an amino group to benzylpenicillin. Amoxicillin differs from ampicillin by the presence of a hydroxyl group on the phenyl side chain. The aminopenicillins were the first penicillins that had activity against some gram-negative organisms, including *H. influenzae, Escherichia coli, Proteus mirabilis, Salmonella* species, and *Shigella* species, while retaining activity against penicillin-susceptible, gram-positive bacteria.[134]

Compared with penicillin G, aminopenicillins are significantly more active against *Listeria monocytogenes;* slightly more active against enterococci; equally active against *Actinomyces, N. meningitidis,* and clostridial and corynebacteria species; and slightly less active against group A streptococci, group B streptococci, and pneumococci. The aminopenicillins are the drugs of choice for treatment of infections caused by *L. monocytogenes* and enterococci. Other organisms susceptible in vitro to ampicillin and amoxicillin include non–penicillinase-producing strains of *H. influenzae, M. catarrhalis, N. gonorrhoeae, S. aureus, E. coli, Salmonella,* and *Shigella.* The in vitro spectrum of activity for amoxicillin and ampicillin is identical, except that amoxicillin is two times less active against *Shigella* and is two to four times more active against enterococci and *Salmonella* than is ampicillin.[134]

As seen with penicillin G, the primary means of acquired resistance to aminopenicillins is β-lactamase production. However, organisms that are resistant to penicillin G or to methicillin because of altered PBPs—*S. pneumoniae* and *S. aureus,* respectively—also are resistant to aminopenicillins.

The broad-spectrum activity of ampicillin and amoxicillin provides the basis for their use for acute infections of the respiratory tract, including otitis media and pneumonia; as a single agent for treatment of acute bacterial meningitis caused by susceptible bacteria (ampicillin only in the United States) and acute and chronic infections of the urinary tract; and for treatment of acute diarrheal disease (when the organisms are susceptible and when therapy is indicated for shigellosis or salmonellosis). By bacteriologic and clinical measures, amoxicillin is significantly less effective than is ampicillin for treatment of shigellosis.[132]

Both drugs are available for oral administration; ampicillin alone is available in a parenteral form. Amoxicillin provides higher and more prolonged serum concentrations than those achieved with equivalent dosages of ampicillin; thus, amoxicillin can be given in lower dosage and three times a day rather than four times as required for ampicillin. An additional advantage of amoxicillin is that absorption is not altered when the antibiotic is administered with food, whereas absorption of ampicillin is decreased significantly when it is given with food. Ampicillin is associated more frequently with diarrhea than is amoxicillin.

EXTENDED-SPECTRUM PENICILLINS. These are semisynthetic derivatives of ampicillin that, because of higher affinity for the PBPs and because of greater penetration through the gram-negative outer membrane, have better activity against gram-negative organisms. Carbenicillin and ticarcillin, the carboxypenicillins, have a carboxyl group replacing the amino group side chain of ampicillin, whereas the acylureidopenicillins have a ureido (urea) side chain (mezlocillin) or ureido and piperazine side chains (piperacillin). Their pharmacologic properties are similar, including the susceptibility to hydrolysis by staphylococcal penicillinases and, to a lesser extent, the β-lactamases of gram-negative bacteria. They differ somewhat in their toxicities and their spectrum of activity.

The activity of carbenicillin is equivalent to or slightly less active than that of ampicillin against *N. gonorrhoeae, N. meningitidis, H. influenzae, E. coli, P. mirabilis, Salmonella* species, and *Shigella* species. It is less active than ampicillin against group A streptococci, pneumococci, and enterococci.[136] Its activity is variable against many *Bacteroides fragilis, Enterobacter,* and *Serratia* organisms, and it is not active against *Klebsiella.* Synergistic activity has been demonstrated when combined with an aminoglycoside; however, caution must be exercised when administering both agents because carbenicillin and other penicillins can inactivate aminoglycosides.

The activity of ticarcillin is similar to that of carbenicillin but is greater against some strains of *P. aeruginosa* and lesser against gram-positive cocci. Because of its increased activity, smaller doses of ticarcillin may be used than with carbenicillin for treatment of disease caused by gram-negative organisms.

Piperacillin and mezlocillin are parenteral penicillins with a spectrum of activity similar to ticarcillin but greater activity in vitro against some gram-negative bacilli and anaerobic bacteria.[49] Piperacillin is more active than is carbenicillin, ticarcillin, or mezlocillin against *P. aeruginosa.* Piperacillin and mezlocillin are more active in vitro than are carbenicillin or ticarcillin against susceptible strains of *E. coli, Klebsiella, Enterobacter,* and *Serratia.*[200] Combination therapy with an aminoglycoside results in synergy against some gram-negative enteric bacilli.[63]

The intravenous preparation of carbenicillin no longer is marketed in the United States; however, an oral preparation, indanyl carbenicillin, is available but seldom used. The oral carbenicillin provides low serum concentrations but sufficient urinary concentrations for treatment of some urinary tract infections caused by bacteria that are resistant to other available oral drugs. The low serum concentrations preclude the use of oral carbenicillin for systemic infection. The other extended-spectrum penicillins are available in parenteral formulations only.

Ticarcillin, a disodium salt, contains 5.2 mEq (120 mg) of sodium per gram. The acylureidopenicillins are monosodium salts and have a lower sodium content than do the carboxypenicillins. The amount of sodium administered may be of concern in treatment of certain patients with renal or cardiac disease. Hypokalemia with metabolic alkalosis occasionally occurs with administration of extended-spectrum penicillins, especially the carboxypenicillins. The penicillin acts as a nonreabsorbable anion in the distal renal tubules, affecting normal hydrogen exchange and secondarily resulting in potassium loss.[28] These extended-spectrum penicillins can bind to platelet adenosine diphosphate receptors, resulting in abnormal platelet aggregation and prolonged bleeding times.[24] This dose-related phenomenon occurs more frequently with administration of ticarcillin than of the acylureidopenicillins. The effects on platelet function may be a consideration when choosing empiric therapy for the thrombocytopenic patient with suspected gram-negative infection.

Piperacillin, mezlocillin, and ticarcillin are effective for treatment of infections caused by susceptible strains of *Klebsiella, Enterobacter, Citrobacter, Serratia,* indole-positive *Proteus, Providencia,* and *Pseudomonas aeruginosa.* Ticarcillin can be used for infections caused by susceptible strains of *Acinetobacter,* and mezlocillin and piperacillin can be used for some infections caused by *B. fragilis.*

These penicillins (usually combined with an aminoglycoside) have been used in adults for treatment of intra-abdominal, gynecologic, and urinary tract infections and sepsis in patients with altered host defenses. Patients with susceptible organisms causing urinary tract infections or sepsis had a better clinical response to ticarcillin than those with lower respiratory tract infections caused by ticarcillin-susceptible bacteria.[146] Because of limited clinical experience in infants and children, piperacillin has not been approved for use in patients younger than 12 years of age.

β-LACTAM/β-LACTAMASE INHIBITOR COMBINATIONS. β-lactamase inhibitors are compounds that have weak antibacterial activity but that can bind irreversibly to many β-lactamases, rendering them inactive.[163] The inhibitors currently in use are clavulanic acid, sulbactam (penicillanic acid sulfone), and tazobactam, the latter of which are halogenated penicillanic acid derivatives. Although these β-lactamase inhibitors are capable of inactivating many β-lactamases, they are not effective against Bush group 1–inducible chromosomal β-lactamases and some plasmid-mediated enzymes, and clavulanate actually can induce group 1 enzymes.[205] These inhibitors have been formulated in a fixed ratio with a β-lactam antibiotic. The spectrum of activity of each combination primarily is determined by the spectrum of activity of the β-lactam. However, many determinants of the inhibitor influence its activity, including its affinity for the β-lactamase and its ability to traverse the gram-negative cell wall to bind to periplasmic β-lactamases.[102]

Amoxicillin–Clavulanic Acid. Amoxicillin combined with potassium clavulanate (Augmentin) was introduced in 1984 for oral administration. The pharmacokinetics of the two drugs is similar; both are absorbed rapidly and are not affected when taken with meals. Gastrointestinal side effects, including nausea, vomiting, and diarrhea, are more common with administration of Augmentin than with amoxicillin alone.[182]

The combination drug is equivalent to amoxicillin alone in activity against amoxicillin-susceptible organisms. The addition of clavulanic acid extends the in vitro activity of amoxicillin to include β-lactamase–producing strains of *S. aureus* (but not methicillin-resistant strains), *H. influenzae, M. catarrhalis, N. gonorrhoeae, E. coli, Proteus* species, and some anaerobic bacteria, including *B. fragilis.* Recently, some β-lactamase–producing strains of *E. coli* were isolated that are resistant to amoxicillin–clavulanic acid because of either hyperproduction of the β-lactamase or production of a β-lactamase that is not susceptible to clavulanate.[183]

Ampicillin or amoxicillin alone is considered preferred therapy for children with mild to moderately severe disease of the respiratory tract, including otitis media and pneumonia. Alternative therapy, including amoxicillin–clavulanic acid, should be considered if a β-lactamase–producing organism is known or suspected to be the cause of the disease. The combination drug is useful in areas where the proportion of β-lactamase–producing strains of *H. influenzae* is large

(≥30 per cent) and where *M. catarrhalis* organisms (the majority of which are β-lactamase producers) are identified more frequently as pathogens in otitis media, sinusitis, and other respiratory tract infections.

Ampicillin-Sulbactam. Ampicillin was combined with sulbactam (Unasyn) to have a parenteral β-lactam/β-lactamase inhibitor combination. The spectrum of activity of ampicillin-sulbactam is similar to that of amoxicillin-clavulanate. It is most useful for monotherapy of potential polymicrobial infections, such as intra-abdominal, gynecologic, and soft tissue infections. The safety and efficacy of ampicillin-sulbactam have not been determined for children younger than 12 years of age.

Ticarcillin–Potassium Clavulanate. Ticarcillin combined with potassium clavulanate (Timentin) extends the spectrum of activity of ticarcillin to include β-lactamase–producing strains of *S. aureus, H. influenzae, E. coli, Klebsiella pneumoniae,* and *B. fragilis.*[35] Because clavulanic acid does not inhibit Bush group 1–inducible chromosomal β-lactamases, derepressed mutant strains of *P. aeruginosa* that are resistant to ticarcillin because of inducible cephalosporinases also are resistant to ticarcillin–potassium clavulanate. Although ticarcillin–potassium clavulanate has not been approved for use in children younger than 12 years of age, the drug has been used frequently in hospital settings and found to be safe and effective for infections caused by susceptible organisms.

Piperacillin-Tazobactam. Piperacillin combined with tazobactam (Zosyn) extends the spectrum of activity of piperacillin to include β-lactamase–producing strains of methicillin-susceptible *S. aureus* and many members of Enterobacteriaceae. Although studies have shown piperacillin-tazobactam to be safe and effective in the treatment of lower respiratory tract infections, intra-abdominal infections, and skin and skin-structure infections in adults,[127] the experience in children is limited. The safety and efficacy of piperacillin-tazobactam have not been established for children.

Adverse Effects and Sensitization

The penicillins are unique among antimicrobial agents in having little dose-related toxicity (Table 231–4). Seizures may occur under circumstances that result in high concentrations of penicillin in nervous tissues: rapid intravenous infusion of single large dosages, substantial dosages for prolonged periods in patients with impaired renal function, high concentrations given by an intrathecal route, or direct application of penicillin to brain tissue, as might occur inadvertently during a neurosurgical procedure. Confusion, dizziness, seizures, and psychosis due to toxic concentrations of procaine have been associated with administration of procaine penicillin G.[176] Nephritis has been associated with administration of some penicillins, most frequently after use of methicillin. Bleeding because of drug-induced platelet aggregation has been noted after administration of carbenicillin and penicillin G.

Although toxicity may not be a significant concern with the penicillins, sensitization is an important factor.[101] Penicillins are haptens—that is, they are low-molecular-weight compounds too small to elicit an immune response alone, but when bound to a carrier molecule (such as host tissues or proteins), they are highly immunogenic in humans. The native penicillin molecule can bind to a protein, as can its penicilloyl and penicillanic metabolites, the major and minor determinants, respectively. Four types of immune-mediated reactions can occur after administration of a penicillin (or any drug or antigen) as described in the following list: immediate hypersensitivity (IgE-mediated) reactions, cytotoxic antibody reactions, immune complex reactions (Arthus reaction), and delayed (cell-mediated) hypersensitivity.[208] It has been estimated that an immediate serious reaction occurs with 2 of every 10,000 courses and fatal reactions occur in 1 of 100,000 treatment courses.[170]

TABLE 231–4. Adverse Reactions to Penicillins*

Type of Reaction	Frequency (%)	Most Frequent*
Electrolyte disturbance		
Sodium overload	Variable	Ticar
Hypokalemia	Variable	Ticar
Hyperkalemia, acute	Rare	PCN G
Gastrointestinal		
Diarrhea	2–5	Amp
Enterocolitis	<1	Amp
Hematologic		
Hemolytic anemia	Rare	PCN G
Neutropenia	1–4	PCN G, Naf, Ox, Pip
Platelet dysfunction	3	Carben, Ticar
Hepatic		
Elevated AST	1–4	Ox, Naf, Carben
Neurologic		
Seizures	Rare	PCN G
Bizarre sensations		Procaine PCN
Renal		
Interstitial nephritis	1–2	Meth
Hemorrhagic cystitis	Rare	Meth
Allergic		
IgE-mediated	0.004–0.4	PCN G
Cytotoxic antibody	Rare	PCN G
Immune complexes	Rare	PCN G
Delayed hypersensitivity	4–8	Amp
Idiopathic	4–8	Amp

*All reactions can occur with any penicillin.

Amp, ampicillin; Carben, carbenicillin; Meth, methicillin; Naf, nafcillin; Ox, oxacillin; PCN G, penicillin G; Ticar, ticarcillin; Pip, piperacillin.

Modified from Chambers, H. F., and Neu, H. C.: Penicillins. *In* Mandell, G. L., Bennett, J. E., and Dolin, R. (eds.): Mandell, Douglas and Bennett's Principles and Practice of Infectious Diseases. 4th ed. New York, Churchill-Livingstone, 1995.

1. *Type 1 immediate hypersensitivity reactions* usually occur within 30 minutes after administration and are a life-threatening event. The interaction of preformed mast cell–bound IgE antibody to the antigenic determinants of penicillin results in release of mast cell mediators.[20] Clinical signs include hypotension or shock, urticaria, laryngeal edema, and bronchospasm. Acute anaphylaxis is rare after administration of penicillin, but a significant number of fatalities occur each year because of the extensive use of these drugs. Children are believed to have fewer systemic reactions than adults, presumably because of less previous exposure to penicillin antigens. Oral preparations are less likely to result in an immediate reaction than are parenteral forms, perhaps because antigens are altered in the gastrointestinal tract, absorption is slower, dosages are smaller, or a combination of these factors.

2. *Type 2 cytotoxic antibody reactions* after passive absorption of the penicilloyl hapten to the membrane of circulating

blood cells or to renal interstitial cells can occur, especially when high dosages of penicillins are used for prolonged periods. IgM antibody, IgG antibody, or both antibodies to the penicilloyl antigen bind to the altered cell surface; complement can be activated; and damage to the cell ensues. Cytotoxic antibody reactions usually manifest more than 72 hours after initiation of antibiotic therapy and include hemolytic anemia, leukopenia, thrombocytopenia, and drug-induced nephritis.

3. *Type 3 immune complex (Arthus) reactions* occur after the formation of immune complexes between soluble penicillin antigens and IgG and IgM antibodies. The complexes lodge in the skin, joints, kidney, or other tissue sites. Complement activation occurs, and the clinical manifestations of serum sickness ensue: cutaneous symptoms (urticaria, maculopapular rash, erythema multiforme), polyarthralgia, and fever. Onset typically is 7 to 21 days after initiation of penicillin therapy but can occur after the antibiotic has been discontinued. Although serum sickness has been associated with administration of penicillins, it occurs more frequently after cefaclor use.

4. *Type 4 delayed hypersensitivity reactions* involve cellular rather than humoral immunity. Thymus-derived lymphocytes react to penicillin haptens bound to host tissue after topical administration of penicillins. Contact dermatitis is rare now that topical penicillins are used no longer.

Idiopathic reactions are those for which an immune-mediated mechanism has not been proved. Included in this category are the morbilliform exanthems, erythema multiforme, photosensitivity reactions, exfoliative dermatitis, and pruritus. Approximately 4 per cent of courses of penicillin and up to 9 per cent of ampicillin or amoxicillin courses of therapy are associated with a maculopapular rash. In some of these patients, the rash is a manifestation of a primary viral infection for which the penicillin inappropriately was prescribed.

Identification of the patient who will have a significant reaction if penicillin is administered still is difficult. Serologic assays (radioallergosorbent tests) for detection of IgE antibodies to major and minor penicillin determinants are available but are time-consuming, expensive, and less sensitive than skin testing. Because the immediate reaction is mediated largely by IgE reagin or skin-sensitizing antibody, the patient who is likely to respond subsequently with a life-threatening reaction can be identified by use of intradermal tests with appropriate antigens. Selection of the most appropriate antigens to be used for skin testing, however, has been problematic because many different antigens may play roles in the allergic reaction. At least 10 metabolic breakdown products of the penicillin nucleus have been identified. Other potential antigens include macromolecular impurities present in solutions of the drug, high-molecular-weight penicillin polymers found in poorly buffered penicillin solutions standing for prolonged periods, side chains of the various penicillins, and bacterial enzymes (amidases) used to prepare semisynthetic penicillins. Thus, investigators have had difficulty in choosing sensitive and specific antigens to use for skin-testing purposes.

The most promising studies of skin-test antigens have been those of Levine,[98] who identified two antigens, penicilloyl polylysine (PRE-PEN, Taylor Pharmacal, Decatur, IL) and a "minor determinant mixture," a preparation of a dilute solution of aqueous crystalline penicillin G that includes metabolic breakdown products. Only the PRE-PEN reagent is commercially available in the United States; a solution of benzylpenicillin has been used as a less effective minor determinant skin-test reagent. The CDC recommends use of major and minor determinants, a positive control (histamine), and a negative control (diluent, phenol saline) after a protocol prepared by Beall.[13, 31] A prick test is performed first. If the patient's penicillin allergy was that of a mild reaction, the skin-test reagent can be used at full strength; however, if the previous history was suggestive of anaphylaxis, a 1:100 dilution of the reagent should be used for the first prick test followed by a full-strength test if there was no reaction with the diluted reagent. An intradermal test is placed and observed for 20 minutes if the prick test result was negative. A positive result is indicated by a wheal-and-flare reaction in 10 to 15 minutes and suggests a significant chance of reaction on subsequent administration of a penicillin. A negative result suggests that a significant allergic reaction will not take place. Although much effort has gone into clinical tests of these antigens, the predictive value of positive and negative results in children still is uncertain. Because there is a risk of severe life-threatening reactions when performing a skin test, it would be prudent to have a physician present and resuscitation equipment and medications readily available.

At present, the physician must rely on the patient's history of an adverse reaction after administration of a penicillin to identify the patient who is likely to be allergic. If the reaction appears to be related to the administration of a penicillin, the drug should be avoided for minor infections. Because no proven alternative therapies to penicillin are recommended for treating patients with neurosyphilis or syphilis in pregnancy, the CDC recommends skin testing and desensitization of patients considered to react positively to the skin-test antigens.[31] If a life-threatening infection should occur and penicillin clearly is the drug of choice, the physician may choose to administer the drug under carefully controlled conditions after desensitization. All penicillins are cross-reactive in regard to sensitization; allergy to any one implies sensitization to all, although cross-sensitivity is considerably less than 100 per cent.

Cephalosporins

The cephalosporins have a broad range of activity that includes gram-positive cocci, gram-negative enteric bacilli, and anaerobic bacteria. Most cephalosporins are relatively resistant to hydrolysis by β-lactamases produced by *S. aureus,* but many are susceptible to gram-negative β-lactamases. Unlike other antimicrobial agents, this group has a high therapeutic-to-toxic index. For simplicity, the cephalosporins have been categorized as first-, second-, and third-generation (Table 231–5) based on the pattern of in vitro activity.

Pharmacokinetics

The cephalosporins are available as parenteral and oral products (Table 231–6). Most of the parenteral drugs can be administered by the intravenous or intramuscular routes. Most of the oral products are absorbed well from the gastrointestinal tract. Esterification of the base compounds of cefuroxime and cefpodoxime is required to enhance gastrointestinal absorption. The presence of food does not alter absorption and, for some antibiotics, even can enhance absorption. Cephalosporins penetrate well into most tissues and body fluids except for cerebrospinal fluid. The first- and second-generation cephalosporins, other than cefuroxime, do not achieve adequate cerebrospinal fluid concentrations. Cerebrospinal fluid penetration of third-generation drugs varies. Because glomerular filtration and tubular secretion are the major modes of excretion, urinary concentrations achieved are sufficient for therapy of urinary tract infections. Ceftriaxone has dual excretion via the kidneys and the biliary tract and achieves high concentration in bile. The presence

TABLE 231–5. Classification Scheme for Cephalosporins

Generic Name	Trade Name	Route
First-generation		
Cephalexin	Keflex, Keftab	PO
Cefadroxil	Duricef, Ultracef	PO
Cephradine	Anspor, Velosef	PO, IM, IV
Cephalothin	Keflin	IV
Cefazolin*	Ancef, Kefzol	IM, IV
Cephapirin	Cefadyl	IM, IV
Second-generation		
Cefaclor*	Ceclor	PO
Cefuroxime axetil	Ceftin	PO
Cefprozil†	Cefzil	PO
Cefamandole*	Mandol	IM, IV
Cefonicid§	Monocid	IM, IV
Ceforanide	Precef	IM, IV
Cefuroxime‡	Zinacef, Kefurox	IM, IV
Cephamycins		
Cefoxitin‡	Mefoxin	IM, IV
Cefotetan§	Cefotan	IM, IV
Cefmetazole§	Zefazone	IV
Third-generation		
Cefixime†	Suprax	PO
Cefpodoxime proxetil†	Vantin	PO
Ceftizoxime†	Cefizox	IM, IV
Cefotaxime	Claforan	IM, IV
Ceftriaxone	Rocephin	IM, IV
Ceftazidime	Fortaz, Tazicef, Tazidime	IM, IV
Cefoperazone§	Cefobid	IM, IV

*Safety and efficacy have not been determined for infants younger than 1 month of age.
†Safety and efficacy have not been determined for infants younger than 6 months of age.
‡Safety and efficacy have not been established for infants younger than 3 months of age.
§Not approved for use in children.
IM, intramuscularly; IV, intravenously; PO, orally.

of moderate to severe renal insufficiency may require dosage or dosing interval adjustments for all cephalosporins except those with biliary excretion. Hepatic insufficiency can affect the metabolism of cephalosporins that undergo biliary excretion; however, ceftriaxone dosage or dosing interval adjustments are required only in the presence of both hepatic and renal insufficiency.

The therapeutic advantages of cephalosporins include concentration-independent bactericidal activity, broad-spectrum antibacterial activity, lack of significant dose-related toxicity, and relative stability against staphylococcal β-lactamases. Certain cautions must be kept in mind when prescribing cephalosporins: none is effective against enterococci, methicillin-resistant staphylococci, and *L. monocytogenes;* resistance may develop rapidly in closed communities, such as neonatal or pediatric intensive care units, because of inducible chromosomal β-lactamases produced by gram-negative bacteria; new products may cause unexpected reactions, such as the serum sickness–like disease described with cefaclor and the bile sludge attributed to ceftriaxone[97]; and, finally, all new products are expensive, especially when compared with generic preparations.

Specific Agents

FIRST-GENERATION CEPHALOSPORINS. The first-generation cephalosporins are effective against gram-positive cocci, including β-lactamase–producing *S. aureus,* and have variable activity against gram-negative enteric bacilli. Six first-generation cephalosporins currently are available for infants and children: the parenteral drugs cephapirin, cephalothin, and cefazolin; the oral products cephalexin and cefadroxil; and cephradine, which is available in both oral and parenteral forms. Because cephalothin and cephapirin are painful in intramuscular injection, the intravenous route is preferred. Cefazolin produces higher concentrations in blood than do the other parenteral first-generation drugs. Cefadroxil can be administered in twice-daily dosing because of its longer serum half-life. None of these agents attain appreciable concentrations in the central nervous system.

These drugs are of value as alternatives to penicillin for disease caused by *S. aureus, S. pyogenes,* and *S. pneumoniae* and are active against some strains of community-acquired gram-negative enteric bacilli, such as *E. coli, P. mirabilis,* and *K. pneumoniae.*[122] The three oral preparations have comparable activity in vitro and in vivo.[122] Both cefazolin and cephalexin are active against methicillin-susceptible *S. aureus;* however, cefazolin is less stable with staphylococcal β-lactamases than is cephalothin,[58] the clinical significance of which has not been established. The antibacterial activity against gram-negative bacteria is similar for all first-generation cephalosporins, except for cefazolin, which has slightly increased gram-negative activity.[165] First-generation cephalosporins are not the drug of choice for any pediatric infection but are of value for children who have a history of minor allergy to penicillin. They have been used to treat staphylococcal and streptococcal skin and skin-structure infections, bone and joint infections, pharyngitis, and uncomplicated community-acquired urinary tract infections caused by susceptible bacteria. Cefadroxil is effective for treatment of streptococcal pharyngitis in a once-a-day dosage schedule. Cephalexin has been used for sequential parenteral-oral treatment of staphylococcal osteomyelitis and arthritis after surgical intervention and an initial period of parenteral antibiotic therapy. Cefazolin has been used for perioperative prophylaxis in selected surgical procedures. Because first-generation cephalosporins have minimal if any activity against *H. influenzae* and *M. catarrhalis,* they should not be used for empiric treatment of respiratory tract infections. Empiric therapy for suspected gram-negative nosocomial infections would be covered better with a third-generation cephalosporin, an aminoglycoside, or both.

SECOND-GENERATION CEPHALOSPORINS. The second-generation cephalosporins consist of three parenteral drugs (cefamandole, cefuroxime, and ceforanide) and three oral preparations (cefaclor, cefuroxime axetil, and cefprozil). Also classified with the second-generation cephalosporins are the cephamycins, of which only one, cefoxitin, is approved for use in children. Compared with the first-generation cephalosporins, the true second-generation agents have similar or somewhat less activity against gram-positive cocci but better activity against *H. influenzae, M. catarrhalis, N. meningitidis, N. gonorrhoeae,* and some members of Enterobacteriaceae. The cephamycins are more active than the first- or true second-generation cephalosporins against gram-negative enteric bacteria and *B. fragilis* but have poor activity against gram-positive cocci.

Cefoxitin. Cefoxitin has excellent activity against anaerobic organisms and is the most active cephalosporin against *B. fragilis.*[16] It has selective activity against gram-negative enteric bacilli but is never active against *Enterobacter* or *Pseudomonas.* Cefoxitin is resistant to hydrolysis by β-lactamases produced by gram-positive bacteria and to some of the gram-negative β-lactamases. Because it is a potent inducer of Bush group 1 chromosomal β-lactamases,[160] indiscriminate use

TABLE 231–6. Pharmacokinetics of Cephalosporins

Antibiotic	Bioavailability* (%)	Protein Binding (%)	Metabolized (%)	Urinary Recovery (%/hours)	Approximate Half-Life† (hours)
First-generation					
Cephalexin	95	10–15	0	90/8	0.9–1.2
Cefadroxil	95	15–20	0	93/24	1.2–1.5
Cephradine	95	8–17	0	60–80/6	0.8–1.3
Cephalothin		70	20–30	60–70/6	0.5–1.0§
Cefazolin		85	0	80–100/24	1.4–1.8§
Cephapirin		44–50	40	70/6	0.5–0.8
Second-generation					
Cefaclor	95	25	0	60–85/8	0.6–0.9
Cefuroxime axetil	37/52	50	0‡	32–48/12	1.3§
Cefprozil	95	36	0	60/8	1.3
Cefamandole		70–80	0	60–85/8	0.5–1.2
Cefonicid		>90	0	99/24	4.5
Cefuroxime		50	0	89/8	1.3–1.7
Cefoxitin		70–80	<5	85/6	0.7–1.1
Third-generation					
Cefixime	40–50	65–70	0	50/24	3–4
Cefpodoxime proxetil	50/>50	40	0‡	29–33/12	2.1–2.8
Ceftizoxime		30	0	85–95/24	1.7
Cefotaxime		38	30–50	60/6	1.0
Ceftriaxone		85–95	0	33–67¶/24	4.3–8.7
Ceftazidime		<10	0	80–90/24	1.9

*Fasting/nonfasting.
†Normal renal function.
‡Prodrug rapidly metabolized to active drug; otherwise, no significant metabolism.
§Elimination half-life prolonged in neonates.
¶Forty to 75 per cent eliminated unchanged in bile.
Modified from *USP DI®, Volume I, Information for the Health Care Professional.* Copyright 1996, The USP Convention, Inc. Permission granted.

should be avoided. Cefoxitin has been shown to be effective for infections involving facultative gram-negative bacilli and anaerobes, such as intra-abdominal, pelvic, and gynecologic infections.[137] Combined with doxycycline, cefoxitin is the drug of choice for treatment of pelvic inflammatory disease.[31] Use of β-lactam/β-lactamase inhibitor combinations or metronidazole rather than cefoxitin should be considered for empiric treatment of patients with life-threatening anaerobic infections, because up to 15 per cent of *B. fragilis* organisms can be resistant to cephamycins. The safety and efficacy of cefoxitin have not been established for infants younger than 3 months of age.

Cefuroxime. Compared with first-generation cephalosporins, cefuroxime is slightly less active against staphylococci but is more active against group A streptococci and pneumococci. Cefuroxime has excellent activity against many members of Enterobacteriaceae.[139] Its stability to β-lactamases is greater than that of first-generation agents or cefamandole, and it is the only first- or second-generation antibiotic that achieves adequate cerebrospinal fluid concentrations, except against *H. influenzae* in some patients. Cefuroxime has been approved for treatment of skin and skin-structure infections, lower respiratory tract infections, bone and joint infections, uncomplicated gonorrhea, and uncomplicated urinary tract infections caused by susceptible bacteria. Cefuroxime is most useful for treatment of infections in which both *S. aureus* and *H. influenzae* type b are likely pathogens—that is, septic arthritis, orbital cellulitis, and severe pneumonias. Cefuroxime offers the advantage of single-drug therapy of these diseases, whereas a combination of a penicillinase-resistant penicillin plus chloramphenicol was required previously. Because of persistently positive 24-hour cerebrospinal fluid cultures in some infants and children with *H. influenzae* meningitis treated with cefuroxime, third-generation cephalosporins (cefotaxime and ceftriaxone) are preferred for therapy of known or suspected meningitis or invasive bacterial disease that may progress to meningitis.[173] With the dramatic reduction in the incidence of invasive *H. influenzae* type b infection in the United States after the introduction of *H. influenzae* type b vaccination, it is no longer imperative to use an antibiotic that provides coverage against both *S. aureus* and *H. influenzae* type b. The safety and efficacy of cefuroxime have not been established for infants younger than 3 months of age.

Cefamandole. Cefamandole is active against gram-positive cocci, including β-lactamase–producing *S. aureus,* and some gram-negative enteric bacteria, and it was the first cephalosporin to be effective for infections caused by *H. influenzae,* including β-lactamase–producing strains.[62, 121] Before the development of cefuroxime, cefamandole was used for respiratory tract, skin, and soft tissue infections in infants and children.[8, 162] Once cefuroxime was approved for use, cefamandole seldom was used because although its spectrum of activity was comparable with that of cefuroxime, some of its pharmacologic features made it less favorable. Cefamandole does not penetrate well into the cerebrospinal fluid, and, because it contains a methylthiotetrazole side chain, altered hemostasis is possible. Clinical and microbiologic failure in cases of meningitis caused by *H. influenzae* (despite in vitro susceptibility and evidence of cerebrospinal fluid penetration) has limited use of cefamandole to disease in which sepsis is not a concern.[184] There is no reason to use this agent in pediatric patients.

Ceforanide. Ceforanide has an antibacterial spectrum similar to that of cefamandole and cefuroxime, but it is less active against *H. influenzae.* Altered hemostasis is a potential adverse effect because of its methylthiotetrazole side chain. Ceforanide has been used for perioperative prophylaxis in adults. Experience in children is limited, and safety and effectiveness have not been established for children younger than 1 year of age.

Cefuroxime Axetil. Cefuroxime axetil is an oral form of cefuroxime with a similar spectrum of activity. It is an ester prodrug of cefuroxime that is metabolized to the active drug by intestinal esterases. Oral absorption is increased by the presence of food. When crushed, the tablet has a bitter taste that makes it unpalatable. The suspension has an unpleasant flavor that makes it difficult for some children to tolerate. The drug may be considered a suitable alternative to amoxicillin for treatment of otitis media and sinusitis when coverage must include β-lactamase–producing bacteria. It has been approved for treatment of uncomplicated urinary tract infections, skin and soft tissue infections, and lower respiratory tract infections caused by susceptible bacteria. Cefuroxime axetil can be used as an alternative to penicillin for the treatment of group A streptococcal pharyngitis.

Cefaclor. Cefaclor is more active than cephalexin against *H. influenzae, M. catarrhalis, E. coli,* and *P. mirabilis* and has activity against staphylococci similar to that of cephalexin. Cefaclor is an unstable compound and is destroyed within 2 hours in human plasma. It is susceptible to hydrolysis by β-lactamases produced by some strains of *Haemophilus* and *M. catarrhalis.* It is effective therapy for otitis media, sinusitis, and mild to moderate cases of pneumonia. Cefaclor is a suitable alternative to amoxicillin for treatment of the child with infections caused by susceptible organisms and suspected allergy to penicillin or when a β-lactamase–producing strain of *H. influenzae* is known or suspected to be a cause of disease. The rare but potential risk of serum sickness as well as its variable stability to some β-lactamases has limited its use. The safety and efficacy of cefaclor have not been established for infants younger than 1 month of age, although it has been used successfully to treat neonatal otitis media.

Cefprozil. Cefprozil has a similar structure to the first-generation cephalosporin, cefadroxil. It is more active than the oral first-generation agents against *Neisseria, H. influenzae,* group A *Streptococcus,* pneumococcus, *E. coli, P. mirabilis, Klebsiella,* and to a lesser extent staphylococci. It has relatively poor activity against *H. influenzae.* Compared with cefaclor, cefprozil is more stable against many β-lactamases. Because of its relatively long serum half-life, cefprozil can be dosed twice daily. Cefprozil is comparable with penicillin, cefaclor, and erythromycin for the treatment of pharyngitis[116] and is equal or superior to cefaclor and erythromycin for the treatment of mild to moderate skin and skin-structure infections.[142] It is approved for use in treatment of upper respiratory tract, mild lower respiratory tract, skin, and skin-structure infections. The safety and efficacy of cefprozil have not been established for infants younger than 6 months of age.

THIRD-GENERATION CEPHALOSPORINS. The third-generation cephalosporins approved for use in children include the parenteral agents cefotaxime, ceftizoxime, ceftriaxone, and ceftazidime and the oral agents cefixime and cefpodoxime proxetil. They are the most potent cephalosporins against gram-negative enteric bacteria.[192] Most of them have excellent activity against *H. influenzae, M. catarrhalis, N. gonorrhoeae, N. meningitidis,* group A streptococci, and penicillin-susceptible pneumococci but relatively poor activity against staphylococci. Ceftazidime is the only agent with activity against *P. aeruginosa.* Increasing resistance to third-generation cephalosporins by members of Enterobacteriaceae on the basis of plasmid-mediated production of extended-spectrum β-lactamases is of concern.[85] The parenteral cephalosporins provide high concentrations of drug in serum and adequate concentrations in cerebrospinal fluid.

Cefotaxime. Cefotaxime has excellent activity against group A streptococci, penicillin-susceptible pneumococci, *H. influenzae, N. meningitidis,* and *N. gonorrhoeae.* Because cefotaxime can be hydrolyzed by Bush group 1–inducible chromosomal β-lactamases and by extended-spectrum β-lactamases, it is not active against those strains of Enterobacteriaceae that produce these β-lactamases. Cefotaxime is metabolized in the liver to desacetyl cefotaxime, a less active metabolite that may act synergistically with cefotaxime. Although metabolized in the liver, cefotaxime is excreted by the kidneys. High serum and tissue concentrations of cefotaxime can be achieved at recommended dosages. The rapid development of resistance of gram-negative enteric bacilli when cefotaxime was used extensively for initial therapy of neonatal sepsis raised concern that extensive use of newer cephalosporins in the nursery or intensive care units might lead to more rapid emergence of drug-resistant bacteria than had been identified with the traditional regimens of a penicillin and an aminoglycoside. Because of its broad spectrum of activity against many of the common pathogens causing pediatric infections, cefotaxime is used widely for inpatient therapy of lower respiratory tract infections, urinary tract infections, sepsis, intra-abdominal infections, bone and joint infections, and meningitis or ventriculitis caused by susceptible organisms.

Ceftizoxime. Ceftizoxime is a parenteral agent with a spectrum of activity similar to that of cefotaxime, except it has better activity against *B. fragilis.* Its safety and efficacy have not been established for infants younger than 6 months of age.

Ceftriaxone. The antibacterial spectrum of ceftriaxone is similar to that of cefotaxime, with activity against group A streptococci, penicillin-susceptible pneumococci, *H. influenzae, Neisseria* species, and many members of Enterobacteriaceae. The activities of ceftriaxone and cefotaxime against methicillin-susceptible *S. aureus* are inconsistent; neither should be used for empiric monotherapy of infections presumed to be caused by staphylococci. Ceftriaxone is not active against most strains of *Pseudomonas.* Ceftriaxone differs from cefotaxime in its pharmacokinetic properties. Ceftriaxone undergoes extensive protein binding and has a long serum half-life. Because of its broad spectrum of activity against many of the pathogens that commonly cause sepsis, meningitis, and respiratory tract infections in older infants and children along with its unique pharmacokinetic features, ceftriaxone has been used excessively for outpatient management of febrile infants and young children who are being evaluated for possible systemic bacterial infection.

Ceftriaxone is effective for various sexually transmitted diseases, including chancroid, proctitis, epididymitis (in combination with doxycycline), and different forms of gonococcal disease (neonatal ophthalmia); uncomplicated urethral, endocervical, rectal, or pharyngeal gonorrhea (in combination with doxycycline for treatment of possible coexisting chlamydial infection); and disseminated gonococcal infection, meningitis, or endocarditis.[31] Ceftriaxone therapy for 5 days is comparable in effectiveness with conventional chloramphenicol therapy for typhoid fever in children.[128] Although third-generation cephalosporins have been used for empiric therapy of nosocomial pneumonia, wound infections, or urinary tract infections caused by gram-negative bacteria, it often is prudent to administer an aminoglycoside instead of or in addition to a third-generation cephalosporin because of the risk of resistance from extended-spectrum β-lactamases.

For infections requiring prolonged therapy (e.g., septic arthritis, osteomyelitis, brain abscess) and caused by susceptible organisms, ceftriaxone therapy is cost-effective for use outside of the hospital. Once the acute signs of disease have diminished and the child remains in the hospital only for parenteral therapy, discharge and once-daily administration of ceftriaxone in the home or clinic can be considered.

Because of its extensive protein binding, ceftriaxone can displace bilirubin from albumin-binding sites, although to date there is no evidence of adverse clinical effects. Cefotaxime is administered to neonates more often than is ceftriaxone because there is considerably more information about its safety and because of the potential but unproven risk of kernicterus. Ceftriaxone is excreted and concentrated in the bile. Gallbladder "sludge" diagnosed by abdominal sonography (and not identifiable by other radiographic techniques) has been demonstrated in some patients who received ceftriaxone. The material appears to be a calcium-ceftriaxone complex and resolves with cessation of the drug.[47] Most patients with ceftriaxone-associated "sludge" are asymptomatic, but occasionally patients have symptoms of gallbladder disease, and there are reports of acute cholecystitis in a few children.

Ceftazidime. Compared with cefotaxime and ceftriaxone, ceftazidime has poor antibacterial activity against *S. aureus*, is less active against penicillin-susceptible *S. pneumoniae*, is slightly less active against group A streptococci, but is more active against *P. aeruginosa*. On a weight basis, ceftazidime is the most effective of all β-lactam antimicrobial agents in vitro against *P. aeruginosa*. It frequently is active in vitro against *P. aeruginosa* strains that are resistant to antipseudomonal penicillins. Gram-negative bacteria can develop resistance to ceftazidime by production of extended-spectrum β-lactamases or because of decreased bacterial cell permeability, as seen with *P. aeruginosa, Acinetobacter*, and some *Serratia* strains. Ceftazidime is indicated for use in infections that are suspected to be caused by *Pseudomonas*, including acute exacerbations of chronic pulmonary infections in cystic fibrosis patients, chronic suppurative otitis media, and febrile illnesses in neutropenic cancer patients.

Cefixime. Cefixime contains a vinyl group instead of a chlorine atom at position 3 of the cephem nucleus and has an aminothiazole oxime group rather than a phenyl glycine side chain. These biochemical changes result in potent gram-negative activity. Cefixime was introduced in 1989 as an oral third-generation cephalosporin with a broad spectrum of activity, including activity against group A streptococci, *H. influenzae, M. catarrhalis*, penicillin-susceptible *S. pneumoniae*, and many members of Enterobacteriaceae, including *Shigella, Salmonella, E. coli, Klebsiella*, and *P. mirabilis*.[10] It is not active against *S. aureus, P. aeruginosa, Serratia, Enterobacter*, or *Citrobacter freundii*. Although cefixime has in vitro activity against penicillin-susceptible pneumococci, lower bacteriologic cures occurred with cefixime when compared with amoxicillin for children with pneumococcal acute otitis media.[81] Cefixime is highly resistant to degradation by β-lactamases. Administration of cefixime is facilitated by once-daily dosing,[53] pleasant taste, and stability of the suspension at room temperature. Cefixime is effective therapy for uncomplicated gonorrhea, uncomplicated urinary tract infections caused by *E. coli* or *P. mirabilis*, shigellosis, and acute otitis media or sinusitis caused by *H. influenzae* or *M. catarrhalis*.[19] It is not recommended for treatment of infections frequently caused by staphylococci, such as skin or soft tissue infections, and is not the most effective agent for treatment of pneumococcal infections. The safety and efficacy of cefixime have not been established for infants younger than 6 months of age.

Cefpodoxime Proxetil. The antibacterial activity of cefpodoxime proxetil is similar to that of cefixime, with the exception of improved activity against staphylococci. Cefpodoxime is active against group A streptococci; penicillin-susceptible pneumococci; β-lactamase–producing strains of *N. gonorrhoeae, H. influenzae*, and *M. catarrhalis*; methicillin-susceptible *S. aureus*; and many members of Enterobacteriaceae. It is not active against *Enterobacter, Pseudomonas, Serratia*, or *Morganella*. Cefpodoxime proxetil, the ester prodrug of cefpodoxime, is cleaved by intestinal esterases to the active drug. Oral absorption is increased by the presence of food. Because of its longer serum half-life, cefpodoxime proxetil can be administered in twice-daily dosing intervals. Cefpodoxime is hydrolyzed by some extended-spectrum β-lactamases.

Cefpodoxime proxetil can be used as an alternative to penicillin or erythromycin for treatment of group A streptococcal pharyngitis.[41] It is comparable with amoxicillin-clavulanate, cefaclor, and cefixime for the treatment of acute otitis media.[36] It is not likely to be effective for treatment of acute otitis media caused by penicillin-resistant pneumococci because it does not penetrate well into the middle ear. It has been approved for outpatient treatment of community-acquired respiratory tract infections, uncomplicated urinary tract infections, and mild skin and skin-structure infections. The safety and efficacy of cefpodoxime proxetil have not been established for infants younger than 6 months of age.

Adverse Effects

The cephalosporins, like the penicillins, are safe for children and have almost no dose-related toxicity. The most common reactions are local ones, including pain at the injection site or thrombophlebitis with parenteral administration, and mild gastrointestinal complaints with oral dosing. Hypersensitivity reactions occur in approximately 1 to 3 per cent of treatment courses and include morbilliform rash, urticaria, and pruritus. Anaphylaxis is uncommon. Drug fever has been associated with cephalosporin administration. Nonspecific, antibiotic-associated diarrhea and, less commonly, *Clostridium difficile* toxin–mediated colitis can occur after cephalosporin use.

Other adverse effects are rare, some of which are unique to one or a few cephalosporins. Physicians should be alert for the uncommon reactions, including reversible neutropenia that can follow prolonged use of high-dosage cephalosporins, Coombs-positive hemolytic anemia, and bleeding. Altered hemostasis because of hypoprothrombinemia can result when using any cephalosporin that contains a methylthiotetrazole side chain (cefamandole, cefoperazone, cefotetan, moxalactam, cefmetazole, and cefmenoxime). These agents act as competitive inhibitors of vitamin K–dependent carboxylase, which converts clotting factors II, VII, IX, and X to their active forms. These methylthiotetrazole antibiotics also have been associated with a disulfiram-like (Antabuse) response in patients drinking alcoholic beverages. Dose-dependent nephrotoxicity occurred with cephaloridine, a first-generation agent that no longer is marketed. Nephrotoxicity has been reported in adults who received cephalothin combined with gentamicin[11]; however, it remains uncertain whether cephalosporins can potentiate aminoglycoside nephrotoxicity.[111] Nephrotoxicity is rare in currently available cephalosporins. Gallbladder sludging, biliary pseudolithiasis, and symptomatic obstructive biliary disease rarely have been associated with ceftriaxone administration.[214]

The cephalosporins may produce allergic reactions similar to those caused by the penicillins. There is cross-sensitization among the cephalosporins, and allergy to one cephalosporin implies allergy to all. Various degrees of immunologic cross-reaction of penicillins and cephalosporins have been demonstrated in vitro and in animal models.[148] Previously quoted studies suggested that the frequency of allergic reactions to cephalosporins ranged from 5.4 to 16.5 per cent in patients with a history of penicillin allergy and from 1 to 2.5 per cent in those without a history of penicillin allergy. The incidence of hypersensitivity to unrelated drugs is increased in some patients who are allergic to penicillin, suggesting that excipients in antibiotic preparations may be responsible for these reactions. Thus, it is uncertain whether the penicillin-allergic patient reacts to a cephalosporin because of cross-allergenicity.[169] Most patients who are believed to be allergic to penicillin receive cephalosporins without adverse reaction. Although a cephalosporin may be used with caution as an alternative to penicillin in children who have an ambiguous history of skin rash, the cephalosporins should be avoided for the patient with a known immediate or accelerated reaction to a penicillin. Currently, skin testing to evaluate for cephalosporin hypersensitivity is not possible because the potential cephalosporin haptens are unknown and no standardized antigen exists.[169]

An unusual serum sickness–like reaction has been reported in children who received cefaclor. The children developed a generalized pruritic rash, similar to erythema multiforme, in some cases accompanied by fever, purpura, and arthritis with pain and swelling in knees and ankles. The signs appeared 5 to 19 days after the start of therapy and generally disappeared within 4 to 5 days after discontinuing the drug. The children had no prior history of allergy to a penicillin or a cephalosporin.[129] Three hundred eleven cases, including 289 children, were reported to the manufacturer by 1982. At that time, approximately 3 million courses of cefaclor had been administered, which suggested a minimal (considering the likelihood of underreporting) incidence of 1 reaction per 10,000 courses.* Levine[99] compared adverse reactions in children who received cefaclor (1017 patients, 2513 courses) or amoxicillin (1009 patients, 2358 courses). Serum sickness (defined as arthritis/arthralgia plus a rash or urticaria) or erythema multiforme occurred in 11 children (1.1 per cent) who received cefaclor but in none of those who received amoxicillin. Recent studies suggest that serum sickness–like reactions to cefaclor are associated with lymphocyte sensitization.[88]

Carbacephems

Carbacephems have a carbon atom at position 1 of the cephem (cephalosporin) nucleus rather than a sulfur atom. The only carbacephem currently available is loracarbef. Loracarbef is similar structurally to cefaclor but has greater chemical stability in solution. The antibacterial spectrum of loracarbef is similar to that of second-generation cephalosporins. Compared with cefaclor, loracarbef has similar activity against penicillin-susceptible pneumococci, group A streptococci, and methicillin-susceptible *S. aureus* and has greater activity against *H. influenzae* and *M. catarrhalis,* including β-lactamase–producing strains.[46] Loracarbef is not active against *P. aeruginosa, Enterobacter, Citrobacter,* indole-positive *Proteus,* or *B. fragilis.*

Loracarbef is more stable than is cefaclor to hydrolysis by β-lactamases but can be hydrolyzed by extended-spectrum β-lactamases. Loracarbef is available for oral administration only. It is absorbed rapidly and well; however, absorption is decreased when taken with food. It has a longer serum half-life than some of the penicillins and can be given twice daily. It is excreted by the kidneys. Loracarbef is relatively well tolerated. Gastrointestinal complaints, including diarrhea, nausea, and vomiting, are the most frequently reported adverse effects but occur with less than 5 per cent of treatment courses. The safety and efficacy of loracarbef have not been established for infants younger than 6 months of age.

Loracarbef can be used as an alternative to penicillin or erythromycin for treatment of group A streptococcal pharyngitis.[45] The effectiveness of loracarbef is similar to that of amoxicillin and amoxicillin-clavulanate for treatment of acute otitis media caused by susceptible bacteria.[59] For treatment of mild to moderate skin and skin-structure infections, the efficacy of loracarbef is comparable with that of cefaclor.[75] It has been approved for use in the treatment of uncomplicated urinary tract infections caused by susceptible bacteria.

β-Lactam Antibiotics Not Approved for Use in Children

Several β-lactam antibiotics are available in the United States but not approved for use in children. Imipenem-cilastatin and meropenem (pending FDA approval), the carbapenems, are agents with broad-spectrum activity that includes gram-positive and gram-negative aerobic bacteria and many anaerobes. Aztreonam, a monobactam, has gram-negative antibacterial activity similar to that of ceftazidime but has no significant gram-positive activity. Although it is a β-lactam, aztreonam is not very immunogenic and can be used in patients with minor forms of β-lactam allergy. Cephalosporins that are not approved for use in children include the second-generation cephalosporin, cefonicid; the cephamycins, cefotetan and cefmetazole; and the third-generation cephalosporin, cefoperazone. Numerous cephalosporins, including ceftibuten and several "fourth"-generation cephalosporins, such as cefpirome and cefipime, still are undergoing investigation.

Vancomycin

Vancomycin, first isolated from *Amycolatopsis orientalis* (formerly called *Streptomyces,* then *Nocardia)* in soil samples from Borneo, is a high-molecular-weight, complex, soluble glycopeptide.[149] Because of the lack of adequate therapy for penicillinase-producing staphylococci, it expeditiously was approved for use by the FDA in 1956 before exhaustive pharmacologic and toxicologic studies had been performed. Once the penicillinase-resistant penicillins were developed, vancomycin was no longer indispensable until the emergence of methicillin-resistant staphylococci in the late 1970s.

Mechanism of Action

Vancomycin is bactericidal against most susceptible gram-positive bacteria except for enterococci, for which it is bacteriostatic. Its major mechanism of action involves prevention of polymerization of the phosphodisaccharide-pentapeptide-lipid complex during the second stage of peptidoglycan cell wall synthesis. Its site of action is distinct from that of β-lactam antibiotics. Additionally, vancomycin alters cytoplasmic membrane permeability and impairs RNA synthesis. In vitro studies suggest that it exhibits concentration-independent/time-dependent bactericidal activity against susceptible organisms, similar to that of β-lactams.[48, 100] A lag phase before onset of rapid killing has been demonstrated in serum-killing studies.[3]

Mechanisms of Resistance

Resistance can be categorized into three types: tolerance, acquired resistance, and inherent resistance. Some susceptible gram-positive bacteria, especially enterococci, are tolerant to

*Data provided by J. Getty, Marketing Plans Manager, Eli Lilly Co., and published in *Pediatric Infectious Disease Newsletter,* edited by J. D. Nelson and G. H. McCracken, Jr., May/June 1982, vol. 8, no. 3.

the bactericidal activity of vancomycin; that is, vancomycin inhibits but does not kill the bacteria (MBC/MIC ratio ≥32). Staphylococci tolerant to vancomycin can have autolysin deficiencies. Although most resistance to vancomycin by gram-positive bacteria is acquired, there are four genera of gram-positive organisms that inherently are resistant to vancomycin: *Erysipelothrix, Lactobacillus, Leuconostoc,* and *Pediococcus.* At least three genes code for acquired vancomycin resistance in enterococci: *VanA, VanB,* and *VanC.*[210] The bacterial target for vancomycin is the D-alanyl-D-alanine group at the end of the pentapeptide side chain produced by D-ala-D-ala ligase. The vancomycin resistance genes encode for ligases that, because of altered substrate specificities, produce a modified peptidoglycan side chain, to which glycopeptides are unable to bind.[159] *VanA* resistance, the phenotype most commonly encountered, is plasmid-mediated and can be induced by either vancomycin or teicoplanin, another glycopeptide that has not been approved for use in the United States. Although vancomycin resistance can affect susceptibility to other investigational glycopeptides, there is no cross-resistance between other unrelated antibiotics. Resistance to vancomycin rarely develops during appropriate therapy, perhaps because of its multiple mechanisms of action, but prolonged or indiscriminate use can contribute to selective pressure resulting in development of vancomycin-resistant enterococci colonizing the gut. Of greatest concern is emergence of enterococci resistant to all currently available antibiotics (vancomycin, ampicillin, and high-level aminoglycoside) and spread of vancomycin resistance to pneumococci and staphylococci.

In Vitro Activity

The in vitro spectrum of activity for vancomycin is limited to gram-positive bacteria with little if any activity against aerobic or anaerobic gram-negative bacilli.[204] Group A streptococci, pneumococci, *Corynebacteria* species, and *C. difficile* are highly susceptible to vancomycin, whereas *L. monocytogenes,* microaerophilic and anaerobic streptococci, enterococci, staphylococci, *Bacillus anthracis,* and other *Clostridium* species have higher MIC values that still are in the susceptible range. The bactericidal activity of vancomycin combined with gentamicin has been shown to be synergistic in vitro against enterococci.[203] Although vancomycin has activity against many gram-positive bacteria, it is not the most active agent for these organisms, except for multiply drug-resistant bacteria, such as methicillin-resistant staphylococci and highly penicillin- and cephalosporin-resistant pneumococci. Clinical studies indicate that vancomycin is safe and effective therapy for staphylococcal infections in children.[172]

Pharmacokinetics

Intravenous administration of vancomycin is preferred because intramuscular injection causes pain and tissue necrosis.[125] Intravenous preparations must be diluted further in normal saline or dextrose solution before slow infusion. Vancomycin is approximately 55 per cent bound to serum proteins and diffuses well into most body tissues with adequate concentrations achieved in pericardial, pleural, ascitic, and synovial fluids. Vancomycin does not diffuse well into cerebrospinal fluid in the absence of inflamed meninges, but adequate cerebrospinal fluid concentrations can be achieved during therapy for meningitis when higher dosages (15 mg/kg every 6 hours) are administered. Intrathecal or intraventricular administration has been used infrequently for central nervous system infections that are difficult to eradicate.[71, 106] Vancomycin is not metabolized significantly and is excreted by glomerular filtration. The mean serum elimination half-life in adults with normal renal function is 6 hours. For children, this ranges from 5 to 10 hours in newborns, 4 hours in older infants, and 2 to 3 hours in children.[172] In anephric patients, the elimination half-life extends to 7 or more days. Vancomycin is not removed effectively by either peritoneal dialysis or hemodialysis, although there have been reports of increased clearance with recently developed hemodialysis filters. Nomograms[126] and patient-individualized Bayesian dosing regimens[92] have been employed for vancomycin dosing in renal failure.

Indications for Use

Because of the possibility of toxicity and the potential for development of resistance, administration of vancomycin should be reserved for patients with moderate to severe infections caused by vancomycin-susceptible bacteria that are resistant to other antibiotics. Vancomycin can be used for treatment of infections caused by β-lactam– and vancomycin-susceptible bacteria in patients with hypersensitivity reactions to β-lactam antimicrobial agents. Empiric therapy of patients with catheter-associated infections frequently includes vancomycin to provide activity against coagulase-negative staphylococci. Although nonabsorbable oral vancomycin is effective therapy for *C. difficile* colitis, oral metronidazole represents first-line therapy; vancomycin should be given only for metronidazole treatment failures to limit the development of vancomycin-resistant enterococci.

Adverse Effects

The purification of recent preparations of vancomycin allegedly has decreased the frequency of adverse reactions. The most common adverse effect is "red man" or "red neck" syndrome, or glycopeptide-induced anaphylactoid reaction,[150] manifested by flushing of the face and upper trunk and pruritus during vancomycin infusion. Vancomycin directly causes release of histamine from mast cells by non–immune-mediated mechanisms. Because it is a dose- and rate-dependent reaction, administering doses less than 500 mg, prolonging the infusion period to at least 1 hour, or doing both decreases the risk of occurrence. Pretreatment with H1-receptor antagonists (diphenhydramine, hydroxyzine) prevents its development, and symptoms usually resolve promptly after discontinuation of the infusion. The spectrum of severity ranges from pruritus with macular rash to hypotension.

Controversy surrounds the issue of vancomycin-induced ototoxicity and nephrotoxicity.[25] Such toxicity has not been demonstrated in experimental animal models. Although there have been numerous case reports of toxicity in humans, the literature is difficult to interpret because of confounding variables, including recent or concurrent use of aminoglycosides or other ototoxic or nephrotoxic agents, lack of identification of antecedent otologic or renal disease, and inconsistencies in sampling methods when measuring serum vancomycin concentrations. Tinnitus and high-tone hearing loss have been associated with vancomycin administration but generally are reversible after discontinuation. If vancomycin is ototoxic, it certainly is not clear whether toxic peak or toxic trough serum concentrations are responsible. Several studies suggest an increased risk of nephrotoxicity when aminoglycosides are used concurrently with vancomycin, especially when administered for longer than 21 days.[68] Other adverse effects seen occasionally with vancomycin use include reversible neutropenia, thrombocytopenia, macular rash, and, rarely, cardiovascular collapse.

The usefulness of serum vancomycin concentration determinations has been argued because a definitive relationship between vancomycin concentration and either adverse effects or clinical outcome has not been proved.[29, 124] Until the significance of vancomycin serum concentration determinations has been clarified, monitoring has been suggested for the following clinical situations only: (1) patients with rapid changes in renal function, (2) patients receiving larger than normal dosages, (3) anephric patients undergoing hemodialysis (to avoid subtherapeutic vancomycin concentrations during prolonged dosing intervals), and (4) patients receiving concomitant therapy with nephrotoxic agents.[124] Further studies evaluating the relationship between serum vancomycin concentrations and clinical outcome and adverse effects are warranted.

Aminoglycosides

Aminoglycosides are natural and semisynthetic compounds that consist of at least two amino sugars bound by a glycosidic linkage to a hexose nucleus, the aminocyclitol ring. A more appropriate name would be aminoglycosidic aminocyclitols. Streptomycin, isolated from *Streptomyces griseus*, was the first aminoglycoside available for use in 1944. Many aminoglycosides have been isolated or developed since that time. The suffix denotes the origin of the aminoglycoside: those ending with the suffix *-mycin* were derived from *Streptomyces* species, whereas those ending with *-micin* were derived from *Micromonospora* species. Currently, eight aminoglycosides are approved for use in the United States (Table 231–7), and several more are available in other countries. Despite the development of less toxic antibiotics with broad-spectrum activity, aminoglycosides continue to fulfill an essential role in the treatment of severe infections caused by aerobic gram-negative bacilli and enterococci.

Mechanism of Action

Against susceptible bacteria, aminoglycosides demonstrate rapid, concentration-dependent bactericidal activity.[48, 100] They exert their effect by binding irreversibly to the 30S subunit of the bacterial ribosome,[179] resulting in inhibition of protein synthesis and induction of translational errors. Bacterial uptake of aminoglycosides can be facilitated by concomitant therapy with cell wall–active antibiotics, such as vancomycin or β-lactams, but transport into the cytoplasm requires two energy- and oxygen-dependent steps, EDP I and EDP II, that use an electrochemical proton gradient. Unlike other protein synthesis inhibitors that usually are bacteriostatic, aminoglycosides are bactericidal. The exact mechanism of bactericidal activity remains elusive, but removal of amino and hydroxyl groups from the aminoglycoside results in loss of antibacterial activity and toxic potential.

TABLE 231–7. Classification Scheme for Aminoglycosides

Aminocyclitol Ring	Family	Member
Streptidine	Streptomycin	Streptomycin
2-Deoxystreptamine	Kanamycin	Kanamycin Amikacin Tobramycin
2-Deoxystreptamine	Gentamicin	Gentamicin Netilmicin
2-Deoxystreptamine	Neomycin	Neomycin Paromomycin

Mechanisms of Resistance

The prevalence of acquired aminoglycoside resistance is relatively low, and its development during therapy is unusual. Bacteria can acquire resistance to aminoglycosides because of alterations in the bacterial target, reduced bacterial cell permeability or uptake, or modification of the antibiotic by bacterial enzymes, the latter being most significant clinically.[42] Mutations in the aminoglycoside-binding site of the 30S ribosome have been associated with high-level resistance to streptomycin but not to other aminoglycosides, possibly because, unlike streptomycin, they bind to multiple sites on the ribosome. Facultative aerobic bacteria causing infection in sites with reduced oxygen tension, anaerobic bacteria, and such fermentative bacteria as streptococci inherently are resistant to aminoglycosides because they are unable to generate an electrochemical proton gradient sufficient for aminoglycoside transport into the cytoplasm. Other bacteria can acquire resistance because of reduced permeability or lack of transport, as demonstrated in staphylococci that quickly develop resistance to aminoglycosides when monotherapy is administered. *P. aeruginosa* and, less frequently, members of Enterobacteriaceae can acquire cross-resistance to all aminoglycosides because of various mechanisms that interfere with uptake or cytoplasmic transport. Least common are altered outer-membrane porins in gram-negative bacteria, and most common are mutations in the lipopolysaccharide, as manifested by a rough colony morphology, resulting in fewer external binding sites for the positively charged aminoglycoside. Plasmid-mediated production of aminoglycoside-modifying enzymes is the most common mechanism of acquired resistance. There are many enzymes with different substrate specificities, several of which can be elaborated simultaneously in the same bacterium. These acetyltransferases, adenylyltransferases, and phosphotransferases interact with amino or hydroxyl groups on the aminoglycoside and modify the aminoglycoside so that it binds poorly to the 30S ribosome.

In Vitro Activity

The in vitro antibacterial spectrum of aminoglycosides includes a wide range of aerobic gram-negative bacilli, many methicillin-susceptible staphylococci, and some mycobacteria.[123] Some gram-negative bacilli, including *Burkholderia cepacia* and *Stenotrophomonas maltophilia*, consistently are resistant to all aminoglycosides. The spectra of activity of gentamicin, tobramycin, and netilmicin are similar, and strains resistant to one usually are resistant to the others. The major advantage of tobramycin is its activity against some strains of *P. aeruginosa* that are resistant to gentamicin and netilmicin. Because many aminoglycoside-modifying enzymes are active against gentamicin, tobramycin, and netilmicin but inactive against amikacin, amikacin frequently is prescribed for empiric therapy of nosocomial gram-negative bacillary infections. Amikacin also has activity against *Mycobacterium avium-intracellulare* complex, some rapidly growing mycobacteria, and *Nocardia asteroides*. Netilmicin is less active than other aminoglycosides against *P. aeruginosa* but can have activity against some gentamicin-resistant aerobic gram-negative bacilli. Although gentamicin, tobramycin, amikacin, and netilmicin have similar spectra of activity, susceptibility testing is recommended because of geographic and interhospital variation in resistance patterns. Lack of activity against *P. aeruginosa*, *Klebsiella* species, and *Serratia* species has limited the use of kanamycin. Streptomycin is inactive against many gram-negative enteric bacilli but does have activity against *Francisella tularensis*, *Yersinia pestis*, and *Mycobacterium tuberculosis*.

Pharmacokinetics

Aminoglycosides have in common many pharmacokinetic characteristics. They are highly polar, water-soluble compounds that are positively charged cations at neutral pH. Their antibacterial activity is pH-dependent, with increased activity at higher pH. They are relatively resistant to degradation at various temperatures and pH values, but in vitro inactivation after exposure to extended-spectrum penicillins, particularly ticarcillin and carbenicillin, has been described.[202] After parenteral administration, aminoglycosides distribute rapidly in extracellular body water, with slow accumulation in tissues. The volume of distribution is decreased (with respect to total body weight) in obese patients and increased in patients with illnesses associated with edema, such as severe infections, burns, and ascites. With the exceptions of proximal renal tubular cells and possibly inner ear hair cells, penetration into other body compartments is impaired because of lipid insolubility, polycationic charge, and size of the aminoglycoside. Proximal renal tubular cells absorb aminoglycosides via carrier-mediated pinocytosis, resulting in renal cortical concentrations exceeding those in plasma. Aminoglycosides do not penetrate the blood-brain barrier in the absence of meningeal inflammation, but with inflammation approximately 20 to 25 per cent of the serum concentration penetrates into cerebrospinal fluid. Because of the narrow therapeutic/toxic index, monotherapy for gram-negative bacillary meningitis with aminoglycosides is not recommended. Aminoglycosides are not metabolized and, after parenteral administration, are excreted unchanged in the kidney by glomerular filtration, with approximately 5 per cent of excreted drug reabsorbed in the proximal tubular cells. Minimal amounts are excreted in saliva and feces. Urine concentrations exceed those in plasma by 25 to 100 times.

After intramuscular injection, aminoglycosides are absorbed completely and peak serum concentrations are achieved within 90 minutes, except in some disease states, such as hypotension, that interfere with tissue perfusion. When administered intravenously, the infusion should be given slowly over 30 to 60 minutes to avoid potential adverse effects. Peak serum concentrations are achieved within 30 to 60 minutes after infusion. Because of their polar nature, absorption after oral administration is insignificant and inadequate to treat systemic infections, but aminoglycosides can accumulate in the presence of renal failure, resulting in concentrations sufficient to cause toxicity. Although they are nonirritating when instilled into pleural or peritoneal spaces, absorption of aminoglycosides is rapid and can result in significant toxicity. In contrast, instillation into the lateral ventricles or irrigation of the bladder has not been associated with significant systemic absorption. Compared with parenteral administration, aerosol administration of aminoglycoside results in higher concentrations in bronchial secretions and less toxicity.[157] Aminoglycosides should not be used topically as ointments or creams because of the rapid development of resistant strains after extensive topical use.

Antimicrobial dosing in newborns and young infants differs from that in older children and adults because of developmental changes in renal function and increased total body water composition. Neonates and young infants have a larger volume of distribution and a reduced glomerular filtration rate; these differences are more pronounced in very low birth weight premature neonates.[152] Aminoglycoside dosing protocols that incorporate these pharmacokinetic variabilities have been developed, with dosage and dosing intervals based on postconceptual age (gestational age plus postnatal age) rather than postnatal age.[104]

The aminoglycoside dosing schedule currently approved for use in older children and adults incorporates a twice- (streptomycin) or three-times-daily regimen. Several pharmacodynamic features of aminoglycosides may work in concert to allow once-daily dosing. Because aminoglycosides demonstrate concentration-dependent bactericidal activity, higher peak serum concentrations result in more extensive and more rapid killing.[201] Aminoglycosides also demonstrate a postantibiotic effect against susceptible aerobic gram-negative bacilli in vitro and in vivo,[39, 213] and the duration of postantibiotic effect is longer the higher the peak serum concentration.[84] When the entire daily dosage of aminoglycoside is administered at one time, a peak serum concentration in the range of 15 to 20 μg/mL can be achieved. In the presence of normal renal function, the serum concentration is low or undetectable before the next dose, but antibacterial activity continues because of the postantibiotic effect. In vitro studies,[18] experimental animal models, and clinical studies in adults suggest that once-daily aminoglycoside dosing may be at least as efficacious as traditional dosing for treatment of some aerobic gram-negative infections.[65] Ototoxicity and nephrotoxicity were less frequent in experimental animal models when daily dosing was administered.[65] Few clinical studies of once-daily aminoglycoside dosing in children exist, but data from the small studies available suggest that efficacy and toxicity are comparable with those seen with traditional dosing schedules.[51] Further clinical studies are necessary before this dosing regimen can be recommended, especially in infants and children.

Indications for Use

The major use of aminoglycosides in children is for serious infections caused by gram-negative enteric bacilli, including neonatal sepsis, sepsis in the child with malignancy or an immunologic defect, abdominal and systemic infections associated with spillage of fecal contents into the peritoneum, and complicated urinary tract infections. Because gentamicin is the least expensive aminoglycoside and the one with which there is the most experience, it often is considered the first-line agent for empiric therapy of suspected aerobic gram-negative bacillary infections in institutions with minimal background resistance. Combinations of an aminoglycoside and a cell wall–active antibiotic have been used for synergistic bactericidal activity. Gentamicin has been administered with penicillin G, ampicillin, or vancomycin for the treatment of enterococcal or viridans streptococcal endocarditis, and gentamicin or tobramycin combined with ceftazidime or an acylureidopenicillin has been used to treat serious infections caused by *P. aeruginosa*. Amikacin often is used for empiric therapy of nosocomial aerobic gram-negative bacillary infections in institutions with significant resistance to gentamicin. Streptomycin is indicated for use alone or in combination with other antibiotics for the treatment of tularemia and plague and combined with other agents for treatment of tuberculosis, brucellosis, and enterococcal endocarditis. Paromomycin is too toxic for parenteral use but when administered orally has been useful for treatment of asymptomatic intestinal amebiasis[1] or for cryptosporidiosis in patients with AIDS.[56]

Adverse Effects

Although aminoglycosides have intrinsic toxicity, allergic reactions are uncommon. All aminoglycosides can injure the proximal renal tubules, the cochlea, the vestibular apparatus, or a combination thereof and can cause neuromuscular blockade, but the risk varies with each agent. Because aminoglycosides do not induce a significant inflammatory response, pain at intramuscular injection sites and phlebitis at intravenous infusion sites are unusual. Hypersensitivity reactions and drug fever are rare.

Many theories have been postulated regarding the mechanism of nephrotoxicity,[66] including inhibition of lysosomal phospholipases within the proximal renal tubules.[198] Clinical findings include a mild, nonoliguric decrease in the glomerular filtration rate that typically is reversible. Compared with traditional dosing, once-daily dosing was less nephrotoxic in experimental animal models.[14] Some studies suggest that neomycin is the most nephrotoxic and streptomycin the least nephrotoxic aminoglycoside. In humans, nephrotoxicity has been associated with prolonged duration of therapy with high dosages, previous aminoglycoside therapy, administration of drugs to critically ill patients with intravascular volume depletion or hyponatremia and to those with impaired kidney function, and concomitant administration of other potentially nephrotoxic agents, such as amphotericin B and loop diuretics.[43] Debate continues regarding the causal association of these factors to nephrotoxicity and the risk of toxicity with each aminoglycoside.[120] Clearly, factors that increase renal cortical uptake of aminoglycoside, such as duration of therapy and dosage regimen, influence the risk of nephrotoxicity.[114]

The mechanism by which aminoglycosides cause vestibular and cochlear ototoxicity has not been elucidated fully. Cochlear damage presents as tinnitus or high-frequency hearing loss, whereas vestibular toxicity manifests as vertigo, nystagmus, and ataxia.[7] Damage can be unilateral or bilateral. Occasionally, ototoxicity is reversible, but permanent damage is more common. Mild cochlear damage may not be recognized because high-frequency hearing range is affected first. Conventional audiograms that do not test high-frequency ranges may not detect cochlear injury. Data from experimental animal models suggest a latent onset of ototoxic symptoms after discontinuation of aminoglycoside therapy, an increased risk of toxicity with concomitant loop diuretic therapy, and variation in ototoxic potential of each aminoglycoside. Delayed onset of high-frequency hearing loss has been confirmed in humans. Factors that increase the risk of aminoglycoside ototoxicity in humans include impaired renal function and prolonged duration of treatment. Although not proved, some studies suggest that streptomycin, gentamicin, and tobramycin are more likely to affect vestibular function and amikacin and kanamycin are more likely to damage the cochlear apparatus, but both functions may be affected by each drug. Animal studies suggest that netilmicin is the least ototoxic aminoglycoside. Although elevated serum peak and trough concentrations are thought to contribute to ototoxicity, a specific threshold for peak or trough concentrations has not been established. Some studies suggest that children are less susceptible to aminoglycoside-induced ototoxicity, but this has not been proved.[7]

Neuromuscular blockade can occur after rapid intravenous infusion, after extensive peritoneal irrigation, or during routine parenteral aminoglycoside administration in patients with underlying conditions that affect the neuromuscular junction, such as myasthenia gravis and botulism, or during concomitant administration of agents that act on the neuromuscular junction, such as succinylcholine.

To avoid toxicity and to ensure therapeutic values, concentrations of aminoglycosides in serum should be monitored in all patients with impaired renal function. Additionally, serum concentrations should be measured in patients who receive treatment for longer than 2 or 3 days (empiric therapy of suspected sepsis); this particularly is relevant to preterm, low birth weight infants. Monitoring also should be considered in obese and undernourished children and in those with chronic disease, for which the volume of distribution of the drug can be altered (e.g., cystic fibrosis).

Macrolides

Erythromycin, isolated from *Streptomyces erythreus* found in a soil sample in the Philippines, was the first macrolide available for use in 1952. Many natural and semisynthetic erythromycin derivatives have been developed since then, three of which are approved for use in pediatrics: erythromycin, clarithromycin, and azithromycin. Macrolide antibiotics consist of a large lactone ring attached by a glycosidic bond to one or more amino or neutral sugar moieties. Erythromycin and clarithromycin have 14-membered lactone rings, whereas azithromycin, an azalide antibiotic that is grouped with the macrolides, has a tertiary amino group inserted in its 15-membered ring. In addition to the similarities in chemical structure, these macrolides have similar antibacterial spectra, mechanisms of action, and mechanisms of resistance, but they differ in their pharmacokinetic characteristics.

Mechanism of Action

Macrolide antibiotics reversibly bind to the 50S ribosomal subunit, inhibiting protein synthesis. Initial studies suggested that antibacterial activity of erythromycin usually was bacteriostatic, but against some actively growing susceptible bacteria, large concentrations of erythromycin were bactericidal.[72, 73] As Mazzei and colleagues[115] noted, the specific interaction resulting in inhibition of protein synthesis is uncertain but thought to involve the dissociation of peptidyl-t-RNA from the ribosomes during the elongation step. Although the exact target or targets are controversial, several studies suggest that macrolides bind to 23S ribosomal RNA and several ribosomal proteins. Erythromycin interferes with binding to the 50S ribosome by chloramphenicol and clindamycin, suggesting common or overlapping binding sites for these agents.

Mechanisms of Resistance

Many gram-negative bacteria inherently are resistant to macrolides because of relative impermeability of their outer membrane. Other bacteria can acquire resistance because of production of enzymes that modify the macrolide, active efflux of the antibiotic, and altered ribosomal targets, the latter occurring most frequently.[94, 95, 206, 207] Two mechanisms by which bacteria can alter their ribosomes and develop macrolide resistance have been identified. High-level resistance because of an altered protein component of the 50S ribosomal subunit has occurred after a one-step chromosomal mutation. This has been demonstrated in *Bacillus subtilis*, *E. coli*, and group A streptococci. Plasmid-mediated MLS_B resistance occurs when adenine residues on the 23S RNA component of the 50S ribosomal subunit are methylated, resulting in an altered target that confers cross-resistance to macrolides, lincosamides, and streptogramin B. This resistance can be constitutive or inducible. When bacteria with inducible MLS_B resistance are exposed to subinhibitory concentrations of erythromycin, production of adenine methylase is turned on and resistance is induced, but when they are exposed to higher concentrations, protein synthesis is inhibited and induced resistance is blocked. This variable response is called dissociated resistance and can be seen in staphylococci, streptococci, and *Bacteroides* species. Less commonly, bacteria produce enzymes that inactivate the macrolide, including esterases, phosphorylases, or glycosylases found in some strains of Enterobacteriaceae. An MS pattern of resistance that is plasmid-mediated results in macrolide resistance because of active efflux. Isolates with this resistance are resistant to erythromycin and to streptogramin B but not to clindamycin.

In Vitro Activity

Erythromycin is effective in vitro against a diverse group of microorganisms, including *Bordetella pertussis*, the bacterium of legionnaires disease *(Legionella pneumophila)*, *Corynebacterium diphtheriae*, spirochetes *(Treponema pallidum)*, mycoplasmas *(Mycoplasma pneumoniae* and *Ureaplasma urealyticum)*, chlamydiae, and gram-positive cocci *(S. pneumoniae, S. pyogenes*, and penicillinase-producing and non–penicillinase-producing strains of methicillin-susceptible *S. aureus)*. Although methicillin-susceptible staphylococci and many streptococci frequently are susceptible, erythromycin-resistant group A streptococci have been reported in Scandinavian countries, France, and Japan.[174] Resistance in these countries occurred in association with increased use of erythromycin by the general population. Penicillin-resistant pneumococci frequently are resistant to macrolides. Erythromycin is highly active against *Campylobacter jejuni* and has adequate activity against *N. meningitidis* and *N. gonorrhoeae* and less activity against *H. influenzae*.

The newer macrolides have spectra of activity similar to that of erythromycin. Compared with erythromycin, clarithromycin has equivalent activity against *M. catarrhalis, H. influenzae, M. pneumoniae, Chlamydia pneumoniae*, and *L. pneumophila*. Clarithromycin is more active than erythromycin against *Chlamydia trachomatis* and *U. urealyticum* and is two to four times more active against most erythromycin-susceptible streptococci and staphylococci. The active metabolite of clarithromycin, 14-hydroxyclarithromycin, is more active than clarithromycin against *H. influenzae* and *M. catarrhalis*, and when combined with clarithromycin, their activities are additive or synergistic.[76, 103] Clarithromycin also has activity against organisms that are resistant to erythromycin, including *Toxoplasma gondii, Mycobacterium leprae*, and *M. avium-intracellulare* complex.

Compared with erythromycin, azithromycin has less activity against gram-positive bacteria but better activity against gram-negative bacteria, including some Enterobacteriaceae, although the clinical importance of the latter is uncertain. The in vitro activity of azithromycin is similar to that of erythromycin and clarithromycin against *M. pneumoniae, C. pneumoniae*, and *L. pneumophila*. Azithromycin is more active than erythromycin against *C. trachomatis* and *U. urealyticum* and more active than erythromycin or clarithromycin against *M. catarrhalis* and *H. influenzae*.[9] Azithromycin has activity against *T. gondii* and, although less than that of clarithromycin, against *M. avium-intracellulare* complex. Azithromycin and clarithromycin are highly effective in vitro against *Borrelia burgdorferi*.[151]

Pharmacokinetics

The macrolides differ in pharmacokinetic properties (Table 231–8). Clarithromycin[64, 70] and azithromycin[131] are gastric-acid–stable and fairly well absorbed from the gastrointestinal tract, whereas erythromycin is acid-labile and absorption varies with the oral preparation. Macrolides undergo metabolism by the hepatic microsomal cytochrome P450 system. Most of the metabolites are inactive with the exception of 14-(R)-hydroxyclarithromycin, an active metabolite that can act additively or synergistically with clarithromycin. The lipophilic macrolides distribute well into tissues and fluids with the exception of cerebrospinal fluid. High intracellular concentrations are achieved, but, with the exception of azithromycin, the macrolides rapidly diffuse out of cells when extracellular concentrations are low. Clarithromycin and azithromycin are transported actively into leukocytes and macrophages. High concentrations of clarithromycin are present in nasal mucosa, tonsils, and pulmonary epithelial lining fluid and alveolar cells.[37] Tissue concentrations of clarithromycin and azithromycin exceed those found in plasma by 2 to 20 times and 10 to 100 times, respectively. Isolated cases of intravascular bacterial infections developing during macrolide therapy for focal infections have been reported,[158] evoking concern that despite elevated tissue concentrations, low serum concentrations may not consistently treat systemic infections. Erythromycin and azithromycin are eliminated primarily by biliary excretion, whereas clarithromycin is excreted predominantly by the kidneys. Reduction in clarithromycin dosage may be required in patients with moderate to severe renal insufficiency. Because of their longer serum half-life values, azithromycin and clarithromycin can be dosed in a once- and twice-daily regimen, respectively, compared with three- or four-times-daily dosing necessary for erythromycin.

TABLE 231–8. Pharmacokinetics of Macrolide Antibiotics

	Erythromycin	Clarithromycin[a]	Azithromycin[b]
Bioavailability (%)	[c]	55	37
Protein binding (%)	70–90	65–75	50[d]
Half-life (hours)	1.4–2	Nonlinear[e]	11–14 (48–96)
C_{max} (μg/mL)[f]	0.8–3[c]	3–7 (1–2)[g] 2–3 (≤1)[h]	0.4 (0.25)
Elimination route			
Biliary excretion	Majority	Minimal	>50%
Renal excretion (%)	2–15	20–40 (10–15)	4.5

[a]Values in parentheses are for active metabolite, 14-OH-clarithromycin.
[b]After one 500-mg dose; values in parentheses are at steady state after 500 mg × 1 day, then 250 mg/day.
[c]Varies with oral preparation and with the presence of food.
[d]Protein binding decreases to 7% at concentrations ≥1 μg/mL.
[e]Varies with dosing; 250 mg twice a day: clarithromycin = 3–4 hours, 14-OH-C = 5–6 hours; 500 mg twice a day: clarithromycin = 5–7 hours, 14-OH-C = 7 hours.
[f]C_{max} = peak serum concentration.
[g]In children given clarithromycin suspension 7.5 mg/kg twice a day.
[h]In adults given clarithromycin tablets 500 mg twice a day.
Modified from *USP DI®, Volume I, Information for the Health Care Professional.* Copyright 1996, The USP Convention, Inc. Permission granted.

Because erythromycin base is unstable at the low pH of the stomach, better-absorbed products were prepared by addition of protective enteric coating or by alteration of the chemical structure through formations of salts and esters. The salt and ester derivatives include the ethylsuccinate or propionate (esters), the stearate (a salt), and the estolate (salt of an ester). The estolate provides the highest concentration of antimicrobial activity in serum, but there still is controversy about which preparation provides the most biologically active drug at the site of infection. Because the base is the active component, all the erythromycin preparations must be hydrolyzed to the base after absorption. Formulations of erythromycin base include tablets, delayed-release tablets, and capsules. Erythromycin estolate is marketed in capsule form, suspension, tablets, and chewable tablets. Erythromycin ethylsuccinate is available in suspension and tablet form. Parenteral preparations of erythromycin include the lactobionate and the gluceptate. Intramuscular administration of these forms is painful and should be avoided. Only oral preparations of the newer macrolides are available. Clarithromycin is available in suspension (125 mg/5 mL and 250 mg/5 mL) and in tablet (250 and 500 mg) form. Azithromycin is manufactured in 250-mg capsules and in suspension (100 mg/5 mL and 200 mg/5 mL).

Indications for Use

Erythromycin is the drug of choice for therapy of chlamydial conjunctivitis, pneumonia, and urethritis; mycoplasmal and *Legionella* pneumonia; and pertussis. It also is approved for use as a preoperative bowel preparation, for treatment of group A streptococcal sinusitis and pharyngitis and for mild pneumococcal pneumonia, uncomplicated skin and soft tissue infections caused by susceptible organisms, diphtheria, and erythrasma. It is approved for use in penicillin-allergic persons as prophylaxis for bacterial endocarditis and rheumatic fever and for treatment of syphilis.

In adults, azithromycin is approved for treatment of bacterial exacerbations of bronchitis, chlamydial cervicitis and urethritis, streptococcal tonsillitis and pharyngitis, uncomplicated skin and soft tissue infections caused by susceptible bacteria, and pneumonia caused by *H. influenzae* and *S. pneumoniae*. Pediatric indications include group A streptococcal pharyngitis[185] and acute otitis media caused by *H. influenzae, M. catarrhalis,* and *S. pneumoniae*.[119] For both conditions, a 5-day regimen has been approved. The safety and efficacy of azithromycin have not been determined for infants younger than 6 months of age.

Clarithromycin is approved for therapy of bacterial exacerbations of bronchitis, streptococcal pharyngitis, mycoplasmal and pneumococcal pneumonia, acute maxillary sinusitis, and uncomplicated skin and soft tissue infections caused by susceptible bacteria. Clinical studies suggest that clarithromycin is as safe and effective as amoxicillin for treatment of acute otitis media in children[153] and is as safe and effective as cefadroxil for treatment of skin infections.[78] The safety and efficacy of clarithromycin have not been established for infants younger than 6 months of age.

Adverse Effects

The macrolides usually are well tolerated and fairly safe. The most common adverse effect is gastrointestinal disturbances that can occur with administration of any macrolide but are associated most commonly with erythromycin use.[30] This is a dose-related phenomenon. Because it acts as a motilin receptor agonist, gastrointestinal symptoms (nausea, vomiting, diarrhea, flatulence, and abdominal cramps) can occur with orally or parenterally administered erythromycin. Enteric coating of erythromycin does not decrease the incidence. Rapid intravenous infusions of erythromycin can result in thrombophlebitis. Cholestatic hepatitis is an unusual but serious macrolide toxicity. It occurs more commonly in adults and possibly in pregnant women and is associated most commonly with the estolate preparation.[22] Onset typically begins about 16 days after beginning therapy and manifests as fever, pruritus, jaundice, elevated liver function tests, and occasionally rash, leukocytosis, and eosinophilia. Signs and symptoms resolve after discontinuation of the macrolide but recur with subsequent therapy. Other adverse reactions are uncommon. Manifestations of hypersensitivity, including rash, fever, and eosinophilia, rarely occur. Transient hearing loss has been described after administration of large dosages of erythromycin lactobionate. Torsades de pointes is an uncommon reaction to intravenous infusions of erythromycin and occasionally occurs during concomitant therapy with cisapride. Gastrointestinal overgrowth of *Candida* is an infrequent occurrence. Gastrointestinal disturbances occur less frequently with clarithromycin[38] and azithromycin, principally because lower dosages are required for effective therapy.

A common and potentially serious toxicity is that of drug interactions.[67, 147] Macrolides are metabolized by hepatic microsomal cytochrome P450 enzymes. Drug interactions can occur during concomitant therapy with two or more drugs that undergo hepatic microsomal P450 metabolism. One proposal for this drug interaction suggests that the macrolide is N-demethylated to a nitrosoalkane that interacts with and inactivates the microsomal enzyme. Toxicity can occur because of interference with metabolism, resulting in accumulation of the second drug. The ability to inactivate the enzyme varies with each macrolide; troleandomycin (a macrolide rarely used) is the most potent inhibitor, followed by erythromycin, then clarithromycin. Azithromycin has not been associated yet with nitrosoalkane formation and resulting drug interactions, but caution should be exercised with concomitant administration of other drugs known to interact with macrolides. Drugs with which macrolides can interact include astemizole, carbamazepine, cisapride, cyclosporin, digoxin, methylprednisolone, terfenadine, theophylline, triazolam, valproate, and warfarin.

Miscellaneous Antibiotics

Lincosamides

Lincosamide antibiotics consist of an amino acid linked to an amino sugar. Lincomycin, elaborated by *Streptomyces lincolnensis* variety *lincolnensis* originally isolated from a soil sample near Lincoln, Nebraska, was the first lincosamide available for use. Clindamycin, a semisynthetic derivative of lincomycin produced by the substitution of a chlorine atom for a hydroxyl group at position 7,[109] was available for use in the early 1970s. Because clindamycin has increased antibacterial activity and better oral absorption than does lincomycin, lincomycin rarely is used.

Mechanism of Action

Lincosamides bind to the 50S subunit of susceptible bacterial ribosomes, inhibiting protein synthesis. The exact mechanism of action is not known but probably involves interference with transpeptidation.[52] Because the ribosomal binding sites for lincosamides overlap with those of chloramphenicol and erythromycin, concurrent use of these agents can result in antagonism and should be avoided. Lincosamides usually are bacteriostatic but can be bactericidal against highly susceptible microorganisms in the presence of high lincosamide concentrations. Even subinhibitory concentrations can potentiate opsonization and phagocytosis of bacteria.

Mechanisms of Resistance

Some bacteria, including members of Enterobacteriaceae, *Pseudomonas,* and *Acinetobacter* species, inherently are resistant to lincosamides, most likely because of relative impermeability of the outer membrane of the cell wall. Acquired resistance can develop because of altered ribosomal target and, less commonly, lincosamide inactivation, whereas resistance because of reduced lincosamide uptake has not been described.[94, 95] Two mechanisms by which bacteria can alter their ribosomes and develop lincosamide resistance have been identified. High-level resistance because of an altered protein component of the 50S ribosomal subunit following a one-step chromosomal mutation confers resistance to erythromycin and often to the lincosamides. Plasmid-mediated MLS_B resistance occurs when adenine residues on the 23S RNA component of the 50S ribosomal subunit are methylated, resulting in an altered target that confers cross-resistance to macrolides, lincosamides, and streptogramin B. This resistance can be constitutive or inducible and can be seen in staphylococci, streptococci, and *Bacteroides* species. Erythromycin is the most potent inducer of MLS_B resistance in staphylococci, whereas any macrolide, lincosamide, or streptogramin B can be inducers in streptococci. Some strains of *B. fragilis* can have inducible MLS_B resistance not easily detected by disk agar diffusion susceptibility testing[186] but recognizable because of frequently concurrent high-level erythromycin resistance. Rarely, staphylococci produce a plasmid-mediated, nonconjugative nucleotidyltransferase that inactivates lincosamides, resulting in high-level resistance to lincomycin and tolerance to clindamycin (MBC/MIC ratio >32).

In Vitro Activity

Both lincosamides are effective in vitro against gram-positive cocci, whereas clindamycin also is active against a wide range of anaerobic bacteria. Clindamycin is many times more active than is lincomycin[118] and as active as or slightly more active than erythromycin against staphylococci, pneumococci, group A streptococci, and viridans streptococci. Unlike erythromycin, the lincosamides do not have clinically significant activity against *H. influenzae, M. pneumoniae,* or *Neisseria* species. Clindamycin is active against many gram-positive cocci, including penicillinase- and nonpenicillinase-producing staphylococci and groups A, B, C, and G beta-hemolytic streptococci and pneumococci, but is not active against enterococci or most methicillin-resistant staphylococci.[44] Many erythromycin-resistant *S. aureus* organisms are resistant to clindamycin, and those that are not often rapidly develop resistance during clindamycin therapy. Erythromycin and lincosamide resistance in pneumococci and group A streptococci has been increasing. Clindamycin has been shown to be active against most penicillin-resistant pneumococci. Most facultative gram-negative bacilli inherently are resistant to clindamycin with the exceptions of *Campylobacter* species (including *C. jejuni* and *C. fetus)* and *Helicobacter pylori.* Anaerobes frequently susceptible to clindamycin include the anaerobic gram-negative bacilli *Bacteroides, Fusobacterium, Prevotella,* and *Porphyromonas* species; the non–spore-forming gram-positive bacilli *Propionibacterium, Eubacterium,* and actinomyces; the anaerobic gram-positive cocci *Peptococcus, Peptostreptococcus,* and microaerophilic streptococci; and many *Clostridia* organisms, excluding *C. difficile, C. sporogenes,* and *C. tertium.* Clindamycin resistance does occur, especially in *Fusobacterium varium,* the non-*fragilis Bacteroides* group, up to 7 per cent of *B. fragilis,* and up to 20 per cent of anaerobic gram-positive cocci. When combined with other agents, clindamycin is active against some protozoa, such as *Babesia* species, *Plasmodium* species, *Pneumocystis carinii,* and *T. gondii.*

Pharmacokinetics

Oral absorption of lincosamides is rapid. The presence of food delays but does not decrease the absorption of clindamycin but does reduce lincomycin absorption. Concomitant administration of kaolin- or attapulgite-containing antidiarrheal agents can decrease absorption; therefore these agents should not be administered within 2 hours before or 3 to 4 hours after oral lincosamides are given. Lincosamides are distributed rapidly and widely to most tissues and fluids, including saliva, sputum, respiratory tissue, pleural fluid, soft tissues, bones and joints, prostate, semen,[145] appendix, and peritoneal fluid.[130] Lincosamides are transported actively into macrophages and polymorphonuclear leukocytes, and high concentrations are achieved in bile, urine, and bone. Penetration into cerebrospinal fluid is limited, even in the presence of inflammation. In experimental pneumococcal meningitis, concentrations of clindamycin in cerebrospinal fluid were about 10 per cent of corresponding serum values. Lincosamides are highly protein bound, with values ranging from 70 to 75 per cent for lincomycin and 92 to 94 per cent for clindamycin. The inactive palmitate and phosphate esters are hydrolyzed in the liver to clindamycin, the active agent. Clindamycin undergoes hepatic biotransformation to active and inactive metabolites. Ten per cent of absorbed lincomycins is excreted unchanged in the urine, 3 per cent is excreted unchanged in the feces, and the remainder is excreted as inactive metabolites primarily in the biliary system. Elimination is delayed in the presence of severe hepatic insufficiency alone or severe concurrent renal and hepatic impairment and can necessitate dosage adjustments. Formulations of lincosamides available for use include lincomycin hydrochloride in 250- and 500-mg capsules and in solution for parenteral use. Clindamycin phosphate, a water-soluble ester of clindamycin and phosphoric acid, is available for parenteral use. Oral formulations include clindamycin palmitate hydrochloride granules reconstituted to 75 mg base per 5 mL and clindamycin hydrochloride capsules in 75, 150, and 300 mg of the base compound. Clindamycin also is available in topical solution, gel, lotion, and vaginal cream.

Indications for Use

Lincomycin can be used for treatment of serious infections caused by susceptible strains of staphylococci, pneumococci, or other streptococci but seldom is used because of the availability of more effective agents. Clindamycin is effective against and has been approved for therapy of staphylococcal bone and joint infections[54]; anaerobic pelvic infections, including pelvic inflammatory disease, nongonococcal tubo-ovarian abscess, and postsurgical vaginal cuff infections; anaerobic intraabdominal infections, including peritonitis and abscesses; pneumonitis, empyema, and lung abscesses caused by anaerobes and as a second-line agent for those infections caused by pneumococci and staphylococci; anaerobic septicemia; and skin and soft tissue infections caused by anaerobes, staphylococci, and streptococci. It also is effective and has been approved as a topical agent for acne vulgaris. Other infections for which clindamycin may be effective but has not been approved for therapy include chronic suppurative otitis media or chronic sinusitis for which anaerobes may play a role, chronic pharyngeal carriers of group A streptococci,[188] odontogenic infections, combined with pyrimethamine for toxoplasmosis of the central nervous system, combined with quinine for uncomplicated falciparum malaria[91] or babesiosis, and combined with primaquine for mild-to-moderate *P. carinii* pneumonia in patients with AIDS.[17] Because of poor penetration into cerebrospinal fluid, it is not approved for therapy of meningitis. Clindamycin is a third-line agent for endocarditis prophylaxis for upper respiratory tract, dental, or oral procedures in persons allergic to or intolerant of amoxicillin and erythromycin.

Adverse Effects

The most frequent side effects include generalized morbilliform-like rash and mild, self-limited diarrhea occurring in up to 10 per cent and in 2 to 20 per cent of patients, respectively. Other gastrointestinal disturbances include anorexia, nausea, vomiting, flatulence, abdominal pain, and a metallic taste. Pseudomembranous colitis, a serious and sometimes fatal illness, is the most concerning adverse event. Most antibiotics have been associated with pseudomembranous colitis, but those most frequently implicated include ampicillin, lincosamides, and cephalosporins. The incidence of lincosamide-associated pseudomembranous colitis varies from 0.1 to 10 per cent. Antibiotic-associated pseudomembranous colitis is caused by overgrowth of toxin-producing strains of *C. difficile*[189]; at least two extracellular toxins are elaborated: toxin A or D-1, a potent enterotoxin, and toxin B or D-2, a cytotoxin.[177] The risk of disease is increased in elderly patients and those with chronic debilitating disease. It is unrelated to total dosage, duration of therapy, route of administration, or underlying disease. Onset most frequently occurs between days 4 and 9 of therapy, but one-third of patients develop signs and symptoms from 2 to 10 weeks after discontinuation of the antibiotic. More than 80 per cent of patients manifest fever, leukocytosis, crampy abdominal pain, and watery diarrhea, and 5 to 10 per cent have bloody diarrhea. Sigmoidoscopic findings include plaque-like lesions on colonic or rectal mucosa consisting of polymorphonuclear leukocytes, chronic inflammatory cells, fibrin, and epithelial debris. Treatment includes prompt discontinuation of the antibiotic, avoidance of antiperistaltic agents, and oral administration of metronidazole or vancomycin.

Other less common adverse events include hypersensitivity reactions, such as urticarial rash, drug fever, and eosinophilia; transient neutropenia, agranulocytosis, or thrombocytopenia; and mild, reversible elevation in hepatic transaminases. Hypotension and cardiac arrest have been reported after rapid intravenous infusion of lincomycin. Caution must be exercised when administering lincosamides to newborns; fatal gasping syndromes have been described, possibly related to the presence of the preservative benzyl alcohol.

Drug interactions include incompatibility with many agents in solution, including aminophylline, ampicillin, barbiturates, calcium gluconate, diphenylhydantoin, and magnesium sulfate, and interaction with hydrocarbon-containing inhalational anesthetics. Lincosamides are weak neuromuscular blockers[178] and can enhance neuromuscular blockade when administered concurrently with neuromuscular blockers. Chloramphenicol and macrolides can have an antagonistic effect when administered concurrently with lincosamides because of competition for ribosomal binding sites.

Chloramphenicol

Chloramphenicol, originally derived from *Streptomyces venezuela* obtained from soil near Caracas, Venezuela, in 1947, now is prepared synthetically. It is a chemically unique agent, containing an aromatic nitro group, an N-dichloroacetyl substituent, and two chiral centers. The availability of less toxic and equally or more effective agents has limited the usefulness of chloramphenicol in the United States.

Mechanism of Action

Chloramphenicol reversibly binds to the 50S subunit of 70S bacterial ribosomes, inhibiting protein synthesis. The exact mechanism remains uncertain but most likely involves suppression of peptidyltransferase activity resulting in inability to form peptide bonds.[211] Because the ribosomal binding sites of chloramphenicol overlap with those of macrolides and clindamycin, concomitant use with a macrolide or clindamycin can result in antagonism and should be avoided. Chloramphenicol usually is bacteriostatic but can be bactericidal when high concentrations are achieved against highly susceptible organisms.

Mechanisms of Resistance

The most common mechanism of acquired resistance is plasmid-mediated production of chloramphenicol acetyltransferase, which acetylates chloramphenicol, rendering it unable to bind to the ribosomal target.[211] This has been documented in many different genera of bacteria, including *H. influenzae,* members of Enterobacteriaceae, *Neisseria,* streptococci, and *S. aureus.* Less commonly, chromosomal or plasmid-mediated alterations in permeability have been a cause of chloramphenicol resistance in *E. coli, H. influenzae, P. aeruginosa,* and *B. cepacia.* Isolated cases of resistance in *B. subtilis* because of altered ribosomes and in anaerobes because of inactivation of chloramphenicol by nitroreduction have been reported.

In Vitro Activity

Chloramphenicol has broad-spectrum activity against aerobic and anaerobic gram-positive and gram-negative bacteria, chlamydiae, mycoplasmas, spirochetes, and rickettsiae.[161] It is bactericidal against susceptible strains of *H. influenzae, N. meningitidis,* and penicillin-susceptible *S. pneumoniae,* whereas it is bacteriostatic against most other susceptible microorganisms.[155] Frequently susceptible aerobic gram-positive cocci include groups A and B beta-hemolytic streptococci, viridans streptococci, and penicillin-susceptible pneumococci. Because penicillin-resistant pneumococci may be tolerant to chloramphenicol in vitro,[61] it is prudent to verify chloramphenicol susceptibility by MBC testing, especially when treating meningitis. Usually, chloramphenicol is active against methicillin-susceptible *S. aureus,* but susceptibility patterns vary with use of chloramphenicol and there are more suitable alternatives for therapy. Susceptible gram-positive bacilli include *Bacillus* species, *L. monocytogenes, C. diphtheriae, Clostridium* species, and *Eubacterium.* Most *N. meningitidis* and *N. gonorrhoeae* organisms are susceptible. The susceptibility of Enterobacteriaceae is variable, including that for *Salmonella* species and *Shigella* species. Other gram-negative bacilli frequently susceptible to chloramphenicol include *H. influenzae, Brucella, B. pertussis, P. multocida, Y. pestis, F. tularensis, Pseudomonas pseudomallei, B. cepacia, Vibrio cholerae,* and *C. jejuni.* Virtually all obligate anaerobes are susceptible.

Pharmacokinetics

After oral administration, absorption of chloramphenicol is rapid and complete. Bioavailability is approximately 80 per cent after oral administration but only 70 per cent after an intravenous dose because approximately 30 per cent of the parenterally administered dose is excreted in the urine before hydrolysis of the succinate ester to the active form. Intramuscular injection results in peak serum concentrations comparable with those achieved after intravenous infusion. Because of its lipid solubility, chloramphenicol diffuses rapidly and widely into tissues and fluids.[161] The highest concentrations are achieved in the liver and kidneys, with high concentrations present in the urine, and therapeutic concentrations are achieved in aqueous and vitreous humor. Cerebrospinal fluid concentrations range from 21 to 50 per cent and from 45 to 89 per cent of serum values in the presence of uninflamed and inflamed meninges, respectively. Brain tissue concentrations exceed those in plasma. Chloramphenicol also distributes into pleural, ascitic, and synovial fluids, saliva, and breast milk. Protein binding ranges from 32 per cent in premature newborns to 50 to 60 per cent in adults. Chloramphenicol palmitate and chloramphenicol sodium succinate are esterified prodrugs of chloramphenicol. Orally administered chloramphenicol palmitate is hydrolyzed to active drug by pancreatic esterases in the small intestines before absorption. After intravenous infusion, chloramphenicol sodium succinate is hydrolyzed rapidly to active drug in the kidneys, liver, and lungs. Ninety per cent of active chloramphenicol is conjugated to the inactive glucuronide primarily by the liver. Immature metabolic functions of the liver in the fetus and newborn result in inadequate conjugation of chloramphenicol, leading to accumulation of toxic concentrations of active drug. Peak serum concentrations in children after a dose of 25 mg/kg range from 19 to 28 μg/mL, whereas in adults receiving doses of 12.5 mg/kg, peak serum values of 11 to 18 μg/mL can be achieved. Although metabolized to inactive metabolites by the liver, chloramphenicol is excreted by the kidneys: 5 to 10 per cent as active drug and 80 per cent as inactive metabolites. Elimination half-life is significantly longer but variable, and serum concentrations are unpredictable in the neonate.[161] Dosage adjustments should be considered in persons with severe hepatic insufficiency or combined hepatic and renal insufficiency and in those patients receiving drugs that compete for hepatic P450 cytochrome oxidases, such as phenytoin, phenobarbital, and rifampin. Chloramphenicol is not removed by peritoneal dialysis or hemodialysis, but charcoal hemoperfusion may lower serum concentrations.

Formulations of chloramphenicol available include the palmitate in an oral suspension of 150 mg base/5 mL, 250-mg capsules of chloramphenicol base, and chloramphenicol sodium succinate for parenteral use. Other formulations include 1 per cent cream for topical use, 0.5 per cent otic solution, 0.5 per cent ophthalmic solution, and 1 per cent ophthalmic ointment.

Indications for Use

Because of its low therapeutic/toxic index, use of chloramphenicol should be reserved for serious infections for which less toxic agents are ineffective or contraindicated. In developed countries, chloramphenicol has been replaced by third-generation cephalosporins for treatment of bacterial meningitis and by clindamycin or metronidazole for therapy of anaerobic infections. Ceftriaxone is a safe and effective alternative to chloramphenicol for therapy of acute typhoid fever.[128] Infections for which chloramphenicol may be indicated include pneumococcal, meningococcal, or *H. influenzae* meningitis in β-lactam–allergic persons, brain abscesses caused by susceptible anaerobic bacteria resistant to other agents, acute typhoid fever, and rickettsial infections (typhus, Q fever, Rocky Mountain spotted fever), and ehrlichiosis in young patients in whom there is a relative contraindication to using tetracyclines. Chloramphenicol is not indicated for treatment of trivial infections, prophylaxis of infections, or treatment of typhoid carrier states.

Adverse Effects

Hematologic adverse events associated with chloramphenicol use include hemolytic anemia in patients with the Mediterranean type of glucose-6-phosphate dehydrogenase deficiency, reversible bone marrow suppression, and aplastic anemia. Reversible bone marrow suppression is a dose-related phenomenon. It usually occurs when serum concentrations exceed 25 μg/mL, as can be seen when administering large dosages, during prolonged therapy, or in patients with impaired liver function. Although mammalian cells contain 80S ribosomes rather than the 70S ribosomes found in procaryotes, mitochondria possess 70S ribosomes. A proposed mechanism of myelosuppression involves inhibition of host mitochondrial protein synthesis.[211] Dose-related bone marrow suppression presents with a peripheral anemia with or without reticulocytopenia, leukopenia, and thrombocytopenia and bone marrow findings of increased cellularity, cytoplasmic vacuolization, and maturation arrest of erythroid and myeloid precursors. In contrast, aplastic anemia is a rare, often fatal idiosyncratic reaction that is unrelated to dosage, duration, or route of therapy.[209] The pathogenesis is understood less well but possibly is related to DNA damage from toxic metabolites of chloramphenicol produced by nitroreduction.[211] Incidence ranges from 1 in 25,000 to 1 in 40,000 courses. Onset can begin during therapy but typically occurs weeks to months or rarely years after therapy has been discontinued. Manifestations include peripheral pancytopenia and hypoplastic or aplastic marrow.

Gray syndrome or gray baby syndrome is a rare but serious and potentially fatal adverse event that usually occurs in newborns but has been described in older children and adults with hepatic insufficiency. Most often it occurs when serum chloramphenicol concentrations exceed 40 μg/mL and is thought to be a result of inhibition of mitochondrial electron transport in liver, skeletal muscle, and myocardium. Onset typically begins 2 to 9 days after initiating therapy. Manifestations include hypothermia, tachypnea, blue-gray skin color (cyanosis), abdominal distention, emesis, unresponsiveness, and refractory metabolic acidosis that can progress to vasomotor collapse and death within 2 days.

Uncommon side effects include hypersensitivity reactions, such as drug fever, rash, urticaria, anaphylaxis, and a Herxheimer-like reaction during therapy of syphilis, typhoid fever, and brucellosis; gastrointestinal symptoms, including nausea, emesis, diarrhea, and an unpleasant taste; and neurologic symptoms, such as peripheral neuritis, headache, mental confusion, and optic neuritis,[156] the latter of which may not be reversible entirely.

Chloramphenicol can inhibit the metabolism of other drugs metabolized by hepatic microsomal cytochrome P450 system, resulting in accumulation of alfentanil, barbiturates, cyclophosphamide, phenytoin, antidiabetic sulfonylureas (more commonly with chlorpropamide and tolbutamide than with glyburide and glipizide), and warfarin during concomitant therapy.[4] Because some agents, such as rifampin,[89] phenobarbital, and phenytoin, are potent inducers of hepatic microsomal enzymes, when they are given concomitantly with chloramphenicol, metabolism is enhanced and serum concentrations of active chloramphenicol are reduced. Other drug interactions include reduction in the effectiveness of estrogen-containing oral contraceptives when used concurrently with chloramphenicol and delay in the response to vitamin B_{12}, folic acid, and iron. A mild disulfiram-like reaction can occur when alcohol is ingested during chloramphenicol therapy. Both cimetidine and chloramphenicol have rare associations with aplastic anemia; a few reports of concomitant use resulting in aplastic anemia have been documented, suggesting a potential for additive or synergistic risk.[209] Concomitant acetaminophen therapy has been the subject of controversy; some studies suggest that co-administration can prolong the elimination half-life of chloramphenicol, but other reports suggest no effect or enhanced metabolism of chloramphenicol. Lincosamides and macrolides can have an antagonistic effect when administered concurrently with chloramphenicol because of competition for ribosomal binding sites. Chloramphenicol can inhibit the in vitro bactericidal activity of cefotaxime and ceftriaxone against susceptible strains of gram-negative bacilli, group B streptococci, and *S. aureus*.[6] Chloramphenicol physically is incompatible in solution with many drugs, including carbenicillin, tetracyclines, and vancomycin.

Because of considerable variability of serum chloramphenicol concentrations, the narrow therapeutic/toxic index, and the potential for drug interactions, it is prudent to monitor serum concentrations of chloramphenicol and peripheral blood counts during therapy.

Sulfonamides

Sulfachrysoidine (Prontosil), discovered in the 1930s, was the first sulfonamide developed. Sulfonamides are broad-spectrum antimicrobial agents derived from sulfanilamide (para-aminobenzene sulfonamide) that are structural analogs of para-amino benzoic acid (PABA) and compete with PABA, resulting in interference with nucleotide synthesis. Sulfanilamide was manipulated to form other compounds with expanded antimicrobial activity and reduced toxicity. Sulfonamides are distributed widely in fluids and tissues. Currently available preparations have greater solubility and are less likely to cause crystalluria than were earlier compounds. Sulfonamides available for single-agent use include sulfacytine (Renoquid), sulfadiazine, sulfamethizole (Thiosulfil Forte), SMX (Gantanol), and sulfisoxazole (Gantrisin). Sulfonamide combinations, including TMP-SMX and erythromycin ethylsuccinate-sulfisoxazole, frequently are used in pediatrics.

Trimethoprim-Sulfamethoxazole

TMP is a diaminopyrimidine antibiotic available for single-agent use. Synergistic antibacterial activity was demonstrated with combinations of TMP and sulfonamides in the late 1960s. Because SMX has rates of absorption and elimination similar to those of TMP, it was the sulfonamide selected for combination.

MECHANISM OF ACTION. SMX competitively inhibits dihydropteroate synthetase, the bacterial enzyme that assimilates PABA into dihydrofolic acid, resulting in reduction in dihydrofolic acid synthesis and therefore reduction in the amount of tetrahydrofolic acid, a cofactor for nucleotide synthesis.[80] Only those bacteria that must synthesize folic acid potentially are susceptible. SMX is bacteriostatic when used alone and can be inhibited by PABA and its derivatives (procaine and tetracaine). TMP reversibly binds and inhibits dihydrofolate reductase, an enzyme that reduces dihydrofolic acid to tetrahydrofolic acid, resulting in diminished amounts of folic acid, an essential cofactor in nucleic acid production.[26] TMP is bacteriostatic when used alone, but in combination with SMX against susceptible bacteria, bactericidal activity can be achieved because of blockade of sequential steps in folic acid metabolism. The effect of sulfonamide in bacteria is circumvented in the mammal, which obtains folate from food sources. The reaction inhibited by TMP is similar in bacteria and mammals but differs quantitatively in the extent of binding of the drug to the enzyme; mammalian dihydrofolate reductase is 60,000 times less sensitive to TMP than is the enzyme in susceptible bacteria.

MECHANISMS OF RESISTANCE. Bacteria inherently can be resistant to either agent or can acquire resistance to TMP or SMX or both agents. Resistance to SMX and other sulfonamides is associated with hyperproduction of PABA, as demonstrated in strains of *Neisseria* species and staphylococci, or because of an altered dihydropteroate synthase enzyme with lower affinity for sulfonamides, as found in *E. coli*.[191] *P. aeruginosa* inherently is resistant to TMP because of cell wall impermeability, whereas *Nocardia* and many anaerobes are resistant because of a TMP-insensitive dihydrofolate reductase. Acquired resistance to TMP can be plasmid-mediated or chromosomal and occurs in members of Enterobacteriaceae, staphylococci, and streptococci. Mechanisms of acquired TMP resistance include cell wall impermeability, thymine auxotrophy, resistant dihydrofolate reductase, and overproduction of dihydrofolate reductase,[83] the most common being plasmid-mediated production of dihydrofolate reductases that are resistant to TMP. Bacteria can develop resistance to both TMP and SMX because of altered cell wall permeability or alternative metabolic pathways (e.g., thymine auxotrophy), whereby they obtain thymine or thymidine from the environment.[191]

IN VITRO ACTIVITY. TMP-SMX has significant activity against a broad spectrum of gram-positive cocci and gram-negative enteric pathogens. TMP is more active than is the sulfonamide, but the mixture is significantly more effective than either drug alone. Synergism is more likely if the bacteria are susceptible to both drugs but can occur even when bacteria are resistant to one agent. Those bacteria with potential susceptibility to the combination include *Brucella, B. cepacia, E. coli, Haemophilus, M. catarrhalis, N. gonorrhoeae, Nocardia, Proteus, Salmonella, Shigella, Serratia marcescens,* methicillin-susceptible *S. aureus, Stenotrophomonas maltophilia,* penicillin-susceptible *S. pneumoniae,* some environmental mycobacteria, *Yersinia enterocolitica,* and the protozoan parasite, *P. carinii.*

PHARMACOKINETICS. Optimal synergistic activity occurs when a 1:20 ratio of TMP and SMX serum concentrations is attained, which can be achieved after administration of a fixed 1:5 ratio of TMP to SMX. Both agents are absorbed rapidly and fairly well when administered alone and in combination. Both penetrate most body fluids and tissues, although TMP frequently penetrates extravascular tissues to a greater degree than does SMX. Both agents cross the placenta, are excreted in breast milk, and diffuse into pleural, peritoneal, synovial, and cerebrospinal fluid. Protein binding varies from 40 to 60 per cent for TMP and from 60 to 70 per cent for SMX. Both are metabolized in the liver to inactive metabolites. The primary route of elimination is by the kidneys, with small amounts excreted in the bile and feces. Dosage adjustments are required for renal impairment.

Available preparations include an oral suspension containing 40 mg of TMP and 200 mg of SMX per 5 mL, tablets containing 80 mg of TMP and 400 mg of SMX, double-strength tablets consisting of 160 mg of TMP and 800 mg of SMX, and a parenteral solution.

INDICATIONS FOR USE. TMP-SMX is approved for therapy of acute exacerbations of chronic bronchitis in adults, enterocolitis caused by susceptible *Shigella* organisms, acute otitis media caused by *H. influenzae* or pneumococcus, *P. carinii* pneumonia, traveler's diarrhea caused by *Shigella* and enterotoxigenic *E. coli,* and acute or chronic urinary tract infections. Although not approved for use and not usually prescribed as a first-line antibiotic, TMP-SMX has been effective therapy for typhoid fever, brucellosis, nocardiosis, sinusitis, biliary tract infections, and bone and joint infections caused by susceptible organisms. It also has been used for *P. carinii* pneumonia prophylaxis in immunosuppressed children with cancer and patients infected with HIV and for prophylaxis of recurrent bacterial urinary tract infections. Because early studies did not evaluate the effect of prolonged or recurrent therapy on somatic growth or bone marrow function in children, TMP-SMX was not approved for prophylaxis or prolonged treatment of otitis media. It is not recommended for therapy of group A streptococcal tonsillopharyngitis because it does not eradicate the organism or prevent the nonsuppurative sequelae reliably.

ADVERSE EFFECTS. Most of the side effects occurring during administration of TMP-SMX are caused by the sulfonamide. Gastrointestinal disturbances and hypersensitivity reactions are the most commonly observed adverse events. Anorexia, nausea, vomiting, diarrhea, drug eruption, and photosensitivity reactions can occur in 1 to 4 per cent of patients. Less frequent hypersensitivity reactions include erythema nodosum, erythema multiforme (including Stevens-Johnson syndrome), urticaria, anaphylaxis, and thyroid damage. Drug-induced hepatitis has been described but is unusual. Central nervous system side effects include vertigo, ataxia, headache, and aseptic meningitis. TMP-SMX can affect renal function when administered to persons with underlying renal disease, but it usually is reversible after discontinuation of therapy. Crystalluria was more common with earlier preparations because of low solubility. SMX has a greater tendency to cause crystalluria than do other currently available sulfonamides because of slower absorption and excretion, but with adequate fluid intake, alkalinization of the urine usually is unnecessary. Interstitial nephritis and tubular necrosis seldom are associated with TMP-SMX use. Blood dyscrasias can be a limiting factor to administration of TMP-SMX. Acute hemolytic anemia has been described after TMP-SMX use in patients with glucose-6-phosphate dehydrogenase deficiency. Although uncommon in patients with normal hematopoietic systems, aplastic anemia, agranulocytosis, leukopenia, and thrombocytopenia can occur. Prolonged use can result in megaloblastic anemia because of impaired folate utilization. Sulfonamide administration can trigger an acute attack of porphyria. Sulfonamides can displace bilirubin from albumin binding sites. Neonates, especially premature infants, can have increased activity of sulfonamides because of reduced conjugation by the immature liver. Because of the increased risk of kernicterus from sulfonamide displacement of bilirubin, use of sulfonamides during the last month of pregnancy and in neonates is discouraged.

Drug-drug interactions with TMP-SMX are numerous. Sulfonamides can displace other drugs from albumin-binding sites, resulting in increased effective activity of the second drug, as can be seen with concurrent administration of methotrexate,[55] phenytoin, sulfonylurea hypoglycemic agents, thiazide diuretics, and warfarin. Drugs that when co-administered can displace sulfonamides from binding sites and lead to increased effective sulfonamide activity include indomethacin, phenylbutazone, probenecid, salicylates, and sulfinpyrazone. Agents that reduce the effect of sulfonamides include methenamine, which results in insoluble urinary precipitates of the sulfonamide, and derivatives of PABA. Sulfonamides physically are incompatible with many drugs, among them aminoglycosides, chloramphenicol, insulin, lincomycin, methicillin, tetracycline, and vancomycin.

Erythromycin Ethylsuccinate-Sulfisoxazole Acetyl

The combination of erythromycin ethylsuccinate and sulfisoxazole acetyl (EES-SSX) in a fixed ratio expands the spectrum of antibacterial activity. The mechanism of action, mechanisms of resistance, pharmacokinetics, and adverse events for EES-SSX are the same as those for each individual drug. Because EES-SSX is effective in vitro against common pathogens causing otitis media in children,[21] it was approved for therapy of acute otitis media. Although not approved for use, it can be effective for therapy of sinusitis caused by *H. influenzae,* pneumococci, and *M. catarrhalis.*

Tetracyclines

Chlortetracycline, also known as Aureomycin, was the first natural tetracycline discovered when isolated from *Streptomyces aureofaciens* in 1948.[57] Many tetracyclines have been developed since then. Those currently marketed include the natural agents tetracycline, oxytetracycline, and demeclocycline and the semisynthetic agents doxycycline and minocycline. Their basic structure consists of a hydronaphthacene nucleus with four fused rings. They differ from each other biochemically by substituent variations at carbons 5, 6, or 7. Their mechanism of action and mechanisms of resistance as well as their spectra of activity are similar, but the analogs differ in degree of activity and in pharmacokinetic properties. Glycylcyclines, a new generation of tetracyclines with improved activity against drug-resistant bacteria, are in phase I clinical studies.[187]

Mechanism of Action

Tetracyclines are bacteriostatic agents that reversibly bind to the 30S subunit of 70S bacterial ribosomes, inhibiting protein synthesis. Because attachment of aminoacyl-tRNA to the ribosome acceptor site is prevented, the bacteria are unable to add amino acids to the growing peptide chain. According to studies of tetracycline in *E. coli,* tetracyclines passively diffuse through outer-membrane porins and then traverse the cytoplasmic membrane by energy-independent and energy-dependent mechanisms; the precise molecular nature of the latter is inconclusive.[34]

Mechanisms of Resistance

Many bacteria, including members of Enterobacteriaceae, *P. aeruginosa,* staphylococci, streptococci, and *Bacteroides,* have developed resistance to tetracyclines. Resistance most often is carried on plasmids but can be chromosomal. The genes encoding for resistance are called *tet,* or tetracycline resistance determinants. Resistance to one tetracycline usually implies resistance to all; however, many tetracycline-resistant bacteria are susceptible to doxycycline, minocycline, or both. The most common mechanism of resistance results from active efflux. *Tet* genes encode for membrane proteins that mediate energy-dependent efflux. These proteins are different in gram-positive and gram-negative bacteria. Efflux has been found in Enterobacteriaceae, enterococci, streptococci, staphylococci, *V. cholerae, Bacteroides, Peptostreptococcus, Eubacterium,* and others. Less commonly, resistance from altered ribosomal targets encoded by different *tet* genes has been found in *N. gonorrhoeae, Mycoplasma,* and *Ureaplasma,* as well as in periodontal isolates of *Veillonella, Fusobacterium nucleatum, Peptostreptococcus,* and *Prevotella* species.[144] Enzymatic inactivation of tetracycline, encoded for by another *tet* gene, has been demonstrated in in vitro studies of aerobically grown *E. coli,* but the clinical significance has not been established.

IN VITRO ACTIVITY

The tetracyclines are broad-spectrum antibiotics with activity against aerobic and anaerobic gram-positive and gram-negative bacteria, chlamydiae, mycoplasmas, rickettsiae, and spirochetes. Activity against gram-negative bacteria has been limited by emergence of tetracycline-resistant strains. Most *P. aeruginosa* and many *Shigella* and *Salmonella* organisms are resistant. Penicillin-susceptible strains of *N. gonorrhoeae* and *N. meningitidis* usually are susceptible to tetracyclines, but penicillin-resistant strains of *N. gonorrhoeae* are not. Gram-negative organisms with continued susceptibility to tetracyclines include *Aeromonas hydrophila, Brucella, Campylobacter,* some *Haemophilus* organisms, *Helicobacter, P. multocida, Plesiomonas shigelloides,* and *Vibrio.* Tetracyclines are active against some gram-positive bacilli, including *Actinomyces israelii, Bacillus anthracis,* many clostridia, *Listeria,* and *Nocardia.* Tetracyclines have excellent activity against *Chlamydia, M. pneumoniae,* and rickettsiae. Other organisms for which tetracyclines have activity include *Mycobacterium marinum* and *B. burgdorferi.* The more lipophilic agents, doxycycline and minocycline, usually are more active than the others. Minocycline has excellent activity against staphylococci, and both doxycycline and minocycline are more active than tetracycline against *S. aureus* and some streptococci but have no activity against enterococci and group B streptococci. Because of extensive plasmid-mediated resistance in pneumococci, therapy with tetracycline should be avoided. Doxycycline and minocycline are more active than the other agents against anaerobic bacteria.

PHARMACOKINETICS

The five tetracycline compounds available for systemic use can be classified by duration of activity: tetracycline and oxytetracycline are short-acting agents, demeclocycline is intermediate-acting, and doxycycline and minocycline are long-acting agents (Table 231–9). Oral administration is the preferred route because of thrombophlebitis associated with intravenous infusion and pain associated with intramuscular injections. Oral absorption ranges from 58 per cent for the short-acting agents to 100 per cent for the long-acting ones. The presence of food decreases the absorption of demeclocycline, oxytetracycline, and tetracycline. Because tetracyclines form insoluble complexes in the gut with aluminum, calcium, iron, magnesium, zinc, and other bivalent and trivalent cations, co-administration with milk and other dairy products, antacids, calcium or iron supplements, cathartics, and other agents can reduce absorption and should be avoided. The differences in lipid solubility affect tissue penetration of the various tetracyclines. All agents readily penetrate many tissues and fluids, among which are pleural, ascitic, and synovial fluids, sinus secretions, sputum, bone, teeth, and breast milk. Tetracyclines can cross the placenta. Highest concentrations are achieved in the bile and can exceed serum concentrations by 5 to 20 times. Therapeutic concentrations of doxycycline can be achieved in tonsillar and pulmonary tissues, the eye, and the prostate,[40] and high concentrations are achieved in myometrial and endometrial tissue[167] and kidney. Minocycline penetrates into sputum, saliva, and tears and into cells of the vestibular apparatus.[86] Minocycline is biotransformed to inactive metabolites by the liver; the other tetracyclines are not metabolized, although it is not clear whether doxycycline is metabolized. Oxytetracycline, demeclocycline, and tetracycline are eliminated unchanged in the urine. Approximately 10 per cent of minocycline is excreted unchanged in the urine, 20 to 35 per cent is excreted unchanged in the feces, and the remainder is excreted as inactive metabolites in the urine and feces. Thirty to forty per cent of doxycycline is excreted in the urine; the remainder is excreted by the biliary tract and by diffusion through the intestinal wall, where some of it is chelated and prevented from reabsorption and enterohepatic cycling. Dosing of short- and intermediate-acting tetracyclines must be adjusted for renal failure.

Systemic formulations available in the United States include tablets, capsules, delayed-release capsules, and suspension for many of the tetracyclines, as well as parenteral preparations of doxycycline, minocycline, and oxytetracycline. Ophthalmic and topical preparations also are available.

INDICATIONS FOR USE

With few exceptions, tetracyclines no longer are the drug of choice for many infections because of the availability of cephalosporins and semisynthetic penicillins with equivalent or greater activity and less frequent side effects. Because of the potential for dental toxicity, tetracyclines are not recommended for use in children younger than 9 years of age, except for specific infections for which alternative therapy potentially is more toxic, such as chloramphenicol for Rocky Mountain spotted fever[2] and ehrlichiosis. Approved indications in the United States include treatment of actinomycosis, anthrax, brucellosis, inclusion conjunctivitis,[168] psittacosis, Q fever, rickettsial pox, Rocky Mountain spotted fever, typhus,

TABLE 231–9. Pharmacokinetics of Tetracyclines

Drug	Oral Absorption (%)	Protein Binding (%)	Primary Route of Excretion	Approximate Half-Life* (hours)
Short-acting				
Oxytetracycline	58	35	Renal	6–10
Tetracycline	75	65	Renal	6–11
Intermediate-acting				
Demeclocycline	66	91	Renal	10–17
Long-acting				
Doxycycline	90–100	93	Gastrointestinal	12–22
Minocycline	90–100	76	Biliary	11–23

*Normal renal function.
Modified from *USP DI®, Volume I, Information for the Health Care Professional.* Copyright 1996, The USP Convention, Inc. Permission granted.

relapsing fever, syphilis, trachoma,[168] yaws, Vincent necrotizing gingivostomatitis caused by *Fusobacterium,* and infections caused by *Bacteroides* species, *Bartonella bacilliformis, C. fetus, F. tularensis, M. pneumoniae, V. cholerae, Y. pestis,* and others. Because of its excellent tissue penetration and spectrum of activity, doxycycline is the preferred tetracycline for therapy of atypical pneumonias caused by *M. pneumoniae* and *C. pneumoniae,* intra-abdominal or pelvic infections, and several sexually transmitted diseases, including granuloma inguinale, chlamydial infections, *U. urealyticum* infection, nongonococcal urethritis, pelvic inflammatory disease (plus cefoxitin), proctitis (plus ceftriaxone), and prostatitis. Doxycycline is an alternative drug for (nonpregnant) penicillin-allergic patients with primary, secondary, or late latent syphilis. Although minocycline is effective for eradicating nasopharyngeal carriage of meningococcus, its potential for vestibular toxicity precludes its use for this purpose. Topical tetracyclines have been used extensively for treatment of acne vulgaris and other dermatologic illnesses.[82]

ADVERSE EFFECTS

Gastrointestinal disturbances are the most common side effect associated with tetracycline use and include anorexia, nausea, emesis, flatulence, and diarrhea. These symptoms occur less frequently with minocycline. Esophageal ulceration had been associated with oral administration of tetracyclines.[60] All tetracyclines except doxycycline can cause a negative nitrogen balance with an elevation in blood urea nitrogen that usually is not significant except in the presence of underlying renal insufficiency. Demeclocycline can cause nephrogenic diabetes insipidus and, for this reason, has been used for treatment of the syndrome of inappropriate antidiuretic hormone secretion. Rarely, tetracyclines have been associated with hepatic injury manifested by elevated transaminases and diffuse vacuolar fatty metamorphosis on biopsy, with or without pancreatitis. It is dose-related, and the risk is increased with pregnancy, malnutrition, and preexisting renal or hepatic disease and in patients receiving other hepatotoxic agents. There is a relative contraindication for use of tetracyclines in children younger than 9 years of age because tetracyclines chelate with calcium and can deposit in developing bones and teeth, leading to transient decrease in bone growth, permanent tooth discoloration, and enamel hypoplasia. The risk of these side effects with one course using appropriate dosages is low; the degree of tooth discoloration is associated with total dosage administered.[69] Minocycline has been associated with reversible vestibular toxicity. All tetracyclines have been associated with pseudotumor cerebri, a benign elevation in intracranial pressure that is reversible after discontinuation of the drug. Some data suggest that there could be an increased risk with concurrent use of tetracycline and isotretinoin.[96] Tetracyclines have been associated with an exaggerated sunburn reaction with sun exposure. This occurs most frequently with demeclocycline and rarely with minocycline. Hypersensitivity reactions are infrequent and include morbilliform rash, urticaria, exfoliative dermatitis, and rarely anaphylaxis. Hyperpigmentation of mucosal membranes, skin, and nails has been noted with tetracycline use, particularly with minocycline.

Drug-drug interactions are numerous. Decrease in absorption of tetracyclines can occur with co-administration of oral antacids, bismuth subsalicylate, iron, kaolin or pectin, zinc sulfate, and other divalent or trivalent cations that chelate the antibiotic. Reduced effect of tetracyclines because of increased metabolism is associated with concomitant use of doxycycline with barbiturates, carbamazepine, phenytoin, rifampin, and alcohol in heavy drinkers. Co-administration with tetracyclines can increase the effect of oral anticoagulants, digoxin, lithium, and theophylline and can decrease the effect of oral contraceptive agents and oral iron. Tetracyclines can inhibit the in vitro bactericidal activity of penicillins and aminoglycosides. Other drug-drug interactions include benign intracranial hypertension with concomitant administration of vitamin A, severe nephrotoxicity with co-administration of methoxyflurane and tetracycline, and localized hemosiderosis with amitriptyline and minocycline.

Fluoroquinolones

Fluoroquinolone antibiotics are derivatives of nalidixic acid. Compared with nalidixic acid, fluoroquinolones have a broader spectrum of activity that includes gram-negative enterics, *P. aeruginosa,* staphylococci, but not all streptococci; better penetration into tissues; and rapid bactericidal activity. They have been used extensively in adults for treatment of skin and soft tissue infections, skeletal infections, and infections of the urinary and respiratory tracts. Use in pediatric patients has been limited because of the potential for induction of arthropathy, as demonstrated in juvenile animal studies. Fluoroquinolones are not approved for use in children but have been used in certain settings, primarily because they are the only oral antibiotics with activity against *P. aeruginosa.* They have been used to treat exacerbations of chronic pseudomonal pulmonary infections in patients with cystic fibrosis, complicated urinary tract infections caused by multiple drug-resistant bacteria, chronic suppurative otitis media, and multidrug-resistant bacterial meningitis.[171] In vitro studies of investigational fluoroquinolones against penicillin- and cephalosporin-resistant pneumococci look promising. Further clinical studies of the safety and efficacy of fluoroquinolones in children are warranted.

SELECTED ASPECTS OF THE ADMINISTRATION OF ANTIMICROBIAL AGENTS

Dosage Schedules for Infants and Children

Dosage schedules of antimicrobial agents commercially available in the United States for infants (beyond the newborn period) and children are listed in Table 231–10. The list is subdivided into dosage schedules for mild to moderate and for severe disease. Oral regimens are used for mild to moderate infections caused by susceptible organisms in areas that are well vascularized and in which adequate concentrations of drug are achieved at the site of infection. Parenteral administration should be considered for severe infections, especially those caused by less susceptible organisms producing disease in areas in which diffusion of drug is limited.

Dosage Schedules for Newborn Infants

The clinical pharmacology of antimicrobial agents administered to the newborn infant is unique and cannot be extrapolated from data in older children or adults.[166] Physiologic and metabolic processes that affect the distribution, metabolism, and excretion of drugs undergo rapid changes during the first few weeks of life. The increased efficiency of kidney function after the first 7 days requires an increase in dosage and a decrease in interval between doses of penicillins and aminoglycosides for maintaining therapeutic concentrations of drug in the blood and tissues. Thus, different dosage schedules are provided for the first week of life and for the subsequent weeks of the neonatal period (Tables 231–11 and 231–12). With survival of very low birth weight, premature

TABLE 231–10. Daily Dosage Schedules for Antimicrobial Agents in Pediatric Patients Beyond the Newborn Period

Agent, Generic (Trade name)	Route	Mild to Moderate Infections	Severe Infections
Penicillin G, crystalline (numerous)	IV, IM	25,000–50,000 units ÷ into four doses	100,000–250,000 units ÷ into six doses
Penicillin G, procaine (numerous)	IM	25,000–50,000 units ÷ into one to two doses	Inappropriate
Penicillin G, benzathine (Bicillin)	IM	<30 lb = 600,000 units; 30–60 lb = 1,200,000 units; >60 lb = 2,400,000 units	Inappropriate
Penicillin G, potassium (numerous)	PO	25–50 mg ÷ into three to four doses	Inappropriate
Penicillin V, phenoxymethyl penicillin (numerous)	PO	25–50 mg ÷ into three to four doses	Inappropriate
Penicillinase-resistant penicillins			
Methicillin (Staphcillin)	IV, IM	100–200 mg ÷ into four doses	200–300 mg ÷ into four to six doses
Oxacillin (Prostaphlin, Bactocill)	IV, IM	50–100 mg ÷ into four doses	150–200 mg ÷ into four to six doses
Nafcillin (Nafcil, Unipen)	IV, IM	50–100 mg ÷ into four doses	100–200 mg ÷ into four to six doses
Cloxacillin (Cloxapen, Tegopen)	PO	50–100 mg ÷ into four doses	Inappropriate
Dicloxacillin (Dycill, Dynapen, Pathocil)	PO	12–25 mg ÷ into four doses	Inappropriate
Aminopenicillins			
Ampicillin (numerous)	IV, IM	100–200 mg ÷ into four doses	200–400 mg ÷ into four doses
	PO	50–100 mg ÷ into four doses	Inappropriate
Ampicillin + sulbactam (Unasyn)	IV	Inappropriate	100–200 mg of ampicillin ÷ into four doses
Amoxicillin (Amoxil, Larotid, Polymox, Trimox, Wymox)	PO	20–40 mg ÷ into three doses	Inappropriate
Amoxicillin + clavulanate (Augmentin)	PO	20–40 mg ÷ into three doses	Inappropriate
Extended-spectrum penicillins			
Carbenicillin indanyl (Geocillin)	PO	30–50 mg ÷ into four doses	Inappropriate
Ticarcillin (Ticar)	IV	50–100 mg ÷ into four doses	200–300 mg ÷ into four to six doses
Ticarcillin + clavulanate (Timentin)	IV	Inappropriate	200–300 mg ÷ into four to six doses
Mezlocillin (Mezlin)	IV	Inappropriate	200–300 mg ÷ into four to six doses
Piperacillin (Pipracil)	IV	Inappropriate	200–300 mg ÷ into four to six doses
Cephalosporins			
Cephalothin (Keflin)	IV, IM	50–100 mg ÷ into four doses	100–125 mg ÷ into four to six doses
Cefazolin (Ancef, Kefzol)	IV, IM	50 mg ÷ into four doses	50–100 mg ÷ into three to four doses
Cephalexin (Keflex, Keftab)	PO	25–50 mg ÷ into four doses	Inappropriate
Cefadroxil (Duricef)	PO	30 mg ÷ into two doses	Inappropriate
Cefaclor (Ceclor)	PO	40 mg ÷ into three doses	Inappropriate
Cefprozil (Cefzil)	PO	30 mg ÷ into two doses	Inappropriate
Loracarbef (Lorabid)	PO	15–30 mg ÷ into two doses	Inappropriate
Cefuroxime axetil (Ceftin)	PO	30–40 mg ÷ into two doses	Inappropriate
Cefuroxime (Kefurox, Zinacef)	IV, IM	Inappropriate	100–200 mg ÷ into three doses
Cefoxitin (Mefoxin)	IV	Inappropriate	80–160 mg ÷ into four to six doses
Cefixime (Suprax)	PO	8 mg ÷ into one to two doses	Inappropriate
Cefpodoxime proxetil (Vantin)	PO	10 mg ÷ into two doses	Inappropriate
Cefotaxime (Claforan)	IV, IM	Inappropriate	100–200 mg ÷ into three to four doses
Ceftriaxone (Rocephin)	IV, IM	Inappropriate	75–100 mg ÷ into one or two doses
Ceftazidime (Fortaz, Tazicef, Tazidime)	IV, IM	Inappropriate	100–150 mg ÷ into three doses
Macrolides			
Erythromycin glucoheptonate (Ilotycin Gluceptate)	IV	Inappropriate	20–50 mg ÷ into four doses

Table continued on following page

TABLE 231–10. Daily Dosage Schedules for Antimicrobial Agents in Pediatric Patients Beyond the Newborn Period *Continued*

Agent, Generic (Trade name)	Route	Mild to Moderate Infections	Severe Infections
Macrolides *(Continued)*			
Erythromycin lactobionate (Erythrocin Lactobionate)	IV	Inappropriate	20–50 mg ÷ into four doses
Erythromycin base (numerous)	PO	20–40 mg ÷ into four doses	Inappropriate
Erythromycin ethylsuccinate (EES, EryPed, Wyamycin E)	PO	20–40 mg ÷ into four doses	Inappropriate
Erythromycin stearate (Erythrocin Stearate, Wyamycin S)	PO	20–40 mg ÷ into four doses	Inappropriate
Erythromycin estolate (Ilosone)	PO	30–40 mg ÷ into four doses	Inappropriate
Clarithromycin (Biaxin)	PO	15 mg ÷ into two doses	Inappropriate
Azithromycin (Zithromax)	PO	10 mg on day 1, then 5 mg thereafter	Inappropriate
Lincosamides			
Lincomycin (Lincocin)	IV, IM	10 mg ÷ into two to three doses	20 mg ÷ into two to three doses
Clindamycin (Cleocin)	IV, IM	Inappropriate	25–40 mg ÷ into four doses
	PO	20–30 mg ÷ into four doses	Inappropriate
Vancomycin (Vancocin)	IV	Inappropriate	30–60 mg ÷ into four doses
Aminoglycosides			
Amikacin (Amikin)	IV, IM	Inappropriate	15–22 mg ÷ into three doses
Gentamicin (Garamycin)	IV, IM	Inappropriate	5–7.5 mg ÷ into three doses
Kanamycin (Kantrex)	IV, IM	Inappropriate	15–30 mg ÷ into three doses
Netilmicin (Netromycin)	IV, IM	Inappropriate	3–7.5 mg ÷ into three doses
Paromomycin (Humatin)	PO	30 mg ÷ into three doses	Inappropriate
Streptomycin (numerous)	IM	Inappropriate	20–40 mg ÷ into two doses
Tobramycin (Nebcin)	IV, IM	Inappropriate	3–6 mg ÷ into three doses
Tetracyclines			
Tetracycline (numerous)	PO	25–50 mg ÷ into four doses	Inappropriate
Doxycycline (Doryx, Vibramycin, Vibratabs)	PO	4 mg ÷ into two doses, then 2 mg once daily	Inappropriate
	IV	Inappropriate	2–4 mg once daily
Chloramphenicol (Chlormycetin)	IV	Inappropriate	50–100 mg ÷ into three to four doses
	PO	Inappropriate	50–75 mg ÷ into three to four doses
Sulfonamides			
Sulfadiazine	IV, SC	Inappropriate	100 mg ÷ into four doses
Sulfisoxazole (Gantrisin)	PO	120 mg ÷ into 4 doses	Inappropriate
Trimethoprim-sulfamethoxazole (Bactrim, Septra, Sulfatrim)	PO	8 mg trimeth/40 mg sulfa ÷ into two doses	Inappropriate
	IV	Inappropriate	10–20 mg trimeth/50–100 mg sulfa ÷ into four doses
Erythromycin ethylsuccinate-sulfisoxazole (Pediazole, Eryzole)	PO	40 mg erythro/120 mg sulfa ÷ into four doses	Inappropriate

*For larger children, maximum dosages may apply.
PO, orally; IV, intravenously; IM, intramuscularly; SC, subcutaneously.

infants, more data are needed about use of antimicrobial agents in these infants with immature metabolic and physiologic mechanisms.[152, 166]

Should Dosages Be Determined by Weight or by Surface Area?

In most standard pediatric texts and in the package inserts prepared by manufacturers, dosages of antibiotics for children are based on body weight. Body surface area correlates more closely with extracellular fluid volume. Some investigators suggest that more predictable serum concentrations can be achieved by use of calculations of dosages based on surface area[77] than by use of those based on weight.[176] This method may be more reliable for drugs that are distributed in extracellular fluid, such as aminoglycosides, especially when prescribed for obese or malnourished children. Currently, however, the convenience of calculating dosage on the basis of weight appears to be the more important consideration.

Use of Oral Preparations for Serious Infections

Oral preparations of antimicrobial agents vary in their degree of absorption from individual to individual and

TABLE 231–11. Dosage Schedules for Antimicrobial Agents Frequently Used in Neonates

Antibiotic	Route	Dosage (mg/kg) and Interval of Administration				
		Weight <1200 g	*Weight 1200–2000 g*		*Weight >2000 g*	
		Age 0–4 Weeks	*Age 0–7 Days*	*Age >7 Days*	*Age 0–7 Days*	*Age >7 Days*
Penicillin G, crystalline (units)	IV	25,000 q 12h	25,000 q 12h	25,000 q 8h	25,000 q 8h	25,000 q 6h
Penicillin G, procaine (units)	IM		50,000 q 24h	50,000 q 24h	50,000 q 24h	50,000 q 24h
Penicillin G, benzathine (units)	IM		50,000 once	50,000 once	50,000 once	50,000 once
Penicillinase-resistant penicillins						
Methicillin	IV, IM	25 q 12h	25 q 12h	25 q 8h	25 q 8h	25 q 6h
Oxacillin	IV, IM	25 q 12h	25 q 12h	25 q 8h	25 q 8h	37.5 q 6h
Nafcillin	IM	25 q 12h	25 q 12h	25 q 8h	25 q 8h	37.5 q 6h
Broad-spectrum penicillins						
Ampicillin	IV, IM					
Meningitis		50 q 12h	50 q 12h	50 q 8h	50 q 8h	50 q 6h
Other infections		25 q 12h	25 q 12h	25 q 8h	25 q 8h	25 q 6h
Ticarcillin	IV	75 q 12h	75 q 12h	75 q 8h	75 q 8h	75 q 6h
Cephalosporins						
Cefazolin	IV, IM	20 q 12h	20 q 12h	20 q 12h	20 q 12h	20 q 8h
Cefotaxime	IV, IM	50 q 12h	50 q 12h	50 q 8h	50 q 12h	50 q 8h
Ceftriaxone	IV, IM	50 q 24h	50 q 24h	50 q 24h	50 q 24h	75 q 24h
Ceftazidime	IV, IM	50 q 12h	50 q 12h	50 q 8h	50 q 8h	50 q 8h
Chloramphenicol*	IV	25 q 24h	25 q 24h	25 q 24h	25 q 24h	25 q 12h
Clindamycin	IV, IM	5 q 12h	5 q 12h	5 q 8h	5 q 8h	5 q 6h
Erythromycin	PO	10 q 12h	10 q 12h	10 q 8h	10 q 12h	10 q 8h

IM, intramuscularly; IV, intravenously; PO, orally.
Modified from Sáez-Llorens, X., and McCracken, G. H., Jr.: Clinical pharmacology of antibacterial agents. *In* Remington, J. S., and Klein, J. O. (eds.): Infectious Diseases of the Fetus and Newborn Infant. 4th ed. Philadelphia, W. B. Saunders, 1995, p. 1325.
*Use with caution in neonates. Appropriate dosage schedule should be based on serum concentration measurements.

within an individual, depending on the illness being treated and the formulation used. Because higher and more consistent serum concentrations of drug are achieved after parenteral administration, the parenteral routes are preferable for serious infections. Sequential parenteral-oral antimicrobial therapy may be an option in patients with uncomplicated pneumonia, pyelonephritis, and suppurative skeletal infections.[117] Results of studies[133, 190] of orally administered antibiotics in children with skeletal infections indicate that this mode of administration can be used successfully for a portion of the therapeutic course.

Specific guidelines for oral therapy of serious infections are recommended: (1) the patient is able to swallow and retain the medication, (2) the dosage is large enough to provide adequate bactericidal concentrations of drug at the site of infection, and (3) the hospital laboratory can perform serum antimicrobial concentration determinations or the serum minimal inhibitory and minimal bactericidal titers to ensure therapeutic values.

Oral therapy can be considered for osteomyelitis and suppurative arthritis only after an initial period of parenteral therapy (5 to 7 days), after results are available from cultures and susceptibility tests, and after there are definite signs of resolution of inflammation. Oral therapy should be initiated before discharge from the hospital in order to ascertain compliance, to determine serum antimicrobial concentrations, and to observe for significant side effects that would preclude use of the oral antibiotic.

Food Interferes with the Absorption of Some Oral Antibiotics

The absorption of some oral antimicrobial agents is decreased significantly when the drug is taken with food or

TABLE 231–12. Dosage Schedule for Antibiotics Based on Postconceptual Age

Antibiotic	Route	Dosage (mg/kg) and Interval of Administration: Gestational Age Plus Weeks of Life			
		≤26	*27–34*	*35–42*	*≥43*
Amikacin	IV, IM	7.5 q 24h	7.5 q 18h	10 q 12h	10 q 8h
Gentamicin	IV, IM	2.5 q 24h	2.5 q 18h	2.5 q 12h	2.5 q 8h
Tobramycin	IV, IM	2.5 q 24h	2.5 q 18h	2.5 q 12h	2.5 q 8h
Vancomycin	IV	15 q 24h	15 q 18h*	15 q 12h*	15 q 8h*

*At 28 days of life, vancomycin is dosed at 20 mg/kg/dose; the interval remains the same.
IM, intramuscularly; IV, intravenously.

near mealtime. These drugs include unbuffered penicillin G, penicillinase-resistant penicillins (nafcillin, oxacillin, cloxacillin, and dicloxacillin), ampicillin, and lincomycin. Dairy products and other foods or medications containing calcium or magnesium salts interfere with absorption of tetracyclines. Absorption of penicillin V, buffered penicillin G, amoxicillin, cephalexin, cefaclor, chloramphenicol, erythromycin, and clindamycin is affected only slightly by food. When absorption is affected by concurrent administration of food, antibiotics should be taken 1 or more hours before or 2 or more hours after meals. A four-times-daily dosage schedule, rarely used for common infections, can be arranged for the drug to be given on arising, 1 hour before lunch and supper, and at bedtime. Most orally administered antibiotics can be administered twice or thrice daily, a schedule that is accommodated easily by most parents.

Intravenous versus Intramuscular Administration

Although after intravenous administration of an antimicrobial agent there is a brief period when the serum antimicrobial concentration is higher than that after intramuscular administration, no therapeutic advantage of intravenous as opposed to intramuscular administration has been demonstrated. Intravenous administration should be used if the patient is in shock or suffers from bleeding diathesis. If prolonged parenteral therapy is anticipated, the pain of injection and the small muscle mass of infants and young children preclude the intramuscular route and make intravenous therapy preferable. The physician must be alert for thrombophlebitis, which can result from prolonged intravenous administration, and for sterile abscesses, which can follow intramuscular administration.

Chloramphenicol, tetracyclines, erythromycin, and vancomycin should be administered intravenously rather than intramuscularly. Chloramphenicol was thought to be absorbed poorly from intramuscular sites, although recent data suggest that this is not the case. Intramuscular injection of parenteral tetracyclines and erythromycin causes local irritation and pain, and intramuscular injection of vancomycin causes tissue necrosis. Care should be given to the administration of intramuscular injections.[15, 105] Sites that minimize the risk of local neural, vascular, or tissue injury should be selected. The preferred site varies with age of the child: the upper anterolateral thigh in infants, the ventrogluteal area in children older than 2 years of age, and the deltoid area for older children. Inadvertent intra-arterial injection of benzathine penicillin G can cause tissue damage.

"Push" versus "Continuous" or "Steady Drip" Intravenous Administration

Antimicrobial agents can be administered intravenously by the "push" method, in which the drug is infused in 5 to 15 minutes; by "steady drip" in 1 to 2 hours; or by "continuous drip," whereby the drug is given throughout the period of administration. The push method results in high antibacterial activity in serum for short periods, whereas the steady and continuous drip methods produce lower but more sustained activity. The risk of adverse effects influences whether an antimicrobial agent should be administered by push or by steady drip. Recent pharmacodynamic studies suggest optimization of bactericidal activity when aminoglycosides are given by push or steady drip once daily and when β-lactams are given in many small, frequent doses or by a continuous drip to maintain concentrations of drug at the infection site that exceed the MIC of the pathogen for much of the dosing interval. Rapid administration (<5 minutes) of large intravenous doses of penicillin should be avoided because of possible adverse central nervous system effects. Aminoglycosides given by the intravenous route should be infused in 20 to 60 minutes rather than as a bolus because high concentrations of drug can cause eighth nerve toxicity. Antimicrobial activity, especially for penicillins, can deteriorate if drugs are kept in solution at room temperature for prolonged periods, as might occur with the use of the continuous drip method. Fresh solutions of penicillins should be administered every 6 to 8 hours when the continuous drip method is used.

Diffusion of Antimicrobial Agents Across Biologic Membranes

Diffusion of any drug across a biologic membrane depends on the molecular size of the drug, the degree of protein binding (only the unbound portion of the drug crosses), the degree of ionization at physiologic pH (only the un-ionized portion is available for equilibration), and solubility in lipids. Thus, the lipid solubility of the un-ionized and unbound fraction of an antimicrobial agent determines the capability of the drug to diffuse to the site of infection. Antibiotics usually are not distributed evenly throughout the body.[140, 141]

Diffusion of antimicrobial agents from the blood into joint space, pleural and pericardial fluid, and middle ear fluid is relatively unimpeded, and high concentrations of many drugs are achieved in these sites after systemic administration. More than 60 per cent of the peak serum concentration of various penicillins and cephalosporins is present in the inflamed joint space.[133] Loculations of fluid in the presence of fibrous adhesions may limit the passage of antimicrobial agents into infected areas.

Diffusion of antibiotics from the blood into cerebrospinal fluid or into the aqueous humor of the eye is more limited. Drugs that are highly soluble in lipids, un-ionized, and minimally bound to proteins (e.g., isoniazid, chloramphenicol, sulfonamides) pass into the cerebrospinal fluid in high concentrations even in the absence of inflammation, whereas drugs such as the macrolides diffuse into cerebrospinal fluid little, if at all. Penicillins, cephalosporins, and aminoglycosides pass into cerebrospinal fluid only when the membrane is inflamed; variable but often low concentrations of drug in cerebrospinal fluid can be present even in the early stages of meningitis. The β-lactams are pumped actively out of the cerebrospinal fluid space by the choroid plexus, a process that partially is inhibited by inflammation.

Duration of Therapy

Physicians must rely on empirically derived schedules of therapy for rapid and complete resolution of disease and minimal risk in terms of clinical or microbiologic failure or drug toxicity. Numerous studies evaluating duration of therapy have been performed for streptococcal pharyngitis; the results are consistent in suggesting that 10 days of oral therapy with penicillin V, erythromycin, or cefadroxil; 5 days of azithromycin; or a single intramuscular dose of benzathine penicillin G is appropriate. Opinions vary and data are conflicting regarding duration of treatment for diseases such as osteomyelitis, suppurative arthritis, and infections of the urinary tract. Radetsky[154] has written an enlightening history of the recommendations for duration of treatment in bacterial meningitis, pointing out that "Even in the absence of specific data certain numbers have an unaccountable power to satisfy and reassure . . . 7, 10, 14 and 21 days have consistently appeared. Even in the trials performed at the dawn of the antimicrobial era, these numbers were chosen."

Dosage Schedules in Children with Renal or Hepatic Insufficiency

The kidneys are the major organs of excretion for most antimicrobial agents, including penicillins, cephalosporins, aminoglycosides, and tetracyclines (with the exception of doxycycline). Because impaired excretion can result in high and possibly toxic serum and tissue antimicrobial concentrations, alterations in dosage schedules should be considered in children with diminished renal function. Antibiotics that require careful adjustment of dosage in renal impairment include imipenem-cilastatin, ticarcillin, aminoglycosides, tetracyclines, and vancomycin. Agents requiring dosage adjustments only when renal failure is severe include most penicillins, cephalosporins, and clindamycin. Drugs that are eliminated by nonrenal mechanisms and therefore do not require adjustment of the dosage schedule in renal impairment include chloramphenicol, cloxacillin, dicloxacillin, doxycycline, erythromycin (including the newer macrolides), metronidazole, nafcillin, oxacillin, and rifampin.

The dosage schedules for patients with renal insufficiency can be altered by administering the usual dosage for the initial dose, then by increasing the interval between doses or decreasing individual dosages (or both in the case of renal shutdown). Although numerous guidelines have been developed to assist the physician,[108, 181] these formulas have been generated from studies of adults with renal impairment, and pediatricians must be cautious in adapting the formulas for use in infants and young children. Serum antimicrobial concentrations should be monitored when aminoglycosides, vancomycin, and other drugs of potential toxicity are administered to children with renal insufficiency. Serum specimens are obtained at the time of the anticipated peak and trough concentrations on the first day and repeated on subsequent days to ensure a safe and effective dosage schedule.[79]

Hepatic disorders can alter plasma protein binding, tissue binding, hepatic metabolism, and distribution of antimicrobials that are metabolized or excreted by the liver.[197] Few data exist regarding adjustment of dosage schedules for antibiotics that are metabolized by the liver in patients with hepatic insufficiency.[93] It would be prudent to avoid the use of tetracyclines and to exercise caution when prescribing macrolides, chloramphenicol, clindamycin, rifampin, and metronidazole to patients with underlying hepatic disease.

Topical Use of Antimicrobial Agents

Topical antimicrobial agents[199] are used for a variety of indications: silver nitrate drops or either erythromycin or tetracycline ointments are used for prevention of gonococcal ophthalmia in newborn infants; bacitracin or polymyxin ointments are available (in many cases without prescription) for first aid of minor cuts, abrasions, and burns; tetracycline, erythromycin, and clindamycin have been used for treatment of pustular acne; and erythromycin, chloramphenicol, sulfonamide, gentamicin, tobramycin, tetracycline, and a combination of TMP and polymyxin B ointments or drops are used for treatment of conjunctivitis, sties, and other minor infections of the eye. The effectiveness of topical antibiotics for prophylaxis of gonococcal ophthalmia is unquestioned; the other uses are of less certain efficacy. Mupirocin is effective in vitro against *S. aureus* (including methicillin-resistant strains) and group A streptococci and is approved for therapy of impetigo but may be of particular value for eradicating nasal carriage of methicillin-resistant staphylococci. Most antibiotics used topically, such as bacitracin, neomycin, and polymyxin B, are of limited use as systemic agents.

Absorption after application to the conjunctivae or large areas of denuded skin can be significant, but application to normal skin does not result in detectable concentrations of antimicrobial activity in blood or urine. Sensitization does not appear to be an important problem with most topical antibiotics, although some patients with chronic dermatoses may react to certain agents, such as neomycin. Antimicrobial agents of value for systemic use should not be applied extensively to the surface of the body or used routinely in closed units (e.g., burn units) because of the risk of inducing resistance.

The Committee on Drugs of the American Academy of Pediatrics concluded that topical antimicrobial agents may prevent infection after minor cuts, abrasions, and burns but that in most instances, gentle cleansing of minor wounds and burns is sufficient antisepsis.[5] Systemic antibiotics rather than topical drugs are recommended for chronic pyodermas, including impetigo, especially when there are more than several lesions.

Current Use of Antimicrobial Agents for Prophylaxis

Chemoprophylaxis refers to use of drugs to prevent infection. Antimicrobial treatment refers to use of drugs after infection has taken place or when early signs of infectious disease are present or infection is suspected. Use of antimicrobial agents for prophylaxis has proved to be of value in many circumstances (Table 231–13) and currently is considered of probable value or is investigational for prevention of infections in many other situations. Prophylaxis is of greatest value when the following criteria are met: use of a single drug with a narrow spectrum of activity; use of a drug with limited side effects or toxicity; and prevention of colonization by an organism of known susceptibility and one that is unlikely to become resistant during the period of drug use.

Use of Antimicrobial Agents for Children in School or Group Day Care

Infants and children usually return to the school or day care during a course of antimicrobial therapy. Because of the problems with administration of drugs outside the home, physicians should prescribe medications that are given infrequently, are relatively stable at ambient temperatures, and need only simple directions. Drugs that are administered in once- or twice-daily schedules are preferred. Chewable tablets, when available, may be of value in reducing the need for the school or day care provider to measure specific amounts of liquid suspension and to refrigerate suspensions. Single-dosage regimens, such as intramuscular benzathine penicillin G for group A streptococcal infections, may be advantageous. Guidelines for administration of medications in school have been published by the Committee of School Health of the American Academy of Pediatrics and should be useful to the physician for prescribing drugs to young children in day care.[212]

TABLE 231–13. Antimicrobial Prophylaxis in Children

Prevention of Infection in Certain Patients	Antimicrobial Agent
Group A streptococcal infection in patients with a history of rheumatic fever	Benzathine penicillin G IM, penicillin G or V PO
Bacterial endocarditis in patients at risk during surgical procedures	
Dental procedures, surgery of upper respiratory tract	Amoxicillin PO; erythromycin or clindamycin in penicillin-allergic patients
Gastrointestinal or genitourinary tract surgery or instrumentation	Penicillin G or ampicillin IM, + streptomycin or gentamicin
Neonatal sepsis caused by group B *Streptococcus*	Ampicillin, IM or IV
Staphylococcal disease in newborn infants	Hexachlorophene
Gonococcal ophthalmia in newborn infants	Silver nitrate or erythromycin ophthalmic ointment
Malaria in travelers to endemic areas	Chloroquine
Meningococcal disease in contacts	Rifampin, ceftriaxone (for serogroup A)
Haemophilus influenzae disease in contacts	Rifampin
Recurrent episodes of acute otitis media	Amoxicillin, sulfisoxazole
Postoperative infections	Penicillinase-resistant penicillins or first- or second-generation cephalosporins
Tuberculosis infections in household contacts	Isoniazid
Recurrent urinary tract infections	Trimethoprim-sulfamethoxazole, nitrofurantoin
Pneumocystis carinii pneumonia in immunosuppressed transplant recipients or patients with AIDS	Trimethoprim-sulfamethoxazole
Influenza A	Amantadine
Sepsis in patients with functional asplenia	Penicillin, amoxicillin, trimethoprim-sulfamethoxazole

IM, intramuscularly; IV, intravenously; PO, orally.

Restriction on Use of Antimicrobial Agents for Infants and Children

Many antimicrobial agents are approved for use in adults but have not been approved by the FDA for use in infants and children. The reasons for lack of approval include recently released drugs with insufficient experience in children—parenteral ampicillin-sulbactam (Unasyn), piperacillin-tazobactam (Zosyn), imipenem-cilastatin (Primaxin), aztreonam (Azactam), and cefmetazole (Zefazone); agents with real or suspected toxicity in children (e.g., damage to articular cartilage in juvenile animals associated with administration of the fluoroquinolones) that preclude use; and antibiotics for which the manufacturers have chosen not to submit data on use in children to the FDA—metronidazole (Flagyl), cefoperazone (Cefobid), piperacillin (Pipracil), and cefotetan (Cefotan). Although a drug that has been approved in adults may be used in children at the discretion of the physician, the prudent physician chooses to use such a drug only when it uniquely is appropriate for the infectious illness and records the basis for choice of the unapproved drug.

The spectrum of activity of the fluoroquinolones against *P. aeruginosa*, methicillin-resistant staphylococci, *H. influenzae* (including β-lactamase–producing strains), and various gram-negative enteric bacilli is ideal for treatment of some difficult pediatric infectious diseases, including acute and chronic pulmonary infection in children with cystic fibrosis, nosocomial staphylococcal infections, meningitis with resistant bacteria, and prophylaxis in leukemic and immunocompromised children.[47] Until the concern for damage to developing joint cartilage is resolved, the quinolones can be used in children only when other agents have been ineffective or are likely to fail and when the parent has given informed consent.

Home Intravenous Antibiotic Therapy

Home intravenous antibiotic therapy now is available in most communities and enables discharge from the hospital earlier than in the past. The safety, effectiveness, and cost-efficiency of such a program have been proved and are of particular value for children who require 4 to 6 weeks of therapy for osteomyelitis or septic arthritis or who have chronic disease, such as cystic fibrosis or malignancy, that can be managed in the home. In many cases, home care enables the patient to resume normal activities, including return to school. The following are factors that are necessary before consideration of home care:

1. Availability of a team including the physician, the pharmacist, a vendor who will supply the drug and supplies, and an intravenous specialty nurse
2. A disease that is stable and requires only continued antimicrobial therapy
3. Unavailability of a suitable oral antibacterial agent and availability of a parenteral antibiotic with low toxicity that the patient can tolerate (as demonstrated in the hospital) and preferably with long half-life to allow infrequent dosing
4. A member of the household is able to administer the antibiotic and provide aseptic care of the venous access device
5. Appropriate follow-up can be maintained for monitoring safety and effectiveness

If problems with venous access arise and ceftriaxone is appropriate therapy, the drug can be administered in the home once a day by a nurse via the intramuscular route with success.[164]

Drug-Drug Interactions

Drug-drug interactions can lead to therapeutic failure because of lack of effective activity of one or both drugs or to serious adverse events because of toxic serum concentrations of one or both drugs.[67] Most children do not require daily medications for chronic diseases; thus, drug-drug interactions are less common in pediatric than geriatric patients, but the potential for interactions exists and must be considered when prescribing antibiotics. Because drug-drug interactions are not limited to prescription medications, inquiries into over-the-counter medication use should be made. Mechanisms for drug-drug interactions are physiochemical, whereby one drug is incompatible physically in solution with another;

pharmacokinetic, whereby one drug interferes with the absorption, distribution, metabolism, or excretion of the other; and pharmacodynamic, whereby one drug affects the activity of a second drug. Examples of each mechanism include inactivation of aminoglycosides by extended-spectrum penicillins, decreased absorption of tetracyclines with co-administration of antacids, and antagonism of sulfonamide activity by procaine because of competition for PABA binding sites.

SUMMARY AND CONCLUSIONS

A summary of the information contained in this chapter is presented in a format of questions that the physician must consider for appropriate use of antimicrobial agents in children.

1. Before the drug is administered:
   a. Have appropriate cultures been obtained for specific microbiologic diagnosis?
   b. Has the patient received the drug previously? If so, did the patient tolerate the drug? Were there any signs of toxicity or sensitization?
   c. Does the patient have a condition that requires exclusion of some drugs? For example, children with glucose-6-phosphate dehydrogenase deficiency may have induced hemolysis when sulfonamides, nitrofurantoin, or primaquine is administered.
2. Factors to be considered when writing orders for administration of antimicrobial agents in a hospital:
   a. If the drug is given by mouth, will co-administration with food interfere with absorption, or is there diarrhea?
   b. If a parenteral route is used, should the drug be administered by the intravenous or the intramuscular route?
   c. If the drug is administered by the intravenous route, is push, steady drip, or continuous drip preferred?
   d. Should the drug be instilled directly at the site of infection?
   e. Will the drug diffuse to the site of infection?
   f. Should incision and drainage of the infected area be performed before or after beginning therapy? Incision and drainage should be considered whenever there is a significant collection of pus. If the drainage procedure is performed before administration of the antibiotic, material can be obtained for culture and susceptibility testing.
   g. Does the patient have renal or hepatic insufficiency that requires alteration of dosage schedule?
   h. Are any special precautions required for household contacts? Prophylaxis may be warranted in special circumstances of infection occurring in the household, day care center, or nursery school.
3. Use of antimicrobial agents in children who are treated as outpatients[113]:
   a. Have the names and functions of the drugs been communicated to the patient and the parent? Do any of the drugs prescribed interact with each other?
   b. Is the dosage schedule simple and satisfactory for the family circumstances (e.g., the child's school schedule, the schedule of the working parents)?
   c. Does the child have an adequate supply of the drug until it can be purchased? If not, use of starter packages is of value. Administration of the first dose in the clinic is advantageous because it provides knowledge of acceptance and tolerability of the drug by the child.
   d. Are parents given instructions for reporting the clinical course by telephone? Is an appointment made for the next visit?
   e. Does the patient or parent know how to assess adequacy of response to the drug? Does the parent know how to take the child's temperature?
   f. Is the total amount of drug prescribed adequate for the course? Will there be need for refill of the prescription?
   g. Is the drug provided in a convenient dosage form? Will the package be provided with an adequate means of measuring the drug? Does the agent require refrigeration?
   h. Has the patient or parent been informed of signs of side effects or toxicity?
   i. Are generic equivalents of the drug adequate?
   j. Will the patient be able to pay for the drug if it is purchased elsewhere (away from the clinic)? If applicable, will a third party pay for this prescription? (In some states, prescription by brand name may not be filled because reimbursement by the third-party payer, such as Medicaid, is insufficient.)
4. After the patient's course:
   a. How long should the patient take the drug?
   b. When should the initial choice of antimicrobial agents be reconsidered? When the results of cultures and appropriate susceptibility tests are available, the initial choice should be reevaluated and altered, if necessary.
   c. What studies should be performed to monitor the safety and adequacy of the regimen? Hematologic indices must be measured during the administration of chloramphenicol to detect any adverse reaction.
   d. Are repeated cultures necessary? In certain cases, the most appropriate criterion of efficacy is evaluation of the results of cultures. Thus, sterilization of the urine by an antimicrobial agent is the definitive test of susceptibility of the organisms to the agent, and urine should be cultured 24 to 48 hours after the onset of treatment for urinary tract infection to define the effectiveness of the drug.
   e. What clinical and laboratory signs of efficacy should be followed? Signs may differ for different diseases and various drugs but should be considered by the physician when the course of therapy is designed.
5. What factors should be considered if the patient fails to respond to the antimicrobial agent? If the patient does not respond appropriately to the course of therapy, various factors must be considered, including those that are related to the disease, host, drug, or organism (Table 231–14).

TABLE 231–14. Factors Contributing to Antimicrobial Failure

Host-related
Foreign body present
Anatomic defect
Defect in immune response to infection
Disease-related
Antibiotic inappropriate for disease
Ancillary therapy not instituted
Sequestered focus of infection (undetected or inaccessible)
Organism-related
Acquired resistance to antimicrobial agent
Superinfection with resistant bacteria
Drug-related
Inadequate compliance
Improper dosage schedule—route, dose, or duration
Inadequate diffusion to site of infection
Drug-drug interactions—antibiotic inactivation or antagonism
Deterioration of drug on storage

Acknowledgments

We would like to acknowledge the contribution of Dr. Jerome Klein, who wrote the previous edition of this chapter. Many of his sections remain intact or have been modified to reflect recently published information or the availability of new antimicrobial agents.

References

1. Abramowicz, M.: Drugs for parasitic infections. Med. Lett. *37*:99–108, 1995.
2. Abramson, J. S., and Givner, L. B.: Should tetracycline be contraindicated for therapy of presumed Rocky Mountain spotted fever in children less than 9 years of age? Pediatrics *86*:123–124, 1990.
3. Ackerman, B. H., Vannier, A. M., and Eudy, E. B.: Analysis of vancomycin time-kill studies with *Staphylococcus* species using a curve stripping program to describe the relationship between concentration and pharmacodynamic response. Antimicrob. Agents Chemother. *36*:1766–1769, 1992.
4. Ambrose, P. J.: Clinical pharmacokinetics of chloramphenicol and chloramphenicol succinate. Clin. Pharmacokinet. *9*:222–238, 1984.
5. American Academy of Pediatrics, Committee on Drugs: Topical antibiotics. Pediatrics *59*:1041–1042, 1977.
6. Asmar, B. I., Prainito, M., and Dajani, A. S.: Antagonistic effect of chloramphenicol in combination with cefotaxime or ceftriaxone. Antimicrob. Agents Chemother. *32*:1375–1378, 1988.
7. Assael, B. M., Parini, R., and Rusconi, F.: Ototoxicity of aminoglycoside antibiotics in infants and children. Pediatr. Infect. Dis. J. *1*:357–365, 1982.
8. Azimi, P. H.: Clinical and laboratory investigation of cefamandole therapy of infections in infants and children. J. Infect. Dis. *137*(Suppl.):S155–S160, 1978.
9. Bahal, N., and Nahata, M. C.: The new macrolide antibiotics: Azithromycin, clarithromycin, irithromycin, and roxithromycin. Ann. Pharmacother. *26*:46–55, 1992.
10. Barry, A. L., and Jones, R. N.: Cefixime: Spectrum of antibacterial activity against 16,016 clinical isolates. Pediatr. Infect. Dis. J. *6*:954–957, 1987.
11. Barza, M.: The nephrotoxicity of cephalosporins: An overview. J. Infect. Dis. *137*(Suppl.):S60–S73, 1978.
12. Bass, J. W., Crast, F. W., Knowles, C. R., et al.: Streptococcal pharyngitis in children: A comparison of four treatment schedules with intramuscular penicillin G benzathine. J. A. M. A. *235*:1112–1116, 1976.
13. Beall, G. N.: Penicillins. *In* Saxon, A. (moderator): Immediate hypersensitivity reactions to β-lactam antibiotics. Ann. Intern. Med. *107*:204–215, 1987.
14. Bennett, W. M., Plamp, C. E., Gilbert, D. N., et al.: The influence of dosage regimen on experimental gentamicin nephrotoxicity: Dissociation of peak serum levels from renal failure. J. Infect. Dis. *140*:576–580, 1979.
15. Bergeson, W. S., Singer, S. A., and Kaplan, A. M.: Intramuscular injections in children. Pediatrics *70*:944–948, 1982.
16. Birnbaum, J., Stapley, E. O., Miller, A. K., et al: Cefoxitin, a semi-synthetic cephamycin: A microbiological overview. J. Antimicrob. Chemother. *4*(Suppl B):S15–S32, 1978.
17. Black, J. R., Feinberg, J., Murphy R. L., et al.: Clindamycin and primaquine therapy for mild-to-moderate episodes of *Pneumocystis carinii* pneumonia in patients with AIDS: AIDS Clinical Trials Group 044. Clin. Infect. Dis. *18*:905–913, 1994.
18. Blaser, J.: Efficacy of once- and thrice-daily dosing of aminoglycosides in in-vitro models of infection. J. Antimicrob. Chemother. *27*(Suppl. C):21–28, 1991.
19. Blumer, J. L.: Cefixime. Drug Ther. *November*:60–84, 1989.
20. Boguniewicz, M., and Leung, D. Y. M.: Hypersensitivity reactions to antibiotics commonly used in children. Pediatr. Infect. Dis. J. *14*:221–231, 1995.
21. Bonacorsi, S., and Bingen, E.: Bactericidal activity of erythromycin associated with sulphasoxazole against the infectious agents most frequently responsible for acute otitis media. J. Antimicrob. Chemother. *33*:885–886, 1994.
22. Braun, P.: Hepatotoxicity of erythromycin. J. Infect. Dis. *119*:300–306, 1969.
23. Breiman, R. F., Butler, J. C., Tenover, F. C., et al.: Emergence of drug-resistant pneumococcal infections in the United States. J. A. M. A. *271*:1831–1835, 1994.
24. Brown, C. H., III, Natelson, E. A., Bradshaw, M. W., et al.: Study of the effects of ticarcillin on blood coagulation and platelet function. Antimicrob. Agents Chemother. *7*:642–657, 1975.
25. Brummett, R. E.: Ototoxicity of vancomycin and analogues. Otolaryngol. Clin. North Am. *26*:821–828, 1993.
26. Burchall, J. J.: Mechanism of action of trimethoprim-sulfamethoxazole-II. J. Infect. Dis. *128*(Suppl.):S437–S441, 1973.
27. Bush, K., Jacoby, G. A., and Medeiros, A. A.: A functional classification scheme for β-lactamases and its correlation with molecular structure. Antimicrob. Agents Chemother. *39*:1211–1233, 1995.
28. Cabizuca, S. V., and Desser, K. B.: Carbenicillin-associated hypokalemic alkalosis. J. A. M. A. *236*:956–957, 1976.
29. Cantú, T. G., Yamanaka-Yuen, N. A., and Lietman, P. S.: Serum vancomycin concentrations: Reappraisal of their clinical value. Clin. Infect. Dis. *18*:533–543, 1994.
30. Carter, B. L., Woodhead, J. C., Cole, K. J., et al.: Gastrointestinal side effects with erythromycin preparations. Drug Intell. Clin. Pharm. *21*:734–738, 1987.
31. Centers for Disease Control: 1993 sexually transmitted diseases treatment guidelines. M. M. W. R. *42*(RR-14):27–44, 44–46, 56–67, 75–81, 1993.
32. Chambers, H. F., and Sachdeva, M.: Binding of β-lactam antibiotics to penicillin-binding proteins in methicillin-resistant *Staphylococcus aureus*. J. Infect. Dis. *161*:1170–1176, 1990.
33. Chesney, P. J., Davis, Y., English, B. K., et al.: Occurrence of *Streptococcus pneumoniae* meningitis during vancomycin and cefotaxime therapy of septicemia in a patient with sickle cell disease. Pediatr. Infect. Dis. J. *14*:1013–1015, 1995.
34. Chopra, I., Hawkey, P. M., and Hinton, M.: Tetracyclines, molecular and clinical aspects. J. Antimicrob. Chemother. *29*:245–277, 1992.
35. Clarke, A. M., and Zemcov, S. J. V.: Clavulanic acid in combination with ticarcillin: An in-vitro comparison with other β-lactams. J. Antimicrob. Chemother. *13*:121–128, 1984
36. Cohen, R.: Clinical experience with cefpodoxime proxetil in acute otitis media. Pediatr. Infect. Dis. J. *14*(Suppl.):S12–S18, 1995.
37. Conte, J. E., Jr., Golden, J. A., Duncan, S., et al.: Intrapulmonary pharmacokinetics of clarithromycin and of erythromycin. Antimicrob. Agents Chemother. *39*:334–338, 1995.
38. Craft, J. C., and Siepman, N.: Overview of the safety profile of clarithromycin suspension in pediatric patients. Pediatr. Infect. Dis. J. *12*(Suppl. 3):S142–S147, 1993.
39. Craig, W. A., and Ebert, S. C.: Killing and regrowth of bacteria in vitro: A review. Scand. J. Infect. Dis. *74*(Suppl.):63–70, 1991.
40. Cunha, B. A., Sibley, C. M., and Ristuccia, A. M.: Doxycycline. Therap. Drug Monitor *4*:115–135, 1982.
41. Dajani, A. S.: Pharyngitis/tonsillitis: European and United States experience with cefpodoxime proxetil. Pediatr. Infect. Dis. J. *14*(Suppl.):S7–S11, 1995.
42. Davies, J. E.: Resistance to aminoglycosides: Mechanisms and frequency. Rev. Infect. Dis. *5*(Suppl. 2):S261–S266, 1983.
43. DeBroe, M. E., Giuliano, R. A., and Verpooten, G. A.: Choice of drug and dosage regimen: Two important risk factors for aminoglycoside nephrotoxicity. Am. J. Med. *80*(Suppl. 6B):S115–S118, 1986.
44. Dhawan, V. K., and Thadepalli, H.: Clindamycin: A review of 15 years of experience. Rev. Infect. Dis. *4*:1133–1153, 1982.
45. Disney, F. A., Hanfling, M. J., and Hausinger, S. A.: Loracarbef (LY 163892) vs. penicillin VK in the treatment of streptococcal pharyngitis and tonsillitis. Pediatr. Infect. Dis. J. *11*(Suppl.):S20–S26, 1992.
46. Doern, G.: In vitro activity of loracarbef and effects of susceptibility test methods. Am. J. Med. *92*(Suppl. 6A):7S–15S, 1992.
47. Douidar, S. M., and Snodgrass, W. R.: Potential role of fluoroquinolones in pediatric infections. Rev. Infect. Dis. *11*:878–889, 1989.
48. Drusano, G. L.: Role of pharmacokinetics in the outcome of infections. Antimicrob. Agents Chemother. *32*:289–297, 1988.
49. Drusano, G. L., Schimpff, S. C., and Hewitt, W. L.: The acylampicillins: Mezlocillin, piperacillin, and azlocillin. Rev. Infect. Dis. *6*:13–32, 1984.
50. Ebert, S. C., and Craig, W. A.: Pharmacodynamic properties of antibiotics: Application to drug monitoring and dosage regimen design. Infect. Control Hosp. Epidemiol. *11*:319–326, 1990.
51. Elhanan, K., Siplovich, L., and Raz, R.: Gentamicin once-daily versus thrice-daily in children. J. Antimicrob. Chemother. *35*:327–332, 1995.
52. Falagas, M. E., and Gorbach, S. L.: Clindamycin and metronidazole. Med. Clin. North Am. *79*:845–867, 1995.
53. Faulkner, R. D., Yacobi, A., Barone, J. S., et al.: Pharmacokinetic profile of cefixime in man. Pediatr. Infect. Dis. J. *6*:963–970, 1987.
54. Feigin, R. D., Pickering, L. K., Anderson, D., et al.: Clindamycin treatment of osteomyelitis and septic arthritis in children. Pediatrics *55*:213–223, 1975.
55. Ferrazzini, G., Klein, J., Sulh, H., et al.: Interaction between trimethoprim-sulfamethoxazole and methotrexate in children with leukemia. J. Pediatr. *117*:823–826, 1990.
56. Fichtenbaum, C. J., Ritchie, D. J., and Powderly, W. G.: Use of paromomycin for treatment of cryptosporidiosis in patients with AIDS. Clin. Infect. Dis. *16*:298–300, 1993.
57. Finland, M.: Twenty-fifth anniversary of the discovery of Aureomycin: The place of the tetracyclines in antimicrobial therapy. Clin. Pharmacol. Ther. *15*:3–8, 1974.
58. Fong, I. W., Engelking, E. R., and Kirby, W. M.: Relative inactivation by *Staphylococcus aureus* of eight cephalosporin antibiotics. Antimicrob. Agents Chemother. *9*:939–944, 1976.
59. Foshee, W. S., and Qvarnberg, Y.: Comparative United States and European trials of loracarbef in the treatment of acute otitis media. Pediatr. Infect. Dis. J. *11*(Suppl.):S12–S19, 1992.
60. Foster, J. A., and Sylvia, L. M.: Doxycycline-induced esophageal ulceration. Ann. Pharmacother. *28*:1185–1187, 1994.
61. Friedland, I. R., Shelton, S., and McCracken, G. H., Jr.: Chloramphenicol in penicillin-resistant pneumococcal meningitis. Lancet *342*:240–241, 1993.
62. Fu, K. P., and Neu, H. C.: A comparative study of the activity of cefaman-

dole and other cephalosporins and analysis of the β-lactamase-stability and synergy of cefamandole with aminoglycosides. J. Infect. Dis. *137*(Suppl.):S38–S48, 1978.
63. Fu, K. P., and Neu, H. C.: Piperacillin, a new penicillin active against many bacteria resistant to other penicillins. Antimicrob. Agents Chemother. *13*:358–367, 1978.
64. Gan, V. N., Chu, S.-Y., Kusmiesz, H. T., et al.: Pharmacokinetics of a clarithromycin suspension in infants and children. Antimicrob. Agents Chemother. *36*:2478–2480, 1992.
65. Gilbert, D. N.: Aminoglycosides. *In* Mandell, G. L., Bennett, J. E., and Dolin, R. (eds.): Mandell, Douglas, and Bennett's Principles and Practice of Infectious Disease. 4th ed. New York, Churchill-Livingstone, 1995, pp. 279–306.
66. Gilbert, D. N.: Once-daily aminoglycoside therapy. Antimicrob. Agents Chemother. *35*:399–405, 1991.
67. Gillum, J. G., Israel, D. S., and Polk, R. E.: Pharmacokinetic drug interactions with antimicrobial agents. Clin. Pharmacokinet. *25*:450–482, 1993.
68. Goetz, M. B., and Sayers, J.: Nephrotoxicity of vancomycin and aminoglycoside therapy separately and in combination. J. Antimicrob. Chemother. *32*:325–334, 1993.
69. Grossman, E. R., Walchik, A., and Freedman, H.: Tetracyclines and permanent teeth: The relation between dose and tooth color. Pediatrics *47*:567–570, 1971.
70. Guay, D. R. P., and Craft, J. C.: Overview of the pharmacology of clarithromycin suspension in children and a comparison with that in adults. Pediatr. Infect. Dis. J. *12*(Suppl.):S106–S111, 1993.
71. Gump, D. W.: Vancomycin for treatment of bacterial meningitis. Rev. Infect. Dis. *3*(Suppl.):S289–S292, 1981.
72. Haight, T. H., and Finland, M.: Antibacterial action of erythromycin. Proc. Soc. Exp. Biol. Med. *81*:175–183, 1952.
73. Haight, T. H., and Finland, M.: Observations on mode of action of erythromycin. Proc. Soc. Exp. Biol. Med. *81*:188–193, 1952.
74. Handwerger, S., and Tomasz, A.: Antibiotic tolerance among clinical isolates of bacteria. Rev. Infect. Dis. *7*:368–386, 1985.
75. Hanfling, M. J., Hausinger, S. A., and Squires, J.: Loracarbef vs. cefaclor in pediatric skin and skin-structure infections. Pediatr. Infect. Dis. J. *11*(Suppl.):S27–S30, 1992.
76. Hardy, D. J., Swanson, R. N., Rode, R. A., et al.: Enhancement of the in vitro and in vivo activities of clarithromycin against *Haemophilus influenzae* by 14-hydroxy-clarithromycin, its major metabolite in humans. Antimicrob. Agents Chemother. *34*:1407–1413, 1990.
77. Haycock, G. B., Schwartz, G. J., and Wisotsky, D. H.: Geometric method for measuring body surface area: A height-weight formula validated in infants, children, and adults. J. Pediatr. *93*:62–66, 1978.
78. Hebert, A. A., Still, J. G., and Reuman, P. D.: Comparative safety and efficacy of clarithromycin and cefadroxil suspensions in the treatment of mild to moderate skin and skin structure infections in children. Pediatr. Infect. Dis. J. *12*(Suppl. 3):S112–S117, 1993.
79. Hewitt, W. L., and McHenry, M. C.: Blood level determinations of antimicrobial drugs: Some clinical considerations. Med. Clin. North Am. *62*:1119–1140, 1978.
80. Hitchings, G. H.: Mechanism of action of trimethoprim-sulfamethoxazole-I. J. Infect. Dis. *128*(Suppl.):S433–S436, 1973.
81. Howie, V. M., and Owen, M. J.: Bacteriologic and clinical efficacy of cefixime compared with amoxicillin in acute otitis media. Pediatr. Infect. Dis. J. *6*:989–991, 1987.
82. Humbert, P., Treffel, P., Chapuis, J.-F., et al.: The tetracyclines in dermatology. J. Am. Acad. Dermatol. *25*:691–697, 1991.
83. Huovinen, P.: Trimethoprim resistance. Antimicrob. Agents Chemother. *31*:1451–1456, 1987.
84. Isaksson, B., Nilsson, L., Maller, R., et al.: Postantibiotic effect of aminoglycosides on gram-negative bacteria evaluated by a new method. J. Antimicrob. Chemother. *22*:23–33, 1988.
85. Jacoby, G. A., and Medeiros, A. A.: More extended-spectrum β-lactamases. Antimicrob. Agents Chemother. *35*:1697–1704, 1991.
86. Jonas, M., and Cunha, B. A.: Minocycline. Ther. Drug Monit. *4*:137–145, 1982.
87. Jorgenson, J. H., Doern, G. V., Maher, L. A., et al.: Antimicrobial resistance among respiratory isolates of *Haemophilus influenzae, Moraxella catarrhalis,* and *Streptococcus pneumoniae* in the United States. Antimicrob. Agents Chemother. *34*:2075–2080, 1990.
88. Kearns, G. L., Wheeler, J. G., Childress, S. H., et al.: Serum sickness-like reactions to cefaclor: Role of hepatic metabolism and individual susceptibility. J. Pediatr. *125*:805–811, 1994.
89. Kelly, H. W., Couch, R. C., Davis, R. L., et al.: Interaction of chloramphenicol and rifampin. J. Pediatr. *112*:817–820, 1988.
90. Klein, J. O., and Finland, M.: The new penicillins. N. Engl. J. Med. *269*:1019–1025, 1963.
91. Kremsner, P. G., Winkler, S., Brandts, C., et al.: Clindamycin in combination with chloroquine or quinine is an effective therapy for uncomplicated *Plasmodium falciparum* malaria in children from Gabon. J. Infect. Dis. *169*:467–470, 1994.
92. Leader, W. G., Chandler, M. H. H., and Castiglia, M.: Pharmacokinetic optimisation of vancomycin therapy. Clin. Pharmacokinet. *28*:327–342, 1995.
93. Lebel, M. H.: Pharmacology of antimicrobial agents in children with hepatic dysfunction. Pediatr. Infect. Dis. J. *5*:686–690, 1986.
94. Leclercq, R., and Courvalin, P.: Bacterial resistance to macrolide, lincosamide, and streptogramin antibiotics. Antimicrob. Agents Chemother. *35*:1267–1272, 1991.
95. Leclercq, R., and Courvalin, P.: Intrinsic and unusual resistance to macrolide, lincosamide, and streptogramin antibiotics in bacteria. Antimicrob. Agents Chemother. *35*:1273–1276, 1991.
96. Lee, S. P., Lipsky, B. A., and Teefey, S. A.: Gallbladder sludge and antibiotics. Pediatr. Infect. Dis. J. *9*:422–423, 1990.
97. Lee, A. G.: Pseudotumor cerebri after treatment with tetracycline and isotretinoin for acne. Cutis *55*:165–168, 1995.
98. Levine, B. B.: Immunologic mechanisms of penicillin allergy: A haptogenic model system for the study of allergic diseases of man. N. Engl. J. Med. *275*:1115–1125, 1966.
99. Levine, L. R.: Quantitative comparison of adverse reactions to cefaclor vs. amoxicillin in a surveillance study. Pediatr. Infect. Dis. J. *4*:358–361, 1985.
100. Levison, M. E.: Pharmacodynamics of antimicrobial agents: Bactericidal and postantibiotic effects. Infect. Dis. Clin. North Am. *9*:483–495, 1995.
101. Lin, R. Y.: A perspective on penicillin allergy. Arch. Intern. Med. *152*:930–937, 1992.
102. Livermore, D. M.: Determinants of the activity of β-lactamase inhibitor combinations. J. Antimicrob. Chemother. *31*(Suppl.):9–21, 1993.
103. Logan, M. N., Ashby, J. P., Andrews, J. M., et al.: The in-vitro and disc susceptibility testing of clarithromycin and its 14-hydroxy metabolite. J. Antimicrob. Chemother. *27*:161–170, 1991.
104. Lopez-Samblas, A. M., Torres, C. L., Wang, H., et al.: Effectiveness of a gentamicin dosing protocol based on postconceptual age: Comparison to published neonatal guidelines. Ann. Pharmacother. *26*:534–538, 1992.
105. Losek, J. D., and Gyuro, J.: Pediatric intramuscular injections: Do you know the procedure and complications? Pediatr. Emerg. Care *8*:79–81, 1992.
106. Luer, M. S., and Hatton, J.: Vancomycin administration into the cerebrospinal fluid: A review. Ann. Pharmacother. *27*:912–921, 1993.
107. Lyon, B. R., and Skurray, R.: Antimicrobial resistance of *Staphylococcus aureus:* Genetic basis. Microbiol. Rev. *51*:88–134, 1987.
108. Maderazo, E. G.: Antibiotic dosing in renal failure. Med. Clin. North Am. *79*:919–931, 1995.
109. Magerlein, B. J.: Modification of lincomycin. Adv. Applied Microbiol. *14*:185–229, 1971.
110. Marcy, S. M., and Klein, J. O.: The isoxazoyl penicillins: Oxacillin, cloxacillin, and dicloxacillin. Med. Clin. North Am. *5*:1127–1143, 1970.
111. Marsh, F. P.: Do cephalosporins potentiate or antagonize aminoglycoside nephrotoxicity? J. Antimicrob. Chemother. *4*:103–106, 1978.
112. Mason, E. O., and Kaplan, S. L.: Penicillin-resistant pneumococci in the United States. Pediatr. Infect. Dis. J. *14*:1017–1018, 1995.
113. Mattar, M. E., Markello, J., and Yaffe, S. J.: Inadequacies in the pharmacologic management of ambulatory children. J. Pediatr. *87*:137–141, 1975.
114. Mattie, H., Craig, W. A., and Pechere, J. C.: Determinants of efficacy and toxicity of aminoglycosides. J. Antimicrob. Chemother. *24*:281–293, 1989.
115. Mazzei, T., Mini, E., Novelli, A., et al.: Chemistry and mode of action of macrolides. J. Antimicrob. Chemother. *31*(Suppl.):1–9, 1993.
116. McCarty, J. M., and Renteria, A.: Treatment of pharyngitis and tonsillitis with cefprozil: Review of 3 multicenter trials. Clin. Infect. Dis. *14*(Suppl.):S224–S230, 1992.
117. McCracken, G. H., Jr.: New era for orally administered antibiotics: Use of sequential parenteral-oral antibiotic therapy for serious infectious diseases of infants and children. Pediatr. Infect. Dis. J. *6*:951–953, 1987.
118. McGehee, R. F., Jr., Smith, C. B., Wilcox, C., et al.: Comparative studies of antibacterial activity in vitro and absorption and excretion of lincomycin and clindamycin. Am. J. Med. Sci. *256*:279–292, 1968.
119. McLinn, S.: Double blind and open label studies of azithromycin in management of acute otitis media in children: A review. Pediatr. Infect. Dis. J. *14*(Suppl.):S62–S66, 1995.
120. Meyer, R. D.: Risk factors and comparisons of clinical nephrotoxicity of aminoglycosides. Am. J. Med. *80*(Suppl.):S119–S125, 1986.
121. Meyers, B. R., and Hirschman, S. Z.: Antibacterial activity of cefamandole in vitro. J. Infect. Dis. *137*(Suppl.):S25–S31, 1978.
122. Moellering, R. C., Jr.: A symposium on piperacillin/tazobactam: A new dimension in antibiotic therapy. Infect. Dis. Clin. Pract. *4*(Suppl.):S1–S36, 1995.
123. Moellering, R. C., Jr.: In vitro antibacterial activity of the aminoglycoside antibiotics. Rev. Infect. Dis. *5*(Suppl.):S212–S231, 1983.
124. Moellering, R. C., Jr.: Monitoring serum vancomycin levels: Climbing the mountain because it is there? Clin. Infect. Dis. *18*:544–546, 1994.
125. Moellering, R. C., Jr., Krogstad, D. J., and Greenblatt, D. J.: Vancomycin therapy in patients with impaired renal function: A nomogram for dosage. Ann. Intern. Med. *94*:343–346, 1981.
126. Moellering, R. C., Jr., Krogstad, D. J., and Greenblatt, D. J.: Pharmacokinetics of vancomycin in normal subjects and in patients with reduced renal function. Rev. Infect. Dis. *3*(Suppl.):S230–S235, 1981.
127. Moellering, R. C., Jr., and Swartz, M. N.: The newer cephalosporins. N. Engl. J. Med. *294*:24–28, 1976.
128. Moosa, A., and Rubidge, C. J.: Once daily ceftriaxone vs. chloramphenicol

for treatment of typhoid fever in children. Pediatr. Infect. Dis. J. *8*:696–699, 1989.

129. Murray, D. L., Singer, D. A., and Singer, A. B.: Cefaclor: A cluster of adverse reactions. N. Engl. J. Med. *303*:1003, 1980.
130. Nagar, H., Berger, S. A., Hammar, B., et al.: Penetration of clindamycin and metronidazole into the appendix and peritoneal fluid in children. Eur. J. Clin. Pharmacol. *37*:209–210, 1989.
131. Nahata, M. C.: Pharmacokinetics of azithromycin in pediatric patients: Comparison with other agents used for treating otitis media and streptococcal pharyngitis. Pediatr. Infect. Dis. J. *14*(Suppl.):S39–S44, 1995.
132. Nelson, J. D., and Haltalin, K. C.: Amoxicillin is less effective than ampicillin against *Shigella* in vitro and in vivo: Relationship of efficacy to activity in serum. J. Infect. Dis. *129*(Suppl.):S222–S227, 1974.
133. Nelson, J. D., Howard, J. B., and Shelton, S.: Oral antibiotic therapy for skeletal infections of children. I. Antibiotic concentrations in suppurative synovial fluid. J. Pediatr. *29*:131–134, 1978.
134. Neu, H. C.: Antimicrobial activity and human pharmacology of amoxicillin. J. Infect. Dis. *129*(Suppl.):S123–S131, 1974.
135. Neu, H. C.: Antistaphylococcal penicillins. Med. Clin. North Am. *66*:51–60, 1982.
136. Neu, H. C.: Cefoxitin: An overview of clinical studies in the United States. Rev. Infect. Dis. *1*:233–239, 1979.
137. Neu, H. C.: Carbenicillin and ticarcillin. Med. Clin. North Am. *66*:61–77, 1982.
138. Neu, H. C.: The crisis in antibiotic resistance. Science *257*:1064–1073, 1992.
139. Neu, H. C., and Fu, K. P.: Cefuroxime, a beta-lactamase-resistant cephalosporin with a broad spectrum of gram-positive and gram-negative activity. Antimicrob. Agents Chemother. *13*:657–664, 1978.
140. Nix, D. E., Goodwin, S. D., Peloquin, C. A., et al.: Antibiotic tissue penetration and its relevance: Impact of tissue penetration on infection response. Antimicrob. Agents Chemother. *35*:1953–1959, 1991.
141. Nix, D. E., Goodwin, S. D., Peloquin, C. A., et al.: Antibiotic tissue penetration and its clinical relevance: Models of tissue penetration and their meaning. Antimicrob. Agents Chemother. *35*:1947–1952, 1991.
142. Nolen, T. M.: Clinical trials of cefprozil for treatment of skin and skin structure infections: Rev. Clin. Infect. Dis. *14*(Suppl.):S255–S263, 1992.
143. Nord, C. E.: Mechanisms of resistance in anaerobic bacteria. Rev. Infect. Dis. *8*(Suppl.):S543–S548, 1986.
144. Olsvik, B., and Tenover, F. C.: Tetracycline resistance in periodontal pathogens. Clin. Infect. Dis. *16*(Suppl.):S310–S313, 1993.
145. Panzer, J. D., Brown, D. C., Epstein, W. L., et al.: Clindamycin levels in various body tissues and fluids. J. Clin. Pharmacol. *12*:259–262, 1972.
146. Parry, M. F., and Neu, H. C.: Ticarcillin for treatment of serious infections with gram-negative bacteria. J. Infect. Dis. *134*:476–485, 1976.
147. Periti, P., Mazzei, T., Mini, E., et al.: Pharmacokinetic drug interactions of macrolides. Clin. Pharmacokinet. *23*:106–131, 1992.
148. Petz, L. D.: Immunologic cross-reactivity between penicillins and cephalosporins: A review. J. Infect. Dis. *137*(Suppl.):S74–S79, 1978.
149. Pfeiffer, R. R.: Structural features of vancomycin. Rev. Infect. Dis. *3*(Suppl.):S205–S209, 1981.
150. Polk, R. E.: Anaphylactoid reactions to glycopeptide antibiotics. J. Antimicrob. Chemother. *27*(Suppl.):17–29, 1991.
151. Preac-Mursic, V., Wilske, B., Schierz, G., et al.: Comparative antimicrobial activity of the new macrolides against *Borrelia burgdorferi*. Eur. J. Clin. Microbiol. Infect. Dis. *8*:651–653, 1989.
152. Prober, C. G., Stevenson, D. K., and Benitz, W. E.: The use of antibiotics in neonates weighing less than 1200 grams. Pediatr. Infect. Dis. J. *9*:111–121, 1990.
153. Pukander, J. S., Jero, J. P., Kaprio, E. A., et al.: Clarithromycin vs amoxicillin suspensions in the treatment of pediatric patients with acute otitis media. Pediatr. Infect. Dis. J. *12*(Suppl.):S118–S121, 1993.
154. Radetsky, M.: Duration of treatment in bacterial meningitis: A historical inquiry. Pediatr. Infect. Dis. J. *9*:2–9, 1990.
155. Rahal, J. J., Jr., and Simberkoff, M. S.: Bactericidal and bacteriostatic action of chloramphenicol against meningeal pathogens. Antimicrob. Agents Chemother. *16*:13–18, 1979.
156. Ramilo, O., Kinane, B. T., and McCracken, G. H., Jr.: Chloramphenicol neurotoxicity. Pediatr. Infect. Dis. J. *7*:358–359, 1988.
157. Ramsey, B. W., Dorkin, H. L., Eisenberg, J. D., et al.: Efficacy of aerosolized tobramycin in patients with cystic fibrosis. N. Engl. J. Med. *328*:1740–1746, 1993.
158. Reid, R., Jr., Bradley, J. S., and Hindler, J.: Pneumococcal meningitis during therapy of otitis media with clarithromycin. Pediatr. Infect. Dis. J. *14*:1104–1105, 1995.
159. Rice, L. B., and Shlaes, D. M.: Vancomycin resistance in the enterococcus: Relevance in pediatrics. Pediatr. Clin. North Am. *42*:601–618, 1995.
160. Richards, G. A., and Klugman, K. P.: Implications of bacterial resistance for the use of beta-lactam agents in clinical practice. S. Afr. Med. J. *83*:163–164, 1993.
161. Ristuccia, A. M.: Chloramphenicol: Clinical pharmacology in pediatrics. Ther. Drug Monit. *7*:159–167, 1985.
162. Rodriguez, W. J., Ross, S., Khan, W. N., et al.: Clinical and laboratory evaluation of cefamandole in infants and children. J. Infect. Dis. *137*(Suppl.):S150–S154, 1978.
163. Rolinson, G. N.: Evolution of β-lactamase inhibitors. Rev. Infect. Dis. *3*(Suppl.):S727–S732, 1991.
164. Russo, T. A., Cook, S., and Gorbach, S. L.: Intramuscular ceftriaxone in home parenteral therapy. Antimicrob. Agents Chemother. *32*:1439–1440, 1988.
165. Sabath, L. D., Wilcox, C., Garner, C., et al.: In vitro activity of cefazolin against recent clinical bacterial isolates. J. Infect. Dis. *128*(Suppl.):S320–S326, 1973.
166. Sáez-Llorens, X., and McCracken, G. H., Jr.: Clinical pharmacology of antibacterial agents. *In* Remington, J. S., and Klein, J. O. (eds.): Infectious Diseases of the Fetus and Newborn Infant. 4th ed. Philadelphia, W. B. Saunders, 1995, pp. 1287–1336.
167. Saivin, S., and Houin, G.: Clinical pharmacokinetics of doxycycline and minocycline. Clin. Pharmacokinet. *15*:355–366, 1988.
168. Salaman, S. M.: Tetracyclines in ophthalmology. Surv. Ophthalmol. *29*:265–275, 1985.
169. Saxon, A.: Immediate hypersensitivity reactions to β-lactam antibiotics. Rev. Infect. Dis. *5*(Suppl.):S368–S379, 1983.
170. Saxon, A., Beall, G. N., Rohr, A. S., et al.: Immediate hypersensitivity reactions to β-lactam antibiotics. Ann. Intern. Med. *107*:204–215, 1987.
171. Schaad, U. B., McCracken, G. H., Jr., and Nelson, J. D.: Clinical pharmacology and efficacy of vancomycin in pediatric patients. J. Pediatr. *96*:119–126, 1980.
172. Schaad, U. B., Salam, M. A., Aujard, Y., et al.: Use of fluoroquinolones in pediatrics: Consensus report of an International Society of Chemotherapy commission. Pediatr. Infect. Dis. J. *14*:1–9, 1995.
173. Schaad, U. B., Suter, S., Gianella-Borradori, A., et al.: A comparison of ceftriaxone and cefuroxime for the treatment of bacterial meningitis in children. N. Engl. J. Med. *322*:141–147, 1990.
174. Seppälä, H., Nissinen, A., Järvinen, H., et al.: Resistance to erythromycin in group A streptococci. N. Engl. J. Med. *326*:292–297, 1992.
175. Siber, G. R., Smith, A. L., and Levin, M. J.: Predictability of peak serum gentamicin concentration with dosage based on body surface area. J. Pediatr. *94*:135–138, 1979.
176. Silber, T. J., and D'Angelo, L.: Psychosis and seizures following the injection of penicillin G procaine: Hoigne's syndrome. Am. J. Dis. Child. *139*:335–337, 1985.
177. Silva, J., Jr.: Update on pseudomembranous colitis. West. J. Med. *151*:644–648, 1989.
178. Snavely, S. R., and Hodges, G. R.: The neurotoxicity of antibacterial agents. Ann. Intern. Med. *101*:92–104, 1984.
179. Spotts, C. R., and Stanier, R. Y.: Mechanism of streptomycin action on bacteria: A unitary hypothesis. Nature *192*:633–637, 1961.
180. Spratt, B. G.: Distinct penicillin binding proteins involved in the division, elongation, and shape of *Escherichia coli* K12. Proc. Natl. Acad. Sci. U. S. A. *72*:2999–3003, 1975.
181. Staniforth, D. H., Lillystone, R. J., and Jackson, D.: Effect of food on the bioavailability and tolerance of clavulanic acid/amoxicillin combination. J. Antimicrob. Chemother. *10*:131–139, 1982.
182. Stapleton, P., Wu, P.-J., King, A., et al.: Incidence and mechanisms of resistance to the combination of amoxicillin and clavulanic acid in *Escherichia coli*. Antimicrob. Agents Chemother. *39*:2478–2483, 1995.
183. Steinberg, E. A., Overturf, G. D., Wilkins, J., et al.: Failure of cefamandole in treatment of meningitis due to *Haemophilus influenzae* type b. J. Infect. Dis. *137*(Suppl.):S180–S186, 1978.
184. Still, J. G.: Management of pediatric patients with group A beta-hemolytic streptococcal pharyngitis: Treatment options. Pediatr. Infect. Dis. J. *14*(Suppl.):S57–S61, 1995.
185. St. Peter, W. L., Redic-Kill, K. A., and Hultstenson, C. E.: Clinical pharmacokinetics of antibiotics in patients with impaired renal function. Clin. Pharmacokinet. *22*:169–210, 1992.
186. Tally, F. P., Cuchural, G. L., Jr., and Malamy, M. H.: Mechanisms of resistance and resistance transfer in anaerobic bacteria: Factors influencing antimicrobial therapy. Rev. Infect. Dis. *6*(Suppl.):260–269, 1984.
187. Tally, F. T., Ellestad, G. A., and Testa, R. T.: Glycylcyclines: A new generation of tetracyclines. J. Antimicrob. Chemother. *35*:449–452, 1995.
188. Tanz, R. R., Poncher, J. R., Corydon, K. E., et al.: Clindamycin treatment of chronic pharyngeal carriage of group A streptococci. J. Pediatr. *119*:123–128, 1991.
189. Tedesco, F. J.: Pseudomembranous colitis: Pathogenesis and therapy. Med. Clin. North Am. *66*:655–664, 1982.
190. Tetzlaff, T. R., McCracken, G. H., Jr., and Nelson, J. D.: Oral antibiotic therapy for skeletal infections of children. II. Therapy of osteomyelitis and suppurative arthritis. J. Pediatr. *92*:485–490, 1978.
191. Then, R. L.: Mechanisms of resistance to trimethoprim, the sulfonamides, and trimethoprim-sulfamethoxazole. Rev. Infect. Dis. *4*:261–269, 1982.
192. Thornsberry, C.: Review of in vitro activity of third-generation cephalosporins and other newer beta-lactam antibiotics against clinically important bacteria. Am. J. Med. *79*(Suppl.):14–20, 1985.
193. Tipper, D. J.: Mode of action of β-lactam antibiotics. Pharmacol. Ther. *27*:1–35, 1985.
194. Tipper, D. J., and Strominger, J. L.: Biosynthesis of the peptidoglycan of bacterial cell walls. J. Biol. Chem. *243*:3169–3179, 1968.
195. Tipper, D. J., and Strominger, J. L.: Mechanism of action of penicillins: A

proposal based on their structural similarity to acyl-D-alanyl-D-alanine. Proc. Nat. Acad. Sci. U. S. A. *54*:1133–1141, 1965.
196. Tomasz, A.: From penicillin-binding proteins to the lysis and death of bacteria: A 1979 view. Rev. Infect. Dis. *1*:434–467, 1979.
197. Tschida, S. J., Vance-Bryan, K., and Zaske, D. E.: Anti-infective agents and hepatic disease. Med. Clin. North Am. *79*:895–917, 1995.
198. Tulkens, P. M.: Experimental studies on nephrotoxicity of aminoglycosides at low doses. Am. J. Med. *80*(Suppl.):S105–S114, 1986.
199. Tunkel, A. R.: Topical antibacterials. *In* Mandell, G. L., Bennett, J. E., and Dolin, R. (eds.): Mandell, Douglas, and Bennett's Principles and Practice of Infectious Disease. 4th ed. New York, Churchill-Livingstone, 1995, pp. 381–389.
200. Verbist, L.: Comparison of the activities of the new ureidopenicillins piperacillin, mezlocillin, azlocillin, and Bay k 4999 against gram-negative organisms. Antimicrob. Agents Chemother. *16*:115–119, 1979.
201. Vogelman, B., and Craig, W. A.: Kinetics of antimicrobial activity. J. Pediatr. *108*:835–840, 1986.
202. Wallace, S. M., and Chan, L. Y.: In vitro interaction of aminoglycosides with β-lactam penicillins. Antimicrob. Agents Chemother. *28*:274–281, 1985.
203. Watanakunakorn, C., and Bakie, C.: Synergism of vancomycin-gentamicin and vancomycin-streptomycin against enterococci. Antimicrob. Agents Chemother. *4*:120–124, 1973.
204. Watanakunakorn, C.: The antibacterial action of vancomycin. Rev. Infect. Dis. *3*(Suppl.):S210–S215, 1981.
205. Weber, D. A., and Sanders, C. C.: Diverse potential of β-lactamase inhibitors to induce class 1 enzymes. Antimicrob. Agents Chemother. *34*:156–158, 1990.
206. Weisblum, B.: Erythromycin resistance by ribosome modification. Antimicrob. Agents Chemother. *39*:577–585, 1995.
207. Weisblum, B.: Insights into erythromycin action from studies of its activity as inducer of resistance. Antimicrob. Agents Chemother. *39*:797–805, 1995.
208. Weiss, M. E., and Adkinson, N. F., Jr.: β-lactam allergy. *In* Mandell, G. L., Bennett, J. E., and Dolin, R. (eds.): Mandell, Douglas, and Bennett's Principles and Practice of Infectious Disease. 4th ed. New York, Churchill-Livingstone, 1995, pp. 272–278.
209. West, B. C., DeVault, G. A., Jr., Clement, J. C., et al.: Aplastic anemia associated with parenteral chloramphenicol: Review of 10 cases including the second case of possible increased risk with cimetidine. Rev. Infect. Dis. *10*:1048–1051, 1988.
210. Woodford, N., and Johnson, A. P.: Glycopeptide resistance in gram-positive bacteria: From black and white to shades of grey. J. Med. Microbiol. *40*:375–378, 1994.
211. Yunis, A. A.: Chloramphenicol: Relation of structure to activity and toxicity. Ann. Rev. Pharmacol. Toxicol. *28*:83–100, 1988.
212. Zanga, J., Donland, M. A., Newton, J., et al.: Administration of medication in school. Pediatrics *74*:433–438, 1984.
213. Zhanel, G. G., and Craig, W. A.: Pharmacokinetic contributions to postantibiotic effects: Focus on aminoglycosides. Clin. Pharmacokinet. *27*:377–392, 1994.
214. Zinberg, J., Chernaik, R., Coman, E., et al.: Reversible symptomatic obstruction associated with ceftriaxone pseudolithiasis. Am. J. Gastroenterol. *86*:1251–1254, 1991.

232

ANTIMICROBIAL PROPHYLAXIS

Adnan S. Dajani and Walid Abuhammour

Antimicrobial prophylaxis is the practice of administering an antimicrobial agent(s) with the intent of preventing an infection. Prevention, rather than treatment, always is preferred, provided the means are available and the risk-benefit and cost-benefit ratios are acceptable. This chapter focuses on the prevention of morbidity and mortality from bacterial infections through the prophylactic, and often empiric, use of antimicrobial agents.

GENERAL PRINCIPLES OF PROPHYLAXIS

Several factors that influence prophylaxis efficacy are related to the potential pathogen, the prophylactic agent, the host, and the disease to be prevented (Table 232–1). Failure to consider all of these factors will lead to ineffective prophylaxis, overuse of antimicrobial agents, promotion of resistant microorganisms, economic waste, and risk of toxicity or side effects. These factors are discussed here in general and more specifically in the latter sections.

The Bacterial Pathogen

Prophylaxis is more effective when a single pathogen, as opposed to multiple pathogens, is targeted. In general, the greater the number of targeted pathogens, the less effective, the more toxic, and the more expensive the regimen becomes. Ideally, prophylaxis should be administered at the time of exposure to the potential pathogen or shortly thereafter. If exposure is prolonged or continuous, prophylaxis becomes less effective and less desirable. Bacteria that are not endogenous to the host (i.e., not part of the host normal flora) generally are targeted more effectively if exposure is known and identified.

The Disease

Severity of the disease to be prevented is a major consideration. Potentially fatal infections (e.g., meningococcemia) or infections that result in high morbidity (e.g., endocarditis) are justifiably targeted diseases. On the other hand, prophylaxis usually is not required for minor illnesses (e.g., cuts, abrasions). The site of infection to be prevented also is important. Adequate concentrations of antimicrobials in organs that are highly vascular and with no barriers readily are achieved, whereas infections in compartments (e.g., middle ear) or involving prosthetic materials may require special considerations.

TABLE 232–1. Factors Influencing Effective Prophylaxis

Single versus multiple potential pathogens
Time of exposure to pathogen
Source of pathogens
Severity of the disease to be prevented
Targeted organ(s) that could get infected
Spectrum of activity of antimicrobial agent
Pharmacokinetics and pharmacodynamics of selected agent
Duration of chemoprophylaxis
Cost, toxicity, side effects, and acceptability of agent
Likelihood and consequences of emerging resistance

The Antimicrobial Agent

The most desirable prophylactic agent is narrow spectrum, inexpensive, easily administered, and well tolerated and has minimal side effects. The less frequently an agent is given, the more reliable is the adherence (compliance) of the patient.[63] Situations in which prophylaxis can be achieved effectively with a single administration of the antimicrobial agent are ideal.

PROPHYLAXIS IN NEWBORN INFANTS

Ophthalmia Neonatorum

Prophylaxis is targeted against *Neisseria gonorrhoeae* and *Chlamydia trachomatis*. Ideally, prophylaxis should be directed at infants who are exposed to these two pathogens; however, it is impossible to identify this group with certainty. Routine prophylaxis has been discontinued in some countries (United Kingdom, Sweden)[22]; however, it is required in the United States.

Topical 1 per cent silver nitrate solution in single-dose ampules or single-dose tubes of an ophthalmic ointment containing 0.5 per cent erythromycin or 1 per cent tetracycline are available. All agents are effective and recommended for prophylaxis of gonococcal ophthalmia neonatorum.[57] Silver nitrate has been in use for such prophylaxis for more than 100 years. Because silver nitrate frequently causes chemical conjunctivitis, its use has been challenged and alternate regimens have been sought. Erythromycin and tetracycline ophthalmic ointments appear to be as effective as silver nitrate solution for routine prophylaxis against gonococcal ophthalmia[74, 119]; however, silver nitrate probably is the most effective agent against penicillinase-producing *N. gonorrhoeae*. The effectiveness of erythromycin or tetracycline in the prevention of ophthalmia caused by penicillinase-producing *N. gonorroheae* has not been established. No topical regimen has proven efficacy against *Chlamydia* conjunctivitis.[10, 23, 58] Furthermore, topical regimens do not eliminate *C. trachomatis* from the nasopharynx and do not prevent pneumonia.

Prophylaxis should be administered as soon as possible after birth. Each eyelid should be wiped gently with sterile cotton before administering local prophylaxis. Care must be exercised to ensure that the solution or ointment is in the conjunctival sac and that it is not flushed from the eye after instillation.

Group B *Streptococcus* Infections

Prophylaxis is aimed at prevention of early-onset neonatal group B *Streptococcus* (GBS) infections.[2, 12, 24, 89, 98, 100] There are no existing recommendations for prophylaxis against late-onset infections.

Several regimens have been attempted to reduce vertical transmission of GBS. Multiple studies employing oral antimicrobial agents to eradicate GBS colonization prepartum (antepartum chemoprophylaxis) have not been successful, even when sexual partners were treated concurrently.[89] Prophylaxis of newborn infants with penicillin G or ampicillin soon after birth (postnatal chemoprophylaxis) is ineffective in preventing early-onset GBS disease, primarily because in most patients infection occurs in utero and the infants are asymptomatic at or within a few hours after birth.

Current recommendations focus on targeting colonized women who fall into special-risk categories (selective intrapartum maternal chemoprophylaxis).[1, 2, 24] The American Academy of Pediatrics recommends that cultures of the lower vagina and anorectum (single swab) be obtained at 26 to 28 weeks' gestation, placed into selective broth medium, transported, and subcultured onto solid media.[24] Women who have no prenatal GBS culture results available and who present in labor with an identified risk factor (Table 232–2) may be tested for GBS by rapid antigen test or by culture. Maternal GBS carriers, identified prepartum or intrapartum, with one or more risk factors should be given intrapartum intravenous ampicillin (2 g initially, then 1 to 2 g every 4 to 6 hours) or penicillin G (5 million units every 6 hours) until delivery.[24] Penicillin-allergic women may be given clindamycin or erythromycin intravenously. Previous delivery of an infant with invasive GBS disease warrants intrapartum maternal chemoprophylaxis for each subsequent pregnancy, regardless of maternal colonization.

TABLE 232–2. Risk Factors for Early-Onset Group B *Streptococcus* (GBS) Infection

Maternal Risk Factors
Premature onset of labor at <37 weeks' gestation
Premature rupture of membranes at <37 weeks' gestation
Rupture of membranes (>18 hours) at any gestation
Maternal fever during labor
Multiple births
High GBS genital inoculum
GBS bacteriuria
Low type-specific GBS capsular polysaccharide antibody
Maternal age <20 years
Black race
Diabetes mellitus
Infant Risk Factors
Low birth weight
Prematurity

Intrapartum antibiotic prophylaxis will prevent substantial numbers but not all cases of early-onset GBS neonatal infections and will decrease the incidence of maternal GBS postpartum endometritis.[77, 84] Although many obstetric care providers take some measure to prevent GBS disease, reported practices often are inconsistent with the existing recommendations.[64] The major contended issue is timing of the antepartum screening cultures.[77]

Management of infants whose mothers received intrapartum chemoprophylaxis remains empiric and should be based on clinical manifestations and gestational age. If indicated, appropriate cultures should be obtained and antimicrobial therapy initiated, pending culture results.[24]

Necrotizing Enterocolitis

Bacterial proliferation and invasion of the intestinal wall are part of the pathogenesis of necrotizing enterocolitis (NEC). Therefore, suppression of the gastrointestinal flora with nonabsorbable oral antimicrobials was attempted in an effort to prevent NEC in premature infants. Administration of oral kanamycin or gentamicin prophylactically in the first few hours of life generated contradictory data. Furthermore, selective overgrowth of resistant organisms in the bowel and significant systemic absorption of aminoglycosides from the injured mucosa are potential risk factors. Currently, oral aminoglycosides are not recommended in the prophylaxis of NEC.

One report[88] suggests that oral vancomycin given for 48 hours before introduction of oral feeds may be beneficial in preventing NEC. These observations have not been confirmed, and such prophylaxis is not practiced routinely or recommended.

Intravascular Catheter Insertions

Infection with coagulase-negative staphylococci, primarily *Staphylococcus epidermidis*, is likely to occur in premature infants or infants who have indwelling vascular catheters. Low-grade sepsis is the most common clinical manifestation; however, meningitis, endocarditis, omphalitis, cellulitis, and other focal infections may occur. Two randomized trials of low-dose vancomycin added to total parenteral nutrition fluids (25 μg of vancomycin per mL of fluid) suggested that such a prophylactic regimen significantly reduced coagulase-negative staphylococcal infections in small premature infants in neonatal intensive care units.[67, 111] Widespread use of this regimen will not be recommended until more data are collected and the issue of emergence of vancomycin-resistant organisms is addressed adequately.[6]

DISEASE-TARGETED PROPHYLAXIS

Rheumatic Fever

Group A *Streptococcus* (GAS) infections of the pharynx are the precipitating cause of rheumatic fever. Appropriate antibiotic treatment of streptococcal pharyngitis prevents acute rheumatic fever in most cases.[37] Because at least one third of episodes of acute rheumatic fever result from inapparent streptococcal infections[30] and some symptomatic patients do not seek medical care, not all instances of rheumatic fever are preventable. Prevention of first attacks (primary prevention) is accomplished by proper identification, adequate antibiotic treatment, and eradication of this streptococcal infection. The individual who has suffered an attack of rheumatic fever is at very high risk to develop recurrences after subsequent GAS pharyngitis and needs continuous chemoprophylaxis to prevent such recurrences (secondary prevention).[32]

Primary Prevention

In selecting a regimen for the treatment of GAS pharyngitis, physicians should consider various factors, including bacteriologic and clinical efficacy, ease of adherence to the recommended regimen (frequency of daily administration, duration of therapy, palatability), cost, spectrum of activity of the selected agent, and potential side effects. No single regimen eradicates GAS from the pharynx in 100 per cent of treated patients.

Penicillin is the antimicrobial agent of choice for the treatment of GAS,[7, 25, 32] except in penicillin-allergic individuals (Table 232–3). Penicillin has a narrow spectrum of activity, has a long-standing proven efficacy, and is the least expensive regimen. GAS that are resistant to penicillin have not been documented. Even when started as long as 9 days after onset of acute illness, penicillin effectively prevents primary attacks of rheumatic fever.[21] Therefore, a brief delay for processing the throat culture (24 to 48 hours) before antibiotic therapy is started does not increase the risk of rheumatic fever. Patients are considered noncontagious 24 hours after initiation of therapy.[110]

Intramuscular benzathine penicillin G is preferred to oral penicillin, particularly for patients who are unlikely to complete a 10-day course of oral therapy and patients with a personal or family history of rheumatic fever or rheumatic heart disease or other environmental factors that place them at substantial risk for the development of rheumatic fever.[32] Benzathine penicillin injections should be given as a single dose in a large muscle mass. This formulation is painful; injections that contain procaine penicillin in addition to benzathine penicillin G are less painful. The combination of 900,000 units of benzathine penicillin G and 300,000 units of procaine penicillin G is satisfactory therapy for most children.[8] The efficacy of this combination for heavier patients, such as teenagers and adults, requires further study. Less discomfort is associated with intramuscular benzathine penicillin G if the medication is warmed to room temperature before administration.

The oral antibiotic of choice is penicillin V (phenoxymethyl penicillin) (see Table 232–3). All patients should continue to

TABLE 232–3. Prevention of Rheumatic Fever

Agent	Dose	Mode	Duration
	Primary Prevention		
Benzathine penicillin G	600,000 units for patients ≤27 kg 1,200,000 units for patients >27 kg	Intramuscularly	Once
Penicillin V	Children: 250 mg 2–3 times daily Adolescents and adults: 500 mg 2–3 times daily	Orally	10 days
	For Individuals Allergic to Penicillin		
Erythromycin	40 mg/kg/day 2–4 times daily (maximum, 1 g/day)	Orally	10 days
	Secondary Prevention		
Benzathine penicillin G	1,200,000 units every 3–4 weeks *or*	Intramuscularly	See text
Penicillin V	250 mg twice daily *or*	Orally	See text
Sulfadiazine	0.5 g once daily for patients ≤27 kg (60 lb) 1.0 g once daily for patients >27 kg (60 lb)	Orally	See text
	For Individuals Allergic to Penicillin and Sulfadiazine		
Erythromycin	250 mg twice daily	Orally	See text

take oral penicillin regularly for an entire 10-day period, even though they likely will be asymptomatic after the first few days. Penicillin V is preferred to penicillin G because it is more resistant to gastric acid. Although the broader spectrum penicillins, ampicillin and amoxicillin, often are used for treatment of GAS pharyngitis, they offer no microbiologic advantage over penicillin.

Oral erythromycin is acceptable for patients allergic to penicillin.[32] Treatment also should be prescribed for 10 days. Erythromycin estolate (20 to 40 mg/kg/day in two to four divided doses) or erythromycin ethyl succinate (40 mg/kg/day in two to four divided doses) is effective in treating streptococcal pharyngitis; however, the efficacy of a twice-daily regimen in adults requires further study. The maximum dose of erythromycin is 1 g/day. Although strains of GAS resistant to erythromycin are prevalent in some areas of the world and have resulted in treatment failures,[103] they are uncommon in most parts of the United States.[27]

The new macrolide azithromycin has a similar susceptibility pattern to that of erythromycin against GAS but may cause less frequent gastrointestinal side effects. Azithromycin can be administered once daily and produces high tonsillar tissue concentrations.[113] A 5-day course of azithromycin is approved by the Food and Drug Administration as a second-line therapy for the treatment of individuals 16 years of age or older with GAS pharyngitis. The recommended dosage is 500 mg as a single dose on the first day followed by 250 mg once daily for 4 days.[62]

A 10-day course of an oral cephalosporin is an acceptable alternative, particularly for penicillin-allergic individuals. Narrower spectrum cephalosporins, such as cefadroxil and cephalexin, probably are preferable to the broader spectrum cephalosporins, such as cefaclor, cefuroxime, cefixime, and cefpodoxime.[32] Some penicillin-allergic persons (<15 per cent) also are allergic to cephalosporins, and these agents should not be used in patients with immediate (anaphylactic-type) hypersensitivity to penicillin. Several reports indicate that a 10-day course with an oral cephalosporin is superior to 10 days of oral penicillin in eradicating GAS from the pharynx.[11, 31, 52, 93] Recent reports suggest that a 5-day course with selected oral cephalosporins is comparable to a 10-day course of oral penicillin in eradicating GAS from the pharynx.[3, 33, 94, 113] Such regimens currently are not approved by the Food and Drug Administration, and further studies are warranted to expand and confirm these observations.

Secondary Prevention

An individual with a previous attack of rheumatic fever who develops streptococcal pharyngitis is at high risk for a recurrent attack of rheumatic fever. A GAS infection need not be symptomatic to trigger a recurrence. Furthermore, rheumatic fever recurrence can occur even when a symptomatic infection is treated optimally. For these reasons, prevention of recurrent rheumatic fever requires continuous antimicrobial prophylaxis rather than recognition and treatment of acute episodes of streptococcal pharyngitis.[32] Continuous prophylaxis is recommended for patients with a well-documented history of rheumatic fever (including cases manifested solely by Sydenham chorea) and those with definite evidence of rheumatic heart disease. Such prophylaxis should be initiated as soon as acute rheumatic fever or rheumatic heart disease is diagnosed. A full therapeutic course of penicillin should be given first to patients with acute rheumatic fever to eradicate residual GAS, even if a throat culture is negative at that time. Streptococcal infections occurring in family members of rheumatic patients should be treated promptly.

An injection of 1,200,000 units of benzathine penicillin G every 4 weeks is the recommended regimen for secondary prevention in most circumstances in the United States (see Table 232–3). In countries where the incidence of rheumatic fever particularly is high, in special circumstances, or in certain high-risk individuals, such as patients with residual rheumatic carditis, the administration of benzathine penicillin G every 3 weeks is justified and recommended.[79, 80] Long-acting penicillin is of particular value in patients with a high risk of rheumatic fever recurrence, especially those with rheumatic heart disease in whom recurrence is very serious. The advantages of benzathine penicillin G must be weighed against inconvenience to the patient and pain of injection, which causes some individuals to discontinue prophylaxis.

Successful oral prophylaxis (penicillin V or sulfadiazine, Table 232–3) depends primarily on patient adherence to prescribed regimens.[34] Patients need detailed, careful, and repeated instructions about the importance of continuing prophylaxis. Most failures of prophylaxis occur in nonadherent patients. Even with optimal patient adherence, risk of recurrence is higher in individuals receiving oral prophylaxis compared with those receiving intramuscular benzathine penicillin G.[45] Oral agents are more appropriate for patients at lower risk for rheumatic recurrence. Accordingly, some physicians elect to switch patients to oral prophylaxis when they have reached late adolescence or young adulthood and have remained free of rheumatic attacks for at least 5 years.

Although sulfonamides are not effective in the eradication of GAS, they do prevent infection. Sulfonamide prophylaxis is contraindicated in late pregnancy because of transplacental passage of the drugs and potential competition with bilirubin for albumin-binding sites.

For the patient who is allergic to penicillin and sulfisoxazole, erythromycin is recommended. There are no published data about the use of other penicillins, macrolides, or cephalosporins for the secondary prevention of rheumatic fever.

Appropriate duration of prophylaxis must be determined for each individual situation.[32] Patients who have had rheumatic carditis are at a relatively high risk for recurrences of carditis and are likely to sustain increasingly severe cardiac involvement with each recurrence. Therefore, patients who have had rheumatic carditis should receive long-term antibiotic prophylaxis, perhaps for life. Prophylaxis should continue, even after valve surgery, including prosthetic valve replacement. Patients who have had rheumatic fever without rheumatic carditis are at considerably less risk of cardiac involvement with a recurrence. Therefore, a physician may consider discontinuing prophylaxis in these individuals after several years.[9] In general, prophylaxis should continue until 5 years have elapsed since the last rheumatic fever attack or age 21 years, whichever is longer.[32]

The decision to discontinue prophylaxis or reinstate it should be made after discussion with the patient of potential risks and benefits and careful consideration of various epidemiologic risk factors.[32] Risk of recurrence increases with multiple previous attacks, whereas the risk decreases as the interval since the most recent attack lengthens. In addition, the likelihood of acquiring a streptococcal upper respiratory tract infection is an important consideration. Individuals with increased exposure to streptococcal infections include children and adolescents, parents of young children, teachers, physicians, nurses and allied health personnel in contact with children, military recruits, and others living in crowded situations. A higher risk of recurrences in economically disadvantaged populations has been demonstrated.

Bacterial Endocarditis

Prophylactic antibiotics are recommended for children who are at risk to develop endocarditis when they undergo proce-

TABLE 232–4. Relative Risk of Endocarditis for Various Conditions

High Risk

Prosthetic valves
Previous episode of endocarditis
Surgically constructed systemic artery to pulmonary artery shunts
Intravenous drug abuse
Indwelling central venous catheters
Complex cyanotic congenital heart disease

Moderate Risk

Uncorrected patent ductus arteriosus
Ventricular septal defect
Uncorrected atrial septal defect (other than secundum)
Bicuspid aortic valve
Mitral valve prolapse with regurgitation and/or dysplastic leaflets
Rheumatic mitral or aortic valve disease
Other acquired valvar diseases
Hypertrophic cardiomyopathy

dures that may induce bacteremia with organisms likely to cause endocarditis. Recommended prophylaxis regimens are based primarily on in vitro studies, data collected from experimental animal models, epidemiologic observations, and clinical experiences. There are no adequate controlled clinical trials to validate the efficacy of such prophylaxis. Prevention of all episodes of bacteremia is impossible, and endocarditis may occur, despite appropriate antimicrobial prophylaxis.[29]

The relative risk of endocarditis varies, depending on the underlying condition (Table 232–4). Although intravenous drug abuse and indwelling central venous catheters are high-risk situations, prophylaxis in these situations is not practical. In general, dental or surgical procedures that induce bleeding from the gingiva or from the mucosal surfaces of the oral, respiratory, gastrointestinal, and genitourinary tracts may cause bacteremia and require prophylaxis (Table 232–5).

Poor dental hygiene and periodontal or periapical infections may produce bacteremia even in the absence of dental or oral procedures. Maintenance of optimal dental care and oral hygiene is important for the prevention of endocarditis in children with underlying cardiac disease. Patients in

TABLE 232–5. Dental and Surgical Procedures for Which Prophylaxis Is Recommended

- Dental procedures known to induce gingival or mucosal bleeding
  - Gingival surgery
  - Subgingival scaling or polishing
  - Subgingival orthodontic banding
  - Extractions
  - Matrix retainers and wedges
  - Periodontal surgery
  - Prophylactic teeth cleaning
- Tonsillectomy and/or adenoidectomy
- Bronchoscopy with rigid bronchoscope
- Esophageal stricture dilatation
- Cystoscopy
- Urethral dilatation
- Urethral catheterization if urinary tract infection is present*
- Urinary tract surgery if urinary tract infection is present*
- Incision and drainage of infected tissue*

*Antibiotic therapy should be directed against the most likely bacterial pathogen.

TABLE 232–6. Recommended Prophylaxis for Dental, Oral, Respiratory Tract, and Esophageal Procedures

Standard General Prophylaxis	
Amoxicillin	50 mg/kg (maximum, 2 g) orally 1 hour before procedure
Unable to Take Oral Medications	
Ampicillin	50 mg/kg (maximum, 2 g) intravenously or intramuscularly within ½ hour before procedure
Penicillin-Allergic	
Clindamycin	20 mg/kg (maximum, 300 mg) orally 1 hour before procedure
or	
Azithromycin	15 mg/kg (maximum, 500 mg) orally 1 hour before procedure
or	
Clarithromycin	
Penicillin-Allergic and Unable to Take Oral Medications	
Clindamycin	20 mg/kg (maximum, 600 mg) intravenously within ½ hour before procedure

For patients in the high-risk category for endocarditis, half the dose may be repeated 6 hours after the initial dose (except for azithromycin; a second dose is not necessary).

whom prosthetic valves or other devices are to be placed should undergo needed dental procedures to establish optimal oral hygiene before cardiac surgery. Prophylaxis is most effective when given perioperatively, starting shortly before a procedure and maintaining prophylaxis for about 10 hours. Doses should ensure adequate serum concentrations during and after a particular procedure.

Alpha-hemolytic streptococci are the most common cause of endocarditis after dental, oral, upper respiratory tract, or esophageal procedures.[29] Prophylaxis after such procedures should be directed specifically against these organisms, which generally are very susceptible to penicillin, ampicillin, or amoxicillin (Table 232–6). The standard general prophylaxis regimen is recommended, even in patients who are at high risk to develop endocarditis. For penicillin-allergic patients, clindamycin is recommended. Azithromycin and clarithromycin also are acceptable alternatives.

Bacterial endocarditis after genitourinary or gastrointestinal tract surgery or instrumentation primarily is caused by enterococci.[29] Bacteremia after gastrointestinal endoscopy in children is very rare,[19, 41] but is more common after genitourinary tract procedures. Gram-negative bacilli may induce bacteremia after such procedures; however, endocarditis rarely is caused by these organisms. Therefore, prophylaxis is directed primarily against enterococci (Table 232–7).

There are special situations in which the aforementioned recommendations may not apply. Surgical procedures through infected tissues require antimicrobial therapy directed against the most likely pathogen. Children who are receiving penicillin prophylaxis for prevention of recurrences of rheumatic fever may have alpha-hemolytic streptococci in their oral cavities that are relatively resistant to penicillins. In such cases, an agent other than amoxicillin (e.g., clindamycin) should be selected for endocarditis prophylaxis. Finally, prophylaxis is recommended for patients who undergo open heart surgery, but such prophylaxis should be aimed primarily against *Staphylococcus aureus* and coagulase-negative staphylococci (see section on cardiovascular surgery later). A first-generation cephalosporin or vancomycin is a reasonable choice and should be used only perioperatively and for no more than 48 hours.

TABLE 232–7. Recommended Prophylaxis for Genitourinary or Gastrointestinal Tract Procedures in Children

High-Risk	
Ampicillin *plus*	50 mg/kg (maximum, 2 g) intravenously or intramuscularly within ½ hour before procedure
Gentamicin	2 mg/kg (maximum, 80 mg) intravenously or intramuscularly within ½ hour before procedure (6 hours later, may use ampicillin, 25 mg/kg intravenously or intramuscularly, or amoxicillin, 25 mg/kg orally)
High-Risk, Penicillin-Allergic	
Vancomycin *plus*	20 mg/kg (maximum, 1 g) intravenously over 1 hour. Complete infusion within ½ hour before procedure
Gentamicin	2 mg/kg (maximum, 80 mg) intravenously or intramuscularly. Complete infusion/injection within ½ hour before procedure
Moderate-Risk	
Amoxicillin *or*	50 mg/kg (maximum, 2 g) orally 1 hour before procedure
Ampicillin	50 mg/kg (maximum, 2 g) intravenously or intramuscularly within ½ hour before procedure
Moderate-Risk, Penicillin-Allergic	
Vancomycin	20 mg/kg (maximum, 1 g) intravenously over 1 hour. Complete infusion within ½ hour before procedure

Recurrent Otitis Media

Acute otitis media is one of the most common infections in infants and children and is characterized by a tendency to recur, particularly during the first few years of life. In addition to tympanostomy tube placement and adenoidectomy, antimicrobial prophylaxis is one of the options recommended for the management of recurrent otitis media.[20, 97]

Antimicrobial prophylaxis currently is recommended for a child who has had three or more episodes of acute otitis media in 6 months or four episodes within a year, with the last episode occurring during the previous 6 months.[51, 91] Prophylaxis is directed against the most common potential pathogens that cause otitis media: *Streptococcus pneumoniae*, *Moraxella catarrhalis*, and nontypable *Haemophilus influenzae*. Amoxicillin, at a dose of 20 mg/kg, or sulfisoxazole, at a dose of 50 mg/kg, may be given orally each evening for a period of 3 to 6 months or during the winter months. Although many other antimicrobial agents are used in the treatment of otitis media, only amoxicillin and sulfisoxazole currently are recommended as prophylactic agents. Antimicrobial prophylaxis must be used with great caution and balanced against the potential for increasing the emergence of resistant organisms, particularly *S. pneumoniae*. If prophylaxis does not prevent recurrent infections, referral to an otolaryngologist is recommended for evaluation and possible tympanostomy tube placement and/or adenoidectomy.

Recurrent Urinary Tract Infection

Urinary tract infection (UTI) occurs in about 5 per cent of females and 1 to 2 per cent of males.[122] Recurrent UTIs are noted in approximately 30 to 50 per cent of children with UTIs, with most recurrences occurring within 3 months after the initial episode. Eighty per cent of recurrences are new infections caused by different colonic bacterial species that have become resistant to recently administered antibiotics. The recurrence rate is not altered by extending the duration of treatment.

Renal parenchymal infections and renal scarring are well-recognized complications of UTI in children.[61, 83, 106] Parenchymal scarring is found in 10 to 15 per cent of children with UTI,[109, 122] and it is estimated that about 10 per cent of children with this complication will develop hypertension and a smaller number may develop renal insufficiency.[65] Vesicoureteral reflux is noted in 30 to 50 per cent of children with UTI,[83] the frequency being directly related to the number of UTI episodes and inversely related to age. Children with reflux have a much higher incidence (30 to 60 per cent) of pyelonephritic scarring than children without reflux. More than 90 per cent of children with renal parenchymal scarring have had vesicoureteral reflux and a history of UTI.[109, 122]

Children who have three or more UTIs in a 12-month period may benefit from suppressive antibiotic therapy for up to 6 months to allow repair of intrinsic bladder defense mechanisms.[122] In children with anatomic defects or reflux, suppressive therapy may be needed for as long as the underlying defect exists.

Appropriate prophylactic agents should result in low serum but high urinary levels of the medication, have a minimal effect on the fecal flora, be well tolerated, and be inexpensive. Methenamine mandelate (75 mg/kg divided every 12 hours) is a suitable agent for prophylaxis because it releases formaldehyde in an acid medium. A pH of 5.5 or lower must be maintained in the urine to obtain optimal results. Ascorbic acid or other acidifying agents should be used to achieve the desired urine acidity. Other useful agents for prophylaxis in children with normal renal function are trimethoprim-sulfamethoxazole (TMP-SMX), nitrofurantoin, and nalidixic acid.[14, 59, 65, 83, 104] TMP-SMX can be given at 2 mg of TMP and 10 mg of SMX per kg in a single daily dose or at 5 mg of TMP and 25 mg of SMX per kg twice a week. TMP has the additional unique characteristic of diffusing into the vaginal and urethral fluids, therefore decreasing bacterial colonization with members of Enterobacteriaceae and diminishing ascending reinfection.[59, 112] Nitrofurantoin is recommended at 1 to 2 mg/kg taken each night. It has been used effectively as prophylaxis for recurrent UTI in infants and children. Pulmonary, neurologic, and hepatic adverse effects have been reported but are rare.[83] Nalidixic acid (not recommended for children) is administered at 30 mg/kg divided every 12 hours. It is a bactericidal agent for most of the common gram-negative uropathogens.

POSTEXPOSURE PROPHYLAXIS

Prophylaxis targeted against specific organisms after an individual is exposed will be discussed in this section.

Pertussis

When a case of pertussis is identified, prompt use of erythromycin prophylaxis in close contacts is effective in limiting secondary transmission. Close contacts are household members, child care attendees, and other individuals who are in contact with the index case for 4 or more hours a day. Chemoprophylaxis is recommended irrespective of age or vaccination status because immunity after pertussis immunization is not absolute and may not prevent infection.[25] The recommended dose of erythromycin is 40 to 50 mg/kg/day (maximum, 2 g/day) to be given orally in four divided doses for 14 days. Individuals who are allergic to erythromycin or cannot tolerate it may be given TMP-SMX, although the efficacy of this regimen has not been documented. The dose is 8 mg/kg/day (TMP) and 40 mg/kg/day (SMX) orally in two divided doses for 14 days.

Persons who have been in contact with an infected individual should be monitored closely for respiratory symptoms for 2 weeks after last contact with the index case. The risk of pertussis in adults providing medical care to children should be recognized. Symptoms may be mild and not readily recognized as pertussis; however, such individuals can transmit the infection.

Meningococcal Infections

Close contacts of patients with invasive disease due to *Neisseria meningitidis* (meningococcemia and/or meningitis) are at higher risk of developing infection than the general population. Secondary cases and outbreaks may occur in households, child care centers, nursery schools, colleges, and military camps.[25] The attack rate for household contacts is 0.3 to 1.0 per cent (300 to 1000 times the rate in the general population). Spread from patients to medical care providers is infrequent unless there is intimate contact (e.g., mouth-to mouth resuscitation, intubation, suctioning). Respiratory tract cultures are not recommended and are not of value in deciding who should receive prophylaxis.[25]

Chemoprophylaxis should be administered as soon as possible, preferably within 24 hours of identifying the index case.[25] Systemic antimicrobial therapy of meningococcal disease does not eradicate nasopharyngeal carriage of *N. meningitidis* reliably; therefore, antimicrobial chemoprophylaxis should be administered to the index patient before discharge from the hospital. The antibiotic of choice in most instances is rifampin. The recommended regimen is 10 mg/kg (maximum, 600 mg) every 12 hours for a total of four doses in 2 days. A liquid preparation can be formulated, or the powder can be mixed with applesauce or a similar vehicle. Rifampin prophylaxis regimen recommended for *H. influenzae* type b disease (see later) also is effective for meningococcal prophylaxis.

Rifampin prophylaxis has several shortcomings.[101] It fails to eradicate *N. meningitidis* in 10 to 20 per cent of pharyngeal carriers.[86] It is not recommended for pregnant women. Side effects are frequent and include headache, dizziness, gastrointestinal symptoms, discoloration of body secretions (saliva, tears, urine), staining of contact lenses, and hepatotoxicity. Finally, several studies have documented the emergence of resistant meningococcal strains after rifampin prophylaxis.[101]

If the meningococcal isolate is known to be susceptible to sulfonamides, sulfisoxazole is recommended. The dose is 500 mg/day for infants, 500 mg every 12 hours for children 1 to 12 years of age, and 1 g every 12 hours for children older than 12 years of age and adults. The duration of prophylaxis is 2 days.

In one study,[101] a single intramuscular injection of ceftriaxone was compared with oral rifampin in eradicating pharyngeal carriage of group A *N. meningitidis* during an outbreak. Ceftriaxone was significantly more effective than rifampin in eradicating meningococci at 1 week (97 per cent vs. 75 per cent) and at 2 weeks (97 per cent vs. 81 per cent) after prophylaxis. Ceftriaxone was administered as a single intramuscular dose (125 mg for children younger than 15 years of age and 250 mg for adults). Although at this stage ceftriaxone is not recommended for routine prophylaxis, it has the advantages of ease of administration, possible greater efficacy, and safety in pregnancy.

Haemophilus influenzae Type b Infections

The risk of secondary invasive disease with *H. influenzae* type b is age-dependent.[5] Household contacts younger than 1 year of age have the highest risk (6 per cent) of developing secondary illness; the risk in children 4 years of age or younger remains high (2.1 per cent). Children older than 6 years of age and adults are at little or no risk. The risk for children attending child care centers may be increased but appears to be less than that for household contacts.[16, 46, 82, 87, 90] Exposed hospital personnel do not require antimicrobial prophylaxis.

Prophylaxis currently is recommended to all household contacts, regardless of age, if at least one of the contacts is younger than 4 years of age and not immunized completely.[25] Complete immunization is defined as having received a conjugate vaccine: (1) at least one dose at 15 months of age or older, (2) two doses between 12 and 14 months of age, or (3) two or more doses when younger than 12 months of age with a booster at 12 months of age or older.

Prophylaxis for nursery and day care center contacts is less well defined, and definitive recommendations are lacking. In general, prophylaxis is recommended for child care centers in the same regimen as recommended for households if (1) the center is attended by unvaccinated or incompletely vaccinated children younger than 2 years of age where contact is 25 hours per week or more or (2) two or more cases of invasive *H. influenzae* type b disease occur among attendees within 60 days and unvaccinated or incompletely vaccinated children attend the facility.[25] In facilities where all contacts are older than 2 years of age, prophylaxis need not be given, regardless of vaccination status.

Rifampin, in a single dose of 20 mg/kg/day (maximum, 600 mg) for 4 days, effectively eliminates the oropharyngeal carriage of *H. influenzae* type b in 95 per cent of treated individuals.[25] This regimen has been shown to be effective in preventing secondary cases of invasive *H. influenzae* type b disease in household members, day care settings, and classroom contacts.[5, 16, 25] Prophylaxis should be initiated as soon as possible because most secondary cases occur during the first week after identification of the index case.[5] The index case also should receive rifampin prophylaxis, usually initiated during hospitalization and just before discharge.

If prophylaxis is given to limit secondary spread to a cohort (household or day care), children vaccinated with any *H. influenzae* type b vaccine and unvaccinated susceptible children should receive prophylaxis.[25] Prophylaxis is not recommended for pregnant women.

Tuberculosis

There are three goals of preventive therapy for tuberculosis: (1) to prevent asymptomatic (latent) infection from progressing to clinical (active) disease, (2) to prevent recurrence of past disease, and (3) to prevent initial infection in individuals who have negative tuberculin skin tests. The first two goals are covered in detail elsewhere. Prevention of initial infection will be addressed here; chemoprophylaxis is given in an attempt to prevent the establishment of infection, and the recipient is protected only as long as antituberculous therapy is continued.

In the United States, isoniazid is the only drug approved by the Food and Drug Administration for chemoprophylaxis against *Mycobacterium tuberculosis*. The recommended dose is 10 to 15 mg/kg/day (maximum, 300 mg/day) to be given as a single dose.

Persons exposed to an infectious case of tuberculosis should undergo tuberculin skin testing, have a chest roentgenogram, and receive isoniazid prophylaxis.[25] If the tuberculin test and chest roentgenogram are negative and the individual is not anergic, isoniazid should be administered for 12 weeks and contact with the index case should be broken. Isoniazid may be discontinued if a repeat skin test after 12 weeks of prophylaxis remains negative. If the skin test becomes positive, isoniazid is continued for a total of 9 months. Candidates for prophylaxis include persons with impaired immunity; household contacts and particularly children younger than 4 years of age; recent contacts, especially HIV-positive contacts; and persons known to be anergic from populations with a high prevalence of tuberculosis.

The newborn infant whose mother or other household contact has tuberculosis should be managed based on individual considerations.

HOST-TARGETED PROPHYLAXIS

Human and Animal Bites

Human and animal bites are relatively common. According to the Centers for Disease Control and Prevention, more than 1 million animal bites that occur each year require medical attention.[115] Human bites accounted for 1 in 600 pediatric emergency visits and dog bites for 1 per cent of all such visits.[102] Dog bites account for 80 to 90 per cent of animal bites that require medical care.[15] The most frequently isolated organisms in human bites are *S. aureus*, gamma-hemolytic streptococci, *Bacteroides* species, *Eikenella corrodens*, and *Fusobacterium* species. In animal bites, *Pasteurella multocida*, *S. aureus*, and anaerobic cocci are the main pathogens.

Data for the use of prophylactic antimicrobials after bites are sparse, and the role of prophylaxis for patients who present early with bite wounds is uncertain.[4, 39, 102, 108] However, because these wounds usually are contaminated with potential pathogens, it is advisable to administer prophylaxis to patients who have the following risk factors: delay of 18 hours or more between the time of injury and the time of initial physician assessment, facial and hand bites, deep puncture wounds, bites that are difficult to irrigate and cleanse adequately prior to repair, delay in primary closure of wound, and wounds in immune-compromised individuals.[4, 15, 38, 81, 102, 123]

Because most human and animal bites result in polymicrobial aerobic and anaerobic infections, prophylaxis should target these organisms. For initial prophylaxis, amoxicillin–clavulanic acid (30 to 50 mg/kg/day) probably is optimal therapy.[13, 15, 44, 108] Prophylaxis is recommended for 3 to 5 days. Combination therapy with penicillin and cephalexin or dicloxacillin has been suggested by some authorities. Although it is only moderately active against *P. multocida*, erythromycin (30 to 50 mg/kg/day) is an accepted alternative in penicillin-allergic children.

Asplenia

The spleen constitutes about 25 per cent of the lymphoid mass. It filters blood at a rate of 150 mL/minute and plays an important role in the primary defense against bacteria that gain access to the circulation.[114] The spleen has an active role in phagocytosis, is a major source of T lymphocytes, and produces IgM antibodies, complement, opsinons, and "tuftsin" (a phagocytosis-promoting tetrapeptide).

Asplenia may be congenital or acquired. Splenectomy is not an uncommon operation and is performed for a variety of indications. Overwhelming and often fatal septicemia and meningitis occur with increased frequency in asplenic individuals.[121] The frequency of sepsis is 60 times greater in children who undergo splenectomies than in normal children. Fatality from sepsis in splenectomized individuals is 200 times more common than death due to sepsis in the normal population.[114] The risk of sepsis is greatest in patients who have undergone splenectomies for underlying immunologic or reticuloendothelial disorders, and the risk is lowest in children after splenectomy for trauma.[71] In all categories, the risk is highest in young infants and children, but it extends to teenagers and adults as well. The period of heightened susceptibility to infection is the initial 1 to 2 years after splenectomy; however, fulminant infection has been reported up to 25 years after splenectomy.

S. pneumoniae is the most common cause of septicemia in splenectomized individuals. Despite prompt diagnosis and treatment, pneumococcal septicemia is associated with a fatality rate as high as 50 per cent. Overall, 80 per cent of postsplenectomy infections are due to bacteria with capsular polysaccharides: *S. pneumoniae*, *H. influenzae*, and *N. meningitidis*.[107, 114]

To reduce the likelihood of serious infections after splenectomy, several measures are advisable. Splenectomy should be performed only when absolutely indicated. If possible, it is best to delay the surgical intervention until 5 or 6 years of age. Although multivalent pneumococcal polysaccharide vaccine provides incomplete protection for patients undergoing splenectomy, especially infants and young children, it should be administered to all these patients, ideally 2 weeks prior to splenectomy.[107] Vaccination against *H. influenzae* type b and *N. meningitidis* types A and C also should be provided. For antibiotic prophylaxis, penicillin is the agent of choice. Penicillin V given twice daily significantly decreases the frequency of invasive pneumococcal infections. Erythromycin or TMP-SMX is an alternate option in patients with documented hypersensitivity to penicillin. The duration of prophylactic coverage remains controversial; current practice is to employ penicillin prophylaxis indefinitely in immunocompromised patients.[107]

Hemoglobinopathies

Functional asplenia is the primary reason for susceptibility to pneumococcal infection in children with sickle-cell anemia. Serum immunoglobulins are normal or increased in these children; however, they have a dysfunctional alternate complement pathway and a decreased opsonic activity (which is mediated by both the alternate and the classical component) against *S. pneumoniae*. Leukocyte function also is defective in patients with sickle-cell anemia; intracellular production of hydrogen peroxide, respiratory stimulation, and hexose monophosphate shunt activity are inadequate during phagocytosis. In contrast, leukocytes from splenectomized patients without sickle-cell anemia exhibit normal phagocytic function accompanied by adequate metabolic stimulation. Immunologic dysfunction is less rapid and less common in children with hemoglobin C–sickle-cell anemia and hemoglobin C–beta-thalassemia.[75]

Patients with sickle-cell disease are at risk of overwhelming infection (septicemia and meningitis) due to encapsulated bacteria, including *S. pneumoniae*, *H. influenzae* type b, and *N. meningitidis*. *S. pneumoniae* is the most important and frequent cause of septicemia and meningitis in these patients.[117] The risk is particularly high in very young children younger than 3 years of age.[49] There also is a trend toward increased frequency of invasive disease in the first 2 to 5 years after splenectomy. Unlike very young children, preschool children appear to be less vulnerable to develop pneumococcal invasive infections, even though they remain functionally asplenic.[50, 117, 120]

The efficacy of penicillin prophylaxis in preventing pneumococcal infection in infants and young children with sickle-cell disease has been well documented in several reports.[42, 49, 50, 92, 120] The recommended dose for penicillin V is 125 mg twice daily in children younger than 5 years of age and 250 mg twice daily in children 5 years of age or older. Some recommend amoxicillin (20 mg/kg/day) or TMP-SMX (4 mg TMP plus 20 mg SMX/kg/day) for children younger than 5 years of age to include coverage against *H. influenzae* type b, which is less likely to be a concern in patients who are immunized adequately.

Because overwhelming infection can occur as early as 3 months of age, detection of sickle-cell anemia should be made in the neonatal period. Babies diagnosed to have sickle-cell anemia should be started on a prophylactic antibiotic regimen no later than 3 to 4 months of age.[50] The optimum duration of prophylaxis is not defined clearly, and the age at which prophylactic penicillin safely can be discontinued is determined arbitrarily. There is a concern that penicillin prophylaxis may decrease the development of natural immunity against pneumococcal infection in children receiving prophylaxis, thus making them more prone to infection after discontinuing the prophylaxis.[17] Another concern is the accelerated development of penicillin-resistant strains of *S. pneumoniae*.[43, 117] A multicenter study by the Prophylactic Penicillin Study II group suggests that in children with sickle-cell anemia who have not had a previous severe pneumococcal infection or a surgical splenectomy and are receiving comprehensive care, prophylaxis safely may be stopped at 5 years of age.[43] Continuous prophylaxis has limitations, and serious overwhelming infection can occur while on prophylaxis. Patients and/or parents should be aware that any febrile illness potentially is serious and that immediate medical attention should be sought.[28, 92]

Cerebrospinal Fluid Leakage

The value of antibiotic prophylaxis in patients with cerebrospinal fluid leakage is debatable.[47, 85] In the absence of meningeal inflammation, many antibiotics do not penetrate the blood-brain barrier and do not attain adequate levels in the cerebrospinal fluid. Antibiotic prophylaxis often fails and frequently alters the normal flora of the respiratory tract, resulting in colonization with resistant bacteria. Prophylaxis may be considered for a short duration while surgical repair is being planned.[85]

SURGICAL PROPHYLAXIS

General Surgical Procedures

Postoperative infection always has been a feared complication of surgical procedures. Skin incision, organ manipulation, and surgical trauma increase the likelihood of local infection. Surgical procedures traditionally are classified as clean, clean-contaminated, and contaminated (Table 232–8). Prophylactic antibiotics are effective in reducing postoperative infections after contaminated and clean-contaminated surgical procedures, whereas their efficacy is more controversial for clean surgical procedures. Clean surgical procedures generally carry a risk of postoperative wound infection that is less than 5 per cent and in many hospitals less than 1 per cent.

TABLE 232–8. Surgical Procedures and Likely Pathogens

Surgical Category	Most Likely Pathogens
Clean	
Neurosurgical	CNS, *Staphylococcus aureus*
Cardiovascular	CNS, *S. aureus*
Orthopedics	CNS, *S. aureus*
Clean-Contaminated	
Burn	Group A streptococci, *S. aureus*, GNB
Gastrointestinal	GNB, anaerobes, enterococci
Urogenital	GNB, enterococci
Respiratory	Alpha-hemolytic streptococci, anaerobes
Contaminated	
Ruptured viscera	GNB, anaerobes, enterococci
Traumatic wounds	*S. aureus*, group A streptococci, clostridia

CNS, coagulase-negative staphylococci; GNB, gram-negative bacilli.

The critical period for development of infection is short, and it is well recognized that optimal prophylaxis should be restricted to the perioperative period. Antibiotic prophylaxis of less than 24 hours' duration is effective both clinically and experimentally. Antibiotic administration should be started at the time of anesthesia induction or immediately before the surgical incision is made and discontinued within 24 hours.

It is beyond the scope of this chapter to address all situations of surgical prophylaxis, and the reader is referred to several recent publications and reviews on the subject.[35, 60, 66, 68, 95, 116]

Neurosurgical Procedures

The use of prophylactic antibiotics for clean neurosurgical procedures still is controversial.[48, 54, 85, 96] However, because of the suggested benefit of prophylactic antibiotics in uncontrolled trials involving a large number of patients, of whom adults were the majority, and in view of the scarcity of definitive studies, the literature supports the use of a short-course prophylactic regimen.[18, 40, 55, 118] Prophylaxis for clean neurosurgical procedures particularly is valuable for high-risk groups (e.g., patients undergoing operative procedures in excess of 4 hours or craniotomies or patients with major underlying pathology).[36, 105]

Placement of cerebrospinal fluid shunts is one of the most common neurosurgical procedures in pediatric patients. An estimated 10,000 new shunt insertions and 6000 revisions are performed annually in the United States. The frequency of shunt infection varies from 1.5 to 39 per cent (average, 10 to 15 per cent).[72, 99] The major route of infection is colonization of the device or the operative wounds during placement.[53] Retrograde spread from the distal end of the catheter or hematogenous seeding accounts for some instances of infection.

Most infections present within 15 days to 2 months of shunt placement.[76, 99] Commensal skin flora are the predominant pathogens. Coagulase-negative staphylococci are the most common pathogens and account for about 70 per cent of shunt infections. *S. aureus* is less common. Gram-negative bacilli are the least common and often are the result of retrograde infection from the peritoneum.[72, 99]

The role of prophylactic antibiotics for placement of cerebrospinal fluid shunts has been controversial. A meta-analysis of 1359 patients in 12 randomized, controlled trials indicated that short-term perioperative antimicrobial prophylaxis at the time of cerebrospinal fluid shunt placement significantly decreases the risk of subsequent device-related infection.[76] Various antimicrobial regimens were used in these trials, including antistaphylococcal penicillins, cephalosporins, TMP-SMX, vancomycin, gentamicin, and combinations. The choice of an appropriate prophylactic regimen in a particular setting should be based on local epidemiology of suspected pathogens, local patterns of antimicrobial susceptibility, cost, and expected toxicity. Duration of perioperative prophylaxis should not exceed 48 hours.[70, 76] Longer duration of prophylaxis increases cost and the risk of adverse reactions and promotes alteration of the normal flora and the emergence of resistant bacteria.

Cardiovascular Surgery

Infectious complications of cardiovascular surgery can be very serious and life-threatening, and antimicrobial prophylaxis commonly is used in most medical centers.[69, 73] The majority of available data are based on reports from adult patients[26, 56]; there is little specific information on prophylactic antibiotic usage in pediatric patients. The goal of prophylactic therapy is the prevention of wound infection, mediastinitis, and endocarditis. A survey of 43 North American academic centers with pediatric cardiovascular surgery programs indicated that all centers use prophylactic antibiotics for all operative procedures.[78] Monotherapy prophylaxis was used by 91 per cent of respondents and consisted almost exclusively of a first- or second-generation cephalosporin. In 95 per cent of centers, prophylaxis was started just before surgery or intraoperatively. Prophylaxis was continued for 48 hours or less in the majority (68 per cent) of instances. Prophylactic antibiotics often were continued while thoracostomy tubes, mediastinal tubes, or transthoracic vascular catheters were in place but usually not for endotracheal tubes, arterial or percutaneous central venous catheters, or temporary pacing wires.

References

1. Allen, U. D., Navas, L., and King, S. M.: Effectiveness of intrapartum penicillin prophylaxis in preventing early-onset group B streptococcal infection: Results of a meta-analysis. Can. Med. Assoc. J. *149*:1659–1665, 1993.
2. American College of Obstetricians and Gynecologists: Group B streptococcal infections in pregnancy. ACOG Technical Bulletin No. 170, Washington, D.C., 1992.
3. Aujard, Y., Boucot, I., Brahimi, N., et al.: Comparative efficacy and safety of four-day cefuroxime axetil and ten-day penicillin treatment of group A beta-hemolytic streptococcal pharyngitis in children. Pediatr. Infect. Dis. J. *14*:295–300, 1995.
4. Baker, D. M., and Moore, S. E.: Human bites in children: A six-year experience. Am. J. Dis. Child. *141*:1285–1290, 1987.
5. Band, J. D., Fraser, D. W., Ajello, G., et al.: Prevention of *Haemophilus influenzae* type B disease. J. A. M. A. *251*:2381–2386, 1984.
6. Barefield, E. S., and Philips, J. B., III: Vancomycin prophylaxis for coagulase-negative staphylococcal bacteremia. J. Pediatr. *125*:230–232, 1994.
7. Bass, J. W.: Antibiotic management of group A streptococcal pharyngotonsillitis. Pediatr. Infect. Dis. J. *10*:S43–S49, 1991.
8. Bass, J. W., Crast, F. W., Knowles, C. R., et al.: Streptococcal pharyngitis in children: A comparison of four treatment schedules with intramuscular penicillin G benzathine. J. A. M. A. *235*:1112–1116, 1976.
9. Berrios, X., del Campo, E., Guzman, B., et al.: Discontinuing rheumatic fever prophylaxis in selected adolescents and young adults. Ann. Intern. Med. *118*:401–406, 1993.
10. Black-Payne, C., Bocchini, J. A., Jr., and Cedotal, C.: Failure of erythromycin ointment for postnatal ocular prophylaxis of chlamydial conjunctivitis. Pediatr. Infect. Dis. J. *8*:491–498, 1989.
11. Block, S. L., Hedrick, J. A., and Tyler, R. D.: Comparative study of the effectiveness of cefixime and penicillin V for the treatment of streptococcal pharyngitis in children and adolescents. Pediatr. Infect. Dis. J. *11*:919–925, 1992.
12. Boyer, K. M., and Gotoff, S. P.: Prevention of early-onset neonatal group B streptococcal disease with selective intrapartum chemoprophylaxis. N. Engl. J. Med. *314*:1665–1669, 1986.
13. Brakenbury, P. H., and Muwanga, C.: A comparative double blind study of amoxicillin/clavulanate vs. placebo in the prevention of infection after animal bites. Arch. Emerg. Med. *6*:251–256, 1989.
14. Brendstrup, L., Hjelt, K., Petersen, K. E., et al.: Nitrofurantoin versus trimethoprim prophylaxis in recurrent urinary tract infection in children: A randomized, double blind study. Acta Paediatr. Scand. *79*:1225–1234, 1990.
15. Brook, I.: Microbiology of human and animal bite wounds in children. Pediatr. Infect. Dis. J. *6*:29–32, 1987.
16. Broome, C. V., Mortimer, E. A., Katz, S. L., et al.: Use of chemoprophylaxis to prevent the spread of *Hemophilus influenzae* B in day-care facilities. N. Engl. J. Med. *316*:1226–1228, 1987.
17. Buchanan, G. R., and Smith, S. J.: Pneumococcal septicemia despite pneumococcal vaccine and prescription of penicillin prophylaxis in children with sickle cell anemia. Am. J. Dis. Child. *140*:428–432, 1986.
18. Bullock, R., Van Dellen, J. R., Ketelbey, W., et al.: A double-blind placebo-controlled trial of perioperative prophylactic antibiotics for elective neurosurgery. J. Neurosurg. *69*:687–691, 1988.
19. Byrne, W., Euler, A., Campbell, M., et al.: Bacteremia in children following upper gastrointestinal endoscopy or colonoscopy. J. Pediatr. Gastroenterol. Nutr. *1*:551–553, 1982.
20. Casselbrant, M. L., Kaleida, P. H., Rockette, H. E., et al.: Efficacy of antimicrobial prophylaxis and of tympanostomy tube insertion for prevention of recurrent acute otitis media: Results of a randomized clinical trial. Pediatr. Infect. Dis. J. *11*:278–286, 1992.
21. Catanzaro, F. J., Stetson, C. A., Morris, A. J., et al.: Symposium on rheumatic fever and rheumatic heart disease. Am. J. Med. *17*:749–756, 1954.
22. Chandler, J. W.: Controversies in ocular prophylaxis of newborns. Arch. Ophthalmol. *107*:814–815, 1989.
23. Chen, J. Y.: Prophylaxis of ophthalmia neonatorum: Comparison of silver nitrate, tetracycline, erythromycin and no prophylaxis. Pediatr. Infect. Dis. J. *11*:1026–1030, 1992.
24. Committee on Infectious Diseases and Committee on Fetus and Newborn: Guidelines for prevention of group B streptococcal (GBS) infection by chemoprophylaxis. Pediatrics *90*:775–778, 1992.
25. Committee on Infectious Diseases, American Academy of Pediatrics: 1994 Red Book: Report of the Committee on Infectious Diseases. Elk Grove Village, IL, American Academy of Pediatrics, 1994.
26. Conte, J. E., Jr., Cohen, S. N., Roe, B. B., et al.: Antibiotic prophylaxis and cardiac surgery: A prospective double-blind comparison of single-dose versus multiple-dose regimens. Ann. Intern. Med. *76*:943–949, 1972.
27. Coonan, K. M., and Kaplan, E. L.: In vitro susceptibility of recent North American group A streptococcal isolates to eleven oral antibiotics. Pediatr. Infect. Dis. J. *13*:630–635, 1994.
28. Cummins, D., Heuschkel, R., and Davies, S. C.: Penicillin prophylaxis in children with sickle cell disease in Brent. Br. Med. J. *302*:989–990, 1991.
29. Dajani, A. S., Bisno, A. L., Chung, K. J., et al.: Prevention of bacterial endocarditis: Recommendations by the American Heart Association. J. A. M. A. *264*:2919–2922, 1990.
30. Dajani, A. S.: Current status of nonsuppurative complications of group A streptococci. Pediatr. Infect. Dis. J. *10*:S25–S27, 1991.
31. Dajani, A. S., Kessler, S. L., Mendelson, R., et al.: Cefpodoxime proxetil vs. penicillin V in pediatric streptococcal pharyngitis/tonsillitis. Pediatr. Infect. Dis. J. 275–279, 1993.
32. Dajani, A., Taubert, K., Ferrieri, P., et al.: Treatment of acute streptococcal pharyngitis and prevention of rheumatic fever: A statement for health professionals. Pediatrics *96*:758–764, 1995.
33. Dajani, A. S.: Pharyngitis/tonsillitis: European and United States experience with cefpodoxime proxetil. Pediatr. Infect. Dis. J. *14*:S7–S11, 1995.
34. Dajani, A. S.: Adherence to physicians' instructions as a factor in managing streptococcal pharyngitis. Pediatrics *97*:976–980, 1996.
35. Dellinger, E. P., Gross, P. A., Barrett, T. L., et al.: Quality standard for antimicrobial prophylaxis in surgical procedures. Clin. Infect. Dis. *18*:422–427, 1994.
36. Dempsey, R., Rapp, R. P., Young, B., et al.: Prophylactic parenteral antibiotics in clean neurosurgic procedures: A review. J. Neurosurg. *69*:52–57, 1988.
37. Denny, F. W., Wannamaker, L. W., Brink, W. R., et al.: Prevention of rheumatic fever: Treatment of the preceding streptococcal infection. J. A. M. A. *143*:151–153, 1950.
38. Dire, D. J.: Cat bite wounds: Risk factors for infection. Ann. Emerg. Med. *20*:973–979, 1991.

39. Dire, D. J., Hogan, D. E., and Walker, J. S.: Prophylactic oral antibiotics for low-risk dog bite wounds. Pediatr. Emerg. Care *8*:194–199, 1992.
40. Djindjian, M., Lepresel, E., and Homs, J. B.: Antibiotic prophylaxis during prolonged clean neurosurgery. J. Neurosurg. *73*:383–386, 1990.
41. El-Baba, M., Tolia, V., Lin, C., et al.: Absence of bacteremia after gastrointestinal procedures in children. Gastrointest. Endosc. *44*:378–381, 1996.
42. El-Hazmi, M. A. F., Bahakim, H. M., Babikar, M. A., et al.: Symptom-free intervals in sicklers: Does pneumococcal vaccination and penicillin prophylaxis have a role? J. Trop. Pediatr. *36*:56–62, 1990.
43. Falletta, J. M., Woods, G. M., Verter, J. I., et al.: Discontinuing penicillin prophylaxis in children with sickle cell anemia. J. Pediatr. *127*:685–690, 1995.
44. Feder, H., Jr., Shanley, J. D., and Barbera, J. A.: Review of 59 patients hospitalized with animal bites. Pediatr. Infect. Dis. J. *6*:24–28, 1987.
45. Feinstein, A. R., Harrison, F. W., Epstein, J. A., et al.: A controlled study of three methods of prophylaxis against streptococcal infection in a population of rheumatic children. N. Engl. J. Med. *260*:697–702, 1959.
46. Fleming, D. W., Leibenhaut, M. H., Albanes, D., et al.: Secondary *Haemophilus influenzae* type B in day-care facilities. J. A. M. A. *254*:509–514, 1985.
47. Frazee, R. C., Mucha, P., Jr., Farnell, M. B., et al.: Meningitis after basilar skull fracture: Does antibiotic prophylaxis help? Postgrad. Med. *83*:267–274, 1988.
48. Gardner, B. P., and Gordon, D. S.: Postoperative infection in shunts for hydrocephalus: Are prophylactic antibiotics necessary? Br. Med. J. *284*:1914–1915, 1982.
49. Gaston, M. H., and Verter, J.: Sickle cell anaemia trial. Stat. Med. *9*:45–51, 1990.
50. Gaston, M. H., Verter, J. I., Woods, G., et al.: Prophylaxis with oral penicillin in children with sickle cell anemia. N. Engl. J. Med. *314*:1593–1599, 1986.
51. Giebink, G. S.: Preventing otitis media. Ann. Otol. Rhinol. Laryngol. *103*:20–23, 1994.
52. Gooch, W. M., McLinn, S. E., Aronovitz, G. H., et al.: Efficacy of cefuroxime axetil suspension compared with that of penicillin V suspension in children with group A streptococcal pharyngitis. Antimicrob. Agents Chemother. *37*:159–163, 1993.
53. Guevara, J. A., Zuccaro, G., Trevisan, A., et al.: Bacterial adhesion to cerebrospinal fluid shunts. J. Neurosurg. *67*:438–445, 1987.
54. Haines, S. J., and Goodman, M. L.: Antibiotic prophylaxis of postoperative neurosurgical wound infection. J. Neurosurg. *56*:103–105, 1982.
55. Haines, S. J.: Efficacy of antibiotic prophylaxis in clean neurosurgical operations. Neurosurgery *24*:401–405, 1989.
56. Hall, J. C., Christiansen, K., Carter, M. J., et al.: Antibiotic prophylaxis in cardiac operations. Ann. Thorac. Surg. *56*:916–922, 1993.
57. Hammerschlag, M. R.: Neonatal ocular prophylaxis. Pediatr. Infect. Dis. J. *7*:81–82, 1988.
58. Hammerschlag, M. R., Cummings, C., Roblin, P., et al.: Efficacy of neonatal ocular prophylaxis for the prevention of chlamydial and gonococcal conjunctivitis. N. Engl. J. Med. 320:769–772, 1989.
59. Hanson, E., Hansson, S., and Jodol, U.: Trimethoprim-sulfadiazine prophylaxis in children with vesicoureteral reflux. Scand. J. Infect. Dis. *21*:201–204, 1989.
60. Hirschmann, J. V., and Inui, T. S.: Antimicrobial prophylaxis: A critique of recent trials. Rev. Infect. Dis. *2*:1–23, 1980.
61. Holland, N. H., Jackson, E. C., Kazee, M., et al.: Relation of urinary tract infection and vesicoureteral reflux to scars: Follow-up of thirty-eight patients. J. Pediatr. *116*(Suppl.):65–71, 1990.
62. Hooton, T. M.: A comparison of azithromycin and penicillin V for the treatment of streptococcal pharyngitis. Am. J. Med. *91*:23S–30S, 1991.
63. Hussar, D. A.: Importance of patient compliance in effective antimicrobial therapy. Pediatr. Infect. Dis. J. *6*:971–975, 1987.
64. Jafari, H. S., Schuchat, A., Hilsdon, R., et al.: Barriers to prevention of perinatal group B streptococcal disease. Pediatr. Infect. Dis. J. *14*:662–667, 1995
65. Jodal, U., Koskimies, O., Hanson, E., et al.: Infection pattern in children with vesicoureteral reflux randomly allocated to operation or long-term antibacterial prophylaxis. J. Urol. *148*:1650–1652, 1992.
66. Jones, R. N., Wojeski, W., Bakke, J., et al.: Antibiotic prophylaxis of 1,036 patients undergoing elective surgical procedures: A prospective, randomized comparative trial of cefazolin, cefoxitin, and cefotaxime in a prepaid medical practice. Am. J. Surg. *153*:341–346, 1987.
67. Kacica, M. A., Horgan, M. J., Ochoa, L., et al.: Prevention of gram-positive sepsis in neonates weighing less than 1500 grams. J. Pediatr. 125:253–258, 1994.
68. Kaiser, A.B.: Antimicrobial prophylaxis in surgery. N. Engl. J. Med. 315:1129–1138, 1986.
69. Kaiser, A. B., Petracek, M. R., Lea, J. W., Jr., et al.: Efficacy of cefazolin, cefamandole, and gentamicin as prophylactic agents in cardiac surgery. Ann. Surg. *206*:791–797, 1987.
70. Kestle, J. R. W., Hoffman, H. J., Soloniuk, D., et al.: A concerted effort to prevent shunt infection. Childs Nerv. Syst. *9*:163–165, 1993.
71. Konradsen, H. B., and Henrichsen, J.: Pneumococcal infections in splenectomized children are preventable. Acta Paediatr. Scand. *80*:423–427, 1991.
72. Kontny, U., Hofling, B., Gutjahr, P., et al.: CSF shunt infections in children. Infection *21*:89–92, 1993.
73. Kreter, B., and Woods, M.: Antibiotic prophylaxis for cardiothoracic operations: Metaanalysis of thirty years of clinical trials. J. Thorac. Cardiovasc. Surg. *104*:590–599, 1992.
74. Laga, M., Plummer, F. A., Piot, P., et al.: Prophylaxis of gonococcal and chlamydial ophthalmia neonatorum: A comparison of silver nitrate and tetracycline. N. Engl. J. Med. *318*:653–657, 1988.
75. Lane, P. A., Rogers, Z. R., Woods, G. M., et al.: Fatal pneumococcal septicemia in hemoglobin SC disease. J. Pediatr. *124*:859–862, 1994.
76. Langley, J. M., LeBlanc, J. C., Drake, J., et al: Efficacy of antimicrobial prophylaxis in placement of cerebrospinal fluid shunts: Meta-analysis. Clin. Infect. Dis. *17*:98–103, 1993.
77. Larsen, J. W., and Dooley, S. L.: Group B streptococcal infections: An obstetrical viewpoint. Pediatrics *91*:148–149, 1993.
78. Lee, K. R., Ring, J. C., and Leggiadro, R. J.: Prophylactic antibiotic use in pediatric cardiovascular surgery: A survey of current practice. Pediatr. Infect. Dis. J. *14*:267–269, 1995.
79. Lue, H. C., Wu, M. H., Hsieh, K. H., et al.: Rheumatic fever recurrences: Controlled study of a 3-week versus 4-week benzathine penicillin prevention program. J. Pediatr. *108*:299–304, 1986.
80. Lue, H. C., Wu, M. H., Wang, J. K., et al.: Long-term outcome of patients with rheumatic fever receiving benzathine penicillin G prophylaxis every three weeks versus every four weeks. J. Pediatr. *125*:812–816, 1994.
81. Maimaris, C., and Quinton, D. N.: Dog-bite lacerations: A controlled trial of primary wound closure. Arch. Emerg. Med. *5*:156–161, 1988.
82. Makintubee, S., Istre, G. R., and Ward, J. I.: Transmission of invasive *Haemophilus influenzae* type B disease in day care settings. J. Pediatr. *111*:180–186, 1987.
83. McCracken, G. H., Jr.: Options in antimicrobial management of urinary tract infections in infants and children. Pediatr. Infect. Dis. J. *8*:552–555, 1989.
84. Mohle-Boetani, J. C., Schuchat, A., Plikaytis, B., et al.: Comparison of prevention strategies for neonatal group B streptococcal infection: A population-based economic analysis. J. A. M. A. *270*:1442–1448, 1993.
85. Mollman, D. H., and Haines, S. J.: Risk factors for postoperative neurosurgical wound infection: A case-control study. J. Neurosurg. *64*:902–906, 1986.
86. Munford, R. S., Vasconcelos, Z. J. S., Phillips, C. J., et al.: Eradication of carriage of *Neisseria meningitidis* in families: A study in Brazil. J. Infect. Dis. *129*:644–649, 1974.
87. Murphy, T. V., Clements, J. F., Breedlove, J. E., et al.: Risk of subsequent disease among day-care contacts of patients with systemic *Hemophilus influenzae* type B disease. N. Engl. J. Med. *316*:5–10, 1987.
88. Ng, P. C., Dear, P. R. F., and Thomas, D. F. M.: Oral vancomycin in prevention of necrotising enterocolitis. Arch. Dis. Child. *63*:1390–1393, 1988.
89. Noya, F. J. D., and Baker, C. J.: Prevention of group B streptococcal infection. Infect. Dis. Clin. North Am. *6*:41–54, 1992.
90. Osterholm, M. T., Pierson, L. M., White, K. E., et al.: The risk of subsequent transmission of *Hemophilus influenzae* type B disease among children in day care. N. Engl. J. Med. *316*:1–5, 1987.
91. Paradise, J. L.: Antimicrobial prophylaxis for recurrent acute otitis media. Ann. Otol. Rhinol. Laryngol. *155*:33–36, 1992.
92. Pegelow, C. H., Armstrong, F. D., Light, S., et al.: Experience with the use of prophylactic penicillin in children with sickle cell anemia. J. Pediatr. *118*:736–738, 1991.
93. Pichichero, M. E., and Margolis, P. A.: A comparison of cephalosporins and penicillin in the treatment of group A streptococcal pharyngitis: A meta-analysis supporting the concept of microbial copathogenicity. Pediatr. Infect. Dis. J. *10*:275–281, 1991.
94. Pichichero, M. E., Gooch, W. M., Rodriguez, W., et al.: Effective short-course treatment of acute group A beta-hemolytic streptococcal tonsillopharyngitis: Ten days of penicillin V vs. 5 days or 10 days of cefpodoxime therapy in children. Arch. Pediatr. Adolesc. Med. *148*:1053–1060, 1994.
95. Platt, R.: Methodologic aspects of clinical studies of perioperative antibiotic prophylaxis. Rev. Infect. Dis. *13*:S810–S814, 1991.
96. Pons, V. G., Denlinger, S. L., Guglielmo, B. J., et al.: Ceftizoxime versus vancomycin and gentamicin in neurosurgical prophylaxis: A randomized, prospective, blinded clinical study. Neurosurgery *33*:416–423, 1993.
97. Principi, N., Marchisio, P., Massironi, E., et al.: Prophylaxis of recurrent acute otitis media and middle-ear effusion. Am. J. Dis. Child. *143*:1414–1418, 1989.
98. Pylipow, M., Gaddis, M., and Kinney, J. S.: Selective intrapartum prophylaxis for group B *Streptococcus* colonization: Management and outcome of newborns. Pediatrics *93*:631–635, 1994.
99. Schoenbaum, S. C., Gardner, P., and Shillito, J.: Infections of cerebrospinal fluid shunts: Epidemiology, clinical manifestations, and therapy. J. Infect. Dis. *131*:543–551, 1975.
100. Schuchat, A., Oxtoby, M., Cochi, S., et al.: Population-based risk factors for neonatal group B streptococcal disease: Results of a cohort study in metropolitan Atlanta. J. Infect. Dis. *162*:672–677, 1990.
101. Schwartz, B., Al-Ttobaiqi, A., and Al-Ruwais, A.: Comparative efficacy of ceftriaxone and rifampicin in eradicating pharyngeal carriage of group A *Neisseria meningitidis*. Lancet *1*:1239–1242, 1988.
102. Schweich, P., and Fleisher, G.: Human bites in children. Pediatr. Emerg. Care *1*:51–53, 1985.

103. Seppala, H., Nissinen, A., Jarvinen, H., et al.: Resistance to erythromycin in group A streptococci. N. Engl. J. Med. *326*:292–297, 1992.
104. Shapiro, E. D.: Infections of the urinary tract. Pediatr. Infect. Dis. J. *11*:165–168, 1992.
105. Shapiro, M.: Prophylaxis in otolaryngologic surgery and neurosurgery: A critical review. Rev. Infect. Dis. *13*(Suppl. 10):S858–S868, 1991.
106. Shortliffe, L. M. D.: The management of urinary tract infections in children without urinary tract abnormalities. Urol. Clin. North Am. *22*:67–73, 1995.
107. Siddins, M., Downie, J., and Wise, K.: Prophylaxis against postsplenectomy pneumococcal infection. Aust. N. Z. J. Surg. *60*:183–187, 1990.
108. Skurka, J., Willert, C., and Yogev, R.: Wound infection following dog bite despite prophylactic penicillin. Infection *14*:134–135, 1986.
109. Smellie, J. M., and Normand, I. C. S.: Urinary infections in children, 1985. Postgrad. Med. J. *61*:895–905, 1985.
110. Snellman, L. W., Stang, H. J., Stang, J. M., et al.: Duration of positive throat cultures for group A streptococci after initiation of antibiotic therapy. Pediatrics *91*:1166–1170, 1993.
111. Spafford, P. S., Sinkin, R. A., Cox, C., et al.: Prevention of central venous catheter-related coagulase-negative staphylococcal sepsis in neonates. J. Pediatr. *125*:259–263, 1994.
112. Stamay, T. A., Condy, M., and Mibara, G.: Prophylactic efficacy of nitrofurantoin macrocrystals and trimethoprim-sulfamethoxazole in urinary infections: Biologic effect on the vaginal and rectal flora. N. Engl. J. Med. *296*:780–783, 1977.
113. Still, J. G.: Management of pediatric patients with group A beta-hemolytic *Streptococcus pharyngitis*: Treatment options. Pediatr. Infect. Dis. J. *14*:S57–S61, 1995.
114. Terezhalmy, G. T., and Hall, E. H.: The asplenic patient: A consideration for antimicrobial prophylaxis. Oral Surg. *57*:114–117, 1984.
115. U.S. Public Health Service: Annual Summary 1976, Publication No. CDC 77-8241. M. M. W. R. 25:43, 1977.
116. Waldvogel, F. A., Vaudaux, P. E., Pittet, D., et al.: Session I. Theoretical and preclinical experimental bases of prophylaxis: Perioperative antibiotic prophylaxis of wound and foreign body infections: Microbial factors affecting efficacy. Rev. Infect. Dis. *13*:S782–S789, 1991.
117. Wong, W. Y., Overturf, G. D., and Powars, D. R.: Infection caused by *Streptococcus pneumoniae* in children with sickle cell disease: Epidemiology, immunologic mechanisms, prophylaxis, and vaccination. Clin. Infect. Dis. *14*:1124–1136, 1992.
118. Young, R. F., and Lawner, P. M.: Perioperative antibiotic prophylaxis for prevention of postoperative neurosurgical infections: A randomized clinical trial. J. Neurosurg. *66*:701–705, 1987.
119. Zanoni, D., Isenberg, S., and Apt, L.: A comparison of silver nitrate with erythromycin for prophylaxis against ophthalmia neonatorum. Clin. Pediatr. *31*:295–298, 1992.
120. Zarkowsky, H. S., Gallagher, D., Gill, F. M., et al.: Bacteremia in sickle hemoglobinopathies. J. Pediatr. *109*:579–585, 1986.
121. Zarrabi, M. H., and Rosner, F.: Serious infections in adults following splenectomy for trauma. Arch. Intern. Med. *144*:1421–1424, 1984.
122. Zelikovic, I., Adelman, R. D., and Nancarrow, P. A.: Urinary tract infections in children: An update. West. J. Med. *157*:554–561, 1992.
123. Zubowicz, V. N., and Gravier, M.: Management of early human bites of the hand: A prospective randomized study. Plast. Reconstr. Surg. *88*:111–114, 1991.

233

ANTIVIRAL AGENTS

Yvonne J. Bryson

Antiviral therapy has come of age and is a rapidly developing field. We have reached the era of clinically useful antiviral compounds, and dozens of compounds are available to treat viral infections. Compared with antibacterial agents, the development of safe and effective antiviral agents initially was slow owing to the close relationship of viral replication and host-cell metabolism. Many potentially effective antiviral substances, unfortunately, inhibited both viral and host-cell functions equally. Toxicity in animals and humans depends on the relative ability of a substance specifically to inhibit viral function without affecting host-cell function. Advances in molecular biology and the understanding of events in viral replication have made it feasible to design specific antiviral agents.

The currently available antiviral agents have been found to inhibit virus-specific functions at the cellular level. This is a basic requirement for all effective antiviral substances. For successful treatment of viral disease with antiviral substances, it is necessary also to understand viral pathogenesis and the relationships of viruses and host cells. Intervention by inhibition of viral replication may be successful only early in acute infections or in those chronic infections involving persistent viral replication, such as that of hepatitis B virus (HBV) or HIV-1 infection. The effect of antiviral agents on recovery and the other outcomes of infection, including latency, oncogenicity, persistence, and resistance to the effects of antiviral agents, also must be considered.

Another requirement for use of antiviral agents is the development of measures that predict successful therapy. Potential antiviral agents currently are evaluated for antiviral activity and toxicity in tissue culture systems, animal models, and, finally, human clinical trials. Although many substances have been shown to have viral inhibitory effects in tissue culture systems, only a minority have progressed to clinical testing. Further development of screening tests for useful antiviral in vitro assays[101] and animal models that may have predictive value for human disease, such as the rabbit eye–herpes simplex virus (HSV) system and the simian immunodeficiency virus (SIV) primate severe combined immunodeficiency hu mouse model for HIV, is necessary.

Correlation of in vitro inhibitory concentrations with achievable levels of these antiviral agents in various target tissues, both intracellularly and extracellularly, as well as with clinical outcome, is important. The pharmacokinetics of various antiviral agents and routes of administration already have proved to be important, as evidenced early on by the lack of idoxuridine (IDUR) penetration into the spinal fluid of patients with fatal herpes encephalitis.[213]

During the past few years, it increasingly has become evident to investigators that the natural history of viral diseases is variable and ill defined. Carefully controlled, double-blind clinical trials for evaluation of antiviral agents are critical.[5, 373] Lack of such trials in the past resulted in the initial systemic use of toxic and ineffective substances, such as cytarabine (Ara-C) and IDUR in herpesvirus infections.[8, 341] With the current licensing of many new effective antiviral agents, newer agents now must be compared with standard therapy. Evaluation of combined therapies may become more complicated and mimic the cancer model for certain diseases, such as HIV-1 infection.

Finally, improved methods of rapid viral diagnosis and the monitoring of antiviral effects are necessary for early and effective treatment of disease.

In this chapter, the basic strategy of antiviral therapy in terms

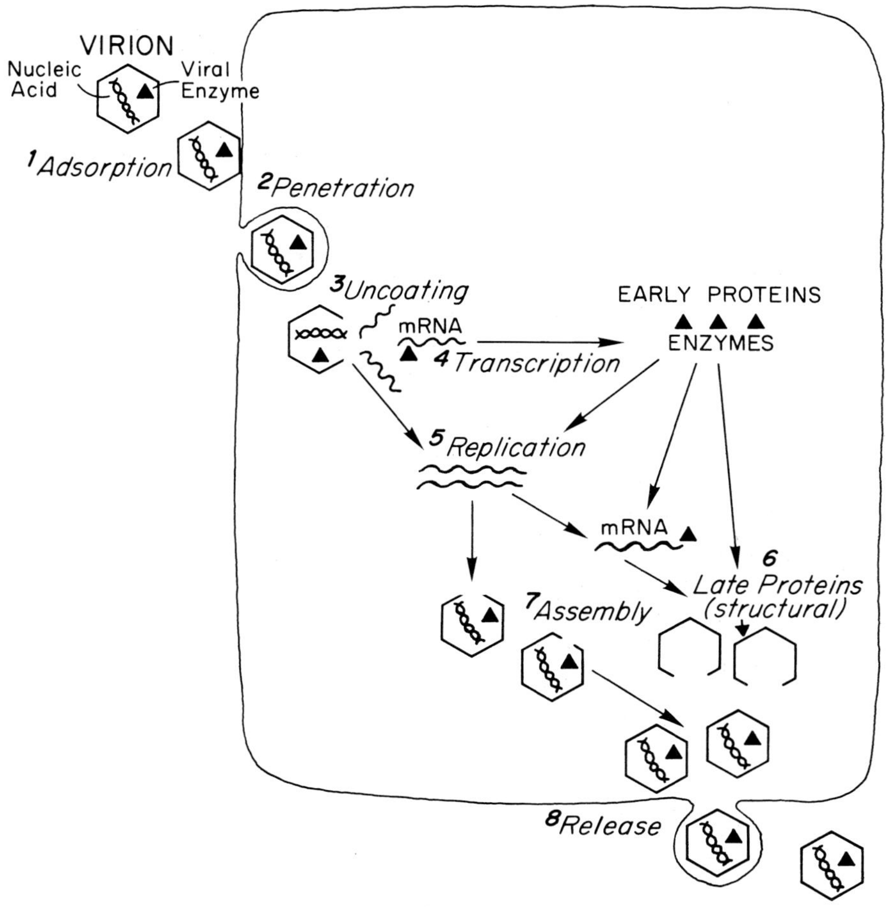

FIGURE 233–1. *Basic steps in intracellular (DNA) viral replication. 1, Adsorption of virion to cell membrane. 2, Penetration. 3, Uncoating, removal of protein coat. 4, Early gene expression, transcription of viral proteins. 5, Replication, synthesis of DNA strands. 6, Late gene expression, transcription of messenger RNA, and translation of late protein synthesis. 7, Maturation and assembly of virions. 8, Release.*

of the potential selective sites of action of antiviral drugs is discussed briefly. There already have been major advances in this area with the use of enzyme-linked immunosorbent assay (ELISA) techniques, monoclonal antibodies, DNA hybridization, and polymerase chain reaction (PCR). The advances in quantitation of virus, including measurements of cytomegalovirus (CMV) viremia by DNA PCR and of HIV by HIV RNA PCR—as both tools for disease prognosis and monitoring of antiviral effect—have revolutionized the current clinical management of these infections. Several review articles provide a more detailed discussion.[55, 86, 91, 108, 149, 159–161, 189, 256, 257, 288, 352, 360, 370]

VIRAL REPLICATION AND SELECTIVE SITES OF ACTION

A rational approach to therapeutic intervention in viral disease first requires some understanding of the basic metabolic processes that distinguish animal virus types from one another and from the host organism. Specific antiviral chemotherapy must be directed to selective sites of action against virus-specific processes.

Viruses contain either DNA or RNA, which is either single- or double-stranded. In addition to the nucleic acid genome, all viruses contain proteins as structural and, many times, as enzymatic components. The protein structural determinants of the virus make up the capsid, which can protect the nucleic acid genome from destructive environments. The capsid also may determine the host range.

The virus codes for viral proteins; however, the host cell provides the machinery to synthesize these proteins. The virus redirects the metabolic activities of the host toward expression and replication of viral genetic information.

The basic steps in viral replication at the cellular level are diagrammed in Figure 233–1 for DNA viruses. Retroviruses differ from DNA viruses in that the former can integrate their genome into the cellular DNA and maintain latency in this form. Theoretically, antiviral intervention is possible at any one of the depicted sites. The major sites of antiviral action of current and potentially clinically useful antiviral agents are listed in Table 233–1.

Figure 233–2 shows a diagram of the replicative cycle of HIV-1 and the major sites of action of antiviral agents, including the potential and currently clinically useful compounds.

Adsorption—Attachment

Virions first must attach to the susceptible cell. This may involve specific cellular receptor sites, as with poliovirus, or a less specific interaction, as occurs with some enveloped viruses. HIV-1 specifically attaches to the CD4 receptor on susceptible cells, although other mechanisms also may be important in virus entry. A second important coreceptor for entry of HIV-1 into cells has been identified and is a major topic of current research.[6, 260] Polyanions, including heparin, have been shown to inhibit adsorption of HSV in vitro.[357]

Penetration and Uncoating

Penetration involves the uptake of virions by the cell by a variety of mechanisms, including pinocytosis, phagocytosis,

TABLE 233–1. Major Sites of Action of Antiviral Agents with Clinical Potential

Site of Action	Substance		Major Viruses Inhibited
Direct inactivation	Ultraviolet light		All
Viral entry	Soluble CD4		HIV-1
Adsorption (attachment)	Heparin		HSV
Penetration	Amantadine*		Influenza A
Uncoating	Rimantadine*		
Viral synthesis			
Transcription			
Replication	Idoxuridine*		HSV
Inhibition of viral enzymes	Trifluorothymidine*		HSV
Viral DNA polymerase	Ara-A vidarabine*		DNA, VZV, EBV, CMV, poxviruses
	Ganciclovir*		CMV, EBV, HSV
	Foscarnet*		DNA, HIV-1
Virus-specific enzymes			
Viral thymidine kinase	Acyclovir*	Valacyclovir*	DNA, HSV, VZV, EBV, CMV
	BVDU	Famciclovir*	DNA, HSV-1, VZV
Reverse transcriptase	Ribavirin*		DNA and RNA, RSV, influenza A and B, Lassa fever, HIV-1
	Zidovudine* (ZDV)		HIV-1
	ddI*		HIV-1
	ddC*		HIV-1
	Stavudine* (d4T)		HIV-1
	Lamivudine* (3TC)		HIV-1, hepatitis B
	Nevirapine*/delaviridine		HIV-1
Viral protein synthesis	Methisazone		Vaccinia, variola
Assembly and release	Protease inhibitors*		HIV-1, some retroviruses
	Interferon*		DNA and RNA
	2-deoxy-D-glucose		HSV
	Interferon		RNA tumor

*Currently licensed antiviral agents.
HSV, herpes simplex virus; VZV, varicella-zoster virus; EBV, Epstein-Barr virus, CMV, cytomegalovirus; RSV, respiratory syncytial virus.

and direct entry. Some enveloped viruses gain access to the cell by fusion with the host membrane. A single virus may use different mechanisms of penetration in the same cell type.

Uncoating is the removal of the protective outer coat of a virus, including the capsid or envelope or both, to expose the viral nucleic acid. This can be a relatively simple event, as with poliovirus, or a complicated two-stage process, as with vaccinia virus.[178]

The major site of action of amantadine hydrochloride and its conjugate rimantadine hydrochloride is here, by inhibition of viral penetration and uncoating.[184, 222, 258]

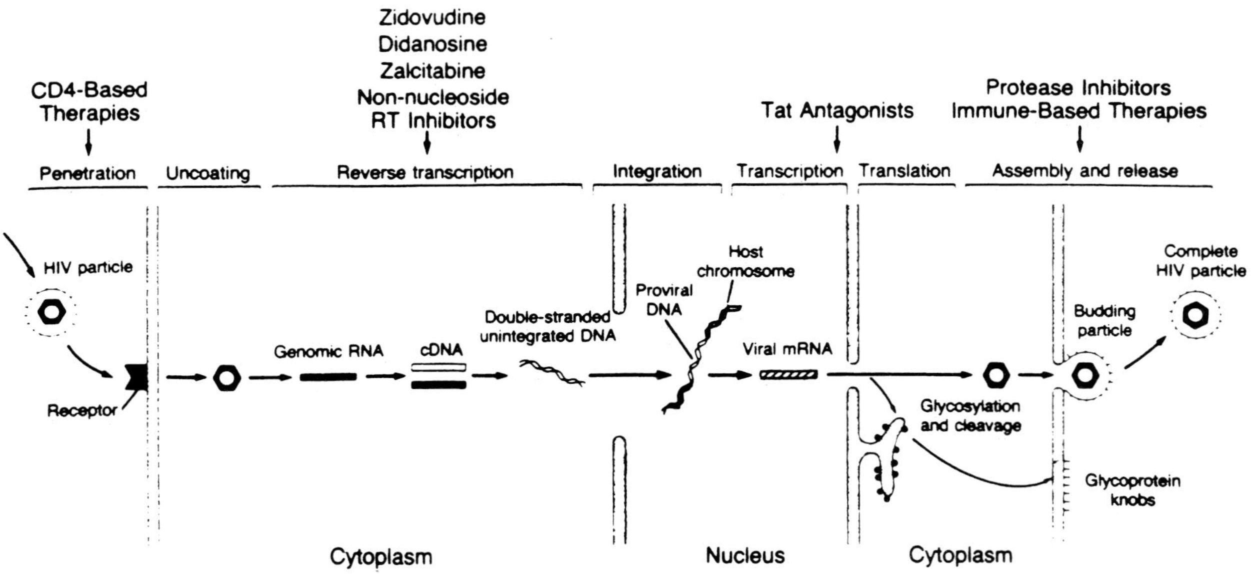

FIGURE 233–2. *Diagram of the replicative cycle of HIV-1, showing the site of action of antiviral agents. Various antiviral agents are shown at the top. RT denotes reverse transcriptase, cDNA denotes complementary DNA, and mRNA denotes messenger RNA. (From Hirsch, M. S., and D'Aquila, R. T.: Therapy for human imunodeficiency virus infection. N. Engl. J. Med. 328:1686–1695, 1993. Reprinted with permission from the New England Journal of Medicine. © 1993, Massachusetts Medical Society.)*

Viral Synthesis

Transcription

Early gene expression involves the transcription of mRNA. The DNA of the DNA viruses serves as a template for transcription of the genetic message to viral mRNA. This is accomplished by parvoviruses, papovaviruses, and some herpesviruses by use of preexisting host enzymes. Alternatively, some DNA viruses, including poxviruses, reoviruses, and most RNA viruses (myxoviruses, paramyxoviruses, rhabdoviruses, bunyaviruses), have virion-coded enzymes that are packaged with the virus.

Replication

Replication of DNA viruses may be catalyzed by virus-coded enzymes (i.e., DNA polymerases) that are different from the host's cellular DNA polymerases. This is the basis for the antiviral activity of some nucleosides. The relative selectivity of a drug on specific viral functions determines its usefulness in terms of viral inhibition versus cell toxicity. Vidarabine (Ara-A) inhibits viral DNA polymerase more than cellular DNA polymerase does.[101]

Acyclovir (ACV), an acyclic guanine derivative, requires a virus-specific thymidine kinase for phosphorylation to ACV triphosphate. This ACV triphosphate then acts as a specific inhibitor of viral DNA polymerase.[107] The selective site of action of this compound on viral processes may account for its lack of cellular toxicity. Inhibition of cellular growth requires a 3000-fold greater drug concentration than that required for viral inhibition. IDUR exerts some of its antiviral effect by incorporation into DNA in place of thymidine, thus causing faulty DNA strands. The nonspecific inhibitory activity of IDUR against both viral and cellular enzymes may account for its low therapeutic ratio in vivo. Inhibition of DNA viruses by trifluorothymidine probably involves a similar mechanism. Ara-C acts as an antimetabolite for DNA viruses. It is incorporated into DNA strands and inhibits both viral and cellular DNA polymerases.

Viral genomes containing RNA must be capable of replication. Replication of viral RNA is catalyzed by virion-coded enzymes that are distinct from the DNA-dependent RNA polymerases in animal cells. In the retrovirus group, the RNA genome is transcribed by a unique virus-coded enzyme, *reverse transcriptase,* into DNA copies. These two viral processes have been observed only in infected cells and, therefore, may be important sites of antiviral action. This is important for potential antiviral activity against the retrovirus HIV-1 associated with AIDS. The current antiviral agents used to treat HIV-1 infection, including zidovudine (ZDV), didanosine (ddI), zalcitabine (ddC), stavudine (d4T), lamivudine (3TC), and non-nucleoside reverse transcriptase inhibitors (nevirapine [NEV] and delaviradine), inhibit reverse transcriptase of HIV-1 as a major mechanism of action.

Inhibition of integration of HIV-1 genome also is a major target of antiviral therapy. However, there are no current clinically useful antiviral agents in this category to date.

Late Viral Expression

Late viral expression involves the synthesis of viral mRNA and proteins after genome replication has begun. Much of the protein synthesized in this instance is used for production of structural virus protein. The process of translating the mRNA into protein synthesis can be interrupted by derivatives of the thiosemicarbazones, such as methisazone, which has been shown to inhibit poxvirus "late protein" synthesis.[384]

Interferon acts on the host cell by producing an "antiviral protein" that can inhibit both early and late translation of viral mRNA directives into viral proteins.

Virus Assembly, Maturation, and Release

Virus assembly, maturation, and release involve assembly of the genome pool and viral structural proteins, which may or may not require specific enzyme action. A glucose analogue, 2-deoxy-D-glucose, seems to exert its antiviral effect by interfering with viral membrane formation.[79] Interferon has been reported to interfere with release of murine leukemia virions from chronically infected cells.[128]

Productive infections may or may not be associated with release of progeny virions from infected cells. When progeny virions are released from cells, spread by extracellular or hematogenous routes may result. In contrast, other viruses may spread by cell-to-cell contact. Several animal viruses form syncytia or fusion of adjacent cells, which may facilitate cell-to-cell transmission. In some cases, this mode of spread obviates the need for maturation of complete virions, and infectious viral genetic material or subviral structures may propagate infection. The new protease inhibitor group of potent antiviral agents for HIV-1 infection, including ritonavir, saquinavir, crixivan, and viracept, inhibit virus assembly and release of HIV virions.

CLINICAL USE OF ANTIVIRAL AGENTS

Antiviral therapy initially was directed to severe, life-threatening illnesses, such as HSV encephalitis, neonatal HSV infections, or infections in the immunocompromised host. However, with the recent development of substances with a selective mechanism of action, the targets of prophylaxis or therapy can be expanded to include diseases with excess morbidity or potential long-term complications (Table 233–2). This list may be expanded as new knowledge develops in the future about potential risks of other viral diseases.

The current status of clinically useful antiviral drugs is outlined in Table 233–3. The growing group of potential agents includes the new protease inhibitors for inhibition of HIV-1 that will be used in combination with other drugs. Recombinant interferons and numerous nucleoside and non-nucleoside inhibitors of HIV-1 are available or will be licensed in the near future. Current strategies for treatment of HIV infection include a combination of potent agents to enhance efficacy and reduce toxicity by using smaller doses of each substance. The goals of treatment of HIV-1 are aimed at reducing virus replication to its lowest level and thereby potentially reducing the rate of mutation. Treatment early during primary infection in both adults and children may be most beneficial.

AMANTADINE HYDROCHLORIDE (SYMMETREL)

Background

If safe, effective vaccines always were available and produced long-lasting immunity against influenza, there would be no interest in the development of chemoprophylactic and chemotherapeutic drugs for this illness. Although several compounds have been found to have anti-influenzal activity in vitro, only amantadine hydrochloride and, recently, its derivative, rimantadine hydrochloride, have had antiviral activity against influenza when used in human beings. Ribavi-

TABLE 233–2. Targets of Antiviral Therapy

DNA Viruses

- Herpes simplex virus type 1
  - Oral stomatitis
  - Keratitis,* severe facial herpes simplex
  - Eczema, burns, whitlow
  - Immunocompromised—mucocutaneous*
  - Encephalitis*
- Herpes simplex virus type 2
  - Neonatal herpes simplex*
  - Genital herpes simplex*
- Varicella-zoster virus
  - Immunocompromised*
  - Chickenpox, varicella-zoster*
  - Young adults—pneumonitis*
  - Varicella-zoster—elderly adults*
- Cytomegalovirus
  - Congenital, perinatal (?)
  - Immunocompromised—AIDS
  - Pneumonitis, retinitis,* gastrointestinal mono-syndrome
- Epstein-Barr virus
  - Mononucleosis,* chronic Epstein-Barr virus infection (mild–severe)
  - Lymphoproliferative syndrome
- Adenovirus
  - Immunocompromised
  - Pneumonia in children
  - Conjunctivitis (?)
- Others
  - Hepatitis B—acute, fulminant hepatitis; chronic*
  - Papillomavirus—warts,* laryngeal warts, condyloma acuminatum*
  - Polyoma-papova—Jakob-Creutzfeldt virus
    - SV40—progressive multifocal leukoencephalopathy

RNA Viruses

- Myxoviruses
  - Influenza A† and B*†
- Paramyxoviruses
  - Respiratory syncytial (immunocompromised)*†
  - Parainfluenza—children
  - Subacute panencephalitis—measles encephalitis, measles pneumonia, measles in immunocompromised
- Togavirus
  - Dengue, equine encephalitis, Japanese B encephalitis
- Enterovirus
  - Enteroviral meningitis (infants), pericarditis
- Arenavirus
  - Lassa fever†
- Retrovirus
  - HTLV-I, HTLV-II—T-cell leukemia, hairy-cell leukemia
  - HIV-1*†
  - HIV-2

*Current therapy available.
†Infants and adults.

rin has been found to have antiviral activity against influenza A and B when given by aerosol.[197, 233]

Although licensed in 1966 for prophylaxis against Asian influenza (H2N2), amantadine has not been used widely by physicians.[300] During the years since licensure, a considerable body of data has accumulated, demonstrating that both amantadine and rimantadine are effective antiviral compounds and should be used more widely for both prevention and treatment of influenza A.[173]

Structure and Mechanism of Action

Amantadine hydrochloride (1-adamantanamine) is a crystalline primary amine with a cage structure as shown in Figure 233–3. Rimantadine hydrochloride has a similar structure. Amantadine does not inactivate virus directly or prevent its adsorption to the cell, and it has no effect on the synthesis of viral components or viral assembly or release.[165, 184] The compound appears to act by interfering with virus penetration of the host cell.[87] Observations on the effect of amantadine on fowl plague virus[184] and more recently on influenza A virus suggest a primary effect on viral uncoating.[219, 322] This unique mechanism of action on a virus-specific process helps explain its lack of toxicity to host cells.

In Vitro and Animal Studies

Antiviral activity of amantadine was demonstrated in tissue culture systems against influenza A virus strains and influenza C, Sendai, pseudorabies, and rubella viruses. No antiviral activity was found against influenza B, Newcastle, parainfluenza 2 and 3, and mumps viruses.[258] Inhibiting concentrations for influenza A virus strains range from 0.05 to 15 µg/mL (mean, 0.1 µg/mL).[150, 236] The antiviral effect against influenza A virus is additive to antibody.[64]

In mice inoculated intranasally with influenza A virus, amantadine administration prevented death in some animals and delayed it in others.[140] Efficacy was greatest in mice treated at the time of infection, but antiviral effect still was evident when treatment was delayed 72 hours after infection. Mice surviving infection as a result of amantadine treatment were immune to subsequent challenge with the same virus as a result of antibody formation.[88]

Resistance to amantadine hydrochloride can be produced in tissue culture systems and in mice by serial passage of influenza virus in the presence of the drug.[64, 267] Resistance to amantadine has not been found in wild strains of influenza A virus.

Although amantadine hydrochloride has been found to have antiviral activity against rubella virus in tissue culture, no antiviral activity was found in rhesus monkeys, hamsters, and rabbits experimentally infected with this virus.[268, 269, 340]

Metabolism and Clinical Pharmacology in Humans

Amantadine is absorbed rapidly and completely from the gastrointestinal tract.[28] The drug is excreted unchanged in the urine, with 56 per cent of a dose excreted within 24 hours and 86 per cent in 4 days; the half-life is 12 to 36 hours. Blood levels range from 0.25 to 1.01 µg/mL in volunteers given 200 to 300 mg of amantadine daily. Because amantadine is excreted in the urine, it is important to adjust the dosage when renal impairment is present to avoid drug accumulation and toxic side effects. This particularly is important in the elderly patient, in whom it is recommended that dosage intervals be adjusted when the creatinine clearance is less than 60 mL/min/1.73 m^2.[166, 253]

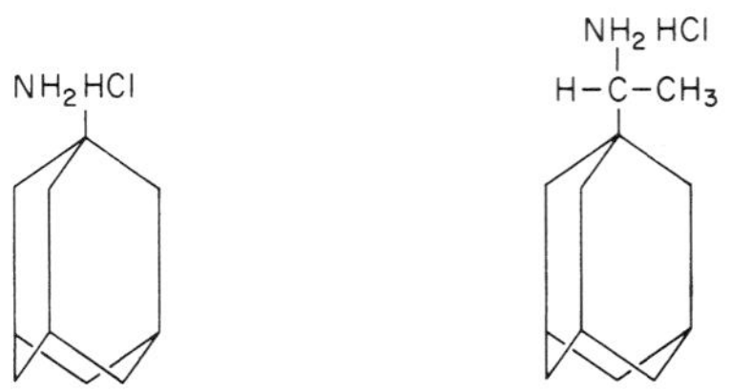

FIGURE 233–3. *The structures of amantadine hydrogen chloride and rimantadine hydrogen chloride.*

TABLE 233–3. Summary of Clinically Useful Antiviral Agents

Antiviral Agent	Indications	Dosage
Amantadine HCl (Symmetrel)	Prophylaxis and treatment of influenza A virus infections in adults and children	Adults: 100–200 mg/day p.o. Children: 4 mg/kg/day p.o.
Adenine arabinoside (Vidarabine)	Treatment of HSV encephalitis in adults and children	15 mg/kg/day over 12 hours constant IV infusion × 10 days
	Treatment of neonatal HSV infections	30 mg/kg/day over 12 hours constant IV infusion × 10 days
	Treatment of mucocutaneous HSV infections in immunocompromised patients	10 mg/kg/day over 12 hours constant IV infusion × 7 days
	Treatment of varicella-zoster virus infections in immunocompromised patients, adults, and children	10–15 mg/kg/day over 12 hours constant IV infusion × 5–7 days
	Treatment of HSV eye infections	Topical ointment
Acyclovir (Zovirax)	Prophylaxis and treatment of mucocutaneous HSV infections in immunocompromised patients	250 mg/kg/dose divided q 8 hr IV × 5 weeks for prophylaxis and 7 days for treatment 400 mg/kg/dose divided 5 times daily p.o.
	Treatment of varicella-zoster virus infections in immunocompromised adults and children	500 mg/kg/dose divided q 8 hr IV × 7 days
	Treatment of HSV encephalitis in adults and children	30 mg/kg/day divided q 8 hr IV × 14 days
	Treatment of neonatal HSV infections	30 mg/kg/day divided q 8 hr IV × 14 days
	Treatment of HSV eye infections (HSV keratitis)	Topical ophthalmic solution
	Treatment of genital HSV infections	
	First episode	5 mg/kg/dose q 8 hr IV × 5 days *or* 250 mg 5 times daily p.o. × 10 days *or* Topical ointment × 10 days
	Recurrent: intermittent treatment	250 mg 5 times daily p.o. × 5 days
	Suppression treatment of very frequent recurrences	250 mg t.i.d. or 400 mg b.i.d. p.o. × 6–12 months
	Treatment of normal adults with varicella-zoster	800 mg 5 times daily p.o. × 7–10 days
	Treatment of normal children with chickenpox	20 mg/kg/dose q 6 hr p.o. × 5–7 days
Valacyclovir	Treatment of herpes zoster	1000 μg t.i.d. × 7–14 days
	Treatment of genital HSV infection	250–500 μg b.i.d. × 5 days
	Prophylaxis of CMV infection	?
Famciclovir	Treatment of herpes zoster	500 μg t.i.d. p.o. × 7–10 days
	Treatment of genital HSV infection	250 μg b.i.d. p.o. × 5–7 days
Ganciclovir	Treatment of CMV infection	5 mg/kg q 12 hr IV × 2–3 weeks
	Prophylaxis of CMV infection in adults	5–6 mg/kg/day IV or 1000 mg t.i.d. p.o.
Foscarnet	Treatment of CMV infection	60 mg/kg q 8 hr IV × 14 days
	Prophylaxis of CMV infection	90 μg/kg/day IV
Ribavirin	Treatment of RSV infections in hospitalized infants	Aerosol for 8–18 hours daily
Rimantidine	Prophylaxis and treatment of influenza A virus infection in adults and children	100–200 mg daily p.o.
Trifluorothymidine	Treatment of HSV eye infection and HSV keratitis	Topical 1% ophthalmic solution
Zidovudine	Treatment of symptomatic adults and children with HIV-1 infection	Adults: 100 mg 5 times daily p.o. or 200 mg t.i.d. p.o. Children: 120–180 mg/kg/dose q 6 hr daily
	Treatment of asymptomatic adults with $\leq$500 CD_4 cells/mm^3	100 mg 5 times daily p.o.
	Prophylaxis of maternal-fetal HIV-1 transmission	100 μg 5 times daily p.o.; mother: constant IV infusion—labor: 2 μg/kg, loading: 1 μg/kg/hr; infant: 2–4 μg/kg q 6 hr daily × 6 weeks
Didanosine	Treatment of HIV infection in adults and children	Adults: 200 μg b.i.d. p.o. Children: 200 mg/kg/day divided q 12 hr b.i.d. p.o.
Zalcitabine	Treatment of HIV infection in adults and children	Adults: 2.25 μg divided t.i.d. p.o. Children: 0.005–0.01 μg/kg q 8 hr p.o.
Stavudine	Treatment of HIV infection in adults and children	Adults: 40 μg b.i.d. p.o. Children: 1 μg/kg q 12 hr p.o. (<40 kg), 40 μg/kg q 12 hr p.o. (>40 kg)

Table continued on following page

TABLE 233–3. Summary of Clinically Useful Antiviral Agents *Continued*

Antiviral Agent	Indications	Dosage
Lamivudine	Treatment of HIV infection in adults and children	Adults: 150 µg b.i.d. p.o. Children: 4 µg/kg q 12 hr p.o.
Nevirapine	Treatment of HIV infection in adults and children	Adults: 200 µg b.i.d. p.o. × 2 weeks followed by 400 µg b.i.d. p.o. Children: 200 µg/kg b.i.d. p.o. (2 months to 9 years of age), 120 µg/kg b.i.d. p.o. (older than 9 years of age)
Protease inhibitors*		
Ritonavir	Treatment of HIV infection in adults	600 µg b.i.d. p.o.
Saquinavir	Treatment of HIV infection in adults	600 µg t.i.d. p.o.
Indinavir (Crixivan)	Treatment of HIV infection in adults	800 µg t.i.d. p.o.
Nelfinavir	Treatment of HIV infection in adults and children	Adults: 750 µg t.i.d. p.o. Children: 25–30 µg/kg t.i.d. p.o.

*Studies not complete in children.

Clinical Studies

Prophylaxis

CHALLENGE STUDIES. Amantadine first was tested prophylactically in 1963 in volunteers challenged with influenza A2 (H2N2) virus by Jackson and associates.[172] Subjects were randomized to receive amantadine, 100 mg twice daily, or placebo; administration was begun 18 hours before infection. Patients receiving amantadine experienced a 50 per cent reduction of infection compared with those receiving placebo ($p < .01$). Tyrrell and associates[356] were unable to confirm this; however, their study showed a low infection rate in the placebo group. Subsequent challenge studies with influenza A H2N2 and H3N2 virus strains confirmed the findings of Jackson and colleagues.[172] These are recorded in Table 233–4. These studies indicated a 50 per cent reduction of infection and a decrease in the symptoms and severity of clinical influenza.

NATURAL INFLUENZA STUDIES. Wendel and associates,[366] in a double-blind trial using 200 mg of amantadine daily, found that 5 of 439 (1.1 per cent) treated subjects developed clinical influenza, compared with 15 of 355 (4.1 per cent) volunteers who received a placebo. In antibody-free, susceptible subjects, 27 per cent of those who received amantadine had a fourfold rise in antibody titer, whereas 48 per cent in the placebo group had antibody titer rise. A summary of prophylactic trials of amantadine against natural outbreaks of influenza A virus infections is presented in Table 233–5. Among unselected drug-treated subjects, fourfold or greater titer rises occurred in 30 per cent fewer subjects than in the placebo group, indicating a 52 per cent protection rate.

Generally, most studies revealed that amantadine resulted in a 50 to 70 per cent reduction in the incidence of clinical cases of influenza. The severity of clinical illness also was reduced. This has been confirmed for H2N2, H3N2, and H1N1 strains of influenza A virus.[254] Efficacy also was demonstrated in a family prophylactic study in England during an epidemic of Asian influenza (H2N2).[131] Household contacts of index cases of active influenza were given either amantadine, 200 mg, or placebo for 10 days at the time the index case was seen. During a 10-day observation period, 2 of 55 (3.6 per cent) drug-treated subjects versus 12 of 85 (14.1 per cent) placebo recipients developed clinical influenza. If only serologically confirmed cases are included, none of the amantadine group and 10 of 69, or 14.5 per cent, of the placebo group had serologic evidence of influenza A virus infection ($p < .01$).

O'Donoghue and associates[261] showed the efficacy of amantadine in prevention of hospital-acquired influenza virus infection. Influenza virus infection occurred in 12 of 61 patients given placebo, 7 of whom were clinically ill, whereas only 2 subclinical infections occurred among 50 patients given amantadine ($p < .01$). A double-blind study compared prophylaxis of amantadine, 200 mg daily, with rimantadine, 200 mg daily, in young college students during an influenza A outbreak. In this trial, both compounds reduced the inci-

TABLE 233–4. Efficacy of Amantadine Hydrochloride Administered Prophylactically Against Influenza A Virus Infection in Challenged Adult Volunteers

Reference	Year	Virus Subtype	Amantadine*	Placebo*	Decreased Viral Isolation and Severity of Illness
143	1963	H2N2			+
306	1965	H2N2	4/14	4/13	−
261	1966	H2N2	0/9	4/9	+
302	1968		8/29	18/29	+
283	1970	H2N2	56/122	106/166	+
284	1970	H3N2	6/17	13/16	+
186	1970	H3N2	2/66	12/75	+
285	1972	H2N2	121/307	227/355	+
		H3N2			+
52	1976	H3N2	6/10	8/104	+

*Number of subjects infected/number in group.

TABLE 233–5. Prophylactic Studies of Amantadine Hydrochloride in Natural Influenza Outbreaks

			Number with Respiratory Illness						
Reference	**Year**	**Population**	***Drug-Treated***	*%*	***Dose***	***Placebo***	*%*	**Decrease in Respiratory Illness**	**Efficacy (%)**
317	1966	Prisoners 17–54 years of age	5/439	1.1	200 mg	15/355	4.2	+	74
244	1966	Children mentally retarded, average age, 8 years	12/126	9	2.6–3.8 mg/kg	13/43	30	+	68
94	1967	Mentally retarded children, 8–19 years of age	1/104	9	60–100 mg; 1–2.5 mg/kg	11/133	8	+	80
39	1968	Adults	33/48	68	200 mg	31/48	64		6
107	1969	Family contacts, variable age	2/55	3.6	200 mg	12/85	14	+	74
89	1969	19–22 years of age	59/2530	2.3	200 mg	220/2210	9.9	+	77
108	1969	Family contacts	5/44	11	200 mg, 100 mg in children	6/42	14	−	20
283	1970	Schoolchildren; 18–30 years of age, male	156/3885	4		192/2498	7.6	+	58
194	1970	Military units; 18–21 years of age	173/2435	7.1	200 mg	129/2127	6	−	18
218	1970	3–50 years of age	2/112	1.7	200 mg	20/103	19	+	91
221	1970	Medical students, 22 years of age	27/192	14	200 mg	57/199	28	+	58
220	1972	Hospitalized patients	0/50	0	200 mg	7/61	11.4	+	100
215	1979	College students, 18–26 years of age	18/136	13	200 mg	45/139	32.4	+	70

dence of influenza illness with equal efficacy. This study also showed that rimantadine was better tolerated and had fewer side effects than amantadine.[96] The reasons for the reduced side effects with rimantadine are unclear; however, rimantadine is an attractive agent for prophylactic use and has been used for years in the former Soviet Union.[387]

Rimantadine also was found to be well tolerated in elderly subjects in nursing homes, and prophylactic effects were enhanced in patients who also received influenza vaccine.[94]

Amantadine currently is recommended for prophylaxis in selected populations when outbreaks of influenza A virus infections occur in a community. These high-risk populations include unvaccinated children and adults with cardiac, pulmonary, and immunodeficient states. Amantadine prophylaxis also should be considered for unvaccinated adults in critical service positions: hospital personnel, police, and firefighters. In addition, unvaccinated persons older than 65 years of age or those living in semiclosed institutional facilities also are at high risk for influenza virus infections and may benefit from amantadine use.[78, 153]

Therapy of Influenza A

Early therapeutic studies of amantadine treatment of acute influenza A virus infection induced in volunteers failed to show any serologic, virologic, or symptomatic clinical benefit.[329] However, other studies of the treatment of natural influenza A did show some therapeutic benefit when treatment was begun within 48 hours of the onset of infection. In a study of prisoners, Wendel and associates[366] found no therapeutic effect of amantadine; however, initiation of treatment was delayed. Wingfield and associates[379] conducted a double-blind study of the therapeutic efficacy of amantadine or rimantadine treatment (200 mg daily) of prisoners during an outbreak of Asian influenza. Statistically significant increases in the rate of overall clinical improvement and the rate of defervescence were noted in the amantadine and rimantadine group, compared with placebo recipients. No differences were noted in the frequency of viral isolation or serologic changes in the two groups. Hayden and associates[150] conducted a double-blind trial of amantadine, rimantadine, and placebo therapy of acute influenza due to an H1N1 influenza A virus strain in 54 college students. Amantadine, rimantadine, or placebo, 100 mg twice daily for 5 days, was given within 48 hours of onset of clinical symptoms. Statistically significant effects were found for reduction of fever (mean, 1 day), respiratory tract symptoms, and return to classes in both amantadine and rimantadine treatment groups, compared with placebo controls.[150, 152] Other studies have confirmed an effect of amantadine treatment in influenza A (H3N2) virus infections; the mean duration of fever has been shortened by approximately 24 hours. However, effects on other clinical symptoms have not been dramatic. Little and associates[218] found that pulmonary function studies improved faster in amantadine-treated patients than in those not so treated. Rimantadine also has been shown to have similar therapeutic effects in uncomplicated influenza in young adults.[386] In children with uncomplicated influenza A virus infection, two studies compared the efficacy of rimantadine to acetaminophen for treatment. The results showed that rimantadine was either superior or equivalent to acetaminophen in clinical effectiveness.[142]

It seems clear that amantadine and rimantadine have some therapeutic role; however, their true use for treatment of influenza remains to be defined. Important questions remain unanswered: whether early treatment with amantadine or its analogue rimantadine prevents the complications of influenza in high-risk populations and whether these drugs are effective in influenza pneumonia. Other possible approaches to the therapy of influenza have included attempts to maximize delivery of the drug to the respiratory tract by aerosol; this is effective in the mouse model.[363] Initial studies by Hayden and associates,[150] using intermittent aerosol administration of amantadine for 5 days to treat acute influenza in young adults, showed a mild reduction in respiratory symptoms but no effect on fever or systemic toxicity. This mode of therapy for uncomplicated acute influenza seems to be too cumbersome for general use. As discussed later in this chapter, ribavirin given by aerosol has proved to be efficacious in the treatment of influenza A in young adults.

Dosage, Toxicity, and Side Effects

The usual dosage of amantadine or rimantadine in adults is 100 to 200 mg orally daily in one or two divided doses, and in children it is 4 to 6 mg/kg/day.

The reported side effects of amantadine hydrochloride seem to be dose-related and include central nervous system effects of insomnia, nervousness, dizziness, depression, inability to concentrate, feelings of personal detachment, and lethargy. Ataxia, nausea, vomiting, dryness of mouth, edema, and livedo reticularis occur occasionally.[279] At current recommended doses of 200 mg daily for influenza prophylaxis in adults, reported side effects have been few, transient, and reversible.[206] In long-term studies by Schwab and colleagues[308] of amantadine in elderly patients with Parkinson disease, side effects were observed in 22 per cent of those who received a dose of 200 mg daily. Jackson and colleagues[174] reported a 20 per cent incidence of side effects in healthy volunteers receiving 200 mg daily and an incidence of up to 40 per cent when the dose was increased to 400 mg daily. There are few data on the use or toxicity of amantadine in children.

Because amantadine is excreted unchanged in the urine, the drug should be administered with caution to patients with renal impairment. In a patient with chronic renal failure, administration of amantadine was associated with acute neurotoxic effects, tremors, bizarre behavior, and hallucinations. Studies in college students during outbreaks due to H1N1 influenza A virus revealed a variable incidence of mild side effects ranging from 6 to 33 per cent, with the usual range of 6 to 10 per cent.[43, 206, 254] The use of antihistamines combined with amantadine may potentiate the anticholinergic and central nervous system side effects of amantadine.[247]

Rimantadine hydrochloride has been reported to have fewer central nervous system side effects than amantadine in several studies.[95]

ANTIVIRAL NUCLEOSIDES

Background

Since the early 1970s, a large amount of effort was directed to the synthesis of analogues of nucleic acid components for use in cancer chemotherapy. Several of the agents proved to be disappointing as antitumor agents but were noted to inhibit DNA viral replication. Because the major mechanism of action of the nucleosides is to inhibit DNA synthesis, cellular DNA synthesis and host enzymes also can be affected. Therefore, the antiviral action of these drugs is nonspecific, and the limit of clinical applicability is related to the therapeutic-toxic ratio. IDUR and the purine analogue cytosine arabinoside have proved to be too toxic for systemic use. However, IDUR ophthalmic ointment has proved to be useful as topical therapy for HSV keratoconjunctivitis and was the first antiviral agent licensed for this use.

Ara-A was one of the first nucleosides with proven efficacy in the treatment of HSV ocular disease, encephalitis, and neonatal infection and varicella-zoster virus (VZV) infection in the immunosuppressed patient. Effective agents such as ACV have been compared with Ara-A as standard therapy. The development of Ara-A and ACV as antiviral agents may be used as models for future antiviral substances.

Other clinically useful nucleosides have been developed, including ganciclovir and foscarnet for the treatment of CMV infection and other proacyclovir-like drugs, such as valaciclovir (VACV) and famciclovir for oral outpatient treatment of VZV infection. There has been significant development of numerous clinically useful compounds, including azidothymidine (ZDV), ddI, ddC, d4T, and 3TC, which currently are licensed for the treatment of HIV-1 infection. Other investigational compounds include the nucleoside 1592 by Glaxo-Wellcome, which has a significant effect on reducing HIV virus load and is in clinical trials.

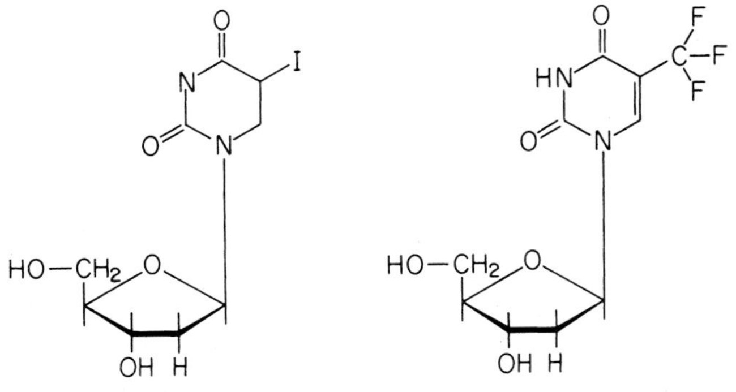

FIGURE 233–4. *The structures of idoxuridine and trifluorothymidine.*

Idoxuridine (Stoxil)

Structure and Mechanism of Action

IDUR (5-iodo-2′-deoxyuridine) is a synthetic nucleoside, an analogue of thymidine with a structure as shown in Figure 233–4. The compound is soluble in water with a maximum solubility of 8 mg/mL in 0.45 per cent sodium chloride or 5 per cent glucose solutions. Studies on the mechanism of antiviral action have been summarized by Prusoff and Goz.[288] IDUR triphosphate is incorporated into DNA and reduces the incorporation of thymidine into DNA.[106] IDUR triphosphate competes with thymidine triphosphate as a substrate for DNA polymerase and is incorporated into both viral and mammalian DNA. This viral DNA may be faulty, with increased susceptibility to strand breakage and subsequent errors in RNA and protein synthesis. Studies of viral replication in the presence of IDUR suggest that nonfunctional viral proteins are produced.[182]

In Vitro and Animal Studies

Herrmann[155] first observed that IDUR inhibited the growth of vaccinia virus and HSV in tissue culture. Antiviral activity has been demonstrated in vitro against the following DNA viruses: HSV, pseudorabies virus, H-1 (hamster osteolytic) virus, equine herpesvirus, CMV, vaccinia virus, polyoma virus, simian virus 4C, simian virus 15, adenoviruses, and bovine rhinotracheitis virus. It also has been reported active against several oncogenic RNA viruses, including Rous sarcoma virus and murine leukemia virus. Inhibitory concentrations for HSV-1 and HSV-2 in tissue culture studies ranged from 0.62 to 2 μg/mL and 0.25 to 75 μg/mL, respectively.[215, 220] IDUR-resistant strains of HSV and vaccinia viruses have developed in the laboratory and have been found in human eye infections with HSV.[273]

IDUR was found to have antiviral activity against a variety of DNA viral infections in animal models. This includes successful topical treatment of HSV keratitis of the rabbit cornea[185, 188, 293] and vaccinial skin and eye infections of rabbits.[185]

Metabolism

IDUR is metabolized rapidly to iodouracil, which has no antiviral activity after systemic administration in people. Approximately 89 per cent of the drug and its metabolite was excreted in the urine by 24 hours.[364] In dogs given intravenous radioactive-labeled IDUR, only small amounts were detectable in the cerebrospinal fluid.[63] Using a microbiologic assay, Lerner and Bailey[215] found minimal antiviral activity in the serum or cerebrospinal fluid of patients given intravenous IDUR. Studies of absorption of IDUR given locally in the rabbit eye reveal peak levels of 12.6 μg/mL in the cornea at 1 hour and persistence for 4 hours.[229]

Clinical Studies and Side Effects

IDUR has been shown in several controlled double-blind studies to be effective in the treatment of acute HSV destructive keratitis in humans.[45, 185, 203] The drug is administered topically and is supplied in 0.5 per cent ointment form. IDUR is licensed for the treatment of HSV keratoconjunctivitis. The overall efficacy rate is 75 per cent. Topical IDUR is not beneficial in HSV stromal eye infections.[272] This probably is due to inadequate penetration to deeper sites of infection. The initial success in treating ocular disease led to the systemic use of IDUR for several life-threatening DNA viral infections, including VZV infection and HSV encephalitis. Uncontrolled and anecdotal studies of IDUR treatment of HSV encephalitis claimed therapeutic benefit. This led to the widespread use of IDUR in this illness until a controlled, double-blind study comparing IDUR, Ara-A, and placebo in the treatment of HSV encephalitis revealed that IDUR was ineffective and had considerable toxicity (i.e., five of six patients whose disease was confirmed by examination of brain biopsy specimens died while receiving IDUR therapy). At autopsy, the brains of several patients contained HSV. Complications of IDUR treatment at the recommended dosage included thrombocytopenia and neutropenia, with problems of secondary infection and bleeding.[8]

As a result of the lack of therapeutic benefit and the profound toxicity of IDUR noted in this study, no further use of it as a systemic antiviral agent is planned.

In a blind controlled study, British investigators reported efficacy of IDUR in dimethyl sulfoxide (DMSO) applied topically to HSV skin infections.[181, 223] The encouraging results obtained in this study suggest that DMSO enhances penetration of the nucleoside through the skin. This mode of therapy merits further consideration.

Vidarabine (Adenine Arabinoside, Ara-A)

Structure and Mechanism of Action

Ara-A (9-β-D-arabinofuranosyladenine), a purine nucleoside, originally was synthesized as an antitumor agent[214] and can be produced by fermentation of *Streptomyces antibioticus*. The structures of Ara-A, its deaminated metabolite arahypoxanthine (Ara-Hx), and the phosphorylated form Ara-A 5′-monophosphate are shown in Figure 233–5. Ara-A is a white crystalline powder with a maximum solubility in water or intravenous solutions of 500 μg/mL. In contrast, Ara-A 5′-monophosphate is water-soluble.

Although certain aspects of the mechanism of action are not known, studies show that Ara-A exerts antiviral activity by inhibition of viral DNA synthesis. It is transported intracellularly and phosphorylated to the monophosphate and triphosphate active forms.[34, 39, 316, 317] Ara-A triphosphate acts as a competitive inhibitor of DNA polymerase with a probable preferential inhibition of viral DNA polymerase, compared with cellular DNA polymerase. Drach and Shipman[101] have postulated that this selective activity against viral DNA polymerase explains the high therapeutic index of Ara-A. There is evidence that Ara-A may act as a chain terminator in HSV DNA strands, thus creating faulty single viral DNA strands.[256, 257]

In Vitro and In Vivo Antiviral Activity

Antiviral activity of Ara-A against HSV and vaccinia virus first was reported by Privat de Garilhe and Rudder[286] in 1964. The spectrum of antiviral activity of Ara-A includes the following DNA viruses: HSV-1 and HIV-2, CMV, VZV, pseudorabies virus, herpesvirus simiae, Epstein-Barr virus (EBV), and vaccinia virus. Rous sarcoma and Shope papilloma virus are sensitive RNA viruses.[65, 310]

In vitro sensitivities of HSV, VZV, and vaccinia viruses to Ara-A have been observed to vary with assay method and cell line used. Minimal 50 per cent inhibitory concentrations range from 8 to 24 μg/mL.[39, 246, 278, 303, 310, 315] Ara-A constantly is being deaminated to the less active Ara-Hx metabolite by tissue culture cells and serum in the growth medium. Differences in in vitro sensitivity values can be explained by the rate of this deamination during the assay incubation. With the use of adenosine deaminase inhibitors in the assay system, constant drug concentrations can be ensured; the 50 per cent plaque inhibition (ED_{50}) concentration of Ara-A for HSV and VZV is reduced to a range of 0.15 to 1.5 μg/mL. Vaccinia virus is even more sensitive to Ara-A, with an ED_{50} value of 0.01 μg/mL. Ara-Hx has antiviral activity approximately 1/30 to 1/50 of that of Ara-A for vaccinia virus, HSV, and VZV.[37, 39, 74] CMV is relatively less sensitive to Ara-A in tissue culture, with 50 per cent inhibitory levels of greater than or equal to 13 μg/mL.

Comparison of in vitro sensitivities of HSV to Ara-C, IDUR, and Ara-A reveals that Ara-C is the most potent inhibitor of DNA. However, it also is the most potent inhibitor of cellular DNA synthesis. There is no evidence for the development of drug resistance to Ara-A in in vitro or animal studies.[246] Ara-A also inhibits acyclovir-resistant strains of HSV and VZV in vitro.[27, 117]

Studies of the combined antiviral effects of interferon with Ara-A, Ara-A 5′-monophosphate, or Ara-Hx against HSV or vaccinia virus revealed additive effects. Ara-A or its deriva-

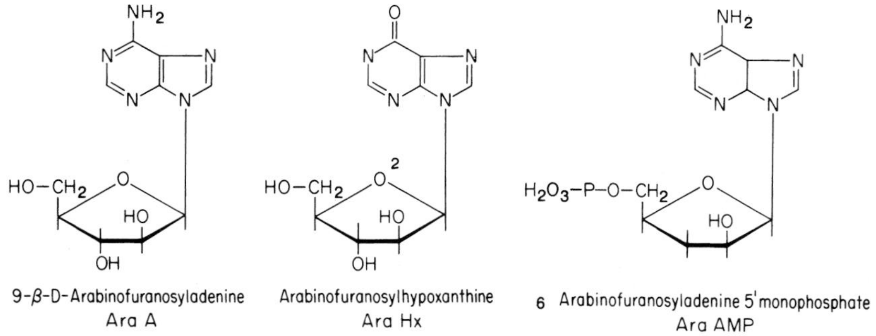

FIGURE 233–5. *The structures of adenine arabinoside, its deaminated metabolite hypoxanthine arabinoside, and the phosphorylated form adenine arabinoside 5′-monophosphate.*

tives did not diminish the antiviral state previously induced by interferon or affect the induction of interferon by virus or poly I:poly C, a synthetic double-stranded RNA.[42]

Ara-A has been evaluated extensively for antiviral activity in a variety of animal systems. Activity has been found against experimental vaccinia and HSV keratitis, vaccinia and HSV-1 and HSV-2 encephalitis, and Shope fibroma virus tumor formation.[192, 319, 325]

Metabolism and Pharmacology

Ara-A is deaminated rapidly by the enzyme adenosine deaminase to the less active metabolite Ara-Hx[54, 196] in vitro[349] and in vivo in higher animals, including simians and humans.

Studies using tritiated labeled Ara-A given intravenously to adults revealed that approximately 60 per cent of the dose was recovered in the urine as Ara-Hx within 24 hours. In similar tracer studies, the half-life of Ara-A was estimated at 4 hours.[194] Initial studies using high-pressure liquid chromatography showed that during constant 12-hour Ara-A infusions in patients, Ara-Hx levels gradually increased with time to peak at 4 to 10 μg/mL.[194] In contrast, levels of Ara-A were at or below limits of detection (≥0.2 μg/mL) by high-performance liquid chromatography methods.[58] Further studies using a sensitive bioassay system (limit of detection, ≥0.004 μg/mL) revealed that Ara-A levels were a low 0.020 to 0.300 μg/mL and were related to the dose and rate of infusion.[44] Mean plasma levels in adults obtained after intravenous doses of 10 and 15 mg/kg/24 hours over 12 hours were 38 and 109 ng/mL, respectively. Similar results were found for neonates, and the plasma-to-cerebrospinal fluid ratio was noted to be 1:1 or 2:1.[38]

In vitro studies indicate that extracellular levels of Ara-A correlate directly with intracellular levels of Ara-A triphosphates, which is presumed to be the active form.[314] There are no in vivo data relating to intracellular concentrations of Ara-A and its derivatives after multiple doses in humans. Comparison of achievable plasma Ara-A levels in patients reveals a marginal overlap with the minimal ED_{50} concentrations of Ara-A against HSV and VZV isolates in tissue culture (Table 233–6).[38] Achievable plasma and cerebrospinal fluid levels of Ara-Hx are far below the in vitro sensitivities for these viruses. Therefore, it is likely that Ara-A rather than Ara-Hx is the active antiviral substance in vivo. Further correlation of extracellular and intracellular drug concentrations, in vitro sensitivities, and clinical outcome may be important in developing a rational approach to effective antiviral therapy.

Observations of penetration of 3 per cent Ara-A ointment applied topically to rabbit eyes revealed that only Ara-Hx entered the aqueous humor. Ara-A was detected in the aqueous humor in two patients with large epithelial defects.[274, 283]

Clinical Studies

Initial clinical trials with Ara-A were targeted for patients with severe or life-threatening DNA viral infections. Promising results were found for treatment of life-threatening HSV infection in normal and immunocompromised hosts and in VZV infections in immunocompromised hosts.[4, 57, 58, 134, 177, 272, 273, 374] These studies were followed up with placebo-controlled trials.

Intravenously administered Ara-A in doses of 15 mg/kg/24 hours was noted to reduce successfully the number of Dane particles and DNA polymerase in chronic HBV infections in two patients. Unexpected mild toxicity was noted in these patients, with transient suppression of granulocytes and platelets.[284] Lower doses of Ara-A (5 mg/kg/24 hours) seem to be equally effective against HBV infection without undue toxicity.[297] These findings suggest that the liver may be an important site for deamination of Ara-A.

Trials of Ara-A in congenital CMV infection and CMV infection in immunosuppressed patients have been less encouraging. This is not surprising because of the high in vitro sensitivities of CMV strains and therapeutic failures in animal model studies.[265] Although urinary and pharyngeal viral shedding transiently can be suppressed provided the initial concentration of virus is not too high, viral replication resumes once treatment is stopped. The natural history of congenital CMV disease is variable and chronic, and therefore efficacy studies of antiviral agents are difficult. Conceivably, even a virostatic antiviral agent could play a role in the treatment of acutely infected infants by lowering the viral load and therefore allowing the host to respond. Studies of CMV infection in renal transplant patients revealed only transient suppression of viruria with little effect on viremia. In addition, further problems were encountered because of the excess fluid requirement due to the insolubility of Ara-A.[53, 299] These problems and the minimal antiviral effect of Ara-A against CMV discouraged further investigation.

Controlled Trials

HERPETIC KERATITIS. Several drugs have proven efficacy against ocular HSV infection. Ara-A (3 per cent vidara-

TABLE 233–6. Comparison of Vidarabine (Ara-A) Plasma Levels with In Vitro Sensitivity Values of Viral Isolates in Clinical Infections[32, 34, 35]

Clinical Category	Number of Viral Strains	In Vitro Sensitivity* Ara-A (ng/mL)‡ Mean	Range	Dose (mg/kg)	Plasma Concentration† Ara-A (ng/mL) Mean	Range
Herpes simplex virus type 1 encephalitis	10	700	300–1200	15	109	31–500
Disseminated herpes simplex virus type 2 neonatal infection	10	690	250–350	15	93	55–171
			600–1600	30–35	217	62–706
Varicella-zoster virus infection in immunosuppressed patients	9	300	150–500	10	38	8–124

*Plaque-reduction assay in human skin fibroblasts.
†Measured by bioassay sensitivity ≥ 4 ng/mL Ara-A.
‡Fifty per cent plaque inhibitory concentration.

bine ointment) has been shown to be effective in the topical treatment of HSV keratoconjunctivitis in blind trials. Toxic reactions to Ara-A occur in 10 per cent of patients. Other alternatives with equivalent or greater efficacy include topical acyclovir (3 per cent ointment) and 1 per cent trifluorothymidine.[71, 77]

The more water-soluble Ara-5′-monophosphate compound also was ineffective against orolabial HSV infections in controlled studies.[334]

VARICELLA-ZOSTER VIRUS INFECTIONS IN IMMUNOCOMPROMISED HOSTS. Ara-A, ACV, VACV, and interferon have been shown to be efficacious in the treatment of VZV infections in immunocompromised hosts.[373] Intravenous Ara-A and ACV or oral ACV and VACV currently are available for treatment. Interferon is not used because of its more toxic side effects. The initial cross-over controlled trial of Ara-A in VZV infections in 87 immunocompromised patients revealed that Ara-A at 10 mg/kg/day intravenously decreased pain and accelerated the healing of mucocutaneous lesions. This study had some inherent limitations due to the cross-over design (5 days of drug or placebo followed by the alternative).[373] A second controlled trial was initiated to evaluate the effect of early Ara-A therapy (within 72 hours) on localized zoster and chickenpox in immunocompromised patients for the prevention of complications (including skin or visceral dissemination, progression in the dermatome, and postherpetic neuralgia). This study showed that Ara-A–treated subjects, compared with placebo-treated subjects, had a decreased incidence of visceral involvement (5 vs. 19 per cent), cutaneous dissemination (i.e., >50 vesicles outside dermatome) (8 vs. 24 per cent), and reduced pain and the time to healing. The total duration of postherpetic neuralgia also was reduced, although the incidence was not affected.[375] Similar results were observed in children with primary chickenpox, with a decrease in morbidity and mortality in the treated group (see Table 233–7 for summary of results).[368]

The dosage used in these studies was 10 mg/kg/day given over 12 hours for 5 to 7 days. Side effects were minimal, with a few patients reporting nausea and vomiting. ACV now is the first drug of choice for treatment of severe VZV infection because of its superiority in blinded trials. The emerging problem of resistance to ACV in immunocompromised patients, however, particularly in those with AIDS, may renew interest in use of Ara-A as a salvage therapy.

HERPES SIMPLEX VIRUS ENCEPHALITIS. Ara-A proved to be the first effective in the treatment of HSV encephalitis and reduced the mortality rate from 70 per cent in a 10-patient placebo group to 28 per cent in 18 treated patients within 1 month and 44 per cent at 6 months of follow-up ($p < .01$).[376] The mortality rate was related directly to the level of consciousness at the initiation of therapy—that is, the earlier the therapy (lethargy state), the better the outcome, as shown in Figure 233–6. The incidence of neurologic sequelae also was reduced in the treated group, with the majority of survivors returning to functional life. Brain biopsy was associated with a low rate of complications and still is recommended in many cases, although newer techniques using HSV PCR on spinal fluid are promising.[377]

A study from Sweden compared Ara-A and ACV in a randomized trial of 53 confirmed HSV encephalitis cases and found a lower mortality rate in the ACV-treated group (19 per cent) versus the Ara-A–treated group (50 per cent). Long-term sequelae also were fewer in the ACV-treated group.[323] These findings were confirmed in the United States by the NIAID National Cooperative Antiviral Group in a study of

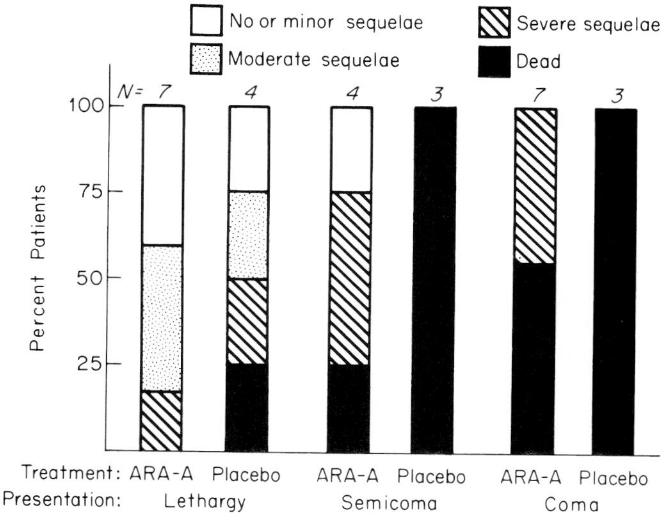

FIGURE 233–6. *A comparative trial of adenine arabinoside or placebo in 28 patients with herpes simplex encephalitis. (From Whitley, R. J., Soong, S. J., Dolin, R., et al.: Adenine arabinoside therapy of biopsy-proved herpes simplex encephalitis: National Institute of Allergy and Infectious Diseases Collaborative Antiviral Study. N. Engl. J. Med 297:289–294, 1977. Reprinted with permission from the New England Journal of Medicine.)*

TABLE 233–7. Effect of Vidarabine Treatment on Clinical Course and Complications of Herpes-Zoster or Chickenpox in Immunocompromised Patients

	Chickenpox			Herpes Zoster		
	Placebo (N = 15)	*Ara-A (N = 19)*	*p Value*	*Placebo (N = 58)*	*Ara-A (N = 63)*	
Percentage patients afebrile on day 5	38%	70%	<.066	—	—	
New vesicle formation	5.6	3.8	<.015	—	—	
Uveitis	—	—		3	1	
Neuropathy	—	—		2	0	
Hepatitis resolved	4	0		3	0	
Pneumonitis resolved	0	1		—	0	
Pneumonitis and hepatitis	2	0		0	0	
Vidarabine	0	0		3	2	
Encephalitis and deaths	2	0		0	0	
Total complications	8	1	<.01	11	3	*p* <.015

From Whitley, R. J., Ch'ien, L. T., Dolin, R., et al.: Adenine arabinoside therapy of herpes zoster in the immunosuppressed. N. Engl. J. Med. *294*:1193–1199, 1976. Reprinted, by permission, from the New England Journal of Medicine.

biopsy-proven cases (see Acyclovir). ACV is the current drug of choice for HSV encephalitis, although Ara-A still may have a role for salvage therapy or if viral resistance to ACV becomes a problem. Further improvement in the outcome of HSV encephalitis will depend on advances in noninvasive diagnostic techniques to allow earlier diagnosis and treatment.

NEONATAL HERPES SIMPLEX VIRUS INFECTION. Ara-A was the first effective drug against neonatal HSV. Intravenous Ara-A treatment at 15 mg/kg/12 hours reduced the mortality of infants with central nervous system disease due to neonatal HSV alone from 50 per cent (placebo recipients) to 10 per cent ($p < .01$). Likewise, the neurologic sequelae in survivors were fewer in the drug-treated versus placebo recipients.[371]

Infants with localized skin lesions and no other manifestations also showed some benefit; however, the outcome in disseminated disease (viremia, hepatitis, pneumonitis) was poor.

Increasing the dose to 30 mg/kg/day in an additional number of infants did not improve morbidity or mortality in disseminated central nervous system disease; however, progression of skin lesions to disseminated or central nervous system disease while receiving therapy was decreased with the higher dose.[372] Seventy per cent of untreated infants with skin lesions progressed to more severe disease, in contrast with approximately 8 per cent of those receiving low-dosage therapy (15 mg/kg/day) and none on high-dosage therapy (30 mg/kg/day) without significant toxicity. This again points out the importance of early diagnosis and treatment of babies with localized skin lesions only. Analysis of the comparative trial of Ara-A at 30 mg/kg/day versus ACV at 30 mg/kg/day shows similar mortality and morbidity figures and a low progression rate of localized skin lesions to invasive disease (4 per cent) with either Ara-A or ACV.[369] ACV, because of the ease of administration, is considered the drug of choice of treatment of neonatal HSV infection.

Dosage, Toxicity, and Side Effects

Side effects attributable to Ara-A have been minimal at the current recommended dose of 5 to 15 mg/kg/day over a 12-hour infusion. In infants with neonatal HSV infection, the dose is higher (30 mg/kg/day). Adverse effects seem to be dose-related and include nausea and vomiting in 16 per cent and mild diarrhea in 5 per cent of patients receiving a dose of 5 to 10 mg/kg/day.[190] At a higher dosage (20 mg/kg/day) in adults, tremors, electroencephalographic abnormalities, megaloblastic bone marrow changes, and weight loss have been reported in a small percentage of patients. These abnormalities did not cause significant morbidity and were reversed when the drug was stopped. However, owing to this potential toxicity, the highest recommended dose for Ara-A in adults is 15 mg/kg/day.[56, 298]

Ara-A was found to be nontoxic to postnatal brain development in the rat, compared with severe inhibition of brain growth by IDUR and Ara-C.[74, 124] It was found to have no adverse effects in studies of cell-mediated immunity.[339] Treatment of chronic hepatitis B with Ara-A at doses of 15 mg/kg/day was associated with some unexplained toxicity with transient thrombocytopenia and leukopenia.[284] Because Ara-A is excreted in the urine, patients with renal insufficiency may have an increased incidence of central nervous system side effects. There are no data at this time relating to dose adjustment in renal failure.[225]

TRIFLUOROTHYMIDINE (5-TRIFLUOROMETHYL-2′-DEOXYURIDINE; F_3TdR)

Trifluorothymidine (F_3TdR) is a halogenated pyrimidine with a structure similar to that of IDUR and thymidine. F_3TdR has a mechanism of action similar to that of IDUR; however, it is incorporated into viral DNA more than into cellular DNA.[129] This selective site of action may account for its more potent activity, compared with that of IDUR, against HSV keratitis in rabbits.[187]

Comparative clinical studies of HSV keratitis treatment with IDUR and F_3TdR revealed more rapid healing of corneal ulcers with F_3TdR. F_3TdR also has been found to be effective in treating patients with keratouveitis.[365] Strains presently resistant to IDUR are sensitive to F_3TdR.

F_3TdR is licensed and can be used for local treatment of HSV eye infections along with Ara-A and IDUR. Because of rapid inactivation and some toxicity when it is administered systemically to people, it is limited to topical use.

ACYCLOVIR

ACV (acycloguanosine; 9-2-hydroxyethoxymethyl) is a guanine derivative with an acyclic side chain and a chemical structure as shown in Figure 233–7. ACV has proven clinical efficacy in a variety of herpesvirus infections. Its unique selective mechanism of action helps explain its general lack of toxicity in clinical trials. The compound requires a virus-specific thymine kinase for phosphorylation to ACV triphosphate, which then preferentially inhibits viral DNA polymerase.[107]

Viral inhibition of HSV occurs at a concentration 3000 times less than that required to inhibit host cellular growth. This property gives the compound a high in vitro therapeutic ratio. The antiviral spectrum of ACV is relatively small and includes HSV-1, HSV-2, VZV, CMV, HBV, and EBV.[67, 68, 82, 304] The minimal 50 per cent inhibitory concentrations of ACV for HSV-1 and HSV-2 are 0.15 μM and 1.62 μM, respectively. The VZV mean 50 per cent inhibitory concentration is 2 to 7 μM, and levels of 25 to 300 μM are necessary to inhibit CMV.[26, 41] Although EBV is not believed to specify thymidine kinase, the sensitivity of the virus to the inhibitory actions of ACV is thought to be due to the greater affinity of EBV-specified DNA polymerase.[270]

ACV has been evaluated in animal model infections. Systemic treatments with ACV of mice with HSV superficial ear infection resulted in local improvement and prevention of establishment of latent infection in the ganglion.[117] Pharmacologic studies reveal high plasma levels after parenteral administration of ACV, with serum peaks of 10 to 60 μM. The plasma half-life after intravenous ACV administration is 3 hours, with 75 per cent of ACV recovered unchanged in the urine and the remainder excreted as the metabolite 9-carboxymethoxymethyl guanine. These serum levels are con-

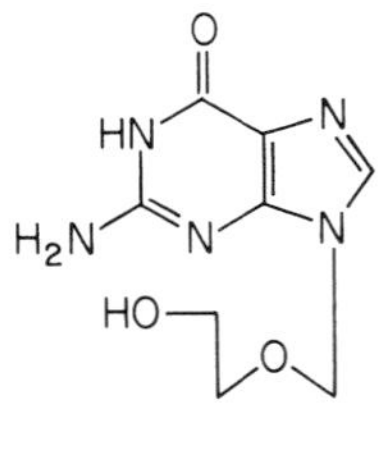

9-(2-hydroxyethoxymethyl) guanine
Acyclovir

FIGURE 233–7. *The structure of acyclovir.*

siderably greater than concentrations required for viral inhibition in vitro for HSV and VZV but less than most in vitro inhibitory concentrations for clinical CMV isolates.[354] In patients with renal impairment, plasma half-life increases with falling creatinine clearance, and dosage should be adjusted when the creatinine clearance falls below 30 μL/min.[29, 212] ACV also is absorbed after oral administration, with achievable plasma levels in the range of 1 to 10 μM.[350] Dosage of ACV for intravenous preparation ranges from 5 to 15 mg/kg body weight given over 1 hour every 8 hours for 5 to 10 days. In neonatal herpes and HSV encephalitis, the dose is 30 mg/kg/day given every 8 hours for 14 to 21 days.[157] Oral dosage ranges between 200 and 400 mg given five times daily for adults; in children, the dosage is 10 mg/kg/dose given every 6 hours orally for HSV and 20 mg/kg/dose given orally every 6 hours for treatment of varicella. ACV now is available in a liquid formulation for children. The prodrug of ACV, VACV, differs from ACV in that it lacks an oxo group at the sixth position and is oxidized to ACV by the enzyme xanthine oxidase.[200] Pharmacokinetic studies using this drug reveal serum levels 10 times higher than those produced by standard oral administration of ACV.[367]

Clinical Trials

Herpes Simplex Virus Infections

HERPES SIMPLEX VIRUS OPHTHALMIC INFECTION. Double-blind studies using ACV administered topically have shown efficacy comparable with that of Ara-A and F_3TdR in the treatment of HSV keratitis.[202] Systemic antiviral agents need to be administered for deeper eye infections or uveitis.

MUCOCUTANEOUS HERPESVIRUS INFECTION IN THE IMMUNOCOMPROMISED HOST. In the immunocompromised host, HSV infections can be severe and chronic and cause significant morbidity, even though they are a rare cause of dissemination and death. Both intravenous and oral ACV given prophylactically to bone marrow transplant patients have been shown to prevent reactivation of mucocutaneous herpes after transplantation. In a study by Saral and colleagues,[302] 70 per cent of placebo recipients and none of the ACV recipients experienced HSV reactivation after transplantation. ACV administered orally in a similar trial was efficacious despite lower plasma levels.[133] Other studies have demonstrated that ACV given intravenously prevents HSV reactivation in seropositive leukemic patients undergoing induction chemotherapy.[285] Further studies are refining the use of ACV for prophylactic administration in certain immunocompromised patients as to dosage and length of therapy. ACV treatment also shortened the clinical course of established mucocutaneous HSV infections, compared with placebo controls, by reducing viral shedding, which enhanced healing of lesions.[245, 362] Oral ACV has been shown to be of similar benefit in treatment of established mucocutaneous disease.[313] Prophylaxis can be of significant benefit to patients who have a high likelihood of reactivation after transplantation or induction chemotherapy. If the HSV antibody titer is positive, the risk of reactivation is 60 to 80 per cent.

Ara-A also has been shown to be effective in the treatment of mucocutaneous HSV infection in immunocompromised patients in a double-blind treatment trial. Virologic and clinical results, however, were substantially less than those obtained with ACV treatment.[378] Therefore, ACV remains the drug of choice for HSV infection in immunocompromised hosts, although Ara-A still may be useful if viral resistance becomes a problem.[362]

HERPES SIMPLEX VIRUS ENCEPHALITIS. Since the initial observation of efficacy of Ara-A for treatment of HSV encephalitis, cooperative multicenter studies of the comparison of standard Ara-A therapy with ACV have been conducted over the last several years in 208 patients who underwent brain biopsy. Results from these studies reveal that ACV treatment has decreased the mortality and morbidity rate of HSV encephalitis, compared with Ara-A treatment.[372] The mortality rate was 54 per cent in the Ara-A recipients, compared with 28 per cent in ACV recipients ($p < .008$) (Fig. 233–8). The mortality rate was higher with either treatment in patients with poorer Glasgow Coma scores (i.e., >10 score, Ara-A 42 per cent vs. ACV 0 per cent; ≤6 score, Ara-A 67 per cent vs. ACV 25 per cent). Long-term morbidity at 6 months also was reduced in the ACV-treated group; 12 of 32 patients (38 per cent) were functioning normally, compared with 5 of 37 patients (14 per cent) in the Ara-A group. As seen in Figure 233–9, patients younger than 30 years and those with a Glasgow Coma score higher than 10 had the best outcome with ACV treatment.[372] These results are similar to those of a randomized study from Sweden comparing the efficacy of Ara-A at 15 mg/kg with ACV at 30 mg/kg daily for 10 days in 59 cases of HSV encephalitis. The authors reported a reduced mortality rate of 19 per cent and subsequent sequelae in 33 per cent of ACV-treated recipients, compared with a mortality rate of 50 per cent with 76 per cent sequelae in Ara-A recipients.[323]

ACV therefore is the drug of choice for the treatment of HSV encephalitis. Further advances in the therapy of HSV encephalitis will derive from the prompt initiation of therapy and accurate noninvasive diagnostic techniques. Newer studies are addressing whether larger doses of ACV, 45 to 60 mg/kg daily, would improve the outcome without increasing toxicity. Unfortunately, brain biopsy still is considered the most definitive method of diagnosis, and this frequently is delayed by reluctance on the part of the physicians and surgeons to perform an invasive technique or lack of response to ACV treatment. Detection of HSV in spinal fluid by HSV PCR may be of help; however, HSV encephalitis cannot be ruled out in cases in which the HSV PCR results are negative. The majority of clinicians usually base the start of ACV treatment on clinical presentation electroencephalography and magnetic resonance imaging scans without a bi-

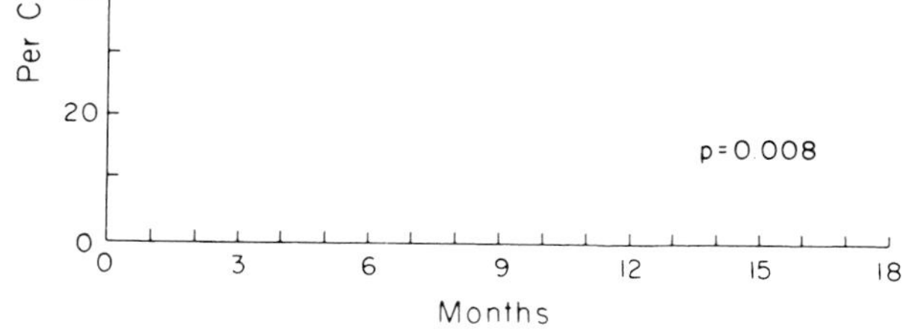

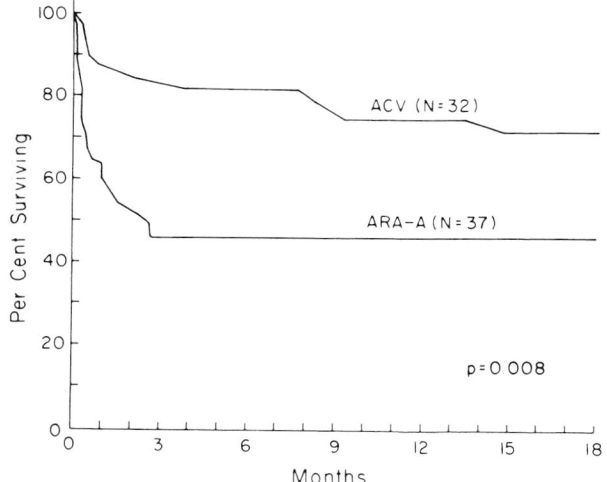

FIGURE 233–8. *Comparison of survival in patients with biopsy-proven herpes simplex encephalitis treated with vidarabine (ARA-A) or acyclovir (ACV); p <.008. (From Whitley, R. J., Alford, C. A., Hirsch, M. S., et al.: Vidarabine versus acyclovir therapy in herpes simplex encephalitis. N. Engl. J. Med. 314:144–149, 1986. Reprinted with permission from the New England Journal of Medicine.)*

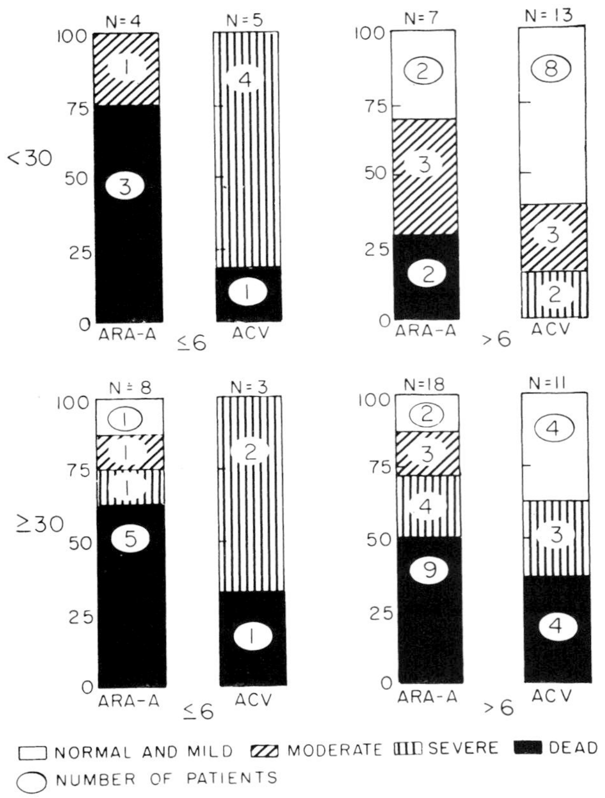

FIGURE 233–9. *Morbidity after vidarabine (Ara-A) or acyclovir (ACV) treatment of biopsy-proven herpes simplex encephalitis, according to age (<30 vs. ≥30) and the Glasgow Coma score (≤6 vs. >6). The scale at the left side of each column indicates percentages (0 to 100). (From Whitley, R. J., Alford, C. A., Hirsch, M. S., et al.: Vidarabine versus acyclovir therapy in herpes simplex encephalitis. N. Engl. J. Med. 314:144–149, 1986. Reprinted with permission from the New England Journal of Medicine.)*

opsy. In the absence of HSV detection by HSV PCR on spinal fluid, diagnosis by brain biopsy still should be considered in cases of focal encephalitis. Up to 50 per cent of biopsied cases prove not to be due to HSV, and in 30 per cent another etiologic factor is identified.[377]

NEONATAL HERPES. The comparative multicenter trial by NIAID of ACV at 30 mg/kg/day versus Ara-A at 30 mg/kg/day in the treatment of neonatal herpes showed similar efficacy for both drugs. There is a modest improvement in the overall mortality rate for neonates with HSV, compared with rates in previous studies. Studies show that progression of localized skin lesions to more invasive central nervous system or disseminated disease is decreased with therapy, with both 30 mg/kg of Ara-A and 30 mg/kg of ACV, whereas untreated, the progression is approximately 70 per cent. In patients treated with either ACV or Ara-A, the rate is reduced to between 0 and 4 per cent.[369] The mortality rate in those with disseminated disease appears to be similar to that found in other studies. The efficacy and safety of ACV are comparable with Ara-A treatment, and ACV is considerably easier to administer. Early diagnosis and prompt institution of therapy seem to be the most critical factors in outcome. The outcome for infants with skin disease only is extremely good if they are treated early because progression to severe forms of the disease can be prevented in most cases. It was observed that infants with three or more skin recurrences of HSV during the first 6 months after treatment of neonatal HSV had a higher rate of mental retardation, perhaps reflecting progressive subclinical central nervous system disease. This has prompted a controlled trial of long-term oral ACV suppression of HSV outbreaks in these infants.

The prophylactic use of ACV in babies exposed to herpes generally is not recommended at this time; however, future studies will assess the benefit of prophylactic antiviral agents in babies at risk of infection. A pediatric suspension of ACV now is available for these studies.

GENITAL HERPESVIRUS INFECTION. Numerous controlled trials of ACV treatment of normal hosts with genital herpesvirus infections have been completed. Topical application of ACV in polyethylene glycol was found to shorten the clinical course of first episodes of genital herpes, although no clinical benefit was demonstrated in those patients with recurrent episodes.[76] Similarly, topical ACV was ineffective in the treatment of recurrent oral HSV infection (fever blisters) in normal hosts.[333] This has been thought to be due to the generally poor skin absorption of ACV when it is administered in a polyethylene glycol base. Controlled studies from England suggest efficacy for treatment of oral HSV when ACV is administered in a cream base. In double-blind trials, systemic therapy with intravenous or orally administered ACV has been shown to be efficacious for first episodes of genital herpes (Table 233–8). Treatment shortened the clini-

TABLE 233–8. First Episode of Genital Herpes Simplex Virus Infection: Duration (Mean Number of Days and Range) of Virus Shedding and the Period from Entry to Crusting and Healing of All Lesions

	Women (N = 31)*			Men (N = 17)*		
	Acyclovir (N = 16)	*Placebo (N = 15)*	p *Value*	*Acyclovir (N = 7)*	*Placebo (N = 10)*	p *Value*
Duration of shedding						
Primary cases	4.9 (2–6)†	14.7 (8–26)	.001	6 (3–11)	15 (12–21)	.02
All cases	3.9 (2–6)	13.4 (2–28)	.0002	4 (1–11)	8 (2–21)	.07
Time to crusting						
Primary cases	8.8 (4–17)	15 (7–25)	.01	5 (4–6)	15 (11–20)	.01
All cases	8.5 (3–21)	12.2 (3–25)	.05	4 (2–6)	8.4 (3–20)	.107
Time to healing						
Primary cases	10 (5–17)	16.2 (9–24)	.015	12 (12–14)	21 (4–29)	.05
All cases	9.5 (3–21)	13.7 (4–25)	.05	12 (10–17)	15 (8–29)	.23

*Primary infection was present in 17 women (10 given drug and 7 given placebo) and 6 men (3 given drug and 3 given placebo).
†Mean number of days (range).
From Bryson, Y. J., Dillon, M., Lovett, M., et al.: Successful treatment of initial genital herpes infection with oral acyclovir. N. Engl. J. Med. *308*:916–921, 1983. Reprinted, by permission, from the New England Journal of Medicine.

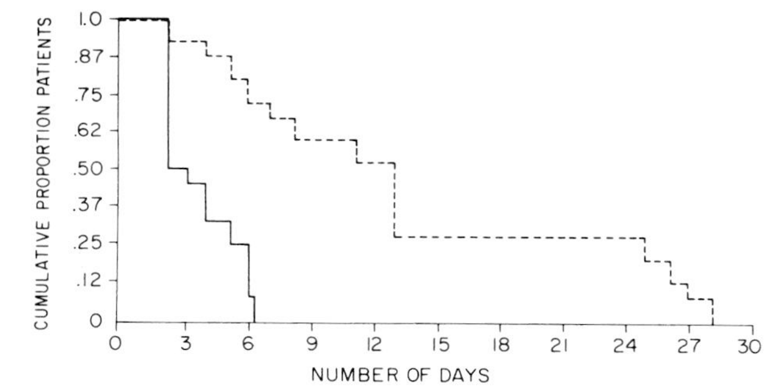

FIGURE 233–10. *Duration of shedding of herpes simplex virus in women treated with acyclovir (---) or placebo (- - -). Shedding from all lesions except those of the cervix was evaluated in 16 acyclovir recipients and 15 placebo recipients from the time of entry until the first negative culture. Survivorship analysis showed that shedding lasted significantly longer in placebo recipients (p = .0002). (From Bryson, Y. J., Dillon, M., Lovett, M., et al.: Treatment of first episodes of genital herpes simplex virus infection with oral acyclovir: A randomized double-blind controlled trial in normal subjects. N. Engl. J. Med. 308:916–921, 1983. Reprinted with permission from the New England Journal of Medicine.)*

cal course of infection by a minimum of a week and reduced the duration of viral shedding, new lesion formation, and systemic symptoms (Fig. 233–10). Cervical virus excretion in women also was reduced significantly.[40, 75]

The goals of treatment of first episodes of primary genital HSV were not only to reduce the clinical course and symptoms of herpes but also to see if early treatment possibly could prevent or affect ganglionic infection and thus reduce long-term recurrence rates.[36]

In one study, preliminary analysis after 2 years of follow-up of patients with primary genital herpes revealed a similar number of patients with recurrences during the first 6 months; however, there was a decrease in long-term recurrence rates after 6 months' follow-up in ACV-treated patients, compared with those who received placebo.[40] Other studies, however, did not include long-term follow-up because of the subsequent licensing of ACV. These data suggest that early limitation of the primary infection may decrease the quantity of latent virus by decreasing the magnitude of ganglionic infection. Oral therapy with ACV is considered the standard of care, allowing outpatient management. Oral therapy is more effective than topical treatment in reducing new lesion formation and systemic symptoms. Therapy of first episodes of genital herpes should be started early in the clinical course (i.e., within 6 days) for the best clinical results.

In double-blind trials using oral ACV given intermittently to patients with recurrent HSV infection, ACV treatment was shown to reduce the duration of each attack, compared with placebo-treated patients.[291] Treatment had no effect on the subsequent rate of recurrences, and clinical benefit was greatest when patients initiated treatment themselves orally within a few hours of onset of clinical symptoms. The duration of viral shedding and lesions was reduced by approximately 2 days in the ACV-treated group, compared with the placebo-treated group. In the subpopulation of patients with chronic and frequently recurrent disease (defined as more than six recurrences per year), daily oral administration of ACV prevented or reduced the frequency of recurrences in approximately 60 to 70 per cent of patients. Subjects who experienced recurrences on prophylaxis had decreased clinical severity and tended to have negative viral cultures.[97, 211, 345] Prophylaxis has been given in dosages of two, three, and five tablets a day and two tablets twice daily, all with similar efficacy. Several studies have examined prophylaxis for up to 5 years, and there seems to be little effect on the frequency of subsequent recurrences. Long-term toxicity studies for more than 5 years of continual administration of ACV revealed no significant side effects in a large cohort of patients. Minor side effects, such as headache, nausea, and diarrhea, were reported in some subjects. Currently, ACV is licensed for use in treatment and suppression of genital herpes.

VARICELLA-ZOSTER VIRUS INFECTION. VZV infections are common and sometimes severe in immunocompromised patients. Primary varicella (chickenpox) and varicella-zoster (shingles) can complicate the course of cancer chemotherapy or organ transplantation in children and adults.[96] Even with the use of passive prophylaxis with zoster immunoglobulin, varicella still may occur in many immunocompromised children. Disseminated disease can result from a primary VZV infection or recurrent infection presenting as herpes zoster and can be associated with a significant mortality rate as high as 17 per cent. Ara-A, interferon, and ACV all have been shown to have therapeutic efficacy for the treatment of VZV infections in the immunocompromised host.[13, 240, 375] However, ACV has proved to be the current primary drug of choice. Several multicenter studies have shown that early intravenous treatment (within 72 hours) with ACV for VZV infection in immunocompromised patients reduces dermatomal spread and decreases complications, including cutaneous and visceral dissemination (only 1 of 52 ACV recipients vs. 11 of 42 placebo recipients had continuation of cutaneous dissemination or development of visceral involvement during the study [$p < .0005$]). In one study, the incidence of visceral dissemination was reduced significantly even when therapy was started after 72 hours. Patients were given 1-hour infusions of 500 mg of ACV per square meter every 8 hours for 7 days. Intravenous ACV also has been shown to be of benefit for treatment of varicella (chickenpox) in immunocompromised children, particularly when therapy was instituted within 72 hours of onset of disease.[12]

As in other studies, instituting therapy early rather than waiting for the development of dissemination or other complications is important.[12, 287]

A prospective randomized trial comparing intravenous ACV with Ara-A in the treatment of VZV infection in severely immunocompromised bone marrow transplant patients who presented within 72 hours of onset of infection showed ACV to be superior to Ara-A treatment.[312] Cutaneous dissemination occurred in none of the ACV recipients and 5 of 10 Ara-A recipients who had localized dermatomal disease ($p < .016$) (Table 233–9). ACV-treated patients had a shortened period of viral shedding, 3 versus 6 days ($p < .013$), and formed fewer new lesions, compared with Ara-A recipients. ACV also significantly shortened the duration of pain, the time to pustulation and crusting of lesion, and the time of complete healing of lesions, 17 versus 28 days ($p < .003$), compared with Ara-A. ACV also reduced the incidence of fever, two versus eight patients ($p < .015$). Because of the severity of the VZV infection in this severely immunocompromised patient population, the difference in the efficacy of these two antiviral agents was demonstrated clearly despite the small number of patients enrolled in the study.[245] ACV now is the drug of choice for treatment of immunocompromised patients with herpes zoster and varicella. In addition, oral ACV given prophylactically to patients after bone marrow transplantation appears to decrease the frequency of zoster during that time[277, 309] in antiviral therapy.[20]

Another target of treatment of VZV infections is the elderly because of chronic pain and postherpetic neuralgia. Early studies showed that intravenous ACV effectively reduced the severity and duration of acute zoster in otherwise normal

TABLE 233–9. Complications Occurring During Treatment of Varicella-Zoster Virus Infection with Acyclovir and Vidarabine

	Treatment Group		
Complication	*Acyclovir*	*Vidarabine*	p *Value**
Cutaneous dissemination†	0/10	5/10	.016
Treatment failure	0/11	4/11	.05
Fever ≥38.5° C	2/11	8/11	.015
Additional therapy required‡	2/11	7/11	.04

*By one-tailed Fisher exact test.
†One patient in each group had a cutaneously disseminated rash at study entry.
‡More than 7 days.
From Shepp, D., Dandliker, R. N., and Meyers, J.: Treatment of varicella-zoster virus infection in severely immunocompromised patients. N. Engl. J. Med. *314*:208–212, 1986. Reprinted, by permission, from the New England Journal of Medicine.

adults.[22] However, outpatient oral treatment is more practical for most patients and now is the standard of care.

Oral ACV at higher doses (800 mg) given five times daily for 7 to 10 days significantly reduces the acute pain and duration of varicella-zoster, compared with placebo. Several studies also have shown that zoster-associated postherpetic neuralgia is reduced significantly in ACV recipients, compared with placebo recipients.[21, 168] Other choices for outpatient treatment of acute zoster in adults include VACV and famciclovir, which both have been proved efficacious.

Controlled studies have shown that oral ACV suspension effectively reduces the severity of chickenpox in normal children. ACV suspension given orally every 6 hours significantly reduced the fever and duration and severity (number of lesions) of disease, compared with placebo.[14] The dose is higher than that required for treatment of HSV infections, 20 mg/kg/dose given in four divided doses in children 5 to 7 years of age. The use of ACV routinely in all children still is controversial; however, the antibody titers to varicella-zoster at 1 year were not affected by therapy, thus ensuring immunity to VZV in these children.

Numerous other drugs, including the ACV-like prodrugs (e.g., VACV, famciclovir), may be of benefit in treatment of varicella in children, and studies are in progress to determine pharmacokinetics and tolerance.

Cytomegalovirus Infection

Although human CMV does not have a virus-specific thymidine kinase, ACV may inhibit CMV in vitro at concentrations between 10 and 25 mg/mL. In vitro, the inhibitory effect of ACV can be increased further by the presence of small amounts of human interferon-α or interferon-β. In clinical trials using intravenous ACV for treatment of CMV infections in immunocompromised hosts, there has been no consistent clinical benefit, although reductions in viremia and viral titers in the urine and in the lung have been observed in some patients. ACV in doses of 400 to 1200 mg/m^2 and interferon in doses of 2 to 40 $\times$ 10^5 units/kg/day alone and in combination were used for treatment of CMV interstitial pneumonia in bone marrow transplant recipients. Although the virus titer was reduced in paired lung specimens, no consistent clinical benefit was seen.[244] In contrast, ACV did show some benefit in reducing the frequency of CMV infection given suppressively in the peritransplantation period for both renal and bone marrow transplant recipients.[21, 26, 359] Although ACV still is used prophylactically in some transplant patients, ganciclovir has been shown to be superior for both prophylaxis and treatment of CMV infections, overall.

Epstein-Barr Virus Infection

ACV has been tried in severe life-threatening EBV infections without a clinical response. A controlled trial of intravenous ACV treatment of 10 mg/kg every 8 hours for 7 days in a double-blind trial of acute mononucleosis showed that pharyngeal shedding of oral EBV was inhibited reversibly ($p < .001$). In 31 patients studied, there was no significant difference in individual symptoms or laboratory parameters between the two groups. However, when data concerning the combined symptoms, such as pharyngitis, swelling, weight loss, and fever, were assessed, ACV significantly reduced these symptoms, compared with placebo-treated patients ($p < .01$). This study was performed in severely sick but otherwise normal patients with infectious mononucleosis.[7] Numerous reports have described failure of ACV treatment of EBV-associated lymphoproliferative diseases after transplantation.[66, 105, 132] Oral ACV has been shown to produce regression of EBV-related oral leukoplakia in HIV-infected patients.[292] However, the lesions recur if treatment is stopped.

Other Infections

ACV also has been shown to be of benefit in primary oral gingivostomatitis, a common infection in children and young adults that can be debilitating and sometimes requires hospitalization for rehydration. There also are anecdotal reports of successful treatment of HSV infections in children with burns, eczema, and other skin disorders.[348] In the absence of controlled studies and because these infections can be life-threatening, I believe that ACV therapy should be given early to reduce potential complications and dissemination.[125] Oral ACV treatment of herpes labialis (cold sores) has been shown to shorten the course of illness in patients who have severe outbreaks and promptly initiate treatment.[337] In subjects who were exposed to sun (skiers) or artificial ultraviolet light, oral ACV decreased the frequency of HSV outbreaks occurring within 2 to 7 days.[335, 336] Topical ACV treatment is of little benefit in otherwise healthy patients with cold sores.[385]

Resistance to Acyclovir

Numerous studies have addressed the potential problem of the development of ACV-resistant strains of HSV or VZV. This problem has been observed in vitro with HSV-1, HSV-2, and VZV strains.[13, 81] Thymidine kinase–negative HSV strains have been reported in clinically immunodeficient subjects, although these strains seem to be less virulent.[86, 318] In other clinical situations, such as recurrent genital herpes simplex, this has not proved to be a major problem to date; however, continued surveillance is important. ACV should be prescribed for approved indications only and at appropriate doses.

Problems with resistant HSV are most common in adult AIDS patients. The lesions can be large, persistent, and disfiguring, and treatment with foscarnet has been successful. Interestingly, once the original lesions cleared, the subsequent recurrences showed the HSV isolates to be sensitive to ACV.[321]

VALACYCLOVIR

Background

VACV, or valacyclovir hydrochloride, is the hydrochloride salt of the L-valine ester of ACV. This antiviral drug significantly increases oral ACV bioavailability. It is absorbed rapidly by the intestines and undergoes cleavage of the ester, resulting in rapid and almost complete conversion to ACV. The bioavailability of ACV from oral VACV is three to five times that of the high-dose oral ACV. The mechanism of action of VACV essentially is the same as that of ACV. The improved pharmacokinetic profile achieved with VACV makes this compound a suitable choice for treatment of herpesvirus infections, in which sustained high plasma concentrations of ACV are desirable.[23]

The spectrum of antiviral activity of VACV essentially is that of ACV and includes herpes group DNA viruses, such as HSV-1, HSV-2, VZV, EBV, human CMV, human herpesvirus–6, and HBV. The basis of resistance of HSV and VZV to ACV also would apply to VACV. Pharmacokinetics of VACV showed that plasma concentrations usually were greater than or equal to 0.5 mg/mL (1.54 μm) at all sampling times for all dose levels and that the drug is detectable 3 hours after administration. Mean peak ACV concentrations achieved from single doses of VACV of 250 mg or higher range from 2.15 to 5.65 mg/mL or 9.5 to 25 μm. These values are higher than values of 1.6 mg/mL or 7.1 μm achieved with high-dose oral ACV administration of 800 mg five times daily. The half-life or T1/2 of ACV after oral administration with VACV ranges from 2.8 to 3 hours. The ACV area under the curve obtained after 1000 mg of VACV is 19.5 hours/mg/mL, which is similar to the 5 mg/kg of ACV administered intravenously.[24]

Clinical Trials

Clinical trials with VACV include the treatment of herpes zoster, suppression of initial and recurrent genital herpes, and suppression of CMV disease. Several studies have compared the efficacy of VACV with that of ACV or placebo for the treatment of herpes zoster in immunocompetent patients who are 50 years of age or older with acute disease and posthepatic neuralgia. One study that compared treatment with VACV (1000 mg three times a day for 7 days vs. 14 days) with treatment with ACV (800 mg orally five times a day for 7 days) found that use of VACV for 7 or 14 days significantly accelerated the resolution of pain compared with ACV. Zoster-associated pain resolved 1.2 to 1.3 times faster in either the 7- or 14-day VACV groups compared with the ACV group. The median time to cessation of pain was 38 and 44 days in the VACV groups and 51 days in the ACV group. When all patients were analyzed, treatment with VACV significantly reduced the duration of posthepatic neuralgia, whether defined as pain after healing or pain after 30 days.[25] There were no significant side effects in this study. VACV should be considered for initial treatment of herpes zoster in adults older than 50 years of age because it is easier to administer three times daily and also has improved results compared with ACV.

A similar study in immunocompetent patients younger than 50 years of age found that VACV reduced the duration of new lesion formation faster during the acute disease compared with ACV, and there was no significant difference in the zoster-associated pain. However, there was a low incidence of zoster-associated pain in this younger group.[327]

There have been several studies for the treatment of first-episode and recurrent genital herpes. One study compared VACV with ACV for primary genital herpes and found that no significant difference in the speed of lesion healing or duration of viral shedding. There also were no differences in rates of resolution of pain or genital symptoms or other signs and symptoms, and the safety profiles were similar for the two drugs. In recurrent genital herpes studies, suppression with VACV compared with ACV treatment showed similar results. There was a slight advantage in terms of median length of episodes of herpes in the VACV group and a slight increase in the number of patients whose lesions were prevented or aborted with treatment in the VACV group. Other studies of herpes showed similar results for VACV and for ACV.[327, 338] There seems to be no added advantage of use of VACV in genital HSV, most probably because HSV is so sensitive to ACV in vitro.

Studies of Cytomegalovirus Clinical Trials

There have been series of studies using VACV for prophylaxis and treatment of CMV in immunocompromised and immunosuppressed patients. These include patients with HIV infection and kidney, heart, lung, and bone marrow transplant recipients. A prophylaxis study for CMV in HIV-infected patients who had low CD4 counts (<100) evaluated oral VACV at 2 g four times a day or ACV at two different doses, 800 or 400 mg two or four times a day. In this study, there was a lower incidence (12 per cent) of confirmed CMV end-points in the VACV arm, compared with 17 per cent in the high-dose ACV arm and 18 per cent in the low-dose ACV arm. The relative risk of developing CMV disease seemed to be reduced for the VACV group compared with the pooled ACV groups.

Side Effects of Valacyclovir

In general, in normal immunocompetent patients, side effects are mild and include gastrointestinal disturbances, nausea, and vomiting. A number of patients with advanced HIV disease who received prolonged high-dose prophylaxis developed thrombotic microangiopathy with features of thrombotic thrombocytopenic purpura or hemolytic uremic syndrome.[227] This was characterized by thrombocytopenia and anemia, fragmented red cells, and elevated serum creatinine. This occurred more frequently in the VACV arm in these HIV-infected patients than in the ACV arms and occurred a median of 59 weeks on study. In this group of patients who received prolonged VACV, there was a shorter time to death compared with the ACV group, and this mainly was due to the side effect of thrombotic thrombocytopenic purpura or hemolytic uremic syndrome. This side effect only has been seen in patients with advanced HIV infection who received long-term high doses of oral VACV. Prolonged treatment of this group of patients with VACV should be considered only with great caution.

FAMCICLOVIR

Famciclovir is the oral prodrug of penciclovir, an antiviral agent that has potent activity against VZV, HSV-1, and HSV-2. Famciclovir is well absorbed orally and is converted to penciclovir. The mechanism of action is similar to that of ACV in that within herpesvirus-infected cells, the viral enzyme thymidine kinase efficiently converts penciclovir to the monophosphate form, which is the active inhibitor of HSV thymidine kinase.

Famciclovir has a prolonged intracellular half-life of approximately 9 to 10 hours in VZV-infected cells and 10 to 20 hours in cells infected with HSV-1 or HSV-2. It has 77 per cent bioavailability and produces higher levels of drug in plasma compared with ACV.[62]

Clinical Trials

Clinical trials of this drug have shown that famciclovir effectively speeds the healing of acute VZV infection, and in a placebo-controlled trial, it reduced the duration of posthepatic neuralgia in elderly patients.[355] Famciclovir also has been studied in the treatment of recurrent genital herpes and showed reduction in times to cessation of virus shedding, complete healing, and loss of symptoms.[301] Famciclovir also was used for suppressive therapy and effectively reduced recurrent genital herpes in patients with frequent recurrences.

Famciclovir currently is licensed for treatment of herpes zoster and HSV genitalis. The dose used for HSV genitalis in adults is 250 mg given twice daily. The dosing for acute herpes zoster in adults is 500 mg given three times a day. Famciclovir also has in vitro activity against HBV and currently is in clinical trials for chronic HBV infection. Virus resistance to famciclovir varies, and cross-resistance of both varicella and herpes simplex to famciclovir and ACV are common. However, some virus strains are resistant to ACV and still are sensitive to famciclovir.

GANCICLOVIR (DHPG)

Ganciclovir (9-[1,3-dihydroxy-2-propoxymethyl] guanine deoxyguanosine; DHPG) is a nucleoside analogue of ACV and has activity in vitro against HSV-1, HSV-2, VZV, CMV, and EBV.[326] The structure is shown in Figure 233–11. The major potential advantage of ganciclovir over other antiviral agents is its potent activity against CMV. It is the first antiviral agent to be effective in treating CMV in humans. The mechanism of action is not fully understood; however, it is a competitive inhibitor of human CMV polymerase and preferentially is activated to the triphosphate form in human CMV-infected fibroblasts.[27, 290] Pharmacokinetics reveal peak plasma ganciclovir levels of 18 to 24 μg after doses of 2.5 mg/kg/8 hours, with cerebrospinal fluid levels of 2 to 2.7 μg at peak plasma levels, and 30 to 40 μg/mL at doses of 5 mg/kg/8 hours. These levels exceed in vitro 50 per cent plaque inhibitory concentration levels for most CMV isolates.[290, 351, 354] The plasma half-life is 2.9 hours, and 12 hours after infusion, serum concentrations are less than 0.5 g/mL. The typical regimen of ganciclovir is a dose of 7.5 to 10 mg/kg/day given intravenously in two divided doses. After oral administration of 1000 mg of ganciclovir three times a day, the maximal and minimal serum concentrations were 1.2 and 0.2 μg/mL, respectively, in adults. The oral bioavailability is about 6 to 9 per cent. However, the serum concentrations achievable after oral ganciclovir are close to the ED_{50} of most clinical CMV isolates (0.2 to 1.6 μg/mL). Ganciclovir has been shown in animal studies to have effects against HSV encephalitis in mice, ocular HSV-1 infection in rabbits, genital HSV infection in guinea pigs, and skin infection in mice.[353] Ganciclovir also has been found to be of benefit in studies of CMV in mice, both in lethal disease and in pneumonitis.

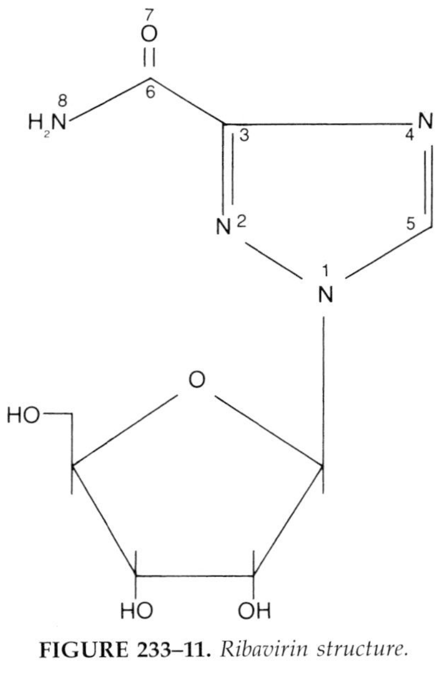

FIGURE 233–11. *Ribavirin structure.*

Ganciclovir has been proved effective in the treatment of several types of CMV infections and also is effective for maintenance and prophylactic therapy. Studies of ganciclovir in immunocompromised patients with CMV infections, including bone marrow transplant recipients with CMV interstitial pneumonia and AIDS patients with CMV gastrointestinal disease and pneumonitis, all have shown some benefit. Patients treated with ganciclovir have variable clinical responses; although ganciclovir is indicated for certain infection, there is definite evidence that treatment has arrested CMV retinitis in AIDS patients, and CMV viral titers have been reduced in plasma and sperm samples in several studies. The treatment involved induction and maintenance therapy, and once the drug is stopped, the disease can flare again. Maintenance therapy is used at a smaller dose of ganciclovir required for inducing a remission, usually 5 to 6 mg/kg/day.[114] A direct comparison of ganciclovir and foscarnet in a multicenter trial of CMV retinitis in AIDS patients showed similar efficacy in preventing disease progression. Combination treatment with foscarnet and ganciclovir for CMV retinitis was found to be superior to either alone.[80] Ganciclovir treatment also reduced the frequency of colonic disease due to CMV in AIDS patients and other immunocompromised patients.[93] Oral ganciclovir therapy has been approved as another option to intravenous maintenance therapy for CMV retinitis and has had equivalent efficacy.[102, 103, 331] Intraocular sustained release ganciclovir implants and ganciclovir injections into the vitreous of the eye also have shown benefit. However, local delivery of drug does not protect against systemic disease. Ganciclovir treatment of primary CMV pneumonia has been most successful with renal transplant recipients. However, efficacy in bone marrow transplants is limited. In one study of 10 bone marrow transplant patients with biopsy-proven CMV infection, Shepp and associates[311] observed a decrease in viruria and viremia, elimination of CMV from respiratory secretions, and a decrease in CMV viral titers in the lung. However, despite this treatment and viral efficacy, 9 of 10 patients died. This group of bone marrow transplant recipients may represent a severe form of CMV infection, and there may be confounding factors such as total body irradiation and the immune response. Studies of prophylactic ganciclovir given shortly after bone marrow engraftment but prior to isolation of virus have shown a significant reduction in the incidence of CMV interstitial pneumonia. Studies in heart, liver, and kidney transplanting showed ganciclovir to be effective prophylaxis.[135, 241, 306, 382]

Ganciclovir also has a more narrow range of therapeutic index than does ACV. There is a dose-related depressive effect on the white blood cell count and number of platelets. Oral ganciclovir therapy has a lower incidence of hematologic side effects. There also is a potential for testicular toxicity and azoospermia, which has been seen in animal studies. The major target for treatment and prophylaxis of CMV infection is the severely immunocompromised patients, including those with AIDS. Studies in children with symptomatic congenital CMV infection are ongoing but suggest that ganciclovir may benefit children with central nervous system disease and reduce hearing defects. Unfortunately, ganciclovir-resistant CMV isolates have been found in immunocompromised patients, particularly adults with AIDS. Foscarnet or a combined therapy is the alternative treatment choice. Cidofovir is a nucleotide that also inhibits CMV replication and has been useful for the treatment of CMV retinitis and maintenance to prevent relapse (see Table 233–2).[80, 204]

RIBAVIRIN

Mechanism of Action and In Vitro Sensitivity Spectrum

Ribavirin (1-β-D-ribofuranosyl-1,2,4-triazole-3-carboxamide) is a synthetic nucleoside with a structure similar to that of guanosine (Fig. 233–12), with broad-spectrum antiviral activity against both DNA and RNA viruses in tissue culture systems. Activity has been demonstrated in vitro against many viruses, including HSV-1 and HSV-2, vaccinia virus, some adenoviruses, parainfluenza virus, influenza A and B viruses, coxsackievirus B, polioviruses, measles virus, members of *Arenaviridae* (including Lassa fever virus), togaviruses, and HIV-1.[320]

Ribavirin is phosphorylated and acts as a competitive inhibitor of inosine 5′-phosphate dehydrogenase, which interferes with guanosine synthesis by depletion of deoxyguanosine triphosphate and guanosine triphosphate pools.[346] Ribavirin also inhibits reverse transcriptase enzyme.

Ribavirin has been reported to inhibit influenza A virus in cell culture without significant inhibition of host-cell protein or RNA synthesis. In cell-free studies, ribavirin 5′-triphosphate has been reported selectively to inhibit influenza A virus RNA-dependent RNA polymerase.[111, 266]

In contrast with these findings, studies of ribavirin treatment of influenza A virus–infected MDCK cells suggest a nonspecific mechanism of antiviral action.[35] Ribavirin has demonstrated significant antiviral activity in infections due to influenza A and B viruses, murine hepatitis virus, parainfluenza viruses, vaccinia viruses, and HSV in various animal model systems.[100, 116, 193, 210] In monkeys infected with Lassa fever virus, ribavirin treatment reduced viremia and increased the survival rate.

Pharmacology and Toxicity

Pharmacokinetic studies showed that ^{14}C-labeled ribavirin given orally had peak plasma levels of 4 to 8 μM at 1 to 1.5 hours. Urinary excretion averaged 33 per cent of the dose over 24 hours and 53 per cent at 72 hours, and radioactive concentrations of ribavirin or its metabolites (<5 per cent of total dose) were detected in red blood cells over about 40 days.[346] With use of a sensitive radioimmunoassay developed by Connor and coworkers,[74] peak plasma levels in children treated with aerosolized ribavirin D averaged 3.5 μM, with much higher levels achieved in respiratory secretions, with a range of 1250 to 28,000 μM. Plasma concentrations increased with the increasing duration of aerosol exposure to an average of 0.8 to 8 μM for administration of aerosol from 2.5 to 20 hours. The plasma T½ averaged approximately 9 hours after cessation of aerosol administration. The mean peak plasma level in adults given 1000 mg/day in three divided doses orally was 3.1 μM. In adults with Lassa fever after intravenous administration of 1000-mg or 500-mg doses, peak plasma levels were 94 μM and 68 μM, respectively. These plasma levels were several times the minimal inhibitory concentration of Lassa fever virus (4 to 40 μM). With short-term administration of doses of 800 to 1000 mg/day in adults, serum bilirubin and serum iron may increase mildly in about one-fourth of patients. Mild anemia may be seen only after prolonged administration (>1 month) but is reversible when the drug is stopped. Animals experience dose-dependent microcytic anemia after prolonged administration. In pregnant rodents treated with higher dose ribavirin, skeletal defects in the developing embryo, as well as fetal resorptions, have been seen.[198] Ribavirin is contraindicated during pregnancy, and pregnant health care workers should take precautions when administering aerosol ribavirin to patients, although the risk of absorbing any significant amount of ribavirin by this route is small. Aerosol ribavirin in both adults and children seems to be well tolerated without specific pulmonary toxic effects with short-term administration.

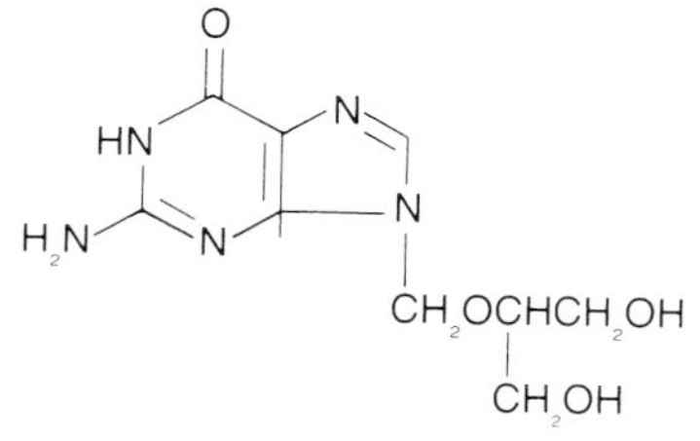

FIGURE 233–12. *DHPG (ganciclovir) structure.*

Clinical Studies

Ribavirin has been given orally, intravenously, and by aerosol in clinical studies of treatment of several viral infections. Studies of prophylactic oral administration of ribavirin to volunteers challenged with influenza A virus revealed a mild diminution in symptoms in drug recipients; other studies reported no benefit. In a prophylactic study, some protection was noted against influenza B virus in adults; however, a later study showed that an oral dose of 1000 mg/day had no clinical or antiviral activity in naturally occurring influenza A outbreaks in adults.[328] In an uncontrolled study, oral ribavirin at 600 mg/day for 14 days reportedly had some clinical benefit in patients with acute hepatitis in which they showed more rapid resolution of bilirubin and liver enzyme elevations. Some studies have suggested some clinical benefit of oral ribavirin in patients with recurrent genital herpes. Further study in these areas would be necessary to assess efficacy.

After encouraging results with aerosol administration of ribavirin in infected animal models, several blinded controlled studies of aerosol administration of ribavirin for both influenza A virus and respiratory syncytial virus (RSV) were completed. In a study of young adults with naturally acquired influenza A or B virus infection, treated within 24 hours of infection, small-particle aerosol given for an average of 23 to 39 hours over a 3-day period was associated with reduction of fever, systemic illness, and influenza virus titer, compared with placebo-treated subjects.[328] In experimental RSV infection of young adults in a placebo-controlled, blinded study, aerosol ribavirin reduced fever and systemic symptoms, compared with controls.[144] Although these studies showed some benefit, the lack of practicality of this approach has limited enthusiasm for developing the drug for treatment.

Controlled studies conducted by Hall and coworkers[144] found that aerosol ribavirin given for an average of 20 hours per day for 3 to 6 days had a significant clinical benefit in the treatment of hospitalized infants with lower respiratory tract infection with RSV. The treated group had a shortened duration of viral shedding and improved clinical status, including respiratory rate, fever, arterial oxygen saturation, and lower respiratory tract signs. In this study, no significant side effects or toxic effects were associated with aerosol therapy, and the resistant pattern of these isolates to ribavirin did not change. The children included in this study had no underlying disease but were moderately or markedly ill. These studies have been expanded to other institutions with similar results. However, because ribavirin is expensive and many children have mild self-limited disease, therapy is not indicated in all infants with RSV. Preliminary results from studies in infants with underlying diseases such as congenital heart disease and bronchopulmonary dysplasia who are at high risk for fatal RSV infection also showed significant clinical benefit from administration of aerosol ribavirin, compared with placebo-treated subjects.[143] The use of respiratory syncytial immunoglobulin given prophylactically to infants with underlying diseases at high risk of developing infection also should be considered prior to the RSV season.

There are several reports of ribavirin administered by aerosol to infants with severe combined immunodeficiency who may have prolonged overwhelming infection with respiratory viruses, particularly RSV, parainfluenza virus, and influenza virus. Patients with both parainfluenza virus and RSV infection reportedly benefited while ribavirin was being administered; however, once the drug was discontinued, viral infection reappeared, and repeated courses were necessary.[235]

Aerosol administration of ribavirin is performed with a Collison generator, which produces an aerosol with a mass median diameter of 1.4 μm with a concentration in the reservoir of 20 mg/mL. The concentrations in secretions are highest when the drug is administered by endotracheal tube, compared with oxygen hood, mask, or tent. Ribavirin accumulates when the length of treatment per day exceeds 8 hours, with a peak level increasing with each subsequent day of therapy. The mean inhibitory concentration of ribavirin for RSV usually is in the range of 10 to 40 μM, whereas the tracheal secretions have concentrations exceeding 4000 μM.

Lassa fever has been reported to be a severe and often fatal disease, caused by an arenavirus, that occurs in Africa (Nigeria, Liberia, and Sierra Leone). The usual symptoms of Lassa fever are fever, sore throat, cough, and abdominal and back pain, which last from 1 to 4 weeks. Gastrointestinal hemorrhage may be seen in severe cases, with death from irreversible hypovolemic shock in 15 to 20 per cent of hospitalized patients. This study was conducted in a selected group of hospitalized patients in Sierra Leone who had an aspartate aminotransferase level of greater than 150 IU/L at the time of hospital admission, which was associated with a case-fatality rate of 55 per cent in a previous phase I study.[234] Patients were separated randomly into two groups, with a group of 29 patients receiving intravenous ribavirin and a second group of 33 patients receiving intravenous ribavirin and 1 unit (300 mL) of convalescent Lassa fever plasma. The dose of ribavirin given was a 2-g loading dose followed by 1 g every 6 hours for 4 days and 0.5 g given intravenously every 8 hours for another 6 days. The case-fatality rate in patients who had met the entry criteria and who were treated for 10 days with intravenous ribavirin begun within the first 6 days of onset of fever was 5 per cent, 1 of 20 ($p < .002$), compared with untreated subjects with similar risk factors. The case-fatality rate in patients in whom ribavirin treatment was begun 7 or more days after onset of fever was 26 per cent, 11 of 43 ($p < .01$). Patients who had high levels of viremia on entry (>10 TIC/mL) had even higher mortality (case-fatality rate of 76 per cent). The case-fatality rate in patients with this risk factor who were treated with intravenous ribavirin within the first 6 days was reduced at 9 per cent, 1 of 11 ($p < .0006$), whereas the case-fatality rate in those treated after 7 or more days of illness was 47 per cent, 9 of 19. In a subgroup of pregnant patients who received Lassa convalescent plasma, mortality was not reduced significantly in any of the high-risk groups. In patients at high risk who were treated with ribavirin and lived, the viral titer in the serum was reduced. This also was observed in patients who lived after plasma therapy.

Although the number of treated cases employing it is lower, oral ribavirin also seems to be effective in reducing the overall mortality of patients with Lassa fever in these high-risk groups. Oral ribavirin was given in a 2-g loading dose followed by 1 g/day every 8 hours for 10 days (Table 233–10). The major side effect was hemolysis with a drop of approximately 20 per cent in hematocrit in some patients; however, this was reversible once the drug was stopped, with no significant changes in white blood cell count, platelet count, liver function, or renal function.

Ribavirin has been approved by the Food and Drug Administration in the United States for aerosol administration for RSV infection in infants. Other potential targets for ribavirin therapy include treatment of common viral encephalitides caused by bunyaviruses.[21, 51, 169] The licensing of ribavirin for aerosol use in RSV infections in infants was a big advance in antiviral chemotherapy. Other antiviral agents with this mode of administration may be useful in the future for treatment of other RSV infections.

ANTIRETROVIRAL THERAPY

Zidovudine (ZDV; Azidothymidine)

ZDV (3′-azido-3′-deoxythymidine) is a nucleoside analogue of thymidine that first was demonstrated to have anti-

TABLE 233–10. Outcome of Lassa Fever in Patients Admitted with Serum Virus Levels $\geq 10^{3.6}$ $TCID_{50}$/mL, According to Type of Therapy and Day of Illness When Therapy Was Initiated

	Treatment Within 6 Days		Treatment at 7 Days or Later	
	Lived	*Died (%)*	*Lived*	*Died (%)*
No treatment	5	15 (75)	6	21 (78)
IV ribavirin*	10	1 (9)	10	9 (47)
Oral ribavirin†	4	1 (20)	3	2 (40)
Plasma	4	5 (56)	5	7 (58)

*The case-fatality rate when treatment was given at ≤6 days was significantly lower than when treatment was given at ≥7 days (p = .026 by Fisher exact test). The case-fatality rate when treatment was given at ≤6 days was significantly lower than in the untreated group (p = .006). The case-fatality rate when treatment was given at ≥7 days was also significantly lower than in the untreated group (p = .035).

†The case-fatality rate when treatment was given at ≤6 days was significantly lower than in the untreated group (p = .04).

From McCormick, J. B., King, I. J., Webb, P. A., et al.: Lassa fever. Effective therapy with ribavirin. N. Engl. J. Med. *314*:20–26, 1986. Reprinted, by permission, from the New England Journal of Medicine.

viral activity against Friend murine leukemia virus and later to HIV-1 in vitro as well as other animal retroviruses.[249, 264] ZDV is converted by cellular thymidine kinase to a monophosphate and by cellular thymidylate kinase into a diphosphate and then by other cell enzymes to the active triphosphate form. ZDV triphosphate then inhibits HIV-1 reverse transcriptase approximately 100 times more than it does the cellular polymerases. ZDV inhibits replication of HIV-1 by at least two mechanisms, including chain termination and competitive inhibition of cellular nucleoside 5′-triphosphates of ZDV.[105] ZDV inhibits HIV-1 replication in vitro at levels greater than 0.1 μM, compared with uninfected lymphocytes at greater than 1 μM. ZDV also has some antibacterial effects against Enterobacteriaceae and *Vibrio* bacteria without effect against gram-positive or most other gram-negative bacteria or mycobacteria.[108]

Pharmacology

ZDV has been used intravenously and orally and is licensed for use in the oral and intravenous formulation. In clinical pharmacology studies, ZDV is absorbed well orally; peak serum concentrations are reached at about 30 to 90 minutes after dose, with a half-life in adults of approximately 1 hour. It has good oral bioavailability, with approximately 65 per cent penetration of the blood-brain barrier at a 1:2 ratio.[30] Children have been included in the evaluation of continuous intravenous ZDV infusion given by a programmable infusion pump and a Hickman catheter. This was designed to achieve a steady-state concentration of 1 μM ZDV plasma level in children. ZDV was administered at various dose levels from 0.5 to 1.8 mg/kg body weight per hour, and plasma concentrations varied with the dose given from 1.9 to 4.5 μM concentration. Oral ZDV, 180 mg/kg given every 6 hours in children, showed peak ZDV levels and a half-life that were similar to those seen in adults.[281] ZDV also has been evaluated in newborns at birth to 3 months of age with a dose of 2 to 4 mg/kg administered intravenously and orally every 6 hours. The clearance of ZDV was increased in children younger than 30 days of age, with a concomitant decrease in plasma concentrations.[15]

ZDV also has been evaluated in third-trimester HIV-1–seropositive pregnant women and their infants in a phase I safety and tolerance trial. This study showed that ZDV was absorbed well at a dose of 200 mg every 6 hours, with plasma concentrations similar to those in nonpregnant adults. ZDV given intravenously during labor and delivery intermittently or by constant infusion resulted in cord plasma ZDV levels in newborns that were identical to the mothers' plasma concentrations at delivery. The serum ZDV half-life in infants was prolonged for the first day of life, compared with older infants. ZDV was tolerated well without any evidence of significant hematologic or other toxic effects in both mothers and infants. All mothers received ZDV from 28 to 36 weeks' gestation through term.[262] These studies provided the basis for the efficacy trial of ZDV for prevention of maternal-fetal HIV-1 infection (AIDS Clinical Trials Group [ACTG] 076). Current pharmacokinetic studies are evaluating the comparison of frequent oral ZDV administration to the constant intravenous infusion for the mother during labor and delivery. Preliminary data suggest that PK levels may be similar, and oral treatment would be more adaptable to clinical settings in the United States and abroad.

Clinical Studies

ADULT TRIALS. ZDV has been studied in numerous well-controlled clinical trials of treatment in adults with HIV infection as monotherapy and in combination with other antiviral agents. Several studies using ZDV alone or in combination also have been completed in HIV-1–infected children. The first study, completed in 1986, enrolled 282 adult patients with AIDS or AIDS-related complex who were ill and within 4 months of their first attack of *Pneumocystis carinii* pneumonia in a multicenter trial. ZDV was administered alone at a dose of 250 mg given every 4 hours; 145 patients received ZDV, and 137 received placebo. This study showed for the first time that ZDV had efficacy for this disease: 19 patients—12 with AIDS and 7 with AIDS-related complex in the placebo group—died, compared with only 1 who received ZDV. In addition, ZDV significantly reduced the number of opportunistic infections; improved functional capacity, weight gain, and neuropsychologic testing; and resulted in a decrease in plasma p24 antigen and a transient increase in CD4 cells.[120] Survival rates also were improved compared with those from natural history studies.[119] The major side effects included toxicity with anemia, requiring transfusions and neutropenia in approximately 16 per cent of patients. Other minor symptoms also included nausea, myalgia, headache, and insomnia.[294]

This study resulted in the licensure of ZDV for treatment of symptomatic HIV-1 infection in adults in 1987.[158] Since then, ZDV has undergone a series of trials and now is used in combination with other antiretroviral agents. Several large blinded clinical trials sponsored by ACTG evaluated the use of ZDV in mildly symptomatic patients (ACTG 016) and asymptomatic adults (ACTG 019), compared with ddI (ACTG 116, 117b).[121] In the 016 protocol, patients were randomized to receive either placebo or ZDV at a total daily dose of 1200 mg. The results showed that in the 710 evaluable subjects, there was a significant reduction in progression rates in subjects in the ZDV arm, compared with those assigned placebo. In addition, it was found that patients who had higher entry levels of CD4 cells did better than did those who had lower CD4 numbers.

In one of the largest studies, ACTG 019, 3200 subjects were enrolled and stratified by baseline CD4 counts of less than 500/mm^3 or greater than 500/mm^3. Subjects received either placebo, 500 mg, or 1500 mg total daily dose of ZDV. Evaluable patients (N = 1338) with less than 500 CD4 cells showed significantly less progression to symptoms or AIDS in both ZDV groups, compared with the placebo group. There was no significant advantage of the larger ZDV dose in efficacy and the lower dose had significantly less toxicity, both hematologically and with other minor toxic effects.[361] Although these early studies showed initial benefit of ZDV therapy, monotherapy with ZDV proved to have no significant long term effects on survival as evidenced by several studies, including the Concorde and Delta trials. In retrospect, this is most likely due to the modest antiviral effect of ZDV and the development of viral resistance to ZDV. ZDV still has a major role in therapy when used in combination and particularly may be important in the treatment of central nervous system disease due to HIV-1. ZDV has had a major impact on the prevention of maternal-fetal HIV-1 transmission (see Zidovudine and Other Strategies for the Prevention of Maternal-Fetal HIV-1 Transmission).

CLINICAL TRIALS IN CHILDREN. Early ZDV trials in children established the pharmacokinetics and safety of intravenous infusions of both ZDV and oral ZDV for children with advanced disease.[281] These studies showed the improvement of neurodevelopmental abnormalities, as measured by an increase in IQ, increases in appetite and weight gain, and a decrease in hepatosplenomegaly and immunoglobulin levels. A study by McKinney and associates of ZDV given at 180 mg/m^2 orally four times daily to severely symptomatic children showed significant clinical improvements in weight gain, neurodevelopmental testing, and laboratory parameters, including a transient increase in CD4 cell count and a decrease in serum p24 antigen in those in whom such findings initially were positive. One of the most interesting findings in this study was the observed reduction in cerebrospinal fluid p24 antigen and the number of positive HIV cerebrospinal fluid cocultures after 8 weeks of ZDV therapy. This is the first direct proof of ZDV's antiviral effect on central nervous system disease.

Several clinical trials sponsored by the NIH Pediatric ACTG further have defined the use of ZDV in children. The ACTG 128 study showed that doses of 120 and 180 mg/kg were similar in efficacy. Most recently, the ACTG 152 study showed that ddI or a combination of ddI and ZDV were superior to ZDV monotherapy in the treatment of children with HIV infection. Further studies of combined therapy of ZDV with other antiretroviral agents, including d4T, 3TC, and NEV, are under way. Triple combination therapy with ZDV, ddI, and NEV early in primary infection have shown dramatic effects on reduction in HIV virus load and preservation of immune response in a small number of children.[221] A double-blind, placebo-controlled study of intravenous gammaglobulin (IVIG) showed efficacy in reduction in the number of days of hospitalization and the number of severe bacterial infections in children. There was no difference in mortality rates, and children who were less severely sick seemed to benefit the most.[250, 251] A follow-up study (ACTG 051) of IVIG versus placebo in children who were receiving antiviral therapy with ZDV showed that IVIG significantly reduced bacterial infections, but the results were similar to those of children receiving Bactrim prophylaxis.[330] IVIG should be considered in children who have repeated serious bacterial infections. Prophylactic ZDV also has been studied in the prevention of occupational exposure to HIV by needlesticks in health care workers, although the risk of transmission by this route is low and seroconversion still can occur despite prompt treatment. ZDV should be administered with other antiviral agents, according to the latest recommendation of the Centers for Disease Control and Prevention. Treatment should be instituted immediately upon knowledge of a needlestick, preferably started within 4 hours and continued for 2 to 6 weeks.[1, 2, 154]

Zidovudine and Other Strategies for the Prevention of Maternal-Fetal HIV-1 Transmission

Over the past few years, there have been major advances in the area of perinatal HIV-1 transmission that have brought new hope for the prevention of pediatric HIV infection. Knowledge of the risk factors associated with transmission has increased, and a landmark study by Connor and associates[73] (ACTG 076) has shown that perinatal transmission could be reduced by approximately 70 per cent by the use of ZDV when given to HIV-infected, drug-naive women during gestation and delivery and for 6 weeks to the infant after birth. ZDV has become the standard of care for prevention of perinatal transmission in HIV-infected pregnant women in the United States and also has had worldwide implications.[52] The results of this study have proved the concept that antiretroviral therapy significantly can reduce perinatal transmission. On the basis of these findings and the recent availability of potent new antiviral compounds, most investigators believe that perinatal transmission further can be reduced to less than 2 per cent.

The treatment regimen used in the ACTG 076 trial was targeted to cover all potential transmission, including in utero with prepartum oral maternal treatment (from 14 weeks onward) and intrapartum by a constant infusion, and to provide prophylaxis for the infant by oral treatment for 6 weeks. The significant reduction from 25 per cent transmission in the placebo recipients to 8 per cent in the ZDV-treated mother-infant pairs also has been reported from some studies in the general population.[123] However, in an inner-city population in the Bronx, New York, only 49 of 125 HIV-infected women were identified before delivery and fewer than half of these women received ZDV therapy,[383] underscoring the difficulty of translating scientific advances into clinical practice.

The relative protective role of the various components of the 076 trial regimen and whether this regimen can be simplified or reduced further is unclear. Several studies have observed a decreased transmission rate when mothers but not newborns received ZDV.[32, 92, 126] This would suggest that the prenatal treatment would be the most important factor in the regimen. However, this does not rule out the possibility that treatment during labor and postpartum of the infant also would not have a prophylactic protective effect on the infant. The question of whether this regimen can be simplified to make it more practical in both developed and developing countries and the relevance and importance of each of the arms is being addressed in further trials in developing countries.

Antiviral therapy results in a reduction of maternal plasma viral load,[92] and preliminary analysis of the virus load in mothers included in the 076 trial showed a 1.7-fold (0.24 log) reduction of HIV RNA in these women with CD4 counts higher than 200 cells/mm^3. Although transmission risk was associated with an increased level of maternal viral load, the use of ZDV was associated with a reduced transmission rate at all levels of maternal HIV RNA. This suggests that the mechanism of protection by ZDV may include both reduction of maternal virus load and prophylaxis of the fetus/newborn because the drug readily crosses the placenta and is present in the amniotic fluid in high concentrations.[262, 332]

The efficacy of ZDV in women with advanced disease, CD4 counts lower than 200, prior antiretroviral drug use, a high virus load, or virus that is ZDV-resistant or who present late in pregnancy or at the time of delivery is limited.[52, 231] Studies in adults have shown that double and triple antiretroviral therapy combinations, including the use of protease inhibitors, can significantly reduce plasma viral load. Carefully controlled trials to address the potential efficacy of drug combinations in reducing vertical transmission designed maximally to reduce maternal virus load are planned. The design of these efficacy trials will include the use of various combinations of antiretroviral drugs initiated as early as 16 to 34 weeks of pregnancy to provide maximum antiretroviral activity through the latter part of pregnancy and delivery and will include administration of these antiretroviral agents to the newborns for a short time. However, this approach may not be practical, feasible, or affordable in many countries.

Frequently, women only come to medical attention when they already are in labor, and an important question is whether intervention strategies initiated at this time could prevent or modify intrapartum transmission. The non-nucleoside reverse transcriptase inhibitors (including NEV, which passes easily through the placenta to the fetus and which has a prolonged half-life after single-dose oral administration) may be ideal candidates for use at the time of delivery.

The safety of drugs during pregnancy and the potential effects on the developing fetus are critical in determining risk versus benefit. Preclinical studies of various antiretroviral agents include studies of reproductive toxicity. Because many women will require combined antiretroviral therapy for their own health, phase I studies are important to establish safety and dose. Phase I studies either have been completed or are ongoing for NEV, ddI, d4T, 3TC, 1592 (Glaxo), and the protease inhibitors. Several of these studies will evaluate these drugs in combinations for both safety and pharmacokinetics. An efficacy trial of the ability of NEV to reduce vertical transmission, wherein NEV is initiated at the time of labor and given to the infant in a single dose at 2 to 3 days of age for women who present after 34 weeks' gestation, is under way. An efficacy trial of a combination of antiretroviral drugs will be initiated late in 1997, and the choice of the best combination will be based on safety, pharmacokinetics, relative antiretroviral activity, and ability of the drugs to cross the placenta. The rapidly changing antiviral therapy in HIV-infected adults will influence the future approaches to prevention of vertical transmission.

In addition, numerous studies are either ongoing or planned in many countries around the world, in both breast feeding and non–breast feeding populations.[84, 113] Trials in Africa, Thailand, and Haiti include comparisons of regimens of reduced ZDV courses in mother and infant, mother only, infant only, and mother postpartum in breast-feeding populations. A World Health Organization trial has started in African countries using a reduced course of combined antiretroviral agents with ZDV and 3TC.

Combination Therapy for HIV Infection

Combination therapy for HIV-1 for patients with less than 500 CD4 counts now is considered the standard of care for adults and most probably will be recommended for all children. New guidelines for the treatment of adults with HIV-1 were published in the *Journal of the American Medical Association* in June of 1996. Advances in quantitation of HIV using HIV RNA PCR have shown that the level of HIV replication measured in HIV RNA copy/mL in plasma is prognostic for long-term outcome and can be used for the monitoring of antiviral effect.[239] Current pediatric trials include triple combination of ZDV, ddI, NEV or a protease inhibitor for the treatment of children with symptomatic HIV infection[282] and for early therapy in newly diagnosed infection.

Further evaluation of the potential synergistic activity of combinations of antiviral agents will be an exciting and rapidly changing avenue for therapeutics for HIV infection.

Antiviral Resistance to Zidovudine

There is laboratory evidence that HIV may become resistant to ZDV in vitro. In patients who had received ZDV for more than 30 months, a significant number of their HIV isolates were resistant to ZDV in vitro. Larder and Kemp[208] published several distinct mutations in the *pol* gene encoding for viral reverse transcriptase that pinpoint several genetic changes in these isolates. The resistant isolates were found to be sensitive to other nucleosides (ddC, ddI, d4T), nonnucleoside reverse transcriptase inhibitors, protease inhibitors (indinavir, saquinavir, ritonavir, viracept), and foscarnet.[207] Important questions remain as to whether resistance develops at the same rate in patients who are given ZDV while they are asymptomatic as in those who are later in the disease process. It also is important whether resistance occurs at the same rate or more rapidly in children infected perinatally who may have a higher viral load and therefore a higher rate of mutations. Because ZDV treatment of HIV-infected pregnant women for the prevention of perinatal transmission is considered the standard of care, there may be more potential transmission of ZDV-resistant virus to newborns. In vitro resistance to ZDV has been associated with clinical disease progression in several studies in children.[259, 263] The treatment with other nucleosides such as 3TC may reverse these mutations when used in combination.[209] It will be important to determine whether initial potent combination therapy reduces the emergence of resistant isolates to antiviral drugs. The reduction of viral replication to undetectably low levels by potent therapy, and therefore potentially reducing the chance of HIV mutation, now potentially is achievable.

Didanosine (Dideoxyinosine; ddI)

ddI, which is similar to ddC, also has in vitro activity against HIV-1. ddI has been shown to be efficacious as monotherapy and in combination with other antiviral agents in adults and children. A phase I pharmacokinetic and safety study was performed in 80 children with HIV infection in six dosage levels varying from 20 to 180 mg/m^2 administered every 8 hours orally. There was evidence of antiretroviral activity as seen by decreases in p24 antigenemia and a transient increase in CD4 counts over time. The children were noted to have improved neurodevelopmental function, and pharmacokinetic analysis revealed that drug levels were obtainable in the cerebrospinal fluid at a ratio of 1:2 or 1:4. Potential side effects include peripheral neuropathy, which has not been observed in any children to date. Several children who received large doses of ddI (315 mg/kg) developed clinical and laboratory evidence of acute pancreatitis. In adults, there also have been reported cases of pancreatitis with some deaths out of more than 9000 adult patients treated. Current trials in pediatrics will include a combination of ddI and ZDV therapy in an effort to reduce the dose necessary for efficacy, to reduce side effects, and to inhibit the emergence of resistant isolates. As previously mentioned, ddI was evaluated in HIV-infected children in a randomized study as monotherapy or combined with ZDV compared with ZDV alone (ACTG 152). This study showed that the children who received ddI alone or a combination of ddI and ZDV had fewer clinical end-points and less disease progression than did children who received ZDV monotherapy. The results of this study have changed initial clinical management of HIV-infected children to include ddI with or without ZDV. Although the efficacy was similar for both monotherapy and combined therapy, the use of ZDV may have an additional advantage for the prevention or treatment of central nervous system disease in these children. This study did not have enough central nervous system end-points to show a significant difference. ddI is known to have poor penetration to the central nervous system compared with ZDV. Overall, ddI has been well tolerated in children at doses starting at 200 mg/kg/day given in two divided doses on an empty stomach.[46]

Side Effects

The major adverse events associated with ddI (Videx) include pancreatitis and peripheral neuropathy, which are more common in patients with advanced disease. In adults, the incidence of peripheral neuropathy is approximately 16 per cent and in children is 3 per cent. The peripheral neuropathy syndrome consists of bilaterally symmetric sensory disturbance in feet, legs, or hands, and this also was uncommon in children. Both pancreatitis and peripheral neuropathy generally are reversible when the drug is stopped.

Zalcitabine (ddC)

ddC has been evaluated in adults and children in clinical trials and has been shown to be efficacious. ddC is a nucleoside that has in vitro effects against HIV that are 100 times higher than those of ZDV in both macrophages and T cells.[248] Studies in adults have shown that ddC can decrease p24 antigenemia in patients with AIDS and AIDS-related complex without suppression of the bone marrow. Side effects observed in phase I studies in adults revealed skin rashes and stomatitis with large doses of ddC. However, the most severe side effect observed was painful peripheral neuropathy that was dose-related.[243] In adults with low CD4 counts (≤300) who were intolerant or whose ZDV treatment had failed, it was found that there was no difference in disease progression or death between the groups.[3] The ACTG 175 and the Delta trial evaluated combinations of ZDV and ddI and of ZDV and ddC versus ddI or ZDV alone and found that either ddI alone or one of the combinations was superior to ZDV monotherapy in adults in terms of disease progression or death.[145] ddC was evaluated in children over an 8-week period in pilot phase I trials using doses from 0.015 to 0.04 mg/kg given every 6 hours. Fifteen children were studied, and no peripheral neuropathy was observed during the 8 weeks; however, skin rashes and mouth sores occurred at the larger doses. There was a transient increase in the CD4 count by week 8 in all patients and a decrease in p24 antigenemia in six of the nine children who had elevated p24 antigen at entry.[59] Additional trials showed that alternating schedules of ddI and ZDV also were well tolerated.[280] The results of the ACTG 138 trial of ddC given at two different doses (0.01 or 0.005 mg/kg) in pediatric patients whose ZDV therapy failed by evidence of intolerance or progression of disease showed that ddC was well tolerated, that peripheral neuropathy occurred infrequently (5 per cent) in children, and that no serious manifestations were associated with neuropathy. Both doses of ddC had equal effects on reducing virus load (p24AG) and increasing weight and growth measures in these children with advanced disease.[330] Another study of combined therapy with ZDV (ACTG 190) showed that the combination was well tolerated. The children on combined therapy had a slower loss of CD4 cells and lower quantitation of HIV in peripheral blood mononuclear cells at all times. Currently, ddC is a useful drug for the treatment of children with HIV-1 and seems to be well tolerated at an initial dose of 0.01 mg/kg.[122]

Stavudine (d4T)

Background

d4T is a thymidine nucleoside analogue with a structure similar to ZDV in which the 3′ hydroxyl group is replaced by a double bond between the 2′ and 3′ carbons of the pentose ring. d4T enters cells via nonfacilitated diffusion and is phosphorylated by cellular kinases to the active triphosphate form. The intracellular half-life of d4T triphosphate is approximately 3.5 hours. d4T inhibits reverse transcriptase via competitive inhibition with deoxythymidine triphosphate and by DNA chain termination.[16, 167, 183]

The 50 per cent inhibitory concentrations for HIV-1 are between 0.01 and 4.1 μm. d4T is active against ZDV-resistant HIV-1 strains. No cross-resistance has been noted for other drugs, such as ddI, ddC, and 3TC. Some in vitro studies showed antagonism between ZDV and d4T, whereas others showed synergy. ACTG 190 showed that adults receiving combined treatment with ZDV and d4T had greater losses of CD4 cells than did those in other arms of the trial. d4T readily is absorbed and has 80 per cent oral bioavailability. Peak serum concentrations are around 1.2 mg/L and are achieved within 1 hour of a 0.67-mg/kg dose with a plasma half-life of 1 to 1.6 hours. Limited data show that d4T crosses the cerebrospinal fluid.[104] d4T also has been shown to cross the placenta.[20] The dosage should be adjusted to 50 per cent in patients who have significant renal impairment (creatinine clearance <50/mL/minute). The current recommended dose in adults is 1 mg/kg/day or 40 mg orally twice a day for patients with an average body weight greater than 60 kg.

Clinical Trials

d4T has been significantly effective in reducing HIV virus load by p24 antigen assay and in reducing disease progression in adults. In one study of 822 subjects with prior ZDV exposure who were randomized to receive either d4T (40 mg twice daily) or ZDV (200 mg three times a day), the authors found a decreased risk of disease progression in the d4T-treated group.[136, 238, 275, 324] d4T also has been studied in pediatric patients in a randomized study of d4T versus ZDV (ACTG 240).[196] Because the results of the ACTG 152 trial showed that ZDV monotherapy was inferior, these children either are continuing on d4T alone or now are receiving combinations of d4T and ZDV or d4T and ddI and are continuing to be evaluated. d4T was well tolerated in these children and now is licensed for use in children. The arm involving ZDV and d4T has been stopped.

d4T also is being investigated in a phase I trial for use alone or in combination with 3TC for prevention of maternal-fetal HIV transmission. Other studies include combinations of d4T with nucleosides and protease inhibitors.[33] Other trials directly are comparing the use of d4T and ddI (alone or in combination with each other) for initial therapy.

Side Effects

The major side effect of d4T was dose-limiting peripheral neuropathy in phase I/II studies. An open study of adults with severe disease whose treatment had failed or who were intolerant to ZDV and received d4T reported a 24 per cent incidence of mild peripheral neuropathy. In further studies of patients who had higher CD4 counts, the incidence of peripheral neuropathy was less (8 per cent). The peripheral neuropathy usually is reversible within 2 weeks, and many patients resumed treatment at a lower dose. Other minor side effects include a mild increase in hepatic transaminases in some patients. Children in general have fewer side effects while receiving d4T than do adults and still are being monitored in several studies.

Overall, d4T seems to be a well-tolerated drug and has a definitive use as an alternative agent in patients who have been on prolonged ZDV treatment or who are intolerant of ZDV. The advantage of d4T over some other nucleosides may be its ability to pass to the central nervous system. Further studies will define better its role in combination with other antiviral agents.

Lamivudine (3TC, Epivir)

3TC (2′-deoxy-3′-thlacytidine) is a reverse transcriptase inhibitor nucleoside that has antiviral activity against HIV-1. It inhibits reverse transcriptase, and once incorporated into viral DNA, it acts as a chain terminator. 3TC has less pronounced inhibition of mammarian DNA polymerases. Multiple laboratory and clinical strains of HIV-1, including ZDV-resistant HIV, have been found to be inhibited by 3TC with an IC_{50} of 0.003 to 1.14 μm. 3TC is more active than ddI by a factor of 10 to 170 times. It has 80 per cent oral bioavailability and is cleared primarily by the kidney. 3TC is synergistic in vitro in combination with ZDV and ddI and is a potent inhibitor of HBV in vitro (IC_{50}, up to 0.1 μm) in HBV-transfected cells and in vivo in chimpanzees chronically infected with HBV.[47]

3TC has undergone pharmacokinetic evaluation in both adults and children and has been shown to produce a sharp decline in virus load (1 to 2 logs) within a week. However, there is rapid selection of resistant virus when 3TC is used as monotherapy due to resistance at the reverse transcriptase codon 184, which confers high-level resistance. When used in combination with ZDV, 3TC can increase the sensitivity to ZDV even if the HIV isolate previously was resistant to ZDV.[217]

Clinical Trials

Several studies in adults using combined therapy of 3TC and ZDV or 3TC and ddC showed significant clinical benefit compared with ZDV monotherapy. Patients were noted to have increases in CD4 counts and decreases in p24AG and, more recently, HIV RNA plasma levels. The combined treatment with ZDV and 3TC showed a significant and more sustained reduction in plasma HIV RNA of over 1.2 logs.[19, 112, 183, 358] Recently, the results of a large, multicenter, double-blind controlled study (CAESAR) with more than 1800 patients entered and randomized to receive 3TC or placebo in addition to either ZDV and ddI or ZDV and ddC showed a significant reduction of disease progression and death in the 3TC combination arms. This study continues to be analyzed. The dose of 3TC used in these studies is 150 mg given two times daily.

Studies in children also have shown that 3TC is well tolerated in children alone and in combination with other nucleosides. Virus load markers, including p24AG and HIV RNA, showed a log drop greater than or equal to 0.71.[217] A large multicenter trial, ACTG 300, currently is in progress to evaluate combined ZDV and 3TC and standard therapy (ddI or ddI and ZDV).

Pharmacokinetic, safety, and tolerance phase I studies of 3TC and ZDV use in HIV-infected pregnant women and their infants revealed that 3TC was well absorbed in pregnancy and crossed the placenta. The newborns also tolerated 3TC during the first 2 weeks of life. It is expected that further efficacy studies will examine ZDV and 3TC alone or in combination with protease inhibitors for prevention of maternal-fetal transmission.

Tolerance and Side Effects

3TC seems to be extremely well tolerated, with minor reports of nausea, headaches, and fatigue. The convenience of twice-a-day dosing also is an attractive feature. Overall, the combination of 3TC and ZDV is one of the most potent of the nucleosides against HIV-1. The addition of protease inhibitors to this combination enhances activity even further and currently is being evaluated in numerous clinical trials. 3TC also is being evaluated in a series of clinical trials for treatment and suppression of chronic HBV infection and shows promising results.

NON-NUCLEOSIDE REVERSE TRANSCRIPTASE INHIBITORS: NEVIRAPINE (NEV)

NEV is a benzodiazepine with specific inhibitory activity against HIV-1 reverse transcript. In vitro, the IC_{50} in human peripheral blood mononuclear cell cultures is 40 mm (0.011 mg/mL). NEV is active against ZDV-resistant viruses and synergistically inhibits HIV-1 replication when used in combination with ZDV. NEV inhibits HIV reverse transcriptase enzyme and does not inhibit human DNA polymerase. NEV and other non-nucleoside reverse transcriptase inhibitors are not active against HIV-2 or other animal lentiviruses.

Pharmacokinetic studies demonstrated high oral bioavailability and passage to the central nervous system in animal studies. Pharmacokinetic studies in adults and children have shown that NEV is well tolerated. Mean steady-state levels were achieved at doses of 200 mg/day in adults; in children, doses of 240 mg/kg/day divided into two individual doses resulted in target steady-state NEV trough concentrations in the range of 3 to 5 mg/mL. NEV has a rapid effect on reduction of virus load of at least a log. However, resistance can develop rapidly because of a single amino-acid change, resulting in a high-level resistance phenotype when used as monotherapy. Adult clinical studies have shown durable reductions in plasma viremia as measured by immune complex–dissociated p24 antigen or HIV RNA when doses of NEV were started at 200 mg and increased to 400 mg daily.[146, 147]

Combined therapy with NEV and other nucleoside drugs, such as ZDV and ddI, has resulted in prolonged antiviral activity in adults and children.[60, 83, 221] NEV is available in both tablet and liquid forms.

The major side effects of NEV may be a potential sedative effect or fatigue in some patients, headache, diarrhea, nausea, fever, and rash. Rash occurs in approximately 4 per cent of patients and can be severe in a small number of patients with Stevens-Johnson–like syndrome. The incidence of rashes was reduced significantly with the use of an induction period of 200 mg of NEV given daily for 2 weeks followed by 400 mg daily. In phase I trials in children, rash was rare and mild. NEV now is licensed for use in combination therapy for treatment of HIV infection in adults. NEV is an excellent potential candidate for interventions in perinatal transmission of HIV, and studies are under way showing that NEV can be given in single dose to a mother during labor with antiviral activity present in the infant for up to 3 days because of the prolonged half-life (ACTG 250). In the Pediatric ACTG, an efficacy trial using NEV at delivery to reduce intrapartum transmission of HIV is under way. This may be a particularly important, practical, and inexpensive way of approaching interruption of transmission in underdeveloped countries because this can be given as a single oral administration to the mother and to the infant.

PROTEASE INHIBITORS

As a class of drugs, the protease inhibitors are the most potent antiretroviral agents yet developed. This group of drugs, when used alone, can suppress viral replication by 100 times or more, and when used in combination with other drugs, such as reverse transcriptase inhibitors, ZDV or 3TC, or ddI, they can reduce viral burden by as much as 1000 times, or 3 logs. In comparison, other nucleoside drugs, such as ZDV and ddC, when used alone achieve reductions in viral load of approximately 10 times, or 1 log.[50]

HIV Protease

The basic mechanism of action of the protease inhibitors is inhibition of HIV protease, which is a product of the *pol* gene of HIV and is required for the processing of initial *gag-pol* or *gag* polypeptide. HIV protease cleaves the polypeptide into eight proteins, one of which is the protease itself. This cleavage allows the processing of polypeptide into mature functional and structural proteins that are required for assembly and pathogenicity of HIV-1.[199]

The protease is a homodymer of two 99-aminoacid chains, with each chain containing one conserved aspartic tripeptide. There are five relatively conserved regions within protease, including the substrate binding domain. The HIV proteases of 1 and 2 have about 50 per cent homology. Although the HIV protease originally was thought to be highly conserved, some data indicate a natural polymorphism in wild-type strains that might result in natural resistance.[296] The majority of protease inhibitors act by binding to their substrates with numerous hydrogen bonds. By acting at the postintegration step of the HIV life cycle, protease inhibitors can inhibit HIV replication in both acute and chronically infected lymphocytes and macrophages. This is different than the reverse transcriptase inhibitors, which can inhibit acute HIV infection of CD4 lymphocytes but not necessarily of macrophages. The protease inhibitors are highly active against HIV-1 at nanomolar concentrations and are synergistic with reverse transcriptase inhibitors in vitro. Protease inhibitors have variable activity against HIV-2 but generally no activity against other retroviruses.[10, 205, 305, 380, 381]

The currently clinically useful protease inhibitors include saquinavir, indinavir, ritonavir, nelflinavir, and several other protease inhibitors that are in phase I studies.

Saquinavir

Saquinavir was the first protease inhibitor to enter clinical development. In vitro activity against HIV-1 shows that a 90 per cent inhibitory concentration is achieved at 6 nm/L. Saquinavir was found to be well tolerated in clinical trials when patients were given up to 600 mg three times daily, including in combination with various reverse transcriptase inhibitors.[195] As with other protease inhibitors, resistance develops after about 16 weeks when saquinavir is used alone, and the advances are short-lived.[205, 305] The reduction in viral burden is moderate for saquinavir. Saquinavir has a lower bioavailability (4 per cent) than some of the other protease inhibitors but has synergistic activity in vivo with other reverse transcriptase inhibitors. Patient response was most prolonged when this drug was used in combination.[69]

Ritonavir

Ritonavir was developed by Abbott Laboratories and is highly active in vitro, with 90 per cent inhibitory concentration between 8 and 40 nm/L. It is protein-bound, but it has a good oral bioavailability.[191] Ritonavir produces a mean 2-log reduction in circulating HIV load, as measured by HIV RNA, 2 to 8 weeks after initiation of treatment.[85, 226] When used in combination with ZDV and 3TC, ritonavir showed a significant and prolonged reduction in HIV viral load from 2.5 to 1.8 logs, with an increase in CD4 counts and, in a significant number of patients, undetectable virus load by HIV RNA PCR (<400 HIV RNA copies per milliliter).[232] Studies in children are in progress to determine safety and pharmacokinetics. Ritonavir also will be studied in phase I trials in combination with ZDV and 3TC in HIV-infected pregnant women for safety and pharmacokinetics.

Safety, Tolerability, and Metabolism

The side effects of protease inhibitors most commonly are nausea, vomiting, and diarrhea. In addition, ritonavir, especially with the liquid formulation, has a bitter metallic taste. Ritonavir is metabolized by cytochrome p-450, 3A4, and 2D6. At therapeutic concentrations, ritonavir also is an inhibitor of p450, 3A4, and other cytochromes. This allows the possibility of interactions with other drugs that similarly are metabolized, which would either increase or decrease the plasma levels of both drugs. Important potential interactions can occur with rifampicin, rifabutin, phenytoin, ketoconazole, itraconazole (but not fluconazole), codeine, piroxicam, terfenadine, astemizole, cimetidine, and some benzodiazepines.

In clinical studies of ritonavir in combination, 1000 subjects who previously received ZDV were administered ritonavir, and after a median 6-month follow-up, 17 per cent discontinued therapy because of adverse reactions versus the 6 per cent who received placebo. The usual adverse events included nausea, vomiting, diarrhea, dysesthesias, and mild general weakness, which usually occurred during the first few weeks.

Indinavir

Indinavir is similar to ritonavir in terms of preferential activity against HIV-1 but is less protein-bound (60 per cent), and animal studies show that it may penetrate the central nervous system to some degree. Indinavir has a mean reduction of viral burden of around 2 logs, with a corresponding increase in CD4 cells. The initial response to triple therapy using ZDV, 3TC, and indinavir showed a significant reduction of viral load to undetectable levels in 86 per cent of the study subjects at the end of 24 weeks. In adults, the current dose is 800-mg tablets given three times daily on an empty stomach.[228] Adverse events of indinavir are slightly different than those of the other protease inhibitors and include dose-related mild indirect hyperbilirubinemia that does not always include an increase in serum transaminases. This hyperbilirubinemia may be similar to Gilbert syndrome. At higher doses of indinavir, there have been reports of nephrolithiasis that is believed to be crystallization of indinavir in the kidney tubules because of its lower solubility. The nephrolithiasis occurred in about 4 per cent of patients, who generally did not require permanent discontinuation of therapy. However, good hydration is important to help avoid this side effect. Indinavir seems to require fewer dose modifications or drug substitutions because of drug interactions, compared with the other two protease inhibitors.

Nelfinavir

Nelfinavir (Agouron Pharmaceuticals) is a protease inhibitor that has significant in vitro activity and similar antiviral activity in vivo, with a mean log reduction greater than or equal to 1.5 in viral load when used alone and synergistic activity when used in combination.[224, 255] The side effects of nelfinavir are similar to those observed with ritonavir and seem to be gastrointestinal (e.g., mild diarrhea and nausea). Nelfinavir has the advantage of having less of a metallic taste than the other protease inhibitors. It currently is undergoing phase I studies in children for tolerance and pharmacokinetics. It recently has been licensed for use in both children and adults in combination with other nucleosides.

Resistance to Protease Inhibitors

Because of the rapid turnover of plasma virions in HIV-1 infection, the protease inhibitors when used alone soon will select for drug-resistant strains, which rapidly may replace drug-sensitive strains; in some instances, drug-sensitive wild-type viral strains will be replaced almost totally by resistant variants in as little as 14 days.[70, 162, 175] The resistance is related more to the number of mutations than to a specific mutation. Several different protease inhibitors have shown different mutations for resistance.[70, 72, 237, 252]

Because HIV replicates at such a high rate, mutations can accumulate rapidly unless there is absolute suppression of all viral replication. When a patient is receiving monotherapy with a protease inhibitor, there seems to be loss of virologic and immunologic activity by the development of both genotypic and phenotypic resistance. The number of mutations observed with dosing with a single protease inhibitor include up to 15 point mutations both in vitro and in vivo.[72, 252] Not all mutations affect in vitro sensitivity. In vitro mutations include areas immediately adjacent to the substrate binding region, and particular mutations at codon 82 appear to be important in causing reduced sensitivity to both indinavir and ritonavir. Other mutations in association with this also seem to be necessary for high-level resistance. Other point mutations at codons 48 and 90 have been seen for saquinavir, which may develop resistance a little more slowly than may ritonavir or indinavir.

The current known patterns of genotypic resistance are not identical for all protease inhibitors, which allows the possibility that two or more non–cross-resistant protease inhibitors could be used effectively in combination for greater or more sustained antiviral effect.

Summary

Overall, there is considerable optimism regarding the use of protease inhibitors in combination with other antiviral agents, resulting in profound and sustained reductions in HIV replication as measured by HIV RNA in plasma. Long-term studies are under way to see whether the in vitro and in vivo results will maintain clinical benefit. The new antiviral agents represent a rapidly growing and exciting area of research whose study will result in the development of new options for therapeutic choices for patients with HIV infection.

SOLUBLE RECOMBINANT CD4

Recombinant CD4 is a unique molecule developed to interact with HIV by preventing the attachment of the virus to cells by inhibition of the GP120 receptor site. Although studies of recombinant CD4 in the laboratory revealed inhibition of HIV, studies in patients have shown, disappointingly, no antiviral effects. Recombinant CD4 seems to be safe and tolerated well in both children and adults. Variations of this molecule may be evaluated further for inhibition of other clinical isolates of HIV.

INTERFERON

Background

Interferon is a natural product with antimicrobial activity and is secreted by vertebrate cells in response to virus infection or stimulation by various nonviral materials. Interferon first was discovered by Isaacs and Lindenmann[171] as a soluble extracellular mediator of virus interference. In addition, many nonantimicrobial actions have been ascribed to it, including inhibition of induction of growth and metastasis of tumors; inhibition of embryogenesis, organ growth, and regeneration; and immunoregulatory activity and enhancement of pathogenesis of certain infections in vitro and in vivo.[176]

Interferon is produced by infection with a variety of viruses or by exposure to double-stranded RNA of natural or synthetic origin. "Immune interferon" is produced by lymphocytes in response to mitogens (phytohemagglutination) or specific antigens to which the lymphocytes are sensitized (e.g., HSV, *Candida*). Interferon comprises a family of glycoproteins that all have antiviral effects but differ physiochemically and antigenically according to the cell of origin and inducers. Cultured human fibroblast diploid cells produce a single interferon species that is distinct from a second species produced by leukocytes in response to viral or double-stranded RNA inducers. These species are distinct from immune interferon produced by lymphocytes in response to mitogens or antigens.[110, 343] The interferon response is an important part of the host's early antiviral defense and therefore is being evaluated in prophylaxis and therapy for a variety of viral diseases. Recombinant interferon-α has been cloned, and large amounts of this substance are available. Numerous clinical trials have been instituted, with several showing clinical efficacy. Immune interferon, or interferon-γ, also has been cloned and should be in clinical trials in the near future. Further detailed information on interferon is the subject of several review articles.[17, 18, 118]

Mechanisms of Action and In Vitro Antiviral Activity

The action of the interferon proteins from a given species is greater in cells of biologically or genetically related species.[216] Interferons are active against a wide range of viruses, which include both DNA and RNA viruses and other microbial pathogens. Interferons do not inactivate viruses directly but instead act on host cells that subsequently become resistant to virus infection. Interferon does not block adsorption or uncoating of viruses. Because interferon is active against both RNA and DNA viruses, a unified mechanism of action would require that interferon act on a process common to both types of viruses. Much evidence indicates that the synthesis of viral proteins is inhibited in interferon-treated cells. Interferon treatment also has been reported to result in inhibition of synthesis and transcription of viral messenger RNA and, in some cases, viral release. Because antagonists of RNA and protein synthesis lack the development of the antiviral state, it has been inferred that interferons are regulatory proteins that induce the synthesis of a second cellular protein, "the antiviral protein," that actually interferes with viral replication.[127, 178, 295] Because interferon-α and interferon-γ have been purified to relative homogeneity, future studies of the mechanism of action or actions of interferon will be performed more easily.[342]

Although most viruses are inhibited by interferon, the in vitro sensitivities vary. For example, myxoviruses are sensitive to interferon, but adenoviruses are relatively resistant. This is important in consideration of therapy. Interferon has been reported to inhibit oncogenic transformation by retroviruses (sarcoma virus, leukemia viruses, and papovaviruses).[128]

Pharmacology

The pharmacokinetics of human leukocyte interferon have been studied in animals and people and have been reviewed by Ho and Armstrong[163] and Merigan and associates.[242]

Clearance of interferon from the circulation is rapid, and kinetics were comparable in several animal species. Similar findings were observed for both leukocyte and fibroblast interferon administered to rabbits.[48] Jordan and associates[180] found that interferon has a half-life in the circulation of 2 to 4 hours after a 24-hour intravenous infusion in humans. Peak levels were obtained 5 to 8 hours after intramuscular injection and 8 to 10 hours after subcutaneous injection.[109] Peak serum levels of 100 units can be obtained. Penetration to the respiratory tract, cerebrospinal fluid, brain, and eye has been poor in animals.[49] Human studies reveal similarly poor penetration to the cerebrospinal fluid, with levels being up to 30 times lower than serum concentrations. This may be a problem in achieving therapeutic levels of interferon for treatment of central nervous system infections without causing systemic toxicity.

Experimental studies in animals revealed that interferon could be administered intracisternally, with a half-life of approximately 60 minutes and a persistence of activity of up to 24 hours.[164] Intrathecal administration has been accomplished in a few isolated instances without known toxicity in humans.[89, 242] Even though interferon seems to be cleared rapidly from the circulation, presumably the antiviral state induced in the tissue lasts longer.[164] Further work is needed to establish the relationships of systemic interferon concentrations, antiviral effects, and clinical outcome. This information greatly would enhance a rational approach to future therapy.

Clinical Studies

The characteristics of interferon, including its occurrence as a natural cell product with broad-spectrum antiviral activity, make it an attractive substance for possible therapeutic use. Its use can be approached in either of two ways. Interferon could be induced to be produced endogenously by host cells, or it could be administered exogenously in a purified form. The effectiveness and the applicability of these methods in clinical situations depend on several factors. First, the virus must be sensitive to the dose of the interferon employed. Second, the ability of the infected host to produce significant amounts of endogenous interferon either by inducers or by specific viral infection is an important variable in the effectiveness of any interferon therapy. Third, interferon must either penetrate or be induced in the infected target organ.

Interferon Inducers

The inducers of interferon include natural and synthetic nucleic acids, microbial products, and low-molecular-weight substances. These inducers have given some excellent results in both prophylactic and therapeutic studies in animals.[138, 139] Unfortunately, results have not been similar in human clinical trials. When given parenterally to humans, the inducers have been toxic and pyrogenic or, as in the case of tilorone hydrochloride, poor inducers of interferon.[90, 138] Some of the systemic toxicity can be avoided by topical administration to superficial infections of the eyes, skin, and respiratory system.[186] In trials, poly I:poly C, a synthetic, double-stranded RNA homopolymer of inosine and cytosine, given intranasally, was reported to reduce respiratory symptoms in rhinovirus type 13 challenge in volunteers.[156]

A less toxic interferon inducer, a substituted propane-diamine, showed some success in alleviating symptoms of infection with rhinovirus type 21 when administered prophylactically. Further study of experimental rhinovirus infections in volunteers with use of a suspension formulation of propanediamine resulted in more marked effects on the frequency and severity of illness and virus shedding.[271] Studies of the effect of poly I:poly C on influenza A/Hong Kong/68 (H3N2) infection in volunteers revealed that symptoms were decreased, compared with those in subjects receiving placebo. However, the duration of viral shedding, antibody responses, and interferon titers in nasal secretions was not affected.[156] A major problem with this approach to therapy is the phenomenon of hypoactivity on repeated exposure to the inducer. In other words, the subject may produce interferon upon first administration of an artificial inducer but, upon repeated administration, does not produce any further interferon for a certain period.[347]

Exogenous Interferon

In contrast with the equivocal results with interferon inducers, prospects for successful use of exogenously administered interferon are better. The major limiting factor in the clinical use of interferon is the potential side effects, which also have been reported with pure recombinant interferon. Interferon has been approved for use in the treatment of chronic granulomatous disease and can be used for treatment of human papillomavirus infection. Initial studies were limited because of the lack of supply of natural interferon; however, the availability of recombinant interferon has opened up the opportunity for a broadened range of clinical trials. The majority of clinical trials have used human leukocyte interferon, interferon-γ, or recombinant interferon-α, although a few trials are using human fibroblast interferon.

In clinical trials, exogenously administered interferon has demonstrated some efficacy against infections due to influenza, papillomavirus, rhinoviruses, rubella, HBV, CMV, HSV, VZV, and vaccinia viruses.[130, 163] Results of selected trials with either prophylactic or therapeutic interferon are summarized in Table 233–11. Topical therapy has been shown to be efficacious in controlled trials of rhinovirus respiratory tract infections and herpesvirus eye infections. Intranasal large-dose leukocyte interferon (14 million units) given in 39 doses before and for 4 days after rhinovirus challenge resulted in reduced severity of illness and viral shedding in a treatment group, compared with placebo recipients.[230] Two double-blind, placebo-controlled studies of prophylactic administration of large-dose (5 million units) intranasal interferon-α_2 against naturally acquired respiratory tract infections showed clinical efficacy in reducing rhinovirus infections. These studies used a family setting in which subjects were administered interferon or placebo intranasally for 7 days when respiratory symptoms developed in another person in the family over a 6-month period. Rhinovirus colds were prevented, with an efficacy of 78 and 79 per cent, respectively, in both studies; however, only 39 and 41 per cent, respectively, of all colds were prevented.[99] This short-term course of interferon generally was well tolerated, with a 10 per cent risk of minor nasal bleeding.[148] This contrasts with the more pronounced local intolerance observed in previous trials using more prolonged administration (28 days).[98, 151]

Daily topical interferon administration for 10 days accelerated healing of herpetic dendritic ulcers and reduced early recurrences.[179] Further trials for substantiating these findings are in progress.

Controlled trials of early treatment of localized herpes zoster in immunosuppressed patients with intramuscular large-dose interferon (5×10^3 units/kg/24 hours) revealed a decreased progression of lesions in the primary dermatome and a reduced incidence of dissemination and postherpetic neuralgia.[240] Similarly, a controlled study of interferon treatment of primary varicella in 18 children with cancer revealed a decrease in complications.[9] Prophylactic studies have indi-

TABLE 233–11. Summary of Selected Clinical Trials of Human Leukocyte Interferon

Therapy	Virus; Type of Study or Illness	Prophylactic	Therapeutic	Results	Reference
Local	Rhinovirus; challenged volunteers	+	+	Decreased symptoms and viral shedding	242
Local	Rhinovirus; natural infections (recombinant interferon-α)	+		Decreased incidence of rhinovirus infections	148
Local	Herpes simplex keratitis (dendritic ulcer)		+	Accelerated healing, reduced recurrences	179
Local injection	Condyloma acuminatum		+	Decreased size of warts	170, 262, 307
Systemic	Condyloma acuminatum		+		
Systemic	Laryngeal warts		+	Regression of warts	31
Systemic	Frequently recurrent genital herpes simplex virus infection	+		Modest suppression of clinical outbreaks over 3-month treatment	201
Systemic	Herpes zoster in adult cancer patients		+	Decreased progression in primary dermatome, decreased dissemination and postherpetic neuralgia	240
Systemic	Varicella in children		+	Decreased visceral dissemination	9
Systemic	Herpes simplex virus reactivation; in normal patients after trigeminal nerve decompression	+		Decreased clinical illness	276
Systemic	Cytomegalovirus infection in renal transplant patients	+		Decreased viremia and length of viral shedding	61
Systemic	Hepatitis B virus infection with chronic active hepatitis		+	Decreased Dane particle–DNA polymerase and hepatitis B core antigenemia	137

cated efficacy in the prevention of reactivation of HSV infections after surgical trigeminal nerve decompression in normal patients. Double-blind, placebo-controlled clinical trials of recombinant interferon-α treatment of genital HSV infections showed a modest suppression of frequently recurrent genital HSV over a 3-month treatment period in interferon recipients compared with placebo recipients.[201] However, there were no beneficial clinical effects when interferon in small (3 million units) and large (50 million units) doses was given intramuscularly during prodromal symptoms of recurrent genital HSV infection.[289] Reduction of CMV viremia and viruria in renal transplant patients has been reported.[61, 276] A follow-up study using a longer course of interferon prophylaxis (14 weeks) (3×10^6 units three times weekly) in renal transplant recipients revealed a reduction in clinical signs of CMV infection, 7 of 22 placebo versus 1 of 20 interferon recipients ($p < .03$), and a reduction in superinfections and CMV-associated glomerulopathy. Interferon was well tolerated in this group, with minimal toxicity. Interferon therapy also has been shown to have clinical benefit in patients with laryngeal papillomas, with regression of lesions, growth control of lesions, or both.[31, 141] Further clinical trials of treatment of genital warts with various dosages, routes of administration, and forms of interferon are ongoing. Several studies also show clinical regression of condylomata acuminata when interferon was given topically and by intramuscular injections.[170, 307]

Greenberg and associates[137] reported that subcutaneous or intramuscular administration of small-dose human leukocyte interferon reduced Dane particle–associated DNA polymerase activity and hepatitis B core antigenemia in patients with chronic HBV infection. Patients in this study did not experience significant toxicity, but there was a mild suppressive effect on the hematologic system, with transient depression in white blood cell and platelet counts that were dose-related and reversible. Whether the effect of interferon in chronic HBV infection is a direct antiviral one, an immune-mediated one, or a combination of both remains to be elucidated. Whether interferon treatment alone or in combination with other antiviral agents can ameliorate or eliminate the disease process in the liver still is under study.

Further potential uses of interferon include treatment of severe viral infections, such as St. Louis encephalitis, Lassa fever, subacute sclerosing panencephalitis, and rabies. Postexposure treatment of rabies in animals by interferon or interferon inducers can prevent fatal disease.[11, 115]

Interferon seems to be most effective when it is used prophylactically, when it is used early in the disease process, or when prolonged viral replication occurs. Clinical successes suggest that interferon still may have important potential in the control of viral disease. The clinical use of interferon products, however, is limited.

Side Effects

The side effects of human leukocyte interferon seem to be related to both the dose and the purity of the preparation used.[344] Fever has been observed frequently in patients given 4×10^4 units/kg/24 hours.[180] In doses of 1.7×10^5 units/kg/24 hours administered intramuscularly, some patients have nausea, vomiting, myalgia, chills, lassitude, and malaise. These effects seem to occur less frequently with more purified preparations.[242] Hematologic effects have been observed, including depression of leukocytes, platelets, and reticulocytes in patients receiving doses of 0.8×10^4 to 5×10^3 units after 3 to 5 days of treatment. These effects readily are reversible and have not proved to be serious. Infants treated with interferon had decreased weight gain and transient liver enzyme elevations, which were reversible. With the experience in the use of the cloned interferons, it now is more clear that interferon itself may be responsible for some of the observed side effects. Therefore, clinical use of interferon is limited by a delicate balance between therapeutic efficacy and tolerable side effects.

References

1. Update: Universal precautions for prevention of transmission of human immunodeficiency virus, hepatitis B virus, and other bloodborne pathogens in health-care settings. M. M. W. R. *37*(24):377–382, 387–388, 1988.
2. Update: Provisional public health service recommendations for chemoprophylaxis after occupational exposure to HIV. M. M. W. R. *45*(22):468–472, 1996.
3. Abrams, D. I., Goldman, A. I., Launer, C., et al.: A comparative trial of didanosine or zalcitabine after treatment with zidovudine in patients with human immunodeficiency virus infection: The Terry Beirn Community Programs for Clinical Research on AIDS [see comments]. N. Engl. J. Med. *330*(10):657–662, 1994.
4. Adams, H. G., Benson, E. A., Alexander, E. R., et al.: Genital herpetic infection in men and women: Clinical course and effect of topical application of adenine arabinoside. J. Infect. Dis. *133*(Suppl.):A151–A159, 1976.
5. Alford, C. A., Jr., and Whitley, R. J.: Treatment of infections due to herpesvirus in humans: A critical review of the state of the art. J. Infect. Dis. *133*(Suppl.):A101–A108, 1976.
6. Alkhatib, G., Combadiere, C., Broder, C. C., et al.: CC CKR5: A RANTES, MIP-1alpha, MIP-1beta receptor as a fusion cofactor for macrophage-tropic HIV-1. Science *272*(5270):1955–1958, 1996.
7. Andersson, J., Britton, S., Ernberg, I., et al.: Effect of acyclovir on infectious mononucleosis: A double-blind, placebo-controlled study. J. Infect. Dis. *153*(2):283–290, 1986.
8. Anonymous: Failure of high dose 5-iodo-2′-deoxyuridine in the therapy of herpes simplex virus encephalitis: Evidence of unacceptable toxicity. N. Engl. J. Med. *292*:599–603, 1975.
9. Arvin, A. M., Feldman, S., and Merigan, T. C.: Human leukocyte interferon in the treatment of varicella in children with cancer: A preliminary controlled trial. Antimicrob. Agents Chemother. *13*(4):605–607, 1978.
10. Ashorn, P., McQuade, T. J., Thairsrivongs, S., et al.: An inhibitor of the protease blocks maturation of human and simian immunodeficiency viruses and spread of infection. Proc. Natl. Acad. Sci. U. S. A. *87*:7472–7476, 1990.
11. Baer, G. M., Shaddock, J. H., Moore, S. A., et al.: Successful prophylaxis against rabies in mice and rhesus monkeys: The interferon system and vaccine. J. Infect. Dis. *136*(2):286–291, 1977.
12. Balfour, H. H., Jr.: Intravenous acyclovir therapy for varicella in immunocompromised children. J. Pediatr. *104*:134–136, 1984.
13. Balfour, H. H., Jr., Bean, B., Laskin, O. L., et al.: Acyclovir halts progression of herpes zoster in immunocompromised patients. N. Engl. J. Med. *308*:1448–1453, 1983.
14. Balfour, H. H., Kelly, J. M., Suarez, C. S., et al.: Acyclovir treatment of varicella in otherwise healthy children. J. Pediatr. *116*:663–669, 1990.
15. Balis, F. M., Pizzo, P. A., Eddy, J., et al.: Pharmacokinetics of zidovudine administered intravenously and orally in children with human immunodeficiency virus infection. J. Pediatr. *114*(5):880–884, 1989.
16. Balzarini, J., Herdewijn, P., and De Clercq, E.: Differential patterns of intracellular metabolism of 2′,3′-didehydro-2′,3′-dideoxythymidine and 3′-azido-2′,3′-dideoxythymidine, two potent anti-human immunodeficiency virus compounds. J. Biol. Chem. *264*(11):6127–6133, 1989.
17. Baron, S., Brunell, P. A., and Grossberg, S. E.: Mechanisms of action and pharmacology: The immune and interferon systems. *In* Galasso, G. J., et al. (eds.): Antiviral Agents and Viral Diseases on Man. New York: Raven Press, 1979, pp. 151–208.
18. Baron, S., and Dianzani, F.: General considerations of the interferon system. Tex. Rep. Biol. Med. *35*:1–10, 1977.
19. Bartlett, J. A., Benoit, S. L., Johnson, V. A., et al.: Lamivudine plus zidovudine compared with zalcitabine plus zidovudine in patients with HIV infection: A randomized, double-blind, placebo-controlled trial. North American HIV Working Party. Ann. Intern. Med. *125*(3):161–172, 1996.
20. Bawdon, R. E., Kaul, S., and Sobhi, S.: The ex vivo transfer of the anti-HIV nucleoside compound d4T in the human placenta. Gynecol. Obstet. Invest. *38*(1):1–4, 1994.
21. Bean, B.: Antiviral therapy: Current concepts and practices. Clin. Microbiol. Rev. *5*(2):146–182, 1992.
22. Bean, B., Aeppli, D., and Balfour, H. H., Jr.: Acyclovir in shingles. J. Antimicrob. Chemother. *12*(Suppl. B):123–127, 1983.
23. Beauchamp, L. M., Orr, G. F., de Miranda, P., et al.: Amino acid ester prodrugs of acyclovir. Antiviral Chem. Chemother. *3*(3):157–164, 1992.
24. Beutner, K. R.: Valacyclovir: A review of its antiviral activity, pharmacokinetic properties, and clinical efficacy. Antiviral Res. *28*(4):281–290, 1995.
25. Beutner, K. R., Friedman, D. J., Forszpaniak, C., et al.: Valaciclovir compared with acyclovir for improved therapy for herpes zoster in immunocompetent adults. Antimicrob. Agents Chemother. *39*(7):1546–1553, 1995.
26. Biron, K. K., and Elion, G. B.: Sensitivity of varicella-zoster virus in vitro to acyclovir. 19th Interscience Conference on Antimicrobial Agents and Chemotherapy, Boston, 1979.
27. Biron, K. K., Stanat, S. C., Sorrell, J. B., et al.: Metabolic activation of the nucleoside analog 9-[(2-hydroxy-1-(hydroxymethyl)ethoxy]methyl)guanine] in human diploid fibroblasts infected with human cytomegalovirus. Proc. Natl. Acad. Sci. U. S. A. *82*(8):2473–2477, 1985.
28. Bleidner, W. E., Harmon, J. B., Hewes, W. E., et al.: Absorption, distribution and excretion of amantadine hydrochloride. J. Pharmacol. Exp. Ther. *150*:484–490, 1965.
29. Blum, M. R., Liao, S. H., and de Miranda P.: Overview of acyclovir pharmacokinetic disposition in adults and children. Am. J. Med. *73*(1A):186–192, 1982.
30. Blum, M. R., Liao, S. H., Good, S. S., et al.: Pharmacokinetics and bioavailability of zidovudine in humans. Am. J. Med. *85*(2A):189–194, 1988.
31. Bomholt, A.: Interferon therapy for laryngeal papillomatosis in adults. Arch. Otolaryngol. *109*(8):550–552, 1983.
32. Boyer, P. J., Dillon, M., Navaie, M., et al.: Factors predictive of maternal-fetal transmission of HIV-1: Preliminary analysis of zidovudine given during pregnancy and/or delivery. J. A. M. A. *271*(24):1925–1930, 1994.
33. Brankovan, V., Tarantini, K., Datema, R., et al.: Strong synergistic anti-HIV activity of a purine and a pyrimidine nucleoside analog, ddI and d4T. V International Conferencea on AIDS, Montreal, 1989.
34. Brink, J. J., and LePage, G. A.: Metabolic effects of 9-D-arabinosylpurines in ascites tumor cells. Cancer Res. *24*:312–318, 1964.
35. Browne, M. J.: Mechanism and specificity of action of ribavirin. Antimicrob. Agents Chemother. *15*(6):747–753, 1979.
36. Bryson, Y. J.: Current status and prospects for oral acyclovir treatment of first episode and recurrent genital herpes simplex virus. J. Antimicrob. Chemother. *12*(Suppl. B):61–65, 1983.
37. Bryson, Y. J., and Connor, J. D.: In vitro susceptibility of varicella zoster virus to adenine arabinoside and hypoxanthine arabinoside. Antimicrob. Agents Chemother. *9*(3):540–543, 1976.
38. Bryson, Y. J., Connor, J. D., and Hebblewaite, D.: Pharmacology and efficacy of Ara-A in neonates and adults. 19th Interscience Conference on Antimicrobial Agents and Chemotherapy, Boston, 1979.
39. Bryson, Y. J., Connor, J. D., Sweetman, L., et al.: Determination of plaque inhibitor activity of adenine arabinoside (9-β-D-arabinofuranosyladenine) for herpes viruses using an adenosine deaminase inhibitor. Antimicrob. Agents Chemother. *6*:98–101, 1974.
40. Bryson, Y. J., Dillon, M., Lovett, M., et al.: Treatment of first episodes of genital herpes simplex virus infection with oral acyclovir: A randomized double-blind controlled trial in normal subjects. N. Engl. J. Med. *308*(16):916–921, 1983.
41. Bryson, Y. J., and Hebblewaite, D.: The in vitro sensitivity of clinical isolate of varicella-zoster to virostatic and virocidal concentrations of acyclovir. International Conference on Human Herpesviruses, Atlanta, 1980.
42. Bryson, Y. J., and Kronenberg, L. H.: Combined antiviral effects of interferon, adenine, arabinoside, hypoxanthine arabinoside, and adenine arabinoside-5′-monophosphate in human fibroblast cultures. Antimicrob. Agents Chemother. *11*(2):299–306, 1977.
43. Bryson, Y. J., Monahan, C., Pollack, M., et al.: A prospective double-blind study of side effects associated with the administration of amantadine for influenza A virus prophylaxis. J. Infect. Dis. *141*(5):543–547, 1980.
44. Bryson, Y. J., Sweetman, L., and Connor, J. D.: Simple sensitive microbioassay for adenine arabinoside and hypoxanthine arabinoside in human plasma. Antimicrob. Agents Chemother. *14*(6):909–915, 1978.
45. Burns, J. P.: A double-blind study of IDU in human herpes simplex keratitis. Arch. Ophthalmol. *70*:381, 1963.
46. Butler, K. M., Husson, R. N., Balis, F. M., et al.: Dideoxyinosine in children with symptomatic human immunodeficiency virus infection. N. Engl. J. Med. *324*:137–144, 1991.
47. Cameron, G. M., Collis, P., Daniel, M., et al.: Lamivudine. Drugs Future *18*:319–323, 1993.
48. Cantell, K., and Pyhala, L.: Pharmacokinetics of human leukocyte interferon. J. Infect. Dis. *133*(Suppl.):A6–A12, 1976.
49. Cantell, K., Pyhala, L., and Strander, H.: Circulating human interferon after intramuscular injection into animals and man. J. Gen. Virol. *25*(3):453–455, 1974.
50. Carr, A., and Cooper, D. A.: HIV protease inhibitors. AIDS *10*(Suppl. A):S151–S157, 1996.
51. Cassidy, L. F., and Patterson, J. L.: Mechanism of La Crosse virus inhibition by ribavirin. Antimicrob. Agents Chemother. *33*(11):2009–2011, 1989.
52. Centers for Disease Control and Prevention: Recommendations of the U.S. Public Health Service Task Force on the use of zidovudine to reduce perinatal transmission of human immunodeficiency virus. M. M. W. R. *43*(RR-11):1–20, 1994.
53. Ch'ien, L. T., Cannon, N. J., Whitley, R. J., et al.: Effect of adenine arabinoside on cytomegalovirus infections. J. Infect. Dis. *130*(1):32–39, 1974.
54. Ch'ien, L. T., Glazko, A. J., Buchanan, R. A., et al.: Human metablolic disposition of 9-β-D-arabinofuranosyladenine (Ara-A). Interscience Conference on Antimicrobial Agents and Chemotherapy, 1971, p. 47.
55. Ch'ien, L. T., Schabel, F. M., Jr., and Alford, C. A., Jr.: Arabinosyl nucleosides and nucleotides. *In* Carter, W. A. (ed.): Selective Inhibitors of Viral Functions. Cleveland, CRC Press, 1973, pp. 227–258.
56. Ch'ien, L. T., Whitley, R. J., Alford, C. A., Jr., et al.: Adenine arabinoside

for therapy of herpes zoster in immunosuppressed patients: Preliminary results of a collaborative study. J. Infect. Dis. *133*(Suppl.):A184–A191, 1976.

57. Ch'ien, L. T., Whitley, R. J., Charamella, L. J., et al.: Clinical and virologic studies with systemic administration of adenine arabinoside in severe progressive, mucocutaneous herpes simplex virus infections. *In* Pavan-Langston, D., Buchanan, R. A., and Alford, C. A., Jr. (eds.): Adenine Arabinoside: An Antiviral Agent. New York, Raven Press, 1975, pp. 205–224.
58. Ch'ien, L. T., Whitley, R. J., Nahmias, A. J., et al.: Antiviral chemotherapy and neonatal herpes simplex virus infecition: A pilot study—Experience with adenine arabinoside (ARA-A). Pediatrics *55*(5):678–685, 1975.
59. Chadwick, E. G., Nazareno, L. A., Nieuwenhuis, T. J., et al.: Phase I evaluation of zalcitabine administered to human immunodeficiency virus-infected children. J. Infect. Dis. *172*(6):1475–1479, 1995.
60. Cheeseman, S. H., Havlir, D., McLaughlin, M. M., et al.: Phase I/II evaluation of nevirapine alone and in combination with zidovudine for infection with human immunodeficiency virus. J. Acquir. Immune Defic. Syndr. Hum. Retrovirol. *8*(2):141–151, 1995.
61. Cheeseman, S. H., Rubin, R. H., Stewart, J. A., et al.: Controlled clinical trial of prophylactic human-leukocyte interferon in renal transplantation: Effects on cytomegalovirus and herpes simplex virus infections. N. Engl. J. Med. *300*(24):1345–1349, 1979.
62. Cirelli, R., Herne, K., McCrary, M., et al.: Famciclovir: Review of clinical efficacy and safety. Antiviral Res. *29*:141–151, 1996.
63. Clarkson, D. R., Oppelt, W. W., and Byvoet, P.: The fate of 5-iodo-2'-deoxyuridine (IUdR) in plasma and cerebrospinal fluid of dogs. J. Pharmacol. Exp. Ther. *157*(3):581–588, 1967.
64. Cochran, W., Maassab, H. F., Tsunoda, A., et al.: Studies on the antiviral activity of amantadine hydrochloride. Ann. N. Y. Acad. Sci. *130*:432–439, 1965.
65. Coker-Vann, M., and Dolin, R.: Effect of adenine arabinoside on Epstein-Barr virus in vitro. J. Infect. Dis. *135*(3):447–453, 1977.
66. Colby, B. M., Shaw, J. E., Elion, G. B., et al.: Effect of acyclovir [9-(2-hydroxyethoxymethyl)guanine] on Epstein-Barr virus DNA replication. J. Virol. *34*(2):560–568, 1980.
67. Colby, B. M., Shaw, J. E., Furman, P. A., et al.: Effect of acycloguanosine on Epstein-Barr virus DNA replication. Herpesvirus Workshop, Cambridge, England, 1978.
68. Colby, B. M., Shaw, J. E., and Pagano, J. S.: Effects of acycloguanosine on Epstein-Barr virus-infected lymphoblastoid cells. Interscience Conference on Antimicrobial Agents and Chemotherapy, Atlanta, 1978.
69. Collier, A. C., Coombs, R. W., Schoenfeld, D. A., et al.: Treatment of human immunodeficiency virus infection with saquinavir, zidovudine, and zalcitabine: AIDS Clinical Trials Group. N. Engl. J. Med. *334*(16):1011–1107, 1996.
70. Collin, G., Dussaix, E., Krivine, A., et al.: Sensitivity to zidovudine and saquinavir in phase I/II dose ranging saquinavir trial. 4th International Workshop on HIV Drug Resistance, Sardinia, 1995.
71. Collum, L. M., Benedict-Smith, A., and Hillary, I. B.: Randomised double-blind trial of acyclovir and idoxuridine in dendritic corneal ulceration. Br. J. Ophthalmol. *64*(10):766–769, 1980.
72. Condra, H. J., Schleif, W. A., Blahy, O. M., et al.: In vivo emergence of HIV-2 variants resistant to multiple protease inhibitors. Nature *374*:569–571, 1995.
73. Connor, E. M., Sperling, R. S., Gelber, R., et al.: Reduction of maternal-infant transmission of human immunodeficiency virus type 1 with zidovudine treatment: Pediatric AIDS Clinical Trials Group Protocol 076 Study Group [see comments]. N. Engl. J. Med. *331*(18):1173–1180, 1994.
74. Connor, J. D., Sweetman, L., Carey, S., et al.: Susceptibility in vitro of several large DNA viruses to the antiviral activity of adenine arabinoside and its metabolite, hypoxanthine arabinoside: Relation to human pharmacology. *In* Pavan-Langston, D., Buchanan, R. A., and Alford, C. A., Jr. (eds.): Adenine Arabinoside: An Antiviral Agent. New York: Raven Press, 1975, pp. 177–196.
75. Corey, L., Fife, K. H., Benedetti, J. K., et al.: Intravenous acyclovir for the treatment of primary genital herpes. Ann. Intern. Med. *98*(6):914–921, 1983.
76. Corey, L., Nahmias, A. J., Guinan, M. E., et al.: A trial of topical acyclovir in genital herpes simplex virus infections. N. Engl. J. Med. *306*(22):1313–1319, 1982.
77. Coster, D. J., McKinnon, J. R., McGill, J. I., et al.: Clinical evaluation of adenine arabinoside and trifluorothymidine in the treatment of corneal ulcers caused by herpes simplex virus. J. Infect. Dis. *133*(Suppl.):A173–A177, 1976.
78. Couch, R. B., and Jackson, G. G.: Antiviral agents in influenza: Summary of Influenza Workshop VIII. J. Infect. Dis. *134*(5):516–527, 1976.
79. Courtney, R. J., Steiner, S. M., and Benyesh-Melnick, M.: Effects of 2-deoxy-D-glucose on herpes simplex virus replication. Virology *52*(2):447–455, 1973.
80. Crumpacker, C. S.: Ganciclovir. N. Engl. J. Med. *335*(10):721–729, 1996.
81. Crumpacker, C. S., Schnipper, L. E., Marlowe, S. I., et al.: Resistance to antiviral drugs of herpes simplex virus isolated from a patient treated with acyclovir. N. Engl. J. Med. *306*(6):343–346, 1982.
82. Crumpacker, C. S., Schnipper, L. E., Zaia, J. A., et al.: Growth inhibition by acycloguanosine of herpesviruses isolated from human infections. Antimicrob. Agents Chemother. *15*(5):642–645, 1979.
83. D'Aquila, R. T., Hughes, M. D., Johnson, V. A., et al.: Nevirapine, zidovudine, and didanosine compared with zidovudine and didanosine in patients with HIV-1 infection: A randomized, double-blind, placebo-controlled trial. National Institute of Allergy and Infectious Diseases AIDS Clinical Trials Group Protocol 241 Investigators. Ann. Intern. Med. *124*(12):1019–1030, 1996.
84. Dabis, F., Msellati, P., Newell, M., et al.: Methodology of intervention trials to reduce mother to child transmission of HIV with special reference to developing countries. AIDS *9*(Suppl. A):S67–S74, 1995.
85. Danner, S. A., Carr, A., Leonard, J. M., et al.: Safety, pharmacokinetics and preliminary efficacy of ritonavir, an inhibitor of HIV-1 protease. N. Engl. J. Med. *333*:1534–1539, 1995.
86. David-West, T. S.: Antiviral chemotherapy. Afr. J. Med. Sci. *1*(1):85–107, 1970.
87. Davies, W. L., Grunert, R. R., Haff, R. E., et al.: Antiviral activity of 1-adamantanamine (amantadine). Science *144*:862–863, 1964.
88. Davies, W. L., Grunert, R. R., and Hoffmann, C. E.: Influenza virus growth and antibody response in amantadine-treated mice. J. Immunol. *95*(6):1090–1094, 1966.
89. De Clercq, E., Edy, V. G., De Vlieger, H., et al.: Intrathecal administration of interferon in neonatal herpes. J. Pediatr. *86*(5):736–739, 1975.
90. De Clercq, E., and Merigan, T. C.: Bis-DEAE-fluorenone: Mechanism of antiviral protection and stimulation of interferon production in the mouse. J. Infect. Dis. *123*(2):190–199, 1971.
91. de Jong, M. D., Boucher, C. A., Galasso, G. J., et al.: Consensus symposium on combined antiviral therapy: International Society for Antiviral Research and the National Institutes of Allergy and Infectious Diseases. Antiviral Res. *29*(1):5–29, 1996.
92. Dickover, R. E., Garratty, E. M., Herman, S. A., et al.: Identification of levels of maternal HIV-1 RNA associated with risk of perinatal transmission: Effect of maternal zidovudine treatment on viral load. J. A. M. A. *275*(8):599–605, 1996.
93. Dietrich, D. T., Kotler, D. P., Busch, D. F., et al.: Ganciclovir treatment of cytomegalovirus clitis in AIDS: A randomized, double-blind, placebo-controlled multicenter study. J. Infect. Dis. *167*:278–282, 1992.
94. Dolin, R., Betts, R. R., Treanor, J. J., et al.: Rimantadine prophylaxis of influenza in the elderly. 23rd Interscience Conference on Antimicrobial Agents and Chemotherapy, 1983, Abstract No. 691.
95. Dolin, R., Reichman, R. C., Madore, H. P., et al.: A controlled trial of amantadine and rimantadine in the prophylaxis of influenza A infection. N. Engl. J. Med. *307*(10):580–584, 1982.
96. Dolin, R., Reichman, R. C., Mazur, M. H., et al.: NIH conference: Herpes zoster-varicella infections in immunosuppressed patients. Ann. Intern. Med. *89*(3):375–388, 1978.
97. Douglas, R. G., Critchlow, C., Benedetti, J., et al.: Double-blind placebo-controlled trial of prophylactic oral acyclovir for frequent recurrences of genital herpes. International Society for STD Research, Seattle, 1983.
98. Douglas, R. M., Albrecht, J. K., Miles, H. B., et al.: Intranasal interferon-alpha 2 prophylaxis of natural respiratory virus infection. J. Infect. Dis. *151*(4):731–736, 1985.
99. Douglas, R. M., Moore, B. W., Miles, H. B., et al.: Prophylactic efficacy of intranasal alpha 2-interferon against rhinovirus infections in the family setting. N. Engl. J. Med. *314*(2):65–70, 1986.
100. Dowling, J. N., Postic, B., and Guevarra, L. O.: Effect of ribavirin on murine cytomegalovirus infection. Antimicrob. Agents Chemother. *10*(5): 809–813, 1976.
101. Drach, J. C., and Shipman, C., Jr.: The selective inhibition of viral DNA synthesis by chemotherapeutic agents: An indicator of clinical usefulness? Ann. N. Y. Acad. Sci. *284*:396–409, 1977.
102. Drew, W. L., Ives, D., Lalezari, J. P., et al.: Oral ganciclovir as maintenance treatment for cytomegalovirus retinitis in patients with AIDS: Syntex Cooperative Oral Ganciclovir Study Group [see comments]. N. Engl. J. Med. *333*(10):615–620, 1995.
103. Drew, W. L., Miner, R. C., Busch, D. F., et al.: Prevalence of resistance in patients receiving ganciclovir for serious cytomegalovirus infection. J. Infect. Dis. *163*(4):716–719, 1991.
104. Dudley, M. N., Graham, K. K., Kaul, S., et al.: Pharmacokinetics of stavudine in patients with AIDS or AIDS-related complex. J. Infect. Dis. *166*(3):480–485, 1992.
105. Dummer, J. S., Bound, L. M., Singh, G., et al.: Epstein-Barr virus-induced lymphoma in a cardiac transplant recipient. Am. J. Med. *77*(1):179–184, 1984.
106. Eidinoff, M. L., Cheong, L., and Rich, M. A.: Incorporation of unnatural phyrimidine bases into deoxyribonucleic acid of mammalian cells. Science *129*:1550–1551, 1959.
107. Elion, G. B., Furman, P. A., Fyfe, J. A., et al.: Selectivity of action of an antiherpetic agent, 9-(2-hydroxyethoxymethyl) guanine. Proc. Natl. Acad. Sci. U. S. A. *74*(12):5716–5720, 1977.
108. Elwell, L. P., Ferone, R., Freeman, G. A., et al.: Antibacterial activity and mechanism of action of 3'-azido-3'-deoxythymidine (BW A509U). Antimicrob. Agents Chemother. *31*(2):274–280, 1987.
109. Emodi, G., Rufli, T., Just, M., et al.: Human interferon therapy for herpes zoster in adults. Scand J. Infect. Dis. *7*(1):1–5, 1975.

110. Epstein, L. B.: Mitogen and antigen induction of interferon in vitro and in vivo. *In* Baron, S., and Dianzani, F. (eds.): The Interferon System: A Current Review to 1978. Galveston, TX, University of Texas Medical Branch, 1977, pp. 42–56. (Texas Reports on Biology and Medicine, vol. 35.)
111. Erikson, B. E., Helgstrand, N. G., Johansson, A., et al.: Inhibition of influenza virus ribonucleic acid polymerase by ribavirin triphosphate. Antimicrob. Agents Chemother. *11*:946–951, 1977.
112. Eron, J. J., Benoit, S. L., Jemsek, J., et al.: Treatment with lamivudine, zidovudine, or both in HIV-positive patients with 200 to 500 CD4+ cells per cubic millimeter: North American HIV Working Party [see comments]. N. Engl. J. Med. *333*(25):1662–1669, 1995.
113. Fast, P., Newell, M., Mofenson, L., et al.: Strategies for prevention of perinatal transmission of HIV infection: Report of a Consensus Workshop (II), Siena, Italy, June 3–6, 1993. J. Acquir. Immune Defic. Syndr. Hum. Retrovirol. *8*:161–175, 1995.
114. Felsenstein, D., D'Amico, D. J., Hirsch, M. S., et al.: Treatment of cytomegalovirus retinitis with 9-[2-hydroxy-1-(hydroxymethyl)ethoxymethyl]guanine. Ann. Intern. Med. *103*(3):377–380, 1985.
115. Fenje, P., and Postic, B.: Protection of rabbits against experimental rabies of poly I-poly C. Nature *226*(241):171–172, 1970.
116. Fenton, R. J., and Potter, C. W.: Dose-response activity of ribavirin against influenza virus infection in ferrets. J. Antimicrob. Chemother. *3*(3):263–271, 1977.
117. Field, H., McMillan, A., and Darby, G.: The sensitivity of acyclovir-resistant mutants of herpes simplex virus to other antiviral drugs. J. Infect. Dis. *143*(2):281–285, 1981.
118. Finter, N. B.: Interferons and Interferon Inducers. New York, American Elsevier, 1973.
119. Fischl, M. A., Richman, D. D., Causey, D. M., et al.: Prolonged zidovudine therapy in patients with AIDS and advanced AIDS-related complex. AZT Collaborative Working Group. J. A. M. A. *262*(17):2405–2410, 1989.
120. Fischl, M. A., Richman, D. D., Grieco, M. H., et al.: The efficacy of azidothymidine (AZT) in the treatment of patients with AIDS and AIDS-related complex: A double-blind, placebo-controlled trial. N. Engl. J. Med. *317*(4):185–191, 1987.
121. Fischl, M. A., Richman, D. D., Hansen, N., et al.: The safety and efficacy of zidovudine (AZT) in the treatment of subjects with mildly symptomatic human immunodeficiency virus type 1 (HIV) infection: A double-blind, placebo-controlled trial. The AIDS Clinical Trials Group [see comments]. Ann. Intern. Med. *112*(10):727–737, 1990.
122. Fischl, M. A., Stanley, K., Collier, A. C., et al.: Combination and monotherapy with zidovudine and zalcitabine in patients with advanced HIV disease: The NIAID AIDS Clinical Trials Group. Ann. Intern. Med. *122*(1):24–32, 1995.
123. Fiscus, S. A., Adimora, A. A., Schoenbach, V. J., et al.: Perinatal HIV infection and the effect of zidovudine therapy on transmission in rural and urban counties [see comments]. J. A. M. A. *275*(19):1483–1488, 1996.
124. Fishaut, J. M., Connor, J. D., and Lampert, P. W.: Comparative effects of arabinosyl nucleosides upon the postnatal growth and development of the rat. Pediatr. Res. *8*(10):825–829, 1974.
125. Foley, F. D., Greenawald, K. A., Nash, G., et al.: Herpesvirus infection in burned patients. N. Engl. J. Med. *282*(12):652–656, 1970.
126. Frenkel, L. M., Wagner, L. E., Demeter, L. M., et al.: Effects of zidovudine use during pregnancy on resistance and vertical transmission of human immunodeficiency virus type 1. Clin. Infect. Dis. *20*(5):1321–1326, 1995.
127. Friedman, R. M., Metz, D. H., Esteban, R. M., et al.: Mechanism of interferon action: Inhibition of viral messenger ribonucleic acid translation in L-cell extracts. J. Virol. *10*(6):1184–1198, 1972.
128. Friedman, R. M., and Ramseur, J. M.: Inhibition of murine leukemia virus production in chronically infected AKR cells: A novel effect of interferon. Proc. Natl. Acad. Sci. U. S. A. *71*(9):3542–3544, 1974.
129. Fujiwara, Y., and Heidelberger, C.: Fluorinated pyrimidines. 38. The incorporation of 5-trifluoromethyl-2'-deoxyuridine into the deoxyribonucleic acid of vaccinia virus. Mol. Pharmacol. *6*(3):281–291, 1970.
130. Galasso, G. J., and Dunnick, J. K.: Interferon, an antiviral drug for use in man. *In* Baron, S., and Dianzani, F. (eds.): The Interferon System: A Current Review to 1978. Galveston, TX, University of Texas Medical Branch, 1977, pp. 478–482.
131. Galbraith, A. W., Oxford, J. S., Schild, G. C., et al.: Study of 1-adamantanamine hydrochloride used prophylactically during the Hong Kong influenza epidemic in the family environment. Bull. W. H. O. *41*(3):677–682, 1969.
132. Garnier, J. L., Berger, F., Betuel, H., et al.: Epstein-Barr virus associated lymphoproliferative diseases (B cell lymphoma) after transplantation. Nephrol. Dial. Transplant. *4*(9):818–823, 1989.
133. Gluckman, E., Lotsberg, J., Devergie, A., et al.: Oral acyclovir prophylactic treatment of herpes simplex infection after bone marrow transplantation. J. Antimicrob. Chemother. *12*(Suppl. B):161–167, 1983.
134. Goodman, E. L., Luby, J. P., and Johnson, M. T.: Prospective double-blind evaluation of topical adenine arabinoside in male herpes progenitalis. Antimicrob. Agents Chemother. *8*(6):693–697, 1975.
135. Goodrich, J. M., Mori, M., Gleaves, C. A., et al.: Early treatment with ganciclovir to prevent cytomegalovirus disease after allogeneic bone marrow transplantation. N. Engl. J. Med. *325*:1601–1607, 1991.
136. Gottlieb, M., Peterson, D., Adler, M., et al.: Comparison of safety and efficacy of two doses of stavudine (Zerit, d4T) in a large simple trial in the US Parallel Track Program. 35th Interscience Conference on Antimicrobial Agents and Chemotherapy, San Francisco, 1995.
137. Greenberg, H. B., Pollard, R. B., Lutwick, L. I., et al.: Effect of human leukocyte interferon on hepatitis B virus infection in patients with chronic active hepatitis. N. Engl. J. Med. *295*(10):517–522, 1976.
138. Grossberg, S. E.: The interferons and their inducers: Molecular and therapeutic considerations. 3. N. Engl. J. Med. *287*(3):122–128, 1972.
139. Grossberg, S. E.: Nonviral interferon inducers: Natural and synthetic products. *In* Baron, S., and Dianzani, F. (eds.): The Interferon System: A Current Review to 1978. Galveston, TX, University of Texas Medical Branch, 1977, pp. 111–116. (Texas Reports on Biology and Medicine, vol. 35.)
140. Grunert, R. R., McGahen, J. W., and Davies, W. L.: The in vivo antiviral activity of 1-adamantanamine (amantadine). 1. Prophylactic and therapeutic activity against influenza viruses. Virology *26*:262–269, 1965.
141. Haglund, S., Lundquist, P. G., Cantell, K., et al.: Interferon therapy in juvenile laryngeal papillomatosis. Arch. Otolaryngol. *107*(6):327–332, 1981.
142. Hall, C. B., Dolin, R., Gala, C., et al.: Rimantadine treatment of influenza A in children. Pediatr. Res. *18*:1084, 1984.
143. Hall, C. B., McBride, J. T., Gala, C. L., et al.: Ribavirin treatment of respiratory syncytial viral infection in infants with underlying cardiopulmonary disease. J. A. M. A. *254*:3047–3051, 1985.
144. Hall, C. B., Walsh, E. E., Hruska, J. F., et al.: Ribavirin treatment of experimental respiratory syncytial viral infection: A controlled double-blind study in young adults. J. A. M. A. *249*(19):2666–2670, 1983.
145. Hammer, S. M., Katzenstein, D. A., Hughes, M. D., et al.: A trial comparing nucleoside monotherapy with combination therapy in HIV-infected adults with cD4 cell counts from 200 to 500 per cubic millimeter. N. Engl. J. Med. *335*(15):1081–1090, 1996.
146. Havlir, D., Cheeseman, S. H., McLaughlin, M., et al.: High-dose nevirapine: Safety, pharmacokinetics, and antiviral effect in patients with human immunodeficiency virus infection. J. Infect. Dis. *171*(3):537–545, 1995.
147. Havlir, D., McLaughlin, M. M., and Richman, D. D.: A pilot study to evaluate the development of resistance to nevirapine in asymptomatic human immunodeficiency virus-infected patients with CD4 cell counts of >500/mm3: AIDS Clinical Trials Group Protocol 208. J. Infect. Dis. *172*(5):1379–1383, 1995.
148. Hayden, F. G., Albrecht, J. K., Kaiser, D. L., et al.: Prevention of natural colds by contact prophylaxis with intranasal alpha 2-interferon. N. Engl. J. Med. *314*(2):71–75, 1986.
149. Hayden, F. G., and Douglas, R. G., Jr.: Antiviral Agents. *In* Mandell, G. L., Douglas, R. G., Jr., and Bennett, J. E. (eds.): Principles and Practices of Infectious Diseases. New York, John Wiley & Sons, 1979, pp. 353–369.
150. Hayden, F. G., Douglas, R. G., Jr., and Simons, R.: Enhancement of activity against influenza viruses by combinations of antiviral agents. Antimicrob. Agents Chemother. *18*(4):536–541, 1980.
151. Hayden, F. G., and Gwaltney, J. M., Jr.: Intranasal interferon alpha 2 for prevention of rhinovirus infection and illness. J. Infect. Dis. *148*(3):543–550, 1983.
152. Hayden, F. G., Hall, W. J., Douglas, R. G., Jr., et al.: Amantadine aerosols in normal volunteers: Pharmacology and safety testing. Antimicrob. Agents Chemother. *16*(5):644–650, 1979.
153. National Institutes of Health: Consensus Development Conference Summary: Amantadine: Does it have a role in the prevention and treatment of influenza? Consensus Development Conference, Washington, D.C., 1979.
154. Henderson, D. K., and Gerberding, J. L.: Prophylactic zidovudine after occupational exposure to the human immunodeficiency virus: An interim analysis. J. Infect. Dis. *160*(2):321–327, 1989.
155. Herrmann, E. C.: Plaque inhibition test for detection of specific inhibitors of DNA-containing viruses. Proc. Soc. Exp. Biol. Med. *107*:142–145, 1961.
156. Hill, D. A., Baron, S., Perkins, J. C., et al.: Evaluation of an interferon inducer in viral respiratory disease. J. A. M. A. *219*(9):1179–1184, 1972.
157. Hintz, M., Connor, J. D., Spector, S. A., et al.: Neonatal acyclovir pharmacokinetics in patients with herpes virus infections. Am. J. Med. *73*(1A):210–214, 1982.
158. Hirsch, M. S.: AIDS commentary: Azidothymidine. J. Infect. Dis. *157*(3):427–431, 1988.
159. Hirsch, V. M., Dapolito, G., Johnson, P. R., et al.: Induction of AIDS by simian immunodeficiency virus from an African green monkey: Species-specific variation in pathogenicity correlates with the extent of in vivo replication. J. Virol. *69*(2):955–967, 1995.
160. Hirsch, V. M., Fuerst, T. R., Sutter, G., et al.: Patterns of viral replication correlate with outcome in simian immunodeficiency virus (SIV)-infected macaques: Effect of prior immunization with a trivalent SIV vaccine in modified vaccinia virus Ankara. J. Virol. *70*(6):3741–3752, 1996.
161. Hirschman, S. Z.: Approaches to antiviral chemotherapy. Am. J. Med. *51*(6):699–703, 1971.
162. Ho, D. D., Neumann, A. U., Perelson, A. S., et al.: Rapid turnover of plasma virions and CD4 lymphocytes in HIV-1 infection [see comments]. Nature *373*(6510):123–126, 1995.
163. Ho, J., and Armstrong, J. A.: Interferon. Ann. Rev. Microbiol. *29*:131–161, 1975.

164. Ho, M.: Pharmaco-kinetics of interferon. *In* Finter, N. B. (ed.): Interferons and Interferon Inducers. New York, American Elsevier, 1973, pp. 241–249.
165. Hoffman, C. E., Neumayer, E. M., Haff, R. F., et al.: Mode of action of the antiviral activity of amantadine in tissue culture. J. Bacteriol. *90*:623–628, 1965.
166. Horadam, V. W., Sharp, J. G., Smilack, J. D., et al.: Pharmacokinetics of amantadine hydrochloride in subjects with normal and impaired renal function. Ann. Intern. Med. *94*(4 Part 1):454–458, 1981.
167. Huang, P., Farquhar, D., and Plunkett, W.: Selective action of 2′,3′-didehydro-2′,3′-dideoxythymidine triphosphate on human immunodeficiency virus reverse transcriptase and human DNA polymerases. J. Biol. Chem. *267*(4):2817–2822, 1992.
168. Huff, J. C., Bean, B., Balfour, H. H., Jr., et al.: Therapy of herpes zoster with oral acyclovir. Am. J. Med. *85*(2A):84–89, 1988.
169. Huggins, J. W.: Prospects for treatment of viral hemorrhagic fevers with ribavirin, a broad-spectrum antiviral drug. Rev. Infect. Dis. *11*(Suppl. 4):S750–S761, 1989.
170. Ikic, D., Bosnic, N., Smerdel, S., et al.: Double-blind clinical study with human leukocyte interferon in the therapy of condyloma acuminata. Proceedings of the Symposium on the Clinical Use of Interferon, Zagreb, 1975, p. 223.
171. Isaacs, A., and Lindenmann, J.: Virus interference. I. The interferon. Proc. R. Soc. Lond. (Biol.) *147*:258–273, 1957.
172. Jackson, G. G., Muldoon, R. L., and Akers, L. W.: Serologic evidence for prevention of influenzal infection in volunteers by an anti-influenzal drug, amantadine hydrochloride. Antimicrob. Agents Chemother. *3*:703–707, 1963.
173. Jackson, G. G., and Stanley, E. D.: Prevention and control of influenza by chemoprophylaxis and chemotherapy: Prospects from examination of recent experience. J. A. M. A. *235*:2739–2742, 1976.
174. Jackson, G. G., Stanley, E. D., and Muldoon, R. L.: Chemoprophylaxis of viral respiratory diseases. Pan-American Health Organization Scientific Publication *147*:595–603, 1967.
175. Jacobsen, H., Haenggi, M., Ott, M., et al.: Reduced sensitivity to saquinavir: An update on genotyping from phase I/II trials. Antiviral Res. *29*(1):95–97, 1996.
176. Johnson, H. M., and Baron, S.: The nature of the suppressive effect of interferon and interferon inducers on the in vitro immune response. Cell Immunol. *25*(1):106–115, 1976.
177. Johnson, M. T., Buchanan, R. A., Luby, J. P., et al.: Treatment of varicella-zoster virus infections with adenine arabinoside. J. Infect. Dis. *131*(3):225–229, 1975.
178. Joklik, W. K., and Becker, Y.: The replication and coating of vaccinia DNA. J. Mol. Biol. *10*:452–474, 1964.
179. Jones, B. R., Coster, D. J., Falcon, M. G., et al.: Topical therapy of ulcerative herpetic keratitis with human interferon. Lancet *2*(7977):128, 1976.
180. Jordan, G. W., Fried, R. P., and Merigan, T. C.: Administration of human leukocyte interferon in herpes zoster. I. Safety, circulating, antiviral activity, and host responses to infection. J. Infect. Dis. *130*(1):56–62, 1974.
181. Juel-Jensen, B. E., and MacCallum, R. W.: Herpes simplex lesions of face treated with idosuridine applied by spray gun: Results of a double-blind controlled trial. B. M. J. *1*:901–903, 1965.
182. Kaplan, A. S., and Ben-Porat, T.: Mode of antiviral action of 5-iodouracil deoxyriboside. J. Mol. Biol. *19*(2):320–332, 1966.
183. Katlama, C., Ingrand, D., Loveday, C., et al.: Safety and efficacy of lamivudine-zidovudine combination therapy in antiretroviral-naive patients: A randomized controlled comparison with zidovudine monotherapy. Lamivudine European HIV Working Group. J. A. M. A. *276*(2):118–125, 1996.
184. Kato, N., and Eggers, H. J.: Inhibition of uncoating of fowl plague virus by l-adamantanamine hydrochloride. Virology *37*(4):632–641, 1969.
185. Kaufman, H. E.: Clinical cure of herpes simplex keratitits by 5-iodo-2′-deoxyuridine. Proc. Soc. Exp. Biol. Med. *109*:251–252, 1962.
186. Kaufman, H. E., Ellison, E. D., and Waltman, S. R.: Double-stranded RNA, an interferon inducer in herpes simplex keratitis. Am. J. Ophthalmol. *68*:486–491, 1977.
187. Kaufman, H. E., and Heidelberger, C.: Therapeutric antiviral action of 5-trifluormethyl-2′-deoxyuridine in herpes simplex keratitis. Science *145*:585–586, 1964.
188. Kaufman, H. E., and Maloney, E. D.: IDU and cytosine arabinoside in experimental herpetic keratitis. Arch. Opthalmol. *69*:126–129, 1963.
189. Keating, M. R.: Antiviral agents. Mayo Clin. Proc. *67*(2):160–178, 1992.
190. Keeny, R. E.: Human tolerance of adenine arabinoside. *In* Pavan-Langston, D., Buchanan, R. A., and Alford, C. A., Jr. (eds.): Adenine Arabinoside: An Antiviral Agent. New York, Raven Press, 1975, pp. 265–274.
191. Kempf, D. J., Marsh, K. C., Denissen, J. F., et al.: ABT-538 is a potent inhibitor of human immunodeficiency virus protease and has high oral bioavailability in humans. Proc. Natl. Acad. Sci. U. S. A. *92*(7):2484–2488, 1995.
192. Kern, E. R., Richards, J. T., Overall, J. C., Jr., et al.: Alteration of mortality and pathogenesis of three experimental herpesvirus hominis infections of mice with adenine arabinoside 5′-monophosphate, adenine arabinoside, and phosphonoacetic acid. Antimicrob. Agents Chemother. *13*(1):53–60, 1978.
193. Khare, G. P., Sidwell, R. W., Witkowski, J. T., et al.: Suppression by 1-beta-D-ribofuranosyl-1,2,4-triazole-3-carboxamide (virazole, ICN 1229) of influenza virus-induced infections in mice. Antimicrob. Agents Chemother. *3*(4):517–522, 1973.
194. Kinkel, A. W., and Buchanan, R. A.: Human pharmacology. *In* Pavan-Langston, D., Buchanan, R. A., and Alford, C. A., Jr. (eds.): Adenine Arabinoside: An Antiviral Agent. New York, Raven Press, 1975, pp. 197–204.
195. Kitchen, V. S., Skinner, C., Ariyoshi, K., et al.: Safety and activity of saquinavir in HIV infection. Lancet *345*:952–955, 1995.
196. Kline, M. W., Fletcher, C. V., Federici, M. E., et al.: Combination therapy with stavudine and didanosine in children with advanced human immunodeficiency virus infection: Pharmacokinetic properties, safety, and immunologic and virologic effects. Pediatrics *97*(6 Part 1):886–890, 1996.
197. Knight, V., McClung, H. W., Wilson, S. Z., et al.: Ribavirin small particle aerosol treatment of influenza. Lancet *2*:945–249, 1981.
198. Kochhar, D. M., Penner, J. D., and Knudsen, T. B.: Embryotoxic, teratogenic, and metabolic effects of ribavirin in mice. Toxicol. Appl. Pharmacol. *52*(1):99–112, 1980.
199. Kramer, R. A., Schaber, M. D., Skalka, A. M., et al.: HTLV-III gag protein is processed in yeast cells by the virus pol protease. Science *231*:1580–1584, 1986.
200. Krenitsky, T. A., Hall, W. W., de Miranda, P., et al.: 6-Deoxyacyclovir: A xanthine oxidase-activated prodrug of acyclovir. Proc. Natl. Acad. Sci. U. S. A. *81*(10):3209–3213, 1984.
201. Kuhls, T. L., Sacher, J., Wiesmeiner, E., et al.: Double-blind study of suppression of recurrent genital HSV infections by recombinant alpha 2 interferon. Interscience Conference of Antimicrobial Agents and Chemotherpy, 1985.
202. La Lau, C., Oosterhuis, J. A., Versteeg, J., et al.: Multicenter trial of acyclovir and trifluorothymidine in herpetic keratitis. Am. J. Med. *73*(1A):305–306, 1982.
203. Laibson, P. R., and Leopold, I. H.: An evaluation of double-blind IDU therapy in 100 cases of herpetic keratitis. Trans. Am. Acad. Ophthalmol. Otolaryngol. *68*:22, 1964.
204. Lalezari, J., Holland, G., Stagg, R., et al.: A randomized, controlled study of cidofovir (CDV) for relapsing cytomegalovirus retinitis (CMV-R) in patients with AIDS. 35th Interscience Conference on Antimicrobial Agents and Chemotherapy, San Francisco, September 17–20, 1995.
205. Lambert, D. M., Petteway, S. R., Jr., McDanal, C. E., et al.: Human immunodeficiency virus type 1 protease inhibitors irreversibly block infectivity of purified virions from chronically infected cells. Antimicrob. Agents Chemother. *36*:982–988, 1992.
206. LaMontagne, J. R., and Galasso, G. J.: Report of a workshop on clinical studies on the efficacy of amantadine and rimantadine against influenza virus. J. Infect. Dis. *138*:928–931, 1978.
207. Larder, B. A., Darby, G., and Richman, D. D.: HIV with reduced sensitivity to zidovudine (AZT) isolated during prolonged therapy. Science *243*(4899):1731–1734, 1989.
208. Larder, B. A., and Kemp, S. D.: Multiple mutations in HIV-1 reverse transcriptase confer high-level resistance to zidovudine (AZT). Science *246*(4934):1155–1158, 1989.
209. Larder, B. A., Kemp, S. D., and Harrigan, P. R.: Potential mechanism for sustained antiretroviral efficacy of ACT-3TC combination therapy. Science *269*:696–699, 1995.
210. Larson, E. W., Stephen, E. L., and Walker, J. S.: Therapeutic effects of small-particle aerosols of ribavirin on parainfluenza (sendai) virus infections of mice. Antimicrob. Agents Chemother. *10*(4):770–772, 1976.
211. Larson, T., Dillon, M., Goldman, L., et al.: Double-blind, placebo-controlled study of acyclovir prophylaxis in frequently recurrent genital herpes simplex virus infections. Interscience Conference on Antimicrobial Agents and Chemotherapy, 1983.
212. Laskin, O. L., Longstreth, J. A., Whelton, A., et al.: Effect of renal failure on the pharmacokinetics of acyclovir. Am. J. Med. *73*(1A):197–201, 1982.
213. Lauter, C. B., Bailey, E. J., and Lerner, A. M.: Absence of idoxuridine and persistence of herpes simplex virus in brains of patients being treated for encephalitis. Proc. Soc. Exp. Biol. Med. *150*:23, 1975.
214. Lee, W. W., Benitez, A., Goodman, L., et al.: Potential anticancer agents. XL. Synthesis of the β-anomer of 9-(D-arabinofuranosyl) adenine. J. Am. Chem. Soc. *82*:2648–2649, 1960.
215. Lerner, A. M., and Bailey, E. J.: Concentrations of idoxuridine in serum, urine, and cerebrospinal fluid of patients with suspected diagnoses of herpesvirus hominis encephalitis. J. Clin. Invest. *51*(1):45–49, 1972.
216. Levy-Koenig, R. E., Golgher, R. R., and Paucker, K.: Immunology of interferons. II. Heterospecific activities of human interferons and their neutralization by antibody. J. Immunol. *104*(4):791–797, 1970.
217. Lewis, L. L., Venzon, D., Church, J., et al.: Lamivudine in children with human immunodeficiency virus infection: A phase I/II study. The National Cancer Institute Pediatric Branch-Human Immunodeficiency Virus Working Group. J. Infect. Dis. *174*(1):16–25, 1996.
218. Little, J. W., Hall, H. J., Douglas, R. G., Jr., et al.: Amantiadine effect on peripheral airways abnormalities in influenza. Ann. Intern. Med. *85*:177, 1976.
219. Long, W. F., and Olusanya, J.: Adamantanamine and early events following influenza virus infection. Arch. Gesamte Virusforsch. *36*(1):18–22, 1972.

220. Lowry, S. P., Melnick, J. L., and Rawls, W. E.: Investigation of plaque formation in chick embryo cells as a biological marker for distinguishing herpes virus type 2 from type 1. J. Gen. Virol. *10*(1):1–9, 1971.
221. Luzuriaga, K., Bryson, Y., McSherry, G., et al.: Pharmacokinetics, safety, and activity of nevirapine in human immunodeficiency virus type 1-infected children. Infect. Dis. *174*:713–721, 1996.
222. Maassab, H. F., and Cochran, K. W.: Rubella virus: Inhibition in vitro by amantadine hydrochloride. Science *145*:1443–1444, 1964.
223. MacCallum, F. O., and Juel-Jensen, B. E.: Herpes simplex virus skin infection in man treated with idoxuridine in dimethyl sulphoxide: Results of double-blind controlled trial. B. M. J. *2*(517):805–807, 1966.
224. Mackowitz, M., Conant, M., Hurley, A., et al.: Phase I/II dose range finding study of the HIV protease inhibitor AG1343. 35th Interscience Conference on Antimicrobial Agents and Chemotherapy, San Francisco, 1995.
225. Marker, S. C., Groth, K. W., Howard, R. J., et al.: Neurological deterioration and lack of therapeutic efficacy in cytomeglovirus-infected renal transplant patients treated with adenine arabinoside. 18th Interscience Conference on Antimicrobial Agents and Chemotherapy, Atlanta, 1978. Abstract No. 519.
226. Markowitz, M., Saag, M., Powderly, W. G., et al.: A preliminary study of ritonavir, an inhibitor of HIV-1 protease, to treat HIV-1 infection. N. Engl. J. Med. *333*(23):1534–1539, 1995.
227. Maslo, C., Peraldi, M. N., Desenclos, T. C., et al.: Evidence for the role of cytomegalovirus in thrombotic microangiopathy in HIV-infected patients. Second National Conference on Human Retroviral and Related Infections, Washington, D.C., 1995.
228. Massari, F., Staszewski, S., Berry, P., et al.: A double-blind, randomized trial of indinavir (MK-639) alone or with zidovudine vs. zidovudine alone in zidovudine naive patients. 35th Interscience Conference on Antimicrobial Agents and Chemotherapy, San Francisco, 1995.
229. Mastan, P. F., and Henderson, J. W.: Penetration of idoxuridine into the anterior segment after transdermal subconjunctival injection. Invest. Ophthalmol. *5*:320–321, 1966.
230. Mate, J., Simon, M., Juvancz, I., et al.: Prophylactic use of amantadine during Hong Kong influenza epidemic. Acta Microbiol. Acad. Sci. Hung. *17*(3):285–296, 1970.
231. Matheson, P. B., Abrams, E. J., Thomas, P. A., et al.: Efficacy of antenatal zidovudine in reducing perinatal transmission of human immunodeficiency virus type 1: The New York City Perinatal HIV Transmission Collaborative Study Group. J. Infect. Dis. *172*(2):353–358, 1995.
232. Mathez, D., De Truchis, P., Gorin, I., et al.: Ritonavir, AZT and ddC as a triple combination in AIDS patients. 3rd Conference on Retroviruses and Opportunistic Infections, Washington, D.C., 1996.
233. McClung, H. W., Knight, V., Gilbert, B. E., et al.: Ribavirin aerosol treatment of influenza B virus infection. J. A. M. A. *249*(19):2671–2674, 1983.
234. McCormick, J. B., King, I. J., Webb, P. A., et al.: Lassa fever: Effective therapy with ribavirin. N. Engl. J. Med. *314*:20–26, 1986.
235. McIntosh, K., Kurachek, S. C., Cairns, L. M., et al.: Treatment of respiratory viral infection in an immunodeficient infant with ribavirin aerosol. Am. J. Dis. Child. *138*(3):305–308, 1984.
236. McLaren, C., and Potter, C. W.: In-vitro inhibition of influenza virus A-Mill Hill 1-72 by amantadine. Lancet *1*(813):1157, 1973.
237. Mellors, J., McMahon, D. K., Chodakewitz, J. A., et al.: Correlation between genotypic evidence of HIV-1 resistance to the protease inhibitor MK-639 and loss of antiretroviral effect in treated patients. Fourth International Workshop on HIV Drug Resistance, Sardinia, Italy, 1995.
238. Mellors, J., Stool, E., Group, B.-S., et al.: Safety and tolerability of Zerit (stavudine, d4T) versus Retrovir (zidovudine, ZDV) in HIV-infected adults with < 500 CD4 cells/mm^3 after at least 6 months of ZDV treatment. 35th Interscience Conference on Antimicrobial Agents on Chemotherapy, San Francisco, 1995.
239. Mellors, J. W., Rinaldo, C. R., Jr., Gupta, P., et al.: Prognosis in HIV-1 infection predicted by the quantity of virus in plasma [see comments]. Science *272*(5265):1167–1170, 1996.
240. Merigan, T. C., Rand, K. H., Pollard, R. B., et al.: Human leukocyte interferon for the treatment of herpes zoster in patients with cancer. N. Engl. J. Med. *298*(18):981–987, 1978.
241. Merigan, T. C., Renlund, D. G., Keay, S., et al.: A controlled trial of ganciclovir to prevent cytomegalovirus disease after heart transplantation. N. Engl. J. Med. *326*:1182–1186, 1992.
242. Merigan, T. C., Skowron, G., Bozette, S. A., et al.: Pharmacokinetics and side effects of interferon in man. *In* Baron, S., and Dianzani, F. (eds.): The Interferon System: A Current Review to 1978. Galveston, TX, University of Texas Medical Branch, 1977, pp. 541–549. (Texas Reports on Biolgy and Medicine, vol. 35.)
243. Merigan, T. C., Skowron, G., Bozzette, S. A., et al.: Circulating p24 antigen levels and responses to dideoxycytidine in human immunodeficiency virus (HIV) infections: A phase I and II study. Ann. Intern. Med. *110*(3):189–194, 1989.
244. Meyers, J. D., McGuffin, R. W., Bryson, Y. J., et al.: Treatment of cytomegalovirus pneumonia after marrow transplant with combined vidarabine and human leukocyte interferon. J. Infect. Dis. *146*(1):80–84, 1982.
245. Meyers, J. D., Wade, J. C., Mitchell, C. D., et al.: Multicenter collaborative trial of intravenous acyclovir for treatment of mucocutaneous herpes simplex virus infection in the immunocompromised host. Am. J. Med. *73*(1A):229–235, 1982.
246. Miller, F. A., Sloan, B. J., and Silverman, C. A.: Antiviral activity of 9-beta-D-arabinofuranosyladenine. VI. Effect of delayed treatment on herpes simplex virus in mice. Antimicrob. Agents Chemother. *9*:192–195, 1969.
247. Millet, V. M., Dreisbach, M., and Bryson, Y. J.: Double-blind controlled study of central nervous system side effects of amantadine, rimantadine, and chlorpheniramine. Antimicrob. Agents Chemother. *21*(1):1–4, 1982.
248. Mitsuya, H., and Broder, S.: Inhibition of the in vitro infectivity and cytopathic effect of human T-lymphotrophic virus type III/lymphadenopathy-associated virus (HTLV-III/LAV) by 2′,3′-dideoxynucleosides. Proc. Natl. Acad. Sci. U. S. A. *83*(6):1911–1915, 1986.
249. Mitsuya, H., Weinhold, K. J., Furman, P. A., et al.: 3′-azido-3′-deoxythymidine (BW A509U): An antiviral agent that inhibits the infectivity and cytopathic effect of human T-lymphotropic virus type III/lymphadenopathy-associated virus in vitro. Proc. Natl. Acad. Sci. U. S. A. *82*(20):7096–7100, 1985.
250. Mofenson, L. M., Bethel, J., Moye, J. J., et al.: Effect of intravenous immunoglobulin (IVIG) on CD4+ lymphocyte decline in HIV-infected children in a clinical trial of IVIG infection prophylaxis: The National Institute of Child Health and Human Development Intravenous Immunoglobulin Clinical Trial Study Group. J. Acquir. Immune Defic. Syndr. *6*(10):1103–1113, 1993.
251. Mofenson, L. M., Moye, J. J., Bethel, J., et al.: Prophylactic intravenous immunoglobulin in HIV-infected children with CD4+ counts of 0.20 × 10(9)/L or more: Effect on viral, opportunistic, and bacterial infections. The National Institute of Child Health and Human Development Intravenous Immunoglobulin Clinical Trial Study Group. J. A. M. A. *268*(4):483–488, 1992.
252. Molla, A., Boucher, C., Korneyeva, M., et al.: Evolution of resistance to the protease inhibitor ritonavir (ABT-538) in HIV-infected patients. 4th International Workshop on HIV Drug Resistance, Sardinia, Italy, 1995.
253. Montanaki, C., Farrari, P., and Bavazzand, A.: Urinary excretion of amantiadine by the elderly. Eur. J. Clin. Pharmacol. *8*:349–356, 1975.
254. Monto, A. S., Gunn, R. A., Bandyk, M. G., et al.: Prevention of Russian influenza by amantadine. J. A. M. A. *241*:1003–1007, 1979.
255. Moyle, C., Youle, M., Chapman, S., et al.: A phase II dose escalation study of the Agouron protease inhibitor AG1343. 35th Interscience Conference on Antimicrobial Agents and Chemotherapy, San Francisco, 1995.
256. Muller WEG, Zahn, R. K., Beyer, R., et al.: 9-beta-D-arabinofuranosyladenine as a tool to study herpes simplex virus DNA replication in vitro. Virology *76*:787–796, 1977.
257. Muller WEG, Zahn, R. K., Bittlingmaier, K., et al.: Inhibition of herpesvirus DNA synthesis by 9-beta-D-arabinofuranosyladenine in vitro and in vivo. Ann. N. Y. Acad. Sci. *284*:34–48, 1977.
258. Neumayer, E. M., Haff, R. F., and Hoffman, C. E.: Antiviral activity of amantadine hydrochloride in tissue culture and in ovo. Proc. Soc. Exp. Biol. Med. *119*:393–396, 1965.
259. Nielsen, K., Wei, L. S., Sim M.-S., et al.: Correlation of clinical progression in human immunodeficiency virus infected children with in vitro zidovudine resistance measured by a direct quantitative peripheral blood lymphocyte assay. J. Infect. Dis. *172*:359–364, 1995.
260. O'Brien, W. A.: HIV-1 entry and reverse transcription in macrophages. J. Leukoc. Biol. *56*(3):273–277, 1994.
261. O'Donoghue, J. M., Ray, C. G., Terry, D. W., Jr., et al.: Prevention of nosocomial influenza infection with amantadine. Am. J. Epidemiol. *97*(4):276–282, 1973.
262. O'Sullivan, M. J., Boyer, P. J., Scott, G. B., et al.: The pharmacokinetics and safety of zidovudine in the third trimester of pregnancy for women infected with human immunodeficiency virus and their infants: Phase I Acquired Immunodeficiency Syndrome Clinical Trials Group study (protocol 082). Zidovudine Collaborative Working Group. Am. J. Obstet. Gynecol. *168*(5):1510–1516, 1993.
263. Ogino, M. T., Dankner, W. M., and Spector, S. A.: Development of zidovudine resistance in children infected with human immunodeficiency virus. J. Pediatr. *123*(1):1–8, 1993.
264. Ostertag, W., Roesler, G., Krieg, C. J., et al.: Induction of endogenous virus and of thymidine kinase by bromodeoxyuridine in cell cultures transformed by Friend virus. Proc. Natl. Acad. Sci. U. S. A. *71*(12):4980–4985, 1974.
265. Overall, J. C., Jr., Kern, E. R., and Glasgow, L. A.: Effective antiviral chemotherapy in cytomegalovirus infection of mice. J. Infect. Dis. *133*(Suppl.):A237–A244, 1976.
266. Oxford, J. S.: Effects of 1-β-D-ribofuranosyl 1,2,4-triazole-3-carboxamide on influenza virus replication and polypeptide synthesis. J. Antimicrob. Chemother. *1*(Suppl.):71–76, 1973.
267. Oxford, J. S., Logan, I. S., and Potter, C. W.: In vivo selection of an influenza A2 strain resistant to amantadine. Nature *226*(240):82–83, 1970.
268. Oxford, J. S., and Schild, G. C.: In vitro inhibition of rubella virus by 1-adamantanamine hydrochloride. Arch. Gesamte Virusforsch. *17*:313–329, 1965.
269. Oxford, J. S., and Schild, G. C.: The evaluation of antiviral compounds for rubella virus using organ cultures. Arch. Gesamte Virusforsch. *22*(3):349–356, 1967.

270. Pagano, J. S., and Datta, A. K.: Perspectives on interactions of acyclovir with Epstein-Barr and other herpes viruses. Am. J. Med. *73*(1A):18–26, 1982.
271. Panusarn, C., Stanley, E. D., Dirda, V., et al.: Prevention of illness from rhinovirus infection by a topical interferon inducer. N. Engl. J. Med. *291*(2):57–61, 1974.
272. Pavan-Langston, D.: Clinical evaluation of adenine arabinoside and idoxuridine in treatment of routine and idoxuridine-complicated herpes simplex keratitis. *In* Pavan-Langston, D., Buchanan, R. A., and Alford, C. A., Jr. (eds.): Adenine Arabinoside: An Antiviral Agent. New York, Raven Press, 1975, pp. 345–356.
273. Pavan-Langston, D., and Dohlman, C. H.: A double-blind clinical study of adenine arabinoside therapy of viral keratoconjunctivitis. Am. J. Ophthalmol. *74*(1):81–88, 1972.
274. Pavan-Langston, D., Dohlman, C. H., Geary, P., et al.: Intraocular penetration of Ara A and idu-therapeutic implications in clinical herpetic uveitis. Trans. Am. Acad. Ophthalmol. Otolaryngol. *77*(4):OP455–OP466, 1973.
275. Pavia, A. T., Gathe, J., and Group B.-S.: Clinical efficiacy of stavudine (d4T, Zerit) compared with zidovudine (ZDV, Retrovir) in ZDV-pretreated HIV-positive patients. 35th Interscience Conference on Antimicrobial Agents and Chemotherapy, San Francisco, 1995.
276. Pazin, G. J., Lam, M. T., Armstrong, J. A., et al.: Interferon prevention of HSV reactivation. 18th Interscience Conference on Antimicrobial Agents and Chemotherapy, Atlanta, 1978.
277. Perren, T. J., Powles, R. L., Easton, D., et al.: Prevention of herpes zoster in patients by long-term oral acyclovir after allogeneic bone marrow transplantation. Am. J. Med. *85*(2A):99–101, 1988.
278. Person, D. A., Sheridan, P. J., and Herrmann, E. C., Jr.: Sensitivity of type 1 and 2 herpes simplex virus to 5-ido-2′-deoxyuridine and 9-β-D-arabinofuranosyladenine. Infect. Immun. *2*:815–820, 1970.
279. Pharmaceuticals D.: Symmetrel (Amantadine Hydrochloride) and Influenza A. Garden City, NY, Physician's Monograph, 1977.
280. Pizzo, P. A., Butler, K., Balis, F., et al.: Dideoxycytidine alone and in an alternating schedule with zidovudine in children with symptomatic human immunodeficiency virus infection. J. Pediatr. *117*(5):799–808, 1990.
281. Pizzo, P. A., Eddy, J., Falloon, J., et al.: Effect of continuous intravenous infusion of zidovudine (AZT) in children with symptomatic HIV infection [see comments]. N. Engl. J. Med. *319*(14):889–896, 1988.
282. Pizzo, P. A., and Wilfert, C. M.: Treatment considerations for children with human immunodeficiency virus infection. Pediatr. Infect. Dis. J. *9*(10):690–699, 1990.
283. Poirier, R. H., Kinkel, A. W., Ellison, A. C., et al.: Intraocular penetration of topical 3 per cent adenine arbinoside. *In* Pavan-Langston, D., Buchanan, R. A., and Alford, C. A., Jr. (eds.): Adenine Arabinoside: An Antiviral Agent. New York, Raven Press, 1975, pp. 307–312.
284. Pollard, R. B., Smith, J. L., Neal, A., et al.: Effect of vidarabine on chronic hepatitis B virus infection. J. A. M. A. *239*(16):1648–1650, 1978.
285. Prentice, H. G.: Use of acyclovir for prophylaxis of herpes infections in severely immunocompromised patients. J. Antimicrob. Chemother. *12*(Suppl. B):153–159, 1983.
286. Privat de Garilhe, M., and Rudder, J. D.: Effet de deux nucl éosides de l'arbinose sur la multiplication des virus de l'herpés et de la vaccine en culture cellulaire. C. R. Acad. Sci. (Paris) *259*:2725–2728, 1964.
287. Prober, C. G., Kirk, L. E., and Keeney, R. E.: Acyclovir therapy of chickenpox in immunosuppressed children: A collaborative study. J. Pediatr. *101*(4):622–625, 1982.
288. Prusoff, W. H., and Goz, B.: Potential mechanisms of action of antiviral agents. Fed. Proc. *32*(6):1679–1687, 1973.
289. Radolf, J., Wofsy, C., Nyland, N., et al.: Recombinant leukocyte interferon A treatment during prodromal symptoms of recurrent herpes genitalis. Interscience Conference on Antimicrobial Agents and Chemotherapy, 1985.
290. Rasmussen, L., Chen, P. T., Mullenax, J. G., et al.: Inhibition of human cytomegalovirus replication by 9-(1,3-dihydroxy-2-propoxymethyl)guanine alone and in combination with human interferons. Antimicrob. Agents Chemother. *26*(4):441–445, 1984.
291. Reichman, R. C., Badger, G. J., Mertz, G. J., et al.: Treatment of recurrent genital herpes simplex infections with oral acyclovir: A controlled trial. J. A. M. A. *251*(16):2103–2107, 1984.
292. Resnick, L., Herbst, J. S., Ablashi, D. V., et al.: Regression of oral hairy leukoplakia after orally administered acyclovir therapy. J. A. M. A. *259*(3):384–388, 1988.
293. Ribeiro do Valle, L. A., Resposo de Melo, P., de Salles Gomez, L. F., et al.: Methisazone in prevention of variola minor among contacts. Lancet *2*:976–978, 1965.
294. Richman, D. D., Fischl, M. A., Grieco, M. H., et al.: The toxicity of azidothymidine (AZT) in the treatment of patients with AIDS and AIDS-related complex. A double-blind, placebo-controlled trial. N. Engl. J. Med. *317*(4):192–197, 1987.
295. Riley, R. L., and Levy, H. B.: Effect of interferon on cellular RNA synthesis and structure. *In* Baron, S., and Dianzani, F. (eds.): The Interferon System: A Current Review to 1978. Galveston, TX, University of Texas Medical Branch, 1977, pp. 239–246. (Texas Reports on Biology and Medicine, vol. 35.)
296. Roberts, N. A., Martin, J. A., Kinchington, D., et al.: Rational design of peptide-based HIV proteinase inhibitors. Science *28*:358–361, 1990.
297. Robinson, W.: Personal communication.
298. Ross, A. H., Julia, A., and Balakrishnan, C.: Toxicity of adenine arabinoside in humans. J. Infect. Dis. *133*(Suppl.):A192–A198, 1976.
299. Rytel, M. W., and Kauffman, H. M.: Clinical efficacy of adenine arabinoside in therapy of cytomegalovirus infections in renal allograft recipients. J. Infect. Dis. *133*(2):202–205, 1976.
300. Sabin, A. B.: Amantadine hydrochloride: Analysis of data related to its proposed use for prevention of A2 influenza virus disease in human beings. J. A. M. A. *200*(11):943–950, 1967.
301. Sacks, S. L., Aoki, F. Y., Diaz-Mitoma, F., et al.: Patient-initiated, twice-daily oral famciclovir for early recurrent genital herpes: A randomized, double-blind multicenter trial. Canadian Famciclovir Study Group. J. A. M. A. *276*(1):44–49, 1996.
302. Saral, R., Burns, W. H., Laskin, O. L., et al.: Acyclovir prophylaxis of herpes-simplex-virus infections. N. Engl. J. Med. *305*(2):63–67, 1981.
303. Schabel, F. M., Jr.: The antiviral activity of 9-beta-D-arabinofuranosyladenine (ARA-A). Chemotherapy *13*(6):321–338, 1968.
304. Schaeffer, H. J., Beauchamp, L., de Miranda, P., et al.: 9-(2-hydroxyethoxymethyl) guanine activity against viruses of the herpes group. Nature *272*(5654):583–585, 1978.
305. Schapiro, J. M., Winters, M. A., Kozal, M. J., et al.: Saquinavir monotherapy trial: Prolonged suppression of viral load and resistance mutations with higher dosage. 35th Interscience Conference on Antimicrobial Agents and Chemotherapy, San Francisco, 1995.
306. Schmidt, G. M., Horack, D. A., Niland, J. C., et al.: A randomized, controlled trial of prophylactic ganciclvoir for cytomegalovirus pulmonary infection in recipients of allogeneic bone marrow transplants. N. Engl. J. Med. *324*:1005–1011, 1991.
307. Schonfeld, A., Nitke, S., Schattner, A., et al.: Intramuscular human interferon-beta injections in treatment of condylomata acuminata. Lancet *1*(8385):1038–1042, 1984.
308. Schwab, R. S., England, A. C., Jr., Poskanzer, D. C., et al.: Amantadine in the treatment of Parkinson's disease. J. A. M. A. *209*:1168–1170, 1969.
309. Selby, P. J., Powles, R. L., Easton, D., et al.: The prophylactic role of intravenous and long-term oral acyclovir after allogeneic bone marrow transplantation. Br. J. Cancer *59*(3):434–438, 1989.
310. Shannon, W. M.: Antiviral activity in vitro. *In* Pavan-Langston, D., Buchanan, R. A., and Alford, C. A., Jr. (eds.): Adenine Arabinoside: An Antiviral Agent. New York, Raven Press, 1975, pp. 1–43.
311. Shepp, D. H., Dandliker, P. S., de Miranda, P., et al.: Activity of 9-[2-hydroxy-1-(hydroxymethyl)ethoxymethyl]guanine in the treatment of cytomegalovirus pneumonia. Ann. Intern. Med. *103*(3):368–373, 1985.
312. Shepp, D. H., Dandliker, P. S., and Meyers, J. D.: Treatment of varicella-zoster virus infection in severely immunocompromised patients: A randomized comparison of acyclovir and vidarabine. N. Engl. J. Med. *314*(4):208–212, 1986.
313. Shepp, D. H., Newton, B. A., Dandliker, P. S., et al.: Oral acyclovir therapy for mucocutaneous herpes simplex virus infections in immunocompromised marrow transplant recipients. Ann. Intern. Med. *102*(6):783–785, 1985.
314. Shipman, C., Jr.: Unpublished results.
315. Shipman, C., Jr., MacCallum, D. K., and Drach, J. C.: Antiviral activity of arabinosyladenine (Ara-A) and arabinosylhypoxanthine (Ara-Hx) on herpes simplex virus type I. Interscience Conference on Antimicrobial Agents and Chemotherapy, 1974, p. 34.
316. Shipman, C., Jr., Smith, S. H., Carlson, R. H., et al.: Antiviral activity of arabinosyladenine and arabinosylhypoxanthine in herpes simplex virus-infected KB cells: Selective inhibition of viral deoxyribonucleic acid synthesis in synchronized suspension cultures. Antimicrob. Agents Chemother. *9*(1):120–127, 1976.
317. Shipman, C., Jr., Smith, S. H., and Drach, J. C.: Selective inhibition of nuclear DNA synthesis by 9-D-arabinofuranosyl adenine in rat cells transformed by Rous sarcoma virus. Proc. Natl. Acad. Sci. U. S. A. *69*(7):1753–1757, 1972.
318. Sibrack, C. D., Gutman, L. T., Wilfert, C. M., et al.: Pathogenicity of acyclovir-resistant herpes simplex virus type 1 from an immunodeficient child. J. Infect. Dis. *146*(5):673–682, 1982.
319. Sidwell, R. W., Dixon, G. J., Schabel, F. M., Jr., et al.: Antiviral activity of 9-beta-D-arabinofuranosyladenine. II. Activity against herpes simplex keratitis in hamsters. Antimicrob. Agents Chemother. *8*:148–154, 1968.
320. Sidwell, R. W., Huffman, J. H., Khare, G. P., et al.: Broad-spectrum antiviral activity of virazole: 1-beta-D-ribofuranosyl-1,2,4-triazole-3-carboxamide. Science *177*(50):705–706, 1972.
321. Siegal, F. P., Lopez, C., Hammer, G. S., et al.: Severe acquired immunodeficiency in male homosexuals, manifested by chronic perianal ulcerative herpes simplex lesions. N. Engl. J. Med. *305*(24):1439–1444, 1981.
322. Skehel, J. J., Hay, A. J., and Armstrong, J. A.: On the mechanism of inhibition of influenza virus replication by amantadine hydrochloride. J. Gen. Virol. *38*:97–110, 1977.
323. Skoldenberg, B., Forsgren, M., Alestig, K., et al.: Acyclovir versus vidarabine in herpes simplex encephalitis: Randomised multicentre study in consecutive Swedish patients. Lancet *2*(8405):707–711, 1984.
324. Skowron G.: Biologic effects and safety of stavudine: Overview of phase I and II clinical trials. J. Infect. Dis. *171*(Suppl. 2):S113–S117, 1995.

325. Sloan, B. J.: Chemotherapy studies in animals. *In* Pavan-Langston, D., Buchanan, R. A., and Alford, C. A., Jr. (eds.): Adenine Arabinoside: An Antiviral Agent. New York, Raven Press, 1975, pp. 45–94.
326. Smee, D. F., Martin, J. C., Verheyden, J. P., et al.: Anti-herpesvirus activity of the acyclic nucleoside 9-(1,3-dihydroxy-2-propoxymethyl)guanine. Antimicrob. Agents Chemother. *23*(5):676–682, 1983.
327. Smiley, M. L., et al.: The efficacy and safety of valaciclovir for the treatment of herpes zoster. *In* Program and Abstracts of the 33rd Interscience Conference on Antimicrobial Agents and Chemotherapy, New Orleans, Louisiana, 1993.
328. Smith, C. B., Charette, R. P., Fox, J. P., et al.: Double-blind evaluation of ribavirin in naturally occurring influenza. *In* Smith, R. A., and Kilpatrick, W. (eds.): Ribavirin: A Broad-spectrum Antiviral Agent. New York, Academic Press, 1980, pp. 147–164.
329. Smorodintsev, A. A., Zlydnikov, D. M., Romanov I, A., et al.: Effectiveness of amantadine hydrochloride (midantane) in prevention of artificially induced influenza. Vopr. Virusol. *17*(2):152–156, 1972.
330. Spector, S. A., Gelber, R. D., McGrath, N., et al.: A controlled trial of intravenous immune globulin for the prevention of serious bacterial infections in children receiving zidovudine for advanced human immunodeficiency virus infection: Pediatric AIDS Clinical Trials Group [see comments]. N. Engl. J. Med. *331*(18):1181–1187, 1994.
331. Spector, S. A., McKinley, G. F., Lalezari, J. P., et al.: Oral ganciclovir for the prevention of cytomegalovirus disease in persons with AIDS: Roche Cooperative Oral Ganciclovir Study Group. N. Engl. J. Med. *334*(23):1491–1497, 1996.
332. Sperling, R. S., Stratton, P., O'Sullivan, M. J., et al.: A survey of zidovudine use in pregnant women with human immunodeficiency virus infection [see comments]. N. Engl. J. Med. *326*(13):857–861, 1992.
333. Spruance, S. L., and Crumpacker, C. S.: Topical 5 percent acyclovir in polyethylene glycol for herpes simplex labialis: Antiviral effect without clinical benefit. Am. J. Med. *73*(1A):315–319, 1982.
334. Spruance, S. L., Crumpacker, C. S., Haines, H., et al.: Ineffectiveness of topical adenine arabinoside 5'-monophosphate in the treatment of recurrent herpes simplex labialis. N. Engl. J. Med. *300*(21):1180–1184, 1979.
335. Spruance, S. L., Freeman, D. J., Stewart, J. C., et al.: The natural history of ultraviolet radiation-induced herpes simplex labialis and response to therapy with peroral and topical formulations of acyclovir. J. Infect. Dis. *163*(4):728–734, 1991.
336. Spruance, S. L., Hamill, M. L., Hoge, W. S., et al.: Acyclovir prevents reactivation of herpes simplex labialis in skiers. J. A. M. A. *260*(11):1597–1599, 1988.
337. Spruance, S. L., Stewart, J. C., Rowe, N. H., et al.: Treatment of recurrent herpes simplex labialis with oral acyclovir. J. Infect. Dis. *161*(2):185–190, 1990.
338. Spruance, S. L., Tyring, S. K., DeGregorio, B., et al.: A large-scale, placebo-controlled, dose-ranging trial of peroral valaciclovir for episodic treatment of recurrent herpes genitalis: Valaciclovir HSV Study Group. Arch. Intern. Med. *156*(15):1729–1735, 1996.
339. Steele, R. W., Chapa, I. A., Vincent, M. M., et al.: Effects of adenine arabinoside on cellular immune mechanisms in humans. Antimicrob. Agents Chemother. *7*(2):203–207, 1975.
340. Stephenson, J. A., Artenstein, M. S., Parkman, P. D., et al.: Effect of amantadine hydrochloride on rubella virus infection in the rhesus monkey. Antimicrob. Agents Chemother. *5*:548–552, 1965.
341. Stevens, D. A., Jordan, G. W., Waddell, T. F., et al.: Adverse effect of cytosine arabinoside on disseminated zoster in a controlled trial. N. Engl. J. Med. *289*(17):873–878, 1973.
342. Stewart, W. E., II: The Interferon System. New York, Springer-Verlag, 1979.
343. Stewart, W. E. D., and Desmyter, J.: Molecular heterogeneity of human leukocyte interferon: Two populations differing in molecular weights, requirements for renaturation, and cross-species antiviral activity. Virology *67*(1):68–73, 1975.
344. Strander, H., Cantell, K., Carlstrom, G., et al.: Clinical and laboratory investigations on man: Systemic administration of potent interferon to man. J. Natl. Cancer Inst. *51*(3):733–742, 1973.
345. Straus, S. E., Seidlin, M., Takiff, H., et al.: Oral acyclovir to suppress recurring herpes simplex virus infections in immunodeficient patients. Ann. Intern. Med. *100*(4):522–524, 1984.
346. Streeter, D. G., Witkowski, J. T., Khare, G. P., et al.: Mechanism of action of 1-D-ribofuranosyl-1,2,4-triazole-3-carboxamide (Virazole), a new broad-spectrum antiviral agent. Proc. Natl. Acad. Sci. U. S. A. *70*(4):1174–1178, 1973.
347. Stringfellow, D. A.: Production of the interferon protein: Hyporesponsiveness. *In* Baron, S., and Dianzani, F. (eds.): The Interferon System: A Current Review to 1978. Galveston, TX, University of Texas Medical Branch, 1977, pp. 126–131.
348. Swart, R. N., Vermeer, B. J., van Der Meer, J. W., et al.: Treatment of eczema herpeticum with acyclovir. Arch. Dermatol. *119*(1):13–16, 1983.
349. Sweetman, L., Connor, J. D., Seshamani, R., et al.: Deamination of adenine arabinoside in cell cultures used for in vitro viral inhibition studies. *In* Pavan-Langston, D., Buchanan, R. A., and Alford, C. A., Jr. (eds.): Adenine Arabinoside: An Antiviral Agent. New York, Raven Press, 1975, pp. 134–144.
350. Tavares, L., Roneker, C., Johnston, K., et al.: 3'-Azido-3'-deoxythymidine in feline leukemia virus–infected cats: A model for therapy and prophylaxis of AIDS. Cancer Res. *47*(12):3190–3194, 1987.
351. Tocci, M. J., Livelli, T. J., Perry, H. C., et al.: Effects of the nucleoside analog 2'-nor-2'-deoxyguanosine on human cytomegalovirus replication. Antimicrob. Agents Chemother. *25*(2):247–252, 1984.
352. Torrence, P. F., Huang, G. F., Edwards, M. W., et al.: 5-Substituted uracil arabinonucleosides as potential antiviral agents. J. Med. Chem. *22*:316–319, 1979.
353. Trousdale, M. D., Nesburn, A. B., Willey, D. E., et al.: Efficacy of BW759 (9-[[2-hydroxy-1(hydroxymethyl)ethoxy]methyl]guanine) against herpes simplex virus type 1 keratitis in rabbits. Curr. Eye Res. *3*(8):1007–1015, 1984.
354. Tyms, A. S., Davis, J. M., Jeffries, D. J., et al.: BWB759U, an analogue of acyclovir, inhibits human cytomegalovirus in vitro. Lancet *2*(8408):924–925, 1984.
355. Tyring, S., Barbarash, R. A., Nahlik, J. E., et al.: Famciclovir for the treatment of acute herpes zoster: Effects on acute disease and postherpetic neuralgia. Ann. Intern. Med. *123*(2):89–96, 1995.
356. Tyrrell, D. A. J., Bynce, M. L., and Hoorn, B.: Studies on the antiviral activity of 1-adamantanamine. Br. J. Exp. Pathol. *46*:370–375, 1965.
357. Vaheri, A.: Heparin and related polyionic substances as virus inhibitors. Acta Pathol. Microbiol. Scand. *171*(Suppl.):1–98, 1964.
358. van Leeuwen, R., Katlama, C., Kitchen, V., et al.: Evaluation of safety and efficacy of 3TC (lamivudine) in patients with asymptomatic or mildly symptomatic human immunodeficiency virus infection: A phase I/II study. J. Infect. Dis. *171*(5):1166–1171, 1995.
359. Van Rooyen, C. E., Casey, J., Lee, S. H., et al.: Vaccinia gangrenosa and 1-methylisatin 3-thiosemicarbazone (methisazone). Can. Med. Assoc. J. *97*(4):160–165, 1967.
360. Vilcek, J.: Fundamentals of virus structure and replication. *In* Galasso, G. J. (ed.): Antiviral Agents and Viral Disease of Man. New York, Raven Press, 1979, pp. 1–38.
361. Volberding, P. A., Lagakos, S. M., Koch, M. A., et al.: Zidovudine in asymptomatic human immunodeficiency virus infection: A controlled trial in persons with fewer than 500 CD4-positive cells per cubic millimeter. N. Engl. J. Med. *322*:941–949, 1990.
362. Wade, J. C., McLaren, C., and Meyers, J. D.: Frequency and significance of acyclovir-resistant herpes simplex virus isolated from marrow transplant patients receiving multiple courses of treatment with acyclovir. J. Infect. Dis. *148*(6):1077–1182, 1983.
363. Walker, J. S., Stephen, E. L., and Spertzel, R. O.: Small particle aerosols of antiviral compounds in treatment of type A influenza pneumonia in mice. J. Infect. Dis. *133S*:A140–A144, 1976.
364. Welch, A. D., Jaffe, J. J., Cardoso, S. S., et al.: Studies on the pharmacology of iododeoxyuridine in animals and man. Proc. Am. Assoc. Cancer Res. *3*:161, 1960.
365. Wellings, P. C., Awdry, P. N., Bors, F. H., et al.: Clinical evaluation of trifluorothymidine in the treatment of herpes simplex corneal ulcers. Am. J. Ophthalmol. *73*(6):932–942, 1972.
366. Wendel, H. A., Snyder, M. T., and Pell, S.: Trial of amantadine in epidemic influenza. Clin. Pharmacol. Ther. *7*(1):38–43, 1966.
367. Whiteman, P. D., Bye, A., Fowle, A. S., et al.: Tolerance and pharmacokinetics of A515U, an acyclovir analogue, in healthy volunteers. Eur. J. Clin. Pharmacol. *27*(4):471–475, 1984.
368. Whitley, R., Hilty, M., Haynes, R., et al.: Vidarabine therapy of varicella in immunosuppressed patients. J. Pediatr. *101*(1):125–131, 1982.
369. Whitley, R. J.: Interim summary of mortality in herpes simplex encephalitis and neonatal herpes simplex virus infections: Vidarabine versus acyclovir. J. Antimicrob. Chemother. *12*(Suppl. B):105–112, 1983.
370. Whitley, R. J.: Antiviral therapy: The time has come. J. Med. Virol. *1*(Suppl.):1, 1993.
371. Whitley, R. J., et al.: Unpublished results, 1980.
372. Whitley, R. J., Alford, C. A., Hirsch, M. A., et al.: Vidarabine versus acyclovir therapy in herpes simplex encephalitis. N. Engl. J. Med. *314*:144–149, 1986.
373. Whitley, R. J., Ch'ien, L. T., Dolin, R., et al.: Adenine arabinoside therapy of herpes zoster in the immunosuppressed. N. Engl. J. Med. *294*:1193–1199, 1976.
374. Whitley, R. J., Ch'ien, L. T., Nahmias, A. J., et al.: Adenine arabinoside therapy of neonatal herpetic infections. *In* Pavan-Langston, D., Buchanan, R. A., and Alford, C. A., Jr. (eds.): Adenine Arabinoside: An Antiviral Agent. New York, Raven Press, 1975, pp. 225–235.
375. Whitley, R. J., Soong, S. J., Dolin, R., et al.: Early vidarabine therapy to control the complications of herpes zoster in immunosuppressed patients. N. Engl. J. Med. *307*(16):971–975, 1982.
376. Whitley, R. J., Soong, S. J., Dolin, R., et al.: Adenine arabinoside therapy of biopsy-proved herpes simplex encephalitis: National Institute of Allergy and Infectious Diseases Collaborative Antiviral Study. N. Engl. J. Med. *297*(6):289–294, 1977.
377. Whitley, R. J., Soong, S. J., Hirsch, M. S., et al.: Herpes simplex encephalitis: Vidarabine therapy and diagnostic problems. N. Engl. J. Med. *304*(6):313–318, 1981.
378. Whitley, R. J., Spruance, S., Hayden, F. G., et al.: Vidarabine therapy for

mucocutaneous herpes simplex virus infections in the immunocompromised host. J. Infect. Dis. *149*(1):1–8, 1984.
379. Wingfield, W. L., Pollack, D., and Grunert, R. R.: Therapeutic efficacy of amantadine HCl and rimantadine HCl in naturally occurring influenza A2 respiratory illness in man. N. Engl. J. Med. *281*(11):579–584, 1969.
380. Winslow, D. L., and Otto, M. J.: HIV protease inhibitors. AIDS *9*(Suppl. A):S183–S192, 1995.
381. Winslow, D. L., Stack, S., King, R., et al.: Limited sequence diversity of the HIV type 1 protease gene from clinical isolates and in vitro susceptibility to HIV protease inhibitors. AIDS Res. Hum. Retroviruses *11*(1):107–113, 1995.
382. Winston, D. J., Wirin, D., Shaked, A., et al.: Randomized comparison of ganciclovir and high-dose acyclovir for long-term cytomegalovirus prophylaxis in liver transplant recipients. Lancet *346*:69–74, 1995.
383. Wiznia, A. A., Crane, M., Lambert, G., et al.: Zidovudine use to reduce perinatal HIV type 1 transmission in an urban medical center. J. A. M. A. *275*:1504–1506, 1996.
384. Woodson, B., and Joklik, W. K.: The inhibition of vaccinia virus multiplication by isatin-β-thiosemicarbazone. Proc. Natl. Acad. Sci. U. S. A. *54*:946–953, 1965.
385. Worral, G.: Topical acyclovir for recurrent herpes labialis in primary care. Can. Fam. Physician *37*:92–98, 1991.
386. Younsin, S. W., Betts, R. F., Roth, F. K., et al.: Reduction in fever and symptoms in young adults with influenza A/Brazil/78 H1N1 infection after treatment with aspirin or amantadine. Antibicrob. Agents Chemother. *23*:577–582, 1983.
387. Zlydnikov, D. M., Kubar, O. I., and Kovaleva, R. P.: Study of rimantadine in the USSR: A review of the literature. Rev. Infect. Dis. *3*:408–421, 1981.

234

ANTIFUNGAL AGENTS

Michael G. Rinaldi

In parallel with the increase in significance and numbers of mycotic infections in contemporary medicine has been an equal ascension of interest in and numbers of new and investigative antifungal drugs. It seems likely that modern practitioners will have at their disposal more antifungal agents than ever before in the history of medicine. In addition to continuing development of new drugs, there also has been renewed examination of older agents employed in newer ways (e.g., various lipid formulations of polyene antimycotics) and combination antifungal therapy, as well as consideration of employing combinations of antifungal drugs with immunomodulating entities.

There are several reasons for the escalation of attention to antifungal agent development: (1) more serious infections caused by fungi (particularly in the host with abrogated immunity); (2) better mycologic acumen by both the clinician and laboratorian as training in medical mycology has improved and become recognized increasingly as important subject matter for health care professionals; (3) and the favorable economic outlook for pharmaceutical manufacturers selling such compounds. However, it seems clear that one major factor has contributed more than all others to the increase in antifungal agents and interest in them. That factor is the pandemic of AIDS and acquisition of disease incited by HIV.

I believe that AIDS/HIV has been responsible mainly for the tremendous and renewed interest in antifungal drug development and use. With the advent of the HIV epidemic came a patient population in which mycoses were prominent, frequent, frustrating, and serious (often fatal), mycoses that simply could not be neglected by the medical world at virtually all levels. Persons with AIDS experience oral-pharyngeal candidiasis (OPC), cryptococcosis, histoplasmosis, coccidioidomycosis, penicillosis, aspergillosis, and a smattering of various other infections caused by both yeasts and molds. If one ascribes to recent molecular evidence and scientific thought that *Pneumocystis carinii* is a fungus,[66] then early in the AIDS epidemic, fungi were a critical component of management of opportunistic infections in this patient group. Cryptococcosis and histoplasmosis became defining opportunistic infections of those infected with HIV, and the majority of AIDS patients continue to experience chronic infections of the oral cavity incited by *Candida* species. As the epidemic progressed and became a pandemic, it became very clear that these mycoses were not dissipating but were becoming major problems for the patients and those caring for them.

At the same time that fungal infections were of major import in those with AIDS and HIV disease, modern medical technology continued its advancement of newer procedures, technologies, and methods to combat human disease. Hence, increased transplantation of organs; use of cytotoxic therapeutic modalities for cancer and various immune system dysfunctions; and widespread and continued injudicious use of antibiotics, steroids, and greatly sophisticated surgical techniques (particularly those involving the gastrointestinal tract) all contributed to an increase of what may be termed "living Petri dishes," patients whose underlying disease, therapy, or both, resulted in a significantly escalating population of individuals with altered immune status. Such patients have been and remain at high risk for development of opportunistic infections, whereby normally harmless microbes (or, for that matter, well-recognized pathogens) may incite disease. Such microorganisms take advantage of the "opportunity" afforded by an immunocompromised host, hence, the term *opportunistic*. It is in such settings that fungal infections have assumed great prominence in contemporary medicine.[49] The need for more efficacious, less toxic, antimycotic agents was and still is evident, and the response has been the introduction of more antifungal drugs than ever before. It also seems apparent that the means by which patients become immunosuppressed are not going to disappear, and it is likely that mycoses will continue to be important infectious disorders in this group. Accordingly, the development and use of new antifungal agents will continue, hopefully to the benefit of all.

Although superficial fungal infections are numerous and of significance in children, this discussion involves those antifungal agents employed to treat invasive or deep fungal infections. Antimycotic agents may be classified in several ways, but the approach followed here is based on their chemical formulations: polyenes (and their various lipid formulations), azoles, 5-fluorocytosine, echinocandins, chitin inhibitors, and others.

POLYENES

Nystatin

One of the first of developed antifungal drugs still employed today is nystatin (NYS). This tetraene was developed mainly as a result of the pioneering work of Hazen and Brown while employed by the New York State Health Department; hence, the compound was named after New York State. NYS remains one of the most powerful of the polyene antifungal drugs due to its antifungal activity and fungicidal nature. It turned out to be too toxic to administer parenterally, and its use has been overwhelmingly topical. It frequently is used to treat fungal infections of the mucous membranes and sometimes skin and has become a widely employed therapy to treat OPC in the patient with HIV disease. Some practitioners also use NYS as an ingested suspension to treat gastrointestinal candidiasis. NYS currently is relatively inexpensive and easily obtainable and so has been used worldwide as an agent to treat superficial and mucocutaneous mycoses. Patients complain of the taste of NYS, and so compliance is not always high if prolonged therapy is necessary, such as with thrush. The OPC problem in cancer patients after and during chemotherapy, those with fungal mucous membrane involvement associated with diabetes and other endocrine disorders, and, most recently, HIV patients has resulted in widespread use of NYS, often with good to excellent results. However, it is important to note that, particularly in AIDS patients, outcomes following NYS therapy for OPC have not been uniformly successful, with patients often being refractory, especially after repeated treatment episodes and as CD4 cell counts diminish.[40]

Interestingly, one report indicated that 15 of 21 fungemias in patients in a burn unit were caused by a relatively rare species of *Candida*, *C. rugosa*, in which the patients were receiving prophylaxis with NYS, compared with none of 18 fungemias that occurred during the period prior to NYS use.[17] Because the burn unit isolates had a common pattern of antifungal drug susceptibility that was different from that of *C. rugosa* isolates from other sources, it was judged that a single strain was likely responsible for the cluster. Further analysis of burn unit isolates employing molecular techniques demonstrated genetic relatedness of the isolates from the original study.[16, 54] Taken together, these results suggest that clonal strain transmission of *C. rugosa* can occur and that serious invasive infection due to this yeast species may be an important clinical consequence of topical NYS prophylaxis. These findings, along with NYS resistance in OPC in AIDS patients, point out that clinical resistance to NYS is possible.

An additional, potentially exciting development with NYS concerns formulation inside liposomes as liposomal NYS (Nyotran). This form of NYS offers the theoretical and potential value of much lesser toxicity to human hosts, compared with the parent compound.[42] Early studies suggest that Nyotran is efficacious and acceptably nontoxic against certain mycoses. Should such investigations be supported by further studies that reflect the safety of this formulation of NYS, the most powerful polyene on the market well could see much broader use in the treatment of invasive mycoses.

Natamycin (Pimaricin)

Natamycin (NATA; pimaricin) is another of the initially developed polyenes. As with NYS, NATA is too toxic for systemic use in humans and has gained a therapeutic niche mainly in the treatment of mycotic infections of the cornea.[59] Topically employed NATA is felt by many ophthalmologists to be first-line therapy for mycotic keratitis caused by a variety of fungal species but most often those of *Candida*, *Fusarium*, and *Aspergillus*. Although not uniformly successful, there is little doubt that NATA has salvaged many people's eyesight in a mycosis that otherwise would haved proved devastating to the cornea.

Amphotericin B

Amphotericin B (AMB) was approved for clinical use in the mid-1950s and quickly became the mainstay of antifungal therapy for deep mycoses.[24] It remains today the "gold standard" in the eyes of many clinicians and is the drug with which all newly developed agents inevitably are compared for efficacy, safety, and spectrum of activity. It is intriguing that despite almost 40 years of use, and as with all polyenes, the precise mechanism of action of AMB still is not resolved completely. Most investigators have shown that polyenes influence the integrity of the fungal (and mammalian) cell membrane. Although grossly oversimplified and incomplete, the mechanism of action according to most scientists involves the binding of AMB to a sterol located in the cell membrane. In the case of fungi, the main sterol involved in such interaction is ergosterol, whereas in humans it is cholesterol. In either case, AMB binds to the sterol in an undoubtedly complex stereochemical fashion, and the resultant binding appears to cause pores, channels, or holes to be produced through the membrane. As a consequence of the pores or holes, essential metabolites of the fungus (or animal or human) "leak" through the openings and the organism dies; hence, the supposed fungicidal nature of AMB. It is important to note that not all investigators believe AMB is fungicidal to all fungi at each exposure. There is no question that fungal-antifungal interactions are complex processes, nor that outcomes of therapy often depend more on the immune status of the host than on the effectiveness of the antifungal drug, but there clearly are situations both in vitro and in vivo whereby AMB does not "kill" each fungal cell it contacts. Obviously, AMB does not kill every mycotic organism it encounters in the infected host, as evidenced by the distressingly dismal mortality rate of some mycoses, such as aspergillosis, whose therapy of choice is AMB. It well may be that in some instances AMB is fungistatic and in others fungicidal. What seems very clear, however, is that AMB exerts its effects very quickly, at least in the test tube. Time-kill curves reflect that AMB and fungal membranes interact within minutes.

AMB is very broad-spectrum in its antifungal activity, which covers the taxonomic gamut of the fungal world. When encountering a life-threatening mycosis caused by almost any fungus, many clinicians still employ AMB as first-line therapy. Although developments of late with new antimycotic agents well may alter the aforementioned view, I find that clinicians generally prefer to commence therapy with AMB and then switch to one of the newer agents after response and stabilization of their patients, if that should occur. There are certain mycoses, such as zygomycosis, in which AMB offers the only current mode of therapeutic intervention.

As surely as AMB has saved many lives, there also is no doubt as to its toxicity. The main problems with this agent involve its toxicity to human cells as well as to those of fungi. Problems with AMB range from administration sequelae to its well-known nephrotoxicity. Individuals receiving AMB therapy may experience infusion-related reactions, blood dyscrasias, chilling and sweating, and other adverse events. Should the drug be given long enough, frequently at high doses (up to 1.2 mg/kg/day), as often is necessary in life-threatening mycotic infections, for example, aspergillal infection of the central nervous system, resultant renal toxicity may ensue. This seems mainly to involve the renal tubular apparatus. The toxicity may be reversible when AMB therapy is terminated or reduced in dose, but often effective treatment requires long-term, high-dose drug with resultant kidney damage that may be permanent. The toxicity of AMB has prompted the ongoing search for antifungal agents that are equally efficacious but whose toxicity is diminished significantly.

It also is notable that physicians who routinely employ AMB (i.e., infectious diseases specialists, hematologists-oncologists, and those who primarily take care of AIDS patients) have "learned" to deal with the toxicities and idiosyncracies of AMB. Perhaps an entire chapter could be devoted to all the various means by which clinicians have attempted to reduce the toxicity of AMB and yet administer effective doses. Numerous paradigms have been published and developed over many years in an effort to administer AMB safely. These involve premedications of various types, salt loading, mannitol infusion, and many alternative strategies. The bottom line seems to be that AMB is, indeed, a very toxic agent, but if administered by knowledgeable, experienced medical personnel, this drug can be lifesaving. It appears that young children and infants experience much less azotemia than adults when receiving AMB, and so saline has not been recommended.[38]

Over the past several years, papers have appeared in the literature involving the dissolution of AMB in various lipid formulations. There have been three major commercial formulations: Abelcet (AMB lipid complex), Ambisome (liposomal AMB), and Amphotec (AMB colloidal dispersion). The basic premise behind the development of each variant is that a lipid-encased/enclosed/bound formulation of AMB results in lesser toxicity with apparent equal efficacy. Indeed, the literature supports the findings of lesser nephrotoxicity of all three agents compared with AMB, and it also seems clear that much higher doses of these agents may be given (up to 8 mg/kg/day, with 5 mg/kg/day being the normal dose).[5] Clinicians who have used these agents indicate that they are not without some of the toxicities associated with AMB intravenous infusion, such as chilling and rigors, but generally concur that kidney toxicity may be less. Few published studies compare the lipid formulations head-to-head with AMB, and none compare one with the other. Increasing numbers of published papers do, however, attest to the relative safety and therapeutic activity of these agents.[7, 13] The companies producing these compounds have decided upon differing marketing strategies; for example, Abelcet is to be used after failure or intolerance of AMB, and Ambisome likely will be marketed as a replacement for and equivalent to AMB but with lesser toxicity.

Finally, several papers and some global anecdotal reports (although most are from France and the United States) have appeared in which AMB has been suspended in Intralipid, a product normally used for parenteral nutritional supplementation. The concept is that AMB in Intralipid is considerably cheaper to formulate than each of the aforementioned three commercial lipid-AMB preparations, which are very costly, but would offer the same benefits, particularly lessened nephrotoxicity. There is difficulty in such approaches, however, in that various groups have formulated the AMB-Intralipid in different ratios (there is no standardized preparation), the optimal ratio of AMB:lipid remains unknown (even for the commercial preparations), and it has been reported and observed that AMB-Intralipid preparations also demonstrate infusion-related toxicities.[64] At this point, the commercial formulations may offer a more prudent approach if one elects to engage in therapy with a lipid-AMB product.

Of note, there are additional nuances to be aware of when treating mycoses with AMB or its lipid variants (or, for that matter, any antifungal drug). Not all fungi are susceptible to AMB, and as always is the case in medicine, there is no substitute for good microbiology. It is critical that the clinician learn the identity of the offending fungal organism. Although it is important to recognize that an organism will not always grow out in the laboratory from patient specimens or that, at times, the only materials available from which to base therapeutic decisions are histopathologic tissue sections, it always is crucial when possible to learn the identity of the etiologic agent. With the ever escalating number of fungal organisms able to incite infections, as well as the expanding list of antifungal drugs demonstrating varying activities against different fungi, serious therapeutic errors may ensue if the organism is misidentified or remains unknown. For example, in a child with leukemia, all the correct predisposing factors of immunosuppression, an evolving pulmonary infiltrate unresponsive to antibacterial therapy, negative cultures, but respiratory specimens showing parallel-walled, branching, septate hyphal elements, it certainly is likely and appropriate to entertain a diagnosis of invasive pulmonary aspergillosis. In such a case, there would be few clinicians who would hestitate in commencing therapy with AMB. However, in this same patient population has been documented infection with exactly the same scenario down to the appearance of septate, branching hyphae in tissue, in which the causative agent turned out to be *Pseudallescheria boydii* (asexual form name, *Scedosporium apiospermum*). In tissue, this fungus virtually is identical to any species of *Aspergillus*. Short of seeing fruiting of the fungus in tissue or employing an immunochemical means to identify the organism, *Pseudallescheria* is identical morphologically to the aspergilli. Perhaps more important, this fungal species innately is resistant to AMB, and optimal therapy likely may be miconazole or better itraconazole (ITRA). It is important to accomplish sound microbiology when possible.

Other fungal species also are well documented as resistant, in vitro and in vivo, to AMB. Such organisms (e.g., species of the mold *Fusarium* and the yeast *Trichosporon ashii*) most often incite disease in the severely immunocompromised patient, and mortality rates are unacceptably high.[69] About 20 per cent of isolates of the yeast *Candida lusitaniae* may exhibit resistance to AMB.[44] Most disturbingly, the recent literature attests to strains, albeit rare, of both *Cryptococcus neoformans* variety *neoformans* and *Candida albicans* resistant to AMB.[51, 52] It has been accepted generally that such common fungal pathogens uniformly were susceptible to AMB. Because standardization of antifungal susceptibility testing is imminent, a case well could be made for its use in selected mycotic cases in which optimal therapy does not appear to be effective or to assist in the explanation of situations as described earlier.[56]

AZOLES

The azole antimycotics have become well entrenched in the therapy of mycotic infections. The development of these compounds dates back to the 1970s with the first-generation imidazoles, which contained an azole ring incorporating two nitrogen molecules. We are entering the "third-generation" azole period. The first imidazole agents appeared to offer an alternative to AMB for the therapy of deep mycoses. At the time, these agents were chemically unique antifungals and exhibited a broad spectrum of activity both in vitro and in vivo.

Imidazoles

Clotrimazole and Miconazole

Such initial agents appeared relatively nontoxic, and so the introduction of clotrimazole and miconazole generated much excitement for potential therapy of serious infections such as coccidioidomycosis. Many of the first azoles were not soluble in water, and so formulation problems for effective and safe administration to humans became apparent. In the case of clotrimazole, it became clear that when the drug was introduced systemically into mammals, including humans, the hepatic microsomal enzymes rapidly degraded the drug to inactive metabolites.[58] Attempts to find a safe vehicle in which to deliver miconazole were fraught with difficulties. The vehicle finally employed, Cremaphor EL, was involved in several literature-reported cardiorespiratory adverse events. Lastly, it was observed that these agents demonstrated fungistatic, rather than fungicidal, effects, and that if therapy was not maintained or was stopped too early, the mycosis recurred because it really had not been eliminated.[31] The early imidazoles did not turn out to be viable replacements for AMB. Such agents did not, however, die; in fact they are used widely in modern medicine as therapeutic modalities for the treatment of superficial mycoses and fungal infections of the mucous membranes. In contemporary practice, gynecologists, dermatologists, family practitioners, and those taking care of patients with HIV disease often employ imidazole antimycotics quite successfully. These drugs are inexpensive and widely available, in some cases over the counter.

Ketoconazole

The next imidazole effort related to invasive mycoses was far more successful and consequential. Ketoconazole (KETO) was introduced clinically at the end of the 1970s and did offer a genuine alternative to AMB for certain mycoses. Until the advent of KETO, therapy of chronic mucocutaneous candidiasis mainly in children and teenagers had been dismal. KETO offered the first therapy with meaningful effect on this particular yeast infection and immune dysfunctional condition. As with previous imidazoles, KETO was remarkably broad-spectrum in vitro and in vivo, including against the agents causing deep fungal diseases. KETO was used to treat many invasive fungal disorders, such as histoplasmosis and coccidioidomycosis. Results with KETO were impressive for some patients and some mycoses. Generally for non–life-threatening diseases and some cases of uncomplicated pulmonary mycoses, KETO performed well and offered an additional strategy for directed therapy.[29] However, as time passed and KETO was used more widely, it became apparent there were some dilemmas with this drug. KETO was available in tablet form only, and if a patient was unable to swallow or was comatose, for example, KETO was not an option for therapy. Investigators began to document various drug-drug interactions between KETO and other drugs, including non–antiinfective agents, in which KETO or the other drug would be rendered inactive or levels would become unacceptably high. This same problem has plagued all azole antimycotics agents in varying degrees. It was noted that KETO had influences upon certain endocrine functions that could result in impotence in males and the development of excess hair in females. Later, the association of KETO and endocrine function became advantageous when it was observed that KETO might be useful as augmentative therapy for prostatic cancer. Most troublesome, however, was the occurrence in approximately 1 of every 100,000 patients of hepatotoxicity caused by KETO, which was implicated in the deaths of a small number of individuals. When using KETO, it is prudent to obtain a pretherapy baseline liver enzyme panel so that comparisons may be made should hepatic dysfunction result during therapy. Finally, it became clear that as with the previous imidazoles, KETO also was fungistatic and, again, when treatment was terminated, the mycosis often recurred.

KETO nevertheless became a very successful agent because it offered the first real alternative to AMB in certain situations of deep fungal infection. KETO is used worldwide to treat a plethora of skin, mucous membrane, and sometimes deep mycotic infections. It is cheap, easily obtainable, and often used to treat OPC in AIDS patients. It was during the KETO era that the first-documented azole resistance problems surfaced and were reported. Patients with chronic mucocutaneous candidiasis from the United Kingdom and Denver, Colorado, became refractory during therapy, and investigators saved both pre- and posttreatment isolates of *C. albicans*.[32] In vitro studies of these strains (which were distributed widely among the global scientific community) demonstrated in vitro resistance of the posttreatment isolates when tested in many laboratories by several different methods. At that time and since, KETO resistance problems have remained rare, but the foundations of azole resistance were laid. KETO really did not replace AMB as first-line therapy for deep mycoses, but the road was paved for the next generation of azole drugs.

Triazoles

The next generation of azole antifungals has turned out to be, thus far, the most important scientifically and therapeutically. Such compounds possess the azole ring in their structure, but, as their name implies, the ring contains three nitrogen molecules rather than the two characteristic of their predecessors. The triazole antimycotic drugs have come to be among the most important developments in the therapy of fungal infections, both deep and superficial. These agents have offered, in some specific mycoses and situations, genuine alternative therapy to AMB and for certain mycotic infections have become the drugs of choice.[9] We are approaching the threshold of the next generation of triazole antifungal agents.

Fluconazole (Diflucan)

This triazole has become one of the most rapidly successful antibiotics ever produced and certainly a major player among antifungal drugs. Fluconazole (FLU) is a low-molecular-weight, water-soluble triazole that readily crosses the blood-brain barrier, gains excellent access to biologic fluids, and is available as both oral and intravenous preparations. The pharmacokinetics of the oral and intravenous preparations essentially are identical, and, thus, if the patient can swallow and absorb the drug, the tablet form renders equal efficacy to the much more expensive intravenous formulation. Although there are some drug-drug interactions between FLU and other agents, they have been lesser in frequency and clinical importance than those associated with other azoles.[26]

FLU's rapid approval (one of the most rapid ever) by the Food and Drug Administration in 1990 coincided with a substantial amount of OPC and cryptococcal meningitis among those with AIDS and HIV disease. It was for these two main conditions that the drug was marketed. The drug was easy to take, worked remarkably well in these two mycoses, and was readily attainable despite its expense. FLU also was remarkably nontoxic and free of side effects. In a relatively short time, virtually all OPC and most cryptococcal meningitis in those with AIDS were being treated with FLU. Initially, the manufacturer's recommended package insert doses were low (50 to 100 mg/day). Investigators recognized early on that this agent likely would be safe and more effective in higher doses. However, recognizing the toxicities of the prior imidazoles, clinicians generally employed low doses of FLU, which appeared to work well. FLU also had been approved for use against invasive candidiasis (candidemia) and increasingly was used by surgeons, particularly after gastrointestinal procedures. Again, doses generally were (and often still are) low. More recently, FLU was approved to treat candidal vaginitis as a one-time 150-mg pill. Most recently, FLU has gained favor as effective therapy for a notoriously difficult-to-treat mycosis, coccidioidal meningitis.[22] FLU also demonstrates good activity in histoplasmosis and blastomycosis.

As the 1990s progressed, it became noticeable to practitioners that AIDS patients being treated with FLU for OPC were experiencing breakthrough disease while on therapy. These observations prompted use of higher doses of FLU, which also worked well for awhile. Eventually, patients on higher doses (200 mg/day) also were observed to have recurrent OPC disease while on therapy. Doses were increased ultimately to 800 mg/day, but breakthrough disease continued to appear. This did not occur with every patient, and many individuals remained disease-free while receiving low-dose FLU. However, it was becoming abundantly clear that the resistance issue with FLU and OPC needed to be examined. Since 1994, many papers have documented scenarios of FLU-resistant strains of *Candida*.[57] Many of these studies were quite thorough and involved susceptibility testing of pre- and posttherapy isolates (i.e., genetic characterization of all strains isolated from particular patients and from all patients in any given study). Results of such studies have been most intriguing. One good example of the development of FLU resistance by *C. albicans* was documented in a series of 17 isolates from a single patient over a 2-year period.[53] During this time, the patient experienced 14 bouts of oral candidiasis and was treated with increasing doses of FLU. Molecular and biochemical analyses confirmed that the isolates were the same strain of *C. albicans* and that the resistance in the isolates was stable over 500 generations of growth in the absence of FLU. This strongly suggests that the changes in this strain are genetic in nature. Additionally, the development of resistance was correlated with the identification of a substrain or variant of the original strain (as identified by restriction length polymorphism analysis with a moderately repetitive probe, Ca3). These analyses demonstrate that azole drug resistance is associated with several small genetic changes, each of which contributes to the overall resistance of the strain. It seems clear that continual use of FLU (and perhaps other triazoles) can result in genetic changes that render OPC refractory to treatment (White and colleagues, unpublished data, 1996).

The development of resistance to FLU has engendered tremendous interest in this area, and it is well to bear in mind definitions employed for resistance. There may be microbiologic resistance in which the fungus actually is resistant to the antifungal agent in the test tube, and there may be clinical resistance in which the patient does not respond to a therapeutic dose of a drug that should be efficacious. Microbiologic and clinical resistance do not correlate necessarily. As with most scientific endeavors, this area is complex and involves the fungus, the host and his/her immunity, the antifungal drug, the dose, the duration of therapy, previous therapy, and compliance.[57]

A very recent study at the time of this writing places the FLU resistance issue in perspective. A cohort of 50 patients with advanced HIV disease and recurrent OPC were assessed prospectively as to the epidemiology and clinical significance of FLU resistance. Resistant yeasts, defined as having minimum inhibitory concentrations (MICs) of greater than 8 μg/mL, were detected in 32 per cent of 50 patients: 14 per cent had resistant *C. albicans*, 14 per cent had resistant non–*C. albicans*, and 4 per cent had mixed resistant yeasts. MICs were above 32 μg/mL in 11 of 16 isolates. Previous FLU use and severe immunosuppression were risk factors for resistance. However, 5 of 25 patients had resistant isolates with no prior FLU use, and all were severely immunosuppressed. Despite the high prevalence of resistance, 48 patients clinically responded to FLU. FLU-resistant *C. albicans* and non–*C. albicans* yeast infections are common in patients with advanced immunodeficiency, but the clinical efficacy of FLU remains high.[55]

Studies conducted by the Centers for Disease Control and Prevention examined FLU resistance patterns of yeast isolates from HIV-positive women. Oropharyngeal and vaginal yeast cultures were obtained from 175 women, 97 of whom were HIV-positive and 78 of whom were HIV-negative. Sixty-seven per cent of HIV-positive and 63 per cent of HIV-negative women had positive oral cultures, and 29 per cent of HIV-positive and 19 per cent of HIV-negative women had positive vaginal cultures (neither contrast being statistically significant). For *C. albicans* isolated from the oral cavity, 13 per cent of strains from HIV-positive women and 3 per cent from HIV-negative women were FLU-resistant (MIC > 64 μg/mL). Ten and zero per cent of isolates from the vagina of HIV-positive and HIV-negative women, respectively, were resistant to FLU. These data may reflect that the pattern of FLU resistance observed in OPC isolates from AIDS patients is occurring in the vagina of HIV-positive women as well.[19]

Another thread of contemporary thought involving FLU advises caution when employing this triazole for the therapy of non–*C. albicans* yeast infections. Infections caused by *Candida glabrata, Candida lusitaniae,* or *Candida parapsilosis* are increasing in the blood and often incite breakthrough fungemia in those already receiving systemic antifungal agents, including FLU and AMB. In particular, *C. glabrata* is an especially important and emerging pathogenic yeast that may demonstrate elevated MICs to both FLU and AMB. Should a patient be infected with *Candida krusei,* FLU should be avoided because this species innately is resistant.[45]

One report documents *C. albicans*–caused fungemia in two patients with leukemia that demonstrated in vitro resistance after FLU prophylaxis (400 mg/day) and empiric AMB therapy (0.5 mg/kg of body weight per day) were administered. The candidal isolates also were resistant in vitro to other azoles and exhibited membrane sterol changes consistent with a mutation in the $\Delta^{5,6}$-sterol desaturase gene. The lack of ergosterol in the cytoplasmic membrane of the FLU-resistant strains also imparted resistance to AMB. Both patients were treated successfully with high-dose AMB (1 to 1.25 mg/kg/day) and flucytosine (150 mg/kg/day).[46] The reader can ascertain that resistance problems with antifungal drugs are not limited then to those with HIV disease and oral, esophageal, or vaginal infections caused by yeasts.

Essentially, the fungi are every bit as "smart" as the bacteria, and if we continue to use FLU injudiciously (at low doses) to treat any real or potential mycosis, particularly in those patients who are immunocomprised and in AIDS patients with low CD4 counts, then we will have no cause for when antifungal resistance, be it microbiologic or clinical or both, emerges. Because there exists documented cross-resistance to azole antimycotics, the concerns with FLU could translate to other triazoles as well, especially if their use is analogous to that of FLU.

Itraconazole (Sporanox)

ITRA is the next-generation compound following in the footsteps of KETO. It is a triazole antifungal agent that was studied and used widely in Europe before its approval in the United States. It has become clear that ITRA may be viewed as the agent of choice for histoplasmosis (both in AIDS and non-AIDS patients), blastomycosis, sporotrichosis, and phaeohyphomycosis (those fungal infections incited by darkly pigmented, or dematiaceous, fungi). It also is the only approved alternative therapy for invasive aspergillosis (aside from the lipid formulations of AMB). In some instances, ITRA also has been effective in the terrible infections caused by *P. boydii*. Generally, ITRA exhibits a greater and more potent spectrum of activity than does FLU in vitro.[63]

Unlike FLU, ITRA is not soluble in water and so does not achieve the high levels seen in biologic fluids with FLU. It is, however, very soluble in lipid and, hence, gains entrance to tissue, which is not bad because that often is where the infecting fungus lives! ITRA is available only as an orally administered capsule, although clinical trials are under way of an oral suspension that offers an alternative, and possibly better, means of delivery and absorption.[50] An intravenous preparation is not available. As with KETO, if a patient is unable to swallow or is unresponsive, there is difficulty in administration of ITRA. Furthermore, ITRA is absorbed better if taken in an acidic environment, that is, with orange juice or cola and meals. Again, as with all azoles, there exists for ITRA the potential for drug-drug interactions when administered with several different compounds, such as rifampin, phenytoin, and carbamazepine. Such drug interactions may have significant consequences for either the ITRA or the other drug, and clinicians carefully should ascertain pertinent drug-drug potential interactions before using ITRA.[8, 9, 35]

The mechanism of action of azole antimycotic agents appears to be the prevention of the synthesis of the main fungal cell membrane sterol, ergosterol, via inhibition of the enzyme lanosterol demethylase, which catalzyes the conversion of lanosterol to ergosterol. As with FLU and the imidazoles discussed previously, ITRA exhibits fungistatic activity at concentrations relevant to therapy. Current approved indications for ITRA in the United States include histoplasmosis, blastomycosis, and aspergillosis (as well as onychomycosis due to dermatophytic fungi), but, as noted earlier, clinicians have employed this agent, successfully and unsuccessfully, for other mycoses. Clinical trials of ITRA to treat OPC in the HIV population are under way.

Because ITRA has not been employed with anywhere near the frequency as has FLU to treat OPC infections in the HIV-positive patient, resistance issues have not been a major topic with this drug. However, azole cross-resistance in vitro is well documented[3] and should promote watchful scrutiny in patients. Additionally, doses of ITRA to treat invasive mycoses have been generally higher than those initially used with FLU. Most investigators now expound that successful triazole therapy for invasive mycoses should commence at a minimum of 400 mg/day. FLU has been given at doses as high as 2000 mg/day, with 800 mg/day being widely employed, but ITRA may engender gastrointestinal upset when the dose exceeds 600 mg/day.[25] ITRA generally does not exhibit the toxicity observed with KETO involving the liver, but it nevertheless has been reported that elevated liver enzyme values do occur, and many practitioners follow similar guidelines as with KETO for monitoring liver function while ITRA is being administered.

Of particular note is the use of ITRA to treat invasive aspergillosis.[14] Many clinicians still believe that the recommended primary therapy for this disease is AMB. There is no "good" invasive aspergillosis, but should infection manifest in the central nervous system or as endocarditis, as opposed to pulmonary disease, outcomes especially are dismal and it is unlikely that most physicians would commence initial therapy with ITRA. There are, however, reports in the literature of successful therapy for invasive disease with ITRA as first-line therapy. Most clinicians likely would commence therapy with AMB, then switch at a later (almost always undefined) time if the patient is felt to be stable and not experiencing progressive disease. The reality of this fungal infection, as with many of the opportunistic mycoses, is that without return of immune function, the outcomes are terrible no matter what therapeutic maneuvers are used.[15]

Combination Therapy

A question arising frequently is that of therapy of invasive mycoses with a combination of AMB (or lipid-associated AMB) and a triazole. On the basis of work by Schaffner and Frick,[61] in which a murine model of aspergillosis was treated with a combination of AMB and KETO, there has been great hesitation in using AMB with an azole. This work showed that the combination of drugs engendered antagonism in this animal model. This was explained partially by consideration of the theoretic mechanisms of action of the two antifungal agents. If KETO prevents synthesis of ergosterol and AMB acts by binding to ergosterol, then it could be postulated that KETO prevents AMB activity by preventing synthesis of its target attachment entity. One also could suggest that if one were to employ this combination, it would be prudent to administer AMB first, followed by KETO, or give the two at the same time; otherwise, KETO would remove the binding site for AMB if administered prior to AMB. Dr. Schaffner recently indicated the same views regarding combinations of AMB plus ITRA and AMB plus FLU for invasive aspergillosis.

On the other hand, other investigators examining this question have not arrived at the same conclusions, at least for a combination of AMB plus FLU for murine candidiasis.[67, 68] These researchers found no antagonism between the two agents in any in vivo experiments and at least additive effects in others. Clearly this area requires further study because it portends important clinical implications in mycoses that often may be fatal despite the best current single-agent therapy.

New, Investigational Triazoles

Clinical trials and preclinical testing are focusing on several other next-generation triazoles. These agents are better than FLU and ITRA in that their activities are enhanced against a broader spectrum of fungi, they are targeted at fungal species that have demonstrated resistance problems with FLU, and, in one case, claim to be fungicidal at concentrations relevant to human therapy. Of course, the quest will continue for triazoles that demonstrate maximum safety profiles as well.

VORICONAZOLE (UK-109,496)

Voriconazole (VOR) is a novel, wide-spectrum triazole derivative whose structure is derived via a chemical modification of FLU by replacement of one triazole moiety with a fluoropyrimidine group and an α-methylation. This compound is different from FLU in several ways: It is not soluble in water, it has a much broader spectrum of activity (including against aspergilli), and it reportedly is fungicidal rather than fungistatic, which most of the other triazoles and imidazoles are. VOR is active against *C. krusei* and *C. glabrata*, a major improvement over FLU. Chemically, VOR is more analogous to ITRA than FLU in that VOR and ITRA must be dissolved in vehicles such as polyethylene glycol or cyclodextrin formulations before delivery to humans or animals.[41]

VOR is exciting in several ways and has undergone clinical trials in Europe evaluating its efficacy and safety in OPC in AIDS patients as well as in invasive aspergillosis. VOR should circumvent the problems of *Candida* resistance to FLU and exert activity against yeast species for which FLU was not active; *C. glabrata* may be the most clinically significant of such species. Perhaps the most exciting aspect of VOR, however, is the fungicidal activity demonstrated with aspergilli and the treatment of aspergillosis. If these findings are confirmed in human clinical trials, this drug could represent a major and significant treatment alternative for this devastating mycosis. Additionally, abstracts indicate that VOR may exhibit activity against other particularly difficult-to-treat opportunistic fungi, such as *Fusarium*.[30, 33] High doses of VOR have been associated with visual aberration problems, but reportedly these are reversible upon cessation of therapy and are not observed in every subject or at lower doses. The medical community eagerly awaits further studies and data involving this next-generation triazole.

D0870

D0870 is another new, investigational triazole that is the (+)enantiomer of a previous nondeveloped triazole, ICI 195, 739. Numerous studies have reported the in vitro and in vivo activity of D0870 versus other triazoles. Generally, D0870 seems more active than FLU against FLU-resistant yeast fungi and also demonstrates good activity against the agents of histoplasmosis, coccidioidomycosis, blastomycosis, and several non–*C. albicans* yeasts. Although D0870 demonstrates in vitro and in vivo activity against species of *Aspergillus*, the data reflect lesser activity than ITRA or AMB, and it is unlikely that this agent would be useful against aspergillosis. The main niche of this agent well may be against yeasts that are considered resistant to FLU.[4, 70]

SCH 56592

Over the years, several azole compounds have been developed, of which the latest is SCH 56592. Unfortunately, mainly due to varying toxicities, none of these compounds came to fruitition. SCH 56592 has entered clinical trials, appears to be safe, and may offer advantages over its previous analog SCH 51048, which exhibited in vitro and in vivo activity against a broad range of pathogenic fungi, including *C. krusei, Coccidioides immitis*, and *Blastomyces dermatitidis*. Studies have demonstrated in vitro activity of SCH 56592 against an even broader spectrum of fungi than its predecessors, including most of the medically significant yeasts as well as aspergilli and the agents of endemic systemic mycoses.[23] Global studies evaluating the efficacy of this compound in OPC also are under way. Should safety profiles hold up, it is likely that this triazole will allow yet another therapeutic option for the treatment of some mycoses for which current therapy is problematic or nonexistent (e.g., infections caused by *Fusarium, P. boydii*, aspergilli, and FLU-resistant yeasts).

Additional new and experimental triazoles are under evaluation, such as T-8581, another compound that is soluble in water and demonstrates pharmacokinetic properties similar to those of FLU but unlike FLU is active against FLU-resistant yeasts and aspergilli.[71]

FLUCYTOSINE (5-FLUOROCYTOSINE)

Introduced in the late 1970s, flucytosine (5-FC) originally was intended as an antineoplastic agent. This compound structurally is an analog of the pyrimidine base cytosine that has been fluorinated. It is soluble in water and crosses the blood-brain barrier. It became clear that this agent was not a fruitful anticancer drug but exhibited excellent in vitro antifungal activity, especially against yeast-fungi. It was, therefore, developed and marketed as an antimycotic agent. 5-FC demonstrates excellent activity in vitro against most of the pathogenic yeasts, including cryptococci, *Candida* species, and *Trichosporon* species. Early on there was some feeling that 5-FC also had the potential to treat aspergillosis. This compound exerts its activity in susceptible fungi via conversion of 5-FC to 5-fluorouracil to 5-fluorouradylic acid; it then is incorporated into RNA or metabolized to 5-fluorodeoxyuradylic acid monophosphate. This latter compound stops synthesis of DNA because of its ability to inhibit thymidylate synthetase.[21, 38]

5-FC may be administered both orally and intravenously, although the intravenous preparation no longer is available from its U.S. manufacturer. 5-FC is absorbed completely, and most is secreted unchanged in urine. In patients with azotemia, it is very important to monitor levels of 5-FC because once serum levels exceed approximately 100 μg/mL, there is danger of marrow toxicity. In fact, it is this potential toxicity that has prompted the most caution in using 5-FC in HIV-positive and HIV-negative patients. With use of 5-FC monotherapy, it also became clear that the drug engendered very rapid development of resistance. Hence, it has come to be common practice that use of 5-FC inevitably is in combination with another antifungal drug. The most widely published and utilized combination therapy is that of AMB plus 5-FC. This combination often is used to treat cryptococcal meningitis and some invasive candidal infections. Although the combination also has shown some evidence of effectiveness against experimental aspergillosis, this has not translated well to humans with this infection.

The combination of AMB plus 5-FC has been described as synergistic in treating cryptococcal meningitis. Yet in animal models of this disease and other mycoses, the combination has been, at best, additive. The combination has never been shown to be better than optimal doses of AMB alone as relates to efficacy. However, the benefit of the combination lies in the reduction of AMB toxicity because a lower dose of the polyene may be employed. Of equal merit, the combination prevents the development of secondary drug resistance to 5-FC. With careful monitoring of 5-FC levels, therefore, the combination results in therapy that is at least as effective and less nephrotoxic as AMB alone. Many clinicians employ this combination as first-line therapy for cryptococcosis of the central nervous system.[38]

Enthusiasm has been generated for combination therapy using 5-FC plus FLU, again, mainly for cryptococcal meningitis in the patient with AIDS. The combination of 5-FC plus FLU is an attractive therapeutic option, given the benign side effects associated with FLU and the ease of oral administration of both agents. The differing mechanisms of action suggest that synergy is possible theoretically; FLU acts by damaging the fungal cell membrane, thereby allowing greater intracellular penetration of 5-FC. In vitro studies convincingly demonstrated the excellent synergistic effects of this combination. More recent in vivo investigations suggest that the combination should be employed for cryptococcal meningitis by exploiting the use of higher doses of FLU and lesser doses of 5-FC; this tactic allows excellent efficacy yet lowered toxicity potential associated with 5-FC.[39, 43] Two factors regarding clinical use of 5-FC remain constant: (1) monitoring of drug levels is required to assist in the prevention of potential bone marrow–associated toxicities, and (2) this agent should never be used as monotherapy because resistance likely will follow soon thereafter; it always is used in combination with another antifungal agent.

ECHINOCANDINS

Although considered the newest entries into the antifungal arena, the echinocandin drugs actually are not "new." The congeners of the compounds currently under development were reported many years ago in the plant pathology literature as inhibitors of cell wall synthesis in fungi causing plant-associated diseases. Two pharmaceutical companies are developing echinocandin-based compounds for the treatment of invasive mycoses. One early candidate of this class of agents, cilofungin, actually came to clinical testing in the early 1990s. However, difficulties with toxicity of the delivery vehicle in which cilofungin was administered and the limited spectrum of activity (active only against *C. albicans* and *C. tropicalis*) prevented further development.[28]

The current compounds are semisynthetic derivatives of the natural product class of antifungal echinocandins and are noncompetitive inhibitors of (1,3)-β-D-glucan synthase, which produces glucan polymers, a major component of fungal cell walls. These lipopeptide antifungal drugs essentially are inhibitors of synthesis of the fungal cell wall and thus unique among currently available antifungal drugs. In some ways, echinocandin derivatives may be viewed as the "penicillins" of antifungal agents, and theoretically these drugs should demonstrate tremendous selective toxicity because humans do not possess such a cell wall.[11]

L-743,872 is water-soluble and has demonstrated potent in vitro fungicidal activity against aspergilli, *Histoplasma capsulatum* variety *capsulatum, Candida* species (including triazole-resistant strains), and some other fungi. L-743,872 is the first in a new family of echinocandins, the pneumocandins, that is under development and blocks synthesis of glucans, which are essential components of fungal cell walls, hence, its fungicidal activity. If this compound reaches the marketplace, it will be one of the first fungicidal agents developed for use in humans since AMB and 5-FC. Animal efficacy studies showed that the compound had potent activity against systemic candidal infections in both immunocompetent and neutropenic mice. The compound exhibited excellent efficacy in both systemic and pulmonary models of aspergillosis as well as activity against the cyst form of pneumocystosis. L-743,872 is administered intravenously once daily and generally has been well tolerated in phase I clinical studies. The low oral absorption of this compound limits the use of L-743,872 to parenteral therapy. The compound is in phase II human clinical trials and has been well tolerated by patients.[1, 6]

The other echinocandin compound, LY-303366, demonstrates analogous properties to L-743,872 with some notable exceptions. This agent also prevents cell-wall (1,3)-β-D-glucan synthesis and also is fungicidal. Unlike L-743,872, however, this compound is not soluble in water and must be prepared for delivery or testing in a suitable vehicle. LY-303366 demonstrates in vitro activity against *Candida* species and in vivo activity against candidiasis, aspergillosis, and pneumocystosis. It is interesting that its in vitro activity against aspergilli is poor, at least as measured by current standardized methods, but that its in vivo activity is very good. It has been suggested that in vitro testing of compounds demonstrating such a discrepancy perhaps could be accomplished by examining effects of the antifungal lipopeptide upon alterations in fungal morphology rather than by measuring traditional MICs.[37] LY-303366 also is undergoing initial clinical trials, and it seems the compound will be delivered orally and topically rather than parenterally, as with L-743,872.[12] These echinocandin compounds merit close observation by the medical community as they undergo further development and testing. Should they prove to be safe and efficacious, these agents have great potential to alter current thinking about antifungal therapy because of their unique mode of action. If truly fungicidal and selectively toxic to only fungi, such drugs could be of immense benefit.

CHITIN INHIBITORS

Another biologic target unique to the fungal cell wall and lacking in humans is the N-acetylglucosamine polymer chitin. Chitin is an important cell wall constituent in many fungi, including many pathogenic for humans. Hence, there has been interest in seeking drugs that inhibit or prevent the synthesis of chitin as antifungal agents for human mycoses. The chemical classes of polyoxins and nikkomycins prevent synthesis of chitin via inhibition of chitin synthase, an enzyme crucial for this component of fungal cell wall building.[10] Early investigations of these two classes demonstrated that activity was present and effective in preventing chitin synthesis but was limited because of unfavorable pharmacokinetics.[28]

The nikkomycin class has received the bulk of attention, with nikkomycin Z (NKZ, SP-920704) currently undergoing clinical development. NKZ is a chemically modified nucleoside dipeptide obtained from secondary metabolites produced by the actinomycetous bacterium *Streptomyces tendae*. In vitro and in vivo studies have shown that NKZ is highly active and most effective against highly chitinous-containing fungi, such as *C. immitis* and *B. dermatitidis*, with lesser activity against yeasts and virtually no activity against aspergilli.[27] It also was reported that NKZ when combined with echinocandins demonstrated synergy, supporting the case for combining NKZ and some azole drugs. More recent in vitro studies of NKZ combined with FLU or ITRA have shown synergy with clinical isolates of *C. albicans, C. parapsilosis*, and some strains of *C. neoformans* variety *neoformans*. Very striking synergy between NKZ and the triazoles was noted with *C. immitis* as well as *Aspergillus fumigatus* and *Aspergillus flavus*. Interestingly, a similar effect was not observed with other species of *Aspergillus* (Li and associates, unpublished data, 1996).

The major hurdle for using NKZ to treat human infections most likely will be pharmacokinetic limitations. If current clinical trials demonstrate that these chitin inhibitors remain available in tissue and/or biologic fluids at sufficient levels and for enough time to exert their antifungal activity, then these agents also offer exciting possibilities for the future treatment of fungal infections.

OTHER ANTIFUNGAL AGENTS

Other agents for treating deep mycoses are being examined, and the interest in this area, as noted at the onset, is intense and ongoing. For example, an antifungal agent long used in Europe and approved only recently for use in the United States is terbinafine (Lamisil). This drug has been embraced widely by the global dermatological community for treating dermatophytic infections in general and onychomycosis in particular.[2, 65] This agent belongs to a class of drugs called the allylamines, is given both orally and topically, and has been very effective in these superficial mycoses, with the target sites being the stratum corneum and the nail plate. Terbinafine primarily has fungicidal action against many fungi as a result of its specific mechanism of squalene epoxidase inhibition. Treated fungi accumulate squalene while becoming deficient in membrane ergosterol. The cidal action is associated closely with the development of high intracellular squalene concentrations, which are believed to interfere with fungal membrane function and cell wall synthesis. In the case of *C. albicans*, it appears that growth inhibition with terbinafine results from ergosterol deficiency, with the filamentous form of the fungus being more susceptible than the yeast form.[60]

Many published studies involve the use of terbinafine to treat dermatophytoses,[18] but papers also suggesting efficacy in cases of chromoblastomycosis,[20] in nonimmunocomprised patients with bronchopulmonary aspergillosis,[62] and in candidiasis of the skin[34] but not in OPC in AIDS or HIV-positive patients. The manufacturer has instituted a systemic mycoses program in which clinical trials are planned to determine the effectiveness of terbinafine in the treatment of oral candidiasis, sporotrichosis, and invasive aspergillosis. Hence, this drug ultimately may be used to treat deep mycoses as well as dermatophytic fungal infections.

A final note involves the interest of combining immunomodulating agents with antifungal drugs in the hope of gaining better outcomes in those individuals with nonfunctional immunity and whose outcomes after infection with mycotic agents all too often are death. Various investigators have described administration of various cytokines and/or white blood cell–stimulating factors along with antifungal therapy to treat those patients who otherwise most certainly would die of their infection.[47, 48] Although there seems to be little doubt that some immunomodulating agents do, indeed, stimulate immune cells, enhanced survival from the fungal infections has not been demonstrated. Intense investigation will continue in this area, aided by the technologies of modern molecular genetics, with the expectation that the future may bring clinical successes in situations whose outcomes almost uniformly have been fatal.[36]

As revealed each month in the medical literature, more and more investigators are interested in and seeking means for more effective and safer therapy for mycotic infections. Furthermore, the pharmaceutical industry is expending more resources and demonstrating more interest in antimycotic drug development than ever before. It is, of course, hoped that research and development will continue to escalate with better and safer drugs.

PEDIATRICS AND ANTIFUNGAL DRUGS

Unfortunately, and far too often, antifungal drugs and guidelines for use, including recommended doses, pharmacokinetics, monitoring measures, safety, and toxicity profiles, are not available for infants or children. Human studies almost always are accomplished in normal adult volunteers and adults with mycotic infections. Pharmaceutical companies often have little or no information about their drugs as relates to appropriate and safe use in children. Pediatric clinicians often must make therapeutic decisions based on review of the adult literature and make adjustments based upon the physical attributes, mycosis, and nature of their patient's total medical picture. To be sure, there are some notable differences between drug administration and effects in children versus adults; such information is simply not always available for antifungal agents. Although some papers cover the use of some of the antifungal agents in children, there is, generally speaking, a genuine dearth of information.

The pediatric infectious diseases community, hematology-oncology clinicians, and those who care for children with HIV disease often gain "on-the-job" training in using these antifungal agents and, fortunately, share such knowledge with the broad pediatric community. It most certainly would be prudent and appropriate to seek collegial and drug company advice and to review the recent literature to ascertain proper dosing, possible drug-drug interactions, side effects and toxicities, and any contraindications or restrictions in a given patient-mycosis scenario. It is hoped that the future development of new antifungal drugs will include some consideration for pediatric use.

Contemporary medical practitioners are in the midst of a "golden age of medical mycology" in that mycoses and the drugs used to treat them have never been more important. It seems very likely that medicine will continue its onward advance of new therapies, diagnostic procedures, techniques, and technologies. With these positive events, however, it also seems very likely that we will continue to produce escalating numbers of "living Petri dishes," including children. This is, indeed, an exciting and challenging time for clinical mycology. The successful management of patients, particularly those with defective immunity, experiencing invasive fungal infections promises to be equally challenging.

References

1. Abruzzo, G., Flattery, A. M., Gill, C. J., et al.: Evaluation of water-soluble pneumocandin analogs L-733560, L-705589, and L-731373 with mouse models of disseminated aspergillosis, candidiasis, and cryptococcosis. Antimicrob. Agents Chemother. *39*:1077–1081, 1995.
2. Balfour, J. A., and Faulds, D.: Terbinafine: A review of its pharmacodynamic and pharmacokinetic properties, and therapeutic potential in superficial mycoses. Drugs *43*:259–284, 1992.
3. Barchiesi, F., Colombo, A. L., McGough, D. A., et al.: In vitro activity of itraconazole against fluconazole-susceptible and -resistant *Candida albicans* isolates from oral cavities of patients infected with human immunodeficiency virus. Antimicrob. Agents Chemother. *38*:1530–1533, 1994.
4. Barchiesi, F., Colombo, A. L., McGough, D. A., et al.: In vitro activity of a new antifungal triazole, D0870, against *Candida albicans* isolates from oral cavities of patients infected with human immunodeficiency virus. Antimicrob. Agents Chemother. *38*:2553–2556, 1994.
5. Brajtburg, J., and Bolard, J.: Carrier effects on biological activity of amphotericin B. Clin. Microbiol. Rev. *9*:512–531, 1996.
6. Bartizal, K., Scott, G., Abruzzo, G. K., et al.: In vitro evaluation of the pneumocandin antifungal agent L-733560, a new water-soluble hybrid of L-705589 and L-731373. Antimicrob. Agents Chemother. *39*:1070–1076, 1995.
7. Bowden, R. A., Cays, M., Gooley, T., et al.: Phase I study of amphotericin B colloidal dispersion for the treatment of invasive fungal infections after marrow transplant. J. Infect. Dis. *173*:1208–1215, 1996.
8. Brodell, R. T., and Elewski, B. E.: Clinical pearl: Systemic antifungal drugs and drug interactions. J. Am. Acad. Dermatol. *33*:259–260, 1995.
9. Como, J. A., and Dismukes, W. E.: Drug therapy: Oral azole drugs as systemic antifungal therapy. N. Engl. J. Med. *330*:263–272, 1994.
10. Decker, H., Zahner, H., Heitsch, H., et al.: Structure-activity relationships of the nikkomycins. J. Gen. Microbiol. *137*(Pt. 8):1805–1813, 1991.
11. Debono, M., and Gordee, R. S.: Antibiotics that inhibit fungal cell wall development. Ann. Rev. Microbiol. *48*:471–497, 1994.
12. Debono, M., Turner, W. W., LaGrandeur, L., et al.: Semisynthetic chemical modification of the antifungal lipopeptide echinocandin B (ECB): Structure-activity studies of the lipophilic and geometric parameters of polyarylated acyl analogs of ECB. J. Medicinal Chem. *38*:3271–3281, 1995.
13. de Marie, S.: Liposomal and lipid-based formulations of amphotericin B. Leukemia *10*(Suppl. 2):S93–S96, 1996.
14. Denning, D. W., Lee, J. Y., Hostetler, J. S., et al.: NIAID Mycoses Study Group multicenter trial of oral itraconazole therapy for invasive aspergillosis. Am. J. Med. *97*:135–144, 1994.
15. Denning, D. W.: Therapeutic outcome in invasive aspergillosis. Clin. Infect. Dis. *23*:608–615, 1996.
16. Dib, J. C., Dubé, M., Kelly, C., et al.: Evaluation of pulsed-field gel electrophoresis as a typing system for *Candida rugosa*: Comparison of karyotype and restriction fragment length polymorphisms. J. Clin. Microbiol. *34*:1494–1496, 1996.
17. Dubé, M. P., Heseltine, P. N. R., Rinaldi, M. G., et al.: Fungemia and colonization with nystatin-resistant *Candida rugosa* in a burn unit. Clin. Infect. Dis. *18*:77–82, 1994.

18. Elewski, B. E.: Cutaneous mycoses in children. Br. J. Dermatol. *134*(Suppl. 46:7–11; discussion 37–38), 1996.
19. Ellerbrock, T., Wright, T., Fothergill, A., et al.: Fluconazole resistance of yeast isolates from HIV+ women. Abstract presented at the 4th Conference on Retroviruses and Opportunistic Infections, January 22–26, 1997, Washington, D.C.
20. Esterre, P., Inzan, C. K., Ramarcel, E. R., et al.: Treatment of chromomycosis with terbinafine: Preliminary results of an open pilot study. Br. J. Dermatol. *134*(Suppl. 46:33–36; discussion 40), 1996.
21. Francis, P., and Walsh, T. J.: Evolving role of flucytosine in immunocompromised patients: New insights into safety, pharmacokinetics, and antifungal therapy. Clin. Infect. Dis. *15*:1003–1018, 1992.
22. Galgiani, J. N., Catanzaro, A., Cloud, G. A., et al.: Fluconazole therapy for coccidioidal meningitis. Ann. Intern. Med. *119*:28–35, 1993.
23. Galgiani, J. N., and Lewis, M. L.: In vitro studies of activities of the antifungal triazoles SCH56592 and itraconazole against *Candida albicans, Cryptococcus neoformans,* and other pathogenic yeasts. Antimicrob. Agents Chemother. *41*:180–183, 1997.
24. Gallis, H. A., Drew, R. H., and Pickard, W. W.: Amphotericin B: 30 years of clinical experience. Rev. Infect. Dis. *12*:308–329, 1990.
25. Graybill, J. R.: The future of antifungal therapy. Clin. Infect. Dis. *22*:S166–S178, 1996.
26. Hay, R. J.: Antifungal drugs. Q. J. Med. *88*:681–684, 1995.
27. Hector, R. F., Zimmer, B. L., and Pappagianis, D.: Evaluation of nikkomycins X and Z in murine models of coccidioidomycosis, histoplasmosis, and blastomycosis. Antimicrob. Agents Chemother. *34*:587–593, 1990.
28. Hector, R. F.: Compounds active against cell walls of medically important fungi. Clin. Microbiol. Rev. *6*:1–21, 1993.
29. Heit, M. C., and Riviere, J. E.: Antifungal therapy: Ketoconazole and other azole derivatives. Compend. Contin. Educ. Pract. Vet. *17*:21–34, 1995.
30. Hitchcock, C. A., Pye, G. W., Oliver, G. P., et al.: UK-109,496, a novel, wide-spectrum triazole derivative for the treatment of fungal infections: Antifungal activity and selectivity in vitro. Abstract F72, p. 125, Program and Abstracts of the 35th Interscience Conference on Antimicrobial Agents and Chemotherapy, September 17–20, San Francisco, CA, 1995.
31. Hoeprich, P. D.: Chemotherapy for systemic mycoses. Prog. Drug. Res. *33*:317–351, 1989.
32. Horsburgh, C. R., and Kirkpatrick, C. H.: Long-term therapy of chronic mucocutaneous candidiasis with ketoconazole: Experience with twenty-one patients. Am. J. Med. *74*:23–29, 1983.
33. Jezeequel, S. G., Clark, M., Cole, S., et al.: UK-109,496, a novel, wide-spectrum triazole derivative for the treatment of fungal infections: Preclinical pharmacokinetics. Abstract F76, p. 126, Program and Abstracts of the 35th Interscience Conference on Antimicrobial Agents and Chemotherapy, September 17–20, San Francisco, CA, 1995.
34. Jung, E. G., Haas, P. J., Brautigam, M., et al.: Systemic treatment of skin candidosis: A randomized comparison of terbinafine and ketoconazole. Mycoses *37*:361–365, 1994.
35. Kahn, G.: Systemic antifungal drugs and drug interactions. J. Am. Acad. Dermatol. *35*:134–135, 1996.
36. Kibbler, C. C., and Prentice, H. G.: What is the risk of infection in patients undergoing peripheral blood stem cell transplantation? Curr. Opin. Infect. Dis. *9*:215–217, 1996.
37. Kurtz, M. B., Heath, I. B., Marrinan, J., et al.: Morphological effects of lipopeptides against *Aspergillus fumigatus* correlate with activities against (1,3)-beta-D-glucan synthase. Antimicrob. Agents Chemother. *38*:1480–1489, 1994.
38. Kwon-Chung, K. J., and Bennett, J. E.: Medical Mycology. Philadelphia, Lea & Febiger, 1992, pp. 81–102.
39. Larsen, R. A., Bauer, M., Weiner, J. M., et al.: Effect of fluconazole on fungicidal activity of flucytosine in murine cryptococcal meningitis. Antimicrob. Agents Chemother. *40*:2178–2182, 1996.
40. MacPhail, L. A., Hilton, J. F., Dodd, C. L., et al.: Prophylaxis with nystatin pastilles for HIV-associated oral candidiasis. J. Acquir. Immune Defic. Syndr. Hum. Retrovirol. *12*:470–476, 1996.
41. Martin, M. V., Yates, J., and Hitchcock, C. A.: Comparison of voriconazole (UK-109,496) and itraconazole in prevention and treatment of *Aspergillus fumigatus* endocarditis in guinea pigs. Antimicrob. Agents Chemother. *41*:13–16, 1997.
42. Mehta, R. T., Hopfer, R. L., Gunner, L. A., et al.: Formulation, toxicity, and antifungal activities in vitro of liposome-encapsulated nystatin as a therapeutic agent for systemic candidiasis. Antimicrob. Agents Chemother. *31*:1897–1900, 1987.
43. Nguyen, M. H., Barchiesi, F., McGough, D. A., et al.: In vitro evaluation of combination of fluconazole and flucytosine against *Cryptococcus neoformans* var. *neoformans*. Antimicrob. Agents Chemother. *39*:1691–1695, 1995.
44. Nguyen, M. H., Morris, A. J., Dobson, M. E., et al.: *Candida lusitaniae*: An important emerging cause of candidemia. Infect. Dis. Clin. Prac. *5*:273–278, 1996.
45. Nguyen, M. H., Peacock, J. E., Morris, A. J., et al.: The changing face of candidemia: Emergence of non-*Candida albicans* species and antifungal resistance. Am. J. Med. *100*:617–623, 1996.
46. Nolte, F. S., Parkinson, T., Falconer, D. J., et al.: Isolation and characterization of fluconazole and amphotericin B-resistant *Candida albicans* from blood of two patients with leukemia. Antimicrob. Agents Chemother. *41*:196–199, 1997.
47. Pagano, L., Morace, G., Barbera, E. O.-L., et al.: Adjuvant therapy with rhGM-CSF for the treatment of *Blastoschizomyces capitatus* systemic infection in a patient with acute myeloid leukemia. Ann. Hematol. *73*:33–34, 1996.
48. Peters, B. G., Adkins, D. R., Harrison, B. R., et al.: Antifungal effects of yeast-derived rhu-GM-CSF in patients receiving high-dose chemotherapy given with or without autologous stem cell transplantation: A retrospective analysis. Bone Marrow Transplant. *18*:93–102, 1996.
49. Pfaller, M. A.: Epidemiology and control of fungal infections. Clin. Infect. Dis. 19(Suppl. 1):S8–S13, 1994.
50. Phillips, P., Zemcov, I., Mahmood, W., et al.: Itraconazole cyclodextrin solution for fluconazole-refractory oropharyngeal candidiasis in AIDS: Correlation of clinical response with in vitro susceptibility. AIDS *10*:1369–1376, 1996.
51. Powderly, W. G., Kobayashi, G. S., Herzig, G. P., et al.: Amphotericin B-resistant yeast infection in severely immuno-compromised patients. Am. J. Med. *84*:826–832, 1988.
52. Powderly, W. G., Keath, E. J., Sokol-Anderson, M., et al.: Amphotericin B-resistant *Cryptococcus neoformans* in a patient with AIDS. Infect. Dis. Clin. Prac. *1*:314–316, 1992.
53. Redding, S., Smith, J., Farinacci, G., et al.: Resistance of *Candida albicans* to fluconazole during treatment of oropharyngeal candidiasis in a patient with AIDS: Documentation of in vitro susceptibility testing and DNA subtype analysis. Clin. Infect. Dis. *18*:240–242, 1994.
54. Redkar, R. J., Dubé, M. P., McCleskey, F. K., et al.: DNA fingerprinting of *Candida rugosa* via repetitive sequence-based PCR. J. Clin. Microbiol. *34*:1677–1681, 1996.
55. Revankar, S. G., Kirkpatrick, W. R., McAtee, R. K., et al.: Detection and significance of fluconazole resistance in oropharyngeal candidiasis in human immunodeficiency virus-infected patients. J. Infect. Dis. *174*:821–827, 1996.
56. Rex, J. H., Pfaller, M. A., Rinaldi, M. G., et al.: Antifungal susceptibility testing. Clin. Microbiol. Rev. *6*:367–381, 1993.
57. Rex, J. H., Rinaldi, M. G., and Pfaller, M. A.: Resistance of *Candida* species to fluconazole. Antimicrob. Agents Chemother. *39*:1–8, 1995.
58. Rinaldi, M. G., and Hoeprich, P. D.: Murine adaptive catabolism of clotrimazole. Abstract 123, Annual Meeting of the American Society for Microbiology, May, Minneapolis, MN, 1972.
59. Rosa, R. H., Jr., Miller, D., and Alfonso, E. C.: The changing spectrum of fungal keratitis in south Florida. Ophthalmology *101*:1005–1013, 1994.
60. Ryder, N. S.: Terbinafine: Mode of action and properties of the squalene epoxidase inhibition. Br. J. Dermatol. *126*(Suppl. 39:2–7), 1992.
61. Schaffner, A., and Frick, P. G.: The effect of ketoconazole on amphotericin B in a model of disseminated aspergillosis. J. Infect. Dis. *151*:902–910, 1985.
62. Schiraldi, G. F., Colombo, M. D., Harari, S., et al.: Terbinafine in the treatment of non-immunocompromised compassionate cases of bronchopulmonary aspergillosis. Mycoses *39*:5–12, 1996.
63. Schutze, G. E.: Oral azole drugs as systemic antifungal therapy. N. Engl. J. Med. *330*:1759–1760, 1994.
64. Sievers, T. M., Kubak, B. M., and Wong-Beringer, A.: Safety and efficacy of intralipid emulsions of amphotericin B. J. Antimicrob. Chemother. *38*:333–347, 1996.
65. Smith, E. B.: Terbinafine: A new topically and systemically effective allylamine antifungal. Introduction. J. Am. Acad. Dermatol. *23*:775–776, 1990.
66. Stringer, J. R.: *Pneumocystis carinii*: What is it, exactly? Clin. Microbiol. Rev. *9*:489–498, 1996.
67. Sugar, A. M., Hitchcock, C. A., Troke, P. F., et al.: Combination therapy of murine invasive candidiasis with fluconazole and amphotericin B. Antimicrob. Agents Chemother. *39*:598–601, 1995.
68. Sugar, A. M.: Use of amphotericin B with azole antifungal drugs: What are we doing? Antimicrob. Agents Chemother. *39*:1907–1912, 1995.
69. Walsh, T. J., Melcher, G. P., Rinaldi, M. G., et al.: *Trichosporon beigelii*, an emerging pathogen resistant to amphotericin Br. J. Clin. Microbiol. *28*:1616–1622, 1990.
70. Wardle, H. M., Law, D., Moore, C. B., et al.: In vitro activity of D0870 compared with those of other azoles against fluconazole-resistant *Candida* spp. Antimicrob. Agents Chemother. *39*:868–871, 1995.
71. Yotsuji, A., Shimizu, K., Araki, H., et al.: T-8581, a new orally and parenterally active triazole antifungal agent: In vitro and in vivo evaluations. Antimicrob. Agents Chemother. *41*:30–34, 1997.

235

Drugs for Parasitic Infections

The Medical Letter

Parasitic infections are found throughout the world. With increasing travel, immigration, use of immunosuppressive drugs, and the spread of AIDS, physicians anywhere may see infections caused by previously unfamiliar parasites. The table below lists first-choice and alternative drugs for most parasitic infections.

From the Medical Letter on Drugs and Therapeutics, Volume 37, Issue 961, November 10, 1995. Material is reprinted by special permission of the publisher.

Drugs for Treatment of Parasitic Infections

Infection		Drug	Adult Dosage	Pediatric Dosage*
AMEBIASIS *(Entamoeba histolytica)*[1]				
Asymptomatic				
Drug of choice:		Iodoquinol[2]	650 mg tid × 20 d	30–40 mg/kg/d in 3 doses × 20 d
	OR	Paromomycin	25–35 mg/kg/d in 3 doses × 7 d	25–35 mg/kg/d in 3 doses × 7 d
Alternative:		Diloxanide furoate[3]	500 mg tid × 10 d	20 mg/kg/d in 3 doses × 10 d
Mild to moderate intestinal disease				
Drug of choice[4]:		Metronidazole	750 mg tid × 10 d	35–50 mg/kg/d in 3 doses × 10 d
	OR	Tinidazole[5]	2 g/d × 3 d	50 mg/kg (max. 2 g) qd × 3 d
Severe intestinal disease, hepatic abscess				
Drug of choice:		Metronidazole	750 mg tid × 10 d	35–50 mg/kg/d in 3 doses × 10 d
	OR	Tinidazole[5]	600 mg bid or 800 mg tid × 5 d	50 mg/kg or 60 mg/kg (max. 2 g) qd × 3 d
AMEBIC *(Acanthamoeba)* keratitis				
Drug of choice:		See footnote 6		
AMEBIC MENINGOENCEPHALITIS, PRIMARY				
Naegleria				
Drug of choice:		Amphotericin B[7, 8]	1 mg/kg/d IV, uncertain duration	1 mg/kg/d IV, uncertain duration
Acanthamoeba				
Drug of choice:		See footnote 9		
ANCYLOSTOMA *caninum* (Eosinophilic enterocolitis)				
Drug of choice:		Mebendazole	100 mg bid × 3 d	100 mg bid × 3 d
	OR	Pyrantel pamoate[8]	11 mg/kg (max. 1 g) × 3 d	11 mg/kg (max. 1 g) × 3 d
	OR	Albendazole	400 mg once	400 mg once
Ancylostoma duodenale, see HOOKWORM				
ANGIOSTRONGYLIASIS				
Angiostrongylus cantonensis				
Drug of choice[10]:		Mebendazole[8]	100 mg bid × 5 d	100 mg bid × 5 d
Angiostrongylus costaricensis				
Drug of choice:		Thiabendazole[8]	75 mg/kg/d in 3 doses × 3 d (max. 3 g/d)[11]	75 mg/kg/d in 3 doses × 3 d (max. 3 g/d)[11]
Alternative:		Mebendazole	200–400 mg tid × 10 d	200–400 mg tid × 10 d
ANISAKIASIS *(Anisakis)*				
Treatment of choice:		Surgical or endoscopic removal		
ASCARIASIS *(Ascaris lumbricoides, roundworm)*				
Drug of choice:		Mebendazole	100 mg bid × 3 d	100 mg bid × 3 d
	OR	Pyrantel pamoate	11 mg/kg once (max. 1 g)	11 mg/kg once (max. 1 g)
	OR	Albendazole	400 mg once	400 mg once

Table continued on following page

Drugs for Treatment of Parasitic Infections *Continued*

Infection	Drug	Adult Dosage	Pediatric Dosage*
BABESIOSIS (*Babesia* species)			
Drugs of choice[12]:	Clindamycin[8]	1.2 grams bid IV or 600 mg tid PO × 7 d	20–40 mg/kg/d in 3 doses × 7 d
	plus quinine	650 mg tid PO × 7 d	25 mg/kg/d in 3 doses × 7 d
BALANTIDIASIS (*Balantidium coli*)			
Drug of choice:	Tetracycline[8]	500 mg qid × 10 d	40 mg/kg/d in 4 doses × 10 d (max. 2 g/d)[13]
Alternatives:	Iodoquinol[2, 8]	650 mg tid × 20 d	40 mg/kg/d in 3 doses × 20 d
	Metronidazole[8]	750 mg tid × 5 d	35–50 mg/kg/d in 3 doses × 5 d
BAYLISASCARIASIS (*Baylisascaris procyonis*)			
Drug of choice:	See footnote 14		
BLASTOCYSTIS *hominis* infection			
Drug of choice:	See footnote 15		
CAPILLARIASIS (*Capillaria phillippinensis*)			
Drug of choice:	Mebendazole[8]	200 mg bid × 20 d	200 mg bid × 20 d
Alternatives:	Albendazole	200 mg bid × 10 d	200 mg bid × 10 d
	Thiabendazole[8]	25 mg/kg/d in 2 doses × 30 d	25 mg/kg/d in 2 doses × 30 d
Chagas' disease, see TRYPANOSOMIASIS			
Clonorchis sinensis, see FLUKE infection			
CRYPTOSPORIDIOSIS (*Cryptosporidium*)			
Drug of choice[16]:	Paromomycin	500–750 mg qid	
CUTANEOUS LARVA MIGRANS (creeping eruption, dog and cat hookworm)			
Drug of choice[17]:	Thiabendazole	Topically ± 50 mg/kg/d PO in 2 doses (max. 3 g/d) × 2–5 d[11]	Topically ± 50 mg/kg/d PO in 2 doses (max. 3 g/d) × 2–5 d[11]
OR	Ivermectin	150–200 μg/kg once	150–200 μg/kg once
OR	Albendazole	200 mg bid × 3 d	200 mg bid × 3 d
CYCLOSPORA infection			
Drug of choice:	Trimethoprim-sulfamethoxazole[18]	TMP 160 mg, SMX 800 mg bid × 7 d	TMP 5 mg/kg, SMX 25 mg/kg bid × 7 d
CYSTICERCOSIS, see TAPEWORM infection			
DIENTAMOEBA *fragilis* infection			
Drug of choice:	Iodoquinol[2]	650 mg tid × 20 d	40 mg/kg/d in 3 doses × 20 d
OR	Paromomycin	25–30 mg/kg/d in 3 doses × 7 d	25–30 mg/kg/d in 3 doses × 7 d
OR	Tetracycline[8]	500 mg qid × 10 d	40 mg/kg/d (max. 2 g/d) in 4 doses × 10 d[13]
Diphyllobothrium latum, see TAPEWORM infection			
DRACUNCULUS *medinensis* (guinea worm) infection			
Drug of choice:	Metronidazole[8, 19]	250 mg tid ×10 d	25 mg/kg/d (max. 750 mg/d) in 3 doses × 10 d
Alternative:	Thiabendazole[8, 19]	50–75 mg/kg/d in 2 doses × 3 d[11]	50–75 mg/kg/d in 2 doses × 3 d[11]
Echinococcus, see TAPEWORM infection			
Entamoeba histolytica, see AMEBIASIS			
ENTAMOEBA *polecki* infection			
Drug choice:	Metronidazole[8]	750 mg tid × 10 d	35–50 mg/kg/d in 3 doses × 10 d
ENTEROBIUS *vermicularis* (pinworm) infection			
Drug of choice:	Pyrantel pamoate	11 mg/kg once (max. 1 g); repeat after 2 wk	11 mg/kg once (max. 1 g); repeat after 2 wk
OR	Mebendazole	A single dose of 100 mg; repeat after 2 wk	A single dose of 100 mg; repeat after 2 wk
OR	Albendazole	400 mg once; repeat in 2 wk	400 mg once; repeat in 2 wk
Fasciola hepatica, see FLUKE infection			

Drugs for Treatment of Parasitic Infections *Continued*

Infection	Drug	Adult Dosage	Pediatric Dosage*
FILARIASIS			
Wuchereria bancrofti, Brugia malayi			
Drug of choice[20]:	Diethylcarbamazine[21]	Day 1: 50 mg PC Day 2: 50 mg tid Day 3: 100 mg tid Days 4 through 21: 6 mg/kg/d in 3 doses[22]	Day 1: 1 mg/kg PC Day 2: 1 mg/kg tid Day 3: 1–2 mg/kg tid Days 4 through 21: 6 mg/kg/d in 3 doses[22]
Loa loa			
Drug of choice[23]:	Diethylcarbamazine[21]	Day 1: 50 mg PO or PC Day 2: 50 mg tid Day 3: 100 mg tid Days 4 through 21: 9 mg/kg/d in 3 doses[22]	Day 1: 1 mg/kg PO or PC Day 2: 1 mg/kg tid Day 3: 1–2 mg/kg tid Days 4 through 21: 9 mg/kg/d in 3 doses[22]
Mansonella ozzardi			
Drug of choice:	See footnote 24		
Mansonella perstans			
Drug of choice:	Mebendazole[8]	100 mg bid × 30 d	
Tropical pulmonary eosinophilia			
Drug of choice:	Diethylcarbamazine	6 mg/kg/d in 3 doses × 21 d	6 mg/kg/d in 3 doses × 21 d
Onchocerca volvulus			
Drug of choice:	Ivermectin[3]	150 μg/kg once, repeated every 3 to 12 mo	150 μg/kg once, repeated every 3 to 12 mo
FLUKE, hermaphroditic, infection			
Clonorchis sinensis (Chinese liver fluke)			
Drug of choice:	Praziquantel	75 mg/kg/d in 3 doses × 1 d	75 mg/kg/d in 3 doses × 1 d
OR	Albendazole	10 mg/kg × 7 d	
Fasciola hepatica (sheep liver fluke)			
Drug of choice[25]:	Bithionol[3]	30–50 mg/kg on alternate days × 10–15 doses	30–50 mg/kg on alternate days × 10–15 doses
Fasciolopsis buski (intestinal fluke)			
Drug of choice:	Praziquantel[8]	75 mg/kg/d in 3 doses × 1 d	75 mg/kg/d in 3 doses × 1 d
Heterophyes heterophyes (intestinal fluke)			
Drug of choice:	Praziquantel[8]	75 mg/kg/d in 3 doses × 1 d	75 mg/kg/d in 3 doses × 1 d
Metagonimus yokogawai (intestinal fluke)			
Drug of choice:	Praziquantel[8]	75 mg/kg/d in 3 doses × 1 d	75 mg/kg/d in 3 doses × 1 d
Nanophyetus salmincola			
Drug of choice:	Praziquantel[8]	60 mg/kg/d in 3 doses × 1 d	60 mg/kg/d in 3 doses × 1 d
Opisthorchis viverrini (liver fluke)			
Drug of choice:	Praziquantel	75 mg/kg/d in 3 doses × 1 d	75 mg/kg/d in 3 doses × 1 d
Paragonimus westermani (lung fluke)			
Drug of choice:	Praziquantel[8]	75 mg/kg/d in 3 doses × 2 d	75 mg/kg/d in 3 doses × 2 d
Alternative[26]:	Bithionol[3]	30–50 mg/kg on alternate days × 10–15 doses	30–50 mg/kg on alternate days × 10–15 doses
GIARDIASIS *(Giardia lamblia)*			
Drug of choice:	Metronidazole[8]	250 mg tid × 5 d	15 mg/kg/d in 3 doses × 5 d
Alternatives[27]:	Tinidazole[5]	2 g once	50 mg/kg once (max. 2 g)
	Furazolidone	100 mg qid × 7–10 d	6 mg/kg/d in 4 doses × 7–10 d
	Paromomycin[28]	25–35 mg/kg/d in 3 doses × 7 d	
GNATHOSTOMIASIS *(Gnathostoma spinigerum)*			
Treatment of choice[29]:	Surgical removal **plus** albendazole[30]	400–800 mg qd × 21 d	
HOOKWORM infection *(Ancyclostoma duodenale, Necator americanus)*			
Drug of choice:	Mebendazole	100 mg bid × 3 d	100 mg bid × 3 d
OR	Pyrantel pamoate[8]	11 mg/kg (max. 1 g) × 3 d	11 mg/kg (max. 1 g) × 3 d
OR	albendazole	400 mg once	400 mg once
Hydatid cyst, see TAPEWORM infection			
Hymenolepis nana, see TAPEWORM infection			
ISOSPORIASIS *(Isospora belli)*			
Drug of choice:	Trimethoprim-sulfamethoxazole[8, 31]	160 mg TMP, 800 mg SMX qid × 10 d, then bid × 3 wk	

Table continued on following page

Drugs for Treatment of Parasitic Infections *Continued*

Infection	Drug	Adult Dosage	Pediatric Dosage*
LEISHMANIASIS *(Leishmania mexicana, L. tropica, L. major, L. braziliensis, L. donovani* [kala-azar])			
Drug of choice:	Sodium stibogluconate[3]	20 mg Sb/kg/d IV or IM × 20–28 d[32]	20 mg Sb/kg/d IV or IM × 20–28 d[32]
OR	Meglumine antimonate	20 mg Sb/kg/d × 20–28 d[32]	20 mg Sb/kg/d × 20–28 d[32]
Alternatives[33]:	Amphotericin B[8]	0.25 to 1 mg/kg by slow infusion daily or every 2 d for up to 8 wk	0.25 to 1 mg/kg by slow infusion daily or every 2 d for up to 8 wk
	Pentamidine isethionate[8]	2–4 mg/kg daily or every 2 d IM for up to 15 doses[32]	2–4 mg/kg daily or every 2 d IM for up to 15 doses[32]
LICE infestation *(Pediculus humanus, capitis, Phthirus pubis)*[34]			
Drug of choice:	1% permethrin[35]	Topically	Topically
OR	0.5% malathion	Topically	Topically
Alternative:	Pyrethrins with piperonyl butoxide	Topically[36]	Topically[36]
Loa loa, see FILARIASIS			
MALARIA, Treatment of *(Plasmodium falciparum, P. ovale, P. vivax,* and *P. malariae)*			
Chloroquine-resistant *P. falciparum*[37]			
ORAL			
Drugs of choice:	Quinine sulfate **plus**	650 mg q8h × 3–7 d[38]	25 mg/kg/d in 3 doses × 3–7 d[38]
	pyrimethamine-sulfadoxine[39]	3 tablets at once on last day of quinine	<1 yr: ¼ tablet 1–3 yr: ½ tablet 4–8 yr: 1 tablet 9–14 yr: 2 tablets
OR	**plus** tetracycline[8]	250 mg qid × 7 d	20 mg/kg/d in 4 doses × 7 d[13]
OR[40]	**plus** clindamycin[8]	900 mg tid × 3–5 d	20–40 mg/kg/d in 3 doses × 3–5 d
Alternatives[41]:	Mefloquine[42, 43]	1250 mg[44]	25 mg/kg once[45] (<45 kg)
	Halofantrine[46]	500 mg q6h × 3 doses; repeat in 1 wk	8 mg/kg q6h × 3 doses (<40 kg); repeat in 1 wk
PARENTERAL			
Drug of choice[47, 48]:	Quinidine gluconate[49, 50]	10 mg/kg loading dose (max. 600 mg) in normal saline slowly over 1 to 2 hr, followed by continuous infusion of 0.02 mg/kg/min until oral therapy can be started	Same as adult dose
OR	Quinine dihydrochloride[50, 51]	20 mg/kg loading dose in 10 mg/kg 5% dextrose over 4 hr, followed by 10 mg/kg over 2–4 hr q8h (max. 1800 mg/d) until oral therapy can be started	Same as adult dose
All *Plasmodium* except chloroquine-resistant *P. falciparum*[37]			
ORAL			
Drug of choice:	Chloroquine phosphate[52, 53]	1 g (600 mg base), then 500 mg (300 mg base) 6 hr later, then 500 mg (300 mg base) at 24 and 48 hr	10 mg base/kg (max. 600 mg base), then 5 mg base/kg 6 hr later, then 5 mg base/kg at 24 and 48 hr
PARENTERAL			
Drug of choice[48]:	Quinidine gluconate[49, 50]	Same as above	Same as above
OR	Quinine dihydrochloride[50, 51]	Same as above	Same as above
Prevention of relapses: *P. vivax* and *P. ovale* only			
Drug of choice:	Primaquine phosphate[54, 55]	26.3 mg (15 mg base)/d × 14 d or 79 mg (45 mg base)/wk × 8 wk	0.3 mg base/kg/d × 14 d
MALARIA, Prevention of[56, 57]			
Chloroquine-sensitive areas			
Drug of choice:	Chloroquine phosphate[58]	500 mg (300 mg base), once/wk[59]	5 mg/kg base once/wk, up to adult dose of 300 mg base
Chloroquine-resistant areas[37]			
Drug of choice[60]:	Mefloquine[43, 58, 61]	250 mg once/wk[59]	15–19 kg: ¼ tablet 20–30 kg: ½ tablet 31–45 kg: ¾ tablet >45 kg: 1 tablet
OR	Doxycycline[58, 62]	100 mg daily[62]	>8 yr: 2 mg/kg/d, up to 100 mg/d

Drugs for Treatment of Parasitic Infections *Continued*

Infection	Drug	Adult Dosage	Pediatric Dosage*
MALARIA *(Continued)*			
Alternatives:	Chloroquine phosphate[58] **plus** pyrimethamine-sulfadoxine[39] for presumptive treatment	Same as above Carry a single dose (3 tablets) for self-treatment of febrile illness when medical care is not immediately available	Same as above <1 yr: ¼ tablet 1–3 yr: ½ tablet 4–8 yr: 1 tablet 9–14 yr: 2 tablets
	OR **plus** proguanil[63] (in Africa south of the Sahara)	200 mg daily	<2 yr: 50 mg daily 2–6 yr: 100 mg daily 7–10 yr: 150 mg daily >10 yr: 200 mg daily
MICROSPORIDIOSIS			
Ocular *(Encephalitozoon hellem, Vittaforma corneae [Nosema corneum])*			
Drug of choice:	See footnote 64		
Intestinal *(Enterocytozoon bieneusi, Septata [Encephalitozoon] intestinalis)*			
Drug of choice:	See footnote 65		
Disseminated (*Encephalitozoon hellem, Encephalitozoon cuniculi, Pleistophora* species)			
Drug of choice:	See footnote 66		
Mites, see SCABIES			
MONILIFORMIS *moniliformis* infection			
Drug of choice:	Pyrantel pamoate[8]	11 mg/kg once, repeat twice, 2 wk apart	11 mg/kg once, repeat twice, 2 wk apart
***Naegleria* species,** see AMEBIC MENINGOENCEPHALITIS, PRIMARY			
Necator americanus, see HOOKWORM infection			
OESOPHAGOSTOMUM *bifurcum*			
Drug of choice:	See footnote 67		
Onchocerca volvulus, see FILARIASIS			
Opisthorchis viverrini, see FLUKE infection			
Paragonimus westermani, see FLUKE infection			
Pediculus capitis, humanus, Phthirus pubis, see LICE			
Pinworm, see ENTEROBIUS			
PNEUMOCYSTIS *carinii* pneumonia[68]			
Drug of choice:	Trimethoprim-sulfamethoxazole	TMP 15 mg/kg/d, SMX 75 mg/kg/d PO or IV in 3 or 4 doses × 14–21 d[69]	Same as adult dose
Alternatives[70]:	Pentamidine	3–4 mg/kg IV qd × 14–21 d[69]	Same as adult dose
	Trimetrexate	45 mg/m² IV qd × 21 d	
	plus folinic acid	20 mg/m² PO or IV q6h × 21 d	
	Trimethoprim[8]	5 mg/kg PO tid × 21 d	
	plus dapsone[8]	100 mg PO qd × 21 d	
	Altovaquone suspension	750 mg bid PO × 21 d	
	Primaquine[8, 55]	15 mg base PO qd × 21 d	
	plus clindamycin[8]	600 mg IV q6h × 21 d, or 300–450 mg PO q6h × 21 d	
Primary and secondary prophylaxis			
Drug of choice:	Trimethoprim-sulfamethoxazole	1 dissolved tablet PO qd or 3×/wk	TMP 150 mg, SMX 750 mg in 2 doses PO 3×/wk
Alternatives:	Dapsone[8]	50–100 mg PO qd or 100 mg PO 2×/wk	2 mg/kg PO qd
	± pyrimethamine[71]	50 mg PO 2×/wk	
	Aerosol pentamidine	300 mg inhaled monthly via *Respirgard II* nebulizer	>5 yr: same as adult dose
Roundworm, see ASCARIASIS			
SCABIES *(Sarcoptes scabiei)*			
Drug of choice:	5% permethrin	Topically	Topically
Alternatives:	Ivermectin	200 μ/kg PO once	200 μg/kg PO once
	10% crotamiton	Topically	Topically

Table continued on following page

Drugs for Treatment of Parasitic Infections *Continued*

Infection	Drug	Adult Dosage	Pediatric Dosage*
SCHISTOSOMIASIS *(Bilharziasis)*			
Schistosoma haematobium			
Drug of choice:	Praziquantel	40 mg/kg/d in 2 doses × 1 d	40 mg/kg/d in 2 doses × 1 d
S. japonicum			
Drug of choice:	Praziquantel	60 mg/kg/d in 3 doses × 1 d	60 mg/kg/d in 3 doses × 1 d
S. mansoni			
Drug of choice:	Praziquantel	40 mg/kg/d in 2 doses × 1 d	40 mg/kg/d in 2 doses × 1 d
Alternative:	Oxamniquine[72]	15 mg/kg once[73]	20 mg/kg/d in 2 doses × 1 d[73]
S. mekongi			
Drug of choice:	Praziquantel	60 mg/kg/d in 3 doses × 1 d	60 mg/kg/d in 3 doses × 1 d
Sleeping sickness, see TRYPANOSOMIASIS			
STRONGYLOIDIASIS *(Strongyloides stercoralis)*			
Drug of choice[74]:	Thiabendazole	50 mg/kg/d in 2 doses (max. 3 g/d) × 2 d[11, 75]	50 mg/kg/d in 2 doses (max. 3 g/d) × 2 d[11, 75]
OR	Ivermectin[76]	200 μg/kg/d × 1–2 d	200 μg/kg/d × 1–2 d
TAPEWORM infection			
Adult (intestinal stage) *Diphyllobothrium latum* (fish), *Taenia saginata* (beef), *Taenia solium* (pork), *Dipylidium caninum* (dog)			
Drug of choice:	Praziquantel[8]	5–10 mg/kg once	5–10 mg/kg once
Hymenolepis nana (dwarf tapeworm)			
Drug of choice:	Praziquantel[8]	25 mg/kg once	25 mg/kg once
Larval (tissue stage)			
Echinococcus granulosus (hydatid cyst)			
Drug of choice:	Albendazole[77, 78]	400 mg bid × 28 days, repeated as necessary	15 mg/kg/d × 28 days, repeated as necessary
Echinococcus multilocularis			
Treatment of choice:	See footnote 79		
Cysticercus cellulosae (cysticercosis)			
Drug of choice[80]:	Albendazole[81]	15 mg/kg/d in 2–3 doses × 8–28 d, repeated as necessary	15 mg/kg/d in 2–3 doses × 8–28 d, repeated as necessary
OR	Praziquantel[8]	50 mg/kg/d in 3 doses × 15 d	50 mg/kg/d in 3 doses × 15 d
Alternative:	Surgery		
Toxocariasis, see VISCERAL LARVA MIGRANS			
TOXOPLASMOSIS *(Toxoplasma gondii)*[82]			
Drugs of choice[83]:	Pyrimethamine[71]	25–100 mg/d × 3–4 wk	2 mg/kg/d × 3 d, then 1 mg/kg/d (max. 25 mg/d) × 4 wk[84]
	plus sulfadiazine	1–1.5 g qid × 3–4 wk	100–200 mg/kg/d × 3–4 wk
Alternative:	Spiramycin[85]	3–4 g/d	50–100 mg/kg/d × 3–4 wk
TRICHINOSIS *(Trichinella spiralis)*			
Drugs of choice:	Steroids for severe symptoms **plus** mebendazole[8, 86]	200–400 mg tid × 3 d, then 400–500 mg tid × 10 d	
TRICHOMONIASIS *(Trichomonas vaginalis)*			
Drug of choice[87]:	Metronidazole	2 g once or 250 mg tid or 375 mg bid PO × 7 d	15 mg/kg/d orally in 3 doses × 7 d
OR	Tinidazole[5]	2 g once	50 mg/kg once (max. 2 g)
TRICHOSTRONGYLUS infection			
Drug of choice:	Pyrantel pamoate[8]	11 mg/kg once (max. 1 g)	11 mg/kg once (max. 1 g)
Alternative:	Mebendazole[8]	100 mg bid × 3 d	100 mg bid × 3 d
OR	Albendazole	400 mg once	400 mg once
TRICHURIASIS (*Trichuris trichiura,* whipworm)			
Drug of choice:	Mebendazole	100 mg bid × 3 d	100 mg bid × 3 d
OR	Albendazole	400 mg once[88]	400 mg once[88]
TRYPANOSOMIASIS			
Trypanosoma cruzi (American trypanosomiasis, Chagas' disease)			
Drug of choice:	Nifurtimox[3, 89]	8–10 mg/kg/d in 4 doses × 120 d	1–10 yr: 15–20 mg/kg/d in 4 doses × 90 d; 11–16 yr: 12.5–15 mg/kg/d in 4 doses × 90 d
Alternative:	Benznidazole[90]	5–7 mg/kg/d × 30–120 d	

Drugs for Treatment of Parasitic Infections *Continued*

Infection		Drug	Adult Dosage	Pediatric Dosage*
T. brucei gambiense; T. b. rhodesiense (African trypanosomiasis, sleeping sickness)				
TRYPANOSOMIASIS *(Continued)*				
Hemolymphatic stage				
Drug of choice:		Suramin[3]	100–200 mg (test dose) IV, then 1 g IV on days 1, 3, 7, 14, and 21	20 mg/kg on days 1, 3, 7, 14, and 21
	OR	Eflornithine	See footnote 91	
Alternative:		Pentamidine isethionate[8]	4 mg/kg/d IM × 10 d	4 mg/kg/d IM × 10 d
Late disease with central nervous system involvement				
Drug of choice:		Melarsoprol[3, 92]	2–3.6 mg/kg/d IV × 3 d; after 1 wk, 3.6 mg/kg per day IV × 3 d; repeat again after 10–21 d	18–25 mg/kg total over 1 mo; initial dose of 0.36 mg/kg IV, increasing gradually to max. 3.6 mg/kg at intervals of 1–5 d for total of 9–10 doses
	OR	Eflornithine	See footnote 91	
Alternatives: *(T. b. gambiense only)*		Tryparsamide	One injection of 30 mg/kg (max. 2 g) IV every 5 d to total of 12 injections; may be repeated after 1 mo	
		plus suramin[3]	One injection of 10 mg/kg IV every 5 d to total of 12 injections; may be repeated after 1 mo	
VISCERAL LARVA MIGRANS[93] (toxocariasis)				
Drug of choice:		Diethylcarbamazine[8]	6 mg/kg/d in 3 doses × 7–10 d	6 mg/kg/d in 3 doses × 7–10 d
Alternatives:		Albendazole	400 mg bid × 3–5 d	400 mg bid × 3–5 d
		Mebendazole[8]	100–200 mg bid × 5 d	100–200 mg bid × 5 d
Whipworm, see TRICHURIASIS				
Wuchereria bancrofti, see FILARIASIS				

1. *Entamoeba histolytica* and *E. dispar,* until recently termed "pathogenic" and "nonpathogenic" *E. histolytica,* respectively, are indistinguishable morphologically.
2. Dosage and duration of administration should not be exceeded because of possibility of causing optic neuritis; maximum dosage is 2 g/day.
3. In the USA, this drug is available from the CDC Drug Service, Centers for Disease Control and Prevention, Atlanta, Georgia 30333; telephone: 404-639-3670 (evenings, weekends, and holidays: 404-639-2888).
4. Treatment should be followed by a course of iodoquinol or one of the other intraluminal drugs used to treat asymptomatic amebiasis.
5. A nitro-imidazole similar to metronidazole, but not marketed in the USA; tinidazole appears to be at least as effective as metronidazole and better tolerated. Ornidazole, a similar drug, also is used outside the USA. Higher dosage is for hepatic abscess.
6. Trophozoites and cysts of *Acanthamoeba* from infected corneas, contact lenses, and their cases are susceptible in vitro to chlorhexidine, polyhexamethylene biguanide, propamidine, pentamidine, diminazine, and neomycin and, especially, to combinations of these drugs (J Hay et al, Eye, 8:555, 1994). For treatment of keratitis caused by *Acanthamoeba,* concurrent topical use of 0.1% propamidine isethionate (*Brolene*–Rhône-Poulenc Rorer, Canada) plus neomycin and oral itraconazole plus topical miconazole have been successful (MB Moore et al, Br J Ophthalmol, 73:271, 1989; Y Ishabashi et al, Am J Ophthalmol, 109:121, 1990). Recently, 0.02% topical polyhexamethylene biguanide (PHMB) has been used successfully in a large number of patients (MJ Elder et al, Lancet, 345:791, 1995). PHMB is available as *Baquacil* (ICI America), a swimming pool disinfectant (E Yee and TK Winarko, Am J Hosp Pharm, 50:2523, 1993).
7. *Naegleria* infections have been treated successfully with amphotericin B, rifampin, and chloramphenicol (A Wang et al, Clin Neurol Neurosurg, 95:249, 1993), amphotericin B, oral rifampin, and oral ketoconazole (N Poungvarin et al, J Med Assoc Thailand, 74:112, 1991), and amphotericin B alone (RL Brown, Arch Intern Med, 152:1330, 1992).
8. An approved drug but considered investigational for this condition by the Food and Drug Administration (FDA).
9. Strains of *Acanthamoeba* isolated from fatal granulomatous amebic encephalitis usually are susceptible in vitro to pentamidine, ketoconazole *(Nizoral),* flucytosine, and (less so) to amphotericin B. One patient with disseminated infection was treated successfully with intravenous pentamidine isethionate, topical chlorhexidine, and 2% ketoconazole cream, followed by oral itraconazole (CA Slater et al, N Engl J Med, 331:85, 1994).
10. Most patients recover spontaneously without antiparasitic drug therapy. Analgesics, corticosteroids, and careful removal of cerebrospinal fluid at frequent intervals can relieve symptoms (J Koo et al, Rev Infect Dis, 10:1155, 1988). Albendazole, levamisole *(Ergamisol),* or ivermectin also has been used successfully in animals.
11. This dose is likely to be toxic and may have to be decreased.
12. Atovaquone suspension, 750 mg bid, plus azithromycin, 500–1000 mg daily, may be effective when quinine and clindamycin fail. Exchange transfusion has been used in severely ill patients with high (>10%) parasitemia (V Iacopino and T Earnhart, Arch Intern Med, 150:1527, 1990). One report indicates that azithromycin *(Zithromax),* 500–1000 mg daily, plus quinine also may be effective (LM Weiss et al, J Infect Dis, 168:1289, 1993). Concurrent use of pentamidine and trimethoprim-sulfamethoxazole has been reported to cure an infection with *B. divergens* (D Raoult et al, Ann Intern Med, 107:944, 1987).
13. Not recommended for use in children younger than 8 years of age.
14. Drugs that could be tried include albendazole, mebendazole, thiabendazole, levamisole *(Ergamisol),* and ivermectin. Steroid therapy may be helpful, especially in eye and central nervous system infections. Ocular baylisascariasis has been treated successfully using laser photocoagulation therapy to destroy the intraretinal larvae.
15. Clinical significance of these organisms is controversial, but metronidazole, 750 mg tid × 10 d, or iodoquinol, 650 mg tid × 20 d, anecdotally has been reported to be effective (PFL Boreham and D Stenzel, Adv Parasitol, 32:2, 1993; JS Keystone; EK Markell, Clin Infect Dis, 21:102 and 104, July 1995).
16. Infection is self-limited in immunocompetent patients. In HIV-infected patients, paromomycin has limited effectiveness (AC White et al, J Infect Dis, 170:419, 1994; F Bissuel, Clin Infect Dis, 18:447, 1994). In unpublished clinical trials, azithromycin, 1250 mg daily for 2 weeks followed by 500 mg daily, apparently has been effective in some patients.

Table continued on following page

17. E Caumes et al, Am J Trop Med Hyg, 49:641, 1993; P Wolf et al, Hautarzt, 44:462, 1993; HD Davies et al, Arch Dermatol, 129:588, 1993.
18. HIV-infected patients may need higher dosage and long-term maintenance (JW Pape et al, Ann Intern Med, 121:654, 1994).
19. Not curative but decreases inflammation and facilitates removing the worm. Mebendazole, 400–800 mg/d for 6 d, has been reported to kill the worm directly.
20. A single dose of ivermectin, 20–200 μg/kg, has been reported to be effective for treatment of microfilaremia (SK Kar et al, Southeast Asian J Trop Med Public Health, 24:80, 1993).
21. Antihistamines or corticosteroids may be required to decrease allergic reactions due to disintegration of microfilariae in the treatment of filarial infections, especially those caused by *Loa loa.*
22. For patients with no microfilariae in the blood, full doses can be given from day 1.
23. Diethylcarbamazine should be administered with special caution in heavy infections with *Loa loa* because rapid killing of microfilariae can provoke an encephalopathy. Ivermectin or albendazole has been used to reduce microfilaremia (Y Martin-Prevel et al, Am J Trop Med Hyg, 48:186, 1993; AD Klion et al, J Infect Dis, 168:202, 1993). Apheresis has been reported to be effective in lowering microfilarial counts in patients heavily infected with *Loa loa* (EA Ottesen, Infect Dis Clin North Am, 7:619, 1993). Diethylcarbamazine, 300 mg once weekly, has been recommended for prevention of loiasis (TB Nutman et al, N Engl J Med, 319:752, 1988).
24. Diethylcarbamazine has no effect. Ivermectin, 150 μg/kg, may be effective (TB Nutman et al, J Infect Dis, 156:622, 1987).
25. Unlike infections with other flukes, *F. hepatica* infections may not respond to praziquantel. Recent data indicate that triclabendazole *(Fasinex),* a veterinary fasciolide, is safe and effective in a single oral dose of 10 mg/kg (W Apt et al, Am J Trop Med Hyg, 52:532, 1995).
26. Unpublished data indicate triclabendazole *(Fasinex),* a veterinary fasciolide, may be effective in a dosage of 5 mg/kg once daily for 3 days or 10 mg/kg twice in 1 day.
27. Fuirazolidone has been reported to be mutagenic and carcinogenic. Albendazole, 400 mg daily × 5 d, may be effective (A Hall and Q Nahar, Trans R Soc Trop Med Hyg, 87:84, 1993). Bacitracin zinc or bacitracin, 120,000 U bid for 10 days, also may be effective (BJ Andrews et al, Am J Trop Med Hyg, 52:318, 1995).
28. Not absorbed and not highly effective but may be useful for treatment of giardiasis in pregnancy.
29. Ivermectin has been reported to be effective in animals (MT Anantaphruti et al, Trop Med Parasitol, 43:65, 1992).
30. P Kraivichian et al, Trans R Soc Trop Med Hyg, 86:418, 1992.
31. In sulfonamide-sensitive patients, such as some HIV-infected patients, pyrimethamine, 50–75 mg daily, has been effective (LM Weiss et al, Ann Intern Med, 109:474, 1988). In immunocompromised patients, it may be necessary to continue therapy indefinitely.
32. May be repeated or continued. A longer duration may be needed for some forms of visceral leishmaniasis.
33. Limited data indicate that ketoconazole *(Nizoral),* 400–600 mg daily for 4 to 8 weeks, may be effective for treatment of cutaneous leishmaniasis (RE Saenz et al, Am J Med, 89:147, 1990). Some studies indicate that *L. donovani* resistant to sodium stibogluconate or meglumine antimonate may respond to recombinant human gamma interferon in addition to antimony (R Badaro and WD Johnson, J Infect Dis, 167 suppl 1:S13, 1993) or pentamidine followed by a course of antimony (CP Thakur et al, Am J Trop Med Hyg, 45:435, 1991). Liposomal encapsulated amphotericin B *(AmBisome,* Vestar, San Dimas, CA) has been used successfully to treat multi-drug-resistant visceral leishmaniasis (RN Davidson et al, Q J Med, 87:75, 1994; R Dietze et al, Clin Infect Dis, 17:981, 1993). Recently, the combination of aminosidine (chemically identical to paromomycin) and sodium stibogluconate has been used to decrease the time to clinical cure of kala-azar (CP Thakur et al, Trans R Soc Trop Med Hyg, 89:219, 1995) and to cure diffuse cutaneous leishmaniasis caused by *L. aethiopica* (S Teklemariam et al, Trans R Soc Trop Med Hyg, 88:334, 1994). In addition, preliminary studies suggest that aminosidine ointment appears to be effective in the treatment of cutaneous Old World leishmaniasis (ADM Bryceson et al, Trans R Soc Trop Med Hyg, 88:226, 1994).
34. For infestation of eyelashes with crab lice, use petrolatum.
35. FDA-approved only for head lice.
36. Some consultants recommend a second application 1 week later to kill hatching progeny.
37. Chloroquine-resistant *P. falciparum* infections occur in all malarious areas except Central America west of the Panama Canal Zone, Mexico, Haiti, the Dominican Republic, and most of the Middle East (chloroquine resistance has been reported in Yemen, Oman, and Iran).
38. In Southeast Asia and possibly in other areas, such as South America, relative resistance to quinine has increased and the treatment should be continued for 7 days.
39. *Fansidar* tablets contain 25 mg of pyrimethamine and 500 mg of sulfadoxine. Resistance to pyrimethamine-sulfadoxine has been reported from Southeast Asia, the Amazon basin, East Africa, Bangladesh, and Oceania.
40. In pregnancy.
41. For treatment of multi-drug-resistant *P. falciparum* infection in Southeast Asia, especially Thailand, where resistance to mefloquine and halofantrine frequently occurs, a 7-day course of quinine and tetracycline is recommended (G Watt et al, Am J Trop Med Hyg, 47:108, 1992). Combinations of artesunate plus mefloquine (C Luxemburger et al, Trans R Soc Trop Med Hyg, 88:213, 1994), artemether plus mefloquine (J Karbwang et al, Trans R Soc Trop Med Hyg, 89:296, 1995), and mefloquine plus tetracycline also are used to treat multi-drug-resistant *P. falciparum* infection.
42. At this dosage, adverse effects, including nausea, vomiting, diarrhea, dizziness, disturbed sense of balance, toxic psychosis, and seizures, can occur. Mefloquine is teratogenic in animals, and it has not been approved for use in pregnancy, but mefloquine prophylaxis has been reported to be safe and effective when used during the second half of pregnancy (F Nosten et al, J Infect Dis, 169:595, 1994). Limited studies also have demonstrated its efficacy in treating *P. falciparum* malaria during pregnancy (K Na Bangchang et al, Trans R Soc Trop Med Hyg, 88:321, 1994). It should not be given together with quinine or quinidine, and caution is required in using quinine or quinidine to treat patients with malaria who have taken mefloquine for prophylaxis. The pediatric dosage has not been approved by the FDA. Resistance to mefloquine has been reported in some areas, such as the Thailand-Myanmar border and the Amazon region, where 25 mg/kg should be used.
43. In the USA, a 250-mg tablet of mefloquine contains 228 mg of mefloquine base. Outside the USA, each 275-mg tablet contains 250 mg of base.
44. 750 mg followed 6–8 hours later by 500 mg.
45. NJ White, Eur J Clin Pharmacol, 34:1, 1988.
46. May be effective in multi-drug-resistant *P. falciparum* malaria, but treatment failures and resistance have been reported, and the drug causes consistent dose-related lengthening of the PR and QTc intervals (A Castot et al, Lancet, 341:1541, 1993). Several patients have developed first-degree block (F Nosten et al, Lancet 341:1054, 1993). The micronized form of halofantrine has improved its bioavailability, but variability in absorption remains an important problem (J Karbwang et al, Clin Pharmacokinet, 27:104, 1994). It should not be taken 1 hour before to 3 hours after meals and should not be used for patients with cardiac conduction defects. Cardiac monitoring is recommended.
47. One study found artemether, a Chinese drug, effective for parenteral treatment of severe malaria in children (NJ White et al, Lancet, 339:317, 1992).
48. Exchange transfusion has been helpful for some patients with high-density (>10%) parasitemia, altered mental status, pulmonary edema, or renal complications (JR Zucker and CC Campbell, Infect Dis Clin North Am, 7:547, 1993).
49. Continuous electrocardiogram, blood pressure, and glucose monitoring are recommended.
50. Quinidine may have greater antimalarial activity than quinine. The loading dose should be decreased or omitted in those patients who have received quinine or mefloquine. If more than 48 hours of parenteral treatment is required, the quinine or quinidine dose should be reduced by one-third to one-half.
51. Not available in the USA. With intravenous administration of quinine dihydrochloride, monitoring of electrocardiogram and blood pressure is recommended. Use of parenteral quinine or quinidine also may lead to severe hypoglycemia; blood glucose should be monitored.
52. If chloroquine phosphate is not available, hydroxychloroquine is as effective; 400 mg of hydroxychloroquine sulfate is equivalent to 500 mg of chloroquine phosphate.
53. In *P. faciparum* malaria, if the patient has not shown a response to conventional doses of chloroquine in 48–72 hours, parasitic resistance to this drug should be considered. *P. vivax* with decreased susceptibility to chloroquine has been reported from Papua-New Guinea, Brazil, Myanmar, India, Colombia, and Indonesia; a single dose of mefloquine, 15 mg/kg, has been recommended to treat these infections.
54. Some relapses have been reported with this regimen; relapses should be treated with chloroquine plus primaquine, 22.5–30 mg base/d × 14 days.

55. Primaquine phosphate can cause hemolytic anemia, especially in patients whose red blood cells are deficient in glucose-6-phosphate dehydrogenase. This deficiency is most common in African, Asian, and Mediterranean peoples. Patients should be screened for glucose-6-phosphate deficiency before treatment. Primaquine should not be used during pregnancy.
56. No drug regimen guarantees protection against malaria. If fever develops within a year (particularly within the first 2 months) after travel to malarious areas, travelers should be advised to seek medical attention. Insect repellents, insecticide-impregnated bed nets, and proper clothing are important adjuncts for malaria prophylaxis.
57. In pregnancy, chloroquine prophylaxis has been used extensively and safely, but the safety of other prophylactic antimalarial agents in pregnancy is unclear. Therefore, travel during pregnancy to chloroquine-resistant areas should be discouraged. (See footnote 42.)
58. For prevention of attack after departure from areas where *P. vivax* and *P. ovale* are endemic, which includes almost all areas where malaria is found (except Haiti), some experts prescribe in addition primaquine phosphate, 15 mg base (26.3 mg)/d, or, for children, 0.3 mg base/kg/d, during the last 2 weeks of prophylaxis. Others prefer to avoid the toxicity of primaquine and rely on surveillance to detect cases when they occur, particularly when exposure was limited or doubtful. See footnotes 54 and 55.
59. Beginning 1 week before travel and continuing weekly for the duration of stay and for 4 weeks after leaving.
60. A recent study has shown that daily primaquine provides effective prophylaxis against chloroquine-resistant *P. falciparum* (WR Weiss et al, J Infect Dis, 171:1569, 1995).
61. The pediatric dosage has not been approved by the FDA, and the drug has not been approved for use during pregnancy. Women should take contraceptive precautions while taking mefloquine and for 2 months after the last dose. Mefloquine is not recommended for patients with cardiac conduction abnormalities. Patients with a history of seizures or psychiatric disorders and those whose occupation requires fine coordination or spatial discrimination probably should avoid mefloquine (Medical Letter, 32:13, 1990). Resistance to mefloquine has been reported in some areas, such as Thailand; in these areas, doxycycline should be used for prophylaxis.
62. Beginning 1 day before travel and continuing for the duration of stay and for 4 weeks after leaving. Use of tetracyclines is contraindicated in pregnancy and in children younger than 8 years of age. Doxycycline can cause gastrointestinal disturbances, vaginal moniliasis, and photosensitivity reactions.
63. Proguanil (*Paludrine*–Ayerst, Canada; ICI, England), which is not available in the USA but is widely available overseas, is recommended mainly for use in Africa south of the Sahara. Prophylaxis is recommended during exposure and for 4 weeks afterwards. Failures in prophylaxis with chloroquine and proguanil have been reported in travelers to Kenya (AJ Barnes, Lancet, 338:1338, 1991).
64. Ocular lesions due to *E. hellem* in HIV-infected patients have responded to fumagillin eyedrops prepared from *Fumidil-B*, a commercial product used to control a microsporidial disease of honey bees, available from Mid-Continent Agrimarketing, Inc., Lenexa, Kansas 66215 (MC Diesenhouse, Am J Ophthalmol, 115:293, 1993). Fumagillin from other sources also has been used successfully (DF Rosberger et al, Cornea, 12:261, 1993). In one report, a keratopathy due to *E. hellem* in an HIV-infected patient was treated successfully with surgical débridement, topical antibiotics, and itraconazole (RW Yee et al, Ophthalmology, 98:196, 1991). For lesions due to *V. corneae*, topical therapy generally is not effective and keratoplasty may be required (RM Davis et al, Ophthalmology, 97:953, 1990).
65. Albendazole, 400 mg bid, may be effective for *S. intestinalis* infections (C Blanshard et al, AIDS, 6:311, 1992) and may be helpful for *E. bieneusi* infections (DT Dieterich et al, J Infect Dis, 169:178, 1994). Octreotide (*Sandostatin*) has provided symptomatic relief in some patients with large-volume diarrhea.
66. Albendazole, 400 mg bid, may be effective for *E. hellem* and *E. cuniculi*. There is no established treatment for *Pleistophora* infection.
67. Albendazole or pyrantel pamoate may be effective (HP Krepel et al, Trans R Soc Trop Med Hyg, 87:87, 1993).
68. In severe disease with room air $PO_2 \leq 70$ mm Hg or Aa gradient ≥ 35 mm Hg, prednisone also should be used (Medical Letter, 37:89, 1995).
69. HIV-infected patients should be treated for 21 days.
70. For patients who have failed or are intolerant to trimethoprim-sulfamethoxazole.
71. Plus folinic acid, 10 mg, with each dose of pyrimethamine.
72. Neuropsychiatric disturbances and seizures have been reported in some patients (H Stokvis et al, Am J Trop Med Hyg, 35:330, 1986).
73. In East Africa, the dose should be increased to 30 mg/kg, and in Egypt and South Africa, 30 mg/kg/d $\times$ 2 d. Some experts recommend 40–60 mg/kg over 2–3 days in all of Africa (KC Shekhar, Drugs, 42:379, 1991).
74. In immunocompromised patients, it may be necessary to prolong therapy or use other agents.
75. In disseminated strongyloidiasis, thiabendazole therapy should be continued for at least 5 days.
76. C Naquira et al, Am J Trop Med Hyg, 40:304, 1989; M Lyagoubi et al, Trans R Soc Trop Med Hyg, 86:541, 1992; PH Gann et al, J Infect Dis, 169:1076, 1994.
77. Albendazole should be taken with a fatty meal to enhance absorption. Some patients may benefit from or require surgical resection of cysts (RK Tompkins, Mayo Clin Proc, 66:1281, 1991). Praziquantel also may be useful preoperatively or in case of spill during surgery.
78. Percutaneous drainage with ultrasound guidance plus albendazole therapy has been effective for management of hepatic hydatid cyst disease (MS Khuroo et al, Gastroenterology, 104:1452, 1993).
79. Surgical excision is the only reliable means of treatment, although some reports have suggested use of albendazole or mebendazole (W Hao et al, Trans R Soc Trop Med Hyg, 88:340, 1994).
80. Corticosteroids should be given for 2–3 days before and during drug therapy for neurocysticercosis. Any cysticercocidal drug may cause irreparable damage when used to treat ocular or spinal cysts, even when corticosteroids are used.
81. Albendazole should be taken with a fatty meal to enhance absorption.
82. In ocular toxoplasmosis, corticosteroids also should be used for an anti-inflammatory effect on the eyes.
83. To treat central nervous system toxoplasmosis in HIV-infected patients, some clinicians have used pyrimethamine, 50–100 mg daily, after a loading dose of 200 mg with a sulfonamide and, when sulfonamide sensitivity developed, have given clindamycin, 1.8–2.4 g/d, in divided doses instead of the sulfonamide (JS Remington et al, Lancet, 338:1142, 1991; BJ Luft et al, N Engl J Med, 329:995, 1993). Atovaquone plus pyrimethamine appears to be an effective alternative in sulfa-intolerant patients (JA Kovacs et al, Lancet, 340:637, 1992). Dapsone-pyrimethamine can prevent first episodes of toxoplasmosis (P-M Girard et al, N Engl J Med, 328:1514, 1993).
84. Congenitally infected newborns should be treated with pyrimethamine every 2 or 3 days and a sulfonamide daily for about 1 year (JS Remington and G Desmonts in JS Remington and JO Klein, eds, *Infectious Disease of the Fetus and Newborn Infant*, 4th ed, Philadelphia: W.B. Saunders, 1995, page 140).
85. For use during pregnancy, continue the drug until delivery. If it has been determined that transmission has occurred in utero, then therapy with pyrimethamine and sulfadiazine should be started.
86. Albendazole or flubendazole (not available in the USA) also may be effective.
87. Sexual partners should be treated simultaneously. Outside the USA, ornidazole also has been used for this condition. Metronidazole-resistant strains have been reported: higher doses of metronidazole for longer periods sometimes are effective against these strains (J Lossick, Rev Infect Dis, 12:S665, 1990). Experimental studies suggest that bacitracin and bacitracin zinc have microbicidal activity against multiple isolates of *T. vaginalis* (BJ Andrews et al, Trans R Soc Trop Med Hyg, 88:704, 1994).
88. In heavy infection, it may be necessary to extend therapy for 3 days.
89. The addition of gamma interferon to nifurtimox for 20 days in a limited number of patients and in experimental animals appears to have shortened the acute phase of Chagas' disease (RE McCabe et al, J Infect Dis, 163:912, 1991).
90. Limited data.
91. In *T. b. gambiense* infections, eflornithine is highly effective in both the hemolymphatic and central nervous system stages. Its effectiveness in *T. b. rhodesiense* infections has been variable. Some clinicians have given 400 mg/kg/d intravenously in four divided doses for 14 days, followed by oral treatment with 300 mg/kg/d for 3–4 wks (F Milord et al, Lancet, 340:652, 1992).
92. In frail patients, begin with as little as 18 mg and increase the dose progressively. Pretreatment with suramin has been advocated for debilitated patients. Corticosteroids have been used to prevent arsenical encephalopathy (J Pepin et al, Trans R Soc Trop Med Hyg, 89:92, 1995).
93. For severe symptoms or eye involvement, corticosteroids can be used in addition.

Manufacturers of Antiparasitic Drugs

Albendazole—*Zentel* (SmithKline Beecham)*
Aminosidine (paromomycin)**

Atovaquone—*Mepron* (Glaxo-Wellcome)
Bacitracin—many manufacturers
Bacitracin-zinc (Apothekernes Laboratorium A.S., Oslo, Norway)**
Benznidazole—*Rochagan* (Roche, Brazil)**

Bithionol—*Bitin* (Tanabe, Japan)†
Chloroquine—*Aralen* (Sanofi Winthrop), others
Crotamiton—*Eurax* (Westwood-Squibb)
Dapsone (Jacobus)

Diethylcarbamazine—*Hetrazan* (Wyeth-Ayerst)*
Diloxanide furoate—*Furamide* (Boots, England)†

Eflornithine (difluoromethylornithine, DFMO)—*Ornidyl** (Merrell Dow)
Flubendazole—(Janssen)**
Furazolidone—*Furoxone* (Roberts)
Halofantrine—*Halfan* (SmithKline Beecham)**
Hydroxychloroquine—*Plaquenil* (Sanofi Winthrop)

Iodoquinol (diiodohydroxyquin)—*Yodoxin* (Glenwood), others
Ivermectin—*Mectizan* (Merck)†
Malathion—*Prioderm***
Mebendazole—*Vermox* (Janssen)
Mefloquine—*Lariam* (Roche)
Meglumine antimonate—*Glucantime* (Rhône-Poulenc Rorer, France)**
Melarsoprol—*Arsobal* (Rhône-Poulenc Rorer, France)†
Metronidazole—*Flagyl* (Searle), others

Nifurtimox—*Lampit* (Bayer, Germany)†
Ornidazole—*Tiberal* (Hoffman-LaRoche, Switzerland)**
Oxamniquine—*Vansil* (Pfizer)
Paromomycin—*Humatin* (Parke-Davis)
Pentamidine isethionate—*Pentam 300* (Fujisawa), *NebuPent* (Fujisawa)
Permethrin—*Nix* (Glaxo-Wellcome), *Elimite* (Herbert), *Lyclear* (Canada)

Praziquantel—*Biltricide* (Miles)
Primaquine phosphate—(Sanofi Winthrop)
Proguanil—*Paludrine* (Ayerst, Canada, ICI, England)**
Pyrantel pamoate—*Antiminth* (Pfizer)
Pyrethrins and piperonyl butoxide—*RID* (Pfizer), others
Pyrimethamine—*Daraprim* (Glaxo-Wellcome)
Pyrimethamine-sulfadoxine—*Fansidar* (Roche)
Quinidine gluconate—(Lilly)
Quinine dihydrochloride**
Quinine sulfate—many manufacturers
Sodium stibogluconate (antimony sodium gluconate)—*Pentostam* (Glaxo-Wellcome, England)†
Spiramycin—*Rovamycine* (Rhône-Poulenc Rorer)*

Sulfadiazine—(Eon Labs, and others)
Suramin—(Bayer, Germany)†
Thiabendazole—*Mintezol* (Merck)
Tinidazole—*Fasigyn* (Pfizer)**
Triclabendazole (Ciba-Geigy)**
Trimetrexate—*Neutrexin* (US Bioscience)
Tryparsamide**

*Available in the USA only from the manufacturer.
**Not available in the USA.
†Available from the CDC Drug Service, Centers for Disease Control and Prevention, Atlanta, Georgia 30333; 404-639-3670 (evenings, weekends, and holidays: 404-639-2888).

Adverse Effects of Some Antiparasitic Drugs*

ALBENDAZOLE *(Zentel)*
Occasional: diarrhea, abdominal pain, migration of *Ascaris* through mouth and nose
Rare: leukopenia, alopecia, increased serum transaminase activity

AMINOSIDINE—see Paromomycin

ATOVAQUONE *(Mepron)*
Frequent: rash, nausea
Occasional: diarrhea

BACITRACIN
Frequent: nephrotoxicity
Occasional: rash
Rare: anaphylaxis

BENZNIDAZOLE *(Rochagan)*
Frequent: allergic rash, dose-dependent polyneuropathy, gastrointestinal disturbances, psychic disturbances

BITHIONOL *(Bitin)*
Frequent: photosensitivity reactions, vomiting, diarrhea, abdominal pain, urticaria
Rare: leukopenia, toxic hepatitis

CHLOROQUINE HYDROCHLORIC ACID and CHLOROQUINE PHOSPHATE (*Aralen* and others)
Occasional: pruritus; vomiting; headache; confusion; depigmentation of the hair; skin eruptions; corneal opacity; weight loss; partial alopecia; extraocular muscle palsies; exacerbation of psoriasis, eczema, and other exfoliative dermatoses; myalgias; photophobia
Rare: irreversible retinal injury (especially when total dosage exceeds 100 g), discoloration of nails and mucus membranes, nerve-type deafness, peripheral neuropathy and myopathy, heart block, blood dyscrasias, hematemesis

Adverse Effects of Some Antiparasitic Drugs* *Continued*

CROTAMITON *(Eurax)*
Occasional: rash, conjunctivitis

DAPSONE
Frequent: rash, transient headache, gastrointestinal irritation, anorexia, infectious mononucleosis-like syndrome
Occasional: cyanosis due to methemoglobinemia and sulfhemoglobinemia; other blood dyscrasias, including hemolytic anemia; nephrotic syndrome; liver damage; peripheral neuropathy; hypersensitivity reactions; increased risk of lepra reactions; insomnia; irritability; uncoordinated speech; agitation; acute psychosis
Rare: renal papillary necrosis, severe hypalbuminemia, epidermal necrolysis, optic atrophy, agranulocytosis, neonatal hyperbilirubinemia after use in pregnancy

DIETHYLCARBAMAZINE CITRATE USP *(Hetrazan)*
Frequent: severe allergic or febrile reactions in patients with microfilariae in the blood or the skin, gastrointestinal disturbances
Rare: encephalopathy

DILOXANIDE FUROATE *(Furamide)*
Frequent: flatulence
Occasional: nausea, vomiting, diarrhea
Rare: diplopia, dizziness, urticaria, pruritus

EFLORNITHINE (difluoromethylornithine, DFMO, *Ornidyl*)
Frequent: anemia, leukopenia
Occasional: diarrhea, thrombocytopenia, seizures
Rare: hearing loss

FLUBENDAZOLE—similar to mebendazole

FURAZOLIDONE *(Furoxone)*
Frequent: nausea, vomiting
Occasional: allergic reactions, including pulmonary infiltration, hypotension, urticaria, fever, vesicular rash; hypoglycemia; headache
Rare: hemolytic anemia in glucose-6-phosphate deficiency and neonates, disulfiram-like reaction with alcohol, monoamine oxidase–inhibitor interactions, polyneuritis

HALOFANTRINE *(Halfan)*
Occasional: diarrhea, abdominal pain, pruritus, prolongation of QTc and PR interval

IODOQUINOL *(Yodoxin)*
Occasional: rash, acne, slight enlargement of the thyroid gland, nausea, diarrhea, cramps, anal pruritus
Rare: optic neuritis, optic atrophy, loss of vision, peripheral neuropathy after prolonged use in high dosage (for months), iodine sensitivity

IVERMECTIN *(Mectizan)*
Occasional: Mazzotti-type reaction seen in onchocerciasis, including fever, pruritus, tender lymph nodes, headache, and joint and bone pain
Rare: hypotension

MALATHION *(Prioderm)*
Occasional: local irritation

MEBENDAZOLE *(Vermox)*
Occasional: diarrhea, abdominal pain, migration of *Ascaris* through mouth and nose
Rare: leukopenia, agranulocytosis, hypospermia

MEFLOQUINE *(Lariam)*
Frequent: vertigo, lightheadedness, nausea, other gastrointestinal disturbances, nightmares, visual disturbances, headache
Occasional: confusion
Rare: psychosis, hypotension, convulsions, coma, paresthesias

MEGLUMINE ANTIMONATE *(Glucantime)*—similar to sodium stibogluconate

MELARSOPROL *(Arsobal)*
Frequent: myocardial damage, albuminuria, hypertension, colic, herxheimer-type reaction, encephalopathy, vomiting, peripheral neuropathy
Rare: shock

METRONIDAZOLE (*Flagyl* and others)
Frequent: GI nausea, headache, dry mouth, metallic taste
Occasional: vomiting, diarrhea, insomnia, weakness, stomatitis, vertigo, tinnitus, paresthesias, rash, dark urine, urethral burning, disulfiram-like reaction with alcohol
Rare: seizures, encephalopathy, pseudomembranous colitis, ataxia, leukopenia, peripheral neuropathy, pancreatitis

Table continued on following page

Adverse Effects of Some Antiparasitic Drugs* *Continued*

NIFURTIMOX *(Lampit)*
Frequent: anorexia, vomiting, weight loss, loss of memory, sleep disorders, tremor, paresthesias, weakness, polyneuritis
Rare: convulsions, fever, pulmonary infiltrates and pleural effusion

ORNIDAZOLE *(Tiberal)*
Occasional: dizziness, headache, gastrointestinal disturbances
Rare: reversible peripheral neuropathy

OXAMNIQUINE *(Vansil)*
Occasional: headache, fever, dizziness, somnolence, nausea, diarrhea, rash, insomnia, hepatic enzyme changes, electrocardiogram changes, electroencephalogram changes, orange-red discoloration of urine
Rare: seizures, neuropsychiatric disturbances

PAROMOMYCIN (aminosidine, *Humatin)*
Frequent: disturbances with oral use
Occasional: eighth-nerve damage (mainly auditory) and renal damage when aminosidine is given intravenously, vertigo, pancreatitis

PENTAMIDINE ISETHIONATE *(Pentam 300, NebuPent)*
Frequent: hypotension, hypoglycemia often followed by diabetes mellitus, vomiting, blood dyscrasias, renal damage, pain at injection site, gastrointestinal disturbances
Occasional: may aggravate diabetes, shock, hypocalcemia, liver damage, cardiotoxicity, delirium, rash
Rare: Herxheimer-type reaction, anaphylaxis, acute pancreatitis, hyperkalemia

PERMETHRIN *(Nix, Elimite)*
Occasional: burning, stinging, numbness, increased pruritus, pain, edema, erythema, rash

PRAZIQUANTEL *(Biltricide)*
Frequent: malaise, headache, dizziness
Occasional: sedation, abdominal discomfort, fever, sweating, nausea, eosinophilia, fatigue
Rare: pruritus, rash

PRIMAQUINE PHOSPHATE USP
Frequent: hemolytic anemia in glucose-6-phosphate deficiency
Occasional: neutropenia, gastrointestinal disturbances, methemoglobinemia
Rare: central nervous system symptoms, hypertension, arrhythmias

PROGUANIL *(Paludrine)*
Occasional: oral ulceration, hair loss, scaling of palms and soles, urticaria
Rare: hematuria (with large doses), vomiting, abdominal pain, diarrhea (with large doses), thrombocytopenia

PYRANTEL PAMOATE *(Antiminth)*
Occasional: gastrointestinal disturbances, headache, dizziness, rash, fever

PYRETHRINS and PIPERONYL BUTOXIDE (*RID*, and others)
Occasional: allergic reactions

PYRIMETHAMINE USP *(Daraprim)*
Occasional: blood dyscrasias, folic acid deficiency
Rare: rash, vomiting, convulsions, shock, possibly pulmonary eosinophilia, fatal cutaneous reactions with **pyrimethamine-sulfadoxine** *(Fansidar)*

QUININE DIHYDROCHLORIDE and SULFATE
Frequent: cinchonism (tinnitus, headache, nausea, abdominal pain, visual disturbance)
Occasional: deafness, hemolytic anemia, other blood dyscrasias, photosensitivity reactions, hypoglycemia, arrhythmias, hypotension, drug fever
Rare: blindness, sudden death if injected too rapidly

SODIUM STIBOGLUCONATE *(Pentostam)*
Frequent: muscle and joint pain, fatigue, nausea, transaminase elevations, T-wave flattening or inversion, pancreatitis
Occasional: weakness, abdominal pain, liver damage, bradycardia, leukopenia, thrombocytopenia, rash, vomiting
Rare: diarrhea, pruritus, myocardial damage, hemolytic anemia, renal damage, shock, sudden death

SPIRAMYCIN *(Rovamycine)*
Occasional: gastrointestinal disturbances
Rare: allergic reactions

SURAMIN SODIUM
Frequent: vomiting, pruritus, urticaria, paresthesias, hyperesthesia of hands and feet, photophobia, peripheral neuropathy
Occasional: kidney damage, blood dyscrasias, shock, optic atrophy

THIABENDAZOLE *(Mintezol)*
Frequent: nausea, vomiting, vertigo, headache, drowsiness, pruritus
Occasional: leukopenia, crystalluria, rash, hallucination and other psychiatric reactions, visual and olfactory disturbance, erythema multiforme
Rare: shock, tinnitus, intrahepatic cholestasis, convulsions, angioneurotic edema, Stevens-Johnson syndrome

Adverse Effects of Some Antiparasitic Drugs* *Continued*

TINIDAZOLE *(Fasigyn)*
Occasional: metallic taste, nausea, vomiting, rash

TRIMETREXATE (with "leucovorin rescue")
Occasional: rash, peripheral neuropathy, bone marrow depression, increased serum aminotransferase activity

TRYPARSAMIDE
Frequent: nausea, vomiting
Occasional: impaired vision, optic atrophy, fever, exfoliative dermatitis, allergic reactions, tinnitus

*Drug interactions generally are not included here, see the current edition of *The Medical Letter Handbook of Adverse Drug Interactions.*

236

IMMUNOMODULATING AGENTS

Timothy R. La Pine, K. Lynn Cates, and Harry R. Hill

Over the past decade, there has been an explosion of basic science research and clinical interest in the functional mechanisms of the immune response and the specific biologic factors that modulate this response. This research has established that a critical and delicate balance in the regulation of both cellular and humoral function is essential for complete immunologic responsiveness to invasive pathogens and that alterations in this regulation may have potential clinical significance. Attempts to augment immune function in the challenged host or during specific immunodeficiency states have focused on a number of immune biologic response modifiers. This, in combination with the advances in recombinant technology, has led to several clinical trials exploring the therapeutic utility of immunomodulating agents in the treatment of specific human disease states.

We review the biologic agents used to manipulate immune regulation for the prevention and management of infectious diseases in infants and children and introduce the actions of potentially useful immunomodulators from in vitro and/or animal model experiments to be seen in future human clinical trials. This review will focus on the cytokine family of recombinant molecules, which plays many key roles in the orchestration of immune regulation. These molecules include lymphokines and monokines (interleukins [ILs] and tumor necrosis factor–alpha [TNF-α], as well as the hematopoietic growth factors); colony-stimulating factors (CSFs); and interferons -alpha, -beta, and -gamma (IFN-α, IFN-β, and IFN-γ). In addition, we will discuss the clinically important activities of intravenous immunoglobulin (IVIG) as well as the integrins and selectins, platelet-activating factor (PAF), and nitric oxide, which are emerging as important immunoregulators of the acute inflammatory response.

CYTOKINES

Lymphokines and Monokines

The cytokines are a family of small soluble protein molecules responsible for cell-to-cell communication. They are produced by several cell types and play crucial roles in many biologic processes, including inflammation, immunity, and hematopoiesis. During infection, genes for nearly all the cytokines are expressed. The biologic activities of the prototype cytokines, the lymphokines and monokines, include ILs and TNF-α; these molecules along with the granulocyte CSFs have received considerable attention as potential immunomodulatory agents. In response to pathogen invasion, these cytokines perform a complex series of interactions to initiate a cascade of biologic events resulting in the propagation and subsequent regulation of the inflammatory response, leading to pathogen alienation, while maintaining host preservation. Thus, the cytokine family, through a complex web of interactions, functions to initiate and then both up-regulate and down-regulate inflammatory responses. Based on their roles of either up-regulating or down-regulating immune responsiveness, the cytokines generally have been classified as either proinflammatory or anti-inflammatory molecules. Although a number of the cytokines, either directly or indirectly, have the potential to perform dual functions, their proinflammatory or anti-inflammatory properties are of considerable basic science and clinical therapeutic interest.[14, 27, 39, 51, 93, 95, 100]

The proinflammatory cytokines and their cellular source are listed in Table 236–1. TNF-α and IL-1 generally are considered to be prominent early proinflammatory mediators. They induce gene expression of other proinflammatory cytokines, including IL-8 and IL-9 leading to neutrophil activation, recruitment, and degranulation. TNF-α and IL-1 also activate a secondary cascade of inflammatory mediators, including the arachidonic acid–derived prostaglandin I_2, thromboxane A_2, prostaglandin E_2, PAF, and complement. The CSFs and IL-3 also are proinflammatory cytokines, which induce bone marrow stem cell production of granulocytes and monocytes in addition to activating neutrophils and inducing IL-1 and TNF-α production.[14, 27, 39, 51, 93, 95, 100]

Prominent among the anti-inflammatory cytokines (Table 236–2) are IL-4, IL-6, IL-10, IL-13 and transforming growth factor-β. These cytokines block endotoxin induction of IL-1 and TNF-α and suppress lymphocyte and monocyte function. IL-1 receptor antagonist (IL-1ra) blocks the proinflammatory action of IL-1 by binding its receptor.[14, 27, 39, 51, 93, 95, 100]

Considerable experimental and clinical interest has focused on the proinflammatory cytokines TNF-α and IL-1 as important early mediators in the pathogenesis of sepsis and

TABLE 236–1. Proinflammatory Cytokines

Cytokine	Function	Predominant Cell Source
Tumor necrosis factor–α	Stimulates IL-6, CSF. Depresses erythropoiesis. Stimulates IL-8, IL-9. Promotes tumor necrosis, endotoxic shock.	Monocytes, macrophages
IL-1	Stimulates proliferation and differentiation of T and B lymphocytes. Stimulates T lymphocytes to produce IL-2. Promotes CSF, IL-8, IL-9 production, endotoxic shock.	Macrophages, astrocytes, monocytes, fibroblasts, keratinocytes, B cells, corneal epithelium, other cell types
IL-2	Stimulates growth of T lymphocytes. Stimulates B lymphocyte, monocyte differentiation. Increases cytotoxicity of T lymphocytes, natural killer cells.	Activated T lymphocytes
IL-3	Is a multipotential hematopoietic cell growth factor. Stimulates early B and T lymphocytes. Is a mast cell growth factor.	Activated T lymphocytes, natural killer cells
IL-5	Stimulates eosinophil formation, differentiation. Augments T-lymphocyte cytotoxicity, proliferation of B lymphocytes.	T lymphocytes, mast cells
IL-7	Supports growth of pre-B lymphocytes. Stimulates T lymphocytes.	B lymphocytes, bone marrow fibroblasts, monocytes
IL-8	Stimulates neutrophil, monocyte, lymphocyte activation chemotaxis.	Monocytes
IL-9	Stimulates neutrophil monocyte, lymphocyte activation chemotaxis. Stimulates erythroid progenitors, helper T lymphocyte growth factor.	T lymphocytes
IL-11	T-lymphocyte–dependent stimulator of B lymphocytes.	Bone marrow fibroblasts
IL-12	Stimulates helper T-lymphocyte differentiation, IL-2 production. Increases cytotoxicity of natural killer cells.	T and B lymphocytes, lymphoblastoid cells
IL-14	Stimulates proliferation of activated B lymphocytes. Inhibits immunoglobulin secretion from B lymphocytes.	T lymphocytes
IL-15	Stimulates T lymphocyte function, proliferation. Enhances natural killer cell function.	Monocytes, macrophages
IL-16	Promotes migration of T lymphocytes.	T lymphocytes
IL-17	Stimulates IL-6, IL-8 production.	T lymphocytes
Granulocyte CSF	Stimulates neutrophil colony formation.	Monocytes, fibroblasts
Granulocyte-macrophage CSF	Stimulates granulocyte, monocyte formation. Induces tumor necrosis factor–α.	T lymphocytes, natural killer cells, endothelial cells, fibroblasts, keratinocytes
Macrophage CSF	Activates monocytes, granulocytes. Stimulates macrophage colony formation. Induces IL-1, tumor necrosis factor–α.	Fibroblasts, monocytes, endothelial cells

CSF, colony-stimulating factor; IL, interleukin.

septic shock syndrome. The basis for the potential therapeutic utility of these two cytokines in human disease states involves two clinically distinct hypotheses: (1) excessive cytokine production results in host immune injury leading to severe shock, and (2) deficient cytokine production renders a host susceptible to infection by invasive pathogens.[93]

The hypothesis that cytokine overproduction can lead to severe lethal shock is demonstrated in several animal models and is suggested in patients with overwhelming sepsis. The outer membranes of gram-negative bacteria contain lipopolysaccharide (LPS) or endotoxin, which induces the early proinflammatory cytokines TNF-α and IL-1. Although these cytokines may protect the host from infection, if expressed in excessive amounts they can lead to multiple organ failure and death. During severe sepsis, the levels of both TNF-α and IL-1 increase proportionately with the degree of hypotension and organ failure. The combination of these two cytokines can result in synergism over their individual effects by several-fold, leading to lethal septic shock syndrome.[19, 20] In animal models of shock and gram-negative sepsis, TNF-α levels rise rapidly after bacterial or endotoxin injection, reaching peak concentrations at 60 to 90 minutes, whereas IL-1 levels rise more slowly, peaking at 180 minutes. A similar time course response has been observed in human subjects injected with endotoxin.[20, 115] Children with septicemia and purpura fulminans and children with meningococcal disease demonstrated a correlation between morbidity and mortality and high serum levels of TNF-α and IL-1.[55, 124] These studies and others implicate TNF-α and IL-1 as prominent modulators in the development of the septic shock syndrome and suggest that a potential therapeutic benefit may be obtained by inhibiting the production of these cytokines and reducing their proinflammatory effects.

The experimental attempts to attenuate the excessive proinflammatory cytokine activity of TNF-α and IL-1 have focused on (1) inhibition of endotoxin release, (2) blocking

TABLE 236–2. Anti-inflammatory Cytokines

Cytokines	Function	Predominant Cell Source
IL-4	Stimulates proliferation of T and B lymphocytes, megakaryocytes. Is a growth factor for mast cells, erythroid precursors.	T lymphocytes
IL-6	Blocks endotoxin induction of IL-1, tumor necrosis factor–α. Stimulates B- and T-lymphocyte–stimulating activity.	Monocytes, T and B lymphocytes, fibroblasts, epithelial and endothelial cells
IL-10	Blocks production of IL-1, tumor necrosis factor–α. Inhibits primary allogenic T-lymphocyte responses. Inhibits IL-2, IL-8, granulocyte-macrophage CSF.	T and B lymphocytes, macrophages, monocytes
IL-13	Blocks production of IL-1, tumor necrosis factor–α, IL-8. Suppresses nitric oxide formation.	T lymphocytes
IL-1 receptor antagonist	Binds IL-1 receptors, blocks IL-1 effects.	Monocytes, macrophages
Transforming growth factor–β	Reduces endotoxin-induced IL-1, tumor necrosis factor–α production.	Monocytes, macrophages

CSF, colony-stimulating factor; IL, interleukin.

endotoxin–target cell binding and preventing the transmembrane signaling mechanisms leading to TNF-α and IL-1 production, (3) controlling the synthesis of TNF-α and IL-1 by inhibiting or suppressing specific cytokine gene transcription and translation, (4) inhibition of TNF-α and IL-1 release, (5) administration of TNF-α and IL-1 neutralizing antibodies and soluble receptors, (6) production and administration of TNF-α and IL-1 receptor antagonists that block specific cytokine binding to target cell receptors, and (7) blockage of TNF-α or IL-1 intracellular transmembrane signaling mechanisms, preventing their action on target cells.[95]

The use of monoclonal antiendotoxin antibodies to inhibit the binding of endotoxin to its target cells has received considerable attention. Numerous in vitro and in vivo animal experiments have suggested that blocking endotoxin leads to improved survival by inhibiting proinflammatory cytokine production and expression.[125] The initial clinical studies in patients with gram-negative bacteremia treated with immunoglobulin preparations directed against endotoxin demonstrated a significant reduction in mortality.[7, 145] Further studies suggest a reduction of septic shock in similarly treated high-risk surgical patients.[7] These observations led to the development of several clinical trials using human monoclonal anti-endotoxin antibodies. HA-1A is a human monoclonal antibody against the lipid A moiety of bacterial endotoxin. The mechanism of HA-1A action is to block endotoxin triggering of the intracellular events leading to proinflammatory cytokine synthesis. In placebo-controlled clinical trials of HA-1A, either HA-1A or placebo was infused over 20 minutes to patients with severe sepsis. These patients received cardiopulmonary support and antibacterial therapy. The etiologic agents of sepsis included *Escherichia coli*, *Pseudomonas*, and *Klebsiella* and *Enterobacter* species. The authors report that HA-1A significantly reduced mortality in adults with septic shock and gram-negative bacteremia. Those patients who were in severe shock before HA-1A administration had a 42 per cent reduction in mortality.[167] Although these early clinical studies using HA-1A were encouraging, a protective role for antiendotoxin antibodies has not been established in subsequent clinical trials.[103] Antiendotoxin therapy may be more effective if given earlier during the sepsis syndrome prior to the development of shock, and because bacterial lysis by antibiotics is an ongoing process and results in further endotoxin release, multiple dosing of antiendotoxin antibodies also may prove beneficial during sepsis syndromes. The future clinical use of antiendotoxin antibodies may be in combination immunomodulation therapies directed at simultaneously blocking several steps in both the propagation and action of proinflammatory cytokines.

Studies of cytokine inhibition have focused on controlling IL-1 and TNF-α with anti–TNF-α antibodies and their soluble receptors and with IL-1 receptor blockers. Control of proinflammatory cytokine synthesis is specific for each individual cytokine and requires an understanding of the unique temporal relationships these molecules have during the propagation of inflammatory responses. A critical aspect of IL-1 and TNF-α gene expression in a variety of cell types has been the reported exquisite sensitivity these cytokines have to bacterial endotoxin.[27, 39, 93, 95] Human blood monocytes synthesize IL-1 and TNF-α in the presence of endotoxin. In the absence of endotoxin, however, gene expression occurs but protein translation does not take place.[147] Thus, these cells may be viewed as being primed for bacterial endotoxin exposure. IL-1 and TNF-α transcription is suppressed by the anti-inflammatory cytokines IL-4, IL-10, IL-13, and transforming growth factor–β, but the clinical therapeutic benefit these cytokines have in treating septic shock remains to be defined.[29, 66, 117, 146] Agents blocking the lipo-oxygenase pathway of arachidonate metabolism also have been implicated in the reduction of TNF-α and IL-1 synthesis, and corticosteroids have been shown to suppress both TNF-α and IL-1 transcription and synthesis, but only when administered before transcription has been initiated.[50, 144] The use of corticosteroids in infants and children with bacterial meningitis has demonstrated that treatment with a combination of dexamethasone and antibiotics results in lower cerebral spinal fluid levels of TNF-α than does treatment with placebo and antibiotics.[124] In addition, corticosteroid-treated patients had fewer neurologic symptoms.[81] Subsequent multicenter trials, however, have failed to establish a protective effect of corticosteroid use in the treatment of children with meningitis.[159] One possible explanation for this discrepancy may be that corticosteroids almost exclusively suppress endotoxin-induced proinflammatory cytokine gene transcription but have little or no effect on proinflammatory cytokine translation.[39, 150] Thus, it has been suggested that the early administration of corticosteroids before transcription has been initiated would block cytokine synthesis. Timing of corticosteroid administration, therefore, may account for some of the clinical variability seen with its use in children with meningitis. Current clinical trials are focusing on TNF-α and IL-1 synthesis with the administration of corticosteroids either before or during antibiotic administration. Similarly, the temporal use of antibiotics, corticosteroids, and antiendotoxin therapy may result in an additive therapeutic benefit.

Neutralizing monoclonal antibodies against murine or human TNF-α have been shown to decrease mortality in several experimental animal models of sepsis.[12, 108, 155] Studies with soluble TNF-α receptors or their immunoadhesion constructs also have demonstrated an immunoprotective effect of TNF-α blockade in animal models of endotoxemia or bacteremia.[10] Although anti–TNF-α antibodies are being used with caution in humans, anti–TNF-α treatment in a limited number of patients with established septic shock resulted in increased vascular hemodymatics and in left ventricular stroke volume.[61] The in vitro use of free soluble TNF-α receptors to bind TNF-α results in a 10- to 50-fold increase in binding affinity over anti–TNF-α monoclonal antibodies.[62] Results from phase II clinical trials using soluble TNF-α receptors, however, have not shown improvement in survival; moreover, high doses actually increased mortality.[142] Antibodies to IL-1 have demonstrated limited clinical utility.[62]

There are naturally occurring substances that inhibit IL-1 synthesis and action, but they also have effects on many of the other cytokines. Specific inhibitors of IL-1, however, have been identified. Most prominent of these is the IL-1 receptor inhibitor that competes with the binding of IL-1 to its cell surface receptor. Recombinant IL-1ra that blocks IL-1 effects has been studied in various animal models.[1, 130] For instance, IL-1ra prevents death from endotoxic shock in rabbits.[130] The therapeutic use of IL-1ra in treating septic shock in early phase II clinical trials showed improved survival at 28 days.[52] The subsequent randomized phase III trials, however, failed to show improvement in patients with severe shock.[50] Further clinical studies are being conducted. IL-1ra also has been used in acute myelogenous leukemia patients. It is proposed that the uncontrolled production of IL-1 by leukemic blasts results in the continued proliferation of these cells and the development of acute myelogenous leukemia. Studies have shown that IL-1ra blocks the spontaneous proliferation and production of granulocyte-macrophage CSF (GM-CSF), IL-1, and IL-6 in the peripheral blood and bone marrow cells of these patients.[137] The potential clinical use of IL-1ra currently is being investigated in patients with psoriasis, rheumatoid arthritis, and myelogenous leukemia.[63] Similarly, combination therapies with the simultaneous blockade of both TNF-α and IL-1 are under investigation in endotoxin models of shock and a number of clinical disease states.[141]

Another promising approach to attenuate an excessive proinflammatory cytokine response is the use of pharmacologic agents. Salyer and associates[143] demonstrated that pentoxifylline, a methylxanthine derivative that blocks TNF-α transcription and production, could override some of the effects of TNF-α on polymorphonuclear leukocytes (PMNs). In their study, the profound decrease in human PMN chemotactic ability caused by excessive TNF-α was restored to normal by treatment with pentoxifylline. The specific mechanisms of pentoxifylline's effect are not known, but it has been shown to restore PMN membrane fluidity inhibited by TNF-α that is critical for cell movement.[129] Furthermore, pentoxifylline can block PMN adhesion to endothelium and result in decreased PMN respiratory burst activity, which effects are thought to be responsible for the improved survival seen in pentoxifylline-treated animal models of endotoxin-induced septic shock.[131] Currently, clinical trials using pentoxifylline in postcardiac surgery patients with early evidence of systemic inflammation suggest a cardioprotective effect with pentoxifylline use.[47] Thus, this and other pharmacologic agents may be useful in preventing or reducing some of the diverse and even fatal effects that are mediated by proinflammatory cytokines.

IVIG may have a potential inhibitory effect on proinflammatory cytokine activity. Patients in the active phase of Kawasaki disease have increased levels of IL-1 and TNF-α. These cytokines may stimulate local inflammatory responses by regulating leukocyte adherence and activation, leading to the vascular damage that is a critical clinical aspect of this disease. It has been suggested further that the effects of IVIG in Kawasaki disease, and perhaps other diseases, may be by attenuating production of the proinflammatory cytokines TNF-α and IL-1.[2, 4, 97] Animal models of LPS-induced TNF-α and IL-1 synthesis demonstrate a suppression of mononuclear cell synthesis of these proinflammatory cytokines when treated with IVIG.[6] The peripheral blood mononuclear cell production of TNF-α and IL-1, however, in Kawasaki disease patients receiving IVIG showed decreased synthesis of IL-1 but not TNF-α.[96] The role of IVIG as an immunomodulator has been suggested in an ever-growing number of clinical disease states because of its broad immunoregulatory potential.[4, 67] Its specific role in arresting proinflammatory cytokine activity, either directly or indirectly, warrants further clinical investigation.

The hypothesis that diminished levels of cytokines may render a host susceptible to infection was introduced by Weatherstone and Rich.[160] They suggested that the increased susceptibility to infection observed in premature neonates may be secondary to deficient proinflammatory cytokine production. In their study, they measured cord blood monocyte secretion of TNF-α and IL-1 with and without LPS stimulation. IL-1 activity by stimulated preterm monocytes did not differ from that observed by LPS-stimulated adult monocytes. TNF-α activity, however, in the LPS-stimulated monocytes from preterm neonates was significantly lower than that in both stimulated and unstimulated adult monocytes. Thus, they concluded that diminished production of TNF-α may predispose the preterm infant to infection. This has not been supported by the studies of infected animals that show markedly elevated TNF-α levels, and subsequent studies in preterm infants have not established a deficiency in TNF-α.[163] Williams and associates[163] and Peat and coworkers[132] have, in contrast, shown that mononuclear cells from term newborns produced enhanced levels of TNF-α in response to group B streptococci or endotoxin. A deleterious role resulting in diminished TNF-α or other proinflammatory cytokines in the premature human infant has yet to be defined, and individuals with specific cytokine deficiencies have yet to be described.

The proinflammatory cytokine IL-2 acts on activated T cells and to some extent on B cells and natural killer cells and causes them to proliferate or differentiate. IL-2 is synthesized by both T cells and natural killer cells.[116, 119] Decreased IL-2 production or IL-2 receptor expression have been noted in a number of clinical disease states, most notably in cases of severe combined immunodeficiency disease. Lesser degrees of abnormalities may occur in AIDS, type 1 diabetes mellitus, systemic lupus erythematosus, and hypogammaglobulinemia.[93, 95, 100] The most important potential for IL-2 in the treatment of disease involves its use in tumor therapy.[140] IL-2 currently is approved for the treatment of metastatic renal carcinoma. Use of IL-2–activated natural killer cells results in a decrease in tumor burden in about 20 per cent of patients, although serious side effects occur. In addition to its potential role as an antitumor agent, IL-2 shares many of the same effects as IFN-γ and may, someday, function as a therapeutic agent in infection, autoimmunity, and immunodeficiency.[95, 140]

Both IL-8 and IL-9 are being investigated in various human disease states, primarily because of their powerful role in stimulating neutrophil function, including activation and chemotaxis. Patients with cystic fibrosis, bronchiectasis, and chronic bronchitis have demonstrated elevated levels of IL-8 in their sputum.[138] The sputum from these patients is highly chemotactic to neutrophils but when treated with monoclonal antibodies to IL-8, this chemotactic effect was inhibited. Aerosolized IL-8 inhibitors have been used in patients with cystic fibrosis and result in decreased inflammation in these patients.[110, 138] IL-8 inhibitors currently are being evaluated in infants with bronchopulmonary dysplasia. It is speculated that the persistently elevated levels of IL-8 seen in the tracheal fluid of ventilated preterm infants lead to neutrophil accumulation and the development of pulmonary fibrosis, which may be reduced by IL-8 inhibitors.[80, 86] Similar studies are being conducted with IL-9 inhibitors. Thus, these cytokines may play an important role in the acute inflammatory response leading to chronic disease states, and blocking this response may be of therapeutic benefit. The proinflammatory cytokine IL-5 has not been implicated in a specific human disease state, but its strong B-cell proliferative effects suggest its role in the pathogenesis of immunodeficiency. Its potent effects on eosinophil production, activation, and migration implicate its action in allergic responses.[16] The other proinflammatory cytokines also are in various developmental stages of clinical investigation. As we learn more about their specific actions, we will be able better to determine their use as potential immunomodulating agents.

There is limited clinical use of the anti-inflammatory cytokines. IL-4 and IL-6 can block both IL-1 and TNF-α transcription.[66, 146] IL-4 has been shown to inhibit human neutrophil adhesion to human endothelial cells while enhancing the adhesion of eosinophils.[121] These effects have not been implicated in specific human disease, but IL-4 action is suggested in allergic responses. Although IL-6 has both anti-inflammatory and proinflammatory effects, the levels of this cytokine were found to correlate with mortality in children with gram-negative and gram-positive sepsis, suggesting that monitoring IL-6 levels may be of prognostic value.[158] Similarly, IL-10 has been shown to block production of IL-1, IL-6, IL-8, IL-12, TNF, and GM-CSF in animal models.[41, 106] It also has effects on mast cells, T cells, and natural killer cells and inhibits primary allogenic T-cell responses. Thus, IL-10 may have a potential role in treating acute and chronic inflammation and may be effective in suppressing transplant rejection.[8, 41] Studies examining the safety and immunomodulatory effects of the intravenous injection of IL-10 in humans demonstrate that it is well tolerated and results in decreased production of both TNF-α and IL-1.[14] Additional clinical studies are being conducted on the potential immunoregulatory effects of the anti-inflammatory cytokines, which may indicate their therapeutic use in human disease states.

Colony-Stimulating Factors

CSFs are involved principally in the production of neutrophils and monocytes. They were discovered because of their ability to stimulate the formation of colonies of granulocytes and monocytes-macrophages in cultured bone marrow cells and were named according to the primary cell colony type that they elicited. GM-CSF induces peripheral blood macrophages and granulocytes. It also has other pleiotropic effects, including stimulation of precursors of megakaryocytes, mast cells, and eosinophils. In addition, GM-CSF affects neutrophil migration and phagocytosis. Granulocyte CSF (G-CSF) induces peripheral blood granulocytes. Its actions are on both the production and function of neutrophils, including migration, phagocytosis, and superoxide generation. Macrophage CSF (M-CSF) induces peripheral mononuclear phagocytes. IL-3 increases mast cell populations as well as the induction of granulocytes, macrophages, eosinophils, and megakaryocytes.[17, 40, 60, 95, 99, 114]

Clinical studies with GM-CSF and G-CSF as adjuvant therapy have been performed in individuals with distinct hematopoietic disorders (congenital agranulocytosis, cyclic neutropenia, or consequences of cytotoxic chemotherapy, AIDS, and aplastic anemia). The CSFs can stimulate granulocyte and monocyte populations in these individuals, but the response is restricted to the number of available stem cells for stimulation. CSF treatment can reverse congenital neutropenia partially or completely and has shown great promise in the regeneration of hematopoietic cells after cytotoxic chemotherapy and high-dose chemotherapy followed by autologous bone marrow transplantation. Recombinant human GM-CSF also has been shown to be beneficial in patients with aplastic anemia.[3, 156] Hammond and associates[64] demonstrated a dramatic increase in neutrophil counts in children with cyclic neutropenia treated with recombinant human G-CSF. Cyclic neutropenia is a rare disorder characterized by regular 21-day cyclic fluctuations in the number of blood neutrophils, monocytes, eosinophils, lymphocytes, platelets, and reticulocytes. Although the exact mechanism of this disorder is not known, it is attributed to a regulatory abnormality affecting stem cell proliferation. These infants have recurrent aphthous stomatitis, pharyngitis, lymphadenopathy, fever, and numerous infections during the periods of neutropenia. The length of cycling in treated infants decreased from 21 days to 1 day, and the neutrophil turnover rate increased nearly fourfold, significantly reducing the frequency of infection. Recombinant G-CSF also has shown promise for infants and children with neutrophil production disorders. Infants with congenital agranulocytosis, Kostmann syndrome, a disorder characterized by severe, persistent absolute neutropenia, show a dramatic increase in neutrophil count after treatment with recombinant human G-CSF.[13] In addition, recombinant human G-CSF and GM-CSF have been used in neutropenic patients with AIDS. Although there is concern that the effects of GM-CSF to activate macrophages in turn may promote HIV replication, current studies are defining the role of recombinant human GM-CSF and G-CSF in AIDS patients.[59, 99]

Thus, CSFs are emerging as significant modulators of human immune function and hematopoiesis. Recombinant G-CSF and GM-CSF have demonstrated promising effects in clinical trials, and the utility of M-CSF and IL-3 currently is being investigated. Because the CSFs also functionally can activate mature granulocytes and monocytes, considerable attention has focused on their future extension in treating individuals at risk for infection. English and colleagues[42] reported decreased GM-CSF production by neonatal T cells. Because a major factor contributing to the increased susceptibility of human neonates to severe infections is their inability to produce adequate numbers of neutrophils in response to bacterial infections, these neonates may benefit from CSF treatment during severe infection. Similar treatment in immunologically stressed burn and trauma patients also may prove beneficial.[34, 128]

INTERFERONS

Interferon-α and Interferon-β

IFNs are glycoproteins that were discovered because of their antiviral properties. They are known to possess antitumor and immunomodulatory activities in addition to their antiviral effects. IFNs have been classified into three major groups: α, β, and γ. IFN-α and IFN-β previously were known as type I IFN, have similar protein structures, and bind the same receptor. IFN-γ, formerly type II interferon, has a much different structure and its own receptor.[5] IFN-α is produced by leukocytes. The earliest demonstration of its clinical usefulness was in the treatment of AIDS-related Kaposi sarcoma (KS). In these initial studies, a KS tumor response occurred in 30 to 50 per cent of the patients treated with recombinant IFN-α.[58, 90, 118, 123] It is speculated that IFN-α exerts its antitumor effect by activating cytotoxic T cells. Since then, placebo-controlled clinical trials have shown that IFN-α also may have a significant antiretroviral effect in HIV-infected patients.[88, 94] Clinical trials are under way to determine the effect of early treatment with IFN-α in reducing HIV disease progression and to determine the therapeutic effect of IFN-α in combination with other drugs in the treatment of HIV and HIV-related diseases.[89]

IFN-α also has been used in varying parts of the world for the treatment of chronic myeloid leukemia, hairy-cell leukemia, basal-cell carcinoma, multiple myeloma, hepatitis B and C, and condylomata acuminata. In chronic myeloid leukemia, early treatment with IFN-α has been reported to elicit complete hematologic remission in more than 70 per cent of the patients treated. Many of these patients had total elimination of the Philadelphia chromosome, which is a hallmark of the disease.[152–154] Eighty per cent to complete remission also has been reported in the treatment of hairy-cell leukemia.[136] Intralesional injection of IFN-α into basal-cell carcinoma of the skin resulted in 81 per cent tumor remission as determined by biopsy.[32, 77] Despite the variability among reports on the use of IFN-α in the treatment of multiple myeloma, it has been approved as a therapy for these patients in a number of European countries.[107]

IFN-α also is used for the treatment of hepatitis B and C.[17] Clinical responses have been reported to be of long duration, with often complete loss of both hepatitis B surface antigen and evidence of viral replication. In chronic hepatitis C, reports of complete responses to therapy determined by the decline of serum aspartate aminotransferase to normal levels have been observed in 50 to 70 per cent of the patients treated. Although serum aspartate aminotransferase levels in one-half of the patients who had improved returned to pretreatment levels within 6 to 12 months after discontinuation of therapy, nearly 20 per cent achieved sustained remission.[35, 38, 72, 87, 133] Studies also have shown that IFN-α is useful in treating genital warts, condylomata acuminata caused by papillomaviruses.[15] Intralesional injections of IFN-α completely eliminated warts in more than 50 per cent of the patients treated. IFN-α also is suggested to reduce the number of lesions in juvenile laryngeal papillomatosis after systemic use.[104] Thus, IFN-α has therapeutic potential as both an antitumor and an antiviral agent.

IFN-β also has received attention as an antiviral and antitumor agent. Its clinical usefulness as a single-agent therapy is suggested in relapsing multiple sclerosis. The mechanisms of IFN-β therapeutic action in multiple sclerosis are unknown.[78] Current studies are investigating IFN-β in combination with IFN-α in the treatment of various malignancies.

Interferon-γ

IFN-γ is produced by CD4 and CD8 cells as well as by natural killer cells.[70] Investigators have reported that circulating mononuclear cells and T lymphocytes from neonates are deficient markedly in their ability to produce IFN-γ in response to a variety of stimuli, compared with adult cells.[98, 149, 164] Studies comparing the relative ability of neonatal and adult mononuclear cells to generate IFN-γ versus IL-2 have shown that neonatal mononuclear cells produce less IFN-γ and generate more IL-2 than do adult cells.[164] Thus, one of the major abnormalities of the neonatal leukocyte is its relatively deficient production of IFN-γ. Subsequent studies using recombinant IFN-γ markedly enhanced the chemotactic response of PMNs from term neonates to levels that were not significantly different from that of PMNs from healthy adults after preincubation with IFN-α.[70] These findings suggest that there is a potential role for using IFN-γ to enhance neonatal host defense mechanisms and thus reduce or prevent the life-threatening systemic, pulmonary, or cutaneous infections commonly observed in neonates.

Job syndrome first was described by Davis and associates in 1965[36] in two patients with recurrent staphylococcal abscesses. Patients with this syndrome often develop chronic sinopulmonary infections and mucocutaneous *Candida* infections. Hill and coworkers[68] observed that the patients with Job syndrome also have a profound defect in neutrophil chemotactic responsiveness along with extreme hyper-IgE. This defect in neutrophil chemotaxis is intermittent and occurs predominantly when the patient is symptomatic.[33, 68, 69] Because IFN-γ production by mononuclear leukocytes in patients with hyper-IgE is deficient markedly or absent, in vitro studies were conducted to determine the effect of recombinant IFN-γ on the chemotactic responsiveness of neutrophils from patients with this syndrome. After pretreatment with IFN-γ, the chemotactic response of the neutrophils from Job syndrome patients increased significantly, with an average enhancement of 300 per cent above baseline to levels not significantly different from matched healthy controls.[79] Preliminary trials of IFN-γ therapy in four patients with Job syndrome of hyper-IgE suggested clinical benefit in three, with a significant decrease in eczema, pulmonary symptoms, and secretions.

Patients with chronic granulomatous disease (CGD) have an inherited deficiency in the proteins required for nicotinamide-adenine dinucleotide phosphate oxidase activity. Phagocytes with this enzymatic defect are able to engulf bacteria but cannot generate the respiratory burst necessary to kill the organisms. Consequently, patients with CGD suffer severe chronic, recurring, and life-threatening infections. The usefulness of treating CGD patients with IFN-γ was suggested by studies showing that this lymphokine can stimulate the respiratory burst of normal phagocytes. Results of studies by Ezekowitz and associates[45] and Sechler and colleagues[148] showed that when macrophages from patients with CGD were treated with IFN-γ in vitro, a respiratory burst occurred and superoxide anion was generated. Sechler and colleagues[148] further demonstrated a partial correction in neutrophils and monocytes from patients with CGD after subcutaneous treatment with recombinant IFN-γ. These initial results suggested that recombinant IFN-γ partially could correct the defective ability of phagocytes to kill bacteria when administered in vivo to patients with CGD. Ezekowitz and associates[46] extended these findings in a double-blind, placebo-controlled trial. They showed that recombinant IFN-γ significantly decreased the relative risk of serious infection in patients with CGD. Patients who received IFN-γ had a 70 per cent reduction in the risk of serious infection compared with controls. Overall, IFN-γ decreases the risk of infection and length of hospitalization in patients with CGD. It is well tolerated, and adverse effects usually easily are alleviated with acetaminophen. When IFN-γ is administered with prophylactic antibiotics, an additive effect occurs, proucing a nearly 20 per cent increase in the infection-free rate of CGD patients compared with IFN-γ alone.[46] IFN-γ was licensed by the Food and Drug Administration in December 1990 for the treatment of patients with CGD. The authors of the collaborative studies recommended its use with the addition of prophylactic antibiotics for treatment of children diagnosed with CGD.[54]

OTHER IMMUNOMODULATING AGENTS

Integrins and Selectins

Recruitment of neutrophils from the blood stream to extravascular sites of inflammation is a critical event in host defense against bacterial infection and in the repair of the tissue damage. Under certain circumstances, neutrophil accumulation may contribute to vascular and tissue injury. Thus, the regulatory mechanisms involved in neutrophil activation, recruitment, and subsequent degranulation are of potential clinical significance. Neutrophil adherence to and migration through capillary endothelium is a critical early event in the acute inflammatory response. The adhesive interactions between leukocytes and endothelial cell surfaces are regulated by two novel families of glycoproteins: the integrins and the selectins. The β-2 integrins are membrane-bound glycoprotein receptors found on the surface of PMNs. The β-2 integrins CD11/CD18 are required for PMN adherence to endothelial cell surfaces. The selectins also are membrane-bound glycoproteins that mediate neutrophil adhesion to endothelial cells. These include L-selectin, which is found on the surface of PMNs, and P-selectin and E-selectin, which are expressed on the surface of activated endothelial cells.[11, 26, 151, 168]

The interaction between the β-2 integrins and the selectins serves to regulate PMN responses during inflammation. In general, P-selectin and E-selectin on the activated endothelial cell surface and L-selectin on the PMN cell surface function to facilitate PMN rolling and tethering to activated capillary endothelium. Once this tethering has occurred and the PMN itself is activated, the β-2 integrin CD11/CD18 receptors on the PMN form a tight adhesion with the endothelial cell surface that facilitates PMN polarization, leading to migration.[11, 26, 151, 168] Congenital β-2 integrin CD11/CD18 deficiency states have been described (leukocyte adhesion deficiency type I [LAD-I]). These patients have profound PMN adhesion and motility defects and recurrent life-threatening infections along with delayed separation of the umbilical cord and juvenile periodontitis.[44, 53] A second type of LAD, LAD-II, has been described due to a deficiency of Sialyl Lewis X, the PMN ligand for E-selectin on endothelial cells.[134] It also has been shown that the tethering of PMNs to P-selectin on activated endothelial cells is critical for PMN priming by PAF and that monoclonal antibodies to P-selectin can block this response.[101] Monoclonal antibodies to P-selectin have been used in animal models of ischemia and reperfusion injury and have been shown to reduce significantly the severe edema and endothelial cell injury observed after reperfusion.[165] Similarly, monoclonal antibodies to P-selectin have resulted in significant endothelial cell preservation in animal models of lung injury and cardiac ischemia.[122, 161] Monoclonal antibodies to E-selectin and L-selectin also are being tested in animal models.[111] With the rapid advancements in identifying new molecules that influence endothelial cell–leukocyte interactions, we will gain greater understanding of the complexity of cellular communication during inflammation.

Platelet-Activating Factor

PAF is a potent phospholipid inflammatory mediator with many biologic effects. Its synthesis is regulated by phospholipase A_2, an enzyme associated with the arachidonic acid pathway. PAF has a very short half-life in vivo because of its rapid degradation by PAF acetylhydrolase. PAF is synthesized by many cell types, including macrophages, neutrophils, platelets, eosinophils, endothelial cells, and hepatocytes.[162] Intravenous infusion of PAF into animals results in pulmonary hypertension, bronchoconstriction, neutropenia, thrombocytopenia, and ischemic bowel necrosis.[9, 28, 65] PAF production is stimulated in a number of clinical disease states, including hypoxia and ischemia, and after administration of biologic agents, such as LPS, CM-CSF, TNF-α, IL-1, bradykinin, and thrombin.[48, 91, 113, 135, 139, 166] Corticosteroids decrease PAF levels by the induction of its natural inhibitor PAF-acetylhydrolase.[57] PAF has been shown to stimulate the production of many other mediators of inflammation, including TNF-α, complement breakdown products, oxygen radicals, catecholamines, prostaglandins, thromboxane, and the leukotrienes.[74, 91, 139, 157, 169] It also activates endothelial cells and neutrophils and monocytes, leading to their adherence and migration.[112] Thus, PAF is a ubiquitous phospholipid mediator with biologic effects and interactions within the inflammatory cascade.

The regulation of PAF has been studied in a number of potential clinical disease states, including sepsis and septic shock.[73] The clinical phase III trials in septic patients and patients in septic shock who received a PAF antagonist did not have a significant reduction in mortality.[37] The role of PAF, however, in the pathogenesis of necrotizing enterocolitis (NEC) has received considerable attention.[22, 25] NEC is an often fatal gastrointestinal disease that predominantly affects premature infants. Exogenous administration of PAF into rat mesenteric circulation causes ischemic bowel necrosis and pathology similar to neonatal NEC.[75] Endotoxin-induced intestinal injury is associated with increased PAF levels, and the infusion of high doses of endotoxin into animals produces a similar pathologic model of NEC that can be prevented by administration of dexamethasone, PAF acetylhydrolase, or PAF receptor antagonists.[24, 76] These animal studies suggest a link between PAF and its regulation and the development of NEC as well as implicate PAF as a potential endogenous inflammatory mediator in the pathogenesis of neonatal NEC.

There is evidence in humans to support an association between PAF and human neonatal NEC. PAF levels are higher in infants with NEC versus controls, and PAF acetylhydrolase activity is lower in infants with NEC.[23] PAF acetylhydrolase is suppressed with prematurity.[21] Because enteral feedings are necessary for the development of NEC, PAF levels were measured in feeding premature infants. In these studies, feedings alone increased circulating PAF levels but not PAF acetylhydrolase and infants fed human breast milk had lower PAF levels and a lower incidence of NEC, suggesting a protective effect of human milk through PAF regulation.[105] Human milk is known to have number of factors protective against infectious disease, including PAF acetylhydrolase.[18, 56] Because PAF acetylhydrolase activity is present in human milk and absent in formulas, it has been suggested that the protective activity observed in human milk against the development of NEC may result from blocking of PAF-related inflammatory responses.[18] The modulation of the many interactions of PAF within the inflammatory cascade may have future clinical potential in regulating neonatal NEC and other infectious disease states.

Nitric Oxide

Nitric oxide is a membrane-permeable gas that functions in the regulation of vascular tone and the inhibition of platelet aggregation and leukocyte adhesion. In addition, nitric oxide has been shown to have antitumor as well as antimicrobial activity. Under normal conditions, nitric oxide synthase induces endothelial cell production of nitric oxide. The signal transduction pathway for nitric oxide is linked to pathways involving vasodilation. There is evidence for activation of the L-arginine–nitric oxide pathway in sepsis, in which the effects of nitric oxide on the vasculature are associated with the severe vascular failure observed during septic shock.[30, 85, 120, 126, 127] Thus, inhibition of nitric oxide production has been proposed as a novel approach for the treatment of the severe hypotension associated with septic shock.

The increased production of nitric oxide observed during septic shock may have several harmful effects. Nitric oxide may be largely responsible for sepsis-induced hypotension. In vitro studies implicate nitric oxide in sepsis-induced myocardial depression, although nitric oxide synthase inhibitors have not been shown to prevent endotoxin-induced myocardial depression in vivo. Nitric oxide also has direct cytotoxic effects, and its overproduction in septic shock can lead to tissue injury and organ failure.[31, 49, 83] In addition, in vitro experiments suggest that nitric oxide may enhance the release of proinflammatory cytokines during septic shock.[43, 126] Nitric oxide production may, however, have some beneficial effects during septic shock. It is implicated in maintaining visceral and other microvasculature blood flow, both as a counterregulatory mechanism to the vasoconstrictive mediators released during sepsis and by its ability to block platelet adhesion, reducing potential microvasculature stasis and thrombosis.[84, 109] In addition, high levels of nitric oxide have antimicrobial activity and enhance LPS-induced cytokine production,[92] although it has yet to be determined if these levels of nitric oxide reflect actual physiologic states.

Because hypotension during sepsis is an important predictor of organ injury and death, use of nitric oxide synthase inhibitors may improve survival in severe septic shock by increasing mean arterial pressure. Nitric oxide synthase inhibitors have been shown to restore vascular responsiveness to catecholamines in animal models of endotoxin-induced septic shock.[71] In addition, nitric oxide synthase inhibition has been shown to normalize mean arterial pressure in anesthetized animals challenged with endotoxin or TNF-α without causing hypertension.[83] These considerations have led to the use of nitric oxide synthase inhibitors to treat hypotension in patients with sepsis and in those receiving cytokine therapy for cancer.[82, 102] Although these agents can alter mean arterial pressure, beneficial effects on clinical outcomes, including survival, only are suggested in human clinical trials.[126] Studies of endotoxin-challenged rats showed that partial nitric oxide synthase inhibition improved survival but that complete inhibition of nitric oxide production clearly is harmful, suggesting a beneficial effect with selective nitric oxide inhibition. More selective studies of nitric oxide inhibition are being conducted, and nitric oxide eventually may have clinical utility in the treatment of infectious disease states.

CONCLUSION

Attempts to augment immune function in infants or children with overwhelming sepsis or immunodeficiency over the past decade have focused on the cytokine family of recombinant molecules that includes the lymphokines and monokines (ILs and TNF-α as well as the hematopoietic growth factors), CSFs, and IFN-α, IFN-β, and IFN-γ. The advances in basic science research and clinical trials have demonstrated that the cytokines play many crucial roles in the pathogenesis of human disease. The interaction among the cytokines initiates the development of a cascade of biologic events leading to the propagation and regulation of inflammation, resulting in host defense against pathogen invasion. Although the cytokines are effective in augmenting immune responses, the overexpression of certain proinflammatory cytokines can lead to severe tissue injury. This has been demonstrated by many animal models of septic shock, in which suppression of the proinflammatory cytokines TNF-α and IL-1 reduces morbidity and mortality. The use of neutralizing antibodies to endotoxin, anti–TNF-α antibodies, and soluble TNF-α and IL-1 receptors, as well as IL-1 receptor antagonists in human clinical trials of sepsis, however, has shown limited therapeutic potential. The future clinical use of cytokine inhibition likely will include a combination of a number of both recombinant and pharmacologic agents that regulate multiple proinflammatory cytokine-mediated steps in the development of inflammation. The proinflammatory and anti-inflammatory effects of the ILs show promise in regulating acute inflammatory responses. The hematopoietic growth factors have demonstrated considerable clinical effect, especially in individuals with distinct hematopoietic disorders and in patients receiving immunosuppressive chemotherapy. IFN-α, IFN-β, and IFN-γ have received considerable attention over the last decade as potential immunomodulators. IFN-α has shown broad clinical application as an antitumor as well as an antiviral agent. IFN-β is being used with some success in patients with relapsing multiple sclerosis, and the stimulatory effects of IFN-γ on human neutrophils suggest its therapeutic use in children with specific neutrophil dysfunction. Investigations defining the actions of the integrins and selectins, PAF, and nitric oxide may provide novel future clinical therapeutic approaches to attenuate acute inflammatory responses. As we learn more about the complexity of intracellular and extracellular interactions and the delicate balance these molecules have in regulating immune responses, we will be able better to implement their clinical use in regulating infectious disease states in infants and children.

References

1. Alexander, H. R., Doherty, G. M., Buresh, C. M., et al.: A recombinant human receptor antagonist to interleukin-1 improves survival after lethal endotoxemia in mice. J. Exp. Med. *173*:1029, 1991.
2. Anderson, J. P., and Anderson, U. G.: Human intravenous immunoglobulin modulates monokine production in vitro. Immunology *71*:372, 1990.
3. Antman, K. S., Griffin, J. D., Elias, A., et al.: Effect of recombinant human granulocyte-macrophage colony-stimulating factor on chemotherapy induced myelosuppression. N. Engl. J. Med. *319*:593, 1988.
4. Ballow, M.: Mechanisms of action of intravenous immune serum globulin therapy. Pediatr. Infect. Dis. J. *13*:806, 1994.
5. Baron, S., Tyring, S. K., Fleischmann, R. W., et al.: The interferons: Mechanism of action and clinical applications. J. A. M. A. *266*:1375, 1991.
6. Basta, M., Kirshborn, P., Frank, M. M., et al.: Mechanisms of therapeutic effects of high-dose intravenous immunoglobulin: Attenuation of acute complement-dependent immune damage in a guinea pig model. J. Clin. Invest. 84:1974, 1989.
7. Baumgartner, J. D., Glauser, M. P., McCutchan, J. A., et al.: Prevention of gram-negative shock and death in surgical patients by antibody to endotoxin core glycolipid. Lancet *2*:59, 1985.
8. Berg, D. J., Kühn, R., and Rajewsky, K.: Interleukin-10 is a central regulator of the response to LPS in murine models of endotoxic shock and the Shwartzman reaction but not endotoxin tolerance. J. Clin. Invest. *96*:2339, 1995.
9. Bernat, A., Herbert, J. M., Salel, V., et al.: Protective effect of SR-27417, a novel PAF antagonist, on PAF-induced or endotoxin-induced hypotension in the rat and the guinea-pig. J. Lipid Mediat. *5*:41, 1992.
10. Bertini, R., Delgado, R., Faggioni, R., et al.: Urinary TNF-binding protein (TNF soluble receptor) protects mice against the lethal effect of TNF and endotoxin shock. Eur. Cytokine Network *4*:39, 1993.
11. Beuilacqua, M. P., and Nelson, M. P.: Selectins. J. Clin. Invest. *91*:379, 1993.
12. Beutler, B., Milsark, I. W., and Cerami, A.: Passive immunization against cachectin/tumor neurosis factor protects mice from lethal effect of endotoxin. Science *229*:869, 1985.

13. Bonilla, M. A., Gillio, A. P., Ruggeno, M., et al.: Effect of recombinant human granulocyte colony-stimulating factor on neutropenia in patients with congenital agranulocytosis. N. Engl. J. Med. *320*:1574, 1989.
14. Borish, L., and Rosenwasser, L. J.: Update on cytokines. J. Allergy Clin. Immunol. *97*:719, 1996.
15. Brodell, R. T.: The use of natural alpha interferon in the treatment of condyloma acuminata. Infect. Med. *13*:56, 1996.
16. Broide, D. H., Paine, M. M., and Firestein, G. S.: Eosinophils express interleukin-5 and granulocyte macrophage-colony stimulating factor mRNA at sites of allergic inflammation in asthmatics. J. Clin. Invest. *90*:1414, 1992.
17. Brou, A. S., Lehman, D., Geertsma, F. R., et al.: Biology and therapeutic uses of myeloid hematopoietic growth factors and interferons. Pediatr. Infect. Dis. J. *15*:563, 1996.
18. Buescher, E. S.: Host defense mechanisms of human milk and their relations to enteric infections and necrotizing enterocolitis. *In* Stoll, B. J., and Kliegman, R. M. (eds.): Clin. Perinatol. *21*:247–262, 1994.
19. Calandra, T., Baumgartner, J. D., Guam, E. G., et al.: Prognostic values of tumor necrosis factor/cachectin, interleukin-1, interferon-alpha, interferon-gamma in the serum of patients with septic shock. J. Infect. Dis. *161*:982, 1990.
20. Cannon, J. G., Tompkins, R. G., Gelfand, J. A., et al.: Circulating interleukin-1 and tumor necrosis factor in septic shock and experimental endotoxin fever. J. Infect. Dis. *161*:79, 1990.
21. Caplan, M. S., Hsueh, W., Kelly, A., et al.: Serum PAF acetylhydrolase increases during neonatal maturation. Prostaglandins *39*:705, 1990.
22. Caplan, M. S., Sun, X. M., and Hsueh, W.: Hypoxia, PAF and necrotizing enterocolitis. Lipids *26*:1340, 1991.
23. Caplan, M. S., Sun, X. M., Hsueh, W., et al.: Role of platelet-activating factor and tumor necrosis factor-alpha in neonatal necrotizing enterocolitis. J. Pediatr. *116*:960, 1990.
24. Caplan, M. S., Kelly, A., and Hsueh, W.: Endotoxin and hypoxia induced intestinal necrosis in rats: The role of platelet activating factor. Pediatr. Res. *31*:428, 1992.
25. Caplan, M. S., and MacKendrick, W.: Inflammatory mediators and intestinal injury. *In* Stoll, B. J., and Kliegman, R. M. (eds.): Clin. Perinatol. *21*:235–246, 1994.
26. Carlos, T. M., and Harlan, J. M.: Leukocyte-endothelial adhesion molecules. Blood *84*:2068, 1994.
27. Cerami, A.: Inflammatory cytokines. Clin. Immunol. Pathol. *62*:53, 1992.
28. Chang, S. W., Feddersen, C. O., Henson, P. M., et al.: Platelet activating factor mediates hemodynamic changes and lung injury in endotoxin-treated rats. J. Clin. Invest. *79*:1498, 1987.
29. Chantry, D., Turner, M., Abrey, E., et al.: Modulation of cytokine production by transforming growth factor-beta. J. Immunol. *142*:4295, 1989.
30. Cobb, J. P., Cunnion, R. E., and Danner, R. L.: Nitric oxide as a target for therapy in septic shock. Crit. Care Med. *21*:1261, 1993.
31. Cobb, J. P., Natanson, C., Banks, S. M., et al.: N-amino-L-arginine, an inhibitor of nitric oxide synthase, raises vascular resistance but increases mortality rates in awake canines challenged with endotoxin. J. Exp. Med. *176*:1175–1182, 1992.
32. Cornell, R. C., Greenway, H. T., Tucker, S. B., et al.: Intralesional interferon therapy for basal cell carcinoma. J. Am. Acad. Dermatol. *23*:694, 1990.
33. Dahl, M. V., Greene, W. H., Quie, P. G.: Infection, dermatitis, increased IgE, and impaired neutrophil chemotaxis. Arch. Dermatol. *112*:1387, 1976.
34. Dale, D. C.: Potential role of colony-stimulating factors in the prevention and treatment of infectious diseases. Clin. Infect. Dis. *18*:S180, 1994.
35. Davis, G. L., Balart, L. A., Shiff, E. R., et al.: Treatment of chronic hepatitis C with recombinant interferon alpha: A multicenter randomized controlled trial. N. Engl. J. Med. *321*:1501, 1989.
36. Davis, D. S., Schaller, J., and Wedgwood, R. J.: Recurrent "cold" staphylococcal abscesses. Lancet *1*:1013, 1965.
37. Dhainaut, J. F., Tenaillon, A., Tulzo, Y., et al.: Platelet-activating factor receptor antagonist BN52021 in the treatment of severe sepsis: A randomized, double-blind, placebo-controlled, multicenter clinical trial. Crit. Care Med. *22*:1720, 1994.
38. DiBisceglie, A. M., Martin, P., Kassianides, C., et al.: Recombinant interferon alpha therapy for chronic hepatitis C: A randomized, double-blind, placebo-controlled trial. N. Engl. J. Med. *321*:1506, 1989.
39. Dinarello, C. A.: The proinflammatory cytokines, interleukin-1 and tumor necrosis factor and the treatment of the septic shock syndrome. J. Infect. Dis. *163*:1177, 1991.
40. Donahue, R. E.: Colony-stimulating factors: Their biological activities and clinical promise. Adv. Vet. Sci. Comp. Med. *36*:291, 1991.
41. D'Andrea, A., Aste-Amezaga, M., Vaiante, N. M., et al.: Interleukin-10 (IL-10) inhibits human lymphocyte interferon-γ production by suppressing natural killer cell stimulatory factor IL-12 synthesis in accessory cells. J. Exp. Med. *178*:1041, 1993.
42. English, K. B., Hammond, W. P., Lewis, D. B., et al.: Decreased granulocyte-macrophage colony stimulating factor production by human neonatal blood mononuclear cells and T cells. Pediatr. Res. *31*:211, 1992.
43. Estrada, C., Gomez, C., Martin, C., et al.: Nitric oxide mediates tumor necrosis factor alpha cytotoxicity in endothelial cells. Biochem. Biophys. Res. Commun. *186*:475, 1992.
44. Etzloni, A., Frydman, M., Pollack, S., et al.: Recurrent severe infections caused by a novel leukocyte adhesion deficiency. N. Engl. J. Med. *327*:1789, 1992.
45. Ezekowitz, R. A. B., Dinauer, M. C., Jaffe, H. S., et al.: Partial correction of the phagocytic defect in patients with X-linked chronic granulomatous disease by subcutaneous interferon gamma. N. Engl. J. Med. *319*:146, 1988.
46. Ezekowitz, R. A. B., and the International Collaborative Study Group to Assess the Efficiency of rIFN-gamma in CGD: Clinical efficacy of recombinant human interferon-gamma (rIFN-gamma) in chronic granulomatous disease (CGD). Clin. Res. *38*:465A, 1990.
47. Falst, E., Schinkel, C., and Zimmer, S.: Update on the mechanisms of immune suppression of injury and immune modulation. World J. Surg. *20*:454, 1996.
48. Feuerstein, G., and Hallenbeck, J. M.: Prostaglandins, leukotrienes and platelet activating factor in shock. Ann. Rev. Pharmacol. Toxicol. *27*:301, 1987.
49. Finkel, M. S., Oddis, C. V., Jacob, T. D., et al.: Negative inotropic effects of cytokines on the heart mediated by nitric oxide. Science *257*:387, 1992.
50. Fisher, C. J., Dhainaut, J.-F. A., Opal, S. M., et al.: Recombinant human interleukin 1 receptor antagonist in the treatment of patients with sepsis syndrome. J. A. M. A. *271*:1836, 1994.
51. Fisher, C. J., Jr., and Zheng, Y.: Potential strategies for inflammatory mediator manipulation: Retrospect and prospect. World J. Surg. *20*:447, 1996.
52. Fisher, C. J., Slotman, G. J., Opal, S. M., et al.: Initial evaluation of human recombinant interleukin-1 receptor antagonist in the treatment of sepsis syndrome: A randomized, open label, placebo controlled muticentric trial. Crit. Care Med. *22*:12, 1994.
53. Frydman, M., Etzioni, A., Eidlitz-Markus, I., et al.: Rambam-Hasharon syndrome of psychomotor retardation, short stature, defective neutrophil motility, and Bombay phenotype. Am. J. Med. Genet. *44*:297, 1992.
54. Gallin, J. I.: Interferon-gamma in the management of chronic granulomatous disease: The evolving use of biologicals in the treatment and prevention of infectious diseases. Rev. Infect. Dis. *13*:3, 1991.
55. Girardin, E., Grau, G., Dayer, J. M., et al.: Tumor necrosis factor and interleukin-1 in the serum of children with severe infectious purpura. N. Engl. J. Med. *319*:397, 1988.
56. Goldman, A. S.: The immune system of human milk: Antimicrobial antiinflammatory and immunomodulating properties. Pediatr. Infect. Dis. J. *12*:664, 1993.
57. Goppelstruebe, M., and Rehfeldt, W.: Glucocorticoids inhibit TNF alpha induced cytosolic phospholipase A2 activity. Biochem. Biophys. Acta *1127*:163, 1992.
58. Groopman, J. E., Gottlieb, M. S., Goodman, J., et al.: Recombinant alpha-2b interferon therapy for Kaposi's sarcoma associated with acquired immune deficiency syndrome. Ann. Intern. Med. *100*:671, 1984.
59. Groopman, J. E., Mitsuyasu, R. T., DeLeo, M. J., et al.: Effect of recombinant human granulocyte-macrophage colony-stimulating factor on myelopoiesis in the acquired immunodeficiency syndrome. N. Engl. J. Med. *317*:593, 1987.
60. Grosh, W. W., and Quesenberry, P. J.: Recombinant human hematopoietic growth factors in the treatment of cytopenias. Clin. Immunol. Immunopathol. *62*:S25, 1992.
61. Guirao, X., and Lowry, S. F.: Biological control of injury and inflammation: Much more than too little or too late. World J. Surg. *20*:437, 1996.
62. Haak-Frendsho, M., Marseters, S. A., Mordenti, J., et al.: Inhibition of TNF by a TNF receptor immunoadhesin: Comparison to an anti-TNF monoclonal antibody. J. Immunol. 152:1347, 1994.
63. Hammerberg, C., Arend, W. P., Fischer, G. J., et al.: Interleukin-1 receptor agonist in normal and psoriatic epidermis. J. Clin. Invest. *90*:571, 1992.
64. Hammond, W. P., Price, T. H., Souza, L. M., et al.: Treatment of cyclic neutropenia with granulocyte colony-stimulating factor. N. Engl. J. Med. *320*:1306, 1989.
65. Hanahan, D. J.: Platelet activating factor: A biologically active phosphoglyceride. Ann. Rev. Biochem. *55*:483, 1986.
66. Hart, P. H., Vitti, G. F., Burgess, D. R., et al.: Potential antiinflammatory effects of interleukin-4: Suppression of human monocyte tumor necrosis factor, interleukin-1 and prostaglandin E2. Proc. Natl. Acad. Sci. U. S. A. *86*:3803, 1984.
67. Hill, H. R.: Intravenous immunoglobulin use in the neonate: Role in prophylaxis and therapy of infection. Pediatr. Infect. Dis. J. *12*:549, 1993.
68. Hill, H. R., Quie, P. G., Ochs, H. D., et al.: Defect in neutrophil granulocyte chemotaxis in Job's syndrome of recurrent "cold" staphylococcal abscesses. Lancet *2*:617, 1974.
69. Hill, H. R., Estensen, R. D., Hogan, N. A., et al.: Severe staphylococcal disease associated with allergic manifestations, hyperimmunoglobulin E, and defective neutrophil chemotaxis. J. Lab. Clin. Med. *112*:1387, 1976.
70. Hill, H. R., Augustine, N. H., and Jaffe, H. S.: Human recombinant interferon enhances neonatal polymorphonuclear leukocyte activation and movement, and increases free intracellular calcium. J. Exp. Med. *173*:767, 1991.
71. Hollenberg, S. M., Cunnion, R. E., and Zimmerberg, J.: Nitric oxide synthase inhibition reverses arteriolar hyporesponsiveness to catecholamines in septic rats. Am. J. Physiol. *264*:660, 1993.
72. Hoofnagle, J. M.: Chronic hepatitis B. N. Engl. J. Med. *323*:337, 1990.

73. Hosfard, D., Koltai, M., and Braquet, P.: Platelet activating factor in shock, sepsis, and organ failure. *In* Schlag, G., and Redl, H. (eds.): Pathophysiology of Shock, Sepsis and Organ Failure. Heidelberg, Springer-Verlag, 1993, pp. 502–517.
74. Hsueh, W., Gonzalez-Crussi, F., and Arroyaue, J. L.: Sequential release of leukotrienes and norepinephrine in rat bowel after platelet-activating factor. Gastroenterology *94*:1412, 1988.
75. Hsueh, W., Gonzalez-Crussi, F., and Arroyaue, J. L.: Platelet-activating factor: An endogenous mediator for bowel necrosis in endotoxemia. FASEB J. *1*:403, 1987.
76. Israel, E. J., Schiffrin, E., Carter, E. A., et al.: Prevention of necrotizing enterocolitis in the rat with prenatal cortisone. Gastroenterology *99*:1333, 1990.
77. Itri, L. M.: The interferons. Cancer *70*:940, 1992.
78. Jacobs, L. D., Cookfair, D. L., Rudick, R. A., et al.: Intramuscular inteferon beta-1a for disease progression in relapsing multiple sclerosis: The Multiple Sclerosis Collaborative Research Group (MSCRG). Ann. Neurol. *39*:285, 1996.
79. Jeppson, J. D., Jaffe, H. S., and Hill, H. R.: Use of recombinant human interferon gamma to enhance neutrophil chemotactic responses in Job's syndrome of hyperimmunoglobulinemia E and recurrent infections. J. Pediatr. *118*:383, 1991.
80. Jones, C. A., Cayabyab, R. B., Kwong, Y. C., et al.: Undetectable interleukin IL-10 and persistent IL-8 expression early in hyaline membrane disease: A possible developmental basis for the predisposition to chronic lung inflammation in preterm newborns. Pediatr. Res. *39*:966, 1996.
81. Kennedy, W. A., Hoyt, J. M., and McCracken, G. H., Jr.: The role of corticosteroid therapy in children with pneumococcal meningitis. Am. J. Dis. Child. *145*:1374, 1991.
82. Kilbourn, R. G., and Griffith, O. W.: Overproduction of nitric oxide in cytokine-mediated septic shock. J. Natl. Cancer Inst. *84*:827, 1992.
83. Kilbourn, R. G., Gross, S. S., Jubran, A., et al.: N-methyl-L-arginine inhibits tumor necrosis factor induced hypotension: Implications for the involvement of nitric oxide. Proc. Natl. Acad. Sci. U. S. A. *87*:3629, 1990.
84. Klabunde, R. E., and Helgren, M. C.: Cardiovascular actions of N-methyl-L-arginine are abolished in a canine shock model using high dose endotoxin. Res. Comm. Chem. Pathol. Pharmacol. *78*:57, 1992.
85. Knowles, R. G., and Moncada, S.: Nitric oxide synthases in mammals. Biochem. J. *298*:249–257, 1994.
86. Kotecha, S., Wilson, K., Wangoo, A., et al.: Increased interleukin IL-13 and IL-6 in bronchiolar lavage fluid obtained from infants with chronic lung disease of prematurity. Pediatr. Res. *40*:250, 1996.
87. Kovenman, J., Baker, B., Waggoner, J., et al.: Long term remission of chronic hepatitis B after alpha-interferon therapy. Ann. Intern. Med. *114*:629, 1991.
88. Krown, S. E., Gold, J. W. M., and Niedzwiecki, D.: Interferon-alpha with zidovudine: Safety, tolerance, and clinical and virological effect in patients with Kaposi's sarcoma associated with the acquired immunodeficiency syndrome (AIDS). Ann. Intern. Med. *112*:812, 1990.
89. Krown, S. E.: Approaches to interferon combination therapy in the treatment of AIDS. Semin. Oncol. *17*:11, 1990.
90. Krown, S. E., Real, F. X., Cunningham-Rundles, C., et al.: Preliminary observations on the effect of recombinant leukocyte A interferon in homosexual men with Kaposi's sarcoma. N. Engl. J. Med. *308*:1071, 1983.
91. Kubes, P., Artovs, K. E., and Granger, D. N.: Platelet-activating factor induced mucosal dysfunction-role of oxidants and granulocytes. Am. J. Physiol. *260*:G965, 1991.
92. Kubes, P., Suzuki, M., and Granger, D. N.: Nitric oxide: An endogenous modulator of leukocyte adhesion. Proc. Natl. Acad. Sci. U. S. A. *88*:4651, 1991.
93. La Pine, T. R., and Hill, H. R.: Immunomodifiers applicable to the prevention and management of infectious diseases in children. Adv. Pediat. Infect. Dis. *9*:37–58, 1994.
94. Lane, H. C., Davey, V., Kovacs, J. A., et al.: Interferon alpha in patients with asymptomatic human immunodeficiency virus (HIV) infection: A randomized, placebo-controlled trial. Ann. Intern. Med. *112*:805, 1990.
95. Lau, A. S.: Cytokines in the pathogenesis and treatment of infectious diseases. Adv. Pediat. Infect. Dis. *9*:211–236, 1994.
96. Leung, D. Y. M., Kurt-Jones, E., Newberger, J. W., et al.: Endothelial cell activation and high interleukin-1 secretion in the pathogenesis of acute Kawasaki disease. Lancet *1*:1298, 1989.
97. Leung, D. Y.: The immunoregulatory effects of IVIG in Kawasaki disease and other autoimmune diseases. *In* Ballow, M. (ed.): IVIG Therapy Today. Totowa, NJ, Humana Press, 1992, pp. 93–104.
98. Lewis, D. D., Weaver, M., Prickett, K., et al.: Restricted production of IL-4 compared to IFN-gamma by human T cells during post natal development. J. Cell. Biochem. *13*:233, 1989.
99. Lieschke, G. J., and Burgess, A. W.: Granulocyte colony-stimulating factor and granulocyte-macrophage colony-stimulating factor. N. Engl. J. Med. *327*:28, 1992.
100. Liles, W. C., and Voorhis, W. C.: Nomenclature and biological significance of cytokines involved in inflammation and host immune response. J. Infect. Dis. *172*:1573, 1995.
101. Lorant, D. E., Topham, M. K., Whatley, R. E., et al.: Inflammatory roles of P-selectin. J. Clin. Invest. *92*:559, 1993.
102. Lorente, J. A., Landin, L., De Pablo, R., et al.: L-arginine pathway in the sepsis syndrome. Crit. Care Med. *21*:1287, 1993.
103. Luce, J. M.: Introduction of new technology into critical care practice: A history of HA-1A human monoclonal antibody against endotoxin. Crit. Care Med. *21*:1233, 1993.
104. Lusk, R. P., MaCabe, B. F., and Mixon, J. H.: Three-year experience of treating recurrent respiratory papilloma with interferon. Ann. Otol. Rhinol. Laryngol. *19*:158, 1987.
105. MacKendrick, W., Hill, N., Hseuh, W., et al.: Increase in plasma platelet activating factor levels in enterally fed premature infants. Biol. Neonate *64*:89, 1993.
106. Malefyt, R. W., Yssel, H., Roncarolo, M. G., et al.: Interleukin-10. Curr. Opin. Immunol. *4*:314, 1992.
107. Mandell, F., Avvisati, G., Amadori, S., et al.: Maintenance treatment with recombinant interferon alpha-2b in patients with multiple myeloma responding to conventional induction chemotherapy. N. Engl. J. Med. *322*:1430, 1990.
108. Mathison, J. C., Wolfson, E., and Uleuitch, R. J.: Participation of tumor necrosis factor in the mediation of gram-negative bacteria lipopolysaccharide-induced injury in rabbits. J. Clin. Invest. *81*:1925, 1988.
109. May, G. R., Crook, P., Moore, P. K., et al.: The role of nitric oxide as an endogenous regulator of platelet neutrophil activation within the pulmonary circulation of the rabbit. Br. J. Pharmacol. *102*:759, 1991.
110. McElvaney, N. G., Nakamura, H., Birrer, P., et al.: Modulation of airway inflammation in cystic fibrosis: In vivo suppression of interleukin-8 levels on the respiratory epithelial surface by aerosolization of recombinant secretory leukoprotease inhibitor. J. Clin. Invest. *90*:1296, 1992.
111. McEver, R. P.: Selectins. Curr. Opin. Immunol. *6*:75, 1994.
112. McIntyre, T. M., Zimmerman, G. A., and Prescott, S. M.: Leukotrienes C4 and D4 stimulate human endothelial cells to synthesize platelet activating factor and bind neutrophils. Proc. Natl. Acad. Sci. U. S. A. *83*:2204, 1986.
113. McIntyre, T. M., Zimmerman, G. A., Satoh, K., et al.: Cultured endothelial cells synthesize both platelet activating factor and prostacyclin in response to histamine, bradykinin, and adenosine triphosphate. J. Clin. Invest. *76*:271, 1985.
114. Metcalf, D.: Control of granulocytes and macrophages: Molecular cellular and clinical aspects. Science *254*:529, 1991.
115. Michie, H. R., Manoque, K. R., Spriggs, D. R., et al.: Detecting circulating tumor necrosis factor after endotoxin administration. N. Engl. J. Med. *318*:1481, 1988.
116. Minami, Y., Kono, T., Miyazaki, T., et al.: The IL-2 receptor complex: Its structure function and target genes. Annu. Rev. Immunol. *11*:245, 1993.
117. Minty, A., Chalon, P., Derocq, J. M., et al.: Interleukin-13 is a new human lymphokine regulating inflammation and immune responses. Nature *362*:248, 1993.
118. Mitsuyasu, R. T.: Use of recombinant interferons and hematopoietic growth factors in patients with human immunodeficiency virus: The evolving use of biologicals in the treatment and prevention of infectious diseases. Rev. Infect. Dis. *13*:9, 1991.
119. Mochizuki, W. J.: Interleukin 2: A class of T cell growth factors. Immunol. Rev. *51*:257, 1980.
120. Moncada, S., Palmer, R. M., and Higgs, E. A.: Nitric oxide: Physiology, pathophysiology, and pharmacology. Pharmacol. Rev. *43*:109–142, 1991.
121. Moser, R., Fehr, J., and Bruijnzeel, P. L. B.: IL-4 controls the selective endothelium driven transmigration of eosinophils from allergic individuals. J. Immunol. *149*:1432, 1992.
122. Mulligan, M. S., Polley, M. J., Bayer, R. J., et al.: Neutrophil-dependent acute lung injury. Requirement for P-selectin (GMP-140). J. Clin. Invest. *90*:1600, 1992.
123. Murray, H. W.: Interferon gamma therapy in AIDS for mononuclear phagocyte activation. Biotherapy *2*:149, 1990.
124. Mustafa, M. M., Lebel, M. H., Ramilo, O., et al.: Correlation of interleukin-1 beta and cachectin concentration in cerebrospinal fluid and outcome from bacterial meningitis. J. Pediatr. *115*:208, 1989.
125. Natanson, C., Eichenholz, P. W., Danner, R. L., et al.: Endotoxin and tumor necrosis factor challenges in dogs stimulate the cardiovascular profile of human septic shock. J. Exp. Med. *169*:823, 1989.
126. Natanson, C., and Hoffman, W. D.: Selected treatment strategies for septic shock based on proposed mechanisms of pathogenesis. Ann. Intern. Med. *120*:771, 1994.
127. Nathan, C., and Hibbs, J. B.: Role of nitric oxide synthesis in macrophage antimicrobial activity. Curr. Opin. Immunol. *3*:65, 1991.
128. Nelson, S.: Role of granulocyte colony-stimulating factor in the immune response to acute bacterial infection in the nonneutropenic host: An overview. Clin. Infect. Dis. *18*:S197, 1994.
129. Newton, A. J., Ashwood, E. R., Yang, K. D., et al.: Effect of pentoxifylline on developmental changes in neutrophil cell surface mobility and membrane fluidity. J. Cell. Physiol. *140*:427, 1989.
130. Ohlsson, K., Bjork, P., Bergenfeldt, M., et al.: Interleukin-1 receptor antagonist reduces mortality from endotoxin shock. Nature *346*:550, 1990.
131. Olsmüller, C., Mayer, N., Micksche, M., et al.: In-vivo modulation of human neutrophil function by pentoxifylline in patients with septic syndrome. Shock *4*:161, 1995.
132. Peat, E. B., Augustine, N. H., Drummond, W. K., et al.: Effects of fibronec-

tin and group B streptococci on tumor necrosis factor-α production by human culture-derived macrophages. Immunology *84*:440, 1995.
133. Perrillo, R. P.: Treatment of chronic hepatitis B with interferon: Experience in western countries. Semin. Liver Dis. *9*:240, 1989.
134. Phillips, M. L., Schwartz, B. R., Etzioni, A., et al.: Neutrophil adhesion in leukocyte adhesion deficiency syndrome type 2. J. Clin. Invest. *96*:2898, 1995.
135. Prescott, S. M., Zimmerman, G. A., and McIntyre, T. M.: Human endothelial cells in culture produce platelet-activating factor when stimulated with thrombin. Proc. Natl. Acad. Sci. U. S. A. *81*:3534, 1984.
136. Quesada, J. R., Reuben, J. R., Manning, J. T., et al.: Alpha interferon for induction of remission in hairy cell leukemia. N. Engl. J. Med. *310*:15, 1984.
137. Rambaldi, A., Torcia, M., Bettoni, S., et al.: Modulation of cell proliferation and cytokine production in acute myeloblastic leukemia by interleukin-1 receptor antagonists and lack of its expression by leukemic cells. Blood *76*:114A, 1990.
138. Richman-Eisenstat, J., Jorens, P. G., Veki, I., et al.: Interleukin-8 an important chemoattractant in the sputum of patients with chronic inflammatory airway disease. Clin. Res. *41*:56A, 1993.
139. Rola-Pleszczynski, M., and Stankova, J.: Differentiation-dependent modulation of TNF production by PAF in human HL-60 myeloid leukemia cells. J. Leukoc. Biol. *51*:609, 1992.
140. Rosenberg, S. A., Lotze, M. T., Muul, L. M., et al.: A progress report on the treatment of 157 patients with advanced cancer using lymphocyte-activated killer cells and interleukin-2 or high doses of interleukin-2 alone. N. Engl. J. Med. *316*:884, 1987.
141. Russell, D., Tucken, K. K., Chinookoswoung, N., et al.: Combined inhibition of interleukin-1 and tumor necrosis factor in rodent endotoxemia: Improved survival and organ function. J. Infect. Dis. *171*:1538, 1995.
142. Sadoff, J. C.: Soluble TNF receptors. Presented at the Third International Congress of the Immune Consequences of Trauma, Shock and Sepsis: Mechanisms of Therapeutic Approaches, Munich, 1994.
143. Salyer, J. L., Bohnsack, J. F., Knape, W. A., et al.: Mechanisms of tumor necrosis factor alpha alteration of PMN adhesion and migration. Am. J. Pathol. *136*:831, 1990.
144. Schade, U. F., Burmeister, I., and Engel, R.: Increased 13-hydroxyoctadienoic acid content in lipopolysaccharide stimulated macrophages. Biochem. Biophys. Res. Comm. *147*:695, 1987.
145. Schedel, I., Driekhausen, U.., Nentwig, B., et al.: Treatment of gram-negative septic shock with an immunoglobulin preparation: A prospective, randomized clinical trial. Crit. Care Med. *19*:1104, 1991.
146. Schindler, R., Mancilla, J., Endes, S., et al.: Correlations and interactions in the production of interleukin-6, IL-1, and tumor necrosis factor in human blood mononuclear cells. Blood *75*:40, 1990.
147. Schindler, R., Clark, B. D., and Dinarello, C. A.: Dissociation between interleukin 1B mRNA and protein synthesis in peripheral blood mononuclear cells. J. Biol. Chem. *265*:10232, 1990.
148. Sechler, J. M. G., Malech, H. L., White, C. J., et al.: Recombinant human interferon-gamma reconstitutes defective phagocyte function in patients with chronic granulomatous disease of childhood. Proc. Natl. Acad. Sci. U. S. A. *85*:4874, 1988.
149. Seki, H., Taga, K., Matsoda, N., et al.: Phenotypic and functional characteristics of active suppressor cells against IFN-gamma production in PHA-stimulated cord blood lymphocytes. J. Immunol. *137*:3158, 1986.
150. Sirko, S., Weisman, S., and Dinarello, C. A.: Transcription, translation and secretion of IL-1 and TNF: Effect of dual cyclooxygenase and lipooxygenase inhibitor. Eur. J. Immunol. *21*:243, 1991.
151. Springer, T. A.: Traffic signals for lymphocyte recirculation and leukocyte migration: The multistep paradigm. Cell *76*:301–314, 1994.
152. Talpaz, M. N., Kantarjian, H. M., Kurzrock, R., et al.: Interferon alpha produces sustained cytogenic responses in chronic myelogenous leukemia: Philadelphia chromosome positive patients. Ann. Intern. Med. *114*:532, 1991.
153. Talpaz, M., Kantarjian, H. M., McCredie, K. B., et al.: Hematologic remission and cytogenic improvement induced by recombinant interferon alpha in chronic myelogenous leukemia. N. Engl. J. Med. *314*:1065, 1986.
154. Talpaz, M., Kantarjian, H. M., McCredie, K. B., et al.: Clinical investigation of human alpha interferon in chronic myelogenous leukemia. Blood *69*:1280, 1987.
155. Tracey, K., Fong, Y., Messe, D. G., et al.: Anti-cachectin/TNF monoclonal antibodies prevent septic shock during lethal bacteremia. Nature *330*:662, 1987.
156. Vadhan-Raj, S., Buescher, S., Broxmeyer, H. E., et al.: Stimulation of myelopoiesis in patients with aplastic anemia by recombinant human granulocyte-macrophage colony-stimulating factor. N. Engl. J. Med. *319*:1628, 1988.
157. Valone, F. H., and Ruis, N. M.: Stimulation of tumor necrosis factor release by cytotoxic analogues of platelet-activating factor. Immunology *76*:24, 1992.
158. Van Deventer, S. J. H., Buller, H. R., Sturk, A., et al.: Endotoxin induced chain reactions. Circ. Shock *31*:246, 1995.
159. Wald, E. R., Kaplan, S. L., Mason, E. O., et al.: Dexamethasone therapy for children with bacterial meningitis. Pediatrics *95*:21, 1995.
160. Weatherstone, K. B., and Rich, E. A.: Tumor necrosis factor/cachectin and interleukin-1 secretion by cord blood monocytes from premature infants. Pediatr. Res. *25*:342, 1989.
161. Weyrich, A. S., Ma, X. L., Lefer, D. J., et al.: In vivo neutralization of P-selectin protects feline heart and endothelium in myocardial ischemia and reperfusion injury. J. Clin. Invest. *91*:2620, 1993.
162. Whatley, R. E., Zimmerman, G. A., McIntyre, T. M., et al.: Production of platelet-activating factor by endothelial cells. Semin. Thromb. Hemost. *13*:445, 1987.
163. Williams, P. A., Bohnsack, J. F., Augustine, N. H., et al.: Production of tumor necrosis factor by human cells in vitro and in vivo induced by group B streptococci. J. Pediatr. *123*:292, 1993.
164. Wilson, C. B., Westall, J., Johnston, L., et al.: Decreased production of interferon gamma by human neonatal cells: Intrinsic and regulatory deficiencies. J. Clin. Invest. *77*:860, 1986.
165. Winn, R. K., Vedder, N. B., Paulson, J. C., et al.: Monoclonal antibodies to P-selectin are effective in preventing reperfusion injury to rabbit ears. Circulation *86*:316, 1992.
166. Wirthmueller, U., De Weck, A. L., and Dahinden, C. A.: Platelet activating factor production in human neutrophils by sequential stimulation with granulocyte-macrophage colony-stimulating factor and chemotactic factors C5A or formyl-methionyl-leucyl-phenylalanine. J. Immunol. *142*:3213, 1989.
167. Ziegler, E. J., Fischer, C. J., Jr., Sprung, C. L., et al.: Treatment of gram-negative bacteremia in septic shock with HA-1A human monoclonal antibody against endotoxin: A randomized, double-blind placebo-controlled trial. N. Engl. J. Med. *324*:429, 1991.
168. Zimmerman, G. A., Prescott, S. M., and McIntyre, T. M.: Endothelial cell interactions with granulocytes: Tethering and signaling molecules. Immunol. Today *13*:93, 1992.
169. Zimmerman, G. A., McIntyre, T. M., and Prescott, S. M.: Production of platelet-nactivating factor by human vascular endothelial cells: Evidence for a requirement for specific agonists and modulation by prostacyclin. Circulation *72*:718, 1985.

PART 6

PREVENTION OF INFECTIOUS DISEASES

237

Active Immunizing Agents

Penelope H. Dennehy, Erica E. Jost, and Georges Peter

The prevention of infectious diseases in children by immunization is one of the outstanding accomplishments of medical science. Children enjoy better health today because of effective immunization programs that in many countries have diminished markedly the morbidity and mortality of once-common contagious diseases. The marked decline in the United States in vaccine-preventable childhood diseases is demonstrated in Table 237–1.[87] The success of immunizations is illustrated further by the 1977 eradication of smallpox achieved after a 10-year effort directed by the World Health Organization (WHO) and the extraordinary progress in global elimination of poliomyelitis in the 1990s.[106, 312] To achieve this progress in child health, scientific technology and medical practice have combined efforts to (1) understand the biology of causal infectious agents, (2) purify these agents and, in some cases, their components, (3) develop and test safe and effective vaccines, (4) manufacture and administer these vaccines to appropriate segments of the population, (5) develop appropriate indications and implement resulting schedules for immunizations, and (6) identify necessary contraindications.

Infectious diseases can be prevented through immunization by (1) stimulating an active immunologic defense (such as from humoral antibody) through the administration of antigens, usually prior to natural exposure to an infectious agent (i.e., active immunization), or (2) temporarily supplying preformed human or animal antibody to persons prior to, or soon after, exposure to certain infectious agents (i.e., passive immunization). Active immunizations, including the currently available vaccines, are discussed in this chapter. Major vaccines (i.e., those discussed in this chapter), their composition, and their routes of administration are listed in Table 237–2.

ACTIVE IMMUNOPROPHYLAXIS: CONSIDERATIONS AND RECOMMENDATIONS

Vaccines

An ideal immunizing agent should include the following characteristics: (1) the agent should be easy to produce in well-standardized preparations that readily are quantifiable and stable in immunobiologic potency, (2) it should be easy to administer, (3) it should not produce disease in the recipient or susceptible contacts, (4) it should induce long-lasting (ideally permanent) immunity that is measurable by available and inexpensive techniques, (5) it should be free of contaminating and potentially toxic substances, and (6) adverse reactions should be minimal and minor in consequences. All of these objectives rarely, if ever, are met with currently available vaccines because they are neither completely safe nor completely effective. Partial immunity and undesirable side effects or reactions, including rare severe reactions, can occur. Nevertheless, vaccines in current use are highly effective and safe.

All active immunizing agents (vaccines) contain one or more antigens that stimulate a protective immunologic response. Some are live-attenuated viruses or bacteria; other vaccines consist of killed microorganisms or contain inactivated components, such as exotoxins (toxoids). In some, the antigen is a highly defined, single constituent, such as the pneumococcal polysaccharides, but in other vaccines, the antigen component is less well defined, such as live virus or whole-cell pertussis vaccines composed of killed *Bordetella pertussis* organisms. Immunizing agents are administered in suspending fluids, such as sterile water, saline, or complex tissue culture fluid, which can contain proteins or other constituents derived from the medium from which the vaccine was produced (e.g., serum proteins, egg antigens, other tissue culture–derived antigens). With some vaccines, certain preservatives, stabilizers, or antibiotics are added (and in some cases have resulted in hypersensitivity reactions). To enhance immunogenicity, particularly for those vaccines containing inactivated microorganisms or their extracted components, adjuvants such as specifically aluminum compounds may be added.

Immunization Schedules

The age and timing of immunization are critical for the success of vaccination. The schedule by which a vaccine is provided is based on multiple factors, including the epidemiology of naturally occurring disease, the age-specific risk of complications due to the natural disease, the anticipated immunologic response of the host to the antigens, the duration of immunity that can be induced, and often recommended ages of routine health care visits. In general, vaccines are recommended at the youngest age at which significant risk for the natural disease and its complications exist and at which a protective immunologic response to the vaccine will occur. An example is measles vaccine, which in the United States routinely is recommended at 12 to 15 months of age because many children have residual transplacentally acquired maternal measles serum antibody in the first year of life that interferes with the antibody response. However,

TABLE 237–1. Reduction in Morbidity of Some Vaccine-Preventable Diseases in the United States[87]

	Maximum Cases (Yr)	1979	1996†
Diphtheria	206,939 (1921)	59	1
Measles	894,134 (1941)	13,597	494
Mumps*	152,209 (1968)	14,225	666
Pertussis	265,269 (1934)	1623	6911
Polio (paralytic)	21,269 (1952)	26	1
Rubella‡	57,686 (1969)	11,795	210
Congenital rubella syndrome	20,000 (1964–1965)	62	2
Tetanus§	601 (1948)	81	28

*First reportable in 1968.
†Suspected cases (vaccine-associated) have been reported and are under investigation.
‡First reportable in 1966.
§First reportable in 1947.

TABLE 237–2. Available Vaccines in the United States for Use in Children and Their Routes of Administration[a]

Vaccine[b]	Type	Recommended Route[c]
BCG	Live bacteria	ID
DTP	Toxoids and inactivated bacteria	IM
DTaP	Toxoids and inactivated bacterial components	IM
Hepatitis A	Inactivated virus	IM
Hepatitis B	Inactivated viral antigen yeast-derived recombinant	IM
Hepatitis B and Hib (combination)	See hepatitis B and Hib	IM
Hib	Polysaccharide-protein conjugate	IM
Hib and DTaP (combination)	See Hib and DTaP	IM
Hib and DTP (combination)	See Hib and DTP	IM
Influenza	Inactivated virus (whole-virus); viral components (split-virus or purified antigens)	IM
Japanese encephalitis	Inactivated virus	SC
Measles	Live virus	SC
Meningococcal	Polysaccharide	SC
MMR	Live viruses	SC
Mumps	Live virus	SC
Pneumococcal	Polysaccharide	IM or SC
Poliovirus (trivalent):		
OPV	Live viruses	PO
IPV	Inactivated virus	SC
Rabies	Inactivated viruses	IM (or ID in some circumstances[d])
Rubella	Live virus	SC
Td and DT (adsorbed)	Toxoids	IM
Typhoid		
Parenteral	Inactivated bacteria	SC (booster may be ID)
Parenteral	Capsular polysaccharide	IM
Oral	Live bacteria	PO
Varicella	Live virus	SC
Yellow fever	Live virus	SC

[a]Only major childhood vaccines and selective others are included.

[b]BCG, bacillus Calmette-Guérin (tuberculosis); DTP, diphtheria and tetanus toxoids and pertussis vaccine; DTaP, diphtheria and tetanus toxoids and acellular pertussis vaccine; Hib, *Haemophilus influenzae* type b conjugate vaccine; MMR, live measles, mumps, and rubella viruses vaccine; OPV, oral poliovirus vaccine; IPV, inactivated poliovirus vaccine; Td, tetanus and diphtheria toxoids (for children 7 years of age or older and adults); DT, diphtheria and tetanus toxoids (for children younger than 7 years of age).

[c]SC, subcutaneous; ID, intradermal; IM, intramuscular; PO, oral.

[d]Human diploid cell rabies vaccine for intradermal use is different in constitution and potency from the intramuscular vaccine; it should be used for preexposure immunization only. Rabies vaccine, absorbed (RVA), should not be used intradermally.

during measles outbreaks in preschool children, measles vaccination is recommended for infants as young as 6 months of age because the risk of complications for measles is high among children younger than 1 year of age.[13, 51] These infants should be vaccinated subsequently at 12 to 15 months of age. Similarly, in countries where measles causes significant morbidity and mortality in infants younger than 9 months of age, the Global Advisory Group of WHO's Expanded Programme on Immunization (EPI) has recommended measles vaccine as early as at 6 months of age.[159]

The recommended doses of vaccine are determined by the number necessary to achieve a uniform and predictable immunologic response and to sustain protection. Some immunizing agents require administration of more than one dose for development of an adequate antibody response and require a reinforcing booster dose to maintain protection; examples are pertussis, diphtheria, and tetanus vaccines. Intervals between doses are based on the kinetics of primary and secondary antibody responses.

Route of Administration

An example of the effect of route of administration on immunologic response is provided by poliomyelitis vaccines. Inactivated poliovirus vaccine given intramuscularly induces systemic immunity through serum antibody production; however, it does not evoke local secretory IgA antibody in the intestinal tract consistently and thereby effectively prevent subsequent transmission of the wild-type virus. Because live-attenuated oral poliovirus vaccine (OPV) induces optimal intestinal as well as systemic antibody, immunization by the oral route was the preferred vaccine for routine immunization against poliomyelitis of children in the United States for three decades and remains the WHO-recommended vaccine for global eradication.[312]

Vaccines containing adjuvants must be injected deep into the muscle mass because if they are administered subcutaneously or intradermally, they can cause local irritation, inflammation, granuloma formation, or necrosis.[5, 70]

Injectable vaccines should be administered in areas unlikely to cause local neural, vascular, or tissue injury.[5, 70] Although the upper, outer quadrant of the buttocks has been used as a frequent site for immunization, this area ordinarily should not be used because the gluteal region consists mostly of fat in young children and because of potential injury to the sciatic nerve. Ideally, intramuscular injections should be given in the anterolateral aspect of the upper thigh or deltoid muscle of the upper arm. The anterolateral aspect of the thigh is preferred for infants because of its muscle mass relative to other sites. For older children, the deltoid muscle usually is sufficiently large for intramuscular injection. The incidence of significant pain in 18-month-old children injected intramuscularly in the thigh is greater than that of deltoid injections and can result in transient limping.[177] The deltoid generally is the preferred site for intramuscular administration of vaccines in children 18 months of age or older, although some physicians prefer the anterolateral thigh for toddlers.[5, 70] Subcutaneous inoculations also usually should be given in the thigh of infants and the deltoid area of older children. Intradermal vaccines usually should be administered on the volar aspect of the forearm.

Recommended routes for administration of vaccines are provided in their package inserts and are summarized in recommendations for immunizations by the Committee on Infectious Diseases (CID) of the American Academy of Pediatrics (AAP)[5] and the Advisory Committee on Immunization Practices (ACIP) of the Centers for Disease Control and Prevention (CDC).[70]

Vaccine Dose

The recommended dose of each immunizing agent is derived from theoretic considerations and vaccine trials. Because inactivated immunizing agents cannot replicate in the host, these vaccines must contain an adequate antigenic mass to stimulate the desired immunologic response. Long-lasting immunity with such vaccines requires repeated doses.

Exceeding the recommended dose can be hazardous because of excessive local or systemic concentrations of immunizing agents, whereas administration of doses smaller than those recommended may result in inadequate responses and protection.[5, 70]

Lapsed Immunizations

In general, intervals between multiple doses of an antigen that are longer than those recommended do not affect the antibody responses achieved, provided the immunization series is completed. Thus, restarting the series after interruption of the vaccine schedule or giving additional doses is not necessary.

Simultaneous Administration of Multiple Vaccines

Because most vaccines can be given simultaneously without impairment of effectiveness or safety, multiple vaccines are given to children concurrently.[190] Simultaneous administration of vaccines particularly is important for the inadequately immunized child whose return for further immunization is doubtful or for the patient for whom travel is imminent. An inactivated vaccine and a live-virus vaccine can be administered simultaneously at different sites without interference with immune response. The exceptions are yellow fever and cholera vaccines because, if administered simultaneously, antibody responses are diminished. Administration of these vaccines, if possible, should be separated by an interval of at least of 3 weeks.[70]

In the case of live-virus vaccines, theoretic considerations indicate that the immune response to one live-virus vaccine might be impaired if given within 4 weeks of another.[70, 241] Thus, whenever possible, live-virus vaccines not administered on the same day should be given at least 1 month (4 weeks) apart. This consideration is the basis of the recommended minimal interval of 1 month (defined as 4 weeks) between doses of measles vaccine, such as would be the case for a previously unimmunized person entering college. However, recent receipt of OPV is not considered a contraindication to measles and other live-virus vaccines given parenterally.

Guidelines for spacing live and killed antigen vaccines are given in Table 237–3.

TABLE 237–3. Guidelines for Spacing the Administration of Live and Killed Antigens[70]

Antigen Combination	Recommended Minimum Interval Between Doses
≥2 killed antigens	None. May be administered simultaneously or at any interval between doses*
Killed and live antigens	None. May be administered simultaneously or at any interval between doses†
≥2 live antigens	4-week minimum if not administered simultaneously.‡ However, oral polio vaccine can be administered at any time before, with, or after measles-mumps-rubella vaccine, if indicated

*If possible, vaccines associated with local or systemic side effects (e.g., cholera, parenteral typhoid, plague vaccines) should be administered on separate occasions to avoid accentuated reactions.

†Cholera vaccine with yellow fever vaccine is the exception. If time permits, these antigens should not be administered simultaneously, and at least 3 weeks should elapse between administration of yellow fever vaccine and cholera vaccine. If the vaccines must be administered simultaneously or within 3 weeks of each other, the antibody response may not be optimal.

‡If oral live typhoid vaccine is indicated (e.g., for international travel undertaken on short notice), it can be administered before, simultaneously with, or after oral polio vaccine.

Record Keeping, Patient Information, Informed Consent, and Reporting

Accurate record keeping by physicians is required, and parents should keep up-to-date immunization records for their children. The 1986 National Childhood Vaccine Injury Act required childhood-mandated vaccines, as of the date of enactment (i.e., those against diphtheria, tetanus, pertussis, polio, measles, mumps, and rubella), that health care providers record in the child's permanent medical record the date of administration of the vaccine, manufacturer name, lot number, and name of the health care provider administering the vaccines.[5]

As a general principle, all children and their parents or caregivers should be informed about the benefits and risks of any vaccines to be administered. For vaccines specified as of 1996 in the Vaccine Injury Act (i.e., diphtheria and tetanus toxoids and pertussis vaccine [DTP] or diphtheria and tetanus toxoids and acellular pertussis vaccine [DTaP], measles, mumps, and rubella vaccine [MMR] or component vaccines, and polio virus vaccines), the CDC has prepared revised and greatly shortened vaccine information statements that must be used by vaccine administrators. For all other vaccines, such as those for *Haemophilus influenzae* type b (Hib), hepatitis B, and varicella, patients, parents, and caregivers also should be informed about benefits and risks. Materials on these other routine childhood vaccines are available from the CDC and AAP. These other vaccines most likely will be added to the National Vaccine Injury Compensation Program in 1997, at which time the use of vaccine information statements prepared by the CDC for these vaccines will be required.

Informed consent should be obtained before administration of vaccines. Some physicians and other health care providers may choose to obtain a parent's signature, but written consent is not required by current law. An appropriate alternative to written consent is to note in the patient's record that the vaccine information statements have been provided and discussed with the parent, patient, or legal guardian.

To increase knowledge about adverse reactions, all temporally associated events severe enough to require the patient to seek medical attention should be reported to the Vaccine Adverse Events Reporting System (VAERS). Because a temporal relationship alone does not indicate causation necessarily, cause-and-effect relationships often are impossible to establish. Epidemiologic and related studies are necessary to ascertain the incidence and nature of adverse reactions to vaccines and are important in ensuring a scientific rationale for vaccine use recommendations and optimal public and professional vaccine acceptance. Health care providers who administer vaccines are required in the United States to report to the VAERS specific adverse events in recipients of those vaccines covered by the Act (Table 237–4). This system for reporting of adverse events associated with vaccination was established by the Department of Health and Human Services to foster the recognition of vaccine-related reactions and further study, as indicated, to establish possible causation. VAERS forms can be obtained by calling 800-822-7967.

The decrease in the occurrence of vaccine-preventable infectious diseases has resulted in a greater number of adverse events temporally related to immunization than cases of disease. Although in some cases, such as vaccine-associated paralytic poliomyelitis, vaccine has been established to be the cause, in other circumstances, such as brain damage alleged to be attributed to whole-cell pertussis vaccine, causation by vaccine has not been proved.[28]

Increased public visibility of vaccine reactions contributed to a marked increase in vaccine litigation in the 1980s as compensation was sought through the judicial system by those alleged to suffer serious vaccine-related sequelae. A marked increase in the manufacturers' actual and anticipated liability costs and subsequent escalating increases in the price of vaccines occurred concomitantly. These and other developments, such as threats to vaccine supply, concerns by parents about vaccine safety, and recognition of the benefits from improved coordination and planning of vaccine programs, led to the passage of the 1986 Vaccine Injury Act and the Compensation Program, a no-fault system to compensate victims of certain presumed vaccine-related events.

The Compensation Program is administered by the Department of Health and Human Services. Decisions on compensation are made by the U.S. Court of Federal Claims and are based on the Vaccine Injury Table, which has been revised since passage of the original legislation in response to new findings and analyses by the several Institute of Medicine committees. Compensation for injuries occurring after the Program's effective date of October 1, 1988, is provided by excise taxes on each vaccine. After initial administrative and financial difficulties at its inception, the program has been successful in reducing vaccine-related litigation, stabilizing vaccine prices, and creating a favorable environment for the introduction of new vaccines.[125]

Vaccine Recommendations and Schedules

In developing recommendations for immunization, multiple factors are considered, including vaccine characteristics, scientific knowledge about the principles of immunization, assessment of the benefits of the vaccine, risk of the disease and its complications, vaccine costs, and risks of adverse reactions. Changes in relative benefits and risks necessitate continued review of recommendations. In the United States, recommendations for immunization of infants and children are made by two different committees, the ACIP of the CDC and the CID of the AAP. These committees work closely together, and, in most circumstances, recommendations are similar. Since 1995, these two committees and the American Academy of Family Practice have issued a single vaccine schedule at least once a year.[82] The 1997 schedule for routine administration of childhood vaccines is given in Figure 237–1.[96a]

A major change in 1996 was the establishment of a routine preadolescent immunization visit at 11 to 12 years of age.[85] The first booster dose of adult tetanus and diphtheria toxoids (Td) should be given at that time, rather than at 14 to 16 years of age, as previously was the case. In addition, at this preadolescent visit, children not previously vaccinated with hepatitis B, varicella (if susceptible), or the second dose of measles-containing vaccine should be given necessary immunizations and scheduled for future visits to receive any vaccines not administered during this visit.

Other countries have similar national processes for formulating immunization schedules and recommendations, based on local epidemiology of diseases and available vaccines. In developing countries, practices are guided by the recommendations of WHO. Current recommendations are listed in Table 237–5.

As new vaccines and scientific knowledge become available, vaccine recommendations and schedules are modified and changed. Examples of changes in this decade include use of Hib conjugate vaccine beginning at 2 months of age, universal infant and adolescent hepatitis B immunization, recommendations for administration of varicella vaccine, and introduction of acellular pertussis vaccine for infants.

Implementation of Vaccine Programs

In addition to availability of safe and effective vaccines and appropriate schedules for their use, effective means of implementation and delivery are necessary for the success of vaccine programs. In the United States, high rates of immunization in school age children have been achieved, in part because of public health programs for vaccine administration, government support for vaccine purchase, and state laws requiring immunization for school entry. In contrast with rates of approximately 95 per cent or higher in school age children, however, immunization rates in infants and young children in the 1980s were significantly lower.[316] In a survey of 21 primarily urban areas throughout the United States, 11 to 58 per cent (median, 44 per cent) of children by their second birthday who entered school in 1991 and 1992 were vaccinated fully. The failure to immunize young children was a major factor in the 1989 to 1991 outbreaks of measles in major urban areas in the United States.[281]

This epidemic and the recognition of low immunization rates prompted a national campaign to achieve the United States Public Health Service's goal of 90 per cent vaccine coverage rate in children by 2 years of age. Initiatives have included improved access to vaccines, education of health care providers in the community, and the development of standards for pediatric immunization practice.[19] These standards serve as guidelines to be followed in improving the delivery of vaccines and include evaluation of the immunization status of patients at all medical visits, use of valid contraindications, simultaneous administration of all indi-

TABLE 237–4. Reportable Events Following Immunization, as Required by the National Childhood Vaccine Injury Act*

Vaccine/Toxoid	Adverse Event	Interval from Vaccination
Tetanus in any combination: DTaP, DTP, DTP-Hib, DT, Td, TT	Anaphylaxis or anaphylactic shock	7 days
	Brachial neuritis	28 days
	Any sequela (including death) of above events	No limit
	Events described in manufacturer's package insert as contraindications to additional doses of vaccine	See package insert
Pertussis in any combination: DTaP, DTP, DTP-Hib, P	Anaphylaxis or anaphylactic shock	7 days
	Encephalopathy (or encephalitis)	7 days
	Any sequela (including death) of above events	No limit
	Events described in manufacturer's package insert as contraindications to additional doses of vaccine	See package insert
Measles, mumps, and rubella in any combination: MMR, MR, M, R	Anaphylaxis or anaphylactic shock	7 days
	Encephalopathy (or encephalitis)	15 days
	Any sequela (including death) of above events	No limit
	Events described in manufacturer's package insert as contraindications to additional doses of vaccine	See package insert
Rubella in any combination: MMR, MR, R	Chronic arthritis	42 days
	Any sequela (including death) of above events	No limit
	Events described in manufacturer's package insert as contraindications to additional doses of vaccine	See package insert
Measles in any combination: MMR, MR, M	Thrombocytopenic purpura	30 days
	Vaccine-strain measles virus infection in an immunodeficient recipient	6 months
	Any sequela (including death) of above events	No limit
	Events described in manufacturer's package insert as contraindications to additional doses of vaccine	See package insert
Oral poliovirus (OPV)	Paralytic polio	
	In a nonimmunodeficient recipient	30 days
	In an immunodeficient recipient	6 months
	In a vaccine-associated community case	No limit
	Vaccine-strain poliovirus infection	
	In a nonimmunodeficient recipient	30 days
	In an immunodeficient recipient	6 months
	In a vaccine-associated community case	No limit
	Any sequela (including death) of above events	No limit
	Events described in manufacturer's package insert as contraindications to additional doses of vaccine	See package insert
Inactivated poliovirus (IPV)	Anaphylaxis or anaphylactic shock	7 days
	Any sequela (including death) of the above events	No limit
	Events described in manufacturer's package insert as contraindications to additional doses of vaccine	See package insert
Hepatitis B	Anaphylaxis or anaphylactic shock	7 days
	Any sequela (including death) of the above events	No limit
	Events described in manufacturer's package insert as contraindications to additional doses of vaccine	See package insert
Haemophilus influenzae type b (Hib)	Early-onset Hib disease	7 days
	Any sequela (including death) of the above events	No limit
	Events described in manufacturer's package insert as contraindications to additional doses of vaccine	See package insert

*Effective March 24, 1997.

The Reportable Events Table (RET) gives adverse events reportable by law to the Vaccine Adverse Event Reporting System (VAERS), including conditions found in the manufacturer's package insert. In addition, individuals are encouraged to report any clinically significant or unexpected events (even if you are not certain the vaccine caused the event) for any vaccine, whether or not it is listed on the RET. Manufacturers also are required by regulation to report to the VAERS program all adverse events made known to them for any vaccine.

Recommended Childhood Immunization Schedule United States, January - December 1997

Vaccines[1] are listed under the routinely recommended ages. Bars indicate range of acceptable ages for vaccination. Shaded bars indicate *catch-up vaccination:* at 11-12 years of age, hepatitis B vaccine should be administered to children not previously vaccinated, and Varicella vaccine should be administered to children not previously vaccinated who lack a reliable history of chickenpox.

Age ► / Vaccine ▼	Birth	1 mo	2 mos	4 mos	6 mos	12 mos	15 mos	18 mos	4-6 yrs	11-12 yrs	14-16 yrs
Hepatitis B[2,3]	Hep B-1 (bar: Birth–2 mos)									Hep B[3] (shaded)	
		Hep B-2 (bar: 1 mo–4 mos)			Hep B-3 (bar: 6 mos–18 mos)						
Diphtheria, Tetanus, Pertussis[4]			DTaP or DTP	DTaP or DTP	DTaP or DTP		DTaP or DTP[4] (bar: 15–18 mos)		DTaP or DTP	Td (bar: 11-12–14-16 yrs)	
H. influenzae type b[5]			Hib	Hib	Hib[5]	Hib[5] (bar: 12–15 mos)					
Polio[6]			Polio[6]	Polio		Polio[6] (bar: 12–18 mos)			Polio		
Measles, Mumps, Rubella[7]						MMR (bar: 12–15 mos)			MMR[7] or	MMR[7]	
Varicella[8]						Var (bar: 12–18 mos)				Var[8] (shaded)	

Approved by the Advisory Committee on Immunization Practices (ACIP), the American Academy of Pediatrics (AAP), and the American Academy of Family Physicians (AAFP).

IS 5081

[1] This schedule indicates the recommended age for routine administration of currently licensed childhood vaccines. Some combination vaccines are available and may be used whenever administration of all components of the vaccine is indicated. Providers should consult the manufacturers' package inserts for detailed recommendations.

[2] **Infants born to HBsAg-negative mothers** should receive 2.5 µg of Merck vaccine (Recombivax HB) or 10 µg of SmithKline Beecham (SB) vaccine (Engerix-B). The 2nd dose should be administered ≥ 1 mo after the 1st dose.
Infants born to HBsAg-positive mothers should receive 0.5 mL hepatitis B immune globulin (HBIG) within 12 hrs of birth, and either 5 µg of Merck vaccine (Recombivax HB) or 10 µg of SB vaccine (Engerix-B) at a separate site. The 2nd dose is recommended at 1-2 mos of age and the 3rd dose at 6 mos of age.
Infants born to mothers whose HBsAg status is unknown should receive either 5 µg of Merck vaccine (Recombivax HB) or 10 µg of SB vaccine (Engerix-B) within 12 hrs of birth. The 2nd dose of vaccine is recommended at 1 mo of age and the 3rd dose at 6 mos of age. Blood should be drawn at the time of delivery to determine the mother's HBsAg status; if it is positive, the infant should receive HBIG as soon as possible (no later than 1 wk of age). The dosage and timing of subsequent vaccine doses should be based upon the mother's HBsAg status.

[3] Children and adolescents who have not been vaccinated against hepatitis B in infancy may begin the series during any childhood visit. Those who have not previously received 3 doses of hepatitis B vaccine should initiate or complete the series during the 11-12 year-old visit. The 2nd dose should be administered at least 1 mo after the 1st dose, and the 3rd dose should be administered at least 4 mos after the 1st dose and at least 2 mos after the 2nd dose.

[4] DTaP (diphtheria and tetanus toxoids and acellular pertussis vaccine) is the preferred vaccine for all doses in the vaccination series, including completion of the series in children who have received ≥1 dose of whole-cell DTP vaccine. Whole-cell DTP is an acceptable alternative to DTaP. The 4th dose of DTaP) may be administered as early as 12 months of age, provided 6 months have elapsed since the 3rd dose, and if the child is considered unlikely to return at 15-18 mos of age. Td (tetanus and diphtheria toxoids, absorbed, for adult use) is recommended at 11-12 years of age if at least 5 years have elapsed since the last dose of DTP, DTaP, or DT. Subsequent routine Td boosters are recommended every 10 years.

[5] Three *H. influenzae* type b (Hib) conjugate vaccines are licensed for infant use. If PRP-OMP (PedvaxHIB [Merck]) is administered at 2 and 4 mos of age, a dose at 6 mos is not required. After completing the primary series, any Hib conjugate vaccine may be used as a booster.

[6] Two poliovirus vaccines are currently licensed in the US: inactivated poliovirus vaccine (IPV) and oral poliovirus vaccine (OPV). The following schedules are all acceptable by the ACIP, the AAP, and the AAFP, and parents and providers may choose among them:
1. IPV at 2 and 4 mos; OPV at 12-18 mos and 4-6 yr
2. IPV at 2, 4, 12-18 mos, and 4-6 yr
3. OPV at 2, 4, 6-18 mos, and 4-6 yr

The ACIP routinely recommends schedule 1. IPV is the only poliovirus vaccine recommended for immunocompromised persons and their household contacts.

[7] The 2nd dose of MMR is routinely recommended at 4-6 yrs of age or at 11-12 yrs of age, but may be administered during any visit, provided at least 1 month has elapsed since receipt of the 1st dose and that both doses are administered at or after 12 months of age.

[8] Susceptible children may receive Varicella vaccine (Var) at any visit after the first birthday, and those who lack a reliable history of chickenpox should be immunized during the 11-12 year-old visit. Children ≥ 13 years of age should receive 2 doses, at least 1 mos apart.

FIGURE 237–1. *Recommended childhood immunization schedule: United States, January–December 1997.*

TABLE 237–5. Schedule of the Expanded Programme on Immunization, World Health Organization

	Vaccines‡			
		Hepatitis B (HB)*		
Age		A	or	B
Birth	BCG, OPV	HB-1		
6 weeks	DTP, OPV	HB-2		HB-1
10 weeks	DTP, OPV			HB-2
14 weeks	DTP, OPV	HB-3		HB-3
9 months	Measles, yellow fever†			

*Schedule A is recommended in countries where perinatal transmission of hepatitis B virus is important (e.g., Southeast Asia) and B in countries where perinatal transmission is less important (e.g., sub-Saharan Africa).

†In countries where yellow fever poses a risk.

‡BCG, bacillus Calmette-Guérin; DTP, diphtheria-tetanus-pertussis; HB, hepatitis B; OPV, oral poliovirus.

cated vaccines, and routine audits by providers of the immunization status of their patients. These and other initiatives have resulted in increasing immunization rates of young children in recent years. According to the National Immunization Survey, coverage rates among children 19 to 35 months of age from April 1994 to March 1995 were 75 per cent for completion of the four doses of DTP, three doses of OPV, and one dose of MMR.[88] These vaccination coverage rates were the highest ever recorded in the United States for preschool age children.

Vaccine Contraindications, Precautions, and Use in Special Circumstances

Recommendations for use of specific vaccines include contraindications and use in special circumstances, such as the immunocompromised patient (from underlying disease or therapy, such as high-dose steroids) and pregnancy.[13, 51] Established, generic contraindications are moderate or severe illness, a previous anaphylactic reaction to the specific vaccine, and a severe hypersensitivity reaction, such as anaphylaxis, to a vaccine constituent.

The decision to defer immunization in the febrile child should be based on the physician's assessment of the severity of the illness rather than the degree of fever. Children with minor illness and low-grade fever generally should be vaccinated, especially if a child is unlikely to return promptly for the deferred immunization.

Administration of live-virus vaccines, such as OPV and MMR, generally is contraindicated in patients with altered immunity. However, the morbidity and mortality of measles and lack of complications from vaccination of HIV-infected children have led to recommendations that these children, unless significantly immunocompromised, should receive MMR.[86]

Because of theoretic risk to the developing fetus, live-virus vaccines in most cases are not recommended for pregnant women.[11, 70] However, inadvertent vaccination is not necessarily a reason for termination of the pregnancy, and some live-virus vaccines, such as those for yellow fever and poliomyelitis, can be given safely to pregnant women. Inactivated bacterial and viral vaccines, composed of antigenic components or killed organisms, such as tetanus toxoids, hepatitis B virus (HBV), and influenza viruses, can and should be given during pregnancy if indicated.

Vaccines can cause severe reactions in some recipients, which may constitute contraindications or precautions to subsequent administration of the specific vaccine. An example is a child with a high fever of 40.5° C or greater after DTP (or DTaP) administration, for whom further doses of pertussis vaccine are not indicated in most cases. This recommendation is based on the unproven but reasonable presumption that children who experience adverse reactions after DTP administration risk having similar reactions of equal or greater magnitude on subsequent DTP administration.[101]

Anaphylactic reactions caused by allergenic components of a vaccine, such as gelatin or egg protein (in vaccine prepared in embryonated chicken eggs), are rare. Vaccines of potential risk for egg-sensitive persons include those against measles, mumps, inactivated influenza, and yellow fever. Before administering vaccines in persons with possible hypersensitivity to vaccine constituents, current recommendations for these vaccines should be reviewed.

In other circumstances, specific immunizations may be contraindicated, based on prior reactions and the child's past history, such as with DTP (e.g., evolving neurologic disorders) and MMR (e.g., immune thrombocytopenia occurring in temporal association with vaccination).[94]

Misconceptions

Appropriate and safe use of vaccines requires knowledge of the patient's relevant medical history, adverse reactions associated with prior receipt of vaccines, and specific indications and contraindications. Without this information, vaccines may be administered inadvertently or not given in circumstances in which immunization is indicated, resulting in missed opportunities for recommended immunization and resulting susceptibility of the child to a preventable disease. Examples of common misconceptions concerning contraindication to vaccines are given in Table 237–6.

International Travel

Foreign travel often is an indication for vaccines not routinely given to children.[11] The risk of exposure to certain vaccine-preventable diseases may be increased relative to that in the United States, and travelers may be exposed to infections that are uncommon or do not occur in this country. Examples include vaccines against hepatitis A, influenza, typhoid fever, yellow fever, and Japanese encephalitis (Table 237–7), depending on the location and circumstances of the person's visit. Some countries may require yellow fever vaccination for entry. The second dose of measles vaccine should be given to children and adolescents who have received only one dose irrespective of age (provided 4 weeks or more have elapsed since the first dose) because the risk of exposure to cases of measles may be substantial in some foreign countries. In addition, children and adolescents should have received all routinely recommended vaccines for their age. Information on vaccine requirements for international travel to different countries is provided in *Health Information for International Travel,* a publication of the CDC.[76] It is revised annually and can be obtained from the Superintendent of Documents, United States Government Printing Office, Washington, DC, 20402-9235. Information also is available from the CDC's International Travelers Hotline by calling 404-332-4559.

TABLE 237–6. Misconceptions Concerning Vaccine Contraindications

Mild acute illness with low-grade fever or mild diarrheal illness in an otherwise well child
Current antimicrobial therapy or the convalescent phase of illness
Reaction to previous diphtheria-tetanus-pertussis vaccine dose that involved only soreness, redness, or swelling in the immediate vicinity of the vaccination site or temperature of less than 105° F (40.5° C)
Prematurity. The appropriate age for initiating most immunization in the prematurely born infant is the usual recommended chronologic age. Vaccine doses should not be reduced for preterm infants.
Pregnancy of mother or other household contact
Recent exposure to an infectious disease
Breast feeding. The only vaccine virus that has been isolated from breast milk is rubella vaccine virus. No evidence indicates that breast milk from women immunized against rubella is harmful to infants.
A history of nonspecific allergies or relatives with allergies
Allergies to penicillin or any other antibiotic, except anaphylactic reactions to neomycin or streptomycin. These reactions occur rarely, if ever. None of the vaccines licensed in the United States contains pencillin.
Allergies to duck meat or duck feathers. No vaccine available in the United States is produced in substrates containing duck antigens.
Family history of convulsions in persons considered for pertussis or measles vaccination
Family history of sudden infant death syndrome in children considered for diphtheria-tetanus-pertussis vaccination.
Family history of an adverse event, unrelated to immunosuppression after vaccination
Malnutrition

Used with permission of the American Academy of Pediatrics: Active immunization. *In* Peter, G. (ed.): 1997 Red Book: Report of the Committee on Infectious Diseases. 24th ed. Elk Grove Village, American Academy of Pediatrics.

Reference Sources

Several comprehensive sources of information about pediatric vaccines are available. The AAP publishes *The Red Book: The Report of the Committee on Infectious Diseases* every 3 years. The current edition is to be published in 1997. In the interval between editions, the AAP publishes recommendations in its newsletter, *AAP News*, and subsequently in *Pediatrics.* The ACIP issues vaccine recommendations and relevant information in *Morbidity and Mortality Weekly Report.* Manufacturers provide product information for each vaccine in the Food and Drug Administration (FDA)-approved package inserts.

TABLE 237–7. Immunization for Foreign Travel

In addition to the routine recommended childhood vaccines (e.g., those against diphtheria, measles, and poliomyelitis), vaccines against the following diseases should be considered, depending on the geographic area and circumstances of the visit:

Cholera
Hepatitis A
Influenza
Japanese encephalitis
Meningococcal disease
Plague
Rabies
Typhoid fever
Yellow fever

VACCINES RECOMMENDED FOR ROUTINE ADMINISTRATION

Diphtheria Toxoid

Introduction of diphtheria toxoid in the 1940s led to a dramatic reduction in the incidence of diphtheria in the United States. However, diphtheria still is a potentially significant public health problem because of two factors. First, serologic surveys in the United States and England have suggested that many adults are not immunized.[58, 114, 208] However, a recent study suggests that, in the United States, most adults in recent years do have protective concentrations of serum antitoxin.[154] Second, adequate immunization has not eliminated completely the potential for transmission of *Corynebacterium diphtheriae* because immunization does not prevent carriage of *C. diphtheriae* in the nasopharynx or on the skin.[58, 219] As a result of an inadequate immunity in adults as well as infants and children, an epidemic of diphtheria in the 1990s has occurred in Russia and other countries of the former Soviet Union, such as Ukraine and the Central Asian republics, causing nearly 48,000 cases in 1994.[137, 162] Case-fatality rates have ranged from 2.8 to 23 per cent in the different states and countries. In addition, diphtheria continues to cause significant morbidity and mortality in developing countries.[136]

Preparations

Diphtheria toxoid is prepared by formaldehyde treatment of *C. diphtheriae* toxin. It is available in combination with tetanus toxoid and either whole-cell or acellular pertussis vaccine (DTP and DTaP, respectively) for routine immunization of infants and children. It also is produced in combination with tetanus toxoid (DT and Td). For children younger than 7 years of age, DT is given if pertussis vaccine is contraindicated, whereas Td, which contains only 15 to 20 per cent (2 Lf maximum) of the diphtheria toxoid in DT (6.7 to 12.5 Lf), is recommended for older children and adults because of adverse reactions related to dose and age.[8, 58] Diphtheria vaccines are adsorbed to an aluminum salt adjuvant.

Adverse Events

Other than local reactions of pain and swelling at the site of the vaccine injection, immunization does not cause significant adverse events. These local reactions have been attributed to hypersensitivity reactions but do not contraindicate further vaccination if otherwise indicated.

Indications

For primary immunization, doses of diphtheria toxoid are given at 2, 4, and 6 months of age. A fourth dose is given 6 to 12 months after the third dose (i.e., at 12 to 18 months of age) to maintain adequate antibody concentrations for the ensuing preschool years. For those not immunized in infancy, the first dose is followed by doses 2 and 8 to 14 months later. A single booster dose at 4 to 6 years of age prior to school entry is indicated, unless the preceding dose was given after the fourth birthday. Interruption of the recommended schedule or delay in administrating subsequent doses during primary immunization does not necessitate restarting the series.

After the 4- to 6-year-old dose, booster doses of diphtheria toxoid (as Td) should be given beginning at the preadolescent immunization visit at 11 to 12 years of age and thereafter every 10 years to maintain immunity.[85] To ensure adequate immunity, children and adults receiving tetanus toxoid for wound management should be given age-appropriate preparations of vaccines containing diphtheria as well as tetanus toxoid.[20]

Patients recovering from diphtheria infection should be immunized because infection does not confer immunity.

Precautions and Contraindications

The only contraindication to diphtheria toxoid is a history of a severe hypersensitivity after the previous dose. Vaccination with either this or tetanus toxoid is not known to be associated with increased risk of convulsions. Local reactions alone do not preclude continued use.

Haemophilus influenzae Type b Vaccine

Prior to the introduction of routine infant and childhood vaccination against this pathogen, Hib was a major cause of invasive bacterial infections in young children in the United States. It was the most common cause of bacterial meningitis and epiglottitis and a significant cause of septic arthritis, occult febrile bacteremia, and pneumonia in children younger than 5 years of age, causing an estimated 12,000 cases of meningitis and 8000 additional cases of invasive Hib disease annually.[105] The cumulative risk of Hib disease was approximately 1 in every 200 American children in the first 5 years of life, with the peak incidence of Hib meningitis occurring between 6 and 12 months of age. In high-risk populations, such as Native Americans, rates of disease in the absence of immunizations were higher and a greater proportion of cases of meningitis occurred in the first year of life than in populations not at high risk.[105, 166, 300]

Because the majority of cases of Hib disease occur in infancy, vaccines that induce protection by 6 months of age are necessary for effective control of Hib disease. Realization of this goal was made possible by the development of conjugate vaccines, in which the capsular polysaccharide of Hib, its major virulence factor, and the antigen against which protective antibodies are directed, are linked to a protein carrier chemically. Whereas the purified capsular polysaccharide, polyribosylribitol phosphate (PRP), is a poor immunogen in children younger than 18 months of age, PRP conjugated to a protein carrier has the antigenic properties of the protein carrier and, as a result, induces protective antibody in infants and young children and significantly greater concentrations of circulating anti-PRP at all ages than does the unconjugated polysaccharide.[252, 300] This age-dependent immunogenic characteristic of purified PRP (and other polysaccharide antigens) is that of a T-cell–independent antigen to which humoral responses are mediated by B-cell lymphocytes alone without T-helper lymphocytes. In contrast, the polysaccharide-protein conjugate vaccines are T-cell–dependent antigens in which T-helper lymphocyte activation as well as B-cell mediation of the humoral antibody response occurs. T-cell–dependent antigens also elicit booster responses, which are important to the effectiveness of polysaccharide vaccines.

The first conjugate vaccine, PRP-D (Table 237–8), was licensed in the United States in 1987 for use in 18-month-old children. Subsequently, the efficacy of several conjugate Hib vaccines in the prevention of invasive Hib disease was demonstrated, leading to routine Hib vaccination of infants in the United States and Western Europe. In the 1990s, as a result, the incidence of Hib invasive disease has been reduced dramatically.[2, 81, 262]

Preparations

All Hib vaccines contain the organism's polysaccharide capsular antigen, PRP. The first vaccine licensed was purified PRP, which was recommended for administration to children 18 to 24 months of age or older in 1985. These products have been replaced by the conjugate polysaccharide-protein vaccines for use in infants. Four conjugate vaccines have been licensed in the United States (see Table 237–8). Each conjugate vaccine is composed of PRP antigen conjugated to a protein carrier and differ in the protein carrier, size of the saccharide component, and chemical linkage. Three of these vaccines, HbOC, PRP-OMP, and PRP-T, are licensed for use in early infancy; PRP-D is approved by the FDA for children 15 months of age or older. Of these products, HbOC and PRP-T either are combined with DTP or can be mixed with DTP (see Table 237–8).

Immunogenicity and Efficacy

Purified PRP vaccine is poorly immunogenic in nearly all children younger than 16 months of age and is not effective until 18 to 24 months of age.[238] Serologic studies indicated that a serum anti-PRP concentration of 1.0 μg/mL or greater 3 weeks after vaccination correlated with protection.[186] For

TABLE 237–8. *Haemophilus influenzae* Type b (Hib) Conjugate Vaccines

Manufacturer	Abbreviation (Trade Name)	Carrier Protein
Connaught Laboratories, Inc.	PRP-D* (ProHIBit)	Diphtheria toxoid
Wyeth-Lederle Laboratories	HbOC† (HIBTITER)	CRM197 (a nontoxic mutant diphtheria toxin)
Merck & Co.	PRP-OPM (PedvaxHIB)	OMP (an outer-membrane protein complex of *Neisseria meningitidis*)
Pasteur-Mérieux-Connaught (distributed by Connaught Laboratories, Inc., and by SmithKline Beecham)	PRP-T‡ (ActHIB, OmniHIB)	Tetanus toxoid

*PRP-D is approved for children 15 months of age or older. HbOC, PRP-OMP, and PRP-T are recommended for infants beginning at approximately 2 months of age.

†HbOC also is available as a combination vaccine with DTP (TETRAMUNE).

‡PRP-T may be reconstituted with DTP or DTaP manufactured by Connaught Laboratories. Other licensed formulations of DTP have not been approved by the Food and Drug Administration for reconstitution and may not be used for this purpose. The combination of PRP-T and DTaP, as of March 1997, is approved only for the fourth doses of DTaP and Hib vaccination.

Used with permission of the American Academy of Pediatrics: *Haemophilus influenzae* infections. *In* Peter, G. (ed.): 1997 Red Book: Report of the Committee on Infectious Diseases. 24th ed. Elk Grove Village, American Academy of Pediatrics.

the conjugate vaccine, the applicability of this antibody concentration as a serologic surrogate of protection from immunization with conjugate vaccines has not been proved, and lower concentrations of anti-PRP after immunization may confer protection.[300]

In contrast with PRP, the conjugate vaccines are immunogenic in infants and young children.[119, 146, 300] Children 15 months of age or older respond well to a single dose of any of the four conjugate vaccines. In infants, the immunogenicity of the conjugate vaccines differs according to the product, age of vaccination, and number of doses.[119, 146, 300] Whereas PRP-OMP induces a significant increase in antibody concentration after a single injection at 2 months of age, the other three do not. For all three vaccines licensed for use in infants, two or three doses in the first 6 months of life result in high rates of seroconversion.[39, 119, 146]

Placebo-controlled field trials in the United States of both HbOC and PRP-OMP in infants demonstrated nearly 100 per cent protection and provided the basis for the initial approval of these vaccines for use in this country. In a study in northern California of HbOC, vaccine efficacy was 100 per cent for infants receiving the three-dose schedule at 2, 4, and 6 months of age.[39] In a Navajo population of infants at high risk of Hib disease who were vaccinated at 2 and 4 months of age with either PRP-OMP or placebo, vaccine efficacy was 100 per cent at 1 year of age and 93 per cent in total.[259] Randomized, placebo-controlled trials of PRP-T were terminated before completion when the FDA approved HbOC and PRP-OMP for use in infants.[135] Licensure of PRP-T was based on the comparable immunogenicity in a three-dose schedule to that of the other two products. In addition, an efficacy trial in Great Britain and the lack of cases in the terminated trials indicate comparable efficacy of PRP-T with that of HbOC and PRP-OMP.[41, 289]

Adverse Events

Hib vaccines are well tolerated. Mild local reactions occur in approximately 25 per cent of recipients but typically are mild and last less than 24 hours.[119, 300] Systemic reactions, such as fever and irritability, are infrequent. When conjugate vaccines are administered concurrently with DTP or DTaP, the incidence of systemic reactions is similar to that observed when only DTP is given.[119]

Whereas cases of invasive Hib disease in the 2 weeks after PRP vaccine indicate an increased risk of disease in the early postvaccination period, risk of disease immediately after conjugate vaccination is not increased.[174] Other serious adverse events, such as anaphylaxis, have not been reported with Hib conjugate vaccines.

Indications[25, 59, 68]

Routine vaccination against Hib disease is recommended for all children beginning at approximately 2 months of age. Three vaccines, HbOC, PRP-T, and PRP-OMP, are licensed in the United States for use in infants. Several of these products can be given with DTP or DTaP, either as a combination vaccine (i.e., HbOC-DTP) or mixed in the same syringe (i.e., PRP-T with DTP or DTaP). One product, PRP-OMP, has been combined with hepatitis B vaccine; this Hib-hepatitis B vaccine now is licensed for use beginning at 6 months of age (Table 237–9). When feasible, the conjugate vaccine product used for the first dose should be used for subsequent doses in children younger than 12 months of age. When sequential doses of different products are given in the first year of life, three doses of any conjugate product are sufficient. A final dose of any product, irrespective of the prior vaccines received, is acceptable at 12 to 15 months of age for completion of the Hib immunization schedule.

For those children in whom Hib immunization has not been initiated by 7 months of age, schedules recommended differ according to the child's age and choice of the conjugate vaccine (see references 25 and 59 for further information). Previously unimmunized children who are 15 months of age or older should be immunized with a single dose of any licensed conjugate *Haemophilus* vaccine. For previously unimmunized children 5 years of age or older, immunization is only indicated if they have an underlying condition predisposing to Hib disease, such as asplenia or HIV infection.

Hepatitis B Vaccine

HBV infection is a major public health problem of global importance. Its incidence especially is high in many Asian and African countries. HBV is a leading cause of acute hepatitis, and those who develop chronic infection are at risk for chronic hepatitis, cirrhosis, and primary hepatocellular carcinoma. In the United States, approximately 300,000 persons are infected each year and 2 million persons are estimated to be chronically infected.[157] These persons not only are at increased risk for chronic and malignant liver disease

TABLE 237–9. Recommendations for *Haemophilus influenzae* Type b Vaccination in Children Immunized Beginning at 2 to 6 Months of Age

Vaccination Product at Initiation*	Total Number of Doses to Be Administered	Recommended Vaccine Regimens*
HbOC or PRP-T	4	3 doses at 2-month intervals; when feasible, same vaccine for doses 1–3; fourth dose at 12 to 15 months of age; any conjugate vaccine for dose 4†
PRP-OMP	3	2 doses at 2-month intervals; when feasible, same vaccine for doses 1 and 2; third dose at 12 to 15 months of age; any conjugate vaccine for dose 3†

*HbOC, PRP-T, or PRP-OMP should be given in a separate syringe and at a separate site from other immunizations, unless specific combinations are approved by the Food and Drug Administration. HbOC also is available as a combination vaccine with DTP (HbOC-DTP). This combination can be used in infants scheduled to receive separate injections of DTP and HbOC. PRP-T may be reconstituted with DTP manufactured by Connaught Laboratories; other licensed formulations of DTP may not be used for this purpose. PRP-T may be reconstituted with DTaP manufactured by Connaught Laboratories for the fourth dose of both vaccines.

†The safety and efficacy of PRP-OMP, PRP-D, PRP-T, and HbOC are likely to be equivalent in children 12 months of age or older.

Used with permission of the American Academy of Pediatrics: *Haemophilus influenzae* infections. *In* Peter, G. (ed.): 1997 Red Book: Report of the Committee on Infectious Diseases. 24th ed. Elk Grove Village, American Academy of Pediatrics.

but also as chronic carriers serve as the reservoir for HBV transmission.

The initial strategies for prevention of hepatitis B through vaccination reflect the varying epidemiology of HBV infection in different areas of the world.[60] In the United States, for example, infection is of comparatively low endemicity and occurs primarily in adolescents and adults. The risk of infection, however, is much greater in certain populations. Examples include those born and living in areas or among groups in which HBV is highly endemic and those with lifestyles predisposing to HBV acquisition, such as male homosexual activity, intravenous drug abuse, and promiscuous heterosexual activity.[3] Consequently, the original strategy of hepatitis B prevention in this country was selective vaccination based on risk factors. In contrast, in geographic areas in which HBV infection is highly endemic, infection usually is acquired at birth or during childhood, resulting in the recommendation for universal vaccination of infants. In the United States, because of the continuing occurrence of hepatitis B despite the availability of a highly effective and safe vaccine, universal infant immunization has been recommended since 1991.[24, 60]

Prevention of acute and chronic HBV infection has become a global priority. WHO recommends that all countries by 1997 routinely vaccinate infants against HBV infection.[97]

Preparations

Hepatitis B vaccines consist of purified hepatitis B surface antigen (HBsAg) prepared either from the plasma of HBsAg chronic carriers or from yeast in which a plasmid containing the gene for HBsAg has been inserted (i.e., through recombinant DNA technology). In the United States, only the recombinant vaccines are available, but plasma-derived vaccines still are used widely in other areas of the world. In addition, a combination Hib–hepatitis B vaccine now is available.

Immunogenicity and Efficacy[10, 97]

The recommended series of three doses of vaccine induces a protective antibody response in more than 95 per cent of infants, children, adolescents, and adults younger than 40 years of age. In field trials, efficacy has been 80 to 95 per cent and generally correlates with immunogenicity. Protection against disease virtually is 100 per cent for persons who develop adequate serum antibody concentrations (anti-HBs ≥10 mIU/mL) after vaccination. Active immunization combined with passive immunoprophylaxis with hepatitis B immunoglobulin (HBIG) administered shortly at birth to infants born of HBsAg-positive mothers is more than 90 per cent effective in preventing HBV transmission and infection of the infant.

Vaccine-induced protection against symptomatic infection in normal hosts is prolonged and correlates with immunologic memory, which has been demonstrated in immunized children and adults for at least 12 years after vaccination. Children immunized at birth are protected for at least 10 years. Thus, the need for routine booster doses has not been demonstrated. Exceptions are hemodialysis patients and possibly other immunocompromised patients in whom protection may persist only as long as adequate serum antibody concentrations persist.

Adverse Events

Other than soreness at the injection site, reactions to hepatitis B vaccine are rare. Postvaccination surveillance after licensure of the plasma-derived vaccine indicated a possible association between Guillain-Barré syndrome (GBS) and receipt of the first vaccine dose, but no evidence indicates an association of GBS with recombinant vaccine.[97] Anaphylaxis has been estimated to occur in 1 in 600,000 doses distributed.[97] Several nonfatal cases have been reported in children.

Indications[10, 83, 97]

Hepatitis B vaccine is recommended for all infants in the United States in a three-dose schedule administered by 18 months of age or earlier. However, in populations in whom childhood HBV infection is highly endemic, such as Alaskan natives, Pacific Islanders, and infants in immigrant or refugee families from countries in which HBV is of intermediate or high endemicity, the schedule should be completed by 12 months of age.

The first dose is recommended shortly after birth but may be given at any time in the first 2 months of life, except in infants of HBsAg-positive mothers. These infants should receive the first dose within the first 12 hours of birth in conjunction with HBIG in order to prevent HBV transmission. Subsequent doses then are given at 1 to 2 and 6 months of age. For infants weighing less than 2 kg who are born to HBsAg-negative mothers, initiation of vaccine should be delayed until just before hospital discharge if the infant weighs 2 kg or more or until approximately 2 months of age when other routine immunizations are given.

For infants of non–HBV-infected mothers, the second dose of vaccine is recommended 1 to 2 months after the first dose followed by a third dose at 6 to 18 months of age.

Universal HBV immunization is recommended in the United States for all 11- and 12-year-old children who have not been immunized previously. In addition, vaccination is indicated for all unvaccinated children younger than 11 years of age who are Pacific Islanders or who reside in households of first-generation immigrants from countries where HBV is of high or intermediate endemicity. Vaccination also is recommended for the following persons:

- Sexually active heterosexual adolescents and adults who have a recently acquired sexually transmitted disease, are identified as prostitutes, or have had one or more sex partners in the previous 6 months
- Homosexual males
- Household contacts of sexual partners of HBsAg-positive persons
- Injecting drug users
- Persons at occupational risk of infection through exposure to blood or blood-contaminated body fluids, such as health care workers and public safety workers
- Residents and staff members of institutions for the developmentally disabled
- Hemodialysis patients (vaccination of those with early renal failure is encouraged before they require hemodialysis)
- Patients who receive clotting factor concentrates
- Members of households with international adoptees who are HBsAg-positive
- Travelers, especially children, to areas with high and intermediate rates of HBV infection who have close contact with the local population or are likely to have contact with blood, such as in a medical setting, or sexual contact with residents
- Inmates in long-term correctional facilities

In addition to active and passive immunoprophylaxis of infants of HBsAg-positive mothers, postexposure prophylaxis is recommended in the following circumstances:

- Sexual partner of an HBsAg-positive person. A single dose of HBIG within 14 days of the last sexual contact and initiation of the three-dose hepatitis B vaccination is recommended for susceptible persons.
- Household exposure of an unvaccinated infant younger than 12 months of age to a primary caregiver who has acute hepatitis B. Infants in this circumstance should receive both HBIG and should be vaccinated.
- Accidental percutaneous or permucosal exposure to HBsAg-positive blood of a susceptible person. This indication is exemplified by a needle stick or other accident involving blood in a hospital. Another example is an injury caused by a bite of an HBsAg-positive child. For this indication, HBIG as well as vaccine is given. Recommendations in these circumstances are complex and are based on the availability of the blood source for HBsAg testing and the hepatitis B vaccination status of the exposed person.

Recommended vaccine dosage differs according to the age of the recipient, product, and status of the host, and the package insert should be consulted before vaccine administration. Booster doses are not recommended, except in the case of hemodialysis and possibly other immunocompromised patients in whom the need should be assessed by annual antibody testing. An additional dose is indicated for those whose serum anti-HBsAg concentration is less than 10 mIU/mL.

Contraindications

The only contraindication is a history of anaphylaxis to a previous dose of vaccine. Although data on the safety of HBV vaccines are not available for pregnant women, these vaccines contain only HBsAg and not live virus and should not be deleterious to the developing fetus. Because HBV infection during pregnancy can result in transmission to the newborn, susceptible women at increased risk of infection should be vaccinated during pregnancy.

Inadvertent vaccination of HBsAg-positive persons has no deleterious effects.

Measles Vaccine

Since the introduction of both an inactivated and a live-virus, attenuated measles vaccine (Edmonston B strain) in the United States in 1963, the reported incidence of measles has decreased by more than 99 per cent. Although the incidence of measles has declined in all age groups, the decline has been greatest in children 5 to 14 years of age.

Measles was targeted for elimination in the United States by 1982. The efforts to eliminate measles were not successful because of two factors. The first was vaccine failure. Prior to 1989, outbreaks occurred in older children in schools in which immunization rates usually were greater than 95 per cent.[155, 211, 226] Attack rates were 1 to 5 per cent, reflecting the accumulation of measles-susceptible persons resulting from vaccine failure. Vaccine failures may be either primary (i.e., failure to develop protective antibody after the initial vaccination) or secondary (i.e., adequate response to vaccine occurred, but immunity was lost subsequently). Measles vaccine is at least 95 per cent effective for children vaccinated at 15 months of age or older. Most evidence has suggested that the majority of cases are primary failures. The waning of immunity appears to be responsible for measles cases in only a small percentage of children.[210, 213, 317] The accumulation of cases due to primary vaccine failure led to the adoption of a routine two-dose measles vaccination schedule in 1989.[23, 51] The purpose of the two-dose schedule was to produce measles immunity in persons with primary vaccine failure. Studies in several age groups indicate that more than 90 per cent of those who fail to respond to the first dose of measles vaccine respond to a second dose.[230]

The second factor was the failure to implement current immunization strategies, especially in the inner cities, where a high proportion of preschool children (≥15 months of age) had not been vaccinated. From 1989 through 1991, the proportion of unvaccinated persons with measles increased, reflecting outbreaks among unvaccinated inner-city preschool aged children. Since 1991, the number of cases in preschool age children has declined because of increased efforts to improve vaccine coverage in inner city areas.

In 1994, the AAP and ACIP recommended routine vaccination with measles vaccine at 12 to 15 months of age. The decision to lower the routine age for primary vaccination to 1 year was based on the observation that most children are susceptible to measles by 12 months of age because of waning transplacental immunity.[207, 209] Most mothers now have vaccine-induced immunity rather than immunity conferred by infection with wild virus. The antibody concentrations induced by measles vaccination generally are lower than those induced by natural measles. Therefore, measles-specific antibodies acquired transplacentally are lower in infants of vaccinated mothers, causing these infants to be susceptible at an earlier age than those whose mothers acquired immunity from natural infection.

Preparations

The live measles virus vaccine (Moraten strain) available in the United States is prepared in chick fibroblast cell culture. Each dose of vaccine contains neomycin, sorbitol, and hydrolyzed gelatin as a stabilizer. Preparations available include a monovalent (measles only) vaccine and two combinations, measles-rubella and MMR. MMR is the vaccine of choice for use in routine vaccination programs for children and adults. In all situations in which measles vaccine is to be used, MMR should be given if the recipient is likely to be susceptible to rubella or mumps.[13]

Inadequate protection against measles can result from the administration of improperly stored vaccine. Prior to reconstitution, measles vaccine must be stored at a temperature between 2° and 8° C (35.6° to 46.4° F) or colder and must be protected from light, which may inactivate the virus. Reconstituted vaccine should be stored in a refrigerator and discarded if not used within 8 hours.

Immunogenicity and Efficacy

Immunization produces a mild or inapparent, noncommunicable infection. Measles antibodies develop in approximately 93 per cent of children vaccinated at 12 months of age and 98 per cent of children vaccinated at 15 months of age.[209] Studies indicate that more than 99 per cent of persons who receive two doses of measles vaccine, separated by at least 1 month, on or after their first birthday develop serologic evidence of measles immunity.[102, 109] Although vaccine-induced antibody titers are lower than those present after natural disease, persistence of protective titers for as long as 16 years after vaccine administration has been demonstrated.[196, 210] Most vaccinated persons who appear to lose antibody have an anamnestic response upon revaccination, indicating that they most likely still are immune.[230] A small percentage of vaccinated persons may lose protection after several years, resulting in secondary vaccine failure.[213, 317]

Adverse Events

Vaccine-associated symptoms, consisting of fever higher than 39.4° C (102.9° F) occurring 5 to 10 days after immunization or transient rash, occur in 5 to 15 per cent of recipients.[237] Serious complications related to vaccine use occur far less frequently than after natural measles.

Thrombocytopenia occurs at a rate of one case for every 30,000 to 40,000 doses distributed. Using data from Sweden and Finland, the Institute of Medicine has concluded that MMR is related causally to thrombocytopenia.[175] The decrease in platelet count presumably is due to the measles component and usually is not apparent clinically. However, thrombocytopenic purpura after vaccination has been reported.

Central nervous system disease, specifically encephalitis or encephalopathy, is reported at a rate of less than one case per 1 million doses of vaccine administered. Because the incidence of encephalitis or encephalopathy after measles vaccination in healthy children is lower than the observed incidence of encephalitis of unknown etiology, some or most of the reported severe neurologic disorders may be related only temporally, rather than causally, to measles immunization. The risk of subacute sclerosing panencephalitis (SSPE) in vaccinated children is extremely low and is estimated to be approximately one-twelfth the risk of SSPE occurring after natural measles (0.7 SSPE cases per million vaccine doses, compared with 8.5 cases per million natural measles infections).[40, 47] Whether measles vaccine causes SSPE is unclear. Some cases of SSPE occur in children with no history of measles or measles vaccination.[13]

Reactions to measles vaccine are not age-related and occur only in susceptible vaccinees. After revaccination, reactions should be expected only in those who failed to respond to the first immunization.

Indications[13, 51]

Measles vaccine is indicated for persons susceptible to measles, unless otherwise contraindicated. The first dose of measles vaccine is recommended at 12 to 15 months of age. The initial dose should be administered at 12 months of age in high-risk areas, such as those with recurrent measles transmission. The second dose is given routinely at 4 to 6 years and no later than 11 to 12 years of age. Both doses of measles vaccine preferably should be given as MMR. The minimum interval between the two doses is 4 weeks.

Adults born prior to 1957 generally may be considered immune to measles because of previous natural infection. Those born after 1956 in whom immunoprophylaxis is indicated should receive two doses of vaccine.

During outbreaks, when the likelihood of exposure is high, measles vaccine should be given to infants as young as 6 months of age. Seroconversion rates to vaccine are significantly less in children vaccinated prior to 1 year of age, compared with those in older children. Children immunized prior to their first birthday then should be revaccinated with MMR at 15 months of age, with a third dose given according to local policy.

Measles still is endemic in many areas of the world. Although vaccination against measles is not a requirement for entry into any country, susceptible children, adolescents, and adults born after 1956 should be offered measles vaccination (usually as MMR) before international travel. Infants 6 months of age or older traveling to areas where measles is endemic or epidemic should be vaccinated before departure. Children 12 to 14 months of age should be given a dose of MMR before departure. Infants 6 to 11 months of age should be vaccinated before departure and revaccinated at 12 to 15 months of age. Vaccination of infants younger than 6 months of age is not necessary because most are protected by maternally derived antibodies.

Exposure to measles in susceptible persons is not a contraindication to vaccination; vaccine given within 72 hours of exposure may provide protection. If exposure does not result in infection, immunization protects against future infection.

Precautions and Contraindications[13, 51]

Immunocompromised patients with conditions such as lymphoreticular or other generalized malignancy and primary or secondary immunodeficiency states should not be given live-virus attenuated measles vaccine. An exception is asymptomatic and mildly symptomatic HIV-infected patients, in whom measles vaccination, given as MMR, is recommended at 15 months of age. This recommendation is based on reports of severe and even fatal measles disease in these children and lack of severe or unusual adverse events associated with vaccination.[49, 194, 215] A report of a young adult with symptomatic HIV infection who was immunized against measles with MMR and developed fatal measles pneumonia has indicated the need for caution in vaccinating symptomatic HIV-infected children who are significantly immunocompromised.[86, 307]

Measles vaccine should not be administered if the person is receiving immunosuppressive doses of systemic corticosteroids. The effects of corticosteroids vary, but many clinicians consider a dose equivalent to either 2 mg/kg of body weight or 20 mg/day of prednisone sufficiently immunosuppressive to raise concerns about the safety of vaccination with live-virus vaccines.

The live-attenuated measles virus used for immunization is not communicable. Therefore, contacts of immunocompromised patients should be vaccinated to prevent the spread of natural measles to such patients.

After cessation of immunosuppressive therapy, measles vaccine generally is withheld for at least 3 months. Because the intensity and type of immunosuppressive therapy, radiation therapy, underlying disease, and other factors determine how quickly immunologic responsiveness is restored, however, a definitive recommendation for an interval after cessation of immunosuppressive therapy when measles vaccine can be administered safely and effectively often is not possible.

Although no direct evidence demonstrates that measles vaccine is harmful to the pregnant female or her fetus, it should not be administered to women known to pregnant or who are considering becoming pregnant within the next 3 months because of the theoretic risk of fetal infection associated with a live-virus vaccine. Women vaccinated with MMR should avoid conception for 3 months after vaccination.

Because measles vaccination temporarily may diminish cutaneous manifestations of cell-mediated immunity, a tuberculin test performed several days to 6 weeks after immunization may yield a false-negative result. Although natural measles virus infection can exacerbate tuberculosis, no evidence indicates that measles vaccination is associated with such an effect. Therefore, tuberculin skin testing is not a prerequisite for measles immunization. If a tuberculin test is indicated, it should be performed on the day of immunization or postponed for 4 to 6 weeks because measles vaccination may suppress tuberculin reactivity temporarily.

Measles vaccine contains chick fibroblast tissue culture protein. Hypersensitivity reactions after measles vaccination are rare. Most are minor and consist of a wheal and flare or urticaria at the injection site. Vaccine guidelines recommend that patients with a history of anaphylactic reaction to egg ingestion be vaccinated only with caution after skin testing, using established desensitization protocols.[148, 164, 199] However, some studies strongly suggest that skin testing to egg protein is not predictive of life-threatening reactions to MMR.[182] Anaphylactic reactions to MMR are extremely rare; only 20 to 30 cases have been reported in the literature.[175] Some reactions have been due to components in the vaccine other than egg protein, such as the gelatin stabilizer or neomycin.[187] Most cases of MMR-associated anaphylactic reactions have occurred in children not identified as allergic to eggs.[182] The recommendation to skin-test egg-allergic children has been modified to cautious immunization without prior testing followed by at least 20 minutes of observation in a setting equipped to deal with immediate hypersensitivity reactions.[13] Persons with histories of nonanaphylactic reactions to egg ingestion or allergies to chicken or feathers are not at increased risk of vaccine-associated reactions.

Children with a previous history of thrombocytopenic purpura or thrombocytopenia may be at risk for developing clinically significant thrombocytopenia after immunization with MMR.[37, 175] The decision to vaccinate should be based on the benefits of immunity to measles, mumps, and rubella and the risk of reoccurrence or exacerbation of the thrombocytopenia after vaccination or from natural infections with measles or rubella. For children who develop thrombocytopenia in the month after a dose of measles-containing vaccine, withholding the second dose of measles vaccine is prudent if the incidence of measles remains low.

Receipt of antibody-containing blood products (whole blood, plasma, or parenteral immunoglobulin) may interfere with seroconversion to measles vaccine. High doses of immunoglobulin preparations can inhibit the immune response to measles vaccine for 3 or more months, depending on the dosage.[269] The length of time that such passively acquired antibody persists depends on the concentration and quantity of the blood product received (Table 237–10).[13]

As in any condition that induces fever during the second year of life, children predisposed to febrile seizures may experience seizures after measles vaccination. Most convulsions after measles immunization are simple febrile seizures and occur in children without known risk factors. Febrile seizures after vaccinations do not increase the risk of subsequent epilepsy or other neurologic disorders.[22] The risk of seizures following measles vaccination may increase among children with a prior history of convulsions or those with a history of convulsions in first-degree family members. Although the exact risk cannot be determined, it appears to be low. The recommendation to immunize children with a personal history of seizures or those with a history of seizures in first-degree family members is based on factors indicating that the benefits greatly outweigh the risks. Prophylactic use of anticonvulsants usually is not feasible because therapeutic concentrations of many currently prescribed anticonvulsants are not achieved for some time after the initiation of therapy.

Mumps Vaccine

Live-virus mumps vaccine became available in the United States in 1967 and was recommended for routine use in 1977. After vaccine licensure, reported mumps cases decreased rapidly. A relative resurgence of mumps occurred in 1986 and 1987. In 1989, the ACIP and AAP implemented a two-dose combined MMR schedule given at 4 to 6 years or at 11 to 12 years of age. After the introduction of the two-dose schedule,

TABLE 237–10. Suggested Intervals Between Immunoglobulin Administration and Measles Vaccination (MMR or Monovalent Measles Vaccine)*

Indication for Immunoglobulin	Route	Dose: U or mL	Dose: mg IgG/kg	Interval (Month)†
Tetanus (as TIG)	IM	250 U	~10	3
Hepatitis A prophylaxis (as IG)				
Contact prophylaxis	IM	0.02 mL/kg	3.3	3
International travel	IM	0.06 mL/kg	10	3
Hepatitis B prophylaxis (as HBIG)	IM	0.06 mL/kg	10	3
Rabies prophylaxis (as RIG)	IM	20 IU/kg	22	4
Measles prophylaxis (as IG)				
Standard	IM	0.25 mL/kg	40	5
Immunocompromised host	IM	0.50 mL/kg	80	6
Varicella prophylaxis (as VZIG)	IM	125 U/10 kg (maximum 625 U)	20–39	5
Blood transfusion				
Washed RBCs	IV	10 mL/kg	Negligible	0
RBCs, adenine-saline added	IV	10 mL/kg	10	3
Packed RBCs	IV	10 mL/kg	20–60	5
Whole blood	IV	10 mL/kg	80–100	6
Plasma/platelet products	IV	10 mL/kg	160	7
Replacement (or therapy) of immune deficiencies (as IGIV)	IV	—	300–400	8
ITP (as IGIV)	IV	—	400	8
RSV-IGIV	IV	—	750	9
ITP	IV	—	1000	10
ITP or Kawasaki disease	IV	—	1600–2000	11

*IG indicates immune globulin; TIG, tetanus IG; IM, intramuscular; HBIG, hepatitis B IG; RIG, rabies IG; VZIG, varicella-zoster IG; IV, intravenous; IGIV, intravenous IG; ITP, immune (formerly termed "idiopathic") thrombocytopenic purpura; and RSV-IGIV, respiratory syncytial virus IGIV.

†These intervals should provide sufficient time for decreases in passive antibodies in all children to allow for an adequate response to measles vaccine. Physicians should not assume that children are fully protected against measles during these intervals. Additional doses of IG or measles vaccine may be indicated after exposure to measles.

Used with permission of the American Academy of Pediatrics: Measles. *In* Peter, G. (ed.): 1997 Red Book: Report of the Committee on Infectious Diseases. 24th ed. Elk Grove Village, American Academy of Pediatrics.

mumps cases declined, reaching a record low in 1993 of 1692 cases.[290]

Prior to vaccine licensure and during the early years of vaccine use, the majority of reported mumps cases occurred in the 5- to 9-year-old age group and 90 per cent of cases occurred in children younger than 15 years of age. A shift in peak incidence from the 5- to 9-year-olds to older age groups was noted from 1985 to 1992, with marked increases among the 10- to 14- and 15- to 19-year-olds. Mumps outbreaks occurred in high schools, on college campuses, and in the work place during 1986 and 1987.[184, 273, 302] The shift in risk to older children and adolescents and the resurgence of mumps in 1986 and 1987 are attributable to the underimmunized cohort of children born between 1967 and 1977, before vaccine came into general use. Since 1992, the proportion of cases occurring among school age children has increased and peak incidence again occurs in the 5- to 9-year-olds.[290]

No evidence indicates waning immunity in vaccinees. The risk of mumps is highest in states without comprehensive school vaccination requirements, providing further evidence that a failure to vaccinate rather than vaccine failure primarily is responsible for the continued occurrence of mumps.[98, 107] Primary vaccine failures do occur, as evidenced by outbreaks in highly vaccinated populations.[43, 99, 165]

Preparations

The live-virus attenuated mumps virus vaccine (Jeryl-Lynn strain) in current use is prepared in chick embryo cell culture and is available individually (monovalent, mumps only) and in combination as mumps-rubella vaccine and MMR. Each dose of vaccine contains neomycin, sorbitol, and hydrolyzed gelatin as stabilizers. Prior to reconstitution, mumps vaccine must be stored at 2° to 8° C (35.6° to 46.4° F) or colder and protected from the light to avoid inactivation. After reconstitution, the vaccine should be used within 8 hours or discarded.

Immunogenicity and Efficacy

The vaccine induces an asymptomatic, noncommunicable infection. More than 97 per cent of susceptible recipients develop protective antibody titers, albeit lower than that after natural infection.[299] Reported clinical vaccine efficacy has ranged from 75 to 95 per cent.[98, 188] The duration of vaccine immunity is unknown, but serologic data indicate that antibody persists for more than 10 years.[297]

Adverse Events

The use of mumps vaccine is associated with few side effects. Parotitis and fever have been reported rarely. Hypersensitivity reactions, including rash, pruritus, and purpura, have been associated temporally with vaccination but are transient and generally mild. Administration of MMR is not harmful if given to a person already immune to one or more of the viruses.[14, 52]

The frequency of reported central nervous system dysfunction after vaccination is not greater than the observed background rate in unimmunized persons.[52] The Institute of Medicine concluded that evidence is inadequate to establish a causal relationship between the Jeryl-Lynn strain of mumps vaccine used in the United States and aseptic meningitis, encephalitis, or sensorineural deafness.[175]

Indications[14, 52]

Routine active immunization with MMR at 12 to 15 months of age is recommended. Most children receive a second dose of mumps vaccine during childhood as a result of the recommendation for routine measles revaccination with MMR. Mumps revaccination is justified by the occurrence of mumps in highly vaccinated populations because substantial numbers of cases have occurred in persons with a history of mumps vaccination.[43, 99, 165]

Susceptible older children, adolescents, and adults also should be vaccinated against mumps. Adults born prior to 1957 generally may be considered immune to mumps as the result of previous natural infection.

Mumps still is endemic throughout most of the world. Although vaccination against mumps is not a requirement for entry into any country, susceptible children, adolescents, and adults born after 1956 should be offered mumps vaccination (usually as MMR) before international travel.

Mumps vaccine is of no proven value in the prevention of disease in susceptible persons after exposure to mumps, probably because the time required to develop protective antibody titers after immunization exceeds the incubation period of clinical mumps. However, if the exposure did not result in infection, the vaccine confers subsequent immunity.

Precautions and Contraindications[14, 52]

Recent vaccine guidelines recommend that patients with a history of anaphylactic reaction to egg ingestion be vaccinated only with caution after skin testing, using established desensitization protocols.[148, 164, 199] However, studies strongly suggest that skin testing to egg protein is not predictive of life-threatening reactions to MMR.[182] Anaphylactic reactions to MMR are extremely rare; only 20 to 30 cases have been reported in the literature.[175] Some reactions have been due to components in the vaccine other than egg protein, such as the gelatin stabilizer or neomycin.[187] Most cases of MMR-associated anaphylactic reactions have occurred in children not identified as allergic to eggs.[182] The recommendation to skin-test egg-allergic children has been modified to cautious immunization without prior testing followed by 20 minutes of observation in a setting equipped to deal with immediate hypersensitivity reactions.[13]

Because of the theoretic risk of fetal damage, mumps vaccine should not be administered to women known to be pregnant or who are considering becoming pregnant within the next 3 months. Women vaccinated with MMR should avoid conception for 3 months after vaccination.

Lymphoreticular or other generalized malignancy and primary or secondary immunodeficiency states are contraindications to the use of mumps vaccine. The exceptions are children with HIV infection who are immunized against measles with MMR (see Measles Vaccine). Because infection after vaccination is noncommunicable, susceptible close contacts of immunosuppressed patients should be vaccinated to avoid mumps exposure in such patients.

After cessation of immunosuppressive therapy, live mumps vaccine generally is withheld for at least 3 months. Because the intensity and type of immunosuppressive therapy, radiation therapy, underlying disease, and other factors determine how quickly immunologic responsiveness is restored, however, a definitive recommendation for an interval after cessation of immunosuppressive therapy when mumps vaccine can be safely and effectively administered often is not possible.

The effect of immunoglobulin preparations on the response to mumps vaccine is unknown. High doses of immunoglobulin preparations can inhibit the immune response to measles vaccine for 3 or more months, depending on the dosage.[269] If mumps vaccine is given as combined MMR, then recommendations for measles vaccine should be followed (see Table 237–10).

Administration of mumps vaccine should be avoided if the person is receiving immunosuppressive dosages of systemic corticosteroids. The effects of corticosteroids vary, but many clinicians consider a dose equivalent to either 2 mg/kg of body weight or 20 mg/day of prednisone sufficiently immunosuppressive to raise concerns about the safety of vaccination with live-virus vaccines.

Pertussis Vaccine

Pertussis (whooping cough) continues to cause significant morbidity and mortality worldwide among young children.[223] In the absence of vaccination, WHO has estimated that approximately 1 million deaths would have occurred from the disease and its complications. In the United States, the number of cases has been reduced by approximately 95 per cent during the vaccine era. Nevertheless, approximately 4000 reported cases of pertussis still occur each year, and the reported incidence has increased since the early 1980s.[79] Relatively large outbreaks of 100 or more cases also have occurred.[103, 126]

The experiences of countries where rates of pertussis vaccination have declined markedly provide strong support for continued routine immunization of infants and young children.[101] For example, in the United Kingdom as a result of adverse publicity about pertussis vaccination, a decrease in immunization rates in 2-year-old children from 77 per cent in 1974 to 30 per cent in 1978 was followed by an epidemic of 102,500 cases of pertussis. A similar experience occurred in Japan when 13,105 cases and 41 deaths occurred in 1979 after routine immunization had been suspended temporarily in 1975.

In the United States, publicity about alleged serious reactions to pertussis vaccine led in the 1980s to public controversy about the risk of pertussis vaccine, costly litigation, escalating vaccine costs, and potential jeopardization of vaccine supply and development.[222, 240] The experience in countries such as England and Japan, the severity of pertussis in young infants, and the usually benign or self-limited sequelae of pertussis vaccination clearly justify continuation of routine childhood immunization. Several risk-benefit analyses have provided additional evidence in support of the benefits of vaccination compared with the risks.[101, 167]

Effective primary preventive programs necessitate immunization of young infants, beginning usually at 2 months of age, because the morbidity and mortality of pertussis are greatest in infants, especially for those younger than 6 months of age.[79, 101] Approximately 35 per cent of reported cases in the United States occur in infants younger than 6 months of age. In this age group, the case-fatality rate for 1992 to 1994 was 0.6 per cent; 71 per cent were hospitalized; and complications, such as pneumonia (14.8 per cent), seizures (1.9 per cent), and encephalopathy (0.2 per cent), were frequent.[79] High rates of immunization in children beyond infancy further may reduce the risk of infection in infants by decreasing the incidence of infection in older family members and resulting transmission of *B. pertussis* within the household.

Preparations

Whole-cell pertussis vaccine, which has been in use for many years, is a suspension of inactivated *B. pertussis* and is combined with diphtheria and tetanus toxoids (DTP). To reduce the incidence of local and systemic reactions caused by these vaccines, acellular vaccines composed of one or more purified components of *B. pertussis* components have been developed and combined with diphtheria and tetanus toxoids (DTaP). Multiple acellular vaccines have been formulated from the different components and methods of production and have been tested in children. All vaccines contain detoxified pertussis toxin (i.e., pertussis toxoid).[118] In addition, vaccines may have one or more of the following *B. pertussis* antigens: filamentous hemagglutinin, pertactin (a 69-kDa outer-membrane protein), and fimbrial proteins, which are agglutinogens. In the United States in the early 1990s, two acellular vaccines were approved for use in children 15 months of age or older (see Indications). As of early 1997, three acellular pertussis vaccines have been approved for primary vaccination during infancy, and licensure of additional products for use in infants is anticipated.

Efficacy

Studies in the United States of household contacts exposed to pertussis indicate that the efficacy of whole-cell vaccine is 80 per cent or greater.[79, 101, 229] Studies reporting lower rates of vaccine efficacy often reflect different criteria for the diagnosis of pertussis and lesser effectiveness of the vaccine in protecting against mild infection than against severe disease.[129] Vaccine-induced immunity persists for at least 3 years and subsequently diminishes with time. Pertussis in those previously vaccinated is less severe than in unvaccinated persons.

The efficacy in infants of eight acellular pertussis vaccines has been evaluated in some studies.[1, 122, 147, 156, 261, 283] Rates of prevention of pertussis with these vaccines have ranged from 58 to 93 per cent. Comparison of efficacy between the different products, however, often is not possible because of differences in study design, vaccine schedule (specifically, the number of doses and age of administration), case definitions for pertussis, and other confounding variables. In general, these acellular vaccines appear to be similar or nearly so in efficacy to most whole-cell vaccines. Whereas in two large trials in Sweden and Italy several acellular vaccines demonstrated substantially greater efficacy compared with that of an approved United States whole-cell vaccine, other whole-cell vaccines appeared slightly more effective than acellular vaccines in other trials.[122] In addition, vaccines in these Swedish and Italian trials were given in a three-dose schedule, in contrast with the four-dose primary schedule for vaccination of young children in the United States.

For both whole-cell and acellular vaccines, serologic correlates of immunogenicity have not been established for assessing efficacy. As a result, field and other epidemiologic studies are necessary to demonstrate efficacy.

Adverse Events

Local and febrile reactions to whole-cell vaccines are common, occurring in more than half of DTP recipients.[108] These manifestations usually develop within the first 24 hours and are brief. The incidence of these reactions after administration of acellular vaccine is significantly less.[1, 118, 147, 156, 283] Comparison of the rates with different acellular vaccines has demonstrated similar safety profiles for each of these vaccines.

More serious reactions to whole-cell vaccines are uncommon. They include prolonged crying of 3 hours or more (occurring in 3 per cent of DTP recipients in a large study); unusual, distinctive, and high-pitched crying (0.1 per cent); high fever of 40.5° C or higher (0.3 per cent); hypotonic-hyporesponsive episodes; and seizures.[108] The incidence of convulsions and hypotonic-hyporesponsive episodes is estimated to be 1 in 1750 immunizations.[108] Most post-DTP seizures are brief, self-limited, and generalized; occur in association with fever; and usually reflect an underlying febrile convulsive disorder.[15] These seizures have not been demonstrated to result in subsequent development of epilepsy or other neurologic sequelae. Predisposing factors include an underlying convulsive disorder, a personal history of prior convulsion, and a family history of convulsions.

Severe reactions to acellular vaccines are rare.[1, 118, 147, 156, 283] As with local and febrile reactions, their occurrence with acellular pertussis vaccination is significantly less likely than that after whole-cell vaccination.

Serious Neurologic Illness

In a large case-control study in Great Britain, the National Childhood Encephalopathy Study, the estimated occurrence of acute neurologic illness resulting in hospitalization was 1 in 140,000 DTP vaccinations.[217] Neurologic sequelae have been reported to be common in a 10-year follow-up study, but no more so than in children with unrelated, acute, neurologic illness in infancy,[216] and reviews of the data have disputed the conclusion that pertussis vaccine can cause neurologic sequelae.[28, 94, 277] The role of whole-cell pertussis vaccine, if any, in causing brain damage remains unproven.[15, 58]

Indications[15, 58, 63, 80]

Vaccination against pertussis is recommended routinely for children at 2, 4, and 6 months of age, followed by a fourth dose at 12 to 18 months of age and a fifth dose at 4 to 6 years of age. Immunization can be started as early as 4 weeks of age if pertussis is prevalent in the community. The interval between doses of the initial series of three doses can be as short as 4 weeks.

For the initial three doses and the fourth dose if given before 15 months of age, only whole-cell vaccine was recommended in the United States until recently. Acellular vaccines had been approved only for the fourth and fifth doses of the pertussis immunization series in children 15 months to 7 years of age. Although either DTaP or DTP may be used for these doses, DTaP is preferred because it has the advantage of lower rates of local reactions, fever, and other common systemic reactions.

Based on the demonstrated efficacy and safety of acellular vaccines in some trials, acellular pertussis vaccine (DTaP) is recommended in infants as the preferred vaccine for all doses, thus replacing whole-cell vaccines in the United States. However, in many countries, including several in Europe as well as developing countries, whole-cell vaccine remains the recommended product.

Pertussis immunization is not indicated for children after 6 years of age because of the diminished risk of pertussis and its complications. Future possible strategies for enhanced control of pertussis, however, include periodic revaccination of adolescents and adults with an acellular vaccine in order to reduce the reservoir of infections in these age groups.

Contraindications and Precautions[15, 58, 63, 80]

Adverse events temporally related to pertussis immunization that contraindicate further administration of either DTP or DTaP are as follows:

- An immediate anaphylactic reaction
- Encephalopathy within 7 days, defined as severe, acute, central nervous system disorder unexplained by another cause; it may be manifested by major alterations of consciousness or by generalized or focal seizures that persist for more than a few hours without recovery within 24 hours

Postvaccination reactions constituting precautions are as follows:

- A convulsion, with or without fever, occurring within 3 days of DTP or DTaP administration
- Persistent, severe, inconsolable screaming or crying for 3 or more hours within 48 hours
- Hypotonic-hyporesponsive episode within 48 hours
- Temperature of 40.5° C (104.9° F) or higher, unexplained by another cause, within 48 hours

With these adverse events occurring in temporal association with DTP or DTaP administration, the decision to administer additional doses of pertussis vaccine carefully should be considered. These events previously were considered to be contraindications to DTP but now are considered precautions. In circumstances such as a pertussis outbreak in which the potential benefits of pertussis immunization outweigh the possible risks, vaccination is indicated, particularly because these events have not been proved to cause permanent sequelae. In addition, the risk of these reactions from DTaP is substantially less than that from DTP.

In children with an evolving neurologic disorder, pertussis immunization should be deferred until the nature and cause of the disorder have been established. A personal history of prior convulsion unrelated to DTP or a family history of convulsions (in the absence of a possible evolving neurologic disorder) is not a contraindication. DTaP strongly is recommended for children who have had febrile or afebrile seizures temporally not associated with pertussis vaccination and for those who have immediate family members with histories of seizure disorders. These children are at increased risk for seizures after receiving DTP as a result of pyrogenic reactions to the whole-cell pertussis vaccine. However, although the risk of seizures is increased, these seizures do not affect the neurologic prognosis of the child. If DTP (i.e., whole-cell vaccine) is given, administration of an antipyretic, such as acetaminophen, at the time of immunization and 4 and 8 hours later reduces the incidence of febrile and local reactions[178] and, thus, may decrease the risk of a postvaccination seizure.

These contraindications and precautions are based on adverse reactions associated with whole-cell vaccine. Although reactions occurring after DTaP administration are much less common than those associated with DTP, at present the contraindications and precautions for DTaP are the same.

Poliomyelitis Vaccine

The widespread implementation of poliovirus vaccine programs has resulted in dramatic reduction in the incidence of paralytic poliomyelitis throughout the world. In contrast with the prevaccine era, when more than 18,000 cases of paralytic disease occurred in the United States annually, the last known case in this country due to indigenous wild-type virus occurred in 1979.[278] Other than rare imported cases, the only cases of paralytic poliomyelitis in the United States since then have been vaccine-related.

This effectiveness of vaccination has led to major and successful initiatives by the Pan American Health Organization and WHO for regional and global, respectively, eradication of poliovirus infections. The last case of poliomyelitis from the Americas was reported in August 1991 from Peru, and the Western Hemisphere in 1994 was certified by an international commission to be free of indigenous wild-type poliovirus.[64, 69] The global eradication initiative also has been successful, resulting in an 80 per cent reduction in the number of reported cases worldwide since the mid-1980s and optimism for worldwide eradication by 2000.[106, 312]

These accomplishments in the elimination of poliovirus

infection have been achieved primarily through the use of OPV. This product has been the vaccine of choice for children in the United States since the early 1960s because it (1) induces optimal intestinal immunity, (2) is painless to administer, (3) secondarily immunizes some contacts by fecal-oral spread of the vaccine virus, therefore contributing to the immunity of the population, and (4) successfully has eliminated disease due to wild-type poliovirus in this country.[46] For these reasons, global eradication necessitates the continued use of OPV.[312] However, because inactivated poliovirus vaccine (IPV) also is highly effective and does not cause vaccine-associated paralytic poliomyelitis (VAPP), IPV has been used for routine immunization in several European countries that have controlled or eliminated poliomyelitis, including Finland, France, and the Netherlands. In Canada, IPV has replaced OPV as the vaccine of choice.[242] Denmark, Israel, and the province of Prince Edward Island in Canada have used sequential schedules of IPV followed by OPV in order to reduce the risk of VAPP and to maintain the aforementioned benefits of OPV. Because in the United States, 8 to 10 cases of VAPP occur annually and the risk of exposure to wild-type polio virus has been reduced markedly or eliminated, the CDC has recommended expanded use of IPV beginning in 1997.[96] Although the ACIP of the CDC recommends a sequential regimen of two doses of IPV followed by two doses of OPV, regimens of OPV only and IPV only also remain acceptable alternatives according to both the ACIP and AAP.[29, 96] The implementation of an IPV only schedule to replace OPV only and sequential schedules will be fostered by the development of combination vaccines, which will reduce the number of necessary injections to complete the immunization schedule for young children and by continuing progress in global eradication of poliomyelitis.

Assuming that global eradication is achieved, eventual discontinuation of poliomyelitis vaccination can be anticipated. However, for the foreseeable future, immunity to poliomyelitis needs to be maintained by widespread implementation of vaccination programs.

Preparations[96]

Two types of poliovirus vaccine currently are licensed in the United States, OPV and IPV. Both vaccines are trivalent, consisting of serotypes 1, 2, and 3. The attenuated strains of poliovirus in OPV are propagated in monkey-kidney tissue. For IPV, the vaccine virus is propagated in either monkey-kidney cells or human diploid (MRC-5) cell cultures before purification and formaldehyde inactivation. These IPV products are enhanced-potency vaccines, which became available in the United States in 1988 and replaced previously available IPV preparations.

Immunogenicity and Efficacy

Both OPV and IPV given in the recommended three-dose series result in immunity to all three polioviruses in nearly 100 per cent of recipients.[96] No evidence suggests waning immunity with either vaccine. Most children seroconvert after two doses and often only after one. Vaccination with either vaccine results in diminished circulation of wild-type poliovirus in the community as the result of induction of mucosal immunity.[228, 242] In contrast with IPV, OPV results in not only pharyngeal immunity but also a high degree of intestinal immunity and provides a substantial degree of resistance to reinfection, which limits circulation of poliovirus from fecal-oral transmission. Intestinal immunity from IPV is incomplete.

The sequential schedule of two doses of IPV followed by two doses of OPV induces excellent humoral and intestinal immunity.[96] At least two doses of IPV are necessary to ensure adequate humoral immunity to protect against VAPP from OPV.

Adverse Events

The only major adverse events associated with poliomyelitis immunization is VAPP resulting from OPV. This is exceedingly rare.[278] Based on the occurrence of 8 to 10 cases yearly in the United States and the number of OPV doses distributed, the risk for infants receiving the first dose of OPV is estimated to be 1 in 1.4 million doses.[96] Of cases of VAPP, approximately 40 per cent occur in otherwise healthy recipients, approximately 80 per cent of which follow the first dose and 90 per cent of which occur in the first year of life.[279] Cases in contacts account for a similar proportion, but three-fourths of these cases are in adults. Nonimmune adults and children who reside in a household with a child who receives OPV or who are otherwise in contact with young children who have received OPV are at risk as the result of possible fecal-oral acquisition and reversion to virulence of the vaccine virus. The remaining cases occur in immunodeficient persons, in whom the risk is 3200 to 6800 times higher. The majority of the cases in this category occur in infants and young children who have disorders of humoral immunity.

In a review of vaccine adverse events by the Institute of Medicine, an increased risk of GBS after OPV administration was observed in studies in Finland.[176] However, reanalysis of this data and a subsequent study in the United States did not demonstrate a causal relationship between GBS and OPV administration.[94, 247] No causal or temporal association of IPV with GBS has been noted.

Indications[29, 96]

Primary immunization against poliovirus is initiated at 2 months of age. As of 1997, three schedules are considered acceptable in the United States: sequential (two doses of IPV followed by two doses of OPV), OPV only, and IPV only. The ACIP recommends the sequential schedule as the preferred choice in many circumstances. The exception is persons who are immunodeficient or who live in households with immunosuppressed persons, such as those with HIV infection, in which only IPV is indicated. In each schedule, doses are given at 2, 4, 12 to 18 months, and 4 and 6 years of age at school entry; in the OPV only schedule, however, the third dose may be given as early as 6 months of age. Whereas with earlier IPV preparations (i.e., nonenhanced formulations) booster doses every 5 years were recommended, booster doses are not recommended for the current enhanced-potency IPV or vaccine schedules utilizing OPV. In the immunization schedule of WHO, doses are recommended at birth and 6, 10, and 14 weeks of age.[5] In geographic areas with endemic polio, a dose may be given when the newborn is discharged from the hospital. Supplementary doses often are given during mass community programs in these areas. Breast feeding does not interfere with successful immunization with OPV.

Routine immunization for adults (18 years of age or older) residing in the United States is not recommended because wild poliovirus no longer is transmitted in this country. However, previously unimmunized persons traveling to countries where poliomyelitis is epidemic or endemic, members of communities of specific population groups experiencing wild-type poliovirus disease, health care workers in close contact with patients who may be excreting wild-type poliovirus, and laboratory workers in contact with specimens that may contain wild-type poliovirus should be vaccinated. Because the risk of VAPP from OPV in adults is higher than in children, IPV is recommended. Those who are immunized incompletely should complete the primary series with either IPV or OPV, irrespective of which vaccine previously had been given. Previously immunized adults who are at increased risk of exposure to poliomyelitis, such as those traveling to countries where poliomyelitis still is endemic, should receive a single dose of either IPV or OPV.

Precautions and Contraindications[17, 96]

OPV is contraindicated in persons with immunodeficiency disorders, such as suspected or proven cellular or humoral immunodeficiency, HIV infection, and malignancy, and in those receiving immunosuppressive therapy (e.g., corticosteroids, cytotoxic agents, radiation therapy). Because of the risk of fecal-oral spread of vaccine virus, OPV also should not be given to household contacts of persons with altered immunity, including those with HIV infection, or to members of households with a family history of immunodeficiency until the immune status of the recipient and other children in the family has been assessed. IPV is indicated for vaccination of these persons.

IPV is contraindicated in persons who have experienced an anaphylactic reaction after a previous dose of IPV or an anaphylactic reaction to one of the antibiotics in the vaccine preparation (i.e., streptomycin, polymyxin B, or neomycin). OPV is contraindicated in persons who have suffered an anaphylactic reaction to either streptomycin or neomycin because the vaccine contains trace amounts of these antibiotics.

Poliomyelitis vaccination generally is contraindicated in pregnant woman because of the theoretic risk of harm to the fetus. However, no deleterious effects from either OPV or IPV administered during pregnancy have been demonstrated, and if immediate protection against poliomyelitis is needed, either OPV or IPV may be given.

Rubella Vaccine

After the licensure of rubella vaccine in 1969, rubella incidence declined from a peak of 57,686 cases in 1969 to a record low of 160 cases in 1992. In the prevaccine era, epidemics of rubella occurred every 6 to 9 years, with the last major United States epidemic occurring in 1964 and 1965. No large epidemics have occurred since the vaccine was licensed in 1969. Limited outbreaks, however, continue to occur among groups of susceptible people with close contact.[73]

Unlike measles and varicella, rubella is reported among several age groups. From 1982 through 1992, approximately 30 per cent of cases occurred in each of three age groups (younger than 5, 5 to 19, and 20 to 39 years of age). Adults older than 40 years of age typically account for less than 10 per cent of reported cases. Some data suggest that the rates of rubella susceptibility are highest among young adults. From 1992 to 1994, 57 per cent of reported rubella cases occurred among persons 20 years of age or older.[73] As was true in the era before vaccination, 10 to 20 per cent of women in the childbearing age group remained susceptible, and efforts to immunize this group were intensified in 1985 in order to prevent congenital rubella. Seronegative rates in postpubertal women appear to have diminished to 6 to 11 per cent.[55]

The incidence of congenital rubella in the United States has paralleled the rise and decline of rubella from 1989 to 1993. Sixty-seven cases, the largest annual reported number of cases since vaccine licensure, occurred in 1970. Although fewer than 5 cases of congenital rubella were reported annually in the 1980s, a moderate resurgence of rubella occurred in 1990 and 1991, with a resultant increase in congenital rubella cases to 25 and 33, respectively. More recently, cases have declined, with no indigenous cases of congenital rubella reported in 1993.[73]

Preparations

Since 1979, RA 27/3 (rubella abortus, twenty-seventh specimen/third extract) vaccine, prepared in human diploid tissue culture, has been the only vaccine available in the United States, replacing the earlier HPV-77 and Cendehill vaccines. RA 27/3 induces higher antibody titers, more closely paralleling the immune response after natural infection than did previous vaccines.[201, 231] In addition to MMR vaccine, monovalent rubella and combinations of measles-rubella and rubella-mumps vaccines are available.

MMR generally is used for routine infant immunization programs. Rubella vaccine should be kept at 2° to 8° C (35.6° to 46.4° F) or colder during storage and should be protected from light to avoid virus inactivation. Once reconstituted, the vaccine should be used within 8 hours.

Immunogenicity and Efficacy

At least 98 per cent of susceptible vaccinees 12 months of age or older develop protective antibody titers.[218] Vaccine-induced rubella antibodies have persisted in more than 90 per cent of vaccinees 16 years after receiving the RA 27/3 vaccine.[104] Lifelong protection against clinical reinfection, asymptomatic viremia, or both usually results from a single dose of vaccine early in childhood.

In some cases, vaccinees exposed to natural rubella developed a rise of antibody titer unassociated with clinical symptoms. Reinfection is associated only rarely with viremia. Significant pharyngeal shedding also is infrequent. Person-to-person transmission, however, has not been reported. Reinfection caused by wild-type rubella virus also may be observed in persons with previous natural rubella. The risk of congenital rubella syndrome from rubella virus reinfection during pregnancy is extremely low.[55]

Adverse Events

Rubella vaccines generally are well tolerated. The most frequent complaints after vaccination are fever, lymphadenopathy, and rash, which occur in 5 to 15 per cent of children 5 to 12 days after vaccination.[18] Transient peripheral neuritis (paresthesia and pain in the arms and legs) has been observed uncommonly, primarily in older age groups.[260]

Approximately 3 per cent of children develop transient joint manifestations, including arthralgia and, less commonly, arthritis 1 to 3 weeks after immunization. Although 25 per cent of adult women report joint pain after vaccination, arthritis with objective clinical findings lasting less than 10 days occurs in 13 to 15 per cent. Cases of persistent or recurrent joint symptoms have been reported but are rare. The Institute of Medicine reviewed all available data on rubella and adverse joint events and concluded that the available evidence was consistent with a causal relationship between the rubella vaccination and chronic arthritis in adult women, although available data on current vaccine strains are limited.[169] The incidence of joint manifestations after immunization is lower than that after natural infection at the corresponding age.

Rubella revaccination is well tolerated, even among college-age and older vaccinees, and is associated with a much lower incidence of adverse reactions than that reported after primary rubella immunization of young adult populations. Reported rates of joint-related complaints of 4 to 18 per cent after revaccination are lower than those reported after primary vaccination.[100, 263]

Indications[18, 55]

Live rubella vaccine generally is recommended for all children at 12 months of age or older; it is given as MMR at 12 to 15 months of age. A second dose of MMR is given at the recommended age for measles revaccination. The vaccine should be provided to previously unimmunized preschool or older school children despite a history of clinical rubella unless serologic tests confirm immunity.

Emphasis should be placed on the immunization of postpubertal males and females, especially college students and those in the military. Rubella vaccine also should be administered to adolescent and adult females of childbearing age who lack a history of prior vaccination. Settings such as premarital screening, routine gynecologic examinations, visits for newborn infants and well-child care, or other medical visits provide opportunities for immunization. The immediate postpartum period also is an excellent time for immunization. Rubella vaccine may be given after anti-Rho(D) immunoglobulin administration, but serologic testing to determine whether seroconversion has occurred should be performed at least 8 weeks after vaccination. When practical, potential vaccinees may be screened for susceptibility. However, vaccination of females of child-bearing age is justifiable, and may be preferable, without prior serologic testing in women not known to be pregnant.

Precautions and Contraindications[18, 55]

Specific contraindications to live rubella vaccine administration include the following: (1) pregnancy, (2) severe febrile illness, (3) known history of anaphylactic reaction to neomycin, which is contained in the vaccine, and (4) immunodeficiency states (malignancy, primary immunodeficiency disease, immunosuppressive or corticosteroid therapy, and radiation therapy).

Postpubertal women of child-bearing age who state that they are pregnant or plan to become pregnant within the next 3 months should not be vaccinated. Vaccinated women should be counseled about the need to avoid pregnancy for 3 months after vaccination.

Although pregnancy is a contraindication to rubella vaccination, the maximal theoretic risk to the fetus is estimated to be 1.6 per cent. From 1979 until 1989, the CDC registered 321 susceptible women who inadvertently had received RA 27/3 rubella vaccine within 3 months before or after conception and carried their pregnancy to term. None of their infants had defects compatible with congenital rubella syndrome, although 2 per cent had serologic evidence of intrauterine infection.[54] Because rubella virus has been isolated from the products of conception of women vaccinated during pregnancy, continued caution with respect to vaccination during pregnancy should be advised. However, the available evidence indicates that inadvertent rubella vaccination during pregnancy ordinarily is not a reason to consider interruption of pregnancy.

Although vaccine virus may be isolated from the pharynx, vaccinees do not transmit rubella to others except in the case of the vaccinated breast-feeding mother. In this situation, the infant may be infected through breast milk and may develop a mild rash illness, but serious adverse effects have not been noted. Infants infected through breast feeding respond normally to rubella vaccination at 15 months of age. Breast feeding is not a contraindication to rubella vaccination.

Concerns about potential transmission of disease from immunized children to susceptible contacts (including pregnant women) have not been supported by studies of susceptible household contacts. Therefore, susceptible children whose household contacts are pregnant may be vaccinated.

Rubella vaccine should not be given during an interval beginning 2 weeks prior to and extending 3 months after administration of immunoglobulin or blood transfusion. Because rubella vaccine usually is given as MMR and recent evidence suggests that high doses of immunoglobulin preparations can inhibit the immune response to measles vaccine for 3 or more months depending on the dosage, rubella vaccination with MMR necessitates deferral for longer periods (see Measles Vaccine).[18, 269]

Tetanus Toxoid

The efficacy of active immunization against tetanus was demonstrated most dramatically in military personnel during World War II, when tetanus toxoid virtually eliminated tetanus in injured servicemen.[205] Since the 1940s, routine immunization of civilians in the United States with tetanus toxoid has been similarly successful in preventing tetanus. In nearly all cases, disease has been reported only in unimmunized or inadequately immunized persons.[56] The potential for occurrence of tetanus, however, is indicated by the significant number of adults in the United States who lack protective concentrations of serum antibody.[138] Although neonatal tetanus nearly has been eliminated in the United States, it is a leading cause of morbidity in newborns in developing countries. As a result, global elimination of neonatal tetanus is a goal of WHO.[71]

Preparations[58]

Tetanus toxoid is prepared by formaldehyde treatment of *Clostridium tetani* toxin. It is provided as both fluid and aluminum salt–adsorbed preparations, but in the United States only the latter is available. Tetanus toxoid is available in combination with diphtheria toxoid and pertussis vaccine, either whole-cell or acellular, for routine administration to infants and children. For children in whom pertussis vaccine is contraindicated, for children 7 years of age or older who have not been immunized, and for booster doses, it is combined with diphtheria toxoid as either DT or Td (see Diphtheria Toxoid). These preparations are identical in the amounts of tetanus toxoid but differ in the quantity of diphtheria toxoid. Fluid toxoid preparations result in a significantly shorter duration of immunity than that induced by aluminum-adsorbed antigens; therefore, adsorbed antigens are recommended.

Immunogenicity and Efficacy

Adequate primary immunization provides sufficient protective titers of antitoxin for at least 10 years and ensures prompt, anamnestic responses to booster injections for several years longer.

Adverse Events

Local reactions of pain, swelling, and induration can occur, but in children these reactions usually are attributable to the whole-cell pertussis vaccine that is combined with tetanus toxoid. In adolescents and adults, hypersensitivity reactions rarely are severe.

Neurologic reactions after administration of tetanus toxoid are rare. These reactions include brachial neuritis and GBS.

Indications: Pre-exposure

For primary immunization, doses of tetanus toxoid should be given at 2, 4, and 6 months of age. A fourth dose is given 6 to 12 months after the third dose (i.e., at 12 to 18 months of age) to maintain adequate serum antibody concentrations for the ensuing preschool years. For those not immunized in infancy, DTP is given at 0 (initial dose), 2, 4, and 10 to 16 months later, followed by a single booster dose at 4 to 6 years of age just prior to school entry. If pertussis vaccine is contraindicated, DT should be used. For persons 7 years of age or older, a primary series of Td given at 0, 2, and 8 to 14 months later is recommended. Interruption of the recommended schedule or delay in administering subsequent doses during primary immunization does not reduce immunity. After completion of early childhood immunization, including a dose of tetanus toxoid at 4 to 6 years of age, booster doses of Td are recommended every 10 years beginning at the 11- to 12-year-old preadolescent immunization visit.

Antepartum[144]

In those areas of the world where the risk of neonatal tetanus is significant, previously unimmunized, pregnant women should receive two antepartum doses, properly spaced, and should complete the three-dose series subsequently. Women immunized more than 10 years previously should receive a booster dose.

Postexposure: Wound Management

The possible need for immunoprophylaxis is an integral aspect of wound management at the time of trauma or injury. The recommended use of tetanus toxoid (as Td) in addition to tetanus immunoglobulin at the time of injury is given in Table 237–11. Specific recommendations depend on the person's immunization status, the nature of the wound, and the duration of time after the injury and prior to evaluation and treatment. After prophylaxis, primary immunization subsequently should be completed in those lacking the recommended number of doses. This conservative approach to the frequency of booster doses of tetanus toxoid in wound management in previously immunized persons is supported by the prolonged immunity from tetanus vaccination and the increased incidence of hypersensitivity reactions associated with frequent booster injections.[121, 236]

Patients convalescing from tetanus infection should complete active immunization because infection often does not confer immunity.

TABLE 237–11. Recommended Tetanus Prophylaxis in Wound Management

History of Tetanus Toxoid (Number of Doses)	Clean, Minor Wounds		All Other Wounds (Tetanus-Prone Wounds)[a]	
	Td[b]	*TIG*	*Td*[b]	*TIG*
Unknown or <3	Yes	No	Yes	Yes
≥3	No[c]	No	No[d]	No

[a]Such as, but not limited to, wounds contaminated with dirt, feces, soil, and saliva; puncture wounds; avulsions; and wounds resulting from missiles, crushing, burns, and frostbite.

[b]For children younger than 7 years of age; DTaP, DTP, or DT (depending on vaccine status of patient) is preferred to tetanus toxoid alone.

[c]Yes, if more than 10 years since last dose.

[d]Yes, if more than 5 years since last dose. More frequent boosters are not needed and can accentuate side effects.

Used with permission of the American Academy of Pediatrics: Tetanus. *In* Peter, G. (ed.): 1997 Red Book: Report of the Committee on Infectious Diseases. 24th ed. Elk Grove Village, American Academy of Pediatrics.

Precautions and Contraindications

A history of an immediate, severe hypersensitivity reaction to tetanus toxoid–containing preparations that is severe or anaphylactic is a contraindication to further vaccination.[58] Persons who experience Arthus-type hypersensitivity reactions after tetanus toxoid administration usually have high serum tetanus antitoxin concentrations and should not be given doses of Td more frequently than every 10 years, even if they have a tetanus-prone wound. If an anaphylactic reaction to a previous dose of tetanus toxoid is suspected, intradermal skin testing may be helpful in determining whether to discontinue tetanus toxoid vaccination.[181] Because in rare cases, tetanus toxoid administration has been associated with recurrence of GBS,[173] the decision to give additional doses in persons with a previous history of this syndrome within 6 weeks after receipt of tetanus toxoid should be based on consideration of the benefits of revaccination and the comparative risk of recurrence of GBS.[94]

Varicella Vaccine

Varicella currently is the most common childhood infectious disease in the United States. Although varicella usually is a benign, self-limited disease in healthy children, recent surveys indicate that the complication rate in varicella is appreciable in healthy children. Approximately 100 deaths from varicella are reported each year.[246] In children between 1 and 14 years of age, complications are unusual and include bacterial superinfection of skin, Reye syndrome, pneumonitis, and encephalitis.[134] Almost 2 of every 1000 children with varicella are hospitalized.[153]

Varicella potentially is severe in children with malignancies and may be fatal in as many as 4 per cent of cases, despite the use of prophylactic immunoglobulin and antiviral therapy.[127] Other high-risk groups of children include those with HIV and other immunocompromising conditions and those receiving high doses of systemic corticosteroids.

Varicella also may cause more severe disease in adults. Although rare, congenital varicella syndrome occurs in approximately 2 per cent of infants born to women who contract varicella in the first or second trimester of pregnancy.[123]

Preparations

Varicella vaccine is a preparation of the Oka strain of varicella virus obtained from the vesicle fluid of a healthy child with varicella that has been attenuated by serial propagation in human embryo lung fibroblasts, guinea pig embryonic cells, and human diploid cell cultures. The vaccine contains trace amounts of neomycin, fetal bovine serum, sucrose, residual components of human diploid (MRC-5) cells, and gelatin. The vaccine does not contain preservatives.

Varicella vaccine is lyophilized and is stored frozen at

−15° C or colder until reconstituted. Any freezer that reliably maintains an average temperature of −15° C and has a separate sealed freezer door is acceptable for storing vaccine. The vaccine also may be stored at refrigerator temperature (2° to 8° C) for as long as 72 hours prior to reconstitution. Vaccine stored at 2° to 8° C that is not used within 72 hours should be discarded. Reconstituted vaccine should be stored at room temperature and discarded if not used within 30 minutes.

Immunogenicity and Efficacy

Varicella vaccine is highly immunogenic in susceptible children. Seroconversion has occurred in greater than 96 per cent of children 12 months to 12 years of age after one dose of vaccine.[303] Preexisting antibody, if present at 12 months of age, does not appear to interfere with antibody response. As with other viral vaccines, the antibody response after immunization is lower than that from natural disease.

Adolescents and adults have age-related decreases in the ability to develop a primary response to varicella virus.[139] Seroconversion rates of 78 to 82 per cent after one dose and 99 per cent after two doses have been reported in those older than 12 years of age.[139, 303]

In ongoing studies in the United States and Japan, serum antibodies to varicella have been detected for as long as 8 to 20 years after immunization in more than 95 per cent of immunized children.[35, 197] Antibody concentrations have persisted for at least 1 year in 97 per cent of adults and adolescents who were administered two doses of vaccine 4 to 8 weeks apart.[139]

Varicella vaccine has been demonstrated to be highly effective in preventing varicella in children and in reducing the severity of infection if they do become infected. In a double-blind, placebo-controlled trial using a vaccine with a higher potency than the currently licensed vaccine, efficacy was an estimated 95 per cent after 7 years.[197] Based on available data, varicella vaccine provides protective efficacy rates of 70 to 90 per cent in children against infection and 95 per cent protection against severe disease.[32] In follow-up studies, less than 1 to 4.4 per cent of vaccinated children per year have developed chickenpox in the 9 years after vaccination. These vaccine-failure cases are mild with fewer skin lesions, lower rates of fever, and more rapid recovery.[38, 295]

Varicella vaccine provides protective efficacy rates of approximately 70 per cent in adults and adolescents who have seroconverted against infection after household exposure. The remaining 30 per cent develop attenuated disease with fewer skin lesions and little or no systemic toxicity, as in children.[139]

Current estimates of vaccine efficacy and antibody persistence in vaccinees are based on observations made when natural varicella infection has been highly prevalent. The extent to which boosting from exposure to natural varicella has affected the efficacy of vaccine or duration of immunity is not known.

Adverse Events

Varicella vaccine has relatively few adverse reactions in children. Local reactions, rashes, and low-grade fevers occur in as many as 10 per cent of vaccine recipients,[32] but rates of rash and fever have been similar in placebo groups in several studies.[124, 298]

A major concern has been whether vaccination would increase the risk of zoster. However, in both healthy and leukemic children, the rate of zoster has been similar to or lower than that expected after chickenpox.[200, 243]

The vaccine strain of virus rarely is transmissible and only from vaccinees with rash.[285] No evidence indicates reversion to virulence of the vaccine strain during transmission; persons acquiring vaccine virus have mild rashes in 75 per cent of cases and have symptomless seroconversion in 25 per cent.[32]

Indications[26, 92]

Varicella vaccine was licensed by the FDA in 1995 for use in persons 12 months of age or older who have not had varicella. One dose of varicella vaccine is recommended for immunization of susceptible healthy children from 12 to 18 months of age. The vaccine may be given concurrently with MMR but at separate sites. In addition, one dose of vaccine is recommended for immunization of all children from age 19 months to the 13th birthday who lack a reliable history of varicella infection and who have not been vaccinated previously. Susceptible healthy adolescents who have reached their 13th birthday should be immunized with two doses of varicella vaccine 4 to 8 weeks apart. If more than 8 weeks elapse after the first dose, the second dose can be administered without restarting the schedule. In adolescents and young adults who do not have a reliable history of varicella, serologic testing for immunity before vaccination is likely to be cost-effective.[204]

No data exist regarding postexposure efficacy of the currently licensed varicella vaccine. Protective efficacy rates are greater than 90 per cent if children are vaccinated within 3 days of exposure in studies of postexposure prophylaxis of children in Japan and the United States using prelicensure formulations of varicella vaccine.[32, 34]

Precautions and Contraindications[26, 92]

Specific contraindications to varicella vaccine administration include the following: (1) pregnancy, (2) severe febrile illness, (3) known history of anaphylactic reaction to vaccine components, and (4) immunodeficiency states (malignancy, primary immunodeficiency disease, immunosuppressive or corticosteroid therapy, and radiation therapy).

Immunocompromised patients with conditions such as lymphoreticular or other generalized malignancy and primary or secondary immunodeficiency conditions should not be given live-virus attenuated varicella vaccine. An exception is patients with acute lymphocytic leukemia in remission in which case a research protocol is available for immunization.[65] This recommendation is based on the successful immunization of children with leukemia with varicella vaccine under carefully controlled circumstances.

Administration of varicella vaccine should be avoided if the patient is receiving immunosuppressive doses of systemic corticosteroids. The effects of corticosteroids vary, but many clinicians consider a dose equivalent to either 2 mg/kg of body weight or 20 mg/day of prednisone to be sufficiently immunosuppressive to raise concerns about the safety of vaccination with live-virus vaccines.

After cessation of immunosuppressive therapy, varicella vaccine generally is withheld for at least 3 months. Because the intensity and type of immunosuppressive therapy, radiation therapy, underlying disease, and other factors determine when immunologic responsiveness will be restored, however, a definitive recommendation for an interval after cessation of immunosuppressive therapy when varicella vaccine can be administered safely and effectively often is not possible.

Transmission of the live-attenuated varicella vaccine virus used for immunization has been documented rarely. Therefore, contacts of immunocompromised patients should be vaccinated to prevent the spread of natural varicella to such patients. Vaccinees who develop a rash in the month after immunization should avoid direct contact with immunocompromised, susceptible persons for the duration of the rash.

Receipt of antibody-containing blood products (whole blood, plasma, or parenteral immunoglobulin) may interfere with seroconversion to varicella vaccine. Varicella vaccine should not be given within at least 5 months after administration of immunoglobulin or blood transfusion.

Although no direct evidence demonstrates that varicella vaccine is harmful to the pregnant female or her fetus, it should not be administered to women known to be pregnant or who are considering becoming pregnant within the month because of the theoretic risk of fetal infection associated with a live-virus vaccine. Vaccinated women should avoid conception for 1 month after vaccination.

Varicella vaccine may be considered for a nursing mother. Although most live-virus vaccines are not secreted in breast milk, whether varicella vaccine virus is excreted in human milk and, if so, whether the infant can be infected are unknown.

Reye syndrome has occurred in children infected with varicella who receive salicylates. Whether varicella vaccine might induce Reye syndrome is not known, but the vaccine manufacturer recommends that salicylates not be given within at least 6 weeks after administration of varicella vaccine.

VACCINES WITH SELECTIVE INDICATIONS

Bacillus Calmette-Guérin Vaccine

Effective control of tuberculosis in the United States has been achieved by the early identification and treatment of cases followed by surveillance of household and other close contacts and institution of appropriate preventive measures for those at high risk of developing disease. In the United States, the mainstay of preventive therapy is isoniazid chemoprophylaxis, which is used in asymptomatically infected people to prevent the progression of infection to disease. In selected instances, however, potential for disease, poor compliance in contacts instructed to take chemoprophylaxis, or failure of chemoprophylaxis may justify immunoprophylaxis.[88] Elsewhere in the world, bacillus Calmette-Guérin (BCG) vaccine is used widely and is recommended routinely at birth by WHO (see Table 237–5). Of primary concern to the pediatrician is the risk to the infant born to a tuberculous mother or living within a household with other identified tuberculous persons.[21]

Preparations

BCG is a live-attenuated strain derived from *Mycobacterium bovis.* All presently available BCG vaccines are derived from the original strain at the Pasteur Institute but have been propagated by different methods in many laboratories and, therefore, vary in their immunogenic and reactogenic properties. BCG vaccine is administered either percutaneously or intradermally. BCG vaccine preparations instilled in the treatment of bladder cancer are not intended to be used as vaccines.[93]

Immunogenicity and Efficacy

Efficacy trials of BCG vaccines available prior to 1955 demonstrated variable efficacy ranging from 0 to 80 per cent[112, 113, 234, 275, 286, 287] Possible explanations for this range in efficacy have included failure to protect against the local strain of *Mycobacterium tuberculosis,* varying potency of vaccine, genetic alterations over time in the local strain, and repeated superinfection with *M. tuberculosis* as a booster.[93, 220] Observational studies in areas where BCG vaccination is performed at birth have demonstrated a 52 to 100 per cent decrease in the incidence of tuberculous meningitis and miliary tuberculosis, as well as a 2 to 80 per cent decrease in pulmonary tuberculosis in vaccinated children younger than 15 years of age.[233, 254, 265, 271, 282, 313] In adolescents and young adults, protective efficacy of BCG vaccine is not so reliable, and in children and adults infected with HIV, efficacy has not been determined.[110, 253]

Adverse Events

BCG vaccination usually results in scarring at the site of injection. BCG vaccine preparations have been associated with localized reactions, including ulceration, lymphadenitis, or both, in 1 to 10 per cent of vaccine recipients. Osteomyelitis, especially of the long bones, occurs in 1 per 1 million vaccinees. The rate may be higher in newborns. Fatal or disseminated BCG infection occurs rarely (0.1 to 1 case per million vaccinees) and almost exclusively in immunocompromised children.[93, 195, 206, 276]

Indications[93]

In the United States, BCG vaccination is recommended for children in the following selected circumstances:

- Tuberculin skin test–negative infants and children who are likely to have repeated exposure to untreated or ineffectively treated sputum-positive pulmonary tuberculosis, who cannot be separated from the source of the exposure, and who cannot be placed on long-term preventive therapy
- Tuberculin skin test–negative infants and children who have or are likely to have repeated exposure to patients with organisms resistant to isoniazid and rifampin

Skin Test Reactivity

Recipients of BCG vaccine should undergo repeat tuberculin skin tests 2 to 3 months after immunization to establish that tuberculin cellular reactivity has developed. Failure to react dictates the need for a repeat BCG vaccination followed by repeat tuberculin test.[93] The tuberculin reaction to BCG vaccine available in the United States generally results in 7 to 15 mm of induration after vaccination and diminishes gradually during subsequent years; without revaccination or repeated exposure to *M. tuberculosis,* reactivity usually disappears within 10 years.[93] Size of the area of induration may be correlated with the number of doses of BCG vaccine.[171] However, tuberculin skin test sensitivity does not correlate with BCG vaccine efficacy.[163] In BCG vaccine recipients, differentiation between a tuberculin reaction representing acquired tuberculous infection and persisting postvaccination reactivity is difficult. Because the degree and duration of protection against tuberculous disease afforded by BCG vaccine are uncertain, a positive tuberculin reaction always must be suspected to indicate disease.

Precautions and Contraindications

BCG vaccine should not be administered to persons with burns or disseminated skin infections or to those whose immune responses are impaired because of congenital immunodeficiency, leukemia, lymphoma, or other generalized malignancy or by immunosuppressive therapy with cytotoxic agents, corticosteroids, or radiation.

In the United States, where the risk of tuberculosis is low, BCG vaccine should not be administered to children with known or suspected asymptomatic HIV infection.[93, 227] However, in populations in whom the risk of tuberculosis is high, WHO has recommended that asymptomatic HIV-infected children receive BCG vaccine at birth or shortly thereafter.[309]

Although no harmful effects of BCG vaccine on the fetus have been documented, women should avoid vaccination during pregnancy.

Cholera Vaccine

Fewer than 300 cases of cholera have been recognized in the United States since the mid-1980s.[75] Most cases have occurred among travelers to cholera-affected areas or persons who have eaten contaminated food brought or imported from these areas.[75] Although cholera remains a significant public health concern in African, South American, and Asian countries, even in these countries the risk to U.S. travelers is low. Persons following the usual tourist itinerary who use standard accommodations in countries reporting cholera are at virtually no risk of infection.[76]

Preparations

The only vaccine currently available in the United States is prepared from a combination of phenol-inactivated whole-cell suspensions of classic Inaba and Ogawa strains of *Vibrio cholerae* O1 and is administered parenterally.[50]

Since 1980, a number of new oral cholera vaccines have been developed. Investigational oral vaccines currently in clinical trials consist of killed whole-cell *Vibrio* preparations or live-attenuated bacterial strains.[202]

Immunogenicity and Efficacy

In field trials conducted in cholera-endemic regions, currently available cholera vaccines have been only approximately 50 per cent effective in reducing the incidence of clinical illness from *V. cholerae* O1 during the 6-month period after vaccination.[50] Illness caused by the recently discovered *V. cholerae* O139 probably is unaffected by currently available vaccines.[76]

Investigational oral vaccines have better efficacy in field trials than do parenteral killed vaccine presently in use and give promise for the availability of more effective vaccines.

Adverse Events

Common vaccine side effects include localized pain, erythema, and induration for 1 to 2 days at the site of injection. The local reaction may be accompanied by fever, malaise, and headache.[50]

Indications

Cholera vaccination is indicated only for travelers to countries that require for entry a valid international certificate of vaccination. However, WHO no longer recommends cholera vaccination for any travelers, and vaccination is not required for entry into or return to the United States.[76, 310]

Travelers to countries with entry requirements should obtain a validated international certificate of vaccination documenting receipt of vaccine 6 days to 6 months prior to entry. Most city, county, and state health departments can validate certificates. Only a single dose is needed to satisfy international health regulations and to allow entry into most countries. A full primary series, recommended only for special high-risk groups working and living in endemic areas, includes two doses administered 1 week to 1 month or more apart. Booster doses are recommended at 6 months after primary immunization and at 6-month intervals thereafter when necessary. Vaccine is not recommended for infants younger than 6 months of age.[7, 50] Cholera and yellow fever vaccinations should be separated by at least 3 weeks; if precluded by time constraints, they may be given simultaneously at separate sites.

Precautions and Contraindications

Extremely rare serious reactions, including neurologic reactions, have been observed and are contraindications to revaccination.[50] The safety of immunization with cholera vaccine during pregnancy has not been established, and, therefore, it should not be used except in the case of substantial risk of infection.[50]

Hepatitis A Vaccine

The occurrence of hepatitis A is highest in developing countries, reflecting the primary route of transmission of fecal-oral, person-to-person spread. Hepatitis A virus (HAV) remains the most common cause of acute viral hepatitis in the United States and continues to cause substantial morbidity and associated costs.[90, 192]

The incidence of disease varies considerably among different populations in the United States.[90, 192, 274] Community-wide outbreaks recurring every 3 to 10 years in high-risk communities account for much of disease occurrence and are a primary target for control by vaccination. Rates of infection are highest among Alaskan Natives and other Native Americans. Other groups at increased risk include travelers to developing countries, homosexual and bisexual men, and users of illicit drugs.

Outbreaks among children attending day care and the staff are common and have been associated with community outbreaks.[158] However, the prevalence of hepatitis A in day care center staffs and among children and adolescents who previously attended day care is not increased and suggests that infections within day care settings most commonly reflect transmission within the community extending to these settings.[90, 179] HAV transmission can occur in institutions for the developmentally disabled. In addition to these examples of direct person-to-person transmission, infection also can be acquired by ingestion of contaminated food or water.

Disease in the United States is most common in children 5 to 14 years of age.[90] Infection rates are appreciable in younger children in whom infection usually is asymptomatic and who serve as a silent reservoir. Thus, control of hepatitis A by active immunization likely will necessitate universal childhood immunization. The finding that 45 per cent of reported cases have no identifiable risk factor indicates that selective immunization is unlikely to have a major effect on the control of hepatitis A.

Preparations

Both inactivated and attenuated HAV vaccines have been developed.[116] Only inactivated vaccines are commercially available. They have been licensed in more than 40 countries, including Canada and the United States.

Inactivated HAV vaccine is prepared by methods similar to those used for inactivated poliomyelitis vaccine. Virus is propagated in human diploid fibroblast cell cultures, formalin-inactivated, and adsorbed to aluminum hydroxide adjuvant.[30, 90]

The two products currently licensed in the United States have two formulations, an adult and a pediatric product, of different antigen content. The pediatric formulation is indicated for persons 2 to 18 years of age. As of March 1997, no vaccine has been approved by the FDA for children younger than 2 years of age.

Immunogenicity and Efficacy

Inactivated viral vaccine is highly immunogenic. After a single dose, 95 per cent of children and nearly all adults seroconvert within 1 month.[30, 90] After a second dose, seroconversion approximates 100 per cent.

Concurrent administration of immunoglobulin and vaccine inhibits the peak serum antibody concentration achieved but not the rate of seroconversion.[293] Because the antibody concentrations are well above the protective concentration, this inhibition is not considered to be clinically significant and supports passive-active immunoprophylaxis when indicated.

Limited data indicate that most infants seroconvert after a three-dose schedule.[90] However, antibody concentrations in those infants with passively acquired maternal anti-HAV are relatively low.

In two large clinical trials of inactivated HAV vaccine in children, protective efficacy has been greater than 90 per cent.[172, 301] In a double-blind, placebo-controlled, randomized study in Thailand involving approximately 34,000 vaccinees, the protective efficacy against clinical hepatitis A was 94 per cent after two doses given 1 month apart; it was 100 per cent after a subsequent 12-month booster dose.[172] Vaccination also has been demonstrated to be effective in controlling outbreaks in communities with a high rate of disease.[90] For example, in a New York State community, in which hepatitis A is highly endemic in children, a single dose of vaccine was 100 per cent effective beginning 3 weeks after immunization in preventing symptomatic disease.[301]

The duration of protection after vaccination is likely to be prolonged. Although the data on persistence of serum antibody and protection against infection are limited to approximately 5 years of experience, adults have been demonstrated to maintain protective antibody concentrations for at least 4 years, and kinetic models of antibody decline indicate possible antibody persistence for 20 years.[291] Data in children are not available to determine if and when booster doses would be indicated.

Adverse Events

Except for rare reports of anaphylaxis and anaphylactoid reaction in adults in Europe and Asia, serious reactions to inactivated HAV vaccine have not been reported.[90] Pain, tenderness, and infection at the injection site can occur.[172]

Indications[30, 90]

HAV vaccine is recommended for persons 2 years of age or older who are at increased risk of infection. The indications are as follows:

- Travel to or work in a country with a high or intermediate incidence of hepatitis A. Immunoglobulin given intramuscularly also is effective, but vaccination is preferred for persons who plan to travel repeatedly or will reside for an extensive period in a high-risk area.
- Children in communities with high rates of hepatitis A and with periodic outbreaks, beginning at 2 years of age
- Susceptible persons with chronic liver disease, including liver transplant recipients
- Sexually active homosexual and bisexual males
- Users of illicit drugs, including "street" drugs
- Occupational risk of hepatitis A. The only group proved to be at increased risk are those working with infected primates or with HAV in a laboratory.

In addition, vaccination should be considered for control of hepatitis A outbreaks in communities in which the rate of infection is increased. However, because the effectiveness of vaccination has not been demonstrated in localized outbreaks, such as in institutions for the developmentally disabled, day care centers, schools, and prisons, intramuscular immunoglobulin currently is recommended for close contact of infected persons in these circumstances. Another possible indication for vaccination is hemophilia because cases of hepatitis A have been reported in patients receiving factor VIII concentrate.[84] At present, HAV vaccination is not indicated routinely for day care attendees and staff or for food handlers.

In the future, licensure of HAV vaccine for infants and development of combination products containing this and other vaccines may lead to inclusion of HAV vaccine in the routine childhood immunization program to control the significant public health burden of hepatitis A.

Influenza Vaccine

Influenza outbreaks occur each year in the United States, and the potential for epidemic (pandemic) spread of this disease in susceptible human populations is well recognized. The impact of influenza on both normal children and those with underlying high-risk conditions is appreciable. Attack rates in normal children have been estimated at 10 to 40 per cent each year, and approximately 1 per cent of these influenza infections result in hospitalization.[142] Periodic minor antigenic changes in influenza A or B virus account for most influenza disease. Although these outbreaks generally are limited in magnitude, the morbidity and mortality of influenza remain discouragingly high. Major antigenic changes of influenza A virus, as occurred in 1957 to 1958 (Asian strain) and again in 1968 to 1969 (Hong Kong variant), account for pandemic spread of disease associated with greater overall morbidity and mortality in highly susceptible human populations. Major difficulties have been encountered in the development and provision of satisfactory immunizing agents for the prevention of influenzal disease because of the antigenic variation in these viruses.

Preparations

Because protective influenza vaccines must contain strains antigenically similar to those strains expected to be prevalent during a given respiratory season, the formulation of vaccines is changed periodically. Each year's influenza vaccine contains three virus strains (usually two subtype A and one subtype B) representing the influenza viruses that are likely to circulate in the United States in the subsequent winter. As a result of rapid and repeated changes in vaccine formulation and resultant recommendations, the CDC issues new guidelines each year. These guidelines should be consulted each fall in anticipation of yearly winter outbreaks of influenza.

TABLE 237–12. Influenza Vaccine Dosage by Patient Age

Age Group	Product[a]	Dosage	No. of Doses[b]
6–35 mo	Split virus only	0.25 mL	1 or 2
3–8 yr	Split virus only	0.50 mL	1 or 2
9–12 yr	Split virus only	0.50 mL	1
>12 yr	Whole or split virus	0.50 mL	1

[a]Because of the lower potential for causing febrile reactions, only split-virus vaccines should be used in children.

[b]Because split-virus vaccine may be less immunogenic than whole-virus vaccine, two doses are recommended for children younger than 9 years of age who are receiving influenza vaccine for the first time.

Adapted from Centers for Disease Control and Prevention: Prevention and control of influenza: Recommendations of the Advisory Committee on Immunization Practices (ACIP). M. M. W. R. *45*(No. RR-15):1–24, 1996.

Only inactivated vaccines are licensed for the prevention of influenza. Vaccines are prepared from virus grown in the allantoic sac of the chick embryo. The virus is purified by ultracentrifugation before inactivation with formalin. Presently available inactivated vaccines include (1) whole-intact virus particles, (2) subvirion preparations derived by disrupting whole virus with organic solvents, and (3) purified surface antigens. To minimize febrile reactions, only subvirion or purified surface antigen preparations should be used for children (younger than 13 years of age); any of the preparations may be used for adolescents and adults. The recommended dosage of influenza vaccine for children is listed in Table 237–12.[89]

Although live influenza virus vaccines are not licensed presently, investigational cold-adapted virus vaccines have been demonstrated to be safe, immunogenic, and protective in pediatric patients.[152, 258, 270]

Immunogenicity and Efficacy

After parenteral administration, nearly all vaccinated children and young adults develop hemagglutinin-inhibition antibody titers that are likely to be protective against infection by strains antigenically similar to those present in the preparation. However, the seroresponse of high-risk children younger than 5 years of age, even with two properly spaced doses of split-virus vaccine, may be erratic.[149, 150]

If provided under optimal conditions (i.e., at an appropriate time and against the appropriate prevailing influenza strain), influenza vaccines can reduce the incidence of disease by 70 per cent in healthy children and younger adults.[89] Unfortunately, protection afforded by inactivated vaccine is transient and yearly immunization is necessary, irrespective of whether significant antigenic changes of a prevailing influenza strain have occurred. Immunogenicities of split- and whole-virus vaccines have been demonstrated to be similar in adults.[89] However, field studies of the efficacy of split-product vaccines in children are lacking.

As determined in clinical trials with swine influenza vaccines in 1976, adequate protection generally is achieved in immunologically primed, healthy persons given a single dose of whole-virus or split-product vaccine. In previously unimmunized populations, such as children younger than 9 years of age, a single dose of split-product vaccine may be significantly less immunogenic than a single dose of whole-virus preparation, and two doses may be required for a satisfactory serum antibody response.[89]

Variable immunogenicity of influenza vaccine has been reported among immunocompromised persons, including those with malignancy. Successful immunologic responses in these populations are most likely to occur when immunized individuals previously have been primed by exposure to antigenically similar influenza strains.[151, 198] The optimal time to immunize children with malignancies who still must undergo chemotherapy is 3 to 4 weeks after chemotherapy has been discontinued and the peripheral granulocyte and lymphocyte counts are greater than 1000/mm^3.[12]

In a study examining the reactogenicity and immunogenicity of two doses of the split-product vaccine in high-risk children 3 to 5 months of age, reactogenicity was low but seroresponse rates were variable with poor responses to most immunizing antigens.[150] No information is available about the efficacy of the influenza vaccines in infants younger than 6 months of age. In addition, the effect of influenza antigens in an inactivated-virus vaccine on the infant's future immune response to influenza is not known.[12]

Adverse Events

Current influenza vaccines contain only noninfectious viruses and cannot cause influenza. Respiratory disease after vaccination represents coincidental illness unrelated to influenza vaccination. Influenza vaccines generally are well tolerated. Less than one-third of vaccinees have been reported to develop local redness or induration for 1 to 2 days at the site of injection. In addition, two types of systemic reactions have occurred. Fever, chills, headache, and malaise, although infrequent, most often affect children who have had no previous exposure to the influenza virus antigens contained in the vaccine. These reactions, which are attributed to influenza antigens, generally begin 6 to 12 hours after vaccination and persist for only 1 to 2 days.[89] The second type of reaction is immediate, presumably is allergic, and may involve hives, angioedema, allergic asthma, or systemic anaphylaxis. These reactions are rare and probably are the result of hypersensitivity to a vaccine component, most likely residual egg protein.

Despite previous concerns about a theoretic risk of vaccine-associated GBS, no increased risk of the syndrome has been observed in association with use of current vaccines in children or adolescents.[89]

Indications

Influenza vaccine is recommended annually for patients 6 months of age or older who are at high risk for disease, for medical care personnel, and for those who wish to decrease their risk of illness due to influenza. Vaccine is most effective when it precedes exposure by no more than 2 to 4 months.

High-risk children are those at increased risk of lower respiratory tract complications or death after influenza infection and include the following[12, 89]:

- Children with chronic disorders of the pulmonary system, including children with asthma
- Children with hemodynamically significant cardiac disease
- Residents of institutions with patients of any age with chronic medical conditions
- Children who have required regular medical follow-up or hospitalization during the preceding year because of chronic metabolic diseases (including diabetes mellitus), renal dysfunction, sickle-cell anemia and other hemoglobinopathies, or immunosuppression (including HIV disease and immunosuppression caused by medications)

- Children and teenagers (6 months to 18 years of age) who are receiving long-term aspirin therapy and therefore might be at risk for developing Reye syndrome after influenza

Medical personnel can transmit influenza to their high-risk patients while they are incubating an infection, experiencing mild or unrecognized infection, or working despite the existence of symptoms, and they can cause nosocomial outbreaks of influenza.[143, 161] In view of the potential for introducing influenza to high-risk groups, such as patients with compromised cardiopulmonary or immune systems or infants in neonatal intensive care units, annual influenza vaccination of physicians, nurses, and other personnel who have extensive contact with these high-risk patient groups is recommended. Vaccination also is indicated for employees of nursing homes and chronic care facilities who have contact with high-risk children and for providers of home care and household members of high-risk patients, including infants with bronchopulmonary dysplasia or congenital heart disease.[89]

Other groups for whom vaccination may be beneficial include the following[89]:

- Students or other persons in institutional settings who reside in dormitories
- Women who would be in the third trimester of pregnancy or early puerperium during the influenza season
- Pregnant women who have medical conditions that increase their risk of complications from influenza should be vaccinated before the influenza season, regardless of the stage of pregnancy
- Foreign travelers, especially those at risk for influenza complications

Precautions and Contraindications

Current influenza vaccines contain only a small quantity of egg protein. Severe hypersensitivity reactions attributable to sensitivity to residual egg protein are rare. Children who have developed hives and who have had swelling of the lips and tongue or experienced acute respiratory distress or collapse after eating eggs should not be given influenza vaccine. Children with documented IgE-mediated hypersensitivity to eggs also may be at increased risk for reactions from influenza vaccine.[89] Children with hypersensitivity to egg proteins and medical conditions placing them at high risk for influenza have been immunized with influenza vaccine using a desensitization protocol.[225] However, because amantadine or rimantadine is effective, these children generally should not receive vaccine.[12]

Pregnancy is not a contraindication to influenza vaccine administration, and vaccination is advised for pregnant women who have an underlying high-risk condition. To avoid concern about the theoretic possibility of teratogenicity, vaccination after the first trimester may be prudent.[89]

Japanese Encephalitis Vaccine

Japanese encephalitis (JE) virus, the most important cause of epidemic arboviral encephalitis in Asia, has a wide clinical spectrum ranging from asymptomatic infection to permanent neurologic sequelae with a high case-fatality rate of 30 to 70 per cent.[221, 288] A mouse-brain vaccine successfully has controlled JE virus infection among human populations in Japan, Korea, and Taiwan since 1968.[232] An investigational vaccine was available in the United States from 1983 through 1987 through travel clinics in collaboration with the CDC. In December 1992, a JE vaccine was licensed in the United States for use in persons living in or traveling to Asia.

Preparations

The JE vaccine licensed in the United States is a formalin-inactivated virus derived from purified infected mouse brain.[67] The vaccine contains gelatin as a stabilizer and thimerosal as a preservative.

Immunogenicity and Efficacy

Immunogenicity studies in the United States indicate that three doses are needed to provide protective concentrations of serum neutralizing antibody in greater than 80 per cent of vaccinees.[244] Protective concentrations have been defined by animal challenge experiments.[232] The longevity of neutralizing antibody after the primary vaccination series is not known. In one Japanese study, protective antibody titers persisted for 3 years after a booster dose.[189]

A field trial conducted in Thai children comparing the efficacy of two inactivated JE vaccines, a monovalent vaccine containing the currently licensed JE vaccine strain and a bivalent vaccine with an additional inactivated JE strain, demonstrated an efficacy of 91 per cent for both vaccines when compared with placebo.[168] Efficacy for a single year for a prototype of the currently licensed vaccine, field tested in Taiwanese children, was 80 per cent.[170]

Adverse Reactions

JE vaccination is associated with a moderate frequency of local and mild systemic side effects. Local reactions occur in about 20 per cent of vaccinees, and approximately 10 per cent have reported systemic side effects, such as fever, headache, malaise, and rash.[67]

The neural tissue substrate of the vaccine has raised concerns about the possibility of vaccine-related neurologic side effects. Rates of JE vaccine-related neurologic complications, including encephalitis, encephalopathy, seizures, and peripheral neuropathy, in Japan are 1 to 2.3 per million vaccinees.[191] However, a causal relationship has not been established between JE vaccine and temporally related neurologic events.

Hypersensitivity-type reactions have been reported. These reactions are characterized by urticaria and angioedema of the extremities, face, and oropharynx, especially of the lips. They occur a median of 12 hours after the first dose of vaccine. The interval between administration of a second dose and onset of symptoms generally is longer, with a median of 3 days and possibly as long as 2 weeks. Reactions have occurred after a second or third dose when preceding doses did not cause symptoms. The reaction rates are similar after both first and second doses: approximately 15 to 62 per 10,000 immunizations among U.S. citizens. The vaccine component responsible for these adverse events has not been identified.[67]

Indications[67]

The JE vaccine is recommended for persons (except infants) who will be residing in areas where JE is endemic or epidemic. Risk for acquiring JE varies highly within endemic regions. Therefore, the incidence of JE in the area of residence, conditions of housing, nature of activities, and the possibility of unexpected travel to high-risk areas are factors that should be considered in the decision to vaccinate.

JE vaccine is *not* recommended for all travelers to Asia. The vaccine should be offered to persons spending a month or longer in endemic areas during the transmission season, especially if travel will include rural areas.

The decision to use JE vaccine should balance the risks for

exposure to the virus and for developing illness, the availability and acceptability of mosquito repellents and other alternative protective measures, and the side effects of vaccination.

The recommended primary immunization series is three doses administered on days 0, 7, and 30. An abbreviated schedule of days 0, 7, and 14 can be used when a longer schedule is impractical because of time constraints. Two doses administered 1 week apart confer short-term immunity in 80 per cent of vaccines. However, this schedule should be used only under unusual circumstances. The last dose should be administered at least 10 days before travel commences to ensure an adequate immune response and access to care if a delayed adverse reaction occurs. No data on vaccine safety and efficacy in infants are available.[6]

The duration of protection is unknown, and definitive recommendations on the timing of booster doses cannot be given. Booster doses may be administered after 2 years.

Precautions and Contraindications

Because generalized urticaria and angioedema can occur within minutes to as long as 2 weeks after vaccination, epinephrine, other medications, and equipment to treat anaphylaxis should be available. Vaccinees should be observed for 30 minutes after vaccination and should be warned about the possibility of delayed urticaria and angioedema, which can occur as long as 2 weeks after vaccination. Vaccinees should be advised to remain in areas with ready access to medical care for 10 days after receiving a dose of JE vaccine.

Hypersensitivity to proteins of rodent or neural origin, to thimerosal, or to a previous dose of JE vaccine is a contraindication to vaccination.

A study in United States military personnel found an association between reactions to JE vaccine and a past history of urticaria. History of urticaria should be considered when weighing risks and benefits of vaccination.

No specific information is available on the safety of JE vaccine in pregnancy. Limited data suggest that the vaccine can be given to patients with altered immune status. Little information is available on how concurrent administration of other vaccines affects the safety and immunogenicity of JE vaccine.

Meningococcal Vaccine

Routine immunization against meningococcal disease is not recommended in the United States because the risk of acquiring meningococcal disease usually is low. Furthermore, no vaccine currently is available for serogroup B, which accounts for nearly one-half of cases in the United States, and the group C vaccine is poorly immunogenic in children 2 years of age or younger, a group accounting for 46 per cent of the cases in recent surveillance data.[180]

Preparations

A quadrivalent vaccine containing serogroups A, C, Y, and W135 currently is licensed for use in the United States. Each vaccine dose contains 50 mg of each of the four purified bacterial capsular polysaccharides.[95] No vaccine is available for use in prevention of group B disease because unconjugated group B polysaccharide is poorly immunogenic in humans. Investigational protein-conjugated meningococcal polysaccharide vaccines that may be protective in children younger than 2 years of age and against group B disease are under study.

Immunogenicity and Efficacy

A single subcutaneous injection is recommended. The vaccine may be administered concurrently with other vaccines but at a different anatomic site. Protective antibody concentrations are achieved within 10 to 14 days after vaccination.

The antibody responses to each of the four polysaccharides in the vaccine are serogroup-specific and independent. The group A polysaccharide induces antibody in some children as young as 3 months of age, although a response comparable with that in adults is not achieved until 4 to 5 years of age.[239] The serum antibody response to serogroup C is age-dependent, with poor response in children younger than 2 years of age.[145] Serum concentrations of antibodies against groups A and C polysaccharides decrease markedly during the first 3 years after a single dose of vaccine. The decrease in antibody occurs more rapidly in infants and young children than in adults.[185, 315]

Field trials of groups A and C meningococcal vaccines in Europe and Africa have demonstrated efficacy rates against serogroup A of 85 to 95 per cent 1 year after vaccination.[239, 294] After 3 years, efficacy rates were 67 per cent in older children but only 10 per cent in children younger than 4 years of age at the time of immunization with serogroup A vaccine.[248] In an epidemic, the serogroup C vaccine demonstrated clinical efficacy rates similar to those of the serogroup A vaccine.[280]

Serogroups Y and W135 antigens are immunogenic and safe in children older than 2 years of age. However, the clinical efficacy of these preparations has not been demonstrated.[4, 33, 292]

Persons with deficiencies of the terminal components of serum complement and those with anatomic or functional splenia have antibody responses to quadrivalent meningococcal vaccines consistent with protection.[256, 257] However, the clinical efficacy of vaccination has not been evaluated in these persons.

Adverse Events

Untoward reactions have been reported infrequently and consist primarily of localized erythema and tenderness. As many as 2 per cent of young children develop fever transiently after immunization.[27, 95]

Indications[27, 95]

Currently, immunization is recommended only for certain high-risk groups, including adults and children older than 2 years of age with deficiencies of the terminal components of serum complement (C5 through C8) or properdin and those with anatomic or functional asplenia. Immunization also may be considered for travelers to countries in which epidemic or hyperendemic meningococcal disease is present and for Americans living in these areas.

When evidence suggests that an outbreak or cluster of meningococcal cases in a defined population is occurring and when the etiologic serogroup is represented in the vaccine, local or state public health authorities may recommend immunization of persons at risk. For close contacts, chemoprophylaxis also must be given because immunization does not prevent early-onset disease.

Little information is available to determine the need or timing for revaccination when persons are at continued risk. A study in adult military personnel demonstrated that antibodies persisted for as long as 10 years after immunization, suggesting that revaccination in adults before 5 years may not be necessary.[315] Because of the possibility of poor response to vaccine in a child immunized before 4 years of age, revaccination should be considered after 1 year if the child first was immunized before he or she was 4 years of age and after 5 years if he or she first was immunized at 4 years of age or older.

Precautions and Contraindications

Because of theoretic considerations, meningococcal polysaccharide vaccines should not be administered to pregnant women unless the risk of disease is substantial. However, evaluation of pregnant women immunized during an epidemic in Brazil demonstrated no adverse effects.[214]

Plague Vaccine

Plague is a potentially epidemic disease caused by *Yersinia pestis* and acquired by humans from contact with infected rodents and bites of their fleas. It occurs in certain regions of Africa, Asia, and South America.[311] In the United States, however, disease is rare; in the past decade, only 10 to 15 cases were reported yearly to the CDC.[91] The most important prevention programs against human plague in the United States involve identification and control of epizootic plague and measures to control the flea vector. Active immunization is of additional protective value in select high-risk persons in this country and for travelers to areas with endemic plague.

Preparations

The plague vaccine presently licensed in the United States consists of formaldehyde-inactivated *Y. pestis*.[91]

Immunogenicity and Efficacy

Field trials in adults have demonstrated serologic responses in 60 to 90 per cent of volunteers after multiple doses of vaccine.[91] Although the efficacy of immunization has not been determined in controlled trials, a retrospective study of United States military personnel in Vietnam suggests a reduced incidence of plague in vaccinated persons. No data on either immunogenicity or safety are available in children.

Adverse Events

Primary immunization can result in mild systemic symptoms, such as malaise, headache, fever, mild lymphadenopathy, and local erythema or induration at the injection site.[212] Reactions can increase in frequency and severity with repeated vaccinations. Severe reactions include marked local inflammation at the injection site and rarely anaphylaxis.[91] They occur most often in persons receiving repeat doses. Vaccine safety has not been evaluated in persons younger than 18 years of age.

Indications[91]

Immunization in the United States is indicated only for persons at high risk of acquiring disease. The indications primarily are persons working routinely with *Y. pestis* organisms and those whose vocation results in regular contact with wild rodents or their fleas in areas in which plague is endemic in these rodents. Vaccination also should be considered for persons traveling, living, or working in such areas and who are likely to be in contact with these hosts, including their fleas.

Primary immunization consists of three doses of vaccine given according to the product circular of the vaccine. Because the vaccine is only approved for persons 18 years of age or older, the manufacturer should be consulted if the vaccine is considered for use in children.

Precautions and Contraindications

Plague vaccine should not be administered to persons with a known hypersensitivity to the vaccine or any of the constituents. Because the safety of immunization with plague vaccine during pregnancy has not been established, immunization should be undertaken only if the risk of infection is substantial.[91]

Pneumococcal Vaccine

Streptococcus pneumoniae is a leading bacterial pathogen, especially among young children, the elderly, and persons with predisposing conditions. In children, it is the most common cause of otitis media, occult bacteremia, and bacterial pneumonia requiring hospitalization. Since the widespread introduction of conjugate Hib vaccination and resulting marked decline in the occurrence of Hib meningitis, *S. pneumoniae* has become a leading cause of bacterial meningitis in children in the United States. In some populations, such as Native Alaskans, the incidence of bacteremia is markedly higher than that reported in other geographic areas of the United States.[117] High-risk groups include children with sickle-cell disease, asplenia, Hodgkin disease, congenital humoral immunodeficiency, HIV infection, and nephrotic syndrome, as well as recipients of organ transplants. Other chronic diseases associated with increased risk of severe pneumococcal disease include chronic cardiovascular and pulmonary diseases, diabetes mellitus, and renal failure. The role of these chronic diseases in predisposing to pneumococcal infection, however, has been demonstrated primarily in adults. Mortality is highest in those who have bacteremia or meningitis, the elderly, and patients with impaired humoral immunity or certain chronic diseases.

Morbidity and mortality of pneumococcal infection appear to be particularly high in developing countries. Development of an effective pneumococcal vaccine for infants in these areas has been given highest priority in an analysis by the Institute of Medicine of needs for vaccine development.[264] The increasing incidence of antimicrobial-resistant pneumococci further underscores the need for effective pneumococcal vaccines for young children.[42]

The benefit of the currently available pneumococcal vaccines in childhood is limited by their poor immunogenicity in children younger than 2 years of age. However, the development of pneumococcal polysaccharide-protein conjugate vaccines that are immunogenic in infancy is in progress and provides promise for more effective pneumococcal immunoprophylaxis.[272]

Preparations

Currently available vaccines are composed of purified, capsular polysaccharide antigens of 23 pneumococcal serotypes. Although 90 different serotypes have been identified, vaccine serotypes account for 88 per cent of bacteremic pneumococcal disease in adults and nearly 100 per cent in children in the United States.[53, 140] The current formulation was licensed in 1983 and replaced the earlier 14-serotype vaccine that was licensed in 1977.

Immunogenicity and Efficacy

Vaccination results in serologic type-specific antibody in most healthy adults and older children. Immunocompromised patients may respond less well. In children younger than 2 years of age, antibody response to most serotypes is poor, including those most likely to cause infection, such as types 6A and 14.[53, 140] Patients with AIDS have impaired antibody responses to vaccination, but asymptomatic HIV-infected adults do respond.[53]

Vaccine efficacy in preventing serious pneumococcal infections has been demonstrated primarily in immunocompetent adults, including the elderly and those with chronic diseases that predispose to pneumococcal infections, such as chronic pulmonary and cardiac disorders and diabetes mellitus. Efficacy against vaccine serotypes ranges from 61 to 75 per cent in adults.[45, 266] Investigations in adults in which vaccine protection against pneumococcal infection has been substantially less have been criticized for methodologic problems.[53] Efficacy in the limited studies of children has been consistent with that in adults. In children with sickle-cell disease or anatomic asplenia, an octavalent vaccine was highly effective in preventing bacteremic infection.[31] In trials in New Guinea children younger than 5 years of age, deaths from pneumonia were reduced by 59 per cent in vaccinated children compared with unvaccinated controls.[251] Although a bacteriologic etiology of pneumonia was not demonstrated in this study, the findings support vaccine efficacy in the prevention of pneumococcal infections in children because pneumococcal infections are major causes of death in developing countries.

Adverse Events

Local reactions at the injection site, such as erythema and pain, are reported in approximately 50 per cent of vaccine recipients.[16] However, more severe local and systemic reactions, such as fever and myalgia, are rare, occurring in less than 1 per cent of vaccine recipients. Severe systemic reactions, such as anaphylaxis, rarely have been reported.

In adults who are revaccinated within 1 to 2 years in early studies, local reactions were more common than those occurring after initial immunization.[53] However, subsequent studies, including those in children, indicate no increase in the incidence or severity of local or systemic reactions following revaccination after longer intervals.[193, 250]

Indications[16]

Pneumococcal vaccine indications are based on risk factors for disease and the age-related immunogenicity of the current purified polysaccharide vaccine formulations. Vaccine is recommended by the AAP for children 2 years of age or older who have one or more of the following risk factors:

- Sickle-cell disease
- Functional or anatomic asplenia
- Nephrotic syndrome or chronic renal failure
- Immunosuppression, such as from chemotherapy, organ transplantation, or malignancy
- Cerebrospinal fluid leak
- HIV infection, symptomatic or asymptomatic

Revaccination

For previously vaccinated children 10 years of age or younger at high risk of severe pneumococcal infection, revaccination after 3 to 5 years is recommended.[16, 53] Such children include those who have functional (e.g., sickle-cell disease) or anatomic asplenia and those who have rapid antibody decline (e.g., nephrotic syndrome, renal failure, organ transplantation).[141] Revaccination should be considered for high-risk older children and adults who were vaccinated 6 years or more earlier.

Contraindications[53]

No contraindications to initial vaccination exist. The safety of pneumococcal vaccine in pregnant women has not been evaluated, but adverse consequences to the fetus have not been observed among newborns whose mothers were vaccinated inadvertently during pregnancy. Ideally, women at high risk of pneumococcal disease should be vaccinated before pregnancy. In persons who have had a severe reaction, such as anaphylaxis or a localized, severe hypersensitivity response, revaccination should be avoided.

Rabies Vaccine

Although human rabies in the United States is rare, rabies in animals remains common, and rabies postexposure prophylaxis frequently is given. Carnivorous wild animals, especially skunks, foxes, coyotes, raccoons, and bats, are a continuing potential source of rabies, accounting for most cases of animal rabies and the few cases of human rabies in the United States. Furthermore, the prevalence of rabies in these animal populations has increased in recent years, and at present an epizootic of raccoon rabies has extended from West Virginia through the Mid-Atlantic states northward through New England.[66, 77, 78] Domestic animals (dogs and cats) account for only a small proportion of proven rabid animals, but as the primary interface between the sylvan reservoir and human beings, they account for most post-exposure immunoprophylaxis against rabies. Rodents (squirrels, hamsters, gerbils, rats, and mice) and lagomorphs (rabbits and hares) rarely are infected; the exception is wood-chucks.[62, 72, 130, 131]

Preparations

Human diploid-cell vaccine (HDCV) has been licensed in the United States since 1980. Another vaccine preparation, rabies vaccine, adsorbed (RVA), derived from a different strain of rabies virus cultured in fetal rhesus lung diploid cells, was licensed in the United States in 1988. Duck embryo rabies vaccine has not been available in the United States since 1981; allergic reactions were common with this vaccine.

Immunogenicity and Efficacy

Essentially all HDCV recipients develop protective antibody titers that persist for at least 2 years. The immunogenicity of RVA is only slightly less than that of HDCV.

The paucity of human cases attests to the efficacy of postexposure prophylaxis using the presently recommended vaccine and immunoglobulin preparations. To date, rabies has not been reported in the United States in any patient who received the currently recommended postexposure measures. However, cases of human rabies after postexposure prophylaxis have resulted from failure to adhere to established guidelines, such as those of the CDC and WHO, and may have been associated with injection of HDCV into the gluteal muscle with resulting decreased immunogenicity.[61, 120, 132, 267, 296]

Adverse Events

Local reactions of pain, erythema, and swelling occur in 25 per cent of HDCV recipients; mild systemic reactions of nausea, abdominal pain, headache, and myalgia occur in approximately 20 per cent. Systemic allergic reactions are reported at a rate of 1 per 1000 vaccinees.[48] Transient neuroparalytic reactions have been observed even less frequently (1 per 170,000 vaccinees).[133] Although the experience with RVA is less, its safety is similar to that of HDCV.

Indications and Precautions

Postexposure Prophylaxis (Table 237–13)

Recommendations for the management of persons with possible exposure to rabies include meticulous attention to thorough cleansing of the wound with soap and water in addition to active immunization and possible immunoglobulin administration. The decision to give rabies immunoprophylaxis depends on the circumstances precipitating the exposure, the species and condition of the animal inflicting the wound, and the prevalence of rabies in local animal populations. Bites or nonbite exposures (scratches, abrasions, open wounds, or mucous membranes contaminated with saliva) are considered significant. Because the need for preventive measures is based on these specific circumstances, including the risk of rabies in the area, the local department of health should be consulted promptly concerning the necessity for postexposure prophylaxis.

A combination of active and passive immunization is indicated for the treatment of all bites and all nonbite exposures inflicted by animals suspected of being or proved to be rabid. When possible, the brains of wild animals (skunks, foxes, coyotes, raccoons, and bats), stray dogs or cats, or symptomatic animals implicated in an exposure should be examined for evidence of rabies in certified laboratories. Immunization always should be initiated promptly and discontinued only if laboratory results are negative. Persons exposed to healthy dogs or cats that are available for observation do not require immediate prophylactic treatment. Implicated healthy domestic dogs or cats should be quarantined and observed for at least 10 days. If symptoms develop that suggest rabies, the exposed person should begin postexposure prophylaxis and the brain of the animal should be examined. An unknown (escaped) animal must be regarded as potentially rabid.

Postexposure prophylaxis should include human rabies immunoglobulin (HRIG). One-half of the dose should be infiltrated locally around the wound, and the other half should be administered intramuscularly. Equine antirabies serum, a serum concentrated and refined from hyperimmune horses, also is effective and may be used when HRIG is not available. It rarely is associated with serum sickness when recipients are screened properly with a skin test prior to administration.[304–306]

Active immunization with HDCV or RVA should be provided as early as possible after exposure, preferably within 48 hours. Either is injected into the deltoid muscle. Four additional intramuscular doses into the deltoid muscle are given 3, 7, 14, and 28 days after the first dose. Death from rabies has been described in a patient given adequate postexposure prophylaxis but in whom HDCV was injected in the gluteal muscle.[267] Because all persons who have been given the five-dose course of HDCV or RVA and then have been serologically tested have demonstrated adequate concentrations of antibody, routine serologic testing is not indicated after postexposure prophylaxis and is reserved for those whose immune response may be impaired by primary disease or by immunosuppressive therapy, such as corticosteroids. Because rabies almost universally is fatal, pregnancy is not a contraindication to rabies prophylaxis.

TABLE 237–13. Rabies Postexposure Prophylaxis for Persons Not Previously Immunized

Animal	Evaluation of Animal at Time of Exposure*	Treatment of Exposed Patient
Wild		
Skunk Fox Raccoon Coyote Bat Woodchuck	Regard as rabid	HRIG and HDCV†
Exotic		
Ferret		Consider individually; need for treatment should be based on local and state public health recommendations
Domestic		
Dogs and cats	Healthy‡	Consider individually; need for treatment should be based on local and state public health recommendations
	Escaped (unknown)	HRIG and HDCV
	Rabid or suspect rabid	HRIG and HDCV†
Other		
Livestock Rodent (except woodchuck) Lagomorph (rabbit and hare)		Consider individually; need for treatment should be based on local and state public health recommendations; bites of squirrels, hamsters, guinea pigs, gerbils, chipmunks, rats, mice, and other rodents (except woodchucks), rabbits, and hares almost never require antirabies prophylaxis

These recommendations are only a guide. They should be used in conjunction with knowledge of the animal species involved, circumstance of the bite or other exposure, vaccination status of the animal, and the presence of rabies in the region.

HDCV, human diploid-cell rabies vaccine; HRIG, human rabies immunoglobulin

*An exposure is considered to be a bite or contamination with saliva on mucosal surfaces or skin that has been cut or abraded.

†Discontinue vaccine if fluorescent antibody test results of the animal are negative.

‡Begin HRIG and HDCV at the first sign of rabies in the biting dog or cat during the observation period (10 to 14 days).

Adapted from Centers for Disease Control: Rabies prevention: United States, 1991. Recommendations of the Immunization Practices Advisory Committee (ACIP). M. M. W. R. *40*(No. RR-13):1–19, 1991.

PRE-EXPOSURE PROPHYLAXIS

Active immunization should be considered for high-risk groups (i.e., veterinarians, animal handlers and control officers, selected laboratory workers, persons visiting countries where rabies is hyperendemic, and persons whose pursuits may involve frequent contact with rabid animals, such as spelunkers). Persons whose risk of exposure is less but whose access to immediate competent medical care is restricted also should be considered for pre-exposure prophylaxis. The primary series consists of three doses at 0, 7, and 28 days given intramuscularly in the deltoid area. The primary series also may be given intradermally and consists of three doses at 0, 7, and 28 days administered in the area over the deltoid (lateral aspect of the upper arm). RVA should not be given by the intradermal route.

Routine postvaccination serologic testing for antirabies antibody after pre-exposure prophylaxis is necessary only for those suspected to be immunosuppressed. In circumstances of continued exposure, however, booster doses of rabies vaccine or serologic testing should be performed.[61] Persons undergoing pre-exposure prophylaxis for rabies and concurrent chloroquine phosphate malaria prophylaxis should not receive HDCV intradermally because chloroquine phosphate has been implicated in reduced antirabies antibodies after intradermal injection.[235]

In patients who have received adequate pre-exposure prophylaxis, postexposure prophylaxis consists of two doses of HDCV, given 3 days apart. HRIG is not recommended under these circumstances. Serum for antibody testing should be obtained from persons whose prophylaxis history or immune status is uncertain, and the course of postexposure active and passive immunoprophylaxis as described for nonimmune persons should be begun immediately. If serologic testing demonstrates adequate antirabies antibody, postexposure prophylaxis may be discontinued.

Typhoid Vaccine

The public health importance of effective typhoid vaccination is substantial in the developing world. In contrast, the incidence of the disease in the United States is low. The majority of reported cases occur among travelers in developing countries.[74] Hence, the primary indication for typhoid vaccination in this country is foreign travel. However, in developing countries without safe water and sanitation for the control of diarrheal diseases, mass immunization potentially is effective in the control of typhoid fever.

Preparations

Three vaccines currently are available for civilians in the United States.[74, 160] A parenteral heat-phenol–inactivated vaccine has been used widely for many years. The two new products are an oral live-attenuated vaccine consisting of a stable mutant, Ty21a, developed by chemical mutagenesis of a pathogenic *Salmonella typhi* strain, and a recently licensed capsular polysaccharide of *S. typhi,* the purified Vi (virulence) antigen, given parenterally. A fourth vaccine, an acetone-inactivated formulation of *S. typhi* for parenteral administration, is available only to the military.

Efficacy

Although field trials have demonstrated the efficacy of each vaccine, no comparative studies have been performed, and the efficacy in children younger than 5 years of age or for travelers to countries with endemic disease has not been determined.[74] Furthermore, no vaccine approaches 100 per cent efficacy, and vaccine immunity can be overcome by a large inoculum of *S. typhi.* In trials of the Ty21a vaccine, efficacy has ranged from 17 to 66 per cent. The efficacy of the capsular polysaccharide vaccine (ViCPS) in two different trials was 74 and 55 per cent, respectively. For the heat-phenol–inactivated vaccine, efficacy has been 51 to 77 per cent. Duration of protection ranges from 2 years for the ViCPS to 5 years for the oral Ty21a vaccine, after which booster doses are necessary.

Adverse Events

Reactions to the oral Ty21a vaccine are mild, consisting of only fever or headache, and occur in less than 5 per cent of recipients. Reactions to the ViCPS vaccine also are infrequent; erythema and induration at the injection site have been reported in approximately 7 per cent of recipients.[74] In contrast, reactions to the inactivated, whole-cell vaccine are more common and severe and include fever in as many as 24 per cent of recipients, headache, and severe local pain or swelling in 3 to 35 per cent of vaccinees.

Indications[74, 160]

Typhoid vaccination in the United States is recommended only for the following groups:

- Travelers to areas where typhoid fever is endemic and in whom risk of exposure is likely
- Persons with intimate exposure to a documented typhoid fever carrier, such as occurs with continuing household contact
- Laboratory workers with frequent contact with *S. typhi*

Vaccination is not recommended for persons attending summer camp, for those in areas of natural disaster, or for control of common-source outbreaks.

In most circumstances, either oral Ty21a or parenteral ViCPS is the preferred vaccine because of the substantially higher rate of adverse reactions with the parenteral inactivated vaccine and similar effectiveness of the three vaccines. However, the parenteral heat-phenol–inactivated vaccine is the only vaccine approved for children between 6 months and 2 years of age. Doses and schedules for the different typhoid vaccines are given in the recommendations of the CDC.[74]

Contraindications

Because the oral vaccine is a live-attenuated vaccine, it should not be given to immunocompromised patients, including those with HIV infection.[74] The vaccine manufacturer also advises that Ty21a vaccine not be administered to persons receiving antimicrobial agents within 24 hours. The only contraindication to vaccination with either ViCPS or parenteral heat-phenol–inactivated vaccine is a history of severe local or systemic reactions after a previous dose.

Yellow Fever Vaccine

Yellow fever presently occurs only in South America and Africa, with recent epidemics in Nigeria and Kenya. Immunization is considered only for persons living in or traveling to areas of yellow fever endemicity.

Preparations

The yellow fever vaccine presently licensed in this country is made from a live-attenuated virus derived from a viral strain (17D) that is prepared in chick embryos.[57] Primary immunization consists of a single, subcutaneous injection of reconstituted, freeze-dried vaccine for both adults and children.

Immunogenicity and Efficacy

Seroconversion rates of 93 per cent have been documented in young children receiving yellow fever vaccine.[314] Immunity after immunization with the 17D strain virus has been demonstrated to persist for more than 10 years.[57, 255, 308] Revaccination is required no more frequently than every 10 years.[255]

Adverse Events

The 17D strain has been associated only rarely with significant neurologic complications. Only 18 cases of postvaccination encephalitis have been recorded since 1945, most in children younger than 4 months of age. Mild side effects, including low-grade fever, headache, and myalgia, have been observed in 2 to 5 per cent of recipients 5 to 10 days after vaccination. Immediate hypersensitivity reactions, including rash, urticaria, and reactive airway symptoms, are extremely uncommon (occurring in fewer than 1 per 1 million doses) and occur primarily in persons with histories of egg allergy.[57]

Indications

Yellow fever vaccine is recommended for persons 9 months of age or older traveling to or residing in areas of yellow fever endemicity. Because of the increased risk of neurologic complications, infants 4 to 8 months of age should be considered for vaccination only when travel to high-risk areas is required and high-level protection against mosquito exposure is not feasible. Vaccination for international travel is required by local health regulations in individual countries. To obtain an international certificate of vaccination, a yellow fever vaccine approved by WHO and administered at a designated yellow fever vaccine center is required. Yellow fever vaccine centers in the United States can be identified by contacting state or local health departments.[76]

Precautions and Contraindications

No adverse effects of yellow fever vaccine on the developing fetus have been demonstrated. However, vaccine administration to pregnant women generally is not indicated because the vaccine contains a live virus. Pregnant women should be considered for vaccination only when travel to high-risk areas is required and protection against mosquito exposure is not feasible.

Children younger than 4 months of age should not receive yellow fever vaccine because of the increased risk of encephalitis in this group.[6]

Yellow fever vaccine poses a theoretic risk to patients with altered immunity as a result of underlying disease or immunosuppressive therapy. However, no anecdotal reports or systematically collected data have linked immunosuppression with adverse events in a vaccine recipient. The decision to immunize immunocompromised patients should be based on evaluation of the patient's degree of immunosuppression weighed against the risk of exposure to the virus. Family members of immunosuppressed persons, who themselves have no contraindications, may receive yellow fever vaccine.[76]

Documented hypersensitivity to eggs is a contraindication to vaccination. However, experience in the military suggests that allergy severe enough to preclude vaccination is uncommon and occurs only in those persons who actually are unable to eat eggs. If international quarantine regulations are the only reason to immunize a patient known to be hypersensitive to eggs, attempts should be made to obtain a waiver. If immunization of a person with a questionable history of egg hypersensitivity is considered essential because of a high risk of exposure, an intradermal skin test may be given as directed in the vaccine package insert.[57]

Simultaneous Administration of Other Vaccines and Drugs

In preparation for imminent travel, other live-virus vaccines may be given at a different site simultaneously with yellow fever vaccine; if not given on the same day, multiple live-virus vaccines, if feasible, should be separated by at least 4 weeks. Cholera and yellow fever vaccine administration, if possible, should be separated by at least 3 weeks.[128] If time constraints preclude this schedule, they may be given simultaneously. Studies have indicated no interference between yellow fever and measles, BCG, or hepatitis B vaccines. However, no data are available on possible interference between yellow fever vaccine and typhoid, plague, rabies, or JE vaccines.[76]

A prospective study of persons given yellow fever vaccine and commercially available immunoglobulin indicated no alteration of the immune response to yellow fever vaccine, compared with controls.[183] Although chloroquine inhibits the replication of yellow fever virus in vitro, it does not affect adversely the antibody response to yellow fever vaccine in persons receiving the drug for antimalarial prophylaxis.[284]

INVESTIGATIONAL VACCINES

Routine immunizations for children virtually have eliminated many infectious diseases from the United States. These successes have encouraged research into vaccines to prevent other serious viral and bacterial diseases affecting children. Current vaccines, although effective, are not ideal and have some distinct disadvantages, including adverse reactions to vaccine components, possible virulence in immunocompromised persons, expensive transport and storage conditions, and the need for multiple injections to complete immunization schedules. The development of new vaccines that bypass these difficulties is a major goal of biomedical and public health researchers.

In 1985, a report by the Institute of Medicine of the National Academy of Sciences reviewed the benefits to the United States that would be associated with the development and use of new and improved vaccines.[111] The report listed 12 diseases for which vaccines were possible, and the direct costs associated with treatment of each disease exceeded 100 million dollars a year. Diseases affecting children targeted on this list for which vaccines are not available included infections with cytomegalovirus (CMV), group B *Streptococcus*, herpes simplex virus (HSV), parainfluenza viruses, respiratory syncytial virus (RSV), and rotavirus.

The approaches to development of new vaccines against childhood pathogens are varied and include molecular biologic approaches, such as microbial component vaccines, vaccines with mutated antigens and reassortant vaccines, and the conventional approaches, such as live-attenuated vaccines.

In microbial component vaccines, purified bacterial or viral components, such as proteins, carbohydrates, peptides, or DNA, induce immune responses. HSV and RSV vaccines consisting of glycoprotein subunits produced by conventional or recombinant techniques are being tested in target populations.[44, 115] A conjugated polysaccharide group B *Streptococcus* vaccine for use in pregnant women is undergoing trials for immunogenicity, and conjugated polysaccharide vaccines for *S. pneumoniae* and *Neisseria meningitidis* are in clinical trials in children.[36, 203, 268]

Reassortant vaccines take advantage of the natural ability of some viruses to exchange genetic material. The most promising rotavirus vaccines are reassortants between animal and human viruses. These vaccines have been tested in large trials in children and have been demonstrated to be safe, immunogenic, and protective.[249]

Cold-adapted, live-virus vaccines are mutated viruses that do not replicate well at body temperature. Investigational cold-adapted vaccines have been developed for RSV, influenza viruses, and parainfluenza virus type 3. Cold-adapted influenza virus vaccines have been demonstrated to be safe, immunogenic, and protective in both adult and pediatric patients.[224] Clinical trials of cold-adapted live parainfluenza virus type 3 and RSV vaccines are just beginning.[115]

Live-attenuated viral vaccines produced by conventional means of attenuation include vaccines against CMV, parainfluenza virus type 3, and RSV. Clinical trials of CMV vaccine are in progress, although development of this vaccine has been slowed by concerns over possible oncogenicity of vaccine virus and the potential for reactivation causing perinatal symptomatic CMV infection.[245]

References

1. Trial synopses. International Symposium on Pertussis Vaccine Trials, Rome, October 30–November 1, 1995, Istituto Superiore di Sanità.
2. Adams, W. G., Deaver, K. A., Cochi, S. L., et al.: Decline of childhood *Haemophilus influenzae* type b (Hib) disease in the Hib vaccine era. J. A. M. A. *269*:221–226, 1993.
3. Alter, J. J., Hadler, S. C., Margolis, H. S., et al.: The changing epidemiology of hepatitis B in the United States. J. A. M. A. *263*:1281–1222, 1990.
4. Ambrosch, F., Wiedermann, G., Crooy, P., et al.: Immunogenicity and side-effects of a new tetravalent meningococcal polysaccharide vaccine. Bull. W. H. O. *61*:317–323, 1983.
5. American Academy of Pediatrics: Active immunization. *In* Peter, G. (ed.): 1997 Red Book: Report of the Committee on Infectious Diseases. 24th ed. Elk Grove Village, American Academy of Pediatrics (in press).
6. American Academy of Pediatrics: Arboviruses. *In* Peter, G. (ed.): 1997 Red Book: Report of the Committee on Infectious Diseases. 24th ed. Elk Grove Village, American Academy of Pediatrics (in press).
7. American Academy of Pediatrics: Cholera. *In* Peter, G. (ed.): 1997 Red Book: Report of the Committee on Infectious Diseases. 24th ed. Elk Grove Village, American Academy of Pediatrics (in press).
8. American Academy of Pediatrics: Diphtheria. *In* Peter, G. (ed.): 1997 Red Book: Report of the Committee on Infectious Diseases. 24th ed. Elk Grove Village, American Academy of Pediatrics (in press).
9. American Academy of Pediatrics: *Haemophilus influenzae* infections. *In* Peter, G. (ed.): 1997 Red Book: Report of the Committee on Infectious Diseases. 24th ed. Elk Grove Village, American Academy of Pediatrics (in press).
10. American Academy of Pediatrics: Hepatitis B. *In* Peter, G. (ed.): 1997 Red Book: Report of the Committee on Infectious Diseases. 24th ed. Elk Grove Village, American Academy of Pediatrics (in press).
11. American Academy of Pediatrics: Immunizations in special circumstances. *In* Peter, G. (ed.): 1997 Red Book: Report of the Committee on Infectious Diseases. 24th ed. Elk Grove Village, American Academy of Pediatrics (in press).
12. American Academy of Pediatrics: Influenza. *In* Peter, G. (ed.): 1997 Red Book: Report of the Committee on Infectious Diseases. 24th ed. Elk Grove Village, American Academy of Pediatrics (in press).
13. American Academy of Pediatrics: Measles. *In* Peter, G. (ed.): 1997 Redbook: Report of the Committee on Infectious Diseases. 24th ed. Elk Grove Village, American Academy of Pediatrics (in press).
14. American Academy of Pediatrics: Mumps. *In* Peter, G. (ed.): 1997 Redbook: Report of the Committee on Infectious Diseases. 24th ed. Elk Grove Village, American Academy of Pediatrics (in press).
15. American Academy of Pediatrics: Pertussis. *In* Peter, G. (ed.): 1997 Red Book: Report of the Committee on Infectious Diseases. 24th ed. Elk Grove Village, American Academy of Pediatrics (in press).
16. American Academy of Pediatrics: Pneumococcal infections. *In* Peter, G. (ed.): 1997 Red Book: Report of the Committee on Infectious Diseases. 24th ed. Elk Grove Village, American Academy of Pediatrics (in press).
17. American Academy of Pediatrics: Poliovirus infections. *In* Peter, G. (ed.): 1997 Red Book: Report of the Committee on Infectious Diseases. 24th ed. Elk Grove Village, American Academy of Pediatrics (in press).
18. American Academy of Pediatrics: Rubella. *In* Peter, G. (ed.): 1997 Redbook: Report of the Committee on Infectious Diseases. 24th ed. Elk Grove Village, American Academy of Pediatrics (in press).
19. American Academy of Pediatrics: Standards for pediatric immunization practices. *In* Peter, G. (ed.): 1997 Red Book: Report of the Committee on Infectious Diseases. 24th ed. Elk Grove Village, American Academy of Pediatrics (in press).
20. American Academy of Pediatrics: Tetanus. *In* Peter, G. (ed.): 1997 Red Book: Report of the Committee on Infectious Diseases. 24th ed. Elk Grove Village, American Academy of Pediatrics (in press).
21. American Academy of Pediatrics: Tuberculosis. *In* Peter, G. (ed.): 1997 Red Book: Report of the Committee on Infectious Diseases. 24th ed. Elk Grove Village, American Academy of Pediatrics (in press).
22. American Academy of Pediatrics, Committee on Infectious Diseases: Personal and family history of seizures and measles immunization. Pediatrics *80*:741–742, 1987.
23. American Academy of Pediatrics, Committee on Infectious Diseases: Measles: Reassessment of the current immunization policy. Pediatrics *84*:1110–1113, 1989.
24. American Academy of Pediatrics, Committee on Infectious Diseases: Universal hepatitis B immunization. Pediatrics *89*:795–800, 1992.
25. American Academy of Pediatrics, Committee on Infectious Diseases: *Haemophilus influenzae* type B conjugate vaccines: Recommendations for immunization with recently and previously licensed vaccines. Pediatrics *92*:480–488, 1993.
26. American Academy of Pediatrics, Committee on Infectious Diseases: Recommendations for the use of live attenuated varicella vaccine. Pediatrics *95*:791–796, 1995.
27. American Academy of Pediatrics, Committee on Infectious Diseases: Meningococcal disease prevention and control strategies for practice-based physicians. Pediatrics *97*:404–411, 1996.
28. American Academy of Pediatrics, Committee on Infectious Diseases: The relationship between pertussis vaccine and central nervous system sequelae: Continuing assessment. Pediatrics *97*:279–281, 1996.
29. American Academy of Pediatrics, Committee on Infectious Diseases: Poliomyelitis prevention: Recommendations for use of inactivated poliovirus vaccine (IPV) and live oral poliovirus vaccine (OPV). Pediatrics *99*:300–305, 1997.
30. American Academy of Pediatrics, Committee on Infectious Diseases: Prevention of hepatitis A infections: Guidelines for use of hepatitis A vaccine and immune globulin. Pediatrics *98*:1207–1215, 1996.
31. Ammann, A. J., Addiego, J., Wara, D. W., et al.: Polyvalent pneumococcal-polysaccharide immunization of patients with sickle-cell anemia and patients with splenectomy. N. Engl. J. Med. *297*:897–900, 1977.
32. Arbeter, A. M., Starr, S. E., and Plotkin, S. A.: Varicella vaccine studies in healthy children and adults. Pediatrics *78*(Suppl.):748–756, 1986.
33. Armand, J., Arminjon, F., Mynard, M. C., et al.: Tetravalent meningococcal polysaccharide vaccine groups A, C, Y, W135: Clinical and serological evaluation. J. Biol. Stand. *10*:335–339, 1982.
34. Asano, Y., Hirose, S., Iwayama, S., et al.: Protective effect of immediate innoculation of a live varicella vaccine in household contacts in relation to viral dose and interval between exposure and vaccination. Biken J. *25*:43–45, 1982.
35. Asano, Y., Nagai, T., Miyata, T., et al.: Long-term protective immunity of recipients of the OKA strain of live varicella vaccine. Pediatrics *75*:667–671, 1985.
36. Baker, C. J.: Immunization to prevent group B streptococcal disease: Victories and vexations. J. Infect. Dis. *161*:917–921, 1990.
37. Beeler, J., Varricchio, F., and Wise, R.: Thrombocytopenia after immunization with measles vaccines: Review of the vaccine adverse events reporting system (1990 to 1994). Pediatr. Infect. Dis. J. *15*:88–90, 1996.
38. Bernstein, H. H., Rothstein, E. P., Watson, B. M., et al.: Clinical survey of natural varicella compared with breakthrough varicella after immunization with live attenuated Oka/Merck varicella vaccine. Pediatrics *92*:833–837, 1993.
39. Black, S. B., Shinefield, H. R., Fireman, B., et al.: Efficacy in infancy of oligosaccharide conjugate *Haemophilus influenzae* type b (HbOC) vaccine in a United States population of 61,080 children. Pediatr. Infect. Dis. J. *10*:97–104, 1991.
40. Bloch, A. B., Orenstein, W. A., Stetler, H. C., et al.: Health impact of measles vaccination in the United States. Pediatrics *76*:524–532, 1985.
41. Booy, R., Moxon, E. R., Macfarlane, J. A., et al.: Efficacy of *Haemophilus influenzae* type b conjugate vaccine in Oxford region. Lancet *340*:847, 1992.
42. Breiman, R. F., Butler, J. C., Tenover, F. C., et al.: Emergence of drug-resistant pneumococcal infections in the United States. J. A. M. A. *271*:1831–1835, 1994.

43. Briss, P. A., Fehrs L. J., Parker, R. A., et al.: Sustained transmission of mumps in a highly vaccinated population: Assessment of primary vaccine failure and waning vaccine-induced immunity. J. Infect. Dis. *169*:77–82, 1994.
44. Burke, R. L.: Development of a herpes simplex virus subunit glycoprotein vaccine for prophylactic and therapeutic use. Rev. Infect. Dis. *13*(Suppl. 11):S906–S911, 1991.
45. Butler, J. C., Breiman R. F., Campbell, J. F., et al.: Pneumococcal polysaccharide vaccine efficacy: An evaluation of current recommendations. J. A. M. A. *270*:1826–1831, 1993.
46. Centers for Disease Control: Poliomyelitis prevention: Recommendations of the Immunization Practices Advisory Committee (ACIP). M. M. W. R. *31*:22–26, 31–34, 1982.
47. Centers for Disease Control: Subacute sclerosing panencephalitis surveillance: United States. M. M. W. R. *31*:585–588, 1982.
48. Centers for Disease Control: Systemic allergic reactions following immunization with human diploid cell rabies vaccine. M. M. W. R. *33*:185–187, 1984.
49. Centers for Disease Control: Immunization of children infected with human immunodeficiency virus: Supplementary ACIP statement. M. M. W. R. *37*:181–183, 1988.
50. Centers for Disease Control: Recommendations of the Immunization Practices Advisory Committee (ACIP): Cholera vaccine. M. M. W. R. *37*:617–624, 1988.
51. Centers for Disease Control: Measles prevention: Recommendations of the Immunization Practices Advisory Committee (ACIP). M. M. W. R. *38*(No. S-9):1–18, 1989.
52. Centers for Disease Control: Mumps prevention: Recomendations of the Immunization Practices Advisory Committee (ACIP). M. M. W. R. *38*:388–400, 1989.
53. Centers for Disease Control: Pneumococcal polysaccharide vaccine: Recommendations of the Advisory Committee on Immunization Practices (ACIP). M. M. W. R. *38*:64–68, 73–76, 1989.
54. Centers for Disease Control: Rubella vaccination during pregnancy: United States, 1971–1988. M. M. W. R. *38*:289–293, 1989.
55. Centers for Disease Control: Rubella prevention: Recommendations of the Immunization Practices Advisory Committee (ACIP). M. M. W. R. *39*(RR-15):1–18, 1990.
56. Centers for Disease Control: Tetanus: United States, 1987 and 1988. M. M. W. R. *39*:37–41, 1990.
57. Centers for Disease Control: Yellow fever vaccine: Recommendations of the Immunization Practices Advisory Committee (ACIP). M. M. W. R. *39*(RR-6):1–6, 1990.
58. Centers for Disease Control: Diphtheria, tetanus, and pertussis: Recommendations for vaccine use and other preventive measures. Recommendations of the Immunization Practices Advisory Committee (ACIP). M. M. W. R. *40*(RR-10):1–28, 1991.
59. Centers for Disease Control: *Haemophilus* b conjugate vaccines for prevention of *Haemophilus influenzae* type b disease among infants and children two months of age and older: Recommendations of the Immunization Practices Advisory Committee (ACIP). M. M. W. R. *40*(RR-1):1–7, 1991.
60. Centers for Disease Control: Hepatitis B virus: A comprehensive strategy for eliminating transmission in the United States through universal childhood vaccination. Recommendations of the Immunization Practices Advisory Committee (ACIP). M. M. W. R. *40*(RR-13):1–25, 1991.
61. Centers for Disease Control: Rabies prevention: United States, 1991. Recommendations of the Immunization Practices Advisory Committee (ACIP). M. M. W. R. *40*(RR-3):1–19, 1991.
62. Centers for Disease Control: Compendium of animal rabies control, 1992. M. M. W. R. *41*(RR-7):1–8, 1992.
63. Centers for Disease Control: Pertussis vaccination: Acellular pertussis vaccine for the fourth and fifth doses of the DTP series. Update to supplementary ACIP statement. Recommendations of the Immunization Practices Advisory Committee (ACIP). M. M. W. R. *41*(RR-16):1–5, 1992.
64. Centers for Disease Control and Prevention: Update: Eradication of paralytic poliomyelitis in the Americas. M. M. W. R. *41*:681–683, 1992.
65. Centers for Disease Control and Prevention: Change in source of information: Availability of varicella vaccine for children with acute lymphocytic leukemia. M. M. W. R. *42*:499, 1993.
66. Centers for Disease Control and Prevention: Human rabies: New York. M. M. W. R. *42*:799–806, 1993.
67. Centers for Disease Control and Prevention: Inactivated Japanese encephalitis virus vaccine: Recommendations of the Advisory Committee on Immunization Practices (ACIP). M. M. W. R. *42*(RR-1):1–15, 1993.
68. Centers for Disease Control and Prevention: Recommendations for use of *Haemophilus influenzae* b conjugate vaccines and a combined diphtheria, tetanus, pertussis, and *Haemophilus* b vaccine: Recommendations fo the Advisory Committee on Immunization Practices (ACIP). M. M. W. R. *42*(RR-13):1–15, 1993.
69. Centers for Disease Control and Prevention: Certification of poliomyelitis eradication: The Americas. M. M. W. R. *43*:720–722, 1994.
70. Centers for Disease Control and Prevention: General recommendations on immunizations: Recommendations of the Advisory Committee on Immunization Practices (ACIP). M. M. W. R. *43*(No. RR-1):1–38, 1994.
71. Centers for Disease Control and Prevention: Progress toward the global elimination of neonatal tetanus, 1989–1993. M. M. W. R. *43*:885–887, 893–894, 1994.
72. Centers for Disease Control and Prevention: Raccoon rabies epizootic: United States, 1993. M. M. W. R. *43*:269–273, 1994.
73. Centers for Disease Control and Prevention: Rubella and congenital rubella syndrome: United States, January 1, 1991–May 7, 1994. M. M. W. R. *43*:391–401, 1994.
74. Centers for Disease Control and Prevention: Typhoid immunization: Recommendations of the Advisory Committee on Immunization Practices (ACIP). M. M. W. R. *43*(RR-14):1–7, 1994.
75. Centers for Disease Control and Prevention: Cholera associated with food transported from El Salvador: Indiana, 1994. M. M. W. R. *44*:385–386, 1995.
76. Centers for Disease Control and Prevention: Health Information for International Travel. Washington, D.C., U.S. Government Printing Office, 1995.
77. Centers for Disease Control and Prevention: Human rabies: West Virginia, 1994. M. M. W. R. *44*:86–93, 1995.
78. Centers for Disease Control and Prevention: Mass treatment of humans exposed to rabies: New Hampshire, 1994. M. M. W. R. *44*:484–486, 1995.
79. Centers for Disease Control and Prevention: Pertussis: United States, January 1992–June 1995. M. M. W. R. *44*:525–529, 1995.
80. Centers for Disease Control and Prevention: Pertussis vaccination: Acellular pertussis vaccine for reinforcing and booster use. Supplementary ACIP statement. Recommendations of the Immunization Practices Advisory Committee (ACIP). M. M. W. R. *41*(RR-1):1–10, 1992.
81. Centers for Disease Control and Prevention: Progress toward elimination of *Haemophilus influenzae* type b disease among infants and children: United States, 1993–1994. M. M. W. R. *44*:545–550, 1995.
82. Centers for Disease Control and Prevention: Recommended childhood immunization schedule: United States, 1995. M. M. W. R. *44*(RR-5):1–9, 1995.
83. Centers for Disease Control and Prevention: Update: Recommendations to prevent hepatitis B virus transmission: United States. M. M. W. R. *44*:574–575, 1995.
84. Centers for Disease Control and Prevention: Hepatitis A among persons with hemophilia who received clotting factor concentrate: United States, September–December 1995. M. M. W. R. *45*:29–32, 1996.
85. Centers for Disease Control and Prevention: Immunization of adolescents: Recommendations of the Advisory Committee on Immunization Practices, the American Academy of Pediatrics, the American Academy of Family Physicians and the American Medical Association. M. M. W. R. *45*(RR-13):1–16, 1996.
86. Centers for Disease Control and Prevention: Measles pneumonitis following measles-mumps-rubella vaccination of a patient with HIV infection, 1993. M. M. W. R. *45*:603–606, 1996.
87. Centers for Disease Control and Prevention: Monthly immunization table. M. M. W. R. *46*:88, 1997.
88. Centers for Disease Control and Prevention: National, state, and urban area vaccination coverage levels among children aged 19–35 months: United States, April 1994–March 1995. M. M. W. R. *45*:145–150, 1996.
89. Centers for Disease Control and Prevention: Prevention and control of influenza: Recommendations of the Advisory Committee on Immunization Practices (ACIP). M. M. W. R. *45*(No. RR-5):1–24, 1996.
90. Centers for Disease Control and Prevention: Prevention of hepatitis A through active and passive immunization: Recommendations of the Immunization Practices Advisory Committee (ACIP). M. M. W. R. *45*(RR-15):1–30, 1996.
91. Centers for Disease Control and Prevention: Prevention of plague: Recommendations of the Advisory Committee on Immunization Practices (ACIP). M. M. W. R. *45*(RR-14):1–15, 1996.
92. Centers for Disease Control and Prevention: Prevention of varicella: Recommendations of the Advisory Committee on Immunization Practices (ACIP). M. M. W. R. *45*(RR-11):1–36, 1996.
93. Centers for Disease Control and Prevention: The role of BCG vaccine in the prevention and control of tuberculosis in the United States: A joint statement by the Advisory Council for the Elimination of Tuberculosis and the Advisory Committee on Immunization Practices. M. M. W. R. *45*(RR-4):1–18, 1996.
94. Centers for Disease Control and Prevention: Update: Vaccine side effects, adverse reactions, contraindications, and precautions. Recommendations of the Advisory Committee on Immunization Practices (ACIP). M. M. W. R. *45*(RR-12):1–35, 1996.
95. Centers for Disease Control and Prevention: Control and prevention of meningococcal disease and control and prevention of serogroup C meningococcal disease: Evaluation and management of suspected outbreaks. Recommendations of the Advisory Committee on Immunization Practices (ACIP). M. M. W. R. *46*(RR-5):1–21, 1997.
96. Centers for Disease Control and Prevention: Poliomyelitis prevention in the United States: Introduction of a sequential schedule of inactivated poliovirus vaccine followed by oral poliovirus vaccine. Recommendations of the Advisory Committee for Immunization Practices (ACIP). M. M. W. R. *46*(RR-3):1–25, 1997.
96a. Centers for Disease Control and Prevention: Recommended childhood immunization schedule, 1997. M. M. W. R. *46*:35–40, 1997.
97. Centers for Disease Control and Prevention: Hepatitis B virus infection:

A comprehensive immunization strategy to eliminate transmission in the United States, 1997 update. M. M. W. R. (in press).

98. Chaiken, B. P., Williams, N. M., Preblud, S. R., et al.: The effect of a school entry law on mumps activity in a school district. J. A. M. A. *257*:2455–2458, 1987.
99. Cheek, J. E., Baron, R., Atlas, H., et al.: Mumps outbreak in a highly vaccinated school population: Evidence for large-scale vaccine failure. Arch. Pediatr. Adolesc. Med. *149*:774–778, 1995.
100. Chen, R. T., Moses, J. M., Markowitz, L. E., et al.: Adverse events following measles-mumps-rubella and measles vaccinations in college students. Vaccine *9*:297–299, 1991.
101. Cherry, J. D., Brunell, P. A., Golden, G. S., et al.: Report of the task force on pertussis and pertussis immunization: 1988. Pediatrics *81*:939–977, 1988.
102. Christenson, B., and Bottiger, M.: Measles antibody: Comparison of long-term vaccination titres, early vaccination titres and naturally acquired immunity to and booster effects on the measles virus. Vaccine *12*:129–133, 1994.
103. Christie, C. D. C., Marx, M. L., Marchant, C. D., et al.: The 1993 epidemic of pertussis in Cincinnati: Resurgence of disease in a highly immunized population of children. N. Engl. J. Med. *331*:16–21, 1994.
104. Chu, S. Y., Bernier, R. H., Stewart, J. A., et al.: Rubella antibody persistence after immunization. J. A. M. A. *259*:3133–3136, 1988.
105. Cochi, S. L., Broome, C. V., and Hightower, M. S.: Immunization of US children with *Haemophilus influenzae* type b polysaccharide vaccine. J. A. M. A. *253*:521–529, 1985.
106. Cochi, S. L., Hull, H. F., and Ward, N. A.: To conquer poliomyelitis forever. Lancet *345*:1589–1590, 1995.
107. Cochi, S. L., Preblud, S. R., and Orenstein, W. A.: Prespectives on the relative resurgence of mumps in the United States. Am. J. Dis. Child. *142*:499–507, 1988.
108. Cody, C. L., Baraff, L. J., Cherry, J. D., et al.: Nature and rates of adverse reactions associated with DTP and DT immunizations in infants and children. Pediatrics *68*:650–660, 1981.
109. Cohn, M. L., Robinson, E. D., Faerber, M., et al.: Measles vaccine failures: Lack of sustained measles-specific immunoglobulin G responses in revaccinated adolescents and young adults. Pediatr. Infect. Dis. J. *13*:34–38, 1994.
110. Colditz G., Berkey C., Mosteller F., et al.: The efficacy of bacillus Calmette-Guérin vaccination of newborns and infants in the prevention of tuberculosis: Meta-analyses of the published literature. Pediatrics *96*:29–35, 1995.
111. Committee on Issues and Priorities for New Vaccine Development, Institute of Medicine: New Vaccine Develoment: Establishing Priorities. Washington, D.C., National Academy Press, 1985.
112. Comstock, G. W., and Palmer, C. E.: Long-term results of BCG vaccination in the southern United States. Am. Rev. Respir. Dis. *93*:171–183, 1966.
113. Comstock, G. W., and Webster, R. G.: A twenty-year evaluation of BCG vaccination in a school population. Am. Rev. Respir. Dis. *100*:839–845, 1969.
114. Crossley, K., Irving, P., Warren, J. B., et al.: Tetanus and diphtheria immunization in urban Minnesota adults. J. A. M. A. *242*:2298–2300, 1979.
115. Crowe, J. E., Jr.: Current approaches to the development of vaccines against disease caused by respiratory syncytial virus (RSV) and parainfluenza virus (PIV): A meeting report of the WHO Programme for Vaccine Development. Vaccine *13*:415–421, 1995.
116. D'Hondt, E.: Possible approaches to develop vaccines against hepatitis A. Vaccine *10*:S48–S52, 1992.
117. Davidson, M., Schraer, C. D., Parkinson, A. J., et al.: Invasive pneumococcal disease in an Alaska native population, 1980 through 1986. J. A. M. A. *261*:715–718, 1989.
118. Decker, M. D., and Edwards, K. M.: Report of the nationwide multicenter acellular pertussis trial. Pediatrics *96*:547–603, 1995.
119. Decker, M. D., Edwards, K. M., Bradley, R., et al.: Comparative trial in infants of four conjugate *Haemophilus influenzae* type b vaccines. J. Pediatr. *120*:184–189, 1992.
120. Duvriendt, J., Staroukine, M. M., Costy, F., et al.: Fatal encephalitis apparently due to rabies: Occurrence after treatment with human diploid cell vaccine but not rabies immune globulin. J. A. M. A. *248*:2304–2306, 1982.
121. Edsall, G., Elliott, M. W., Peebles, T. C., et al.: Excessive use of tetanus toxoid boosters. J. A. M. A. *202*:17–19, 1967.
122. Edwards, K. M., and Decker, M. D.: Acellular pertussis vaccines for infants. N. Engl. J. Med. *334*:391–392, 1996.
123. Enders, G., Miller, E., Cradock-Watson, J., et al.: Consequences of varicella and herpes zoster in pregnancy: Prospective study of 1739 cases. Lancet *343*:1547–1550, 1994.
124. Englund, J. A., Suarez, C. S., Kelly, J., et al.: Placebo-controlled trial of varicella vaccine given with or after measles-mumps-rubella vaccine. J. Pediatr. *114*:37–44, 1989.
125. Evans, G., and Marcuse, E. K.: Vaccine Injury Compensation Program update. The Report on Pediatric Infectious Diseases *4*:22–23, 1994.
126. Farizo, K. M., Cochi, S. L., Zell, E. R., et al.: Epidemiological features of pertussis in the United States, 1980–1989. Clin. Infect. Dis. *14*:708–719, 1992.
127. Feldman, S., and Lott, L.: Varicella in children with cancer: Impact of antiviral therapy and prophylaxis. Pediatrics *80*:465–472, 1987.
128. Felsenfeld, O., Wolf, R. H., Gyr, K., et al.: Simultaneous vaccination against cholera and yellow fever. Lancet *1*:457–458, 1973.
129. Fine, P. E. M., and Clarkson, J. A.: Reflections on the efficacy of pertussis vaccine. Rev. Infect. Dis. *9*:866–883, 1987.
130. Fishbein, D. B., Belotto, A. J., Pacer, R. E., et al.: Rabies in rodents and lagomorphs in the United States, 1971–1984: Increased cases in the woodchuck *(Marmota monax)* in mid-Atlantic states. J. Wild. Dis. *22*:151–155, 1986.
131. Fishbein, D. B., and Robinson, L. E.: Rabies. N. Engl. J. Med. *329*:1632–1638, 1993.
132. Fishbein, D. B., Sawyer, L. A., Reid-Sanden, F. L., et al.: Administration of human diploid-cell rabies vaccine in the gluteal area. N. Engl. J. Med. *318*:124–125, 1988.
133. Fishbein, D. B., Yenne, K. M., Dreesen, D. W., et al.: Risk factors for systemic hypersensitivity reactions after booster vaccinations with human diploid cell rabies vaccine: A nationwide prospective study. Vaccine *11*:1390–1394, 1993.
134. Fleischer, G. W., Henry, W., McSorley, M., et al.: Life-threatening complications of varicella. Am. J. Dis. Child. *135*:896–899, 1981.
135. Fritzell, B., and Plotkin, S.: Efficacy and safety of a *Haemophilus influenzae* type b capsular polysaccharide-tetanus protein conjugate vaccine. J. Pediatr. *121*:355–362, 1992.
136. Galazka, A. M., and Robertson, S. E.: Diphtheria: Changing patterns in the developing world and the industrial world. Eur. J. Epidemiol. *11*:107–117, 1995.
137. Galazka, A. M., Robertson, S. E., and Oblapenko, G. P.: Resurgence of diphtheria. Eur. J. Epidemiol. *11*:95–105, 1995.
138. Gergen, P. J., McQuillan, G. M., Kiely, M., et al.: A population-based serologic survey of immunity to tetanus in the United States. N. Engl. J. Med. *332*:761–766, 1995.
139. Gershon, A. A., Steinberg, S. P., LaRussa, P., et al.: Immunization of healthy adults with live attenuated varicella vaccine. J. Infect. Dis. *158*:132–137, 1988.
140. Giebink, G. S.: Preventing pneumococcal disease in children: Recommendations for using pneumococcal vaccine. Pediatr. Infect. Dis. *4*:343–348, 1985.
141. Giebink, G. S., Le, C. T., and Schiffman, G.: Decline of serum antibody in splenectomized children after vaccination with pneumococcal capsular polysaccharides. J. Pediatr. *105*:576–582, 1984.
142. Glezen, W., Six, H., Frank, A., et al.: Impact of epidemics upon communities and families. *In* Kendal, A., and Patriaca, P. (eds.): Options for the Control of Influenza. New York, Alan R. Liss, 1986, pp. 63–73.
143. Glezen, W. P.: Consideration of the risk of influenza in children and indications for prophylaxis. Rev. Infect. Dis. *2*:408–420, 1980.
144. Global Advisory Group Expanded Program on Immunization World Health Organization: Achieving the major disease control goals. Wkly. Epidemiol. Rec. *69*:29–31, 34–35, 1994.
145. Gold, R., Lepow, M. L., Goldschneider, I., et al.: Kinetics of antibody production to group A and group C meningococcal polysaccharide vaccines administered during the first six years of life: Prospects for routine immunization of infants and children. J. Infect. Dis. *140*:690–697, 1979.
146. Granoff, D. M., Anderson, E. L., Osterholm, M. T., et al.: Differences in the immunogenicity of three *Haemophilus influenzae* type b conjugate vaccines in infants. J. Pediatr. *121*:187–194, 1992.
147. Greco, D., Salmaso, S., Mastrantonio, P., et al.: A controlled trial of two acellular vaccines and one whole-cell vaccine against pertussis. N. Engl. J. Med. *334*:341–348, 1996.
148. Greenberg, M. A., and Birx, D. L.: Safe administration of mumps-measles-rubella vaccine in egg-allergic children. J. Pediatr. *113*:504–506, 1988.
149. Groothuis, J. R., Levin, M. J., Lehr, M. V., et al.: Immune response to split-product influenza vaccine in preterm and full-term young children. Vaccine *10*:221–225, 1992.
150. Groothuis, J. R., Levin, M. J., Rabalais, G. P., et al.: Immunization of high-risk infants younger than 18 months of age with split-product influenza vaccine. Pediatrics *87*:823–828, 1991.
151. Gross, P. A., Lee, H., Wolff, J. A., et al.: Influenza immunization in immunosuppressed children. J. Pediatr. *92*:30–35, 1978.
152. Gruber, W. C., Taber, L. H., Glezen, W. P., et al.: Live attenuated and inactivated influenza vaccine in school-age children. Am. J. Dis. Child. *144*:595–600, 1990.
153. Guess, H. A., Broughton, D. D., Melton, L. J., III, et al.: Population-based studies of varicella complications. Pediatrics *78*(Suppl.):723–727, 1986.
154. Gupta, R. K., Griffin, P. J., Xu, J., et al.: Diphtheria antitoxin levels in US blood and plasma donors. J. Infect. Dis. *173*:1493–1497, 1996.
155. Gustafson, T. L., Brunnell, P. A., Lievens, A. W., et al.: Measles outbreak in a "fully immunized" secondary school population. N. Engl. J. Med. *316*:771–774, 1987.
156. Gustafsson, L., Hallander, H. O., Olin, P., et al.: A controlled trial of a two-component acellular, a five-component acellular, and a whole-cell pertussis vaccine. N. Engl. J. Med. *334*:349–355, 1996.
157. Hadler, S. C., and Margolis, H. S.: Hepatitis B immunization: Vaccine types, efficacy, and indications. *In* Remington, J. S., and Swartz, M. N. (eds.): Current Clinical Topics in Infectious Diseases. Boston, Blackwell Scientific, 1992, pp. 282–308.

158. Hadler, S. C., and McFarland, L.: Hepatitis in day care centers: Epidemiology and prevention. Rev. Infect. Dis. *8*:548–557, 1986.
159. Hall, A. J., and Greenwood, B. M.: Modern vaccines: Practice in developing countries. Lancet *335*:774–777, 1990.
160. Hall, C. B.: A single shot at *Salmonella typhi:* A new typhoid vaccine with pediatric advantages. Pediatrics *96*:348–350, 1995.
161. Hall, C. B., and Douglas, R. G., Jr.: Nosocomial influenza infection as a cause of intercurrent fevers in infants. Pediatrics *55*:673–677, 1975.
162. Hardy, I. R. B., Dittmann, S., and Sutter, R. W.: Current situation and control strategies for resurgence of diphtheria in newly independent states of the former Soviet Union. Lancet *347*:1739–1744, 1996.
163. Hart, P. D. A., Sutherland, I., and Thomas, J.: The immunity conferred by effective BCG and vole bacillus vaccines, in relation to individual variations in induced tuberculin sensitivity and to technical variations in the vaccines. Tubercle *48*:201–210, 1967.
164. Herman, J. J., Radin, R., and Schneiderman, R.: Allergic reactions to measles (rubeola) vaccine in patients hypersensitive to egg protein. J. Pediatrics *102*:196–199, 1983.
165. Hersh, B. S., Fine, P. E. M., Kent, W. K., et al.: Mumps outbreak in a highly vaccinated population. J. Pediatr. *119*:187–193, 1991.
166. Hetherington, S., and Lepow, M. L.: Epidemiology and immunology of *Hemophilus influenzae* type b infections in childhood: Implications for chemoprophylaxis and immunization. Adv. Pediatr. Infect. Dis. *2*:1–18, 1987.
167. Hinman, A. R., and Koplan, J. P.: Pertussis and pertussis vaccine: Reanalysis of benefits, risks and costs. J. A. M. A. *251*:3109–3113, 1984.
168. Hoke, C., Nisalak, A., Sangawhipa, N., et al.: Protection against Japanese encephalitis by inactivated vaccines. N. Engl. J. Med. *319*:608–614, 1988.
169. Howson, C. P., Katz, M., Johnston, R. B., Jr., et al.: Chronic arthritis after rubella vaccination. Clin. Infect. Dis. *15*:307–312, 1992.
170. Hsu, T. C., Chow, L. P., Wei, H. Y., et al.: A completed field trial for an evaluation of the effectiveness of mouse-brain Japanese vaccine. *In* McDHammon, W., Kitaoka, M., and Downs, W. G., (eds.): Immunization for Japanese encephalitis. Amsterdam, Excerpta Medica, 1972, pp. 285–291.
171. Ildirim, I., Hacimustafaoglu, M., and Ediz B.: Correlation of tuberculin induration with the number of bacillus Calmette-Guérin vaccines. Pediatr. Infect. Dis. J. *14*:1060–1063, 1995.
172. Innis, B. L., Snitbhan, R., Kunasol, P., et al.: Protection against hepatitis A by an inactivated vaccine. J. A. M. A. *271*:1328–1334, 1994.
173. Institute of Medicine, Vaccine Safety Committee: Diphtheria and tetanus toxoids. *In* Stratton, K. R., Howe, C. J., and Johnston, R. B., Jr. (eds.): Adverse Events Associated with Childhood Vaccines. Washington, D.C., National Academy Press, 1994, pp. 67–117.
174. Institute of Medicine, Vaccine Safety Committee: *Haemophilus influenzae* type b vaccines. *In* Stratton, K. R., Howe, C. J., and Johnston, R. B., Jr. (eds.): Adverse Events Associated with Childhood Vaccines. Washington, D.C., National Academy Press, 1994, pp. 236–273.
175. Institute of Medicine, Vaccine Safety Committee: Measles and mumps vaccine. *In* Stratton, K. R., Howe, C. J., and Johnston, R. B., Jr. (eds.): Adverse Events Associated with Childhood Vaccines. Washington, D.C., National Academy Press, 1994, pp. 118–186.
176. Institute of Medicine, Vaccine Safety Committee: Polio vaccines. *In* Stratton, K. R., Howe, C. J., and Johnston, R. B., Jr. (eds.): Adverse Events Associated with Childhood Vaccines. Washington, D.C., National Academy Press, 1994, pp. 187–210.
177. Ipp, M. M., Gold, R., Goldbach, M., et al.: Adverse reactions to diphtheria, tetanus, pertussis-polio vaccination at 18 months of age: Effect of injection site and needle length. Pediatrics *83*:679–682, 1989.
178. Ipp, M. M., Gold, R., Greenberg, S., et al.: Acetaminophen prophylaxis of adverse reactions following vaccination of infants with diphtheria-pertussis-tetanus toxoids-polio vaccine. Pediatr. Infect. Dis. J. *6*:721–725, 1987.
179. Jackson, L. A., Stewart, L. K., Solomon, S. L., et al.: Risk of infection with hepatitis A, B or C, cytomegalovirus, varicella or measles among child care providers. Pediatr. Infect. Dis. J. *15*:584–589, 1996.
180. Jackson, L. A., and Wenger, J. D.: Laboratory-based surveillance for meningococcal disease in selected areas, United States 1989–1991. M. M. W. R. *42*(SS-2):21–30, 1993.
181. Jacobs, R. L., Lowe, R. S., and Lanier, B. Q.: Q: Adverse reactions to tetanus toxoid. J. A. M. A. *247*:40–42, 1982.
182. James, J. M., Burks, A. W., Roberson, P. K., et al.: Safe administration of the measles vaccine to children allergic to eggs. N. Engl. J. Med. *332*:1262–1266, 1995.
183. Kaplan, J. E., Nelson, D. B., Schonberger, L. B., et al.: The effect of immune globulin on trivalent oral polio and yellow fever vaccinations. Bull. W. H. O. *62*:585–590, 1984.
184. Kaplan, K. M., Marder, D. C., Cochi, S. L., et al.: Mumps in the workplace: Further evidence of the changing epidemiology of a childhood vaccine-preventable disease. J. A. M. A. *260*:1434–1438, 1988.
185. Käyhty, H., Karanko, V., Peltolta, H., et al.: Serum antibodies to capsular polysaccharide vaccine of group A *Neisseria meningitidis* followed for three years in infants and children. J. Infect. Dis. *142*:861–868, 1980.
186. Käyhty, H., Peltola, H., Karanko, V., et al.: The protective level of serum antibodies to the capsular polysaccharide of *Haemophilus influenzae* type b. J. Infect. Dis. *147*:1100, 1983.
187. Kelso, J. M., Jones, R. T., and Yunginger, J. W.: Anaphylaxis to measles, mumps, and rubella vaccine mediated by IgE to gelatin. J. Allergy Clin. Immunol. *91*:867–872, 1993.
188. Kim-Farley, R., Bart, S., Stetler, H., et al.: Clinical mumps vaccine efficacy. Am. J. Epidemiol. *121*:593–597, 1985.
189. Kinamitsu, M.: A field trial with an improved Japanese encephalitis vaccine in a nonendemic area of disease. Biken J. *13*:313–328, 1970.
190. King, G. E., and Hadler, S. C.: Simultaneous administration of childhood vaccines: An important public health policy that is safe and efficacious. Pediatr. Infect. Dis. J. *13*:394–407, 1994.
191. Kitaoka, M.: Follow-up on use of vaccine in children in Japan. *In* Hammon W. McD., Kitaoka, M., and Downs, W. G. (eds.): Immunization for Japanese Encephalitis. Amsterdam, Excerpta Medica, 1972, pp. 275–277.
192. Koff, R. S.: Seroepidemiology of hepatitis A in the United States. J. Infect. Dis. *171*:S19–S23, 1995.
193. Konradsen, H. B., Pedersen, F. K., and Henrichsen, J.: Pneumococcal revaccination of splenectomized children. Pediatr. Infect. Dis. J. *9*:258–263, 1990.
194. Krasinski, K., and Borkowsky, W.: Measles and measles immunity in children infected with human immunodeficiency virus. J. A. M. A. *261*:2512–2516, 1989.
195. Kröger, L., Korppi, M., Brander, E., et al.: Osteitis caused by bacille Calmette-Guérin vaccination: A retrospective analysis of 222 cases. J. Infect. Dis. *172*:574–576, 1995.
196. Krugman, S.: Further attenuated measles vaccine: Characteristics and use. Rev. Infect. Dis. *5*:477–481, 1983.
197. Kuter, B. J., Weibel, R. E., Guess, H. A., et al.: Oka/Merck varicella vaccine in healthy children: Final report of a 2-year efficacy study and 7-year follow-up studies. Vaccine *9*:643–647, 1991.
198. Lange, B., Shapiro, S. A., Waldman, M. T. G., et al.: Antibody responses to influenza immunization of children with acute lymphoblastic leukemia. J. Infect. Dis. *140*:402–406, 1979.
199. Lavi, S., Zimmerman, B., Koren, G., et al.: Administration of measles, mumps and rubella virus vaccine (live) to egg-allergic children. J. A. M. A. *263*:269–271, 1990.
200. Lawrence, R., Gershon, A. A., Holzman, R., et al.: The risk of zoster after varicella vaccination in children with leukemia. N. Engl. J. Med. *318*:543–548, 1988.
201. Lerman, S. J., Bollinger, M., and Brunken, J. M.: Clinical and serological evaluation of measles, mumps, and rubella (HPV-77:DE-5 and RA27/3) virus vaccines, singly and in combination. Pediatrics *68*:18–22, 1981.
202. Levine, M. M., and Pierce N. F.: Immunity and vaccine development. *In* Barua, D., and Greenough, W. B., III (eds.): Cholera. New York, Plenum Medical, 1992, pp. 285–327.
203. Lieberman, J. M., Chiu, S. S., Wong, V. K., et al.: Safety and immunogenicity of a serogroups A/C *Neisseria meningiditis* oligosaccharide-protein conjugate vaccine in young children: A randomized controlled trial. J. A. M. A. *275*:1499–1503, 1996.
204. Lieu, T. A., Finkler, L. J., Sorel, M. E., et al.: Cost-effectiveness of varicella serotesting versus presumptive vaccination of school-age children and adolescents. Pediatrics *95*:632–638, 1995.
205. Long, A. P., and Sartwell, P. E.: Tetanus in the United States Army in World War II. Bull. U. S. Army Med. Dept. *7*:371–385, 1947.
206. Lotte, A., Wasz-Hockert, O., Poisson, N., et al.: BCG complications: Estimates of the risks among vaccinated subjects and statistical analysis of their main characteristics. Adv. Tuberc. Res. *21*:107–193, 1984.
207. Maldonado, Y. A., Lawrence, E. C., DeHovitz, R., et al.: Early loss of passive measles antibody in infants of mothers with vaccine-induced immunity. Pediatrics *96*:447–450, 1995.
208. Maple, P. A., Efstratiou, A., George, R. C., et al.: Diphtheria immunity in UK blood donors. Lancet *345*:963–965, 1995.
209. Markowitz, L. E., Albrecht, P., Rhodes, P., et al.: Changing levels of measles antibody titers in women and children in the United States: Impact on response to vaccination. Pediatrics *97*:53–58, 1996.
210. Markowitz, L. E., Preblud, S. R., Fine, P. E., et al.: Duration of live measles vaccine-induced immunity. Pediatr. Infect. Dis. J. *9*:101–110, 1990.
211. Markowitz, L. E., Preblud, S. R., Orenstein, W. A., et al.: Patterns of transmission in measles outbreaks in the United States, 1985–1986. N. Engl. J. Med. *320*:75–81, 1989.
212. Marshall, J. D., Jr., Bartelloni, P. J., Cavanaugh, D. C., et al.: Plague immunization. II. Relationship of adverse clinical reactions to multiple immunizations with killed vaccine. J. Infect. Dis. *129*:S19–S25, 1974.
213. Mathias, R. G., Meekison, W. G., Arcand, T. A., et al.: The role of secondary vaccine failures in measles outbreaks. Am. J. Public Health *79*:475–478, 1989.
214. McCormick, J. B., Gusmao, H. H., Nakamura, S., et al.: Antibody response to serogroup A and C meningococcal polysaccharide vaccines in infants born of mothers vaccinated during pregnancy. J. Clin. Invest. *65*:1141–1144, 1980.
215. McLaughlin, P., Thomas, P., Onorato, I., et al.: Live virus vaccine in human immunodeficiency virus-infected children: A retrospective survey. Pediatrics *82*:229–233, 1988.
216. Miller, D., Madge, N., Diamond, J., et al.: Pertussis immunisation and serious acute neurological illnesses in children. B. M. J. *307*:1171–1176, 1993.

217. Miller, D., Wadsworth, J., Diamond, J., et al.: Pertussis vaccine and whooping cough and risk factors in acute neurological illness and death in young children. Dev. Biol. Stand. *61*:389–394, 1985.
218. Miller, E., Hill, A., Morgan-Capner, P., et al.: Antibodies to measles, mumps and rubella in UK children 4 years after vaccination with different MMR vaccines. Vaccine *13*:799–802, 1995.
219. Miller, L. W., Older, J. J., Drake, J., et al.: Diphtheria immunization: Effect upon carriers and the control of outbreaks. Am. J. Dis. Child. *123*:197–199, 1972.
220. Milstien, J. B., and Gibson, J. J.: Quality control of BCG vaccine by WHO: A review of factors that may influence vaccine effectiveness and safety. Bull. W. H. O. *68*:93–108, 1990.
221. Monath, T. P.: Flaviviruses. *In* Fields, B. N., and Knipe, D. M. (eds.): Virology. New York, Raven Press, 1990, pp. 763–814.
222. Mortimer, E. A., Jr.: Pertussis and pertussis vaccine. *In* Aronoff S. C., (ed.): Advances in Pediatric Infectious Diseases. Chicago, Year Book Medical, 1990, pp. 1–27.
223. Moxon, E. R., and Rappuoli, R.: Modern vaccines: *Haemophilus influenzae* infections and whooping cough. Lancet *335*:1324–1329, 1990.
224. Murphy, B.: Use of live attenuated cold-adapted influenza A reassortant virus vaccines in infants, children, young adults and elderly adults. Infect. Dis. Clin. Pract. *2*:174–181, 1993.
225. Murphy, K., and Strunk, R.: Safe administration of influenza vaccine in asthmatic children hypersensitive to egg proteins. J. Pediatr. *106*:931–933, 1985.
226. Nkowane, B. M., Bart, K. J., Orenstein W. A., et al.: Measles outbreak in a vaccinated school population: Epidemiology, strains of transmission and the role of vaccine failures. Am. J. Public Health *77*:434–438, 1987.
227. O'Brien, K., Ruff, A., Louis, M., et al.: Bacillus Calmette-Guérin complications in children born to HIV-1-infected women with a review of the literature. Pediatrics *95*:414–418, 1995.
228. Onorato, I. M., Modlin, J. F., McBean, A. M., et al.: Mucosal immunity induced by enhanced-potency inactivated and oral polio vaccines. J. Infect. Dis. *163*:1–6, 1991.
229. Onorato, I. M., Wassilak, S. G., and Meade, B.: Efficacy of whole-cell pertussis vaccine in preschool children in the United States. J. A. M. A. *267*:2745–2749, 1992.
230. Orenstein, W. A., Albrecht, P., Herrmann, K. L., et al.: The plaque-neutralization test as a measure of prior exposure to measles virus. J. Infect. Dis. *155*:146–149, 1987.
231. Orenstein, W. A., Bart, K. J., Hinman, H. R., et al.: The opportunity and obligation to eliminate rubella from the United States. J. A. M. A. *251*:1988–1994, 1984.
232. Oya, A.: Japanese encephalitis vaccine. Acta Pediatr. Jpn. *30*:175–184, 1988.
233. Padungchan, S., Konjanart, S., Kasiratta, S., et al.: The effectiveness of BCG vaccination of the newborn against childhood tuberculosis in Bangkok. Bull. W. H. O. *64*:247–258, 1986.
234. Palmer, C. E., Shaw, L. W., and Comstock, G. W.: Community trials of BCG vaccination. Am. Rev. Tuberculosis *177*:877–907, 1958.
235. Pappaioneau, M., Fishbein, D. B., Dreesen, D. W., et al.: Antibody response to preexposure human diploid-cell rabies vaccine given concurrently with chloroquine. N. Engl. J. Med. *314*:280–284, 1986.
236. Peebles, T. C., Levine, L., Eldred, M. C., et al.: Tetanus toxoid emergency bosters: A reappraisal. N. Engl. J. Med. *280*:575–580, 1969.
237. Peltola, H., and Heinonen, O.: Frequency of true adverse reactions to measles-mumps-rubella vaccine. Lancet *1*:939–942, 1986.
238. Peltola, H., Käyhty, H., Viortanen, M., et al.: Prevention of *Hemophilus influenzae* type b. N. Engl. J. Med. *310*:1561–1566, 1984.
239. Peltola, H., Mäkelä, P. H., Käyhty, H., et al.: Clinical efficacy of meningococcus group A capsular polysaccharide vaccine in children three months to five years of age. N. Engl. J. Med. *297*:686–691, 1977.
240. Peter, G.: Vaccine crisis: An emerging societal problem. J. Infect. Dis. *151*:981–983, 1985.
241. Petralli, J. K., Merigan, T. C., and Wilbur, J. R.: Action of endogenous interferon against vaccinia infection in children. Lancet *2*:401–405, 1965.
242. Plotkin, S. A.: Inactivated polio vaccine for the United States: A missed vaccination opportunity. Pediatr. Infect. Dis. J. *14*:835–839, 1995.
243. Plotkin, S. A., Starr, S. E., Connor, K., et al.: Zoster in normal children after varicella vaccine. J. Infect. Dis. *159*:1000–1001, 1989.
244. Poland, J. D., Cropp, C. B., Craven, R. B., et al.: Evaluation of the potency and safety of inactivated Japanese encephalitis vaccine in US inhabitants. J. Infect. Dis. *161*:878–882, 1990.
245. Porath, A., McNutt, R. A., Smiley, L. M., et al.: Effectiveness and cost benefit of a proposed live cytomegalovirus vaccine in the prevention of congenital disease. Rev. Infect. Dis. *12*:31–40, 1990.
246. Preblud, S. R.: Varicella: Complications and costs. Pediatrics *78*(Suppl.): 728–735, 1986.
247. Rantala, H., Cherry, J. D., Shields, W. D., et al.: Epidemiology of Guillain-Barré syndrome in children: Relationship of oral polio vaccine administration to occurrence. J. Pediatr. *124*:220–223, 1994.
248. Reingold, A. L., Hightower, A. W., Bolan, G. A., et al.: Age-specific differences in duration of clinical protection after vaccination with meningococcal polysaccharide A vaccine. Lancet *2*:114–118, 1985.
249. Rennels, M. B., Glass, R. I., Dennehy, P. H., et al.: Safety and efficacy of high-dose rhesus-human reassortant rotavirus vaccines: Report of the National Multicenter Trial. United States Rotavirus Vaccine Efficacy Group. Pediatrics *97*:7–13, 1996.
250. Rigau-Perez, J. G., Overturf, G. D., Chan, L. S., et al.: Reactions to booster pneumococcal vaccination in patients with sickle cell disease. J. Pediatr. Infect. Dis. *2*:199–202, 1983.
251. Riley, I. D., Lehmann, D., Alpers, M. P., et al.: Pneumococcal vaccine prevents death from acute lower-respiratory-tract infections in Papua New Guinean children. Lancet *2*:877–881, 1986.
252. Robbins, J. B., and Schnerson, R.: Polysaccharide-protein conjugates: A new generation of vaccines. J. Infect. Dis. *161*:821–832, 1990.
253. Rodrigues, L., Diwan, V., and Wheeler, J.: Protective effect of BCG against tuberculous meningitis and miliary tuberculosis: A meta-analysis. Int. J. Epidemiol. *22*:1154–1158, 1993.
254. Romanus, V.: Tuberculosis in bacillus-Calmette-Guérin-immunized and unimmunized children in Sweden: A ten-year evaluation following the cessation of general bacillus Calmette-Guérin immunization of the newborn in 1975. Pediatr. Infect. Dis. *6*:272–280, 1987.
255. Rosenzweig, E. C., Babione, R. W., and Wisseman, C. L., Jr.: Immunological studies with group B arthropod-borne viruses. IV. Persistence of yellow fever antibodies following vaccination with 17D strain yellow fever vaccine. Am. J. Trop. Med. Hyg. *12*:230–235, 1963.
256. Ross, S. C., and Densen, P.: Complement deficiency states and infection: Epidemiology, pathogenesis and consequences of neisserial and other infections in an immune deficiency. Medicine *63*:243–273, 1984.
257. Ruben, F. L., Hankins, W. A., Zeigler, Z., et al.: Antibody responses to meningococcal polysaccharide vaccine in adults without a spleen. Am. J. Med. *76*:115–121, 1984.
258. Rudenko, L. G., Slepushkin, A. N., Monto, A. S., et al.: Comparison of live attenuated and inactivated influenza vaccines in schoolchildren in Russia: Safety and efficacy in two Moscow schools, 1987/88. Vaccine *11*:3230–328, 1993.
259. Santosham, M., Wolff, M., Reid, R., et al.: The efficacy in Navajo infants of a conjugate vaccine consisting of *Haemophilus influenzae* type b polysaccharide and *Neisseria meningitidis* outer-membrane protein complex. N. Engl. J. Med. *324*:1767–1772, 1991.
260. Schaffner, W., Fleet, W. F., Kilroy, A. W., et al.: Polyneuropathy following rubella immunization: A follow-up and review of the problem. Am. J. Dis. Child. *127*:684-688, 1974.
261. Schmitt, H. J., Wirsing von König, C. H., Neiss, A., et al.: Efficacy of acellular pertussis vaccine in early childhood after household exposure. J. A. M. A. *275*:37–41, 1996.
262. Schoendorf, K. C., Adams, W. G., Kiely, J. L., et al.: National trends in *Haemophilus influenzae* meningitis mortality and hospitalization among children, 1980 through 1991. Pediatrics *93*:663–668, 1994.
263. Seager, C., Moriarity, J., Ngai, A., et al.: Low incidence of adverse experiences after measles or measles-rubella mass revaccination at a college campus. Vaccine *12*:1018–1020, 1994.
264. Shann, F.: Modern vaccines: Pneumococcus and influenza. Lancet *335*: 898–901, 1990.
265. Shapiro, C., Cook, N., Evans, D., et al.: A case-control study of BCG and childhood tuberculosis in Cali, Colombia. Int. J. Epidemiol. *14*:441–446, 1985.
266. Shapiro, E. D., Berg, A. T., Austrian, R., et al.: The protective efficacy of polyvalent pneumococcal polysaccharide vaccine. N. Engl. J. Med. *325*:1453–1460, 1991.
267. Shill, M., Baynes, R. D., and Miller, S. D.: Fatal rabies encephalitis despite appropriate post-exposure prophylaxis: A case report. N. Engl. J. Med. *316*:1257–1258, 1987.
268. Siber, G. R.: Pneumococcal disease: Prospects for a new generation of vaccines. Science *265*:1385–1387, 1994.
269. Siber, G. R., Werner, B. G., Halsey, N. A., et al.: Interference of immune globulin with measles and rubella immunization. J. Pediatr. *122*:204–211, 1993.
270. Slepushkin, A. N., Obrosova-Serova, N. P., Burtseva, E. I., et al.: Comparison of live attenuated and inactivated influenza vaccines in schoolchildren in Russia: Safety and efficacy in two Moscow schools, 1987/88. Vaccine *11*:323–328, 1993.
271. Smith, P. B.: Case-control studies of the efficacy of BCG against tuberculosis. Proceedings of the XXVIth IUAT World Conference on Tuberculosis and Respiratory Diseases. Singapore and Japan, Professional Postgraduate Services, International, 1987, pp. 73–79.
272. Sniadack, D. H., Schwartz, B., Lipman, H., et al.: Potential interventions for the prevention of childhood pneumonia: Geographic and temporal differences in serotype and serogroup distribution of sterile site pneumococcal isolates from children: Implications for vaccine strategies. Pediatr. Infect. Dis. J. *14*:503–510, 1995.
273. Sosin, D. M., Cochi, S. L., Gunn, R. A., et al.: The changing epidemiology of mumps and its impact on university campuses. Pediatrics *84*:779–784, 1989.
274. Steffen, R., Kane, M. A., Shapiro, C. N., et al.: Epidemiology and prevention of hepatitis A in travelers. J. A. M. A. *272*:885–889, 1994.
275. Stein, S. C., and Aronson, J. D.: The occurrence of pulmonary lesions in BCG-vaccinated and unvaccinated persons. Am. Rev. Tuberculosis *68*:695–712, 1953.
276. Stone, M., Vannier, A., Storch, S., et al.: Brief report: Meningitis due to

iatrogenic BCG infection in two immunocompromised children. N. Engl. J. Med. *333*:561–563, 1995.
277. Stratton, K. R., Howe, C. J., and Johnston, R. B., Jr. (eds.): DPT Vaccine and Chronic Nervous System Dysfunction: A New Analysis. Washington, D.C., National Academy Press, 1994.
278. Strebel, P. M., Sutter, R. W., Cochi, S. L., et al.: Epidemiology of poliomyelitis in the United States one decade after the last reported case of indigenous wild virus-associated disease. Clin. Infect. Dis. *14*:568–579, 1992.
279. Sutter, R. W., and Prevots, D. R.: Vaccine-associated paralytic poliomyelitis among immunodeficient persons. Infect. Med. *426*:429–430, 435–438, 1994.
280. Taunay, A. d. E., Galvao, P. A., deMorais, J. S., et al.: Disease prevention by meningococcal serogroup C polysaccharide vaccine in preschool children: Results after eleven months in Sao Paulo, Brazil. Pediatr. Res. *8*:429A, 1974.
281. The National Vaccine Advisory Committee: The measles epidemic: The problems, barriers, and recommendations. J. A. M. A. *266*:1547–1552, 1991.
282. Tidjani, O., Amedome, A., and ten Dam, H. G.: The protective effect of BCG vaccination of the newborn against childhood tuberculosis in an African community. Tubercle *67*:269–281, 1986.
283. Trollfors, B., Taranger, J., Lagergard, T., et al.: A placebo-controlled trial of a pertussis-toxoid vaccine. N. Engl. J. Med. *333*:1045–1050, 1995.
284. Tsai, T. F., Bolin, R. A., Lazuick, J. S., et al.: Chloroquine does not adversely affect the antibody response to yellow fever vaccine. J. Infect. Dis. *154*:726–727, 1986.
285. Tsolia, M., Gershon, A. A., Steinberg, S. P., et al.: Live attenuated varicella-vaccine: Evidence that the virus is attenuated and the importance of skin lesions in transmission of varicella-zoster virus. J. Pediatr. *116*:184–189, 1990.
286. Tuberculosis Prevention Trial: Trial of BCG vaccines in South India for tuberculosis prevention: First report. Bull. W. H. O. *57*:819–827, 1979.
287. Tuberculosis Prevention Trial: Trial of BCG vaccines in South India for tuberculosis prevention. Indian J. Med. Res. *72*(Suppl.):1–74, 1980.
288. Umenai, T., Krzysko, R., Bektimirov, T. A., et al.: Japanese encephalitis: Current worldwide status. Bull. W. H. O. *63*:625–631, 1985.
289. Vadheim, C. M., Greenberg, D. P., Partridge, S., et al.: Effectiveness and safety of an *Haemophilus influenzae* type b conjugate vaccine (PRP-T) in young infants. Pediatrics *92*:272–279, 1993.
290. van Loon, F. P. L., Holmes, S. J., Sirotkin, B., et al.: Mumps surveillance: United States, 1988–1993. M. M. W. R. *44*(SS-3):1–14, 1995.
291. VanDamme, P., Thoelen, S., Cramm, M., et al.: Inactivated hepatitis A vaccine: Reactogenicity, immunogenicity, and long-term antibody persistence. J. Med. Virol. *44*:446–451, 1994.
292. Vodopija, I., Baklaic, Z., Hauser, P., et al.: Reactivity and immunogenicity of bivalent (AC) and tetravalent (ACW135Y) meningococcal vaccines containing O-acetyl-negative or O-acetyl-positive group C polysaccharide. Infect. Immun. *42*:599–604, 1983.
293. Wagner, G., Lavanchy, D., Darioli, R., et al.: Simultaneous active and passive immunization against hepatitis A studied in a population of travelers. Vaccine *11*:1027–1032, 1993.
294. Wahdan, M. H., Rizk, F., El-Akkad, A. M., et al.: A controlled field trial of a serogroup A meningococcal polysaccharide vaccine. Bull. W. H. O. *48*:667–673, 1973.
295. Watson, B. M., Piercy, S. A., Plotkin, S. A., et al.: Modified chickenpox in children immunized with the Oka/Merck varicella vaccine. Pediatrics *91*:17–22, 1993.
296. Wattanasri, S., Boonthai, P., and Prasert, T.: Human rabies after late administration of human diploid cell vaccine without hyperimmune serum. Lancet *2*:870, 1982.
297. Weibel, R. E., Buynak, E. B., McLean, A. A., et al.: Pesistence of antibody in human subjects for 7 to 10 years following the administration of combined live attenuated measles, mumps and rubella virus vaccines. Proc. Soc. Exp. Biol. Med. *165*:260–263, 1980.
298. Weibel, R. E., Neff, B. J., Kuter, B. J., et al.: Live attenuated varicella vaccine: Efficacy trial in healthy children. N. Engl. J. Med. *310*:1409–1415, 1984.
299. Weibel, R. E., Stokes, J., Jr., Buynak, E. B., et al.: Live attenuated mumps vaccine. III. Clinical and serologic aspects in a field evaluation. N. Engl. J. Med. *276*:245–251, 1967.
300. Wenger, J. D., Ward, J. I., and Broome, D. V.: Prevention of *Haemophilus influenzae* type b disease: Vaccines and passive prophylaxis. *In* Remington, J. S., and Swartz, M. N. (eds.): Current Clinical Topics in Infectious Diseases. Boston, Blackwell Scientific, 1989, pp. 306–339.
301. Werzberger, A., Mensch, B., Kuter, B., et al.: A controlled trial of a formalin-inactivated hepatitis A vaccine in healthy children. N. Engl. J. Med. *327*:453–457, 1992.
302. Wharton, M., Cochi, S. L., Hutcheson, R. H., et al.: A large outbreak of mumps in the post-vaccine era. J. Infect. Dis. *158*:1253–1260, 1988.
303. White, C. J., Kuter, B. J., Hildebrand, C. S., et al.: Varicella vaccine (VARIVAX) in healthy children and adolescents: Results from 1987–1989 clinical trials. Pediatrics *87*:604–610, 1991.
304. Wilde, H., Chomchey, P., Sompob, P., et al.: Safety of equine rabies immune globulin. Lancet *2*:1275, 1987.
305. Wilde, H., Chomchey, P., Sompob, P., et al.: Adverse effects of equine rabies immune globulin. Vaccine *7*:10, 1989.
306. Wilde, H., and Chutivongse, S.: Equine rabies immune globulin: A product with an undeserved poor reputation. Am. J. Trop. Med. Hyg. *42*:175–178, 1990.
307. Wilfert, C., and Halsey, N.: Immunocompromised might face vaccine risks. AAP News June 1996, p. 12.
308. Wisseman, C. L., Jr., and Sweet, B. H.: Immunological studies with group B arthropod-borne viruses. III. Response of human subjects to revaccination with 17D strain yellow fever vaccine. Am. J. Trop. Med. Hyg. *11*:570–575, 1962.
309. World Health Organization: Special Programme on AIDS and Expanded Programme on Immunization: Joint statement: Consultation on human immunodeficiency virus (HIV) and routine childhood immunization. Wkly. Epidemiol. Rec. *62*:297–299, 1987.
310. World Health Organization: Guidelines for Cholera Control: Programme for Control of Diarrheal Disease. Geneva, World Health Organization, 1991.
311. World Health Organization: Human plague in 1993. Wkly. Epidmiol. Rec. *7*:45–48, 1994.
312. World Health Organization: Expanded programme on immunization: Statement on poliomyelitis eradication. Wkly. Epidemiol. Rec. *70*:345–347, 1995.
313. Young, T. K., and Hershfield, E. S.: A case-control study to evaluate the effectiveness of mass neonatal BCG vaccination among Canadian Indians. Am. J. Public Health *76*:783–786, 1986.
314. Yvonnet, B., Coursaget, P., Deubel, V., et al.: Simultaneous administration of hepatitis B and yellow fever vaccines. J. Med. Virol. *19*:307–311, 1986.
315. Zangwill, K. M., Stout, R. W., Carlone, G. M., et al.: Duration of antibody response after meningococcal polysaccharide vaccination in U.S. Air Force personnel. J. Infect. Dis. *169*:847–852, 1994.
316. Zell, E. R., Dieta, V., Stevenson, J., et al.: Low vaccination levels of US preschool and school-age children: Retrospective assessments of vaccination coverage, 1991–1992. J. A. M. A. *271*:833–834, 1994.
317. Zhuji Measles Vaccine Study Group: Epidemiologic examination of immunity period of measles vaccine. Chin. Med. J. *67*:19–22, 1987.

238

PASSIVE IMMUNIZATION

E. Richard Stiehm

Passive immunization is the administration of antibodies from an immune subject to provide temporary protection against a microbial agent, poison, or cell. Generally, passive immunization is used to provide temporary immunity in an unimmunized subject exposed to an infectious disease when active immunization is unavailable (e.g., respiratory syncytial virus infection), is contraindicated (e.g., varicella in an immunocompromised child), or has not been given prior to exposure (e.g., tetanus, rabies).

Passive immunization also is used in the management of certain disorders associated with toxins (e.g., diphtheria), in certain bites (e.g., snake, spider), as a specific (e.g., Rho[D]

TABLE 238–1. Antibody Preparations Available for Passive Immunity in the United States

Product	Abbreviations or Brand Names	Principal Use
Standard human immune serum globulins	HISG, Gamma Globulin	
Intravenous immunoglobulin	IVIG, IGIV	Treatment of antibody deficiency, immune thrombocytopenic purpura, Kawasaki disease, other immunoregulatory and inflammatory diseases
Intramuscular immunoglobulin	ISG, IG	Treatment of antibody deficiency, prevention of measles, hepatitis A
Special human immune serum globulins*		
Hepatitis B immunoglobulin	HBIG	Prevention of hepatitis B
Varicella-zoster immunoglobulin	VZIG	Modification or prevention of chicken pox
Rabies immunoglobulin	RIG	Prevention of rabies
Tetanus immunoglobulin	TIG	Prevention or treatment of tetanus
Vaccinia immunoglobulin†	VIG	Prevention or treatment of smallpox, vaccinia
Western equine encephalitis immunoglobulin†	WEE-IG	Prevention, after laboratory accident with WEE virus
Rho(D) immunoglobulin	RhoGAM	Prevention of Rh hemolytic disease
Cytomegalovirus immunoglobulin	CMV-IVIG	Prevention and treatment of cytomegalovirus infections
Animal serums and globulins		
Tetanus antitoxin (equine)	TAT	Prevention or treatment of tetanus (when TIG unavailable)
Diphtheria antitoxin (equine)	DAT	Treatment of diphtheria
Botulism antitoxin (equine)		Treatment of botulism
Lactrodectus mactans antivenin (equine)		Treatment of black widow spider bites
Crotalidae polyvalent antivenin (equine)		Treatment of most snake bites
Micrurus fulvius antivenin (equine)		Treatment of coral snake bites
Digoxin immune Fab fragments (ovine)	Digibind	Digoxin or digitoxin overdose
Anti-CD3 monoclonal antibody (murine)	OKT3 Muromonab-CD3	Immunosuppresion
Lymphocyte immunoglobulin, antithymocyte Globulin (equine)	ATG, Atgam	Immunosuppression

*All but cytomegalovirus intravenous immunoglobulin are for intramuscular or subcutaneous use.
†Available through the Centers for Disease Control and Prevention, Atlanta, GA, telephone 404–639–3670.

immunoglobulin [IG]) or nonspecific (e.g., antilymphocyte serum) immunosuppressant, and in treatment of certain infectious diseases.

Three types of preparations are used in passive immunization: (1) standard human immune serum globulin for general use; this is available in two forms—intramuscular IG and intravenous IG (IVIG); (2) special IGs with a known antibody content for specific illnesses; and (3) animal serums and antitoxins. These are listed in Table 238–1. Most of the licensed special IGs are for intramuscular use only. Whole blood, plasma, or serum also can be used in passive immunization.

Passive immunization is not always effective; the duration is short and variable (1 to 6 weeks), and undesirable reactions may occur, especially if the antiserum is of nonhuman origin. Immune serum globulin and special IGs are identical, except that the latter are derived from patients hyperimmunized or convalescing from a specific infection and the antibody content to the specific antigen is assayed; they are useful in several disorders in which IG is of little or no value.

ANIMAL SERUMS AND ANTITOXINS

Animal serums and antitoxins are derived from the serum of immunized animals, usually horses (equine). Because these serums are foreign proteins, they carry a significant risk. Thus, they should be administered only when specifically indicated, after sensitivity tests, and by a physician prepared to deal with a hypersensitivity reaction.

A careful history must be taken before an animal serum is injected. Inquiry must be made about asthma, hay fever, urticaria, and previous injections of animal serums. Patients with a history of asthma, allergic rhinitis, or other allergic symptoms on exposure to horses may be dangerously sensitive to the corresponding serum and should receive it only with the utmost caution.

Sensitivity Tests for Animal Serum

A scratch, prick, or puncture skin test, followed by an intradermal skin test, always should be performed before any injection of animal serum, whether or not the patient has received the serum previously. A scratch, prick, or puncture test is performed by applying a drop of 1:100 dilution in saline of the serum to the site of a superficial scratch, prick, or puncture on the volar aspect of the forearm and observing it for 20 minutes. A positive control (histamine phosphate 0.1 per cent) and negative control (saline) also should be applied. A positive reaction consists of erythema or wheal formation 3 mm greater than the control. (Note: Prior use of antihistaminics may render these test results negative.)

If the scratch, prick, or puncture test result is negative, an intradermal test is performed by injecting 0.5 mL of a 1:100 saline dilution. The reaction is read after 10 to 30 minutes and is positive if a wheal appears that is 3 mm greater than the control. In persons with a history of allergy, the initial test dose is reduced to 0.05 mL of a 1:1000 dilution. Again, positive (histamine phosphate 0.01 per cent) and negative control tests should be done.

Although intradermal skin tests have resulted in fatalities, scratch, prick, and puncture tests have not. Therefore, a skin test never should be performed (nor a serum injected) unless a syringe containing 1 mL of 1:1000 epinephrine is within immediate reach.

Skin tests can indicate the probability of sensitivity. However, a negative skin test result is not an absolute guarantee of absence of sensitivity. Therefore, either a specific history of allergy or a positive skin test result with horse serum is sufficient reason for special caution. A positive history of sensitivity to horse dander indicates the need for extreme caution.

Administration of Animal Serum

If the history and sensitivity test results are negative, the indicated dose of serum may be given intramuscularly with epinephrine at hand. The patient should be watched closely for an hour for adverse reaction.

Intravenous injection may be indicated if a high concentration of circulating antibody is required rapidly, as in severe tetanus or diphtheria. In such instances, a preliminary dose of 0.5 mL of serum should be diluted in 10 mL of either physiologic saline or 5 per cent glucose solution. This preparation should be given intravenously over 5 minutes, and the patient should be watched for 30 minutes for reactions. If no reaction occurs, the remainder of the serum, diluted 1:20, may be given at a rate not to exceed 1 mL/minute.

If the skin test result is positive or a history of allergy to animal serum is present and the need for the serum is unquestioned (and epinephrine is at hand), a procedure commonly called desensitization can be undertaken, but it is unlikely that any significant desensitization occurs. This procedure merely results in establishing temporary tolerance level to the serum. Desensitization should be performed by trained personnel with the necessary emergency equipment and drugs immediately available.

Desensitization consists of periodic (at 15-minute intervals) injection or infusion of progressively larger doses of the serum, starting at a low dose, until tolerance is achieved. Schedules for intravenous and intradermal-subcutaneous-intramuscular desensitization are given in the *1994 Red Book.*[7] Administration of sera after desensitization must be continuous; protection from desensitization is lost rapidly.

Hypersensitivity Reactions to Animal Serum

Hypersensitivity reactions to animal serum may be of four general types: (1) anaphylactic reactions consisting of urticaria, dyspnea, cyanosis, shock, and unconsciousness occurring seconds to minutes after an injection, (2) acute febrile reactions consisting of moderate or severe hyperpyrexia within 2 hours after an injection, (3) serum sickness reactions consisting of urticaria, arthritis, adenopathy, and fever occurring hours to days after an injection, depending on the dose and the presence or degree of prior sensitization (serum sickness occurs within hours or a few days after the second injection and within 7 to 12 days after the first injection), and (4) various delayed reactions, including peripheral neuritis (serum neuritis).

Treatment of Hypersensitivity Reactions to Animal Serum

For anaphylactic reactions, epinephrine 1:1000 at a dose of 0.01 mL/kg immediately is given subcutaneously or intramuscularly. If there is not immediate improvement, epinephrine 1:1000 at a dose of 0.01 mL/kg, maximum dose of 0.5 mL, is given intravenously. The 1:1000 epinephrine must be diluted 1:10 in physiologic saline and injected slowly. Epinephrine may be repeated in 5 to 15 minutes if the response is not satisfactory. Vasopressors and positive-pressure oxygen are helpful. For severe urticaria or edema, particularly edema of the larynx, intramuscular injections of antihistamines and corticosteroids are indicated. Serum therapy (if necessary) should be resumed 6 to 8 hours later or until all visible signs of reaction have subsided.

Mild febrile reactions (≤38.9° C [102° F]) are treated with aspirin or acetaminophen. Severe febrile reactions can cause convulsions and death and should be treated rigorously with sponge baths or other cooling means to reduce the temperature promptly. Serum sickness and serum neuritis generally are treated with corticosteroids.

HUMAN IMMUNE SERUM GLOBULIN (GAMMA-GLOBULIN)

Human immune serum globulin (gamma-globulin) for general use is available in two forms, the intramuscular preparation (IG) and the intravenous preparations (IVIG). IG is used for both the treatment of antibody immunodeficiencies and the prevention of certain infectious disorders, as outlined in Table 238–2, whereas IVIG is used primarily in the treatment of primary and secondary antibody deficiencies and immunoregulatory disorders (e.g., immune thrombocytopenic purpura, Kawasaki disease). Although intravenous preparations theoretically could be manufactured and substituted for the high-titered intramuscular preparations, their greater expense and their limited use have inhibited this development. However, cytomegalovirus IVIG (CMV-IVIG)[308, 309] and respiratory syncytial virus IVIG (RSV-IVIG)[130a, 131] are available.

TABLE 238–2. Advantages and Disadvantages of Intravenous Immunoglobulin (IVIG) Compared with Intramuscular Immunoglobulin

Advantages of IVIG
Less painful
No pooling within tissues
No sterile abscesses
No mercury exposure
No volume limitation
Rapid attainment of blood levels
Less frequent injections
High levels feasible
Half-life studies feasible
Useful in other disorders
Daily treatment feasible
Disadvantages of IVIG
More expensive
Venous access necessary
Longer time of administration
More frequent side effects (5 to 15%)
More severe side effects
Hepatitis (a few cases)
Aseptic meningitis (a few cases)
Renal insufficiency (a few cases)

Intramuscular Immunoglobulin

Pharmacology

IG is prepared from pooled human serum by the Cohn alcohol fractionation procedure (thus deriving its alternative name of Cohn Fraction II). This procedure removes most other serum proteins, hepatitis viruses, HIV-1, and HIV-2, thus providing a safe product for intramuscular injection. It is reconstituted as a sterile 16.5 per cent solution (165 mg/mL) with thimerosal as a preservative. It contains a wide spectrum of antibodies to viral and bacterial antigens.

IG is 95 per cent IgG, but trace quantities of IgM and IgA and other serum proteins are present. The IgM and IgA are insignificant therapeutically because of their rapid half-lives (about 7 days) and their low concentrations in IG. IG contains all IgG allotypes (Gm and Km types).

IG is approved only for intramuscular or subcutaneous use, and intravenous injection of IG is contraindicated. It aggregates in vitro to complexes of high molecular weight (9.5S to 40S), which are strongly anticomplementary. These aggregates probably are responsible for the occasional systemic reactions to IG. The incidence of these reactions is increased if the recipient has received IG previously or if it inadvertently is given intravenously. Agammaglobulinemic boys with affected male relatives (suggesting X-linked inheritance) may have a lower incidence of reactions.[225] Small intradermal injections of IG are not of value (except as a placebo), and they are contraindicated.

Immunoglobulin in Antibody Immunodeficiencies

The usual dosage of IG for antibody immunodeficiency is 100 mg/kg/month, about equivalent to 0.7 mL/kg/month of the commercially available 16.5 per cent (165 mg/mL) product. A double or triple dose is given at the onset of therapy, often over a 3- to 5-day period. The maximum dosage should not exceed 20 or 30 mL per week. Few studies of the optimal dosage are available; however, the Medical Research Council Working Party[225] found that 25 mg/kg/week (100 mg/kg/month) was equivalent therapeutically to 50 mg/kg/week but that 10 mg/kg/week was inadequate.

IG should be given at multiple sites in order to avoid giving more than 5 mL at any one site (10 mL in a large adult). The buttocks are the preferred sites, but the anterior thighs also can be used. Tenderness, sterile abscesses, fibrosis, and sciatic nerve injury may result from these injections. The danger of sciatic nerve injury especially is great in a small malnourished infant with inadequate muscle and fat in the gluteal regions. Large doses of IG should not be given to patients with severe thrombocytopenia because of the risk of hematoma and infection.

The injections initially are given at monthly intervals. If the patient continues to have infection or if a characteristic symptom recurs at the end of the injection period (such as cough, conjunctivitis, diarrhea, arthralgia, or purulent nasal discharge), the interval between doses is decreased to 3 or 2 weeks. Older patients often report that they can tell when their IgG level is low and when they need another injection. During acute infections, IgG catabolism increases, so extra injections of IG often are given.

Because no specific serum level of IgG must be maintained, serial IG assays are unnecessary in assessing the effectiveness of treatment. The maximum increase of the serum IgG level after a standard IG injection varies from patient to patient and from dose to dose because of different rates of absorption, local proteolysis at the injection site, and distribution within the tissues. An intramuscular injection of 100 mg/kg of IG usually raises the IgG serum level by 100 mg/dL after 2 to 4 days.[323] Thus, a recent IG injection usually does not obscure the diagnosis of hypogammaglobulinemia.

Adverse Effects of Immunoglobulin

Although IG is one of the safest biologic products available, rare anaphylactic reactions to intramuscular injections have been reported, particularly in patients requiring repeat injections.[101] The Medical Research Council Working Party[225] noted such reactions in 33 of 175 patients (19 per cent) treated over a 10-year period. In all, there were 85 reactions to about 40,000 injections; in eight patients, the injections were stopped as a result of these adverse effects, and one death was recorded. Such reactions occurred at any stage of treatment and were unrelated to any particular lot number of IG or its anticomplementary activity. The symptoms include anxiety, nausea, vomiting, malaise, flushing, facial swelling, cyanosis, and loss of consciousness. Immediate treatment with epinephrine and antihistamines is indicated.

Persons who experience such reactions should be evaluated before a repeat injection. Skin should be tested using several lots of IG.[101] A skin test result that is positive for an old but not a new lot of IG may indicate a particular idiosyncratic reaction to a particular lot. Under these circumstances, incremental doses of IG from a new lot are recommended. Other patients develop IgE antibodies to IgG, which results in positive immediate skin test results to all IG lots. In many others, no cause of the reactions can be found. Some of these patients tolerate gradually increasing doses of IG, particularly if they are premedicated with aspirin, diphenhydramine, or corticosteroids. Finally, a few patients have developed antibodies to the IgA present in minute quantities in IG; these IgA antibodies can be detected serologically in several laboratories.[363]

Patients with antibodies to IgA may have a reaction to gamma-globulin as a result of the trace quantities of IgA in IG or IVIG.[363] IVIG low in IgA or IgA-deficient plasma can be used under these circumstances.

Administration of exogenous gamma-globulin may inhibit the endogenous synthesis of gamma-globulin. In immunodeficiency with hyper-IgM, IG injections result in diminution of IgM levels, suggesting feedback inhibition of endogenous IgM synthesis.[321] We have noted depressed IgG levels in a few patients given IG from early infancy that return to normal when the injections are stopped.

IG injections or infusions may inhibit antibody responses to vaccine antigens, such as measles or varicella. Siber and associates[296] recommend an interval of 3 months between IVIG or IG therapy and vaccine administration after IG doses of less than 40 mg/kg, 6 months for doses of 40 to 80 mg/kg, 8 months for doses of 80 to 400 mg/kg, and 12 months for large doses (1 to 2 g/kg).

Late side effects to IG injections are uncommon; however, some patients develop fibrosis of the buttocks or localized subcutaneous atrophy at the site of repeated injections. Repeated injections of IG may result in high levels of mercury as a result of the thimerosal preservative. Although one patient developed symptoms of acrodynia (mercury toxicity) as a result of such therapy,[219] most remained asymptomatic.

Subcutaneous Immunoglobulin Infusions

As an alternative to intramuscular injections, IG can be given to immunodeficient patients by slow (0.05 to 0.2 mL/kg/hour) subcutaneous injections.[30] These injections, which are self-administered into the abdominal wall with the use of a battery-operated pump (Auto syringe), are well tolerated and enable patients to receive increased quantities of IG and maintain higher serum levels of IgG. This therapy is in general use in several European countries because of the high cost of IVIG.[114] The usual dose is 100 mg/kg/week. We have used this route successfully in immunodeficient patients with poor venous access, aseptic meningitis, or anaphylactic reactions to IVIG.[371] Gardulf and associates[114] have shortened the administration time of subcutaneous IG by using a rate of 10 mL/hour with only minimal adverse reactions.

Use of Immunoglobulin in Other Conditions

Use of the special IGs listed in Table 238–1 is discussed later in the chapter under the specific disease for which the IGs are prepared. This section reviews some other uses of standard IG.

ASTHMA AND ALLERGIES. Several studies reviewed by Thomas and McGovern[347] have claimed a beneficial effect of IG in asthma and other allergic conditions. Even 0.1-mL intradermal doses have been recommended.[265] However, two double-blind studies could not find significant benefit from such therapy.[1, 148] Thus, IG should not be used in these disorders.

ACUTE INFECTIONS. Monthly IG (0.15 to 0.4 mL/lb) did not help in the prevention of upper respiratory tract infection, otitis, skin infection, gastrointestinal tract upset, or fever in children.[23] Finkel and Haworth[109] found that 0.4 mL/kg of IG given to children younger than 2 years of age with acute respiratory tract infection was of no clinical benefit.

Others have shown that IG[165] or IVIG[169] is of no value in the prevention of recurrent acute otitis media.

BURNS. Kefalides and associates[174] were able to reduce the mortality rate of severely burned children by administering plasma (1 mL/kg body weight for each 1 per cent of surface area burned) or IG (1 mL/kg on days 1, 3, and 5) from 40 to 20 per cent. They concluded that solutions containing antibodies (plasma or IG) were more effective in reducing infection complications than were other colloids. However, Stone and associates[331] could not achieve any clinical benefit from IG therapy (0.4 mL/kg every third day until skin coverage) in 60 burned subjects compared with 40 controls.

Convalescent plasma, special IG with high antibody titer to *Pseudomonas,* and *Pseudomonas* vaccines also have been used in burn patients in attempts to reduce infections but without proof of efficacy.[85, 234] The use of IVIG in burns is discussed later in the chapter.

MALARIA. Cohen and associates[80] showed that hyperimmune IG from convalescing adults given to young children 4 months to 2.5 years of age in doses of 1.2 to 2.5 g significantly reduced their blood trophozoite count compared with untreated patients or patients treated with IG from normal adults. These children remained protected for a period of 3 months, at which time they were susceptible to reinfection. These studies suggest that humoral antibody exerts a beneficial effect in malaria and that a vaccine against malaria may be efficacious.[168]

SEVERE BACTERIAL INFECTIONS. Case studies suggest that in certain refractory infections, the addition of IG to the antibiotic regimen has provided some therapeutic benefit. In some, there is dramatic improvement on the addition of IG to a long, unsuccessful course of antibiotic therapy.[285] Waisbren[364] found that IG improved therapy when added to a long, unsuccessful course of antibiotic therapy in 6 of 46 patients with refractory infections, most due to *Staphylococcus.* These patients did not have hypogammaglobulinemia and were given IG in doses of 0.7 to 1.0 mL/kg.

Bodey and associates[41] could not demonstrate any therapeutic benefit of IG in the treatment of infection in acute leukemia. All patients received antibiotics. Many of the fevers were unexplained and may have been due to the underlying disease.

PREMATURITY. Premature infants have significantly lower levels of IgG at birth, have a more severe and prolonged period of physiologic hypogammaglobulinemia, and are more susceptible to infectious diseases and sudden infant death syndrome.[227] Further, they have a transient opsonic deficiency, partly correctable with IG.[110] Thus, IG in the prophylaxis of infection in these infants has considerable theoretic justification.

In 1960, Steen[317] gave IG (80 mg/kg) every 2 weeks to 10 premature infants who weighed between 1000 and 2000 g for 2 to 4 months and compared them with 10 untreated infants; no differences in rates of infection or levels of gamma-globulin were noted.

In 1963, Amer and colleagues[6] gave 92 premature infants IG and 68 control premature infants 5 per cent human albumin for the first 8 months of life. The dosage of IG was 240 mg/kg/month (double dose at onset of therapy). No differences were noted in the gamma-globulin levels of the treatment and the control groups during the study period, but when the infants were 12 months of age (after IG injections had been discontinued for several months), the gamma-globulin levels were significantly *higher* in the control infants (720 ± 270 mg/dL) than in the IG-treated infants (620 ± 220 mg/dL, $p < .01$). In the IG-treated group, fewer episodes of exanthems developed (13 per cent vs. 33.8 per cent); fewer deaths occurred during the first month of life (one vs. five); the hospital stay was shorter (7.8 days vs. 12.4 days); a larger number of infants were free of infections during the study period (43 per cent vs. 12 per cent); and fewer multiple infections occurred (11 per cent vs. 56 per cent). In all, six of the infants in the IG-treated group died (one from infection) and nine in the control group died (six from infection), a difference that was not significant. This study provides only suggestive evidence for efficacy of IG in the first year of life.

In 1966, Diamond and associates[92] gave 165 mg of IG to 241 premature infants upon their admission to the nursery and again when they were discharged and compared them with 135 untreated controls with regard to infections, morbidity, and mortality. The frequency, type, and severity of infections were similar in the two groups for the 6 weeks of the study.

In 1987, Conway and colleagues[82] reported a trial of IG (50 mg/kg/week) in 120 premature infants less than 32 weeks of gestation during their stay in the premature unit. IG was given to 59 infants; 61 infants matched for gestational age were left untreated. The level of IgG was about 100 mg/dL greater in the IG-treated group than in the untreated group. Among 62 episodes of proved or probable infections in the two groups, 40 (70 per cent) of 62 occurred in the untreated group. Twenty-one (34 per cent) of 61 of the infants in the untreated group and 13 (22 per cent) of 59 of those in the IG-treated group had at least one infection. No deaths due to infection occurred in the IG-treated group, and three deaths due to infection occurred in the control group. The authors concluded that IG had some protective value, despite the modest increase in IgG levels.

These mixed results indicate that IG is of limited and unproven value and is not indicated in the routine management of low birth weight infants. The use of IVIG in premature infants is discussed later in the chapter.

BACTERIAL POLYSACCHARIDE IMMUNOGLOBULIN. Santoshan and associates[281] administered human IG prepared from the sera of donors immunized with pneumococcal, meningococcal, and *Haemophilus influenzae* type b polysaccharide vaccines (bacterial polysaccharide IG) to Apache Indian infants living on reservations in Arizona. The 222 infants in the study group received 80 mg/kg of bacterial polysaccharide IG at 2, 6, and 10 months of age, and the 218 infants in the control group received saline injections at the same times. The infants were followed for 18 months. The levels of *H. influenzae* type b polysaccharide antibody were nonprotective in 55 to 66 per cent of the placebo recipients and in 3 to 14 per cent of the bacterial polysaccharide IG recipients. During the period of the study, seven cases of invasive *H. influenzae* type b disease and four cases of invasive pneumococcal disease occurred in the control group, compared with one and two cases, respectively, in the bacterial polysaccharide IG–treated group. The rate of *H. influenzae* type b infection significantly was reduced, and the subsequent ability to respond to *H. influenzae* type b vaccine was not lost.

Bacterial polysaccharide IG also was studied as a prophylactic agent for acute otitis media.[294] Ninety-one children older than 2 years of age with one episode of acute otitis media in the first 6 months of life or two or three episodes in the first 24 months of life were given bacterial polysaccharide IG at 0.5 mL or placebo on days 1 and 30 and studied for 120 days. The frequency of acute otitis media due to *S. pneumoniae* during 120 days was decreased significantly (7 episodes vs. 17 episodes), but the total number of episodes of acute otitis media was similar in the two groups. The investigators concluded that bacterial polysaccharide IG might be of value in children or groups of children (e.g., HIV-infected children) with susceptibility to recurrent *S. pneumoniae* acute otitis media. Bacterial polysaccharide IG is not licensed.

PERTUSSIS IMMUNOGLOBULIN. Pertussis IG (human) formerly was available for treatment, but studies, including a placebo-controlled trial,[15] showed little or no benefit and the product was removed from the United States market. Swedish investigators[124] developed a lot of high-titered pertussis IG from donors immunized with acellular pertussis vaccines and used a dose of 8 mL (a larger dose than that used in the previous trial) in a small, controlled trial of 47 infants with pertussis, 33 of whom received the IG preparation. Their was a significantly shorter duration of whoop (8.7 days vs. 20.6 days) but no differences in coughing or vomiting in the treated group compared with the placebo group. Further trials are in progress.

Ichimaru and associates[153] successfully treated a 1-year-old child with severe pertussis with an IVIG preparation selected for its high titers to pertussis toxin and filamentous hemagglutinin antibody. A dose of 350 mg/kg/day for 3 days was used.

Intravenous Immunoglobulin

IVIG is further treated human immune serum globulin that has been rendered free of complexes and thus safe for intravenous infusion. This product can be given in large quantities for antibody deficiencies[53] and several autoimmune and inflammatory disorders.[97] Several methods to treat Cohn Fraction II have been used to eliminate high-molecular-weight complexes: these include treatment with proteolytic enzymes, ultracentrifugation, and reduction of sulfhydryl bonds followed by alkylation and incubation at low pH. Solvent and detergent treatment or pasteurization also is used to ensure viral inactivation. Although these additional procedures increase its production cost, IVIG has several advantages over intramuscular immune serum globulin: (1) larger quantities of IgG can be given, (2) high levels of serum IgG can be achieved rapidly, (3) painful, intramuscular injections are avoided, (4) tissue pooling or proteolysis is avoided, and (5) self-administration is possible (see Table 238–2).

Pharmacology

The first IVIG produced in the United States in 1981 was Gamimune (Cutter Biological, Miles, Berkeley, CA), a reduced and alkylated 5 per cent solution containing 10 per cent maltose (Table 238–3). The second IVIG produced was prepared by acidification and treatment with pepsin; the lyophilized powder could be reconstituted as a 3, 6, or 12 per cent solution (Sandoglobulin, Sandoz Pharmaceuticals Corp., East Hanover, NJ). Since then, several other IVIGs have been introduced by different manufacturers (see Table 238–3). Some are 5 to 10 per cent solutions; others are lyophilized powders that are reconstituted as 3 to 12 per cent solutions.

Although these products vary slightly,[304] they generally are therapeutically equivalent and usually are selected on the basis of cost and convenience. There are minor IgA and IgG subclass differences.[10, 304] Antibody titers also may vary from lot to lot, as well as among different IVIGs.[73] Products low in IgA content, such as Gammagard or Polygam (Baxter Healthcare, Glendale, CA), are used to minimize reactions in patients with hypogammaglobulinemia and concurrent IgA deficiency or when anti-BIgA antibodies are present in the recipient. Very sensitive patients may not tolerate any IVIG. Premixed liquids have the advantage of convenience because the reconstitution step is not required; however, most must be kept refrigerated.

All currently available IVIG products have adequate serum half-lives (15 to 25 days), have a wide spectrum of antibody activity, have minimal anticomplementary activity, and are free of bacterial and viral contamination.

Administration of Intravenous Immunoglobulin

IVIG administration requires venous access, which sometimes is a problem in small children. It also requires close monitoring during the infusion. Adverse reactions to IVIG tend to be more frequent and more severe than with IG injections.

IVIG is contraindicated in patients who have had an anaphylactic reaction to IVIG or other blood products. It is given with great caution in patients who have IgG subclass deficiencies with IgA deficiency or anti-IgA antibodies.[88]

Typically, an IVIG infusion requires 2 to 4 hours to administer. The initial rate is 0.01 mL/kg/minute, but this can be doubled at 20- to 30-minute intervals if there are no side effects to a maximal rate of 0.08 mL/kg/minute. Adverse effects tend to be associated with rapid infusion rates in patients with concurrent acute infections, in previously untreated patients, or when significant time between infusions has transpired (intervals >6 weeks). Immediate minor reactions can be avoided or diminished by slowing the infusion rate. Patients experiencing minor side effects, such as headaches, shaking chills, nausea and vomiting, and myalgia/arthralgia, can be pretreated with aspirin, diphenhydramine (Benadryl), or hydrocortisone (1 hour before infusion). Occasionally, switching to a different product (generally one available as a solution) alleviates the reactions.

A few investigators have given high concentrations (9 and 12 per cent solutions) infused rapidly over a period of 20 to 40 minutes; this rapid rate can be tolerated by some patients.[284] However, this should not be performed except by experienced personnel equipped to manage adverse reac-

TABLE 238–3. Intravenous Immunoglobulin (IVIG) Preparations Used in the United States

Name of Preparation, Year Released, and Manufacturer	Isolation Method	Product Form (Stabilizers)	Comments
Sandoglobulin (1984) Sandoz Pharmaceuticals, East Hanover, NJ	Acid and pepsin	Lyophilized. Reconstitute as 3, 6, 9, or 12% solution. Available in 1-, 3-, and 6-g bottles (5% sucrose)	Reaction rates may be somewhat higher than other IVIG products. *Storage:* Room temperature
Gammagard (1986)* Gammagard S/D (1995) Baxter Healthcare Co., Hyland Division, Glendale, CA	Polyethylene glycol (PEG) and ultrafiltration; solvent-detergent treatment	Lyophilized. Reconstitute as 5% or 10% solution. 2.5-, 5-, and 10-g bottles (3% albumin and glycine)	A number of hepatitis C cases reported. Withdrawn from the market in 1994. Recommended for patients with absent IgA. *Storage:* Room temperature
Gamimune-N (1986—5%) (1992—10%) Miles/Cutter Laboratories Berkeley, CA	Acid and diafiltration	Liquid. 5% or 10% solution. Available in 0.5-, 2.5-, 5-, and 12.5-g bottles (10% maltose)	Low rate of side effects. *Storage:* Refrigerated
Iveegam (1988) Immuno-US, Rochester, MI	Trypsin and PEG	Lyophilized. Reconstitute as 5% solution. Available in 0.5-, 1-, 2.5-, and 5-g bottles (5% glucose)	First used in Kawasaki disease trials. *Storage:* Refrigerated
Venoglobulin-I (1988) Alpha Therapeutics Corp., Los Angeles, CA	PEG-DEAE-sephadex fractionation	Lyophilized. Reconstitute as 5% solution. Available in 0.5-, 2.5-, 5-, and 10-g bottles (albumin and 2% mannitol)	*Storage:* Room temperature
Polygam (1988)* Polygam S/D (1995) American Red Cross, Washington, D.C.	PEG and ultrafiltration; solvent-detergent treatment	Lyophilized. Reconstitute as 5% or 10% solution. Available in 2.5-, 5-, and 10-g bottles (3% albumin and glycine)	Manufactured for the American Red Cross by Baxter Pharmaceuticals from volunteer donors. Withdrawn from market in 1994 along with Gammagard. Reintroduced as Polygam S/D. *Storage:* Room temperature
Gammar-IV (1989) Armour Pharmaceuticals, Kankakee, IL	Low–ionic-strength ethanol fractionation	Lyophilized. Reconstitute as 5% solution. Available in 1-, 2.5-, 5- and 10-g bottles (albumin and 5% sucrose)	*Storage:* Room temperature
CytoGam (1991) Med Immune, Inc., Gaithersburg, MD	PEG and ultrafiltration; solvent-detergent treatment	Lyophilized. Reconstitute as 5% solution. Available in 2.5-g bottles (albumin and 5% sucrose)	Enriched for cytomegalovirus antibodies. Manufactured by the Massachusetts Public Health Biologic Laboratories for Med Immune. *Storage:* Refrigerated
Venoglobulin-S (1992) Alpha Therapeutics, Los Angeles, CA	PEG and DEAE-Sephadex fractionation; solvent-detergent treatment	Liquid. 5% solution. Available in 2.5-, 5-, and 10-g bottles (5% D-sorbitol)	Reaction rates may be somewhat higher than other IVIG products. *Storage:* Room temperature
Venoglobulin-S (1995) Alpha Therapeutics, Los Angeles, CA	PEG and DEAE-Sephadex fractionation; solvent-detergent treatment	Liquid. 10% solution. Available in 5-, 10-, and 20-g bottles (5% D-sorbitol)	Reaction rates may be somewhat higher than other IVIG products. *Storage:* Refrigerated
Gammar-P (1995) Armour Pharmaceuticals, Kankakee, IL	Low–ionic-strength ethanol fractionation; pasteurization	Lyophilized. Reconstitute as 5% solution. Available in 1-, 2.5-, 5-, and 10-g bottles (albumin and 5% sucrose)	*Storage:* Room temperature
Respiratory Syncytial Virus Immune Globulin Intravenous RespiGam (1996) Med Immune, Inc., Gaithersburg, MD	Ethanol fractionation; solvent-detergent treatment	Lyophilized. Reconstitute as 5% solution. Available in 2.5-g bottles.	Enriched for respiratory syncytial virus (RSV) antibodies for prevention of RSV infections in high-risk infants. Manufactured by the Massachusetts Public Health Laboratories for Med Immune. *Storage:* Refrigerated

*No longer available.

tions. In responsible, older patients receiving infusions without adverse effects, infusion by self-administration at home can be accomplished at great cost savings.[11, 185, 314] However IVIG infusions usually are performed in the clinic setting or by home infusion teams.

Adverse Effects of Intravenous Immunoglobulin

Between 5 and 15 per cent of IVIG infusions are associated with adverse reactions; typically, these include headaches, nausea and vomiting, flushing, chills, myalgia, arthralgia, and abdominal pain. Occasionally, chest tightness, hives, and anaphylactoid reactions occur. Severe life-threatening anaphylactic reactions are rare. Certain brands of IVIG may be more reactogenic; in one study in Kawasaki disease, the two IVIGs used were equivalent therapeutically, but one had a 12-fold (2 per cent vs. 25 per cent) increase in side effects.[272] Serious, late (but rare) side reactions[95] include aseptic meningitis,[173, 359] cerebral thrombosis,[381] renal insufficiency,[263] and hemolytic anemia.[49] Thus, IVIG infusions should be supervised by persons with the experience as well as the skill and knowledge to handle these reactions. Nurses or parents or others who perform home infusions must be taught to recognize and treat adverse reactions.

Hepatitis C Virus Contamination of Intravenous Immunoglobulin

Hepatitis C has been transmitted through certain experimental IVIG lots,[207, 242] in some European preparations,[35, 36, 203, 373] and in commercially available United States lots.[71, 283] Bjoro and associates[36] reported that immunocompromised patients had a severe and rapidly progressive course of hepatitis C infection and that the responses to interferon were poor.

Until the report of an outbreak of hepatitis C in 1994,[71] there had never been a United States report of hepatitis associated with a commercially available IVIG. As of October 1994, there were reports of 137 suspected cases, 88 of which were confirmed.[71, 283] Fifty-one of the 88 patients (58 per cent) had primary immunodeficiencies, and 63 per cent eventually became symptomatic. The Gammagard involved in the outbreak has been replaced with Gammagard-SD, the preparation of which includes solvent-detergent treatment to inactivate hepatitis C virus and other membrane-enveloped viruses.

Manufacturers of other preparations also have incorporated procedures to inactivate hepatitis C virus and most other viruses. Each of the various methods seems effective, but none can guarantee the total absence of infectious virus. However, no cases of HIV transmission have ever been reported with IVIG administration.[145, 155, 283]

Intravenous Immunoglobulin in Primary Immunodeficiencies

IVIG is indicated in patients with profound primary antibody deficiency (quantitative and qualitative), in patients with combined immunodeficiencies, and in those with secondary immunodeficiency with significant antibody deficiency (Table 238–4). Regular infusion of IVIG can keep patients with primary antibody immunodeficiencies free from infections for long periods or lessen the severity and frequency of chronic infections. Patients with X-linked agammaglobulinemia, common variable immunodeficiency, and the hyper-IgM syndrome clearly benefit from replacement therapy. In disorders characterized by combined antibody and cellular defects and in those with secondary immunodeficiencies, IVIG serves as an important ancillary treatment but does not correct the associated T-cell defect or underlying cause of the secondary immunodeficiency.

TABLE 238–4. Some Immunodeficiencies in Which Human Intravenous Immunoglobulin May be Beneficial

Antibody deficiencies
X-linked agammaglobulinemia
Common variable immunodeficiency
Immunodeficiency with hyper-IgM
Transient hypogammaglobulinemia of infancy (sometimes)
IgG subclass deficiency IgA deficiency (sometimes)
Antibody deficiency with normal immunoglobulins
Combined deficiencies
Severe combined immunodeficiencies (all types)
Wiskott-Aldrich syndrome
Ataxia-telangiectasia
Short-limbed dwarfism
X-linked lymphoproliferative syndrome
Secondary immunodeficiencies
Malignancies with antibody deficiencies; multiple myeloma, chronic lymphocytic leukemia, other cancers
Protein-losing enteropathy with hypogammaglobulinemia
Nephrotic syndrome with hypogammaglobulinemia
Pediatric AIDS
Intensive care patients: trauma, surgery, or shock
Post-transplantation period
Post bone marrow transplantation
Burns
Prematurity

Given at equivalent doses (100/mg/kg/month), IVIG infusions were as effective as IG injections in antibody immunodeficiency.[9] Other studies utilizing IVIG at larger doses (150 to 200 mg/kg every 3 to 4 weeks) demonstrated its therapeutic superiority over IG.[33, 87, 231, 241] Subsequent studies have suggested that patients receiving high IVIG doses (500 mg/kg/month) had fewer sinopulmonary infections than those receiving conventional doses (150 mg/kg/month).[31] When patients have chronic lung disease or continued infection despite usual doses of IVIG, higher doses (400 to 600 mg/kg/month) may result in improved pulmonary function and fewer infections.[31, 271]

These large doses of IVIG are not warranted in patients who do well on conventional doses because of the increased costs. Our practice is to administer between 300 and 400 mg/kg of IVIG per month to keep the serum IgG trough level above 500 mg/dL (near-normal levels) or 300 mg/dL above the pretreatment level. Some patients with severe disease do not respond to higher doses or more frequent infusions because of permanent tissue damage or deep-seated chronic infection.

IVIG also is used in patients with recurrent infections with antibody deficiency and normal or near-normal IG levels. Rarely, IVIG is indicated in infants with transient hypogammaglobulinemia with persistent infection nonresponsive to antibiotics. It also has been used in patients with IgG subclass deficiencies, but controlled studies demonstrating efficacy are lacking.[34, 184, 300]

A syndrome of polymyositis, chronic encephalitis, or both caused by persistent enteroviral infection of the central nervous system in patients with agammaglobulinemia has been treated successfully with very high doses of IVIG containing specific antibody to the virus.[104, 224] However, some patients have not responded.[86]

Intravenous Immunoglobulin in Secondary Immunodeficiencies

Some patients with secondary immunodeficiencies have low levels of immunoglobulins, poor antibody responses to antigenic challenge, and low levels of natural antibodies. This may result from loss of immunoglobulin, loss of immune cells, or the toxic effect of therapy or infection on the immune system. Table 238–4 includes those diseases and conditions where secondary immunodeficiency can occur. Laboratory criteria that support the use of IVIG include (1) significant hypogammaglobulinemia (serum IgG <200 mg/dL or total immunoglobulin level [IgG + IgM + IgA] <400 mg/dL); (2) absent or low natural antibodies; (3) absent or poor response to antigenic challenge (e.g., tetanus, pneumococcal vaccines); and (4) lack of an antibody response to the infecting organism.[325]

HEMATOLOGIC/ONCOLOGIC DISEASES. Antibody deficiencies can occur with multiple myeloma, chronic lymphocytic leukemia, lymphomas, and advanced cancer. A double-blind, multicenter study concluded that the prophylactic infusion of 400 mg/kg of IVIG every 3 weeks reduced the incidence of bacterial infections in patients with chronic lymphocytic leukemia.[83] The treatment group had fewer infections with *S. pneumoniae* and *H. influenzae,* but there was no difference in infections due to other gram-negative bacteria, fungi, or viruses. This beneficial effect was confirmed in a subsequent study,[113] although concerns have been raised about its cost-effectiveness in this setting.[368] IVIG also has been shown to reduce the incidence of infections in patients with multiple myeloma[72] and patients with lung cancer receiving chemotherapy.[287]

PROTEIN-LOSING ENTEROPATHY AND NEPHROTIC SYNDROME. Some pediatric patients develop antibody deficiency associated with massive proteinuria (nephrosis) or diarrhea (protein-losing enteropathy) and accelerated IgG catabolism. Many of these patients have minimal trouble with recurrent infection, probably because antibody synthesis is intact and probably is accelerated; however, if the IG loss exceeds the synthetic capacity, severe hypogammaglobulinemia may result. IVIG can be used diagnostically in such cases; a large intravenous infusion followed by serial measurements of serum IgG levels can document an accelerated IgG half-life (i.e., less than 10 days). These patients are candidates for IVIG therapy if they have recurrent infections and low IgG levels (<200 mg/dL). Large and repeated doses are necessary. Occasionally, antibody infusions help control the severe diarrhea of protein-losing enteropathy.[62]

INTENSIVE CARE PATIENTS: TRAUMA/SURGERY/SHOCK. Patients undergoing severe stress associated with trauma or extensive surgery have profound exposure and susceptibility to infection and a spectrum of immune deficiencies, including cutaneous anergy, leukocyte dysfunction, hypogammaglobulinemia, and transiently impaired antibody synthesis.[118, 233, 374] Bowel stasis and hypotension may promote gram-negative sepsis, endotoxemia, or both with development of severe and often irreversible shock. Studies by Ziegler and associates[385] and Baumgartner and associates[25] suggested that when antisera to a mutant J5 *Escherichia coli* endotoxin with anti–lipid A activity was used in bacteremic or surgical intensive care unit patients, the incidence and severity of severe shock could be reduced. However, Calandra and colleagues,[60] who utilized a human IVIG to J5 *E. coli* in 71 patients with gram-negative infections and shock, could not confirm their results. They gave a single infusion of 200 mg/kg; a control group received a similar dose of regular IVIG. There was no difference in mortality, onset of time to shock, or complications.

Several monoclonal antibody preparations to endotoxin are under study, and one, HA-IA, a human monoclonal IgM antibody, has been used with mixed results in the treatment of patients with sepsis and gram-negative bacteremia.[333, 384]

Just and coworkers[167] utilized regular IVIG and antibiotics in 50 intensive care unit patients suspected of having infections and compared their outcome with that of 54 control patients who received antibiotics alone. Although there was no difference in survival, there was a trend to indicate that the IVIG-antibiotic group had a shortened intensive care unit stay, a shorter period in which respirator therapy was necessary, and improved renal function and that there was a favorable effect on infection (i.e., infections were a less likely cause of death in these patients). A multicenter study of 352 postsurgical patients confirmed the observation that standard IVIG (400 mg/kg at weekly intervals) reduced the incidence of infections and shortened the stay in the intensive care unit compared with placebo-treated or hyperimmune core-lipopolysaccharide IG–treated patients.[157]

Other studies of IVIG in trauma/surgery patients[90, 118] and head trauma patients[120] have shown questionable efficacy. In sum, these studies provide no compelling evidence for the routine use of IVIG in trauma/surgical/intensive care unit patients.

PREMATURITY. All premature infants have low levels of maternally derived IgG at birth, and most develop IgG levels approaching 100 mg/dL in the first months of life.[19] These IgG levels may be depressed further by pulmonary disease (with transudation into the lung), stress (with increased IgG catabolism), and multiple blood drawing.[278] In addition, their sluggish antibody responses; their concurrent IgM and IgA deficiency; and their immature complement, phagocytic, and T-cell systems make them extraordinarily susceptible to infection.[227] Although routine use of IG in premature infants (reviewed earlier) has been of doubtful value, the availability of IVIG and the increasing number of surviving premature infants have reawakened interest in the routine use of IVIG in all tiny premature infants.

The results of six single-institution, controlled studies[58, 75, 78, 141, 181, 316] on the use of IVIG in prevention of infection are shown in Table 238–5. All enrolled premature newborns within the first 48 hours of life, but the definition of sepsis, the rate of infection in the controls, and the dosage and brand of IVIG varied. Four of six studies showed a statistically significant benefit in the prevention of sepsis, and two studies showed diminished mortality.

Based on these encouraging results, four groups undertook larger, multicenter studies,[14, 106, 217, 370] also summarized in Table 238–5. Only one of these studies[14] showed a significant benefit in decreasing bacterial infections; even in this study, there was no significant difference in survival or duration of hospitalization. In one study,[217] IVIG was associated with a higher incidence of infection, possibly associated with the very large dose of IVIG employed, with resultant development of reticuloendothelial blockade and immune system inhibition.

Thus, the evidence to date supports the National Institutes of Health Consensus Statement (1990) that concluded that IVIG should not be given routinely to infants of low birth weight.[240]

However, IVIG may be of benefit in selected septic newborns not responding to antibiotics, particularly in the presence of neutropenia and possibly with the concomitant use of granulocyte colony–stimulating factor or granulocyte-macrophage colony–stimulating factor. The future use of monoclonal antibodies or high-titered IVIGs to specific infectious agents (e.g., group B streptococci) also may be forthcoming.[147]

POST TRANSPLANTATION. Conditioning regimens to

TABLE 238–5. Results of 10 Studies of the Use of IVIG in Prevention of Sepsis in Noninfected Low Birth Weight Infants

	Birth Weight or Gestational Age	IVIG Dose and Frequency	Number of Patients/Controls	Septic Episodes Patients/Controls	Deaths: Patients/Controls	Efficacy
Single-Center Studies						
Haque et al., 1986[141] (Saudi Arabia)	900 to 1500 g	120 mg/kg on day 1 Repeated on day 8 in 1/2 of patients	100/50	4 (4%)/8 (16%)	0/2 (4%)	Yes
Chirico et al., 1987[75] (Italy)	<1400 g	500 mg/kg/week × 4	43/40	2 (5%)/8 (20%)	7 (16%)/13 (32%)	Yes
Stabile et al., 1988[316] (Italy)	<1790 g	500 mg/kg on days 1, 2, 3, 7, 14, 21, and 28	40/40	5 (13%)/3 (8%)	7 (18%)/7 (18%)	No
Clapp et al., 1988[78] (U.S.A.)	<2000 g	Repeated infusions to keep IgG level >700 mg/dL	56/144	0/16 (11%)	3 (5%)/10 (7%)	Yes
Bussel, 1990[58] (U.S.A.)	700 to 1300 g	1000 mg on days 1, 2, 3, 4, and 15	61/65	9 (15%)/16 (25%)	NA*	Yes†
Kinney et al., 1991[181] (U.S.A.)	<1000 g, 1000–1500 g <1500 g	750 mg/kg within 72 hours, then every 14 days	82/88	5 (6%)/5 (6%)	4 (5)/4 (%)	No
TOTALS			**382/427**	**25 (65%)/56 (13%)**	**21 (6%)/36 (8%)**	
Multicenter Studies						
Magny et al., 1991[217] (France)	<32 weeks' gestation	500 mg/kg on days 0, 1, 2, 3, 17, and 31	120/115	25 (21%)/12 (10%)	7 (6%)/5 (4%)	No
Baker et al., 1992[14] (U.S.A.)	500 to 1700 g	500 mg/kg on days 3–7, 1 week later, and then every 14 days	287/297	70 (24%)/104 (35%)	10 (3%)/5 (4%)	Yes
Weisman et al., 1994[370] (U.S.A.)	500 to 2000 g ≤34 weeks' gestation	500 mg/kg on day 1	372/381	40 (11%)/38 (10%)	48 (13%)/50 (13%)	No
Fanaroff et al., 1994[106] (U.S.A.)	500 to 1500 g	700–900 mg/kg on days 1–4, repeated every 14 days	1204/1212	186 (16%)/209 (17%)	136 (11%)/130 (11%)	No
TOTALS			**1983/2005**	**321 (15%)/363 (18%)**	**201 (10%)/199 (10%)**	

*Not available.
†Significant in first 30 days; by day 70, there was no difference in the two groups.

eliminate or reduce the host's hematopoietic and immune systems during transplantation (bone marrow and solid organ) render these patients extremely susceptible to infection.[351]

The use of IVIG to prevent these infections, particularly sepsis, pneumonia, or gastrointestinal infections, has met with limited success,[123, 334, 336] with the exception of preventing complications from CMV infection (discussed in the next section).

One report did demonstrate some benefit from infusions of IVIG in a controlled trial on 382 bone marrow recipients.[336] The study patients received 500 mg/kg of IVIG weekly for 90 days, then monthly for 1 year, with a resultant decrease in the number of infections, number of platelet transfusions, and incidence of graft-versus-host disease. A recent review from the same group of investigators concluded that IVIG has shown benefit by reducing septicemia, interstitial pneumonia, fatal CMV disease, acute graft-versus-host disease, and transplant-related mortality in adult recipients of related marrow transplants.[335] Thus, IVIG has been recommended for allogeneic marrow transplant recipients[175, 274] but not for autologous transplantation.[133, 379]

BURNS. Bacterial sepsis, particularly *Pseudomonas* and *E. coli* sepsis, is the leading cause of death in the 300,000 patients hospitalized annually in the United States for burns.[232] These patients develop hypogammaglobulinemia due to protein loss in proportion to the severity of the burn. High-dose IVIG prolonged survival in experimentally burned mice infected with *Pseudomonas,* and preliminary studies of IG and plasma in human burn patients were encouraging.[164, 174, 293] IVIG with high titers against *Pseudomonas* has been prepared and is under evaluation; proof of efficacy is lacking.[253, 293]

Intravenous Immunoglobulin in Viral Infections

The availability of IVIG permits the administration of large quantities of specific antibody to a virus either in prevention or in treatment of a specific infection. Promising results of IVIG treatment have led to the development and testing of high-titered, special IVIGs for certain viral infections, including CMV-IVIG and RSV-IVIG.

CYTOMEGALOVIRUS INFECTIONS. The most extensive use of IVIG for a specific infectious disorder is for prevention of CMV infections in bone marrow transplant patients at high risk for disseminated infection and pneumonia.[378] These trials were prompted by the former ineffectiveness of antiviral therapy in CMV,[378] certain animal studies that indicated a beneficial effect of passive immunization in CMV,[289] and a more favorable outcome in CMV infections if CMV antibody is synthesized by the patient.[238, 302] Currently available IVIG preparations contain antibody to CMV at varying titers; a high-titered CMV-IVIG also is available (see Table 238–3).

Cytomegalovirus Infection Prevention. Winston[377] has summarized six early studies of the efficacy of preventing CMV infection or pneumonia by the use of CMV antibody (as CMV immune plasma, high-dose IVIG, or high-titered CMV-IVIG). The incidence of CMV infection was 35 per cent (45 of 130 patients) in antibody-treated patients compared with 51 per cent (68 of 133 patients) in control, untreated patients. More significantly, CMV pneumonia was reduced from 23 per cent in the control group to 8 per cent in the antibody-treated group. These combined results suggest that immunoglobulin or plasma, although not necessarily preventing CMV infection, modifies the severity of infection and prevents CMV pneumonia in bone marrow transplant patients. The magnitude of this effect depends on whether the recipient or donor has had a previous CMV infection; in CMV-negative donors and recipients given CMV-negative blood products, the use of CMV antibody may be unnecessary.[45]

Other studies have shown benefit of IVIG or CMV-IVIG in preventing CMV infection in CMV-negative kidney transplant recipients[310, 312, 319] and liver transplant recipients.[28, 79, 308] In CMV-seronegative heart transplant patients given a heart from a CMV-positive donor, CMV-IVIG alone did not prevent seroconversion or CMV disease.[17] In CMV-positive heart transplant patients, ganciclovir was more effective than CMV-IVIG in preventing CMV disease. Neither regimen prevents seroconversion of a recipient given a heart from a CMV-positive donor.[5] The combination of CMV-IVIG and ganciclovir probably is best in reducing the risk of both primary CMV infection and associated mortality.[79, 256, 286] Optimal dose and dose-scheduling regimens for both IVIG and CMV-IVIG are yet to be established but are likely to involve high and frequent doses and, thus, to be expensive.

Cytomegalovirus Infection in Newborns. Snydman and associates[309] gave two doses of CMV-IVIG to 82 multiply transfused premature newborns (within 24 hours of the first infusion and 10 days later) and placebo infusion to 89 control infusions. The rate of CMV infection did not vary between the IG recipients (8 of 82, 10 per cent) and placebo recipients (10 of 89, 11 per cent). However, among the 31 infants receiving CMV-IVIG whose mothers were CMV-seropositive, there was one episode of acute CMV syndrome, compared with five episodes in the 40 infants of CMV-seropositive women who received placebo infusions. This study suggests but does not prove a role for CMV-IVIG in infants at risk for CMV infection.

Treatment of Cytomegalovirus Infection. In addition to prophylaxis, IVIG rich in CMV antibodies may be beneficial in the treatment of established CMV infections.[102, 266, 376] Although the use of IVIG alone in established CMV infection is of no or marginal value,[266] two studies indicate that CMV antibody (as CMV-IVIG or high-dose IVIG) combined with the antiviral drug ganciclovir was effective in the treatment of CMV pneumonia in bone marrow transplant recipients. Recipients of ganciclovir or IG alone had a combined survival rate of 13 per cent (13 of 100), compared with a survival rate of 60 per cent (20 of 35) in recipients of both drugs.[102, 376]

HIV INFECTION. There is considerable rationale for the use of IVIG in patients with advanced HIV disease (particularly children), including their increased susceptibility to common bacterial and viral infections, poor primary antibody responses to vaccine antigens despite hypergammaglobulinemia, and, in children, a limited antibody spectrum to common bacterial pathogens. Although the central immune defect in AIDS is a loss of helper T-cell (CD4) numbers and function, the polyclonal B-cell activation and defective T-cell helper function result in a significant B-cell deficiency.[32, 243] Thus, in children with AIDS, bacterial infections are more common than opportunistic infections. Patients with AIDS also may develop immune-mediated thrombocytopenic purpura and viral diseases (e.g., RSV, parainfluenza, and CMV infections) amenable to IVIG therapy.

Preliminary studies in symptomatic HIV pediatric patients suggest a beneficial effect of IVIG in HIV-infected children. Calvelli and Rubinstein[61] reported that among 14 patients given regular IVIG infusions over a 2-year period (in addition to antibiotics when necessary), 1 patient developed sepsis and only 2 died; among 28 untreated controls (antibiotics only), 18 developed sepsis and 14 died. Siegel and Oleske[298] reported 10 deaths in 12 untreated controls and only 3 deaths in 19 IVIG-treated children with AIDS from 1981 to 1983. The overall mortality rate over a 4-year period was 50 per cent for untreated patients and 35 per cent for IVIG-treated patients.

However, these observations were uncontrolled. Accordingly, two National Institutes of Health multicenter, double-blind studies were undertaken to determine the efficacy of IVIG in decreasing infections and improving survival in children with AIDS.[158, 315] The 372 children in the first study received 400 mg/kg of IVIG every 4 weeks or an albumin control for 2 years.[158] Thirty per cent of all children in the IVIG-treated group had serious infections, compared with 42 per cent of the children in the placebo group. Fewer ill children (those with CD4 lymphocyte counts >200 cells/mm^3) benefited in particular from IVIG. Children in this category had fewer serious infections and were hospitalized less than the placebo group, and their CD4 counts dropped less rapidly than those of the placebo group.[228] The mortality rate in both groups, however, was identical. The children with CD4 counts less than 200 cells/mm^3 (i.e., those with severely impaired immunity) who were given IVIG had no significant decrease in infections, days of hospitalization, or mortality rate, compared with their counterparts in the placebo group. The authors concluded that IVIG significantly reduces the risk of infections in some children with symptomatic HIV infection, primarily those with CD4 counts between 200 and 500 CD4 cells/mm^3. In a follow-up study, the placebo group was allowed to cross-over to receive IVIG with a drop in the rate of serious infection and hospitalizations.[229]

In a subsequent National Institutes of Health controlled trial of IVIG in which all of the children received zidovudine, there again was a significant decrease in serious bacterial infections, but this benefit was limited to children who did not receive trimethoprim-sulfamethoxazole prophylaxis for *Pneumocystis carinii* pneumonia.[315] The consensus of an HIV working group was that HIV-infected children with significant hypogammaglobulinemia or documented poor antibody formation may be candidates for IVIG therapy. We also use IVIG in HIV-infected children whose recurrent infections are not controlled by antibiotics and who have chronic nonspecific diarrhea with failure to thrive.

IVIG in large doses (0.5 to 1.0 g/kg for 3 to 5 days) has been shown to be effective in HIV-infected adults[55, 198, 252] and children[198] with thrombocytopenia. Regular IVIG infusion also improved left ventricular function in HIV-infected children with dilated cardiac myopathy.[209] Kiehl and colleagues[178a] showed that regular IVIG infusions every 21 days decreased the frequency and severity of serious infections in adults with advanced HIV infection.

HIV Intravenous Immunoglobulin and HIV Immune Plasma. Current lots of IVIG contain no HIV antibodies because HIV-seropositive donors are excluded from the donor pool. The use of antibody to HIV (obtained from asymptomatic, HIV-seropositive donors, available experimentally as HIV immune plasma or HIV-IVIG) in prevention and treatment of HIV is being explored.

These products are treated with low temperature, alcohol, heat, or beta-propiolactone to render them free of live HIV or other viruses and are employed to (1) prevent infection of acutely infected animals inoculated with HIV,[257] (2) improve the clinical status of patients with advanced AIDS,[172] and (3) prevent maternal-fetal transmission (by administering HIV-IVIG to the pregnant woman and her newborn infant).

Three single-institution, controlled[160, 208, 362] therapeutic trials of HIV immune plasma have been completed. Two showed encouraging results, with reduction of the rate of opportunistic infections and maintenance of CD4 counts[208, 362]; the patients most likely to benefit had moderately advanced disease and a high viral burden but maintained some T-cell immunity (CD4 >50 cells/mm^3). A study of the use of HIV-IVIG in the treatment of children is pending.

A double-blind, multicenter, controlled trial of HIV-IVIG (vs. standard IVIG) for the prevention of maternal-fetal HIV transmission is being conducted through the National Institutes of Health AIDS Clinical Trial Group. Pregnant HIV-positive women, all of whom are on antiretroviral therapy, receive HIV-IVIG (or IVIG) every 4 weeks during pregnancy, and their newborn infants receive an infusion of HIV-IVIG (or IVIG) at birth (plus zidovudine for 6 weeks). The rationale is that transmitting women may lack neutralizing antibody to their predominant HIV strain, and HIV-IVIG may provide this antibody to them and their infants, reduce their viral burdens, and intercept virus entering their infants.

ENTEROVIRUS ENCEPHALITIS AND POLYMYOSITIS. Chronic meningoencephalitis and polymyositis due to enterovirus (usually echovirus) characteristically occur in patients with X-linked agammaglobulinemia.[86, 224] Treatment with high doses of IVIG may modify the severity of infection and improve survival. A review of published reports[86, 104, 138, 163, 201, 224, 255] shows that 8 of 11 patients treated with IVIG survived, compared with only 2 of 10 patients given intramuscular IG or immune plasma and 0 of 4 patients who received no treatment. Two patients who received intraventricular IG as well as IVIG had resolution of cerebrospinal fluid pleocytosis with eradication of the echovirus from the cerebrospinal fluid.[138] However, most other patients, including two others given intraventricular IG,[104, 255] had a chronic fluctuating course with persistent cerebrospinal fluid pleocytosis and positive cerebrospinal fluid cultures.[86, 201, 255]

EPSTEIN-BARR VIRUS INFECTION. IVIG has been advocated for the treatment of chronic Epstein-Barr virus infection.[108, 348] In uncontrolled studies, 8 of 12[108] and 19 of 29[348] patients showed clinical improvement. John Sullivan, M.D., suggests the prophylactic use of IVIG in Epstein-Barr virus–seronegative male infants and children with the X-linked lymphoproliferative syndrome to prevent Epstein-Barr virus infection. These boys develop severe and sometimes fatal complications from this virus. However, an Epstein-Barr virus–seronegative college student with X-linked lymphoproliferative syndrome died of overwhelming Epstein-Barr virus infection, despite monthly IVIG infusions.[244]

The use of IVIG in combination with interferon-α has been reported to be of benefit in the Epstein-Barr virus–induced lymphoproliferative disorder that results from the immunosuppression used in transplantation procedures.[290, 341]

RESPIRATORY SYNCYTIAL VIRUS INFECTION. In animal models, the administration of IVIG modifies the severity of RSV infection,[143, 259, 260] with significant reduction of viral shedding from the lungs and nose. A double-blind, multicenter, placebo-controlled trial of high-dose IVIG rich in RSV antibody (RSV-IG) in the prevention of RSV infection in 249 high-risk infants and young children with prematurity, bronchopulmonary dysplasia, or congenital heart disease was conducted.[131] Subjects were randomized to receive 750 mg/kg of RSV-IG (high-dose), 150 mg/kg of RSV-IG (low-dose), or no treatment monthly during the respiratory virus season. Recipients of high-dose RSV-IG had a significant (75 per cent) reduction of RSV lower respiratory tract infection compared with the control group, particularly severe lower respiratory tract infections. The high-dose subjects experienced a significant reduction in number and days of hospitalizations and the need for ribavirin. Low-dose recipients had no clinically significant benefit over the control group. Although the study suggested safety and efficacy, study design problems identified by the United States Food and Drug Administration initially postponed licensing this product[100] but it finally was licensed in 1996.

In a subsequent placebo-controlled, double-blind study, RSV-IVIG (750 mg/kg/month) reduced the incidence and severity of RSV infection of infants younger than 24 months of age who were born prematurely (less than 35 weeks' gestation) or who had bronchopulmonary dysplasia, particularly those receiving oxygen therapy within the preceding 6 momths. Thus, in early 1996, RSV-IVIG was licensed for use in the prevention of lower respiratory tract infection in these two groups of high-risk infants during the respiratory virus season (October to May). Fluid overload with the infusion may be a problem for some infants with pulmonary disease because the recommended dose is 15 mL/kg (750 mg/kg of a 5 per cent solution). RSV-IVIG is not recommended for infants with cardiac disease or in the treatment of RSV infections.[130a]

RSV-IVIG at a dose of 750 mg/kg also was found to reduce the incidence of acute otitis media in the treated infants, including episodes of RSV otitis and bacterial otitis.[302a]

RSV-IVIG also is recommended for immunodeficient infants in the first 2 years of life who are receiving IVIG infusions or are undergoing transplantation procedures. RSV-IVIG can be given instead of regular IVIG during the respiratory virus season.

RSV-IVIG treatment is expensive and cumbersome and because of the large volume of fluid administered, it often is associated with side effects. Mumps-measles-rubella and varicella vaccines should not be given until 9 months after RSV-IVIG therapy. Routine vaccination for diphtheria-pertussis-tetanus, polio, hepatitis B, and *Haemophilus influenzae* type B polysaccharide can be given, but an extra dose is recommended for these vaccines to ensure an adequate immune response.

Monoclonal antibody agent RSV is being tested as a treatment modality.

Aerosolized IVIG with a significant RSV antibody titer has been used in the therapy of acute RSV infection.[269]

OTHER RESPIRATORY TRACT VIRAL INFECTIONS. IVIG preparations contain antibodies to several common respiratory tract viral pathogens, including adenoviruses, influenza viruses, and parainfluenza viruses. Clinical data from controlled trials on the efficacy of IVIG for these viral lower respiratory tract infections are not available. Adenovirus pneumonia has occurred in immunodeficient children lacking neutralizing antibody to adenovirus, and one child recovered after receiving intramuscular IG.[89] In contrast, IVIG failed to eradicate parainfluenza in a child with severe combined immunodeficiency[322] and one child with advanced HIV disease.

PARVOVIRUS INFECTIONS. Parvovirus B19 can cause transient aplastic anemia (and thrombocytopenia) in sickle-cell disease patients and chronic aplastic anemia in immunodeficient or severely immunosuppressed patients.[186] High-dose IVIG can cure parvovirus B19 infection with reversal of the anemia.[156, 199, 343] However, failures of IVIG have been reported,[46] and, for patients unable to make antibody, continuous IVIG may be necessary to prevent recurrence.[130, 239]

OTHER VIRAL AND PROTOZOAL INFECTIONS. IVIG or high-titered maternal plasma has been used to treat neonatal enteroviral infection.[161, 262] However, a small, double-blind trial in neonates showed no clinical benefit of IVIG infusion.[3] An immunosuppressed adult with disseminated central nervous system echovirus infection was treated successfully with IVIG.[306] One study suggested that IVIG reduced recurrences of genital herpes simplex virus infections.[218] Lassa fever has been treated with immune plasma with anecdotal benefit.[204, 230] IVIG was of no benefit in cerebral malaria.[346]

Intravenous Immunoglobulin in Bacterial Infections

Antibody therapy has an important historic niche in the treatment of bacterial infections.[64] Immune serum was used successfully in the preantibiotic era for the treatment of *H. influenzae* meningitis, whooping cough, and meningococcal meningitis. Antibody therapy remains an essential part of the treatment of bacterial infections in which toxins are produced; optimal treatment of both tetanus and diphtheria includes the use of concomitant antitoxin (human or equine) and antibiotics.

Antibody has several modes of action in the treatment of bacterial disease. It provides opsonins for enhanced phagocytosis that may be absent or depleted during acute infection. Antibody attachment to organisms or infected cells may promote complement lysis or antibody-dependent cellular cytotoxicity. In infection in which toxins are elaborated, antibody provides antitoxic activity. Finally, antibody enhances leukocyte mobility and prevents neutrophil depletion, possibly by release of chemotactic factors and agglutination of organisms for phagocytosis.

Animal studies also indicate that combination antibiotic and antibody therapy sometimes is superior to either alone. For example, the survival of neutropenic mice with experimental *Pseudomonas* infection is 25 per cent with antibiotics, 21 per cent with IVIG, and 62 per cent with the combination.[81] Experimental infections with other organisms, including group B streptococci, *Staphylococcus aureus, E. coli,* and *Klebsiella,* also suggest that antibiotics and IG may be synergistic.[180] In contrast, it was shown that when using an animal model of group B streptococcal infection, IVIG given in conjunction with penicillin significantly increased the rate of mortality.[179] There also are a few reports of septic deaths in humans associated with IVIG therapy, possibly through the occurrence of reticuloendothelial blockade.[180]

GRAM-NEGATIVE INFECTIONS. The most extensive use of IG for infections in adults has involved the trauma/shock/postoperative patients suspected of having gram-negative infections as reviewed earlier under secondary immunodeficiency.[25, 60, 90, 118, 157, 167, 384, 385] There is some evidence that IVIG has therapeutic potential in the prevention of infection in some patients, but routine use is not indicated.

CYSTIC FIBROSIS. Winnie and associates[375] suggested that IVIG may improve pulmonary function in pulmonary exacerbations of cystic fibrosis. All subjects received antibiotics, were older than 12 years of age, and had no long-term benefit from the IVIG. Van Wye and coworkers[358] had similar results using hyperimmune *Pseudomonas* IVIG in cystic fibrosis patients.

SEPTIC PREMATURE INFANTS. Premature infants are exceptionally susceptible to bacterial sepsis, and clinical signs of sepsis, such as fever and leukocytosis, may not be apparent in these newborns. Thus, IVIG, in conjunction with antibiotics, has been advocated in the early management of proven or suspected sepsis of the newborn. However, only a few studies are available. Sidiropoulos and coworkers[297] treated successive infants suspected of having neonatal sepsis with antibiotics or antibiotics plus IVIG (0.5 to 1.0 g/day for 6 days). Four of 15 of the infants in the group treated with antibiotics alone died, compared with 2 of 20 of the infants in the group treated with antibiotics plus IVIG. Among premature infants who weighed less than 2500 g, the mortality rate was 44 per cent (four of nine) among those who received only antibiotics and 9 per cent (1 of 11) among those who received antibiotics plus IVIG, a significant difference.

Haque and associates[140] treated preterm infants (28 to 37 weeks of gestation) suspected of having bacterial sepsis with antibiotics alone (30 infants) or antibiotics plus an IgM-enriched IVIG preparation (30 infants). The daily dose of IVIG administered was 190 mg/kg of IgG and 30 mg/kg of IgM and was continued for 4 days. The mortality rate was 20 per cent (6 of 30) in the group that received antibiotics alone and

3.3 per cent (1 of 30) in the group that received antibiotics plus IVIG, a significant difference.

These studies suggest but do not prove that IVIG is of some value in septic premature newborns. Of particular concern are possible long-term adverse effects. These and other studies[58, 75, 78, 141, 278] indicate minimal side effects or complications of IVIG.

When IVIG is used, it seems reasonable to normalize the IgG level between 600 and 1000 mg/dL; this requires frequent infusions and determination of IgG levels.[78] In general, a dose of 100 mg/kg raises the serum IgG level about 100 mg/dL. The National Institutes of Health IVIG consensus conference of May 1990 concluded that IVIG as adjunct therapy in preterm infants with infections is not supported by the current data and that additional trials, especially involving the use of high-titer preparation, are indicated.[240] Nothing in the ensuing years negates this conclusion.

Intravenous Immunoglobulin in Immunoregulatory Disorders

High-dose IVIG has immunosuppressive and anti-inflammatory effects that make it a valuable agent in the treatment of several autoimmune or inflammatory disorders[97] (see Table 238–6). High-dose IVIG (1 to 2 g/kg/week) may work by the following mechanisms[18, 97, 301, 342]:

1. Inhibiting antibody synthesis (possibly by a direct effect on proliferating B cells)
2. Combining directly with autoimmune antibodies (because it contains anti-idiotypic antibodies)
3. Blocking the uptake of antibody-coated cells in the spleen and liver (Fc-receptor blockade of antibody-dependent cellular cytotoxicity)
4. Down-regulating immune activation by decreasing inflammatory cytokine release or action
5. Combining with bacterial superantigens that may be present in certain inflammatory disorders (e.g, toxic shock syndrome)
6. Inhibiting complement-mediated tissue injury

The best-documented uses of high-dose IVIG as an immunoregulator are in the treatment of Kawasaki disease and immune thrombocytopenic purpura. In most other disorders, the reports of efficacy are based on small, uncontrolled studies or case studies.

KAWASAKI DISEASE. Kawasaki disease is an acute, inflammatory, febrile childhood disorder of unknown cause.[206] Generalized vasculitis is common, but coronary artery obstruction or aneurysm can cause long-term morbidity and, on occasion, death. The major goal of therapy is to reduce the rate of coronary artery disease. IVIG initially was shown to reduce coronary artery complications and to shorten the febrile period.[112] A large Unites States multicenter study compared aspirin alone with high-dose IVIG (400 mg/kg/day for 4 days) plus aspirin.[237] The IVIG-aspirin combination was superior to aspirin alone in preventing coronary artery abnormalities. A subsequent controlled study showed that a single 2-g/kg dose of IVIG was superior to four daily 400-mg/kg doses (both groups received aspirin) in reducing the rate of coronary artery disease.[236] Thus, current optimal treatment includes a single high dose of IVIG (1 to 2 g/kg) together with aspirin.

IMMUNE THROMBOCYTOPENIC PURPURA. High-dose IVIG (1 to 2 g over 1 to 4 days) rapidly reverses the thrombocytopenia in pediatric patients with acute immune thrombocytopenic purpura, probably by interfering with reticuloendothelial uptake of antibody-coated platelets.[154, 324] It is at least as effective as corticosteroid therapy and has a more rapid onset of action. Because acute immune thrombocytopenic purpura in children is a self-limiting disorder, IVIG probably does not affect the basic cause of the disease or decrease the likelihood of chronic immune thrombocytopenic purpura.

IVIG is less effective in chronic immune thrombocytopenic purpura but may be of special value for the short-term correction of thrombocytopenia during emergencies. Other forms of immune thrombocytopenia have been managed with IVIG, including postinfectious thrombocytopenia, the thrombocytopenia of AIDS, and autoimmune and isoimmune thrombocytopenia of newborns.[135]

IVIG also has been used in the treatment of immune neutropenia[56] and autoimmune hemolytic anemia.[56, 216, 254]

GUILLAIN-BARRÉ SYNDROME. IVIG is effective in the treatment of Guillain-Barré syndrome, possibly by interfering with the action or the synthesis of antineuronal antibodies.[182, 361] A large Dutch study compared plasmapheresis (n = 73) with IVIG (n = 74) in moderate to severely affected adult patients.[357] Both treatment groups improved, but those treated with IVIG responded faster and had greater improvement. A similar result was achieved in a smaller pediatric study.[353] Because IVIG is much easier to use and less expensive than plasmapheresis, a trial of IVIG should be used before plasmapheresis is undertaken.

OTHER IMMUNOREGULATORY DISORDERS. High-dose IVIG has been used in a number of other disorders associated with the presence of harmful autoantibodies or chronic inflammation[97] (see Table 238–6). Particularly convincing is its value in chronic inflammatory demyelinating polyneuropathy and myasthenia gravis. The reported benefit of IVIG in other diseases (see Table 238–6) is based on anecdotal reports on small studies.

Immunoglobulin Use by Unusual Routes (Oral, Intrathecal, Aerosol)

The action of oral IG administered to provide antimicrobial activity to the gastrointestinal tract mimics that of antibody-rich colostrum and breast milk. In humans, little or no ingested IG is absorbed intact into the systemic circulation.[8] Some oral IG traverses the entire gastrointestinal tract undigested, particularly in premature infants.[40] Oral IG may neutralize microorganisms, inhibit their colonization, and prevent their attachment to the gastrointestinal mucosa.

Rotavirus Infection

Barnes and colleagues[22] fed human IG for 7 days or a placebo to premature infants in a nursery in which rotavirus was endemic. Rotavirus-associated diarrhea developed in 6 of 11 babies given placebo and in 1 of 14 given oral gammaglobulin.

Prevention of rotavirus also has been reported with oral cow colostrum[98] and infant formula supplemented with bovine antibodies.[350] Losonsky and coworkers[211] used oral human IG successfully to interrupt the excretion of rotavirus in immunodeficient patients chronically infected with rotavirus. Kanfer and associates[171] used oral human IG to treat rotavirus infection after bone marrow transplantation.

Necrotizing Enterocolitis

Eibl and colleagues[99] were able to prevent necrotizing enterocolitis in all 90 infants given oral IG rich in serum IgA. There were six cases among 91 control infants. Similar results

TABLE 238–6. Noninfectious Uses of Human Intravenous Immunoglobulin

Proven benefit*	
	Kawasaki disease
	Immune thrombocytopenic purpura
	Guillian-Barré syndrome
	Dermatomyositis
	Chronic inflammatory demyelinating polyneuropathy
Probable benefit†	
	Neonatal isoimmune or autoimmune thrombocytopenic purpura
	Postinfectious thrombocytopenic purpura
	Immune neutropenia (including neonatal)
	Autoimmune hemolytic anemia
	Myasthenia gravis
	Multifocal motor neuropathy
Possible benefit‡	
	Anticardiolipin antibody syndrome
	Toxic shock syndrome
	Coagulopathy with factor VIII inhibitor
	Bullous pemphigoid
	Churg-Strauss vasculitides
	Other vasculitides
	Graves ophthalmopathy
Unproven benefit§	
	Intractable epilepsy
	Steroid-dependent asthma
	Eczema (atopic dermatitis)
	Juvenile rheumatoid arthritis
	Lupus erythematosus
	Recurrent abortion
	Hemolytic-uremic syndrome
	Multiple sclerosis
	Viral myocarditis
	Chronic fatigue syndrome
	Rasmussen encephalitis
	Sydenham chorea
	Type I diabetes mellitis
	Inflammatory bowel disease

*Controlled studies demonstrate efficacy.
†Several case reports or uncontrolled series are convincing.
‡Preliminary studies are encouraging but incomplete.
§Preliminary studies are limited or equivocal.

in necrotizing enterocolitis were obtained with oral monomeric IgG by Rubaltetti and colleagues[275] in Italy.

Cryptosporidia Infection

Bovine colostrum was used successfully to treat cryptosporidia diarrhea in HIV infection.[291a] Borowitz and Saulsbury[44] used oral IG to treat cryptosporidia infection successfully in a child with acute leukemia. A clinical trial in HIV patients is under way.

Diarrhea

Oral human IG has been used in the period after bone marrow transplantation to prevent viral gastroenteritis[84] and to treat nonspecific diarrhea in immunodeficient subjects.[226]

Other Uses

Human IG has been used intrathecally in the treatment of viral encephalomyelitis in antibody deficiency[104] and as a respiratory aerosol in RSV infection.[269] Use of antitoxin intrathecally in tetanus is discussed in the section on tetanus.

PASSIVE IMMUNITY IN SPECIFIC DISEASES

Botulism and Botulinum Antitoxin

Botulism, a severe paralytic poisoning, results from the ingestion or absorption of the neurotoxin from *Clostridium botulinum.* Three clinical variants are recognized: food poisoning from ingestion of contaminated canned food; wound botulism from a contaminated local infection; and infant botulism, presumably from ingestion of *C. botulinum* spores, their multiplication in the gastrointestinal tract, elaboration of toxin, and subsequent absorption.[29, 66] Seven immunologic types of *C. botulinum* have been identified, designated A through G, each elaborating an immunologically distinct toxin. Almost all human botulism has resulted from ingestion of toxins A, B, and E, the latter usually associated with fish and marine mammal products.[187, 188]

Japanese studies, reviewed by Dolman and Hda,[93] indicate that antitoxin therapy is effective in type-E botulism; the mortality rate of type-E botulism was 49 per cent in 135 untreated cases and 3.5 per cent in 85 antitoxin-treated cases.

Tacket and associates[339] noted that 46 patients who had type-A, food-borne botulism and who received trivalent antitoxin had a lower mortality rate (27 per cent) than 13 patients who did not receive antitoxin (46 per cent). Early antitoxin administration resulted in a shorter clinical course.

The presence of toxin in the blood long after the appearance of clinical symptoms or toxin ingestion gives theoretic support to the use of antitoxin to prevent further binding of toxin to tissue. Some antitoxin remains in the circulation for more than 30 days, indicating that a single initial dose is adequate therapy.

Equine antitoxin to types A, B, and E is the primary antitoxin available in the United States. The decision to use antitoxin is complicated by its unknown efficacy and its side effects.

Recommendations

Antitoxins to A, B, and E (collectively called trivalent antitoxins) should be administered to symptomatic patients as soon as possible after testing for sensitivity to horse serum.[66] These are made by Connaught Laboratories (Willowdale, Ontario; 717-839-7187) and distributed by the state health departments or the United States Centers for Disease Control and Prevention in Atlanta (404-639-3670 or -2888). One vial of each antitoxin is given intravenously, and an additional vial of each antitoxin is given intramuscularly. In severe wound infections, higher doses may be needed, guided by antibody titers after the initial antitoxin dose. Antitoxin is not indicated in infant botulism.

Antitoxin can be given prophylactically to persons known to have ingested contaminated food. The risks of serum reactions (about 25 per cent) must be weighed against the risk of contracting the disease.

A controlled trial of human botulism IG (BIG) in the treatment of infant botulism is under way by the State of California Department of Health Service. Only infants in California can enter the trial. The phone number for the California BIG Hotline is 510-540-2646.

Diphtheria and Diphtheria Antitoxin

Much of the damaging effect of diphtheria results from the *Corynebacterium diphtheriae* toxin elaborated and absorbed at the site of the diphtheritic membrane. This toxin not only has a local effect to perpetuate membrane formation but also is distributed via the blood to the heart, nervous system, kidney, and other organs. The larger the membrane, the more toxin elaborated; in addition, more toxin is elaborated from a membrane involving the pharynx and tonsils compared with that involving the larynx and trachea.

Diphtheria toxin is present in three forms: (1) circulating and unbound, (2) loosely bound to the tissues, and (3) firmly bound to the tissues. Antitoxin neutralizes circulating toxin and competes with and partially neutralizes loosely bound toxin but has no effect on tissue-bound toxin. Thus, optimal passive immunity must be initiated at an early stage of the disease via the intravenous route, so as to intercept toxin before it becomes tissue-bound.

Antitoxin of animal origin remains the mainstay of treatment, as it was in the preantibiotic era. Diphtheria was the first illness in which antiserum was used as standard therapy; Fibiger[107] proved its efficacy in 1898 when he showed that 5 of 204 patients given horse antitoxin died, whereas 14 of 201 not given antiserum died. Paschlau[250] demonstrated the importance of early administration of antitoxin in 1949; the fatality rate of 197 cases treated within 48 hours was 1.96 per cent, compared with 8.9 per cent when treatment was delayed until the fourth or fifth day. Other authors have noted similar findings.[344]

Tasman and associates[345] have emphasized the importance of intravenous administration of antitoxin because rapid achievement of high blood levels results in rapid neutralization of antitoxin and the appearance, within 30 minutes, of antitoxin in the saliva. They showed that the mortality rate and the severity of the myocarditis and neuritis in experimental diphtheria in guinea pigs could be reduced by giving antitoxin intravenously rather than intramuscularly.

McCloskey and Smilack[220] determined the antitoxin content of standard human IG. None of the lots tested contained diphtheria antitoxin in sufficient concentration to allow use of IG for antitoxic therapy. They suggested that an IVIG with high-titer antitoxin activity be developed to eliminate the risk of giving horse serum intravenously.

Recommendations

Diphtheria antitoxin of equine origin is indicated in all suspected or proven cases of diphtheria. It is available in vials containing 20,000 U from Connaught Laboratories. Prior to its administration, it is necessary to perform skin tests for sensitivity. If there is a previous history of serum reactions or these test results are positive, a schedule of desensitization must be followed.

The amount of antitoxin given depends on the location and the extensiveness of the membrane, the degree of systemic toxicity, and the duration of illness. In severe and late cases, intravenous use is indicated; in mild forms, intramuscular administration will suffice. In all cases, diphtheria antitoxin should be given promptly rather than delayed while waiting for bacterial confirmation of the diagnosis.

In cutaneous diphtheria, antitoxin is of uncertain value; when used, the dose is 20,000 to 40,000 U intramuscularly to prevent toxic sequelae. In pharyngeal or laryngeal disease, 20,000 to 40,000 U are given intramuscularly; in nasopharyngeal disease, 40,000 to 80,000 U are given intramuscularly; and in extensive disease with neck edema of more than 3 days' duration, 80,000 to 120,000 U are given intravenously. Although antimicrobial therapy is a valuable aid in the treatment of diphtheria, it is not a substitute for antitoxin therapy.

Routine use of antitoxin in asymptomatic, exposed susceptible persons is not recommended. With heavy exposure or an extremely susceptible host, antitoxin 5000 to 10,000 U intramuscularly can be given in addition to antibiotics and diphtheria immunization; proof of efficacy is lacking.

Hepatitis A

Human IG has been used most widely for the prevention of hepatitis A. This need may be decreased by the widespread use of hepatitis-A vaccine. The efficacy of IG was demonstrated by the 1945 studies of Stokes and Neefe[327] aborting an epidemic in a children's summer camp, of Havens and Paul[142] controlling an institutional epidemic, and of Gellis and associates[115] preventing hepatitis A in the Mediterranean theater of operations at the close of World War II. The combined use of IG, use of the new vaccine, and scrupulous cleanliness can interrupt the intestinal-oral circuit of transmission and abort an incipient epidemic.

IG is efficacious in hepatitis A if given any time during the incubation period up until 6 days before the onset of disease. The protection persists for a period of 6 to 8 weeks. Stokes and associates[328] noted that a single small dose of IG (0.02 mL/kg) provided a degree of protection for up to 9 months for persons residing at an institution in which hepatitis A was endemic.

The effectiveness of IG in hepatitis A varies from 80 to 95 per cent, depending on how soon it is administered after exposure and the severity of the exposure.[365] IG suppresses the clinical manifestations of the disease, but anicteric hepatitis is not prevented, and the ratio of anicteric hepatitis to icteric hepatitis may be as high as 12:1.[196] Because the period of protection exceeds the expected duration of the IG, the concept of passive-active immunity has emerged, in which, as a result of continuous exposure, a mild illness ensues and, in turn, confers long-lasting immunity.[196, 328, 365]

The initial studies of Stokes and Neefe[327] employed an IG dose of 0.15 mL/lb. Other early workers used doses of 0.06 to 0.12 mL/lb.[115, 142] In 1951, Stokes and associates[328] showed that doses as small as 0.01 mL/lb were effective in limiting spread but not totally preventing hepatitis. Hsia and associates[152] in 1954 also noted that a dose of 0.01 mL/lb was effective in preventing hepatitis among family contacts. However, Ward and associates[366] in 1958 were able to reduce the incidence of hepatitis in institutional patients from 19.5 cases per 1000 to 7.4 cases per 1000 with 0.01 mL/kg and to 1.7 cases per 1000 with 0.06 mL/kg. The larger dose may be particularly important in adults because their disease is more severe.

The use of serologic tests for hepatitis A provides a way to determine the (1) immunity of a subject, (2) presence of inapparent infection, (3) titer of hepatitis A virus in lots of IG, and (4) validity of the passive-active immunity concept.[365, 366] In earlier studies, Krugman[191] showed that an IG preparation with a titer of 1:3200 by an immune adherence test was effective in neutralizing the infectivity of MS-1 serum, a serum known to contain hepatitis A virus. Among seronegative children who received the IG–hepatitis A mixture, six remained seronegative and two became seropositive; one became ill. In contrast, 8 of 14 children who received MS-1 serum without IG developed hepatitis.

Most current lots of IG have antibodies to hepatitis A virus by a competitive-inhibition radioimmunoassay. Titers greater than 1:100 are protective.[305]

Recommendations

HOUSEHOLD OR SEXUAL CONTACTS. Adults or children with a known intimate exposure to hepatitis A, such as a household or sexual contact, should be given a single IG dose of 0.02 mL/kg as soon as possible after exposure. Serologic testing for hepatitis A is unnecessary and may delay administration of IG. The use of IG after 2 weeks of exposure is not indicated.

IG usually is unnecessary for children and their teachers exposed to hepatitis A at day school. However, IG prophylaxis is recommended for children and staff exposed at a boarding school or in a school for retarded children, where the opportunities for fecal-oral route transmission are increased. Hospitalized children exposed to another child with hepatitis A in the hospital ward need not be given IG.

INSTITUTIONAL OUTBREAKS. Institutional hepatitis A outbreaks, such as in boarding schools, day care centers, facilities for the mentally retarded, and prisons, require aggressive action. Other cohorts, employees, and adult members of the households of infants who wear diapers and who attend these facilities should be treated immediately with 0.02 mL/kg of IG. If recognition of the initial case is delayed 3 or more weeks or if there is spread to other cohorts, staff, or household contacts, all personnel (staff and children) should be given IG. If an outbreak of hepatitis A is traced to a food handler, IG should be given to his or her close contacts and other restaurant employees.[63]

FOREIGN TRAVEL. Ordinary tourist travel does not require IG prophylaxis or hepatitis A vaccine. However, persons traveling to developing countries should receive vaccine 1 month prior to departure. If the departure date is less than 1 month away, 0.02 mL/kg of IG and vaccine can be used. The IG provides immediate protection and does not interfere with the efficacy of the vaccine.

PRIMATE EXPOSURE. Certain subhuman primates, such as chimpanzees, may carry hepatitis A virus. Animal handlers should observe scrupulous hygiene and be given hepatitis A vaccine. If bitten and unimmunized, they should receive 0.06 mL/kg of IG and vaccine.

NEEDLE EXPOSURE. IG is indicated for susceptible persons accidentally inoculated with blood or serum from a patient with hepatitis A. The recommended dose is 0.02 mL/kg. Pregnancy is not a contraindication for IG administration.

NEWBORN INFANTS OF INFECTED MOTHERS. Unless the mother is jaundiced at the time of delivery, no special care of the infant is necessary, such as IG administration or recommendations against breast feeding. If the mother is jaundiced, the infant can be given 0.02 mL/kg of IG; efficacy is not established.

Hepatitis B and Hepatitis B Immunoglobulin

Immunoglobulin in Hepatitis B

In contrast with its proven efficacy in the prophylaxis of hepatitis A, IG was not able to prevent posttransfusion hepatitis or hepatitis B ("serum hepatitis") reliably. This inconsistency derived from the fact, not appreciated initially, that most (up to 80 per cent) cases of posttransfusion hepatitis were not caused by the hepatitis B virus.

The initial study of IG in hepatitis B was conducted in 1945 by Grossman and associates,[132] who treated alternate battle casualties given whole blood or plasma with two 10-mL injections of IG 1 month apart. The incidence of icteric hepatitis was 1.3 per cent in 384 IG-treated patients and 9.9 per cent in 384 control patients, a highly significant difference that suggested a beneficial effect of IG. In 1947, Duncan and associates[96] reported the results from a similar study, although they gave only one 10-mL injection; hepatitis occurred in 1.2 per cent of 2406 patients in the IG-treated group and 0.9 per cent of patients in the control group, an insignificant difference. The mean incubation period in the IG-treated group was prolonged significantly (to 103 days) over that in the control group (87 days). Drake and associates[94] could not demonstrate a beneficial effect of IG derived from convalescent hepatitis patients when given to volunteers deliberately inoculated with blood or serum from an infected patient. The IG was ineffective given intramuscularly or when mixed with the infective serum prior to its injection.

Holland and associates[150] could not alter the incidence or severity of post-transfusion hepatitis in 84 open-heart surgery patients compared with 83 controls by giving IG in two 10-mL doses 1 month apart. These findings were confirmed in a large cooperative study of 5189 transfused cardiovascular patients given 10 mL of IG during the first, fourth, and seventh postoperative weeks.[122] Redeker and associates[264] could not demonstrate that IG protected spouses of persons with hepatitis B. Similarly, Kuhns and associates[197] could not reduce the incidence of post-transfusion hepatitis B with 20 mL of IG. Both of these latter studies used IG with low hepatitis B surface antigen antibody (anti-HBs) titers.

Several factors probably are responsible for the variation of effectiveness of IG in hepatitis B. One is the variable degree of exposure to the hepatitis B virus, which can be massive (as with a blood transfusion) or minimal (as with a casual sexual partner or household contact). A second factor is the variable level of anti-HBs in various lots of IG. Because IG is not titered for anti-HBs, it no longer is recommended for hepatitis B prophylaxis.

Hepatitis B Immunoglobulin

Soon after the identification of hepatitis B surface antigen (HBsAg) and its antibody (anti-HBs), it became evident that measurement of the antibody content of IG would permit selection of lots (or donors) with high titers of anti-HBs; such selection results in IG lots with anti-HBs titers of at least 1:100,000 by radioimmunoassay. This product (hepatitis B IG [HBIG]) has been licensed since 1978 for the prevention of hepatitis B.[67, 69]

Krugman and associates[192, 194] in 1971 evaluated high-titered HBIG in institutionalized children injected with the infective serum MS-2. All 11 children exposed to MS-2 serum developed hepatitis; two became icteric, and five remained HBsAg carriers after 320 days. Among five children given MS-2 serum and standard IG, three developed hepatitis; two were icteric, but none became a carrier. Among 10 children exposed to MS-2 serum and HBIG, 6 were protected completely, 1 had a transient infection, and 3 developed classic hepatitis. The researchers concluded that HBIG was 70 per cent effective under these circumstances. Their later studies confirmed that HBIG could reduce significantly the incidence, severity, and carrier rate of HBsAg after parenteral exposure to hepatitis B virus.[191]

Szmuness and associates[337] tested the efficacy of HBIG compared with IG by giving either standard IG or HBIG to retarded, institutionalized children at admission and at 4-month intervals for 1.5 to 2 years and comparing the incidence of hepatitis with that of untreated subjects. Both globulin-treated groups had a lower attack rate (11 per cent vs. 25 per cent) and lower incidence of chronic antigenemia (0 per cent vs. 13.5 per cent). Thus, both IG and HBIG were effective in preventing or modifying nonparenterally transmitted hepatitis B in an endemic setting. Of note is that 55 per cent of the patients treated with standard IG developed anti-HBs, whereas only 23 per cent of the patients treated with HBIG developed antibody, suggesting that passive-active immunity occurred more frequently in the group that received standard IG than in the group that received HBIG.

Seeff and associates[288] gave either HBIG or standard IG to 302 persons accidentally exposed to material infectious for hepatitis B. The incidence of both clinical and subclinical hepatitis during the first 6 months was 0.7 per cent in the HBIG-treated group and 6.1 per cent in the IG-treated group. At 6 months, 32 per cent of the IG recipients and 6 per cent of the HBIG recipients had antibody, indicating minimal passive-active immunity in the HBIG-treated group; Grady[121] reported similar results with HBIG after accidental exposure. The incidence of hepatitis at 6 months was 7 per cent (of 251 patients) with standard IG, 5 per cent (of 208 patients) with intermediate-titer HBIG, and 2 per cent (of 253 patients) with high-titer HBIG. This protection waned after 6 months, and differences in the groups became less apparent after 9 months, possibly because of re-exposure, delayed onset of infection, or failure of passive-active immunity.

Two studies in renal dialysis units also support the effectiveness of HBIG. Desmyter and associates[91] found that HBsAg antigenemia occurred at 16 months in 10 of 14 patients on dialysis given standard IG every 6 months, but in only 2 of 15 patients on dialysis given HBIG on a similar schedule. Prince and associates[258] gave standard IG or HBIG to 318 new dialysis patients and 296 staff members every 4 months; they reduced the incidence of hepatitis B from 23.1 per cent in the IG patients to 7.9 per cent in the HBIG patients. There was only a slight decrease in incidence of hepatitis in the HBIG–treated staff members (11.1 vs. 6.9 per cent).

Redeker and associates[264] found that HBIG was effective in preventing hepatitis B after 150 days in spouses of patients with hepatitis B. Nine of 33 spouses treated with standard IG developed hepatitis, whereas only 1 of 25 spouses receiving HBIG developed hepatitis B.

Prevention of Vertical Transmission

Beasley and associates[26, 27] studied the efficacy of HBIG in preventing perinatal transmission of the hepatitis B virus carrier state from a mother to her newborn infant. HBIG or placebo was given at birth to the infants of the hepatitis B e antigen–positive, HBsAg-carrier mothers, and the infants were followed for at least 15 months. Among 61 placebo recipients, 92 per cent became carriers; among 67 infants who received 1.0 mL of HBIG at birth, 54 per cent became carriers; among 57 infants who received 0.5 mL of HBIG at birth and at 3 and 6 months, 26 per cent became carriers. Passive-active immunization, indicated by the presence of anti-HBs, occurred in 27 per cent of the single-dose group and in 61 per cent of the three-dose group.

Based on these and other studies[162, 268] that suggested that multiple HBIG doses were more effective in interrupting vertical transmission of the HBsAg-carrier state than a single HBIG dose, advisory committees in 1981 recommended that all infants of HBsAg-positive mothers be given HBIG (0.5 mL) immediately after birth and again at 3 and 6 months. However, a number of these infants became infected sometime after their last HBIG dose (i.e., in the second or third year of life), indicating a need for more durable active immunity.

Wong and associates[380] studied the efficacy of hepatitis B vaccine given in conjunction with HBIG in the prevention of vertical transmission of the carrier state from mother to infant. They gave hepatitis B vaccine (36 infants), hepatitis B vaccine plus one dose of HBIG (35 infants), hepatitis B vaccine plus seven monthly HBIG doses (35 infants), or placebo (35 infants) to infants of HBsAg-positive mothers. In all vaccine groups, development of the persistent carrier state significantly was reduced compared with the placebo group (21 per cent, 2.9 per cent, and 6.8 per cent, respectively, vs. 73.2 per cent). All infants of the treatment groups developed anti-HBs, indicating that HBIG did not interfere with active immunization.

This and other studies[76, 170, 340] indicate that HBIG given at the time of birth followed by hepatitis B vaccine provides optimal passive-active immunity for long-lasting prevention of the carrier state, and this is the current recommendation. Studies in adults also confirm that HBIG given before or simultaneously with the first dose of hepatitis B vaccine does not interfere with the antibody response to hepatitis B vaccine.[338, 382]

HBIG is not of value in the treatment of either acute[4] or chronic[267] hepatitis B virus infection.

Hepatitis B Immunoglobulin Use in Liver Transplantation

Liver transplantation in a hepatitis B virus–infected patient is associated with a high rate of recurrence in the new liver (about 50 per cent in 3 years) and subsequent mortality. HBIG, given intravenously(!) or by the usual intramuscular route, has been used to prevent hepatitis B recurrence.[279] In a retrospective analysis of 359 transplants, hepatitis B recurrence was 74 ± 6 per cent among 67 patients given no HBIG, 74 ± 5 per cent among 83 patients given HBIG for 2 months, and 36 ± 4 per cent among the 209 patients given HBIG for 6 months or longer. The exact dose, frequency, and duration of therapy have not been established. Because lifelong therapy may be necessary, an intravenous form of HBIG is under development.

Recommendations

HBIG is recommended after parenteral or mucous membrane (oral, sexual, ophthalmic) contact with persons with hepatitis B virus infection or with HBsAg-positive materials (e.g., blood, plasma) and for neonates born to HBsAg-positive mothers (Table 238–7). It is available in 0.5-mL, prefilled syringes and in 1-mL and 5-mL vials.

EXPOSURE TO BLOOD PRODUCTS CONTAINING HEPATITIS B SURFACE ANTIGEN. No prospective studies have tested the efficacy of a combination of HBIG and hepatitis B vaccine in preventing hepatitis B after accidental exposure. This includes exposure by the percutaneous, ocular, and mucous membrane routes as well as by human bites that penetrate the skin. Because health care workers at risk for such accidents are hepatitis B vaccine candidates and because combination HBIG and hepatitis B vaccine is more effective than HBIG alone in perinatal exposure, this combination also is recommended after accidental exposure.

If the blood or secretions come from a person known to be HBsAg-positive or if the status of the exposure donor is unknown, immediate prophylaxis is indicated. A single dose of HBIG (0.06 mL/kg or 5 mL for adults) should be given as soon as possible, preferably within 24 hours of exposure. Hepatitis B vaccine should be given simultaneously at a different site and repeated after 1 and 6 months (see Table 238–7).

After massive exposure (i.e., via a blood transfusion), much larger doses of HBIG probably are indicated.

If a person has received at least two doses of hepatitis B vaccine before accidental exposure, HBIG is unnecessary if serologic tests show adequate anti-HBs titers (>10 mIU by radioimmunoassay). If hepatitis B vaccine is not given, two

TABLE 238–7. Hepatitis B Postexposure Recommendations for Hepatitis B Immunoglobulin (HBIG) and Hepatitis B Vaccine

Exposure	HBIG		Vaccine	
	Dose	*Recommended Timing*	*Dose*	*Recommended Timing*
Perinatal				
Infant of HBsAg† mother	0.5 mL, IM	Within 12 hours of birth	0.5 mL*	First dose within 12 hours, repeat 2 or 3 times
Infant of mother whose HBsAg status is unknown	0.5 mL, IM	Within 7 days if mother is found to be HBsAg†	0.5 mL*	First dose within 12 hours, repeat 2 or 3 times
Percutaneous (known exposure)				
Nonvaccinated	0.06 mL/kg, IM	Immediately	1.0 mL†	First dose immediately, repeat 2 times
Previously vaccinated	0.06 mL/kg, IM	Test patient for anti-HBs; if anti-HBs >10 mIU/mL, omit HBIG	1.0 mL Booster	Test patient for anti-HBs; if anti-HBs >10 mIU/mL, omit booster
Sexual				
Nonvaccinated	0.06 mL/kg IM	Immediately, not later than 14 days	1.0 mL	First dose immediately, repeat 2 times
Vaccinated	—	—	—	—

*High-risk infant dose (Merck)
†Adult dose (Merck)
HBsAG, hepatitis B surface antigen; anti-HBs, antibody to HBsAg.

doses of HBIG should be used, the second given 1 month after the first.

PERINATAL EXPOSURE OF INFANTS. If the mother is HBsAg- and hepatitis B e antigen–positive, 85 per cent of her untreated offspring will become infected and will become chronic carriers, some of whom will develop chronic hepatitis, cirrhosis, or hepatic cancer. If the mother is HBsAg-positive only, the risk of her offspring becoming carriers is less but still significant. Accordingly, these infants also are candidates for prophylaxis.

Infants Born to Hepatitis B Surface Antigen–Positive Women. For optimal passive-active immunity, HBIG (0.5 mL) is given to the newborn at birth (preferably in the delivery room but within 12 hours at the latest). Hepatitis B vaccine (at a dose twice that used for unexposed infants) is begun simultaneously and repeated at 1 and 6 months (see Table 238–7). This combination is only about 90 per cent effective in preventing the carrier state because intrauterine infection is not prevented.

Infants Born to Mothers Not Tested for Hepatitis B Surface Antigen. If the HBsAg status of the mother is unknown, hepatitis B vaccine should be given within 12 hours at the higher dose recommended for infants of carrier mothers, and HBIG (0.5 mL) should be given immediately (no later than 7 days) if the mother is shown to be a carrier. If the mother is seronegative, vaccine is continued at the smaller dose for unexposed infants.

HBIG effectiveness is diminished markedly if administration is delayed beyond 48 hours. Nevertheless, if the mother is found to be HBsAg-positive at birth, HBIG and hepatitis B vaccine should be given to her infant, even if there has been a significant delay. In this situation, the infant can be tested for HBsAg and anti-HBs at 12 to 15 months to determine the success of the HBIG and vaccine regimen. If HBsAg is present, the infant probably is a carrier; if anti-HBs is present, the child was immunized successfully. HBIG administration at birth should not interfere with polio, diphtheria-pertussis-tetanus, or other vaccines given at 2 months of age.

SEXUAL EXPOSURE TO HEPATITIS B OR A CARRIER OF HEPATITIS B. Sexual exposure to a person who has hepatitis B or is a carrier is an indication for HBIG (0.06 mL/kg, 5 mL maximum) and the initiation of hepatitis B vaccine. These should be given as soon as possible but not after 14 days of the exposure. If only HBIG is given, a second HBIG dose is recommended after 30 days.

With sexually exposed persons (including rape victims) for whom the HBsAg status of the contact is not known, HBIG (0.06 mL/kg, 5 mL maximum) is given and hepatitis B vaccine started. Alternatively, the vaccine can be given and the HBsAg status of the contact determined; if positive, HBIG can be given within 7 days and the vaccine schedule continued.

POSSIBLE EXPOSURES. After possible exposures (percutaneous, ingestion, sexual) to an unidentified person or body fluid in which the HBsAg status is unknown, a decision to treat with HBIG must be made individually, based on the likelihood that the source is HBsAg–positive and the seriousness of the exposure. Hepatitis B vaccine should be initiated immediately.

Ideally, the source should be tested for HBsAg positivity; if the results are available within 7 days, HBIG (0.06 mL/kg) can be given immediately and again at 1 month if the source is HBsAg-positive. When the source cannot be tested or when the source is likely to be HBsAg-positive, HBIG is given immediately and again at 1 month.

If the exposed person is a high-risk patient (e.g., immunodeficient, immunosuppressed, institutionalized, afflicted with Down syndrome, Asian, or undergoing hemodialysis) or is in a unit for which past environmental control measures have been ineffective, HBIG should be given.

HBIG is not indicated routinely after blood transfusions. A school or hospital exposure is not an indication for HBIG.

Hepatitis C

Several studies prior to 1990 suggested that the incidence or seriousness of non-A, non-B (presumably hepatitis C), post-transfusion hepatitis could be decreased by the administration of IG at the time of transfusion.[183, 280, 303] Since that time, IG and IVIG donors have been screened for antibody to hepatitis C virus and, if positive, eliminated from the donor pool. This eliminated hepatitis C virus antibody activity from IG preparations. This in turn may have facilitated the transmission of hepatitis C by certain lots of IVIG (see earlier) because the presence of hepatitis C virus antibodies might neutralize live virus surviving the fractionation process. Development of a hepatitis C virus IVIG is under consideration for use after liver transplantation for chronic hepatitis C.

In sum, IG or IVIG is of no value in hepatitis C prophylaxis.

Measles

Cenci[65] reported the first successful prophylaxis of measles with convalescent serum in 1907. Serum first was used in the United States in 1916 by Park and Freeman[247] and Zingher,[386] who gave either 4 or 8 mL of convalescent serum to 41 recently exposed children at New York Metropolitan Hospital. None of the 20 children receiving the 8-mL dose and 3 of the 20 children receiving the 4-mL dose developed measles. Park and Freeman[247] in 1926 found that 6 to 10 mL of convalescent serum was 92 per cent efficacious in preventing measles in recently exposed persons, a finding confirmed and extended by Stillerman and associates.[326] Placental extracts containing serum antibodies also were used in the prevention and modification of measles.[223]

Studies by Stokes and associates[330] and Ordman and associates[245] in 1944 established that (1) large doses (0.05 mL/kg) of IG given immediately after exposure could prevent measles, (2) lesser doses (0.01 mL/kg) given immediately after exposure could modify measles, and (3) large doses (0.05 mL/kg) given in the early stages of clinical illness could lessen the severity of measles. Greenberg and associates[127] conclusively demonstrated that IG was superior to placental extract in the prevention and modification of measles.

Black and Yannet[37] in 1960 observed that 19 of 38 children given IG (0.1 mL/lb) during a measles epidemic at a mental institution developed antibodies but had no clinical evidence of disease, suggesting passive-active immunity. Greenberg and associates[128] in 1955 noted that there was a lower incidence of measles encephalitis in IG-modified measles.

The next use of IG in measles was in diminishing side effects of the Edmonston strain of attenuated measles vaccine. Krugman and associates[195] in 1962 noted that the simultaneous administration of 0.02 mL/lb of IG and Edmonston measles vaccine, compared with the vaccine alone, reduced the incidence of high fever from 40 to 14 per cent and the incidence of rash from 10 to 2 per cent. The mean titer of measles antibody achieved was somewhat reduced by the IG, and there was a slight decrease in the rate of seroconversion; nevertheless, the vaccine-IG combination was 95 per cent effective.[329] The use of further attenuated measles vaccine has eliminated the necessity for concomitant IG injections. Furthermore, the widespread use of measles vaccine greatly has reduced the need for IG for measles.

The antibody titers achieved by immunization are less than those achieved by natural infection, with the result that (1) some immunized subjects are susceptible, (2) infants of immunized mothers have less passively acquired maternal antibody,[205] and (3) the titer of measles antibody in IG and IVIG is not as high as formerly found (although it must have a minimal titer of measles to pass government standards). Indeed, Subbarro and associates,[332] investigating the measles serostatus of the staff and patients in a neonatal intensive care unit after measles exposure by a house officer, noted that 3 of 41 (71 per cent) of the staff members were seronegative and that 15 of 21 infants (71 per cent) were seronegative; the latter finding correlated with the degree of prematurity and older age (because of metabolism of maternal antibody).

Recommendations

NORMAL INFANTS AND CHILDREN. In nonvaccinated normal children older than 15 months of age and exposed to measles, measles vaccine should be given; a preventive dose of IG (0.25 mL/kg intramuscularly) should be given as soon as possible after exposure but no later than 6 days after exposure. Five to 6 months later, measles vaccine should be given for permanent immunity. Alternatively, an attenuating dose of IG can be given at a lower dose (0.05 mL/kg). Exposed infants younger than 15 months of age (including infants of immunized mothers) should be given IG at 0.25 mL/kg. Infants younger than 6 months of age traveling to a country in which measles is endemic should be given 0.25 mL/kg of IG. Such infants between 6 and 15 months of age should be given measles vaccine.

HIGH-RISK CHILDREN. High-risk children (those with leukemia, lymphoma, malignancy, immunodeficiency [including HIV], or taking immunosuppressive drugs) exposed to measles should be given a double IG dose (0.5 mL/kg, maximum 15 mL), even if they have been immunized previously. Immunodeficient children receiving regular IVIG doses of 200 mg/kg/month or greater do not require additional IG upon measles exposure.

OTHERS. Unimmunized children of mothers who develop measles should be given 0.25 mL/kg of IG. Exposed, susceptible, pregnant women should be given IG at 0.25 mL/kg, maximum 15 mL, because measles vaccine is contraindicated during pregnancy.

Poliomyelitis

Before the development of poliomyelitis vaccines in the mid-1950s, IG was used extensively in the prevention of poliomyelitis. Bodian[42, 43] showed that Red Cross IG had neutralizing antibody to all three strains of poliovirus in approximately equal titers and that rhesus monkeys given intramuscular poliovirus could be protected against disease by subcutaneous administration of IG.

Bloxsom,[39] in an uncontrolled study during a 1948 Texas epidemic, gave 841 contacts an average dose of 2 mL of IG and noted only four cases at 1, 2, 3, and 42 days after the IG injection. He suggested that the IG was given too late to prevent the first three cases and that protection had worn off in the fourth case.

A committee on immunization of the National Foundation for Infantile Paralysis recommended in March 1951 that a controlled study be conducted on the efficacy of IG in the prevention of poliomyelitis during epidemics. Hammon and associates[139] subsequently undertook a massive field study in communities in three states during poliomyelitis epidemics. Fifty-five thousand children(!), 1 to 11 years of age, received either IG (average dose 0.14 mL/lb) or gelatin in a double-blind fashion. During the first week after injection, 12 cases occurred among the IG recipients and 16 cases occurred among the gelatin recipients. In the second week, there were 3 and 23 cases in the two groups, respectively, and, in the third to fifth weeks, there were 6 and 38 cases in the two groups, respectively. When protection was incomplete, there was some alteration of severity. Protection waned by 6 weeks and disappeared by 8 weeks. These clinical results were confirmed by virus isolation or rise in antibody titers in affected patients.

IG is an inefficient method of poliomyelitis prophylaxis, preventing only one case for every 500 to 2000 injections and then only for a brief time. Its chief value was in close family contacts of affected children and in aborting severe local epidemics.

Recommendations

The use of IG rarely is indicated in the prevention of poliomyelitis. An exposed unimmunized subject can be given 0.15 mL/kg of IG. An unimmunized patient who is traveling to an endemic or epidemic area and who cannot have vaccine also can be given this dose of IG for temporary protection.

Rabies, Rabies Immunoglobulin, and Hyperimmune Rabies Serum

Rabies is the ideal disease for passive immunization because the exact moment, the exact source, and the exact location of exposure are known. Furthermore, the long incubation period and the fact that the virus remains localized to the wound for several days enhance the effectiveness of passive immunization.

Rabies serum first was prepared in 1889 by Babes and Lepp.[13] However, variable experimental results, difficulty in interpreting field results, and the development of rabies vaccine led to a loss of interest in passive immunity. Habel[137] in 1945 conducted a series of studies in experimental rabies in mice, guinea pigs, and monkeys, using rabbit hyperimmune serum. He showed that antibody worked by two mechanisms: (1) neutralizing the virus while still in the tissues and (2) retarding the spread of virus within the nervous system, thus prolonging the incubation period and permitting active immunity by vaccine to become established. Serum prophylaxis alone gave consistently better results than vaccine alone, was effective when given up to 3 days after infection, and was more effective when given locally at the site of virus inoculation.

On the basis of these studies, the World Health Organization Expert Committee in 1950 recommended that a field trial of the efficacy of hyperimmune rabies serum, in conjunction with vaccine, be conducted.[105] This was undertaken in Iran because multiple bites by a single rabid wolf coming into isolated villages were not uncommon and this severe exposure was associated with a 40 to 50 per cent mortality rate. In 1954, a single rabid wolf bit 27 persons, 17 of whom were bitten on the head. These 17 were divided into three groups: five received vaccine alone, seven received vaccine and one dose of antirabies serum, and five received vaccine and two doses of antirabies serum.[20] Three of five persons treated with vaccine alone died of rabies, one of seven in the one-dose antiserum group died, and none of five in the two-dose antiserum group died. Antibody studies conducted on these patients indicated that a single or a double dose of antiserum, followed by 14 to 21 daily doses of vaccine, results in significant levels of circulating antibody for as long as 50 days.[136] The antibody found early is supplied passively; after the tenth day, the antibody present is a result of the vaccine. Thus, optimal treatment requires both passive and active immunization.

Prior to 1971, the only available antiserum was of equine origin. It still is the only product available in some countries. Since 1971, human rabies IG has been available in the United States and many other countries and is preferred because of the lessened risk of serum reactions.[299] Furthermore, the human antibody has a half-life in the circulation twice that of equine antibody, with the result that higher levels of passive antibody are maintained. However, the antibody response to the vaccine given concomitantly is suppressed more effectively.[210] Accordingly, smaller quantities of rabies IG must be given to achieve passive-active immunity (20 IU/kg); when larger doses (40 IU/kg) are given, active immunity is depressed significantly.[59]

Two vaccines are available for rabies: the human diploid-cell rabies vaccine and rhesus diploid-cell vaccine, absorbed. The use of these vaccines does not lessen the need for simultaneous passive immunity at the time of exposure; indeed, two cases[367] of fatal rabies have been reported after rabies exposure in which diploid-cell vaccine but no rabies IG was given.

A case of fatal rabies was reported in a 19-year-old man bitten on the finger by a rabid mongoose, despite the recommended postexposure prophylaxis (rabies IG and five doses of human diploid-cell vaccine).[292] Possible reasons for failure included (1) inadequacy of the recommended dose of rabies IG, (2) vaccine injection into the gluteal region where there is more fat than in the recommended deltoid region, and (3) decreased antibody response to the vaccine as a result of a possible immunodeficiency state.

Recommendations

Rabies IG or rabies antiserum is recommended in nonimmunized persons for *all bites by animals in which rabies cannot be ruled out* and for nonbite exposure to animals proved or suspected of being rabid.[68] Such treatment should be given as early as possible after exposure but should be used regardless of the interval between exposure and treatment. Half of the rabies IG (or equine rabies antiserum) should be injected locally at the wound site (if anatomically feasible) and the rest given intramuscularly in the deltoid area. If the wound is extensive, the rabies IG intended for local use can be diluted to facilitate multiple injections.[372] Vaccine then should be given at a different site with a different needle and syringe. This regimen has been used successfully during pregnancy.[77]

Rabies IG (or rabies antiserum) should not be administered after rabies exposure if the person (1) has had adequate pre- or postexposure prophylaxis with rabies vaccine or (2) has a known protective antirabies titer after another vaccine regimen. These persons are given two booster doses of rabies vaccine only, one on the day of exposure and the other on day 3.

If rabies IG is unavailable, equine rabies antiserum should be used, preceded by skin testing. If a person is known to be allergic to horse serum, rabies IG must be used or a schedule of desensitization employed.

The recommended dose is 20 IU/kg of rabies IG or 40 IU/kg of equine rabies antiserum. Rabies IG (or antiserum) is given as soon after exposure as possible. If rabies IG inadvertently was not given as soon as possible, it should be given immediately regardless of the time elapsed. If vaccine has been started, rabies IG still should be given for up to 8 days after the onset of the first dose of vaccine.

Rabies IG is supplied in 2- and 10-mL vials containing 150 IU/mL. Equine rabies antiserum is supplied in 5-mL vials containing 200 IU/mL but is not available in the United States. Because rabies IG and rabies antiserum may inhibit the immune response to simultaneously administered rabies vaccine, it is necessary to give five doses of vaccine rather than the three recommended for pre-exposure primary immunization. After possible exposure to rabies, rabies vaccine is recommended at 0, 3, 7, 14, and 28 days when rabies IG is given at day 0. Antibody testing should be done 2 to 3 weeks after the last injection to ensure an adequate antibody response.

Rabies IG is not used simultaneously when rabies vaccine is given prophylactically to unexposed high-risk persons.

Rabies IG and rabies antiserum are of no value in the treatment of established rabies infection.

Rubella

Rubella prevention by IG rarely is used because of its unreliable efficacy. Early studies, such as those of Greenberg[129] in 1947, suggested some prophylactic benefit. He gave 20 children exposed to rubella 5 mL of IG; none developed rubella, whereas 6 of 20 noninjected controls developed rubella. Korns[190] in 1952 showed that one lot of IG at a dose of 0.1 mL/lb partially protected mentally retarded institutionalized subjects against epidemic rubella. Nine of 45 IG-injected subjects developed rubella compared with 35 of 60 uninjected controls, a significant difference. However, another IG lot was ineffective and a third was only slightly effective, suggesting that their titers of rubella antibodies varied significantly.

Grayston and Watten[125] studied the efficacy of IG during a rubella epidemic in Taiwan in 1958. They found that 5 mL of IG could reduce the incidence of clinical rubella from 20.4 to 8.5 per cent. Lower doses were not effective. The period of protection lasted from 1 to 12 weeks after inoculation. There was no evidence of modification of infection. Brody and associates[47] carried out similar studies during an epidemic in Alaska in 1964. IG (0.55 mL/kg) resulted in an attack rate of 18 per cent in school age boys; in uninjected girls, the attack rate was 89 per cent. Fifteen of 40 boys who were given IG and who did not develop clinical rubella had a rise in antibody, indicating subclinical infection. The IG protection lasted for 1 month.

Houser and Schalet[151] were able to prevent rubella completely with doses of 15 mL of IG given to military recruits *prior* to exposure to rubella. Thus, passive immunity is achieved best by early administration of large doses.

Green and associates[126] and Krugman and colleagues[193] conducted the most extensive studies on IG prophylaxis in rubella, aimed at answering the question of its value in the prevention of congenital rubella syndrome when given to exposed expectant mothers in the first trimester of pregnancy. They deliberately exposed 200 children to rubella virus (as infected serum) by intramuscular injection or aerosol into the pharynx; this was respectively 100 per cent and 80 per cent effective in transmitting infection. IG containing neutralizing antibody at titers of 1:32 to 1:64 given at doses of 0.12 to 0.2 mL/lb had no demonstrable effect in preventing rubella in experimentally inoculated subjects or in patients exposed to rubella. Viremia was not prevented, although the duration of viremia was shortened. The IG dose was selected to approximate the 20-mL dose generally given to exposed pregnant women.

Lundstrom and associates[213] gave 251 exposed pregnant Swedish women 4 mL of convalescent rubella IG and 28 exposed pregnant women 24 mL of standard IG. Six of 251 (2.4 per cent) developed rubella; three of these six women aborted, and one had a child with probable congenital rubella. None of the 28 women given 24 mL of IG contracted rubella. The researchers believed that this low incidence represented a significant protective effect. Their later studies demonstrated that convalescent rubella IG given to women with manifest rubella did not protect against congenital rubella or lessen the probability of fetal damage.[214]

Recommendations

The use of IG to prevent rubella in nonpregnant females and males is not indicated because of the mildness of disease and the possible interference with active immunity.

IG is not recommended in most exposed pregnant women because the clinical syndrome may be masked and congenital rubella not reliably prevented. However, for exposed pregnant women who for religious or other reasons will not consider therapeutic abortion, a large dose of IG may be of some value. After possible exposure, an antibody test should be performed immediately. Several assays (latex or enzyme-linked immunosorbent assay) are available for rapid determination of rubella antibody. If antibody is present, the woman is not susceptible and she can be reassured. If antibody is absent or there will be a significant delay in obtaining the result, the woman is considered susceptible. Then IG can be given in a total dose of 0.55 mL/kg at several sites. The antibody test is repeated after 1 month. A negative result indicates that rubella was prevented or exposure did not occur. A positive result (when the preinjection antibody test was negative) indicates that infection has occurred despite IG.

Tetanus, Tetanus Immunoglobulin, and Tetanus Antitoxin

Antitoxin in the treatment of tetanus was introduced in medicine by Behring and Kitasato[251] in 1890; large doses (50 to 100 mL) of serum from horses immunized with tetanus toxin were used. The dose gradually was increased to 300 to 500 mL, equivalent to 300 to 500 U of antitoxin. As means to increase the production and concentration of antitoxin developed and a high mortality rate persisted, the dosage of antitoxin was increased until doses as high as 200,000 IU, repeated at weekly intervals, were recommended.[251] Despite such heroic therapy, there was no solid proof of efficacy.

However, in 1960, Brown and colleagues,[48] using sequential analysis, found that the mortality rate was 49 per cent among 41 tetanus patients receiving 200,000 U of antitoxin and 76 per cent in 38 patients not receiving antitoxin, a statistically significant difference that established therapeutic efficacy. Extensive controlled studies established that mortality rates did not improve when doses of 10,000 to 500,000 U were used.[212, 352, 354, 355, 356] Similarly, Patel and associates[251] could find no difference in the mortality of tetanus using doses of antitoxin from 5000 to 60,000 U. Adequate blood levels of antitoxin were noted in all cases, even in fatal cases, with a dose of 10,000 U. In mild cases, no antitoxin was necessary. They and others have reported considerable differences in mortality rates, ranging from 0 to 98 per cent; this primarily depends on the severity rather than the dose of antitoxin.

Athavale[12] established that antitoxin was of benefit in tetanus neonatorum and in tetanus in children up to 12 years of age. Antitoxin affected the mortality rate in mild and moderate cases but not in severe cases. A dose of 10,000 IU was as effective as one of 30,000 IU.

The mechanism of action of antitoxin is to neutralize toxin prior to its arrival in the nervous system via the circulation. It also can neutralize toxin locally and prevent its systemic absorption. Thus, antitoxin should be given at the site of toxin production (e.g., at the site of a wound) and intravenously (in severe cases) or intramuscularly, the latter being reserved for less severe cases.

It was estimated that 750,000 annual doses of tetanus antitoxin were needed in the United Kingdom, which is equivalent to 2 million doses in the United States.[277] Serum sickness occurs in 6 to 14 per cent and fatal anaphylaxis in 1 of every 100,000 injections. Thus, hyperimmune human tetanus IG, first available in the early 1960s, gradually has replaced equine tetanus antitoxin.

Rubbo and Suri[276] and Rubinstein[277] showed that human tetanus IG given intramuscularly (5 to 10 U/kg) provides adequate circulating antitoxin levels and is maintained in the circulation for a considerably longer time than is equine tetanus antitoxin.

The efficacy of human tetanus IG is equivalent to that of equine tetanus antitoxin. McCracken and associates[222] compared the results of 500 U of tetanus IG with 10,000 U of tetanus antitoxin in the treatment of tetanus neonatorum. Among the 65 infants in each treatment group, there was no difference in severity, length of hospital stay, need for sedation or gavage feeding, or mortality rate (43 and 42 per cent, respectively). Blake and associates[38] analyzed 545 tetanus cases reported to the Centers for Disease Control and Prevention from 1965 to 1971 and could find no difference in outcome between those patients treated with equine tetanus antitoxin and those treated with tetanus IG.

Gupta and associates[134] gave tetanus IG intrathecally to alternate patients with early tetanus. Among 49 patients given intrathecal tetanus IG (250 U), three got worse and one died; among 48 patients given intramuscular tetanus IG (1000 U), 15 got worse and 10 died. There were no side effects. However, Herrero and associates[146] could not prove a benefit of intrathecal antitoxin in tetanus neonatorum. A meta-analysis of intrathecal therapy also cast doubt on its efficacy.[2]

Tetanus IG can be given along with tetanus toxoid (10 Lf U) for passive-active immunization. A dose of 250 U of tetanus IG given intramuscularly at a site different from that of the toxoid does not interfere with the active antibody response.[221]

Lee and Lederman[202] measured the antitetanus toxoid IgG in 29 lots of IVIG and showed considerable variability, although all lots had titers greater than 4 lu/mL (mean was 21 lu/mL). All lots would provide sufficient tetanus antibody if used at doses of 100 mg/kg as an alternative to tetanus IG or tetanus antitoxin.

Recommendations

PROPHYLAXIS. If a nonimmunized person sustains a serious injury or a bite, 250 to 500 U of tetanus IG should be given intramuscularly as soon as possible. The larger dose should be used if there is an extensive wound or delay in treatment. Alum-precipitated toxoid to initiate active immunity is given at a different site, using a separate syringe. If tetanus IG is unavailable, 3000 to 5000 U of tetanus antitoxin (equine) is given (after screening and testing the patient for serum sensitivity). Tetanus IG is available in individual vials containing 250 units each. Tetanus antitoxin is available in vials containing 1500 or 20,000 units each.

TREATMENT. In addition to antibiotics and wound management, tetanus IG in doses of 300 to 6000 U should be given, part infiltrated near the wound and the rest given intramuscularly.

If tetanus IG is unavailable, equine tetanus antitoxin should be given in a single dose of 50,000 to 100,000 U with 20,000 U given intravenously (after appropriate testing for sensitivity). In severe cases, 20,000 U of tetanus antitoxin should be given intravenously. Intrathecal tetanus IG or tetanus antitoxin usually is unnecessary and is not recommended. Upon recovery, primary immunization should be undertaken. In tetanus neonatorum, McCracken and associates[222] found that 500 IU of tetanus IG intramuscularly or 10,000 U of equine antitoxin were equally efficacious.

IVIG can be used as an alternative to tetanus IG or tetanus antitoxin. A minimal dose of 100 mg/kg is suggested.[202, 261]

Vaccinia, Smallpox, and Vaccinia Immunoglobulin

Although smallpox has been eradicated from the globe since 1979, the virus exists in government laboratories in the United States and Russia and vaccination still is being used on a limited basis (including in the United States military and individuals utilizing vaccinia vectors in research laboratories). Accordingly, passive immunization occasionally is necessary after laboratory accidents, after inadvertent vaccination of high-risk persons, or after exposure of high-risk persons to recently vaccinated persons.

Passive immunization against vaccinia was used as early as 1895, when Hlava and Honl[149] showed that school children could be protected from vaccinia by the injection of 3 to 10 mL of immune calf serum. At the same time, protective antibodies after vaccination and passive transmission of these antibodies from mothers to infants were demonstrated.[318] Thereafter, the effective prevention of smallpox by well-organized mass vaccine campaigns diminished interest in passive immunization.

Janeway, quoted by Enders,[103] in 1944 found neutralizing vaccinia antibody in IG, and Verlinde and Spaander[360] in 1966 found high titers of such antibodies in convalescent IG from recently vaccinated persons. Gispen and associates[117] in 1956 developed a human vaccinia IG that was shown not to interfere with active immunity, and they proposed its use with vaccine as prophylaxis against vaccinia encephalitis.

The value of human vaccinia IG in smallpox or disseminated vaccinia is based on the presence of viremia, which leads to secondary dissemination; administration of neutralizing antibody prevents or limits the spread of infection and thus modifies the clinical expression of the disease.

In 1955, Kempe and colleagues[21, 177] initiated a series of studies on the efficacy of human vaccinia IG in smallpox and vaccinia complications. They used a human vaccinia IG that was prepared from recently vaccinated donors with a neutralizing titer of 1:256 to 1:512, compared with the titers of 1:16 or 1:32 in standard IG. The households of new admissions to the Madras (India) Smallpox Hospital were visited, and alternate family contacts received human vaccinia IG (1.0 g in adults, 0.5 g in children).[176] After 25 days, eight cases of smallpox developed in 75 contacts not given human vaccinia IG and two cases developed in 56 contacts given human vaccinia IG, a significant difference. A similar, more extensive study disclosed 21 cases of smallpox (four severe) among 379 contacts serving as controls and five cases of smallpox (none severe) among 326 contacts given human vaccinia IG.[177]

Kempe[178] also reported the results of 300 cases of smallpox vaccination (vaccinia) complications treated with human vaccinia IG; these included 62 cases of generalized vaccinia, 132 cases of eczema vaccinatum, 23 cases of vaccinia necrosum, 12 cases of vaccinia encephalitis, and 28 cases of autoinoculation. In addition, human vaccinia IG was given prophylactically to 44 eczematoid children requiring smallpox vaccine (0.6 to 1.2 mL/kg). Human vaccinia IG did not affect the course of vaccinia encephalitis. Twenty-seven of 28 patients with autoinoculation who received human vaccinia IG did well. There were nine deaths among 132 patients with eczema vaccinatum given human vaccinia IG; this 7 per cent mortality rate compares favorably with the usual mortality rate of 30 to 40 per cent with supportive care only. All 62 patients with generalized vaccinia given human vaccinia IG did well, although four children required a second course. Among 23 patients with vaccinia necrosum who received human vaccinia IG, there were seven deaths (30 per cent); however, this is a generally fatal disease, and most of these patients had immune defects.[21] These results strongly supported the efficacy of human vaccinia IG and were confirmed subsequently by studies in Sweden[215] and the United Kingdom.[291]

Nanning[235] studied the effect of human vaccinia IG on postvaccinia encephalitis. He gave a placebo or 2 mL of human vaccinia IG to Dutch military recruits at the time of primary vaccination; there were three cases of encephalitis among 43,630 vaccinated recruits given human vaccinia IG, compared with 13 cases among 53,044 recruits in the control group. This 77 per cent reduction is statistically significant.

Recommendations

Nonimmunized patients exposed to smallpox virus should be given human vaccinia IG to prevent or modify the disease; it should be given intramuscularly at a dose of 0.3 mL/kg 12 to 24 hours after concomitant smallpox vaccine.[177] Human vaccinia IG no longer is manufactured in the United States but still is available from the Centers for Disease Control and Prevention.

Eczematous children who must be vaccinated should be given human vaccinia IG (0.3 mL/kg) intramuscularly simultaneously at another site. Eczematous children or other persons with extensive dermatitis inadvertently exposed to a recently vaccinated person also should receive human vaccinia IG (0.3 mL/kg).

Accidental vaccination or autoinoculation of the eye, eczema vaccinatum, severe generalized vaccinia, and vaccinia necrosum are all indications for human vaccinia IG. The initial dose is 0.6 mL/kg, but repeat doses may be necessary.

Human vaccinia IG is not indicated for established smallpox infections, postvaccinia encephalitis, or hypersensitivity and toxic rashes after vaccination.

Varicella, Herpes Zoster, and Varicella-Zoster Immunoglobulin

Immunoglobulin in Varicella

After the success of IG in the prevention of measles and hepatitis, IG was evaluated for the prevention of varicella. Although Funkhauser[111] in 1948 showed some beneficial effects of standard IG in prevention of varicella in an uncontrolled study, Greenberg[129] and Schaeffer and Toomey[282] were unable to prevent chickenpox in exposed children using doses of 2.5 to 20 mL.

Others reported anecdotal evidence for the efficacy of IG in large doses during the early stages of chickenpox and herpes zoster. These claims included prompt relief of pain in zoster[369] and rapid resolution of skin lesions.[200, 270] However, even high-titered IG (zoster IG) does not prevent dissemination of herpes zoster.[320]

Ross[273] in 1962 gave 242 children IG in doses of 0.1 to 0.6 mL/lb within 3 days of exposure to chickenpox; 209 similarly exposed, uninjected children were used as controls. The attack rate was the same (97 per cent) in both groups, indicating that IG does not prevent varicella under these conditions. However, with doses of IG above 0.2 mL/kg, the severity of the disease was reduced, as indicated by a decreased number of pox and lessened temperature. Children receiving the largest dose of IG (0.6 mL/lb) had maximal temperatures of 38.9° C (102° F), compared with 41.1° C (106° F) for the controls, and 40 pox versus 207 for the controls. Others also have reported similar but uncontrolled observations that IG modifies the severity of chickenpox.[159, 349]

Varicella-Zoster Immunoglobulin in Varicella

The prophylactic value of large IG doses in decreasing the incidence and severity of varicella led to the trial of high-titered plasma or IG preparations to prevent varicella.[16] These preparations include zoster IG and zoster immune plasma from convalescing zoster patients and varicella-zoster IG (VZIG) prepared from high-titered normal adults.

Brunell and associates[52] in 1969 selected convalescing zoster patients whose complement-fixing antibody titers were 1:256 or greater and prepared zoster IG from their plasma; this material had titers considerably higher than did standard IG. Exposed children from six families in which chickenpox was occurring were given zoster IG or IG at doses of 2 mL. None of six children receiving zoster IG developed chickenpox, whereas all six children given IG developed chickenpox. No antibody developed in the zoster IG–treated group, indicating that the disease was prevented.

Because this dose did not prevent varicella in leukemic children or other high-risk patients, a larger dose (5 mL) was used in a later study to modify or prevent varicella in eight of nine high-risk children successfully.[50, 51] Severe varicella developed in one child given a less-potent preparation of zoster IG. These observations were confirmed in two later studies. Judelsohn and associates[166] gave zoster IG to 56 exposed high-risk children; mild varicella occurred in seven patients and was prevented in the others, most of whom were susceptible as determined by absence of serum antibody. Gershon and associates[116] gave zoster IG to 15 seronegative high-risk exposed children; varicella was severe in 1, mild in 9, and subclinical in 5. Subclinical infection was determined by the acquisition of membrane antibody, detected by fluorescent microscopy. Orenstein and associates[246] studied 553 exposed, high-risk patients who received zoster IG of two different titers (1:1280 vs. 1:2560 or greater). They found that the clinical attack rate after zoster IG correlated with the type of exposure (36 per cent with a household exposure, 7.7 per cent with a hospital exposure, and 0 per cent with a school exposure developed varicella), the rise in antibody titer (45 per cent of patients without a fourfold titer increase became ill, compared with 22 per cent of patients with a fourfold or greater rise in titer), and the titer of the administrated zoster IG (there were significantly more complications and deaths among recipients of the lower-titer zoster IG).

Because of the limited supply of zoster IG and zoster immune plasma, VZIG from normal adults has become the commercially available product in the United States. Zaia and associates[383] compared the efficacy of zoster IG and VZIG in immunocompromised children exposed to varicella. The varicella attack rates and clinical severity of the recipients did not differ significantly. There was a higher incidence of subclinical infection, as indicated by a rise in antibody titer in the zoster IG recipients (31.3 per cent), than in the VZIG recipients (16 per cent). A larger dose of VZIG (2.5 mL/10 kg vs. 1.25 mL/10 kg) reduced the frequency of subclinical infection (from 20 to 4.3 per cent). Several high-risk patients with demonstrable serum antibody at exposure developed varicella, indicating that history-negative seropositive patients are at risk for clinical varicella-zoster virus infection and should be given zoster IG, regardless of antibody titer.

Intravenous Immunoglobulin in Varicella

Paryani and associates in 1984[248, 249] observed that eight patients given IVIG at standard doses (200 to 300 mg/kg) achieved varicella-zoster virus antibody titers comparable with those achieved by persons given intramuscular VZIG at standard doses, despite the lower titer of antibody in the IVIG. This is because of the large quantity of antibody administered and the complete availability of the IVIG. Chen and Liang[74] successfully prevented chickenpox in children with leukemia by a single dose of 200 mg/kg of IVIG. This experience suggests that IVIG can be used prophylactically instead of intramuscular VZIG, particularly in situations in which intramuscular injections are contraindicated because of thrombocytopenia.

Immunodeficient patients (including HIV-infected patients) receiving regular infusions of IVIG (>200 mg/kg/month) rarely get chickenpox after exposure. When chickenpox does occur, the onset is delayed or the severity is modified.

Recommendations

For normal children exposed to varicella, standard IG can be expected to modify the disease and VZIG to prevent it.[50] However, because varicella is a mild disease in most children, prophylaxis usually is not indicated. If the child is older than 12 months of age, varicella vaccine can be given.

In high-risk immunocompromised children and in high-risk adults, the decision to administer VZIG is based on the likelihood of susceptibility, the nature of the exposure (Table 238–8), and the risk of developing varicella (Table 238–9). VZIG is expensive ($100 for 125 IU; up to $500 for an adult weighing more than 40 kg), and the modified infection that ensues may not lead to lifelong immunity and may increase the risk of developing zoster later in life.

DETERMINATION OF SUSCEPTIBILITY. Susceptibility usually is determined from historic information elicited by an experienced interviewer. Varicella-zoster virus antibody tests to determine varicella susceptibility are not widely available and are often unreliable. Complement fixation, fluorescent antibody, enzyme-linked immunosorbent assay, and neutralizing antibody tests are available, but their results may be negative despite immunity and, when positive, may not indicate immunity, particularly in neonates and immunocompromised subjects. Table 238–10 summarizes the determination of susceptibility.

TABLE 238–8. Exposure Criteria for Which Varicella-Zoster Immunoglobulin (VZIG) Is Indicated*

1. One of the following type of exposures to persons with chicken pox or zoster:
   - a. *Household*—residing in the same household
   - b. *Playmate contact*—>1 hour of play indoors
   - c. *Hospital*
     - **Varicella:**
       - a. In same 2- to 4-bed room or adjacent beds in a large ward
       - b. Face-to-face contact with an infectious staff member or patient
       - c. Visit by a patient deemed contagious
     - **Zoster:** Intimate contact (e.g., touching, hugging) with a person deemed contagious
   - d. *Newborn infant*—onset of varicella in mother 5 days or less before delivery or within 48 hours after delivery

   and
2. Time elapsed after exposure is such that VZIG can be administered within 96 hours but preferably sooner

*Patients should meet both criteria.

From Centers for Disease Control: Varicella zoster immune globulin for the prevention of chickenpox: Recommendations of the Immunization Practices Advisory Committee. Ann. Intern. Med. *100*:859–865, 1984.

TABLE 238–9. Candidates for Varicella-Zoster Immunoglobulin (VZIG) Provided Significant Exposure* Has Occurred

- Immunocompromised children without history of chicken pox*
- Susceptible, pregnant women
- Newborn infant whose mother had onset of chicken pox within 5 days before delivery or 48 hours after delivery
- Hospitalized premature infants (≥28 weeks' gestation) whose mother has no history of chicken pox
- Hospitalized premature infants (<weeks' gestation or ≤1000 g), regardless of maternal history

*Immunocompromised adolescents and adults are likely to be immune, but if they are susceptible, they also should receive IVIG.

With the exception of bone marrow transplant recipients, healthy and immunocompromised persons who by history have had prior varicella infection are considered immune. Healthy adults and children 15 years of age and older with a negative or uncertain history generally are considered immune; however, those who are immunocompromised are considered susceptible. Approximately 85 to 95 per cent of adults and children 15 years of age or older with a negative or uncertain history of prior varicella are immune, particularly those who are older siblings in large families and those whose children have had varicella. Children who are younger than 15 years of age and do not have a history of varicella are considered susceptible, unless proven otherwise using a sensitive serologic assay; however, results of these assays must be interpreted cautiously in immunocompromised children. Children or adults who have received bone marrow transplants should be considered susceptible to varicella, regardless of prior history of the disease in the donor or recipient. Bone marrow transplant recipients who develop varicella or herpes zoster after transplantation subsequently can be considered immune.

NORMAL CHILDREN. As noted, prophylaxis for most normal children is not indicated, particularly with the availability of vaccine for prevention and acyclovir for treatment. However, special circumstances (e.g., future travel, surgery, risk of exposure of an immunocompromised sibling) may require its use; the dose is identical to that for immunocompromised children.

IMMUNOCOMPROMISED CHILDREN. The principal use of VZIG is after exposure to zoster or chickenpox (see Table 238–8) of susceptible immunocompromised children. This includes children with primary and secondary immunodeficiencies (including symptomatic HIV infection), with neoplastic diseases, and receiving immunosuppressive therapy (including systemic [not aerosolized] corticosteroids at a dose of 1 mg/kg/day or greater).[189] VZIG only may modify varicella rather than prevent it. Although children with neoplastic disease and children receiving immunosuppressive therapy and with definitive history of varicella are considered immune, patients with primary antibody or cellular immunodeficiency or children receiving bone marrow transplants should be considered susceptible, regardless of prior history.

NEWBORNS. VZIG is recommended for all newborns whose mother develops varicella within 5 days before or 48 hours after delivery, regardless of whether the mother received VZIG. Varicella is life-threatening in these newborns, and VZIG may be expected to modify but not prevent the disease. VZIG probably is unnecessary for term newborns whose mothers develop varicella more than 5 days before

TABLE 238–10. Determination of Susceptibility to Varicella in Some Selected Situations*

Group	Immune Status	Carefully Obtained Prior History of Varicella	Detectable Varicella Antibody by a Reliable Test	Susceptibility Status
Children (<15 years of age)	Immunocompromised	Yes →	Unnecessary to perform →	Immune
		No or unknown† →	† →	Susceptible
Adolescents and adults (≥15 years of age)	Normal	Yes →	Unnecessary to perform →	Immune
		No or unknown →	Not performed →	Generally consider immune‡
			Yes →	Immune
			No →	Susceptible
	Immunocompromised	Yes →	Unnecessary to perform →	Immune
		No or unknown† →	† →	Consider susceptible‡

*This table provides general guidelines for determining susceptibility in frequently encountered situations. Not all potential scenarios are considered. In all situations, individual judgment also should be used. See text for details.

†Some immunocompromised persons with detectable antibody before varicella-zoster immunoglobulin administration, presumably passively transferred by recent transfusions, have developed clinical varicella. Until further evaluation of serologic tests in the immunocompromised has been completed, one may have to rely on a carefully obtained clinical history by an experienced interviewer to determine susceptibility (i.e., the absence of a history of clinical varicella).

‡More than 85 per cent and probably more than 95 per cent of such persons are immune.

From Centers for Disease Control: Varicella zoster immune globulin for the prevention of chickenpox: Recommendations of the Immunization Practices Advisory Committee. Ann. Intern. Med. *100*:859–865, 1984.

delivery, inasmuch as they will receive some transplacental antibody and will be protected from severe disease.

Postnatal exposure to varicella usually does not represent a threat to normal infants, particularly if the mother has had varicella, because transplacental antibodies will modify or protect the infant. However, for exposed infants born at less than 28 weeks' gestation or weighing less than 1000 g, VZIG is recommended because transplacental passage of IgG is lessened significantly and the infant's cellular immune system is immature. In larger exposed premature infants, VZIG is recommended for those whose mothers do not have a history of varicella.

Neonates exposed by a staff member in the neonatal intensive care unit should be tested for varicella antibodies and given VZIG if susceptible. Many such infants, despite maternal seropositivity, are seronegative, particularly premature infants who are several weeks old.[119]

IMMUNOCOMPROMISED ADULTS. Exposed immunocompromised adults who are believed susceptible should receive VZIG. Most probably are immune, but, in this high-risk situation, prophylaxis is justified.

NORMAL ADULTS. Adults are more susceptible to severe varicella than are children; the death rate from varicella in adults is 50 per 100,000 compared with 2 per 100,000 in children, and the complication rate is increased by 9 to 25 times. Accordingly, some exposed adults, depending on their health and the need to avoid or modify varicella, are candidates for VZIG. Although the cost of VZIG is substantial, under certain circumstances, the benefits clearly outweigh this expense. Other options are to give varicella vaccine immediately, acyclovir prophylactically, or acyclovir at the first onset of infection.

PREGNANT WOMEN. Exposed pregnant women should be considered the same as other normal exposed adults. There is no evidence that VZIG given during pregnancy prevents intrauterine, congenital, or neonatal varicella. It is unlikely that VZIG given to a pregnant woman with varicella within 5 days of delivery will result in sufficient transplacental passage to modify or prevent varicella in her infant. Accordingly, the infant should be given VZIG regardless of whether the mother has received VZIG prenatally.

DOSAGE. VZIG should be given as soon as possible after exposure but probably is effective if given within 4 or 5 days after exposure. It is of no value in the treatment of varicella or zoster. It probably confers protection for 3 weeks. Antibody determinations before and 2 months after administration may help to determine the immune status of the individual and whether subclinical or modified infection has resulted.

VZIG is supplied in vials of 125 units (about 1.25 mL). The recommended dose is 125 units/10 kg, up to a maximum of 625 units (five vials). The minimum dose is 125 units. The necessity for higher doses in adults weighing more than 50 kg is not established. The cost is about $100 per vial. The product is prepared by the Massachusetts Public Health Biologic Laboratories and is distributed through pharmacies and regional distribution centers of the American Red Cross.[70] If VZIG is unavailable or unaffordable, IVIG or IG at 200 mg/kg can be substituted.

SPECIAL ANTIBODY PREPARATIONS FOR NONINFECTIOUS USE

Rho(D) Immunoglobulin

Rho(D) IG (anti-D IG, RhoGAM) is high-titer human anti-rhesus immune serum globulin used in the prevention of Rh and hemolytic disease of newborns. It is given to Rh-negative mothers after delivery of an Rh-positive infant or after miscarriage or abortion. It also should be used after inadvertent transfusion of an Rh-negative person with Rh-positive blood.

Anti-D IG has been used successfully in the treatment of immune thrombocytopenic purpura in Rh-positive persons.[57] The anti-D IG coats the red blood cells, which in turn causes reticuloendothelial blockade, similar to the effect of high-dose IVIG in this disorder.

Immunosuppressive Antibodies

Two antibodies—one a mouse monoclonal antibody directed against human CD3 lymphocytes (OKT3-Muromonab) and another, antithymocyte globulin (Atgam), a polyclonal equine preparation—are used for immunosuppression, particularly for transplantation procedures.

Antivenins

Three equine antivenins are commercially available for bites by black widow spiders and coral snakes and other poisonous snakes in the United States. Antivenins for other creature bites (e.g., of scorpions) are available in other countries.[313]

Digoxin Antibody

An ovine (sheep) antibody fragment (Fab portion of IgG) binds to digoxin and digitoxin (Digibind) and is of value in the treatment of digitalis toxicity or accidental ingestion.[307] Fragmentation of the antibody results in a rapid catabolism; after its intravenous infusion, it combines with the drug and removes it rapidly from the serum. A goat Fab fragment to colchicine was used successfully to treat a woman with colchicine overdose.[24]

FUTURE DIRECTIONS IN PASSIVE IMMUNITY

Several high-titered human IGs are being tested for clinical efficacy; these include a group B streptococcal IVIG (for premature infants), a bacterial polysaccharide IG (for high-risk infants), a *Pseudomonas* IVIG (for burn patients), and an HIV-IVIG (for HIV treatment and prevention). RSV-IVIG was discussed previously.

The use of monoclonal antibodies, both human and murine, to treat specific infections should be forthcoming. These monoclonal antibodies may be used alone or added to polyvalent IVIG to increase the titer to a specific microorganism.

The use of monoclonal antibodies to neutralize cells, bind to receptors, and detoxify certain drugs is expected. Monoclonal anti-idiotypic antibodies also may be used to suppress autoimmune disease or inhibit a specific harmful autoantibody.

The use of monoclonal antibodies directed to specific tumor cells or organs to deliver radioisotopes or chemotherapeutic agents is feasible. Such antibodies also could be used diagnostically for tumor cell or infection localization.

Chimeric antibodies containing the antigen-reactive site of a mouse monoclonal antibody attached to the constant regions of a human antibody can be made; these "humanized" monoclonals have a longer half-life and better complement-fixation ability than the intact mouse monoclonal antibody.

Engineered antibodies, made by DNA recombinational techniques from selected light and heavy chain genes, may permit the synthesis of very high-titered therapeutic antibodies.[54]

References

1. Abernathy, R. S., Strem, E. L., and Good, R. A.: Chronic asthma in childhood: Double blind controlled study of treatment with gamma globulin. Pediatrics *21*:980–993, 1958.
2. Abrutyn, E., and Berlin, J. A.: Intrathecal therapy in tetanus: A meta-analysis. J. A. M. A. *266*:2262–2267, 1991.
3. Abzug, M. G., Keyserling, H. L., Lee, M. L., et al.: Neonatal enterovirus infection: Virology, serology, and effects of intravenous immune globulin. Clin. Infect. Dis. *20*:1201–1206, 1995.
4. Acute Hepatic Failure Study Group: Failure of specific immunotherapy in fulminant type B hepatitis. Ann. Intern. Med. *86*:272–277, 1977.
5. Aguado, J. M., Gomez-Sanchez, M. A., Lumbreras, C., et al.: Prospective randomized trial of efficacy of ganciclovir versus that of anti-cytomegalovirus (CMV) immunoglobulin to prevent CMV disease in CMV-seropositive heart transplant recipients treated with OKT3. Antimicrob. Agents Chemother. *39*:1643–1645, 1995.
6. Amer, J., Ott, E., Ibbott, F. A., et al.: The effect of monthly gamma globulin administration on morbidity and mortality from infection in premature infants during the first year of life. Pediatrics *32*:4–9, 1963.
7. American Academy of Pediatrics: Active and passive immunization. *In* Peter, G. (ed.): 1994 Red Book: Report of the Committee on Infectious Diseases. 23rd ed. Elk Grove Village, IL, American Academy of Pediatrics, 1994, pp. 7–71.
8. Ammann, A. J., and Stiehm, E. R.: Immune globulin levels in colostrum and breast milk, and serum from formula and breast fed newborns. Proc. Soc. Exp. Biol. Med. *122*:1098–1100, 1966.
9. Ammann, A. J., Ashman, R. F., Buckley, R. H., et al.: Use of intravenous gamma globulin in antibody immunodeficiency: Results of a multicenter controlled trial. Clin. Immunol. Immunopathol. *22*:60–67, 1982.
10. Apfelzweig, R., Piszkiewicz, D., and Hooper, J. A.: Immunoglobulin A concentrations in commercial immune globulins. J. Clin. Immunol. *7*:46–50, 1987.
11. Ashida, E. R., and Saxon, A.: Home intravenous immunoglobulin infusion by self-infusion. J. Clin. Immunol. *6*:306–309, 1986.
12. Athavale, V. B.: Role of tetanus antitoxin in the treatment of tetanus in children. J. Pediatr. *68*:289–293, 1966.
13. Babes, V., and Lepp, M.: Recherches sur la vaccination antirabique. Ann. Inst. Pasteur *3*:385–390, 1889.
14. Baker, C. J., Melish, M. E., Hall, R. T., et al.: Intravenous immune globulin for the prevention of nosocomial infection in low-birth-weight neonates. N. Engl. J. Med. *327*:213–219, 1992.
15. Balagtos, R. C., Nelson, K. E., Levin, S., et al.: Treatment of pertussis with pertussis immune globulin. J. Pediatr. *79*:203–208, 1971.
16. Balfour, H. H., Jr., Groth, K. E., McCullough, J., et al.: Prevention or modification of varicella using zoster immune plasma. Am. J. Dis. Child. *131*:693–696, 1977.
17. Balk, A. H. W., Weimar, P. H., Rothbarth, K., et al.: Passive immunization against cytomegalovirus in allograft recipients: The Rotterdam Heart Transplant Program experience. Infection *21*:195–200, 1993.
18. Ballow, M.: Mechanisms of action of intravenous immune globulin. Pediatr. Infect. Dis. J. *13*:806–811, 1994.
19. Ballow, M., Cates, K. L., Rowe, J. C., et al.: Development of the immune system in very low birth weight (less than 1500 g) premature infants: Concentrations of plasma immunoglobulins and patterns of infections. Pediatr. Res. *20*:899–904, 1986.
20. Baltazard, M., and Bahmanyar, M.: Essai pratique du sérum antirabique chez les mordus par loups enragés. Bull. W. H. O. *13*:747–772, 1955.
21. Barbero, G. J., Gray, A., Scott, T. F. M., et al.: Vaccinia gangrenosa treated with hyperimmune vaccinial gamma globulin. Pediatrics *16*:609–618, 1955.
22. Barnes, G. L., Doyle, L. W., Hewson, P. H., et al.: A randomised trial of oral gammaglobulin in low birth weight infants infected with rotavirus. Lancet *1*:1371–1373, 1982.
23. Baron, S., Barnett, E. V., Goldsmith, R. S., et al.: Prophylaxis of infections by gamma globulin. Am. J. Hyg. 79:186–195, 1964.
24. Baud, F. J., Sabouraud, A., Vicaut, E., et al.: Treatment of severe colchicine overdose with colchicine-specific Fab fragments. N. Engl. J. Med. *332*:642–645, 1995.
25. Baumgartner, J. D., Glauser, M. P., McCutchan, J. A., et al.: Prevention of gram negative shock and death in surgical patients by antibody to endotoxin core glycolipid. Lancet *2*:59–63, 1985.
26. Beasley, R. P., Hwang, L. Y., Stevens, C. E., et al.: Efficacy of hepatitis B immune globulin for prevention of perinatal transmission of the hepatitis B virus carrier state: Final report of a randomized double blind, placebo controlled trial. Hepatology *3*:135–141, 1983.
27. Beasley, R. P., Lin, C. C., Wang, K. Y., et al.: Hepatitis B immune globulin (HBIG) efficacy in the interruption of perinatal transmission of hepatitis B virus carrier state. Lancet *2*:388–392, 1981.
28. Bell, R., Shei, A., McDonald, J. A., et al.: The role of CMV immune prophylaxis in patients at risk for primary CMV infection following orthoptic liver transplantation. Transplant. Proc. *21*:3781–3782, 1989.
29. Berg, B. O.: Syndrome of infant botulism. Pediatrics *59*:321–322, 1977.
30. Berger, M., Cupps, T. R., and Fauci, A.: Immunoglobulin replacement therapy by slow subcutaneous infusion. Ann. Intern. Med. *93*:55–56, 1980.
31. Bernatowska, E., Madalinski, K., Janowicz, W., et al.: Results of a prospective controlled two dose crossover study with intravenous immunoglobulin and comparison (retrospective) with plasma treatment. Clin. Immunol. Immunopathol. *43*:153–162, 1987.
32. Bernstein, L. J., Krieger, B. Z., Novic, B. et al.: Bacterial infections in acquired immunodeficiency syndrome of children. Pediatr. Infect. Dis. *4*:472–475, 1985.

33. Björkander, J., Hammarstrom, L., Smith, C. I. E., et al.: Immunoglobulin prophylaxis in patients with antibody deficiency syndromes and anti IgA antibodies. J. Clin. Immunol. *7*:8–15, 1987.
34. Björkander, J., Bengtsson, U., Oxelius, V. A., et al.: Symptoms and efficacy of intravenous immunoglobulin prophylaxis in patients with low serum levels of IgG subclasses. J. Allergy Clin. Immunol. *77*:124–127, 1986.
35. Björkander, J., Cunningham-Rundles, C., and Ludon, P.: Intravenous immunoglobulin prophylaxis causing liver damage in 16 of 77 patients with hypogammaglobulinemia or IgG subclass deficiency. Am. J. Med. *84*:107–111, 1988.
36. Bjoro, K., Froland, S. S., Yun, Z., et al.: Hepatitis C infection in patients with contaminated immune globulin. N. Engl. J. Med. *331*:1607–1611, 1994.
37. Black, F. L., and Yannet, H.: Inapparent measles after gamma globulin administration. J. A. M. A. *173*:87–92, 1960.
38. Blake, P. A., Feldman, R. A., Buchanan, T. M., et al.: Serologic therapy of tetanus in the United States, 1965–1971. J. A. M. A. *235*:42–44, 1976.
39. Bloxsom, A.: Use of immune serum globulin (human) as prophylaxis against poliomyelitis. Texas Med. *74*:468–470, 1949.
40. Blum, P. M., Phelps, D. L., Ank, B. J., et al.: Survival of oral human immune serum globulin in the gastrointestinal tract of low birth weight infants. Pediatr. Res. *15*:1256–1260, 1981.
41. Bodey, G. P., Nies, B. A., Mohberg, N. R., et al.: Use of gamma globulin in infection in acute leukemia patients. J. A. M. A. *190*:1099–1102, 1964.
42. Bodian, D.: Experimental studies on passive immunization against poliomyelitis. I. Protection with human gamma globulin against intramuscular inoculation and combined passive and active immunization. Am. J. Hyg. *54*:132–143, 1951.
43. Bodian, D.: Neutralization of three immunological types of poliomyelitis virus by human gamma globulin. Proc. Soc. Exp. Biol. Med. *72*:259–261, 1949.
44. Borowitz, S. M., and Saulsbury, F. T.: Treatment of chronic cryptosporidial infection with orally administered human serum immune globulin. J. Pediatr. *119*:593–595, 1991.
45. Bowden, R. A., Sayers, M., Flournoy, N., et al.: Cytomegalovirus immune globulin and seronegative blood products to prevent primary cytomegalovirus infection after marrow transplantation. N. Engl. J. Med. *314*:1006–1010, 1986.
46. Bowman, C. A., Cohen, B. J., Norfolk, D. R., et al.: Red cell aplasia associated with human parvovirus B19 and HIV infection: Failure to respond clinically to intravenous immunoglobulin. AIDS *4*:1038–1039, 1990.
47. Brody, J. A., Sever, J. L., and Schiff, G. M.: Prevention of rubella by gamma globulin during an epidemic in Barrow, Alaska, in 1964. N. Engl. J. Med. *272*:127–129, 1965.
48. Brown, A., Mohamed, S. D., Montgomery, R. D., et al.: Value of a large dose of antitoxin in clinical tetanus. Lancet 2:227–230, 1960.
49. Brox, A. G., Courmoyer, D., Sternbach, M., et al.: Hemolytic anemia following intravenous immunoglobulin administration. Am. J. Med. *83*:633–635, 1987.
50. Brunell, P. A., and Gershon, A. A.: Passive immunization against varicella zoster infections. J. Infect. Dis. *127*:415–423, 1973.
51. Brunell, P. A., Gershon, A. A., Hughes, W. T., et al.: Prevention of varicella in high risk children: A collaborative study. Pediatrics *50*:718–722, 1972.
52. Brunell, P. A., Ross, A., Miller, L. H., et al.: Prevention of varicella by zoster immune globulin. N. Engl. J. Med. *280*:1191–1194, 1969.
53. Buckley, R. H., and Schiff, R. I.: The use of intravenous immune globulin in immunodeficiency diseases. N. Engl. J. Med. 325:110–117, 1991.
54. Burton, D. R., Pyati, J., Koduri, R., et al.: Efficient neutralization of primary isolates of HIV-1 by a recombinant human monoclonal antibody. Science *266*:1024–1027, 1994.
55. Bussel, J. B., and Himi, J. S.: Isolated thrombocytopenia in patients infected with HIV: Treatment with intravenous gammaglobulin. Am. J. Hematol. *28*:79–84, 1988.
56. Bussel, J. B., Lalezari, P., Hilgartner, M., et al.: Reversal of neutropenia with intravenous immunoglobulin in autoimmune hemolytic anaemia. Br. J. Haematol. *60*:387–388, 1985.
57. Bussel, J. B., Graziano, J. N., Kimberly, R. P., et al.: Intravenous anti-D treatment of immune thrombocytopenic purpura: Analysis of efficacy, toxicity, and mechanism of effect. Blood *77*:1884–1893, 1991.
58. Bussel, J. B.: Intravenous gammaglobulin in the prophylaxis of late sepsis in very low birth weight infants: Preliminary results of a randomized, double blind, placebo controlled trial. Rev. Infect. Dis. *12*:S457–S462, 1990.
59. Cabasso, V. J., Loofbourow, J. C., Roby, R. E., et al.: Rabies immune globulin of human origin: Preparation and dosage determination in non exposed volunteer subjects. Bull. W. H. O. *45*:303–315, 1971.
60. Calandra, T., Glauser, M. P., Schellekens, J., et al.: Treatment of gram negative septic shock with human IgG antibody to *Escherichia coli* J5: A prospective, double blind, randomized trial. J. Infect. Dis. *158*:312–319, 1988.
61. Calvelli, T. A., and Rubinstein, A.: Intravenous gamma globulin in infant acquired immunodeficiency syndrome. Pediatr. Infect. Dis. *5*:S207–S210, 1986.
62. Cannon, R. A., Blum, P. M., Ament, M. E., et al.: Reversal of enterocolitis associated combined immunodeficiency by plasma therapy. J. Pediatr. *101*:711–717, 1982.
63. Carl, M., Francis, D. P., and Maynard, J. E.: Food borne hepatitis A: Recommendations for control. J. Infect. Dis. *148*:1133–1135, 1983.
64. Casadevall, A., and Scharff, M. D.: Return to the past: The case for antibody-based therapies in infectious diseases. Clin. Infect. Dis. *21*:150–161, 1995.
65. Cenci, F.: Alcune esperienze di sieroimmunizzazione e sieroterapia nel morbillo. Riv. Clin. Pediatr. *5*:1017–1025, 1907.
66. Centers for Disease Control: Botulism in the United States, 1899–1977. Handbook for Epidemiologists, Clinicians and Laboratory Workers. May 1979.
67. Centers for Disease Control: Postexposure prophylaxis of hepatitis B. M. M. W. R. *33*:285–290, 1984.
68. Centers for Disease Control: Rabies prevention in the United States 1984: Recommendations of the Immunization Practices Advisory Committee. M. M. W. R. *33*:393–402, 1984.
69. Centers for Disease Control: Recommendations for protection against viral hepatitis. M. M. W. R. *34*:313–324, 329, 335, 1985.
70. Centers for Disease Control: Varicella zoster immune globulin for the prevention of chickenpox: Recommendations of the Immunization Practices Advisory Committee. Ann. Intern. Med. *100*:859–865, 1984.
71. Centers for Disease Control: Outbreak of hepatitis C associated with intravenous immunoglobulin adminstration: United States, October 1993–June 1994. M. M. W. R. *43*:505–508, 1994.
72. Chapel, H. M., Lee, M., Hargreaves, R., et al.: Randomized trial of intravenous immunoglobulin as prophylaxis against infection in plateau-phase multiple myeloma. Lancet *343*:1059–1063, 1994.
73. Chehimi, H., Peppard, J., and Immanuel, D.: Selection of an intravenous immunoglobulin for immunoprophylaxis of cytomegalovirus infections: An in vitro comparison of currently available and previously effective immune globulins. Bone Marrow Transplant. *2*:395–402, 1987.
74. Chen, S. H., and Liang, D. C.: Intravenous immunoglobulin prophylaxis in children with acute leukemia following exposure to varicella. Pediatr. Hematol. Oncol. *9*:347–351, 1992.
75. Chirico, G., Rondini, G., Plebani, A., et al.: Intravenous gammaglobulin therapy for prophylaxis of infection in high risk neonates. J. Pediatr. *110*:437–442, 1987.
76. Chung, W. K., Yoo, J. Y., Sun, H. S., et al.: Prevention of perinatal transmission of hepatitis B virus: A comparison between the efficacy of passive and passive active immunization in Korea. J. Infect. Dis. *151*:280–286, 1985.
77. Chutivongse, S., and Wilde, H.: Postexposure rabies vaccination during pregnancy: Experience with 21 patients. Vaccine *7*:546–548, 1989.
78. Clapp, D. W., Kliegman, R. M., Baley, J. E., et al.: Use of intravenously administered immune globulin to prevent nosocomial sepsis in low birth weight infants: Report of a pilot study. J. Pediatr. *115*:973–978, 1989.
79. Cofer, J. B., Morris, C. A., Sutker, W. L., et al.: The effect of prophylactic immune globulin on cytomegalovirus infection and liver transplants. *In* Imbach, P. (ed.): Immunotherapy with IVIG. London, Academic Press, 1991, pp. 229–235.
80. Cohen, S., McGregor, I. A., and Carrington, S.: Gamma globulin and acquired immunity to human malaria. Nature *192*:733–737, 1961.
81. Collins, M. S., Tasy, G. C., Hector, R. F., et al.: Immunoglobulin G: Potentiation of tobramycin and azlocillin in the treatment of *Pseudomonas aeruginosa* sepsis in neutropenic mice and neutralization of exotoxin A in vivo. Rev. Infect. Dis. *8*:S420–S425, 1986.
82. Conway, S. P., Gillies, D. R. N., and Docherty, A.: Neonatal infection in premature infants and use of human immunoglobulin. Arch. Dis. Child. *62*:1252–1256, 1987.
83. Cooperative Group for the Study of Immunoglobulin in Chronic Lymphocytic Leukemia: Intravenous immunoglobulin for the prevention of infection in chronic lymphocytic leukemia. N. Engl. J. Med. *319*:902–907, 1988.
84. Copelon, E. A., and Tutschka, P. J.: Immunoglobulin in bone marrow transplantation. *In* Morell, A., and Nydegger, U. E. (eds.): Clinical Use of Intravenous Immunoglobulins. New York, Academic Press, 1986, pp. 117–121.
85. Craig, R. D. P.: Immunotherapy for severe burns in children. Plast. Reconstr. Surg. *35*:263–270, 1965.
86. Crennan, J. M., Van Scoy, R. E., McKenna, C. H., et al.: Echovirus polymyositis in patients with hypogammaglobulinemia: Failure of high dose intravenous gammaglobulin therapy and review of the literature. Am. J. Med. *81*:35–42, 1986.
87. Cunningham-Rundles, C., Siegal, F. P., Smithwick, E. M., et al.: Efficacy of intravenous immunoglobulin in primary humoral immunodeficiency disease. Ann. Intern. Med. *101*:435–439, 1984.
88. Cunningham-Rundles, C., Bjorkander, J., and Hanson, L. A.: Therapeutic use of an IgA depleted intravenous immunoglobulin patient. *In* Morell, A., and Nydegger, U. E. (eds.): Clinical Use of Intravenous Immunoglobulin. London, Academic Press, 1986, pp. 87–96.
89. Dagan, R., Schwartz, R. H., Insel, R. A., et al.: Severe diffuse adenovirus 7a pneumonia in a child with combined immunodeficiency: Possible therapeutic effect of human immune serum globulin containing specific neutralizing antibody. Pediatr. Infect. Dis. *3*:246–251, 1984.
90. DeSimone, C., Delogu, G., and Corbetta, G.: Intravenous immunoglobu-

lins in association with antibiotics: A therapeutic trial in septic intensive care unit patients. Crit. Care Med. *16*:23–26, 1988.

91. Desmyter, J., Bradburne, A. F., Vermylen, C., et al.: Hepatitis B immunoglobulin in prevention of HBs anti genemia in haemodialysis patients. Lancet *2*:377–379, 1975.
92. Diamond, E. F., Purugganan, H. B., and Choi, H. J.: Effect of prophylactic administration on infection morbidity in premature infants. Illinois Med. J. *130*:668–670, 1966.
93. Dolman, C. E., and Hda, H.: Type E botulism: Its epidemiology, prevention and specific treatment. Can. J. Public Health *54*:293–308, 1963.
94. Drake, M. E., Barondess, J. A., Bashe, W. J., Jr., et al.: Failure of convalescent gamma globulin to protect against homologous serum hepatitis. J. A. M. A. *152*:690–693, 1953.
95. Duhem, C., Dicato, M. A., and Ries, F.: Side-effects of intravenous immune globulins. Clin. Exp. Immunol. *97*:79–83, 1994.
96. Duncan, G. G., Christian, H. A., and Stokes, J., Jr.: An evaluation of immune serum globulin as a prophylactic agent against homologous serum hepatitis. Am. J. Med. Sci. *213*:53–57, 1947.
97. Dwyer, J. M.: Manipulating the immune system with immune globulin. N. Engl. J. Med. *326*:107–116, 1992.
98. Ebina, T., Umezu, K., Ohyama, S., et al.: Prevention of rotavirus infection by cow colostrum containing antibody against human rotavirus. Lancet *2*:1029–1030, 1983.
99. Eibl, M. M., Wolf, H. M., Furnkranz, H., et al.: Prevention of necrotizing enterocolitis in low birth weight infants by IgA-IgG feeding. N. Engl. J. Med. *319*:1–7, 1988.
100. Ellenberg, S. S., Epstein, J. S., Fratantoni, J. C., et al.: A trial of RSV immune globulin in infants and young children: The FDA's view. N. Engl. J. Med. *331*:203–204, 1994.
101. Ellis, E. F., and Henney, C. S.: Adverse reactions following administration of human gamma globulin. J. Allergy *43*:45–54, 1969.
102. Emanuel, D., Cunningham, I., Jules Elysee, K., et al.: Cytomegalovirus pneumonia after bone marrow transplantation successfully treated with the combination of ganciclovir and high dose intravenous immune globulin. Ann. Intern. Med. *109*:777–782, 1988.
103. Enders, J. F.: Chemical, clinical, and immunological studies on the products of human plasma fractionation. X. The concentrations of certain antibodies in globulin fractions derived from human blood plasma. J. Clin. Invest. *23*:510–530, 1944.
104. Erlendsson, K., Swartz, T., and Dwyer, J. M.: Successful reversal of echovirus encephalitis in X-linked hypogammaglobulinemia by intraventricular administration of immunoglobulin. N. Engl. J. Med. *312*:351–353, 1985.
105. Expert Committee on Rabies: Hyperimmune antirabies serum. W. H. O. Tech. Rep. Ser. *28*:23–25, 1950.
106. Fanaroff, A. A., Korones, S. B., Wright, L. L., et al.: A controlled trial of intravenous immune globulin to reduce nosocomial infections in very low-birth-weight infants. N. Engl. J. Med. *330*:1107–1113, 1994.
107. Fibiger, J.: Om serum behandling af difteri. Hospitalstidende *6*:337–339, 1898.
108. Finberg, R. W.: Immunology of infection. Immunol. Allergy Clin. North Am. *8*:137–144, 1988.
109. Finkel, K. C., and Haworth, J. C.: Clinical trial to assess the effectiveness of gamma globulin in acute infections in young children. Pediatrics *25*:798–806, 1960.
110. Forman, M. L., and Stiehm, E. R.: Impaired opsonic activity but normal phagocytosis in low birth weight infants. N. Engl. J. Med. *281*:926–931, 1969.
111. Funkhauser, W. L.: The use of gamma globulin antibodies to control chickenpox in a convalescent hospital for children. J. Pediatr. *32*:257–259, 1948.
112. Furusho, K., Kamiya, T., Nakano, H., et al.: High dose intravenous gamma globulin for Kawasaki disease. Lancet *1*:1055–1058, 1984.
113. Gamm, H., Huber, C. H., Chapel, H., et al.: Intravenous immune globulin in chronic lymphocytic leukemia. Clin. Exp. Immunol. *97*(Suppl.):17–20, 1994.
114. Gardulf, A., Hammarstrom, L., and Smith, C. I. E.: Home treatment of hypogammaglobulinaemia with subcutaneous gammaglobulin by rapid infusion. Lancet *338*:162–166, 1991.
115. Gellis, S. S., Stokes, J., Jr., Brother, G. M., et al.: The use of human immune serum globulin (gamma globulin) in infectious (epidemic) hepatitis in the Mediterranean theater of operations. I. Studies on prophylaxis in two epidemics of infectious hepatitis. J. A. M. A. *128*:1062–1063, 1945.
116. Gershon, A. A., Steinberg, S., and Brunell, P. A.: Zoster immune globulin: A further assessment. N. Engl. J. Med. *290*:243–245, 1974.
117. Gispen, R., Lansberg, H. P., and Nanning, W.: The effect of antivaccinia gamma globulin on smallpox vaccination in view of a proposed attempt to prevent postvaccinal encephalitis. Antonie van Leeuwenhoek *22*:89–102, 1956.
118. Glinz, W., Grob, P. V. J., Nydegger, U. E., et al.: Polyvalent immunoglobulins for prophylaxis of bacterial infections in patients following multiple trauma. Intensive Care Med. *11*:288–294, 1985.
119. Gold, W. L., Boulton, J. E., Goldman, C., et al.: Management of varicella exposure in the neonatal intensive care unit. Pediatr. Infect. Dis. J. *12*:954–955, 1993.
120. Gooding, A. M., Bastian, J. F., Peterson, B. M., et al.: Safety and efficacy of intravenous immunoglobulin prophylaxis in pediatric head trauma patients: A double-blind controlled trial. J. Crit. Care *4*:212–216, 1993.
121. Grady, G. F.: Hepatitis B immune globulin prevention of hepatitis from accidental exposure among medical personnel. N. Engl. J. Med. *293*:1067–1070, 1975.
122. Grady, G. F.: Prevention of post transfusion hepatitis by gamma globulin: Preliminary report: A cooperative study. J. A. M. A. *214*:140–142, 1970.
123. Graham-Pole, J., Camitta, B., Casper, J., et al.: Intravenous immunoglobulin may lessen all forms of infection in patients receiving allogeneic bone marrow transplantation for acute lymphoblastic leukemia: A Pediatric Oncology Group study. Bone Marrow Transplant *3*:559–566, 1988.
124. Granstrom, M., Olinder-Nielsen, A. M., Holmblad, P., et al.: Specific immunoglobulin for treatment of whooping cough. Lancet *338*:1230–1233, 1991.
125. Grayston, J. T., and Watten, R. H.: Epidemic rubella in Taiwan, 1957–1958. III. Gamma globulin in the prevention of rubella. N. Engl. J. Med. *261*:1145–1150, 1959.
126. Green, R. H., Balsamo, M. R., Giles, J. P., et al.: Studies of the natural history and prevention of rubella. Am. J. Dis. Child. *110*:348–365, 1965.
127. Greenberg, M., Frant, S., and Rutstein, D. D.: "Gamma globulin" and "placental globulin": A comparison of their effectiveness in the prevention and modification of measles. J. A. M. A. *126*:944–947, 1944.
128. Greenberg, M., Pellitteri, O., and Eisenstein, D. T.: Measles encephalitis. I. Prophylactic effect of gamma globulin. J. Pediatr. *46*:642–647, 1955.
129. Greenberg, M.: Gamma globulin in pediatrics. Med. Clin. North Am. *May*:602–608, 1947.
130. Griffin, T. C., Squires, J. E., Timmons, C. F., et al.: Chronic human parovirus B19-induced erythroid hypoplasia as the initial manifestation of human immunodeficiency virus infection. J. Pediatr. *118*:899–901, 1991.

130a. Groothius, J. R., Somoes, E. A. F., Hemming, V. G., et al.: Respiratory syncytial virus (RSV) infection in preterm infants and the protective effects of RSV immune globulin (RSVIG). Pediatrics *95*:463–467, 1995.

131. Groothuis, J. R., Simoes, E. A. F., Levin, M. J., et al.: Prophylactic administration of respiratory syncytial virus immune globulin to high-risk infants and young children. N. Engl. J. Med. *329*:1524–1530, 1993.
132. Grossman, E. B., Stewart, S. G., and Stokes, J. P.: Post-transfusion hepatitis in battle casualties. J. A. M. A. *129*:991–994, 1945.
133. Guglielmo, B. J., Wong-Beringe, R. A., and Linker, C. A.: Immune globulin therapy in allogeneic bone marrow transplant: A critical review. Bone Marrow Transplant. *13*:499–510, 1994.
134. Gupta, P. S., Kapoor, R., Goyal, S., et al.: Intrathecal human tetanus immunoglobulin in early tetanus. Lancet *2*:439–440, 1980.
135. Haas, A.: Use of intravenous immunoglobulin in immunoregulatory disorders. *In* Stiehm, E. R. (moderator): Intravenous immunoglobulins as therapeutic agents. Ann. Intern. Med. *107*:367–382, 1987.
136. Habel, K., and Koprowski, H.: Laboratory data supporting the clinical trial of antirabies serum in persons bitten by a rabid wolf. Bull. W. H. O. *13*:773–779, 1955.
137. Habel, K.: Seroprophylaxis in experimental rabies. Public Health Rep. *60*:545–560, 1945.
138. Hadfield, M. G., Seidlin, M., Houff, S. A., et al.: Echovirus meningoencephalitis with administration of intrathecal immunoglobulin. J. Neuropathol. Exp. Neurol. *44*:520–529, 1985.
139. Hammon, W. McD., Coriell, L. L., Stokes, J., Jr., et al.: Evaluation of Red Cross gamma globulin as a prophylactic agent for poliomyelitis (5 parts). J. A. M. A. *150*:739–760, 1950; *151*:1272–1285, 1953; *156*:21–27, 1954.
140. Haque, K. N., Zaidi, M. H., and Bahakim, H.: IgM enriched intravenous immunoglobulin therapy in neonatal sepsis. Am. J. Dis. Child. *142*:1293–1296, 1988.
141. Haque, K. N., Zaidi, M. H., Haque, S. K., et al.: Intravenous immunoglobulin for prevention of sepsis in preterm and low birthweight infants. Pediatr. Infect. Dis. *5*:622–625, 1986.
142. Havens, W. P., Jr., and Paul, J. R.: Prevention of infectious hepatitis with gamma globulin. J. A. M. A. *129*:270–271, 1945.
143. Hemming, V. G., and Prince, P. G.: Intravenous immunoglobulin G in viral respiratory infections for newborns and infants. Pediatr. Infect. Dis. *5*(Suppl. 13):S204–S206, 1986.
144. Hemming, V. G., Prince, P. G., Horswood, R. L., et al.: Studies of passive immunotherapy for infections of respiratory syncytial virus in the respiratory tract of a primate model. J. Infect. Dis. *152*:1083–1087, 1985.
145. Henin, Y., Marechal, V., Barre, F., et al.: Inactivation and partition of HIV during Kistler and Nitschmann fractionation of human blood plasma. Vox Sang *54*:78–83, 1988.
146. Herrero, J. I. H., Beltrán, R. R., and Sánchez, A. M. M.: Failure of intrathecal tetanus antitoxin in the treatment of tetanus neonatorum. J. Infect. Dis. *164*:619–620, 1991.
147. Hill, H. R.: Intravenous immunoglobulin use in the neonate: Role in prophylaxis and therapy of infection. Pediatr. Infect. Dis. J. *12*:549–558, 1993.
148. Hilman, B. C., Triplett, F., Crawford, L. V., et al.: Intracutaneous immune serum globulin therapy in allergic children. J. A. M. A. *207*:902–906, 1969.
149. Hlava, J., and Honl, I.: Serum vaccinicum und seine wirkungen. Wien. Klin. Rundschau *9*:625–627, 1895.
150. Holland, P. V., Rubenson, R. M., Morrow, A. G., et al.: Gamma globulin

in the prophylaxis of post transfusion hepatitis. J. A. M. A. *196*:471–474, 1966.
151. Houser, H. B., and Schalet, N.: Prevention of rubella with gamma globulin. Clin. Res. *6*:281–282, 1958.
152. Hsia, D. Y., Lonsway, M., Jr., and Gellis, S. S.: Gamma globulin in the prevention of infectious hepatitis: Studies on the use of small doses in family outbreaks. N. Engl. J. Med. *250*:417–419, 1954.
153. Ichimaru, T., Ohara, Y., Hojo, M., et al.: Treatment of severe pertussis by administration of specific gamma globulin with high titers anti-toxin antibody. Acta Paediatr. *82*:1076–1078, 1993.
154. Imbach, P., Barundun, S., d' Apuzzo, V., et al.: High-dose intravenous gammaglobulin for idiopathic thrombocytopenic purpura in childhood. Lancet *1*:1228–1231, 1981.
155. Imbach, P., Perret, B., Babington, R., et al.: Safety of intravenous immunoglobulin preparations. Vox Sang *61*:1–4, 1991.
156. Inoue, S., Kinra, N. K., Mukkamala, S. R., et al.: Parvovirus B19 infection: Aplastic crisis, erythema infectiosum and idiopathic thrombocytopenic purpura. Pediatr. Infect. Dis. J. *10*:251–253, 1991.
157. Intravenous Immunoglobulin Collaborative Study Group: Prophylactic intravenous administration of standard immune globulin as compared with core-lipopolysaccharide immune globulin in patients at high risk of postsurgical infection. N. Engl. J. Med. *327*:234–240, 1991.
158. Intravenous Immunoglobulin Study Group: Intravenous immune globulin for the prevention of bacterial infections in children with symptomatic human immunodeficiency virus infection. N. Engl. J. Med. *325*:73–80, 1991.
159. Iriarte, P. V., Tangco, A., Jagasia, K. H., et al.: Effect of gamma globulin on modification of chickenpox in children with malignant disease. Cancer *18*:112–116, 1965.
160. Jacobson, J. M., Colman, N., Ostrow, N. A., et al.: Passive immunotherapy in the treatment of advanced human immunodeficiency virus infection. J. Infect. Dis. *168*:298–305, 1993.
161. Jantausch, B. A., Luban, N. L. C., Duffy, L., et al.: Maternal plasma transfusion in the treatment of disseminated neonatal echovirus 11 infection. Pediatr. Infect. Dis. J. *14*:154–155, 1995.
162. Jhaveri, R., Rosenfeld, W., Salazar, D., et al.: High titer multiple dose therapy with HBIG in newborn infants of HBsAg positive mothers. J. Pediatr. *97*:305–308, 1980.
163. Johnson, P. R., Jr., Edwards, K. M., and Wright, P. F.: Failure of intraventricular gamma globulin to eradicate echovirus encephalitis in a patient with X linked agammaglobulinemia. N. Engl. J. Med. *313*:1546–547, 1985.
164. Jones, R. J., Roe, E. A., and Gupta, J. L.: Controlled trial of *Pseudomonas* immunoglobulin and vaccine in burn patients. Lancet *2*:1263–1265, 1980.
165. Jorgensen, F., Andersson, B., Hanson, L. A., et al.: Gamma-globulin treatment of recurrent acute otitis media in children. Pediatr. Infect. Dis. J. *9*:389–394, 1990.
166. Judelsohn, R. G., Meyers, J. D., Ellis, R. J., et al.: Efficacy of zoster immune globulin. Pediatrics *53*:476–480, 1974.
167. Just, H. M., Voge, W., Metzger, M., et al.: Treatment of intensive care unit patients with severe nosocomial infections. *In* Morell, A., and Nydegger, U. E. (eds.): Clinical Use of Intravenous Immunoglobulins. New York, Academic Press, 1986, pp. 346–352.
168. Kabat, E. A.: Uses of hyperimmune human gamma globulin. N. Engl. J. Med. *269*:247–254, 1963.
169. Kalm, O., Prellner, K., and Chrisensen, P.: The effect of intravenous immunoglobulin treatment in recurrent acute otitis media. Int. J. Pediatr. Otorhinolaryngol. *11*:237–246, 1986.
170. Kanai, K., Takehiro, A., Noto, H., et al.: Prevention of perinatal transmission of hepatitis B virus (HBV) to children of e antigen positive HBV carrier mothers by hepatitis B immune globulin and HBV vaccine. J. Infect. Dis. *151*:287–290, 1985.
171. Kanfer, E. J., Abrahamson, G., Taylor, J., et al.: Severe rotavirus-associated diarrhoea following bone marrow transplantation: Treatment with oral immunoglobulin. Bone Marrow Transplant. *14*:651–652, 1994.
172. Karpas, A., Hill, F., Youle, M., et al.: Effects of passive immunization in patients with the acquired immunodeficiency syndrome related complex and acquired immunodeficiency syndrome. Proc. Natl. Acad. Sci. U. S. A. *85*:9234–9237, 1988.
173. Kato, E., Shindo, S., Eto, Y., et al.: Administration of immune globulin associated with aseptic meningitis. J. A. M. A. *259*:3267–3271, 1988.
174. Kefalides, N. A., Arana, J. A., Bazan, A., et al.: Role of infection in mortality from severe burns: Evaluation of plasma, gamma globulin, albumin, and saline solution therapy in a group of Peruvian children. N. Engl. J. Med. *267*:317–323, 1962.
175. Keller, T., McGrath, K., Newland, A., et al.: Indications for use of intravenous immunoglobulin: Recommendations of the Australasian Society of Blood Transfusion consensus symposium. Med. J. Aust. *159*:204–206, 1993.
176. Kempe, C. H., Berge, T. O., and England, B.: Hyperimmune vaccinial gamma globulin: Source, evaluation, and use in prophylaxis and therapy. Pediatrics *18*:177–188, 1956.
177. Kempe, C. H., Bowles, C., Meiklejohn, G., et al.: The use of vaccinia hyperimmune gamma globulin in the prophylaxis of smallpox. Bull. W. H. O. *25*:41–48, 1961.
178. Kempe, C. H.: Studies on smallpox and complications of smallpox vaccination. Pediatrics *26*:176–189, 1960.
178a. Kiehl, M. G., Stoll, R., Broder, M., et al.: A controlled trial of intravenous immune globulin for the prevention of serious infections in adults with advanced human immunodeficiency virus infection. Arch. Intern. Med. *156*:2545–2550, 1996.
179. Kim, K. S.: High dose intravenous immune globulin impairs antibacterial activity of antibiotics. J. Allergy Clin. Immunol. *84*:588–594, 1989.
180. Kim, K. S.: Use of intravenous immunoglobulins in bacterial diseases. *In* Stiehm, E. R. (moderator): Intravenous Immunoglobulins as Therapeutic Agents. Ann. Intern. Med. *107*:367–382, 1987.
181. Kinney, J., Mundorf, L., Gleason, C., et al.: Efficacy and pharmacokinetics of intravenous immune globulin administration to high-risk neonates. Am. J. Dis. Child. *145*:1233–1238, 1991.
182. Kleyweg, R. P., VanDerMeche, F. G., and Meulstee, J.: Treatment of Guillain-Barré syndrome with high-dose gamma-globulin. Neurology *38*:1639–1641, 1988.
183. Knodell, R. G., Ginsberg, A. L., Conrad, A. L., et al.: Efficacy of prophylactic gamma-globulin in preventing non-A non-B post transfusion hepatitis. Lancet *1*:557–561, 1976.
184. Knudson, A. P.: Patients with IgG subclass and/or selective antibody deficiency to polysaccharide antigens: Initiation of a controlled clinical trial of intravenous immunoglobulin. J. Allergy Clin. Immunol. *84*:640–647, 1989.
185. Kobayashi, R. H., Kobayashi, A. D., Lee, N., et al.: Home self administration of intravenous immunoglobulin therapy in children. Pediatrics *85*:705–709, 1990.
186. Koch, W. C., Massey, G., Russel, C. E., et al.: Manifestations and treatment of human parvovirus B19 infection in immunocompromised patients. J. Pediatr. *116*:335–359, 1990.
187. Koenig, M. G., Drutz, D. J., Mushlin, A. I., et al.: Type B botulism in man. Am. J. Med. *42*:208–219, 1967.
188. Koenig, M. G., Spickard, A., Cardella, M. A., et al.: Clinical and laboratory observations on type E botulism in man. Medicine *43*:517–545, 1964.
189. Kohl, S: Risk of chickenpox in asthmatic children receiving inhalation steroids and therapeutic recommendations. Pediatr. Infect. Dis. J. *12*:174–175, 1993.
190. Korns, R. F.: Prophylaxis of German measles with immune serum globulin. J. Infect. Dis. *90*:183–192, 1952.
191. Krugman, S.: Effect of human immune serum globulin on infectivity of hepatitis. J. Infect. Dis. *134*:70–74, 1976.
192. Krugman, S., and Giles, J. P.: Viral hepatitis, type B (MS 2 strain): Further observations in natural history and prevention. N. Engl. J. Med. *288*:755–760, 1973.
193. Krugman, S., and Ward, R.: Demonstration of neutralizing antibody in gamma globulin and re-evaluation of the rubella problem. N. Engl. J. Med. *259*:16–19, 1958.
194. Krugman, S., Giles, J. P., and Hammond, J.: Viral hepatitis, type B (MS 2 strain): Prevention with specific hepatitis B immune serum globulin. J. A. M. A. *218*:1665–1670, 1971.
195. Krugman, S., Giles, J. P., Jacobs, A. M., et al.: Studies with live attenuated measles virus vaccine. Am. J. Dis. Child. *103*:353–363, 1962.
196. Krugman, S., Ward, R., Giles, J. P., et al.: Infectious hepatitis: Studies on the effectiveness of gamma globulin and on the incidence of inapparent infection. J. A. M. A. *174*:823–830, 1960.
197. Kuhns, W. J., Prince, A. M., Brotman, B., et al.: A clinical and laboratory evaluation of immune serum globulin from donors with a history of hepatitis: Attempted prevention of post transfusion hepatitis. Am. J. Med. Sci. *272*:255–261, 1976.
198. Kurtzberg, J., Friedman, H. S., Kinney, P. R., et al.: Management of human immunodeficiency virus-associated thrombocytopenia with intravenous gammaglobulin. Am. J. Pediatr. Hematol. Oncol. *9*:299–301, 1987.
199. Kurtzman, G., Frickhofen, N., Kimball, J., et al.: Pure red cell aplasia of 10 years' duration due to persistent parvovirus B19 infection and its cure with immunoglobulin therapy. N. Engl. J. Med. *321*:519–523, 1989.
200. Lea, W. A., Jr., and Taylor, W. B.: Gamma globulin in the treatment of herpes zoster. Texas Med. *54*:594–596, 1958.
201. Lederman, H. M., and Winkelstein, J. A.: X-linked agammaglobulinemia: An analysis of 96 patients. Medicine *64*:145–146, 1985.
202. Lee, D. C., and Lederman, H. M.: Anti-tetanus toxoid antibodies in intravenous gamma globulin: An alternative to tetanus immune globulin. J. Infect. Dis. *166*:642–645, 1992.
203. Lehner, P. J., Webster, A. D.: Hepatitis C from immunoglobulin infusion. B. M. J. *306*:1541–1542, 1993.
204. Leifer, E., Gocke, D. J., and Borne, H.: Lassa fever, a new virus disease from West Africa. II. Report of a laboratory-acquired infection treated with plasma from a person recently recovered from the disease. Am. J. Trop. Med. Hyg. *19*:677–679, 1970.
205. Lennon, J. L., and Black, F. I.: Maternally derived measles immunity in era of vaccine-protected mothers. J. Pediatr. *108*:671–676, 1986.
206. Leung, D. Y., Burns, J., Newberger, J., et al.: Reversal of immunoregulatory abnormalities in Kawasaki syndrome by intravenous gammaglobulin. J. Clin. Invest. *79*:468–472, 1987.
207. Lever, A. M., Webster, A. D. B., Brown, D., et al.: Non A, non B hepatitis occurring in agammaglobulinaemic patients after intravenous immunoglobulin. Lancet *2*:1062–1064, 1984.
208. Levy, J., Youvan, T., Lee, M. L., et al.: Passive hyperimmune plasma

therapy in the treatment of acquired immunodeficiency syndrome: Results of a 12-month multicenter double-blind controlled trial. Blood *4*:2130–2135, 1994.
209. Lipshultz, S. E., Orav, E. J., Sanders, S. P., et al.: Immunoglobulins and left ventricular structure and function in pediatric HIV infection. Circulation *92*:2220–2225, 1995.
210. Loofbourow, J. C., Cabasso, V. J., Roby, R. E., et al.: Rabies immune globulin (human): Clinical trials and dose determination. J. A. M. A. *217*:1825–1831, 1971.
211. Losonsky, G. A., Johnson, J., Winkelstein, J. A., et al.: Oral administration of human serum immunoglobulin in immunodeficient patients with viral gastroenteritis: A pharmacokinetic and functional analysis. J. Clin. Invest. *76*:2362–2367, 1985.
212. Lucas, A. O., Willis, A. J., Mohamed, S. D., et al.: A comparison of the value of 500,000 I.U. tetanus antitoxin with 200,000 I.U. in the treatment of tetanus. Clin. Pharmacol. Ther. *6*:592–597, 1965.
213. Lundström, R., Thorén, C., and Blomquist, B.: Gamma globulin against rubella in pregnancy. I. Prevention of maternal rubella by gamma globulin and convalescent gamma globulin: A follow up study. Acta Paediatr. *50*:444–452, 1961.
214. Lundström, R., Thorén, C., and Blomquist, B.: Gamma globulin against rubella in pregnancy. II. Manifest maternal rubella in early pregnancy treated with convalescent gamma globulin: A follow up study. Acta Paediatr. *50*:453–456, 1961.
215. Lundström, R.: Complications of smallpox vaccination and their treatment with vaccinia immune globulin. J. Pediatr. *49*:129–140, 1956.
216. MacIntyre, E. A., Linch, D. C., Macy, M. G., et al.: Successful response to intravenous immunoglobulin in autoimmune hemolytic anemia. Br. J. Haematol. *60*:387–388, 1985.
217. Magny, J. F., Bremard Oury, C., Brault, D., et al.: Intravenous immunoglobulin therapy for prevention of infection in high risk premature infants: Report of a multicenter, double blind study. Pediatrics *88*:437–443, 1991.
218. Masci, S., De Simone, C., Famularo, G., et al.: Intravenous immunoglobulins suppress the recurrences of genital herpes simplex virus: A clinical and immunological study. Immunopharmacol. Immunotoxicol. *17*:33–47, 1995.
219. Matheson, D. S., Clarkson, T. W., and Gelfand, E. W.: Mercury toxicity (acrodynia) induced by long term injection of gamma globulin. J. Pediatr. 97:153–155, 1980.
220. McCloskey, R. V., and Smilack, J.: Diphtheria antitoxin content of human immune serum globulins. Ann. Intern. Med. *77*:757–758, 1972.
221. McComb, J. A., and Dwyer, R. C.: Passive active immunization with tetanus immune globulin (human). N. Engl. J. Med. *268*:857–862, 1963.
222. McCracken, G. H., Jr., Dowell, D. L., and Marshall, F. N.: Double blind trial of equine antitoxin and human immune globulin in tetanus neonatorum. Lancet *1*:1146–1149, 1971.
223. McKhann, C. F., Green, A. A., and Coady, H.: Factors influencing the effectiveness of placental extract in the prevention and modification of measles. J. Pediatr. *6*:603–614, 1935.
224. Mease, P. J., Ochs, H. D., and Wedgwood, R. J.: Successful treatment of echovirus meningoencephalitis and myositis fasciitis with intravenous immune globulin therapy in a patient with X-linked agammaglobulinemia. N. Engl. J. Med. *304*:1278–1281, 1981.
225. Medical Research Council Working Party: Hypogammaglobulinemia in the United Kingdom. Lancet *1*:163–169, 1969.
226. Melamed, I., Griffiths, A. M., and Roifman, C. M.: Benefit of oral immune globulin therapy in patients with immunodeficiency and chronic diarrhea. J. Pediatr. *3*:486–489, 1991.
227. Miller, M. E.: The immunodeficiencies of immaturity. *In* Stiehm, E. R. (ed.): Immunologic Disorders in Infants and Children. 3rd ed. Philadelphia, W. B. Saunders, 1989, pp. 196–225.
228. Mofenson, L. M., Bethel, J., Moye, J., et al.: Effect of intravenous immunoglobulin (IVIG) on CD4$^+$ lymphocyte decline in HIV-infected children in a clinical trial of IVIG infection prophylaxis. J. AIDS *6*:1103–1113, 1993.
229. Mofenson, L. M., Moye, J., Korelitz, J., et al.: Crossover of placebo patients to intravenous immunoglobulin confirms efficacy for prophylaxis of bacterial infections and reduction of hospitalizations in human immunodeficiency virus-infected children. Pediatr. Infect. Dis. J. *13*:477–484, 1994.
230. Monath, T. P., and Casals, J.: Diagnosis of Lassa fever and the isolation and management of patients. Bull. W. H. O. *52*:707–715, 1975.
231. Montanaro, A., and Pirofsky, B.: Prolonged intervals of high dose IVIG in patients with primary immune deficiency states. Am. J. Med. *76*(Suppl. 3A):67–72, 1984.
232. Munster, A. M.: Immunologic response of trauma and burns. Am. J. Med. *7*:142–145, 1984.
233. Munster, A. M.: Infections in burns. *In* Morell, A., and Nydegger, U. E. (eds.): Clinical Use of Intravenous Immunoglobulins. New York, Academic Press, 1986, pp. 339–344.
234. Nance, F. C., Hines, J. L., Fulton, R. E., et al.: Treatment of experimental burn wound sepsis by post burn immunization with polyvalent *Pseudomonas* antigen. Surgery *68*:248–253, 1970.
235. Nanning, W.: Prophylactic effect of anti-vaccinia gamma globulin against post vaccinial encephalitis. Bull. W. H. O. *27*:317–324, 1962.
236. Newburger, J. W., Takahashi, M., Beiser, A. S., et al.: A single intravenous infusion of gamma globulin as compared with four infusions in the treatment of acute Kawasaki syndrome. N. Engl. J. Med. *324*:1633–1639, 1991.
237. Newburger, J. W., Takahashi, M., Burns, J. C., et al.: The treatment of Kawasaki syndrome with intravenous gamma globulin. N. Engl. J. Med. *315*:341–347, 1986.
238. Nieman, P. E., Reeves, W., Ray, G., et al.: A prospective analysis of interstitial pneumonia and opportunistic viral infection among recipients of allogeneic bone marrow grafts. J. Infect. Dis. *136*:754–767, 1977.
239. Nigro, G., D'Eufemia, P., Zerbini, M., et al.: Parvovirus B19 infection in a hypogammaglobulinemic infant with neurologic disorders and anemia: Successful immunoglobulin therapy. Pediatr. Infect. Dis. J: *13*:1019–1021, 1994.
240. NIH Consensus Development Conference: Diseases, doses, recommendations for intravenous immunoglobulin: HLB Newsletter. Natl. Inst. Heart Lung Blood Dis. *6*:73–78, 1990.
241. Nolte, N. T., Pirofsky, B., Gerritz, G. A., et al.: Intravenous immunoglobulin therapy for antibody deficiency. Clin. Exp. Immunol. *36*:237–243, 1979.
242. Ochs, H. D., Fischer, S. H., Virant, F. S, et al.: Non-A non-B hepatitis and intravenous immunoglobulin. Lancet *1*:404–405, 1985.
243. Ochs, H. D.: Intravenous immunoglobulin in the treatment and prevention of acute infections in pediatric acquired immunodeficiency syndrome patients. Pediatr. Infect. Dis. *6*:509–511, 1987.
244. Okano, M., Bashir, R. M., Davis, J. R., et al.: Detection of primary Epstein-Barr virus infection in a patient with X-linked lymphoproliferative disease receiving immunoglobulin prophylaxis. Am. J. Hematol. *36*:294–296, 1991.
245. Ordman, C. W., Jennings, C. G., Jr., and Janeway, C. A.: Chemical, clinical and immunological studies on the products of human plasma fractionation. XII. The use of concentrated normal human serum gamma globulin (human immune serum globulin) in the prevention and attention of measles. J. Clin. Invest. *23*:541–549, 1944.
246. Orenstein, W. A., Heymann, D. L., Ellis, R. J., et al.: Prophylaxis of varicella in high risk children: Dose response effect of zoster immune globulin. J. Pediatr. *98*:368–373, 1981.
247. Park, W. H., and Freeman, R. G., Jr.: The prophylactic use of measles convalescent serum. J. A. M. A. *87*:556–558, 1926.
248. Paryani, S. G., Arvin, A. M., Koropchak, C. M., et al.: Comparison of varicella zoster antibody titers in patients given intravenous immune serum globulin or varicella zoster immune globulin. J. Pediatr. *105*:200–205, 1984.
249. Paryani, S. G., Arvin, A. M., Koropchak, C. M., et al.: Varicella zoster antibody titers after the administration of intravenous immune serum globulin or varicella zoster immune globulin. Am. J. Med. *76*:124–127, 1984.
250. Paschlau, V. A.: Zur umstrittenen wirksamkeit des diphtherie heilserums. Dtsch. Med. Wochenschr. *74*:1569–1573, 1949.
251. Patel, J. C., Mehta, B. C., Nanavati, B. H., et al.: Role of serum therapy in tetanus. Lancet *1*:740–743, 1963.
252. Pollach, A. N., Janinis, J., and Green, D.: Successful intravenous immunoglobulin therapy for human immunodeficiency virus-associated thrombocytopenia. Arch. Intern. Med. *148*:695–697, 1988.
253. Pollack, M.: Antibody activity against *Pseudomonas aeruginosa* in immune globulins prepared for intravenous use in humans. J. Infect. Dis. *147*:1090–1098, 1983.
254. Pollack, S., Cunningham Rundles, C., Smithwick, E. M., et al.: High dose intravenous gamma globulin for autoimmune neutropenia. N. Engl. J. Med. *307*:253, 1982.
255. Prentice, R. L., Dalgleish, A. G., Gatenby, P. A., et al.: Central nervous system echovirus infection in Bruton's X-linked hypogammaglobulinemia. Aust. N. Z. J. Med. *15*:443–445, 1985.
256. Prian, G. W., and Koep, L. J.: Elimination of cytomegalovirus disease in liver transplant patients treated prophylactically with combination cytomegalovirus hyperimmune globulin and ganciclovir. Transplant. Proc. *26*(Suppl. 1):54–55, 1994.
257. Prince, A. M., Horowitz, B., Baker, L., et al.: Failure of a human immunodeficiency virus (HIV) immune globulin to protect chimpanzees against experimental challenge with HIV. Proc. Natl. Acad. Sci. U. S. A. *85*:6944–6948, 1988.
258. Prince, A. M., Szmuness, W., Mann, M. K., et al.: Hepatitis B "immune" globulin: Effectiveness in prevention of dialysis associated hepatitis. N. Engl. J. Med. *293*:1063–1067, 1975.
259. Prince, G. A., Hemming, V. G., and Chanock, R. M.: The use of purified immunoglobulin in the therapy of respiratory syncytial virus infection. Pediatr. Infect. Dis. *5*:S201–S203, 1986.
260. Prince, G. A., Hemming, V. G., Horswood, R. L., et al.: Immunoprophylaxis and immunotherapy of respiratory syncytial virus infection in the cotton rat. Virus Res. *3*:193–206, 1985.
261. Ranki, A.: Intravenous immune globulin for passive tetanus prophylaxis. J. Infect. Dis. *167*:498–499, 1993.
262. Rao, S. P., Teitlebaum, J., and Miller, S. T.: Intravenous immune globulin and aseptic meningitis. Am. J. Dis. Child. *146*:539–540, 1992.
263. Rault, R., Piraino, B., Johnston, J. R., et al.: Pulmonary and renal toxicity of intravenous immunoglobulin. Clin. Nephrol. *36*:83–86, 1991.
264. Redeker, A. G., Mosley, J. W., Gocke, D. J., et al.: Hepatitis B immune

globulin as a prophylactic measure for spouses exposed to acute type B hepatitis. N. Engl. J. Med. *293*:1055–1059, 1975.

265. Redner, B., and Markow, H.: Effects of minute doses of gamma globulin in children with active allergic manifestations. J. A. M. A. *185*:692–695, 1963.
266. Reed, E. C., Bowden, R. A., Dandliker, P. S., et al.: Treatment of cytomegalovirus pneumonia with ganciclovir and intravenous cytomegalovirus immunoglobulin in patients with bone marrow transplants. Ann. Intern. Med. *109*:783–788, 1988.
267. Reed, W. D., Eddleston, A. L. W. F., Cullens, H., et al.: Infusion of hepatitis B antibody in antigen positive active chronic hepatitis. Lancet 2:1347–1351, 1973.
268. Reesink, H. W., Reerink Brongers, E. E., Lafeber Schut, B. J. T., et al.: Prevention of chronic HBsAg carrier state in infants by HBsAg positive mothers by hepatitis B immunoglobulin. Lancet 2:436–438, 1979.
269. Rimensberger, P. C., and Schaad, U. B.: Clinical experience with aerosolized immunoglobulin treatment of respiratory syncytial virus infection in infants. Pediatr. Infect. Dis. J. *13*:328–330, 1994.
270. Rodarte, J. G., and Williams, B. H.: Treatment of herpes zoster and chickenpox with immune globulin. Arch. Dermatol. *73*:553–556, 1956.
271. Roifman, C. M., Livison, H., and Gelfand, E. W.: High dose vs low dose intravenous immunoglobulin in hypogammaglobulinemia and chronic lung disease. Lancet *1*:1075–1077, 1987.
272. Rosenfeld, E. A., Shulman, S. T., Corydon, K. E., et al.: Comparative safety and efficacy of two immune globulin products in Kawasaki disease. J. Pediatr. *126*:1000–1003, 1995.
273. Ross, A. H.: Modification of chickenpox in family contacts by administration of gamma globulin. N. Engl. J. Med. *267*:369–376, 1962.
274. Rowe, J. M., Ciobanu, N., Ascensao, J., et al.: Recommended guidelines for the management of autologous and allogeneic bone marrow transplantation. Ann. Intern. Med. *120*:143–158, 1994.
275. Rubaltelli, F., Benini, F., and Sala, M.: Prevention of necrotizing enterocolitis in neonates at risk by oral administration of monomeric IgG. Dev. Pharmacol. Ther. *17*:138–143, 1991.
276. Rubbo, S. D., and Suri, J. C.: Passive immunization against tetanus with human immune globulin. B. M. J. *2*:79–81, 1962.
277. Rubinstein, H. M.: Studies on human tetanus antitoxin. Am. J. Hyg. *76*:276–292, 1962.
278. Ruderman, J. W., Peter, J. B., Gall, R. C., et al.: Prevention of hypogammaglobulinemia of prematurity with intravenous immune globulin. J. Perinatol. *10*:150–155, 1988.
279. Samuel, D., Muller, R., Alexander, G., et al.: Liver transplantation in European patients with the hepatitis B surface antigen. N. Engl. J. Med. *329*:1842–1847, 1993.
280. Sanchez Quijano, A., Pireda, J. A., Lissen, E., et al.: Prevention of post transfusion non A, non B hepatitis by non specific immunoglobulin in heart surgery patients. Lancet *1*:1245–1249, 1988.
281. Santoshan, M., Reid, R., Ambrosino, D. N., et al.: Prevention of *Haemophilus influenzae* type b infections in high risk infants treated with bacterial polysaccharide immune globulin. N. Engl. J. Med. *317*:923–929, 1987.
282. Schaeffer, M., and Toomey, J. A.: Failure of gamma globulin to prevent varicella. J. Pediatr. *33*:749–752, 1948.
283. Schiff, R. I.: Transmission of viral infections through intravenous immune globulin. N. Engl. J. Med. *331*:1649–1650, 1994.
284. Schiff, R. I., Sedlak, D., and Buckley, R. H.: Rapid infusion of Sandoglobulin in patients with primary humoral immunodeficiency. J. Allergy Clin. Immunol. *88*:61–67, 1991.
285. Schless, A. P., and Harell, G. S.: Human gamma globulin in the treatment of bacterial infections. Am. J. Med. *44*:325–329, 1968.
286. Schmidt, G. M., Kovacs, A., Zaia, J. A., et al.: Ganciclovir/immunoglobulin combination therapy for the treatment of human cytomegalovirus-associated interstitial pneumonia in bone marrow allograft recipients. Transplantation *46*:905–907, 1988.
287. Schmidt, R. E., Hartlapp, J. H., Niese, D., et al.: Reduction of infection frequency by intravenous gammaglobulins during intensive induction therapy for small cell carcinoma of the lung. Infection *12*:167–170, 1984.
288. Seeff, L. B., Zimmerman, H. J., Wright, E. C., et al.: Efficacy of hepatitis B immune serum globulin following "needlestick" exposure: A preliminary report of the Veterans Administration Cooperative Study. Lancet *2*:939–941, 1975.
289. Shanley, J. D., Jordan, M. C., and Stevens, J. G.: Modification by adoptive humoral immunity of murine cytomegalovirus infection. J. Infect. Dis. *143*:231–237, 1981.
290. Shapiro, R. S., Chavenet, A., MucGuire, W., et al.: Treatment of B-cell lymphoproliferative disorders with interferon-alpha and intravenous gammaglobulin. N. Engl. J. Med. *318*:1334, 1988.
291. Sharp, J. C. M., and Fletcher, W. B.: Experience of antivaccinia immunoglobulin in the United Kingdom. Lancet *1*:656–659, 1973.
291a. Shield, J., Melville, C., Novelli, V., et al.: Bovine colostrum immunoglobulin concentrate for cryptosporidiosis in AIDS. Arch. Dis. Child. *69*:451–453, 1993.
292. Shill, M., Baynes, R. D., and Miller, S. D.: Fatal rabies encephalitis despite appropriate post exposure prophylaxis. N. Engl. J. Med. *316*:1257–1258, 1987.
293. Shirani, K. Z., Vaughan, G. M., McManus, A. T., et al.: Replacement therapy with modified immunoglobulin G in burn patients: Preliminary kinetic studies. Am. J. Med. *76*:175–180, 1984.
294. Shurin, P. A., Rehmus, J. M., Johnson, C. E., et al.: Bacterial polysaccharide immune globulin for prophylaxis of acute otitis media in high-risk children. J. Pediatr. *123*:801–810, 1993.
295. Siadak, M. F., Kopecky, K., and Sullivan, K. M.: Reduction in transplant-related complications in patients given intravenous immune globulin after allogeneic marrow transplantation. Clin. Exp. Immunol. *97*(Suppl. 1):53–57, 1994.
296. Siber, G. R., Werner, B. G., Halse, N. A., et al.: Interference of immune globulin with measles and rubella immunization. J. Pediatr. *122*:204–211, 1993.
297. Sidiropoulos, D., Boehme, U., Von Muralt, G., et al.: Immunoglobulin supplementation in prevention or treatment of neonatal sepsis. Pediatr. Infect. Dis. *5*:S193–S194, 1986.
298. Siegel, F. P., and Oleske, J.: Management of the acquired immune deficiency syndrome: Is there a role for immune globulins? *In* Morell, A., and Nydegger, U. E. (eds.): Clinical Use of Intravenous Immunoglobulins. New York, Academic Press, 1986, pp. 373–384.
299. Sikes, R. K.: Human rabies immune globulin. Public Health Rep. *84*:797–801, 1969.
300. Silk, H., and Geha, R. S.: Intravenous immunoglobulin prophylaxis in children with IgG subclass 2 deficiency. J. Allergy Clin. Immunol. *79*:188–192, 1987.
301. Silvestris, F., Cafforio, P., and Dammacco, F.: Pathogenic anti-DNA idiotype-reactive IgG in intravenous immunoglobulin preparations. Clin. Exp. Immunol. *97*:19–25, 1994.
302. Simmons, R. L., Matas, A. J., Rattazzi, L. C., et al.: Clinical characteristics of the lethal cytomegalovirus infection following renal transplantation. Surgery *82*:537–546, 1977.
302a. Simoes, E. A. F., Groothuis, J. R., Tristram, D. A., et al.: Respiratory syncytial virus–enriched globulin for the prevention of acute otitis media in high-risk children. J. Pediatr. *129*:214–219, 1996.
303. Simon, N.: Prevention of non A, non B hepatitis in haemodialysis patients by hepatitis B immunoglobulin. Lancet *2*:1047, 1984.
304. Skavaril, F., and Gardi, A.: Differences among available immunoglobulin preparations for intravenous use. Pediatr. Infect. Dis. *7*(Suppl.):43–48, 1988.
305. Smallwood, L. A., Tabor, E., Finlayson, J. S., et al.: Antibodies to hepatitis A virus in immune serum globulin. J. Med. Virol. *7*:21–27, 1981.
306. Smith, J. K., Chi, D. S., Guarderas, J., et al.: Disseminated echovirus infection in a patient with multiple myeloma and a functional defect in complement. Arch. Intern. Med. *149*:1455–1457, 1989.
307. Smith, T. W., Haber, E., Yeatman, L., et al.: Reversal of advanced digoxin intoxication with Fab fragments of digoxin-specific antibodies. N. Engl. J. Med. *294*:797–800, 1976.
308. Snydman, D. R., Werner, B. G., Doughtery, N. N., et al.: A further analysis of the use of cytomegalovirus immune globulin in orthotopic liver transplant patients at risk for primary infection. Transplant. Proc. *26*(Suppl. 1):23–27, 1994.
309. Snydman, D. R., Werner, B. G., Meissner, H. C., et al.: Use of cytomegalovirus immunoglobulin in multiply transfused premature neonates. Pediatr. Infect. Dis J. *14*:34–40, 1995.
310. Snydman, D. R.: Cytomegalovirus immunoglobulins in the prevention and treatment of cytomegalovirus disease. Rev. Infect. Dis. *12*(Suppl. 7):839–848, 1990.
311. Snydman, D. R., Werner, B. G., and Tilney, N. L.: Final analysis of primary cytomegalovirus disease prevention in renal transplant recipients with a cytomegalovirus immune globulin: Comparison of the randomized and open label trials. Transplant. Proc. *23*:1357–1360, 1991.
312. Snydman, D. R., Werner, B. G., Heinze Lacey, B., et al.: Use of cytomegalovirus immune globulin to prevent cytomegalovirus disease in renal transplant recipients. N. Engl. J. Med. *317*:1049–1054, 1987.
313. Sofer, S., Shahak, E., and Gueron, M.: Scorpion envenomation and antivenom therapy. J. Pediatr. *124*:973–978, 1994.
314. Sorensen, R. U., Kallick, M. D., and Berger, M.: Home treatment of antibody deficiency syndromes with intravenous immunoglobulin. J. Allergy Clin. Immunol. *80*:810–815, 1987.
315. Spector, S. A., Gelber, R. D., McGrath, N., et al.: A controlled trial of intravenous immune globulin for the prevention of serious bacterial infections in children receiving zidovudine for advanced human immunodeficiency virus infection. N. Engl. J. Med. *331*:1181–1187, 1994.
316. Stabile, A., Sopo, S. M., Romanelli, V., et al.: Intravenous immunoglobulin for prophylaxis of neonatal sepsis in premature infants. Arch. Dis. Child. *63*:441–443, 1988.
317. Steen, J. A.: Gamma globulin in preventing infections in prematures. Arch. Pediatr. *77*:291–294, 1960.
318. Steinberg, G. M.: Wissenschaftliche untersuchungen hber das spezifische Infektionsagens der blattern und die erzeugung kunstlicher immunitat gegen diese. Krankheit. Zentralbl. Bakt. I. *19*:857–868, 1896.
319. Steinmueller, D. R., Graneto, D., Swift, C., et al.: Use of intravenous immunoglobulin prophylaxis for primary cytomegalovirus infection post living-related-donor renal transplantation. Transplant. Proc. *21*:2069–2071, 1989.
320. Stevens, D. A., and Merigan, T. C.: Zoster immune globulin prophylaxis of disseminated zoster in compromised hosts. Arch. Intern. Med. *140*:52–54, 1980.

321. Stiehm, E. R., and Fudenberg, H. H.: Clinical and immunologic features of dysgammaglobulinemia type I: Report of a case diagnosed in the first year of life. Am. J. Med. *40*:805–815, 1966.
322. Stiehm, E. R., Chin, T. W., Haas, A., et al.: Infectious complications of the primary immunodeficiencies. Clin. Immunol. Immunopathol. *40*:69–86, 1986.
323. Stiehm, E. R., Vaerman, J. P., and Fudenberg, H. H.: Plasma infusions in immunologic deficiency states: Metabolic and therapeutic studies. Blood *28*:918–938, 1966.
324. Stiehm, E. R.: The use of human intravenous immune globulin in immunoregulatory disorders and in the newborn period. Immunol. Allergy Clin. North Am. *8*:39–50, 1988.
325. Stiehm, E. R.: Recent progress in the use of intravenous immunoglobulin. Curr. Probl. Pediatr. *22*:335–348, 1992.
326. Stillerman, M., Marks, H. H., and Thalhimer, W.: Prophylaxis of measles with convalescent serum. Am. J. Dis. Child. *67*:1–14, 1944.
327. Stokes, J., Jr., and Neefe, J. R.: The prevention and attenuation of infectious hepatitis by gamma globulin. J. A. M. A. *127*:144–145, 1945.
328. Stokes, J., Jr., Farquhar, J. A., Drake, M. E., et al.: Infectious hepatitis: Length of protection of immune serum globulin (gamma globulin) during epidemics. J. A. M. A. *147*:714–719, 1951.
329. Stokes, J., Jr., Hilleman, M. R., Weibel, R. E., et al.: Efficacy of live, attenuated measles virus vaccine given with human immune globulin. N. Engl. J. Med. *265*:507–513, 1961.
330. Stokes, J., Jr., Maris, E. P., and Gellis, S. S.: Chemical, clinical and immunological studies on the products of human plasma fractionation. XI. The use of concentrated normal human serum in the prophylaxis and treatment of measles. J. Clin. Invest. *23*:531–540, 1944.
331. Stone, H. H., Graber, C. D., Martin, J. D., Jr., et al.: Evaluation of gamma globulin for prophylaxis against burn sepsis. Surgery *58*:810–814, 1965.
332. Subbarao, E. K., Andrews-Mann, L., Amin, S., et al.: Postexposure prophylaxis for measles in a neonatal intensive care unit. J. Pediatr. *117*:782–785, 1990.
333. Suffredini, A. F.: Current prospects for the treatment of clinical sepsis. Crit. Care Med. *22*:S12–S18, 1994.
334. Sullivan, K. M.: Immunoglobulin therapy in bone marrow transplantation. Am. J. Med. *83*(Suppl. 4A):34–35, 1987.
335. Sullivan, K. M., Kopecky, K. J., Jocom, J., et al.: Immunomodulatory and antimicrobial efficacy of intravenous immunoglobulin in bone marrow transplantation. N. Engl. J. Med. *323*:705–712, 1990.
336. Sullivan, K. M.: Intravenous immune globulin prophylaxis in recipients of a marrow transplant. J. Allergy Clin. Immunol. *84*:632–639, 1989.
337. Szmuness, W., Prince, A. M., Goodman, M., et al.: Hepatitis B immune serum globulin in prevention of non parenterally transmitted hepatitis B. N. Engl. J. Med. *290*:701–706, 1974.
338. Szmuness, W., Stevens, C. E., Oleszko, W. R., et al.: Passive active immunisation against hepatitis B: Immunogenicity studies in adult Americans. Lancet *1*:575–577, 1981.
339. Tacket, C. O., Shandera, W. X., Mann, J. M., et al.: Equine antitoxin use and other factors that predict outcome in type A foodborne botulism. Am. J. Med. *76*:794–798, 1984.
340. Tada, H., Yanagida, M., Mishina, J., et al.: Combined passive and active immunization for preventing perinatal transmission of hepatitis B virus carrier state. Pediatrics *70*:613–619, 1982.
341. Taguchi, Y., Purtilo, D. T., and Okano, M.: The effect of intravenous immunoglobulin and interferon-alpha on Epstein-Barr virus-induced lymphoproliferative disorder in a liver transplant recipient. Transplantation *57*:1813–1815, 1994.
342. Takei, S., Arora, Y. K., and Walker, S. M.: Intravenous immunoglobulin contains specific antibodies inhibitory to activation of T cells by staphylococcal toxin superantigens. J. Clin. Invest. *91*:602–607, 1993.
343. Tang, M. L., Kemp, A. S., and Moaven, L. D.: Parvovirus B19-associated red blood cell aplasia in combined immunodeficiency with normal immunoglobulins. Pediatr. Infect. Dis. J. *13*:539–541, 1994.
344. Tasman, A., and Landsberg, H. P.: Problems concerning the prophylaxis, pathogenesis and therapy of diphtheria. Bull. W. H. O. *16*:939–973, 1957.
345. Tasman, A., Minkenhof, J. E., Vink, H. H., et al.: Importance of intravenous injection of diphtheria antiserum. Lancet *1*:1299–1304, 1958.
346. Taylor, T. E., Molyneux, M. E., Wirima, J. J., et al.: Intravenous immunoglobulin in the treatment of paediatric cerebral malaria. Clin. Exp. Immunol. *90*:357–362, 1992.
347. Thomas, O. C., and McGovern, J. P.: The gamma globulins with special reference to the controversy concerning their use for asthmatic children. South. Med. J. *57*:498–504, 1964.
348. Tobi, M., and Straus, S. E.: Chronic Epstein Barr virus disease: A workshop held by the National Institute of Allergy and Infectious Diseases. Ann. Intern. Med. *103*:951–953, 1985.
349. Trimble, G. X.: Attenuation of chickenpox with gamma globulin. Can. Med. Assoc. J. *77*:697–699, 1957.
350. Turner, R. B., and Kelsey, D. K.: Passive immunization for prevention of rotavirus illness in healthy infants. Pediatr. Infect. Dis. J. *12*:718–722, 1993.
351. Tutscha, P. J.: Diminishing morbidity and mortality of bone marrow transplantation. Vox Sang *51*(Suppl. 2):87–94, 1986.
352. Vaishnava, H., Goyal, R. K., Neogy, C. N., et al.: A controlled trial of antiserum in the treatment of tetanus. Lancet *2*:1371–1374, 1966.
353. Vajsar, J., Sloane, A., Wood, E., et al.: Plasmapheresis vs. intravenous immunoglobulin treatment in childhood Guillain-Barré syndrome. Arch. Pediatr. Adolesc. Med. *148*:1210–1212, 1994.
354. Vakil, B. J., Tulpule, T. H., Armitage, P., et al.: A comparison of the value of 200,000 I.U. of tetanus antitoxin (horse) with 10,000 I.U. in the treatment of tetanus. Clin. Pharmacol. Ther. *9*:465–471, 1968.
355. Vakil, B. J., Tulpule, T. H., Armitage, P., et al.: A comparison of the value of 200,000 I.U. tetanus antitoxin (horse) with 20,000 I.U. in the treatment of tetanus. Clin. Pharmacol. Ther. *5*:695–698, 1964.
356. Vakil, B. J., Tulpule, T. H., Armitage, P., et al.: A comparison of the value of 200,000 I.U. tetanus antitoxin with 50,000 I.U. in the treatment of tetanus. Clin. Pharmacol. Ther. *4*:182–187, 1963.
357. Van Der Meche, F. G., and Schmitz, P. I.: A randomized trial comparing intravenous immune globulin and plasma exchange in Guillain-Barré syndrome. N. Engl. J. Med. *326*:1123–1129, 1992.
358. Van Wye, J. E., Collins, M. S., Baylor, M., et al.: *Pseudomonas* hyperimmune globulin passive immunotherapy for pulmonary exacerbations in cystic fibrosis. Pediatr. Pulmonol. *9*:7–18, 1990.
359. Vera-Ramirez, M., Charlet, M., and Parry, G. J.: Recurrent aseptic meningitis complicating intravenous immunoglobulin therapy for chronic inflammatory demyelinating polyradiculoneuropathy. Neurology *42*:1636–1637, 1992.
360. Verlinde, J. D., and Spaander, J.: Neutralisatie van vaccine virus door gamma globuline. Ned. Tijdschr. Geneesk. *93*:2958–2962, 1949.
361. Vermeulen, M., VanDerMeche, F. G., Steelman, J. D. et al.: Plasma and gammaglobulin infusion in chronic inflammatory polyneuropathy. J. Neurol. Sci. *70*:317–326, 1985.
362. Vittecoq, D., Chevret, S., Morand-Joubert, L., et al.: Passive immunotherapy in AIDS: A double-blind randomized study based on transfusions of plasma rich in anti-human immunodeficiency virus 1 antibodies vs. transfusions of seronegative plasma. Proc. Natl. Acad. Sci. U. S. A. *92*:1195–1199, 1995.
363. Vyas, G. N., Perkins, H. A., and Fudenberg, H. H.: Anaphylactoid transfusion reactions associated with anti IgA. Lancet *2*:312–315, 1968.
364. Waisbren, B. A.: The treatment of bacterial infections with the combination of antibiotics and gamma globulin. Antibiot. Chemother. *7*:322–333, 1957.
365. Ward, R., and Krugman, S.: Etiology, epidemiology and prevention of viral hepatitis. Prog. Med. Virol. *4*:87–118, 1962.
366. Ward, R., Krugman, S., Giles, J. P., et al.: Infectious hepatitis: Studies of its natural history and prevention. N. Engl. J. Med. *258*:407–416, 1958.
367. Wattanasri, S., Boonthai, P., and Thongcharoen, P.: Human rabies after late administration of human diploid cell vaccine without hyperimmune serum. Lancet *2*:870, 1982.
368. Weeks, J. C., Tierney, M. R., and Weinstein, M. C.: Cost-effectiveness of prophylactic intravenous immune globulin in chronic lymphocytic leukemia. N. Engl. J. Med. *325*:81–86, 1991.
369. Weintraub, I.: Treatment of herpes zoster with gamma globulin. J. A. M. A. *157*:1611, 1955.
370. Weisman, L. E., Stoll, B. J., Kueser, T. J., et al.: Intravenous immune globulin prophylaxis of late-onset sepsis in premature neonates. J. Pediatr. *125*:922–930, 1994.
371. Welch, M. J., and Stiehm, E. R.: Slow subcutaneous immunoglobulin therapy in a patient with reactions to intramuscular immunoglobulin. J. Clin. Immunol. *3*:285–286, 1983.
372. Wilde, H., Khawplot, P., Benjavongkulchai, M., et al.: Method of administration of rabies immune globulin. Vaccine *12*:1150–1151, 1994.
373. Williams, P. E., Yap, P. L., Gillon, J., et al.: Transmission of non-A or non-B hepatitis by pH4 treated intravenous immunoglobulin. Vox Sang *57*:15–18, 1989.
374. Wilson, N. W., Ochs, H. D., Peterson, B., et al.: Abnormal primary antibody responses in pediatric trauma patients. J. Pediatr. *115*:424–427, 1989.
375. Winnie, G. B., Cowan, R. G., and Wade, N. A.: Intravenous immune globulin treatment of pulmonary exacerbations in cystic fibrosis. J. Pediatr. *114*:309–314, 1989.
376. Winston, D. J., Ho, W. G., and Chaplin, R. E.: Ganciclovir and intravenous immunoglobulin in bone marow transplantation. *In* Champlin, R. E., and Gale, R. P. (eds.): New Strategies in Bone Marrow Transplantation. New York, Wiley-Liss, 1991, pp. 337–348.
377. Winston, D. J.: Use in viral infections. *In* Stiehm, E. R. (moderator): Intravenous Immunoglobulins as Therapeutic Agents. Ann. Intern. Med. *107*:367–382, 1987.
378. Winston, D. H., Ho, W. G., Gale, R. P., et al.: Treatment and prevention of interstitial pneumonia after bone marrow transplantation. *In* Gale, R. P., and Champlin, R. E. (eds.): Progress in Bone Marrow Transplantation. New York, Alan R. Liss, 1987, p. 52.
379. Wolff, S. N., Fay, J. W., Herzig, R. H., et al.: High-dose weekly intravenous immunoglobulin to prevent infections in patients undergoing autologous bone marrow transplantation or severe myelosuppressive therapy: A study of the American Bone Marrow Transplant Group. Ann. Intern. Med. *118*:937–942, 1993.
380. Wong, V. C., Ip, H. M. H., Reesink, H. W., et al.: Prevention of the HBsAg carrier state in newborn infants of mothers who are chronic carriers of HBsAg and HBeAg by administration of hepatitis B vaccine and hepatitis B immunoglobulin. Lancet *1*:921–926.

381. Woodruff, R. K., Griff, A. P., Firkin, F. L., et al.: Fatal thrombotic events during treatment of autoimmune thrombocytopenia with intravenous immunoglobulins in elderly patients. Lancet *2*:217–219, 1986.
382. Zachoval, R., Jilg, W., Lorbeer, B., et al.: Passive/active immunization against hepatitis B. J. Infect. Dis. *150*:112–117, 1984.
383. Zaia, J. A., Levin, M. J., Preblud, S. R., et al.: Evaluation of varicella zoster immune globulin: Protection of immunosuppressed children after household exposure to varicella. J. Infect. Dis. *147*:737–743, 1983.
384. Ziegler, E. J., Fisher, C. J., Jr., Sprung, C. L., et al.: Treatment of gram negative bacteremia and septic shock with HA 1A human monoclonal antibody against endotoxin. N. Engl. J. Med. *324*:429–436, 1991.
385. Ziegler, E. J., McCutchan, J. A., Fierer, J., et al.: Treatment of gram negative bacteremia and shock with human antiserum to a mutant *Escherichia coli*. N. Engl. J. Med. *307*:1225–1230, 1982.
386. Zingher, A.: Convalescent whole blood, plasma, and serum in prophylaxis of measles. J. A. M. A. *82*:1180–1187, 1924.

OTHER PREVENTIVE CONSIDERATIONS

❑ ❑ ❑

239

PUBLIC HEALTH CONSIDERATIONS

Steven L. Solomon and David W. Fraser

Public health can be defined as those aspects of health and disease that are determined by the interaction of people and their environment, including but not limited to circumstances in which the condition of one person or group of persons affects that of others. These diseases may be nutritional, toxic, or infectious, but they are alike in that they all have an exogenous source. Because the source is exogenous, cases of diseases that fall under public health tend to occur in clusters, patterns of which are determined by the interplay of exposure and susceptibility. The main thrusts of disease control in public health are (1) prevention of additional cases by identification and elimination of the source of exposure or prevention of transmission from it and (2) identification of the high-risk susceptible group and reduction of its susceptibility.

The tools for control of public health problems fall into two categories: recognition/evaluation and intervention. Foremost among the tools for recognition and evaluation is surveillance, which can be defined as the systematic collection of information about the occurrence of disease in a community.[140] When, through surveillance or serendipity, an unusual cluster of disease is recognized, an epidemic investigation is required, to include the description of the disease, determination of the pattern of its occurrence in the community, formulation of hypotheses of the cause of the unusual frequency, testing of the hypotheses, and framing of control methods. Of assistance in both surveillance and epidemic investigation is the recognition of common patterns of disease spread either within groups of people or from the environment to people.

There are many tools for intervention. Two important categories are not considered in this chapter because they are addressed at length elsewhere in this book; one is immunization (active and passive) (Chapters 237 and 238), and the other is treatment of individual patients. Tools that are discussed here include isolation, chemoprophylaxis, water and food sanitation (including the special situation of international travel), and vector control.

SURVEILLANCE

The primary purpose of surveillance is to permit the timely recognition of new public health problems through the monitoring of the pattern of disease occurrence in the community, with the ultimate aim to effect early control of these problems.[140] A secondary purpose is to answer defined questions about the pattern of disease occurrence, but the ultimate goal is the same.

Surveillance involves the collection of data, collation and analysis, and feedback of information. When used properly, this information helps in the directing of disease control activities and evaluation of their impact. In the primary collection of information, three major factors must be defined.[24] The first is the population to be surveyed, which may be circumscribed geographically (e.g., the United States) or may be restricted to a certain age group (e.g., infants, for the surveillance of birth defects) or to a certain institution (e.g., a school, a hospital, the army). Second, the data to be monitored can be as crude as the number of cases of disease or deaths from a disease. Additional information that could be collected and be useful epidemiologically includes the characteristics of ill persons with regard to age, sex, place of residence, occupation, and so on, or detailed characteristics of the organisms involved, such as antibiotic sensitivity, serogroup, or site of the body from which an isolate was made. The third and most important element of the reporting system is the primary reporting source. Unless a report of disease is initiated—by a physician, infection control practitioner, or laboratory—no information is generated. Incentives to the primary reporting source to maintain good reporting are essential for the maintenance of a useful surveillance system.

In each state, the reporting of specified infectious diseases is required by law. However, state laws vary with regard to the persons who are responsible for reporting, the diseases or conditions that are reportable, and the circumstances under which reporting is to occur.[39, 80] Specific information generally is available upon request from state or local health agencies.

The collection of surveillance information on disease occurrence is pointless unless the data are used to initiate or modify control actions. The first step is the collation and analysis, which may be done at the level of the local health department, the state health department, or the federal government. If this is done in a timely fashion, problems can be recognized early and a response made.

After this information is collated and analyzed, the results are fed back to the primary reporting source as well as to others interested in the data. This feedback serves to maintain interest in the reporting system and thus maintain the quality of data obtained and continuously to update persons at each level of the surveillance system about the changing patterns of disease occurrence and new strategies for disease control.

One vehicle for the feedback of national surveillance information is the *Morbidity and Mortality Weekly Report*, which is published by the Centers for Disease Control and Prevention (CDC). Also published by the CDC are periodic summaries of surveillance activities relating to specific diseases. Regular summaries of surveillance activities also are published by the World Health Organization and by many state health departments.

The identification of a disease problem in the course of surveillance should prompt an attempt to control the problem. This may involve the initiation of an epidemic investigation if surveillance data suggest an unusual frequency of occurrence of a disease or the adjustment in a public health program if, for example, surveillance data suggest that vaccine is not being given to a particular age group of susceptible people.

EPIDEMIC INVESTIGATION

When faced with a possible outbreak, it is useful for the investigator to approach the inquiry systematically.

1. *Verify the diagnosis.* Review of available clinical and laboratory information and examination of a few patients will permit creation of a list of possible diagnoses and will suggest additional diagnostic specimens that may be needed to secure the diagnosis. The investigation may proceed without a microbiologic diagnosis if a clearly defined clinical syndrome can be identified. With or without microbiologic confirmation, a firm case definition is needed.
2. *Confirm the existence of an epidemic.* Through use of the objective case definition, the baseline incidence of the illness before the apparent epidemic should be determined by review of appropriate microbiologic, serologic, or clinical records. Armed with these data, the investigator can decide whether recent events indicate an unusual clustering of illness, that is, whether an epidemic exists.
3. *Describe the time, place, and person.* Graphic display of the distribution of cases in time not only confirms the existence of an epidemic but also indicates whether the outbreak is waxing or waning. It may permit judgment about whether the outbreak is spread from person to person or from a common source of exposure and an estimate of the incubation period. Comparison of the characteristics of cases in regard to age, sex, geographic location, and other relevant factors with those of persons who reasonably might have been considered to have been at risk but who did not become ill forms the basis for making epidemiologic hypotheses. The attack rate, (number ill/number ill + number well), is a useful method of describing the risk of illness in various groups.
4. *Frame an epidemiologic hypothesis.* Using the diagnosis (presumed or confirmed) and the pattern of disease occurrence, the investigator may hypothesize one or several possible common sources of infection and one or more modes of spread (food- or water-borne, airborne, vector-borne, or by a particular therapeutic or diagnostic procedure). Alternatively, the hypothesis may be of person-to-person spread.
5. *Identify the control group(s).* Central to the epidemiologic process is the identification of a group of persons who might have developed illness but who did not.[52] The activities and exposures that set the well persons apart from the sick persons often point to the source of the outbreak. For gastroenteritis occurring after a church supper, one control group might be those who went to the supper but did not get sick; another control group might be residents of the same community who did not attend the supper. For histoplasmosis in schoolchildren occurring after a school clean-up program, controls might be the well children.
6. *Test the hypothesis epidemiologically.* The attack rates of illness among persons exposed or not exposed to a hypothesized source then are compared using the number of cases and controls in each group. A true common source should be associated with a higher attack rate among those exposed to it than among those not so exposed. Statistical tests are useful to assess the significance of differences observed in attack rates of those exposed and not exposed.
7. *Explain the outliers.* Any case that occurs in a person not apparently exposed to an implicated common source needs to be explained. As an example, if vanilla ice cream were implicated as the common source in a food-borne outbreak and ill persons are found who only ate chocolate ice cream, one might hypothesize reasonably cross-contamination of the ice cream scoop. Faulty memory of exposure to a common source and the simultaneous occurrence of endemic cases unrelated to the outbreak may complicate this stage of the investigation.
8. *Confirm the hypothesis microbiologically.* Cultures of the implicated common-source material may permit recovery of the infectious agent. When a microorganism is isolated, typing methods may be used to support the epidemiologic hypothesis by demonstrating that the same strain was responsible for disease in all affected patients and can be recovered from the common source. Traditional methods for typing microorganisms—serotyping, biotyping, antimicrobial sensitivity testing, and immunoblotting—remain very useful. In recent years, these techniques have been supplemented and in some settings replaced by DNA-based typing methods, such as plasmid profile analysis, pulsed-field gel electrophoresis of chromosomal DNA, and the use of polymerase chain reaction for identifying DNA segments.[97, 139] However, culturing the agent from a particular site without epidemiologic implication of that site as a source of infection provides little or no information needed to direct control measures.
9. *Implement control measures.* Knowledge of the agent, source, and mode of spread permits drafting of control measures and their implementation. Without careful attention to this step, the investigation is an academic exercise only.
10. *Measure the impact of control measures.* This step doubles as the ultimate testing of the epidemiologic hypothesis and as an assessment of the design and implementation of the control measures. Surveillance for the occurrence of disease in groups shown to be at high risk is the most common technique used for this measurement, and a decrease in the attack rate to zero or to the baseline incidence is the measure of success.

An example of the process is the investigation of an epidemic of postoperative group A streptococcal wound infections. In November 1970, the CDC was informed by the staff of a 140-bed hospital that a large number of streptococcal wound infections had occurred in the preceding 2 weeks and that two patients had died. In his subsequent investigation, Conrad Fulkerson determined that group A streptococci had been isolated (step 1) and that the number of patients in the hospital with group A streptococcal isolates from wounds increased from two in September to seven in October and to four in the first 10 days of November. Earlier months had averaged one case per month (step 2). He found that the 13 infected patients came from six preoperative wards in the hospital, had widely ranging ages, had a variety of surgical procedures, and included members of both sexes. The interval from operation to onset of wound infection was 0.5 to 2 days for 10 patients; two of the three patients who had intervals greater than 2 days had been given prophylactic systemic antibiotics at surgery (step 3).

Because group A streptococci almost invariably are spread from person to person, because patients came from many wards, and because most cases occurred shortly after surgery, Dr. Fulkerson hypothesized that spread had occurred from one of the operating room personnel to the patients during

TABLE 239–1. Operating Room Log Excerpt from Epidemiologic Investigation

Surgical Case No.	Sex	Surgeon	Assistant	Anesthesiologist	Circulating Nurse	Scrub Nurse
1709	F	Zellner	Pane	Mutsen	Land	Roman
1719	F	Wilson	Toulson	Sutterfield	Roman	Bartt
1726*	F	Dryden	Zellner	Sutterfield	Grasser	Bartt
1733	F	Dryden	Walker	Taylor	Hodge	Roman
1744	M	Wilson	—	—	Peak	Bartt
1760	F	Polson	Riley	Mutsen	Jones	Land
1773	F	Martin	Riley	Sutterfield	Hodge	Roman
1788	F	Stein	Wilson	Mutsen	Hodge	Bartt
1795	F	Polson	Pane	Mutsen	Jones	Bartt
1807	M	Dryden	Riley	Sutterfield	Jones	Roman
1831	F	Kirk	Toulson	Taylor	Peak	Land
1847	F	Martin	Wright	Mutsen	Peak	Roman
1865	F	Wilson	Dryden	Taylor	Hodge	Roman
1874	F	Bear	Zellner	Taylor	Swift	Roman
1895	F	Berger	Sartorius	Sutterfield	Swift	Hodge
1905*	F	Zellner	Ballson	Sutterfield	Jones	Roman
1918	M	Wilson	Toulson, Martin	Sutterfield	Jones	Hodge
1938	F	Berger	Toulson	Sutterfield	Jones	Hodge
1942*	M	Berger	Caroll	Sutterfield	Jones	Hodge
1953	F	Kirk	Toulson	Taylor	Peak	Roman
1964*	F	Bear	Dryden	Sutterfield	Hodge	Roman
1968	F	Berger	—	Mutsen	Peak	Land
1982	F	Stein	Toulson	Sutterfield	Peak	Grasser
1996*	M	Ballson	Inger	Sutterfield	Hodge	Roman
1999	F	Martin	Pane	Taylor	Peak	Roman
2017*	F	Zellner	Bear	Sutterfield	Jones	Roman
2019*	F	Zellner	Bear	Sutterfield	Jones	Roman
2023	F	Martin	Able	Sutterfield	Swift	Roman
2039	M	Ballson	Dryden	Sutterfield	Swift	Peak
2050	F	Martin	Toulson	Sutterfield	Jones	Bartt
2069*	F	Dryden	Martin	Sutterfield	Jones	Peak
2074	F	Zellner	Bear	Taylor	Jones	Land
2083	F	Wilson	—	—	Land	—
2093*	F	Bear	Caroll	Mutsen	Hodge	Roman
2101	M	Martin	Toulson	Sutterfield	Peak	Roman
2119	F	Bear	Zellner	Taylor	Hodge	Peak
2134	F	Avis	—	Sutterfield	Peak	—
2148	M	Kirk	Pool	Sutterfield	Peak	Swift
2162*	F	Martin	Riley	Taylor	Swift	Bartt
2166	F	Bear	Zellner	Taylor	Land	Peak
2173	M	Martin	Ballson	Taylor	Jones	Land
2183	F	Wilson	Toulson	Taylor	Land	Roman
2194*	F	Berger	Wilson	Taylor	Peak	Roman
2200*	F	Polson	Dryden	Sutterfield	Jones	Roman
2202*	F	Wilson	—	Taylor	Hodge	Bartt
2208	F	Martin	Pool	Sutterfield	Land	—
2224	F	Bear	Caroll	—	Land	Bartt

*Patients who developed postoperative streptococcal wound infection.

surgery (step 4). Dr. Fulkerson chose as the control group all persons who underwent major operations during the epidemic period (step 5). These were listed in the operating room log in chronologic order. To reduce this list to a more workable size, Table 239–1 includes only every fifth member of the actual control group as well as the 13 cases. You may wish to execute step 6 yourself, using the data in Table 239–1. Once convinced that you have identified the source using epidemiologic methods, you may wish to speculate on step 7 and design an investigation to satisfy step 8 before turning to the Appendix at the end of this chapter for the dénouement.

COMMON PATTERNS OF DISEASE SPREAD

Disease Spread from Animals to People

Many infectious diseases are transmitted from other animals to humans. The physician who routinely inquires about animal contacts as part of the clinical and epidemiologic history of an ill patient frequently finds valuable clues to an obscure diagnosis. Table 239–2 lists infectious disease agents for which there is some suggestive or definitive evidence that disease can be spread from animal to human, either directly or via a vector. A distinctive disease name associated with the organism also is listed, as are the various animal groups that have been suggested or shown to act as sources of transmission to humans. The frequency with which an animal group serves as a source of infection for humans and the frequency with which a vector is involved are indicated in a semiquantitative fashion. Omitted are many species that may be infected with the organism but do not appear to act as a source of human infection. Also omitted are certain rare or accidental infectious diseases. The complex life cycles of some parasites are difficult to display in tabular form; intermediate animal hosts are designated in Table 239–2 to facilitate interpretation. Details of the clinical presentation,

Text continued on page 2813

TABLE 239–2. Infectious Disease Spread from Animals to Humans*

		Animal Source†															
Organism	**Disease**	***Vector-borne‡***	***Dogs***	***Cats***	***Cattle***	***Horses***	***Swine***	***Sheep, Goats***	***Domestic Fowl***	***Pigeons***	***Parrots, Parakeets***	***Mice, Rats***	***Rabbits***	***Fish***	***Shellfish***	***Turtles***	***Nonhuman Primates***	***Other***
Bacterial Diseases																		
Spirochetes and Curved Bacteria																		
Borrelia species	Relapsing fever	++			?	?						2					?	Opossums ? Squirrels 2 Small rodents 2 Armadillos ?
Borrelia burgdorferi	Lyme disease	++	?	?	?							2	?					Deer 2 Birds ? Other rodents 2 Other carnivores?
Leptospira interrogans	Leptospirosis		2	1	2	1	2	1				2	?					Skunks 1 Squirrels 1 Raccoons 1 Many animals 2
Spirillum minus	Rat-bite fever											3						Carnivores 1 Other rodents ?
Gram-Negative Rods																		
Pseudomonas pseudomallei	Melioidosis	?	?			?												
Pseudomonas mallei	Glanders		?			3		?										Mules 3 Wolves ? Asses 3
Brucella abortus	Brucellosis				3													
Brucella suis					2		3											
Brucella melitensis								3										
Brucella canis			3															
Bordetella bronchiseptica			2	1								?	2					Guinea pigs 2
Francisella tularensis	Tularemia	+							2			2	2					Muskrats 2 Beaver 1 Other rodents 1 Squirrels 1 Hamsters 2
Campylobacter species			1	1	2			1	3			1						
Salmonella species			1	1	1	1	1	1	3	1	1	1	1	1	1	2	2	Many 1,2
Shigella species																	2	
Yersinia pestis	Plague	++	1	2								2	1					Ground squirrels 2 Prairie dogs 2 Wild carnivores 1 Tree squirrels 1 Other rodents 1
Yersinia pseudotuberculosis			1	1									?					Canary 1 Hamster ? Guinea pig ?
Yersinia enterocolitica			1				3											
Vibrio parahaemolyticus															?			
Vibrio vulnificus															3			
Pasteurella multocida			2	2	2	1	2		1				1					Opossum 1
Pasteurella haemolytica																		Deer 1

TABLE 239–2. Infectious Disease Spread from Animals to Humans* *Continued*

Organism	Disease	Animal Source† Vector-borne‡	Dogs	Cats	Cattle	Horses	Swine	Sheep, Goats	Domestic Fowl	Pigeons	Parrots, Parakeets	Mice, Rats	Rabbits	Fish	Shellfish	Turtles	Nonhuman Primates	Other
Pasteurella pneumotropica			2	2														
Capnocytophaga canimorsus			2															Coyotes ? Bears ? Tigers ?
Streptobacillus moniliformis	Rat-bite fever											2						
Bartenella henselae	Bacillary angiomatosis, ? cat-scratch disease			3														
Gram-Positive Cocci																		
Staphylococcus aureus							?							?				
Streptococcus group A				1														
Streptococcus group B				?														
Streptococcus group C						2												
Streptococcus group R							2											
Streptococcus group S							2											
Gram-Positive Rods																		
Bacillus anthracis	Anthrax				2	2		2										
Clostridium tetani	Tetanus				?	?												
Listeria monocytogenes					1			1	1									Whales 1
Erysipelothrix insidiosa							3		2			?		2	2			Seals 1
Corynebacterium equi					?		?	?										
Corynebacterium pyogenes								?										
Corynebacterium pseudotuberculosis								?										
Mycobacterium tuberculosis	Tuberculosis		1	1	1												2	
Mycobacterium bovis			1	1	3													
Mycobacterium ovium							?											
Mycobacterium marinum														2				Dolphins 1 Poikilotherms 1
Mycobacterium leprae	Leprosy	?																Armadillo ?
Dermatophilus congolensis					?	?		?										
Rickettsiae																		
Ehrlichia chaffeensis	Human ehrlichiosis	+ +																?
Rickettsia prowazekii	Louse-borne typhus	+ +			?	?	?	?										
Rickettsia typhi	Murine typhus	+ +		1								3						
Rickettsia ricketsii	Rockey Mountain spotted fever	+ +	2	2								2	2					Other rodents 2 Birds ?
Rickettsia siberica	North Asian tick typhus	+ +										3						Birds ?

Table continued on following page

TABLE 239–2. Infectious Disease Spread from Animals to Humans* *Continued*

Organism	Disease	Animal Source†																
		Vector-borne‡	Dogs	Cats	Cattle	Horses	Swine	Sheep, Goats	Domestic Fowl	Pigeons	Parrots, Parakeets	Mice, Rats	Rabbits	Fish	Shellfish	Turtles	Nonhuman Primates	Other
Rickettsia conorii	Fièvre boutonneuse	+ +	2									2						Birds ?
Rickettsia australis	Queensland tick typhus	+ +										2						Small marsupials 2
Rickettsia akari	Rickettsialpox	+ +										3						
Rickettsia tsutsugamushi	Scrub typhus	+ +										3						Birds ?
Coxiella burnetii	Q fever	+			2			3										Small mammals 2 Birds ?
Chlamydiae																		
Chlamydia psittaci	Psittacosis	?		1	?				2	2	2							Other birds 2 Muskrats ?
Fungal Diseases																		
Microsporum canis	Ringworm		2	2														
Microsporum equinum	Ringworm					2												
Microsporum nanum	Ringworm						2											
Trichophyton equinum	Ringworm					2												
Microsporum gallinae	Ringworm								2									
Trichophyton mentagrophytes var. *quinckeanum*												2						
Trichophyton mentagrophytes var. *erinacei*	Ringworm																	Hedgehogs 2
Trichophyton mentagrophytes var. *mentagrophytes*	Ringworm		2									2						
Trichophyton verrucosum	Ringworm				2													
Parasitic Diseases																		
Helminths																		
Angiostrongylus species												2		3	*3*§			Amphibians 3 Reptiles 3
Capillaria hepatica			1	1								2						
Capillaria philipinensis														3				
Dioctophyma renale														2				Mink and other fish-eating mammals 2
Trichinella spiralis			?				3											Bears 1, Seals 1 Walruses 1, Whales 1
Filaria																		
Brugia malayi	Filariasis	+ +		2													2	Other carnivores 2
Dirofilaria immitis	Heartworm	+ +	3															
Dirofilaria tenuis		+ +																Raccoons 3
Dirofilaria repens		+ +	2	2														
Nematodes																		
Ascaris lumbricoides							1											
Ascaris suum							1											

TABLE 239–2. Infectious Disease Spread from Animals to Humans* *Continued*

Organism	Disease	Animal Source†: Vector-borne‡	Dogs	Cats	Cattle	Horses	Swine	Sheep, Goats	Domestic Fowl	Pigeons	Parrots, Parakeets	Mice, Rats	Rabbits	Fish	Shellfish	Turtles	Nonhuman Primates	Other
Ancylostoma braziliense	Cutaneous larva migrans		2	3														
Ancylostoma caninum	Cutaneous larva migrans		2															
Ancylostoma ceylonicum	Cutaneous larva migrans		2	2														
Uncinaria stenocephala	Cutaneous larva migrans		2	2														Foxes 1
Gnathostoma spinigerum	Visceral and cutaneous larva migrans		2	2					2					2				Frogs 1 Snakes 1 Raccoons 2
Toxocara canis	Visceral larva migrans		3															Other canids 2
Toxocara cati	Visceral larva migrans			3														
Anisakis species														*3*				Marine mammals 2
Strongyloides stercoralis			2	2												?		
Trichostrongylus species					2	2		2										Donkeys 2
Trematodes																		
Schistosoma hoematobium															*3*		3	
Schistosoma japonicum			2	2	2	2	2	2				2			*3*			
Schistosoma mansoni												?			*3*			Baboons 2
Clinostomum complanatum														2				
Clonorchis sinensis	Oriental liver fluke		2	2										*3*	*3*			
Dicrocoelium dendriticum					2			2							*2*			Ants *2*
Dicrocoelium hospes					2			2							*2*			Ants *2*
Echinostoma species			1	1			1			2	2	1		*1*	*2*			
Fasciola gigantica	Liver fluke				2	2		2							*2*			
Fasciola hepatica	Liver fluke				2			2							*2*			
Fasciolopsis buski	Liver fluke						2								*2*			
Gastrodiscoides hominis							2								*2*	*3*		
Haplorchis species			2											*3*	*2*			Numerous birds and mammals 2
Heterophyes species			2	*2*								2		*3*	*3*			Other birds 2 Other carnivores 2
Metagonimus species															*3*	*2*		Numerous birds and mammals 2
Opisthorchis felineus				2										*3*	*2*			Numerous other birds, reptiles, and mammals 2
Paragonimus species															*3*			Numerous mammals 2
Heterophids																		
Centrocestus formosanum			2	2								2		*3*	*2*			Other birds 2

Table continued on following page

TABLE 239–2. Infectious Disease Spread from Animals to Humans* *Continued*

Organism	Disease	Animal Source†															
		Vector-borne‡	*Dogs*	*Cats*	*Cattle*	*Horses*	*Swine*	*Sheep, Goats*	*Domestic Fowl*	*Pigeons*	*Parrots, Parakeets*	*Mice, Rats*	*Rabbits*	*Fish*	*Shellfish*	*Turtles*	*Nonhuman Primates*	*Other*
Stellantchasmus species			2	2										*3*	*2*			
Cestodes																		
Taenia saginata	Taeniasis				3													
Taenia solium	Taeniasis/ Cysticercosis		2				3											
Echinococcus granulosus	Hydatid disease		3				*3*											Other carnivores 2
Echinococcus multilocularis	Hydatid disease		3	2								*2*						Foxes 2
Bertiella species	Tapeworm	+ +															1	
Diphyllobothrium latum	Fish tapeworm													*3*				Other carnivores 2
Dipylidium caninum	Tapeworm	+ +	3	2														
Hymenolepis diminuta	Tapeworm	+ +										2						
Hymenolepis nana	Tapeworm	?										2						Hamsters ?
Mesocestoides species	Tapeworm	?	2	2														Snakes *1* Birds *1* Other carnivores *2*
Spirometra species	Sparginosis		1	1			1		1			*1*						Frogs *2* Copepods *1* Snakes *1*
Protozoa																		
Trypanosoma cruzi	Chagas disease	+ +	2	2									2					Raccoons 2 Guinea pigs 2 Opossum ? Armadillo ? Numerous small mammals 2
Trypanosoma gambiense	Gambian sleeping sickness	+ +	1				1											
Trypanosoma rhodesiense	Rhodesian sleeping sickness	+ +			2													Bushbuck 2
Leishmania brasiliensis	Espundia, uta, etc.	+ +										2						Other rodents 2 Sloths ? Anteater ?
Leishmania mexicana	Espundia, uta, etc.	+ +										2						Small mammals 2
Leishmania donovani	Kala-azar	+ +	2	?	?	?		?				2						Jackals 2 Foxes 2
Leishmania chagasi	Kala-azar	+ +	2									2						Foxes Other rodents 2
Leishmania tropica	Oriental sore	+ +	2									2						Gerbils 2 Other rodents 2
Leishmania major	Oriental sore, etc.	+ +																Gerbils 2 Other rodents 2
Leishmania aethiopica	Oriental sore, etc.	+ +																Hyrax 2 Other rodents 2
Plasmodium knowlesi	Malaria	+ +															2	
Plasmodium simium	Malaria	+ +															?	

TABLE 239–2. Infectious Disease Spread from Animals to Humans* *Continued*

		Animal Source†																
Organism	**Disease**	***Vector-borne‡***	***Dogs***	***Cats***	***Cattle***	***Horses***	***Swine***	***Sheep, Goats***	***Domestic Fowl***	***Pigeons***	***Parrots, Parakeets***	***Mice, Rats***	***Rabbits***	***Fish***	***Shellfish***	***Turtles***	***Nonhuman Primates***	***Other***
Babesia divergens	Babesiosis	+ +			2													
Babesia microti	Babesiosis	+ +										2						Deer 2
Pneumocystis carinii												?						
Sarcocystis species					?		?	?									1	
Toxoplasma gondii		?		2	2		2	2	?			?						
Cryptosporidium species	Cryptosporidiosis		?	?	2	?	?	?	?		?	?	?	?			?	Deer ?
Viral Diseases																		
Herpesvirus simiae	Monkey B encephalitis																3	
Cowpox					3													
Pseudocowpox	Milker's nodule				3													
Orf								3										
Bovine papular stomatitis					3													
Monkeypox																	3	
Vesicular stomatitis		?			2													
Junin fever	Argentine hemorrhagic fever											3						
Machupo	Bolivian hemorrhagic fever											3						
Hantaan	Korean hemorrhagic fever											3						Shrews 1, Voles 1 Other rodents 1
Sin Nombre	Hantavirus pulmonary syndrome											3						
Lassa												3						
Lymphocytic choriomeningitis												2						Hamsters 2
Hepatitis A															2		2	
Influenza A/swine	Swine influenza						2											
Newcastle									3									
Foot and mouth disease					1			1										
Marburg																	2	
Ebola																	1	
Rabies			2	1	1													Wolf 2 Bat 1, Fox 1 Skunk 1 Mongoose 1 Raccoon 1 Jackal 1
Arboviruses																		
Chikungunya		+ +															2	
O'nyong nyong		+ +															?	

Table continued on following page

TABLE 239–2. Infectious Disease Spread from Animals to Humans* *Continued*

		Animal Source†																	
Organism	Disease	*Vector-borne‡*	*Dogs*	*Cats*	*Cattle*	*Horses*	*Swine*	*Sheep, Goats*	*Domestic Fowl*	*Pigeons*	*Parrots, Parakeets*	*Mice, Rats*	*Rabbits*	*Fish*	*Shellfish*	*Turtles*	*Nonhuman Primates*	*Other*
Sindbis		+ +							?	?								Other birds 2
Eastern equine encephalitis		+ +																Other birds 3
Western equine encephalitis		+ +																Other birds 3
Venezuelan equine encephalitis		+ +				2						2						
Yellow fever		+ +															2	
Japanese encephalitis		+ +				?	2											Other birds 2
Murray Valley encephalitis		+ +																Other birds 3
Wesselsbron		+						3										
West Nile		+ +								?								Other birds 3
Zika		+ +															2	
St. Louis encephalitis		+ +							?	?								Other birds 3
Ilheus		+ +																Other birds ?
Kyasanur Forest disease		+ +										2					2	
Louping ill		+ +							3									Other birds ?
Omsk hemorrhagic fever		+ +			?							?						Muskrat ?
Powassan		+ +										?						Birds ? Squirrels ? Woodchucks ?
Tick-borne encephalitis		+ +			2			2				2						Other birds 2
Dengue		+ +															?	
Bwamba		+ +															?	
LaCrosse		+ +																Chipmunks 2 Foxes 2 Squirrels 2
California encephalitis		+ +											?					Squirrels 2
Oropouche		+ +															?	Other birds ? Sloth ?
Kemerovo		+ +			2	?						2						Other birds ?
Congo/CHF	Crimean hemorrhagic fever	+ +			2	2						2	2					Other birds 2
Colorado tick fever		+ +										1						Ground squirrels 3 Porcupines ?
Nairobi sheep disease		+ +						3										
Rift Valley fever		+ +			2			2				?						
Ross River		+ +					?	?										Kangaroos ?*
Mayaro		+ +																Other mammals ?
Group C fevers		+ +										3					1	Other birds ?

*Certain rare or accidental infectious diseases omitted.

†Animal species that seem to be sources, either directly or through a vector, of microbial agents that infect humans: 3, typical source of human infection; 2, common source of human infection; 1, rare source of human infection; ?, speculative source of human infection. Many diseases and many animal species are omitted for which evidence is lacking that infection is transmitted from lower animals to humans.

‡Disease acquired through bites from, contact with, or ingestion of insects or arachnids; + +, disease typically vector-borne; +, disease occasionally vector-borne; ?, speculation that disease occasionally may be vector-borne.

§Numbers in italics indicate intermediate hosts for certain parasitic diseases.

differential diagnosis, and treatment of the zoonoses are found in the appropriate chapters elsewhere in this book. For a complete description of the circumstances under which each agent is spread from animal to person, consult a textbook of zoonoses.[1, 14]

Excluded from Table 239–2 are several interesting groups of infectious diseases in which human beings and animals appear to interact but in which infection does not spread from animals to people. The first group includes organisms that infect both animals and humans from a common source in nature. These include *Pseudomonas pseudomallei, Blastomyces dermatitidis,* and *Aspergillus* species, which, from soil or other inanimate sources, can infect a wide variety of animal species, including humans.

A few diseases typically are spread from humans to animals. Perhaps the most prominent example of this is *Herpesvirus hominis,* which can cause a fatal encephalitis in nonhuman primates when spread from humans. Tuberculosis also can spread from humans to nonhuman primates, as well as the reverse.

Cryptococcus neoformans lives in animal feces but does not infect animals. From the fecal material, these organisms may spread to infect people.

Some organisms can be transmitted by fomites of animal origin. These act as mechanical carriers, and the process does not involve infection of the animals. Examples include *Histoplasma capsulatum,* which has been observed to be spread by chicken feathers, and *Coccidioides immitis,* which can be spread in bales of wool contaminated with fungus-laden dust.

Another group of diseases are spread from person to person but through an insect vector, either typically or on occasion. Filariasis caused by *Wuchereria bancrofti* is a prime example of a disease in which vector-borne person-to-person spread is the rule. Typhoid and yaws have been shown to be spread by vectors on occasion. There is evidence that *Mycobacterium leprae* can be recovered from mosquitoes that have fed on patients with lepromatous leprosy, and there has been speculation that such mosquitoes may serve as vectors of transmission.

Disease Spread from Person to Person

As members of groups—including the family, school, camp, day care center, and church—children are at risk of acquiring or spreading infectious agents that are transmitted from person to person. Knowledge of the typical patterns of spread can be useful in planning surveillance or in designing control measures. For example, recognition that diarrhea commonly results from person-to-person spread in day care centers and that it can indicate inadequate hygienic practices may justify specific surveillance for diarrhea in that setting. Documentation of secondary cases in various categories of contacts of cases of meningococcal disease permits focusing the delivery of chemoprophylaxis on just the high-risk groups.

In this section, spread in the family and the school is discussed, but several groups of interest are omitted. The important areas of disease transmission within day care centers and within hospitals are discussed in separate chapters. Maternal transmission of specific infections to the fetus or neonate also is reviewed elsewhere in this book. Spread, especially of enteric diseases, within institutions for the mentally retarded is recognized widely as an important problem, but it does not impinge directly on the practice of most pediatricians.

The Family

Spread of disease agents in the family can be considered in two stages: introduction of the agent into the family, usually by a single member ("index case" or "index carrier") and the spread to other family members. The spread to other members can be described in terms of rapidity and intensity, the latter commonly measured by the secondary infection rate (or secondary attack rate), which is defined as the proportion of the contacts of the index carrier or index case who become infected (or ill) in a given interval after the introduction. The secondary infection rate varies from agent to agent and may be affected by the age and sex of the introducer, size of the family, crowding, age of household contacts, prior immunity, and intervention attempted, including isolation, treatment, and chemoprophylaxis. The ratio of the secondary attack rate to the incidence of disease in the community is a measure of the importance of the family as a focus of disease.[62]

Of the bacteria spread by the respiratory route, pneumococci, group A streptococci, meningococci, and *Haemophilus influenzae* have been studied most completely. In a study of English families of five persons each (mother, father, and three children, the youngest of whom was younger than 5 years of age), type-specific introductions of pneumococci were made most frequently by the middle child.[16] The oldest and middle children were the most efficient spreaders of pneumococci to other family members. Among household contacts, children were more likely than their parents to become infected. The overall secondary infection rate was 9 per cent. Children with group A streptococcal infection in members of families in Cleveland, Ohio, were even more important than children with pneumococcal infection as introducers and as recipients of intrafamilial transmission.[83] The pattern for meningococcal infection has been reported to be strikingly different. The most common introducers of meningococci into families are men, followed distantly and in decreasing order of frequency by women, girls, and boys.[68] Once meningococci are introduced, all family members may become infected, although studies of carriers in household contacts of cases of meningococcal disease in Brazil suggest that spread may proceed from an adult to older children and only thereafter to infants.[111]

Children younger than 5 years of age have the greatest risk of serious disease from *H. influenzae* type b infection. Overall carriage rates are less than 5 per cent, although high rates of colonization have been reported in settings such as day care where young children are in close contact and in families with a child with invasive *H. influenzae* type b disease.[105] Among unvaccinated contacts of cases of *H. influenzae* type b disease, children younger than 5 years of age have the highest carriage rates (30 to 40 per cent); carriage rates drop progressively with increasing age.[7] However, the epidemiology of *H. influenzae* type b disease has been changed markedly by the use of vaccines; annual disease incidence among children younger than 5 years of age fell 71 per cent (from 37/100,000 to 11/100,000) from 1989 to 1991, after the introduction of conjugate vaccines.[2] Unlike earlier polysaccharide vaccines, conjugate vaccines appear to prevent colonization as well as disease; one study using a matched case-control analysis showed that conjugate vaccines had an 81 per cent efficacy of decreasing colonization.[112]

Bordetella pertussis spreads easily within families. In a study of 21 families in Finland, 83 per cent of family members of primary cases showed serologic evidence of secondary infection.[104] Secondary attack rates for symptomatic disease were lower among older children and adults. Children 2 to 15 years of age were more likely to introduce pertussis into the family than were younger children or family members older than 15 years of age. Adults may be of increasing importance as reservoirs of *B. pertussis* leading to infection in infants.[92, 113] A study in Germany of 122 households with an index case of pertussis showed that index cases who were adults were as likely to spread pertussis within the family as were index cases who were children. Fourteen (78 per cent) of 18 adults and 74 (71 per cent) of 104 children spread pertussis to at least one other family member.[147] Outbreaks have been reported in which an adult with persistent bronchitis acted as a source of pertussis for children.[88, 93]

Both tuberculosis and leprosy usually are acquired by children from adults who introduce the mycobacteria into the household. These introducers typically shed large numbers of bacteria from the respiratory tract (especially from the nose in lepromatous leprosy) for months or years. Secondary attack rates are similar for the two diseases and are highest for tuberculosis in children younger than 5 years of age.[127] For leprosy, children of all ages beyond the neonatal period are at significant risk.

Introducers who are ill tend to be more efficient spreaders of bacteria in the respiratory tract. In the Cleveland study, spread of group A streptococci was 2.7 times as frequent when the introducer was symptomatic as when the introducer was asymptomatic. Spread of group A streptococci was observed among Egyptian families particularly frequently if the person who introduced the strain into the household was ill enough to seek medical care or if the strain persisted in the respiratory tract of the introducer for 3 or more months.[53] Nasal shedders have been shown to be more efficient spreaders,[98] and nasal shedding commonly is found early in illness. In 14 (56 per cent) of the 25 episodes of transfer of pneumococci observed in Virginia families, the spreader had sneezing, rhinorrhea, nasal congestion, or cough during the 2-week period in which transfer occurred, whereas such symptoms were present in 159 (37 per cent) of the other 423 2-week periods of observation.[69] Again, this may relate to higher rates of recovery of pneumococci from the nose during symptoms of upper respiratory tract infection.[137]

Crowding has been observed inconsistently to affect spread of pneumococci. English families living in only two rooms had a secondary infection rate of 16.0 per cent, whereas those living in four or more rooms had an 11.2 per cent secondary infection rate.[16] Floor space was not shown to affect spread in Syracuse, New York, families.[49] Limited ventilation of houses seems to promote spread of meningococci in the meningitis belt in Africa.[65] In a population-based case-control study, household crowding was shown to be a risk factor for *H. influenzae* disease.[40] Ill children were 2.6 times more likely to live in households containing one or more persons per room than were well children in control families. The magnitude of risk associated with crowding increased as the extent of crowding increased.

Carriage may persist for many months for meningococci[68] and group A streptococci[83] and may result in multiple cases of disease in a family widely separated in time. Typically, however, half of the secondary cases of meningococcal and *H. influenzae* type b disease occur within 5 days of the index case.[60, 67, 111]

The changing epidemiology of measles and mumps demonstrates the impact of vaccines on the transmission of viral diseases spread by the respiratory route. The age at which a person is most at risk for one of these diseases is determined largely by the communicability of the virus and the completeness of immunity. Hope-Simpson[77] calculated that 75 per cent of susceptible family contacts exposed to a case of measles developed that disease, whereas the corresponding figures for varicella and mumps were 61 per cent and 31 per cent, respectively. In that study, the mean ages at which infection occurred were 5.6, 6.7, and 11.5 years for measles, varicella, and mumps, respectively, typical of figures obtained in the prevaccine era. Spread of measles prior to the introduction of vaccine occurred primarily among younger schoolchildren (5 to 9 years of age) within the community, with secondary spread to siblings within the family. From 1960 to 1964, 53 per cent of all measles cases occurred in children 5 to 9 years of age and 37 per cent in children younger than 5 years of age.[58] However, transmission now is most likely to occur among older schoolchildren and college students, whereas preschoolers, especially those too young to receive vaccine, constitute a continuing pool of susceptible persons.[96] In 1994, only 10 per cent of measles cases were reported in children 5 to 9 years of age; 40 per cent occurred among children and adolescents 10 to 19 years of age, and 26 per cent were in children younger than 5 years of age.[36] A comparable change has been seen in the epidemiology of mumps, with a decreasing proportion of cases in younger schoolchildren and an increasing proportion among older children, adolescents, and young adults.[41, 142]

For respiratory syncytial virus, the secondary attack rates of infants have been estimated at 45 per cent, higher than the corresponding rate of 27 per cent for all family contacts.[70] The infant's older sibling is the most frequent introducer of respiratory syncytial virus into the family. In the study of Cleveland families, common respiratory diseases (including the common cold, rhinitis, laryngitis, and bronchitis) occurred more often in young schoolchildren than in preschool children and, among the latter, more frequently in siblings of schoolchildren than in preschool children without such siblings.[47] Secondary attack rates of common respiratory diseases averaged 25 per cent, were highest in children younger than 5 years of age (37 to 49 per cent), and were similar in preschool children with or without siblings in school.

The epidemiology of some acute respiratory diseases also may be changing. Transmission varies both with levels of immunity and opportunities for exposure of susceptible persons. A comparison of the Cleveland family study data with data from a more recent longitudinal study of children in day care suggested that out-of-home child care may be lowering the age of first exposure to and infection with acute respiratory pathogens.[46] In a study of lower respiratory tract infections in children younger than 2 years of age, children hospitalized with lower respiratory tract infections were three times more likely to have received care in a day care center attended by six or more children.[6] Crowding in the child's home also was observed to be an independent factor increasing the risk of respiratory disease in that study.

In the Seattle Virus Watch study of family spread of influenza virus, schoolchildren were the most likely family members to develop community-acquired infection and then introduce the infection into the household; they also were most at risk for spread from other family members (57 to 63 per cent secondary attack rate).[57] However, secondary attack rates among all household members were highest (70 to 75 per cent) when the introducer was younger than 5 years of age.

Parvovirus B19 infection appears to be transmitted effectively within families with a secondary attack rate of 50 per cent among close contacts[25]; risk of transmission appears to decrease with advancing age.[85] Preschool-age children, especially those in day care, may introduce cytomegalovirus into the family, infecting seronegative mothers and posing a risk to the fetus if the mother is pregnant.[119] The risk of transmission from child to mother is greatest if the child is younger than 20 months of age.[3]

The spread of some enteric diseases within the family also has been studied. In two community outbreaks of shigellosis,

Weissman and associates[144] found that in 86 per cent of families the bacterium was introduced by a child younger than 10 years of age. The secondary attack rate averaged 31 per cent and was highest in children younger than 5 years of age. The secondary attack rate was significantly higher in families with an initial case in a preschool-age child than in those with an initial case in an older person. Spread within the family did not correlate with family size or household crowding but appeared to be highly dependent on whether or not there was an ill preschool-age child in the family.

After a food-borne outbreak of Norwalk gastroenteritis associated with a school cafeteria, secondary transmission occurred in 44 per cent of households with a primary case. In households with a primary case, the risk of secondary illness was twice as high among preschool-age children (70 per cent attack rate) as among adults (31 per cent).[75]

Poliovirus seems to spread more readily than *Shigella* in families. Gelfand and associates[63] studied household contacts of children found to have wild poliovirus infection. Among household contacts, evidence of recent infection, usually no later than 1 month after that in the index child, was found in 73 per cent of adults, 96 per cent of older siblings, and 84 per cent of younger siblings. Studying spread of live poliomyelitis vaccine virus strains in families, they found a secondary infection rate among susceptibles of 53 per cent in a lower economic group and 9 per cent in a higher economic group.[64] Secondary infection rates were higher with type 3 (77 per cent) than with types 1 (47 per cent) or 2 (36 per cent). Virus appeared to spread more readily from those with pharyngeal excretion and less readily from adults than from children.

In the study of Cleveland families, "infectious gastroenteritis" was found to be introduced most commonly by children younger than 6 years of age.[47] The secondary attack rate averaged 11 per cent and was highest in children younger than 8 years of age. The secondary attack rate was related directly to the number of major gastrointestinal symptoms (vomiting, diarrhea, and abdominal pain) suffered by the index case: 10 per cent for contacts of those with one symptom, 16 per cent for contacts of those with two, and 32 per cent for contacts of those with all three.

Helicobacter pylori infections cluster within families.[50] The families of children with *H. pylori* infection identified in the gastric antrum after endoscopy were studied for positive serology to *H. pylori* antibody. Seventy-four per cent of parents of infected children were seropositive, compared with 24 per cent of parents of uninfected children; 82 per cent of siblings of infected children also were positive. A study of 215 adults in England found an association between seropositivity for *H. pylori* antibodies and a history of crowded living conditions in childhood.[102]

In a community-wide study of rotavirus transmission, children younger than 2 years of age were most likely to introduce the infection into the family.[86] Persons living in households with a child younger than 2 years of age had a risk of becoming infected that was 2.9 (for adults) to 3.5 times (for children 10 to 17 years of age) higher than persons of comparable age in other families.

Young children attending day care also are likely to introduce into their families infections associated with parasitic enteropathogens. A study in Houston, Texas, found a 17 per cent secondary attack rate for *Giardia* enteritis in families with a child who became infected in day care.[120] At least one secondary case of giardiasis was identified in 47 per cent of all households with a *Giardia*-infected child during an outbreak at a Washington, D.C., day care center.[123] During an outbreak of diarrheal disease at a day care center in Oklahoma, stool samples were positive for *Cryptosporidium* in 23 per cent of household contacts of children with confirmed *Cryptosporidium* infection.[73]

International adoptees may introduce infectious diseases that are endemic in the child's country of origin into families that might otherwise not be at risk. In one study, parents of hepatitis B surface antigen (HBsAg)–seropositive adopted children were five times more likely to have serologic evidence of hepatitis B virus infection than parents of HBsAg-seronegative adoptees.[61] Children from various countries also have been shown to have tuberculosis, cytomegalovirus infection, congenital syphilis, and enteric pathogen infections when joining their adopted families.[78] Careful screening has been recommended for such children to identify and treat these infections.

Schools

In general, infectious disease agents spread much less readily from child to child in schools than in day care centers. Jacobson and associates[82] showed during an epidemic of meningococcal disease in Brazil that young elementary school classmates of a case of meningitis seemed not to be placed at increased risk of meningitis. Low carriage and acquisition rates for classroom contacts of meningococcal carriers similarly were demonstrated during a study of primary schoolchildren in England.[22] However, small outbreaks can occur in schools. A review of serogroup C meningococcal outbreaks in the United States found four outbreaks that occurred in elementary or junior high schools in the period from 1980 to 1993.[81] The number of cases involved in each outbreak, ranging from 3 to 7, generally was less than in community outbreaks, although attack rates (233 to 1028/100,000 students) generally were higher than in community outbreaks. The relatively high attack rates and the short interval between cases in these outbreaks led to rapid institution of vaccination programs, which may have had a role in limiting spread.

Attack rates of shigellosis during a group of outbreaks in elementary schools ranged from 0.4 to 1.1 per cent; the higher values occurred in schools with larger numbers of children younger than 8 years of age.[141] Enforced handwashing and disinfection of items potentially contaminated with feces have been associated with control of a shigellosis outbreak in an elementary school.[11]

Typically, spread in schools is less than that in families. In a measles outbreak that involved children in 20 of 26 classrooms in one school, the attack rate in unimmunized pupils with no history of measles was only 16 per cent.[44] Landrigan[89] observed in a community outbreak that measles spread most quickly in situations in which unvaccinated children were brought together for the first time; in urban areas this occurred in day care centers and nursery schools, whereas in rural areas, where day care was unusual, this occurred in elementary schools.

Schools may serve to spread infection from family to family. In recent outbreaks of measles, mumps, and pertussis, children infected within classroom settings appear to have spread disease to younger siblings at home. These outbreaks have occurred in school settings in which a high proportion of students have been immunized previously.[17, 96, 99, 107] In outbreaks of measles and mumps, failure of the vaccine to evoke a protective immunologic response (primary vaccine failure) has been a more significant factor resulting in susceptibility to infection than waning immunity from prior successful vaccination (secondary vaccine failure). Waning immunity has been shown to be a particular problem leading to susceptibility to pertussis in adolescents and adults.

Occasionally, person-to-person spread in the school appears to be very efficient. Miller and associates[106] described a diphtheria outbreak in an elementary school in which 34 per cent of all students were found to be infected and 30 per cent of unimmunized students developed clinical diphtheria. The reason for the intense spread was not found. In a measles outbreak in a high school, 69 secondary cases occurred in a single generation; aerosolization of virus by a vigorously coughing index case and inadequate levels of immunity among a cohort of students were identified as probable factors leading to a high level of transmission.[38]

Since 1965, 28 outbreaks of tuberculosis in children have been reported.[84] More than 70 per cent of these outbreaks occurred in schools. In one outbreak in an elementary school, a physical education teacher with cavitary pulmonary tuberculosis was identified as the source case.[76] Of 343 students in the school, 176 were found to be skin test–positive. Infection was associated with frequency of contact with the teacher. Abnormal chest radiographs were found in 32 children, and active disease was associated with having a low body mass index. Although occasional outbreaks of tuberculosis can occur in schools and in day care homes,[84, 114] children younger than 12 years of age rarely spread the infection and are more likely to be sentinels of infection in the adults with whom they are in contact. Widespread tuberculin skin test screening of schoolchildren has been shown not to be cost-effective[108]; screening is recommended only for groups of children considered to be at high risk for infection.[42]

Settings that result in a greater level of person-to-person contact than found in typical classroom settings, such as participation in school sports[10, 110] or attendance at a boarding school (or summer camp), also can result in more efficient disease transmission.[18, 132]

CONTROL METHODS

Isolation

The indications for isolation of patients with infectious diseases have changed greatly in this century with increasing knowledge of the modes of spread and with antimicrobial therapy, which rapidly renders cases of many diseases noninfectious. The value of isolation of diphtheria patients was shown in Providence, Rhode Island, in 1904 to 1913 and probably still is of some value. The attack rate among family contacts of diphtheria patients treated at home was 6.5 per cent, whereas among contacts of patients treated in the hospital it was 4.3 per cent; adjusting for the ages of contacts in the two groups, hospitalization was associated with a 43 per cent decrease in cases of household contacts.[48] Specific therapy has made such institutional isolation unnecessary for some diseases. Isolation of bacilliferous leprosy patients, which once was a central part of leprosy control, no longer is necessary because dapsone and rifampin quickly kill most *M. leprae;* therapy rapidly prevents any further risk of transmission.

The indications for and techniques of isolation of patients in hospitals to prevent nosocomial transmission are discussed elsewhere in this book. An extensive, practical discussion of disease control strategies, including isolation, is available readily in *Control of Communicable Diseases Manual*,[13] which can be purchased in paperback from the American Public Health Association, 1015 15th Street, N.W., Washington, D.C., 20005. Mostly, the need for isolation of children without hospitalization is occasioned by bacterial respiratory disease, diarrhea, acute viral diseases of childhood, conjunctivitis, contagious skin diseases, and arthropod-borne diseases.

For those bacterial respiratory diseases for which therapy rapidly and consistently renders a patient noninfectious, isolation of infected children may be as brief as 1 or 2 days (as for group A streptococcal pharyngitis). Isolation of patients known to have whooping cough still is recommended for at least 5 days after the initiation of erythromycin therapy. For patients with diphtheria, two negative nose and throat cultures 1 day or more apart, taken at least 24 hours after completing antimicrobial therapy, are urged prior to lifting quarantines; this may be prudent, even though erythromycin given for 7 days in appropriate doses makes pharyngeal carriers of *Corynebacterium diphtheriae* culture-negative in 92 per cent of patients.[100]

An attempt should be made to limit contamination with feces of children with diarrhea. Careful handwashing is of great importance, both for the children and those who take care of them. Clothing and linen contaminated with excreta should be laundered. Adults who are infected with, and may be excreting, *Salmonella, Shigella, Yersinia enterocolitica,* hepatitis A virus, or other enterically transmitted pathogens should be excluded from food preparation or direct care of young children.

Indications for isolation of patients with acute viral diseases of childhood depend on the severity of illness and the degree of contagiousness. There is no established value of isolation for the common acute viral respiratory diseases. For rubella, isolation is recommended only from women in early pregnancy. Isolation of poliomyelitis patients within the home is of little value because spread occurs most commonly during the prodrome. The same holds true for measles, which spreads efficiently, although the period of communicability can extend until 4 days after the onset of rash and children with measles should be kept home from school at least that long. Attempts are made to isolate children with varicella and mumps from school for 7 and 9 days, respectively, after onset of typical illness; these diseases spread less efficiently than measles.[77]

Children with conjunctivitis caused by transmissible agents should be excluded from school during the acute phase of illness. This form of isolation may help limit spread of *H. influenzae* biogroup *aegyptius*, pneumococcus, picornavirus, adenovirus, or *Chlamydia trachomatis*.

Children with contagious skin diseases should avoid skin contact with other children outside their family. Those with molluscum contagiosum, herpes simplex, or impetigo should avoid wrestling or other contact sports.[10] Those with scabies should be excluded from school until the day after treatment. Children with tinea corporis should avoid gymnasia, swimming pools, and contact sports.

Children in the early phases of arthropod-borne diseases, when the infecting organism still may be in the blood, should avoid bites by the vector. A wide variety of illnesses are included: arboviral diseases, bartonellosis, leishmaniasis, microfilarial infections, malaria, and African trypanosomiasis.

Chemoprophylaxis

The word *chemoprophylaxis* is used loosely in this section to describe the use of antimicrobial drugs to (1) prevent infection (as with falciparum malaria), (2) treat asymptomatic infection and thereby prevent disease (as with isoniazid treatment of tuberculin skin test–positive children), and (3) treat disease and thereby prevent complications of the disease (as with primary prevention of acute rheumatic fever). In each situation, however, the primary purpose is to prevent a disease by administering an antimicrobial agent that affects the causative microorganism.

The decision to initiate chemoprophylaxis and the choice and dosage of agents require careful consideration of both the child's clinical status and the epidemiologic factors that may place the child at risk for disease. Local health departments should be notified of exposures to communicable diseases; they often can provide useful additional information on recommended treatment regimens. In addition, they may need to conduct an investigation to ensure that all exposed persons have been identified and, when necessary, treated or placed under observation.

A summary of 13 diseases for which chemoprophylaxis may be administered to children is given in Table 239–3. Some special situations, such as chemoprophylaxis of immunodeficient children and mass prophylaxis to abort epidemics, are omitted from the discussion. For a more detailed discussion of antimicrobial drug usage in disease prevention, the regularly updated *Red Book: Report of the Committee on Infectious Diseases* of the American Academy of Pediatrics should be consulted.[43]

Acute rheumatic fever after streptococcal pharyngitis can be prevented in 90 per cent of patients, despite delay in drug administration of as much as 9 days after onset of sore throat.[23] Success rates are related directly to the eradication of the streptococci and are highest with repository penicillin. Provision of neighborhood health centers (and presumably delivery of primary prophylaxis) has been associated with a significant decrease in acute rheumatic fever in an urban population.[66] Secondary prophylaxis also can be as much as 90 per cent effective and depends largely on the faithfulness with which an effective drug is taken.

One study has suggested that antibiotics will prevent acute glomerulonephritis following group A streptococcal pharyngitis,[126] but the apparent reduction was not statistically significant.[143] There is no evidence that antibiotics will prevent acute glomerulonephritis following streptococcal skin infection. Studies to determine the effectiveness of chemoprophylaxis and optimal drug regimens are needed.

Among untreated household contacts of endemic meningococcal cases, 0.4 per cent develop secondary cases; in epidemics, the figure may rise to 5 per cent.[103] Day care center and other intimate contacts also are at risk. Rifampin is the drug of choice for treatment of contacts. However, rifampin is associated with adverse side effects, is teratogenic, and may not eliminate carriage.[130] Ceftriaxone recently has been recommended as an alternative agent. Because of the emergence of sulfonamide-resistant strains of *Neisseria meningitidis*, the use of sulfadiazine as a prophylactic agent now is limited to outbreaks in which the causal microorganism is known to be sulfonamide-susceptible.

Gonococcal ophthalmia can be contracted by the infant from an infected mother during birth. Silver nitrate, erythromycin, or tetracycline instilled into the eyes is effective in preventing this potential cause of corneal ulceration and blindness.[34, 71] Silver nitrate, in use since the nineteenth century, is less costly than the antibiotics but may be associated with a higher incidence of chemical conjunctivitis. These agents do not appear to be effective in preventing neonatal conjunctivitis caused by *C. trachomatis*, although some studies have produced contradictory results. In one study, the incidence of neonatal chlamydial ophthalmia among infants born to mothers with chlamydial infection was 20 per cent in those who received silver nitrate prophylaxis and 14 per cent and 11 per cent in those receiving erythromycin and tetracycline, respectively.[71] Despite appropriate prophylaxis, 0.06 per cent of the infants born in that hospital during the study period developed gonococcal ophthalmia. A recent study of 3117 infants in Kenya showed that use of a 2.5 per cent solution of povidone-iodine as prophylaxis against ophthalmia neonatorum resulted in fewer infections (13.1 per cent of treated infants) than either 0.5 per cent erythromycin ointment (15.2 per cent) or 1 per cent silver nitrate solution (17.5 per cent).[79] As demonstrated in previous studies, the presence of maternal vaginal infection was correlated highly with infectious conjunctivitis. Screening for and treatment of gonococcal and chlamydial infections in pregnant women are the best ways to prevent neonatal disease.[34]

Isoniazid prophylaxis can prevent infection in uninfected tuberculin-negative contacts of tuberculosis cases.[4, 133, 135] Children usually are infected as a result of exposure to an adult with infectious tuberculosis. Skin test–negative children who have been close contacts of infectious persons (e.g., household contacts) should receive preventive therapy for a minimum of 12 weeks after the last contact with the infectious source. If a repeat skin test remains negative, preventive therapy may be discontinued, unless there is a continuing exposure to the infectious source. If the repeat skin test is positive, therapy should be continued for 9 months.[4] Isoniazid prophylaxis also has been shown to decrease disease incidence in tuberculin-positive children.[54] Compared with adults or older children, young children have a greater risk of developing tuberculous disease when infected, are more likely to develop disseminated disease, and are less likely to develop isoniazid hepatitis when treated with that drug. Thus, young children generally have a high priority for receipt of isoniazid prophylaxis.

The risk of leprosy in children who are household contacts of a lepromatous patient was shown in one double-blind trial to be halved by 3 years of dapsone prophylaxis.[115] Community-wide prophylaxis in hyperendemic areas also has been successful.

In a study of 37 households with a primary case of pertussis during a community outbreak, administration of erythromycin prophylaxis to contacts was associated with a decreased likelihood of secondary cases.[134] Delays in beginning erythromycin treatment of primary cases and prophylaxis of contacts were associated with increased secondary spread. Similarly, in a study of a pertussis outbreak in an institutionalized population, erythromycin was shown to be effective in reducing the attack rate and severity of disease among exposed persons.[136] Because the disease may be fatal in infants, it is this group that is most in need of effective prophylaxis.

Erythromycin and benzathine penicillin G have been shown to be effective in eliminating pharyngeal carriage of *C. diphtheriae* in 92 and 84 per cent, respectively, of those treated.[100] The effectiveness of these drugs as chemoprophylaxis against diphtheria has not been studied. However, the high incidence of diphtheria in nonimmune household contacts of cases,[48] the side effects of diphtheria antitoxin, and delay associated with and possible false negativity of cultures are points in favor of giving chemoprophylaxis. Because the vaccine is directed against the toxin, immunized persons still may be carriers and become infected; thus, chemoprophylaxis should be administered to all close contacts regardless of immunization status. All close contacts should be cultured and kept under surveillance for 7 days. Patients with positive cultures should complete a full course of antimicrobial treatment. Previously immunized contacts should receive a booster dose of vaccine. Active immunization should be initiated for those who have not been immunized fully in the past.

Cases of primary or secondary pneumonic plague are potential sources of person-to-person spread. Tetracycline, sulfonamides (including sulfadiazine and trimethoprim-sulfamethoxazole), streptomycin, and chloramphenicol all have been used in treatment and variously suggested as agents for prophylaxis.[122, 145, 146] Tetracycline is the drug of choice for contacts older than 9 years of age. Chemoprophylaxis of

TABLE 239–3. Chemoprophylaxis Against Communicable Disease in Children

Disease	Target Group	Value for Chemoprophylaxis	Recommended Drug*	Regimen*	Vaccine for Target Group	Ref.
Acute glomerulonephritis	Those with group A streptococcal infection in nephritis outbreak	Proposed	Benzathine penicillin G IM	≤27 kg: 600,000 units >27 kg: 1,200,000 units	No	45, 143
			Penicillin V PO	Children: 250 mg 2–3 times daily × 10 days Adolescents: 500 mg 2–3 times daily × 10 days		
			Erythromycin estolate PO	20–40 mg/kg/day in 2–4 divided doses (not to exceed 1 g/day) × 10 days		
			Erythromycin ethyl succinate PO	40 mg/kg/day in 2–4 divided doses (not to exceed 1 g/day) × 10 days		
Acute rheumatic fever (ARF)	Those with group A streptococcal infection (not impetigo)	Shown	See above	See above	No	45
	Those with previous ARF	Shown	Benzathine penicillin G IM	1,200,000 units every 3–4 weeks		
			Penicillin V PO	250 mg twice a day		
			Sulfadiazine PO	≤27 kg: 0.5 g daily >27 kg: 1 g daily		
			Erythromycin PO	250 mg twice a day		
Cholera	Household contacts of a case	Shown	Tetracycline PO	≥9 years: 50 mg/kg/day in 4 divided doses × 3 days	No	13, 43, 138
			Doxycycline PO	≥9 years: 6 mg/kg in a single dose		
			Trimethoprim-sulfamethoxazole PO	8–10 mg/kg/day trimethoprim, 40–50 mg/kg/day sulfamethoxazole in 2 divided doses × 3 days		
Diphtheria	Household, day care center, or other close contacts of a case	Proposed	Erythromycin PO	40–50 mg/kg/day in divided doses (not to exceed 2 g/day) × 7 days	Yes	43, 100
			Benzathine penicillin G IM	<30 kg: 600,000 units ≥30 kg: 1,200,000 units		
Gonorrhea	Neonates	Shown	Silver nitrate Erythromycin Tetracycline All instilled into the eye	1% aqueous solution 0.5% ophthalmic ointment 1% ophthalmic ointment	No	34
Haemophilus influenzae disease	Household contacts of a case when ≥1 susceptible contact is <4 years old	Shown	Rifampin PO	<1 month: 10–20 mg/kg/day once daily × 4 days ≥1 month: 20/mg/kg/day once daily × 4 days (maximum dose 600 mg/day)	Yes	7, 43
	Day care center contacts of a case	Proposed	Rifampin PO	<1 month: 10–20 mg/kg/day once daily × 4 days ≥1 month: 20 mg/kg/day once daily × 4 days (maximum dose 600 mg/day)		
Leprosy	Household contacts of lepromatous and dimorphous cases	Shown	Dapsone PO	1 mg/kg/day	Yes	43
Malaria	Travelers to malarious areas without chloroquine-resistant strains	Shown	Chloroquine phosphate PO	5 mg/kg base (8.3 mg/kg salt) once/week (not to exceed 300 mg base/week); start 1–2 weeks before entering malarious area, continue during travel and for 4 weeks after leaving such areas	No	27, 30
			Hydroxychloroquine sulfate PO	5 mg/kg base (6.5 mg/kg salt) once/week (not to exceed 310 mg base/week); start 1–2 weeks before entering malarious area, continue during travel and for 4 weeks after leaving such areas		

TABLE 239–3. Chemoprophylaxis Against Communicable Disease in Children *Continued*

Disease	Target Group	Value for Chemoprophylaxis	Recommended Drug*	Regimen*	Vaccine for Target Group	Ref.
	Travelers to malarious areas with chloroquine-resistant strains		Mefloquine PO	15–19 kg: 1/4 tablet/week 20–30 kg: 1/2 tablet/week 31–45 kg: 3/4 tablet/week >45 kg: 1 tablet/week; start 1–2 weeks before entering malarious area, continue during travel and for 4 weeks after leaving such areas		
			Doxycycline PO	>8 years: 2 mg/kg of body weight/day (not to exceed 100 mg/day); start 1–2 days before entering malarious area, continue during travel and for 4 weeks after leaving such areas		
			Chloroquine PO plus Proguanil PO	See above <2 years: 50 mg/day 2–6 years: 100 mg/day 7–10 years: 150 mg/day >10 years: 200 mg/day; take daily during exposure and continue for 4 weeks after last exposure		
Meningococcal disease	Household, day care center, nursery school, or other close contacts of a case	Suggested	Rifampin PO	<1 month: 5–10 mg/kg twice a day × 2 days ≥1 month: 10 mg/kg (not to exceed 600 mg/day) twice a day × 2 days	Yes (if group A, C, or Y or W-135)	43, 130
			Ceftriaxone IM	<12 years: 125 mg in a single dose ≥12 years: 250 mg in a single dose		
			Sulfadiazine PO (if organism is sensitive)	125–150 mg/kg/day in 2–4 divided doses × 2 days; up to 1 g twice daily for older children and adolescents		
Pertussis	Close contacts irrespective of vaccine status	Proposed	Erythromycin PO	40–50 mg/kg/24 hours (not to exceed 2 g) in 4 divided doses × 14 days	Yes	43, 134
Plague	Contacts of pneumonic cases	Proposed	Tetracycline PO	≥9 years: 15–20 mg/kg/24 hours in 4 divided doses × 7 days	No	122, 145
			Trimethoprim-sulfamethoxazole PO	8 mg/kg/day trimethoprim, 40 mg/kg/day sulfamethoxazole in 2 divided doses × 7 days		
Tuberculosis	Exposed, skin test–negative	Shown	Isoniazid PO	10–15 mg/kg daily (maximum 300 mg); continue for 12 weeks after last contact with infectious source; may discontinue if skin test remains negative after 12 weeks	BCG?	4
	Skin test–positive	Shown	Isoniazid PO	10–15 mg/kg daily (maximum 300 mg) for 9 months		
	Skin test–positive contacts of cases with isoniazid-resistant, rifampin-susceptible organisms	Proposed	Rifampin PO	10–20 mg/kg daily (maximum 600 mg) for 9 months		
Yaws	Close contacts of a case	Shown	Benzathine penicillin G IM	<10 years: 600,000 units ≥10 years: 1,200,000 units	No	19

*Some recommended drugs and dosages are subject to change.
IM, intramuscularly; PO, orally; BCG, bacille Calmette-Guérin.

contacts generally is practiced and in recent experience in the United States has not been associated with failure; however, the efficacy of chemoprophylaxis has not been measured.[122, 146]

Cholera typically is not spread from person to person in households. However, in developing countries, if the household secondary attack rate is known to be high, family contacts may be treated prophylactically with tetracycline or doxycycline to prevent illness.[138] In the United States, prophylactic treatment is not recommended unless there is a high likelihood of secondary transmission caused by unusually poor sanitary or hygienic conditions. After the first day of prophylaxis, tetracycline prophylaxis for 5 days is associated with a decrease in cases in contacts from 12.6 to 0.3 per cent.[101] Some strains of cholera are tetracycline-resistant; alternative drugs include trimethoprim-sulfamethoxazole, erythromycin, and furazolidone. Tetracyclines cause staining of developing teeth and should not be used in children younger than 9 years of age.

Mass campaigns of treatment of patients with yaws and their community contacts have been successful in decreasing the prevalence of the disease markedly, although transmission has not been stopped completely.[19] Similar campaigns have been even more effective in control of hyperendemic nonvenereal syphilis.

Chloroquine is effective prophylaxis against malarial parasitemia caused by *Plasmodium vivax, P. ovale, P. malariae,* and chloroquine-sensitive strains of *P. falciparum*; however, chloroquine resistance of *P. falciparum* has spread to most areas of the world with malaria.[27, 37] Mefloquine is an effective prophylactic agent against drug-resistant *P. falciparum,* but it is not recommended for children weighing less than 15 kg or for pregnant women. Alternative regimens, including doxycycline and proguanil, are contraindicated in small children and in pregnancy or are incompletely effective. Thus, persons anticipating travel to areas with chloroquine-resistant *P. falciparum* must weigh carefully the risks of acquiring disease and the problems associated with prophylaxis for small children and pregnant women.[27, 30, 37]

P. vivax and *P. ovale,* which have an extraerythrocytic form, may relapse after chloroquine has been stopped. Primaquine, taken as terminal prophylaxis after leaving the malarious area, decreases the risk of relapses; however, it may cause severe hemolysis in persons with G-6-PD deficiency.[27, 37] Deciding whether or not to give terminal prophylaxis with primaquine depends on individual factors, including the degree of the traveler's risk of acquiring *Plasmodium* with an extraerythrocytic form and the potential for adverse reactions; primaquine generally is indicated for persons who have had prolonged exposure in endemic areas.

Water Purification

The average per capita use of water in the United States is about 600 liters per day. The provision of a safe and plentiful water supply is a major factor in prevention of some communicable diseases. Purification of water occurs both naturally and through human intervention. Natural methods include evaporation and condensation, filtration through the earth, and a series of processes acting during the flow of a stream or on standing: aeration, light-accelerated plant growth, gravity, and oxidation and reduction of organic material by bacteria.[117] Municipal water-treatment programs use a variety of measures to ensure the safety of community water supplies, including protection of the watershed, chemical disinfection, and filtration of surface water supplies such as lakes and rivers.[35] A failure in one of these systems can result in a widespread risk of water-borne disease. Although many such outbreaks involve a few dozen to a few hundred persons, more than 400,000 cases of illness may have resulted from an outbreak of cryptosporidiosis in Milwaukee, Wisconsin, in 1993.[94] The outbreak was associated with a marked increase in turbidity of the water supply and the failure of coagulation and filtration at the water treatment plant to remove oocysts of *Cryptosporidium* from the treated water.

Since 1971, the CDC and the Environmental Protection Agency have maintained a voluntary surveillance system for the reporting of water-borne disease outbreaks. Figure 239–1 shows the annual number of disease outbreaks associated with water intended for drinking reported from 1971 to 1992 in the United States.[28, 74, 109] From 1986 to 1992, 114 outbreaks were reported, for which a cause was found in 51: *Giardia lamblia* (20), chemicals (7), *Shigella* (7), Norwalk agent (4), hepatitis A virus (4), *Cryptosporidium* (4), and other specific pathogens (5), including *Salmonella, Campylobacter,* and *Escherichia coli.* The factors apparently resulting in these outbreaks were treatment deficiencies (57), untreated ground water (32), deficiencies in the distribution system (14), untreated surface water (4), and unknown or multiple factors (7). Outbreaks more commonly occurred in the summer; 25 per cent of the outbreaks occurred in the month of July.

An increasingly important problem is the occurrence of water-borne disease outbreaks associated with recreational

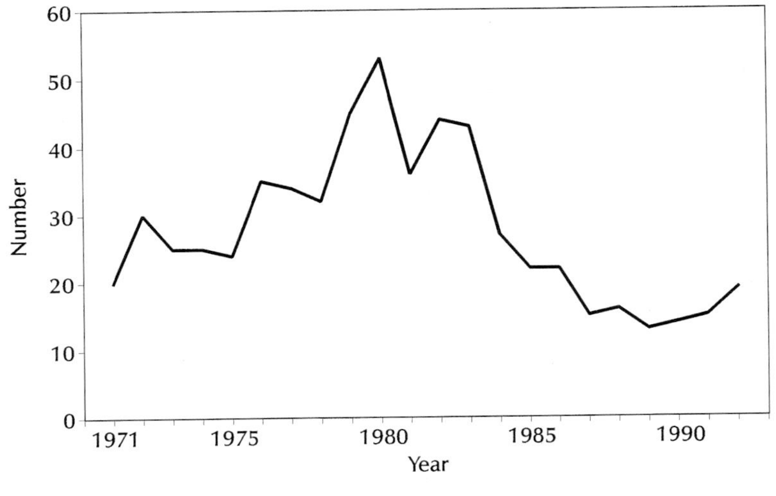

FIGURE 239–1. *Average annual number of water-borne disease outbreaks reported, United States, 1971–1992. (Adapted from Moore, A. C., Herwaldt, B. L., Craun, G. F., et al.: Surveillance for waterborne disease outbreaks: United States, 1991–1992. In CDC Surveillance Summaries, November 19, 1993. M. M. W. R. 42(SS-5):1–22, 1993.)*

water use, as for swimming or wading and in hot tubs or spas.[109] From 1986 to 1992, 101 such outbreaks were reported; diseases transmitted in this manner include shigellosis, cryptosporidiosis, Norwalk virus diarrhea, viral conjunctivitis, giardiasis, legionellosis, and *Pseudomonas* dermatitis.[21, 26, 95, 124] Nine deaths were reported, all associated with cases of primary amebic meningoencephalitis due to *Naegleria* infections in persons who recently had been swimming.[32]

Milk Sanitation

Milk has been demonstrated as the vehicle for transmission in outbreaks of brucellosis, tuberculosis, and diphtheria, as well as outbreaks caused by group A streptococci, *Salmonella, Shigella, Campylobacter, Listeria, Y. enterocolitica,* and staphylococcal toxin.[125] Although the quality of milk has improved steadily in the United States—largely through mechanization and sanitation of milking operations, pasteurization, and cold storage—the use of raw milk as a "health food" continues to account for outbreaks of disease, particularly those caused by *Salmonella* and *Campylobacter.*[125] Children sometimes drink raw milk while visiting dairy farms on school field trips or other youth activities; a retrospective survey of state health departments identified 20 outbreaks involving a total of 458 cases of *Campylobacter* enteritis occurring as a result of such activities during the period of 1981 to 1990.[148]

The quality of milk is monitored by a standard bacterial plate count, the phosphatase test (an assay for prior pasteurization), and measurement of the density of coliform organisms.[59] Nonetheless, pasteurized milk has been associated with outbreaks of enteric disease.[56, 128] Both postpasteurization contamination at the dairy[128] and intrinsic contamination with survival of organisms despite adequate pasteurization[56] have been suggested as possible mechanisms of transmission.

The incidence of milk-borne outbreaks has decreased greatly in the past 40 years in the United States. From 1917 to 1941, 168 outbreaks (7 per year) were traced to raw milk in New York State alone.[51] From 1983 to 1991, fewer than three milk-borne outbreaks per year were reported for the entire country.[9, 29] The most common etiologies were *Campylobacter* and *Salmonella.* One of these outbreaks, caused by antimicrobial-resistant *Salmonella typhimurium* that contaminated pasteurized 2 per cent milk, was the largest *Salmonella* infection outbreak ever identified in the United States, affecting an estimated 200,000 people.[128]

Food Sanitation

Foods other than milk have been shown to be the vehicle of transmission in outbreaks caused by 10 or more genera of bacteria, hepatitis A virus, Norwalk-like viruses, and a variety of parasites, in addition to a wide range of toxic chemicals. Major public health programs in the United States relating to inspection of meat and poultry, shellfish sanitation, and inspection of public eating and drinking places have had significant impact, notably in reduction of tuberculosis and brucellosis in cattle and limitation of spread of typhoid and hepatitis A by contaminated shellfish. Significant problem areas remain, however. Contamination of meat, poultry, and eggs with *Salmonella, Yersinia, E. coli* O157:H7, *Listeria,* and other pathogens and deficiencies in food storage and preparation both in eating establishments and in the home still contribute to outbreaks and sporadic cases.[12, 29, 90, 129, 131] In addition, new problems can result from changes in the food industry and in patterns of food consumption.[72] In recent years, several large outbreaks of salmonellosis have been associated with the widespread distribution of fresh produce, a previously rare vehicle of *Salmonella* transmission. These outbreaks have occurred after notable increases over the past two decades in the per capita consumption of fresh fruits and vegetables in the United States.[31, 72] Larger, centralized production and processing facilities with extensive distribution networks may increase the number of persons affected when commercial products do become contaminated.[12, 29, 91, 128] Adequate cooking of foods, proper canning techniques (both commercial and home), and refrigeration are major contributors to control of food-borne outbreaks. In about half of the food-borne disease outbreaks, one or more food preparation practices are reported to be contributing factors; improper storage or holding temperature is reported in about two-thirds of these outbreaks and poor personal hygiene of the food handler in about two-fifths.[9, 29]

Although the number of outbreaks reported to public health authorities represents only a small fraction of those that occur, these reports can provide important insights into the epidemiology of food-borne disease. From 1983 to 1991, the number of outbreaks and the number of cases reported annually remained relatively constant (Table 239–4).[9, 29] The specific cause is confirmed in about 40 per cent of all outbreaks, and of these, bacterial pathogens, particularly *Salmonella,* account for the majority. Other infectious etiologies include *Clostridium botulinum, Clostridium perfringens, Campylobacter, Shigella, Vibrio cholera,* hepatitis A virus, *Giardia,* and *Trichinella spiralis.* In recent years, *Salmonella enteritidis* has become the most commonly isolated cause of food-borne outbreaks and, when identified, is most likely to have been associated with consumption of eggs or foods containing eggs.

Health Information for International Travel

International travel, whether by child or adult, necessitates preparation beforehand to obtain the proper immunizations, contingency plans for the possibility of meeting with unsanitary food or water during the travel, and the realization that illnesses acquired abroad may not be manifested until return home with consequent diagnostic difficulties.[8]

Needs for active and passive immunization are covered elsewhere in this book and are summarized fully in two continuously updated CDC publications to which the reader is referred: *Health Information for International Travel*[37] (which can be purchased from the Superintendent of Documents, U.S. Government Printing Office, Washington, D.C., 20402) and the *Morbidity and Mortality Weekly Report.*

Safe water may be found in many hotels in large cities throughout the world, but only water from adequately chlorinated sources can be considered truly safe. Where chlorinated water is not available, canned or bottled carbonated beverages and beverages made from boiled water (as well as beer or wine) may be safe. Transmission of cholera by uncarbonated bottled mineral water has been described.[15] Ice made from unchlorinated water may contaminate an otherwise safe beverage, either directly or by leaving contaminated water on the outside of the container. Although heat treatment by boiling is the most reliable method to render questionable water potable, chemical treatment also can be used.[37]

Heat:

1. Bring the water to a vigorous boil. Allow to cool at room temperature—do not add ice. At very high altitudes, for an extra margin of safety, boil for several minutes or use chemical disinfection.

TABLE 239–4. Food-borne Disease Outbreaks and Cases Reported in the United States, 1983–1991, by Etiology

	1983	1984	1985	1986	1987	1988	1989	1990	1991
Total number of outbreaks/cases reported	505/ 14,898	543/ 16,420	495/ 31,079	467/ 12,781	387/ 16,500	451/ 15,732	505/ 15,867	532/ 19,883	528/ 14,76
Total number of reported outbreaks with a confirmed cause	187	185	220	181	136	183	221	237	214
Per cent of all reported outbreaks with a confirmed cause	37	34	44	39	35	41	44	45	41
Number of outbreaks/cases caused by bacterial diseases	127/7082	128/7307	143/ 22,132	119/4855	83/8928	139/7156	171/6557	196/9002	173/6335
Number of outbreaks/cases caused by *Salmonella*	72/2427	78/4479	79/ 19,660	61/2833	52/1846	94/2987	117/4920	136/6290	122/4146
Per cent of all bacterial outbreaks caused by *Salmonella*	57	61	55	51	63	68	68	69	71
Number of outbreaks/cases caused by chemical agents	45/264	42/216	58/392	48/215	39/157	29/139	37/153	27/270	31/159
Number of outbreaks/cases caused by viral diseases	11/550	4/610	10/411	8/68	10/552	12/795	8/379	9/452	7/114
Number of outbreaks/cases caused by parasitic diseases	4/8	11/60	9/52	6/666	4/15	3/34	5/36	5/234	3/73

Adapted from Bean, N. H., Goulding, J. S., Lao, C., et al.: Surveillance for foodborne-disease outbreaks: United States, 1988–1992. M. M. W. R. *45*(SS-5):1–66, 1996, and Centers for Disease Control: Foodborne disease outbreaks, 5-year summary, 1983–1987. M. M. W. R. *39*(SS-1):15–57, 1990.

2. Adding a pinch of salt to each quart or pouring the water from one clean container to another several times will improve the taste.

Chemicals:

1. Tincture of iodine. Follow directions in Table 239–5. Let stand for at least 30 minutes.

2. Tetraglycine hydroperiodide tablets (can be purchased at pharmacies and sporting goods stores). The manufacturer's instructions should be followed. If water is cloudy, the number of tablets should be doubled; if water is extremely cold, an attempt should be made to warm the water, and the recommended contact time should be increased to achieve reliable disinfection.

Cloudy water should be strained through a clean cloth into a container to remove any sediment or floating matter prior to treatment with heat or iodine. Although chlorine has been used for chemical disinfection, its germicidal activity varies greatly with pH, temperature, and the organic content of the water to be purified and thus is less reliable than iodine.

Food should be selected carefully. In areas of the world where hygiene and sanitation are poor, the traveler should avoid salads, uncooked vegetables, unpasteurized milk, and milk products such as cheese and eat only food that can be peeled by the traveler or has been cooked and still is hot.

TABLE 239–5. Treatment of Water with Tincture of Iodine

Tincture of Iodine	Drops* to be Added per Quart or Liter of: *Clean Water*	*Cold or Cloudy Water*†
2%	5	10
1. Let stand for 30 minutes.		
2. Water is safe to use.		

*1 drop is 0.05 mL.

†Very turbid or very cold water may require prolonged contact time; let stand up to several hours prior to use, if possible.

Adapted from Centers for Disease Control and Prevention: Health Information for International Travel 1995. HHS Publication No. (CDC) 95-8280, 1995.

Children 0 to 2 years of age have a high risk of acquiring traveler's diarrhea.[37, 121] Immediate medical attention should be sought for the infant or child with blood or mucus in the stool, fever with rigors, or persistent vomiting or diarrhea with dehydration. Because infants and small children especially are at risk for dehydration, parents need to be aware of the signs of dehydration (Table 239–6) and be prepared to use oral rehydration therapy as a preventive measure while medical attention is being obtained. Replacing fluid losses may be achieved best by use of an oral rehydration solution containing appropriate concentrations of electrolytes and glucose.[33, 37, 118] Oral rehydration solution packets are available at stores or pharmacies in almost all developing countries. Oral rehydration solution is prepared by adding one packet to the appropriate volume of boiled or treated water.[37]

Although prophylaxis with several different agents, including trimethoprim-sulfamethoxazole, doxycycline, fluoroquinolone antibiotics, and bismuth subsalicylate, may prevent some cases of traveler's diarrhea in adults, no drug has been shown to be both safe and effective for this purpose in children.[37] Diiodohydroxyquin (Entero-Vioform) especially is dangerous because of its association with subacute myelo-optic neuropathy.[116] Administration of bismuth subsalicylate may lead to salicylate toxicity.

Vector Control

Techniques of environmental control of vectors responsible for disease transmission have included eradication of habitats for mosquito larvae, construction of rat-proof houses, and elimination of rodent habitats.[149] In some instances, dam construction, large-scale irrigation projects, and deforestation have led to increases in densities of vectors responsible for transmission of schistosomiasis, onchocerciasis, and mosquito-borne diseases.

TABLE 239–6. Assessment of Dehydration Levels in Infants

	Signs of Dehydration		
	Mild	*Moderate*	*Severe*
General Condition	Thirsty, restless, agitated	Thirsty, restless, irritable	Withdrawn, somnolent, or comatose
Pulse	Normal	Rapid and weak	Rapid and weak
Anterior fontanelle	Normal	Sunken	Very sunken
Eyes	Normal	Sunken	Very sunken
Tears	Present	Absent	Absent
Urine	Normal	Reduced and concentrated	None for several hours
Weight loss	4–5%	6–9%	≥10%

Adapted from Centers for Disease Control and Prevention: Health Information for International Travel 1995. HHS Publication No. (CDC) 95-8280, 1995.

Chemical control of vectors, which seemed so attractive a few years ago, has been complicated by environmental contamination by undegraded chemicals and by the appearance of vectors resistant to the organochlorine insecticides (DDT, dieldrin), organophosphorus insecticides (malathion, fenitrothion), and carbonates (propoxur, carbaryl). The persistence of DDT and dieldrin in the environment has resulted in their being banned in some countries and their use being severely restricted in others. The use of ultralow-volume spraying, as with malathion in the control of malaria, has permitted use of minimal amounts of insecticide while still effecting a decrease in disease incidence over a considerable area.[87]

The rising incidence of tick-borne diseases, especially Lyme disease, has led to an increased interest in methods for the control of ticks and their animal hosts. Area-wide spraying of pesticides in residential areas may reduce tick populations but also may pose health or environmental risks if these chemicals are applied improperly. Personal protection includes avoiding vector-infested areas, wearing protective clothing, using insect repellents applied to skin (e.g., N,N-diethyl-meta-toluamide) or to clothing (permethrin), and frequently inspecting for and prompt removal of attached ticks. These individual preventive measures can be practiced in any circumstance where exposure to infected ticks may occur.[5]

Experimental work with genetic and biologic control of vectors has had limited success, as with the use of larvivorous fish, chemosterilized male mosquitoes, or parasites that attack the vector.[5, 20]

APPENDIX

The attack rate was considerably higher among those patients attended by any of eight people (four surgeons, an anesthesiologist, and three nurses) than among patients who were not. Only for Sutterfield, the anesthesiologist, however, was the difference so marked that the probability of the association occurring by chance alone was less than 0.05 (Table 239–7). The attack rate for patients for whom Sutterfield was listed in the operating room log as the anesthesiologist was 43 per cent (10/23) in comparison with an attack rate of 13 per cent (3/24) for those for whom Sutterfield was not listed. (Note that these attack rates are artificially high because four fifths of the actual controls have been omitted, but the comparison still is valid.) This finding appears to implicate Sutterfield as the source of infection (step 6).

TABLE 239–7. Recorded Intraoperative Care by Anesthesiologist Sutterfield Among Cases of Group A Streptococcal Wound Infection and Controls

		Cases	Controls	Total
Recorded contact with Sutterfield	Yes	10	13	23
	No	3	21	24
	Total	13	34	47

χ^2 is 5.63, 1 d.f.; p is .018.

The three patients who became ill but for whom Sutterfield's name did not appear in their record must be explained. Interviews with the anesthesiology staff determined that it was not uncommon for one anesthesiologist to spell another for brief periods on a long case without recording the fact on the operating room log; this may explain the three outliers (step 7).

To confirm the hypothesis microbiologically, cultures were made from throat, nose, skin, and anus specimens from two surgeons, Sutterfield, and three nurses. Only from Sutterfield, and only from his anus, were group A streptococci recovered; the strain was M nontypable T 28, the same strain isolated from the cases (step 8). Subsequently, Sutterfield was treated with antibiotics, and his streptococcal carriage was eradicated (step 9). Prospective surveillance for group A streptococcal wound infections of the hospital showed none in the subsequent several months (step 10).

References

1. Acha, P. N., and Szyfres, B.: Zoonoses and Communicable Diseases Common to Man and Animals. 2nd ed. Washington, D.C., Pan American Health Organization, 1987.
2. Adams, W. G., Deaver, K. A., Cochi, S. L., et al.: Decline of childhood *Haemophilus influenzae* type b (Hib) disease in the Hib vaccine era. J. A. M. A. *269*:221–226, 1993
3. Adler, S. P.: Cytomegalovirus transmission and child day care. Adv. Pediatr. Infect. Dis. *7*:109–122, 1992.
4. American Thoracic Society: Treatment of tuberculosis and tuberculosis infection in adults and children. Am. J. Respir. Crit. Care Med. *149*:1359–1374, 1994.
5. Anderson, J. F.: Preventing Lyme disease. Rheum. Dis. Clin. North Am. *15*:757–766, 1989.
6. Anderson, L. J., Parker, R. A., Strikas, R. A., et al.: Day-care center attendance and hospitalization for lower respiratory tract illness. Pediatrics *82*:300–308, 1988.
7. Band, J. D., Fraser, D. W., and Ajello, G.: *Hemophilus influenzae* disease study group: Prevention of *Hemophilus influenzae* type b disease. J. A. M. A. *251*:2381–2386, 1984.
8. Barry, M.: Medical considerations for international travel with infants and older children. Infect. Dis. Clin. North Am. *6*:389–404, 1992.
9. Bean, N. H., Goulding, J. S., Lao, C., et al.: Surveillance for foodborne-disease outbreaks: United States, 1988–1992. M. M. W. R. *45*(SS-5):1–66, 1996.
10. Becker, T. M., Kodsi, R., Bailey, P., et al.: Grappling with herpes: Herpes gladiatorum. Am. J. Sports Med. *16*:665–669, 1988.
11. Beer, B., O'Donnell, G. M., and Henderson, R. J.: A school outbreak of

Sonne dysentery controlled by hygienic measures. Monthly Bull. Ministry Health (Lond.) *25*:36–41, 1966.
12. Bell, B. P., Goldoft M., Griffin P. M., et al.: A multistate outbreak of *Escherichia coli* O157:H7–associated bloody diarrhea and hemolytic uremic syndrome from hamburgers: The Washington experience. J. A. M. A. *272*:1349–1353, 1994.
13. Benenson, A. S. (ed.): Control of Communicable Diseases Manual. 16th ed. Washington, D.C., American Public Health Association, 1995.
14. Beran, G. W. (ed.-in-chief): Handbook of Zoonoses. 2nd ed. Boca Raton, CRC Press, 1994.
15. Blake, P. A., Rosenberg, M. L., Florencia, J., et al.: Cholera in Portugal, 1974. II. Transmission by bottled mineral water. Am. J. Epidemiol. *105*:344–348, 1977.
16. Brimblecombe, F. S. W., Cruickshank, R., Masters, P. L., et al.: Family studies of respiratory infections. Br. Med. J. *1*:119–128, 1958.
17. Briss, P. A., Fehrs, L. J., Parker, R. A., et al.: Sustained transmission of mumps in a highly vaccinated population: Assessment of primary vaccine failure and waning vaccine-induced immunity. J. Infect. Dis. *169*:77–82, 1994.
18. Broome, C. V., LaVenture, M., Kaye, H. S., et al.: An explosive outbreak of *Mycoplasma pneumoniae* infection in a summer camp. Pediatrics *66*:884–888, 1980.
19. Brown, S. T.: Therapy for nonvenereal treponematoses: Review of the efficacy of penicillin and consideration of alternatives. Rev. Infect. Dis. *7*:S318–S326, 1985.
20. Bruce-Chwatt, L. J.: Malaria and its control: Present situation and future prospects. Annu. Rev. Public Health *8*:75–110, 1987.
21. Caldwell, G. G., Lindsey, N. J., Wulff, H., et al.: Epidemic of adenovirus type 7 acute conjunctivitis in swimmers. Am. J. Epidemiol. *99*:230–234, 1974.
22. Cann, K. J., Rogers, T. R., Jones, D. M., et al.: *Neisseria meningitidis* in a primary school. Arch. Dis. Child. *62*:1113–1117, 1987.
23. Catanzaro, F. J., Stetson, C. A., Morris, A. J., et al.: The role of *Streptococcus* in the pathogenesis of rheumatic fever. Am. J. Med. *17*:749–756, 1954.
24. Centers for Disease Control: Guidelines for evaluating surveillance systems. M. M. W. R. *37*(Suppl. S-5):1–18, 1988.
25. Centers for Disease Control: Risks associated with human parvovirus B19 infection. M. M. W. R. *38*:81–88, 93–97, 1989.
26. Centers for Disease Control: Swimming-associated cryptosporidiosis: Los Angeles County. M. M. W. R. *39*:343–345, 1990.
27. Centers for Disease Control: Recommendations for the prevention of malaria among travellers. M. M. W. R. *39*(RR-3):1–10, 1990.
28. Centers for Disease Control: Water-related disease outbreaks, 1986–1988. M. M. W. R. *39*(SS-1):1–14, 1990.
29. Centers for Disease Control: Foodborne disease outbreaks, 5-year summary, 1983–1987. M. M. W. R. *39*(SS-1):15–57, 1990.
30. Centers for Disease Control: Change of dosing regimen for malaria prophylaxis with mefloquine. M. M. W. R. *40*:72–73, 1991.
31. Centers for Disease Control: Multistate outbreak of *Salmonella poona* infections: United States and Canada, 1991. M. M. W. R. *40*:549–552, 1991.
32. Centers for Disease Control: Primary amebic meningoencephalitis: North Carolina, 1991. M. M. W. R. *41*:437–440, 1992.
33. Centers for Disease Control and Prevention: The management of acute diarrhea in children: Oral rehydration, maintenance, and nutritional therapy. M. M. W. R. *41*(RR-16):1–20, 1992.
34. Centers for Disease Control and Prevention: 1993 sexually transmitted diseases treatment guidelines. M. M. W. R. *42*(RR-14):1–99, 1993.
35. Centers for Disease Control and Prevention: Assessment of inadequately filtered public drinking water: Washington, D.C., December 1993. M. M. W. R. *43*:661–663,669, 1994.
36. Centers for Disease Control and Prevention: Health Information for International Travel 1995. HHS Publication No. (CDC) 95-8280, 1995.
37. Centers for Disease Control and Prevention: Summary of notifiable diseases, United States, 1994. M. M. W. R. *43*(53):1–12, 1994.
38. Chen, R. T., Goldbaum, G. M., Wassilak, S. G. F., et al.: An explosive point-source measles outbreak in a highly vaccinated population. Am. J. Epidemiol. *129*:173–182, 1989.
39. Chorba, T. L., Berkelman, R. L., Safford, S. K., et al.: Mandatory reporting of infectious diseases by clinicians. J. A. M. A. *262*:3018–3026, 1989.
40. Cochi, S. L., Fleming, D. W., Hightower, A. W., et al.: Primary invasive *Haemophilus influenzae* type b disease: A population-based assessment of risk factors. J. Pediatr. *108*:887–896, 1986.
41. Cochi, S. L., Preblud, S. R., and Orenstein, W. A.: Perspectives on the relative resurgence of mumps in the United States. Am. J. Dis. Child. *142*:499–507, 1988.
42. Committee on Infectious Diseases, American Academy of Pediatrics: Screening for tuberculosis in infants and children. Pediatrics *93*:131–134, 1994.
43. Committee on Infectious Diseases, American Academy of Pediatrics: 1994 Red Book: Report of the Committee on Infectious Diseases. 23rd ed. Elk Grove Village, IL, American Academy of Pediatrics, 1994.
44. Currier, R. W., Hardy, G. E., Jr., and Conrad, J. L.: Measles in previously vaccinated children: Evaluation of an outbreak. Am. J. Dis. Child. *124*:854–857, 1972.
45. Dajani, A. S., Taubert, K., Ferrieri, P., et al.: Treatment of acute streptococcal pharyngitis and prevention of rheumatic fever: A statement for health professionals. Pediatrics *96*:758–764, 1995.
46. Denny, F. W., Collier, A. M., and Henderson, F. W.: Acute respiratory infections in day care. Rev. Infect. Dis. *8*:527–532, 1986.
47. Dingle, J. H., Badger, G. F., and Jordan, W. S., Jr.: Illness in the Home: A Study of 25,000 Illnesses in a Group of Cleveland Families. Cleveland, Western Reserve University, 1964.
48. Doull, J. A.: Factors influencing selective distribution in diphtheria. Prev. Med. *4*:371–404, 1930.
49. Dowling, J. N., Sheehe, P. R., and Feldman, H. A.: Pharyngeal pneumococcal acquisition in "normal" families: A longitudinal study. J. Infect. Dis. *124*:9–17, 1971.
50. Drumm, B., Perez-Perez, G. I., Blaser, M. J., et al.: Intrafamilial clustering of *Helicobacter pylori* infection. N. Engl. J. Med. *322*:359–363, 1990.
51. Dublin, T. D., Rogers, E. F. H., Perkins, J. E., et al.: Milkborne outbreaks due to serologically typed hemolytic streptococci. Am. J. Public Health *33*:157–166, 1943.
52. Dwyer, D. M., Strickler, H., Goodman, R. A., et al.: Use of case-control studies in outbreak investigations. Epidemiol. Rev. *16*:109–123, 1994.
53. El Kholy, A., Fraser, D. W., Guirguis, N., et al.: A controlled study of penicillin therapy of group A streptococcal acquisitions in Egyptian families. J. Infect. Dis. *141*:759–771, 1980.
54. Ferebee, S. H.: Controlled chemoprophylaxis trials in tuberculosis: A general review. Adv. Tuberc. Res. *17*:38–106, 1970.
55. Filice, G. A., and Fraser, D. W.: Management of household contacts of leprosy patients. Ann. Intern. Med. *88*:538–542, 1978.
56. Fleming, D. W., Cochi, S. L., MacDonald, K. L., et al.: Pasteurized milk as a vehicle of infection in an outbreak of listeriosis. N. Engl. J. Med. *312*:404–407, 1985.
57. Fox, J. P., Cooney, M. K., Hall, C. E., et al.: Influenza virus infections in Seattle families, 1975–1979. II. Pattern of infection in invaded households and relation of age and prior antibody to occurrence of infection and related illness. Am. J. Epidemiol. *116*:228–242, 1982.
58. Frank, J. A., Jr., Orenstein, W. A., Bart, K. J., et al.: Major impediments to measles elimination: The modern epidemiology of an ancient disease. Am. J. Dis. Child. *139*:881–888, 1985.
59. Frank J. F., and Barnhart M. H.: Food and dairy sanitation. *In* Last, J. M., and Wallace R. B. (eds.): Maxcy-Rosenau-Last, Public Health and Preventive Medicine. 13th ed. Norwalk, Appleton & Lange, 1992, pp. 589–618.
60. Fraser, D. W.: *Haemophilus influenzae* in the community and the home. *In* Sell, S. H., and Wright, P. F. (eds.): *Haemophilus influenzae:* Epidemiology, Immunology and Prevention of Disease. New York, Elsevier Biomedical, 1982.
61. Friede, A., Harris, J. R., Kobayashi, J. M., et al.: Transmission of hepatitis B virus from adopted Asian children to their American families. Am. J. Public Health *78*:26–29, 1988.
62. Frost, W. H.: The familial aggregation of infectious diseases. Am. J. Public Health *28*:7–13, 1938.
63. Gelfand, H. M., LeBlanc, D. R., Fox, J. P., et al.: Studies on the development of natural immunity to poliomyelitis in Louisiana. II. Description and analysis of episodes of infection observed in study group households. Am. J. Hyg. *65*:367–385, 1957.
64. Gelfand, H. M., Potash, L., LeBlanc, D. R., et al.: Intrafamilial and interfamilial spread of living vaccine strains of polioviruses. J. A. M. A. *170*:2039–2048, 1959.
65. Ghipponi, P., Darrigol, J., Skalova, R., et al.: Study of bacterial air pollution in an arid region of Africa affected by cerebrospinal meningitis. Bull. W. H. O. *45*:95–101, 1971.
66. Gordis, L.: Effectiveness of comprehensive-care programs in preventing rheumatic fever. N. Engl. J. Med. *289*:331–335, 1973.
67. Granoff, D. M., and Daum, R. S.: Spread of *Haemophilus influenzae* type b: Recent epidemiologic and therapeutic considerations. J. Pediatr. *97*:854–860, 1980.
68. Greenfield, S., Sheehe, P. R., and Feldman, H. A.: Meningococcal carriage in a population of "normal" families. J. Infect. Dis. *123*:67–73, 1971.
69. Gwaltney, J. M., Jr., Sande, M. A., Austrian, R., et al.: Pneumococcal spread in families. II. Transfer colds and serum antibody. J. Infect. Dis. *132*:62–68, 1975.
70. Hall, C. B., Geiman, J. M., Biggar, R., et al.: Respiratory syncytial virus infections within families. N. Engl. J. Med. *294*:414–419, 1976.
71. Hammerschlag, M. R., Cummings, C., Roblin, P. M., et al.: Efficacy of neonatal ocular prophylaxis for the prevention of chlamydial and gonococcal conjunctivitis. N. Engl. J. Med. *320*:769–772, 1989.
72. Hedberg, C. W., MacDonald, K. L., and Osterholm, M. T.: Changing epidemiology of food-borne disease: A Minnesota perspective. Clin. Infect. Dis. *18*:671–682, 1994.
73. Heijbel, H., Slaine, K., Seigel, B., et al.: Outbreak of diarrhea in a day care center with spread to household members: The role of *Cryptosporidium*. Pediatr. Infect. Dis. J. *6*:532–535, 1987.
74. Herwaldt, B. L., Craun, G. F., Stokes, S. L., et al.: Waterborne-disease outbreaks, 1989–1990. *In* CDC Surveillance Summaries, December 1991. M. M. W. R. *40*(SS-3):1-21, 1991.
75. Heun, E. M., Vogt, R. L., Hudson, P. J., et al.: Risk factors for secondary transmission in households after a common-source outbreak of Norwalk gastroenteritis. Am. J. Epidemiol. *126*:1181–1186, 1987.

76. Hoge, C. W., Fisher, L., Donnell, H. D., Jr., et al.: Risk factors for transmission of *Mycobacterium tuberculosis* in a primary school outbreak: Lack of racial difference in susceptibility to infection. Am. J. Epidemiol. *139*:520–530, 1994.
77. Hope-Simpson, R. E. H.: Infectiousness of communicable diseases in the household (measles, chicken pox, and mumps). Lancet *2*:549–554, 1952.
78. Hostetter, M. K., Iverson, S., Dole, K., et al.: Unsuspected infectious diseases and other medical diagnoses in the evaluation of internationally adopted children. Pediatrics *4*:559–564, 1989.
79. Isenberg, S. J., Apt, L., and Wood, M.: A controlled trial of povidone-iodine as a prophylaxis against ophthalmia neonatorum. N. Engl. J. Med. *332*:562–566, 1995.
80. Istre, G. R.: Disease surveillance at the state and local level. *In* Halperin, W., Baker, E. L., and Monson, R. R. (eds.): Public Health Surveillance. New York, Van Nostrand Reinhold, 1992, pp. 42–55.
81. Jackson, L. A., Schuchat, A., Reeves, M. W., et al.: Serogroup C meningococcal outbreaks in the United States: An emerging threat. J. A. M. A. *273*:383–389, 1995.
82. Jacobson, J. A., Camargos, P. A. M., Ferreira, J. T., et al.: The risk of meningitis among classroom contacts during an epidemic of meningococcal disease. Am. J. Epidemiol. *104*:552–555, 1976.
83. James, W. E. S., Badger, G. F., and Dingle, J. H.: A study of illness in a group of Cleveland families. XIX. The epidemiology of the acquisition of group A streptococci and of associated illnesses. N. Engl. J. Med. *262*:687–694, 1960.
84. Jereb, J. A., Kelly, G. D., and Porterfield, D. S.: The epidemiology of tuberculosis in children. Semin. Pediatr. Infect. Dis. *4*:220–231, 1993.
85. Koch, W. C., and Adler, S. P.: Human parvovirus B19 infections in women of childbearing age and within families. Pediatr. Infect. Dis. *8*:83–87, 1989.
86. Koopman, J. S., Monto, A. S., and Longini, I. M.: The Tecumseh study. XVI. Family and community sources of rotavirus infection. Am. J. Epidemiol. *130*:760–768, 1989.
87. Krogstad, D. J., Joseph, V. R., and Newton, L. H.: A prospective study of the effects of ultralow volume (ULV) aerial application of malathion on epidemic *Plasmodium falciparum* malaria. Am. J. Trop. Med. Hyg. *24*:199–205, 1975.
88. Kurt, T. L., Yeager, A. S., Guenette, S., et al.: Spread of pertussis by hospital staff. J. A. M. A. *221*:264–267, 1972.
89. Landrigan, P. J.: Epidemic measles in a divided city. J. A. M. A. *221*:567–570, 1972.
90. Lee, L. A., Gerber, A. R., Lonsway, D. R., et al.: *Yersinia enterocolitica* 0:3 infections in infants and children, associated with the household preparation of chitterlings. N. Engl. J. Med. *322*:984–987, 1990.
91. Linnan, M. J., Mascola, L., Lou, X. D., et al.: Epidemic listeriosis associated with Mexican-style cheese. N. Engl. J. Med. *319*:823–829, 1988.
92. Linnemann, C. C., Jr., and Nasenbeny, J.: Pertussis in the adult. Annu. Rev. Med. *28*:179–185, 1977.
93. Linnemann, C. C., Jr., Perlstein, P. H., Ramundo, N., et al.: Use of pertussis vaccine in an epidemic involving hospital staff. Lancet *2*:540–541, 1975.
94. MacKenzie W. R., Hoxie N. J., Proctor, M. E., et al.: A massive outbreak in Milwaukee of *Cryptosporidium* infection transmitted through the public water supply. N. Engl. J. Med. *331*:161–167, 1994.
95. Makintubee, S., Mallonee, J., and Istre, G. R.: Shigellosis outbreak associated with swimming. Am. J. Public Health *77*:166–168, 1987.
96. Markowitz, L. E., Preblud, S. R., Orenstein, W. A., et al.: Patterns of transmission in measles outbreaks in the United States, 1985–1986. N. Engl. J. Med. *320*:75–81, 1989.
97. Maslow, J. N., Mulligan, M. E., and Arbeit, R. D.: Molecular epidemiology: Application of contemporary techniques to the typing of microorganisms. Clin. Infect. Dis. *17*:153–164, 1993.
98. Master, P. L., Brumfitt, W., and Mendez, R. L.: Bacterial flora of the upper respiratory tract in Paddington families, 1952–1954. Br. Med. J. *1*:1200–1205, 1958.
99. Matson, D. O., Byington, C., Canfield, M., et al.: Investigation of a measles outbreak in a fully vaccinated school population including serum studies before and after revaccination. Pediatr. Infect. Dis. J. *12*:292–299, 1993.
100. McCloskey, R. V., Green, M. J., Eller, J., et al.: Treatment of diphtheria carriers: Benzathine penicillin, erythromycin, and clindamycin. Ann. Intern. Med. *81*:788–791, 1974.
101. McCormack, W. M., Chowdhury, A. M., Hahangir, N., et al.: Tetracycline prophylaxis in families of cholera patients. Bull. W. H. O. *38*:787–792, 1968.
102. Mendall, M. A., Goggin, P. M., Molineaux, N., et al.: Childhood living conditions and *Helicobacter pylori* seropositivity in adult life. Lancet *339*:896–897, 1992.
103. Meningococcal Disease Surveillance Group: Meningococcal disease secondary attack rate and chemoprophylaxis in the United States, 1974. J. A. M. A. *235*:261–265, 1976.
104. Mertsola, J., Ruuskanen, O., Eerola, E., et al.: Intrafamilial spread of pertussis. J. Pediatr. *103*:359–363, 1983.
105. Michaels, R. H., and Norden, C. W.: Pharyngeal colonization with *Haemophilus influenzae* type b: A longitudinal study of families with a child with meningitis or epiglottitis due to *H. influenzae* type b. J. Infect. Dis. *136*:222–228, 1977.
106. Miller, L. W., Older, J. J., Drake, J., et al.: Diphtheria immunization: Effect upon carriers and the control of outbreaks. Am. J. Dis. Child. *123*:197–199, 1972.
107. Mink, C. A., Sirota, N. M., and Nugent, S.: Outbreak of pertussis in a fully immunized adolescent and adult population. Arch. Pediatr. Adol. Med. *148*:153–157, 1994.
108. Mohle-Boetani, J. C., Miller, B., Halpern, M., et al.: School-based screening for tuberculous infection: A cost-benefit analysis. J. A. M. A. *274*:613–619, 1995.
109. Moore, A. C., Herwaldt, B. L., Craun, G. F., et al.: Surveillance for waterborne disease outbreaks: United States, 1991–1992. *In* CDC Surveillance Summaries, November 19, 1993. M. M. W. R. *42*(SS-5):1–22, 1993.
110. Moore, M., Baron, R. C., Filstein, M. R., et al.: Aseptic meningitis and high school football players. J. A. M. A. *249*:2039–2042, 1983.
111. Munford, R. S., Taunay, A. E., Morais, J. S., et al.: Spread of meningococcal infection within households. Lancet *1*:1275–1278, 1974.
112. Murphy, T. V., Pastor, P., Medley, F., et al.: Decreased *Haemophilus* colonization in children vaccinated with *Haemophilus influenzae* type b conjugate vaccine. J. Pediatr. *122*:517–523, 1993
113. Nelson, J. D.: The changing epidemiology of pertussis in young infants: The role of adults as reservoirs of infection. Am. J. Dis. Child. *132*:371–373, 1978.
114. Nolan, C. M., Barr, H., Elarth, A. M., et al.: Tuberculosis in a day-care home. Pediatrics *79*:630–632, 1987.
115. Noordeen, S. K.: Chemoprophylaxis in leprosy. Lepr. India *41*:247–254, 1969.
116. Oakley, G. P., Jr.: The neurotoxicity of the halogenated hydroxyquinolines. J. A. M. A. *225*:395–397, 1973.
117. Okun D. A.: Water quality management. *In* Last J. M., and Wallace R. B. (eds.): Maxcey-Rosenau-Last Public Health and Preventive Medicine. 13th ed. Norwalk, Appleton & Lange, 1992, pp. 619–648.
118. Oral rehydration solutions. Med. Lett. Drugs Ther. *25*:19–20, 1983.
119. Pass, R. F., Little, E. A., Stagno, S., et al.: Young children as a probable source of maternal and congenital cytomegalovirus infection. N. Engl. J. Med. *316*:1366–1370, 1987.
120. Pickering, L. K., Evans, D. G., DuPont, H. L., et al.: Diarrhea caused by *Shigella* rotavirus and *Giardia* in day-care centers: Prospective study. J. Pediatr. *99*:51–56, 1981.
121. Pitzinger, B., Steffen, R., and Tschopp, A.: Incidence and clinical features of traveler's diarrhea in infants and children. Pediatr. Infect. Dis. J. *10*:719–723, 1991.
122. Poland, J. D., Quan, T. J., and Barnes, A. M.: Plague. *In* Beran, G. W. (ed.-in-chief): Handbook of Zoonoses. 2nd ed. Boca Raton, CRC Press, 1994, pp. 93–112.
123. Polis, M. A., Tuazon, C. U., Alling, D. W., et al.: Transmission of *Giardia lamblia* from a day care center to the community. Am. J. Public Health *76*:1142–1144, 1986.
124. Porter, J. D., Ragazzoni, H. P., Buchanon, J. D., et al.: *Giardia* transmission in a swimming pool. Am. J. Public Health *78*:659–662, 1988.
125. Potter, M. E., Kaufmann, A. F., Blake, P. A., et al.: Unpasteurized milk: The hazards of a health fetish. J. A. M. A. *252*:2050–2054, 1984.
126. Rammelkamp, C. H., Jr.: Epidemic nephritis. Trans. Assoc. Am. Physicians *67*:276–282, 1954.
127. Rees, R. J. W., and Meade, T. W.: Comparison of the modes of spread and the incidence of tuberculosis and leprosy. Lancet *1*:47–49, 1974.
128. Ryan, C. A., Nickels, M. K., Hargrett-Bean, N. T., et al.: Massive outbreak of antimicrobial-resistant salmonellosis traced to pasteurized milk. J. A. M. A. *258*:3269–3274, 1987.
129. St. Louis, M. E., Morse, D. L., Potter, M. E., et al.: The emergence of grade A eggs as a major source of *Salmonella enteritidis* infections: New implications for the control of salmonellosis. J. A. M. A. *259*:2103–2107, 1988.
130. Schwartz, B.: Chemoprophylaxis for bacterial infections: Principles of and application to meningococcal infections. Rev. Infect. Dis. *13*(Suppl. 2):S170–S173, 1991.
131. Schwartz, B., Broome, C. V., Brown, G. R., et al.: Association of sporadic listeriosis with consumption of uncooked hot dogs and undercooked chicken. Lancet *2*:779–782, 1988.
132. Schwartz, B., Harrison, L. H., Motter, J. S., et al.: Investigation of an outbreak of *Moraxella* conjunctivitis at a Navajo boarding school. Am. J. Ophthalmol. *107*:341–347, 1989.
133. Snider, D. E., Rieder, H. L., Combs, D., et al.: Tuberculosis in children. Pediatr. Infect. Dis. *7*:271–278, 1988.
134. Sprauer, M. A., Cochi, S. L., Zell, E. R., et al.: Prevention of secondary transmission of pertussis in households with early use of erythromycin. Am. J. Dis. Child. *146*:177–181, 1992.
135. Starke, J. R., Jacobs, R. F., and Jereb, J.: Resurgence of tuberculosis in children. J. Pediatr. *120*:839–855, 1992.
136. Steketee, R. W., Wassilak, S. G. F., Adkins, W. N., et al.: Evidence for a high attack rate and efficacy of erythromycin prophylaxis in a pertussis outbreak in a facility for the developmentally disabled. J. Infect. Dis. *157*:434–440, 1988.
137. Straker, E., Hill, A. B., and Lovell, R.: A study of the nasopharyngeal bacterial flora of different groups of persons observed in London and southeast England during the years 1930 to 1937. Reports on Public

Health and Medical Subjects 90. London, His Majesty's Stationery Office, 1939, pp. 7–51.
138. Swerdlow, D. L., and Ries, A. A.: Cholera in the Americas: Guidelines for the clinician. J. A. M. A. *267*:1495–1499, 1992.
139. Tenover, F. C., Arbeit, R., Archer, G., et al.: Comparison of traditional and molecular methods of typing isolates of *Staphylococcus aureus*. J. Clin. Microbiol. *32*:407–415, 1994.
140. Thacker, S. B., and Berkelman, R. L.: Public health surveillance in the United States. Epidemiol. Rev. *10*:164–190, 1988.
141. Thomas, M. E. M., and Tillett, H. E.: Sonne dysentery in day schools and nurseries: An eighteen-year study in Edmonton. J. Hyg. *71*:593–602, 1973.
142. Van Loon, F. P. L., Holmes, S. J., Sirotkin, B. I., et al.: Mumps surveillance: United States, 1988–1993. *In* CDC Surveillance Summaries, August 11, 1995. M. M. W. R. *44*(SS-3):1–14, 1995.
143. Weinstein, L., and LeFrock, J.: Does antimicrobial therapy of streptococcal pharyngitis or pyoderma alter the risk of glomerulonephritis? J. Infect. Dis. *124*:229–231, 1971.
144. Weissman, J. B., Schmerler, A., Weiler, P., et al.: The role of preschool children and day-care centers in the spread of shigellosis in urban communities. J. Pediatr. *84*:797–802, 1974.
145. Werner, S. B., Weidmer, C. E., Nelson, B. C., et al.: Primary plague pneumonia contracted from a domestic cat at South Lake Tahoe, Calif. J. A. M. A. *251*:929–931, 1984.
146. White, M. E., Gordon, D., Poland, J. D., et al.: Recommendations for the control of *Yersinia pestis* infections. Infect. Control *1*:326-329, 1980.
147. Wirsing von König, C. H., Postels-Multani, S., Bock, H. L., et al.: Pertussis in adults: Frequency of transmission after household exposure. Lancet *346*:1326–1329, 1995.
148. Wood, R. C., MacDonald, K. L., and Osterholm, M. T.: *Campylobacter* enteritis outbreaks associated with drinking raw milk during youth activities: A 10-year review of outbreaks in the United States. J. A. M. A. *268*:3228–3230, 1992.
149. World Health Organization: Ecology and Control of Vectors in Public Health. Geneva, Technical Report Series No. 561, 1975.

240

Infections in Day Care Environments

Ellen R. Wald

An ever-increasing number of young women in the work force have contributed to the large number of infants and toddlers receiving out-of-home care. Current estimates are that about 75 per cent of the mothers of children younger than 5 years of age work outside the home, accounting for 13 million children receiving some form of child day care. About one-half of these children receive care in their own homes provided by parents or relatives. Twenty per cent receive care in family day care and 28 per cent in day care centers. As children grow older, families increasingly rely on center care and decrease use of parental care.[20]

The term *day care* is used to describe a variety of different options for the supervision of children in the absence of their parents. Types of day care include (1) large day care centers that are housed in nonresidential settings and provide care for at least seven children in one location (included here are situations in which the parental employer is the sponsor of the day care, frequently at the site of employment, and also preschool and nursery schools in which child care is provided in a structured, primarily educational setting); (2) day care homes in which care is provided in a residential setting for six or fewer children; (3) before- and after-school care designed to bridge the gaps between organized schools (such as preschool or public or private school) and parental departure for or return from work, and (4) cooperatives in which child care is rendered by parents who alternate in caring for their own children as well as other enrolled children.

The quality of care provided to children attending various day care facilities varies widely. Although day care centers are licensed in most states, only 23 per cent of children in out-of-home care are enrolled in these facilities.[164] State regulations vary from state to state; some are quite lenient in setting suggested ratios for staff to child, while others have no regulations governing group size. Even if there were impeccable regulations and well-trained caregivers, the regulations would not protect the vast majority of children who are in unlicensed facilities.

Many factors contribute to the transmission of infectious agents in the day care setting (Table 240–1). Most important are host factors relating to the immunologic susceptibility of young children. Once infection is established, it is transmitted easily because of the natural tendency for intimacy in an age group that has not established acceptable toileting practices and is ignorant of basic hygienic practices. Respiratory and gastrointestinal pathogens frequently contaminate toys.

Caregivers may have received insufficient training in infection control practices. A lack of policy regarding immunization and health care screening for employees may contribute to the spread of infection. In addition, overcrowding, understaffing, and poorly designed physical environments foster transmission of infectious agents in day care. A lack of or inadequate number of hand washing facilities for both children and providers creates an almost insurmountable barrier to infection control.

Major risk factors for spread of infection relate to the age

TABLE 240–1. Risk Factors for Infectious Disease in Day Care

Children
1. Immunologic susceptibility to infectious agents
2. Lack of toilet training
3. Natural tendency to intimacy
4. Frequent oral contact with environment
5. Lack of awareness and practice of good hygiene

Caregivers
1. Insufficient training in infection control
2. Lack of policy regarding immunization
3. Inadequate screening for infectious diseases

Environmental and Economic Problems
1. Inappropriate staff:child ratios
2. Overcrowding
3. Failure to separate age groups
4. Poorly designed physical plant
   a. Inadequate or poorly placed sinks
   b. Failure to separate toilet areas from areas of food preparation
5. Parental pressure to admit sick children to day care

of the participants, the number of children, and ratio of staff to children. The last is determined in part by the age of the children and the experience of the day care provider. In overcrowded situations with inadequate staff, infection easily is spread because of inadequate hand washing and attention to other facets of infection control.

Factors identified as particularly important in the spread of gastrointestinal organisms are large numbers of diaper-age children in centers where staff members who diaper children also are responsible for food preparation.[12, 57] It is important to separate diaper-age children from those who are older to limit spread of enteric illness. If meals are prepared in the day care setting, it is essential to separate this activity from toilet areas. If food is brought from home, it should be transported properly and stored to avoid spoilage. Lack of attention to this issue may result in additional illness. Day care centers that operate for profit also are at higher risk for infectious disease outbreaks, probably reflecting lower staff-to-children ratios.[93] Finally, parents may not withdraw ill children from attendance at day care voluntarily because of the expense and inconvenience of creating alternate child care arrangements.

MODES OF TRANSMISSION OF INFECTIOUS DISEASES

The most important pathogens and their modes of transmission of infection in day care are shown in Table 240–2. Respiratory infections by far are the most common cause of illness in infants, toddlers, and preschoolers, regardless of whether they attend day care.

Respiratory

For some microbiologic species causing infection, the mode of transmission is the airborne route. The organism is aerosolized and remains in the air like cigarette smoke. Direct contact with the infected individual is not necessary for spread of the infection. Illnesses known to be transmitted this way include measles, varicella, pertussis, and tuberculosis.

Most commonly, respiratory organisms are spread by the production of droplets that are laden with infective particles. These droplets may be transmitted directly from mucosa to mucosa when there is close physical contact. More often, droplets land on nonporous surfaces (e.g., cribs, tables, chairs) or on clothes and paper (fomites) and remain infective for minutes to hours. Hand contact with contaminated surfaces and fomites can result in infection if the hands touch the nasal or conjunctival mucosa.[60] Agents that can be transmitted by droplet spread (mucosa-to-mucosa), from finger to mucosa, or by fomites include most respiratory viruses (respiratory syncytial, rhinovirus, influenza, parainfluenza, adenovirus, parvovirus B19, measles, mumps, rubella, and varicella), *Haemophilus influenzae* type b (Hib), *Neisseria meningitidis,* and *Streptococcus pyogenes.*[49, 51, 56, 59] Finger-to-mucosa spread of respiratory pathogens is the most important and common mechanism for transmission of viral and bacterial infections.[65] Consequently, hand washing is an essential element of preventing spread of infection.

Gastrointestinal

Spread of gastrointestinal organisms is by fecal-oral transmission. The number of organisms required to produce infection will determine if infection occurs by person-to-person spread or if a food or fluid intermediary is required. For example, rotavirus, *Giardia lamblia,* and *Shigella* species are transmitted readily by very small numbers of organisms found on the hands (without obvious gross contamination) after person-to-person contact or by touching infected surfaces. In contrast, *Salmonella,* rarely a cause of diarrheal outbreaks in the day care setting, requires large numbers of organisms to produce infection. Accordingly, an intermediary

TABLE 240–2. Pathogens and Modes of Transmission of Infection in Day Care

Mode of Transmission	Bacteria	Viruses	Parasites
Respiratory	*Haemophilus influenzae* type b *Streptococcus pneumoniae* *Neisseria meningitidis* *Streptococcus pyogenes* *Bordetella pertussis* *Mycobacterium tuberculosis*	Adenovirus Influenzae A & B Measles Mumps Parainfluenza Parvovirus B19 Respiratory syncytial Rhinovirus Rubella Varicella	
Fecal-oral	*Campylobacter jejuni* *Salmonella* species *Shigella* species *Clostridium difficile* *Escherichia coli* O157:H7	Enteroviruses Hepatitis A Rotavirus Calicivirus	*Cryptosporidium* *Giardia lamblia* *Enterobius vermicularis*
Person-to-person via skin contact	*Streptococcus pyogenes* *Staphylococcus aureus*	Herpes simplex	*Pediculus capitis* *Sarcoptes scabei* *Tricophyton* species *Microsporum* species
Contact with blood, urine, or saliva		Cytomegalovirus Hepatitis B Herpes simplex HIV	

Used with permission of the American Academy of Pediatrics and Peter, G. (eds.): 1994 Red Book: Report of the Committee on Infectious Diseases. 23rd ed. Elk Grove Village, American Academy of Pediatrics, 1994, p. 82.

step of food or beverage contamination is required to allow organisms to replicate up to the necessary inocula.

Numerous studies have demonstrated fecal organisms on day care center environmental surfaces, with which infants and toddlers have had contact, and on the hands of care providers.[40, 82, 165, 171] The contamination of the environment is highest when the day care children are younger than 3 years of age. This age predilection correlates with the number of children still wearing diapers.[166] Important pathogens, including fecal bacteria, rotavirus, hepatitis A virus, and *G. lamblia* cysts, are able to survive on environmental surfaces for periods ranging from hours to weeks.[27, 89]

Skin

Bacterial, viral, and parasitic infections of the skin can be transmitted from person to person by direct contact. Bacterial pathogens, such as *S. pyogenes* and *Staphylococcus aureus*, usually are not primarily invasive unless there is a break in the integument, such as might occur with minor trauma (e.g., insect bites). Herpes simplex virus may be transmitted from skin or mucosa to skin by direct contact, again only if the skin is broken. Infestations, such as scabies and lice, are transmitted from person to person by mobile parasites. The superficial dermatophytes responsible for tinea infections (trichophyton, microsporum, and epidermophyton) are transmitted from person to person or by contact with infected fomites, such as combs, hairbrushes, and hats.

Blood, Urine, and Saliva

Hepatitis B virus (HBV), HIV, and cytomegalovirus (CMV) theoretically can be transmitted by blood, urine, and saliva. For HBV, HIV, and CMV, transmission by blood and sexual activity (presumably resulting in mild trauma, thereby leading to blood exposure) is the rule in adults. Although both HBV and HIV can be demonstrated in urine and saliva, exchange of these body fluids is very unlikely to transmit infection. At day care, transmission of CMV probably occurs between attendees by contamination of toys with saliva. Mothers and day care providers can become infected with CMV by the finger-to-mucosa route after hand contamination by urine or saliva.

PATTERNS OF INFECTION IN DAY CARE

Children in day care experience several different patterns of occurrence of infection (Table 240–3).[54] Most of the increased infectious disease burden found in day care centers is experienced by the children themselves. They have an excess of respiratory and gastrointestinal infections compared with children who are in home care.[168] Certain specific infections, such as Hib, rotavirus, and respiratory syncytial virus (RSV), are shouldered almost exclusively by the children. However, on occasion, adult personnel working as providers will experience some of the same respiratory and gastrointestinal infections as the children. Examples of infections for which day care attendees and staff share an increased burden include shigellosis, giardiasis, and invasive meningococcal disease.

Several infections barely recognizable in the day care child (because they are mild or asymptomatic) cause significant repercussions when they are spread to adults—either parents or day care providers. The most notable of these is hepatitis A, which in adults tends to be an illness of moderate severity often leading to extended absences from work.

TABLE 240–3. Patterns of Occurrence of Infections Experienced in Day Care

Patterns of Occurrence	Examples
1. Clinical manifestation of infection primarily in children	*Haemophilus influenzae* type b infection Respiratory syncytial virus, rotavirus infections
2. Infection affects children, day care staff, and close family members	Shigellosis, giardiasis *Neisseria meningitidis* infection
3. Inapparent infection in children with clinically important infection in adult contacts	Hepatitis A
4. Inapparent or mild infection in children and adults but may have serious consequences for fetus in pregnant contact	Cytomegalovirus infection Rubella Parvovirus B19 infection Coxsackievirus A16 infection

Modified from Goodman, R. A., Osterholm, M. T., Granoff, D. M., et al.: Infectious diseases and child day care. Reproduced by permission of Pediatrics *74*:134–139, Copyright 1984.

Lastly, for some infections, clinical manifestations in adults are mild, but there is concern regarding potential effects of the infection on the fetus if the child care provider or mother of a day care attendee is pregnant. CMV and rubella virus are associated with severe birth defects if infection occurs in the first trimester. Infection with parvovirus B19 during pregnancy poses a risk for nonimmune hydrops in the fetus.

INFECTIOUS AGENTS IN DAY CARE

Infections Spread by the Respiratory Route

Viral Upper Respiratory Infections

Respiratory viruses (rhinovirus, RSV, parainfluenza, influenza, adenoviruses, and Epstein-Barr) are the most common cause of infection in preschool children.[14, 36, 49] The range of clinical manifestations includes asymptomatic infection, simple upper respiratory infections (rhinitis), acute otitis media, pharyngitis, croup, tracheitis, bronchiolitis, and pneumonitis. Disease may be mild or severe and involve single or multiple levels of the respiratory tree. Children may experience multiple infections with each agent because of (1) antigenic diversity within virus subtypes (e.g., influenza A virus), (2) multiple subtypes (e.g., rhinoviruses), and (3) failure to develop immunity after a single exposure (e.g., RSV). Viruses are shed from the site of infection (conjunctiva, nose, throat), even before clinical symptoms develop, thereby making it difficult to control the spread of these infections in day care. There is ample documentation that children in day care (family or large day care centers) experience more respiratory infections than children in home care.[37, 45, 70, 95, 147, 150, 168] The risk of infection for children in group or family care is intermediate between that for large day care centers and home care.[168]

The most common bacterial complication of viral upper respiratory infections is acute otitis media. The peak age incidence of otitis media is between 6 and 18 months, paralleling the incidence of viral upper respiratory tract infections.

TABLE 240–4. Comparisons of Annualized Rates of Acute Respiratory Tract Infections, Otitis Media, and Antibiotic Treatment Among Children in Various Modes of Child Care

Study	Length of Time Observed	Annual Rate of Acute Respiratory Infection (per Child-Year)	Annual Rate of Otitis Media (per Child-Year)	Annual Rate of Antibiotic Treatment (per Child-Year)
Wald et al.[168]*				
DCC (n = 33)	12–18 months	6.3		
DCH (n = 23)	12–18 months	5.1		
HC (n = 97)	12–18 months	3.9		
Strangert[150]†				
DCC (n = 108)	8 months	7.5	1.2	1.9
DHC (n = 42)	8 months	7.5	1.3	1.6
HC (n = 57)	8 months	3.0	0.5	0.8
Stahlberg[147]‡				
DCC (n = 23)	8 weeks	13.8	2.3	4.8
DCC (n = 23)	8 weeks	12.0	0.9	2.8
HC (n = 23)	8 weeks	9.9	1.1	1.4
Reves and Jones[131]§				
DCC (n = 42)	8 weeks	8.1	6.0	9.1
DCH (n = 72)	8 weeks	2.6	1.6	2.7
HC (n = 156)	8 weeks	3.0	1.6	2.5

*Telephone interview every 2 weeks.
†Active surveillance in DCC; telephone call every 4 months for children in DCH and HC.
‡Daily diary in all groups.
§Health maintenance organization abstraction covering an 8-week period for each child.
DCC, day care center; DCH, day care home; HC, cared for at home.
Modified from Reves, R. R., and Jones, J. A.: Antibiotic use and resistance patterns in day care centers. Semin. Pediatr. Infect. Dis. 1:212–221, 1990.

The majority of children have had at least one episode of acute otitis media by the time they reach their second birthday, and approximately one-third will have had at least three episodes of acute otitis media by that time.[159] Not surprisingly, as the frequency of viral respiratory infections is increased in children attending day care, these children experience a notable increase in the frequency of otitis media.[131, 147, 150, 151, 168] Table 240–4 shows a comparison of the annualized rates of acute respiratory tract infections, otitis media, and antibiotic treatment among children in various modes of child care. Wald and collegues[168] provided data indicating that the risk of hospitalization for performance of myringotomy with tube placement was highest for children in large day care. Likewise, the risk for recurrent acute otitis media and persistent middle ear effusion also is higher for children in day care compared with those cared for at home.[31, 44, 148, 162]

It is not recommended that children with mild respiratory infections be excluded from day care or separated from the group of well children because this strategy has not been shown to achieve an overall reduction of infections for children in day care.

Systemic Viral Infections

Cytomegalovirus

CMV is a common cause of infection in preschool children. Most often the infection completely is asymptomatic.[71] Rarely, the child may experience a febrile illness with lymphadenopathy and hepatosplenomegaly. The sources of CMV in the day care setting are infants and children who have been infected by their mothers via vertical transmission either in utero (1 to 2 per cent), perinatally (2 to 3 per cent), or postpartum through breast feeding (about 6 per cent). Strangert[150] reported the isolation of CMV from 7 of 10 children between 21 and 30 months of age in one day care center. Strom[153] found that 13 of 18 (72 per cent) children between 24 and 36 months of age in a single nursery excreted CMV. Urine cultures frequently persistently were positive for CMV for many months. Other investigators demonstrated that peak rates of infection occur between 1 and 3 years of age, when viral excretion may be documented in up to 70 per cent of children in day care, as shown in Table 240–5.[1, 72, 79, 104, 115, 117]

Infection in the preschool child leads to viral shedding documented by positive CMV cultures obtained from swabs of the throat (thereby contaminating saliva) and urine. Transmission probably occurs through fomites (toys and blankets) contaminated with saliva rather than by respiratory droplets.[145] Shedding of CMV is as chronic among infected toddlers in day care centers as it is for children with perinatal or congenital infection.[116, 117]

CMV is a problem if acquisition of infection occurs during early pregnancy in day care providers or mothers of children attending day care.[1–4] This may lead to clinically evident congenital CMV infection (microcephaly, hepatosplenomegaly, chorioretinitis, psychomotor retardation, and deafness) in approximately 5 per cent of infected children. Another 10 to 15 per cent of infants experience occult but potentially damaging infection, which results in milder degrees of hearing loss and learning disabilities.[146]

Parvovirus B19

Parvovirus B19, the etiologic agent of erythema infectiosum, or fifth disease, is spread by the respiratory route. Viral replication, viremia, and nasopharyngeal shedding occur approximately 1 week before the development of clinical symptoms. This is a benign disease of childhood (in a normal host) that may occur in preschool and school children. The clinical illness is characterized by an erythematous rash on

TABLE 240–5. Excretion of Cytomegalovirus (CMV) in Urine from Children in Day Care

Study	No. of Day Care Centers Studied	Age of Children Studied (Months)	No. of Children Studied	No. (%) with CMV in Urine
Strangert[150]	1	21–30	10	7 (70)
	13	6–36	40	9 (23)
Strom[153]	1	24–36	18	13 (72)
Pass et al.[115]	1	3–12	11	1 (9)
		13–24	18	15 (83)
		25–36	16	10 (63)
		36–60	25	10 (40)
Pass et al.[117]	1	0–60	103	59 (57)
Hutto et al.[72]	3	<12	10	0 (0)
		12–24	38	14 (37)
		25–36	35	27 (77)
		38–48+	143	36 (25)
Jones et al.[79]	11	<12	33	8 (21)
		12–24	51	15 (29)
		25–48	52	9 (17)
Adler[1]	1	0–24	31	8 (25)
		24–60	34	7 (20)
Murph et al.[104]	1	0–9	8	2 (25)
		12–24	12	8 (67)
		25–36	14	4 (29)
		37–48+	39	3 (8)

the face, giving a "slapped cheek" appearance. Patients usually do not have fever or other constitutional symptoms. The rash progresses after the first day and spreads as a maculopapular eruption beginning on the proximal extremities and extending to the distal parts and trunk. After several days, these lesions develop into a lacy reticular pattern on the proximal extremities and then fade. Unrecognized in the immunocompetent host is an infection of the erythrocyte precursor, which leads to a transient red blood cell aplasia.

In adults, parvovirus B19 infection frequently causes arthralgias and arthritis. Its clinical importance in the context of day care infections is transmission from an infected preschool child to a pregnant mother or day care provider.[51] In a large outbreak of erythema infectiosum in Connecticut, 19 per cent of susceptible adult school personnel became infected; the highest rates of seroconversion were observed in personnel in contact with large numbers of young children. Infection of the fetus may lead to nonimmune hydrops secondary to infection of the erythrocyte progenitor cells. Estimates for fetal loss when a pregnant woman of unknown antibody status is exposed to parvovirus are 2.5 per cent after household exposure and 1.5 per cent after occupational exposure in school or day care.[9]

Coxsackievirus A16

Epidemics of coxsackievirus A16 infection cause hand, foot, and mouth disease, a clinical syndrome characterized by a vesicular exanthem on the distal extremities and mild stomatitis. Two outbreaks have been reported in children attending day care.[42, 43] The disease is mild in children but has a high attack rate. Its importance relates to the possibility of infection during pregnancy, which may lead to spontaneous abortion.[42, 108]

Streptococcus pyogenes or Group A *Streptococcus*

Group A *Streptococcus* (GAS) is a common cause of respiratory and skin infections. The most common expression of infection with GAS is the development of pharyngitis and fever in an elementary school child. Usually, the throat infection is accompanied by tender anterior cervical nodes. In classic infection, none of the usual signs of viral upper respiratory disease—coryza, cough, and conjunctivitis—is present. Illness peaks in the late winter and spring. In contrast, streptococcal infection of the preschool child or child in day care takes the form of a protracted upper respiratory infection. Specifically, these patients present with low-grade fever, persistent nasal discharge, anorexia, and cervical adenopathy.

Although it can be assumed that exposure of day care children to an index case of streptococcal pharyngitis would result in secondary cases, few epidemics of GAS have been reported in day care.[41, 143] However, a recent outbreak was reported from a day care center in which preschool children shared facilities with kindergarten children in an "after" school program.[143] During a 3-month period, 47 per cent of the day care population had positive cultures for GAS or a rapid antigen detection test. Children with GAS infections of their throat or skin should be excluded from day care for 24 hours after the initiation of appropriate antibiotic treatment.

Invasive Bacterial Disease

Haemophilus Influenzae Type b

Hib used to be the major bacterial pathogen of childhood, causing meningitis, epiglottitis, pneumonia, facial cellulitis, and septic arthritis. These infections occurred in children between 2 months and 5 years of age, with a peak between 6 and 18 months of age. The organism colonizes the nasopharynx before becoming blood-borne; hematogenous dissemination results in a distant focus of infection. Infected children usually have a several-day history of mild upper respiratory symptoms followed by the abrupt onset of high fever and localized symptoms indicating the site of infection (e.g., irritability or seizures in central nervous system infection, cutaneous findings in cellulitis). Colonized individuals who lack anticapsular antibody are susceptible to the development of invasive disease.[55]

In the 1980s, there was considerable debate regarding whether children in day care had a higher risk than those in home care for primary episodes of infection with Hib. The risk for primary disease in an individual child is defined as the risk of disease with Hib for that child in the absence of a known contact with another case in the previous 60 days. Many cases of infection due to Hib have occurred in children attending day care.[26, 53, 74, 129, 156] In several studies, it has been estimated that between 28 and 40 per cent of infections due to Hib have occurred in children attending day care.[74, 129] However, there has been significant variation in the presence and magnitude of the increased risk dependent on the age of the child, type and size of the day care facility, and geographic location of the facility. In general, studies have shown that the risk of primary Hib infection is highest in younger children (≤23 months of age) during their first month of enrollment in day care and among children attending a larger day care center as opposed to a day care home.[74, 129]

An additional concern was whether there was a significantly elevated risk of secondary cases of Hib infection in the day care setting. Although several studies have substantiated an increased risk of secondary cases of invasive Hib infection in day care attendees exposed to another attendee with infection due to Hib,[10, 45, 97] others have not.[105, 112] Based on available data,[10, 45, 97, 105, 112] the risk of secondary disease among day care classroom contacts of a child with invasive Hib probably was higher than among children of similar age in the general population; however, the magnitude was not well defined and varied depending on day care center characteristics and geographic location. The management of day care attendees younger than 2 years of age who were exposed to a case of invasive infection caused by Hib was controversial.[32]

The availability and universal use (in infancy) of effective vaccines for the prevention of Hib infections dramatically have changed the epidemiology of infections caused by this pathogen. Schulte and coworkers[136] recently reviewed the pattern of invasive infections caused by Hib occurring in New York State. They demonstrated a dramatic decline in the incidence of Hib disease in children younger than 5 years of age, both those in day care and in home care. The decrease in cases of infection attributable to Hib occurred among children attending day care centers before being observed in non–day care attendees, perhaps reflecting the requirement for Hib vaccine before enrollment in day care. The virtual disappearance of this once common and serious problem and the high immunization rates with Hib vaccine obviate a lengthy discussion regarding the need for rifampin prophylaxis after exposure to cases of invasive disease. In the rare instance of a case of invasive Hib disease in a family day care center housing other susceptible children (<4 years of age), all day care contacts (adults and children) should receive rifampin, at 20 mg/kg/day, once daily for 4 days.

Neisseria meningitidis

N. meningitidis is a gram-negative, polysaccharide-encapsulated diplococcus found colonizing the nasopharynx. It is the second leading cause of meningitis in the United States. Other manifestations of infection include pericarditis, sepsis, and pneumonia. Similar to that among patients experiencing infection with Hib, the attack rate is highest among children between 2 months and 5 years of age, with a peak between 6 and 12 months of age. The pathogenesis is hematogenous dissemination from the nasopharynx as a site of colonization. Household contacts exposed to patients with meningococcal disease are at a significantly higher risk of developing that disease than is the general population.[33, 101, 103]

Secondary spread of infection with *N. meningitidis* has been recognized as a potential risk, especially in situations of crowding, such as in military barracks and college dormitories. In addition, reports suggest that the risk of secondary disease due to *N. meningitidis* is increased in the day care setting.[35, 76, 91, 134] In a Belgian report,[35] exposure in a day care nursery during a prolonged meningococcal epidemic conferred a 76 times greater risk of infection compared with similarly aged children cared for at home. Prompt institution of rifampin prophylaxis is the recommended strategy for management of all intimate contacts of a person with invasive disease due to *N. meningitidis* in order to prevent secondary or associated illness. It is not recommended that throat cultures be performed to identify those who require rifampin prophylaxis. The cultures may be insensitive, and waiting for results will delay appropriate management.

Streptococcus pneumoniae

Pneumococci are the most common cause of bacterial infections of the upper and lower respiratory tract, including otitis media, sinusitis, and pneumonia.[137] As respiratory pathogens, they also cause other upper respiratory tract infections, such as conjunctivitis, and important systemic illnesses, including occult bacteremia, bacteremic periorbital cellulitis, and meningitis.

Although one might expect transmission of *Streptococcus pneumoniae* in the day care setting to be similar to that of Hib and *N. meningitidis*, there has been relatively little systematic study of this phenomenon. Multiply antibiotic-resistant *S. pneumoniae*, a problem that began in the 1970s, now is widespread in South Africa and large parts of Europe. It is increasing as a problem in the United States.

Although *S. pneumoniae* is the most common cause of otitis media and otitis media is the most common infection caused by *S. pneumoniae*, the rarity of performance of tympanocentesis (despite the frequency of otitis media in children in day care) indicates delayed appreciation of the fact that *S. pneumoniae* is spread easily in the day care setting. The ease of transmission of penicillin-resistant *S. pneumoniae* (the resistance providing a readily recognizable marker) in the day care setting has been demonstrated amply.[64, 126, 127] In addition, although the risk of secondary cases of pneumococcal disease for children in day care compared with those in home care is unknown, an outbreak of invasive disease[127] caused by *S. pneumoniae* in a day care has brought increased attention to this issue. Investigation of the outbreak in Houston failed to demonstrate that carriage of multiply antibiotic-resistant *S. pneumoniae* differed significantly between children who had or had not been taking antibiotics recently; however, a study of children in an Ohio day care[130] showed that prophylactic doses of antibiotics and frequent use of antibiotics were risk factors for nasopharyngeal carriage of antibiotic-resistant *S. pneumoniae*. The most recent cluster of cases of invasive pneumococcal disease occurring in young children in child care[25] involved a 12F serotype of pneumococcus that was penicillin-sensitive; three of six children in the day care experienced bacteremic infections.

Several reports claim that rifampin is ineffective or only partially effective in eradicating carriage of *S. pneumoniae*.[127, 130] However, this may be explained by inadequacy of the dose of rifampin,[127] lack of compliance with drug administration, or inappropriate timing for test-of-cure cultures.

Mycobacterium tuberculosis

Reported cases of tuberculosis have been on the incline in the United States since 1987, including an increase in the number of infected children. Children with tuberculosis generally are not infectious. Rather, an adult in the environment invariably has active disease. Three clusters of cases of tuberculosis in children have been traced to attendance at day care.[81, 92, 107] Screening of all day care personnel, both staff and volunteers, with tuberculin skin testing is essential to eliminate this problem.

Infections of the Gastrointestinal Tract

Giardia lamblia

G. lamblia is one of the most common causes of diarrhea in the day care setting.[17] Infection can result from ingestion of as few as 10 cysts. Transmission most commonly results from person-to-person spread, although water-borne outbreaks have been documented. Parents of day care attendees are at risk for infection.[122] Demonstration of *G. lamblia* cysts on environmental surfaces indicates additional potential for transmission.[27] Infection with this parasite causes infestation of the duodenum and proximal jejunum and results in asymptomatic carriage more often than it causes clinical disease.[73] After an incubation period of approximately 2 weeks, the symptomatic patient experiences diarrhea, intermittent abdominal pain, anorexia, and flatulence. The most notable feature of the infection is its tendency to become protracted, thereby leading to weight loss, failure to thrive, and anemia. Diagnosis is made by recovery of the organism from stool specimens or occasionally by examination of a sample of a duodenal aspirate or an intestinal biopsy.[77, 160] After resolution of symptoms, either by virtue of treatment or spontaneous cure, the patient may continue to shed cysts for a very long time.[73] Treatment is not recommended for asymptomatic individuals shedding *G. lamblia* cysts. For symptomatic individuals, treatment may be undertaken with metronidazole, furazolidone, or quinacrine. Relapses occur in approximately 15 per cent of patients.

Cryptosporidium

Cryptosporidium is a cause of severe diarrhea in immunocompromised hosts but usually causes self-limited illness in immunocompetent children or adults.[29] The parasite may be spread from person to person or via food or water. The usual clinical symptoms are watery diarrhea and low-grade fever with abdominal pain and weight loss. Vomiting occurs in approximately 30 per cent of patients.

Cryptosporidium, like *G. lamblia*, has a very low infectious dose for humans. Ninety per cent of infant nonhuman primates will become infected with 10 to 50 oocysts.[102] Spread of infection is facilitated in the day care center because oocysts shed in the feces of infected persons are highly resistant to common disinfectants. Many outbreaks of diarrhea caused by *Cryptosporidium* have been reported from day care centers.[5, 6, 28, 30, 63, 158] Asymptomatic children and adults shed oocysts for weeks after infection.[29]

Diagnosis is made by examination of the stool for oocysts using special stains. Treatment is supportive. Exclusion from day care is recommended until the patient is asymptomatic.

Shigella

Infection with *Shigella* species causes illness of variable severity but easy transmissibility. Accordingly, *Shigella* is one of the most common causes of diarrhea outbreaks in the day care population,[21, 119, 121, 155, 169, 170] and *Shigella* infection was among the first enteric diseases recognized to be spread in day care. Infection can be caused by as few as 10 to 100 organisms. Although a low inoculum is sufficient to cause infection, the organism does not survive well outside of the human host. Person-to-person transmission is considered more important than environmental contamination.[169] Although infection with *Shigella* may be caused by one of four species (*S. sonnei*, *S. flexneri*, *S. dysenteriae*, and *S. boydii*), *S. sonnei* and *S. flexneri* are the most common.

Shigellosis primarily is a disease of young children. In outbreaks, younger children have the highest attack rate and are the most effective transmitters of infection.[161] Day care personnel and family contacts also experience high attack rates.[68, 157] After an incubation period of several days, the patient with classic disease develops fever and watery diarrhea, followed by crampy abdominal pain, tenesmus, and mucoid bloody stools. In many cases, the illness is mild and indistinguishable from other causes of gastroenteritis. The presence of fecal leukocytes upon examination of the stool provides supportive information; stool culture is diagnostic.

Treatment of shigellosis with an appropriate antimicrobial effectively terminates the illness. Susceptibilities vary, but sulfamethoxazole-trimethoprim for 5 days most often is effective in the United States. Antimicrobial treatment decreases the duration of symptoms and fecal shedding. Untreated persons continue to excrete organisms for several weeks.

Campylobacter jejuni

Campylobacter jejuni is a more common cause of diarrhea in children than *Shigella* species but is less likely than *Shigella* to cause outbreaks of diarrheal disease in day care centers.[75, 90, 114] Most often, a high inoculum of *Campylobacter* is required to produce infection, thereby necessitating a food or water vehicle. Less often, transmission can occur by person-to-person spread of smaller numbers of organisms. The clinical presentation is variable, but the usual onset is with fever, abdominal pain, and diarrhea. Many cases resemble classic shigellosis. Watery diarrhea and low-grade fever with only modest constitutional signs of illness also may be observed. The illness usually lasts between 3 and 7 days. The diagnosis can be made by culture of the stool; examination of the stool by darkfield or direct smear may be very informative if performed by an experienced observer.

Treatment with erythromycin is effective in terminating excretion of the infective organism; this may be important in controlling epidemics or outbreaks. The impact of erythromycin on the clinical course of disease is variable.

Salmonella

Salmonella is the most common cause of bacterial diarrhea in many parts of the United States, but it is an uncommon cause of gastroenteritis outbreaks in day care.[94] Because the organism is widespread in nature, it has been very difficult to control. There are 2200 different serotypes of *Salmonella*. Infection usually occurs after ingestion of contaminated food or beverages. Person-to-person spread is very uncommon, except in infancy when the infective dose is low.[174]

The most common expression of infection with *Salmonella* is uncomplicated gastroenteritis. The illness begins approximately 12 to 36 hours after exposure and often is characterized initially by vomiting and subsequently by diarrhea. Abdominal pain and fever are frequent accompaniments; occasionally, stools will contain mucus and blood. Although most cases are self-limited, *Salmonella* can be distinguished from other causes of gastroenteritis by its occasionally protracted course. Diagnosis is made by culture of the stool. In general, antimicrobials are not recommended unless bacteremia is documented. Management of special hosts, such as neonates and immunocompromised patients, is controversial.

Although some authors recommend antimicrobial therapy for these groups, few data support this recommendation. Exclusion from day care is recommended until the diarrhea resolves. Once stools are normal, there is little reason to restrict attendance. Stool cultures from household contacts, day care contacts, or the index case in convalescence rarely are indicated.[161]

Clostridium difficile

Clostridium difficile is the classic cause of pseudomembranous colitis in patients who have received or are receiving antimicrobial agents and rarely causes disease unassociated with antimicrobial use. The organism, a gram-positive spore-forming rod, is distributed widely in soil and in the gastrointestinal tract of humans. It frequently is found colonizing asymptomatic newborns. Disease is a consequence of the elaboration of toxin(s) by vegetative organisms. Hospital environments and day care facilities are a reservoir for the organism.[84, 85] During outbreaks of *C. difficile* diarrhea in day care centers, environmental contamination is increased, as is the recovery of *C. difficile* from the hands of children and staff.[85]

Clinical symptoms include fever, diarrhea, and abdominal cramps. Stools may contain blood and mucus. The illness varies in severity from mild to life-threatening. The diagnosis of *C. difficile* gastroenteritis is made by recovery of the toxin from a stool sample. Treatment includes cessation of antibiotics and supportive care. Specific antimicrobial therapy with oral vancomycin or metronidazole may be necessary to achieve a clinical cure. Metronidazole is favored in an era of concern regarding the development of vancomycin-resistant enterococci after the use of oral vancomycin. Children and personnel should be excluded from day care until they are asymptomatic.

Escherichia coli

Several outbreaks of diarrhea due to various *Escherichia coli* strains have been associated with significant morbidity and mortality in the child care setting. In 1986, an outbreak of diarrhea caused by *E. coli* O157:H7 was reported from a day care attended by 107 children.[144] Thirty-four per cent of attendees became ill, with a significant increase in risk for younger children. Approximately one-third of the children with diarrhea had bloody stools, and three children developed hemolytic-uremic syndrome. Although infection with *E. coli* O157:H7 usually occurs after ingestion of contaminated beef, person-to-person spread of infection was most likely in this epidemic. The diarrheal illness also was documented in family members of ill children. Subsequent epidemiologic studies in Minnesota have confirmed the mode of transmission for *E. coli* O157:H7 to be person-to-person in the day care setting.[15] Accordingly, symptomatic children should be excluded until stools are formed and culture-negative for *E. coli* O157:H7.

E. coli O157:H7 are recovered from stool samples after being plated on MacConkey-sorbitol agar. Sorbitol-negative colonies of *E. coli* are picked and screened with 0157 antisera by tube agglutination. Antibiotic treatment is not recommended for persons with diarrhea caused by *E. coli* O157:H7. Approximately 5 to 10 per cent of children infected with *E. coli* O157:H7 develop hemolytic-uremic syndrome.

Outbreaks of diarrhea due to enteropathogenic *E. coli* in the child care setting have been characterized by chronic, often relapsing diarrhea in infants and toddlers.[19, 118] The diarrheal illness has had a high attack rate (56 to 90 per cent) and led to prolonged hospitalizations in 8 to 30 per cent of affected children.

Rotavirus

Rotavirus is the most common etiology for gastroenteritis in infants and children and the leading cause of hospitalization due to gastroenteritis in industrialized countries, including the United States.[18, 98] It is an important cause of diarrhea in developing countries as well and contributes substantially to the worldwide mortality figures for gastroenteritis.

Rotavirus frequently is recovered from asymptomatic hosts, especially neonates and infants.[24] It is shed in large numbers in the stool of symptomatic patients, thereby contributing to the high prevalence of the virus on environmental surfaces during outbreaks.[173] Viral shedding occurs both before and after symptoms have appeared[120]; a low inoculum is required to cause infection.

Most illnesses due to rotavirus occur in the winter in temperate climates but year-round in tropical areas. The peak attack rate is in the age group of 6 to 24 months. After a brief incubation period of 2 to 3 days, patients may have prodromal respiratory symptoms (coryza and cough) and then present with varying combinations of vomiting, diarrhea, and low-grade fever that last 3 to 5 days. The range of severity is broad; dehydration occasionally may be profound. Spread of rotavirus infections is extremely common in the hospital; not surprisingly, transmission within a day care center is very rapid, and many outbreaks have been reported in this setting.[13, 109, 110, 120, 121, 132] In prospective studies of diarrheal illness in children attending day care, rotavirus was implicated in 6 to 24 per cent of cases of gastroenteritis[12, 67, 154] and in 20 to 40 per cent of outbreaks.[13, 121] Day care workers and family contacts are at risk for rotavirus infection.

Rotavirus cannot be cultivated easily in tissue culture in a viral diagnostic laboratory. Diagnosis is made with an antigen detection method used on a stool specimen. Treatment is supportive, and exclusion is recommended until diarrhea resolves.

Hepatitis A Virus

Hepatitis A virus (HAV), an enterovirus, is the most common cause of acute hepatitis in children. As with other enteric pathogens, this organism is transmitted by the fecal-oral route. Manifestations of infection vary remarkably according to age. In small children, infection with HAV may be entirely asymptomatic or associated with relatively mild and nonspecific symptoms, such as low-grade fever, anorexia, nausea, vomiting, and diarrhea. Jaundice, a more specific marker of liver disease, occurs in less than 10 per cent of children younger than 6 years of age.[52, 149] In contrast, adults with hepatitis A often are icteric in conjunction with other gastrointestinal symptoms. Infection, when symptomatic, usually lasts several weeks but occasionally can become protracted.

HAV is shed in the stool of infected persons, in high density, from 2 weeks before until 1 week after the onset of clinical symptoms. Transmission primarily is person-to-person, but fomites may play an important role because the organism can persist and remain infective in the dried state for months.[99] Diagnosis usually is made with serologic evidence of marker antibodies against HAV (IgM anti-HAV). Treatment is symptomatic. Prevention of illness in contacts can be accomplished with intramuscular immune serum globulin and most recently with hepatitis A vaccine.[172] A recent study[113] conducted among children residing in a Hasidic Jewish community in New York State demonstrated the efficacy of the inactivated hepatitis A vaccine in preventing hepatitis A during 7 months of follow-up after vaccination. Further study is under way to determine duration of immunity and need for boosters.

HAV can be spread easily in day care centers with diaper-age children because of the facility of person-to-person transmission.[58, 149] Spread of infection barely is noticeable, until an adult contact (usually a parent or day care worker) develops symptomatic infection with HAV. Other contacts, including siblings, extended family members, and babysitters, also are affected frequently. Clusters of cases of hepatitis A in communities have been traced to a single day care center. The risk of a hepatitis outbreak in a day care center has been shown to be related directly to the number and age of children in attendance and the hours that the center is open. Larger centers with longer hours and diaper-age children have the highest rates of infection and greatest spread to the community.[57]

Infections Spread by Skin Contact

Group A Streptococcus

GAS has become a less common cause of impetigo and pyoderma in children over the last decade with a concomitant rise in cases caused by *S. aureus*. Nonetheless, the organism still can cause superficial infections of traumatized skin (insect bites, scratches), erysipelas, and cellulitis. The latter infections can result in the abrupt onset of fever and dramatic cutaneous erythema and tenderness often accompanied by regional adenopathy. Diagnosis can be made by careful performance of wound cultures (obtained after careful cleansing of the periwound area) or tissue aspirates. Spread of typical impetigo is common within families and presumably also would occur within day care centers. Children should be excluded from day care until 24 hours of appropriate antimicrobial therapy (of a 10-day course) has been completed.

Scabies

Scabies is an infection of the skin caused by infestation with the female mite *Sarcoptes scabiei*. Transmitted person-to-person by an infested individual, the mite buries itself beneath the strateum corneum and burrows along for its 30-day life span, laying two to three eggs per day. The larval and nymphal mites scatter after hatching to embed themselves in skin at distant sites. Some 3 to 6 weeks later, a pruritic eruption (worse at night) develops, leading to excoriation, bleeding, and crusting. The distribution of lesions varies with age. In adults and older children, the eruption, consisting of papules, vesicles, and nodules, is common in the interdigital spaces of the hands, on the extensor surface of the elbow, and around the umbilicus, waist, axillary line, and genital area. In infants and young children, vesicular and eczematous lesions are found on the hands and feet, as well as the face and head.

Diagnosis is made by scraping the lesions and demonstrating the mite, ova, or mite feces. Treatment of the index case should be undertaken with a scabicide, preferably 5 per cent permethrin, applied to the entire body. Alternative less desirable drugs are lindane and crotamiton. Asymptomatic contacts should be treated simultaneously because they unknowingly may be infected and capable of transmitting the mite during this asymptomatic period. Clothing and bed linens should be washed, dry-cleaned, or stored for a week to ensure their noninfectivity.

Although scabies is spread primarily by intimate personal contact, skin-to-skin transmission can occur after prolonged casual contact, as occurs in institutional settings, nursing homes, and day care.[135] Mites can survive for 2 to 3 days on inanimate surfaces, which permits transmission via fomites, such as clothes, bed linens, and furniture. An outbreak of scabies recently was reported in a hospital-affiliated day care facility.[135] Elimination of the problem required a coordinated effort with simultaneous treatment of all potentially infected individuals. An infected child should be excluded from day care for 24 hours after treatment is undertaken. More commonly, transmission occurs within the family setting.

Head Lice

Head lice infestation is common in day care and school-aged children consequent to infection with *Pediculus capitis*. The insect, a hemophagic ectoparasite, obtains nourishment by sucking capillary blood from the scalp. Female lice attach egg cases (nits) to the hair shafts at or very near the scalp. The eggs hatch 8 to 11 days later, releasing three louse nymphs.

The diagnosis is made when the symptoms of scalp pruritus, excoriation, pyoderma, and regional lymphadenopathy cause one to inspect the scalp closely. Nits are observed readily, although live lice may be difficult to see, especially in light infestations. Transmission is by direct contact with or spread by fomites of live lice. The latter is facilitated when there is common storage of hats and coats.

Treatment is with permethrin shampoos to eradicate the lice. Nits can be removed mechanically with spiral combs after preparation of the hair with vinegar soaks or a commercially prepared rinse. All clothing and infested bedding can be disinfected by machine washing or drying (using temperatures of at least 128.3° F [53.5° C]), dry cleaning, or storing in plastic bags for about 10 days.

Infections Spread by Contact with Blood, Urine, and Saliva

Hepatitis B Virus

HBV is a DNA-containing virus that causes a wide range of clinical manifestations from asymptomatic seroconversion to fatal hepatitis. Infection in children is more likely to be asymptomatic than that in adults.[100] Common symptoms include fever, fatigue, anorexia, malaise, and jaundice. Other gastrointestinal symptoms, such as nausea, vomiting, and diarrhea, may be prominent. Joint symptoms (arthritis and arthralgias) and cutaneous lesions (papular acrodermatitis) may be observed early in the illness.

The most common modes of transmission of HBV in adults are contact with blood and sexual activity. Young children usually acquire infection with HBV by vertical transmission from their mother at delivery. The maternal infection may be acute or chronic. Infection acquired vertically by the infant usually is asymptomatic, but it leads to chronic carriage of hepatitis B surface antigen in most cases. With increasing immigration and adoption of infants from HBV-endemic areas, more HBV-carrier children will be identified.[61]

Transmission of HBV within the day care setting has been documented only twice in the United States.[34, 139] In one case, the probable source was a bite by a child who was a carrier of HBV.[139] In the other, a day care worker with chapped hands was exposed to the blood of a child who was a HBV carrier.[34] Three other investigations have failed to demonstrate transmission in day care, despite long-term contact, including one situation with a high potential for blood exposure.[34, 139, 140] The most recent surveillance activity showed only 1 of 496 children in day care to be infected with HBV without a family member as a potential source.[48] In Japan, where the background prevalence of hepatitis B surface antigen carriage is higher than in the United States, data suggest that transmission of HBV most probably occurs among children in nursery schools.[62] The current recommendation to screen all parturients for HBV and to undertake universal immunization against hepatitis B in infancy should curtail spread of this infection in the future. Because of the low risk of transmission within the day care setting, the American Academy of Pediatrics, the American Public Health Association, and the Centers for Disease Control and Prevention do not recommend exclusion of HBV-infected children from day care or HBV screening of children as a criterion for entry.[7]

Cytomegalovirus

CMV can be transmitted by blood, urine, and saliva, as described earlier.

HIV

To date, HIV infection has not been reported to be transmitted in a day care center. In light of its rare horizontal transmission to nonsexual contacts within households with an infected member, HIV would not be expected to spread in day care.[50, 78] The risk of transmission of HIV is less than 1 in 500 exposures, even when there is direct inoculation with HIV-infected blood by needlestick injury to a health care worker. The risk of exposures other than by direct inoculation is far less than 1 in 500. The risk in day care is even lower. Potential high-risk situations might involve HIV-positive children who are persistent biters or who have extensive weeping skin lesions.

One example of possible transmission of HIV between siblings was reported from Germany.[167] In this case, a bite may have been the source, although complete information on other interactions between the brothers was not available. Other reports have indicated a lack of transmission to 35 individuals bitten or scratched by an HIV-infected person.[39, 142, 163] In addition, a study of family members of HIV-infected children reported no seroconversions to HIV in nine contacts bitten by HIV-infected children and seven uninfected children who bit HIV-infected children.[133] These studies support the lack of evidence for transmission of HIV in the day care setting.

VACCINE-PREVENTABLE DISEASES

Diphtheria

Diphtheria now is a very rare disease in the United States; fewer than five cases a year have been observed recently. The infection can present with nasal symptoms, as membranous pharyngitis, as obstructive laryngotracheitis, or with skin manifestations. The prominent symptoms usually are a severe sore throat and croup accompanied by toxemia.

Corynebacterium diphtheriae is spread by droplets from people with infection or carriers after intimate contact. Individuals are susceptible if they have not been immunized or have been immunized only partially. Treatment is with antitoxin and antibiotics (erythromycin or penicillin). Prophylaxis can be accomplished with erythromycin or penicillin if an individual is found to be a carrier. Immunization with diphtheria-tetanus-pertussis or diphtheria-tetanus vaccine is effective in preventing disease and spread of infection.

Varicella-Zoster

Varicella-zoster, or chicken pox, is a common, highly contagious infection of childhood affecting more than 80 per cent of the population by the time they reach 10 years of age. The infection easily is spread by the airborne route and by respiratory droplets. The infection is characterized by a pruritic, generalized, vesicular rash that occurs in one to six crops, each crop separated by 24 to 36 hours. Fever usually is mild. The most common complication is secondary bacterial pyoderma. The varicella-zoster virus remains latent in the body after primary infection but can reactivate as herpes zoster or "shingles," manifesting as a vesicular eruption involving one to three sensory dermatomes. If infection is acquired in early pregnancy, a varicella embryopathy (limb bands or amputation) has been noted in a small fraction of offspring.

More than one-third of the cases of varicella in the United States are estimated to occur in persons younger than 5 years of age.[124] Data on the relative risk of children in day care developing varicella are minimal.[80] However, outbreaks of varicella in day care centers are known to be common, and the prevalence of varicella in children who attend day care appears to be higher than that documented for the general population.[47] Children with varicella are excluded from day care and may return 6 days after onset of rash or when all their lesions are crusted.

The newly available varicella vaccine is recommended to be given to all children between 12 and 15 months of age. The availability of this vaccine should alter dramatically the epidemiology of varicella in the future, both within and outside of the day care situation.[87]

Measles

Measles (rubeola) is a highly contagious respiratory infection. After many years of decline, it again reached epidemic proportions in impoverished and medically underserved inner-city areas in the United States between 1989 and 1992. Although susceptibility to measles virus infection occurs when maternal antibody wanes, the peak age group for measles in the preimmunization era was school age children between 5 and 9 years of age. More recently, outbreaks have involved preschool children, setting the stage for day care outbreaks.

Measles virus is spread by droplets, hand transmission, and the airborne route. The illness usually is moderate to severe; a high fever and prominent respiratory symptoms (cough, coryza, and conjunctivitis) are present for several days before the onset of the rash. Diarrhea occasionally may be a prominent feature. After the rash erupts, the fever and respiratory symptoms persist for several more days. Pneumonia and encephalitis are complications of measles virus infection; each occurs with an incidence of 1 per 1000 cases.

Measles is prevented effectively by immunization. Current recommendations are to immunize twice: once between 12 and 15 months of age and again at 4 to 6 years or 10 to 14 years of age.[7, 22] In epidemic situations, a primary immunization may be given before a child is 12 months of age. In that case, another vaccination is given between 12 and 15 months of age, and the first is not counted toward the two required for full protection.

When measles is diagnosed in a child attending day care after several days of illness, intramuscular immune serum globulin is the most effective way to prevent secondary cases in susceptible contacts. When there has been a single recent exposure to a case of measles, administration of measles-mumps-rubella vaccine within 3 days of exposure should be effective in preventing natural infection.

Rubella

Rubella, another exanthematous disease of childhood, is much milder than rubeola but attacks a similar age group. As with measles, rubella until recently nearly had been eradicated by routine universal immunization with the measles-mumps-rubella vaccine.

Clinically, rubella is characterized by mild fever, lymphadenopathy (postauricular and occipital), and rash. The illness is difficult to distinguish from other viral exanthems. Infection may be completely asymptomatic. The child with documented rubella should be excluded from day care until 5 days after onset of illness.

If rubella is contracted during the first or early second trimester of pregnancy, a severe fetal infection resulting in microcephaly, deafness, congenital heart defects, eye disorders, and psychomotor retardation may result. Acquisition of infection during pregnancy may be a potential hazard for day care personnel or mothers of children who attend day care.

Congenital rubella syndrome can be eliminated by appropriate immunization of preschoolers and personnel. There are no specific recommendations for care after exposure of a susceptible pregnant adult.

Pertussis

Pertussis, or whooping cough, is a highly communicable respiratory disease caused by *Bordetella pertussis*. The attack rate and severity of disease are highest in the first year of life. The illness classically is divided into three phases: catarrhal, paroxysmal, and convalescent. In the first stage, the child has no fever but has symptoms, primarily rhinorrhea and a cough. When the nasal symptoms resolve, however, the cough becomes and remains very prominent for many weeks. The cough is characterized by paroxysms that are followed by an inspiratory effort (whoop) or leave the child exhausted and occasionally apneic. The convalescent stage is the many weeks necessary for complete recovery. Treatment with erythromycin is effective in decreasing the shedding of organisms, but it does not alter the course of the disease.

Complete immunization with sequential use of whole killed pertussis vaccine and acellular pertussis vaccine or a five-dose series of acellular pertussis vaccine is effective in preventing most cases of pertussis, although illness does occur in partially and occasionally fully immunized children. After exposure to a case, erythromycin for 14 days provides effective prophylaxis, despite its negligible clinical effect after the paroxysmal stage begins. This is recommended for exposure in day care.[11] If appropriate, booster doses of whole cell or acellular diphtheria-tetanus-pertussis vaccine should be given to exposed children in a day care or household setting. A child with pertussis should be excluded from day care until 7 days of a 14-day course of erythromycin has been received.

Poliomyelitis

Poliovirus is an enterovirus that now rarely causes disease in the United States. Although most infections with poliovirus are subclinical, in the preimmunization era, polio was the major cause of acquired paralytic disease, especially among older children and young adults. In some developing countries, it still is a major health problem.

Poliomyelitis is prevented effectively by the use of either the live oral poliovirus vaccine or inactivated enhanced-potency parenteral vaccine. From a public health point of view, the oral vaccine is effective in protecting the individual and the community because oral poliovirus vaccine is the only vaccine in use that provides herd immunity. The development of secretory and humoral antibodies in the vaccinee and shedding of the live virus result from an immunization strategy that mimics the natural route of infection. New recommendations from the Advisory Committee on Immunization Practices of the Centers for Disease Control and Prevention are supporting the use of sequential inactive enhanced-potency parenteral vaccine and oral poliovirus vaccine in the future.[7a, 125] Alternatively, continued use of either oral poliovirus vaccine or the inactivated vaccine for all four doses is acceptable.[7a]

Mumps

Mumps is a relatively benign infection of childhood that often is asymptomatic. The most prominent clinical feature is parotitis. Occasionally, a clinically significant central nervous system infection causes unilateral sensorineural deafness. This infection virtually has been eliminated by widespread use of the mumps-measles-rubella vaccine. Children with mumps should be excluded from the day care setting until parotid swelling subsides or, if swelling is prolonged, until 9 days after onset of swelling.

Hepatitis B

HBV is a vaccine-preventable infection that is spread by contact with blood, urine, and saliva, as described earlier.

MANAGEMENT OF INFECTIONS

Exclusion Policy

The American Academy of Pediatrics and the American Public Health Association have reached a consensus regarding exclusion policies for children attending day care.[8] The recommendations reflect the understanding that when children have moderate to severe illnesses, they should not be allowed to participate in usual activities or may require more individualized care than is available and that the spread of certain communicable diseases within the day care center will be reduced by the exclusion of people with infections. Accordingly, children known to have highly infectious illnesses should not be allowed to attend day care until treatment is initiated (as for head lice or GAS infections) or symptoms have resolved (diarrhea due to *Shigella*, rotavirus, or *Giardia*) or until transmissibility has waned, as in pertussis, varicella, measles, and mumps. In addition, children should be excluded if the contagiousness of their illness is uncertain (e.g., if a child has a high fever and a rash). A complete list of recommendations for exclusions is shown in Table 240–6.

Important conditions that do not require necessarily exclusion from day care include (1) asymptomatic excretion of an enteropathogen, (2) nonpurulent conjunctivitis, (3) a rash without a fever or behavioral change, (4) CMV infection, (5) the carrier state of HBV, and (6) HIV infection. Any exceptions to this statement are found in the individual discussions of the infectious agents. For many infections, the highest risk of disease transmission occurs prior to the appearance of recognizable symptoms. Once illness occurs, other children already have been exposed and exclusion is a less-effective

TABLE 240–6. Recommendations for Exclusion from Day Care

Symptoms

- The illness prevents the child from participating comfortably in program activities.
- The illness results in a greater care need than the child care staff can provide without compromising the health and safety of the other children.
- The child has any of the following conditions: fever, unusual lethargy, irritability, persistent crying, difficulty breathing, or other signs of possible severe illness.
- Diarrhea (defined as an increased number of stools compared with the child's normal pattern, with increased stool water and/or decreased form) that is not contained by diapers or toilet use.
- Vomiting two or more times in the previous 24 hours, unless the vomiting is determined to be due to a noncommunicable condition and the child is not in danger of dehydration.
- Mouth sores associated with an inability of the child to control his/her saliva, unless the child's physician or local health department authority states that the child is noninfectious.
- Rash with fever or behavior change, until a physician has determined the illness not to be a communicable disease.

Specific Diseases

- Purulent conjunctivitis (defined as pink or red conjunctiva with white or yellow eye discharge, often with matted eyelids after sleep and eye pain or redness of the eyelids or skin surrounding the eye), until examined by a physician and approved for readmission, with or without treatment.
- Tuberculosis, until the child's physician or local health department authority states that the child is noninfectious.
- Impetigo, until 24 hours after treatment has been initiated.
- Ringworm, until the morning after topical or systemic therapy has been started.
- Streptococcal pharyngitis, until 24 hours after treatment has been initiated and until the child has been afebrile for 24 hours.
- Pinworms, until the morning after therapy has been given.
- Head lice (pediculosis), until the morning after the first treatment.
- Scabies, until after treatment has been completed.
- Varicella, until the sixth day after onset of rash or sooner if all lesions have dried and crusted.
- Pertussis (which is confirmed by laboratory or suspected based on symptoms of the illness or because of cough onset within 14 days of having face-to-face contact with a person in a household or classroom who has a laboratory-confirmed case of pertussis), until 5 days of appropriate antibiotic therapy (currently, erythromycin) has been completed (total course of treatment is 14 days).
- Measles, until 5 days after the onset of rash.
- Mumps, until 9 days after the onset of parotid gland swelling.
- Hepatitis A virus infection, until 1 week after onset of illness and jaundice, if present, has disappeared or until passive immunoprophylaxis (immune serum globulin) has been administered to appropriate children and staff in the program, as directed by the responsible health department.

Used with permission of the American Academy of Pediatrics and Peter, G. (eds.): 1994 Red Book: Report of the Committee on Infectious Diseases. 23rd ed. Elk Grove Village, American Academy of Pediatrics, 1994, p. 82.

strategy. This explains why exclusion has not been shown to be effective in reducing the frequency of viral upper respiratory tract infections.

Prophylaxis of Infection

Prophylaxis is a strategy that may be helpful in the management of some infections that occur in day care centers. For example, if a child has had invasive disease caused by *N. meningitidis*, rifampin prophylaxis for all day care contacts may prevent secondary or associated cases. If a child has pertussis, exposed children may be protected by a booster immunization if appropriate and prescription of erythromycin for prophylaxis. Intramuscular immune serum globulin may be used to protect susceptible contacts after exposure to measles or hepatitis A.

Vaccination

Vaccination can be used as a strategy to prevent infection during epidemics in a community. For example, immunization with measles-mumps-rubella vaccine is successful in terminating epidemics of measles in elementary or high school. Varicella vaccine also can be used community-wide to curtail the spread of chickenpox. The newly available hepatitis A vaccine is an appropriate intervention for controlling the outbreak of hepatitis A in day care centers and other settings.[69]

HBV rarely has been reported to be transmitted in a day care setting in the United States. Hepatitis B vaccine, now recommended for universal use in infancy, protects against transmission of infection if a carrier of HBV is identified.

PREVENTION OF INFECTIONS

Vaccination

There currently are 11 vaccine-preventable diseases for a preschool child: diphtheria, tetanus, pertussis, polio, measles, mumps, rubella, varicella, Hib infection, hepatitis A, and hepatitis B. The timely and appropriate use of these immunizations successfully will eliminate these problems from the day care setting. Recommendations for the use of hepatitis A vaccine in children are awaited. Studies have shown that children who attend registered day care facilities are more likely to be up-to-date in their immunizations than children cared for at home.[66] Laws requiring the age-appropriate vaccination of children attending licensed child day care programs exist in almost all states.[23]

Education

An integral part of the control of infection within a day care center is education of staff and families. The staff must understand the general principles of infection transmission and control. Education before job placement and frequent inservice seminars reinforce the importance of some basic techniques, especially hand washing. Supervision is essential to ensure compliance with policies.[86]

Parents should be educated regarding recognition of illness, especially illnesses that are best cared for at home. The rationale and importance of compliance with center rules should be emphasized. The child care program should inform parents of the need to share information about communicable illnesses in the child or a family member.

TABLE 240–7. Immunizations for Day Care Employees

Vaccine	Personnel	Schedule
Diphtheria, tetanus	All	Every 10 years
Measles-mumps-rubella	All	If born after 1955, evidence of prior infection or two doses at least 1 month apart
Varicella	Nonimmune	Two doses 1 month apart
Polio	All	Primary immunization with inactivated polio virus vaccine if needed. Consider booster if previously immunized.
Influenza A/B	If older than 55 years of age	Annually
Hepatitis B	Advised	0, 1, and 6 months
Hepatitis A	All	Two doses 1 month apart

Written Policies

Each day care facility should have written policies for managing child and employee illness.[8] There should be written procedures for hand washing, personal hygiene policies, environmental sanitation policies and procedures, and policies for filing and updating immunization records. Employees should be screened for tuberculosis by skin testing when hired and annually if initially the skin test is negative. If the skin test is positive, a chest radiograph should be performed. Other recommendations regarding immunization of day care employees are shown in Table 240–7. There is no need to screen day care attendees or employees for HIV, HBV, or CMV.

Physical Plant Characteristics

In the planning of day care facilities, areas for infants and toddlers should be separated from those for older children. Because fecal contamination is related strongly and inversely to age, it is important to have a physical plant large enough to separate children younger than 3 years of age from older children. If this is not possible, an age restriction should be placed on admission. The kitchen and food storage areas should be separated from the toilet space. Because hand contamination represents the most critical factor in transmission of infection, hand washing facilities must be available to staff and children. This especially is important in the diaper changing and food preparation areas. The hand washing facility preferably is pedal-operated and in easy reach of soap and towel dispensers.

When construction materials are selected, the choice should be based on durability and ease of cleaning. Diaper changing areas should be cleaned easily and light-colored so soilage can be detected. A pedal-operated, closed receptacle is ideal for the disposal of soiled diapers. Only paper diapers should be used. The toddler area should be equipped with training toilets and junior-sized toilets. The use of potty chairs should be discouraged. If they are used, they should be emptied into the toilet, cleaned in a utility sink, and disinfected after each use.[8] These areas must be cleaned frequently.

Hygienic Standards

The key factor in disease prevention in the day care setting is the maintenance of optimal hygienic standards based on recognized mechanisms of transmission of infection. Hand washing is considered the single most important preventive measure,[11, 16, 54, 86, 122] in recognition of the fact that both respiratory and enteric pathogens are spread by contaminated hands.

References

1. Adler, S. P.: The molecular epidemiology of cytomegalovirus transmission among children attending a day care center. J. Infect. Dis. *152*:760–768, 1985.
2. Adler, S. P.: Molecular epidemiology of cytomegalovirus: Evidence for viral transmission to parents from children infected at a day care center. Pediatr. Infect. Dis. J. *5*:315–318, 1986.
3. Adler, S. P.: Cytomegalovirus transmission among children in day care, their mothers and caretakers. Pediatr. Infect. Dis. J. *7*:279–285, 1988.
4. Adler, S. P.: Molecular epidemiology of cytomegalovirus: Viral transmission among children attending a day care center, their parents, and caretakers. J. Pediatr. *112*:366–372, 1988.
5. Albert, G., Bell, L. M., Kirkpatrick, C. E., et al.: Cryptosporidiosis in a day care center. N. Engl. J. Med. *311*:860–861, 1984.
6. Alpert, G., Bell, L. M., Kirkpatrick, C. E., et al.: Outbreak of cryptosporidiosis in a day-care center. Pediatrics *77*:152–157, 1986.
7. American Academy of Pediatrics and Peter, G. (eds.): 1994 Red Book: Report of the Committee on Infectious Diseases. 23rd ed. Elk Grove Village, IL, American Academy of Pediatrics, 1994, p. 82.
7a. American Committee on Immunization Practices: Poliomyelitis prevention in the United States: Introduction of a sequential vaccination schedule of inactivated poliovirus vaccine followed by oral poliovirus vaccine. M. M. W. R. *46*:1–22, 1997.
8. American Public Health Association and American Academy of Pediatrics: Caring for our children. *In* National Health and Safety Performance Standards: Guidelines for Out-of-Home Child Care Programs. Washington, DC, and Elk Grove Village, IL, APHA/AAP, 1992.
9. Anderson, L. J.: Human parvoviruses. J. Infect. Dis. *161*:603–608, 1990.
10. Band, J. D., Fraser, D. W., and Ajello, G.: *Haemophilus influenzae* disease study group: Prevention of *Haemophilus influenzae* type b disease by rifampin prophylaxis. J. A. M. A. *251*:2381–2386, 1984.
11. Bartlett, A. V., Broome, C. V., Hadler, S. C., et al.: Public health considerations of infectious diseases in child day care centers. J. Pediatr. *105*:683–701, 1984.
12. Bartlett, A. V., Moore, M., Gary, G. W., et al.: Diarrheal illness among infants and toddlers in child day care centers. J. Pediatr. *107*:495–502, 1985.
13. Bartlett, A. V., Reves, R. R., and Pickering, L. K.: Rotavirus in infant-toddler day care centers: Epidemiology relevant to disease control strategies. J. Pediatr. *113*:435–441, 1988.
14. Beem, M. O.: Acute respiratory illness in nursery school children: A longitudinal study of the occurrence of illness and respiratory viruses. Am. J. Epidemiol. *90*:30–44, 1969.
15. Belongia, E. A., Osterholm, M. T., Soler, J. T., et al.: Transmission of *Escherichia coli* O157:H7 infection in Minnesota child day care facilities. J. A. M. A. *269*:883–888, 1993.
16. Black, R. E., Dykes, A. C., Anderson, K. E., et al.: Handwashing to prevent diarrhea in day-care centers. Am. J. Epidemiol. *113*:445–451, 1981.
17. Black, R. E., Dykes, A. C., Sinclair, S. P., et al.: Giardiasis in day-care centers: Evidence of person-to-person transmission. Pediatrics *60*:486–491, 1977.
18. Blacklow, N., and Greenberg, H. B.: Medical progress: Viral gastroenteritis. N. Engl. J. Med. *325*:252–264, 1991.
19. Bower, J. R., Congeni, B. L., Cleary, T. G., et al.: *Escherichia coli* O114: Nonmotile as a pathogen in an outbreak of severe diarrhea associated with a day care center. J. Infect. Dis. *160*:243–247, 1989.
20. Cain, V. S.: Child care and child health: Use of population surveys. Pediatrics *94*:1096–1098, 1994.
21. Centers for Disease Control: Multiply-resistant shigellosis in a day-care center: Texas. M. M. W. R. *35*:753–755, 1986.
22. Centers for Disease Control: Recommendations of the Immunization Practice's Advisory Committee (ACIP): Measles prevention. M. M. W. R. *38*(Suppl. S–9):1–18, 1989.
23. Centers for Disease Control: State Immunization Requirements, 1991–1992. Washington, DC, U. S. Department of Health and Human Services, CDC, 1992.
24. Champsaur, H., Questiaux, E., Prevot, J., et al.: Rotavirus carriage, asymptomatic infection and disease in the first two years of life. 1. Virus shedding. J. Infect. Dis. *149*:667–673, 1984.
25. Cherian, T., Steinhoff, M. C., Harrison, L. H., Rohn et al.: A cluster of

invasive pneumococcal disease in young children in child care. J. A. M. A. *271*:695–697, 1994.

26. Cochi, S. L., Fleming, D. W., Hightower, A. W., et al.: Primary invasive *Haemophilus influenzae* type b disease: A population-based assessment of risk factors. J. Pediatr. *108*:887–896, 1986.
27. Cody, M. M., Sottnek, H. M., and O'Leary, V. S.: Recovery of *Giardia lamblia* cysts from chairs and tables in child day care centers. Pediatrics *94*(Suppl.):1006–1008, 1994.
28. Combee, C. L., Collinge, M. L., and Britt, E. M.: Cryptosporidiosis in a hospital associated day care center. Pediatr. Infect. Dis. J. *5*:528–532, 1986.
29. Cordell, R. L., and Addiss, D. G.: Cryptosporidiosis in child care settings: A review of the literature and recommendations for prevention and control. Pediatr. Infect. Dis. J. *13*:310–317, 1994.
30. Crawford, F. G., Vermund, S., Ma, J. Y., et al.: Asymptomatic cryptosporidiosis in a New York City day care center. Pediatr. Infect. Dis. J. *7*:806–807, 1988.
31. Daly, K., Giebink, S., Le, C. T., et al.: Determining risk for chronic otitis media with effusion. Pediatr. Infect. Dis. J. *7*:471–475, 1988.
32. Dashefsky, B., Wald, E., and Li, K.: Commentary: Management of contacts of children in day care with invasive *Haemophilus influenzae* type b disease. Pediatrics *78*:939, 1986.
33. DeMaeyer-Aeempoel, S., Reginster-Hancuse, G., Dachy, A., et al.: Meningococcal disease in Belgium: Secondary attack rate among household, day-care nursery, and pre-elementary school contacts. J. Infect. *3*(Suppl. 1):63–70, 1981.
34. Desoda, C. C., Shapiro, C. N., Carroll, K., et al.: Hepatitis B virus transmission between a child and staff member at a day care center. Pediatr. Infect. Dis. J. *13*:828–830, 1994.
35. DeWals, P., Hertoghe, L., Borlée-Grimée, I., et al.: Meningococcal disease in Belgium: Secondary attack rates among household, day-care nursery and pre-elementary school contacts. J. Infect. *1*(Suppl.):53–61, 1981.
36. Dingle, J. H., Badger, G. F., and Jordan, W. S., Jr.: Illness in the Home. Cleveland, Press of Western Reserve University, 1964.
37. Doyle, A. B.: Incidence of illness in early group and family day-care. Pediatrics *58*:607–613, 1976.
38. Doyle, M. G., Van, R., and Pickering, L. K.: Penicillin-resistant *Streptococcus pneumoniae* in children in home care and day care. Pediatr. Infect. Dis. J. *11*:831–835, 1992.
39. Drummond, J. A.: Seronegative 18 months after being bitten by a patient with AIDS. J. A. M. A. *256*:2342–2343, 1986.
40. Ekanem, E. E., DuPont, H. L., Pickering, L. K., et al.: Transmission dynamics of enteric bacteria in day-care centers. Am. J. Epidemiol. *118*:562–572, 1983.
41. Falck, G., and Kjellander, J.: Outbreak of group A streptococcal infection in a day care center. Pediatr. Infect. Dis. J. *11*:914–919, 1992.
42. Ferson, M. J., and Bell, S. M.: Outbreak of coxsackie A16 hand, foot and mouth disease in a child day care center. Am. J. Public Health *81*:1675–1676, 1991.
43. Ferson, M. J.: Infections in day care. Curr. Opin. Pediatr. *5*:35–40, 1993.
44. Fiellau-Nikolajsen, M.: Tympanometry in 3-year old children. ORL J. *41*:193–205, 1979.
45. Fleming, D. W., Cochi, S. L., Hightower, A. W., et al.: Childhood upper respiratory tract infections: To what degree is incidence affected by day care attendance? Pediatrics *79*:55–60, 1987.
46. Fleming, D. W., Leibenhaut, M. H., Albanea, D., et al.: Secondary *Haemophilus influenzae* type b in day care facilities: Risk factors and prevention. J. A. M. A. *254*:509–514, 1985.
47. Foscarelli, P.: Infectious conditions in day care: There is more than enteritis and rhinitis. Am. J. Dis. Child. *144*:955–956, 1990.
48. Foy, H. M., Swenson, P. D., and Freitag-Koontz, M. J., et al.: Surveillance for transmission of hepatitis B in child day care. Pediatrics *94*(Suppl.):1002–1004, 1994.
49. Frenck, R. W., and Glezen, W. P.: Respiratory tract infections in children in day care. Semin. Pediatr. Infect. Dis. *1*:234–244, 1990.
50. Friedland, G. H., Saltzman, B. R., Rogers, M. F., et al.: Lack of transmission of HTLV-III/LAV infection to household contacts of patients with AIDS or AIDS-related complex with oral candidiasis. N. Engl. J. Med. *314*:344–349, 1986.
51. Gillespie, S. M., Cartter, M. L., Asch, S., et al.: Occupational risk of human parvovirus B19 infection for school and day care personnel during an outbreak of erythema infectiosum. J. A. M. A. *263*:2061–2065, 1990.
52. Gingrich, G. A., Hadler, S. C., Elder, H. A., et al.: Serologic investigation of an outbreak of hepatitis A in a rural day care center. Am. J. Public Health *73*:1190–1193, 1983.
53. Ginsburg, C. M., McCracken, G. H., Jr., Rae, S., et al.: *Haemophilus influenzae* type b disease: Incidence in a day-care center. J. A. M. A. *238*:604–607, 1977.
54. Goodman, R. A., Osterholm, M. T., Granoff, D. M., et al.: Infectious diseases and child day care. Pediatrics *74*:134–139, 1984.
55. Granoff, D. M., Gilsdorf, J., Gessert, C. E., et al.: *Haemophilus influenzae* type b in a day care center: Relationship of nasopharyngeal carriage to development of anticapsular antibody. Pediatrics *65*:65–68, 1980.
56. Gwaltney, J. M., Moskalski, P. B., and Hendley, J. O.: Hand-to-hand transmission of rhinovirus colds. Ann. Intern. Med. *88*:463–467, 1978.
57. Hadler, S. C., Erben, J. J., Francis, D. P., et al.: Risk factors for hepatitis A in day-care centers. J. Infect. Dis. *145*:255–261, 1982.
58. Hadler, S. C., Webster, H. M., Erbin, J. J., et al.: Hepatitis A in day-care centers: A community-wide assessment. N. Engl. J. Med. *302*:1222–1227, 1980.
59. Hall, C. B., and Douglas, R. G.: Modes of transmission of respiratory syncytial virus. J. Pediatr. *99*:100–103, 1981.
60. Hall, C. B., Douglas, R. G., and Geimann, J. M.: Possible transmission by fomites of respiratory syncytial virus. J. Infect. Dis. *141*:98–102, 1980.
61. Hayani, K. C., and Pickering, L. K.: Screening of immigrant children for infectious diseases. Adv. Pediatr. Infect. Dis. *6*:91–110, 1990.
62. Hayashi, J., Kashiwagi, S., Nomura, H., et al.: Hepatitis B transmission in nursery schools. Am. J. Epidemiol. *125*:492–498, 1987.
63. Heijbel, H., Slaine, K., Seigel, B., et al.: Outbreak of diarrhea in a day care center with spread to household members: The role of *Cryptosporidium*. Pediatr. Infect. Dis. J. *6*:744–749, 1987.
64. Henderson, F. W., Gilligan, P. H., Wait, K., et al.: Nasopharyngeal carriage of antibiotic resistant pneumococci by children in group day care. J. Infect. Dis. *157*:256–263, 1988.
65. Hendley, J. O., Wenzel, R. P., and Gwaltney, J. M.: Transmission of rhinovirus colds by self-inoculation. N. Engl. J. Med. *288*:1361–1364, 1973.
66. Hinman, A. R.: Vaccine-preventable diseases and child day care. Rev. Infect. Dis. *8*:573–583, 1986.
67. Hjelt, K., Paerregaard, A., Nielson, O. H., et al.: Acute gastroenteritis in children attending day care centers with special reference to rotavirus infections. I. Aetiology and epidemiology aspects. Acta Paediatr. Scand. *76*:754–762, 1987.
68. Hoffman, R. E., and Shillam, P. J.: The use of hygiene, cohorting, and antimicrobial therapy to control an outbreak of shigellosis. Am. J. Dis. Child. *144*:219–221, 1990.
69. Hurwitz, E. S., Desada, C. C., Shapiro, C. N., et al.: Hepatitis infections in the day care setting. Pediatrics *94*(Suppl.):1023–1024, 1994.
70. Hurwitz, E. S., Gunn, W. J., Pinsky, P. F., et al.: A nationwide study of the risk of respiratory illness associated with day care attendance. Pediatrics *87*:62–69, 1991.
71. Hutto, C., Little, E. A., Ricks, R., et al.: Isolation of cytomegalovirus from toys and hands in a day care center. J. Infect. Dis. *154*:527–530, 1986.
72. Hutto, C., Ricks, R., Garvie, M., et al.: Epidemiology of cytomegalovirus infections in young children: Day care vs. home care. Pediatr. Infect. Dis. J. *4*:149–152, 1985.
73. Ish-Horowicz, M., Korman, S. H., Shapiro, M., et al.: Asymptomatic giardiasis in children. Pediatr. Infect. Dis. J. *8*:773–779, 1989.
74. Istre, G. R., Conner, J. S., Broome, C. V., et al.: Risk factors for primary invasive *Haemophilus influenzae* disease: Increased risk from day-care attendance and school age household members. J. Pediatr. *106*:190–195, 1985.
75. Itoh T., Saito K., Maruyama T., et al.: An outbreak of enteritis due to *Campylobacter fetus* subspecies *jejuni* at a nursery school in Tokyo. Microbiol. Immunol. *24*:371–379, 1980.
76. Jacobson, J. A., Filice, G. A., and Holloway, J. T.: Meningococcal disease in day-care centers. Pediatrics *59*:299–300, 1977.
77. Janoff, E. N., Craft, J. C., Pickering, L. K., et al.: Diagnosis of *Giardia* infections by detection of parasite specific antigens. J. Clin. Microbiol. *27*:431–435, 1989.
78. Jones, D. S., and Rogers, M. F.: Human immunodeficiency virus infection in children in day care. Semin. Pediatr. Infect. Dis. *1*:280–286, 1990.
79. Jones, L. A., Duke-Duncan, P. M., and Yeager, A. S.: Cytomegalovirus infections in infant-toddler centers: Centers for development delay versus regular day care. J. Infect. Dis. *151*:953–955, 1985.
80. Jones, S. E. E., Armstrong, C. B., Bland, C., et al.: Varicella prevalence in day care centers. Pediatr. Infect. Dis. J. *14*:404, 1995.
81. Kaupas, V.: Tuberculosis in a family day-care home: Report of an outbreak and recommendations for prevention. J. A. M. A. *228*:851–854, 1974.
82. Keswick, B. H., Pickering, L. K., DuPont, H. L., et al.: Survival and detection of rotavirus on environmental surfaces in day care centers. Appl. Environ. Microbiol. *46*:813–816, 1983.
83. Keystone, J. S., Krayden, S., and Warren, M. R.: Person-to-person transmission of *Giardia lamblia* in day care nurseries. Can. Med. Assoc. J. *119*:241–242, 247–248, 1978.
84. Kim, K., Dupont, H. L., and Pickering, L. K.: Outbreaks of diarrhea associated with *Clostridium difficile* and its toxin in day care centers: Evidence of person-to-person spread. J. Pediatr. *102*:376–382, 1983.
85. Kim, K. H., Fekety, R., Batts, D. H., et al.: Isolation of *Clostridium difficile* from the environment and contact of patients with antibiotic-associated colitis. J. Infect. Dis. *143*:42–46, 1981.
86. Kotch, J. B., Weigle, K. A., Weber, D. J., et al.: Evaluation of a hygienic intervention in child day care centers. Pediatrics *94*(Suppl.):991–994, 1994.
87. Krause, P. R., and Klinman, D. M.: Efficacy, immunogenicity, safety and use of live attenuated chickenpox vaccine. J. Pediatr. *127*:518–525, 1995.
88. Krugman, S., Katz, S., Gershon, A. A., et al.: Infectious Diseases of Children. 5th ed. St. Louis, C. V. Mosby, 1985, pp. 71–73.
89. Laborde, D. J., Weigle, K. A., Weber, D. J., et al.: The frequency, level, and distribution of fecal contamination in day care center classrooms. Pediatrics *94*(Suppl.):1008–1011, 1994.

90. Lauwers, W., DeBoeck, S. M., and Butzler, J. P.: *Campylobacter* enteritis in Brussels. Lancet *1*:604–605, 1978.
91. Leggiadro, R. J., Baddour, L. M., Frasch, C. E., et al.: Invasive meningococcal disease: Secondary spread in a day care center. South. Med. J. *82*:511–513, 1989.
92. Leggiadro, R. J., Callery, B., Dowdy, S., et al.: An outbreak of tuberculosis in a family day care home. Pediatr. Infect. Dis. J. *8*:52–54, 1989.
93. Lemp, G. F., Woodward, W. E., Pickering, L. K., et al.: The relation of staff to the incidence of diarrhea in day care centers. Am. J. Epidemiol. *120*:750–758, 1984.
94. Lieb, S., Gunn, R. A., and Taylor, D. N.: Salmonellosis in a day care center. J. Pediatr. *100*:1004, 1982.
95. Loda, F. W., Glezen, W. P., and Clyde, W. A., Jr.: Respiratory disease in group day care. Pediatrics *49*:428–437, 1972.
96. Lundgren, K., Ingvarsson, L., and Olofsson, B.: Epidemiologic aspects in children with recurrent otitis media. *In* Lim, D. J., Bluestone, C. D., Klein, J. O., et al. (eds.): Recent Advances in Otitis Media with Effusion. Philadelphia, B. C. Decker, 1984, pp. 22–25.
97. Makintubee, S., Istre, G. R., and Ward, J. I.: Transmission of invasive *Haemophilus influenzae* type b disease in day care settings. J. Pediatr. *111*:180–186, 1987.
98. Matson, D. O., and Estes, M. K.: Impact of rotavirus infection at a large pediatric hospital. J. Infect. Dis. *162*:598–604, 1990.
99. McCaustland, K. A., Bond, W. W., Bradley, D. W., et al.: Survival of hepatitis A virus in feces after drying and storage for 1 month. J. Clin. Microbiol. *16*:957–958, 1982.
100. McMahon, B. J., Alward, W. L. M., Hall, D. B., et al.: Acute hepatitis B virus infection: Relation of age to the clinical expression of disease and subsequent development of the carrier state. J. Infect. Dis. *151*:599–603, 1985.
101. The Meningococcal Disease Surveillance Group: Meningococcal disease secondary attack rate and chemoprophylaxis in the United States, 1974. J. A. M. A. *235*:261–265, 1976.
102. Miller, R. A., Bronsdon, M. A., and Morton, W. R.: Experimental cryptosporidiosis in a primate model. J. Infect. Dis. *161*:312–315, 1990.
103. Munford, R. S., de Morais, J. S., Tauney, A. E., et al.: Spread of meningococcal infection in households. Lancet *1*:1275–1278, 1974.
104. Murph, J. R., Bale, J. F., Murray, J. C., et al.: Cytomegalovirus transmission in a Midwest day care center: Possible relationship to child care practices. J. Pediatr. *109*:35–39, 1986.
105. Murphy, T. V., Clements, J. F., Breedlove, J. S., et al.: Risk of subsequent disease among day-care contacts of patients with systemic *Haemophilus influenzae* type b disease. N. Engl. J. Med. *316*:5–10, 1987.
106. Murphy, T. V., Osterholm, M. T., and Granoff, D. M.: Risk of *H. influenzae* type b (HIB) disease (DIS) in children attending day care in Dallas County, Texas (DAL), and Minnesota (MN). Pediatr. Res. *25*:103A, 1989.
107. Nolan, C. M., Barr, H., Elarth, A. M., et al.: Tuberculosis in a day-care home. Pediatrics *79*:630–631, 1987.
108. Ogilvie, M. M., and Tearne, C. F.: Spontaneous abortion after hand-foot-and-mouth disease caused by coxsackie virus A16. Br. Med. J. *281*:1627–1628, 1980.
109. O'Ryan, M., and Matson, D. O.: Viral gastroenteritis pathogens in the day care center setting. Semin. Pediatr. Infect. Dis. *1*:252–262, 1990.
110. O'Ryan, M., Matson, D. O., Estes, M. K., et al.: Molecular epidemiology of rotaviruses in children attending day care centers in Houston. J. Infect. Dis. *162*:810–816, 1990.
111. Osterholm, M. T.: Lack of efficacy of *Haemophilus* b polysaccharide vaccine in Minnesota. J. A. M. A. *260*:1423–1428, 1988.
112. Osterholm, M. T., Pierson, L. M., White, K. E., et al.: The risk of subsequent transmission of *Haemophilus influenzae* type b disease among children in day care. N. Engl. J. Med. *316*:1–5, 1987.
113. Osterholm, M. T., Reves, R. R., Murph, J. R., et al.: Infectious diseases and child day care. Pediatr. Infect. Dis. J. *11*:531–541, 1992.
114. Pai, C. H., Sorger, S., Lackman, L., et al.: *Campylobacter* enteritis in children. J. Pediatr. *94*:589–91, 1979.
115. Pass, R. F., August, A., Dworsky, M. E., et al.: Cytomegalovirus infection in a day-care center. N. Engl. J. Med. *307*:477–479, 1982.
116. Pass, R. F., and Hutto, C.: Group day care and cytomegalovirus infections of mothers and children. Rev. Infect. Dis. *8*:599–605, 1986.
117. Pass, R. F., Hutto, S. C., Reynolds, D., et al.: Increased frequency of cytomegalovirus infection in children in group day care. Pediatrics *74*:121–126, 1984.
118. Paulozi, L. J., Johnson, K. E., Komahele, L. M., et al.: Diarrhea associated with adherent enteropathogenic *Escherichia coli* in an infant and toddler center, Seattle, Washington. Pediatrics *77*:296–300, 1986.
119. Pickering, L. K.: Bacterial and parasitic enteropathogens in day care. Semin. Pediatr. Infect. Dis. *1*:263–269, 1990.
120. Pickering, L. K., Bartlett, A. V., Reves, R. R., et al.: Asymptomatic excretion of rotavirus before and after rotavirus diarrhea in children in day care centers. J. Paediatr. *112*:361–365, 1988.
121. Pickering, L. K., Evans, D. G., Dupont, H. L., et al.: Diarrhea caused by *Shigella*, rotavirus, and *Giardia* in day-care centers: Prospective study. J. Pediatr. *99*:51–56, 1981.
122. Pickering, L. K., and Woodward, W. E.: Diarrhea in day care centers. Pediatr. Infect. Dis. J. *1*:47–52, 1982.
123. Pickering, L. K., Woodward, W. E., Dupont, H. L., et al.: Occurrence of *Giardia lamblia* in children in day care centers. J. Pediatr. *104*:522–526, 1984.
124. Preblud, S. R.: Age-specific risks of varicella complications. Pediatrics *68*:14–17, 1981.
125. Plotkin, S. A.: Inactivated polio vaccine for the United States: A missed vaccination opportunity. Pediatr. Infect. Dis. J. *14*:835–839, 1995.
126. Radetsky, M. S., Istre, G. R., Johansen, T. L., et al.: Multiply-resistant pneumococcus causing meningitis and its epidemiology within a day care center. Lancet *2*:771–773, 1981.
127. Rauch, A. M., O'Ryan, M., Van, R., et al.: Invasive disease due to multiply resistant *Streptococcus pneumoniae* in a Houston, Texas, day-care center. Am. J. Dis. Child. *144*:923–927, 1990.
128. Rauch, A. M., Van, R., Bartlett, A. V., et al.: Longitudinal study of *Giardia lamblia* infection in a day care center population. Pediatr. Infect. Dis. J. *9*:186–189, 1990.
129. Redmond, S. R., and Pichichero, M. E.: *Haemophilus influenzae* type b disease: An epidemiologic study with special reference to day-care centers. J. A. M. A. *252*:2581–2584, 1984.
130. Reichler, M. R., Allphin, A. A., Breiman, R. F., et al.: The spread of multiply resistant *Streptococcus pneumoniae* at a day care center in Ohio. J. Infect. Dis. *166*:1346–1353, 1992.
131. Reves, R. R., and Jones, J. A.: Antibiotic use and resistance patterns in day care centers. Semin. Pediatr. Infect. Dis. *1*:212–221, 1990.
132. Rodriguez, W. J., Kim, H. W., Brandt, C. D., et al.: Common exposure outbreak of gastroenteritis due to type 2 rotavirus with high secondary attack rate within families. J. Infect. Dis. *140*:353–357, 1979.
133. Rogers, M. F., White, C. R., Sanders, R., et al.: Lack of evidence of transmission of human immunodeficiency virus from infected children to their household contacts. Pediatrics *85*:210–214, 1990.
134. Saez-Nieto, J. A., Perucha, M., Casamayor, H., et al.: Outbreak of infection caused by *Neisseria meningitidis* group C type 2 in a nursery. J. Infect. *8*:49–55, 1984.
135. Sargent, S. J., and Martin, J. T.: Scabies outbreak in a day-care center. Pediatrics *94*(Suppl.):1012–1013, 1994.
136. Schulte, E. E., Birkhead, G. S., Kondraki, S. F., et al.: Patterns of *Haemophilus influenzae* type b invasive disease in New York State, 1987 to 1991: The role of vaccination requirements for day-care attendance. Pediatrics *94*(Suppl.):1014–1015, 1994.
137. Schwartz, B., Giebink, G. S., Henderson, F. G. W., et al.: Respiratory infections in day care. Pediatrics *94*(Suppl.):1018–1020, 1994.
138. Sealy, D. P., and Schuman, S. H.: Endemic giardiasis and day care. Pediatrics *72*:154–158, 1983.
139. Shapiro, C. N., McCaig, L. F., Gensheimer, K. F., et al.: Hepatitis B virus transmission between children in day care. Pediatr. Infect. Dis. J. *8*:870–875, 1989.
140. Shapiro, E. D.: Lack of transmission of hepatitis B in a day care center. J. Pediatr. *110*:90–92, 1987.
141. Shapiro, E. D., Murphy, T. V., Wald, E. R., et al.: The protective efficacy of *Haemophilus* b polysaccharide vaccine. J. A. M. A. *269*:1419–1422, 1988.
142. Shirley, L. R., and Rokss, S. A.: Risk of transmission of human immunodeficiency virus by bite of an infected toddler. J. Pediatr. *114*:425–427, 1989.
143. Smith, T. D., Wilkinson, V., and Kaplan, E. L.: Group A *Streptococcus*–associated upper respiratory tract infections in a day care center. Pediatrics *83*:380–384, 1989.
144. Spika, J. S., Parson, J. E., Nordenberg, D., et al.: Hemolytic uremic syndrome and diarrhea associated with *Escherichia coli* O157:H7 in a day care center. J. Pediatr. *109*:287–291, 1986.
145. Stagno, S., and Cloud, G. A.: Working parents: The impact of day care and breast feeding on cytomegalovirus infections in offspring. Proc. Natl. Acad. Sci. U. S. A. *91*:2384–2389, 1994.
146. Stagno, S., Pass, R. F., Cloud, G., et al.: Primary cytomegalovirus infection in pregnancy: Incidence, transmission to fetus and clinical outcome. J. A. M. A. *256*:1904–1908, 1986.
147. Stahlberg, M. R.: The influence of form of day care on occurrence of acute respiratory tract infections among young children. Acta Pediatr. Scand. *282*(Suppl. 1):1–87, 1980.
148. Stahlberg, M. R., Ruuskanen, O., and Virolainen, E.: Risk factors for recurrent otitis media. Pediatr. Infect. Dis. J. *5*:30–32, 1986.
149. Storch, G., McFarland, L. M., Kelso, K., et al.: Viral hepatitis associated with day-care centers. J. A. M. A. *242*:1514–1581, 1979.
150. Strangert, K.: Respiratory illness in preschool children and different forms of day care. Pediatrics *57*:191–196, 1976.
151. Strangert, K., Carlstrom, G., Jeansson, S., et al.: Infections in preschool children in group day care. Acta Paediatr. Scand. *65*:455–463, 1976.
152. Strangert, K.: Otitis media in young children in different types of day care. Scand. J. Infect. Dis. *9*:119–123, 1977.
153. Strom, J.: Study of infections and illnesses in a day nursery based on inclusion-bearing cells in the urine and infectious agent in faeces, urine and nasal secretion. Scand. J. Infect. Dis. *11*:265–269, 1979.
154. Sullivan, P., Woodward, W. E., Pickering, L. K., et al.: Longitudinal study of occurrence of diarrheal disease in day care centers. Am. J. Public Health *74*:987–991, 1984.
155. Tacket, C. O., and Cohen, M. L.: Shigellosis in day care centers: Use

of plasmid analysis to assess control measures. Pediatr. Infect. Dis. J. *2*:127–130, 1983.
156. Takala, A. K., Eskola, J., Palmgren, J., et al.: Risk factors of invasive *Haemophilus influenzae* type b disease among children in Finland. J. Pediatr. *115*:694–701, 1989.
157. Taute, R. V., Johnson, K. E., Boase, J. C., et al.: Control of day care shigellosis: A trial of convalescent day care in isolation. Am. J. Public Health *76*:627–630, 1986.
158. Taylor, J. P., Perdue, J. N., Dinley, D., et al.: Cryptosporidiosis outbreak in a day care center. Am. J. Dis. Child. *39*:1023–1025, 1985.
159. Teele, D. W., Klein, J. D., Rosner, B., et al.: Epidemiology of otitis media during the first seven years of life in children in greater Boston: A prospective cohort study. J. Infect. Dis. *160*:83–94, 1989.
160. Thompson, S. C.: *Giardia lamblia* in children and the child care settings: A review of the literature. J. Paediatr. Child. Health *30*:202–209, 1994.
161. Thompson, S. C.: Infectious diarrhea in children: Controlling transmission in the child care setting. J. Paediatr. Child. Health *30*:210–219, 1994.
162. Tos, M., Poulsen, G., and Borch, J.: Tympanometry in 2-year-old children. ORL J. *40*:77–85, 1978.
163. Tsoukas, C., Hadjis, T., Shuster, J., et al.: Lack of transmission of HIV through human bites and scratches. J. Acq. Immune Defic. Synd. *1*:505–507, 1988.
164. U. S. Bureau of the Census: Who's Minding the Kids? Child Care Arrangements: Winter 1984–85. Current Population Reports. Series P-70, No. 9. Washington, DC, U. S. Government Printing Office, 1987.
165. Van, R., Morrow, A. L., Reves, R. R., et al.: Environmental contamination in child day care centers. Am. J. Epidemiol. *133*:460–470, 1991.
166. Van, R., Wun, C. C., Morrow, A. L., et al.: The effect of diaper type and overclothes on fecal contamination in day care centers. J. A. M. A. *265*:1840–1844, 1991.
167. Wahn, V., Kramer, H. H., Voit, T., et al.: Horizontal transmission of HIV infection between two siblings. Lancet *2*:694, 1986.
168. Wald, E. R., Dashefsky, B., Byers, C., et al.: Frequency and severity of infections in day care. J. Pediatr. *112*:540–546, 1988.
169. Weissman, J. B., Gangarosa, E. J., Schmerler, A., et al.: Shigellosis in day care centers. Lancet *1*:88–90, 1975.
170. Weissman, J. B., Schmerler, A., Weiler, P., et al.: The role of preschool children and day care centers in the spread of shigellosis in urban communities. J. Pediatr. *84*:797–802, 1974.
171. Weniger, B. G., Ruttenber, J., Goodman, R. A., et al.: Fecal coliforms on environmental surfaces in two day care centers. Appl. Environ. Microbiol. *45*:733–735, 1983.
172. Werzberger, A., Meusch, B., Kuter, B., et al.: A controlled trial of formalin inactivated hepatitis A vaccine in healthy children. N. Engl. J. Med. *327*:453–457, 1992.
173. Wilde, J., Van, R., Pickering, L., et al.: Detection of rotaviruses in the day care environment by reverse transcriptase polymerase chain reaction. J. Infect. Dis. *166*:507–511, 1992.
174. Wilson, R., Feldman, R. A., Davis, J., et al.: Salmonellosis in infants: The importance of intrafamilial transmission. Pediatrics *69*:436–438, 1982.

241

HUMAN BITES

Ellie J. C. Goldstein

Human bites have been recorded since the biblical era and currently are a common cause of serious medical and surgical disease. They are the third most frequent type of bite after dog and cat bites. Reports of secondary infections after a human bite in children have been noted in the United States since at least 1910.[39] Approximately 30 per cent of human bites are accidental, resulting from injuries that are self-inflicted (such as bitten lips and nail biting) or resulting from injuries suffered while playing sports or games, during falls, during dental therapy, and during treatment of seizures. They also may be intentional, with 70 per cent resulting from aggressive behavior. Fighting is the primary cause of human bites, but aggressive bites also may occur during play (especially in the day care setting). Bite wounds also may be incurred in the course of restraining impaired patients, as a consequence of criminal or police activities, or from child abuse and child battering.[23] Sexual bites or "love nips" account for 5 to 20 per cent of human bite wounds and either may be intentional or accidental and occur in children of all ages.[1, 57, 68, 69]

INCIDENCE AND EPIDEMIOLOGY

In 1977, the New York City Department of Health altered its reporting system to include human bites. From that year's data of 892 reports, Marr and colleagues[46] noted an incidence of 10.7 human bites/100,000 population/year with a range of 0.9 to 60.9/100,000 population for different geographic areas. Although there was a bias that median income, population density, and younger age might have been factors in this geographic variance, it could not be substantiated. Human bites have their peak incidence in the spring and early summer for both children[3] and adults[46] and on Saturdays, especially within the 15- to 30-year-old age group. Alcohol and drug abuse may play a role in some of these instances. For children[13] and adults,[46] bites are more common in males than females (1.35 to 1.5 to 1), except for the 15- to 20-year-old and the 55- to 60-year-old age groups, in which females are bitten more frequently; human bites are most frequent in men 20 to 25 years of age. Most bites in teenagers are associated with aggressive behavior. This pattern was documented in 1936 by Welch,[67] who reported that teenagers accounted for 5 of 13 human bite cases, some of which resulted in amputations. Farmer and Mann[18] noted that 12 per cent of their bite patients at a large urban hospital were younger than 20 years of age. Bites to the lip occurred most often in women (78 per cent women vs. 22 per cent men) and to the lower lip (65 per cent) more often than to the upper lip (35 per cent).[64] Baker and Moore[3] reported that of 322 children who suffered human bites, 21 per cent were younger than 5 years of age, 21 per cent were 5 to 10 years of age, and 58 per cent were older than 10 years of age. When corrected for sex, 64 per cent of the girls and 39 per cent of the boys were 12 years of age or older.

Biting is common in the day care center and is the third most commonly reported injury. The incidence peaks in the middle morning and during the early school year in September. Toddlers from 13 to 30 months of age are bitten more often than infants and other preschoolers,[62] and males are bitten more frequently than females.[22] Bites account for 3 and 6 per cent of reported injuries in boys and girls, respectively,[20] and may be self-inflicted in many cases.[13] Others have noted that approximately 50 per cent of all children enrolled in day care suffer bite wounds, with a rate of 3.9 bites/child/year in general but 9.4 bites/male child/year for full-time enrollees.[22, 60] Garrard and colleagues[22] reported that 104 of 224 children (46 per cent) experienced 347 bites in a single year, and Solomons and Elardo[60] noted that 66 of 133 children

(50 per cent) experienced 224 bites in a 42-month period. Fortunately, most of these bites are minor and do not break the skin. A higher proportion of bites in younger children (such as preschoolers) are to the face, whereas the majority of bites to adolescents are on the upper extremities and hands.

Paronychial infections are not actual bites, but when infection occurs, it is related to oral flora contamination when children bite or suck their fingers. Brook[10] noted children from 2 to 9 years of age (mean age, 5 years, 8 months) who were treated at a children's hospital for paronychial infection and reported the bacteriology and presentations of these infections.

Bites as harbingers or signs of child abuse are more common in the 0- to 4-year-old age group[63]; the age of abusing parents was younger than 20 years for mothers and younger than 22 years for fathers. An attempt should be made to identify the biter and measure distances between circular bite marks to ascertain the spread. In addition, biting children may have learned this behavior from abusive adults and themselves be victims of human bites.

BACTERIOLOGY

The bacteriology of these wounds, including those of occlusional bites, clenched-fist injuries, and paronychia, reflects the human oral flora of the biter and has been the focus of various studies.[5, 11, 24, 25, 27, 30, 36] Human saliva and dental plaque can contain more than 42 different species of bacteria in concentrations of 10^8 colony-forming units per milliliter. Table 241–1 lists common human bite wound isolates and their relative frequency of isolation. The alpha-hemolytic streptococci are the most frequent isolates. Other common bacterial isolates include *Streptococcus pyogenes, Staphylococcus aureus, Haemophilus* species, *Eikenella corrodens,* and oral anaerobes, especially *Prevotella* and *Porphyromonas* species. Cultures of virtually all infected bite wounds grow bacterial pathogens; wound cultures of patients who present less than 8 hours after injury before the development of clinical infection yield potential bacterial pathogens in 85 per cent of cases.[24, 33] The bacteriology of the early-presenting, colonized wounds is remarkably similar to the bacteria isolated from those presenting later with established infection. The average bite wound yields between 3.4 and 5.4 bacterial isolates per wound, composed of 1.7 to 2.4 aerobes and 1.7 to 3.0 anaerobes.[11, 24] Anaerobes were recognized as important pathogens and markers for serious bite infections, especially those involving the hand, as early as 1936.[4, 9, 29, 51, 52, 67] Anaerobes are isolated from more than 50 per cent of human bite wounds, almost always in mixed culture with aerobes, and are associated more often with more serious infections, amputation, and the presence of abscesses.[24, 29] Many of the anaerobes isolated from human bite wounds, especially the *Prevotella* and *Porphyromonas* species, are β-lactamase producers.[11, 30]

E. corrodens, a capnophilic, gram-negative rod that is part of the normal human oral flora, has been recognized as an important pathogen in approximately 20 per cent of clenched-fist injuries.[25, 27] It has an unusual antimicrobial susceptibility pattern, being susceptible to penicillin but resistant to first-generation cephalosporins, β-lactamase–stable penicillins (such as oxacillin), and erythromycin.[26, 28] When unrecognized or treated with the incorrect antibiotic, *E. corrodens* has been associated with therapeutic failure.[27] Usually isolated in mixed culture, it may be missed by microbiologists because of its slow growth characteristics and by overgrowth of other bacterial colonies. *E. corrodens* produces a small colony that "pits" or "corrodes" the agar surface and has a light yellow pigment and a smell like hypochlorite bleach.

The bacteriology of paronychial infections is similar to that of other human bite infections, except that aerobes and anaerobes each have been isolated in pure culture in 27 per cent of cases.[10] Brook[10] found a total of 3.6 isolates per specimen composed of 1.4 aerobes, 2.0 anaerobes, and 0.2 *Candida albicans;* β-lactamase–producing organisms were found in 45 per cent of wounds, including isolates of *Prevotella melaninogenica* and *Prevotella oralis.*

In addition to oral bacterial infection, human bites have been associated with viral infection, such as herpes simplex virus,[21, 47] cytomegalovirus,[47] hepatitis B virus,[12, 15] hepatitis C virus,[17] and possibly HIV,[1, 47, 56, 59] as well as syphilis,[19] tuberculosis,[33] actinomycosis,[8] and tetanus.[49, 55]

CLINICAL PRESENTATION

Human bites may be categorized into three groups: (1) bites resulting in paronychial infections, (2) occlusional bites, and (3) clenched-fist injuries. Patients in the latter two categories may present early (<8 hours after injury) for wound care or tetanus boosters or late (>8 hours after injury), usually because of established infection or infectious complications. All share the predominance of oral aerobic and anaerobic bacteria as primary etiologic pathogens. Noninfectious complications may include injury to tendons and nerves or fractures. Potential complications of human bites are noted in Table 241–2. Table 241–3 lists some of the diseases acquired as a result of human bites. The incidence of infection after human bites is estimated to be from 10 to 30 per cent. Because of the typically superficial nature of the human bite wound injury to children, the infection rate in children is estimated to be approximately 10 per cent.

Bites Resulting in Paronychial Infections

Paronychia are infections (inflammation) of the structures of the distal phalanx, either those surrounding the nail or the bone itself. Most are due to finger sucking in younger children but may be due to accidental biting. The area is red, tender, and swollen and may have some underlying purulence.

Occlusional Bites

Occlusional bites occur when the teeth actually contact any part of the human anatomy. Human bite wounds occur most often in the upper extremity (18 to 71 per cent), the head and neck (4 to 33 per cent), the thorax and abdomen (6 to 25 per cent), the breasts or genitals (3 to 25 per cent), and the lower extremity (3 to 11 per cent).[3, 22, 24, 46, 65] Vale and Noguchi[65] reported the anatomic distribution of bite marks in 67 forensically evaluated cases, including 13 (19 per cent) cases in children younger than 15 years of age. They noted more than one bite mark in 40 per cent of victims and that female victims were bitten most frequently on the breasts, arms, and legs, whereas bites to males more often were on the upper extremities and shoulders. Marr and colleagues[46] did not differentiate the location of bites by sex of the victim but noted that 15 per cent were to the head and neck, 12 per cent were to the thorax and abdomen, 61 per cent were to the upper extremities, 4 per cent were to the lower extremities, and 9 per cent were to unknown locations. My experience with teenagers and adults is similar to that of Marr and colleagues,[46] perhaps because of the selection bias of those patients who seek medical care or come to the attention of

TABLE 241–1. Approximate Prevalence and Bacteriology of Isolates from Human Bite Wound Infections

Isolate	Prevalence	Present in: OB*	Present in: CFI*
Aerobes			
Streptococci			
Alpha-hemolytic	28–90%	+	+
Beta-hemolytic			
Group A	17–26%	+	+
Other	12%	+	+
Gamma-hemolytic	3–33%	+	–
Enterococci	11%	–	+
Staphylococcus aureus	13–50%	+	+
Staphylococcus, coagulase-negative	11–53%	+	+
Haemophilus influenzae	6%	+	+
Haemophilus species (other)	11–20%	+	+
Eikenella corrodens	10–29%	+	+
Micrococcus species	3–5%	–	+
Moraxella species	3%	+	–
Neisseria species	11–15%	+	+
Corynebacterium species	28–41%	+	+
Acinetobacter calcoaceticus	4–6%	–	+
Escherichia coli	6%	+	–
Klebsiella pneumoniae	3–6%	+	+
Enterobacter species	3–4%	+	–
Nocardia species	3%	–	+
Anaerobes			
Acidaminococcus species	2%	+	+
Actinomyces species	4%	+	+
Bacteroides ovatus	6%	–	+
Bacteroides ureolyticus	3–11%	+	–
Bacteroides species (unspeciated)	12–33%	+	+
Bifidobacterium species	11%	–	+
Clostridium perfringens	4%	+	–
Prevotella (*Bacteroides*) *melaninogenica*	15–22%	+	+
Prevotella (*Bacteroides*) *intermedia*	11–26%	+	+
Prevotella (*Bacteroides*) *oralis*	6–17%	+	+
Prevotella buccae	15%	+	+
Prevotella disiens	3%	–	+
Prevotella loeschii	3%	+	+
Eubacterium species	3–11%	+	+
Fusobacterium nucleatum	12–33%	+	+
Fusobacterium necrophorum	6%	–	+
Fusobacterium species	17%	–	+
Peptostreptococcus anaerobius	3%	+	–
Peptostreptococcus asaccharolyticus	22%	+	+
Peptostreptococcus intermedius	3%	+	–
Peptostreptococcus magnus	3–17%	+	+
Peptostreptococcus micros	12%	+	+
Gamella (Peptostreptococcus) morbillorum	3%	+	–
Peptostreptococcus prevotii	3%	+	–
Peptostreptococcus species	3–22%	+	+
Veillonella parvula	9–11%	+	+
Veillonella species	6–18%	+	+
Spirochetes	5–30%	+	+

*OB, occlusional bite wounds; CFI, clenched-fist injuries.
+, present; –, absent.
Based on a compilation of data from references 5, 11, 24, 36, and 54.

infectious disease consultants. When the hand is involved, wounds tend to occur most frequently on the terminal phalanx of the middle (long) finger of the dominant hand.[2, 6, 16, 24] Bites to the upper extremities are most frequent in toddlers (66 per cent), infants (71 per cent), and preschoolers (46 per cent)[22] and in children overall (42 per cent).[3]

Most wounds are minor and require routine care with cleansing and bandaging. The infection rate after occlusional bite wounds has been estimated to be 10 to 30 per cent, of which 87 per cent may require hospitalization.[3, 41] Those wounds to the hand and with any edema or crush injury and those that involve a bone or a joint have a greater potential for infection. Infections, when they occur, usually present as cellulitis. If the child presents to medical or school officials early,[16, 41] these injuries rarely result in serious complications. Patients in whom presentation is delayed (>12 hours after injury) probably have preselection bias because they usually seek attention because of an already established infection. These infections usually spread proximally and not distally and in less than 5 per cent of cases have associated fever, lymphangitis, or lymphadenopathy. There may be a malodorous discharge or abscess formation if anaerobes are involved.

TABLE 241–2. Potential Complications of Human Bite Wounds

Abscess
Cellulitis
Compartment syndrome
Fracture
Necrotizing fasciitis
Nerve severance/injury
Osteomyelitis
Scarlet fever
Sepsis
Septic arthritis
Tendon severance/injury
Tenosynovitis
Toxic shock syndrome

Complications may be limited to skin defects (when there are skin avulsions), but septic arthritis and osteomyelitis may occur if the joint or bone is involved. In immunocompromised hosts, such as those with hematologic malignancy or neutropenia, sepsis may occur. Amputation may occur as a result of the initial bite in approximately 2 to 5 per cent of cases or as a result of serious, chronic infection in 0 to 18 per cent of cases.[4, 16, 41, 43, 48, 50, 67] Tendon injury, primary nerve injury and tenosynovitis, compartment syndrome, and resultant secondary nerve damage may occur.[53]

Clenched-Fist Injuries

Clenched-fist injuries are the most serious of human bite wounds and occur when the closed fist of one person strikes another in the teeth and there is a break in the skin. The most common cause is a fight, although cases can occur during contact sports or boxing, if gloves are not worn. The metacarpal phalangeal joint (knuckle) of the middle (long) finger of the dominant hand most frequently is involved.[25, 27, 58] The break in the skin may be only 2 to 5 mm in length but often results in penetration into the joint or even the bone. Patients and physicians may underestimate the potentially serious nature of these wounds. During the initial contact, bacteria penetrate the knuckle area and upon relaxation of the hand are carried by the tendons further back into the potential spaces of the hand. Infection may spread laterally, between the collateral and accessory ligaments, or dorsally into the thin-walled bursa overlying the metacarpal head or into the palmar space deep spaces of the hand. The typical patient avoids seeking attention because of the circumstances surrounding the injury (fight) and often wakes up 6 to 8 hours later with a painful, throbbing, swollen, infected hand and then seeks medical attention. Often, there is a purulent exudate, which may be foul if *P. melaninogenica* or other anaerobes are present, emanating from the injury, and the patient comes to the physician with the hand elevated to diminish the pain. The swelling usually spreads proximally and not distally from the site of injury. The physician should take both aerobic and anaerobic cultures and secure the assistance of a surgeon experienced in hand cases. Chuinard and D'Ambrosia[14] and others[44, 45, 54] have outlined the surgical management of these wounds; this includes the determination, under a bloodless field, of whether or not there has been penetration of the joint capsule or if there is only localized cellulitis. Complications are frequent, and in my experience, these have a 50 per cent chance of developing septic arthritis, osteomyelitis, or both. The range of motion of the hand usually is limited by swelling and edema but also may be limited as a result of tendon injury or severance or as a result of nerve injury or severance. Permanent limitation of the range of motion and joint stiffness are frequent results of osteomyelitis to the affected joints. Osteomyelitis, which usually involves the small bones of the hand, often is manifested by continued pain, swelling, and erythema with or without drainage at 10 days to 3 weeks after injury.[18] Osteomyelitis and septic arthritis due to *E. corrodens,* often in association with alpha-hemolytic streptococci, often are insidious and persistent and may lead to amputation, especially if treated with the wrong antibiotics.[27] Other complications include fracture, color-button abscess, and muscle atrophy.

TABLE 241–3. Diseases Transmitted by Human Bite Wounds

Actinomycosis
Cytomegalovirus infection
Hepatitis B virus infection
Hepatitis C virus infection
Herpesvirus infection
HIV infection
Invasive group A *Streptococcus* infection
Syphilis
Tetanus
Toxic shock syndrome
Tuberculosis
Whitlow

HIV TRANSMISSION POTENTIAL

Reports[2, 59] have noted the transmission of HIV from biter to victim. HIV is isolated uncommonly from the saliva of infected persons, and when recovered it has been in low numbers. Consequently, the possibility of HIV transmission is considered unlikely, although possible.[56] Richman and Rickman[56] reviewed instances of reported HIV transmission via human bites and concluded that "no well documented case of HIV transmission through bites exists"; the risk of HIV transmission is possible biologically but appears to be negligible. A review and commentary of professional sports–related injuries also noted the unlikely possibility of HIV transmission via sporting events and outlined similar, common-sense control measures.[47] Opinions vary widely about whether children with HIV should be permitted to attend school,[7] especially children in preschool. Most schools allow attendance, unless significant, real risk exists in an individual's behavior or hygienic habits.

TREATMENT

Basic elements of management are outlined in Table 241–4. These include a complete history of the circumstances of the occurrence, with an attempt to identify the biter. If the biter is identified, some questions about the presence of herpes and other potentially orally transmitted viral diseases should be asked. Awareness of the potential for child abuse or battering must be considered, and a search should be carried out for other associated injuries. The examination must include evaluation of range of motion if a hand or joint is involved, determination of the integrity of tendons and nerves and of the vascular supply, and a diagram of the location of the bite marks. Because most victims have multiple wounds, a thorough search should be made covering the entire body, and the wounds should be measured. Special attention must

TABLE 241–4. Management Procedures for Human Bite Wounds

- Obtain history from patient
  - Situation leading to injury
  - Place of occurrence
  - Patient allergy
  - Other medications (potential interactions)
- Perform evaluation of patient
  - Nerve function
  - Tendon function
  - Vascular integrity
  - Range of motion
  - Potential bone and joint involvement
- Diagram or photograph wound
- Mark leading edge of cellulitis
- Culture wound (if infected)
- Irrigate wound
- Débride wound cautiously
- Drain abscess
- Administer antimicrobial agents
  - Prophylactic therapy, 3 to 5 days
  - Longer duration for established infection
- Elevate injured area
- Immobilize wound area (3 days for hands)
- Have the patient exercise the injured area (if previously immobilized)
- Close the wound
  - Primary for face and head
  - Delayed for early wounds
  - Secondary intent for infected wounds
- Administer tetanus toxoid
- Obtain radiograph (if indicated)
- Submit Health Department report (if required)

be paid to any wound close to bones or joints, especially when involving the hands, and the possibility of bone or joint penetration should be considered. Radiographic studies of the hand should be obtained for all clenched-fist injuries or in any situation if there is suspicion of fracture or the potential for osteomyelitis. Magnification radiography may be helpful in identifying bone penetration. If tetanus immunization is not current, a toxoid booster should be given. If there is no record of immunization, tetanus immunoglobulin and tetanus toxoid should be given.

The wound should be cleansed with normal saline, and any foreign body or debris and necrotic tissue should be removed. Cautious débridement is indicated for some wounds, with care not to create a potential skin defect. The wound then is irrigated using a syringe and needle/catheter tip as a high-pressure jet to diminish the bacterial inoculum. Aerobic and anaerobic cultures should be obtained and Gram stain performed if infection is present. In cases of clenched-fist injury, a hand surgeon should examine the patient to determine if the joint capsule or bone has been compromised.[14] With many hand infections, especially after exploration of clenched-fist injuries, immobilization using a plaster splint is employed. Elevation of a swollen or inflamed part is crucial to healing. Elevation should be to above the level of the heart. Promises by patients or family to "keep the hand up" should not be believed unless a properly fitting sling is issued or made from a scarf; tubular stockinet and an intravenous pole also may be used. Legs and hands also can be elevated using pillows. The use and value of topical agents have not been studied, although most patients have applied them prior to seeking medical attention.[24]

Antimicrobial agents should be selected empirically according to the most likely pathogens and their usual susceptibility patterns to antimicrobial agents.[32, 34, 35, 37, 38] If cultures are performed, therapy should be adjusted according to the organisms isolated and their specific susceptibility to antimicrobial agents. The activity of commonly used antibiotics against usual human bite wound pathogens is outlined in Table 241–5. Common pathogens that need to be considered in the selection of antimicrobial therapy include streptococci, *S. aureus, Haemophilus* species, *E. corrodens,* and β-lactamase–producing oral anaerobes. A potentially useful oral agent is amoxicillin–clavulanic acid; otherwise, combinations, such as cefuroxime plus clindamycin or metronidazole, can be substituted. A variety of other combination regimens may be employed. Potentially useful intravenous agents include ampicillin-sulbactam, ticarcillin–clavulanic acid, cefoxitin, cefotetan, imipenem, and combinations of such agents as cefuroxime or cefotaxime plus clindamycin or metronidazole. First-generation cephalosporins are of limited utility because of poor activity against *E. corrodens* and some anaerobes[26, 28] and should not be used as empirical monotherapy. Erythromycin also has poor activity against *E. corrodens* and *Fusobacterium nucleatum,*[31] and its use as monotherapy can lead to therapeu-

TABLE 241–5. Comparative In Vitro Antimicrobial Activity of Selected Oral Antimicrobial Agents Against Common Human Bite Wound Pathogens

Agent	*Staphylococcus aureus*	Streptococci	*Haemophilus*	*Eikenella corrodens*	Anaerobes
Amoxicillin	−	+	v	+	v
Amoxicillin–clavulanic acid	+	+	+	+	+
Cephalexin	+	+	−	−	−
Cefaclor	+	+	+	−	−
Cefuroxime	+	+	+	+	−
Cefprozil	+	+	+	−	−
Loracarbef	+	+	+	−	−
Dicloxacillin	+	+	−	−	−
Erythromycin	v	+	v	−	−
Azithromycin	+	+	+	+	v
Clarithromycin	+	+	+	−	−
Trimethoprim-sulfamethoxazole	+	v	+	+	−
Chloramphenicol	v	v	v	+	+

Note: because of contraindications in pediatric patients, tetracyclines and fluoroquinolones are not included.
+, active; −, poorly active or inactive; v, variable.

tic failure. Newer macrolides, including azithromycin, show improved activity against the spectrum of bite wound pathogens compared with erythromycin, but *F. nucleatum* remains relatively resistant.[34, 35] Once patient-specific cultures return, antimicrobial therapy should be adjusted for the patient's individual isolates and susceptibility pattern. The duration of antimicrobial therapy is determined by the type and severity of infection. Prophylactic antimicrobial agents typically are given for 3 to 5 days, whereas the course for established infection usually is longer, such as 10 to 14 days for cellulitis and 4 to 6 weeks for septic arthritis and osteomyelitis. If there is any question about the prompt filling of a prescription because of financial or other concerns, a dose of intramuscular or intravenous antibiotics should be administered and hospitalization should be considered.

Patients' wounds should be re-examined within 24 to 48 hours. If outpatient therapy is initiated and the cellulitis advances, hospitalization is indicated. Table 241–6 lists the reasons for hospitalization of patients with human bite wounds. These include patient noncompliance and virtually all clenched-fist injuries.

Infected wounds should not be closed. However, the value and risks of primary closure for patients who present less than 8 hours after injury and without any symptoms or signs of established infection have never been studied in a prospective or randomized manner. Exceptions are wounds to the face and neck and losses of the lip, for which early primary closure has been successful.[64, 66] However, the information about those wounds probably is not applicable to bite wounds to the hands or other parts of the body for several reasons: (1) head and face wounds are débrided and copiously irrigated with up to a liter of normal saline, which diminishes the bacterial inoculum, (2) most surgeons give a course of 5 or more days of antibiotic, (3) the blood supply to the head and face area is superior to that to most other anatomic areas, and (4) these areas rarely are dependent, and therefore edema and swelling resolve more rapidly or do not develop. Using primary wound closure in early presenting, uninfected wounds remains at the physician's discretion. Wounds to the hands should be observed and left open for either delayed primary or secondary closure.

TABLE 241–6. Indications for Hospitalization of a Victim of a Human Bite Injury

Clenched-fist injury
Immunocompromised host
Asplenia (diagnostic or traumatic)
Cirrhosis
Leukemia
Lupus/steroids
Mastectomy (radical or modified radical)
Crush injury
Edema
Preexisting to injured area or developed during therapy
Cirrhosis
Mastectomy
Malnutrition
Congestive heart failure
Fever (>100.5° F)
Lymphadenopathy
Patient noncompliance
Failure to take medication
Failure to elevate injured area
Osteomyelitis
Septic arthritis
Advance of infection despite outpatient therapy

In general, hyperbaric oxygen therapy of human bite wounds remains of unproven benefit. Lehman and colleagues[40] prospectively studied the use a portable hyperbaric oxygen chamber in 16 of 43 patients admitted to the hospital for human bite infections of the hand, almost all due to clenched-fist injuries. They found that there was no benefit for mild or moderate infections, but hospital stay was shortened (4.7 vs. 11.2 days) in patients with severe infections. Although the authors felt that the return of function was more rapid in the hyperbaric group, there were limitations in follow-up that precluded evaluation, and the institution of an early, aggressive exercise program may have been an important factor.

PREVENTION

Mast and colleagues[47] reviewed both risk and prevention strategies for the transmission of blood-borne pathogens during sports. Prevention strategies include appropriate infection control measures in the sports setting and education of young athletes, as well as their coaches and trainers. Bites may occur in the day care setting, even "when caregivers are vigilant." The use of "disciplinary techniques," including the use of a developmentally appropriate curriculum ("busy, happy children are less likely to get into serious mischief"), avoidance of too much open space in classrooms, and discipline that pays attention to redirected positive behavior, has been advocated.[60, 62] More attention should be given to the victim than to the aggressor; teachers should work with the biter on behavior modification with reinforcement, extinction, and punishment strategies, which should be limited to "time-out" procedures.

References

1. Al Fallouji, M.: Traumatic love bites. Br. J. Surg. *77*:100–101, 1990.
2. Anonymous: Transmission of HIV by human bite. Lancet 2:522, 1987.
3. Baker, M. D., and Moore, S. E.: Human bites in children. Am. J. Dis. Child. *41*:1285–1290, 1987.
4. Barnes, M. N., and Bibby, B. G.: A summary of reports and a bacteriologic study of infections caused by human tooth wounds. J. Am. Dent. Assoc. *26*:1163–1170, 1939.
5. Barnham, I.: Once bitten, twice shy: Microbiology of bites. Rev. Med. Microbiol. 2:31–6, 1991.
6. Bassadre, J. O., and Parry, S. W.: Indications for surgical debridement in 125 human bites to the hands. Arch. Surg. *126*:65–67, 1991.
7. Blackman, J. A., and Appel, B. R.: Epidemiologic and legal considerations in the exclusion of children with acquired immunodefficiency syndrome, cytomegalovirus or herpes simplex infection from group care. Pediatr. Infect. Dis. J. *6*:1011–1015, 1987.
8. Blinkhorn, R. J., Strimbu, V., Effron, D., et al.: "Punch" actinomycosis causing osteomyelitis of the hand. Arch. Intern. Med. *148*:2668–2670, 1988.
9. Boland, F. K.: Morsus humanus: Sixty cases of human bites in Negroes. J. A. M. A. *116*:127–131, 1941.
10. Brook, I.: Bacteriologic study of paronychia in children. Am. J. Surg. *141*:703–705, 1981.
11. Brook, I.: Microbiology of human and animal bite wounds in children. Pediatr. Infect. Dis. J. *6*:29–32, 1987.
12. Cancio-Bello, T. P., deMedina. M., Shorey, P., et al.: An institutional outbreak of hepatitis B related to a human biting carrier. J. Infect. Dis. *146*:652–656, 1982.
13. Chang, A., Lugg, M. M., and Nebedum, A.: Injuries among preschool children enrolled in day-care centers. Pediatrics *83*:272–277, 1989.
14. Chuinard, R. G., and D'Ambrosia, R. D.: Human bite infections of the hand. J. Bone Joint Surg. [Am.] *59*:416–418, 1977.
15. Davis, L. G., Weber, D. J., and Kemon, S. M.: Horizontal transmission of hepatitis B virus. Lancet *1*:889–893, 1989.
16. Dreyfuss, U. Y., and Singer, M.: Human bites of the hand: A study of one hundred and six patients. J. Hand Surg. [Am.] *10*:884–889, 1985.
17. Dusheiko, G. M., Smith, M., and Schever, P. F.: Hepatitis C virus transmitted by human bite. Lancet *336*:503–504, 1990.
18. Farmer, C. B., and Mann, R. J.: Human bite infections of the hand. South. Med. J. *59*:515–518, 1966.

19. Fiumara, N. J., and Exnor, J. H.: Primary syphilis following a human bite. Sex. Transm. Dis. *8*:21–82, 1981.
20. Fuller, E. M.: Injury-prone children. Am. J. Orthopsychiatry *18*:708–723, 1948.
21. Fuortes, L., and Melson, E.: Brief report: Primary and recurrent herpes simplex infection in a pediatric nurse resulting from a human bite. Infect. Control Hosp. Epidemiol. *10*:120, 1989.
22. Garrard, J., Leland, N., and Smith, D. K.: Epidemiology of human bites to children in a day-care center. Am. J. Dis. Child. *142*:643–650, 1988.
23. Gold, M. H., Roenigk, H. H., Jr., Smith, E. S., et al.: Evaluation and treatment of patients with human bite marks. Am. J. Forens. Med. Pathol. *10*:140–143, 1989.
24. Goldstein, E. J. C., Citron, D. M., Wield, B., et al.: Bacteriology of human and animal bite wounds. J. Clin. Microbiol. *8*:667–672, 1978.
25. Goldstein, E. J. C., Miller, T. A., Citron, D. M., et al.: Infections following clenched-fist injury: A new perspective. J. Hand Surg. *3*:455–457, 1978.
26. Goldstein, E. J. C., Gombert, M. E., and Agyare, E. O.: Susceptibility of *Eikenella corrodens* to newer beta-lactam antibiotics. Antimicrob. Agents Chemother. *18*:832–833, 1980.
27. Goldstein, E. J. C., Barones, M. F., and Miller, T. A.: *Eikenella corrodens* in hand infections. J. Hand Surg. *8*:563–566, 1983.
28. Goldstein, E. J. C., and Citron, D. M.: Susceptibility of *Eikenella corrodens* to penicillin, apalcillin, and twelve cephalosporins. Antimicrob. Agents Chemother. *26*:947–948, 1984.
29. Goldstein, E. J. C., Citron, D. M., and Finegold, S. M.: Role of anaerobic bacteria in bite wound infections. Rev. Infect. Dis. *6*:S177–S783, 1984.
30. Goldstein, E. J. C., Reinhardt, J. F., Murray, P. M., et al.: Animal and human bite wounds: A comparative study of augmentin vs. penicillin +/− dicloxacillin. Postgrad. Med. J. Special Suppl.:105–110, 1984.
31. Goldstein, E. J. C., Citron, D. M., Vagvolgyi, A. E., et al.: Susceptibility of bite wound bacteria to seven oral antimicrobial agents, including RU-985, a new erythromycin: Considerations in choosing empiric therapy. Antimicrob. Agents Chemother. *29*:556–559, 1986.
32. Goldstein, E. J. C., and Citron, D. M.: Comparative activities of cefuroxime, amoxicillin–clavulanic acid, ciprofloxacin, enoxacin, and ofloxacin against aerobic and anaerobic bacteria isolated from bite wounds. Antimicrob. Agents Chemother. *32*:1143–1148, 1988.
33. Goldstein, E. J. C.: Bite wounds and infection. Clin. Infect. Dis. *14*:633–640, 1991.
34. Goldstein, E. J. C., and Citron, D. M.: Comparative susceptibilities of 173 aerobic and anaerobic bite wound isolates to sparfloxacin, temafloxacin, clarithromycin and older agents. Antimicrob. Agents Chemother. *37*:1150–1153, 1993.
35. Goldstein, E. J. C., Nesbit, C. A., and Citron, D. M.: Comparative in vitro activities of azithromycin, Bay y 3118, levofloxacin, sparfloxacin, and 11 other oral antimicrobial agents against 194 aerobic and anaerobic bite wound isolates. Antimicrob. Agents Chemother. *39*:1097–1100, 1995.
36. Gonzalez, M. N., Papierski, P., and Hal, R., Jr.: Osteomyelitis of the hand after a human bite. J. Hand Surg. [Am.] *18*:520–522, 1993.
37. Guba, A. M., Mulliken, J. B., and Hoopes, J. E.: The selection of antibiotics for human bites of the hand. Plast. Reconstr. Surg. *56*:538–541, 1975.
38. Haughey, R. E., Lammers, R. L., and Wagner, D. K.: Use of antibiotics in the initial management of soft-tissue hand wounds. Ann. Emerg. Med. *10*:187–192, 1981.
39. Hultgen, J. D.: Partial gangrene of the left index finger caused by symbiosis of the fusiform *Bacillus* and the *Spirochaeta denticola*. J. A. M. A. *10*:887–890, 1910.
40. Lehman, W. L., Jr., Jones, W. W., Allo, M. D., et al.: Human bite infections of the hand: Adjunct treatment with hyperbaric oxygen. Infect. Surg. *14*:460–465, 1985.
41. Lindsey, D., Christopher, M., Hollenbach, J., et al.: Natural course of human bite wound: Incidence of infection and complications in 434 bites and 803 lacerations in the same group of patients. J. Trauma *27*:45–48, 1987.
42. Long, W. T., Filler, B., Cox, E., et al.: Toxic shock syndrome after a human bite to the hand. J. Hand Surg. [Am.] *13*:957–959, 1988.
43. Loro, A., and Franceschi, F.: Human bites and finger infections: A survey at Dodoma Regional Hospital, Tanzania. Trop. Doctor *22*:24–26, 1992.
44. Malinowski, R. W., Strate, R. G., Perry, J. F., Jr., et al.: The management of human bite injuries of the hand. J. Trauma *19*:655–659, 1979.
45. Mann, R. J., Hoffeld, T. A., and Farmer, C. B.: Human bites of the hand: Twenty years of experience. J. Hand Surg. *2*:97–104, 1977.
46. Marr, J. S., Beck, A. M., and Lugo, J. A., Jr.: An epidemiologic study of the human bite. Public Health Rep. *94*:514–521, 1979.
47. Mast, E. E., Goodman, R. A., Bond, W. W., et al.: Transmission of blood-borne pathogens during sports: Risk and prevention. Ann. Intern. Med. *122*:283–285, 1995.
48. Mennen, U., and Howells, C. J.: Human fight-bite injuries of the hand: A study of 100 cases within 18 months. J. Hand Surg. [Br.] *16*:431–435, 1991.
49. Muguti, G. I., and Dixon, M. S.: Tetanus following human bite. Br. J. Plast. Surg. *45*:614–615, 1992.
50. Muguti, G. I., Zvomuya-Ncube, M., and Bvuma, E. T.: Experiences with human bites in Zimbabwe. Central African J. Med. *37*:294–298, 1991.
51. Murphy, R., Katz, S., and Massaro, D.: *Fusobacterium* septicemia following a human bite. Arch. Intern. Med. *111*:97–99, 1963.
52. Narsete, T. A., Omer, G. E., and Moneim, M. S.: Hand infections from human saliva. Orthop. Rev. *12*:81–84, 1983.
53. Nunley, D. L., Sasaki, T., Atkins, A., et al.: Hand infections in hospitalized patients. Am. J. Surg. *140*:374–376, 1980.
54. Peeples, E., Boswick, J. A., Jr., and Scott, F. A.: Wounds of the hand contaminated by human and animal saliva. J. Trauma *20*:383–389, 1980.
55. Prevots, R., Sutter, R. W., Strebel, P. M., et al.: Tetanus surveillance—United States, 1989–1990. M. M. W. R. *41*(SS-8):1–9, 1992.
56. Rickman, K. M., and Richman, L. S.: The potential for transmission of human immunodeficiency virus through human bites. J. AIDS *6*:402–406, 1993.
57. Schweich, P., and Fleisher, G.: Human bites in children. Pediatr. Emerg. Care *1*:51–53, 1985.
58. Shields, C., Patzakis, M. J., Meyers, M. H., et al.: Hand infections secondary to human bites. J. Trauma *15*:235–236, 1975.
59. Shirley, L. R., and Ross, S. A.: Risk of transmission of human immunodeficiency virus by bite of an infected toddler. J. Pediatr. *114*:425–427, 1989.
60. Solomons, H. C., and Elardo, R.: Bite injuries at a day care center. Early Child. Res. Q. *4*:89–96, 1989.
61. Solomons, H. C., Lakin, J. A., Snider, B. C., et al.: Is day care safe for children? Accident records reviewed. Child. Health Care *10*:90–93, 1982.
62. Solomons, H. C., and Elardo, R.: Biting in day care centers: Incidence, prevention and intervention. J. Pediatr. Health Care *5*:191–196, 1991.
63. Sperber, N. D.: Bite marks, oral and facial injuries: Harbingers of severe child abuse. Pediatrician *16*:207–211, 1989.
64. Uchendu, B. O.: Primary lip closure of human bite losses of the lip. Plast. Reconstr. Surg. *90*:841–845, 1992.
65. Vale, G. L., and Noguchi, T. T.: Anatomical distribution of human bite marks in a series of 67 cases. J. Forens. Sci. *28*:61–69, 1983.
66. Weinstein, R. A., Stephen, R. J., Morof, A., et al.: Human bites: Review of the literature and report of a case. J. Oral Surg. *31*:792–794, 1973.
67. Welch, C. E.: Human bite infections of the hand. N. Engl. J. Med. *215*:901–908, 1936.
68. Wolf, J. S., Gomez, R., and McAninch, J. W.: Human bites to the penis. J. Urol. *147*:1265–2067, 1992.
69. Wolf, J. S., Turzan, C., Cattolica, E. V., et al.: Dog bites to the male genitalia: Characteristics, management and comparison with human bites. J. Urol. *149*:286–289, 1993.

242

ANIMAL BITES

Morven S. Edwards

Many children delight in teasing dogs, and without caution go too near them, by which they get miserably torn and mangled. . . . What these boys had been doing to enrage the dog we cannot tell, but suspect they had been tormenting him in some way, thinking that as he was chained he could not injure them. But they were mistaken in this, and one of them is likely to be bitten very severely.[5]

Author unknown, 1830

HISTORICAL ASPECTS

Although the agents causing infection were undefined, the consequences to children of bites resulting from "worrying" dogs, noted in the opening quotation, were of concern in the nineteenth century just as they are today.[35] As early as 1933, it was recognized that human bites were more likely to result in infectious processes than those of animals, such as dogs, horses, mules, or bears, the exception being cats.[40] In early reports concerning bite wound infections, the wounds were found to contain fusiform bacilli and spirochetal organisms.[69, 75, 121] More recently, it has become evident that a vast array of both aerobic and anaerobic organisms making up the normal flora of the biting animal must be considered potential pathogens in the infected bite wound.

The importance of surgical débridement and drainage in the treatment of infected bite wounds was well-recognized in the era before antibiotics. However, in spite of this mode of treatment, wound infections were associated with high morbidity.[120] In one report from 1936, amputation was required in one-third of cases in which treatment was delayed for 24 hours or more.[146] Adjuncts to cleansing, such as electrocauterization[96] and even radiation therapy, were employed in an effort to prevent or treat infection, but it was not until the introduction of penicillin that the outcome of bite wound infection was improved over that achieved by symptomatic therapy alone.[120]

EPIDEMIOLOGY

Approximately 108 million cats and dogs are kept as pets in the United States.[61] The estimated annual incidence of animal bites is 1 to 2 million dog bites, 400,000 cat bites, and 45,000 snake bites, which incur an estimated 30 million dollars in annual health care costs.[51, 60, 67, 88, 144] Species of animals that have been reported to cause at least 1 per cent of bite injuries are rabbits, skunks, squirrels, horses, rats, hogs, and monkeys.[30, 43, 140, 141] A number of severe facial injuries have been inflicted because of unprovoked pet ferret attacks.[115] Considered together, however, bites from nondomestic animals, generally thought to pose a higher risk for rabies transmission, constitute less than 1 per cent of reported bites.[136] The most frequently bitten site is the right arm, presumably because of attempts by bite victims to use their dominant arm for defense, and at least three-quarters of all bites are located on the extremities.[71, 94, 141] Facial bites account for only 10 per cent of bites, but the majority of these (58 to 64 per cent) are sustained by children younger than 10 years of age.[71, 88]

Children are the most common victims of reported animal bites.[90] From one-half to three-fourths of dog bites are reported in persons younger than 20 years of age.[71, 136] The peak incidence is among children from 5 to 14 years of age.[13, 136] It is estimated that nearly 2 per cent of children 5 to 9 years of age are bitten annually. In one survey, 15.4 per cent of 531 children by 1 year of age had, at some time, been bitten by a mammal.[30] Many of these bites did not require a physician visit and were not reported. Among cases that are reported, the number of children bitten exceeds the rate of all reportable childhood diseases.[18] Thus, it is not surprising that as many as 1 per cent of all pediatric emergency room visits during the summer months are for the treatment of animal bites.[41, 83, 88] Most bites occur during the late afternoon and early evening hours.[71, 88] Boys sustain dog bites twice as often as girls, but girls are bitten more frequently by cats.[71, 88, 103]

Large dogs with an average weight of 50 pounds or more account for the majority of animal bites[71] and are implicated most frequently in bites with a fatal outcome. Of 157 dog bite–related fatalities that occurred in the United States from 1979 through 1988, pit bull breeds were implicated most frequently. Other purebreds, including German shepherds, chow chows, rottweilers, and Dobermans, also have been identified as perpetrators.[57, 61] The proportion of deaths attributable to pit bull terriers has increased from 20 per cent in 1979 and 1980 to 62 per cent in 1987 and 1988.[128] These animals can exert a biting force (1500 pounds per square inch) several times that of a German shepherd. The severity of wounds inflicted by this breed also is due to the tendency to inflict multiple bites and to bite and grind the molars into tissue. Ninety-four per cent of pit bull injuries in one study were the consequence of unprovoked attacks.[9] In most instances (75 per cent), the dog's owner is known by the victim, although only a small percentage of bites are caused by a family-owned dog.[71] Stray dogs account for only 10 per cent of bites inflicted.[71, 88] When circumstances are known, the majority of mammalian bites are provoked, although the victim may not have agitated the animal intentionally.[30, 88, 132]

Infection is a common complication of animal bites. Between 3 and 20 per cent of dog bites and 20 to 50 per cent of cat bites for which medical care is sought develop infections.[1, 26, 61, 88, 95, 144] With the exception of monkey bites, which have a high (25 per cent) infection rate, infection after other mammalian bites is uncommon.[1, 43] Factors influencing the risk for infection include patient age, wound type, wound location, and length of time between the bite and initiation of treatment.[17, 24] Children younger than 4 years of age have been reported to have an increased incidence of wound infection by some but not all investigators, and infection is more common in patients older than 50 years of age.[24] Wounds of the hand are more likely to become infected (30 to 36 per cent) than are those of the arm (17 to 27 per cent), leg (15 to 17 per cent), or face (4 to 11 per cent).[24, 26] Puncture wounds are more likely to become infected than lacerations, superficial wounds, or wounds with skin and soft tissue defects.[1, 24, 26, 140] Infection is likely when wounds are repaired surgically or when care is delayed more than 24 hours after injury.[24, 140]

MICROBIOLOGY

It has been suggested that the mammalian mouth can be viewed as a microbial incubator supporting the growth of some 200 species of facultative organisms and obligate anaerobes.[45] The normal oral flora of the animal rather than the skin flora of the victim is the source of most bacteria isolated from bite-wound cultures,[66, 103] but each may be viewed as a potential source of infection. Infections usually are polymicrobial and contain mixed aerobic-anaerobic isolates. When carefully sought, anaerobes may be isolated from approximately 40 per cent of animal bite wounds.[64] Table 242–1 enumerates the bacterial isolates from 83 dog bite victims who were assessed at the time bite-wound infection was evident.[26, 64, 95, 120] Frequent isolates from infected wounds include streptococci (particularly viridans streptococci and non–group A beta-hemolytic streptococci), coagulase-positive and -negative staphylococci, *Pasteurella multocida,* and, among anaerobes, various *Bacteroides* species. *Staphylococcus intermedius* is a frequent isolate from canine gingiva that has been implicated in bite wound infections.[138] No significant difference in the prevalence of various isolates has been shown in studies comparing the flora from noninfected and infected dog bite wounds.[27, 66] Although similar data for cats and other mammals are not available, the high incidence of *P. multocida* infections after cat bites and the known high prevalence of this organism in the normal feline oral flora suggest that mouth flora are the usual source of these infections.

P. multocida carrier rates range as high as 66 per cent for dogs and 90 per cent for cats, and this organism is associated with 25 to 50 per cent of dog and 80 per cent of cat bite infections.[7] Infection is not restricted to the bite of house cats; infection also has been reported after lion,[23, 137] cougar,[89] and tiger bites.[23] The type of wound commonly inflicted (i.e., puncture by cats vs. laceration by dogs) might explain the species-specific disparity in infection rates. There is no conclusive evidence that the biotypes A and B commonly associated with cat bites are more virulent than the more varied biotypes associated with dog bites.[113]

Another group of significant canine pathogens are the gram-negative rods that have been classified under the Centers for Disease Control and Prevention alphanumeric system. Among these, dysgonic fermenter 2 (DF-2) has been classified as *Capnocytophaga canimorsus*[21] and is a common isolate from the canine mouth. The former Iij, which has been recovered from the oral flora in 90 per cent of normal dogs, now is named *Weeksella zoohelcum.*[79] M-5 is speciated as *Neisseria weaveri.*[4] The majority of infections reported in association with these species occurs in splenectomized persons or in those with conditions of host immunocompromise. However, infections also may occur in patients with no predisposing conditions.[80]

Among persons sustaining alligator bite wounds, infection most commonly is due to *Aeromonas hydrophila.* A report of mixed infection with *A. hydrophila, Enterobacter agglomerans,* and *Citrobacter diversus* and the frequency with which *Proteus vulgaris* and *Pseudomonas* species are isolated from alligator mouths suggests that the treatment of alligator bites should be directed at gram-negative species.[55] *Vibrio* infection should be suspected as a complication of shark bite, as well as of all wounds exposed to salt water.[119] Animal bites have been implicated as the vehicles for transmission of an extensive array of systemic infectious diseases caused by viruses, fungi, and mycobacteria, in addition to bacteria (Table 242–2).[49] For some of these infections, the list of "other animals" that may transmit the infection via biting is extensive. For example, tularemia may be transmitted by the bite of the wild boar, coyote, hog, lamb, muskrat, opossum, raccoon, rat, skunk, squirrel, snapping turtle, and weasel.[82]

TABLE 242–1. Aerobic and Anaerobic Bacteria Isolated from 83 Infected Dog Bites[26, 52, 64, 95, 120, 133]

Isolate	Number of Positive Cultures (% of Infections)
Gram-Positive Aerobes	
Corynebacterium species	7 (8)
Diphtheroids	2 (2)
Micrococcus species	3 (4)
Staphylococcus aureus	19 (23)
Staphylococcus epidermidis	12 (14)
Streptococcus species*	25 (30)
Gram-Negative Aerobes	
Acinetobacter species	4 (5)
Actinobacillus species	3 (4)
Chromobacterium species	1 (1)
Eikenella corrodens	1 (1)
Escherichia coli	1 (1)
Haemophilus species	2 (2)
Klebsiella-Enterobacter	4 (5)
Neisseria species	1 (1)
Pasteurella multocida	34 (41)
Proteus mirabilis	1 (1)
Pseudomonas species	5 (6)
Unclassified rods	2 (2)
Unspecific	2 (2)
Anaerobes†	
Bacteroides species	15 (65)
Clostridium species	1 (4)
Eubacterium species	2 (9)
Fusobacterium species	1 (4)
Fusobacterium nucleatum	2 (9)
Fusobacterium russii	1 (4)
Leptothrix buccalis	1 (4)
Peptococcus species	3 (13)
Peptostreptococcus species	2 (9)
Propionibacterium species	4 (17)
Veillonella species	1 (4)

*Includes alpha, beta, and nonhemolytic isolates.
†Percentages based on assessment of 23 infections.

CLINICAL MANIFESTATIONS

Signs of bacterial infection after animal bites develop within hours to several days after injury. As noted by Goldstein and associates,[63] infection usually is why patients seek medical attention more than 12 hours after injury, whereas those presenting earlier are more concerned with prophylaxis or surgical repair. Signs suggestive of wound infection include localized swelling, erythema, and pain with or without serosanguineous or purulent drainage (Fig. 242–1). The clinical signs vary with the infecting organism, site of injury, and type of bite.

In patients with *P. multocida* infection, the characteristic clinical syndrome of intense pain, swelling, and erythema develops rapidly, often within hours after injury.[97] Intense cellulitis usually is evident within 24 to 36 hours after the bite[7, 38, 78, 97] but occasionally may be delayed for 3 to 5 days.[38, 78] Despite these intense local symptoms, patients usually are afebrile and less than 20 per cent have lymphangitis and

TABLE 242–2. Systemic Infections Transmissible by Animal Bites

Infection	Type of Bite*	Representative References
Viral		
Arbovirus (Rio Bravo infection)†	Bat	82
Cytomegalovirus	Chimpanzee	111
Hemorrhagic fever with renal syndrome‡	Rodent	44
Monkey pox	Chimpanzee	112
Rabies	C, D, O	30, 45, 139
B virus (herpesvirus simiae) encephalitis	Monkey	82
Venezuelan equine encephalitis‖	Bat	139
Bacterial		
Brucellosis	D	124
Cat-scratch disease	C, D, monkey	27
Leptospirosis	D, mouse, rat	82, 98, 118
Plague	C	32
Rat-bite fever§	D, rat, mouse, squirrel, weasel, gerbil	58, 82, 149
Tetanus	D	136
Tularemia	C, D, O	29, 50, 82, 101, 122
Mycobacterial		
M. marinum	Dolphin	56
M. fortuitum	D	6
Fungal		
Blastomycosis	D	59, 77, 85
Parasitic		
Trypanosomiasis‖	Bat	139

*D is dog, C is cat, O is other mammals.
†Due to California bat salivary gland virus.
‡Murine virus nephropathy.
§Both Haverhill fever due to *Streptobacillus moniliformis* and sodoku, caused by *Spirillum minus*.
‖Possible or questionable transmission.

regional adenitis. In contrast, patients with wound infection due to staphylococci or streptococci generally experience less intense pain, have a delay between injury and onset of symptoms of days rather than hours, and may present with a more diffuse, less fiery cellulitis. Extensive gas in the tissues of the forearm clinically suggestive of clostridial gas gangrene has been described from infection due to *S. anginosus* and *Streptococcus mutans* after horse bite lacerations.[105] Wound infection clinically resembling that due to *P. multocida* from which the related but more unusual gram-negative rod *Actinobacillus lignieresii* was isolated has been reported in a child who sustained a facial bite by a horse.[39]

"Seal finger," an entity probably due to an as yet undefined infectious agent, deserves mention because failure to initiate appropriate therapy may result in permanent sequelae. Infection may result from contact through a skin laceration with the skin of the seal or from a seal tooth or claw-associated puncture wound.[104, 108] The incubation period averages 4 to 8 days, and infection is characterized by severe pain and often massive swelling, moderate erythema, and, in some cases, regional adenopathy and ascending lymphangitis. There is a predilection for involvement of the joint closest to the inoculation site.[104] Once the diagnosis is made, treatment should be initiated with tetracycline, which is the drug of choice.[104, 108] The use of other antibiotics, including ampicillin, erythromycin, and cephalosporins, produces no effect and has been associated with progression of infection and joint destruction.[108]

Among patients with systemic infections transmitted by an animal bite, the incubation period and clinical manifestations vary with the causative agent. For example, streptobacillary rat-bite fever occurs after an incubation period of less than 1 week, whereas spirillary rat-bite fever, or sodoku, has a 2-week asymptomatic interval from bite. It should be noted, however, that rat-bite fever due to *Spirillum minor* and *S. moniliformis* can occur together. The term squirrel-bite fever has been suggested for a syndrome, clinically similar to streptobacillary rat-bite fever, that has been described after the bite of the ground squirrel *Xerus erythropus*.[109] For most of the infections listed in Table 242–2, the bite wound serves as the site of inoculation and has healed completely during the incubation period. For example, fatal encephalitis has resulted from the bite or scratch of a monkey that actively is shedding B virus (herpesvirus simiae). Institution of acyclovir treatment intravenously at the time of injury may abort disease progression.[11, 33] The systemic symptoms heralding the onset of systemic infections due to animal bite do not depend on the mode of transmission and are discussed in their respective chapters. A high index of suspicion may be required to trace the infection to the animal source. However, with tularemia, an ulcerative[122] or pustular[50] lesion develops at the bite site 4 to 7 days after injury in association with fever, chills, and painful regional adenopathy. In a case of *Mycobacterium marinum* infection after a dolphin bite, one of several discrete fluctuant masses containing the isolate developed in an area just proximal to the original wound.[56] With cat-scratch disease due to *Bartonella henselae*, a papule or pustule may be present at the original bite site when systemic signs develop.

The jaws and teeth of dogs are likely to produce multiple puncture wounds as well as jagged lacerations with devitalized tissue. These lesions may be associated with depressed skull fractures, which may be present in more than one cranial region.[148] Puncture wounds, particularly those inflicted by cat bites, often are deceptively innocuous.[148] Inoculation of organisms deep into poorly vascularized areas, such as tendon sheaths, fascia, joints, and bones, is likely to result in an infected wound.[20]

Some of the complications that have resulted from direct extension or generalized spread of infection due to animal

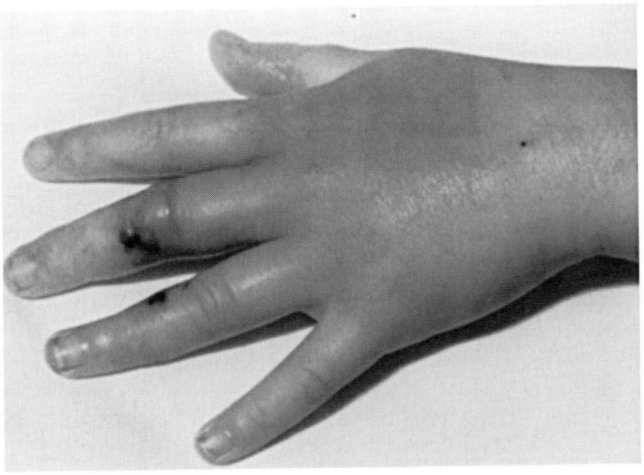

FIGURE 242–1. *Dog bite wound–associated tenosynovitis in a 4-year-old girl. Group D* Streptococcus *was isolated from the wound culture.*

TABLE 242–3. Some Infectious Complications of Animal Bites

Complications	Isolates	Type of Bite*	Representative References
Direct Extension			
Arthritis	*Pasteurella multocida*	D, C, lion	23, 51
Brain abscess	*Peptococcus*	D	3
	P. multocida	D	91
	Streptococcus bovis	Rooster	12
	Clostridium tertium		
	Aspergillus niger		
	Capnocytophaga canimorsus‖	D	81
Endophthalmitis	*P. multocida*	C	152
Orbital cellulitis	Not specified	Rat	42
Osteomyelitis	*Haemophilus hemoglobinophilus*	D	93
	P. multocida	D, C, lion	2, 7, 15, 23, 38, 51, 84, 97, 99
	VE-2, EF-4,† *P. multocida*	D	84
	Acinetobacter calcoaceticus	D	52
	Acinetobacter anitratus	Hamster	106
	Enterococcus	Monkey	52
Synovitis	*Mycobacterium fortuitum*	D	6
Tendonitis, tenosynovitis	*Pseudomonas aeruginosa*	D	52
	P. multocida	C, D	20, 72
Generalized			
Endocarditis	*P. multocida*	D	129
	Pasteurella spp.	C	70
	Erysipelothrix rhusiopathiae	D	14
	P. multocida	C	147
	Unclassified, GNR‡	D	86, 130
Generalized Schwartzman reaction	*P. multocida*†	D	110
Meningitis ± sepsis§	Unclassified, GNR	D	16, 19
	P. multocida	D, tiger	10, 23
	Streptobacillus moniliformis	D	58
Mycotic aneurysm	*P. multocida*	C	68
Pneumonia	*P. multocida*	C	74
Sepsis ± coagulopathy	*Bacteroides* spp.	D	53
	P. multocida	D, C	87, 151
	C. canimorsus	D	86
Sepsis, infected knee joint prostheses	*P. multocida, P. aeruginosa*	C	114
Sepsis, postsplenectomy	Unclassified GNR, including *C. canimorsus*	D	54, 80, 107

*C is cat, D is dog.
†Isolates possibly associated with infection.
‡GNR is gram-negative rods.
§Includes some probable direct extension cases.
‖Formerly dysgonic fermenter type 2, DF-2.

bites are summarized in Table 242–3. Tenosynovitis due to *P. multocida* may be apparent within hours after injury,[20] or the diagnosis may be delayed for days to weeks after the bite until the persistence of swelling, tenderness of pain with motion, and mass overlying the involved tendon sheath suggest the diagnosis.[97] The occurrence of *Pasteurella* osteomyelitis after cat bites was reported first in 1942.[2] Both acute[84, 97] and chronic[7, 15, 38, 84, 97] disease subsequently have been described, and each is characterized by pain, swelling, and tenderness over the involved bone. In patients with chronic infection, draining sinuses or a persistently draining wound is a frequent presenting sign. When the periosteum has been entered, osteomyelitis may develop, despite early local care and treatment with penicillin. Although combined osteomyelitis and septic arthritis have been reported, septic arthritis alone shows a predilection for previously damaged joints.[48] Although feline incisors are more likely to penetrate the periosteum than are canine incisors, osteomyelitis may occur as a complication of dog as well as cat bites.[84, 99]

Bites to the cranium occur with relative frequency in small children because their heads are at the level of the mouth of medium to large dogs. The complications of perforating cranial bites that have been described in children include compound depressed skull fractures, dural lacerations, and extensive intracerebral injuries, which may prove fatal.[23, 148] Both brain abscess and meningitis may occur as complications of these injuries (Table 242–3).

Generalized or systemic complications from animal bites occur usually, but not exclusively, in hosts with altered immune status. For example, the three most common underlying findings in *C. canimorsus*–associated infections are splenectomy, alcoholism, and chronic lung diseases.[54, 86, 107] Disseminated intravascular coagulation, hypotension, cutaneous gangrene, and renal failure also have been described in patients with leukemia or lymphoma and in association with steroid therapy.[86, 153] Symptoms ensue 1 day to 2 weeks after dog or, occasionally, cat bites; the overall mortality rate from *C. canimorsus* septicemia exceeds 20 per cent.[31, 37, 76] However, bacteremia and fatal endocarditis due to this organism have occurred in immunocompetent patients.[37, 96] Although removal of bilaterally affected knee joint prostheses was required to achieve cure of infection due to *P. multocida* and *Pseudomonas aeruginosa* in one report,[114] cure also has been achieved with antibiotics and drainage with the prosthesis remaining in situ.[51]

DIAGNOSIS AND TREATMENT

The most important principle in the diagnosis of infection from animal bite wounds is the proper use of the wound culture. A culture need not be obtained from children presenting in the immediate postinjury period (the first 12 hours) unless the bite is located on the face or hand or there are signs of infection. The isolates from an uninfected but contaminated wound reflect the normal flora of the biting animal and do not predict the future development of infection.[17, 24] Routine determination of the microorganisms colonizing bites on the face or hands is a useful precaution because of the potentially devastating consequences of infection at these locations. After cleansing, wound culture should be obtained routinely when patients present at an interval exceeding 12 hours from the time of injury, unless there are no signs of infection.

When a wound culture is obtained, the microbiology laboratory should be informed that the source of the culture is an animal bite wound. This should optimize accuracy because *P. multocida* may be mistaken morphologically for *Neisseria* or *Haemophilus influenzae*,[97, 141] appropriate media must be employed for the isolation of anaerobes, and gram-negative rods should be considered pathogens. A blood culture should be obtained when temperature elevation is substantial (greater than 38.9° C [102° F] rectally) or if systemic toxicity is evident, although associated bacteremia is rare.[52] Radiographic evaluation of the bite-injured area is indicated when possible or if the periosteum definitely has been penetrated. A computerized tomographic study may be an aid to detecting periosteal defects, particularly in children with cranial bite wounds. For patients in whom a wound infection has extended locally, sutures, if present, should be removed and material from the involved tissue compartment should be obtained for study. Material should be aspirated from areas of cellulitis or drained from areas of frank abscess formation. If osteomyelitis is suspected, a diagnostic bone biopsy should be submitted for Gram stain, culture, and histopathologic evaluation. If the course of wound infection is indolent, acid-fast stains and mycobacterial cultures should be performed. Serum for serologic testing should be obtained from patients with symptoms suggesting hepatitis B, tularemia, syphilis, or blastomycosis. The details of the indicated diagnostic evaluation for systemic infections transmissible by animal bite (see Table 242–2) are specified in the appropriate chapters.

The first step in wound care is to cleanse the wound and surrounding area.[73] Visible dirt should be sponged away gently to avoid further damage to traumatized tissue. The wound should be irrigated copiously using 150 to 200 mL of normal saline. Cleansing by high-pressure syringe irrigation using a 25-mL syringe and 19-gauge needle is effective.[25, 135, 143] This method of irrigation decreased the incidence of dog bite wound–associated infection fivefold, from 69 to 12 per cent.[24] A 1 per cent povidone-iodine solution has been suggested as an alternative irrigant to saline, although it has not been proved to have antiseptic activity.[27] More concentrated solutions should not be employed because they may damage tissues and delay wound healing.[27] Alternatively, irrigation may be carried out using the nonionic surfactant Pluronic F-68, which does not harm tissues but has been shown to prevent development of infection in the experimental situation.[73, 125] If rabies is considered a risk, the use of 1 per cent benzalkonium chloride for possible virucidal activity followed by irrigation with saline has been suggested.[27] Puncture wounds should be cleansed but not irrigated because irrigation further may damage tissues.

Devitalized tissues should then be débrided. Callaham[24] has shown that further careful trimming of the wound edge in nonpuncture wounds is associated with a significant decrease in the rate of infection. Others believe that wound excision should not be considered standard treatment.[46] The issue of bite wound closure has been controversial. In the series published by Lee and associates[95] in 1960, sutured wounds had an infection rate twice that of unsutured wounds. More recently, in a retrospective study, Callaham[25] found that infection rates were significantly lower in sutured than in nonsutured wounds. However, the same investigator demonstrated no difference in the infection rate among 57 patients assessed prospectively, with the exception of those suffering hand bites, which were more likely to become infected when sutured.[26] After appropriate cleansing and débridement, it appears that most nonpuncture animal bite wounds except those involving the hand can be treated by primary closure without influencing significantly the incidence of infection.[24, 25, 88, 102, 140]

The data with which to assess the use of prophylactic antibiotics after animal bites are sparse. One investigator found that oxacillin did not reduce the incidence of infection after dog bite wounds[47] but did after cat bites.[48] In another study, a trend toward a reduced infection rate, particularly for hand wounds, was shown for patients receiving penicillin prophylactically after dog bites.[26] In a well-designed, prospective study limited to children with nonfacial dog bites that did not require closure, prophylactic penicillin at a dose of 250 mg four times daily for 5 days did not affect significantly the rate of infection.[17] Among 58 patients, the infection rate was 3.6 per cent in both the treatment and the placebo groups. Prophylactic dicloxacillin, cephalexin, or erythromycin was not beneficial for low-risk dog bite wounds in another prospective study. The wound infection rates for the antibiotic and control groups were 1.1 and 5.1 per cent, respectively.[41]

A meta-analysis of eight randomized trials totaling 783 patients with dog bite wounds found that prophylactic antibiotics did reduce the incidence of infection.[36] The estimated cumulative incidence of infection was 16 per cent in controls, and the relative risk was 0.56 (95 per cent confidence interval, 0.38 to 0.82) in patients given antibiotics compared with controls. Treatment of about 14 patients was required to prevent one infection. Thus, one view is that prophylaxis has a role, but it should be employed selectively.[28] Alternatively, some consider antibiotic use therapeutic rather than prophylactic in this setting and suggest antibiotic therapy in all dog bites except those that present more than 24 hours after injury with no clinical signs of infection.[147]

Until additional data are available, it would appear reasonable to use prophylactic antibiotics in the following circumstances: (1) all cat bites, (2) dog bites more than 8 hours old, (3) moderate to severe dog bites less than 8 hours old, especially if edema or crush injury is present, (4) deep puncture wounds (especially if bone or joint penetration may have occurred), (5) facial wounds, (6) all hand bites, (7) wounds in the genital area, and (8) wounds in immunocompromised persons.[61, 103, 143, 145]

Empiric treatment should be directed toward the most common infecting organisms, *P. multocida*, staphylococci, streptococci, and anaerobes.[103] Amoxicillin–clavulanic acid (Augmentin) is active against almost all species of bacteria found in bite wounds and may be considered the drug of choice for empiric oral treatment.[22, 62] The recommended dosage is 40 mg/kg/day administered at 8-hour intervals. Erythromycin is only moderately active against *P. multocida*.[103, 134] Oral alternatives for the penicillin-allergic child include trimethoprim-sulfamethoxazole (10 and 50 mg/kg/day) plus clindamycin (30 mg/kg/day) or cefuroxime axetil (30 mg/kg/day) plus metronidazole (30 mg/kg/day). For hospitalized patients requiring prophylaxis, ampicillin-sulbactam (Unasyn) (200 mg/kg/day), ticarcillin–clavulanic acid (Timentin) (200 mg/kg/day), or the combination of penicillin G (200,000 units/kg/day) and a penicillinase-resistant penicillin (150 mg/kg/day) at 6-hour intervals is suggested.[8] Imipenem (60 mg/kg/day) is an alternative choice.

Penicillin is the drug of choice for *P. multocida* infection. This organism has a median minimal inhibitory concentration to penicillin G of 0.1 to 0.8 μg/mL.[51, 52] Other active antibiotics in vitro are ampicillin, carbenicillin, tetracycline, chloramphenicol, cephalothin,[134] trimethoprim-sulfamethoxazole, and third-generation cephalosporins.[52] Cefuroxime is potentially useful and is more active than cephalexin.[62] Antibiotics with poor activity against *P. multocida* include the penicillinase-resistant penicillins, clindamycin, and aminoglycosides.[134]

As a general guideline, a suggested duration of therapy, assuming proper drainage has been established, is 10 days for cellulitis or localized abscess, 2 to 3 weeks for tenosynovitis, and 3 to 4 weeks for osteomyelitis. When improvement is evident, treatment can be completed orally. At least 4 weeks of intravenous therapy should be employed for patients with endocarditis. Although there are too few patients to establish the required dosage with certainty, ampicillin (400 mg/kg/day) has been employed successfully for the treatment of *P. multocida* meningitis.[10] The antimicrobial therapy for wound infections caused by organisms other than *P. multocida* or unclassified gram-negative rod isolates or those with mixed flora should be guided initially by the findings on Gram stain and ultimately by susceptibility studies.

In every child sustaining a bite wound, the immunization status should be determined to assess the need for tetanus prophylaxis and whether rabies prophylaxis should be undertaken (see appropriate chapters).

SNAKE BITES

Approximately 8000 people are bitten yearly by poisonous snakes in the United States.[142] Among these, some 49 per cent of bites occur in people younger than 20 years of age. The curiosity of children may contribute to this exposure because many are bitten while handling poisonous snakes.[116] Between 9 and 15 persons die yearly from snake bites.[92]

Venomous snakes are divided into four families, of which two, the Crotalidae (rattlesnakes, copperheads, and water moccasins) and the Elapidae (coral snakes), are found in the United States.[126] Snake venoms are among the most complex of proteins. The local effects of the venom of pit vipers (Crotalidae), which are rich in proteolytic activity, include swelling, pain, edema, ecchymosis, and tissue necrosis with bulla formation.[126] The venom of the eastern coral snake causes minimal local tissue destruction. Systemic effects of Crotalid envenomation result from increased blood vessel permeability and hemolysis and may include hematuria, hematemesis, and disseminated intravascular coagulopathy.[126] The venom of the eastern coral snake is a neurotoxin that produces paresthesia of the involved extremity followed by involvement of the cranial nerves and bulbar paralysis.

Since the preantibiotic era, it has been recognized that the oral flora of snakes' mouths frequently harbor multiple organisms, particularly gram-negative bacilli, staphylococci, and anaerobes.[117, 150] Goldstein and associates[65] isolated 58 aerobic and 28 anaerobic organisms upon culturing the venom from 15 rattlesnakes. The most commonly isolated aerobes were *P. aeruginosa, Proteus* species, and *S. epidermidis*. Among the anaerobes, *Clostridium* species were the most frequent isolates; *Bacteroides fragilis* also was recovered. It has been suggested that the defecation of prey during ingestion is responsible for this preponderance of gastrointestinal flora.[65] Goldstein and associates,[65] by cleansing the fangs carefully before collection, demonstrated that the venom itself is sterile, indicating that bacterial isolates potentially contaminating snake bite wounds are a reflection of the oral flora.

The role of empiric antibiotics after snake bite wounds is undefined, as is the incidence of infection and subsequent complications. Definition of the incidence of infection is compounded by the fact that the inflammatory changes of envenomation may be difficult to differentiate from those of infection.[94] At least one instance of osteomyelitis as a complication of infected snake bite has been documented.[127] Russell[127] suggests that a broad-spectrum antibiotic, such as ampicillin, be employed for injuries with severe tissue involvement but not for cases with minor or minimal envenomation. Other experts suggest that antibiotics should be withheld *unless* evidence of bacterial infection develops and that treatment should be guided by the results of Gram stain and susceptibility testing.[142]

References

1. Aghababian, R. V., and Conte, J. E.: Mammalian bite wounds. Ann. Emerg. Med. *9*:79–83, 1980.
2. Allin, A. E.: Cat-bite wound infection. Can. Med. Assoc. J. *46*:48–50, 1942.
3. Alpert, G., and Sutton, L. N.: Brain abscess following cranial dog bite. Clin. Pediatr. *23*:580, 1984.
4. Andersen, B. M., Steigerwalt, A. G., O'Conner, S. P., et al.: *Neisseria weaveri* sp. nov., formerly CDC group M-5, a gram-negative bacterium associated with dog bite wounds. J. Clin. Microbiol. *31*:2456–2466, 1993.
5. Anonymous: The Book of Accidents: Designed for Young Children. New Haven, Sidney's Press, 1830.
6. Ariel, H., Haas, H., Weinberg, H., et al.: *Mycobacterium fortuitum* granulomatous synovitis caused by a dog bite. J. Hand Surg. *8*:342–343, 1983.
7. Arons, M. S., Fernando, L., and Polayes, I. M.: *Pasteurella multocida*: The major cause of hand infections following domestic animal bites. J. Hand Surg. *7*:47–52, 1982.
8. August, J. R.: Dog and cat bites. J. Am. Vet. Met. Assoc. *193*:1394–1398, 1988.
9. Avner, J. R., and Baker, M. D.: Dog bites in urban children. Pediatrics *88*:55–57, 1991.
10. Belardi, F. G., Pascoe, J. M., and Beegle, E. D.: *Pasteurella multocida* meningitis in an infant following occipital dog bite. J. Fam. Pract. *14*:778–782, 1982.
11. Benson, P. M., Malane, S. L., Banks, R., et al.: B virus (*Herpesvirus simiae*) and human infection. Arch. Dermatol. *125*:1247–1248, 1989.
12. Berkowitz, F. E., and Jacobs, D. W. C.: Fatal case of brain abscess caused by rooster pecking. Pediatr. Infect. Dis. *6*:941–942, 1987.
13. Berzon, D. R., and DeHoff, J. D.: Medical cost and other aspects of dog bites in Baltimore. Public Health Rep. *89*:377–381, 1974.
14. Bibler, M. R.: *Erysipelothrix rhusiopathiae* endocarditis. Rev. Infect. Dis. *10*:1062–1063, 1988.
15. Bjorkhölm, B., and Tönnes, E.: *Pasteurella multocida* osteomyelitis caused by cat bite. J. Infect. *6*:175–177, 1983.
16. Bobo, R. A., and Newton, E. J.: A previously undescribed gram-negative bacillus causing septicemia and meningitis. Am. J. Clin. Pathol. *65*:546–569, 1976.
17. Boenning, D. A., Fleisher, G. R., and Campos, J. M.: Dog bites in children: Epidemiology, microbiology, and penicillin prophylactic therapy. Am. J. Emerg. Med. *1*:17–21, 1983.
18. Borchelt, P. L., Lockwood, R., Beck, A. M., et al.: Attacks by packs of dogs involving predation of human beings. Public Health Rep. *98*:57–66, 1983.
19. Bracis, R., Seibers, K., and Julien, R. M.: Meningitis caused by group II J following a dog bite. West. J. Med. *131*:438–440, 1979.
20. Branson, D., and Bunkfeldt, F., Jr.: *Pasteurella multocida* in animal bites of humans. Am. J. Clin. Pathol. *48*:552–555, 1967.
21. Brenner, D. J., Hollis, D. G., Fanning, G. R., et al.: *Capnocytophaga canimorsus* sp. nov. (formerly CDC group DF-2), a cause of septicemia following dog bite, and *C. cynodegmi* sp. nov., a cause of localized wound infection following dog bite. J. Clin. Microbiol. *27*:231–235, 1989.
22. Brook, I.: Human and animal bites. J. Fam. Pract. *28*:713–718, 1989.

23. Burdge, D. R., Scheifele, D., and Speert, D. P.: Serious *Pasteurella multocida* infections from lion and tiger bites. J. A. M. A. *253*:3296–3297, 1985.
24. Callaham, M.: Treatment of common dog bites: Infection risk factors. J. Am. Coll. Emerg. Phy. *7*:83–87, 1978.
25. Callaham, M.: Dog bite wounds. J. A. M. A. *244*:2327–2328, 1980.
26. Callaham, M.: Prophylactic antibiotics in common dog bite wounds: A controlled study. Ann. Emerg. Med. *9*:410–414, 1980.
27. Callaham, M.: Human and animal bites. Top. Emerg. Med. *4*:1–15, 1982.
28. Callaham, M.: Prophylactic antibiotics in dog bite wounds: Nipping at the heels of progress. Ann. Emerg. Med. *23*:577–579, 1994.
29. Capellan, J., and Fong, I. W.: Tularemia from a cat bite: Case report and review of feline-associated tularemia. Clin. Infect. Dis. *16*:472–475, 1993.
30. Carithers, H. A.: Mammalian bites of children. Am. J. Dis. Child. *95*:150–156, 1958.
31. Carpenter, P. D., Heppner, B. T., and Gnann, J. W., Jr.: DF-2 bacteremia following dog bites: Report of two cases. Am. J. Med. *82*:621–623, 1987.
32. Centers for Disease Control: Plague: United States. M. M. W. R. *26*:337, 1977.
33. Centers for Disease Control: B-virus infection in humans: Pensacola, Florida. J. A. M. A. *257*:3192–3193, 3198, 1987.
34. Chretien, J. H., and Garagusi, V. F.: Infections associated with pets. Am. Fam. Physician *41*:831–845, 1990.
35. Cone, T. E., Jr.: Book of accidents. Excerpt VIII. Worrying dogs. Pediatrics *47*:460, 1971.
36. Cummings, P.: Antibiotics to prevent infection in patients with dog bite wounds: A meta-analysis of randomized trials. Ann. Emerg. Med. *23*:535–540, 1994.
37. Dankner, W. M., Davis, C. E., and Thompson, M. A.: DF-2 bacteremia following a dog bite in a 4-month-old child. Pediatr. Infect. Dis. *6*:695–696, 1987.
38. DeBoer, R. G., and Dumler, M.: *Pasteurella multocida* infections: A report of six cases. Am. J. Clin. Pathol. *40*:339–344, 1963.
39. Dibb, W. L., Digranes, A., and Tønjum, S.: *Actinobacillus lignieresii* infection after a horse bite. B. M. J. *283*:583–584, 1981.
40. Dimtza, A.: Ueber Bissverletzungen. Schweiz. Med. Wochenschr. *63*:505, 1933.
41. Dire, D. J., Hogan, D. E., and Walker, J. S.: Prophylactic oral antibiotics for low-risk dog bite wounds. Pediatr. Emerg. Care *8*:194–199, 1992.
42. Diwan, R., Sen, D. K., and Sood, G. C.: Rat bite orbital cellulitis. Br. J. Ophthal. *54*:211, 1970.
43. Douglas, L. G.: Bite wounds. Am. Fam. Physician *11*:93–99, 1975.
44. Dournon, E., Moriniere, B., Matheron, S., et al.: HFRS after a wild rodent bite in the Haute-Savoie: And risk of exposure to hantaan-like virus in a Paris laboratory. Lancet *1*:676–677, 1984.
45. Edlich, R. F., Spengler, M. D., and Rodeheaver, G. T.: Mammalian bites. Compr. Ther. *9*:41–47, 1983.
46. Elenbaas, R. M., McNabney, W. K., and Robinson, W. A.: Prophylactic antibiotics and dog bite wounds. J. A. M. A. *246*:833–834, 1981.
47. Elenbaas, R. M., McNabney, W. K., and Robinson, W. A.: Prophylactic oxacillin in dog bite wounds. Ann. Emerg. Med. *11*:248–251, 1982.
48. Elenbaas, R. M., McNabney, W. K., and Robinson, W. A.: Evaluation of prophylactic oxacillin in cat bite wounds. Ann. Emerg. Med. *13*:155–157, 1984.
49. Elliot, D. L., Tolle, S. W., Goldberg, L., et al.: Pet-associated illness. N. Engl. J. Med. *313*:985–995, 1985.
50. Evans, M. E., McGee, Z. A., Hunter, P. T., et al.: Tularemia and the tomcat. J. A. M. A. *246*:1343, 1981.
51. Ewing, R., Fainstein, V., Musher, D. M., et al.: Articular and skeletal infections caused by *Pasteurella multocida*. South. Med. J. *73*:1349–1352, 1980.
52. Feder, H. M., Shanley, J. D., and Barbera, J. A.: Review of 59 patients hospitalized with animal bites. Pediatr. Infect. Dis. *6*:24–28, 1987.
53. Fiala, M., Bauer, H., Khaleeli, M., et al.: Dog bite, *Bacteroides* infection, coagulopathy, renal microangiopathy. Ann. Intern. Med. *87*:248–249, 1977.
54. Findling, J. W., Pohlmann, G. P., and Rose, H. D.: Fulminant gram-negative bacillemia (DF-2) following a dog bite in an asplenic woman. Am. J. Med. *68*:154–156, 1980.
55. Flandry, F., Lisecki, E. J., Domingue, G. J., et al.: Initial antibiotic therapy for alligator bites: Characterization of the oral flora of *Alligator mississippiensis*. South. Med. J. *82*:262–266, 1989.
56. Flowers, D. J.: Human infection due to *Mycobacterium marinum* after a dolphin bite. J. Clin. Pathol. *23*:475–477, 1970.
57. Gershman, K. A., Sacks, J. J., and Wright, J. C.: Which dogs bite? A case-control study of risk factors. Pediatrics *93*:913–917, 1994.
58. Gilbert, G. L., Cassidy, J. F., and Bennett, N. M.: Rat-bite fever. Med. J. Aust. *2*:1131–1134, 1971.
59. Gnann, J. W., Jr., Bressler, G. S., Bodet C. A., III, et al.: Human blastomycosis after a dog bite. Ann. Intern. Med. *98*:48–49, 1983.
60. Goldstein, E. J. C.: Management of human and animal bite wounds. J. Am. Acad. Dermatol. *21*:1275–1279, 1989.
61. Goldstein, E. J. C.: Bite wounds and infection. Clin. Infect. Dis. *14*:663–640, 1992.
62. Goldstein, E. J. C., and Citron, D. M.: Comparative activities of cefuroxime, amoxicillin-clavulanic acid, ciprofloxacin, enoxacin, and ofloxacin against aerobic and anaerobic bacteria isolated from bite wounds. Antimicrob. Agents Chemother. *32*:1143–1148, 1988.
63. Goldstein, E. J. C., Citron, D. M., and Finegold, S. M.: Dog bite wounds and infection: A prospective clinical study. Ann. Emerg. Med. *9*:508–512, 1980.
64. Goldstein, E. J. C., Citron, D. M., and Finegold, S. M.: Role of anaerobic bacteria in bite-wound infections. Rev. Infect. Dis. *6*:S177–S183, 1984.
65. Goldstein, E. J. C., Citron, D. M., Gonzalez, H., et al.: Bacteriology of rattlesnake venom and implications for therapy. J. Infect. Dis. *140*:818–821, 1979.
66. Goldstein, E. J. C., Citron, D. M., Wield, B., et al.: Bacteriology of human and animal bite wounds. J. Clin. Microbiol. *8*:667–672, 1978.
67. Goldstein, E. J. C., and Richwald, G. A.: Human and animal bite wounds. Am. Fam. Physician *36*:101–109, 1987.
68. Goldstein, R. W., Goodhart, G. L., and Moore, J. E.: *Pasteurella multocida* infection after animal bites. N. Engl. J. Med. *315*:460, 1986.
69. Guba, A. M., Jr., Mulliken, J. B., and Hoopes, J. E.: The selection of antibiotics for human bites of the hand. Plast. Reconstr. Surg. *56*:538–541, 1975.
70. Gump, D. W., and Holden, R. A.: Endocarditis caused by a new species of *Pasteurella*. Ann. Intern. Med. *76*:275–278, 1972.
71. Harris, D., Imperato, P. J., and Oken, B.: Dog bites: An unrecognized epidemic. Bull. N. Y. Acad. Med. *50*:981–1000, 1974.
72. Hawkins, L. G.: Local *Pasteurella multocida* infections. J. Bone Joint Surg. [Am.] *51*:363–365, 1969.
73. Hawkins, J., Paris, P. M., and Stewart, R. D.: Mammalian bites: Rational approach to management. Postgrad. Med. *73*:52–64, 1983.
74. Henderson, J. A. M., and Rowsell, H. C.: Fatal *Pasteurella multocida* pneumonia in an IgA-deficient cat fancier. West. J. Med. *150*:208–210, 1989.
75. Hennessy, P. H., and Fletcher, W.: Infection with the organisms of Vincent's angina following man-bite. Lancet *2*:127–128, 1920.
76. Hicklin, H., Verghese, A., and Alvarez, S.: Dysgonic fermenter 2 septicemia. Rev. Infect. Dis. *9*:884–890, 1987.
77. Hiemenz, J. W., Coccari, P. J., and Macher, A. M.: Human blastomycosis from dog bites. Ann. Intern. Med. *98*:1030, 1983.
78. Holloway, W. J., Scott, E. G., and Adams, Y. B.: *Pasteurella multocida* infection in man: Report of 21 cases. Am. J. Clin. Pathol. *51*:705–708, 1969.
79. Holmes, B., Steigerwalt, A. G., Weaver, R. E., et al.: *Weeksella zoohelcum* sp. nov. (formerly group II-J) from human clinical specimens. Syst. Appl. Microbiol. *8*:191–196, 1986.
80. Howard, A. J., Hughes, M., Parry, H., et al.: Dog bites and dysgonic fermenting organisms. Lancet *2*:1022–1023, 1983.
81. Hsu, H.-W., and Finberg, R. W.: Infections associated with animal exposure in two infants. Rev. Infect. Dis. *11*:108–115, 1989.
82. Hubbert, W. T., McCulloch, W. F., and Schnurrenberger, P. R. (eds.): Diseases Transmitted from Animals to Man. 6th ed. Springfield, IL, Charles C Thomas, 1975, pp. 1117–1128.
83. Jaffe, A. C.: Animal bites. Pediatr. Clin. North Am. *30*:405–413, 1983.
84. Jarvis, W. R., Banko, S., Snyder, E., et al.: *Pasteurella multocida* osteomyelitis following dog bites. Am. J. Dis. Child. *135*:625–627, 1981.
85. Jaspers, R. H.: Transmission of blastomyces from animals to man. J. Am. Vet. Med. Soc. *164*:8, 1974.
86. Job, L., Horman, J. T., Grigor, J. K., et al.: Dysgonic fermenter-2: A clinico-epidemiologic review. J. Emerg. Med. *7*:185–192, 1989.
87. Jones, A. G. H., and Lockton, J. A.: Fatal *Pasteurella multocida* septicaemia following a cat bite in a man without liver disease. J. Infect. *15*:229–235, 1987.
88. Kizer, K. W.: Epidemiologic and clinical aspects of animal bite injuries. J. Am. Coll. Emerg. Phy. *8*:134–141, 1979.
89. Kizer, K. W.: *Pasteurella multocida* infection from a cougar bite: A review of cougar attacks. West. J. Med. *150*:87–90, 1989.
90. Klein, D.: Friendly dog syndrome. N. Y. State J. Med. *66*:2306–2309, 1966.
91. Klein, D. M., and Cohen, M. E.: *Pasteurella multocida* brain abscess following perforating cranial dog bite. J. Pediatr. *92*:588–589, 1978.
92. Kurecki, B. A., III, and Brownlee, H. J., Jr.: Venomous snake bites in the United States. J. Fam. Pract. *25*:386–392, 1987.
93. Lavine, L. S., Isenberg, H. D., Rubins, W., et al.: Unusual osteomyelitis following superficial dog bite. Clin. Orthop. *98*:251–253, 1974.
94. Ledbetter, E. O., and Kutscher, A. E.: The aerobic and anaerobic flora of rattlesnake fangs and venom: Therapeutic implications. Arch. Environ. Health *19*:770–778, 1969.
95. Lee, M. L. H., and Buhr, A. J.: Dog-bites and local infection with *Pasteurella septica*. B. M. J. *1*:169–171, 1960.
96. Lowry, T. M.: The surgical treatment of human bites. Ann. Surg. *104*:1103–1111, 1936.
97. Lucas, G. L., and Bartlett, D. H.: *Pasteurella multocida* infection in the hand. Plast. Reconstr. Surg. *67*:49–53, 1981.
98. Luzzi, G. A., Milne, L. M., and Waitkins, S. A.: Rat-bite acquired leptospirosis. J. Infect. *15*:57–60, 1987.
99. Maccabe, A. F., and Conn, N.: The isolation of *Pasteurella septica* following dog and cat bites: A report of 5 cases. Scott. Med. J. *13*:242–244, 1968.
100. MacQuarrie, M. B., Forghani, B., and Wolochow, D. A.: Hepatitis B transmitted by a human bite. J. A. M. A. *230*:723–724, 1974.
101. Magee, J. S., Steele, R. W., Kelly, N. R., et al.: Tularemia transmitted by a squirrel bite. Pediatr. Infect. Dis. *8*:123–125, 1989.

102. Maimaris, C., and Quinton, D. N.: Dog-bite lacerations: A controlled trial of primary wound closure. Arch. Emerg. Med. *5*:156–161, 1988.
103. Marcy, S. M.: Special Series: Management of pediatric infectious diseases in office practice. Infections due to dog and cat bites. Pediatr. Infect. Dis. *1*:351–356, 1982.
104. Markham, R. B., and Polk, B. F.: Seal finger. Rev. Infect. Dis. *1*:567–579, 1979.
105. Marrie, T. J., Bent, J. M., West, A. B., et al.: Extensive gas in tissues of the forearm after horsebite. South. Med. J. *72*:1473–1474, 1979.
106. Martin, R. W., Martin, D. L., and Levy, C. S.: *Acinetobacter* osteomyelitis from a hamster bite. Pediatr. Infect. Dis. J. *7*:364–365, 1988.
107. Martone, W. J., Zuehl, R. W., Minson, G. E., et al.: Postsplenectomy sepsis with DF-2: Report of a case with isolation of the organism from the patient's dog. Ann. Intern. Med. *93*:457–458, 1980.
108. Mass, D. P., Newmeyer, W. L., and Kilgore, E. S., Jr: Seal finger. J. Hand Surg. *6*:610–612, 1981.
109. McMillan, B., and Boulger, L. R.: Squirrel-bite fever. Trans. R. Soc. Trop. Med. Hyg. *62*:567, 1968.
110. Meyers, B. R., Hirschman, S. Z., and Sloan, W.: Generalized Shwartzman reaction in man after a dog bite: Consumption coagulopathy, symmetrical peripheral gangrene, and renal cortical necrosis. Ann. Intern. Med. *73*:433–438, 1970.
111. Muchmore, E.: Possible cytomegalovirus infection in man following chimpanzee bite. Lab. Anim. Sci. *21*:1080–1081, 1971.
112. Mutombo, M. W., Arita, I., and JeZek, Z.: Human monkey pox transmitted by a chimpanzee in a tropical rain forest area of Zaire. Lancet *1*:735–737, 1983.
113. Oberhofer, T. R.: Characteristics and biotypes of *Pasteurella multocida* isolated from humans. J. Clin. Microbiol. *13*:566–571, 1981.
114. Orton, D. W., and Fulcher, W. H.: *Pasteurella multocida*: Bilateral septic knee joint prostheses from a distant cat bite. Ann. Emerg. Med. *13*:1065–1067, 1984.
115. Paisley, J. W., and Lauer, B. A.: Severe facial injuries to infants due to unprovoked attacks by pet ferrets. J. A. M. A. *259*:2005–2006, 1988.
116. Parrish, H. M.: Analysis of 460 fatalities from venomous animals in the United States. Am. J. Med. Sci. *245*:129–141, 1963.
117. Parrish, H. M., MacLaurin, A. W., and Tuttle, R. L.: North American pit vipers: Bacterial flora of the mouths and venom glands. Va. Med. *83*:383–385, 1956.
118. Parry, W. H., and Seymour, M. W.: An unusual case of leptospirosis. Practitioner *210*:791–793, 1973.
119. Pavia, A. T., Bryan, J. A., and Maher, K. L.: *Vibrio carchariae* infection after a shark bite. Ann. Intern. Med. *111*:85–86, 1989.
120. Peeples, C., Boswick, J. A., Jr., and Scott, F. A.: Wounds of the hand contaminated by human or animal saliva. J. Trauma *20*:383–389, 1980.
121. Peters, W. H.: Hand infection apparently due to *Bacillus fusiformis*. J. Infect. Dis. *8*:455–462, 1911.
122. Quenzer, R. W., Mostow, S. R., and Emerson, J. K.: Catbite tularemia. J. A. M. A. *238*:1845, 1977.
123. Richman, K. M., and Rickman, L. S.: The potential for transmission of human immunodeficiency virus through human bites. J. Acquir. Immune Defic. Syndr. Hum. Retrovirol. *6*:402–406, 1993.
124. Robertson, M. G.: *Brucella* infection transmitted by dog bite. J. A. M. A. *225*:750–751, 1973.
125. Rodeheaver, G. T., Kurtz, L., Kircher, B. J., et al.: Pluronic F-68: A promising new skin wound cleanser. Ann. Emerg. Med. *9*:572–576, 1980.
126. Russell, F. E.: Venomous animal injuries. Curr. Probl. Pediatr. *3*:1–47, 1973.
127. Russell, F. E.: Snake venom poisoning in the United States. Ann. Rev. Med. *31*:247–259, 1980.
128. Sacks, J. J., Sattin, R. W., and Bonzo, S. E.: Dog bite–related fatalities from 1979 through 1988. J. A. M. A. *262*:1489–1492, 1989.
129. Sannella, N. A., Tavano, P., McGoldrick, D. A., et al.: Aortic graft sepsis caused by *Pasteurella multocida*. J. Vasc. Surg. *5*:887–888, 1987.
130. Shankar, P. S., Scott, J. H., and Anderson, C. L.: Atypical endocarditis due to gram-negative bacillus transmitted by dog bite. South. Med. J. *73*:1640–1641, 1980.
131. Shirley, L. R., and Ross, S. A.: Risk of transmission of human immunodeficiency virus by bite of an infected toddler. J. Pediatr. *114*:425–427, 1989.
132. Spence, G.: A review of animal bites in Delaware, 1989 to 1990. Del. Med. J. *62*:1425–1429, 1990.
133. Spencer, R. D., Matta, H., Ferguson, D. G., et al.: Routine culture of dog bites. Ann. Emerg. Med. *16*:730, 1987.
134. Stevens, D. L., Higbee, J. W., Oberhofer, T. R., et al.: Antibiotic susceptibilities of human isolates of *Pasteurella multocida*. Antimicrob. Agents Chemother. *16*:322–324, 1979.
135. Stevenson, T. R., Thacker, J. G., Rodeheaver, G. T., et al.: Cleansing the traumatic wound by high pressure syringe irrigation. J. Am. Coll. Emerg. Phys. *5*:17–21, 1976.
136. Strassburg, M. A., Greenland, S., Marron, J. A., et al.: Animal bites: Patterns of treatment. Ann. Emerg. Med. *10*:193–197, 1981.
137. Swartz, M. N., and Kunz, L. J.: *Pasteurella multocida* infections in man. Report of two cases: Meningitis and infected cat bite. N. Engl. J. Med. *261*:889–893, 1959.
138. Talan, D. A., Staatz, D., Staatz, A., et al.: *Staphylococcus intermedius* in canine gingiva and canine-inflicted human wound infections: Laboratory characterization of a newly recognized zoonotic pathogen. J. Clin. Microbiol. *27*:78–81, 1989.
139. Thomas, J. G., Jr., and Harlan, H. J.: Vampire bat bites seen in humans in Panama: Their characterization, recognition, and management. Milit. Med. *146*:410–412, 1981.
140. Thomson, H. G., and Svitek, V.: Small animal bites: The role of primary closure. J. Trauma *13*:20–23, 1973.
141. Tindall, J. P., and Harrison, C. M.: *Pasteurella multocida* infections following animal injuries, especially cat bites. Arch. Dermatol. *105*:412–416, 1972.
142. Treatment of snakebite in the USA. Med. Lett. Drugs Ther. *24*:87–89, 1982.
143. Trott, A.: Care of mammalian bites. Pediatr. Infect. Dis. *6*:8–10, 1987.
144. Underman, A. E.: Bite wounds inflicted by dogs and cats. Vet. Clin. North Am. *17*:195–207, 1987.
145. Weber, D. J., and Hansen, A. R.: Infections resulting from animal bites. Infect. Dis. Clin. North Am. *5*:663–680, 1991.
146. Welch, C. E.: Human bite infections of the hand. N. Engl. J. Med. *215*:901–908, 1936.
147. Wiggins, M. E., Akelman, E., and Weiss, A.-P. C.: The management of dog bites and dog bite infections to the hand. Orthopedics *17*:617–623, 1994.
148. Wilberger, J. E., Jr., and Pang, D.: Craniocerebral injuries from dog bites. J. A. M. A. *249*:2685–2688, 1983.
149. Wilkins, E. G. L., Millar, J. G. B., Cockcroft, P. M., et al.: Rat-bite fever in a gerbil breeder. J. Infect. *16*:177–180, 1988.
150. Williams, F. E., Freeman, M., Kennedy, E.: The bacterial flora of the mouths of Australian venomous snakes in captivity. Med. J. Aust. *2*:190–193, 1934.
151. Williams, E.: Septicaemia caused by an organism resembling *Pasteurella septica* after a dog-bite. B. M. J. *2*:169–171, 1960.
152. Yokoyama, T., Hara, S., Funakubo, H., et al.: *Pasteurella multocida* endophthalmitis after a cat bite. Ophthalmic Surg. *18*:520–522, 1987.
153. Zumla, A., Lipscomb, G., Corbett, M., et al.: Dysgonic fermenter-type 2: An emerging zoonosis: Report of two cases and review. Q. J. Med. *257*(New Series 68):741–752, 1988.

PART 7

GUIDES TO THE DIAGNOSIS OF INFECTION

243

Use of the Bacteriology, Mycology, and Parasitology Laboratories

Sheldon L. Kaplan and Edward O. Mason, Jr.

An efficient and proficient bacteriology laboratory is of preeminent importance in the care of patients with infection. Well-trained personnel and a laboratory supervisor or director with expertise in microbiology, mycology, and serology are more important than expensive equipment and a large armamentarium of tests and services. The laboratory should strive continually to meet the needs of patients and physicians by producing prompt and accurate data. This goal requires cooperation and communication between the physician and laboratory personnel.

SPECIMEN COLLECTION

The physician, after evaluating the clinical and epidemiologic circumstances of a given infection, usually suspects various etiologic possibilities. Appropriate cultures should be obtained and submitted promptly to the laboratory along with relevant clinical and epidemiologic data.

Whenever possible, specimens should be obtained before the initiation of antibiotic therapy and directly from the site of infection, even if an invasive procedure, needle aspiration, or surgical drainage is required. Surface cultures obtained from the general area of a deep infection seldom are helpful. For example, throat and nasopharyngeal cultures are of no real value in establishing the etiologic agent of otitis media or sinusitis, and sinus tract isolates may not reflect the primary etiologic agent of osteomyelitis or deep-seated abscesses.

When the transport of specimens to the laboratory could be delayed, carrier media should be employed. If unusual or fastidious microorganisms are suspected, the laboratory should be notified in advance so that appropriate materials or media can be made available for specimen collection, for example, Thayer-Martin medium for gonococci or prereduced media for anaerobes.

The attending physician as well as the laboratory director must insist that specimens submitted to the laboratory be of sufficient quality and quantity for adequate evaluation. Sputum specimens that do not contain purulent material should not be processed. The time of collection of clean voided urine specimens should be recorded so that if their arrival at the laboratory is delayed unduly, repeat specimens can be requested. In most instances, stool specimens are preferable to rectal swabs for isolation of enteric pathogens. If purulent material is drained or aspirated, a volume of the material should be submitted rather than swab specimens. Surgical specimens should be submitted in sterile bottles without fixative. In some instances, it is preferable for the attending physician or laboratory director to obtain cultures personally and to transport them to the laboratory. If an unusual microorganism is suspected, the laboratory should be notified so that the specimen can be placed on appropriate media (e.g., cysteine nutrient agar of *Francisella tularensis).*

SPECIMEN INSPECTION AND STAINING

Laboratory personnel should inspect specimens carefully before proceeding with culturing and staining. Sputum specimens must contain purulent material. Stool specimens should be inspected for gross evidence of blood, mucus, and pus. Body fluids should be examined for turbidity. Purulent material and exudates should be inspected for color, consistency, odor, and evidence of granules (e.g., sulfur granules).

Gram Stain, Procedure, and Interpretation

The Gram-stained smear probably is the single most important laboratory procedure in infectious disease diagnosis. Virtually all clinical specimens should be Gram stained as a routine part of the laboratory evaluation. This procedure serves three functions: (1) it further documents the quality of the specimen, (2) it alerts laboratory personnel to the presence of microorganisms that might require special media for isolation, and (3) it provides the physician with clues about the etiologic agent so that initial antibiotic therapy can be selected intelligently.

The specimen is applied to a clean, glass microscope slide with a loop or swab and allowed to air-dry. It then is heat-fixed by passage once or twice through a burner flame. Overheating must be avoided because it causes morphologic distortion of bacteria and cellular elements and may cause crystallization of the dye, obscuring interpretation. One or two extra slides should be prepared and saved to be available for staining if the initial procedure is inadequate technically.

A variety of Gram-staining methods have been described. An adequate procedure is:

1. Air-dry and *lightly* heat-fix.
2. Flood slide with crystal violet. Allow to stand 30 seconds.
3. Wash with tap water.
4. Flood slide with iodine. Allow to stand 30 seconds.
5. Wash with tap water.
6. Destain with acetone-alcohol mixture until dye ceases to run from the edge of a thin part of the specimen.
7. Wash with tap water.
8. Counterstain with safranin for 30 seconds.
9. Wash with tap water and blot dry.

Interpretation of the Gram-stained smear requires some skill and practice. When the procedure is performed properly, background material and cellular elements stain red or pink. If they stain blue or purple, the smear has not been decolorized adequately. If microorganisms that morphologically resemble staphylococci or streptococci stain red rather than dark blue, the smear probably has been over-decolorized. Bizarre morphologic forms may result from too much heat fixation as well as from prior antibiotic therapy.

Interpretation of the Gram-stained smear includes noting the quantity and characteristics of cellular elements, estimating the overall number of microorganisms, and judging the predominant microorganism. Gram-positive bacteria are seen easily, and one must take care to search the background for gram-negative organisms, especially intracellular organisms.

However, the Gram stain can be misinterpreted by inexperienced observers; a common error is to think that deposits of crystal violet are gram-positive cocci. False-positive results also may be due to contaminating viable or nonviable microorganisms in the materials used for the procedure or in specimen tubes. Morphologic terms should be used to describe what is seen on the smear instead of attempting species designations. It is impossible to distinguish among *Streptococcus* species, between *Staphylococcus aureus* and *S. epidermidis*, among *Neisseria* species, and among various gram-negative enteric bacteria on the Gram-stained smear. If the initial smear reveals no bacteria, it is helpful to centrifuge the specimen and stain a thick smear of the sediment.

The Gram stain remains one of the most important techniques by which to identify a bacterial pathogen rapidly in a patient specimen. Although the Gram stain does not provide definite proof that a particular microorganism is present, when the technique is performed and interpreted properly, the probable causative agent is demonstrated in many cases. This particularly is true for the examination of cerebrospinal fluid in children with bacterial meningitis. For instance, in *Streptococcus pneumoniae* meningitis, the cerebrospinal fluid Gram stain is reported positive in up to 79 per cent of patients in most studies.[79, 89]

The greater the density of microorganisms in the cerebrospinal fluid (>10^5 colony-forming units [CFU]/mL), the more likely that the Gram stain is positive. Prior antimicrobial therapy may decrease the cerebrospinal fluid density of *Haemophilus influenzae* type b or *Neisseria meningitidis* and, thus, render the Gram stain negative.[44] There also is a tendency for gram-positive organisms to appear gram-negative in selected cases in which antibiotics have been administered before lumbar puncture.

Gram stain of urine can detect significant bacteriuria rapidly, with approximately 90 per cent accuracy. Two or more gram-negative rods per high-power field of unspun urine are associated with quantitative urine cultures exceeding 10^5 CFU/mL.[48]

Typical morphologic features of *Campylobacter* (slender curved rods, "sea gull" or "equivalent sign" appearance) may be observed in stool specimens by Gram or carbolfuchsin stain.[154] Gram-stain of undiluted blood drawn back through a central catheter may permit a presumptive diagnosis of catheter-related sepsis.[106] These are just a few examples of how the Gram stain can provide valuable information inexpensively and rapidly.

Acridine Orange Stain

Acridine orange is a fluorochrome that stains the nucleic acids of bacteria, other microorganisms, and background material in clinical specimens, and this stain can be an important aid for rapidly discerning the presence of bacteria in specimens in low numbers. The stain is simple and rapid but requires the use of a fluorescent microscope. In practice, the specimen is scanned at low power, and the presence of brightly fluorescing bacteria is seen easily against the yellow to pale-green appearance of human cells under a fluorescent microscope. The shape but not the Gram stain reaction then is confirmed at higher magnification. The procedure especially is useful when the specimen background is high, as often is encountered with gram-negative bacteria in low numbers in thick exudates or in blood-culture bottles. Also, intracellular bacteria are detected more readily by acridine orange than by Gram stain. Kleiman and associates[85] noted that the acridine orange stain was superior to the Gram stain in detecting bacteria in cerebrospinal fluid, including specimens collected from children who had been receiving antibiotics. The acridine orange stain especially is valuable for examining clinical specimens that are negative by Gram stain. The acridine orange stain also has proved valuable in detecting bacteria in buffy coats in neonates with septicemia.[84] As with the Gram stain technique, experience in the interpretation of the acridine orange stain is required for an accurate result.

Acid-Fast Stain, Procedure, and Interpretation

Acid-fast stains of sputum or cerebrospinal fluid should be performed if pulmonary tuberculosis or tuberculous meningitis is suspected. Because gastric contents and urine often are contaminated by saprophytic mycobacteria, acid-fast smears of these specimens are of little value. The procedure for the Ziehl-Neelsen acid-fast stain is as follows:

1. Cover the smear with filter paper and flood the slide with carbolfuchsin.
2. Steam (do not boil) the slide for 5 minutes, adding more carbolfuchsin as necessary.
3. Rinse the slide with a gentle stream of tap water.
4. Decolorize with acid alcohol until no more color appears in the washings; rinse with tap water.
5. Counterstain with aqueous methylene blue for 30 seconds, rinse with tap water, and air dry.

Mycobacterium species and *Nocardia* species stain red, whereas other organisms and background material stain blue. *Mycobacterium* species sometimes have a beaded appearance, and *Nocardia* species often stain unevenly.[9] For *Nocardia*, destaining with acid alcohol should *not* exceed 5 to 10 seconds; as an alternative, 2 per cent sulfuric acid should be used in place of acid alcohol and allowed to stand on the smear for 1 minute. The laboratory always should be informed of the suspicion of *Nocardia* infection when stains are requested, and the physician should be assured that the proper destaining procedure was used if the acid-fast stain is reported as negative and the clinical picture is one of *Nocardia* infection.

Many laboratories use fluorescence microscopy with auramine-rhodamine stain for the detection of *Mycobacterium* species in clinical specimens because of the ease and speed of the technique.

Microscopic Examination for Fungi

Unfixed specimens of pus, sputum, or tissue scrapings may be examined as a wet mount in a drop of 10 per cent potassium hydroxide. This procedure cleans the specimen, leaving the more resistant fungal structures intact. Caution is necessary to avoid confusing artifacts with fungi; however, the procedure may give the physician rapid presumptive information.

Specimens from suspected fungal infections also should be fixed and stained with procedures that distinguish fungi specifically. The hematoxylin and eosin stain is not suitable as a fungal stain, although careful examination may demonstrate hyphal elements in tissues. More suitable fungal stains are the periodic acid–Schiff stain and Gomori methenamine silver stain. The former stains fungal elements purple-red; the latter stains them black. One or both should be requested when fungal disease is suspected.

Calcofluor white specifically binds to chitin or cellulose and is brightly fluorescent when viewed by ultraviolet light, which makes the stain useful for detecting fungi in tissues and wet mount specimens.[60] It can be used with 10 per cent potassium hydroxide to view yeasts and hyphal elements in skin scrapings. Another advantage is that it can be used on specimens previously stained by the periodic acid–Schiff or methenamine silver techniques if those stains require confirmation.

COUNTERCURRENT IMMUNOELECTROPHORESIS

Countercurrent immunoelectrophoresis demonstrates bacterial antigens most successfully in the rapid detection of the capsular polysaccharides of *H. influenzae* type b, *S. pneumoniae, N. meningitidis,* and group B *Streptococcus.* Countercurrent immunoelectrophoresis is predicated on the principle that when placed in agar of correct pH and ionic strength, polysaccharide antigens are charged negatively and antibodies are charged less negatively. When an electric current is passed through the agar, the antigen migrates toward the anode and the antibody diffuses to the cathode by endosmosis (carried along by buffer ions). If an antibody is directed against an antigen, a line of precipitation forms between the antibody- and antigen-containing wells. This technique has been replaced by latex agglutination in most laboratories.

LATEX AGGLUTINATION

Latex agglutination is a popular technique for detecting antigens from many microorganisms because of the ease and speed of the method and its greater sensitivity than that of countercurrent immunoelectrophoresis, as well as the fact that additional laboratory equipment is unnecessary. A number of latex agglutination kits are commercially available either in a combination form or for individual antigens. Antiserum to specific antigen is adsorbed onto latex particles of uniform diameter, usually 0.8 μm. After washing, the coated latex particles are resuspended to a proper dilution. Control latex particles are prepared similarly, but serum from an unimmunized animal (same species from which the specific antiserum was obtained) is used. When the antigen to which the antiserum is directed on the latex particles is added to the latex particles, visible agglutination of latex particles occurs. Control latex particles should not agglutinate. Both positive and negative control specimens should be included with each patient specimen. Sera containing rheumatoid factor are associated with false-positive latex agglutination tests. The optimal fluid for latex agglutination testing is cerebrospinal fluid because nonspecific agglutination of latex particles is rare with cerebrospinal fluid. However, urine and sera have been associated with nonspecific agglutination, noted by agglutination of the control latex particles, which prevents interpretation of the test. In addition, agglutination of more than one type of antiserum may occur and also results in an uninterpretable test. Heating and diluting sera and urine avoid some of these nonspecific reactions, and the manufacturers of the commercial latex agglutination kits recommend various means by which to avoid nonspecific reactions for their products. It is important to note that filtration of urine through polysulfone, but not nitrocellulose or cellulose acetate, may be associated with false-positive latex agglutination for *H. influenzae* type b.[187]

Latex agglutination has been found to be a sensitive method by which to detect *H. influenzae* type b, *S. pneumoniae, N. meningitidis,* group B *Streptococcus,* and *Cryptococcus neoformans* in cerebrospinal fluid. Latex particles coated with either monoclonal (Directogen, Hynson, Westcott and Dunning, Baltimore, MD) or equine (Bactigen, Wampole Laboratories, Cranbury, NJ) antisera to *N. meningitidis* group B are commercially available, but experience with the group B serotype is not extensive, and further study is necessary before the reliability of these reagents is known. In almost all of the comparative studies, latex agglutination is superior to countercurrent immunoelectrophoresis for detecting the capsular polysaccharide antigen of the three major meningeal pathogens in cerebrospinal fluid. In an infant primate model, Scheifele and associates[151] consistently found positive latex agglutination tests with as few as 10^2 CFU/mL of *H. influenzae* type b and antigenemia was detected significantly earlier ($p < .001$) by latex agglutination than by countercurrent immunoelectrophoresis. Latex agglutination revealed antigen in all cerebrospinal fluid specimens greater than or equal to 10^3 CFU/mL and in five of seven with 10^2 CFU/mL. Sensitivity of latex agglutination for purified group B streptococcal polysaccharide is 63 ng/mL, compared with 500 ng/mL for countercurrent immunoelectrophoresis.[5]

Latex agglutination tests for *C. difficile* (actually detect glutamate dehydrogenase produced by toxigenic and nontoxigenic *C. difficile*) are not sufficiently sensitive to be used alone.[128]

COAGGLUTINATION OF *STAPHYLOCOCCUS AUREUS*

The Cowan strain of *S. aureus* contains in its outer-membrane protein A, which binds the Fc portion of IgG, thus leaving the Fab fragment free to bind with antigen. In the presence of homologous antigen, antibody-coated *S. aureus* visibly agglutinates. *S. aureus* protein A coagglutination requires the same controls as latex agglutination does—that is, *S. aureus* coated with normal sera from the same animal used to develop specific antisera to serve as a control suspension as well as positive and negative control specimens. As with latex agglutination, coagglutination has been evaluated mainly for detecting antigen in the cerebrospinal fluid for the major pathogens causing bacterial meningitis in children. Nonspecific agglutination with uninterpretable tests also occurs with the coagglutination test.

SELECTED STUDIES USED IN THE DIAGNOSIS OF MENINGITIS

Tables 243–1 through 243–4 compare selected studies using the techniques described in the preceding sections for the detection of the three major meningeal pathogens in cerebrospinal fluid. In general, latex agglutination is more sensitive than is countercurrent immunoelectrophoresis. With all these methods, urine is an excellent source for antigen detection and may give positive results when the cerebrospinal fluid and sera results are negative. Furthermore, the urine may remain positive for several days after the initiation of large-dose antibiotics, thus allowing identification of a causative agent, even when all cultures are negative. Urine is the best antigen source for bacteremic nonmeningitis infections such as pneumonia, for cellulitis due to *H. influenzae* type b and *S. pneumoniae,* or for sepsis due to group B streptococci.[25, 177] However, *H. influenzae* type b capsular polysaccharide can be detected in urine by latex agglutination for several days after immunization with certain *H. influenzae* type b protein-conjugate vaccines.[100, 161] Thus, a history for recent *H. influenzae* type b immunization should be sought to exclude this possibility. Because children with anatomic or functional asplenia may develop high densities of bacteremia during

TABLE 243–1. Cerebrospinal Fluid Findings in *Haemophilus influenzae* Type b Meningitis

Author	Number of Patients	Culture +	Gram Stain +	CIE +	LPA +	Coagglutination +	Gram Stain − CIE +	Gram Stain + CIE −	Gram Stain + LPA + CIE −
Feigin et al. 1976[43]/Kaplan et al. 1984[78]	218	209	185/216 (86%)	178/209 (85%)		—	18	19	8
Olcen 1978[120]	30	30	25	24		20			
Dirks-Go and Zanen 1978[30]	60	60	—	55	64	34			
Colding and Lind 1977[23]	30	30	25	23			1	3	
Wasilauskas and Hampton 1982[183]	17	17	17	15	—	17	0	2	
Bortolussi et al. 1982[15]	—	—	19/25	19/23	26/29				
Ingram et al. 1983[73]	—	39	35/38	32	32 Bactogen 36 Wellcogen				
Tilton et al. 1984[175]	18	17	—	17	14/18 Directogen 14/14 Bactogen				

+, positive; −, negative.
CIE, countercurrent immunoelectrophoresis; LPA, latex particle agglutination.

TABLE 243–2. Cerebrospinal Fluid Findings in *Streptococcus pneumoniae* Meningitis

Author	Number of Patients	Culture +	Gram Stain +	CIE +	LA +	Coagglutination +	Gram Stain − CIE +	Gram Stain + CIE −
Kaplan 1983[79]	35	32	28/34	20/33	—	—	0	7
Olcen 1978[120]	15	14	13	8	—	—	—	—
Dirks-Go and Zanen 1978[30]	73	73	—	47	57	54	—	—
Colding and Lind 1977[23]	32	32	29	14	—	—	2	16
Wasilauskas and Hampton 1982[183]	11	10	8	7	—	11	—	—
Ingram et al. 1983[73]	—	16	12/14	9	11	4	—	—
Drow et al. 1983[33]	—	28	—	16	—	16	—	—
Tilton et al. 1984[175]	7	6	—	5/7	7/7	6/7	—	—

+, positive, −, negative.
CIE, countercurrent immunoelectrophoresis; LA, latex agglutination.

TABLE 243–3. Cerebrospinal Fluid Findings in *Neisseria meningitidis* Meningitis

Author	Number of Patients	Culture +	Gram Stain +	CIE +	LA +	Coagglutination +	Gram Stain − CIE +	Gram Stain + CIE −
Kaplan 1983[79]	26	23	15	8/25	—	—	2	8
Olcen 1978[120]	30	25	18	9	—	10	—	—
Dirks-Go and Zanen 1978[30]	68	68	—	50	48	33	—	—
Colding and Lind 1977[23]	64	64	50	35	—	—	2	17
Bortolussi et al. 1982[15]	—	—	10/11	7/10	11/11	—	—	—
Ingram et al. 1983[73]	—	19	10/12	6/17	13	—	—	—
Drow et al. 1983[33]	—	22	—	8	—	13 (3/9 for group B)	—	—
Tilton et al. 1984[175]	9	9	—	4	7 4/5+ Directogen for group B 4/6+ Bactogen for group B	4/8 for group B		

+, positive; − negative.
CIE, countercurrent immunoelectrophoresis; LA, latex agglutination.

TABLE 243–4. Cerebrospinal Fluid Findings in Group B Streptococcal Meningitis

Author	Number of Patients or Specimen	Culture +	Gram Stain +	CIE +	LA +	Coagglutination +	Gram Stain − CIE +	Gram Stain + CIE −	False-Positive
Edwards et al. 1979[36]	12	12 11/26	—	11	12 14/26 subsequent samples	—			One CSF w/*S. pneumoniae* + by LA
Stechenberg et al. 1979[164]	27	27	—	17	—	—		3	
Webb and Baker 1980[185]	28	28	—	23	22	—			
Webb et al. 1980[186]	23	23	—	20	—	19			
Baker et al. 1980[6]	26	24	25	23	—	—			
Baker and Rench 1983[5]	24	24	—	21	22	—			

+, positive; −, negative.
CIE, countercurrent immunoelectrophoresis; CSF, cerebrospinal fluid; LA, latex agglutination.

overwhelming sepsis, these immunologic techniques may detect antigen in sera from such patients.

The routine use of rapid antigen-detection techniques for cerebrospinal fluid from children with suspected bacterial meningitis is not warranted, although in selected circumstances this test can be useful.[104] If a child with bacterial meningitis has been treated with an oral or parenteral agent prior to a lumbar puncture, in some patients the Gram stain and culture of the cerebrospinal fluid may be negative for the causative pathogen. In children who are severely ill and too unstable for a lumbar puncture, several days of parenteral antibiotics are likely to render the cerebrospinal fluid sterile on culture. In such cases, antigen detection can be helpful. However, in the vast majority of children with suspected bacterial meningitis, the initial antibiotic therapy is not influenced or changed as a result of an antigen-detection test.

ANTIGEN QUANTITATION

The presence or quantity of antigen in sera or cerebrospinal fluid of patients with bacterial meningitis correlates with severity of illness and prognosis. In patients with meningitis due to group A *N. meningitidis*, positive serum countercurrent immunoelectrophoresis was associated with a greater incidence of petechiae and neurologic sequelae.[58, 192] In another study, Hoffman and Edwards[69] noted that high concentrations of group C meningococcal antigen in cerebrospinal fluid were associated with prolonged coma and clinical evidence of markedly increased intracranial pressure. In addition, decreased platelet counts, fibrinogen, complement, and prolongation of prothrombin and partial thromboplastin times were more common in patients with detectable antigen in serum.

H. influenzae type b meningitis has been studied the most carefully in terms of quantitation of antigen and prognosis. In two prospective studies of *H. influenzae* type b meningitis, children with greater than 1.28 μg/mL of polyribosylribitol phosphate antigen in the cerebrospinal fluid specimen obtained on admission had a significantly increased incidence ($X^2 = 18.7$; $p < .00002$) of neurologic sequelae or death, compared with children with lower values.[78, 79]

Stechenberg and associates[164] noted that the mortality rate associated with group B streptococcal infections was significantly higher ($p < .001$) in infants with positive than in those with negative serum countercurrent immunoelectrophoresis. Baker and associates[6] found that in neonates with meningitis due to group B *Streptococcus*, antigen concentration in admission cerebrospinal fluid was significantly less ($p < .05$) in patients with normal developmental and neurologic examinations than in infants who were abnormal neurologically or who died.

In patients with cryptococcal meningitis, the titer of cryptococcal antigen by latex agglutination in cerebrospinal fluid or serum may provide prognostic information. Diamond and Bennett[29] found that patients who died with active disease during therapy had significantly higher titers ($p < .001$) of cryptococcal antigen in cerebrospinal fluid and serum than did patients who were cured. Furthermore, a high antigen titer in cerebrospinal fluid at the beginning of therapy as well as a failure of a positive antigen titer to decrease or turn negative was correlated with treatment failure. Similarly, Bennett and associates,[11] in a large, collaborative study, noted that the geometric mean cryptococcal antigen titer in cerebrospinal fluid was higher in unsuccessfully treated patients than in improved or cured patients at the beginning of therapy (1:676 vs. 1:95; $p < .01$) and at the completion of treatment (1:137 vs. 1:12; $p < .02$).

ENZYME IMMUNOASSAYS

Enzyme immunoassay has been developed for the detection of a wide variety of microbial antigens in clinical material, although it currently is in use in clinical microbiology laboratories for the detection of only a few selected bacteria. The advantages of enzyme immunoassay include (1) sensitivity with in vitro standards that is superior to other immunologic techniques (however, this may not translate into superior performance with clinical specimens), (2) use of diluted reagents that are relatively cheap (expensive equipment and radioactive material are unnecessary), and (3) the ability to be automated.

Most types of enzyme-linked immunosorbent assays are the direct or indirect variety and are based on the fact that when an antibody and enzyme are linked covalently, their respective immunologic and enzymatic activities are retained. Enzyme-linked immunosorbent assay takes advantage of the ability of a single enzyme molecule to catalyze the alteration of many molecules of substrate, which can intensify an antibody-antigen reaction.[199] Antibody to a specific antigen is bound to a solid phase, such as a polyvinyl microtitration plate or plastic bead, usually by absorption. Unbound antibody is removed, and the solid phase either can be used immediately or can be stored until needed. The clinical specimen containing the microbial antigen is placed in the well and incubated for a variable period, during which antigen is bound to the solid-phase antibody. The wells are washed, and in the direct enzyme-linked immunosorbent assay, an enzyme-labeled antibody to the same antigen is applied. With the indirect method, unlabeled antibody from an animal species different from the solid-phase antibody is applied. Then enzyme-linked antibody directed against the globulin of the second antibody is applied. The plates are washed, and the substrate for the enzyme is added. The substrate is catalyzed by the linked enzymes, and the rate of reaction, usually monitored by a color change, depends on the amount of enzyme-labeled antibody, which is related directly to the quantity of antigen in the clinical specimen. The color change can be read visually or quantitated with a spectrophotometer. The indirect technique avoids the need for a separate enzyme-linked antibody for each antigen and is somewhat more sensitive than is the direct method, but it adds another step to the procedure. Alkaline phosphatase and horse-radish peroxidase are just two of the enzymes that are suitable for enzyme-linked immunosorbent assay. Membrane-bound antigen capture simplifies these techniques, which can be performed in minutes in a self-contained disposable device. In an excellent review, Yolken[199] described the different variations of enzyme immunoassay that are intended to increase the sensitivity and specificity as well as decrease the time restraints of enzyme immunoassay.

Selected antigens for which enzyme-linked immunosorbent assay has been described are outlined in Table 243–5. Perhaps the enzyme-linked immunosorbent assay technique will have its greatest application for the rapid detection of viral and fungal infections.[138] Enzyme immunoassay for bacterial detection are commercially available for *N. gonorrhoeae, Chlamydia trachomatis,* and group A *Streptococcus.*

IMMUNOFLUORESCENCE

Immunofluorescent techniques have been employed for several years for the rapid detection of viral and bacterial infections. This procedure requires high-quality antisera, fluorescein conjugates, a fluorescent microscope, and, most important, an experienced microscopist in order for reliable and reproducible results to be achieved. The immunofluorescence procedure is not well suited for large volumes of specimens but has been used successfully in both clinical and research laboratories for rapid diagnosis of selected bacterial pathogens.

Bordetella pertussis infection can be diagnosed tentatively by immunofluorescence procedures rapidly on nasopharyngeal swabs.[101] However, as with any immunofluorescence technique, the source of antibody and the experience of the observer greatly influence the reliability of the results. In many instances, the immunofluorescence test result is positive but cultures are negative for *B. pertussis* in children with suspected whooping cough. Unfortunately, *B. pertussis* may be difficult to isolate, even when a nasopharyngeal swab is streaked immediately on appropriate media at the patient's bedside.

Fluorescent-antibody stains of sputum, pleural fluid, or lung tissue for *Legionella pneumophila* or skin biopsy material for *Rickettsia rickettsii* have been applied successfully to the diagnosis of these infections in children.[17, 46] Immunofluorescent stains have been developed for rapid identification of *Pneumocystis carinii,*[174] *Escherichia coli* 0157:H7,[125] and *Shigella dysenteriae.*[1]

TABLE 243–5. Selected Microbial Antigens Detectable by Enzyme Immunoassay

Bacteria
Haemophilus influenzae type b[26, 127]
Streptococcus pneumoniae[58, 63, 126, 158]
Neisseria meningitidis A[158]
Neisseria gonorrhoeae[124, 129, 162]
Group A *Streptococcus*[30, 31, 73, 80]
Group B *Streptococcus*[109, 134, 159]
Mycobacterium tuberculosis[146, 184]
Staphylococcus aureus[92]
Chlamydia trachomata[99]
Vibrio cholerae 01[65]
Clostridium difficile[56]
Mycoplasma pneumoniae[102]
Escherichia coli 0157[35]
Fungi
Candida albicans[2, 93, 122, 155]
Aspergillus fumigatus[145]
Coccidioides immitis[181]
Histoplasma capsulatum[200]
Parasites
Giardia lamblia[142, 150]
Taenia solium[42]
Cryptosporidium parvum[141]
Entamoeba histocystica[195]

DNA HYBRIDIZATION

DNA technology has been applied to the rapid identification of a number of different microorganisms by detecting specific segments of microbial DNA in clinical specimens.[133, 152] This technique is based on homologous DNA-DNA binding, in which a single-stranded, cloned DNA probe generally is labeled with a radioactively labeled nucleotide. Biotin-labeled DNA probes or other nonradioactive labels avoid the use of radioactive material. Clinical specimens are treated to free nucleic acids and then placed on nitrocellulose paper and allowed to dry (dot blot). The nitrocellulose paper is incubated with the labeled probe DNA for hybridization. The paper is subjected to autoradiography to expose radiographic film for radiolabeled probes or other detector systems, depending on the label employed. DNA probes are available for *N. gonorrhoeae,*[22] *C. trachomatis,*[28, 71] *L. pneumophila,*[126] *Mycoplasma pneumoniae,*[66] and *Mycobacterium tuberculosis.*[38] *Listeria monocytogenes* also has been detected using DNA probes.[27]

POLYMERASE CHAIN REACTION

Amplifying sequences of target DNA for detecting the presence of specific microorganisms is an incredibly powerful and sensitive tool.[39, 133, 152] The techniques are well established, and the reagents and instrumentation are widely available. The one major requirement for polymerase chain reaction is the need for specific oligonucleotides to act as primers for the DNA amplification. The synthesis of these oligonucleotides requires detection of a well-characterized region of the genetic sequence of the microorganism. Oligonucleotides from a wide variety of microorganisms have been synthesized, and new applications are being introduced with extraordinary speed (Table 243–6). Because the technique is so sensitive, any slight contamination may lead to false-positive results. Thus, great care must be taken during the procedure so that foreign DNA is not introduced into the assay. Further evaluation and perhaps modification of polymerase chain reaction are necessary before it can be applied routinely in clinical practice.

TABLE 243–6. Detection of Pathogens by Polymerase Chain Reaction

Bordetella pertussis[94]
Borrelia burgdorferi[140]
Chlamydia trachomatis[122]
Enteroinvasive *Escherichia coli*[49]
Legionella pneumophila[163]
Leptospira species[8]
Mycobacterium leprae[193]
Mycobacterium tuberculosis[37]
Mycoplasma pneumoniae[13]
Neisseria meningitidis[117]
Pneumocystis carinii[21]
Rickettsia rickettsii[178]
Shigella[49]
Streptococcus pneumoniae[144]
Toxoplasma gondii[20]
Treponema pallidum[59]
Trypanosoma cruzi[110]

IDENTIFICATION-SPECIATION

Most diagnostic bacteriology laboratories now use one of the multitest systems for microbial identification, which, by a variety of methods, correctly and consistently allows rapid identification to the genus and species level. Smaller laboratories that do not or cannot provide this information routinely should have arrangements with a qualified reference laboratory capable of identification to this level. More specific identification, such as phage typing, serotyping, plasmid typing, and chromosomal restriction-enzyme analysis, seldom is necessary for the treatment of the individual patient but may be important for hospital epidemiology.[180] Thus, a system whereby isolates from significant infections, or isolates with unexpected susceptibility patterns, are retained for a reasonable amount of time in the event that further identification is required would seem a prudent practice.

Individual laboratories define significant isolates that they routinely report from nonsterile sites differently, depending on agreements reached between the laboratory director and the medical staff. In general, only group A streptococci are reported from throat cultures. If infections caused by *Corynebacterium diphtheriae* or *B. pertussis* are suspected, the physician must notify the laboratory so that appropriate culture media and identification techniques can be employed. Other similar potential sources of confusion exist and can be averted consistently through communication with the laboratory.

Bacterial taxonomy is changing continually to reflect advances in technology, which allows the more precise definition in the relationships between the genera and species of bacteria. Recently, for example, the group D streptococci were deemed sufficiently independent from the genus *Streptococcus* to be removed and placed in their own genus, *Enterococcus*. Microbiology laboratories must adjust to name changes to remain current with the identification schema, and the physician must be made aware of these changes. Examples of some changes are listed in Table 243–7.[18, 168]

SELECTED ORGANISMS OR INFECTIONS

Bacteria

Neisseria gonorrhoeae

Gram stain of a urethral discharge in a male with urethritis is highly specific (>90 per cent) and sensitive (96 to 98 per cent) for the diagnosis of *N. gonorrhoeae* infections. In females and asymptomatic males, the usefulness of the Gram stain is not as great. Several investigators have evaluated a commercially produced enzyme immunoassay for detecting *N. gonorrhoeae* antigen (Gonozyme, Abbott Laboratories). The assay can be performed in 2 hours, and urethral or endocervical specimens can be stored for as long as 30 days without affecting the results.[124, 162] Antigen can be detected in the face of negative cultures due to previous or concurrent administration of antibiotics. Stamm and associates[162] found the Gonozyme test to be 94 per cent sensitive and 98 per cent specific, compared with culture results in men, but it was no better than Gram stain in diagnosing gonorrhea. On the other hand, in women, the enzyme immunoassay was 78 per cent sensitive and 98 per cent specific, compared with cervical culture, but had a significantly better sensitivity than did cervical Gram stain (78 per cent vs. 40 per cent, $p < .001$).

Detection of *N. gonorrhoeae* by DNA probe has been reported by several groups.[22, 71] A commercially available probe assay has a sensitivity exceeding 90 per cent, which culture does not. Positive predictive values approach 90 per cent as well. This test requires about 2 hours to complete. Costs for this test may be less than for standard cultures. Because viable organisms need not be present for a positive result, DNA probe for *N. gonorrhoeae* should be the test for documenting eradication of the organism unless at least 10 days have elapsed since the treatment was administered.[22]

Group A Beta-Hemolytic Streptococcus

Throat culture is the time-honored manner by which to confirm group A streptococcal pharyngitis, despite the variables that may affect culture results.[81] Cultures require 36 to 48 hours for final identification, and the clinician frequently feels obligated to administer antibiotics before knowing culture results. Techniques for the rapid identification of group A *Streptococcus* in the throat employ nitrous acid extraction of the throat swabs followed by incubation of the extracted fluid with the test reagents. Tests that employ latex agglutination and enzyme immunoassay technology are available. Many different rapid streptococcal antigen tests are available that have been compared with blood-agar culture of throat swabs.[31, 53–55, 80] In general, the sensitivity of the rapid tests varies between 70 and 90 per cent, compared with that of blood-agar cultures. The specificity of the tests is excellent. Thus, for any of the tests, a positive result is a reliable indicator of group A streptococcal pharyngitis. However, a routine throat culture should be performed when the rapid test result is negative. Which test to use in the office or laboratory setting is an individual decision based on personal experience, cost, and need for other equipment, as well as the sensitivity and specificity of the technique. The accuracy of the test results when the test is performed by properly trained nurses is equivalent to that of laboratory technologist in a pediatric satellite laboratory setting.[32] A commercially produced chemiluminescent DNA probe for group A *Streptococcus* appears to be more sensitive than the other rapid detection tests but is more time-consuming and labor-intensive.[67]

Group B Streptococcus

Latex agglutination tests for group B *Streptococcus* are most useful in the cerebrospinal fluid of babies with suspected meningitis but in most instances do not influence the selection of the initial empiric antibiotics. If the cerebrospinal fluid culture is negative because of prior parenteral therapy,

TABLE 243–7. Bacterial Name Changes

New Terminology	Older Terminology
Enterococcus faecalis	*Streptococcus faecalis*
Enterococcus faecium	*Streptococcus faecium*
Gardnerella vaginalis	*Haemophilus vaginalis*
Helicobacter pylori	*Campylobacter pylori*
Branhamella catarrhalis	*Moraxella catarrhalis*
	Neisseria catarrhalis
Morganelli morgani	*Proteus morgani*
Pantoea agglomerans	*Enterobacter agglomerans*
Plesiomonas shigelloides	*Aeromonas shigelloides*
Prevotella melaninogenicus	*Bacteroides melaninogenicus*
Staphylococcus saprophyticus	*Micrococcus*
Pediococcus equinus	*Streptococcus equinus*
Streptococcus adjacens	Nutritionally variant streptococci
Streptococcus defectivus	Nutritionally variant streptococci
Actinomyces pyogenes	*Corynebacterium pyogenes*
Arcanobacterium haemolyticum	*Corynebacterium haemolyticum*
Corynebacterium jeikeium	*Corynebacterium* group JK
	CDC group JK
Agrobacterium tumefaciens	*Agrobacterium radiobacter*
Burkholderia cepacia	*Pseudomonas cepacia*
Burkholderia mallei	*Pseudomonas mallei*
Burkholderia pickettii	*Pseudomonas pickettii*
Burkholderia pseudomallei	*Pseudomonas pseudomallei*
Chryseobacterium meningosepticum	*Flavobacterium meningosepticum*
Comamonas acidovorans	*Pseudomonas acidovorans*
Stenotrophomonas maltophilia	*Xanthomonas maltophilia*
	Pseudomonas maltophilia

antigen detection may be the only method by which an etiologic diagnosis is established.

One of the most difficult problems is determining the clinical significance of a latex agglutination test result positive for group B *Streptococcus* in the urine of a baby with negative blood cultures, cerebrospinal fluid cultures, or both.[50, 136] In some neonates, this may be due to cross-reacting bacteria, such as group G *Streptococcus* causing sepsis, or prior treatment of the mother that has led to sterile cultures in the newborn.[64] In others, perineal colonization or contamination of urine specimens with group B *Streptococcus* may explain the "false-positive" latex agglutination results.[148] In experimental animals, ingestion of group B streptococci can result in positive latex agglutination reactions in the urine, suggesting gastrointestinal absorption of the antigen.[3] For some babies, no reason for the false-positive test can be identified. Some investigators suggest repeating the latex agglutination test with use of urine collected under sterile conditions; if the test still is positive, true antigenuria is suggested. Interpretation of a positive group B *Streptococcus* latex agglutination test in the urine of a baby with negative cultures relies on the clinical judgment of the physician, who must account for all the known data regarding the baby and not just the latex agglutination test results.

Group B streptococcal antigen-detection tests cannot be used as the exclusive means to screen for group B streptococcal carriage of the genital tract of women at delivery. "Heavily colonized" women are more likely to be identified[157, 198] than women colonized with a low concentration of group B streptococci. The role of group B streptococcal rapid antigen tests in the strategies for preventing early-onset group B streptococcal infection in the neonate has been outlined by the American Academy of Pediatrics.[24]

Mycobacterium tuberculosis

The diagnosis of tuberculous meningitis in children frequently is based on typical cerebrospinal fluid (pleocytosis, mononuclear predominance, depressed glucose concentrations) and clinical findings. In many instances, an acid-fast stain and culture of cerebrospinal fluid are negative or the culture does not become positive until many weeks after therapy has been initiated. A rapid method for detecting mycobacterial antigens in cerebrospinal fluid could be extremely beneficial when one encounters a child in whom tuberculous meningitis is suspected. Enzyme-linked immunosorbent assay and other techniques to detect mycobacterial antigen in cerebrospinal fluid have not proved satisfactory. Adenosine deaminase activity may be increased in the cerebrospinal fluid of patients with tuberculous meningitis, but this is not a specific test.

Numerous laboratories have described polymerase chain reaction assays for diagnosis of tuberculosis from sputum specimens.[47, 118, 149] The sensitivity, specificity, false-positive, and false-negative rates are not known, and these tests are not approved yet for commercial diagnostic evaluation.[107] In pediatrics, the value of polymerase chain reaction for *M. tuberculosis* from gastric aspirates is unknown. Several laboratories using different polymerase chain reaction strategies and DNA sequences for probes have reported the detection of *M. tuberculosis* products in cerebrospinal fluid from patients with tuberculosis meningitis.[90, 96] This application would be a valuable addition to routine diagnostic studies for rapid diagnosis because only a minority of children with tuberculosis meningitis have positive acid-fast bacteria stains of cerebrospinal fluid.

Urinary Tract Infections

Since the 1980s, automated methods have been available to detect bacteriuria more quickly and perhaps more cheaply than with the conventional agar plate culture technique.[130, 131] In several studies, urine specimens with 10^5 CFU/mL of a single pathogen could be identified within 5 hours. The negative predictive value for the automated urine screening methods is close to 100 per cent for greater than 10^5 CFU/mL; however, the positive predictive value is only between 20 and 40 per cent. Thus, a negative automated urine screen virtually eliminates the possibility of bacteriuria exceeding 10^5 CFU/mL. These automated techniques generally require expensive equipment and are practical only for screening large numbers of urine specimens.

Strips for indicating nitrites (product of bacterial metabolism) or leukocyte esterase are available for screening urine for infection.[176] Urine is screened best for nitrate on the first morning void. Leukocyte esterase strips may not be as sensitive in febrile children as in adult women. Bacteria noted on Gram stain of uncentrifuged urine (any bacteria per oil immersion field) plus 10 or more white blood cells/mm^3 in urine obtained using a catheter in febrile children younger than 2 years of age was found to be an excellent predictor of urine cultures containing greater than or equal to 50,000 CFU/mL.[68]

Fungi

One of the most difficult and perplexing problems for the clinician is the decision of when to initiate therapy for fungal infections, such as candidiasis or aspergillosis, in the immunocompromised host. Frequently, there are no clinical signs or laboratory evidence of disseminated fungal infection, and yet fungi are demonstrated throughout the body at necropsy. Even when cultures are positive for these ubiquitous fungi, their meaning is unclear. Positive cultures simply may represent surface colonization. Because the diagnosis of fungal infections is so difficult, antifungal treatment is delayed commonly and thereby frequently ineffective. Serologic techniques that demonstrate serum antibodies or precipitins to *Candida* or *Aspergillus* are not reliable and are difficult to interpret. Furthermore, the very patients in whom these tests would be most valuable may be unable to mount an antibody response because of immunosuppression.

Candida

As a result of the problems with rapid serodiagnosis of fungal infections, several investigators have developed methods to detect fungal antigens, such as *Candida* mannan.[74] *Candida* mannan has been detected by countercurrent immunoelectrophoresis,[82] enzyme immunoassay,[155] radioimmunoassay,[188] and latex agglutination[52] in the sera of patients with invasive candidiasis. Antibody to *Candida* antigens was produced in rabbits by the individual laboratories in each case. In general, these procedures are specific when positive but lack sensitivity (mannan was detected in the sera of 50 to 60 per cent of patients with proven disseminated *Candida* infection). A commercially produced latex agglutination kit is available for detecting *Candida* antigens of unknown composition (Cand-Tec, Ramco Laboratories, Houston, TX). Initial studies of this test appeared promising; however, subsequent evaluations have reported unacceptably low sensitivity and specificity for the diagnosis of invasive candidiasis.[4, 41, 51, 91, 115] There virtually is no information on the value of the Cand-Tec test in children, and this test cannot be recommended for the rapid or early diagnosis of invasive candidiasis in immunocompromised children.[153]

Walsh and associates[182] have described a double-sandwich liposomal immunoassay to detect circulating *Candida* enolase, a 48-kd cytoplasmic antigen. They used multiple serum samples and detected enolase in 11 of 13 cases of deep-tissue infection and in 7 of 11 cases of fungemia, all occurring in neutropenic cancer patients. Specificity of the test was 96 per cent. Other immunoassays developed for cytoplasmic antigens of *Candida* have been evaluated, and initial studies suggest that this approach may be suitable for further study in the neutropenic cancer patient.[108] Polymerase chain reaction technology for detecting *Candida* species has been applied by several groups, and preliminary results are encouraging.[77]

Cryptococcus neoformans

The latex agglutination test has been a valuable method by which to detect and quantitate cryptococcal polysaccharide in cerebrospinal fluid and sera. In comparative evaluations, certain commercial *Cryptococcus* latex agglutination kits were more reliable than were others.[171, 197] When proper controls are included, latex agglutination for cryptococcal antigen is highly specific and sensitive (100 per cent), although, as with latex agglutination tests in general, rheumatoid factor and other interfering proteins may cause false-positive results. Dithiothreitol, EDTA-heat extraction, or protease treatment of serum or cerebrospinal fluid can eliminate these interfering factors without affecting the cryptococcal antigen titer significantly.[165] Some experts warn that cryptococcal antigen titers of less than or equal to 1:8 in cerebrospinal fluid should be interpreted cautiously.[70] Furthermore, false-negative results appear to be more common in the normal compared with the immunocompromised host with cryptococcal meningitis.[12] False-positive latex agglutination tests are rare (<0.3 per cent) but have been reported as a result of contamination of cerebrospinal fluid with surface condensation from agar (syneresis fluid).[14] India ink mount can detect *C. neoformans* in cerebrospinal fluid, rapidly and conveniently, and is positive in about 60 per cent of patients with cryptococcal meningitis. However, this technique requires experienced laboratory personnel in order to distinguish the cryptococcal organism from mononuclear white blood cells. Both the India ink preparation and the latex agglutination test may remain positive after the cerebrospinal fluid is culture-negative and even subsequent to apparent cure of cryptococcal meningitis.

Aspergillosis

Invasive aspergillosis is a fungal infection, predominantly of the immunocompromised host, that has approximately an 80 per cent mortality rate. As in systemic candidiasis, early diagnosis and treatment are mandatory if outcome is to be favorable. Antibody determination for invasive aspergillosis also is unreliable in immunocompromised patients, and antigen-detection techniques hold the greatest promise for rapid early diagnosis. Radioimmunoassay, countercurrent immunoelectrophoresis, and enzyme-linked immunosorbent assay techniques have been used to detect galactomannan antigen in the serum and urine of patients with invasive or disseminated aspergillosis.[34, 88, 156] In general, these procedures have been 100 per cent specific and 50 to 100 per cent sensitive for *Aspergillus* infections, although multiple specimens may be required and antisera directed against *Aspergillus fumigatus* cross-react with *A. flavus.* Weiner and associates[189] described a radioimmunoassay for *Aspergillus* carbohydrate that prospectively detected antigen in the sera of four of six patients with invasive aspergillosis for 8 to 75 days after the onset of pulmonary infiltrates. These investigations of laboratory techniques employed rabbit antisera. Several groups have developed polymerase chain reaction techniques to detect *Aspergillus* species.[105] In small clinical studies, polymerase chain reaction–positive bronchoalveolar lavage fluid was correlated with invasive aspergillosis, but positive results also were reported in patients whose respiratory tracts probably only were colonized.[170] Large prospective studies are necessary to define the value of detecting *Aspergillus* by polymerase chain reaction.

Histoplasma capsulatum

Wheat and associates[191, 200] have developed radioimmunoassay and enzyme-linked immunosorbent assay techniques for detecting the polysaccharide antigen of *H. capsulatum*. Antibody to *H. capsulatum* was produced by immunizing rabbits with formalinized live yeast cells. Antigen was detected in serum and urine (90 per cent of patients tested) obtained from persons with disseminated histoplasmosis. When the test was evaluated in patients with AIDS and disseminated histoplasmosis, high levels of antigen were detected in the urine of 97 per cent of patients and in the sera of 79 per cent of patients.[190] Antigen levels decreased during and after antifungal therapy. Widespread availability of this test should lead to earlier diagnosis and perhaps superior monitoring of disseminated histoplasmosis, especially for patients with AIDS.

Parasites

Pneumocystis carinii

The most reliable method by which to diagnose *P. carinii* pneumonitis is lung biopsy. Obviously, this invasive procedure is considered cautiously in terms of its risk-to-benefit ratio when the physician is faced with an immunocompromised patient with interstitial pneumonitis. A rapid method for the reliable detection of circulating antigen from *P. carinii* possibly could avoid the necessity for lung biopsy in patients but, to date, is not available. Two groups have used rabbit antisera to detect *P. carinii* antigen in sera by countercurrent immunoelectrophoresis, but this approach has not been perfected further.[132]

Stains of induced sputum or fluid obtained by bronchoalveolar lavage may demonstrate *P. carinii* cysts in patients with AIDS and *P. carinii* pneumonia.[119] Immunofluorescent stain of these specimens with monoclonal antibodies enhances the detection of cysts, compared with Giemsa-like (Diff-Quick) or toluidine blue D stains.[87] Calcofluor white staining of respiratory specimens is quick but not as sensitive as the immunofluorescent stain.[167, 174] However, with the immunofluorescent stain, *P. carinii* cysts may be detected in asymptomatic patients with AIDS; thus, the laboratory and clinical findings must be considered together carefully.[116]

Polymerase chain reaction can detect *P. carinii* in bronchoalveolar lavage fluid, induced sputum, and even blood.[95, 143] In one study, polymerase chain reaction was more sensitive than conventional staining techniques for induced sputum but was not superior to conventional stain for bronchoalveolar lavage fluid.[143] As with immunofluorescent staining, some asymptomatic carriage of *P. carinii* may be identified by polymerase chain reaction. *P. carinii* was detected by nested polymerase chain reaction in blood specimens, which might suggest disseminated infection. Polymerase chain reaction of blood especially is of interest in the young infant with suspected *P. carinii* infection in whom an induced sputum sample is difficult to obtain.

Chlamydia trachomatis

Bell and associates[10] found a direct fluorescent monoclonal-antibody stain to be specific and sensitive for establishing the diagnosis of *C. trachomatis* conjunctivitis. Fluorescing elementary bodies were seen within the epithelial cells, and the procedure required about an hour to complete. Positive immunofluorescent smears were found in specimens from all 21 infants who were culture-positive when inflamed eyes were examined. Other investigators have documented the excellent sensitivity and specificity of commercially available fluorescent monoclonal-antibody stains for detecting *C. trachomatis* in conjunctival specimens obtained from infants with conjunctivitis.[137, 139] Paisley and associates[123] reported that this technique correlated well with culture results in nasopharyngeal secretions obtained from infants younger than 6 months of age with pneumonitis.

Enzyme immunoassays also are available for the rapid identification of *C. trachomatis* in conjunctival and nasopharyngeal specimens.[61, 62] For both enzyme immunoassay and fluorescent antibody tests, specimens that are rapid test–positive but culture-negative have been reported. However, these do not seem to be false-positive results but, rather, instances in which the rapid tests are more sensitive than the culture techniques are. Care must be taken in the proper use of these commercially available laboratory tests. The tests appear to be good for the respiratory specimens but lack specificity for chlamydial infection of the vagina in prepubertal girls and thus should not be used in the evaluation of sexual abuse.[135]

In recent years, a number of techniques have been applied successfully to the rapid identification of microorganisms causing a wide variety of infections. In the future, we can look forward to the rapid detection of virtually any microbial antigen and, it is hoped, as a result be able to provide optimal therapy and the most advantageous outcome for the patient.

ANTIBIOTIC SUSCEPTIBILITY TESTING

Antibiotic susceptibility testing is an important function of the microbiology laboratory and should be performed on all bacteria isolated from serious infections. Instances in which the susceptibility of an isolate can be predicted accurately without susceptibility testing are, unfortunately, diminishing to the point that *S. pyogenes* alone remains predictably susceptible to all of the agents prescribed most often. This worldwide emergence of antibiotic resistance in previously susceptible bacteria creates problems for physicians and the laboratory alike.[172] Prior to 1979, reports of antibiotic-resistant *S. pneumoniae* were sporadic.[86] Subsequently, pneumococci resistant to penicillin, the third-generation cephalosporins, erythromycin, trimethoprim-sulfamethoxazole, and chloramphenicol have been reported increasingly and associated with treatment failures using these agents.[16, 86, 103, 160] Delayed responses to penicillin therapy in patients with meningitis caused by *N. meningitidis* have been reported from Spain and the United States and linked to strains with modified penicillin-binding proteins.[19, 179, 196] Multiply antibiotic-resistant enterococci rapidly are becoming resistant to vancomycin, seriously diminishing the ability to treat nosocomial infections caused by these organisms.[111, 173] Thus, emerging antibiotic resistance makes the selection of empiric antibiotics more difficult, increases the cost of therapy, and forces the microbiology laboratory to test more bacteria to an increasing number of antibiotics in an effort accurately to determine effective antibiotic therapy.

Selection of one of the several methods available for susceptibility testing varies with such factors as the size of the hospital, the patient population, and the laboratory budget.[75, 147] The agar diffusion test, or Kirby-Bauer test, is one of the oldest and most standardized methods of susceptibility testing and probably will remain a reliable primary as well as backup system for several reasons.[45, 147] It is cost-efficient; it is easy to perform, control, and interpret; and it allows customized selection of antimicrobials tested to reflect physician preferences, hospital formulary, and changing resistance patterns. The results of disk diffusion reported as susceptible, intermediate, and resistant are qualitative, but the interpretations of susceptibility and resistance are defined clearly by published guidelines and well understood by all physicians. Quantitative methods or tube dilution procedures (macro and micro) give more precise results in the form of a minimum inhibitory concentration but generally are needed only for difficult infections, such as meningitis, osteomyelitis, or endocarditis, and the results are interpreted best by physicians with infectious disease training (Fig. 243–1). Automated versions of the microbroth procedure are restricted further by the inability to specify antibiotics included in the commercial panels and the lack of clinically useful end-points applicable to all pathogens and antibiotic-bacterial species combinations for which results can be unreliable.[45] All antibiotic susceptibility test results are influenced by a number of factors, including growth media, cation content, inoculum concentration, antibiotic concentration, incubation time, and incubation temperature. Standardization of these factors is addressed for disk diffusion and microbroth dilution procedures in methods recommended by the Subcommittee on Antimicrobial Susceptibility Testing of the National Committee for Clinical Laboratory Standards.[113] The proper performance of the procedure with an appropriate control strain of known susceptibility should be adhered to strictly for accurate reproducible results and is required by all of the laboratory accrediting agencies.

Automated quantitative antibiotic susceptibility systems are becoming more available and affordable. The cost-effectiveness of these systems often is increased by combining identification and antibiotic susceptibility on the same test plate and by freeze-drying the contents of the plates, thus significantly increasing their shelf life. Instrument failure can occur, requiring back-up systems for both identification and antibiotic susceptibility. In addition to the benefits of automation, these systems often provide same-day susceptibility results, which some claim leads to more effective antibiotic management, although this remains controversial.[45] Major deficiencies of the automated systems are the limitation of the numbers of antibiotics and concentration ranges of the antibiotics tested. Custom-prepared panels with specified concentrations of antibiotics are available but are more expensive. Additionally, automated systems often deliver erroneous results for nutritionally fastidious bacteria or with difficult-to-detect resistance mechanisms, such as methicillin-resistant *S. aureus* and the newly emerging vancomycin-resistant strains of enterococci. Media supplements provided by the manufacturers to correct these deficiencies often are inadequate, and *S. aureus, S. pneumoniae, Enterococcus* species, and *Haemophilus* species require manual systems for accurate testing.

E-test

The E-test (AB Biodisk, Solna, Sweden) is performed as a disk diffusion test is, but, by placing an antibiotic concentration gradient on a plastic strip, the resulting elliptical zone of inhibition is interpreted as a quantitative minimum inhibitory concentration (Fig. 243–2). The advantage is a quantitative result with a diffusion test that allows any antibiotic to be tested on media containing nutritional supplements that allows testing of fastidious as well as nonfastidious bacteria and anaerobes.[121] Studies have verified the accuracy of the procedure with most bacteria,[7] including *S. pneumoniae,*[97] *H. influenzae,*[76] and *N. meningitidis.*[57, 72] Although the E-test is relatively expensive, judicious selection of relevant antibiotics by the physician should allow this procedure to become a useful tool in antibiotic susceptibility testing.

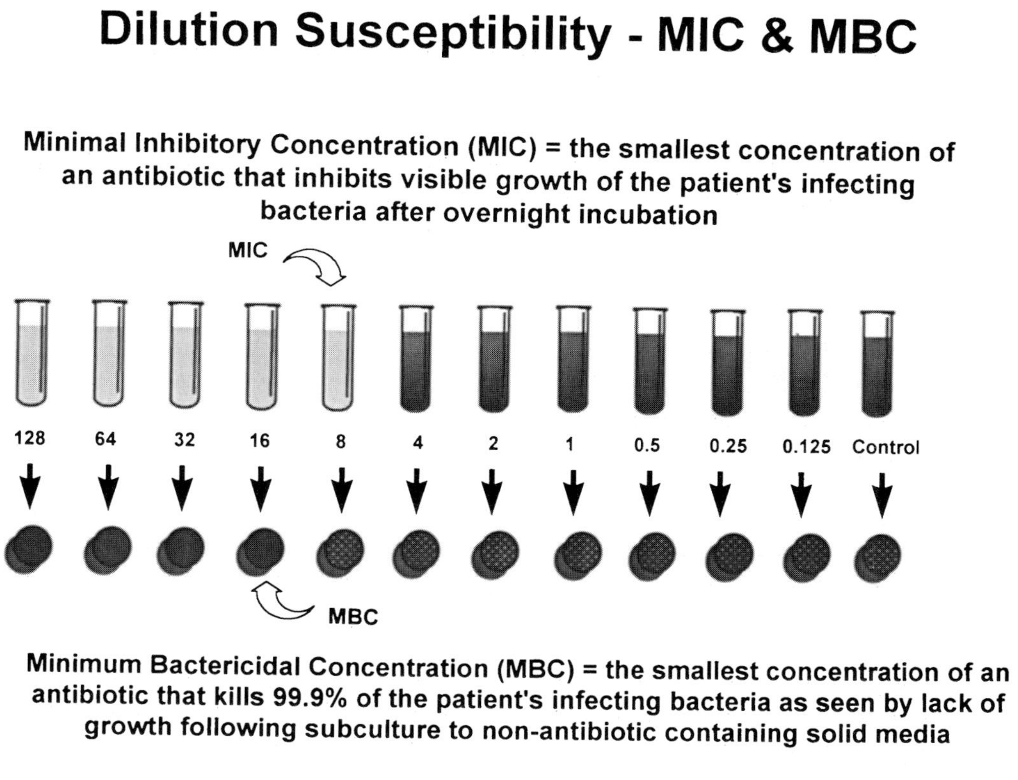

Dilution Susceptibility - MIC & MBC
Minimal Inhibitory Concentration (MIC) = the smallest concentration of an antibiotic that inhibits visible growth of the patient's infecting bacteria after overnight incubation
MIC
128
64
32
16
8
4
2
1
0.5
0.25
0.125
Control
MBC
Minimum Bactericidal Concentration (MBC) = the smallest concentration of an antibiotic that kills 99.9% of the patient's infecting bacteria as seen by lack of growth following subculture to non-antibiotic containing solid media

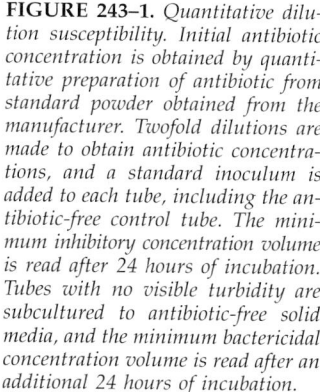

FIGURE 243–1. *Quantitative dilution susceptibility. Initial antibiotic concentration is obtained by quantitative preparation of antibiotic from standard powder obtained from the manufacturer. Twofold dilutions are made to obtain antibiotic concentrations, and a standard inoculum is added to each tube, including the antibiotic-free control tube. The minimum inhibitory concentration volume is read after 24 hours of incubation. Tubes with no visible turbidity are subcultured to antibiotic-free solid media, and the minimum bactericidal concentration volume is read after an additional 24 hours of incubation.*

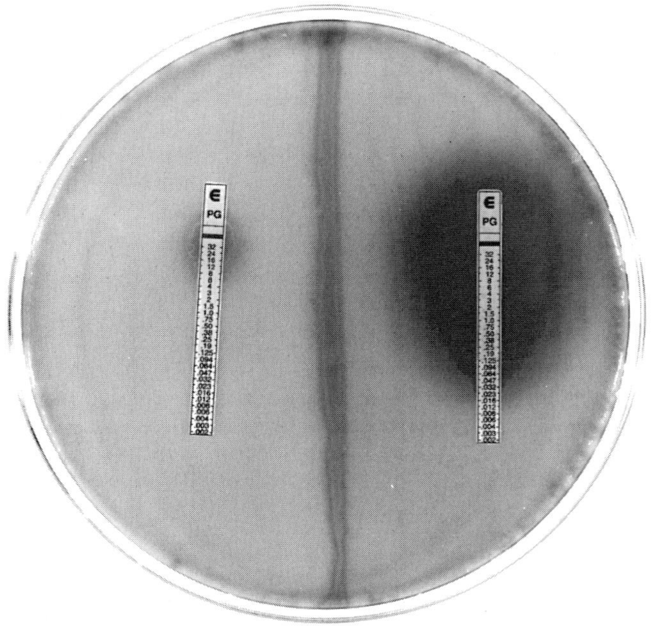

FIGURE 243–2. *E-test. Plastic strips containing an antibiotic gradient are placed on a lawn of bacterial inoculum, and the plate is incubated for 24 hours. In this figure, two pneumococcal strains are tested for susceptibility to penicillin. The strain on the right is susceptible with a minimum inhibitory concentration value of .032 μg/mL. The strain on the left is resistant with a minimum inhibitory concentration value of 16 μg/mL.*

β-Lactamase Test

The detection of the β-lactamase enzyme responsible for the inactivation of ampicillin, penicillin, and other β-lactam antibiotics affords a rapid method for assessing the susceptibility of several bacteria to these compounds. In the microbiology laboratory, the detection of the β-lactamase has clinical value in the prediction of resistance by *H. influenzae, N. gonorrhoeae, M. catarrhalis, S. aureus, Enterococcus* species, and *Bacteroides* species. These rapid tests (1 to 60 minutes) can be accomplished using acidometric, iodometric, or chromogenic cephalosporin methods (nitrocefin). The latter is commercially available and is useful for all the species listed (it is the only reliable method for testing *M. catarrhalis).* When testing this group of bacteria, a positive test signifies resistance to penicillin, ampicillin, and other aminopenicillins. It does not imply resistance to the β-lactamase–stable penicillins (oxacillin, nafcillin, methicillin) for *S. aureus* or for the extended spectrum cephalosporins for *H. influenzae* and *N. gonorrhoeae.* Also, although β-lactamase is the primary mechanism of resistance for most *H. influenzae* and *N. gonorrhoeae* organisms, there are rare reports of resistance to these compounds by mechanisms involving the modification of the penicillin-binding proteins that this test does not detect. β-Lactamase results do not predict always susceptibility or resistance to the penicillin-class antibiotics in Enterobacteriaceae and *Pseudomonas* species,[169] with which enzymes may be detected only after induction with subinhibitory concentrations of antibiotic.

Chloramphenicol Acetyltransferase

Resistance to chloramphenicol can be predicted rapidly by detecting the enzyme chloramphenicol acetyltransferase in an assay similar to the nitrocefin β-lactamase test. It has been used for testing *H. influenzae* and *S. pneumoniae* but, because of the decline in the use of chloramphenicol in clinical therapy, may not be available readily in all clinical laboratories.

SPECIAL STUDIES

A variety of specialized antibiotic-related studies may be offered by the microbiology or infectious disease laboratory or may be available through a reference laboratory. Most are expensive to perform and labor-intensive, and some may be influenced by concurrent antibiotic therapy. Request for and interpretation of these tests should be limited in most cases to the physician with special infectious disease training.

Antibiotic Assay

Assay procedures for determining blood levels of potentially toxic antibiotics should be available in or accessible to all hospital bacteriology laboratories. This information is vital in the management of infections in patients with compromised renal function. Standardized immunologic and radiometric assays are available for determining levels of the aminoglycosides and vancomycin. Bioassay procedures based on diffusion of the antibiotic in agar seeded with an indicator organism are available in reference or research laboratories for unique instances when antibiotic levels are needed and no commercial assay kit is available. Often, these assays are restricted by being valid only if the patient is receiving no other antibiotic concurrently.

Serum Bactericidal Test

The serum bactericidal test is performed by diluting the patient's serum and determining the minimal dilution that has inhibitory and bactericidal activity against the bacteria isolated from the infection (Fig. 243–3). In practice, it is much like performing quantitative susceptibility studies on that patient's infecting bacteria, except that in addition to measuring total metabolized antibiotics, it also measures the effects of serum factors in the blood. The test is easy to perform in that only a sample of serum, usually obtained at the nadir (trough) and the peak of the anticipated dose cycle, and the infecting bacteria from the patient are all that are required.[114, 129] There is, however, substantial controversy regarding the performance, interpretation, and relevance of the bactericidal titer.[98, 166] Until recently, there were no standard procedures for the performance of bactericidal titers similar to the standards developed for quantitative susceptibility, and inter- as well as intralaboratory variations were significant. The National Center for Clinical Laboratory Standards has published guidelines for the performance, which include the use of 50 per cent serum in the broth media to simulate more closely in vivo conditions.[112, 114] Whereas these efforts are necessary to minimize variations, some question remains as to how the addition of a serum source different from the patient's truly reflects individual patient serum. In addition, this requirement adds to the logistics and expense of performing the test. Alternative guidelines for the procedure omit the use of a serum diluent. Interpretation of the test results also is controversial.[98] There is disagreement as to how much the peak or trough level must exceed the minimal inhibitory concentration/minimal bactericidal concentration of the bacteria to be optimally therapeutic and whether it is more advantageous to maintain the peak or the trough above a given level.[194] As one would suspect, clinical data to support

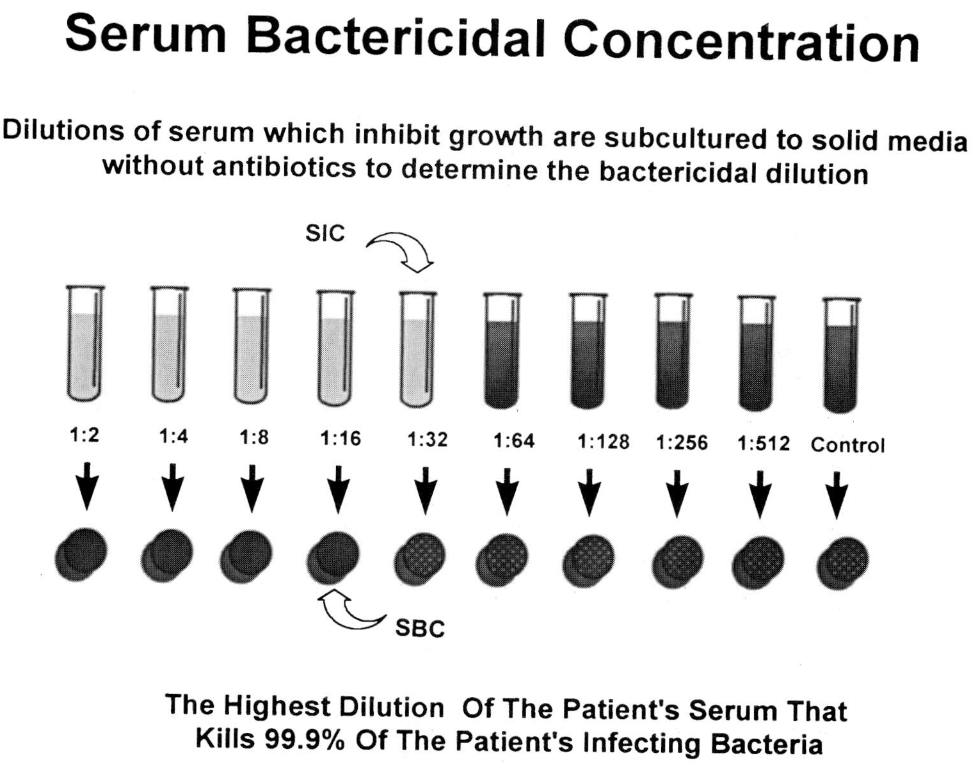

FIGURE 243–3. *Serum bactericidal concentration (SBC). Serum obtained from the patient while on antibiotic therapy is diluted by two times to obtain concentration ranges. A carefully controlled bacterial inoculum is added to all tubes and incubated for 24 hours. The serum inhibitory concentration (SIC) is the greatest dilution that inhibits growth, judged by the lack of visible turbidity. Tubes with no visible growth are subcultured to antibiotic-free solid media, and the serum bactericidal concentration is read after an additional 24 hours of incubation.*

all of these variables are difficult to obtain. Finally, it is important to realize that the bactericidal titer reflects conditions in the serum, and data to guide the interpretation of the results when the site of infection is other than blood are incomplete.

Synergy

In special instances, combinations of antibiotics may be tested in vitro to confirm synergy or to detect antagonistic activity between two antibiotics. All of these tests are labor-intensive and require special expertise in design and interpretation; furthermore, the therapeutic value remains questionable. Thus, they should be performed only in carefully selected circumstances.[40, 83] Several methods are available.

Fixed Combinations

Several compounds are tested regularly in combination (sulfamethoxazole-trimethoprim, erythromycin-sulfisoxazole, amoxicillin– and ticarcillin–clavulanic acid, piperacillin-tazobactam, and ampicillin-sulbactam). Standard disks are available for testing these compounds by disk-diffusion methods. Quantitative susceptibility testing is performed best by a reference laboratory regularly engaged in testing these compounds.

Checkerboard

One method of obtaining quantitative assessment of antibiotic activity in the presence of another antibiotic is the broth dilution method, most often with use of microdilution plates. The tests are labor-intensive and require experienced personnel and proper controls. The results of these tests are expressed as fractional inhibitory concentrations of one drug in the presence of the other. In general, a combination is considered synergistic if the fractional inhibitory concentration is less than or equal to 0.5 and is antagonistic if the fractional inhibitory concentration is greater than or equal to 4.0.[83]

Growth Curve

Growth curve also is a labor-intensive method of assessing the effects of antibiotic combinations in vitro. The bacteria are grown in broths containing appropriate dilutions of the antibiotics, alone and in combination. Viable cells are counted at the beginning and at several points during the experiment. Increased killing in the presence of the combination is considered synergistic, and decreased killing is considered antagonistic. Again, there are several controversial issues in regard to this method of testing: (1) the concentration of the antibiotics to be tested, (2) the length of time for the test, and (3) the similarity of test conditions and in vivo conditions.

Screening (Enterococcus)

Synergy between β-lactam antibiotics and the aminoglycosides may be of significant therapeutic benefit in infections caused by enterococci. This synergy with β-lactam antibiotics is not universal among strains of enterococci but is predictable by demonstrating the absence of high-level aminoglycoside resistance.[113] This demonstration can be made by using a single tube containing 500 μg/mL of gentamicin and 1000 μg/mL of streptomycin and observing the presence or absence of growth. Although synergy with a β-lactam is ruled out by the determination of high-level aminoglycoside resistance (growth in the screen tube), synergy with that aminoglycoside cannot be assumed universally.

References

1. Albert, M. J., Ansaruzzaman, M., Abu, R. M. A., et al.: Fluorescent antibody staining test for rapid diagnosis of *Shigella dysenteriae* 1 infection. Diagn. Microbiol. Infect. Dis. *15*:359–361, 1992.
2. Araj, G. F., Hopfer, R. L., Chestnut, S., et al.: Diagnostic value of the enzyme-linked immunosorbent assay for detection of *Candida albicans* cytoplasmic antigen in sera of cancer patients. J. Clin. Microbiol. *16*:46–52, 1982.
3. Ascher, D. P., Wilson, S., Mendiola, J., et al.: Group B streptococcal latex agglutination testing in neonates. J. Pediatr. *119*:458–461, 1991.
4. Bailey, J. W., Sada, E., Brass, C., et al.: Diagnosis of systemic candidiasis by latex agglutination for serum antigen. J. Clin. Microbiol. *21*:749–752, 1985.
5. Baker, C. J., and Rench, M. A.: Commercial latex agglutination for detection of group B streptococcal antigen in body fluids. J. Pediatr. *102*:393–395, 1983.
6. Baker, C. J., Webb, B. J., Jackson, C. V., et al.: Countercurrent immunoelectrophoresis in the evaluation of infants with group B streptococcal disease. Pediatrics *65*:1110–1114, 1980.
7. Baker, C. N., Stocker, S. A., Culver, D. H., et al.: Comparison of the E test to agar dilution, broth microdilution, and agar diffusion susceptibility testing techniques by using a special challenge set of bacteria. J. Clin. Microbiol. *29*:533–538, 1991.
8. Bal, A. E., Gravekamp, C., Hartskeerl, R. A., et al.: Detection of leptospires in urine by PCR for early diagnosis of leptospirosis. J. Clin. Microbiol. *32*:1894–1898, 1994.
9. Beaman, B. L., Saubolle, M. A., and Wallace, R. J.: *Nocardia*, *Rhodococcus*, *Streptomyces*, *Oerskovia*, and other aerobic actinomycetes of medical importance. *In* Murray, P. R., Baron, E. J., Pfaller, M. A., et al.: (eds.): Manual of Clinical Microbiology. 6th ed. Washington, D.C., American Society for Microbiology, 1995, pp. 379–399.
10. Bell, T. A., Kuo, C.-C., Stamm, W. E., et al.: Direct fluorescent monoclonal antibody stain for rapid detection of infant *Chlamydia trachomatis* infections. Pediatrics *74*:224–228, 1984.
11. Bennett, J. E., Dismukes, W. E., Duma, R. J., et al.: A comparison of amphotericin B alone and combined with flucytosine in the treatment of cryptococcal meningitis. N. Engl. J. Med. *301*:126–131, 1979.
12. Berlin, L., and Pincus, J. H.: Cryptococcal meningitis: False-negative antigen test results and cultures in nonimmunosuppressed patients. Arch. Neurol. *46*:1312–1316, 1989.
13. Bernet, C., Garret, M., Barbeyrac, B. D., et al.: Detection of *Mycoplasma pneumoniae* by using the polymerase chain reaction. J. Clin. Microbiol. *27*:2492–2496, 1989.
14. Boom, W. H., Piper, D. J., Ruoff, K. L., et al.: New cause for false-positive results with the cryptococcal antigen test by latex agglutination. J. Clin. Microbiol. *22*:856–857, 1985.
15. Bortolussi, R., Wort, A. J., and Casey, S.: The latex agglutination test versus counterimmunoelectrophoresis for rapid diagnosis of bacterial meningitis. Can. Med. Assoc. J. *127*:489–493, 1982.
16. Bradley, J. S., and Connor, J. D.: Ceftriaxone failure in meningitis caused by *Streptococcus pneumoniae* with reduced susceptibility to beta-lactam antibiotics. Pediatr. Infect. Dis. J. *11*:871–873, 1991.
17. Brady, M. T.: Nosocomial legionnaires disease in a children's hospital. J. Pediatr. *115*:46–50, 1989.
18. Bruckner, D. A., and Cikibba, P.: Nomenclature for aerobic and facultative bacteria. Clin. Infect. Dis. *21*:263–272, 1995.
19. Buck, G. E., and Adams, M.: Meningococcus with reduced susceptibility to penicillin isolated in the United States. Pediatr. Infect. Dis. J. *13*:156–157, 1994.
20. Burg, J. L., Grover, C. M., Pouletty, P., et al.: Direct and sensitive detection of a pathogenic protozoan, *Toxoplasma gondii*, by polymerase chain reaction. J. Clin. Microbiol. *27*:1787–1792, 1989.
21. Cartwright, C. P., Nelson, N. A., and Gill, V. J.: Development and evaluation of a rapid and simple procedure for detection of *Pneumocystis carinii* by PCR. J. Clin. Microbiol. *32*:1634–1638, 1994.
22. Chapin-Robertson, K., Reece, E. A., and Edberg, S. C.: Evaluation of the Gen-Probe PACE II assay for the direct detection of *Neisseria gonorrhoeae* in endocervical specimens. Diagn. Microbiol. Infect. Dis. *15*:645–649, 1992.
23. Colding, H., and Lind, I.: Counterimmunoelectrophoresis in the diagnosis of bacterial meningitis. J. Clin. Microbiol. *5*:405–409, 1977.
24. Committee on Infectious Diseases and Committee on Fetus and Newborn: Guidelines for prevention of group B streptococcal (GBS) infection by chemoprophylaxis. Pediatrics *90*:775–778, 1992.
25. Coonrod, J. D.: Urine as an antigen reservoir for diagnosis of infectious diseases: Infectious Diseases Symposium. Am. J. Med. *75*(Suppl. 1B):85–92, 1983.
26. Crosson, F. J., Winkelstein, J. A., and Moxon, E. R.: Enzyme-linked immunosorbent assay for detection and quantitation of capsular antigen of *Haemophilus influenzae* type b. Infect. Immun. *22*:617–619, 1978.
27. Datta, A. R., Wentz, B. A., and Hill, W. E.: Detection of hemolytic *Listeria monocytogenes* by using DNA colony hybridization. Appl. Environ. Microbiol. *53*:2256–2259, 1987.
28. Dean, D., Palmer, L., Pant, C. R., et al.: Use of a *Chlamydia trachomatis* DNA probe for detection of ocular chlamydia. J. Clin. Microbiol. *27*:1062–1067, 1989.
29. Diamond, R. D., and Bennett, J. E.: Prognostic factors in cryptococcal meningitis. Ann. Intern. Med. *80*:176–181, 1974.
30. Dirks-Go, S. I. S., and Zanen, H. C.: Latex agglutination, counterimmunoelectrophoresis, and protein A co-agglutination in diagnosis of bacterial meningitis. J. Clin. Pathol. *31*:1167–1171, 1978.
31. Dobkin, D., and Shulman, S. T.: Evaluation of an ELISA for group A streptococcal antigen for diagnosis of pharyngitis. J. Pediatr. *110*:566–569, 1987.
32. Donatelli, J., Macone, A., Goldmann, D. A., et. al.: Rapid detection of group A streptococci: Comparative performance by nurses and laboratory technologists in pediatric satellite laboratories using three test kits. J. Clin. Microbiol. *30*:138–142, 1992.
33. Drow, D. L., Welch, D. F., Hensel, D., et al.: Evaluation of the Phadebact CSF test for detection of the four most common causes of bacterial meningitis. J. Clin. Microbiol. *18*:1358–1361, 1983.
34. Dupont, B., Huber, M., Kim, S. J., et al.: Galactomannan antigenemia and antigenuria in aspergillosis: Studies in patients and experimentally infected rabbits. J. Infect. Dis. *155*:1–11, 1987.
35. Dylla, B. L., Vetter, E. A., Hughes, J. G., et al.: Evaluation of an immunoassay for direct detection of *Escherichia coli* 0157 in stool specimens. J. Clin. Microbiol. *33*:222–224, 1995.
36. Edwards, M. S., Kasper, D. L., and Baker, C. J.: Rapid diagnosis of type III group B streptococcal meningitis by latex particle agglutination. J. Pediatr. *95*:202–205, 1979.
37. Eisenach, K. D., Cave, M. D., Bates, J. H. et al.: Polymerase chain reaction amplification of a repetitive DNA sequence for *Mycobacterium tuberculosis*. J. Infect. Dis. *161*:977–981, 1990.
38. Eisenach, K. D., Crawford, J. T., and Bates, J. H.: Repetitive DNA sequences as probes for *Mycobacterium tuberculosis*. J. Clin. Microbiol. *26*:2240–2245, 1988.
39. Eisenstein, B. I.: New molecular techniques for microbial epidemiology and the diagnosis of infectious diseases. J. Infect. Dis. *161*:592–602, 1990.
40. Eliopoulos, G. M., and Eliopoulos, C. T.: Antibiotic combinations: Should they be tested? Clin. Microbiol. Rev. *1*:139–156, 1988.
41. Escuro, R. S., Jacobs, M., Gerson, S. L., et al.: Prospective evaluation of a candida antigen detection test for invasive candidiasis in immunocompromised adult patients with cancer. Am. J. Med. *87*:621–627, 1989.
42. Estrada, J. J., and Kuhn, R. E.: Immunochemical detection of antigens of larval *Taenia solium* and anti-larval antibodies in the cerebrospinal fluid of patients with neurocysticercosis. J. Neurol. Sci. *71*:39–48, 1985.
43. Feigin, R. D., Stechenberg, B. W., Chang, M. J., et al.: Prospective evaluation of treatment of *Haemophilus influenzae* meningitis. J. Pediatr. *88*:542–548, 1976.
44. Feldman, W. E.: Effect of prior antibiotic therapy on concentrations of bacteria in CSF. Am. J. Dis. Child. *132*:672–674, 1978.
45. Ferraro, M. J.: Automated antimicrobial susceptibility testing: What the infectious diseases subspecialist needs to know. Curr. Clin. Top. Infect. Dis. *14*:103–119, 1994.
46. Fleisher, G., Lennette, E. T., and Honig, P.: Diagnosis of Rocky Mountain spotted fever by immunofluorescent identification of *Rickettsia rickettsii* in skin biopsy tissue. J. Pediatr. *95*:63–65, 1979.
47. Forbes, B. A., and Hicks, K. E. S.: Direct detection of *Mycobacterium tuberculosis* in respiratory specimens in a clinical laboratory by polymerase chain reaction. J. Clin. Microbiol. *31*:1688–1694, 1993.
48. Forbes, B. A., and Granato, P. A.: Processing specimens for bacteria. *In* Murray, P. R., Baron, E. J., Pfaller, M. A., et al. (eds.): Manual of Clinical Microbiology. 6th ed. Washington, D.C., American Society for Microbiology, 1995, pp. 265–281.
49. Frankel, G., Riley, L., Giron, J. A., et al.: Detection of *Shigella* in feces using DNA application. J. Infect. Dis. *161*:1252–1256, 1990.
50. Friedman, C. A., Wender, D. F., and Rawson, J. E.: Rapid diagnosis of group B streptococcal infection utilizing a commercially available latex agglutination assay. Pediatrics *73*:27–30, 1984.
51. Fung, J. C., Donta, S. T., and Tilton, R. C.: *Candida* detection system (CAND-TEC) to differentiate between *Candida albicans* colonization and disease. J. Clin. Microbiol. *24*:542–547, 1986.
52. Gentry, L. O., Wilkinson, I. D., Lea, A. S., et al.: Latex agglutination test for detection of *Candida* antigen in patients with disseminated disease. Eur. J. Clin. Microbiol. *2*:122–128, 1983.
53. Gerber, M. A., Randolph, M. F., Chantry, J., et al.: Antigen detection test for streptococcal pharyngitis: Evaluation of sensitivity with respect to true infection. J. Pediatr. *108*:654–658, 1986.
54. Gerber, M. A., Spadaccini, L. J., Wright, L. L., et al.: Latex agglutination tests for rapid identification of group A streptococci directly from throat swabs. J. Pediatr. *105*:702–705, 1984.
55. Gerber, M. A.: Comparison of throat cultures and rapid strep tests for diagnosis of streptococcal pharyngitis. Pediatr. Infect. Dis. J. *8*:820–824, 1989.
56. Girolami, P. C. D., Hanff, P. A., Eichelberger, K., et al.: Multicenter evaluation of a new enzyme immunoassay for detection of *Clostridium difficile* enterotoxin A. J. Clin. Microbiol. *30*:1085–1088, 1992.
57. Gomez-Herruz, P., Gonzalez-Palacios, R., Romanyk, J., et al.: Evaluation of the Etest for penicillin susceptibility testing of *Neisseria meningitidis*. Diagn. Microbiol. Infect. Dis. *21*:115–117, 1995.
58. Greenwood, B. M., Whittle, H. C., and Dominic-Rajkovic, O.: Countercur-

rent immunoelectrophoresis in the diagnosis of meningococcal infections. Lancet 2:519–521, 1971.
59. Grimprel, E., Sanchez, P. J., Wendel, G. D., et al.: Use of polymerase chain reaction and rabbit infectivity testing to detect *Treponema pallidum* in amniotic fluid, fetal and neonatal sera, and cerebrospinal fluid. J. Clin. Microbiol. *29*:1711–1718, 1991.
60. Hageage, G. J., and Harrington, B. J.: Use of calcofluor white in clinical mycology. Lab. Med. *15*:109–112, 1984.
61. Hammerschlag, M. R., Gelling, M., Roblin, P. M., et al.: Comparison of Kodak Surecell *Chlamydia* Test Kit with culture for the diagnosis of chlamydial conjunctivitis in infants. J. Clin. Microbiol. *28*:1441–1442, 1990.
62. Hammerschlag, M. R., Roblin, P. M., Cummings, C., et al.: Comparison of enzyme immunoassay and culture for diagnosis of chlamydial conjunctivitis and respiratory infections in infants. J. Clin. Microbiol. *25*:2306–2308, 1987.
63. Harding, S. A., Scheld, W. M., McGowan, M. D., et al.: Enzyme-linked immunosorbent assay for detection of *Streptococcus pneumoniae* antigen. J. Clin. Microbiol. *10*:339–342, 1979.
64. Harris, M. C., Deuber, C., Polin, R. A., et al.: Investigation of apparent false-positive urine latex particle agglutination tests for the detection of group B *Streptococcus* antigen. J. Clin. Microbiol. *27*:2214–2217, 1989.
65. Hasan, J. A. K., Huq, A., Tamplin, M. L., et al.: A novel kit for rapid detection of *Vibrio cholerae* 01. J. Clin. Microbiol. *32*:249–252, 1994.
66. Hata, D., Kuze, F., Mochizuki, Y., et al.: Evaluation of DNA probe test for rapid diagnosis of *Mycoplasma pneumoniae* infections. J. Pediatr. *116*:273–276, 1990.
67. Heiter, B. J., and Borubeau, P. P.: Comparison of the Gen-Probe group A streptococcus direct test with culture and a rapid streptococcal antigen detection assay for diagnosis of streptococcal pharyngitis. J. Clin. Microbiol. *31*:2070–2073, 1993.
68. Hoberman, A., Wald, E. R., Reynods, E. A., et al.: Pyuria and bacteriuria in urine specimens obtained by catheter from young children with fever. J. Pediatr. *124*:513–519, 1994.
69. Hoffman, T. A., and Edwards, E. A.: Group-specific polysaccharide antigen and humoral antibody response in disease due to *Neisseria meningitidis*. J. Infect. Dis. *126*:636–644, 1972.
70. Hopfer, R. L., Perry, E. V., and Fainstein, V.: Diagnostic value of cryptococcal antigen in the cerebrospinal fluid of patients with malignant disease. J. Infect. Dis. *145*:915, 1982.
71. Hosein, I. K., Kaunitz, A. M., and Craft, S. J.: Detection of cervical *Chlamydia trachomatis* and *Neisseria gonorrhoeae* with deoxyribonucleic acid probe assays in obstetric patients. Am. J. Obstet. Gynecol. *167*:588–591, 1992.
72. Hughes, J. H., Biedenbach, D. J., Erwin, M. E., et al.: E test as susceptibility test and epidemiologic tool for evaluation of *Neisseria meningitidis* isolates. J. Clin. Microbiol. *31*:3255–3259, 1993.
73. Ingram, D. L., Pearson, A. W., and Occhiuti, A. R.: Detection of bacterial antigens in body fluids with the Wellcogen *Haemophilus influenzae* b, *Streptococcus pneumoniae*, and *Neisseria meningitidis* (ACYW135) latex agglutination tests. J. Clin. Microbiol. *18*:1119–1121, 1983.
74. Jones, J. M.: Laboratory diagnosis of invasive candidiasis. Clin. Microbiol. Rev. *3*:32–45, 1990.
75. Jorgensen, J. H.: Antimicrobial susceptibility testing of bacteria that grow aerobically. Infect. Dis. Clin. North Am. *7*:393–409, 1993.
76. Jorgensen, J. H., Howell, A. W., and Maher, L. A.: Quantitative antimicrobial susceptibility testing of *Haemophilus influenzae* and *Streptococcus pneumoniae* by using the E-test. J. Clin. Microbiol. *29*:109–114, 1991.
77. Kan, V. L.: Polymerase chain reaction for the diagnosis of candidemia. J. Infect. Dis. *168*:779–783, 1993.
78. Kaplan, S. L., Mason, E. O., Mason, S. K., et al.: Prospective comparative trial of moxalactam versus ampicillin or chloramphenicol for treatment of *Haemophilus influenzae* type b meningitis in children. J. Pediatr. *104*:447–453, 1984.
79. Kaplan, S. L.: Antigen detection in cerebrospinal fluid: Pros and cons: Infectious Diseases Symposium. Am. J. Med. *75*(Suppl. 1B):109–118, 1983.
80. Kellogg, J. A., Landis, R. C., Nussbaum, A. S., et al.: Performance of an enzyme immunoassay test and anaerobic culture for detection of group A streptococci in a pediatric practice versus a hospital laboratory. J. Pediatr. *111*:18–21, 1987.
81. Kellogg, J. A.: Suitability of throat culture procedures for detection of group A streptococci and as reference standards for evaluation of streptococcal antigen detection kits. J. Clin. Microbiol. *28*:165–169, 1990.
82. Kerkering, T. M., Espinel-Ingroff, A., and Shadomy, S.: Detection of candida antigenemia by counterimmunoelectrophoresis in patients with invasive candidiasis. J. Infect. Dis. *140*:659–664, 1979.
83. King, T. C., Schlessinger, D., and Krogstad, D. J.: The assessment of drug combinations. Rev. Infect. Dis. *3*:627–633, 1981.
84. Kleiman, M. B., Reynolds, J. K., Schreiner, R. L., et al.: Rapid diagnosis of neonatal bacteremia with acridine orange–stained buffy coat smears. J. Pediatr. *105*:419–421, 1984.
85. Kleiman, M. B., Reynolds, J. K., Watts, N. H., et al.: Superiority of acridine orange stain versus Gram stain in partially treated bacterial meningitis. J. Pediatr. *104*:401–404, 1984.
86. Klugman, K. P.: Pneumococcal resistance to antibiotics. Clin. Microbiol. Rev. *3*:171–196, 1990.
87. Kovacs, J. A., Ng, V. L., Masur, H., et al.: Diagnosis of *Pneumocystis carinii* pneumonia: Improved detection in sputum with use of monoclonal antibodies. N. Engl. J. Med. *318*:589–593, 1988.
88. Kurup, V. P., and Kumar, A.: Immunodiagnosis of aspergillosis. Clin. Microbiol. Rev. *4*:439–456, 1991.
89. Laxer, R. M., and Marks, M. I.: Pneumococcal meningitis in children. Am. J. Dis. Child. *131*:850–853, 1977.
90. Lee, B. W., Tan, J. A., Wong, S. C., et al.: DNA amplification by the polymerase chain reaction for the rapid diagnosis of tuberculous meningitis: Comparison of protocols involving three mycobacterial DNA sequences, IS6110, 65kDa antigen, and MPB64. J. Neurol. Sci. *123*:173–179, 1994.
91. Lemieux, C., St.-Germain, G., Vincelette, J., et al.: Collaborative evaluation of antigen detection by a commercial latex agglutination test and enzyme immunoassay in the diagnosis of invasive candidiasis. J. Clin. Microbiol. *28*:249–253, 1990.
92. Lentino, J. R., and Rytel, M. W.: Detection of circulating free and complexed staphylococcal antigens by enzyme-linked immunosorbent assay. J. Clin. Microbiol. *16*:1019–1024, 1982.
93. Lew, M. A., Siber, G. R., Donahue, D. M., et al.: Enhanced detection with an enzyme-linked immunosorbent assay of *Candida* mannan in antibody-containing serum after heat-extraction. J. Infect. Dis. *145*:45–56, 1982.
94. Li, Z., Jansen, D. L., Finn, T. M., et al.: Identification of *Bordetella pertussis* infection by shared-primer PCR. J. Clin. Microbiol. *32*:783–789, 1994.
95. Lipschick, G. Y., Gill, V. J., Lundgren, J. D., et al.: Improved diagnosis of *Pneumocystis carinii* infection by polymerase chain reaction on induced sputum and blood. Lancet *340*:203–206, 1992.
96. Liu, P. Y.-F., Shi, Z.-Y., Lau, Y.-J., et al.: Rapid diagnosis of tuberculous meningitis by a simplified nested amplification protocol. Neurology *44*:1161–1164, 1994.
97. Macias, E. A., Mason, E. O., Jr., Ocera, H. Y., et al.: Comparison of E test with standard broth microdilution for determining antibiotic susceptibilities of penicillin-resistant strains of *Streptococcus pneumoniae*. J. Clin. Microbiol. *32*:430–432, 1994.
98. MacLowry, J. D.: Perspective: The serum dilution test. J. Infect. Dis. *160*:624–626, 1989.
99. Magder, L. S., Klotz, K. C., Bush, L. H., et al.: Effect of patient characteristics on performance of an enzyme immunoassay for detecting cervical *Chlamydia trachomatis* infection. J. Clin. Microbiol. *28*:781–784, 1990.
100. Marchant, C. D., Band, E., Froeschle, J. E., et al.: Depression of anticapsular antibody after immunization with *Haemophilus influenzae* type b polysaccharide-diphtheria conjugate vaccine. Pediatr. Infect. Dis. J. *8*:508–511, 1989.
101. Marcon, M. J.: *Bordetella*. *In* Murray, P. R., Baron, E. J., Pfaller, M. A., et al. (eds.): Manual of Clinical Microbiology. 6th ed. Washington, D.C., American Society for Microbiology, 1995, pp. 566–573.
102. Marmion, B. P., Williamson, J., Worswick, D. A., et al.: Experience with newer techniques for the laboratory detection of *Mycoplasma pneumoniae* infection: Adelaide, 1978–1992. Clin. Infect. Dis. *17*(Suppl. 1):90–99, 1993.
103. Mason, E. O., Jr., Kaplan, S. L., Lamberth, L. B., et al.: Increased rate of isolation of penicillin-resistant *Streptococcus pneumoniae* in a children's hospital and in vitro susceptibilities to antibiotics of potential therapeutic use. Antimicrob. Agents Chemother. *36*:1703–1707, 1992.
104. Maxson, S., Lewno, M. J., and Schutze, G. E.: Clinical usefulness of cerebrospinal fluid bacterial antigen studies. J. Pediatr. *125*:235–238, 1994.
105. Melchers, W. J. G., Verweij, P. E., Hurk, P., et al.: General primer-mediated PCR for detection of *Aspergillus* species. J. Clin. Microbiol. *32*:1710–1717, 1994.
106. Moonens, F., El Alami, S., Gossum, A. V., et al.: Usefulness of Gram staining of blood collected from total parenteral nutrition catheter for rapid diagnosis of catheter-related sepsis. J. Clin. Microbiol. *32*:1578–1579, 1994.
107. Morbidity and Mortality Weekly Report: Diagnosis of tuberculosis by nucleic acid amplification methods applied to clinical specimens. M. M. W. R. *42*:686, 1993.
108. Morhart, M., Rennie, R., Ziola, B., et al.: Evaulation of enzyme immunoassay for *Candida* cytoplasmic antigen in neutropenic cancer patients. J. Clin. Microbiol. *32*:766–776, 1994.
109. Morrow, D. L., Kline, J. B., Douglas, S. D., et al.: Rapid detection of group B streptococcal antigen by monoclonal antibody sandwich enzyme assay. J. Clin. Microbiol. *19*:457–459, 1984.
110. Moser, D. R., Kirchhoff, L. V., and Donelson, J. E.: Detection of *Trypanosoma cruzi* by DNA amplification using the polymerase chain reaction. J. Clin. Microbiol. *27*:1477–1482, 1989.
111. Murray, B. E.: The life and times of the *Enterococcus*. Clin. Microbiol. Rev. *3*:46–65, 1990.
112. National Committee for Clinical Laboratory Standards: Methodology for the Serum Bactericidal Test: Tentative Guideline. NCCLS Document M21-T. Villanova, PA, NCCLS, 1992.
113. National Committee for Clinical Laboratory Standards: Methods for Dilution Antimicrobial Susceptibility Tests for Bacteria That Grow Aerobically. 3rd ed. Approved Standard. NCCLS Document M7-A3. Villanova, PA, NCCLS, 1993.
114. National Committee for Clinical Laboratory Standards: Methods for De-

termining Bactericidal Activity of Antimicrobial Agents: Tentative Guideline. NCCLS Document M26-T. Villanova, PA, NCCLS, 1992.
115. Ness, M. J., Vaughan, W. P., and Woods, G. L.: *Candida* antigen latex test for detection of invasive candidiasis in immunocompromised patients. J. Infect. Dis. *159*:495–502, 1989.
116. Ng, V. L., Yajko, D. M., McPhaul, L. W., et al.: Evaluation of an indirect fluorescent-antibody stain for detection of *Pneumocystis carinii* in respiratory specimens. J. Clin. Microbiol. *28*:975–979, 1990.
117. Ni, H., Knight, A. I., Cartwright, K., et al.: Polymerase chain reaction for diagnosis of meningococcal meningitis. Lancet *340*:1432–1434, 1992.
118. Nolte, F. S., Metchock, B., McGowan, J. E., Jr., et al.: Direct detection of *Mycobacterium tuberculosis* in sputum by polymerase chain reaction and DNA hybridization. J. Clin. Microbiol. *31*:1777–1782, 1993.
119. Ognibene, F. P., Gill, V. J., Pizzo, P. A., et al.: Induced sputum to diagnose *Pneumocystis carinii* pneumonia in immunosuppressed pediatric patients. J. Pediatr. *115*:430–433, 1989.
120. Olcen, P.: Serological methods for rapid diagnosis of *Haemophilus influenzae, Neisseria meningitidis,* and *Streptococcus pneumoniae* in cerebrospinal fluid: A comparison of co-agglutination, immunofluorescence, and immunoelectroosmophoresis. Scand. J. Infect. Dis. *10*:283–289, 1978.
121. Olsson-Liljequist, B., and Nord, C. E.: Methods for susceptibility testing of anaerobic bacteria. Clin. Infect. Dis. *18*(Suppl. 4):S293–S296, 1994.
122. Ostergaard, L., Birkelund, S., and Christiansen, G.: Use of polymerase chain reaction for detection of *Chlamydia trachomatis.* J. Clin. Microbiol. *28*:1254–1260, 1990.
123. Paisley, J. W., Lauer, B. A., Melinkovich, P., et al.: Rapid diagnosis of *Chlamydia trachomatis* pneumonia in infants by direct immunofluorescence microscopy of nasopharyngeal secretions. J. Pediatr. *109*:653–655, 1986.
124. Papasian, C. J., Bartholomew, W. R., and Amsterdam, D.: Validity of an enzyme immunoassay for detection of *Neisseria gonorrhoeae* antigens. J. Clin. Microbiol. *19*:347–350, 1984.
125. Park, C. H., Hixon, D. L., Morrison, W. L., et al.: Rapid diagnosis of enterohemmorrhagic *Escherichia coli* 0157:H7 directly from fecal specimens using immunofluorescence stain. Am. J. Clin. Pathol. *101*:91–94, 1994.
126. Pasculle, A. W., Veto, G. E., Krystofiak, S., et al.: Laboratory and clinical evaluation of a commercial DNA probe for the detection of *Legionella* spp. J. Clin. Microbiol. *27*:2350–2358, 1989.
127. Pepple, J., Moxon, E. R., and Yolken, R. H.: Indirect enzyme-linked immunosorbent assay for the quantitation of the type-specific antigen of *Haemophilus influenzae* b: A preliminary report. J. Pediatr. *97*:233–237, 1980.
128. Peterson, L. R., and Kelly, P. J.: The role of the clinical microbiology laboratory in the management of *Clostridium difficile*–associated diarrhea. Infect. Dis. Clin. North Am. *7*:277–293, 1993.
129. Peterson, L. R., and Shanholtzer, C. J.: Tests for bactericidal effects of antimicrobial agents: Technical performance and clinical relevance. Clin. Microbiol. Rev. *5*:420–432, 1992.
130. Pezzlo, M. T., Wetkowski, M. A., Peterson, E. M., et al.: Evaluation of a two-minute test for urine screening. J. Clin. Microbiol. *18*:697–701, 1983.
131. Pezzlo, M. T.: Automated methods for detection of bacteriuria. Am. J. Med. *75*:71–78, 1983.
132. Pifer, L. L., Hughes, W. T., Stagno, S., et al.: *Pneumocystis carinii* infection: Evidence for high prevalence in normal and immunosuppressed children. Pediatrics *61*:35–41, 1978.
133. Podzorski, R. P., and Persing, D. H.: Molecular detection and identification of microorganisms. *In* Murray, P. R., Baron, E. J., Pfaller, M. A., et al. (eds.): Manual of Clinical Microbiology. 6th ed. Washington, D.C., ASM Press, 1995, pp. 130–134.
134. Polin, R. A., and Kenneth, R.: Use of monoclonal antibodies in an enzyme-linked inhibition assay for rapid detection of streptococcal antigen. J. Pediatr. *97*:540–544, 1980.
135. Porder, K., Sanchez, N., Roblin, P. M., et al.: Lack of specificity of chlamydiazyme for detection of vaginal chlamydial infection in prepubertal girls. Pediatr. Infect. Dis. J. *8*:358–360, 1989.
136. Rabalais, G. P., Bronfin, D. R., and Daum, R. S.: Evaluation of a commercially available latex agglutination test for rapid diagnosis of group B streptococcal infections. Pediatr. Infect. Dis. J. *6*:177–181, 1987.
137. Rapoza, P. A., Quinn, T. C., Kiessling, L. A., et al.: Assessment of neonatal conjunctivitis with a direct immunofluorescent monoclonal antibody stain for chlamydia. J. A. M. A. *255*:3369–3373, 1986.
138. Richman, D. D., Cleveland, P. H., Redfield, D. C., et al.: Rapid viral diagnosis. J. Infect. Dis. *149*:298–310, 1984.
139. Roblin, P. M., Hammerschlag, M. R., Cummings, C., et al.: Comparison of two rapid microscopic methods and culture for detection of *Chlamydia trachomatis* in ocular and nasopharyngeal specimens from infants. J. Clin. Microbiol. *27*:968–970, 1989.
140. Rosa, P. A., and Schwan, T. G.: A specific and sensitive assay for the Lyme disease spirochete *Borrelia burgdorferi* using the polymerase chain reaction. J. Infect. Dis. *160*:1018–1029, 1989.
141. Rosenblatt, J. E., and Sloan L. M.: Evaluation of an enzyme-linked immunosorbent assay for detection of *Cryptosporidium* spp. in stool specimens. J. Clin. Microbiol. *31*:1468–1471, 1993.
142. Rosenblatt, J. E., Sloan, L. M., and Schneider, S. K.: Evaluation of an enzyme-linked immunosorbent assay for the detection of *Giardia lamblia* in stool specimens. Diagn. Microbiol. Infect. Dis. *16*:337–341, 1993.
143. Rowx, P., Laxrard, I., Poirot, J. L., et al.: Usefulness of PCR for detection of *Pneumocystis carinii* DNA. J. Clin. Microbiol. *32*:2324–2326, 1994.
144. Rudolph, K. M., Parkinson, A. J., Black, C. M., et al.: Evaluation of polymerase chain reaction for diagnosis of pneumococcal pneumonia. J. Clin. Microbiol. *31*:2661–2666, 1993.
145. Sabetta, J. R., Miniter, P., and Andriole, V. T.: The diagnosis of invasive aspergillosis by an enzyme-linked immunosorbent assay for circulating antigen. J. Infect. Dis. *152*:946–953, 1985.
146. Sada, E., Lopez-Vidal, Y., Ruiz-Palacios, G. M., et al.: Detection of mycobacterial antigens in cerebrospinal fluid of patients with tuberculous meningitis by enzyme-linked immunosorbent assay. Lancet *11*:651–652, 1983.
147. Sahm, D. F., Neuman, M. A., Thornsberry, C., et al.: Cumitech 25: Current concepts and approaches to antimicrobial agent susceptibility testing. *In* McGowan, J. E., Jr. (ed.): Washington, D.C., American Society for Microbiology, 1988.
148. Sanchez, P. J., Siegel, J. D., Cushion, N. B., et al.: Significance of a positive urine group B streptococcal latex agglutination test in neonates. J. Pediatr. *116*:601–606, 1990.
149. Savic, B., Sjöbring, V., Alugupalli, S., et al.: Evaluation of polymerase chain reaction, tuberculostearic acid analysis, and direct microscopy for the detection of *Mycobacterium tuberculosis* in sputum. J. Infect. Dis. *166*:1177–1180, 1992.
150. Scheffer, E. H., and Van Etta, L. L.: Evaluation of rapid commercial enzyme immunoassay for detection of *Giardia lamblia* in formalin-preserved stool specimens. J. Clin. Microbiol. *32*:1807–1808, 1994.
151. Scheifele, D. W., Daum, R. S., Syriopoulou, V. P., et al.: Comparison of two antigen detection techniques in a primate model of *Haemophilus influenzae* type b infection. Infect. Immun. *23*:827–831, 1979.
152. Schochetman, G., Ou, C.-Y., and Jones, W. K.: Polymerase chain reaction. J. Infect. Dis. *158*:1154–1157, 1988.
153. Schreiber, J. R., Maynard, E., and Lew, M. A.: *Candida* antigen detection in two premature neonates with disseminated candidiasis. Pediatrics *74*:838–841, 1984.
154. Schwartz, R. H., Bryan, C., Rodriguez, W. J., et al.: Experience with the microbiologic diagnosis of *Campylobacter* enteritis in an office laboratory. Pediatr. Infect. Dis. *2*:298–301, 1983.
155. Segal, E., Berg, R. A., Pizzo, P. A., et al.: Detection of *Candida* antigen in sera of patients with candidiasis by an enzyme-linked immunosorbent assay: Inhibition technique. J. Clin. Microbiol. *10*:116–118, 1979.
156. Shaffer, P. J., Kobayashi, G. S., and Medoff, G.: Demonstration of antigenemia in patients with invasive aspergillosis by solid phase (protein A–rich *Staphylococcus aureus)* radioimmunoassay. Am. J. Med. *67*:627–630, 1979.
157. Simpson, A. J. H., Mawn, J. A., and Heard, S. R.: Assessment of two methods for rapid intrapartum detection of vaginal group B streptococcal colonisation. J. Clin. Pathol. *47*:752–755, 1994.
158. Sippel, J. E., Prato, C. M., Girgis, N. I., et al.: Detection of *Neisseria meningitidis* group A, *Haemophilus influenzae* type b, and *Streptococcus pneumoniae* antigens in cerebrospinal fluid specimens by antigen capture enzyme-linked immunosorbent assays. J. Clin. Microbiol. *20*:259–265, 1984.
159. Skoll, M. A., Mercer, B. M., Baselski, V., et al.: Evaluation of two rapid group B streptococcal antigen tests in labor and delivery patients. Obstet. Gynecol. *77*:322–326, 1991.
160. Sloas, M. M., Barrett, F. F., Chesney, P. J., et al.: Cephalosporin treatment failure in penicillin- and cephalosporin-resistant *Streptococcus pneumoniae* meningitis. Pediatr. Infect. Dis. J. *11*:662–666, 1992.
161. Sood, S. K., Ballanco, G. A., Mather, F. J., et al.: Distribution and excretion of capsular antigen after immunization with *Haemophilus infuenzae* type b polysaccharide–*Neisseria meningitidis* outer membrane protein conjugate vaccine. J. Infect. Dis. *161*:574–577, 1990.
162. Stamm, W. E., Cole, B., Fennell, C., et al.: Antigen detection for the diagnosis of gonorrhea. J. Clin. Microbiol. *19*:399–403, 1984.
163. Starnbach, M. N., Falkow, S., and Tompkins, L. S.: Species-specific detection of *Legionella pneumophila* in water by DNA amplification and hybridization. J. Clin. Microbiol. *27*:1257–1261, 1989.
164. Stechenberg, B. W., Schreiner, R. L., Gross, S. M., et al.: Countercurrent immunoelectrophoresis in group B streptococcal disease. Pediatrics *64*:632–634, 1979.
165. Stockman, L., and Roberts, G. D.: Specificity of latex test for cryptococcal antigen: A rapid, simple method for eliminating interference factors. J. Clin. Microbiol. *16*:965–967, 1982.
166. Stratton, C. W.: Serum bactericidal test. Clin. Microbiol. Rev. *1*:19–26, 1988.
167. Stratton, N., Hryniewicki, J., Aarnoes, S. L., et al.: Comparison of monoclonal antibody and calcaflour white stains for the detection of *Pneumocystis carinii* from respiratory specimens. J. Clin. Microbiol. *29*:645–647, 1991.
168. Summanen, P.: Microbiology terminology update: Clinically significant anaerobic gram-positive and gram-negative bacteria (excluding spirochetes). Clin. Infect. Dis. *21*:273–276, 1995.
169. Swenson, J. M., Hindler, J. A., and Peterson, L. R.: Special tests for detecting antibacterial resistance. *In* Murray, P. R., Baron, E. J., Pfaller, M. A., et al. (eds.): Manual of Clinical Microbiology. 6th ed. Washington, D.C., American Society for Microbiology, 1995, pp. 1356–1367.
170. Tang, C. M., Holden, D. W., Aufauvre-Brown, A., et al.: The detection of

Aspergillus spp. by the polymerase chain reaction and its evaluation in brochoalveolar lavage fluid. Am. Rev. Respir. Dis. *148*:1313–1317, 1993.
171. Tanner, D. C., Weinstein, M. P., Fedozciw, B., et al.: Comparison of commercial kits for detection of cryptococcal antigen. J. Clin. Microbiol. *32*:1680–1684, 1994.
172. Tenover, F. C.: Novel and emerging mechanisms of antimicrobial resistance in nosocomial pathogens. Am. J. Med. *91*(Suppl. 3B):76S–81S, 1991.
173. Tenover, F. C., Tokars, J., Swenson, J., et al.: Ability of clinical laboratories to detect antimicrobial agent–resistant enterococci. J. Clin. Microbiol. *31*:1695–1699, 1993.
174. Tiley, S. M., Marriott, D. J. E., and Harkness, J. L.: An evaluation of four methods for the detection of *Pneumocystis carinii* in clinical specimens. Pathology *26*:325–328, 1994.
175. Tilton, R. C., Dias, F., and Ryan, R. W.: Comparative evaluation of three commercial products and counterimmunoelectrophoresis for the detection of antigens in cerebrospinal fluid. J. Clin. Microbiol. *20*:231–234, 1984.
176. Todd, J. K.: Management of urinary tract infections: Children are different. Pediatr. Rev. *16*:190–196, 1995.
177. Turner, R. B., Hayden, F. G., and Hendley, J. O.: Counterimmunoelectrophoresis of urine for diagnosis of bacterial pneumonia in pediatric outpatients. Pediatrics *71*:780–783, 1983.
178. Tzianabos, T., Anderson, B. E., and McDade, J. E.: Detection of *Rickettsia rickettsii* DNA in clinical specimens by using polymerase chain reaction technology. J. Clin. Microbiol. *27*:2866–2868, 1989.
179. van Esso, D., Fontanls, D., Uriz, S, et al.: *Neisseria meningitidis* strains with decreased susceptibility to penicillin. Pediatr. Infect. Dis. J. *6*:438–439, 1987.
180. Wachsmuth, K.: Molecular epidemiology of bacterial infections: Examples of methodology and of investigations of outbreaks. Rev. Infect. Dis. *8*:682–692, 1986.
181. Wack, E. E., Dugger, K. O., and Galgiani, J. N.: Enzyme-linked immunosorbent assay for antigens of *Coccidioides immitis:* Human sera interference corrected by acidification–heat extraction. J. Lab. Clin. Med. *111*:560–565, 1988.
182. Walsh, T. J., Hathorn, J. W., Sober, J. D., et al.: Detection of circulating candida enolase by immunoassay in patients with cancer and invasive candidiasis. N. Engl. J. Med. *324*:1026–1031, 1991.
183. Wasilauskas, B. L., and Hampton, K. D.: Determination of bacterial meningitis: A retrospective study of 80 cerebrospinal fluid specimens evaluated by four in vitro methods. J. Clin. Microbiol. *16*:531–535, 1982.
184. Watt, G., Zaraspe, G., Bautista, S., et al.: Rapid diagnosis of tuberculous meningitis by using an enzyme-linked immunosorbent assay to detect mycobacterial antigen and antibody in cerebrospinal fluid. J. Infect. Dis. *158*:681–686, 1988.
185. Webb, B. J., and Baker, C. J.: Commercial latex agglutination test for rapid diagnosis of group B streptococcal infection in infants. J. Clin. Microbiol. *12*:442–444, 1980.
186. Webb, B. J., Edwards, M. S., and Baker, C. J.: Comparison of slide coagglutination test and countercurrent immunoelectrophoresis for detection of group B streptococcal antigen in cerebrospinal fluid from infants with meningitis. J. Clin. Microbiol. *11*:263–265, 1980.
187. Weinberg, G. A., and Storch, G. A.: Preparation of urine samples for use in commercial latex agglutination tests for bacterial meningitis. J. Clin. Microbiol. *21*:899–901, 1985.
188. Weiner, M. H., and Coats-Stephen, M.: Immunodiagnosis of systemic candidiasis: Mannan antigenemia detected by radioimmunoassay in experimental and human infections. J. Infect. Dis. *140*:989–993, 1979.
189. Weiner, M. H., Talbot, G. H., Gerson, S. L., et al.: Antigen detection in the diagnosis of invasive aspergillosis: Utility in controlled, blinded trials. Ann. Intern. Med. *99*:777–782, 1983.
190. Wheat, L. J., Connolly-Stringfield, P., Kohler, R. B., et al.: *Histoplasma capsulatum* polysaccharide antigen detection in diagnosis and management of disseminated histoplasmosis in patients with acquired immunodeficiency syndrome. Am. J. Med. *87*:396–400, 1989.
191. Wheat, L. J., Kohler, R. B., and Tervari, R. P.: Diagnosis of disseminated histoplasmosis by detection of *Histoplasma capsulatum* antigen in serum and urine specimens. N. Engl. J. Med. *314*:83–88, 1986.
192. Whittle, H. C., Greenwood, B. M., Davidson, N. M., et al.: Meningococcal antigen in diagnosis and treatment of group A meningococcal infections. Am. J. Med. *58*:823–828, 1975.
193. Williams, D. L., Gillis, T. P., Booth, R. J., et al.: The use of a specific DNA probe and polymerase chain reaction for the detection of *Mycobacterium leprae*. J. Infect. Dis. *162*:193–200, 1990.
194. Wolfson, J. S., and Swartz, M. N.: Serum bactericidal activity as a monitor of antibiotic therapy. N. Engl. J. Med. *312*:968–975, 1985.
195. Wonsit, R. N., Thammapalerd, N., Tharavanij, S., et al.: Enzyme-linked immunosorbent assay based on monoclonal and polyclonal antibodies for the detection of *Entamoeba histolytica* antigen in faecal specimens. Trans. R. Soc. Trop. Med. Hyg. *86*:166–169, 1992.
196. Woods, C. R., Smith, A. L., Wasilauskas, B. L., et al.: Invasive disease caused by *Neisseria meningitidis* relatively resistant to penicillin in North Carolina. J. Infect. Dis. *170*:453–456, 1994.
197. Wu, T. C., and Koo, S. Y.: Comparison of three commercial cryptococcal latex kits for detection of cryptococcal antigen. J. Clin. Microbiol. *18*:1127–1130, 1983.
198. Yancey, M. K., Armer, T., Clark, P., et al.: Assessment of rapid identification tests for genital carriage of group B streptococci. Obstet. Gynecol. *80*:1038–1047, 1992.
199. Yolken, R. H.: Enzyme immunoassays for the detection of infectious antigens in body fluids: Current limitations and future prospects. Rev. Infect. Dis. *4*:35–68, 1982.
200. Zimmerman, S. E., Stringfield, P. C., Wheat, R. B., et al.: Comparison of sandwich solid-phase radioimmunoassay and two enzyme-linked immunosorbent assays for detection of *Histoplasma capsulatum* polysaccharide antigen. J. Infect. Dis. *160*:678–685, 1989.

244

USE OF THE DIAGNOSTIC VIROLOGY LABORATORY

Marjorie J. Miller and James D. Cherry

In the present era of readily available, sophisticated, and complex equipment to aid in medical diagnosis and of exciting new therapeutic programs, it is sad to note that practical, clinical, and diagnostic virologic services are available in only a modest number of hospitals and, where available, frequently are not used appropriately by physicians. Because of the present renewed interest in useful viral diagnosis, several innovative methods for the rapid identification of viral infections have been developed. However, laboratories have been supplying useful clinical and viral diagnostic services for more than 25 years. The major problem during the last two-and-a-half decades has been the lack of positive attitude and indoctrination, not lack of adequate methods.

Clinical bacteriology and mycology evolved slowly over a span of more than a century, whereas virology made a comparable advance in a 10-year period with the advent of tissue culture techniques. Initially, virology developed as a tool of the researcher; during the decade of 1950 to 1960, many of the major virus-disease associations that we know today were made, and both polioviruses and measles virus were attenuated for vaccine development. During this period of rapid development, research funds were readily available, so young persons with an interest in virology gravitated to investigative endeavors. Also, hospital clinical microbiology laboratories were operated primarily by persons trained as bacteriologists and pathologists, who felt in general that because the new virologic techniques were so different, it would be impractical to introduce them into the setting of a hospital laboratory. This idea also was fostered by epidemiologists and researchers. Because of the lack of diagnostic services locally, then, state and federal facilities instituted viral diagnostic services. In addition, many research programs offered limited diagnostic services for special cases.

Although the services of state laboratories and the research units contributed to our understanding of the spectrum of viral illness, their methods of operation did much to hinder the ultimate development of useful clinical viral diagnostic laboratory services. Because these units were directed by epidemiologists and others interested in the dynamics of disease rather than in individual patients, services were not geared to the welfare of the patient. It was routine to collect specimens from patients but to perform viral diagnostic procedures only if the physician provided acute and convalescent-phase sera. This always led to such a delay that most physicians lost interest; they directed their concerns to more pressing problems.

Progress in virology continued at a remarkable rate. However, by the mid-1960s, the major share of research in virology shifted from epidemiologic considerations and clinical disease associations to more basic laboratory virology. With this change in research emphasis, the attitude that we have learned all there is to know about clinical diseases associated with viral infections prevailed. More alarming is the fact that few medical school departments of microbiology presently staff persons qualified to teach clinical aspects of virology. The result is that few students today receive any practical training in this sphere.

Another aspect that contributes greatly to the lack of and the failure to use viral diagnostic services relates to medical economics and the delivery of health care. At present, major research efforts are directed to health care systems. Although these programs are necessary, all seem flawed. No research program takes into consideration the fact that even the simplest aspect of clinical medicine (such as respiratory infection) is dynamic and not static; most health care evaluation systems seem to assume that we know all there is to know about routine medical problems. This attitude is deplorable because, of course, there still is much to learn about "simple" problems such as upper respiratory infections. Even more important, care suffers when physicians are denied the chance to be inquisitive about the problems they confront.

Because diagnosis is the foundation of all medical care, it should be unnecessary to justify accurate diagnosis of specific viral disease. However, it is apparent from the preceding discussion that the values of viral diagnosis need emphasis. Specific reasons why clinical virologic laboratory services should be available routinely are listed in Table 244–1. Routine viral diagnostic laboratories should be similar to bacteriology laboratories and specialize in the identification of specific etiologic agents as rapidly as possible. Serologic study in cases of possible viral disease often can be relegated to reference laboratories, as is done when serologic studies are carried out in possible bacterial and fungal infections. At present, some laboratories routinely provide effective viral diagnostic services; laboratory reports of viral isolates reach physicians almost as rapidly as do bacterial reports, and charges are similar to those for conventional bacteriologic procedures.[88, 89, 146, 176]

This chapter presents general aspects of viral diagnosis, including specimen selection, collection, and transport; conventional and modified culture for virus isolation and identification; and rapid detection of viral antigens and nucleic acids directly in specimens. Specific aspects of viral diagnosis are presented in the respective chapters covering the particular agents.

TABLE 244–1. Why Clinical Virologic Laboratory Services Should Be Available on a Routine Basis

Knowledge of etiology in the clinical setting tunes the physician's interest, leading to better care.
Knowledge of viral infection reduces inappropriate antibiotic administration.
Knowledge of viral etiology reduces costs and discomfort of unnecessary diagnostic procedures and lengthy hospital stays.
Virologic diagnosis is critical for the use of presently available antiviral drugs. As new drugs are developed, this becomes even more important.
Wider use of viral diagnostic services leads to a better understanding of disease processes: viral-bacterial interactions and relationship of viruses to "noninfectious diseases," such as myocardial infarctions and pancreatitis.
Success and failure of viral vaccines are monitored more accurately.
Better patient awareness results from specific viral study. Patients like to know their illness, and this can be useful historically when future medical illnesses occur.
More accurate prognosis of disease outcome is made when the specific etiologic agent is known.
The routine availability and use of viral diagnostic services make the physician more aware of priorities in medical research. The morbidity and mortality due to specific viral agents, such as respiratory syncytial virus, should lead to interest in development of new vaccines.

SPECIMEN COLLECTION AND TRANSPORT

Currently, many well-equipped state public health laboratories use traditional as well as more recently developed technologies that should ensure the successful recovery of viruses from a high percentage of submitted specimens. However, the isolation rates in these facilities frequently are poor because of suboptimal collection and transport of specimens. In contrast, some small hospital-based laboratories offering a limited variety of procedures frequently have high isolation rates because of efficient, rapid collection and transport of specimens.

Specimen Collection Sites

The selection of appropriate sites for specimen collection as early in the acute phase of the illness as possible is critical to the recovery of viruses. A guide to recommended collection sites for specific viral syndromes is presented in Table 244–2. In general, the extent of the diagnostic investigation should be dictated by the characteristics of the illness being studied. For example, in common respiratory illnesses, such as pharyngitis or croup, the collection of a single specimen from the throat is all that usually is necessary. In other situations in which an illness is severe or unique, the collection of specimens from multiple sites is important. In addition, in the unusual case, serum should be obtained for frozen storage in case subsequent serologic studies are required.

In unusual and severe illnesses, it frequently is necessary to use invasive procedures (e.g., brain, cardiac, liver, lung biopsies; needle aspiration of body fluids) to obtain material for laboratory study. Many medical specialists argue against these invasive procedures because little can be done to treat viral illnesses. However, in our experience, the knowledge gained from a positive viral identification justifies some risk in specimen collection. At present, antiviral drugs are similar to antibacterial and antifungal agents in that they usually can be used effectively only after definitive identification of the etiologic agent. The demonstration of a viral etiologic agent in diseases such as encephalitis, pneumonia, or cardiac disease can prevent the unnecessary administration of antibiotics and steroids. In many cases, overutilization of services, patient trauma, and overall cost can be reduced when a viral etiologic agent is confirmed. Finally, the prognosis of a particular illness is more accurate when the specific etiologic agent is known.

Collection of Specimens

Specimens for virus culture or direct examination generally are obtained as for other microbiologic study. The primary purpose of a transport medium is to provide a protective protein, neutral pH, and antibiotics for control of microbial contamination and, most importantly, to prevent desiccation. Many viral transport and storage media are commercially available or are prepared readily in the laboratory; their utility has been reviewed.[104] Convenient and practical collection devices, such as the Culturette (Becton-Dickinson, Cokeysville, MD) or Virocult (Medical Wire and Equipment Co., Victory Gardens, NY), consist of a swab, usually Dacron or rayon, on a plastic or aluminum shaft accompanied by a self-contained transport medium (Stuart or Amies) and are routinely available in most hospitals for bacteriologic culture. Calcium alginate swabs, which are toxic to herpes simplex virus and wooden shafts, which may be toxic for viruses as well as the cell culture system itself, should not be used. Saline or holding media that contain serum also should be avoided. Useful liquid transport media (2-mL aliquots in screw-capped vials) consist of tryptose phosphate broth with 0.5 per cent bovine albumin; Hanks balanced salt solution with 5 per cent gelatin or 10 per cent bovine albumin; or buffered sucrose phosphate (0.2 M, 2-SP),[92, 104] which has been used as a combined transport for viral, chlamydial, and mycoplasmal culture requests[16] and is appropriate for long-term frozen storage of specimens and isolates.[8]

Some of these transport media also have been evaluated and found acceptable for use in rapid methods, such as enzyme-linked immunosorbent assay (ELISA)[166, 252] and polymerase chain reaction (PCR).[153]

Throat

Specimens from the throat should be obtained with a swab in a manner similar to that employed for bacterial culture. The posterior pharyngeal wall and tonsillar surfaces, any inflamed or erythematous areas, and any visible lesions are swabbed firmly without contact with the tongue and anterior oral cavity.

Nose and Nasopharyngeal

Specimens should be collected with nasopharyngeal swabs (with thin, flexible wire shafts) by inserting the swab into the nasopharynx and rotating to obtain the maximum number of ciliated, columnar epithelial cells and then placing the swab in transport medium. Alternatively, a flexible nasal probe with a cupped tip may be used (Rhinoprobe, Rhinotechnics, San Diego, CA).[101] Nasopharyngeal cultures can be obtained from infants by the wash technique described by Hall and Douglas.[84] With this method, a small amount of sterile phosphate-buffered saline (3 to 7 mL) is squeezed into the nose with a nasal bulb aspirator (1-oz. tapered) and then immediately withdrawn and placed in a sterile screw-capped container. Alternatively, nasopharyngeal aspirates may be obtained using a mucus collection device. An appropriately sized catheter is inserted nasally into the posterior nasopharynx; intermittent suction is applied as the catheter is withdrawn. Aspirate is washed through the tubing with 5 to 8 mL of transport medium or sterile phosphate-buffered saline. Washes and aspirates (vs. swabs) are preferred for direct antigen detection because more epithelial cells are obtained with this method.[3]

Other Respiratory (Sputum, Tracheal Aspirates, Bronchial Washings, Bronchoalveolar Lavage)

Collection depends on the volume obtained. Volumes of greater than or equal to 0.5 mL should be placed in a sterile container and sealed tightly. If the volume is less than 0.5 mL, the specimen is placed in 2 mL of transport medium.

Eye

Exudate or pus should be removed first with a sterile swab. Conjunctival specimens may be obtained by pressing a swab premoistened with sterile saline firmly against the inflamed areas. The swab is returned to the self-contained transport device or the tip is broken off into 2 mL of transport medium. Corneal scrapings should be obtained by an ophthalmologist or other trained person and placed in transport medium immediately.

Body Fluids Other Than Blood

Body fluids such as urine (clean-voided, 10 to 20 mL), cerebrospinal fluid (2 to 5 mL), pleural effusion, and peritoneal, pericardial, or joint fluids should be collected under sterile conditions and placed in securely sealed sterile containers. For small volumes (<0.5 mL), the specimen may be placed in transport medium.

Lesions

Select fresh vesicles because virus recovery from older lesions decreases significantly. Gently swab the area with sterile saline. Rupture the vesicle and collect both fluid and cells from the base of the lesion. Material obtained from several lesions may be pooled. Desiccation must not occur; swabs should be submitted moistened with their self-contained transport medium or, if that is unavailable, placed in 2 mL of transport medium. Specimens may be collected with a swab or aspirated with a 26-gauge needle attached to a tuberculin syringe. Aspirated fluid should be rinsed into 1 to 2 mL of transport medium.

For direct antigen detection by immunofluorescence (IF) (direct fluorescent antibody, or DFA), the vesicle is ruptured as previously described and epithelial cells are collected by firmly swabbing the base of the lesion. Cells are transferred to a clean glass slide by firmly rolling the swab back and forth over a 5- to 10-mm area (dime-size); for differentiation of herpes simplex virus types 1 and 2 (HSV-1 and HSV-2) and varicella-zoster virus (VZV), prepare three areas.

Stool and Rectal

Because of initial studies with polioviruses and other enteroviruses, the culture of fecal material has been overemphasized in virology. Both enteroviruses and adenoviruses can be recovered readily from stool, but because these agents are

TABLE 244–2. Specimen Collection Guide for the Diagnosis of Viral Infections Based on Viral Syndrome and Etiologic Agent Suspected

Main Location or Category of Illness	Clinical Diagnosis	Specimen Collection Source: *Most Practical*	Specimen Collection Source: *Most Definitive*	Other Sources	Etiologic Agent Suspected*
Upper respiratory tract	Common cold, nasopharyngitis	Nasopharynx/nose	Nasopharynx/nose	Nasal wash, stool, blood	Rhinoviruses, coronaviruses, parainfluenza viruses, respiratory syncytial virus, enteroviruses, adenoviruses
	Pharyngitis	Throat	Throat	Stool, blood	Adenoviruses, enteroviruses, Epstein-Barr virus, influenza viruses, parainfluenza viruses
	Herpangina, other enanthems	Throat	Lesions	Stool, blood	Enteroviruses, herpes simplex virus
	Laryngitis, laryngotracheitis	Throat	Larynx or trachea	Nasal wash	Parainfluenza viruses, influenza viruses
	Parotitis, other salivary gland enlargement	Throat	Stensen duct	Urine, blood, cerebrospinal fluid	Mumps virus, enteroviruses
Lower respiratory tract	Bronchitis, bronchiolitis, pneumonia	Throat	Bronchoalveolar lavage, bronchial washing, biopsy	Stool, blood	Respiratory syncytial virus, parainfluenza viruses, adenoviruses, influenza viruses
	Pleurodynia	Throat	Throat	Stool	Enteroviruses
	Pleural effusion	Pleural fluid	Pleural fluid	Throat, stool, blood	Enteroviruses, adenoviruses
Heart	Myocarditis, pericarditis, conduction defects	Throat	Pericardial fluid, biopsy	Stool, blood, urine	Enteroviruses, influenza viruses
Central nervous system	Meningitis	Throat	Cerebrospinal fluid	Stool, blood, urine	Enteroviruses, mumps virus, arboviruses, herpes simplex virus type 2, lymphocytic choriomeningitis virus
	Encephalitis	Throat	Brain biopsy	Cerebrospinal fluid, stool, blood, urine	Arboviruses, mumps virus, enteroviruses, herpes simplex virus type 1, influenza viruses
	Guillain-Barré syndrome, cerebellar ataxia, transverse myelitis, poliomyelitis	Throat	Throat	Stool, blood, cerebrospinal fluid	Influenza viruses, arboviruses, enteroviruses, Epstein-Barr virus
Genital tract	Orchitis, epididymitis	Throat	Testicular biopsy	Stool, blood, urine	Mumps, enteroviruses, lymphocytic choriomeningitis virus
	Herpes genitalis	Lesions	Lesions	Vagina, cervix, urethra	Herpes simplex virus
Urinary tract	Cytomegalovirus infection	Urine	Urine	Throat, blood	Cytomegalovirus
	Hematuria and/or pyuria	Throat, urine	Urine	Blood, stool	Arboviruses, enteroviruses, mumps virus, adenoviruses

Gastrointestinal tract	Nausea and/or vomiting	Throat	Throat	Stool, blood	Enteroviruses, influenza viruses, Norwalk-like agents
	Diarrhea	Stool	Stool	Throat	Rotaviruses, Norwalk-like agents, enteroviruses, adenoviruses
	Abdominal pain	Throat	Throat	Stool, blood	Enteroviruses, adenoviruses
	Acute abdomen, mesenteric adenitis	Throat	Mesenteric lymph node biopsy, peritoneal fluid	Stool, blood	Enteroviruses, adenoviruses
	Hepatitis	Throat	Liver biopsy	Stool, blood	Hepatitis A, B, C, E, and G viruses, Epstein-Barr virus, adenoviruses, enteroviruses
	Pancreatitis	Throat	Duodenal fluid	Stool, blood	Enteroviruses
	Reye syndrome	Throat	Liver biopsy	Blood	Influenza viruses, varicella virus
Reticuloendothelial system	Hepatosplenomegaly	Throat	Blood, liver biopsy	Stool, urine	Adenoviruses, enteroviruses, Epstein-Barr virus, cytomegalovirus
	Generalized lymphadenopathy	Throat	Blood, lymph node biopsy	Stool, urine	Adenoviruses, enteroviruses, Epstein-Barr virus, cytomegalovirus
	Immune deficiency	Blood	Blood	Lymph nodes	HIV
Bone or joints	Osteomyelitis	Bone	Bone	Throat, blood, urine, skin lesion	Rubella virus, vaccinia virus
	Arthritis	Joint fluid	Joint fluid	Throat, blood, urine	Rubella virus, arboviruses
Muscle	Myositis	Throat	Muscle biopsy	Stool, blood	Influenza viruses, enteroviruses
Skin	Exanthematous disease	Throat	Vesicular fluid, skin biopsy	Stool, blood, urine, eye	Measles virus, rubella virus, varicella virus, enteroviruses, common respiratory viruses
Eye	Conjunctivitis including pharyngoconjunctival fever	Eye	Eye	Throat, stool	Adenoviruses, enteroviruses
Fever	Nonspecific febrile illness (human-to-human transmission)	Throat	Blood	Stool, urine, cerebrospinal fluid	Enteroviruses, influenza viruses, adenoviruses, cytomegalovirus
	Nonspecific febrile illness (arthropod vector)	Blood	Blood	Throat, urine, cerebrospinal fluid	Arboviruses
	Fever of unknown origin	Blood	Blood	Urine, stool, throat	Hepatitis A, B, C, E, and G viruses, cytomegalovirus, herpes simplex virus, Epstein-Barr virus, adenoviruses
Congenital infection	Rubella virus, cytomegalovirus infections	Throat	Blood	Urine, nasopharynx, biopsy material, cerebrospinal fluid	Rubella virus, cytomegalovirus
Perinatal and neonatal infections	HIV infection	Blood	Blood	Lymph node	HIV
	Herpes simplex virus, cytomegalovirus, enterovirus infections	Throat	Blood	Urine, nasopharynx, stool, skin lesions, cerebrospinal fluid	Enteroviruses, respiratory syncytial virus, influenza viruses, herpes simplex virus, cytomegalovirus

*This listing includes only the more commonly associated agents; it is likely that with more general use of viral diagnostic services, new virus-disease associations will be made.

carried in the lower gastrointestinal tract for considerable periods after acute infection, the use of this source for diagnosis of specific illnesses is limited. A specimen of fecal material is practical only when the specific primary diagnosis is diarrhea or when concomitant serologic study with paired sera can be performed.

For the recovery of enteroviruses, fresh stool specimens are better than rectal swabs; transfer 2 to 5 g (2 to 3 tsp) of formed or liquid specimen to a sterile, leak-proof container. However, from a practical point of view, the rectal swab is the simplest method of specimen collection. A rectal swab can be obtained immediately, whereas the collection of a stool specimen usually entails considerable delay. It is important that the swab contain visible stool; insert the swab 3 to 5 cm into the rectum, roll the swab against the mucosa, and then transport in a Culturette or similar device.

Blood

Some viruses can be recovered from the serum or red blood cells, but in general, the leukocytes are a better source of virus. Fresh blood (optimally 5 mL) is collected in a suitable anticoagulant (heparin, ethylene diamine tetraacetic acid, acid citrate dextrose) and transported to the laboratory for processing by density gradient centrifugation[9] or other methods to enrich for leukocytes. Edetic acid is the anticoagulant of choice because this is an acceptable transport for culture as well as molecular methods such as hybridization and PCR.

Bone Marrow

Aspirate about 2 mL into a tube or syringe containing heparin anticoagulant, mix thoroughly to prevent clotting, and transport without further additives or diluents.

Biopsy Specimens

For biopsies, fresh tissue obtained from the affected site should be placed in 2 mL of transport medium to prevent desiccation.

Autopsy Specimens

Most postmortem specimens are almost useless for viral cultivation because of the manner in which autopsies usually are performed. If labile agents are to be recovered, the autopsy should be performed within 4 hours of death. All tissues (1- to 2.5-cm cubes) for study should be obtained aseptically, and individual tissue should be collected with sterile instruments and placed in separate sterile containers. Because the usual autopsy routine employs the fixation of specimens, it is vital that specimens for viral isolation are not placed in containers with fixatives such as formalin or other preservatives.

Transport to the Laboratory

The method of specimen handling from the time of collection to laboratory processing is critical for preservation of virus infectivity and subsequent recovery in culture. In general, the less time between collection and inoculation into cell culture, the greater the chance of virus recovery. Specimens should not be frozen or exposed to temperatures greater than 22° C. For short-term storage (≤5 days) of most viruses, the specimen should be held at 4° C until it can be processed in the laboratory. For transport to the laboratory, this temperature can be achieved with the use of cold packs or simply by placing one ice cube next to the specimen container within an aluminum foil wrapping.

Although the degree of sensitivity varies, all viruses are inactivated by ultraviolet light. Therefore, it is important to shield specimens from sunlight. This can be accomplished by the use of opaque transport boxes or the wrapping of individual specimens in aluminum foil or opaque paper.

When considerable delay between collection and culture will occur (transport to other laboratories, holiday schedules, and so on), special preparation is necessary. This preparation needs to be individualized and based on the most likely viral cause of a particular illness. For example, when an enteroviral etiologic agent is suspected, freezing of the specimen (−70° C) and shipping with dry ice are satisfactory. In contrast, a urine specimen from a patient with possible cytomegalovirus (CMV) infection should not be frozen. It should be shipped under wet ice at 4° C; CMV in the urine is stable for several days at 4° C. In addition, media are available for transport as well as long-term storage that protects virus against the deleterious effects of temperature fluctuations, particularly freeze-thawing.[92] For specific characteristics of individual viruses, see Chapters 157 to 192 and the general references at the end of this chapter.[129, 159, 209, 220]

LABORATORY DIAGNOSIS OF VIRAL INFECTIONS

Previously, the perception that virus isolation was difficult, nonproductive, and too slow to be of clinical utility combined with the lack of consistently available reliable reagents discouraged the use of diagnostic virology services. Since the mid-1980s, there has been a dramatic increase in the quality and availability of diagnostic reagents, primarily monoclonal antibodies, which has significantly improved the turnaround time to reporting of virology results. Direct detection of viral antigens in clinical specimens—for example, the herpes group viruses (HSV, VZV, CMV), respiratory syncytial virus (RSV), influenza viruses, adenoviruses, and rotaviruses, usually by IF, an immunoperoxidase (IP) test, or ELISA—has become routine and has made same-day results a reality. In addition, detection of viral antigens in cell culture by application of IF/IP staining or ELISA, before the appearance of cytopathic effect (CPE), has reduced greatly the time to reporting of a positive result. More recently, molecular techniques for the direct detection and quantitation of viral nucleic acids in specimens[48, 99, 172] have begun the transition from research tool to routine use in the clinical laboratory as commercial reagents become readily available, methods are simplified and standardized, and some assays are manufactured in kit format. Methods for the laboratory diagnosis of specific viral infections are presented in Chapters 157 to 192, and detailed methods are provided in the general references at the end of this chapter.[99, 129, 159, 192, 209, 220] Table 244–3 summarizes specific methods for the laboratory identification of viruses in addition to indications for serologic study for selected viruses.

VIRUS ISOLATION

Despite technologic advances and innovations, culture remains the cornerstone of the diagnostic virology laboratory. Culture still is among the most sensitive of diagnostic methods because theoretically a single infectious virus can be detected. Unlike rapid methods, which are limited to the detection of a specific viral antigen or nucleic acid, culture is open-ended and permits the detection of unexpected viruses,

TABLE 244–3. Common Laboratory Methods for Virus Isolation, Identification, and Direct Detection and Most Useful Method for Diagnosis of Specific Viral Illnesses

	Culture/Direct Detection	Identification of Isolates	Serology	Most Useful Method for Diagnosis of Specific Viral Illness
Adenoviruses	Primary HEK, A549, WI-38, HEp-2, HeLa, KB cell culture/FA, ELISA	Group identified by characteristic CPE and/or FA; type identified by neutralization with specific antiserum	CF on paired sera, ELISA, HAI	Virus isolation
Arboviruses of North America	Suckling mouse intracerebral inoculation, Vero, BHK-21, LLC-MK2 cell culture	Neutralization with specific antiserum	CF on paired sera, HAI, indirect FA, IgM antibody capture ELISA	CF on paired sera
Coronaviruses	Human embryo tracheal organ culture, HEK	Neutralization with specific antiserum	Neutralization, CF, HAI on paired sera	No practical method presently available
Rhinoviruses	WI-38, MRC-5 cell culture	Characteristic CPE; stability on exposure to lipid solvents and inactivation at pH 3	Neutralization on paired sera	Virus isolation
Enteroviruses	MK, WI-38 cell culture, suckling mouse inoculation (intracerebral and intraperitoneal)	Group identified by characteristic CPE in cell culture or illness or pathology in mice; type identified by neutralization with specific antiserum; FA for some serotypes	Neutralization, CF, HAI on paired sera	Virus isolation
Cytomegalovirus	WI-38, MRC-5, foreskin cell culture/FA, IP	Characteristic CPE, FA/IP for definitive identification	CF on paired sera, ELISA, LA, indirect FA	Virus isolation
Epstein-Barr virus (EBV)	Practical method not available	Practical method not available	Indirect FA against viral capsid antigen on paired sera; indirect FA against early antigen in single serum	Infectious mononucleosis rapid slide tests; rarely EBV-specific FA test
Herpes simplex viruses	WI-38, MRC-5, primary RK cell culture/FA, IP, ELISA	Characteristic CPE; FA, IP, ELISA for definitive identification	CF on paired sera, ELISA, indirect FA	Virus isolation; antigen detection by FA, ELISA
HIV	ELISA, PCR, bDNA	ELISA, Western blot	ELISA, Western blot, indirect FA	ELISA
Influenza viruses	MK, LLC-MK2, MDCK cell culture and chicken embryo (amniotic sac and allantoic cavity) inoculation/FA, ELISA	HA or hemadsorption of guinea pig or chicken erythrocytes and inhibition with specific antiserum for type/strain identification; FA for identification of type	CF, HAI; ELISA on paired sera	Virus isolation; antigen detection by FA, ELISA
Measles virus	Primary MK, HEK cell culture/FA	Hemadsorption and HA of monkey erythrocytes and inhibition with specific antiserum or identification by FA	CF, HAI on paired sera; identification of measles-specific IgM antibody by ELISA, indirect FA	Identification of measles-specific IgM antibody by ELISA, indirect FA or CF/HAI antibody titer rise
Parainfluenza viruses, mumps virus	Primary MK, LLC-MK2, HEK cell culture/FA	Hemadsorption and HA of guinea pig erythrocytes; specific identification by FA	CF, HAI on paired sera, ELISA, indirect FA	Virus isolation
Respiratory syncytial virus	HEp-2, WI-38 cell culture/FA, ELISA	Characteristic CPE in absence of hemadsorption; specific identification by FA	CF on paired sera, ELISA, indirect FA	Detection of viral antigen by FA/ELISA; virus isolation
Rabies virus (animal infections)	Demonstration of Negri bodies by microscopic examination of brain or demonstration of viral antigen by FA, mouse inoculation	Demonstration of Negri bodies or antigen by FA	Neutralization, ELISA	Antigen detection by FA

Table continued on following page

TABLE 244–3. Common Laboratory Methods for Virus Isolation, Identification, and Direct Detection and Most Useful Method for Diagnosis of Specific Viral Illnesses *Continued*

	Culture/Direct Detection	Identification of Isolates	Serology	Most Useful Method for Diagnosis of Specific Viral Illness
Reoviruses	Primary MK, HEK, HeLa cell culture/EM	CPE; neutralization with specific antiserum; HAI, FA	Neutralization, HAI on paired sera	Virus isolation
Rubella virus	African green monkey kidney cell culture	Interference of enteroviral CPE, neutralization with specific antiserum	HAI on paired sera; identification of rubella-specific IgM antibody by ELISA, indirect FA	Identification of rubella-specific IgM antibody by ELISA, indirect FA or HAI antibody titer rise
Poxviruses	MK, WI38 cell culture/FA, EM	Characteristic CPE; FA or appearance on EM	Not useful for diagnosis	Antigen detection by FA, EM
Varicella-zoster virus	WI-38, MRC-5 cell culture/FA	Characteristic CPE; FA for definitive identification	CF on paired sera, EIA, LA, IHA, IAHA, ACIF, FAMA	Detection of viral antigen by FA; virus isolation
Hepatitis A virus	Demonstration of antigen by ELISA, IEM, RIA	ELISA, IEM, RIA	ELISA, RIA, HAI	Identification of HAV specific IgM by ELISA, RIA
Hepatitis B virus	Demonstration of antigen by ELISA, RIA, HA; demonstration of DNA hybridization, PCR	ELISA, RIA, HA	ELISA, RIA, HA	Demonstration of antigen, nucleic acid
Hepatitis C virus	Demonstration of RNA by PCR or bDNA	Practical method not available	ELISA, RIBA	ELISA, RIBA, demonstration of viral RNA
Norwalk-like agents	Demonstration of antigen by IEM, RIA	IEM, RIA	ELISA, RIA-BL; serology not used routinely	Demonstration of antigen
Rotavirus	Demonstration of antigen by ELISA, LA, EM	EM, ELISA	ELISA; serology not used routinely	Demonstration of antigen
Adenovirus 40/41	Demonstration of antigens by ELISA	ELISA	CF, ELISA on paired sera; serology not used routinely	Demonstration of antigen

For details, see Section 17.

ACIF, anticomplement immunofluorescence; A549, human lung carcinoma; BHK-21, continuous baby hamster kidney cell line; bDNA, branched DNA; CF, complement fixation; CPE, cytopathic effect; ELISA, enzyme-linked immunosorbent assay; EM, electron microscopy; FA, immunofluorescent antibody; FAMA, fluorescent antibody to membrane antigen; HA, hemagglutination; HAI, hemagglutination inhibition; HEK, human embryonic kidney; HEp-2, human laryngeal carcinoma cells; IAHA, immune adherence hemagglutination assay; IHA, indirect hemagglutination; IEM, immune electron microscopy; IP, immunoperoxidase test; KB, oral cavity carcinoma; LA, latex agglutination; LLC-MK2, continuous line of rhesus MK; MDCK, Madin-Darby canine kidney; MK, monkey kidney; PCR, polymerase chain reaction; RIA, radioimmunoassay; RIA-BL, radioimmunoassay blocking test; RIBA, recombinant immunoblot assay; RK, rabbit kidney; Vero, continuous line of African green MK; WI-38, MRC-5, human fetal diploid lung fibroblasts.

new viruses, or multiple viruses within the same specimen. In addition, a broad range of specimens can be evaluated, whereas rapid methods usually are approved or licensed for use with specimens collected from specific sites. Viruses that can be isolated and identified readily include adenoviruses, HSV, VZV, CMV, enteroviruses, rhinoviruses, influenza and parainfluenza viruses, RSV, rubella virus, mumps virus, and measles virus. The number and type of isolates encountered depends on the patient population, season, and type of specimens submitted. For optimal laboratory diagnosis, it is important to indicate the virus suspected on the requisition because some viruses require specific cell lines, procedures for identification, or both. Cultures are maintained for different time frames before finalizing a report of negative results, depending on the virus being sought; for example, HSV cultures usually are observed for 5 to 7 days, CMV for 1 month, and all others for 2 to 4 weeks. Improvements and modifications in culture methods have resulted in more rapid identification of isolates, with greater than 70 per cent being reported within 5 days.[46, 95]

Traditional Culture

Although animals such as suckling mice and chicken embryos originally were the only means of isolating viruses, most laboratories now use cell culture exclusively. A variety of cell lines capable of supporting the growth of a broad spectrum of viruses can be obtained fresh weekly from commercial sources. After specimen inoculation, cultures are observed at regular intervals for evidence of viral infection characterized by the appearance of CPE or the ability to hemadsorb or hemagglutinate red blood cells. Adenoviruses, CMV, HSV, VZV, rhinoviruses, and enteroviruses can be identified and reported by their characteristic CPE. The mean time between specimen inoculation and the appearance of

CPE usually is 1 week or less for most of this group except CMV and some adenoviruses, which may require longer incubation. Cultures containing HSV and enteroviruses often are positive within 1 to 2 and 3 to 5 days, respectively. In the event of atypical or questionable CPE, IF using monoclonal antibodies can be used specifically to identify CMV, VZV, HSV-1, HSV-2, adenoviruses, enteroviruses, and some select coxsackieviruses and echoviruses in infected cell culture. Although rarely performed, the neutralization test is used definitively to identify adenoviruses and enteroviruses if serotyping is requested for epidemiologic or other reasons.[99, 209]

The respiratory viruses, including the parainfluenza and influenza viruses, which may or may not produce CPE, usually can be detected within 5 to 7 days of specimen inoculation with use of the traditional hemadsorption method in which a suspension of guinea pig red blood cells is added to the cell culture. The red blood cells are observed to adhere to tissue culture cells infected with these viruses, usually 3 to 5 days after inoculation of specimens for most isolates.[157] An adaptation of this method uses cell culture medium and guinea pig red blood cells in a microtiter plate format to detect viral hemagglutinins in suspension. Results are similar to those observed with hemadsorption but are more rapid and simple to perform when screening numerous specimens.[106] RSV presumptively is identified, usually within 3 to 5 days of specimen inoculation, by its typical CPE (syncytium formation) and inability to hemadsorb/hemagglutinate guinea pig red blood cells. This group of viruses is identified definitively by IF using monoclonal antibodies.[99, 209]

Finally, the traditional method for isolation and identification of rubella virus employs primary African green monkey kidney cells in conjunction with the interference assay. After specified intervals following inoculation, cultures are challenged with a second virus, usually echovirus 11, incubated for an additional 3 to 4 days, and examined for CPE. The presence of rubella virus interferes with the growth of the challenge virus, and no CPE is observed; on the other hand, if challenge virus grows and produces CPE, the specimen is considered negative for rubella virus. Final identification of the isolate requires neutralization of the interference with specific rubella antibody.[159, 209]

Serologic diagnosis is recommended for those viruses that are difficult or impossible to isolate in commonly available cell cultures or that require special techniques for detection of their presence. For instance, in most cases of arbovirus infection, the study of paired sera for antibody development is the most rewarding for diagnosis. HIV infection usually is identified best by the demonstration of serum antibody or antigen with the use of ELISA. Measles virus is relatively difficult to grow, and its identification can take considerable time; when measles is suspected, the diagnosis is confirmed most easily by serologic study. Paired sera collected 1 week apart usually reveal a fourfold antibody titer rise. Alternatively, the demonstration of specific IgM antibody allows diagnosis with use of a single serum sample. Similarly, serology is useful for the diagnosis of mumps virus. Although mumps virus can be isolated in the same cell lines used for other paramyxoviruses and detected by hemadsorption/hemagglutination as previously described, such requests are rare. Rubella virus requires 2 or more weeks for isolation and specific identification. Because of this delay, rubella virus infection, other than that acquired congenitally, is confirmed best by serologic study. In all instances of suspected congenital rubella, virus isolation should be attempted.

Modified Culture

A variety of physical and chemical methods have been evaluated for their ability to enhance the rapid detection of virus in culture.[95] These include the effect of low- and high-speed rolling of cultures, centrifugation, chemicals such as dimethylsulfoxide, hormones such as dexamethasone, and enzymes such as trypsin on the isolation of viruses. Early detection of viral antigens in culture by IF and an IP test, prior to the appearance of CPE, also has been evaluated.[61, 154, 177, 198] A technique that employs the physical method of centrifugation with early antigen detection in cell culture and is called variously the shell vial assay (SVA), spin amplified technique, or culture amplified antigen detection is used routinely in most laboratories to decrease the time to detection of a positive culture. Cell lines are propagated on 12-mm round coverslips in 1-dram shell vials. An aliquot of specimen is inoculated into the vial, centrifuged at $700 \times g$ for 1 hour, and incubated 1 to 3 days, depending on the virus being sought. Antigen typically is detected by IF or occasionally by IP staining using monoclonal antibodies directed against a specific virus.

SVA was described initially and evaluated extensively for HSV[57, 75, 135, 175, 180, 201] and CMV,[62, 70, 74, 76, 128, 170, 171, 185] and its use since has been extended to the rapid identification of VZV,[73, 205] adenovirus,[8, 59, 136, 236] RSV,[14, 218] influenza virus,[60, 155, 213, 225] parainfluenza virus,[206] and measles virus[156] antigens in culture. Pooled antibodies directed against seven commonly isolated respiratory viruses (adenovirus, influenza viruses A and B, parainfluenza virus types 1, 2, and 3, and RSV) also have been evaluated.[142, 167, 184] SVA also has been applied to the detection of enteroviruses[113] and human herpesvirus type 6.[150]

Although rapid, sensitive, and specific, SVA is an adjunct to and not a substitute for traditional culture. Its sensitivity compared with that of traditional culture averages around 85 per cent (range, 70 to 100 per cent) and depends on a number of variables, including cell line,[275] age of cells,[62] virus concentration,[275] type of specimen,[128, 170] number of vials inoculated,[170] and type of reagents employed.[58, 75, 154, 175, 201] Table 244–4 summarizes typical time to detection of a positive result in traditional culture and SVA, sensitivity of SVA versus culture, and turnaround time for each.

Other culture modifications include hybridization[58, 65] and ELISA[8, 43, 149, 250, 258] for rapid detection of viruses. A modification of cell culture for the rapid detection of HSV is ELVIS (enzyme-linked virus-inducible system).[222, 223] This system consists of a mixture of modified baby hamster kidney cells and MRC5 cells. The modified baby hamster kidney cells

TABLE 244–4. Detection of Virus in Traditional Culture and Shell Vial Assay

	Traditional Culture		Shell Vial Assay	
Virus	*Usual Day Positive, Range*	*Negative Turnaround Time*	*Day Stained (Range)*	*% Sensitivity vs. Culture*
Adenovirus	4–10	2–3 wk	2 (1–3)	50–100
CMV	7–14	1 mo	2 (1–3)	75–100
Enterovirus	1–7	2–3 wk	3	93
HSV	1–3	5–7 d	1	70–100
HHV-6	NA	2–3 wk	3 (2–3)	86
Influenza	3–7	2–3 wk	2 (1–3)	56–100
Parainfluenza	3–7	2–3 wk	2 (1–3)	80–100
RSV	3–7	2–3 wk	2 (1–3)	73–100
VZV	5–10	2–3 wk	3 (2–5)	80–100

CMV, cytomegalovirus; HHV-6, human herpesvirus type 6; HSV, herpes simplex virus; RSV, respiratory syncytial virus; VZV, varicella-zoster virus.

contain an HSV-inducible promoter and an *Escherichia coli LacZ* reporter gene that produces β-galactosidase only when cells are infected with HSV. After the addition of a substrate for the β-galactosidase, infected cells stain blue while uninfected cells remain colorless. ELVIS appears to be comparable with culture for the detection of HSV-positive specimens (95 to 100 per cent sensitivity) in a similar time frame, 1.4 to 1.7 days.[139] This system may have future application to antiviral susceptibility testing.[211]

DIRECT DETECTION

Cytology

Historically, rapid detection of viral infection relied on light microscopy and evaluation of tissue and exfoliated cells for viral inclusions or other CPEs. Cytologic identification of virus is most useful in illnesses with vesicular exanthems, such as HSV or VZV infections. A scraping of the base of a lesion (Tzanck smear, Fig. 163–18) due to HSV or VZV reveals multinucleated giant and balloon cells when stained with hematoxylin and eosin, Wright, or Giemsa stain. In contrast, vesicular lesions due to enteroviral infections do not contain giant or balloon cells, and allergy-related lesions contain eosinophils. Cytologic study of urine in congenital CMV infection occasionally reveals cells with the characteristic "owl's eye" intranuclear inclusions in 25 to 50 per cent of cases, and nasal or pharyngeal smears in measles may reveal typical giant cells (Fig. 183–5). These types of stains no longer are performed routinely in most diagnostic virology laboratories, having been replaced by IF, which is more sensitive and specific.[28, 29] Whereas the Tzanck smear cannot differentiate HSV from VZV and the presence of multinucleated giant cells is necessary to make the diagnosis, IF can identify specifically the causative agent, and the presence of viral antigen in balloon or giant cells is diagnostic.

Antigen Detection

Antigen detection methods are available for the majority of commonly isolated viruses. Advantages of these methods include speed; the use of standardized reagents and kits; the ability to detect nonviable, nonculturable, or difficult-to-grow viruses; and the ability to detect antigen when culture may be negative late in the course of infection. Generally, for viruses that can be cultured, these methods are not as sensitive as optimized culture; thus, culture backup is recommended. These tests also are approved for specific specimen types. DFA, indirect immunofluorescent assay (IFA), and ELISA are used most commonly for antigen detection in the clinical laboratory.

Immunofluorescence

Antigen detection by IF requires the collection of the appropriate cell types (i.e., those in which the virus propagates) in adequate numbers for evaluation. In some cases, the specimen is placed on the slide directly (e.g., HSV or VZV detection), but usually the sample is transported to the laboratory for processing and slide preparation (e.g., for respiratory virus detection).

DFA methods use a virus-specific monoclonal antibody labeled with fluorescein dye to detect antigen and usually require approximately 30 to 45 minutes to complete. If specimen processing is required and slides are prepared in the laboratory, additional time is necessary. For IFA, unlabeled monoclonal antibody is added to the sample and incubated for 30 minutes followed by a wash and the addition of fluorescein-labeled anti-mouse immunoglobulin. After an additional 30 minutes, incubation, and a wash step, the slide can be examined for typical fluorescence (for excellent photographic examples, see reference 192). IFA can be completed in 2 to 3 hours, depending on specimen processing requirements and the number of viral antigens being sought. The advantage of DFA or IFA is the ability to determine specimen adequacy and to perform small batch and demand testing. A high-quality microscope and skilled, experienced personnel for optimal specimen preparation and evaluation are required.

The first DFA reagent available for use in the diagnostic laboratory was for the detection of HSV[77] in genital, dermal, oral, and anal lesions. The test has not been validated for the detection of HSV in cerebrospinal fluid (CSF), asymptomatic genital or tracheal aspirates, and bronchoalveolar lavage (BAL) specimens from immunocompromised patients. The sensitivity of DFA versus culture for HSV detection ranges from 72 to 92 per cent[120, 179] and like culture depends on the stage of the lesion.[28, 29] The ability to detect HSV by DFA or culture decreases with the stage and age of the lesion. DFA or culture detected HSV in 96.7 per cent of vesicles, 79.2 per cent of pustules, 44.7 per cent of ulcers, and 16.7 per cent of crusts; HSV was detected in 82 per cent of lesions less than 24 hours of age, in 77 per cent of lesions 25 to 72 hours of age, in 50 per cent of lesions 73 to 121 hours of age, and in 15 per cent of lesions older than 122 hours of age.[28]

DFA is an excellent method for the detection of VZV in lesion material, and because the virus is labile, sensitivity is superior to that of culture.[24, 47, 73, 205, 210] In a comparison of DFA and culture for the detection of VZV in skin lesions, the sensitivity and negative predictive values were 97.5 and 96.8 per cent for DFA and 49.4 and 60.4 per cent for culture, respectively. This is the exception to the usual culture backup recommendation for most antigen detection methods.

Rapid detection of CMV antigen in lung tissue or BAL specimens[51, 83, 137, 253, 260] and liver tissue[169] for diagnosis of CMV pneumonia or hepatitis also has been examined. Sensitivity is less than that of culture or SVA, ranging from 56 to 100 per cent, and results were best when a mixture of antibodies directed against early and late viral antigens was used.[253] Sensitivity may be reduced further because BAL specimens virtually have replaced lung biopsy for diagnosis of CMV pneumonia. A comparison of the cellular portion, supernate, and whole BAL for isolation of CMV in culture suggested that in most BAL specimens, CMV is associated with the cell-free rather than the cellular component.[23]

The antigenemia assay[248, 249] is a sensitive, specific, and rapid method for the detection of CMV viremia. Antigenemia has been used for early diagnosis of CMV infection[53, 54, 122]; to monitor patients at high risk for CMV disease, including bone marrow,[13] heart transplant,[68] renal transplant,[247] liver transplant,[246] and AIDS patients[144]; and to monitor treatment of severe disease after organ transplantation.[68, 245] Clinically, it has been useful in detecting infection before the onset of symptoms, and through quantitation of viral load it has enabled the differentiation of disease from asymptomatic infection.[69, 123, 233] The assay consists of the separation of leukocytes from whole blood, spotting or cytocentrifuging cells onto microscope slides, fixation and permeabilization, staining with monoclonal antibodies, and detection by fluorescein- or peroxidase-labeled secondary antibodies. Antigen-positive leukocytes are quantitated. Once the assay was optimized,[12, 67, 69] standardized IFA[122] and IP[53, 54] kits became commercially available. Antigenemia is more sensitive than traditional culture or SVA for detecting CMV viremia. Antigenemia results were positive in 91 per cent (90 of 99) of confirmed active CMV infections, compared with 34 per cent (34 of 99) for culture[122]; another study yielded similar antigenemia results: 91 per cent sensitivity versus 66 per cent and 57 per cent sensitivity for culture and SVA, respectively.[53] Disadvantages of the assay are that it is labor-intensive, time-consuming, and subjective; the leukocyte suspension must be adjusted to 10^6/mL; and the specimen must be processed quickly because storage for longer than 6 hours results in inaccurate quantitation of positive cells.[12, 123]

Finally, DFA and IFA are useful for the rapid detection of common respiratory virus antigens[145, 147, 186, 219, 227, 255, 256, 266] in nasopharyngeal washes, aspirates, and suctions. DFA for RSV has been evaluated extensively,[18, 109, 145, 158, 186, 227, 234] and its sensitivity compared with that of optimized culture ranges from 80 to 97 per cent. As is the case for VZV, RSV is relatively labile and antigen detection actually may be more sensitive than culture; thus, culture backup usually is not required. However, culture still may be advisable because 5 to 25 per cent of specimens submitted for diagnosis of RSV contain other viruses.[11] Sensitivity of IFA for detection of influenza virus A and B, parainfluenza virus, and adenovirus antigens varies when compared with that of culture, ranging from 29 to 100 per cent,[8, 142, 145, 219, 227] and culture must be performed for optimal diagnosis.

Enzyme-Linked Immunosorbent Assay

Standardized, well-characterized commercial kits for the detection of viral antigen by ELISA are available for HSV, RSV, influenza virus A, rotavirus, adenovirus, and hepatitis B virus (HBV). Intracellular as well as extracellular antigen can be detected, the method is simple technically, and suboptimal specimen handling still may yield positive results. ELISAs come in two basic formats, either a classic microtiter/tube system or the more recently developed self-contained membrane assays. The microtiter/tube format uses antibodies lining the surface of the solid phase to capture viral antigen, which in turn is reacted with an enzyme-labeled secondary antibody followed by detection with the addition of substrate and color development. Results are read spectrophotometrically and thus are objective, eliminating some of the difficulties inherent in microscopic techniques that require technical skill and expertise for evaluation of specimens. These tests are relatively inexpensive, are automatable, are suitable for processing large numbers of specimens, and usually can be completed within 2 to 4 hours. Specimens normally are batched and cannot be tested on demand as previously described for IF. In addition, the adequacy of the specimen cannot be ascertained. The membrane assays use the membrane as the solid support, which retains viral antigen. Enzyme-labeled antibodies are added to react with trapped antigen, and antigen-antibody complexes are detected via a chromogenic substrate. The results are read visually. Although rapid (15 to 20 minutes) and simple to perform, these tests are more expensive, require more hands-on time, and do not result in objective end-points. False-positive results and interpretation can be a problem.

Numerous studies have evaluated the performance of ELISA for HSV detection in genital, dermal, oral, and ocular specimens.[27, 35, 71, 78, 107, 166, 214, 251, 252] Herpchek (DuPont Pharmaceuticals, Wilmington, DE) has been investigated most frequently and compared with culture yields sensitivities and specificities ranging from 72 to 99 per cent and 92 to 100 per cent, respectively (average sensitivity is approximately 90 per cent). An automated system, VIDAS (Vitek), also has shown promise with sensitivity, specificity, positive predictive value (PPV), and negative predictive value (NPV) of 92, 89, 83, and 95 per cent, respectively.[107] Results obtained with another assay (Ortho ELISA) yielded an unacceptably low sensitivity of 35 per cent, but specificity, PPV, and NPV were 100, 100, and 85 per cent, respectively,[78] illustrating the substantial differences among assays and the need for evaluation and validation by the laboratory. Membrane assays are less sensitive than microwell ELISA, with a reported sensitivity, specificity, PPV, and NPV of 73, 99, 97, and 84 per cent, respectively, and thus infrequently are used.[45, 276]

Detection of RSV antigen in nasopharyngeal aspirates, washes, suctions, and swabs, like HSV, also has been evaluated extensively in standard[63, 85, 108, 124, 234, 244] and membrane[44, 85, 115, 140, 151, 196, 229, 234, 244, 268] ELISA formats. Reported sensitivity, specificity, PPV, and NPV for standard ELISA ranged from 71 to 91, 87 to 100, 95, and 94 per cent, respectively, and for membrane enzyme immunoassay (EIA) from 57 to 94, 73 to 100, 38 to 100, and 75 to 97 per cent, respectively. When results of TestPack (Abbott Diagnostics, North Chicago, IL) and Directigen Flu A (Becton-Dickinson) membrane EIAs are compared, TestPack appears more sensitive and specific for detection of RSV antigen; mean sensitivity, specificity, PPV, and NPV for TestPack and Directigen were 87, 93, 89, and 92 per cent and 76, 81, 63, and 89 per cent, respectively. In many of these studies, antibody-blocking assays confirmed the specificity of ELISA. Manufacturers also have exhibited interest in developing ELISA for detection of influenza virus A antigen both in standard[130] and in membrane format (Directigen Flu A).[105, 130, 199, 257] Sensitivity and specificity for membrane EIA are similar to those reported for RSV, 62 to 100 and 92 to 94 per cent, respectively. In a comparison of IFA, membrane EIA, standard EIA, and culture for the diagnosis of influenza virus A in institutionalized patients, sensitivity and specificity were 93 and 97, 87 and 99, 93 and 98, and 87 and 100 per cent, respectively.

For diagnosis of rotavirus and adenovirus 40/41 infections, ELISA is the only rapid test available in the clinical laboratory. Rotavirus antigen detection by standard ELISA has been studied thoroughly.[32, 37, 116, 141, 235] Many of the assays have excellent sensitivity (93 to 100 per cent) and specificity (98 to 100 per cent) when compared with those of electron microscopy (EM), although best results were obtained with monoclonal (vs. polyclonal) antibody-based kits (see references 37 and 141 for a review of available tests). Some assays can be read either visually or spectrophotometrically so that instrumentation is not always necessary. A membrane EIA also is available for rotavirus antigen detection (TestPack, Abbott) and, as is typical of this format, is somewhat less sensitive than standard ELISA, requiring approximately 2 to 4 $\times$ 10^7 virions/mL (vs. 10^6/mL) for detection of a positive culture. Reported sensitivity and specificity compared with those of EM are 95 to 100 per cent and 90 to 100 per cent, respectively.[15, 20] An excellent ELISA for detection of adenovirus 40/41 in stool specimens is available, yielding reported sensitivity, specificity, PPV, and NPV of 96, 96, 95, and 96 per cent, respectively.[90, 103, 267]

Latex Agglutination

Latex agglutination (LA) has been used primarily to diagnose rotavirus infection,[37, 141, 168, 202, 203] although assays also are available for detection of adenovirus[81] and HSV[226] antigens. LA is the least technically demanding of the tests described thus far, is rapid (2 to 5 minutes for rotavirus, 25 minutes for HSV), and is adequate for testing specimens collected early in the course of infection but is not as sensitive as standard ELISA, requiring 10^7 virions/mL for detection of a positive specimen. Sensitivity, specificity, PPV, and NPV for detection of rotavirus antigen by LA range from 70 to 93, 80 to 100, 76 to 100, and 85 to 95 per cent, respectively (see references 37 and 141 for review); those for HSV were 73, 89, 89, and 72 per cent, respectively.[226] Adenovirus LA sensitivity and specificity compared with EM were 95 and 100 per cent, respectively.[81]

Nucleic Acid Detection

Molecular methods for the detection, identification, and characterization of microorganisms increasingly are being adapted for use in the clinical laboratory.[114, 172, 173, 178, 231, 232, 261, 263, 264] There are two broad categories for detecting nucleic acids: direct detection using labeled DNA or RNA probes and hybridization or amplification of selected nucleic acid targets followed by amplified product detection. Direct hybridization formats include solid-phase (slot/spot/dot blot, microwell/bead capture, Southern/Northern blots), solution-phase, and in situ hybridization.[52, 114, 172, 232, 264] Nucleic acid amplification techniques are characterized as target (PCR), probe (ligase chain reaction), or signal (branched-chain DNA [bDNA]) amplification types.[52, 172, 231, 264] Some of this methodology is moving from the research to the clinical laboratory for the following reasons: (1) replacement of radio labels with enzyme, chemiluminescent, or affinity labels (e.g., biotin), (2) replacement of more cumbersome, labor-intensive detection methods with simplified, objective ELISA-like formats, (3) simplified specimen preparation methods for releasing and exposing target nucleic acid, (4) the availability of standardized, optimized, and quality-controlled reagents and kits, and (5) the publication of guidelines and recommendations for use of molecular testing in infectious disease diagnosis.[52] A few of these techniques with respect to their application for diagnosis and monitoring of select viral infections are described in the following section. Table 244–5 lists various methods and their relative analytic sensitivity for the detection of viruses, viral antigen, or viral nucleic acid.

In Situ Hybridization

In situ hybridization is a type of solid-phase hybridization assay in which whole cells or tissue sections fixed to microscope slides are taken through the hybridization process within the morphologic context of infected tissue. Cell suspensions, fresh-frozen, and formalin-fixed paraffin-embedded tissue sections have been used as the starting material for hybridization. The target nucleic acid is made accessible for hybridization via proteases and heat to increase availability of the target while preserving cellular architecture and morphology through the use of fixatives such as formalin, paraformaldehyde, or glutaraldehyde.[172] Detection systems include radiolabeled as well as enzyme-, biotin-, and digoxigenin-labeled probes. Some commercial kits are available, but methods often are optimized individually, leading to variations in sensitivity among laboratories. In situ hybridization has been applied to the study and diagnosis of numerous infections,[172, 239, 241] particularly CMV viremia,[34, 224] pneumonia,[72, 160, 260] hepatitis,[56, 169] and HSV infection.[64, 124, 187, 228] In some cases, culture,[72] immunocytochemistry,[228] and histopathology[56] had equivalent or superior sensitivity compared with hybridization. Although in situ hybridization probably is one of the first molecular techniques applied to the diagnosis of viral infections, lack of sensitivity, cost, and complexity have precluded its widespread use in diagnostic virology laboratories. In addition, the technique is related more closely to routine histologic staining and immunocytochemistry and thus is suited better to other areas of the pathology laboratory.[240, 241]

TABLE 244–5. Comparison of Analytic Sensitivities

Detection Method	Approximate Detection Limit of Assay (Copies/mL)
Culture	1–10
Antigen	
IF-, IP-stained cells	1–10
Microwell ELISA	10^3 to 10^6
Membrane ELISA	10^7
Latex agglutination	10^7
Electron microscopy	10^6 to 10^7
Nucleic acid	
Radiolabeled oligonucleotide probes	10^6
Radiolabeled full-length probes	10^4
Enzyme-labeled probes	10^4
Chemiluminescent probes	10^4
Compound or branched probes	10^4
Nucleic acid amplification	≤ 10 to 10^3

ELISA, enzyme-linked immunosorbent assay; IF, immunofluorescent; IP, immunoperoxidase.

Signal Amplification

In signal amplification, target nucleic acid is hybridized with complementary DNA or RNA probes, captured onto a solid surface such as a microtiter well or test tube, and, in an assay similar to ELISA, detected after the addition of enzyme-labeled probes and substrate. The attachment of multiple enzyme-labeled probes to each captured target molecule allows for the amplification of the signal rather than the target nucleic acid itself. Thus, the signal generated is approximately proportional to the quantity of target nucleic acid in the sample, which is determined from a standard curve. Two signal amplification systems that have become commercially available are bDNA (Quantiplex, Chiron Corp., Emeryville, CA) and Hybrid Capture System (HCS) (Digene Corp., Silver Spring, MD) assays.

bDNA

Quantiplex assays have been developed for the detection of HBV,[19, 87, 273] hepatitis C virus (HCV),[38, 133, 165] and HIV[40, 188] viremia. Virus is concentrated from plasma or serum; target nucleic acid is released by disruption, hybridized with target and capture probes, and incubated overnight. Captured complex is hybridized with bDNA, incubated and washed, hybridized with alkaline phosphatase–labeled probes, and detected via a chemiluminescent substrate.[38] As many as 3000 alkaline phosphatase–labeled probe molecules can be incorporated onto each target molecule, thereby amplifying the signal and increasing the sensitivity of detection.[172] Because the signal is proportional to the quantity of nucleic acid in the specimen, the assay can be used to quantitate viral burden. Although the analytic sensitivity of bDNA is less than that obtained with PCR (10^4 to 10^6 copies/mL compared with 10^2 to 10^3 copies/mL, respectively), bDNA's ability to quantitate viral burden using a relatively simple and reproducible method has made it useful in the diagnosis and prognosis of HBV,[19, 87, 94, 273] HCV,[38, 94, 165] and HIV[38, 188] infections, as well as in monitoring the response to antiviral therapy.

Hybrid Capture System

HCS assays have been developed for the detection of human papilloma virus, HBV,[7] HSV,[132] and CMV[96, 97, 126, 127, 134, 143, 152] infections. Briefly, specimens are treated to release viral DNA, target DNA combines with specific RNA probes creating RNA:DNA hybrids, hybrids are captured onto a test tube coated with capture antibody specific for RNA:DNA hybrids, and captured hybrids are detected with multiple antihybrid antibodies conjugated to alkaline phosphatase. The bound alkaline phosphatase is detected with a chemiluminescent substrate. Similar to the case with bDNA, up to 3000 alkaline phosphatase molecules can bind to each captured hybrid, and the signal generated is proportional to the quantity of nucleic acid in the original sample.

HCS has been evaluated for the detection and quantitation of CMV viremia; correlation to symptomatic infection; and response to therapy in renal,[96, 126, 127] liver,[126, 127, 134] heart,[126, 127] and bone marrow transplant[126] and HIV-positive patients.[97, 143, 152] HCS was more sensitive than traditional tube culture, SVA, or both, and it was useful for the early detection of CMV infections. Higher DNA concentrations correlated with clinically significant disease or progression, and quantitative DNA was useful in monitoring antiviral therapy. As with all quantitative methods, there is a need to determine the threshold levels that predict disease in various patient populations. For CMV, the lower limit of accurate quantitation is 5000 copies/mL, although the presence of DNA below this level can be identified; future improvements include quantitation to 500 copies/mL, levels similar to those detected by PCR.

Target Amplification—Polymerase Chain Reaction

Of the molecular techniques developed recently, probably none has had a greater impact on basic and clinical research than PCR. PCR has been applied to the detection and study of numerous if not most bacteria, fungi, parasites, and viruses. PCR is a target amplification technique in which a specific nucleic acid sequence is replicated by repeated cycles of denaturation, annealing, and extension directed by an oligonucleotide primer pair that defines the region of interest.[172, 264] Target nucleic acid is produced in sufficient quantities to render it detectable by a variety of methods. The most practical and adaptable detection methods use an ELISA-like format with 96-well microtiter plates. These methods employ biotinylated primers in the amplification step, which are incorporated into the PCR product and subsequently detected via avidin-biotin interaction. In one scheme (Roche Diagnostic Systems, Branchburg, NJ), the biotinylated PCR product is captured through hybridization with a specific probe attached to the microwell and detected with avidin-horseradish peroxidase conjugate. This system also employs enzymatic prevention of carryover contamination.[110, 118, 133, 165, 188, 195, 212, 259, 272] Another system (Digene Corp.) uses solution hybridization with specific RNA probes to form RNA:DNA hybrids that are captured onto streptavidin-coated microwells. Bound PCR product then is detected by the addition of alkaline phosphatase conjugated antibodies directed against RNA:DNA hybrids. This is a universal product detection system that has been used to detect amplified CMV,[55, 119] HBV,[243] and HIV[131] and can be adapted for the detection of numerous targets using specific primer/probe sets. Issues that surround the implementation of PCR diagnostics include the production of diagnostic kits, the availability of standardized kits approved by the Food and Drug Administration, guidelines for use and interpretation, standardization and quality control of test procedures and specimen preparation, qualitative versus quantitative PCR, validation of test protocols, participation in proficiency surveys such as the College of American Pathologists survey, and re-evaluation of the gold standard. Although PCR is a powerful and sensitive technique, as with all other diagnostic tests, interpretation of results must integrate clinical presentation, patient history, supporting laboratory data, and treatment records. PCR is a rapid, sensitive, and specific tool that clinically is useful for the diagnosis of particular viral infections in select situations. PCR is useful (1) when culture is too insensitive, lengthy, expensive, difficult, impractical, or unavailable, (2) for confirmation of infection, (3) for early detection of infection, (4) for detection late in disease, (5) for resolution of indeterminate serology results, (6) to monitor the status of disease, and (7) to monitor response to therapy (Table 244–6). Use of PCR for the diagnosis of select viral infections is addressed later.

TABLE 244–6. Clinical Use of Polymerase Chain Reaction for the Diagnosis of Selected Viral Infections

Virus	Clinical Utility
CMV	Diagnosis of CNS infection; diagnosis of neonatal/congenital infection; diagnosis of ocular infections; diagnosis and monitoring of active infection/viral load in immunocompromised hosts
EBV	Diagnosis of active EBV infection; diagnosis of CNS infection; diagnosis and monitoring of EBV-related lymphoproliferative disorders in liver and bone marrow transplants undergoing suppression
Enteroviruses	Rapid diagnosis of CNS infection
HBV	Early detection of infection; confirmation of infectivity; monitoring of viral load and therapeutic efficacy in chronic hepatitis
HCV	Detection before seroconversion; resolution of indeterminate or ambiguous serology; monitoring of viral load and therapeutic efficacy in chronic infection
HHV-6	Confirmation of infection
HIV	Detection before seroconversion; resolution of indeterminate immunoblot results; evaluation of suspected prenatal and intrapartum HIV infection; monitoring of viral load to evaluate therapeutic efficacy and disease progression
HSV	Diagnosis of HSV encephalitis; confirmation of neonatal HSV infection; detection of virus in late lesions; diagnosis of ocular infections
HTLV I/II	Detection of HTLV-I in adult T-cell leukemia and lymphoma and tropical spastic paraparesis/HTLV-I–associated myelopathy (TSP/HAM)
Parvovirus B19	Detection of infection; early detection prior to seroconversion
VZV	Diagnosis of CNS infection; detection of virus in late or atypical lesions; diagnosis of ocular infections

CMV, cytomegalovirus; CNS, central nervous system; EBV, Epstein-Barr virus; HBV, hepatitis B virus; HCV, hepatitis C virus; HHV-6, human herpesvirus type 6; HIV, human immunodeficiency virus; HSV, herpes simplex virus; HTLV I/II, human T-cell lymphotropic virus types I and II; VZV, varicella-zoster virus.

PCR has been used to detect HSV DNA in a variety of clinical specimens, including CSF and brain biopsy material,[4, 39, 82, 112, 121, 181, 182, 197, 207, 237, 242, 262] skin lesions,[161, 162] genital lesions,[27, 41, 86] and ocular samples.[100, 270] The application of PCR to CSF specimens for the diagnosis of HSV encephalitis (HSE) has received a great deal of emphasis. Brain biopsy remains the gold standard for diagnosis. However, it rarely is performed, and patients are treated empirically. Traditional laboratory methods, including culture, antigen detection, intrathecal antibody production, CSF and serum antibodies, and serum/CSF antibody ratio, lack sensitivity or specificity or are too slow and most useful for retrospective diagnosis. Numerous reports have documented the utility of CSF PCR for diagnosing HSE in a timely manner with sensitivity and specificity greater than 95 and 100 per cent, respectively.[4, 39, 82, 112, 121, 181, 182, 197, 207, 237, 242, 262] Most of these studies have used some combination of traditional methods along with clinical observation and radiodiagnostic studies for case definition. Lakeman and Whitley[121] compared CSF PCR and brain biopsy in 101 patients, 54 with biopsy-proven HSE and 47 who were biopsy culture–negative. CSF PCR sensitivity and specificity were 98 per cent (53 of 54) and 94 per cent (44 of 47), respectively. The PCR-positive, biopsy-negative specimens remained PCR-positive in repeat assays with two different primer pairs and were considered true-positive; culture failures perhaps were due to sampling problems. The PCR-negative, biopsy-positive sample remained PCR-negative after DNA extraction and was not inhibitory to PCR. Patients also were followed after acyclovir treatment; 100, 98, 47, and 21 per cent of CSF specimens were PCR-positive at times 0, 0 to 7, 8 to 14, and greater than 15 days, respectively, after brain biopsy and initiation of therapy. The authors concluded that PCR should be the standard for diagnosis of HSE because sensitivity and specificity were adequate for the diagnosis of focal biopsy-proven HSE; its usefulness for defining the spectrum of HSV infection of the central nervous system (CNS) continues to be investigated. Detection of HSV DNA in skin and genital lesions has shown that PCR is more sensitive than culture, is able to identify asymptomatic HSV, detects the presence of HSV over a longer period (in older lesions and even fixed tissue), and has greater diagnostic value than culture and clinical observations for assessing genital HSV and treatment efficacy in patients with recurrent genital HSV.[27, 41, 86, 161, 162] PCR also is useful for the diagnosis of ocular infections due to specific viruses or as supporting information in the clinical diagnosis of specific ocular disease syndromes.[100, 270]

PCR has been used to diagnose cutaneous,[42, 111, 117, 161, 162] ocular,[164, 270] CNS,[183, 216] and congenital VZV infections[98] and as a tool for studying the natural history of primary and reactivated disease.[42, 111, 117] The primary clinical utility of PCR is for diagnosis of VZV CNS infections because virus isolation rarely is successful and intrathecal antibodies cannot be used as an early diagnostic tool.[183, 216]

Significant morbidity and mortality are associated with CMV infection primarily in organ transplant recipients and patients with AIDS, requiring surveillance and monitoring for infection or disease by culture or antigenemia. Increasingly, PCR is being used to detect CMV DNA in blood,[16, 49, 50, 66, 79, 102, 153, 163, 215, 221, 259, 277] CSF,[2, 5, 22, 80, 265] urine,[36, 153] and the same spectrum of specimens submitted for culture.[153] Whole blood, peripheral blood leukocytes, serum, and plasma have been evaluated extensively for detection of infection, association with clinical disease, and therapeutic monitoring. Although PCR was positive earlier and remained positive longer and was more sensitive than culture or antigenemia for detection of CMV infection using whole blood or peripheral blood leukocytes, in the absence of a positive culture or antigenemia, PCR was not associated always with clinical symptoms and did not predict necessarily or correlate with appearance of clinical disease, although it did predict a risk of relapse.[50, 68, 102, 277] Detection of CMV DNA in serum or plasma, however, correlated with viremia, clinical disease, or both in patients with CMV infections,[16, 221, 259] including congenital CMV infection.[163] Detection of mRNA in peripheral blood leukocytes by reverse transcriptase PCR also has been used to assess active productive CMV infection and identification of patients at risk of developing symptomatic infection.[10, 79] Detection of CMV viremia by PCR also is useful for monitoring antiviral therapy, both for the early initiation of treatment and as a predictor of treatment efficacy.[49, 68, 259, 277] In addition, commercial kits (Roche) for the qualitative and quantitative detection of CMV DNA from plasma are under evaluation.[259] PCR also is useful for the diagnosis of CMV CNS infections, primarily in AIDS patients,[5, 22, 80, 265] with reported sensitivity ranging from 79 to 100 per cent.[5]

Conventional diagnostic methods usually are not useful in the evaluation of Epstein-Barr virus (EBV)-related disorders in immunosuppressed patients. Culture is not practical or useful, and serology is difficult to interpret in the setting of immunosuppression. PCR offers the possibility of rapid detection of EBV in a variety of clinical specimens and allows a semiquantitative or quantitative estimate of viral load. PCR has been used for the diagnosis of AIDS-related CNS lymphoma,[6] EBV-related lymphoproliferative disorders,[30, 138, 230] and other EBV-associated diseases (e.g., infectious mononucleosis, fatal infectious mononucleosis, chronic-active EBV infection, and EBV-associated hemophagocytic syndromes) in which increased DNA concentrations were associated with more severe clinical categories.[269] PCR particularly is useful for early identification and diagnosis of lymphoproliferative disorders in pediatric patients after liver transplantation for monitoring EBV levels so that immunosuppression can be adjusted and as a prognostic marker.[30, 138]

PCR is useful for early detection of HIV infection, resolution of indeterminate Western blot results, evaluation of suspected prenatal and intrapartum infection, and monitoring viral load for prognosis and evaluation of therapeutic efficacy.[91, 110, 118, 148, 188, 189] Qualitative[110, 118] (for detection of proviral DNA in peripheral blood leukocytes) and quantitative[188, 200] (for detection of viral RNA in plasma) kits are commercially available (Roche), and the quantitative assay has Food and Drug Administration approval. Quantitative PCR is useful for correlating RNA levels to disease stage, predicting clinical outcome, and monitoring response to therapy.[91, 148] However, guidelines for optimal use of PCR and other quantitative assays (bDNA, nucleic acid sequence–based amplification [NASBA]) still are evolving.[200] In a comparison of PCR, NASBA, and bDNA,[188] no significant differences in sensitivity were found for baseline measurement of HIV-1 RNA levels among the three assays. In addition, changes in RNA levels in response to therapy were comparable. The lower limit of detection for PCR, NASBA, and bDNA was 200 copies/mL, 4000 copies/mL, and 10,000 copies/mL, respectively; turnaround time was 6 hours, 5 hours, and 1.5 days, respectively. Commercial kits (Roche) also are available for detection of HCV RNA in plasma.[133, 165, 195, 212, 274] Detection of HCV RNA is useful in the diagnosis of acute hepatitis prior to seroconversion, for detection of chronic HCV in seronegative patients, for resolution of indeterminate serologic tests, and to monitor patients receiving therapy. PCR was more sensitive than bDNA,[133, 165] with approximately 11 per cent of true-positives undetected by bDNA.[165] The analytical sensitivity of PCR and bDNA was 400 copies/mL and 3.5×10^5 copies/mL, respectively.[165]

With regard to enteroviruses, PCR has been used to diagnose enteroviral CNS[17, 190, 191, 193, 194, 204, 208, 272] and neonatal infections[1, 33, 191] and to identify vaccine[271] and wild-type[21] poliovirus infections. Major emphasis, however, has been placed on developing a rapid, sensitive method for diagnosing aseptic meningitis because up to 25 to 35 per cent of specimens from patients with characteristic enterovirus infection are negative, and when positive, require an average of 4 to 8 days for detection in culture.[193, 204, 272] CSF evaluation for pleocytosis is not always reliable because specimens with no pleocytosis also may be culture- or PCR-positive.[190, 204] PCR for diagnosis of enteroviral CNS infections has sensitivity, specificity, PPV, and NPV of 95 to 100, 97 to 100, approximately 98, and 98 per cent, respectively.[190, 191, 193, 194, 204, 208] Commercial kits (Roche) also have become available, yielding rapid (<6 hours), sensitive, and specific results.[194, 204, 272] Rapid diagnosis by PCR also will have an effect on patient management with regard to days of hospitalization, antibiotic treatment, and therefore overall cost.[190, 208]

SUMMARY

Methods for the laboratory diagnosis of viral infections have been reviewed, including culture, SVA, antigen detection, and molecular diagnostic methods. The use of these tests in some combination is most useful because a single test may not yield a diagnosis. For many viruses, culture has been the gold standard or reference method for evaluation of the new, rapid tests. However, culture is not 100 per cent sensitive nor always diagnostic of symptomatic infection. With the newer methods, particularly molecular diagnostic methods, the gold standard is changing and evaluation of new techniques must be compared against a spectrum of laboratory and clinical data. Standards for performance and guidelines for use and interpretation of molecular techniques are becoming available. Quantitative (vs. qualitative) viral results may be useful in interpretation of tests, particularly with regard to viruses causing latent infection, or to monitor therapy or disease progression. Finally, interpretation of any result requires integration of clinical history and presentation, a variety of laboratory data, treatment records, and observation of trends over time.

References

1. Abzug, M. J., Loeffelholz, M., and Rotbart, H. A.: Diagnosis of neonatal enterovirus infection by polymerase chain reaction. J. Pediatr. *126*:447–450, 1995.
2. Achim, C. L., Nagra, R. M., Wang, R., et al.: Detection of cytomegalovirus in cerebrospinal fluid autopsy specimens from AIDS patients. J. Infect. Dis. *169*:623–627, 1994.
3. Ahluwalia, G., Embree, J., McNicol, P., et al.: Comparison of nasopharyngeal aspirate and nasopharyngeal swab specimens for respiratory syncytial virus diagnosis by cell culture, indirect immunofluorescence assay, and enzyme-linked immunosorbent assay. J. Clin. Microbiol. *25*:763–767, 1987.
4. Ando, Y., Kimura, H., Miwata, H., et al.: Quantitative analysis of herpes simplex virus DNA in cerebrospinal fluid of children with herpes simplex encephalitis. J. Med. Virol. *41*:170–173, 1993.
5. Arribas, J. R., Storch, G. A., Clifford, D. B., et al.: Cytomegalovirus encephalitis. Ann. Intern. Med. *125*:577–587, 1996.
6. Arribas, J. R., Clifford, D. B., Fichtenbaum, C. J., et al.: Detection of Epstein-Barr virus DNA in cerebrospinal fluid for diagnosis of AIDS-related central nervous system lymphoma. J. Clin. Microbiol. *33*:1580–1583, 1995.
7. Aspinall, S., Steele, A. D., Peenze, I., et al.: Detection and quantitation of hepatitis B virus DNA: Comparison of two commercial hybridization assays with polymerase chain reaction. J. Viral Hepatol. *2*:107–111, 1995.
8. August, M. J., and Warford, A. L.: Evaluation of a commercial monoclonal antibody for detection of adenovirus antigen. J. Clin. Microbiol. *25*:2233–2235, 1987.
9. Bettoli, E. J., Brewer, P. M., Oxtoby, M. J., et al.: The role of temperature and swab materials in the recovery of herpes simplex virus from lesions. J. Infect. Dis. *145*:399, 1982.
10. Bitsch, A., Kirchner, H., Dupke, R., et al.: Cytomegalovirus transcripts in peripheral blood leukocytes of actively infected transplant patients detected by reverse transcription-polymerase chain reaction. J. Infect. Dis. *167*:740–743, 1992.
11. Blanding, J. G., Hoshiko, M. G., and Stutman, H. R.: Routine viral culture for pediatric respiratory syncytial specimens submitted for direct immunofluorescence testing. J. Clin. Microbiol. *27*:1438–1440, 1989.
12. Boeckh, M., Woogerd, P. M., Stevens-Ayers, T., et al.: Factors influencing detection of quantitative cytomegalovirus antigenemia. J. Clin. Microbiol. *32*:832–834, 1994.
13. Boeckh, M., Bowden, R. A., Goodrich, J. M., et al.: Cytomegalovirus antigen detection in peripheral blood leukocytes after allogeneic marrow transplantation. Blood *80*:1358–1364, 1992.
14. Bromberg, K., Tannis, G., and Daldone, B.: Early use of indirect immunofluorescence for the detection of respiratory syncytial virus in HEp-2 cell culture. Am. J. Clin. Pathol. *96*:127–129, 1991.
15. Brooks, R. G., Brown, L., and Franklin, R. B.: Comparison of a new rapid test (TestPack Rotavirus) with standard enzyme immunoassay and electron microscopy for the detection of rotavirus in symptomatic hospitalized children. J. Clin. Microbiol. *27*:775–777, 1989.
16. Brytting, M., Xu, W., Wahren, B., et al.: Cytomegalovirus DNA detection in sera from patients with active cytomegalovirus infections. J. Clin. Microbiol. *30*:1937–1941, 1992.
17. Casas, I., Klapper, P. E., Cleator, G. M., et al.: Two different PCR assays to detect enteroviral RNA in CSF samples from patients with acute aseptic meningitis. J. Med. Virol. *47*:378–385, 1995.
18. Cheeseman, S. H., Pierik, L. T., Leombruno, D., et al.: Evaluation of a commercially available direct immunofluorescence staining reagent for the detection of respiratory syncytial virus in respiratory secretions. J. Clin. Microbiol. *24*:155–156, 1986.
19. Chen, C. H., Wang, J. T., Lee, C. Z., et al.: Quantitative detection of hepatitis B virus DNA in human sera by branched-DNA signal amplification. J. Virol. Methods *53*:131–137, 1995.
20. Chernesky, M., Castriciano, S., Mahony, J., et al.: Ability of TESTPACK ROTAVIRUS enzyme immunoassay to diagnose rotavirus gastroenteritis. J. Clin. Microbiol. *26*:2459–2461, 1988.
21. Chezzi, C.: Rapid diagnosis of poliovirus infection by PCR amplification. J. Clin. Microbiol. *34*:1722–1725, 1996.
22. Cinque, P., Vago, L., Brytting, M., et al.: Cytomegalovirus infection of the central nervous system in patients with AIDS: Diagnosis by DNA amplification from cerebrospinal fluid. J. Infect. Dis. *166*:1408–1411, 1992.
23. Clarke, L. M., Daidone, B. J., Inghida, R., et al.: Differential recovery of cytomegalovirus from cellular and supernatant components of bronchoalveolar lavage specimens. Am. J. Clin. Pathol. *97*:313–317, 1992.
24. Coffin, S. E., and Hodinka, R. L.: Utility of direct immunofluorescence and virus culture for detection of varicella-zoster virus in skin lesions. J. Clin. Microbiol. *33*:2792–2795, 1995.
25. Cole, L. J., Campbell, M. B., and Gleaves, C. A.: Detection of HSV from clinical specimens using the ELVIS™ tube culture test as compared to standard cell culture. 12th Annual Clinical Virology Symposium, 1996, Clearwater, Florida. Abstract M20.
26. Cone, R. W., Swenson, P. D., Hobson, A. C., et al.: Herpes simplex virus detection from genital lesions: A comparative study using antigen detection (HerpChek) and culture. J. Clin. Microbiol. *31*:1774–1776, 1993.
27. Cone, R. W., Hobson, A. C., Palmer, J., et al.: Extended duration of herpes simplex virus DNA in genital lesions detected by the polymerase chain reaction. J. Infect. Dis. *164*:757–760, 1991.
28. Corey, L.: Laboratory diagnosis of herpes simplex virus infections: Principles guiding the development of rapid diagnostic tests. Diagn. Microbiol. Infect. Dis. *4*:111S–119S, 1986.
29. Corey, L., and Spear, P. G.: Infections with herpes simplex viruses. N. Engl. J. Med. *314*:686–691, 749–757, 1986.
30. Cox, K. L., Lawrence-Miyasaki, L. S., Garcia-Kennedy, R., et al.: An increased incidence of Epstein-Barr virus infection and lymphoproliferative disorder in young children on FK506 after liver transplantation. Transplantation *59*:524–529, 1995.
31. Crane, L. R., Gutterman, P. A., Chapel, T., et al.: Incubation of swab materials with herpes simplex virus. J. Infect. Dis. *141*:531, 1980.
32. Cromien, J. L., Himmelreich, C. A., Glass, R. I., et al.: Evaluation of new commercial enzyme immunoassay for rotavirus detection. J. Clin. Microbiol. *25*:2359–2362, 1987.
33. Dagan, R.: Nonpolio enteroviruses and the febrile young infant: Epidemiologic, clinical and diagnostic aspects. Pediatr. Infect. Dis. J. *15*:67–71, 1996.
34. Dankner, W. M., McCutchan, J. A., Richman, D. D., et al.: Localization of human cytomegalovirus in peripheral blood leukocytes by in situ hybridization. J. Infect. Dis. *161*:31–36, 1990.
35. Dascal, A. J., Chan-Thim, J., Morahan, M., et al.: Diagnosis of herpes simplex virus infection in a clinical setting by a direct antigen detection enzyme immunoassay. J. Clin. Microbiol. *27*:700–704, 1989.
36. Demmler, G. J., Buffone, G. J., Schimbor, C. M., et al.: Detection of cytomegalovirus in urine from newborns by using polymerase chain reaction DNA amplification. J. Infect. Dis. *158*:1177–1184, 1988.

37. Dennehy, P. H., Gauntlett, D. R., and Tenle, W. E.: Comparison of nine commercial immunoassays for the detection of rotavirus in fecal specimens. J. Clin. Microbiol. *26*:1630, 1988.
38. Detmer, J., Lagier, R., Flynn, J., et al.: Accurate quantification of hepatitis C virus (HCV) RNA from all HCV genotypes by using branched-DNA technology. J. Clin. Microbiol. *34*:901–907, 1996.
39. DeVincenzo, J. P., and Thorne, G.: Mild herpes simplex encephalitis diagnosed by polymerase chain reaction: A case report and review. Pediatr. Infect. Dis. J. *13*:662–664, 1994.
40. Dewar, R. L., Highbarger, H. C., Sarmiento, M. D., et al.: Application of branched DNA signal amplification to monitor human immunodeficiency virus type 1 burden in human plasma. J. Infect. Dis. *170*:1172–1179, 1994.
41. Diaz-Mitoma, F., Ruben, M., Sacks, S., et al.: Detection of viral DNA to evaluate outcome of antiviral treatment of patients with recurrent genital herpes. J. Clin. Microbiol. *34*:657–663, 1996.
42. Dlugosch, D., Eis-Hubinger, A. M., Kleim, J. P., et al.: Diagnosis of acute and latent varicella-zoster virus infections using the polymerase chain reaction. J. Med. Virol. *35*:136–141, 1992.
43. Döller, G., Schuy, W., Tjhen, K. Y., et al.: Direct detection of influenza virus antigen in nasopharyngeal specimens by direct enzyme immunoassay in comparison with quantitating virus shedding. J. Clin. Microbiol. *30*:866–869, 1992.
44. Dominguez, E. A., Taber, L. H., and Couch, R. B.: Comparison of rapid diagnostic techniques for respiratory syncytial and influenza A virus respiratory infections in young children. J. Clin. Microbiol. *31*:2286–2290, 1993.
45. Dorian, K. J., Beatty, E., and Atterbury, K. E.: Detection of herpes simplex virus by Kodak SureCell herpes test. J. Clin. Microbiol. *28*:2117–2119, 1990.
46. Drew, W. L.: Controversies in viral diagnosis. Rev. Infect. Dis. *8*:814–824, 1986.
47. Drew, W. L., and Mintz, L.: Rapid diagnosis of varicella-zoster virus infection by direct immunofluorescence. Am. J. Clin. Pathol. *73*:699–701, 1980.
48. Ehrlich, G. D., and Greenberg, S. J.: PCR-Based Diagnostics in Infectious Disease. Boston, Blackwell Scientific, 1994.
49. Einsele, H., Ehninger, G., Steidle, M., et al.: Polymerase chain reaction to evaluate antiviral therapy for cytomegalovirus disease. Lancet *338*:1170–1172, 1991.
50. Einsele, H., Steidle, M., Vallbracht, A., et al.: Early occurrence of human cytomegalovirus infection after bone marrow transplantation as demonstrated by the polymerase chain reaction technique. Blood *77*:1104–1110, 1991.
51. Emmanuel, D., Peppard, J., Gold, J., et al.: Rapid immunodiagnosis of cytomegalovirus pneumonia by bronchoalveolar lavage using human and murine monoclonal antibodies. Ann. Intern. Med. *104*:476–481, 1986.
52. Enns, R. K., Bromley, S. E., Day, S. P., et al.: Molecular Diagnostic Methods for Infectious Diseases: Approved Guideline. NCCLS Document MM3-A, NCCLS, Villanova, PA, 1995.
53. Erice, A., Holm, M. A., Sanjuan, M. V., et al.: Evaluation of CMV-vue antigenemia assay for rapid detection of cytomegalovirus in mixed-leukocyte blood fractions. J. Clin. Microbiol. *33*:1014–1015, 1995.
54. Erice, A., Holm, M. A., Gill, P. C., et al.: Cytomegalovirus (CMV) antigenemia assay is more sensitive than shell vial cultures for rapid detection of CMV in polymorphonuclear blood leukocytes. J. Clin. Microbiol. *30*:2822–2825, 1992.
55. Espy, M. J., and Smith, T. F.: Comparison of SHARP signal system and southern blot hybridization analysis for detection of cytomegalovirus in clinical specimens by PCR. J. Clin. Microbiol. *33*:3028–3030, 1995.
56. Espy, M. J., Paya, C. V., Holley, K. E., et al.: Diagnosis of cytomegalovirus hepatitis by histopathology and in situ hybridization in liver transplantation. Diagn. Microbiol. Infect. Dis. *14*:293–296, 1991.
57. Espy, M. J., Wold, A. D., Jesperson, D. J., et al.: Comparison of shell vials and conventional tubes seeded with rhabdomyosarcoma and MRC-5 cells for the rapid detection of herpes simplex virus. J. Clin. Microbiol. *29*:2701–2703, 1991.
58. Espy, M. J., and Smith, T. F.: Detection of herpes simplex virus in conventional tube cell cultures and in shell vials with a DNA probe kit and monoclonal antibodies. J. Clin. Microbiol. *26*:22–24, 1988.
59. Espy, M. J., Hierholzer, J. C., and Smith, T. F.: The effect of centrifugation on the rapid detection of adenovirus in shell vials. Am. J. Clin. Pathol. *88*:358–360, 1987.
60. Espy, M. J., Smith, T. F., Harmon, M. W., et al.: Rapid detection of influenza virus by shell vial assay with monoclonal antibodies. J. Clin. Microbiol. *24*:677–679, 1986.
61. Fayram, S. L., Aarnaes, S., and de la Maza, L. M.: Comparison of CultureSet to a conventional tissue culture fluorescent antibody technique for isolation and identification of herpes simplex virus. J. Clin. Microbiol. *18*:215–216, 1983.
62. Fedorko, D. P., Ilstrup, D. M., and Smith, T. F.: Effect of age of shell vial monolayers on detection of cytomegalovirus from urine specimens. J. Clin. Microbiol. *27*:2107–2109, 1989.
63. Flander, R. T., Lindsay, P. D., Chairez, R., et al.: The evaluation of clinical specimens for the presence of respiratory syncytial virus antigen using an enzyme immunoassay. J. Med. Virol. *19*:1–9, 1986.
64. Forghani, B., Dupuis, K. W., and Schmidt, N. J.: Rapid detection of herpes simplex virus DNA in human brain tissue by in situ hybridization. J. Clin. Microbiol. *22*:656–658, 1985.
65. Forman, M. C., Merz, C. S., and Charache, P.: Detection of herpes simplex virus by a nonradiometric spin-amplified in situ hybridization assay. J. Clin. Microbiol. *30*:581–584, 1992.
66. Gerdes, J. C., Spees, E. K., Fitting, K., et al.: Prospective study utilizing a quantitative polymerase chain reaction for detection of cytomegalovirus DNA in the blood of renal transplant patients. Transplant. Proc. *25*:1411–1413, 1993.
67. Gerna, G., Revello, M. G., Percivalle, E., et al.: Comparison of different immunostaining techniques and monoclonal antibodies to the lower matrix phosphoprotein (pp65) for optimal quantitation of human cytomegalovirus antigenemia. J. Clin. Microbiol. *30*:1232–1237, 1992.
68. Gerna, G., Zipeto, D., Parea, M., et al.: Monitoring of human cytomegalovirus infections and ganciclovir treatment in heart transplant recipients by determination of viremia, antigenemia and DNAemia. J. Infect. Dis. *164*:488–498, 1991.
69. Gerna, G., Revello, M. G., Percivalle, E., et al.: Quantification of human cytomegalovirus viremia by using monoclonal antibodies to different viral proteins. J. Clin. Microbiol. *28*:2681–2688, 1990.
70. Gleaves, C. A., Hursh, D. A., and Meyers, J. D.: Detection of human cytomegalovirus in clinical specimens by centrifugation culture with a nonhuman cell line. J. Clin. Microbiol. *30*:1045–1048, 1992.
71. Gleaves, C. A., Rice, D. H., and Lee, C. F.: Evaluation of an enzyme immunoassay for the detection of herpes simplex virus (HSV) antigen from clinical specimens in viral transport media. J. Virol. Methods *28*:133–139, 1990.
72. Gleaves, C. A., Myerson, D., Bowden, R. A., et al.: Direct detection of cytomegalovirus from bronchoalveolar lavage samples by using a rapid in situ DNA hybridization assay. J. Clin. Microbiol. *27*:2429–2432, 1990.
73. Gleaves, C. A., Lee, C. F., Bustamante, C. I., et al.: Use of murine monoclonal antibodies for laboratory diagnosis of varicella-zoster virus infection. J. Clin. Microbiol. *26*:1623–1625, 1988.
74. Gleaves, C. A., Smith, T. F., Shuster, E. A., et al.: Comparison of standard tube and shell vial cell culture techniques for detection of cytomegalovirus in clinical specimens. J. Clin. Microbiol. *21*:217–222, 1985.
75. Gleaves, C. A., Wilson, D. J., Wold, A. D., et al.: Detection and serotyping of herpes simplex virus in MRC-5 cells by use of centrifugation and monoclonal antibodies 16 h postinoculation. J. Clin. Microbiol. *21*:29–32, 1985.
76. Gleaves, C. A., Smith, T. F., Shuster, E. A., et al.: Rapid detection of cytomegalovirus in MRC-5 cells inoculated with urine specimens by using low speed centrifugation and monoclonal antibody to an early antigen. J. Clin. Microbiol. *19*:917–919, 1984.
77. Goldstein, L. C., Corey, L., McDougall, J. K., et al.: Monoclonal antibodies to herpes simplex viruses: Use in antigenic typing and rapid diagnosis. J. Infect. Dis. *147*:829–837, 1983.
78. Gonik, B., Seibel, M., Berkowitz, A., et al.: Comparison of two enzyme-linked immunosorbent assays for detection of herpes simplex virus antigen. J. Clin. Microbiol. *29*:436–438, 1991.
79. Gozlan, J., Saloed, J. M., Chouaid, C., et al.: Human cytomegalovirus (HCMV) late mRNA detection in peripheral blood of AIDS patients: Diagnostic value for HCMV disease compared with those of viral culture and HCMV DNA detection. J. Clin. Microbiol. *31*:1943–1945, 1993.
80. Gozlan, J., Salord, J. M., Roullet, E., et al.: Rapid detection of cytomegalovirus DNA in cerebrospinal fluid of AIDS patients with neurologic disorders. J. Infect. Dis. *166*:1416–1421, 1992.
81. Grandien, M., Pettersson, C. A., Svensson, L., et al.: Latex agglutination test for adenovirus diagnosis in diarrheal disease. J. Med. Virol. *23*:311, 1987.
82. Guffond, T., Dewilde, A., Lobert, P. E., et al.: Significance and clinical relevance of the detection of herpes simplex virus DNA by the polymerase chain reaction in cerebrospinal fluid from patients with presumed encephalitis. Clin. Infect. Dis. *18*:744–749, 1994.
83. Hackman, R. C., Myerson, D., Meyers, J. D., et al.: Rapid diagnosis of cytomegalovirus pneumonia by tissue immunofluorescence with a murine monoclonal antibody. J. Infect. Dis. *151*:325, 1985.
84. Hall, C. B., and Douglas, R. G., Jr.: Clinically useful method for the isolation of respiratory syncytial virus. J. Infect. Dis. *131*:1–10, 1975.
85. Halstead, D. C., Todd, S., and Fritch, G.: Evaluation of five methods for respiratory syncytial virus detection. J. Clin. Microbiol. *28*:1021–1025, 1990.
86. Hardy, D. A., Arvin, A. M., Yasukawa, L. L., et al.: The successful identification of asymptomatic genital herpes simplex infection at delivery using the polymerase chain reaction. J. Infect. Dis. *162*:1031–1035, 1990.
87. Hendricks, D. A., Stowe, B. J., Hoo, B. S., et al.: Quantitation of HBV DNA in human serum using a branched DNA (bDNA) signal amplification assay. Am. J. Clin. Pathol. *104*:537–546, 1995.
88. Hermann, E. C., Jr.: The tragedy of viral diagnosis. Postgrad. Med. J. *46*:545–550, 1970.
89. Hermann, E. C., Jr.: Experience in providing a viral diagnostic laboratory compatible with medical practice. Mayo Clin. Proc. *42*:112–123, 1967.
90. Herrmann, J. E., Perron-Henry, D. M., and Blacklow, N. R.: Antigen detection with monoclonal antibodies for the diagnosis of adenovirus gastroenteritis. J. Infect. Dis. *155*:1167–1171, 1987.

91. Ho, D. D.: Viral counts count in HIV infection. Science *272*:1124–1125, 1996.
92. Howell, C. L., and Miller, M. J.: Effect of sucrose phosphate and sorbitol on infectivity of enveloped viruses during storage. J. Clin. Microbiol. *18*:658–662, 1983.
93. Howell, C. L., Miller, M. J., and Martin, W. J.: Comparison of rates of virus isolation from leukocyte populations separated from blood by conventional and Ficoll-Paque/Macrodex methods. J. Clin. Microbiol. *10*:533–537, 1979.
94. Hu, K.-Q., and Vierling, J. M.: Molecular diagnostic techniques for viral hepatitis. Gastroenterol. Clin. North Am. *23*:479–537, 1994.
95. Hughes, J. H.: Physical and chemical methods for enhancing rapid detection of viruses and other agents. Clin. Microbiol. Rev. *6*:150–175, 1993.
96. Imbert-Marcille, B.-M., Cantarovich, D., Boedec, S., et al.: Evaluation of a new quantification method for cytomegalovirus DNA in leucocytes: Clinical value in renal transplant recipients. Scand. J. Infect. Dis. *99*(Suppl.): 15–16, 1995.
97. Isada, C., Kohn, D., Lazar, J. G., et al.: Rapid diagnosis of cytomegalovirus (CMV) using the Digene Hybrid Capture System: A comparison with tissue culture and polymerase chain reaction (PCR). 12th Annual Clinical Virology Symposium, 1996, Clearwater, FL. Abstract S19.
98. Isada, N. B., Paar, D. P., Johnson, M., et al.: In utero diagnosis of congenital varicella zoster infection by chorionic villus sampling and polymerase chain reaction. Am. J. Obstet. Gynecol. *165*:1727–1730, 1991.
99. Isenberg, H. D. (ed.): Clinical Microbiology Procedure Handbook. Washington, D. C., American Society for Microbiology, 1992, Supplement No. 1, 1994.
100. Jackson, R., Morris, D. J., Cooper, R. J., et al.: Multiplex polymerase chain reaction for adenovirus and herpes simplex virus in eye swabs. J. Virol. Methods *56*:41–48, 1996.
101. Jalowayski, A. A., Walpita, P., Puryear, B. A., et al.: Rapid detection of respiratory syncytial virus in nasopharyngeal specimens obtained with the rhinoprobe scraper. J. Clin. Microbiol. *28*:738–741, 1990.
102. Jiwa, N. M., van Gemert, G. W., Raap, A. K., et al.: Rapid detection of human cytomegalovirus DNA in peripheral blood leukocytes of viremic transplant recipients by the polymerase chain reaction. Transplantation *48*:72–76, 1989.
103. Johansson, M. E., Uhnoo, I., Svensson, L., et al.: Enzyme-linked immunosorbent assay for detection of enteric adenovirus 41. J. Med. Virol. *17*:19–27, 1985.
104. Johnson, F. B.: Transport of viral specimens. Clin. Microbiol. Rev. *3*:120–131, 1990.
105. Johnston, S. L. G., and Bloy, H.: Evaluation of a rapid enzyme immunoassay for detection of influenza A virus. J. Clin. Microbiol. *31*:142–143, 1993.
106. Johnston, S. L. G., Wellens, K., and Siegel, C.: Comparison of hemagglutination and hemadsorption tests for influenza detection. Diagn. Microbiol. Infect. Dis. *15*:363–365, 1992.
107. Johnston, S. L. G., Hamilton, S., Bindra, P., et al.: Evaluation of an automated immunodiagnostic assay system for direct detection of herpes simplex virus antigen in clinical specimens. J. Clin. Microbiol. *30*:1042–1044, 1992.
108. Johnston, S. L. G., and Siegel, C. S.: Evaluation of direct immunofluorescence, enzyme immunoassay, centrifugation culture, and conventional culture for the detection of respiratory syncytial virus. J. Clin. Microbiol. *28*:2394–2397, 1990.
109. Kellog, J. A.: Culture vs. direct antigen assays for detection of microbial pathogens from lower respiratory tract specimens suspected of containing the respiratory syncytial virus. Arch. Pathol. Lab. Med. *115*:451–458, 1991.
110. Khadir, A., Coutlee, F., Saint-Antoine, P., et al.: Clinical evaluation of Amplicor HIV-1 test for detection of human immunodeficiency virus type 1 proviral DNA in peripheral blood mononuclear cells. J. AIDS Hum. Retrovirol. *9*:257–263, 1995.
111. Kido, S., Ozaki, T., Asada, H., et al.: Detection of varicella-zoster virus DNA in clinical samples from patients with VZV by the polymerase chain reaction. J. Clin. Microbiol. *29*:76–79, 1991.
112. Kimura, H., Futamura, M., Kito, H., et al.: Detection of viral DNA in neonatal herpes simplex virus infections: Frequent and prolonged presence in serum and cerebrospinal fluid. J. Infect. Dis. *164*:289–293, 1991.
113. Klespies, S. L., Cebula, D. E., Kelley, C. L., et al.: Detection of enteroviruses from clinical specimens by spin amplification shell vial culture and monoclonal antibody assay. J. Clin. Microbiol. *34*:1465–1467, 1996.
114. Kohne, D. E.: The use of DNA probes to detect and identify microorganisms. Adv. Exptl. Med. Biol. *263*:11–35, 1990.
115. Kok, T. W., Barancek, K., and Burrell, C. J.: Evaluation of the Becton Dickinson Directigen Test for respiratory syncytial virus in nasopharyngeal aspirates. J. Clin. Microbiol. *28*:1458–1459, 1990.
116. Kok, T. W., and Burrell, C. J.: Comparison of five enzyme immunoassays, electron microscopy and latex agglutination for detection of rotavirus in fecal specimens. J. Clin. Microbiol. *27*:364, 1989.
117. Koropchak, C. M.: Investigation of varicella-zoster virus by polymerase chain reaction in the immunocompromised host with acute varicella. J. Infect. Dis. *163*:1016–1022, 1990.
118. Kovacs, A., Xu, J., Rasheed, S., et al.: Comparison of a rapid nonisotopic polymerase chain reaction assay with four commonly used methods for the early diagnosis of human immunodeficiency virus type 1 infection in neonates and children. Pediatr. Infect. Dis. J. *14*:948–954, 1995.
119. Krajden, M., Shankaran, P., Bourke, C., et al.: Detection of cytomegalovirus in blood donors by PCR using the Digene SHARP signal system assay: Effects of sample preparation and detection methodology. J. Clin. Microbiol. *34*:29–33, 1996.
120. Lafferty, W. E., Kroftt, S., Remington, M., et al.: Diagnosis of herpes simplex virus by direct immunofluorescence and viral isolation from samples of external genital lesions in a high prevalence population. J. Clin. Microbiol. *25*:323, 1987.
121. Lakeman, F. D., and Whitley, R. J.: Diagnosis of herpes simplex encephalitis: Application of polymerase chain reaction to cerebrospinal fluid from brain-biopsied patients and correlation with disease. J. Infect. Dis. *171*:856–863, 1995.
122. Landry, M. L., Ferguson, D., Stevens-Ayers, T., et al.: Evaluation of CMV Brite kit for detection of cytomegalovirus pp65 antigenemia in peripheral blood leukocytes by immunofluorescence. J. Clin. Microbiol. *34*:1337–1339, 1996.
123. Landry, M. L., and Ferguson, D.: Comparison of quantitative cytomegalovirus antigenemia assay with culture methods and correlation with clinical disease. J. Clin. Microbiol. *31*:2851–2856, 1993.
124. Langenberg, A., Zbanysek, R., Dragavon, J., et al.: Detection of herpes simplex virus DNA from genital lesions by in situ hybridization. J. Clin. Microbiol. *26*:933–937, 1988.
125. Lauer, B. A., Masters, H. A., Wren, C. G., et al.: Rapid detection of respiratory syncytial virus in nasopharyngeal secretions by an enzyme-linked immunosorbent assay. J. Clin. Microbiol. *22*:782, 1985.
126. Lazar, J., Salim, H., Scearce, L., et al.: Improved detection of CMV viremia: A multicenter trial of the Hybrid Capture™ CMV DNA assay. San Diego Nucleic Acids Conference, American Association of Clinical Chemistry, 1995.
127. Lazzarotto, T., Campisi, B., Galli, S., et al.: A quantitative test (HCMV Hybrid Capture™) to detect human cytomegalovirus DNA in the blood of immunocompromised patients compared with antigenemia and polymerase chain reaction. Fifth International Cytomegalovirus Conference, Stockholm, 1995.
128. Leland, D. S., Hansing, R. L., and French, M. L. V.: Clinical experience with cytomegalovirus isolation using both conventional cell cultures and rapid shell vial techniques. J. Clin. Microbiol. *27*:1159–1162, 1989.
129. Lennette, E. H. (ed.): Laboratory Diagnosis of Viral Infections. 2nd ed. New York, Marcel Dekker, 1992.
130. Leonardi, G. P., Leib, H., Birkhead, G. S., et al.: Comparison of rapid detection methods for influenza A virus and their value in health care management of institutionalized geriatric patients. J. Clin. Microbiol. *32*:70–74, 1994.
131. Lin, H. J., Haywood, M., and Hollinger, F. B.: Application of a commercial kit for detection of PCR products to quantification of human immunodeficiency virus type 1 RNA and proviral DNA. J. Clin. Microbiol. *34*:329–333, 1996.
132. Long, C., Cullen, A., Cox, T., et al.: Rapid detection and typing of herpes simplex virus using the Hybrid Capture™ system. 12th Annual Clinical Virology Symposium, 1996, Clearwater, FL. Abstract M25.
133. Lunel, F., Mariotti, M., Cresta, P., et al.: Comparative study of conventional and novel strategies for the detection of hepatitis C virus RNA in serum: Amplicor, branched-DNA, NASBA and in-house PCR. J. Virol. Methods *54*:159–171, 1995.
134. Macartney, M., Gane, E., and Williams, R.: Comparison of Hybrid Capture (TM) CMV DNA assay with PCR, IgM detection, cell culture and DEAFF test in liver transplant patients. Fifth International Cytomegalovirus Conference, Stockholm, 1995.
135. MacDonald, R. L., Hughes, B. L., Aarnaes, S. L., et al.: Evaluation of a shell vial centrifugation method for the detection of herpes simplex virus. Diagn. Microbiol. Infect. Dis. *9*:51, 1988.
136. Mahafzah, A. M., and Landry, M. L.: Evaluation of immunofluorescent reagents, centrifugation, and conventional cultures for the diagnosis of adenovirus infection. Diagn. Microbiol. Infect. Dis. *12*:407–411, 1989.
137. Martin, W. J., II, and Smith, T. F.: Rapid detection of cytomegalovirus in bronchoalveolar lavage specimens by a monoclonal antibody method. J. Clin. Microbiol. *23*:1006–1008, 1986.
138. Martinez, O. M., Villanueva, J. C., Lawrence-Miyasaki, L., et al.: Viral and immunologic aspects of Epstein-Barr virus infection in pediatric liver transplant recipients. Transplantation *59*:519–524, 1995.
139. Mason, T., Bloom, G., and Leland, D.: Evaluation of ELVIS™ HSV Gold, a commercially available tube culture system featuring a genetically engineered cell line and a histochemical assay for detection of herpes simplex virus (HSV). 12th Annual Clinical Virology Symposium, 1996, Clearwater, FL. Abstract M24.
140. Masters, H. B., Bate, B. J., Wren, C., et al.: Detection of respiratory syncytial virus antigen in nasopharyngeal secretions by Abbott Diagnostics enzyme immunoassay. J. Clin. Microbiol. *26*:1103–1105, 1988.
141. Mathewson, J. J., Winsor, D. K., DuPont, H. L., et al.: Evaluation of assay systems for the detection of rotavirus in stool specimens. Diagn. Microbiol. Infect. Dis. *12*:139–141, 1989.
142. Matthey, S., Nicholson, D., Ruhs, S., et al.: Rapid detection of respiratory

viruses by shell vial culture and direct staining by using pooled and individual monoclonal antibodies. J. Clin. Microbiol. 30:540–544, 1992.
143. Mazzulli, T., Wood, S., Chua, R., et al.: Evaluation of the Digene Hybrid Capture™ system for the detection and quantitation of human cytomegalovirus viremia in human immunodeficiency virus–infected patients. J. Clin. Microbiol. 34:2959–2962, 1996.
144. Mazzulli, T., Rubin, R. H., Ferraro, M. J., et al.: Cytomegalovirus antigenemia: Clinical correlations in transplant recipients and in persons with AIDS. J. Clin. Microbiol. 31:2824–2827, 1993.
145. McDonald, J. C., and Quennec, P.: Utility of a respiratory virus panel containing a monoclonal antibody pool for screening of respiratory specimens in nonpeak respiratory syncytial virus season. J. Clin. Microbiol. 31:2809–2811, 1993.
146. McIntosh, K.: Recent advances in viral diagnosis. Arch. Pathol. Lab. Med. 104:3–6, 1980.
147. McQuillin, J., Madeley, C. R., and Kendal, A. P.: Monoclonal antibodies for the rapid diagnosis of influenza A and B virus infections by immunofluorescence. Lancet 2:911, 1985.
148. Mellors, J. W., Rinaldo, C. R., Jr., Gupta, P., et al.: Prognosis in HIV-1 infection predicted by the quantity of virus in plasma. Science 272:1167–1176, 1996.
149. Michalski, F. J., Shaikh, M., Sahraie, F., et al.: Enzyme-linked immunosorbent assay spin amplification technique for herpes simplex virus antigen detection. J. Clin. Microbiol. 24:310–311, 1986.
150. Milburn, G. L., Carrigan, D., Dienglewicz, R., et al.: Diagnosis of active human herpesvirus six (HHV-6) infection in immunocompromised patients with a rapid shell vial assay. 96th General Meeting of the American Society of Microbiology, New Orleans, 1996. Abstract C136.
151. Miller, H., Milk, R., and Diaz-Mitoma, F.: Comparison of the VIDAS RSV assay and the Abbott Testpack RSV with direct immunofluorescence for detection of respiratory syncytial virus in nasopharyngeal aspirates. J. Clin. Microbiol. 31:1336–1338, 1993.
152. Miller, M. J., Wagar, E. A., Moe, A. A., et al.: Comparison of nucleic acid hybridization, culture, and shell vial assay for detection of CMV in blood. 96th General Meeting of the American Society of Microbiology, New Orleans, 1996. Abstract C89.
153. Miller, M. J., Bovey, S., Pado, K., et al.: Application of PCR to multiple specimen types for diagnosis of cytomegalovirus infection: Comparison with cell culture and shell vial assay. J. Clin. Microbiol. 32:5–10, 1994.
154. Miller, M. J., and Howell, C. L.: Rapid detection and identification of herpes simplex virus in cell culture by a direct immunoperoxidase staining procedure. J. Clin. Microbiol. 18:550–553, 1983.
155. Mills, R. D., Cain, K. J., and Woods, G. L.: Detection of influenza virus by centrifugal inoculation of MDCK cells and staining with monoclonal antibodies. J. Clin. Microbiol. 27:2505–2508, 1989.
156. Minnich, L. L., Goodenough, F., and Ray, C. G.: Use of immunofluorescence to identify measles virus infection. J. Clin. Microbiol. 29:1148–1150, 1991.
157. Minnich, L. L., and Ray, C. G.: Early testing of cell culture for detection of hemadsorbing viruses. J. Clin. Microbiol. 25:421–422, 1987.
158. Minnich, L. L., and Ray, C. G.: Comparison of direct and indirect immunofluorescence staining of clinical specimens for detection of respiratory syncytial virus antigen. J. Clin. Microbiol. 15:969, 1982.
159. Murray, P. R., Baron, E. J., Pfaller, M. A., et al. (eds.): Manual of Clinical Microbiology. 6th ed. Washington, D. C., American Society for Microbiology, 1995.
160. Myerson, D., Hackman, R. C., and Meyers, J. D.: Diagnosis of cytomegalovirus pneumonia by in situ hybridization. J. Infect. Dis. 150:272–277, 1984.
161. Nahass, G. T., Mandel, M. J., Cook, S., et al.: Detection of herpes simplex and varicella zoster infection from cutaneous lesions in different clinical stages with the polymerase chain reaction. J. Am. Acad. Dermatol. 32:730–733, 1995.
162. Nahass, G. T., Goldstein, B. A., Zhu, W., et al.: Comparison of Tzanck, viral culture, and DNA diagnostic methods in detection of herpes simplex and varicella zoster infection (PCR). J. A. M. A. 268:2541–2544, 1992.
163. Nelson, C. T., Istas, A. S., Wilkerson, M. K., et al.: PCR detection of cytomegalovirus DNA in serum as a diagnostic test for congenital cytomegalovirus infection. J. Clin. Microbiol. 33:3317–3318, 1995.
164. Nishi, M., Hanashiro, R., Mori, S., et al.: Polymerase chain reaction for the detection of the varicella zoster genome in ocular samples from patients with acute retinal necrosis. Am. J. Ophthalmol. 114:603–609, 1992.
165. Nolte, F. S., Thurmond, C., and Fried, M. W.: Preclinical evaluation of AMPLICOR hepatitis C virus test for detection of hepatitis C virus RNA. J. Clin. Microbiol. 33:1775–1778, 1995.
166. Ogburn, J. R., Hoffpauir, J. T., Cole, E., et al.: Evaluation of new transport medium for detection of herpes simplex virus by culture and direct enzyme-linked immunosorbent assay. J. Clin. Microbiol. 32:3082–3084, 1994.
167. Olsen, M. A., Shuch, K. M., Sambol, A. R., et al.: Isolation of seven respiratory viruses in shell vials: A practical and highly sensitive method. J. Clin. Microbiol. 31:422–425, 1993.
168. Pai, C. H., Shahrabad, M. S., and Ince, B.: Rapid diagnosis of rotavirus gastroenteritis by a commercial latex agglutination test. J. Clin. Microbiol. 22:846–850, 1985.
169. Paya, C. V., Holley, K. E., and Wiesner, R. H.: Early diagnosis of cytomegalovirus hepatitis in liver transplant recipients: Role of immunostaining, DNA hybridization, and culture of hepatic tissue. Hepatology 12:119, 1990.
170. Paya, C. V., Wold, A. D., Ilstrup, D. M., et al.: Evaluation of number of shell vial cell cultures per clinical specimen for rapid diagnosis of cytomegalovirus infection. J. Clin. Microbiol. 26:198–200, 1988.
171. Paya, C. V., Wold, A. D., and Smith, T. F.: Detection of cytomegalovirus infections in specimens other than urine by the shell vial assay and conventional tube cell cultures. J. Clin. Microbiol. 25:755–757, 1987.
172. Persing, D. H., Smith, T. F., Tenover, F. C., et al. (eds.): Diagnostic Molecular Microbiology, Principles and Applications. Washington, D. C., American Society for Microbiology, 1993.
173. Persing, D. H.: Polymerase chain reaction: Trenches to benches. J. Clin. Microbiol. 29:1281–1285, 1991.
174. Peter, J. B.: The polymerase chain reaction: Amplifying our options. Rev. Infect. Dis. 13:166–171, 1991.
175. Peterson, E. M., Hughes, B. L., Aarnaes, S. L., et al.: Comparison of primary rabbit kidney and MRC-5 cells and two stain procedures for herpes simplex virus detection by a shell vial centrifugation method. J. Clin. Microbiol. 26:222–224, 1988.
176. Peterson, L. R., Moore, B. M., Edelman, C. K., et al.: Primary virus isolation by a satellite laboratory. Arch. Pathol. Lab. Med. 104:9–10, 1980.
177. Phillips, L. E., Magliola, R. A., Stehlik, M. L., et al.: Retrospective evaluation of the isolation and identification of herpes simplex virus with CultureSet and human fibroblasts. J. Clin. Microbiol. 22:255–258, 1985.
178. Podzorski, R. P., and Persing, D. H.: PCR: The next decade. Clin. Microbiol. Newsl. 15:137–143, 1993.
179. Pouletty, P., Chomel, J. J., Thourvenot, D., et al.: Detection of herpes simplex virus in direct specimens by immunofluorescence assay using a monoclonal antibody. J. Clin. Microbiol. 25:958–959, 1987.
180. Pruneda, R. C., and Almanza, I.: Centrifugation-shell vial technique for rapid detection of herpes simplex virus cytopathic effect in Vero cells. J. Clin. Microbiol. 25:423–424, 1987.
181. Puchhammer-Stockl, E., Heinz, F. X., and Kunz, C.: Evaluation of three nonradioactive DNA detection systems for identification of herpes simplex DNA amplified from cerebrospinal fluid. J. Virol Methods 43:257–266, 1993.
182. Puchhammer-Stockl, E., Heinz, F. X., Kundi, M., et al.: Evaluation of the polymerase chain reaction for diagnosis of herpes simplex virus encephalitis. J. Clin. Microbiol. 31:146–148, 1993.
183. Puchhammer-Stockl, E., Popow-Kraupp, T., Heinz, F., et al.: Detection of varicella-zoster virus DNA by polymerase chain reaction in the cerebrospinal fluid of patients suffering from neurological complications associated with chicken pox or herpes zoster. J. Clin. Microbiol. 29:1513–1516, 1991.
184. Rabalais, G. P., Stout, G. G., Ladd, K. L., et al.: Rapid diagnosis of respiratory viral infections by using a shell vial assay and monoclonal antibody pool. J. Clin. Microbiol. 30:1505–1508, 1992.
185. Rabella, N., and Drew, W. L.: Comparison of conventional and shell vial cultures for detecting cytomegalovirus infection. J. Clin. Microbiol. 4:806–807, 1990.
186. Ray, C. G., and Minnich, L. L.: Efficiency of immunofluorescence for rapid detection of common respiratory viruses. J. Clin. Microbiol. 25:355, 1987.
187. Redfield, D. C., Richman, D. D., Albanil, S., et al.: Detection of herpes simplex virus in clinical specimens by DNA hybridization. Diagn. Microbiol. Infect. Dis. 1:117–128, 1983.
188. Revets, H., Marissens, D., DeWit, S., et al.: Comparative evaluation of NASBA HIV-1 RNA QT, AMPLICOR-HIV Monitor, and QUANTIPLEX HIV RNA assay, three methods for quantification of human immunodeficiency virus type 1 RNA in plasma. J. Clin. Microbiol. 34:1058–1064, 1996.
189. Rogers, M. F., Ou, C. Y., Rayfield, M., et al.: Use of the polymerase chain reaction for early detection of the proviral sequences of human immunodeficiency virus in infants born to seropositive mothers. N. Engl. J. Med. 320:1649, 1989.
190. Romero, J. R., Hinrichs, S. H., Cavalieri, S. J., et al.: Potential health care cost saving from PCR based-rapid diagnosis of enteroviral meningitis. Abstract. Society of Pediatric Research Annual Meeting, Washington, D.C., May 6–10, 1996.
191. Romero, J. R., and Rotbart, H. A.: PCR based strategies for the detection of human enteroviruses. *In* Ehrlich, G. D., and Greenberg, S. J. (eds.): PCR-Based Diagnostics in Infectious Disease. Boston, Blackwell Scientific Publications, 1994, pp. 341–374.
192. Rossier, E., Miller, H. R., and Phipps, P. H.: Rapid Viral Diagnosis by Immunofluorescence: An Atlas and Practical Guide. Ottawa, University of Ottawa Press, 1989.
193. Rotbart, H. A.: Enteroviral infections of the central nervous system. Clin. Infect. Dis. 20:971–981, 1995.
194. Rotbart, H. A., Sawyer, M. H., Fast, S., et al.: Diagnosis of enteroviral meningitis by using PCR with a colorimetric microwell detection assay. J. Clin. Microbiol. 32:2590–2592, 1994.
195. Roth, W. K., Lee, J. H., Ruster, B., et al.: Comparison of two quantitative hepatitis C virus reverse transcriptase PCR assays. J. Clin. Microbiol. 34:261–264, 1996.
196. Rothbarth, P. H., Hermus, M. C., and Schrijnemakers, P.: Reliability of two

new test kits for rapid diagnosis of respiratory syncytial virus infection. J. Clin. Microbiol. *29*:824–826, 1991.
197. Rowley, A. H., Whitley, R. J., Lakeman, F. D., et al.: Rapid detection of herpes simplex virus DNA in cerebrospinal fluid of patients with herpes simplex encephalitis. Lancet *335*:440–441, 1990.
198. Rubin, S. J., and Rogers, S.: Comparison of Culture Set and primary rabbit kidney cell culture for the detection of herpes simplex virus. J. Clin. Microbiol. *19*:920–922, 1984.
199. Ryan-Poirier, K. A., Katz, J. M., Webster, R. G., et al.: Application of Directigen Flu-A for the detection of influenza A virus in human and nonhuman specimens. J. Clin. Microbiol. *30*:1072–1075, 1992.
200. Saag, M. S., Holodniy, M., Kuritzkes, D. R., et al.: HIV viral load markers in clinical practice. Nature Med. *2*:625–629, 1996.
201. Salmon, V. C., Turner, R. B., Speranza, M. J., et al.: Rapid detection of herpes simplex virus in clinical specimens by centrifugation and immunoperoxidase staining. J. Clin. Microbiol. *23*:683–686, 1986.
202. Sambourg, M. A., Goudeau, A., Courant, C., et al.: Direct appraisal of latex agglutination testing, a convenient alternative to enzyme immunoassay for the detection of rotavirus in childhood gastroenteritis, by comparison of two enzyme immunoassays and two latex tests. J. Clin. Microbiol. *21*:622–625, 1985.
203. Sanders, R. C., Campbell, A. D., and Jenkins, M. F.: Routine detection of human rotavirus by latex agglutination: Comparison with enzyme-linked immunosorbent assay, electron microscopy, and polyacrylamide gel electrophoresis. J. Virol. Methods *13*:285, 1986.
204. Sawyer, M. H., Holland, D., Aintablian, N., et al.: Diagnosis of enteroviral central nervous system infection by polymerase chain reaction during a large community outbreak. Pediatr. Infect. Dis. J. *13*:177–182, 1994.
205. Schirm, J., Meulenberg, J., Pastoor, G., et al.: Rapid detection of varicella zoster virus in clinical specimens using monoclonal antibodies on shell vials and smears. J. Med. Virol. *28*:1–6, 1989.
206. Schirm, J., Luijt, D. S., Pastoor, G. W., et al.: Rapid detection of respiratory viruses using mixtures of monoclonal antibodies on shell vial cultures. J. Med. Virol. *38*:147–151, 1992.
207. Schlesinger, Y., Buller, R. S., Brunstrom, J. E., et al.: Expanded spectrum of herpes simplex encephalitis in childhood. J. Pediatr. *126*:234–241, 1995.
208. Schlesinger, Y., Sawyer, M. H., and Storch, G. A.: Enteroviral meningitis in infancy: Potential role for polymerase chain reaction in patient management. Pediatrics *94*:157–162, 1994.
209. Schmidt, N. J., and Emmons, R. W. (eds.): Diagnostic Procedures for Viral, Rickettsial, and Chlamydial Infections. 6th ed. Washington, D.C., American Public Health Association, 1989.
210. Schmidt, N. J., Gallo, D., Devlin, V., et al.: Direct immunofluorescence staining for detection of herpes simplex and varicella zoster virus antigens in vesicular lesions and certain tissue specimens. J. Clin. Microbiol. *12*:651–655, 1980.
211. Scholl, D. R., Dul, J. C., McHard, K. D., et al.: ELVIRA (TM) HSV promoter cell clone for rapid antiviral resistance testing. 12th Annual Clinical Virology Symposium, Clearwater, FL, 1996. Abstract M29.
212. Seme, K., and Poljak, M.: Use of a commercial PCR kit for detection of hepatitis C virus. Eur. J. Clin. Microbiol. Infect. Dis. *14*:549–552, 1995.
213. Seno, M., Kanamoto, Y., Takao, S., et al.: Enhancing effect of centrifugation on isolation of influenza virus from clinical specimens. J. Clin. Microbiol. *28*:1669–1670, 1990.
214. Sewell, D. L., and Horn, S. A.: Evaluation of a commercial enzyme linked immunosorbent assay for the detection of herpes simplex virus. J. Clin. Microbiol. *21*:457–458, 1985.
215. Shibata, D., Martin, W. J., Appleman, M. D., et al.: Detection of cytomegalovirus DNA in peripheral blood of patients infected with human immunodeficiency virus. J. Infect. Dis. *158*:1185–1192, 1988.
216. Shoji, H., Honda, Y., Murai, I., et al.: Detection of varicella zoster virus DNA by polymerase chain reaction in cerebrospinal fluid of patients with herpes simplex meningitis. J. Neurol. *239*:69–70, 1992.
217. Smith, T. F., Weed, L. A., Pettersen, G. R., et al.: Recovery of *Chlamydia* and genital *Mycoplasma* transported in sucrose phosphate buffer and urease colortest medium. Health Lab. Sci. *14*:30–34, 1977.
218. Smith, M. C., Creutz, C., and Huang, Y. T.: Detection of respiratory syncytial virus in nasopharyngeal secretions by shell vial technique. J. Clin. Microbiol. *29*:463–465, 1991.
219. Spada, B., Biehler, K., Chegas, P., et al.: Comparison of rapid immunofluorescence assay to cell culture isolation for the detection of influenza A and B viruses in nasopharyngeal secretions from infants and children. J. Virol. Methods *33*:305–310, 1991.
220. Specter, S., and Lancz, G. J. (eds.): Clinical Virology Manual. 2nd ed. New York, Elsevier, 1992.
221. Spector, S. A., Merrill, R., Wolf, D., et al.: Detection of human cytomegalovirus in plasma of AIDS patients during acute visceral disease by DNA amplification. J. Clin. Microbiol. *30*:2359–2365, 1992.
222. Stabell, E. C., O'Rourke, S. R., Storch, G. A., et al.: Evaluation of a genetically engineered cell line and a histochemical β-galactosidase assay to detect herpes simplex virus in clinical specimens. J. Clin. Microbiol. *31*:2796–2798, 1993.
223. Stabell, E. C., and Olivo, P. D.: Isolation of a cell line for rapid and sensitive histochemical assay for the detection of herpes simplex virus. J. Virol. Methods *38*:195–204, 1992.
224. Stockl, E., Popow-Kraupp, T., Heinz, F. X., et al.: Potential of in situ hybridization for early diagnosis of productive cytomegalovirus infection. J. Clin. Microbiol. *26*:2536–2540, 1988.
225. Stokes, C. E., Bernstein, J. M., Kyger, S. A., et al.: Rapid diagnosis of influenza A and B by 24-h fluorescent focus assays. J. Clin. Microbiol. *26*:1263–1266, 1988.
226. Storch, G. A., Reed, C. A., and Dula, Z. A.: Evaluation of a latex agglutination test for herpes simplex virus. J. Clin. Microbiol. *26*:787, 1988.
227. Stout, C., Murphy, M. D., Lawrence, S., et al.: Evaluation of a monoclonal antibody pool for rapid diagnosis of respiratory viral infections. J. Clin. Microbiol. *27*:448–452, 1989.
228. Strickler, J. G., Manivel, J. C., Copenhaver, C. M., et al.: Comparison of in situ hybridization and immunohistochemistry for detection of cytomegalovirus and herpes simplex virus. Hum. Pathol. *21*:443, 1990.
229. Swierkosz, E. M., Flander, R., Melvin, L., et al.: Evaluation of the Abbott TEST PACK RSV enzyme immunoassay for detection of respiratory syncytial virus in nasopharyngeal swab specimens. J. Clin. Microbiol. *27*:1151–1154, 1989.
230. Telenti, A., Marshall, W. F., and Smith, T. F.: Detection of Epstein-Barr virus by polymerase chain reaction. J. Clin. Microbiol. *28*:2187–2190, 1990.
231. Templeton, N. S.: The polymerase chain reaction: History, methods, and applications. Diagn. Mol. Pathol. *1*:58–72, 1992.
232. Tenover, F. C.: Diagnostic deoxyribonucleic probes for infectious diseases. Clin. Microbiol. Rev. *1*:82–101, 1988.
233. The, T. H., van der Ploeg, M., van der Berg, A. P., et al.: Direct detection of cytomegalovirus in peripheral blood leukocytes: A review of the antigenemia assay and the polymerase chain reaction. Transplantation *54*:193–198, 1992.
234. Thomas, E. E., and Book, L. E.: Comparison of two rapid methods for detection of respiratory syncytial virus (TestPack RSV and Ortho ELISA) with direct immunofluorescence and virus isolation for the diagnosis of pediatric RSV infection. J. Clin. Microbiol. *29*:632–635, 1991.
235. Thomas, E. E., Puterman, M. L., Kawano, E., et al.: Evaluation of several immunoassays for detection of rotavirus in pediatric stool samples. J. Clin. Microbiol. *26*:1189–1193, 1988.
236. Trabelsi, A., Pozzetto, B., Mbida, A. D., et al.: Evaluation of four methods for rapid detection of adenovirus. Eur. J. Clin. Microbiol. Infect. Dis. *11*:535–539, 1992.
237. Troendle-Atkins, J., Demmler, G. J., and Buffone, G. J.: Rapid diagnosis of herpes simplex virus encephalitis by using the polymerase chain reaction. J. Pediatr. *123*:376–380, 1993.
239. Unger, E. R.: In situ and northern hybridizations: Technical considerations guiding clinical application. Cancer *69*:1532–1535, 1992.
240. Unger, E. R., and Brigati, D. J.: Colorimetric in situ hybridization in clinical virology: Development of automated technology. Curr. Top. Microbiol. Immunol. *143*:21–31, 1989.
241. Unger, E. R., Budgeon, L. R., Myerson, D., et al.: Viral diagnosis by in situ hybridization: Description of a rapid simplified colorimetric method. Am. J. Surg. Pathol. *10*:1–8, 1986.
242. Uren, E. C., Johnson, P. D. R., Montanaro, J., et al.: Herpes simplex virus encephalitis in pediatrics: Diagnosis by detection of antibodies and DNA in cerebrospinal fluid. Pediatr. Infect. Dis. J. *12*:1001–1006, 1993.
243. Valentine-Thon, E.: Evaluation of SHARP signal system for enzymatic detection of amplified hepatitis B virus DNA. J. Clin. Microbiol. *33*:477–480, 1995.
244. Van Beers, D., DeFoor, M., DiCesare, L., et al.: Evaluation of a commercial enzyme and immunomembrane filter assay for detection of respiratory syncytial virus in clinical specimens. Eur. J. Clin. Microbiol. Infect. Dis. *10*:1073–1076, 1991.
245. Van den Berg, A. P., Tegzass, A. M., Scholten-Sampson, A., et al.: Monitoring antigenemia is useful in guiding treatment of severe cytomegalovirus disease after organ transplantation. Transplant. Infect. *5*:101–107, 1992.
246. Van den Berg, A. P., Klompmaker, I. J., Haagsma, E. B., et al.: Antigenemia in the diagnosis and monitoring of active cytomegalovirus infection after liver transplantation. J. Infect. Dis. *164*:265–270, 1991.
247. Van den Berg, A. P., van der Bij, W., van Son, W. J., et al.: Cytomegalovirus antigenemia as a useful marker of symptomatic cytomegalovirus infection after renal transplantation: A report of 130 consecutive patients. Transplantation *48*:991–995, 1989.
248. Van der Bij, W., Schirm, J., Torensma, R., et al.: Comparison between viremia and antigenemia for detection of cytomegalovirus in blood. J. Clin. Microbiol. *26*:2531–2535, 1988.
249. Van der Bij, W., Torensma, R., van Son, W. J., et al.: Rapid immunodiagnosis of active cytomegalovirus infection by monoclonal antibody staining of blood leukocytes. J. Med. Virol. *25*:179–188, 1988.
250. Verano, L., and Michalski, F. J.: Spin-amplified culture followed by enzyme immunoassay for detection of herpes simplex virus in patient specimens: A comparative study. Clin. Diagn. Virol. *1*:23–28, 1993.
251. Verano, L., and Michalski, F. J.: Comparison of direct antigen enzyme immunoassay, HerpChek, with cell culture for detection of herpes simplex virus from clinical specimens. J. Clin. Microbiol. *33*:1378–1379, 1995.
252. Verano, L., and Michalski, F. J.: Herpes simplex virus antigen direct detection in standard virus transport medium by DuPont HerpChek enzyme-linked immunosorbent assay. J. Clin. Microbiol. *28*:2555–2558, 1990.

253. Volpi, A., Whitley, R. J., Ceballos, R., et al.: Rapid diagnosis of pneumonia due to cytomegalovirus with specific monoclonal antibodies. J. Infect. Dis. *147*:1119–1120, 1983.
254. Waecker, N. J., Jr., Shope, T. R., Weber, P. A., et al.: The Rhino-Probe® nasal culturette for detecting respiratory syncytial virus in children. Pediatr. Infect. Dis. J. *12*:326–329, 1993.
255. Walls, H. H., Harmon, M. W., Slagle, J. J., et al.: Characterization and evaluation of monoclonal antibodies developed for typing influenza A and influenza B viruses. J. Clin. Microbiol. *23*:240–245, 1986.
256. Waner, J. L., Whitehurst, N. J., Downs, T., et al.: Production of monoclonal antibodies against parainfluenza 3 virus and their use in diagnosis by immunofluorescence. J. Clin. Microbiol. *22*:535, 1985.
257. Waner, J. L., Todd, S. J., Shalaby, P., et al.: Comparison of Directigen Flu–A with viral isolation and direct immunofluorescence for the rapid detection and identification of influenza A virus. J. Clin. Microbiol. *29*:479–482, 1991.
258. Warford, A. L., Chung, J. W., Drill, A. E., et al.: Amplification techniques for detection of herpes simplex virus in neonatal and maternal genital specimens obtained at delivery. J. Clin. Microbiol. *27*:1324–1328, 1989.
259. Warford, A. L., Kao, S. Y., Valantine, H., et al.: Evaluation of CMV plasma PCR for monitoring of heart transplant recipients receiving both gancyclovir and cytogam prophylaxis. 12th Annual Clinical Virology Symposium, Clearwater, FL, 1996. Abstract S18.
260. Weiss, R. L., Snow, G. W., Schumann, G. B., et al.: Diagnosis of cytomegalovirus pneumonitis on bronchoalveolar lavage fluid: Comparison of cytology, immunofluorescence, and in situ hybridization with viral isolation. Diagn. Cytopathol. *7*:243–247, 1990.
261. White, T. J., Madej, R., and Persing, D. H.: The polymerase chain reaction: Clinical applications. Adv. Clin. Chem. *29*:161–196, 1992.
262. Whitley, R. J., and Lakeman, F.: Herpes simplex virus infections of the central nervous system: Therapeutic and diagnostic considerations. Clin. Infect. Dis. *20*:414–420, 1995.
263. Williams, S. D., and Kwok, S.: Polymerase chain reaction: Applications for viral detection. *In* Lennette, E. H. (ed.): Laboratory Diagnosis of Viral Infections. 2nd ed. New York, Marcel Dekker, 1992, pp. 147–173.
264. Wolcott, M. J.: Advances in nucleic acid based detection methods. Clin. Microbiol. Rev. *5*:370–386, 1992.
265. Wolf, D. G., and Spector, S. A.: Diagnosis of human cytomegalovirus central nervous system disease in AIDS patients by DNA amplification from cerebrospinal fluid. J. Infect. Dis. *166*:1412–1415, 1992.
266. Wong, D. T., Welliver, R. C., Riddlesberger, K. R., et al.: Rapid diagnosis of parainfluenza virus infection in children. J. Clin. Microbiol. *16*:164–167, 1982.
267. Wood, D. J., Bijlsma, K., de Jong, J. C., et al.: Evaluation of a commercial monoclonal antibody-based enzyme immunoassay for detection of adenovirus types 40 and 41 in stool specimens. J. Clin. Microbiol. *27*:1155–1158, 1989.
268. Wren, C. G., Bate, B. J., Masters, H. B., et al.: Detection of respiratory syncytial virus antigen in nasal washings by Abbott TestPack enzyme immunoassay. J. Clin. Microbiol. *28*:1395–1397, 1990.
269. Yamamoto, M., Kimura, H., Hironaka, T., et al.: Detection and quantification of virus DNA in plasma of patients with Epstein-Barr virus–associated diseases. J. Clin. Microbiol. *33*:1765–1768, 1995.
270. Yamamoto, S., Pavan-Langston, D., Kinoshita, S., et al.: Detecting herpes virus DNA in uveitis using the polymerase chain reaction. Br. J. Ophthalmol. *80*:465–468, 1996.
271. Yang, C. F., De, L., Holloway, B. P., et al.: Detection and identification of vaccine-related polioviruses by the polymerase chain reaction. Virus Res. *20*:159–179, 1991.
272. Yerly, S., Gervaix, A., Simonet, V., et al.: Rapid and sensitive detection of enteroviruses in specimens from patients with aseptic meningitis. J. Clin. Microbiol. *34*:199–201, 1996.
273. Zaaijer, H. L., ter Borg, F., Cuypers, H. T. M., et al.: Comparison of methods for detection of hepatitis B virus DNA. J. Clin. Microbiol. *32*:2088–2091, 1994.
274. Zeuzem, S., Ruster, B., and Roth, W. K.: Clinical evaluation of a new polymerase chain reaction assay (Amplicor HCV) for detection of hepatitis C virus. Z. Gastroenterol. *32*:342–347, 1994.
275. Zhao, L., Landry, M. L., Balkovic, E. S., et al.: Impact of cell culture sensitivity and virus concentration on rapid detection of herpes simplex virus by cytopathic effects and immunoperoxidase staining. J. Clin. Microbiol. *25*:1401–1405, 1987.
276. Zimmerman, S. J., Moses, E., and Sofat, N.: Evaluation of a visual, rapid, membrane enzyme immunoassay for the detection of herpes simplex virus antigen. J. Clin. Microbiol. *29*:842–845, 1991.
277. Zipeto, D., Revello, M. G., Silini, E., et al.: Development and clinical significance of a diagnostic assay based on the polymerase chain reaction for detection of human cytomegalovirus DNA in blood samples from immunocompromised patients. J. Clin. Microbiol. *30*:527–530, 1992.

245

USE OF THE SEROLOGY LABORATORY

Edward O. Mason, Jr.

Serologic diagnosis of infectious diseases may be accomplished either by the demonstration of a specific antibody response in the patient's serum or by the demonstration of the presence of antigens of the infecting agent in tissue or body fluids with the use of hyperimmune sera of known specificity. These two diagnostic approaches often are used simultaneously and may be performed in the same laboratory. This chapter, however, is concerned primarily with the interpretation of the serologic response of the patient in order to diagnose infectious diseases. Appropriate use and interpretation of antigen detection tests are presented in Chapters 243 and 244.

Selection of optimal serologic procedures for the diagnosis of an infectious agent involves considerations of sensitivity, specificity, antigen availability, time, and cost. A variety of techniques have been developed and applied to the serologic diagnosis of infectious diseases. Before any one procedure is adopted, the advantages, disadvantages, and performance of each of the many tests (Table 245–1) should be considered carefully. Evaluation of new procedures begins with comparison of the sensitivity and specificity of the proposed assay with results obtained by testing the same samples by established serologic techniques. Once the reliability and reproducibility of the new assay have been determined, the value of the new procedure in predicting the presence or absence of disease must be determined by prospective clinical trials.

Serologic diagnoses are made either by demonstrating a fourfold rise in the antibody titer between the acute and convalescent serum samples or by detecting specific IgM antibodies (indicating a recent infection) elicited by the infecting agent. The laboratory must be prepared to document accurately the time of collection of serum samples and to preserve them adequately until companion samples can be obtained and tested together. Interfering substances caused by improper handling and storage of the samples can be minimized by prompt removal of the serum from the clot and by storage at $-20°$ C or below. Even when circumstances do not permit immediate freezing, separation of the serum often allows future analysis. Likewise, the samples must be protected adequately from further deterioration of the antibody content when they are referred to outside laboratories.

The purity of any serologic reagent is a limiting factor in the usefulness of any assay. The availability of specific monoclonal antiglobulin for use in indirect fluorescent antibody (IFA) tests, enzyme-linked immunosorbent assays (ELISAs), and radioimmunoassays (RIAs) has permitted the stan-

TABLE 245–1. Serologic Procedures

Agglutination reactions
Bacterial
Latex
Hemagglutination
Hemagglutination inhibition
Precipitin reactions
Tube precipitation
Gel immunodiffusion
Countercurrent immunoelectrophoresis
Immunofluorescence
Indirect immunofluorescence
Indirect complement fixation
Enzyme-linked immunosorbent assay
Radioimmunoassay
Complement fixation
Neutralization
Viral
Toxin
Western blot (immunoblot)

dardization of many procedures that quantitate the primary IgM antibody response, which allows rapid diagnosis of infection with only a single determination. The availability and interpretation of serologic tests for the diagnosis of bacterial, fungal, parasitic, and viral infections are discussed in the paragraphs that follow.

SERODIAGNOSIS OF BACTERIAL INFECTIONS

Borrelia Serology

Infection caused by *Borrelia burgdorferi* (Lyme borreliosis, Lyme disease, erythema chronicum migrans, and others) remains a clinical diagnosis. After the identification and isolation of the spirochetal etiologic agent in 1982, an IFA method for serologic diagnosis was developed and reported to be both specific and sensitive.[15, 158] Experience with the test, however, has revealed that there are cross-reactions in sera of patients with other spirochetal and tick-borne diseases.[107] Results of the test often are negative in early primary Lyme disease, and the antibody response to different antigens varies with the stage of infection.[105, 107] Interlaboratory reproducibility was shown to be poor when serum specimens from 17 asymptomatic workers in an endemic area were sent to four different laboratories, and 6 tested positive in at least one laboratory and none tested positive in all four laboratories.[70] Subsequently, ELISA was reported to be more specific, sensitive, and less dependent on subjective variables inherent in the IFA test.[30, 106] ELISA has become the test of choice in most laboratories, yet this test also is subject to problems of cross-reactivity with antibodies from other diseases[105] and interlaboratory variability.[103] In one study, two identical serum specimens from nine patients, representing a spectrum of Lyme disease symptoms, were sent to nine different laboratories 2 weeks apart. The wide variability in the reported results ranged from the detection of antibody in 18 of 18 specimens in one laboratory to only 8 of 18 in another laboratory. With either procedure, false-negative reactions are common early in the course of Lyme borreliosis and in patients treated with antibiotics during the first stage of the disease.[6] Immunoblotting of extracts of *B. burgdorferi* allows analysis of the immunologic response to the individual components of the spirochete and has been shown to be the most sensitive method for detecting antibody responses during the early stages of infection.[46, 61] There also is evidence that serologic responses vary as a result of antigenic differences in *Borrelia* antigens from organisms from different geographic regions.[14] Other investigators have proposed the use of flagellar antigens in the diagnosis of Lyme disease, especially in the early stages of the disease.[64] The flagellar antigens show no variation among strains and are easy to prepare and purify, which makes them attractive candidates for standardized antigens. ELISA methodology using recombinant p83 antigen appears to be a specific test for determination of late-stage Lyme disease.[140] Children with well-documented, resolved Lyme arthritis remain seropositive for at least 6 months after therapy, making borreliosis a tempting diagnosis for many unexplained symptoms.[144] Thus, consensus remains that until the testing procedure is standardized and reference materials are universally available, the results of serologic testing should not be used as the sole criterion for the diagnosis of infection with *B. burgdorferi*.[69]

Brucella Serology

Serodiagnosis of brucellosis is useful because members of the genus *Brucella* often cause insidious infections and are difficult to culture in the laboratory. The first antibody response to infection with *Brucella* is by IgM, followed by an IgG response.[48] The standardized tube agglutination test can demonstrate reliably both of these antibodies separately or together when it is performed according to a strictly standardized protocol. *Brucella* antigen obtained from the United States Department of Agriculture National Animal Disease Center in Ames, Iowa, is prepared with a single strain of *Brucella abortus* but reacts with antibodies to *Brucella suis* and *Brucella melitensis*, as well as *B. abortus*.[155] A tube agglutination titer of greater than or equal to 1:160 or a fourfold rise in the agglutination titer is diagnostic of brucellosis.[191] Vaccination to or natural disease caused by *Vibrio cholerae*, *Francisella tularensis*, or *Yersinia enterocolitica* evokes cross-reacting antibodies; however, the titers are not usually as high as those encountered in brucellosis. The agglutination procedure outlined by the National Research Council Committee on the Public Aspects of Brucellosis requires the dilution scheme to be carried out at least to a titer of 1:320 in order to avoid false-negative reactions caused by a "prozone" effect due to the presence of heat-labile blocking substances.[191]

In contrast with serologic responses in other diseases, the IgM antibody induced by infection with *Brucella* may persist indefinitely.[188] The IgG antibody, which appears later in the course of the disease, declines rapidly with appropriate antibiotic therapy. The presence of IgG antibody in the serum therefore signifies present or recent infection.[188] Persistence of or increase in the IgG antibody is correlated with inadequate treatment and is highly prognostic.[141] The standard tube agglutination test measures both IgG and IgM responses. Treatment of the serum with 2-mercaptoethanol dissociates IgM and permits the measurement of the IgG response alone[12] but lowers the sensitivity of the test. Use of 2-mercaptoethanol to measure IgG antibody should be considered as a secondary procedure after a positive titer is obtained by the standard agglutination test.[12]

Efforts to establish the utility of ELISA for the diagnosis of human brucellosis have found that although the results are encouraging, the technique requires further study in prospective trials to establish the confidence retained by the older tube agglutination techniques.[33] Differentiation of relapsing and chronic disease, which is difficult to discern with standard agglutination tests, seems to be detected more readily by ELISA measurement of rises in IgA and IgG antibodies, however.[129, 189]

Infection of humans by a fourth species of *Brucella, Brucella canis,* is rare; however, at least 30 cases (2 in children) have been reported since 1967.[170, 188] Standard *Brucella* antibody tests do not detect infection with *B. canis.* When such an infection is suspected, serum should be referred to a state reference laboratory. Infection with *B. canis* in humans usually results in antibody titers greater than 1:100.[21]

Leptospira Serology

The definitive serologic test for leptospirosis is the microagglutination test performed with live leptospire antigens representing 12 to 16 individual serotypes.[161] Maintaining viable stock cultures of these organisms is difficult, which makes the test impractical for all but large reference or research facilities. Antibodies elicited in response to acute leptospiral infection do not appear until day 6 to 12 after infection and reach their peak by week 3 to 4 of infection.[186] The following points should be considered in the interpretation of serologic results:

1. There may not be a fourfold rise in the titer if the serum sample is obtained late in the course of disease and the titer has reached a peak.
2. Negative titers do not rule out leptospirosis because the infecting strain may not be represented in the antigen panel used to screen for antibody.
3. Prompt initiation of antibiotic therapy can suppress the serologic response.

Many laboratories perform leptospiral serologic testing by the macroagglutination technique using four pools containing three serotypes each of killed antigen preparation. This slide agglutination test is easy to perform and rapid but unfortunately is of very low specificity.[162] The slide agglutination test is hampered further by the inconsistent quality of the killed antigens available and cross-reactions among these antigens.

An indirect hemagglutination assay (IHA) for the detection of leptospiral antibodies, which uses an alcohol extract of a single leptospiral strain as a sensitizing antigen, has been reported.[162] The sensitivity of IHA was 92 per cent, compared with 69 per cent for the macroagglutination test. The specificity of IHA was 95 per cent, whereas the specificity of the macroagglutination test was 83 per cent. Although IHA seems to offer improved serologic testing for leptospirosis, it does not reliably detect antibodies late in the course of disease.[162]

Two procedures, the IgM-specific dot-ELISA, modified from the original procedure described by Pappas and colleagues,[127] and the genus-specific microscopic agglutination test, have been found comparable in sensitivity and specificity to the classic macroagglutination procedure for the diagnosis of leptospirosis. A modification of this procedure by Ribeiro and colleagues[142] found that the dot-ELISA using a proteinase K-resistant antigen detected antibody activity in 43 per cent of acute-phase sera that were missed by the microscopic agglutination test. Both tests use a single, broadly reactive antigen derived from the nonpathogenic strain of *Leptospira biflexa* serovar Patoc 1 to replace the battery of serotype antigens used in the macroagglutination procedure.[176]

Mycoplasma Serology

Detection of infection caused by *Mycoplasma pneumoniae* often is based on clinical symptoms rather than on isolation of the pathogen.[19] The presence of serum cold agglutinins is a nonspecific indication of *Mycoplasma* infection.[58, 165] Because *Mycoplasma* has a long incubation period, serum cold agglutinins appear earlier than more specific complement-fixation (CF) titers do and often are elevated by the first week after the development of symptoms. Cold agglutinins also may be elicited in several viral diseases, as well as in noninfectious illnesses.[50] Thus, a serum cold agglutinin titer of greater than 1:64 is only suggestive of *Mycoplasma* infection. The severity of the infection also is reflected in the magnitude of the serum cold agglutination response, and mild infections may not elicit an increase in the cold agglutinin titer.

Screening serum for cold agglutinins before titration for quantitation eliminates the need to evaluate negative samples.[58] A rapid method of qualitative screening of cold agglutinins can be performed away from the laboratory by using a few drops of capillary blood (finger-stick) and a small citrated collection tube. Positive results, seen by clumping of the red blood cells when the tube is placed on ice and dissolution of the clumps when the tube is warmed, should be confirmed by quantitative determination of the titer in the laboratory.[58]

Although there are several specific serologic tests for *M. pneumoniae* (growth inhibition test, immunofluorescence, IHA, and RIA), the only test available in nonresearch laboratories is the CF test using a glycolipid antigen. A single titer of greater than 1:256 is only suggestive evidence of a recent infection, and a fourfold rise is required for a definitive diagnosis of *Mycoplasma* infection.[19] Because the CF antibody titers rise slowly and peak 1 month after infection, it may be necessary to repeat titers on paired specimens at weekly intervals.

Evidence provided by retrospective analysis of a small group of patients with both clinical and CF titer evidence of *Mycoplasma* disease demonstrated IgM antibodies in 70 per cent of acute and 100 per cent of convalescent sera with use of urease-conjugated ELISA.[26] Two rapid qualitative assays are commercially available that detect IgM antibodies. One, an enzyme-linked immunobinding assay using a protein antigen, was as sensitive as the CF test but currently is recommended only as a rapid screening procedure.[168]

Rickettsia Serology

The Weil-Felix test is a nonspecific serologic test that uses *Proteus vulgaris* strains OX-19, OX-2, and OX-K to detect agglutinins in the serum of patients who may have one of several rickettsial diseases.[65] *Proteus* agglutination is easy to perform, and the reagents are readily available commercially. Although clinical suspicion together with high (>1:160) OX-19 or OX-2 titers is highly suggestive of a diagnosis of Rocky Mountain spotted fever, the results of the Weil-Felix test should be confirmed by other specific rickettsial serologic procedures.[67] Conversely, negative Weil-Felix test results do not rule out rickettsial infection because antibody titers may not appear for 2 to 3 weeks, especially in cases in which antibiotic therapy was instituted promptly. Low Weil-Felix titers can be evoked in response to infections caused by *Proteus, Leptospira,* and other rickettsiae or in severe hepatitis.[67]

The CF test uses group-specific rickettsial antigens to distinguish between the typhus group and the spotted fever group of diseases. The CF test lacks sensitivity, and detection of antibody also can be delayed by antibiotic therapy.[95] In addition, because the Centers for Disease Control and Prevention have stopped distribution of the CF antigen, performance and standardization of the CF test are in jeopardy.[173]

The microindirect IFA test is reported to be as specific as and more sensitive than the CF test.[68, 134] By spotting four different antigens on the same circle of an immunofluorescence slide, the test can measure specifically the antibody titer to four rickettsial antigens simultaneously with the same drop of diluted serum.[66] Latex-agglutination (LA) tests using *Rickettsia rickettsii* antigens are as specific and sensitive as the microindirect IFA test is.[65] LA test materials are commercially available, and a rapid enzyme immunoassay kit for the detection of IgG and IgM antibodies to *Rickettsia typhi* is being evaluated.[93] IFA testing for rickettsial disease is limited to public health, research, or reference laboratories.[173]

Salmonella Serology

Improvements in the ability to isolate *Salmonella* have reduced the importance of detecting *Salmonella* agglutinins (Widal test). Many variables that affect this test (stage of disease, effects of antibiotics, normal agglutinins, and previous vaccinations) make interpretation and definition of a diagnostic Widal titer difficult. No single titer can be considered diagnostic, and a fourfold rise between acute and convalescent sera should be interpreted as diagnostic only if the sera are tested together.[53]

The original Widal test is a tube agglutinin test that uses commercially available O (somatic) and H (flagellar) *Salmonella* antigens.[185] The slide agglutination test cannot replace the tube agglutination procedure, although some manufacturers of antigen preparations describe this rapid modification as an alternative procedure.[53] Testing for antibodies to both the O and H antigens is necessary for proper interpretation. Tests using antigens other than *Salmonella typhi* or *Salmonella enteritidis* bioserotypes A, B, or C should not be performed because (1) salmonellae other than these rarely are associated with enteric fever illness and (2) gastrointestinal infections alone rarely evoke antibody responses.[53]

Demonstration of antibody to the capsular polysaccharide Vi antigen has been associated with carrier states after infection with *S. typhi*.[185] Agglutination tests for Vi antibodies, however, are of low specificity and sensitivity.[10] The use of purified Vi antigen[121] in ELISA[7] may improve serologic identification of typhoid carriers.

Staphylococcus Serology

The diagnosis of endocarditis, osteomyelitis, and other systemic infections caused by *Staphylococcus aureus* often can be aided by the availability of a reliable serologic procedure. The detection of teichoic acid antibodies by agar gel diffusion in the serum of patients has been reported to be specific for systemic *S. aureus* infection.[183] Unfortunately, the sensitivity of the procedure is only 36 per cent.[118] The use of counterimmunoelectrophoresis (CIE) to detect teichoic acid antibodies improves the sensitivity but lowers the specificity of the assay.[118] ELISA is reported to be a specific and sensitive method for detection of antibodies to teichoic acid in *S. aureus* systemic infections. Thisyakorn and associates[169] reported that a serum ELISA titer of greater than 1:3200 has a sensitivity of 93 per cent and a specificity of 89 per cent in children with culture-proven *S. aureus* infection.

The teichoic acid antigen is either a sonicate or an extract of the Lafferty strain of *S. aureus*, and variations in preparations have hampered comparisons of results among laboratories.[182] This single antigen preparation detects all strains of *S. aureus*.[150] One commercially available preparation (Endo-Staph, Meridian Diagnostics) with a standardized teichoic acid antigen is reported to be reliable.[182] Regardless of the test used, an antibody response only is detected 10 to 14 days after infection and may not be detected at all in immunocompromised patients. Studies have shown that immunodiffusion tests and ELISA show higher immune response to teichoic acid in patients with endocarditis and bacteremia caused by *S. aureus*, compared with control sera from patients without staphylococcal disease.[9] The serologic response does not, however, distinguish between endocarditis and bacteremia caused by *S. aureus*. Likewise, attempts to use antibody responses to another *S. aureus* surface antigen, protein A, were not sensitive or specific enough for diagnosis.[56]

Streptococcus Serology

Infection by *Streptococcus pyogenes* (group A *Streptococcus*) may elicit antibodies to different bacterial extracellular enzymes, depending on the *Streptococcus* strain, the age of the host, the site of the infection, and the duration of the antigenic stimulus.[132] The most frequent measure of antibody response to *S. pyogenes* infection is the antistreptolysin O (ASO) reaction. Antibody to streptolysin O, an oxygen-labile extracellular hemolysin, can be detected within 2 to 4 weeks in 85 per cent of patients after pharyngeal streptococcal infection.[87] However, ASO antibodies are elevated only slightly or undetected after pyodermal streptococcal infection.[175] Thus, serologic responses to other streptococcal antigens (DNase B, hyaluronidase, NADase, and streptokinase) are necessary to document antecedent streptococcal disease and nonsuppurative complications. Because assessment of antibodies to these individual antigens is costly and laborious, a screening procedure (Streptozyme, Wampole Laboratories, Stamford, CT) often is used to detect elevation of antibodies to any one of these several antigens. The Streptozyme test is an IHA that uses erythrocytes that have been sensitized to several extracellular enzymes of a strain of *S. pyogenes*. The test is not quantitative, and positive results should be confirmed by determining antibodies to the individual antigens. Mild elevations of individual antibody titers may not be detected by the Streptozyme test.[71] The Streptozyme test is the only commercially available test that is sufficiently sensitive (100 per cent in this case) to detect anti-ASO elevations but is less sensitive (22 per cent) in detecting anti–DNase B antibodies.[84] Different lots of erythrocyte antigens used in the Streptozyme procedure may vary in strength, and other streptococci may produce identical enzymes. Thus, when strong clinical suspicion of streptococcal disease is not supported by Streptozyme screening tests, the individual antibody determinations must be performed.[89] The significance of single titers should be established by each laboratory after analysis of baseline values for noninfected children of different age groups in that area. In any test, however, a rise of two (0.3 log) or more dilutions between acute and convalescent sera is significant.

Syphilis Serology

Nontreponemal serologic tests for syphilis are the CF tests described by Wasserman and Kolmer and the newer Venereal Disease Research Laboratory (VDRL) and rapid plasma reagin (RPR) flocculation tests. The nontreponemal tests are sensitive, rapid, and suited for mass screening procedures but have a high percentage of false-positive results. For this reason, positive results by one of the nontreponemal tests should be confirmed by a treponemal test, such as the *Treponema pallidum* immobilization test, the fluorescent treponemal antibody test, the fluorescent treponemal antibody-absorption (FTA-ABS) test, or the microhemagglutination *T. pallidum* (MHA-TP) antibody test.

Nontreponemal Tests

Most laboratories now perform either a VDRL or an RPR test rather than a CF test because of the ease and ready commercial availability of the former test reagents. The results of both tests are comparable and both can be quantitated, but only the VDRL test is suitable for detecting antibody in the cerebrospinal fluid for the diagnosis of neurologic syphilis. The antibody titers measured by the VDRL and RPR tests decrease with the institution of proper antibiotic therapy and revert to negative when the patient has completed successful therapy. The antigen used in these tests is a cardiolipin-lecithin-cholesterol complex that detects antibody elicited by infections caused by other bacterial or viral pathogens, by collagen vascular disease, by hepatitis, or by drug addiction.[131] These biologic false-positive titers usually are less than or equal to 1:8 and usually disappear in 6 months. In contrast, false-positive titers in sera may persist longer than 6 months in certain chronic diseases, such as autoimmune disorders and connective tissue disease.[184] The specific treponemal antibody test results usually are negative in these cases.

Treponemal Tests

FTA-ABS and MHA-TP tests are specific tests whose technical difficulty and cost make them unsuitable for routine screening.[96] The primary function of the FTA-ABS test is to confirm the specificity of the nontreponemal test; quantitation of the FTA-ABS test has not proved prognostic in that the antibody titer does not decrease with treatment. Also, the value of the FTA-ABS in the detection of antibody in the cerebrospinal fluid has not been established. Lack of sensitivity has hampered the development of FTA-ABS-IgM test that exclusively detects IgM antibody to *T. pallidum*. The diagnosis of congenital syphilis is complicated further by maternal IgG crossing the placental barrier and reacting with VDRL and RPR tests, which detect primarily IgG antibodies. The low sensitivity of the FTA-ABS-IgM test makes the confirmation of congenital syphilis especially difficult in asymptomatic neonates. Fractionation of *T. pallidum* antigens and use of polyacrylamide gel electrophoresis with Western blotting to nitrocellulose has shown that neonatal IgM directed against a 47-kd antigen of *T. pallidum* may be a better diagnostic predictor of congenital syphilis.[100, 146] IgM-capture ELISA has been found to be more sensitive than the FTA-ABS test for the diagnosis of congenital syphilis when interpreted along with the mother's clinical history.[96, 99] This same commercially available system using IgG capture also has been found to be as sensitive and specific as the RPR test for syphilis screening.[152]

The MHA-TP test is a treponemal test with a specificity similar to that of the FTA-ABS test. The MHA-TP test is easier to perform technically, and the interpretation of the end-point is less subjective. Although the MHA-TP test is slightly less sensitive in detecting antibodies in early primary syphilis, it appears to be a reasonable alternative to the technically more demanding FTA-ABS test.[42] None of the treponemal tests distinguishes between syphilis and other treponematoses (yaws, pinta, and bejel).

SERODIAGNOSIS OF FUNGAL INFECTIONS

Aspergillus Serology

Invasive aspergillosis is almost exclusively a disease of the immunocompromised patient. Diagnosis is difficult, and tissue for culture often requires a biopsy. Because these patients often are the least able to tolerate such invasive procedures, numerous serologic methods have been developed in an attempt to lessen the risk associated with biopsy. Antibodies to *Aspergillus* antigens rarely are found in the serum of healthy persons, even though species of *Aspergillus* are abundant in the environment.[102] Immunodiffusion (ID) tests and more sensitive ELISAs reliably can demonstrate antibodies to *Aspergillus* with 70 to 90 per cent sensitivity in nonimmunocompromised patients with either aspergilloma or allergic aspergillosis.[102, 130] However, the value of serodiagnosis of invasive aspergillosis remains controversial.[34] Young and Bennett[190] reported the complete lack of a serologic response to *Aspergillus* antigens in 16 patients with histologically confirmed aspergillosis. However, Holmberg and associates[78] have shown that a CIE procedure could detect 70 per cent and ELISA could detect 80 per cent of episodes of subsequently proven invasive aspergillosis. Unfortunately, the purified antigens required for these tests must be prepared in research laboratories and thus have restricted availability.

Blastomyces Serology

The CF test using yeast-phase antigen was the first test used in serodiagnosis of infection by *Blastomyces dermatitidis*. Although this test still is widely available in clinical laboratories, it is of little diagnostic or prognostic value in this disease.[147, 148] CF test results are positive (>1:8) in only 50 per cent of patients with histologically proven blastomycosis, and there are significant cross-reactions in serum from patients with confirmed histoplasmosis and coccidioidomycosis.[16] Although there are few reports of blastomycosis in pediatric patients, one study found that similar to the findings in infected adults, only 5 of 12 children infected with *B. dermatitidis* had a positive CF response.[136]

Kaufman and associates[91] have described an ID test for blastomycosis that relies on the presence of specific precipitin bands (A and B) as a more sensitive and specific indication of active infection by this fungus. The A band alone or together with the B band was present in 79 per cent of sera from persons with proven blastomycosis. There are no reports of false-positive results, and the disappearance of the bands may correlate with successful therapy. The detection of this A band depends on carefully prepared antigens and the use of control sera containing the A and B precipitins. These are not often available, and at least one commercially available kit has been found unreliable.[147, 148]

Candida Serology

Methods other than culture would be useful to distinguish invasive candidiasis from colonization with *Candida albicans* in that 15 to 40 per cent of cases of disseminated candidiasis diagnosed at necropsy cannot be confirmed by culture before the death of the patient.[45] Tests for invasive candidiasis must detect antibody responses to antigens that distinguish between colonized and infected persons.[137] Measurement of antibody to a variety of *Candida* antigens includes whole-cell agglutination, gel diffusion, LA, CIE, and, more recently, RIA and ELISA.[35] Comparisons of the efficacy and usefulness of these procedures are difficult because (1) investigators are not consistent in their definition of invasive candidiasis, (2) a majority of patients are immunosuppressed, making antibody detection unreliable, (3) many antigen preparations are undefined, and (4) different experimental methods and study designs make comparisons difficult.

CIE, ID, and LA tests for antibody to *C. albicans* were compared in a collaborative, nonclinical study of immunocompetent patients with systemic candidiasis and were shown to have sensitivities of 80 per cent or greater.[113, 171] These tests can be of value in the diagnosis of invasive candidal disease but rely heavily on the use of standardized reagents that are not yet commercially available. Furthermore, studies using more sensitive RIA and ELISA techniques have shown that cell-wall mannan antibodies are a consistent component of human serum in immunocompetent persons.[57] Immunoblot analysis of cell-wall mannan-free protein extracts of *C. albicans,* using sera from neutropenic patients, detected these proteins in 25 to 70 of the sera tested.[111] A study in Sweden found elevated IgG, IgM, and IgA to three different antigens in 10 of 10 children actively infected with *C. albicans* and little response in 280 healthy control children. In addition to the small number of infected children studied, the report did not include any clinical information on which the value of the findings could be judged.[94] Thus, because of technical inadequacies in antigen purity, availability, and specificity, as well as the absence of antibody response in the patient population most at risk of invasive candidiasis, use of antibody tests for the diagnosis of systemic candidiasis appears to be of little clinical value.[88]

Coccidioides Serology

Unlike their use in many of the other mycoses, serologic procedures in the diagnosis and prognosis of disease caused by *Coccidioides immitis* are of established value. Two antigens, coccidioidin (a mycelial-phase antigen) and spherulin (an endospore antigen), are detected in response to infection by this fungus. The most useful tests are tube precipitin (TP) tests, LA tests, CF tests, and gel ID using coccidioidin antigen.[124] Both TP and LA tests measure IgM, but the LA test is more sensitive, detecting 71 per cent versus 13 per cent[85, 86] of positive specimens. The LA test, however, does have a 6 to 10 per cent false-positive rate.[27] Many patients with asymptomatic pulmonary disease may never have a positive TP test result, which may explain the added sensitivity of these LA test results. It also is possible that the testing of sera from patients in the later stages of disease results in false-negative reactions in both of these tests because of the disappearance of IgM antibodies. Neither test is quantitative. The LA test is commercially available, is easy to perform, and is faster than the TP test (4 minutes vs. 3 days). Because the low protein content of cerebrospinal fluid (CSF) destabilizes the latex/coccidioidin particles, causing nonspecific agglutination,[123] the LA test is not suitable for detecting antibody in spinal fluid. Neither the LA nor the TP test should ever be used in the diagnosis of coccidioidal meningitis.[40]

If the coccidioidin antigen is heated and used in the ID test, it is known as the IDTP test. It detects IgM antibody, as in the LA and TP tests, and is of intermediate sensitivity between these two tests. The LA test and the IDTP test are considered screening tests, and positive results should be confirmed with a standard TP test or followed with a CF test.

Both the CF test and the ID tests (using unheated, ultrafiltered coccidioidin-IDCF) detect IgG responses to infection by *C. immitis.* The CF test is both diagnostic and prognostic and, despite its difficulty in performance, is invaluable in the management of symptomatic coccidioidomycosis. As many as 60 per cent of patients with asymptomatic pulmonary coccidioidomycosis may fail to develop CF antibodies.[40] In those patients who do develop antibodies, a low and stable titer may indicate mild morbidity, and a declining titer usually is associated with clinical improvement or favorable response to therapy.[153, 154] A rising CF titer is associated with dissemination and has a poor prognosis.[124] In cases in which rising or declining titers may be of clinical importance, it has been suggested that aliquots of serum from each serologic determination be frozen and all specimens be retested together to avoid the variations inherent in CF test procedures.[40, 125]

Detection of antibody to *C. immitis* by CF, IDTP, or IDCF tests in CSF is specific for coccidioidal meningitis. Previous studies showed that the CF test detects antibodies in the CSF of 76 per cent of 92 patients with coccidioidal meningitis.[125] Overnight incubation of the antigen-antibody complex at 4° C (39.2° F) improved the sensitivity of the CF test. This modification allowed the detection of *C. immitis* antibodies in the CSF of 96 per cent of 265 patients with culture-proven meningitis.[126]

ELISA using both TP and CF antigens has been approved by the Food and Drug Administration and is commercially available. It has been shown to be reliable and rapid and overcomes problems encountered with serum that is anticomplementary. The test can be used to detect antibody in both serum and CSF. Because it uses specific anti-IgG and anti-IgM, the results are more specific than ID and CF tests. At present, it is approved only for qualitative results from serum, but the optical density units correlate well with CF titer antibody levels.[109]

Cryptococcus Serology

Cryptococcosis is diagnosed rapidly and accurately by the detection of cryptococcal capsule polysaccharide in CSF or serum by the LA test.[92] Although there are several methods for the detection of the serologic response of patients to *Cryptococcus neoformans,* they are of little use in the clinical diagnosis or prognosis of the disease.[37]

Histoplasma Serology

In cases of primary acute pulmonary *Histoplasma capsulatum,* serologic evidence of infection often is all that is available to the clinician. Unfortunately, serodiagnosis is not completely specific or sensitive enough to be of unrestricted usefulness. The CF test can be performed with two antigens: a yeast-phase extract and a filtrate of the mycelial phase (histoplasmin).[91] Antibodies to the yeast antigen usually are positive (≥1:32) in patients with uncomplicated histoplasmosis within 4 weeks of exposure to the agent.[91] The CF test using the yeast-phase antigen has been reported to have a specificity and sensitivity of 90 to 94 per cent.[8, 90] Use of the mycelial antigen in CF tests, on the other hand, has a specificity of 99 per cent but with a greatly reduced sensitivity of 68 to 80 per cent.[8, 90] Titers of 1:8 and 1:16 are difficult to interpret and often are found in patients with other pulmonary mycoses.[91]

The ID test, first described by Heiner,[72] has advantages over the CF test in that anticomplementary sera can be tested and the technical difficulties of the CF test are avoided. The ID test is less sensitive than the CF test and is not quantitative, but it is specific. Original studies found six precipitin bands in serum from patients with histoplasmosis by using the histoplasmin (mycelial) antigen. Two of these bands, designated M and H, were found to be of diagnostic significance. The H band is specific for active histoplasmosis and is unaffected by skin testing. Unfortunately, it may not be present in the serum of many patients with active histoplasmosis.[72] The M band appears before the H band in patients with histoplasmosis, persists after recovery, and also may appear as the result of prior application of skin-test antigen. The presence of M and H bands together is highly suggestive of active histoplasmosis (sensitivity 90 per cent, specificity 94 per cent) and is comparable with a CF yeast antigen titer of 1:32 or greater.[181] Current recommendations are that the CF test using the yeast-phase antigen and the ID test using histoplasmin be used together in serodiagnosis of histoplasmosis.[8] Contrary to serologic titers in coccidioidomycosis, persistence of elevated titers to *Histoplasma* antigens does not correlate with disseminated disease.[181] Lack of specificity, caused by cross-reactions with antibodies present in other fungal and bacterial diseases, has been a major problem in the reliable serodiagnosis of histoplasmosis. Studies have demonstrated a wider range of cross-reactions than was recognized previously, which makes proper interpretation more difficult.[180] CF test results were positive for histoplasmosis in 18 per cent of patients with other fungal infections and in 34 per cent of patients with tuberculosis. These false-positive reactions were even greater with use of an RIA procedure that previously was shown to be more sensitive than CF or ID reaction in detecting early histoplasmosis.[179] As with serologic tests for most mycoses, especially in immunocompromised patients, lack of an immune response does not rule out histoplasmosis.[130]

There is evidence that both the CF test and the ID test are useful in detecting antibody in the CSF of patients with disseminated histoplasmosis and meningitis.[135] This antibody appears to be produced locally in the central nervous system. Three patients with disseminated histoplasmosis but without meningitis did not have detectable antibody to *H. capsulatum* in the CSF by any test. It would seem reasonable to perform CF and ID tests for histoplasmosis on the CSF of patients with suspected histoplasmosis and clinical signs of meningitis.

Paracoccidioides Serology

Serodiagnostic tests of infections caused by *Paracoccidioides brasiliensis* are as specific and sensitive as those tests used to diagnose coccidioidomycosis. Tests available include CF and agar gel diffusion and a highly sensitive and specific ELISA. ID tests, using the E_2 antigen, and ELISAs, using either the E_2 antigen or the absorbed whole filtrate antigen, have sensitivities and specificities between 94 and 100 per cent.[112] Immunoblot testing using a purified gp43 antigen treated with sodium metapeiodate had a sensitivity and a specificity of 100 per cent.[167]

SERODIAGNOSIS OF PARASITIC INFECTIONS

Serodiagnosis of parasitic infections is of less value than are similar diagnostic procedures for viral, bacterial, and fungal pathogens. Primary reasons for this are the complex nature and multiplicity of parasite antigens. Because of this, sensitive and specific serologic tests have been difficult to develop. Interpretation of tests is difficult because most parasitic diseases are chronic, making precise stages of illness difficult to identify. The development of newer serologic methods as well as the availability of chemically defined antigens has enhanced the reliability of the serodiagnosis in several parasitic diseases. Most of these serologic tests are available only through research/reference laboratories or the Centers for Disease Control and Prevention laboratory. Table 245–2 lists the serologic methods available for selected parasitic diseases.

TABLE 245–2. Recently Described Serologic Procedures that May Be Adjuncts in the Diagnosis of Parasitic Infections

	IFA	RIA	ELISA	CIE
Amebiasis	R (54)		R (110)	A (3)
Cryptosporidiosis	A (17)			
Cysticercosis		A (115)	A (117)	
Malaria	A (29)			
*Pneumocystis**			R (104)	
Strongyloidiasis			R (18)	
Toxocariasis (visceral larva migrans)			R (32)	

Abbreviations: CIE, counterimmunoelectrophoresis; ELISA, enzyme-linked immunosorbent assay; IFA, indirect fluorescent antibody assay; RIA, radioimmunoassay.

R, reported in literature; A, available in research/reference laboratories.

*Phylogeny of *Pneumocystis carinii* not determined; may be more related to the fungi.

Toxoplasma Serology

The Sabin-Feldman dye test remains the standard technique for demonstrating antibodies elicited by infection with *Toxoplasma gondii*.[145] Unfortunately, it is technically difficult and time consuming, and it requires live trophozoites, which must be propagated biweekly in mice. Introduction of the IFA test for toxoplasmosis led to ease of performance and good correlation with dye test titers. Killed whole *Toxoplasma* trophozoites fixed on microscope slides (commercially available) are exposed to dilutions of the test serum. After incubation, unreacted serum is removed by washing, and fluorescein-tagged antihuman globulin is allowed to incubate on the cells. After removal of any unreacted antiglobulin, the slides are examined with an ultraviolet light microscope. The presence of antibody to *Toxoplasma* is demonstrated by observing a smooth ring of fluorescence surrounding the crescent-shaped *Toxoplasma* trophozoite. A minor difficulty in the interpretation of some reactions by the IFA technique is the occasional instance of "polar" fluorescence caused by the nonspecific binding of immunoglobulin to the Fc receptors found on the surface of the parasite.[13]

The dye test is reliable, specific, and extremely sensitive; however, the titer peaks in 6 to 8 weeks and can remain high for life. Rising titers seldom can be demonstrated, and the test is suitable only for the detection of previous infection.[178] The IFA test using anti-IgG or antiglobulins also is useful in detecting previous infection, and a titer of greater than or equal to 1:256 is highly suggestive of recent or current infection.

The IFA-IgM test is useful and reliable in predicting recent or ongoing infection with *T. gondii*.[119] IgM titers may rise with the onset of symptoms and begin to disappear in 4 to 6 months.[120] Thus, demonstration of an IgM response of greater than or equal to 1:64 is evidence of recent infection. ELISA also has been shown to be useful in the diagnosis of recent *Toxoplasma* infection and additionally is more sensitive and specific than the IFA procedure. An ELISA-IgM titer of greater than or equal to 1:256 is equivalent to an IFA-IgM titer of 1:64 and is highly indicative of recent infection.[36] Use of a "double sandwich" technique to IgM ELISA further improves sensitivity and avoids problems of interference from other globulins in serum.[151] Demonstration of anti-*Toxoplasma* IgM in the umbilical cord serum or serum of neonates by either procedure is diagnostic of congenital toxoplasmosis.

However, failure to demonstrate IgM titers does not rule out congenital infection.

Demonstration of anti-*Toxoplasma* IgA and IgE using ELISA is a reliable indication of acute infection or congenital infection in the fetus or infant. It does not identify patients with chronic infection or patients with AIDS and toxoplasmic encephalitis.[159, 187]

SERODIAGNOSIS OF VIRAL INFECTIONS

Because of the acute nature of most viral infections, serologic testing generally is helpful in the diagnostic setting in confirming the specific agent responsible after resolution of the disease. Rapid and reliable methods of determining serologic evidence of past infections by a variety of agents are essential in blood transfusions and organ transplantation. As vaccines against such viruses as hepatitis A and B virus and varicella become available, the immune status of potential vaccine recipients will be important in developing a cost-effective strategy for immunization programs. Adequate quantities of acute and convalescent sera always should be obtained and held for future viral serologic study. It is important that those responsible for saving this sera understand that it must be separated promptly from the clot, carefully labeled, and stored at −20° C or below. Failure to care for the samples properly may make subsequent serologic examinations impossible.

Because of the multiple serotypes found in many viral groups, neutralization titers against the patient's isolate often are the only means of confirming that the virus isolated was responsible for the illness. For neutralization tests, the viral isolate and the acute and convalescent sera must be forwarded to a laboratory capable of performing such procedures. Viral diseases that require confirmation by neutralization are infections with rhinovirus, echovirus, and coxsackievirus. Other viral diseases can be diagnosed either by neutralization tests or by serologic tests using antigens that are commercially available or prepared in the laboratory (Table 245–3).

TABLE 245–3. Commonly Available Viral Serologic Tests

	CF	HAI	NEUT	IFA	RIA	ELISA	Immunoblot
Adenovirus	X		X				
Arbovirus	X	X	X	X			
Coxsackievirus			X				
Cytomegalovirus	X	X	X	X			
Echovirus			X				
Epstein-Barr virus				X			
Hepatitis A virus					X	X	
Hepatitis B virus					X	X	
Hepatitis C virus						X	X
Herpes simplex virus	X		X				
Influenza virus	X	X	X				
Measles virus	X	X					
Mumps virus	X	X					
Poliovirus	X		X				
Rabies virus			X				
Respiratory syncytial virus	X	X	X	X		X	
Rhinovirus			X				
Rubella virus	X	X	X				
Smallpox virus	X	X					
Varicella-zoster virus	X						
Yellow fever virus	X	X	X		X		

Abbreviations: CF, complement-fixation test; ELISA, enzyme-linked immunosorbent assay; HAI, hemagglutination-inhibition test; IFA, indirect fluorescent antibody assay; NEUT, neutralization test; RIA, radioimmunoassay.

Cytomegalovirus Serology

Techniques for the detection of antibodies to cytomegalovirus (CMV) include neutralization tests, CF tests, IHAs, ELISAs, RIAs, immunoprecipitation tests, immunofluorescence tests, and anticomplement immunofluorescence tests.[81, 82] The use of 9 serologic techniques and 14 different antigen preparations makes interpretation of serologic data in the diagnosis of CMV infection difficult. Interpretation is hampered further by the difficulty in correlating the time the serum sample was obtained with the precise stage of the disease process. Although CF tests are the basis for much of the data, ELISAs are more sensitive and are being accepted as routine laboratory procedures.[11, 114]

Conclusive diagnosis of congenital CMV is made by culture of the virus from urine or other body fluids during the newborn period. Although this is a reliable procedure, results may not be known for 1 to 3 weeks. Rapid serodiagnosis of infection in these patients is difficult. CF antibody titers (with CMV strain AD 169 antigen) for detecting IgG often are the only tests performed. IgG antibodies to CMV in the newborn are unreliable in predicting congenital infections because these titers may represent transplacentally acquired maternal IgG elicited by previous exposure. Thus, serodiagnosis of congenital infection requires demonstration of the persistence of CF antibody after the loss of maternal IgG at 3 to 6 months of age. Alternatively, demonstration of specific IgM antibody in a single serum specimen is diagnostic of congenital CMV.[73] The effectiveness of IFA techniques, however, is hampered by the inconsistent quality of commercial anti-IgM sera, the lower sensitivity of the IFA procedure (due partly to the subjectiveness of reading the results), and the high prevalence of false-positive results due to interference by antinuclear antibody.[97, 156, 157] Infection of test cells with CMV in the preparation of antigen slides for use in the IFA test causes the induction of Fc receptors on the surface of the cells, which then can bind IgG nonspecifically. This nonspecific interference can be avoided in IFA tests by using an anticomplement immunofluorescence procedure[39] or ELISA.[43] The use of antigens derived by recombinant technology may be helpful in the standardization of antigens and lead to more useful serologic assays.[172] Use of RIA for CMV IgM antibody (RIA-IgM) increases the sensitivity of IgM detection to 89 per cent, and detection of RIA-IgM in the umbilical cord serum is diagnostic of congenital CMV infection.[59] There also is evidence that elevated RIA-IgM titers are correlated with more severe symptoms. Unfortunately, rheumatoid factor present in serum often interferes with the detection of CMV-specific antibodies in the RIA-IgM test. Removal of this rheumatoid factor by adsorption or fractionation of the serum is time-consuming, restricting this test to research laboratories.

Primary CMV infection is accompanied by the transient production of CMV-specific IgM antibody, which persists for as long as 4 months. Detection of this IgM by RIA is diagnostic of a primary infection.[60] The IgM response is specific for primary infection; however, it is speculated that IgM may persist as a result of reactivation of CMV, continual exposure to different strains of the virus, or both.[38] Seroconversion (as demonstrated by tests that measure IgG) also is evidence of a primary infection with CMV. The IgM response is specific for primary infection and has not been demonstrated in patients who are known to have been infected with CMV previously. No serologic procedure was found that could differentiate active from chronic infection as measured by viral culture or antigen detection in patients with acquired immunodeficiency syndrome.[98] Thus, the presence of an antibody titer to CMV of the IgG class with the absence of an IgM response indicates past exposure to CMV.

Epstein-Barr Virus (Infectious Mononucleosis) Serology

Infectious mononucleosis can be serodiagnosed by demonstration of specific antibodies to Epstein-Barr virus (EBV) or by demonstration of nonspecific heterophile antibodies. Heterophile antibodies may appear in the course of mononucleosis or serum sickness or can occur idiopathically, and they can be demonstrated by the agglutination of sheep erythrocytes.[128] This agglutination is nonspecific and without diagnostic significance unless the serum is adsorbed first with beef erythrocyte antigen and guinea pig kidney antigen. After adsorption with guinea pig kidney, serum from patients with infectious mononucleosis continues to agglutinate the sheep cells, whereas adsorption of the same serum with beef-cell antigen abolishes the agglutination reaction. The Monospot test, a commercial modification of the heterophile test, improves the sensitivity of heterophile antibody testing by using horse erythrocytes. Nonetheless, serum used in Monospot tests also must be adsorbed to be specific for mononucleosis. Newer commercially available tests based on immunochromatographic assay and LA are rapid and simple to perform and have sensitivities between 91 and 96 per cent, respectively, and specificities of 99 per cent.[47] Heterophile antibodies, however, do not appear in the serum of 10 to 15 per cent of patients with typical mononucleosis syndromes, and further testing is indicated.

EBV can infect cells in tissue culture, and the growth of the cells can be stopped at different stages of the infective process. By manipulating the expression of the antigens present in the cell cultures, one can use IFA testing to demonstrate antibodies to at least three important antigens that are useful in determining the stage of illness.[55] IgG antibodies to the viral capsid (EBV-VCA) appear with the onset of symptoms and persist for life.[74] Presence of IgG anti-VCA represents past exposure to EBV and is of little diagnostic significance. IgM anti-VCA, in the absence of rheumatoid factor, usually suffices for the diagnosis of acute EBV infection.[163] This diagnosis is reinforced by the absence of an antibody titer to the nuclear antigen and the presence of antibodies to the D component of the EBV early antigen, although these antibodies cannot be detected in 10 to 20 per cent of children with acute EBV infection.[163] Primary infection also is indicated by finding a titer against IgG antinuclear antigen because antibodies to this antigen do not appear until late in the course of mononucleosis (Table 245–4).[4, 52, 75]

Hepatitis Virus Serology

Hepatitis A Virus

Antibody to hepatitis A virus (HAV) can be detected accurately by RIA, a hemagglutination inhibition (HAI) test, or ELISA. These tests are commercially available and can detect either total immunoglobulin or IgM antibody alone. Infection with HAV produces lifelong immunity, as evidenced by a persistent IgG antibody titer.[25] Detection of IgG alone is useful to determine individual immunity to HAV in cases in which immunoglobulin prophylaxis is to be administered after exposure of susceptible persons or to selected candidates to receive vaccine. Acute HAV infection can be diagnosed by detecting anti-HAV IgM in a single serum sample.[41, 51] IgM antibody appears 12 to 15 days after infection and often is elevated at the time of the onset of symptoms. IgG rises later in the course of illness and peaks while the IgM is declining. A newly developed solid-phase antibody capture hemadsorption assay for IgM antibody is reported to be equally or more sensitive and specific than RIA, can produce results in 6 hours, and can be read visually as agglutination of goose red blood cells.[164]

TABLE 245–4. Interpretation of Epstein-Barr Virus Serology

	IgM-VCA	IgG-VCA	Anti-NA	Anti-EA
Current infection	+	+	−	−/+
Recent infection	−/+	+	−/+	+
Past infection	−	+	+	−

+, antibody present; −, antibody absent; −/+, no antibody or seroconversion.
Abbreviations: EA, early antigen; NA, nuclear antigen; VCA, viral capsid antibody.

TABLE 245–5. Markers of Hepatitis Type B Virus (HBV) Infection

Marker	Acute HBV	Chronic: *Active*	Chronic: *Persistent*	Chronic: *Carrier*	Vaccinated
HBsAg	+	+	+	+	−
HBeAg	+	+/−	+/−	+/−	−
Anti-HBs	+/−	−	−	−	+
Anti-HBc	+	+	+	+	−
Anti-HBe	+	+/−	+/−	+/−	−
Symptoms	+	+	−	−	−

+, detectable in serum; −, not detectable in serum; +/−, detection depends on stage of illness.

Hepatitis B Virus

Tests for hepatitis B virus (HBV) antigen and antibody are used to monitor the course and prognosis of HBV infection and to determine postexposure immune status; they also are used as cost-effective guides to immunization (Table 245–5).[25] Three antigens may be detected during the course of illness in patients infected with HBV:

1. The surface antigen (HBsAg), formerly known as the Australia antigen, is the outer envelope protein of the virus particle. It can be detected in the blood during the incubation period before symptoms appear and during acute infection.[174] HBsAg disappears during recovery, but it does so at variable rates in individual cases.[80]
2. The core antigen (HBcAg) is the nucleocapsid of the virion. This antigen can be detected in the hepatocytes of patients with HBV infection by using immunofluorescent techniques. HBcAg is not detected in serum and is thus of little diagnostic importance.[143]
3. The e antigen (HBeAg) is a soluble protein component of the nucleocapsid. Its presence in blood is correlated with large quantities of circulating virus, greater infectivity, and more active liver disease. Persistence of circulating HBeAg is prognostic of chronic hepatitis.[79, 80]

Antibody to these antigens can be detected by RIA and ELISA systems and also is useful in the diagnosis and prognosis of HBV infection.

1. Anti-HBs (antibody to the surface antigen) is present during all acute and chronic hepatic disease as well as in most patients who have recovered from HBV infection. Chronic HBV carriers may have both HBsAg and anti-HBs

circulating simultaneously. Vaccination with HBsAg gives rise to anti-HBs alone and indicates immunity to HBV.[166]

2. Anti-HBc (antibody to the core antigen) IgM is present in high titer in acute disease and in lower titer in chronic disease, which makes distinction between these two manifestations of disease possible.[28]

3. Anti-HBe (antibody to the e antigen) may be prognostic in that its early appearance (before 6 weeks) is correlated with uncomplicated recovery. Delay in the appearance of anti-HBe may be prognostic of developing chronic hepatitis.[2]

Hepatitis C Virus

Detection of infection with hepatitis C virus (HCV) is important in screening blood donors and management of patients with HCV. Serologic procedures are performed with cloned antigens and are referred to as first-, second-, and third-generation ELISAs or immunoblot tests.[31] First-generation EIAs detected antibody in a majority of non-A, non-B posttransfusion patients with hepatitis but lacked sensitivity in early stages of disease and gave false-positive reactions when used in blood donor screening programs. Development of second-generation EIAs permitted earlier detection of infection and resulted in greater specificity.[108] The third-generation EIAs incorporate additional recombinant antigens but with only minor improvements in sensitivity and specificity.[108] Immunoblot assays are useful in the analysis of cross-reactions seen with other infections and results that are interpreted as indeterminate by EIA.[44] Detection of IgM antibodies in patients with HCV does not differentiate acute from chronic infections.[192] In many cases, it is necessary to perform serologic tests sequentially over time for accurate assessment of disease.[149]

HIV-1 Serology

ELISAs for antibody to HIV-1, originally developed in 1985 for blood-donor screening,[22] now have been modified to screen for both HIV-1 and HIV-2 alone or together for clinical diagnosis of AIDS.[76, 101] The significance of the detection of antibody without clinical symptoms and in patients without obvious risk factors requires careful clinical correlation and additional confirmatory testing. The ability to culture the virus and to find viral products via polymerase chain reaction technology also is of value in the interpretation and prognosis of the infection.

An ELISA using inactivated, disrupted whole virus now is licensed to several commercial sources. The sensitivity of this test has been determined to be between 93 and 95 per cent, and it has a demonstrated specificity greater than 99 per cent.[133, 177] Newer ELISA reagents containing specific viral protein antigens derived from recombinant gene technology have been reported to be more specific and now are commercially available. Repeatedly positive ELISA results must be confirmed by Western blot analysis.[23, 160] Patients with negative ELISA results who are symptomatic or who have one or more risk factors, regardless of symptoms, should undergo serum testing by Western blot analysis and procedures to isolate the virus or its products. In Western blotting, the proteins of the disrupted virus are separated by molecular weight electrophoretically and transferred from polyacrylamide gel to nitrocellulose paper. These discrete protein bands are reacted first with the patient's serum and then reacted with enzymatically labeled anti-immunoglobulins and visualized by the addition of an enzyme substrate to produce colored bands on the nitrocellulose.[77] Interpretation of the results has been the subject of some confusion in that the opinions of at least four agencies or committees and the one licensed manufacturer differ on the significance of the reactive proteins in a positive test result. The World Health Organization has made recommendations on the interpretation of Western blot analysis for HIV-1.[5] Among these recommendations are that (1) laboratories should report test results as positive, indeterminate, or negative, (2) negative results are those that detect *no* bands, (3) positive results detect any two of the proteins labeled p24, gp41, and gp120/gp160, and (4) patients with results interpreted as indeterminate must undergo repeat testing at intervals determined by the physician, who must evaluate the indeterminate results as a part of the entire clinical history of the patient. It probably is prudent for the laboratory report to list the individual bands detected so that the physician is aware of the criteria used in the interpretation of the test.

Measles Virus Serology

Evidence of acute measles virus infection in the form of a fourfold rise in IHA or CF antibody titer between acute and convalescent sera often is useful in distinguishing among diseases causing similar exanthems. Likewise, immunity to measles virus is confirmed by either IHA or CF testing. The plaque reduction neutralization (PRN) assay has been reported to be more sensitive than standard neutralization, IHA, and CF tests, but it is labor-intensive and technically difficult.[1] Chen and colleagues[24] found that PRN titers between 128 and 1052 are partially protective and that titers greater than 1052 definitely are protective against classic measles. Using these values, Ratnam and colleagues[139] compared four commercial ELISA kits and found comparable results when PRN titers were either less than 8 (negative) or greater than 1052 (strongly positive). The lack of sensitivity of these assays in detecting measles antibody at low levels could be important in epidemiologic surveys because these tests most often are used in routine serology laboratories.

Subacute sclerosing panencephalitis, a severe manifestation of persistent measles virus infection, can be diagnosed accurately by detecting measles antibody in the CSF by either CF or IHA procedures. In this disease, measles antibody titer in the CSF often exceeds 1:1280.[83]

Rubella Virus Serology

The HAI test is the standard procedure used to document either active infection with or susceptibility to rubella virus. The test is based on the ability of immune serum to prevent the agglutination of chick erythrocytes by rubella virus. Properly performed, the test is sensitive and specific.[122] However, serum samples may contain nonspecific inhibitors that must be removed by adsorption of the serum with kaolin, heparin/manganese chloride, or dextran sulfate before testing.[49] The time-consuming preparation of the sample diminishes the suitability of this test as a rapid screening procedure. Thus, other tests (passive hemagglutination, ELISA, and IFA) have been developed, are commercially available, and do not require adsorption or treatment of sera. All are suitable for determining immunity status, and a significant titer rise must be observed between acute and convalescent sera to diagnose infection. Rubella virus titers are variable, and it is imperative that paired sera be tested together using the same assay. Congenital infection can be diagnosed by testing serum for IgM-specific antibody.[62, 138]

The performance results of 11 commercially available rubella kits have been reported by Castellano and associates.[20]

As in most serologic tests, the sensitivity and specificity vary inversely. Thus, it is necessary for the laboratory to investigate the various procedures and select the serologic test that offers the best compromise between sensitivity and specificity and that fulfills the needs of the type of rubella testing to be performed. It also has been reported that whole-virus ELISAs may not correspond to results obtained by HAI tests in congenitally infected infants.[63, 116]

References

1. Albrecht, P., Herrmann, K., and Burns, G. R.: Role of virus strain in conventional and enhanced measles plaque neutralization test. J. Virol. Method. *3*:251–260, 1981.
2. Aldershvile, J., Frosner, G. G., Nielsen, J. O., et al.: Hepatitis B e antigen and antibody measured by radioimmunoassay in acute hepatitis B surface antigen–positive hepatitis. J. Infect. Dis. *141*:293–298, 1980.
3. Alper, E. L., Littler, C., and Monroe, L. S.: Counterelectrophoresis in the diagnosis of amebiasis. Am. J. Gastroenterol. *65*:63–67, 1976.
4. Andiman, W. A.: Epstein-Barr virus-associated syndromes: A critical reexamination. J. Pediatr. Infect. Dis. *3*:198–203, 1984.
5. Anonymous: AIDS: Proposed WHO criteria for interpreting Western blot assays for HIV-1, HIV-2, and HTLV-1/HTLV-II. Bull. W. H. O. *69*:127–133, 1991.
6. Barbour, A. G.: Laboratory aspects of Lyme borreliosis. Clin. Microbiol. Rev. *1*:399–414, 1988.
7. Barrett, T. J., Snyder, J. D., Blake, P. A., et al.: Enzyme-linked immunosorbent assay for detection of *Salmonella typhi* Vi antigen in urine from typhoid patients. J. Clin. Microbiol. *15*:235–237, 1982.
8. Bauman, D. S., and Smith, C. D.: Comparison of immunodiffusion and complement fixation tests in the diagnosis of histoplasmosis. J. Clin. Microbiol. *2*:77–80, 1975.
9. Bayer, A. S., Lam, K., Ginzton, L., et al.: *Staphylococcus aureus* bacteremia: Clinical, serologic, and echocardiographic findings in patients with and without endocarditis. Arch. Intern. Med. *147*:457–462, 1987.
10. Bokkenheuser, V., Smity, P., and Richardson, N.: A challenge to the validity of the Vi test for the detection of chronic typhoid carriers. Am. J. Public Health *54*:1501–1503, 1964.
11. Booth, J. C., Hannington, G., Bakir, T. M. F., et al.: Comparison of enzyme-linked immunosorbent assay, radioimmunoassay, complement fixation, anticomplement immunofluorescence and passive haemagglutination techniques for detecting cytomegalovirus IgG antibody. J. Clin. Pathol. *35*:1345–1348, 1982.
12. Buchanan, T. M., and Faber, L. C.: 2-mercaptoethanol brucella agglutination test: Usefulness for predicting recovery from brucellosis. J. Clin. Microbiol. *11*:691–693, 1980.
13. Budzko, D. B., Tyler, L., and Armstrong, D.: Fc receptors on the surface of *Toxoplasma gondii* trophozoites: A confounding factor in testing for anti-*Toxoplasma* antibodies by indirect immunofluorescence. J. Clin. Microbiol. *27*:959–961, 1989.
14. Bunikis, J., Olsen, B., Westman, G., et al.: Variable serum immunoglobulin responses against different *Borrelia burgdorferi* sensu lato species in a population at risk for and patients with Lyme disease. J. Clin. Microbiol. *33*:1473–1478, 1995.
15. Burgdorfer, W., Barbour, A. G., Hayes, S. F., et al.: Lyme disease: A tick-borne spirochetosis? Science *216*:1317–1319, 1982.
16. Busey, J. F.: North American blastomycosis. Gen. Pract. *30*:88–95, 1964.
17. Campbell, P. N., and Current, W. L.: Demonstration of serum antibodies to *Cryptosporidium* sp. in normal and immunodeficient humans with confirmed infections. J. Clin. Microbiol. *18*:165–169, 1983.
18. Carroll, S. M., Karthigasu, K. T., and Grove, D. I.: Serodiagnosis of human strongyloidiasis by an enzyme-linked immunosorbent assay. Trans. R. Soc. Trop. Med. Hyg. *75*:706–709, 1981.
19. Cassell, G. H., and Cole, B. C.: Mycoplasmas as agents of human disease. N. Engl. J. Med. *304*:80–89, 1981.
20. Castellano, G. A., Madden, D. L., Hazzard, G. T., et al.: Evaluation of commercially available diagnostic test kits for rubella. J. Infect. Dis. *143*:578–584, 1981.
21. Centers for Disease Control: Brucellosis surveillance: 1975. Surveillance Annual Summary, 1975. Atlanta, U.S. Department of Health, Education, and Welfare, 1975. Atlanta, July 1976, p. 14.
22. Centers for Disease Control: Provisional Public Health Service inter-agency recommendations for screening donated blood and plasma for antibody to the virus causing acquired immunodeficiency syndrome. M. M. W. R. *34*:1–5, 1985.
23. Centers for Disease Control: Recommendation for assisting in the prevention of perinatal transmission of human T-lymphotropic virus type III/lymphadenopathy-associated virus and acquired immunodeficiency syndrome. M. M. W. R. *34*:721–732, 1985.
24. Chen, R. T., Markowitz, L. E., Albrecht, P., et al.: Measles antibody: Reevaluation of protective titers. J. Infect. Dis. *162*:1036–1042, 1990.
25. Chernesky, M. A., Escobar, M. R., Swenson, P. D., et al.: Laboratory diagnosis of hepatitis viruses. *In* Specter, S. (ed.): Cumitech 18. Washington, D.C., American Society for Microbiology, 1984, pp. 1–12.
26. Chia, W. K., Spence, L., Dunkley, L., et al.: Development of urease conjugated enzyme-linked immunosorbent assays (ELISA) for the detection of IgM and IgG antibodies against *Mycoplasma pneumoniae* in human sera. Diagn. Microbiol. Infect. Dis. *11*:101–107, 1988.
27. Chick, E. W., Baum, G. L., Furcolow, M. L., et al.: Scientific assembly statement: The use of skin tests and serologic tests in histoplasmosis, coccidioidomycosis, and blastomycosis. Am. Rev. Respir. Dis. *108*:156–159, 1973.
28. Cohen, B. J.: The IgM antibody response to the core antigen of hepatitis B virus. J. Med. Virol. *3*:141–150, 1978.
29. Collins, W. E., and Skinner, J. C.: The indirect fluorescent antibody test for malaria. Am. J. Trop. Med. Hyg. *21*:690–695, 1972.
30. Craft, J. E., Grodzicki, R. L., and Steere, A. C.: The antibody response in Lyme disease: Evaluation of diagnostic tests. J. Infect. Dis. *149*:789–795, 1984.
31. Cuthbert, J. A.: Hepatitis C: Progress and problems. Clin. Microbiol. Rev. *7*:505–532, 1994.
32. Cypess, R. H., Karol, M. H., Zidian, J. L., et al.: Larva-specific antibodies in patients with visceral larva migrans. J. Infect. Dis. *135*:633–640, 1977.
33. De Klerk, E., and Anderson, R.: Comparative evaluation of the enzyme-linked immunosorbent assay in the laboratory diagnosis of brucellosis. J. Clin. Microbiol. *21*:381–386, 1985.
34. de Repentigny, L.: Serodiagnosis of candidiasis, aspergillosis, and cryptococcosis. Clin. Infect. Dis. *14*:S11–S22, 1992.
35. de Repentigny, L., and Reiss, E.: Current trends in immunodiagnosis of candidiasis and aspergillosis. Rev. Infect. Dis. *6*:301–312, 1984.
36. Desmonts, G., Naot, Y., and Remington, J. S.: Immunoglobulin M-immunosorbent agglutination assay for diagnosis of infectious diseases: Diagnosis of acute congenital and acquired *Toxoplasma* infections. J. Clin. Microbiol. *14*:486–491, 1981.
37. Diamond, R. D., and Bennett, J. E.: Prognostic factors in cryptococcal meningitis. Ann. Intern. Med. *80*:176–181, 1974.
38. Drew, W. L., Sweet, E., Miner, R. C., et al.: Multiple infections with cytomegalovirus in patients with acquired immunodeficiency syndrome: Documentation by Southern blot hybridization. J. Infect. Dis. *150*:952, 1984.
39. Drew, W. L.: Diagnosis of cytomegalovirus infection. Rev. Infect. Dis. *10*:S468–S476, 1988.
40. Drutz, D. J., and Catanzaro, A.: Coccidioidomycosis: Part 1. Am. Rev. Respir. Dis. *117*:559–585, 1978.
41. Duermeyer, W., Wielaard, F., and van der Veen, J.: A new principle for the detection of specific IgM antibodies applied in an ELISA for hepatitis. Am. J. Med. Virol. *4*:25–32, 1979.
42. Dyckman, J. D., Storms, S., and Huber, T. W.: Reactivity of microhemagglutination, fluorescent treponemal antibody absorption, and Venereal Disease Research Laboratory tests in primary syphilis. J. Clin. Microbiol. *12*:629–630, 1980.
43. Dylewski, J. S., Rasmussen, L., Mills, J., et al.: Large-scale serological screening for cytomegalovirus in homosexual males by enzyme-linked immunosorbent assay. J. Clin. Microbiol. *19*:200–203, 1984.
44. Ebeling, F., Naukkarianen, R., and Leikola, J.: Recombinant immunoblot assay for hepatitis C virus antibody as predictor of infectivity. Lancet *335*:982–983, 1990.
45. Edwards, J. E., Lehrer, R. I., Stiehm, E. R., et al.: Severe candidal infections: Clinical perspective, immune defense mechanisms, and current concepts of therapy. Ann. Intern. Med. *89*:91–106, 1978.
46. Engstrom, S. M., Shoop, E., and Johnson, R. C.: Immunoblot interpretation criteria for serodiagnosis of early Lyme disease. J. Clin. Microbiol. *33*:419–427, 1995.
47. Farhat, S. E., Finn, S., Chua, R., et al.: Rapid detection of infectious mononucleosis–associated heterophile antibodies by a novel immunochromatographic assay and a latex agglutination test. J. Clin. Microbiol. *31*:1597–1600, 1993.
48. Farrell, I. D., Robertson, L., and Hinchliffe, P. M.: Serum antibody response in acute brucellosis. J. Hyg. *74*:23–28, 1975.
49. Feldman, H. A.: Removal by heparin-$MnCL_2$ of nonspecific rubella hemagglutinin serum inhibitor. Proc. Soc. Exp. Biol. Med. *127*:570–573, 1968.
50. Finland, M., Peterson, O. L., Allen, E., II, et al.: Cold agglutinins. I. Occurrence of cold isohemagglutinins in various conditions. J. Clin. Invest. *24*:451, 1945.
51. Flehmig, G., Ranke, M., Berthold, H., et al.: A solid-phase radioimmunoassay for detection of IgM antibodies to hepatitis A virus. J. Infect. Dis. *140*:169–175, 1979.
52. Fleisher, G., Henle, W., Henle, G., et al.: Primary infection with Epstein-Barr virus in infants in the United States: Clinical and serologic observations. J. Infect. Dis. *139*:553–558, 1979.
53. Freter, R.: Agglutinin titration (Widal) for the diagnosis of enteric fever and other enterobacterial infections. *In* Rose, N. R., and Friedman, H. (eds.): Manual of Clinical Immunology. Washington, D.C., American Society for Microbiology, 1976, pp. 285–288.
54. Garcia, L. S., Bruckner, D. A., Brewer, T. C., et al.: Comparison of indirect fluorescent-antibody amoebic serology with counterimmunoelectrophore-

sis and indirect hemagglutination amoebic serologies. J. Clin. Microbiol. *15*:603–605, 1982.

55. Ginsburg, C. M., Henle, W., Henle, G., et al.: Infectious mononucleosis in children: Evaluation of Epstein-Barr virus–specific serological data. J. A. M. A. *237*:781–785, 1977.
56. Greenberg, D. P., Bayer, A. S., Turner, D., et al.: Antibody responses to protein A in patients with *Staphylococcus aureus* bacteremia and endocarditis. J. Clin. Microbiol. *28*:458–462, 1990.
57. Greenfield, R. A., Bussey, M. J., Stephens, J. L., et al.: Serial enzyme-linked immunosorbent assays for antibody to *Candida* antigens during induction chemotherapy for acute leukemia. J. Infect. Dis. *148*:275–283, 1983.
58. Griffin, J. P.: Rapid screening for cold agglutinins in pneumonia. Ann. Intern. Med. *70*:701–705, 1969.
59. Griffiths, P. D., Stagno, S., Pass, R. F., et al.: Congenital cytomegalovirus infection: Diagnostic and prognostic significance of the detection of specific immunoglobulin M antibodies in cord serum. Pediatrics *69*:544–549, 1982.
60. Griffiths, P. D., Stagno, S., Pass, R. F., et al.: Infection with cytomegalovirus during pregnancy: Specific IgM antibodies as a marker of recent primary infection. J. Infect. Dis. *145*:647–652, 1982.
61. Grodzicki, R. L., and Steere, A. C.: Diagnosing early Lyme disease by immunoblotting: Comparison with indirect ELISA using different antigen preparations. J. Infect. Dis. *157*:790–797, 1988.
62. Gupta, J. D., Peterson, V., Stout, M., et al.: Single-sample diagnosis of recent rubella by fractionation of antibody on Sephadex G-200 column. J. Clin. Pathol. *24*:547–550, 1971.
63. Hancock, E. J., Pot, K., Pterman, M. L., et al.: Lack of association between titers of HAI antibody and whole-virus ELISA values for patients with congenital rubella syndrome. J. Infect. Dis. *154*:1031–1032, 1986.
64. Hansen, K., Hindersson, P., and Pedersen, N. S.: Measurement of antibodies to the *Borrelia burgdorferi* flagellum improves serodiagnosis in Lyme disease. J. Clin. Microbiol. *26*:338–346, 1988.
65. Hechemy, K. E., Anacker, R. L., Philip, R. N., et al.: Detection of Rocky Mountain spotted fever antibodies by a latex agglutination test. J. Clin. Microbiol. *12*:144–150, 1980.
66. Hechemy, K. E., and Michaelson, E. E.: Rocky Mountain spotted fever: A resurgent problem. Lab. Management *Oct.*:29–40, 1981.
67. Hechemy, K. E., Stevens, R. W., Sasowski, S., et al.: Discrepancies in Weil-Felix and microimmunofluoresence test for Rocky Mountain spotted fever. J. Clin. Microbiol. *9*:292–293, 1979.
68. Hechemy, K. E.: Laboratory diagnosis of Rocky Mountain spotted fever. N. Engl. J. Med. *300*:859–860, 1979.
69. Hedberg, C. W., and Osterholm, M. T.: Serologic tests for antibody to *Borrelia burgdorferi:* Another Pandora's box for medicine? Arch. Intern. Med. *150*:732–733, 1990.
70. Hedberg, C. W., Osterholm, M. T., MacDonald, K. I., et al.: An interlaboratory study of antibody to *Borrelia burgdorferi*. J. Infect. Dis. *155*:1325–1327, 1987.
71. Hederstedt, B., Holm, S. E., and Wadstrom, T.: Discrepancy between results of the Streptozyme test and those of the antideoxyribonuclease B and antihyaluronidase tests. J. Clin. Microbiol. *8*:50–53, 1978.
72. Heiner, D. C.: Diagnosis of histoplasmosis using precipitin reactions in agar gel. Pediatrics *22*:616–627, 1958.
73. Hekker, A. C., Brand-Saathof, B., Vis, J., et al.: Indirect immunofluorescence test for detection of IgM antibodies to cytomegalovirus. J. Infect. Dis. *140*:596–600, 1979.
74. Henle, G., Henle, W., and Horwitz, C. A.: Antibodies to Epstein-Barr virus–associated nuclear antigen in infectious mononucleosis. J. Infect. Dis. *130*:231–239, 1974.
75. Henle, W., Henle, G., and Horwitz, C. A.: Epstein-Barr virus–specific diagnostic tests in infectious mononucleosis. Hum. Pathol. *5*:551–565, 1974.
76. Hess, G., Avillez, F., Lourenco, M. H., et al.: Diagnosis of human immunodeficiency virus (HIV) infection: Multicenter evaluation of a newly developed anti-HIV 1 and 2 enzyme immunoassay. J. Clin. Microbiol. *32*:403–406, 1994.
77. Hirsch, M. S., Wormser, G. P., Schooley, R. T., et al.: Risk of nosocomial infection with human T-cell lymphotropic virus III (HTLV-III). N. Engl. J. Med. *312*:1–4, 1985.
78. Holmberg, K., Berdischewsky, M., and Young L. S.: Serologic immunodiagnosis of invasive aspergillosis. J. Infect. Dis. *141*:656–664, 1980.
79. Hoofnagle, J. H., Dusheiko, G. M., Seeff, L. B., et al.: Seroconversion from hepatitis B e antigen to antibody in chronic type B hepatitis. Ann. Intern. Med. *94*:744–748, 1981.
80. Hoofnagle, J. H.: Serological markers of hepatitis B virus infection. Annu. Rev. Med. *32*:1–11, 1981.
81. Hopson, D. K., Niles, A. C., and Murray, P. R.; Comparison of the Vitek Immunodiagnostic Assay System with three immunoassay systems for detection of cytomegalovirus-specific immunoglobulin G. J. Clin. Microbiol. *30*:2893–2895, 1993.
82. Horodniceanu, F., and Michelson, S.: Assessment of human cytomegalovirus antibody detection techniques. Arch. Virol. *64*:287–301, 1980.
83. Horta-Barbosa, L., Krebs, H., Ley, A., et al.: Progressive increase in cerebrospinal fluid measles antibody levels in subacute sclerosing panencephalitis. Pediatrics *47*:782–783, 1971.
84. Hostetler, C. L., Sawyer, K. P., and Nachamkin, I.: Comparison of three rapid methods for detection of antibodies to streptolysin O and DNase B. J. Clin. Microbiol. *26*:1406–1408, 1988.
85. Huppert, M.: Serology of coccidioidomycosis. Mycopathol. Mycol. Appl. *41*:107–113, 1970.
86. Huppert, M., Pererson, E. T., Sun, S. H., et al.: Evaluation of a latex particle agglutination test for coccidioidomycosis. Am. J. Clin. Pathol. *49*:96–102, 1968.
87. Janef, J., Janeff, D., Taranta, A., et al.: A screening test for streptococcal antibodies. Lab. Med. *2*:38–40, 1971.
88. Jones, J. M.: Laboratory diagnosis of invasive candidiasis. Clin. Microbiol. Rev. *3*:32–45, 1990.
89. Kaplan, E. L., and Huwe, B. B.: The sensitivity and specificity of an agglutination test for antibodies to streptococcal extracellular antigens: A quantitative analysis and comparison of the Streptozyme test with the anti-streptolysin O and anti-deoxyribonuclease B tests. J. Pediatr. *96*:367–372, 1980.
90. Kaufman, L.: Laboratory methods for the diagnosis and confirmation of systemic mycoses. Clin. Infect. Dis. *14*:S14–S29, 1992.
91. Kaufman, L., McLaughlin, D. W., Clark, M. J., et al.: Specific immunodiffusion test for blastomycosis. Appl. Microbiol. *26*:244–247, 1973.
92. Kaufman, L.: Serodiagnosis of fungal disease. *In* Rose, N. R., and Friedman, H. (eds.): Manual of Clinical Immunology. Washington, D.C., American Society for Microbiology, 1976, pp. 363–381.
93. Kelly, D. J., Chan, C. T., Paxton, H., et al.: Comparative evaluation of a commercial enzyme immunoassay for the detection of human antibody to *Rickettsia typhi*. Clin. Diagn. Immunol. 2:355–360, 1995.
94. Klingspor, L., Eberhared, T. H., Stintzing, G., et al.: Antibody response to *Candida* and its use in clinical practice. Mycoses *37*:199–204, 1994.
95. Lackman, D. B., and Gerloff, R. K.: The effect of antibiotic therapy upon diagnostic and serologic tests for Rocky Mountain spotted fever. Public Health Lab. *11*:97–99, 1953.
96. Larsen, S. A., Steiner, B. M., and Rudolph, A. H.: Laboratory diagnosis and interpretation of tests for syphilis. Clin. Microbiol. Rev. *8*:1–21, 1995.
97. Lazzarotto, T., Casa, B. D., Campisis, B., et al.: Enzyme-linked immunosorbent assay for detection of cytomegalovirus-IgM: Comparison between eight commercial kits, immunofluorescence, and immunoblotting. J. Clin. Lab. Analysis *6*:216–218, 1992.
98. Lazzarotto, T., Dal Monte, P., Boccuni, M. C., et al.: Lack of correlation between virus detection and serologic tests for diagnosis of active cytomegalovirus infection in patients with AIDS. J. Clin. Microbiol. *30*:1027–1029, 1992.
99. Lefebre, J. Bertrand, M., and Bauriaud, R. Evaluation of the Captia enzyme immunoassays for detection of immunoglobulins G and M to *Treponema pallidum* in syphilis. J. Clin. Microbiol. *28*:1704–1707, 1990.
100. Lewis, L. L., Taber, L. H., and Baughn, R. E.: Evaluation of immunoglobulin M Western blot analysis in the diagnosis of congenital syphilis. J. Clin. Microbiol. *28*:296–302, 1990.
101. Lin, H. J.: Laboratory tests for human immunodeficiency viruses. J. Int. Fed. Clin. Chem. *7*:61–66, 1995.
102. Longbottom, J. L.: Immunologic aspects of infection and allergy due to *Aspergillus* species. Mykosen *116*:207–217, 1978.
103. Luger, S. W., and Krauss, E.: Serologic tests for Lyme disease: Interlaboratory variability. Arch. Intern. Med. *150*:761–763, 1990.
104. Maddison, S. E., Hayes, G. V., Slemenda, S. B., et al.: Detection of specific antibody by enzyme-linked immunosorbent assay and antigenemia by counterimmunoelectrophoresis in humans infected with *Pneumocystis carinii*. J. Clin. Microbiol. *15*:1036–1043, 1982.
105. Magnarelli, L. A., Anderson, J. F., and Johnson, R. C.: Cross-reactivity in serological tests for Lyme disease and other spirochetal infections. J. Infect. Dis. *156*:183–188, 1987.
106. Magnarelli, L. A., Meegan, J. M., Anderson J. F., et al.: Comparison of an indirect fluorescent-antibody test with an enzyme-linked assay for serological studies of Lyme disease. J. Clin. Microbiol. *20*:181–184, 1984.
107. Magnarelli, L. A., Dumler, J. S., Anderson, J. F., et al.: Coexistence of antibodies to tick-borne pathogens of babesiosis, ehrlichiosis, and Lyme borreliosis in human sera. J. Clin. Microbiol. *33*:3054–3057, 1995.
108. Marcellin, P., Martino-Peignoux, M., Gabriel, F., et al.: Chronic non-B, non-C hepatitis among blood donors assessed with HCV third generation tests and polymerase chain reaction. J. Hepatol. *19*:167–170, 1993.
109. Martins, T. B., Jaskowski, T. D., Mouritsen, C. L., et al.: Comparison of commercially available enzyme immunoassay with traditional serological tests for detection of antibodies to *Coccidioides immitis*. J. Clin. Microbiol. *33*:940–943, 1995.
110. Mathews, H. M., Walls, K. W., and Huong, A. Y.: Microvolume, kinetic-dependent enzyme-linked immunosorbent assay for amoeba antibodies. J. Clin. Microbiol. *19*:221–224, 1984.
111. Matthews, R. C., Burnie, J. P., and Tabaqchali, S.: Immunoblot analysis of the serological response in systemic candidosis. Lancet *2*:1415–1418, 1984.
112. Mendes-Giannini, M. J. S., Camargo, M. E., Lacaz, C. S., et al.: Immunoenzymatic absorption test for serodiagnosis of paracoccidioidomycosis. J. Clin. Microbiol. *20*:103–108, 1984.
113. Merz, W. G., Evans, G. L., Shadomy, S., et al.: Laboratory evaluation of serological tests for systemic candidiasis: A cooperative study. J. Clin. Microbiol. *5*:596–603, 1977.

114. Middeldorp, J. M., Johgsma, J., ter Haar, A., et al.: Detection of immunoglobulin M and G antibodies against cytomegalovirus early and late antigens by enzyme-linked immunosorbent assay. J. Clin. Microbiol. *20*:763–771, 1984.
115. Miller, B., Goldberg, M. A., Heiner, D., et al.: A new immunologic test for CNS cysticercosis. Neurology *34*:695, 1984.
116. Mitchell, L. A., Zhang, T., Ho, M., et al.: Characterization of rubella virus-specific antibody responses by using a new synthetic peptide-base enzyme-linked immunosorbent assay. J. Clin. Microbiol. *30*:1841–1847, 1992.
117. Mohammad, I. N., Heiner, D. C., Miller, B. L., et al.: Enzyme-linked immunosorbent assay for the diagnosis of cerebral cysticercosis. J. Clin. Microbiol. *20*:775–779, 1984.
118. Nagel, J. G., Tuazon, C. U., Cardella, T. A., et al.: Teichoic acid serologic diagnosis of staphylococcal endocarditis. Ann. Intern. Med. *82*:13–17, 1975.
119. Naot, Y., and Remington, J. S.: An enzyme-linked immunosorbent assay for detection of IgM antibodies to *Toxoplasma gondii:* Use for diagnosis of acute acquired toxoplasmosis. J. Infect. Dis. *142*:757–766, 1980.
120. Naot, Y., Guptill, D. R., and Remington, J. S.: Duration of IgM antibodies to *Toxoplasma gondii* after acute acquired toxoplasmosis. J. Infect. Dis. *145*:770, 1982.
121. Nolan, C. M., Feeley, J. C., White, P. C., Jr., et al.: Evaluation of a new assay for Vi antibody in chronic carriers of *Salmonella typhi.* J. Clin. Microbiol. *12*:22–26, 1980.
122. Palmer, D. F., Cavallaro, J. J., and Herrmann, K. L.: A Procedural Guide to the Performance of Rubella Hemagglutination-Inhibition Tests. Atlanta, Centers for Disease Control, 1977, p. 88.
123. Pappagianis, D., and Crane, R.: Survival in coccidioidal meningitis since introduction of amphotericin B. *In* Ajello, L. (ed.): Coccidioidomycosis: Current Clinical and Diagnostic Status. Miami, Symposia Specialists Medical Books, 1977, pp. 223–237.
124. Pappagianis, D., and Zimmer, B. L.: Serology of coccidioidomycosis. Clin. Microbiol. Rev. *3*:247–268, 1990.
125. Pappagianis, D., Krasnow, R. I., and Beall, S.: False-positive reactions of cerebrospinal fluid and diluted sera with the coccidioidal latex-agglutination test. Am. J. Clin. Pathol. *66*:916–921, 1976.
126. Pappagianis, D.: Coccidioidomycosis. *In* Samter, M. (ed.): Immunological Diseases. Boston, Little, Brown, 1978, p. 652.
127. Pappas, M. G., Ballou, W. R., Gray, M. R., et al.: Rapid serodiagnosis of leptospirosis using the IgM-specific dot-ELISA: Comparison with the microscopic agglutination test. Am. J. Trop. Med. Hyg. *34*:346–354, 1985.
128. Paul, J. R., and Bunnell, W. W.: The presence of heterophile antibodies in infectious mononucleosis. Am. J. Med. Sci. *183*:90–104, 1932.
129. Pellicer, T., Ariza, J., Foz, A., et al.: Specific antibodies detected during relapse of human brucellosis. J. Infect. Dis. *157*:918–924, 1988.
130. Penn, R. L., Lambert, R. S., and George, R. B.: Invasive fungal infections: The use of serologic tests in diagnosis and management. Arch. Intern. Med. *143*:1215–1220, 1983.
131. Peter, C. R., Thompson, M. A., and Wilson, D. L.: False-positive reactions in the Rapid Plasma Reagin-Card, fluorescent treponemal antibody-absorbed, and hemagglutination treponemal syphilis serology tests. J. Clin. Microbiol. *9*:369–372, 1979.
132. Peter, G., and Smith, A. L.: Group A streptococcal infections of the skin and pharynx. N. Engl. J. Med. *297*:311–317, 1977.
133. Petricciani, J. C.: Licensed tests for antibody to human T-lymphotropic virus type III: Sensitivity and specificity. Ann. Intern. Med. *103*:726–729, 1985.
134. Philip, R. N., Casper, E. A., Ormsbee, R. A., et al.: Microimmunofluorescence test for the serological study of Rocky Mountain spotted fever and typhus. J. Clin. Microbiol. *3*:51–61, 1976.
135. Plouffe, J. F., and Fass, R. J.: *Histoplasma* meningitis: Diagnostic value of cerebrospinal fluid serology. Ann. Intern. Med. *92*:189–191, 1980.
136. Powell, D. A., and Schuit, K. E.: Acute pulmonary blastomycosis in children: Clinical course and follow-up. Pediatrics *63*:736–740, 1979.
137. Preisler, H. D., Hasenclever, H. F., Levitan, A. A., et al.: Serologic diagnosis of disseminated candidiasis in patients with acute leukemia. Ann. Intern. Med. *70*:19–30, 1969.
138. Punnarugsa, V., and Mungmee, V.: Detection of rubella virus immunoglobulin G (IgG) and IgM antibodies in whole blood on Whatman paper: Comparison with detection in sera. J. Clin. Microbiol. *29*:2209–2212, 1991.
139. Ratnam, S., Gadag, V., West, R., et al.: Comparison of commercial enzyme immunoassay kits with plaque reduction neutralization test for detection of measles virus antibody. J. Clin. Microbiol. *33*:811–815, 1995.
140. Rauer, S., Kayser, M., Neubert, U., et al.: Establishment of enzyme-linked immunosorbent assay using purified recombinant 83-kilodalton antigen of *Borrelia burgdorferi* sensu stricto and *Borrelia afzelli* for serodiagnosis of Lyme disease. J. Clin. Microbiol. *33*:2596–2600, 1995.
141. Reddin, J. L., Anderson, R. K., Jenness, R., et al.: Significance of 7S and macroglobulin *Brucella* agglutinins in human brucellosis. N. Engl. J. Med. *272*:1263–1267, 1965.
142. Ribeiro, M. A., Souza, C. C., and Almeida, S. H. P.: Dot-ELISA for human leptospirosis employing immunodominant antigen. J. Trop. Med. Hyg. *98*:452–456, 1995.
143. Rizzetto, M., Shih, J. W. K., Verme, G., et al.: A radioimmunoassay for HBcAg in the sera of HBsAg carriers: Serum HBcAg, serum DNA polymerase activity, and liver HBcAg immunofluorescence as markers of chronic liver disease. Gastroenterology *80*:1420–1427, 1981.
144. Rose, C. D., Fawcett, P. T., Gibney, K. M., et al.: Residual serologic reactivity in children with resolved Lyme arthritis. J. Rheumatol. *23*:367–369, 1996.
145. Sabin, A. E., and Feldman, H. A.: Dyes as microchemical indicators of a new immunity phenomenon affecting protozoan parasite *(Toxoplasma).* Science *108*:660–663, 1948.
146. Sanchez, P. J., McCracken, G. H., Jr., Wendel, G. D., et al.: Molecular analysis of the fetal IgM response to *Treponema pallidum* antigens: Implications for improved serodiagnosis of congenital syphilis. J. Infect. Dis. *159*:508–517, 1989.
147. Sarosi, G. A., and Davies, S. F.: Blastomycosis. Am. Rev. Respir. Dis. *120*:911–938, 1979.
148. Sarosi, G. A., Davies, S. F., Klein, B., et al.: Recent developments in blastomycosis. Am. Rev. Respir. Dis. *134*:817–818, 1986.
149. Schneider, L., and Geha, R.: Outbreak of hepatitis C associated with intravenous immunoglobulin administration: United States, October 1993–June 1994. M. M. W. R. *43*:505–509, 1994.
150. Sheagren, J. N., Menes, B. I., Han, D. P., et al.: Technical aspects of the *Staphylococcus aureus* teichoic acid antibody assay: Gel diffusion and counterimmunoelectrophoretic assays, antigen preparation, antigen selection, concentration effects, and cross-reactions with other organisms. J. Clin. Microbiol. *13*:293–300, 1981.
151. Siegel, J. P., and Remington, J. S.: Comparison of methods for quantitating antigen-specific immunoglobulin M antibody with a reverse enzyme-linked immonosorbent assay. J. Clin. Microbiol. *18*:63–70, 1983.
152. Silletti, R. P.: Comparison of Captia syphilis G enzyme immunoassay with rapid plasma reagin test for detection of syphilis. J. Clin. Microbiol. *33*:1829–1831, 1995.
153. Smith, C. E., Saito, M. N. T., and Simons, S. A.: Pattern of 39,500 serologic tests in coccidioidomycosis. J. A. M. A. *160*:546–552, 1956.
154. Smith, C. E.: Coccidioidomycosis. Pediatr. Clin. North Am. *2*:109–125, 1955.
155. Spink, W. W., McCullough, N. B., Hutchings, L. M., et al.: A standardized antigen and agglutination technique for human brucellosis: Report No. 3 of the National Research Council Committee on Public Aspects of Brucellosis. Am. J. Clin. Pathol. *24*:496–498, 1954.
156. Stagno, S., Pass, R. F., Reynolds, D. W., et al.: Comparative study of diagnostic procedures for congenital cytomegalovirus infection. Pediatrics *65*:251–257, 1980.
157. Stagno, S., Reynolds, D. W., Tsiantos, A., et al.: Comparative serial virologic and serologic studies of symptomatic and subclinical congenitally and natally acquired cytomegalovirus infections. J. Infect. Dis. *132*:568–577, 1975.
158. Steere, A. C., Grodzicki, R. L., Kornblatt, A. N., et al.: The spirochetal etiology of Lyme disease. N. Engl. J. Med. *308*:733–740, 1983.
159. Stepick-Bick, P., Thulliez, P., Araujo, F. G., et al.: IgA antibodies for diagnosis of acute congenital and acquired toxoplasmosis. J. Infect. Dis. *162*:270–273, 1990.
160. Sullivan, M. T., Jucke, H., Kadey, S. D., et al.: Evaluation of an indirect immunofluorescence assay for confirmation of human immunodeficiency virus type 1 antibody in U.S. blood donor sera. J. Clin. Microbiol. *30*:2509–2510, 1992.
161. Sulzer, C. R., and Jones, W. L.: Leptospirosis: Methods in Laboratory Diagnosis. Publ. No. (CDC) 74–8275. Centers for Disease Control, U.S. Department of Health, Education, and Welfare, 1974.
162. Sulzer, C. R., Glosser, J. W., Rogers, F., et al.: Evaluation of an indirect hemagglutination test for the diagnosis of human leptospirosis. J. Clin. Microbiol. *2*:218–221, 1975.
163. Sumaya, C. V.: Epstein-Barr virus serologic testing: Diagnostic indications and interpretations. Pediatr. Infect. Dis. J. *5*:337–342, 1986.
164. Summers, P. L., Dubois, D. R., Cohen, W. H., et al.: Solid-phase antibody capture hemadsorption assay of detection of hepatitis A virus immunoglobulin M antibodies. J. Clin. Microbiol. *31*:1299–1302, 1993.
165. Sussman, S. J., Magoffin, R. L., Lennette, E. H., et al.: Cold agglutinins, Eaton agent, and respiratory infections of children. Pediatrics *38*:571–577, 1966.
166. Szmuness, W., Stevens, C. E., Harley, E. J., et al.: Hepatitis B vaccine: Demonstration of efficacy in a controlled clinical trial in a high-risk population in the United States. N. Engl. J. Med. *303*:833–841, 1980.
167. Taborda, C. P., and Camargo, Z. P.: Diagnosis of paracoccidioidomycosis by dot immunobinding assay for antibody detection using the purified and specific antigen gp43. J. Clin. Microbiol. *32*:554–556, 1994.
168. Thacker, W. L., and Talkington, D. F.: Comparison of two rapid commercial tests with complement fixation for serologic diagnosis of *Mycoplasma pneumoniae* infections. J. Clin. Microbiol. *33*:1212–1214, 1995.
169. Thisyakorn, U., Shelton, S., Lin, T., et al.: Detection of teichoic acid antibodies in children with staphylococcal infections. Pediatr. Infect. Dis. *3*:222–225, 1984.
170. Tosi, M. F., and Nelson, T. J.: *Brucella canis* infection in a 17-month-old child successfully treated with moxalactam. J. Pediatr. *101*:725–727, 1982.
171. van Deventer, A. J., van Vliet, H. J., Voogd, L., et al.: Increased specificity of antibody detection in surgical patients with invasive candidiasis with

cytoplasmic antigens depleted of mannan residues. J. Clin. Microbiol. *31*:994–997, 1993.
172. Vornhage, R., Plachter, B., Hinderer, W., et al.: Early serodiagnosis of acute human cytomegalovirus infection by enzyme-linked immunosorbent assay using recombinant antigens. J. Clin. Microbiol. *32*:981–986, 1994.
173. Walker, D. H.: Diagnosis of rickettsial diseases. Pathol. Annu. *23*:69–96, 1988.
174. Wands, J. R., Bruns, R. R., Carlson, R. I., et al.: Monoclonal IgM radioimmunoassay for hepatitis B surface antigen: High binding activity in serum that is unreactive with conventional antibodies. Proc. Natl. Acad. Sci. U. S. A. *79*:1277–1281, 1982.
175. Wannamaker, L.: Differences between streptococcal infections of the throat and of the skin. N. Engl. J. Med. *282*:23–31, 1970.
176. Watt, G., Alquiza, L. M., Padre, L. P., et al.: The rapid diagnosis of leptospirosis: A prospective comparison of the dot enzyme-linked immunosorbent assay and the genus-specific microscopic agglutination test at different stages of illness. J. Infect. Dis. *157*:840–842, 1988.
177. Weiss, S. H., Goedert, J. J., Sarngadharan, M. G., et al.: Screening test for HTLV-III (AIDS agent) antibodies. J. A. M. A. *253*:221–225, 1985.
178. Welch, P. C., Masur, H., Jones, T. C., et al.: Serologic diagnosis of acute lymphadenopathic toxoplasmosis. J. Infect. Dis. *142*:256–264, 1980.
179. Wheat, J. J., Kohler, R. B., French, M. L. V., et al.: IgM and IgG histoplasmal antibody response in histoplasmosis. Am. Rev. Respir. Dis. *128*:65–70, 1983.
180. Wheat, J., French, M. L. V., Kamel, S., et al.: Evaluation of cross-reactions in *Histoplasma capsulatum* serologic tests. J. Clin. Microbiol. *23*:493–499, 1986.
181. Wheat, J., French, M. L. V., Kohler, R. B., et al.: The diagnostic laboratory tests for histoplasmosis: Analysis of experience in a large urban outbreak. Ann. Intern. Med. *97*:680–685, 1982.
182. Wheat, J., Kohler, R. B., Garten, M., et al.: Commercially available (Endo-Staph) assay for teichoic acid antibodies: Evaluation in patients with serious *Staphylococcus aureus* infections and in controls. Arch. Intern. Med. *144*:261–264, 1984.
183. Wheat, L. J., and White, A. C.: Rapid diagnosis of staphylococcal infections. *In* Rytel, M. W. (ed.): Rapid Diagnosis in Infectious Diseases. Boca Raton, FL, CRC Press, 1979, pp. 115–124.
184. Wilfert, C., and Gutman, L.: Genitourinary tract infections: Syphilis. *In* Feigin, R. D., and Cherry, J. D. (eds.): Textbook of Pediatric Infectious Diseases. Philadelphia, W. B. Saunders, 1981, pp. 388–400.
185. Wilson, G. S., and Miles, A. A. (eds.): Enteric infections. *In* Topley and Wilson's Principles of Bacteriology and Immunity. Baltimore, Williams & Wilkins, 1975, pp. 2005–2039.
186. Wong, M. L., Kaplan, S., Dunkle, L. M., et al.: Leptospirosis: A childhood disease. J. Pediatr. *90*:532–537, 1977.
187. Wong, S. Y., Hajdu, M. P., Ramirez, R., et al.: Role of specific immunoglobulin E in diagnosis of acute toxoplasma infection and toxoplasmosis. J. Clin. Microbiol. *31*:2952–2959, 1993.
188. Young, E. J.: Human brucellosis. Rev. Infect. Dis. *5*:821–842, 1983.
189. Young, E. J.: An overview of human brucellosis. Clin. Infect. Dis. *21*:283–290, 1995.
190. Young, R. C., and Bennett, J. E.: Invasive aspergillosis: Absence of detectable antibody reponse. Am. Rev. Respir. Dis. *104*:710–716, 1971.
191. Yow, M. D.: Brucellosis. *In* Feigin, R. D., and Cherry, J. D. (eds.): Textbook of Pediatric Infectious Diseases. Philadelphia, W. B. Saunders, 1981, pp. 828–833.
192. Zaaijer, H. L., Mimms, L. T., Cuyers, H. T., et al.: Variability of IgM response in hepatitis C virus infection. J. Med. Virol. *40*:184–187, 1993.

PART 8

Biostatistics Applicable to the Subspecialty of Infectious Diseases

246

EPIDEMIOLOGY AND BIOSTATISTICS

Eugene D. Shapiro

Clinicians care for individual patients, each of whom has certain unique problems. Clinicians base their decisions on a panoply of factors that include features of the acute and chronic medical problems of the patients as well as features of both their personalities (e.g., How likely are they to comply with a certain therapeutic regimen?) and their private lives (e.g., Can they afford a certain medication? Are they planning to travel out of the country in the next few days?).

In contrast, epidemiologists study groups of people. They draw conclusions from studies of large numbers of patients and usually base conclusions on probabilities and biostatistical analyses of average (mean) outcomes.

Fortunately, these two approaches—the individualistic approach of the clinician and the probabilistic approach of the classic epidemiologist—are not incompatible. Indeed, each can illuminate the other. So it is that a chapter on epidemiology and biostatistics is included in a clinical textbook of pediatric infectious diseases. The goal of this chapter is not to make the reader an expert in these fields—there are courses and textbooks designed for that purpose.[5, 8–11, 18–20] The goal is to summarize how selected key aspects of epidemiology and biostatistics can be applied to understand studies that will improve our abilities to evaluate and to treat children with infectious diseases.

EPIDEMIOLOGY

Design of Studies

Overview

Epidemiologic studies generally are designed to be either descriptive or analytic. In *descriptive* studies, the goal is to describe a population (e.g., the clinical manifestations of and the prognosis of children with tuberculosis). In *analytic* studies, the goal is to assess associations among two or more variables (e.g., Are children who received an experimental vaccine less likely than controls to develop the infection that the vaccine is intended to prevent?). Indeed, analytic studies usually are designed to assess whether there is a causal association between the variables (e.g., Is a vaccine efficacious? Do children who attend day care centers have a higher risk of infections caused by certain bacteria or viruses?). Of course, it may not be possible to categorize a study so easily. In a primarily descriptive study, causal associations within subgroups may be assessed (e.g., in a study of the clinical epidemiology of tuberculosis in children, the investigators may compare the mortality rates of younger children with those of older children or of children with tuberculous meningitis with those of children with infection at other sites).

Most studies, whether descriptive or analytic, seek to reach conclusions about the particular group that is being assessed (e.g., children with tuberculosis). However, because it is not possible to study all persons with the condition of interest, investigators inevitably study a *sample* of persons and hope that the conclusions that are drawn from studying the sample apply to the entire population of interest (the *target population*). The *validity* of a study refers to the extent to which the results are true (accurate). The extent to which the conclusions drawn from the study sample (e.g., children with tuberculosis at Bellevue Hospital in New York City) are valid for the target population (e.g., all children with tuberculosis in New York City) is a measure of the study's *internal validity*. The extent to which the conclusions drawn from the study sample are valid for a less restrictively defined, larger population (e.g., all children with tuberculosis in the United States) is a measure of the study's *external validity*, which also is called its *generalizability*. To ensure that a study is both valid and generalizable, investigators must take steps to protect against a variety of potential biases (discussed later) that may distort the results of a study.

Elements of an Analytic Study

Epidemiologists refer to the major elements of an analytic study as the *exposure* and the *outcome*. The *exposure* is the factor that the investigator hypothesizes is related causally to the outcome of interest. In this context, the term *exposure* is not used in the classic sense of potential contact with an infectious agent; rather, it is any factor (e.g., living at a certain altitude, race, receipt of either a vaccine or a medication, smoking cigarettes) that may be associated causally with the outcome. The *outcome* is the effect (e.g., disease caused by a particular bacterium) that putatively is related causally to the exposure. The putative association may be one in which the exposure either causes or prevents the outcome of interest.

Before the specific type of study is defined, several additional elements of a study must be considered. One is how the *sample* for the study is selected. In general, investigators select a sample of the population based either on exposure (e.g., patients who either received or did not receive a vaccine, or who either attend or do not attend group day care) or on outcome (e.g., patients who either had or did not have pneumococcal bacteremia, patients who either died or survived). Another key element is the *timing* of the study in relation to the timing of exposure and outcome. In studies in which the timing is *historical*, both the exposure and the outcome occurred before the study was initiated (e.g., a case-control study of a vaccine's efficacy in which cases with disease are identified from historical logbooks and antecedent receipt of the vaccine is determined from medical records). Timing may be concurrent—that is, both the exposure and the outcome occur after the study is initiated (e.g., a randomized clinical trial of the efficacy of a new antibiotic). Timing may be a mixture of historical and concurrent (e.g., a study of the current IQ of children who previously had aseptic meningitis).

A final important element of a study is its *direction*. Direction is used to describe the order in which outcome and exposure are assessed. This may be done in a *forward* direction, from exposure to outcome (e.g., in a clinical trial of a vaccine's efficacy, the exposure [receipt or nonreceipt of the experimental vaccine] occurs first, and the occurrence of the outcome [the infection that the vaccine is designed to prevent] is determined subsequently). Alternatively, a study's direction may be *backward*, from outcome to exposure (e.g., in a case-control study, the outcome [e.g., pneumococcal bacteremia] is determined first, and exposure [e.g., prior receipt of pneumococcal vaccine] is determined subsequently). Or, exposure and outcome may be determined simultaneously (e.g., a survey in which determination of both whether subjects have sickle-cell disease and whether they were taking penicillin occurs at the same time). A study's direction can have important implications for inferences about causal associations; for example, even though there may be a strong statistical association between sickle-cell disease and use of penicillin, it would be erroneous to conclude that the penicillin caused the sickle-cell disease. Although such an inference obviously is not plausible in this instance, the dangers of making erroneous inferences about causality are very real when exposures and outcomes that are less well understood are studied.

Although the terms *prospective* and *retrospective* are used widely, there is substantial variability in how they are applied. The term *prospective* is used to describe studies in which selection of the sample is based on the exposure, in which the timing is concurrent, or in which the direction of the study is forward (from exposure to outcome). The term *retrospective* is used to describe studies in which the selection of the sample is based on the outcome, in which the timing is historical, or in which the direction of the study is backward (from outcome to exposure). It is preferable to refer to the specific elements of the study rather than to use the terms *prospective* and *retrospective* that are applied so imprecisely.

Types of Studies

Epidemiologic studies may be classified as either experimental or observational. In *experimental studies,* the exposure is assigned by the investigators (e.g., in a clinical trial of an experimental vaccine, the investigator assigns subjects to receive either the experimental vaccine or a placebo). In *observational studies,* the exposure occurs naturally (e.g., rainfall in a study that assesses the effect of the amount of rainfall on rates of mosquito-borne infections), is selected by the subjects or their parents (e.g., attendance of group day care in a study that assesses the frequency of infectious illnesses among children who attend and others who do not attend group day care), or is assigned in the course of regular medical care (e.g., receipt of a licensed vaccine in a case-control study of the protective efficacy of the vaccine). Observational studies also are called *surveys.*

Experimental Studies

The paradigm for an experimental study is the *randomized clinical trial,* which is a special type of a *longitudinal cohort study* in which the exposure is assigned randomly to the subjects by the investigators. In randomized trials, the direction of the study always is forward, selection (or categorization) of subjects always is based on exposure (i.e., exposure is determined at the time of randomization), and timing always is concurrent (both exposure and outcome are determined during the real period of the study). Randomized trials are the sine qua non for evaluating the effect of new agents designed either to prevent (e.g., vaccines, prophylactic drugs) or to treat (e.g., antimicrobials) diseases. By randomly allocating subjects to receive or not receive the agent that is being tested, potential bias is minimized. Theoretically, if the size of the sample is adequate, the only difference between the groups is whether they received the experimental agent. Consequently, if the study is conducted properly, it is reasonable to infer that statistically significant differences in outcomes between the groups were related causally to the experimental agent. For this reason, in most instances the efficacy of new therapeutic agents or of new vaccines must be demonstrated in clinical trials before the Food and Drug Administration will license them (although in some instances new products are licensed if criteria for safety and for some surrogate end-point, such as a serologic correlate of immunity, are met).

TABLE 246–1. Randomized Clinical Trials

Advantages
1. Gold standard for scientific validity
   a. Randomization ensures unbiased allocation of the exposure (e.g., a new drug or an experimental vaccine)
   b. Blinding ensures unbiased assessment of outcomes

Disadvantages
1. Poor statistical power for rare diseases
   a. Requires large samples
2. Requires longitudinal follow-up
3. Logistically complex and expensive
4. Impaired generalizability when the study population differs from the ultimate target population
5. Ethical issues
   a. Requires informed consent
   b. Difficult to use to evaluate licensed (presumably efficacious) products

The advantages and disadvantages of randomized trials are summarized in Table 246–1. Although clinical trials are the gold standard for investigators who wish to design a scientifically valid study, they do have a number of limitations. A major problem is that clinical trials usually are expensive. Subjects need to be selected, enrolled, and followed longitudinally to detect the outcomes. When the outcome is a disease that is relatively rare (e.g., pneumococcal bacteremia), large samples are needed to provide adequate statistical power. Because sponsors of clinical trials usually want to test a new drug or an experimental vaccine under conditions that will maximize the chance that it will be found to be efficacious, patients with co-morbid conditions (e.g., sickle-cell disease, asplenia, metastatic cancer) that might affect their responses to the new agent often are excluded from the study. If the subjects who are excluded are an important part of the target population for the new agent (e.g., the patients with the co-morbid conditions are likely to be at high risk of serious complications of the disease and so potentially could benefit greatly from an effective new intervention), the generalizability of the results of the clinical trial may be impaired.

Most randomized clinical trials are conducted in a double-blind manner; that is, neither the investigators nor the subjects know whether they received the experimental intervention (e.g., a new drug) or the comparison agent (e.g., a placebo, a standardly used agent). Double blinding helps to ensure lack of bias in the ascertainment of the outcome because neither the subject nor the investigator can be influenced to (or not to) either seek medical care or undergo diagnostic tests based on which of the interventions was received.

Randomized clinical trials may pose difficult ethical problems because the new (and potentially efficacious) agent is not given to the controls. By the time that clinical trials are begun, usually there already is some evidence to suggest that the agent is efficacious (e.g., preliminary studies that show that a new vaccine induces antibodies). Consequently, some patients and patient advocates might suggest that it is not ethical to withhold a potentially efficacious therapeutic agent or a vaccine from persons at risk (e.g., it may be difficult to have persons agree to be potential controls in studies of a promising new therapy).

Problems also may arise when the licensing of a product for the target population is based on studies that are conducted in a different population. For example, polyvalent pneumococcal polysaccharide vaccine was licensed in the United States for the elderly and for adults with chronic conditions, such as chronic obstructive pulmonary disease and congestive heart failure, that put them at increased risk of serious pneumococcal infections. However, the data on which licensure was based were from clinical trials conducted among young goldminers in South Africa who were at risk not because of their age or underlying illnesses but because of the conditions in which they lived and worked. Reports of vaccine failures and of poor antibody responses to the vaccine in the target population in the United States led to questions about the vaccine's efficacy.[4] However, once the vaccine was licensed, it was difficult ethically to conduct a randomized clinical trial in the target population because it would mean withholding, on a random basis, a licensed (and presumably efficacious) vaccine from patients at risk. Consequently, all but one of the postlicensure studies of this vaccine's efficacy were observational studies.

It is possible to conduct an experimental study in which the exposure is not assigned randomly. For example, one might conduct an experimental cohort study in which volunteers receive a certain intervention (e.g., a new drug) while controls receive no intervention. Both groups would be followed forward in time while undergoing surveillance for the outcome event. Although such a study incorporates some of the features of a randomized clinical trial, because the intervention is not assigned randomly, such studies are subject to significant biases.

Observational Studies

Observational Cohort Studies

The direction of cohort studies always is forward, and the selection (or categorization) of subjects always is based on exposure, but the timing may be concurrent, historical, or mixed. Thus, a cohort study may identify a cohort of subjects at a point (or at several points) in time in the recent or remote past, categorize them as to their status with regard to the exposure (e.g., receipt of either a vaccine or a drug), and then follow them forward in time for the occurrence of the outcome event (e.g., an infection) until a certain point in time, which could be in the past, present, or future. As in a clinical trial, subjects must not have the outcome at the onset of the study.

Cohort studies share many of the disadvantages of randomized clinical trials (see Table 246–1) but have the additional disadvantage that, because they are not experimental, they are subject to many potential biases. On the other hand, cohort studies have many practical advantages (e.g., the timing can be historical, so it is possible to conduct a 30-year follow-up study in just months), and because they are observational studies, there usually are fewer potential ethical problems than in a randomized trial. In addition, for rare exposures it is critical to be able to base selection of subjects on exposure.

Case-Control Studies

In both clinical trials and observational cohort studies, the selection of subjects is based on their exposure and they are followed in a forward direction until the outcome is determined. In *case-control studies,* the process is reversed. Subjects are selected on the basis of an outcome. The cases have the outcome, usually a disease; the controls do not have the outcome. The direction of the study is backward—the prior exposure is ascertained after the subjects are selected. The timing of case-control studies usually is historical, but it may be mixed; the timing of the exposure always is historical, but the timing of the outcome may be either historical or concurrent. For example, an investigator may conduct a case-control study of a vaccine's efficacy in which persons who are infected (cases) are identified concurrently through active surveillance of a microbiology laboratory. Because case-control studies are nonexperimental and the exposure (and, sometimes, the outcome) occurred in the past, there is great potential for bias both in the selection of the sample and in the ascertainment of both the exposure and the outcome. The advantages and the disadvantages of case-control studies are shown in Table 246–2.

TABLE 246–2. Case-Control Studies

Advantages
1. Statistically powerful method to assess outcomes that are rare or delayed
2. Logistically easier and more efficient than large experimental or observational cohort studies
3. No longitudinal follow-up, so it can be completed relatively quickly and inexpensively
4. Ethically acceptable because it is an observational study

Disadvantage
1. Subject to many potential biases

Cross-Sectional Studies

Unlike in cohort studies (both experimental and observational), in which subjects are followed forward from exposure to outcome, and case-control studies, in which subjects are followed backward from outcome to exposure, in cross-sectional studies, outcome and exposure are determined at the same point in time. In cohort studies, causal inference is made from cause to effect, whereas in case-control studies, causal inference is made from effect to cause. In cross-sectional studies, it may not be possible to determine whether the exposure preceded the outcome. Consequently, it may not be possible to make valid causal inferences from a cross-sectional study.

The selection of subjects for a cross-sectional study may be based on outcome, exposure, or neither. However, because cross-sectional studies include only persons with prevalent outcomes, they particularly are problematic for studies of infectious diseases because patients whose illnesses (outcomes) either resolved or resulted in death before the point in time at which the study is conducted are not counted as having the outcome. Consequently, cross-sectional studies are more suitable to the study of chronic conditions and rarely are used in studies of infectious diseases.

Analysis of Epidemiologic Studies

The results of epidemiologic studies with dichotomous exposures and outcomes often are displayed in a 2 × 2 *contingency table.* However, the way the results are analyzed statistically depends on the type of study.

TABLE 246–3. Analysis of Experimental or Observational Cohort Studies

	Outcome Present	Outcome Absent	Total
Exposed	a	b	a + b
Unexposed	c	d	c + d
Total	a + c	b + d	

Risk in exposed subjects: a/(a + b)
Risk in unexposed subjects: c/(c + d)
Relative risk: (a/a + b) ÷ (c/c + d)
Attributable risk: (a/a + b) − (c/c + d)

Cohort Studies

The analysis of longitudinal cohort studies (both experimental trials and observational studies) is shown in Table 246–3. The measure of association between the exposure and the outcome is the *relative risk* (sometimes called the *risk ratio),* which is an expression of the *magnitude* of this association in the study sample and represents an *estimate* of the association in the population from which the study sample was drawn. A relative risk of 1 indicates that there is no association between the exposure and the outcome, a relative risk greater than 1 indicates that the exposure is associated with an increased risk of the outcome, and a relative risk less than 1 indicates that the exposure is associated with a decreased risk of the outcome. The *attributable risk* (the risk of the outcome that is attributable to the exposure) is calculated as the risk in exposed subjects minus the risk in the unexposed subjects. Of course, it is necessary to test the statistical significance of any association because the relative risk could be greater than 1 or less than 1 by chance (see later sections on stochastic statistics and on confidence intervals).

These analyses assume that there is no attrition among the subjects in the study. However, because of death, migration out of the study area, and loss to follow-up as well as variation in the time of enrollment (enrollment in either a clinical trial or an observational cohort study may occur over a prolonged period or, indeed, throughout a study), there virtually always is variation among the subjects in the duration of time that they are at risk of developing the outcome. If the average time at risk among the exposed and the unexposed subjects is equal, the analysis shown in Table 246–3 is likely to be valid. However, if there is a great deal of irregular attrition or new enrollment during the study, the denominator is expressed better as person-time at risk (e.g., person-months, person-years) rather than as the number of persons in the group. When this method is used, the rate then is called the *incidence density rate* and the index of comparison is called the *incidence density ratio.*

In studies of infectious diseases, the outcome event often is the occurrence of an infection. Frequently, persons who become infected recover and may remain at risk of developing the outcome event again. Nevertheless, a subject usually should be *censored* (i.e., removed from the study) once the outcome event occurs. The fact that the outcome occurred may indicate that the subject is at increased risk of the outcome, independent of the exposure that is being assessed. For example, consider a study of the protective efficacy of a conjugate pneumococcal vaccine's efficacy in which one of the subjects (it does not matter whether the subject is a vaccinee or a control) develops three or four episodes of invasive infections caused by pneumococci (perhaps because the subject has a previously unrecognized underlying condition, such as AIDS or an immunoglobulin deficiency). It would distort the estimate of the vaccine's efficacy substantially if each of the outcome events was counted. Certainly, in a primary analysis, only the initial event should be counted. Another reason to censor the subject is that, in some instances, the outcome event may be fatal. If some subjects die of the outcome (and therefore must be censored), not censoring subjects with the outcome who survive is, in effect, incorporating an assessment of the exposure's effect on prognosis and not just on the risk of the outcome event.

It may be necessary to use a different method to adjust for unequal durations of follow-up in a study, particularly when there is a long latent period between exposure and outcome (a condition that often is met when the study is of the effect of a potential carcinogen, for example). In such instances, it may be misleading simply to sum the total person-times of exposure, because the outcome is more likely to occur many years after exposure. For example, although the total person-time at risk would be the same, the risk of developing an outcome clearly may be substantially different for 500 persons, each of whom is followed for 2 years after exposure, than it may be for 40 persons, each of whom is followed for 25 years. For such situations, the analyses must be adjusted for variation in the length of follow-up. This can be done with the use of *survival analysis* (also known as *life-table analysis).* The two basic methods of survival analysis, the *actuarial* method and the *Kaplan-Meier (product-limit)* method, are described in detail elsewhere.[12]

Case-Control and Cross-Sectional Studies

The analysis of a case-control study (with dichotomous outcomes and exposures) is shown in Table 246–4. Because selection of subjects is based on their outcomes, one cannot calculate the risk of developing the outcome, as one would in a longitudinal study (such as a clinical trial). Instead, one calculates the proportion of each group (cases and controls) that is exposed. The measure of association in a case-control study is the *odds ratio.* The *odds* of some occurrence is the probability that it will occur divided by the probability that it will not occur. In a case-control study, we are interested in the odds of exposure. The odds ratio is the ratio of the odds of exposure among cases (a/c) divided by the odds of exposure among controls (b/d). For rare events, the odds ratio closely approximates the relative risk of exposure that would be found in a longitudinal study of the same association. Cross-sectional studies are analyzed either like a case-control study (if the selection of subjects was based on their outcomes) or like a cohort study (if the selection of subjects was based on their exposures).

Bias

Bias occurs when the estimate of the association between the exposure and the outcome in the sample differs systemat-

TABLE 246–4. Analysis of Case-Control Studies

	Cases (Outcome Present)	Controls (Outcome Absent)
Exposed	a	b
Unexposed	c	d

Proportion of exposed cases: a/(a + c)
Proportion of exposed controls: b/(b + d)
Odds of exposure among cases: a/c
Odds of exposure among controls: b/d
Odds ratio: (a/c) ÷ (b/d) or (ad) ÷ (bc)

ically from the true value in the population. Bias in the estimate of the association is different than bias in the measurement of individual variables. The latter bias (which may occur, for example, if an instrument, such as a thermometer, is calibrated incorrectly) may or may not affect the estimate of association in an epidemiologic study. Biased measurements usually affect the exposed and the unexposed groups equally. By contrast, *analytic bias* is the effect of *differential error* (*nonrandom error)* on the assessment of the relationship between exposure and outcome. Analytic bias can occur because of *information bias* (as a result of differential error in the ascertainment of either the exposure or the outcome), *sample distortion bias* (because the joint distribution of the exposure and the outcome in the sample chosen for the study is not representative of the distribution of these factors in the target population), and *confounding bias* (because the joint distribution of one or more variables that independently are related both to the exposure and to the outcome is distributed unequally in the groups that are being compared). Ensuring that bias does not affect a study is critical to its validity. Furthermore, although it sometimes is possible to use statistical methods to adjust for certain sources of bias (particularly for confounding bias) in the analysis of the results of a study, adjustment for bias after the fact may be impossible.

An example of information bias is *detection bias,* which occurs when there is differential detection of the outcome in the exposed and the unexposed groups. For example, there have been a number of studies in which clinical scales to assess whether children with fever have a serious illness have been developed.[13] Often, however, the "serious illness" may include certain abnormal laboratory tests (such as an abnormal radiograph of the chest or a low concentration of sodium in the serum). Because children with high scores on these scales were more likely to undergo diagnostic tests, detection bias may have occurred because similar abnormalities (such as a "silent" pneumonia or a mildly depressed concentration of sodium in the serum) might go undetected in the "unexposed" group (children with lower scores on the clinical scale), a much smaller proportion of whom underwent a diagnostic test to detect a possible outcome. The best way to avoid information bias is to use standardized, consistent methods to ascertain both the exposure and the outcome and to blind subjects and investigators to ensure that there is not differential ascertainment of either the outcome (in longitudinal studies) or of the exposure (in case-control studies).

Sample distortion bias occurs when the sample in a study is not representative of the target population. However, a nonrepresentative sample does not lead to bias necessarily; bias in the assessment of the association between exposure and outcome occurs only if there is differential distribution of the exposure (or differential risk of the outcome) in the subjects who are selected for the study compared with the overall target population. This can be the result of *selection bias*. For example, consider a case-control study of the protective efficacy of a licensed vaccine in which the control subjects (the uninfected patients) were chosen from private practices in affluent suburbs, whereas the case subjects (the infected patients) were any patients who developed a serious infection and were hospitalized. It is likely that the association between antecedent vaccination and infection is biased because the controls are not a representative sample of the population from which the cases emerged, and a higher proportion of them are likely to have been vaccinated compared with all uninfected persons in the population. Another possible source of sample distortion bias is differential loss to follow-up in a longitudinal study. The potential for sample distortion bias can be minimized by maximizing the probability that a representative sample will be selected, ideally by random sampling (or some other kind of unbiased sampling) and by minimizing loss to follow-up in longitudinal studies.

Confounding bias occurs when the association between exposure and outcome is distorted by a variable (a *confounder)* that is distributed unequally between the groups, is associated independently with both the exposure and the outcome, and is not in the causal pathway from exposure to outcome. One example of confounding bias is *susceptibility bias,* which occurs when the risk of the subjects (to developing the outcome) differs in the exposed and the unexposed groups, independent of the exposure. For example, imagine a longitudinal study of the protective efficacy of a vaccine against *Haemophilus influenzae* type b in infants. It would be important to ensure that an equal proportion of subjects in the vaccinated and the unvaccinated groups attended group day care because attendance of group day care is associated with an increased risk of developing infection with *H. influenzae* type b. If a substantially higher proportion of vaccinees than of controls attended group day care, it might confound the assessment of the vaccine's efficacy and result in a biased (lower) estimate of the effect of a vaccine. By contrast, if a disproportionate number of controls attended group day care, the estimate of the vaccine's efficacy might be biased in the opposite direction (it would be erroneously high because controls would have a disproportionately higher risk of developing infection with *H. influenzae* type b than would vaccinees).

In the previous example, it might be possible to adjust for the effect of the confounder by either stratification or multivariable analysis (see later). However, it may not always be possible to identify confounders. Random allocation of subjects probably is the best strategy to protect against confounding, especially against potential confounders that cannot be identified.

STATISTICS

Summary Statistics

Perhaps the most basic use of statistical analysis is to summarize data. This type of statistical analysis often is called either *summary* or *descriptive* statistics. The specific summary measures that are used depend, in part, on whether the variables being summarized are *continuous* (variables with equal distance between intervals) or *categorical* (variables with two or more discrete categories). Age, weight, height, temperature, concentration of creatinine in the serum, and the number of hours spent in group day care all are examples of continuous variables (sometimes called *dimensional* or *quantitative* variables). Race, sex, country of residence, and whether a patient is being ventilated artificially are examples of categorical variables (sometimes called *discrete* variables). Of course, continuous variables can be analyzed categorically (e.g., age can be divided into either a *dichotomous* variable [$<$45 years or $\geq$45 years] or a *polychotomous* variable [20 to 44 years, 45 to 59 years, or $\geq$60 years]).

Continuous Variables

A *frequency distribution* is the classification of the values of a sample of continuous variables into successive categories (e.g., for a sample of different ages, one might place each value into different 5-year [0 to 4 years, 5 to 9 years, etc.], 3-year [0 to 2 years, 3 to 5 years, etc.], or 1-year [0 years, 1 year, 2 years, 3 years, etc.] categories) and expression of the frequency of values within each category.

A sample of values of a continuous variable also can be summarized mathematically by describing its central tendency, shape, and spread. The *central tendency* can be expressed as a *mean* (or *average*), a *median* (the middle value of the sample), or a *mode* (the most frequent value in the sample). The mean value is calculated by summing all of the individual values in the sample and dividing by the number of individual values. Thus, for a sample that is composed of subjects aged 1, 1, 2, 2, 2, 3, 3, 4, 10, and 12 years, the mean age is 4 years (40/10), the median age (the age for which half of the subjects are older than and half are younger than its value—if there are an even number of subjects, the median is the mean of the two middle values) is 2.5 years [(2+3)/2], and the mode is 2 years. These summary measures provide only a limited view of the data. For example, the mean of a distribution can be shifted in the direction of extreme outlying values; in the example, the mean is 4 years even though 70 per cent of the subjects are younger than 4 years of age. Likewise, from the median value alone, one would not know whether there were outlying values. Consequently, it is important to describe the spread of a distribution.

The *spread* of a sample may be expressed by its *range* and by its *standard deviation*. The range of a sample is the interval between the highest and the lowest value in its distribution. In the example, the range is from 1 to 12 years. Another useful way of mathematically summarizing the spread of a distribution is to express the interval between each individual value and the mean value of the sample. To summarize these values, one cannot simply sum all of the differences because the sum always equals zero (the sum of the positive differences equals the sum of the negative differences). To avoid this problem, the standard deviation of a sample is used. This parameter is calculated by taking the square root of the *variance* of the sample. The variance is the sum of the squares of the differences from the mean of each individual value, divided by the number of *degrees of freedom* of the sample (which is equal to the number of values in the sample minus one, or $N-1$). The sum of squares is divided by the number of degrees of freedom of the sample (N−1), rather than by N (the actual number in the sample), because this calculation is thought more accurately to represent the true variance of the population from which a sample is taken.

To calculate the standard deviation of the sample in the example, one must determine the variance, which is the sum of the squares of the difference of each individual value from the mean of the sample:

$$(2[4-1]^2 + 3[4-2]^2 + 2[4-3]^2 + [4-4]^2 + [4-10]^2 + [4-12]^2) \div (10-1)$$

Which equals 132/9, or 14.6667 years. The standard deviation simply is the square root of the variance, which is 3.8297 years.

In the medical literature, investigators often use the *standard error of the mean* (which is the variance divided by the square root of the number in the sample) to express the spread of the frequency distribution of a sample. However, the standard error actually is designed to be a measure of the standard deviation of the means of repeated samples from a single source population. Because the standard error always is smaller than the standard deviation of a single sample, it gives the erroneous impression that the spread of a sample is smaller than it actually is. A large sample with a large spread (and a large standard deviation) may have a small standard error. The standard error should not be used to describe the spread of a single sample.

The general shape of the frequency distribution can be inferred from the parameters given earlier. The characteristics of the most important distribution in statistics, the familiar bell-shaped curve of the normal distribution, are shown in Figure 246–1 and are discussed in a later section about diagnostic tests. The peak value of any distribution is the mode. A distribution may be bimodal, trimodal, etc., if there are two or more modes. A frequency distribution may be asymmetric, or *skewed*. If the mean is greater than the median (as in the example), the distribution is skewed to the right. If the mean is less than the median, the distribution is skewed to the left.

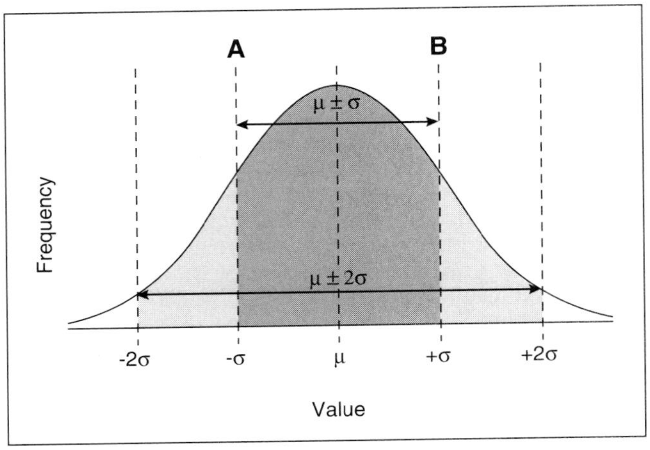

FIGURE 246–1. *Theoretic normal (gaussian) distribution showing where 1 and 2 standard deviations above and below the mean would fall. The Greek letter* mu (μ) *stands for the mean in the theoretic distribution, and the Greek letter* sigma (σ) *stands for the standard deviation in the theoretic population. (The italic Roman letters* x̄ *and* s *apply to an observed [sample] population.) In this figure, the area under the curve represents all of the observations in the distribution. One standard deviation above and below the mean, shown in dark gray and represented by the distance from point A to point B, is equivalent to 68 per cent of the area under the curve, and therefore 68 per cent of the observations in a normal distribution fall within this range. Two standard deviations above and below the mean, represented by the areas shown in dark and light gray, are equivalent to 95.4 per cent of the area of the curve or 95.4 per cent of the observations in a normal distribution. (From Jekel, J. F., Elmore, J. G., and Katz, D. L.: Epidemiology, Biostatistics, and Preventive Medicine. Philadelphia, W. B. Saunders, 1996, p. 118.)*

An investigator may want to summarize the relationship between two different continuous variables. This can be done with the use of linear regression, in which a straight line is constructed to represent the relationship between a continuous *dependent variable* (y) and a continuous *independent variable* (x). An equation ($y=a+bx$) can be created that represents the best "fit" to describe the relationship between the actual values of y and of x, in which a (the *intercept*) is the value of y when x equals zero and b (the *regression coefficient*) is the slope of the line. Such an equation allows us to summarize the relationship between these variables and to extrapolate the value of each variable for conditions that may not have been observed in the sample. For example, one can calculate the incremental value of y for each interval change in the value of x.

Categorical Variables

The measure usually used to summarize categorical data is called a *rate* or a *proportion*. Rates consist of a numerator and a denominator. The numerator represents the actual number of persons in the sample that have the characteristic of interest (e.g., those with fever, those with tuberculosis, those who received a vaccine), and the denominator is the total number of persons in the sample. The persons in the numerator must be included in the group that the denominator represents, and it must be possible for the persons in the denominator to have the characteristic that the numerator represents. For example, if one were interested in the rate of testicular cancer in the population, women should not be included in the denominator because it is not possible for them to have testicular cancer. Some experts believe that rates should include a time factor and should express a change over time. However, the term is widely used to refer to a proportion of a sample, as described earlier.

One of the most important rates that is calculated in epidemiologic studies is the *incidence rate,* which is the number of persons who develop a certain outcome divided by the number of persons who could have developed the outcome during a specified period. For example, a comparison may be made of the incidence rates of an infection over time in two groups in which the interventions given to prevent an infection differed (e.g., a vaccine and a placebo).

Another important rate, the *prevalence rate,* is the number of persons who develop a certain outcome divided by the total number of persons in the group at a specific point in time. In the calculation of the incidence rate, persons who, at *zero time* (before the study begins), already developed the outcome (e.g., prevalent cases) are excluded from both the numerator and the denominator. At time zero, the numerator of the incidence rate is zero. Thus, if one were interested in the incidence rate of lung cancer, persons who had lung cancer at the beginning of the study period would be excluded. The prevalence rate, by contrast, is measured at one point in time, and the numerator includes all persons with the outcome at that time.

Certain features of many infectious diseases affect both the prevalence rate and the incidence rate as measures of the occurrence of disease. The prevalence rate of any condition is related to its chronicity and the mortality rate associated with it; conditions that are common and chronic but that are not associated necessarily with immediate mortality (e.g., atherosclerotic heart disease) have a relatively high prevalence rate. On the other hand, the prevalence rates of conditions that either have a low mortality rate and resolve completely (such as many infectious illnesses) or have a high short-term mortality rate are relatively low. To get a reliable estimate of the importance of such conditions, it is necessary to determine their incidence rates.

Stochastic Statistics

Statistical Significance

Stochastic statistics deals with probability. Most readers are familiar with the use of "p values" to assess the *statistical significance* of a finding from a study. Usually, the threshold used to separate "significant" from "nonsignificant" results in a probability (p value) of less than 0.05. This means that (arbitrarily, by convention) if a result is likely to be observed by chance fewer than 1 in 20 times, the finding is considered to be "statistically significant." It must be emphasized, however, that statistical significance and clinical significance are very different. A statistically significant result means that the result is considered unlikely to be attributable to chance alone. As we shall see, the p value is related not only to the magnitude of the difference between the things that are being compared (e.g., a characteristic either of the exposed and the unexposed groups in a longitudinal study or of the cases and the controls in a case-control study) but also to the size of the sample. Consequently, differences that are clinically unimportant (e.g., a difference in mean weight of 0.2 kg between two groups, a difference of 4 per cent in the distribution of whites between two groups) can be statistically significant if the size of the sample is large. It is important to remember that a statistically significant finding may be of no clinical significance.

By the same token, the "magic" p value of 0.05 itself may be misleading because it is an arbitrary threshold; in fact, there usually is little difference in the results associated with a p value of 0.04 and one associated with a p value of 0.06. If the size of a sample is small, a large, clinically important difference may not be statistically significant. One should not dismiss automatically the importance of a finding for which the p value is greater than or equal to 0.05.

Hypothesis Testing

In most epidemiologic studies, stochastic tests are used to test the validity of a hypothesis. By convention, one tests the validity of the *null hypothesis* that there is no difference in either the mean value of the characteristic (for continuous variables) or in the frequency distribution of the characteristic (for categorical values) between the groups being compared. In essence, one is testing the probability that the two samples that are being compared (exposed subjects vs. unexposed subjects or cases vs. controls) emerged from the same population—that is, whether a difference between the groups could have been the result of chance if the two samples were selected randomly from the same population or whether the difference is so great that it is unlikely (less than 1 chance in 20, or a p value of <0.05) that the difference could have occurred by chance; if so, it is likely that the samples actually represent a true difference in the populations either of exposed subjects versus unexposed subjects or of cases versus controls.

Hypotheses can be either *bidirectional (nondirectional)* or *unidirectional (directional).* A nondirectional hypothesis asks whether there is an association between exposed and unexposed subjects, but it does not assume in which direction the association will occur. For example, one might ask whether there is an association between the height of fever and the outcomes of children with typhoid fever without specifying whether the association would be in the direction of better or worse outcomes (perhaps high fever indicates a more severe infection, or perhaps it indicates a more vigorous immune response). In such instances, the associated p value should be interpreted in a bidirectional, or *two-tailed,* manner because the distribution of the test statistic contains two "tails," one at either end of the curve; the p value represents the sum of the area under the two tails of the curve. In effect, one is specifying that for a result to be statistically significant, there must be a less than 2.5 per cent probability of the result being in a positive direction and a less than 2.5 per cent probability of the result being in a negative direction. Most tables of p values provide results that are to be interpreted in a two-tailed manner (because this is the most conservative approach to testing a hypothesis), so the p value for a given test statistic can be read directly from the table.

In some instances, however, one might have good reason to suspect that an exposure is associated with an outcome in a unidirectional manner (e.g., that possession of a handgun is associated with an increased risk of sustaining a gunshot wound). If, in advance, the investigator decides to test this hypothesis in a unidirectional manner (the null hypothesis for which would be that ownership of a gun is not associated with an increased risk of a gunshot wound), it might be appropriate to interpret the results of a test statistic in a unidirectional, or *one-tailed,* manner. To derive a one-tailed p value, the two-tailed value is divided by 2. Thus, if the two-tailed p value is 0.06, the one-tailed value for the same result is 0.03. Clearly, it is easier to obtain statistically significant results by testing hypotheses in a unidirectional manner. However, it is important to specify before the study is conducted the a priori plan as to how the results of statistical tests will be interpreted. Furthermore, although it might seem that many hypotheses would lend themselves to unidirectional analyses (e.g., one might think that an experimental vaccine that has been shown to be immunogenic could only be beneficial), in fact unidirectional analyses only rarely are used. First, the possibility that an exposure may have an effect opposite to that which is expected usually cannot be ruled out in advance. For example, it was found that persons who were immunized with a vaccine composed of inactivated respiratory syncytial virus had an increased risk of symptomatic infection with the virus. In addition, because two-tailed interpretation of data is more conservative, many authorities (such as editors of journals and such licensing agencies as the Food and Drug Administration) demand two-tailed analyses.

Type I Error, Type II Error, and Statistical Power

There are two types of errors that can be made when testing the validity of a null hypothesis. The first occurs when the null hypothesis is true but is rejected erroneously, which leads to an erroneous conclusion that there is a difference between the exposed and unexposed subjects; this kind of mistake is termed *type I error,* or *alpha error.* If a test statistic with a p value of less than 0.05 is accepted as statistically significant (and the null hypothesis is rejected on that basis), approximately 5 per cent of the time a type I error is made because, if there really is no difference between the groups, that result will occur by chance 1 in 20 times. By contrast, if the p value is less than 0.001, a type I error will occur fewer than 1 in 1000 times if the null hypothesis is rejected.

The other kind of error, *type II error,* or *beta error,* occurs when the null hypothesis erroneously is not rejected even though there truly is a difference between the two groups. If the p value associated with the result is greater than or equal to 0.05, the probability that the null hypothesis is false is not sufficiently low to reject it (even though there may be only a 6 per cent probability that the observed result could have occurred by chance).

Type I and type II errors are mutually exclusive. If one rejects the null hypothesis, one risks committing a type I error, the probability of which is equal to the p value. In such instances, a type II error cannot occur. If one accepts (i.e., fails to reject) the null hypothesis, one may commit a type II error (in which case a type I error cannot occur). The probability of committing a type II error is not related directly to the observed p value. Instead, one can estimate the probability of committing a type II error (beta error) before the study begins based on an assumed (clinically important) degree of association between the exposure and the outcome. Certain assumptions also must be made about the magnitude of the effect among the exposed subjects and about the frequency of the outcome in the unexposed subjects. One is calculating a unidirectional probability that, by chance, the study will fail to detect an association equal to or greater than the magnitude that is specified for what is, in effect, an *alternative hypothesis* (i.e., that there truly is an association between the exposure and the outcome). The *statistical power* of a study (the unidirectional probability that the null hypothesis will be rejected given a specified degree of type I error—usually <5 per cent) is equal to 1 minus beta.

In designing a study, adequate statistical power is critical to ensure that a true association between the exposure and the outcome is not missed erroneously. The probability of type II error depends on the size of the sample, the degree of variance within the sample, and the magnitude of the association that one wants to be able to detect: the smaller the sample, the larger the variance, and the smaller the magnitude of the association that one wants to detect, the larger the beta error (type II error) will be and the lower the statistical power of the study to detect an association will be. Of these factors, the investigator usually has control only over the size of the sample (because the variance generally is a relatively fixed attribute in the population of the characteristic being measured and the magnitude of association that is chosen usually is the minimum association that is clinically meaningful; for example, it would not make sense to design a study of an experimental vaccine so that it could detect as little as 30 per cent efficacy because in most instances, such a product would not be licensed unless the magnitude of its effect was much greater).

Exactly what constitutes adequate power is debatable. Because it often is expensive and time-consuming to enroll a large number of subjects in a study, the power a study is designed to have often depends on both the financial resources and the time available to conduct the study. A statistical power of 80 per cent often is chosen as a reasonable compromise between ensuring that there are enough subjects to answer the research hypothesis and the realities of logistical and financial exigencies. On the other hand, if a pharmaceutical company has invested many years and millions of dollars to develop a new drug or a new vaccine, they may demand that a pivotal clinical trial of the product have greater than or equal to 90 per cent power to detect a clinically meaningful effect to try to ensure that it will be licensed if it is efficacious.

Multiple Comparisons

Another more subtle problem in interpreting results arises when more than one hypothesis is assessed in a single study. If multiple tests of statistical significance are performed in a study, the probability that, by chance alone, the p value associated with any one variable will be less than 0.05 is substantially greater than 5 per cent. In fact, the probability that by chance at least one test will be associated with a p value of less than 0.05 is equal to $1-(0.95)^k$, with k equal to the number of independent tests of statistical significance that are performed. Thus, if 10 different hypotheses are tested, there is a 40 per cent probability that at least one of them will be statistically significant (i.e., that at least one of the tests will have a p value of <0.05). Of course, this violates the arbitrary rule that we only consider a finding to be statistically significant if it is likely to have occurred by chance less than 5 per cent of the time. If multiple different associations in a study have associated p values of less than 0.05, it is difficult to know which occurred by chance and which truly are statistically significant.

On the other hand, studies often are expensive, time-consuming, and logistically difficult to conduct. Therefore, it sometimes is reasonable to try to increase efficiency by assessing more than one hypothesis in a single study. To address this problem, one can specify in advance the *primary hypothesis* and the *secondary* and *tertiary hypotheses.* One then might give most credence to the statistical test of the primary hypothesis. Another approach is to lower the threshold used to define statistical significance by dividing 0.05 by the number of different tests that are performed. Thus, if five independent hypotheses are tested, any one would have to be associated with a p value of less than 0.01 before the null hypothesis would be rejected. However, this approach might be too stringent because the different hypotheses that are being tested often are not truly independent, and the probability that two or more associations will be statistically significant may be greater than the product of their individual probabilities. For example, one might assess whether infection is associated both with diarrhea and with vomiting; if it is associated with one of these, there usually is a higher than chance probability that it also is associated with the other. At the least, an investigator should acknowledge this potential problem and its consequences before drawing conclusions from the study.

Tests of Statistical Significance

It is beyond the scope of this chapter to go into detail about the many different stochastic tests that are available. However, several general comments as well as descriptions of a few commonly used tests are in order.

Tests of statistical significance are either parametric or nonparametric. The test statistic of a *parametric* test is based on the assumption that the frequency distribution of the characteristic being assessed in the source population follows certain parameters. For example, for certain tests it is assumed that the characteristic in the population has a normal distribution. If the assumption is violated (e.g., the characteristic is not distributed normally), the statistical test will not be valid. In such instances, it might be appropriate to use a test based on a different, skewed distribution, such as the *Poisson distribution* for rare events, that might reflect more accurately the distribution of the characteristic in the population.

Alternative approaches to assess the statistical significance of differences between groups, if it is known that the distribution of the characteristic in the population is highly skewed, include transforming the data so that they are normalized, usually by converting the values to their logarithmic equivalent or by using a *nonparametric* test.[21] Nonparametric tests, such as the *Mann-Whitney U-test* and the *Wilcoxon ranked sum test*, do not depend directly on the numerical values of the data; instead, the individual values are ranked in order of their values, and the statistical analyses are based on the relative ranks of the values in the different groups, rather than on an assumed distribution in the population or in the sample.

For large samples, parametric tests usually are valid and often are easier to calculate than nonparametric tests. For smaller samples and for samples with highly skewed distributions, nonparametric tests or tests that use log-transformed data may be preferable.

Continuous Variables

To test the statistical significance of differences between groups in continuous variables (such as degree of fever, IQ, age, or a score on a standardized questionnaire), the mean values of the different groups can be compared.[22] The tests of statistical significance use the magnitude of the difference of the means and the variance in the sample to assess the probability that the difference could occur by chance. If more than two groups are being compared for a single variable, this procedure is called *one-way analysis of variance*. The null hypothesis is that the mean values from each group are the same (i.e., that the different groups are random samples from the same population). The total variance in all of the subjects is separated into the amount that is attributable to differences between the groups of subjects (the *intergroup variance)* and the amount that is attributable to differences among the subjects within each group (the *intragroup variance)*. The greater the quotient of the intergroup variance divided by the intragroup variance (the *F-ratio)*, the more likely it is that the differences between the groups are statistically significant (i.e., that they are not due to chance variation). The statistical significance of the F-ratio can be determined from the *F-test* table of p values. When this type of test is performed to assess the statistical significance of the simultaneous effects of two factors (by stratifying into additional groups), the test is called *two-way analysis of variance*.

The familiar *t-test* is just a special form of one-way analysis of variance in which the means of just two groups are compared. A *one-sample t-test* assesses whether the mean value of the study sample is statistically significantly different than the mean value in the source population. It assumes that the mean value in the source population is known. It is calculated by dividing the difference of the mean of the sample minus the mean of the population by the quotient of the variance of the sample divided by the square root of the number in the sample.

A more common use of the t-test is to assess the statistical significance of the difference between the mean values of either a characteristic or an outcome of subjects in two different samples (e.g., of the exposed and the unexposed groups in a study). The null hypothesis of this *two-sample t-test* is that the mean values of the two samples are not statistically significantly different (i.e., that they could be random samples from the same population). The t-test statistic is equal to the difference in the mean values of the two samples divided by the square root of the pooled variance of the samples (the standard error of the difference of the means of the two groups). The p value of the result (t) is read from the table of the t distribution with the degrees of freedom equal to the sum of the number of subjects in each sample minus 2.

Categorical Values

The chi-square statistic (χ^2) commonly is used to assess the statistical significance of differences in categorical values between groups.[6] Most often, proportions of two different groups (e.g., the proportions of the exposed and of the unexposed group that developed the outcome) are compared. Typically, the data are displayed in a *2 × 2 contingency table* (Table 246–5). The null hypothesis is that there is no association between the exposure and the outcome (or whatever the rows and columns represent), that is, that the two groups could be random samples from the same population. This is tested statistically by comparing the number of subjects that would be expected to be in a given cell by chance to the actual frequency (the observed frequency). The expected frequency can be calculated from the total number of subjects in the rows and the columns (the marginal totals) and is equal to the product of the number of subjects in the row times the number of subjects in the column divided by the total number of subjects in the sample.

The value of χ^2 (with N equal to the total number of subjects) is shown in Table 246–5. The statistical significance

TABLE 246–5. 2 × 2 Contingency Table

	Outcome Present	Outcome Absent	Total
Exposed	a	b	a + b
Unexposed	c	d	c + d
Total	a + c	b + d	N

$\chi^2 = [(ad - bc)^2N] \div [(a+b)(a+c)(b+d)(c+d)]$

of χ^2 can be determined by reading the *p* values from a table of the χ^2 distribution. The larger the value of χ^2, the less likely it is that the observed proportions could have occurred by chance. Unfortunately, the assumption that the probability that the observed proportions of a random sample of subjects will follow the χ^2 distribution is not necessarily accurate if the expected frequency of any cell is small. Consequently, many experts use a *continuity correction* (sometimes called the *Yates correction)* to adjust for the deviation from the smooth, continuous theoretic distribution of χ^2 when the discrete values of small numbers of expected subjects disrupt the validity of the assumed distribution. The equation for χ^2 with the continuity correction is

$$\chi_c^2 = [(|ad - bc| - (N/2))^2\, N] \div [(a + b)(a + c)(c + d)(b + d)]$$

If the expected frequency in any cell is very small (often defined as <5), the χ^2 test, even with the continuity correction, is not a valid estimate of the probability that the observed values could have occurred by chance. In such instances, the *Fisher exact test*, which is based on a hypergeometric distribution, should be used to assess the statistical significance of differences in categorical values.

Confidence Intervals

Although the validity of a null hypothesis typically is tested by stochastic tests and the use of *p* values, construction of a *confidence interval* (usually a *95 per cent confidence interval)* has the advantage of providing information about both the *precision* of the estimate of the association (the narrower the confidence interval, the more precise the estimate) and its statistical significance.[3] Confidence intervals have become a standard component of reports of the results of epidemiologic studies. Although the term *confidence limit* sometimes is used, *confidence interval* is preferred because the former term erroneously suggests that there is a limit to the range of possible values.

Analyses of studies are concerned with both estimation (of the "true" value of the association between the exposure and the outcome in the population) and hypothesis testing (i.e., What is the probability that any association that is observed could have occurred by chance alone?). A sample of the population is enrolled in any study. It is hoped that the association observed in the study is an accurate estimate of the true value of the association in the entire population. However, if an unbiased study were repeated many times, by chance alone the results will vary (because of random *sampling error)*. A confidence interval is a range of values, based on the estimate and the spread of the data from a single study, within which the true value of the association in the population is likely to lie with a specified probability (e.g., 95 per cent of the time for a 95 per cent confidence interval, 99 per cent of the time for a 99 per cent confidence interval). Confidence intervals provide information about both the magnitude of associations (so that the clinical significance of the estimate can be assessed) and its statistical significance. If the confidence interval is calculated for a single outcome and if the 95 per cent confidence interval for the difference between two groups does not include zero, the outcome is statistically significant (i.e., there is <5 per cent probability that the null hypothesis of no difference between the groups is true). If the confidence interval is for a risk ratio or an odds ratio, the association will be statistically significant if the 95 per cent confidence interval for the association does not include one (i.e., there is <5 per cent probability that the null hypothesis of no association is true). Confidence intervals can be calculated with both continuous and categorical data, as well as for estimates of a single proportion and for differences (or associations) between two groups.

Adjustment for Potential Confounding Variables

The effect of confounding variables on the associations between exposure and outcome may be controlled in either the design or the analysis of a study. Random allocation of subjects to the exposed and the unexposed groups is a common strategy to avoid the effect of confounding in longitudinal studies. Although randomization actually ensures only lack of bias if a confounding variable is distributed unevenly between the groups (because an uneven distribution is as likely to favor the exposed group as the unexposed group), randomization is likely to be effective in preventing confounding if the size of the sample is large (which makes substantial inequalities between groups in the distribution of an independent variable unlikely). Nevertheless, an investigator must check to ensure that confounding does not occur, even in a randomized clinical trial.

Another way to ensure that a potential confounding variable does not affect the results of a study is to *match* on that variable. Subjects in the exposed and the unexposed groups (or, in a case-control study, the cases and the controls) can be matched on certain variables that are known to be associated independently with both the exposure and the outcome. This can be done either by matching subjects individually or by *frequency matching* (i.e., ensuring that the overall frequency distribution of the potential confounder is the same among the cases and the controls). Matching can ensure that the matched variable (e.g., race, age) does not affect the observed association between exposure and outcome.

One disadvantage of matching is that the effect of the matched variable on the association between exposure and outcome cannot be assessed as it might be if either stratification or multivariable analysis were used to control for confounding. If matching is used in the design of the study, it is necessary to analyze the data using special tests for matched designs. For example, in a matched-pairs case-control study, only discordant pairs (matched pairs in which the cases and controls differ in their exposure status) provide information. The calculation of the matched odds ratio and the associated test of statistical significance *(McNemar* χ^2) are shown in Table 246–6.

It also is possible to adjust for the effect of potential confounders in the analyses. One way to accomplish this is with *stratification*. This is performed by dividing the data into different groups, or *strata,* according to the potential confounder. For example, a study may indicate that children whose parents both work were three times more likely to develop fever during the course of a study than were children whose parents both do not work. We may suspect,

TABLE 246–6. Analysis of a Matched Case-Control Study

	Cases	
Controls	***Exposed***	***Unexposed***
Exposed	a	b
Unexposed	c	d

Matched odds ratio: b/c
McNemar χ^2: $(b - c)^2/(b + c)$
McNemar χ^2 (with continuity correction: $(|b - c| - 1)^2/(b + c)$

however, that it is not having both parents at work, per se, that results in this increased risk of fever; rather, it is likely that it is another factor independently related to the risk of fever and to the probability that both parents work. Attendance at group day care is such a factor. If we stratified the results of the study by whether the children attended group day care, we most likely would find that a disproportionate number of children whose parents both work also attended group day care. When the risk ratios in the two different strata were combined (using the *Mantel-Haenszel technique*), we probably would find that the apparent association between having parents who both work and the risk of fever disappears when the effect of attendance at group day care is controlled by stratification.

The advantages of stratification are that it can be understood easily and it can be performed without changing the design of the study after it is completed. One disadvantage is that it is necessary to be able to identify and to measure accurately potential confounders (which is not necessary if one allocates subjects to different groups randomly). In addition, if there are several different potential confounders, it may be difficult and time-consuming to perform the calculations, and the size of the individual strata may be so small that the ability to make statistical inferences is poor.

Finally, one can adjust for confounding with the use of one of many *multivariable statistical techniques*, such as *multiple linear regression* (if both the dependent and the independent variables are continuous) or *logistic regression* (if the dependent variable is dichotomous and the independent variables are either categorical or continuous). Detailed description of multivariable techniques is beyond the scope of this chapter. However, in general, these techniques involve creating a mathematical model that fits the data and then using that model to analyze various associations.[1, 2, 5, 20] Although multivariable techniques are a powerful tool to try to assess the effects of and to control for potential confounding variables, they depend on mathematical assumptions that may not be valid always and use techniques that are not intuitively obvious.

Meta-analysis

The term *meta-analysis* refers to a number of different types of analyses. The common feature of all meta-analyses is that they summarize the results of two or more different studies. The term often is used to refer to a quantitative technique in which the results of different studies are combined after they are weighted in the calculations according to the size of their samples and the variance of their results. The term also sometimes refers to a qualitative analysis of a group of studies, including critical analyses that rate the methodologic soundness of different studies but do not combine their results quantitatively. For example, one might review a group of studies that reached different conclusions about a topic. If the methodologically rigorous studies had similar results that differed from those of the weaker studies, one might conclude that the results of the better studies were more likely to be valid.

The concept of producing a single, statistically valid result by combining the results of different, often contradictory studies has great appeal. However, quantitative meta-analysis has many shortcomings. Perhaps chief among them is that no distinction is made between studies that are sound methodologically and those that are not. Thus, the results of a meta-analysis may be dominated by a large but methodologically questionable study, whereas a superbly done but smaller study may fail to override the impact of the larger study in the meta-analysis. Another major problem is the selection of studies to include in a meta-analysis. Should only published, peer-reviewed studies be included (although there clearly is a bias that studies with a positive result are more likely to be published than are studies with a negative result)? Should the analysis be limited only to studies that meet certain basic criteria for methodologic rigor (and who should decide on the criteria and whether they are met), or should only randomized clinical trials be included? What formula should be used to weight the different studies? Is it valid to combine the results of methodologically different studies? Results of meta-analyses should be interpreted with great circumspection.[23]

DIAGNOSTIC TESTS

Although clinicians typically order diagnostic tests many times each day, misinterpretation and misuse of diagnostic tests are extremely common.[17] The widespread practice of interpreting continuous values (e.g., the total white blood cell count) in a dichotomous manner (so that the result is either "normal" or "abnormal") and the failure fully to appreciate the difference between the accuracy of a diagnostic test (i.e., its sensitivity and specificity) and its predictive value are major factors in the misuse of diagnostic tests.

What Is Normal?

In most instances, the "cutoff" for an abnormal test of a continuous variable, such as the total white blood cell count or the concentration of antibodies against an infectious agent, is based on the distribution of the results of the test in the population. It usually is assumed that the distribution of most such results in the population will follow a Gaussian (or "normal") distribution, which is illustrated by the bell-shaped curve in Figure 246–1. Gauss and other statisticians used the term *normal* to refer to the shape of this curve. However, in medicine, the term *normal* long has been used to mean something very different—the dichotomy between a state of health (*normal*) and one of disease (*abnormal*). Unfortunately, the different meanings of these terms often have been used interchangeably, which has added to confusion in the interpretation of diagnostic tests.

In a normal distribution, the mode (the most frequent value) is the mean value, and 68.3 per cent, 95.4 per cent, and 99.7 per cent of the values lie within (plus or minus) one, two, and three standard deviations from the mean value, respectively. The cutoff for an abnormal test result often arbitrarily is defined as any value that is more than two standard deviations from the mean of a normally distributed population; thus, 5 per cent (actually 4.6 per cent) of the population would be categorized as abnormal. Half of the people with abnormal results will be two standard deviations below the mean, and half will be two standard deviations above the mean. Thus, 2.5 per cent (actually 2.3 per cent) of the population will have abnormally high values. In some instances, three standard deviations (or some other arbitrary parameter) are used to determine the cutoff. However, it is important to realize that these definitions of normal and abnormal merely are statistical models that should not be translated necessarily to mean that 2.5 per cent of the population is "diseased." As noted earlier, with this kind of statistical logic, the diagnosis of disease may be related to the number of tests that are performed because if multiple tests are performed, there is an increased likelihood that any one will be abnormal. If 15 independent tests are performed on

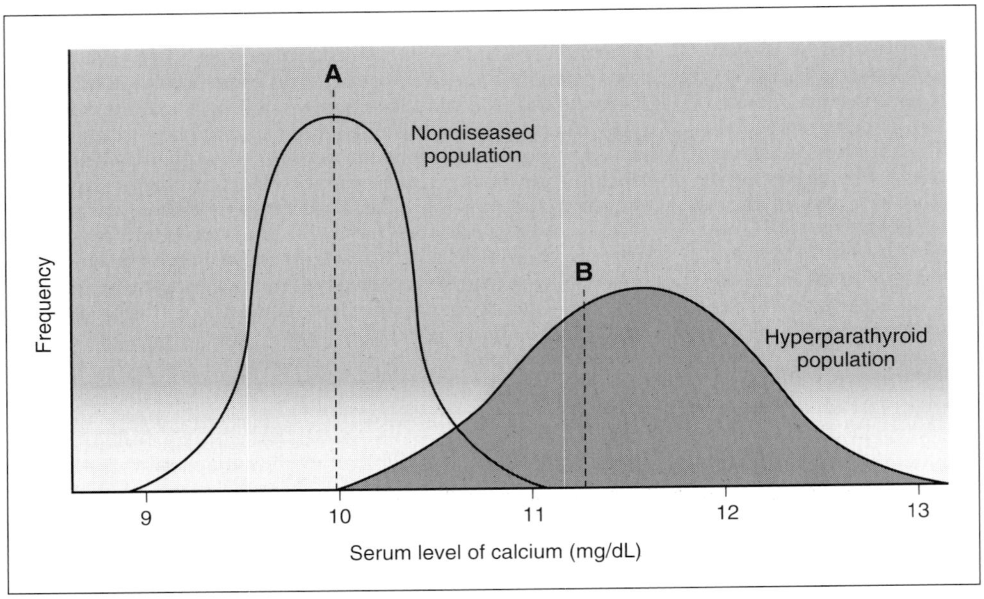

FIGURE 246–2. *Overlap in values of randomly taken tests in a population in which most of the people are healthy (curve on the left) but some of the people are diseased (curve on the right). A person with a level of calcium below point A would be unlikely to have hyperparathyroidism. A person with a level of calcium above point B would be likely to have an abnormality of calcium metabolism, possibly hyperparathyroidism. A person with a level of calcium between point A and point B may or may not have an abnormality of calcium metabolism. (Note: The normal range of calcium depends on the method used in a specific laboratory. In some laboratories, the range is from 8.5 to 10.5 mg/dL. In others, as in this illustration, it is from 9 to 11 mg/dL.) (From Jekel, J. F., Elmore, J. G., and Katz, D. L.: Epidemiology, Biostatistics, and Preventive Medicine. Philadelphia, W. B. Saunders, 1996, p. 88.)*

a patient, the probability that any one of the test results will be abnormal by chance is 54 per cent.

There are other statistical models that might be more appropriate for assessing a diagnostic test. For example, interpreting diagnostic tests would be relatively easy if there were two separate, nonoverlapping normal distributions of diseased and disease-free patients. Unfortunately, although this model may apply for some rare conditions (such as genetic disorders in which affected persons are missing an enzyme that metabolizes certain substances, which leads to uniquely high concentrations of the substance in persons with the disorder), the model rarely is applicable. A model that is more appropriate for most infectious illness is shown in Figure 246–2. In this model (the example of which uses levels of serum calcium), there are diseased and nondiseased populations with separate, partially overlapping distributions. The specificity of a diagnostic test is related directly to the degree to which the two distributions overlap.

Accuracy of a Diagnostic Test

Two important characteristics of a diagnostic test—its *reproducibility* and its *validity*—are the key components of its accuracy. The reproducibility (sometimes called *reliability* or *precision)* of a test simply is the degree to which retesting yields the same result. A test that is not reproducible is of little diagnostic value. The validity of a test may be divided into two components: *sensitivity* and *specificity* (Table 246–7).

TABLE 246–7. Statistical Indices of a Diagnostic Test

Result of Test	Disease	No Disease
Positive	a	b
Negative	c	d
True positives: a	Sensitivity = a/(a + c)	
False positives: b	Specificity = d/(b + d)	
True negatives: d	Positive predictive value = a/(a + b)	
False negatives: c	Negative predictive value = d/(c + d)	

The *sensitivity* of a test is the proportion of persons with disease that is identified accurately by the test as having disease (true positives/[true positives + false negatives]). The *specificity* of a test is the proportion of persons without disease that is identified accurately by the test as not having disease (true negatives/[true negatives + false positives]). The ideal test has both a specificity and a sensitivity of 1. Of course, no diagnostic tests are that accurate. Indeed, there is a tradeoff between sensitivity and specificity—usually, the more sensitive a test is, the less specific it is, and vice versa.

Although the sensitivity and specificity of a given test often are considered to be absolute characteristics of a test, in fact these characteristics do depend on the types of patients included in the studies in which the indices of the test were developed. Indeed, it is common for tests that appear to be highly sensitive and specific in preliminary studies to prove to be much less so when used in actual clinical practice. This is because the preliminary studies that establish a test's sensitivity and specificity frequently are affected by problems of spectrum and bias.[16] If the patients enrolled in studies used to assess the test (both those with disease and those without disease) have a relatively narrow spectrum of clinical manifestations, both the sensitivity and the specificity of a diagnostic test may appear to be better than they actually are. For example, if one were to assess the sensitivity of a differential heterophile test to diagnose infection with Epstein-Barr virus (EBV), its sensitivity would appear far better if all of the subjects infected with EBV were teenagers with severe pharyngitis (a high proportion of whom will have a positive heterophile test result) than if it included subjects with a broader spectrum of manifestations of EBV infection (such as toddlers with symptoms of an infection of the upper respiratory tract, who are much less likely to have a positive heterophile test result when infected with EBV). Likewise, the specificity of a diagnostic test may appear to be better when only asymptomatic, healthy persons are used as nondiseased subjects instead of including patients with other illnesses that produce symptoms similar to those of the target illness.

In addition, it is important to realize that the cutoffs for classifying results as either normal or abnormal usually are somewhat arbitrary and may depend on how the test is used as well as on the nature of the disease that one is trying to detect. If a diagnostic test is being used to screen a population for a relatively mild disorder with a low prevalence, one would want to use a cutoff that results in high specificity to avoid having a large number of false-positive results, even at the expense of lower sensitivity. On the other hand, if the diagnostic test is for a serious disorder or is used not for screening but for diagnosis in a targeted population with at least a moderate prevalence of the disorder (e.g., a white blood cell count in cerebrospinal fluid to detect possible bacterial meningitis in febrile children), one might want to err on the side of overdiagnosis and therefore use a cutoff with a high sensitivity at the expense of lower specificity.

Predictive Value of a Diagnostic Test

Sensitivity and specificity are important characteristics of a diagnostic test, but to calculate them one must know whether the patients do or do not have the disease; clearly, if a physician already had this knowledge, he or she would not need to perform the test in the first place. From the perspective of a clinician who is caring for an individual patient, the key characteristic of a diagnostic test is its *predictive value* (Table 246–7). That is, if a test result is positive, what is the probability that the patient has the disease *(positive predictive value)*? Conversely, if a test result is negative, what is the probability that a patient does not have the disease *(negative predictive value)*? However, unlike sensitivity and specificity, the predictive value of a test depends critically on the prevalence of the disease among the subjects who are tested.

This is illustrated by the example in Table 246–8. In example *a*, the prevalence of the disease in the sample is 1 per cent and the positive predictive value of a positive test result is only 8.8 per cent. By contrast, as shown in examples *b* and *c*, when the prevalence of disease in the sample rises to 10 per cent and to 50 per cent, respectively, the positive predictive value of a positive test result rises to 51.4 per cent and to 90.5 per cent, respectively, even though the sensitivity and the specificity of the test are constant. By the same token, as the prevalence of disease in the sample that is tested rises, the predictive value of a negative test result falls, although the negative predictive value remains reasonably good unless the prevalence of disease approaches 90 per cent or more.

It is important for clinicians to be aware of these epidemiologic truths when ordering diagnostic tests for patients. Sometimes a physician orders tests to "rule out" the possibility that a patient's symptoms are due to a disease that, based on the patient's history, physical examination, and prior laboratory tests, is unlikely to be the cause of the problem (i.e., the "prior probability" that the patient has the disease is low). Unless the specificity of such tests approaches 100 per cent (which is unlikely for most serologic tests), in such situations the great majority of positive test results will be falsely positive; the physician then will find himself in the unfortunate position of ignoring the result, ordering additional diagnostic tests, or treating the patient for a disease that likely is not the cause of the patient's symptoms. Consequently, clinicians should be selective in ordering diagnostic tests.

ASSESSMENT OF THE PROTECTIVE EFFICACY OF A VACCINE

The protective efficacy of a vaccine may be assessed with either experimental or observational studies. The classic way to assess a vaccine's efficacy is in an experimental, randomized, double-blind clinical trial. The major observational designs available are cohort studies and case-control studies, although there are a large variety of hybrid designs, such as household-exposure studies and indirect cohort studies, complete descriptions of which are beyond the scope of this chapter.[14, 15] Table 246–9 illustrates the calculation of the protective efficacy of a pneumococcal vaccine with data from clinical trials, cohort studies, and case-control studies.

Clinical Trials

In a randomized clinical trial, subjects at risk of the infection in question would be assigned randomly either to re-

TABLE 246–8. Predictive Value of a Diagnostic Test with 95% Sensitivity and 90% Specificity with Different Prevalences of Disease in the Sample

	Test	Disease	No Disease	Total
a*				
	Positive	95	990	1085
	Negative	5	8910	8915
	Total	100	9900	10,000
	Positive predictive value = 8.8%		Negative predictive value = 99.9%	
b†	**Test**	**Disease**	**No Disease**	**Total**
	Positive	950	900	1850
	Negative	50	8100	8150
	Total	1000	9000	10,000
	Positive predictive value = 51.4%		Negative predictive value = 99.4%	
c‡	**Test**	**Disease**	**No Disease**	**Total**
	Positive	4750	500	5250
	Negative	250	4500	4750
	Total	5000	5000	10,000
	Positive predictive value = 90.5%		Negative predictive value = 94.7%	

*Prevalence of disease: 1%.
†Prevalence of disease: 10%.
‡Prevalence of disease: 50%.

TABLE 246–9. Calculation of Protective Efficacy (PE) of Pneumococcal Vaccine

Clinical Trial or Cohort Study	Pneumococcal Infection	No Pneumococcal Infection	Total
Vaccinated	a	b	a + b
Not vaccinated	c	d	c + d
PE = [(c/c + d) − (a/(a + b)] ÷ (c/c + d) = 1 − [(a/(a + b) ÷ (c/c + d)]*			
Case-Control Study	**Pneumococcal Infection (Cases)**	**No Pneumococcal Infection (Controls)**	
Vaccinated	a	b	
Not vaccinated	c	d	
	PE = 1 − [(ad) ÷ (bc)]†		

*The expression [(a/(a + b) ÷ (c/c + d)] also is known as the relative risk of infection in vaccinated versus unvaccinated persons.
†The expression [(ad) ÷ (bc)] is the odds ratio relating vaccination to infection. In a case-control study, the odds ratio approximates the relative risk if the outcome is rare.

ceive the vaccine (vaccinees) or not to receive the vaccine (controls). After receipt of the vaccine, all subjects would be observed for the occurrence of the infection during an appropriate period of follow-up. At the conclusion of the study, the *protective efficacy* (PE) of the vaccine, an index devised by Greenwood and Yule[7] to indicate the proportionate reduction in the frequency of disease attributable to the vaccine, would be calculated. PE is defined as follows:

$$\text{PE} = \frac{(\text{risk of infection in controls}) - (\text{risk of infection in vaccinees})}{(\text{risk of infection in controls})}$$

A PE of 100 per cent indicates complete protection against infection, a PE of 0 per cent indicates no protection, and negative values indicate that there was a greater risk of infection among vaccinees than among controls. By rearranging terms, PE equals 1 minus the risk of infection in vaccinees divided by the risk of infection in controls. Because the ratio in this equation is the relative risk of infection in vaccinees compared with controls, PE is, by definition, equal to 1 minus the relative risk.

Observational Cohort Studies

In a cohort study, subjects at risk would be selected on the basis of whether they had been vaccinated or had been left unvaccinated during routine clinical care. The vaccinated and unvaccinated groups then would be followed longitudinally to assess the frequencies of infection. The analysis of cohort studies of a vaccine's PE is similar to that for clinical trials, but because the study is nonexperimental, the results are more subject to bias than are those of a well-conducted, randomized clinical trial.

Case-Control Studies

In a case-control study, patients with antecedent conditions that place them at high risk of pneumococcal infection would be eligible to be subjects. Patients with serious pneumococcal infections would be selected as subjects in the case group. The control group would consist of subjects with similar high-risk conditions but without pneumococcal infections. The two groups then would be compared for the frequencies of antecedent vaccination with pneumococcal vaccine.

In a case-control study, the strength of the relationship between vaccination and subsequent infection also is measured by an odds ratio (the ratio of the odds of vaccination in the case-subjects to the odds of vaccination in the controls). Because the odds ratio in a case-control study closely approximates the relative risk of pneumococcal infection in a longitudinal study and because PE is defined as 1 minus the relative risk, the value (1 − odds ratio) closely approximates the PE that would be calculated from a longitudinal study.

References

1. Breslow, N. E., Day, N. E. and Davis, W. (eds.): Statistical Methods in Cancer Research. Volume I. The Analysis of Case-Control Studies. Lyon, International Agency for Research on Cancer, 1980.
2. Breslow, N. E., Day, N. E., and Heseltine, E. (eds.): Statistical Methods in Cancer Research. Vol. II: The Design and Analysis of Cohort Studies. Lyon, International Agency for Research on Cancer, 1987.
3. Bulpitt, C. J.: Confidence intervals. Lancet *1*:494–497, 1987.
4. Clemens, J. D., and Shapiro, E. D.: The pneumococcal vaccine controversy: Are there alternatives to randomized clinical trials: Rev. Infect. Dis. *6*:589–600, 1984.
5. Feinstein, A. R.: Clinical Epidemiology: The Architecture of Clinical Research. Philadelphia, W. B. Saunders, 1985.
6. Fleiss, J.: Statistical Methods for Rates and Proportions. 2nd ed. New York, John Wiley & Sons, 1981.
7. Greenwood, M., and Yule, U. G.: The statistics of anti-typhoid and anti-cholera inoculations, and the interpretation of such statistics in general. Proc. R. Soc. Med. *8*:113–194, 1915.
8. Jekel, J. F., Elmore, J. G., and Katz, D. L.: Epidemiology, Biostatistics and Preventive Medicine. Philadelphia, W. B. Saunders, 1996.
9. Kahn, H. A., and Sempos, C. T.: Statistical Methods in Epidemiology. Monographs in Epidemiology and Biostatistics. Vol. 12. New York, Oxford University Press, 1989.
10. Kelsey, J. L., Thompson, W. D., and Evans, A. S.: Methods in Observational Epidemiology. Monographs in Epidemiology and Biostatistics. Vol. 10. New York, Oxford University Press, 1986.
11. Kleinbaum, D. G, Kupper, L. L., and Morgenstern, H.: Epidemiologic Research: Principles and Quantitative Methods. Belmont, Lifetime Learning Publications Division, Wadsworth, 1982.
12. Lee, E. T.: Statistical Methods for Survival Data Analysis. Belmont, Lifetime Learning Publications Division, Wadsworth, 1980.
13. McCarthy, P. L., Sharpe, M. R., Spiesel, S. Z., et al.: Observation scales to identify serious illness in febrile children. Pediatrics *70*:802–809, 1982.
14. Orenstein, W. A., Bernier, R. H., Dondero, T. J., et al.: Field evaluation of vaccine efficacy. Bull. W. H. O. *63*:1055–1068, 1985.
15. Orenstein, W. A., Bernier, R. H., and Hinman, A. R.: Assessing vaccine efficacy in the field: Further observations. Epidemiol. Rev. *10*:212–241, 1988.
16. Ransahoff, D. F., and Feinstein, A. R.: Problems of spectrum and bias in evaluating the efficacy of diagnostic tests. N. Engl. J. Med. *299*:926–930, 1978.
17. Riegelman, R. K., and Hirsch, R. P.: Studying a Study and Testing a Test: How to Read the Medical Literature. 2nd ed. Boston, Little, Brown, 1989.
18. Sackett, D. L., Haynes, R. B., Guyatt, G. H., et al.: Clinical Epidemiology:

A Basic Science for Clinical Medicine. 2nd ed. Boston, Little, Brown, 1991.

19. Schlesselman, J. J.: Case-Control Studies: Design, Conduct, Analysis. Monographs in Epidemiology, New York, Oxford University Press, 1982.
20. Selvin, S.: Statistical analysis of epidemiologic data. *In* Kelsey, J. L., Marmot, M. G., Stolley, P. D., et al. (eds.): Monographs in Epidemiology and Biostatistics. Vol. 17. New York, Oxford University Press, 1991.
21. Siegel, S.: Nonparametric Statistics for the Behavioral Sciences. McGraw-Hill Series in Psychology. New York, McGraw-Hill, 1956.
22. Snedecor, G. W., and Cochran, W. G.: Statistical Methods. 7th ed. Ames, The Iowa State University Press, 1980.
23. Thompson, S. G., and Pocock, S. J.: Can meta-analyses be trusted? Lancet *338*:1127–1130, 1991.

INDEX

❏ ❏ ❏

Note: Page numbers in *italics* refer to illustrations; page numbers followed by t refer to tables.

ISBN 0-7216-7163-2

90071

9 780721 671635